The Physiology of Reproduction

SECOND EDITION

The Physiology of Reproduction

SECOND EDITION

Volume 1

Editors-in-Chief

Ernst Knobil
The H. Wayne Hightower Professor
in the Medical Sciences and
Director, Laboratory for Neuroendocrinology
The University of Texas
Health Science Center at Houston—Medical School
Houston, Texas

Jimmy D. Neill
Professor and Chairman
Department of Physiology and Biophysics
The University of Alabama at Birmingham
Birmingham, Alabama

Associate Editors

Gilbert S. Greenwald
Distinguished Professor
Department of Physiology
University of Kansas Medical Center
Kansas City, Kansas

Clement L. Markert
University Research Professor
Department of Animal Sciences
North Carolina State University
School of Agriculture and Life Sciences
Raleigh, North Carolina

Donald W. Pfaff
Professor
Laboratory of Neurobiology and Behavior
Rockefeller University
New York, New York

Raven Press New York

Raven Press, Ltd., 1185 Avenue of the Americas, New York, New York 10036

Made in the United States of America

Library of Congress Cataloging-in-Publication Data

The Physiology of reproduction/editors-in-chief, Ernst Knobil, Jimmy D. Neill:
associate editors, Gilbert S. Greenwald, Clement L. Markert, Donald W. Pfaff.
—2nd ed.
p. cm.
Includes bibliographical references and index.
ISBN 0-7817-0086-8
1. Reproduction. 2. Mammals—Physiology. I. Knobil, Ernst.
II. Neill, Jimmy D.
[DNLM: 1. Reproduction. WQ 205 P5784 1993]
QP251.P525 1993
599'.016—dc20
DNLM/DLC
for Library of Congress 93-853
CIP

The material contained in this volume was submitted as previously unpublished material, except in the instances in which some of the illustrative material was derived. Chapters 11, by Gore-Langton and Armstrong, 20, by Bardin et al., and 25, by Everett, were reprinted from the first edition of this volume (Raven Press, 1988).

Great care has been taken to maintain the accuracy of the information contained in the volume. However, neither Raven Press nor the editors can be held responsible for errors or for any consequences arising from the use of the information contained herein.

Materials appearing in this book prepared by individuals as part of their official duties as U.S. Government employees are not covered by the above-mentioned copyright.

9 8 7 6 5 4 3 2 1

Contents

VOLUME 2

Reproduction Behavior and Its Control

Reproductive Processes and Their Control

Contributors

Eli Y. Adashi
Department of Obstetrics & Gynecology and Physiology
Division of Reproductive Endocrinology
University of Maryland School of Medicine
405 West Redwood Street, Third Floor
Baltimore, Maryland 21201

David F. Albertini
Department of Anatomy and Cellular Biology
Tufts University School of Medicine
Boston, Massachusetts 02111

David T. Armstrong
Medical Research Council Group in Reproductive Biology
Department of Physiology and Obstetrics & Gynecology
The University of Western Ontario
London, Ontario N6A 5A5
Canada

C. Wayne Bardin
Center for Biomedical Research
The Population Council
1230 York Avenue
New York, New York 10021

George S. Benson
Department of Surgery
Division of Urology
University of Texas Medical School at Houston
6431 Fannin, Suite 6018
Houston, Texas 77030

Louise M. Bilezikjian
Peptide Biology Laboratory
Salk Institute
San Diego, California 92138

George R. Bousfield
Department of Biological Sciences
Wichita State University
1845 N. Fairmount
Wichita, Kansas 67260

Robert D.H. Boyd
Department of Child Health
University of Manchester, St. Mary's Hospital
Hathersage Road
Manchester M13 OJH
United Kingdom

Robert M. Brenner
Division of Reproductive Sciences
Oregon Regional Primate Research Center
505 N.W. 185th Avenue
Beaverton, Oregon 97006

Franklin H. Bronson
Department of Zoology
University of Texas at Austin
28 Patterson Laboratory
Austin, Texas 78712

D. E. Brooks (Deceased)
Department of Animal Sciences
Waite Agricultural Research Institute
University of Adelaide
Adelaide, South Australia

Carol A. Burdsal
Laboratory of Radiobiology and Environmental Health
University of California, San Francisco
San Francisco, California 94143

Graham J. Burton
Department of Anatomy
University of Cambridge
Downing Street
Cambridge CB2 3DY
England

Anne Grete Byskov
Laboratory of Reproductive Biology II
University Hospital of Copenhagen
Rigshospitalet Section 5821
Blegdamsvej 9
DK-2100 Copenhagen
Denmark

John R. G. Challis
Department of Obstetrics and Gynecology
St. Josephs Hospital
268 Grosvenor Street
London, Ontario N6A 4VA
Canada

C. Yan Cheng
The Population Council
1230 York Avenue
New York, New York 10021

James H. Clark
Department of Cell Biology
Baylor College of Medicine
One Baylor Plaza
Houston, Texas 77074

G. Clarke
Department of Anatomy
The School of Medical Sciences
University of Bristol
University Walk
Bristol, Avon B517 2HT
United Kingdom

Donald S. Coffey
James Buchanan Brady Urological Institute
Research Laboratories
The Johns Hopkins University
Baltimore, Maryland 21205

P. Michael Conn
Department of Pharmacology
University of Iowa College of Medicine
Bowen Science Building
Iowa City, Iowa 52242

Alan C. Dalkin
Department of Internal Medicine
Division of Endocrinology
University of Virginia Health Sciences Center
Charlottesville, Virginia 22908

Sophie V. Drouva
Department of Neuroendocrinology
INSERM U-159
2ter Rue d'Alesia
75014 Paris
France

E. M. Eddy
Gamete Biology Section
Laboratory of Reproductive & Developmental Toxicology
National Institute of Environmental Health Sciences
National Institutes of Health
Research Triangle Park, North Carolina 27709

Lawrence L. Espey
Department of Biology
Trinity University
715 Stadium Drive
San Antonio, Texas 78212

John W. Everett (Deceased)
Department of Neurobiology
Duke University School of Medicine
Durham, North Carolina 27710

Deborah Fairchild-Benyo
Department of Obstetrics & Gynecology
Magee Women's Hospital
Pittsburgh, Pennsylvania 15213

Caleb E. Finch
Department of Biological Sciences
Andrus Gerontology Center
University of Southern California
P.O. Box 77912
University Park
Los Angeles, California 90081

Douglas L. Foster
Department of Developmental and Reproductive Biology
University of Michigan
300 N. Ingalls Building, Room 1101
Ann Arbor, Michigan 48109

Marc E. Freeman
Department of Biological Science
Florida State University
Tallahassee, Florida 32306

Harold Gainer
Laboratory for Neurochemistry
National Institute of Neurological Disorders and Stroke
National Institutes of Health
Building 36, Room 4D-20
Bethesda, Maryland 20892

Frederick W. George
Department of Internal Medicine
University of Texas Southwestern Medical Center at Dallas
5323 Harry Hines Boulevard
Dallas, Texas 75235

Thomas J. Gill III
Department of Pathology
University of Pittsburgh
School of Medicine
716A Scaife Hall
Pittsburgh, Pennsylvania 15261

Robert L. Goodman
Department of Physiology and Biophysics
West Virginia University
Morgantown, West Virginia 26506

Robert E. Gore-Langton
Department of Physiology and Obstetrics & Gynecology
The University of Western Ontario
London, Ontario N6A 5A5
Canada

Roy O. Greep
Oakwood
135 Oak Street
Foxboro, Massachusetts 02035

Gilbert S. Greenwald
Department of Physiology
University of Kansas Medical Center
39th Street and Rainbow Boulevard
Kansas City, Kansas 66103

Glen L. Gunsalus
The Population Council
1230 York Avenue
New York, New York 10021

Raphael Guzman
Cancer Research Laboratory
Department of Molecular and Cell Biology
University of California at Berkeley
491 Life Sciences Addition
Berkeley, California 94720

Daniel J. Haisenleder
Department of Internal Medicine
Division of Endocrinology
University of Virginia Health Sciences Center
Charlottesville, Virginia 22908

Peter F. Hall
Department of Endocrinology
Prince of Wales Hospital
Avoca Street
Randwick, Sydney, N.S.W. 2031
Australia

Michael J. K. Harper
Department of Obstetrics and Gynecology
Baylor College of Medicine
One Baylor Plaza
Houston, Texas 77030

Paul D. Heideman
Department of Zoology
Institute of Reproductive Biology
University of Texas
Austin, Texas 78712

Julane Hotchkiss
Laboratory for Neuroendocrinology
University of Texas Health Science Center at Houston
The University of Texas Medical School
6431 Fannin Street
Houston, Texas 77030

Poul Erik Høyer
Institute of Medical Anatomy A
The Panum Institute
University of Copenhagen
Blegdamsvej 3
DK-2200 Copenhagen
Denmark

Walter Imagawa
Cancer Research Laboratory
Department of Molecular and Cell Biology
University of California at Berkeley
491 Life Sciences Addition
Berkeley, California 94720

Peter Kaufmann
Institut fur Anatomie
Rheinisch Westfalische Technische Hochschule Aachen
Melatener Strasse 211
Wendlingweg 2
D 5100 Aachen
Germany

J. B. Kerr
Department of Anatomy
Institute of Reproduction and Development
Monash University
Melbourne, Victoria 3168
Australia

Ernst Knobil
Laboratory for Neuroendocrinology
The University of Texas Health Science Center at Houston
The University of Texas Medical School
P.O. Box 20708
Houston, Texas 77225

Claude Kordon
Department of Neuroendocrinology
INSERM U-159
2ter Rue d'Alesia
75014 Paris
France

Lee-Ming Kow
Laboratory of Neurobiology and Behavior
The Rockefeller University
1230 York Avenue
New York, New York 10021

D. M. de Kretser
Department of Anatomy
Institute of Reproduction and Development
Monash University
Melbourne, Victoria 3168
Australia

Harry Lipner
Department of Biological Sciences
Florida State University
Tallahassee, Florida 32306

Izhar Livne
Department of Anatomy and Cell Biology
College of Physicians and Surgeons of Columbia University
630 East 168th Street
New York, New York 10032

Markham C. Luke
James Buchanan Brady Urological Institute
Research Laboratories
The Johns Hopkins Hospital
Baltimore, Maryland 21205

Stephen J. Lye
Samuel Lumenfeld Research Institute
Mount Sinai Hospital
Toronto, Ontario M5G 1X5
Canada

S. Maddocks
Department of Animal Sciences
Waite Agricultural Research Institute
University of Adelaide
South Australia

Dhushy Mahendran
Department of Child Health
University of Manchester, St. Mary's Hospital
Hathersage Road
Manchester M13 OJH
United Kingdom

Shailaja K. Mani
Department of Cell Biology
Baylor College of Medicine
One Baylor Plaza
Houston, Texas 77030

Peter Marler
Department of Animal Physiology and Department of Psychology
University of California, Davis
Davis, California 95616

John C. Marshall
Department of Internal Medicine
University of Virginia Health Sciences Center
Box 511
Charlottesville, Virginia 22908

Gonzalo Martinez de la Escalera
Instituto de Investigaciones Biomedicas
Departamento de Fisiologia
Universidad Nacionale Autonoma de Mexico
Mexico

Margaret M. McCarthy
Laboratory of Neurobiology and Behavior
The Rockefeller University
1230 York Avenue
New York, New York 10021

Alan S. McNeilly
MRC Reproductive Biology Unit
University of Edinburgh
Centre for Reproductive Biology
37 Chalmers Street
Edinburgh EH3 9EW
Scotland

Robert L. Meisel
Department of Psychological Sciences
Purdue University
West Lafayette, Indiana 47907

James M. Metcalfe
Veterans' Affairs Medical Center
Vancouver Division
P.O. Box 1035 (II-V)
Portland, Oregon 97201

Frank H. Morriss, Jr.
Department of Pediatrics
The University of Iowa College of Medicine
University of Iowa Hospitals and Clinics
200 Hawkins Drive
Iowa City, Iowa 52242

Neil A. Mustow
The Population Council
1230 York Avenue
New York, New York 10021

György M. Nagy
Second Department of Anatomy
Semmelweis University Medical School
Hungary H–1450

Satyabrata Nandi
Department of Molecular & Cell Biology and Cancer Research Laboratory
491 Life Sciences Addition
University of California, Berkeley
Berkeley, California 94720

Jimmy D. Neill
Department of Physiology and Biophysics
University of Alabama School of Medicine
UAB Station
Birmingham, Alabama 35294

James F. Nelson
Department of Physiology
Health Science Center
7703 Floyd Curl Drive
University of Texas at San Antonio
San Antonio, Texas 78284

Terry M. Nett
Department of Physiology
Colorado State University
Fort Collins, Colorado 80523

Gordon D. Niswender
Department of Physiology
Colorado State University
Fort Collins, Colorado 80523

Michael Numan
Department of Psychology
Boston College
140 Commonwealth Avenue
McGuinn Hall
Chestnut Hill, Massachusetts 02167

Deborah A. O'Brien
Gamete Biology Section
Laboratory of Reproductive and Developmental Toxicology
National Institute of Environmental Health Sciences
National Institutes of Health
Research Triangle Park
North Carolina 27709
and
Laboratories for Reproductive Biology
Departments of Pediatrics and Cell Biology and Anatomy
The University of North Carolina at Chapel Hill
Chapel Hill, North Carolina 27599

Sergio R. Ojeda
Division of Neuroscience
Oregon Regional Primate Research Center
505 N.W. 185th Avenue
Beaverton, Oregon 97006

Linda Ogren
Biology Board of Studies
Thimann Laboratories
University of California, Santa Cruz
Santa Cruz, California 95064

Robert B. Page
Department of Surgery
Division of Neurosurgery
Penn State College of Medicine
University Hospital
The Milton S. Hershey Medical Center
P.O. Box 850
Hershey, Pennsylvania 17033

Roger A. Pedersen
Laboratory of Radiobiology and Environmental Health (LR-102)
University of California, San Francisco
San Francisco, California 94143

W. Michael Perry
Department of Biological Sciences
Wichita State University
1845 N. Fairmount
Wichita, Kansas 67260

Donald W. Pfaff
Laboratory of Neurobiology and Behavior
The Rockefeller University
1230 York Avenue
New York, New York 10021

Tony M. Plant
Department of Cell Biology and Physiology
University of Pittsburgh School of Medicine
W1451 Biomedical Science Tower
Pittsburgh, Pennsylvania 15261

Victor D. Ramirez
Department of Physiology and Biophysics
University of Illinois
425 Burrill Hall
407 S. Goodwin Avenue
Urbana, Illinois 61801

Catherine Rivier
Peptide Biology Laboratory
Salk Institute
San Diego, California 92138

Shyamal K. Roy
Department of Obstetrics & Gynecology and Physiology & Biophysics
University of Nebraska School of Medicine
Omaha, Nebraska 68198

Benjamin D. Sachs
Department of Psychology
University of Connecticut
Storrs, Connecticut 06269

Susan Schwartz-Giblin
Laboratory of Neurogenetics
NIPAA
National Institutes of Health
12501 Washington Place
Rockville, Maryland 20852

Brian P. Setchell
Department of Animal Sciences
Waite Agricultural Institute
University of Adelaide
Waite Road
Urrbrae, 5064
South Australia

Richard M. Sharpe
MRC Reproductive Biology Unit
University of Edinburgh
Centre for Reproductive Biology
37 Chalmers Street
Edinburgh EH3 9EW
Scotland

O. David Sherwood
University of Illinois College of Medicine
Department of Physiology and Biophysics
Urbana, Illinois 61801

Ann-Judith Silverman
Department of Anatomy and Cell Biology
College of Physicians and Surgeons of Columbia University
630 West 168th Street
New York, New York 10032

Ov Daniel Slayden
Division of Reproductive Sciences
Oregon Regional Primate Research Center
505 N.W. 185th Avenue
Beaverton, Oregon 97006

Samuel Solomon
Endocrine Laboratory
Royal Victoria Hospital
687 Pine Avenue West
Montreal, Quebec H3A 1A1
Canada

W. Lin Soufi
Duke University Medical Center
Durham, North Carolina 27710

Michael K. Stock
Heart Research Laboratory L-464
Oregon Health Sciences University
3181 S.W. Sam Jackson Park Road
Portland, Oregon 97201

Alastair J. S. Summerlee
Department of Biomedical Sciences
Ontario Veterinary College
University of Guelph
Guelph, Ontario N16 2W1
Canada

Frank Talamantes
Biology Board of Studies
Thimann Laboratories
University of California, Santa Cruz
Santa Cruz, California 95064

Andrée Tixier-Vidal
Groupe de Neuroendocrinologie Cellulaire et Molecularie
College de France
11 Place Marcelin Berthelot
75231 Paris Cedex 05
France

Claude Tougard
Groupe de Neuroendocrinologie Cellulaire et Molecularie
College de France
11 Place Marcelin Berthelot
75231 Paris Cedex 05
France

Alex Tsafriri
Department of Hormone Research
The Weizmann Institute of Science
Rehovot 76100
Israel

H. Allen Tucker
Department of Animal Science
Michigan State University
230 Anthony Hall
East Lansing, Michigan 48824

Fred W. Turek
NSF Center for Biological Timing
Department of Neurobiology and Physiology
Northwestern University
2153 North Campus Drive
Evanston, Illinois 60208
and
Department of Psychiatry
Free University of Brussels
808 Route de Lennik
B-1070 Brussels
Belgium

Henryk F. Urbanski
Division of Neuroscience
Oregon Regional Primate Research Center
505 N.W. 185th Avenue
Beaverton, Oregon 97006

Eve Van Cauter
Department of Medicine
University of Chicago
MC 1027
Chicago, Illinois 60637

John G. Vandenbergh
Department of Zoology
North Carolina State University
Box 7617
Raleigh, North Carolina 27695

Wylie W. Vale
Clayton Foundation Laboratories for Peptide Biology
Salk Institute
10010 North Torrey Pines Road
La Jolla, California 92037

Frederick S. vom Saal
Division of Biological Sciences
John M. Dalton Research Center
University of Missouri
114 Lefevre Hall
Columbia, Missouri 65211

Jonathan B. Wakerley
Department of Anatomy
University of Bristol
School of Medical Sciences
University Walk
Bristol BS8 1TD
United Kingdom

Darrell N. Ward
Department of Biochemistry and Molecular Biology
University of Texas
M.D. Anderson Cancer Center
1515 Holcombe Boulevard
Box 36
Houston, Texas 77030

Paul M. Wassarman
Department of Cell Biology
Roche Institute of Molecular Biology
Roche Research Center
340 Kingsland Street
Nutley, New Jersey 07110

Richard I. Weiner
Department of Obstetrics, Gynecology, and Reproductive Sciences
University of California, San Francisco
School of Medicine
San Francisco, California 94143

H. M. Weitlauf
Department of Cell Biology and Anatomy
Texas Tech University Health Sciences Center
3601 4th Street
Lubbock, Texas 79430

Carol S. Whaling
Animal Communication Laboratory
University of California, Davis
Davis, California 95616

Jean D. Wilson
Department of Internal Medicine
University of Texas Southwestern Medical Center at Dallas
5323 Harry Hines Boulevard
Dallas, Texas 75235

John C. Wingfield
Department of Zoology
NJ-15
University of Washington
Seattle, Washington 98195

Joan W. Witkin
Department of Anatomy and Cell Biology
College of Physicians and Surgeons of Columbia University
630 West 168th Street
New York, New York 10032

Susan Wray
Laboratory of Neurochemistry
National Institute of Neurological Disorders and Stroke
National Institutes of Health
Building 36, Room 4D-12
Bethesda, Maryland 20892

R. Yanagimachi
Department of Anatomy and Reproductive Biology
University of Hawaii School of Medicine
Honolulu, Hawaii 96822

Jason Yang
Cancer Research Laboratory
Department of Molecular and Cell Biology
University of California at Berkeley
491 Life Sciences Addition
Berkeley, California 94720

Anthony J. Zeleznik
Department of Obstetrics and Gynecology
Magee Women's Hospital
Pittsburgh, Pennsylvania 15213

Foreword

I am pleased and honored to have been asked to prepare the Foreword to this volume of work depicting the progress in research on the physiology of reproduction as well as the resulting gains in understanding made over the past few years. The expertise that is represented by the numerous contributors to this work is so impressive that I am humbled even to contemplate adding anything of note. It is only by virtue of having personally witnessed a very large segment of twentieth century research on reproduction that I am emboldened to reflect on the byways and the trail blazings that have brought this field to its present proud state of enlightenment with regard to the long sought-after means of controlling the procreative process in humankind. Clearly, there are many important and knotty problems yet to be resolved, but the pace of progress over the past several years has quickened to the extent that one is left in expectant wonderment as to where and when the next revolutionizing development will occur.

The experimental method of studying reproduction was initiated in 1849 with Berthold's discovery of a blood-borne activity that came from the testis and stimulated growth of distant organs such as the comb and wattles. In so doing he utilized one of the most fundamental means of demonstrating the function of an endocrine organ, namely, surgical removal to determine what deficiencies follow, coupled with implantation or transplantation to ascertain whether the deficiencies were repaired. At that time it was not possible to take the next step, namely, preparation of an active extract of the testes, because nothing was known about the nature of the bioactivity. Forty years later, Brown-Sequard claimed to have prepared an active extract of dog testes; however, as is well known, his enthusiastic claims for restoration of his own sexual activity at an advanced age were not substantiated. Actually, these simple means of studying reproductive physiology persisted well into the twentieth century, including the studies of such pioneering stalwarts as Marshall, Heape, Prenant, Bouin, Ancel, Loeb, Cushing, and Aschner. Observations otherwise were limited to cyclic and seasonal changes in sexual behavior among common laboratory and small domestic animals. This type of eyeball research remained in vogue through the early 1920s and overlapped the extension of visualization to the microscopic level. The latter revealed, for the first time, the precise timing of events in the ovarian cycle through microscopically observable cellular changes in the vaginal fluid. My point in mentioning these early studies is to emphasize that although the tools and techniques were inordinately primitive by present standards, the results established a firm base of knowledge on which to build.

The study of cyclic changes in the vaginal smear in rats and the findings of estrogenic activity in follicular fluid during the early 1920s led to an explosion of interest in the study of reproduction. The field was fortunate in attracting to its ranks a small band of exceedingly able biologists and biochemists who, in 1932, were to become authors of the classic first edition compendium, *Sex and Internal Secretions,* a volume overwhelmingly devoted to reproductive endocrinology. It was this landmark of progress that finally gave propriety to the study of reproduction and put it on a par with the study of other major bodily systems. Incredible as it may seem, it was only a decade earlier that a distinguished panel of the National Research Council had declared that sex research was not a fitting topic for scientific study.

Lest our pride in today's spectacular pace of progress unduly bedazzle the mind, it should not be overlooked that the developments recorded in the ten-year span from 1926 to 1936 may never be equaled. Among those monumental achievements, all of the native sex steroid hormones were brought to light, their structures were determined, their functions were defined, and they were made available in pure form for research and therapy. Similarly, all of the pituitary, placental, and urinary tropic hormones were identified, and their functions were defined. Like today's competition for priority rights, publicity, and potential financial gain, these earlier periods also were times for intense rivalries, but rarely with prospects for financial rewards. It would be difficult to overstate the boost that was given to basic and clinical research in reproduction as a result of the availability of estradiol-17B, testosterone, and progesterone in pure form and of known potency. The replacement of homemade extracts and such elastic entities as rat units, mouse units, capon units, and so forth, with micrograms of pure hormone was revolutionizing and allowed the study of reproduction on a quantitative basis.

Prior to World War II the thrust of research on reproduction dealt predominantly with the steroid hormones. This was the heyday of steroid biochemistry. After World War II the emphasis shifted to the protein and peptide hormones, where it still remains strong. This prolonged and difficult effort yielded many biochemical triumphs. Most notable among these were the isolation of the pituitary, placental, and urinary gonadotropins, as well as the determination of their primary structure as glycoproteins comprised of two dissimilar and covalently bonded subunits, the isolation and synthesis of the gonadotropin-releasing hormone (GnRH) of hypothalamic origin, and the isolation and structural characterization of relaxin.

The availability of pure protein and polypeptide hormones made possible the production of hormone-specific antibodies as well as the application of immunological techniques to the study of reproduction. An outcome of great consequence was the development of radioimmunoassay as the new means of measuring all of the hormones relating to reproduction. The sensitivity of this new technique was so great that it made possible, for the first time, the measurement of all these hormones in the body fluids. It had the further distinct advantage of requiring such a small amount of fluid that the monitoring of blood levels of the hormones of reproduction could be done throughout an estrous or menstrual cycle by close serial sampling. This revealed still another and most unexpected finding, the pulsatile pattern of secretion.

Identifying the homeostatic mechanism(s) responsible for maintaining a steady state in various physiologic systems of the body has been fraught with many challenging problems, but these pale in comparison with the difficulties encountered in trying to elucidate the mechanisms maintaining a constantly changing system, a characteristic of the reproductive system of female mammals. The earliest piece of evidence suggested the existence of a "push-pull" mechanism that later came to be known as *negative feedback*. It was based on the demonstration that an estrogenic extract administered to immature rats would maintain the ovaries in an infantile state. This was quickly followed by conclusive evidence that estrogen acted to inhibit pituitary follicle-stimulating hormone (FSH) stimulation of follicular growth and maturation; however, the effect on luteinizing hormone (LH), ovulation, and luteinization remained unsettled. Gaps continued to exist in all proposed explanations of reproductive cycles. None of these explanations took into account the influence of photoperiodicity on seasonal breeders, nor did they account for the role of the stimulus of mating in nonspontaneous ovulators. Following the discovery of the hypothalamic control of pituitary function, estrogen was shown to exert its action on both the pituitary and the hypothalamus; however, the problem of accounting for cyclicity remained. Adding to the complexity, radioimmunoassay revealed an unexpectedly high level of blood estrogen just prior to ovulation, an event not in keeping with the negative feedback concept.

Finally, after many years of searching for a way out of this frustrating situation, a glimmer of light appeared at the end of this long dark tunnel—light that soon turned to brilliance. In 1969, Goding and associated found that the administration of large doses of estrogen to ewes at the time of estrus did not block, but instead entrained, ovulation. Shortly thereafter, in more elaborate examination of the relationship of blood estrogen levels and ovulation in rhesus monkeys in Knobil's laboratory, it was revealed that elevated estrogen levels preceded and appeared to trigger ovulation. On further examination, Knobil and colleagues found that when blood estrogen reached a critical level the feedback mechanism switched from a negative to a positive, or stimulative, action. This utterly new finding greatly advanced our understanding of the endocrine mechanism governing reproductive cycles. There still remain, however, some uncertainties: Why does the switch in feedback action occur; to what extent and at what stage of the cycle does estrogen act at the level of the pituitary or the hypothalamus, or both; and lastly, what role, if any, do the ovarian peptides, especially inhibin, play in controlling reproductive cycles?

The progress of research on reproduction has been chronicled in numerous review articles by individual authors. Many have appeared in *Recent Progress in Hormone Research, Volumes 1 to 42.* Other major sources include the multiple editions of such titles as: *Marshall's Physiology of Reproduc-*

tion, now being produced in its fourth edition; *Sex and Internal Secretions,* whose third and last edition was issued in 1961; two volumes on the *Female Reproductive System* (1973), and one on the *Male Reproductive System* (1975) in *Section 7 of the Handbook of Physiology,* published by the American Physiological Society; and four serial volumes on reproductive physiology in the *International Review of Physiology,* the last one being issued in 1983. The present volume will provide comprehensive coverage and meet the current needs of the field of reproductive physiology, a field that is rapidly gathering momentum from the application of new and highly sophisticated tools and techniques.

In viewing the vast literature dealing with research on the male and female reproductive systems and considering the rate at which it is accumulating, one might ask whether this staggering proliferation of books and articles is essential to progress; the answer is an emphatic "Yes!" The yardstick by which progress is measured in this or any other field is not in number of articles published or amount of financial support but in improved understanding. Such gains are generally marked by sharp peaks at indeterminate intervals, separated by avalanches of incremental gains, as recorded in an ever-growing list of journals. The point to remember is that without this persistent chipping away at a major problem there would be no solutions and no quantum leaps forward. In research very little comes from out of the blue. Part of the driving force in research is its adventuresome nature and ever-present possibility that one's efforts will pay off in an important manner. It may not be entirely fair, but in research (as in most human activities), the spoils go to the victor in the form of kudos, prizes, awards, public attention, and, increasingly in the present technological age, monetary gains—sometimes of great magnitude. What effect this latter may have, if any, on the long-cherished sanctity of science has not been determined, but it has become a matter of concern.

This volume bears the title *The Physiology of Reproduction.* Physiology, by traditional consensus, is that branch of science which studies the functions of a living organism or any of its parts and includes the basic underlying processes. It will be understood that most of the studies reviewed here will be based more on holistic research than on research at the submicroscopic or molecular level. It is unfortunate that the excitement generated by recent fantastic advances in molecular biology and development has tended to downgrade the value of whole-animal research, and physiology in particular is sometimes looked upon as passé. Actually, the two categories of research are complementary, and both are essential for maximal advancement of knowledge. Whole-animal research cannot become outdated because it is the quintessence of biological relevance and the means by which molecular findings must ultimately be evaluated.

In the same vein, no one immersed in reproductive endocrinology can be unaware of the current tendency to regard research at the molecular level as representative of exceptional scientific talent. This is a common consequence of the opening of a new arena of investigation. I recall an incident that happened at a scientific meeting back in the 1930s. The first three papers in a session chaired by an eminent embryologist were on endocrine topics—mine was the third. That being ended, the chairman took pains to assure the audience that the meeting could now turn to considerations of more fundamental nature. One of the other three papers was given by Herbert M. Evans, who bristled noticeably but held his fire. There was also an earlier period when one either worked on steroid biochemistry or something of lesser appeal like biology. Anyone who remembers the 1950s will recall a flash-in-the-pan ignited by cybernetics, a study of automatic control systems both neural and physical. The gurus of cybernetics captured the attention of the press and of audiences throughout the land, but eventually this obsession suffered the fate of other passing preoccupations. My own observation is that the closer one approaches the molecular level of research, the more one becomes dependent on highly sophisticated instrumentation to make the observations and to read out results that are often quite free of extraneous variables. Toward the obverse situation, one's dependence on an extensive background of experience and physiological insight increases as does the unavoidable complex of *in vivo* variables that must be taken into account. In either case we have today the availability of far more diverse approaches to a given problem in any field of biomedical research than has ever existed before. In Berthold's day there was only one experimental method available; today's number is untold but is probably in the hundreds, perhaps thousands. That is an exceedingly promising situation and one to which investigators of all persuasions must adjust. Open minds will experience exhilaration over substantive achievements at any point on this observational spectrum.

One of the major factors influencing research on reproduction has been the availability of funds or lack thereof. Prior to the institution of federal funding (i.e., prior to the middle of the twentieth century), reproductive research was sparsely supported by university departmental funds, industry, small grants from the Committee for Research in Problems of Sex within the National Research Council, and some aid from the Rockefeller Foundation. The National Institutes of Health were slow in providing significant support of research on reproduction because of restrictions on the support of work related in any way to birth control. This occurred despite the simultaneous postwar baby boom. What kept research afloat during this critical period was major support by the Ford Foundation plus lesser contributions by other major foundations. It was not until the establishment in 1968 of the Center for Population Research in the NICHD that major governmental funding in this area became available, but the boost was short-lived. As a result of the imposition of fiscal restraints in the early 1970s, federal support dwindled and has remained at a minimal level ever since. Support from all sources is woefully incommensurate with the distressing expansion of the human population and the need for safe, effective, economical, and readily available means of limiting human fertility.

The physiology of reproduction is predominantly under hormonal control. The first essential step in studying reproduction was identification of the hormones involved and the functions they serve. This having been accomplished, efforts turned to a detailed analysis as to how hormones act within the body. During the past decade there has been a rising tide of interest in the binding of steroid, protein, or peptide hormones to receptors on specific target cells. Much effort is currently being directed toward the isolation and chemical characterization of these receptors. They are known to be composed of a protein or proteins, and some information has already been gained as to their partial or provisional structure. This, however, is only a preliminary step in the complex process whereby hormone action results in an end response such as growth, secretion of a target cell hormone, or altered behavior. The curtain has already been raised on the climatic and final chapter of the story on how hormones act. This involves linkage of the hormone-receptor complex with the nuclear genetic apparatus leading through a now well-defined series of processes to the manifestation of a physiological response in the living organism. Genes that bring about the expression of certain hormonal signals are being isolated, modified, transferred between species, and also inserted into bacteria where they direct the biosynthesis of specific hormones in large quantity. Thus genes are being manipulated in ways that raise the potential of altering the reproductive process. It is largely as a result of developments in endocrinology at the molecular level that bewildering possibilities loom on the horizons of reproductive research—they are within reach; they are science, not fiction; and they stagger the imagination.

It being granted that nothing succeeds like success, then a new edition of this highly successful two-volume compendium on *The Physiology of Reproduction* is destined for an illustrious fate. This second edition will maintain the same high standards of the first and again fulfill an existing need in a field that is experiencing rapid growth and exhilarating progress. Like the first edition, this one will provide a critical assessment of the state-of-the-art in every aspect of research on the physiology of reproduction by eminent authorities.

In the years intervening between this edition and the last, notable changes have taken place in the study of reproduction. These stem largely from major advances in technology. Remarkable new instruments, techniques, and methods have enabled investigators to probe ever deeper into the interaction between hormones and genes, thereby eliciting *in vivo* responses. New parameters are being added to the target tissues of the classical reproductive hormones as revealed by the presence of receptor sites in tissues, the physiologic significance of which often remains tantalizingly obscure. Similarly, newly identified substances of endocrine or paracrine nature are being added to this domain of research with persisting frequency. Some of these substances—the endothelins, interleukins, activins, inhibins and prorenin, to name a few—also exhibit a puzzling array of effects on extraneous tissues. Their study is being aided by the fact that their structure is known and, though rare, they are available.

Great strides are also being made in many other aspects of research on reproduction. Much work is being done on the structure of receptors and the loci of binding sites on segments of the folded gonadotropic molecules. A full-scale effort is underway seeking an elucidation of the neural mechanism underlying pulsatile secretion. Neuroendocrinologists are closing in on an elusive pulse generator located in the central nervous system. This looms as another landmark discovery in reproductive biology.

Research on reproduction is flourishing and the future appears bright. The taboos are gone. All aspects of the reproductive process are an open book. One area that has taken a quantum leap forward is the clinical application of an important body of relevant new knowledge gained in both basic and clinical spheres. Expanded opportunities have been opened by greatly improved diagnostic procedures, more effective treatment of disorders, and new methods of controlling fertility. Contributing greatly to this explosive development is the dissemination of information on reproductive matters to the lay public by the mass media. Concerned individuals have been made aware of the existing new means of manipulating the male and female reproductive systems for enhancement or inhibition of fertility. The joys and comforts that accrue respectively to these opposing modes of fertility control have enriched the lives of a grateful public. To that end I may note that it was by virtue of these frontier reproductive measures that my own progeny includes a new grandson and namesake.

Roy O. Greep

Preface to the First Edition

This work was undertaken, after much deliberation, in an attempt to fill a need for a comprehensive, scholarly treatise on the physiology of mammalian reproduction. A major inspiration for this effort has been the volume *Sex and Internal Secretions,* a factual and conceptual beacon which guided generations of reproductive biologists from the time of its first publication in 1932 to the appearance of its last edition over a quarter of a century ago.

The book is divided into five major sections, and these, in turn, are loosely arrayed in two domains. The first covers the components of the reproductive system, and the second discusses reproductive processes and their physiological control. In the latter, we have included reproductive behavior in the conviction that this fundamental aspect of reproduction clearly belongs in the physiological realm and will remain a demanding challenge long after all the other mysteries in the field have been resolved.

In our discussion of reproductive systems, we have been aware of the profound differences among mammals in the way some fundamental processes, such as the ovarian cycle, are controlled. We have addressed this issue, in part, by providing separate coverage of major mammalian groups where this seemed appropriate. It has been left to the reader to ascertain the similarities and differences among them. In any case, we must ever be mindful in considering reproductive processes, from the control of ovulation to the initiation of parturition, not to extrapolate from one species to another without due reflection.

It is hoped that this book will be useful to all serious students of reproductive physiology be they scientists, teachers, or physicians.

THE EDITORS

Preface

The second edition of this work represents the labor of some 61 groups of authors and is, therefore, marked by inevitable redundancies and lacunae. The six years that have elapsed between the first and second editions have seen dramatic and often unanticipated developments in some aspects of reproductive biology, with only little new understanding in others. But, as expected, the quantity and difficulty of the questions raised has increased manifold. We remain markedly ill-informed of the complex control systems that govern reproductive processes and surprised by the striking species differences in the accomplishment of common, fundamental reproductive tasks. The control of ovulation, the advent of puberty, and the initiation of parturition are but three cases in point.

We are deeply saddened by the untimely loss of Larry L. Ewing who contributed so much to the construction of the first edition with his wisdom and good humor, to say nothing of his hard work and devotion to the enterprise.

As these volumes were in the final stages of completion, the field also lost one of its great pioneers and most sagacious contributors, John W. Everett. We are privileged to count one of his last publications among the chapters of this work.

We hope that our expectations for the first edition have also been achieved in the second: scholarly, comprehensive examinations of the principal issues in reproductive physiology that will remain useful for a decade, at least, to all serious students of reproductive physiology.

THE EDITORS

The Gametes, Fertilization, and Early Embryogenesis

The Physiology of Reproduction, Second Edition,
edited by E. Knobil and J.D. Neill,
Raven Press, Ltd., New York © 1994.

CHAPTER 1

Sex Determination and Differentiation

Frederick W. George and Jean D. Wilson

Sexual differentiation in the eutherian mammal is a sequential process beginning with the establishment of chromosomal sex at fertilization, followed by the development of gonadal sex, and culminating in the formation of the sexual phenotypes (Fig. 1). Each step in this process is dependent on the preceding one, and under normal circumstances, chromosomal sex agrees with phenotypic sex. Occasionally, however, chromosomal sex and phenotypic sex do not agree, or the sexual phenotype is ambiguous. Although abnormalities of sexual development occur at many different levels, they are rarely life-threatening. Consequently, the overall process of sexual differentiation has been carefully studied and is probably understood in greater detail than any other embryonic system. In many cases, disorders of sexual differentiation are inherited as single gene mutations, and the analysis of these disorders has been especially informative in defining the molecular and genetic determinants in sexual development. The principal focus of this chapter is on the development of sex in humans; however, animal studies are discussed when they provide important insight.

Department of Internal Medicine, The University of Texas Southwestern Medical Center at Dallas, Dallas, Texas 75235

CHROMOSOMAL SEX

Early genetic studies in *Drosophila* documented that sex determination in the fly is controlled by the number of X chromosomes and that the Y chromosome plays no role in the process except for a contribution to male fertility (reviewed in ref. 1). This paradigm was also thought to apply to mammalian sex determination, but when karyotyping techniques for mammalian chromosomes were developed in the 1960s, it became apparent that the presence of the Y chromosome in the mammal correlates with male development. Indeed, no matter how many X chromosomes are present in the genome of the conceptus, the presence of a single Y chromosome (as in 47,XXY, 48,XXXY, 48,XXYY, etc.) dictates formation of a testis and, therefore, male development (2). Two X chromosomes appear to be necessary for normal ovarian development, and the presence of a second X chromosome in men (as in 47,XXY) impairs spermatogenesis. A likely explanation for the infertility in the

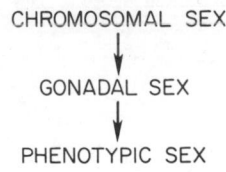

CHROMOSOMAL SEX
↓
GONADAL SEX
↓
PHENOTYPIC SEX

FIG. 1. Jost paradigm.

47,XXY state is the inactivation of the X chromosome during pairing of the X and Y chromosomes spermatogenesis (2) (see below). In other words, some X-encoded gene product must impair male germ-cell development (3). This concept is in keeping with the fact that balanced translocations of X chromosomes to autosomes that prevent complete inactivation of X-chromosomal genes in mice (4) and humans (5) also cause male infertility. Furthermore, in the creeping vole (6), the X chromosome is eliminated from the testicular germ cell line, implying that a single X chromosome is not essential for either testicular differentiation or spermatogenesis.

The Y Chromosome

The Y chromosome is one of the smallest of the human chromosomes, although its size can vary considerably because of variation in length of the long arm (Fig. 2). The Y chromosomes of virtually all species, including the human, contain "satellites" of deoxyribonucleic acid (DNA) that are visible under certain staining procedures. However, because the Y chromosome-associated satellite DNA of one species does not cross-hybridize with that of other species, it is unlikely that these satellites play a fundamental role in the function of the chromosome (1).

Homologous single-copy regions of DNA on the human X and Y chromosomes have been identified by restriction endonuclease techniques. These sequences of DNA appear to be unique to the human and different from homologous regions on the sex chromosomes in other species. Consequently, although the regions are specific to the sex chromosomes, they are also thought not to play a role in sex determination (7). Some of the homologous regions are on the tips of the short arms of the X and Y chromosomes (the pseudoautosomal region) (8) and are responsible for pairing of the two chromosomes during meiosis (see below).

About 70% of the DNA of the human Y consists of repeated sequences on the long arm (9). These sequences are related, in an evolutionary sense, to sequences on the human X. Hence, no perceptible phenotypic effect is apparent when the long arm of the Y is translocated onto an autosome. These repetitive fragments are present in such diverse species as *Drosophila,* mouse, and human and are composed of two repeating base quadruplets (GATA and GACA). In the human, these repetitive fragments are thought to be responsible for much of the variability in length among normal Y chromosomes and for fluorescence of the long arm. Two fluorescent bands are clearly visible in interphase nuclei (Fig. 2).

A map of the entire euchromatic region (short arm, centromere, proximal long arm) of the human Y chromosome has been constructed by analyzing the DNA of individuals with partial Y chromosomes (10). The Y-specific genes are interspersed among regions of DNA that are homologous to sequences on the X chromosome (11).

Testis-Determining Gene

Cytologic analyses of structural abnormalities of the Y chromosome in humans provided the first clue as to the location of the testis determinant. Loss of the fluorescent segment of the long arm (Yq−) (Fig. 2) or formation of a Y "ring" chromosome (which involves loss of the distal-most segments of both the long and short arms) does not interfere with formation of a normal testis (2). Furthermore, male development is normal when the Y chromosome consists of a duplicated short arm [i(Y_p)] with no long arm. However, isochromosomes for the long arm of the Y in which there is loss of the short arm [i(Y_q)] (Fig.

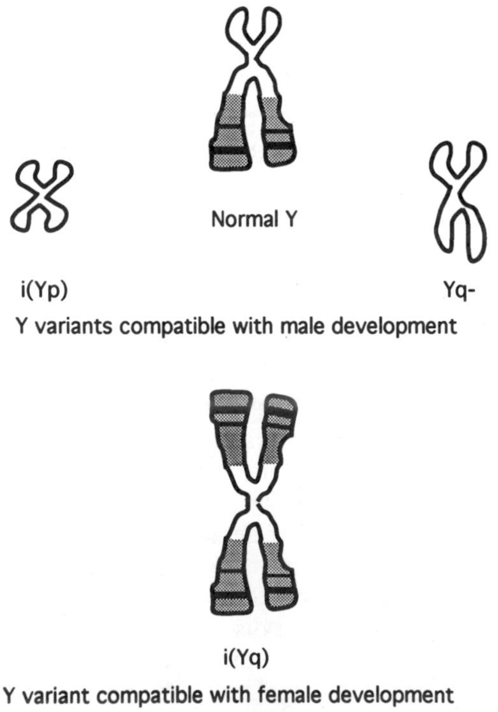

FIG. 2. Normal and variant Y chromosomes. *Shading* indicates quinacrine-bright region of long arm (Yq). Three abnormal types are depicted: i(Yp), isochrome of short arm; i(Yq), isochrome of long arm; Yq−, fragment arising as result of loss of distal long arm.

2) result in failure of testicular development and formation of a female phenotype (12–14). On the basis of such studies, it was deduced that the testis-determining region of the Y chromosome is located near the centromere on the short arm (15). Additional genes on the short or long arms appear to be essential for normal spermatogenesis and hence for male fertility (8).

A theory that gained much attention during the 1970s and early 1980s was that the primary inducer of testicular differentiation is a histocompatibility antigen (H-Y) encoded on the short arm (16). However, there is now considerable evidence that the relationship between the expression of the H-Y antigen and testicular development is not one of cause and effect (17–21). The discovery of male mice with testes that were H-Y antigen negative effectively ruled out the H-Y antigen as a candidate for the primary testis inducer (22). In fact, the gene encoding the H-Y antigen is located on the long arm of the human Y chromosome (23).

The study of XX males and XY females has been invaluable in identifying the testis-determining gene. Initially, Page et al. (24), using deletion analyses focused on region 1A2 of the human Y chromosome because it was apparently the sole region of the Y chromosome present in an XX male and absent in an XY female. All 140 kb of this region were cloned, and a gene that encodes a zinc-finger-containing protein (ZFY) was located and postulated as the testis determinant (24). However, three complicating issues argued against a role for ZFY as the primary testis determinant. First, the gene has a nearly identical homologue on the X chromosome (ZFX) (25–27). Second, homologous sequences to ZFY are found on autosomes in marsupials despite the fact that male differentiation in the marsupial is Y determined (28). Third, the ZFY gene is absent in most true hermaphrodites and in many 46,XX males (29–31).

The fact that the XX males described by Palmer et al. (31) lacked the ZFY but were positive for markers in the 1A1 region of the Y chromosome focused the search for the testis determinant on the region distal to the ZFY gene. A single-copy gene, SRY, was identified in the 35 kb of DNA in the distal half of region 1A1 (32) (Fig. 3). Although the position of this gene in region 1A1 of the Y was in conflict with the original proposal that the testis-determining region had been isolated to region 1A2 of the Y, the apparent paradox was resolved when Page et al. (33) subsequently reported that there is an additional deletion in region 1A1 of the XY female they studied. A similar gene, *Sry,* was mapped in the *Sxr* region of the mouse, was deleted in an XY female mouse, and is expressed in supporting cells of the testis (34,35).

Direct evidence that SRY is the primary testis determinant was obtained when the mouse *Sry* gene was introduced as a partial transgene into mouse embryos and was shown to cause testicular development in chromosomally female transgenic mice (36).

Ovary-Determining Genes

Many genes are involved in gonadal differentiation, and it is likely that the SRY gene on the Y chromosome

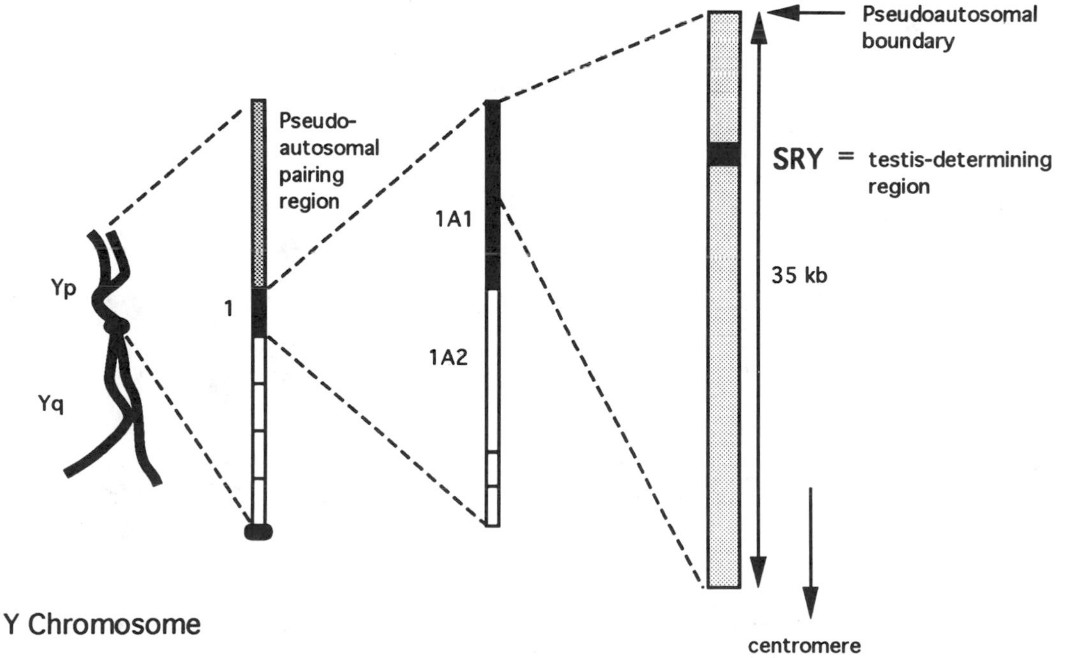

FIG. 3. Location of sex-determining region (SRY) on Y chromosome. (Adapted from ref. 283.)

acts as a switch to direct the expression of a genetic cascade that results in testicular development. Eicher and Washburn (37) reported that genotypic male mice carrying a Y chromosome derived from a *Mus domesticus* strain on the genetic background of an inbred *Mus musculus* strain (C57BL/6J) develop ovaries or ovotestes. Ovarian development in these animals is apparently due to interaction between an autosomal recessive gene carried by C57BL/6J and the Y chromosome of *Mus domesticus.* Other autosomal testis-determining loci have subsequently been identified (38,39). Based on these results, Eicher and colleagues have proposed that, besides the testis-determining gene(s) on the Y chromosome and the autosomal genes necessary for testicular differentiation, ovary-determining genes are essential for ovarian embryogenesis. Burgoyne (40) also postulated the existence of specific ovary-determining genes. According to his formulation, the testis-determining genes in normal XY males are activated before, and neutralize, ovary-determining gene(s). XX individuals lack the initial testis-determining gene, and hence the ovary-determining gene(s) is free to act. Mutations within the testis-determining loci that interfere with the timely and coordinate expression of these genes may prevent suppression of ovarian determinants, with subsequent development of ovarian tissue in XY individuals (41).

Pairing of the X and Y Chromosomes; Pseudoautosomal Inheritance

The two X chromosomes in females pair at the centromere and segregate during the first meiotic division of oogenesis by a mechanism analogous to the pairing of the autosomes. The X and Y chromosomes also pair during meiosis to ensure appropriate segregation. However, the pairing of X and Y does not occur at the centromere but rather at a region of homology on the distal, short arms of the two chromosomes (42) (Fig. 4). In this way, the chromosomes duplicate and partition properly on the spindle. Thus, two types of spermatozoa are produced at the second meiotic division, those containing a single X chromosome and those containing a single Y.

The first genetic evidence that crossing-over is a regular feature of X and Y pairing was provided by Keitges et al. (43), who demonstrated that the mouse steroid sulfatase (*STS*), which appeared to be inherited autosomally, is in fact encoded on either the X or Y chromosome. This observation suggested that obligatory crossover of the X and Y proximal to the *STS* locus accounts for the presence of X or Y linkage. Pseudoautosomal loci have also been reported in the human (44,45). Because the sex-determining region of the Y chromosome is located near (within 20 kb) the region of X-Y pairing and obliga-

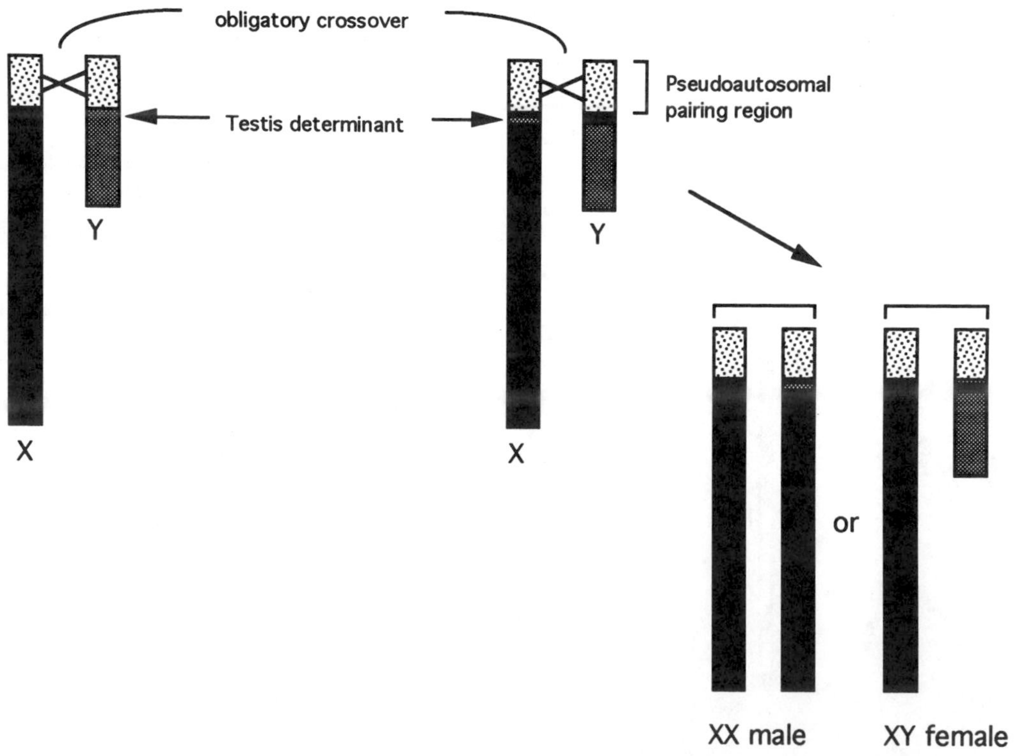

FIG. 4. Sex chromosome pairing and aberrant transfer of testis-determining region of Y to X chromosome. (Adapted from ref. 283.)

tory crossover, it is not surprising that the testis determinant, on occasion, is transferred to the X chromosome or that the gametes thus formed may transmit information for sex determination that is apparently contradictory to the sex chromosome composition (Fig. 4).

Anomalies of Sex Determination

The XX_{Sxr} Male Mouse

The sex-reversal mutation in the mouse (*Sxr*), causes $X_{Sxr}X$ females to develop as phenotypic (albeit infertile) males (46). On the basis of lineage studies, this trait was originally assumed to be caused by an autosomal mutation. In 1966, Ferguson-Smith (47) proposed that sex reversal could be explained by an abnormal exchange of genetic material during meiosis that resulted in the transfer of the testis-determining gene to the X chromosome and deletion of this corresponding region from the paired Y chromosome.

In keeping with this formulation, a Y-specific DNA fragment was detected on the distal end of an X chromosome in XX_{Sxr} mice in 1982 (48,49). This finding, coupled with the formulation of Ferguson-Smith (47) and Burgoyne (50) that crossing-over occurs in the pairing region of the X and Y chromosomes during meiosis, provided an explanation for both the apparent (pseudo) autosomal inheritance of the Sxr mutation and for testicular development in the absence of a Y chromosome (51). The testis determinant is present as a duplicated element on the distal pairing region of the Y chromosome of male mice carrying the *Sxr* gene on the Y chromosome. Translocation of this duplicated testis-determining region to the X chromosome during meiosis and transmission of the "mutant" X chromosome to XX offspring causes testicular differentiation. Although XY males carrying the duplicated testis-determining region on the distal X chromosome are fertile, $X_{Sxr}X$ males are not. In this sense, this disorder is a phenocopy of the 47,XXY Klinefelter's syndrome in humans involving only a fragment of, rather than the entire, Y chromosome.

Sex Reversal in Man

Sex reversal also occurs in humans. The incidence of a 46,XX karyotype in phenotypic men is approximately one in 20,000 to 24,000 births (52). Clinical features include small, firm testes, normal male wolffian duct derivatives, and male external genitalia. Azoospermia, and hence infertility, are invariably present (53,54).

These 46,XX men resemble those with Klinefelter's syndrome (55). Today, most cases of human sex reversal are considered to be the result of transfer of the testis-determining gene on the Y chromosome to the X chromosome during an abnormal crossover event in meiosis, analogous to the situation in the *Sxr* mouse, and many XX males, like the XX_{Sxr} mouse, contain Y-specific DNA on the tip of an X chromosome (15,56–58). Additional genes encoded on the human X and Y chromosomes are also inherited pseudoautosomally (59–61), and at least one of these genes, MIC2, is sufficiently close to the testis-determining region on the short arm of the Y to be a potential marker for the testis determinant(s) (62).

True Hermaphroditism

True hermaphroditism is a condition in which both an ovary and testis, or a gonad with histologic features of both ovary and testis (ovotestis), are present (63). To justify the diagnosis, both types of germ cells must be present; the presence of ovarian stroma without oocytes is not sufficient. True hermaphroditism is actually several different disorders (64). About two-thirds of human subjects have a 46,XX karyotype, one-tenth have a 46,XY karyotype, and the remainder are chromosomal mosaics (i.e., either 46,XX/46,XY or 45,X/46,XY chimeras). Instances of true hermaphroditism associated with mosaicism are generally assumed to be clonal in origin, with the X- or XX-containing cells giving rise to ovarian cell lines and the Y-containing cell lines giving rise to testicular elements. 46,XY true hermaphroditism is assumed to be caused by a mutation in the testis-determining gene(s) that impairs suppression of the ovarian determinants (37,38,65).

Hermaphroditism in the presence of a 46,XX karyotype, like the XX male syndrome, is an apparent contradiction to the axiom that a Y chromosome is necessary for testicular differentiation. Although several family aggregates of 46,XX true hermaphroditism have been reported (66–70), most cases are sporadic in occurrence. The available data in the familial cases are compatible either with autosomal dominant mutations or translocation of a fragment of the Y chromosome in a parental cell line. Indeed, approximately one-fourth of 46,XX true hermaphrodites harbor genetic sequences indicative of Y to X translocations. Also, two families have been reported in which one affected member was a 46,XX male and the other was a 46,XX true hermaphrodite (71,72). The cause of the remaining instances of 46,XX true hermaphroditism is unknown.

At a theoretical level, the same type of situation, namely, duplication of the testis-determining region on the Y chromosome and translocation of these genes onto the X chromosome, could explain the development of the XX male and the XX true hermaphrodite, depending on the completeness and frequency of the inactivation of such testis-determining genes during the embryogenesis of the XX individual carrying such a translocation. This model has two implications for the human disorder: First, the testis-determining region, and hence Y chromosome fragments, should be detectable in all cells from 46,XX true hermaphrodites and from 46,XX men. Second, if the translocation is to an X chromosome and not to an autosome, it explains why the XX male is more common than the XX true hermaphrodite. It has yet to be proven if this model can explain the potential fertility of the XX true hermaphrodite.

X Chromosome Inactivation

According to the Lyon (73) hypothesis, extragonadal cells in the female have only one active X chromosome; additional X chromosomes are inactivated and form the sex chromatin bodies in the nuclei of somatic cells in females. The mechanism of inactivation of the X chromosome differs in the ovary and in peripheral tissues. In women heterozygous for polymorphisms of the X-linked gene for glucose-6-phosphate dehydrogenase, oocytes express both alleles of this enzyme (74,75). Although both X chromosomes appear to be active in germ cells before they enter meiosis (76); Kratzer and Chapman (77) have shown that only one X chromosome is active in the ovary up to day 10 of embryogenesis in the mouse and that the inactive X is reactivated as the germ cells enter meiosis. Thus, although random X inactivation occurs in ovarian germ cells, the inactive X is reactivated during oogenesis. In testicular development, the single X chromosome appears to be inactivated as a part of the XY body. Random X inactivation in somatic cells involves a chemical modification of the DNA and is thought to be fundamentally different than the X chromosome inactivation in the formation of the XY body (78,79).

X/autosome translocations have been described in mice in which the normal X (the one not involved in the translocation) is preferentially inactivated (80). When female mice carrying such an X/autosome translocation (the translocated X is designated X_T) are mated with males carrying the sex-reversal mutation ($X_{Sxr}Y$), the $X_{Sxr}X_T$ offspring can develop as infertile males, fertile females, or hermaphrodites (81–83). One explanation for this finding is that the region of the X chromosome that carries the *Sxr* gene (or testis-determining region) may be inactivated in some cells but not others. The inactivation process is conceived as spreading to a variable extent from the inactive X chromatin to the *Sxr* fragment, and it is assumed that the extent of inactivation is transmitted to progeny cells after the time of X chromosome inactivation during embryogenesis. In effect, such XX individuals are mosaics, with some cell lines expressing *Sxr* and some not. Gonadal sex (and hence the aggregate sex of the individual) depends on the proportion of cells expressing *Sxr* in the gonadal primordia. If 30% or more of the cells in a gonadal primordia are XY, a testis usually develops. When the X chromosome containing the *Sxr* gene is paired with an X chromosome carrying the autosomal translocation (X_TX_{Sxr}), most embryos develop as females, and hermaphrodites occur at a low, but measurable, frequency. However, when an X chromosome bearing the Sxr locus is paired with a normal X chromosome (XX_{Sxr}), half of the cells express *Sxr,* and most individuals will be infertile males; females and hermaphrodites are rare.

GONADAL SEX

Embryonic Development

The gonads develop as stratifications of the coelomic epithelium on the medial aspect of the mesonephric kidney (the urogenital ridge) around the fourth week of human gestation. Most cell types of the gonads are derived from the mesoderm of the urogenital ridges. The primordial germ cells originate, however, outside the area of the presumptive gonad and are initially identifiable in the entoderm of the yolk sac; they are derived from the primitive ectodermal cells of the inner cell mass (84) and are distinguishable from other cells of the developing embryo because of their large size, large, round nuclei and clear cytoplasm. Histochemically, they contain high alkaline phosphatase and glycogen (85). The mechanism by which the germ cells differentiate is not understood, but the process begins early so that primordial germ cells can be recognized in the 4.5-day-old human blastocyst (86,87). At the beginning of the fourth week of development, the germ cells begin to migrate by amoeboid movement (88–90) through the gut entoderm and into the mesoderm of the mesentery, finally ending up in the coelomic epithelium of the gonadal ridges. It is not known what entices the primordial germ cells to migrate to this area. However, once the gonadal ridges are reached, the gonocytes move from the epithelium into the parenchyma and lose their motile characteristics (91). Closely attached epithelial cells move with them into the underlying mesenchyme. The formation of the gonadal blastema is completed during the fifth week of human embryogenesis, and at this time, the primitive, "indifferent" gonad is composed of three distinct cell types: germ cells, supporting cells of the coelomic epithelium of the gonadal ridge that either give rise to the Sertoli cells of the testis or the granulosa cells of the ovary, and stromal (interstitial) cells derived from the mesenchyme of the gonadal ridge.

Histologic Differentiation of the Fetal Gonad

The first sign of sexual dimorphism of the gonads is the development of the primordial Sertoli cells and their aggregation into spermatogenic cords in the fetal testis (92). In the human, this occurs during the sixth week of gestation (93). The fetal ovary, however, shows no characteristic development until months later in embryogenesis and initially is identified histologically only by exclusion. At about the sixth month, the primitive granulosa cells begin to organize around the dividing oocytes to form single layers characteristic of primordial follicles (94). Gonadogenesis in other mammalian species is similar to that in humans in that histologic differentiation of the fetal testis precedes that of the ovary by days to weeks.

It seems unlikely that gonadal differentiation is totally dependent on the presence or type of germ cell that migrates into the coelomic epithelium of the gonadal ridge. Neither selective destruction of germ cells with drugs (95) nor surgical excision of primordial germ cells in the anterior germinal crest before they complete migration to the gonadal primordium (96) inhibits gonadal development. Furthermore, mutant mice homozygous for the atrichosis gene are genetically deficient in germ cells, yet the Sertoli cells differentiate and aggregate into tubules devoid of germ cells (97). Thus, the somatic cells of the primitive gonad alone can organize into an ovary or a testis irrespective of the presence or absence of the germ cells.

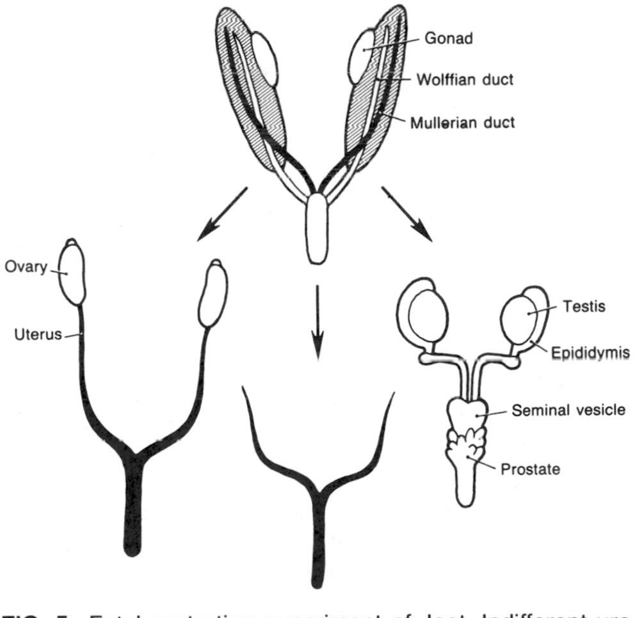

FIG. 5. Fetal castration experiment of Jost. Indifferent urogenital tract (*top*) undergoes male differentiation (*bottom right*) if a testis develops or female differentiation (*bottom left*) if an ovary develops. Embryos castrated before sexual differentiation develop as phenotypic females (*bottom middle*). (Adapted from ref. 99.)

Endocrine Differentiation of the Testis

By demonstrating that castration of sexually indifferent rabbit embryos of either sex results in female development (Fig. 5), Jost (98,99) established that the induced phenotype in eutherian mammals is male and that secretion from the fetal testes are necessary for male development. Development of the female urogenital tract occurs in the absence of gonads. Furthermore, Jost deduced that two hormones from the fetal testes are essential for male development: a peptide hormone that acts ipsilaterally to cause regression of the mullerian duct (mullerian-inhibiting hormone), and an androgenic steroid responsible for virilization of the wolffian duct, urogenital sinus, and urogenital tubercle.

Mullerian-Inhibiting Hormone

Mullerian-inhibiting hormone is a large (approximately 140 kDa) dimeric glycoprotein formed by the Sertoli cells of the fetal and newborn testis (100–105). It is thought to act locally to suppress mullerian duct development rather than as a circulating hormone (however, see ref. 106). The fetal mullerian duct is sensitive to the action of the hormone for only a short period during embryogenesis (107). Monoclonal antibodies to mullerian-inhibiting hormone (108,109) block mullerian duct regression in a species-specific manner in *in vitro* (110) and *in vivo* bioassays (111). Although mullerian duct regression begins in the male embryo shortly after formation of the spermatic cords in the fetal testis (107), the secretion of mullerian-inhibiting hormone is independent of spermatogenic tubule formation (112).

The cDNAs for the bovine and human mullerian-inhibiting hormones have been cloned (113–115). The longest cDNA isolated hybridizes to a 2000 nucleotide transcript expressed exclusively in gonadal tissues. Cate et al. (113) identified genomic clones from human and bovine cosmid libraries and established the identity of the cloned human gene by transfection/expression studies. The gene for human mullerian-inhibiting hormone has 78% homology with the bovine gene. The amino acid sequence in the carboxy terminus of the bovine and human polypeptides is extremely high, and both hormones contain two potential *N*-linked glycosylation sites (115). The human gene for mullerian-inhibiting hormone is located on chromosome 19 (116) and contains five coding exons, separated by relatively short introns, so that the total size of the gene is only 28 kb (107).

The concept that mullerian duct regression in the male is an active process is supported by studies of the persistent mullerian duct syndrome (117–120). In this disorder, genetic and phenotypic males have fallopian tubes and a uterus besides normal wolffian duct-derived structures. Indeed, two types of mutations have been described in this disorder. In one, nucleotide substitutions within the coding sequence of the gene either cause a premature stop codon so that no protein is formed (121) or cause an amino acid substitution so that an unstable protein is synthesized (122). In these varieties, no mullerian-inhibiting hormone can be assayed in the testis. In the other type of mutation, defects in action of the hormone are presumed to be responsible; for example, the testes of newborn dogs with this disorder secrete biologically active mullerian-inhibiting hormone, suggesting that the underlying mutation causes resistance to the action of the hormone (123).

Besides its role in causing regression of the mullerian duct in the male embryo, several types of evidence suggest that this hormone influences the histologic and endocrine differentiation of the gonad. First, the addition of purified mullerian-inhibiting hormone causes development of cord-like structures in cultured, 14-day fetal ovaries, suggesting that it may promote testicular differentiation (124). Second, the hormone induces endocrine sex reversal of fetal rat ovaries in culture (125). Third, female transgenic mice that express human mullerian-inhibiting hormone not only have complete failure of development of the mullerian-derived structures but also have gonads with testicular features, namely, the organization of somatic cells into cord-like structures (126).

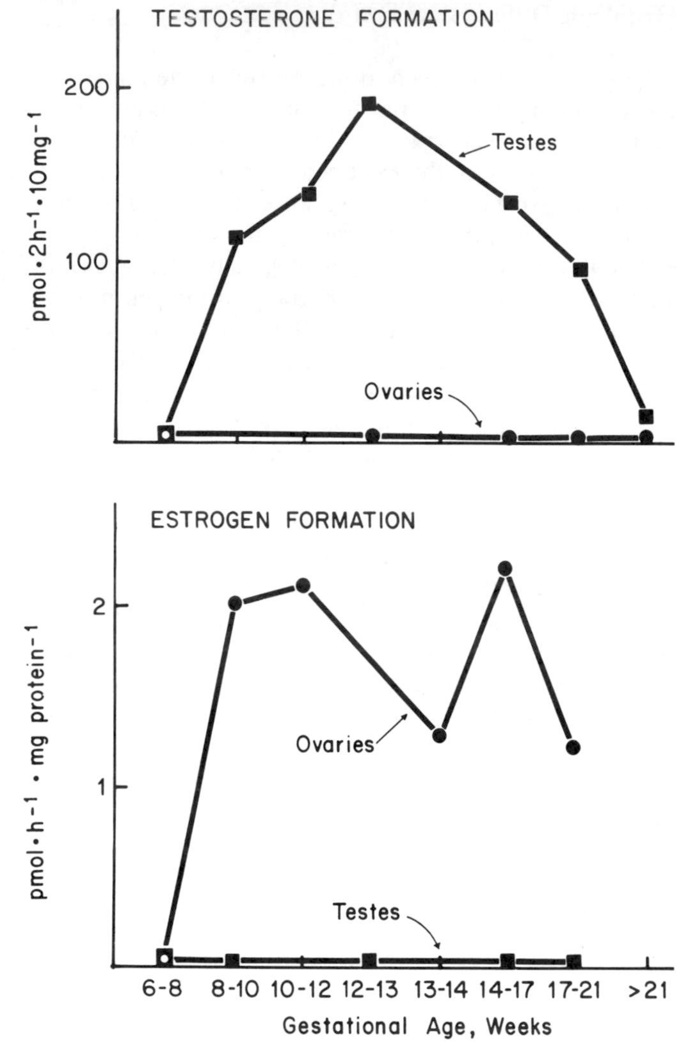

FIG. 6. Enzymatic differentiation of human fetal gonad. (Adapted from refs. 128 and 153.)

Androgen

The second developmental hormone of the fetal testis was deduced by Jost (98) to be an androgenic steroid. Testosterone, the principal testicular androgen in postnatal life, is also the androgenic steroid formed by the testes of rabbit and human embryos during male phenotypic development (127–129). Testosterone formation in the testis begins shortly after the onset of differentiation of the spermatogenic cords and is coincident with the histologic differentiation of the fetal Leydig cells (130).

The critical role of testosterone in the development of the male urogenital tract was deduced from three types of embryologic and endocrinologic evidence. First, as shown in Fig. 6, the fact that testosterone synthesis immediately precedes the initiation of virilization of the urogenital tract in a variety of species suggested a cause-and-effect relationship between the two events (127–129,131,132). Second, the administration of androgens to female embryos at the appropriate time in fetal development causes male development of the internal and external genitalia (133,134). Third, administration of pharmacologic agents that specifically inhibit the synthesis or action of androgens impairs male development (135,136).

This concept has been substantiated by genetic studies. For example, in the human, single-gene defects in androgen biosynthesis cause inadequate testosterone synthesis by the testis and incomplete virilization of the male embryo (137,138). Severely affected men may develop as phenotypic women, with complete failure of virilization of the wolffian ducts, urogenital sinus, and external genitalia. At the other extreme, mildly affected men appear normal, except for developmental abnormalities such as hypospadias. The fact that the fallopian tubes and uterus are absent in such patients indicates that regression of the mullerian ducts takes place normally under such circumstances and that mullerian duct regression is not primarily dependent on testosterone biosynthesis or action.

Regulation of Testosterone Synthesis in the Fetal Testis

The enzymatic differentiation of the fetal gonads that underlies the onset of endocrine function has been characterized in detail in the rabbit embryo. Endocrine differentiation of ovaries and testes in this species is apparent between days 17 and 18 of gestation and is manifested by an increase in the rate of 3β-hydroxysteroid dehydrogenase activity in the fetal testis and by an increase in aromatase (estrogen synthetase) in the fetal ovary (139). At this time of development, activities of all other enzymes in the pathway of steroid hormone synthesis are similar in ovaries and testes (140) (Fig. 7). Thus, in the rabbit, changes in the rates of only a few enzymatic reactions in the gonads at a critical time in embryonic development have profound consequences for sexual differentiation. Furthermore, this enzymatic differentiation appears to be an autonomous function of the steroidogenic cells, because it occurs at the appropriate time in fetal testes that are cultured in defined medium without hormones (141,142) and in testes that fail to develop spermatogenic cords (143).

Whether the actual rate of testosterone production in the fetal rabbit testis is regulated by fetal and/or maternal (placental) gonadotropins at the onset of testosterone synthesis is less clear. On the one hand, receptors for luteinizing hormone (LH) are present in the fetal rabbit testis at the time of initial testosterone synthesis (144): furthermore, these LH receptors are functional, as evidenced by the enhancement of testicular cyclic adenosine monophosphate (AMP) formation (142) and of cholesterol side-chain cleavage activity (140) by human chorionic gonadotropin. On the other hand, basal, unstimulated cholesterol side-chain cleavage activity in fetal rabbit testes in the absence of gonadotropin stimulation appears to be sufficient to provide enough steroid substrate to support maximal testosterone synthesis during the initial period of male phenotypic development. As a consequence, the onset of testosterone synthesis and the resulting differentiation of the male urogenital tract in rabbits may be independent of gonadotropin control. Later in embryogenesis, when sexual differentiation is far advanced, testosterone synthesis is regulated by gonadotropin (140).

It is uncertain whether these findings are applicable to the onset of fetal testosterone synthesis in other species. In the human, the situation is complicated by the fact that the placenta synthesizes and secretes large amounts of chorionic gonadotropin with potent LH activity during the time of embryonic sexual differentiation (145). Although LH receptors are present in the fetal testis as early as the twelfth week of gestation (146–148), it is not clear whether the addition of human chorionic gonadotropin *in vitro* is able to stimulate either basal cyclic AMP formation or testosterone synthesis during the critical initial phase (146,149,150). However, the report that male pseudohermaphroditism can result from a defect in testicular gonadotropin receptors is in keeping with a role for regulation of testosterone synthesis by gonadotropin at the time of male phenotypic differentiation (151). Until direct studies are performed in the human fetal testis between 8 and 12 weeks of gestation, it will not be possible to resolve the question of whether gonadotropin is critical for the initiation of testosterone synthesis in the human fetal testis. Because testosterone synthesis is gonadotropin-dependent during the latter two-thirds of human gestation, analogous to the situation in the rabbit embryo, it follows that those aspects of male sexual development that take place during this time—growth of the penis and descent of the testes—are probably gonadotropin-dependent in all species (152).

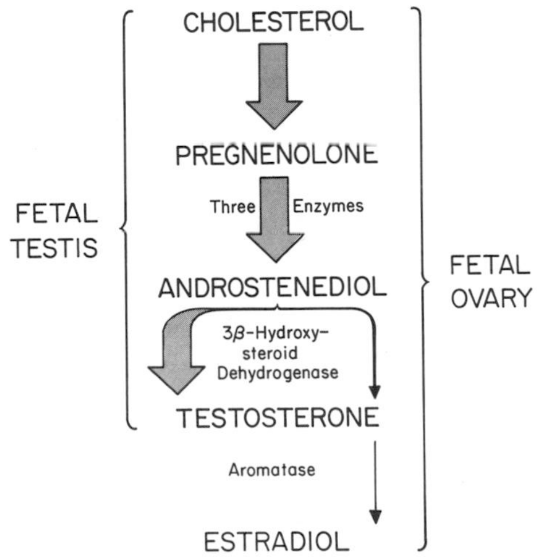

FIG. 7. Enzymatic differentiation of fetal rabbit ovaries and testes on day 18 of gestation.

Endocrine Differentiation of the Ovary

In many species, endocrine differentiation of the fetal ovary, as evidenced by the onset of the capacity to synthesize estrogen, occurs simultaneously with the development of the ability of the fetal testis to synthesize testosterone (139,153) (Fig. 6). Although estrogen formation does not appear to be essential for normal development of the female phenotype (98), estrogen may play a role in the development of the ovary itself (154).

Possible Role of Steroid Hormones in Gonadal Differentiation

In some species, it is possible to influence gonadal differentiation with sex hormones (reviewed in ref. 155). For example, in the embryonic male (ZZ) bird, treatment with estrogens during embryonic development leads to the development of an ovotestis. In amphibians and fish, treatment with steroid hormones of the opposite sex can lead to sex reversal of the gonads. In contrast with the striking effects of sex hormones on the differentiation of the gonads of birds and amphibians is the failure to obtain similar effects in mammalian embryos (156–161). Nevertheless, transplantation experiments suggest that the indifferent mammalian gonad has, at least, limited bipotentiality. Although the testicular primordium appears to be stable in its development, fetal ovarian development is more pliant. For example, fetal rodent ovaries develop "testis-like" structures when transplanted into male hosts (162–167), and these grafted ovaries secrete testosterone *in vitro* (168). Thus, in some situations, mammalian gonadal differentiation is influenced by the endocrine environment.

PHENOTYPIC SEX

Urogenital Tract Development During the Indifferent Phase

Before the eighth week of human development, the urogenital tract is identical in the two sexes. The internal accessory organs of reproduction develop from a dual duct system (wolffian and mullerian) that forms a part of the mesonephric kidney early in embryogenesis (Fig. 8, top). Within the substance of the mesonephros, tubules connect primitive capillary networks with a longitudinal mesonephric (wolffian) duct. The wolffian duct extends caudally to the primitive urogenital sinus. At about 6 weeks, the development of the paramesonephric (mullerian) ducts begins in embryos of both sexes as an evagination in the coelomic epithelium just lateral to the wolff-

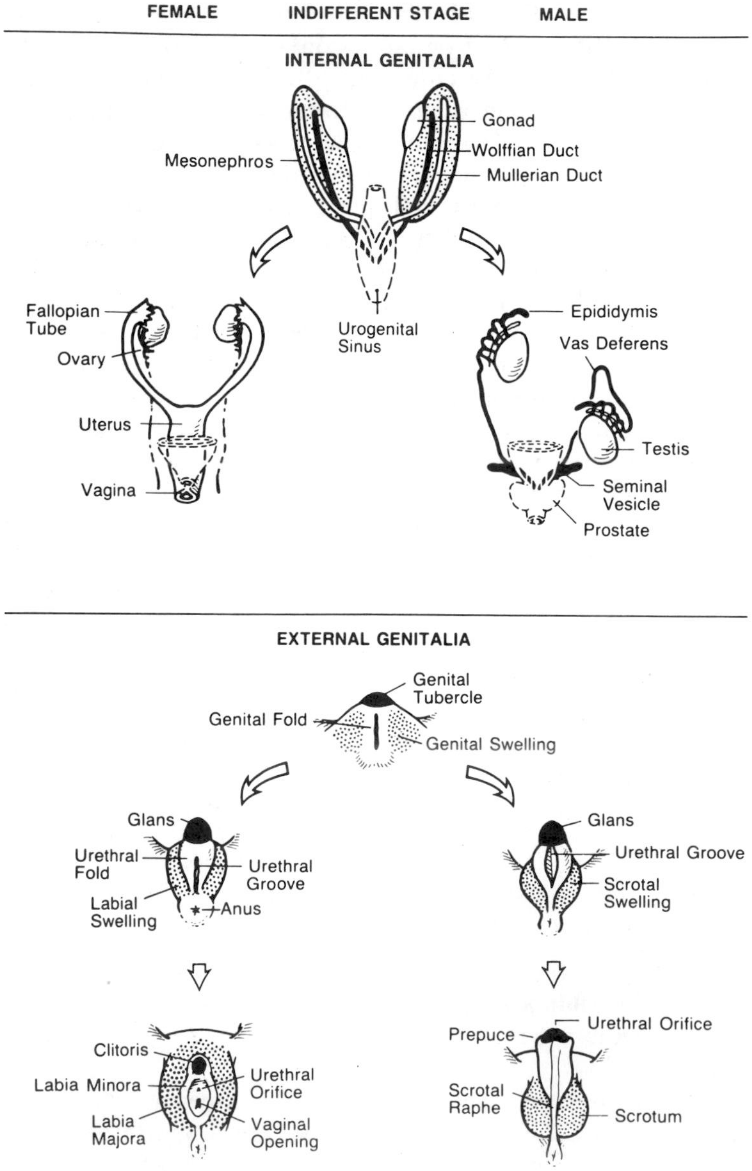

FIG. 8. Differentiation of internal and external genitalia.

ian ducts. This evagination develops into a tubular structure, the caudal end of which becomes intimately associated with the wolffian duct (i.e., no basement membrane separates their epithelia) (169). Whether the mullerian duct "splits off" from the wolffian duct in its later caudal development to become an independent duct system emptying into the urogenital sinus or whether the wolffian duct simply acts as a guide for the formation of the mullerian duct from the coelomic epithelium is uncertain. However, mullerian duct development does not take place in the absence of the wolffian duct (169). At the end of the indifferent phase of phenotypic sexual differentiation (before the eighth week of human gestation), the two ducts (wolffian and mullerian) begin to develop into the internal accessory organs of reproduction (Fig. 8). The termination of the mesonephric ducts in the urogenital sinus divides the sinus into an upper and lower portion. The upper portion, the vesicourethral canal, is involved in the development of the bladder and the urethra. The lower portion contributes to the development of the lower urogenital tract.

Before the eighth week of gestation, the anlagen of the external genitalia are also indistinguishable in the two sexes. The genital eminence is a rounded mass between the umbilicus and the tail (170) and is composed of a genital tubercle flanked by prominent genital swellings. The opening of the urogenital sinus between the genital swellings (the urethral groove) is surrounded by genital folds (Fig. 8, bottom). Around the start of week 7 of gestation in the human, the genital tubercle elongates somewhat; a shallow, circular depression defines the glans of the tubercle. At this stage of development, the external genitalia of male and female embryos are indistinguishable.

Male Development

The first sign of male differentiation of the urogenital tract is degeneration of the mullerian ducts adjacent to the testes, a process that begins just after the formation of the spermatogenic cords in the fetal testis. Eventually, the mullerian ducts of the male almost completely disappear.

The transformation of the wolffian ducts into the male ejaculatory system begins subsequent to the onset of mullerian duct regression. The portion of the wolffian duct adjacent to the testis becomes convoluted to form the epididymis; the central portion of the duct becomes the vas deferens. The seminal vesicles develop as buds off the lower portions of the wolffian ducts just before they enter into the urogenital sinus. The prostatic and membranous portions of the male urethra develop from the pelvic portion of the urogenital sinus. The prostate originates as a series of endodermal buds in the wall of this portion of the urogenital sinus beginning at about the tenth week of gestation (171–174). These prostatic buds rapidly form canalized ducts, and by the thirteenth week of gestation, functionally differentiated cells line these rudimentary ducts. Differentiation of the fetal prostate and virilization of the wolffian duct system are dependent on androgen production by the testis, which begins during the eighth week of gestation.

The external genitalia of the male begin to develop shortly after the onset of virilization of the wolffian ducts and urogenital sinus (Fig. 8, bottom). The genital tubercle elongates, and the urethral folds begin to fuse over the urethral groove from posterior to anterior so that the urogenital cleft closes to form the penile urethra. The fusion of the urethral folds brings the two genital swellings together to form the scrotum (Fig. 8, bottom). These early events in male development are completed relatively early (by the end of week 12) in human fetal development and are dependent on androgen secretion by the testis.

Two aspects of male phenotypic development take place during the latter phases of gestation. The first involves growth of the male phallus. Just after closure of the male urethra is complete, there is little difference in the size of the genital tubercle in the two sexes, but the male phallus grows during the latter phases of fetal development under the influence of androgens from the fetal testis and by the time of birth is larger than the urogenital tubercle of the female.

Testicular descent (Fig. 9) also occurs late (175), and for the purpose of discussion, we have divided this complex process into three phases. The first (transabdominal movement) involves, at a minimum, degeneration of the peritoneal fold that anchors the cranial part of the gonad to the abdominal wall, shortening of the caudal gonadal ligament (gubernaculum), and rapid growth of the abdominal-pelvic region of the fetus. As a result, the testis comes to rest against the anterior abdominal wall in the inguinal region. The second phase involves the formation of the processus vaginalis and development of the inguinal canal and scrotum. Increasing intraabdominal pressure is believed to cause a herniation in the abdominal wall (the processus vaginalis) along the course of the inguinal portion of the gubernaculum. Continued pressure causes enlargement of the processus vaginalis around the gubernaculum and leads to formation of the inguinal canal. The gubernaculum increases in size until the diameter of the inguinal canal approaches that of the testis. In the final stage of testicular descent, the abdominal testis traverses the inguinal canal and comes to rest in the scrotum. Descent of the testis into the scrotum probably involves a progressive degeneration of the proximal portion of the gubernaculum. The overall process is, at least in part, regulated by androgens (152,176–179), especially during the stage of gubernacular outgrowth

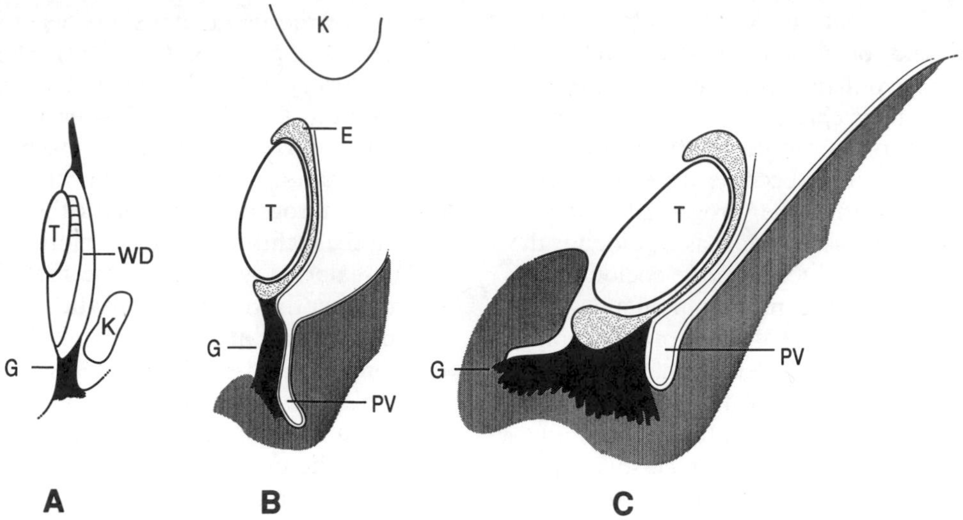

FIG. 9. Testicular descent. **A:** Before transabdominal descent; **B:** Formation of the processus vaginalis; **C:** Transinguinal descent. *T*, testis; *WD*, wolffian duct; *K*, kidney; *E*, epididymis; *G*, gubernaculum; *PV*, processus vaginalis.

(180,181). The first stage, involving transabdominal movement of the testis, may be mediated by mullerian-inhibiting hormone (182).

Female Development

The internal reproductive tract of the female is formed from the mullerian ducts; the wolffian ducts persist only in remnant form. The cephalic ends of the mullerian ducts (the portions derived from the coelomic epithelium) are the anlagen for the fallopian tubes, and the caudal portions of the ducts fuse to form the uterus (Fig. 10). Contact of the mullerian ducts with the urogenital sinus induces an intense proliferation of endodermal cells that results in the formation of the uterovaginal plate between the mullerian ducts and the urogenital sinus (183). Although the mullerian ducts and wolffian ducts both contribute to the formation of the uterovaginal plate, the relative degree to which they contribute is unknown (169,184–186). The cells of the uterovaginal plate proliferate, thus increasing the distance between the developing uterus and the urogenital sinus (Fig. 10). Later, the plate canalizes to form the lumen of the vagina.

In contrast to the male, in which the phallic and pelvic portions of the urogenital sinus are enclosed by fusion of the genital folds, most of the urogenital sinus of the female remains exposed on the surface as a cleft into which the vagina and urethra open (Fig. 8). The urogenital tubercle of the female undergoes limited growth and development to form the clitoris.

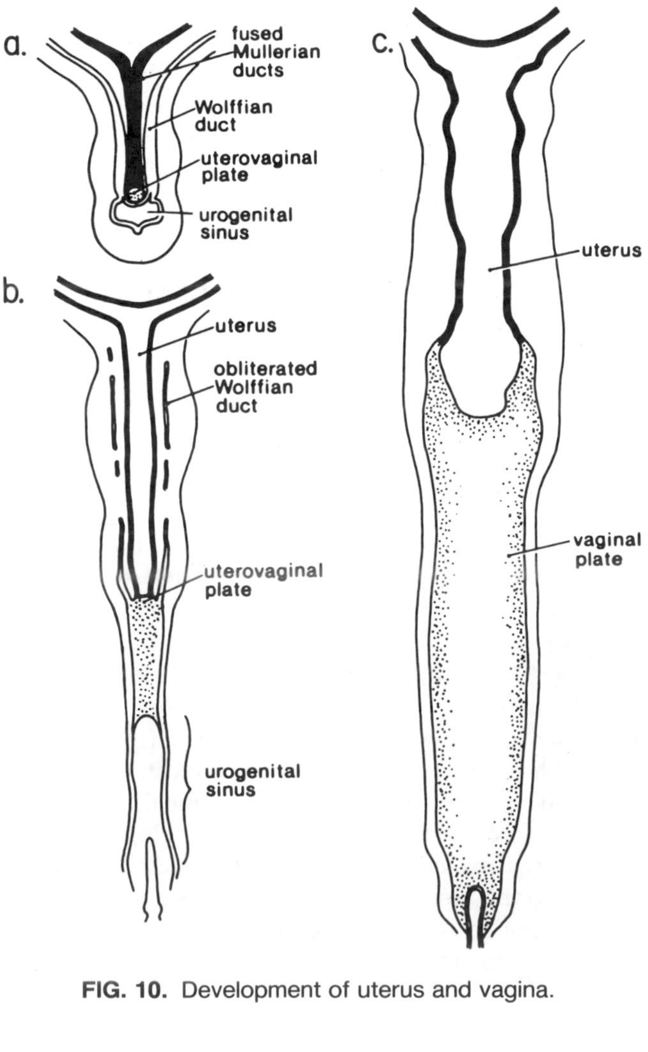

FIG. 10. Development of uterus and vagina.

Breast Development in Both Sexes

The breasts develop along "mammary lines," which are bilateral epidermal thickenings that extend from the forelimbs to the hindlimbs on the ventral surface of the embryo. In human development, these mammary lines largely disappear except for a small portion on each side of the thoracic region that condenses and penetrates the underlying mesenchyme. This single pair of mammary buds undergoes little change until the fifth month of development, when secondary epithelial buds begin to appear and nipples develop. Proliferation of the rudimentary ducts occurs throughout the remainder of gestation so that, by the time of birth, 15 to 25 separate glands are connected to the exterior through the nipple. In some species, breast development in males is inhibited by androgens during embryogenesis (187–189), but this does not occur in humans; the development of the breast in boys and girls is identical before puberty (190).

Endocrine Control of Male Phenotypic Development

By demonstrating that castration of sexually indifferent rabbit embryos invariably results in female phenotypic development (Fig. 5), Jost (98,191) established that the induced phenotype in mammalian embryos is male and that secretions from the fetal testis are necessary for male phenotypic development. Formation of the female urogenital tract does not require secretions from the fetal ovaries, because female phenotypic development occurs in the absence of gonads. Furthermore, Jost deduced that two substances from the fetal testes are essential for male development: the polypeptide mullerian-inhibiting hormone that acts ipsilaterally to cause regression of the mullerian ducts, and the androgenic steroid testosterone that is responsible for virilization of the wolffian ducts, urogenital sinus, and genital tubercle.

Mechanism of Action of Mullerian-Inhibiting Hormone

The initial endocrine function of the fetal testis is probably secretion of mullerian-inhibiting hormone. Although the hormone has been purified and much is known about its structure (192–194) and about the gene that encodes it (195,196), the mechanism of its action is poorly understood. The hallmarks of mullerian duct regression are dissolution of the basement membrane of the epithelial cells lining the duct and subsequent condensation of mesenchymal cells around the duct (197–200). A model, based largely on indirect evidence, proposes that mullerian-inhibiting substance acts by blocking phosphorylation of tyrosine residues on membrane proteins, possibly antagonizing the action of growth factors, such as epidermal growth factor (115,201–204).

Even though they are not primarily responsible for mullerian duct regression, androgens and estrogens appear to influence the process. For example, regression of rat mullerian ducts in organ culture is enhanced by testosterone, although testosterone alone is inactive (205,206). Interestingly, neither 5α-dihydrotestosterone (DHT) nor estradiol affects mullerian duct regression in this system. In other systems, estrogens interfere with mullerian duct regression (207–210). The finding that partially purified mullerian-inhibiting hormone is cytotoxic to a human ovarian cancer-derived cell line but not to cell lines derived from adenocarcinoma of the colon raises the possibility that mullerian-inhibiting hormone may also inhibit growth of malignant tumors of the female genital tract (211–213).

Mechanism of Androgen Action

Basic Model

The current concept of how androgens act within target cells is schematically depicted in Fig. 11. Testosterone, the main androgen secreted by the fetal and adult testes and the major circulating androgen in males, is thought to enter target cells passively by diffusion. In some cells, testosterone is converted to the potent androgen DHT by steroid 5α-reductase within the cells. In androgen target tissues, testosterone or DHT binds to the same specific, high-affinity, intranuclear receptor protein, thereby activating the receptor such that it acquires a high affinity for binding to specific acceptor sites on the DNA. This activated, hormone-receptor complex then acts as a regulator of transcription in androgen target tissues, enhancing the transcription of some genes and inhibiting expression of others. DHT has a higher affinity for the androgen receptor than does testosterone (214–217), and the DHT-receptor complex activates reporter genes at lower concentration (218). Because of its higher (approximately 10-fold) affinity for the androgen receptor, DHT formation probably acts primarily to amplify the regulatory signal for most androgen-responsive genes. Also, formation of the DHT-receptor complex may be absolutely required for the regulation of some gene networks (219).

Role of Dihydrotestosterone in Virilization

Separate roles for testosterone and DHT in male differentiation were postulated on the basis of studies of androgen metabolism in embryos (128,220). In rat, rabbit, guinea pig, and human embryos, 5α-reductase is expressed in the urogenital sinus and urogenital tubercle

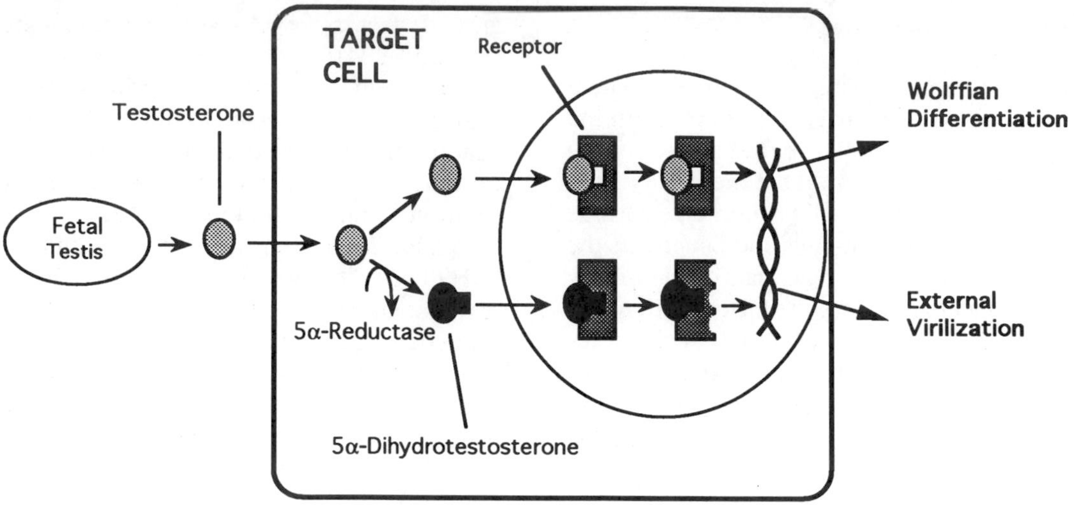

FIG. 11. Androgen action.

before virilization takes place; however, the enzyme is virtually undetectable in the wolffian duct derivatives until after virilization is advanced. Therefore, it was postulated that testosterone mediates virilization of the wolffian ducts, whereas DHT is responsible for differentiation of the male urethra, prostate, and external genitalia (220).

This hypothesis was substantiated by studies of patients with a deficiency of the 5α-reductase enzyme, steroid 5α-reductase deficiency. This disorder, in which affected men develop as phenotypic females or as severely undervirilized males, is caused by a rare, autosomal recessive mutation (221–224). Affected 46,XY individuals have a predominantly female habitus in association with bilateral testes. The internal urogenital tract, which is derived from the wolffian duct (epididymis, vas deferens, seminal vesicle, and ejaculatory duct), is virilized normally, however, and terminates in a pseudovagina. At the time of expected puberty, testosterone production increases into the male range, and the external genitalia may virilize to a limited extent. Axillary and pubic hair develop normally; the breasts remain undeveloped. There is considerable heterogeneity in the mutant 5α-reductases among different families with the disorder (221,224,225).

Complementary DNAs have been cloned for two human isozymes of steroid 5α-reductase (226–228) that have distinct biochemical and pharmacologic properties. The genes that encode these isozymes have similar intron-exon structures, and the proteins encoded by these genes are of similar length (Fig. 12). One of these genes is located on chromosome 5 and encodes the type 1 isozyme, which has a basic pH optimum and a relatively high Km for testosterone. The other gene encodes the type 2 isozyme, which has an acidic pH optimum, a low Km for testosterone, and a low K_i (3 to 5 nM) for the 5α-reductase inhibitor finasteride (228) and maps to human chromosome 2 (229). The type 1 isozyme is expressed in skin and, at very low levels, in the prostate; its role in androgen physiology is not defined. The type 2 isozyme is the main form expressed in the urogenital tract, and mutations in the gene encoding this enzyme cause 5α-reductase deficiency (230). The substrate and cofactor binding sites are tentatively assigned to exon 1 and exons 4 and 5, respectively, based on studies of mutant enzymes with abnormal substrate or cofactor binding kinetics (230).

The rat also has two genes that encode 5α-reductase, but because a mutation that causes decreased DHT formation has not been described in an animal species, ge-

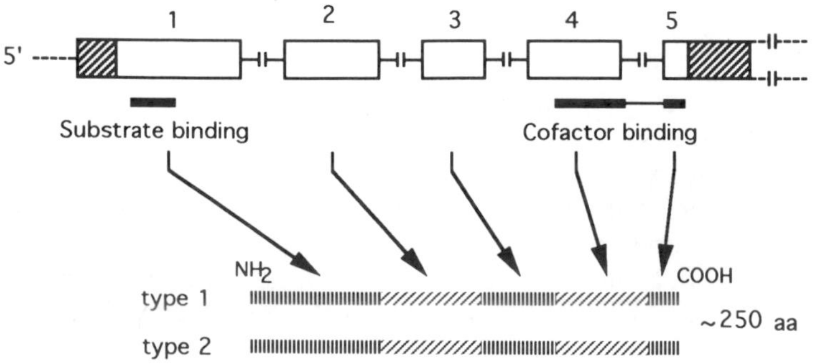

FIG. 12. Human 5α-reductase genes and predicted proteins. There are two human (and rat) genes with similar structures that code for separate 5α-reductases. Type 1 gene is located on chromosome 5, and type 2 gene is located on chromosome 2. Mutations in type 2 gene cause 5α-reductase deficiency.

netic studies of the separate roles for testosterone and DHT in formation of the male phenotype are not possible. However, the administration to pregnant rats of 5α-reductase inhibitors, in amounts sufficient to inhibit both isozymes during the period of embryonic sexual differentiation reproduces many of the characteristics of the human 5α-reductase deficiency phenotype in the male offspring. Namely, the inhibitors impair virilization of the external genitalia but have no effect on the virilization of wolffian duct structures (134,188,231–233). Because the androgen receptor of wolffian duct-derived structures, like androgen receptors from the external genitalia and prostate, appears to bind DHT preferentially (214), it is not clear how testosterone mediates wolffian duct differentiation but does not virilize the urogenital sinus and external genitalia. One possible explanation is that the local concentration of testosterone in the wolffian duct may be exceptionally high because of direct secretion from the testis into the lumen of the wolffian duct and that the high concentration of testosterone compensates for its relative ineffectiveness as an androgen. Two types of evidence are in keeping with this theory. First, active immunization of pregnant rabbits against testosterone reduces circulating androgen and causes selective impairment of external virilization in male offspring, similar to the phenotype in males with 5α-reductase deficiency (234), suggesting that androgens that are not exposed to antibody (androgens within the lumen of the wolffian ducts) may remain effective. Second, a heritable trait in the rat that causes unilateral hypoplasia of the testis in 50% of males (235) also causes ipsilateral hypoplasia of the epididymis and vas deferens despite the fact that prostate development and virilization of the external genitalia are normal, presumably mediated by plasma androgens derived from the normal testis. This finding is consistent with the concept that a noncirculating factor from the testis (testosterone) causes virilization of the adjacent wolffian duct.

A perplexing aspect of 5α-reductase deficiency is that partial virilization occurs in some patients at the time of expected puberty (222). Late virilization in these patients may be due to some combination of (a) higher levels of plasma testosterone at puberty than during embryogenesis, (b) the presence of some residual 5α-reductase 2 activity in all patients with this defect, or (c) enhancement of the activity of 5α-reductase 1 at puberty (236).

Role of the Androgen Receptor in Male Development

A specific, high-affinity receptor protein mediates the action of both testosterone and DHT in androgen-dependent tissues. Androgen receptors in the fetus have characteristics similar to those in adult androgen-dependent tissues and are believed to mediate virilization of the fetus by the same mechanisms as in postnatal life (214). Studies of single-gene mutations that impair function of the androgen receptor are in keeping with this concept.

The essential role of the androgen receptor in the embryonic action of androgens was initially established as the result of studies of the testicular feminization (*Tfm*) mutation in the mouse. In this X-linked disorder, affected males have testes and normal testosterone production but are profoundly resistant to endogenous and exogenous androgens and develop as phenotypic females (237–239). DHT formation in peripheral tissues is normal, but the androgen receptor within the cell is not detectable because of a mutation in the gene on the X chromosome that encodes the receptor (240–242). Consequently, the hormone fails to elicit a response, and androgen-mediated virilization of the wolffian ducts, urogenital sinus, and external genitalia does not take place. However, because mullerian duct derivatives (fallopian tubes and uterus) are not present, the mullerian-inhibiting function of the fetal testis is presumed to be normal.

Studies of subjects with the human counterpart of the *Tfm* mutation have provided additional insight into the role of the androgen receptor in embryonic virilization (225). Defects of the human androgen receptor cause a spectrum of abnormalities in 46,XY men that vary in severity from men with mild defects in androgen action to phenotypic women with the syndrome of testicular feminization. Women with testicular feminization usually come to the attention of the physician when they are evaluated for primary amenorrhea. The karyotype is 46,XY, but the general habitus is female. Axillary, facial, and pubic hair is absent or scanty. The external genitalia are unambiguously female, and the vagina is short and blind-ending. All internal genitalia are absent except testes, which may be located in the abdomen, along the course of the inguinal canal, or in the labia majora. Female breast development at the time of expected puberty is due to increased estrogen synthesis by the testis (243). A small percentage of women with the phenotype of *incomplete testicular feminization* have axillary and pubic hair, as well as a modest degree of virilization (244). Men with Reifenstein's syndrome (most commonly men with hypospadias, azoospermia, and gynecomastia; see ref. 225), phenotypically normal men with infertility (245,246), and rare undervirilized but fertile men complete the spectrum of disorders of the androgen receptor.

The molecular defect in some patients is similar to that in the *Tfm* mouse (i.e., no high-affinity androgen receptor can be detected in tissue homogenates; 247–249). Other patients with *testicular feminization* have either diminished amount or qualitative abnormalities of the receptor (250–255). In still other patients, androgen resistance occurs despite the fact that the androgen binding is apparently normal.

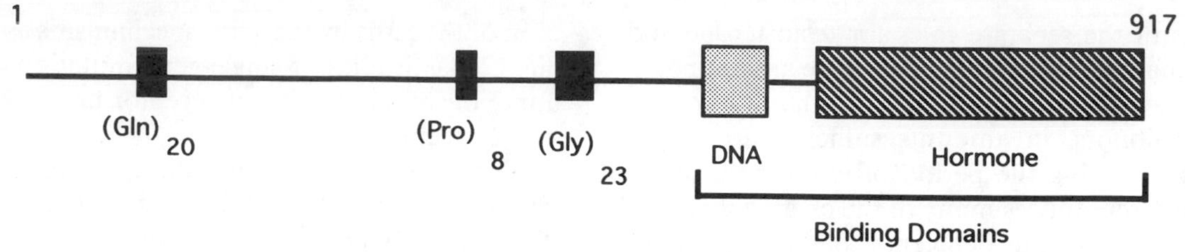

FIG. 13. Human androgen receptor.

The primary structure of the human androgen receptor was inferred from sequences of cDNA clones (256–259). The full-length cDNA for the human androgen receptor predicts a protein of 917 amino acids and a molecular weight of 99 kD (Fig. 13). The androgen receptor shares structural similarities with other members of the steroid–thyroid hormone–retinoid class of transcription regulatory factors (260). A centrally located DNA-binding domain is highly conserved among these receptors, and the hormone-binding domain is located in the carboxy terminal region (Fig. 13). The amino terminal segment of the androgen receptor contains three separate homopolymeric segments of unknown function, namely, repeats of glutamine, proline, and glycine.

Sequencing of the androgen receptor cDNA in unrelated subjects with syndromes of androgen resistance indicates that most of the defects are due to mutations that cause a premature termination codon or a single amino acid substitution within the open reading frame of the gene (261). Most of these mutations, furthermore, are within the DNA-binding or androgen-binding domains of the receptor. Less frequently, partial or complete gene deletions are present (262,263). Functional studies and immunoblot assays of the receptor in these patients indicate that impairment of androgen action (and hence the phenotypic abnormalities) is either the result of defects that cause decreased abundance or decreased function of the receptor, or both.

Role of the Mesenchyme in Androgen Action

In many tissues, the embryonic mesenchyme (stroma) appears to control the differentiation of the associated epithelium (reviewed in ref. 264). A compelling case for stromal–epithelial interactions in androgen action comes from the use of tissue recombinant techniques for study of the development of the urogenital sinus. When mesenchyme from the urogenital sinus of embryonic mouse is recombined with homotypic urogenital sinus epithelium and grown as intraocular grafts in intact male animals, the epithelium acquires the characteristics of the glandular epithelium of the prostate (265,266). In contrast, heterotypic recombinants of epithelium from urogenital sinus and mesenchyme of integumental origin are incapable of glandular (prostatic) development under the same circumstances but instead form the keratinized epithelium characteristic of skin (Fig. 14). Furthermore, mesenchyme from the urogenital sinus of

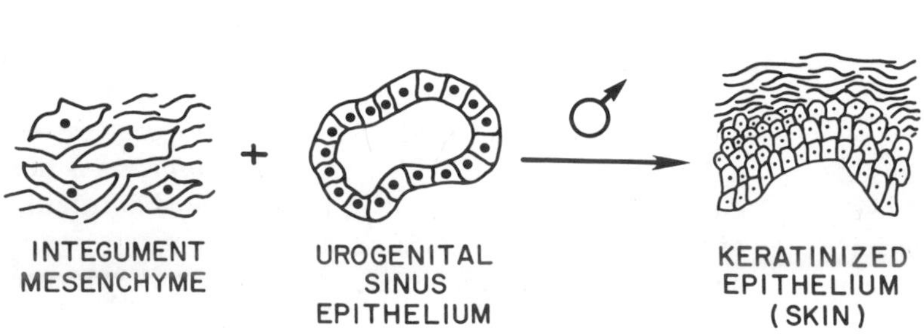

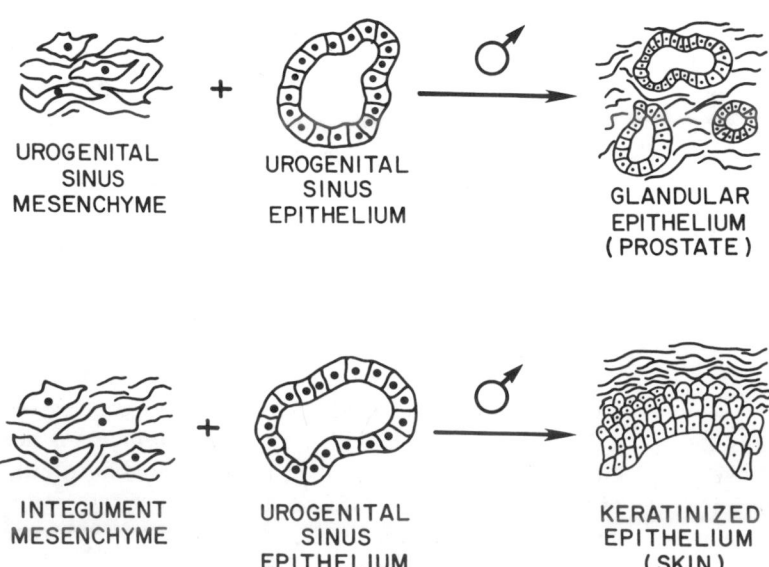

FIG. 14. Tissue recombinant experiments of Cunha et al. (264).

androgen-resistant (*Tfm*/Y) mice is incapable of mediating prostatic differentiation when recombined with normal urogenital sinus epithelium and exposed to androgen. However, when reciprocal recombinants (*Tfm*/Y epithelium with normal mesenchyme) are made, prostatelike development occurs (267,268).

Autoradiographic studies of androgen binding in urogenital sinus of developing rats (269) provide additional insight into the role of the mesenchyme in morphogenesis of the prostate. At the time of prostatic bud formation, androgen binding is located predominantly in the mesenchymal cells that surround the developing buds. Mesenchymal cells of the urogenital sinus of female embryos also have androgen binding. In contrast, the epithelial cells of the fetal urogenital sinus do not bind androgen. After postnatal day 10, androgen binding is detectable in the epithelial cells of the prostate, and labeling of the surrounding mesenchyme becomes less prominent. These findings suggest that during morphogenesis of the male urogenital tract, androgen action is initiated through the mesenchyme, whereas androgen response of the prostate after differentiation is mediated primarily in the epithelium.

A similar system is responsible for androgen-mediated regression of the embryonic mammary bud in the mouse (270,271). However, in this tissue, the response to androgen requires specific interaction of mammary mesenchyme with mammary epithelium (272), suggesting that in some cases the epithelium may also play a role in the differentiation process. The epithelium of mesodermal origin, when recombined with androgen-responsive mesenchyme, may also respond differently than does epithelium of endoderm (264). Elucidating the nature of these mesenchymal-epithelial interactions is of critical importance in understanding androgen-mediated differentiative processes.

Despite the fact that a great deal of information has accumulated concerning the hormones involved in differentiation of the urogenital tract and about the cellular sites of their initial actions, little is known about the specific gene products synthesized in response to the hormones or how such products direct cellular organization during embryogenesis.

Effects of Androgens in Female Embryos

Female embryos have the same androgen receptor system in the urogenital tract as do male embryos (214). For example, androgen receptor levels are similar in analogous regions of the female and male urogenital tracts (Fig. 15). Therefore, it is not surprising that administration of androgens at the appropriate time during embryogenesis causes profound virilization of female offspring (133). The anatomic consequences of such an

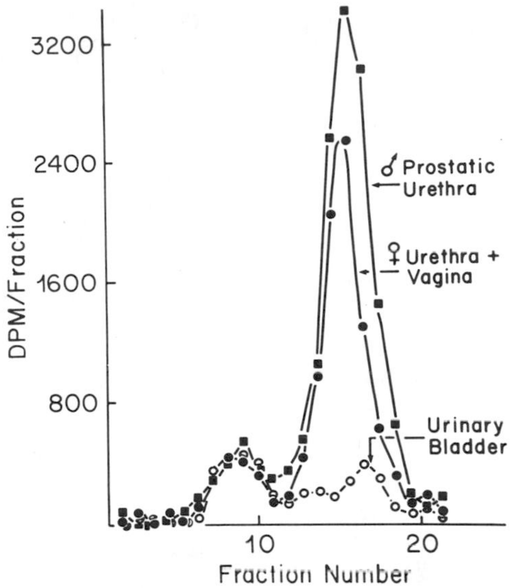

FIG. 15. Sucrose gradient analysis of [^{3}H] DHT binding in cytosol of urogenital sinuses and bladder of fetal rabbits on day 28 of gestation.

experiment in rats are illustrated in Fig. 16. Figure 16A and B show urogenital tracts dissected from female and male newborn rats whose mother had been treated with oil (control) from day 14 through day 21 of gestation. Figure 16C shows a urogenital tract from a newborn female exposed *in utero* to an inactive androgen analog (5β-DHT). Figure 16D shows a urogenital tract from a female exposed to 5α-DHT. In this female embryo, DHT caused differentiation of the wolffian ducts into prominent epididymides, vasa deferentia, and seminal vesicles. Furthermore, the urogenital sinuses from DHT-treated females contained prostatic buds and male-type urethras and exhibited no vaginal development. The fact that females virilize in response to androgen indicates that differences in anatomic development between males and females depend on the hormonal signals themselves and not on differences in the hormone receptors in target tissues. It also follows that the sexual fate of the normal embryo is determined largely by whether testosterone production commences in the fetal testis at the precise time in embryonic development.

The most common cause of virilization of human female embryos is congenital adrenal hyperplasia (273). Inherited mutations that result in decreased synthesis of cortisol in the adrenal gland lead to a compensatory increase in adrenocorticotropic hormone (ACTH) secretion by the pituitary. This, in turn, leads to an increase in the secretion of adrenal androgens that virilize the external genitalia of the female. The internal genitalia are, however, not virilized, and wolffian duct remnants are normal in women with congenital adrenal hyperplasia. It is likely that the degeneration of the wolffian ducts occurs before the onset of adrenal androgen synthesis.

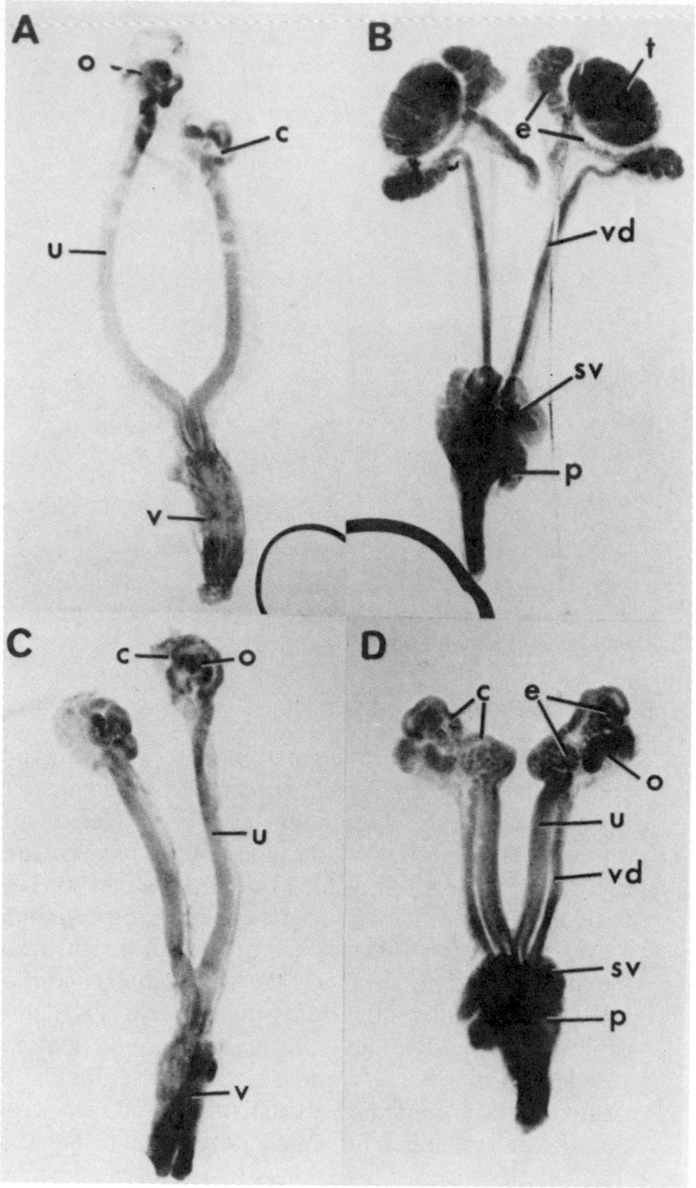

FIG. 16. Virilization of female rat urogenital tract caused by 5α-DHT administration to mother. **A** and **B**, respectively: Female and male urogenital tracts of newborn rat from a mother given oil from days 14 to 21 of gestation. **C:** Female urogenital tracts after administration of 5β-DHT. **D:** Female urogenital tract after administration of 5α-DHT. *o*, ovary; *u*, uterus; *c*, coils of the oviduct; *v*, vagina; *t*, testis; *e*, epididymis; *vd*, vas deferens; *sv*, seminal vesicle; *p*, prostate. (From ref. 133, with permission.)

DO HORMONES PLAY A ROLE IN FEMALE DEVELOPMENT?

In the eutherian mammal, embryogenesis takes place in a virtual "sea" of hormones (steroidal and nonsteroidal) derived from the placenta, the maternal circulation, the fetal adrenal, the fetal testis, and possibly from the fetal ovary. It is not known whether any of these substances influence female phenotypic differentiation or development. It is conceivable that estrogens or progestogens, or both, are involved in the growth and maturation of the female urogenital tract during the latter part of embryonic development, even if they are not required for their differentiation. Presumably, fetal castration experiments (such as those performed by Jost [98] to elucidate the role of the fetal testis in male differentiation) would be uninformative, because removal of fetal ovaries would not remove main sources of female hormones. Experimental agents that block estrogen synthesis or action interfere with placental function and precipitate abortion. Furthermore, no mutations have been identified that result in resistance to estrogen action. This is in contrast to the situation in regard to testosterone synthesis and action in which single-gene mutations that interfere with hormone action have been characterized in many species (225). In the rabbit, estrogen synthesis is temporarily activated in both male and female embryos at the time the blastocyst implants in the uterine wall between days 6 and 7 of gestation (274) (Fig. 17). Later in rabbit embryogenesis, estrogen synthesis

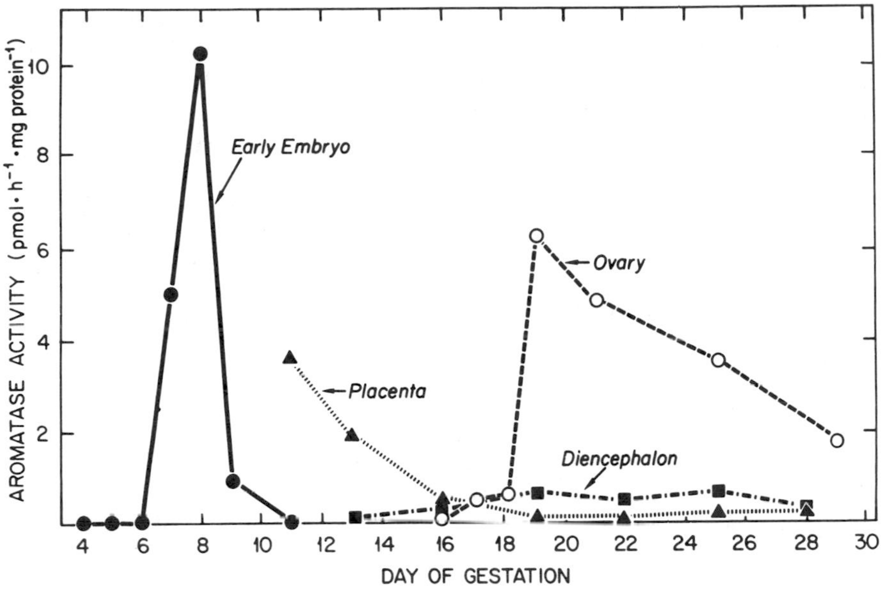

FIG. 17. Distribution of aromatase activity in developing rabbit embryo. (Composite of data in refs. 139, 274, and 275.)

(aromatase activity) is activated in placenta (transiently), brain (275), and ovary (139), but aromatase activity in these tissues is never as high as in the implanting blastocyst (Fig. 17). Estrogens may be necessary for implantation and survival of the blastocyst (276,277), suggesting that estrogen action is essential for life in eutherian mammals. If this is true, mutations that prevent the response to estrogens may be lethal at an early stage of development by preventing implantation of the blastocyst.

In many species, estradiol formation is initiated in the ovary before definitive histologic differentiation has occurred; it is possible that the cellular organization of the ovary may be mediated, in part, by estrogens formed locally (154), analogous to the postulated role of testosterone in maturation of the spermatogenic cords of the testis.

SEX DIFFERENTIATION IN THE MARSUPIAL

In contrast to eutherian mammals in which sexual differentiation occurs *in utero,* marsupial young show little evidence of sexual differentiation at the time of birth. Development of the sexual phenotypes takes place in the pouch, independent of the maternal milieu, and the pouch young are accessible for experimentation throughout sexual development. Marsupials, therefore, represent an important model system for studying the hormonal factors that control sexual differentiation. Burns (278) studied the effects of the administration of androgen or estrogen on the development of the sexual phenotypes in newborn opossums (*Didephis virginiana*). Although these steroids influenced development of the external genitalia in the pouch young of both sexes, their administration from the day of birth does not accelerate the time of sexual differentiation or influence the development of the pouch or scrotum (155,278–280). Furthermore, the scrotal bulges and the mammary anlagen can be identified in the fetus before birth (280), and pouch development is the first evidence of sexual dimorphism in marsupials that can be identified grossly after birth. In the Tammar Wallaby, differentiation of the pouch and scrotum commences before the onset of testosterone synthesis in the testis (281), and studies of chromosomal dismutation states indicate that scrotal development in marsupials occurs when only one X chromosome (XY or XO) is present, whereas two X chromosomes (XX or XXY) are necessary for pouch formation (280).

These different types of evidence imply that development of the androgen receptor or some other rate-limiting process in androgen action, other than the onset of testicular testosterone secretion, determines the timing of virilization of the urogenital sinus and urogenital tubercle. It also implies that the differentiation of the scrotum and the pouch in the marsupial is controlled by nonhormonal processes. Thus, phenotypic development in marsupials differs in several respects from the process in eutherian mammals.

SUMMARY

Jost's formulation has proved to be a powerful paradigm for understanding normal and abnormal sexual differentiation in the eutherian mammal. Chromosomal sex determines gonadal sex, and gonadal sex determines phenotypic sex. Although the gene responsible for initiating the entire process has been localized on the Y chromosome, a minimum of 19 genes, some with autosomal and some with X-chromosomal loci, have been implicated in sex differentiation. The expression of many, if not all, of these "secondary" genes occurs in both male and female embryos and in differentiation of the functional fetal testis that determines phenotypic sex in the eutherian mammal.

Much of our understanding of the process of sex determination and differentiation is because, unlike most developmental systems, abnormalities of sex are not lethal, and affected individuals come to the attention of physicians and scientists and are systematically studied. Many of the abnormalities are due to single-gene defects, and analysis of these disorders in humans and animals has provided insight into the endocrine, molecular, and genetic determinants that regulate sexual differentiation.

Determinants on the Y chromosome cause the indifferent gonad to develop into a testis. Two hormonal secretions from the fetal testis, mullerian-inhibiting hormone and testosterone, then transform the indifferent urogenital tract into one that is characteristic of the male. Mullerian-inhibiting hormone, secreted by the fetal Sertoli cells, causes regression of the female (mullerian) duct system in the male embryo. Testosterone, secreted by the fetal Leydig cells, is responsible for the remainder of male development, including stabilization and differentiation of the wolffian ducts into the male accessory organs of reproduction and formation of the male external genitalia and prostate.

A major portion of androgen action in the fetus and in postembryonic life is mediated by the 5α-reduced metabolite of testosterone, DHT. Genetic deficiency of the steroid 5α-reductase 2 enzyme in humans impairs androgen action and causes a specific form of male pseudohermaphroditism in which external virilization is impaired but wolffian duct development is normal. Abnormalities of the common androgen receptor that mediates the action of both testosterone and DHT impairs all androgen action during embryogenesis, the completeness of impairment depending on the specific mutation.

The role of hormones in female development is less clear. In the eutherian mammal, it has not been possible to design experiments to determine whether hormones from the placenta, the maternal circulation, or the fetal ovary play an essential role in female development.

Although the hormonal and genetic factors responsible for mammalian sexual differentiation are understood in considerable detail, many fundamental issues in embryonic development of the urogenital tract remain poorly understood. What, for instance, is the mechanism by which the same hormonal signal is translated into different physiologic effects in different tissues? What molecular and cellular changes cause these diverse differentiative events? What causes the tissue-specific expression of the androgen receptor and steroid 5α-reductase 2 in tissue of the urogenital tract? Ultimately, these fundamental issues of embryogenesis will have to be clarified before it will be possible to understand the entire program by which the myriad of genetic determinants and hormones interact to cause sexual development.

REFERENCES

1. Vogel F, Motulsky AG. *Human Genetics,* Ed 2. Berlin: Springer-Verlag, 1986.
2. Davis RM. Localisation of male determining factors in man: a thorough review of structural anomalies of the Y chromosome. *J Med Genet* 1981;18:161–195.
3. McLaren A, Monk M. X chromosome activity in the germ cells of sex-reversed mouse embryos. *J Reprod Fertil* 1982;63: 533–537.
4. Forejt J. Meiotic studies of translocations causing male sterility in the mouse. II. Double heterozygotes for Robertsonian translocations. *Cytogenet Cell Genet* 1979;19:159–179.
5. Madan K. Balanced structural changes involving the human X: effect on sexual phenotype. *Hum Genet* 1983;63:216–221.
6. Ohno S, Jainchill J, Stenius C. The creeping vole (*Microtus oregoni*) as a gonosomic mosaic. The OY/XY constitution of the male. *Cytogenetics* 1963;2:232–239.
7. Page D, de Martinville B, Barker D, et al. Single-copy sequence hybridizes to a polymorphic and homologous loci on human X and Y chromosomes. *Proc Natl Acad Sci USA* 1982;79: 5352–5356.
8. Goodfellow P, Darling S, Wolfe J. The human Y chromosome. *J Med Genet* 1985;22:329–344.
9. Cooke HJ, Fantes J, Green D. Structure and evolution of human Y chromosome DNA. *Differentiation* 1985;23:S48–S55.
10. Vollrath D, Foote S, Hilton A, et al. The human Y chromosome: a 43-interval map based on naturally occurring deletions. *Science* 1992;258:52–59.
11. Foote S, Vollrath D, Hilton A, Page DC. The human Y chromosome: overlapping DNA clones spanning the euchromatic region. *Science* 1992;258:60–66.
12. Book JA, Eilon B, Halbrecht I, Komlos L, Shabtay F. Isochromosome Y [46, X, i(Yq)] and female phenotype. *Clin Genet* 1973;41:410–414.
13. Gordon JW, Ruddle FH. Mammalian gonadal determination and gametogenesis. *Science* 1981;211:1265–1271.
14. Jacobs PA, Ross A. Structural abnormalities of the Y chromosome in man. *Nature* 1966;210:352–354.
15. Vergnaud G, Page DC, Simmler MC, et al. A deletion map of the human Y chromosome based on DNA hybridization. *Am J Hum Genet* 1986;38:109–124.
16. Wachtel S. *H-Y Antigen and the Biology of Sex Determination.* New York: Grune & Stratton, 1983.
17. Crichton DN, Steel CM. Serologically detectable H-Y ("male") antigen: Mr or myth? *Immunol Today* 1985;6:202–203.
18. Gore-Langston RE, Tung PS, Fritz IB. The absence of specific interaction of Sertoli-cell-secreted proteins with antibodies directed against H-Y antigen. *Cell* 1983;32:289–301.
19. Jones HW Jr, Rary JM, Rock JA, Cummings D. The role of H-Y antigen in human sexual development. *Johns Hopkins Med J* 1979;145:33–43.
20. Wolfe J, Goodfellow PN. The elusive testis determining factor. *Trends Genet* 1985;1:3–4.
21. Zenzes MT, Reed TE. Variability in serologically detected male antigen titer and some resulting problems: a critical review. *Hum Genet* 1984;66:103–109.
22. McLaren A, Simpson E, Tomonari K, Chandler P, Hogg H. Male sexual differentiation in mice lacking H-Y antigen. *Nature* 1984;312:552–555.

23. Cantrell MA, Bogan JS, Simpson E, et al. Deletion mapping of H-Y antigen to the long arm of the human Y chromosome. *Genomics* 1992;13:1255–1260.
24. Page DC, Mosher R, Simpson EM, et al. The sex-determining region of the human Y chromosome encodes a finger protein. *Cell* 1987;51:1091–1104.
25. Palmer M, Berta P, Sinclair A, Pym B, Goodfellow P. Comparison of ZFY and ZFX transcripts. *Proc Natl Acad Sci USA* 1990;87:1681–1685.
26. Affara NA, Chambers D, O'Brien J, et al. Evidence for distinguishable transcript of the putative testis-determining gene (ZFY) and mapping of homologous cDNA sequences to chromosomes X, Y, and 9. *Nucleic Acids Res* 1989;17:2987–2999.
27. North M, Sargent C, O'Brien J, et al. Comparison of ZFY and ZFX gene structure and analysis of alternative 3′ untranslated regions of ZFY. *Nucleic Acids Res* 1991;19:2579–2586.
28. Sinclair AH, Foster JW, Spencer JA, et al. Sequences homologous to ZFY, a candidate human sex-determining gene, are autosomal in marsupials. *Nature* 1988;336:780–783.
29. Ferguson-Smith MA, Affara NA. Accidental X-Y recombination and the aetiology of XX males and true hermaphrodites. *Philos Trans R Soc Lond B* 1988;322:133–144.
30. Ferguson-Smith MA, Cooke A, Affara NA, Boyd E, Tolmie JL. Genotype-phenotype correlations in XX males and their bearing on the current theories of sex determination. *Hum Genet* 1990;84:198–202.
31. Palmer M, Sinclair AH, Berta P, et al. Genetic evidence that ZFY is not the testis-determining factor. *Nature* 1989;342:937–939.
32. Sinclair AH, Berta P, Palmer M, et al. A gene from the human sex-determining region encodes a protein with homology to a conserved DNA-binding motif. *Nature* 1990;346:240–244.
33. Page DC, Fisher E, McGillivry B, Brown LG. Additional deletion in the sex-determining region of the human Y chromosome resolves paradox of X,t(Y;22) female. *Nature* 1990;346:279–281.
34. Gubbay J, Collignon J, Koopman P, et al. A gene mapping to the sex-determining region of the mouse Y chromosome is a member of a novel family of embryonically expressed genes. *Nature* 1990;346:245–250.
35. Koopman P, Munsterberg A, Capel B, Vivian N, Lovell-Badge R. Expression of a candidate sex-determining gene during mouse testis differentiation. *Nature* 1990;348:450–452.
36. Koopman P, Gubbay J, Vivian N, Goodfellow PN, Lovell-Badge R. Male development of chromosomally female mice transgenic for Sry. *Nature* 1991;351:117–121.
37. Eicher EM, Washburn LL. Inherited sex reversal in mice: identification of a new primary sex-determining gene. *J Exp Zool* 1983;228:297–304.
38. Eicher EM, Washburn LL. Genetic control of primary sex determination in mice. *Annu Rev Genet* 1986;20:327–360.
39. Eicher EM. Autosomal genes involved in mammalian primary sex determination. *Philos Trans R Soc Lond B* 1988;322:109–118.
40. Burgoyne PS. Role of mammalian Y chromosome in sex determination. *Philos Trans R Soc Lond B* 1988;322:63–72.
41. Palmer SJ, Burgoyne PS. The *Mus musculus domesticus Tdy* allele acts later than the *Mus musculus musculus* Tdy allele: a basis for XY sex-reversal in C57BL/6-Y^{pos} mice. *Development* 1991;113:709–714.
42. Burgoyne PS. Mammalian X and Y crossover. *Nature* 1986;319:258–259.
43. Keitges E, Rivest M, Siniscalo M, Gartler SM. X-linkage of steroid sulphatase in mouse is evidence for a functional Y-linked allele. *Nature* 1985;315:226–227.
44. Rouyer F, Simmler M-C, Johnsson C, Vergnaud G, Cooke HJ, Weissenbach J. A gradient of sex linkage in the pseudoautosomal region of the human sex chromosomes. *Nature* 1986;319:291–295.
45. Levilliers J, Quack B, Weissenbach J, Petit C. Exchange of terminal portions of X- and Y-chromosomal short arms in human XY females. *Proc Natl Acad Sci USA* 1989;86:2296–2300.
46. Cattanach BM, Pollard CE, Hawkes SG. Sex-reversed mice: XX and XO males. *Cytogenetics* 1971;10:318–337.
47. Ferguson-Smith MA. X-Y chromosomal interchange in the aetiology of true hermaphroditism and of XX Klinefelter's syndrome. *Lancet* 1966;ii:475–476.
48. Singe L, Jones KW. Sex reversal in the mouse (*Mus musculus*) is caused by a recurrent non-reciprocal crossover involving the X and the aberrant Y chromosome. *Cell* 1982;28:205–216.
49. Evans EP, Burtenshaw MD, Cattanach BH. Meiotic crossing-over between the X and Y chromosomes of male mice carrying the sex-reversing (Sxr) factor. *Nature* 1982;300:443–445.
50. Burgoyne PS. Genetic homology and crossing over in the X and Y chromosomes of mammals. *Hum Genet* 1982;61:85–90.
51. McLaren A. Sex reversal in the mouse. *Differentiation* 1983;23:S93–S98.
52. de la Chapelle A. The etiology of maleness in XX men. *Hum Genet* 1981;58:105–116.
53. Perez-Palacios G, Medina M, Ullao-Aguirre A, et al. Gonadotropin dynamics in XX males. *J Clin Endocrinol Metab* 1981;53:254–257.
54. Schweikert HU, Weissbach L, Leyendecker G, Schwinger E, Wartenberg H, Kruck F. Clinical, endocrinological, and cytological characterization of two 46,XX males. *J Clin Endocrinol Metab* 1982;54:745–752.
55. Roe TF, Alfi OS. Ambiguous genitalia in XX male children: report of two infants. *Pediatrics* 1977;60:55–59.
56. Andersson M, Page DC, de la Chapelle A. Chromosome Y-specific DNA is transferred to the short arm of the X chromosome in human XX males. *Science* 1986;233:786–788.
57. de la Chapelle A, Tippett PA, Wetterstrand G, Page D. Genetic evidence of X-Y interchange in a human XX male. *Nature* 1984;307:170–171.
58. Guellaen G, Casanova M, Bishop C, et al. Human XX males with single-copy DNA fragments. *Nature* 1984;307:172–173.
59. Cooke HJ, Brown WRA, Rappold GA. Hypervariable telomeric sequences from the human sex chromosomes are pseudoautosomal. *Nature* 1985;317:687–692.
60. Rouyer F, Simmler MC, Johnsson C, Vergnaud G, Cooke HJ, Weissenbach J. A gradient of sex linkage in the pseudoautosomal region of the human sex chromosomes. *Nature* 1986;319:291–295.
61. Simmler MC, Rouyer F, Vergnaud G, et al. Pseudoautosomal DNA sequences in the pairing region of the human sex chromosomes. *Nature* 1985;317:692–697.
62. Goodfellow PJ, Darling SM, Thomas NS, Goodfellow PN. A pseudoautosomal gene in man. *Science* 1986;234:740–743.
63. van Niekerk WA. True hermaphroditism. *Pediatr Adolesc Endocrinol* 1981;8:80–99.
64. Simpson JL. True hermaphroditism: etiology and phenotypic considerations. *Birth Defects* 1978;14:9–35.
65. Eicher EM, Washburn LL, Whitney JB III, Morrow KE. *Mus poschiavinus* Y chromosome in the C57BL/6J murine genome causes sex reversal. *Science* 1982;217:535–537.
66. Clayton GW, Smith JD, Rosenberg HS. Familial true hermaphroditism in pre- and postpubertal genetic females. Hormonal and morphologic studies. *J Clin Endocrinol Metab* 1958;18:1349–1358.
67. Gallegos AJ, Guizar E, Cortes-Gallegos V, Cervantes C, Bedolla N, Parra A. Familial true hermaphroditism in three siblings: plasma hormonal profile and *in vitro* steroid biosynthesis in gonadal structures. *J Clin Endocrinol Metab* 1976;42:653–660.
68. Lowry RB, Honore LH, Arnold WJD, Johnson HW, Kliman MR, Marshall RH. Familial true hermaphroditism. *Birth Defects* 1975;11:105–113.
69. Mori Y, Mitzutani S. Familial true hermaphroditism in genetic females. *Jpn J Urol* 1968;59:857–864.
70. Rosenberg HS, Clayton GW, Hsu TC. Familial true hermaphroditism. *J Clin Endocrinol Metab* 1963;23:203–206.
71. Berger R, Abonyi D, Nodot A, Vialatte J, Lejeune J. Hermaphrodisme vrai et "Garcon XX" dans une fratrie. *Rev Eur Etud Clin Biol* 1970;15:330–333.
72. Kasdan R, Nankin HR, Troen P, Wald N, Pan S, Yanaihara T. Paternal transmission of maleness in XX human beings. *N Engl J Med* 1973;288:539–545.
73. Lyon MF. X-chromosome inactivation and the location and expression of X-linked genes. *Am J Hum Genet* 1988;42:8–16.

74. Gartler SM, Liskay RM, Campbell BK, Sparkes R, Gant N. Evidence for two functional X chromosomes in human oocytes. *Cell Differentiation* 1972;1:215–218.
75. Gartler SM, Liskay RM, Gant N. Two functional X chromosomes in human fetal oocytes. *Exp Cell Res* 1973;82:464–465.
76. Migeon BR, Jelalian K. Evidence for two active X chromosomes in germ cells of females before meiotic entry. *Nature* 1977;269: 242–243.
77. Kratzer PG, Chapman VM. X chromosome reactivation in oocytes of *Mus caroli*. *Proc Natl Acad Sci USA* 1981;78:4041–4044.
78. Venolia L, Cooper DW, O'Brien DA, Millette CF, Gartler SM. Transformation of the *Hprt* gene with DNA from spermatogenic cells. *Chromosoma* 1984;90:185–189.
79. Yen PH, Patel P, Chinault AC, Mohandas T, Shapiro LJ. Differential methylation of hypoxanthine phosphoribosyl transferase genes on active and inactive human X chromosomes. *Proc Natl Acad Sci USA* 1984;83:1759–1763.
80. Ohno S, Lyon MF. Cytological study of Searle's X-autosome translocation in *Mus musculus*. *Chromosoma (Berlin)* 1965;16: 90–100.
81. Cattanach BM, Evans EP, Burtenshaw MD, Barlow J. Male, female and intersex development in mice of identical chromosome constitution. *Nature* 1982;300:445–446.
82. McLaren A, Monk M. Fertile females produced by inactivation of the X chromosome of "sex-reversed" mice. *Nature* 1982;300: 446–448.
83. Searle AG. Is sex-linked Tabby really recessive in the mouse? *Heredity* 1962;17:297.
84. Gardner RL, Lyon MF, Evans EP, Burtenshaw MD. Clonal analysis of X-chromosome inactivation and the origin of the germ line in the mouse. *J Embryol Exp Morphol* 1985;88:349–363.
85. MaKay DG, Hertig AT, Adams EC, Danziger S. Histochemical observation on the germ cells of the human embryo. *Anat Rec* 1953;117:201–220.
86. Hertig AT, Adams EC, McKay DG, Rock J, Mulligan WJ, Menkin M. A description of 34 human ova within the first 17 days of development. *Am J Anat* 1956;98:435–493.
87. Ginsburg M, Snow MHL, McLaren A. Primordial germ cells in the mouse embryo during gastrulation. *Development* 1990;110: 521–528.
88. Blandau RJ, White BJ, Rumery RE. Observations on the movements of the living primordial germ cells in the mouse. *Fertil Steril* 1963;14:482–489.
89. Fujimoto T, Miyayama Y, Fuyuta M. The origin, migration and fine morphology of human primordial germ cells. *Anat Rec* 1977;188:315–330.
90. Witschi E. Migration of the germ cells of human embryos from the yolk sac to the primitive gonadal folds. *Contrib Embryol Carnegie Inst Wash* 1948;32:67–80.
91. Donovan PK, Stott D, Cairns LA, Heasman J, Wylie CC. Migratory and postmigratory mouse primordial germ cells behave differently in culture. *Cell* 1986;44:831–838.
92. Jost A, Magre S. Testicular development phases and dual hormonal control of sexual organogenesis. *In:* Serio M ed. *Sexual Differentiation: Basic and Clinical Aspects.* New York: Raven Press, 1984;1–15.
93. Jirasek JE. Principles of reproductive embryology. *In:* Simpson JL, ed. *Disorders of Sexual Differentiation.* New York: Academic Press, 1976;51–110.
94. Gillman J. The development of the gonads in man, with a consideration of the role of fetal endocrines and the histiogenesis of ovarian tumors. *Contrib Embryol Carnegie Inst Wash* 1948;32: 83–131.
95. Merchant H. Rat gonadal and ovarian organ-ogenesis with and without germ cells. An ultrastructural study. *Dev Biol* 1975;44:1–21.
96. McCarrey JR, Abbott UK. Chick gonad differentiation following excision of primordial germ cells. *Dev Biol* 1978;66:256–265.
97. Handel MA, Eppig JJ. Sertoli cell differentiation in the testes of mice genetically deficient in germ cells. *Biol Reprod* 1979;20: 1031–1038.
98. Jost A. Problems in fetal endocrinology: the gonadal and hypophyseal hormones. *Recent Prog Horm Res* 1953;8:379–418.
99. Jost A. A new look at the mechanism controlling sexual differentiation in mammals. *Johns Hopkins Med J* 1972;130:38–53.
100. Donahoe PK, Ho Y, Morikawa Y, Hendren WH. Mullerian inhibiting substance in human testes after birth. *J Pediatr Surg* 1977;12:323–330.
101. Donahoe PK, Ito Y, Price JM, Hendren WH III. Mullerian inhibiting substance activity in bovine fetal, newborn and prepubertal testes. *Biol Rep* 1977;16:238–243.
102. Picard JY, Tran D, Josso N. Biosynthesis of labelled antimullerian hormone by fetal testes: evidence for the glycoprotein nature of the hormone and for its disulfide-bonded structure. *Mol Cell Endocrinol* 1978;12:17–30.
103. Price JM. The secretion of mullerian inhibiting substance by cultured isolated Sertoli cells of the neonatal calf. *Am J Anat* 1979;156:147–157.
104. Tran D, Josso N. Localization of antimullerian hormone in the rough endoplasmic reticulum of the developing Sertoli cell using immunocytochemistry with a monoclonal antibody. *Endocrinology* 1982;111:1562–1567.
105. Vigier B, Picard J-Y, Champargue J, Forest MG, Heyman Y, Josso N. Secretion of anti-mullerian hormone by immature bovine Sertoli cells in primary culture studied by a competition-type radioimmunoassay: lack of modulation by either FSH or testosterone. *Mol Cell Endocrinol* 1985;43:141–150.
106. Hutson JM, Donahoe PK. Is mullerian-inhibiting substance a circulating hormone in the chick-quail chimera? *Endocrinology* 1983;113:1470–1475.
107. Josso N, Boussin L, Knebelmann B, Nihoul-Fekete C, Picard J-Y. Anti-mullerian hormone and intersex states. *Trends Endocrinol Metab* 1991;2:227–233.
108. Mudgett-Hunter M, Budzik GP, Sullivan M, Donahoe PK. Monoclonal antibody to mullerian inhibiting substance. *J Immunol* 1982;128:1327–1333.
109. Vigier B, Legali L, Picard J-Y, Josso N. A sensitive radioimmunoassay for bovine anti-mullerian hormone, allowing its detection in male and freemartin fetal serum. *Endocrinology* 1982;111: 1409–1411.
110. Vigier B, Picard J-Y, Josso N. A monoclonal antibody against anti-mullerian hormone. *Endocrinology* 1982;110:131–137.
111. Tran D, Picard J-Y, Vigier B, Berger R, Josso N. Persistence of mullerian ducts in male rabbit passively immunized against bovine anti-mullerian hormone during fetal life. *Dev Biol* 1986;116:160–167.
112. Magre S, Jost A. Dissociation between testicular organogenesis and endocrine cytodifferentiation of Sertoli cells. *Proc Natl Acad Sci USA* 1984;81:7831–7834.
113. Cate RL, Mattalian RJ, Hession C, et al. Isolation of the bovine and human genes for mullerian inhibiting substance and expression of the human gene in animals cells. *Cell* 1986;45:685–698.
114. Picard J-Y, Benarous R, Guerrier D, Josso N, Kahn A. Cloning and expression of the cDNA for anti-Mullerian hormone. *Proc Natl Acad Sci USA* 1986;83:5464–5468.
115. Donahoe PK, Cate RL, MacLaughlin DT, et al. Mullerian inhibiting substance: gene structure and mechanism of action of a fetal regressor. *Recent Prog Horm Res* 1987;43:431–462.
116. Cohen-Haguenauer O, Picard J-Y, Mattei M-G, et al. Mapping of the gene for anti-mullerian hormone to the short arm of human chromosome 19. *Cytogenet Cell Genet* 1987;44:2–6.
117. Armendares S, Buentello L, Frenk S. Two male sibs with uterus and fallopian tubes. A rare, probably inherited disorder. *Clin Genet* 1973;4:291–296.
118. Brook CGD. Persistent mullerian duct syndrome. *Pediatr Adolesc Endocrinol* 1981;8:100–104.
119. Brook CGD, Wagner H, Zachmann M, et al. Familial occurrence of persistent mullerian structures in otherwise normal males. *Br Med J* 1973;1:771–773.
120. Sloan WR, Walsh PC. Familial persistent mullerian duct syndrome. *J Urol* 1976;115:459–461.
121. Knebelmann B, Boussin L, Guerrier D, et al. Anti-mullerian hormone Bruxelles: a nonsense mutation associated with the persistent mullerian duct syndrome. *Proc Natl Acad Sci USA* 1991;88:3767–3771.
122. Rosenthal IM. Molecular basis for persistent mullerian duct syndrome. *Int Pediatr* 1992;7:9–12.
123. Meyers-Wallen VN, Donahoe PK, Ueno S, Manganaro TF, Patterson DF. Mullerian inhibiting substance is present in testes of

dogs with persistent mullerian duct syndrome. *Biol Reprod* 1989;41:881–888.
124. Vigier B, Watrin F, Magre S, Tran D, Josso N. Purified bovine AMH induces a characteristic freemartin effect in fetal rat prospective ovaries exposed to it *in vitro. Development* 1987;100: 43–55.
125. Vigier B, Forest MG, Eychenne B, et al. Anti-mullerian hormone produces endocrine sex reversal of fetal ovaries. *Proc Natl Acad Sci USA* 1989;86:3684–3688.
126. Behringer RR, Cate RL, Froelick GJ, Palmiter RD, Brinster RL. Abnormal sexual development in transgenic mice chronically expressing mullerian inhibiting substance. *Nature* 1990;345: 167–170.
127. Lipsett MB, Tullner WW. Testosterone synthesis by the fetal rabbit gonad. *Endocrinology* 1965;77:273–277.
128. Siiteri PK, Wilson JD. Testosterone formation and metabolism during male sexual differentiation in the human embryo. *J Clin Endocrinol Metab* 1974;38:113–125.
129. Wilson JD, Siiteri PK. Developmental pattern of testosterone synthesis in the fetal gonad of the rabbit. *Endocrinology* 1973;92:1182–1191.
130. Gondos B. Development and differentiation of the testis and male reproductive tract. *In:* Steinberger A, Steinberger E, eds. *Testicular Development, Structure and Function.* New York: Raven Press, 1980;3–20.
131. Attal J. Levels of testosterone, androstenedione, estrone and estradiol-17β in the testes of fetal sheep. *Endocrinology* 1969;85:280–289.
132. Rigaudiere N. The androgens in the guinea-pig foetus throughout the embryonic development. *Acta Endocrinol* 1979;92:174–186.
133. Schultz FM, Wilson JD. Virilization of the wolffian duct in the rat fetus by various androgens. *Endocrinology* 1974;94:979–986.
134. George FW, Peterson KG. 5α-Dihydrotestosterone formation is necessary for embryogenesis of the rat prostate. *Endocrinology* 1988;122:1159–1164.
135. Goldman AS. Production of hypospadias in the rat by selective inhibition of fetal testicular 17α-hydroxylase and C_{17-20}-lyase. *Endocrinology* 1971;88:527–531.
136. Neumann F, von Berswordt-Wallrabe R, Elger W, Steinbeck H, Hahn JD, Kramer M. Aspects of androgen-dependent events as studied by antiandrogens. *Recent Prog Horm Res* 1970;26: 337–405.
137. Griffin JE, Wilson JD. Hereditary male pseudohermaphroditism. *Clin Obstet Gynecol* 1978;5:457–479.
138. Wilson JD, Goldstein JL. Classification of hereditary disorders of sexual development. *Birth Defects* 1975;11:1–16.
139. Milewich L, George FW, Wilson JD. Estrogen formation by the ovary of the rabbit embryo. *Endocrinology* 1977;100:187–196.
140. George FW, Simpson ER, Milewich L, Wilson JD. Studies on the regulation of steroid hormone biosynthesis in fetal rabbit gonads. *Endocrinology* 1979;105:1100–1106.
141. George FW, Wilson JD. Endocrine differentiation of the rabbit ovary in culture. *Nature* 1980;283:861–863.
142. George FW, Catt KJ, Neaves WB, Wilson JD. Studies on the regulation of testosterone synthesis in the rabbit fetal testis. *Endocrinology* 1978;102:665–673.
143. Patsavoudi E, Magre S, Castanier M, Scholler R, Jost A. Dissociation between testicular morphogenesis and functional differentiation of Leydig cells. *J Endocrinol* 1985;105:235–238.
144. Catt KJ, Dufau ML, Neaves WB, Walsh PC, Wilson JD. LH-hCG receptors and testosterone content during differentiation of the testis in the rabbit embryo. *Endocrinology* 1975;97: 1157–1165.
145. Reyes FI, Boroditsky RS, Winter JSD, Faiman C. Studies on human sexual development. II. Fetal and maternal serum gonadotropin and sex steroid concentrations. *J Clin Endocrinol Metab* 1974;38:612–617.
146. Huhtaniemi IT, Korenbrat CC, Jaffe RB. hCG binding and stimulation of testosterone biosynthesis in the human fetal testis. *J Clin Endocrinol Metab* 1977;44:963–967.
147. Molsberry RL, Carr BR, Mendelson CR, Simpson ER. Human chorionic gonadotropin binding to human fetal testes as a function of gestational age. *J Clin Endocrinol Metab* 1982;55: 791–794.
148. Rabinovici J, Jaffe RB. Development and regulation of growth and differentiated function in human and subhuman primate fetal gonads. *Endocr Rev* 1990;11:532–557.
149. Abramovich DR, Baker TG, Neal P. Effect of human chorionic gonadotrophin on testosterone secretion by the foetal human testis in organ culture. *J Endocrinol* 1974;60:179–185.
150. Word RA, George FW, Wilson JD, Carr BR. Testosterone synthesis and adenylate cyclase activity in the early human fetal testis appear to be independent of human chorionic gonadotropin control. *J Clin Endocrinol Metab* 1989;69:204–208.
151. Schwartz M, Imperato-McGinley J, Peterson RE, et al. Male pseudohermaphroditism secondary to an abnormality in Leydig cell differentiation. *J Clin Endocrinol Metab* 1981;53:123–127.
152. Rajfer J, Walsh PC. Hormonal regulation of testicular descent: experimental and clinical observations. *J Urol* 1977;118: 985–990.
153. George FW, Wilson JD. Conversion of androgen to estrogen by the human fetal ovary. *J Clin Endocrinol Metab* 1978;47: 550–555.
154. Gondos B, George FW, Wilson JD. Granulosa cell differentiation and estrogen synthesis in the fetal rabbit ovary. *Biol Reprod* 1983;29:329–344.
155. Burns RK. Role of hormones in the differentiation of sex. *In:* Young WC, ed. *Sex and Internal Secretions.* Baltimore: Williams & Wilkins, 1961;76–158.
156. Bruner JA, Witschi E. Testosterone-induced modifications of sex development in female hamsters. *Am J Anat* 1946;79:293–320.
157. Greene RR. Hormonal factors in sex inversion: the effects of sex hormones on embryonic sexual structures of the rat. *Biol Symp* 1942;9:105–123.
158. Jost A. Recherches sur la differenciation de l'embyon de lapin. II Action des androgens synthese sur histogenses genitale. *Arch Anat Microscop Morph* 1947;36:242–270.
159. Turner CD. The influence of testosterone propionate upon sexual differentiation in genetic female mice (etc.). *J Exp Zool* 1940;83:1–31.
160. Wells LJ, van Wagenen G. Androgen-induced female pseudohermaphroditism in the monkey (*Macaca mulatta*): anatomy of the reproductive organs. *Contrib Embryol Carnegie Inst Wash* 1954;35:93–106.
161. White MR. Effects of hormones on embryonic sex differentiation in the golden hamster. *J Exp Zool* 1949;110:153–181.
162. Buyse A. The differentiation of transplanted mammalian gonad primordia. *J Exp Zool* 1935;70:1–41.
163. Holyoke EA. The differentiation of embryonic gonads transplanted to the adult omentum in the albino rat. *Anat Rec* 1949;103:675–699.
164. Mangoushi MA. Scrotal allografts of fetal ovaries. *J Anat* 1975;120:595–599.
165. Moore CR, Price D. Differentiation of embryonic gonads transplanted into postnatal hosts. *J Exp Zool* 1942;90:229–265.
166. Taketo T, Merchant-Larios H, Koide SS. Induction of testicular differentiation in fetal mouse ovary by transplantation into adult male mice. *Proc Soc Exp Biol Med* 1984;176:148–153.
167. Torrey TW. Intraocular grafts of embryonic gonads of the rat. *J Exp Zool* 1950;115:37–38.
168. Taketo-Hosotani T, Merchant-Larios H, Thau RB, Koide SS. Testicular differentiation in fetal mouse ovaries following transplantation into adult mice. *J Exp Zool* 1985;236:229–237.
169. Gruenwald P. The relation of the growing mullerian duct to the wolffian duct and its importance for the genesis of malformation. *Anat Rec* 1941;81:1–19.
170. Spaulding MH. The development of the external genitalia in the human embryo. *Contrib Embryol Carnegie Inst Wash* 1921;13: 69–88.
171. Bengmark S. *The Prostatic Urethra and Prostate Glands.* Lund, Sweden: Berlingska Boktryckeriet, 1958.
172. Lowsley OS. The development of the human prostate with reference to the development of other structures of the neck of the urinary bladder. *Am J Anat* 1912;13:299–349.
173. Kellokumpo-Lehtinen P, Santti R, Pelliniemi LJ. Correlation of early cytodifferentiation of the human fetal prostate and Leydig cells. *Anat Rec* 1980;196:263–273.

174. Shapiro E. Embryologic development of the prostate. *Urol Clin North Am* 1990;17:487–493.
175. Gier HT, Marion GB. Development of the mammalian testis and genital ducts. *Biol Reprod* 1969;1:1–23.
176. Elder JS, Isaacs JT, Walsh PC. Androgenic sensitivity of the gubernaculum testis: evidence for hormonal/mechanical interactions in testicular descent. *J Urol* 1982;127:170–176.
177. George FW, Peterson KG. Partial characterization of the androgen receptor of the newborn rat gubernaculum. *Biol Reprod* 1988;39:536–539.
178. George FW. Developmental pattern of 5α-reductase activity in the gubernaculum. *Endocrinology* 1989;124:727–732.
179. Husmann DA, McPhaul MJ. Localization of the androgen receptor in the developing rat gubernaculum. *Endocrinology* 1991;128: 383–387.
180. Spencer JR, Torrado T, Sanchez RS, Vaughan ED Jr, Imperato-McGinley J. Effects of flutamide and finasteride on rat testicular descent. *Endocrinology* 1991;129:741–748.
181. Husmann DA, McPhaul MJ. Time-specific androgen blockade with flutamide inhibits testicular descent in the rat. *Endocrinology* 1991;129:1409–1416.
182. Hutson JM. A biphasic model for the hormonal control of testicular descent. *Lancet* 1985;2:419–421.
183. O'Rahilly R. The development of the vagina in the human. *Birth Defects* 1977;13:123–136.
184. Bok G, Drews U. The role of the wolffian ducts in the formation of the sinus vagina: an organ culture study. *J Embryol Exp Morphol* 1983;73:275–295.
185. Bulmer D. The development of the human vagina. *J Anat* 1957;91:490–509.
186. Lawrence WD, Whitaker D, Sugimura H, Cunha GR, Dickersin R, Robboy SJ. An ultrastructural study of the developing urogenital tract in early human fetuses. *Am J Obstet Gynecol* 1992;167:185–193.
187. Goldman AS, Shapiro BH, Neumann F. Role of testosterone and its metabolites in the differentiation of the mammary gland in rats. *Endocrinology* 1976;99:1490–1495.
188. Imperato-McGinley J, Binienda Z, Gedney J, Vaughan ED. Nipple differentiation in fetal male rats treated with an inhibitor of the enzyme 5α-reductase: definition of a selective role for dihydrotestosterone. *Endocrinology* 1986;118:132–137.
189. Kratochwil K. *In vitro* analysis of the hormonal basis for the sexual dimorphism in the embryonic development of the mouse mammary gland. *J Embryol Exp Morphol* 1971;25:141–153.
190. Pfaltz CR. Das emryonale und postnatale Verholten der mannlichen Brust driise beim menschen. II. Das mammarorgan im Kindes-, Junglings-, Mannes-und Greisenalter. *Acta Anat* 1949;8: 293–328.
191. Jost A. The role of fetal hormones in prenatal development. *Harvey Lect* 1961;55:201–226.
192. Budzik GP, Powell SM, Kamagata S, Donahoe PK. Mullerian-inhibiting substance fractionation by dye affinity chromatography. *Cell* 1983;34:307–314.
193. Donahoe PK, Budzik GP, Trelstad R, et al. Mullerian inhibiting substance: an update. *Recent Prog Horm Res* 1982;38:279–326.
194. Josso N, Picard J-Y, Tran D. The anti-mullerian hormone. *Recent Prog Horm Res* 1977;33:117–167.
195. Cate RL, Mattaliano RJ, Hession C, et al. Isolation of the bovine and human genes for mullerian inhibiting substance and expression of the human gene in animal cells. *Cell* 1986;45:685–698.
196. Picard JY, Benarous R, Guerrier D, Josso N, Kahn A. Cloning and expression of cDNA for anti-mullerian hormone. *Proc Natl Acad Sci USA* 1986;83:5464–5468.
197. Dyche WJ. A comparative study of the differentiation and involution of the mullerian duct and wolffian duct in the male and female fetal mouse. *J Morphol* 1979;162:175–210.
198. Trelstad RL, Hayashi K, Hayashi K, Donahoe PK. The epithelial-mesenchymal interface of the male rat mullerian duct: loss of basement membrane integrity and ductal regression. *Dev Biol* 1982;92:27–40.
199. Price JM, Donahoe PK, Ito Y, Hendren WH III. Programmed cell death in the mullerian duct induced by mullerian inhibiting substance. *Am J Anat* 1977;149:353–376.
200. Trelstad RL, Hayashi A, Hayashi K, Donahoe PK. the epithelial-mesenchymal interface of the male mullerian duct: basement membrane integrity and ductal regression. *Dev Biol* 1982;92: 27–40.
201. Coughlin JP, Donahoe PK, Budzik GP, MacLaughlin DT. Mullerian inhibiting substance blocks autophosphorylation of the EGF receptor by inhibiting tyrosine kinase. *Mol Cell Endocrinol* 1987;49:75–86.
202. Cigarroa FG, Coughlin JP, Donahoe PK, White MF, Uitvlugt N, MacLaughlin DT. Recombinant human mullerian inhibiting substance inhibits epidermal growth factor receptor tyrosine kinase. *Growth Factors* 1989;1:179–191.
203. Donahoe PK, Hutson JM, Fallat ME, Kamagata S, Budzik GP. Mechanism of action of mullerian inhibiting substance. *Annu Rev Physiol* 1984;46:53–65.
204. Hutson JM, Fallat ME, Kamagata S, Donahoe PK, Budzik GP. Phosphorylation events during mullerian duct regression. *Science* 1984;223:586–588.
205. Fallat ME, Hutson JM, Budzik GP, Donahoe PK. Androgen stimulation of nucleotide pyrophosphatase during mullerian duct regression. *Endocrinology* 1984;114:1592–1598.
206. Ikawa H, Hutson JM, Budzik GP, MacLaughlin DT, Donahoe PK. Steroid enhancement of mullerian duct regression. *J Pediatr Surg* 1982;17:453–458.
207. Hutson JM, Donahoe PK, MacLaughlin DT. Steroid modulation of mullerian duct regression in the chick embryo. *Gen Comp Endocrinol* 1985;57:88–102.
208. Hutson JM, Ikawa H, Donahoe PK. Estrogen inhibition of mullerian inhibiting substance in the chick embryo. *J Pediatr Surg* 1982;17:953–959.
209. McLachlan JA. Prenatal exposure to diethylstilbestrol in mice: toxicological studies. *J Toxicol Environ Health* 1977;2:527–537.
210. Teng CS, Teng CT. Prenatal effect of the estrogenic hormone on embryonic genital organ differentiation. *In:* Hamilton TH, Clark JH, Sadler NA, eds. *Ontogeny of Receptors and Reproductive Hormone Action.* New York: Raven Press, 1979;421–440.
211. Donahoe PK, Fuller AF Jr, Sailly RE, Guy SR, Budzik GP. Mullerian inhibiting substance inhibits growth of a human ovarian cancer in nude mice. *Ann Surg* 1981;194:472–480.
212. Donahoe PK, Swann DA, Hayashi A, Sullivan MD. Mullerian duct regression in the embryo correlated with cytotoxic activity against human ovarian cancer. *Science* 1979;205:913–915.
213. Fuller AF Jr, Guy S, Budzik GP, Donahoe PK. Mullerian-inhibiting substance inhibits colony growth of a human ovarian carcinoma cell line. *J Clin Endocrinol Metab* 1982;42:653–660.
214. George FW, Noble JF. Androgen receptors are similar in fetal and adult rabbits. *Endocrinology* 1984;115:1451–1458.
215. Kovacs WJ, Griffin JE, Wilson JD. Transformation of human androgen receptors to the deoxyribonucleic acid-binding state. *Endocrinology* 1983;113:1574–1581.
216. Maes M, Sultan C, Zerhouni N, Rothwell SW, Migeon CJ. Role of testosterone binding to the androgen receptor in male sexual differentiation of patients with 5a-reductase deficiency. *J Steroid Biochem* 1979;11:1385–1390.
217. Wilbert DM, Griffin JE, Wilson JD. Characterization of the cytosol androgen receptor of the human prostate. *J Clin Endocrinol Metab* 1983;56:113–120.
218. Deslypere J-P, Young M, Wilson JD, McPhaul MJ. Testosterone and 5a-dihydrotestosterone interact differently with the androgen receptor to enhance transcription of the MMTV-CAT reporter gene. *Mol Cell Endocrinol* 1992;88:15–22.
219. George FW, Russell DW, Wilson JD. Feed-forward control of prostate growth: dihydrotestosterone induces expression of its own biosynthetic enzyme, steroid 5α-reductase. *Proc Natl Acad Sci USA* 1991;88:8044–8047.
220. Wilson JD, Lasnitzki I. Dihydrotestosterone formation in fetal tissues of the rabbit and rat. *Endocrinology* 1971;89:659–668.
221. Fisher LK, Kogut MD, Moore RJ, et al. Clinical, endocrinological, and enzymatic characterization of two patients with 5α-reductase deficiency. Evidence that a single enzyme is responsible for the 5α-reduction of cortisol and testosterone. *J Clin Endocrinol Metab* 1978;47:653–664.
222. Peterson RE, Imperato-McGinley J, Gautier T, Sturla E. Male

pseudohermaphroditism due to steroid 5α-reductase deficiency. *Am J Med* 1977;62:170–191.
223. Walsh PC, Madden JD, Harrod MJ, Goldstein JL, MacDonald PC, Wilson JD. Familial incomplete male pseudohermaphroditism, type 2. Decreased dihydrotestosterone formation in pseudovaginal perineoscrotal hypospadias. *N Engl J Med* 1974;291: 944–949.
224. Imperato-McGinley J, Guerrero L, Gautier T, Peterson RE. Steroid 5α-reductase deficiency in man: an inherited form of male pseudohermaphroditism. *Science* 1974;186:1213–1215.
225. Griffin JE, Wilson JD. The androgen resistance syndromes: 5α-reductase deficiency, testicular feminization, and related disorders. *In:* Scriver CR, Beaudet AL, Sly WS, Valle D, eds. *The Metabolic Basis of Inherited Disease,* Ed. 6. New York: McGraw-Hill, 1989;1919–1944.
226. Andersson S, Russell DW. Structural and biochemical properties of cloned and expressed human and rat steroid 5α-reductases. *Proc Natl Acad Sci USA* 1990;87:3640–3644.
227. Andersson S, Berman DM, Jenkins EP, Russell DW. Deletion of steroid 5α-reductase 2 gene in male pseudohermaphroditism. *Nature* 1991;354:159–161.
228. Jenkins EP, Andersson S, Imperato McGinley J, Wilson JD, Russell DW. Genetic and pharmacological evidence for more than one human steroid 5α-reductase. *J Clin Invest* 1992;89: 293–300.
229. Jenkins EP, Hsieh CL, Milatovich A, et al. Characterization and chromosomal mapping of a human steroid 5α-reductase gene and pseudogene and mapping of the mouse homologue. *Genomics* 1991;11:1102–1112.
230. Thigpen AE, Davis DL, Milatovich A, et al. Molecular genetics of steroid 5α-reductase 2 deficiency. *J Clin Invest* 1992;90:799–809.
231. Brooks JR, Baptista EM, Berman C, et al. Response of rat ventral prostate to a new and novel 5 alpha-reductase inhibitor. *Endocrinology* 1991;109(3):830–836.
232. Brooks JR, Berman C, Hitchens M, et al. Biological activities of a new steroidal inhibitor of delta 4-5 alpha-reductase. *Proceedings of the Society for Experimental Biology and Medicine.* 1982;169(1):67–73.
233. Anderson CA, Clark RL. External genitalia of the rat: normal development and the histogenesis of 5α-reductase inhibitor-induced abnormalities. *Teratology* 1990;42:483–496.
234. Bidlingmaier F, Knorr D, Neumann F. Inhibition of masculine differentiation in male offspring of rabbits actively immunized against testosterone before pregnancy. *Nature* 1977;226:647–648.
235. Ikadai H, Sakuma Y, Suzuki K, Imamichi T. Congenital abnormalities of the male genital organs in the newly established TW rat strain. *Cong Anom* 1985;25:65–71.
236. Thigpen AE, Silver RI, Guileyardo JM, Casey ML, McConnell JD, Russell DW. Tissue distribution and ontogeny of steroid 5α-reductase isozyme expression. (*in press*)
237. Bardin CW, Bullock LP, Sherins RJ, Mowszowicz I, Blackburn WR. Androgen metabolism and mechanism of action in male pseudohermaphroditism: a study of testicular feminization. *Recent Prog Horm Res* 1973;29:65–105.
238. Goldstein JL, Wilson JD. Studies on the pathogenesis of the pseudohermaphroditism in the mouse with testicular feminization. *J Clin Invest* 1972;51:1647–1658.
239. Lyon MF, Hawkes SG. X-Linked gene for testicular feminization in the mouse. *Nature* 1970;227:1217–1219.
240. Bullock LP, Bardin CW, Ohno S. The androgen insensitive mouse: absence of intranuclear androgen retention in the kidney. *Biochem Biophys Res Commun* 1971;44:1537–1543.
241. Gehring U, Tomkins GM, Ohno S. Effect of the androgen-insensitivity mutation on a cytoplasmic receptor for dihydrotestosterone. *Nature New Biol* 1971;232:106–107.
242. Verhoeven G, Wilson JD. Cytosol androgen binding in submandibular gland and kidney of the normal mouse and the mouse with testicular feminization. *Endocrinology* 1976;99:79–92.
243. MacDonald PC, Madden JD, Brenner PF, Wilson JD, Siiteri PK. Origin of estrogen in normal men and in women with testicular feminization. *J Clin Endocrinol Metab* 1979;49:905–916.
244. Madden JD, Walsh PC, MacDonald PC, Wilson JD. Clinical and endocrinological characterization of a patient with the syndrome of incomplete testicular feminization. *J Clin Endocrinol Metab* 1975;40:751–760.
245. Aiman J, Griffin JE. The frequency of androgen receptor deficiency in infertile men. *J Clin Endocrinol Metab* 1982;54: 725–732.
246. Aiman J, Griffin JE, Gazak JM, Wilson JD, MacDonald PC. Androgen insensitivity as a cause of infertility in otherwise normal men. *N Engl J Med* 1979;300:223–227.
247. Griffin JE, Punyashthiti K, Wilson JD. Dihydrotestosterone binding by cultured human fibroblasts. Comparison of cells from control subject and from patients with hereditary male pseudohermaphroditism due to androgen resistance. *J Clin Invest* 1976;57:1342–1351.
248. Keenan BS, Meyer WJ III, Hadjian AJ, Jones HW, Migeon CJ. Syndrome of androgen insensitivity in man: absence of 5-dihydrotestosterone binding protein in skin fibroblasts. *J Clin Endocrinol Metab* 1974;38:1143–1146.
249. He WW, Kumar MV, Tindall DJ. A frame-shift mutation in the androgen receptor gene causes complete androgen insensitivity in the testicular-feminized mouse. *Nucleic Acids Res* 1991;19: 2373–2378.
250. Griffin JE. Testicular feminization associated with a thermolabile androgen receptor in cultured human fibroblasts. *J Clin Invest* 1979;64:1624–1631.
251. Griffin JE, Durrant JL. Qualitative receptor defects in families with androgen resistance: failure of stabilization of the fibroblast cytosol androgen receptor. *J Clin Endocrinol Metab* 1982;55: 465–474.
252. Kovacs WJ, Griffin JE, Weaver DD, Carlson BR, Wilson JD. A mutation that causes lability of the androgen receptor under conditions that normally promote DNA-binding state. *J Clin Invest* 1984;73:1095–1104.
253. Brown TR, Maes M, Rothwell SW, Migeon CJ. Human complete androgen insensitivity with normal dihydrotestosterone receptor binding capacity in cultured genital skin fibroblasts. Evidence for a qualitative abnormality of the receptor. *J Clin Endocrinol Metab* 1982;55:61–69.
254. Eil C. Familial incomplete male pseudohermaphroditism associated with impaired nuclear androgen retention. *J Clin Invest* 1983;71:850–858.
255. Kaufman M, Pinsky L, Hollander R, Bailey JD. Regulation of the androgen receptor in normal and androgen resistant genital skin fibroblasts. *J Steroid Biochem* 1983;18:383–390.
256. Chang C, Kokontis J, Liao S. Structural analysis of complementary DNA and amino acid sequences of human and rat androgen receptors. *Proc Natl Acad Sci USA* 1988;85:7211–7215.
257. Lubahn DB, Joseph DR, Sar M, et al. The human androgen receptor: complementary deoxyribonucleic acid cloning, sequence analysis, and gene expression in prostate. *Mol Endocrinol* 1988;2(12):1265–1275.
258. Trapman J, Klaassen P, Kuiper GGJM, et al. Cloning and expression of a cDNA encoding the human androgen receptor. *Biochem Biophys Res Commun* 1988;153:241–248.
259. Tilley WD, Marcelli M, Wilson JD, McPhaul MJ. Characterization and expression of a cDNA encoding the human androgen receptor. *Proc Natl Acad Sci USA* 1989;86:327–331.
260. Carson-Jurica MA, Schrader WT, O'Malley BW. Steroid receptor family: structure and functions. *Endocr Rev* 1990;11: 201–220.
261. McPhaul MJ, Marcelli M, Tilley WD, Griffin JE, Wilson JD. Androgen resistance caused by mutations in the androgen receptor gene. *FASEB J* 1991;5:2910–2915.
262. French FS, Lubahn DB, Brown TR, et al. Molecular basis of androgen insensitivity. *Recent Prog Horm Res* 1990;46:1–38.
263. McPhaul MJ, Marcelli M, Zoppi S, Griffin JE, Wilson JD. Genetic basis of endocrine disease. The spectrum of mutations in the androgen receptor gene that cause androgen resistance. *J Clin Endocrinol Metab* 1993;76(1):17–23.
264. Cunha GR, Chung LWK, Shannon JM, Reese BA. Stromal-epithelia; interactions in sex differentiation. *Biol Reprod* 1980;22:19–42.
265. Cunha GR. Epithelial–mesenchymal interactions in primordial

gland structures which become responsive to androgenic stimulation. *Anat Rec* 1972;172:179–196.
266. Cunha GR. Tissue interactions between epithelium and mesenchyme of urogenital and integumental origin. *Anat Rec* 1972;172:529–542.
267. Cunha GR, Chung LWK. Stromal–epithelial interactions. I. Induction of prostatic phenotype in urothelium of testicular feminized (*Tfm*/Y) mice. *J Steroid Biochem* 1981;14:1317–1321.
268. Lasnitzki I, Mizuno T. Prostatic induction: interaction of epithelium and mesenchyme from wild-type and androgen insensitive mice with testicular feminization. *J Endocrinol* 1980;85: 423–428.
269. Takeda H, Mizuno T, Lasnitzki I. Autoradiographic studies of androgen-binding sites in the rat urogenital sinus and postnatal prostate. *J Endocrinol* 1985;104:87–92.
270. Drews U, Drews U. Regression of mouse mammary gland anlagen in recombinants of *Tfm* and wild-type tissues: testosterone acts via the mesenchyme. *Cell* 1977;10:401–404.
271. Kratochwil K, Schwartz P. Tissue interaction in androgen response of embryonic mammary rudiment of mouse: identification of target tissue for testosterone. *Proc Natl Acad Sci USA* 1976;73:4041–4044.
272. Heuberger B, Fritzka I, Wasner G, Kratochwil K. Induction of androgen receptor formation by epithelium–mesenchyme interaction in embryonic mouse mammary gland. *Proc Natl Acad Sci USA* 1982;79:2957–2961.
273. New MI, White PC, Pang S, Dupont B, Speiser PW. The adrenal hyperplasias. In: Scriver CR, Beaudet AL, Sly WS, Valle D, eds. *The Metabolic Basis of Inherited Disease,* Ed 6. New York: McGraw-Hill, 1989;1881–1918.
274. George FW, Wilson JD. Estrogen formation in the early rabbit embryo. *Science* 1978;199:200–202.
275. George FW, Tobelman WT, Milewich L, Wilson JD. Aromatase activity in the developing rabbit brain. *Endocrinology* 1978;102: 86–91.
276. Dickman Z, Dey SK. A new concept: control of early pregnancy by steroid hormones originating in the preimplantation embryo. *Vitam Horm* 1976;34:215–242.
277. Dickman Z, Gupta JS, Dey SK. Does "blastocyst estrogen" initiate implantation? *Science* 1977;195:687–688.
278. Burns RK. The differentiation of the phallus in the opossum and its reaction to sex hormones. *Contrib Embryol Carnegie Inst Wash* 1945;31:147–162.
279. Renfree MB, Short RV, OW-S. Experimental manipulation of sexual differentiation in wallaby pouch young with exogenous steroids. *Development* 1988;104:689–701.
280. Renfree MB. The role of genes and hormones in marsupial sexual differentiation. *J Zool* 1992;226:165–173.
281. Renfree MB, Wilson JD, Short RV, Shaw GS, George FW. Steroid hormone content of the gonads of the Tammar Wallaby during sexual differentiation. *Biol Reprod* 1992;47:644–647.
282. McLaren A. What makes a man? *Nature* 1990;346:216–217.
283. Affara NA. Sex and the single Y. *Bio Essays* 1991;13:475–478.

The Physiology of Reproduction, Second Edition,
edited by E. Knobil and J.D. Neill,
Raven Press, Ltd., New York © 1994.

CHAPTER 2

The Spermatozoon

E. M. Eddy[1] and Deborah A. O'Brien[2]

The spermatozoon is the end product of the process of gametogenesis in the male, which occurs within the seminiferous tubules of the testis (1). This process involves a series of mitotic divisions of spermatogonial stem cells, two meiotic divisions by spermatocytes, extensive morphological remodeling of spermatids during spermiogenesis, and the release of free cells into the lumen of the seminiferous tubules by spermiation. These events are probably the result of overlapping developmental programs of gene expression (2,3). It is an interesting paradox that the process of spermatogenesis produces a cell that is both highly differentiated in structure and function and, at the same time, developmentally totipotent, being able to combine with the egg and thereby begin the process that gives rise to a new individual (4,5).

The mammalian spermatozoon has two main components, the *head* and the *flagellum* or tail, which are joined at the neck (Fig. 1). The head consists of the acrosome, the nucleus, and small amounts of cytoskeletal structures and cytoplasm. The *acrosome* is surrounded by a membrane and contains hydrolytic enzymes. It overlies the anterior end of the nucleus. The sperm *nucleus* contains only one member of each chromosome pair, and the chromatin is highly condensed. The flagellum contains a central *axoneme* surrounded by *outer dense fibers* extending from the head to near the posterior end. In addition, the anterior part of the flagellum contains mitochondria wrapped in a tight helix around the dense fibers, and the posterior part of the tail contains a *fibrous sheath* surrounding the outer dense fibers. The outer dense fibers and the fibrous sheath form the cytoskeleton of the flagellum. These cytoskeletal features may have evolved with the development of internal fertilization (6). The flagellum, like the head, is closely wrapped by the plasma membrane and contains little cytoplasm. Although all mammalian spermatozoa have these general characteristics, there are species-specific differences in the size and shape of the head and the length and relative size of the components of the flagellum.

Nonmammalian species show greater variation in sperm structure than mammals. Although sperm in

[1] Gamete Biology Section, Laboratory of Reproductive and Developmental Toxicology, National Institute of Environmental Health Sciences, National Institutes of Health, Research Triangle Park, North Carolina 27709

[2] Gamete Biology Section, Laboratory of Reproductive and Developmental Toxicology, National Institute of Environmental Health Sciences, National Institutes of Health, Research Triangle Park, North Carolina 27709; and Laboratories for Reproductive Biology, Departments of Pediatrics and Cell Biology and Anatomy, The University of North Carolina at Chapel Hill, Chapel Hill, North Carolina 27599

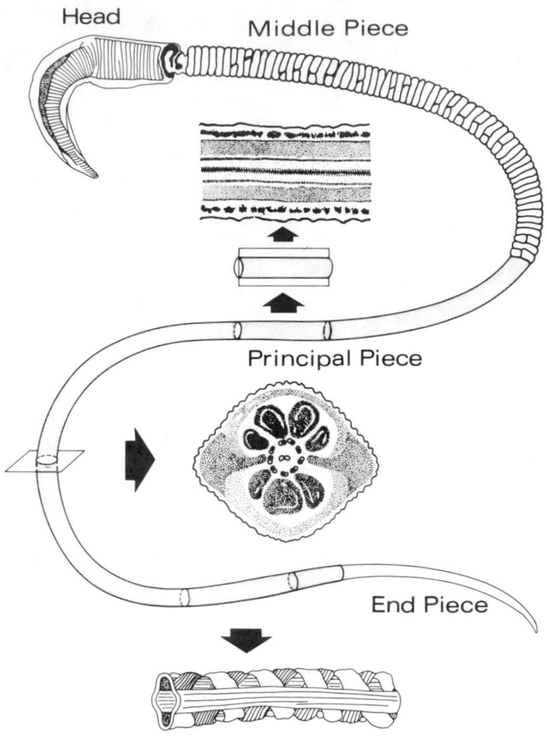

FIG. 1. General features of the mammalian spermatozoon. The head of the sperm is attached to the connecting piece of the flagellum. The other regions of the flagellum are the middle piece, the principal piece, and the end piece. The middle piece contains the mitochondrial sheath, and the principal piece contains the fibrous sheath. Longitudinal and cross-sectional views of the principal piece and a segment of fibrous sheath are indicated by *arrows;* the internal components of the flagellum are identified in Figs. 8 and 9.

most invertebrates and nonmammalian vertebrates have an acrosome, they often contain few mitochondria, and the flagellum usually consists only of an axoneme. In some species, spermatozoa are amoeboid cells lacking an acrosome and a flagellum (7,8).

The specialized structural features of the spermatozoon are a reflection of its unique functional activities. The acrosome contains enzymes essential for fertilization, and the flagellum contains the energy sources and machinery necessary to produce motility. The roles of these components are to ensure delivery of the genetic material contained in the sperm nucleus to the egg, where combination of the haploid male and female pronuclei occurs, producing the zygote. In most vertebrates, the sex chromosome carried in the haploid sperm nucleus determines the sex of the resulting animal (9). Both a maternal and a paternal genome are required for development to proceed to term, probably because of differential imprinting of genes during gametogenesis in males and females (10,11).

This chapter examines the characteristics of the mammalian spermatozoon, with particular attention to the molecules currently known to contribute to its structures and functions. The major topics considered are: the organization of the sperm plasma membrane into domains, changes in the composition and function of the domains during the life of the cell, the structural components of the head of the sperm, and the features of the flagellum. Other chapters in this volume are concerned with the formation of the male gamete (1), the participation of the spermatozoon in fertilization (5), and the subsequent development of a new individual (4). They should be consulted for additional information necessary for understanding the structure and function of the spermatozoon and its role in the reproductive process.

THE PLASMA MEMBRANE

Surface Domains

A unique feature of the spermatozoon is that the plasma membrane is subdivided into well-delineated regional domains that differ in composition and function. The heterogeneous nature of the sperm surface is shown by studies of surface charge, lectin binding to specific sugar moieties, freeze-fracture patterns, and antibody labeling. The evidence that the organization and composition of the plasma membrane vary between different regions of the sperm surface has led to the concept that the sperm plasma membrane is a mosaic of restricted domains that reflect the specialized functions of surface and cytoplasmic components of the spermatozoon (12–16). These domains are dynamic features that undergo changes in organization and composition during the life of the cell (17).

The major domains of the plasma membrane on the sperm head of most mammals are the *acrosomal region* (anterior head) and the *postacrosomal region* (posterior head) (Fig. 2). The plasma membrane of the acrosomal region can usually be subdivided into (a) the *marginal segment* (apical segment, anterior band, peripheral rim) domain over the anterior margin of the acrosome, (b) the *principal segment* (acrosomal segment) domain over the major portion of the acrosome, and (c) the *equatorial segment* (posterior acrosome) domain over the posterior part of the acrosome (18). The marginal and principal segment domains together are frequently referred to as the *anterior acrosome* or the *acrosomal cap.* These two domains are separated by the central crescent in guinea pig sperm and possibly other species (17).

The *postacrosomal region* (posterior head, postacrosomal segment) domain includes the plasma membrane between the posterior margin of the acrosome and the neck. The marginal and principal segment domains of the acrosomal cap in guinea pig sperm and possibly other species are separated by the *central crescent* (17). The margin between the acrosomal and postacrosomal

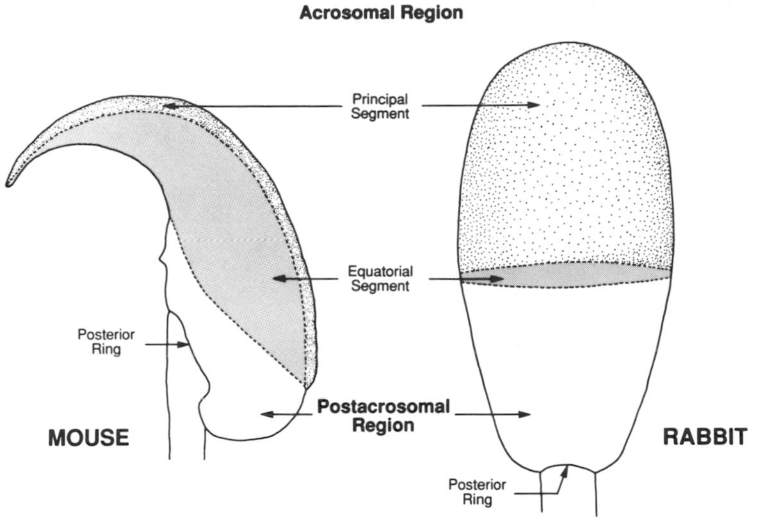

FIG. 2. Plasma membrane domains on the surface of the head of mouse and rabbit spermatozoa. The major domains on the sperm head are the acrosomal region (acrosomal cap) and postacrosomal region (posterior head). In many species, the acrosomal region can be further subdivided into the marginal segment (apical segment), the principal segment (acrosomal segment), and the equatorial segment (posterior acrosome). The acrosomal region domain is more extensive on sperm with a spatulate head, such as those of the rabbit, whereas the equatorial segment domain is larger on sperm with a falciform head. The posterior ring defines the boundary between the postacrosomal domain of the head and the middle piece domain of the flagellum. The distribution of the domains of sperm from these and other species are compared in Fig. 3.

regions may be delimited by the *serrated band* (subacrosomal ring), which girdles the sperm head at the posterior margin of the equatorial segment (Table 1).

The *posterior ring* (nuclear ring, striated ring) is at the junction between head and tail and apparently forms a tight seal between the cytoplasmic compartments of the two main portions of the spermatozoon. The plasma membrane of the flagellum is separated into the *middle piece* domain overlying the mitochondrial sheath and the *posterior tail* (principal piece, distal tail) domain. These domains are separated by the *annulus,* a fibrous ring that is a component of the flagellar cytoskeleton and appears to adhere to the inner surface of the plasma membrane.

The Mosaic Sperm Surface

The first observations to suggest heterogeneity of the sperm plasma membrane came from studies of surface charge (Table 1). When spermatozoa from the ram, rabbit, or bull are suspended between oppositely charged electrodes, they are drawn tail first by electrophoresis toward the anode. This suggests that sperm have a net negative charge and that more of this charge is associated with the tail than with the head (19–21). Other studies demonstrate that at least some of the moieties responsible for the net negative charge are on the sperm surface and that there are regional differences in the distribution of surface charge. In electron microscopic studies of rabbit and stallion sperm, the binding of positively charged colloidal iron hydroxide to the surface is greater on the flagellum than on the head (22–24).

Additional evidence that the sperm surface is heterogeneous is provided by studies using lectins as impermeant probes. Lectins bind particular saccharide molecules with relatively high specificity (25,26). They are often multimeric, may bind simultaneously to more than one saccharide ligand on a given cell, and can cause agglutination by linking adjacent cells. Lectins can be conjugated with fluorescent markers, enzymes, radioactive labels, or tags visible in the electron microscope. Agglutination assays carried out with spermatozoa from multiple species demonstrate that regional differences occur in the location and amount of specific saccharides on the sperm surface (Table 1). Soybean agglutinin (SBA; recognizing α-D-GalNAc, D-Gal) causes bull sperm to agglutinate tail to tail (27). Concanavalin A (Con A; recognizing α-D-Glc, α-D-Man) and wheat-germ agglutinin (WGA; recognizing $[\beta(1\text{–}4)\text{D-GalNAc}]_2$) have a similar effect on hamster sperm (28). Agglutination does not appear to result from more lectin-binding sites being present on the tail than on the head (29,30). Quantitative studies using iodinated lectins indicate that 1 to 3×10^7 Con-A- and WGA-binding sites are present per rabbit or hamster epididymal sperm (31). However, approximately ten times more Con A binding sites are present per square micrometer on the mouse sperm head than on the flagellum (30). The greater surface area and motion of the tail, compared to the head, apparently lead to tail-to-tail agglutination in the presence of lectins.

The use of lectins conjugated with fluorescent labels or ultrastructural markers demonstrates that different saccharides are heterogeneously distributed on the sperm surface (Table 1). These studies also verify that lectin-binding sites are generally present in higher density on the head than on the tail (32). Con A binds predominantly to saccharides present on the anterior acrosome of mouse sperm (33,34), and WGA binds mainly to the head of mouse sperm and the anterior acrosome of guinea pig and goat sperm (35–37). Soybean agglutinin binds to the principal segment of the anterior acrosome of guinea pig sperm (30), and peanut agglutinin (PNA; recognizing D-Gal, β[1–3]-GalNAc) binds to the same

TABLE 1. *Regional heterogeneity of the sperm plasma membrane*

Characteristics	References
Surface charge distribution	
Sperm drawn tail first toward the anode in electrophoretic field	19–21
Positively charged colloidal iron hydroxide particle binding greater on the tail than on the head	22–24
Surface saccharide distribution	
Sperm agglutinated tail to tail following lectin treatment	27,28
Different lectins bind to specific regions of the sperm surface	32–41
Intramembranous particle distribution	
Hexagonal arrays of particles in the plasma membrane overlying the acrosome	14,17,18,42–46
Dense populations of intramembranous particles in the plasma membrane overlying the postacrosomal region	36,42,47,48,52
Oblique strands of particles in plasma membrane of middle piece overlying mitochondria	12,13,18,42,53,62,63
Localized surface features	
Serrated band at posterior margin of equatorial segment of acrosome	13,48–52
Palisades of prominent particles at posterior margin of postacrosomal region	42,53–55
Belt of fine periodicities in plasma membrane over the posterior ring	13,42,48,56–68
Close array of fine particles in plasma membrane over annulus	42,53
Staggered row of large particles running longitudinally on principal piece	42,53,63,66–69
Membrane-intercalating agents	
Filipin-induced complexes with sterols frequent in plasma membrane over acrosome	14,18,55,68,70,71
Polymyxin B binds anionic phospholipids in plasma membrane over anterior acrosome	14,44,72,73
Fluorescent lipid analog integrates preferentially into plasma membrane over acrosome	74
Sperm plasma membrane antigens recognized by antisera	
Antigens shared with other cells in restricted domains on sperm surface	
Principal segment of acrosomal region	78
Equatorial segment of acrosomal region	76
Postacrosomal region	77
Antigens in single domains recognized by antisera to male germ cells	
Acrosomal segment of acrosomal region	79
Postacrosomal region	80
Posterior tail	81
Antigens in multiple domains recognized by antisera to male germ cells	
Equatorial segment of acrosomal region and postacrosomal region	82
Acrosomal region and midpiece	81
Head and midpiece	83
Whole tail	83
Entire sperm surface	85–87

segment on mouse sperm (38). A peroxidase histochemical method detects more intense Con A binding on the head than on the tail of rabbit sperm (39). Electron microscopy of rabbit sperm treated with ferritin-conjugated castor-bean agglutinin (RCA; recognizing β-D-Gal, D-GalNAc) also reveals a greater RCA binding on the head than on the tail (40). Comparable studies on hamster sperm find greater binding of ferritin- or hemocyanin-labeled Con A on the head than on the tail (41). In general, these studies also show that the surface domains recognized by lectins are not often well defined.

Freeze-fracture, freeze-etch, and surface replica studies also demonstrate regional differences in the sperm surface that correspond to domains. Variations occur in the number, size, and patterns of distribution of intramembranous particles and in the presence of other membrane-associated structures associated with different regions of the plasma membrane (Table 1). Particle size and distribution vary between species and change with epididymal maturation, capacitation, and the acrosome reaction. However, characteristic patterns are often associated with the marginal and equatorial segments of the anterior acrosome, the posterior margin of the equatorial segment, and the postacrosomal region of the sperm head. Specializations have also been observed in the plasma membrane overlying the posterior ring and the annulus.

The plasma membrane overlying the anterior acrosome and equatorial segment usually contains randomly distributed intramembranous particles. However, numerous hexagonal arrays of particles are present in these regions in guinea pig sperm, particularly when the sperm are stacked closely together in the epididymis (14,42,43). The particle arrays correspond to a similar quiltlike pattern in the surface coat of guinea pig sperm (17,44). This coating is visible in sections and surface replicas and can be removed from living sperm by treatment with either trypsin or neuraminidase (44). Quiltlike patches of particles are also seen in the anterior acrosome region of sperm from rat (45), boar (46), and golden hamster (18) but not mouse (47). The quiltlike arrays are particularly abundant in the marginal segment of golden hamster sperm (18). The serrated band at the posterior margin of the equatorial segment contains closely packed particles in a saw-toothed pattern (Table 1). The location and general topography of the serrated band can be seen by light microscopy (48), scanning electron microscopy (48–50), or transmission electron microscopy (13,51,52).

The plasma membrane of the postacrosomal region usually contains a denser population of intramembranous particles than the acrosomal region (36,42,48,52, 53), and the particles are sometimes clustered (Table 1). In addition, the plasma membrane at the basal part of the postacrosomal region contains prominent bands or palisades of particles (42,53–55) just anterior to the posterior ring (Table 1).

The plasma membrane over the posterior ring contains a belt of fine periodicities or cords of small particles and is firmly attached to a belt of dense fibrous material associated with the nuclear envelope (13,42,48,51,56, 57). The posterior ring appears to produce a seal between the head and tail cytoplasmic compartments of the spermatozoon, which may allow different ionic and metabolic conditions to be maintained in the head and flagellum (58). The posterior ring is visible by light microscopy (59,60) and in sections (59,60) and replicas of sperm examined by electron microscopy (57).

The plasma membrane of the midpiece region of the flagellum in some species contains strands of particles running in diagonal arrays coinciding in pitch with the underlying helically wound mitochondria (Table 1). The particle strands appear to be present only when the plasma membrane is closely applied to mitochondria; these strands are usually not present in cytoplasmic droplets (13,18,42,53,62,63). It has been suggested (12) that the particle strands might be homologous to the necklace of particles at the base of cilia (64). The strands are particularly prominent in guinea pig sperm. In other species, patches of hexagonally packed particles are present in the midpiece plasma membrane and tend to follow the contour of the mitochondrial helix (58). A different pattern has been reported in opossum spermatozoa, where aggregates of intramembranous particles are longitudinally arranged (65).

The annulus is a dense fibrous ring surrounding the axoneme of the flagellum at the junction between middle piece and posterior tail. The plasma membrane in this area contains a close array of small particles, sometimes in circumferential strands (42). Because the plasma membrane is closely applied to the annulus, these features may represent anchoring of the annulus to proteins within the plasma membrane (53).

The intramembranous particles in the plasma membrane of the posterior tail appear larger than those in the middle piece. In addition, staggered double rows of yet larger particles are present in the plasma membrane of the posterior tail in some species (42,63). They resemble a *zipper* coursing longitudinally over the ribs of the fibrous sheath, opposite outer dense fiber number 1 (42). The zipperlike structure terminates before the posterior end of the posterior tail domain. The large particles that form this structure are seen on surface replicas and are probably part of a transmembrane complex (53,66). The particles are slightly oval with a depression in their center, possibly a pore, suggesting that they may be sites of ion transport (67). It has also been postulated that the zipper is a membrane-anchoring device for axonemal components (66). Treatment of guinea pig sperm with digitonin, a detergent that disrupts cholesterol-rich plasma membranes (68), does not remove the zipper. However, the particles can be removed by subsequent treatment with Triton X-100 (66). The zipper binds the lectins Con A, RCA, and WGA, and the Triton-X-100-soluble fraction contains four polypeptides ranging from 24,000 to 110,000 daltons (69).

Studies using freeze-fracture following treatment with membrane intercalating agents provide additional evidence that the plasma membrane composition differs between domains (Table 1). Guinea pig sperm treated with filipin develop filipin–sterol complexes between plaques of intramembranous particles in the principal segment and equatorial segment domains of the acrosomal region (55,68,70). Filipin is a polyene that complexes β-hydroxysterols with sterol, and the results imply that these domains are sterol-rich. The plasma membrane of the postacrosomal region has less than one-fourth as many filipin–sterol complexes as the acrosomal region, and the pattern produced suggests that sterols are present mainly in the outer half of the bilayer (14,70). The plasma membrane in the acrosomal region of stallion and golden hamster sperm also appears to have significantly higher amounts of sterols than the postacrosomal region (18,71). The area between the principal and equatorial segments of guinea pig sperm often contains circles of membrane cleared of sterols and intramembranous particles (43,67).

The antibiotic polymyxin B binds anionic phospholipids, producing crenelation of anionic phospholipid-rich membranes (72,73). The results of treating guinea pig sperm with polymyxin B indicate that the plasma membrane over the marginal segment of the acrosomal region has a high anionic lipid concentration (72). However, anionic lipids are less abundant in the principal and equatorial segments (14,44,72).

The fluorescent lipid analog, 1,1′-dihexadecyl-3,3′-tetramethyl-indocarbocyanine perchlorate (C_{16}diI) intercalates into the outer leaflet of the plasma membrane. The acrosomal region of ram sperm labels more intensely with this agent than the postacrosomal region (74). The differences in affinity of the probe for these regions apparently result from interactions of the probe with lipids and proteins heterogeneously distributed within the plane of the membrane.

Sperm-Surface Antigens

Antibodies prepared against spermatozoa, germ cells, somatic cells, or isolated molecules have identified distinct surface domains on living sperm (Table 2). Antibodies can be conjugated directly with various labels or detected indirectly with secondary antibodies (75) that carry labels visible by light or electron microscopy. Antibodies can also be used to isolate and identify specific molecules and to test their roles in bioassays. In some cases, it is found that antigens shared with other cell types are restricted to specific regions of the sperm surface. With mouse sperm, (a) an antiserum to the H-Y antigen reacts with the plasma membrane over the equatorial segment (76), (b) an antiserum to F9 teratocarcinoma cells binds to the postacrosomal region (77), and (c) an antiserum to galactosyltransferase binds to the principal segment of the acrosomal region (78). Antisera to sperm or spermatogenic cells can also react with specific regions such as the principal segment of the acrosomal region (79), the postacrosomal region (80), or the posterior tail (81). Other antisera to germ cells react with multiple regions of the sperm surface such as the equatorial segment and postacrosomal region (82), the acrosomal region and middle piece (81), the head and midpiece (83), the whole tail (84), or the entire sperm surface (85–87). The molecules recognized by these antisera have not been identified in most cases. It is tempting to speculate that antisera reacting with specific regions may recognize one or a few antigens, whereas those reacting with the whole surface recognize multiple antigens. However, binding to the whole sperm surface has been seen with an antiserum to a single antigen (86) or to multiple antigens (87).

The multiple and variable specificities of antisera to whole cells or mixtures of antigens limit their usefulness for dissecting the distribution of sperm-surface components and for defining the biochemical characteristics and functional roles of such components. Monoclonal antibodies have been produced against spermatozoa to overcome some of these limitations (Table 2). Although monoclonal antibodies are often specific to particular molecules, they may also recognize epitopes shared by many molecules (88). Furthermore, even monoclonal antibodies that label only one domain on the sperm surface may immunoprecipitate proteins of more than one molecular weight (15). In some cases these proteins are subunits of a molecular complex that coprecipitate under such conditions (89,90), but in other cases they might be functionally unrelated molecules that share a common epitope recognized by the antibody. Monoclonal antibodies have been used to study mouse, rat, guinea pig, human, boar, hamster, and rabbit sperm. Some monoclonal antibodies recognize multiple domains, including those of the whole sperm surface (91–93), the whole head (15,93–97), or the whole tail (15,91,94,98–103). However, other monoclonal antibodies bind to the individual domains of the principal segment, equatorial segment, anterior acrosome, postacrosomal region, middle piece, or posterior tail of living sperm (15,38,88,89,94,96,97, 99,103–126) (Table 2). Other patterns are seen on air-dried or fixed sperm, but these treatments can expose internal antigens (92). In addition, some monoclonal antibodies recognize variable patterns or apparent subdomains on spermatozoa. This might occur as a result of shedding of sperm-surface components during processing or partial masking of components by extrinsic molecules or relocation of components as a consequence of membrane fluidity (127). However, a variety of studies have used monoclonal antibodies of sperm from different species to confirm that the surface consists of well-defined domains and that different proteins and glycoproteins may be either confined to individual domains or shared by multiple domains (Table 2).

Formation of Domains

Most sperm-surface domains probably are established during spermiogenesis as round spermatids are remodeled into spermatozoa. However, spermatozoa undergo additional shape and surface changes during epididymal maturation, and some domains acquire their final form and composition after spermiogenesis. The domains associated with the middle piece and the acrosomal region are most affected by epididymal maturation. The cytoplasmic droplet migrates from the anterior to the posterior end of the middle piece and is usually shed as sperm transit the epididymis. The acrosome can undergo a reduction in size (21,128) and, in some species, most notably the guinea pig, a substantial change in shape in the epididymis (129).

There is also a correlation between the time of appearance of some surface components during guinea pig spermatogenesis and their final localization (130). Whole cell (WC-1) and posterior tail (PT-1, PT-10) antigens appear on the surface in pachytene spermatocytes or earlier. However, anterior tail antigens (AT-1, AT-10) are first detected on early round spermatids, whereas whole head (WH-1, WH-30), anterior head (AH-20), and posterior head (PH-30) antigens are initially seen on acrosome-phase spermatids. It has been hypothesized (130) that the temporal regulation of surface expression of these antigens directs them to their correct surface domains, with newly synthesized proteins being inserted into the anteriormost domain. These antigens do not diffuse into more posterior domains because either they are anchored in the anterior domain or there are barriers to diffusion between domains. Localization of antigens to domains may not require a specific sorting mechanism, although some proteins may contain information or signals that identify them for removal from inappropriate domains (130).

New surface antigens also appear in specific domains during epididymal maturation and may arise through modification or unmasking of preexisting molecules or by attachment of new molecules to acceptor sites already segregated into domains (118,131,132). In addition, redistribution of preexisting surface components from multiple domains to a single domain or from one domain to another can occur in the epididymis. Proteolysis appears to be required for redistribution of some components in the epididymis but not for others. The PH-20, PH-30, and AH-50 antigens of guinea pig sperm are redistributed following proteolysis *in vivo* or *in vitro* (131). PH-20 is present over the entire surface of sperm from the corpus epididymidis but becomes localized to the postacrosomal region in the cauda epididymidis (132). PH-30 and AH-30 are on the whole head of testicular sperm, but PH-30 is localized to the posterior head and AH-30 to the anterior head of sperm from the cauda epididymides (132). In addition, as rat sperm transit the proximal caput epididymidis, the CE9 membrane protein undergoes endoproteolytic cleavage in the extracellular domain and moves from the posterior tail to the middle piece (122,134). However, proteolysis is apparently not involved in redistribution of another rat sperm tail surface component, which moves from the principal segment in the caput epididymidis to the middle piece and principal segment in the corpus and cauda epididymidis (124).

The mechanisms responsible for establishing sperm-surface domains during spermiogenesis are not well defined. Most surface domains overlie distinct cytoplasmic organelles or features, suggesting that morphogenetic processes that establish the shape and organization of the spermatozoon have a major role in determining the location of surface domains. Furthermore, since transmembrane proteins are stabilized by linkage through membrane skeleton proteins to cytoskeletal structures (135,136), such associations may be important for defining the boundaries and contents of different sperm-surface domains. Components of the membrane skeleton complex possibly involved in producing domains include actin, myosin, and spectrin.

The similar temporal and spatial patterns of *actin* distribution during spermiogenesis in several species suggest that actin has a role in sperm head development. Actin has been identified in the subacrosomal space of round spermatids in the rabbit (137), ground squirrel (138), rat (139,140), mouse (141), guinea pig (142), hamster (143), boar (144), monkey, and human (143). It has been suggested that since the location of filamentous actin coincides with the distribution of surface galactosyltransferase in mouse spermatids, actin-containing microfilaments may participate in the redistribution of this enzyme from the whole-cell surface to the principal segment domain of the acrosomal region (141).

There is less similarity between species in actin distribution in spermatozoa than there is spermatids. Actin has been found in the postacrosomal region of rabbit, bull, and boar sperm (137,145–151). It also is present around the connecting piece in the neck region of hamster, rabbit, bull, and human sperm (152). Furthermore, it is seen in the posterior region of the head and in the connecting piece, middle piece, and principal piece of the tail of human sperm (145,153). The localization of actin along the concave margin of the hamster sperm head (148,154) may maintain the close apposition of the plasma membrane to the underlying filament network in this region (148,155).

Myosin is reported to be present in the acrosomal region of human sperm by some investigators (145) and in the neck region by others (145). Vinculin and α-actinin are often components of the membrane skeleton in other cells but are not detected in mouse spermatogenic cells (141). In addition, filamentous structures are observed in association with the plasma membrane on the concave margin of the acrosome in vole spermatozoa (157). These may correspond to the cytoskeletal structure between the plasma membrane and the acrosome in hamster sperm (155).

Spectrin is a major actin- and calmodulin-binding protein that is associated closely with the cytoplasmic surface of the plasma membrane of many cell types (158,159). Spectrin is present in the cytoplasm overlying the acrosome of round spermatids, elongating spermatids, and some testicular sperm in the mouse but is not detected in epididymal sperm (160). In the rat, fodrin (brain spectrin) is associated with the plasma membrane of pachytene spermatocytes and round spermatids, whereas spectrin is present as discrete aggregates in pachytene spermatocytes and associated with the developing acrosome of round spermatids (161). Fodrin is not detected in rat testicular sperm, but spectrin is seen in the middle piece of about 10% of testicular sperm. Neither is present in epididymal sperm (161). Spectrin is not detected in guinea pig sperm (162), but human spermatozoa contain spectrin in the anterior acrosome and principal piece regions (161). Rabbit sperm contain spectrin in the anterior acrosome region and postacrosomal segment of the head and the principal piece of the tail (151). Calmodulin is also present in the subacrosomal area, the anterior part of the postacrosomal region, and the neck and middle piece of the tail of rabbit sperm (151). Protein 4.1 is part of the membrane skeleton of erythrocytes, and a protein-4.1-like component is present in the acrosomal and principal piece regions of rat testicular and epididymal sperm (161).

TABLE 2. *Sperm-surface domains recognized with monoclonal antibodies*

Antibodies	Species	Mass (kD)	References
Antigens restricted to single domains			
Principal segment of acrosomal region			
HS 1A.1	Human	ND[a]	88
MA 1	Human	84	105
MA 2	Human	ND	105
MA 3	Human	240	105
D81,G112,G176,G225[b]	Human	ND	106
H31b	Human	50	125
SMA1	Mouse	ND	94
1B3	Mouse	28	108
MS-1	Mouse	69	107
AMSIV-33[b]	Mouse	200	103
——	Mouse	ND	109
J1,C6	Mouse	ND	28
M5	Mouse	150–160	110,118
M41	Mouse	60,35,21	110,118
M42	Mouse	220–240	110,118
W33	Mouse	27–33	118
W71	Mouse	105	118
AH-1	Guinea pig	52	15,96,97
AH-2	Guinea pig	70,62,46,25,18	15,96,97
AH-3	Guinea pig	62,52,38	15,96,97
AH-4	Guinea pig	38,16	15,96,97
AH-5	Guinea pig	ND	15,96,97
8C10.5	Rabbit	63	111
Equatorial segment			
D3	Human	ND	106
21D3	Human	ND	126
M2[c]	Mouse	44,36	112
M29[c]	Mouse	40	112
Postacrosomal region			
HS 1E.1	Human	73,56,53	88
PH-1	Guinea pig	60	15,96,97
PH-2	Guinea pig	66,48,41	15,96,97
PH-3	Guinea pig	58,48	15,96,97
PH-4	Guinea pig	ND	15,96,97
PH-20	Guinea pig	64	97
PH-30	Guinea pig	60,44	89
1B6	Rat	ND	91
WS 35.22	Hamster	ND	113
Middle piece			
MA 4	Human	30	105
HSA-1	Human	ND	99
AMSIV-25[b]	Mouse	ND	103
Posterior tail			
PT-1	Guinea pig	ND	15,96,97
CE9	Rat	42–48	122
Antigens present in multiple domains			
Whole head			
SMA3	Mouse	ND	94
OBF13	Mouse	ND	95
WH-1	Guinea pig	42	15
WH-2	Guinea pig	89,45	15,96,97
WH-3	Guinea pig	ND	15,96,97
MC31	Rat	26–28	124
HMS3.1	Hamster	ND	93
P86/5	Boar	78,52,45	119
Acrosomal region and midpiece			
G177	Human	ND	106
WH 97.25	Hamster	>500	113

TABLE 2. *Continued.*

Antibodies	Species	Mass (kD)	References
Principal segment of acrosomal region, equatorial segment, whole tail			
W108	Mouse	86,67,62,57	118
Equatorial segment and middle piece			
bF4	Human	ND	106
HS 2M.1	Human	83,32	88
HS 2N.1	Human	105–26	88
Equatorial segment and principal piece			
M2	Mouse	44,36	112
Equatorial segment and whole tail			
MA 5	Human	71	105
MA 6	Human	ND	105
Postacrosomal region and middle piece			
HS-4	Human	130	114
Neck and middle piece			
MS 76.11	Hamster	ND	113
Middle piece and end piece			
WS 64.23	Hamster	23	113
Whole tail			
YWK-1	Human	84	98
HSA-1	Human	ND	99
SP1D1, AP7A7	Human	ND	100
SMA4	Mouse	54	94
T21	Mouse	54	102
AMSIV-54,[b] AMSIV-75[b]	Mouse	ND	103
WT-1	Guinea pig	ND	15
2B1	Rat	40	91,120
Whole sperm			
2D6	Rat	23	92
HMS1.0, HMS2.0	Hamster	ND	92

[a] ND, not determined.
[b] Determined by indirect immunofluorescence on fixed or air-dried sperm.
[c] Determined by indirect immunofluorescence on acrosome-reacted sperm.

Microtubules play an important role in determining cell shape, and microtubules in the manchette may be responsible for the elongation and shaping of the spermatid nucleus (163). The manchette is a sheath of microtubules that assemble as spermatid elongation begins. It attaches to a deposition of dense fibrillar material on the plasma membrane that migrates from the anterior to the caudal end of the nucleus during spermiogenesis (164). This attachment site later becomes the posterior ring, which lies at the junction between head and tail and separates the domains of the postacrosomal region and the middle piece. This suggests that the manchette contributes to the definition of the boundary between the two surface domains. A comparative study of morphogenetic factors influencing the shape of the sperm head concluded that its form is probably a consequence of the aggregation of DNA and protein during condensation of chromatin rather than of forces external to the nucleus (164).

Studies on mice with genetic mutations (*azh*/*azh* or *sys*/*sys*) or treated with cytotoxic agents (vinblastine, taxol, 5-fluorouracil, or cytoxan) support the hypothesis that the manchette is involved in sperm nuclear shaping (165–168). Manchette abnormalities are often related to nuclear abnormalities, suggesting that the manchette may exert pressure to deform the nucleus caudal to the acrosome during the early elongation phase of spermiogenesis.

Although microtubulelike components have been observed in close association with the plasma membrane overlying the postacrosomal region of bull sperm (157,169) and vole sperm (157), they have not been shown to contain tubulin. Such features may represent the periodic densities seen in the postnuclear dense lamina (169,170).

The Sertoli cells may influence the establishment of domains, particularly those on the sperm head. Junctional structures referred to as Sertoli-cell "ectoplasmic specializations" maintain a tight association between Sertoli cells and spermatids (171). The ectoplasmic specializations are prominent in the elongation and maturation phases of spermiogenesis and seem to grasp the spermatid head (172). This association is maintained until near the time of sperm release (173) and apparently holds the spermatid in a recess extending deeply into the surface of the Sertoli cell. The ectoplasmic specialization consists of bundles of actin or actinlike filaments and more deeply placed saccules of endoplasmic reticulum within the Sertoli cell (171). They might aid in shaping the sperm head or in maintaining cell polarity necessary for domain formation. However, sperm head shape is refined and surface antigens are redistributed in the epididymis (132), indicating that Sertoli cells do not impose the final shape and composition of domains.

Another specialized association arises between Sertoli cells and spermatids late in spermiogenesis. The "tubulobulbar complexes" formed as spermatids begin to move from deep recesses in the surface of Sertoli cells toward the lumen of the seminiferous tubule (174). These complexes form around the spermatid head as the ectoplasmic specialization begins to dissociate (171). Successive generations of complexes extend from spermatids into Sertoli cells, where they are actively phagocytosed (175). This process continues until spermiation, and morphometric data indicate that as much as 70% of the cytoplasm of spermatids is eliminated by this mechanism (175). This process may substantially alter the composition and organization of the sperm plasma membrane and could help define the nature and organization of surface domains.

Maintenance of Domains

Sperm-surface domains might be maintained by restriction of mobility of surface molecules in their final domain, by the existence of a membrane barrier to surface component movement at the domain boundary, or through thermodynamic partitioning of molecules into a specific region (97). Restriction of mobility could occur through interactions of intramembranous components with molecules outside or inside the membrane. Although there is no direct evidence that external constraints can be imposed on domains by molecules applied to the sperm surface, capacitation involves loss of extrinsic components and a concomitant increase in membrane mobility in some domains. Also, the glycocalyx between closely stacked sperm heads in the guinea pig has a septate pattern (176) that may be congruent with the quilted pattern of intramembranous particles in that area of the plasma membrane (42). This quilted pattern is diminished by treatments that remove the cell coat (14,43). Furthermore, there is a correlation between the loss of the quilted pattern and changes in the rat sperm glycocalyx in the epididymis (45). Proteolysis-dependent redistribution of surface antigens in the epididymis might involve release of antigens from a restraining surface network, allowing other external or internal localization processes to occur (132).

Internal constraints help to form barriers between sperm plasma membrane domains and to maintain domains. The plasma membrane regions over the annulus and the posterior ring are closely associated with cytoplasmic components forming and stabilizing these specialized regions. Two antigens (2B1, 2D6) present over the whole surface of the flagellum of rat sperm show antibody-induced patching but do not migrate onto the head (91), perhaps because of the posterior ring. The annulus develops during spermiogenesis and initially encircles the axonemal complex near the base of the flagellum. It underlies the plasma membrane, where it is reflected onto the base of the flagellum (177). The annulus remains adherent to the plasma membrane as it moves down the flagellum to take up its final position at the posterior end of the mitochondrial sheath and the anterior end of the fibrous sheath. At this location, the annulus separates the middle piece and posterior tail domains. The PT-1 antigen exhibits free diffusion within the plasma membrane of the distal tail domain but apparently is prevented from migrating into the midpiece by the annulus (178).

However, there may be species-specific differences in the effectiveness of the annulus as a barrier in defining surface domains. Anterior tail and posterior tail surface antigens appear to be constrained by this barrier in the guinea pig (130), but surface antigens migrate between these domains during epididymal maturation in the rat (124,134).

Other structures that may serve as constraints or anchors of plasma membrane domains include components seen as transmembrane particles in freeze-fracture studies. For example, the zipperlike structure of the flagellum appears to attach to the ribs of the fibrous sheath (42). Also, the oblique strands of intramembranous particles in the middle piece are associated with the underlying mitochondria (42). Furthermore, the plasma membrane of the postacrosomal region is apposed to long rodlike structures that form the postnuclear dense lamina (48,179) and may stabilize the plasma membrane of this domain. Finally, the particle-bare and filipin-complex sparse plasma membrane of the anterior crescent overlies a cytoplasmic tuft that may help define a barrier between the anterior acrosome and the equatorial segment domains (48,179).

Although most sperm-surface antigens are unable to migrate into other domains, this is not the case for all membrane components. By fluorescence recovery after photobleaching (FRAP), it is observed that there is free exchange of a lipid analog by lateral diffusion between plasma membrane of head and midpiece regions and between plasma membrane of the midpiece and distal tail (74).

Although lipid is free to diffuse in the plasma membrane of most somatic cells (180), FRAP measurements indicate that a large fraction of the plasma membrane lipids of mammalian sperm is not free to diffuse laterally (74,181). The nondiffusing lipid pool develops during spermiogenesis (182) but can increase to more than 50%

of the lipid during epididymal maturation (74). The diffusion rate is not significantly affected when ram sperm are treated with pronase, suggesting that interactions with surface proteins do not restrict plasma membrane lipids (183). When sperm are subjected to hypoosmotic shock to produce surface blebs, the diffusion rate for lipids is comparable on blebs and on untreated sperm, suggesting that interactions of plasma membrane lipids with underlying cytoskeletal elements do not affect diffusion (183). In addition, when artificial bilayers are formed from sperm plasma membrane lipid extracts, the fraction of nondiffusing lipid is about the same as that on intact sperm, suggesting that lipid–lipid interactions are responsible for restricting lateral lipid movement (183). Differential scanning calorimetry studies indicate that significant amounts of gel-phase lipids are present, which allow sperm plasma membrane lipids to segregate into coexisting fluid and gel domains at physiological temperatures (184). The gel domains may contain the nondiffusing lipid fraction present in the sperm plasma membrane.

The PH-20 guinea pig sperm surface antigen is not an integral membrane protein but is anchored in the plasma membrane by attachment to a glycosyl-phosphatidylinositol lipid (185). The PH-20 protein is localized to the posterior sperm head, but following the acrosome reaction it migrates from the plasma membrane into the inner acrosomal membrane when these membranes become continuous (97). Although it might be expected to behave like a lipid, the PH-20 protein migrates against a concentration gradient rather than by passive diffusion (186). Interactions with unknown extracellular elements on the posterior head domain may account for this restricted motility of PH-20 prior to the acrosome reaction (187), and a change in the distribution of such elements could serve to concentrate PH-20 toward the inner acrosomal membrane after the acrosome reaction (186).

Plasma Membrane Composition

The sperm plasma membrane does not have unusual cholesterol or glycolipid content but contains relatively high amounts of plasmalogens and other ether-linked phospholipids (184,188,189) and of lipids with long, polyunsaturated aliphatic chains (190). Phospholipids make up about 70% of the total plasma membrane lipid in boar sperm (191), and choline phospholipids account for almost two-thirds of phospholipids in the plasma membrane of the anterior head of ram sperm (188). Steroids are the next most abundant lipid, with a cholesterol/phospholipid molar ratio of about 0.12 (191). Freeze-fracture studies with filipin suggest that the amount of sterol in the anterior acrosome is about four times that present in the postacrosomal region in guinea pig and bull spermatozoa (14,43,55). The postacrosomal region contains few sterols or anionic lipids in guinea pig spermatozoa (44), but the cytoplasmic droplet of the middle piece is probably rich in both (14,70). Also, cholesterol sulfate makes up only a small fraction of the total sterol content but is a major component of the plasma membrane over the acrosome of human sperm (192).

Although not abundant, glycolipids unique to sperm are present (191,193–196) and could control lateral domain organization (183). The major glycolipid in spermatogenic cells and sperm is sulfogalactosylglycerolipid (SGG), which is also found to a much lesser extent in brain (197,198). The SGG is present in both the head and tail fractions of spermatozoa (197). A monoclonal antibody to SGG (199) reacts with the equatorial segment and midpiece of living mouse spermatozoa.

Free fatty acid makes up a relatively small amount of the lipid in boar spermatozoa, whereas diacylglycerols are present in about the same amounts as glycolipids (191). The phospholipid/protein ratio is approximately 0.68 on a weight basis in plasma membranes isolated from boar spermatozoa (191), suggesting that the amounts of total lipid and protein are about the same. However, this is for the whole plasma membrane, and the amount and type of lipids and the lipid/protein ratios are probably different in various domains. Furthermore, changes in the lipid content of the spermatozoal plasma membrane occur during maturation and capacitation (5), and these may have substantial effects on the composition and function of the membrane in different domains.

Modifications of the Sperm Plasma Membrane During Epididymal Maturation

When mammalian sperm are released from the seminiferous epithelium, they are still immature and incapable of effective forward motility and lack the ability to fertilize eggs. Sperm acquire these abilities as they pass through the epididymis, where they undergo substantial changes in function, composition, and organization (2,5,200–202). Functional changes occur in metabolic processes (203), the pattern and effectiveness of flagellar activity (201,204,305), and the ability to bind to the zona pellucida (206,207). Changes in plasma membrane composition and organization contribute to these functional modifications. They are reflected by changes in surface charge, lectin binding, intramembranous particle distribution, membrane fluidity, lipid composition, protein composition, and antibody binding as sperm travel through the epididymis (Table 3).

Changes in Surface Charge, Lectin Binding, and Plasma Membrane Structure

The net negative surface charge is greater on sperm from the cauda epididymidis than on sperm from the

TABLE 3. *Sperm-surface modifications during epididymal maturation*

Modification	References
Increase in net negative surface charge	21,208,209
Increase in binding of cationic colloidal iron	22–24,211,212
Changes in lectin-binding properties	37,39,210,213–217
Changes in intramembranous particle distribution	17,18,45,46,218–220
Changes in membrane fluidity	74,235
Decreases in lipid content	221–228
Decreases in cholesterol content	229–231
Increases in sulfoconjugated sterols	230,232
Changes in protein and glycoprotein and glycoprotein composition	
New surface components detected with vectorial labels	241–248
New surface components detected by gel electrophoresis	249–264
New surface components characterized with antisera	270–290
New surface components detected with monoclonal antibodies	91–94,101,108,123,202,291–297
Loss of surface components	38,108,244,245,253,332

caput epididymidis in several species (21,208,209). Alterations in the nature and amounts of saccharides and glycoproteins on the sperm surface are probably responsible for this change. The density of colloidal iron particle binding to the tail is greater on sperm from the cauda epididymidis than on sperm from the corpus epididymidis in the rabbit (22,23), and increases in sialic acid moieties are suggested to cause this change (210). Studies using neuraminidase treatment and colloidal iron staining provide evidence both for (211) and against net changes in sperm surface sialic acids in the epididymis (23,24,212).

Studies with lectin provide additional evidence of changes in sperm surface saccharides during epididymal maturation. Binding of WGA and RCA, but not Con A, decreases as sperm move from caput to cauda epididymidis in the rabbit (210). Decreased binding of WGA to hyrax sperm (213) and of RCA (214) and Con A (215) to ram sperm occurs with maturation. Washing epididymal fluid components away from rabbit sperm appears to increase Con A binding after maturation. Although sperm from the caput epididymidis bind Con A poorly even when washed, sperm from the cauda epididymidis bind substantially more Con A after they have been washed than before washing, particularly over the head (39). This suggests that sperm-coating substances from epididymal fluid mask lectin-binding sites on unwashed sperm. Con A binding to rat spermatozoa increases over the acrosome during maturation (216), and the total amount of material detergent extracted from rat sperm that binds to a Con A affinity column approximately doubles with maturation (217). Binding of Con A over the whole surface and of WGA to the anterior acrosome increases with maturation of goat sperm (37).

Boar sperm are seen by freeze-fracture to have geometric arrays of intramembranous particles over the anterior acrosome in the distal region of the caput epididymidis. A different hexagonal array develops on sperm entering the cauda epididymidis, initially at the margin of the acrosome and then extending to the postacrosomal region (46). Increased filipin incorporation is seen in the plasma membrane of the principal and equatorial segments with maturation in the boar (218). In rat spermatozoa, plaques of parallel rows of particles appear in the plasma membrane of the head in the caput epididymidis but largely disappear by the proximal cauda epididymis (45). However, periodic parallel ridges appear on the surface of the acrosome in the distal part of the cauda epididymidis (219,220). A quiltlike surface pattern overlying a hexagonal array of intramembranous particles appears over much of the guinea pig sperm acrosome during maturation (17). Golden hamster sperm develop a similar quiltlike pattern in the marginal segment of the acrosome in the caput and corpus epididymidis, but this pattern is absent on sperm from the cauda epididymidis and vas deferens (18). At least some of these changes in patterns of surface features and intramembranous particles probably reflect changes in the nature of the sperm glycocalyx during epididymal transit (17,45).

Changes in Lipid Content

The lipid content of whole sperm decreases during epididymal maturation in boar, bull, ram, and rat (221–228), and the cholesterol content decreases in ram, rat, and hamster sperm (229–231). The cholesterol/phospholipid ratio and concentration of phosphatidylserine, phosphatidylethanolamine, cardiolipin, and ethanolamine plasmalogen decrease in whole ram sperm (222,229). However, increases occur in the amount of sulfoconjugated sterols in whole hamster and human sperm (230,232) and in unsaturated fatty acids in whole ram sperm (229). Studies using plasma membranes isolated from boar spermatozoa confirm earlier results with whole sperm that the amount of lipid decreases during epididymal maturation (190). Although there is a decrease in cholesterol, no significant change is seen in the cholesterol/phospholipid ratio. There are also decreases in phosphatidylethanolamine and phosphatidylinositol as well as increases in dermosterol, cholesterol sulfate, phosphatidylcholine, and polyphosphoinositides. There is a decrease in the level of fatty acids and an increase in diacylglycerol but no change in the degree of saturation of fatty acids. Plasma membrane from the anterior head region of ram sperm is particularly rich in ethanolamine and choline phosphoglycerides (188). The amount of dermosterol and ethanolamine in this region of the plasma membrane decreases, whereas the cholesterol-to-phospholipid ratio increases, during epididymal maturation.

Changes in the amount and composition of lipids in the plasma membrane of sperm during maturation are thought to explain why ejaculated sperm are more sensitive to cold shock than are testicular sperm (233,234). These changes may also account for the maturation-dependent decrease in charge density at the phospholipid–water interface of ram spermatozoa, detected by electron spin resonance (233), and the decrease in membrane fluidity of bull spermatozoa, seen by fluorescence polarization spectroscopy (235). Analysis of testicular and ejaculated ram spermatozoa by FRAP indicates that there are regional differences in the decrease of plasma membrane fluidity (74). During maturation, the diffusion rate of a fluorescent lipid analog increases in all regions of the sperm except the midpiece.

Changes in Protein Composition

The sperm plasma membrane also undergoes major changes in protein composition during epididymal maturation (2,236,240). These changes occur by addition of new components to the sperm surface, by unmasking or modification of preexisting sperm-surface moieties, or by loss of sperm-surface components. They have been identified using biochemical approaches and antibodies to sperm-surface components or epididymal fluid components (Table 3). Changes in glycoproteins are probably responsible for most of the modifications in sperm-surface charge and lectin binding during epididymal maturation, although changes in glycolipid composition may also be a factor. Changes involving a particular component often occur within specific regions of the epididymis, suggesting that specializations of epididymal function in these regions play important roles in modifications of the sperm surface during epididymal maturation.

New components that appear on the sperm surface have been detected in biochemical studies using vectorial labeling of sperm from different regions of the epididymis. For example, when galactose oxidase and tritium borohydride are used to tag accessible D-glucose and *N*-acetyl-D-galactosamine residues, a 37,000-dalton glycoprotein is detected on sperm from the cauda epididymidis but not on sperm from the corpus epididymidis of the rat (241). Similar results are seen when lactoperoxidase and iodine are used to label surface tyrosine residues or when fluorescein-conjugated Con A lectin is used to identify glycoprotein-containing bands on polyacrylamide gels (242). Other studies using similar approaches find that the major surface change during rat sperm maturation is the increase in amount of a surface glycoprotein of 31,000 to 37,500 daltons (243–248). Changes in sperm surface proteins during maturation are also seen in gel electrophoresis studies of sperm from mouse (249,250), rat (251–253), ram (254–257), bull (258), rabbit (259), boar (260), chimpanzee (261), and human (262–264).

Changes in Sperm-Surface Antigens

Immunologic approaches are also effective for identifying changes in sperm surface composition during maturation (Table 3). Studies using these approaches complement earlier biochemical studies, and the two procedures are frequently used together. Antisera raised against either spermatozoa or epididymal fluid often react with both, suggesting that an epididymal fluid component binds to the sperm surface. This has given rise to the term "sperm-coating antigens" for components found both in the fluid and on sperm (265–269). Sperm might also shed components into the epididymal fluid during maturation that are recognized by antisera to sperm. However, several studies identify components that are secreted by the epididymis and become bound to the sperm surface.

AEG (acidic epididymal glycoprotein) is a 33,000-dalton glycoprotein from the rat epididymis. Immunohistochemical studies with an antiserum to AEG show that it is secreted by principal cells in the epithelium of the caput and corpus epididymides and binds to sperm as they leave the initial segment of the caput epididymidis (270). AEG has a slight stimulatory effect on sperm motility, but bovine serum albumin and rabbit serum are equally effective (271).

SEP (specific epididymal proteins) are also present in the rat epididymis. Immunohistochemical studies show that these proteins are organ specific (272), and gel electrophoresis studies shown that they are a mixture of proteins. The SEP include the PAS-positive glycoproteins C (22,400 daltons and p*I* 5.35–5.79) and D and E (37,000 daltons and p*I* 5.13 and 4.95, respectively) (273). The SEP are synthesized mainly in the caput epididymidis, and sperm are coated with SEP as they leave the initial segment of the caput epididymidis (274). Proteins D and E bind weakly to sperm and can be removed by a modest increase in ionic strength of the medium (274,275). The antiserum to proteins D and E binds to the head of mature sperm and inhibits fertilization in artificially inseminated animals (276).

Other proteins isolated from the rat caput epididymidis are designated proteins B and C (16,000 daltons), D (27,000 daltons), and E (28,000 daltons) (277–279). Proteins D and E are not detected on sperm from the testis, but they are present on sperm from the cauda epididymidis. Proteins B and C show little if any binding to sperm (280,281). Antisera to proteins D and E bind to the head of sperm from the cauda epididymidis but not to sperm from the testis (281). When proteins B and C are labeled biosynthetically, they and protein G (37,000 daltons) are found to bind to sperm from testis and cauda epididymidis and to erythrocytes to a similar degree, suggesting that the binding of these proteins is not specific to epididymal sperm (278).

The SP sialoprotein (37,500 daltons, p*I* 4.7) from rat epididymis is detected by immunohistochemistry on the apical surface of epithelial cells lining the caput and corpus epididymides, in the cytoplasm of some epididymal epithelial cells, and on sperm in the lumen of the epididymis (248). The antiserum does not cross-react with supernatants of epididymal homogenates from dog, rabbit, guinea pig, or human. Two extrinsic glycoproteins of 100,000 and 50,000 daltons were extracted from cauda sperm in the rat by washing with a high-ionic-strength buffer (282). Antisera to these glycoproteins react with the "periacrosomal" region of the head of cauda sperm, and immunohistochemical studies indicate that the antigens first appear in the cytoplasm of principal cells in the proximal region of the cauda epididymidis. Peptide maps suggest that the two glycoproteins have very similar composition and that the larger molecule may be a dimer of the smaller molecule. The lectins that bind to both glycoproteins on Western blots indicate that their glycoconjugates contain mannose and *N*-acetylglucosamine (282).

Several biochemical and immunologic studies appear to have characterized the same rat sperm-surface glycoproteins (283). Proteins B and C (271,277) are probably the same as those referred to by other investigators as proteins II and III (270). Also, proteins D and E are probably the same as those referred to as AEG (270), protein IV (284), SP (248), and the 32K protein (285). The cDNAs encoding some of these proteins and the predicted primary amino acid sequences for proteins B and C are identical (283,286). The two proteins are probably produced by posttranslational modification of a common precursor. In addition, the cDNA sequences for proteins D and E (283,287) and for AEG (288) encode the same protein.

Although epididymal secretory products that become associated with the sperm surface are best characterized in the rat, studies in other species show that this is a general phenomenon. In the rabbit, epididymal glycoproteins first become associated with spermatozoa in the distal caput and proximal corpus epididymidis (289). In the hamster, epididymal glycoproteins first become associated with the sperm in the proximal caput epididymidis (289,290). In the human, an antiserum to ejaculated spermatozoa reacts specifically with epididymal fluid and with epididymal sperm but not with testicular sperm and apparently identifies an epididymal secretory product that binds to sperm (262).

Several studies have used monoclonal antibodies to examine sperm-surface changes during maturation. They are highly specific probes and often identify antigens restricted to specific domains on the sperm surface. Two rat sperm-surface antigens first appear in the caput epididymis; one is present on the postacrosomal portion of the head (identified with monoclonal antibody 1B6), and the other is uniformly distributed over the entire sperm surface (identified with monoclonal antibody 2D6) (91). The latter antigen is susceptible to antibody-induced patching and is inserted into the egg surface on fertilization (91,92). Two antigens on hamster spermatozoa are modified during maturation (93). An antigen recognized by antibody HM 3.1 is present over the head at a high concentration and on more sperm from the caudia epididymidis than on sperm from the testis (recognized by antibody HM 3.1). The antigen recognized by antibody HM 5.8 is present over the entire tail and appears to be present in higher concentration on sperm from the corpus epididymidis than on sperm from caput or cauda epididymides. Antibody HM 3.1 blocks fertilization *in vitro,* whereas HM 5.8 reduces fertilization *in vitro* through sperm agglutination. A 28,000-dalton antigen (identified with monoclonal antibody 1B3) is present over the entire surface of rat sperm from the testis or caput epididymidis but is present only on the tip of the head of sperm from the cauda epididymidis (108).

Some sperm surface maturation antigens recognized by monoclonal antibodies are secreted by the epididymal epithelium. One antigen carrying the fucosylated lactosaminoglycan SSEA-1 is secreted by the caput epididymidis and absorbed by sperm in mice (291). Another sperm maturation antigen (SMA4) is secreted by the epithelium in the distal caput and proximal corpus epididymides and binds to the whole tail (94,292–295). It is first present as an 85,000-dalton component and apparently is trimmed to a 54,000-dalton component on attachment to the surface of the flagellum. SMA4 binds WGA, and its terminal carbohydrate residues are rich in sialic acids (123,294–297). A primary function of SMA4 may be to prevent tail-to-tail agglutination of sperm during storage in the epididymis (295,296). The binding of SMA4 to the sperm surface appears to be stabilized by a factor present in epididymal fluid (202,293).

The appearance of new antigens on the sperm surface during epididymal maturation might also occur by unmasking or alteration of preexisting sperm-surface proteins. A carbohydrate epitope apparently is unmasked as mouse sperm undergo maturation (123). The 54,000-dalton glycoprotein is recognized by monoclonal antibody T21 and can be unmasked on sperm or the isolated glycoprotein by neuraminidase treatment. Proteases (203,298–302) are present in the epididymis, and β-galactosidase and β-glucuronidase are secreted in substantial amounts by rat epididymal cells in culture (303). In addition, the secretion of glycosidases in the epididymis is reported to be androgen dependent (304,305). Such enzymes might be responsible for unmasking of sperm-surface maturation components by partial degradation of surface glycoproteins. Other sperm antigens undergo endoproteolytic cleavage in the epididymis and subsequently redistribute to different domains (89,132, 134). A proteinase inhibitor has been isolated from the epididymis in the mouse (306), and such activities might be involved in regulating or limiting enzyme-mediated sperm-surface modifications in the epididymis.

Changes in Sperm-Surface Carbohydrates

Another way that sperm-surface components are altered in the epididymis is by glycosylation. Epididymal fluid or homogenates are rich in glycosyltransferases, glycosidases, and dolichol (307). The rat epididymis contains androgen-dependent glucosyl-and mannosyltransferases (308), and the highest β-*N*-glucosaminidase, β-*N*-acetylgalactosaminidase, and β-*N*-galactosidase activities are in the corpus region (302). Also, *N*-acetylneuraminyltransferase activity is higher in caput than in cauda epididymidis (309), although some sialoglycoproteins in the epididymal fluids are produced only in the cauda (243). There is evidence that the increase in negative surface charge by ram and bull spermatozoa in the epididymis results from the addition of sialic acid groups to the sperm surface (16). Other studies have suggested that lactosaminoglycans present on the surface of testicular spermatozoa are fucosylated by an epididymal fucosyltransferase (310).

UDP-galactose:*N*-acetylglucosamine galactosyltransferase activity is detected in fluids from the vas deferens of mice and rats (311–313) and in the rete testis fluid of rats (314). The galactosyltransferase appears to be produced in the testis and concentrated in the caput epididymis (314). Rat sperm incorporate galactose from UDP-[^{12}C]galactose into surface glycoproteins, and the addition of rete testis fluid increases the amount incorporated (315). The major incorporation is into 37,000- and 23,000-dalton proteins, suggesting that sperm-surface components are altered during maturation by galactosylation of exposed *N*-acetylglucosamine residues (315). The 37,000-dalton glycoprotein may be the same maturation-dependent sperm-surface glycoprotein identified in earlier surface-labeling studies (241).

Glycosyltransferase enzymes present on the sperm surface include α-D-mannosidase (316,317) and fucosyltransferase (318,319). In addition, β-1,4-galactosyltransferase is present on spermatogenic cells (141) and sperm (78,320,321) and may be involved in sperm-surface modifications during epididymal maturation. This enzyme appears to be functionally different from the one in epididymal fluid (322). Molecular cloning data indicate that there is a single β-1,4-galactosyltransferase gene but that spermatogenic cells contain unique transcripts (323,324). There is evidence that β-1,4-galactosyltransferase may be regulated by α-lactalbumin present in epididymal fluid (325,326) and on the surface of the sperm flagellum (327,328). However, other studies indicate that the α-lactalbumin activity detected may be an artifact (329,330).

The sperm-surface galactosyltransferase is present over the acrosome in the mouse (78). Galactosyltransferase may bind to oligosaccharide residues in the egg zona pellucida ZP3 glycoprotein as part of the fertilization process (322,331). A mouse strain that has a genetic predisposition for increased fertilizing ability also has elevated sperm-surface galactosyltransferase activity (321). However, sperm from recombinant strains of these mice do not show elevated galactosyltransferase activity or increased fertilizing ability (322).

Loss of Sperm-Surface Components

Sperm-surface glycoproteins are also lost during epididymal maturation (Table 3). However, it is not known in most cases if the glycoproteins are shed from the sperm surface, modified in molecular weight by processes such as limited proteolysis or addition of new moieties, or are still present but no longer accessible to surface labeling because of masking by other moieties. A 110,000-dalton glycoprotein is a major surface component of rat testicular spermatozoa labeled with glucose oxidase and tritium borohydride, but is not labeled on sperm from the cauda epididymidis (244,245). In addition, 94,000-, 72,000-, and 59,000-dalton components are iodinated on rat sperm from the caput epididymidis but not on sperm from the cauda epididymidis (332). A 28,000-dalton antigen is immunostained over the entire surface of mouse sperm from the testis and caput epididymidis, whereas sperm from the cauda epididymidis are labeled only over the anterior acrosome (108). Other immunohistochemical studies have suggested that terminal *N*-acetylglucosamine residues on testicular sperm are lost during epididymal transit, probably as a result of masking by galactosylation (38). Some proteins lost from rat sperm in the epididymis are found in the epididymal fluid. These include a 72,500-dalton protein in the caput epididymidis and two proteins of 115,000 and 70,000 daltons in the cauda epididymidis (253). However, 67,500-, 64,000-, 19,500-, and 18,500-dalton proteins are lost from rat sperm in the cauda epididymidis without appearing in epididymal fluid (253).

Modification of the Sperm Plasma Membrane During Ejaculation

Other alterations in sperm-surface composition result from ejaculation or being in the female reproductive tract (5). Changes resulting from ejaculation occur in surface charge (208,333–335), lectin binding (28,29), and lipid composition (192,334). In addition, blood-group antigens (335,336), histocompatibility antigens (337), and immunosuppressive factors (338) are adsorbed during ejaculation. Sperm also become coated with proteins produced by accessory glands and present in the seminal plasma. Upon ejaculation, human sperm acquire lactoferrin (339,340), ferrisplan (341), PP5 (342), HSP-5 (343), pg12 (344), and a basic 140,000-dalton protein (345), all products of the seminal vesicles. Antibodies to the basic 140,000-dalton protein cross-react immunologically with the rat 17,000-dalton seminal-vesicle protein-IV (RSV-IV) (346). A rat 50,000-dalton seminal-vesicle protein is present on ejaculated but not on epididymal sperm (269). A rabbit 20,000-dalton protein is present on ejaculated but not on epididymal sperm (347). Both 25,000- and 14,000-dalton proteins bind to bull sperm during ejaculation (258). A 34,000-dalton component is present on ejaculated mouse sperm, on sperm from the distal vas deferens, and in seminal-vesicle fluid but not on epididymal sperm (87).

Some of the proteins acquired by sperm during ejaculation bind to specific domains. A 6400-dalton proteinase inhibitor produced by mouse seminal vesicles binds to a 15,000-dalton plasma-membrane component over the acrosome (348). A 30,000-dalton dog prostate protein is a proteolytic enzyme and is present on the tail and post-acrosomal regions (349). Some components in the seminal plasma also appear to interact with each other and the sperm surface. Transglutaminase promotes covalent linking of spermidine to RSV-IV *in vitro,* and the protein is then able to bind to rat sperm (350). During ejaculation, a calcium-dependent transglutaminase from the prostate may modify a seminal-vesicle protein to enhance its binding to the sperm surface (350).

THE SPERM HEAD

The mammalian sperm head contains the nucleus and acrosome surrounded by moderate amounts of cytoskeletal components and cytoplasm (Figs. 3–6). The acrosome is located at the anterior end of the head, close to the underside of the plasma membrane, and is deeply

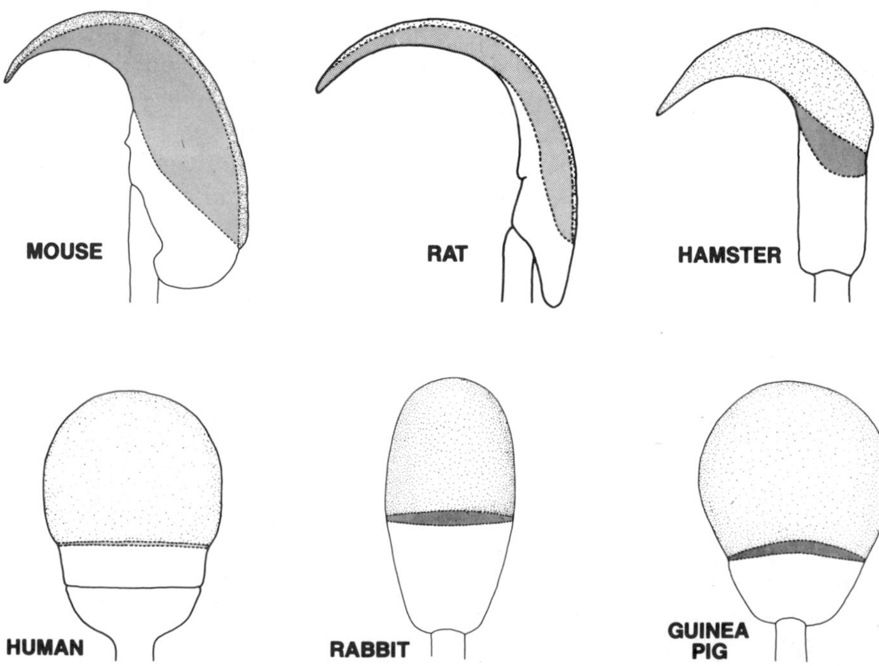

FIG. 3. The shape of the head of spermatozoa from different species. The falciform heads of mouse, rat, and hamster sperm are viewed laterally, whereas the spatulate heads of human, rabbit, and guinea pig sperm are viewed dorsoventrally. The acrosomal region domain is subdivided into the marginal segment (*lighter shading*) and the equatorial segment (*darker shading*). (Adapted from Yanagimachi, ref. 239.)

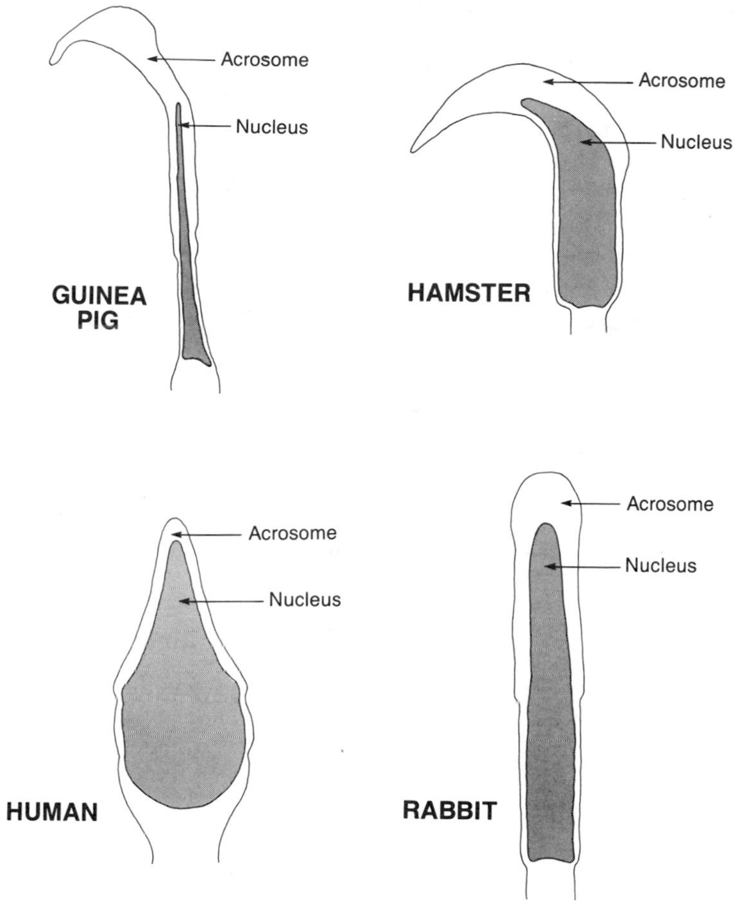

FIG. 4. Cross-sectional views of the heads of spermatozoa from different species. Guinea pig, rabbit, and human sperm heads are seen in the sagittal plane, whereas the hamster sperm head is seen in the coronal plane. The acrosome and nucleus of rabbit and human spermatozoa are relatively symmetrical, but those of guinea pig and hamster are asymmetric in these planes.

indented posteriorly by the nucleus. Cytoskeletal components lie in the narrow space between the acrosome and the nucleus and between the acrosome and the plasma membrane. Sperm of most mammalian species have a spatulate head (Fig. 3), and the nucleus and acrosome are flattened in the plane of the anterior–posterior axis of the sperm. The acrosome and nucleus are usually symmetrical structures. However, in some animals, protrusions of the acrosome extend perpendicular to the flattened plane of the sperm head (Fig. 4). Rodent sperm usually have a falciform-shaped head, with the acrosome overlying the convex margin of the nucleus. Although sperm are uniform in size and shape within most species, there is often variability in the shape and size of the sperm head in humans, even in fertile individuals (351,352).

The Sperm Nucleus

The chromatin of the sperm nucleus is highly condensed, and its volume is significantly less than that of the nucleus of a somatic cell. The organization and amount of DNA and the arrangement and composition of the nucleoproteins are unique features of the sperm nucleus (353). The two meiotic divisions that occur during spermatogenesis result in the sperm containing only one copy of each chromosome.

Nuclear Proteins

The major nuclear proteins associated with mammalian sperm DNA are protamines (354–356). These are relatively small (27–65 amino acids) and highly basic proteins rich in arginine and cysteine. The mRNAs encoding mouse protamines are synthesized in spermatids, indicating that protamines are products of the haploid genome (357). The highly condensed protamine–DNA complex is stabilized by disulfide bonds between the protamines. Most mammals have only one active protamine gene, but mice and humans have two (355,356,358–360). There are two general models for the association of protamines with DNA (361). One suggests that protamines are present in an extended configuration and lie in the major or minor groove of the DNA helix. They are presumed to cross-link the chromatin by forming covalent disulfide linkages with protamines on nearby DNA

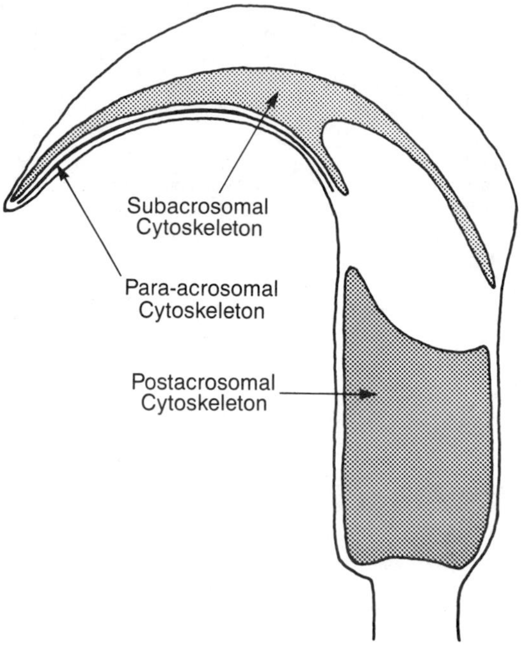

FIG. 5. Cytoskeleton of head of the hamster spermatozoon. The subacrosomal cytoskeleton (perforatorium) lies between the acrosome and the anterior part of the nucleus and extends to the tip of the falciform head. The para-acrosomal cytoskeleton (filamentous cytoskeletal complex) lies between the plasma membrane and the acrosome on the concave margin of the head of hamster sperm and possibly sperm of other species. The postacrosomal cytoskeleton (postacrosomal sheath) surrounds the posterior part of the nucleus, lying between the plasma membrane of the postacrosomal domain and the nuclear envelope of the posterior part of the nucleus.

(363). The other model suggests that protamine is packaged into α-helical cylinders (363). These cylinders are thought to lie in the major or minor DNA groove and to facilitate orderly DNA condensation. They may subsequently cross-link with neighboring cylinders to effect stabilization.

Although both models are based on physical data and presume the lack of nucleosomes in sperm nuclei, some morphological studies have suggested that nucleosomes are present (364,365). In addition, studies using freeze-fracture (42,48,51), birefringence (366), and physical methods (367) suggest that the chromatin in sperm of some mammals is stacked in lamellar plates. However, the chromatin of mouse and human spermatozoa appears to have a random fibrogranular organization (56,368). Additional studies will be required to understand fully how protamines and other nucleoproteins (354,361,369) interact with DNA in sperm nuclei (352).

Nuclear Envelope

The sperm nucleus is enclosed by an unusual nuclear envelope. Over most of the nucleus, nuclear pores are absent, and the inner and outer membranes of the nuclear envelope lie only 7 to 10 nm apart. The two nuclear membranes are 40 to 60 nm apart in most other cells (12,42,48,56,370). Caudal to the posterior ring, in the so-called "redundant nuclear envelope," sperm nuclear pores are abundant and arranged in a hexagonal pattern. The membranes of the anterior part of the nuclear envelope contain a rich array of randomly distributed intramembranous particles (371), whereas the closely ap-

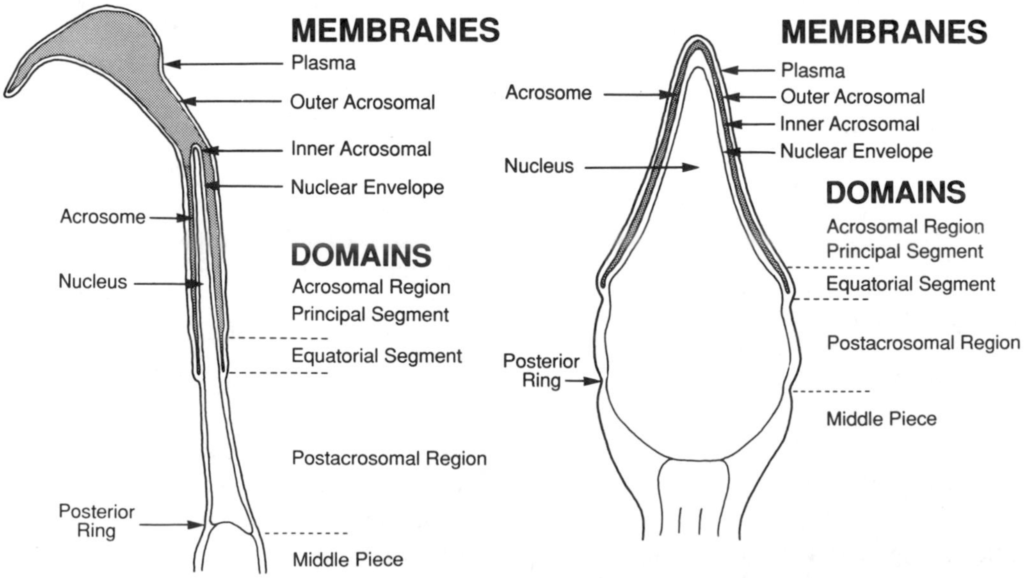

FIG. 6. Structure of the head of guinea pig and human sperm. The plasma membrane of the principal segment domain and equatorial segment domain overlies the outer membrane of the acrosome. The inner acrosomal membrane, in turn, overlies the nuclear envelope. The acrosome is thinner in the equatorial segment region than in the principal segment region.

posed membranes of the nuclear envelope in the implantation fossa contain large, closely packed particles surrounding particle-free areas (42).

Nuclear Lamina

The nuclear lamina is a protein meshwork lining the inner surface of the nuclear envelope and forms part of the nuclear skeletal network anchoring the chromatin (372–376). There are four closely related proteins in the nuclear lamina of somatic cells in mammals: lamins A, B_1, B_2, and C. Lamin A (70,000 daltons) and lamin C (60,000 daltons) have similar peptide maps but different *C*-terminal domains that probably arise by differential splicing of RNA from one gene (377,378). However, lamins B_1 and B_2 are encoded by two different genes (377,378). The lamins have extensive sequence homology with intermediate filament proteins (379,380) and apparently belong to the same family of structural proteins.

Immunohistochemical and Western blotting studies have given contradictory results on whether or not mouse sperm contain lamins (381–385). However, biochemical studies have identified a 60,000-dalton protein present in rat pachytene spermatocyte nuclear matrix, spermatid nuclear lamina, and mature sperm that is not found in somatic cell nuclei (386–388). Peptide mapping and Western blot studies suggest that this germ-cell-specific protein is related to lamin B.

Sequence analysis of a mouse spermatogenic cell cDNA clone indicates that it encodes a unique 54,000-dalton protein referred to as lamin B_3 (389). Lamin B_3 mRNA appears to be generated by differential splicing and alternative polyadenylation of transcripts from the same gene that gives rise to lamin B_2 mRNA. When somatic cells are transfected with a vector expressing lamin B_3, their nuclei become hook-shaped (389). The lamin B_3 mRNA and protein are present in pachytene spermatocytes, but the protein is not detected in sperm (389).

Cytoskeleton of Sperm Head

Cytoskeletal structures are located in three regions of the head of mammalian sperm (Table 4). The *subacrosomal cytoskeleton* is located between the acrosome and nucleus, the *postacrosomal cytoskeleton* lies between the nucleus and the plasma membrane posterior to the acrosome, and the *para-acrosomal cytoskeleton* is present between the anterior tip and convex surface of the acrosome and the plasma membrane of falciform sperm (Fig. 5).

Structure and Composition of the Sperm Head Cytoskeleton

The subacrosomal and postacrosomal cytoskeletons can be isolated together (368) and are referred to as the *perinuclear theca* (361,369). This complex covers the external surface of the nuclear envelope and contains a diverse population of proteins ranging from 8,000 to 80,000 daltons. The major proteins present are 25,000, 16,500, 15,000, and 13,000 daltons (368). The isolated perinuclear theca retains the shape of the sperm nucleus in the absence of DNA and the acrosome. It has been suggested that the perinuclear theca may be an extrinsic determinant of nuclear shape (361).

The *subacrosomal cytoskeleton* (perforatorium, subacrosomal layer, perinuclear material) is composed of amorphous, electron-dense material and occupies the narrow space between the inner acrosomal membrane and the outer membrane of the nuclear envelope (390). It is a prominent feature of rodent sperm with falciform-shaped heads, such as those of rat, mouse, and hamster. In these species, the subacrosomal cytoskeleton is re-

TABLE 4. *Sperm cytoskeletal components*

Component	References
Head	
Subacrosomal cytoskeleton (perforatorium, subacrosomal layer, perinuclear material)	361,368,369,390–405
Postacrosomal cytoskeleton (postacrosomal sheath, postnuclear sheath, postacrosomal dense lamina, postnuclear cap, postnuclear body)	12,42,48,51–54,56,157,219,370,391, 396,399,400,406–417
Para-acrosomal cytoskeleton (filamentous cytoskeletal complex)	155,157,219
Connecting piece	
Capitulum	12,33,42,370,371,534–539
Segmented columns	426,532
Tail	541–544
Axoneme	
Outer dense fibers	12,431,562,573–598
Satellite fibers	12,391,579,599,600
Fibrous sheath	7,12,351,391,396,402,576,578,580, 581,590,603–616

ferred to as the *perforatorium* (391) because of its similarity in appearance to a structure by this name in toads (392) and birds (393). It is thought to have a mechanical role in egg penetration (394,395). In rat sperm, the perforatorium is a curved triangular rod anterior to the apex of the head. It splits into one dorsal and two ventral interconnected prongs, which taper posteriorly to become continuous with the postacrosomal dense lamina (369). However, the subacrosomal cytoskeleton is a minor component of the spatula-shaped heads present in sperm of most mammalian species (396,397).

The perforatorium is first visible in early spermatids as a dense layer between the forming acrosomal granule and the nuclear envelope. It extends over the anterior pole of the nucleus, just ahead of the advancing acrosome, as the sperm head elongates during spermiogenesis (396,399,400). The perforatorium becomes a distinct structure only at the very end of spermiogenesis in the rat (396,400).

The perforatorium becomes more resistant to solubilization during epididymal transit, apparently because of extensive disulfide bond formation (390,397,402). The resistance to solubilization was used to develop a procedure for isolating the perforatorium from mature rat sperm (390,402). Initial studies indicated that it consists primarily of a 13,000-dalton cysteine-rich protein (390). Later studies identified proteins of approximately 43,000, 35,000, 16,000, 13,400, and 13,000 daltons (403). The 16,000-dalton protein is the most abundant of these and probably corresponds to the 13,000-dalton protein seen earlier. Immunohistochemical studies indicate that the 16,000-, 13,400-, and 13,000-dalton proteins are restricted to the thicker apical portion of the rat perforatorium and inner zone of the apical spur, whereas the other proteins are distributed throughout the perforatorium (400,404).

The *postacrosomal cytoskeleton* (postacrosomal sheath, postnuclear sheath, postacrosomal dense lamina, postnuclear cap, postnuclear body) is usually referred to as the *postacrosomal sheath* and lies between the nuclear envelope and the plasma membrane of the postacrosomal segment of the sperm head (12,48,370,391,399,406, 407). It is continuous with the posterior end of the subacrosomal cytoskeleton at the posterior margin of the acrosome and extends caudally to the posterior ring. It is a 10- to 15-nm-thick layer containing an ordered array of filaments (48,52,157,219,370,408). In bull sperm, the postacrosomal sheath is composed of closely associated 10- to 12-nm filaments lying parallel to the long axis of the head (409). The basal region contains coarse striations formed by short rows of large particles (12,42,48, 51,53,54,56,408) and is a zone of close adhesion between the plasma membrane, the postacrosomal cytoskeleton, and the nuclear envelope (409).

Postacrosomal sheath formation begins during spermiogenesis with spermatid elongation (396). Dense material appears just caudal to the posterior margin of the acrosome coincident with the formation of the manchette (410). The postacrosomal cytoskeleton appears to assemble as the manchette moves caudally to form the posterior ring (400,411).

Antibodies have been developed that recognize proteins restricted to the postacrosomal sheath. A 58,000-dalton protein is a major constituent of the postacrosomal sheath of bull sperm (412). This may be the same as a 60,000-dalton protein, termed *calicin,* present in the postacrosomal sheath of bull, rat, human, boar, guinea pig, hamster, and mouse sperm (413,414). In addition, a group of 74,000- to 56,000-dalton proteins, termed *multiple-band polypeptides,* are present in both the subacrosomal cytoskeleton and postacrosomal sheath of bull and rat sperm (413).

Other studies have used monoclonal antibodies to identify proteins that seem to be in the postacrosomal sheath. In mouse sperm, these include *thecins,* three 80,000- to 75,000-dalton proteins that are processed to smaller proteins during epididymal maturation (415), and an antigen that is associated with the outermost layer of the postacrosomal sheath (416). A protein of about 40,000 daltons and several proteins greater than 80,000 daltons is found in the postacrosomal sheath in bull sperm (417).

The *para-acrosomal cytoskeleton* (filamentous cytoskeletal complex) is present in hamster sperm, lying between the acrosome and the plasma membrane (155). It is a tripartite structure, consisting of a cone at the anterior tip and a bifurcated sheet on the convex surface of the head. It is formed of filaments similar in size to intermediate filaments. Filaments have also been seen along the convex side of the acrosome of vole sperm (157), and striations were noted along the ventral surface of the acrosome of rat sperm (219), suggesting that the para-acrosomal cytoskeleton may be present in other species.

Roles of the Sperm-Head Cytoskeleton

Sperm-head cytoskeletal components may have a structural role in defining the shape of the sperm head (394,395) and a functional role in aiding sperm penetration of the egg and its investments at fertilization (409,411). However, the different parts of the perinuclear theca may have different roles. The perforatorium develops as a distinct structure at the very end of spermiogenesis (396,401). Because sperm have largely acquired their final form by that time, the perforatorium probably does not cause sperm to acquire the falciform shape but might provide structural reinforcement to stabilize that shape.

The postacrosomal sheath is slightly more prominent in spatulate sperm than in falciform sperm. It too develops after elongation and flattening of the spermatid head. It might help to maintain the asymmetric shape, but the perinuclear theca can be solubilized without greatly affecting the shape of the sperm nucleus (413). Another possibility is that the perinuclear theca provides stiffening and support for the posterior part of the sperm head to prevent its flexure during sperm motion. An additional role of the perinuclear theca might be to link together and stabilize the association of the acrosome, nucleus, and postacrosomal plasma membrane (361, 396,399,413). Other potential roles of the postacrosomal sheath are to generate or maintain the distinctive properties of the overlying plasma membrane (412) or bind the plasma membrane to the sperm (404). Which of these functions the sperm-head cytoskeleton serves may become known once its composition is more fully defined.

Filamentous actin has been identified by several procedures in the subacrosomal space in spermatids of various species (143). However, actin does not appear to be a component of the sperm head cytoskeleton in mature sperm (137,145,149,418–422). In addition, structures similar in appearance to intermediate filaments are present in the postacrosomal (409) and para-acrosomal (155) cytoskeleton. However, antibodies to intermediate filaments do not react with these regions of the sperm head (156,409). This suggests that the sperm-head cytoskeletal structures are composed of unique proteins or of isoforms of cytoskeletal proteins that are specific to spermatogenic cells and lack antigenic determinants present on related proteins in somatic cells. However, sperm-head cytoskeletal proteins may be related to flagellar cytoskeletal proteins. In sterile mutant mice, both the head and flagellum of sperm often are defectively formed (423,424).

The Acrosome

The acrosome originates from the Golgi complex in the spermatid and contains enzymes necessary for the sperm to penetrate through the investments of the egg to achieve fertilization. This membranous structure sits as a cap over the nucleus in the anterior part of the sperm head.

Structure of Acrosome

The *inner acrosomal membrane* overlies the anterior part of the outer membrane of the nucleus. It is continuous with the *outer acrosomal membrane,* which lies close to the inner surface of the plasma membrane of the anterior sperm head. The acrosome consists of two segments, the *acrosomal cap* (anterior acrosome) and the *equatorial segment* (posterior acrosome), which correspond in distribution to the plasma membrane domains with the same names (Fig. 6). During the acrosome reaction, the outer acrosomal membrane and the plasma membrane fuse and vesiculate, and most of the acrosomal contents are discharged. The inner acrosomal membrane and the equatorial segment persist until sperm–egg fusion in most species (5). Acrosome shape and size vary widely between species (Figs. 3 and 4), and the distribution and relative prominence of these two segments differ accordingly (391).

The equatorial segment forms a band that approximately overlies the equator of the head of spatulate spermatozoa. In sperm possessing a falciform head, the equatorial segment may cover much of the lateral surfaces of the head. However, in species such as the woolly opossum (425), which have a discoid sperm head flattened in the plane perpendicular to the axis of the tail ("carpet-tack-shaped head"), an equatorial segment may not be identifiable. The portion of the acrosomal cap that extends beyond the anterior margin of the nucleus is referred to as the *marginal segment* (apical segment, anterior band, peripheral rim), and the portion overlying the nucleus is referred to as the *principal segment* (acrosomal segment). In the human, monkey, bull, boar, rabbit, and bat the acrosome is relatively small, with no appreciable extension beyond the nucleus, whereas in the guinea pig, chinchilla, and ground squirrel the acrosome has a large apical segment (129,179,391,426).

Electron microscopy reveals that the acrosome, particularly the marginal segment, often has a more complex shape than is obvious by examining sperm smeared onto a slide. The shape of the acrosome is characteristic of the species (391,426). The final shape of the acrosome may be influenced by extrinsic forces generated by cytoskeletal elements in the spermatid and/or Sertoli-cell cytoplasm (155,172) or by forces intrinsic to the nucleus (164,389). However, in some species, it also appears that forces intrinsic to the acrosome may be involved. Acrosomes of guinea pig and chinchilla sperm continue to undergo morphological differentiation after spermatogenesis, and the definitive shape is not achieved until sperm reaches the distal portion of the epididymis (129,426). As might be expected from species differences, genetic factors also influence acrosome formation and shape. Structurally defective acrosomes form in pink-eyed sterile mutant mice (427,428). However, acrosomes fail to form in blind sterile mutant mice, even though proacrosomal granules, the manchette, and flagellar structures form, and some nuclear elongation and chromatin condensation occur (406,424).

The acrosome sometimes shows an internal lamellar or crystalline structure (42), an ordered substructure (429), or a cobblestonelike pattern (54,408). A 4.2-nm periodicity is present in the cortical region of the acrosome of rat sperm, lying just deep to the outer acrosomal membrane on the convex surface (42,439). A similar pattern is also present in the acrosome of human sperm (431). Other evidence that the acrosome has a substructure comes from studies on hamster spermatozoa disrupted by nitrogen cavitation. This treatment results in loss of much of the acrosomal matrix, but components immediately underlying the outer acrosomal membrane remain intact (155). These components are present in two areas: one is a larger and looser layer of fibrous material over the dorsal and lateral surfaces of the acrosome; the other is a more compact fibrous layer adjacent to the anterior margin of the acrosome.

The membrane of the acrosome, particularly the equatorial segment, contains particles that form a crystalline array, giving the membrane a highly regular, granular appearance. These may be an indication of ordered structure in the underlying acrosomal components. Such features have been reported in rabbit (48), bull (408,432), human (56), rat (42,433), mouse (371), guinea pig (42,432,433), degu (432), and rhesus monkey (432). This pattern has been seen by freeze-etch, by freeze-fracture, and on replicas of air-dried and critical-point-dried spermatozoa. Although the outer acrosomal membrane appears to be fragile and easily displaced or disrupted at the time of the acrosome reaction, it also has a thickened appearance because of an electron-dense coating on the inner surface (434–438). This inner surface coat of the outer acrosomal membrane has been isolated from bull sperm and shown to be composed mainly of three high-molecular-weight glycoproteins (290,000, 280,000, and 260,000 daltons) as well as 115,000-, 81,000-, 58,000-, and 46,000-dalton proteins. In addition, there is a set of proteins between 34,000 and 12,000 daltons (438). Lectins bind to the inner surface of the membrane; WGA is observed to bind to the 46,000-dalton component. It was suggested that glycosylated molecules at this site may help to stabilize the membrane or play a functional role in the membrane fusion events of the acrosome reaction (438). The 200,000- and 58,000-dalton components are phosphorylated in a cAMP-independent manner, whereas the proteins between 34,000 and 12,000 daltons appear to include calmodulin-binding proteins (438).

Inner acrosomal membrane development begins in early spermatids when the membrane of the proacrosomal granule abuts and then flattens against the nuclear envelope. The granule spreads over the apical end of the nucleus during acrosomal development and nuclear elongation (392,439). The inner acrosomal membrane is exposed and becomes continuous with the plasma membrane when the acrosome reaction occurs. The inner acrosomal membrane in mouse and rabbit spermatozoa is quite resistant to chemical and physical disruption, including treatment with nonionic detergents and sonication (440,441). However, boar sperm inner acrosomal membrane is sensitive to proteinase treatment (442), and lectins are found to bind to the inner acrosomal membrane of sperm from hamster (41,443) and guinea pig (35), indicating that glycoproteins are present. Bridges 7 nm wide and with 7-nm center-to-center spacing were reported to be present between the inner and outer acrosomal membranes in boar sperm, apparently holding these structures together (442). However, the inner acrosomal membrane appears to be fluid because antigens recognized by monoclonal antibody PH-20 migrate from the plasma membrane of the postacrosomal region of the guinea pig sperm head to the inner acrosomal membrane following the acrosome reaction (121,186,187). It has been suggested that the inner acrosomal membrane is associated with an extensive scaffolding network, possibly transmembrane in nature, in the equatorial segment (397).

Contents of Acrosome

The acrosome is a unique sperm organelle (444) that is required for fertilization in mammals. Multiple enzymes are present in the acrosome, including several acid hydrolases commonly found in lysosomes and other enzymes specific to spermatogenic cells (Table 5). Although it has been described as a specialized lysosome (203,445), the acrosome also has the characteristics of a regulated secretory vesicle. During the acrosome reaction, acrosomal contents are released by calcium-mediated exocytosis in response to specific signals (5). Following the release and activation of acrosomal enzymes, spermatozoa penetrate the zona pellucida surrounding the oocyte, a process that can be blocked by protease inhibitors (446,447).

The best-characterized constituent of the acrosome is proacrosin, a member of the serine protease superfamily that is expressed only in spermatogenic cells. This trypsinlike protease differs from similar enzymes in other tissues in molecular weight, substrate specificity, and inhibitor specificity (448–452). The nucleotide sequences have been determined recently for proacrosin

TABLE 5. *Enzymes in the acrosome*

Enzyme	References
β-*N*-Acetylglucosaminadase	507
Acid phosphatase	506
Acrosin	448–475
Arylamidase	503
Arylsulfatase A	494,505
Aspartylamidase	504
Calpain II	500
Cathepsin-D-like peptidase	496
Collagenase-like peptidase	495
Dipeptidyl peptidase	498,499
Esterases, nonspecific	502
β-Galactosidase	492–494
Hyaluronidase	470,482–491
Neuraminidase	501
Phospholipase A_2	510,511
Phospholipases C	508,509

cDNAs from several mammalian species, including boar (453,454), human (455,456), mouse (457,458), and rat (459).

The amino acid sequences deduced from these cDNAs indicate that proacrosin contains two domains with marked homology to other serine proteases and a COOH-terminal tail domain that is unique in the superfamily (453,460,461). Domain I, the zymogen domain, contains a signal sequence and the light chain portion of the active enzyme. During activation of the precursor, the light chain is cleaved from the heavy chain between arginine and valine at positions 23 and 24 but remains attached to the heavy chain by two disulfide bonds. Domain II, the catalytic domain, contains conserved active-site residues (histidine, aspartate, and serine at positions 70, 124, and 222) and two asparagine-linked glycosylation sites. A carbohydrate-binding region that may play a role in binding of sperm to the zona pellucida has been identified in the catalytic domain of boar proacrosin (460). Twelve cysteine residues in domains I and II are conserved in all proacrosins that have been sequenced, and eight of these are conserved in the serine protease superfamily. Domain III at the COOH-terminal end of proacrosin is a proline-rich segment that is less conserved between species and is not present in other serine proteases. This tail domain is lost during the conversion of proacrosin to the mature enzyme by successive proteolytic cleavages yielding multiple acrosins with intermediate molecular weights (453,462,463).

Although proacrosin synthesis occurs predominantly in round spermatids, proacrosin mRNA or protein has been detected in pachytene spermatocytes in the mouse (464), guinea pig (465), and human (466). Proacrosin is glycosylated and appears to contain both *N*-linked and *O*-linked oligosaccharides (465,467). During epididymal transit of sperm in the guinea pig, the oligosaccharide side chains are modified to produce a smaller proacrosin (468).

Immunolocalization studies suggest that proacrosin is present mainly in the anterior acrosome in human, boar, bull, and rabbit spermatozoa (469), but it is also reported to be localized to the inner acrosomal membrane (470–472). However, since acrosin is rapidly released following the acrosome reaction, the bulk of the proacrosin may be in the soluble acrosomal matrix (239). The conversion of proacrosin from the inactive zymogen to the active enzyme occurs during the acrosome reaction (448–450,452,473). Recent studies suggest that proacrosin is activated prior to its release from the acrosome of guinea pig sperm (474,475).

Other acrosomal constituents may regulate proacrosin activation. Acrosinin, a 32,000-dalton protein that appears to regulate the proacrosin activation sequence, is present in boar spermatozoa (476). In addition, acrosin inhibitors are present both within the acrosome (477) and in seminal plasma (478,479). Sperm-associated inhibitors in the boar resemble the Kazal-type inhibitors present in seminal plasma (480). Another serine protease inhibitor closely related to the plasma protein C inhibitor has been identified in the acrosome of human spermatozoa and perhaps other mammalian species (481).

Hyaluronidase present in the acrosome can be distinguished from the common lysosomal form and, like proacrosin, appears to be a spermatogenic cell-specific isozyme (482–484). This glycosidase is abundant in the acrosome (485) and is located predominantly in the principal segment in bull (486,487) and ram sperm (470). Most of the hyaluronidase of guinea pig sperm is recovered in the soluble acrosome fraction (489). However, ram sperm denuded of the plasma membrane and outer acrosomal membrane still have half the hyaluronidase of sperm with intact acrosomes (488), suggesting that some of the enzyme may be bound to the inner acrosomal membrane (488). Multiple oligomeric forms of hyaluronidase are present in both ram and bull spermatozoa (490). These oligomers appear to be formed by intermolecular disulfide cross-linking between α and β monomers, which may differ in their degree of glycosylation (490).

Two forms of β-galactosidase have been isolated from rat testis and spermatozoa, a lysosomal form and a smaller acrosomal form with distinct physicochemical and enzymatic properties (492,493). A 67,000-dalton β-galactosidase has been identified in rabbit sperm acrosomes, and additional larger species are detected in testis homogenates (494). Although acrosomal β-galactosidase was originally identified as a distinct isozyme (492,493), further studies are needed to determine if the sperm enzyme is derived from the larger form present in the testis. Similarly, β-*N*-acetylglucosaminidase is another acrosomal hydrolase that is smaller than isoforms isolated from the testis (493,494).

Other hydrolytic enzymes have been detected in the acrosome (Table 5). Proteinases reported include a 110,000-dalton collagenaselike peptidase with a pH optimum of 7.5 (495), a cathepsin-D-like protease (496), trypsinlike proteases distinct from acrosin (497), and dipeptidyl peptidase II (498,499). Antiserum to a calcium-activated neutral proteinase, calpain II, reacted with porcine sperm acrosomes by indirect immunofluorescence and recognized an 80,000-dalton subunit of the enzyme on immunoblots (500). In addition, neuraminidase (501), nonspecific esterases (502), arylamidase (503), aspartylamidase (504), arylsulfatase A (494,505), acid phosphatase (506), β-*N*-acetylglucosaminidase (507), phospholipase C (508,509), and possibly phospholipase A_2 (510,511) have been reported to be present in the acrosome.

Other proteins identified as acrosomal constituents may function during the acrosome reaction. Immunocytochemical studies have determined that inhibitory guanine nucleotide-binding regulatory proteins (G_i proteins) are associated with the developing acrosome (512) and are retained in the acrosomal region of mature spermatozoa (513,514). This immunoreactivity is lost following induction of the acrosome reaction (514), consistent with the hypothesis that G_i proteins function as signal-transducing elements mediating this exocytotic event (515). Immunocytochemical methods also indicate that cyclins and *cdc2* serine/threonine protein kinase are localized in the acrosomal region of human spermatozoa (516). Thus far, the acrosomal location of these regulatory proteins has not been confirmed by ultrastructural studies.

Calmodulin has been detected in the acrosomal region of epididymal sperm (517), although immunoelectron microscopic studies suggest that it is localized predominantly in the postacrosomal region (151,518). A spectrinlike protein present in the acrosomal region of human sperm has been identified as the major calmodulin-binding protein in these cells (156). Ultrastructural studies of rabbit sperm indicate that spectrin is a component of the inner and outer acrosomal membranes as well as of the plasma membrane (151).

Acrogranin, a 67,000-dalton glycoprotein, was originally identified as an acrosomal constituent in guinea pig spermatogenic cells and sperm (519). Amino acid sequences deduced from cDNA sequences indicate that mouse and guinea pig acrogranins have extensive homology with granulins and epithelins, growth-modulating peptides previously identified in somatic tissues (520). Other peptides have been localized in the acrosome by immunocytochemical methods, including proenkephalin in rats (521), gastrin in humans (522), and the related cholecystokinin peptide in other mammals (523). The functional roles of these peptides during spermatogenesis or fertilization have not been determined.

Numerous acrosomal antigens of unknown function have been identified with both polyclonal and monoclonal antibodies (524–526). The amino acid sequence has been deduced from the cDNA sequence for human SP-10, an acrosomal antigen that is also present in other primates and pigs (527,528). SP-10 appears to be expressed only in spermatogenic cells and is associated with the inner acrosomal membrane and acrosomal matrix (529). Multiple immunoreactive polypeptides are detected with a monoclonal antibody to SP-10 and may result from endoproteolytic cleavage within the acrosome (530). It has recently been determined that MSA-63, a mouse acrosomal antigen, has a high degree of homology with SP-10 (531).

THE FLAGELLUM

The flagellum of the mammalian spermatozoon consists of four distinct segments: the *connecting piece* (neck), the *middle piece,* the *principal piece,* and the *end piece* (Fig. 1). The main structural components within the flagellum of the mammalian sperm are the *axoneme,* the *mitochondrial sheath,* the *outer dense fibers,* and the *fibrous sheath* (Table 4). The axoneme is composed of a "9 + 2" complex of microtubules that extends the full length of the flagellum. The outer dense fibers are adjacent to the axoneme and extend from the connecting piece to the posterior end of the principal piece. In addition, the middle-piece segment contains the mitochondrial sheath, whereas the principal-piece segment contains the fibrous sheath. The mitochondria lie between the plasma membrane and the outer dense fibers in the middle piece, whereas the fibrous sheath lies between the plasma membrane and the outer dense fibers in the principal piece. The base of the flagellum abuts the nucleus at the junction between connecting piece and head (170,532,533).

The flagellum provides the motile force necessary for the sperm to reach the egg surface and achieve fertilization. The different elements of the flagellum generate and shape the waves of bending that produce this force and propagate the waves from the base to the tip. The human sperm is about 60 μm long, and the flagellum is 55 μm of this length (351). However, sperm vary considerably in length between species. Rabbit sperm are 46 μm long, mouse sperm are 120 μm long, rat sperm are 190 μm long, and Chinese hamster sperm are 250 μm long (430). The flagellum of a human sperm is greater than 1 μm in diameter in the connecting-piece segment and tapers toward the posterior tip (351).

Connecting Piece

The main components of the connecting piece (Fig. 7) are the *capitulum* (the dense fibrous platelike structure that conforms to the shape of the *implantation fossa*) and the *segmented columns* (12) (Table 4). The implantation fossa develops with the apposition of the nuclear envelope and the *basal plate,* a dense plaque of material that is adherent to the outer nuclear membrane of the nuclear envelope. The interspace between the two membranes of the nuclear envelope in this region contains a regular array of periodic densities 6 nm wide and 6 nm apart (12). Freeze-fracture studies indicate that the membrane of the nuclear envelope lining the implantation fossa contains a dense population of large and regularly spaced intramembranous particles surrounding a central particle-free region (42). Fine filaments traversing the narrow region between capitulum and basal plate presumably are responsible for attaching the capitulum of the flagellum to the basal plate of the head (370,371). Trypsin treatment appears to cleave heads from tails at the plane between capitulum and basal plate (33,534), but decapitation of sperm with primary amines or sodium dodecyl sulfate usually results in cleavage between the inner nuclear membrane and the outer nuclear membrane (535). Heads and tails can also be separated

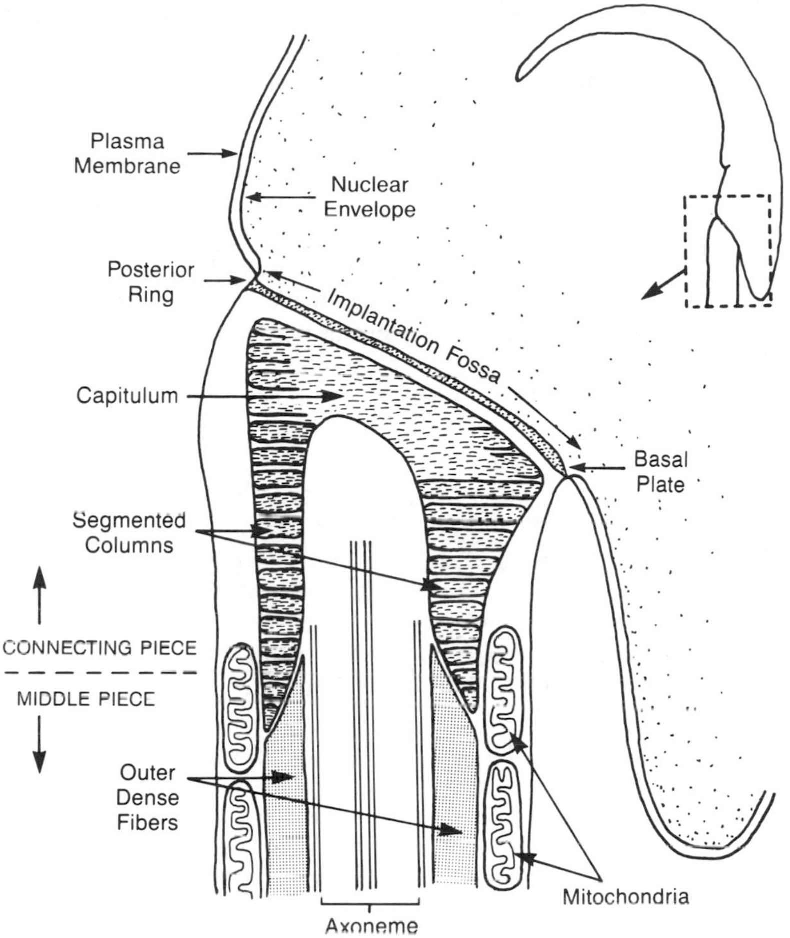

FIG. 7. Connecting piece of the flagellum. The basal plate is adherent to the nuclear envelope, defining the implantation fossa and forming the site of attachment of the flagellum to the sperm head. The connecting piece is topped by the capitulum, with the segmented columns extending from it caudally to fuse with the outer dense fibers. (Modified from Woolley and Fawcett, ref. 541.)

by sonication, but the cleavage site is not predictable (536,537).

The basal plate and capitulum are composed of proteins that are soluble in ionic detergent containing a disulfide-bond-reducing agent (537,538). Although the composition of these structures is not known, they may be related to ciliary rootlets (12), which contain a 250,000- and 230,000-dalton protein dimer called *ankyrin* (351). A genetic defect sometimes occurs in bulls that causes the flagella of most mature sperm to be detached from the heads (203). Detachment begins during late spermatogenesis and continues in the epididymis; the resulting detached flagella are motile, metabolically active, and able to penetrate cervical mucus (539).

Extending posteriorly from the capitulum are usually two major and five minor segmented columns 1 to 2 μm in length. The two major columns split into two columns each and, along with the other five columns, fuse to the nine outer dense fibers extending throughout most of the remaining length of the flagellum (Fig. 8). However, the segmented columns and outer dense fibers have different origins, and the continuity between them develops late in spermiogenesis (426,532). The segmented columns of the connecting piece are cross-striated, with a typical periodicity of 6.65 nm between segments. Each segment, in turn, has nine or ten horizontal bands (426). During development of the flagellum, a transversely or obliquely oriented proximal centriole lies between the longitudinally oriented distal centriole and the depression in the capitulum (426). The distal centriole is continuous with the axoneme and is surrounded by other accessory structures of the connecting piece. In many species, the distal centriole disintegrates late in spermatogenesis, and the proximal centriole is retained (179,370,406,532,540). The proximal centriole has been proposed to be the center of sperm motility (532). However, the proximal centriole disintegrates during the latter part of spermiogenesis in some species with normal motility (426,541), indicating that it is not required for generation of the flagellar beat. It appears that the centrioles serve as organizing centers for the formation of the axoneme and segmented columns but are not required for initiation or propagation of waves bending along the tail (12). The connecting piece terminates distally at the beginning of the mitochondrial sheath and middle piece.

Axoneme

The axoneme or axial filament complex of the mammalian sperm tail (Fig. 9) has the same organization as cilia and flagella of most plants and animals. It consists

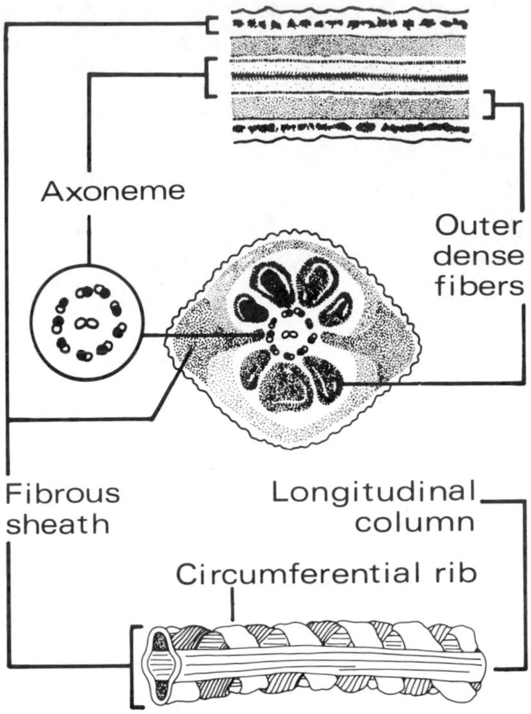

FIG. 8. Cytoskeletal components of the sperm flagellum. The axoneme extends from the connecting piece of the flagellum to the distal tip. In the principal piece of the flagellum the axoneme is surrounded by the fibrous sheath, composed of longitudinal columns connected by circumferential ribs. The outer dense fibers extend from the connecting piece to the posterior part of the principal piece. They lie between the mitochondrial sheath and the axoneme in the middle piece and between the fibrous sheath and the axoneme in the principal piece.

of two central microtubules surrounded by nine microtubule doublets (542). Each doublet consists of a complete A microtubule, onto which is attached a "C-shaped" B microtubule. Two arms extend from the A microtubule toward the B microtubule of the adjacent doublet. When axonemes are viewed from base to tip, the arms project clockwise (543). In the rat spermatozoon, the central pair of microtubules extend into the connecting piece to the capitulum, whereas the other microtubules appear to end on the remnants of the base of the distal centriole (541,544). Spokes radiate helically from the central pair of microtubules to the outer doublets around the central tubules (545). The doublets are numbered 1 through 9, with number 1 being the doublet situated on a plane perpendicular to that bisecting both microtubules of the central pair. Doublet number 2 is adjacent to the arms of doublet number 1, and so on.

The microtubules are composed of α-tubulin and β-tubulin, closely related proteins of approximately 56,000 and 54,000 daltons, respectively (546). New forms of α-tubulin and β-tubulin are synthesized in spermatids (546,547). Multiple α-tubulin and β-tubulin genes may be expressed at different times during spermatogenesis (548), including the postmeiotic phase (357). One spermatid α-tubulin mRNA has been shown to have a unique sequence, suggesting that it is encoded by a different gene than those for other α-tubulin mRNAs and is translated into an isoform that is specific to spermatogenic cells (547). If this tubulin is present in the microtubules of the flagellum, it might be involved in determining some of the special properties of the sperm axoneme.

Proteins that function in association with microtubules in other cells have not yet been shown to have roles in the functions in mammalian sperm. Kinesin is a protein complex that interacts with microtubules to effect movement (549). It is composed of two heavy chains of 124,000 daltons and two light chains of 64,000 daltons (550). Kinesin is a unidirectional motor that moves toward the [+] end of microtubules (549). It requires ATP but differs from myosin or dynein in structural and enzymatic characteristics (549,551). Although kinesin is present in the rat spermatid manchette (552), it is unknown if this protein complex has a role in generating or propa-

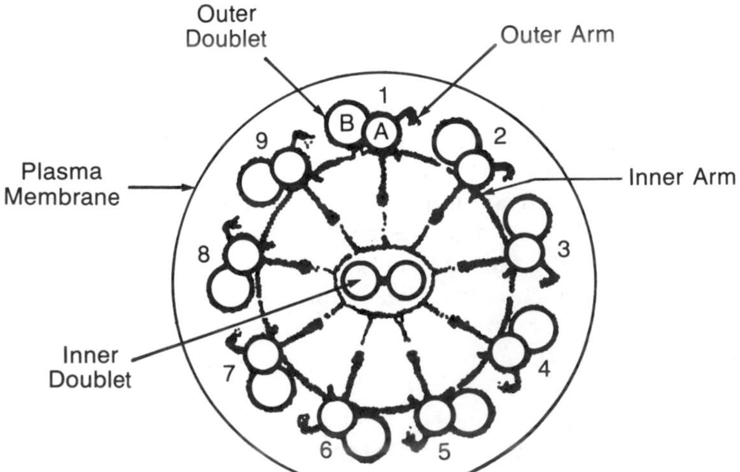

FIG. 9. The axoneme in the end piece of the sperm flagellum. Nine outer doublets of microtubules surround a central pair of microtubules. The outer doublets consist of microtubules A and B. Inner and outer dynein arms extend from the A microtubule toward the B microtubule of the adjacent pair.

gating the flagellar wave during mammalian sperm motility.

Dynein was originally identified in the axoneme of sea urchin sperm (553). It has ATPase activity (554) and moves unidirectionally toward the [−] end of microtubules (555). It is responsible for the sliding forces generated between adjacent doublets of microtubules during flagellar movement (556). ATPase activity has been extracted from mammalian sperm and identified by cytochemistry on the arms of the doublets and at the junction between radial spokes and central tubules in human sperm (351). Although dynein is present in rat spermatids (552), it has not been identified in mammalian sperm.

Sea urchin sperm flagellum can be dissociated with various treatments to release ribbons of two to four protofilaments (557). These ribbons can be further fractionated with chemical agents into filaments 2 to 3 nm in diameter (558). They are highly insoluble and have physical and chemical properties similar to intermediate filaments (559,560). The filaments contain 55,000-, 51,000-, and 47,000-dalton proteins named tektins, and an antiserum to this set of proteins reacts with the entire length of the axoneme (561). The tektins appear to be structural components of the microtubule doublets and may be involved in assembly or function of microtubules in the sea urchin sperm flagellum (561).

Mitochondrial Sheath

The mitochondria are helically wrapped around the outer dense fibers in the middle piece of the sperm tail (Fig. 1). They are generally arranged end to end, but the number of parallel helices, the number of gyres, and the length of the middle piece vary between species. In the mouse, the mitochondria are usually arranged in two parallel helices, with an average of 87 windings around the flagellum (562). The morphogenesis of this arrangement in the spermatid occurs by (a) migration of the annulus from the connecting piece down the flagellum to the beginning of the fibrous sheath, (b) formation of a dextral helix of elongated mitochondria around the flagellum, (c) division of these mitochondria into spherical mitochondria, and, (d) finally, elongation and end-to-end apposition of these mitochondria into two tight sinistral helices (562). In the mouse, the mitochondria are usually of variable length and abut end to end at random along the helix. Genetic selection has been used to produce strains of mice with sperm midpieces longer and shorter than the 21-μm average length (563).

In some species there is a high degree of uniformity in the organization of the mitochondrial sheath. Mitochondrial sheaths composed of a precise number of mitochondria of identical size and shape are present in the little brown bat (170), woolly opossum (564), and Chinese hamster (432). In the common brown bat there are two mitochondria of identical size in each turn of the gyre, and their ends always meet on a plane passing through the central pair of microtubules in the axoneme (170). In the rhesus monkey there is a tendency for the demarcation between mitochondria to occur in longitudinal register in alternate gyres (432).

The length of the middle piece and the disposition of mitochondria in spermatozoa have been determined for several species using surface replica methods (432). The middle piece in bull sperm is 12 μm long, and there are usually three helices of mitochondria organized into about 64 gyres. In addition, some of these mitochondria extend parallel with the long axis of the flagellum into the connecting piece. The rabbit sperm midpiece is 8.5 μm long and contains about 41 gyres of mitochondria in a quadruple or quintuple helix. The middle piece of rhesus monkey spermatozoa is about 10 μm long with 40 gyres of mitochondria arranged in a single or double helix. The middle piece of rat sperm is 64 μm long and contains about 362 mitochondrial gyres. The large outer dense fibers in rat sperm produce a broad middle piece, and the gently spiraling mitochondria fit together in intricate patterns. The middle piece in Chinese hamster sperm is about 100 μm long, with the mitochondria apparently being disposed in a double helix, each wrapping one-third of the circumference of the middle piece. The degu sperm middle piece is 7 μm long, with about 33 gyres of mitochondria forming concentric rows of single or double helices. Finally, the guinea pig spermatozoan middle piece is 9 μm long, and the mitochondria are arranged in irregular concentric patterns (432).

The mitochondrial sheath adheres to an underlying complex of filaments named the submitochondrial reticulum (SMR) (155,565). The SMR complex is a network of ribbons of filamentous material that are laterally interconnected and fuse with the annulus at the junction between the midpiece and the principal piece. Fractions isolated from bull sperm that are enriched for the SMR complex are resistant to solubilization and are enriched for 56,000- and 54,000-dalton proteins (566). The SMR may function in assembling and maintaining the ordered array of mitochondria in the midpiece (565).

Another component of the midpiece is the mitochondrial capsule protein (MCP) (567). This 17,000- to 15,000-dalton fibrous protein binds selenium and forms an insoluble capsule around sperm mitochondria. Selenium deficiency causes abnormal development of the sperm midpiece, leading to disorganization of the mitochondrial sheath (568). The MCP contains an unusually high percentage of proline and cysteine and a low percentage of hydrophobic amino acids (569,570). The MCP protein is synthesized in elongating spermatids in the rat (571), and the mRNA encoding this protein is transcribed in late pachytene spermatocytes and at higher levels in spermatids in the mouse (572).

Outer Dense Fibers

The nine outer dense fibers surround the axoneme, forming a "9 + 9 + 2" complex throughout the length of the middle piece and most of the principal piece of the flagellum of mammalian sperm (Figs. 1 and 8). Although similar structures are present in sperm of nonmammalian species (7), it has not been determined whether these are related in composition or function to the outer dense fibers in mammalian sperm. The basic structural plan of the sperm flagellum shows little variation in mammals, but the outer dense fibers differ considerably in size and shape between species. The fibers are often teardrop-shaped in cross section, with the peripheral margin of the fiber being rounded and the centrally projecting portion tapering toward a doublet of the axoneme (12).

The outer dense fibers also differ among themselves in shape and size, with fibers 1, 5, and 6 (and sometimes 9) being larger than the others. They are numbered corresponding to the adjacent microtubule doublet. The fibers are thickest in the proximal part of the middle piece and gradually taper in size toward the distal tip. They terminate in the proximal half of the principal piece in human, macaque, and bat sperm but extend to near the end of the principal piece in rat, hamster, guinea pig, and ground squirrel sperm (12). In human (573), bull, and rat sperm (574), the outer dense fibers occupy 60% of the length of the principal piece. In most species, fibers 3 and 8 terminate in the first part of the principal piece, and their place is taken by inward extensions of the longitudinal columns of the fibrous sheath. The larger fibers (1, 5, and 6) are usually the last to terminate (575).

The formation of outer dense fibers begins in spermatids, with the appearance of a small dense fiber immediately adjacent to the outer aspect of each microtubule doublet (576–578). In the rat, outer dense fibers first appear in the most proximal part of the future middle piece in step 8 of spermatid development and extend into the principal piece by step 14 (579). During step 15 the outer dense fibers increase in diameter and change shape, with fibers 1, 5, and 6 developing ahead of the other fibers. During step 16 the fibers enlarge rapidly along their entire length and take on their nearly final form, with slight growth continuing during steps 17 to 19 (579). Immunocytochemical studies have confirmed the proximal-to-distal direction of assembly of the outer dense fibers (580,581). Studies using autoradiography to localize metabolically incorporated proline and cysteine suggest that rapid protein synthesis accompanies the growth of the outer dense fibers during step 16 (579).

By electron microscopy, the outer dense fibers usually appear homogeneous, with a slightly less dense cortical layer. This cortical layer stains intensely with phosphotungstic acid (582) and tannic acid (12). When fixed in the presence of ruthenium red, the fibers appear to be composed of a single lamina of 6- to 7-nm globular particles (583). Surface replicas of sperm from rat or mouse outer dense fibers show striations with a periodicity of 40 nm in the outer contour of the cortex (562,583). These striations have the same 70–80° "sinistral obliquity" as the mitochondrial helix in the middle piece (562). The striations appear to be composed of a double linear array of 6- to 8-nm diameter globular subunits (583), and a central depression in each striation probably accounts for an apparent periodicity of 20 nm seen on negatively stained specimens (583,584). In the bull, periodicities of 20 nm (645) and 50 nm (586) are reported, and the outer dense fibers of human sperm have a 16-nm repeat (431). Studies on the rat indicate that the periodic substructure is confined to the cortex (583); however, this substructure is present in both cortical and medullary elements in human and bull sperm (431,584).

The relative insolubility of fibrous components of the flagellum in detergent solutions lacking disulfide-bond-reducing agents has allowed outer dense fibers to be isolated for biochemical analysis. The flagellum is reported to contain keratinlike proteins rich in cysteine (587) that are increasingly cross-linked by disulfide bonds during epididymal maturation (396,538). Rat sperm outer dense fibers contain four to six major proteins between 90,000 and 11,000 daltons (583,588–590), and they are phosphorylated (589). Bull sperm outer dense fibers contain three major proteins between 85,000 and 11,000 daltons (584,586,591). The amino acid composition of bull sperm outer dense fibers is similar to that of rat (591). Two proteins of 67,000 and 55,000 daltons are present in outer dense fibers of human sperm (592).

Two rat testis cDNAs have been isolated (593) that encode proteins similar in size and amino acid content to the 30,400-dalton and 26,000-dalton outer dense fiber proteins in rat sperm (589). The mRNAs are first transcribed in round spermatids and appear to be alternatively spliced products from a single gene (593). The mRNAs encode proteins with homologies to a protein present in *Drosophila melanogaster* spermatocytes (594). Similar mRNAs are also present in testes of human, mouse, bull, boar, and horse (593).

The outer dense fiber proteins have a high cysteine content (583,584,589), but there are differences between individual outer dense fiber proteins in amino acid composition, amino-terminal amino acids, net charge, and phosphorylation (583,584,589,591). The 87,000-dalton protein in rat outer dense fibers contains relatively large amounts of glutamic acid, lysine, alanine, and leucine but has relatively small amounts of serine, glycine, and cysteine. However, the 30,400-, 26,000-, 18,400-, and 11,500-dalton proteins contain high amounts of cysteine, tyrosine, proline, and glycine but less glutamic acid. The 13,000-dalton protein has high glutamic acid content and no histidine (589). The 30,400- and 26,000-dalton proteins have similar amino acid composition, a histidine at the amino-terminal position, and similar peptide maps, suggesting that they are closely related proteins (589).

Other differences have been reported for the proteins of the outer dense fibers. Infrared spectrum analysis suggests that the higher-molecular-weight components have an α-helical configuration (584). The smaller components are capable of binding zinc to their sulfhydryl groups (595). Zinc is required for spermatogenesis (596), is incorporated into the flagellum in late spermatids (597), and is localized in the outer dense fibers (584). Isoelectric focusing studies indicate that the proteins have large charge heterogeneities, probably as a result of posttranslational modifications (589,598). However, other studies indicate that carbohydrates are either absent (583) or barely detectable, suggesting that they may be present as contaminants (589). The major outer dense fiber protein of the rat contains appreciable amounts of phosphoserine, which could account for the charge heterogeneities, particularly for the larger proteins (589). Triglycerides may also be associated with the outer dense fibers (586,588). The structure and composition of outer dense fiber proteins will become better understood as the genes for these proteins are cloned and characterized (593).

Satellite fibers are present in the flagellar matrix between the outer dense fibers (12,391,599). These fibers form in step 19 of spermiogenesis in the rat, just before spermatozoa are released from the seminiferous epithelium (579). They are present in limited number in most species but are highly developed in the ground squirrel (391) and bandicoot (600), which have thick sperm tails (391). They may be accessory tensile elements of the motor apparatus (391). The satellite fibers appear to arise by separating from the edge of the outer dense fibers (12). However, they have not been isolated separately from the outer dense fibers, and their composition is not known.

It has been speculated that the outer dense fibers might be contractile because of their close association with the axoneme, their coincident appearance during phylogeny with internal fertilization, and a concomitant increase in the size of the mitochondrial sheath (391). It has been suggested that outer dense fibers are antigenically similar to actin (582) and that an ATPase is associated with the outer dense fibers (601). However, biochemical studies have not found a similarity in composition of outer dense fibers and actin, myosin, or tubulin (583). Other investigators have been unable to detect ATPase activity associated with outer dense fibers (586,599). This suggests that it is unlikely that the outer dense fibers play an active role in flagellar motion. However, stabilization of outer dense fiber proteins by abundant disulfide cross-linking may give them significant passive elastic properties that serve to stiffen or provide elastic recoil for the sperm tail (12).

High-speed cinematography of mouse, human, rabbit, and opossum sperm indicates that they are relatively flexible, forming arcs with a small radius of curvature as they beat. However, rat and Chinese hamster sperm appear very stiff while beating and have a large radius of curvature (430). There is a correlation between the radius of curvature and the size of the dense fibers in these species, suggesting that the dense fibers might influence the form of the beat by determining the elastic properties of the sperm tail (430). Measurement of the relative tensile strengths of sperm of seven mammalian species indicates that tensile strength correlates with the size of the outer dense fibers (602). It is suggested that the outer dense fibers provide added strength to protect sperm from damage by shear forces encountered during epididymal transit or ejaculation (602).

Fibrous Sheath

The fibrous sheath defines the extent of the principal piece (Figs. 1 and 8), the longest segment of the flagellum (391). This cytoskeletal structure is unique to the flagellum of sperm of mammals and some birds. It closely underlies the plasma membrane but is not directly attached to it (7). The fibrous sheath is a tapering cylinder formed by *two longitudinal columns* connected by *circumferential ribs* (Fig. 9). The columns are formed by longitudinally oriented, loosely packed filamentous structures 15 to 20 nm in diameter. The longitudinal columns run peripheral to microtubule doublets 3 and 8 of the axoneme and are attached to outer dense fibers 3 and 8 in the proximal part of the principal piece (576). Distal to the termination of these two dense fibers, the tapered central edges of the longitudinal columns attach to ridges projecting from microtubule doublets 3 and 8 (391). The columns lie approximately in the plane of the central pair of axoneme microtubules throughout the principal piece segment and have been referred to as *dorsal* and *ventral columns* in sperm containing a falciform head (391). The size and shape of the longitudinal columns vary between species. They are narrow and inconspicuous in the common brown bat and guinea pig but are large in the Chinese hamster and opossum and result in prominent ridges that give the principal piece an elliptical profile in cross section (391).

The ribs of the fibrous sheath are composed of closely packed, circumferentially oriented filaments (391). The ribs broaden toward their ends, where they merge with the longitudinal columns and with each other. They are closely spaced and may bifurcate and anastomose with adjacent ribs. This occurs frequently in the mouse, resulting in broad bands instead of slender separate ribs. The ribs may also vary in shape and size, being broad and flat in the bat and greatly expanded at their ends in the opossum. The thickness of the ribs diminishes toward the distal end of the principal piece, and the ribs end abruptly at the posterior margin of the principal piece (12,391). In human spermatozoa, the ribs are 10 to 20 nm apart and about 50 nm thick (351).

Formation of the fibrous sheath takes place throughout much of spermiogenesis in the rat and proceeds in a distal-to-proximal direction (580,581,603). The longitudinal columns first appear as thin rods joined to microtubule doublets 3 and 8 near the distal end of the flagellum in step 2 of spermiogenesis. The columns increase in length during steps 2 to 10. In step 11, evenly spaced and circumferentially arranged pairs of spines form against the plasma membrane in the distal part of the flagellum. During steps 12 to 14, these structures associate with the columns in a distal-to-proximal direction. In early step 15, additional material is deposited between the pairs of spines to form the definitive ribs, and the longitudinal columns become thickened. During steps 15 to 16, additional ribs are formed from posterior to anterior along the remaining proximal segment of the principal piece (603). Fibrous sheath proteins are synthesized during the entire 15-day period of fibrous sheath formation (603). Filamentous material present in the cytoplasm of earlier-stage spermatids appears to be the rib precursor in human (577,605), marmoset (604), and bandicoot sperm (578).

The fibrous sheath is highly resistant to acid solubilization (606), and the proteins of the fibrous sheath are stabilized by disulfide bonds (396). These characteristics were utilized to develop a procedure for isolating the fibrous sheath from rat sperm (402,607). Isolated rat fibrous sheaths are reported to contain three to seven major proteins from 115,000 to 11,500 daltons (590,607–609). An 80,000-dalton protein is phosphorylated, and peptide map analysis indicates that 80,000- and 11,500-dalton proteins are unrelated to proteins of similar size in the outer dense fibers (608). The major insoluble tail component synthesized during spermiogenesis in the mouse is a 74,000-dalton protein (610) that may be a fibrous sheath component. The isolated mouse sperm fibrous sheath contains five major proteins of 112,000 to 24,000 daltons (609). The major proteins in the isolated human sperm fibrous sheath are 68,000 daltons and 54,000 to 51,000 daltons (611).

Antibodies have been used to characterize some of the fibrous sheath components. Monoclonal antibody K32 (612) first reacts with a component in the cytoplasm of step-14 spermatids, binds to the proximal portion of the principal piece in step-15 spermatids, and recognizes the fibrous sheath in step-16 spermatids (613). The proximal-to-distal appearance of the component is opposite in direction to the general pattern of fibrous sheath formation in the rat (603). The protein recognized by K32 has not been identified. Monoclonal antibody ATC recognizes a 67,000-dalton protein in mouse fibrous sheath, a 65,000-dalton protein in rat fibrous sheath, and a 66,000-dalton protein in hamster fibrous sheath (614). ATC also reacts with late spermatids in these species, but does not react with spermatids or the fibrous sheath of rabbit or guinea pig.

Monoclonal antibody GDA-J/F3 was prepared against nucleated cells in human semen (615). It binds to the fibrous sheath of human sperm, abnormal germ cells in human semen, and the flagellum in sections of the human testis (615,616). GDA-J/F3 does not recognize a protein on Western blots of human fibrous sheaths, suggesting that the epitope is denatured during gel electrophoresis. Monoclonal antibody RT97, originally prepared against a 200,000-dalton neurofilament protein, recognizes a 97,000-dalton protein (AJ-p97) on Western blots of human sperm fibrous sheaths (616). AJ-p97 is not detected in human fibrous sheaths following alkaline phosphatase treatment, indicating that the RT97 epitope contains a phosphorylated amino acid (616). RT97 does not recognize proteins in mouse and rat sperm, suggesting that the epitope is not highly conserved (616). In addition, monoclonal antibodies S69 and S70 recognize proteins of 68,000 daltons and a triplet between 54,000 and 51,000 daltons in human sperm fibrous sheath (611). Proteins of 68,000, 53,000, and 45,000 daltons were recognized by both antibodies on Western blots of nonreduced human sperm extracts.

Antibodies against rat outer dense fibers cross-react with the 14,400-dalton fibrous sheath protein, whereas antibodies against the rat fibrous sheath cross-react with the 14,400-dalton outer dense fiber protein (590). Antibodies affinity purified from the 14,400-dalton outer dense fiber protein cross-react with several fibrous sheath proteins. However, it appears that the 14,400-dalton proteins in the outer dense fibers and fibrous sheath are not identical but share antigenic epitopes, as do some of the other proteins in the outer dense fibers and fibrous sheath (580,590). The mouse fibrous sheath contains proteins that share epitopes with intermediate-filament proteins, but the proteins are distinctly different in size. These fibrous sheath proteins may be products of genes related to those for intermediate-filament proteins but expressed only during spermatogenesis (609).

The function of the fibrous sheath may be to modulate the plane of the flagellar beat. The attachment of doublets 3 and 8 to the longitudinal columns might restrict their participation in microtubule sliding and axoneme binding during flagellar motion. The longitudinal columns themselves might also limit bending of the flagellum in this same plane, whereas flagellar bending perpendicular to this plane would not be restricted by these features (12). Although sperm appear to swim with a planar effective stroke and recovery stroke somewhat like cilia, they also rotate (617), and the propagated waves have a three-dimensional component in the distal portion of the tail (12). However, it is not known how the fibrous sheath might influence flagellar movement in the female reproductive tract.

Abnormal Flagella

Spermatozoa with abnormal flagella are present in low numbers in many mammals but are relatively common in humans. One study indicated that 12.5 ± 5.5% of sperm from 20 fertile men have abnormal flagella and that an even higher number of sperm (24.4 ± 7.7%) have abnormal axonemes, with only 41.6 ± 15.3% of sperm being motile (618). Infertile men are reported to have from 18% (619) to over 30% (620) sperm with abnormal tails. It is generally assumed that abnormal sperm have little chance of achieving fertilization. However, completely immotile human spermatozoa have been reported to undergo capacitation, the acrosome reaction, and fusion with the vitelline membrane of zona-free hamster oocytes *in vitro* (621). Also, a sperm tail lacking four doublets and the outer dense fibers has been observed in the cytoplasm of a fertilized mouse egg (622).

Anecdotal reports of infertile men with sperm that are immotile or have abnormal flagella are not uncommon (623–626). Patients with "dysplasia of the fibrous sheath" syndrome have sperm with short, rigid, thick, and immotile tails and hyperplastic and disorganized fibrous sheaths (627). A hereditary condition referred to as *immotile-cilia syndrome* or *Kartagener's syndrome,* results in male sterility, situs inversus in 50% of cases, and chronic respiratory problems (628). These conditions are directly or indirectly a consequence of an autosomal recessive trait that causes cilia or flagella to fail to perform normal and coordinated movements (629). Men with the syndrome have sperm with defective axonemes having either a partial or complete lack of dynein arms, a lack of outer dynein arms, a lack of inner arms, or abnormally short spokes and a lack of the central sheath (630). Because of the different types of defects seen in sperm and cilia, the failure to locate a single gene by linkage analysis, and the relatively high prevalence of the condition, it has been suggested that the mutation of multiple genes may produce the syndrome (628).

Several mutations that affect formation of the flagellum have been identified in mice. The mutations are pleiotropic, causing defects in tissues in addition to the seminiferous epithelium; most affect formation of the sperm head as well as the flagellum (423,424). Homozygous mice with the Wobbler mutation apparently produce normal numbers of sperm, but few are motile (631). The sperm appear to have average-length tails and normal heads, but 70% of the sperm in the vas deferens have ultrastructural defects in the flagellum. These defects include the absence of one to four outer doublets and the corresponding dense fibers, most commonly those from positions 4 through 7. Other defects seen less frequently are supernumerary microtubules or the absence of central pair tubules in the axoneme (691). Defective sperm are common in *T/t* mice, with the most frequent flagellar defects seen in sterile mice being a lack of four outer dense fibers and doublets (632). The male-sterile mutation hydrocephalic-polydactyl (*hpy*) results in the absence of a flagellum or in partially assembled axonemal structures and/or poorly organized aggregates of other tail components (633). The axoneme is usually absent or abnormally formed, and the outer dense fibers and fibrous sheath are morphologically atypical when present. The axoneme dysgenesis might be caused by failure to form stable structures because of defective subunits (633).

The sperm from infertile men with a condition referred to as flagellar dyskinesia have normal axonemes but abnormal periaxonemal structures. These include abnormal extension of individual dense fibers along the axoneme, altered order of termination of these structures, and a modified number and location of longitudinal columns of the fibrous sheath (573). The outer dense fibers have abnormal positions with respect to each other, being placed symmetrically with respect to a plane that passes through microtubular doublet 1 and between doublets 5 and 6. The most common defect of the longitudinal columns of the fibrous sheath is the presence of only one column adjacent to doublet 3 or 8 (573). These abnormalities might be caused by a defect of the components of the wall of the A microtubules of the outer nine doublets at the site of formation or assembly of the outer dense fibers and longitudinal columns (620).

A common defect seen in an abnormal or degenerating flagellum is the absence of microtubule doublets 4 through 7 and the associated dense fibers (631,632,634). The same alteration is produced by adding ATP to detergent-extracted rat sperm tails. Doublets 8 through 3 and the associated dense fibers appear to remain firmly attached to the fibrous sheath, whereas doublets 4 through 7 are extruded from the sperm tail (544). This suggests that some sperm seen with this defect may be degenerating. In some conditions, the flagellar axoneme may appear to form normally and then to become progressively disorganized. This occurs during spermiogenesis in quaking (635) and in *hpy/hpy* mice (633). However, in Wobbler mice, the percentage of abnormal sperm increases as they transit the male tract. Only about 5% of sperm tails are abnormal in the testis, but nearly 70% of sperm from the vas deferens have abnormal flagella (631).

Flagellar Motion

The flagellar wave is propagated in a plane perpendicular to the central pair of microtubules of the axoneme and passes through doublet 1 and between doublets 5 and 6, with the active stoke being toward doublet 1 (636). The flagellum twists during bend propagation (637,638), with the plane of bending moving toward doublet 2 (637). The part of the axoneme containing doublets 1 through 5 is thought to be active during this phase of flagellar motion (637). The outer dense fibers and fibrous sheath appear to play a passive role in flagellar motion (639–642). The tapering of the dense fibers is believed to decrease local resistance to bending (573,643) and might explain the progressive increase in the amplitude of curvature observed during flagellar wave propagation (641,643,644). The small flagellar amplitude observed in certain abnormal human sperm (645) may result from constraints imposed by the abnormal arrangement of dense fibers in those sperm (573).

Sperm acquire the capacity for progressive motility during epididymal maturation. Sperm from the cauda epididymidis are immotile in epididymal fluid, and it is not until they are diluted into physiological medium that the capacity for motility is expressed. Immotility may be enforced in some species by the viscoelastic drag produced by the high-molecular-weight glycoprotein immobilin present in epididymal fluid (646,647). However, rabbit sperm show motility in their native fluid (648), and epididymal fluid in the bull is not particularly viscous (649). Sperm from the caput epididymidis in most mammals have a vibratory or slow and ineffective beat that often results in circular swimming patterns (230). In contrast, sperm from the cauda epididymidis usually move with a vigorous motion that results in rapid forward movement. In correlation with this change in swimming pattern, the flagellum appears to become more rigid and to beat with a reduced arc of curvature (238). This may be because of the increased disulfide bond formation that occurs in outer dense fibers and the fibrous sheath during epididymal maturation (397). However, cauda sperm from different species show different patterns of motility, flagellar beat, and flagellar rigidity (430). Sperm undergo additional changes in the pattern of motility in the female reproductive tract. They become hyperactivated as capacitation proceeds and move with a vigorous whiplike beating of the flagellum at the time of fertilization (5,239).

A variety of factors appear to be involved in the initiation and regulation of sperm motility (Table 6), but a unifying hypothesis for how these factors interact to produce coordinated flagellar activity is lacking. A key second messenger in this process is cyclic adenosine monophosphate (cAMP). The cAMP levels increase in sperm during epididymal transit (650,651) and phosphodiesterase inhibitors that elevate cAMP levels induce partial motility in caput sperm (652). A more effective pattern of motility is induced in caput sperm by addition of a "forward motility protein" present in epididymal fluid (651,653).

The major role of cAMP in sperm is probably to mediate cAMP-stimulated phosphorylation of proteins essential for initiation or maintenance of motility (654). ATP is converted to cAMP in sperm by a calcium-dependent adenylate cyclase that may be controlled partly by calmodulin (655,656). Multiple genes encoding calmodulin are expressed during spermatogenesis (657). The 55,000- and 49,000-dalton regulatory subunits (RI and RII) and the 40,000-dalton catalytic (C) subunit of cAMP-dependent protein kinase are present in sperm, and most of the cAMP-binding activity is in the tail (658,659). Unique mRNA species for these subunits are present in spermatogenic cells (660–664).

Other enzymes needed for protein phosphorylation and dephosphorylation are also present in sperm, including protein phosphatases (665,666) and cAMP phosphodiesterase (667,668). There are four cAMP phosphodiesterase genes expressed in the rat testis (669), and multiple cAMP mRNAs are present in spermatogenic cells (670). One of the cAMP phosphodiesterase

TABLE 6. *Factors involved in initiation and regulation of sperm motility*

Factor	References
ATP interacts with dynein ATPase to promote sliding of outer doublets of axoneme	675–678
Calcium-dependent and calmodulin-regulated adenylate cyclase converts ATP to cAMP	655,656
Cyclic AMP levels in sperm increase during epididymal transit	650,651
Phosphodiesterase inhibitors elevate cAMP levels and induce partial motility in caput sperm	652
Calmodulin-binding protein that inhibits phosphodiesterase present	671,672
Increase in internal pH and cAMP induces motility	673,674
Cyclic-AMP-dependent protein kinase present	658–664
Cyclic AMP stimulates phosphorylation of sperm protein	687,688
Phosphoprotein phosphatase present	665,666
Cyclic AMP phosphodiesterase present	667–670
Inhibitor of cAMP-dependent protein kinase present	671
Low-molecular-weight factor in seminal plasma stimulates sperm adenylate cyclase	679
Adenosine and analogs elevate cAMP levels and initiate motility in caput sperm in a pH-dependent manner	680
High levels of adenosine inhibit sperm adenylate cyclase activity	681–683
Adenosine increases level of *S*-adenosylhomocysteine, which inhibits sperm motility	694,695
Adenylate cyclase inhibitory guanine-nucleotide-binding protein present	686
Inhibitor of cAMP-independent protein kinase present in seminal plasma	690,691
Inhibitor of calcium uptake present in seminal plasma	693
Forward motility protein in epididymal fluid modulates pattern of sperm motility	651,653
Motility inhibitor present in seminal plasma	589
pH-dependent sperm motility quiescence factor present in epididymal fluid	649,697
Immotility of epididymal sperm enforced by viscoelastic drag produced by high-molecular-weight glycoprotein in epididymal fluid	646,647

genes is expressed at high levels in spermatids (670). In addition, sperm contain an inhibitor of cAMP-dependent protein kinase (671) and calspermin, a 32,000-dalton calmodulin-binding protein that inhibits phosphodiesterase and is expressed specifically in spermatids at high levels (672).

Another change that occurs as sperm transit the epididymis is an increase in internal pH. Bicarbonate ions, in the presence of calcium, markedly elevate cAMP levels in cauda sperm (673), and conditions that elevate both pH and cAMP in caput sperm cause them to swim like cauda sperm (674). ATP is required for motility, and one of its roles is to interact with ATPases associated with the dynein arms to promote sliding of the outer doublets (675). Sperm that are permeabilized by detergent treatment are immotile but can be reactivated with ATP, and subsequent addition of cAMP causes an increase in motility (676–678).

Prostaglandins and steroid hormones alter cAMP levels in other tissues, and the presence of these molecules in seminal plasma might influence motility by affecting sperm cAMP levels and adenylate cyclase activity (654). In addition, a low-molecular-weight factor in porcine seminal plasma stimulates sperm adenylate cyclase activity (679), and adenosine and its analogs elevate cAMP levels to initiate motility in immature caput sperm in a pH-dependent manner (680). Some of the adenosine analogs used do not appear to enter cells, suggesting that adenosine may act on sperm through external adenosine receptors. Furthermore, high levels of adenosine inhibit sperm adenylate cyclase activity, possibly through an inhibitory site associated with the adenylate cyclase catalytic subunit (681–683). Sperm adenylate cyclase is not affected by fluoride, guanine nucleotides, forskolin, or cholera toxin plus NAD (654,684), suggesting that the enzyme is not regulated by guanidine-nucleotide-binding regulatory proteins. This was supported initially by observations that G_s and G_i guanidine-binding proteins could not be detected in sperm (685), but subsequent studies found that the G_i protein α_i subunit and the 35,000-dalton β subunit are present in detergent extracts of mouse, bovine, and human sperm (686). However, G_s is not detected, and adenylate cyclase does not reconstitute with the addition of exogenous G_s regulatory protein (686), suggesting that regulation of adenylate cyclase may be unique in sperm (685).

Adenylate cyclase activation in most cells results in phosphorylation of specific proteins by cAMP-dependent protein kinases (684). Radioactive phosphate is incorporated into a 55,000-dalton protein in sperm from the cauda epididymidis but not into sperm from the caput epididymis of the rat (687). In addition, a 55,000-dalton protein in bull sperm is more heavily phosphorylated in motile than in nonmotile sperm (687). Sperm tubulin is phosphorylated in a cAMP-dependent manner, and the amount of phosphorylation correlates with an increase in sperm motility (671). Tubulin is approximately 55,000 daltons, but the phosphorylated protein in bull sperm does not bind colchicine and is probably not tubulin (687). The stimulatory effect of cAMP on reactivation of detergent-extracted dog, human, and sea urchin sperm requires the phosphorylation of "axokinin," a 56,000-dalton protein synthesized during spermatogenesis (688).

Other modulators of sperm motility have been reported. A motility inhibitor of seminal plasma is highest in the fluid from the seminal vesicles but is also present in prostatic fluid from bull, rat, and rabbit (689). This 15,000-dalton protein inhibits the reactivation of motility in detergent-extracted sperm and reduces the motility of previously reactivated sperm. The motility inhibitor may in turn be regulated by a dialyzable activator (689). An inhibitor of cAMP-independent protein kinase is also present in human seminal plasma (690,691). It is a high-molecular-weight, heat-labile, trypsin-insensitive protein. It does not appear to inhibit motility via an enzymatic mechanism, and its presence in seminal plasma of vasectomized men indicates that it is produced by one of the male accessory glands. Seminal plasma also contains low-molecular-weight components that inhibit the pattern (692) of uptake of calcium by sperm (693), and calcium is important for sperm motility (654,677,678). Adenosine has been shown to increase the level of *S*-adenosylhomocysteine, a competitive inhibitor of *S*-adenosylmethionine protein carboxymethylation (694). Carboxymethylation occurs in motile sperm (695,696), and agents that elevate *S*-adenosylhomocysteine inhibit sperm motility (694). In addition, a pH-dependent sperm motility quiescence factor is present in bovine cauda epididymal fluid (649,697).

SUMMARY

An understanding of the composition, organization, and function of the sperm surface is beginning to emerge. An increasing number of the protein, glycoprotein, and lipid constituents of the sperm plasma membrane have been identified and characterized. A key advance has been the realization that the sperm plasma membrane is a mosaic whose components often are segregated into specific regions or domains. The regional differentiation in composition of the sperm surface correlates with specialized functions that are associated with specific domains. Thus, molecules involved in the acrosome reaction are present over the anterior acrosome (104), molecules involved in fusion of the sperm and egg are present over the posterior acrosome (110), and molecules involved in flagellar activity are associated with the plasma membrane of the flagellum (686).

It is also known that the composition of the plasma membrane is modified after spermatozoa leave the testis. Changes occur during maturation in the epididymis, exposure to accessory gland secretory products during ejaculation, and in the female reproductive tract (5). These changes indicate that although the domains are relatively constant, the components of the sperm surface are dynamic features of the cell.

However, much more remains to be learned about the composition, organization, and function of the sperm surface. Although proteins in specific domains have been identified, the amino acid sequences, native structures, and gene structure and expression remain to be determined for most. Advances in molecular genetics are beginning to allow information gained about functionally significant sperm-surface molecules in laboratory animals to be applied to understanding the roles of comparable proteins in humans. The use of molecular modeling approaches to predict the structure of these proteins will help to determine how they associate with other molecules in the cytoplasm and plasma membrane as well as how they participate in sperm functions. Although progress has occurred in the characterization of the sperm plasma membrane (191), the distribution of specific lipids in different domains and their roles in sperm function remain to be determined. Also, much remains to be learned about how and when sperm surface domains are established, what mechanisms are responsible for targeting or segregating molecules into specific domains, and how the boundaries or domains are maintained.

Careful morphological studies have provided a rich knowledge of the structural architecture of spermatozoa from many different species. In addition, the timing and sequence of formation during spermatogenesis of many of the unique structures of sperm are reasonably well defined. However, relatively little is known about the mechanisms of morphogenesis of spermatozoa, the regulation of these mechanisms, and the composition and function of sperm-specific structures. An example is the cytoskeletal architecture of the head and flagellum (Table 4). The cytoskeleton of the sperm head includes structures lying between the acrosome and the nucleus, between the acrosome and plasma membrane, and surrounding the nucleus posterior to the acrosome. Some of these structures are more distinct in sperm containing a falciform head, whereas others are more obvious in sperm possessing a spatulate head. Several of the proteins in these structures have been partially characterized, but their relationship to structural proteins of other cells, when they are synthesized, and how they interact to form the cytoskeleton of the sperm head are not known. It remains to be learned if these features determine or maintain the shape of the sperm head.

The cytoskeleton of the flagellum includes the axoneme, outer dense fibers, fibrous sheath, and satellite fibers. Little is known about the composition and function of these structures and what regulates their assembly into the complex and highly organized flagellum. Although efforts are under way to identify the proteins in these structural components, the time of synthesis, distribution, organization, and function of specific proteins remain to be determined. When the individual components of the flagellum are characterized, it may be possible to begin to understand how they function together to produce the effective flagellar beat.

These limitations are also true for other components and activities of the spermatozoon. A few of the enzymes of the acrosome have been well characterized *in vitro,* but their function *in vivo* is not well understood. Remarkably little is known about the nature and role of most of the other enzymes reported to be in the acrosome. Changes during epididymal maturation give sperm the ability to perform coordinated flagellar motion. This is likely to involve components of the cAMP-dependent second message system in spermatozoa that are used in other cells to respond to external stimuli (654). However, neither the external stimuli that influence flagellar motion nor the sperm receptor for these stimuli has been identified (686).

The specialized features of sperm give them the ability to deliver new genetic material to the egg. It remains to be determined how chromatin is organized in the mammalian spermatozoon, how paternally derived genes required during development are imprinted during spermatogenesis, and whether sperm have other roles in the initiation of development besides activating the egg and donating a haploid genome to the next generation.

It is apparent that many questions remain about the composition, organization, and function of the spermatozoon. However, many can be answered with the research methods now available in cell and molecular biology. Monoclonal antibodies have already been valuable for determining the structure and function of sperm-surface domains. They are specific, sensitive, and easily used morphological, biochemical, and physiological probes. The tools of molecular genetics are also proving to be extremely valuable for understanding the structure and function of spermatogenic cell constituents. Knowledge of the genes responsible for sperm structure and function should allow sophisticated advances in the diagnosis, treatment, and prevention of male infertility.

Other powerful physical and chemical approaches, such as fluorescent membrane-intercalating agents and FRAP, are providing important new insights into the properties of the plasma membrane and the behavior of specific surface antigens. Because the spermatozoon is highly polarized and can be studied *in vitro,* it is the cell of choice for such investigations. The use of these and other new approaches should continue to provide substantially better knowledge and understanding of the composition, organization, and function of the spermatozoon.

ACKNOWLEDGMENTS

The preparation of this chapter was supported in part by grants HD26485 (DO) and HD18968 (Laboratories for Reproductive Biology) from the National Institutes of Health.

REFERENCES

1. de Kretser DM, Kerr JB. The cytology of the testis. Chapter 21, *this volume.*
2. Eddy EM, O'Brien DA, Welch JE. Mammalian sperm development in vivo and in vitro. In: Wassarman PM, ed. *Elements of mammalian fertilization,* vol 1, *Basic concepts.* Boca Raton: CRC Press; 1991:1–28.
3. Eddy EM, Welch JE, O'Brien DA. Gene expression during spermatogenesis. In: de Kretser DM, ed. *Cellular and molecular mechanisms in male reproduction.* Orlando: Academic Press [*in press*].
4. Pedersen RA. Early mammalian embryogenesis. Chapter 6, *this volume.*
5. Yanagimachi R. Mammalian fertilization. Chapter 5, *this volume.*
6. Baccetti B. Evolutionary trends in sperm structure. *Comp Biochem Physiol* 1986;85A:29–36.
7. Baccetti B, Afzelius BA. *Monographs in developmental biology,* vol 10, *The biology of the sperm cell.* Basel: S Karger; 1976.
8. Roosen-Runge E. *Developmental and cell biology series, vol 10, The process of spermatogenesis in mammals.* Cambridge: Cambridge University Press; 1977.
9. Segal S. Sexual differentiation in vertebrates. In: Halvorson HO, Monroy A, eds. *MBL lectures in biology, vol 7, The origin and evolution of sex.* New York: Alan R Liss; 1985:263–270.
10. Anderegg C, Markert CL. Successful rescue of microsurgically produced homozygous uniparental mouse embryos via production of aggregation chimeras. *Proc Natl Acad Sci USA* 1986; 83:6509–6513.
11. Surani MA, Allen ND, Barton SC, et al. Developmental consequences of imprinting of parental chromosomes by DNA methylation. *Phil Trans R Soc (Lond)* [*Biol*] 1990;326:313–327.
12. Fawcett DW. The mammalian spermatozoon. *Dev Biol* 1975; 44:394–436.
13. Koehler JK. The mammalian sperm surface: Studies with specific labeling techniques. In: Bourne GH, Danielli JF, eds. *International review of cytology, vol 54.* New York: Academic Press; 1978:73–108.
14. Friend DS. Plasma-membrane diversity in a highly polarized cell. *J Cell Biol* 1982;93:243–249.
15. Primakoff P, Myles DG. A map of the guinea pig sperm surface constructed with monoclonal antibodies. *Dev Biol* 1983;98: 417–428.
16. Holt WV. Membrane heterogeneity in the mammalian spermatozoon. In: Bourne GH, Danielli JF, eds. *International review of cytology, vol 87.* New York: Academic Press; 1984:159–194.
17. Bearer EL, Friend DS. Morphology of mammalian sperm membranes during differentiation, maturation, and capacitation. *J Electron Microsc Technol* 1990;16:281–297.
18. Toshimori K, Higashi R, Ōura C. Filipin-sterol complexes in golden hamster sperm membranes with special reference to epididymal maturation. *Cell Tissue Res* 1987;250:673–680.
19. Bangham AD. Electrophoretic characteristics of ram and rabbit spermatozoa. *Proc R Soc Lond* [*Biol*] 1961;155:292–305.
20. Nevo AC, Michaeli I, Schindler H. Electrophoretic properties of bull and of rabbit spermatozoa. *Exp Cell Res* 1961;23:69–83.
21. Bedford JM. Changes in the electrophoretic properties of rabbit spermatozoa during passage through the epididymis. *Nature* 1963;200:1178–1180.
22. Cooper GW, Bedford JM. Acquisition of surface charge by the plasma membrane of mammalian spermatozoa during epididymal maturation. *Anat Rec* 1971;169:300–301.
23. Yanagimachi R, Noda YD, Fujimoto M, Nicolson G. The distribution of negative surface charges on mammalian spermatozoa. *Am J Anat* 1972;135:497–520.
24. Lopez ML, de Souza W, Bustos-Obregon E. Cytochemical analysis of the anionic sites on the membrane of the stallion spermatozoa during the epididymal transit. *Gamete Res* 1987;18:319–332.
25. Sharon N, Lis H. Use of lectins for the study of membranes. In: Korn ED, ed. *Methods in membrane biology, vol 3.* New York: Academic Press; 1974:147–199.
26. Nicolson G. The interactions of lectins with animal cell surfaces. In: Bourne GH, Danielli JF, eds. *International review of cytology, vol 39.* New York: Academic Press; 1974:89–190.
27. Kashiwahara T, Tanaka R, Matsomoto T. Tail to tail agglomeration of bull spermatozoa by phytoagglutinins present in soy beans. *Nature* 1965;207:831–832.
28. Nicolson G, Yanagimachi R. Terminal saccharides on sperm plasma membranes. Identification by specific agglutinins. *Science* 1972;177:276–279.
29. Nicolson G, Poste G, Ji TH. The dynamics of cell membrane organization. In: Poste G, Nicolson G, eds. *Dynamic aspects of cell surface organization.* Amsterdam: North Holland; 1977: 1–73.
30. Koehler JK. Lectins as probes of the spermatozoon surface. *Arch Androl* 1981;6:197–217.
31. Nicolson G, Lacorbiere M, Yanagimachi R. Quantitative determination of plant agglutinin membrane sites on mammalian spermatozoa. *Proc Soc Exp Biol Med* 1972;141:661–663.
32. Lee SH, Ahuja KK. An investigation using lectins of glycocomponents of mouse spermatozoa during capacitation and sperm-zona binding. *J Reprod Fertil* 1987;80:65–74.
33. Edelman GM, Millette CF. Molecular probes of spermatozoon structures. *Proc Nat Acad Sci USA* 1971;68:2436–2440.
34. Millette CF. Distribution and mobility of lectin binding sites on mammalian spermatozoa. In: Edidin M, Johnson MH, eds. *Immunobiology of gametes.* Cambridge: Cambridge University Press; 1977:51–71.
35. Schwarz MA, Koehler JK. Alterations in lectin binding to guinea pig spermatozoa accompanying in vitro capacitation and the acrosome reaction. *Biol Reprod* 1976;21:1295–1307.
36. Koehler JK. The mammalian sperm surface: An overview of structure with particular reference to mouse spermatozoa. In: Amann RP, Seidel GE Jr, eds. *Prospects for sexing mammalian sperm.* Boulder: Colorado Associated University Press; 1982: 23–42.
37. Sarkar M, Majumder GC, Chatterjee T. Goat sperm membrane: Lectin-binding sites of sperm surface and lectin affinity chromatography of the mature sperm membrane antigens. *Biochim Biophys Acta* 1991;1070:198–204.
38. Fenderson BA, O'Brien DA, Millette CF, Eddy EM. Stage-specific expression of three cell surface carbohydrate antigens during murine spermatogenesis detected with monoclonal antibodies. *Dev Biol* 1984;103:117–128.
39. Gordon M, Dandekar PV, Bartoszewicz W. The surface coat of epididymal, ejaculated and capacitated sperm. *J Ultrastruct Res* 1975;50:199–207.
40. Nicolson G, Yanagimachi R. Mobility and restriction of mobility of plasma membrane lectin-binding components. *Science* 1974;184:1294–1296.
41. Kinsey WH, Koehler JK. Fine structural localizations of Concanavalin A binding sites on hamster spermatozoa. *J Supramol Struct* 1976;5:185–189.
42. Friend DS, Fawcett DW. Membrane differentiations in freeze-fractured mammalian sperm. *J Cell Biol* 1974;63:641–664.
43. Friend DS. Freeze-fracture alterations in guinea-pig sperm membrane preceding gamete fusion. In: Gilula NB, ed. *Membrane–membrane interactions.* New York: Raven Press; 1980:153–165.
44. Bearer EL, Friend DS. Modifications of anionic lipid domains preceding membrane fusion in guinea pig sperm. *J Cell Biol* 1982;92:604–615.
45. Suzuki F, Nagano T. Epididymal maturation of rat spermatozoa studied by thin sectioning and freeze-fracture. *Biol Reprod* 1980;22:1219–1231.
46. Suzuki F. Changes in intramembranous particle distribution in

epididymal spermatozoa of the boar. *Anat Rec* 1981;199: 361–376.
47. Toshimori K, Higashi R, Ōura C. Distribution of intramembranous particles and filipin–sterol complexes in mouse sperm membranes: Polyene antibiotic filipin treatment. *Am J Anat* 1985;174:455–470.
48. Koehler JK. A freeze-etch study of rabbit spermatozoa with particular reference to head structures. *J Ultrastruct Res* 1970;33: 598–614.
49. Schulte-Wrede S, Wetzstein R. Raster-Elektronenmikroskopie von Spermien des Hausschaufs (*Ovis ammon aries,* L). *Z Zellforsch* 1972;134:105–127.
50. Eddy EM, Koehler JK. Restricted domains of the sperm surface. In: Johari O, ed. *Scanning electron microscopy, vol 3.* Chicago: SEM Inc, 1982:1313–1323.
51. Koehler JK. Fine structure observations in frozen-etched bovine spermatozoa. *J Ultrastruct Res* 1966;16:359–375.
52. Phillips DM. Surface of the equatorial segment of mammalian acrosome. *Biol Reprod* 1977;16:128–137.
53. Koehler JK. Studies on the structure of the postnuclear sheath of water buffalo spermatozoa. *J Ultrastruct Res* 1973;44:355–368.
54. Fléchon JE. Freeze-fracturing of rabbit spermatozoa. *J Submicrosc Cytol* 1974;19:59–64.
55. Bradley MP, Ryans DG, Forrester IT. Effects of filipin, digitonin, and polymyxin B on plasma membrane of ram spermatozoa—an EM study. *Arch Androl* 1980;4:195–204.
56. Koehler JK. Human sperm head ultrastructure: A freeze-etching study. *J Ultrastruct Res* 1972;39:520–539.
57. Woolley DM. A posterior ring in the spermatozoa of species of muridae. *J Reprod Fertil* 1970;23:361–363.
58. Koehler JK. Structural heterogeneity of the mammalian sperm flagellar membrane. *J Submicrosc Cytol* 1983;15:247–253.
59. Gresson RAR, Zlotnik I. A comparative study of the cytoplasmic components of the male germ-cells of certain mammals. *Proc R Soc Edinb [Biol]* 1945;62:137–170.
60. Hancock JL, Trevan DJ. The acrosome and post-nuclear cap of bull spermatozoa. *J Roy Microsc Soc* 1957;76:77–83.
61. Pikó L. Gamete structure and sperm entry in mammals. In: Metz CB, Monroy A, eds. *Fertilization, vol 2.* New York: Academic Press; 1969:325–403.
62. Friend DS, Rudolf I. Acrosomal disruption in sperm. Freeze-fracture of altered membranes. *J Cell Biol* 1974;63:466–479.
63. Koehler JK, Gaddum-Rosse P. Media induced alterations of the membrane associated particles of the guinea pig sperm tail. *J Ultrastruct Res* 1975;51:106–118.
64. Gilula NB, Satir P. The ciliary necklace: A ciliary membrane specialization. *J Cell Biol* 1972;53:494–509.
65. Olson GE, Lifsics M, Hamilton DW, Fawcett DW. Structural specializations in the flagellar plasma membrane of opossum spermatozoa. *J Ultrastruct Res* 1977;59:207–221.
66. Friend DS, Elias PM, Rudolf I. Disassembly of the guinea-pig sperm tail. In: Fawcett DW, Bedford JM, eds. *The spermatozoon.* Baltimore: Urban & Schwarzenberg; 1979:157–168.
67. Friend DS, Heuser JE. Orderly particle arrays on the mitochondrial outer membrane in rapidly-frozen sperm. *Anat Rec* 1981;159:198–199.
68. Elias PM, Friend DS, Goerke J. Membrane sterol heterogeneity. Freeze-fracture detection with saponins and filipin. *J Histochem Cytochem* 1979;27:1247–1260.
69. Enders GC, Werb Z, Friend DS. Lectin binding to guinea-pig sperm zipper particles. *J Cell Sci* 1983;60:303–329.
70. Friend DS. Membrane organization and differentiation in the guinea-pig spermatozoon. In: Van Blerkom J, Motta PM, eds. *Ultrastructure of reproduction.* The Hague: Martinus Nijhoff; 1984:75–85.
71. Lopez ML, de Souza W. Distribution of filipin–sterol complexes in the plasma membrane of stallion spermatozoa during the epididymal maturation process. *Mol Reprod Dev* 1991;28:158–168.
72. Bearer EL, Friend DS. Anionic lipid domains: Correlation and functional topography in a mammalian cell membrane. *Proc Natl Acad Sci USA* 1980;77:6601–6605.
73. Friend DS, Bearer EL. β-Hydroxysterol distribution as determined by freeze-fracture cytochemistry. *Histochem J* 1981; 13:535–546.
74. Wolf DE, Voglmayr JK. Diffusion and regionalization in membranes of maturing ram spermatozoa. *J Cell Biol* 1984;98: 1678–1684.
75. Sternberger LA. *Immunocytochemistry.* New York: John Wiley & Sons; 1979.
76. Koo GC, Stackpole CW, Boyse EA, Hammerling U, Lardis MP. Topographical location of H-Y antigen on mouse spermatozoa by immunoelectronmicroscopy. *Proc Natl Acad Sci USA* 1973; 70:1502–1505.
77. Fellous M, Gachelin G, Buc-Caron M-H, Dubois P, Jacob F. Similar location of an early embryonic antigen on mouse and human spermatozoa. *Dev Biol* 1974;41:331–337.
78. Lopez LC, Bayna EM, Litoff D, Shaper NL, Shaper JH, Shur BD. Receptor function of mouse sperm surface galactosyltransferase during fertilization. *J Cell Biol* 1985;101:1501–1510.
79. O'Rand MG, Romrell LJ. Appearance of regional surface autoantigens during spermatogenesis: Comparison of anti-testis and anti-sperm antisera. *Dev Biol* 1980;75:431–441.
80. Koehler JK. Studies on the distribution of antigenic sites on the surface of rabbit spermatozoa. *J Cell Biol* 1974;67:647–659.
81. Millette CF, Bellvé AR. Temporal expression of membrane antigens during mouse spermatogenesis. *J Cell Biol* 1977;74:86–97.
82. Koehler JK, Perkins WD. Fine structure observations on the distribution of antigenic sites on guinea pig spermatozoa. *J Cell Biol* 1974;60:789–795.
83. Tung KSK, Han L-BP, Evan AP. Differentiation autoantigen of testicular cells and spermatozoa in the guinea pig. *Dev Biol* 1979;68:224–238.
84. Tung PS, Fritz IB. Specific surface antigens on rat pachytene spermatocytes and successive classes of germinal cells. *Dev Biol* 1978;64:297–315.
85. Koo GC, Boyse EA, Wachtel SS. Immunogenetic techniques and approaches in the study of sperm and testicular cell surface antigens. In: Edidin M, Johnson MH, eds. *Immunobiology of gametes,* Cambridge: Cambridge University Press; 1973:73–80.
86. O'Rand MJ. The presence of sperm-specific isoantigens on the egg following fertilization. *J Exp Zool* 1977;202:267–273.
87. Herr JC, Eddy EM. Identification of mouse sperm surface antigens by a surface labeling and immunoprecipitation approach. *Biol Reprod* 1980;22:1263–1274.
88. Villarroya S, Scholler R. Regional heterogeneity of human spermatozoa detected with monoclonal antibodies. *J Reprod Fertil* 1986;76:435–447.
89. Primakoff P, Cowan A, Hyatt H, Tredick-Kline J, Myles DG. Purification of the guinea pig sperm PH-20 antigen and detection of a site-specific endoproteolytic activity in sperm preparations that cleves PH-20 into two disulfide-linked fragments. *Biol Reprod* 1988;38:921–934.
90. Blobel CP, Myles DG, Primakoff P, White JM. Proteolytic processing of a protein involved in sperm-egg fusion correlates with acquisition of fertilization competence. *J Cell Biol* 1990;111: 69–78.
91. Gaunt SJ, Brown CR, Jones R. Identification of mobile and fixed antigens on the plasma membrane of rat spermatozoa using monoclonal antibodies. *Exp Cell Res* 1983;144:275–284.
92. Jones R, Brown CR, von Glós KI, Gaunt SJ. Development of a maturation antigen on the plasma membrane of rat spermatozoa in the epididymis and its fate during fertilization. *Exp Cell Res* 1985;156:31–44.
93. Moore HDM, Hartman TD. Localization by monoclonal antibodies of various surface antigens of hamster spermatozoa and the effect of antibody on fertilization in vitro. *J Reprod Fertil* 1984;70:175–183.
94. Feuchter FA, Vernon RB, Eddy EM. Analysis of the sperm surface with monoclonal antibodies: Topographically restricted antigens appearing in the epididymis. *Biol Reprod* 1981;24: 1099–1110.
95. Okabe M, Katsuaki T, Adachi T, Kohama T, Mimura T. Inconsistent reactivity of an anti-sperm monoclonal antibody and its relationship to sperm capacitation. *J Reprod Immunol* 1986;9:67–70.
96. Myles DG, Primakoff P, Bellvé AR. Surface domains of the guinea pig sperm defined with monoclonal antibodies. *Cell* 1981;23:433–439.

97. Myles DG, Primakoff P. Sperm surface domains. In: Springer TA, ed. *Hybridoma technology in the biosciences and medicine.* New York: Plenum Press; 1985:239–250.
98. Yan CY, Wang LF, Sato E, Koide SS. Monoclonal antibody inducing human sperm agglutination. *Am J Reprod Immunol* 1983;4:111–115.
99. Herr JC, Fowler JE, Howards SS, Sigman M, Sutherland WM, Koons DJ. Human antisperm monoclonal antibodies constructed postvasectomy. *Biol Reprod* 1985;32:695–712.
100. Glassy MC, Surh CD, Sarkar S. Murine monoclonal antibodies that identify antigenically distinct subpopulations of human sperm. *Hybridoma* 1984;3:363–371.
101. Vernon RB, Muller CH, Eddy EM. Further characterization of a secreted epididymal glycoprotein in mice that binds to sperm tails. *J Androl* 1987;8:123–128.
102. Toshimori K, Araki S, Tanii I, Ōura C. Masking the cryptodeterminant on the 54-kilodalton mouse sperm surface antigen. *Biol Reprod* 1992;47:1161–1167.
103. Schmell ED, Gulyas BJ, Yuan LC, August JT. Identification of mammalian sperm surface antigens: II. Characterization of an acrosomal cap protein and a tail protein using monoclonal anti-mouse sperm antibodies. *J Reprod Immunol* 1982;4:91–106.
104. Saling PM. Mouse sperm antigens that participate in fertilization. IV. A monoclonal antibody prevents zona penetration by inhibition of the acrosome reaction. *Dev Biol* 1986;117:511–519.
105. Isahakia M, Alexander NJ. Interspecies cross-reactivity of monoclonal antibodies directed against human sperm antigens. *Biol Reprod* 1984;30:1015–1026.
106. Hinrichsen-Kohane AC, Hinrichsen MJ, Schill W-B. Analysis of antigen expression on human spermatozoa by means of monoclonal antibodies. *Fertil Steril* 1985;43:279–285.
107. Crichton DN, Cohen BB. Analysis of the murine sperm surface with monoclonal antibodies. *J Reprod Fertil* 1983;68:497–505.
108. Gaunt SJ. A 28K-dalton cell surface autoantigen of spermatogenesis: Characterization using a monoclonal antibody. *Dev Biol* 1982;89:92–100.
109. Lee GC-Y, Wong E, Teh C-Z. Analysis of mouse sperm isoantigens using specific monoclonal antibodies. *Am J Reprod Immunol* 1984;6:37–43.
110. Saling PM, Lakoski KA. Mouse sperm antigens that participate in fertilization. II. Inhibition of sperm penetration through the zona pellucida using monoclonal antibodies. *Biol Reprod* 1985; 33:527–536.
111. Naz RN, Saxe JM, Menge AC. Inhibition of fertility in rabbits by monoclonal antibodies against sperm. *Biol Reprod* 1983;28: 249–254.
112. Saling PM, Irons G, Waibel R. Mouse sperm antigens that participate in fertilization. I. Inhibition of sperm fusion with the egg plasma membrane using monoclonal antibodies. *Biol Reprod* 1985;33:515–526.
113. Ellis DH, Hartman TD, Moore HDM. Maturation and function of the hamster spermatozoon probed with monoclonal antibodies. *J Reprod Immunol* 1985;7:299–314.
114. Wolf DP, Sokoloski JE, Dandekar P, Bechtol KB. Characterization of human sperm surface antigens with monoclonal antibodies. *Biol Reprod* 1983;29:713–723.
115. Naz RK, Alexander NJ, Isahakia M, Hamilton MS. Monoclonal antibody to a human germ cell membrane glycoprotein that inhibits fertilization. *Science* 1984;225:342–344.
116. Bechtol KB, Brown SC, Kennett RH. Recognition of differentiation antigens of spermatogenesis in the mouse by using antibodies from spleen cell-myeloma hybrids after syngeneic immunization. *Proc Natl Acad Sci USA* 1979;76:363–367.
117. Bechtol KB. Characterization of a cell-surface differentiation antigen of mouse spermatogenesis: Timing and localization of expression by immunohistochemistry using a monoclonal antibody. *J Embryol Exp Morphol* 1984;81:93–104.
118. Lakoski K, Williams C, Saling P. Proteins of the acrosome region in mouse sperm: Immunological probes reveal post-testicular modifications. *Gamete Res* 1989;23:21–37.
119. Topfer-Petersen E, Friess AE, Stoffel M, Schill WB. Boar sperm membranes antigens. I. Topography of a mobile glycoprotein of the sperm cell membrane. *Histochemistry* 1990;93:485–490.
120. Jones R, Shalgi R, Hoyland J, Phillips DM. Topographical rearrangement of a plasma membrane antigen during capacitation of rat spermatozoa in vitro. *Dev Biol* 1990;139:349–362.
121. Myles DG, Primakoff P. Localized surface antigens of guinea pig sperm migrate to new regions prior to fertilization. *J Cell Biol* 1984;99:1634–1641.
122. Nehme CL, Cesario MM, Myles DG, Koppel DE, Bartles JR. Breaching the diffusion barrier that compartmentalizes the transmembrane glycoprotein CE9 to the posterior-tail plasma membrane domain of the rat spermatozoon. *J Cell Biol* 1993; 120:687–694.
123. Toshimori K, Araki S, Ōura C. Immunohistochemical localization of 54,000 dalton sialoglycoprotein in the mouse epididymal duct. *Arch Histol Cytol* 1987;53:333–338.
124. Toshimori K, Tanii I, Araki S, Ōura C. A rat sperm flagellar surface antigen that originates in the testis and is expressed on the flagellar surface during epididymal transit. *Mol Reprod Dev* 1992;32:399–408.
125. Anderson DJ, Michaelson JS, Johnson PM. Trophoblast/leukocyte-common antigen is expressed by human testicular germ cells and appears on the surface of acrosome-reacted sperm. *Biol Reprod* 1989;41:285–293.
126. Lee GC-Y, Wong E, Richter DE, Menge AC. Monoclonal antibodies to human sperm antigens-II. *J Reprod Immunol* 1984;6:227–238.
127. Saxena NK, Russell LD, Saxena N, Peterson RN. Immunofluorescence antigen localization on boar sperm plasma membranes: Monoclonal antibodies reveal apparent new domains and apparent redistribution of surface antigens during sperm maturation and at ejaculation. *Anat Rec* 1986;214:238–252.
128. Jones RC. Studies of the structure of the head of boar spermatozoa from the epididymis. *J Reprod Fertil [Suppl]* 1971;13:51–64.
129. Fawcett DW, Hollenberg RD. Changes in the acrosomes of guinea pig spermatozoa during passage through the epididymis. *J Reprod Fertil Suppl* 1963;6:276–292.
130. Cowan AE, Myles DG. Biogenesis of surface domains during spermiogenesis in the guinea pig. *Dev Biol* 1993;155:124–133.
131. Eddy EM, Vernon RB, Muller CH, Hahnel AC, Fenderson BA. Immunodissection of sperm surface modifications during epididymal maturation. *Am J Anat* 1985;174:225–237.
132. Phelps BM, Koppel DE, Primakoff P, Myles DG. Evidence that proteolysis of the surface is an initial step in the mechanism of formation of sperm cell surface domains. *J Cell Biol* 1990;111:1839–1847.
133. Phelps BM, Myles DG. The guinea pig sperm plasma membrane protein, PH-20, reaches the surface via two transport pathways and becomes localized to a domain after an initial uniform distribution. *Dev Biol* 1987;123:63–72.
134. Petruszak JAM, Nehme CL, Bartles JR. Endoproteolytic cleavage in the extracellular domain of the integral plasma membrane protein CE9 precedes its redistribution from the posterior to the anterior tail of the rat spermatozoon during epididymal maturation. *J Cell Biol* 1991;114:917–927.
135. Burridge K, Feramisco JR. α-Actinin and vinculin from nonmuscle cells: Calcium-sensitive interactions with actin. In: *Cold Spring Harbor symposia on quantitative biology, vol XLVI, Part 2.* New York: Cold Spring Harbor Laboratories; 1982:587–597.
136. Marchesi VT. Stabilizing infrastructure of cell membranes. *Annu Rev Cell Biol* 1985;1:531–561.
137. Welch JE, O'Rand MG. Identification and distribution of actin in spermatogenic cells and spermatozoa of the rabbit. *Dev Biol* 1985;109:411–417.
138. Vogl AW, Grove BD, Lew GJ. Distribution of actin in Sertoli cell ectoplasmic specializations and associated spermatids in the ground squirrel testis. *Anat Rec* 1986;215:331–341.
139. Masri BA, Russell LD, Vogl AW. Distribution of actin in spermatids and adjacent Sertoli cell regions of the rat. *Anat Rec* 1987;218:20–26.
140. Russell LD, Weber JE, Vogl AW. Characterization of filaments within the subacrosomal space of rat spermatids during spermiogenesis. *Tissue Cell* 1986;18:887–898.
141. Scully NF, Shaper JH, Shur BD. Spatial and temporal expression of cell surface galactosyltransferase during mouse spermatogenesis and epididymal maturation. *Dev Biol* 1987;124:111–124.
142. Halenda RM, Primakoff P, Myles DG. Actin filaments, localized

to the region of the developing acrosome during early stages, are lost during later states of guinea pig spermiogenesis. *Biol Reprod* 1987;36:491–499.
143. Fouquet J-P, Kann M-L. Species-specific localization of actin in mammalian spermatozoa: Fact or artifact? *Microsc Res Tech* 1992;20:251–258.
144. Camatini M, Anelli G, Casale A. Identification of actin in boar spermatids and spermatozoa by immunoelectron microscopy. *Eur J Cell Biol* 1986;42:311–318.
145. Campanella C, Gabbiani G, Baccetti B, Burrini AG, Pallini V. Actin and myosin in the vertebrate acrosomal region. *J Submicrosc Cytol* 1979;11:53–71.
146. Clarke GN, Yanagimachi R. Actin in mammalian sperm heads. *J Exp Zool* 1978;205:125–132.
147. Greenberg BJ, Tamblyn TM. Actin from mature bovine spermatozoa. *J Cell Biol* 1981;91:191a.
148. Flaherty SP, Winfrey VP, Olson GE. Localization of actin in mammalian spermatozoa: A comparison of eight species. *Anat Rec* 1986;216:504–515.
149. Peterson RN, Russell LD, Bundman D, Freund M. Presence of microfilaments and tubular structure in chemically induced acrosome reactions of boar spermatozoa. *Biol Reprod* 1978;19: 459–465.
150. Tamblyn TM. Identification of actin in boar epididymal spermatozoa. *Biol Reprod* 1980;22:727–734.
151. Camatini M, Colombo A, Bonfanti P. Identification of spectrin and calmodulin in rabbit spermiogenesis and spermatozoa. *Mol Reprod Dev* 1991;28:62–69.
152. Flaherty SP, Winfrey VP, Olson GE. Localization of actin in human, bull, rabbit, and hamster sperm by immunoelectron microscopy. *Anat Rec* 1988;221:599–610.
153. Clarke GN, Clarke FM, Wilson S. Actin in human spermatozoa. *Biol Reprod* 1982;26:319–327.
154. Talbot P, Kleve MG. Hamster sperm cross-react with antiactin. *J Exp Zool* 1978;204:131–136.
155. Olson GE, Winfrey VP. Substructure of a cytoskeletal complex associated with the hamster sperm acrosome. *J Ultrastruct Res* 1985;92:167–179.
156. Virtanen I, Bradley RA, Paasivuo R, Lehto V-P. Distinct cytoskeletal domains revealed in sperm cells. *J Cell Biol* 1984;99: 1083–1091.
157. Koehler JK. Observations on the fine structure of vole spermatozoa with particular reference to cytoskeletal elements in the mature sperm head. *Gamete Res* 1978;1:247–257.
158. Goodman SR, Schiffer K. The spectrin membrane skeleton of normal and abnormal human erythrocytes: A review. *Am J Physiol* 1983;244:C121–C141.
159. Lazarides E, Moon RT. Assembly and topogenesis of the spectrin-based membrane skeleton in erythroid development. *Cell* 1984;37:354–356.
160. Damjanov I, Damjanov A, Lehto V-P, Virtanen I. Spectrin in mouse gametogenesis and embryogenesis. *Dev Biol* 1986;114: 132–140.
161. De Cesaris P, Filippini A, Ziparo E, Russo MA, Stefanini M. Distribution of analogues of spectrin, fodrin and protein 4.1 in rat spermatogenic cells. *Prog Clin Biol Res* 1989;296:149–152.
162. Repasky EA, Granger BL, Lazarides E. Wide-spread occurrence of avian spectrin in nonerythroid cells. *Cell* 1982;29:821–833.
163. McIntosh JR, Porter KR. Microtubules in the spermatids of the domestic fowl. *J Cell Biol* 1967;35:153–173.
164. Fawcett DW, Anderson WA, Phillips DM. Morphogenetic factors influencing the shape of the sperm head. *Dev Biol* 1971;26:220–251.
165. Cole A, Meistrich ML, Cherry LM, Trostle-Weige PK. Nuclear and manchette development of spermatids of normal and *azh/azh* mutant mice. *Biol Reprod* 1988;38:385–401.
166. Meistrich ML, Trostle-Weige PK, Russell LD. Abnormal manchette development in spermatids of *azh/azh* mutant mice. *Am J Anat* 1990;188:74–86.
167. MacGregor GR, Russell LD, Van Beek MEAB, et al. Symplastic spermatids (sys): A recessive insertional mutation in mice causing a defect in spermatogenesis. *Proc Natl Acad Sci USA* 1990;87:5016–5020.
168. Russell LD, Russell JA, MacGregor GR, Meistrich ML. Linkage of manchette microtubules to the nuclear envelope and observations of the role of the manchette in nuclear shaping during spermiogenesis in rodents. *Am J Anat* 1991;192:97–120.
169. Blom E, Birch-Anderson A. The ultrastructure of decapitated sperm defect in Guernsey bulls. *J Reprod Fertil* 1970;23:67–72.
170. Fawcett DW, Ito S. The fine structure of bat spermatozoa. *Am J Anat* 1965;116:567–610.
171. Russell LD. Sertoli-germ cell interactions: A review. *Gamete Res* 1980;3:179–202.
172. Russell LD. Spermiation—the sperm release process: Ultrastructural observations and unresolved problems. In: Van Vlerkom J, Motta PM, eds. *Ultrastructure of reproduction.* The Hague: Martinus Nijhoff; 1984:46–66.
173. Ross MH, Dobler J. The Sertoli cell junctional specializations and their relationship to the germinal epithelium as observed after efferent ductule ligation. *Anat Rec* 1975;183:267–292.
174. Russell LD, Clermont Y. Anchoring device between Sertoli cells and late spermatids in rat seminiferous tubules. *Anat Rec* 1984;185:259–278.
175. Russell LD. Spermatid–Sertoli tubulobulbar complexes as devices for elimination of cytoplasm from the head region of late spermatids of the rat. *Anat Rec* 1979;194:233–246.
176. Burgos MH, Blaquier J, Cameo MS, Gutierrez L. Morphological maturation of spermatozoa in the epididymis. In: Vilardo JT, Kasprow BA, eds. *Biology of reproduction. Symposium III, Pan American Congress of Anatomy.* New Orleans: Pan American Association of Anatomy; 1972:367–371.
177. Fawcett DW, Eddy EM, Phillips DM. Observations on the fine structure and relationships of the chromatoid body in mammalian spermatogenesis. *Biol Reprod* 1970;2:129–153.
178. Myles DG, Primakoff P, Koppel DE. A localized surface protein of guinea pig sperm exhibits free diffusion in its domain. *J Cell Biol* 1984;98:1905–1909.
179. Fawcett DW. The anatomy of the mammalian spermatozoon with particular reference to the guinea pig. *Z Zellforsch* 1965;67:279–296.
180. Edidin M. Molecular motions and membrane organization and function. In: Finian JB, Michell RH, eds. *Comprehensive biochemistry.* Amsterdam: Elsevier/North Holland Biomedical Press; 1981:37–82.
181. Wolf DE, Hagopian SS, Lewis RG, Voglmayr JK, Fairbanks G. Lateral regionalization and diffusion of a maturation dependent antigen in the ram sperm plasma membrane. *J Cell Biol* 1986;102:1826–1831.
182. Wolf DE, Scott BK, Millette CF. The development of regionalized lipid diffusibility in the germ cell plasma membrane during spermatogenesis in the mouse. *J Cell Biol* 1986;103:1745–1750.
183. Wolf DE, Lipscomb AC, Maynard VM. Causes of nondiffusing lipid in the plasma membrane of mammalian spermatozoa. *Biochemistry* 1988;27:860–865.
184. Wolf DE, Maynard VM, McKinnon CA, Melchior DL. Lipid domains in the ram sperm plasma membrane demonstrated by differential scanning calorimetry. *Proc Natl Acad Sci USA* 1990;87:6893–6896.
185. Phelps BM, Primakoff P, Koppel DE, Low MG, Myles DG. Restricted lateral diffusion of PH-20, a PI-anchored sperm membrane protein. *Science* 1988;240:1780–1782.
186. Cowan AE, Myles DG, Koppel DE. Migration of the guinea pig sperm membrane protein PH-20 from one localized surface domain to another does not occur by a simple diffusion-trapping mechanism. *Dev Biol* 1991;144:189–198.
187. Cowen AE, Primakoff P, Myles DG. Sperm exocytosis increases the amount of PH-20 antigen on the surface of guinea pig sperm. *J Cell Biol* 1986;103:1289–1297.
188. Parks JE, Hammerstedt RH. Developmental changes occurring in the lipids of ram epididymal spermatozoa plasma membrane. *Biol Reprod* 1985;32:653–668.
189. Agrawal P, Magargee SF, Hammerstedt H. Isolation and characterization of the plasma membrane of rat cauda epididymal spermatozoa. *J Androl* 1988;9:178–189.
190. Evans RW, Weaver DE, Clegg ED. Diacyl, alkenyl and alkyl ether phospholipids in ejaculated, in utero-, and in vitro-incubated porcine spermatozoa. *J Lipid Res* 1980;21:223–228.
191. Nikolopoulou M, Soucek DA, Vary JC. Changes in the lipid con-

tent of boar sperm plasma membranes during epididymal maturation. *Biochim Biophys Acta* 1985;815:486–498.
192. Langlais J, Zollinger M, Plante L, Chapdelaine A, Bleau G, Roberts KD. Localization of cholesteryl sulfate in human spermatozoa in support of a hypothesis for the mechanism of capacitation. *Proc Natl Acad Sci USA* 1981;78:7266–7270.
193. Parks JE, Arion JW, Foote RH. Lipids of plasma membrane and outer acrosomal membrane from bovine spermatozoa. *Biol Reprod* 1987;37:1249–1258.
194. Nikolopoulou M, Soucek DA, Vary JC. Lipid composition of the membrane released after an in vitro acrosome reaction of epididymal boar sperm. *Lipids* 1986;21:566–570.
195. Nikolopoulou M, Soucek DA, Vary JC. Modulation of the lipid composition of boar sperm plasma membranes during an acrosome reaction in vitro. *Arch Biochem Biophys* 1986;250:30–37.
196. Mack SR, Zaneveld LJ, Peterson RN, Hunt W, Russell LD. Characterization of human sperm plasma membrane: Glycolipids and polypeptides. *J Exp Zool* 1987;243:339–346.
197. Murry RK, Narasimhan R, Levine M, Shirley M, Lingwood CA, Schachter H. Galactoglycerolipids of mammalian testis, spermatozoa and nervous tissues. In: Sweeley C, ed. *ACS Symposium Series no. 128, Cell surface glycolipids.* Washington: American Chemical Society Press; 1980:105–125.
198. Ishizuka I, Yamakawa T. Glycoglycerolipids. In: Wiegandt H, ed. *Glycolipids.* New York: Elsevier; 1985:101–197.
199. Eddy EM, Muller CH, Lingwood CA. Preparation of monoclonal antibody to sulfatoxygalactosylglycerolipid by in vitro immunization with a glycolipid-glass conjugate. *J Immunol Methods* 1985;81:137–146.
200. Robaire B, Hermo L. Efferent ducts, epididymis, and vas deferens: Structure, functions, and their regulation. In: Knobil E, Neill JD, ed. *The Physiology of Reproduction.* New York: Raven Press, 1988:999–1080.
201. Eddy EM, O'Brien DA. Biology of the gamete: Maturation, transport and fertilization. In: Working PK, ed. *Toxicology of the male and female reproductive systems.* New York: Hemisphere; 1989:31–100.
202. Eddy EM, McGee RS, Willis WD, O'Brien DA. Immunodissection of sperm surface modifications during epididymal maturation. *Bull Assoc Anat* 1991;75:139–144.
203. Mann T, Lutwak-Mann C. *Male reproductive function and semen.* New York: Springer-Verlag; 1981.
204. Acott TS, Katz DF, Hoskins DD. Movement characteristics of bovine epididymal spermatozoa: Effects of forward motility protein and epididymal maturation. *Biol Reprod* 1983;29:389–399.
205. Cooper TG, Waites GMH, Nieschlag E. The epididymis and male fertility. A symposium report. *Int J Androl* 1986;9:81–90.
206. Saling PM. Development of the ability to bind zonae pellucidae during epididymal maturation: Reversible immobilization of mouse spermatozoa by lanthanum. *Biol Reprod* 1982;26:429–436.
207. Orgebin-Crist M-C, Fournier-Delpech S. Sperm–egg interaction. Evidence for maturational changes during epididymal transit. *J Androl* 1982;3:429–433.
208. Moore HDM. The net negative surface charge of mammalian spermatozoa as determined by isoelectric focusing. Changes following sperm maturation, ejaculation, incubation in the female tract, and after enzyme treatment. *Int J Androl* 1979;2:244–262.
209. Bedford JM, Calvin HI, Cooper GW. The maturation of spermatozoa in the human epididymis. *J Reprod Fertil [Suppl]* 1973;18:199–213.
210. Nicolson GL, Usui N, Yanagimachi R, Yanagimachi H, Smith JR. Lectin-binding sites on the plasma membranes of rabbit spermatozoa. Changes in surface receptors during epididymal maturation and after ejaculation. *J Cell Biol* 1977;74:950–962.
211. Holt WV. Surface-bound sialic acid on ram and bull spermatozoa: Deposition during epididymal transit and stability during washing. *Biol Reprod* 1980;23:847–857.
212. Fléchon JE. Ultrastructural and cytochemical modifications of rabbit spermatozoa during epididymal transport. In: Hafez ESE, Thibault CG, eds. *The Biology of spermatozoa. Transport, survival and fertilizing ability.* Basel: S Karger; 1975:36–45.
213. Bedford JM, Millar RP. The character of sperm maturation in the epididymis of the ascrotal hyrax, *Procavia capensis* and armadillo, *Dasypus novemcinctus. Biol Reprod* 1978;19:396–406.
214. Hammerstedt RH, Hay SR, Amann RP. Modification of ram sperm membranes during epididymal transit. *Biol Reprod* 1982;27:745–754.
215. Fournier-Delpech S, Courot M. Glycoproteins of ram sperm plasma membrane. Relationship of protein having affinity for Con A to epididymal maturation. *Biochem Biophys Res Commun* 1980;96:756–761.
216. Lewin LW, Weissenberg R, Sobel JS, Marcus Z, Nebel L. Differences in Con-A-FITC binding to rat spermatozoa during epididymal maturation and capacitation. *Arch Androl* 1979;2:279–281.
217. Fournier-Delpech S, Danzo BJ, Orgebin-Crist M-C. Extraction of concanavalin A affinity material from rat testicular and epididymal spermatozoa. *Ann Biol Anim Biochem Biophys* 1977;17:207–213.
218. Seki N, Toyama Y, Nagano T. Changes in the distribution of filipin–sterol complexes in the boar sperm head plasma membrane during epididymal maturation and in the uterus. *Anat Rec* 1992;232:221–230.
219. Phillips DM. Cell surface structure of rodent sperm heads. *J Exp Zool* 1975;191:1–8.
220. Toyama Y, Nagano T. Maturation changes of the plasma membrane of rat spermatozoa observed by surface replica, rapid-freeze and deep-etch, and freeze-fracture methods. *Anat Rec* 1988;220:43–50.
221. Dawson RMC, Scott TW. Phospholipid composition of epididymal spermatozoa prepared by density gradient centrifugation. *Nature* 1964;202:292–293.
222. Quinn PJ, White IG. Phospholipid and cholesterol content of epididymal and ejaculated ram spermatozoa and seminal plasma in relation to cold shock. *Aust J Biol Sci* 1967;20:1205–1215.
223. Grogan DE, Mayer DT, Sikes JD. Quantitative differences in phospholipids of ejaculated spermatozoa and spermatozoa from three different levels of the epididymis of the boar. *J Reprod Fertil* 1966;12:431–436.
224. Poulos A, Voglmayr JK, White IG. Phospholipid changes in spermatozoa during passage through the genital tract of the bull. *Biochim Biophys Acta* 1973;306:194–202.
225. Poulos A, Brown-Woodman PDC, White IG, Cox RI. Changes in phospholipids of ram spermatozoa during migration through the epididymis and possible origin of prostaglandins F_2 in testicular and epididymal fluid. *Biochim Biophys Acta* 1975;388:12–21.
226. Terner C, MacLaughlin J, Smith BR. Changes in lipase and phospholipase activities of rat spermatozoa in transit from the caput to the cauda epididymis. *J Reprod Fertil* 1975;45:1–8.
227. Evans RW, Setchell BP. Lipid changes in boar spermatozoa during epididymal maturation with some observations on the flow and composition of boar rete testis fluid. *J Reprod Fertil* 1979;57:189–196.
228. Aveldano MI, Rotstein NP, Vermouth N. Lipid remodelling during epididymal maturation of rat spermatozoa. *Biochem J* 1992;283:235–241.
229. Scott TW, Voglmayr JK, Stechell BP. Lipid composition and metabolism in testicular and ejaculated ram spermatozoa. *Biochem J* 1967;102:456–461.
230. Bleau G, VandenHeuvel WJA. Desmosteryl sulfate and desmosterol in hamster epididymis. *Steroids* 1974;24:549–556.
231. Legault Y, Bouthillier M, Bleau G, Chapdelaine A, Roberts KD. The sterol and sterol sulfate content of the male hamster reproductive tract. *Biol Reprod* 1979;20:1213–1219.
232. Lalumiere G, Bleau G, Chapdelaine A, Roberts KD. Cholesterol sulfate and sterol sulphatase in the human reproductive tract. *Steroids* 1976;27:247–260.
233. Hammerstedt RH, Keith AD, Hay S, Deluca N, Amann RP. Changes in ram sperm membranes during epididymal transit. *Arch Biochem Biophys* 1979;196:7–12.
234. Voglmayr JK, Scott TW, Setchell BP, Waites GMH. Metabolism of testicular spermatozoa and characteristics of testicular fluid collected from conscious rams. *J Reprod Fertil* 1967;14:87–99.
235. Vijayasarathy S, Balaram P. Regional differentiation in bull sperm plasma membranes. *Biochem Biophys Res Commun* 1982;108:760–764.
236. Orgebin-Crist M-C, Danzo BJ, Davies J. Endocrine control of the

development and maintenance of sperm fertilizing ability in the epididymis. In: Greep RO, ed. *Handbook of physiology, vol 5, Endocrinology, Sect 7, Male reproductive system.* Washington: American Physiological Society; 1975:319–338.
237. Hamilton DW. Structure and function of the epithelium lining the ductuli efferentes, ductus epididymis, and ductus deferens in the rat. In: Greep RO, ed. *Handbook of physiology, vol 5, Endocrinology, Sect 7, Male reproductive system.* Washington: American Physiological Society; 1975:259–301.
238. Bedford JM. Maturation, transport and fate of spermatozoa in the epididymis. In: Greep RO, ed. *Handbook of physiology, vol 5, Endocrinology, Sect 7, Male reproductive system.* Washington: American Physiological Society; 1975:303–317.
239. Yanagimachi R. Mechanisms of fertilization in mammals. In: Mastroianni L, Biggers JD, eds. *Fertilization and embryonic development in vitro.* New York: Plenum Press; 1981:81–182.
240. Austin CR. Sperm maturation in the male and female genital tracts. In: Metz CB, Monroy A, eds. *Biology of fertilization, vol 2, Biology of the sperm.* Orlando: Academic Press; 1985:121–155.
241. Olson GE, Hamilton DW. Characterization of the surface glycoproteins of rat spermatozoa. *Biol Reprod* 1978;19:26–35.
242. Olson GE, Danzo BJ. Surface changes in rat spermatozoa during epididymal transit. *Biol Reprod* 1981;24:431–443.
243. Toowicharanount P, Chulavatnatol M. Characterization of sialoglycoproteins of rat epididymal fluid and spermatozoa by periodate-tritiated borohydride. *J Reprod Fertil* 1983;67: 133–141.
244. Brown CR, von Glós KI, Jones R. Changes in plasma membrane glycoproteins of rat spermatozoa during maturation in the epididymis. *J Cell Biol* 1983;96:256–264.
245. Jones R, Phorpramool C, Setchell BP, Brown CR. Labelling of membrane glycoproteins on rat spermatozoa collected from different regions of the epididymis. *Biochem J* 1981;200:457–460.
246. Jones R, von Glós KI, Brown CR. Characterization of hormonally regulated secretory proteins from the caput epididymidis of the rabbit. *Biochem J* 1981;196:105–114.
247. Zaheb R, Orr GA. Characterization of a maturation-associated glycoprotein on the plasma membrane of rat caudal epididymal sperm. *J Biol Chem* 1984;259:839–848.
248. Faye JC, Duguet L, Mazzuca M, Bayard F. Purification, radioimmunoassay, and immunohistochemical localization of a glycoprotein produced by the rat epididymis. *Biol Reprod* 1980; 23:423–432.
249. Cornwall GA, Vreeburg JT, Holland MK, Orgebin-Crist M-C. Interactions of labeled epididymal secretory proteins with spermatozoa after injection of ^{35}S-methionine in the mouse. *Biol Reprod* 1990;43:121–129.
250. Jimenez C, Lefrancois AM, Ghyselinck NB, Dufaure JP. Characterization and hormonal regulation of 24 kDa protein synthesis by the adult murine epididymis. *J Endocrinol* 1992;133:197–203.
251. Jones R, Brown CR, Cran DG, Gaunt SJ. Surface and internal antigens of rat spermatozoa distinguished using monoclonal antibodies. *Gamete Res* 1983;8:255–265.
252. Sylvester SR, Skinner MK, Griswold MD. A sulfated glycoprotein synthesized by Sertoli cells and by epididymal cells is a component of the sperm membrane. *Biol Reprod* 1984;31: 1087–1101.
253. Kaur J, Ramakrishnan PR, Rajalakshmi M. Alterations in protein profile of rat spermatozoa during maturation. *Andrologia* 1991;23:53–56.
254. Voglmayr JK, Fairbanks G, Jakowitz MA, Colella JR. Post-testicular developmental changes in the ram sperm cell surface and their relationship to luminal fluid proteins of the reproductive tract. *Biol Reprod* 1980;22:655–667.
255. Voglmayr JK, Fairbanks G, Vespa DB, Colella JR. Studies on mechanisms of surface modifications in ram spermatozoa during the final stages of differentiation. *Biol Reprod* 1982;26:483–500.
256. Voglmayr JK, Fairbanks G, Lewis RG. Surface glycoprotein changes in ram spermatozoa during epididymal maturation. *Biol Reprod* 1983;29:767–775.
257. Dacheaux JL, Voglmayr JK. Sequence of sperm cell surface differentiation and its relationship to exogenous fluid proteins in the ram epididymis. *Biol Reprod* 1983;29:1033–1046.
258. Vieurla M, Rajaniemi H. Radioiodination of surface proteins of bull spermatozoa and their characterization by sodium dodecyl sulfate-polyacrylamide gel electrophoresis. *J Reprod Fertil* 1980;58:483–489.
259. Nicolson GL, Bronginski AB, Beattie G, Yanagimachi R. Cell surface changes in the proteins of rabbit spermatozoa during epididymal passage. *Gamete Res* 1979;2:153–162.
260. Russell LD, Peterson RN, Hunt W, Strack LE. Post-testicular surface modifications and contributions of reproductive tract fluids to the surface polypeptide composition of boar spermatozoa. *Biol Reprod* 1980;30:959–978.
261. Young LG, Hinton BT, Gould KG. Surface changes in chimpanzee sperm during epididymal transit. *Biol Reprod* 1985;32: 399–412.
262. Tezón JG, Ramella E, Cameo MS, Vazquez MH, Blaquier JA. Immunochemical localization of secretory antigens in the human epididymis and their association with spermatozoa. *Biol Reprod* 1985;32:591–597.
263. Dacheux JL, Chevrier C, Lanson Y. Motility and surface transformations of human spermatozoa during epididymal transit. *Ann NY Acad Sci* 1987;513:560–563.
264. Ross P, Kan FWK, Antaki P, Vigneault N, Chapdelaine A, Roberts KD. Protein synthesis and secretion in the human epididymis and immunoreactivity with sperm antibodies. *Mol Reprod Dev* 1990;26:12–23.
265. Hunter AG. Differentiation of rabbit sperm antigens from those of seminal plasma. *J Reprod Fertil* 1969;20:413–418.
266. Barker LDS, Amann RP. Epididymal physiology. I. Specificity of antisera against bull spermatozoa and reproductive fluids. *J Reprod Fertil* 1970;22:441–452.
267. Barker LDS, Amann RP. Epididymal physiology. II. Immunofluorescent analysis of epithelial secretion and absorption, and of bovine sperm maturation. *J Reprod Fertil* 1971;26:319–332.
268. Killian GJ, Amann RP. Immunoelectrophoretic characterization of fluid and sperm entering and leaving the bovine epididymis. *Biol Reprod* 1973;9:489–499.
269. Draveland E, Joshi MS. Sperm-coating antigens secreted by the epididymis and seminal vesicle of the rat. *Biol Reprod* 1981;25:649–658.
270. Lea OA, Petrusz P, French F. Purification and localization of acidic epididymal glycoprotein (AEG): A sperm coating protein secreted by the rat epididymis. *Int J Androl* [*Suppl*] 1978;2: 592–607.
271. Cameo MS, Blaquier JA. Androgen-controlled specific proteins in rat epididymis. *J Endocrinol* 1976;69:47–55.
272. Pholpramol C, Lea OA, Burrow PV, Dott HM, Setchell BP. The effects of acidic epididymal glycoprotein (AEG) and some other proteins on the motility of rat epididymal spermatozoa. *Int J Androl* 1983;6:240–248.
273. Garberi JC, Kohane AC, Cameo MS, Blaquier JA. Isolation and characterization of specific rat epididymal proteins. *Mol Cell Endocrinol* 1979;13:73–82.
274. Kohane AC, Gonzáles Echeverría FMC, Piñeiro L, Blaquier JA. Interactions of proteins of epididymal origin with spermatozoa. *Biol Reprod* 1980;23:737–742.
275. Kohane AC, González Echeverría FMC, Piñeiro L, Blaquier JA. Distribution and site of production of specific proteins in rat epididymis. *Biol Reprod* 1980;23:181–187.
276. Cuasnicú PS, Gonzáles Echeverría F, Piazza A, Cameo MS, Blaquier JA. Antibodies against epididymal glycoproteins block fertilizing ability in rat. *J Reprod Fertil* 1984;72:461–471.
277. Brooks DE, Higgins SJ. Characterization and androgen-dependence of proteins associated with luminal fluid and spermatozoa in the rat epididymis. *J Reprod Fertil* 1980;59:262–375.
278. Brooks DE. Secretion of proteins and glycoproteins by the rat epididymis: regional differences, androgen-dependence, and effects of protease inhibitors, procaine, and tunicamycin. *Biol Reprod* 1981;25:1099–1117.
279. Brooks DE. Metabolic activity in the epididymis and its regulation by androgens. *Physiol Rev* 1981;61:515–555.
280. Brooks DE. Selective binding of specific rat epididymal secretory proteins to spermatozoa and erythrocytes. *Gamete Res* 1983;4: 367–376.
281. Brooks DE, Tiver K. Localization of epididymal secretory proteins on rat spermatozoa. *J Reprod Fertil* 1983;69:651–657.

282. Rifkin J, Olson GE. Characterization of maturation-dependent extrinsic proteins of the rat sperm surface. *J Cell Biol* 1985;100:1582–1591.
283. Brooks DE. Developmental expression and androgenic regulation of the mRNA for major secretory proteins of the rat epididymis. *Mol Cell Endocrinol* 1987;53:59–66.
284. Jones R, Brown CR, VonGlos KI, Parker MG. Hormonal regulation of protein synthesis in the rat epididymis. Characterization of androgen-dependent and testicular fluid-dependent proteins. *Biochem J* 1980;188:667–676.
285. Wong PYD, Tsang AYF. Studies of the binding of a 32 K rat epididymal protein to rat epididymal spermatozoa. *Biol Reprod* 1982;27:1239–1246.
286. Brooks DE, Means AR, Wright EJ, Singh SP, Tiver KK. Molecular cloning of the cDNA for two major androgen-dependent secretory proteins of 18.5 kilodaltons synthesized by the rat epididymis. *J Biol Chem* 1986;26:4956–4961.
287. Brooks DE, Means AR, Wright EJ, Singh SP, Tiver KK. Molecular cloning of the cDNA for androgen-dependent sperm-coating glycoproteins secreted by the rat epididymis. *Eur J Biochem* 1986;161:13–18.
288. Charest NJ, Joseph DR, Wilson EM, French FS. Molecular cloning of complementary deoxyribonucleic acid for an androgen-regulated epididymal protein. *Mol Endocrinol* 1988;2:999–1004.
289. Moore HDM. Localization of specific glycoproteins secreted by the rabbit and hamster epididymis. *Biol Reprod* 1980;22: 705–718.
290. González Echiveriá F, Cuasnicú PS, Blaquier JA. Identification of androgen-dependent glycoproteins in the hamster epididymis and their association with spermatozoa. *J Reprod Fertil* 1982;64:1–7.
291. Fox N, Damjanov I, Knowles BB, Solter D. Teratocarcinoma antigen is secreted by epididymal cells and coupled to maturing sperm. *Exp Cell Res* 1982;137:485–488.
292. Vernon RB, Muller CH, Herr JC, Feuchter FA, Eddy EM. Epididymal secretion of a mouse sperm surface component recognized by a monoclonal antibody. *Biol Reprod* 1982;26:133–141.
293. Vernon RB, Hamilton MS, Eddy EM. Effects of in vivo and in vitro fertilization environments on the expression of a surface antigen of the mouse sperm tail. *Biol Reprod* 1985;32:669–680.
294. Eddy EM, McGee RS, Willis WD, O'Brien DA. Immunodissection of sperm maturation. In: Baccetti B, ed. *Serono Symposia Publications from Raven Press, vol 75, Comparative spermatology 20 years after.* New York: Raven Press; 1991:643–646.
295. Feuchter FA, Tabet AJ, Green MF. Maturation antigen of the mouse sperm flagellum. I. Analysis of its secretion, association with sperm, and function. *Am J Anat* 1988;181:67–76.
296. Feuchter FA, Green MF, Tabet AJ. Maturation antigen of the mouse sperm flagellum: II. Origin from holocrine cells of the distal caput epididymis. *Anat Rec* 1987;217:146–152.
297. Toshimori K, Araki S, Ōura C. Cryptodeterminant of a sperm maturation antigen on the mouse flagellar surface. *Biol Reprod* 1990;42:151–160.
298. Jones R. Comparative biochemistry of mammalian epididymal plasma. *Comp Biochem Physiol [B]* 1978;61:365–370.
299. Zaneveld LJD, Chatterton RT. *Biochemistry of mammalian reproduction.* New York: John Wiley & Sons; 1982.
300. Conchie J, Findlay J, Levvy GA. Mammalian glycosidases. Distribution in the body. *Biochem J* 1959;71:318–325.
301. Kemp WR, Killian GJ. Glycosidase activity in epididymal epithelial cells isolated from normal and α-chlorohydrin treated male rats. *Contraception* 1978;17:93–101.
302. Chapman DA, Killian GJ. Glycosidase activities in principal cells, basal cells, fibroblasts and spermatozoa isolated from the rat epididymis. *Biol Reprod* 1984;31:627–636.
303. Skudlarek MD, Orgebin-Christ M-C. Glycosidases in cultured rat epididymal cells: enzyme Activity, synthesis and secretion. *Biol Reprod* 1986;35:167–178.
304. Grandmont A-M, Chapdelaine P, Tremblay RR. Presence of α-glucosidases in the male reproductive system of the rat and hormonal influences. *Can J Biochem Cell Biol* 1983;61:764–769.
305. Jones R. Absorption and secretion in the cauda epididymidis of the rabbit and the effects of degenerating spermatozoa on epididymal plasma after castration. *J Endocrinol* 1974;63:157–165.
306. Poirier GR, Jackson J. Isolation and characterization of two proteinase inhibitors from the male reproductive tract of mice. *Gamete Res* 1981;4:555–569.
307. Wenstrom JC, Hamilton DW. Dolichol concentration and biosynthesis in rat testis and epididymis. *Biol Reprod* 1980;23: 1054–1069.
308. Iusem NB, de Larminant MA, Tezón JG, Blaquier JA, Belocopitow E. Androgen dependence of protein *N*-glycosylation in rat epididymis. *Endocrinology* 1984;114:1448–1458.
309. Bernal A, Torres J, Reyes A, Rosada A. Presence and regional distribution of sialyl transferase in the epididymis of the rat. *Biol Reprod* 1980;23:290–293.
310. Cossu G, Boitani C. Lactosaminoglycans synthesized by mouse male germ cells are fucosylated by an epididymal fucosyltransferase. *Dev Biol* 1984;102:402–408.
311. Letts PJ, Meistrich MR, Bruce WR, Schachter H. Glycoprotein glycosyltransferase levels during spermatogenesis in mice. *Biochim Biophys Acta* 1974;343:192–207.
312. Reddy PRK, Tadolini B, Wilson J, Williams-Ashman HG. Glycoprotein glycosyltransferase in male reproductive organs and their hormonal regulations. *Mol Cell Endocrinol* 1976;5:23–31.
313. Tadolini B, Wilson J, Reddy PRK, Williams-Ashman HG. Characteristics and hormonal control of some glycoprotein glycosyltransferase reactions in male reproductive organs. *Adv Enzymol Regulation* 1977;15:319–336.
314. Hamilton DW. UDP-galactose: *N*-acetylglucosamine galactosyltransferase in fluids from rat testis and epididymis. *Biol Reprod* 1980;23:377–385.
315. Hamilton DW, Gould RP. Preliminary observations on enzymatic galactosylation of glycoproteins on the surface of rat caput epididymal spermatozoa. *Int J Androl [Suppl]* 1982;5:73–80.
316. Tulsiani DRP, Skudlarek MD, Orgebin-Crist M-C. Novel alpha-D-mannosidease of rat sperm plasma membranes: Characterization and potential role in sperm–egg interactions. *J Cell Biol* 1989;109:1257–1267.
317. Tulsiani DRP, Skudlarek MD, Orgebin-Crist M-C. Human sperm plasma membranes possess α-D-mannosidase activity but no galactosyltransferase activity. *Biol Reprod* 1990;42:843–858.
318. Cardullo RA, Armant DR, Millette CF. Characterization of fucosyltransferase activity during mouse spermatogenesis: Evidence for a cell surface fucosyltransferase. *Biochemistry* 1989;28: 1611–1617.
319. Ram PA, Cardullo RA, Millette CF. Expression and topographical localization of cell surface fucosyltransferase activity during epididymal sperm maturation in the mouse. *Gamete Res* 1989;22:321–332.
320. Durr R, Shur B, Roth S. Sperm-associated sialyltransferase activity. *Nature* 1977;265:547–548.
321. Shur BD, Bennett D. A specific defect in galactosyltransferase on sperm bearing mutant alleles of the *T/t* locus. *Dev Biol* 1979;71:243–259.
322. Shur BD, Hall NG. A role for mouse sperm surface galactosyltransferase in sperm binding to the egg zona pellucida. *J Cell Biol* 1982;95:574–579.
323. Shaper NL, Wright WW, Shaper JH. Murine β1,4-galactosyltransferase: Both the amounts and structure of the mRNA are regulated during spermatogenesis. *Proc Natl Acad Sci USA* 1990;87:791–795.
324. Harduin-Lepers A, Shaper NL, Mahoney JA, Shaper JH. Murine β1,4-galactosyltransferase: Round spermatid transcripts are characterized by an extended 5′-untranslated region. *Glycobiology* 1992;2:361–368.
325. Hamilton DW. Evidence for α-lactalbumin-like activity in reproductive tract fluids of the male rat. *Biol Reprod* 1981;25:385–392.
326. Quasba PK, Hewlett IK, Byers S. The presence of the milk protein, α-lacatalbumin and its mRNA in the rat epididymis. *Biochem Biophys Res Commun* 1983;117:306–312.
327. Klinefelter GR, Hamilton DW. Synthesis and secretion of proteins by perfused caput epididymal tubules, and association of secreted proteins with spermatozoa. *Biol Reprod* 1985;33: 1017–1027.
328. Ensrude K, Wenstrom JC, Baker JB, Hamilton DW. A monoclonal antibody against rat epididymal α-lactalbumin-like 24Kd

polypeptide recognizes rat cauda sperm surface. *J Androl* [*Suppl*] 1985;6:54.
329. Walker JE, Jones R, Moore A, Hamilton DW, Hall L. Analysis of major androgen-regulated cDNA clones from the rat epididymis. *Mol Cell Endocrinol* 1990;74:61–68.
330. Holpert M, Cooper TG. Re-examination of the presence of alpha-lactalbumin in the epididymis of the rat. *J Reprod Fertil* 1990;90:503–514.
331. Miller DJ, Macek MB, Shur BD. Complementarity between sperm surface β-1,4-galactosyl-transferase and egg-coat ZP3 mediates sperm-egg binding. *Nature* 1992;357:589–593.
332. Olson GE, Orgebin-Crist M-C. Sperm surface changes during epididymal maturation. *Ann NY Acad Sci* 1982;383:372–390.
333. Vaidya RA, Glass RW, Dandekar P, Johnson K. Decrease in electrophoretic mobility of rabbit spermatozoa following intrauterine incubation. *J Reprod Fertil* 1971;24:299–301.
334. Rosado A, Valezquez A, Lara-Ricalde R. Cell polarography. II. Effect of neuraminidase and follicular fluid upon the surface characteristics of human spermatozoa. *Fertil Steril* 1973;24: 349–354.
335. Edwards RG, Ferguson LC, Coombs RRA. Blood group antigens on human spermatozoa. *J Reprod Fertil* 1964;7:153–161.
336. Boettcher B. Correlation between human ABO blood group antigens in seminal plasma and on seminal spermatozoa. *J Reprod Fertil* 1968;16:49–54.
337. Kerek G, Biberfeld P, Afzelius BA. Demonstration of HL-A antigens, "species," and "semen"-specific antigens on human spermatozoa. *Int J Fertil* 1973;18:145–155.
338. James K, Hargreave TB. Immunosuppression by seminal plasma and its possible clinical significance. *Immunol Today* 1984; 5:357–363.
339. Hekman A, Rumke P. The antigens of human seminal plasma with special reference to lactoferrin, a spermatozoa coating antigen. *Fertil Steril* 1969;20:312–323.
340. Roberts TK, Boettcher B. Identification of human sperm coating antigen. *J Reprod Fertil* 1969;18:347–350.
341. Koyama Y, Takuda Y, Takamura T, Isojima S. Localization of human seminal plasma No. 7 antigen (ferrisplan) in accessory glands of the male genital tract. *J Reprod Immunol* 1983;5: 135–143.
342. Wahlstrom T, Bohn H, Seppala M. Immunohistochemical demonstration of placental protein 5 (PP5)-like material in the seminal vesicle and the ampullar part of the vas deferens. *Life Sci* 1982;31:2723–2725.
343. Evans RJ, Herr JC. Immunohistochemical localization of the MHS-5 antigen in principal cells of human seminal vesicle epithelium. *Anat Rec* 1986;214:372–377.
344. Saji F, Minagawa Y, Ohashi K, Negoro T, Tanizawa O. Further characterization of a human sperm coating antigen (gp12). *Am J Reprod Immunol* 1986;12:13–16.
345. Abrescia P, Lombardi G, De Rosa M, Quagliozzi L, Guardiola J, Metafora S. Identification and preliminary characterization of sperm-binding protein in normal human semen. *J Reprod Fertil* 1985;73:71–77.
346. Ostrowski MC, Kistler MK, Kistler WS. Purification and cell-free synthesis of a major protein from rat seminal vesicle secretion. *J Biol Chem* 1979;254:4007–4021.
347. Oliphant G, Singhas CA. Iodination of rabbit sperm plasma membrane: relationship of specific surface proteins to epididymal function and sperm capacitation. *Biol Reprod* 1979;21: 937–944.
348. Irwin M, Nicholson N, Haywood JT, Pourier GR. Immunofluorescent localization of a murine seminal vesicle proteinase inhibitor. *Biol Reprod* 1983;28:1201–1206.
349. Isaacs W, Coffey DS. The predominant protein of canine seminal plasma is an enzyme. *J Biol Chem* 1984;259:11520–11526.
350. Paonessa G, Metafora G, Tajana G, et al. Transglutaminase-mediated modifications of the rat sperm surface in vitro. *Science* 1984;226:852–855.
351. Baccetti B. The human spermatozoon. In: Van Blerkom J, Motta PM, eds. *Ultrastructure of reproduction.* The Hague: Martinus Nijhoff; 1984:110–126.
352. Wyrobek AJ, Gordon LA, Burkhart JG, et al. An evaluation of human sperm as indicators of chemically induced alterations of spermatogenic function. A report of the U.S. Environmental Protection Agency Gene-Tox Program. *Mutat Res* 1983;115: 73–148.
353. Ward WS, Coffey DS. DNA packaging and organization in mammalian spermatozoa: Comparison with somatic cells. *Biol Reprod* 1991;44:569–574.
354. Grimes SR Jr. Nuclear proteins in spermatogenesis. *Comp Biochem Physiol* 1986;83B:495–500.
355. Hecht NB. Mammalian protamines and their expression. In: Hnilica L, Stein G, Stein J, eds. *Histones and other basic nuclear proteins.* Boca Raton: CRC Press; 1989:347–373.
356. Oliva R, Dixon GH. Vertebrate protamine genes and the histone-to-protamine replacement reaction. In: Cohn ME, Moldave K, eds. *Progress in nucleic acid research and molecular biology, vol 40.* New York: Academic Press; 1991:25–94.
357. Hecht NB, Bower PA, Waters SH, Yelick PC, Distel RJ. Evidence for haploid expression of mouse testicular genes. *Exp Cell Res* 1986;164:183–190.
358. Bellvé AR, Carraway R. Characterization of two basic chromosomal proteins isolated from mouse spermatozoa. *J Cell Biol* 1978;79:177a.
359. Mayer JF, Chang TSK, Zirkin BR. Spermatogenesis in the mouse. 2. Amino acid incorporation into basic nucleoproteins of mouse spermatids and spermatozoa. *Biol Reprod* 1981;25: 1041–1051.
360. Balhorn R, Weston S, Thomas C, Wyrobek AJ. DNA packaging in mouse spermatids. Synthesis of protamine variants and four transition proteins. *Exp Cell Res* 1984;150:298–308.
361. Bellvé AR, O'Brien DA. The mammalian spermatozoon: Structure and temporal assembly. In: Hartmann HF, ed. *Mechanisms and control of animal fertilization.* Orlando: Academic Press; 1983:55–137.
362. Balhorn R. A model for the structure of chromatin in mammalian sperm. *J Cell Biol* 1982;93:298–305.
363. Warrent RW, Kim S-H. α-Helix–double helix interaction shown in the structure of a protamine-transfer RNA complex and a nucleoprotamine model. *Nature* 1978;271:130–135.
364. Gusse M, Chevaillier P. Electron microscopic evidence for the presence of globular structures in different sperm chromatins. *J Cell Biol* 1980;87:280–284.
365. Tsanev R, Avramova Z. Nonprotamine nucleoprotein ultrastructures in mature ram sperm nuclei. *Eur J Cell Biol* 1981;24: 139–145.
366. Bendet IJ, Bearden J Jr. Birefringence of bull sperm. II. Form birefringence of bull sperm. *J Cell Biol* 1972;55:501–510.
367. Sipski MR, Wagner TE. The total structure and organization of chromosomal fibers in eutherian sperm nuclei. *Biol Reprod* 1977;16:428–440.
368. Bellvé AR. Biogenesis of the mammalian spermatozoon. In: Amann RP, Seidel GE Jr, eds. *Prospects for sexing mammalian sperm.* Boulder: Colorado Associated University Press; 1982:69–102.
369. Bellvé AR, Chandrika R, Martinova YS, Barth AH. The perinuclear natrix as a structural element of the mouse sperm nucleus. *Biol Reprod* 1992;47:451–465.
370. Pedersen H. The postacrosomal region of man and *Macaca artoides. J Ultrastruct Res* 1972;40:366–377.
371. Stackpole CW, Devorkin D. Membrane organization in mouse spermatozoa revealed by freeze-etching. *J Ultrastruct Res* 1974;49:167–187.
372. Gerace L, Comeau C, Benson M. Organization and modulation of nuclear lamina structure. *J Cell Sci* [*Suppl*] 1984;1:137–160.
373. Krohne G, Benavente R. The nuclear lamins. A multigene family of proteins in evolution and differentiation. *Exp Cell Res* 1986;162:1–10.
374. Gerace L, Blum A, Blobel G. Immunocytochemical localization of the major polypeptides of the nuclear pore complex lamina fraction. Interphase and mitotic distribution. *J Cell Biol* 1978;79:546–566.
375. Hancock R, Baulikis T. Functional organisation of the nucleus. In: Bourne GH, Danielli JF, eds. *International review of cytology, vol. 79.* New York: Academic Press; 1982:165–214.

376. Lebkowski YS, Laemmli UK. Non-histone proteins and long-range organization of HeLa interphase DNA. *J Mol Biol* 1982;156:121–141.
377. Hoger TH, Krohne G, Franke WW. Amino acid sequence and molecular characterization of murine lamin B as deduced from cDNA clones. *Eur J Cell Biol* 1988;47:283–290.
378. Hoger TH, Zatloukal K, Waizenegger I, Krohne G. Characterization of a second highly conserved B-type lamin present in cells previously thought to contain only a single B-type lamin. *Chromosoma* 1990;99:379–390.
379. McKeon FD, Kirschner MW, Caput D. Homologies in both primary and secondary structure between nuclear envelope and intermediate filament proteins. *Nature* 1986;319:463–468.
380. Fisher DZ, Chaudhary N, Blobel G. cDNA sequencing of nuclear lamins A and C reveals primary and secondary structural homology to intermediate filament proteins. *Proc Natl Acad Sci USA* 1986;83:6450–6454.
381. Stick R, Schwarz H. The disappearance of the nuclear lamina during spermatogenesis: An electron microscopic and immunofluorescence study. *Cell Differ* 1982;11:235–243.
382. Hogner D, Telling A, Lepper K, Jost E. Patterns of nuclear lamins in diverse animal and plant cells and in germ cells as revealed by immunoflourescence microscopy with polyclonal and monoclonal antibodies. *Tissue Cell* 1984;16:693–703.
383. Maul GG, French BT, Bechtol KB. Identification and redistribution of lamins during nuclear differentiation in mouse spermatogenesis. *Dev Biol* 1986;115:68–77.
384. Moss SB, Donovan MJ, Bellvé AR. The occurrence and distribution of lamin proteins during mammalian spermatogenesis and early embryonic development. *Ann NY Acad Sci* 1987;513:74–89.
385. Moss SB, Burnham BL, Bellvé AR. The differential expression of lamin epitopes during mouse spermatogenesis. *Mol Reprod Dev* 1993;34:164–174.
386. Behal A, Prakash K, Rao MR. Identification of a meiotic prophase-specific nuclear matrix protein in the rat. *J Biol Chem* 1987;262:10898–10902.
387. Sudhaker L, Rao MRS. Stage-dependent changes in localization of a germ cell-specific lamin during mammalian spermatogenesis. *J Biol Chem* 1990;265:22526–22532.
388. Sudhakar L, Sivakumar N, Behal A, Rao MRS. Evolutionary conservation of a germ cell-specific lamin persisting through mammalian spermiogenesis. *Exp Cell Res* 1992;198:78–84.
389. Furukawa K, Hotta Y. cDNA cloning of a germ cell specific lamin B3 from mouse spermatocytes and analysis of its function by ectopic expression in somatic cells. *EMBO J* 1993;12:97–106.
390. Olson GE, Hamilton DW, Fawcett DW. Isolation and characterization of the perforatorium of rat spermatozoa. *J Reprod Fertil* 1976;47:293–297.
391. Fawcett DW. A comparative view of sperm ultrastructure. *Biol Reprod [Suppl]* 1970;2:90–127.
392. Burgos MH, Fawcett DW. An electron microscopic study of spermatid differentiation in the toad. *Bufo arenarum* Hensel. *J Biophys Biochem Cytol* 1956;2:223–240.
393. Nagano T. Observations on the fine structure of the developing spermatid in the domestic chicken. *J Cell Biol* 1962;14:193–205.
394. Clermont Y, Einberg E, Leblond CP, Wagner S. The perforatorium—an extension of the nuclear membrane of the rat spermatozoon. *Anat Rec* 1955;121:1–12.
395. Yanagimachi R, Noda YD. Ultrastructural changes in the hamster sperm head during fertilization. *J Ultrastruct Res* 1970;31:465–485.
396. Lalli M, Clermont Y. Structural changes in the head component of the rat spermatid during late spermatogenesis. *Am J Anat* 1981;160:419–434.
397. Calvin HI, Bedford JM. Formatin of disulfide bonds in the nucleus and accessory structures of mammalian spermatozoa during maturation in the epididymis. *J Reprod Fertil* 1971;13:65–75.
398. Huang TTF, Yanagimachi R. Inner acrosomal membrane of mammalian spermatozoa: Its properties and possible functions in fertilization. *Am J Anat* 1985;174:249–268.
399. Courtens JL, Courot M, Fléchon JE. The perinuclear substance of boar, bull, ram and rabbit spermatozoa. *J Ultrastruct Res* 1976;57:54–64.
400. Longo FJ, Cook S. Formation of perinuclear theca in spermatozoa of diverse mammalian species: Relationship of the manchette and multiple band polypeptides. *Mol Reprod Dev* 1991;28:380–393.
401. Oko R, Clermont Y. Origin and distribution of perforatorial proteins during spermatogenesis of the rat: An immunocytochemical study. *Anat Rec* 1991;230:489–501.
402. Austin CR, Bishop MWH. Some features of the acrosome and perforatorium in mammalian spermatozoa. *Proc R Soc (Lond) [Biol]* 1958;149:234–240.
403. Olson GE. Isolation of the fibrous sheath and perforatorium of rat spermatozoa. In: Fawcett DW, Bedford JM, eds. *The spermatozoon.* Baltimore: Urban & Schwarzenberg; 1979:395–400.
404. Oko R, Clermont Y. Isolation, structure and protein composition of the perforatorium of rat spermatozoa. *Biol Reprod* 1988;39:673–687.
405. Oko R, Moussakova L, Clermont Y. Regional differences in composition of the perforatorium and outer periacrosomal layer of the rat spermatozoon as revealed by immunocytochemistry. *Am J Anat* 1990;188:64–73.
406. Fouquet J-P, Valentin A, Kann M-L. Perinuclear cytoskeleton of acrosome-less spermaids in the blind sterile mutant mouse. *Tissue Cell* 1992;24:655–665.
407. Nicander L, Bane A. Fine structure of the sperm head in some mammals with particular reference to the acrosome and subacrosomal substance. *Z Zelforsch* 1966;72:496–515.
408. Plattner H. Bull spermatozoa: A re-investigation by freeze etching using widely different cryofixation procedures. *J Submicrosc Cytol* 1971;3:19–32.
409. Olson GE, Noland TD, Winfrey VP, Garbers DL. Substructure of the postacrosomal sheath of bovine spermatozoa. *J Ultrastruct Res* 1983;85:204–218.
410. Maxwell WL. The acrosomal zonule. *Tissue Cell* 1982;14:283–288.
411. Czaker R. Morphogenesis and cytochemistry of the postacrosomal dense lamina during mouse spermiogenesis. *J Ultrastruct Res* 1985;90:26–39.
412. Olson GE, Winfrey VP. Characterization of the postacrosomal sheath of bovine spermatozoa. *Gamete Res* 1988;20:329–342.
413. Longo FJ, Krohne G, Franke WW. Basic proteins of the perinuclear theca of mammalian spermatozoa and spermatids: A novel class of cytoskeletal elements. *J Cell Biol* 1987;105:1105–1120.
414. Paranko J, Longo F, Potts J, Krohne G, Franke WW. Widespread occurrence of calicin, a basic cytoskeletal protein of sperm cells, in diverse mammalian species. *Differentiation* 1988;38:21–27.
415. Bellvé AR, Chandrika R, Barth A. Temporal expression, polar distribution and transition of an epitope in the perinuclear theca during mouse spermatogenesis. *J Cell Sci* 1990;96:745–756.
416. Toshimori K, Tanii I, Oura C, Eddy EM. A monoclonal antibody, MN13, that recognizes specifically a novel substance between the postacrosomal sheath and the overlying plasma membrane in the mammalian sperm head. *Mol Reprod Dev* 1991;29:289–293.
417. MacRae TH, Lange BMH, Gull K. Production and characterization of monoclonal antibodies to the mammalian sperm cytoskeleton. *Mol Reprod Dev* 1990;25:384–392.
418. Tamblyn TM. Identification of actin in boar epididymal spermatozoa. *Biol Reprod* 1980;22:727–734.
419. Baccetti B, Bigliardi E, Burrini AG. The morphogenesis of the vertebrate perforatorium. *J Ultrastruct Res* 1980;71:272–287.
420. Olson GE, Winfrey VP, Flaherty SP. Cytoskeletal assemblies of mammalian spermatozoa. *Ann NY Acad Sci* 1987;513:222–246.
421. Fouquet J-P, Kann M-L, Dadoune J-P. Immunogold distribution of actin during spermiogenesis in the rat, hamster, monkey, and human. *Anat Rec* 1989;223:35–42.
422. Camatini M, Colombo A, Bonfanti P. Cytoskeletal elements in mammalian spermiogenesis and spermatozoa. *Microsc Res Tech* 1992;20:232–250.
423. Searle AG. The genetics of sterility in the mouse. In: Crosignai PG, Rubin BL, Fraccaro M, eds. *Genetic control of gamete production and function.* New York: Grune & Stratton; 1982:93–114.
424. Sotomayor RE, Handel MA. Failure of acrosome assembly in a male sterile mutant. *Biol Reprod* 1986;34:171–182.
425. Phillips DM. Development of spermatozoa in the wolly opossum

with special reference to the shaping of the sperm head. *J Ultrastruct Res* 1970;33:369–380.
426. Fawcett DW, Phillips DM. Observations on the release of spermatozoa and on changes in the head during passage through the epididymis. *J Reprod Fertil [Suppl]* 1969;6:405–418.
427. Hunt DM, Johnson DR. Abnormal spermiogenesis in two pink-eyed sterile mutants in the mouse. *J Embryol Exp Morphol* 1971;26:111–121.
428. Bryan JHD. Spermatogenesis revisited: III. The course of spermatogenesis in a male-sterile pink-eyed mutant type in the mouse. *Cell Tissue Res* 1977;180:173–186.
429. Wooding FBP. The effect of Triton X-100 on the ultrastructure of ejaculated bovine sperm. *J Ultrastruct Res* 1973;42:502–516.
430. Phillips DM. Substructure of the mammalian acrosome. *J Ultrastruct Res* 1972;38:591–604.
431. Pedersen H. Further observations on the fine structure of the human spermatozoon. *Z Zellforsch* 1972;123:305–315.
432. Phillips DM. Mitochondrial disposition in mammalian spermatozoa. *J Ultrastruct Res* 1977;58:144–154.
433. Koehler JK. Periodicities in the acrosome or acrosomal membrane: Some observations on mammalian spermatozoa. *Biol J Linnean Soc [Suppl]* 1975;1:337–342.
434. Zahler WL, Doak GA. Isolation of the outer acrosomal membrane from bull spermatozoa. *Biochim Biophys Acta* 1975;406:479–488.
435. Russell L, Peterson R, Freund M. Direct evidence for formation of hybrid vesicles by fusion of plasma and outer acrosomal membranes during the acrosome reaction in boar spermatozoa. *J Exp Zool* 1979;208:41–56.
436. Noland TD, Olson GE, Garbers DL. Purification and partial characterization of plasma membranes from bovine spermatozoa. *Biol Reprod* 1983;29:987–998.
437. Topfer-Petersen E, Schill WB. A new separation method of subcellular fractions of boar spermatozoa. *Andrologia* 1981;13: 174–176.
438. Olson GE, Winfrey VP, Garbers DL, Noland TD. Isolation and characterization of a macromolecular complex associated with the outer acrosomal membrane of bovine spermatozoa. *Biol Reprod* 1985;33:761–779.
439. Hermo L, Rambourg LA, Clermont Y. Three-dimensional architecture of the cortical region of the Golgi apparatus in rat spermatids. *Am J Anat* 1980;157:357–373.
440. Thakkar JK, East J, Seyler D, Fanson RC. Surface-active phospholipase A_2 in mouse spermatozoa. *Biochim Biophys Acta* 1983;754:44–50.
441. Rahi H, Sheikhnejade G, Srivastava PN. Isolation of the inner acrosomal-nuclear membrane complex from rabbit spermatozoa. *Gamete Res* 1983;7:215–225.
442. Russell L, Peterson RN, Freund M. On the presence of bridges linking the inner and outer acrosomal membranes of boar spermatozoa. *Anat Rec* 1979;198:449–459.
443. Yanagimachi R. Specificity of sperm–egg interaction. In: Edidin M, Johnson MH, eds. *Immunobiology of gametes.* London: Cambridge University Press; 1981:255–296.
444. Fawcett DW. Morphogenesis of the mammalian sperm acrosome in new perspective. In: Afzelius BA, ed. *The functional anatomy of the spermatozoon.* Oxford: Pergamon Press; 1975:199–210.
445. Allison AC, Hartree EF. Lysosomal enzymes in the acrosome and their possible role in fertilization. *J Reprod Fertil* 1970;21: 501–515.
446. Stambaugh R, Brackett BG, Mastroianni L. Inhibition of in vitro fertilization of rabbit ova by trypsin inhibitors. *Biol Reprod* 1969;1:223–227.
447. Beyler SA, Zaneveld LJD. Inhibition of in vitro fertilization of mouse gametes by proteinase inhibitors. *J Reprod Fertil* 1982;66:425–431.
448. Polakoski KL, Parrish RF. Boar proacrosin. Purification and preliminary activation studies of proacrosin isolated from ejaculated boar sperm. *J Biol Chem* 1977;252:1888–1894.
449. Tobias PS, Schumacher GFB. Observation of two proacrosins in extracts of human spermatozoa. *Biochem Biophys Res Commun* 1977;74:434–439.
450. Brown CR, Harrison RAP. The activation of proacrosin in spermatozoa from ram, bull and boar. *Biochim Biophys Acta* 1978;526:202–217.
451. Mukerji SK, Meizel S. Rabbit testis proacrosin. Purification, molecular weight estimation, and amino acid and carbohydrate composition of the molecule. *J Biol Chem* 1979;254: 11721–11728.
452. Müller-Esterl W, Fritz H. Sperm acrosin. In: Lorand L, ed. *Methods in enzymology, vol 80.* New York: Academic Press; 1981:621–632.
453. Baba T, Kashiwabara S-I, Watanabe K, et al. Activation and maturation mechanisms of boar acrosin zymogen based on the deduced primary structure. *J Biol Chem* 1989;264:11920–11927.
454. Adham IM, Klemm U, Maier W-M, Hoyer-Fender S, Tsaousidou S, Engel W. Molecular cloning of preproacrosin and analysis of its expression pattern in spermatogenesis. *Eur J Biochem* 1989;182:563–568.
455. Baba T, Watanabe K, Kashiwabara S-I, Arai Y. Primary structure of human proacrosin deduced from its cDNA sequence. *FEBS Lett* 1989;244:296–300.
456. Adham IM, Klemm U, Maier W-M, Engel W. Molecular cloning of human preproacrosin cDNA. *Hum Genet* 1990;84:125–128.
457. Kashiwabara S-I, Baba T, Takada M, Wantanabe K, Yano Y, Arai Y. Primary structure of mouse proacrosin deduced from the cDNA sequence and its gene expression during spermatogenesis. *J Biochem* 1990;108:785–791.
458. Klemm U, Maier W-M, Tsaousidou S, Adham IM, Willison K, Engel W. Mouse preproacrosin: cDNA sequence, primary structure and postmeiotic expression in spermatogenesis. *Differentiation* 1990;42:160–166.
459. Klemm U, Flake A, Engel W. Rat sperm acrosin: cDNA sequence, derived primary structure and phylogenetic origin. *Biochim Biophys Acta* 1991;1090:270–272.
460. Töpfer-Petersen E, Čechová D, Henschen A, Steinberger M, Friess AE, Zucker A. Cell biology of acrosomal proteins. *Andrologia* 1990;Suppl 1:110–121.
461. Klemm U, Müller-Esterl W, Engel W. Acrosin, the peculiar sperm-specific serine protease. *Hum Genet* 1991;87:635–641.
462. Baba T, Michikawa Y, Kawakura K, Arai Y. Activation of boar proacrosin is effected by processing at both *N*- and *C*-terminal portions of the zymogen molecule. *FEBS Lett* 1989;244: 132–136.
463. Želenzná B, Čechová D, Henschen A. Isolation of the boar sperm acrosin peptide released during the conversion of α-form into β-form. *Hoppe Seylers Z Biol Chem* 1989;370:323–327.
464. Kashiwabara S-I, Arai Y, Kodaira K, Baba T. Acrosin biosynthesis in meiotic and postmeiotic spermatogenic cells. *Biochem Biophys Res Commun* 1990;173:240–245.
465. Anakwe OO, Sharma S, Hardy DM, Gerton GL. Guinea pig proacrosin is synthesized principally by round spermatids and contains *O*-linked as well as *N*-linked oligosaccharide side chains. *Mol Reprod Dev* 1991;29:172–179.
466. Escalier D, Gallo J-M, Albert M, et al. Human acrosome biogenesis: Immunodetection of proacrosin in primary spermatocytes and of its partitioning pattern during meiosis. *Development* 1991;113:779–788.
467. Moos J, Tesarik J, Leca G, Peknicova J. Mechanism of maturation and nature of carbohydrate chains of boar sperm acrosin. *FEBS Lett* 1991;294:27–30.
468. Anakwe OO, Sharma S, Hoff HB, Hardy DM, Gerton GL. Maturation of guinea pig sperm in the epididymis involves the modification of proacrosin oligosaccharide side chains. *Mol Reprod Dev* 1991;29:294–301.
469. Garner DL, Easton MP. Immunofluorescent localization of acrosin in mammalian spermatozoa. *J Exp Zool* 1977;200:157–162.
470. Morton DB. Acrosomal enzymes: Immunochemical localization of acrosin and hyaluronidase in ram spermatozoa. *J Reprod Fertil* 1975;45:375–378.
471. Morton DB. Lysosomal enzymes in mammalian spermatozoa. In: Edidin M, Johnson MH, eds. *Immunobiology of gametes.* London: Cambridge University Press; 1977:115–155.
472. Green DPL, Hockaday AR. The histochemical localization of acrosin in guinea-pig sperm after the acrosome reaction. *J Cell Sci* 1978;32:177–184.

473. Mukerji SK, Meizel S. The molecular transformation of rabbit testis proacrosin into acrosin. *Arch Biochem Biophys* 1975;168:720–721.
474. Noland TD, Davis LS, Olson GE. Regulation of proacrosin conversion in isolated guinea pig sperm acrosomal apical segments. *J Biol Chem* 1989;264:13586–13590.
475. Nuzzo NA, Anderson RA Jr, Zaneveld LJD. Proacrosin activation and acrosin release during the guinea pig acrosome reaction. *Mol Reprod Dev* 1990;25:52–60.
476. Baba T, Michikawa Y, Kashiwabara S-I, Arai Y. Proacrosin activation in the presence of a 32-kDa protein from boar spermatozoa. *Biochem Biophys Res Commun* 1989;160:1026–1032.
477. Flörke-Gerloff S, Tschesche H, Müller-Esterl W, Engel W. Intra-acrosomally located acrosin-inhibitors: Evolution and developmental patterns in mammals. *Gamete Res* 1984;10:327–337.
478. Möritz A, Lilja H, Fink E. Molecular cloning and sequence analysis of the cDNA encoding the human acrosin-trypsin inhibitor (HUSI-II). *FEBS Lett* 1991;278:127–130.
479. Jonáková V, Čechová D, Töpfer-Petersen E, Calvete JJ, Veselsky L. Variability of acrosin inhibitors in boar reproductive tract. *Biomed Biochim Acta* 1991;50:691–695.
480. Jonáková V, Calvete JJ, Mann K, Schäfer W, Schmid ER, Töpfer-Peterson E. The complete primary structure of three isoforms of a boar sperm-associated acrosin inhibitor. *FEBS Lett* 1992;297:147–150.
481. Moore A, Penfold LM, Johnson JL, Latchman DS, Moore HDM. Human sperm–egg binding is inhibited by peptides corresponding to core region of an acrosomal serine protease inhibitor. *Mol Reprod Dev* 1993;34:280–291.
482. Zaneveld LJD, Polakoski KL, Schumacher GFB. Properties of acrosomal hyaluronidase from bull spermatozoa. Evidence for its similarity to testicular hyaluronidase. *J Biol Chem* 1973; 248:564–570.
483. Yang C-H, Srivastava PN. Purification and properties of hyaluronidase from bull sperm. *J Biol Chem* 1975;250:79–83.
484. Goldberg E. Isozymes in testes and spermatozoa. In: Ratazzi M, Scandalios J, Whitt G, eds. *Isozymes: Current topics in biological and medical research, vol 1.* New York: Alan R Liss; 1977:79–124.
485. Brown CR. Distribution of hyaluronidase in the ram spermatozoon. *J Reprod Fertil* 1981;45:537–539.
486. Mancini RE, Alonso A, Barquet J, Nemirovski B. Histo-immunological localization of hyaluronidase in bull testis. *J Reprod Fertil* 1964;8:325–330.
487. Gould SF, Bernstein MH. Localization of bovine sperm hyaluronidase. *Differentiation* 1975;3:123–132.
488. Hardy DM, Oda MN, Friend DS, Huang TTF Jr. A mechanism for differential release of acrosomal enzymes during the acrosome reaction. *Biochem J* 1991;275:759–766.
489. Brown CR. Distribution of hyaluronidase in the ram spermatozoa. *J Reprod Fertil* 1975;45:537–539.
490. Harrison RAP, Gaunt SJ. Multiple forms of ram and bull sperm hyaluronidase revealed by using monoclonal antibodies. *J Reprod Fertil* 1988;82:777–785.
491. Harrison RAP. Preliminary characterization of the multiple forms of ram sperm hyaluronidase. *Biochem J* 1988;252: 875–882.
492. Majumder GC, Turkington RW. Acrosomal and lysosomal isoenzymes of β-galactosidase and *N*-acetyl-β-glucosaminidase in rat testis. *Biochemistry* 1974;13:2857–2864.
493. Majumder GC, Lessin S, Turkington RW. Hormonal regulation of isoenzymes of *N*-acetyl-β-glucosaminidase and β-galactosidase during spermatogenesis in the rat. *Endocrinology* 1975;96: 890–897.
494. Nikolajczyk BS, O'Rand MG. Characterization of rabbit testis β-galactosidase and arylsulfatase A: Purification and localization in spermatozoa during the acrosome reaction. *Biol Reprod* 1992;46:366–378.
495. Koren E, Milkovic S. "Collagenase-like" peptidase in human, rat and bull spermatozoa. *J Reprod Fertil* 1973;32:349–356.
496. Erickson RP, Martin SR. The relationship of mouse spermatozoal to mouse testicular cathepsins. *Arch Biochem Biophys* 1974;165:114–120.
497. Arboleda CE, Gerton GL. Studies of three major proteases associated with guinea pig sperm acrosomes. *J Exp Zool* 244:277–287.
498. Talbot P, DiCarlantonio G. Cytochemical localization of dipeptidyl peptidase II (DPP II) in mature guinea pig sperm. *J Histochem Cytochem* 1985;33:1169–1172.
499. DiCarlantonio G, Talbot P, Dudenhausen E. Partial purification and characterization of dipeptidyl peptidase II (DPP II) from guinea pig testes. *Gamete Res* 1986;15:161–175.
500. Schollmeyer JE. Identification of calpain II in porcine sperm. *Biol Reprod* 1986;34:721–731.
501. Srivastava PN, Abou-Issa H. Purification and properties of rabbit spermatozoal acrosomal neuraminidase. *Biochem J* 1977; 161:193–200.
502. Bryan JHD, Unithan RR. Non-specific esterase activity in bovine acrosomes. *Histochem J* 1972;4:413–419.
503. Meizel S, Cotham J. Partial characterization of a new bull sperm arylaminidase. *J Reprod Fertil* 1972;28:303–307.
504. Bhalla VK, Tillman WL, Williams WL. Presence of β-aspartyl *N*-acetylglucosamine amido hydrolase in mammalian spermatozoa. *J Reprod Fertil* 1973;34:137–139.
505. Dudkiewicz AB. Purification of boar acrosomal arylsulfatase A and possible role in the penetration of cumulus cells. *Biol Reprod* 1984;30:1005–1014.
506. Gonzales LW, Meizel S. Acid phosphatases of rabbit spermatozoa. II. Partial purification and biochemical characterization of the multiple forms of rabbit spermatozoan acid phosphatase. *Biochim Biophys Acta* 1973;320:180–194.
507. Stambaugh R, Buckley J. Comparative studies of the acrosomal enzymes of rabbit, rhesus monkey and human spermatozoa. *Biol Reprod* 1970;3:275–282.
508. Ribbes H, Plantavid M, Bennet PJ, Chap H, Douste-Blazy L. Phospholipase C from human sperm specific for phosphoinositides. *Biochim Biophys Acta* 1987;919:245–254.
509. Hinkovska-Galchev V, Srivastava PN. Phosphatidylcholine and phosphatidylinositol-specific phospholipases C of bull and rabbit spermatozoa. *Mol Reprod Dev* 1992;33:281–286.
510. Meizel S. The importance of hydrolytic enzymes to an exocytotic event, the mammalian sperm acrosome reaction. *Biol Rev* 1984;59:125–157.
511. Rönkkö S. Immunocytochemical localization of phospholipase A_2 in the bovine seminal vesicle and on the surface of the ejaculated spermatozoa. *Int J Biochem* 1992;24:869–876.
512. Karnik NS, Newman S, Kopf GS, Gerton GL. Developmental expression of G protein α subunits in mouse spermatogenic cells: Evidence that $G_{\alpha i}$ is associated with the developing acrosome. *Dev Biol* 1992;152:393–402.
513. Garty NB, Galiani D, Aharonheim A, et al. G-proteins in mammalian gametes: An immunocytochemical study. *J Cell Sci* 1988;91:21–31.
514. Glassner M, Jones J, Kligman I, Woolkalis MJ, Gerton GL, Kopf GS. Immunocytochemical and biochemical characterization of guanine nucleotide-binding regulatory proteins in mammalian spermatozoa. *Dev Biol* 1991;146:438–450.
515. Kopf GS, Gerton GL. The mammalian sperm acrosome and the acrosome reaction. In: Wassarman PM, ed. *Elements of fertilization, vol 1.* Boca Raton: CRC Press; 1991:153–203.
516. Naz RK, Ahmad K, Kaplan P. Involvement of cyclins and *cdc2* serine/threonine protein kinase in human sperm cell function. *Biol Reprod* 1993;48:720–728.
517. Jones HP, Lenz RW, Palevitz BA, Cormier MJ. Calmodulin localization in mammalian spermatozoa. *Proc Natl Acad Sci USA* 1980;77:2772–2776.
518. Weinman S, Ores-Carton C, Escaig F, Feinberg J, Puszkin S. Calmodulin immunoelectron microscopy: redistribution during ram spermatogenesis and epididymal maturation. II. *J Histochem Cytochem* 1986;34:1181–1193.
519. Anakwe OO, Gerton GL. Acrosome biogenesis during meiosis: Evidence from the synthesis and distribution of an acrosomal glycoprotein, acrogranin, during guinea pig spermatogenesis. *Biol Reprod* 1990;42:317–328.
520. Baba T, Hoff HB III, Nemoto H, et al. Acrogranin, an acrosomal cysteine-rich glycoprotein, is the precursor of the growth-

modulating peptides, granulins, and epithelins, and is expressed in somatic as well as male germ cells. *Mol Reprod Dev* 1993;34:233–243.
521. Kew D, Muffly KE, Kilpatrick DL. Proenkephalin products are stored in the sperm acrosome and may function in fertilization. *Proc Natl Acad Sci USA* 1990;87:9143–9147.
522. Schalling M, Persson H, Pelto-Huikko M, et al. Expression and localization of gastrin messenger RNA and peptide in spermatogenic cells. *J Clin Invest* 1990;86:660–669.
523. Persson H, Rehfeld JF, Ericsson A, Schalling M, Pelto-Huikko M, Hökfelt T. Transient expression of the cholecystokinin gene in male germ cells and accumulation of the peptide in the acrosomal granule: Possible role of cholecystokinin in fertilization. *Proc Natl Acad Sci USA* 1989;86:6166–6170.
524. Marquant-Le Guienne B, De Almeida M. Role of guinea-pig sperm autoantigens in capacitation and the acrosome reaction. *J Reprod Fertil* 1986;77:337–345.
525. Hardy DM, Huang TTF Jr, Driscoll WJ, Tung KSK, Wild GC. Purification and characterization of the primary acrosomal autoantigen of guinea pig epididymal spermatozoa. *Biol Reprod* 1988;38:423–437.
526. Gerton GL, O'Brien DA, Eddy EM. Antigens recognized by monoclonal antibody to mouse acrosomal components differ in guinea pig spermatogenic cells and sperm. *Biol Reprod* 1988;39:431–441.
527. Herr JC, Wright RM, John E, Foster J, Kays T, Flickinger CJ. Identification of human acrosomal antigen SP-10 in primates and pigs. *Biol Reprod* 1990;42:377–382.
528. Wright RM, John E, Klotz K, Flickinger CJ, Herr JC. Cloning and sequencing of cDNAs coding for the human intra-acrosomal antigen SP-10. *Biol Reprod* 1990;42:693–701.
529. Foster JA, Herr JC. Interactions of human sperm acrosomal protein SP-10 with the acrosomal membranes. *Biol Reprod* 1992;46:981–990.
530. Herr JC, Klotz K, Shannon J, Wright RM, Flickinger CJ. Purification and microsequencing of the intra-acrosomal protein SP-10. Evidence that SP-10 heterogeneity results from endoproteolytic processes. *Biol Reprod* 1992;47:11–20.
531. Liu M-S, Aebersold R, Fann C-H, Lee C-YG. Molecular and developmental studies of a sperm acrosome antigen recognized by HS-63 monoclonal antibody. *Biol Reprod* 1992;46:937–948.
532. Zamboni L, Stefanini M. The fine structure of the neck of mammalian spermatozoa. *Anat Rec* 1971;169:155–172.
533. Ōura C. The ultrastructure and development of the neck region of the golden hamster spermatozoon. *Monitore Zool Ital* 1971;5:253–264.
534. Millette CF, Spear PG, Gall WE, Edelman GM. Chemical dissection of mammalian spermatozoa. *J Cell Biol* 1973;58:662–675.
535. Young RJ, Cooper GW. Separation of the head and tail of mammalian spermatozoa by primary amines: Evidence for their junction by Schiff bases. In: Fawcett DW, Bedford JM, eds. *The spermatozoon.* Baltimore: Urban & Schwarzenberg; 1979:391–394.
536. Calvin HI. Isolation and subfractionation of mammalian sperm heads and tails. In: Prescott DM, ed. *Methods in cell biology, vol 13.* New York: Academic Press; 1976:85–104.
537. Bellvé AR, Anderson E, Hanley-Bowdoin L. Synthesis and amino acid composition of basic proteins in mammalian sperm nuclei. *Dev Biol* 1975;47:349–365.
538. Bedford JM, Calvin HI. Changes in the —S—S— linked structures of the sperm tail during epididymal maturation with comparative observations in sub-mammalian species. *J Exp Zool* 1974;187:181–204.
539. Blom E, Birch-Anderson A. The ultrastructure of the bull sperm. *Nord Vet Med* 1970;17:193–212.
540. Illison L. Fine structure of the mature spermatozoan head and neck of the mouse. *J Anat* 1966;100:949–950.
541. Woolley DM, Fawcett DW. The degeneration and disappearance of the centrioles during the development of the rat spermatozoon. *Anat Rec* 1973;177:289–302.
542. Fawcett DW, Porter KR. A study of the fine structure of ciliated epithelia. *J Morphol* 1954;94:221–281.
543. Gibbons IR, Grimstone AV. On flagellar structure in certain flagellates. *J Biophys Biochem Cytol* 1960;7:697–716.
544. Olson GE, Linck RW. Observations of the structural components of flagellar axonemes and central pair microtubules from rat sperm. *J Ultrastruct Res* 1977;61:21–43.
545. Bryan J, Wilson L. Are cytoplasmic microtubules heteropolymers? *Proc Natl Acad Sci USA* 1971;8:1762–1766.
546. Hecht NB, Kleene KC, Distel RJ, Silver LM. The differential expression of the actins and tubulins during spermatogenesis in the mouse. *Exp Cell Res* 1984;153:275–280.
547. Distel RJ, Kleene KC, Hecht NB. Haploid expression of a mouse testis α-tubulin gene. *Science* 224:68–70.
548. Slaughter GR, Meistrich ML, Means AR. Expression of RNAs for calmodulin, actins, and tubulins in rat testis cells. *Biol Reprod* 1989;40:395–405.
549. Vale RD, Reese TS, Sheetz MP. Identification of a novel force generating protein, kinesin, involved in microtubule-based motility. *Cell* 1985;42:39–50.
550. Vale RD, Goldstein LSB. One motor, many tails: An expanding repertoire of force-generating enzymes. *Cell* 1990;60:883–885.
551. Vale RD, Schnapp BJ, Mitchison T, Steuer E, Reese TS, Sheetz MP. Different axoplasmic proteins generate movement in opposite directions along microtubules in vitro. *Cell* 1985;43:623–632.
552. Hall ES, Eveleth J, Jiang C, Redenbach DM, Boekelheide K. Distribution of the microtubule-dependent motors cytoplasmic dynein and kinesin in rat testis. *Biol Reprod* 1992;46:817–828.
553. Pratt MM, Hisanaga S, Begg DA. An improved purification method for cytoplasmic dynein. *J Cell Biochem* 1984;26:19–33.
554. Gibbons IR, Rowe AJ. Dynein: A protein with ATPase activity from cilia. *Science* 1965;149:424–426.
555. Paschal BM, Vallee RB. Retrograde transport by the microtubule-associated protein MAP 1C. *Nature* 1987;330:181–183.
556. Gibbons IR, Fronk E. Some properties of bound and soluble dynein from sea urchin flagella. *J Cell Biol* 1972;54:365–381.
557. Linck RW. Flagellar doublet microtubules: Fractionation of minor components and α-tubulin from specific regions of the A-tubule. *J Cell Sci* 1976;20:405–539.
558. Linck RW, Langevin GL. Structure and chemical composition of insoluble filamentous components of sperm flagellar microtubules. *J Cell Biol* 1982;58:1–22.
559. Linck RW. The structure of microtubules. *Ann NY Acad Sci* 1982;383:98–121.
560. Linck RW, Albertini DF, Kenny DM, Langevin GL. Tektin filaments: Chemically unique filaments of sperm flagellar microtubules. *Cell Motil* 1982;Suppl 1:127–132.
561. Linck RW, Amos LA, Amos WB. Localization of tektin filaments in microtubules of sea urchin flagella by immunoelectron microscopy. *J Cell Biol* 1985;100:126–135.
562. Woolley DM. Striations in the peripheral fibers of rat and mouse spermatozoa. *J Cell Biol* 1971;49:936–939.
563. Woolley DM. Selection for the length of the spermatozoan midpiece in the mouse. *Genet Res* 1970;16:225–228.
564. Phillips DM. Ultrastructure of spermatozoa of the woolly opossum *Caluromys philander. J Ultrastruct Res* 1970;33:381–397.
565. Olson GE, Winfrey VP. Mitochondria—cytoskeletal interactions in the sperm midpiece. *J Struct Biol* 1990;103:13–22.
566. Olson GE, Winfrey VP. Isolation of a cytoskeletal complex associated with sperm mitochondria. *Biol Reprod* 1989;40:142.
567. Calvin HI, Cooper GW, Wallace EW. Evidence that selenium in rat sperm is associated with a cysteine-rich structural protein of the mitochondrial capsule. *Gamete Res* 1981;4:139–149.
568. Calvin HI, Wallace EW, Cooper GW. Role of selenium in the organization of the mitochondrial sheath in the organization of the mitochondrial sheath in rodent spermatozoa. In: Spallholz JE, Martin JL, Ganther HE, eds. *Selenium in biology and medicine.* Westport: AVI; 1981:319–324.
569. Pallini V, Bacci E. Bull sperm selenium is bound to a structural protein of mitochondria. *J Submicr Cytol* 1979;11:165–170.
570. Pallini V, Baccetti B, Burrini AG. A peculiar cysteine-rich polypeptide as related to some unusual properties of mammalian sperm mitochondria. In: Fawcett DW, Bedford JM, eds. *The spermatozoon: Maturation, motility, surface properties and comparative aspects.* Baltimore: Urban & Schwarzenberg; 1979:141–151.

571. Calvin HI, Grosshans K, Musicant-Shikora SR, Turner SI. A developmental study of rat sperm and testis selenoproteins. *J Reprod Fertil* 1987;81:1–11.
572. Kleene KC, Smith J, Bozorgzadeh A, et al. Sequence and developmental expression of the mRNA encoding the seleno-protein of the sperm mitochondrial capsule in the mouse. *Dev Biol* 1990;137:395–402.
573. Serres C, Feneux D, Jouannet P. Abnormal distribution of the periaxonemal structures in a human sperm flagellar dyskinesia. *Cell Motil Cytoskel* 1984;6:68–76.
574. Lindemann CB, Fentie I, Rikmenspoel R. A selective effect of Ni^{2+} on wave initiation in bull sperm flagella. *J Cell Biol* 1980;87:420–426.
575. Telkka A, Fawcett DW, Christensen AK. Further observations on the structure of the mammalian sperm tail. *Anat Rec* 1961;141:231–246.
576. Fawcett DW, Phillips DW. The fine structure and development of the neck region of the mammalian spermatozoon. *Anat Rec* 1969;165:153–184.
577. de Kretser DM. Ultrastructural features of human spermiogenesis. *Z Zellforsch* 1969;98:229–236.
578. Sapsford CS, Rae CA, Cleland KW. Ultrastructural studies on the development and form of the principal piece sheath of the Bandicoot spermatozoon. *Aust J Zool* 1970;8:21–48.
579. Irons MJ, Clermont Y. Formation of the outer dense fibers during spermiogenesis in the rat. *Anat Rec* 1982;202:463–471.
580. Oko R, Clermont Y. Light microscopic immunocytochemical study of fibrous sheath and outer dense fiber formation in the rat spermatid. *Anat Rec* 1989;225:46–55.
581. Clermont Y, Oko R, Hermo L. Immunocytochemical localization of proteins utilized in the formation of outer dense fibers and fibrous sheath in rat spermatids: An electron microscope study. *Anat Rec* 1990;227:447–457.
582. Gordon M, Bensch KG. Cytochemical differentiation of the guinea pig sperm flagellum with phosphotungstic acid. *J Ultrastruct Res* 1968;24:33–50.
583. Olson GE, Sammons DW. Structural chemistry of outer dense fibers of rat sperm. *Biol Reprod* 1980;22:319–332.
584. Baccetti B, Pallini V, Burrini AG. The accessory fibers of the sperm tail. III. High-sulfur and low-sulfur components in mammals and cephalopods. *J Ultrastruct Res* 1976;57:289–308.
585. Pihlaja DJ, Roth LE. Bovine sperm fractionation. II. Morphology and chemical analysis of tail segments. *J Ultrastruct Res* 1973;44:293–309.
586. Baccetti B, Pallini V, Burrini AG. The accessory fibers of the sperm tail. I. Structure and chemical composition of the bull coarse fibers. *J Submicrosc Cytol* 1973;5:237–256.
587. Zittle CW, O'Dell RA. Chemical studies of bull spermatozoa. Lipid, sulfur, cystine, nitrogen, phosphorus, and nucleic acid content of whole spermatozoa and of the parts obtained by physical means. *J Biol Chem* 1941;140:899–907.
588. Price JM. Biochemical and morphological studies of outer dense fibers of rat spermatozoa. *J Cell Biol* 1973;59:272a.
589. Vera JC, Brito M, Zuvic T, Burzio LO. Polypeptide composition of rat sperm outer dense fibers. *J Biol Chem* 1984;259: 5970–5977.
590. Oko R. Comparative analysis of proteins from the fibrous sheath and outer dense fibers of rat spermatozoa. *Biol Reprod* 1988;39:168–182.
591. Brito M, Figueroa J, Vera JC, Cortes P, Hott R, Burzio LO. Phosphoproteins are structural components of bull sperm outer dense fiber. *Gamete Res* 1986;15:327–336.
592. Henkel R, Stalf T, Miska W. Isolation and partial characterization of the outer dense fiber proteins from human spermatozoa. *Hoppe Seylers Z Biol Chem* 1992;373:685–689.
593. Burfeind P, Hoyer-Fender S. Sequence and developmental expression of a mRNA encoding a putative protein of rat sperm outer dense fibers. *Dev Biol* 1991;148:195–204.
594. Kuhn R, Schafer U, Schafer M. *Cis*-acting regions sufficient for spermatocyte-specific transcriptional and spermatid-specific transcriptional and spermatid-specific translational control of the *Drosophila melanogaster* gene mst(3)gl-9. *EMBO J* 1988; 7:447–454.
595. Calvin HI. Electrophoretic evidence for the identity of the major zinc-binding polypeptides in the rat sperm tail. *Biol Reprod* 1979;21:873–882.
596. Gunn SA, Gould TC. Cadmium and other mineral elements. In: Johnson AD, Gomes WR, Vandemark NL, eds. *The testis, vol III*. New York: Academic Press; 1970:377–481.
597. Miller MJ, Vincent NR, Mawson CA. An autoradiographic study of the distribution of zinc-65 in rat tissues. *J Histochem Cytochem* 1961;9:111–125.
598. Bradley FM, Meth BM, Bellvé AR. Structural proteins of the mouse spermatozoan tail: An electrophoretic analysis. *Biol Reprod* 1981;24:691–701.
599. Nagano T. Localization of adenosine triphosphatase activity in the rat sperm tail as revealed by electron microscopy. *J Cell Biol* 1965;25:101–112.
600. Cleland KW, Lord Rothschild. The bandicoot spermatozoon: An electron microscopic study of the tail. *Proc R Soc Lond [Biol]* 1959;150:24–42.
601. Nelson L. Cytochemical studies with the electron microscope. I. Adenosine triphosphatease in the rat spermatozoa. *Biochim Biophys Acta* 1958;27:634–641.
602. Baltz JM, Williams PO, Cone RA. Dense fibers protect mammalian sperm against damage. *Biol Reprod* 1990;43:485–491.
603. Irons MJ, Clermont Y. Formatin of the outer dense fibers during spermiogenesis in the rat. *Anat Rec* 1982;202:463–471.
604. Rattner JB, Brinkley BR. Ultrastructure of mammalian spermiogenesis. I. A tubular complex in developing sperm of the cotton-top marmoset *Sequinus oedipus*. *J Ultrastruct Res* 1970; 32:316–322.
605. Wartenberg H, Holstein AF. Morphology of the "spindle-shaped body" in the developing tail of human spermatids. *Cell Tissue Res* 1975;159:435–443.
606. Bradfield JRG. Fibre patterns in animal flagella and cilia. *Symp Soc Exp Biol* 1955;9:306–334.
607. Olson GE, Hamilton DW, Fawcett DW. Isolation and characterization of the fibrous sheath of rat epididymal spermatozoa. *Biol Reprod* 1976;14:517–530.
608. Brito M, Figueroa J, Maldonado EU, Vera JC, Burzio LO. The major component of the rat sperm fibrous sheath is a phosphoprotein. *Gamete Res* 1989;22:205–217.
609. Eddy EM, O'Brien DA, Fenderson BA, Welch JE. Intermediate filament-like proteins in the fibrous sheath of the mouse sperm flagellum. *Ann NY Acad Sci* 1991;637:224–239.
610. O'Brien DO, Bellvé AR. Protein constituents of the mouse spermatozoon. II. Temporal synthesis during spermatogenesis. *Dev Biol* 1980;75:405–418.
611. Beecher KL, Homyk M, Lee C-YG, Herr JC. Evidence that 68-kilodalton and 54–51-kilodalton polypeptides are components of the human sperm fibrous sheath. *Biol Reprod* 1993;48:154–164.
612. Koyama Y, Shinomiya T, Sakai Y, Shiba T, Yanagisawa KO. Identification of sperm antigenic determinants with phylogenetically diverse and limited distribution using monoclonal antibodies. *J Reprod Immunol* 1984;6:141–150.
613. Sakai Y, Koyama Y-I, Fujimoto H, Nakamoto T, Yamashina S. Immunocytochemical study on fibrous sheath formation in mouse spermiogenesis using a monoclonal antibody. *Anat Rec* 1986;215:119–126.
614. Fenderson BA, Toshimori K, Muller CH, Lane TF, Eddy EM. Identification of a protein in the fibrous sheath of the sperm flagellum. *Biol Reprod* 1987;38:345–357.
615. Jassim A, Auger D, Oliver T, Sachs J. GDA-J/F3 monoclonal antibody as a novel probe for the human sperm tail fibrous sheath and its anomalies. *Hum Reprod* 1990;5:990–996.
616. Jassim A. AJ-p97: A novel antigen of the human sperm tail fibrous sheath detected by a neurofilament monoclonal antibody. *J Reprod Immunol* 1991;20:15–26.
617. Phillips DM. Comparative analysis of mammalian sperm motility. *J Cell Biol* 1972;53:561–573.
618. Hunter DG, Kretzer FL. Abnormal axonemes in sperm of fertile men. *Arch Androl* 1986;16:1–12.
619. Pelfrey RJ, Overstreet JW, Lewis EL. Abnormalities of sperm morphology in cases of persistent infertility after vasectomy reversal. *Fertil Steril* 1982;33:160–166.

620. Escalier D, Serres C. Aberrant distribution of the peri-axonemal structures in the human spermatozoon: possible role of the axoneme in the spatial organization of the flagellar components. *Biol Cell* 1985;53:239–250.
621. Aitken RJ, Ross A, Lees MM. Analysis of sperm function in Kartagener's syndrome. *Fertil Steril* 1983;40:696–698.
622. Smith D, Ōura C, Zamboni L. Fertilizing ability of structurally abnormal spermatozoa. *Nature* 1970;227:79–80.
623. Baccetti B, Burrini AG, Pallini V. Spermatozoa and cilia lacking axoneme in an infertile man. *Andrologia* 1980;12:525–532.
624. Ross A, Christie S, Edmond P. Ultrastructural tail defects in the spermatozoa from two men attending a subfertility clinic. *J Reprod Fertil* 1975;32:243–251.
625. Williamson RA, Koehler JK, Smith WD. Ultrastructural sperm tail defects associated with sperm immotility. *Fertil Steril* 1984;41:103–107.
626. Sauvalle A, Le Bris C, Izard J. Supernumerary microtubules and prolongation of the middle piece in two infertile patients. *Int J Fertil* 1983;28:173–176.
627. Chemes HE, Brugo S, Zanchetti F, Carrere C, Lavieri JC. Dysplasia of the fibrous sheath: An ultrastructural defect of human spermatozoa associated with sperm immotility and primary sterility. *Fertil Steril* 1987;48:664–669.
628. Afzelius BA. Genetical and ultrastructural aspects of the immotile-cilia syndrome. *Am J Hum Genet* 1981;33:852–864.
629. Afzelius BA. A human syndrome caused by immotile cilia. *Science* 1976;193:317–319.
630. Afzelius BA, Eliasson R. Flagellar mutants in man: On the heterogeneity of the immotile-cilia syndrome. *J Ultrastruct Res* 1979;69:43–52.
631. Leestma JE, Sepsenwol S. Sperm tail axoneme alterations in the Wobbler mouse. *J Reprod Fertil* 1980;58:267–270.
632. Olds PJ. Effect of the T locus on sperm ultrastructure in the house mouse. *J Anat* 1971;109:31–37.
633. Bryan JHD. Spermatogenesis revisited: IV. The course of spermiogenesis in mice homozygous for another male-sterility-inducing mutation, hpy (hydrocephalic-polydactyl). *Cell Tissue Res* 1977;180:187–201.
634. Cooper TG, Hamilton DW. Observations on destruction of spermatozoa in the cauda epididymides and proximal vas deferens of non-seasonal male animals. *Am J Anat* 1977;149:93–110.
635. Bennett WI, Gall AM, Southard JL, Sidman RL. Abnormal spermiogenesis in quaking. A myelin-deficient mutant mouse. *Biol Reprod* 1971;5:30–58.
636. Woolley DM. Evidence for twisted plane undulation in golden hamster sperm tails. *J Cell Biol* 1977;67:159–170.
637. Yeung CH, Woolley DM. Three-dimensional bend propagation in hamster sperm models and the direction of roll in free-swimming cells. *Cell Motil* 1984;4:215–226.
638. Woolley DM, Osborn IW. Three-dimensional geometry of motile hamster spermatozoa. *J Cell Sci* 1984;67:159–170.
639. Phillips DM, Olson GE. Mammalian sperm motility. Structure in relation to function. In: Afzelius BA, ed. *The functional anatomy of the spermatozoon.* New York: Pergamon Press; 1975:117–126.
640. Lindemann CB. Requirements for motility in mammalian sperm. In: Steinberger A, Steinberger E, eds. *Testicular development, structure and function.* New York: Raven Press; 1980:473–479.
641. Yeung CH, Woolley DM. A study of bend formation in locally reactivated hamster sperm flagella. *J Muscle Res Cell Motil* 1983;4:625–645.
642. Rikmenspoel R. Movements and active moments of bull sperm flagella as a function of temperature and viscosity. *J Exp Biol* 1984;108:205–230.
643. Serres C, Feneux D, Jouannet P, David G. Influence of the flagellar wave development and propagation on the human sperm movement in seminal plasma. *Gamete Res* 1984;9:183–195.
644. Gray J. The movement of the spermatozoa of the bull. *J Exp Biol* 1958;35:96–108.
645. Feneux D, Serres C, Jouannet P. Sliding spermatozoa: A dyskinesia responsible for human infertility? *Fertil Steril* 1985;44:508–511.
646. Turner TT, Giles RD. A sperm motility inhibiting factor in the rat epididymis. *Am J Physiol* 1982;242:R199–R203.
647. Usselman MC, Cone RA. Rat sperm are mechanically immobilized in the cauda epididymidis by "immobilin," a high molecular weight glycoprotein. *Biol Reprod* 1983;29:1241–1253.
648. Turner TT, Reich GW. Cauda epididymidal sperm motility: A comparison among five species. *Biol Reprod* 1985;32:120–128.
649. Carr DW, Acott TS. Inhibition of bovine spermatozoa by cauda epididymidal fluid: I. Studies of a sperm motility quiescence factor. *Biol Reprod* 1984;30:913–925.
650. Hoskins DD, Stephens DT, Hall ML. Cyclic adenosine 3′,5′-monophosphate and protein kinase levels in developing bovine spermatozoa. *J Reprod Fertil* 1974;37:131–133.
651. Amann RP, Hay SR, Hammerstedt RH. Yield, characteristics, motility and cAMP content of sperm isolated from seven regions of ram epididymis. *Biol Reprod* 1982;27:723–733.
652. Chulavatnatol M, Panyim S, Wititsuwannakul D. Comparison of phosphorylated proteins in intact rat spermatozoa from caput and cauda epididymidis. *Biol Reprod* 1982;26:197–207.
653. Brandt H, Acott TS, Johnson DJ, Hoskins DD. Evidence for the epididymal origin of bovine sperm forward motility protein. *Biol Reprod* 1978;19:830–835.
654. Garbers DL, Kopf GS. The regulation of spermatozoa by calcium and cyclic nucleotides. In: Greengard P, Robison GA, eds. *Advances in cyclic nucleotide research.* New York: Raven Press; 1980:251–306.
655. Hyne RV, Garbers DL. Regulation of guinea pig sperm adenylate cyclase by calcium. *Biol Reprod* 1979;21:1135–1142.
656. Wasco WM, Orr GA. Function of calmodulin in mammalian sperm: Presence of a calmodulin-dependent cyclic nucleotide phosphodiesterase associated with demembranated rat caudal epididymal sperm. *Biochem Biophys Res Commun* 1984;118:632–642.
657. Slaughter GR, Means AR. Analysis of expression of multiple genes encoding calmodulin during spermatogenesis. *Mol Endocrinol* 1989;3:1569–1578.
658. Horowitz JA, Toeg H, Orr GA. Characterization and localization of cAMP-dependent protein kinases in rat caudal epididymal sperm. *J Biol Chem* 1984;259:832–838.
659. Noland TD, Corbin JD, Garbers DL. Cyclic AMP-dependent protein kinase isozymes of bovine epididymal spermatozoa: Evidence against the existence of an ectokinase. *Biol Reprod* 1986;34:681–689.
660. Sandberg M, Tasken K, Oyen O, Hansson V, Jahnsen T. Molecular cloning, cDNA structure and deduced amino acid sequence for A type I regulatory subunit of cAMP-dependent protein kinase from human testis. *Biochem Biophys Res Commun* 1987;149:939–945.
661. Oyen O, Scott JD, Cadd GG, et al. A unique mRNA species for a regulatory subunit of cAMP-dependent protein kinase is specifically induced in haploid germ cells. *FEBS Lett* 1988;229:391–394.
662. Beebe SJ, Oyen O, Sandberg M, Frøysa A, Hansson V, Jahnsen T. Molecular cloning of a tissue-specific protein kinase (Cγ) from human testis—Representing a third isoform for the catalytic subunit of cAMP-dependent protein kinase. *Mol Endocrinol* 1990;4:465–475.
663. Massa JS, Fellows RE, Maurer RA. Rat RIb isoform of type I regulatory subunit of cyclic adenosine monophosphate-dependent protein kinase: cDNA sequence analysis, mRNA tissue specificity, and rat/mouse difference in expression in testis. *Mol Reprod Dev* 1990;26:129–133.
664. Oyen O, Myklebust F, Scott JD, et al. Subunits of cyclic adenosine 3′,5′-monophosphate-dependent protein kinase show differential and distinct expression patterns during germ cell differentiation: Alternative polyadenylation in germ cells gives rise to unique smaller-sized mRNA species. *Biol Reprod* 1990;43:46–54.
665. Tang FY, Hoskins DD. Phosphoprotein phosphatase of bovine epididymal spermatozoa. *Biochem Biophys Res Commun* 1976;62:328–335.
666. Kitagawa Y, Sasaki K, Shima H, Shibuya M, Sugimura T, Nagao

M. Protein phosphatases possibly involved in rat spermatogenesis. *Biochem Biophys Res Commun* 1990;171:230–235.
667. Tash JS. Investigations on adenosine 3′,5′-monophosphate phosphodiesterase in ram semen and initial characterization of a sperm-specific enzyme. *J Reprod Fertil* 1976;47:63–67.
668. Stephens DT, Wang JL, Hoskins DD. The cyclic AMP phosphodiesterase of bovine spermatozoa: Multiple forms, kinetic properties, and changes during development. *Biol Reprod* 1979; 20:483–491.
669. Swinnen JV, Joseph DR, Conti M. Molecular cloning of rat homologues of the *Drosophila melanogaster* dunce cAMP phosphodiesterase: Evidence for a family of genes. *Proc Natl Acad Sci USA* 86:5325–5329.
670. Welch JE, Swinnen JV, O'Brien DA, Eddy EM, Conti M. Unique adenosine 3′,5′ cyclic monophosphate phosphodiesterase messenger ribonucleic acids in rat spermatogenic cells: Evidence for differential gene expression during spermatogenesis. *Biol Reprod* 1992;46:1027–1033.
671. Tash JS, Means AR. Regulation of protein phosphorylation and motility of sperm by cyclic adenosine monophosphate and calcium. *Biol Reprod* 1982;26:745–763.
672. Ono T, Koide Y, Arai Y, Yamashita K. Establishment of an efficient purification method and further characterization of 32K calmodulin-binding protein in testis. *J Biochem* 1985;98: 1455–1461.
673. Garbers DL, Tubb DJ, Hyne RV. A requirement of bicarbonate for Ca^{2+}-induced elevation of cyclic AMP in guinea pig spermatozoa. *J Biol Chem* 1982;257:8980–8984.
674. Vijayaraghavan S, Critchlow LM, Hoskins DD. Evidence for a role for cellular alkalinization in the cyclic adenosine 3′,5′-monophosphate-mediated initiation of motility in bovine caput spermatozoa. *Biol Reprod* 1985;32:489–500.
675. Gibbons IR. Cilia and flagella of eukaryotes. *J Cell Biol* 1981;91:107s–124s.
676. Lindemann CB. A cAMP-induced increase in the motility of demembranated bull sperm models. *Cell* 1978;13:9–18.
677. Mohri H, Yanagimachi R. Characteristics of motor apparatus in testicular, epididymal and ejaculated spermatozoa. A study using demembranated sperm models. *Exp Cell Res* 1980;127:191–196.
678. White IG, Voglmayr JK. ATP-induced reactivation of ram testicular, cauda epididymal, and ejaculated spermatozoa extracted with Triton X-100. *Biol Reprod* 1986;34:183–193.
679. Okamura N, Sugita Y. Activation of spermatozoan adenylate cyclase by a low molecular weight factor in porcine seminal plasma. *J Biol Chem* 1983;258:13056–13062.
680. Vijayaraghavan S, Hoskins DD. Regulation of bovine sperm motility and cyclic adenosine 3′,5′-monophosphate by adenosine and its analogues. *Biol Reprod* 1986;34:468–477.
681. Hyne RV, Lopata A. Calcium and adenosine affect human sperm adenylate cyclase activity. *Gamete Res* 1982;6:81–89.
682. Brown MA, Casillas ER. Bovine sperm adenylate cyclase inhibition by adenosine and adenosine analogs. *J Androl* 1984; 5:361–368.
683. Henry D, Ferino F, Tomova S, Ferry N, Stengel D, Hanoune J. Inhibition of the catalytic subunit of ram sperm adenylate cyclase by adenosine. *Biochem Biophys Res Commun* 1986;137: 970–977.
684. Krebs EG, Beavo JA. Phosphorylation-dephosphorylation of enzymes. *Annu Rev Biochem* 1979;48:923–956.
685. Hildebrandt JD, Codina J, Tash JS, et al. The membrane-bound spermatozoal adenyl cyclase system does not share coupling characteristics with somatic cell adenyl cyclases. *Endocrinology* 1985;116:1357–1366.
686. Kopf GS, Woolkalis MJ, Gerton GL. Evidence for a guanine nucleotide-binding regulatory protein in invertebrate and mammalian sperm. Identification by islet-activating protein-catalyzed ADP-ribosylation and immunochemical methods. *J Biol Chem* 1986;261:7327–7331.
687. Brandt H, Hoskins DD. A cAMP-dependent phosphorylated motility protein in bovine epididymal sperm. *J Biol Chem* 1980;255:982–987.
688. Tash JS, Kakar SS, Means AR. Flagellar motility requires the cAMP-dependent phosphorylation of a heat-stable NP-40-soluble 56 kd protein, axokinin. *Cell* 1984;38:551–559.
689. de Lamirande E, Gagnon C. Origin of a motility inhibitor within the male reproductive tract. *J Androl* 1984;5:269–276.
690. Freedman MF, Kopf GS. Characterization of a seminal plasma-associated inhibitor of human seminal plasma protein kinase. *Biol Reprod* 1985;32:322–332.
691. Pliego JF, Van-Arsdalen K, Kopf GS. Distribution of a seminal plasma-associated protein kinase inhibitor in normal, oligozoospermic, and vasectomized men. *Biol Reprod* 1986;34:885–893.
692. Byrd W, Sokoloski JE, Wolf DP. Analysis of calcium uptake during incubation of human spermatozoa. *Biol Reprod* [*Suppl*] 1983;28:103.
693. Rufo GA, Singh JP, Babcock DF, Lardy HA. Purification and characterization of a calcium transport inhibitor from bovine seminal plasma. *J Biol Chem* 1982;257:4627–4632.
694. Goh P, Hoskins DD. The involvement of methyl transfer reactions and *S*-adenosylhomocysteine in the regulation of bovine sperm motility. *Gamete Res* 1985;12:399–409.
695. Bouchard P, Penningroth SM, Cheung A, Gagnon C, Bardin CW. Erythro-9-[3-(2-hydroxynonyl)] adenine is an inhibitor of sperm motility that blocks dynein ATPase and protein carboxymethylase activities. *Proc Natl Acad Sci USA* 1981;78: 1033–1036.
696. Gagnon C, Sherins RJ, Phillips DM, Bardin CW. Deficiency of protein carboxymethylase in immotile spermatozoa of infertile men. *N Engl J Med* 1982;306:821–825.
697. Acott TS, Carr DW. Inhibition of bovine spermatozoa by cauda epididymal fluid: II. Interaction of pH and a quiescence factor. *Biol Reprod* 1984;30:926–935.

The Physiology of Reproduction, Second Edition,
edited by E. Knobil and J.D. Neill,
Raven Press, Ltd., New York © 1994.

CHAPTER 3

The Mammalian Ovum

Paul M. Wassarman[1] and David F. Albertini[2]

GENERAL INTRODUCTION

The mammalian ovum, or egg, is the link between one generation and the next. In 1880, Nussbaum (235) recognized that "The fertilized egg, accordingly, divides into cells that constitute the individual and cells for maintenance of the species." This concept was expanded insightfully by Wilson (381), who in 1925 explained that the differences in form and function between sperm and egg are attributable to "a physiological division of labor between the gametes of the two sexes." Continuing this theme, Wilson explained:

> The ovum has to supply most of the material for the body of the embryo, and often also to provide for its protection and maintenance during development. For this service it prepares by extensive growth, accumulat-

[1] Roche Institute of Molecular Biology, Roche Research Center, Nutley, New Jersey 07110
[2] Department of Anatomy and Cellular Biology, Tufts University School of Medicine, Boston, Massachusetts 02111

ing a large amount of protoplasm, commonly laden with reserve food matter (yolk or deutoplasm), and in many cases becoming surrounded by membranes or other protective envelopes. During its early history, therefore, the ovum is characterized by predominance of the constructive or anabolic process of metabolism (381).

Herein lies the origin of the concept that there is not only a genetic but also a biochemical basis for the phrase "embryogenesis begins during oogenesis." Today, there is overwhelming experimental evidence that the zygote inherits from the egg an extensive reserve of macromolecules and organelles that, to varying degrees, supports the nutritional, synthetic, energetic, and regulatory requirements of the early embryo (13,60,101). This is as true for mammals as it is for lower vertebrates and invertebrates, despite the obvious enormous differences in both reproductive and developmental behavior of mammals and nonmammals.

Here, many of the features of mammalian egg development are reviewed. Although emphasis is placed on mouse egg development in order to increase the clarity of the presentation, most of the principles discussed can be applied to other mammals. Furthermore, in the interest of clarity and brevity, some important contributions are not cited, and specific points of view are adopted on issues that may be the subject of some controversy among workers in the field. It is hoped that because of these and other shortcomings the reader will be stimulated to refer to other detailed accounts of research on mammalian egg development (12,14,40,60,127,129, 160,172,180,252,306,307,350,393–395,360) as well as technical aspects of this research (99,100,160,172,278,365).

THE MAMMALIAN OVUM: A CHRONOLOGICAL PERSPECTIVE

Although the ovary was recognized as an anatomic entity by Herophilus of Alexandria in ca. 300 B.C. and described in some detail by Soranus of Ephesus in ca. A.D. 50, the mammalian ovum or egg was not identified until early in the 19th century by Karl Ernst von Baer. Earlier, de Graaf (ca. 1670) had recognized that eggs came from the ovary but concluded incorrectly that the entire follicle (Graafian follicle) was an egg. This misconception was rectified somewhat by Cruickshank (ca. 1795) and others; however, it remained for von Baer (ca. 1825) to elucidate the exact anatomic relationship between egg and follicle in mammals (Fig. 1). Nearly 150 years, then, separated identification of spermatozoa by Leeuwenhoek (ca. 1675) and eggs by von Baer.

Waldeyer (ca. 1870) is credited with championing the concept that, in mammals, the sexually mature female possesses a finite stock of oocytes that is drawn upon throughout her reproductive life. However, the alternative view, that generation of oocytes is a continual process throughout a female's reproductive life (i.e., similar to spermatogenesis), although based on subjective interpretation of relevant observations, prevailed during the first half of this century. Not until the early 1950s was this controversial issue finally put to rest and Waldeyer's tenet accepted, essentially because of the work of Zuckerman and colleagues. Goette (ca. 1875) and Nussbaum (ca. 1880) were among the first to recognize that primordial germ cells, destined to give rise to oocytes and eggs, arise from undifferentiated cells located some distance away from, and appearing before the formation of, the genital ridges. Appreciation for the subsequent organogenesis of the mammalian ovary came about primarily as a result of the work of de Winiwarter and Sainmont in 1910, and by the 1920s, a great deal of cytological information about oocyte development was already available.

In the 1920s it was recognized that the ovary is under functional control of the anterior hypophysis, and, by the late 1920s and early 1930s, the relationship between oocyte and follicle development began to be appreciated as a result of work by Brambell, Parkes, Zuckerman,

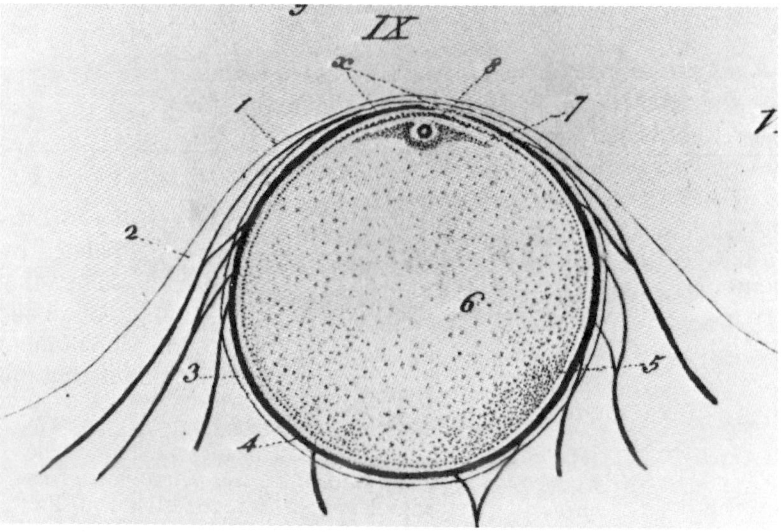

FIG. 1. Drawing of the mammalian egg within the Graafian follicle by von Baer, *De Ovi Mammalium et Hominis Genesi* (1827). Vesicula Graafiana (mediae magnitudinis) scrofae, decies aucta ad axin dissecta (IX). (*1*) Epithelium peritoneale; (*2*) tela formativa (stroma); (*3*) stratum externum (thecae); (*4*) stratum internum (thecae); (*5*) membrana granulosa (nuclei); (*6*) fluidum contentum; (*7*) discus proligerus (nuclei); (*8*) ovulum (nuclei); (*x*) stigma. (From ref. 318.)

Pincus, and colleagues. Particularly important work during this period, primarily from Pincus's laboratory, involved comparison of mammalian egg behavior *in vivo* and *in vitro.* In the late 1930s, the principal ovarian steroids were isolated and characterized, and by the early 1950s, much of the endocrinological basis of pituitary–ovarian interaction affecting oogenesis and ovulation was appreciated. By the 1960s, *in vitro* culture of mammalian eggs and biochemical investigation of their metabolism became a reality as a result of work by Mintz, Biggers, McLaren, Epstein, Brinster, Graham, Piko, and others. This brief history has been drawn from discussions found in the literature (10,235,280,318,381,393,395).

DEVELOPMENT OF THE OVUM

Oogenesis: From Primordial Germ Cells to Eggs

In mammals, oogenesis begins relatively early in fetal development and ends, months to years later, in the sexually mature adult (27,28,55–57,138,155,172,180,252, 259,291,320,385,393,395). Oogenesis begins with primordial germ cell formation and encompasses a series of cellular transformations, from primordial germ cells to oogonia (fetus), from oogonia to oocytes (fetus), and from oocytes to eggs (adult) (Fig. 2). This exquisitely orchestrated process results in a cell uniquely able to give rise to a new individual that expresses and maintains characteristics of the species. A description of oogenesis in mammals follows.

Origin and Behavior of Primordial Germ Cells

Eggs originate from a small number of stem cells, the *primordial germ cells,* that have an extragonadal origin (65,69,88,120,121,138,155,164,172,180,217,224,385). Formation of these cells in presomite embryos signals the beginning of oogenesis. In 8-day mouse embryos (four pairs of somites), as few as 15 and as many as 100 primordial germ cells are recognizable because of their

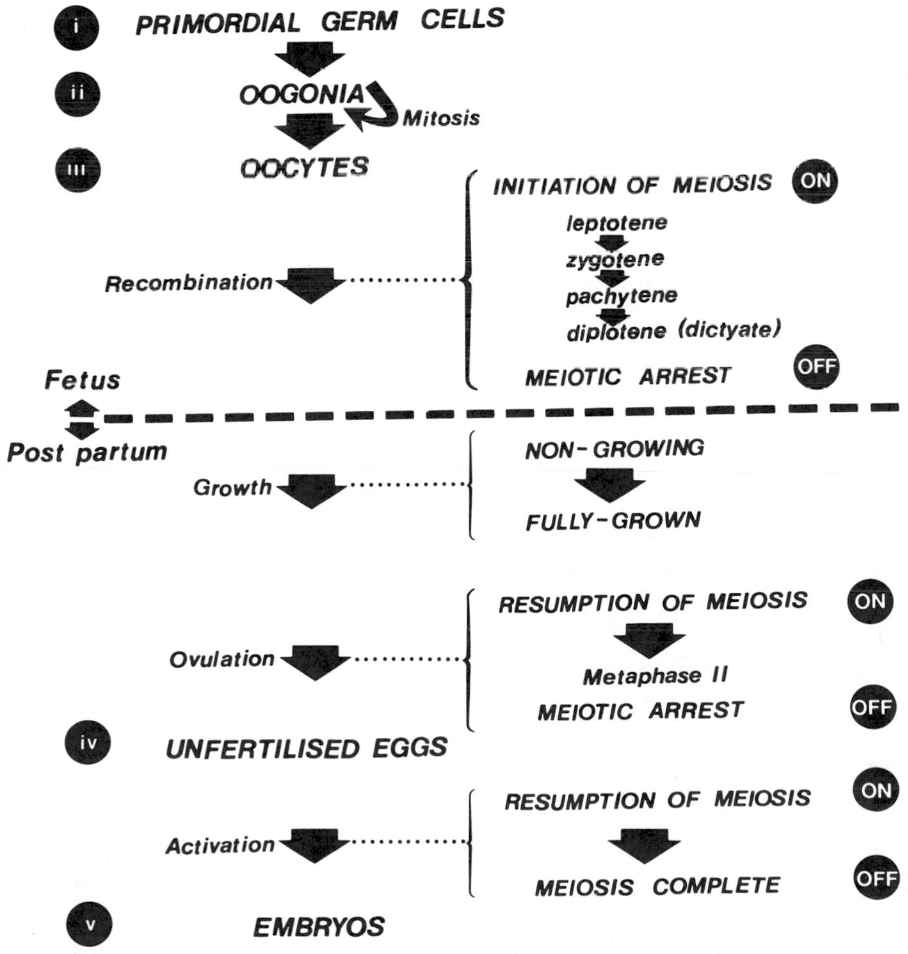

FIG. 2. Landmarks of oogenesis in the mouse. Progression from primordial germ cells to nongrowing oocytes during fetal development, as well as from nongrowing oocytes to fertilized eggs in sexually mature adults.

size, distinctive morphology, and characteristic cytochemical staining properties. These large cells (~12 μm in diameter) are found in the yolk sac endoderm and in that region of the allantois arising from the primitive streak. Several lines of evidence suggest that the embryonic rudiment of the allantois and caudal end of the primitive streak may be considered regions of primordial germ cell formation. In this context, it has been found that primitive ectoderm, taken from the caudal end of 7- to 7.5-day egg cylinders and cultured *in vitro,* differentiates into cells having properties characteristic of primordial germ cells. Subsequently, primordial germ cells migrate, first by passive transfer into the endodermal epithelium of the hindgut (170–350 primordial germ cells are found in or near the hindgut epithelium in 9-day embryos) and then by ameboid movement along the dorsal mesentery of the genital ridges (present in 10- to 11-day embryos) found in the roof of the coelom, the site of gonad development. It appears likely that chemotactic mechanisms operate during migration of primordial germ cells from extraembryonic sites to the presumptive gonad. As a result of continuous mitotic activity, the number of primordial germ cells increases to approximately 5,000 in 11- to 12-day embryos and to more than 20,000 by the time genital ridges of 13- to 14-day embryos are fully colonized. (This represents a doubling of the number of primordial germ cells every 18 hours or so between day 8 and day 14 of embryogenesis; it is estimated that they divide seven to eight times during the 4-day migration period.) Primordial germ cells proliferate for only 2 to 3 days after migrating to the genital ridges; fewer than 1% of the germ cells exhibit an S phase in 16- to 17-day embryos. These primordial germ cells are the sole source of adult germ cells. It is noteworthy that both the origin and migration of primordial germ cells to the genital ridges are the same in males and females; gonadal sex differentiation, to either testis or ovary, occurs in the 12- to 13-day embryo. In summary, the germ cell line originates before or during primitive streak formation (~7-day embryo), but precisely where, when, and how is still not clear. Mouse primordial germ cells are found sequentially in four different sites as embryogenesis proceeds: (a) First, they appear in the extraembryonic tissues of the yolk sac and allantois of 8- to 9-day embryos. (b) Then they appear in the hindgut epithelium of 9- to 10-day embryos. (c) Then they are found in the dorsal mesentery of the gut of 10- to 12-day embryos. (d) Finally they are found in the developing gonads of 10.5- to 11-day embryos. These primordial germ cells are the sole source of adult germ cells.

From Primordial Germ Cells to Oogonia

Upon reaching the surface epithelium of the gonad, primordial germ cells move into the cortex and, together with supporting epithelial cells, give rise to the cortical sex cords (138,154,180,394). The somatic components of the ovary arise from coelomic epithelium and mesenchyme of the dorsal body wall, and the mesonephros probably makes a contribution. In 13-day mouse embryos (52–60 pairs of somites) containing a differentiated ovary, migration of primordial germ cells is complete, with virtually all of the cells converted to actively dividing *oogonia* in the sex cords. Oogonia exhibit a characteristic morphology (including the presence of intercellular bridges connecting adjacent germ cells) and a high frequency of mitotic division.

From Oogonia to Nongrowing Oocytes

As early as day 12 of embryogenesis, a few oogonia (~5%) enter the preleptotene, and then leptotene, stage of the first meiotic prophase (27,28,69,138,154,180, 259,394). Once meiotic prophase commences, apparently there is no endocrine requirement for continued meiotic progression. Furthermore, since germ cells, either cultured *in vitro* or located at ectopic sites, enter and progress through meiosis, a gonadal environment is not required for the progress of meiosis (102,345).

It is during preleptotene (interphase following the last mitotic division of oogonia) that the final DNA replication takes place in preparation for *meiosis.* This synthetic activity signals transformation of oogonia into *oocytes.* It is possible that a factor originating from the rete ovarii, or simply contact with the rete ovarii, induces oogonia to enter meiosis. In 14-day mouse embryos (61–62 pairs of somites), the germ cell population is about equally divided between oogonia and oocytes, and by day 17 (full quota of 65 pairs of somites), the ovary contains only oocytes at various stages of the first meiotic prophase (20,27,28,30–34,137,162,327). Oocytes progress through leptotene in 3 to 6 hours and then take 12 to 40 hours to complete zygotene. During zygotene, homologous chromosomes pair and synapse to form what appear to be single chromosomes but are actually bivalents composed of four chromatids. In 16-day embryos, nearly all oocytes are in pachytene of the first meiotic prophase, a stage that lasts about 60 hours and involves genetic crossing-over and recombination. Therefore, it takes approximately 4 days to complete nuclear progression from leptotene through pachytene. By day 18 of embryogenesis, the first oocytes are seen in diplotene of the first meiotic prophase, with their chromosomes exhibiting chiasmata that result from crossing-over. By parturition, a majority of oocytes have entered late diplotene ("diffuse diplotene"), or the so-called dictyate stage, and by day 5 post-partum, nearly all oocytes have reached the dictyate stage, where they will remain until stimulated to resume meiosis at the time of ovulation. This pool of small (~12–15 μm in diameter), nongrowing oocytes is the sole source of unfertilized eggs in the sexually mature adult.

From Nongrowing to Fully Grown Oocytes

Shortly after birth, the mouse ovary is populated with approximately 8000 nongrowing oocytes arrested in meiosis and enclosed within several squamous follicular cells (27,28,57,180,259,394). Approximately 50% of these oocytes are lost during the first 2 weeks following birth; this is attributable, in large measure, to oocytes leaving the ovary through the surface epithelium. However, during this same period, more oocytes begin to grow (~5%) than at any other period in the lifetime of the mouse.

Commencement of oocyte growth is apparently regulated within the ovary, with the number of oocytes entering the growth phase being a function of the size of the pool of nongrowing oocytes (189). The oocyte and its surrounding follicle grow coordinately, progressing through a series of definable morphological stages (255–260). In sexually mature mice, oocytes complete growth before formation of a follicular antrum, consequently, the vast majority of follicle growth occurs after the oocyte has stopped growing. Growth is continuous, ending in either ovulation of a matured oocyte (unfertilized egg) or degeneration (atresia) of the oocyte and its follicle.

Completion of oocyte growth in the mouse takes 2 to 3 weeks, a relatively short period of time in comparison to the months or years required for completion of oocyte growth in many nonmammalian species (12,14,28,101, 180,257,259,267,355,393,395). The oocyte grows from a diameter of about 12 μm (volume ~0.9 pl) to a final diameter of about 80 μm (volume ~270 pl), not including the zona pellucida (discussed in the sections on structural and biochemical aspects of oocyte growth). Therefore, during its growth phase, while continually arrested in dictyate of the first meiotic prophase, the mouse oocyte undergoes a roughly 300-fold increase in volume and becomes one of the largest cells of the body. Each oocyte is contained within a cellular follicle (~17 μm in diameter) that grows concomitantly with the oocyte, from a single layer of a few flattened cells to three layers of cuboidal *granulosa cells* (~900 cells; ~125 μm diameter follicle) by the time the oocyte has completed its growth (9,28,43,57,68,138,170,171,173,180,243,255,260, 355,393–395). The *theca* is first distinguishable, outside of and separated by a basement membrane from the granulosa cells, when the granulosa region is two cell layers thick (~400 cells; ~100 μm diameter follicle). During a period of several days, while the oocyte remains a constant size, the follicular cells undergo rapid division, increasing to more than 50,000 cells and resulting in a *Graafian follicle* greater than 600 μm in diameter. The follicle exhibits an incipient *antrum* when it is several layers thick (~6000 cells; ~250 μm diameter follicle), and, as the antrum expands, the oocyte takes up an acentric position surrounded by two or more layers of granulosa cells. The innermost layer of granulosa cells becomes columnar in shape and constitutes the *corona radiata;* these cells form specialized intercellular junctions, called *gap junctions,* with the oolemma.

From Fully Grown Oocytes to Unfertilized Eggs

In sexually mature mice, fully grown oocytes in Graafian follicles resume meiosis and complete the first meiotic reductive division just prior to ovulation (discussed in the sections on structural, regulatory, and biochemical aspects of oocyte maturation). Resumption of meiosis can be mediated by a hormonal stimulus *in vivo* or simply by the release of oocytes from their ovarian follicles into a suitable culture medium *in vitro* (27,28,127, 336,337,373). Oocytes undergo nuclear progression from dictyate of the first meiotic prophase (four times the haploid DNA complement) to metaphase II (two times the haploid DNA complement). They remain at this stage of meiosis in the oviduct, or in culture, until stimulated to complete meiosis when either fertilization or parthenogenetic activation occurs. Progression from the dictyate stage (*oocyte*) to metaphase II (*egg*) of meiosis is called *meiotic maturation.* Meiotic maturation is characterized by dissolution of the oocyte's nuclear (germinal vesicle) membrane, condensation of chromatin into distinct bivalents, separation of homologous chromosomes, emission of the first polar body, and arrest of meiosis with chromosomes aligned on the metaphase II spindle (discussed in the section on structural aspects of oocyte maturation). These ovulated eggs complete meiosis, with separation of chromatids and emission of a second polar body (second reductive division), upon fertilization.

Summary

It should be apparent that the process of oogenesis in mammals includes several noteworthy features, including (a) extraembryonic and extragonadal origin of germ cells, (b) migration of germ cells to presumptive gonads, (c) sexual differentiation of germ cells into oogonia or spermatogonia, (d) cessation of mitosis (oogonia) and initiation of meiosis (oocytes), (e) prolonged cessation of meiosis in the dictyate stage, (f) oocyte growth, (g) reinitiation of meiosis (meiotic maturation; first meiotic reduction) and ovulation (eggs), and (h) completion of meiosis (second meiotic reduction) in response to fertilization. From the appearance of primordial germ cells during fetal development until ovulation of unfertilized eggs in sexually mature adults, oogenesis represents one of the most highly specialized and regulated biological processes in mammals.

GROWTH OF THE OOCYTE: STRUCTURAL ASPECTS

Oocyte Growth: General Features

Throughout the reproductive life of mammals, ovaries contain pools of nongrowing and growing oocytes arrested in dictyate of the first meiotic prophase. Only fully grown oocytes resume meiosis and are ovulated during each reproductive (estrous) cycle. Recruitment of oocytes into the growing pool is apparently under control of pituitary gonadotropins, although oocyte growth, without follicle development, does occur in hypophysectomized animals and during culture *in vitro* in the absence of hormones. The volume of a mouse oocyte increases nearly 300-fold during its 2- to 3-week growth phase. This tremendous enlargement of the cell is indicative of a period of intense metabolic activity (discussed in the section on biochemical aspects of oocyte growth), which, in turn, is reflected in marked changes in oocyte ultrastructure, including the appearance (biogenesis) of some novel organelles (2,15,42,180,242,326,332,350, 367,374,387,388). For example, cortical granules and the zona pellucida, both involved in regulating fertilization, first appear in oocytes during their growth phase. A description of certain of the ultrastructural changes accompanying oocyte growth follows.

Nucleus (Germinal Vesicle)

The nucleus, or germinal vesicle (GV), of growing mouse oocytes increases in diameter, from 9 to 10 μm in small (~20 μm) oocytes to 20 to 22 μm in fully grown (~80 μm) oocytes (87,367). Consequently, growth of mouse oocytes results in a marked change in the ratio of cytoplasmic to nucleoplasmic volume, increasing from about 8:1 in small oocytes to about 64:1 in fully grown oocytes. Concomitant with nuclear enlargement, the nucleolus and extranucleolar bodies undergo progressive, characteristic ultrastructural changes, while chromosomes remain as highly diffuse bivalents. However, once growth is completed, the chromatin assumes a more condensed appearance, especially in the immediate vicinity of the nucleolus. This transformation in chromatin organization is characterized by a progressive envelopment of the nucleolus by heterochromatin. The change is initiated at the time of antrum formation in the mouse (212), but it commences at somewhat later stages of folliculogenesis in other mammals (214).

Nucleolus

The nucleus (GV) of growing mouse oocytes contains a single large nucleolus and, frequently, one or two smaller nucleoli. Throughout oocyte growth, the nucleolus enlarges, increasing in diameter from 2 to 3 μm in small (~20 μm) oocytes to 9 to 10 μm in fully grown (~80 μm) oocytes (85,86,367) (Fig. 3). This enlargement is accompanied by progressive changes in nucleolar fine structure, indicative of a period of intense ribosomal-RNA synthesis (18,29,85,86,165,220,221,241,251,306). The nucleolus undergoes a transition during oocyte growth, from a diffuse, reticulated type of structure, composed primarily of a fibrillogranular network (small oocytes), to a dense, uniform mass, exclusively fibrillar in nature (fully grown oocytes).

Mitochondria

Oocyte growth is accompanied not only by a substantial increase in the number of mitochondria present but also by marked changes in mitochondrial ultrastructure (328,332,367,382,388) (Fig. 4). Small (~20 μm) oocytes contain elongated (~1.5 μm long) mitochondria with numerous transversely oriented cristae in the so-called orthodox configuration and, in most cases, contain a single vacuole. Continued oocyte growth is accompanied by accumulation of round and oval-shaped mitochondria, which are vacuolated and beginning to display columnar-shaped arched cristae. Throughout this growth period, mitochondria are closely associated with smooth endoplasmic reticulum and are present in increasing numbers. Many dumbbell-shaped mitochondria are found, indicative of extensive mitochondrial growth and division. Fully grown oocytes (~80 μm) contain round or oval (~0.5 μm diameter), highly vacuolated mitochondria (~10^5 per oocyte) (219,266) that have arched and concentrically arranged cristae. Consequently, the morphology of mitochondria in fully grown oocytes is radically different than that of mitochondria in nongrowing and small oocytes.

Golgi Complex

As in the case of mitochondria, the Golgi complex undergoes dramatic ultrastructural changes during oocyte growth; these changes are indicative of increasing Golgi activity (332,367,388) (Fig. 5). In small (~20 μm) oocytes, Golgi membranes appear as flattened stacks of arched lamellae and are associated with few, if any, vacuoles or granules. During early stages of oocyte growth, Golgi membranes become more active, as evidenced by lamellae that are spaced further apart (swelling at termini of lamellae), by the appearance of vacuoles, and by the proximity of numerous lipid vesicles. In the middle to late stages of oocyte growth, Golgi membranes exhibit increased numbers of very swollen, stacked lamellae that are associated with numerous vacuoles, granules, coated vesicles, and lipid vesicles. These changes are consistent

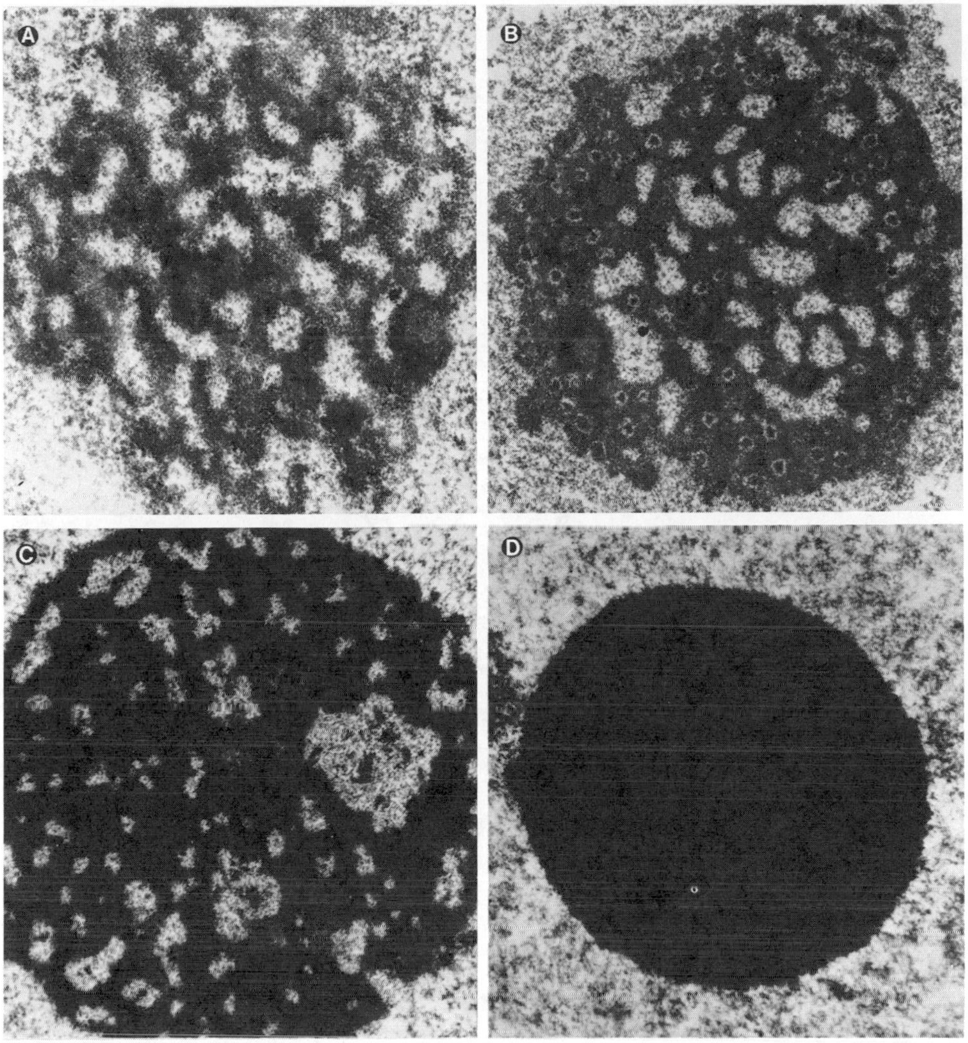

FIG. 3. Transmission electron micrographs comparing nucleolar ultrastructure during growth of the mouse oocyte. Oocytes are isolated from 3- (**A**), 5- (**B**), 10- (**C**), and 14-day-old (**D**) animals and range in diameter from about 20 μm (3 days) to 60 μm (14 days). Note the marked change from a sparse, fibrillogranular (A) to a dense (D) nucleolus during oocyte growth. (From ref. 367.)

with increased participation of the Golgi in processing and concentration of secretory products (e.g., zona pellucida glycoproteins) and cortical granule formation during oocyte growth. It is noteworthy that, concomitant with the conversion of fully grown oocytes to fertilized eggs, there is a dramatic decrease in the amount of recognizable Golgi membrane and an increase in the number of small membrane vesicles.

Cortical Granules

Cortical granules are small, spherical, membrane-bound organelles that are found in the cortical region of unfertilized eggs and are thought to resemble lysosomes (115–118,158,304). These granules fuse with the oolemma at fertilization and, by releasing their contents (including proteinases) into the perivitelline space, alter functional properties of the zona pellucida (secondary block to polyspermy) (117,356–360,370). Mouse eggs contain approximately 4500 cortical granules (ranging in diameter from 200 to 600 nm) within about 2 μm of the plasma membrane (236). Cortical granules first appear during oocyte growth, associated with an expanding Golgi that has moved to the subcortical region of growing oocytes. Although it is clear that cortical granules are derived from Golgi, certain evidence suggests that there is a contribution from multivesicular bodies as well as from granular endoplasmic reticulum. Morphological studies suggest that the cortical granule population is heterogeneous with respect to contents, with some granules even containing ordered crystalline arrays. It is unclear whether this heterogeneity of cortical granule contents reflects functional differences or simply different extents

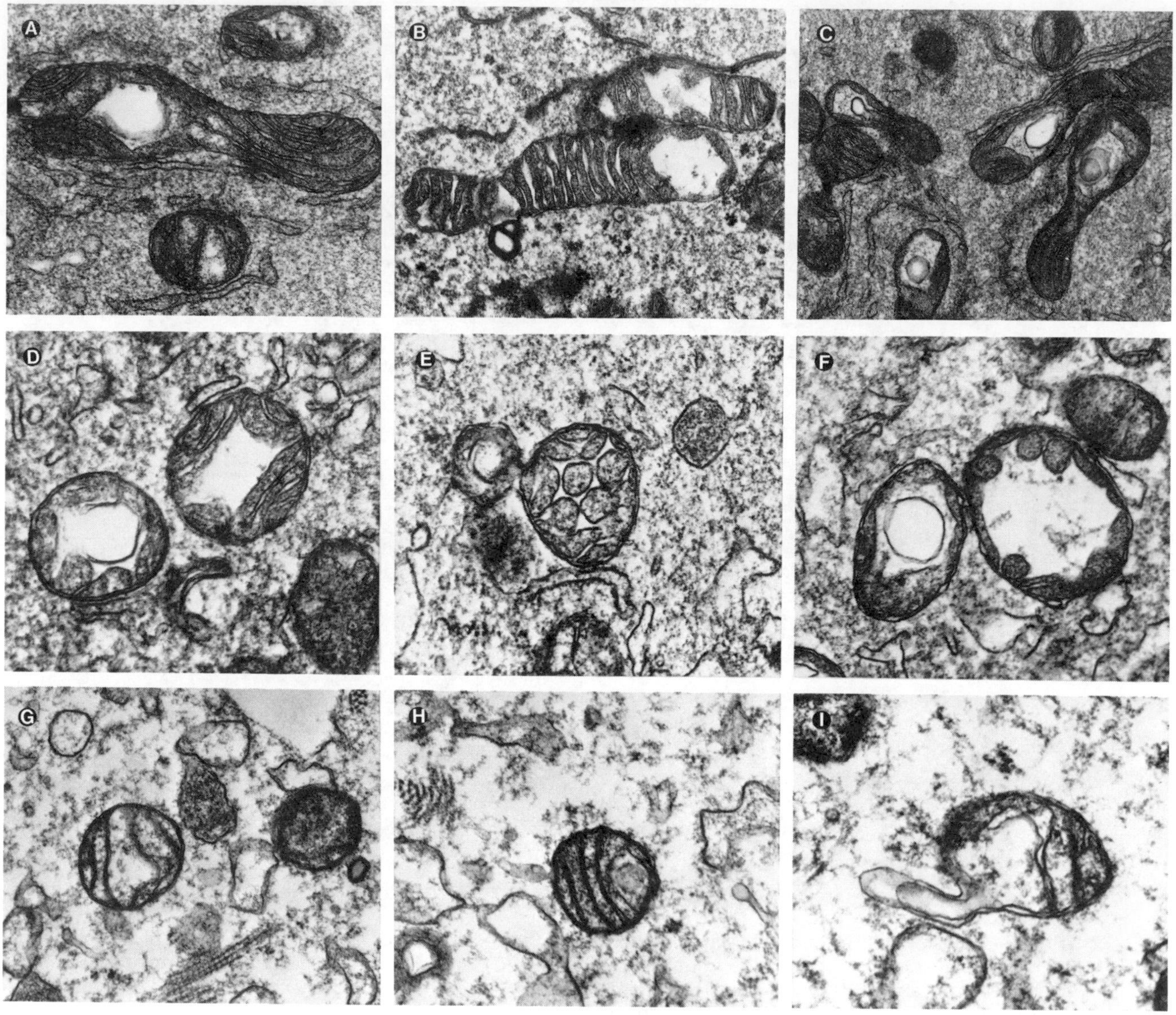

FIG. 4. Transmission electron micrographs comparing mitochondrial ultrastructure during growth of the mouse oocyte. Oocytes are isolated from 5- (**A**), 3- (**B**), 5- (**C**), 10- (**D–F**), and 21-day-old (**G–I**) animals and range in diameter from about 20 μm (3 days) to 85 μm (21 days). Note the marked change from elongated mitochondria with transverse cristae (''orthodox configuration'') (A–C) to round or oval mitochondria with concentric cristae (''unorthodox configuration'') (D–I) during oocyte growth. (From ref. 367.)

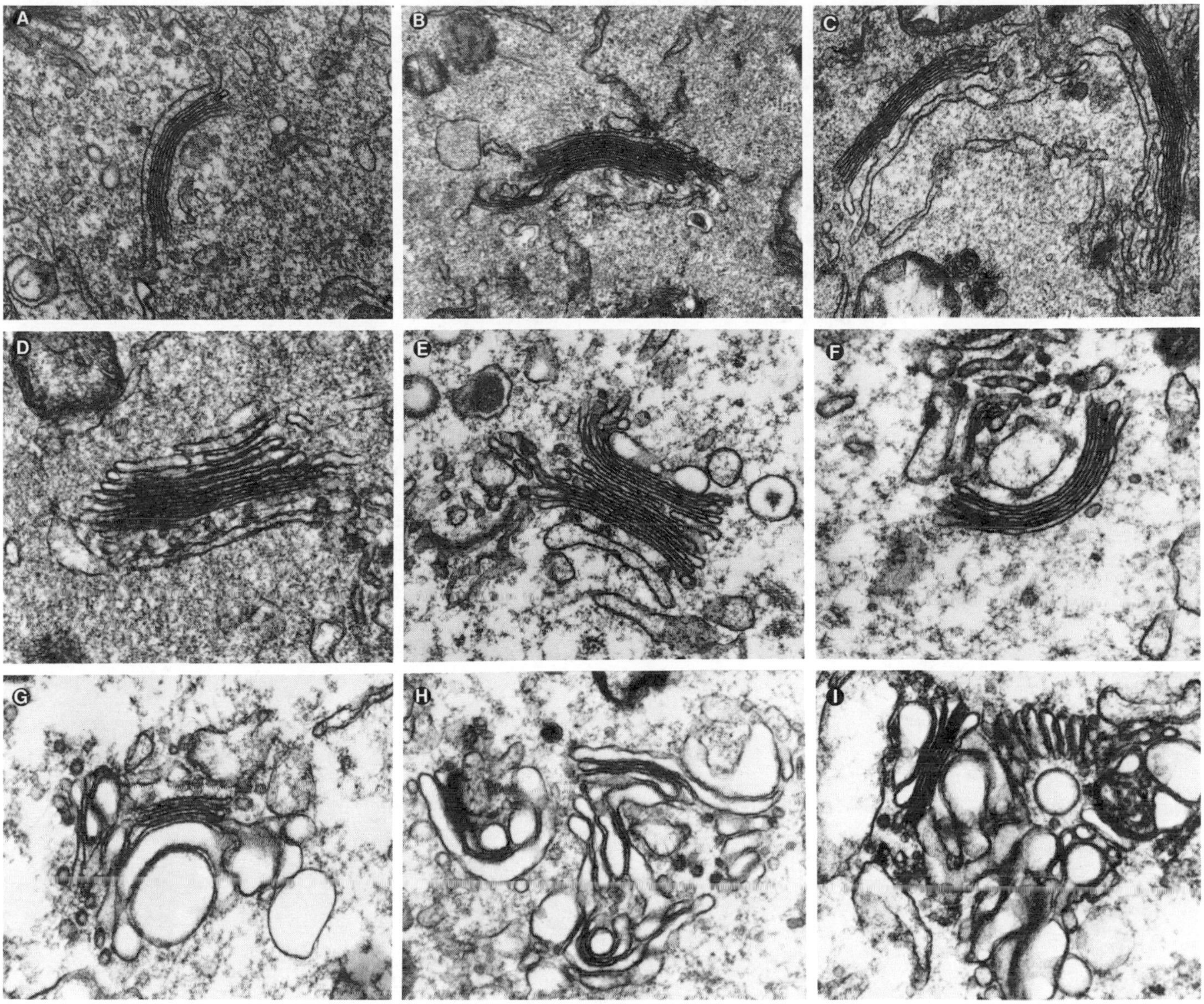

FIG. 5. Transmission electron micrographs comparing Golgi complex ultrastructure during growth of the mouse oocyte. Oocytes isolated from 3- (**A**), 5- (**B**), 8- (**C**), 10- (**D**), 14- (**E,F**), and 21-day-old (**G–I**) animals and ranging in diameter from about 20 μm (3 days) to 85 μm (21 days). Note the marked change from flattened stacks of parallel lamellae (A–D) to swollen, highly vacuolated, granular lamellae (E–I) during oocyte growth. (From ref. 367.)

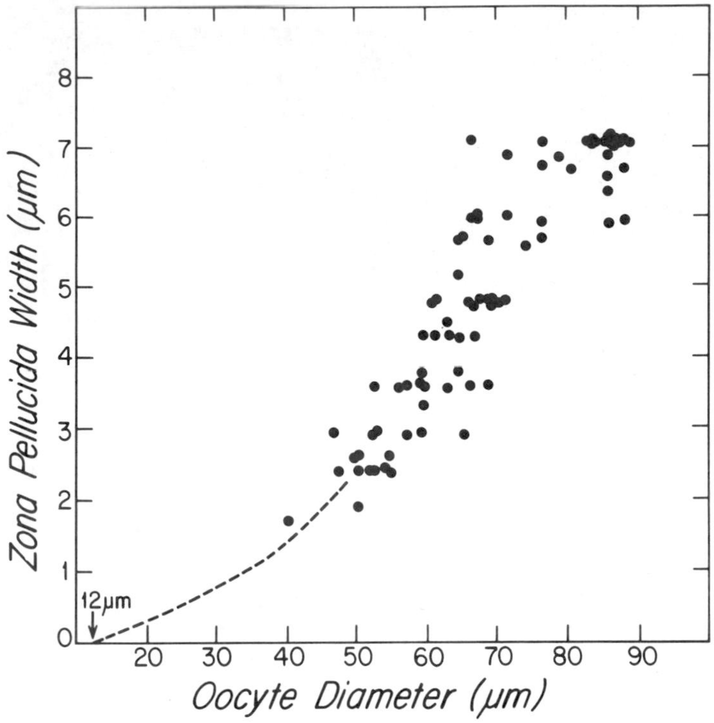

FIG. 6. Relationship between width of zona pellucida and diameter of oocytes during growth of mouse oocytes. Note that as oocytes increase in diameter from about 40 μm to 85 μm the zona pellucida increases in width from about 1.6 to 7 μm (i.e., about 4.5 times). (Data taken from J. M. Greve and P. M. Wassarman, *unpublished results*.)

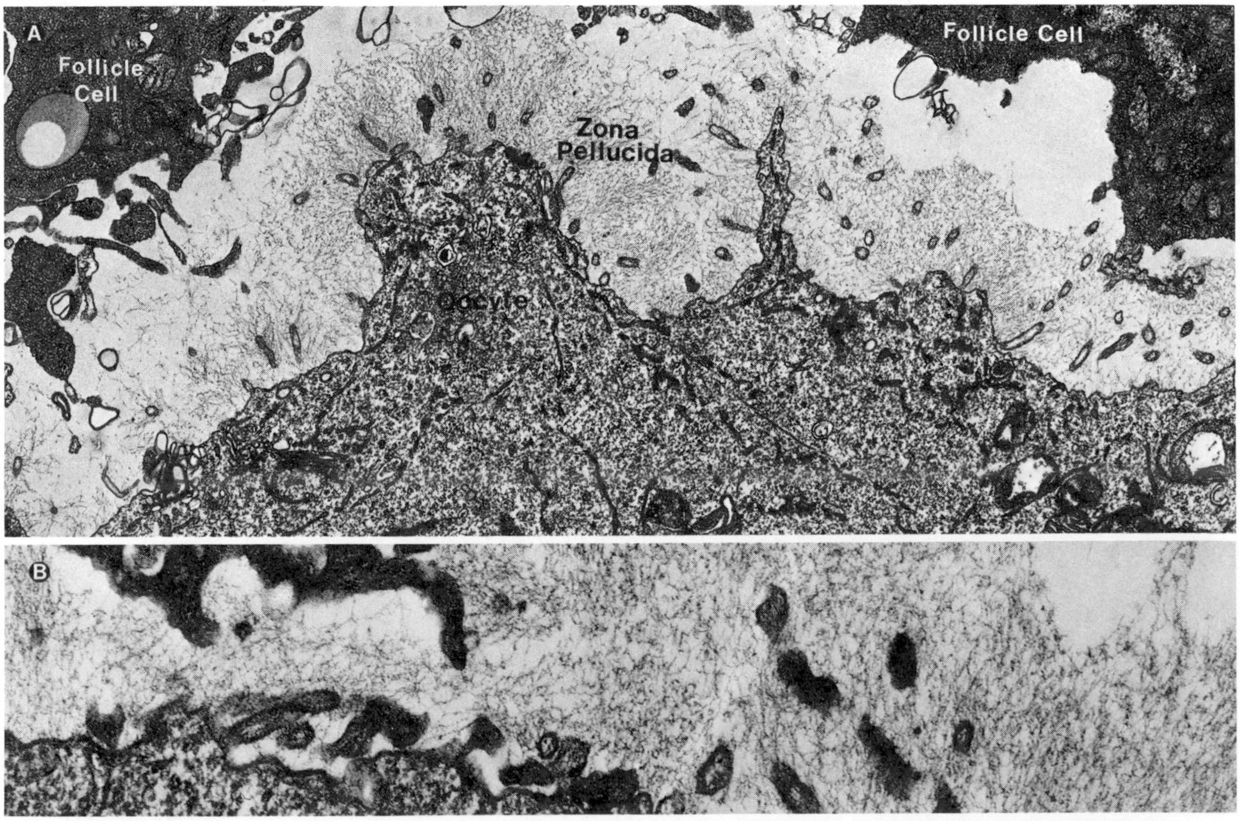

FIG. 7. Transmission electron micrographs of mouse zona pellucida filaments during the early stages of oocyte growth. Shown are stained and sectioned growing oocytes (about 20 μm in diameter) with associated follicle cells and developing zona pellucida (**A,B**). Note the filamentous nature of the nascent zona pellucida and its close apposition to the surface of the growing oocyte.

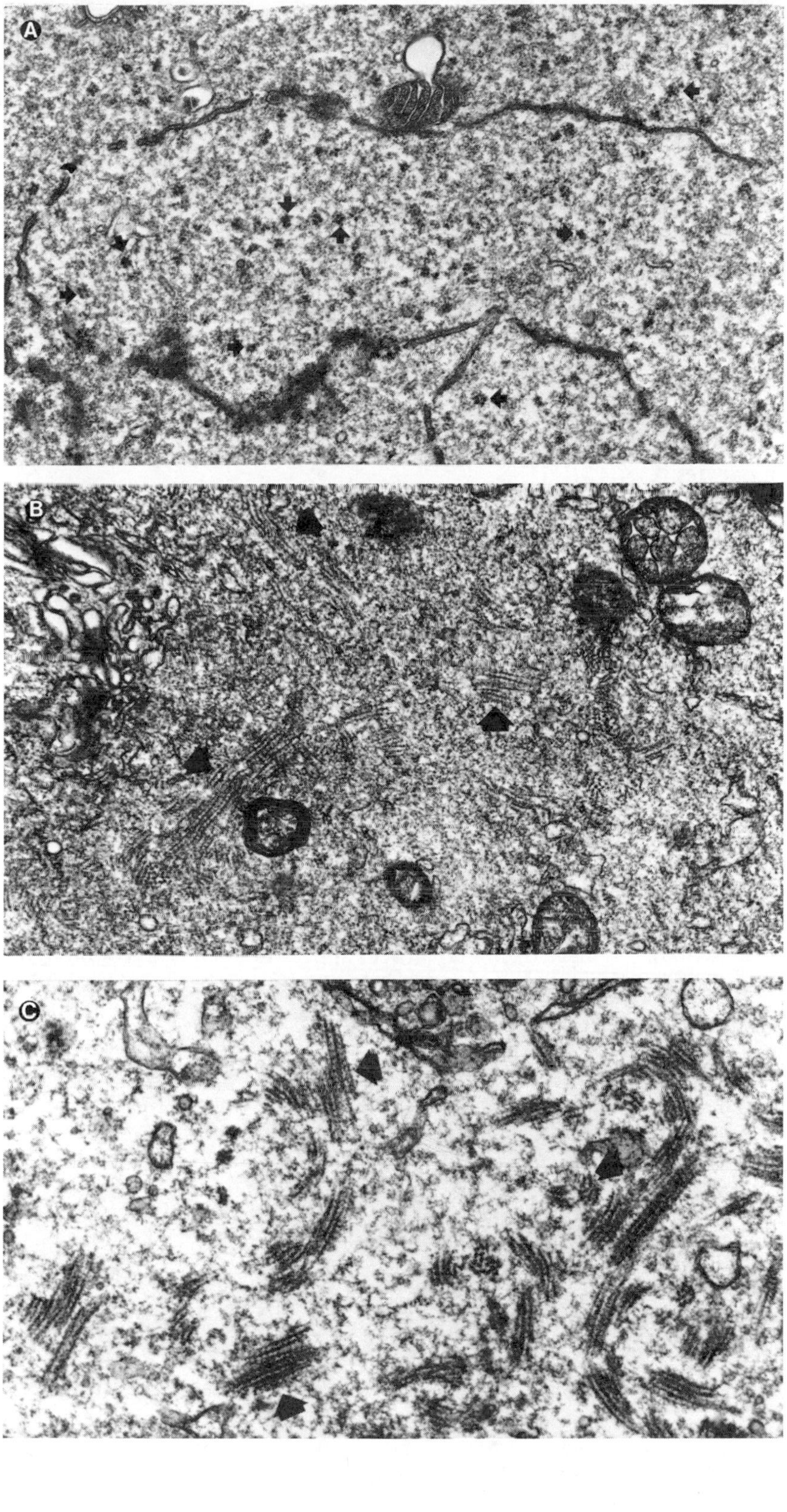

FIG. 8. Transmission electron micrographs comparing oocyte cytoplasm during growth of the mouse oocyte. Oocytes are isolated from 3- (**A**), 10- (**B**), and 21-day-old (**C**) animals and range in diameter from about 20 μm (3 days) to 85 μm (21 days). Note the abundance of clustered ribosomes during the early stages of oocyte growth (A: *arrows*), the appearance of lattice structures during the middle stages of oocyte growth (B: *arrows*), and the considerable accumulation of lattice structures during the late stages of oocyte growth (C: *arrows*). (From ref. 367.)

of granule maturation. In any case, it is clear that oocyte growth is accompanied by formation and accumulation of increasing numbers of cortical granules in anticipation of ovulation and fertilization. Recently, a mouse egg 75-kilodalton cortical granule protein (p75), was identified as a product of growing oocytes, and this identification should lead to new insights into cortical granule biosynthesis during oogenesis (262).

Zona Pellucida

The zona pellucida, a relatively thick extracellular coat that surrounds all mammalian eggs, appears during oocyte growth, increasing in width as oocytes increase in diameter (44,60,82,119,163,181,355,358,367,370) (Fig. 6). In mice, the zona pellucida of fully grown oocytes is about 7 μm thick, contains about 3 ng of protein, and is permeable to both large macromolecules and small viruses. The protein components of zonae pellucidae are synthesized and secreted by growing oocytes, representing a major metabolic activity of the oocyte during this period (discussed in the section on biochemical aspects of oocyte growth). Appearance of zona pellucida material in the perivitelline space correlates with initiation of oocyte growth; nongrowing oocytes do not have a zona pellucida. In early stages of oocyte growth, zona pellucida material appears as patches of fine filaments between the oocyte and follicle cells (Fig. 7). These filaments are of uniform width, can be several microns in length, and exhibit a structural periodicity (157,358,370). As growth continues, the zona pellucida becomes a denser and thicker meshwork of interconnected filaments completely surrounding the oocyte and largely separating it from follicle cells. However, contact between the oocyte and the innermost layer of follicle cells continues via junctional complexes formed between oocyte microvilli and follicle cell extensions that penetrate the zona pellucida (discussed in the section on the role of intercellular communication). As in the case of cortical granules, the zona pellucida is laid down during oocyte growth in anticipation of its roles during and after fertilization (14,159,360,361). The zona pellucida contains sperm receptors that mediate sperm–egg interaction as a prelude to fertilization; it also participates in a secondary block to polyspermy following fertilization of eggs (45,47,134,135,230,356–362,364).

Ribosomes

Ribosomal RNA accumulates through much of mouse oocyte growth (discussed in the section on biochemical aspects of oocyte growth), consistent with changes in nucleolar morphology during this period. It is estimated that the number of ribosomes present in the cytoplasm increases three- to fourfold as the oocyte diameter increases from 20 to 65 μm (143). However, the enormous change in oocyte volume during this period of growth suggests that ribosome density (i.e., number of ribosomes per cubic micrometer of cytoplasm) decreases as much as tenfold. The number of ribosomes present in polysomes also increases severalfold during oocyte growth, with the number of single polysomes, which are abundant in small oocytes (>70% of total), decreasing dramatically (<10% of total) in large oocytes. These changes in the ribosome population during oocyte growth are consistent with changes in overall rates of protein synthesis during this period. For, whereas the rate of protein synthesis per oocyte increases dramatically, the rate per picoliter of cytoplasm actually decreases during oocyte growth (discussed in the section on biochemical aspects of oocyte growth).

Cytoplasmic Lattices

Latticelike structures (placques, lamellae, fibrillar arrays) are found in the cytoplasm of both fully grown mouse oocytes and unfertilized eggs (67,332,374–376,388). Although not present in nongrowing oocytes, these lattices increase in number dramatically throughout oocyte growth and become a dominant feature of the fully grown oocyte. In some cases, the lattices appear as highly ordered aggregates of individual chains (67) (Fig. 8). The chains, in turn, are composed of particles that are connected by bridges, giving rise to a structural periodicity. The individual chains themselves are interconnected, so that lattices appear to form layers of interconnected sheets. The function of this extremely abundant cytoplasmic component is not known, although the possibility that it serves either as yolk (332) or as a storage form of ribosomes (22,25,62,67,264), since it completely disappears during the cleavage stages of early embryogenesis, has been considered.

OOCYTE MATURATION: STRUCTURAL ASPECTS

Meiotic Maturation: General Features

Meiotic maturation specifically refers to the conversion of fully grown oocytes (present in antral follicles) into unfertilized eggs just prior to ovulation, following the preovulatory gonadotropin (follicle-stimulating hormone [FSH] and luteinizing hormone [LH]) surge. In particular, meiotic maturation involves nuclear progression, from dictyate of the first meiotic prophase (late G_2) to metaphase II (first meiotic reduction), as well as metabolic changes necessary for activation of the egg at fertilization. Isolated, fully grown oocytes undergo meiotic

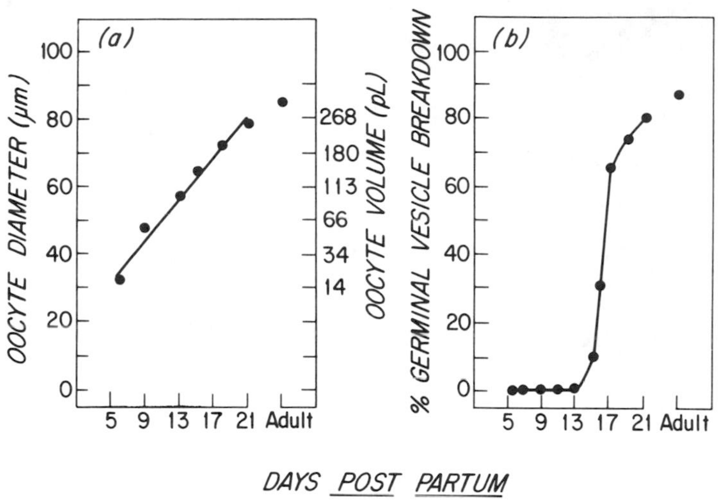

FIG. 9. Relationship between mouse oocyte diameter and ability of oocytes to undergo meiotic maturation *in vitro.* (**a**) Diameter (in microns) of isolated oocytes as a function of the age (days *post-partum*) of the donor mice. (**b**) Percent of isolated oocytes undergoing germinal vesicle breakdown *in vitro* as a function of the age (days *post-partum*) of the donor mice. (Data taken from ref. 325.)

maturation spontaneously during culture *in vitro* in the absence of hormones (79,268,335), thus providing an advantageous experimental system for structural and biochemical studies. The timing of cytological events (e.g., nuclear membrane breakdown, spindle formation) observed with maturing oocytes *in vitro* resembles that observed *in vivo.* Only oocytes that have undergone successful meiotic maturation are capable of being fertilized and developing normally. Mammalian oocytes matured and fertilized *in vitro* exhibit normal preimplantation development *in vitro* (224,349) and develop into viable fetuses following transplantation to the uteri of foster mothers (97,231,303).

Acquisition of Meiotic Competence

Dictyate-stage oocytes acquire the ability to undergo meiotic reduction (*meiotic competence*) during oocyte growth (325,334,336,337). This applies to oocytes *in vivo* as well as to those grown under *in vitro* conditions. Only mouse oocytes larger than about 60 μm in diameter mature *in vitro;* smaller oocytes remain arrested at the dictyate stage (Fig. 9). However, small meiotically incompetent oocytes are able to mature *in vitro* following fusion with large meiotically competent oocytes (35,36,141). The acquisition of meiotic competence apparently occurs in two steps: growing oocytes first acquire the ability to undergo nuclear (GV) envelope breakdown with progression to metaphase I, followed by acquisition of the ability to progress from metaphase I to metaphase II (325). Certain evidence suggests that the acquisition of meiotic competence is time dependent but independent of the presence of follicle cells, heterologous cell contacts, and cell growth (72). In this context, it is evident that mouse oocytes should be included among those meiotic and mitotic cell types for which the transition from G_2 to M phase of the cell cycle is regulated by a cytoplasmic factor, the so-called maturation-promoting factor (MPF). MPF activity appears during meiotic maturation of mouse oocytes (35,324), reaching highest levels at metaphase of meiosis I and II and diminishing at anaphase–telophase of meiosis I or after completion of meiosis (140).

Although a thorough analysis of the regulation of MPF activity during meiotic maturation in mammalian oocytes has not been completed, essential structural events associated with the G_2-to-M cell cycle transition in this meiotic cell type have recently been elucidated (3). During the course of meiotic competence acquisition in the mouse, several important modifications in nuclear and cytoplasmic structure occur indicative of a G_2-to-M cell cycle transition. These changes include the appearance of a perinuclear shell of heterochromatin, the loss of an interphase array of cytoplasmic microtubules, and the appearance of phosphorylated centrosomes (212,380,378) (Fig. 10). Since these changes coincide in the mouse with the formation of the follicular antrum, a process initiated by FSH, it is likely that FSH plays a role in the acquisition of meiotic competence.

Nuclear (Germinal Vesicle) Breakdown

Within a few hours of culture *in vitro,* fully grown mouse oocytes undergo complete nuclear breakdown (GVBD) or dissolution (71,111,323) (Fig. 11). This process begins with slight undulation of the nuclear envelope a few minutes after oocytes are placed in culture, which continues with increasing intensity during the next 1 to 2 hours. These undulations may be related to chromosome condensation that is initiated during this period. Nuclear pores disappear within 1 hour or so of culture; breaks in the nuclear envelope are visible after about 2 hours, on average. After 3 hours of culture, on average, the nuclear envelope is completely dispersed

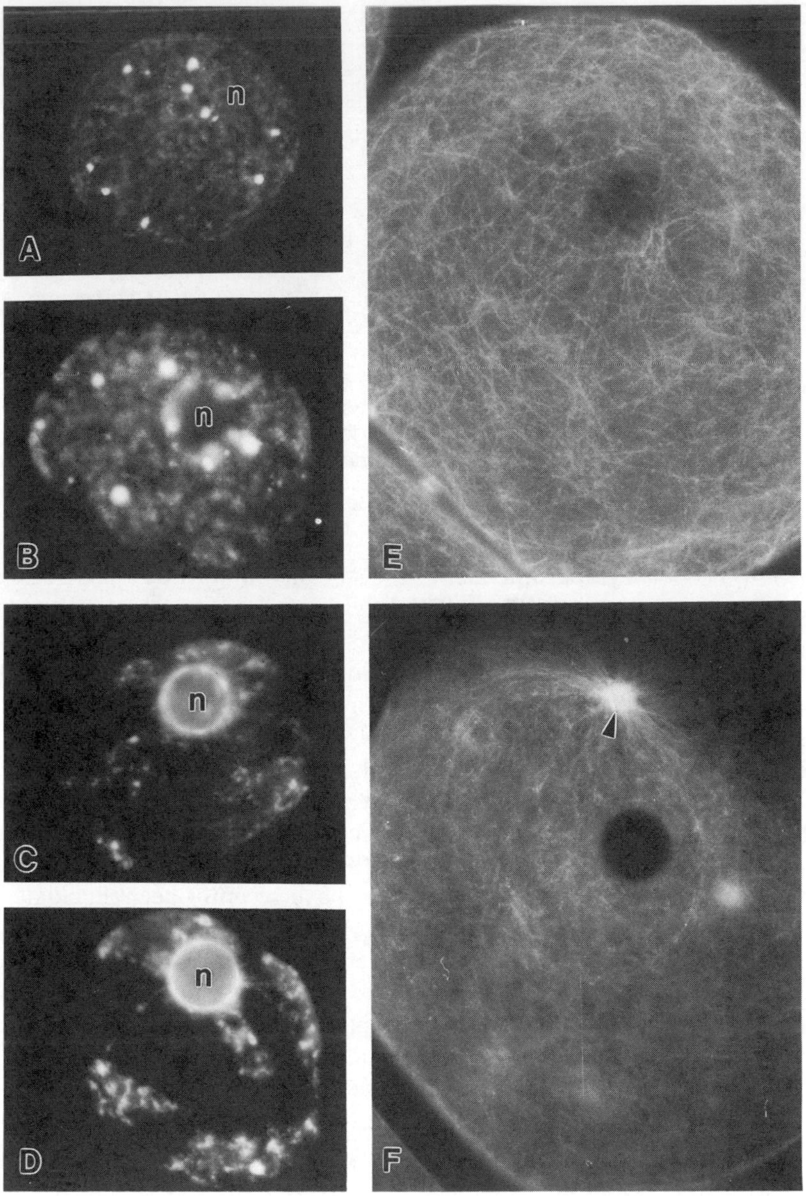

FIG. 10. Mouse oocyte chromatin (**A–D**) and microtubule (**E,F**) staining patterns prior to (**A,B,E**) and following (**C,D,F**) acquisition of meiotic competence. Heterochromatin progressively (**A–D**) accumulates around the nucleolus (n) of the germinal vesicle. Incompetent oocytes display an interphase microtubule network (**E**), whereas competent oocytes contain few microtubules and prominent asters (*arrowhead,* **F**).

into membrane doublets that apparently join the endoplasmic reticulum pool, perhaps to play a subsequent role in pronuclear and nuclear envelope formation (333). The mean time for complete breakdown of the nuclear envelope, measured from the first sign of membrane disintegration to disappearance of the nucleolus, is 11 minutes. Disappearance of the nucleolus occurs shortly after contacting invading cytoplasm (Fig. 12). In contrast, the nuclear lamina, a fibrous mesh comprised of lamins A, B, and C that lines the inner nuclear membrane, persists throughout GV breakdown and appears to disintegrate just prior to metaphase of meiosis I (6). It should also be noted that significant changes in the number and distribution of cortical granules also occur during meiotic maturation of mouse oocytes (116,117).

Chromosome Condensation

During meiotic maturation, oocyte chromosomes (bivalents) pass through metaphase I, anaphase I, and telophase I, arresting at metaphase II without an intervening prophase II (Fig. 13). Diffuse dictyate-stage chromosomes (resembling "lampbrush" chromosomes) undergo significant condensation along the inner margin of the nuclear envelope, concomitant with the envelope's undulatory behavior (71,368). During this period, chiasmata move to the ends of the chromosomes. The chromatin becomes heterochromatic and contains dense granules that increase in number with increasing chromosome condensation. Chromosome condensation occurs within the agranular vestige of the nucleus within 20

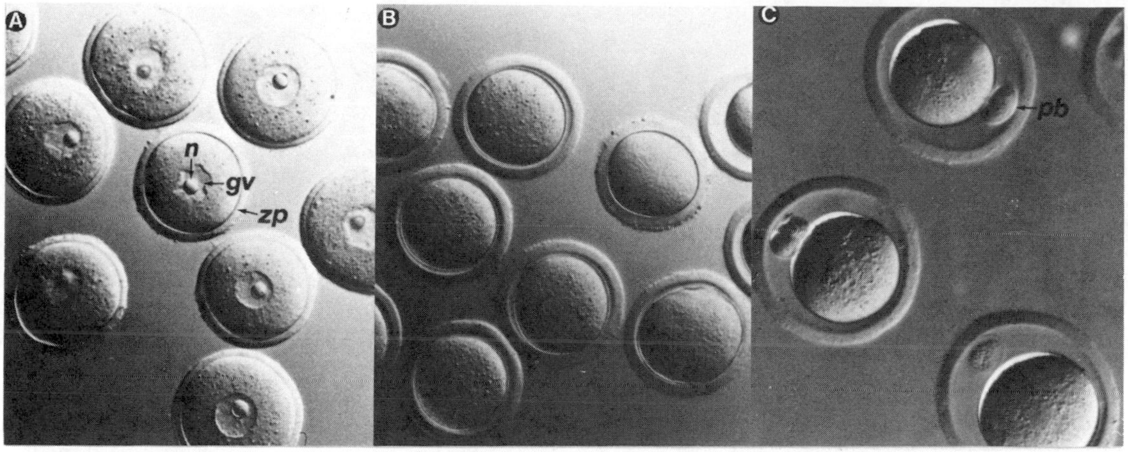

FIG. 11. Light photomicrographs of fully grown mouse oocytes during culture *in vitro.* Photographs were taken using Nomarski differential interference contrast microscopy. **A:** Isolated oocytes arrested in dictyate of the first meiotic prophase. **B:** Isolated oocytes that have undergone germinal vesicle breakdown and chromosome condensation during culture. **C:** Isolated oocytes that have completed meiotic maturation in culture and become unfertilized eggs. Note that they have emitted a polar body and have arrested at metaphase II. (gv) Germinal vesicle; (n) nucleolus; (zp) zona pellucida.

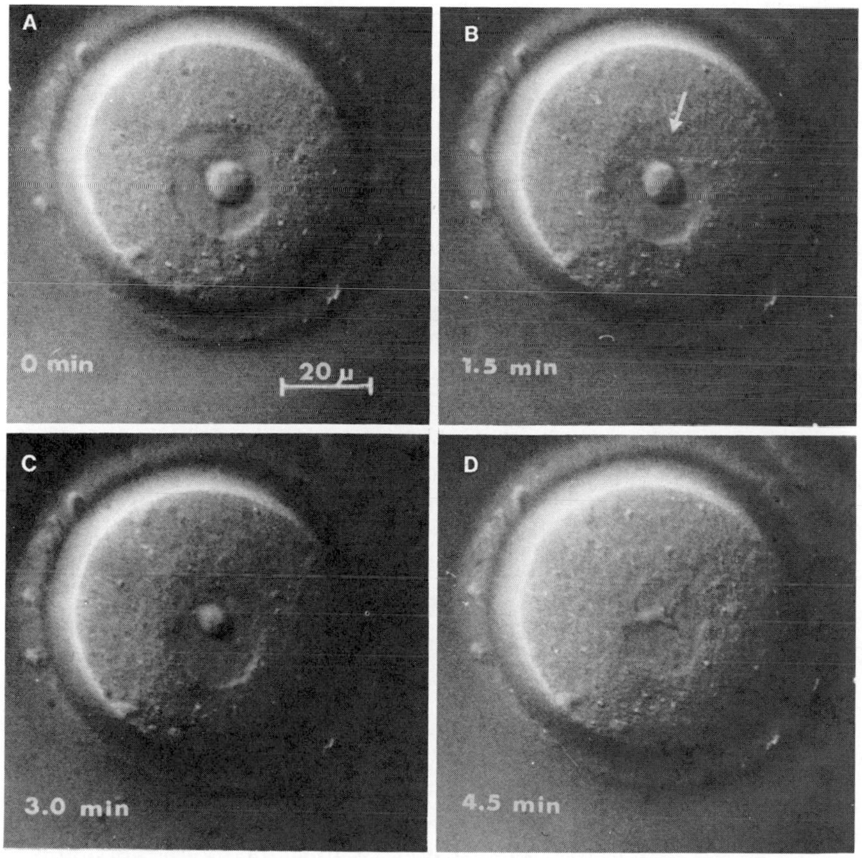

FIG. 12. Light photomicrographs of a fully grown mouse oocyte undergoing germinal vesicle breakdown during culture *in vitro.* Photographs were taken from a cinefilm made using Nomarski differential interference contrast microscopy. Actual time elapsed (in minutes) is recorded. **A:** Intact germinal vesicle with a single prominent nucleolus. **B:** Incipient disintegration of the germinal vesicle membrane with invasion of cytoplasm into the germinal vesicle. **C:** Vestiges of germinal vesicle remain and the nucleolus begins to shrink in size. **D:** Complete dissolution of the germinal vesicle membrane with only a small remnant of the nucleolus remaining; the region occupied by the germinal vesicle remains granular. (From ref. 323.)

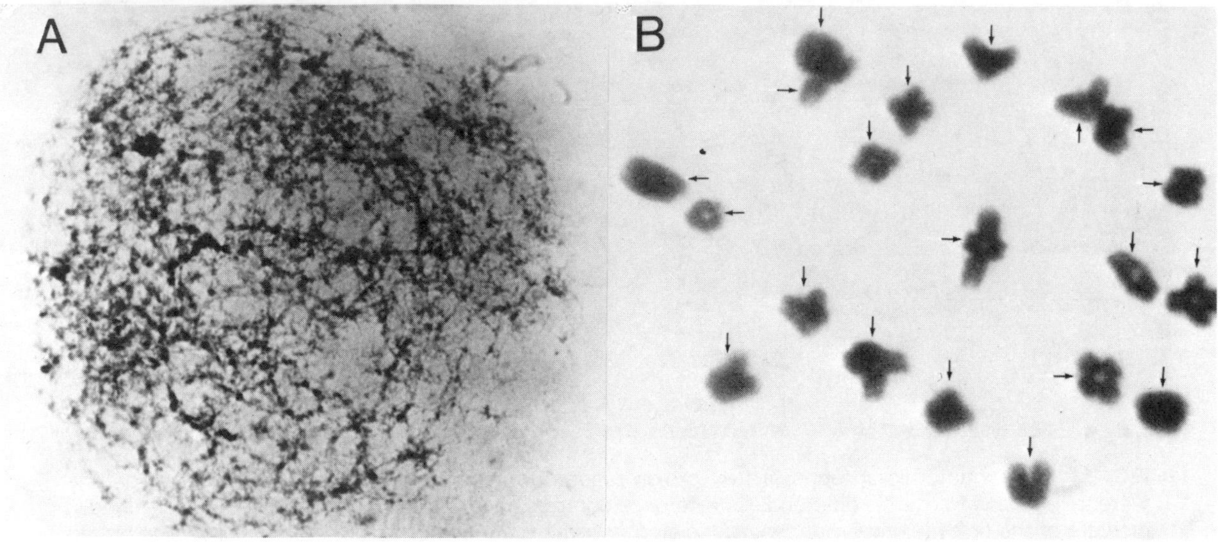

FIG. 13. Chromosome spreads from fully grown mouse oocytes during culture *in vitro*. Shown are Geimsa-stained chromosome spreads from oocytes before (**A**) and after (**B**) germinal vesicle breakdown (i.e., the early stages of meiotic maturation). Note the diffuse state of chromosomes prior to germinal vesicle breakdown (dictyate of the first meiotic prophase) as compared to after germinal vesicle breakdown. Arrows (in part B) indicate 20 bivalents.

minutes of nucleolar dissolution. After 2 to 3 hours of culture, on average, when chromosome condensation is nearly complete (with "lampbrush" loops withdrawn), the bivalents are V-shaped and telocentric and are often associated with fragments of nuclear envelope. Shortly thereafter, highly condensed chromosomes become circularly arranged in the center of the egg, lose their contacts with nuclear envelope fragments, and then (after 6–9 hours of culture) line up on the equator of the metaphase I spindle.

Spindle Formation

During the period of nuclear envelope breakdown (GVBD) and chromosome condensation, kinetochores with associated microtubules, as well as other microtubule-organizing centers, appear; microtubules extend from these centers, through breaks in the nuclear envelope, into the nucleoplasm (70,71). Apparently, there is a kinetochore associated with each chromatid of each chromosomal homolog. A small but morphologically identifiable meiotic spindle appears after about 6 hours of culture and is clearly recognizable by 9 hours (Fig. 14). Unlike the situation in most cells, the poles of the oocyte spindle lack centrioles and are composed solely of bands of so-called pericentriolar material. Pericentriolar material becomes associated with the forming spindle poles during prometaphase and is highly phosphorylated and condensed at metaphase; it disappears from the spindle poles during telophase. In parallel with these progressive changes in the organization of the pericentriolar material at the spindle poles, cytoplasmic centrosomes, also containing this material and nucleating microtubules, undergo alterations in number and location during meiotic maturation. These structures are most numerous at prometaphase and anaphase of meiosis and are located in the oocyte cortex, except at the site of spindle attachment (218).

The size of the spindle increases progressively, with a fully formed, barrel-shaped metaphase I spindle present within 9 to 10 hours of culture (111,323,366). The pole-to-pole distance of the spindle is about 40 μm, and its width is about 25 μm (Fig. 15). One of the spindle's poles is located near the cortex of the cell; the spindle is surrounded by a dense area composed of mitochondria, vacuoles, and granules. Cortical granules are excluded from the site of spindle attachment where a thick submembranous band of actin filaments is located. As meiosis proceeds to anaphase, bivalents move toward the opposite ends of the spindle, and the spindle rotates through 90°. These movements apparently involve microfilaments. It is noteworthy that maturing oocytes spend about 6 hours in prometaphase I (period from initial chromosome condensation to lineup of bivalents on the metaphase I plate) and about 4 hours in metaphase I. This long period probably reflects the time necessary to synthesize and assemble the spindle apparatus.

Polar Body Emission

Anaphase and telophase figures predominate by 10 to 13 hours of culture *in vitro,* and it is during this period

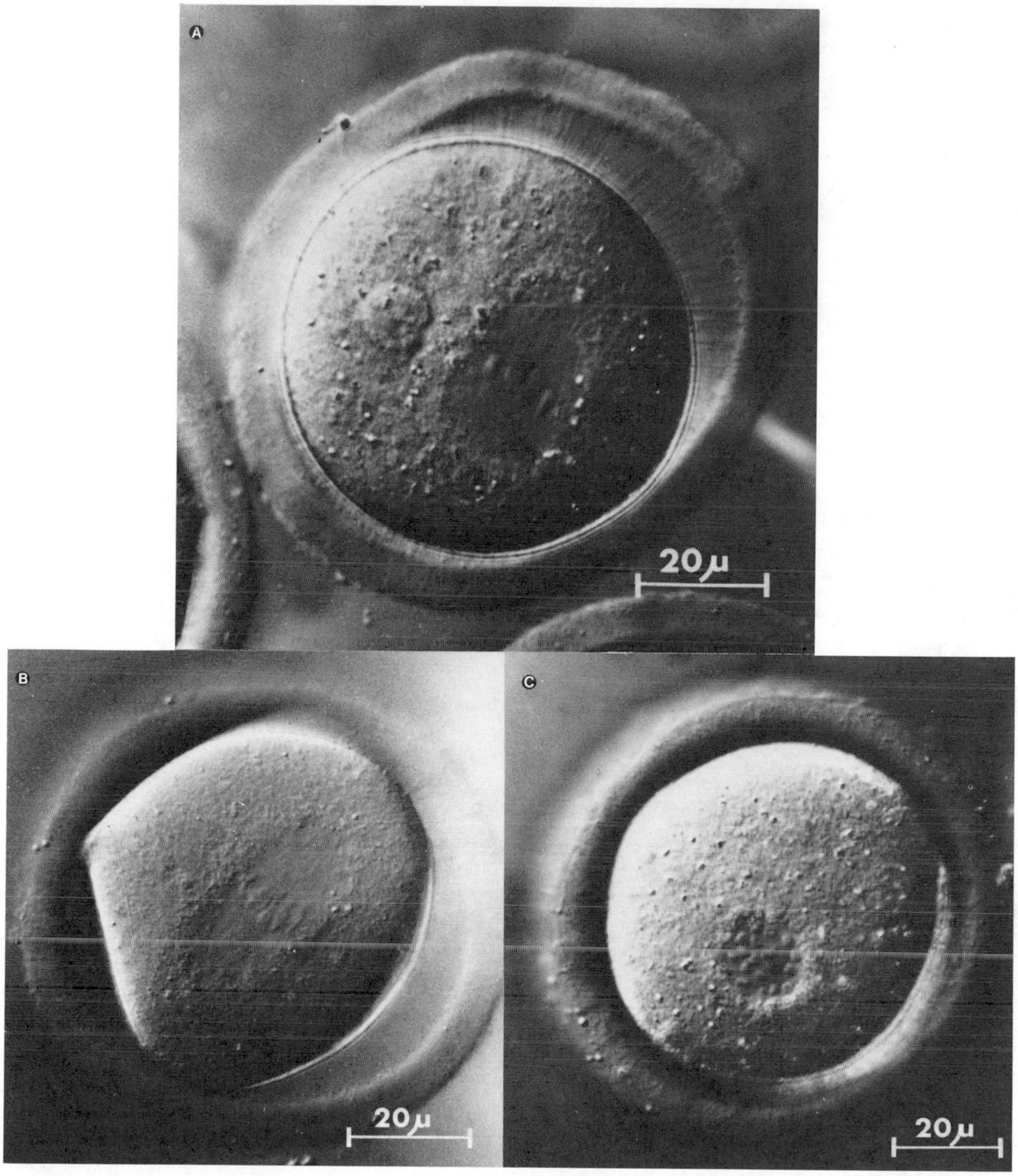

FIG. 14. Light photomicrographs of fully grown mouse oocytes at metaphase I during culture *in vitro*. Photographs were taken from a cinefilm made using Nomarski differential interference contrast microscopy. **A:** Early metaphase-I oocyte with a short, almost spherical, spindle. **B:** Late metaphase-I oocyte with an elongated spindle. Note that the oocyte plasmalemma is still attached to the zona pellucida at one point, causing distortion of the oocyte's shape. **C:** Polar view of a late metaphase-I oocyte with 17 or 18 bivalents seen clearly in the plane of focus. (From ref. 323.)

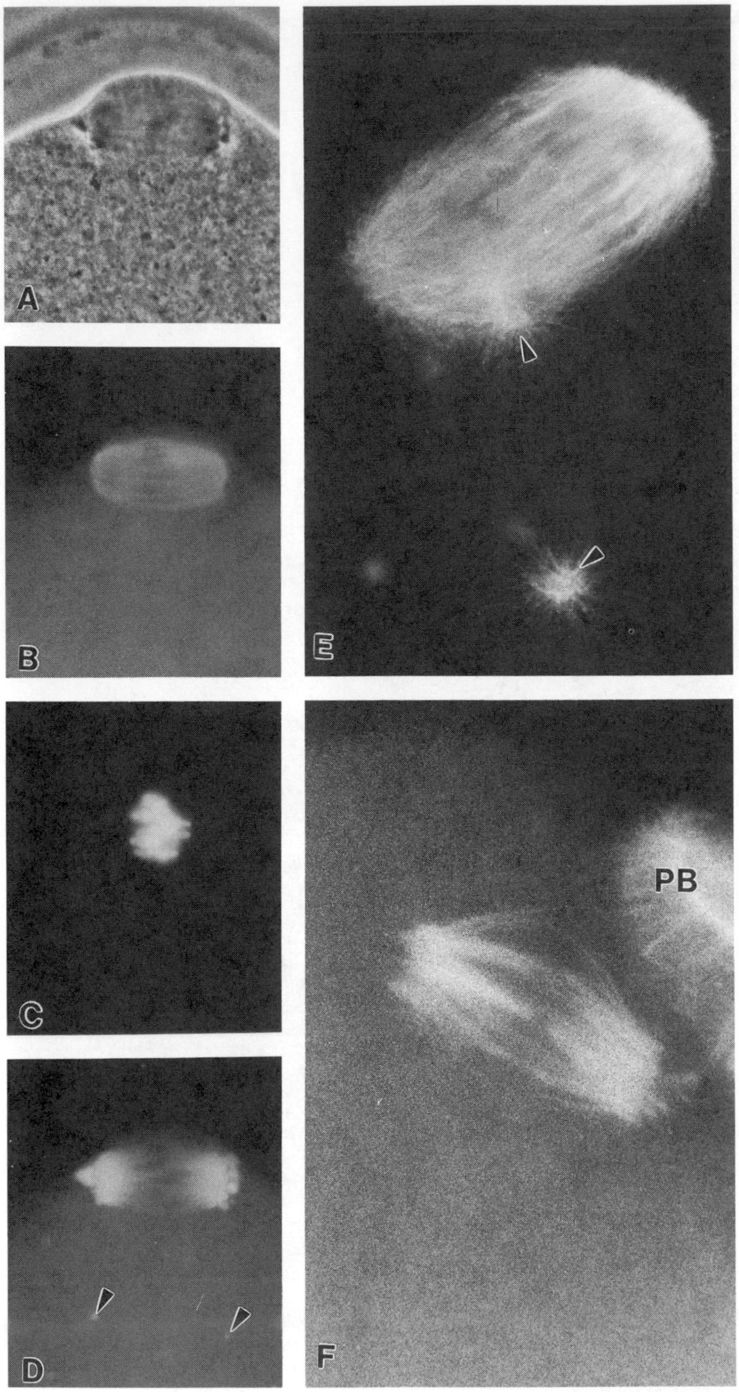

FIG. 15. Progression in mouse oocytes from metaphase I (**A–D**) to anaphase I (**E**) and metaphase II (**F**). **Left panel** illustrates a metaphase I spindle in phase contrast (**A**) and fluorescence after staining from microtubules (**B**), chromatin (**C**), and phosphorylated proteins (**D**); note phosphorylated cytoplasmic foci (*arrowheads*). In **E,** prominent cytoplasmic asters (*arrowheads*) reappear during anaphase but are absent at metaphase II (**F**). Polar body, PB.

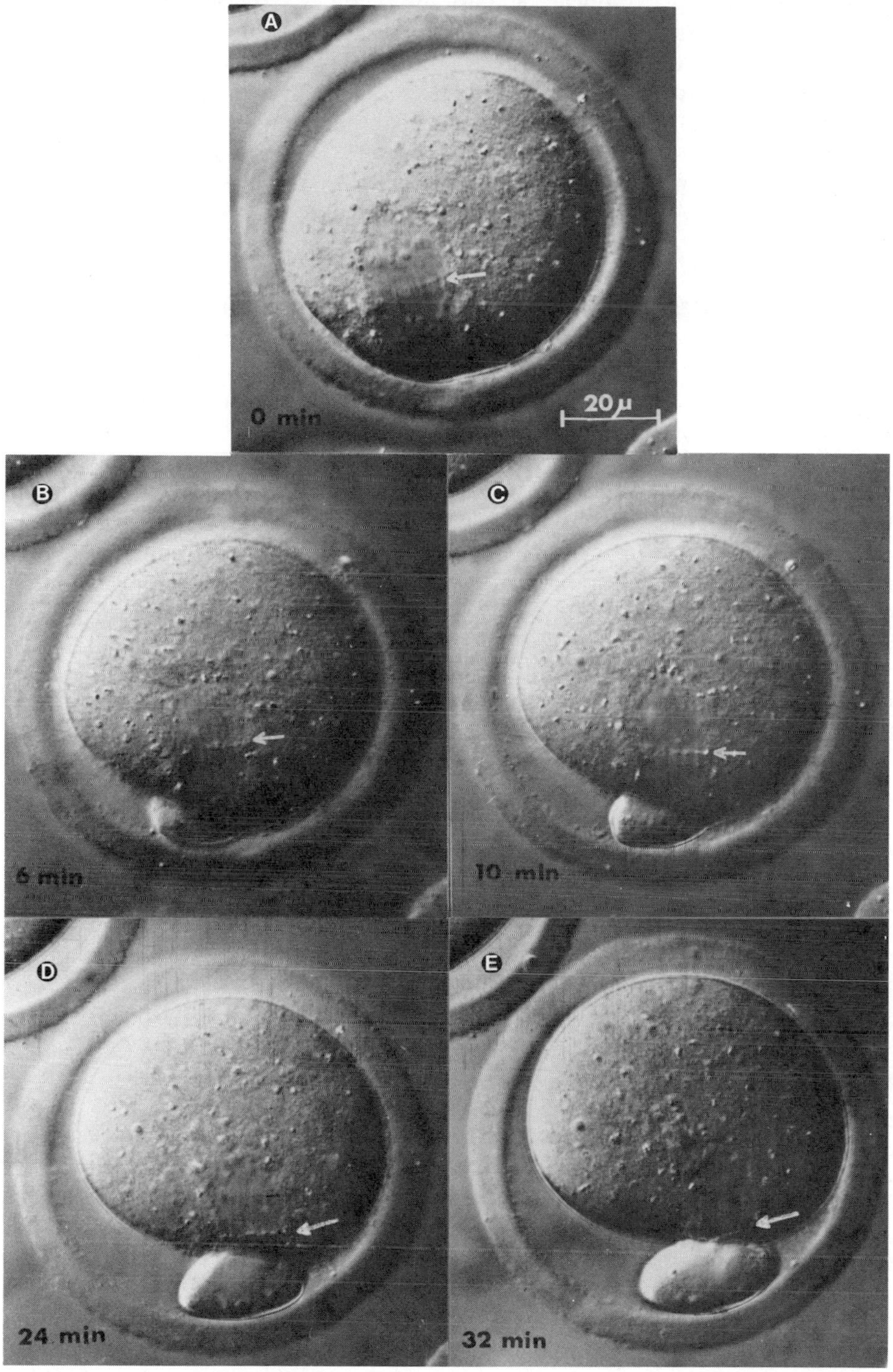

FIG. 16. Light photomicrographs of a fully grown mouse oocyte at anaphase I and telophase I during culture *in vitro.* Photographs were taken from a cinefilm made using Nomarski differential interference contrast microscopy. Actual time elapsed (in minutes) is recorded. **A:** Early anaphase-I oocyte with the midbody forming between the separating groups of chromosomes (*arrow*). Note the slight outpocketing of the oocyte membrane well in advance of the migrating polar-body chromosomes. **B:** Late anaphase I. **C:** Late anaphase I—early telophase I with polar-body chromosomes in the polar body. **D:** Telophase I with the entire spindle moving toward the polar body. **E:** Telophase I with the midbody reaching the boundary separating the oocyte and polar body. (From ref. 323.)

that a bulge, destined to become the first polar body, appears (Fig. 16). During telophase the midbody (a membranous and vacuolar basophilic ring around the central region of the telophase spindle) is formed, and pinching-off of the polar body is initiated (111,323,366). Separation of homologous chromosomes takes place, together with an asymmetric cleavage of oocyte cytoplasm containing one-half of the original chromosomal complement (late telophase). In addition to chromosomes, the first polar body contains a variety of organelles, including mitochondria, ribosomes, and cortical granules, as well as the midbody (387). Although a spindle is occasionally found in the first polar body, it is rarely a well-defined structure, and polar body chromosomes begin to degenerate in late telophase I. An area deficient in organelles such as cortical granules but rich in submembranous microfilamentous actin overlies the metaphase II spindle of unfertilized eggs. Furthermore, plasma membrane overlying the spindle is relatively smooth, whereas the remainder of the egg surface is highly microvillous. Microtubule-organizing centers, not associated with the spindle, are found in the cytoplasm near the cell's cortex. Progression beyond metaphase II, with separation of chromatids and emission of a second polar body, awaits fertilization or parthenogenetic activation of the egg.

OOCYTE MATURATION: REGULATORY ASPECTS

Meiotic Maturation: General Considerations

Mammalian oocytes have the unusual ability to undergo meiotic maturation spontaneously when released from follicles and cultured *in vitro* (127,128,210, 211,267,268,336,337,373). Unlike oocytes from nonmammalian species, no hormonal stimulus is needed for mammalian oocytes to reinitiate meiotic progression and reach metaphase II (i.e., to undergo the transition from oocyte to egg) *in vitro.* It is in this context that regulation of meiotic maturation, including prolonged arrest of oocytes at the dictyate stage and reentry of oocytes into meiotic progression just prior to ovulation, has been considered experimentally.

Inhibitors of Meiotic Maturation

A variety of agents prevent spontaneous meiotic maturation of mouse oocytes *in vitro* at specific stages of nuclear progression. Nuclear (GV) breakdown, the initial morphological feature characteristic of meiotic maturation, is inhibited by dibutyryl cyclic adenosine monophosphate (dbcAMP) and agents that increase intracellular levels of cyclic adenosine monophosphate (cAMP) (127,336,337) (discussed in the section on the role of cAMP). However, even in the presence of dbcAMP, the nuclear membrane becomes extremely convoluted, and chromosome condensation is initiated but aborts at a stage short of compact bivalents (368). Complete chromosome condensation requires breakdown of the nuclear envelope, probably attributable to the multiple associations of dictyate chromosomes with the nuclear envelope (71,333,368). In the presence of puromycin (protein synthesis inhibitor), colcemid (microtubule assembly inhibitor), or cytochalasin B (microfilament assembly inhibitor), nuclear membrane breakdown and chromosome condensation occur in an apparently normal manner (368,373). However, nuclear progression is blocked at the circular bivalent stage when oocytes are cultured continuously in the presence of either puromycin or colcemid, whereas oocytes cultured in the presence of cytochalasin B proceed to metaphase I, form a normal spindle, and arrest (321,368,373). Although this suggests that nascent protein synthesis is not required for nuclear (GV) breakdown and chromosome condensation, it is possible that spontaneous resumption of meiosis *in vitro* is, in fact, dependent on some oocyte proteins with very high turnover rates (122). The effect of cytochalasin on meiotic maturation suggests that microfilaments are involved in events following metaphase I spindle formation (e.g., separation of homologous chromosomes). Emission of a polar body is inhibited by all of these drugs, suggesting that cytokinesis is blocked when any one of the earlier events of maturation fails to take place (368,373). In this context, it has been found that activators of protein kinase C (e.g., phorbol esters; see below), but not dbcAMP, inhibit polar body emission by oocytes that had already undergone nuclear (GV) breakdown *in vitro* (51).

Role of cAMP

Spontaneous maturation of mouse oocytes does not occur *in vitro* when oocytes are cultured in the presence of either membrane-permeable analogs of cAMP, such as dbcAMP and 8-bromo-cAMP, or inhibitors of cyclic nucleotide phosphodiesterase (PDE), such as isobutyl methylxanthine (IBMX) and theophylline (83,105,203, 312,314,368). Similarly, other agents that increase intracellular cAMP levels by activation of adenylate cyclase, such as forskolin, also prevent spontaneous maturation of mouse oocytes *in vitro* (53,104,246,273,298,312,345). Furthermore, microinjection of PDE into oocytes cultured in the presence of IBMX overcomes the inhibitory effect of IBMX on meiotic maturation (50). An oocyte PDE activity has been identified and characterized and has been shown to be membrane-bound and modulated by calmodulin; a calmodulin-dependent step occurs subsequent to, or concurrently with, the decrease in oocyte cAMP levels (see below) during spontaneous maturation (54). The behavior of oocytes under these conditions suggests that cAMP is involved in the maintenance of meiotic arrest at the dictyate stage, such that a fall in intracellular cAMP levels could signal reentry of oocytes into meiotic progression. In fact, a significant decrease in cAMP levels of oocytes does occur just prior to nuclear envelope (GV) breakdown, both *in vitro* and *in vivo* (106,312,368). Therefore, just as cAMP is involved in regulating the G_2-to-M transition during the mitotic cell cycle, it appears to be involved in the reentry of oocytes into meiotic progression. It should be noted that exposure of oocytes to dbcAMP following nuclear envelope (GV) breakdown has no effect on subsequent events of meiotic maturation; polar-body emission with arrest at metaphase II occurs in a normal manner (368,373).

Involvement of cAMP in meiotic maturation implies that, as in many other biological situations, it acts via cAMP-dependent protein kinase (PK), an enzyme consisting of catalytic (C) and regulatory (R) subunits (142, 232). Although the R–C complex is enzymatically inactive, binding of cAMP to the R (inhibitory) subunit results in dissociation of the complex and activation of the C subunit kinase activity. Assuming that continuous phosphorylation of an oocyte protein(s) by PK is essential for maintenance of meiotic arrest, cAMP levels could thereby regulate meiotic maturation by determining the amount of free C subunit available. Under conditions of low levels of free C subunit (low cAMP), the relevant oocyte phosphoprotein(s) would be dephosphorylated, and the meiotic maturation would be initiated. In this context, mouse oocytes microinjected with the C subunit of PK fail to undergo spontaneous meiotic maturation during culture *in vitro* in the absence of dbcAMP and IBMX (50,51). Furthermore, changes in the phosphorylation patterns of oocyte proteins under a variety of experimental conditions are consistent with this proposed regulatory scheme (50,312). However, other evidence suggests that cAMP is only one of the components of a complex system employed in the maintenance of oocytes in the dictyate stage of the first meiotic prophase (discussed in the sections on the roles of calcium, intercellular communication, steroids, and oocyte maturation inhibitor). In particular, it is noteworthy that increasing the levels of cAMP in cumulus cells, in the presence of FSH or cholera toxin, results in inhibition of meiotic maturation without a detectable rise in oocyte cAMP levels (130,313). This suggests the possibility that an inhibitory factor other than cAMP is transferred from cumulus cells to oocytes, resulting in inhibition of meiotic maturation *in vitro* (discussed in the section on the role of oocyte maturation inhibitor).

Finally, phorbol esters and diacylglycerol, known activators of calcium/phospholipid-dependent protein kinase (PK-C), also inhibit spontaneous maturation of oocytes *in vitro* without a decrease in oocyte cAMP levels (51). These PK-C activators also inhibit the changes in oocyte phosphoprotein metabolism associated with spontaneous maturation, suggesting that PK-C activators inhibit resumption of meiosis by acting distal to a decrease in cAMP-dependent PK activity, prior to changes in oocyte phosphoprotein metabolism that are necessary for resumption of meiosis.

Role of Calcium

Involvement of calmodulin during meiotic maturation implies that there is a role for calcium (54,103,196,338). Verapamil and tetracaine, two inhibitors of transmembrane calcium transport, transiently prevent breakdown of the nuclear (GV) envelope *in vitro* (250). Furthermore, increasing extracellular calcium concentrations decreases the effectiveness of dbcAMP as an inhibitor of meiotic maturation, whereas verapamil and tetracaine (which decrease intracellular calcium concentration) increase its effectiveness (269). Therefore, intracellular levels of calcium and cAMP may act synergistically, through a calmodulin-dependent step, to regulate meiotic maturation of mammalian oocytes.

Role of Intercellular Communication

Gap junctions represent regions of physical continuity between cellular membranes. As such, in many biological systems they serve as mediators of intercellular communication and metabolic coupling by permitting passage of small molecules between cells; in this manner, one type of cell can influence the function of another (147,194). Fully grown mouse oocytes are coupled with surrounding cumulus cells by gap junctions (4,5,7,8,146). They are found at areas of contact between the oocyte's plasma membrane and processes that emanate from cumulus cells and traverse the zona pellucida. Furthermore, an extensive network of gap junctions interconnects all follicle cells with the cumulus and, consequently, with the oocyte.

Throughout oocyte growth and folliculogenesis, both *in vivo* and *in vitro,* gap junctions mediate intercellular communication between the oocyte and follicle cells. The cells are both metabolically and ionically coupled, and iontophoretically injected dye is transferred between cumulus cells and oocyte (146,277). However, just prior to ovulation there is a significant decrease in the number of gap junctions, together with a decrease in the extent of ionic coupling, and, following ovulation, the oocyte and surrounding cumulus cells are no longer coupled as a result of mucification and cumulus expansion (108,146, 167,193,223) (Fig. 17). In the latter state, cumulus cell processes are retracted away from the oocyte surface. This behavior suggests that spontaneous meiotic maturation takes place *in vitro* as a result of removing oocytes from the inhibitory influence of follicle cells. In this con-

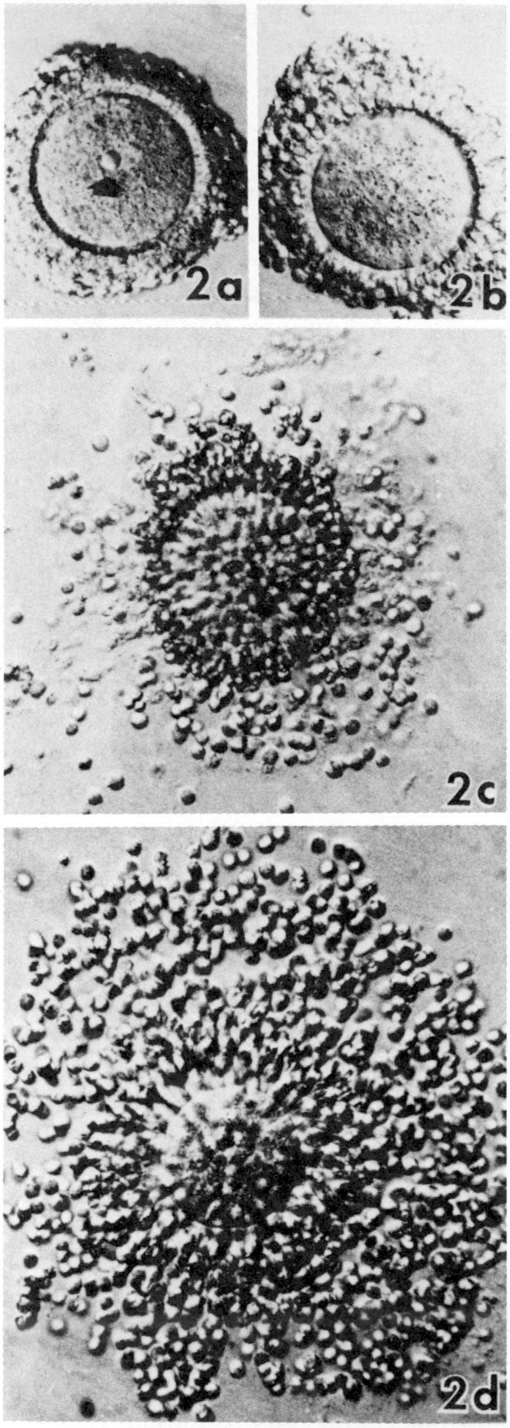

FIG. 17. Light photomicrographs of oocyte-cumulus-cell complexes isolated from control and hCG-injected mice. (**a**) Control; (**b–d**) 3, 6, and 9 hr post-hCG injection. The germinal vesicle is clearly seen (*arrow*) in the oocytes from control mice (a). At 3 hr post-hCG, the germinal vesicle has broken down, but cumulus cells are still tightly packed around the oocytes (b). At 6 hr post-hCG injection, cumulus expansion includes only the outer cumulus cell, while those adjacent to the oocyte are still tightly packed (c). Cumulus expansion appears complete by 9 hr post-hCG (d), and these oocytes show a reduction in intercellular coupling as compared to controls. (From ref. 126.)

text, it has been demonstrated that either grafting oocytes to follicle walls or coculture of oocytes with granulosa cells prevents spontaneous maturation *in vitro.*

Between 2 and 3 hours following administration of an ovulatory stimulus (hCG), there is about a 15-fold decrease in the net area of cumulus cell gap junction membrane (i.e., about 90% of the total gap junction membrane per cumulus cell is lost within an hour) (193) (Fig. 18). The loss of cumulus cell gap junctions is temporally correlated with nuclear envelope (GV) breakdown and cumulus expansion (126,193,296). In this context, the inhibitory effects of both FSH and suboptimal concentrations of dbcAMP are lost when intercellular communication between cumulus cells and the oocyte is disrupted *in vitro.* However, although the coupling of cumulus cells and the oocyte terminates before ovulation, it is not completed until after nuclear envelope (GV) breakdown. Therefore, although it is tempting to attribute the onset of meiotic maturation exclusively to termination of intercellular communication between cumulus cells and the oocyte (e.g., cessation of transfer of an "inhibitory factor" from cumulus cells to the oocyte via gap junctions), there is evidence to the contrary.

Role of Steroids

Although LH induces both maturation of oocytes and progesterone production in intact follicles *in vitro,* LH apparently does not induce maturation via progesterone synthesis (107,109,336,337). Furthermore, it remains problematic whether or not other steroid hormones, such as estradiol and testosterone, play a role in regulation of meiotic maturation. Whereas, a number of steroid hormones potentiate the FSH-induced inhibition of meiotic maturation of cumulus cell-enclosed oocytes *in vitro* (without an increase in oocyte cAMP levels; see section on nuclear [GV] breakdown), they only inhibit maturation of denuded oocytes when their cAMP levels are elevated by exposure to dbcAMP or forskolin (127,130,274,313). On the other hand, at very high nonphysiological concentrations, testosterone, progesterone, prenenolone, as well as other steroids, inhibit meiotic maturation, either alone or in conjunction with dbcAMP or agents that affect intracellular cAMP levels (131,139,195,213,222,276,279,322).

Role of Oocyte Maturation Inhibitor

It has been suggested that oocyte maturation inhibitor (OMI), a product of granulosa cells, maintains oocytes in the dictyate stage of first meiotic prophase (336,337, 339,341,342). This is consistent with the relatively old observation that follicular fluid inhibits oocyte maturation *in vitro* (76,80,81,161,340,341,343). OMI is a poly-

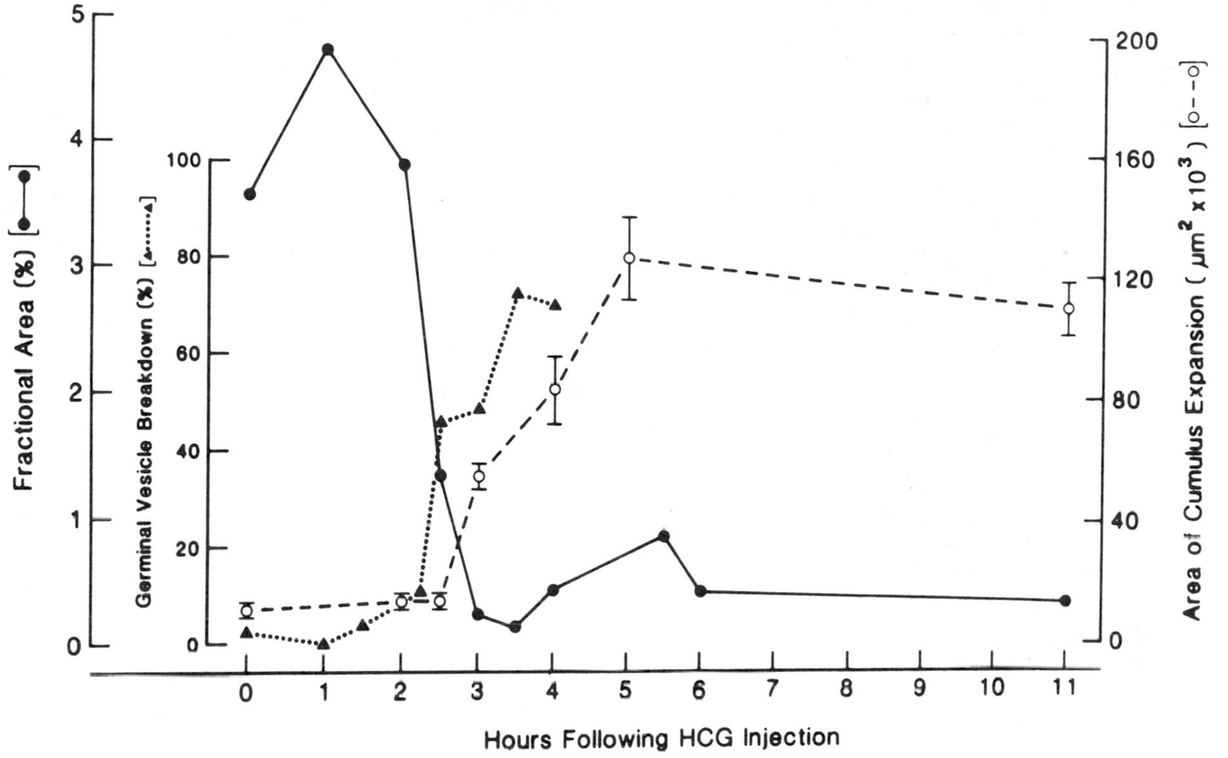

FIG. 18. Changes in gap-junction fractional area, projected cumulus-oocyte area, and fraction of rat oocytes showing no germinal vesicle at varying times after an ovulatory stimulus. (From ref. 193.)

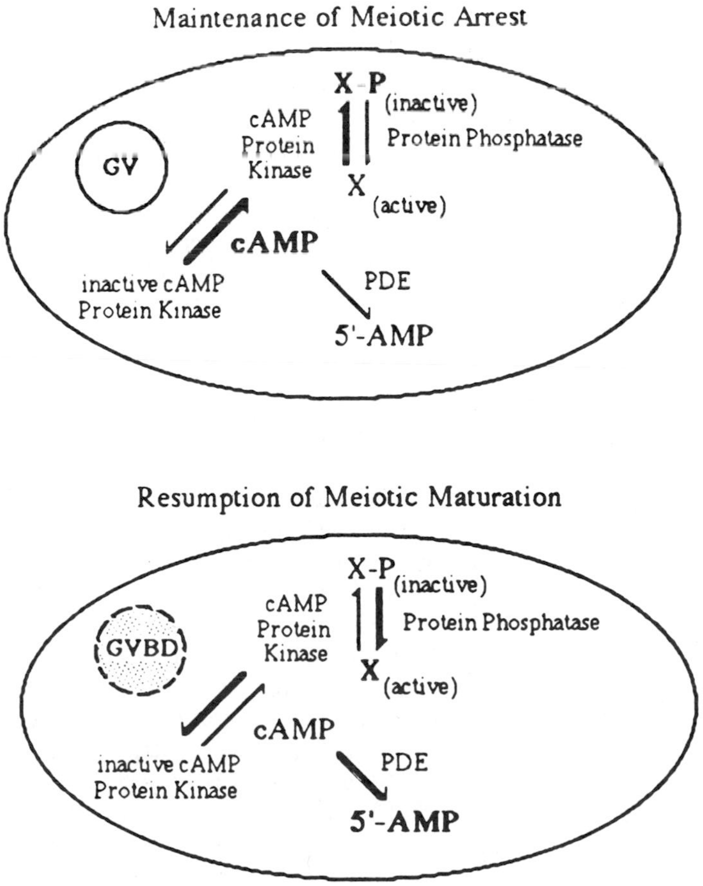

FIG. 19. Model of regulation of meiotic arrest and resumption of meiosis. The model proposes that a phosphoprotein, X-P, maintains meiotic arrest; the dephosphorylated form, X, promotes resumption of meiosis. X is phosphorylated by protein kinase, and X-P is dephosphorylated by phosphoprotein phosphatase; these two enzyme activities determine the steady-state levels of X-P and X in the oocyte. Resumption of meiosis is initiated by a decrease in cAMP, which leads to a decrease in protein kinase activity. Assuming that phosphoprotein phosphatase activity is unchanged, this decrease in protein kinase activity would induce a net dephosphorylation of X-P, triggering resumption of meiosis. It should be noted that although X is depicted as actively promoting GVBD (germinal vesicle breakdown), X-P could just as well actively maintain meiotic arrest; this would not alter the model significantly. Boldface type indicates the putative predominant species. (From ref. 50.)

peptide that has a molecular mass of about 1 to 2 kilodaltons, is found in follicular fluid from ovaries of a variety of mammals, and prevents oocytes from undergoing spontaneous meiotic maturation when cultured *in vitro*. However, OMI apparently exerts its inhibitory action via cumulus cells, since it prevents maturation of oocytes cultured with their cumulus cells but does not interfere with maturation of completely denuded oocytes; in this context, it is likely that OMI is small enough to pass through gap junctions between cumulus cells and the oocyte (336,337,339). Preovulatory follicles have relatively low concentrations of OMI, consistent with its proposed role in regulating meiotic maturation. It is possible that the inhibitory action of OMI is potentiated by cAMP, suggesting that OMI could account for some of the effects of cAMP on cumulus-enclosed oocytes observed *in vitro* (52,114,130,313) (discussed in section on regulatory aspects of oocyte maturation). However, it should be noted that the existence of OMI has been seriously questioned in some quarters and, in the absence of additional biochemical support, remains a highly controversial subject (133,197,198,275). Furthermore, recent evidence suggests that hypoxanthine and/or adenosine are, in fact, the low-molecular-weight components of follicular fluid that prevent spontaneous meiotic maturation of oocytes *in vitro* (112,132).

Summary

Many factors potentially influence the maintenance of mammalian oocytes in the dictyate stage of first meiotic prophase. These include cAMP, as well as enzyme systems involved in regulating intracellular levels of cAMP, calcium, calmodulin, steroids, hypophyseal hormones, purine bases, putative polypeptide inhibitors, and intercellular communication between cumulus cells and between cumulus cells and the oocyte, in the form of gap junctions. At present, the interplay between these factors in regulating meiotic maturation both *in vivo* and *in vitro* is not precisely understood, precluding formulation of a detailed regulatory pathway that satisfies all relevant observations. However, it is clear that such a pathway would include many of the features thought to be involved in regulation of meiotic maturation of amphibian oocytes (205) and would undoubtedly involve cAMP (Fig. 19). Finally, it is apparent that, overall, it is the integrity of the follicle that maintains mammalian oocytes in meiotic arrest.

GROWTH OF THE OOCYTE: BIOCHEMICAL ASPECTS

Oocyte Growth *In Vitro*

The ability to isolate and culture growing mouse oocytes *in vitro* has resulted in significant advances in our understanding of various aspects of the metabolism of oocyte growth. Improving on earlier methods for obtaining growing oocytes from juvenile animals, at least two reliable culture systems are now available that support oocyte growth *in vitro*. In one, follicles obtained from collagenase-treated juvenile ovaries rapidly attach to culture dishes, and, although some granulosa cells leave the follicles, oocytes remain surrounded by at least one layer of granulosa cells (123–125,129,166). These oocytes increase in size at a rate comparable to that observed *in vivo*. In the other system, follicles obtained from Pronase-treated juvenile ovaries rapidly attach to culture dishes and then follicle cells migrate away, liberating oocytes that rest on a monolayer of ovarian cells (19,37). These oocytes grow, but at a rate lower than that observed *in vivo* (19). In both of these systems, oocyte growth is assessed to be normal in that oocytes (a) display increasing levels of CO_2 production from exogenous pyruvate, (b) exhibit appropriate changes in size, morphology, and ultrastructure, (c) express growth-specific, differential regulation of certain isozyme activities (66), (d) exhibit a progressively thickening zona pellucida, and (e) become competent to undergo meiotic maturation during prolonged culture *in vitro*.

Intercellular communication between the oocyte and granulosa cells, via gap junctions, apparently is necessary for oocyte growth *in vitro* (19,125,168). In the absence of gap junctions, oocytes grow very little, if at all, and, after several days in culture, undergo necrosis. It is likely that denuded oocytes will become necrotic because they normally depend on granulosa cells to meet certain of their nutritional demands. In this connection, gap-junction-mediated metabolic cooperativity between oocytes and cumulus cells has been demonstrated in several ways. For example, cumulus-enclosed fully grown oocytes take up significantly more leucine, uridine, choline, and inositol from culture medium than do denuded, fully-grown oocytes (98,167,223,369) (Figs. 20 and 21).

Similarly, follicle-enclosed growing oocytes take up significantly more uridine, guanosine, choline, and deoxyglucose from culture medium than do denuded, growing oocytes (166). Furthermore, differences in the distribution of phosphorylated metabolites of ribonucleosides in oocytes have been noted when investigators have compared denuded with either cumulus or follicle-enclosed oocytes cultured *in vitro* (63,166). The evidence suggests, for example, that oocytes derive most of their ribonucleosides and ribonucleotides from granulosa cells; denuded oocytes are poorly able to take up ribonucleosides and metabolize them to ribonucleotides. In addition, since growing oocytes lack the energy-dependent, so-called A-transport system for uptake of certain amino acids, it is likely that follicle cells provide these amino acids, routing them to oocytes through gap junctions (93). These and other observations strongly suggest that intercellular communication between follicle cells and

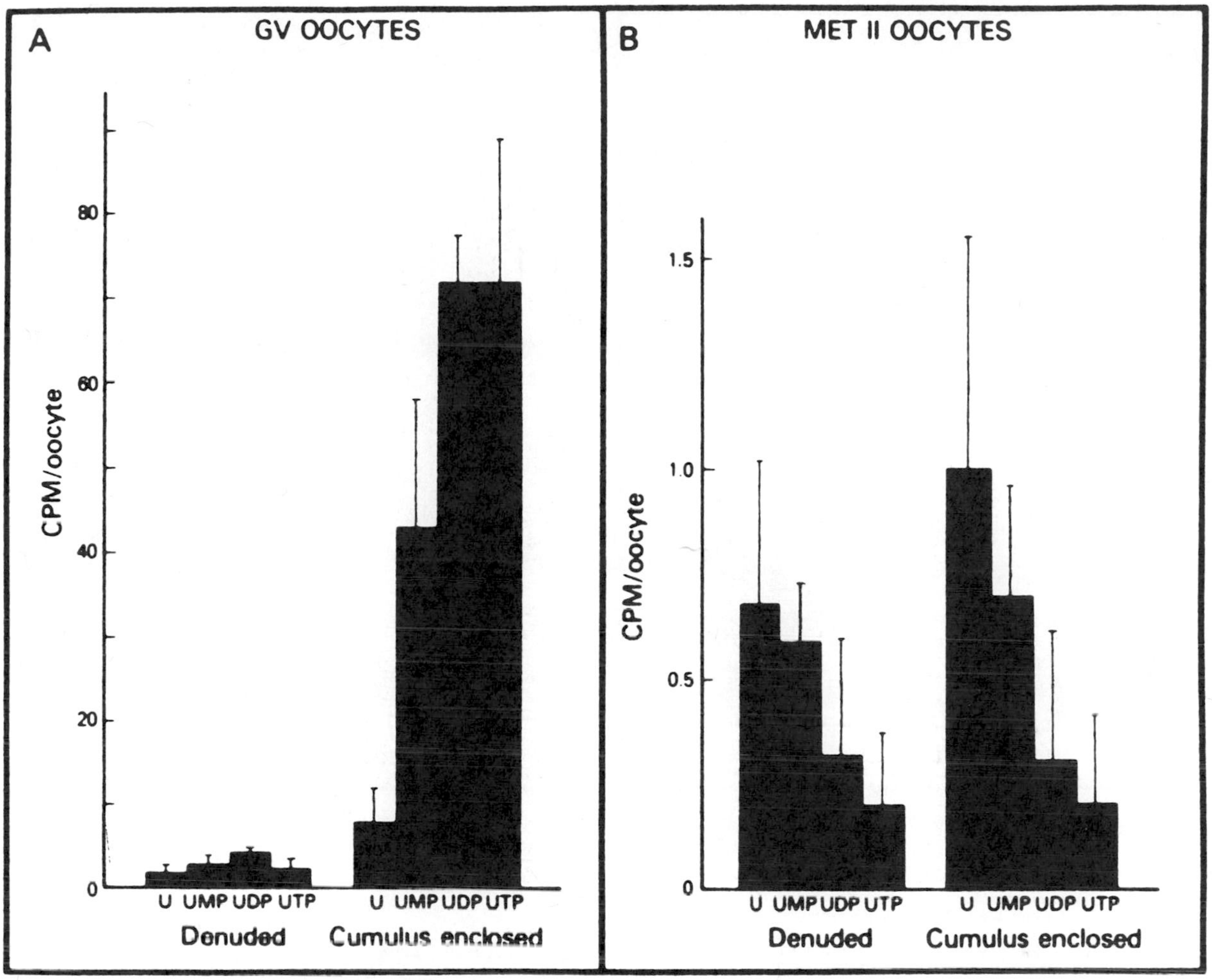

FIG. 20. Distribution of uridine, UMP, UDP, and UTP in denuded and cumulus-enclosed mouse oocytes at two stages of nuclear progression. **A:** Oocytes arrested at the dictyate stage of the first meiotic prophase. **B:** Oocytes arrested at metaphase II (unfertilized eggs). (From ref. 167.)

oocytes plays a vital nutritional role during oocyte growth. Consistent with this role, the extent of metabolic cooperativity increases during oocyte growth *in vivo* and *in vitro,* and the rate of oocyte growth *in vitro* is positively correlated with the extent of intercellular communication (gap junction formation) (63) (Fig. 22). Perhaps, the relationship between oocyte growth and intercellular communication reflects "an economization and compartmentalization of metabolic function, thereby liberating the oocyte from numerous housekeeping functions" (63). Such a division of labor between oocytes and follicle cells would emulate the situation in most nonmammals.

Overall RNA Synthesis

Fully grown mouse oocytes contain about 500 to 600 pg of RNA, or about 200 times the amount found in typical somatic cells (18,182,245,329,355). Of the total, approximately 10% to 15% is polyadenylated RNA (informational RNA), 20% to 25% is transfer RNA, and 60% to 65% is ribosomal RNA (18,329). Virtually all of this RNA is synthesized during the 2- to 3-week period of oocyte growth (discussed in the section on structural aspects of oocyte growth). The RNA content of oocytes increases dramatically during their growth phase, with RNA accumulation exhibiting biphasic kinetics with respect to oocyte volume (182,329). During early and mid-growth stages, changes in nucleolar ultrastructure and in levels of RNA polymerase activity are consistent with high rates of transcription of ribosomal-DNA (136,193, 225–229). Although the rate of RNA synthesis during this period is high with respect to some somatic cells, it does not approach the rates estimated for growing amphibian oocytes, which have bone fide "lampbrush chromosomes," leading some, but not all, investigators to conclude that "true lampbrush chromosomes do not exist at any point in development of mouse oocytes" (18).

When oocytes reach about three-quarters of their final volume, they contain nearly as much RNA as is found in fully grown oocytes (329) (Fig. 23). It can be estimated

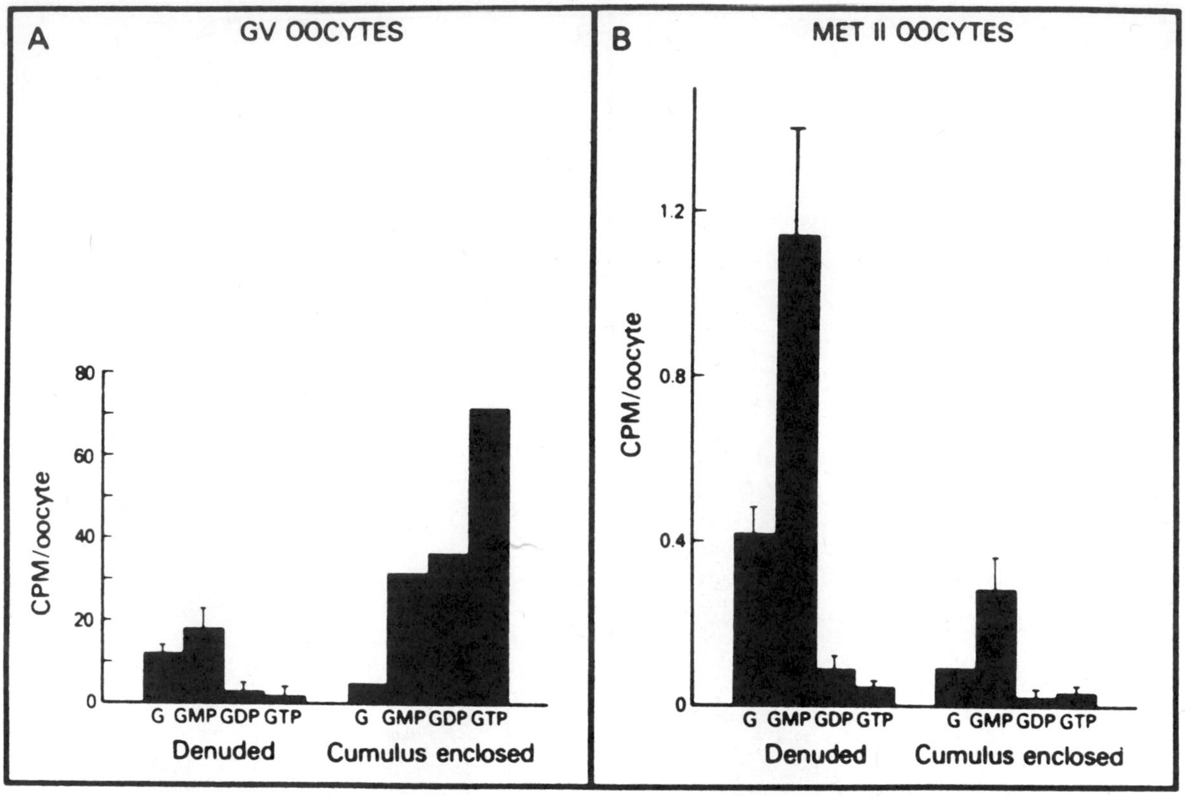

FIG. 21. Distribution of guanosine, GMP, GDP, and GTP in denuded and cumulus-enclosed mouse oocytes at two stages of nuclear progression. **A:** Oocytes arrested at the dictyate stage of the first meiotic prophase. **B:** Oocytes arrested at metaphase II (unfertilized eggs). (From ref. 167.)

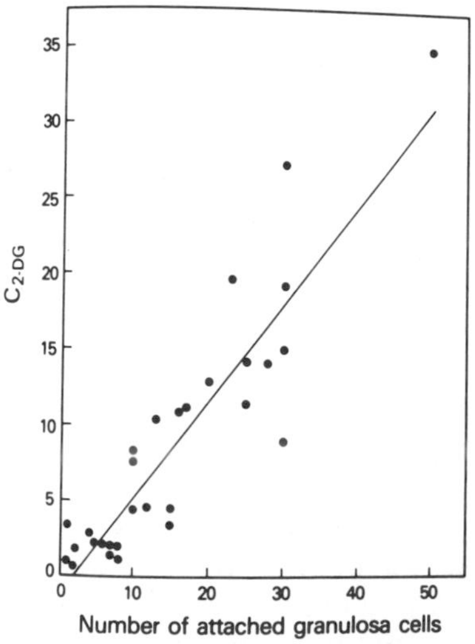

FIG. 22. Intercellular communication as monitored by metabolic cooperativity between granulosa cells and oocytes. Value of $C_{2\text{-DG}}$ (2-deoxyglucose), indicative of intercellular communication, is plotted as a function of the number of granulosa cells attached to oocytes. *C*, a metabolic cooperativity ratio, is defined as $(A - B)/B$, where *A* is the number of cpm/granulosa cell-enclosed oocyte and *B* is the number of cpm/denuded oocyte. Values of *C* greater than 0 indicate the existence of metabolic cooperativity. Each point represents a determination made with a single oocyte–granulosa-cell complex. Note that *C* increases with increasing numbers of attached granulosa cells. (From ref. 63.)

that, overall, there is a 300-fold increase in the RNA content of oocytes during their growth phase, consistent with changes in nuclear and nucleolar sizes as well as in levels of RNA synthesis during this period. Similarly, measurements of endogenous levels of RNA polymerase during oocyte growth are consistent with progressively increasing extents of RNA synthesis until oocytes reach about three-quarters of their final volume (225,228). RNA continues to be synthesized in fully grown oocytes, although at a diminished rate compared to midgrowth oocytes, and declines to barely detectable levels only after the onset of meiotic maturation (ovulation) (48,284,369).

Specific RNA Synthesis

Several experimental approaches have been used to assess synthesis of specific classes of RNA during oocyte growth in mice:

1. A radiolabeled RNA precursor, such as $[^3H]$-uridine/adenosine, is injected into the ovarian bursa. Analyses of radiolabeled RNA in ovulated eggs are then carried out 1 to 24 days after the injection. Since the major growth phase of oocytes occurs between 20 and 6

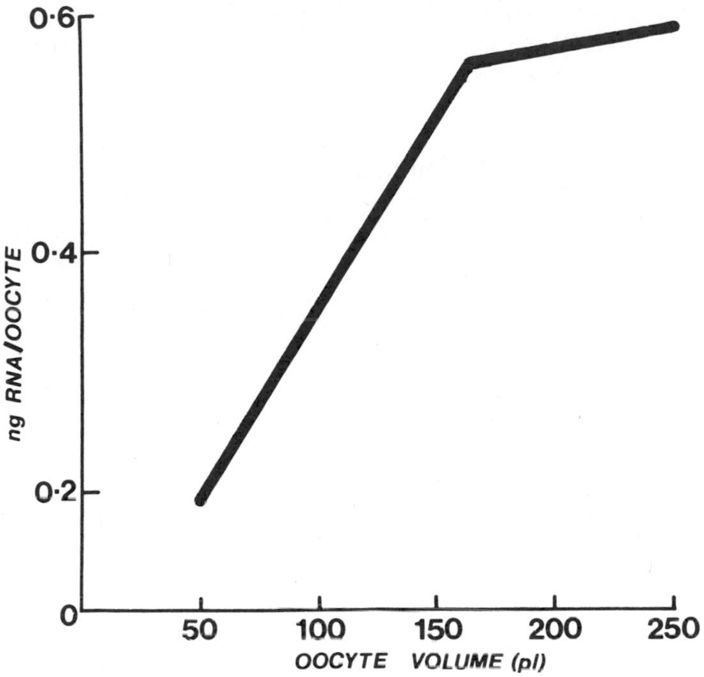

FIG. 23. Relationship between mouse oocyte growth and accumulation of oocyte RNA. Note that, overall, there is nearly a 300-fold increase in RNA content during growth of mouse oocytes, from about 12 to 85 μm in diameter. Here, the smallest oocytes examined were about 40 μm in diameter; the change in RNA content during growth of oocytes from 12 to 40 μm was not determined. (From ref. 329.)

days prior to ovulation, these analyses provide information about kinds of RNA synthesized and their stability *in vivo* (16,18,23,110,178).

The time course of RNA labeling following injection of [^{3}H]uridine/adenosine into the ovarian bursa indicates that significant levels of RNA synthesis occur in growing oocytes during the 2 weeks prior to ovulation. Furthermore, about three-quarters of nascent RNA, synthesized 19 to 43 hours after bursal injection of radiolabel, is retained until ovulation 10 to 20 days later, suggesting that RNA synthesized in growing oocytes is extremely stable. Analyses of the RNA on sucrose gradients and gels indicate that about 65%, 20%, and 15% of the radiolabel is in ribosomal RNA, 5S, transfer RNA, and heterogeneous RNA, respectively, throughout oocyte growth. The average rate of ribosomal RNA synthesis is 15 fg/min during oocyte growth. It is not necessary to propose extensive amplification of the mouse oocyte's ribosomal genes in order to account for this level of ribosomal RNA synthesis, although a fourfold amplification may occur in oocytes from other mammals (383,384). At any time during oocyte growth, from 7 to 19 days prior to ovulation, approximately 10% of radiolabel present in nascent RNA is associated with polyadenylated RNA. Furthermore, 9% to 12% of RNA synthesized at each stage of oocyte growth and conserved in unfertilized eggs is polyadenylated RNA. From such information, one can calculate (a) that enough polyadenylated RNA is made during oocyte growth to account for about 6% to 8% of the mass of egg RNA (~30–45 pg) and (b) that enough polyadenylated RNA is produced to account for virtually all polysomal informational RNA present in mouse eggs. The relatively large amount of informational RNA in eggs is attributable to both high rates of synthesis during oocyte growth and unusual stability of the RNA.

2. Denuded oocytes, cumulus–oocyte complexes, or follicle-enclosed oocytes are incubated in the presence of a radiolabeled RNA precursor in an appropriate culture medium *in vitro*. Analyses of radiolabeled RNA in oocytes are then carried out after various times of culture (17,18,49,61).

Total RNA synthesized by follicle-enclosed growing oocytes is unusually stable (having a half-life of about 28 days) as long as oocytes continue growing *in vitro* (the half-life decreases to about 4 days when oocytes are viable, but the oocytes do not grow *in vitro*). Under conditions of oocyte growth, turnover of ribosomal, 5S, and transfer RNA is barely detectable. On the other hand, polyadenylated RNA turns over slowly (with a half-life of about 10 days) and exhibits kinetics suggestive of a relatively unstable species of high-molecular-weight heterogeneous RNA. As much as one-half of RNA synthesized by follicle-enclosed growing oocytes, 35 to 65 μm in diameter, is polyadenylated, decreasing to as little as one-fifth of the nascent RNA of fully grown oocytes.

The behavior of heterogeneous RNA has been well characterized in denuded oocytes cultured in the presence of ovarian somatic cell monolayers, under conditions that permit oocyte growth *in vitro*. In these growing oocytes, heterogeneous RNA is synthesized at the relatively high rate of 0.6 pg/min and turns over rapidly, with a half-life of 20 minutes. As a result of the high rate of synthesis, the steady-state amount of nuclear, heterogeneous-RNA present in these oocytes is quite large, approximating 15 pg. About 2% of this RNA is conserved, reaches the cytoplasm, and accumulates at the rate of approximately 0.01 pg/min. All of these values are based on the assumption that ribosomal RNA is synthesized at the rate of 0.2 ng/week and is completely stable during the measurements.

3. ^{3}H-labeled poly-(U) is hybridized *in situ* to ovarian sections or fixed oocytes, followed by autoradiography, to estimate relative amounts, as well as intracellular localization, of polyadenylated RNA (18,26,264,329).

By this method, the kinetics of accumulation of polyadenylated RNA are similar to the biphasic kinetics of accumulation of total RNA during oocyte growth. Nearly 95% of the polyadenylated RNA present in fully grown oocytes is found in growing oocytes that have reached about three-quarters of their final volume. There is as much as a two-fold reduction in the amount of cytoplasmic polyadenylated RNA during the interval between completion of oocyte growth and ovulation; however, the relative concentration of polyadenylated RNA in the nucleus remains about two times that in the cytoplasm, suggesting that polyadenylated RNA synthesis continues following completion of oocyte growth. Solution hybridization experiments suggest that, just prior to ovulation, fully grown oocytes contain about 26 pg of polyadenylated RNA but that this falls to about 19 pg in unfertilized eggs.

Finally, it would appear that growing mouse oocytes also synthesize an RNA species resembling Ul-RNA, a small nuclear RNA thought to play a role in processing of heterogeneous nuclear RNA (hnRNA) (183). Similarly, growing oocytes contain intracisternal A-particle-related RNA sequences (IAP RNA), which are found at high levels in fully grown oocytes (~17,000 molecules/oocyte; 61 fg), but at much lower levels in unfertilized eggs (~1,000 molecules/egg; 4 fg) (265). On the other hand, surprisingly, mouse egg RNA is not enriched in Alulike repetitive sequence transcripts, as compared to cytoplasmic RNA from various mammalian tissues (183).

RNA Synthesis: Summary

From the preceding, it should be apparent that RNA synthesis and accumulation are major activities of growing mammalian oocytes. On a per cell basis, the fully grown mouse oocyte contains about 200 times more RNA and 1000 times more ribosomes than does a typical mammalian somatic cell. Especially noteworthy is the large amount of informational RNA in fully grown oocytes, large even in comparison with amphibian oocytes (on a percentage of total RNA basis). It should be realized, however, that on a volume (per picoliter) basis, mouse oocytes are not unlike somatic cells with respect to RNA and ribosome concentration. Therefore, to some extent, it is simply the failure of growing oocytes to undergo cytokinesis that results in unusually large stores of RNA and ribosomes.

Overall Protein Synthesis

Electrophoretic analyses of proteins synthesized by growing and fully grown mouse oocytes reveal a remarkable degree of constancy at the qualitative level (151,314,355). Several hundred discrete species are detected on fluorograms of high-resolution two-dimensional gels containing proteins radiolabeled with [^{35}S]methionine during culture of oocytes *in vitro*. The most intensely radiolabeled proteins are also the most abundant, based on patterns of comparable silver-stained gels. Although changes in overall patterns of protein synthesis occur during oocyte growth, most, but not all, of these can be characterized as quantitative changes. In other words, overall, these analyses suggest that the same proteins are synthesized throughout oocyte growth, but at different relative rates at different times in the growth phase. It is almost certain that stage-specific synthesis of particular proteins occurs during oocyte growth (e.g., proteins involved in regulation of meiotic maturation); however, thus far, these proteins have not been identified. Analysis of cDNA libraries, prepared from messenger RNA purified at different stages of oocyte growth, should lead to identification and characterization of such proteins.

The sizes of endogenous methionine pools and absolute rates of protein synthesis in growing and fully grown mouse oocytes have been determined using isolated oocytes that are denuded of follicle cells and cultured *in vitro* (310,311,355) (Fig. 24). As the oocyte undergoes about a 300-fold increase in volume during its growth phase, a corresponding increase occurs in the size of the oocyte's endogenous methionine pool, from 0.16 to 56 fmole/oocyte. Therefore, each doubling of oocyte volume is accompanied by a doubling of the size of the methionine pool, such that the concentration of intracellular free methionine remains fairly constant at about 170 μM throughout oocyte growth. These analyses also suggest that the entire intracellular methionine pool, not just a smaller compartment of the pool, serves as precursor for protein synthesis. On the other hand, although the absolute rate of protein synthesis increases markedly during oocyte growth, from 1.1 to 41.8 pg/hr per oocyte, the increase is only about 38-fold as compared to the 300-fold increase in oocyte volume. Consequently, the absolute rate of protein synthesis, expressed on a volume (per picoliter) basis, actually decreases during oocyte growth. As a result, it takes about 10 pl of cytoplasm from a fully grown oocyte to synthesize as much as 1 pl of protein from a nongrowing oocyte. Considering that 90% of the cytoplasmic volume of amphibian oocytes consists of yolk platelets, leaving only 10% as active cyto-

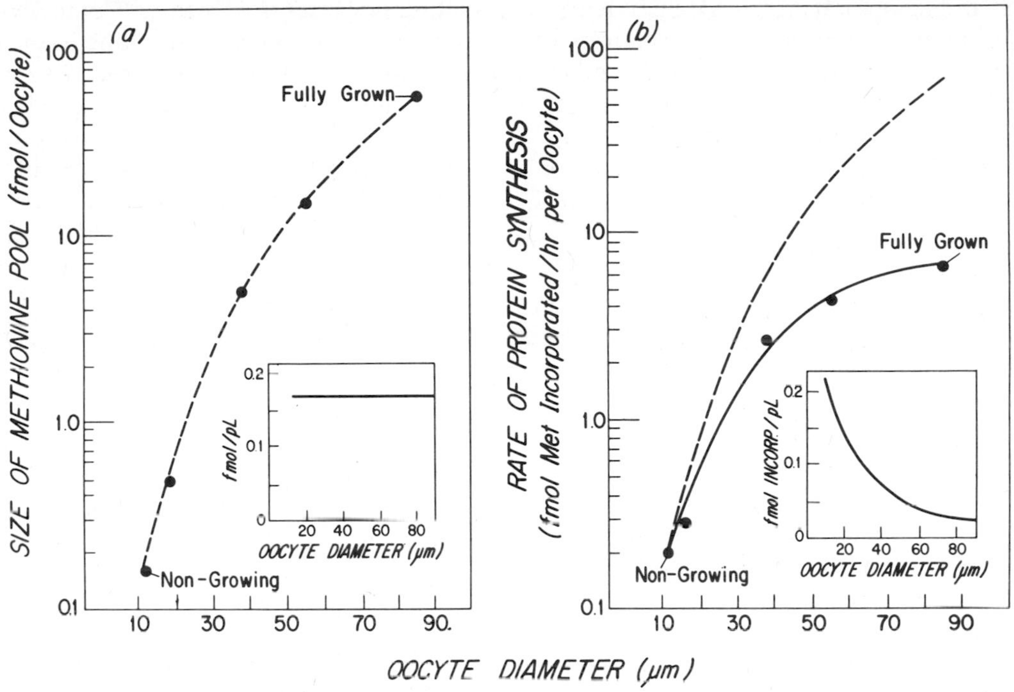

FIG. 24. Relationship between mouse oocyte diameter, sizes of intracellular methionine pools, and absolute rates of protein synthesis. (a) Methionine pool sizes as a function of oocyte diameter. (●) Experimentally determined values for methionine pool sizes. (– – –) Theoretical curve constructed by assuming a simple linear relationship between methionine pool size and oocyte volume, using a value of 56 fmole of methionine per oocyte for the fully grown oocyte. (*Inset*) Data converted to femtomoles of methionine per picoliter as a function of oocyte diameter. (b) Absolute rates of protein synthesis as a function of oocyte diameter. (●) Experimentally determined values for absolute rates of protein synthesis. (– – –) Theoretical curve constructed by assuming a simple linear relationship between absolute rates of protein synthesis and oocyte volume, using a value of 41.8 pg/hr per oocyte for the fully grown oocyte. (*Inset*) Data converted to femtomoles of methionine incorporated per picoliter as a function of oocyte diameter. (From ref. 311.)

plasm, the absolute rate of protein synthesis in fully grown mouse oocytes (~0.17 pg/hr per pl) compares quite favorably with that of amphibian oocytes (~0.34 pg/hr per pl).

Calculations using values for absolute rates of protein synthesis, given above, indicate that only about one-half of the protein present in fully grown mouse oocytes can be accounted for by protein synthesis during oocyte growth (311). This apparent discrepancy may be accounted for by errors in one (or more) of the measurements or by the presence of a yolklike component in oocytes that is synthesized elsewhere and taken up by endocytosis (analogous to the situation in amphibians). The former possibility should be considered seriously in view of the fact that these measurements were made with denuded oocytes. In the presence of follicle cells *in vivo,* the absolute rates of protein synthesis in growing oocytes may be substantially higher than reported for the *in vitro* situation (73,295). Similarly, the presence of a yolklike component in mouse oocytes should be considered seriously, since mammalian oocytes have the capacity to accumulate such a component from the blood (148–150). Therefore, whether or not growing oocytes synthesize all of the protein found in fully grown oocytes remains an open question.

Specific Protein Synthesis

At least three different experimental approaches have been used to identify specific oocyte proteins and examine their synthesis during oocyte growth in mice (355): (a) immunoprecipitation of metabolically radiolabeled proteins with antisera directed against specific proteins; (b) coelectrophoresis of metabolically radiolabeled proteins with purified proteins on high-resolution two-dimensional gels; (c) specific inhibition of the synthesis of particular proteins. Used in combination with absolute rates of protein synthesis, these approaches permit determination of rates of synthesis of specific proteins during oocyte growth.

Mitochondrial Proteins

Growing and fully grown oocytes synthesize several proteins encoded by the mitochondrial genome

(74,263). Overall, mitochondrial protein synthesis represents 1% to 2% of total protein synthesis during oocyte growth, not unlike the percentage estimated for other eukaryotic cells. It is noteworthy that the same spectrum of mitochondrial proteins is synthesized as the mitochondrial undergo morphological transformations during oocyte growth (discussed in the section on structural aspects of oocyte growth).

Ribosomal Proteins

Synthesis of ribosomal proteins occurs throughout oocyte grown and in fully grown oocytes (191,192). It is estimated that ribosomal protein synthesis accounts for 1.5% of total protein synthesis during oocyte growth, resulting in the accumulation of about 200 pg of ribosomal protein in fully grown oocytes. This large store of ribosomal protein reflects the large number of ribosomes ($\sim 10^8$) assembled during oocyte growth (discussed in the section on structural aspects of oocyte growth). It is noteworthy that different ribosomal proteins are synthesized at different rates (i.e., not under tight coordinate control) during oocyte growth, even though the proteins are present in equimolar amounts in ribosomes.

Zona Pellucida Glycoproteins

The mouse oocyte's zona pellucida is composed of three different glycoproteins, all of which are synthesized and secreted by growing oocytes (44,46,156,287,297,317). Synthesis of zona pellucida glycoproteins represents as much as 5% to 10% of total protein synthesis in growing oocytes. Furthermore, zona pellucida glycoproteins are the major class of proteins glycosylated and secreted during oocyte growth. One of the zona pellucida glycoproteins, called ZP3, functions as both sperm receptor and acrosome reaction inducer during fertilization of ovulated eggs (45,47,134,135).

Histones

Histone H4 is synthesized by growing and fully grown oocytes, accounting for about 0.07% and 0.05% of total protein synthesis, respectively (371). It is estimated that synthesis of all four types of histone (H2A, H2B, H3, and H4) represents 0.2% to 0.3% of total protein synthesis during oocyte growth, resulting in the accumulation of about 60 pg of histone in fully grown oocytes.

Tubulin

The α and β subunits of tubulin are synthesized throughout oocyte growth and are among the most abundant proteins in mouse oocytes (310,311). Tubulin synthesis represents 1.5% to 2.0% of total protein synthesis during oocyte growth, resulting in the accumulation of as much as 300 pg of tubulin in fully grown oocytes. Presumably, this tubulin store is recruited to form the relatively large spindles observed during meiotic maturation of fully grown oocytes (discussed in the section on structural aspects of oocyte maturation).

Actin

Synthesis of actin occurs throughout oocyte growth, representing about 1% of total protein synthesis during this period (273). The distribution of synthesis (percent of total) among α (muscle type), β (cytoplasmic type), and γ (cytoplasmic type) actin during oocyte growth is approximately 5%, 80%, and 15%, respectively.

Calmodulin

Although rates of synthesis are not available, it is clear that calmodulin is synthesized and accumulates during oocyte growth, accounting for as much as 0.3% of the total oocyte protein (54).

Lactate Dehydrogenase

"Heart-type" lactate dehydrogenase (LDH-B_4) is synthesized throughout oocyte growth, representing 2% to 5% of total protein synthesis during this period (75,206,207). As a result, 200 to 400 pg of lactate dehydrogenase accumulates in fully grown oocytes.

Creatine Kinase

Although rates of synthesis are not available, it is clear that creatine kinase is synthesized and accumulates throughout oocyte growth, accounting for as much as 1.4% of the total protein in fully grown mouse oocytes (177). Presumably, this relatively large store of creatine kinase is used to maintain the high level of ATP found in fully grown oocytes.

Glucose-6-phosphate Dehydrogenase

Although rates of synthesis are not available, it is clear that glucose-6-phosphate dehydrogenase is synthesized and accumulates throughout oocyte growth, since its specific activity (units/pl) remains constant during this period (206). Presumably, the relatively large store of glucose-6-phosphate dehydrogenase is required to produce NADPH-reducing equivalents.

Finally, it is clear that synthesis of certain proteins is regulated in a posttranscriptional manner during oocyte growth; an example of this is the synthesis of the fertilization proteins (58,75). Messenger-RNA for the fertilization proteins is synthesized throughout oocyte growth but is translated at extremely low rates, in view of its abundance, during this period (2 to 3 weeks). It is only subsequent to fertilization that this particular class of proteins is synthesized at high rates, apparently utilizing messenger RNA transcribed days to weeks earlier during oocyte growth.

Protein Synthesis: Summary

Fully grown mouse oocytes contain about 25 ng of protein, exclusive of the zona pellucida, or about 50 to 60 times more protein than a mammalian liver cell (59,202,314,355). Since the volume of a fully grown oocyte is about 50 to 60 times greater than that of a liver cell, the concentration of protein (pg/pl) is about the same in both cell types. Therefore, as in the case of RNA and ribosomes (discussed in the section on biochemical aspects of oocyte growth), it is apparently the failure of growing oocytes to undergo cytokinesis that results in an unusually large store of protein. Whether or not the growing oocyte itself synthesizes all of this protein remains an open question; the possibility remains that some proteins are synthesized elsewhere and taken up into growing oocytes by endocytosis. It is clear that both structural proteins and enzymes are synthesized and stored throughout oocyte growth. Turnover of nascent protein in growing mouse oocytes, like nascent RNA, occurs at a relatively low rate, partly accounting for the large stores inherited by unfertilized eggs. Some proteins synthesized by growing oocytes, such as zona pellucida and some cortical granule proteins, are essential for development beyond the unfertilized egg stage and may be unique to mammalian oocytes. Regulatory proteins involved in stage-specific transcription and translation, as well as in control of meiosis, undoubtedly are synthesized during oocyte growth and should be identified and characterized in the near future by application of recombinant DNA and immunological technology. Finally, it would appear that translation of some oocyte messenger RNAs is regulated such that translation rates during oocyte growth do not reflect messenger RNA abundance (posttranscriptional control).

OOCYTE MATURATION: BIOCHEMICAL ASPECTS

Meiotic Maturation *In Vitro*

A discussion of morphological and regulatory events that are characteristic of meiotic maturation *in vitro* is presented above (see sections on fully grown oocytes and unfertilized eggs, on structural aspects of oocyte maturation, and on regulatory aspects of oocyte maturation). In particular, it is important to reiterate that mammalian oocytes matured *in vitro,* under appropriate culture conditions, undergo normal development following insemination. Therefore, it is reasonable to assume that biochemical measurements made during this period *in vitro* are physiologically meaningful.

RNA Synthesis

Although RNA continues to be synthesized in fully grown oocytes (discussed in the section on biochemical aspects of oocyte growth), RNA synthesis is barely detectable after breakdown of the nuclear envelope (GV) and chromosome condensation (i.e., after meiotic maturation is initiated) (248,284,369). Cessation of ribosomal RNA synthesis apparently is associated with dissolution of the nucleolus upon mixing of nucleoplasm and cytoplasm. Furthermore, as much as one-half of the polyadenylated RNA accumulated during oocyte growth is either degraded or deadenylated during meiotic maturation (18,24). Therefore, during a period when certain maternal messages are utilized for the first time (see below), there is an overall decrease in levels of total and polyadenylated RNA inherited by the unfertilized egg from the fully grown oocyte.

Protein Synthesis

The sizes of the methionine pool and absolute rates of protein synthesis during meiotic maturation of mouse oocytes *in vitro* have been determined (308,355). As meiotic maturation progresses from the dictyate stage to metaphase II, the size of the intracellular methionine pool decreases from about 56 ($\sim$170 μm) to 35 fmole per oocyte ($\sim$138 μm), and the absolute rate of protein synthesis decreases from about 42 to 33 pg/hr per oocyte. The decrease in absolute rate of protein synthesis during this period is not simply because of the decrease in size of the intracellular methionine pool. Because the absolute rate of protein synthesis in ovulated eggs is nearly identical to that in oocytes matured *in vitro,* the decrease observed during meiotic maturation apparently is of physiological significance. Since the rate of RNA synthesis decreases dramatically following breakdown of the nuclear envelope and chromosome condensation, it is likely that the modest decrease in absolute rate of protein synthesis during meiotic maturation reflects turnover of oocyte RNA (see above) and/or translational control mechanisms.

The decrease in overall protein synthesis during meiotic maturation of oocytes is reflected in the behavior of a variety of specific proteins (346,348,355). For example, the rates of synthesis of tubulin, actin, histones, and ribosomal proteins decrease by 30% to 50%, and the rate of synthesis of lactate dehydrogenase decreases by 80% to 90% during meiotic maturation. Synthesis of zona pellucida glycoproteins decreases to extremely low levels during meiotic maturation. In this context, electrophoretic analyses of nascent proteins have revealed many changes in the overall pattern of protein synthesis during meiotic maturation of oocytes (96,214,215,281,285, 309,315,346,354,372). Both the appearance and disappearance of particular protein species have been noted. Virtually all of the changes observed in protein synthesis occur subsequent to nuclear envelope (GV) dissolution but are not dependent on other events such as spindle formation or polar body emission. Oocytes that remain arrested at the dictyate stage, with an intact nuclear envelope, either in the presence or absence of drugs, do not exhibit these changes in protein synthesis.

It is likely that many of the changes in protein synthesis accompanying meiotic maturation result from mixing of the oocyte's nucleoplasm and cytoplasm and would be expected to participate in the regulation of meiotic cell cycle progression. Candidate proteins whose synthesis and/or degradation have been implicated in cell cycle control include the catalytic and regulatory subunits of MPF, $p34^{cdc2}$ and cyclins, respectively, as well as putative MPF-stabilizing proteins such as cytostatic factor (CSF) and *c-mos* (379). It is becoming increasingly apparent that, in addition to translational control, posttranslational modifications of the cell cycle proteins constitute a critical mechanism by which meiotic progression is regulated (3).

Phosphorylation changes in the $p34^{cdc2}$ protein kinase are now recognized as the basis for regulation of MPF activity during the M phase of the eukaryotic cell cycle. In mouse oocytes, $p34^{cdc2}$ is maximally phosphorylated in immature, GV stage oocytes and becomes dephosphorylated during *in vitro* maturation (84). As in mitotic systems, dephosphorylation of tyrosine-15 on $p34^{cdc2}$ is essential for MPF activation, and this transformation can be inhibited by agents that elevate oocyte cAMP levels. Coupled with the observation that inhibitors of protein phosphatases 1 and 2A can elicit GV breakdown in drug-arrested oocytes, it appears that cytoplasmic factors influencing the phosphorylation status of $p34^{cdc2}$ play pivotal roles in both meiotic arrest and resumption (144).

Summary

Meiotic maturation represents the final stage of preparation of eggs for fertilization and early development (discussed in the sections on fully grown oocytes and unfertilized eggs, on structural aspects of oocyte maturation, and on regulatory aspects of oocyte maturation). Accordingly, biochemical changes occur during this period that are essential for meiotic progression as well as for further development. These changes appear to involve posttranslational modifications in cell cycle control proteins.

EXPRESSION OF SPECIFIC GENES DURING OOGENESIS

c-mos

The *c-mos* proto-oncogene is the cellular homolog of the transforming gene *v-mos* from Moloney murine sarcoma virus (249). It is a member of the serine/threonine protein kinase family. Unlike many proto-oncogenes, expression of *c-mos* in mice is restricted to a few tissues, most notably ovary and testis (271). Results of *in situ* hybridization analyses suggest that *c-mos* expression occurs specifically in growing and fully grown oocytes within the ovary (153,234). Quantification of these results indicates that *c-mos* messenger RNA accumulates to a steady-state level of about 10^5 copies per fully grown oocyte during oocyte growth. *c-mos* is also expressed specifically within the germ cell compartment of the testis.

Northern blot and *in situ* hybridization analyses have revealed the pattern of *c-mos* expression during meiotic maturation of oocytes, as well as during early embryogenesis (152,233). During meiotic maturation (i.e., conversion of fully grown oocytes into unfertilized eggs), the level of *c-mos* transcripts decreases by about 20%. This decrease does not occur until eggs have entered metaphase II and the first polar body has been extruded (233). In addition, the size of *c-mos* transcripts increases from 1.40 kilobases to 1.65 kilobases because of posttranscriptional polyadenylation of preexisting cytoplasmic transcripts (152). The level of *c-mos* transcripts continues to fall following fertilization, such that *c-mos* messenger-RNA is undetectable at the two-cell stage of development and remains undetectable through the blastocyst stage of development. Overall, the pattern of *c-mos* expression described is consistent with the behavior of the bulk of maternal poly-$(A)^+$ RNA in mammalian eggs. Furthermore, cytoplasmic polyadenylation of stored maternal messenger RNA has been reported for a variety of animals, including mice (24,91,101,176,288) and is apparently generally related to temporal translation of processed messenger RNA.

The *c-mos* oncoprotein, $p39^{mos}$, is first synthesized by meiotically arrested, fully grown oocytes having an intact GV, is present during meiotic maturation and in unfertilized eggs (253,390) but cannot be detected in growing oocytes or in fertilized eggs (253). Certain lines of evidence suggest that $p39^{mos}$ plays a role in meiotic maturation. Fully grown oocytes microinjected with *c-mos* antisense RNA (240,253), or exposed to antibodies directed against $p39^{mos}$ (390), undergo GV breakdown and either do not extrude a first polar body (253,390) or fail to enter the second meiotic division (240). Results of analogous experiments carried out in *Xenopus llaevis* (294) suggest that *Xenopus* p39^{mos} is cytostatic factor (CSF) itself, or is an essential component of CSF. Cytostatic factor is an activity in amphibian cells that prevents inactivation of maturation-promoting factor (MPF), and there is evidence to suggest that p39^{mos} may accomplish this by phosphorylation of cyclin (290). Maturation-promoting factor is a key regulatory component of the G_2/M transition in both meiotic and mitotic cells in all eukaryotic organisms (232). Therefore, it seems likely that p39^{mos} plays a similar role in meiotic maturation of mouse oocytes by interacting directly with MPF, with other components of the MPF pathway, and/or with other proteins. For instance, *c-mos* may be involved in regulating spindle formation and/or function during meiotic maturation of mouse oocytes (390). Degradation of p39^{mos} is apparently not involved in the release of ovulated eggs from metaphase II arrest (377). Thus, *c-mos* messenger RNA apparently is a stored maternal message that is polyadenylated and translated in a temporally specific manner during oogenesis, thereby permitting p39^{mos} to play a vital role during meiotic maturation.

oct-3

oct-3 is a maternally expressed octamer-binding protein that is encoded by the murine *oct-3* gene (244,289,302). *oct-3* is a relatively new member of the POU domain family of regulatory genes. Such genes share a region, the POU domain, that consists of a POU-specific domain and a POU homeobox domain, linked by a short variable region (169). Like all other POU domain proteins (293), *oct-3* protein is capable of transactivating promoters containing an octamer motif through the DNA binding properties of its POU domain (199,244,289,300–302).

oct-3 was identified as the first example of a transcription factor that is specific for the earliest stages of mammalian development. Clues to the pattern of *oct-3* expression were provided by studies of *oct-3* binding activity in extracts prepared from both male and female primordial germ cells (PGCs), ovulated eggs, embryonic stem (ES) cells, and embryonic carcinoma (EC) cell lines (199,301). The *oct-3* gene is expressed as both a maternal and embryonic messenger RNA, and *oct-3* expression has been studied by a combination of Northern blot and *in situ* hybridization analyses, as well as by ribonuclease (RNase) protection analyses (289,300,302).

oct-3 messenger-RNA is detected as a 1.55 kilobases transcript in growing mouse oocytes and ovulated eggs but is not found in nongrowing oocytes (289,300). *oct-3* messenger-RNA is also present in fertilized eggs (289). Zygotic expression of *oct-3* is first detected at the morula stage of development, and throughout early embryogenesis *oct-3* expression is detectable in cells that are pluripotent or totipotent (289,300). At day 8.5 of development, expression of *oct-3* is restricted to PGCs. In adult animals, *oct-3* expression is limited to oocytes within the ovary and to testis, but not to sperm (289,300). *oct-3* messenger-RNA is found in RNA prepared from undifferentiated, but not differentiated EC cells, as well as in RNA prepared from ES cells (289). A role for zygotic *oct-3* protein has yet to be described, but it may act in maintaining the differentiation capability of cells that express the protein (289,300). Thus, *oct-3* expression during early mouse development is specific to cells that are either totipotent or pluripotent and, thus, possess the ability to differentiate. *oct-3* expression is specific to cells constituting the germline lineage.

c-kit

The *c-kit* proto-oncogene is the cellular homolog of *v-kit*, an oncogene present in HZ4 feline sarcoma virus (38). *c-kit* is a member of the tyrosine kinase receptor family (38,204,272,386) and its ligand, stem cell factor (SCF) or kit ligand (KL), has been identified (209,391). Interest in *c-kit* and SCF intensified when they were shown to be encoded at the murine genetic loci white-spotting (W) and steel (Sl), respectively (77,145, 238,391). Mutations at both of these loci have been of interest for many years, since they both produce a very similar range of pleiotrophic effects, affecting development of hematopoietic, melanocyte, and germ-cell lineages (292,319).

Embryonic expression of *c-kit* in mice is very complex (247). In this context, it should be noted that, in general, there is good correlation between sites of *c-kit* expression and the three major cell types affected by mutations at the W locus. However, *c-kit* is also expressed in tissues not known to be affected in W mutants (e.g., CNS, craniofacial structures, and intestinal tract). In normal adult mice, *c-kit* messenger RNA (5.5 kilobases) is found in RNA prepared from placenta, brain, bone marrow, lung, ovary, and testis (238).

Sites of *c-kit* expression in mouse ovary have been identified by Northern blot and *in situ* hybridization analyses (208,247). Northern blot hybridization analyses of RNA prepared from growing oocytes, ovulated eggs, two-cell embryos, and blastocysts revealed that *c-kit* transcripts are present in nongrowing oocytes, and their steady-state level increases during oocyte growth. It is estimated that fully grown oocytes contain about 15 fg of *c-kit* messenger-RNA. The level of *c-kit* messenger-RNA declines severalfold following fertilization, and *c-kit* transcripts are undetectable by the blastocyst stage of development (208). *In situ* hybridization analyses of ovarian sections, prepared from prenatal and postnatal mice of various ages, confirmed this pattern of *c-kit* expression and provided additional information. For example, they revealed that *c-kit* expression is first detected in ovarian sections of prenatal mice, specifically within oocytes that have reached diplotene of the first meiotic prophase where they remain throughout growth (208). *c-kit* expression is also detected in interstitial tissue of ovaries from 14- to 17-day animals, but never in follicle cells at any stage of their development (208,247). Spermatogonic cells are a site of *c-kit* expression in the testis (208).

The presence or absence of *c-kit* protein during early mouse development correlates very well with *c-kit* expression during this period. Results of indirect immunofluorescence analyses, using antibodies directed against *c-kit* protein (239), indicate that the protein is present on the surface of oocytes, ovulated eggs, and one- and two-cell embryos but not on blastocysts (208). These findings suggest a role for *c-kit* in postnatal development of female germ cells, in addition to its well-established role in proliferation and migration of primordial germ cells. It has been suggested that *c-kit* plays a role in initiation and/or maintenance of oocyte growth (208) and in meiotic maturation of oocytes (208,247). Phenotypes of certain W and Sl mutations provide a basis for these suggestions. For example, in W/W^v and W^v/W^v mice, the rate of development of oocytes and spermatogenic cells is slower than in wild type mice (95), and in juvenile Sl/Sl^t infertile females, ovaries lack follicles with growing oocytes, despite the presence of abundant primordial follicles (190).

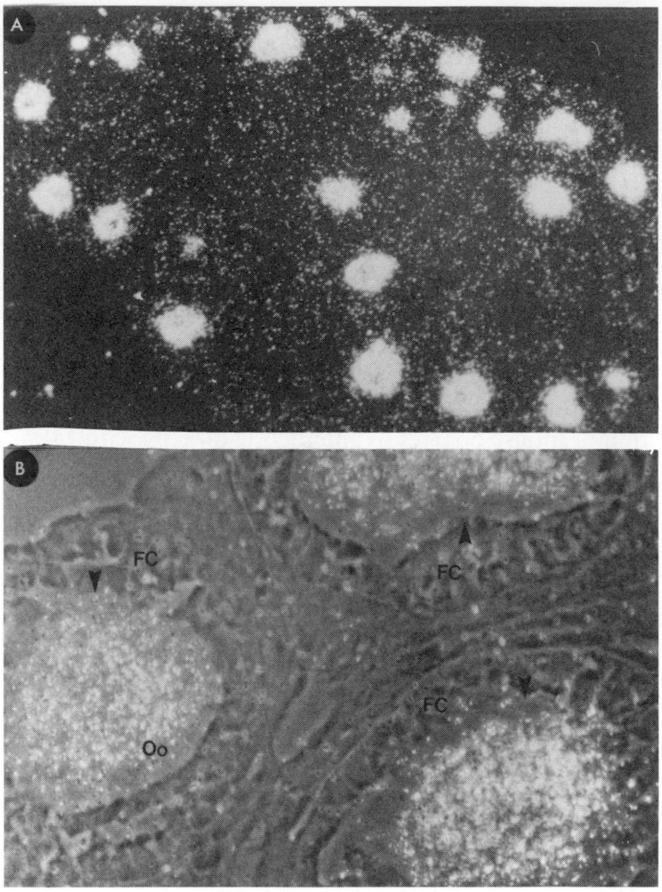

FIG. 25. In situ hybridization analysis of *mZP3* expression in mouse oocytes. Shown are photomicrographs (bright-field, **A**; dark-field, **B**) of the same ovarian section hybridized with a radiolabeled *mZP3* probe and subjected to autoradiography. Follicle cells, FC. Oocyte, Oo.

mZP3

mZP3 is one of three glycoproteins (mZP1-3) that make up the mouse egg extracellular coat, or zona pellucida. mZP3 is an 83-kilodalton glycoprotein that consists of a 44-kilodalton polypeptide (402 amino acids), three or four complex-type, asparagine- (N-)linked oligosaccharides, and an unknown number of serine/threonine- (O-) linked oligosaccharides (44,45,47,134,135, 230,287,358,359,362,364). During initial stages of fertilization, mZP3 serves as both a primary sperm receptor, involved in species-specific binding of sperm to eggs and as inducer of the acrosome reaction, a form of exocytosis in sperm (356–364).

mZP3 is a single-copy gene that encodes a 1.5-kilobase, polyadenylated messenger RNA (184,185,187, 282,283,286). Results of Northern blot and *in situ* hybridization analyses, as well as RNase protection analyses, suggest that *mZP3* is expressed exclusively in growing oocytes (188,261,286) (Fig. 25). In adult female mice, *mZP3* messenger RNA is found only in RNA prepared from ovaries and, within ovaries, it is found only in growing oocytes. RNase protection assays indicate that nongrowing oocytes (12–15 μm diameter) contain undetectable levels of *mZP3* messenger-RNA ($<1 \times 10^3$ copies/oocyte). However, the steady-state level of *mZP3* messenger-RNA increases markedly during oocyte growth (2–3 weeks), reaching 2.5 to 3×10^5 copies per 70 to 80 μm diameter oocyte (188,286). A dramatic fall in *mZP3* messenger-RNA levels occurs during ovulation (meiotic maturation), when as much as 98% of *mZP3* messenger-RNA is destroyed (5×10^3 copies/unfertilized egg). RNase protection assays indicate that unfertilized eggs and cleavage-stage embryos contain undetectable levels of *mZP3* messenger RNA ($<1 \times 10^3$ copies/zygote). These findings are consistent with results of assays of mZP3 synthesis and secretion during oogenesis and early development (46,297,358,364).

Expression of *mZP3* is regulated by *cis*-acting sequence(s) in the 5′-flanking region of the gene, together with oocyte-specific protein(s) (201,299). It has been demonstrated that only 470 base pairs of *mZP3* gene 5′-flanking region are sufficient to target expression of a reporter gene, encoding firefly luciferase, to growing oocytes in transgenic mice. An oocyte-specific protein (~60 kilodaltons) called OSP-1 binds to the sequence 5′-TGATAA-3′ located within the first 100 base pairs of the *mZP3* gene promoter. Changes in levels of this protein during oogenesis and early cleavage are consistent with the pattern of *mZP3* gene expression during these stages of mouse development. Thus, OSP-1 may interact with other ubiquitous or cell-specific proteins to activate *mZP3* gene expression during oocyte growth.

t-PA

Tissue-type plasminogen activator (*t-PA*) (72 kilodaltons) is a member of the family of serine proteases that convert the serum protein, plasminogen, into plasmin (330). Although *t-PA* activity cannot be detected in fully grown mouse oocytes, unfertilized and fertilized eggs exhibit relatively high levels of *t-PA* activity *in vitro* (175). The biological function of such high levels of *t-PA* during these stages of development is not clear. *t-PA* first appears during meiotic maturation of oocytes and is dependent on GV breakdown but not on polar body emission. *t-PA* activity can be detected 5 hours after GV breakdown. Furthermore, the appearance of *t-PA* during meiotic maturation is not dependent on concomitant transcription (i.e., occurs in the presence of either actinomycin D or α-amanitin), suggesting the presence of untranslated *t-PA* messenger RNA in fully grown oocytes.

Several lines of evidence suggest that appearance of *t-PA* activity in unfertilized mouse eggs is regulated posttranscriptionally during oogenesis. Although *t-PA* activity cannot be detected in growing or fully grown oocytes, Northern blot hybridization analyses reveal that *t-PA* messenger RNA is present in growing oocytes (Fig. 26) and accumulates to a steady-state level of about 10^5 copies in the cytoplasm of fully grown oocytes (176). Translation of stored *t-PA* messenger RNA is triggered by meiotic maturation of oocytes. Furthermore, *t-PA* messenger RNA is destroyed during the latter stages of meiotic maturation, such that undetectable levels of the message are found in fertilized eggs.

Concomitant with the appearance of *t-PA* activity in oocytes that have resumed meiosis, *t-PA* messenger-RNA undergoes a substantial increase in size (~400–600 nucleotides) as result of increased polyadenylation at the 3′-end of the molecule (176). This structural change is initiated within 3 hours of GV breakdown. Microinjection of antisense RNAs complementary to 103 nucleotides of the extreme 3′-untranslated region of *t-PA* messenger RNA into fully-grown oocytes leads to hybrid formation and amputation of the 3′-terminal sequences of the message (331). Such modification of *t-PA* messenger RNA in oocytes is sufficient to prevent polyadenylation, translational activation, and destabilization of the message during meiotic maturation of oocytes. These and other observations (352) strongly suggest that cytoplasmic 3′ polyadenylation, regulated by sequences in the 3′-noncoding region of *t-PA* messenger RNA, is necessary and sufficient for translational activation of the message during meiotic maturation of mouse oocytes. (It should be noted that hypoxanthine phosphoribosyltransferase [*HPRT*] messenger RNA in fully grown mouse oocytes undergoes polyadenylation [~150–200 nucleotides] at its 3′-end during meiotic maturation, and this precedes an increase in HPRT activity [254].)

LDH-B

Fully grown mouse oocytes possess unusually high levels of lactate dehydrogenase (LDH) activity, with virtually all of the activity attributable to the "heart-type" isozyme, LDH-B_4 (11,75,206,207). LDH synthesis, which represents as much as 1.8% of total protein synthesis during oocyte growth, decreases about sevenfold during meiotic maturation of oocytes and about 20-fold in fertilized eggs (as compared with fully grown oocytes)

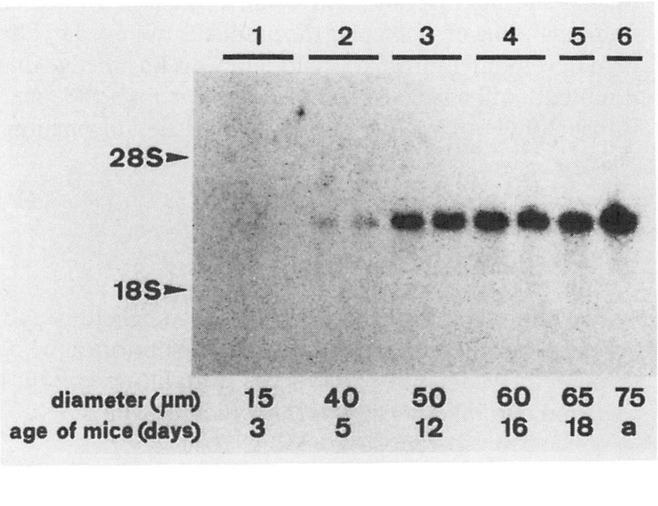

FIG. 26. Accumulation of *t-PA* mRNA during oocyte growth. RNA from primordial, growing, and fully grown primary oocytes was analyzed by Northern blot hybridization using a cRNA probe transcribed from pSP65-MT$_1$. Each lane contains the RNA from 40 oocytes of the indicated size, derived from mice of the indicated age; (a), adult. (From ref. 176.)

(75). Fully grown oocytes possess about 150 fg of *LDH* messenger RNA, or about 2 × 10^5 copies per oocyte (286). During meiotic maturation of oocytes, the steady-state level of *LDH* messenger RNA falls only by about 20%, whereas LDH synthesis falls about sevenfold. A similar discrepancy has been noted for changes in β-actin synthesis and *β-actin* messenger RNA levels during meiotic maturation of mouse oocytes and has been attributed to deadenylation (~200 nucleotides) of *β-actin* messenger RNA (24,254). Similarly, *α-tubulin* messenger RNA undergoes extensive deadenylation and degradation during meiotic maturation (254). In this context, the size of *LDH* messenger RNA decreases in size from about 1.4 kilobases in fully grown oocytes to about 1.3 kilobases in unfertilized eggs (R. Roller and P. Wassarman, unpublished results).

THE UNFERTILIZED EGG: MACROMOLECULAR STORES

The unfertilized mammalian egg, like nonmammalian eggs, contains an extensive store of materials poised to be mobilized following fertilization (18,39,41,89–92,179,200,270,305,355,363). The mouse egg contains about 40 pg of DNA (not including polar body), 500 pg of RNA, 20 to 25 ng of protein (not including zona pellucida), and 150 pg of glycogen. In addition, the egg inherits from the oocyte about 100,000 mitochondria, 100,000,000 ribosomes, 4,500 cortical granules, and a zona pellucida. Each egg has about 800 fmole of ATP, as compared to about 15 to 25 fmole found in a typical somatic cell. Finally, the egg inherits substantial pools of tubulin (250 pg) and actin (100 pg), as well as unusually high levels of a variety of enzymes involved in macromolecular biosynthesis and energy metabolism. Since the unfertilized mouse egg is 60 to 70 times larger (volume) than a typical somatic cell, accumulation of this impressive store is attributable, at least in part, to growth without cytokinesis.

Although cleavage of mouse embryos is extremely slow, relative to amphibian and echinoderm embryos, the mass of nascent proteins synthesized during this period is very small compared to that contributed by the unfertilized egg. For example, during the transition from a one- to eight-cell mouse embryo (~60 hr), about 50 pg of tubulin is synthesized by the cleaving embryo (~6 pg/blastomere); this represents only about 20% of the tubulin pool (~250 pg) inherited by the embryo from the unfertilized egg (1,310,311,355). A similar situation applies for many of the structural proteins and enzymes examined during oogenesis and early embryogenesis in mammals. Furthermore, it is clear that certain organelles, such as cortical granules, zona pellucida, centrosomes, and mitochondria, are made during oogenesis for use during fertilization and early embryogenesis. It is also likely that the large store of ribosomes inherited by the embryo functions during the first two to three cleavage divisions, at which time the rates of synthesis of ribosomal RNA and ribosomal proteins achieve relatively high levels. Finally, unfertilized eggs inherit a store of histones sufficient to support the first few cleavage divisions.

Thus, in the egg, oogenesis achieves several objectives: an increase in genotypic variation, production of a haploid cell, biogenesis of macromolecules and organelles involved in fertilization, and establishment of a store of materials to support and regulate development of the preimplantation embryo. In all of these respects, mammalian eggs resemble their nonmammalian counterpart.

A FINAL WORD

It is hoped that this presentation has conveyed the theme that "animal development is rooted in oogenesis," the process by which eggs are produced. This is as true for mammals as it is for nonmammals. Research in this particular area has a long, illustrious history and continues to reveal principles that underlie not only animal development, but also cellular mechanisms in general. Research on molecular aspects of mammalian egg and embryo development, in particular, has made impressive strides in recent years; this has been made possible largely by important conceptual and technological advances. In many instances, the paucity of biological material available from mammals, a factor that inhibited research on mammalian oogenesis for so long, is no longer as serious a consideration. Perhaps, most exciting, is the prospect that one will soon be able to carry out and investigate the entire process of mammalian oogenesis, from primordial germ cells to unfertilized eggs, in culture *in vitro.* The technology required to fertilize such eggs *in vitro* and produce viable offspring is already available. Consequently, it is to be expected that expanded research on egg and embryo development in mammals during the next decade will achieve a more complete understanding of molecular mechanisms involved in our own development from a single cell. This knowledge undoubtedly will have far-reaching consequences and great impact on both medical and social issues in ensuing years.

ACKNOWLEDGMENTS

The authors are delighted to take this opportunity to acknowledge the members of their laboratories who, through the years, have provided a stimulating, productive, and cordial environment in which to work.

REFERENCES

1. Abreu S, Brinster R. Synthesis of tubulin and actin during the preimplantation development of the mouse. *Exp Cell Res* 1978;114:135–141.
2. Adams E, Hertig A. Studies on guinea pig oocytes. 1. Electron microscopic observations on the development of cytoplasmic organelles in oocytes of primordial and primary follicles. *J Cell Biol* 1964;21:397–427.
3. Albertini DF. Regulation of meiotic maturation in the mammalian oocyte: Interplay between exongenous cues and microtubule cytoskeleton. *BioEssays* 1992;5:100–105.
4. Albertini D, Anderson E. The appearance and structure of the intercellular connections during the ontogeny of the rabbit ovarian follicle with special reference to gap junctions. *J Cell Biol* 1974;2:234–250.
5. Albertini D, Fawcett D, Olds P. Morphological variations in gap junctions of ovarian granulosa cells. *Tissue Cell* 1975;7:389–405.
6. Albertini DF, Wickramasinghe D, Messinger SM, Mattson BA, Plancha CE. Nuclear and cytoplasmic changes during oocyte maturation. In: Barister B, ed. *Preimplantation embryo development.* New York: Springer-Verlag, 1993:3–21.
7. Amsterdam A, Josephs R, Lieberman M, Lindner H. Organization of intramembrane particles in freeze-cleaved gap junctions of rat graafian follicles: Optical diffraction analysis. *J Cell Sci* 1976;21:93–105.
8. Anderson E, Albertini E. Gap junctions between the oocyte and companion follicle cells in the mammalian ovary. *J Cell Biol* 1976;71:680–686.
9. Anderson E, Wilkinson R, Lee G, Meller S. A correlative microscopical analysis of differentiating ovarian follicles of mammals. *J Morphol* 1978;156:339–366.
10. Asdell A. Historical introduction. In: Cole H, Cupps P, eds. *Reproduction in domestic animals.* New York: Academic Press; 1969;1–14.
11. Auerbach S, Brinster R. Lactate dehydrogenase isozymes in mouse blastocyst cultures. *Exp Cell Res* 1968;53:313–315.
12. Austin C. *The mammalian egg* Oxford: Blackwell Science Publications; 1961.
13. Austin C. The egg. In: Austin C, Short R. *Reproduction in mammals, vol 1.* Cambridge: Cambridge University Press; 1982:46–62.
14. Austin C, Short R, eds. *Reproduction in mammals, vol 1, Germ cells and fertilization.* Cambridge: Cambridge University Press; 1982.
15. Baca M, Zamboni L. The fine structure of human follicular oocytes. *J Ultrastruct Res* 1967;19:354–381.
16. Bachvarova R. Incorporation of tritiated adenosine into mouse ovum RNA. *Dev Biol* 1974;40:52–58.
17. Bachvarova R. Synthesis, turnover, and stability of heterogeneous RNA in growing mouse oocytes. *Dev Biol* 1981;86:384–392.
18. Bachvarova R. Gene expression during oogenesis and oocyte development in mammals. In: Browder L, ed. *Developmental biology: A comprehensive synthesis. vol 1, Oogenesis.* New York: Plenum Press; 1985:453–524.
19. Bachvarova R, Baran M, Tejblum A. Development of naked growing mouse oocytes *in vitro. J Exp Zool* 1980;211:159–169.
20. Bachvarova R, Burns J, Speigelman I, Choy J, Chaganti R. Morphology and transcriptional activity of mouse oocyte chromosomes. *Chromosoma* 1982;86:181–196.
21. Bachvarova R, Cohen E, DeLeon V, Tokunaga K, Sakiyama S, Paynton B. Amounts and modulation of actin mRNAs in mouse oocytes and embryos. *Development* 1989;106:561–565.
22. Bachvarova R, De Leon V. Stored and polysomal ribosomes of mouse ova. *Dev Biol* 1977;58:248–254.
23. Bachvarova R, De Leon V. Polyadenylated RNA of mouse ova and loss of maternal RNA in early development. *Dev Biol* 1980;74:1–8.
24. Bachvarova R, De Leon V, Johnson A, Kaplan G, Paynton B. Changes in total RNA, polyadenylated RNA, and actin mRNA during meiotic maturation of mouse oocytes. *Dev Biol* 1985;108:325–331.
25. Bachvarova R, De Leon V, Spiegelman I. Mouse egg ribosomes: Evidence for storage in lattices. *J Embryol Exp Morphol* 1981;62:153–164.
26. Bachvarova R, Moy K. Autoradiographic studies on the distribution of labeled maternal RNA in early mouse embryos. *J Exp Zool* 1985;285:67–76.
27. Baker T. Oogenesis and ovarian development. In: Balin H, Glasser S, eds. *Reproductive biology.* Amsterdam: Excerpta Medica; 1972:398–437.
28. Baker T. Oogenesis and ovulation. In: Austin C, Short R, eds. *Reproduction in mammals, vol 1.* Cambridge: Cambridge University Press; 1982:17–45.
29. Baker T, Beaumont H, Franchi L. The uptake of tritiated uridine and phenylalanine by the ovaries of rats and monkeys. *J Cell Sci* 1969;4:655–675.
30. Baker T, Franchi L. The structure of the chromosomes in human primordial oocytes. *Chromosoma* 1967;22:358–377.
31. Baker T, Franchi L. The fine structure of oogonia and oocytes in human ovaries. *J Cell Sci* 1967;2:213–224.
32. Baker T, Franchi L. The fine structure of chromosomes in bovine primordial oocytes. *J Reprod Fertil* 1967;14:511–513.
33. Baker T, Franchi L. The fine structure of oogonia and oocytes in the rhesus monkey (*Macaca mulatta*). *Z Zellforsch Mikrosk Anat* 1972;126:53–74.
34. Bakken A, McClanahan M. Patterns of RNA synthesis in early meiotic prophase oocytes from fetal mouse ovaries. *Chromosoma* 1978,67:21–40.
35. Balakier H. Induction of maturation in small oocytes from sexually immature mice by fusion with meiotic or mitotic cells. *Exp Cell Res* 1978;112:137–141.
36. Balakier H, Czolowska R. Cytoplasmic control of nuclear maturation in mouse oocytes. *Exp Cell Res* 1977;110:466–469.
37. Baran M, Bachvarova R. *In vitro* culture of growing mouse oocytes. *J Exp Zool* 1977;202:283–289.
38. Besmer P, Murphy J, George P, et al. A new acute transforming feline retrovirus and relationship of its oncogene *v-kit* with the protein kinase gene family. *Nature* 1986;320:415–421.
39. Biggers J. Metabolism of mouse embryos. *J Reprod Fertil (Suppl)* 1971;14.41–54.
40. Biggers J, Schuetz A, eds. *Oogenesis.* Baltimore: University Park Press; 1973.
41. Biggers J, Stern S. Metabolism of the preimplantation mammalian embryo. *Adv Reprod Physiol* 1973;6:1–59.
42. Blanchette E. A study of the fine structure of the rabbit primary oocyte. *J Ultrastruct Res* 1961;5:349–363.
43. Blandau R. Growth of the ovarian follicle and ovulation. *Prog Gynecol* 1970;5:58–76.
44. Bleil J, Wassarman P. Structure and function of the zona pellucida: Identification and characterization of the proteins of the mouse oocyte's zona pellucida. *Dev Biol* 1980;76:185–202.
45. Bleil J, Wassarman P. Mammalian sperm-egg interaction: Identification of a glycoprotein in mouse egg zonae pellucidae possessing sperm receptor activity. *Cell* 1980;20:873–882.
46. Bleil J, Wassarman P. Synthesis of zona pellucida proteins by denuded and follicle-enclosed mouse oocytes during culture *in vitro. Proc Natl Acad Sci USA* 1980;77:1029–1033.
47. Bleil J, Wassarman P. Autoradiographic visualization of the mouse egg's sperm receptor bound to sperm. *J Cell Biol* 1986;102:1363–1371.
48. Bloom A, Mukherjee B. RNA synthesis in maturing mouse oocytes. *Exp Cell Res* 1972;74:577–582.
49. Boreen S, Gizang E, Schultz R. Biochemical studies of mammalian oogenesis: Synthesis of SS and 4S RNA during growth of the mouse oocyte. *Gamete Res* 1983;8:379–383.
50. Bornslaeger E, Mattei P, Schultz R. Involvement of cAMP-dependent protein kinase and protein phosphorylation in regulation of mouse oocyte maturation. *Dev Biol* 1986;114:453–462.
51. Bornslaeger E, Poueymirou W, Mattei P, Schultz R. Effects of protein kinase C activators on germinal vesicle breakdown and polar body emission of mouse oocytes. *Exp Cell Res* 1986;165:507–517.

52. Bornslaeger E, Schultz R. Regulation of mouse oocyte maturation: Effect of elevating cumulus cell cAMP on oocyte cAMP levels. *Biol Reprod* 1985;33:698–704.
53. Bornslaeger E, Schultz R. Adenylate cyclase activity in zona-free mouse oocytes. *Exp Cell Res* 1985;156:277–281.
54. Bornslaeger E, Wilde M, Schultz R. Regulation of mouse oocyte maturation: Involvement of cyclic AMP phosphodiesterase and calmodulin. *Dev Biol* 1984;105:488–499.
55. Brambell F. The development and morphology of the gonads of the mouse. Part 1. The morphogenesis of the indifferent gonad and of the ovary. *Proc R Soc Lond* [*Biol*] 1927;101:391–409.
56. Brambell F. The development and morphology of the gonads of the mouse. Part III. The growth of the follicles. *Proc R Soc Lond* [*Biol*] 1928;103:258–272.
57. Brambell F. Ovarian changes. In: Parkes A, ed. *Marshall's physiology of reproduction, vol 1.* New York: Longmans, Green; 1956:397–542.
58. Braude P, Pelham H, Flach G, Lobatto R. Posttranscriptional control in the early mouse embryo. *Nature* 1979;282:102–105.
59. Brinster R. Protein content of the mouse embryo during the first five days of development. *J Reprod Fertil* 1967;10:227–240.
60. Browder L, ed. *Developmental biology: A comprehensive synthesis, vol 1, Oogenesis* New York: Plenum Press; 1985.
61. Brower P, Gizang E, Boreen S, Schultz R. Biochemical studies of mammalian oogenesis: Synthesis and stability of various classes of RNA during growth of the mouse oocyte *in vitro. Dev Biol* 1981;86:373–383.
62. Brower P, Schultz R. Biochemical studies of mammalian oogenesis: Possible existence of a ribosomal and poly(A)-containing RNA-protein supramolecular complex in mouse oocytes. *J Exp Zool* 1982;220:251–260.
63. Brower P, Schultz R. Intercellular communication between granulosa cells and mouse oocytes: Existence and possible nutritional role during oocyte growth. *Dev Biol* 1982;90:144–153.
64. Buccione R, Banderhyden BC, Caron PJ, Eppig JJ. FSH-induced expansion of the mouse cumulus oophorous *in vitro* is dependent upon a specific factor(s) secreted by the oocyte. *Dev Biol* 1990;138:16–25.
65. Buccione R, Schroeder AC, Eppig JJ. Interactions between somatic cells and germ cells throughout mammalian oogenesis. *Biol Reprod* 1990;43:543–547.
66. Buehr M, McLaren A. Expression of glucose-phosphate isomerase in relation to growth of the mouse oocyte *in vivo* and *in vitro. Gamete Res* 1985;11:271–281.
67. Burkholder G, Comings D, Okada T. A storage form of ribosomes in mouse oocytes. *Exp Cell Res* 1971;69:361–371.
68. Byskov A. Ultrastructural studies on the preovulatory follicle in the mouse ovary. *Z Zellforsch Mikrosk Anat* 1969;100:285–299.
69. Byskov A. Primordial germ cells and regulation of meiosis. In: Austin C, Short R, eds. *Reproduction in mammals, vol 1.* Cambridge: Cambridge University Press; 1982:1–16.
70. Calarco P. The kinetochore in oocyte maturation. In: Biggers J, Schuetz A, eds. *Oogenesis.* Baltimore: University Park Press; 1972;65–86.
71. Calarco P, Donahue R, Szollosi D. Germinal vesicle breakdown in the mouse oocyte. *J Cell Sci* 1972;10:369–385.
72. Canipari R, Palombi F, Riminucci M, Mangia F. Early programming and maturation competence in mouse oogenesis. *Dev Biol* 1984;102:519–524.
73. Canipari R, Pietrolucci A, Mangia F. Increase of total protein synthesis during mouse oocyte growth. *J Reprod Fertil* 1979;57:405–413.
74. Cascio S, Wassarman P. Program of early development in the mammal: Synthesis of mitochondrial proteins during oogenesis and early embryogenesis in the mouse. *Dev Biol* 1981;83: 166–172.
75. Cascio S, Wassarman P. Program of early development in the mammal: Post-transcriptional control of a class of proteins synthesized by mouse oocytes and early embryos. *Dev Biol* 1982;89:397–408.
76. Centola G, Anderson L, Channing C. Oocyte maturation inhibition activity in porcine granulosa cells. *Gamete Res* 1981;4:451–462.
77. Chabot B, Stephenson D, Chapman V, Besmer P, Bernstein A. The proto-oncogene c-*kit* encoding a transmembrane tyrosine kinase receptor maps to the mouse W locus. *Nature* 1988;335:88–89.
78. Chamberlin M, Dean J. Genomic organization of a sex specific gene: The primary sperm receptor of the mouse zona pellucida. *Dev Biol* 1990;131:207–214.
79. Chang M. The maturation of rabbit oocytes in culture and their maturation, activation, fertilization, and subsequent development in the fallopian tubes. *J Exp Zool* 1955;128:378–405.
80. Chari S, Hillensjo T, Magnusson C, Sturm G, Daume E. *In vitro* inhibition of rat oocyte meiosis by human follicular fluid fractions. *Arch Gynecol* 1983;233:155–164.
81. Chiquoine A. The identification, origin and migration of the primordial germ cells in the mouse embryo. *Anat Rec* 1954;118:135–146.
82. Chiquoine A. The development of the zona pellucida of the mammalian ovum. *Am J Anat* 1960;106:149–170.
83. Cho W-K, Stern S, Biggers J. Inhibitory effect of dibutyryl cAMP on mouse oocyte maturation *in vitro. J Exp Zool* 1974;187:383–386.
84. Choi T, Aoki F, Mori M, Yamashita M, Nagahama Y, Kohmoto K. Activation of $p34^{cdc2}$ protein kinase activity in meiotic and mitotic cell cycles in mouse oocytes and embryos. *Development* 1991;113:789–795.
85. Chouinard L. A light- and electron-microscope study of the nucleolus during growth of the oocyte in the prepubertal mouse. *J Cell Sci* 1991;9:637–663.
86. Chouinard L. An electron-microscope study of the extranucleolar bodies during growth of the oocyte in the prepubertal mouse. *J Cell Sci* 1973;12:55–69.
87. Chouinard L. A light- and electron-microscope study of the oocyte nucleus during development of the antral follicle in the prepubertal mouse. *J Cell Sci* 1975;17:589–615.
88. Clark J, Eddy E. Fine structural observations on the origin and association of primordial germ cells of the mouse. *Dev Biol* 1975;47:136–155.
89. Clegg K, Piko L. Size and specific activity of the UTP pool and overall rates of RNA synthesis in early mouse embryos. *Dev Biol* 1977;58:76–95.
90. Clegg K, Piko L. RNA synthesis and cytoplasmic polyadenylation in the one-cell mouse embryo. *Nature* 1982;295:342–345.
91. Clegg K, Piko L. Poly(A) length, cytoplasmic adenylation and synthesis of poly(A)+ RNA in early mouse embryos. *Dev Biol* 1983;95:331–341.
92. Clegg K, Piko L. Quantitative aspects of RNA synthesis and polyadenylation in 1-cell and 2-cell mouse embryos. *J Embryol Exp Morphol* 1983;74:169–182.
93. Colonna R, Cecconi S, Buccione R, Mangia F. Amino acid transport systems in growing mouse oocytes. *Cell Biol Int Rep* 1983;7:1007–1015.
94. Copeland N, Gilbert D, Cho B, et al. Mast cell growth factor maps near the steel locus on mouse chromosome 10 and is deleted in a number of steel alleles. *Cell* 1990;63:175–183.
95. Coulombre J, Russell E. Analysis of the pleiotropism at the W-locus in the mouse. The effects of W and W^v substitution upon postnatal development of germ cells. *J Exp Zool* 1954;126: 277–295.
96. Crosby I, Osborn J, Moor R. Changes in protein phosphorylation during the maturation of mammalian oocytes *in vitro. J Exp Zool* 1984;229:459–466.
97. Cross P, Brinster R. *In vitro* development of mouse oocytes. *Biol Reprod* 1970;3:298–307.
98. Cross P, Brinster R. Leucine uptake and incorporation at three stages of mouse oocyte maturation. *Exp Cell Res* 1974;86:43–46.
99. Daniel J, ed. *Methods in mammalian embryology.* San Francisco: WH Freeman; 1971.
100. Daniel J, ed. *Methods in mammalian reproduction.* New York: Academic Press; 1978.
101. Davidson E. *Gene activity in early development.* Orlando: Academic Press; 1986.
102. De Felici M, McLaren A. Isolation of mouse primordial germ cells. *Exp Cell Res* 1982;142:476–482.

103. De Felici M, Siracusa G. Survival of isolated, fully-grown mouse ovarian oocytes is strictly dependent on external Ca^{2+}. *Dev Biol* 1982;92:539–543.
104. Dekel N, Aberdam E, Sherizly I. Spontaneous maturation *in vitro* of cumulus-enclosed rat oocytes is inhibited by forskolin. *Biol Reprod* 1984;31:244–250.
105. Dekel N, Beers W. Rat oocyte maturation *in vitro:* Relief of cyclic AMP inhibition with gonadotropins. *Proc Natl Acad Sci USA* 1978;75:4369–4373.
106. Dekel N, Beers W. Development of the rat oocyte *in vitro:* Inhibition and induction of maturation in the presence or absence of the cumulus oophorus. *Dev Biol* 1980;75:247–254.
107. Dekel N, Hillensjo T, Kraicer P. Maturational effects of gonadotropins on the cumulus-oocyte complex of the rat. *Biol Reprod* 1979;20:191–197.
108. Dekel N, Kraicer P, Phillips D, Sanchez R, Segal S. Cellular associations in the rat oocyte-cumulus cell complex: Morphology and ovulatory changes. *Gamete Res* 1978;1:47–57.
109. Dekel N, Lawrence T, Gilula N, Beers W. Modulation of cell-to-cell communication in the cumulus-oocyte complex and the regulation of oocyte maturation by LH. *Dev Biol* 1981;80:356–362.
110. DeLeon V, Johnson A, Bachvarova R. Half-lives and relative amounts of stored and polysomal ribosomes and poly(A^+)-RNA in mouse oocytes. *Dev Biol* 1983;98:400–408.
111. Donahue R. Maturation of the mouse oocyte *in vitro.* 1. Sequence and timing of nuclear progression. *J Exp Zool* 1968;169:237–250.
112. Downs S, Coleman D, Ward-Bailey P, Eppig J. Hypoxanthine is the principal inhibitor of murine oocyte maturation in a low molecular weight fraction of porcine follicular fluid. *Proc Natl Acad Sci USA* 1985;82:454–458.
113. Downs SM, Daniel SAJ, Bornslaeger EA, Hoppe PC, Eppig JJ. Maintenance of meiotic arrest in mouse oocytes by purines: Modulation of cAMP levels and cAMP phosphodiesterase activity. *Gamete Res* 1989;23:323–334.
114. Downs S, Eppig J. Cyclic adenosine monophosphate and ovarian follicular fluid act synergistically to inhibit mouse oocyte maturation. *Endocrinology* 1984;114:418–427.
115. Ducibella T. Mammalian egg cortical granules and the cortical reaction. In: Wassarman P, ed. *Elements of mammalian fertilization, vol 1, Basic concepts.* Boca Raton, FL: CRC Press; 1991:205–232.
116. Ducibella T, Anderson E, Albertini DF, Aalberg J, Rangarajan S. Quantitative changes in cortical granule number and distribution in the mouse oocyte during meiotic maturation. *Dev Biol* 1988;130:184–197.
117. Ducibella T, Kurasawa S, Rangarajan S, Kopf GS, Schultz RM. Precocious loss of cortical granules during mouse oocyte meiotic maturation and correlation with an egg-induced modification of the zona pellucida. *Dev Biol* 1990;137:46–55.
118. Ducibella T, Rangarajan S, Anderson E. The development of mouse oocyte cortical granule competence is accompanied by major changes in cortical vesicles and not cortical granule depth. *Dev Biol* 1988;130:789–792.
119. Dunbar B, Wardrip N, Hedrick J. Isolation, physiochemical properties, and macromolecular composition of zona pellucida from porcine oocytes. *Biochemistry* 1980;19:356–365.
120. Eddy E, Hahnel A. Establishment of the germ line in mammals. In: McLaren A, Wylie C, eds. *7th Symposium of British Society for Developmental Biology.* Cambridge: Cambridge University Press; 1983:41–69.
121. Eddy E, Clark J, Gong D, Fenderson B. Origin and migration of primordial germ cells in mammals. *Gamete Res* 1981;4:333–362.
122. Ekholm C, Magnusson C. Rat oocyte maturation: Effects of protein synthesis inhibitors. *Biol Reprod* 1979;21:1287–1293.
123. Eppig J. Analysis of mouse oogenesis *in vitro.* Oocyte isolation and the utilization of exogenous energy sources by growing oocytes. *J Exp Zool* 1976;198:375–382.
124. Eppig J. Mouse oocyte development *in vitro* with various culture systems. *Dev Biol* 1977;60:371–388.
125. Eppig J. A comparison between oocyte growth in coculture with granulosa cells and oocytes with granulosa cell-oocyte junctional contact maintained *in vitro. J Exp Zool* 1979;209:345–353.
126. Eppig J. The relationship between cumulus cell-oocyte coupling, oocyte meiotic maturation, and cumulus expansion. *Dev Biol* 1982;89:268–272.
127. Eppig J. Oocyte–somatic cell interactions during oocyte growth and maturation in the mammal. In: Browder L, ed. *Developmental biology: A comprehensive synthesis, vol 1, Oogenesis.* New York: Plenum Press; 1985:313–347.
128. Eppig J. Intercommunication between mammalian oocytes and companion somatic cells. *BioEssays* 1991;13:569–574.
129. Eppig J. Mammalian oocyte development *in vivo* and *in vitro.* In: Wassarman PM, ed. *Elements of mammalian fertilization, vol 1, Basic concepts.* Boca Raton, FL: CRC Press; 1991:57–76.
130. Eppig J, Freter R, Ward-Bailey P, Schultz R. Inhibition of oocyte maturation in the mouse: Participation of cAMP, steroid hormones, and a putative maturation-inhibitory factor. *Dev Biol* 1983;100:39–49.
131. Eppig J, Koide S. Effects of progesterone and oestradiol-173 on the spontaneous meiotic maturation of mouse oocytes. *J Reprod Fertil* 1978;53:99–101.
132. Eppig J, Ward-Bailey P, Coleman D. Hypoxanthine and adenosine in murine ovarian follicular fluid: Concentrations and activity in maintaining oocyte meiotic arrest. *Biol Reprod* 1985;33:1041–1049.
133. Fleming A, Khalil W, Armstrong D. Porcine follicular fluid does not inhibit maturation of rat oocytes *in vitro. J Reprod Fertil* 1985;69:665–670.
134. Florman H, Bechtol K, Wassarman P. Enzymatic dissection of the functions of the mouse egg's receptor for sperm. *Dev Biol* 1984;106:243–255.
135. Florman H, Wassarman P. O-Linked oligosaccharides of mouse egg ZP3 account for its sperm receptor activity. *Cell* 1985;41:313–324.
136. Fourcroy J. RNA synthesis in immature mouse oocyte development. *J Exp Zool* 1982;219:257–266.
137. Franchi L, Mandl A. The ultrastructure of oogonia and oocytes in the foetal and neonatal rat. *Proc R Soc Lond [Biol]* 1962;157:99–114.
138. Franchi L, Mandl A, Zuckerman S. The development of the ovary and the process of oogenesis. In: Zuckerman S, ed. *The ovary, vol 1.* New York: Academic Press; 1962:1–88.
139. Freter R, Schultz R. Regulation of murine oocyte maturation: Evidence for a gonadotropin-induced, cAMP-dependent reduction in a maturation inhibitor. *J Cell Biol* 1984;98:1119–1128.
140. Fulka J, Jung T, Moor RM. The fall of biological maturation promoting factor (MPF) and histone H1 kinase activity during anaphase and telophase in mouse oocytes. *Mol Reprod Dev* 1992;32:378–382.
141. Fulka J, Motlik J, Fulfa J, Crozet N. Inhibition of nuclear maturation in fully-grown porcine and mouse oocytes after their fusion with growing porcine oocytes. *J Exp Zool* 1985;235:255–259.
142. Garbers DL, Kopf GS. The regulation of spermatoza by calcium and cyclic nucleotides. In: Greengard P, Robison GA, eds. *Advances in cyclic nucleotide research.* New York: Raven Press, 1980:251–306.
143. Garcia R, Pereyra-Alfonso S, Sotelo J. Protein-synthesizing machinery in the growing oocyte of the cyclic mouse. *Differentiation (Berl)* 1979;14:101–106.
144. Gavin A, Tsukitani Y, Schorderet-Slatkine S. Induction of M-phase entry of prophase blocked mouse oocytes through microinjection of okadaic acid, a specific phosphatase inhibitor. *Exp Cell Res* 1991;192:75–81.
145. Geissler E, Ryan M, Housman D. The dominant-white spotting (W) locus of the mouse encodes the *c-kit* proto-oncogene. *Cell* 1988;55:185–192.
146. Gilula N, Epstein M, Beers W. Cell-to-cell communication and ovulation: A study of the cumulus cell-oocyte complex. *J Cell Biol* 1978;78:58–75.
147. Gilula N, Reeves O, Steinbach A. Metabolic coupling, ionic coupling, and cell contacts. *Nature* 1972;235:262–265.
148. Glass L. Localization of autologous and heterologous serum antigens in the mouse ovary. *Dev Biol* 1961;3:797–804.
149. Glass L. Transmission of maternal proteins into oocytes. *Adv Biosci* 1971;6:29–58.

150. Glass L, Cons J. Stage-dependent transfer of systematically injected foreign protein antigen and radiolabel into mouse ovarian follicles. *Anat Rec* 1968;162:139–156.
151. Golbus M, Stein M. Qualitative patterns of protein synthesis in the mouse oocyte. *J Exp Zool* 1976;198:337–342.
152. Goldman D, Kiessling A, Cooper G. Post-transcriptional processing suggests that c-*mos* functions as a maternal message in mouse eggs. *Oncogene* 1988;2:159–162.
153. Goldman D, Kiessling A, Millette C, Cooper G. Expression of c-*mos* RNA in germ cells of male and female mice. *Proc Natl Acad Sci USA* 1987;84:4509–4513.
154. Gondos B. Oogonia and oocytes in mammals. In: Jones R, ed. *The vertebrate ovary.* New York: Plenum Press; 1978:83–120.
155. Green E, ed. *Biology of the laboratory mouse.* New York: Dover Publications; 1975.
156. Greve J, Salzmann G, Roller R, Wassarman P. Biosynthesis of the major zona pellucida glycoprotein secreted by oocytes during mammalian oogenesis. *Cell* 1982;31:749–759.
157. Greve J, Wassarman P. Mouse egg extracellular coat is a matrix of interconnected filaments possessing a structural repeat. *J Mol Biol* 1985;181:253–264.
158. Gulyas B. Cortical granules of mammalian eggs. *Int Rev Cytol* 1980;63:357–392.
159. Gwatkin R. *Fertilization Mechanisms in Man and Mammals.* New York: Plenum Press; 1977.
160. Gwatkin RBL, ed. *Developmental biology: A comprehensive synthesis, vol 4, Manipulation of mammalian development.* New York: Plenum Press; 1986.
161. Gwatkin R, Andersen O. Hamster oocyte maturation *in vitro:* Inhibition by follicular components. *Life Sci* 1976;19:527–536.
162. Habibi B, Franchi L. Fine-structural changes in the nucleus of primordial oocytes in immature hamsters. *J Cell Sci* 1978;34:209–223.
163. Haddad A, Nagai E. Radioautographic study of glycoprotein biosynthesis and renewal in the ovarian follicles of mice and the origin of the zona pellucida. *Cell Tissue Res* 1977;177:347–369.
164. Hardisty M. Primordial germ cells and the vertebrate germ line. In: Jones R, ed. *The vertebrate ovary.* New York: Plenum Press; 1978:1–82.
165. Hartung M, Stahl A. Autoradiographic study of RNA synthesis during meiotic prophase in the human oocyte. *Cytogenet Cell Genet* 1978;20:51–58.
166. Heller D, Cahill D, Schultz R. Biochemical studies of mammalian oogenesis: Metabolic cooperativity between granulosa cells and growing mouse oocytes. *Dev Biol* 1981;84:455–464.
167. Heller D, Schultz R. Ribonucleoside metabolism by mouse oocytes: Metabolic cooperativity between the fully-grown oocyte and cumulus cells. *J Exp Zool* 1980;214:355–364.
168. Herlands R, Schultz R. Regulation of mouse oocyte growth: Probable nutritional role for intercellular communication between follicle cells and oocytes in oocyte growth. *J Exp Zool* 1984;229:317–325.
169. Herr W, Sturm R, Clerc R, et al. The POU domain: A large conserved region in the mammalian *pit*-1, *oct*-1, *oct*-2, and *Caenorhabditis elegans unc*-86 gene products. *Genes Dev* 1988;2:1513–1516.
170. Hertig A, Adams E. Studies on the human oocyte and its follicle. Ultrastructural and cytochemical observations on the primordial follicle stage. *J Cell Biol* 1967;34:647–675.
171. Hisaw F. Development of the Graafian follicle and ovulation. *Physiol Rev* 1947;27:95–119.
172. Hogan B, Costantini F, Lacy E, eds. *Manipulating the mouse embryo. A laboratory manual.* Cold Spring Harbor, NY: Cold Spring Harbor Laboratory; 1986.
173. Hope J. The fine structure of the developing follicle of the rhesus ovary. *J Ultrastruct Res* 1965;12:592–610.
174. Huang E, Nocka K, Beier D, et al. The hematopoietic growth factor KL is encoded by the Sl locus and is the ligand of the c-*kit* receptor, the gene product of the W locus. *Cell* 1990;63:225–233.
175. Huarte J, Belin D, Vassalli J-D. Plasminogen activator in mouse and rat oocytes: Induction during meiotic maturation. *Cell* 1985;43:551–558.
176. Huarte J, Belin D, Vassalli A, Strickland S, Vassalli J-D. Meiotic maturation of mouse oocytes triggers the translation and polyadenylation of dormant tissue-type plasminogen activator mRNA. *Genes Dev* 1987;1:1201–1211.
177. Iyengar M, Iyengar C, Chen H, Brinster R, Bornslaeger E, Schultz R. Expression of creatine kinase isoenzyme during oogenesis and embryogenesis in the mouse. *Dev Biol* 1983;96:263–268.
178. Jahn C, Baran M, Bachvarova R. Stability of RNA synthesized by the mouse oocyte during its major growth phase. *J Exp Zool* 1976;197:161–172.
179. Johnson M, McConnell J, Van Blerkom J. Programmed development in the mouse embryo. *J Embryol Exp Morphol (Suppl)* 1984;83:197–231.
180. Jones R, ed. *The vertebrate ovary.* New York: Plenum Press; 1978.
181. Kang Y. Development of the zona pellucida in the rat oocyte. *Am J Anat* 1974;139:535–566.
182. Kaplan G, Abreu S, Bachvarova R. rRNA accumulation and protein synthetic patterns in growing mouse oocytes. *J Exp Zool* 1982;220:361–380.
183. Kaplan G, Jelinek W, Bachvarova R. Repetitive sequence transcripts and U1 RNA in mouse oocytes and eggs. *Dev Biol* 1985;109:15–24.
184. Kinloch R, Roller R, Fimiani C, Wassarman D, Wassarman P. Primary structure of the mouse sperm receptor's polypeptide chain determined by genomic cloning. *Proc Natl Acad Sci USA* 1988;85:6409–6413.
185. Kinloch R, Roller R, Wassarman P. Organization and expression of the mouse sperm receptor gene. In: Davidson E, Ruderman J, Posakony J, eds. *Developmental biology.* New York: Wiley-Liss; 1990:9–20.
186. Kinloch R, Ruiz-Seiler B, Wassarman P. Genomic organization and polypeptide primary structure of zona pellucida glycoprotein hZP3, the hamster sperm receptor. *Dev Biol* 1990;142:414–420.
187. Kinloch R, Wassarman P. Nucleotide sequence of the gene encoding zona pellucida glycoprotein ZP3—the mouse sperm receptor. *Nucleic Acids Res* 1989;17:2861–2863.
188. Kinloch R, Wassarman P. Profile of a mammalian sperm receptor gene. *New Biol* 1989;1:232–238.
189. Krarup T, Pedersen T, Faber M. Regulation of oocyte growth in the mouse ovary. *Nature* 1969;224:187–188.
190. Kuroda H, Terada N, Nakayama H, Matsumoto K, Kitamura Y. Infertility due to growth arrest of ovarian follicles in Sl/Sl^{t} mice. *Dev Biol* 1988;126:71–79.
191. LaMarca M, Wassarman P. Program of early development in the mammal: Changes in absolute rates of synthesis of ribosomal proteins during oogenesis and early embryogenesis in the mouse. *Dev Biol* 1979;73:103–119.
192. LaMarca M, Wassarman P. Relationship between rates of synthesis and intracellular distribution of ribosomal proteins during oogenesis in the mouse. *Dev Biol* 1984;102:525–530.
193. Larsen W, Wert S, Brunner G. A dramatic loss of cumulus cell gap junctions is correlated with germinal vesicle breakdown in rat oocytes. *Dev Biol* 1986;113:517–521.
194. Lawrence T, Beers W, Gilula N. Transmission of hormonal stimulation by cell-to-cell communication. *Nature* 1978;272:501–506.
195. Lawrence T, Ginzberg R, Gilula N, Beers W. Hormonally induced cell shape changes in cultured rat ovarian granulosa cells. *J Cell Biol* 1979;80:21–36.
196. Leibfried L, First N. Effects of divalent cations on *in vitro* maturation of bovine oocytes. *J Exp Zool* 1979;210:575–580.
197. Leibfried L, First N. Effect of bovine and porcine follicular fluid and granulosa cells on maturation of oocytes *in vitro. Biol Reprod* 1980;23:699–704.
198. Leibfried L, First N. Follicular control of meiosis in the porcine oocyte. *Biol Reprod* 1980;23:705–709.
199. Lenardo M, Staudt L, Robbins P, Kuang A, Mulligan R, Baltimore D. Repression of the IgH enhancer in teratocarcinoma cells associated with a novel octamer factor. *Science* 1989;243:544–546.
200. Levey L, Stull G, Brinster R. Poly(A) and synthesis of polyadenylated RNA in the preimplantation mouse embryo. *Dev Biol* 1978;64:140–148.
201. Lira S, Kinloch R, Mortillo S, Wassarman P. An upstream region of the mouse ZP3 gene directs expression of firefly luciferase spe-

cifically to growing oocytes in transgenic mice. *Proc Natl Acad Sci USA* 1990;87:7215–7219.
202. Lowenstein J, Cohen A. Dry mass, lipid content, and protein content of the intact and zona-free mouse ovum. *J Embryol Exp Morphol* 1964;12:113–121.
203. Magnusson C, Hillensjo T. Inhibition of maturation and metabolism of rat oocytes by cyclic AMP. *J Exp Zool* 1977;201:138–147.
204. Majumder S, Brown K, Qiu F, Besmer P. c-*kit* protein, a transmembrane kinase: Identification in tissues and characterization. *Mol Cell Biol* 1988;8:4896–4903.
205. Maller J. Oocyte maturation in amphibians. In: Browder L, ed. *Developmental biology: A comprehensive synthesis, vol 1, Oogenesis.* New York: Plenum Press; 1985:289–311.
206. Mangia F, Epstein C. Biochemical studies of growing mouse oocytes: Preparation of oocytes and analysis of glucose-6-phosphate dehydrogenase and lactic dehydrogenase activities. *Dev Biol* 1975;45:211–220.
207. Mangia F, Erickson R, Epstein C. Synthesis of LDHI during mammalian oogenesis and early development. *Dev Biol* 1976;54:146–150.
208. Manova K, Nocka K, Besmer P, Bachvarova R. Gonadal expression of c-*kit* encoded at the W locus of the mouse. *Development* 1990;110:1057–1069.
209. Martin F, Suggs S, Langley K, et al. Primary structure and functional expression of rat and human stem cell factors DNAs. *Cell* 1990;63:203–211.
210. Masui Y. Meiotic arrest in animal oocytes. In: Metz C, Monroy A, eds. *Biology of fertilization, vol 1.* New York: Academic Press; 1985:189–220.
211. Masui Y, Clark H. Regulation of oocyte maturation. *Int Rev Cytol* 1979;57:185–282.
212. Mattson BA, Albertini DF. Oogenesis: Chromatin and microtubule dynamics during meiotic prophase. *Mol Reprod Dev* 1990;25:374–383.
213. McGaughey R. The culture of pig oocytes in minimal medium, and the influence of progesterone and estradiol-17β on meiotic maturation. *Endocrinology* 1977;100:39–45.
214. McGaughey R, Montgomery D, Richter J. Germinal vesicle configuration and patterns of polypeptide synthesis of porcine oocytes from antral follicles of different size, as related to their competency for spontaneous maturation. *J Exp Zool* 1979;209: 239–254.
215. McGaughey R, Van Blerkom J. Patterns of polypeptide synthesis of porcine oocytes during maturation *in vitro.* *Dev Biol* 1977;56:241–254.
216. McLaren A. The embryo. In: Austin C, Short R, eds. *Reproduction in mammals, vol 2.* Cambridge: Cambridge University Press; 1982:1–25.
217. McLaren A, Wylie C, eds. *Current problems in germ cell differentiation: 7th symposium British Society of Developmental Biology.* Cambridge: Cambridge University Press; 1983.
218. Messinger SM, Albertini DF. Centrosome and microtubule dynamics during meiotic progression in the mouse oocyte. *J Cell Sci* 1991;100:289–298.
219. Michaels G, Hauswirth W, Laipis P. Mitochondrial DNA copy number in bovine oocytes and somatic cells. *Dev Biol* 1982;94:246–251.
220. Mirre C, Stahl A. Ultrastructure and activity of the nucleolar organizer in the mouse oocyte during meiotic prophase. *J Cell Sci* 1978;31:79–100.
221. Mirre C, Stahl A. Ultrastructural organization, sites of transcription and distribution of fibrillar centers in the nucleolus of the mouse oocyte. *J Cell Sci* 1981;48:53–64.
222. Moor R, Osborn J, Cran D, Walters D. Selective effect of gonadotrophins on cell coupling, nuclear maturation and protein synthesis in mammalian oocytes. *J Embryol Exp Morphol* 1981;61:347–365.
223. Moor R, Smith M, Dawson R. Measurement of intercellular coupling between oocytes and cumulus cells using intracellular markers. *Exp Cell Res* 1980;126:15–29.
224. Moor R, Trounson A. Hormonal and follicular factors affecting maturation of sheep oocytes *in vitro* and their subsequent developmental capacity. *J Reprod Fertil* 1977;49:101–109.
225. Moore G. RNA synthesis in fixed cells by endogenous RNA polymerase. *Exp Cell Res* 1978;111:317–326.
226. Moore G, Lintern-Moore S. A correlation between growth and RNA synthesis in the mouse oocyte. *J Reprod Fertil* 1974;39:163–166.
227. Moore G, Lintern-Moore S. Transcription of the mouse oocyte genome. *Biol Reprod* 1978;18:865–870.
228. Moore G, Lintern-Moore S. Stimulation of endogenous RNA polymerase I activity in the mouse oocyte after PMSG treatment. *Biol Reprod* 1979;21:373–377.
229. Moore G, Lintern-Moore S, Peters H, Faber M. RNA synthesis in the mouse oocyte. *J Cell Biol* 1974;60:416–422.
230. Mortillo S, Wassarman P. Differential binding of gold-labeled zona pellucida glycoproteins mZP2 and mZP3 to mouse sperm membrane compartments. *Development* 1991;113:141–149.
231. Mukherjee A. Normal progeny from fertilization *in vitro* of mouse oocytes matured in culture and spermatozoa capacitated *in vitro.* *Nature* 1972;237:397–398.
232. Murray A, Kirschner M. What controls the cell cycle. *Sci Am* 1991;264(3):56–63.
233. Mutter G, Grills G, Wolgemuth D. Evidence for the involvement of the proto-oncogene *c-mos* in mammalian meiotic maturation and possibly very early embryogenesis. *EMBO J* 1988;7: 683–689.
234. Mutter G, Wolgemuth D. Distinct developmental patterns of c-*mos* protooncogene expression in female and male mouse germ cells. *Proc Natl Acad Sci USA* 1987;84:5301–5305.
235. Needham J. *A history of embryology.* Cambridge: Cambridge University Press; 1959.
236. Nicosia S, Wolf D, Inoue M. Cortical granule distribution and cell surface characteristics in mouse eggs. *Dev Biol* 1977;57:56–74.
237. Nocka K, Buck J, Levi E, Besmer P. Candidate ligand for the c-*kit* transmembrane kinase receptor: KL, a fibroblast derived growth factor stimulates mast cells and erythroid progenitors. *EMBO J* 1990;10:3287–3294.
238. Nocka K, Majumder S, Chabot B, et al. Expression of c-*kit* gene products in known cellular targets of W mutations in normal and W mutant mice—evidence for an impaired c-*kit* kinase in mutant mice. *Genes Dev* 1979;3:816–826.
239. Nocka K, Tan J, Chiu E, et al. Molecular bases of dominant negative and loss of function mutations at the murine c-*kit*/white spotting locus: W37, Wv, W41 and W. *EMBO J* 1990;9: 1805–1813.
240. O'Keefe S, Wolfes H, Kiessling A, Cooper G. Microinjection of antisense c-*mos* oligonucleotides prevents meiosis II in the maturing mouse egg. *Proc Natl Acad Sci USA* 1989;86:7038–7042.
241. Oakberg E. Relationship between stage of follicular development and RNA synthesis in the mouse oocyte. *Mutat Res* 1968;6:155–165.
242. Odor D. Electron microscopic studies on ovarian oocytes and unfertilized tubal ova in the rat. *J Biophys Biochem Cytol* 1960;7:567–574.
243. Odor D. The ultrastructure of unilaminar follicles of the hamster ovary. *Am J Anat* 1965;116:493–522.
244. Okamoto K, Okazawa H, Okuda A, Sakai M, Muramatsu M, Hamada H. A novel octamer binding transcription factor is differentially expressed in mouse embryonic cells. *Cell* 1990;60: 461–472.
245. Olds P, Stem S, Biggers J. Chemical estimates of the RNA and DNA contents of the early mouse embryo. *J Exp Zool* 1973;186:39–46.
246. Olsiewski P, Beers W. cAMP synthesis in the rat oocyte. *Dev Biol* 1983;100:287–293.
247. Orr-Urtreger A, Avivi A, Zimmer Y, Givol D, Yarden Y, Lonai P. Developmental expression of c-*kit*, a proto-oncogene encoded by the W locus. *Development* 1990;109:911–923.
248. Osborn J, Moor R. Time-dependent effects of α-amanitin on nuclear maturation and protein synthesis in mammalian oocytes. *J Embryol Exp Morphol* 1983;73:317–338.
249. Oskarsson M, McClements W, Blair D, Maizel J, Vande Woude G. Properties of a normal mouse cell DNA sequence (sarc) homologous to the src sequence of Moloney sarcoma virus. *Science* 1980;207:1222–1224.
250. Paleos G, Powers R. The effect of calcium on the first meiotic division of the mammalian oocyte. *J Exp Zool* 1981;217: 409–416.

251. Palombi F, Viron A. Nuclear cytochemistry of mouse oogenesis. I. Changes in extranuclear ribonucleoprotein components through meiotic prophase. *J Ultrastruct Res* 1977;61:10–20.
252. Parkes A, ed. *Marshall's physiology of reproduction, vol 1, part 1.* New York: Longmans, Green; 1956.
253. Paules R, Buccione R, Moschel R, Vande Woude G, Eppig J. Mouse *Mos* protooncogene product is present and functions during oogenesis. *Proc Natl Acad Sci USA* 1989;86:5395–5399.
254. Paynton B, Rempel R, Bachvarova R. Changes in state of adenylation and time course of degradation of maternal mRNAs during oocyte maturation and early embryonic development in the mouse. *Dev Biol* 1988;129:304–314.
255. Pedersen T. Follicle growth in the immature mouse ovary. *Acta Endocrinol* (Kbh) 1969;62:117–132.
256. Pedersen T. Follicle kinetics in the ovary of the cyclic mouse. *Acta Endocrinol* (Kbh) 1970;64:304–323.
257. Pedersen T. Follicle growth in the mouse ovary. In: Biggers J, Schuetz A, eds. *Oogenesis.* Baltimore: University Park Press; 1972;361–367.
258. Pedersen T, Peters H. Proposal for the classification of oocytes and follicles in the mouse ovary. *J Reprod Fertil* 1968;17:555–557.
259. Peters H. The development of the mouse ovary from birth to maturity. *Acta Endocrinol* (Kbh) 1969;62:98–116.
260. Peters H. Folliculogenesis in mammals. In: Jones R, ed. *The vertebrate ovary.* New York: Plenum Press; 1978:121–144.
261. Philpott C, Ringuette M, Dean J. Oocyte-specific expression and developmental regulation of ZP3, the sperm receptor of the mouse zona pellucida. *Dev Biol* 1987;121:568–575.
262. Pierce KE, Siebert MC, Kopf GS, Schultz RM, Calarco PG. Characterization and localization of a mouse egg cortical granule antigen prior to and following fertilization or egg activation. *Dev Biol* 1990;141:381–392.
263. Piko L, Chase D. Role of the mitochondrial genome during early development in mice. *J Cell Biol* 1973;58:357–378.
264. Piko L, Clegg K. Quantitative changes in total RNA, total poly(A) and ribosomes in early mouse embryos. *Dev Biol* 1982;89:362–378.
265. Piko L, Hammons M, Taylor K. Amounts, synthesis, and some properties of intracisternal A particle-related RNA in early mouse embryos. *Proc Natl Acad Sci USA* 1984;81:488–492.
266. Piko L, Matsumoto L. Number of mitochondria and some properties of mitochondrial DNA in the mouse egg. *Dev Biol* 1976;49:1–10.
267. Pincus G. *The eggs of mammals.* New York: Macmillan; 1936.
268. Pincus G, Enzmann E. The comparative behavior of mammalian eggs *in vivo* and *in vitro.* 1. The activation of ovarian eggs. *J Exp Med* 1935;62:665–675.
269. Powers R, Paleos G. Combined effects of calcium and dibutyryl cAMP on germinal vesicle breakdown in the mouse oocyte. *J Reprod Fertil* 1982;66:1–8.
270. Pratt H, Bolton V, Gudgeon K. The legacy from the oocyte and its role in controlling early development of the mouse embryo. *Ciba Found Symp* 1983;98:197–227.
271. Propst F, Vande Woude G. Expression of *c-mos* proto-oncogene transcripts in mouse tissues. *Nature* 1985;315:516–518.
272. Qui F, Ray P, Brown K, et al. Primary structure of *c-kit:* Relationship with the CSF-1/PDGF receptor kinase family—Oncogenic activation of *v-kit* involves deletion of extracellular domain and C terminus. *EMBO J* 1988;7:1003–1011.
273. Racowsky C. Effect of forskolin on the spontaneous maturation and cyclic AMP content of hamster oocyte–cumulus complexes. *J Exp Zool* 1985;234:87–96.
274. Racowsky C. Antagonistic actions of estradiol and tamoxifen upon forskolin-dependent meiotic arrest, intercellular coupling, and the cAMP content of hamster oocyte–cumulus complexes. *J Exp Zool* 1985;234:251–260.
275. Racowsky C, McGaughey R. Further studies of the effects of follicular fluid and membrane granulosa cells on the spontaneous maturation of pig oocytes. *J Reprod Fertil* 1982;66:505–512.
276. Racowsky C, McGaughey R. In the absence of protein, estradiol suppresses meiosis of porcine oocytes *in vitro. J Exp Zool* 1982;224:103–110.
277. Racowsky C, Satterlie R. Metabolic, fluorescent dye and electrical coupling between hamster oocytes and cumulus cells during meiotic maturation *in vivo* and *in vitro. Dev Biol* 1985;108:191–202.
278. Rafferty K. *Methods in experimental embryology of the mouse.* Baltimore: Johns Hopkins Press; 1970.
279. Rice C, McGaughey R. Effect of testosterone and dibutyryl cAMP on the spontaneous maturation of pig oocytes. *J Reprod Fertil* 1981;62:245–256.
280. Richards J. Maturation of ovarian follicles: Actions and interactions of pituitary and ovarian hormones on follicular cell differentiation. *Physiol Rev* 1980;60:51–89.
281. Richter J, McGaughey R. Patterns of polypeptide synthesis in mouse oocytes during germinal vesicle breakdown and during maintenance of the germinal vesicle stage by dibutyryl cAMP. *Dev Biol* 1981;83:188–192.
282. Ringuette M, Chamberlin M, Baur A, Sobieski D, Dean J. Molecular analysis of cDNA coding for ZP3, a sperm binding protein of the mouse zona pellucida. *Dev Biol* 1988;127:287–295.
283. Ringuette M, Sobieski D, Chamow S, Dean J. Oocyte-specific gene expression: Molecular characterization of a cDNA coding for ZP3, the sperm receptor of the mouse zona pellucida. *Proc Natl Acad Sci USA* 1986;83:4341–4345.
284. Rodman T, Bachvarova R. RNA synthesis in preovulatory mouse oocytes. *J Cell Biol* 1976;70:251–257.
285. Rodman T, Barth A. Chromosomes of mouse oocytes in maturation: Differential trypsin sensitivity and amino acid incorporation. *Dev Biol* 1979;68:82–95.
286. Roller R, Kinloch R, Hiraoka B, Li SS-L, Wassarman P. Gene expression during mammalian oogenesis and early embryogenesis: Quantification of three messenger RNAs abundant in fully-grown mouse oocytes. *Development* 1989;106:251–261.
287. Roller R, Wassarman P. Role of asparagine-linked oligosaccharides in secretion of glycoproteins of the mouse egg's extracellular coat. *J Biol Chem* 1985;258:13243–13249.
288. Rosenthal E, Ruderman J. Widespread changes in the translation and adenylation of maternal messenger RNAs following fertilization of *Spisula* oocytes. *Dev Biol* 1987;121:237–246.
289. Rosner M, Vigano M, Ozato K, et al. A POU-domain transcription factor in early stem cells and germ cells of the mammalian embryo. *Nature* 1990;345:686–692.
290. Roy L, Singh B, Gauthier J, Arlinghaus R, Nordeen S, Maller J. The cyclin B2 component of MPF is a substrate for the c-*mos* protooncogene product. *Cell* 1990;61:825–831.
291. Rugh R. *The mouse: Its reproduction and development.* Minneapolis: Burgess; 1968.
292. Russell E. Hereditary anemias of the mouse: A review for geneticists. *Adv Genet* 1979;20:357–459.
293. Ruvkun G, Finney M. Regulation of transcription and cell identity by POU domain proteins. *Cell* 1991;64:475–478.
294. Sagata N, Watanabe N, Vande Woude G, Ikawa Y. The *c-mos* proto-oncogene product is a cytostatic factor responsible for meiotic arrest in vertebrate eggs. *Nature* 1989;342:512–518.
295. Salustri A, Martinozzi M. A comparison of protein synthetic activity in *in vitro* cultured denuded and follicle-enclosed oocytes. *Cell Biol Int Rep* 1983;7:1049–1055.
296. Salustri A, Siracusa G. Metabolic coupling cumulus expansion and meiotic resumption in mouse cumuli oophori cultured *in vitro* in the presence of FSH or dbcAMP, or stimulated *in vivo* by hCG. *J Reprod Fertil* 1983;68:335–341.
297. Salzmann G, Greve J, Roller R, Wassarman P. Biosynthesis of the sperm receptor during oogenesis in the mouse. *EMBO J* 1983;2:1451–1456.
298. Sato E, Koide S. Forskolin and mouse oocyte maturation *in vitro. J Exp Zool* 1984;230:125–129.
299. Schickler M, Lira S, Kinloch R, Wassarman P. A mouse oocyte-specific protein that binds to a region of mZP3 promoter responsible for oocyte-specific mZP3 gene expression. *Mol Cell Biol* 1992;12:120–127.
300. Schöler H, Dressler G, Balling R, Rohdewohld H, Gruss P. Oct-4: A germline-specific transcription factor mapping to the mouse *t*-complex. *EMBO J* 1990;9:2185–2195.
301. Schöler H, Hatzopoulos A, Balling R, Suzuki N, Gruss P. A family of octamer-specific proteins present during mouse embryo-

genesis: Evidence for germline-specific expression of an Oct factor. *EMBO J* 1989;8:2543–2550.
302. Schöler H, Ruppert S, Suzuki N, Chowdhury K, Gruss P. New type of POU domain in germ line-specific protein Oct-4. *Nature* 1990;344:435–439.
303. Schroeder A, Eppig J. The developmental capacity of mouse oocytes that matured spontaneously *in vitro* is normal. *Dev Biol* 1984;102:493–497.
304. Schuel H. Functions of egg cortical granules. In: Metz C, Monroy A, eds. *Biology of fertilization, vol 3.* New York: Academic Press; 1985:1–44.
305. Schultz G. Polyadenylic acid-containing RNA in unfertilized and fertilized eggs of the rabbit. *Dev Biol* 1975;44:270–277.
306. Schultz RM. Molecular aspects of mammalian oocyte growth and maturation. In: Rossant J, Pedersen RA, eds. *Experimental approaches to mammalian embryonic development.* Cambridge: Cambridge University Press; 1986:195–238.
307. Schultz RM. Meiotic maturation of mammalian oocytes. In: Wassarman PM, ed. *Elements of mammalian fertilization, vol 1, Basic concepts.* Boca Raton, FL: CRC Press; 1991:77–104.
308. Schultz R, LaMarca M, Wassamman P. Absolute rates of protein synthesis during meiotic maturation of mammalian oocytes *in vitro. Proc Natl Acad Sci USA* 1978;75:4160–4164.
309. Schultz R, Letourneau G, Wassarman P. Meiotic maturation of mouse oocytes *in vitro:* Protein synthesis in nucleate and anucleate oocyte fragments. *J Cell Sci* 1978;30:251–264.
310. Schultz R, Letourneau G, Wassamman P. Program of early development in the mammal: Changes in patterns and absolute rates of tubulin and total protein synthesis during oogenesis and early embryogenesis in the mouse. *Dev Biol* 1979;68:341–359.
311. Schultz R, Letourneau G, Wassarman P. Program of early development in the mammal: Changes in the patterns and absolute rates of tubulin and total protein synthesis during oocyte growth in the mouse. *Dev Biol* 1979;73:120–133.
312. Schultz R, Montgomery R, Belanoff J. Regulation of mouse oocyte meiotic maturation: Implication of a decrease in oocyte cAMP and protein dephosphorylation in commitment to resume meiosis. *Dev Biol* 1983;97:264–273.
313. Schultz R, Montgomery R, Ward-Bailey P, Eppig J. Regulation of oocyte maturation in the mouse: Possible roles of intercellular communication, cAMP, and testosterone. *Dev Biol* 1983;95: 294–304.
314. Schultz R, Wassarman P. Biochemical studies of mammalian oogenesis: Protein synthesis during oocyte growth and meiotic maturation in the mouse. *J Cell Sci* 1977;24:167–194.
315. Schultz R, Wassarman P. Specific changes in the pattern of protein synthesis during meiotic maturation of mammalian oocytes *in vitro. Proc Natl Acad Sci USA* 1977;74:538–541.
316. Schultz R, Wassarman P. Efficient extraction and quantitative determination of nanogram amounts of cellular RNA. *Anal Biochem* 1980;104:328–334.
317. Shimuzu S, Tsuji M, Dean J. *In vitro* biosynthesis of three sulfated glycoproteins of murine zonae pellucidae by oocytes grown in follicle culture. *J Biol Chem* 1983;258:5858–5863.
318. Short R. The discovery of the ovaries. In: *The Ovary, vol 1,* edited by S. Zuckerman and B. Weir, pp. 1–41. Academic Press, New York.
319. Silvers W. *The coat colors of mice.* New York: Springer-Verlag; 1979.
320. Siracusa G, De Felici M, Salustri A. The proliferative and meiotic history of mammalian female germ cells. In: *Biology of Fertilization, vol 1,* edited by C. Metz and A. Monroy, pp. 253–298. Academic Press, New York.
321. Siracusa G, Whittingham D, Molinaro M, Vivarelli E. Parthenogenetic activation of mouse oocytes induced by inhibitors of protein synthesis. *J Embryol Exp Morphol* 1978;43:157–166.
322. Smith D, Tenney D. Effect of steroids on mouse oocyte maturation *in vitro. J Reprod Fertil* 1980;60:331–338.
323. Sorensen R. Cinemicrography of mouse oocyte maturation utilizing Nomarski differential-interference microscopy. *Am J Anat* 1973;136:265–276.
324. Sorensen R, Cyert M, Pedersen R. Active maturation-promoting factor is present in mature mouse oocytes. *J Cell Biol* 1985;100:1637–1640.
325. Sorensen R, Wassarman P. Relationship between growth and meiotic maturation of the mouse oocyte. *Dev Biol* 1976;50:531–536.
326. Sotelo J, Porter K. An electron microscope study of the rat ovum. *J Biophys Biochem Cytol* 1959;5:327–341.
327. Speed R. Meiosis in the foetal mouse ovary. 1. An analysis at the light microscope level using surface-spreading. *Chromosoma* 1982;85:427–437.
328. Stern S, Biggers J, Anderson E. Mitochondria and early development of the mouse. *J Exp Zool* 1971;176:179–192.
329. Sternlicht A, Schultz R. Biochemical studies of mammalian oogenesis: Kinetics of accumulation of total and poly(A) containing RNA during growth of the mouse oocyte. *J Exp Zool* 1981;215:191–200.
330. Strickland S. Plasminogen activator in early development. In: Johnson M, ed. *Development in mammals.* Amsterdam: Elsevier/North Holland; 1980:81–100.
331. Strickland S, Huarte J, Belin D, Vassalli A, Rickles R, Vassalli J-D. Antisense RNA directed against the 3′ noncoding region prevents dormant mRNA activation in mouse oocytes. *Science* 1988;241:680–684.
332. Szollosi D. Changes of some cell organelles during oogenesis in mammals. In: Biggers J, Schuetz A, eds. *Oogenesis.* Baltimore: University Park Press; 1972:47–64.
333. Szollosi D, Calarco P, Donahue R. The nuclear envelope: Its breakdown and fate in mammalian oogonia and oocytes. *Anat Rec* 1972;174:325–340.
334. Szybek K. *In vitro* maturation of oocytes from sexually immature mice. *J Endocrinol* 1972;54:527–528.
335. Thibault C. Final stages of mammalian oocyte maturation. In: Biggers J, Schuetz A, eds. *Oogenesis.* Baltimore: University Park Press; 1972:397–411.
336. Tsafriri A. Oocyte maturation in mammals. In: Jones R, ed. *The vertebrate ovary.* New York: Plenum Press; 1978:409–442.
337. Tsafriri A. The control of meiotic maturation in mammals. In: Metz C, Monroy A, eds. *Biology of fertilization, vol 1.* New York: Academic Press; 1985:221–252.
338. Tsafriri A, Bar-Ami S. Role of divalent cations in the resumption of meiosis in rat oocytes. *J Exp Zool* 1978;205:293–300.
339. Tsafriri A, Bar-Ami S, Lindner H. Control of the development of meiotic competence and of oocyte maturation in mammals. In: Beier H, Lindner H, eds. *Fertilization of the human egg in vitro.* Berlin: Springer-Verlag; 1983:3–17.
340. Tsafriri A, Channing C. An inhibitory influence of granulosa cells and follicular fluid upon porcine oocyte meiosis *in vitro. Endocrinology* 1975;96:992.
341. Tsafriri A, Channing C, Pomerantz S, Lindner H. Inhibition of maturation of isolated rat oocytes by porcine follicular fluid. *J Endocrinol* 1977;75:258–291.
342. Tsafriri A, Dekel N, Bar-Ami S. The role of oocyte maturation inhibitor in follicular regulation of oocyte maturation. *J Reprod Fertil* 1982;64:541–551.
343. Tsafriri A, Pomerantz S, Channing C. Inhibition of oocyte maturation by porcine follicular fluid: Partial characterization of the inhibitor. *Biol Reprod* 1976;14:511–516.
344. Upadhyay S, Zamboni L. Ectopic germ cells: Natural model for the study of germ cell sexual differentiation. *Proc Natl Acad Sci USA* 1982;79:6584–6588.
345. Urner F, Herrmann W, Baulieu E, Schorderet-Slatkine S. Inhibition of denuded mouse oocyte maturation of forskolin, an activator of adenylate cyclase. *Endocrinology* 1983;113:1170–1172.
346. Van Blerkom J. Protein synthesis during oogenesis and early embryogenesis in the mammal. In: Metz C, Monroy A, eds. *Biology of fertilization, vol 3.* New York: Academic Press; 1985:379–401.
347. Van Blerkom J. Structural relationship and posttranslational modification of stage-specific proteins synthesized during early preimplantation development in the mouse. *Proc Natl Acad Sci USA* 1981;78:7629–7633.
348. Van Blerkom J, McGaughey R. Molecular differentiation of the rabbit ovum. I. During oocyte maturation *in vivo* and *in vitro. Dev Biol* 1978;63:139–150.
349. Van Blerkom J, McGaughey R. Molecular differentiation of the rabbit ovum. II. During the preimplantation development of *in vivo* and *in vitro* matured oocytes. *Dev Biol* 1978;63:151–164.

350. Van Blerkom J, Motta P. *The cellular basis of mammalian reproduction.* Baltimore: Urban & Schwarzenberg; 1979.
351. Vanderhyden BC, Caron PJ, Buccione R, Eppig JJ. Developmental pattern of the secretion of cumulus expansion-enabling factor by mouse oocytes and the role of oocytes in promoting granulosa cell differentiation. *Dev Biol* 1990;140:307–317.
352. Vassalli J-D, Huarte H, Belin D, et al. Regulated polyadenylation controls mRNA translation during meiotic maturation of mouse oocytes. *Genes Dev* 1989;3:2163–2171.
353. Vivarelli E, Conti M, De Felici M, Siracusa G. Meiotic resumption and intracellular cAMP levels in mouse oocytes treated with compounds which act on cAMP metabolism. *Cell Differ* 1983;12:271–276.
354. Warnes G, Moor R, Johnson M. Changes in protein synthesis during maturation of sheep oocytes *in vivo* and *in vitro.* *J Reprod Fertil* 1977;49:331–335.
355. Wassarman P. Oogenesis: Synthetic events in the developing mammalian egg. In: Hartmann J, ed. *Mechanism and control of animal fertilization.* New York: Academic Press; 1983:1–54.
356. Wassarman P. Early events in mammalian fertilization. *Annu Rev Cell Biol* 1987;3:109–142.
357. Wassarman P. The biology and chemistry of fertilization. *Science* 1987;235:553–560.
358. Wassarman P. Zona pellucida glycoproteins. *Annu Rev Biochem* 1988;57:415–442.
359. Wassarman P. Profile of a mammalian sperm receptor. *Development* 1990;108:1–17.
360. Wassarman P, ed. *Elements of Mammalian Fertilization, vols 1, 2.* Boca Raton, FL: CRC Press; 1991.
361. Wassarman P. Mouse gamete adhesion molecules. *Biol Reprod* 1992;46:186–191.
362. Wassarman P. Mammalian fertilization: Sperm receptor genes and glycoproteins. *Adv Dev Biochem* 1993;2:155–195.
363. Wassarman P, Bleil J, Cascio S, et al. Programming of gene expression during mammalian oogenesis. In: Jagiello G, Vogel H, eds. *Bioregulators of Reproduction,* New York: Academic Press; 1981:119–150.
364. Wassarman P, Bleil J, Florman H, et al. The mouse egg's receptor for sperm: What is it and how does it work? *Cold Spring Harbor Symp Quant Biol* 1985;50:11–19.
365. Wassarman P, DePamphilis ML, eds. *Guide to techniques in mouse development: Methods in enzymology, vol 225.* Orlando, FL: Academic Press; 1993.
366. Wassarman P, Fujiwara K. Immunofluorescent antitubulin staining of spindles during meiotic maturation of mouse oocytes *in vitro.* *J Cell Sci* 1978;29:171–188.
367. Wassarman P, Josefowicz W. Oocyte development in the mouse: An ultrastructural comparison of oocytes isolated at various stages of growth and meiotic competence. *J Morphol* 1978;156:209–235.
368. Wassarman P, Josefowicz W, Letourneau G. Meiotic maturation of mouse oocytes *in vitro:* Inhibition of maturation at specific stages of nuclear progression. *J Cell Sci* 1976;22:531–545.
369. Wassarman P, Letourneau G. RNA synthesis in fully-grown mouse oocytes. *Nature* 1976;361:73–74.
370. Wassarman P, Mortillo S. Structure of the mouse egg extracellular coat. *Int Rev Cytol* 1991;130:85–110.
371. Wassarman P, Mrozak S. Program of early development in the mammal: Synthesis and intracellular migration of histone H4 during oogenesis in the mouse. *Dev Biol* 1981;84:364–371.
372. Wassarman P, Schultz R, Letourneau G. Protein synthesis during meiotic maturation of mouse oocytes *in vitro.* Synthesis and phosphorylation of a protein localized in the germinal vesicle. *Dev Biol* 1979;69:94–107.
373. Wassarman P, Schultz R, Letourneau G, LaMarca M, Bleil J. Meiotic maturation of mouse oocytes *in vitro.* In: Channing C, Marsh J, Sadler W, eds. *Ovarian follicular and corpus luteum function.* New York: Plenum Press; 1979:251–268.
374. Weakley B. Electron microscopy of the oocyte and granulosa cells in the developing ovarian follicles of the golden hamster (*Mesocricetus auratus*). *J Anat* 1966;100:503–534.
375. Weakley B. Investigations into the structure and fixation properties of cytoplasmic lamellae of hamster oocytes. *Z Zellforsch Mikrosk Anat* 1967;81:91–99.
376. Weakley B. Comparison of cytoplasmic lamellae and membranous elements in oocytes of five mammalian species. *Z Zellforsch Mikrosk Anat* 1968;85:109–123.
377. Weber M, Kubiak J, Arlinghaus R, Pines J, Maro B. *c-mos* proto-oncogene product is partly degraded after release from meiotic arrest and persists during interphase in mouse zygotes. *Dev Biol* 1991;148:393–397.
378. Wickramasinghe D, Albertini DF. Centrosome phosphorylation and the developmental expression of meiotic competence in mouse oocytes. *Dev Biol* 1992;152:62–74.
379. Wickramasinghe D, Albertini DF. Cell cycle control during mammalian oogenesis. *Curr Top Dev Biol* 1993;28:125–153.
380. Wickramasinghe D, Ebert KM, Albertini DF. Meiotic competence acquisition is associated with the appearance of M-phase characteristics in growing mouse oocytes. *Dev Biol* 1991;143: 162–172.
381. Wilson E. *The cell in development and heredity.* New York: Macmillan; 1925.
382. Wischnitzer S. Intramitochondrial transformations during oocyte maturation in the mouse. *J Morphol* 1967;121:29–46.
383. Wolgemuth D, Jagiello G, Henderson A. Quantitation of ribosomal RNA genes in fetal human oocyte nuclei using rRNA: DNA hybridization *in situ.* Evidence for increased multiplicity. *Exp Cell Res* 1979;118:181–190.
384. Wolgemuth D, Jagiello G, Henderson A. Baboon late diplotene oocytes contain micronucleoli and a low level of extra rDNA templates. *Dev Biol* 1980;78:598–604.
385. Wylie C, ed. Germ cell development. *Sem Dev Biol* 4[*in press*].
386. Yarden Y, Kuang W-J, Yang-Feng T, et al. Human proto-oncogene *c-kit:* A new cell surface receptor tyrosine kinase for an unidentified ligand. *EMBO J* 1987;6:3341–3351.
387. Zamboni L. Ultrastructure of mammalian oocytes and ova. *Biol Reprod (Suppl)* 1970;2:44–63.
388. Zamboni L. Comparative studies on the ultrastructure of mammalian oocytes. In: *Oogenesis,* edited by J. Biggers and A. Schuetz, pp. 5–46. University Park Press, Baltimore.
389. Zamboni L, Mastroianni L. Electron microscopy studies on rabbit ova. I. The follicular oocyte. *J Ultrastruct Res* 1966;14:95–117.
390. Zhao X, Singh B, Batten B. The role of *c-mos* proto-oncoprotein in mammalian meiotic maturation. *Oncogene* 1990;6:43–49.
391. Zsebo K, Williams D, Geissler EN, et al. Stem cell factor is encoded at the *Sl* locus of the mouse and is the ligand for the *c-kit* tyrosine kinase receptor. *Cell* 1990;63:213–224.
392. Zsebo K, Wypych J, McNiece I, et al. Identification, purification and biological characterization of hematopoietic stem cell factor from Buffalo rat liver-conditioned medium. *Cell* 1990;63: 195–201.
393. Zuckerman S, ed. *The ovary, vol 1.* New York: Academic Press; 1962.
394. Zuckerman S, Baker T. The development of the ovary and the process of oogenesis. In: Zuckerman S, Weir B, eds. *The ovary, vol 1.* New York: Academic Press; 1977:42–68.
395. Zuckerman S, Weir B, eds. *The ovary.* New York: Academic Press; 1977.

The Physiology of Reproduction, Second Edition,
edited by E. Knobil and J.D. Neill,
Raven Press, Ltd., New York © 1994.

CHAPTER 4

Gamete and Zygote Transport

Michael J. K. Harper

FOREWORD

When the first version of this chapter, entitled "Gamete and Zygote Transport," was written in 1985/86, I concluded with the words "that the approaches of the past have failed to provide us with the correct blueprint for integration of function of this system [i.e., the oviduct as an organ central to gamete and zygote transport] and that new approaches are required" (1). Now, some 6 years later, it is clear that in many areas of reproductive biology tremendous advances have been made, especially with the application of modern techniques of molecular biology. These are powerful techniques, but techniques, nevertheless, to answer specific questions and not ends in themselves. Thus, it is important to frame appropriate questions, bearing in mind that we wish to understand the integration of the system and to eschew a reductionist mentality, as individual parts of a jigsaw puzzle tell us little about the picture as a whole.

Recent studies have provided information on topics such as sperm maturation and binding to the zona pellucida, fertilization, and zygote growth and development, but the question remains whether such information has improved our understanding of the system as a whole. One should not prejudge this issue without a critical assessment of all available evidence, and so in this revision of the original chapter, I have endeavored to present that new information that bears on the processes of "gamete and zygote transport." This provides the readers with a comprehensive look at the "trees," from which they can then stand back and view the "forest." At the end of the chapter, I again attempt to summarize my view of our understanding of these complex processes. The readers must then decide for themselves whether their assessment is the same or different, realizing that the perspective of even a well-defined forest may vary according to the standpoint. Thus, each viewer must make his or her own interpretation of a work of art, no matter how well

Department of Obstetrics and Gynecology, Baylor College of Medicine, Houston, Texas 77030 known and well analyzed. Nevertheless, there will be some congruity between the interpretations of the different viewers, and in the same fashion, it is to be hoped that this will also be true for readers of this chapter.

INTRODUCTION

Gametes are properly defined as mature germ cells possessing a haploid chromosome set capable of initiating formation of a new individual by fusion with another gamete (2). Thus, at the moment of ovulation, the ovum is a gamete because it has already undergone the first meiotic division with extrusion of the first polar body and has reached the metaphase stage of the second meiotic division, where it is arrested until activation occurs. This is generally induced by penetration of a spermatozoon through the vitelline membrane of the ovum, although it can also occur parthenogenetically. The spermatozoon at the moment of ejaculation is also a gamete because it has been produced through the two meiotic divisions that result in four spermatozoa being produced from each primary spermatocyte. Therefore, strictly speaking, the term *gamete* is applicable only up to fertilization. Fertilization is a process that begins with sperm penetration and is completed at syngamy, which is defined as the union of the two sets of haploid chromosomes to form a new diploid fertilized ovum (or egg). Strictly speaking, the correct term for this new structure is *zygote.*

Hence the title of this chapter is somewhat misleading because, although initial transport of sperm and egg deals with them as gametes, after fertilization the further transport should be referred to as *zygote transport.* In modern usage, one finds the terms *ovum, oocyte, egg,* and *zygote* used interchangeably and qualified as fertilized or unfertilized, two-cell, etc. Because an ovum, by definition, is unfertilized, this qualification should be unnecessary. In this chapter, the term *gamete* (ovum or spermatozoon) is used to refer to the haploid chromosomal state, and the term *zygote* is used to refer to the diploid chromosomal state resulting from the union of the two gametes. Later stages are referred to as *embryos.* The term *oviduct(s)* is preferred over the more correct term *fallopian tube(s)* (named after their discoverer, Gabrielle Fallopius, who described them in 1561 [3]) solely because of brevity.

Much of the gamete transport takes place in the oviduct: Spermatozoa are transported upward to the site of fertilization, and ova are transported downward from the ovarian (or distal) end of the oviduct to the uterine (or proximal) end, during which time fertilization and early development as a zygote occur. However, before ova, which enter the oviduct only after ovulation, and spermatozoa, after ejaculation and deposition in the vagina (in primates; in some other species, spermatozoa are deposited into the uterus) can meet, the spermatozoa have to transverse the cervix, the uterus, and the uterotubal junction before reaching the oviduct. Each of these barriers reduces the population of spermatozoa such that, theoretically, only the fittest and most normal ones have the opportunity of fertilizing an ovum. This is one way in which natural selection operates to ensure the survival of the optimal genetic combinations from generation to generation. In this chapter, each of these different events is discussed. There may be some overlap with other chapters; in those cases, the discussion of these duplicated events is limited here to the information necessary to understand the integration of this system.

SPERM TRANSPORT

Sperm Transport in the Male

It has been recently proposed that during spermatogenesis ectoplasmic specializations associated with bundles of microtubules that line Sertoli cell crypts act as vehicles and tracks, respectively, for transport of spermatids through the seminiferous epithelium. The microtubules exhibit uniform polarity, and this appears to provide the basis for the direction of force generation and spermatid transport (4). The importance of the microtubules in spermiation and sperm transport is further shown by the observation that intratesticular injection of taxol, a compound that stabilizes microtubules, inhibits spermatid transport to the rim of the seminiferous tubule and from the rim to the base of the tubule. Similar injections of cytochalasin D, which inhibits actin-related processes, interfered with tubulobulbar complex development and sperm transport through the duct system. Because Sertoli cell fluid secretion was not affected but myoid-cell actin cytoskeletal organization was inhibited, it was concluded that cytoskeletal activity was important for spermiation and sperm transport through the seminiferous tubule (5).

Following the process of spermatogenesis, the spermatozoa, which are almost completely immotile, are transported passively from the seminiferous tubules to the rete testis. The rete testis is a branched reservoir into which both ends of each seminiferous tubule open. The rete testis is linked to the epididymis by the 10 to 20 vasa efferentia that are located near the upper pole of the testis. These efferent ducts become highly convoluted as they reach the epididymis.

The epididymis is a single, long, highly convoluted duct on the posterior border of the testis. It has usually been divided into three regions—the head, the body, and the tail (caput, corpus, and cauda)—but these are rather arbitrary divisions, and the exact proportions of the epididymis contributing to each segment vary between species. In the human, the caput region is comprised largely of the extensive efferent duct system, and unlike in other species, the cauda is inconspicuous.

Sperm transport into and through the epididymis is not due to sperm motility but is thought to be a passive process due initially to secretions flowing from the testis and also assisted by ciliary activity of the luminal epithelium and contractile activity of the smooth-muscle elements of the efferent duct walls (6). Regular peristaltic contractions of the epididymal duct wall propel the spermatozoa from the caput to the cauda. The rate of transport through this organ is not influenced by ligation of the vasa efferentia (7,8), reinforcing the notion of epididymal transport being a local phenomenon. These peristaltic contractions have been observed in both rats and rabbits (9,10) and seem likely to be a general phenomenon. The cauda epididymidis and the vas deferens are richly innervated with sympathetic neurons lying in association with smooth-muscle cells, whereas in the caput of the epididymis, the adrenergic nerve terminals are sparse and are more associated with blood vessels (11–13). As in the female, these neurons are short and postganglionic, originating from ganglia lying near the effector organ (11), and are of special significance in the process of ejaculation.

The significance of the sympathetic nervous system for sperm transport and maturation has been demonstrated by experiments in rats in which the inferior mesenteric plexus was removed. Within a week, the number but not motility of spermatozoa in the cauda epididymis and the initial segment of the vas deferens, and the weight of the epididymis, were significantly increased compared with those of sham-operated controls (14). Sperm transit through the epididymis is relatively slow and fairly constant among different species. In the human, the mean epididymal transport time has been estimated to be 12 days (15), but owing to mixing of epididymal contents of younger and older spermatozoa, the actual transport time of any one sperm may be considerably different from the mean value (16). More accurate estimates can be made in experimental animals. For example, using quantitative light microscopic autoradiography after [^{3}H]thymidine labeling, it has been determined that, in hamsters, spermatozoa are transported through the different sections of the epididymis as follows: caput, corpus, proximal cauda, and distal cauda; 3, 2, 2, and 6 days, respectively. Transport through the proximal ductus deferens takes an extra 2 days (17). Time of transport of spermatozoa through the epididymis can be decreased about 10% to 30% by increased frequency of ejaculation in rams (18). In men, it was claimed that when seminal emission frequency was increased from 3.5 to 8.6 times per week, sperm concentration was decreased 55% (19). No such consistent effect was observed in another study in normal or infertile men who ejaculated twice a day for 3 to 5 days (20,21), although a small drop from the first to the second ejaculation on each day was seen (20). Sperm motility appeared unaffected (20). Although surgical diversion of the epididymis into the abdomen raises the temperature to which spermatozoa are exposed, spermatozoal maturation in the epididymis is not compromised. Transit time through the epididymides is, however, accelerated by 4 to 7 days (22). This lack of effect on spermatozoal maturation is surprising, because intraabdominal placement of both testis and epididymis rapidly leads to sterility (23) that is, however, accompanied by only minor changes in epididymal secretions (24).

Estimates of spermatozoan production, numbers of epididymal spermatozoa, and epididymal transit times have been made using specimens taken from apparently healthy men within 24 h of sudden death (25). There was no difference in epididymal transit time for men aged 20 to 49 years compared with those aged 50 to 79 years, but, interestingly, in men with threefold higher daily sperm production rates, epididymal sperm numbers remained constant. On this basis, it was concluded that epididymal transit time was considerably shortened in the men with higher sperm production rates. The numbers of epididymal spermatozoa were approximately 200 million per side (i.e., 400 million total per individual). These findings are consistent with those of Ammann and Howards (26), who showed that the capacity of the human epididymis to accommodate spermatozoa was much smaller than in other animals (i.e., millions versus billions).

In the normal state, spermatozoa are transported from the epididymis to the vas deferens by a steady flow of secretion through the epididymis and the contractile activity of the lower portion of the epididymis. Although it has been generally held that up to 50% of spermatozoa not ejaculated are reabsorbed by the male reproductive tract, this now seems to be less certain. The current view is that, in many species, excess spermatozoa are voided in the urine and that constant leakage of spermatozoa occurs (27–30). In the human, retrograde ejaculation caused by weak bladder neck function, spinal cord injury, or prostate surgery is well documented, but whether spermatozoa are normally voided in the urine is not certain. However, in rams subjected to electroejaculation during the nonbreeding season, between 4% and 80% of the spermatozoa in the ejaculate were found in the first postejaculation micturition. Similar results were obtained in rams studied during the breeding season. The percentage of spermatozoa found in the urine was significantly greater after ejaculation as compared with before (30). It is known that, after vasectomy or in men with bilateral obstruction of the epididymides, macrophages are involved in phagocytosis of spermatozoa (31). In bulls and boars, the marked reduction of defective sperm (without mitochondrial spirals) in the secretion of the efferent ducts and after passage through the caput epididymidis has been taken as an indication that active phagocytosis of sperm is occurring in these portions of the male reproductive tract (32). In mice, use of radiolabeled spermatozoa showed that a proportion of sperm products (subsequent to phagocytosis?) could be found in the caudal and paraaortic lymph nodes (33). The likelihood is that the human behaves like other species and that excess sperm are lost gradually through leakage down the vas deferens and voiding during urination.

Testicular spermatozoa are functionally immature and cannot fertilize an ovum. During transport through the epididymis, the sperm undergo certain maturational changes, so that at ejaculation, fully functional spermatozoa are released. These changes occur in morphology, motility, and metabolism. In some species, spermatozoa derived from the caput are unable to fertilize ova, but this is not true for a proportion of spermatozoa taken from the corpus. Spermatozoa from the cauda or vas deferens are almost always fully fertile (34). Most of the changes occurring in the epididymis relate to the acquisition of motility. This has been studied extensively in a variety of species (6) but is somewhat different in the human than in rodents, in that there is no circling phase of sperm activity (35).

Sperm from the caput epididymis exhibit varied patterns of motility, ranging from immotility to a vigorous flexing movement of the tail. Rapid forward progression occurs only with a reduced flexing of the tail; this appears first in a few spermatozoa in the corpus and is the general pattern in those from the cauda and vas deferens (35). Thus, acquisition of progressive motility may be largely a function of aging of the spermatozoa. In the hamster, a somewhat different pattern has been described (36). Spermatozoa recovered from the portion of the cauda epididymidis near the corpus exhibited helical, hyperactivated, or a mixed swimming pattern, whereas those recovered from the distal portion of the cauda or the ejaculate showed a low-amplitude planar, flagellar movement. However, incubation *in vitro* under capacitating conditions for 3 to 4 h converted this pattern to the helical or hyperactivated one. The helical pattern was considered to be a transitional phase between the low-amplitude and hyperactivated patterns, and, as such spermatozoa exhibited higher average path velocities, could be of importance for sperm transport through the epididymis. Calcium appears to be an important regulator of spermatozoal motility. In the human, calcium ions stimulate motility of immature epididymal spermatozoa but inhibit motility of ejaculated spermatozoa (37). This suggests that, at least in the human, sperm maturation regulates the response to calcium and that acquisition of progressive motility may be a function of epididymal maturation. Motility is a prerequisite for fertility (38,39). Such maturation is reflected in the many biochemical changes that occur in sperm in the epididymis.

The activity of different enzymes in epididymal spermatozoa has been studied. In rat spermatozoa, mitochondrial malate dehydrogenase decreases during epididymal transit (40), whereas membrane glycosidases (β-glucosidase, β-galactosidase, β-*N*-acetylglucosaminidase and β-*N*-acetylgalactosaminidase) increased from the caput to the corpus and then declined from the corpus to the cauda (41). As a result of the positive correlation between decreasing spermatozoal carbohydrate and protein content and increasing glycosidase activity, it was suggested that these membrane-bound enzymes play a role in modifying the surface of the spermatozoa during epididymal transit. In goat spermatozoa, phosphatidylinositol-specific phospholipase C (another membrane-bound enzyme) increased 6.5-fold during epididymal transit, whereas in epididymal fluid samples it decreased fourfold. Thirty-five percent of this enzyme was in a soluble form and 44% was head-associated (42). A sperm-specific enzyme, lactate dehydrogenase C-4, is important for fertilizing capacity, because immunization of male but not female mice resulted in reduced fertilization, even though sperm transport to the oviduct was not impaired (43).

During epididymal transit, total protein decreased 2.4-fold in spermatozoa and remained unchanged in epididymal fluid (42). In mice, protein synthesis and binding to sperm were studied using injections of [^{35}S]-methionine (44,45). The quantity of labeled proteins in the luminal fluid was two to four times higher in the caput than in the corpus or cauda. Two proteins (25 kDa and 18 kDa) were found in the caput but not in the other regions, whereas another 29-kDa protein was found in high amounts in corpus and cauda fluid (44). Interaction of such proteins with spermatozoa during epididymal transport was, however, variable. The 25-kDa protein remained significantly associated with spermatozoa during transit, whereas the 18-kDa protein did not remain sperm-associated. Proteins of 40 and 35 kDa bound to spermatozoa in increasing amounts during epididymal transport, whereas others (54, 44, and 29 kDa) bound to spermatozoa only in the caput (45). These proteins were not identified, so the significance of these interactions is still speculative, except insofar as they are likely to modify the spermatozoal surface membrane. Examination of surface membrane proteins of boar spermatozoa provided evidence for such complex sequential changes in macromolecular composition and orientation. During epididymal maturation, most of the testicular proteins were removed from the spermatozoal surface, and these were replaced by new low-molecular-weight peptides (46). These new glycopeptides appear simultaneously with the appearance of forward progressive motility, at least in the boar (47). Perhaps as a consequence of such surface changes, the fluidity of the spermatozoal membrane decreases significantly during epididymal maturation (48). One characterized glycoprotein (sulfated glycoprotein-2, clusterin) secreted by Sertoli (49) and principal cells of the caput epididymidis (50) binds to spermatozoa as they transit the epididymis. In the caput, sulfated glycoprotein-2 is not regulated by testicular factors, whereas testosterone can depress its concentration in the corpus and cauda (51). During epididymal transit, spermatozoa undergo not only surface membrane changes but also nuclear changes. Nuclear protamines play a role in morphogenesis and stabilization of the head of the spermatozoon (52,53). Immunocytochemical localization of protamine showed increasing staining from the rete testis to the corpus of the epididymis followed by a sharp decline thereafter (54). These findings were taken to indicate that the corpus is a critical site for the relation between DNA and the nucleoproteins. These different studies underscore the importance of the epididymis for sperm maturation, which is a prerequisite for acquisition of fertilizing capacity.

There is evidence from the rabbit, in which species sperm motility but not fertility can be achieved after ligation of the lower region of the corpus epididymidis, that motility is not necessarily synonymous with fertilizing capacity (55). Although, in the rabbit, fertilizing capacity is acquired during transport through the epididymis, this does not seem to be so clear-cut in the human. In men subjected to epididymovasostomy (where the vas is joined to the caput region of the epididymis to bypass an epididymal blockage), fertility, at least in a proportion of individuals, is restored (56). Although it is claimed that human sperm only need to be exposed to the environment of the caput before passing into the vas deferens to complete maturation and become capable of fertilization, it appears that the more distal the site of anastomosis, the greater the chance of a subsequent pregnancy (57). Because some men after this operation ejaculate normal numbers of sperm, this was adduced as evidence that the caput was the main site of sperm storage in man (57), although, as noted above, the capacity of the human epididymis to store sperm is limited. More recent studies using an improved microsurgical technique in which the vas deferens is attached to a single surface convolution of the ductus epididymidis have led to improved results. In 60% of 102 men, spermatozoa were obtained, and 10% of these men were fertile, as their wives became pregnant (58). In contrast, where infertility cannot be reversed by this procedure and sperm are aspirated from the epididymis and used in an *in vitro* fertilization procedure, success rates are low: Only 18% of ova were fertilized *in vitro* and a pregnancy rate of 3% achieved in each *in vitro* fertilization cycle (58). However, reversal of a simple vasectomy by microsurgical vasovasotomy also leads to restored fertility in only a percentage of men (59), so that the low incidence of fertility after epididymovasostomy may relate to factors other than lack of sperm maturation. Vasectomy, at least in mice, even after a long period, does not affect spermatogenesis and spermatozoal transport to the epididymis (33,60), but it was noted that sperm products could be found in the caudal and paraaortic lymph nodes to a greater degree than in normal mice (33). Nevertheless, the restoration of some degree of fertility after epididymovasovasostomy must indicate that, in men, maturation of spermatozoa can be mostly completed in the caput epididymidis and the vas deferens or *in vitro* and that changes occurring in the corpus or cauda are of lesser importance.

Ejaculation

The process of ejaculation and orgasm in the male can be divided into two component parts—seminal emission and a central excitatory state (61). It is suggested that for orgasm there is a "buildup of excitation in specific centers in the central nervous system" and that when there is a neuroelectrical discharge, the excitation spreads to adjoining regions of the central nervous system (61). The so-called ejaculation can itself be subdivided into seminal emission and ejaculation proper. Seminal emission is defined as a leakage or oozing of spermatozoa from the penis without any pulsatile properties, whereas ejaculation indicates the emission of semen in spurts. Ejaculation usually occurs only in tandem with orgasm.

It is well known from a variety of experimental evidence that α-adrenergic neurons are intimately involved in the process of seminal emission. Patients who have been subjected to surgery to remove lymph glands in the thorax and abdomen as part of the treatment of testicular tumors do not experience seminal emission. That is, they can experience orgasm but have a so-called dry ejaculation. Erection is, however, normal. Semen is not even voided retrogradely into the bladder. This type of surgery unavoidably involves extensive damage to sympathetic nerves from T12 to L3. In contrast, removal of T2 to T11 ganglia by transthoracic sympathectomy does not disturb ejaculation (62,63). As noted above, the male reproductive tract is mainly innervated by short adrenergic neurons, and these are located in the cauda epididymidis and vas deferens (11). Thus, stimulation of these neurons leads to movement of the spermatozoa from the cauda of the epididymis but not from the caput or the corpus. It has been found that repeated ejaculation of rats, which reduced sperm numbers in the ejaculate almost to zero, did not deplete sperm numbers in the upper portions of the epididymis (64). Parasympathetic fibers also innervate the male genital tract, but they probably do not participate in the motor innervation of the longitudinal musculature of the vas deferens (65,66). Experiments with nerve stimulation in dogs indicate that sympathetic pathways from the hypogastric and lumbosacral nerves control seminal emission and that, when the hypogastric nerves are transected, the lumbosacral ones can, after a delay, compensate (67). Further studies on the control of seminal emission by the caudal mesenteric plexus (equivalent to the inferior mesenteric and inferior hypogastric plexuses in the human) have been performed in dogs. Stimulation of a splanchnic nerve group branching at thoracic and L1 ganglia failed to effect emission, whereas stimulation of a group branching at L1-L5 ganglia and descending behind the spermatic arteries was 100% effective (68). Furthermore, stimulation of the end of the severed spermatic vein, which usually caused no or minimal seminal emission, after bilateral transection of the hypogastric nerves and sympathetic trunks and a delay of 1 month, caused seminal emission in all six dogs studied, with normal volumes in four of them. In contrast, stimulation of the tail of the epididymidis resulted in a full volume emission in all dogs, regardless of whether they were transected or not (69). It was found in men undergoing treatment for prostatic carcinoma or testicular biopsy that epididymal stimulation was similarly effective (69).

In men, different ejaculatory disorders have been reported, ranging from unsatisfactory timing of ejaculation (premature and retarded), absence of ejaculation, and ejaculation without pleasure (70). Normal emission and ejaculation require coordinated anatomic, neurophysiologic, and psychological function, and it is only by delineation of the affected component that appropriate treatment can be instituted (71). The whole sequence of events from erection to ejaculation is highly androgen-dependent, and some types of ejaculatory failure can be corrected by androgen treatment (72). Seminal emission can be induced, in the absence of testicular damage, in anejaculatory men who have undergone retroperitoneal lymphadenectomy for cancer of the testis by transrectal electroejaculation (73). Semen characteristics were normal, and seven pregnancies resulted from 74 attempts at artificial insemination with such specimens in 19 patients (73). Similarly, electroejaculation has been used extensively to obtain semen specimens in men with spinal cord injuries. Usually, specimens of acceptable quality can be obtained in antegrade manner, although occasionally retrograde emission into the bladder occurs (74–81). In some studies, the use of penile vibration has been used as an alternative to electroejaculation, but semen quality is inconsistent or poor (77,82). However, semen quality is also only adequate after electroejaculation. In some studies, intrathecal neostigmine or subcutaneous physostigmine has been used as adjunctive therapy, but this has been associated with increased side effects (i.e., nausea, vomiting, elevated blood pressure, and headache) (75). In one study, it was noted that better semen specimens were obtained when the spinal cord injury had occurred more than 6 months previously (77), although this was not observed by others (79). As noted above in the dog studies, a delay after hypogastric nerve injury permits collateral nerves to compensate (67,68).

When a biochemical comparison was performed in men between electroejaculates and normal ejaculates, significantly lower levels of fructose, albumin, glutamic oxaloacetic transaminase, and alkaline phosphatase and higher levels of chloride were noted in the electroejaculates (83). It was speculated that these biochemical abnormalities contributed to the poorer seminal quality of spinal cord-injured men, but whether these changes resulted from the injury or the electroejaculation procedure was not certain (83). Nevertheless, pregnancies have been reported in the spouses of paraplegic men with lesions of T5-6 and T4-5, using semen obtained by electroejaculation (78). It is now suggested that with improved equipment and technique, electroejaculation can be considered as an outpatient procedure (80).

Further evidence that the motor innervation of the ductus deferens is largely α-adrenergic is provided by *in vitro* studies on the human vas deferens (84) and from patients receiving drugs that produce chemical sympathectomy (e.g., guanethidine) (63,85). Similar findings have been reported after treatment with the α-adrenergic blocking drug phenoxybenzamine (86) and with the psychoactive drug thioridazine hydrochloride (a moderate α-adrenergic blocker) (87–89). Indeed, phenoxybenzamine has been recommended as a treatment for premature ejaculation (90,91). This treatment is modestly successful but can lead to "dry" ejaculation, as described above. Understanding of the control of the ejaculatory response by the α-adrenergic system has been further refined by experiments in dogs. It was found that low doses of yohimbine and rauwolscine, both α-2 adrenergic receptor antagonists, stimulated the ejaculatory response, whereas corynanthine, an α-1 adrenergic receptor antagonist, was without effect (92). This suggests that under normal conditions the α-2 system is inhibitory, and this is the effect that clonidine, an α-2 agonist, produces in dogs (93). However, it was also noted that high doses of yohimbine were inhibitory, and this might explain the apparently contradictory effects of clinical treatments with the adrenergic blocker phenoxybenzamine.

The pulsatile forces producing the ejaculatory discharge, although partly caused by the contractile waves along the vas deferens controlled by the α-adrenergic system, are mainly caused by the rhythmic muscular contractions of the ischiocavernosus and bulbospongiosus striated-muscle groups, which surround the urethra in the penis (61). Interestingly, these latter muscles show no electromyographic activity during erection and detumescence cycles produced by visual stimuli (94). Electromyographic bursts of activity in the bulbocavernosus muscles are not always correlated with expulsion of semen, thus implying some redundancy in the system. Phenoxybenzamine treatment in two men did not reduce electromyographic activity or orgasmic pleasure but did reduce seminal volume (94), thus providing a physiologic basis for "dry" ejaculation. It has been proposed that thioridazine inhibits seminal emission because it reduces both phasic and tonic shortening of the longitudinal muscle of the vas deferens. It also enhances the lengthening action of noradrenaline (95). Associated with ejaculation, increased plasma levels of oxytocin have been detected, which may be causally associated with muscular activity of the reproductive tract (96,97). Vasopressin levels are elevated only during sexual arousal and return to baseline by ejaculation (97).

It has been claimed that erection involves inhibition of α-adrenergic and stimulation of β-adrenergic influence, combined with release of a noncholinergic vasodilator, possibly vasointestinal peptide (98). The pumping action in the penis gives rise to ejaculation, which is closely associated with orgasm—the characteristic ejaculatory inevitability that, once started, is hard to stop even with the use of the squeeze technique (99). Thus, premature ejaculation is a cause for distress among a significant proportion of men, although not apparently in nonprimates. This would suggest that there is a distinct psychological component in the etiology of this condition, although no difference has been detected in the ability of premature and nonpremature ejaculators to assess the level of their sexual arousal (100). Measurement of evoked potentials from the perineal and perianal areas indicates the presence of a reflex hyperexcitability in premature ejaculators compared with control men (101), suggesting a physiologic basis for this condition modulated by the higher centers. Intracavernous treatment with phentolamine (an α-adrenergic blocker) and papaverine (a nonspecific smooth-muscle relaxant) has been recommended as a treatment for premature ejaculation in otherwise healthy men. However, this treatment ensures maintenance of an erection for 2 to 4 h, even though ejaculation has occurred, and so, in fact, does not prevent the premature ejaculation (102).

Similarly, other intracavernous treatments with vasoactive intestinal peptide (VIP) or prostaglandin (PG) E_1 have been suggested as treatment for impotence of diabetic, neurogenic, or psychogenic etiology. There is a physiologic reason why VIP might be effective. Immunoreactive VIP and neuropeptide Y nerve fibers have been detected in intracavernous smooth muscles and arterial and venous tunicae in the human penis (103). This distribution of nerve fibers could regulate tone of these muscles and of penile blood supply. However, intracavernous injection of VIP alone, although it causes some tumescence, does not produce adequate penile rigidity for intromission (104,105). A combination of VIP and papaverine gives as good results as phentolamine and papaverine (105). More recently, PGE_1 alone or combined with papaverine has been used for impotence of organic origin with good success (106,107). Reported side effects are minimal, and the occurrence of prolonged erection is low (~4%), thus making treatment with PGE_1 alone suitable for home use (107). Prostaglandin E_1 is a vasodilator, and this factor alone, or when combined with the smooth muscle relaxing effect of papaverine, permits penile engorgement and erection. These treatments, although they induce erection, do not affect the timing of ejaculation, and thus sexual activity can continue after ejaculation.

In certain individuals, retrograde ejaculation into the bladder occurs. This occurs most frequently after prostatectomy, retroperitoneal lymph node dissection, and diabetes (108–110). In such cases, if drug therapy with α-adrenergic stimulators is unsuccessful, surgery is recommended (108–110). In diabetic patients, it has been suggested that retrograde ejaculation occurs because of lack of tone of the inner sphincter of the bladder, and it is certain that after transurethral resection for bladder stenosis, a percentage of patients will experience this condition (111). Bladder neck reconstruction can alleviate this problem (112). Alternatively, for couples wishing to get pregnant, recovery and washing of sperm collected from the urine, followed by luteinizing hormone and timed intrauterine insemination, resulted in seven pregnancies in six patients (113). This is a much simpler solution than bladder neck reconstruction.

During the process of seminal emission and ejaculation, the mature spermatozoa from the epididymis, already suspended in secretions from the testis and epididymis, are, during their transport through the vas deferens and urethra, further joined by the secretions of the different accessory glands [i.e., the ampullary glands, the seminal vesicles, the prostate, and the bulbourethral (Cowper's) and urethral (Littré's) glands] (Fig. 1). Analysis of the different portions of the ejaculate reveals considerable differences in sperm density and biochemical characteristics that can be used to determine the accessory gland from which the main proportion of that sample is derived (115,116). The highest sperm density is usually seen in the third and fourth fractions, with a pro-

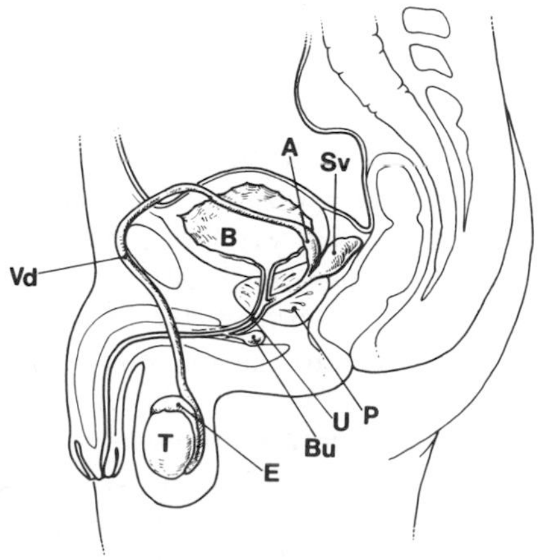

FIG. 1. Lower part of trunk in a man, showing reproductive tract and neighboring organs. (*A*) Ampulla; (*B*) bladder; (*Bu*) bulbourethral glands; (*E*) epididymis; (*P*) prostate; (*Sv*) seminal vesicles; (*T*) testis; (*U*) urethra; (*Vd*) vas deferens. (From ref. 114, with permission.)

gressive decline in subsequent fractions. In most men, the ejaculate cannot be subdivided into more than six fractions. Interestingly, sperm motility is significantly lower in the fractions from the second half of the total ejaculate (116). When split semen samples were obtained from normal and oligospermic infertile men, it was found that motile sperm concentration was significantly higher in the first two fractions than in the rest of the ejaculate in normal men, whereas in the infertile men, the highest percentage of motile sperm was in fraction one. In both groups, motile sperm concentration was significantly correlated with *in vitro* penetration into bovine cervical mucus but not with hamster egg penetration (117).

The bulk of the seminal plasma (fluid portion of the ejaculate) is derived from the seminal vesicles (60%) and the prostate (30%) (118). The pH of semen is basic, lying between 7.2 and 7.8, and reflects the relative contributions of acidic prostatic fluid (pH, 6.5) and the alkaline seminal vesicular secretion. Prostatic fluid is rich in citric acid, acid phosphatase, zinc, and magnesium, whereas the seminal vesicular secretion is rich in fructose (3.2 mg/ml) and 19-hydroxylated prostaglandins (long-chain unsaturated fatty acids derived mainly from arachidonic acid) and contains smaller amounts of inositol and sorbitol (115,119). The essential need of such secretions for fertility is questionable, as microaspirated epididymal sperm can give rise to pregnancy, albeit with a low success rate (58). A similar conclusion can be drawn from experiments in male hamsters, in which complete removal of the accessory sex organs did not affect the fertilization rate, although fewer spermatozoa reached the oviduct (120). However, in mice after removal of the seminal vesicles, a reduction in fertilization rate, attributed to alterations in sperm motility, was seen (121). One explanation for this beneficial effect of seminal vesicle secretion might be provided by the following study. Secretory particles, containing Mg^{2+}, Ca^{2+}-activated ATPase, aminopeptidase A, alanyl aminopeptidase, γ-glutamyl transpeptidase, and dipeptidyl peptidase IV, obtained from bovine seminal vesicle secretion, initiated hyperactivation and the acrosome reaction in bovine epididymal spermatozoa within minutes (122). There is a suggestion that there is a correlation between zinc concentration in seminal plasma and spermatozoal motility; this zinc is largely derived from the prostate (123). It is certain that the spermatozoal nucleus takes up zinc at ejaculation, and this is thought to be important for subsequent spermatozoal chromatin decondensation (124). An organelle, termed the *prostasome,* appears in the prostatic lumen by endocytosis from the prostatic epithelial cells. Prostasomes have a membrane-linked Mg^{2+}, Ca^{2+}-dependent ATPase, Zn^{2+}-dependent aminopeptidase and ATPase, and a protein kinase activity (125–127). Lactic dehydrogenase (LDH) activity in prostasomes has also been described, that in seminal plasma of normal men being predominantly LDH-C4, whereas in infertile men the isoenzymes, LDH-1, 2, and 3, were enriched (128). Human prostasomes contain high amounts of nucleic acid and exhibit a high cholesterol-to-phospholipid ratio (129,130). The function of the prostasomes is unknown, but they exhibit strong immunosuppressive activity, which, combined with that of the 19-hydroxylated PGEs, may neutralize the immune defenses of the female tract, thus permitting alloantigenic spermatozoa a good chance of achieving fertilization (131). Thus, although accessory organ secretions may not be essential, they may improve fertility when this is compromised.

The normal volume of the ejaculate in the human male is between 2 and 6 ml, and a sperm concentration of 40 million to 250 million spermatozoa per milliliter has been considered normal (132). More recently, these parameters have been revised, and sperm counts of 10 million per milliliter or 25 million per ejaculate, provided other factors are not abnormal (e.g., motility or presence of abnormal forms), are considered perfectly compatible with normal fertility (133,134). Indeed, normal pregnancies have occurred in partners of men whose ejaculates had sperm counts of less than 1 million per milliliter, the sperm counts being depressed by hormonal therapy (depomedroxyprogesterone acetate and testosterone) to produce a contraceptive effect (135). Thus, if motility and shape are normal, even very low numbers of spermatozoa can induce pregnancy in a fertile partner. The presence of poor motility and/or the presence of many abnormally formed spermatozoa is usually associated with infertility.

In the human, the ejaculated semen is deposited into the vagina close to the external cervical os. In some other species, notably pigs and horses, spermatozoa are ejaculated directly into the uterine cavity, and thus the cervical canal and its mucoid secretion are not barriers to sperm transport. The vagina is very acid, with a pH of less than 5.0 in normal women. This acidity is maintained by the presence of lactic acid formed by the action of *Doederlein bacilli* on the vaginal secretions. The spermatozoa find this a hostile environment and those that are not rapidly entrapped in the cervical mucus or have progressed to the upper portions of the reproductive tract die and are voided to the exterior. In one normally fertile couple, an immediate change (within 8 sec) in vaginal pH from 4.3 to 7.2 was seen after deposition of the seminal plasma, which has buffering capacity. This provides a temporarily more favorable environment for the spermatozoa. However, vaginal pH reverts to normal within 4 min of ejaculation (136).

Immediately after ejaculation in primates, seminal plasma coagulates (within 1 min); this coagulum is broken down by proteolytic enzymes in the ejaculate within the next 20 to 30 min. Within 1 h, all material should be liquefied and all spermatozoa should be fully motile (132,137). The coagulum probably acts to retain spermatozoa in the vagina close to the cervical canal, thus permitting maximal access for the spermatozoa to become entrapped in the cervical mucus. In infertile couples, there is a significant positive correlation between the degree of coagulation and liquefaction time, spermatozoal numbers, and motility (138).

Coitus in the human is relatively rapid, usually occurring within a few minutes of intromission (139). In other species, the process can be very prolonged (camels and pigs) or very rapid (rabbits and bulls). During intercourse, intravaginal pressure is negative during intromission and male orgasm but becomes positive to 40 cm H_2O during female orgasm, followed by a sharp fall after orgasm to a negative pressure of 26 cm H_2O (140). This may lead to sucking of spermatozoa into the cervical canal. Also, elevated plasma oxytocin levels can be detected in women during orgasm (141), which, through stimulation of smooth-muscle activity, may also cause propulsion of spermatozoa into the cervical canal. Testosterone levels in men have been found not to vary immediately before and after intercourse (142) and thus are not directly involved in the ejaculatory process. Inhibition of androgenic activity with an antiandrogenic drug such as cyproterone acetate, however, causes atrophy of accessory structures and sexual organs, partial failure of spermatogenesis, and loss of libido and potency (143,144). Thus, a continued normal plasma level of androgenic stimulation is essential for the correct functioning of the reproductive tract, sperm maturation, and spermiogenesis.

Sperm Transport Through the Cervix

The role of vaginal and uterine contractions in the transport of spermatozoa from the vagina to the uterus has been well reviewed by Fox and Fox (139). Although there seems to be good evidence that, in some species fluids placed in the vagina can enter the uterus in detectable amounts and relatively rapidly, the situation is much less clear in the human. Particulate material placed in the vagina has been claimed to enter the uterus (145–147). In the best-documented case, carbon particles suspended in 30% dextran were used, but 10 U of oxytocin was given intramuscularly at the same time (147). In contrast, radioopaque fluid failed to enter the uterus from a cervical cap during either coitus or clitoral stimulation (148,149).

It is now well known that human semen contains large quantities of different prostaglandins, mainly the 19-hydroxylated series (150,151). These PGs are less biologically active than the related PGE_2 or $PGF_{2\alpha}$; substantial quantities of the PGE series are also present in the seminal plasma of fertile men. Given that PGs stimulate uterine contractility and thus cause uterine pain, for example in dysmenorrhea (152), it seems unlikely that much seminal fluid *per se* enters the uterus. However, spermatozoa can pass rapidly to the oviducts; within 5 min of artificial insemination, spermatozoa were found within the oviducts of women, but the numbers were small, ranging from 4 to 53 within 5 to 45 min after insemination (153). Spermatozoa migrate through midcycle cervical mucus at a rate of only 2.0 to 3.0 mm/min (154). It is clear that sperm motility alone would be unable to cause sperm passage to the oviducts within 5 min. This suggests that the negative vaginal pressure recorded after orgasm, coupled with the associated increased vaginal and uterine contractions (140), immediately propels the small proportion of the ejaculated spermatozoa not trapped in the coagulum between the cervical mucus and cervical epithelium into the uterus; along with these spermatozoa may be carried a small quantity of seminal fluid. Although PGs are known to cause contractions of both uterine and oviductal musculature, the relationship between levels of seminal plasma PGs and male fertility is tenuous or nonexistent (155). Nonetheless, if $PGF_{2\alpha}$ is added to midcycle cervical mucus at a concentration of 250 ng/ml and the mucus is incubated for 1 h at 37°C, sperm motility and sperm penetration through the mucus are increased significantly (156). Also, human relaxin has been shown to stimulate human sperm movement through bovine cervical mucus (157) and is known to be present in human seminal plasma (158).

Because most spermatozoa that reach the oviducts do so much later after insemination than those discussed above, it seems probable that sperm motility is important in the progression through the cervical mucus lying in the cervical canal. The cervical canal has very thick walls composed mainly of connective tissue and is lined with many deep crypts. These crypts are pockets of columnar epithelium of the cervical mucosa that extend in many different directions and can even be branched (159). The cervical epithelium is composed of both ciliated and nonciliated (presumably secretory) cells covered with microvilli. The secretory cells are filled with cytoplasmic granules, and the intensity of reaction with the periodic acid-Schiff (PAS) reagent is related to the number of these granules. The release of secretory granules seems to be caused by rupture of the cell membrane rather than by an apocrine mechanism (159). Ciliary action does not appear to be important in sperm transport through the cervix but may assist passage of the cervical secretions (mucus) to the vagina. The consensus is that "the rate of mucus secretion is a function of (a) the number of mucus-secretory units in the cervical canal, (b) the percentage of mucus-secreting cells per unit, and (c) the secretory activity and the responsiveness of secretory cells to circulating hormones" (159). Approximately 100 such mucus-secreting units are in the cervical canal, and the mucous secretion varies from 600 mg/day at midcycle to 20 to 60 μg/day at other times in the cycle in normal women of reproductive age (159).

Cervical mucus is comprised of two main elements: cervical mucin and soluble components. The mucin is a glycoprotein rich in carbohydrates (more than 40%), with a fibrillar system of glycoproteins linked either directly by disulfide bonds or through cross-linking polypeptides. Cervical mucin has a polypeptide core rich in hydroxyl amino acids (i.e., threonine and serine), and these constitute one-third of the total polypeptides. Considerable quantities of proline and alanine are also present, but there are only small amounts of basic (e.g., lysine and arginine), sulfur-containing (e.g., cysteine and methionine), and aromatic (e.g., tyrosine and phenylalanine) amino acids. About 70% to 80% of the molecular weight is contributed by the carbohydrate side chains, including galactose (30%), sialic acid (10% to 20%), glucosamine (7% to 10%), galactosamine (7% to 10%), and fucose (5%) (159).

The soluble components of the mucus consist of inorganic salts (e.g., NaCl), proteins, and low-molecular-weight organic compounds (e.g., glucose, mannose, maltose, amino acids, peptides, and lipids). The soluble proteins are dispersed throughout the aqueous phase of the mucous gel. The consistency of this hydrogel (cervical mucus contains 95% water at midcycle) changes in relation to the balance between the secretion of ovarian hormones, mainly estradiol and progesterone. At midcycle, which is under estrogenic dominance, mucus is thin and watery and is composed of macromolecular fibrils arranged to form micelles (parallel chains) with spaces between the micelles large enough to permit the passage of spermatozoa. This has been confirmed by a study of the interaction of spermatozoa with cervical mucus from ovulatory women using transmission electron microscopy, which showed that the microstructure consists of a homogeneous pattern of structural elements with fibrillar and ribbonlike properties (160). In contrast, under the dominance of progesterone (i.e., during the luteal phase of the cycle), cervical mucus contains less water (90%), is thicker, and lacks the micellar structure and hence is unsuitable for sperm migration (159).

The consistency of the mucus has been assessed in terms of consistency, crystallization (ferning), and spinnbarkeit (fibrosity). Observation of these changes in cervical mucus by the individual woman forms the basis for the ovulation method (Billings) of natural family planning (161,162). In one large-scale trial, more than 94% of women of different ethnic backgrounds and economic circumstances were successfully taught this method (163). Unfortunately, the overall cumulative net probability of discontinuation because of pregnancy was 19.6%, although this was mainly a matter of inaccurate application of instructions or lack of motivation, considering that the modified Pearl index for method failure was only 2.8 (164). Thus, the physical changes in the mucus at midcycle (fertile period) are definitive and easily recognized. Spermatozoa can begin to penetrate cervical mucus as early as the ninth day of the cycle; the rate of penetration then increases gradually, reaching a peak at or just before ovulation (the time of the estradiol peak), and is inhibited within 1 to 2 days after ovulation as progesterone levels rise (165) (Fig. 2). The interaction of spermatozoa with cervical mucus has been reviewed relatively recently, and the nonhomogeneity of the mucus has been stressed (167). Thus, spermatozoal pen-

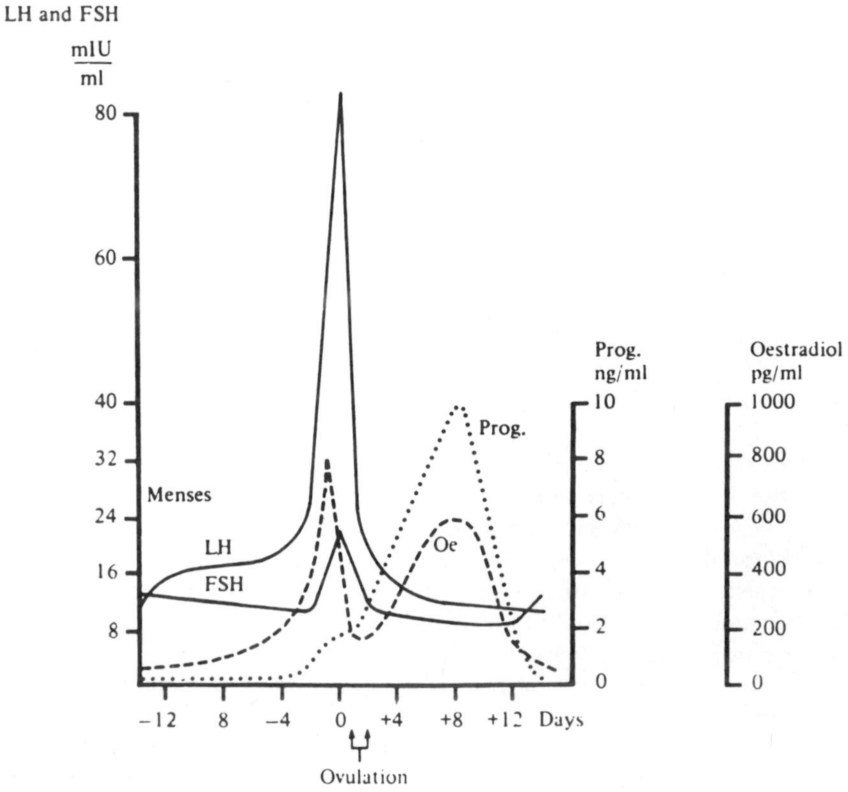

FIG. 2. Plasma levels of gonadotropins (*LH* and *FSH*, —), estradiol (*Oe*, – – –), and progesterone (*Prog.*, · · · · ·) during the human menstrual cycle. The cycle is centered on day 0, the day of the midcycle peak of LH. [Adapted from Speroff L, Vande Wiele RL. Regulation of the human menstrual cycle. *Am J Obstet Gynecol* 1971; 109:234–247. (From ref. 166, with permission.)]

etration through the mucous interior is different from that at the sperm–mucus interphase. These latter authors suggested that three factors contribute to spermatozoal penetration at the sperm–mucus interphase—sperm motility and concentration, seminal enzymes, and contractions of the reproductive tract (167).

Spermatozoa, after entry into the cervical mucus, are not uniformly distributed throughout the mucus but tend to be in the vicinity of the mucosal surface (168). Many spermatozoa are lodged in the cervical crypts, from which they are subsequently released to continue their journey upward through the reproductive tract. Apparently only motile spermatozoa are lodged in these crypts, where they are separated from the leukocytes in the central mass of mucus and thus protected from phagocytosis (168). Dead spermatozoa are eliminated from the tract either by phagocytosis or by the movement of the cervical mucus to the vagina. Thus, it has been suggested that the cervical crypts act as reservoirs to permit a continued release of viable spermatozoa over a period of hours (169). However, a more recent view is that the main site of sperm storage is the isthmic region of the oviduct and that capacitation and the acrosome reaction take place in close proximity to the site of fertilization (170). This seems a more plausible suggestion from a physiologic basis, as it is certain that sperm do not undergo the acrosome reaction while in the cervical mucus (171). The cervix clearly provides a major barrier to sperm ascent to the uterus. In experiments in rabbits in which about 280 million spermatozoa were deposited in the vagina at coitus, only 0.6% were found in the uteri 2 h later, and this increased to a maximum of only 1.74% at 12 h (172). Similar data are not available for women.

Sperm transport through the cervix can therefore be separated into three distinct phases: initial rapid transport, sperm storage in the crypts, and a final prolonged phase. The extent of the final phase is not known precisely, but in well-documented studies, motile spermatozoa have been found in the mucus up to 2 to 3 days after coitus (see ref. 173 for further references). Claims of motile sperm being found up to $3\frac{1}{2}$ weeks after coitus seem less believable (173).

In summary, it seems that four main factors are involved with sperm passage through the cervix: (a) spermatozoal motility; (b) muscular activity of the vagina, cervix, and uterus; (c) structure of the cervical mucus; and (d) the cervical crypts. All play a major role, but in the absence of sperm motility, it seems that few, if any, spermatozoa will reach the uterus.

In view of the importance of sperm motility for progression through cervical mucus, assessment of sperm motility and cervical mucus consistency has become important in determining a possible cause of infertility and the optimal treatment. A mathematical model has been used to study spermatozoal transport through cervical mucus (174). This model considers transverse waves along the tail and transverse and longitudinal motion of the cervical canal. Such transverse waves, along with spermatozoal motility, appear to be important for progression toward the uterus (174). Thus, attempts have been made to establish tests that will define the normality or otherwise of spermatozoa–cervical mucus interaction. Where physicochemical abnormalities of the cervical mucus are detected, treatment with estrogen to restore ovulatory-type mucus can be helpful (175). Another major complicating factor is the presence of antispermatozoal antibodies. Of different tests used, the direct immunobead test gave a positive predictive value of 80% as a screening procedure for sperm-agglutinating antibodies (176). Cervical mucus from infertile women containing cytotoxic antibodies to their husband's spermatozoa inhibited sperm motility, whereas mucus without antibodies was without effect (177). It has also been found that semen specimens from infertile couples with more than 50% abnormal sperm morphology had significantly lower sperm numbers, motility, forward progression, and ability to penetrate cervical mucus (178). In such couples, antisperm antibodies can be detected in the serum of about one-third of the couples, and serum titers are correlated with decreased sperm quality and function (178). Treatment for such conditions can include desensitizing therapy, condoms, and artificial insemination with the husband's sperm (175). One explanation for the interaction between spermatozoa and antisperm antibodies in semen or cervical mucus is an interaction between galactose residues on spermatozoa and galactose recognition sites on the antibodies (179). Indeed, exposure of spermatozoa to D-galactose in the presence of chymotrypsin reduced bound antisperm antibodies and improved the ability of the spermatozoa to penetrate mucus (179). Increased bacterial counts in cervical mucus have also been associated with inhibition of sperm penetration into the mucus (180).

The possibility that the cause of infertility is due to failure of spermatozoa to penetrate the mucus can be assessed *in vitro*. Both bovine and human mucus can be used (181–183). Use of bovine mucus can be substituted for human mucus for some tests of sperm function from oligospermic men but is not so suitable for tests of sperm with antisperm antibodies (182). Because suitable human mucus cannot always be readily obtained, use of a synthetic mucus substitute, a sodium hyaluronate solution, has been examined (184). The results obtained were significantly correlated with those observed using human cervical mucus, but it was concluded that, although use of hyaluronate was a useful adjunctive test for routine screening, it might not necessarily replace that using human mucus for in-depth assessment of the infertile couple. The prognostic value of such tests has been examined. Only sperm motility, assessed as penetration into cervical mucus *in vitro* at 2 to 6 h, had any prognostic success for pregnancy (185,186).

Postcoital tests are often performed to determine the presence of motile spermatozoa in the cervical mucus as a potential indicator of sperm transport through the mucus. The optimal time for performing the test has been variable, although for maximal information, 8 to 10 h after intercourse seems to be preferred, and the number of motile spermatozoa considered adequate varies widely (187). Thus, the usefulness of such tests has been questioned (187). However, a reduced postcoital test sperm count has been shown to be significantly associated with the presence of antibodies in the husband's serum to autologous sperm and a reduced sperm motility to be significantly associated with cytotoxic antibodies in the wife's serum and cervical mucus (188). In couples with unexplained infertility, the correlation between the postcoital test and the chance of conception has been assessed, and classification of the results by sperm movement showed that the best predictor of pregnancy was the presence of at least one spermatozoon with sluggish mobility per high-power field. It was concluded, therefore, that the most efficient form of motility in cervical mucus was slow or sluggish (189). It is clear that cervical mucus can filter out abnormal or defective spermatozoa, especially those with abnormal head shapes (190,191).

Thus, for a variety of reasons (involving both spermatozoal abnormalities and lack of motility, antibodies to spermatozoa secreted in cervical mucus, and/or inappropriate cervical mucus consistency), sperm transport from the vagina to the uterus can be significantly compromised and forms one of the main reasons for failure of fertilization. However, in couples of normal fertility, the filtering action of the cervical mucus provides a mechanism to ensure that only the fittest spermatozoa ascend toward the site of fertilization, thus providing a positive selection pressure for survival of the species.

Sperm Transport Through the Uterus

From the foregoing discussion, it is clear that, if spermatozoa can be found in the oviducts within 5 min of insemination, they cannot have reached there solely through their own motility. This indicates that contractions of the uterine smooth musculature (myometrium) are extremely important in ensuring this rapid propulsion from the internal cervical os to the uterotubal junction. It may be that smooth-muscle contractility is stimulated by substances released at coitus or present in the semen. Oxytocin levels in peripheral plasma of women are elevated at orgasm and afterward (141,192), but the nonpregnant uterus is not responsive to oxytocin (193). Excretion of catecholamines increases in humans during increased emotional and sexual (noncoital) excitement (194).

The presence of PGs in the ejaculate has already been noted (150,151,155). Even if the PGs do not enter the uterus directly, they can be readily absorbed through the vaginal wall (195–197). Prostaglandins can stimulate uterine activity both *in vitro* (198,199) and *in vivo* (200). However, it has been estimated that, on balance, the composition of seminal fluid PGs, if applied directly to uterine strips *in vitro,* would lead to an inhibition of uterine contractility (199). However, administration of pharmacologic doses of prostaglandins *in vivo* usually stimulates endogenous production of PGs, which are known to cause uterine contractions (201). These comments apply to the so-called classical PGs (e.g., $PGF_{2\alpha}$ and PGE_2), but most PGs in seminal plasma are 19-hydroxylated compounds. The activity of 19-hydroxy-$PGF_{1\alpha}$ and PGE_1 on human myometrium *in vitro* has been studied: 19-hydroxy-$PGE_{1\alpha}$ decreased myometrial activity significantly at 10^{-4} M, whereas 19-hydroxy-$PGF_{1\alpha}$ was without effect (202). The interaction between these compounds and the parent PGs was not studied, and so whether the overall effect of seminal plasma is stimulatory or inhibitory on uterine contractility is not known.

Recently, platelet-activating factor (PAF), another lipid capable of stimulating smooth-muscle activity (203) and perhaps sperm motility (204), has been detected both in spermatozoa (205,206) and in uterine tissues (207–209), although not in uterine fluid (208). The spermatozoal PAF can be secreted and can increase fertilization of mouse oocytes *in vitro* (206,210). Spermatozoa-derived PAF might, however, induce increased sperm motility *in vivo* as well as *in vitro.* Platelet-activating factor usually exerts its actions through high-affinity PAF receptors, which have recently been cloned in guinea pig lung and human neutrophils (211–213), and are apparently present in endometrial epithelial (214–216) and myometrial cells (217). No such receptors have yet been reported on spermatozoa. Spermatozoa do not synthesize PGs, and so sperm transport through the uterus may be due to the combined action of spermatozoal PAF and seminal plasma or uterine PGs on uterine contractility, and PAF-induced sperm motility.

When spermatozoa are suspended in uterine fluid, there is no known mechanism to ensure that they will always swim toward the uterotubal junction, so that, in the absence of an external force propelling them in that direction, sperm movement in the uterine cavity is likely to be random. Inert particles have also been shown to be rapidly transported from one end of the uterus to the other (147).

Sperm numbers in the uterus increase with time (up to 6 h) after mating, then remain more or less constant up to 18 h, at least in the rabbit. During this time, the percentage of nonviable sperm in the uterus does not change greatly (218). In contrast, it has been shown that when large numbers of spermatozoa are placed in a rabbit uterine horn with both ends ligated, only 20% of the spermatozoa can be recovered 6 h later. This destruction of spermatozoa is caused by an influx of leukocytes that phagocytose the spermatozoa (172,219). This is one major mechanism by which dead, damaged, or immotile spermatozoa are removed from the reproductive tract.

In some species, especially the bat, spermatozoa can become lodged in a uterine gland and thus perhaps remain protected from phagocytosis for long periods of time (220). However, this is probably not the case in humans. Sperm are found in the uterus consistently up to 24 h after intercourse, but only a few are found thereafter (221). Intensive efforts to locate sperm in the uterus between 25 and 41 h after coitus, at a time when many sperm are still present in cervical mucus, were also relatively unsuccessful, although up to 90% of spermatozoa placed in the uterus could be recovered 30 min later (222). This suggests that destruction or removal of spermatozoa from the uterus increases after 24 h. There is certainly good evidence that there is leukocytic infiltration into the uterus and cervix (223), about 10^9 leukocytes (mainly polymorphonuclear leukocytes and macrophages) being at the cervix within 4 h after insemination, and some evidence for phagocytosis of spermatozoa in humans (224). Thus, spermatozoa are apparently greatly outnumbered by leukocytes. However, accurate estimation of spermatozoal numbers in the uterus in humans is difficult, and the values obtained may well be underestimates. A new technique of ultrasound-guided transfundal spermatozoal recovery has been described in cynomolgus monkeys, and spermatozoa were recovered at both 8 and 24 h after coitus (225). At 6 h, no sperm were detected in two monkeys, whereas in five of the remaining six, sperm numbers in the aspirates ranged from 4.1×10^2 to 3.5×10^5; in the final monkey, the aspirate was thought to have been contaminated with cervical mucus and associated sperm. These estimates are higher than those previously observed in women, but by 24 h, even in these monkeys only few or no spermatozoa were found (225). Consequently, it must be supposed that most spermatozoa pass to the oviduct within a few hours and that those remaining in the uterus are removed by phagocytosis. Evidence supporting this notion is provided by sheep and cattle, in which about 6 to 8 h is required for a functional population of sperm to enter the oviducts from the uterus, and by other species, in which even less time is required for this same process (170).

In infertile patients, especially those with hostile cervical mucus or antisperm antibodies, intrauterine insemination with husband or donor spermatozoa after washing and "swim-up" for selection of the most motile specimens has become a widely used technique to establish pregnancy. The success rate can be improved from 25% (cervical insemination) to 75% by using intrauterine insemination (226). Pregnancies can also be achieved with intrauterine insemination of as little as 1–2 million spermatozoa (227). The factor with the greatest influence on achievement of pregnancy was the degree of spermatozoal motility, especially after the swim-up procedure, rather than sperm numbers (228,229). Indeed, pregnancies have been reported after intrauterine insemination with spermatozoa aspirated from an alloplastic spermatocele in men with vas obstruction (230). These studies confirm the observation that, when fertility is subnormal, the strong filtering action of the cervical mucus is a major factor and that, provided the sperm are motile, even small numbers in the uterus can give rise to pregnancy. Although no direct measurements have been made on transport time through the uterus in humans, such observations have been made in bitches at estrus with a unilateral uterine fistula (231). Spermatozoa reached the end of the fistula within 1 min of natural mating or artificial insemination with the dog in the head-down position and within 2 min after artificial insemination with the dog in the normal position. Also, a certain percentage of spermatozoa after intrauterine insemination will leak back through the cervix, with the greatest number in estrous cows being seen in the first 3 h (232). Passage of the inseminating pipette in this species may, however, stimulate uterine contractions (233).

In rabbits, spermatozoa in the uterus have the greatest flagellar activity $1\frac{1}{2}$ to 16 h after mating. The swimming trajectories of most spermatozoa, which have progressive motility, are linear, but circular movement has also been seen (234). Progressive motility appears to be related to the ability to fertilize ova. There is little information on the changes in pattern of sperm motility within the human uterus, but in mice it has been concluded that hyperactivated flagellar bending is initiated before entry into the oviducts, although sperm recovered from the uterus itself showed straight trajectories with little lateral oscillation (235,236). In one *in vitro* study of human spermatozoal swimming characteristics on epithelial monolayers, it was noted that spermatozoa swimming on monolayers of uterine or oviductal origin exhibited a higher degree of hyperactivation than in control medium or on a kidney cell line (237). Hyperactivation involves an asymmetric flagellar beating with nonprogressive movement, and this condition may give such spermatozoa an advantage in penetrating viscous oviductal fluid and the cumulus mass (238).

At the time of ovulation, the human endometrium is characterized by the following: epithelial glands increased in length and tortuosity, the individual columnar epithelial cells at their greatest height, and maximal pseudostratification of the nuclei. There is also less edema in the stroma than was present during the few days earlier, but there are still many mitoses. It is only after ovulation that intraluminal secretion from these epithelial cells becomes exceptionally abundant (239). At the time of ovulation, endometrial secretions have been found to contain a variety of proteins; in particular, albumin, prealbumin, transferrin, and posttransferrin have been identified (240,241). Zones of precipitation that are not present in serum have also been found in the β-globulin region in uterine washings (242). Total uterine protein, uncontaminated by sperm or blood, is greatest just before ovulation (243). Osmolarity of uterine fluid is about 284 mOsmol/L and does not differ throughout the cycle. Total cation concentration and that of albumin are lower in uterine fluid than in serum. The concentration of potassium is high and that of sodium and calcium is low compared with those of serum. Only potassium and calcium vary throughout the cycle, being lowest at midcycle (244). Uterine fluid volumes are greatest at midcycle, about 83 to 180 μl (245). Human uterine fluid also contains several amino acids, with taurine being predominant, and it has been suggested that taurine might sustain motility of spermatozoa by protecting them from the harmful effect of high potassium concentrations (246). In the female tract, calcium binding substances and calcium transport inhibitors added to spermatozoa from seminal fluid at ejaculation are removed during capacitation (37). Ram spermatozoa experience a partial loss of a major surface component (M_r 97,000) during incubation in uterine fluid and show a shift toward an M_r-24,000 component. Furthermore, selective absorption to the spermatozoal surface of an M_r-16,000 polypeptide from uterine fluid has been observed (247). It was suggested that these changes were related to the capacitation process. It has been noted that seminal plasma levels of ionized calcium in the human are higher than serum and cervical mucus levels, which are similar. Despite this difference or addition of increasing quantities of calcium to human spermatozoa *in vitro,* motility was unaffected, and it was therefore suggested that spermatozoa can maintain an internal ionized calcium level adequate for motility, irrespective of external calcium fluctuations (248).

Changes in the composition of uterine fluid by the presence of a copper-releasing intrauterine device (IUD) may be responsible for the reduced rate of fertilization seen in women wearing such a device (249). Studies on the epithelial cells of the endometrium indicate that, at midcycle, material staining with PAS is present and that ribonucleoprotein and alkaline phosphatase are maximal (250). Lastly, there will be a mixture of cells in uterine fluid, representing the following: migratory cells such as neutrophils, macrophages, and lymphocytes; exfoliated epithelial cells; foreign cells such as bacteria; and nonnucleated portions of epithelial cells. The number of cells present is variable but, in the absence of an IUD, ranges between 10,000 and 100,000 (251). A recent review on the significance of leukocytes in the genital tract sheds little light on their role in the uterus. Three possible roles are suggested—"priming" the tract for fertilization and implantation, preventing infection and removing the products of insemination, and modulating the immune response to spermatozoa (223)—but each of these is still speculative, except for phagocytosis of spermatozoa. Artificial intravaginal insemination, with the balance of the husband's sperm sample, of women undergoing *in vitro* fertilization at the time of oocyte fertilization resulted in a significantly better pregnancy rate after embryo transfer 36 to 48 h later (252). As this effect was observed in women with patent or blocked oviducts, it was suggested that the spermatozoa were inducing some uterine response.

In summary, sperm transport through the uterus depends mainly on uterine contractions and not on sperm motility. The spermatozoa are suspended in the uterine secretions. Owing to the difficulties of collecting human uterine fluid without altering its properties during the collection process, information on composition of such fluid is limited, but this fluid certainly acts to suspend, maintain, and stimulate spermatozoa during the transport process and contains macrophages that remove dead and nonviable spermatozoa.

Sperm Transport Through the Uterotubal Junction

Although the cervical canal acts as a major barrier to sperm ascent, substantial numbers still reach the uterus. In those species in which intrauterine insemination occurs, clearly the numbers in the uterus are very large. Nonetheless, the number of spermatozoa that actually

TABLE 1. *Species variation in number of spermatozoa ejaculated and site of deposition in different animals*[a]

Animal	Average number of sperm/ejaculate (millions)	Site of sperm deposition	Number of sperm in ampulla of oviduct
Mouse	50	Uterus	<100
Rat	58	Vagina	500
Rabbit (buck)	280	Vagina	250–500
Ferret	—	Uterus	18–1,600
Guinea pig	80	Vagina and uterus	25–50
Bull	3,000	Vagina	A few
Ram	1,000	Vagina	600–700
Boar	8,000	Uterus	1,000
Man	280	Vagina	200

From ref. 114, with permission.
[a] Data from various sources.

enter the oviduct remains remarkably constant. It seems that the uterotubal junction forms a further barrier to sperm ascent (Table 1). The anatomic complexity of the junction, which is very complex in some species, such as the pig, and comparatively simple in others, such as the carnivores, does not seem to be related to its ability to impair sperm transport.

Woodruff and Pauerstein (253) reviewed many morphologic studies and concluded that no anatomic sphincter could be demonstrated at the uterotubal junction of the human oviduct. Furthermore, there is no mucosal or capillary structure acting as a valve. The intramural portion of the human oviduct is convoluted and varies in length from 1 to 2 cm. Owing to its tortuosity, it is impossible to pass a probe through the interstitial portion of the human oviduct. The diameter of the lumen in this portion of the oviduct is approximately 0.1 to 1 mm (Fig. 3). Use of the injected latex method showed that the intramural segment of the oviduct has an S-shaped course with double curves and a length of between 0.9 and 1.7 cm (256). The oviductal epithelial folds may continue all the way to the uterine cavity or terminate a few millimeters short of this. There is an increase in cell density and number of ciliated cells as the isthmic region is reached, and at the uterotubal junction the presence of mucosal folds directed toward the oviductal lumen was confirmed (256). The inner longitudinal smooth-muscle layer of the interstitial portion disappears in the isthmus approximately 2.5 cm from the uterotubal junction. The outer smooth-muscle layer continues into the broad ligament (254). Recent studies of the morphology of the uterotubal junction of mice and pigs during the preovulatory period have been made. Although there are significant differences from the human, there are also similarities, which may help to elucidate the physiologic control of this region. In mice, the smooth-muscle cells of the uterotubal junction are similar to those of the myometrium, but only at the junction do the circular layer of such cells form a ring (257). In all regions at estrus and proestrus, the oviductal smooth-muscle cells show increased organelle content, enlargement of contact area, and appearance of myoblasts (257). Whether more extensive investigation of the human oviduct precisely at the time of ovulation would show a similar arrangement

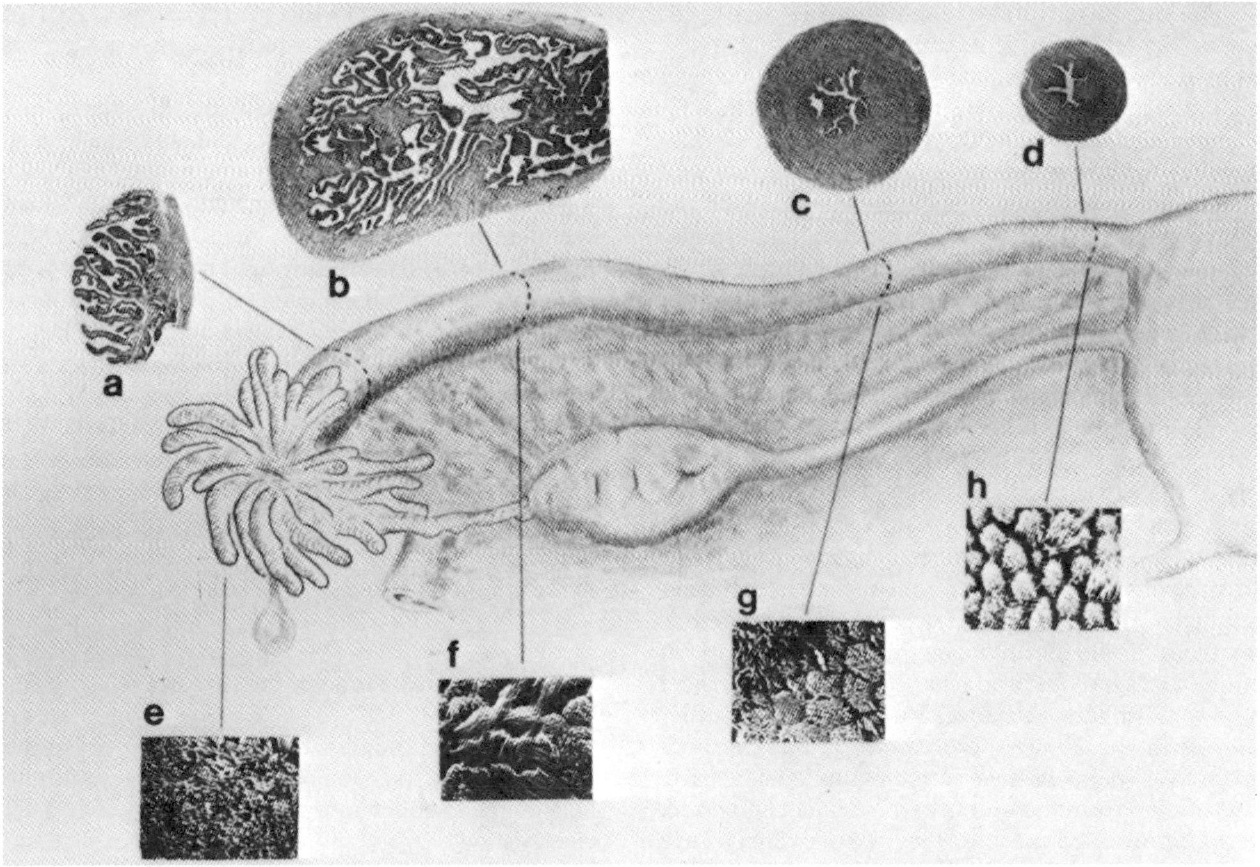

FIG. 3. Anatomy and morphology of human oviduct. **A–D:** Light microscopy photomicrographs depicting cross sections taken at level of distal ampulla, midampulla, distal isthmus, and proximal isthmus, respectively. **E–H:** Scanning electron microscopy photomicrographs depicting surface ultrastructure of oviductal lumen at level of fimbriae, midampulla, distal isthmus, and proximal isthmus, respectively. (From refs. 254 and 255, with permission.)

of smooth muscle cells is uncertain. In preovulatory pigs, both ciliated and nonciliated secretory simple columnar epithelial cells have been seen (258). In the secretory cells, secretory vesicles are present, and these are more abundant in inseminated compared with nonmated animals, as is the presence of lymphocytes, monocytes, and macrophages among the epithelial cells. Interestingly, neutrophils invaded only the uterine epithelium, participating in phagocytosis of epithelial cells and spermatozoa. They were never found in the uterotubal junction, irrespective of whether the gilts had been mated. Spermatozoa remaining in the uterus exhibited damaged plasma membranes, whereas all those in the uterotubal region were ultrastructurally normal (258). In a companion paper, it was noted that the infundibular-cornual ligament, a well-developed muscular structure running under the mesothelium of the uterotubal region, exhibits rhythmic contracts at ovulation that are dependent on local PG production—both PGE_2 and $PGF_{2\alpha}$ are stimulatory (259). Contractions of this ligament may be important, not only for ovum capture from the ovarian surface but also for propulsion of spermatozoa through the uterotubal junction to the site of storage in the isthmus. Whether control of muscular activity by locally produced PGs occurs in humans is not known.

Despite the tortuosity of the human interstitial region of the oviduct, it has been stated that the passage of inert small particles can occur in either direction and at all times in the cycle (253), and there is evidence for oviductal fluid contributing to uterine fluid at midcycle (246). In gilts, although some dead spermatozoa do reach the oviducts, they do so in lesser numbers than do normally motile ones (260). Similarly, in hamsters, spermatozoa of rat, mouse, guinea pig, and rabbit, as well as dead hamster sperm, ascended to the oviduct, although in lesser numbers than motile hamster spermatozoa (261). Furthermore, capacitated spermatozoa penetrated the uterotubal junction less well than uncapacitated ones, because of the hyperactivated (less linear) swimming trajectory of the capacitated spermatozoa (262). In a study of rat reproductive tracts *in vitro,* only motile spermatozoa passed through the uterotubal junction (263). In contrast, several earlier publications suggested that dead spermatozoa and inert particles can be transported as efficiently as motile spermatozoa through the uterotubal junction in rats, rabbits, and pigs (264–267). Thus, there may be some difference between the human and other species, as in the latter, sperm motility may be more important for sperm passage to the oviduct, and clearly passage of fluid from the uterus to the oviduct or oviduct to uterus is prevented except at the time of ovum passage through the uterotubal junction some 3 days after ovulation (268,269).

Although the numbers of spermatozoa found in the oviducts are very similar in different species, despite the differing numbers of spermatozoa ejaculated and the different sites of deposition of the ejaculate, there is evidence, from studies on rabbits, that when inseminations with very small numbers of sperm are performed, fewer spermatozoa reach the oviduct. Inseminations with normal numbers of spermatozoa (200+ million), or even ten times less, have no effect in this regard, but insemination with only 0.5% of the total ejaculate (1.21 million spermatozoa) reduced sperm in the oviduct about 60 times (5,000 to 6,000 down to an average of 88) (270). In the human, where there is no apparent barrier to passage of inert particles through the uterotubal junction (147,253), it is not clear why only 1,000 or so spermatozoa reach the oviduct (271–273), but there is a relationship between the number of spermatozoa inseminated and the number reaching the oviduct during the first 45 min after insemination (274). However, it is clear that spermatozoa do not have to traverse the reproductive tract to be able to fertilize the ova. In rabbits, no difference in fertilization rate or embryo survival is seen between intravaginal or intratubal insemination (275). Similarly, in the human, use of the gamete intrafallopian transfer (GIFT) procedure for infertility, in which both ova and ejaculated spermatozoa (after washing and swim-up) are transferred to the ampullar region of the oviduct by the infundibulum, gives rise to pregnancies (276,277). However, in this procedure, at least 100,000 spermatozoa must be transferred to ensure a pregnancy (277,278).

Thus, it is clear that, while a certain filtering of spermatozoa does occur at the uterotubal junction, presumably to permit the fittest to survive to fertilize the ova in the oviduct, if selection of spermatozoa is performed by other means, fertilization occurs normally. Consequently, sperm passage through the uterotubal junction is not physiologically obligate for fertility, even though it may be helpful in reducing the chance of fertilization by a defective or abnormal spermatozoon. However, if the uterotubal junction is occluded because of pathology or a sterilization procedure, sperm transport will be blocked and pregnancy prevented. Hysteroscopy can be used to assess the degree of mucosal damage at the uterotubal ostium (279) and falloposcopy for exploration of the whole length of the oviduct and treatment of stenosis and intraluminal adhesions (280).

Sperm Transport Through the Oviduct

Spermatozoa progress through the oviduct to the site of fertilization and then onward out of the infundibular end of the oviduct into the peritoneal cavity. This is clearly shown by the pioneering work of Ahlgren (271), in which sperm numbers in the ampullar region of normal human oviducts did not exceed 200 during the period of 2 to 34 h after intercourse; however, in women with oviductal pathology, which involves occlusion of the infundibulum and causes hydrosalpinx, many thousands were seen.

A review, by Ahlgren and collaborators (281), of the many reports on sperm migration in women shows that, in cases in which examination of peritoneal fluid was performed, spermatozoa were usually found. These reports were confirmed by Ahlgren's own observations. Interestingly, the percentage of spermatozoa with normal morphology, which averaged 84% ($n = 8$ patients examined 10 to 60 h postintercourse) in the ejaculate, was much higher in the uterus (96%; $n = 3$ at 11 to 60 h) and oviduct (93%; $n = 8$ at 10 to 60 h) (281). Furthermore, up to 85 h after intercourse, motile spermatozoa could be recovered from the cervix, the uterine cavity, the ampullar region of the oviduct, and the abdominal cavity (271,281). An earlier report had indicated that motile spermatozoa could be found up to at least 60 h after intercourse (282), and there have been many reports of motile sperm in the oviducts at shorter times after intercourse. It is likely that 85 h may be the upper limit of maintenance of sperm motility in the human. Whether this is also the upper limit for fertilizing capacity is not known, but if motility is still present, there would seem to be a chance for fertilization to occur. Thus, when natural family planning methods are to be used, an allowance of up to 4 days for sperm survival should be made.

It was originally thought that spermatozoa moved up the oviduct in a constant progression, with the numbers reaching the ampullar region rising progressively until a constant number was achieved after a few hours (283). This is now known to be incorrect. Spermatozoa, after entry into the oviduct, are distributed in two ways. A few spermatozoa are rapidly transported to the ampullar region, and these are the ones observed by different investigators shortly after mating or intercourse (Table 2). These are not the spermatozoa that generally fertilize ova in species in which mating takes place before ovulation. In species such as the human, in which intercourse may occur before, after, or at the same time as ovulation, it cannot be definitively stated that the first spermatozoa do not normally fertilize the ovum. However, in view of the similarity of the second phase of sperm transport in the oviduct in many species, it is likely that generally the same trend holds true.

TABLE 2. *Time between coitus or artificial insemination and arrival of spermatozoa in oviduct*[a]

Animal	Time	Region of tube
Mouse	15 min	Ampulla
Rat	15–20 min	Ampulla
Hamster	2–60 min	Ampulla
Rabbit (doe)	A few minutes	Ampulla
Guinea pig	15 min	Ampulla
Bitch	2 min–a few hours	Oviducts
Sow	15 min	Ampulla
Cow	2–13 min	Ampulla
Ewe	6 min–5 hr	Ampulla
Woman	5–68 min	Oviducts

From ref. 114, with permission.
[a] Data from various sources.

The second phase of sperm distribution and transport was first observed in small animals [e.g., the mouse (284) and the rabbit (285)]. It was found that, after sperm entry into the oviduct, most of the spermatozoa remained in the proximal isthmus until about the time of ovulation. It is now known that this congregation of spermatozoa in the isthmus occurs in pigs (286,287), sheep (288,289), and cows (290,291). Indeed, in sheep and cows, a minimum period of 6 to 8 h is required for accumulation of a sufficient population of spermatozoa in the oviducts to achieve good fertilization (170). Similarly, the studies of Croxatto and collaborators (272) document that the same trend is seen in the human. They flushed whole oviducts and recovered considerably larger numbers of spermatozoa than had Ahlgren (271), who had flushed only the ampullar region. By analogy with the results of his extensive studies on sperm transport in the oviducts of farm animals, Hunter (170) also concluded that this delay of spermatozoa at the isthmic region of the oviduct occurs in the human (i.e., the "distal portion of the isthmus acts as a functional sperm reservoir") and that capacitation and the acrosome reaction may also be suppressed in this region. This raises the question of what controls the subsequent upward movement of the spermatozoa to achieve fertilization. It was originally suggested that the presence of the products of ovulation in the oviduct might initiate this reaction (292). Several authors working with different species have also suggested that sperm transport in the oviduct is stimulated by the ovulatory process (287,289,291,293,294). In sheep, it was noted that there are larger numbers of spermatozoa present in the oviduct ipsilateral to the ovulating ovary (295). The nature of the stimulatory factor(s) associated with ovulation responsible for the stimulation of sperm movement from the isthmus to the site of fertilization has not been defined. However, recent *in vitro* experiments with human sperm showed that spermatozoal accumulation into follicular fluid is significantly higher than into buffer and that this stimulatory effect of fluid from an individual follicle correlates significantly with the fertilizability of the ovum from the same follicle (294). This finding has now been confirmed by another group of investigators (296). Bovine follicular fluid can induce capacitation and the acrosome reaction, and these effects are concentration-dependent. Spermatozoa exposed to higher concentrations of follicular fluid are better able to fertilize oocytes in a short period than are those exposed to lesser concentrations (297). However, similar effects can be achieved with oviductal fluid, so this effect may not be related to that stimulating sperm movement.

Different mechanisms have been adduced as to why spermatozoa remain in the isthmus and do not continuously migrate toward the infundibulum. It has been suggested that elevated concentrations of steroids (progesterone, androstenedione, and estradiol) and $PGF_{2\alpha}$ in the arterioles supplying the proximal portion of the oviduct, compared with peripheral plasma (which implies a local transfer from ovary to oviduct), may provide a mechanism for regulating isthmic patency and contractility (298). The membrane-bound localization of the enzyme, carbonic anhydrase, in the secretory cells of the uterotubal junction and the isthmus may regulate the acid–base status of the luminal fluid in this region and thus be important for regulation of sperm immotility (299). The local isthmic concentration of potassium and pyruvate may be similarly important, in that potassium is inhibitory and pyruvate is stimulatory to sperm motility (300), and there is also an increasing temperature gradient from the isthmus to the ampulla (301). Luminal concentrations of catecholamines (dopamine, epinephrine, and norepinephrine) are highest at estrus and in the isthmus compared with the ampulla (302). What role such vasoactive and smooth-muscle-stimulating compounds may play in regulation of myosalpingeal activity is unknown.

When the spermatozoa do move onward from the isthmus toward the ampulla, it is clear that sperm motility becomes important. If a 1- to 2-cm segment of the ampulla is microsurgically reversed, oocytes do not traverse the reversed segment but are still fertilized. In the reversed segment, the cilia of the epithelial cells are beating in an adovarian rather than in the usual abovarian direction. This changed direction of beat, in combination with a changed direction of luminal fluid flow, prevents the zygotes from moving toward the ampullar-isthmic junction but does not affect sperm transport, which must be achieved by some combination of motility and fluid flow (303). Such findings are likely to be the same for other species.

One of the main reasons that spermatozoa remain in the isthmus has to do with their motility. This has been extensively studied in the rabbit (234). In the lower isthmus, the percentage of spermatozoa with activated motility was minimal up to 4 h postcoitum, then increased to about 3% at 6 h and remained relatively constant up to 16 h. In contrast, in the ampulla, the percentage of spermatozoa with activated motility was minimal up to 6 h, then rose rapidly and more or less continuously up to 16 h, when it was 35%. In the lower isthmus, flagellar activity and thus progressive movement was low. In contrast, the "activated motility" seen in the ampulla beginning at 6 h postcoitum was characterized by alternating patterns of linear progressive and vigorous nonprogressive movement (234). In the nonprogressive mode, the spermatozoa swam in a tight circle and exhibited whiplike activity of the tail, whereas in the progressive mode they often appeared to "crawl" in the presence of cellular debris, as described by Phillips (304). Owing to the thin wall of the mouse oviduct, *in vivo* observations on sperm movement have been possible. As noted above, spermatozoa in the isthmic region were immotile and attached to the epithelial cells, whereas spermatozoa elsewhere appeared normally motile (305). A significantly higher proportion of spermatozoa in the ampulla were free compared with the isthmus, and it seemed that only spermatozoa showing hyperactivation broke free (306). This change in sperm motility associated with detachment from the isthmic epithelium and progression toward the ampullar region has recently been reviewed extensively (167). The hyperactivation of spermatozoa has been examined by many authors and in different species, perhaps because it is a useful marker related to the process of capacitation and perhaps because it is important for sperm transport and penetration of the oocyte investments (167). In *in vitro* experiments at 37°C, it was noted that human spermatozoa swimming over monolayers of bovine oviductal or human endometrial but not over monkey kidney cells showed high rates of hyperactivation. At room temperature, no difference in swimming pattern was seen (237). Such a temperature-controlled effect could be consistent with the observation of a temperature gradient between the isthmus and ampulla *in vivo* (301). Hyperactivated spermatozoa beat with decreased symmetry and exhibit bends of greater curvature in midpiece and proximal principal piece. As a result, motion may be less progressive, but such extreme curvatures may be essential for penetration of cumulus oophorus and zona pellucida (167).

Many of the motile spermatozoa had cilia attached to their heads, thus suggesting a close apposition to epithelial cells of the isthmus (234), which is perhaps caused by oviductal mucus (307,308). It has recently been shown that the fertilizing capacity of bovine spermatozoa can be maintained for up to 48 h *in vitro* in those binding by the rostral portion of the acrosome to endosalpingeal epithelial cells but not by binding to tracheal epithelial cells or in the absence of cells (309). There is also evidence from experiments in hamsters that spermatozoa in the isthmic region are firmly attached to epithelial cells until their release around the time of ovulation (310). Such a mechanism could be important in maintaining fertilizing capacity *in vitro* during the period of sperm storage in the isthmus. By flushing human oviducts with oil and collecting the aqueous material extruded before the oil, Croxatto (personal communication) calculated that the volume of oviductal secretions at midcycle ranges from 20 to 40 μl. On this basis, he estimated that the *concentration* of spermatozoa in the oviduct can range from 5,000 to 50,000 per milliliter. Even these concentrations are two orders of magnitude lower than those used in *in vitro* fertilization programs, and it is not surprising that excessive numbers of spermatozoa attached to the zona pellucida are common in such *in vitro* fertilized ova (311). This phenomenon is not seen in normally fertilized ova but, provided that polyspermy does not occur, is apparently not deleterious to zygote development.

Studies of polypeptide secretion from epithelial cells of porcine oviducts showed five main bands with M_r of 90, 78, 40, 30, and 14 kDa, with some evidence of binding to spermatozoa. Furthermore, incubation of spermatozoa with such oviductal cell cultures for as little as 2.5 h reduced the incidence of polyspermy of pig oocytes *in vitro* and maintained sperm motility (312). Similarly, in sheep, binding to spermatozoa by 140-, 95-, 78-, and 53-kDa polypeptides secreted by the oviduct and, in humans, binding to the head of spermatozoa by a 54-kDa glycoprotein purified from oviductal fluid, have also been observed (247,313). Scanning electronmicroscopy of bull spermatozoa before ovulation showed that those in the isthmus had droplets of secretory material attached to the anterior portion of the intact head, perhaps acquired in the isthmic lumen, which contained viscous secretory matter (314). Such a mechanism operating *in vivo* could be one way that polyspermy is avoided even if excess numbers of spermatozoa enter the oviduct.

The structure of the oviduct has been the subject of extensive investigation for at least 400 years. A short description is included here to place in perspective the different component parts and structures that play a role in both sperm and, as described below, ovum transport (253) (Fig. 3). The intramural portion (also called *interstitial portion*), which includes the uterotubal junction, has already been described. The isthmus begins at the junction between the uterus and oviduct (uterotubal junction) and extends distally for 2 to 3 cm, ending at the ampullar-isthmic junction. The wall of this segment consists of a very thick layer of smooth musculature, encompassing a narrow lumen of approximately 0.4 mm. Because the musculature is better developed in this region than in the adjacent ones, it can perhaps be classified as a sphincter and is certainly a main factor in controlling ovum transport to the uterus.

The ampulla is the longest portion of the human oviduct and extends from the ampullar-isthmic junction to the infundibulum, a distance of about 5 to 8 cm. The lumen of the ampulla is wider than that of the isthmus, ranging from 1 cm at the infundibular end to 1 mm at the ampullar-isthmic junction. The wall is relatively thin in this region, with a thin musculature and well-developed mucosal surface with many-branched folds.

The infundibulum is the trumpet-shaped organ that comprises the most distal portion of the oviduct and that opens into the peritoneal cavity. It has very thin walls and is covered with densely ciliated, petal-like structures known as *fimbriae.* The fimbriae are partially attached to the ovarian surface, and this arrangement helps to maintain close apposition of the ovary and oviduct, thus facilitating ovum "pick-up" at the time of ovulation.

There are two main types of cells in the oviductal epithelium: ciliated and secretory. The ciliated cells are much more numerous on the fimbriae and in the ampulla. The secretory cells predominate in the isthmus. Both types of cells undergo changes in structure and function under the influence of the ovarian hormones secreted during the menstrual cycle (Fig. 2). These changes have been reviewed in detail by Jansen (315). At midcycle, the epithelium reaches maximal height (30 to 35 μm), and both ciliated and secretory cells are of equal height. The secretory cells form domes among the tufts of cilia, but shortly after ovulation, as the secretory cells shrink in height because of discharge of secretion, the cilia become more prominent. Then, the whole epithelium becomes shorter because of broadening and flattening of the ciliated cells.

At midcycle, the secretory cells of the isthmus appear to be most active, with an apocrine secretion occurring. Serous granules also appear in the apical portion of these secretory cells. The isthmus can be fully filled with secretion at this time. Apocrine secretion does not appear to occur in the ampulla. This secretion continues through the ovulatory period, and some can also be seen in the ampulla.

The fluid in the oviduct is composed of the secretions from these epithelial cells by diffusion of nutrients from plasma. This secretion is stimulated by estrogen (316) and is maximal at midcycle (317,318). Protein concentration is maximal at the time of ovulation and consists predominantly of albumin (33.8%), β-globulin (44.4%), and γ-globulin (1.8%) (318). Potassium and chloride are present in oviductal fluid in higher concentrations than in serum, but calcium concentration is lower. Sodium and magnesium concentrations are similar to those in serum (319). This balance gives rise to a negative potential and can be expected to maintain acidic high-molecular-weight proteoglycans and glycoproteins in an expanded state (315). The enzymes, amylase and lactate dehydrogenase, which are abundant in oviductal fluid (317), can convert the large quantities of glycogen present to pyruvate and glucose. Pyruvate is an essential substrate for early zygote cleavage and growth (320), whereas spermatozoa and later stages of zygote development can use the glucose as an energy source (115,321). As many as 27 amino acids can be detected in mouse oviductal fluid and their concentration changes after fertilization (322). Also, bicarbonate ion concentration is high at midcycle and is accompanied by an increase in the pH of oviductal fluid, from 7.1 to 7.3 in the follicular phase to 7.5 to 7.8 at ovulation, in the monkey (323). There is active secretion of fluid coupled with chloride transport along an electrochemical gradient, which can be inhibited by elevated concentrations of cyclic adenosine monophosphate and calcium ions (324). The formation and function of oviductal fluid in the rabbit have been reviewed (325).

It appears that the secretion in the ampulla will be more watery because of the greater transudation caused by the larger surface area of epithelium, whereas in the isthmus, the secretion will have more mucous consistency for the reverse reasons and because of the larger number of secretory cells in this region (315). The endosalpinx in the ampulla is highly plicated and the branched folds tend to occlude the lumen, whereas in the isthmus, the endosalpinx is much less plicated and the individual folds are much shorter and broader. The cilia on the epithelial surface all beat toward the uterus, do not differ in rhythm among the different portions of the oviduct, and exhibit no greater activity at the time of ovulation than earlier in the cycle (326). This abovarian beat causes a current of oviductal fluid flow over the epithelium in the same direction. Owing to the thicker consistency of the isthmic secretions, the thicker muscular wall not permitting distention, the narrower lumen, and the edema of the wall itself (327), fluid passage through the isthmus and into the uterus is not permitted or is only minimal (at least until the time of ovum passage into the uterus after ovulation). Consequently, the direction of fluid flow is reversed (328), and a flow of fluid in the less-ciliated mucosal crypts develops toward the infundibulum. In this way, excess oviductal secretion is voided through the infundibulum to the peritoneal cavity, carrying with it those spermatozoa that have reached the ampullar region. This is a constant process until all spermatozoa have left the oviduct, or the ovum and oviductal fluid are transported into the uterus. Spermatozoa that have entered the peritoneal cavity can still fertilize oocytes by entry into the contralateral oviduct (329) or either oviduct, in the case of artificial intraperitoneal insemination (330).

During the periovulatory period, the oviductal musculature is not quiescent. Electrophysiologic recording of rabbit oviducts has shown that there are bursts of electrical activity propagating in each direction, with some indication of more propagating toward the ovary at ovulation (331,332). Similar activity has been seen in human oviducts (333). *In vitro,* annular segments and longitudinal strips of human oviduct also show high spontaneous activity in the periovulatory phase (334). The consequence of this muscular activity is to ensure a thorough mixing of the luminal contents, which increases the chance of spermatozoon and ovum meeting and may also hasten sperm transport through the ampulla and into the peritoneal cavity.

During transport through the reproductive tract, the spermatozoa undergo certain maturational changes that are a prerequisite for fertilization. These involve a complex series of events, many of which occur just before fertilization and thus are dealt with in detail in Chapter 5 by Yanagimachi in this volume. Here only an overview is provided to show how these events provide the final scene in the saga of sperm transport from testis to oviduct.

Freshly ejaculated spermatozoa are incapable of fertilization; during their brief stay in the uterus (in some species) and oviduct, they undergo a process known as *capacitation,* which prepares them for the final change before fertilization can begin. Capacitation involves a destabilization of the plasma membrane of the sperm head without any visible morphological changes (335). Capacitation was first described by Austin and Chang independently (336,337). The necessity for capacitation of human sperm has been debated, because fertilization of human ova can be achieved *in vitro* in defined media containing follicular fluid, human blood serum, or fetal cord blood (338–341). Even though no morphologic evidence for capacitation exists, it is known that there is a cholesterol efflux from mammalian spermatozoa that is thought to be one of the early steps in capacitation. At estrus in the bovine, high-density lipoprotein concentration in oviductal fluid increased, and this may serve as an acceptor for sperm cholesterol and thus promote capacitation and the acrosome reaction (342). Capacitation must be a rapid process in the human and easily accomplished *in vitro.* This is not the case for other species, such as the rabbit (343), in which the optimal conditions involve sequential exposure to uterus and oviduct. After capacitation and when the spermatozoa come into close contact with the investments of the ovum (cumulus oophorus and corona radiata cells) in the ampullar region of the oviduct, a final maturational change occurs. This is known as the *acrosome reaction* and involves the fusion of the outer acrosomal membrane and the plasma membrane, thereby permitting release, through the pores thus formed, of certain enzymes involved in the fertilization process, notably hyaluronidase and acrosin (335). If spermatozoa die in the oviduct, the acrosome reaction as described does not occur; instead, the acrosome is lost intact. *In vitro* fertilization experiments using physiologic numbers of spermatozoa (1–20) have confirmed the importance of capacitation. Uncapacitated spermatozoa do not bind to the zona pellucida and mostly do not penetrate the cumulus oophorus cell layer. In contrast, capacitated but acrosome-intact spermatozoa penetrate the cumulus layer but often fail to penetrate the inner corona radiata layer of cells or do so with difficulty (344). These experiments have been used as evidence that the acrosome reaction normally occurs in the vicinity of the zona pellucida.

In most species, fertilization occurs only in the oviduct, but experimentally one can demonstrate that, in limited cases, fertilization can take place in the uterus (e.g., in the rabbit; see ref. 345), but this is not the case in the hamster (346). In the human, uterine fertilization can occur, at least in a limited number of cases (347–349), and this reemphasizes the ease with which capacitation and the acrosome reaction must occur in humans.

In summary, sperm transport through the oviduct consists of a rapid phase and a slow phase. Sperm remaining in the isthmus are mostly immotile and only gradually acquire motility and move up to the site of fertilization. Sperm movement is caused by a combination of sperm motility, fluid flow, and muscular activity of the oviductal musculature.

OVULATION AND OVUM "PICK-UP"

The process of ovulation is discussed in another chapter and so will not be dealt with here, except insofar as it relates to the entry of the ovum into the oviduct. In some species, ovulation is triggered by the act of coitus, as in the rabbit, and in others it is causally linked to a defined estrous period during which the female is receptive to the male. In both of these situations, mating antedates ovulation by a number of hours, and capacitated spermatozoa are already waiting in the oviduct by the time the ovum arrives. The situation can often be different in the human, because intercourse takes place throughout the cycle, not just around the time of ovulation at midcycle. Consequently, spermatozoa may be present in the oviducts at the time of ovulation or may arrive there only after ovulation and ovum "pick-up" have occurred. Thus, there is a greater possibility of an aged ovum being fertilized. However, in couples practicing natural family planning, in which the risk of inadvertent interaction of aged gametes might be higher, generally no increased incidence of fetal anomalies or spontaneous abortions has been noted (350).

It is known that, in many species, aging of the ovum before fertilization as a result of delaying insemination progressively diminishes the number of young born as the delay increases and also increases the percentage of abnormally developing embryos (351). In mice, studies of combinations of *in vitro* aged spermatozoa and/or oocytes have shown that aging of both spermatozoa and oocytes decreases fertilization, but apparently by different mechanisms (352). This type of aging should be distinguished from that resulting from advancing maternal age. In a longitudinal study of aging mice, it was found that the earliest sign of declining reproductive activity was reduced fertilization rate, followed by a reduced ovulation rate, and lastly, by absence of estrous cycles (353). Aging of the mouse zona pellucida owing to increased maternal age results in a concomitant reduction in ability of spermatozoa to penetrate the zona (354). Similarly, in women, reproductive capacity declines with age, and it is for such women that advanced assisted reproduction techniques, such as *in vitro* fertilization or GIFT, are most suitable (355). A recent study of 27 couples (maternal age, 28 to 43 years) in an *in vitro* fertilization program showed that although there was no effect of age on oocyte number, oocyte stage of maturation, or fertilization rate, occurrence of diploid oocytes was confined to older women, and in immature oocytes, abnormalities of sperm chromosome condensation were also seen (356). Other studies have confirmed that poor oocyte quality related to maternal age is the main cause of failure to achieve a pregnancy (357,358), as, when ovum donation is used, the uteri of such older women are perfectly capable of sustaining a normal pregnancy (357). However, in a large series of patients (aged 16 to 76 years) undergoing gynecologic surgery, only aneuploidy in follicular cells but not in oocytes was correlated with advancing maternal age (359). In three women (31 to 39 years of age) with unexplained infertility, it was found that neither the husband's nor donor spermatozoa could achieve fertilization but that the husband's spermatozoa could fertilize donor oocytes (360). This suggests that defective oocytes can exist even in younger women. Although it is known that there is an increased incidence of trisomy 21, an autosomal translocation, with advancing maternal age, there is no information that this occurs as a result of aging of the gametes after ovulation. The fertilizable life of the human oocyte has been estimated as approximately 24 h, but apparently the oocytes remain fertilizable longer than they remain capable of producing normal young (361).

Ovulation occurs a number of hours after the release of a surge of luteinizing hormone (LH) from the anterior pituitary gland. Luteinizing hormone induces a great many changes in the follicle, and among these is the resumption of meiosis in the oocyte. Thus, in most species, at ovulation, ovum development has reached the metaphase stage of the second meiotic division and remains at this stage until fertilization begins. However, it has been claimed that in dogs, oocytes are ovulated still as primary oocytes and are not capable of being fertilized until about 60 h after ovulation, when the first meiotic division occurs (362). The time between the LH surge and ovulation varies among species, being only about 12 to 15 h in rodents but as long as 42 h in the pig (166). In the human, ovulation occurs between 40 and 63 h after the estradiol peak in peripheral serum (363), and the estradiol peak antedates the LH peak by about 24 h (364). This indicates that ovulation occurs between 16 and 39 h after the LH surge. Peters and McNatty (365) have given a figure of 28 to 36 h after the LH surge for the human. As a result of the hormonal changes taking place around the time of ovulation (Fig. 2), changes also occur in the cellular investments surrounding the ovum.

At ovulation, the ovum is surrounded by two distinct arrangements of follicle cells (the cumulus cells). Closely attached to the zona pellucida are the coronal cells, arranged radially and two to three cells thick—the so-called *corona radiata.* Surrounding the corona radiata are more cells—the cumulus oophorus—a sticky gelatinous matrix containing many cumulus cells. The maturity of the oocyte-cumulus complex, which is correlated with a high activity of the enzyme Δ^5, 3β-hydroxysteroid dehydrogenase in the complex, is important for normal ovum pick-up and successful fertilization (366). It may also be important for the early stages of ovum transport. Other factors that may be involved in or correlated with maturation of the oocyte-cumulus complex have been recently reviewed (367).

In animals without a closed bursa at the infundibular end of the oviduct, follicular rupture and extrusion of the ovum are not an explosive process; instead, there is an immediate protrusion of a portion of the cumulus containing the ovum from the ruptured follicle followed by a slow oozing of the remainder of this cumulus oophorus in a strandlike manner (368). It seems that there are four possible mechanisms involved in transfer of the ovum from the ovarian surface across the fimbriae into the oviduct. It has been suggested that there is a region of negative pressure caused by local contractions of the oviductal musculature in the infundibular region (369). Negative pressures within the oviduct have been detected by means of intraluminal catheters (370). Whether these negative pressures do exert any suction effect is questionable, because the soft-walled ampulla would collapse, thereby closing the lumen, and because, at least in the rabbit, ovum pick-up can occur despite the presence of a ligation just below the infundibulum (371). On balance, Blandau (368) thought that it is unlikely that such a phenomenon is involved in ovum pick-up.

A second possibility is that integrated contractions of the oviduct and its accessory membranes, the fimbriae and the ovary, contribute to ensure the mechanical pick-up of the ovum in its cumulus mass. It is known that these structures are active during ovulation in the human (372,373), and similar observations have been made in many other species (368). The smooth musculature of the oviductal and ovarian ligaments contracts, so that these structures are brought into close apposition. They then contract rhythmically so that the folds of fimbriae are swept across the ovarian surface. The fimbriae become engorged with blood and themselves also contract rhythmically (371,374). There is a periovulatory accumulation and depletion of mitochondrial-bound calcium and ciliary cell glycogen and lipid that may be related to the increased metabolic activity of fimbrial epithelial cells at ovulation (375).

A third possibility involves the cilia, which are all beating toward the uterotubal junction, on the fimbriae. Intimate contact of these cilia with the cumulus mass is held to be critical to the process of ovum pick-up. The cilia become attached to the cumulus mass and draw it out into long streamers as they attempt to propel the ovum and its investments into the ostium of the oviduct (374).

Lastly, it has recently been suggested that elastic and filamentous strands of oviductal mucus may become attached to the ovarian surface at the time of ovulation. This hypothesis was advanced on the basis of studies in 11 preovulatory women using a falloposcope to catheterize the oviduct. In four of them, a clear mucous strand could be extruded from the oviduct and attached to the ovarian surface. This contact was not broken until the mucus was stretched to a length of 7 mm. It was believed that such sticky strands could play a large role in ensuring the entry of the ovulated oocytes into the oviduct (376).

Thus, it is likely that ovum pick-up is caused by a combination of factors, the most important being the ciliary beat and the rhythmic sweeping of the ovarian surface by the fimbriae. This can, however, be influenced by external factors. Peritoneal fluid from women with endometriosis contains a large-molecular-weight factor that can inhibit the ability of fimbriae to capture oocytes (377).

Observations on ovum pick-up have been best documented in the rabbit by the pioneering studies of Blandau (368), but it is likely, given the anatomic similarities, that the mechanisms are the same in primates. However, despite the efficiency of this process under optimal circumstances, the close apposition of ovarian surface and fimbriae is not essential for ovum pick-up. Microsurgical removal of the infundibulum and fimbriae and of the first 2 cm of the ampulla does not cause infertility in rabbits (378,379). Transperitoneal migration of ova is known to occur in women with only one ovary and the contralateral oviduct (380,381). However, in five unilaterally ovariectomized monkeys with only a single contralateral oviduct, no pregnancies resulted in 28 cycles, whereas when the single ovaries and oviducts were surgically apposed, three of five monkeys conceived in nine cycles (382). When one ovary was enclosed in a peritoneal bursa in rabbits, only a low incidence of transperitoneal migration of ova to the contralateral tube was seen (383). Similarly, inert particles or spermatozoa placed in the peritoneal cavity can be found in the oviduct (384–388), but owing to their smaller size, this pick-up can probably be accomplished by ciliary action alone. Further evidence as to the efficiency of the pick-up process is provided by experiments in which Silastic hoods were placed over the infundibulum in monkeys in an attempt to prevent ovum pick-up. These hoods were anchored by six inert sutures, but it was found that even small gaps in the suturing of the hood permitted ovum pick-up and pregnancy (389,390). Similar findings were recorded in limited studies in women when plastic hoods were used (391). However, actual extrusion of the oocyte does not always occur at ovulation. Luteinization of unruptured follicles has been recorded in animals (392–395), and there is indirect evidence for the same occurrence in women (396). This syndrome of luteinized unruptured follicle can be a cause for infertility (397) and may even occur in normally fertile women (398). Pharmacologically, this failure of follicular rupture can be induced by inhibition of PG synthesis (392–395,398). This is concordant with the suggestion by Espey (399) that ovulation is similar to an inflammatory reaction, in that the "degradative events of this acute inflammatory response cause the follicle wall to decompose and rupture." The eicosanoids involved seem to be more those of the lipoxygenase pathway than the cyclooxygenase one (400, 401). It has been recently proposed that these degradative events of the ovulatory process are dependent on depolarization of follicular cell membranes (400).

In summary, ovum pick-up is an efficient process in which ciliary activity on the fimbriae as well as the rhythmic contractions of the fimbriated folds, the ampullar smooth musculature, and the ligaments supporting the ovary and the oviduct all participate to differing degrees.

OVUM TRANSPORT

Although the overall transport time is remarkably constant for most mammalian species (3 to 4 days), there are differences in the detailed pattern of transport through the different regions of the oviduct. With the exception of horses and bats, it has always been considered that the transport time in most species is the same whether the oocytes are fertilized or not. More careful measurements of oviductal transport time indicate that this may not be true in some other species. In the horse, unfertilized oocytes remain in the oviducts and the zygote derived from a fertile mating at a subsequent estrous period bypasses the unfertilized oocytes and enters the uterus at the appropriate time (402–406), usually day 5 to 6 after ovulation (407). Similarly, only embryos, not oocytes, are transported to the uterus in bats (408). It has now been shown that the transport of zygotes in pregnant rats and hamsters differs from that of oocytes in nonpregnant animals (409,410), although the differences are much less dramatic than in the horse. Whether such a phenomenon exists in other species, including the human, is not known and may depend on the mechanism(s) regulating such differential transport.

Conventional wisdom has been that the zygote is a passive object progressing through the oviduct solely under the control of oviductal factors. Indeed, in the rat it has been concluded that the differential oviductal transport is controlled by differences in the hormonal milieu between pregnant and cycling animals, although differences in uterine transport were ascribed to some unidentified embryo property (411). It is well known that exogenous steroid hormones, depending on doses, duration of action, and time of administration (relative to ovulation), can change the pattern of zygote transport dramatically (see section on *Steroid Hormones* for discussion). However, it is now clear that the zygote is not a passive object during its growth and development but produces a variety of growth factors and lipids, such as eicosanoids and PAF (see section on *Zygote Factors* for discussion). Horse oviductal embryos have been shown to secrete large amounts of PGE_2, combined with a small amount of $PGF_{2\alpha}$ (412). Administration of PGE_2 by intraoviductal infusion to pregnant mares hastens the transport of both embryos and oocytes to the uterus (413), but neither phenylbutazone nor progesterone had any such action (414). In rats, oviductal embryos produce large amounts of PGE_1 but only small amounts of PGE_2 and $PGF_{2\alpha}$, whereas similar-aged unfertilized oocytes secrete smaller amounts of PGE_1 and similar amounts of the other two PGs (415). Indomethacin treatment apparently accelerates transport of oocytes to the uterus, and so it was concluded that, in this species, PGE_1 inhibits oviductal transport by reducing spontaneous motility of the myosalpinx (415). This implies that zygotes can control their own rate of transport (416). However, Hunter (417) proposed a simple explanation for the differential transport of oocytes and zygotes, at least for the horse. In his opinion, structural alterations in the oocyte and its zona pellucida caused by degeneration make it easily deformable and therefore not so likely to be transported as a more rigid sphere. However, transfer of uterine horse embryos back to the oviducts resulted in arrival of the embryos in the uterus within 48 h, 2 days earlier than the normal time of arrival of horse zygotes into the uterus. This was not the case with sham transfers, which definitely implies that the horse embryo can regulate its own transport (418).

Whether such differential control of oocyte and zygote transport through the oviduct is a more general phenomenon or not, and whatever the mechanism, it is known that in some species, although not necessarily the human, zygotes can survive in the oviduct after fertilization at a time when they cannot survive in the uterus (419). Thus, in these species, a correct programming of the oviduct to retain the ova until they are capable of survival in the uterine environment is essential. The different physiologic components that operate to regulate ovum transport are discussed in separate subsections below.

Zygote Survival

Early mammalian embryogenesis is dealt with fully in another chapter and thus only those aspects of zygote growth and development that are dependent on interaction with the oviductal environment are discussed here. Secretions of the oviductal epithelial cells are important in maintaining growth and well-being of the developing embryo. In nonprimates, premature entry of the ova into the uterus is detrimental to their further development, suggesting either that uterine secretion is hostile at this time or that it lacks some essential nutrient (419). In primates, this seems not to be the case, in that after Estes' operation (347,349,420), ova ovulated into the uterine cavity can become fertilized and undergo complete development without exposure to oviductal secretions. The collected material has been summarized by Adams (421), and although firm data are absent in many reports, it seems that approximately 11% of patients can eventually become pregnant after this procedure (i.e., 29 of 270 patients operated in 11 series). In many reports, there is no indication as to the length of time elapsing between operation and pregnancy. However, in the best-documented cases, Adams (421) estimated that 14 pregnancies in eight patients may have occurred over a period of 267 menstrual cycles. If these estimates are correct, this indicates a pregnancy rate of only 6.78 per 100 women-years. In this situation, not only does the zygote have to survive in the uterus, but also the ovum must be fertilized in the uterus and, as noted above, in other species this process is not optimal (345,346). Thus, a large proportion of the failures to become pregnant may be a reflection of lack of fertilization rather than interference with embryonic survival.

This supposition is made more plausible by the experiments of Marston and collaborators (422) in rhesus monkeys. They transferred two freshly fertilized zygotes from one oviduct to another, which resulted in two successful live births. Six other successful live births also resulted from autotransfers of seven two- to six-cell zygotes from one oviduct to the other, but the transfer of a 22-cell morula failed. In these experiments, the success rate for transfers from one oviduct to another was an astonishing 80% (eight of ten transfers). In these same experiments, autotransfers of two seven- to eight-cell zygotes from the oviduct to the uterus resulted in only a chemical pregnancy (positive pregnancy test). This preliminary work was then continued; successful live births were achieved after transfer of oviductal zygotes at early stages (two to six cells) to the uterus of the same animals, 24 h earlier than they would normally have arrived there without the intervening culture period (423).

In women, the GIFT or zygote intrafallopian transfer (ZIFT) procedures are now well established as alternatives to intrauterine embryo transfer after *in vitro* fertilization (IVF-ET) in infertile patients. However, although clinical pregnancy rates after GIFT are much higher than those after intrauterine transfers (276,277, 424–426), those after ZIFT are not different from those for IVF-ET. The latest figures/retrieval from the registry of US and Canadian clinics for 1991 are 34% (1,515 pregnancies), 20% (442 pregnancies), and 19% (4,017 pregnancies) for GIFT, ZIFT, and IVF-ET, respectively (426). Transfer of two- to four-cell embryos (tubal embryo transfer: TET) gives results as good or better than ZIFT (427). None of these pregnancy rates approaches that reported by Marston and associates in monkeys (422,423), but it must be recognized that the human experience is collected from women who *a priori* had an infertility problem, whereas only normally fertile monkeys were studied. Nevertheless, these results indicate that, even in the infertile woman, oocytes or zygotes placed in the oviducts can become fertilized and/or develop normally. Pregnancies have even resulted from placing immature oocytes in the oviduct, allowing *in vivo* maturation, followed by delayed intrauterine insemination (428). This attests to the robustness of the oviductal system and its ability to function efficiently under abnormal circumstances. The main factors in determining the successful outcome of GIFT are the quality of spermatozoa and oocytes. If three or more fully mature oocytes are transferred, pregnancy is 3.8 times more likely than for a lesser number. Similarly, for spermatozoa, the likelihood of pregnancy is 0.34 and 0.22 for insemination of samples with motility less than 30% or normal morphology less than 50%, respectively (429). At least in the case of ZIFT, fertilization failure cannot account for failure of pregnancy, so other factors, such as abnormal embryo development, transport, growth, or implantation, must be involved.

Early development in embryos of most species appears to take place largely under the control of the maternal genome (see ref. 430 for further references), with the sequential activation and use of components from the oocyte (431). In mouse embryogenesis, DNA replication takes place over a 1- to $1\frac{1}{2}$-h period after the first cleavage division. Two bursts of putative transcription occur immediately before and after DNA replication, and translation products are detectable within 3 to 4 h (432). The entire first cell cycle, from cleavage to the two-cell stage in the mouse, the second round of DNA replication, and the loss of maternal mRNA are all regulated at a post-transcriptional level and are independent of the expression of the embryonic genome (432). A similar sequence of events appears to take place in the human zygote after fertilization, but the embryonic genome is not activated until the four- to eight-cell stage (433,434). In the mouse, the timing of development through this first two-cell stage is controlled by an event associated with sperm penetration rather than germinal vesicle breakdown (435). It is postulated that, after ovulation, development is controlled at two levels. An endogenous program, initiated by oocyte maturation, may regulate the "housekeeping" functions of the zygote, whereas sperm penetration activates a further endogenous program that initiates embryogenesis (435). Evidence that cytoskeletal organization is important is shown by the correlation between its disruption during oocyte aging and the ability of the mouse oocyte to be parthenogenetically activated (436,437). A correlation between the presence of atypical chromatin condensation in spontaneously ovulated oocytes at metaphase II and the level of embryonic death has been observed in rats. This was exacerbated by postovulatory aging of the oocytes (438).

In *in vitro* culture under certain conditions, zygote development blocks at different stages, and this block may be correlated with the change in transcription of the maternal to the embryonic genome (439). *In vitro* cultured mouse embryos grow more slowly, do not develop endoderm or typical abembryonic trophoblast cells, and have reduced DNA polymerase activity compared with *in vivo* grown embryos of the same age (440). This confirms the importance of the oviductal environment for development, at least in the mouse. Transcripts for β-hCG first appear at the eight-cell stage and seem correlated with transcription of the embryonic genome (441), whereas transcripts for different growth factors, platelet-derived growth factor, and transforming growth factor (TGF) -α and -β occur later (442). Transcription of both maternal and paternal contributions to the embryonic genome are important for normal embryonic development. Failure to express the paternal genome leads to defective trophoblast growth and that of the maternal genome can permit trophoblastic growth with embryonic failure (443). Clinically, the latter could result in the condition of hydatidiform mole.

The early one-cell mouse zygote requires pyruvate or oxaloacetate as an energy source; at the two-cell stage, it can also use phosphoenolpyruvate and lactate, and it is only at the eight-cell stage that glucose can be used (see ref. 444 for further references). Thus, the mouse embryo is very dependent on the correct composition of the culture medium for *in vitro* development. The presence of the growth factors, epidermal growth factor and TGF-α or TGF-β_1, in the culture medium promotes mouse embryonic development between the eight-cell and blastocyst stages and increases the rate of hatching (445). Osteonectin, an acid protein rich in cysteine, possibly involved in basement membrane formation and cell migration, appears at the blastocyst stage in the inner cell mass (446). Addition of PAF to the culture medium has been claimed to stimulate cell division in mouse embryos (resulting in blastocysts with more cells than untreated embryos) (447), increase oxidative metabolism of energy substrates (448), promote trophoblastic outgrowth (449), and give rise to an improved implantation rate on retransfer of treated embryos (447). Supplementation of the culture medium with PAF has also been claimed to improve the pregnancy rate in a human *in vitro* fertilization embryo transfer program (450). Such an effect may be mediated through PAF receptors, which, at least in the rabbit, have been shown to be present on the cells of the embryoblast just before implantation (216,451). Also, PAF has been reported to be secreted from early-stage embryos of a variety of species (452), and the presence of this secretion is correlated, at least partially, with the likelihood of that embryo giving rise to pregnancy (453). Although the secretion of PAF or a PAF-like substance by zygotes of different species seems established, the beneficial effect of its addition to cultured embryos awaits confirmation by others.

In the human, a variety of different media, ranging from simple to complex (e.g., Krebs-Ringer bicarbonate, Ham's F10, Earle's, Modified Whitten's, Whittingham's modified, Tyrode's, and Menezeo's B2) have all been used by *in vitro* fertilization programs (311,341,454–457). Many of these media are then supplemented with a serum source, either fetal cord serum or heat-inactivated serum from the ovum donor. Serum can, however, apparently be eliminated, and the bovine serum albumin can be replaced with human serum albumin, with no effect on cleavage *in vitro* or on subsequent survival *in vivo* of *in vitro*-fertilized human ova (456). Thus, it seems that the human zygote is much less dependent on a critical composition of the surrounding medium either *in vivo* or *in vitro* than are those of the mouse and other species.

In vitro-cultured human zygotes reach the one-cell (pronuclear) stage at 12 to 31 h after insemination, the two-cell stage between 27 and 43 h, the four-cell stage between 36 and 65 h, the eight-cell stage between 45 and 73 h, and the 16-cell stage between 68 and 85 h (311). Compaction of the blastomeres occurs between 96 and 120 h at the morula stage of 32 cells, and a blastocoele is visible between 120 and 144 h. Fully expanded blastocysts and those hatched from the zona pellucida have been observed at 140 to 160 h after *in vitro* insemination (311).

The many reports of successful human pregnancies after intrauterine deposition of oocytes fertilized *in vitro* and at an early stage of development confirm that oviductal secretions are not essential for ovum development (311,341,457). However, a higher rate of blastocyst formation has been seen in human embryos cultured in the presence of epithelial cells derived from the ampullar region of the oviduct from women undergoing elective hysterectomy than in control embryos cultured in the presence of serum (458). The percentage of embryos hatching was not different (458), and ultrastructurally both groups of embryos were similar (459). This evidence suggests that some factors secreted by oviductal cells may be beneficial, perhaps only under less than optimal conditions, for embryonic growth. It is certain that oocytes and zygotes of several species take up substances from the oviductal fluid. A 215-kDa glycoprotein is taken up from the ampullary fluid and sequestered in the perivitelline space of mouse embryos. This uptake is specific, as serum albumin is not similarly sequestered (460). In the hamster, glycoconjugates containing terminal *N*-acetyl-*C*-galactosamine residues are secreted by the oviductal isthmic epithelial secretory cells and become associated with the matrix of the zona pellucida during ovum transport. It is suggested that these glycoproteins are a source of zona components (461–463). Similarly, in pigs, the presence in zona pellucida of oocytes of two glycoproteins, 250 and 90 kDa, of oviductal fluid was detected. At the two- to four-cell stage, additional oviductal glycoproteins of 150, 57, 50, and 25 kDa were detected on the zona (464). In sheep, a 92-kDa glycoprotein secreted by the oviductal ampullar but not isthmic epithelium has been found to cover the surface of the zona pellucida and also on the blastomere membranes but not inside the blastomeres (465). The function of these different proteins that bind to the zona is not known, but their presence substantiates the belief that oviductal secretions can be important for embryonic growth and development. In the human, oviductal secretions may, as noted above, be important for sperm transport and maintenance of sperm viability. Their role in ovum transport is questionable. Even if their importance in sperm transport may be overstated, as in experiments in which the isthmic region of the oviduct is resected, fertilization and early cleavage of the zygotes proceed normally. The only abnormality seen is an increased incidence of polyspermy, presumably caused by the loss of filtering function of the isthmus (466,467).

Zygote Factors

Simmen and Simmen (468) reviewed the evidence for the potential role of peptide growth factors and protooncogenes in mammalian conceptus development and implantation. They summarized the available information through 1990 in tabular form, and this is reproduced here as Table 3. Many of the documented interactions are concerned with the uterus and the time of implantation and thus are relevant only after the embryo has reached the uterus. However, there is clear evidence that heparin-binding growth factors, TGF-α and -β, insulin-like growth factors (IGF)-1 and -2, IGF binding proteins, platelet-derived growth factor, and epidermal growth factor are all involved in early embryogenesis. The conclusion drawn by Simmen and Simmen (468) at the time of writing was that, although growth factors are regulators of cellular proliferation, differentiation, and invasiveness, there is no direct evidence for their involvement in embryogenesis. However, Paria and Dey (445) had already shown that epidermal growth factor and TGF-α or -β_1 promoted mouse embryonic growth to the blastocyst stage and promoted hatching *in vitro.* It has now been shown that IGF-1 also stimulates growth of mouse embryos in culture, causing an increase in the number of cells in the inner cell mass but not those of the trophectoderm (502). Insulin itself had already been reported to stimulate metabolism and growth of mouse embryos via receptors present from the eight-cell stage (503–506), and the related growth factor, IGF-1, also stimulates embryonic metabolism (442). mRNA for IGF-1 is present in the mouse embryo (442), as is that for TGF-β_1 at a later stage, but not those for TGF-β_2 or activin β_A, which are expressed only in the decidua. mRNAs for activin β_B and inhibin α were not detected in either embryo or decidua (507). In bovine embryos, transcripts for TGF-α and PDGF-A are detectable at all stages from one-cell to blastocyst as in the mouse. However, transcripts for TGF-β_2 and IGF-2 and receptors for PDGF-α, insulin, IGF-1, and IGF-2 are also detectable during this same period in the cow (508). It was suggested that these transcripts were products of both the maternal and embryonic genome, unlike the situation in the mouse, in which they were products of only the embryonic genome. In the bovine, products of the maternal genome alone (i.e., basic FGF and bovine trophoblast protein) were detected only up to the eight-cell stage, and transcripts for epidermal growth factor and nerve growth factor were not detected at any stage (508). Similarly, in human embryos, TGFα and IGF-2 were detected at the morular stage and could possibly be involved in the transformation from morula to blastocyst. Earlier-stage embryos were not examined (509). Thus, there is abundant evidence for the presence of a variety of growth factors being expressed at different stages of embryonic development and for the presence of growth factor receptors and expressed peptides, and there is even limited evidence for a physiologic role for such factors in embryonic growth and development.

TABLE 3. *Molecular aspects of implantation and potential involvement of peptide growth factors*[a]

	HBGFs	TGF-βs	TGF-α	IGF-1	IGF-2	IGFBPs	PDGF	CSF-I	EGF	References
Early embryogenesis	X	X	X	X	X	X	X			442,445,469–475
Trophoblast growth	X	X	X	X	X	X	X	X	X	476–485
Endometrial cell proliferation, differentiation, turnover	X	X	X	X	X	X			X	480,485,486–491
Modulation of extracellular matrix	X	X								485,492
Conceptus invasiveness					X	X	X			476,478,481
Blood island formation	X									493
Angiogenesis	X		X						X	494–496
Cell migration	X	X					X			497
Cell adhesion	X	X					X			498
Regulation of steroidogenesis	X			X		X				499,500
Protection of fetal allograft		X						X		480,485
Stromal–epithelial interactions		X		X					X	485,486,489,501

From ref. 468, with permission.
[a] X represents postulated functions for the indicated growth factors.

Embryos of different stages have been reported to contain or release other substances, such as steroids, histamine, and PGs, which could all potentially affect the activity of the oviductal musculature. Synthesis of both estrogens and progesterone by mouse embryos (510,511) and estrogens by rabbit (512,513), pig (514), donkey and horse (515), and cow (516) embryos has been reported. However, all these experiments were conducted with late (morula or blastocyst) stages of embryo development, when the embryos would be in the uterus and not the oviduct. Thus, such steroid production is more likely to be associated with uterine spacing, orientation, and implantation than with oviductal transport. Steroid production by earlier-stage embryos may occur, but its detection may be difficult because of the small amounts of protein in such embryos.

Similarly, rabbit blastocysts can synthesize histamine (517) and possess histamine receptors (518). Blastocysts of a variety of species can synthesize PGs (519–532), and at least in the rabbit, there is evidence for PG storage and programed release (533,534). Here again, the blastocyst PGs would appear to be more likely involved in the implantation process. PAF is another lipid but one that has been detected as being secreted from oviductal-stage embryos of mice, sheep, and humans (452,453,535–537), although others have questioned this (538,539). It has been claimed that embryonic PAF is essential for the establishment of pregnancy, because in the mouse, blockade of embryonic PAF but not endometrial receptors by PAF antagonists prevents implantation (449). It is a fact that rabbit blastocysts possess receptors for PAF (216,451), but whether this is true for earlier-stage embryos is not known. Also, PAF receptors have also been described in rabbit oviductal tissue, with significant differences being observed in ampullar binding affinity and isthmic binding capacity between days 3 and 6 of pregnancy, when embryos would be in the oviduct and uterus, respectively (540). PAF is known to induce vascular permeability changes and to cause contraction of smooth muscle (203,541), and thus embryo-derived PAF could conceivably be a factor regulating oviductal function. No studies on the effect of PAF on oviductal transport of zygotes have been reported.

In summary, however, the question remains whether any of the above factors, which certainly act on the embryo, are also acting on the oviductal regulatory systems. At present, there is no good evidence in this regard.

PHYSIOLOGIC CONTROL MECHANISMS

When considering mechanisms that control the function of the oviduct and consequently the transportation of ova and zygotes, it is necessary to consider the contractility of the smooth musculature, the activity of the cilia, and the flow of oviductal secretion. Each of these topics and factors that may influence them are discussed in this section. The nature and extent of oviductal secretions have already been described in the section entitled *Sperm Transport Through the Oviduct.* It was noted that, owing to the larger diameter of the lumen and the thin expandable wall of the ampulla, more secretion remains in the ampulla than in the isthmus, and thus ampullar secretion tends to be more watery.

Steroid Hormones

It is known that receptors for steroid hormones are present in oviductal tissue (542–546) and that steroid concentrations in oviductal tissue are higher than in peripheral plasma (547,548). Both estradiol and progesterone receptor concentrations are highest in the proliferative phase of the cycle (544,549,550). Progesterone binding sites are similar in isthmus and myometrium during follicular, ovulatory, and luteal phases of the cycle, whereas ampullar receptor concentrations are always higher. In all tissues examined during the luteal phase, there was a negative correlation between cytoplasmic but not nuclear receptor levels and plasma progesterone levels (549,550). Estrogen receptors were always higher in the ampulla than in the isthmus (550). Autoradiographic study of localization of both estradiol and progesterone receptors in the ampulla of the human oviduct showed that the epithelial cell binding was always greater than that of the underlying cells, irrespective of the stage of the cycle. Binding of both steroids was much higher during the proliferative than during the secretory phase and was inversely related to serum hormone levels (551). This is in contrast to an earlier report that claimed there was no difference in staining intensity for the estrogen receptor between different parts of the oviduct and only minimal changes during the cycle (552).

In ovariectomized monkeys, all specific estrogen receptor localization in the oviduct was nuclear, but after 14 days' estradiol treatment, higher levels of localization were seen in both cytoplasm and nucleus; a further 14 days' treatment with combined estradiol and progesterone down-regulated receptor levels (553). In ovariectomized rabbits, estradiol treatment differentially regulated progesterone receptor immunoreactivity in the oviduct, increasing it in the stroma and myosalpinx but not in the epithelium of the ampulla and decreasing it in the epithelium of the isthmus (554). Thus, it is clear that there are steroid hormone receptors in the oviduct and that their concentrations and localization can be regulated by hormonal levels.

It is still not certain that the known actions of estrogens and progestins on gamete transport (555–558) are caused by transduction by a receptor-activated mechanism. Several studies have attempted to look at this question directly. The administration to rabbits of clomiphene, an antiestrogen with mixed antagonistic/agonistic properties, accelerated ovum transport and caused changes in nuclear estrogen receptor concentrations. At 24 h after mating, there was a correlation between increased estrogen receptor in the isthmus and a decline in the ampulla and the ampullar-isthmic junction in untreated animals. Isthmic binding then remained constant up to 144 h. Clomiphene treatment decreased isthmic estrogen receptor concentrations, and this was thought to permit the accelerated transport (559). Another study in rabbits, with tamoxifen, a more potent antiestrogen, showed an increase in ampullar cytosolic estrogen receptor up to 34 h, followed by a decline at 48 h. Nuclear receptor levels were not examined (560). In rats, the situation was different. Examination of the temporal relationships between ovum transport and nuclear concentration of oviductal steroid receptor concentrations showed that there was no correlation between plasma hormone levels and tissue nuclear receptor concentrations. Indeed, differences between the rate of ovum transport in pregnant compared with nonpregnant animals occurred during a time of declining oviductal receptor concentrations. Some evidence was obtained to show that there was a transitory increase in oviductal nuclear estrogen receptors in pregnant rats at the time of entry of the zygotes into the uterus (561). Owing to the small size of the rat oviduct, differentiation between different regions could not be made. Furthermore, when accelerated zygote transport was induced by estrogen administration, although the magnitude of the acceleration was positively correlated with the duration of the increase in plasma estradiol levels, this was not accompanied by alterations in tissue levels of the steroid (562). This action of estrogen on ovum transport could be blocked by progesterone treatment, which downregulated the estrogen receptor concentration, an effect mediated by progesterone receptors (563). Although a subcutaneous injection of estradiol can accelerate ovum transport in rats, a short intravenous infusion cannot, and this is because the infusion stimulates an increased secretion of adrenal progesterone, which, like exogenous progesterone, blunts the response to estrogen (564). In pigs, it has, however, been claimed that there is a correlation between changes in estradiol and progesterone levels and oviductal steroid receptor levels (565). Although, clearly, physiologic plasma levels of steroidal hormones exert actions on the oviduct transduced by appropriate receptors, which control many of its functions, the correlation between plasma and tissue levels of hormone or receptor concentration is not that explicit, which suggests that some paracrine interaction between the zygote and the oviductal epithelium may directly regulate the rate of passage through the oviduct.

Many reports in the older literature demonstrate that pharmacologic doses of hormones can affect ovum transport (555–558), but whether these are solely receptor-mediated events is not known. Most such studies have dealt with a variety of laboratory rodents, and the exact effects of estrogens and progestins on the human oviduct are not known. An emergency postcoital contraceptive treatment based on the administration of estrogen (diethylstilbestrol or ethinyl estradiol) (566,567) or a combination of ethinyl estradiol and *dl*-norgestrel (568) is known to prevent pregnancy reliably, provided that treatment is started within 72 h of the unprotected coitus. As the first 72 h after ovulation is the time when ovum transport is occurring, this suggests that estrogens interfere with ovum transport in the same manner as in animals, although whether this is by acceleration into the uterus or retardation in the oviduct is not known. Given the propensity for ectopic pregnancies in the human (253), it seems probable that these steroid treatments cause accelerated transport, because ectopic pregnancy rates are unchanged (although one ectopic pregnancy has been recorded in a woman taking ethinylestradiol-levonorgestrel) (569); these treatments must also accelerate the zygote out of the uterus, or else an intrauterine pregnancy would occur. However, *large* doses of estrogen given during the period of ovum transport can cause an increased incidence of ectopic pregnancies (570,571).

The closest approximation that can be achieved with regard to examining the effects of progestins on the human oviduct is provided by studies in which megestrol acetate was given continuously from an implant, thus causing delayed transport of ovum surrogates (572). In women using such implants for contraception, there was a significant increase in the incidence of ectopic pregnancy (573). Again, this is a result dissimilar to that seen in nonprimates, but the dosing schedule also differed significantly. Continuous low-dose progestins given for oral contraception similarly increase the incidence of ectopic pregnancy (574). These findings definitely imply that progesterone may delay zygote transport in humans. However, a correlation between low serum progesterone levels and incidence of tubal pregnancies has also been noted (575). Low serum progesterone levels are correlated with reduced myoelectrical activity of the oviduct, possibly leading to weak propulsive forces and a greater chance of ectopic pregnancy (576). Lavy and DeCherney (577) argued that either a high estrogenic or progestational environment predisposes to an increased risk of ectopic pregnancy. Thus, an appropriate balance between these opposing hormonal effects or the absence of estrogenic action rather than presence of progestational effect may be a key factor in the etiology of this condition. Support for this latter suggestion is provided by experiments in rats, in which administration of 4-hydroxyandrostenedione, an aromatase inhibitor, reduced estrogen levels without affecting those of progesterone, and caused trapping of the zygotes in the oviduct (578). Conversely, treatment of rats with the antiprogestin, RU 486, had little effect on the rate of ovum transport (579,580). Similarly, reduction of progesterone secretion by cadmium treatment of rats also failed to alter ovum transport (581). These studies all emphasize the key role of estrogen rather than of progesterone in control of ovum transport in the rat. Such control mechanisms may be relevant to the human.

Experiments in rabbits have shown that in the absence of ovarian steroid hormones (e.g., after ovariectomy), ovum transport is extremely irregular, with many ova or ovum surrogates retained in the oviducts (582–584). In such animals, deprived of hormonal support, progesterone alone has little effect on transport of ovum surrogates (584), whereas estrogen alone causes either "locking" of ova in the oviduct or premature expulsion to the uterus, depending on dose and timing of administration relative to entry of ova into the oviducts (556,557, 583,584). Administration of constant combinations of estrogen and progesterone are not more successful in regularizing transport when compared with administration of each one alone (584,585). More normal results have been achieved in long-term ovariectomized animals by use of a regimen of decreasing estrogen and increasing progesterone treatments (586). In rabbits passively immunized with antibodies against estradiol beginning at 24 h before the ovulating injection, ova were trapped in the oviduct at 72 h, whereas if the injections began at 72 h before the hCG, then there was evidence for some degree of accelerated transport at 48 h (587). Administration of the antiestrogens centchroman and clomiphene during the period of ovum transport caused accelerated transport (559,560). Similarly, administration of centchroman to rats at 24 h after mating caused accelerated transport (588). Other experiments in rats have confirmed the hypothesis that estrogen can trap ova in the ampulla or accelerate them through the isthmus, depending on the dose and time of administration (556). Delayed transfers of microspheres showed that at about 34 h after ovulation, the ampullar-isthmic junction, which had permitted passage of the spheres, became closed and the spheres were retained in the ampulla. Estradiol treatment did not affect the opening and closing of the ampullar-isthmic junction but did cause rapid acceleration of microspheres in the isthmus to the uterus (589). This action of estradiol is a local, direct one on the oviduct (590).

In summary, the correct programming of ovum or zygote transport through the oviduct is very dependent on the support provided by the ovarian hormones estradiol and progesterone and, more importantly, on the secretion of these hormones in the correct balance during the first few days after ovulation. It is very probable that ovarian steroidal hormones do affect the human oviduct and can disrupt transport. It is still not clear whether these actions are wholly or partially regulated by hormone receptors in oviductal tissue. As muscular activity of the myosalpinx is certainly involved in regulation of ovum transport, study of nuclear concentrations of hormone receptors in the smooth-muscle cells would seem most relevant for resolving this issue. Such localization can be detected only by immunocytochemical or autoradiographic techniques, as tissue samples will be too small for conventional binding studies to give meaningful results for the different cell types and stages of the cycle. Thus, the studies reported have not proved especially illuminating in this regard.

Catecholamines

Many agents are known to stimulate or relax the musculature of the oviduct. These include the catecholamines, PGs, and peptides. Norepinephrine is the main catecholamine present in the sympathetic nerve endings of the oviduct (334,591,592). The oviduct is supplied with both "long" and "short" adrenergic neurons, and it is the short ones that are important in innervation of the oviductal smooth musculature (334). Both α- and β-adrenergic receptors in smooth musculature have been detected (593,594). The distribution of this innervation in the human oviduct has been described as follows: The thin muscle layer in the ampulla contains relatively few nerves, and these are mainly vasomotor fibers. In the isthmus, the innervation is greatly increased, especially the number of fibers supplying the circular muscle layer. The number of fluorescent nerves then decreases in the portion of the isthmus adjacent to the uterotubal junction and is further decreased in the intramural portion (334,595). In *in vitro* studies, norepinephrine contracts the longitudinal muscle layer of the isthmus, and this activity is particularly intense just before ovulation. The circular muscles contract only at ovulation; otherwise, they relax on administration of norepinephrine (334, 596). As β-adrenergic receptors predominate in the human oviduct throughout the cycle, it has been suggested that adrenergic stimulation would primarily cause relaxation (596). Both norepinephrine and isoproterenol have been reported to decrease the activity of both circular and longitudinal muscle layers of the human ampulla *in vitro* (597). Uptake of tritiated norepinephrine by the oviduct is much higher than by uterus but shows no cyclic variation (598). Adenosine stimulates the response of the human oviductal isthmus to nerve stimulation, especially in the proliferative phase of the cycle, but higher concentrations are inhibitory at all phases. Adenosine exhibits a prejunctional inhibition of norepinephrine release through A_1-receptors and modulates nerve-stimulated contractions through postjunctional effects on stimulatory A_1- and inhibitory A_2-receptors (599). Use of an adenosine antagonist enhanced nerve-stimulated contractile responses and norepinephrine release by human oviduct in both the proliferative and secretory phases (600). This was taken as evidence that endogenous purines were normally inhibiting the oviductal adrenergic system. No role for cholinergic nerves has been defined (596). However, cholinergic nerve fibers have been found in human oviductal musculature at all stages of pregnancy and also in the mucosa during later pregnancy (601). Similar fibers were found in rabbit oviduct, the greatest number being in the isthmus, with only a few in the ampulla. Under progestational influence, the numbers of fibers declined (602).

In cows, the responses of the oviductal circular and longitudinal muscles are mainly mediated by inhibitory β-adrenergic receptors, which mask the stimulatory actions of the α-adrenergic receptors. Thus, the adrenergic innervation of the cow oviduct may be to produce relaxation (603) as in the human (596). In pigs, both estrogen and progesterone, alone or in combination, greatly increased the norepinephrine content of the oviduct (604) but had only a modest effect on acetyl choline activity (605). Injection of immature rats with pregnant mare's serum gonadotropin to induce ovulation, although it reduced ovarian norepinephrine synthesis and content, reduced only synthesis but not content in the oviduct (606). In adult rats, oviductal norepinephrine concentrations are higher at estrus than at diestrus. Both estradiol and reserpine treatment reduced oviductal norepinephrine. The action of estradiol was considered to be due to increased use of norepinephrine. In contrast, although 5-hydroxytryptamine (5-HT) concentrations were also higher in the oviduct at estrus than at diestrus, they were unaffected by either estradiol or reserpine treatment (607).

In rabbits, because of the larger oviduct, information is available on the norepinephrine concentrations in the different regions. Norepinephrine concentrations are always higher in the ampulla than in the isthmus (592). In the ampulla and proximal isthmus (portion nearest the uterus), the norepinephrine concentration was unchanged during the time of ovum transport, but that in the distal isthmus adjacent to the ampullar-isthmic junction showed a sharp decline at 17 h after an ovulating injection. An estrogen treatment that causes "locking" of zygotes at the ampullar-isthmic junction significantly increased norepinephrine concentrations in the ampulla and distal isthmus, whereas a progesterone treatment that causes accelerated transport significantly decreased norepinephrine concentration in the distal isthmus. No specific measurements were made on the ampullar-isthmic junction region (592). A study of rabbit oviduct fluid showed that norepinephrine concentrations were always lower in ampullar than in isthmic fluid (302), which is inconsistent with the tissue concentrations (592). Fluid concentrations of all biogenic amines measured, norepinephrine, dopamine, and epinephrine, all declined between estrus and ovulation (302). When measurements of norepinephrine of the ampullar-isthmic junction were made, it was found that a "tubal-locking" estrogen treatment increased norepinephrine content and decreased the length of electromyographic discharges but increased their frequency. α-Adrenergic blockade significantly reduced electromyographic activity, whereas β-adrenergic blockade was without effect (608). These authors considered adrenergic innervation to play a significant role in oviductal motility. An earlier study by the same group had found no change in norepinephrine content in any region of the oviduct using the same estrogenic treatment and had concluded that "estrogen-induced 'tube locking' of ova was not mediated through the noradrenergic processes" (609).

Some of the above results could be considered evidence for the existence of a noradrenergically regulated isthmic sphincter that would retain the zygotes in the oviduct for the necessary 2 to 3 days after ovulation. However, destruction of these neurons, either by a chemical agent (6-hydroxydopamine) or by surgical denervation, had little disruptive effect on ovum transport in rabbits (610). An alternative approach has been to deplete endogenous stores of norepinephrine with reserpine or to increase them with iproniazid, an inhibitor of monoamine oxidase. Such treatments in rabbits were again ineffective in disrupting transport (611). α-Adrenergic blockade by phenoxybenzamine (612,613), as well as β-adrenergic blockade with propranolol (613), similarly had little effect on transport, although electromyographic activity was reduced by α-adrenergic blockade (608). When the parameter examined was fertility rather than ovum transport, neither reserpine in rabbits nor 6-hydroxydopamine in mice affected the number of live young born (614,615).

It must be concluded that, despite the extensive innervation of the isthmic region of the oviduct, the adrenergic system is not a primary control pathway for modulation of ovum transport. However, it clearly modulates activity of the smooth-muscle layers, and where oviductal function is disrupted because of hydrosalpinx, besides the mucosal changes, adrenergic innervation of the oviduct is greatly reduced (616). Finally, the oviduct is only sparsely innervated by cholinergic fibers, and the parasympathetic system probably plays little role in regulation of ovum transport (253,596,617).

Prostaglandins

Prostaglandin concentrations in oviductal tissue have been shown to vary with the stage of pregnancy in rabbits (618,619) and in hamsters (620). Prostaglandins have also been identified by immunohistology in human oviducts (621) and in oviductal tissue extracts subjected to thin-layer chromatography (622). In these latter experiments, it was suggested that, although $PGF_{2\alpha}$ was consistently found in the isthmic extracts, the ampullar extracts contained mainly only PGE_1. Such regional differences in PG content were not seen in rabbits (618,619) and, in view of the relatively insensitive methods used, may not be correct in the human. Direct measurements by radioimmunoassay of human oviductal tissue concentrations showed that both PGF and PGE decreased from the fimbria to the uterotubal junction. Luteal phase levels of both PGs were about twice those of the follicular phase (623). Oviductal fluid levels of $PGF_{2\alpha}$ rose rapidly after ovulation in the rabbit, and the ratio of $PGF_{2\alpha}/PGE_2$ was 3.7:1 within 24 h of the ovulating injection (624). Ampullar segments of rabbit oviducts removed 24 h after an ovulating injection and suspended *in vitro* released both PGF and PGE into the medium, with a ratio of 1.2:1. Removal of the endosalpinx stimulated release of both PGs, PGF more than PGE (ratio 1.7:1). This stimulated release was inhibited by blockade of PG synthesis (625). Similar results were obtained with isthmic segments (626). It was concluded that spontaneous activity of the smooth muscle might result from PGs produced by the myosalpinx acting on internally or externally directed membrane receptors on these smooth-muscle cells to initiate electrical or mechanical activity (625,626). In isthmic oviductal segments taken from estrous animals, secretion of PGE was not changed by increasing tension in either a circular or longitudinal orientation, but that of PGF was increased significantly by increasing tension in the circular but not in the longitudinal orientation (627). This led to the suggestion that distension of the isthmus *in vivo* could give rise to increased PGF release, which might be important for ovum transport. However, cyclooxygenase is localized only to secretory cells of the oviductal epithelium (628), which could account for the appearance of PGs in oviductal fluid but is not consistent with PG production by the myosalpinx. In the rabbit, significant uptake of radiolabeled PGs by embryos was seen only from day 5 onward, a time when the blastocysts would be in the uterus (629). No uptake of PGE_2 by mouse oviducts was seen under conditions in which significant uterine accumulation occurred (630). The function of this secretion of PGs is not known.

Despite the variations in PG concentrations seen in different portions of the oviduct—ampulla and isthmus—and changing secretion, it is difficult to relate these changes to regulation of ovum transport. Measurements of tissue but not of levels of PGs secreted are subject to artifact (631), which complicates interpretation of the results. However, it is known that PGF- and PGE-series PGs can have differing effects on oviductal musculature *in vitro* and *in vivo*. In the human, PGE_1 and PGE_2 relax the circular muscle layers of the isthmus *in vitro* but contract the longitudinal muscle. $PGF_{2\alpha}$ causes a powerful stimulation of both these muscular layers (597,632). In contrast, PGI_2 has only a weak stimulatory effect on both layers (633). That these differences are not just artifacts of the recording technique has been shown in later experiments, as a high degree of agreement between electrical and mechanical signals was observed (634). Indeed, these differing responses have been used as the basis for a bioassay for detection of these three PGs, or mixtures thereof (635). *In vitro* studies of muscular activity of human oviducts showed the presence of spontaneous prepotentials followed by slow waves that triggered contraction of the tissue. These slow waves were inhibited by PGE_2 and enhanced by $PGF_{2\alpha}$. The ampulla was most sensitive to actions of PGE_2 at ovulation, whereas the isthmus was most sensitive to the actions of $PGF_{2\alpha}$ during the luteal phase (636). Cyclic AMP may act as a second messenger mediating the actions of PGs, because they increase adenylyl cyclase in human oviduct. The greatest response is to PGE_1, but this shows a regional variation, being greater in the ampulla and lower in the isthmus. No such regional difference in response is seen for $PGF_{2\alpha}$ (637).

In vivo recording poses many more problems than the *in vitro* system because it usually entails placing the recording device into the lumen of the oviduct, thus possibly altering the system response as a result of the foreign body. Nonetheless, some idea of the integrated activity of the system can be obtained by use of intraluminal balloons or open-ended catheters. Limited studies in the human have shown that intravenous or topical administration of PGE_2 is inhibitory and that $PGF_{2\alpha}$, administered similarly, stimulates oviductal contractility (638). More extensive *in vivo* studies can be performed only in experimental animals, such as the rabbit. In this species, it was found that intravenous $PGF_{1\alpha}$ and $PGF_{2\alpha}$ increased spontaneous oviductal activity, whereas PGE_1 and PGE_2 suppressed it (639). Injection of high doses of PGEs often caused an initial contraction, which was then followed by relaxation (639). This had previously been reported also in sheep (640). In the rabbit, the actions of one series of PGs can counteract the actions of the other series, but the second PG must be administered intravenously at least 2 min after the first one (641). Similarly, a stimulation of activity caused by norepinephrine can be suppressed by PGEs, and the relaxation induced by β-stimulation (isoproterenol) can be overcome by PGFs (641). However, the actions of the PGs cannot be mediated through the adrenergic system, because the PGs still exert their characteristic effects in the face of α- or β-adrenergic blockade (641). Subcutaneous administration of the PGs produced qualitatively similar results but with a longer period of action than by the intravenous route (639). Also, limited data are available from studies in rhesus monkeys. Intravenous administration of PGEs had little effect on spontaneous activity during the preovulatory period, but some suppression of bursts of activity after ovulation was seen. Prostaglandin $F_{2\alpha}$ caused an increase in amplitude of contractions only just before ovulation (642).

Thus, there is considerable evidence, obtained from several species, that oviductal tissue contains PGs and is sensitive to their actions. It is tempting to hypothesize that the balance between the PGEs and PGFs could provide a control mechanism for the activity of the smooth musculature. If this is the case, one would expect to find distinct binding sites for $PGF_{2\alpha}$ and for PGE_2. Preparations of single smooth-muscle cells have been made from ampulla and distal and proximal isthmic segments from rabbits at different times after an ovulating injection or mating. The binding affinity (equilibrium dissociation constant) for $PGF_{2\alpha}$ was 0.19 nM; that for PGE_2 was 0.55 nM (643). These affinities did not differ at different stages of pregnancy or pseudopregnancy, but the actual number of binding sites/cell was changed (644). The numbers of PGE_2-binding sites measured increases in the distal isthmus at 48 h and in the proximal isthmus at 48 and 72 h after the ovulating injection. The concentration of $PGF_{2\alpha}$-binding sites is high in the distal isthmus up to 48 h and then falls, whereas that in the proximal isthmus does not change between the estrous and 72-h pregnant or pseudopregnant condition (643,644). Furthermore, uptake of radiolabeled calcium [^{45}Ca] was increased when such cells were exposed to 1 nM $PGF_{2\alpha}$ but was decreased after exposure to 1 nM PGE_2. Calcium uptake by the smooth-muscle cells thus paralleled the contractile activity (645). There was no correlation between the numbers of binding sites and oviductal PG concentrations measured previously. However, given the generally relaxing properties of E series and contracting properties of F series PGs, these changes in PG-binding sites in rabbit oviduct would fit with the notion of a progressive relaxation of the isthmic region from the ampullar-isthmic junction to the uterotubal junction during the 24-h period before the zygotes enter the uterus around 72 h after the ovulating stimulus. In contrast, in horses, more PGE_2 bound to the ampulla than to the isthmus and was not different on days 2 and 5 after ovulation (646) [the embryos enter the uterus on day 5 to 6 (403,407)]. Binding of $PGF_{2\alpha}$ was not examined in this study (646). Thus, in this species, although it has been suggested that embryo-derived PGE_2 acts via such receptors to regulate their transport (412), the lack of change in isthmic binding capacity with time after ovulation raises a question about such an interpretation, even though pharmacologic doses of PGE_2 can accelerate embryo transport (413).

Another paradigm that has been used to study the role of PGs as regulators of ovum transport has involved the use of inhibitors of PG synthesis in an attempt to disrupt the transport process. Treatment of rabbits with a variety of inhibitors of PG synthesis, release, or metabolism during the first 24 h after ovulation had only modest effects on the rate of ovum transport, the most effective compound being benzydamine, an inhibitor of thromboxane synthesis; classical inhibitors of cyclooxygenase (e.g., indomethacin and sodium meclofenamate) were without effect (647). No greater effect was seen if reserpine treatment to deplete catecholamines and sodium meclofenamate treatment to deplete PGs were combined (647). Indomethacin treatment was similarly ineffective in hamsters (620). In other experiments in rabbits in which indomethacin was given 11 times during the period of ovum transport, no effect on numbers of implantations was seen (648). The effect on ovum transport in rabbits of a continuous intrauterine infusion of indomethacin or lonazolac, an inhibitor of the key enzyme 15-hydroxy PG dehydrogenase that metabolizes PGs to less active metabolites, thus reducing or increasing PG levels, respectively, has been studied. These infusions began between 60 and 72 h before the ovulating injection and continued up to the time of autopsy at 28 or 52 h after the ovulating injection. Up to 52 h, no acceleration of zygotes to the uterus was seen, but at this time, compared with controls, significantly more zygotes were in the isthmus than in the ampulla. No effect of infusion of lonazolac was detected (649). Field-stimulated contractions of the rabbit isthmus *in vitro* are decreased by PGE_2 and increased by indomethacin, and this was positively correlated with changes in norepinephrine release (650). This again emphasizes the connection between PGs and the adrenergic control of oviductal function. However, taken together, the effect of blockade of PG synthesis on ovum transport has not been impressive. This failure may have several explanations. First, suppression of the cyclooxygenase enzyme will usually inhibit production of all PGE, PGF, and PGI series equally. Thus, if a particular ratio of PGE_2 to $PGF_{2\alpha}$ is important, this may not be altered even though actual PG concentrations may be depressed. Second, indomethacin suppresses mainly cyclooxygenase, and if eicosanoids produced via the lipoxygenase pathway (e.g., leukotrienes, HETES, or lipoxins) are important, in most experiments these would have been little affected. Last, although PGs like the catecholamines can affect myosalpingeal activity, this may be only indirectly responsible for regulation of ovum transport.

Nevertheless, as noted above, there is evidence that embryo-derived PGs may regulate the transport of zygotes but not oocytes in rats and horses (412–416,646). Prostaglandin production by rabbit embryos has also been detected, commencing on day 4 after the ovulating stimulus—a time when they would not be in the oviduct (524,526,533). Examination of earlier-stage embryos for PG production has not been reported, and so whether zygote PGs play a role in this species is questionable. Investigations into the role of PGs on ovum transport have also examined the actions of exogenously administered PGs. In general, systemic administration of such

PGs as PGE_1, PGE_2, and $PGF_{2\alpha}$ has not been very effective (see ref. 642 for further references), perhaps because of rapid metabolism (651–653), except when given in large pharmacologic doses (642). When effects were seen, they depended on the species, the time of administration relative to ovulation, and the dose; thus, generally, an acceleration of transport was seen with both PGE- and PGF-series compounds, but occasionally a delay of transport was recorded. More predictable effects were seen after intraperitoneal administration in hamsters when the PG could act directly on the oviduct. Prostaglandin $F_{2\alpha}$ usually caused accelerated transport (620), but even in these experiments, a luteolytic action on the corpora lutea of pregnancy was seen and a reduction of progesterone secretion may also have been implicated in the results observed. Even in the experiments in horses, in which a positive acceleration of transport was achieved with PGE_2, success was obtained only when PGE_2 was given by continuous oviductal infusion. Administration of PGE_2 by intramuscular or intraperitoneal injection or by a single intraoviductal infusion was without effect. This speaks to the need for continued exposure of the oviductal PG receptors to the PG and for adequate local concentration for a pharmacologic effect to be manifest. There seems a need to reexamine this whole question using local infusions of different PGs in a species such as the rabbit in which a large amount of background information on tissue concentrations, tissue secretion, receptor capacity, and effects of systemically administered PGs and their synthesis inhibitors is available.

In summary, there is some evidence to suggest that PGs may play some role in regulation of ovum transport, the best evidence being the changing binding capacity of the different regions of the oviduct, the occasional experiment showing altered transport resulting from administration of exogenous PGs or PG synthesis inhibitors, and the possibility of embryo PGs regulating their own transport. Nevertheless, there is more negative than positive information, and perhaps for the moment the verdict must be "not proven." Even though there is substantial evidence that there is a physiologic interaction between PG and adrenergic regulation, there are also experiments (641,647) reducing the importance of this connection.

Peptides

Peptidergic neurons have now been described in the female genital tract of a variety of species, including the cat, guinea pig, and rat (654). Vasoactive intestinal peptide, a 28-amino-acid peptide first isolated from porcine duodenum (655,656), has been identified by immunofluorescence in such nerves in uterus, cervix, and prostate (654). Moderate numbers of fine varicose fibers were found in the oviduct of the cat but not in that of the guinea pig or rat (654). In the human, a moderate number of VIP-containing nerves have been found in the isthmic region of the oviduct. These are localized primarily beneath the epithelium but also to a lesser extent in the lamina propria of the mucosa and the smooth musculature (657). This was confirmed in another study in which moderate reactivity was seen in epithelium and both circular and longitudinal muscle layers (658). In contrast, in a further immunocytochemical study, it was claimed that the VIP-containing nerves were especially concentrated in the circular muscle layer of the human oviduct (659). In none of these studies was any indication given if any cyclic variation occurred.

In vitro experiments with the isthmic region of the human oviduct showed that electrical field stimulation reduced the motor activity of the circular muscle layer. This effect was blocked by tetrodotoxin, suggesting neural involvement. It was deduced that VIP was the neural transmitter responsible for this inhibition of activity (660). Vasoactive intestinal peptide is also known to be a potent inhibitor of spontaneous motor activity of the isthmic region of the oviduct, the ED_{50} falling between 25 and 200 ng/ml in the bath fluid (661). Further studies revealed that there was good agreement between immunohistochemical and immunochemical measurements of VIP location and concentration, and VIP was found to inhibit spontaneous activity of the ampulla (both circular and longitudinal muscle layers) and of the isthmus (both circular and longitudinal muscle layers). The ED_{50} for inhibition of circular muscle activity of the isthmus was approximately 10^{-8} M (662). It was suggested that this peptidergic innervation might play a role in control of the sphincter function of the oviduct. To test this hypothesis, experiments were performed in which rabbits were given estrogen alone or in combination with progesterone, and the content of VIP in the oviducts was measured by radioimmunoassay (663). Estrogen treatment increased VIP, but addition of progesterone for the last 3 days of estrogen treatment returned VIP levels to control values. Reduction of both circular and longitudinal muscular spontaneous activity was seen in this species also, with ED_{50} values similar to those for the human (662,663). Levels of VIP have now been measured in human oviducts during the menstrual cycle. The concentration of VIP was about twice as high in the isthmus as in the ampulla in the follicular phase and about fivefold higher in the luteal phase. Concentrations in the ampulla did not vary throughout the cycle, whereas those in the isthmus were somewhat higher at ovulation and significantly higher in the luteal phase than in the follicular phase (664). Mean values in the isthmus ranged from about 1.5 to 3.7 pmol/g wet weight (664). Similar values have been recorded by others (659).

Vasoactive intestinal peptide acts through high-affinity membrane receptors in the uterus (665) and thus probably acts similarly in the oviduct. Activation of these receptors is thought to affect the calcium balance in the cell by causing calcium sequestration or extrusion and to inhibit generator potential, cause hyperpolarization, and increase membrane permeability to potassium (666). These events have been adduced as evidence that VIP is the nonadrenergic, noncholinergic neurotransmitter that causes relaxation of oviductal smooth muscle (667). The presence of such a neurotransmitter had been suggested previously (668). The sensitivity of this action on the putative sphincter in the isthmic region supports a role for VIP in control of ovum transport. It has been previously shown, using doughnut-shaped intraluminal pressure transducers, that the isthmic lumen of the rabbit oviduct is constricted after ovulation (669) and relaxes by 56 h after ovulation, a time when ova normally pass through this region (670).

These data provided significant evidence that VIP indeed could act as an important control mechanism for oviductal function. However, when rabbits were infused with VIP at a rate of 75 pmol/kg/min for 1 h at the time of the preovulatory progesterone surge (i.e., between 2 and 3 h after mating) or for 4 h at the time of ovulation (i.e., 9 to 13 h after mating), no effects on ovum transport were seen. Similarly, fertility was unaffected. This dose of VIP was sufficient to increase plasma progesterone levels, although its action on oviductal musculature was not studied (671). It is likely that the dose administered was not optimal, because *in vitro,* no effects on human oviductal musculature were seen at 10^{-10} M (663), and in previous experiments in the rabbit, only modest *in vivo* inhibition of isthmic motility had been observed at a dose of 7.5×10^{-11} M/kg/min (which equals 1 μg/min) (672). It may be that, like the PGs, VIP needs to be given locally to exert an observable effect.

The presence of other peptides in the oviduct has also been reported. Neuropeptide Y, a 36-amino-acid neuropeptide with a COOH-terminal tyrosine (673), has been described in the rat reproductive tract (674). Fluorescence immunocytochemistry revealed its presence in the ovary, oviduct, uterus, and cervix. The most prominent supply was found in the cervix (674). However, further work revealed that peptide Y immunoreactivity was found in nerve fibers around blood vessels and in the muscle layers of the human oviduct. A few fibers were connected to the isthmic epithelium, but the remaining ones were distributed in a pattern similar to that of adrenergic fibers (658,675–677). Further studies showed that it is unlikely that neuropeptide Y and norepinephrine are colocalized in the same nerves, because there is a discrepancy between the two types of histochemically identified fibers (595); however, in a separate study by the same group, it was claimed on the basis of sequential staining for dopamine β-hydroxylase and neuropeptide Y, combined with destruction of the noradrenergic neurons with 6-hydroxydopamine, that neuropeptide Y might indeed be stored in sympathetic nerves (678). Although the distribution of neuropeptide Y in the oviduct is similar to that of VIP and peptide histidine isoleucine (i.e., in the smooth-muscle layers and subepithelially), the former are the most numerous. Similar patterns of neuropeptide Y have been found in the oviducts of various other species (678,679).

Radioimmunoassay measurements showed that, in the oviducts of rat, mouse, and guinea pig, neuropeptide Y concentrations were always the highest among the peptides. In the rat and mouse, VIP was the next most abundant peptide, but in the guinea pig, large quantities of substance P were seen (680). Neuropeptide Y concentrations were similar in the ampulla and isthmus of the human oviduct, being about 40 pmol/g wet weight of tissue. Neuropeptide Y by itself had no effect on resting tension or on frequency and amplitude of spontaneous contractions of helical strips of human oviduct *in vitro* (676,677,681). Neuropeptide Y inhibited the adrenergic contractile response and [^{3}H]norepinephrine release to field stimulation in the longitudinal muscle layer of the isthmus. Similarly, neuropeptide Y inhibited norepinephrine release in response to field stimulation in the isthmus of both mature and immature rabbits (682). This suggests that the peptide acts through prejunctional adrenergic inhibition (675). However, it was also found that neuropeptide Y inhibited the effects of acetyl choline on helical strips of human oviduct (676,681). Although neuropeptide Y may be involved in regulation of blood flow in the genital tract, its functional significance for regulation of oviductal function is uncertain.

Very few enkephalin-immunoreactive nerve fibers have been found in the cat female reproductive tract, except in the region of the cervix (683). Neither met- nor leu-enkephalin had a stimulatory or inhibitory action on human ampullar or isthmic oviductal contractility (684). Similar findings were recorded in experiments using the same tissues from cats and rabbits. It was, however, observed that leu-enkephalin increased myometrial blood flow in cats (685). In rat and guinea pig, no met-enkephalin immunoreactivity was seen in oviductal tissue, but in pig oviduct, reactivity was seen in the muscular and submucosal layers (686). Assay of met-enkephalin in rabbit oviduct revealed the presence of small amounts, which were not different between the day of the ovulating stimulus or day 3 of pseudopregnancy (687). Leu-enkephalin inhibited norepinephrine release from rabbit oviduct induced by field stimulation (682). Thus, it may be concluded that although endogenous opioid peptides may be important in uterine function, they do not seem to be so in the oviduct.

Substance P was first described in 1931 (688) and identified as an undecapeptide in 1971 (689). Substance P-like immunoreactivity has been described in the female genitourinary tract of guinea pigs and cats but not in the rat. Although such fibers are frequent in the vagina, they are sparse in the uterus and oviducts (690). However, a later paper from the same group claimed that "nerves containing substance P were particularly numerous in the oviducts of both guinea pigs and rats, supplying the muscular wall and blood vessels" (678). Studies using radioimmunoassay showed that substance P was low in the mouse oviduct but relatively more abundant in that of the guinea pig. In this latter species, the concentrations in the uterus, oviduct, and ovary were similar, whereas in the mouse, the highest concentration was in the vagina. In these experiments, the stage of the estrous cycle was not stated (680). Modest immunoreactivity for substance P has been shown in all structures of the human oviduct with the exception of the epithelium (658). Both human and rabbit oviducts have been shown to be sensitive to the action of substance P. The ED_{50} for causing contraction in the human oviduct *in vitro* is only 57 nM (691,692). Further studies revealed that the stimulation of the human oviduct by substance P at a concentration of 10^{-6} M could be antagonized by addition of VIP at a concentration of 6×10^{-7} M (684). Such actions could be modulated through substance P-binding sites, but in the human oviduct, binding of radiolabeled ligand is apparently restricted to the vascular endothelium (693). Such findings are not consistent with the contractile activity of substance P on the oviduct, unless the contractions are caused indirectly by release of another neurotransmitter.

When radioimmunoassay measurements of substance P were made in different portions of the human oviduct, the concentrations were as follows: 3.09 ± 1.40, 1.08 ± 0.30, and 0.74 ± 0.30 pmol/g wet weight of tissue in the uterotubal junction, ampullar-isthmic junction, and ampulla, respectively (694). Both circular and longitudinal muscle preparations from the human ampullar-isthmic junction responded to substance P at 10^{-6} M, but at 10^{-7} M, the longitudinal muscle layer showed a greater stimulation than did the circular layer (694). Removal of calcium from the medium inhibited this stimulation, and VIP (10^{-7} M) significantly decreased the response (694). Substance P also increased uterine blood flow in the cat (685). This peptidergic system seems not to involve either the adrenergic or cholinergic nervous systems, as neither cholinergic nor adrenergic (α- or β-) blockade inhibited the responses of the oviduct to substance P or VIP (685,694).

There are sparse reports of other peptides that have been detected in oviductal tissue. Gastrin-releasing peptide (bombesin) was scarce in the oviducts of several species including humans (678) and localized mainly in the muscle layer, around blood vessels, and in the submucosa (695). Peptide histidine isoleucine was colocalized with VIP in nerve plexuses of the oviductal smooth muscle (678). Peptide histidine methionine was similarly localized (659). Neurotensin was found mainly in circular smooth muscle and the blood vessels of the oviduct (658) and exerted excitatory effects on helical strips of human oviduct, increasing resting tension, and amplitude and frequency of spontaneous contractions (696). Somatostatin immunoreactive nerve fibers have been detected in the mesosalpinx of the pig oviduct (679). Calcitonin gene-related peptide immunoreactive nerves are abundant in both the circular and longitudinal muscle layers of the human oviduct and also around blood vessels and in the submucosa (658,695). In pig oviducts, there was more angiotensin I converting enzyme (ACE) activity in the ampulla than in the isthmus, but the former did not vary during the cycle, whereas the latter was greater at estrus. Prostaglandin synthesis inhibitors had little effect on this activity. It was suggested that the low ACE activity in the isthmus could be responsible for the longer stimulatory effect of bradykinin on the isthmic than on the ampullar musculature. Alternatively, it was suggested that another carboxy-peptidase might be present in the isthmus but not in the ampulla (697).

It is clear that several peptides exert actions on the smooth musculature and blood supply of the oviduct. Information about many of them is insufficient to make any judgments about their regulatory role in oviductal function. However, it has been suggested that, in view of the opposing activities of VIP and substance P, these peptides could provide a peptidergic control mechanism (694). More work is necessary to prove this hypothesis.

Cyclic nucleotides have been thought to be involved in the control of smooth-muscle contractions. Increases in cyclic AMP have been associated with relaxation, whereas increases in cyclic GMP have been associated with contraction (698,699). In the oviduct, cyclic AMP levels are increased by PGE_2 and decreased by $PGF_{2\alpha}$ (700), which fits the general theory regarding cyclic nucleotides and contraction. Such changes could provide a mechanism for regulation of myogenic activity, but in the same series of experiments, it was found that altered tissue cyclic AMP levels were not essential for the actions of adrenergic agonists to be manifest on the oviduct (700). Furthermore, cyclic GMP levels were not decreased, nor were cyclic AMP levels increased, in the isthmic region of rabbit oviducts at 68 h after an ovulating injection and injection of a dose of estrogen that would normally decrease muscular activity. Levels of both cyclic nucleotides were, however, higher in the isthmus than in the ampulla (701).

Cyclic nucleotides are known to exert direct effects on oviducts *in vitro* (702). Dibutyryl cyclic AMP induces relaxation of the isthmus and ampulla in rabbits, guinea pigs, and humans. It also reduces the response to norepinephrine and $PGF_{2\alpha}$. Similarly, theophylline, a phosphodiesterase inhibitor, increases cyclic AMP levels in oviduct tissue and inhibits spontaneous and $PGF_{2\alpha}$-induced activity. Conversely, imidazole, an activator of phosphodiesterase, increases oviductal contractility. Last, in these same experiments, cyclic AMP concentration was found to decrease in the rabbit oviductal isthmus during the first 3 days after ovulation. PGE_2 restored these values to control levels and inhibited isthmic contractions. However, the cyclic AMP values recorded (702) were about five to six times lower than those found by others (701). Thus, whether the changes in cyclic nucleotides are directly responsible for changes in contractility or are simply associated with such changes is not clear. It seems unlikely that, in themselves, the cyclic nucleotides can provide the major control mechanism, although they may act as second messengers for transduction of agonists binding to cell membrane receptors (637).

Gamma-aminobutyric acid (GABA) is a major inhibitory neurotransmitter in the brain, and it has been found in higher concentrations in the oviduct than in the brain of the rat (703,704). When rat oviducts were autotransplanted, there was a much lower concentration of both GABA and the main enzyme involved in its biosynthesis, L-glutamate-1-decarboxylase (GAD), than in control oviducts. This was considered to be evidence for extrinsic GABAergic innervation of the oviduct, probably via the vagus nerve (705). Ovariectomy significantly reduces both GAD activity and GABA concentrations, and although GAD activity is restored by combined estradiol and progesterone treatment, GABA levels are unaffected by any steroid treatment (705–707). Furthermore, the concentration of GABA in rat oviducts does not change during the estrous cycle (708). The enzyme responsible for degradation of GABA is GABA-transaminase, which is mainly located extraneuronally in the epithelial cells of both ampulla and isthmus of the rat oviduct. The activity of this enzyme is changed significantly during pregnancy (709). Depending on whether it is in neural or nonneural tissue, GAD appears in two types; the enzyme in the oviduct is similar to that in brain neurons, and it was thus suggested that GABA in the rat oviduct seems to be synthesized using glutamic acid rather than putrescine as precursor and that these levels are not due to uptake of GABA from serum (710). These latter authors were unable to detect GABA binding to rat oviduct or to observe any effect on spontaneous or electrically stimulated muscular activity and indeed reported a preferential mucosal rather than muscular localization of GABA (710).

Similarly, GABA has been found in the human oviduct, and a single population of high-affinity binding sites has been identified (K_D = 40 nM; B_{max} = 690 fmol/mg protein; nonspecific binding < 20%) (711). In the rat oviduct, similar specific binding was observed (K_D = 52 nM), but the maximum binding site concentration was very low (B_{max} = 17 fmol/mg protein) and nonspecific binding was very high (~50%) (712). For this reason and because of the irreproducibility of the binding studies, others have concluded that GABA binding in this tissue is nonexistent or dependent on an uncontrolled critical variable (713). In the human oviduct, GABA levels are higher in the ampulla than in the isthmus (711,714), but binding capacity is greater in the isthmus and GABA can influence isthmic contractility (711). GABA increases the frequency and decreases the amplitude of spontaneous contractions in both circular and longitudinal layers of human ampulla *in vitro* (715). $GABA_B$ receptors were thought to be involved. *In vitro* studies with estrous rabbit oviducts also showed that high concentrations of GABA (10^{-5} M) increased contraction frequency and elevated basal tone in both longitudinal and circular muscle from ampulla and isthmus. This action was not inhibited by bicuculline, suggesting a $GABA_B$ receptor system. Neither α- nor β-adrenergic blockade inhibited the actions of GABA on the oviduct, thus eliminating involvement of the sympathetic nervous system (716). Further studies showed, however, that stimulus-evoked GABA efflux from rabbit oviduct differs from that of neuronal release (717) and that uptake of [^{3}H]GABA is localized to the oviductal epithelium (718). These findings are consistent with those reported for the rat (710). There is no information on the effects of GABA or of its inhibition on ovum transport, but given the questions regarding the presence of receptors on oviductal smooth muscle and the lack of effect on oviductal contractility except at pharmacologic doses, it seems unlikely that GABA is a major regulatory factor of oviductal function.

Oxytocin has been shown to stimulate oviductal contractility in sheep (719) and in the human (720). However, the stimulatory effect of oxytocin is maximal during menstruation and only minimal at ovulation. In contrast, vasopressin is more effective during the preovulatory period (720). In rats, binding sites for oxytocin have been observed in oviductal homogenates with an apparent K_D of 1.8×10^{-9} M. Binding capacity was 215 fmol/mg protein (721). In contrast, in rabbit oviduct, although low concentrations of binding sites for arginine vasopressin are present under all experimental conditions, sites for oxytocin are detected only after treatment with pharmacologic doses of estrogen (722). In sheep oviducts, however, oxytocin receptors were detected with a K_D of 1.7 nM. Binding capacity was highest at estrus (77.7 fmol/mg protein) and then fell after ovulation. The low binding seen in anestrous animals could be increased by estrogen and progesterone treatment (723). This binding was localized to the smooth-muscle layers of the isthmic region at estrus (724). High-affinity oxytocin receptors in the sheep oviduct were confined to the smooth-muscle layers of both ampulla and isthmus, and their concentration (about 50 pmol/mg protein) was also highest within 2 days of estrus (725,726) and was not detected at other stages of the cycle (726). When oxytocin was infused into the peripheral circulation of ewes in a pulsatile fashion, no significant relationships were observed between plasma concentrations of oxytocin and motility of the cervix or uterus. No observations were made on oviductal contractility in these studies (727). Oxytocin receptors have also been detected in human oviducts; although ampullar receptor concentration does not change during the cycle, receptor concentration is highest in the isthmus during the secretory phase (550). Immunoreactive arginine vasopressin and oxytocin are also greatest in the isthmic region of the human oviduct (728). Although oxytocin receptors have been demonstrated in the muscle layers of the oviduct, appear to be highest at the time of ovulation, and can be altered by hormonal treatment, there does not seem to be any very persuasive evidence that oxytocin regulates ovum transport. Furthermore, in the human, oviductal response to oxytocin is lowest at midcycle, which makes it unlikely that oxytocin is an important regulator of oviductal function.

Apart from the suggestion that VIP and substance P could form the basis for a peptidergic control system for the oviduct, based on the information available, even this hypothesis is not well substantiated but clearly is worthy of further investigation.

Contractility of the Smooth Musculature

The previous sections have identified at least three systems that exhibit positive and negative effects on oviductal contractility and that might be implicated as control systems: the adrenergic system, the PGs, and a peptidergic system (VIP and substance P). Which, if any, is the control system remains unclear, although they all affect contractility. It has always been assumed that change in contractility is the main factor promoting ovum transport to the uterus. Studies on the rapid phase of ovum transport through the ampullar region have certainly demonstrated that waves of contraction are correlated with the movement of the cumulus mass containing the ova (729,730). In the rabbit, the phase of ampullar transport is rapid (731), whereas in other species, such as the human or the rhesus monkey, it can take up to 24 h or longer (732,733). Ova usually pass into the uterus between 96 and 120 h after the LH peak in women, so that the actual total time of transport is about 80 h (734).

It may be that this progression toward the uterus is a result of intrinsic activity of the oviductal musculature. Talo and Brundin (735) devised a technique for recording, in detail, muscular activity of the rabbit oviduct. Spontaneous electrical activity and intraluminal pressure were simultaneously recorded *in vitro* by means of suction electrodes and perfusion at constant flow rates of 1.4, 2, or 5.8 μl/min. Suction electrodes were used to map electrical activity throughout the whole oviduct (736). Using such techniques, it has been reported that the electrical activity of the oviduct varies from that of other structures of the reproductive tract, at least in duration. The duration of bursts is short (a few seconds) and the contractions are of a short phasic type (331). The rabbit oviduct normally exhibits multipacemaker activity with shifting pacemaker location, being highest in the distal isthmus or at the ampullar-isthmic junction. In the isthmus and ampullar-isthmic junction of postovulatory rabbit oviducts, all regions can initiate electrical activity, but certain pacemaker regions may predominate statistically. The frequency of generation may vary in a short segment. Electrical activity often propagates in both directions but over shorter distances in the isthmus than in the ampulla. The speed of propagation is normally low, only a few millimeters per second, but reaches nearly 20 mm/sec in the isthmus of castrated, estrogen-treated rabbits (331). Microelectrodes and isometric tension-recording methods have been used to study the electrical and mechanical properties of longitudinal smooth-muscle cells of the isthmus of the rabbit oviduct. Estrogen treatment depolarized and progesterone treatment repolarized the muscle cell membranes and caused a decrease or an increase in spontaneous activity of the oviduct, respectively (737). Spontaneous burst discharges correlated well with spontaneous contractions. Field stimulation of isthmic preparations showed that the resulting contractions are mediated via the α-adrenergic system, as they are inhibited by the α_1-adrenergic antagonists prazosin and D2343 (738); the α_1- and α_2-adrenergic antagonist phentolamine (739); and PGE_2 acting via inhibition of norepinephrine release (650). Recording of oviductal motility using impedance plethysmography showed that mating caused a characteristic pattern (740). There was initial relaxation of both ampulla and isthmus, followed by increased isthmic motility up to 48 h after mating, and then a final phase with reduction of motility at 72 to 96 h to the basal level seen before mating. It was concluded that the increased isthmic motility acted to retard the transport of zygotes until 72 h, when the decreasing activity permitted their entry to the uterus. Administration of progesterone relaxed both segments of the oviduct and thus permitted accelerated transport (740). Similarly, in cows, in which oviductal motility was assessed by measuring changes in intraluminal diameter, increased frequency and amplitude of motility were seen 3 to 5 days before estrus; the patterns remained similar until they decreased about 3 to 5 days later, thus correlating with entry of ova into the uterus (741). In contrast, in cow oviducts *in vitro*, no difference in frequency of contractions was seen during the estrous cycle, and the adrenergic nerves involved in contraction were of the α_2 subtype, which were masked by the dilating action of the β_2 subtype (603). Taken together, these different studies suggest that the *in vivo* findings may be more relevant to the real physiologic situation.

The frequency of spontaneous contractions of the guinea pig oviduct *in vitro* was higher at estrus than in other phases of the cycle, and these contractions were correlated with the rate of oxidative but not of glycolytic metabolism (742). Also, it was suggested that potassium channels, regulated by intracellular calcium concentrations, were involved in the generation of bursts of action potentials associated with spontaneous activity of the guinea pig oviduct (743). In the human, it was also found that potassium-induced stimulation of both circular and longitudinal muscle layers of the ampullar-isthmic junction were dependent on entry of extracellular calcium via calcium channels (744), and pacemaker activity initiating electrical activity seemed to be higher in the ampulla than in the isthmus (333). When isolated strips of the different muscle layers were studied *in vitro,* it was found that there was good correlation between electrical and mechanical activity and that the external longitudinal muscle layer of the isthmus responded best to stretch (596). Its activity was characterized by slow waves of depolarization, which gave rise to contraction, and prolonged spikes, which were followed by phasic waves. Unlike the other muscle layers, the external longitudinal one of the isthmus was the only one that did not show a significant decrease in activity during the secretory compared with the proliferative phase of the cycle. α-Adrenergic activation predominated in this layer, whereas β-adrenergic inhibition was predominant in the other layers (596). Furthermore, the action of PGs is not the same on both circular and longitudinal layers (597,744,745), and the spontaneous activity of the different layers reacts differently at different phases of the cycle (596,636). In the ampullar region, an increase in intraluminal pressure caused an increase in ampullar diameter and a decrease in the amplitude of the contractions of the circular muscle (746), and strips of circular and longitudinal muscle from the ampulla of women with hydrosalpinx, where the lumen would have been continuously distended for a considerable period, showed reduced frequency of contraction but with a longer duration and higher amplitude (747). In such oviducts, adrenergic innervation is greatly reduced (616). Intraluminal pressure does not vary in the isthmic region of pig oviducts during the time of ovum transport, even though unilateral ovariectomy greatly changes the levels of estradiol and progesterone in the utero-ovarian vein (748). Thus, it seems that intraluminal pressure changes are unlikely to be regulated by local steroid action, and this raises the question whether, in fact, intraluminal pressure changes may not occur as a result of the presence of zygotes and, if so, whether these are sufficient to affect oviductal contractility.

A hypothesis regarding ovum transport, in which ova are propelled by circular muscular contractions whose direction approaches randomness, has been developed (332). In these studies, ova were usually located in a region of inactivity, proximal to the uterus. At the time of uterine entry, this inactive region was short (less than 10% of oviductal length) (332). It is not certain whether uterine entry involves activation of the entire isthmus (which could be brief if contractions are unidirectional) or whether other mechanisms also operate at the uterotubal junction. A computer model of ovum transport suggests that these changes in bias and propagation would promote propulsion toward the uterotubal junction (749).

It has been suggested that, over the 3-day period of transport, a net directional bias toward the uterus develops that causes the ultimate appearance of the ovum or zygote in the uterus (749,750). In the ampulla, this bias is associated with differences in distance traveled by the cumulus masses in each direction, rather than with the number of movements (751). Associated with this bias in movement toward the uterus is a constriction of the circular muscle layer of the isthmus after ovulation, thus producing its sphincter action (670). This sphincteric action does not depend on any active process but is simply due to the contrasting morphology of the ampulla and isthmus and the relative distensibility of these two regions of the oviduct (752).

The most probable explanation for regulation of net movement of zygotes toward the uterus is provided by the myogenic activity of the oviductal musculature and the random walk theory. It seems intuitively that the noradrenergic system interacting with endogenous PGs may be part of the regulatory system, but the role played by peptidergic neurons and factors secreted by zygotes has not been elucidated.

Ciliary Activity

As discussed in the sections entitled *Sperm Transport Through the Oviduct* and *Ovulation and Ovum "Pick-Up,"* the endosalpinx is lined with an epithelial surface that has a variable number of ciliated cells, this number being greatest in the fimbria and least in the isthmus. These cells undergo changes in structure with the cyclic changes in steroid hormone levels. Under progestational influence, ciliated cells tend to dedifferentiate and so be reduced in number (753). Ciliogenesis takes place during the proliferative phase of the cycle, and mature cilia are seen at midcycle (754). In contrast, ciliary activity seems to be increased during the luteal phase of the cycle (755). A similar increase in ciliary activity has been seen in the rabbit oviduct by the third day after mating (756). By this time, the ova or zygotes would be in the sparsely ciliated isthmus, so the significance of this change is unknown. Ciliary activity of rabbit oviduct *in vitro* can be stimulated both by adenosine triphosphate (ATP) and by $PGF_{2\alpha}$, and it has been suggested that ATP acts through a purinergic receptor coupled to influx of extracellular calcium and that $PGF_{2\alpha}$ acts through mobilization of intracellular calcium (757). In the human, the frequency of ciliary activity is highest on the fimbriae, intermediate in the ampulla, and lowest at the isthmic level. However, no significant differences in ciliary activity were detected during the cycle (758).

It has been suggested that ciliary activity can provide some, or perhaps all, of the propulsive force that is required to transport ova along the ampullar region of the oviduct. If a 1-cm (or larger) segment of the oviduct is surgically reversed in rabbits, ova are not transported across the reversed segment in which cilia now beat toward the ovary rather than in the usual orientation toward the uterus (759,760). Similarly, if a polyethylene tube is inserted into the ampulla of the rabbit oviduct, ova can pass through tubes up to 10 mm long but not through those of 15 mm or longer (761). Ciliary activity was clearly not involved in ovum movement through the 10-mm tube. In the human, a correlation has been made between a reduction in the percentage of ciliated cells present on the fimbriae and infertility (762), but this failure to become pregnant may be more a reflection of problems with ovum pick-up after ovulation than with subsequent transport. It has also been recorded that women suffering from the immotile cilia syndrome, in which cilia throughout the body are nonfunctional, are normally fertile (763,764). Although in these particular patients, the absence of ciliary activity in the oviduct was not specifically confirmed, the implication remains that ciliary activity is not essential for ovum transport in the human. This has been refuted on the basis of one woman with Kartagener's syndrome who had absolutely immotile cilia in both respiratory and reproductive tracts and who had primary infertility of 8-years' duration (765). In Kartagener's syndrome, there is a complete absence of dynein arms in the axonemes of all ciliary structures (766). A second case of a 27-year-old sterile woman has now been reported. She also had a total absence of dynein arms in the oviductal cilia (767). In previously reported cases, respiratory ciliary activity was usually abnormal rather than absent, suggesting the possibility of some ciliary activity in the reproductive tract.

It would seem that ciliary activity is at least a contributory factor in the regulation of ovum transport, because in experiments with rabbits, it was found that the rate of transport through the ampullar region was abnormally slow in the absence of the cumulus oophorus (730,768). Retarded or inhibited transport of similar ovum surrogates has also been seen in sheep (769). This suggests that an important interaction between the cumulus and the cilia may occur in these species. In rats, however, when muscular activity of the oviduct is blocked by isoproterenol, transport of ovum surrogates through the ampulla is unchanged (770). In the human, ovum surrogates appear to be transported more readily, and actual size is not so critical until sizes of 600 μm or larger are used (387).

On balance, it must be concluded that in the human, at least, ciliary activity plays little, if any, role in the process of ovum transport through the ampulla, and it plays no role in transport through the isthmus. It is likely to be important in ensuring normal pick-up of ova from the ovarian surface or from the peritoneal cavity at ovulation.

Oviductal Secretions

The nature of the oviductal secretion has already been described in the section entitled *Sperm Transport Through the Oviduct* in connection with its role in sperm transport and in the section entitled *Zygote Survival.* Whether it plays any major role in ovum transport *per se* is questionable. The experiments mentioned above on reversal of ampullar segments and placement of tubes in the ampulla suggest that fluid flow alone is insufficient to transport ova along the ampulla (759–761).

However, it is known that fluid will accumulate in the rabbit oviduct if the fimbriated end is ligated (771) and that this accumulation disappears only at the time the ova usually enter the uterus, approximately 60 to 72 h after mating (268). If a plastic tube is inserted through the ampullar-isthmic junction, the fluid flows through the tube and carries the ova with it into the uterus inappropriately early (771). A similar sphincter mechanism has been shown to operate at the uterotubal junction in the cow (772), sheep (773), and human (774). Yet, it has also been claimed that there is no evidence for a functional sphincter at the uterotubal junction in the human and that small particles pass in either direction through the interstitial portion of the oviduct at any time in the cycle (253). It may be that there is a functional occlusion occurring for only a limited period of 2 to 3 days after ovulation.

It is unusual to find ova in the final 10% of the isthmic region of the oviduct; usually they are clumped just above this final portion and then pass rapidly *en masse* into the uterus (363,585,768). There is little circular muscular activity in this region (268). Recording of electrical activity of the oviduct confirmed that there was a region of inactivity in the isthmus that was reduced to less than 10% of the oviductal length at the time of entry of ova into the uterus (332). Edema of the isthmus occurring around the time of ovulation has been observed in rabbits (327), pigs (775), and humans (326). Reduction of this edema can be produced by progesterone treatment in pigs (776,777), and a similar reduction occurs normally about 68 h after ovulation in the rabbit (327,778).

Thus, the reduction in length of the inactive segment (332), combined with relaxation of isthmic constriction (670) and reduction of edema under the action of progesterone, may be sufficient to permit fluid flow to carry the ova into the uterus.

Oviductal secretions have been claimed to play a role in maintaining ova at the ampullar-isthmic junction for a considerable period during the transport process. Koester (779) proposed that the isthmic constriction is such that fluid flow, back up the ampulla to the infundibulum and thence into the peritoneal cavity, is sufficiently strong to prevent the denuded ova from entering the isthmus until this constriction starts to relax. Whether this is the case or whether the isthmic constriction alone is sufficient to prevent ovum entry is not certain.

Besides the role of oviductal fluid as a transport vehicle, which is to some extent defined by its physical properties, there is also the interaction of the macromolecules in this secretion with the developing zygote. This appears to occur in most species. Some of these substances bind to the zona pellucida, and others may be taken up by the blastomeres. Enzymes involved in ion transport, such as Na^+, K^+-ATPase and carbonic anhydrase, have been detected in epithelial cells of rat and mouse oviducts (780). Calcium concentrations are maximal in bovine isthmic fluid at estrus (781) and are similarly elevated by estrogen in oviductal fluid of sheep (782). In bovine oviductal fluid, magnesium concentrations vary with stage of the cycle but not between oviduct regions. Potassium and sodium concentrations show no variations related to cycle stage or region, but potassium is higher in oviductal fluid than in serum (781). Neither the sodium/potassium nor calcium/magnesium ratios in rabbit oviductal fluid varied during the 48 h after an ovulating injection, but as in cows, the potassium concentration in the oviduct was higher than in serum (624). In rat oviducts, staining for calbindin-D9k, which is thought to be involved in transcellular movement of calcium, has been found in epithelium of both ampulla and isthmus, and its presence can be induced by estrogen (783).

The free surface of both rat ampullar and isthmic epithelial cells reacts with several lectins, and secretory granules containing sialic acid and fucose have been identified (784). Similar studies have been conducted with rabbits, and secretory activity is greater in the isthmus than in the ampulla. Carboxylated and sulfated glycosaminoglycans are localized mainly in the isthmus, whereas glycoconjugates are found in both regions (785). Secretion of sulfated glycoproteins was increased from ampullar explants on days 2 and 3 and from isthmic explants on day 4 by estrogen and progesterone treatment but not by estrogen alone. Maximal secretion of sulfated glycoproteins was some 20 times greater from ampulla than from isthmus (786). Secretion of glycoproteins by the oviduct seems to be a consistent occurrence in many species, having been reported in sheep (465,787), pigs (788), and baboons (789–791). Oviduct-specific proteins in the baboon were in the 100- to 130-kDa range, were estrogen-dependent, and were found in all secretory granules in all regions of the oviduct. Withdrawal of estrogen or the administration of progesterone caused regression of the epithelium, especially the ampulla, and reduction of the glycoproteins (789,791). A glycoprotein of 120 kDa has now been cloned; a single message of 2.8 kb is present in oviducts of estradiol-treated baboons and *in vitro* translation gave rise to a 66-kDa protein with no known homology to other proteins. A similar mRNA has been found in human, hamster, rabbit, and mouse oviducts (792).

In the human oviduct, a glycocalyx covering the cilia of all ciliated cells contained glycoconjugates with fucose residues, sulfate esters, and terminal sialic acid-β-galactose disaccharides. Secretory granules were also seen in some cells (793), some of which may have been glycogen (794,795), which could act as an energy source for ciliary activity. Alternatively, it has been suggested that, as in other metabolically polarized cells, such as spermatozoa, a phosphocreatine shuttle between isozymes of creatine kinase localized at the mitochondrion and flagellum could facilitate energy transport. Such a system has been demonstrated in the ciliated cells of the rabbit oviduct (796).

Endometrial secretory proteins have also been found in the oviduct. Placental protein 5 (PP5), a serine protease inhibitor glycoprotein, has been localized to the oviductal epithelium, and its content is similar in the different regions of the oviduct (797). PP10-immunoreactive material has been identified in monocytic and lymphoid cells of the oviductal mucosa in all phases of the cycle (798), and a β-lactoglobulin homolog (PP14) has been found in ampulla and isthmus of human oviducts throughout the cycle and in approximately equivalent amounts (799). Message levels for this protein and another endometrial protein, IGF binding protein-1 (IGFBP-1), are very low in epithelial cells of the oviduct (800). However, mRNA transcripts for IGFBP-2, -3, and -4 are detectable in human oviductal isthmus, and ampullar epithelial cells secrete IGFBP-2 and -3 *in vitro* (801). Insulinlike growth factors-1 and -2 have been found in porcine oviductal fluid, and their concentration is highest at estrus, whereas plasma levels do not vary (802). Insulinlike growth factor-1 is known to stimulate embryonic metabolism (803). Another endometrial protein, pregnancy-associated plasma protein-A (PAPP-A), has also been detected in all portions of the human oviduct, but there were no differences in concentration between regions and only a slight indication of higher levels in the proliferative compared with the secretory phase (804). The oviduct can mount a secretory immune response, as IgA-secreting cells, T cells, and T-suppressor (CD8+) cells have all been identified in human oviduct (805–807). Blood group antigens ABO (793) and the HLA class II antigens (DR, DP, and DQ in pregnant but only DP and DQ in nonpregnant patients) (808) are expressed on oviductal epithelium. Lymphoid tissue is located in the interstitial portion of the human but not the rabbit oviduct (807).

Thus, the oviductal epithelium is highly metabolically active, but in only a few instances are there significant differences between regions or between phases of the cycle. This raises the question of the function of these secretory products during the phase of zygote transport and early development. Further studies of these secretions may be facilitated by the establishment of *in vitro* cultures of oviductal epithelial cells (809–811). Coculture of mouse embryos with human oviductal epithelial explants has been shown to exert a beneficial effect on early development of mouse embryos (812). Similar beneficial effects have been described for development of bovine embryos cocultured with bovine oviductal epithelial cells (813,814), rabbit embryos cocultured with rabbit oviductal epithelial cells (815,816), and also porcine embryos cultured with porcine oviductal fluid (817). However, these positive results may reflect only the fact that the standard medium used was suboptimal and that, under optimal conditions, defined media can effectively support embryo development for at least a limited period. In the human, the embryos are usually returned to the oviduct or uterine cavity relatively early after fertilization and therefore can still be exposed to the different factors secreted by the maternal environment, many of which are secreted into both the uterine and oviductal lumina. Furthermore, the better pregnancy rates achieved with GIFT versus IVF-ET suggest that the oviductal environment, if not obligate, is at least beneficial, especially under suboptimal conditions.

In summary, oviductal secretions are likely to be important for several reasons. First, they may prevent entry of zygotes into the isthmus because of the force of reverse flow; second, they can assist ovum or zygote entry into the uterus at the appropriate time when the uterotubal junction is relaxed under the influence of progesterone; and, last, they may play a role in early embryonic growth and development.

TIME OF OVUM TRANSPORT THROUGH THE OVIDUCT

Ovum transport in the rabbit ampulla takes only a few minutes—approximately 4 to 15 min (729–731,818–820). This process takes somewhat longer in the pig—about 45 min (821). Transport through the ampulla is much slower in the sheep (769). The situation in primates is not so clear, because observation of transport of newly ovulated or transferred ova to the ampullar region has not been studied, except in *Macaca nemestrina* (the pig-tailed macaque), in which a transit time of 22 min has been recorded (374).

In the rabbit, ova are retained at the ampullar-isthmic junction for approximately 24 h before passing on into the isthmus (585,768). The situation is much different in primates. In baboons (*Papio anubis*), the ova remain in the ampulla for approximately 36 h (half the total transport time) (822); however, in rhesus monkeys (*Macaca mulatta*), ova are found in the ampulla until 48 h after ovulation (two-thirds of total transport time) (733); and in women, ova can be confined to the ampulla for up to 72 h (nine-tenths of total transport time) (732). Ova first appear in the uterus in women about 80 h after ovulation (732). An earlier article had indicated that ova could be found in the uterus as early as 2 days after ovulation, whereas zygotes were observed there on only the fourth and fifth days after ovulation (823). However, timing of ovulation was not so precise in these experiments as in subsequent ones. This raises a question as to whether there really was a significant difference in time of transport between zygotes and oocytes. Previously, conventional wisdom was that this was uncertain, but in the light of new information that differential transport can occur in species other than the horse and the bat and that transport may be influenced by either mechanical factors or paracrine interactions between the developing embryos and the oviduct, this difference may well be real. Nevertheless, the recorded difference is small, and perhaps this question should be reexamined under tightly controlled conditions.

Human zygotes enter the uterus in a relatively immature state compared with those in some other mammals (Table 4). A 12-cell zygote was the youngest one that has been recovered from the human uterus (824), and a seven-cell zygote was the oldest one still found in the human oviduct (572). Thus, uterine entry of zygotes occurs approximately at the seven- to 12-cell stage. This agrees well with the cleavage rates recorded after *in vitro* fertilization, where eight-cell zygotes are seen between 45 and 73 h and 16-cell ones are seen between 68 and 85 h after insemination (311).

During the process of transport through the oviduct, the ova lose the cumulus oophorus. This can occur mechanically in unmated animals or by the action of hyaluronidase released from the sperm heads in mated animals. Usually denudation occurs faster in mated than in unmated animals (Table 4). Whether this is also true of the human is not certain; however, an unfertilized ovum with the corona radiata cells still attached has been recorded at the ampullar-isthmic junction at 72 h after the LH peak (i.e., approximately 56 h after ovulation) (732). In contrast, a two-cell zygote almost completely denuded of cumulus and corona cells was recovered from the oviduct by Hertig and collaborators (824). The age of this latter zygote was presumed to be between $1\frac{1}{2}$ and $2\frac{1}{2}$ days, but dating was estimated from endometrial morphology and menstrual history, so it is only approximate. Nonetheless, this two-cell zygote is unlikely to be older than the unfertilized ovum described by Croxatto et al. (732). In some species, such as the rabbit, the corona radiata cells do not disperse as readily as the cumulus oophorus and may remain attached even after sperm penetration of the ovum has occurred (825). Persistence of the corona cells has also been reported for human ova, even though the cumulus mass has dispersed (826). The corona radiata also persists in the rhesus monkey. One unfertilized ovum still had corona cells present up to approximately 24 to 48 h after ovulation, whereas another ovum was denuded at 12 to 24 h after ovulation. A fertilized two-cell ovum, recovered 23 h after mating (but ovulation had occurred previous to mating), was totally denuded (827). In other studies, six unfertilized monkey ova still were in cumulus at 36 ± 12 h after ovulation (determined by laparoscopy), whereas one seven- to eight-cell zygote, recovered at the same time

TABLE 4. *Time of egg denudation, time of entry into uterus, and cell stage at entry, in relation to ovulation*[a]

Animal	Denudation of eggs after ovulation (h)	Entry into uterus after ovulation (h)	Cell stage at entry
Opossum	—	24	Pronuclear
Shrew	—	87–95	Late morula
Rate	Rapid	95–100	8–16
Mouse	12	72	16–32
Guinea pig	24+	80–85	8
Rabbit (doe)	6	60	Morula
	8–10[b]		
Bitch	48 or more	168–192	16–32
Ferret	$19\frac{1}{2}$–40	$88\frac{1}{2}$–$108\frac{1}{2}$	16–32
Cat	48 or more	121–$161\frac{1}{2}$	Late morula
Mare	<24	120+[c]	16
Sow	<24	24–48	4
Cow	9–14	72	8–16
Goat	<$30\frac{1}{2}$	85–98	12
Ewe	0–5	70–80	8–16
Rhesus monkey	24	72 ± 12	16
	48[b]		
Baboon	48[b]	72	—
Woman	?24	80	7–12

From ref. 114, with permission.
[a] Data from various sources.
[b] Unmated.
[c] Except unfertilized eggs.

interval, was denuded. All four zygotes that were recovered at 48 ± 12 h were denuded (828). The importance of these cellular investments for normal ovum transport in the human is not certain, as transport through the ampulla is slow and denudation has already occurred before passage through the isthmus usually commences.

In summary, ovum transport in the human consists of slow transit through the ampulla, with retention at the ampullar-isthmic junction until 72 h after ovulation, followed by transport through the isthmus and uterotubal junction into the uterus during the subsequent 8 h.

PHARMACOLOGIC ACTIONS ON THE OVIDUCT AND CONTRACEPTIVE POTENTIAL

In the section entitled *Physiologic Control Mechanisms,* a great many agents that affect oviductal motility and sperm transport have been described. These included steroids, cyclic nucleotides, PGs, catecholamines, and assorted peptides. It is clear that when excessive amounts of these drugs are administered exogenously, interference with ovum transport can result. Consequently, synthetic estrogens, antiestrogens, synthetic progestins, and assorted PGs have all been used to accelerate transport of ova through the oviduct in a variety of mammals (see refs. 829–831 for further references). Apart from the use of estrogens and/or progestin combinations for contraceptive purposes (566–568), there is little good evidence for such actions occurring in the human.

Again, in small animals, a variety of substances have been shown to stimulate oviductal contractility. These include angiotensin, bradykinin, epinephrine, norepinephrine, and phenylephrine. Others induce a relaxation of activity (e.g., butanephrine, isoproterenol, and vasopressin) (see ref. 832 for further references). Other substances, such as $PGF_{2\alpha}$ and substance P (which cause contraction) and PGE_2 and VIP (which cause relaxation), have already been discussed (see sections entitled *Prostaglandins* and *Peptides*). Unfortunately, the correlation between changes in oviductal motility and accelerated transport is not well established. On the one hand, increased motility, as seen with high doses of estrogen, can, in the rabbit, accelerate ova from the isthmus or trap them above the ampullar-isthmic junction, whereas on the other hand, as discussed in the section on *Contractility of the Smooth Musculature,* relaxation of the isthmus and uterotubal junction by progesterone treatment can hasten ova in the uterus. Thus, the effect of any given pharmacologic agent may well depend on the time of administration relative to ovulation and whether it is given as a bolus or continuously, systemically, or locally. Furthermore, in the human there is always the risk of ectopic pregnancy if zygotes are trapped in the oviduct. Thus, despite the fact that the action of many of the pharmacologic agents already discussed is similar in primates to that seen in nonprimates, their potential as contraceptive agents seems limited.

It has been reported that an ergot alkaloid, ergonovine maleate, which is not active in rabbits, has a potent stimulatory action on the human oviduct at a dose of 10 μg intravenously. Repeated administration at 4- to 6-h intervals maintained contractility (833). It has been claimed that a daily oral dose of 0.02 mg of ergonovine maleate provides some contraceptive effect, but six pregnancies in 48 women over 262 months of use were nonetheless observed (833). When this drug was given only pre- or postcoitally, pregnancies also occurred. It was therefore suggested that it was necessary to combine ergonovine treatment (to stimulate oviductal contractility) with sparteine sulfate (to stimulate uterine contractility). Sparteine sulfate at a single oral dose of 100 to 200 mg maintains uterine activity for up to 3 h and, given at the same dose every 4 h for 3 days, causes abortion (833). Preliminary clinical trials suggested that the combination could be acceptable and effective (833,834).

Further successful application of this method has not been reported, and there appear to be no other suitable candidates for a contraceptive that would act exclusively by altering oviductal transport time. The difficulties inherent in this approach in the human have already been discussed: Briefly, they involve the possibility of ectopic pregnancy when transport is delayed and the possibility of normal pregnancy even when transport is accelerated, unless the uterus is evacuated. Expulsion of embryos from the oviduct and uterus is not always achieved to the same degree by any particular treatment, and consequently the most effective treatment for accelerating oviductal transport may not be the best for reducing the actual number of implantations. Such a dichotomy has been demonstrated in rats (835), and the experiments with ergonovine maleate and sparteine sulfate in women discussed above provide confirmatory evidence for this dual action. However, uterine evacuation can be more reliably achieved (at the time of a missed menses), either by PGs alone (836,837) or, more acceptably, combined with the antiprogestin mifepristone (RU486) because of the reduced incidence of side effects (838,839). Surgical evacuation of the uterus is also a safe and acceptable procedure.

Thus, although estrogens, progestins, or estrogen–progestin combinations have been used as postcoital contraceptives (566–569,840,841), they are suitable for use only in a single cycle, in which the potential need outweighs the possibility that pregnancy will not in any case ensue because intercourse did not take place at the time of ovulation. Because such treatments work only during the very limited period of 72 h after ovulation (842) and produce significant side effects, they are suitable only as emergency treatments and, without a satisfactory method to predict the time of ovulation, will not be practical during normal cycles with repeated coital exposures. In summary, with the present state of knowledge, it is unlikely that satisfactory contraception can be achieved by accelerating zygote transport from the oviduct to the uterus and thence through the cervical canal.

PATHOLOGY OF THE OVIDUCT

The normal functioning of the oviduct can be disrupted by a variety of pathologic causes. Many of these have been dealt with extensively by Woodruff and Pauerstein (253) and more recently by Clement (843) and are not discussed in detail here. One of the most common is salpingitis (i.e., inflammation of the oviduct). This can arise from an ascending infection through the cervix and endometrium, as a result of puerperal or posttraumatic endometritis or from adjacent or distant inflammation. The morphologic changes that can occur have been described by Clement (843).

The ascending infection is usually associated with a sexually transmitted disease (e.g., gonorrhea or chlamydial infection). Where the salpingitis becomes chronic, the oviduct can fill with pus (pyosalpinx) or fluid secretion (hydrosalpinx). In either case, fertility will be severely compromised or abolished. Genital tuberculosis, secondary to systemic infection, may be one of the greatest causes of infertility in developing countries. Although the result can resemble salpingitis or chronic nontuberculous salpingitis, typically there are granulomatous changes. Last, a variety of oviductal tumors, both benign and neoplastic, that cause luminal occlusion have been recorded (253).

Infertility can be caused by obvious pathologic conditions that occlude the reproductive tract and so prevent normal gamete transport or by more subtle conditions that result in so-called unexplained infertility. In these latter conditions, disruption of oviduct function may occur, but if it does, there seems to be no dominant factor in the etiology of this disease. It has been estimated that, worldwide, 5% to 10% of all married couples may be infertile (844). It was found as a result of further worldwide studies that in 26% of couples enrolled with no demonstrable cause of infertility but in which the cause was subsequently diagnosed, only the female partner was affected, and in 19.4%, both partners were affected. An oviductal factor was identified in 44.6% and 29.6% of these two subsets, respectively (845). A later report indicated that bilateral oviductal occlusion was diagnosed in 14.2% of cases overall, ranging from 42% in Africa to 16% in other developing countries and to 9% in developed countries (846). These differences were ascribed to varying levels of sexually transmitted diseases and the occurrence of postpartum or postabortal infections in these areas. In all countries, the incidence of bilateral occlusion always increased with number of pregnancies, previous abortion, or previous live birth. The usual methods of diagnosis of oviductal occlusion are hysterosalpingography, insufflation, or laparoscopy, with hysterosalpingography being the most reliable, although they may be superceded by the new technique of falloposcopy (280).

Repair of occluded oviducts can be successful, but skilled microsurgical procedures are required to give the best results (847,848). Obviously, where infection is the predisposing cause of the oviductal pathology, its cure must antedate any attempt at reconstructive surgery. It is only relatively recently in developed countries that the role of infection with *Chlamydia trichomatis* has been recognized as a cause of oviductal sterility and failure of tuboplastic repair procedures. In a series of 69 women with oviductal obstruction, 18.8% were found to have positive cultures for *Chlamydia* compared with only 2% in 49 normal controls (849).

An increased risk of pelvic inflammatory disease has been reported to be associated with the use of an IUD (850,851), and at least in nulliparous women, an association with an increased risk for subsequent infertility is also associated with IUD use (852,853). Endometriosis, which involves the implantation of endometrial cells in ectopic locations such as the peritoneal surface or the ovaries, is found in approximately 50% of women presenting with infertility and in about 38% with unexplained infertility (854,855). In many cases, salpingitis can be clinically confirmed in association with histologically proven endometriosis, and in these women, this alone could be the cause of the resulting infertility (856). However, in many instances, no obvious pathology of the oviduct can be seen. In such cases, it has been suggested that inappropriate production of PGs from the endometriotic implants on the peritoneum or ovary could disrupt oviductal function. Excessive PG concentrations have been found in the abdominal fluid of such women (857,858) and in monkeys with artificially induced endometriosis (859). However, in other studies, PG levels have not been elevated (860–862) or were not associated with endometriosis in infertile patients (863). In women with suspected acute pelvic inflammatory disease, there was an association between acute salpingitis, presence of microbes and neutrophils in the peritoneal cavity, and elevated levels of leukotriene B_4 and PGE_2 in peritoneal fluid (864). Thus, if there is any effect of endogenous PGs on oviductal function in infertile patients with endometriosis, the association seems tenuous.

The incidence of ectopic pregnancy has been reported to vary from one in 30 to one in 300 live births, depending on the population surveyed (865). Its incidence in the United States is increasing; the incidence rose from 4.8 per 1,000 live births in 1970 to 14.5 per 1,000 live births in 1980 (866). It has been claimed that ectopic pregnancy does not seem to be associated with coexisting salpingitis (865), but this view may have to be modified. More recent studies have shown that between 29% and 54% of women experiencing ectopic pregnancy exhibit evidence of salpingitis (867,868). Prior salpingitis may give rise to salpingitis isthmica nodosa, which can be associated with an increased incidence of ectopic pregnancy (869,870). There is also a reported association between a prior history of genital herpes and trichomoniasis and an increased incidence of ectopic pregnancy (871), but, in fact, when other confounding factors are controlled for, the increased risk is very slight (872). However, in this latter analysis, it was found that the presence of antibody to *Chlamydia trachomatis* was associated with a twofold increased risk of an ectopic pregnancy in the oviduct (872). Women who had experienced an ectopic pregnancy had significantly elevated IgG but not IgM antibodies to *Chlamydia trachomatis* compared with controls, and the greater antibody titers were associated with greater oviductal mucosal damage (873,874). A mouse model has been developed in which local infection with *Chlamydia trachomatis* gives rise to oviductal pathology, including mucous congestion, edema, and loss of cilia. This pathology was not associated with disrupted ovum transport and fertility in all strains of mice, which suggests a genetic component to the etiology (875,876). This model may prove useful for further studies of the etiology, treatment, and prevention of chlamydia-induced oviductal pregnancies. Nevertheless, in some women there is no obvious reason why the developing embryo implants in an extrauterine site, especially in the oviduct. Certainly, when the oviductal lumen is partially occluded at the uterotubal junction, as when hysteroscopic sterilization using cautery is performed, then the incidence of ectopic pregnancy can be greatly increased (877). Conversely, a markedly decreased incidence of ectopic pregnancies has been noted in patients who were treated with PGs for termination of first-trimester pregnancies (878).

Although IUD use is associated with an increase in the relative incidence of ectopic pregnancies as a result of the prevention of the intrauterine ones, there is actually no increase in absolute numbers of ectopic pregnancies for most IUDs (879–881). However, IUDs releasing progesterone have been associated with a positive increased ectopic pregnancy rate (881,882). Similarly, previous abortion (883) or use of large doses of estrogen as an interceptive agent (570,571) can increase the incidence of ectopic pregnancy. Use of chronic low-dose progestins for contraception (573,574) has also been reported to have a similar effect. It has been suggested that there can be a hormonal basis for ectopic pregnancy (577), and this might have a physiologic basis through the reduced oviductal activity associated with low progesterone levels (576). Ovarian stimulation associated with treatments to stimulate follicular development for an assisted reproductive technology procedure (884–890) caused an increased incidence of ectopic pregnancies. Although there is a clear implication that this increased incidence is caused by the changed hormonal conditions resulting from the ovarian stimulation regimens, at least two groups have suggested that the ectopic pregnancies are associated with preexisting oviductal pathology (888, 890). However, it has been noted that in at least some oviductal pregnancies, there was a changed pattern of myoelectrical activity that could explain the retention of the zygote in the oviduct (891). It must also be remembered that these assisted reproductive technologies are used only for couples who are infertile, although this is not always a female problem. Indeed, there have been several reports of women experiencing simultaneous intrauterine and intraoviductal pregnancies (892–894). Ectopic pregnancies contralateral to the corpus luteum or the side of GIFT have also been reported (867,895,896). The incidence in nonstimulated conception cycles seems to be about 20% to 30% (867,895), but whether this is due to transperitoneal migration of zygotes or retrograde ascent from the uterus is not certain. Taken together, the evidence suggests that interference with the balance of ovarian steroids necessary for normal zygote transport can be a cause of failure of the transport mechanism, especially if there is intercurrent pathology of the oviduct.

Because ectopic pregnancy does not occur naturally in nonprimates, and even when it is induced artificially in sites outside the reproductive tract it gives rise to growth of only trophoblast, no small animal model is available for experimental manipulation. Even in nonhuman primates, the incidence of ectopic pregnancy is extremely rare (253,897,898). The most common locations for pregnancies in the oviduct are the ampulla (60%) and isthmus (30%) (869); presumably the zygotes are trapped either at the ampullar-isthmic or uterotubal junctions. In view of the lack of a suitable animal model, further work on the causality of this condition can be achieved only retrospectively in case control studies or in prospective large-scale epidemiologic studies, and even then interpretation may be difficult because of multiple etiologies. It may be necessary to study each set with a defined etiology separately.

TRANSPORT AND SPACING OF ZYGOTES IN THE UTERUS

Once the developing embryo enters the uterus, it is transported to the site of implantation primarily by muscular activity of the uterine wall. The position that the blastocyst achieves within the uterus is not random but is the same within any major taxonomic group (899). This leads to a fixed placental position. Even in the simplex uterus of the human, in which the uterine lumen is dorsoventrally flattened and implantation occurs most often on the surface of the midportion of the anterior wall of the uterus (900), the site of attachment is still regarded as antimesometrial. However, as Mossman questioned in 1971 (899): "How is orientation brought about, and what is its biological significance to the species?" Twenty years later, we still have no answer to this question.

The regularity of positioning of blastocysts in the uterus suggests that there must be some underlying mechanism. In those polytocous species with multiple embryos within a single uterine horn, the regular spacing along the horn, except in the case of overcrowding, can be explained mainly by muscular activity of the myometrium. In the rabbit, whose blastocysts swell to about 5 mm at implantation (901), the blastocysts act as a focal point for the initiation of waves of muscular contraction. This results in uniform spacing of the blastocysts (902). It is now known that rabbit blastocysts contain and produce PGs (524,526,533), which can be transported from the uterine lumen to the myometrium (903). Prostaglandins can be accumulated by the rabbit blastocyst and released in a site-directed manner (534,629). The release of these PGs could be the trigger to initiate regular spacing in the uterus in this species. Prostaglandin synthesis has also been reported for blastocysts of sheep (521,523), cows (522), and pigs (527). Thus it may be that this is a common mechanism inducing regular spacing. In mice, uterine contractility has been shown to be the overriding cause of blastocyst spacing (904), and in rats, changes in electrical activity of the myometrium have been correlated with blastocyst spacing in the uterus (905). In monotocous species, such as the human, the situation is not so clear. In the luminal epithelium, ciliated cells that might contribute to the orientation in the endometrial cavity have been described in the human (906). The role that other blastocyst factors, such as growth factors, may play in orientation and spacing is unknown. Nevertheless, in the absence of other evidence, it seems likely that myometrial contractions triggered by the presence of the blastocyst play a major role in blastocyst placement in the human as in other species. The process of implantation from apposition, through attachment to invasion and decidualization, is dealt with in another chapter.

CONCLUSIONS

This review has attempted to highlight different processes that have been proposed as control mechanisms for gamete and zygote transport. In most species, the role of the oviduct is central to this phase of the reproductive process. It ensures an environment for maturation of spermatozoa and for fertilization and subsequent zygote development. Clearly, many mechanisms exert actions on oviductal function, although no particular one can be shown to be the controlling factor. It seems that there is a redundancy of mechanisms which can substitute one for another. In the opinion of Jansen (315), the oviduct "has much redundancy in its repertoire of gamete transporting properties," and there is a lack of convincing evidence that any one predominates in regulation of ovum transport. This view, espoused in 1984, has not been altered by any of the new information obtained in the intervening period. It seems that further investigation of the potential peptidergic regulation of oviductal smooth musculature may be warranted, as it is the potential control system that is the least well studied. What has proved most novel and of great potential interest concerns the role of zygote factors in regulation of zygote transport, especially as compared with transport of oocytes. The fact that differential oviductal transport has been documented in several species suggests that further investigation for the presence of a similar phenomenon in primates should have high priority. New information on sperm maturation and transport in the oviduct suggests that this is also a more complex process than simple transport due to oviductal fluid flow or sperm motility, as previously assumed. Oocyte or follicular fluid factors may also be involved in sperm movement to the site of fertilization, and the notion of chemotaxis of sperm to the oocyte surface at fertilization has been lent respectability. Such findings should spur further investigations in this area. Even though much of the present evidence derives from nonprimates, there may be general application to the human. However, it must be remembered that human embryos are hardy [i.e., survive well after removal of a blastomere at the eight-cell stage (907) or freezing (908,909)] and they can implant in either the oviduct or the uterus, without exposure to the other organ, so apparently neither the oviduct nor the uterus is essential for zygote development and implantation. In such exceptional cases, the incidence of successful pregnancy is low, and thus exposure of gametes and zygotes to both uterus and oviduct is beneficial.

Still, the oviduct remains an enigma, and the concerted efforts of many scientists over the past half century have not yet yielded a blueprint for the regulation of the complete system. Recent studies have, however, made great progress toward understanding cellular regulation and function of spermatozoa, oocytes, and zygotes and, to a lesser extent, of the products secreted by the oviduct and uterus, and it is in such efforts that the best hope lies for elucidation of the integration of the system. Similar studies have yielded more information on the male reproductive tract and the transport and maturation of spermatozoa before ejaculation.

Clearly, the use of assisted reproductive technologies has permitted the dissection of components of the reproductive system and resulted in more information on the importance of the different organs, from epididymis to oviduct, for maturation and development, without necessarily elucidating the exact cellular mechanisms. However, such information points the way to the next questions to be posed and studied. Many anomalies are still to be elucidated. For example, if only one spermatozoon is required to fertilize an ovum, why are large numbers in the oviduct important, even when GIFT is performed and both oocytes and spermatozoa are placed in apposition together in the oviduct at the putative site of fertilization? Why does ectopic pregnancy not occur in other species? Is it that the oviduct is hostile to development beyond the morular stage, except in the human? There is some evidence that this may be the case in the rabbit (910), but whether this is due to an inhibitory protein, peptide, or lipid or just a different osmolarity of oviductal compared with uterine fluid has not been resolved. What growth factors are produced by the zygote and what by the oviduct? At what stages are they produced, and on what cells do they act? Are these actions autocrine or paracrine, and is there redundancy in the system?

These are just some of the interesting questions that need to be resolved. In the *Foreword,* I indicated that the readers will have to judge for themselves whether the new information permits a better understanding of the integration of the transport systems for spermatozoa and zygotes. In my judgment, we have not yet reached that stage, but I do believe now that there are promising lines of research that could lead us to that goal. When the previous version of this chapter was written, I was much more pessimistic as to the possibility of making significant progress toward this goal.

ACKNOWLEDGMENTS

The writing of this chapter and some of the work described herein were supported by NIH grant HD14048. Grateful thanks are due to Beverly Evans for typing the first draft and to Gretta Small for production and editorial assistance of the finished version.

REFERENCES

1. Harper MJK. Gamete and zygote transport. In: Knobil E, Neill JC, Ewing LL, Greenwald GS, Markert CL, and Pfaff DW. *The Physiology of Reproduction.* New York: Raven Press, 1988; 103–134.
2. Woolf HB, ed. *Webster's New Collegiate Dictionary.* Springfield, MA: G. C. Merriam Co., 1977;472.
3. Fisher GJ. Historical and biographical notes: V. Gabriel Fallopius, 1523–1562. *Ann Anat Surg Soc* 1880;2:200–204.
4. Redenbach DM, Vogl AW. Microtubule polarity in Sertoli cells: a model for microtubule-based spermatid transport. *Eur J Cell Biol* 1991;54:277–290.
5. Russell LD, Saxena NK, Turner TT. Cytoskeletal involvement in spermiation and sperm transport. *Tissue Cell* 1989;21:361–379.
6. Bedford JM. Maturation, transport and fate of spermatozoa in the epididymis. In: Hamilton DW, Greep RO, eds. *Handbook of Physiology, Section 7: Endocrinology, Vol. 5, Male Reproductive System.* Washington, DC: American Physiological Society, 1975;303–317.
7. MacMillan EW. The mechanical influence of the vasa efferentia

on the transport of radiopaque medium through the ductus epididymidis of the rat. *Stud Fertil* 1957;9:65–71.
8. MacMillan EW, Aukland J. The transport of radiopaque medium through the initial segment of the rat epididymis. *J Reprod Fertil* 1960;1:139–145.
9. Risley PL. Physiology of the male accessory organs. In: Hartman CG, ed. *Mechanisms Concerned with Conception,* New York: Macmillan, 1963;73–133.
10. Cross BA. Hypothalamic influences on sperm transport in the male and female genital tract. In: Lloyd CW, ed. *Recent Progress in the Endocrinology of Reproduction.* New York: Academic Press, 1959;167–177.
11. Sjöstrand NO. The adrenergic innervation of the vas deferens and the accessory male genital glands. *Acta Physiol Scand* 1965; 65(Suppl 257).
12. El-Badawi A, Schenk EA. The distribution of cholinergic and adrenergic nerves in the mammalian epididymis. *Am J Anat* 1967;121:1–14.
13. Baumgarten HG, Holstein AF, Rosengren E. Arrangement, ultrastructure, and adrenergic innervation of smooth musculature of the ductuli efferentes, ductus epididymidis and ductus deferens of man. *Z Mikrosk Anat Forsch* 1971;120:37–79.
14. Billups KL, Tillman S, Chang TS. Ablation of the inferior mesenteric plexus in the rat: alteration of sperm storage in the epididymis and vas deferens. *J Urol* 1990;143:625–629.
15. Rowley M, Teshima JF, Heller CG. Duration of transit of spermatozoa through the human male ductular system. *Fertil Steril* 1970;21:390–396.
16. Orgebin-Crist MC. Passage of spermatozoa labelled with thymidine-^{3}H through the ductus epididymidis of the rabbit. *J Reprod Fertil* 1965;10:241–251.
17. Hikim AP, Hoffer AP. Duration of epididymal sperm transit in hamster: an autoradiographic study. *Gamete Res* 1988;19: 411–416.
18. Amir D, Ortavant R. Influence de la fréquence des collectes sur la duré du transit des spermatozoides dans le canal epididymaire du belier. *Ann Biol Anim Biochim Biophys* 1968;8:195–207.
19. Freund M. Interrelationships among the characteristics of human semen and factors affecting semen-specimen quality. *J Reprod Fertil* 1962;4:143–159.
20. Confino FJ, Friberg J, Dudkiewicz AB, Gleicher N. Effect of ejaculation frequency on sperm quality. *Arch Androl* 1986;16: 203–207.
21. Wilton LJ, Temple-Smith PD, Baker HW, De Kretser DM. Human male infertility caused by degeneration and death of sperm in the epididymis. *Fertil Steril* 1988;49:1052–1058.
22. Bedford JM. Influence of abdominal temperature on epididymal function in the rat and rabbit. *Am J Anat* 1978;152:509–522.
23. Cummins JM, Glover TD. Artificial cryptorchidism and fertility in the rabbit. *J Reprod Fertil* 1970;23:423–433.
24. Jones R. The effects of artificial cryptorchidism on the composition of epididymal plasma in the rabbit. *Fertil Steril* 1975;25: 432–438.
25. Johnson L, Varner DD. Effect of daily spermatozoan production but not age on transit time of spermatozoa through the human epididymis. *Biol Reprod* 1988;39:812–817.
26. Ammann RP, Howards SS. Daily spermatozoal production and epididymal spermatozoal reserves of the human male. *J Urol* 1980;124:211–215.
27. Orbach J. Spontaneous ejaculation in the rat. *Science* 1961; 134:1072–1073.
28. Lino BF, Braden AWH, Turnbull EK. Fate of unejaculated spermatozoa. *Nature* 1967;213:594–595.
29. Martan J. Epididymal histochemistry and physiology. *Biol Reprod* 1969;(suppl)1:134–154.
30. Pineda MH, Dooley MP, Hembrough FB, Hsu WH. Retrograde flow of spermatozoa into the urinary bladder of rams. *Am J Vet Res* 1987;48:562–568.
31. Phadke AM. Fate of spermatozoa in case of obstructive azoospermia and after ligation of vas deferens in man. *J Reprod Fertil* 1964;7:1–12.
32. Kozumplik J. Migration of protoplasmic droplets and phagocytosis of damaged sperm during their passage through the efferent ducts in boars and bulls. *Vet Med (Praha)* 1987;32:343–354.
33. Barratt CL, Cohen J. Fate of superfluous sperm products after vasectomy and in the normal male tract of the mouse. *J Reprod Fertil* 1986;78:1–10.
34. Orgebin-Crist MC. Maturation of spermatozoa in the rabbit epididymis. Fertilizing ability and embryonic mortality in does inseminated with epididymal spermatozoa. *Ann Biol Anim Biochim Biophys* 1967;7:373–389.
35. Bedford JM, Calvin H, Cooper GW. The maturation of spermatozoa in the human epididymis. *J Reprod Fertil (Suppl)* 1973;18:199–213.
36. Suarez SS. Hamster sperm motility transformation during development of hyperactivation *in vitro* and epididymal maturation. *Gamete Res* 1988;19:51–65.
37. Hong CY, Chiang BN, Turner P. Calcium ion is the key regulator of human sperm function. *Lancet* 1984;ii:1449–1451.
38. Escalier D, David G. Pathology of the cytoskeleton of the human sperm flagellum: axonemal and peri-axonemal anomalies. *Biol Cell* 1984;50:37–52.
39. Merlino GT, Stahle C, Jhappan C, Linton R, Mahon KA, Willingham MC. Inactivation of a sperm motility gene by insertion of an epidermal growth factor receptor transgene whose product is overexpressed and compartmentalized during spermatogenesis. *Genes Dev* 1991;5:1395–1406.
40. Matsuzawa T, Sawada H. Histochemical changes in rat sperm malate dehydrogenase activity during passage through epididymis. *Endocrinol Jpn* 1987;34:231–235.
41. Hall JC, Killian GJ. Changes in rat sperm membrane glycosidase activities and carbohydrate and protein contents associated with epididymal transit. *Biol Reprod* 1987;36:709–718.
42. Bansal P, Atreja SK. Phosphoinositide specific phospholipase C activity of goat spermatozoa in transit from the caput to the cauda epididymis. *Indian J Biochem Biophys* 1991;28:307–311.
43. Mahi-Brown CA, VandeVoort CA, McGuiness RP, Overstreet JW, O'Hern P, Golderg E. Immunization of male but not female mice with the sperm-specific isozyme of lactate dehydrogenase (LDH-C4) impairs fertilization *in vivo. Am J Reprod Immunol* 1990;24:1–8.
44. Vreeburg JT, Holland MK, Cornwall GA, Orgebin-Crist M-C. Secretion and transport of mouse epididymal proteins after injection of ^{35}S-methionine. *Biol Reprod* 1990;43:113–120.
45. Cornwall GA, Vreeburg JT, Holland MK, Orgebin-Crist M-C. Interactions of labeled epididymal secretory proteins with spermatozoa after injection of ^{35}S-methionine in the mouse. *Biol Reprod* 1990;43:121–129.
46. Dacheux JL, Dacheux F, Paquignon M. Changes in sperm surface membrane and luminal protein fluid content during epididymal transit in the boar. *Biol Reprod* 1989;40:635–651.
47. Jeulin C, Soufir JC, Marson J, Paquignon M, Dacheux JL. The distribution of carnitine and acetylcarnitine in the epididymis and epididymal spermatozoa of the boar. *J Reprod Fertil* 1987;79:523–529.
48. Rana AP, Majumder GC. Changes in the fluidity of the goat sperm plasma membrane in transit from caput to cauda epididymis. *Biochem Int* 1990;21:797–803.
49. Blaschuk O, Fritz IB. Isoelectric forms of clusterin isolated from ram testis fluid and from secretions of primary cultures of ram and rat Sertoli-cell-enriched preparations. *Can J Biochem Cell Biol* 1984;62:456–461.
50. Hermo L, Wright J, Oko R, Morales CR. Role of epithelial cells of the male excurrent duct system of the rat in the endocytosis or secretion of sulfated glycoprotein-2 (clusterin). *Biol Reprod* 1991;44:1113–1131.
51. Cyr DG, Robaire B. Regulation of sulfated glycoprotein-2 (clusterin) messenger ribonucleic acid in the rat epididymis. *Endocrinology* 1992;130:2160–2166.
52. Bedford JM, Calvin H. Changes in S-S crosslinks in sperm head with particular reference to eutherian mammals. *J Exp Zool* 1974;187:181–204.
53. Loir M, Lanneau M. Structural function of the basic nuclear proteins in ram spermatids. *Ultrastruct Res* 1984;86:262–276.
54. Rodriguez-Martinez H, Courtens JL, Kvist U, Plöen L. Immunocytochemical localization of nuclear protamine in boar spermatozoa during epididymal transit. *J Reprod Fertil* 1990;89: 591–595.

55. Bedford JM. Effect of duct ligation on the fertilizing ability of spermatozoa from different regions of the rabbit epididymis. *J Exp Zool* 1967;166:271–282.
56. Young DH. Surgical treatment of male infertility. *J Reprod Fertil* 1970;23:541–542.
57. Schoysman RJ, Bedford JM. The role of the human epididymis in sperm maturation and sperm storage as reflected in the consequences of epididymovasostomy. *Fertil Steril* 1986;46:293–299.
58. Southwick GJ, Temple-Smith PD. Epididymal microsurgery: current techniques and new horizons. *Microsurgery* 1988;9: 266–277.
59. Silber SJ. Reversal of vasectomy and the treatment of male infertility. *J Androl* 1980;1:261–268.
60. Barratt CL, Cohen J. Quantitative effects of short- and long-term vasectomy on mouse spermatogenesis and sperm transport. *Contraception* 1988;37:415–424.
61. Bancroft J. Human sexual behaviour. In: Austin CR, Short RV, eds. *Reproduction in Mammals, Vol 8: Human Sexuality.* Cambridge, UK: Cambridge University Press, 1980;34–67.
62. Whitelaw GP, Smithwick RH. Some secondary effects of sympathectomy with particular reference to disturbance of sexual function. *N Engl J Med* 1951;245:121–130.
63. Kedia KR, Markland C. The ejaculatory process. In: Hafez ESE, ed. *Human Semen and Fertility Regulation in Men.* St. Louis: CV Mosby, 1976;497–503.
64. Bedford JM. Personal communication. 1986.
65. Ambache N, Zar MA. Evidence against adrenergic motor transmission to the guinea-pig vas deferens. *J Physiol (Lond)* 1971;216:359–389.
66. Furness JB, Iwayama T. The arrangement and identification of axons innervating the vas deferens of the guinea pig. *J Anat* 1972;113:179–196.
67. Kihara K, Sato K, Ando M, Sato T, Oshima H. Lumbosacral sympathetic trunk as a compensatory pathway for seminal emission after bilateral hypogastric nerve transections in the dog. *J Urol* 1991;145:640–643.
68. Kihara K, Sato K, Ando M, Sato T, Oshima H. Ability of each lumbar splanchnic nerve and disability of thoracic ones to generate seminal emission in the dog. *J Urol* 1992;147:260–263.
69. Sato K, Kihara K, Ando M, Sato T, Oshima H. Seminal emission by electrical stimulation of the spermatic nerve and epididymis. *Int J Urol* 1991;14:461–467.
70. Vandereycken W. Towards a better understanding of ejaculatory disorders. *Acta Psychiatr Belg* 1986;86:57–63.
71. Murphy JB, Lipschultz LI. Abnormalities of ejaculation. *Urol Clin North Am* 1987;14:588–596.
72. Yeates WK. Ejaculation and its disorders. *Arch Ital Urol Nefrol Androl* 1990;62:137–148.
73. Ohl DA, Denil J, Bennett CJ, Randolph JF, Menge AC, McCabe M. Electroejaculation following retroperitoneal lymphadenectomy. *J Urol* 1991;145:980–983.
74. Warner H, Martin DE, Perkash I, Speck V, Nathan B. Electrostimulation of erection and ejaculation and collection of semen in spinal cord injured humans. *J Rehabil Res Dev* 1986;23:21–31.
75. Ver Voort SM. Ejaculatory stimulation in spinal-cord injured men. *Urology* 1987;29:282–289.
76. Halstead LS, Ver Voort S, Seager SW. Rectal probe electrostimulation in the treatment of anejaculatory spinal cord injured men. *Paraplegia* 1987;25:120–129.
77. Sarkarati M, Rossier AB, Fam BA. Experiences in vibratory and electro-ejaculation techniques in spinal cord injury patients: a preliminary report. *J Urol* 1987;138:59–62.
78. Bennett CJ, Ayers JWT, Randolph JF Jr, et al. Electroejaculation of paraplegic males followed by pregnancies. *Fertil Steril* 1987;48:1070–1072.
79. Ohl DA, Bennett CJ, McCabe M, Menge AC, McGuire EJ. Predictors of success in electroejaculation of spinal cord injured men. *J Urol* 1989;142:1483–1486.
80. Perkash I, Martin DE, Warner H, Speck V. Electroejaculation in spinal cord injury patients: simplified new equipment and technique. *J Urol* 1990;143:305–307.
81. Lucas MG, Hargreave TB, Edmond P, Creasey GH, McParland M, Seager SW. Sperm retrieval by electro-ejaculation. Preliminary experience in patients with secondary anejaculation. *Br J Urol* 1991;67:191–194.
82. Sønksen JO, Drewes AM, Biering-Sørensen F, Giwercman AJ. Vibration-induced reflex ejaculation in patients with spinal cord injuries. *Ugeskr Laeger* 1991;153:2888–2890.
83. Hirsch IH, Jeyendran RS, Sedor J, Rosencrans RR, Staas WE. Biochemical analysis of electroejaculates in spinal cord injured men: comparison to normal ejaculates. *J Urol* 1991;145:73–76.
84. MacLeod DG, Reynolds DG, Demaree GE. Some pharmacologic characteristics of the human vas deferens. *Invest Urol* 1973;10:338–341.
85. Bauer GE, Hull RD, Stokes GS, Raftos J. The reversibility of side effects of guanethidine therapy. *Med J Aust* 1973;1:930–933.
86. Green M, Berman S. Failure of ejaculation produced by dibenzyline. *Conn State Med J* 1954;18:30–33.
87. Singh H. A case of inhibition of ejaculation as a side effect of mellaril. *Am J Psychiatry* 1961;117:1041–1042.
88. Freyhan FA. Loss of ejaculation during mellaril treatment. *Am J Psychiatry* 1961;118:171–172.
89. Heller J. Another case of inhibition of ejaculation as a side effect of mellaril. *Am J Psychiatry* 1961;118:173.
90. Shilon M, Paz GF, Homonnai ZT. The use of phenoxybenzamine treatment in premature ejaculation. *Fertil Steril* 1984; 42:659–661.
91. Beretta G, Chelo E, Fanciullacci F, Zanollo A. Effect of an alpha-blocking agent (phenoxybenzamine) in the management of premature ejaculation. *Acta Eur Fertil* 1986;17:43–45.
92. Yonezawa A, Kawamura S, Ando R, Tadano T, Nobunaga T, Kimura Y. Biphasic effects of yohimbine on the ejaculatory response in the dog. *Life Sci* 1991;48:PL103–109.
93. Yonezawa A, Ando R, Tadano T, Kisara K, Miyamoto A, Kimura Y. Evidence for central alpha 2-adrenergic mechanism of clonidine-induced ejaculatory disturbance in dogs. *J Pharmacobiodyn* 1986;9:1032–1035.
94. Gerstenberg TC, Levin RJ, Wagner G. Erection and ejaculation in man. Assessment of the electromyographic activity of the bulbocavernosus and ischiocavernosus muscles. *Br J Urol* 1990; 65:395–402.
95. Amobi NIB, Smith ICH. Effects of thioridazine on mechanical responses of human vas deferens induced by noradrenaline or potassium. *J Reprod Fertil* 1992;95:1–10.
96. Carmichael MS, Humbert R, Dixen J, Palmisano G, Greenleaf W, Davidson JM. Plasma oxytocin increases in the human sexual response. *J Clin Endocrinol Metab* 1987;64:27–31.
97. Murphy MR, Seckl JR, Burton S, Checkley SA, Lightman SL. Changes in oxytocin and vasopressin secretion during sexual activity in man. *J Clin Endocrinol Metab* 1987;65:738–741.
98. Segraves RT. Effects of psychotropic drugs on human erection and ejaculation. *Arch Gen Psychiatry* 1989;46:275–284.
99. Masters WH, Johnson VE. Premature ejaculation. In: *Human Sexual Inadequacy.* Boston: Little, Brown, 1970;92–115.
100. Strassberg DS, Kelly MP, Carroll C, Kircher JC. The psychophysiological nature of premature ejaculation. *Arch Sex Behav* 1987;16:327–336.
101. Colpi GM, Fanciullacci F, Beretta S, Negri L, Zanollo A. Evoked sacral potentials in subjects with true premature ejaculation. *Andrologia* 1986;18:583–586.
102. Fein RL. Intracavernous medication for treatment of premature ejaculation. *Urology* 1990;35:301–303.
103. Wespes E, Shiffman S, Schulman CC, Vanderhaeghen JJ. Peptide innervation of the penis. *Acta Urol Belg* 1990;58:29–41.
104. Roy JB, Petrone RL, Said SI. A clinical trial of intracavernous vasoactive intestinal peptide to induce penile erection. *J Urol* 1990;143:302–304.
105. Kiely EA, Bloom SR, Williams G. Penile response to intracavernosal vasoactive intestinal polypeptide alone and in combination with other vasoactive agents. *Br J Urol* 1989;64:191–194.
106. Thiounn N. Intracavernous injections in 1991. *J Urol (Paris)* 1991;97:189–194.
107. Bellorofonte C, Ruoppolo M, Dell'Acqua S, et al. Endocavernous drug infusions revisited. *Arch Ital Urol Nefrol Androl* 1991;63: 475–479.
108. Barth V. Retrograde ejaculation as a cause of aspermia following

retroperitoneal lymph node excision and the effective use of alpha sympathomimmetic drugs. *Z Urol Nephrol* 1990;83:115–119.
109. Ibragimov AZ, Aliev TA, Abdullaev KI, Mirza-Zade VA. The function of the closure apparatus of the bladder in retrograde ejaculation in diabetics. *Urol Nephrol (Mosk)* 1990;3:65–68.
110. Hershlag A, Schiff SF, DeCherney AH. Retrograde ejaculation. *Hum Reprod* 1991;6:255–258.
111. Neĭkov K, Tachev S, Panchev P, Tsvetkov D. Retrograde ejaculation following transurethral surgery for bladder neck sclerosis. *Khirurgiia (Sofia)* 1989;42:53–56.
112. Middleton RG, Urry RL. The Young-Dees operation for the correction of retrograde ejaculation. *J Urol* 1986;136:1208–1209.
113. Urry RL, Middleton RG, McGavin S. A simple and effective technique for increasing pregnancy rates in couples with retrograde ejaculation. *Fertil Steril* 1986;46:1124–1127.
114. Harper MJK. Sperm and egg transport. In: Austin CR, Short RV, eds. *Reproduction in Mammals. I. Germ Cells and Fertilization,* Ed 2. Cambridge, UK: Cambridge University Press, 1982;102–127.
115. Mann T. *The Biochemistry of Semen and of the Male Reproductive Tract.* London: Methuen & Co., 1964.
116. Eliasson R, Lindholmer C. Distribution and properties of spermatozoa in different fractions of split ejaculates. *Fertil Steril* 1972;23:252–256.
117. Sokol RZ, Madding CI, Handelsman JJ, Swerdloff RS. The split ejaculate: assessment of fertility potential using two in vitro test systems. *Andrologia* 1986;18:380–386.
118. Lundquist F. Aspects of the biochemistry of human semen. *Acta Physiol Scand* 1949;19(suppl 66):108.
119. Cavazos LF. The mammalian accessory sex glands: a morphological and functional analysis. In: Greep RO, Koblinsky MA, eds. *Frontiers in Reproduction and Fertility Control. A Review of the Reproductive Sciences and Contraceptive Development.* Cambridge, MA: MIT Press, 1977;402–410.
120. Chow PH, O WS. Effects of male accessory sex glands on sperm transport, fertilization and embryonic loss in hamsters. *Int J Androl* 1989;12:155–163.
121. Peitz B, Olds-Clark P. Effects of seminal vesicle removal on fertility and uterine sperm motility in the house mouse. *Biol Reprod* 1986;35:608–617.
122. Agrawal Y, Vanha-Perttula T. Effect of secretory particles in bovine seminal vesicle secretion on sperm motility and acrosome reaction. *J Reprod Fertil* 1987;79:409–419.
123. Sanada S, Yoshida O. Zinc concentrations and total amount of zinc in seminal plasma of infertile men with special reference to prostatic secretory function. *Hinyokika Kiyo* 1985;31:1971–1987.
124. Björndahl L, Kjellberg S, Roomans GM, Kvist U. The human sperm nucleus takes up zinc at ejaculation. *Int J Androl* 1986;9:77–80.
125. Ronquist G, Brody I. The prostasome: its secretion and function in man. *Biochim Biophys Acta* 1985;822:203–218.
126. Ronquist G, Frithz G, Jansson A. Prostasome membrane associated enzyme activities and semen parameters in men attending an infertility clinic. *Urol Int* 1988;43:133–138.
127. Ronquist G. Zinc ion stimulation of ATP cleavage by prostasomes from human seminal plasma. *Urol Int* 1988;43:334–340.
128. Olsson I, Ronquist G. Isoenzyme pattern of lactate dehydrogenase associated with human prostasomes. *Urol Int* 1990;45: 346–349.
129. Olsson I, Ronquist G. Nucleic acid association to human prostasomes. *Arch Androl* 1990;24:1–10.
130. Arvidson G, Ronquist G, Wikander G, Ojteg AC. Human prostasome membranes exhibit very high cholesterol/phospholipid ratios yielding high molecular ordering. *Biochim Biophys Acta* 1989;984:167–173.
131. Kelly RW, Holland P, Skibinski G, et al. Extracellular organelles (prostasomes) are immunosuppressive components of human semen. *Clin Exp Immunol* 1991;86:550–556.
132. Eliasson R. Parameters of male fertility. In: Hafez ESE, Evans TN, eds. *Human Reproduction. Conception and Contraception.* Hagerstown, MD: Harper & Row, 1973;39–51.
133. Nelson CMK, Bunge RG. Semen analysis: evidence for changing parameters of male fertility potential. *Fertil Steril* 1974; 25:503–507.
134. Zuckerman Z, Rodriguez-Rigau LJ, Smith KD, Steinberger E. Frequency distribution of sperm counts in fertile and infertile males. *Fertil Steril* 1977;28:1310–1313.
135. Barfield A, Melo J, Coutinho E, et al. Pregnancies associated with sperm concentrations below 10 million/ml in clinical studies of a potential male contraceptive method, monthly depot medroxyprogesterone acetate and testosterone esters. *Contraception* 1979;20:121–127.
136. Fox CA, Meldrum SJ, Watson BW. Continuous measurement by radio-telemetry of vaginal pH during human coitus. *J Reprod Fertil* 1973;33:69–75.
137. Dukelow WR. Semen and artificial insemination. In: Hafez ESE, ed. *Comparative Reproduction of Nonhuman Primates.* Springfield, IL: Charles C Thomas, 1971;115–127.
138. Mandal A, Bhattacharyya AK. Relationships between the coagulation-liquefaction property of human ejaculates and their volume, sperm count and motility. *Clin Reprod Fertil* 1987; 5:367–371.
139. Fox CA, Fox B. A comparative study of coital physiology with special reference to the sexual climax. *J Reprod Fertil* 1971;24:319–336.
140. Fox CA, Wolff HS, Baker JA. Measurement of intra-vaginal and intra-uterine pressures during human coitus by radio-telemetry. *J Reprod Fertil* 1970;22:243–251.
141. Carmichael MS, Humbert R, Dixen J, Palmisano G, Greenleaf W, Davidson JM. Plasma oxytocin increases in the human sexual response. *J Clin Endocrinol Metab* 1987;64:27–31.
142. Fox CA, Ismail AAA, Love DN, Kirkham KE, Loraine JA. Studies on the relationship between plasma testosterone levels and human sexual activity. *J Endocrinol* 1972;52:51–58.
143. Neumann F, Von Berswoldt-Wallrabe R, Elger W, Steinbeck H, Hahn JD, Kramer M. Aspects of androgen-dependent events as studied by antiandrogens. *Recent Prog Horm Res* 1970;26: 337–405.
144. Morse HC, Leach DR, Rowley MJ, Heller CG. Effect of cyproterone acetate on sperm concentration, seminal fluid volume, testicular cytology and levels of plasma and urinary ICSH, FSH and testosterone in normal men. *J Reprod Fertil* 1973;32:365–378.
145. Amersbach R. Sterilität und Frigidität. *Münch Med Wochenschr* 1930;77:225–227.
146. Trapl J. Neue Anschauugen über den Ei- und Samentransport in den inneren Geschlechtsteilen der Frau. *Zentralbl Gynakol* 1943;67:547–550.
147. Egli GE, Newton M. The transport of carbon particles in the human female reproductive tract. *Fertil Steril* 1961;12:151–155.
148. Grafenberg E. The role of urethra in female orgasm. *Int J Sex* 1950;3:145–158.
149. Masters WH, Johnson VE. *Human Sexual Response.* Boston: Little, Brown, 1966.
150. Bygdeman M, Samuelsson B. Analysis of prostaglandins in human semen. Prostaglandins and related factors 44. *Clin Chim Acta* 1966;13:465–474.
151. Bygdeman M, Fredericsson B, Svanborg K, Samuelsson B. The relation between fertility and prostaglandin content of seminal fluid in man. *Fertil Steril* 1970;21:622–629.
152. Wiqvist N, Widholm O, Nillius SJ, Nilsson B. Dysmenorrhea and prostaglandins. *Acta Obstet Gynecol Scand* (*Suppl*) 1979;87.
153. Settlage DSF, Motoshima M, Tredway DR. Sperm transport from the external cervical os to the fallopian tubes in women: a time and quantitation study. *Fertil Steril* 1973;24:655–661.
154. Moghissi KS. Sperm migration through the human cervix. In: Elstein M, Moghissi KS, Borth R, eds. *Cervical Mucus in Human Reproduction.* Copenhagen: Scriptor, 1972;128–152.
155. Templeton AA, Cooper I, Kelly RW. Prostaglandin concentrations in the semen of fertile men. *J Reprod Fertil* 1978;52: 147–150.
156. Eskin BA, Azarbal S, Sepic R, Slate WG. *In vitro* responses of the spermatozoa-cervical mucus system treated with prostaglandin $F_{2\alpha}$. *Obstet Gynecol* 1973;41:436–439.
157. Colon JM, Gagliardi C, Schoenfeld C, Amelar RD, Dubin L, Weiss G. Human relaxin stimulates human sperm penetration of bovine cervical mucus. *Fertil Steril* 1989;52:340–342.
158. Weiss G, Goldsmith LT, Schoenfeld C, D'Eletto R. Partial purification of relaxin from human seminal plasma. *Am J Obstet Gynecol* 1986;154:749–755.

159. Elstein M, Moghissi KS, Borth R, eds. *Cervical Mucus in Human Reproduction.* Copenhagen: Scriptor, 1972.
160. Yudin AI, Hanson FW, Katz DF. Human cervical mucus and its interaction with sperm: a fine-structural view. *Biol Reprod* 1989;40:661–671.
161. Billings EL, Billings JJ, Brown JB, Burger HG. Symptoms and hormonal changes accompanying ovulation. *Lancet* 1972;i: 282–284.
162. Flynn AM, Lynch SS. Cervical mucus and identification of the fertile phase of the menstrual cycle. *Br J Obstet Gynaecol* 1976;83:656–659.
163. World Health Organization. A prospective multicentre trial of the ovulation method of natural family planning. I. The teaching phase. *Fertil Steril* 1981;36:152–158.
164. World Health Organization. A prospective multicentre trial of the ovulation method of natural family planning. II. The effectiveness phase. *Fertil Steril* 1981;36:591–598.
165. Moghissi KS. Cyclic changes of cervical mucus in normal and progestin-treated women. *Fertil Steril* 1966;17:663–675.
166. Baker TG. Oogenesis and ovulation. In: Austin CR, Short RV, eds. *Reproduction in Mammals. I. Germ Cells and Fertilization.* Ed 2. Cambridge, UK: Cambridge University Press, 1982;17–45.
167. Katz DF, Drobnis EZ, Overstreet JW. Factors regulating mammalian sperm migration through the female reproductive tract and oocyte vestments. *Gamete Res* 1989;22:443–469.
168. Mattner PE. The distribution of spermatozoa and leucocytes in the female genital tract in goats and cattle. *J Reprod Fertil* 1968;17:253–261.
169. Hafez ESE. The comparative anatomy of the mammalian cervix. In: Blandau RJ, Moghissi KS, eds. *The Biology of the Cervix.* Chicago: University of Chicago Press, 1973;23–56.
170. Hunter RHF. Human fertilization *in vivo,* with special reference to progression, storage and release of competent spermatozoa. *Hum Reprod* 1987;2:329–332.
171. Bielfeld P, Jayendran RS, Zanefeld LJ. Human spermatozoa do not undergo the acrosome reaction during storage in the cervix. *Intl J Fertil* 1991;36:302–306.
172. Chang MC. Reaction of the uterus on spermatozoa in the rabbit. *Ann Ostet Ginecol* 1956;78:74–86.
173. Hafez ESE. Gamete transport. In: Hafez ESE, Evans TN, eds. *Human Reproduction. Conception and Contraception.* Hagerstown, MD: Harper & Row, 1973;85–118.
174. Shukla JB, Chandra P, Sharma R, Radhakrishnamacharya G. Effects of peristaltic and longitudinal wave motion of the channel wall on movement of micro-organisms: application to spermatozoa transport. *J Biomechan* 1988;21:947–954.
175. Krzemiński A, Sikorski R, Bokiniec M. Sperm penetration through cervical mucus in infertile couples in relation to selected cervical factors. *Hum Reprod* 1988;3:353–355.
176. Pretorius E, Franken DR. The immunobead technique: an indicator of disturbed sperm cervical mucus interaction. *Andrologia* 1988;20:5–9.
177. Mathur S, Rosenlund C, Carlton M, et al. Studies on sperm survival and motility in the presence of cytotoxic sperm antibodies. *Am J Reprod Immunol Microbiol* 1988;17:41–47.
178. Menge AC, Beitner O. Interrelationships among semen characteristics, antisperm antibodies, and cervical mucus penetration assays in infertile human couples. *Fertil Steril* 1989;51:486–492.
179. Chantler E, Sharma R, Sharman D. Changes in cervical mucus that prevent penetration by spermatozoa. *Symp Soc Exp Biol* 1989;43:325–336.
180. Tan SL, Scammell G, Houang E. The midcycle cervical microbial flora as studied by the weighed-swab method, and its possible correlation with results of sperm cervical mucus penetration tests. *Fertil Steril* 1987;47:941–946.
181. Keel BA, Webster BW. Correlation of human sperm motility characteristics with an *in vitro* cervical mucus penetration test. *Fertil Steril* 1988;49:138–143.
182. Ikuma K, Saito Y, Takeda M, Koyama K, Isojima S. Bovine cervical mucus as a substitute for human cervical mucus. *Nippon Sanka Fujinka Gakkai Zasshi* 1988;40:888–894.
183. De Geyter C, Bals-Pratsch M, Doeren M, et al. Human and bovine cervical mucus penetration as a test of sperm function for *in-vitro* fertilization. *Hum Reprod* 1988;3:948–954.
184. Mortimer D, Mortimer ST, Shu MA, Swart R. A simplified approach to sperm-cervical mucus interaction testing using a hyaluronate migration test. *Hum Reprod* 1990;5:835–841.
185. Kolodzief FB, Katzorke T, Propping D. Prognostic value of the sperm-penetration-meter test according to Kremer. *Andrologia* 1986;18:539–544.
186. Eggert-Kruse W, Leinhos G, Gerhard I, Tilgen W, Runnebaum B. Prognostic value of *in vitro* sperm penetration into hormonally standardized human cervical mucus. *Fertil Steril* 1989;51: 317–323.
187. Jaffe SB, Jewelewicz R. The basic infertility investigation. *Fertil Steril* 1991;56:599–613.
188. Daru J, Williamson HO, Rust PF, Homm RJ, Mathur S. A computerized postcoital test of sperm motility: comparison with clinical postcoital test and correlations with sperm antibodies. *Arch Androl* 1988;21:189–203.
189. Dunphy BC, Barratt CLR, Kay R, Jones DE, Cooke ID. Postcoital test: which form of spermatozoal motility is associated with a good fertility outcome? *Andrologia* 1990;22:269–273.
190. Freundl G, Grimm HJ, Hofmann N. Selective filtration of abnormal spermatozoa by the cervical mucus. *Hum Reprod* 1988;3: 277–280.
191. Katz DF, Morales P, Samuels SJ, Overstreet JW. Mechanisms of filtration of morphologically abnormal human sperm by cervical mucus. *Fertil Steril* 1990;54:513–516.
192. Fox CA, Knaggs GS. Milk-ejection activity (oxytocin) in peripheral venous blood in man during lactation and in association with coitus. *J Endocrinol* 1969;45:145–146.
193. Kumar D. Hormonal regulation of myometrial activity: clinical implications. In: Wynn RM, ed. *Cellular Biology of the Uterus.* New York: Appleton-Century-Crofts, 1967;449–474.
194. Levi L. The urinary output of adrenalin and noradrenalin during pleasant and unpleasant emotional states. A preliminary report. *Psychosom Med* 1965;27:80–85.
195. Sparks M, Lee CM. Clinical use of PGs in fertility control. *Popul Rep* 1973;G:1–15.
196. Bygdeman M, Bergström S. Clinical use of prostaglandins for pregnancy termination. *Popul Rep* 1976;G:65–75.
197. Gréen K, Bygdeman M. Plasma levels of the methyl ester of 15-methyl $PGF_{2\alpha}$ in connection with intravenous and vaginal administration. *Prostaglandins* 1976;11:879–892.
198. Bygdeman M, Eliasson R. The effect of prostaglandin from human seminal fluid on the motility of the non-pregnant human uterus *in vitro. Acta Physiol Scand* 1963;59:43–51.
199. Bygdeman M, Hamberg M, Samuelsson B. The content of different prostaglandins in human seminal fluid and their threshold dose on the human myometrium. *Mem Soc Endocrinol* 1976;14:49–63.
200. Karim SMM, Sharma SD. Therapeutic abortion and induction of labour by the intravaginal administration of prostaglandins E_2 or $F_{2\alpha}$. *J. Obstet Gynaecol Br Commonw* 1971;78:294–300.
201. Gréen K, Svanborg K. On the mechanism of action of 15-methyl $PGF_{2\alpha}$ as an abortifacient. *Prostaglandins* 1979;17:277–282.
202. Gottlieb C, Andersson E, Fried G. The effect of 19-hydroxy prostaglandins on the human myometrium *in vitro. Prostaglandins* 1991;41:607–613.
203. Braquet P, Touqui L, Shen TY, Vargaftig BB. Perspectives in platelet-activating research. *Pharmacol Rev* 1987;39:97–145.
204. Ricker DD, Minhas BS, Kumar R, Robertson JL, Dodson MG. The effect of platelet-activating factor on the motility of human spermatozoa. *Fertil Steril* 1989;52:655–658.
205. Kumar R, Harper MJK, Hanahan DJ. Occurrence of platelet-activating factor in rabbit spermatozoa. *Arch Biochem Biophys* 1988;260:497–502.
206. Kuzan FB, Geissler FT, Henderson WR Jr. Role of spermatozoal platelet-activating factor in fertilization. *Prostaglandins* 1990; 39:61–74.
207. Yasuda K, Satouchi K, Saito K. Platelet-activating factor in normal rat uterus. *Biochem Biophys Res Commun* 1986;138: 1231–1236.
208. Angle MJ, Jones MA, McManus LM, Pinckard RN, Harper MJK. Platelet-activating factor in the rabbit uterus during early pregnancy. *J Reprod Fertil* 1988;83:711–722.
209. Alecozay AA, Casslén BG, Riehl RM, et al. Platelet-activating

factor (PAF) in the human luteal phase endometrium. *Biol Reprod* 1989;41:578–586.
210. Minhas BS, Kumar R, Ricker DD, Roudebush WE, Dodson MG, Fortunato SJ. Effects of platelet activating factor on mouse oocyte fertilization *in vitro*. *Am J Obstet Gynecol* 1989;161: 1714–1717.
211. Honda Z-i, Nakamura M, Miki I, et al. Cloning by functional expression of platelet-activating factor receptor from guinea pig lung. *Nature* 1991;349:342–346.
212. Nakamura M, Honda Z-i, Izumi T, et al. Molecular cloning and expression of platelet-activating factor receptor from human leukocytes. *J Biol Chem* 1991;266:20400–20405.
213. Ye R, Prossnitz ER, Cochrane CG. Characterization of a human cDNA that encodes a functional receptor for platelet-activating factor. *Biochem Biophys Res Commun* 1991;180:105–111.
214. Kudolo GB, Harper MJK. Characterization of platelet-activating factor binding sites on uterine membranes from pregnant rabbits. *Biol Reprod* 1989;41:587–603.
215. Kudolo GB, Harper MJK. Estimation of platelet-activating factor receptors in the endometrium of the pregnant rabbit: regulation of ligand availability and catabolism by bovine serum albumin. *Biol Reprod* 1990;43:368–377.
216. Kudolo GB, Kasamo M, Harper MJK. Autoradiographic localization of platelet-activating factor (PAF) binding sites in the rabbit endometrium during the peri-implantation period. *Cell Tissue Res* 1991;265:231–241.
217. Zhu Y-p, Word RA, Johnston JM. The presence of high affinity binding sites for platelet-activating factor in human myometrium and its role in uterine contraction (abstract). *Proc Soc Gynecol Invest* 1990;37:161.
218. Overstreet JW, Cooper GW, Katz DF. Sperm transport in the reproductive tract of the female rabbit. II. The sustained phase of transport. *Biol Reprod* 1978;19:115–132.
219. Howe GR. Leukocytic response to spermatozoa in ligated segments of the rabbit vagina, uterus and oviduct. *J Reprod Fertil* 1967;13:563–566.
220. Austin CR. Fate of spermatozoa in the female genital tract. *J Reprod Fertil* 1960;1:151–156.
221. Rubinstein BB, Strauss H, Lazarus ML, Hankin H. Sperm survival in women. Motile sperm in the fundus and tubes of surgical cases. *Fertil Steril* 1951;2:15–19.
222. Moyer DL, Rimdusit S, Mishell DR, Jr. Sperm distribution and degradation in the human female reproductive tract. *Obstet Gynecol* 1970;35:831–840.
223. Barratt CLR, Bolton AE, Cooke ID. Functional significance of white blood cells in the male and female reproductive tract. *Hum Reprod* 1990;5:639–648.
224. Pandya IJ, Cohen J. The leucocytic reaction of the human cervix to spermatozoa. *Fertil Steril* 1985;43:417–421.
225. VandeVoort CA, Tollner TL, Tarantal AF, Overstreet JW. Ultrasound-guided transfundal uterine sperm recovery from *Macaca fascicularis*. *Gamete Res* 1989;24:327–331.
226. Urry RL, Middleton RG, Jones K, Poulson M, Worley R, Keye W. Artificial insemination: a comparison of pregnancy rates with intrauterine versus cervical insemination and washed sperm versus swim-up preparations. *Fertil Steril* 1988;49:1036–1038.
227. DiMarzo SJ, Rakoff JS. Intrauterine insemination with husband's washed sperm. *Fertil Steril* 1986;46:470–475.
228. Arny M, Quagliarello J. Semen quality before and after processing by a swim-up method: relationship to outcome of intrauterine insemination. *Fertil Steril* 1987;48:643–648.
229. Francavilla F, Romano R, Santucci R, Poccia G. Effect of sperm morphology and motile sperm count on outcome of intrauterine insemination in oligozoospermia and/or asthenozoospermia. *Fertil Steril* 1990;53:892–897.
230. Mićič S, Papič N, Mladenovič I, Proročič M, Genbaćev O. Intrauterine insemination with spermatozoa recovered from the aspirate of artificial spermatocele. *Hum Reprod* 1990;5:582–585.
231. Tsutsui T, Kawakami E, Murao I, Ogasa A. Transport of spermatozoa in the reproductive tract of the bitch: observations through the uterine fistula. *Nippon Juigaku Zasshi* 1989;51:560–565.
232. Gallagher GR, Senger PL. Concentrations of spermatozoa in the vagina of heifers after deposition of semen in the uterine horns, uterine body or cervix. *J Reprod Fertil* 1989;86:19–25.
233. Rowson LEA, Bennett JP, Harper MJK. The problem of nonsurgical egg transfer to the cow uterus. *Vet Rec* 1964;76:21–23.
234. Cooper GW, Overstreet JW, Katz DF. The motility of rabbit spermatozoa recovered from the female reproductive tract. *Gamete Res* 1979;2:35–42.
235. Olds-Clarke P. Motility characteristics of sperm from the uterus and oviducts of female mice after mating to congenic males differing in sperm transport and fertility. *Biol Reprod* 1986;34: 453–467.
236. Suarez SS, Osman RA. Initiation of hyperactivated flagellar bending in mouse sperm within the female reproductive tract. *Biol Reprod* 1987;36:1191–1198.
237. Guerin JF, Ouhibi N, Regnier-Vigouroux G, Menezo Y. Movement characteristics and hyperactivation of human sperm on different epithelial cell monolayers. *Int J Androl* 1991;14:412–422.
238. Suarez SS, Katz DF, Owen DH, Andrew JB, Powell RL. Evidence for the function of hyperactivated motility in sperm. *Biol Reprod* 1991;44:375–381.
239. Wynn RM. Histology and ultrastructure of the human endometrium. In: Wynn RM, ed. *Biology of the Uterus*. New York: Plenum Press, 1977;341–376.
240. Beier HM, Beier-Hellwig K. Specific secretory protein of the female genital tract. *Acta Endocrinol (Suppl)* 1973;180:404–422.
241. Beier HM. Oviducal and uterine fluids. *J Reprod Fertil* 1974;37:221–237.
242. Bernstein GS, Aladjem F, Chen S. Proteins in human endometrial washings—a preliminary report. *Fertil Steril* 1971;22: 722–726.
243. Maathius JB, Aitken RJ. Cyclic variation in concentrations of protein and hexose in human uterine flushings collected by an improved technique. *J Reprod Fertil* 1978;52:289–295.
244. Casslén B, Nilsson B. Human uterine fluid examined in undiluted samples for osmolarity and the concentrations of inorganic ions, albumin, glucose and urea. *Am J Obstet Gynecol* 1984;150:877–881.
245. Casslén B. Uterine fluid volume. Cyclic variations and possible extrauterine contributions. *J Reprod Med* 1986;31:506–510.
246. Casslén BG. Free amino acids in human uterine fluid. Possible role of high taurine concentration. *J Reprod Med* 1987;32: 181–184.
247. Voglmayr JK, Sawyer RF Jr. Surface transformation of ram spermatozoa in uterine, oviduct and cauda epididymal fluids *in vitro*. *J Reprod Fertil* 1986;78:315–325.
248. Magnus Ø, Åbyholm T, Kofstad J, Purvis K. Ionized calcium in human male and female reproductive fluids: relationships to sperm motility. *Hum Reprod* 1990;5:94–98.
249. Alvarez F, Diaz S, Croxatto HB. Personal communication. 1985.
250. Wilborn WH, Flowers CE. Histoenzymology of human endometrium during the proliferative and secretory phases. In: Beller FK, Schumacher GFB, eds. *The Biology of the Fluids of the Female Genital Tract*. New York: Elsevier/North Holland, 1979;73–87.
251. Moyer DL, El Sahwi S, Macaulay L, Shaw ST Jr. Cells of the uterine fluid. In: Beller FK, Schumacher GFB, eds. *The Biology of the Fluids of the Female Genital Tract*. New York: Elsevier/ North Holland, 1979;59–71.
252. Bellinge BS, Copeland CM, Thomas TD, Mazzucchelli RE, O'Neill G, Cohen MJ. The influence of patient insemination on the implantation rate in in-vitro fertilization and embryo transfer programme. *Fertil Steril* 1986;46:252–256.
253. Woodruff JD, Pauerstein CJ. *The Fallopian Tube. Structure, Function, Pathology, and Management*. Baltimore: Williams & Wilkins, 1969.
254. Eddy CA, Pauerstein CJ. Tubal reproductive function and the development of reversible sterilization techniques. In: Sciarra JJ, Zatuchni GI, Speidel JJ, eds. *Reversal of Sterilization*. Hagerstown, MD: Harper & Row, 1978;100–116.
255. Eddy CA, Harper MJK. Gamete transport, fertilization, and implantation. In: Shain RN, Pauerstein CJ, eds. *Fertility Control. Biologic and Behavioral Aspects*. Hagerstown, MD: Harper & Row, 1980;32–48.
256. Rocca M, el Habashy M, Nayel S, Madwar A. The intramural segment of the uterotubal junction: an anatomic and histologic study. *Int J Gynaecol Obstet* 1989;28:343–349.
257. Faussone-Pellegrini MS, Bani G. The muscle coat morphology of

the mouse oviduct during the estrous cycle. *Arch Histol Cytol* 1990;53:167–178.

258. Rodriguez-Martinez H, Nicander L, Viring S, Einarsson S. Ultrastructure of the uterotubal junction in preovulatory pigs. *Anat Histol Embryol* 1990;19:16–36.
259. Persson E, Rodriguez-Martinez H. The ligamentum infundibulocornuale in the pig: morphological and physiological studies of the smooth muscle component. *Acta Anat* 1990;138:111–120.
260. Baker RD, Degen AA. Transport of live and dead boar spermatozoa within the reproductive tract of gilts. *J Reprod Fertil* 1972;28:369–377.
261. Smith TT, Koyanagi F, Yanagimachi R. Quantitative comparison of the presence of the passage of homologous and heterologous spermatozoa through the uterotubal junction of the golden hamster. *Gamete Res* 1988;19:227–234.
262. Shalgi R, Smith TT, Yanagimachi R. A quantitative comparison of the passage of capacitated and uncapacitated hamster spermatozoa through the uterotubal junction. *Biol Reprod* 1992;46: 419–424.
263. Gaddum-Rosse P. Some observations on sperm transport through the uterotubal junction of the rat. *Am J Anat* 1981;160:333–341.
264. Howe GR, Black DL. Migration of rat and foreign spermatozoa through the utero-tubal junction of the oestrous rat. *J Reprod Fertil* 1963;5:95–100.
265. Marcus SL. The passage of rat and foreign spermatozoa through the uterotubal junction of the rat. *Am J Obstet Gynecol* 1965;91:985–989.
266. Glover TD, Patterson JA. The passage of ^{131}I-labelled copolymer polystyrene-divinylbenzene microspheres through the reproductive tract of the female rabbit. *J Endocrinol* 1963;26:175–176.
267. First NL, Short RE, Peters JB, Stratman FW. Transport and loss of boar spermatozoa in the reproductive tract of the sow. *J Anim Sci* 1968;27:1037–1040.
268. Black DL, Asdell SA. Transport through the rabbit oviduct. *Am J Physiol* 1958;192:63–68.
269. Black DL, Asdell SA. Mechanism controlling entry of ova into rabbit uterus. *Am J Physiol* 1959;197:1275–1278.
270. Chang MC. Fertilization in relation to the number of spermatozoa in the fallopian tubes of rabbits. *Ann Ostet Ginecol* 1951;73:918–925.
271. Ahlgren M. Sperm transport to and survival in the human fallopian tube. *Gynecol Invest* 1975;6:206–214.
272. Croxatto HB, Faundes A, Medel M, et al. Studies on sperm migration in the human female genital tract. In: Hafez ESE, Thibault CG, eds. *The Biology of Spermatozoa.* Basel: Karger, 1975;56–62.
273. Croxatto HB. Personal communication. 1985.
274. Settlage DSF, Motoshima M, Tredway D. Sperm transport from the vagina to the Fallopian tubes in women. In: Hafez ESE, Thibault CG, eds. *The Biology of Spermatozoa.* Basel: Karger, 1975;74–82.
275. Foldesy RG, Bedford JM, Orgebin-Crist MC. Fertilizing rabbit spermatozoa are not selected as a special population by the female tract. *J Reprod Fertil* 1984;70:75–82.
276. Guastella G, Comparetto G, Gullo D, et al. Gamete intrafallopian transfer (GIFT): a new technique for the treatment of unexplained infertility. *Acta Eur Fertil* 1985;16:311–316.
277. Asch RH, Balmaceda JP, Ellsworth LR, Wong PC. Preliminary experiences with gamete intrafallopian transfer (GIFT). *Fertil Steril* 1986;45:366–371.
278. Matson PL, Blackledge DG, Richardson PA, Turner SR, Yovich YM, Yovich JL. The role of gamete intrafallopian transfer (GIFT) in the treatment of oligospermic infertility. *Fertil Steril* 1987;48:608–612.
279. Vancaillie T, Schmidt EH. The uterotubal junction. A proposal for classifying its morphology as assessed with hysteroscopy. *J Reprod Med* 1988;33:624–629.
280. Kerin J, Daykhovsky L, Segalowitz J, et al. Falloposcopy: a microendoscopic technique for visual exploration of the human fallopian tube from the uterotubal ostium to the fimbria using a transvaginal approach. *Fertil Steril* 1990;54:390–400.
281. Ahlgren M, Boström K, Malmqvist R. Sperm transport and survival in women with special reference to the fallopian tube. In: Hafez ESE, Thibault CG, eds. *The Biology of Spermatozoa.* Basel: Karger, 1973;63–73.
282. Horne HW Jr, Audet C. "Spider cells," a new inhabitant of peritoneal fluid. A preliminary report. *Obstet Gynecol* 1985;11: 421–423.
283. Braden AWH. Distribution of sperms in the genital tract of the female rabbit after coitus. *Aust J Biol Sci* 1953;6:693–705.
284. Zamboni L. Fertilization in the mouse. In: Moghissi KS, Hafez ESE, eds. *Biology of Mammalian Fertilization and Implantation.* Springfield, IL: Charles C Thomas, 1972;213–262.
285. Harper MJK. Relationship between sperm transport and penetration of eggs in the rabbit oviduct. *Biol Reprod* 1973;8:441–450.
286. Hunter RHF. Physiological aspects of sperm transport in the domestic pig, *Sus scrofa*. II. Regulation, survival and fate of cells. *Br Vet J* 1975;131:681–690.
287. Hunter RHF. Pre-ovulatory arrest and peri-ovulatory redistribution of competent spermatozoa in the isthmus of the pig oviduct. *J Reprod Fertil* 1984;72:203–211.
288. Hunter RHF, Barwise L, King R. Sperm transport, storage and release in the sheep oviduct in relation to the time of ovulation. *Br Vet J* 1982;138:225–232.
289. Hunter RHF, Nichol R. Transport of spermatozoa in the sheep oviduct: preovulatory sequestering of cells in the caudal isthmus. *J Exp Zool* 1983;228:121–128.
290. Hunter RHF, Wilmut I. The rate of functional sperm transport into the oviducts of mated cows. *Anim Reprod Sci* 1983;5:167–173.
291. Hunter RHF, Wilmut I. Sperm transport in the cow: periovulatory redistribution of viable cells within the oviduct. *Reprod Nutr Dev* 1984;24:597–608.
292. Harper MJK. Stimulation of sperm movement from the isthmus to the site of fertilization in the rabbit oviduct. *Biol Reprod* 1973;8:369–377.
293. Ito M, Smith TT, Yanagimachi R. Effect of ovulation on sperm transport in the hamster oviduct. *J Reprod Fertil* 1991;93: 157–163.
294. Ralt D, Goldenberg M, Fetterolf P, et al. Sperm attraction to a follicular factor(s) correlates with human egg fertilizability. *Proc Natl Acad Sci USA* 1991;88:2840–2844.
295. Marinov MF, Petkov Z. Sperm forward movement in the female genital tract of sheep. *Vet Med Nauki* 1988;20:28–33.
296. Villanueva-Díaz C, Avias-Martínez J, Bustos-López H, Vadillo-Ortega F. Novel model for study of human sperm chemotaxis. *Fertil Steril* 1992;58:392–395.
297. McNutt TL, Killian GJ. Influence of bovine follicular and oviduct fluids on sperm capacitation in vitro. *J Androl* 1991;12: 244–252.
298. Hunter RHF, Cook B, Poyser NL. Regulation of oviduct function in pigs by local transfer of ovarian steroids and prostaglandins: a mechanism to influence sperm transport. *Eur J Obstet Gynaecol Reprod Biol* 1983;14:225–232.
299. Rodriguez-Martinez H, Ekstedt E, Ridderstråle Y. Histochemical localization of carbonic anhydrase in the female genitalia of pigs during the oestrous cycle. *Acta Anat* 1991;140:41–47.
300. Burkman LJ, Overstreet JW, Katz DF. A possible role for potassium and pyruvate in the modulation of sperm motility in the rabbit oviductal isthmus. *J Reprod Fertil* 1984;71:367–376.
301. Hunter RHF, Nicol R. A pre-ovulatory temperature gradient between the isthmus and ampulla of pig oviducts during the phase of sperm storage. *J Reprod Fertil* 1986;77:599–606.
302. Khatchadourian C, Menezo Y, Gerard M, Thibault C. Catecholamines within the rabbit oviduct at fertilization time. *Hum Reprod* 1987;2:1–5.
303. Nagasaka T. Effect of microsurgical ampullary segmental reversal on fertilization in the rabbit. *Nippon Sanka Fujinka Gakkai Zasshi* 1984;36:2155–2160.
304. Phillips DM. Comparative analysis of mammalian sperm motility. *J Cell Biol* 1972;53:561–573.
305. Suarez SS. Sperm transport and motility in the mouse oviduct: observations in situ. *Biol Reprod* 1987;36:203–210.
306. Demott RP, Suarez SS. Hyperactivated sperm progress in the mouse oviduct. *Biol Reprod* 1992;46:779–785.
307. Jansen RPS. Fallopian tube isthmic mucus and ovum transport. *Science* 1978;201:349–351.

308. Jansen RPS, Bajpai VK. Oviduct acid mucus glycoproteins in the estrous rabbit: ultrastructure and histochemistry. *Biol Reprod* 1982;26:155–168.
309. Pollard JW, Plante C, King WA, Hansen PJ, Betteridge KJ, Suarez SS. Fertilizing capacity of bovine sperm may be maintained by binding to oviductal epithelial cells. *Biol Reprod* 1991;44:102–107.
310. Smith TT, Yanagimachi R. Attachment and release of spermatozoa from the caudal isthmus of the hamster oviduct. *J Reprod Fertil* 1991;91:567–573.
311. Trounson AE, Mohr LR, Wood C, Leeton JF. Effect of delayed insemination on *in vitro* fertilization, culture and transfer of human embryos. *J Reprod Fertil* 1982;64:285–294.
312. Nagai T, Moor RM. Effect of oviduct cells on the incidence of polyspermy in pig eggs fertilized *in vitro. Mol Reprod Dev* 1990;26:377–382.
313. Lippes J, Wagh PV. Human oviductal fluid (hOF) proteins. IV. Evidence for hOF proteins binding to human sperm. *Fertil Steril* 1989;51:89–94.
314. Hunter RHF, Fléchon B, Fléchon JE. Distribution, morphology and epithelial interactions of bovine spermatozoa in the oviduct before and after ovulation: a scanning electron microscope study. *Tissue Cell* 1991;23:641–656.
315. Jansen RPS. Endocrine response in the fallopian tube. *Endocr Rev* 1984;5:525–551.
316. Hammar M, Larsson-Cohn U. Massive enlargement of occluded tubes after postmenopausal treatment with natural estrogens. *Acta Obstet Gynecol Scand* 1978;57:189–190.
317. Lippes J, Enders RG, Pragay DA, Bartholomew WR. The collection and analysis of human fallopian tube fluid. *Contraception* 1972;5:85–103.
318. Lippes J, Kramer J, Alfonso LA, Dacalos ED, Lucero R. Human oviductal fluid proteins. *Fertil Steril* 1981;36:623–629.
319. Borland RM, Biggers JD, Lechene CP, Taymor ML. Elemental composition of fluid in the human fallopian tube. *J Reprod Fertil* 1980;58:479–482.
320. Brinster RL. Studies on the development of mouse embryos *in vitro*. II. The effect of energy source. *J Exp Zool* 1965;158:59–68.
321. Brinster RL. *In vitro* culture of mammalian embryos. *J Anim Sci* 1968;27(suppl 1):1–14.
322. Oshiba Y, Ueno M, Fujiwara T, Hata K, Suzuki S, Iizuka R. Morphology and secretion of the oviduct. *Progr Clin Biol Res* 1989;296:399–404.
323. Maas DHA, Storey BT, Mastroianni L Jr. Hydrogen ion and carbon dioxide content of the oviductal fluid of the Rhesus monkey (*Macaca mulatta*). *Fertil Steril* 1977;28:981–985.
324. Gott AL, Gray SM, James AF, Leese HJ. The mechanism and control of rabbit oviduct fluid formation. *Biol Reprod* 1988; 39:758–763.
325. Leese HJ. The formation and function of oviduct fluid. *J Reprod Fertil* 1988;82:843–856.
326. Weström L, Mårdh P-A, Mecklenberg C, Håkansson CH. Studies on ciliated epithelia of the human genital tract. II. The mucociliary wave pattern of fallopian tube epithelium. *Fertil Steril* 1977;28:955–961.
327. Hodgson BJ. Post-ovulatory changes in the water content and inulin space of the rabbit oviduct. *J Reprod Fertil* 1978; 53:349–351.
328. Blake JR, Vann PG, Winet H. A model of ovum transport. *J Theor Biol* 1983;102:145–166.
329. Brown C, LaVigne WE, Padilla SL. Unruptured pregnancy in a heterotopic fallopian tube: evidence for transperitoneal sperm migration. *Am J Obstet Gynecol* 1987;156:88–90.
330. Turhan NO, Artini PG, D'Ambrogio G, Droghini F, Volpe A, Genazzani AR. Studies on direct intraperitoneal insemination in the management of male factor, cervical factor, unexplained and immunological infertility. *Hum Reprod* 1992;7:66–71.
331. Talo A. Electrophysiology of the oviduct. In: Harper MJK, Pauerstein CJ, Adams CE, Coutinho EM, Croxatto HB, Paton DM, eds. *Ovum Transport and Fertility Regulation.* Copenhagen: Scriptor, 1976;161–167.
332. Talo A, Hodgson BJ. Spike bursts in rabbit oviduct. I. Effect of ovulation. *Am J Physiol* 1978;234:E430–E438.
333. Talo A, Pulkkinen MO. Electrical activity in the human oviduct during the menstrual cycle. *Am J Obstet Gynecol* 1982; 142:135–147.
334. Owman CL, Falck B, Johansson EDB, et al. Autonomic nerves and related amine receptors mediating motor activity in the oviduct of monkey and man. Histochemical, chemical and pharmacological study. In: Harper MJK, Pauerstein CJ, Adams CE, Coutinho EM, Croxatto HB, Paton DM, eds. *Ovum Transport and Fertility Regulation.* Copenhagen: Scriptor, 1976;256–275.
335. Chang MC, Austin CR, Bedford JM, Brackett BG, Hunter RHF, Yanagimachi R. Capacitation of spermatozoa and fertilization in mammals. In: Greep RO, Koblinsky MA, eds. *Frontiers in Reproduction and Fertility Control. A Review of the Reproductive Sciences and Contraceptive Development.* Cambridge, MA: MIT Press, 1977;434–451.
336. Austin CR. Observations on the penetration of sperm into the mammalian egg. *Aust J Sci Res B* 1951;4:581–596.
337. Chang MC. Fertilizing capacity of spermatozoa deposited into the fallopian tubes. *Nature* 1951;168:697–698.
338. Brackett BG, Seitz HM Jr, Rocha G, Mastroianni L Jr. The mammalian fertilization process. In: Moghissi KS, Hafez ESE, eds. *Biology of Mammalian Fertilization and Implantation.* Springfield, IL: Charles C Thomas, 1972;165–184.
339. Edwards RG, Bavister BD, Steptoe PC. Early stages of fertilization *in vitro* of human oocytes matured *in vitro. Nature* 1969;221:632–635.
340. Edwards RG, Steptoe PC, Purdy JM. Fertilization and cleavage *in vitro* of preovulatory human oocytes. *Nature* 1970; 227:1307–1309.
341. Ahuja KK, Smith W, Tucker M, Craft I. Successful pregnancies from the transfer of pronucleate embryos in an outpatient *in vitro* fertilization program. *Fertil Steril* 1985;44:181–184.
342. Ehrenwald E, Foote RH, Parks JE. Bovine oviductal fluid components and their potential role in sperm cholesterol efflux. *Mol Reprod Dev* 1990;25:195–204.
343. Harper MJK, Chang MC. Some aspects of the biology of mammalian eggs and spermatozoa. *Adv Reprod Physiol* 1971; 5:167–218.
344. Corselli J, Talbot P. *In vitro* penetration of hamster oocyte-cumulus complexes using physiological numbers of sperm. *Dev Biol* 1987;122:227–242.
345. Chang MC. Développement de la capacité fertilisatrice des spermatozoïdes du lapin à l'intérieur du tractus génital femelle et fécondabilité des oeufs de lapine. In: *La Fonction Tubaire et Ses Troubles: Physiologie, Explorations, Pathologie, Thérapeutique.* Paris: Masson & Cie, 1955;40–52.
346. Hunter RHF. Attempted fertilization of hamster eggs following transplantation into the uterus. *J Exp Zool* 1968;168:511–516.
347. Estes WL Jr, Heitmeyer PL. Pregnancy following ovarian implantation. *Am J Surg* 1934;24:563–580.
348. Preston PG. Transplantation of the ovary into the uterine cavity for the treatment of sterility in women. *J Obstet Gynaecol Br Emp* 1953;60:862–864.
349. Iklé FA. Schwangerschaft nach Implantation des Ovars in den Uterus. *Gynaecologia* 1961;151:95–99.
350. Simpson JL, Gray RH, Queenan JT, et al. Pregnancy outcome associated with natural family planning (NFP, scientific basis and experimental design for an international cohort study. *Adv Contracept* 1988;4:247–264.
351. Austin CR. Ageing and reproduction: post-ovulatory deterioration of the egg. *J Reprod Fertil (Suppl)* 1970;12:39–53.
352. Smith AL, Lodge JR. Interactions of aged gametes: *in vitro* fertilization using *in vitro*-aged sperm and *in vivo*-aged ova in the mouse. *Gamete Res* 1987;16:47–56.
353. Tappa B, Amao H, Ogasa A, Takahashi KW. Changes in the estrous cycle and number of ovulated and fertilized ova in aging female IVCS mice. *Jikken Dobutsu* 1989;38:115–119.
354. Nogués C, Ponsà M, Vidal F, Boada M, Egozcue J. Effects of aging on the zona pellucida surface of mouse oocytes. *J In Vitro Fertil Embryo Transfer* 1988;5:225–229.
355. Cittadini E, Palermo R. Infertility in advanced reproductive age. Results of *in vitro* fertilization and embryo transfer according to the woman's age. *Acta Eur Fertil* 1989;20:285–297.
356. Zenses MT, de Geyter C, Bordt J, Schneider HP, Nieschlag E. Abnormalities of sperm chromosome condensation in the cyto-

plasm of immature human oocytes. *Hum Reprod* 1990; 5:842–846.
357. Navot D, Bergh PA, Williams MA, et al. Poor oocyte quality rather than implantation failure as a cause of age-related decline in female fertility. *Lancet* 1991;337:1375–1377.
358. Levran D, Ben-Shlomo I, Dor J, Ben-Rafael Z, Nebel L, Mashiach S. Aging of endometrium and oocytes: observations on conception and abortion rates in an egg donation model. *Fertil Steril* 1991;56:1091–1094.
359. Wertheim I, Jagiello GM, Ducayen MB. Aging and aneuploidy in human oocytes and follicular cells. *J Gerontol* 1986;41:567–573.
360. Ezra Y, Simon A, Laufer N. Defective oocytes: a new subgroup of unexplained infertility. *Fertil Steril* 1992;58:24–27.
361. Austin CR. The egg. In: Austin CR, Short RV, eds. *Reproduction in Mammals. I. Germ Cells and Fertilization,* Ed 2. Cambridge, UK: Cambridge University Press, 1982;46–62.
362. Tsutsui T. Gamete physiology and timing of ovulation and fertilization in dogs. *J Reprod Fertil Suppl* 1989;39:269–275.
363. Cheviakoff S, Díaz S, Carril M, et al. Ovum transport in women. In: Harper MJK, Pauerstein CJ, Adams CE, Coutinho EM, Croxatto HB, Paton DM, eds. *Ovum Transport and Fertility Regulation.* Copenhagen: Scriptor, 1976;416–424.
364. Ferin J, Thomas K, Johansson EDB. Ovulation detection. In: Hafez ESE, Evans TN, eds. *Human Reproduction. Conception and Contraception.* Hagerstown, MD: Harper & Row, 1973; 260–283.
365. Peters H, McNatty KP. *The Ovary: A Correlation Between Structure and Function.* Berkeley: University of California Press, 1980.
366. Suchanek E, Grizelj V, Kozaric Z, Simunic V, Casl M-T. Histochemical demonstration of a Δ^5, 3β-hydroxysteroid dehydrogenase activity of cumulus cells related to the maturity and developmental potential of recovered oocytes. *Fertil Steril* 1990; 54:873–878.
367. Urdl W. Criteria of the maturity of follicle and oocyte within the scope of in vitro fertilization. An overview. *Wien Medizin Wochenschr* 1991;141:2–9.
368. Blandau RJ. Gamete transport—comparative aspects. In: Hafez ESE, Blandau RJ, eds. *The Mammalian Oviduct. Comparative Biology and Methodology.* Chicago: University of Chicago Press, 1969;129–162.
369. Westman A. Investigations into the transit of ova in man. *J Obstet Gynaecol Br Emp* 1937;44:821–838.
370. Maia HS, Coutinho EM. Peristalsis and antiperistalsis of the human fallopian tube during the menstrual cycle. *Biol Reprod* 1970;2:305–314.
371. Clewe TH, Mastroianni L Jr. Mechanisms of ovum pickup. I. Functional capacity of rabbit oviducts ligated near the fimbriae. *Fertil Steril* 1958;9:13–17.
372. Doyle JB. Exploratory culdotomy for observation of tubo-ovarian physiology at ovulation time. *Fertil Steril* 1951; 2:475–484.
373. Doyle JB. Ovulation and the effects of selective uterotubal denervation. Direct observations by culdotomy. *Fertil Steril* 1954;5:105–129.
374. Blandau RJ, Verdugo P. An overview of gamete transport—comparative aspects. In: Harper MJK, Pauerstein CJ, Adams CE, Coutinho EM, Croxatto HB, Paton DM, eds. *Ovum Transport and Fertility Regulation.* Copenhagen: Scriptor, 1976;138–146.
375. Lindenbaum ES, Peretz RA, Beach D. Menstrual-cycle-dependent and -independent features of the human fallopian tube fimbrial epithelium: an ultrastructural and cytochemical study. *Gynecol Obstet Invest* 1983;16:76–85.
376. Kerin JF, Williams DB, Serden SP, Daykhovsky L, Grundfest WS, Surrey ES. Falloposcopic identification of a fimbro-ovarian mucus connection as a possible mechanism for tubal oocyte capture. *J Laparoendoscop Surg* 1991;1:97–101.
377. Suginami H, Yano K, Watanabe K, Matsura S. A factor inhibiting ovum capture by the oviductal fimbriae present in endometriosis peritoneal fluid. *Fertil Steril* 1986;46:1140–1146.
378. Beyth Y, Winston RML. Ovum capture and fertility following microsurgical fimbriectomy in the rabbit. *Fertil Steril* 1981; 35:464–466.
379. Ebihara T, Kawakami S, Yoshimura Y, et al. Effects of experimental salpingoplasty on fertility in the rabbit. *Nippon Sanka Fujinka Gakkai Zasshi* 1988;40:847–854.
380. First A. Transperitoneal migration of ovum or spermatozoon. *Obstet Gynecol* 1954;4:431–434.
381. Ben-nun I, Fejgin M, Gruber A, Ben-Aderet N. Transperitoneal ovum migration in women with unilateral congenital ovarian absence. *Acta Obstet Gynecol Scand* 1988;67:665–667.
382. Sopelak VM, Hodgen GD. Contralateral tubal-ovarian apposition and fertility in hemiovariectomized primates. *Fertil Steril* 1984;42:633–637.
383. McComb PF, Coppo ME. The transperitoneal migration of ova in the rabbit. *Acta Eur Fertil* 1986;17:5–7.
384. Heil K. Der Fimbrienstrom und die Überwanderung des Eies vom Ovarium zur Tube. *Arch Gynaekol* 1893;43:503–533.
385. Lode A. Experimentelle Beiträge zur Lehre der Wanderung des Eies von Ovarium zur Tube. *Arhc Gynaekol* 1984;45:293–322.
386. Gyarmati E. Sulla eliminazione transtubarica di sostanze estranee introdotte nella cavità peritoneale. *Riv Ital Ginecol* 1934;16:721–735.
387. Díaz J, Vásquez J, Díaz S, Díaz F, Croxatto HB. Transport of ovum surrogates by the human oviduct. In: Harper MJK, Pauerstein CJ, Adams CE, Coutinho EM, Croxatto HB, Paton DM, eds. *Ovum Transport and Fertility Regulation.* Copenhagen: Scriptor, 1976;404–415.
388. Van Pelt LF. Intraperitoneal insemination of *Macaca mulatta. Fertil Steril* 1970;21:159–162.
389. Laufe LE, Eddy C, Brosens I, Boeckx W. Reversible methods of fimbrial closure. In: Zatuchni GI, Labbok MH, Sciarra JJ, eds. *Research Frontiers in Fertility Regulation.* Hagerstown, MD: Harper & Row, 1980;287–301.
390. Laufe LE. Personal communication. 1985.
391. El Kady AA, Sami G, Lawrence KA, Badawi S. The tubal hood: a potentially reversible sterilization technique. In: Sciarra JJ, Zatuchni GI, Speidel JJ, eds. *Reversal of Sterilization.* Hagerstown, MD: Harper & Row, 1978;232–240.
392. Orczyk GP, Behrman HR. Ovulation blockade by aspirin or indomethacin—*in vivo* evidence for a role of prostaglandin in gonadotrophin secretion. *Prostaglandins* 1972;1:3–20.
393. Armstrong DT, Grinwich DL. Blockade of spontaneous and LH-induced ovulation in rats by indomethacin, an inhibitor of prostaglandin synthesis. *Prostaglandins* 1972;1:21–36.
394. Grinwich DL, Kennedy TG, Armstrong DT. Dissociation of ovulatory and steroidogenic actions of luteinising hormone in rabbits with indomethacin, an inhibitor of prostaglandin biosynthesis. *Prostaglandins* 1972;1:89–96.
395. O'Grady JP, Caldwell BV, Auletta FJ, Speroff L. The effects of an inhibitor of prostaglandin synthesis (indomethacin) on ovulation, pregnancy and pseudopregnancy in the rabbit. *Prostaglandins* 1972;1:97–106.
396. Bateman BG, Kolp LA, Nunley WC Jr, Thomas TS, Mills SE. Oocyte retention after follicle luteinization. *Fertil Steril* 1990;54:793–798.
397. Marik J, Hulka J. Luteinized unruptured follicle syndrome: a subtle cause of infertility. *Fertil Steril* 1978;29:270–274.
398. Killick S, Elstein M. Pharmacologic production of luteinized unruptured follicles by prostaglandin synthetase inhibitors. *Fertil Steril* 1987;47:773–777.
399. Espey LL. Ovulation as an inflammatory reaction—a hypothesis. *Biol Reprod* 1980;22:73–106.
400. Espey LL. A review of factors that could influence membrane potentials of ovarian follicular cells during mammalian ovulation. *Acta Endocrinol (Copenh)* 1992;126:suppl 2:1–32.
401. Yoshimura Y, Nakamura Y, Shiraki M, et al. Involvement of leukotriene B_4 in ovulation in the rabbit. *Endocrinology* 1991;129:193–199.
402. Van Niekerk CH, Gerneke WH. Persistence and parthogenetic cleavage of tubal ova in the mare. *Onderstepoort J Vet Res* 1966;33:195–232.
403. Oguri N, Tsutsumi Y. Non-surgical recovery of equine eggs, and an attempt at non-surgical egg transfer in horses. *J Reprod Fertil* 1972;31:187–195.
404. Steffeenhagen WP, Pineda MH, Ginther OJ. Retention of unfertilized ova in uterine tubes of mares. *Am J Vet Res* 1972;33:2391–2398.

405. Betteridge KJ, Mitchell D. Direct evidence of retention of unfertilized ova in the oviduct of the mare. *J Reprod Fertil* 1974;39:145–148.
406. Flood PF, Jong A, Betteridge KJ. The location of eggs retained in the oviducts of mares. *J Reprod Fertil* 1979;57:291–294.
407. Betteridge KJ, Eaglesome MD, Mitchell D, Flood PF, Beriault R. Development of horse embryos up to 22 days after ovulation: observation on fresh specimens. *J Anat* 1982;135:191–209.
408. Rasweiler JJ. Differential transport of embryos and degenerating ova by the oviducts of the long-tongued bat, *Glossophaga soricina*. *J Reprod Fertil* 1979;55:329–334.
409. Forcedello ML, Vera R, Croxatto HB. Ovum transport in pregnant, pseudopregnant and cyclic rats and its relationship to estradiol and progesterone blood levels. *Biol Reprod* 1981; 24:760–765.
410. Ortiz ME, Bedregal P, Carvajal MI, Croxatto HB. Fertilized and unfertilized ova are transported at different rates by the hamster oviduct. *Biol Reprod* 1986;34:777–781.
411. Villalón M, Ortiz ME, Aguayo C, Muñoz J, Croxatto HB. Differential transport of fertilized and unfertilized ova in the rat. *Biol Reprod* 1982;26:337–341.
412. Weber JA, Freeman DA, Vanderwall DK, Woods GL. Prostaglandin E_2 secretion by oviductal transport-stage equine embryos. *Biol Reprod* 1991;45:540–543.
413. Weber JA, Freeman DA, Vanderwall DK, Woods GL. Prostaglandin E_2 hastens oviductal transport of equine embryos. *Biol Reprod* 1991;45:544–546.
414. Hinrichs K, Watson ED. Effect of administration of phenylbutazone or progesterone on recovery of embryos from the uterus of mares 5 days after ovulation. *Am J Vet Res* 1991;52:678–681.
415. Viggiano M, Cebral E, Gimeno AL, Gimeno MF. Probable influence of ova and embryo prostaglandins in the differential transport in pregnant and cycling rats. *Prostaglandins Leukot Essent Fatty Acids* 1992;45:211–215.
416. Viggiano M, Zicari JL, Gimeno AL, Gimeno MF. Influence of ova within rat oviducts on spontaneous motility and on prostaglandin production. *Prostaglandins Leukot Essent Fatty Acids* 1990;41:13–17.
417. Hunter RHF. Differential transport of fertilised and unfertilised eggs in equine fallopian tubes: a straightforward explanation. *Vet Rec* 1989;125:304.
418. Freeman DA, Woods GL, Vanderwall DK, Weber JA. Embryo-initiated oviductal transport in mares. *J Reprod Fertil* 1992; 95:535–538.
419. Adams CE. Egg survival relative to maternal endocrine status. In: Harper MJK, Pauerstein CJ, Adams CE, Coutinho EM, Croxatto HB, Paton DM, eds. *Ovum Transport and Fertility Regulation*. Copenhagen: Scriptor, 1976;425–440.
420. Estes WL Jr. Ovarian implantation. The preservation of ovarian function after operation for disease of the pelvic viscera. *Surg Gynecol Obstet* 1924;38:394–398.
421. Adams CE. Consequences of accelerated ovum transport, including a re-evaluation of Estes' operation. *J Reprod Fertil* 1979;55:239–246.
422. Marston JH, Penn R, Sivelle PC. Successful autotransfer of tubal eggs in the rhesus monkey (*Macaca mulatta*). *J Reprod Fertil* 1979;49:175–176.
423. World Health Organization. *Special Programme of Research, Development and Research Training in Human Reproduction. Seventh Annual Report*. Geneva: WHO, 1978;88.
424. Nemiro JS, McGaughey RW. An alternative to *in vitro* fertilization-embryo transfer: the successful transfer of human oocytes and spermatozoa to the distal oviduct. *Fertil Steril* 1986;46:644–652.
425. Cefalù E, Cittadini E, Balmaceda JP, et al. Successful gamete intrafallopian transfer following failed artificial insemination by donor: evidence for a defect in gamete transport? *Fertil Steril* 1988;50:279–282.
426. Society for Assisted Reproductive Technology, The American Fertility Society. Assisted reproductive technology in the United States and Canada: 1991 results from the Society for Assisted Reproductive Technology generated from The American Fertility Society Registry. *Fertil Steril* 1993:59:956–962.
427. Asch RH. Uterine versus tubal embryo transfer in the human. Comparative analysis of implantation, pregnancy, and live-birth rates. *Ann NY Acad Sci* 1991;626:461–466.
428. Leung CK, Leong MK, Tucker MJ, et al. Pregnancies from the fallopian replacement of immature eggs with delayed intrauterine insemination. *Hum. Reprod* 1989;4:80–81.
429. Guzick DS, Balmaceda JP, Ord T, Asch RH. The importance of egg and sperm factors in predicting the likelihood of pregnancy from gamete intrafallopian transfer. *Fertil Steril* 1989; 52:795–800.
430. Pratt HPM, Bolton VN, Gudgeon KA. The legacy from the oocyte and its role in controlling early development of the mouse embryo. In: Porter R, Whelan J, eds. *Molecular Biology of Egg Maturation*. Ciba Symposium 98. London: Pitman, 1983; 197–227.
431. Davidson EH. *Gene Activity in Early Development*, Ed 2. New York: Academic Press, 1976.
432. Bolton VN, Oades PJ, Johnson MH. The relationship between cleavage, DNA replication, and gene expression in the mouse 2-cell embryo. *J Embryol Exp Morphol* 1984;79:139–163.
433. Braude P, Bolton V, Moore S. Human gene expression first occurs between the four- and eight-cell stages of preimplantation development. *Nature* 1988;332:459–462.
434. Tesařík KJ, Kopečný V, Plachot M, Mandelbaum J. Early morphological signs of embryonic genome expression in human preimplantation development as revealed by quantitative electron microscopy. *Dev Biol* 1988;128:15–20.
435. Howlett SK, Bolton VN. Sequence and regulation of morphological and molecular events during the first cell cycle of mouse embryogenesis. *J Embryol Exp Morphol* 1985;87:175–206.
436. Webb M, Howlett SK, Maro B. Parthenogenesis and cytoskeletal organization in ageing mouse eggs. *J Embryol Exp Morphol* 1986;95:131–145.
437. Dyban AP, Noniashvili EM. Parthenogenetic development of murine ova activated by heat shock. *Ontogenez* 1986; 17:587–598.
438. Slozina NM, Ponomareva NA, Linskaia MN, Neronova EG, Nikitin AI. Variants of chromosome compaction and the estimation of the capacity of mammalian oocytes for further development. *Tsitologiia* 1990;32:1187–1192.
439. Bolton VN, Hawes SM, Taylor CT, Parsons JH. Development of spare human preimplantation embryos *in vitro*: an analysis of the correlations among gross morphology, cleavage rates, and development to the blastocyst. *J In Vitro Fertil Embryo Transf* 1989;6:30–35.
440. Kiessling AA, Davis HW, Williams CS, Sauter RW, Harrison LW. Development and DNA polymerase activities in cultured preimplantation mouse embryos: comparison with embryos developed *in vivo*. *J Exp Zool* 1991;258:34–47.
441. Bonduelle M-L, Dodd R, Liebars I, Van Steirteghem A, Williamson R, Akhurst R. Chorionic gonadotrophin-β mRNA, a trophoblast marker, is expressed in human 8-cell embryos derived from trinucleate zygotes. *Hum Reprod* 1988;3:909–914.
442. Rappolee DA, Brenner CA, Schultz R, Mark D, Werb Z. Developmental expression of PDGF, TGF-α, and TGF-β genes in preimplantation mouse embryos. *Science* 1988;241:1823–1825.
443. Surani MA, Allen ND, Barton SC, et al. Developmental consequences of imprinting of parental chromosomes by DNA methylation. *Philos Trans R Soc Lond* [*Biol*] 1990;B326:313–327.
444. Biggers JD, Borland RM. Physiological aspects of growth and development of the preimplantation mammalian embryo. *Annu Rev. Physiol* 1976;38:95–119.
445. Paria SC, Dey SK. Preimplantation embryo development *in vitro*: cooperative interactions among embryos and role of growth factors. *Proc Natl Acad Sci USA* 1990;87:4756–4760.
446. Latham KE, Howe CC. SPARC synthesis in pre-implantation and early post-implantation mouse embryos. *Roux's Arch Dev. Biol* 1991;199:364–369.
447. Ryan JP, Spinks NR, O'Neill C, Wales RG. Implantation potential and fetal viability of mouse embryos cultured in media supplemented with platelet-activating factor. *J Reprod Fertil* 1990; 89:309–315.
448. Ryan JP, O'Neill C, Wales RG. Oxidative metabolism of energy substrates by preimplantation mouse embryos in the presence of platelet-activating factor. *J Reprod Fertil* 1990;89:301–307.

449. Spinks NR, Ryan JP, O'Neill C. Antagonists of embryo-derived platelet-activating factor act by inhibiting the ability of the mouse embryo to implant. *J Reprod Fertil* 1990;88:241–248.
450. O'Neill C, Collier M, Ammit AJ, Ryan JP, Saunders DM, Pike IL. Supplementation of *in-vitro* fertilisation culture medium with platelet-activating factor. *Lancet* 1989;ii:769–772.
451. Jones MA, Kudolo GB, Harper MJK. Rabbit blastocysts accumulate platelet-activating factor (PAF) and lyso-PAF *in vitro. Mol Reprod Dev* 1992;32:243–250.
452. O'Neill C. Embryo-derived platelet-activating factor: a preimplantation mediator of maternal recognition of pregnancy. *Domestic Anim Endocrinol* 1987;4:69–85.
453. Collier M, O'Neill C, Ammit AJ, Saunders DM. Measurement of human embryo-derived platelet-activating factor (PAF) using a quantitative bioassay of platelet aggregation. *Hum Reprod* 1990;5:323–328.
454. Wentz AG, Torbit CA, Daniell JF, et al. Combined screening laparoscopy and timed follicle aspiration for human *in vitro* fertilization. *Fertil Steril* 1983;39:270–276.
455. Mahadevan MM, Trounson AO, Leeton JF. Successful use of human cryobanking for *in vitro* fertilization. *Fertil Steril* 1983;40:340–343.
456. Menezeo Y, Testart J, Perrone D. Serum is not necessary in human *in vitro* fertilization, early embryo culture, and transfer. *Fertil Steril* 1984;42:750–755.
457. Veeck OL, Wortham JWE Jr, Witmyer J, et al. Maturation and fertilization of morphologically immature human oocytes in a program of *in vitro* fertilization. *Fertil Steril* 1983;39:594–602.
458. Bongso A, Ng S-C, Sathananthan H, Ng PL, Rauff M, Ratnam S. Improved quality of human embryos when co-cultured with human ampullary cells. *Hum Reprod* 1989;4:706–713.
459. Sathananthan H, Bongso A, Ng S-C, Ho J, Mok H, Ratnam S. Ultrastructure of preimplantation human embryos co-cultured with human ampullary cells. *Hum Reprod* 1989;5:309–318.
460. Kapur RP, Johnson LV. Selective sequestration of an oviductal fluid glycoprotein in the perivitelline space of mouse oocytes and embryos. *J Exp Zool* 1986;238:249–260.
461. Léveillé MC, Roberts KD, Chevalier S, Chapdelaine A, Bleau G. Uptake of an oviductal antigen by the hamster zona pellucida. *Biol Reprod* 1987;36:227–238.
462. Kan FW, Roux E, St.-Jacques S, Bleau G. Demonstration by lectin-gold cytochemistry of transfer of glycoconjugates of oviductal origin to the zona pellucida of oocytes after ovulation in the hamster. *Anat Rec* 1990;226:37–47.
463. Abe H, Oikawa T. Immunocytochemical localization of an oviductal zona pellucida glycoprotein in the oviductal epithelium of the golden hamster. *Anat Rec* 1991;229:305–314.
464. Brown CR, Cheng WK. Changes in composition of the porcine zona pellucida during development of the oocyte to the 2- to 4-cell embryo. *J Embryol Exp Morphol* 1986;92:183–191.
465. Gandolfi F, Modina S, Brevini TA, Galli C, Moor RM, Lauria A. Oviduct ampullary epithelium contributes a glycoprotein to the zona pellucida, perivitelline space and blastomeres membrane of sheep embryos. *Eur. J. Basic Appl. Histochem* 1991;35:383–392.
466. Hunter FHF, Léglise PC. Tubal surgery in the rabbit: fertilization and polyspermy after resection of the isthmus. *Am J Anat* 1971;132:145–152.
467. Hunter RHF, Léglise PC. Polyspermic fertilization following tubal surgery in pigs, with particular reference to the role of the isthmus. *J Reprod Fertil* 1971;24:233–246.
468. Simmen FA, Simmen RCM. Peptide growth factors and proto-oncogenes in mammalian conceptus development. *Biol Reprod* 1991;44:1–5.
469. Kimelman D, Kirschner M. Synergistic induction of mesoderm by FGF and TGF-β and the identification of an mRNA coding for FGF in the early *Xenopus* embryo. *Cell* 1987;51:869–877.
470. Slack JMW, Darlington BG, Heath JK, Godsave SF. Mesoderm induction in early *Xenopus* embryos by heparin-binding growth factors. *Nature* 1987;326:197–200.
471. Kimelman D, Abraham JA, Haaparanta T, Palisi TM, Kirschner MW. The presence of fibroblast growth factor in the frog egg: its role as a natural mesoderm inducer. *Science* 1988;242:1053–1056.
472. Paterno GD, Gillespie LL, Dixon MS, Slack JMW, Heath JK. Mesoderm-inducing properties of *int*-2 and kFGF: two oncogene-encoded growth factors related to FGF. *Development* 1989;106:79–83.
473. Rappolee DA, Sturm KS, Schultz GA, et al. The expression and function of growth factor ligands and receptors during early development of mouse embryos. In: Schomberg D, ed. *Growth Factors in Reproduction.* Serono Symposia. New York: Springer-Verlag, 1990;207–218.
474. Mattson BA, Rosenblum IY, Smith RM, Heyner S. Autoradiographic evidence for insulin and insulin-like growth factor binding to early mouse embryos. *Diabetes* 1988;37:585–589.
475. Heyner S, Smith RM, Schultz GA. Temporally regulated expression of insulin and insulin-like factors and their receptors in early mammalian development. *BioEssays* 1989;11:171–176.
476. Goustin AS, Betscholtz C, Pfeifer-Ohlsson S, et al. Coexpression of the *sis* and *myc* proto-oncogenes in developing human placenta suggests autocrine control of trophoblast growth. *Cell* 1985;41:301–312.
477. Wang C-Y, Daimon M, Shen S.-J, Engelmann GL, Ilan J. Insulin-like growth factor I messenger ribonucleic acid in the developing human placenta and in term placenta of diabetics. *Mol Endocrinol* 1988;2:217–229.
478. Ohlsson R, Larsson E, Nilsson O, Wahlstrom T, Sundstrom P. Blastocyst implantation precedes induction of insulin-like growth factor II gene expression in human trophoblasts. *Development* 1989;106:555–559.
479. Arceci RJ, Shanahan F, Stanley ER, Pollard JW. Temporal expression and location of colony-stimulating factor-I (CSF-I) and its receptor in the female reproductive tract are consistent with CSF-I regulated placental development. *Proc. Natl. Acad. Sci. USA* 1989;86:8818–8822.
480. Pollard JW. Regulation of polypeptide growth factor synthesis and growth factor-related gene expression in the rat and mouse uterus before and after implantation. *J Reprod Fertil* 1990;88:721–731.
481. Rutanen E-M, Pekonen F, Makinen T. Soluble 34K binding protein inhibits the binding of insulin-like growth factor I to its cell receptors in human secretory phase endometrium: evidence for autocrine/paracrine regulation of growth factor action. *J Clin Endocrinol Metab* 1988;66:173–180.
482. Letcher R, Simmen RCM, Bazer FW, Simmen FA. Insulin-like growth factor-I expression during early conceptus development in the pig. *Biol Reprod* 1989;41:1143–1151.
483. Ko Y, Lee CY, Ott TL, et al. Insulin-like growth factors in sheep uterine fluids: concentrations and relationship to ovine trophoblast protein-1 production during early pregnancy. *Biol Reprod* 1990;45:135–142.
484. Geisert RD, Lee C-Y, Simmen FA, et al. Expression of messenger RNAs encoding insulin-like growth factor-I, -II, and insulin-like growth factor binding protein-2 in bovine endometrium during the estrous cycle and early pregnancy. *Biol Reprod* 1991;45:975–983.
485. Tamada H, McMaster MT, Flanders KC, Andrews GK, Dey SK. Cell type-specific expression of transforming growth factor-$\beta 1$ in the mouse uterus during the periimplantation period. *Mol Endocrinol* 1990;4:965–972.
486. Ghahary A, Chakrabarti S, Murphy LJ. Localization of the sites of synthesis and action of insulin-like growth factor-I in the rat uterus. *Mol Endocrinol* 1990;4:191–195.
487. Simmen RCM, Ko Y, Liu XH, Wilde MH, Pope WF, Simmen FA. A uterine cell mitogen distinct from epidermal growth factor in porcine uterine luminal fluids: characterization and partial purification. *Biol Reprod* 1988;38:551–561.
488. Chakraborty C, Tawfik OW, Dey SK. Epidermal growth factor binding in rat uterus during the peri-implantation period. *Biochem Biophys Res Commun* 1988;153:564–569.
489. Huet-Hudson YM, Chakraborty C, De SK, Suzuki Y, Andrews GK, Dey SK. Estrogen regulates the synthesis of epidermal growth factor in mouse uterine epithelial cells. *Mol Endocrinol* 1990;4:510–523.
490. Flanders KC, Marascalco BA, Roberts AB, Sporn MB. Transforming growth factor β: a multifunctional regulatory peptide with actions in the reproductive system. In: Schomberg D, ed.

Growth Factors in Reproduction. New York: Springer-Verlag, 1990;23–38.

491. Simmen RCM, Simmen FA, Hofig A, Farmer SJ, Bazer FW. Hormonal regulation of insulin-like growth factor gene expression in pig uterus. *Endocrinology* 1990;127:2166–2174.
492. Edwards JR, Murphy G, Reynolds JJ, et al. Transforming growth factor beta modulates the expression of collagenase and metalloproteinase inhibitor. *EMBO J* 1987;6:1899–1904.
493. Knochel W, Grunz H, Loppnow-Blinde B, Tiedemann H, Tiedemann H. Mesoderm induction and blood island formation by angiogenic growth factors and embryonic inducing factors. *Blut* 1989;59:207–213.
494. Brigstock DR, Heap RB, Brown KD. Polypeptide growth factors in uterine tissues and secretions. *J Reprod Fertil* 1989; 85:747–758.
495. Millaway DS, Redmer DA, Kirsch JD, Anthony RV, Reynolds LP. Angiogenic activity of maternal and fetal placental tissues of ewes throughout gestation. *J Reprod Fertil* 1989;86:689–696.
496. Milner PG, Li Y-S, Hoffman RM, Kodner CM, Siegel NR, Deuel TF. A novel 17 kD heparin-binding growth factor (HBGF-8) in bovine uterus: purification and *N*-terminal amino acid sequence. *Biochem Biophys Res Commun* 1989;165:1096–1103.
497. Wilkinson DG, Peters G, Dickson C, McMahon AP. Expression of the FGF-related proto-oncogene *int*-2 during gastrulation and neurulation in the mouse. *EMBO J* 1988;7:691–695.
498. Anklesaria P, Teixido J, Laiho M, Pierce JH, Greenberger JS, Massague J. Cell-cell adhesion mediated by binding of membrane-anchored transforming growth factor α to epidermal growth factor receptors promotes cell proliferation. *Proc Natl Acad Sci USA* 1990;87:3289–3293.
499. Nestler JE. Insulin and insulin-like growth factor-I stimulate the 3β-hydroxysteroid dehydrogenase activity of human placental cytotrophoblasts. *Endocrinology* 1989;125:2127–2133.
500. Erickson GF, Garzo VG, Magoffin DA. Insulin-like growth factor-I regulates aromatase activity in human granulosa and granulosa luteal cells. *J Clin Endocrinol Metab* 1989;69:716–724.
501. DiAugustine RP, Petrusz P, Bell GI, et al. Influence of estrogens on mouse uterine epidermal growth factor precursor protein and messenger ribonucleic acid. *Endocrinology* 1988;122:2355–2363.
502. Harvey MB, Kaye PL. Insulin-like growth factor-1 stimulates growth of mouse preimplantation embryos *in vitro. Mol Reprod Dev* 1992;31:195–199.
503. Harvey MB, Kaye PL. Insulin stimulates mitogenesis of the inner cell mass and morphological development of mouse blastocysts. *Development* 1990;110:963–967.
504. Harvey MB, Kaye PL. Mouse blastocysts respond metabolically to short term stimulation by insulin and IGF-1 through the insulin receptor. *Mol Reprod Dev* 1991;29:253–258.
505. Harvey MB, Kaye PL. Visualisation of insulin receptors on mouse preembryos. *Reprod Fertil Dev* 1991;3:9–15.
506. Harvey MB, Kaye PL. IGF-2 receptors are first expressed at the two-cell stage of mouse development. *Development* 1991; 111:1057–1060.
507. Manova K, Paynton BV, Bachvarova RF. Expression of activins and TGFβ1 and β2 RNAs in early postimplantation mouse embryos and uterine decidua. *Mech Dev* 1992;36:141–152.
508. Watson AJ, Hogan A, Hahnel A, Wiemer KE, Schultz GA. Expression of growth factor ligand and receptor genes in the preimplantation bovine embryo. *Mol Reprod Dev* 1992;31:87–95.
509. Hemmings R, Langlais J, Falcone T, Granger L, Miron P, Guyda H. Human embryos produce transforming growth factors α activity and insulin-like growth factors II. *Fertil Steril* 1992; 58:101–104.
510. Wu JT. Changes in the 17β-hydroxysteroid dehydrogenase activity of mouse blastocysts during delayed implantation. *Biol Reprod* 1988;39:1021–1026.
511. Wu JT, Liu ZH. Conversion of pregnenolone to progesterone by mouse morulae and blastocysts. *J Reprod Fertil* 1990;88:93–98.
512. Tanaka T, Fujimoto S, Sakuragi N, Ichinoe K. Estrogen formation from cholesterol in rabbit preimplantation blastocysts and corpora lutea in vitro. *Int. J. Fertil* 1988;33:212–215.
513. Wu JT, Williams KI. Metabolism of estrogens by rabbit blastocysts: formation of estrogen glucosides and preferential conversion of estrone to estradiol-17β. *Steroids* 1989;54:401–419.
514. Chakraborty C, Davis DL, Dey SK. Estradiol-15α-hydroxylation: a new avenue of estrogen metabolism in periimplantation pig blastocysts. *J Steroid Biochem* 1990;35: 209–219.
515. Heap RB, Hamon MH, Allen WR. Oestrogen production by the preimplantation donkey conceptus compared with that of the horse and the effect of between-species embryo transfer. *J Reprod Fertil* 1991;93:141–147.
516. Wilson JM, Zalesky DD, Looney CR, Bondioli KR, Magness RR. Hormone secretion by preimplantation embryos in a dynamic *in vitro* culture system. *Biol Reprod* 1992;46:295–300.
517. Dey SK, Johnson DC, Santos JG. Is histamine production by the blastocyst required for implantation? *Biol Reprod* 1979; 21:1169–1173.
518. Dey SK, Villanueva C, Abdou L. Histamine receptors on rabbit blastocyst and endometrial cell membranes. *Nature* 1979; 278:648–649.
519. Shemesh M, Milaguir F, Ayalon N, Hansel W. Steroidogenesis and prostaglandin synthesis by cultured bovine blastocysts. *J Reprod Fertil* 1979;56:181–185.
520. Chepenik KP, Smith JB. Synthesis of prostaglandins by mouse embryos. *IRCS Med Sci* 1980;8:783.
521. Marcus GJ. Prostaglandin formation by the sheep embryo and endometrium as an indication of maternal recognition of pregnancy. *Biol Reprod* 1981;25:56–64.
522. Lewis GS, Thatcher WW, Bazer FW, Curl JS. Metabolism of arachidonic acid *in vitro* by bovine blastocysts and endometrium. *Biol Reprod* 1982;27:431–439.
523. Hyland HH, Manns JG, Humphrey WD. Prostaglandin production by ovine embryos and endometrium *in vitro. J Reprod Fertil* 1982;65:299–304.
524. Dey SK, Chien SM, Cox CL, Crist RD. Prostaglandin synthesis in the rabbit blastocyst. *Prostaglandins* 1980;19:449–453.
525. Pakrasi PL, Dey SK. Blastocyst is the source of prostaglandins in the implantation site in the rabbit. *Prostaglandins* 1982;24: 73–77.
526. Harper MJK, Norris CJ, Rajkumar K. Prostaglandin release by zygotes and endometria of pregnant rabbits. *Biol Reprod* 1983;28:350–362.
527. Davis DL, Pakrasi PL, Dey SK. Prostaglandins in swine blastocysts. *Biol Reprod* 1983;28:1114–1118.
528. Racowsky C, Biggers JD. Are blastocyst prostaglandins produced endogenously? *Biol Reprod* 1983;29:379–388.
529. Pakrasi PL, Becka R, Dey SK. Cyclo-oxygenase and lipoxygenase pathways in the preimplantation rabbit uterus and blastocyst. *Prostaglandins* 1985;29:481–495.
530. Kasamo M, Ishikawa M, Yamashita Y, Sengoku K, Shimizu T. Possible role of prostaglandin F in blastocyst implantation. *Prostaglandins* 1986;31:321–336.
531. Harper MJK, Jones MA, Norris CJ, Woodard DS. Prostaglandin synthesis by day-6 rabbit blastocysts *in vitro. J Reprod Fertil* 1989;86:315–325.
532. Holmes PV, Sjögren A, Hamberger L. Prostaglandin-E2 released by pre-implantation human conceptuses. *J Reprod Immunol* 1990;17:79–86.
533. Dickman Z, Spilman CH. Prostaglandins in rabbit blastocysts. *Science* 1975;190:997–998.
534. Jones MA, Anderson W, Turner TG, Harper MJK. Storage *in vivo* of [^{3}H]prostaglandins by rabbit blastocysts. *Endocrinology* 1985;116:993–997.
535. Collier M, O'Neill C, Ammit AJ, Saunders DM. Biochemical and pharmacological characterization of human embryo-derived platelet-activating factor. *Hum Reprod* 1988;3:993–998.
536. Adamson LM, Podsiadly B, Smart YC, Stanger JD, Roberts TK. Studies on murine embryo-derived platelet-activating factor (EPAF). *Mol Reprod Dev* 1991;30:207–213.
537. Battye KM, Ammit AJ, O'Neill C, Evans G. Production of platelet-activating factor by the pre-implantation sheep embryo. *J Reprod Fertil* 1991;93:507–512.
538. Smal MA, Dziadek M, Cooney SJ, Attard M, Baldo BA. Examination for platelet-activating factor production by preimplantation mouse embryos using a specific radioimmunoassay. *J Reprod Fertil* 1990;90:419–425.
539. Amiel ML, Duquenne C, Benveniste J, Testart J. Platelet aggre-

gating activity in human embryo culture media free of PAF-acether. *Hum Reprod* 1989;4:327–330.
540. Yang Y-Q, Kudolo GB, Harper MJK. Binding of platelet-activating factor to oviductal membranes during early pregnancy in the rabbit. *J Lipid Med* 1992;5:77–96.
541. Pinekard RN, McManus LM, Hanahan DJ. Chemistry and biology of acetyl glyceryl ether phosphoryleholine (platelet-activating factor). *Adv Inflammation Res* 1982;4:147–180.
542. Verhage HG, Akbar M, Jaffe RC. Cyclic changes in cytosol progesterone receptor of human fallopian tube. *J Clin Endocrinol Metab* 1980;51:776–780.
543. Punnonen R, Lukola A. Binding of estrogen and progestin in the human fallopian tube. *Fertil Steril* 1981;36:610–614.
544. Pollow K, Inthraphuvasak J, Manz B, Grill H-J, Pollow B. A comparison of cytoplasmic and nuclear estradiol and progesterone receptors in human fallopian tube and endometrial tissue. *Fertil Steril* 1981;36:615–622.
545. Pollow K, Inthraphuvasak J, Grill HJ, Manz B. Estradiol and progesterone binding components in the cytosol of normal human fallopian tubes. *J Steroid Biochem* 1982;16:429–435.
546. Pino AM, Devoto L, Soto E, Castro O, Sierraltа W. Changes in cytosolic and nuclear estradiol receptors of normal fallopian tube throughout the menstrual cycle. *J Steroid Biochem* 1982; 16:193–197.
547. Batra S, Helm G, Owman C, Sjöberg N-O, Walles B. Female sex steroid concentrations in the ampullary and isthmic regions of the human fallopian tube and their relationship to plasma concentrations during the menstrual cycle. *Am J Obstet Gynecol* 1980;136:986–991.
548. Devoto L, Soto E, Magofke AM, Sierralta W. Unconjugated steroids in the fallopian tube and peripheral blood during the normal menstrual cycle. *Fertil Steril* 1980;33:613–617.
549. Helm G, Batra S, Owman C. Cytoplasmic and nuclear progesterone receptors in human fallopian tube and their relationship to plasma steroids during the menstrual cycle. *Int J Fertil* 1987;32:162–166.
550. Sato N. Cyclic changes in sex steroids, prostaglandins and oxytocin receptors of normal fallopian tube throughout the menstrual cycle. *Nippon Sanka Fujinka Gakkai Zasshi* 1988;40:1432–1438.
551. Lindenbaum ES, Beach D, Peretz BA. Steroidal binding sites in the ampulla of the human fallopian tube—autoradiographic and biochemical study. *Eur J Obstet Gynecol Reprod Biol* 1987; 24:201–209.
552. Press MF, Nousek-Goebl NA, Bur M, Greene GL. Estrogen receptor localization in the female genital tract. *Am J Pathol* 1986;123:280–292.
553. West NB, McClellan MC, Sternfeld MD, Brenner RM. Immunocytochemistry versus binding assays of the estrogen receptor in the reproductive tract of spayed and hormone-treated macaques. *Endocrinology* 1987;121:1789–1800.
554. Hyde BA, Blaustein JD, Black DL. Differential regulation of progestin receptor immunoreactivity in the rabbit oviduct. *Endocrinology* 1989;125:1479–1483.
555. Burdick HO, Pincus G. The effect of oestrin injections upon the developing ova of mice and rabbits. *Am J Physiol* 1935; 111:201–208.
556. Chang MC, Harper MJK. Effects of ethinyl estradiol on egg transport and development in the rabbit. *Endocrinology* 1966; 78:860–872.
557. Greenwald GS. Species differences in egg transport in response to exogenous estrogen. *Anat Rec* 1967;157:163–172.
558. Chang MC. Effects of progesterone and related compounds on fertilization, transportation and development of rabbit eggs. *Endocrinology* 1967;81:1251–1260.
559. Gupta JS, Roy SK. Effect of clomiphene on nuclear estrogen receptor of the fallopian tube during ovum transport in rabbits. *Endocr Res* 1989;15:339–353.
560. Gupta JS, Roy SK. Effect of tamoxifen on cytosolic estrogen receptor in the different parts of fallopian tube and uterus during ovum transport. *Exp Clin Endocrinol* 1987;90:293–300.
561. Fuentealba B, Nieto M, Croxatto HB. Estrogen and progesterone receptors in the oviduct during egg transport in cyclic and pregnant rats. *Biol Reprod* 1988;39:751–757.
562. Forcedello ML, de la Cerda ML, Croxatto HB. Effectiveness of different estrogen pulses in plasma for accelerating ovum transport and their relation to estradiol levels in the rat oviduct. *Endocrinology* 1986;119:1189–1194.
563. Fuentealba B, Nieto M, Croxatto HB. Progesterone abbreviates the nuclear retention of estrogen receptor in the rat oviduct and counteracts estrogen action on egg transport. *Biol Reprod* 1988;38:63–69.
564. Morãn FM, Forcedello ML, Croxatto HB. Increased secretion of adrenal progesterone explains the lack of response of oviductal embryo transport to a short intravenous infusion of estradiol in the rat. *Arch Biol Med Exp* 1990;23:299–305.
565. Stanchev Ph, Rodriguez-Martinez H, Edqvist LE, Eriksson H. Oestradiol and progesterone receptors in the pig oviduct during the oestrous cycle. *J Steroid Biochem* 1985;22:115–120.
566. Kuchera L. Postcoital contraception with diethylstilbestrol. *JAMA* 1974;218:562–563.
567. Haspels AA. Interception: postcoital estrogens in 3016 women. *Contraception* 1976;14:375–381.
568. Yuzpe AA, Smith RP, Rademaker SW. A multicenter clinical investigation employing ethinyl estradiol combined with *dl*-norgestrel as a postcoital contraceptive agent. *Fertil Steril* 1982;37:508–513.
569. Kubba AA, Guillebaud J. Case of ectopic pregnancy after postcoital contraception with ethinyloestradiol-levonorgestrel. *Br Med J* 1983;287:1343–1344.
570. Morris JM, van Wagenen G. Interception: the use of postovulatory estrogens to prevent implantation. *Am J Obstet Gynecol* 1973;15:101–106.
571. Coutinho EM. In discussion of paper. Tubal and uterine motility. In: Diczfalusy E, Borell U, eds. *Control of Human Fertility.* Nobel Symposium 15. New York: John Wiley & Sons, 1971;97–115.
572. Croxatto HB. The duration of egg transport and its regulation in mammals. In: Coutinho EM, Fuchs F, eds. *Physiology and Genetics of Reproduction, Part B.* New York: Plenum Press, 1974;159–166.
573. Croxatto HB, Díaz S, Atria P, Cheviakoff S, Rosatti S, Oddó H. Contraceptive action of megestrol acetate implants in women. *Contraception* 1971;4:155–167.
574. Liukko P, Erkkola R, Laakso L. Ectopic pregnancies during the use of low-dose progestogens for oral contraception. *Contraception* 1977;16:575–580.
575. Buck RH, Joubert SM, Norman RJ. Serum progesterone in the diagnosis of ectopic pregnancy: a valuable diagnostic test? *Fertil Steril* 1988;50:752–755.
576. Pulkkinen MO, Jaakola UM. Low serum progesterone levels and tubal dysfunction—a possible cause of ectopic pregnancy. *Am J Obstet Gynecol* 1989;161:934–937.
577. Lavy G, DeCherney AH. The hormonal basis of ectopic pregnancy. *Clin Obstet Gynecol* 1987;30:217–224.
578. Forcedello ML, Croxatto HB. Effects of 4-hydroxyandrostenedione and exogenous testosterone on blood concentrations of oestradiol and oviducal embryo transport in the rat. *J Endocrinol* 1988;118:93–100.
579. Psychoyos A, Prapas I. Inhibition of egg development and implantation in rats after post-coital administration of the progesterone antagonist RU 486. *J Reprod Fertil* 1987;80:487–491.
580. Fuentealba B, Nieto M, Croxatto HB. Ovum transport in pregnant rats is little affected by RU 486 and exogenous progesterone as compared to cycling rats. *Biol Reprod* 1987;37:768–774.
581. Paksy K, Varga B, Nãray M, Olajos F, Folly G. Altered ovarian progesterone secretion induced by cadmium fails to interfere with embryo transport in the oviduct of the rat. *Reprod Toxicol* 1992;6:77–83.
582. Adams CE. Egg development in the rabbit: the influence of postcoital ligation of the uterine tube and of ovariectomy. *J Endocrinol* 1958;16:283–293.
583. Noyes RW, Adams CE, Walton A. The transport of ova in relation to the dosage of oestrogen in ovariectomized rabbits. *J Endocrinol* 1959;18:108–117.
584. Harper MJK. The effects of constant doses of oestrogen and progesterone on the transport of artificial eggs through the reproductive tract of ovariectomized rabbits. *J Endocrinol* 1964;30:1–19.
585. Greenwald GS. A study of the transport of ova through the rabbit oviduct. *Fertil Steril* 1961;12:80–95.
586. Harper MJK. The effects of decreasing doses of oestrogen and increasing doses of progesterone on the transport of artificial eggs

through the reproductive tract of ovariectomized rabbits. *J Endocrinol* 1965;31:217–226.

587. Bigsby RM, Duby RT, Black DL. Effects of passive immunization against estradiol on rabbit ovum transport. *Int J Fertil* 1986;31:240–245.
588. Singh MM, Bhalla V, Wadhwa V, Kamboj V. Effect of centchroman on tubal transport and preimplantation embryonic development in rats. *J Reprod Fertil* 1986;76:317–324.
589. Moore GD, Croxatto HB. Effects of delayed transfer and treatment with oestrogen on the transport of microspheres by the rat oviduct. *J Reprod Fertil* 1988;83:795–802.
590. Zenteno J, Silva C, Cãrdenas H, Croxatto HB. Effect of oestradiol delivered from a periovidućal device on ovum transport in mice. *J Reprod Fertil* 1989;86:545–548.
591. Owman Ch, Rosengren E, Sjöberg N-O. Adrenergic innervation of the human female reproductive organs: a histochemical and chemical investigation. *Obstet Gynecol* 1967;30:763–773.
592. Bodkhe RR, Harper MJK. Mechanism of egg transport: changes in amount of adrenergic transmitter in the genital tract of normal and hormone treated rabbits. In: Segal SJ, Crozier R, Corfman PA, Condiffe PG, eds. *The Regulation of Mammalian Reproduction.* NIH Symposium. Springfield, IL: Charles C Thomas, 1973;364–374.
593. Brundin J. Distribution and function of adrenergic nerves in the rabbit fallopian tube. *Acta Physiol Scand* 1965;66(Suppl. 259):57 pp.
594. Marshall JM. Adrenergic innervation of the female reproductive tract: anatomy, physiology and pharmacology. *Ergeb Physiol* 1970;62:6–67.
595. Owman C, Stjernqvist M, Helm G, Kannisto P, Stöberg NO, Sundler F. Comparative histochemical distribution of nerve fibres storing noradrcnalinc and neuropeptide Y (NPY) in human ovary, fallopian tube, and uterus. *Med Biol* 1986;64:57–65.
596. Samuelson UE, Sjöstrand NO. Myogenic and neurogenic control of electrical and mechanical activity in human oviductal smooth muscle. *Acta Physiol Scand* 1986;126:355–363.
597. László A, Nádasy GL, Monos E, Zsolnai B. Effect of pharmacological agents on the activity of the circular and longitudinal smooth muscle layers of human fallopian tube ampullar segments. *Acta Physiol Hung* 1988;72:123–133.
598. Saarikoski S. Adrenoceptor function in female genital tract. *Gynecol Obstet Invest* 1988;26:56–62.
599. Wiklund NP, Samuelson UE, Brundin J. Adenosine modulation of adrenergic neurotransmission in the human fallopian tube. *Eur J Pharmacol* 1986;123:11–18.
600. Samuelson UE, Wiklund NP, Gustafsson LE. Endogenous purines may modulate adrenergic neurotransmission in the human fallopian tube. *Neurosci Lett* 1988;86:51–55.
601. Kraus V, Gombos A. Changes in cholinergic innervation in the human oviduct during pregnancy. *Cesk Gynekol* 1990; 55:741–747.
602. Kraus V, Gombos A, Dusek N. Cholinergic innervation of the oviduct in rabbits. *Vet Med (Praha)* 1991;36:297–302.
603. Isla M, Costa G, García-Pascual A, Triguero D, García-Sacristá NA. Intrinsic spontaneous activity and beta-adrenoceptor-mediated tubal dilatation affect ovum transport in the oviduct of the cow. *J Reprod Fertil* 1989;85:79–87.
604. Lakomy M, Kotwica J, Calka J, Kaleczyc J. The effect of oestradiol benzoate and progesterone on the noradrenalin content in organs of the female reproductive system of sexually immature pigs. *Gegenbaurs Morphol Jahr* 1986;132:129–143.
605. Lakomy M, Kaleczyc J, Calka J. The effect of oestradiol benzoate and progesterone on AChE activity in the nerves of the female reproductive system of immature pigs. *Gegenbaurs Morphol Jahrb* 1986;132:333–348.
606. Arbogast LA, Garris PA, Rhoades TA, Ben-Jonathan N. Changes in ovarian norepinephrine synthesis throughout the follicular and luteal phase. *Biol Reprod* 1987;36:899–906.
607. Juorio AV, Chedrese PJ, Li XM. The influence of ovarian hormones on the rat oviductal and uterine concentration of noradrenaline and 5-hydroxytryptamine. *Neurochem Res* 1989; 14:821–827.
608. Sachy A, Jakubowski A, Bernet F, Verleye M, Rousseau JP. Electromyographic activity and noradrenaline content of the rabbit oviduct under different hormonal states. *Reprod Nutr Dev* 1989;29:171–183.
609. Bernet F, Verleye M, Sachy A. Pre-ovulatory injection of estradiol-17β: effect on noradrenaline activity in different parts of the rabbit oviduct. *Reprod Nutr Dev* 1987;27:791–799.
610. Pauerstein CJ, Hodgson BJ, Fremming BD, Martin JE. Effects of sympathetic denervation of the rabbit oviduct on normal ovum transport and on transport modified by estrogen and progesterone. *Gynecol Invest* 1974;5:121–132.
611. Bodkhe RR, Harper MJK. Changes in the amount of adrenergic neurotransmitter in the genital tract of untreated rabbits, and rabbits given reserpine or iproniazid during the time of egg transport. *Biol Reprod* 1972;6:288–297.
612. Pauerstein CJ, Fremming BD, Martin JE. Estrogen-induced tubal arrest of ovum: antagonism by alpha adrenergic blockade. *Obstet Gynecol* 1970;35:671–675.
613. Polidoro JP, Howe GR, Black DL. The effects of adrenergic drugs on ovum transport through the rabbit oviduct. *J Reprod Fertil* 1973;35:331–337.
614. Hodgson BJ, Eddy CA. The autonomic nervous system and its relationship to tubal ovum transport—a reappraisal. *Gynecol Invest* 1975;6:162–185.
615. Johns A, Chlumecky J, Paton DM. Role of adrenergic nerves in ovulation and ovum transport. *Lancet* 1974;ii:1079.
616. Donnez J, Caprasse J, Casanas-Roux F, Ferin J, Thomas K. Loss of adrenergic innervation in induced rabbit hydrosalpinx. *Gynecol Obstet Invest* 1986;21:213–216.
617. Jordan SM. Adrenergic and cholinergic innervation of the reproductive tract and ovary in the guinea pig and rabbit. *J Physiol (Lond)* 1970;210:115P–117P.
618. Saksena SK, Harper MJK. Relationship between concentration of prostaglandin F (PGF) in the oviduct and egg transport in rabbits. *Biol Reprod* 1975;13:68–76.
619. Rajkumar K, Garg SK, Sharma PI. Relationship between concentration of prostaglandins E and F in the regulation of ovum transport in rabbits. *Prostaglandins Med* 1979;2:445–454.
620. Thomas CMG. Steroid Hormones, Prostaglandins and Ovum Transport: A Study in the Golden Hamster, *Mesocricetus auratus* (Waterhouse). PhD Thesis, Catholic University of Nijmegen, Janssen, Nijmegen, 1978.
621. Ogra SS, Kirton KT, Tomasi TB Jr, Lippes J. Prostaglandins in the human fallopian tube. *Fertil Steril* 1974;25:250–255.
622. Vastik-Fernandez J, Gimeno MF, Lima F, Gimeno AL. Spontaneous motility and distribution of prostaglandins in different segments of human fallopian tubes. *Am J Obstet Gynecol* 1975;122:663–668.
623. Nieder J, Augustin W. Prostaglandin E and F profiles in human fallopian tubes during different phases of the menstrual cycle. *Gynecol Obstet Invest* 1986;21:202–207.
624. Ebihara T, Yoshimura Y, Shiraki M, et al. Role of endosalpinx in the oviductal environment. *Nippon Sanka Fujinka Gakkai Zasshi* 1989;41:881–887.
625. Harper MJK, Coons LW, Radicke DA, Hodgson BJ, Valenzuela G. Role of prostaglandins in contractile activity of the ampulla of the rabbit oviduct. *Am J Physiol* 1980;238:E157–E166.
626. Harper MJK. Prostaglandin (PG) production by rabbit oviduct (abstracts). Fourth International Prostaglandin Conference, Washington, DC, 1979.
627. Rajkumar K, Coons LW, Harper MJK, Johns A. Effects of tension and transmural stimulation on prostaglandin production by estrous rabbit oviductal isthmus. *Prostaglandins* 1981;21:889–897.
628. Van Voorhis BJ, Huettner PC, Clark MR, Hill JA. Immunohistochemical localization of prostaglandin H synthase in the female reproductive tract and endometriosis. *Am J Obstet Gynecol* 1990;163:57–62.
629. Jones MA, Harper MJK. Rabbit blastocysts accumulate [^{3}H]-prostaglandins *in vitro*. *Endocrinology* 1984;115:817–823.
630. Saffaripour S, Jones MA. Prostaglandin (PG) accumulation *in vitro* by mouse ovaries, oviducts, and uteri. *Prostaglandins* 1988;36:229–239.
631. Granström E, Samuelsson B. Quantitative measurement of prostaglandins and thromboxanes: General considerations. *Adv Prostaglandin Thromboxane Leukotriene Res* 1978;5:1–13.
632. Lindblom B, Hamberger L, Wiqvist N. Differentiated contractile effects of prostaglandins E and F on the isolated circular and

longitudinal smooth muscle of the human oviduct. *Fertil Steril* 1978;30:553–559.
633. Lindblom B, Wilhelmsson L, Wiqvist N. The action of prostacyclin (PGI_2) on the contractility of the isolated circular and longitudinal muscle layer of the human oviduct. *Prostaglandins* 1979;17:99–104.
634. Lindblom B, Wikland M. Simultaneous recording of electrical and mechanical activity in isolated smooth muscle of the human oviduct. *Biol Reprod* 1982;27:393–398.
635. Lindblom B. A simple prostaglandin bioassay based on smooth muscle preparations from the human oviduct. *Prostaglandins Leukot Essent Fatty Acids* 1988;31:59–63.
636. Nozaki M, Ito Y. Menstrual cycle and sensitivity of human fallopian tube to prostaglandins. *Am J Physiol* 1986;251: R1126–R1136.
637. Tanbo T, Bjørnerheim R, Abyholm T, Hansson V. Hormone-responsive adenylyl cyclase in the human fallopian tube. *J Clin Endocrinol Metab* 1991;73:335–340.
638. Coutinho EM, Maia HS. The contractile response of the human uterus, fallopian tubes and ovary to prostaglandins *in vivo. Fertil Steril* 1971;22:539–543.
639. Spilman CH, Harper MJK. Effect of prostaglandins on oviduct motility in estrous rabbits. *Biol Reprod* 1973;9:36–45.
640. Horton EW, Main IHM, Thompson CJ. Effects of prostaglandins on the oviduct, studied in rabbits and ewes. *J Physiol (Lond)* 1965;180:514–528.
641. Spilman CH, Harper MJK. Comparison of the effects of adrenergic drugs and prostaglandins on rabbit oviduct motility. *Biol Reprod* 1974;10:549–554.
642. Spilman CH, Harper MJK. Effects of prostaglandins on oviductal motility and egg transport. *Gynecol Invest* 1976;6:186–205.
643. Riehl RM, Harper MJK. Preparation of smooth muscle cell suspensions from the rabbit oviduct and prostaglandin binding analysis. *Endocrinology* 1981;108:18–26.
644. Riehl RM, Harper MJK. Changes in prostaglandin binding capacity of single oviductal smooth muscle cells after ovulation in the rabbit. *Endocrinology* 1981;109:1011–1016.
645. Riehl RM. Prostaglandin Binding Sites in the Rabbit Oviduct: A Dissertation. PhD Thesis, University of Texas Graduate School of Biomedical Sciences at San Antonio, 1980.
646. Weber JA, Woods GL, Freeman DA, Vanderwall DK. Prostaglandin E_2-specific binding to the oviduct. *Prostaglandins* 1992; 43:61–65.
647. Valenzuela G, Ross HD, Hodgson BJ, Harper MJK, Pauerstein CJ. Effect of inhibitors of prostaglandin synthesis and metabolism on ovum transport in the rabbit. *Fertil Steril* 1977; 28:992–997.
648. Hodgson BJ. Effects of indomethacin and ICI 46,474 administered during ovum transport on fertility in rabbits. *Biol Reprod* 1976;14:451–457.
649. Schlegel W, Vancaillie T, Schneider HP. The influence of continuous intrauterine infusion of enzyme-inhibitors of the arachidonic acid cascade on ovulation and tubal ovum transport in the hyperstimulated rabbit. *Horm Metab Res* 1986;18:386–390.
650. Chernaeva L, Charakchieva S. Estradiol effect on indomethacin and prostaglandin E_2-modulation of adrenergic transmission in the rabbit oviduct. *Prostaglandins* 1991;41:571–583.
651. Ånggård E, Samuelsson B. Prostaglandins and related factors 28. Metabolism of prostaglandin E_1 in guinea-pig lung: The structure of two metabolites. *J Biol Chem* 1964;239:4097–4102.
652. Ångåard E, Samuelsson B. The metabolism of prostaglandins in lung tissue. In: Bergström S, Samuelsson B, eds. *Prostaglandins.* Nobel Symposium 2. New York: Interscience, 1967;97–105.
653. Samuelsson B, Granström E, Gréen K, Hamberg M. Metabolism of prostaglandins. *Ann NY Acad Sci* 1971;180:138–161.
654. Alm P, Alumets J, Håkanson R, et al. Origin and distribution of VIP (vasoactive intestinal polypeptide) nerves in the genitourinary tract. *Cell Tissue Res* 1980;205:337–347.
655. Said SI, Mutt V. Polypeptide with broad biological activity: isolation from small intestine *Science* 1970;169:1217–1218.
656. Mutt V, and Said SI. Structure of the porcine vasoactive intestinal octosapeptide. *Eur J Biochem* 1974;42:581–589.
657. Alm P, Alumets J, Håkanson R, et al. Vasoactive intestinal polypeptide nerves in the human female genital tract. *Am J Obstet Gynecol* 1980;136:349–351.
658. Reinecke M, Gauwerky JFH, Schneider K. Peptiderge (NPY, NT, VIP, SP, CGRP) Innervation der funktionellen Systeme des Uterus und der Tube des Menschen. *Arch Gynecol Obstet* 1989;245:399–401.
659. Blank MA, Allen JM, Huang WM, et al. The regional distribution of NPY-, PHM-, and VIP-containing nerves in the human female genital tract. *Int J Fertil* 1986;31:218–222.
660. Helm G, Håkanson R, Leander S, Owman C, Sjöberg N-O, Sporrong B. Neurogenic relaxation mediated by vasoactive intestinal polypeptide (VIP) in the isthmus of the human fallopian tube. *Regul Pept,* 1982;3:145–153.
661. Walles B, Håkanson R, Helm G, Owman Ch, Sjöberg N-O, Sundler F. Relaxation of human female genital sphincters by the neuropeptide vasoactive intestinal polypeptide. *Am J Obstet Gynecol* 1980;138:337–338.
662. Helm G, Ottesen B, Fahrenkrug J, et al. Vasoactive intestinal polypeptide (VIP) in the human female reproductive tract: distribution and motor effects. *Biol Reprod* 1981;25:227–234.
663. Helm G, Ekman R, Rydhstöm H, Sjöberg N-O, Walles B. Changes in oviductal VIP content induced by sex steroids and inhibitory effect of VIP on spontaneous oviductal contractility. *Acta Physiol Scand* 1985;125:219–224.
664. Helm G, Ekman R, Owman C. Cyclic fluctuations of vasoactive intestinal polypeptide measured radioimmunologically in various regions of the human fallopian tube. *Int J Fertil* 1987; 32:467–471.
665. Ottesen B, Larsen J-J, Staun-Olsen P, Gammeltoft S, Fahrenkrug J. Influence of pregnancy and sex steroids on concentration, motor effect and receptor binding of VIP in the rabbit female genital tract. *Regul Pept* 1985;11:83–92.
666. Bolton TB, Lang RJ, Ottesen B. Mechanism of action of vasoactive intestinal polypeptide on myometrial smooth muscle of rabbit and guinea pig. *J Physiol (Lond)* 1981;318:41–56.
667. Fahrenkrug J, Ottesen B, Palle C. Vasoactive intestinal polypeptide and the reproductive system. *Ann NY Acad Sci* 1989;527: 393–404.
668. Lindblom B, Ljung B, Hamberger L. Adrenergic and novel nonadrenergic neuronal mechanisms in the control of smooth muscle activity in the human oviduct. *Acta Physiol Scand* 1979;196: 215–220.
669. Blair WD, Beck L. A system for measurement of oviductal motility and contractility and chronic changes in luminal diameter. In: Harper MJK, Pauerstein CJ, Adams CE, Coutinho EM, Croxatto HB, Paton DM, eds. *Ovum Transport and Fertility Regulation.* Copenhagen: Scriptor, 1976;41–74.
670. Blair WD, Beck L. Demonstration of postovulatory sphincter action by the isthmus of the rabbit oviduct. *Fertil Steril* 1976;27:431–441.
671. Fredericks CM, Lundqvist LE, Mathur RS, Ashton SH, Landgrebe SC. Effects of vasoactive intestinal polypeptide upon ovarian steroids, ovum transport and fertility in the rabbit. *Biol Reprod* 1983;28:1052–1060.
672. Fredericks CM, Ashton SH. Effects of vasoactive intestinal polypeptide (VIP) on the *in vitro* and *in vivo* motility of the rabbit reproductive tract. *Fertil Steril* 1982;37:845–850.
673. Tatemoto K. Neuropeptide Y: complete amino acid sequence of the brain peptide. *Proc Natl Acad Sci USA* 1982;79:5485–5489.
674. Stjernqvist M, Emson P, Owman Ch, Sjöberg N-O, Sundler F, Tatemoto K. Neuropeptide Y in the female reproductive tract of the rat. Distribution of nerve fibers and motor effects. *Neurosci Lett* 1983;39:279–284.
675. Samuelson UE, Dalsgaard C-J. Action and localization of neuropeptide Y in the human fallopian tube. *Neurosci Lett* 1985;58:49–54.
676. Heinrich D, Reinecke M, Gauwerky JF, Forssmann WG. Immunohistochemical and biological evidence for a neuromodulator function of neuropeptide Y in the human oviduct. *Arch Gynecol Obstet* 1987;241:127–132.
677. Jørgensen JC, Sheikh SP, Forman A, Nørgård M, Schwartz TW, Ottesen B. Neuropeptide Y in the human female genital tract: localization and biological action. *Am J Physiol* 1989;257: E220–E227.
678. Kannisto P, Ekblad E, Helm G, et al. Existence and coexistence of peptides in nerves of the mammalian ovary and oviduct dem-

onstrated by immunocytochemistry. *Histochemistry* 1986;86: 25–34.
679. Häppölä O, Lakomy M, Majewski M, Yanaihara N. Distribution of somatostatin- and neuropeptide Y-immunoreactive nerve fibers in the porcine female reproductive system. *Neurosci Lett* 1991;122:273–276.
680. Huang WM, Gu J, Blank MA, Allen JM, Bloom SR, Polak JM. Peptide-immunoreactive nerves in the mammalian female genital tract. *Histochem J.* 1984;16:1297–1310.
681. Gauwerky JFH, Reinecke M, Schneider K. Regulative Peptide in der Tuba uterina des Menschen. *Arch Gynecol Obstet* 1989; 245:401–404.
682. Chernaeva L, Charakchieva S. Leucine-enkephalin- and neuropeptide Y-modulation of [^{3}H]noradrenaline release in the oviduct of mature and juvenile rabbits. *Gen Pharmacol* 1988;19: 137–142.
683. Alm P, Alumets J, Håkanson R, et al. Enkephalin-immunoreactive nerve fibers in the feline genito-urinary tract. *Histochemistry* 1981;72:351–355.
684. Ottesen B, Söndergaard F, Fahrenkrug J. Neuropeptides in the regulation of female genital smooth muscle contractility. *Acta Obstet Gynecol* 1983;62:591–592.
685. Ottesen B, Gram BR, Fahrenkrug J. Neuropeptides in the female genital tract: effect on vascular and non-vascular smooth muscle. *Peptides* 1983;4:387–392.
686. Häppölä O, Lakomy M, Yanaihara N. Met5-enkephalin- and met5-enkephalin-arg6-gly7-leu8-immunoreactive nerve fibers in the pig female reproductive system. *Neurosci Lett* 1989;101: 156–162.
687. Li W-I, Wu H, Kumar AM. Synthesis and secretion of immunoreactive methionine-enkephalin from rabbit reproductive tissues *in vivo* and *in vitro. Biol Reprod* 1991;45:691–697.
688. von Euler US, Gaddum JH. An unidentified depressor substance in certain tissue extracts. *J Physiol (Lond)* 1931;72:74–87.
689. Chang MM, Leeman SE, Niall HD. Amino-acid sequence of substance P. *Nature (New Biol),* 1971;232:86–87.
690. Alm P, Alumets J, Brodin E, et al. Peptidergic (substance P) nerves in the genito-urinary tract. *Neuroscience* 1978;3:419–425.
691. Zetler G, Mönkemeier D, Wiechell H. Stimulation of fallopian tubes by prostaglandin $F_{2\alpha}$, biogenic amines and peptides. *J Reprod Fertil* 1969;18:147–149.
692. Zetler G, Mönkemeier D, Wiechell H. Peptid-Receptoren für Tachykinine in der Tuba uterina des Menschen. *Naunyn Schmiedebergs Arch Pharmacol* 1969;262:97–111.
693. Nimmo AJ, Whitaker EM, Carstairs JR, Morrison JF. The autoradiographic localization of calcitonin gene-related peptide and substance P receptors in human fallopian tubes. *Q J Exp Physiol* 1989;74:955–958.
694. Forman A, Andersson K-E, Maigaard S, Ulmsten U. Concentrations and contractile effects of substance P in the human ampullary-isthmic junction. *Acta Physiol Scand* 1985;124:17–23.
695. Häppölä O, Lakomy M. Immunohistochemical localization of calcitonin gene-related peptide and bombesin/gastrin-releasing peptide in nerve fibers of the rat, guinea pig and pig female genital organs. *Histochemistry* 1989;92:211–218.
696. Reinecke M. Neurotensin in the human fallopian tube: immunohistochemical localization and effects of synthetic neurotensin on motor activity *in vitro. Neurosci Lett* 1987;73:220–224.
697. Fernãndez-Pardal J, Chaud M, Viggiano M, Gimeno MF, Gimeno AL. Converting enzyme activity in sow oviducts at different stages of the sex cycle. Influence of inhibitors of prostaglandin synthesis and its possible role in the inotropic effects of bradykinin. *Pharmacol Res Commun* 1986;18:49–60.
698. Schultz G, Schultz K, Hardman JG. Effects of norepinephrine on cyclic nucleotide levels in the ductus deferens of the rat. *Metabolism* 1975;24:429–437.
699. Johansson S, Andersson RGG. Variations of cyclic nucleotide monophosphate levels during spontaneous uterine contractions. *Experientia* 1975;31:1314–1315.
700. Lindblom B, Hamberger L. Cyclic AMP and contractility of the human oviduct. *Biol Reprod* 1980;22:173–178.
701. Valenzuela G, Antonini R, Hodgson BJ, Jones DJ, Harper MJK. Cyclic nucleotides and prostaglandins (PGs) produced by the rabbit oviduct: effects of estrogen treatment. *Res Commun Chem Pathol Pharmacol* 1977;17:361–364.
702. Maia H Jr, Barbosa I, Coutinho EM. Relationship between cyclic AMP levels and oviductal contractility. In: Harper MJK, Pauerstein CJ, Adams CE, Coutinho EM, Croxatto HB, Paton DM, eds. *Ovum Transport and Fertility Regulation.* Copenhagen: Scriptor, 1976;168–181.
703. Martin del Rio R. γ-Aminobutyric acid system in rat oviduct. *J Biol Chem* 1981;256:9816–9819.
704. Erdö SL, Rosdy B, Szporny L. Higher GABA concentrations in fallopian tube than in brain of the rat. *J Neurochem* 1982;38:1174–1176.
705. Celotti F, Apud JA, Rovescalli AC, Melcangi RC, Negri-Cesi P, Racagni G. The GABAergic extrinsic innervation of the rat fallopian tubes: biochemical evidence and endocrine modulation. In: Racagni G, Donoso AO, eds. *GABA and Endocrine Function.* New York: Raven Press, 1986;251–264.
706. Celotti F, Apud JA, Melcangi RC, Masotto C, Tappaz M, Racagni G. Endocrine modulation of gamma-aminobutyric acidergic innervation in the rat fallopian tube. *Endocrinology* 1986;118:334–339.
707. Celotti F, Apud, JA, Rovescalli AC, Negri-Cesi P, Racagni G. Possible involvement of ovarian mechanisms other than estrogen-progesterone secretion in the regulation of glutamic acid decarboxylase activity of the rat fallopian tubes. *Endocrinology* 1987;120:700–706.
708. Gimeno MF, Fernandez-Pardal J, Viggiano M, Pezzot MD, Gimeno AL. On the presence of GABA in ovarian, tubal and uterine rat tissues. Modification at different stages of the estrous cycle and during pregnancy. In: Racagni G, Donoso AO, eds. *GABA and Endocrine Function.* New York: Raven Press, 1986;275–282.
709. Amenta F, Cavallotti C, Mione MC, Erdö SL. Segmental distribution and gestational changes of GABA-transaminase activity in the rat oviduct. *J Reprod Fertil* 1986;78:593–599.
710. Orensanz LM, Fernández I, Martin del Rio R, Storm-Mathisen J. Gamma-aminobutyric acid in the rat oviduct. In: Racagni G, Donoso AO, eds. *GABA and Endocrine Function.* New York: Raven Press, 1986;265–274.
711. Erdö SL, László A, Szporny L, Zsolnai B. High density of specific GABA binding sites in the human fallopian tube. *Neurosci Lett* 1983;42:155–160.
712. Erdö SL, Lapis E. Presence of GABA receptors in rat oviduct. *Neurosci Lett* 1982;33:275–279.
713. Orensanz LM, Fernández I. On the binding of γ-[^{3}H]aminobutyric acid to the rat oviduct. *Neurosci Lett* 1985;57:213–214.
714. Erdö SL, Kiss B, Szporny L. Comparative characterization of glutamate decarboxylase in crude homogenates of oviduct, ovary and hypothalamus. *J Neurochem* 1984;43:1532–1537.
715. László A, Nádasy GL, Erdö SL, Monos E, Siklósi G, Zsolnai B. Effects of GABA on the spontaneous muscular activity of the human fallopian tube ampullar segments *in vitro. Acta Physiol Hung* 1990;76:123–130.
716. Erdö SL, Riese M, Kärpäti E, and Szporny L. $GABA_B$ receptor-mediated stimulation of the contractility of isolated rabbit oviduct. *Eur J Pharmacol* 1984;99:333–336.
717. Erdö SL, Kiss B, Riesz M, Szporny L. Stimulus-evoked efflux of GABA from preloaded slices of the rabbit oviduct. *Eur J Pharmacol* 1986;130:295–303.
718. Erdö L, Amenta F. Characterization and localization of high-affinity GABA uptake in slices of rabbit oviduct. *Eur J Pharmacol* 1986;130:287–294.
719. Noonan JJ, Adair RL, Halbert SA, Ringo JA, Reeves JJ. Quantitative assessment of oxytocin-stimulated oviduct contractions of the ewe by optoelectronic measurements. *J Anim Sci* 1978;47: 914–918.
720. Coutinho EM, Maia H. The influence of the ovarian steroids on the response of the human fallopian tubes to neurohypophyseal hormones *in vivo. Am J Obstet Gynecol* 1970;108:194–202.
721. Soloff MS. Oxytocin receptors in rat oviduct. *Biochem Biophys Res Commun* 1975;66:671–677.
722. Maggi M, Genazzani AD, Giannini S, et al. Vasopressin and oxytocin receptors in vagina, myometrium, and oviduct of rabbits. *Endocrinology* 1988;122:2970–2980.
723. Ayad VJ, McGoff SA, Wathes DC. Oxytocin receptors in the oviduct during the oestrous cycle of the ewe. *J Endocrinol* 1990;124:353–359.

724. Wallace JM, Helliwell R, Morgan RJ. Autoradiographical localization of oxytocin binding sites on ovine oviduct and uterus throughout the estrous cycle. *Reprod Fertil Dev* 1991;3:127–135.
725. Ayad VJ, Guldenaar SEF, Wathes DC. Characterization and localization of oxytocin receptors in the uterus and oviduct of the nonpregnant ewe using an iodinated receptor antagonist. *J Endocrinol* 1991;128:187–195.
726. Wallace JM, Helliwell R, Morgan PJ. Autoradiographic localization of oxytocin binding sites on ovine oviduct and uterus throughout the oestrous cycle. *Reprod Fertil Dev* 1991;3: 127–135.
727. Garcia-Villar R, Toutain PL, Schams D, Ruckebusch Y. Are regular activity episodes of the genital tract controlled by pulsatile releases of oxytocin? *Biol Reprod* 1983;29:1183–1188.
728. Lundin S, Forman A, Rechberger T, Svane D, Andersson KE. Immunoreactive oxytocin and vasopressin in the non-pregnant human uterus and oviductal isthmus. *Acta Endocrinol (Copenh)* 1989;120:239–244.
729. Harper MJK. Egg movement through the ampullar region of the fallopian tube of the rabbit. In: *Proceedings of the IVth International Congress on Animal Reproduction, The Hague,* 1961; 375–380.
730. Harper MJK. The mechanisms involved in the movement of newly ovulated eggs through the ampulla of the rabbit fallopian tube. *J Reprod Fertil* 1961;2:522–524.
731. Harper MJK. Transport of eggs in cumulus through the ampulla of the rabbit oviduct in relation to day of pseudopregnancy. *Endocrinology* 1965;77:114–123.
732. Croxatto HB, Ortiz ME, Díaz S, Hess R, Balmaceda J, Croxatto H-D. Studies on the duration of egg transport by the human oviduct. II. Ovum location at various intervals following the luteinizing hormone peak. *Am J Obstet Gynecol* 1978;132:629–634.
733. Eddy CA, Garcia RG, Kraemer DC, Pauerstein CJ. Detailed time course of ovum transport in the rhesus monkey (*Macaca mulatta*). *Biol Reprod* 1975;13:363–369.
734. Diaz S, Ortiz ME, Croxatto HB. Studies on the duration of ovum transport by the human oviduct. III. Time interval between the luteinizing hormone peak and recovery of ova by transcervical flushing of the uterus in normal women. *Am J Obstet Gynecol* 1980;137:116–121.
735. Talo A, Brundin J. Muscular activity in the rabbit oviduct: a combination of electric and mechanic recordings. *Biol Reprod* 1971;5:67–77.
736. Talo A, Hodgson BJ. Effect of time after ovulation and estrogen and progesterone on electrical activity of the rabbit oviduct. *Pharmacologist* 1976;18:181 (abstract No. 377).
737. Nozaki M, Ito Y. Changes in physiological properties of rabbit oviduct by ovarian steroids. *Am J Physiol* 1987;252: R1059–R1065.
738. Olsson OA, Gustasson B. The effect of D2343 in transmurally stimulated rabbit isthmus muscle. *Acta Pharmacol Toxicol* 1985;56:427–430.
739. Chernaeva L. Adrenergic mechanisms of the contractile response of rabbit oviduct to electrical stimulation. *Gen Pharmacol* 1988;19:625–630.
740. Singh SB, Manchanda SK, Das M. Coitus induced changes in oviductal motility and effect of progesterone. *Ind J Med Res* 1990;92:260–266.
741. Bennett WA, Watts TL, Blair WD, Waldhalm SJ, Fuquay JW. Patterns of oviducal motility in the cow during the oestrous cycle. *J Reprod Fertil* 1988;83:537–543.
742. Lydrup ML, Hellstrand P. Rate of oxidative and glycolytic metabolism in the guinea-pig oviduct in relation to contractility and hormonal cycle. *Acta Physiol Scand* 1986;128:525–533.
743. Lydrup ML, Hellstrand P. Effects of extracellular K^+ and Ca^{2+} on membrane potential, contraction and $^{86}Rb^+$ efflux in guinea-pig mesotubarium. *Pflugers Arch Eur J Physiol* 1990;451:664–670.
744. Forman A, Andersson KE, Ulmsten U. Effect of calcium and nifedipine on noradrenaline- and PGF2α-induced activity of the ampullary-isthmic junction of the human oviduct *in vitro. J Reprod Fertil* 1983;67:343–349.
745. Lindblom, Andersson A. Influence of cyclooxygenase inhibitors and arachidonic acid on contractile activity of the human fallopian tube. *Biol Reprod* 1985;32:475–479.
746. Nádasy GL, László A, Monos E, Zsolnai B. Spontaneous periodic contraction of the ampullar segment of the human fallopian tube *in vitro. Acta Physiol Hung* 1988;72:13–21.
747. Otubu JA, Winston RM. Spontaneous contractile pattern of isolated circular and longitudinal muscle layers from the ampullae of normal and damaged fallopian tubes. *Afr J Med Med Sci* 1987;16:33–37.
748. Pettersson A, Larsson B, Einarson E. The effect of unilateral ovariectomy on intraluminal pressure in the porcine oviductal isthmus. *Zentralbl Veterinarmed [A]* 1991;38:481–484.
749. Portnow J, Talo A, Hodgson BJ. A random walk model of ovum transport. *Bull Math Biol* 1977;39:349–357.
750. Hodgson BJ, Talo A, Pauerstein CJ. Oviductal ovum surrogate movement: interrelation with muscular activity. *Biol Reprod* 1977;16:394–396.
751. Verdugo P, Blandau RJ, Tam PY, Halbert SA. Stochastic elements in the development of deterministic models of egg transport. In: Harper MJK, Pauerstein CJ, Adams CE, Coutinho EM, Croxatto HB, Paton DM, eds. *Ovum Transport and Fertility Regulation.* Copenhagen: Scriptor, 1976;126–137.
752. Halbert SA, Szal SE, Broderson SH. Anatomical basis of a passive mechanism for ovum retention at the ampulloisthmic junction. *Anat Rec* 1988;221:841–845.
753. Brenner RM, Carlisle KS, Hess DL, Sandow BA, West NB. Morphology of the oviducts and endometria of cynomolgus macaques during the menstrual cycle. *Biol Reprod* 1983;29: 1289–1302.
754. Verhage HG, Bareither ML, Jaffe RC, Akbar M. Cyclic changes in ciliation, secretion and cell height of the oviductal epithelium in women. *Am J Anat* 1979;156:505–511.
755. Critoph FN, Dennis KJ. Ciliary activity in the human oviduct. *Br J Obstet Gynaecol* 1977;84:216–218.
756. Borell U, Nilsson O, Westman A. Ciliary activity in the rabbit fallopian tube during oestrus and after copulation. *Acta Obstet Gynecol Scand* 1957;36:22–28.
757. Villalón M, Hinds TR, Verdugo P. Stimulus-response coupling in mammalian ciliated cells. Demonstration of two mechanisms of control for cytosolic [Ca^{2+}]. *Biophys. J.* 1989;56:1255–1258.
758. Yamaoka S, Cilium movement of human oviduct. *Nippon Sanka Fujinka Gakkai Zasshi* 1987;39:777–784.
759. Eddy CA, Flores JJ, Archer DR, Pauerstein CJ. The role of cilia in fertility: an evaluation by selective microsurgical modification of the rabbit oviduct. *Am J Obstet Gynecol* 1978;132:814–820.
760. McComb PF, Halbert SA, Gomel V. Pregnancy, ciliary transport, and the reversed ampullary segment of the rabbit fallopian tube. *Fertil Steril* 1980;34:386–390.
761. Dickmann Z. The role of the cumulus oophorus and tubal factors in the process of fertilization of the rabbit egg. In: *Proceedings of the IVth International Congress on Animal Reproduction, The Hague* 1961;731–735.
762. Brosens IA, Vasquez G. Fimbrial microbiopsy. *J Reprod Med* 1976;16:171–178.
763. Afzelius BA, Camner P, Mossberg B. On the function of cilia in the female reproductive tract. *Fertil Steril* 1978;29:72–74.
764. Bleau G, Richer C-L, Bousquet D. Absence of dynein arms in cilia of endocervical cells in a fertile woman. *Fertil Steril* 1978;30:362–363.
765. McComb P, Langley L, Villalon M, Verdugo P. The oviductal cilia and Kartagener's syndrome. *Fertil Steril* 1986;46:412–416.
766. Afzelius BA, Eliasson R, Johnsen Ø, Lindholmer C. Lack of dynein arms in immotile human spermatozoa. *J Cell Biol* 1975;66:225–232.
767. Lurie M, Tur-Kaspa I, Weill S, Katz I, Rabinovici J, Goldenberg S. Ciliary ultrastructure of respiratory and fallopian tube epithelium in a sterile woman with Kartagener's syndrome. A quantitative estimation. *Chest,* 1989;95:578–581.
768. Harper MJK, Bennett JP, Boursnell JC, Rowson LEA. An autoradiographic method for the study of egg transport in the rabbit fallopian tube. *J Reprod Fertil* 1960;1:249–267.
769. Bennett JP, Rowson LEA. The use of radioactive artificial eggs in studies of egg transfer and transport in the female reproductive tract. In: *Proceedings of the IVth International Congress on Animal Reproduction, The Hague,* 1961;360–366.
770. Halbert SA, Becker DR, Szal SE. Ovum transport in the rat oviductal ampulla in the absence of muscle contractility. *Biol Reprod.* 1989;40:1131–1136.

771. Black DL, Asdell SA. Transport through the rabbit oviduct. *Am J Physiol* 1958;192:63–68.
772. Black DL, Davis J. A blocking mechanism in the cow oviduct. *J Reprod Fertil* 1962;4:21–26.
773. Edgar DG, Asdell SA. The valve-like action of the utero-tubal junction of the ewe. *J Endocrinol* 1960;21:315–320.
774. Rauscher H. Rundfischgespräch zum III. Hauptthema. Von der Ovulation zur Implantation. *Arch Gynakol* 1969;207:181–182.
775. Hunter RHF. Polyspermic fertilization in pigs after tubal deposition of excessive numbers of spermatozoa. *J Exp Zool* 1973;183:57–64.
776. Day BN, Polge C. Effects of progesterone on fertilization and egg transport in the pig. *J Reprod Fertil* 1968;17:227–230.
777. Hunter RHF. Local action of progesterone leading to polyspermic fertilization in pigs. *J Reprod Fertil* 1972;31:433–444.
778. Seki K, Rawson JMR, Hodgson BJ. Postovulatory changes in cell contacts and intercellular space of rabbit oviductal smooth muscle. *Biol Reprod* 1978;18:679–685.
779. Koester H. Ovum transport. In: Gibian H, Plotz EJ, eds. *Mammalian Reproduction: 21 Colloquium der Geselleschaft für Biologische Chemie.* Heidelberg: Springer-Verlag, 1970;189–228.
780. Ge ZH, Spicer SS. Immunocytochemistry of ion transport mediators in the genital tract of female rodents. *Biol Reprod* 1988;38:439–452.
781. Grippo AA, Henault MA, Anderson SH, Killian GJ. Cation concentrations in fluid from the oviduct ampulla and isthmus of cows during the estrous cycle. *J Dairy Sci* 1992;75:58–65.
782. Ward JP, Watson PF, Noakes DE. Chronic *in situ* monitoring of the free calcium ion concentration in the uterine tubes and horns of the sheep. *Comp Biochem Physiol [A]* 1989,94.765–769.
783. Mathieu CL, Mills SE, Burnett SH, Cloney DL, Bruns DE, Bruns ME. The presence and estrogen control of immunoreactive calbindin-D9k in the fallopian tube of the rat. *Endocrinology* 1989;125:2745–2750.
784. Menghi G, Bondi AM, Materazzi G. Codistribution of lectin reactive glycoderivatives and PA-TCH-SP positive sites in rat oviduct. *Acta Histochem* 1989;86:101–110.
785. Menghi G, Bondi AM, Accili D, Materazzi G. Fine localization of sulphated and non-sulphated glycoconjugates in the rabbit oviduct during the estrous cycle. *Acta Histochem* 1984;74:121–132.
786. Erickson-Lawrence MF, Turner TT, Thomas TS, Oliphant G. Effect of steroid hormones on sulfated oviductal glycoprotein secretion by oviductal explants *in vitro. Biol Reprod* 1989;40: 1311–1319.
787. Gandolfi F, Brevini TA, Richardson L, Brown CR, Moor RM. Characterization of proteins secreted by sheep oviduct epithelial cells and their function in embryonic development. *Development* 1989;106:303–312.
788. Buhi WC, Vallet JL, Bazer FW. *De novo* synthesis and release of polypeptides from cyclic and early pregnant porcine oviductal tissue in explant culture. *J Exp Zool* 1989;252:79–88.
789. Verhage HG, Fazleabas AT. The *in vitro* synthesis of estrogen-dependent proteins by the baboon (*Papio anubis*) oviduct. *Endocrinology* 1988;123:552–558.
790. Verhage HG, Boice ML, Mavrogianis P, Donnelly K, Fazleabas AT. Immunological characterization and immunocytochemical localization of oviduct-specific glycoproteins in the baboon (*Papio anubis*). *Endocrinology* 1989;124:2464–2472.
791. Verhage HG, Mavrogianis PA, Boice ML, Li W, Fazleabas AT. Oviductal epithelium of the baboon: hormonal control and the immuno-gold localization of oviduct-specific glycoproteins. *Am J Anat* 1990;187:81–90.
792. Donelly KM, Fazleabas AT, Verhage HG, Mavrogianis PA, Jaffe RC. Cloning of a recombinant complementary DNA to a baboon (*Papio anubis*) estradiol-dependent oviduct-specific glycoprotein. *Mol Endocrinol* 1991;5:356–364.
793. Schulte BA, Rao KP, Kreutner A, Thomopoulos GN, Spicer SS. Histochemical examination of glycoconjugates of epithelial cells in the human fallopian tube. *Lab Invest* 1985;52:207–219.
794. Schultka R, Cech S. Application of "mild" periodic acid oxidation to the ultrahistochemical detection of sialic-acid containing compounds in human fallopian tube epithelium. *Acta Histochem* 1990;88:65–69.
795. Schultka R, Cech S. Demonstration of glycogen in human oviduct epithelium. *Acta Histochem* 1989;87:137–139.
796. Tombes RM, Shapiro BM. Energy transport and cell polarity: relationship of phosphagen kinase activity to sperm function. *J Exp Zool* 1989;251:82–90.
797. Bützow R. The human fallopian tube contains placental protein 5. *Hum Reprod* 1989;4:17–20.
798. Tiitinen A, Wahlström T, Julkunen M, Seppälä M. The content and immunohistochemical localization of placental protein 10 (PP10) in the fallopian tube. *Br J Obstet Gynaecol* 1986;93: 924–927.
799. Julkunen M, Wahlström T, Seppälä M. Human fallopian tube contains placental protein 14. *Am J Obstet Gynecol* 1986;154: 1076–1079.
800. Julkunen M, Koistinen R, Suikkari AM, Seppälä M, Jänne OA. Identification by hybridization histochemistry of human endometrial cells expressing mRNAs encoding a uterine β-lactoglobulin homologue and insulin-like growth factor-binding protein-1. *Mol Endocrinol* 1990;4:700–707.
801. Giudice LC, Dsupin BA, Irwin JC, Eckert RL. Identification of insulin-like growth factor factor binding proteins in human oviduct. *Fertil Steril* 1992;57:294–301.
802. Wiseman DL, Henricks DM, Eberhardt DM, Bridges WC. Identification and content of insulin-like growth factors in porcine oviductal fluid. *Biol Reprod* 1992;47:126–132.
803. Rappolee DA, Sturm KS, Schultz GA, Pedersen RA, Werb Z. The expression of growth factor ligands and receptors in preimplantation mouse embryos. In: Heyner S, Wiley L, eds. *Early Embryo Development and Paracrine Relationships.* New York: AR Liss, 1990;11–25.
804. Sjöberg J, Wahlström T, Grudzinskas JG, Sinosich MJ. Demonstration of pregnancy-associated plasma protein A (PAPP A) like material in the fallopian tube. *Fertil Steril* 1986;45:517–521.
805. Peters WM. Nature of "basal" and "reserve" cells in oviductal and cervical epithelium in man. *J Clin Pathol* 1986;39:306–312.
806. Kutteh WH, Blackwell RE, Gore H, Kutteh CC, Carr BR, Mestecky J. Secretory immune system of the female reproductive tract. II. Local immune system in normal and infected fallopian tube. *Fertil Steril* 1990;54:51–55.
807. Otsuki Y, Maeda Y, Magari S, Sugimoto O. Lymphatics and lymphoid tissue of the fallopian tube: immunoelectronmicroscopic study. *Anat Rec* 1989;225:288–296.
808. Bulmer JN, Earl U. The expression of class II MHC gene products by fallopian tube epithelium in pregnancy and throughout the menstrual cycle. *Immunology* 1987;61:207–213.
809. Bongso A, Ng S-C, Sathananthan H, Ng PL, Rauff M, Ratnam SS. Establishment of human ampullary cell cultures. *Hum Reprod* 1989;4:486–494.
810. Henriksen T, Tanbo T, Abyholm T, Oppedal BR, Claussen OP. Epithelial cells from human fallopian tube in culture. *Hum Reprod* 1990;5:25–31.
811. Takeuchi K, Maruyama I, Yamamoto S, Oki T, Nagata Y. Isolation and monolayer culture of human fallopian tube epithelial cells. *In Vitro Cell Dev Biol* 1991;27A:720–724.
812. Goldberg JM, Khalifa EA, Friedman CI, Kim MH. Improvement of *in vitro* fertilization and early embryo development in mice by coculture with human fallopian tube epithelium. *Am J Obstet Gynecol* 1991;165:1802–1805.
813. Ellington JE, Farrell PB, Simkin ME, Foote RH, Goldman EE, McGrath AB. Development and survival after transfer of cow embryos cultured from 1-2-cells to morulae or blastocysts in rabbit oviducts or in a simple medium with bovine oviduct epithelial cells. *J Reprod Fertil* 1990;89:293–299.
814. Xu KP, Yadav BR, Rorie RW, Plante L, Betteridge KJ, King WA. Development and viability of bovine embryos derived from oocytes matured and fertilized *in vitro* and co-cultured with bovine oviducal epithelial cells. *J Reprod Fertil* 1992;94:33–43.
815. Carney EW, Tobback C, Foote RH. Co-culture of rabbit one-cell embryos with rabbit oviduct epithelial cells. *In Vitro Cell Dev Biol* 1990;26:629–635.
816. Carney EW, Foote RH. Effects of superovulation, embryo recovery, culture system and embryo transfer on development of rabbit embryos *in vivo* and *in vitro. J Reprod Fertil* 1990;89:543–551.
817. Archibong AE, Petters RM, Johnson BH. Development of porcine embryos from one- and two-cell stages to blastocysts in culture medium supplemented with porcine oviductal fluid. *Biol Reprod* 1989;41:1076–1083.

818. Harper MJK. Hormonal control of transport of eggs in cumulus through the ampulla of the rabbit oviduct. *Endocrinology* 1966;78:568–574.
819. Blandau RJ. Observing ovulation and egg transport. In: Daniel JC Jr, ed. *Methods in Mammalian Embryology.* San Francisco: WH Freeman, 1970;1–14.
820. Boling JF, Blandau RJ. Egg transport through the ampullae of the oviducts of rabbits under various experimental conditions. *Biol Reprod* 1971;4:174–184.
821. Hunter RHF. Chronological and cytological details of fertilization and early embryonic development in the domestic pig, *Sus scrofa. Anat Rec* 1974;178:169–186.
822. Eddy CA, Turner TT, Kraemer DC, Pauerstein CJ. Pattern and duration of ovum transport in the baboon (*Papio anubis*). *Obstet Gynecol* 1976;47:658–664.
823. Croxatto HB, Díaz S, Fuentalba B, Croxatto HD, Carrillo D, Fabres C. Studies on the duration of egg transport in the human oviduct. 1. The time interval between ovulation and egg recovery from the uterus in normal women. *Fertil Steril* 1972;23:447–458.
824. Hertig AT, Rock J, Adams EC. A description of 34 human ova within the first 17 days of development. *Am J Anat* 1956;98: 435–493.
825. Chang MC, Bedford JM. Fertilizability of rabbit ova after removal of the corona radiata. *Fertil Steril* 1962;13:421–425.
826. Allen E, Pratt JP, Newell QU, Bland LJ. Human tubal ova; related early corpora lutea and uterine tubes. *Contrib Embryol Carnegie Inst* 1930;22:45–76.
827. Lewis WH, Hartman CG. Tubal ova of the rhesus monkey. *Contrib Embryol Carnegie Inst* 1941;29:7–14.
828. Eddy CA. Personal communication. 1986.
829. Harper MJK. Pharmacological control of reproduction in women. *Prog Drug Res* 1968;12:47–136.
830. Harper MJK. Agents with antifertility effects during preimplantation stages of pregnancy. In: Moghissi KS, Hafez ESE, eds. *Biology of Mammalian Fertilization and Implantation.* Springfield, IL: Charles C Thomas, 1972;431–492.
831. Harper MJK. Contraception—retrospect and prospect. *Prog Drug Res* 1977;21:293–407.
832. Black DL. Neural control of oviduct musculature. In: Johnson AD, Foley CH, eds. *The Oviduct and Its Functions.* New York: Academic Press, 1974;65–118.
833. Coutinho EM. Interference with ovum transport: implications for fertility control. In: Harper MJK, Pauerstein CJ, Adams CE, Coutinho EM, Croxatto HB, Paton DM, eds. *Ovum Transport and Fertility Regulation.* Copenhagen: Scriptor, 1976;544–556.
834. Coutinho AM, Maia H, Nascimento L. The response of the human fallopian tube to ergonovine and methyl-ergonovine *in vivo. Am J Obstet Gynecol* 1976;126:48–54.
835. Ortiz ME, Bastías G, Darrigrande O, Croxatto HB. Importance of uterine expulsion of embryos in the interceptive mechanism of postcoital oestradiol in rats. *Reprod Fertil Dev* 1991;3:333–337.
836. Bygdeman M, Bremme K, Christensen N, Lundström V, Gréen K. A comparison of two stable prostaglandin E analogues for termination of early pregnancy and for cervical dilatation. *Contraception* 1980;22:471–483.
837. Bygdeman M, Christensen N, Gréen K, Zheng S. Self-administration of prostaglandin for termination of early pregnancy. *Contraception* 1981;24:45–52.
838. Kovacs L, Sas M, Resch BA, et al. Termination of very early pregnancy by RU486—an antiprogestational compound. *Contraception* 1984;29:399–410.
839. Swahn ML, Cekan S, Wang B, Lundström V, Bygdeman M. Pharmacokinetic and clinical studies of RU486 for regulation of fertility. In: Baulieu E-E, Segal SJ, eds. *The Antiprogestin Steroid RU486 and Human Fertility Control.* New York: Plenum Press, 1985;249–258.
840. Farkas M, Apró G, Sas M. Clinico-pharmacological examination of Postinor (0.75 mg *d*-norgestrel). *Ther Hung* 1981;29:22–30.
841. World Health Organization Task Force on Post-Ovulatory Methods for Fertility Regulation. Postcoital contraception with levonorgestrel during the peri-ovulatory phase of the menstrual cycle. *Contraception* 1987;36:275–286.
842. Blye RP. The use of postcoital contraceptive agents. *Am J Obstet Gynecol* 1973;116:1044–1050.
843. Clement PB. Pathology of gamete and zygote transport: cervical, endometrial, myometrial, and tubal factors in infertility. *Monogr Pathol* 1991;33:140–194.
844. World Health Organization. *Special Programme of Research, Development and Research Training in Human Reproduction. Eighth Annual Report.* Geneva: WHO, 1979.
845. World Health Organization. *Special Programme of Research, Development and Research Training in Human Reproduction. Eleventh Annual Report.* Geneva: WHO, 1982.
846. World Health Organization. *Special Programme of Research, Development and Research Training in Human Reproduction. Thirteenth Annual Report.* Geneva: WHO, 1984.
847. Winston, RML. Microsurgery of the fallopian tube: from fantasy to reality. *Fertil Steril* 1980;34:521–533.
848. Wallach EE. Tubal reconstructive surgery—1980. *Fertil Steril* 1980;34:531–533.
849. Henry-Suchet J, Catalan F, Loffredo V, et al. *Chlamydia trachomatis* associated with chronic inflammation in abdominal specimens from women selected for tuboplasty. *Fertil Steril* 1981;36:599–605.
850. Faulkner WL, Ory HW. Intrauterine devices and acute pelvic inflammatory disease. *JAMA,* 1976;235:1851–1853.
851. Weström L, Bengtsson LP, Mårdh P. The risk of pelvic inflammatory disease in women using intrauterine contraceptive devices as compared to non-users. *Lancet* 1976;ii:221–224.
852. Daling JR, Weiss NS, Metch BJ, et al. Primary tubal infertility in relation to the use of an intrauterine device. *N Engl J Med* 1985;312:937–941.
853. Cramer DW, Schiff I, Schoenbaum SC, et al. Tubal infertility and the intrauterine device. *N Engl J Med* 1985;312:941–947.
854. Ben-Nun I, Greenblatt RB. Infertility associated with endometriosis. In: Semm K, Greenblatt RB, Mettler L, eds. *Genital Endometriosis in Infertility.* New York: Thieme-Stratton, 1982;1–10.
855. Friedman J. The incidence of endometriosis in unexplained infertility. In: Semm K, Greenblatt RB, Mettler L, eds. *Genital Endometriosis in Infertility.* New York: Thieme-Stratton, 1982;28–31.
856. Czernobilsky B, Silverstein A. Salpingitis in ovarian endometriosis. *Fertil Steril* 1978;30:45–49.
857. Drake TS, O'Brien WF, Ramwell PW, Metz SA. Peritoneal fluid thromboxane B_2 and 6-ketoprostaglandin $F_{1\alpha}$ in endometriosis. *Am J Obstet Gynecol* 1981;141:401–404.
858. Ylikorkala O, Koskimies A, Laatkainen T, Tenhunen A, Viinikka L. Peritoneal fluid prostaglandins in endometriosis, tubal disorders, and unexplained infertility. *Obstet Gynecol* 1984; 63:616–620.
859. Schenken RS, Asch RH, Williams RF, Hodgen GD. Etiology of infertility in monkeys with endometriosis: measurement of peritoneal fluid prostaglandins. *Am J Obstet Gynecol* 1984;150: 349–353.
860. Rock JA, Dubin NH, Ghodgaonkar RB, Bergquist CA, Erozan YS, Kimball AW Jr. Cul-de-sac fluid in women with endometriosis: fluid volume and prostanoid concentration during the proliferative phase of the cycle—days 8 to 12. *Fertil Steril* 1982;37:747–750.
861. Sgarlata CS, Hertelendy F, Mikhail G. The prostanoid content in peritoneal fluid and plasma of women with endometriosis. *Am J Obstet Gynecol* 1983;147:563–565.
862. Damon M, Thaler H, Mercklein L, Denjean R, Hedon B, Crastes de Paulet A. Prostanoids in the peritoneal fluids of infertile women. In: Raynaud J-P, Ojasoo T, Martini L, eds. *Medical Management of Endometriosis.* New York: Raven Press, 1984;107–124.
863. Badawy SZA, Marshall L, Gabel AA, Nusbaum ML. The concentration of 13,14-dihydro-15-keto prostaglandin $F_{2\alpha}$ and prostaglandin E_2 in peritoneal fluid of infertile patients with and without endometriosis. *Fertil Steril* 1982;38:166–170.
864. Heinonen PK, Aine R, Seppälä E. Peritoneal fluid leukotriene B_4 and prostaglandin E_2 in acute salpingitis. *Gynecol Obstet Invest* 1990;29:292–295.
865. Pauerstein CJ. *The Fallopian Tube: A Reappraisal.* Philadelphia: Lea & Febiger, 1974.
866. Centers for Disease Control. Ectopic pregnancies—United

States, 1979–1980. Centers for Disease Control. *MMWR* 1984;33:201–202.
867. Pauerstein CJ, Croxatto HB, Eddy CA, Ramzy I, Walters MD. Anatomy and pathology of tubal pregnancy. *Obstet Gynecol* 1986;67:301–308.
868. Wagrowska-Danilewicz M, Danilewicz M, Gwóźdź A. Morphological causes of tubal pregnancy. *Wiad Lek* 1990;43:953–958.
869. Persaud V. Etiology of tubal ectopic pregnancy. Radiologic and pathologic studies. *Obstet Gynecol* 1970;36:257–263.
870. Stock RJ. Histopathology of fallopian tubes with recurrent tubal pregnancy. *Obstet Gynecol* 1990;75:9–14.
871. Sherman KJ, Chow WH, Daling JR, Weiss NS. Sexually transmitted diseases and the risk of tubal pregnancy. *J Reprod Med* 1988;33:30–34.
872. Sherman KJ, Daling JR, Stergachis A, et al. Sexually transmitted diseases and tubal pregnancy. *Sex Trnsm Dis* 1990;17:115–121.
873. Walters MD, Eddy CA, Gibbs RS, Schacter J, Holden AE. Antibodies to *Chlamydia trachomatis* and risk for tubal pregnancy. *Am J Obstet Gynecol* 1988;159:942–946.
874. Brunnemann H, Salloum H, Alexander H, Zenner I, Baumann L. Genital *Chlamydia* infections and extrauterine pregnancy. *Geburtshilfe Frauenheilkd* 1989;49:179–182.
875. Tuffrey M, Falder P, Gale J, Quinn R, Taylor-Robinson D. Infertility in mice infected genitally with a human strain of *Chlamydia trachomatis*. *J Reprod Fertil* 1986;78:251–260.
876. Tuffrey M, Alexander F, Inman C, Ward ME. Correlation of infertility with altered tubal morphology and function in mice with salpingitis induced by a human genital-tract isolate of *Chlamydia trachomatis*. *J Reprod Fertil* 1990;88:295–305.
877. Israngkun C, Phaosavasdi S. Hysteroscopic sterilization: complications in 296 cases. In: Sciarra JJ, Droegemueller W, Speidel JJ, eds. *Advances in Female Sterilization Techniques.* Hagerstown, MD: Harper & Row, 1976;148–152.
878. Borten M, Friedman EA. Ectopic pregnancy among early abortion patients: does prostaglandin reduce the incidence? *Prostaglandins,* 1985;30:891–905.
879. Lehfeldt H, Tietze C, Gorstein F. Ovarian pregnancy and the intrauterine device. *Am J Obstet Gynecol* 1970;108:1005–1009.
880. Seward PH, Israel R, Ballard CA. Ectopic pregnancy and intrauterine contraception. A definite relationship. *Obstet Gynecol* 1972;40:214–217.
881. Tatum HJ, Schmidt FH. Contraceptive and sterilization practices and extrauterine pregnancy: a realistic perspective. *Fertil Steril* 1977;28:407–421.
882. Díaz S, Croxatto HB, Pavez M, et al. Ectopic pregnancies associated with low dose progestagen-releasing IUDs. *Contraception* 1980;22:259–269.
883. Panayotou PP, Kaskarelis DB, Miettinen OS, Trichopoulos DB, Kalandidi AK. Induced abortion and ectopic pregnancy. *Am J Obstet Gynecol* 1972;114:507–510.
884. McBain JC, Pepperell RJ, Robinson HP, Smith MA, Brown JB. An unexpectedly high rate of ectopic pregnancy following the induction of ovulation with human pituitary and chorionic gonadotrophin. *Br J Obstet Gynaecol* 1980;87:5–9.
885. Snyder T, del Castillo J, Graff J, Hoxsey R, Hefti M. Heterotopic pregnancy after *in vitro* fertilization and ovulatory drugs. *Ann Emerg Med* 1988;17:846–849.
886. Gamberdella FR, Marrs RP. Heterotopic pregnancy associated with assisted reproductive technology. *Am J Obstet Gynecol* 1989;160:1520–1522.
887. Glasner MJ, Aron E, Eskin BA. Ovulation induction with clomiphene and the rise in heterotopic pregnancies. A report of two cases. *J Reprod Med* 1990;35:175–178.
888. Herman A, Ron-El R, Golan A, Weinraub Z, Bukovsky I, Caspi E. The role of tubal pathology and other parameters in ectopic pregnancies occurring in *in vitro* fertilization and embryo transfer. *Fertil Steril* 1990;54:864–868.
889. Lewin A, Simon A, Rabinowitz R, Schenker JG. Second-trimester heterotopic pregnancy after *in vitro* fertilization and embryo transfer—a case report and review of the literature. *Int J Fertil* 1991;36:227–230.
890. Dubuisson JB, Aubriot FX, Mathieu L, Foulot H, Mandelbrot L, and de Jolière JB. Risk factors for ectopic pregnancy in 556 pregnancies after *in vitro* fertilization: implications for preventive management. *Fertil Steril* 1991;56:686–690.
891. Pulkkinen MO, Talo A. Myoelectrical activity in the human oviduct with tubal pregnancy. *Am J Obstet Gynecol* 1984;148: 151–154.
892. Barash A, Shoham Z, Blickstein I, Yamini M, Borenstein R. Simultaneous tubal and intra-uterine pregnancy following *in vitro* fertilization and embryo transfer. *Acta Obstet Gynecol Scand* 1989;68:643–644.
893. Raccuia JS, Neckles S, Butler D, Kahn M, Ibrahim IM. Synchronous intrauterine and ectopic pregnancy associated with clomiphene citrate. *Surg Gynecol Obstet* 1989;168:417–420.
894. Hanf V, Dietl J, Gagsteiger F, Pfeiffer KH. Bilateral tubal pregnancy with intra-uterine gestation after IVF-ET: therapy by bilateral laparoscopic salpingectomy; a case report. *Eur J Obstet Gynecol Reprod Biol* 1990;37:87–90.
895. Insunza A, de Pablo F, Croxatto HD, Letelier LM, Morante M, Croxatto HB. On the rate of tubal pregnancy contralateral to the corpus luteum. *Acta Obstet Gynecol Scand* 1988;67:433–436.
896. Guirgis RR, Fiamanya W, al-Shawaf T, Craft IL. Left ectopic pregnancy following gamete intra-fallopian transfer into the right fallopian tube: a report on two cases. *Hum Reprod* 1990;5: 1023–1024.
897. Thibault C. Some pathological aspects of ovum maturation and gamete transport in mammals and man. *Acta Endocrinol (Copenh),* 1972;70(suppl 166):59–66.
898. Jerome CP, Hendrickx AG. A tubal pregnancy in a rhesus monkey (*Macaca mulatta*). *Vet Pathol* 1982;19:239–245.
899. Mossman HW. Orientation and site of attachment of the blastocyst: a comparative study. In: Blandau RJ, ed. *The Biology of the Blastocyst.* Chicago: University of Chicago Press, 1971;49–57.
900. Tuchmann-Duplessis H, David G, Haegel P. *Illustrated Human Embryology, Vol 1, Embryogenesis.* New York: Springer-Verlag, 1972.
901. Beatty RA. Variation in the number of corpora lutea and in the number and size of 6-day blastocysts in rabbits subjected to superovulation treatment. *J Endocrinol* 1958;17:248–260.
902. Böving BG. Rabbit blastocyst distribution. *Am J Anat* 1956;98:403–434.
903. Cao Z-D, Jones MA, Harper MJK. Prostaglandin translocation from the lumen of the rabbit uterus *in vitro* in relation to day of pregnancy or pseudopregnancy. *Biol Reprod* 1984;31:505–519.
904. McLaren A, Michie D. The spacing of implantation in the mouse uterus. *Mem Soc Endocrinol* 1959;6:65–75.
905. Legrand C, Banuelos-Nevarez A, Maltier JP. Changes in electrical activity of myometrium during intrauterine distribution of rat blastocysts and after prazosin administration. *J Reprod Fertil* 1989;86:39–49.
906. Hafez ESE, Ludwig H. Scanning electron microscopy of the endometrium. In: Wynn RM, ed. *Biology of the Uterus.* New York: Plenum Press, 1977;309–340.
907. Hardy K, Martin KL, Leese HJ, Winston RML, Handyside AH. Human preimplantation development *in vitro* is not adversely affected by biopsy at the 8-cell stage. *Hum Reprod* 1990;5: 708–714.
908. Cohen J, De Vane GW, Elsner CW, et al. Cryopreservation of zygotes and early cleaved human embryos. *Fertil Steril* 1988;49:283–289.
909. Hartshorne GM, Elder K, Crow J, Dyson H, Edwards RG. The influence of *in-vitro* development upon post-thaw survival and implantation of cryopreserved human blastocysts. *Hum Reprod* 1991;6:136–131.
910. Pauerstein CJ, Eddy CA, Koong MK, Moore GD. Rabbit endosalpinx suppresses ectopic implantation. *Fertil Steril* 1990; 54:522–526.
911. Bedford JM, Yanagimachi R. Initiation of sperm motility after mating in the rat and hamster. *J Androl* 1992;13:444–449.

The Physiology of Reproduction, Second Edition,
edited by E. Knobil and J.D. Neill,
Raven Press, Ltd., New York © 1994.

CHAPTER 5

Mammalian Fertilization

R. Yanagimachi

Fertilization is the process whereby individual gametes from the female and male unite to create offspring whose genetic makeup is different from both parents. This bisexual mode of reproduction via fertilization emerged during evolution and has been maintained in most metazoans including mammals. Although the reason for this is still not clearly understood, this process may accelerate the rate of adaptation in evolution while avoiding irreversible accumulation of detrimental mutations in the face of a competitive and constantly changing environment (1238). From the standpoint of their genomes, eggs and spermatozoa are equal, but their life history and behavior before and during fertilization are quite different. The spermatozoon usually moves and always takes the intuitive in order to fuse with and activate the egg. When activated by the fertilizing spermatozoon, the egg, with a dual complement of the female and male genomes, eliminates all or almost all of the nonnuclear elements of the spermatozoon and starts to develop into a new individual.

Before 1950, much of fertilization research utilized the gametes of invertebrates (e.g., sea urchins) and nonmammalian vertebrates (e.g., fish and frogs), mainly because of the availability of large quantities of gametes. In addition, synchronous fertilization and development in these animals can be achieved very easily in laboratory dishes. In contrast, the number of mammalian eggs available at a particular time is generally "disappointingly" small. Furthermore, even today, fertilization and development of mammalian eggs *in vitro* requires considerable effort by the investigators.

Despite such inherent handicaps, recent advances in our knowledge of mammalian fertilization have been impressive, owing to the endeavor of many investigators. In fact, at present, some areas of mammalian fertilization research are ahead of fertilization research in invertebrates and nonmammalian vertebrates. The rapid progress in research at the frontiers and the publication of a vast number of research papers dealing with a wide variety of animal species (from marsupials to humans) makes it difficult to include all the available information in a single review. Therefore, for important details, readers are referred to individual papers and reviews cited in each section of this review as well as to books covering relatively wide areas of mammalian fertilization research (688,718,899,1022,1130,1641). Other books (1181,1236,1453,1454) emphasize fertilization research in invertebrates and nonmammalian vertebrates, but they include several important chapters on mammalian fertilization as well. Students of fertilization should read, at least once, such classic reviews as those by Austin (20), Austin and Walton (26), Bishop (60), Blandau (63), Hartman (1021a), and Piko (396). Many "treasures" are still hidden therein.

Department of Anatomy and Reproductive Biology, University of Hawaii School of Medicine, Honolulu, Hawaii 96822

EPIDIDYMAL MATURATION OF SPERMATOZOA

Mammalian spermatozoa are highly differentiated by the time they leave the testis. Nonetheless, they do not yet have the ability to move progressively or interact with and fertilize eggs. They gain these abilities while passing through the epididymis. This sperm maturation process has been studied extensively (for reviews, see 22, 53,111,122,144,227,233,362,374,376,734,837a,837b, 908). The need for the epididymal maturation of mammalian spermatozoa contrasts with the situation in most invertebrates and lower vertebrates (such as teleost fish and anuran amphibians) in which the spermatozoa leaving the testis already have full fertilizing capacity.

The Site Where Spermatozoa Acquire Fertilizing Ability

The anatomical location in the epididymis where mammalian spermatozoa begin to acquire their fertilizing ability varies according to species. In some species (e.g., the boar), some fertile spermatozoa first appear at the level of the caput epididymis, whereas in others (e.g., the rat) it occurs in the distal segment of the corpus epididymis (Fig. 1) (122). Apparently, spermatozoa do not gain their fertilizing capacity simultaneously in the same region. Some spermatozoa become able to fertilize much sooner (or in a more proximal region of the epididymis) than others. However, as a general rule, it is not until they reach the proximal cauda epididymis (the major sperm storage site) that the great majority of spermatozoa attain their full fertilizing potential.

Sperm fertility usually refers to the ability of spermatozoa to fertilize physiologically normal and structurally intact eggs either *in vivo* or *in vitro*. Under experimental conditions or after surgical manipulation of the eggs or of the male tract, the spermatozoa, which are otherwise infertile, may become fertile. For instance, mouse spermatozoa collected from the corpus epididymis fertilize only 3% of zona-intact eggs, but they fertilize 51% of the eggs if injected microsurgically into the perivitelline space (1039). What is missing in most of the corpus spermatozoa is the ability to pass through the zona, not the ability to undergo the acrosome reaction (1146). Rabbit spermatozoa in the caput epididymis, which are normally infertile, become fertile there when their downstream migration is prevented by duct ligation (724).

As judged by indirect indices, human spermatozoa in normal epididymis probably do not generally develop the fertilizing ability until they reach the corpus region (729,733). However, when the human epididymis is obstructed in a way analogous to the ligation model in the

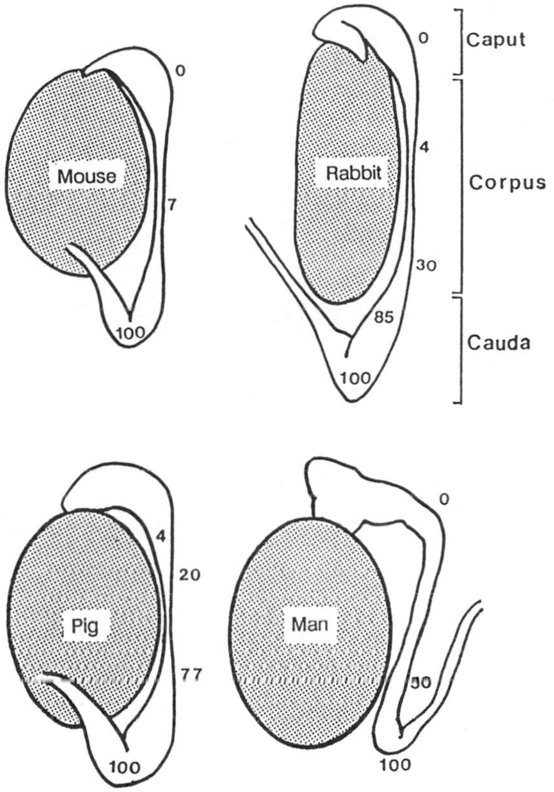

FIG. 1. Development of the fertilizing ability of spermatozoa in the epididymis. The percentage of eggs fertilized by the spermatozoa from the distal cauda epididymis was standardized as 100. Fertility of mouse and rabbit spermatozoa was determined by *in vitro* insemination (mouse, ref. 1043; pig, ref. 1058) or *in vivo* insemination (rabbit, ref. 721). Human sperm fertility was estimated by (i) sperm's ability to fertilize zona-free hamster eggs, (ii) motility patterns, (iii) surface characteristics and (iv) the structural stability of the head and tail (ref. 729).

rabbit, then spermatozoa that can fertilize eggs *in vitro* may sometimes appear in the caput region (1492). Moreover, fertile spermatozoa are often ejaculated after the vas deferens has been linked by anastomosis to the caput of the obstructed human epididymis (1461,1491) and sometimes after anastomosis directly to the vas efferentia (Fig. 2) (1490). Thus, in regard to maturation, the functional relationship between spermatozoa and the successive regions of the human epididymis seems very flexible. At least in man the epididymis does not have an absolutely essential role in the maturation process. The acquisition of fertilizing ability as spermatozoa reach the corpus of the normal epididymis may be partly a matter of time, and it is quite possible that even in the normal tract, as well as in the obstructed tract, the caput and perhaps even the vas deferens secrete the specific components necessary for functional maturation (837,1217). Although the human, with "exceptionally" rapid sperm transport in the epididymis (1094), may be an extreme example in this regard, such a functional flexibility between spermatozoa and the male tract may occur in some other mammals, although not apparently to any degree in murine rodents.

Development of the Sperm's Ability to Move

One of the most prominent changes in the spermatozoa during epididymal maturation is the development of sperm motility. Testicular spermatozoa are either motionless or weakly motile. This is true not only within the testicular environment but also when these spermatozoa are suspended in physiological salt solutions. Fully mature spermatozoa released from the cauda epididymis, on the other hand, begin active, progressive movement upon exposure to physiological salt solutions. The inability of testicular spermatozoa to move appears to be due, at least in part, to the immaturity of the plasma membrane, because these spermatozoa can move almost as actively as mature cauda epididymal spermatozoa if they are demembranated and exposed to adenosine triphosphate (ATP), cyclic adenosine monophosphate (cAMP), and magnesium ions (Mg^{2+}) (Fig. 3) (252,326,512,1076, 1260). However, as demembranated testicular spermatozoa do not respond to ATP/cAMP as quickly as demembranated mature spermatozoa (326,512), some fine adjustment (e.g., modification of dynein ATPase) may be occurring during epididymal maturation (512). Transfer of several substances, such as glycerol-3-phosphorylcholine (250) a forward motility protein (2,3) from the epididymal fluid, an alteration in a cAMP-modulated protein kinase system (1683) and the develop-

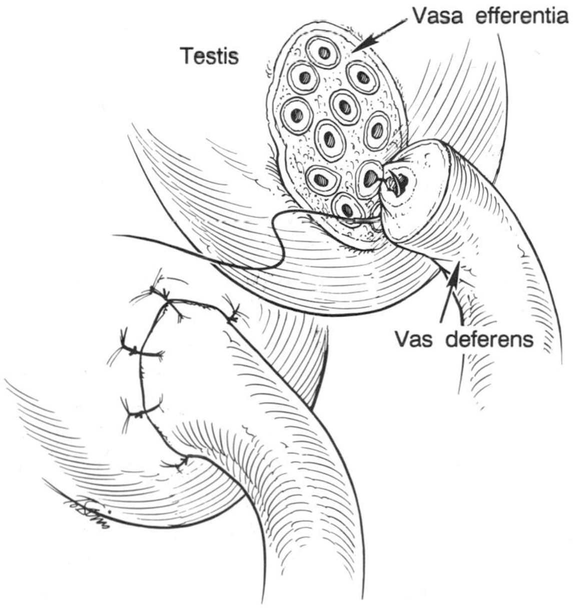

FIG. 2. Microsurgical anastomosis of the vas deferens to one of the vasa efferentia. (From ref. 1490.)

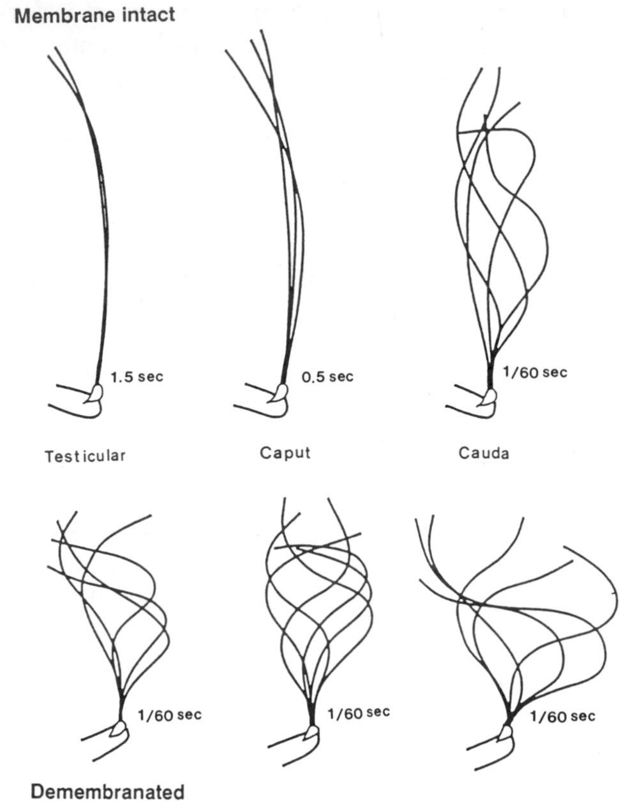

FIG. 3. Comparison of the movement patterns of golden hamster spermatozoa with or without plasma membranes. *Top row,* membrane intact spermatozoa. *Bottom row,* the spermatozoa demembraned with Triton and reactivated by ATP. Each spermatozoon was grasped by its head with a micropipette. Time intervals between successive images are shown next to the head. Note that the testicular spermatozoa become motile when they are demembraned and supplied with exogenous ATP. (From ref. 1260.)

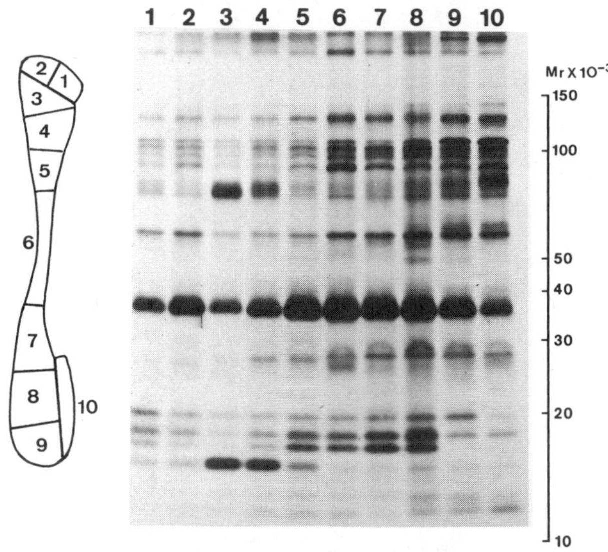

FIG. 4. Polyacylamide gel electrophoresis of proteins secreted by various segments of the rat epididymis. The epididymis is subdivided into ten arbitrary segments: *1–2* is the initial segment, *3–5* is the caput epididymis, *6–7* is the corpus epididymis, and *8–10* is the cauda epididymis. (From ref. 82.)

ment of the mechanism that keeps intracellular calcium ions (Ca^{2+}) low (1628), seem to contribute to the development of the sperm's ability to move properly.

Maturational Changes in the Sperm Plasma Membrane

The epididymis has a very active fluid-absorbing and fluid-secreting activity. The osmolarity (123) and chemical composition (81,236,286,290,1608,1682a) of the fluid-secreting activity. The osmolarity (123) and chemito another (Figs. 4 and 5) (82,1390). Therefore, it is not surprising that the sperm plasma membrane, which is exposed directly to the epididymal fluid, is altered step by step as the spermatozoa pass through the different regions of the epididymis (144,153,234,362).

During epididymal maturation, membrane lipids of spermatozoa undergo distinct physical and chemical alterations (352,384,434,1670,1671). Changes in the distribution pattern of intramembraneous protein (glycoprotein) particles in the sperm plasma membrane during maturation (360,407,464,1539) seem to reflect chemical alterations of both membrane lipids and proteins. The fact that the epididymis displays a high rate of cholesterol synthesis activity (206,209) and that cholesterol (sterol) is transferred into the plasma membrane of ma-

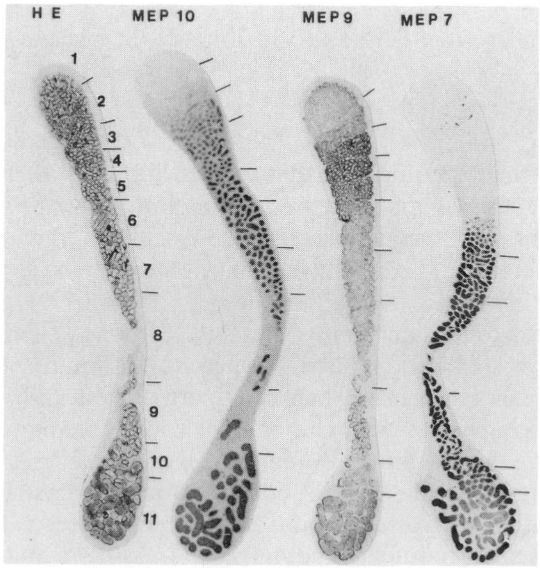

FIG. 5. Longitudinal sections of mouse epididymides, showing immunolocalization of three epididymal proteins, MEP 10 (18 kDa), MEP 9 (25 kDa), and MEP 7 (29 kDa). HE is a hematoxylin-eosin stained section. The numbers to the right of the HE represent the histological divisions of the mouse epididymis. *1,* Proximal caput; *2,* mid-caput; *3–4,* distal caput; *5–9,* corpus; *10–11,* cauda. (From ref. 1390.)

turing spermatozoa (1469,1538,1539) suggests that cholesterol is one of the key molecules that alter the membrane characteristics of spermatozoa during maturation (384). Stabilization of the membrane by cholesterol may be beneficial to spermatozoa, which must travel through various, often hostile, microenvironments within the female tract before reaching the eggs.

The sperm plasma membrane has both membrane-integrated and surface-adsorbed proteins when spermatozoa leave the testis (53,370,418,862). Some of these intrinsic proteins change their location in or on the plasma membrane during sperm maturation. Others are altered, masked, or replaced progressively by new proteins of epididymal origin. The epididymis, in particular its caput and corpus segments, secretes a variety of proteins, and some bind tightly to the spermatozoa (271,1133,1134,1631). Some proteins are modified upon binding to the spermatozoa. Such dynamic membrane modifications occur throughout the male tract, but most actively in the caput and corpus epididymides where the spermatozoa acquire their fertilizing ability (112,143b,144,412,478,517,862,1147,1363,1651).

A steady increase in net negative surface charge (37,147,232,328,544) and dramatic changes in the lectin-binding ability (147,211,351,361,1198,1716) of the sperm surface during epididymal maturation indicate active glycosylation (1011) of sperm surface components. This glycosylation seems to be mediated, at least in part, by galactosyltransferase and sialytransferase in the epididymal fluid (56,207,210,1604) as well as an α-lactalbuminlike substance (208,258). When spermatozoa attain full maturity, some surface glycoproteins, either membrane-integrated or membrane-adsorbed, are located over the entire sperm head, whereas others are restricted to the acrosomal or postacrosomal region of the head (e.g., 412,1358,1359). Some of these glycoproteins and polypeptides stabilize the plasma membrane and may prevent premature acrosome reactions (1401, 1589). Others are believed to mediate interactions between spermatozoa and the zona pellucida (1146,1358, 1359) or the egg plasma membrane (1382) during fertilization. Perhaps, membrane components essential for cell survival (e.g., Na^+–K^+–ATPase) must be in the sperm plasma membrane all the time, but those that will later perform sperm-specific functions (e.g., those assisting sperm survival in the female tract as well as those essential for sperm interactions with egg zona and plasma membrane) may be added to the sperm plasma membrane (or altered to active forms) while spermatozoa are maturing in the epididymis. It is important to note that membrane alterations during epididymal maturation are not limited to the plasma membrane of the sperm head. Adsorption and/or integration of several specific glycoproteins and peptides on or in the plasma membrane of the tail are also well documented (83,88,363,478,932,1042,1325,1599,1623). Some of the surface glycoproteins on the sperm tail may serve to prevent premature hyperactivation.

Maturational Changes in Sperm Structures Other than the Plasma Membrane

Sperm structural components other than the plasma membrane also undergo changes during sperm maturation. Alteration in the distribution pattern of antigens on the outer acrosomal membrane (1363) is one example. This may represent a preparation of the outer acrosomal membrane for subsequent fusion with the overlying plasma membrane during the acrosome reaction. Figure 6 illustrates the distribution of four rat antigens recognized by monoclonal antibodies. Changes in the distribution pattern of these antigens during sperm maturation are well demonstrated. Here, special attention should be directed to the antigen recognized by antibody 2D6. Although it appears as if a single antigen migrated from head to tail during maturation, in reality antibody 2D6 recognizes two separate antigens, one on the outer acrosomal membrane and the other on the tail plasma membrane (1363). As the outer acrosomal membrane and the plasma membrane are not connected, the antigen on the outer acrosomal membrane must be either removed or masked during sperm maturation. Later another antigen appears (or becomes reactive to the antibody) on the plasma membrane of the sperm tail.

The acrosome undergoes gross morphological changes during epididymal maturation of spermatozoa in some species (e.g., the guinea pig, bush baby, pig-tailed monkey, and marsupials) (44a,151,230,734). Molecular configurations of the acrosomal matrix and enzymes may change simultaneously. Sperm nuclei of most eutherian mammals do not undergo gross structural changes during epididymal maturation, but nuclear protamines are extensively cross-linked by disulfide bonds as spermatozoa pass through the epididymis (47,273,386,1139). The resulting rigidity of the nuclei (heads) seems to facilitate sperm passage through the rather "tough" zona pellucida by permitting the tail's thrust to be translated along the axis of the sperm head to the zona quite directly (731). Similarly, disulfide cross-linking of proteins of the outer dense fiber and fibrous sheath during sperm maturation (48) may serve to increase the bending force generated by the axonemmae (734).

CAPACITATION OF SPERMATOZOA

Spermatozoa that have matured in the epididymis are capable of moving actively, yet they do not have the immediate capacity for fertilization. They gain this ability after residing in the female tract for some period of time. The physiological (functional) changes that render the

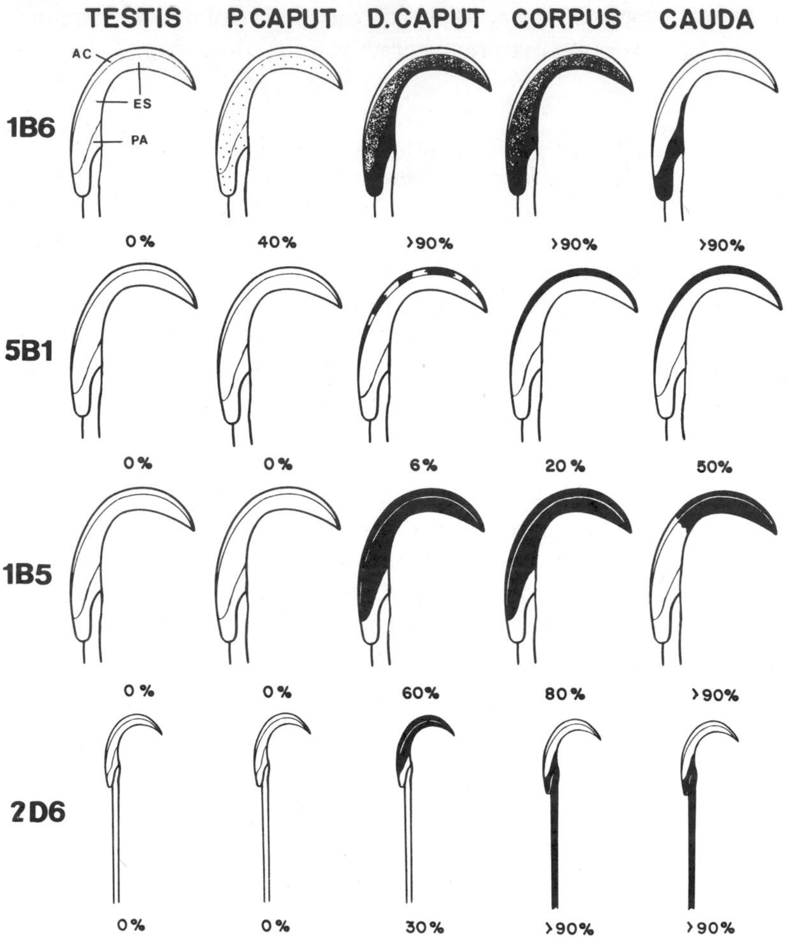

FIG. 6. Diagrams showing changes in the distribution pattern of rat sperm antigens during epididymal maturation. The antigen recognized by monoclonal antibody 1B6 is on the plasma membrane. Those recognized by antibodies 5B1 and 1B5 are on the outer acrosomal membrane. The antigen that binds to the antibody 2D6 is on both the outer acrosomal membrane and the tail plasma membrane. Numbers (percent of sperm showing specific fluorescence) represent averages of four to seven experiments rounded to the nearest factor of 10. (From ref. 1363.)

spermatozoa competent to fertilize are collectively called *capacitation.*

The discovery of capacitation was the result of frustrating attempts by pioneers who tried to fertilize eggs *in vitro* with ejaculated or epididymal spermatozoa. In 1949, Noyes, Finkle, and Rocke found that rabbit spermatozoa collected from either semen or the vas deferens were unable to fertilize eggs in the oviduct, whereas those spermatozoa that had resided in the oviducts of donors for 4 to 8 hr could do so (1298). Perhaps these investigators did not fully realize the implication of their important findings and never published a full paper on this subject. Therefore, the credit for discovering capacitation must go to Chang (811,814) and Austin (17,21), who first documented the experimental evidence of the need for capacitation in the rabbit and rat. It was Thibault and his associates (1584a) who made the first convincing report of successful *in vitro* fertilization (of the rabbit) using capacitated uterine spermatozoa.

Even today, over 40 years since the discovery of capacitation, its molecular basis is not yet fully understood. However, a major event in capacitation is believed to be the removal or alteration of a stabilizer or protective coat from the sperm plasma membrane, which sensitizes the membrane to the specific milieu of fertilization and, more importantly, to the target of spermatozoa—the eggs (375,396,530,723,938,1434).

We are now able to capacitate spermatozoa of a wide variety of mammalian species *in vitro* (see 899), but we must keep in mind that capacitation naturally takes place within the female tract, the physiology of which is under autonomic nerve and hormonal controls.

Sperm Deposition, Storage, and Ascent in the Female Tract

In a majority of eutherian mammals (e.g., cow, sheep, rabbit, and primates), semen is deposited in the anterior vagina during coitus. In others (e.g., pig, horse, dog, and many rodents), the bulk of semen enters the uterus directly or is forced through the cervical canal during coitus (1060). Perhaps this occurs in part because a momentary relaxation of the cervix and vaginal contraction results from the copulatory stimuli. Regardless of the site of semen deposition, the vast majority of spermatozoa are eliminated from the tract sooner or later (888). Only a minute fraction of spermatozoa migrate successfully to the site of fertilization (the ampulla or ampullar-isthmic junction). For instance, in laboratory rodents the live sperm-to-egg ratio in the ampulla during the time of fertilization can be 1:1 or even less (120,552,1477). The female tract at least tends to prevent morphologically abnormal spermatozoa from reaching the site of fertilization (1278,1286,1396), but obviously not all fertilizing spermatozoa are genetically normal.

In species in which most spermatozoa are deposited in the uterus during coitus, the utero–tubal junction is the major barrier for sperm ascent to the ampulla. Numerous mucosal folds and the narrow lumen of the utero–tubal junction permit migration of only a very small fraction of uterine spermatozoa into the oviduct. In the hamster, for example, less than 0.001% of the 10^8 to 10^9 uterine spermatozoa successfully enter each oviduct (1500) even though a thick semen mass is pushed repeatedly against the utero–tubal junction by adoviductal contractions of the uterus (738,1735).

It was once thought that fertilizing spermatozoa quickly reach the site of fertilization and await the arrival of eggs (60). It is now clear that fertilizing spermatozoa are sequestered in the lower part of the oviductal isthmus until ovulation begins. In other words, sperm ascent to the ampulla and egg descent to the ampulla occur synchronously (see 383,1060,1062,1503). In the pig, a sufficient number of spermatozoa to give maximum fertilization are sequestered in the isthmus within 1 to 2 hr of mating (244,1061). The time when spermatozoa are released from the isthmus is influenced by the time of ovulation or the time of mating in relation to ovulation. In the hamster, for example, sperm release begins sooner when animals are mated during or after ovulation compared to mating several hours before ovulation (1500,1700). This makes sense because normal embryonic development is favored when eggs in the oviduct are fertilized soon after ovulation.

In species in which semen is deposited in the vagina at coitus, the spermatozoa must negotiate the highly folded, mucus-filled cervix before entering the uterus. During the periovulatory period the mucus serves to (i) protect spermatozoa from the hostile vaginal environment and phagocytosis by vaginal leucocytes, (ii) prevent entry of seminal plasma into the uterus, (iii) exclude morphologically (possibly functionally) abnormal spermatozoa, and (iv) retain and conserve spermatozoa for later migration to the upper tract (914,1115,1258,1277, 1334,1658). Spermatozoa entering the mucus tend to swim along the longitudinal microstructure of the mucus glycoproteins to reach the surface of the secretory epithelium (1115). Many stay there, but others break away from the epithelium, swim along the longitudinally arranged folds and shallow grooves of the epithelium (1280), and reach the uterus. The release of spermatozoa from the human cervix may continue for days (1015, 1277,1334). Sperm ascent through the uterus seems to be accomplished primarily by the contractile activity of the uterine wall. Sperm motility may only serve the purpose of maintaining the cells in suspension within the uterine fluid (1658). In the sheep and cow, the spermatozoa that pass through the utero–tubal junction are sequestered in the lower segment of the isthmus until the onset of ovulation (1060,1062). Although not yet fully confirmed, the isthmic storage of spermatozoa prior to fertilization could be universal in mammals (899,1060). The relative importance of the cervix and the isthmus as sperm storage sites in animals such as primates is yet to be determined.

The lower segment of the isthmus where the fertilizing spermatozoa are stored is rich in adrenergic receptors (1089) and has a direct supply of blood rich in ovarian hormones (Fig. 7) (1064), suggesting that this particular region of the oviduct could be sensitive to even the slightest changes in ovarian hormone profile. When viewed under the scanning electron microscope, pig and bull spermatozoa in the isthmus and utero–tubal junction are in close contact with the epithelium (935,1065, 1066) (Fig. 8). When hamster oviducts were excised a few hours after mating and the contents of the isthmus were examined through the oviduct's semitransparent wall, spermatozoa were seen attached to the mucosal surface, rocking back and forth with the rostral surface of their heads, occasionally breaking free to swim a short distance before attaching again. Motile spermatozoa in groups were commonly observed in the epithelial crypts (1502) (Fig. 9) as in the case of the mouse (1525). The spermatozoa attached to the epithelium, especially those deep within the furrows of mucosal folds and within the crypts, could not be removed readily by flushing medium through the oviduct. Circumstantial evidence has suggested that these spermatozoa represent a subpopulation which are later released from the isthmus and fertilize the eggs (1502).

Sperm attachment to the isthmic mucosa does not appear to be highly cell-specific because spermatozoa can attach to cells other than the mucosa cells of the isthmus. Interestingly, spermatozoa live longer when they remain attached to cells than when they are free in the medium.

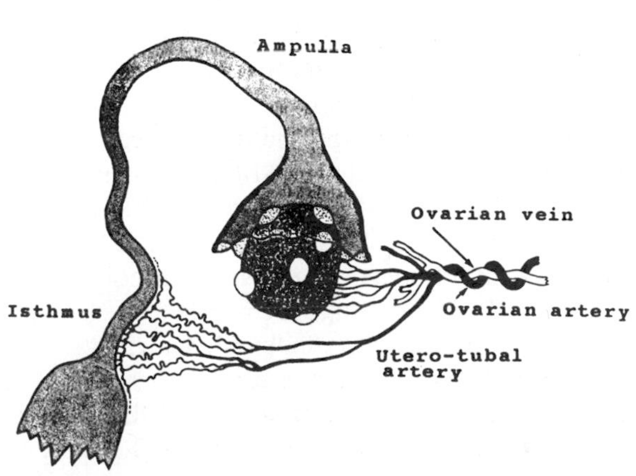

FIG. 7. Representation of the arterial blood supply to the ovary and isthmus of the pig oviduct. (From ref. 1064.)

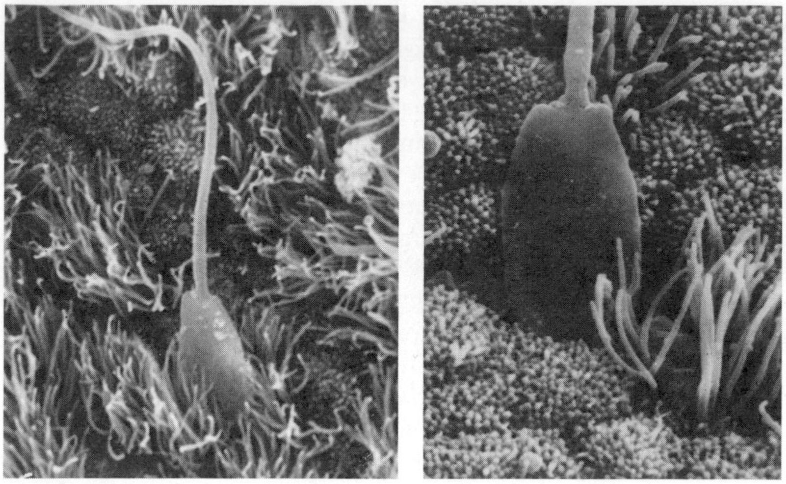

FIG. 8. Scanning electron micrographs of pig spermatozoa in close contact with epithelial cells of the isthmus (*A*) and the utero–tubal junction (*B*). (From ref. 935.)

The cells do not need to be oviductal cells (689,1376), but spermatozoa live (remain fertile) longer on oviductal cells than on nonoviductal cells (1376). The luminal environment of the isthmus may not be as "clean and hospitable" as generally imagined. For example, the lumen of the hamster isthmus is filled with epithelial cell debris as well as dead spermatozoa (1502) that are being pushed back and forth by peristaltic movements of the oviduct. Spermatozoa attached to the sides of mucosal folds or in the crypts are relatively free from such debris, and this could be one of the reasons why epithelium-bound spermatozoa have a better chance of survival than unattached spermatozoa in the lumen, at least in the hamster.

The mechanism by which isthmus-bound spermatozoa are released is not clear but seems to be related to changes in the sperm head plasma membrane associated with capacitation (see below). Hyperactivated motility of spermatozoa may also facilitate sperm release from the isthmus (872,1503). Migration of free spermatozoa from the isthmus to the ampulla seems to be accomplished by both sperm motility and contractile movement of the oviduct (1062,1334). It is unlikely that an adovarian propulsive movement of the oviduct, which becomes distinct during the periovulatory period (713,714), is solely responsible for sperm transport in the oviduct. One possible function of this oviductal movement is orienting randomly moving spermatozoa toward the ampulla. We generally assume that spermatozoa of all eutherian mammals behave similarly within female tracts. It would be interesting to determine whether large spermatozoa in small animals (e.g., mouse with 120 μm long sperm) and small spermatozoa in large animals (e.g., whales with 30–60 μm long sperm; cf. 859,1215) behave in an identical manner in the female tract.

It is tempting to speculate that eggs (or egg-associated substances) attract spermatozoa from a distance as for some invertebrates (1244). Although there have been several claims of sperm chemotaxis in cattle and the human (e.g., 912,981,1073,1389,1466), the evidence is not very convincing (530,1202,1244). Since mammalian spermatozoa move actively within the oviduct and the oviduct itself displays a very active contractile (mixing) movement during the periovulatory period, sperm chemotaxis, if it exists, must be of secondary importance in bringing spermatozoa and egg together. According to Harper (1017), the presence of living eggs in the ampulla of the rabbit oviduct stimulates sperm ascent from the isthmus to the ampulla. However, his conclusion is based on the rate of fertilization, rather than a direct count of spermatozoa in the ampulla. It has been reported that larger numbers of spermatozoa reach the ampullae of superovulated animals compared to control, naturally ovulating animals (1079,1477). The cause of this phenomenon is yet to be investigated.

Capacitation *In Vivo*

Site of Capacitation

The site where fertilizing spermatozoa begin and end capacitation may vary according to species. In species in which semen is deposited in the uterus during coitus, spermatozoa seem to complete all or most parts of capacitation in the lower segment of the isthmus where fertilizing spermatozoa are stored. In the hamster, sperm capacitation within the isthmus progresses faster when females mate after ovulation than when they mate before ovulation (1501). It is unlikely that all the spermatozoa complete capacitation and leave the isthmus simultaneously. Instead, individual spermatozoa seem to be capacitated at different rates (perhaps partly due to physiological differences among individual spermatozoa and the location of spermatozoa within the isthmus) and leave the isthmus, a few at a time, over an extended period. In the pig, this period could be 2 days or more (1063). Perhaps, many spermatozoa die within the isthmus without completing capacitation (1502).

In species in which spermatozoa are deposited in the vagina at coitus, sperm capacitation may begin while

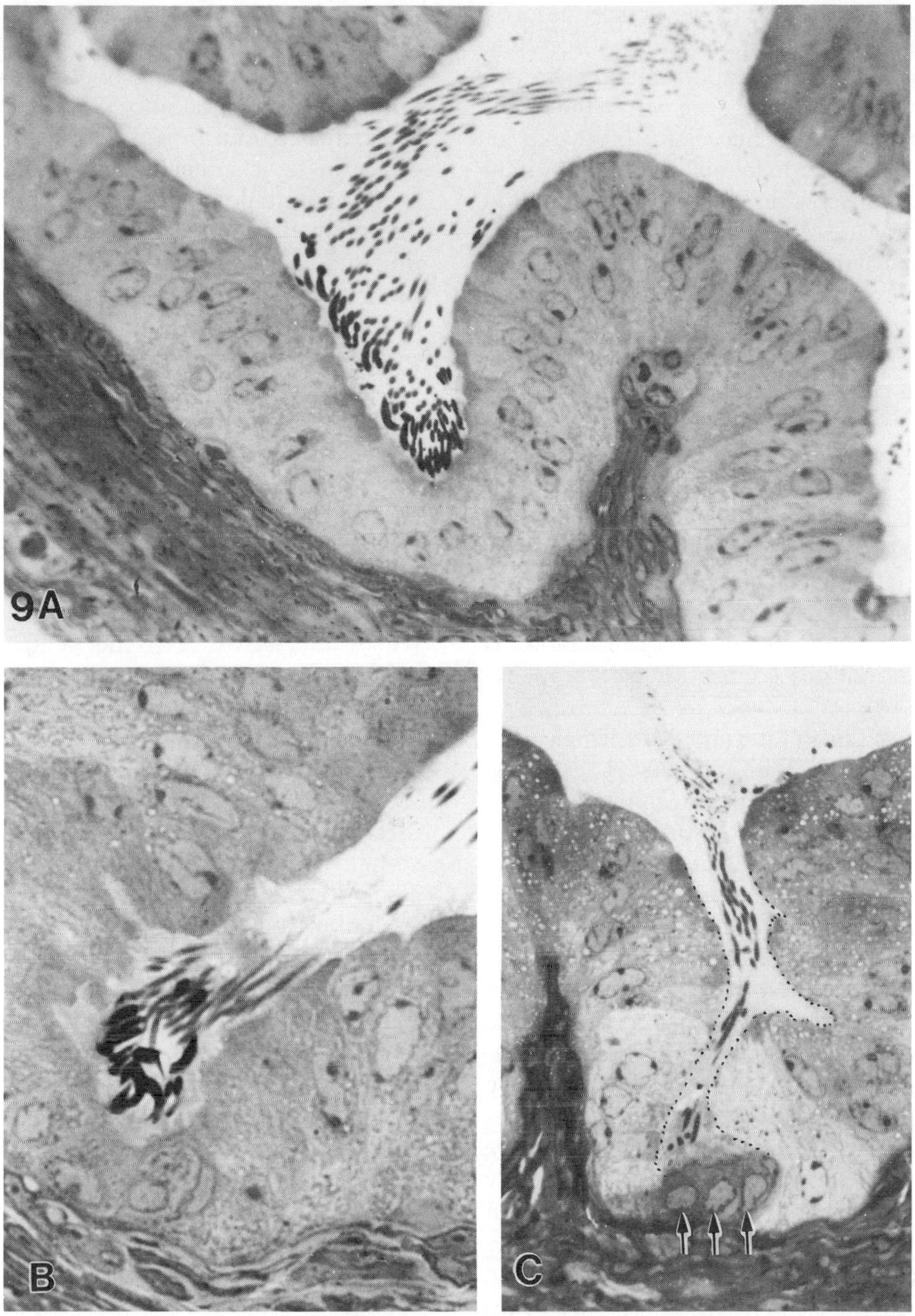

FIG. 9. Cross sections of the isthmus of golden hamster oviduct, approximately 3 hr after mating, showing groups of spermatozoa attached to the mucosal surface of isthmic crypts. *Arrows* in figure C indicate a group of basal cells of the crypt to which spermatozoa commonly attach with their heads (1502).

spermatozoa pass through the cervical mucus. "Rubbing off" sperm–surface-adsorbed materials (including seminal plasma proteins) against the mucus network may facilitate capacitation (990,1115). Although some spermatozoa are certainly in an advanced stage of capacitation after passing through the mucus (1149), it is unknown whether they (and fully capacitated spermatozoa) are able to enter the oviduct to participate in fertilization. In the hamster, fully capacitated spermatozoa are not able to migrate from the uterus to the oviduct efficiently (1479), although the uterus of the hamster functionally corresponds to the vagina of the rabbit as far as sperm deposition in the female tract is concerned.

Specificity and Speciality of the Female Tract in Relation to Capacitation

According to Bedford (722), rabbit spermatozoa are capacitated most efficiently when they sequentially pass through the uterus and oviduct. However, spermatozoa can be fully capacitated in the uterus without ascending to the oviduct (782,813). Capacitation can occur in isolated oviducts slowly (4,725) and even within the rabbit vagina to some extent (722). Successful pregnancy in women following gamete intra fallopian transfer (GIFT) (sperm and egg transfer into the oviduct ampulla) (780,1162,1226) indicates that human spermatozoa do not need to experience the uterus and the isthmic region of the oviduct to become capacitated. Successful pregnancies in women following direct intraperitoneal insemination (DIPI) (945,1164,1225,1425) as well as an almost unbelievable case study published in the *British Journal of Obstetrics and Gynecology* (1622), strongly suggest that sperm capacitation is possible in the peritoneal cavity and/or the ampulla. All these facts suggest that *in vivo* capacitation is not strictly organ-specific. Capacitation in the female tract is not species-specific either because the spermatozoa and eggs of one species can effect fertilization in the female tract of other species (cf. 130,177,229,405,425). It is obvious that capacitation is possible *in vitro* without any contributions from the female tract (see below).

What then is special or unique about the female tract in relation to capacitation? The uniqueness lies in the ability of the tract to deliver enough capacitated spermatozoa to all the ovulated eggs before the eggs age excessively. When a female animal becomes ready to ovulate, she comes in estrus and accepts a male(s). If she mates immediately or soon after the onset of estrus, spermatozoa that have been "selected at" the cervix and/or the utero-tubal junction are stored in the lower segment of the oviductal isthmus, not too far from and not too close to the ampulla (or utero-tubal junction) where fertilization is to take place. The spermatozoa adhering to the epithelium of the isthmus survive and undergo capacitation slowly. Some complete capacitation about the time of ovulation, leave the isthmus, and fertilize the recently ovulated eggs. Other spermatozoa complete capacitation after ovulation and leave the isthmus a few at a time, so that all eggs are fertilized even if the last egg enters the oviduct much later than the first one. If the female cannot mate until after ovulation, capacitation within the isthmus is hastened and the spermatozoa leave the isthmus sooner, before the eggs in the oviduct age excessively. The ability of the female tract to control the speed of capacitation and deliver freshly capacitated spermatozoa to all of the ovulated eggs regardless of the time of mating seems to be beneficial to the reproduction of all mammals, especially those ovulating many eggs over an extended period of time and those without a distinct behavioral estrus.

Capacitation *In Vitro*

Early investigators used various biological fluids (e.g., oviduct fluid, follicular fluid, and blood serum) to capacitate spermatozoa *in vitro*. The composition of these fluids was so complex that it was difficult to determine which components were involved in inducing or supporting capacitation. Since Toyoda et al. (486) reported the first successful *in vitro* fertilization (IVF) of mouse eggs using a "chemically defined medium," analysis of sperm capacitation *in vitro* has become considerably easier. The media commonly used today for *in vitro* fertilization (and *in vitro* sperm capacitation) are modified Tyrode's and Krebs–Ringer's solutions supplemented with the appropriate energy sources (e.g., glucose, lactate, and pyruvate) and albumin. Commercially available tissue culture media (e.g., Ham F10) supplemented with blood serum are also commonly used, particularly for human IVF. So far, no single medium has been found to support *in vitro* sperm capacitation and fertilization in all species. The spermatozoa and eggs of each species seem to require their own specific environment in order to perform their functions most efficiently. This is understandable because gametes and the microenvironment of the female tract have evolved independently in each species.

The primary goal of many investigators who have engaged in the study of *in vitro* fertilization (IVF) was to fertilize eggs, not to analyze the mechanism of sperm capacitation. Although the information obtained by these investigators can be very valuable, caution must be used in interpreting their conclusions, at least with respect to sperm capacitation. For instance, many investigators concluded that certain reagents blocked sperm capacitation completely because fertilization *in vitro* did not occur in the presence of these reagents. Their conclusions may or may not be correct, because capacitation is not the only sperm requirement for successful fertilization. To fertilize the eggs, the spermatozoa must be highly motile as well as capable of undergoing the acrosome reaction, penetrating through the egg investments, and fusing with the egg. Successful fertilization *in vitro* certainly implies that the spermatozoa underwent capacitation. Unsuccessful IVF, on the other hand, does not necessarily mean that the spermatozoa had failed to become capacitated.

Some investigators have used the acrosome reaction as an indicator of the completion of capacitation. Because the spermatozoa do not undergo the acrosome reaction, either spontaneously or mediated by ligands (e.g., zona pellucida), unless they become capacitated, the acrosome reaction certainly can be used as an indicator for the completion of capacitation. We must be careful, however, because unusual conditions or special reagents may induce the acrosome reaction, bypassing capacitation. Conversely, neither does the absence of the acrosome reaction mean that the spermatozoa failed to undergo capacitation. These spermatozoa may well be capacitated but may merely be prevented from undergoing the acrosome reaction.

One might hope for 100% of spermatozoa *in vitro* to survive and complete capacitation simultaneously. In reality, many spermatozoa die before undergoing or completing capacitation. Senescence/death of spermatozoa and capacitation take place side by side even under the most favorable *in vitro* conditions. Unless we monitor the viability of spermatozoa carefully during *in vitro* culture, we may be investigating the results of sperm senescence/death rather than capacitation. Here, I will summarize what we have learned about the conditions or factors that affect or control sperm capacitation *in vitro.* This is not intended to be a complete literature survey. Readers are referred to the following reviews for more detailed information about sperm capacitation (22,41, 42,45,50,104,170,227,283,329,369,410,415,530,734, 899,938,954,955,956,1434,1488,1522,1523).

Some Factors Controlling or Affecting Capacitation as Revealed by *In Vitro* Studies

Temperature

Sperm capacitation is temperature dependent (157, 309). An incubation temperature of 37°C to 38°C, used in most laboratories, is apparently adequate to support *in vitro* capacitation in most cases. However, it is interesting to note that IVF of pig and sheep eggs, once thought to be very difficult, can now be achieved easily by preincubating spermatozoa at 39°C and/or mixing the eggs and freshly ejaculated (washed) spermatozoa at this temperature (cf. 102,113). At least in the sheep and pig, capacitation seems to proceed far more efficiently at the natural body temperature of these animals (38.7°C–39.7°C, mean 39°C) than at 37°C to 38°C (102,1600). Even such a small temperature difference may make a big difference in the physical state of membrane lipids (1041), which is of critical importance for capacitation (see below).

Interspecies and Intraspecies Variations

Spermatozoa of some species are much more difficult to be capacitated *in vitro* than those of others. The difference may not be absolute, but rather a feature of our technique. For example, *in vitro* capacitation of human spermatozoa was thought to be very difficult 20 years ago. It is now one of the easiest among mammals (see 1373). Once we learn the "tricks," anything that is considered difficult becomes easy. Spermatozoa of some species, including the human, do not require any special ingredients in the medium for capacitation. Media based on simple balanced salt solutions (e.g., Tyrode's and Krebs–Ringer's solutions) supplemented with the proper energy sources and proteins (e.g., serum or serum albumin) are sufficient for capacitation. Spermatozoa of some other species require additional (special) substances in the medium for successful capacitation (see below).

The minimum and median times needed for capacitation *in vitro* differ considerably from species to species. The minimum time for capacitation could be less than 1 hr in some species (e.g., mice, cats, and perhaps humans), whereas in some other species it can take several hours (e.g., rabbits). Such variations are likely due to the innate differences in the physical and chemical characteristics of the sperm plasma membrane. It is important to note that the minimum and median time required for capacitation, either *in vivo* or *in vitro,* is not rigidly fixed. Within limits, the time varies depending on the physiological state of the animal and the physical and chemical composition of the medium. Perhaps, conditions that keep the sperm membranes stable prolong capacitation time, whereas those conditions that destabilize membranes shorten the capacitation time (see below).

It is not expected that all the spermatozoa from the same ejaculate capacitate synchronously. Some might capacitate faster than others, even under the same conditions. Furthermore, spermatozoa from some males might capacitate considerably faster (or more easily) than those from some other males of the same species. A minimum capacitation time for a given species determined from experiments that used a small number of individual males should be interpreted with caution. Variations among individual males within species is not negligible (cf. 436 and 534 for the rat and the human, respectively). Genetic influences on sperm capacitation and capacitation time must be considered (235, 1142,1319,1685).

Epididymal Spermatozoa vs. Ejaculated Spermatozoa

Both cauda epididymal and ejaculated spermatozoa are considered equally mature and fertile, but these two types of spermatozoa do not necessarily behave in the same way *in vitro.* According to Shalgi et al. (436), who compared the fertilizing ability *in vitro* of the cauda epididymal and ejaculated spermatozoa from the same male rat, epididymal spermatozoa fertilize more eggs (average 59%) than ejaculated spermatozoa (average 21%) under identical experimental conditions. There are many reports that both epididymal and ejaculated spermatozoa fertilize eggs *in vitro* at the same rate (e.g., see 378) but, in general, epididymal spermatozoa fertilize eggs *in vitro* more easily than ejaculated spermatozoa. Nagai et al. (349) reported that 71% to 75% of pig eggs are fertilized *in vitro* by cauda epididymal spermatozoa, whereas none are fertilized by ejaculated spermatozoa. Interestingly, these epididymal spermatozoa become infertile when they are exposed to the seminal plasma.

The cat is very interesting in terms of sperm capacitation. According to Niwa et al. (353), cat spermatozoa, freshly collected from the cauda epididymis, are capable of penetrating eggs as early as 20 min after insemination. By 30 min after insemination, 100% of the eggs are penetrated. This is the fastest egg penetration by fresh epididymal spermatozoa ever recorded. One may wonder if cat spermatozoa even require capacitation. Incidentally, cats have a very poorly developed cauda epididymis (J. M. Bedford, personal communication). Wildt (1662) found that ejaculated cat spermatozoa do not penetrate eggs as fast as epididymal spermatozoa do. Although some ejaculated spermatozoa penetrate eggs within 30 min after insemination, the maximum level of fertilization (>90%) is not achieved until approximately 3 hr after insemination (985). Thus, cat spermatozoa exposed to the seminal plasma during ejaculation seem to require some time for capacitation.

Why are ejaculated spermatozoa of many species more resistant to *in vitro* capacitation than are epididymal spermatozoa? Perhaps the plasma membrane of ejaculated spermatozoa is more stable than that of epididymal spermatozoa. Although the plasma membrane of the epididymal spermatozoa is already stabilized, to some extent, by adsorption and/or integration of epididymal glycoproteins, it seems to be further "stabilized" upon its contact with the seminal plasma. There is ample evidence that some of the seminal plasma components (e.g., glycoproteins or polypeptides, including the so-called decapacitation factor, and fibronectinlike proteins) bind very firmly to the surface of ejaculated spermatozoa (1,243,269,330,359,420,433,502,539). The binding is so firm that these components may not be readily removed from the sperm surface by repeated washings with ordinary physiological solutions (420, 509). As already stated, the removal or alteration of sperm surface-coating materials is most likely an essential but species variable part of capacitation. Apparently, the genital tract of the estrous female is capable of capacitating both epididymal and ejaculated spermatozoa equally (378), suggesting that it has some very efficient mechanisms to remove or alter sperm surface-coating materials originating from the epididymis (the primary surface coat) and the seminal plasma (the secondary surface coat).

When the epididymides of the rabbit, rat, and hamster are surgically moved into the peritoneal cavity (allowing the testis to remain in the scrotum), sperm transit through the epididymis is accelerated and sperm storage in the epididymis is depressed (730). Hamster spermatozoa collected from such epididymides are capacitated, both *in vivo* and *in vitro,* considerably faster than those from control animals (737). This may be due, in part, to a less complete stabilization of the sperm surface by the primary surface coat.

Composition of the Medium

Table 1 shows the composition of media which are known to support *in vitro* capacitation of mouse and human spermatozoa. The ionic composition of sheep oviductal fluid is also shown in this table for comparison.

TABLE 1. *Concentrations (mM) of the components in media for mouse and human* in vitro *fertilization and in sheep oviductal fluid*

	IVF medium		Oviductal fluid[c] in:	
Components	Mouse[a]	Human[b]	Ampulla	Isthmus
Cation				
Na	141.50	148.33	135.00	141.00
K	6.77	5.06	8.12	6.90
Ca	1.71	2.04	3.80	2.98
Mg	1.19	0.20	0.59	0.54
Anion				
Cl	98.63	110.37	122.00	120.00
HCO_3	25.07	25.00	23.70	27.30
PO_4	1.19	0.37	1.11[d]	
SO_4	1.19	0.20	N.D.[e]	N.D.
Energy substrate				
Lactate	25.00	21.40	5.60	3.40
Pyruvate	1.00	0.33	N.D.	N.D.
Glucose	5.56	2.78	N.D.[f]	N.D.

[a] Data from Inouet and Wolf, ref. 251. This medium is supplemented with bovine serum albumin (3.3 mg/mL) before use.

[b] Data from Quinn et al., ref. 1387. This medium is supplemented with 7.5% to 10% human serum.

[c] Of estrous ewe; data from Table 2 of Restall and Wales, ref. 409.

[d] Site of fluid collection, not identified; data from Table 1 of Restall and Wales, ref. 408.

[e] N.D., no data.

[f] The presence of pyruvate and glucose in oviductal fluids of other species has been reported (see refs. 170 and 212).

One might think that all of the components in sperm-capacitating media must contribute, directly or indirectly, to capacitation. If a particular component in the medium is absolutely necessary for capacitation, deleting this component should render the medium completely incapable of capacitating spermatozoa. It is somewhat surprising to learn that there is no such component. Media free of or deficient in the potassium ion (K^+) are known to capacitate spermatozoa (62,169,338). Although not as efficiently as in complete media, capacitation can proceed in media deficient in Ca^{2+} (168, 547,953,954) HCO_3^- (288), exogenous energy substrates (172,430), albumin (158,171,682,796), or even Na^+ and Cl^- in the case of guinea pig spermatozoa (1735). Thus, the presence or absence of a particular component in the medium may not be critical for capacitation. As long as other medium components and endogenous energy can support sperm viability, capacitation seems to proceed.

The spermatozoa of many mammals can survive and capacitate in artificial media similar to the modified Tyrode's and Krebs–Ringer's solutions shown in Table 1. For the spermatozoa of some other species, additional ingredient(s) is (are) needed. Golden hamster spermatozoa, for example, need a sperm motility factor (SMF) (35,524–526). Without it, spermatozoa simply die in any medium. This factor was identified to be taurine or hypotaurine (110,306,342). No one knows how SMF maintains the viability of hamster spermatozoa. It may prolong the sperm's life by slowing down peroxidation of membrane lipids (12) or by protecting the spermatozoa from free oxygen radicals generated by sperm metabolism (687). Alternatively, it may serve as a membrane-stabilizing osmoregulator (494). Why is it that golden hamster spermatozoa cannot survive in artificial media without SMF, whereas spermatozoa of most other species can do without it? Since the spermatozoa of hamsters, guinea pigs, and humans all contain the factors capable of supporting hamster sperm survival (34), the species difference could be due to the stability of SMF within cells. Hamster spermatozoa probably are unable to maintain an adequate intracellular concentration of SMF unless the surrounding medium contains a high concentration of SMF. Spermatozoa of other species, on the other hand, may be able to maintain an adequate intracellular SMF concentration without extracellular SMF.

In vitro capacitation of bovine spermatozoa is facilitated by the presence of heparin (1343), which may assist the removal of a seminal plasma component from the sperm surface (1241). *In vitro* fertilization of rhesus and squirrel monkey eggs is facilitated by the presence of dibutyryl cAMP and caffeine (716,810,1680), which are known to increase the intensity of sperm tail movement (767). *In vivo* sperm capacitation of these species may be assisted by substances with the same or similar biological activities.

Events that Occur in Spermatozoa during Capacitation

Changes in Intracellular Ions

Like other cells, live spermatozoa must maintain ionic gradients across the plasma membrane; the concentration of K^+ inside the cell is higher than outside, whereas the reverse is true for Na^+ (312). This ionic gradient is believed to be maintained by an ATPase-mediated Na^+/K^+ exchange pump (401,402,488). According to Babcock (27), intracellular concentrations of K^+ and Na^+ in bovine (cauda epididymal) spermatozoa are approximately 120 mM and 14 mM, respectively.

Are the intracellular concentrations of K^+ and Na^+ maintained constant during the entire course of capacitation? Hyne et al. (247) reported that guinea pig spermatozoa incubated in a capacitating medium (consisting of 106 mM NaCl, 1 mM $MgCl_2$, 15 mM $NaHCO_3$, 20 mM Na-lactate, and 0.25 mM Na-pyruvate) reduce their intracellular K^+ concentration significantly (from 3–5 μg to 0.6 $\mu g/10^8$ sperm) by the end of 2 hr incubation when the spermatozoa are ready for the acrosome reaction. Intracellular Na^+ concentration, on the other hand, increases dramatically (from 0.2–0.4 μg to 11–12 $\mu g/10^8$ sperm) during the same period. Although there is no doubt that intracellular concentrations of K^+ and Na^+ are altered in the medium Hyne et al. used, it should be noted that the medium used was lacking or at least deficient in K^+. The drastic ion changes reported by Hyne et al. could be due, in part, to a gradual inactivation of sperm Na^+,K^+-ATPase in the K^+-deficient environment. Mrsny et al. (341) found that Na^+,K^+-ATPase activity of hamster spermatozoa increases significantly during a 2-hr incubation in a normal capacitating medium. Whether intracellular concentrations of Na^+ and K^+ remain unchanged or are altered during capacitation was not reported by these investigators.

It is well established that a massive influx of Ca^{2+} takes place during the acrosome reaction (530,1588,1696), but little is known about the kinetics of intracellular Ca^{2+} during capacitation. Generally, it is agreed that the concentration of intracellular Ca^{2+} in spermatozoa is rather low, in both head and tail regions, because of the presence of an ATPase-mediated Ca^{2+} pump, a Na^+/Ca^{2+} antiporter, and a Ca^{2+}/H^+ exchange system in the plasma membrane (75–80,497,1408,1415) as well as Ca^{2+} sequestering in mitochondria (1074). According to Singh et al. (448), guinea-pig spermatozoa pick up radioactive Ca^{2+} during the first hour of incubation in a capacitating medium. Singh et al. suggested that this is caused by a loose association of Ca^{2+} to the sperm surface, rather than an acute movement of Ca^{2+} into the spermatozoa. Using quin-2, a calcium-selective fluorescent indicator, Mahanes et al. (308) found that the concentration of intracellular free Ca^{2+} in rabbit spermatozoa did not change as the result of *in vitro* capacitation. Since the technique these investigators used allowed them to measure Ca^{2+} in sperm mass, rather than in individual spermatozoa, they suggested that Ca^{2+} concentration might change in discrete, localized regions of the spermatozoon.

Whether intracellular free Ca^{2+} increases (700, 954,960,1316,1530) or does not increase (308,942, 1430) during capacitation is controversial. Perhaps, spermatozoa keep the concentration of intracellular free Ca^{2+} much lower than that in the medium all the time, even after a massive influx of Ca^{2+} has taken place in the acrosomal region during the acrosome reaction. The acrosome reaction is exocytotic and can be considered a well-controlled local cell lysis caused by a massive Ca^{2+} influx. In spermatozoa, some (most?) of the intracellular Ca^{2+} seems to be stored or sequestered in both mitochondria (1074) and calcium-binding proteins (800,930, 946,1269,1296,1649). Whether the sequestering of Ca^{2+} by spermatozoa is to maintain low intracellular Ca^{2+} or a preparation for later events (e.g., the acrosome reaction) remains to be determined.

Changes in Metabolism

There are many reports that spermatozoa exhibit increased metabolism (e.g., glycolytic activity and oxygen consumption) after incubation in the female tract or in media capable of supporting capacitation (see 72, 874,956,959). Boell (72) reported that mouse spermatozoa incubated in a capacitating medium (modified Krebs–Ringer's solution containing albumin and energy substrates) exhibit a constantly high level of respiration from the beginning to the end of a 2.5-hr incubation period. Since the spermatozoa consume oxygen at the same rate in noncapacitating media (e.g., albumin-free Krebs–Ringer's solution or phosphate-buffered sucrose, both containing energy substrates), Boell concluded that "the increased respiration of sperm in a capacitating medium is due to the presence of oxidizable substrates and, as such, is an accompaniment of the process of capacitation rather than a factor in bringing it about."

Changes in Adenylate Cyclase–cAMP Systems

In most species, spermatozoa begin to move actively upon contact with seminal plasma at ejaculation (cf. 738). Although the spermatozoa destined to fertilize may temporarily experience a reduction or loss of motility while they are in certain segments of the female genital tract (380,1525), they are vigorously motile at least at the end of capacitation. In most *in vitro* capacitation systems, spermatozoa keep moving fairly actively throughout the capacitation period.

Undoubtedly, activation of cAMP-dependent protein kinase and phosphorylation of sperm proteins play vital roles in the initiation and maintenance of sperm motility (for reviews, see refs. 216,312,475,734). Are these biochemical events just for sustaining sperm motility or are they actively involved in the advancement of capacitation? There is evidence that sperm adenylate cyclase activity increases during capacitation (55,170,457,458). Increased adenylate cyclase activity probably increases cAMP availability and turnover rate (457), which, in turn, would stimulate cAMP-dependent protein kinase. Stimulated protein kinase may alter the structure of sperm proteins (membrane and/or motor apparatus) through phosphorylation (237,246). A number of investigators have reported significant increases in the cAMP level in spermatozoa during capacitation (954,1630), but others could not confirm this (e.g., 1138,1657).

Several questions remain to be answered. For example, are the cAMP levels found in freshly ejaculated spermatozoa enough to keep spermatozoa alive and moving? Do spermatozoa need to "build up" a cAMP reserve for later events (the acrosome reaction and hyperactivation of spermatozoa)?

Changes in the Nucleus

The nuclei of mature spermatozoa of most eutherian mammals are very stable structures owing to extensive cross-links of nuclear proteins by disulfide (—S—S—) bonds (94). Their stability is maintained throughout capacitation (273,324). The nuclear proteins of human spermatozoa are also cross-linked by —S—S— bonds (49), but less extensively than those of many other species (65). In the seminal plasma, Zn^{2+} (of prostate origin) binds to the free —SH radicals of the nuclear proteins of spermatozoa upon ejaculation (276), thus causing a temporary stabilization of nuclear proteins (275,411). During capacitation, nuclei lose Zn^{2+} and increase in stability, probably by oxidation of released —SH radicals in disulfide bonds (292).

Sperm nuclei of some infertile men partially decondense and their Feulgen DNA concentration increases significantly during incubation in capacitation medium (1427), but this does not occur in the sperm nuclei of fertile men (1067). The nuclei of mouse spermatozoa remain highly stabilized during sperm passage through the female tract; in fact, the nuclei of spermatozoa collected from the uterus and oviduct are more stabilized by —S—S— bonds than those from the cauda epididymis and vas deferens (1349).

Changes in the Acrosome

The form of the acrosome does not change noticeably during capacitation in most species (38,115,465, 481,547). According to Wincek et al. (513), enzymatically inactive proacrosin in the boar sperm acrosome is converted to enzymatically active acrosin by the glycosaminoglycans in uterine fluid. There is no doubt that glycosaminoglycans stimulate the conversion of proacrosin to acrosin in test tubes (385), but how do such large molecules like glycosaminoglycans penetrate into the acrosome through both the plasma and acrosomal membranes of spermatozoa? Whether acrosomal enzymes remain as inactive forms (185) or are converted to active forms during capacitation is still open to debate.

Changes in the Plasma Membrane

Because the plasma membrane is directly exposed to the capacitating environment, it is not surprising that very significant changes take place in this membrane during capacitation. Since Weinman and Williams (510) and Piko (395) postulated that the removal or alteration of coating material from the sperm surface constitutes an important part of capacitation, evidence supporting this view has accumulated (cf. Fig. 10) (104,266,267,359, 530,1488,1696). The coating materials that are known (or believed) to be removed or altered during capacitation include the so-called decapacitation factors (957, 1241,1322–1324), 5 to 10 kDa caltrin (838,938,1153), a 6.4-kDa protein with proteinase-inhibiting activity (769), 15-, 16-, and 23-kDa glycoproteins (1344,1644), and spermine (1428), all of seminal plasma origin, and the acrosome-stabilizing 125- to 259-kDa protein of epididymal origin (1324,1650). Instead of compiling a complete list of publications, only relatively few articles confirming and/or adding new information about the removal or alteration of sperm surface materials during capacitation will be cited here.

According to Okabe et al. (356), an antigen which specifically binds to the monoclonal antibody TSC4 is present on the plasma membrane over the entire acrosome of cauda epididymal spermatozoa of the mouse. This antigen, of corpus epididymis origin, cannot be easily removed from the sperm surface by repeated washings. It disappears by the time spermatozoa enter the perivitelline space of the egg. This antigen must be either removed or altered (masked?) during capacitation. Okabe et al. (357) have reported another interesting mouse sperm antigen. This antigen which binds specifically to the monoclonal antibody OBF13 is not detectable on cauda epididymal spermatozoa. It becomes detectable on the head plasma membrane when the spermatozoa are capacitated *in vitro*. This antigen must be hidden (masked) in fresh epididymal spermatozoa and then exposed during capacitation (Fig. 11).

Other antigens that appear to change their distribution during capacitation include fibronectinlike molecules on the human sperm surface (967), T and S antigens on the guinea pig sperm head (1208), and a 37-kDa protein on the rat sperm head (1412). Shalgi et al. (1474) de-

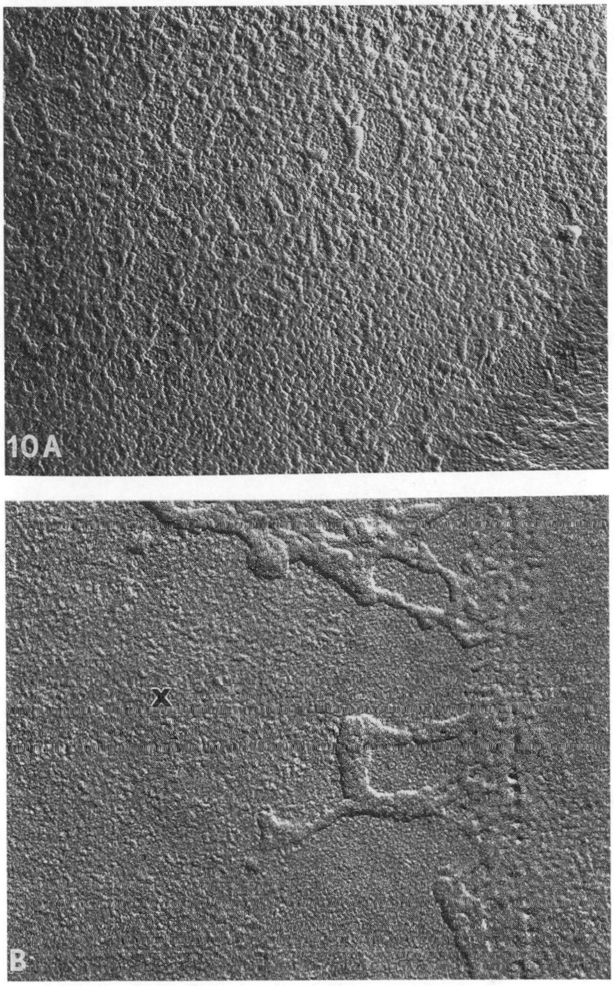

FIG. 10. Surface replicas of the acrosomal region of guinea pig spermatozoa. During incubation in a sperm-capacitating medium, the surface coat is removed or altered, exposing the plasma membrane surface (x). Thirty minutes (**A**) and 24–26 hours (**B**) after the start of sperm incubation in Ca^{2+}-deficient TS medium (Provided by Dr. Daniel S. Friend.)

tected a 40-kDa antigen, 2B1, by immunofluorescence in the tail region of uncapacitated rat spermatozoa. When the spermatozoa were capacitated, the antigen was detected in the acrosomal cap region, no longer in the tail region. We might preliminarily conclude that the antigen in question migrates from the tail to the acrosomal region during capacitation, but serious consideration is needed here. First of all, the immunofluorescence technique used at the light microscopic level cannot detect whether the sperm membranes are intact, broken, or missing at the time of staining. As pointed out by Phillips et al. (1363), one monoclonal antibody may bind to two or more different antigens at different sites on the spermatozoon, one on the outer acrosomal membrane, for example, and the other on the plasma membrane of the sperm tail. These two membranes are not connected during capacitation, and therefore migration of an antigen from one membrane to another cannot

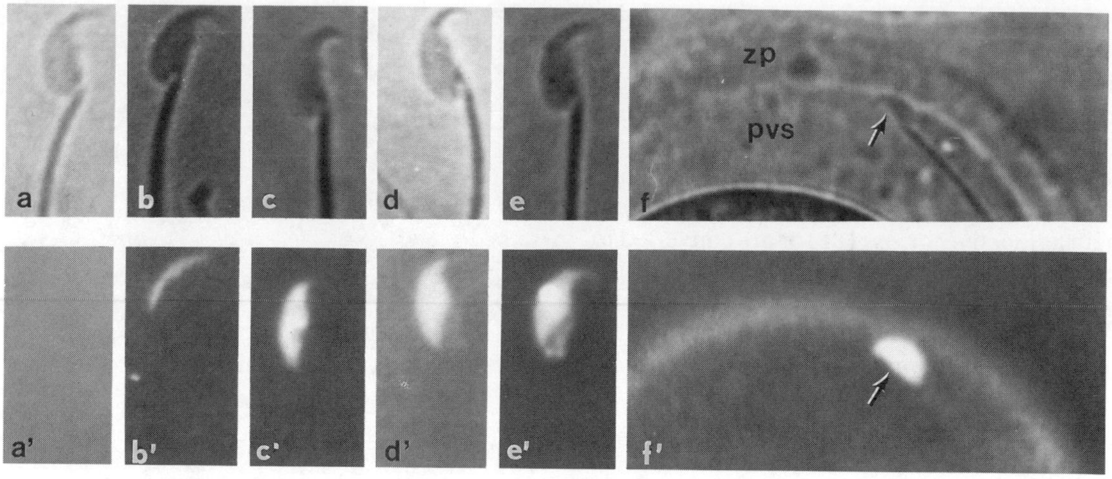

FIG. 11. Photomicrographs of mouse sperm heads showing that an antigen, recognizable by a monoclonal antibody (OBF13), is exposed or becomes reactive during *in vitro* capacitation. *a–f,* phase-contrast micrographs; *a′–f′*, indirect immunofluorescence micrographs. (*pvs*) Perivitelline space; (*zp*) zona pellucida. (From ref. 357.)

occur (1363). Since light microscopy cannot differentiate the plasma membrane over the acrosome from the underlying acrosomal membrane and matrix, very careful interpretation is needed when antigen distibution is altered during capacitation, particularly when it involves the acrosomal region. Antigen SMA (496,1623), which disappears from the tail plasma membrane during capacitation (Fig. 12) (495) may or may not be identical to the tail antigen 2B1 (1103,1474) which "migrates" to the acrosomal region during capacitation.

Voglmayr and Sawyer (503) found that ejaculated ram spermatozoa incubated in uterine fluid release three different glycosylated proteins (65, 41, and 24 kDa) from their surfaces into the fluid. At the same time, the spermatozoa adsorb a 16-kDa protein from the fluid. In the oviductal fluid, they release 97-kDa and 41-kDa proteins from their surfaces. Interestingly, spermatozoa exposed first to uterine fluid and then to oviductal fluid adsorb several components (13–190 kDa) from the latter. Although the uterus is not the likely site of pig sperm capacitation and Voglmayr and Sawyer did not evaluate how the oviductal and uterine fluids were effective in capacitating spermatozoa *in vitro,* their finding nevertheless suggests the possibility that the release of sperm surface components and the simultaneous absorption of exogenous fluid components are integral parts of capacitation *in vivo.*

In the *fluid mosaic model* of biological membranes (447), proteins (or glycoproteins) are noncovalently associated with the lipid bilayers that form the matrix of the membrane. Intrinsic proteins, which are firmly embedded in the bilayer, can be removed only by harsh

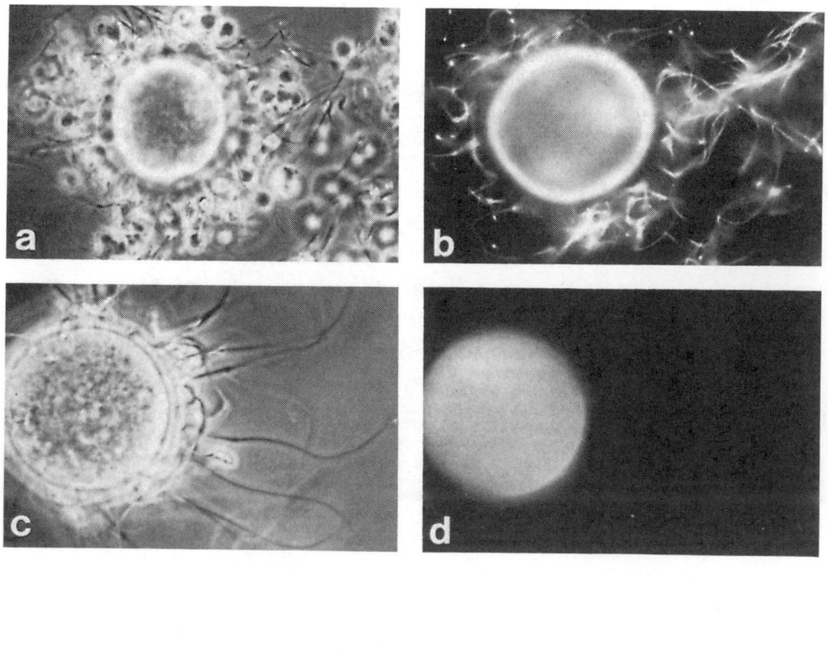

FIG. 12. Photomicrographs of mouse spermatozoa and eggs, showing that a sperm tail antigen is lost or becomes unreactive with a monoclonal antibody (SMA4) during capacitation. Thirty minutes (*a* and *b*) and 4 hr (*c* and *d*) after epididymal spermatozoa were suspended in a sperm-capacitating medium. *a* and *c,* Phase-contrast micrographs; *b* and *d,* immunofluorescence micrographs. (From ref. 495.)

treatments (e.g., detergent), whereas peripheral proteins, which are associated with the membrane primarily through electrostatic interactions, can be liberated by merely adding chelating agents or by increasing the pH or ionic strength (186). Thus, most of the proteins or glycoproteins released from sperm surfaces during capacitation are likely to be peripheral proteins/glycoproteins. Changes in the lectin-binding ability of the sperm plasma membrane during capacitation (265,672,849, 1493,1557) indicate the carbohydrate moiety of the peripheral and integral glycoproteins is altered during capacitation. Removal of terminal sialic acid from the sperm surface glycoproteins during capacitation has been suggested (280,1507).

Freeze-fracture examination of the plasma membranes of hamster and guinea pig spermatozoa incubated in capacitation media revealed that intramembraneous particles (IMPs), which are intrinsic proteins within lipid bilayers, change their distributions in both the head and tail regions (963,1539,1540). Figure 13A shows IMPs that are almost evenly distributed in the plasma membrane over the acrosome of an uncapacitated guinea-pig spermatozoon. The membrane of the same area of a capacitated spermatozoon has many small patches that are free of IMPs (Fig. 13B). IMP-free zones appear in the plasma membrane during capacitation in human spermatozoa as well (476). Whether such capacitation-associated membrane changes are mediated by the sperm cytoskeleton (807) and the phosphorylation/dephosphorylation of membrane proteins by protein kinase (966) is an open question.

Friend (174) and Bearer and Friend (36) found that IMP-free areas, unlike the surrounding IMP-rich areas, have no or very few sterols (e.g., cholesterol) and anionic lipids (e.g., cardiolipin). The plasma membrane covering the middle piece of uncapacitated guinea-pig spermatozoa has concentrically arranged IMPs in close apposition to the underlying mitochondrial helix. This unique arrangement of IMPs disappears when spermatozoa are capacitated (268). All of these changes must be the result of physical and/or chemical alteration of lipid bilayers during capacitation.

Wolf and Gadulo (1669), who assessed the fluidity of the mouse sperm plasma membrane using the fluorescence photobleaching technique, found that membrane fluidity changes most prominently in the principal piece of the tail during capacitation. The relative amounts of various membrane phospholipids may not change during capacitation, but the distribution of each lipid in the outer and inner leaflets may be altered by capacitation (913). There have been several articles reporting or suggesting that the phospholipid composition of the sperm membrane changes during capacitation. According to Snider and Clegg (450), phosphatidyl inositol, which is absent from freshly ejaculated porcine spermatozoa, is synthesized by spermatozoa during incubation (capacitation?) in the female genital tract. Methylation of phospholipids (e.g., conversion of phosphatidyl ethanolamine to phosphatidyl choline) seems to occur during capacitation of hamster spermatozoa (298). Bearer and Friend (36) have postulated that during capacitation of guinea-pig spermatozoa, intracellular phosphatidic acid is converted to cardiolipin, which is then inserted into the outer leaflet of the lipid bilayer of the plasma membrane.

Much attention has been directed toward cholesterol in the sperm membranes (for reviews, see 182,283, 1342). This is reasonable because cholesterol is known to

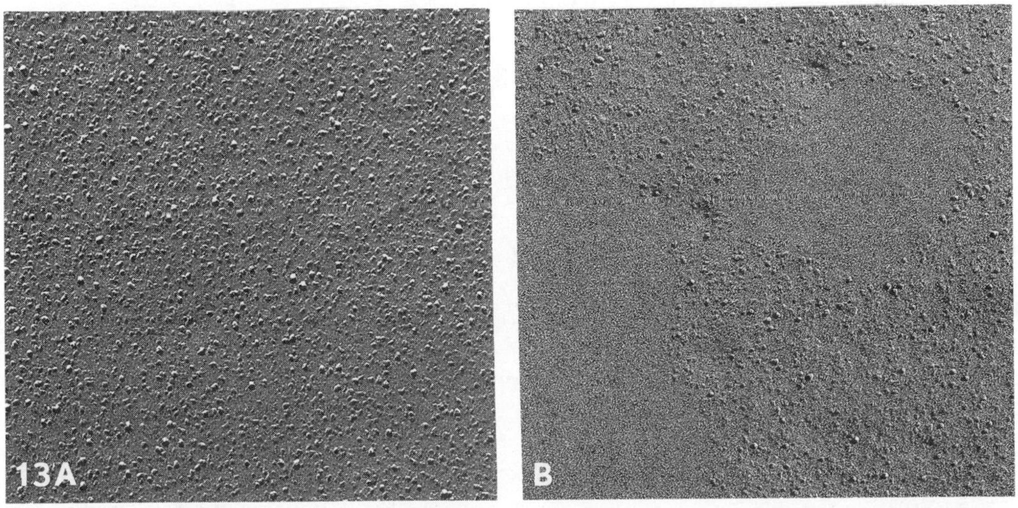

FIG. 13. Intramembranous particles in the plasma membrane of the acrosomal cap region of guinea pig spermatozoa before (**A**) and after (**B**) capacitation *in vitro*. Note the presence of particle-free patches in the plasma membrane of the capacitated spermatozoon. Capacitated spermatozoa were prepared by incubating cauda epididymal spermatozoa for 17 hr in a Ca^{2+}-deficient mT medium. (Provided by Dr. Fumie Suzuki.)

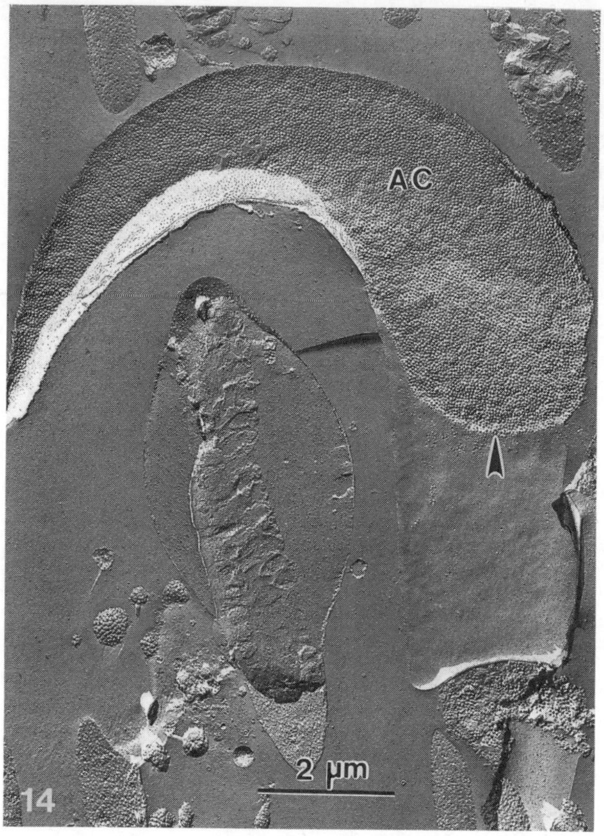

FIG. 14. A mature, uncapacitated golden hamster spermatozoon, freeze-fractured after filipin treatment. Note the densely and evenly distributed filipin-sterol complexes in the plasma membrane of the acrosomal region (*AC*). An arrowhead indicates the posterior boarder of the equatorial segment region. (From ref. 1538.)

exert a variety of profound effects on the characteristics of all biological membranes (e.g., active and passive ion permeability) by regulating orientation, fluidity, and thickness of membrane lipids (99). Figure 14 shows the freeze-fractured plasma membrane of a hamster spermatozoon after treatment with the polyene antibiotic, filipin. When filipin binds to sterols like cholesterol in membranes, the filipin/sterol complexes divert the membrane away from the side of higher sterol concentration (962). When viewed after freeze-fracture, sterol-rich (cholesterol-rich) areas of the membrane appear as small bumps. It will be seen from this figure that sterols are abundant in the plasma membrane over the acrosome. The density of sterols in this area is sharply reduced after capacitation (1540). Albumin and high-density lipoproteins in the female tract are believed to pick up cholesterol from the sperm plasma membrane (129,283,911,1392–1395).

Although the importance of cholesterol removal from the sperm plasma membrane for capacitation has been stressed repeatedly (182,183,283,910,911,1046), it could be the phase separation of the membrane phospholipids and cholesterol (lateral migration of these molecules within the lipid bilayers to form domains), not the complete removal of cholesterol from the membrane, that is more important for capacitation. There are reports that the fluidity of lipids of the sperm head and tail plasma membranes changes as a result of capacitation (367,368,451,514,1669). Cholesterol movement could be responsible, in part, for such changes.

What Happens during Capacitation—Overview

It is beyond any doubt that the sperm plasma membrane undergoes a variety of changes in preparation for fertilization. We may assume that sperm plasma membrane is "biologically frozen" when spermatozoa leave the male's body and its "defrosting" represents capacitation. Although many other changes occur in the sperm's structural and chemical constituents, whether they are essential components of capacitation remains uncertain. The inherent difficulty in studying capacitation lies in the heterogenity of spermatozoa. Even under the most favorable capacitating condition, not all of the spermatozoa survive and capacitate. Many may die without ever starting or completing capacitation, even though the spermatozoa as a whole become functionally capacitated (able to fertilize all or most eggs). Care must be taken to avoid studying the results of sperm senescence/death rather than capacitation. The fact that fresh epididymal spermatozoa of some species (e.g., the cat) are ready for fertilization (353) should not be overlooked. Fresh epididymal spermatozoa of the guinea pig are able to undergo the acrosome reaction without prior *in vitro* incubation (474,752,1693). Should these species be ignored simply as being exceptional? Whether the sperm structures and components, other than the plasma membrane, really do need preparatory changes for fertilization during capacitation is a question that remains to be answered.

ACROSOME AND THE ACROSOME REACTION

Acrosome and Acrosomal Enzymes

The acrosome is a membrane-bound, caplike structure covering the anterior portion of the sperm nucleus. Although the size and shape of the acrosome vary considerably from species to species (24,150), its basic structure is the same in all eutherian mammals. The acrosome consists of the anteriorly located acrosomal cap and the posteriorly located equatorial segment. Figure 15 illustrates the relative size and topographical relationship between these two segments of the acrosome in seven different species. While the acrosomal cap is loaded with hydrolyzing enzymes, the equatorial segment could be enzymatically "empty." The acrosome is believed to be

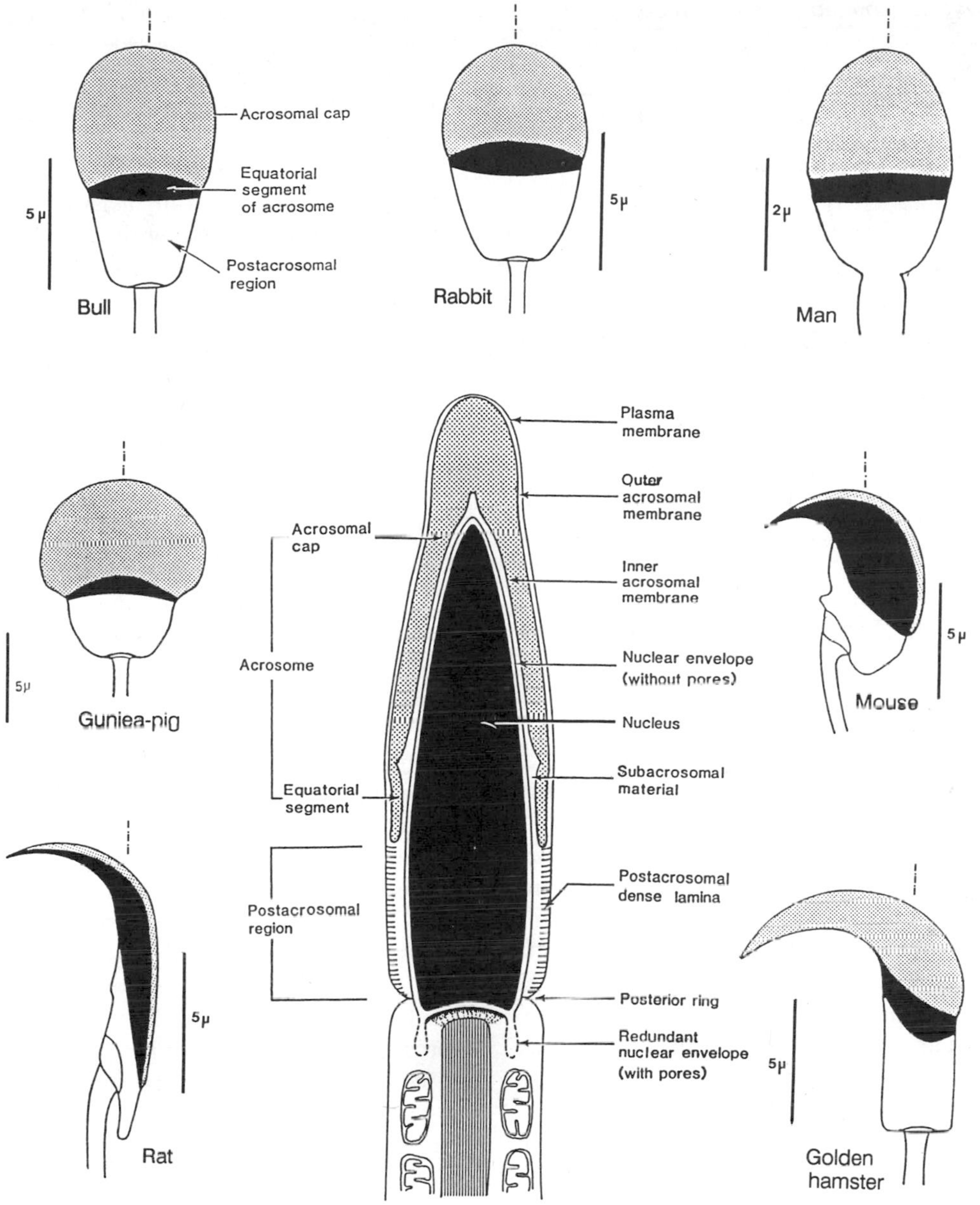

FIG. 15. Diagrams illustrating the relative size and topographical relationship between the acrosomal cap and the equatorial segment of the spermatozoa of seven different species. Although shapes and relative size of these two regions of the acrosome vary from species to species, their basic structures are the same. The central figure is a schematic representation of the sagittal section (– – –) through the head. (Modified slightly from ref. 530.)

analogous to a lysosome (11) or a zymogen granule of pancreatic cells (173). Synthesis of acrosomal enzymes begins as early as the pachytene stage of meiosis when the acrosome vesicle is not yet formed (680). Table 2 lists the enzymes reported to be of acrosomal origin. Although some (e.g., phospholipases) could have been extracted from the acrosomal and/or plasma membranes, rather than the contents of the acrosome, there is no doubt that the acrosome contains a large array of powerful hydrolyzing enzymes (for a recent review, see 1725). Phillips (1362) stated "The distinct shapes of acrosome, arrangement of paracrystalline material, and occurrence of areas of different densities suggest that the acrosome is not simply a bag of enzymes. It seems likely that structural proteins may be involved in maintaining acrosome shape and the positioning of different functional components within the acrosomal matrix. A high degree of acrosome organization may be required to assure the release of acrosome components in a precise order as the spermatozoa traverse the egg vestments."

Hyaluronidase and acrosin are the two acrosomal enzymes that have been most extensively studied and well

TABLE 2. *Enzymes reported to be of acrosomal origin*

First reported before 1980	First reported after 1980 (refs.)
Hyaluronidase	N-Acetylexosaminidase (454)
Acrosin	Galactosidase (454)
Proacrosin	Glucuronidase (454)
Acid proteinase	L-Fucosidase (454)
Esterase	Phospholipase C (453)
Neuraminidase	Cathepsin D (456)
Phosphatase	Cathepsin L (1224)
Phospholipase A	Ornithin decarboxylase (400)
N-Acetylglucosaminidase	Calpain II (435)
Arylsulfatase	Metalloendoprotease (989)
Arylamidase	Caproyl esterase (1633)
Collagenase	Peptidyl peptidase (417b)

characterized (1018,1019,1127,1611,1725). Their presence within the acrosome has been demonstrated convincingly by cytochemical or immunocytochemical techniques at the electron microscopic level (97,192,196, 253,440,504). Although several investigators maintained that a portion of acrosomal hyaluronidase and acrosin is bound tightly to the inner acrosomal membrane and remains there even after the acrosome reaction (e.g., 253,1573), none of the evidence presented at the electron microscopic level is strong enough to verify this yet (for discussion, see ref. 241).

Carbohydrate is a distinct component of the acrosomal matrix (231,270,285). A glycoprotein layer covering the inner surface of the outer acrosomal membrane (152) may serve to hold vesiculated (fenestrated) plasma and outer acrosomal membranes together during the acrosome reaction. Some glycoproteins or carbohydrate-containing materials within the acrosomal matrix may be important in compartmentalization of enzymes within the acrosome. Conversion of proacrosin into enzymatically active acrosin, which occurs just before or during the acrosome reaction (984), may be aided by glycoproteins in the acrosomal matrix.

Functional Significance of the Acrosome Reaction

The eggs of many animals are surrounded by glycoprotein coats through which spermatozoa must pass before reaching the egg plasma membrane. In some invertebrates and nonmammalian vertebrates, acrosomal "lysins" released by (or carried on the surface of) an acrosome-reacted spermatozoon dissolve the coat locally to produce a "hole" through which the spermatozoon then swims (660). The dissolution of the coat by lysins is either enzymatic or stoichiometric (1047).

Eggs of all eutherian mammals are surrounded by a thick glycoprotein coat, the zona pellucida. At ovulation, the zona is further surrounded by the cumulus oophorus, which consists of cumulus cells and their matrix. The main component of the cumulus matrix is polymerized hyaluronic acid. It has been thought for many years that hyaluronidase released from acrosome-reacting spermatozoa digests the cumulus matrix and that acrosin carried on the surface of acrosome-reacted spermatozoa aids in the passage of spermatozoa through the zona. Although this notion must be reevaluated (see below), there is no doubt that only acrosome-reacted spermatozoa are capable of passing through the zona and fusing with the egg plasma membrane (530,660,1696). In other words, the acrosome reaction has at least dual functions: it renders spermatozoa capable of (i) penetrating through the zona and (ii) fusing with the egg plasma membrane.

Morphology, Detection, and Kinetics of the Acrosome Reaction

Distinction Between True and False Acrosome Reactions

Since the acrosome contains a variety of powerful hydrolyzing enzymes, the acrosome may be autodigested in moribund or dead spermatozoa when their membranes loose semipermeability. The outer acrosomal membrane and the overlying plasma membrane may either be destroyed (partially or totally) or become detached from the main body of the spermatozoon. Under the light microscope, spermatozoa with disrupted or missing plasma and outer acrosomal membranes may look like acrosome-reacting or acrosome-reacted spermatozoa. It is very important to distinguish such degenerative acrosomal modifications that begin in moribund and dead spermatozoa from the physiological acrosome reaction that occurs in live, motile spermatozoa. Bedford (41) proposed that the former be called *false* acrosome reactions and the latter *true* acrosome reactions.

Exocytotic Nature of the Acrosome Reaction

The typical, true acrosome reaction involves multiple fusions between the outer acrosomal membrane and the overlying plasma membrane, which enables the contents of the acrosome to escape through the fenestrated membranes (Figs. 16 and 17). Since Barros et al. (29) first demonstrated this membrane "vesication" in the hamster and rabbit, a number of investigators have confirmed this not only in these species, but also in a variety of other mammalian species including the human (Fig. 18).

The site where the point fusions between the plasma membrane and the outer acrosomal membrane first takes place may vary according to species. It could be the frontal or peripheral margin of the acrosomal cap region in the case of the rabbit (cf. refs. 44b and 530). In the golden hamster (133) and ram (154,155,455,508), it could be at or near the border of the acrosomal cap region and the equatorial segment of the acrosome. This is

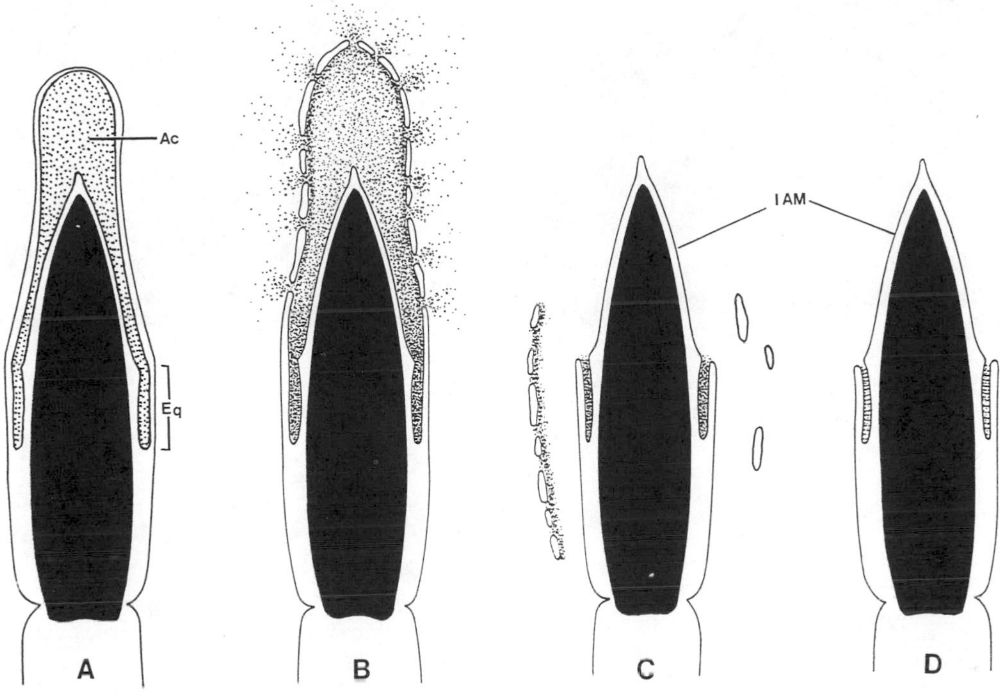

FIG. 16. Diagrams illustrating the progression of the acrosome reaction. (**A**) Before the reaction. (**B**) The reaction in progress; multiple fusions between the plasma and outer acrosomal membrane allow the release or exposure of acrosomal contents (enzymes). (**C–D**) The reaction is completed; vesiculated membranes are held together by a "sticky" acrosomal matrix or disperse. *Ac,* Acrosomal cap; *Eq,* equatorial segment; *IAM,* inner acrosomal membrane. (Modified slightly from ref. 530.)

not surprising because in the spermatozoa of many species, the plasma and outer acrosomal membranes appear to be least stable in this region (179). According to Watson and Plummer (508), the outer acrosomal membrane of this region is very rich in calcium-binding sites. The equatorial segment of the acrosome is not involved in vesication of the membranes during the acrosome reaction (cf. Fig. 16D). This could be due to the presence of calpactin II (749) as well as vimentin and intermediate filaments that act to tightly connect the outer acrosomal and overlying plasma membrane of this region of the spermatozoon (720). However, the equatorial segment

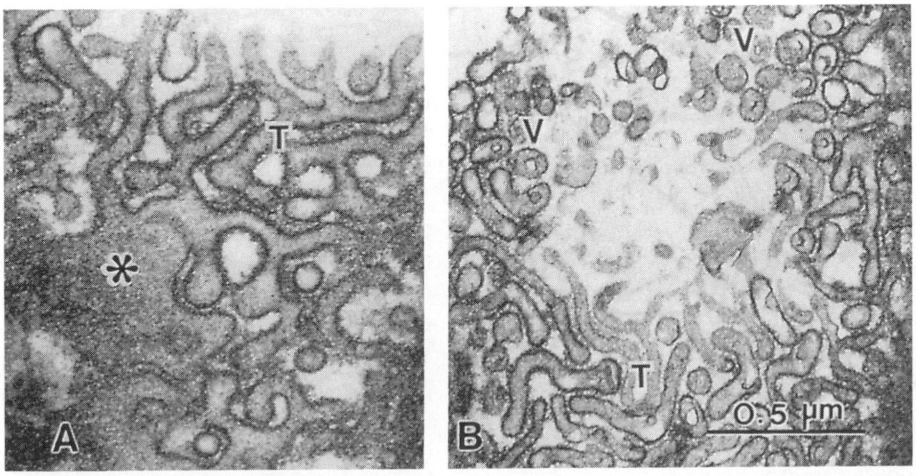

FIG. 17. Grazing sections through "vesiculating" plasma and outer acrosomal membranes of acrosome-reacting guinea pig spermatozoa. **B** shows a more advanced stage of vesiculation than **A.** *V,* Hybrid membrane vesicle; *T,* hybrid membrane tubule; ∗, as-yet-unfused region of the acrosome (ref. 937). (Provided by Dr. Gary E. Olson.)

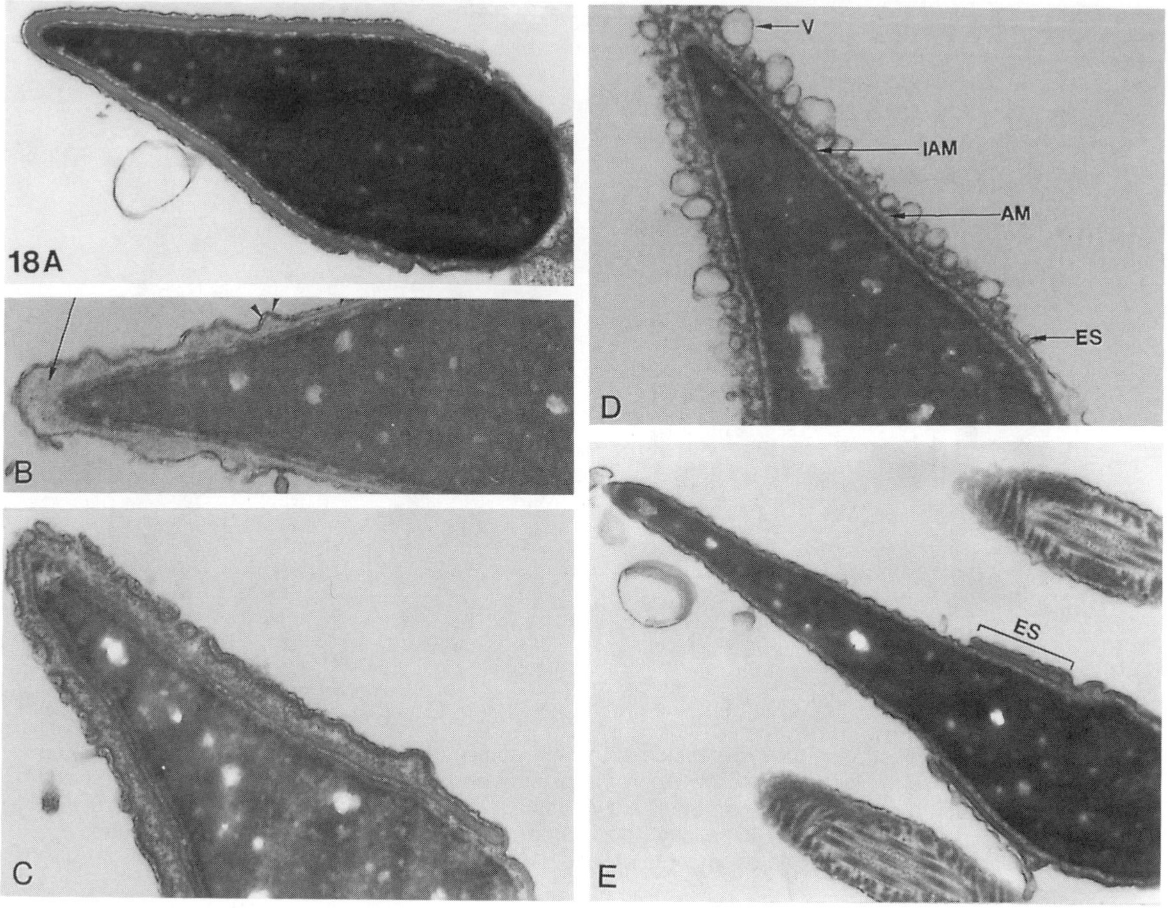

FIG. 18. Progression of the acrosome reaction in human spermatozoa. The reaction was triggered by exposing capacitated spermatozoa to human follicular fluid. **A,** a capacitated, acrosome-intact sperm. **B,** 5 sec after exposure to follicular fluid; the acrosomal matrix (arrow) is swollen; *arrowheads* indicate the plasma and outer acrosomal membranes. **C,** 10 sec after exposure to follicular fluid; the plasma and outer acrosomal membranes begin to fuse at the anterior region of the acrosome. **D,** 20 sec after exposure to follicular fluid; vesicles (*V*) formed by the fusion of the plasma and outer acrosomal membranes; vesicles are embedded in the acrosomal matrix (*AM*); membrane vesiculation is not extended to the equatorial segment (*ES*); *IAM,* the inner acrosomal membrane. **E,** Acrosome-reacted spermatozoon with intact equatorial segment (*ES*). (From refs. 1586,1720.)

may eventually vesiculate and be lost as time passes after the acrosome reaction (710,991,1626).

In some species (e.g., pig, human, possum, flying fox) the outer acrosomal membrane invaginates to form many intraacrosomal vesicles before the contents of the acrosome are released (348,706,858,1216,1421,1520). Such an acrosomal modification should be considered a degenerative change in senescent spermatozoa until its physiological normality is demonstrated unequivocally.

Methods to Assess Acrosomal Status of Spermatozoa: Advantages and Disadvantages

Electron Microscopy

Although it is laborious and time consuming, transmission electron microscopy is still the only technique that allows us to examine in detail the status of the acrosome including the acrosome reaction. If all or the vast majority of spermatozoa are alive at the moment of fixation, it is fairly certain that the ultrastructural pictures will represent acrosomal changes in living spermatozoa. If not, care must be taken in interpreting the results of the observation. When the outer acrosomal membrane is continuous with the overlying plasma membrane and the rest of the plasma membrane is intact, the acrosome reaction we see is most likely the true acrosome reaction. When the plasma membrane is broken or missing at any place, regardless of its extent, the acrosomal modifications we observe should be considered degenerative or the false acrosome reaction. It is possible that the plasma and outer acrosomal membranes of capacitated spermatozoa are much more vulnerable to chemical treatment (fixation) than those of uncapacitated spermatozoa. Poor fixation or improper postfixation handling could cause disruption of sperm membranes. Therefore, every precaution is needed to interpret the observations by electron microscopy. Although scanning electron microscopy gives spectacular images of spermatozoa, its resolution is not high enough to examine details of the sperm membranes. Therefore, it should be used in conjunction with the transmission electron microscopy and/or other means of microscopic assessment.

Phase-Contrast (Interference-Contrast) Microscopy

If spermatozoa have large acrosomes, we can readily detect changes in their acrosomes in living spermatozoa. The acrosomes of musk-shrew (107,264) and guinea-pig (528) spermatozoa, for example, are so large (Fig. 19A) that a low-power objective lens (e.g., 4×) would be sufficient to detect acrosomal modifications in vigorously motile spermatozoa. Although the acrosomes of Chinese hamster (539) and golden hamster (541) spermatozoa are considerably smaller than those of musk-shrew and guinea-pig spermatozoa, we can clearly visualize the acrosome reaction in living spermatozoa of these species using a 40× phase-contrast objective lens (Fig. 19B,C). With some experience, the acrosome reaction (the presence or absence of an acrosomal cap) in moving spermatozoa can be evaluated with ease. When the spermatozoa are moving very vigorously (e.g., hyperactivated), assessing the acrosome reaction can be very difficult or impossible. This difficulty can be overcome by slowing down sperm movement by, for example, (i) cooling the microscope stage, (ii) suspending spermatozoa in a very viscous medium, (iii) minimizing the volume of sperm suspension under the coverslip, or (iv) immobilizing spermatozoa, one by one, by a brief exposure to an ultraviolet spot (119). The acrosomes of rabbit and mouse spermatozoa are thin and tightly fitted to the sperm heads. Detecting the acrosome reaction in live spermatozoa of these species is obviously more difficult, but it is certainly possible (69,382,461,1405). If a large number of live spermatozoa have to be examined for their acrosomal status within a short time, a high resolution video recording is recommended.

Staining

Spermatozoa of many mammals (e.g., the rat, bull, ram, monkey, and human) have either very thin or tightly fitted acrosomes and consequently their acrosome reactions are difficult to detect in the living state. Therefore, many staining techniques have been developed (see 845). Only two of them are considered here. One uses Hoechst 33258 (a fluorescent DNA-binding dye) and specific plant lectins or antiacrosome antibodies. Spermatozoa are first treated in a medium containing Hoechst. Since this dye has limited membrane permeability, only the nuclei of dead spermatozoa pick up the dye, whereas those of living spermatozoa, with intact plasma membranes, do not. Spermatozoa are then fixed and stained with acrosome-affinity lectins (e.g., *Pisum sativum* agglutinin) (847,1234,1578) or antibodies raised against acrosomal contents (516,675,1268) or the acrosomal membrane (931,1441,1595).

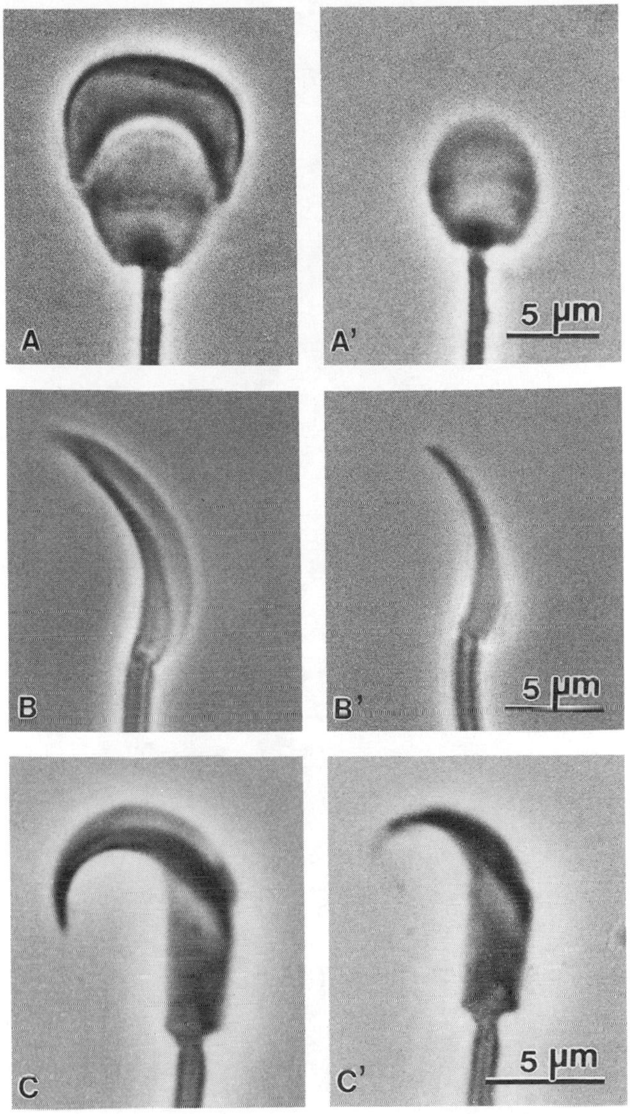

FIG. 19. Phase-contrast micrographs of guinea pig (**A**), Chinese hamster (**B**), and golden hamster (**C**) spermatozoa before and after the acrosome reaction.

Four types of fluorescence patterns can be seen when examined with a fluorescence microscope: (i) the acrosomal cap fluoresces, but not the nucleus, (ii) neither the acrosomal cap nor the nucleus fluoresces, (iii) both the acrosomal cap and the nucleus fluoresce, and (iv) only the nucleus fluoresces. Those spermatozoa exhibiting type (i) pattern are considered live spermatozoa with intact acrosomes or undergoing the acrosome reaction at the time of fixation. Those having pattern (ii) are be-

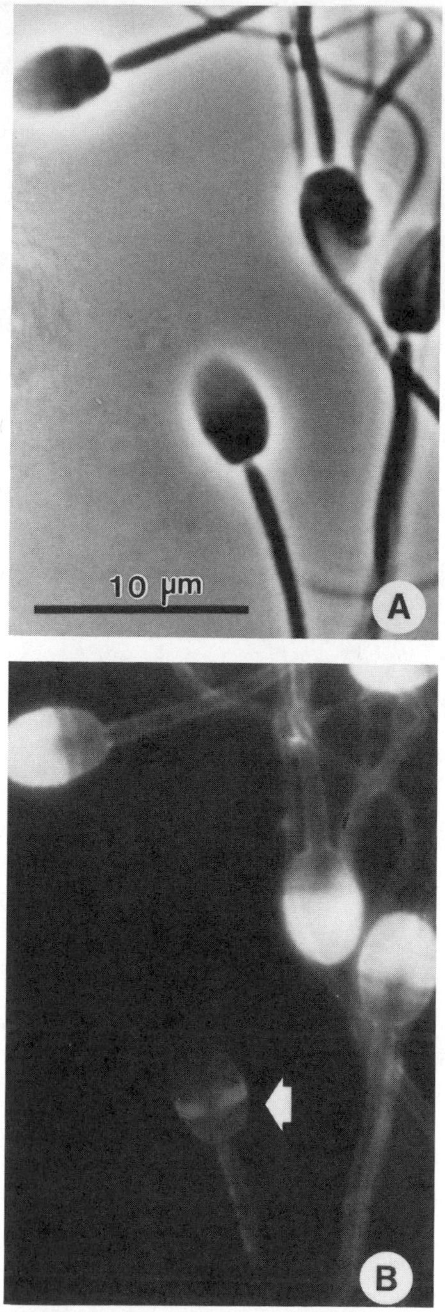

FIG. 20. Cynomolgus monkey spermatozoa stained with FITC-conjugated *Pisum sativum* agglutinin. Phase-contrast microscopy (**A**) cannot differentiate acrosome-reacted spermatozoa from acrosome-intact ones, whereas the lectin-staining method (**B**) is readily able to do so. An acrosome-reacted spermatozoon without acrosomal matrix (*white arrow* in B) does not exhibit FITC fluorescence in the acrosomal cap region. (From ref. 846.).

lieved to be live spermatozoa that have completed true acrosome reaction (Fig. 20) (846). Those having patterns (iii) and (iv) are considered to be spermatozoa that have died after undergoing the acrosome reaction or have died with or without acrosomal degeneration. Techniques using Hoechst dye are relatively simple and also can be applied even when only very few spermatozoa are available for acrosome assessment (1270). If acrosomes are not extremely small (e.g., those of bull spermatozoa), true acrosome reactions can be distinguished from false reactions without the aid of lectins or antibodies: spermatozoa are stained Hoechst first, then fixed, and finally examined using both phase-contrast and fluorescence microscopes. Spermatozoa without acrosomal caps or any nuclear fluorescence are considered to have completed the true acrosome reaction (871).

However, all techniques utilizing Hoechst staining have an inherent problem. The plasma membranes of moribund spermatozoa are often impenetrable to the Hoechst dye, and thus some moribund spermatozoa may be classified as live, potentially fertile spermatozoa. Therefore, it is important to determine the viability of spermatozoa before staining/fixation in order to increase the reliability of the technique. Although fluorescent lectins are readily accessible, most of them cannot be used for examination of spermatozoa on or in eggs, because the zonae and plasma membranes of mammalian eggs have a strong affinity for various lectins (1292,1705). Antiacrosome antibody, now commercially available (845), is better suited for examination of the spermatozoa on or in the zona.

Another technique, developed originally for mouse spermatozoa, uses an antibiotic chlortetracycline (CTC) which stains the sperm surface differently depending on the stage of capacitation and the acrosome reaction (427,1158,1634). The principle of this technique is not very clear. Chlortetracycline may bind to a Ca^{2+}-affinity substance (427) or an anionic peptide on the sperm plasma membrane (957,958). According to Fraser et al. (957,958), this peptide is secreted by the epididymis and has a sperm-decapacitating activity. During capacitation, the CTC-binding pattern changes and, after the acrosome reaction, spermatozoa show no CTC-binding (Fig. 21). This simple technique has been applied to assess the acrosomal status of human (1160) and monkey (1120) spermatozoa. Again, there is room for improvement, because this technique does not allow one to distinguish live spermatozoa from moribund/dead spermatozoa.

Techniques using fluoresceins have a common problem. Spermatozoa must be killed before examining their acrosomes. Once spermatozoa are killed, it cannot be determined with certainty whether the one under observation was vigorous, weakly motile, or totally motionless at the time of fixation unless the same spermatozoon is continuously traced. If some membrane-permeable compounds or fluoresceins are found to have specific affinity to the acrosomal membrane or acrosomal contents, they can be applied for determination of the acrosomal status in living spermatozoa using either a regular microscope or an image-intensified UV microscope.

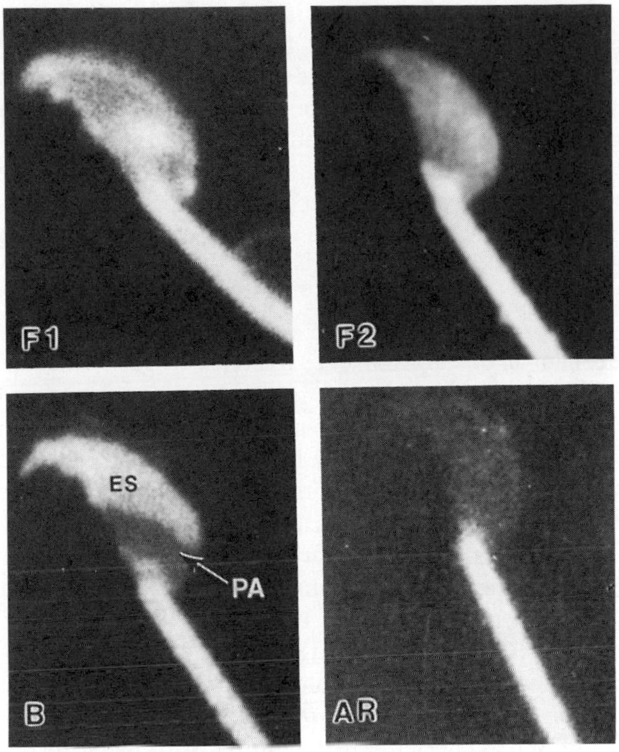

FIG. 21. Mouse spermatozoa stained with chlorotetracycline (CTC), showing changes in the staining pattern of their heads during capacitation and after acrosome reaction. Patterns *F1* and *F2*, uncapacitated. Pattern *B*, capacitated, acrosome-intact. Pattern *AR*, acrosome-reacted. *ES*, equatorial segment, *PA*, postacrosomal region. (From ref. 1634.)

Speed of the Acrosome Reaction

When spermatozoa are fully capacitated and receive the proper stimuli, they initiate and complete the acrosome reaction rather promptly. For example, guinea-pig spermatozoa that have been capacitated in a Ca^{2+}-deficient medium begin the reaction between 30 and 60 sec after exposure to a normal concentration of Ca^{2+} (approximately 2 mM); the reaction is completed by most spermatozoa within the next 5 min (547). Ohzu and Yanagimachi (354) have found that hamster spermatozoa preincubated for 1 to 2 hr in a normal capacitating medium can complete the acrosome reaction within 2 min following exposure to a low concentration of lysolecithin (0.05 mg/mL). Some capacitated monkey spermatozoa are able to complete the acrosome reaction on zonae pellucidae within 1 min (1616). When capacitated human spermatozoa are exposed to human follicular fluid, membrane fusion between the plasma and outer acrosomal membrane is first detected in 5 to 10 sec; the reaction (including dispersion of acrosome matrix) is completed within the next 3 min (1720). According to Lee and Storey (1159), the acrosome reaction of mouse spermatozoa on the zona pellucida occurs gradually within a population, but individual spermatozoa complete the reaction within 2 min.

Acrosome Reaction *In Vivo*

The false acrosome reaction, associated with sperm death, occurs all the time in the female tract. The female tract is by no means hospitable to all spermatozoa. Only those in the right place (microenvironment) at the right time can stay alive within the tract. According to Zinaman et al. (1732), virtually all viable spermatozoa collected from the human cervical mucus had intact acrosomes even 3 days after artificial insemination, indicating that the cervical mucus provides a rather hospitable environment to spermatozoa. Many spermatozoa die in the vagina, uterus, and oviduct, but perhaps all (or virtually all) viable spermatozoa in the uterus (1335) and oviductal isthmus (1501) have intact acrosomes. Although a few may undergo a true acrosome reaction in the ampulla, the great majority of motile spermatozoa, free in the oviductal lumen, seem to retain their acrosomes (24,43,90,120,382,461,540). All motile hamster spermatozoa observed directly through the transparent wall of the oviductal ampulla during the periovulatory period were acrosome-intact (1735). Some spermatozoa may initiate the early stage of the acrosome reaction within the cumulus oophorus (121), but the balance of evidence indicates that fertilizing spermatozoa do not initiate the true acrosome reaction *in vivo* until they come into contact with the zona pellucida (851,853 and see below).

Zona-Mediated Acrosome Reaction vs. Spontaneous Acrosome Reaction

Perhaps in all mammalian species, fertilizing spermatozoa, both *in vivo* and *in vitro,* undergo the acrosome reaction on the surface of the zona pellucida before penetrating into it (cf. 758,1138). In general, the zona-mediated acrosome reaction is species-specific in that the spermatozoa undergo the acrosome reaction most efficiently on the zona of the same species (see ref. 1615). However, the zona-mediated acrosome reaction is not rigidly species-specific. For example, solubilized mouse zonae can induce the acrosome reaction of human spermatozoa (1160). Hamster spermatozoa are not only able to undergo the acrosome reaction on human zonae, but they are also able to penetrate it (1714). Ram spermatozoa are apparently able to undergo the acrosome reaction on the bovine zona before penetrating it (1498).

It is well established that spermatozoa of most species are able to undergo a true acrosome reaction in the absence of the zona. The acrosome reaction in actively motile spermatozoa in sperm capacitation media, without any stimulative reagents, is commonly called the *sponta-*

neous acrosome reaction. The incidence of the spontaneous acrosome reaction seems to depend on various factors including (i) the species (Fig. 22) and strain (1318) of the animal, (ii) the composition of the medium (30,707,839,1332,1521) (guinea pig in Fig. 22), (iii) the state of epididymal storage of spermatozoa (738,855) (hamster in Fig. 22), and perhaps pre- and postejaculation treatments (678) and the immunological condition (1150) of spermatozoa. It is generally assumed that the spontaneous acrosome reaction is an unphysiological or spurious event, because the acrosome reaction in fertilizing spermatozoa normally occurs on the surface of the zona pellucida, not in the medium (1138,1589,1656). At least in the mouse, spermatozoa that have undergone the acrosome reaction in the medium are unable to bind to the zona, and consequently they are unable to fertilize eggs (1138,1434). In this respect, the spontaneous acrosome reaction is certainly unphysiological or even pathological. However, the spermatozoa that have undergone spontaneous acrosome reactions are not totally impotent. Hamster spermatozoa that have undergone the acrosome reaction within the oviduct in the absence of native eggs and their vestments can fertilize zona-free eggs installed in the same oviduct (854). Mouse spermatozoa that have undergone the acrosome reaction in the absence of native zonae are perfectly capable of fertilizing zona-free eggs and producing normal fertile offspring (Fig. 23) (1284).

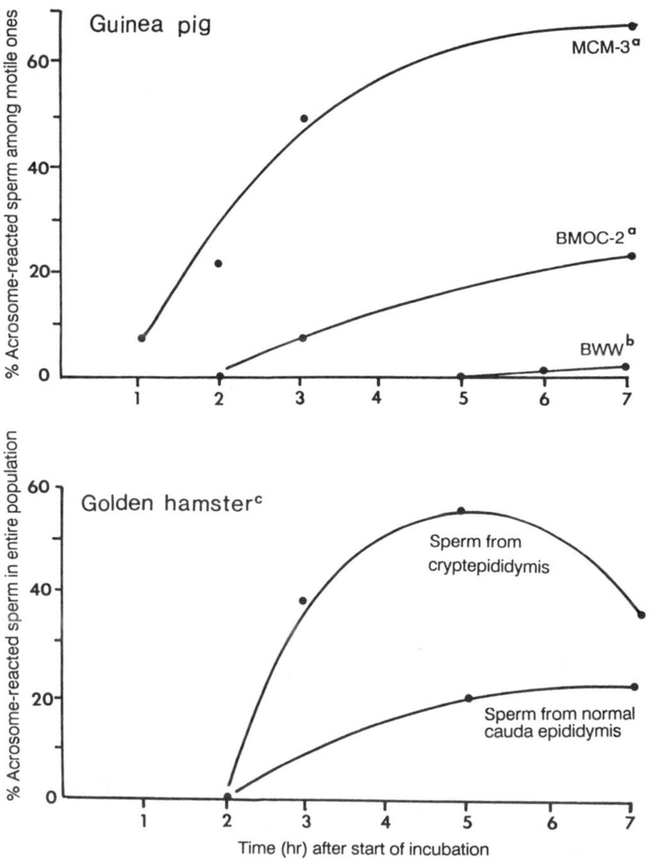

FIG. 22. Spontaneous acrosome reaction in guinea pig and golden hamster spermatozoa. In the guinea pig, the rate of spontaneous acrosome reaction is influenced by the composition of the medium. Hamster spermatozoa from cryptoepididymis undergo the spontaneous acrosome reaction at a considerably higher rate than those from intact epididymis. Males with cryptepididymides are fertile. (From refs. 707 [A], 547 [B], 737 [C].)

Mechanism of the Acrosome Reaction

Since Saling et al. (426) and Bleil and Wassarman (761) reported convincingly that mouse zona pellucida induces the acrosome reaction of capacitated mouse spermatozoa, the ability of the zona to induce the acrosome reaction has been confirmed in a variety of animals including the rat (1478), hamster (103,1615), rabbit (371,1294), cattle (115,941), pig (746,1028), sheep (116), monkey (1616), and human (828,848,1157). The mechanism by which the zona molecules trigger the acrosome reaction has been studied intensively, particularly in the mouse. When I presented a diagram of the possible mechanism of mammalian sperm acrosome reaction about 10 years ago (Fig. 24), G-protein mediated signal transduction systems had not been considered. It is now clear that mammalian spermatozoa share a number of common characteristics within the signal transduction mechanisms that operate in a variety of other cells.

In the case of the mouse, and perhaps in many other mammals, ZP3, one of the zona glycoproteins, acts as a ligand (68) and its binding with the sperm's receptor triggers chain reactions leading to the acrosome reaction. The ZP3 peptide chain must be intact to exert its ligand's activity (163,506,759). The precise oligosaccharide sequence of ZP3 does not seem to be of critical importance for its acrosome reaction-inducing activity (739). The following description is largely based on the information compiled by Saling (1434,1435), Kopf and Gerton (1138), Storey (1522,1523), Harrison and Roldan (1021), and Roldan and Harrison (1417).

Figure 25 by Saling (1434) illustrates the major preparatory changes in the plasma membrane for the acrosome reaction. Uncapacitated spermatozoa (Fig. 25A) are characterized by a nonfluid and nonreactive plasma membrane. These membrane characteristics are due to a high cholesterol concentration in the membrane and the presence of a decapacitation factor (DF) that anchors the zona receptors (R_{zp}) to the membrane. There may be more than one kind of R_{zp}. They are shown here in two different patterns. One R_{zp} has a protein tyrosine kinase activity (1165,1168). When capacitated (Fig. 25B), the plasma membrane becomes more fluid by a cholesterol efflux and the removal of DF, which renders R_{zp} freely movable within the plane of the membrane. ZP3 ligand,

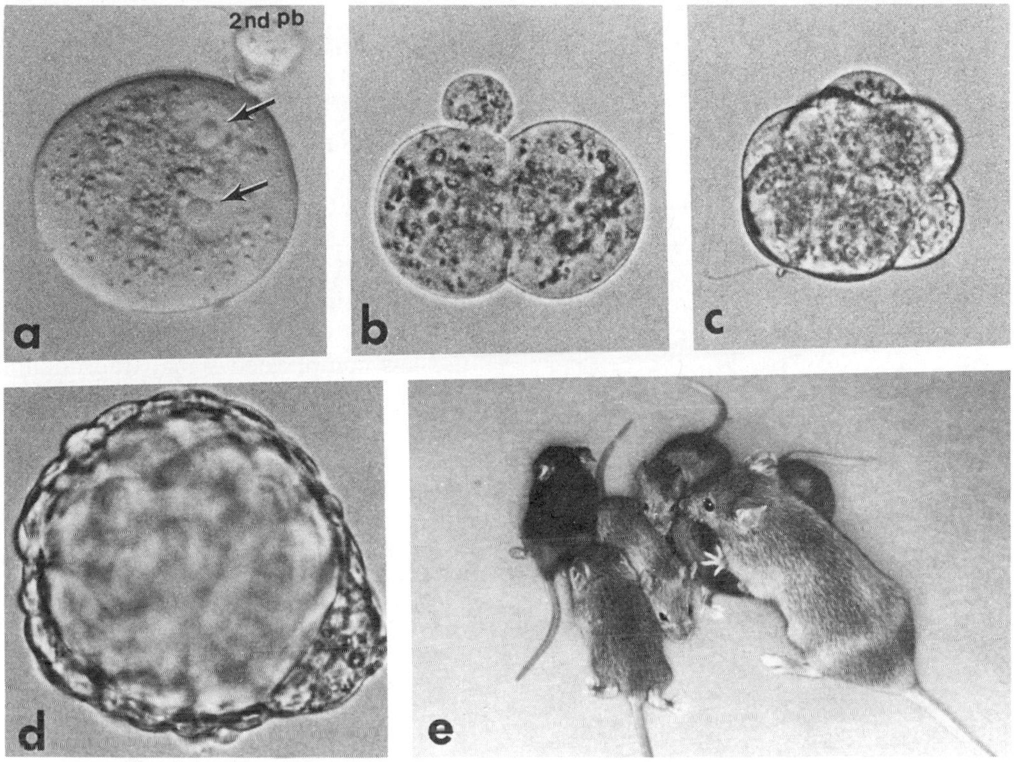

FIG. 23. Production of normal mice from eggs fertilized and developed without zonae pellucidae. Zona-free eggs fertilized *in vitro* (*a*) developed normally (*b–d*); when transplanted into foster mothers, they developed into normal young. (*e*) An adult mouse developed from a zona-free egg, with her own pups. *Arrows* in *a* indicate sperm and egg pronuclei. (From ref. 1284.)

when it binds to the R_{zp} (Fig. 25C), causes an aggregation of the receptors (1167), which activates R_{zp}. Activated R_{zp} triggers the reaction cascade that leads to the acrosome reaction. A tentative model of zona receptor aggregation by ZP3 is shown in Figure 26.

Figure 27 is a diagram largely based on the concept presented by Kopf and Gerton (1138). The R_{zp} activated by ZP3 stimulates a G protein, which in turn stimulates phospholipase C (PLC) activity in the sperm plasma membrane. Phospholipase C cleaves phosphatidylinosi-

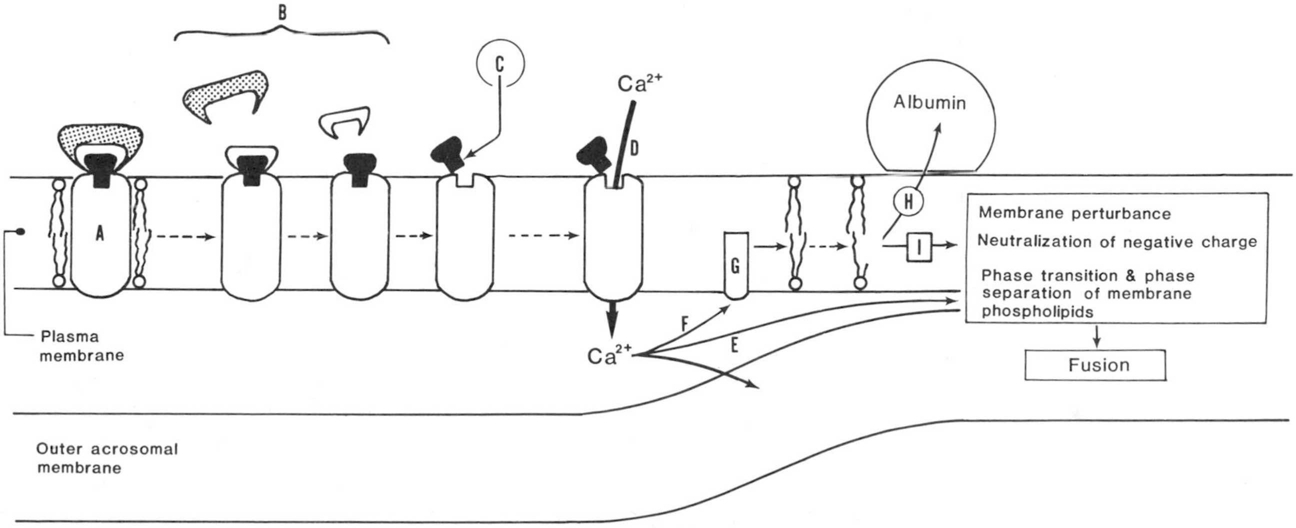

FIG. 24. A hypothetical model for the mechanism of the acrosome reaction, published by this author in 1981 (ref. 530), shows that extracellular Ca^{2+} entering the spermatozoon through Ca^{2+} channels causes the membrane fusion between the plasma and outer acrosomal membranes.

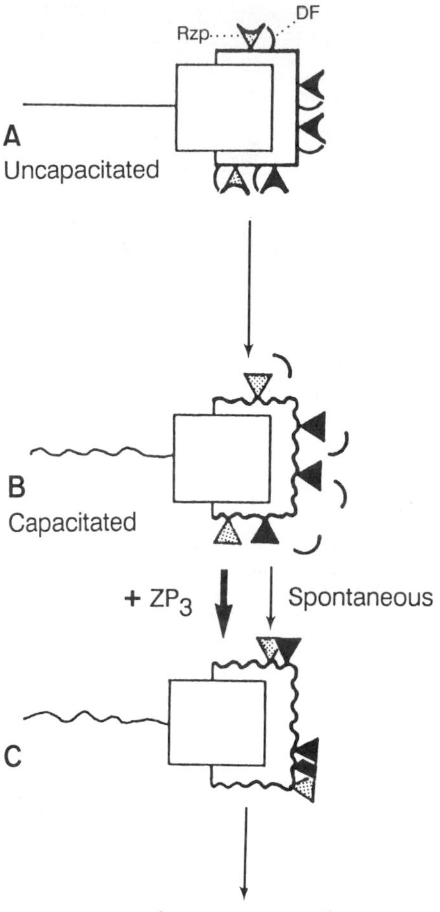

FIG. 25. A proposed model for the relationship between capacitation and the acrosome reaction. (From ref. 1434.) For explanation, see the text.

tol diphosphate (PIP_2) into diacylglycerol (DAG) and inositol triphosphate (IP_3). Inositol triphostate increases intracellular Ca^{2+} concentration by releasing Ca^{2+} from intracellular stores. Diacylglycerol activates Ca^{2+}-dependent protein kinase C (PK-C), which phosphorylates proteins. A part of IP_3 is methylated to become IP_4, which regulates the opening of voltage-dependent Ca^{2+} channels (940), thus allowing a massive influx of extracellular Ca^{2+}. Some of this Ca^{2+} acts on membrane phospholipids directly to facilitate membrane fusion. The activated G protein also stimulates phospholipases A_2 (PLA) which cleaves phosphatidyl choline (PC) into lysophosphatidyl choline (LC) plus arachidonic acid (AA), both known to be highly fusogenic (158,160). Simultaneously, phospholipase D (PLD) activated by G protein cleaves PC to choline and phosphatidic acid (PA), which is also fusogenic. One should realize that Ca^{2+} itself is fusogenic by neutralizing a negative charge of membranes, causing phase transition and phase separation of membrane phospholipids (530). Activated G protein triggers another chain reaction. It activates adenylate cyclase (AC), which in turn stimulates cAMP production. Protein kinase (PK-A) that is cAMP-dependent phosphorylates proteins essential for the acrosome reaction. Some of the cAMP acts on a gated Na^+ channel to allow Na^+ influx and H^+ efflux, bringing a rise in intracellular pH.

Influx of Ca^{2+}, a rise in intracellular pH, and the production of the fusogenic compounds described above are all believed to be essential for the acrosome reaction. However, since the acrosome reaction is a terminal event that occurs very quickly, it is possible that spermatozoa use less complicated signal transduction systems than somatic cells do. In fact, according to Roldan and his associates (1416,1418), ram spermatozoa do not have active protein kinase C, which disagrees with the findings of Endo et al. (915) and Rotem et al. (1423,1423a). Gen-

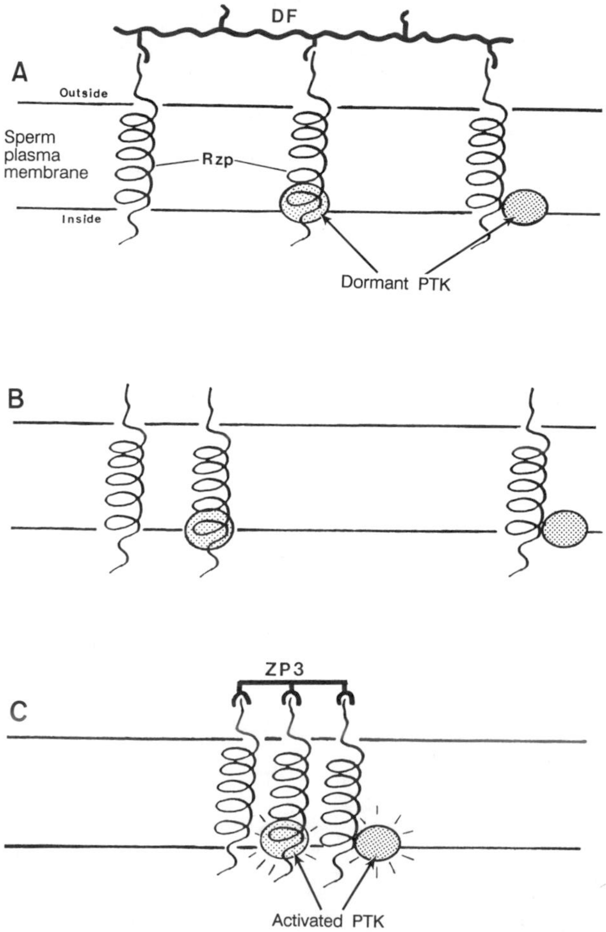

FIG. 26. A model showing activation of protein tyrosine kinase, PTK. (**A**) R_{zp} is originally masked by decapacitation factor, DF. (**B**) When DF is removed after capacitation, receptors are able to move "freely" in the lipid bilayers. (**C**) ZP3 aggregates R_{zp}; aggregated R_{zp} activates PTK which phosphorylate various proteins needed for the acrosome reaction. PTK activity may be in the R_{zp} molecule or in a molecule different from R_{zp} as illustrated in this diagram.

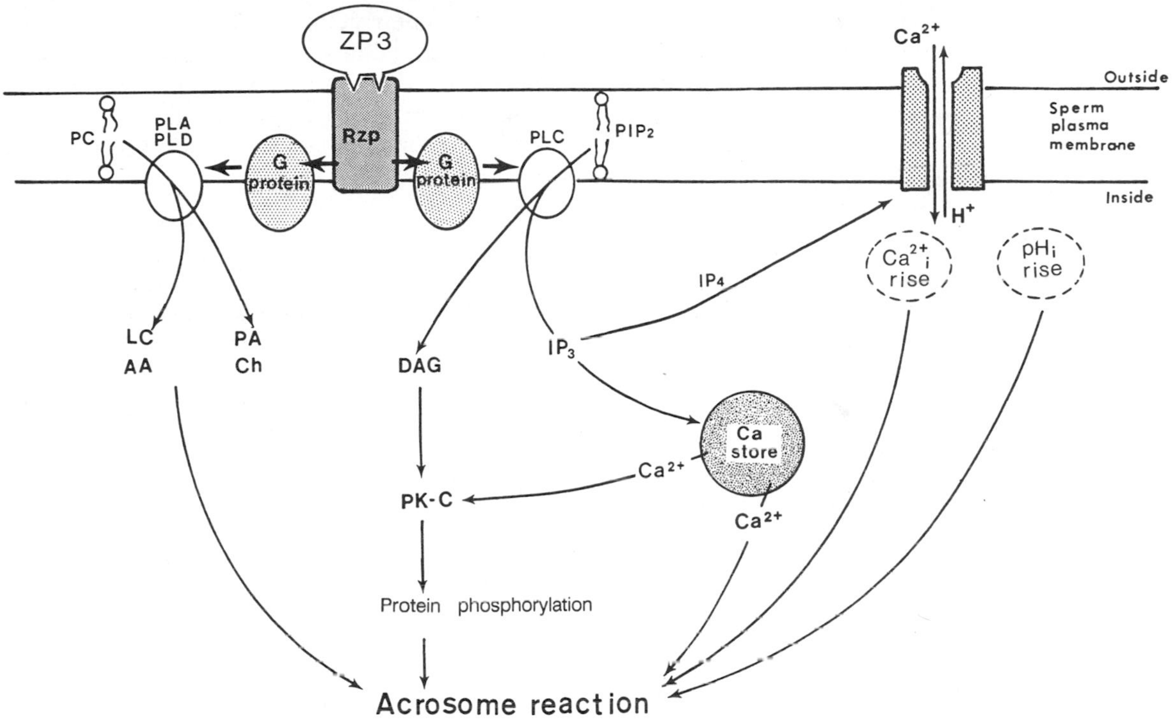

FIG. 27. Hypothetical pathways in zona-induced acrosome reaction. (cf. ref. 1138.) For explanation, see the text.

eration of inositol tetrakis-phosphate (IP_4) from IP_3 and protein phosphorylation, which Kopf and Gerton (1138) thought to be important for the acrosome reaction, was not detected by Roldan (personal communication).

Figure 28 illustrates the pathway proposed by Roldan and Harrison (1021,1417), which is much simpler than the pathway put forward by Kopf and Gerton (1138). According to this model, sperm receptors (R) activated by ligands open gated Ca^{2+} channels, allowing a Ca^{2+} influx. Increased intracellular Ca^{2+} concentration activates PLC, which cleaves PIP_2 into DAG and IP_3. Both DAG and Ca^{2+} stimulate PLA (1418) to produce the

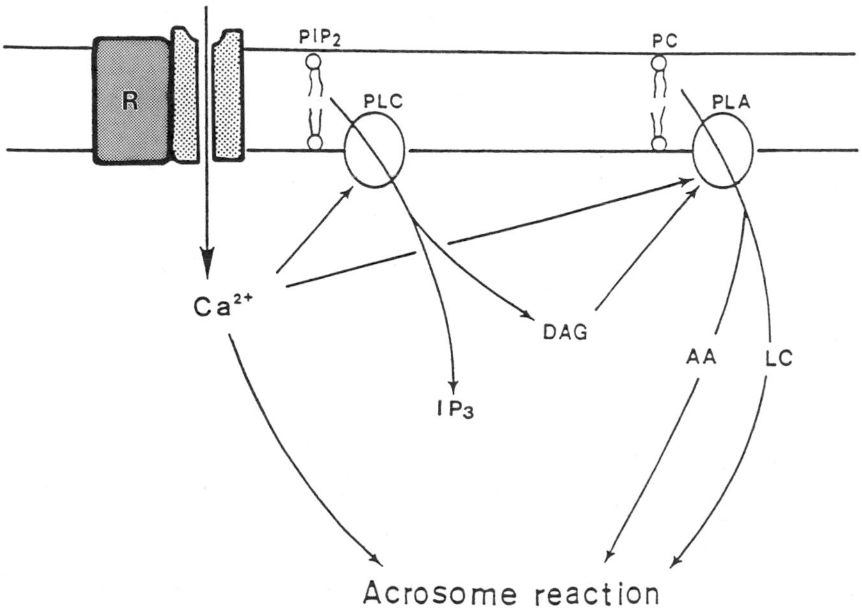

FIG. 28. Another proposed pathway of the acrosome reaction (cf. refs. 1021, 1417). For explanation, see the text.

fusogenic LA and AA. These investigators could not find active protein kinase C in ram spermatozoa (1416) and consider that the DAG–PLA cascade plays a central role in the acrosome reaction. This hypothesis is based on the ram sperm model using Ca^{2+}-ionophore as the acrosome reaction-inducing agent instead of the zona pellucida. One may argue that the acrosome reaction induced by ionophore is unphysiological and the processes involved could be very different from zona-induced reaction. However, the differences could occur in the initial steps of the reaction, not in the downstream cascades of the chain reactions.

Saling (1434) has speculated that R_{zp} in capacitated spermatozoa are able to aggregate by themselves, and this aggregation induces the spontaneous acrosome reaction. Although I agree with this hypothesis, there may be another type of spontaneous acrosome reaction, one that is related to aging of spermatozoa. As spermatozoa age in the female tract or in artificial media, Na^+- and/or Ca^{2+}-pumping mechanisms may become less efficient with time (due to depletion of ATP, for example). This would result in gradual increases in intracellular Ca^{2+} and pH. When intracellular Ca^{2+} and H^+ concentrations reach certain threshold levels, it may be enough to trigger the acrosome reaction without the activation of R_{zp}.

It has been reported that anti-R_{zp} antibodies (1167,1195) and some antibodies against sperm surface components (664,1150) induce the acrosome reaction. This may be explained by the aggregation and activation of R_{zp} by these antibodies. The acrosome reaction induced by electroporation (1338,1592) and calcium ionophore is probably due to a massive influx of extracellular Ca^{2+}. The acrosome reaction induced by lysolecithin (354,1014) may be due to a membrane perturbation followed by Ca^{2+} influx. Progesterone can induce the acrosome reaction of human spermatozoa very efficiently (1233,1333), but the mechanism by which it triggers the acrosome reaction is not clear at present. Progesterone may induce the acrosome reaction by binding to and aggregating steroid receptors in the plasma membrane (1577,1579) and causing Ca^{2+} (790,1586) and Cl^- (1667) influx. The relationship between progesterone receptors and R_{zp} and the physiological significance of the progesterone-induced acrosome reaction in fertilization remains to be determined.

Regardless of the type of stimulus, it is important to note that most of the known stimuli are unable to induce the acrosome reaction unless the spermatozoa have been capacitated (354,474,796,797,1675,1720). Although there are few important exceptions to this rule (e.g., an instantaneous acrosome reaction of guinea pig spermatozoa by physical and chemical stimuli; 474,708,1693), the sperm plasma membrane in an uncapacitated state, in general, appears to be either inaccessible to various stimuli (including the ligand ZP3) or incapable of responding to the stimuli.

Activation of R_{zp} and the subsequent membrane fusion, which were discussed above, are merely a part of the acrosome reaction. Activation release of acrosomal enzymes and the swelling dispersion of the acrosome matrix are also essential parts of the acrosome reaction. Table 3 lists the extracellular and intracellular components that influence the mammalian sperm acrosome

TABLE 3. *Molecules reported to be involved in the acrosome reaction, excluding components of female tract secretory products, cumulus oophorus, zona pellucida, and most of the substances involved in signal transduction systems*

Molecules	Refs[a]
Extracellular[b]	
H^+	245, 249, 338, 346, 519
Ca^{2+}	47, 57, 193, 287, 417, 448, 474, 547, 1713
Na^+	58, 245, 247, 249, 345, 960a, 1713
K^+	62, 245, 247, 338, 519
Cl^-	1667, 1713
HCO_3^-	70, 245, 288, 753, 768, 1506, 1713
Glucose/puruvate/lactate	34, 134, 167, 172, 325, 343
Albumin	183, 255, 283, 303, 304, 1713
Sperm membrane	
Intramembranous proteins	36, 155, 174, 546
SS/SH in proteins	156, 537
Anionic phospholipids	36
Cholesterol	36, 129, 158, 183, 284
Fatty acids (including arachidonic acid)	160, 320, 321
Prostaglandins	320, 1106, 1426
Lysophospholipids	158, 298, 354
Na^+, K^+-ATPase	15, 78, 339, 341
Ca^{2+}/Mg^+-dependent ATPase	547, 1415
Plasmin	1504
Intracellular	
Ca^{2+}	57, 508, 750, 756
Calmodulin	257, 521, 800
Unidentified Ca^+-binding molecule	398, 419, 598
Calpain II	435
Cytoskeletal system (including actin)	364, 435, 473, 501, 805–807
Intraacrosomal[c]	
Proteases (including acrosin)	133, 187, 195, 239, 242, 305, 310, 308, 1174a, 1372, 1587
Cathepsin D	456
H^+	239, 317, 1053
Natural acrosin inhibitor	59, 184, 553

[a] For additional references see Meizel, (refs. 314–316), Fraser (170, 955) and Kopf and Gerton (1138).
[b] Including influx and efflux through the plasma membrane.
[c] Controlling the proacrosin/acrosin status and the dispersion of acrosome matrix.

reaction. Zona glycoproteins and most of the molecules involved in the signal transduction system are not included in this table. It is possible that some of the listed molecules affected capacitation rather than the acrosome reaction. Many articles have reported that certain conditions or compounds enhanced or blocked the acrosome reaction, because the incidence of the acrosome reaction was increased or reduced when spermatozoa were incubated under particular conditions or in the presence of particular compounds. Although the acrosome reaction was surely affected, the particular conditions or compounds may have had effects on the capacitation process preceding the acrosome reaction. This should be kept in mind when reading original reports of *in vivo* and *in vitro* inhibition of the acrosome reaction. For more information about various aspects of the mammalian sperm acrosome reaction, readers are referred to refs. 170,283,313,316,530,899,955,956,1138,1166,1434, 1435,1488,1522–1524, 1696,1725,1726). Of these, refs. 170,965,1725, and 1726 emphasize, among others, the importance of energy substrate and the adenylate cyclase–cAMP–protein kinase system for the acrosome reaction and capacitation.

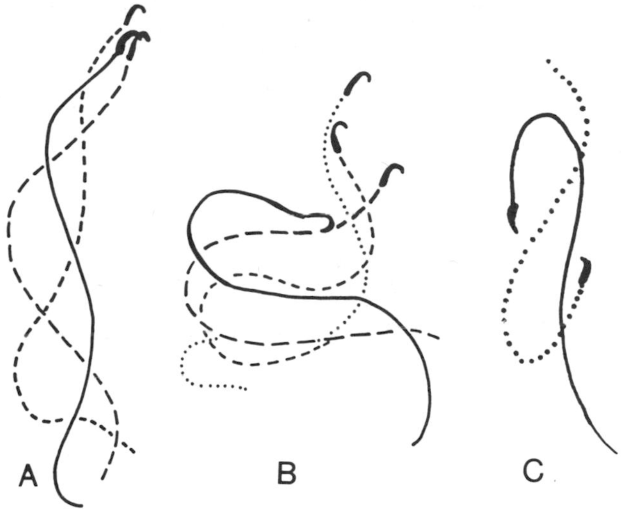

FIG. 29. Movement patterns of golden hamster spermatozoa before and after hyperactivation. (**A**) Spermatozoon immediately after being suspended in a capacitating medium. (**B,C**) Hyperactivated spermatozoa, approximately 4 hr after the start of incubation in the capacitating medium. (A and B from ref. 1528; C from ref. 887.)

HYPERACTIVATION OF SPERMATOZOA

Spermatozoa of some species begin to move frantically before they undergo the acrosome reaction. The term *hyperactivation* has been used (530) to describe this type of motility and to differentiate it from the term *activation,* which had been referred to as the initiation of movement by quiescent epididymal or vas deferens spermatozoa.

General Features of Hyperactivated Motility

The golden hamster was the species in which the phenomenon of hyperactivation was first recognized (524,526). Hamster spermatozoa, like those of most other species, are either motionless or only very weakly motile while they are stored in the epididymis and vas deferens. Upon contact with the capacitation medium, there is an initial burst of sperm motility (Fig. 29A) followed by a relatively quiescent state of motility. During this relatively quiescent state, most spermatozoa agglutinate in a head-to-head fashion (531) and beat their tails rather stiffly. After about 2 hours of relative quiescence, agglutinated spermatozoa begin to break free from each other to swim freely in the medium, which indicates that the surface characteristics of the spermatozoa have changed as they become capacitated. At this time, the spermatozoa begin to move much more actively than ever before. At first they swim in a linear fashion but soon display a characteristic movement seen as a very vigorous, whiplashlike beating of the tail (Fig. 29B), often with the sperm head tracing an erratic figure-eight pattern (Fig. 29C). Nonprogressive (dancing) movements are interspersed with brief episodes of linear (dashing) movements.

These two types of movements are collectively termed hyperactivation. The figure-eight aspect should not be overemphasized. It is just one phase of sperm hyperactivation in some species and does not exist in every species. It may never occur or may occur much less dramatically, for example, in some strains of mice (1524). What is important in hyperactivation is the increased thrust generated by the sperm flagellum, not a particular pattern of movement per se.

As the size, structure, and beat frequency of the sperm flagellum vary greatly from species to species (802,1360), we must expect that the pattern of hyperactivation also varies among species. Figure 30 illustrates the hyperactivated motility patterns of rat, mouse, Chinese hamster, pig, and human spermatozoa. It is important to note that the spermatozoa of a given species change their motility pattern depending on the physical and chemical characteristics of the surrounding medium. Hyperactivation is no exception. Its pattern is influenced greatly by the surrounding microstructure and the viscosity of the medium (Fig. 31) (887,1115,1528,1580). It is unknown at present whether hyperactivation is limited to just certain species or is a general phenomenon in mammals, but the number of species in which sperm hyperactivation has been recognized is increasing steadily. They include golden hamsters, Chinese hamsters, mice, rats, guinea pigs, rabbits, dogs, dolphins, sheep, cattle, pigs, nonhuman primates, and humans (792,887,1115,1696).

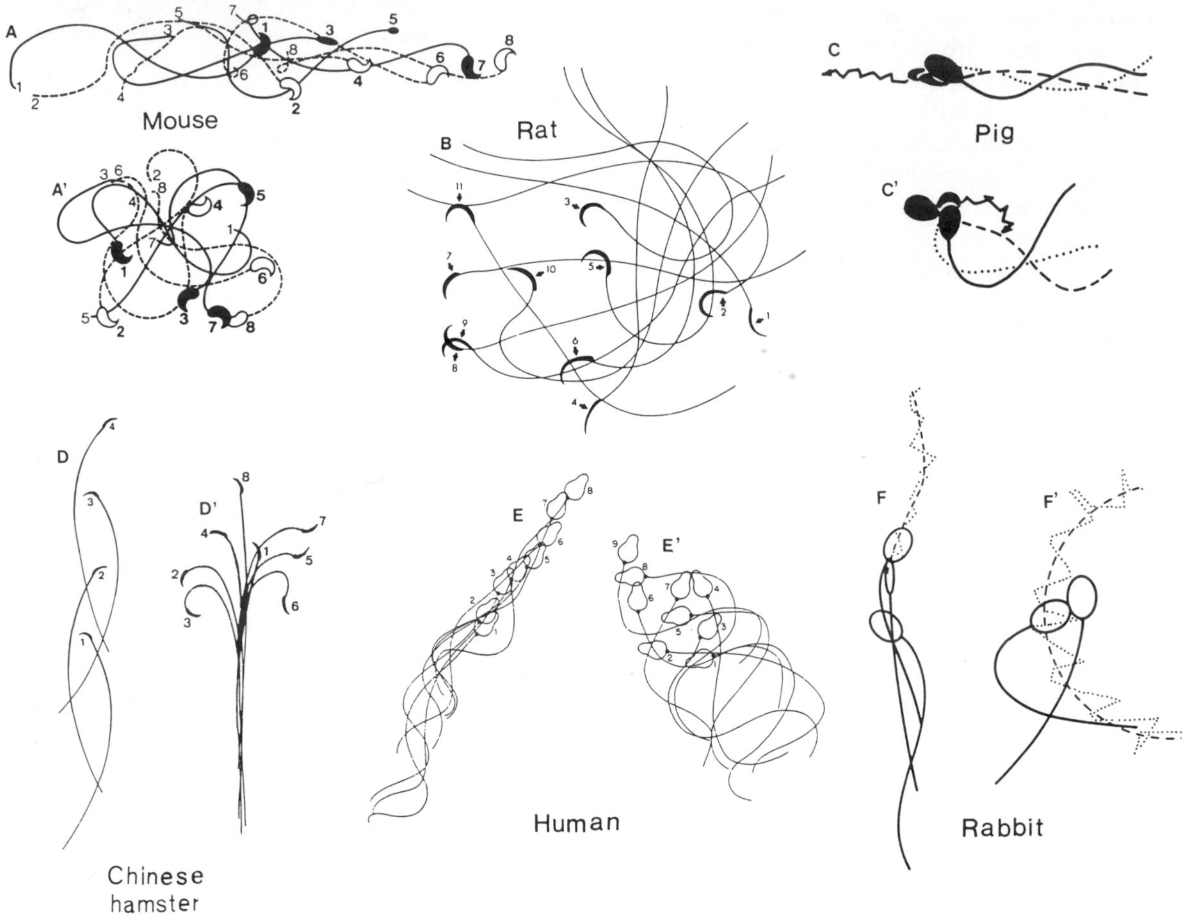

FIG. 30. Diagrams showing patterns of sperm movement before (**A–F**) and during hyperactivation (**A′–F′**). References: mouse (166), rat (1477), pig (1527), Chinese hamster (539), human (1271), and rabbit (461).

The Site where Sperm Hyperactivation Begins *In Vivo*

In the rabbit, all spermatozoa in the oviductal isthmus are weakly motile (93,380), whereas most spermatozoa in the ampulla are hyperactivated (461). This suggests that the hyperactivated motility of rabbit spermatozoa begins sometime before or after they leave the isthmus. In the hamster and mouse, spermatozoa seem to begin hyperactivated motility shortly before they are released from the isthmus. Hyperactivated motility may assist the spermatozoa in breaking free from the isthmus reservoir (872,1503). According to Shalgi et al. (1479) and Olds-Clarke and Sego (1321), hyperactivated hamster and mouse spermatozoa placed in the uteri of estrous females cannot enter the oviducts very efficiently. Apparently, the uterus is not the place for hamster and mouse spermatozoa to initiate their hyperactivated motility.

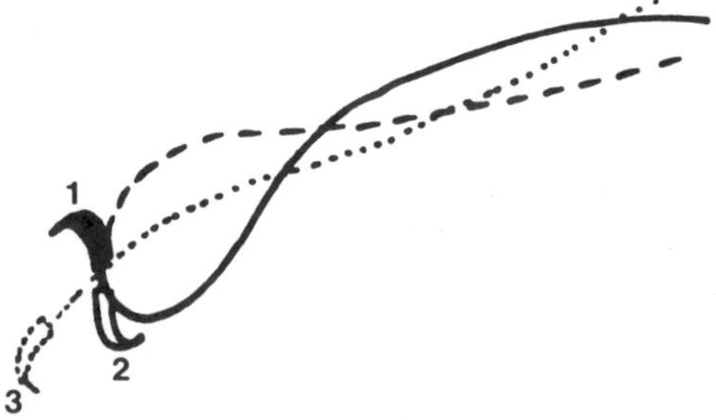

FIG. 31. A hyperactivated golden hamster spermatozoon during penetration through the viscous cumulus oophorus. (Redrawn from video photomicrographs in ref. 1115.)

Physiological Role of Hyperactivation

Some investigators have cast doubt on the physiological role of sperm hyperactivation in fertilization because they have never seen a typical figure-eight movement in the fertilization medium, or saw a figure-eight-like movement in seminal plasma or shortly before sperm death. However, the balance of evidence indicates that there is a close correlation between the ability of spermatozoa to display hyperactivated motility and the ability of spermatozoa to fertilize zona-intact eggs (Fig. 32) (159,

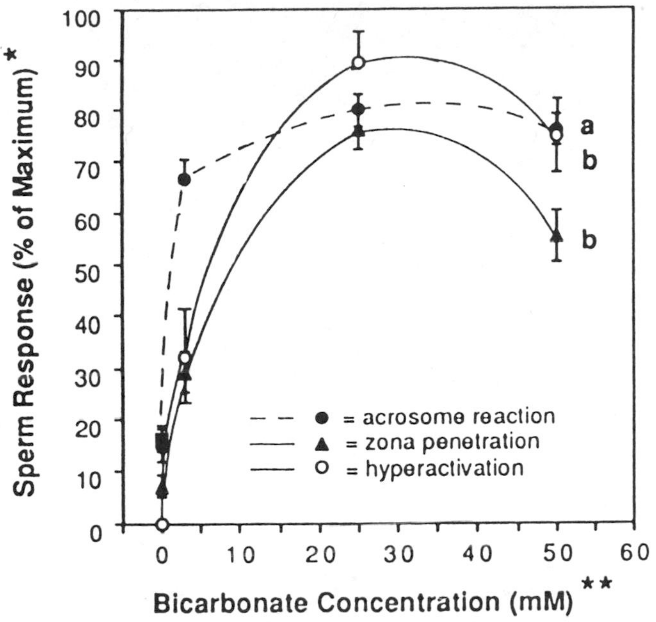

FIG. 32. Effects of extracellular bicarbonate concentration on the acrosome reaction, hyperactivation, and zona penetration by hamster spermatozoa. Note that there is a close correlation between sperm hyperactivation and zona penetration. (From ref. 768, with a slight modification.)

172,532,768,1093). Hyperactivated motility of spermatozoa, as seen *in vitro,* is apparently physiological because spermatozoa displaying hyperactivated motility have also been observed through the semitransparent wall of the ampullae of hamster and mouse oviducts during the periovulatory period (261,527,872,1529). In addition, hyperactivated spermatozoa have been collected from the ampullae of the rat (1477), rabbit (108), guinea pig (540), pig (1527), and sheep (118) about the time of fertilization.

The nondirectional component of hyperactivated motility may assist the spermatozoa in detaching from the epithelium of the inner folds and crypts of the oviductal isthmus where spermatozoa preferentially attach during *in vivo* capacitation (872,1502). The strong thrusting power generated by the vigorous tail movements may also facilitate spermatozoa in swimming through the viscous fluid of the oviduct (872,1526,1528) as well as the egg vestments, particularly the relatively "tough" zona pellucida (262,530,734,1696). As already stated, there is a close correlation between hyperacitvated motility of spermatozoa and the sperm's ability to penetrate the zona. If spermatozoa undergo hyperactivation prematurely in the wrong place in the female tract, it may result in exhaustion of spermatozoa and the failure of these spermatozoa to fertilize (1171,1317,1320). Figure 33 illustrates the possible relationships of sperm hyperactivation with capacitation, acrosome reaction, and other events in fertilization (530,1697).

Mechanism of Sperm Hyperactivation

Background

The physical condition and chemical constitution of the medium markedly influence the initiation and maintenance of hyperactivated motility. Hamster spermatozoa, for example, never initiate hyperactivated motility in Ca^{2+}-free or Ca^{2+}-deficient media (532). When the spermatozoa are first hyperactivated in the regular Ca^{2+}-containing medium and then transferred into a Ca^{2+}-deficient medium, they remain hyperactivated. But, 30 to 60 min later none are hyperactivated. The loss of hyperactivated motility in the Ca^{2+}-deficient medium is reversible as the addition of a normal concentration of Ca^{2+} (about 2 mM) back to the medium restores hyperactivated movement almost instantly (532). The requirement for extracellular Ca^{2+} for hyperactivation has been reported in the mouse (14,109,166,168,1285), guinea pig (547), and pig (1527). The presence of bicarbonate ions in the medium is beneficial for hyperactivation, although perhaps not essential (70,753,768,1285). Potassium ions (93,169) and the types of energy substrates in the medium (93,109,134,172,530) are also important for the initiation and maintenance of hyperactivated motility.

Biochemical Bases of Sperm Activation and Hyperactivation

From the studies on the spermatozoa of various invertebrates and vertebrate species, it is well established that

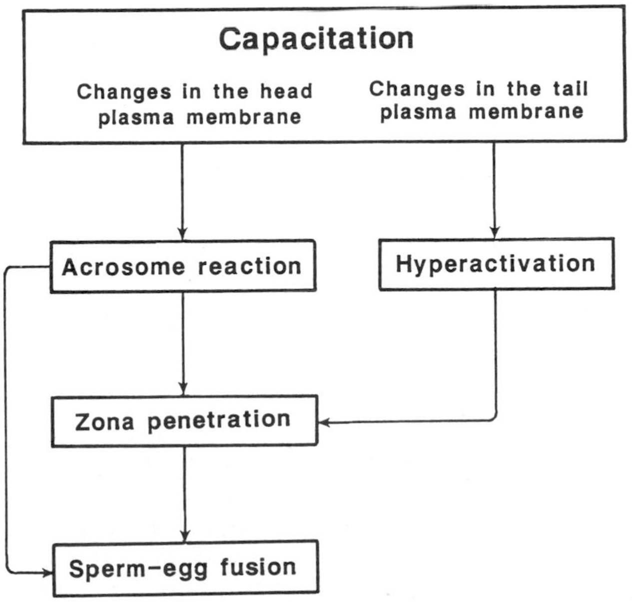

FIG. 33. Possible relationships among sperm capacitation, acrosome reaction, and hyperactivation. (From ref. 1697.)

the activation of quiescent spermatozoa (epididymal/vas deferens spermatozoa in the case of mammals, and testicular spermatozoa in the case of sea urchin and fish) is coupled with a rise in the intracellular cAMP level (for reviews, see 734,1275,1563). In the salmonid fishes, intracellular K^+ fluxes upon exposure of the spermatozoa to fresh water. Concomitantly, Ca^{2+} influxes from the surrounding water (840) or is released from intracellular stores (772). An increase in the intracellular Ca^{2+} level stimulates adenylate cyclase, resulting in a transient increase in intracellular cAMP. The elevated cAMP level stimulates protein kinase A, which subsequently activates trypsin kinase. Activated trypsin kinase phosphorylates tyrosine residues of an axonemal 15-kDa protein. This protein phosphorylation allows the axoneme to slide and bend (1275). Once the axonemal protein is phosphorylated, and as long as it remains phosphorylated, cAMP is unnecessary for sperm movement. The presence of ATP alone is sufficient to maintain the axoneme sliding and bending.

There seems little doubt that in mammals Ca^{2+}, adenylate cyclase, cAMP, protein kinase, and protein phosphorylation are all involved in the initiation of sperm motility (734,1563). The presence of G proteins and protein kinases in the sperm tail has been reported. However, many important questions remain unanswered. For instance, why do (e.g., hamster) spermatozoa show an initial burst of vigorous motility followed by a less vigorous phase of motility before initiation of hyperactivated motility? Are some forms of receptors involved in sperm activation? If so, where do they exist and what are their ligands? Spermatozoa of many mammalian species can initiate motility in the absence of extracellular Ca^{2+}. Does this mean that Ca^{2+} released from intracellular stores is more important in activating adenylate cyclase? What triggers Ca^{2+} release or Ca^{2+} influx? If a Ca^{2+} influx really takes place, where does it occur, along the entire surface of the spermatozoon or in restricted points (Fig. 34)?

The mechanism of motility initiation of quiescent spermatozoa, particularly its triggering mechanism, is not clear. Therefore, it is not surprising that the mechanism of hyperactivation is less well understood. What is fairly certain is that (i) extracellular Ca^{2+} is needed for initiation and maintenance of hyperactivation, (ii) sperm tail contains both G protein (975,980,1034) and protein kinase (1261,1341,1423). Here I propose a working model for the mechanism of sperm hyperactivation (Fig. 35). Hyperactivated motility normally takes place upon completion of capacitation, suggesting that the loss or alteration of the surface coat of the sperm tail during or at the end of capacitation exposes or activates putative receptors (R). The receptors, when activated either spontaneously or by ligands (using some medium component?), stimulate G protein, which in turn activates Ca^{2+} channels allowing a transient Ca^{2+} influx. The Ca^{2+} that

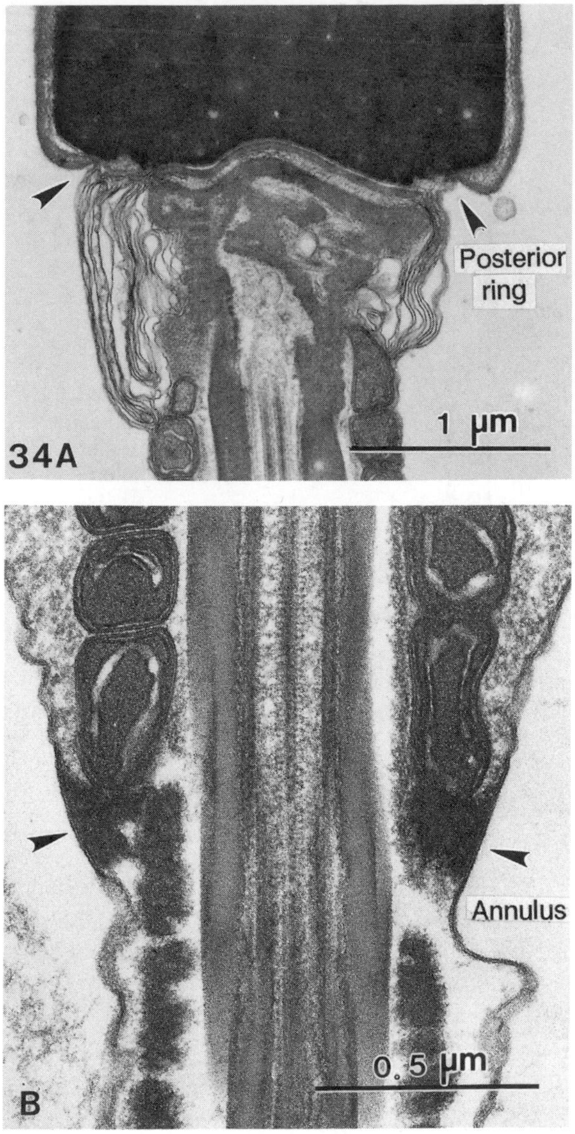

FIG. 34. Posterior ring (**A**) and annulus (**B**) of golden hamster spermatozoon. Like the ciliary necklace and plaque (ref. 1668), these structures may be the sites of Ca^{2+} entry into sperm tail. (B provided by Dr. Gary E. Olson.)

enters then stimulates adenylate cyclase (Ad) to initiate a cAMP-protein kinase cascade. Activated G protein may also activate Na^+/H^+ channels (antiport), allowing a rise in intracellular pH. Studies using demembranated sperm models have revealed that the concentrations of intracellular Ca^{2+}, H^+, and cAMP regulate the wave form of sperm tail (982,1170,1259,1563), whereas the intracellular $MgMg^{2+}$ level influences the stiffness of the axoneme (413).

Lindemann and Kanous (1172) have proposed, based on their studies on demembranated spermatozoa, that sperm quiescence in the epididymis, activation upon ejaculation and hyperactivation of capacitated spermatozoa can all be explained in terms of intracellular centrations of Ca^{2+}, H^+, and cAMP (Table 4). Recently

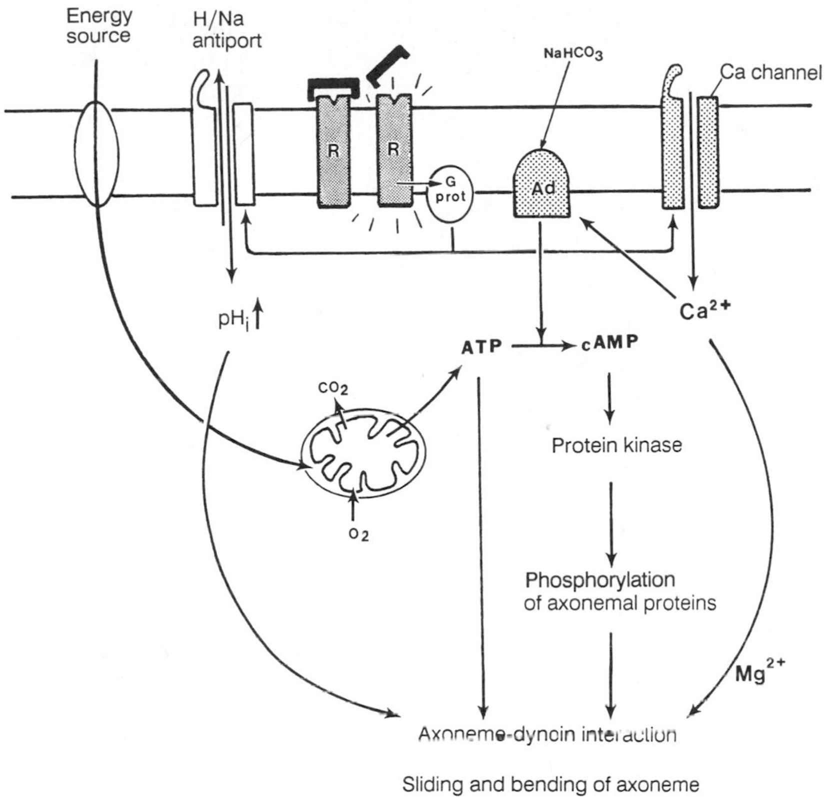

FIG. 35. A hypothetical model of sperm hyperactivation. For explanation, see the text.

Suarez et al. (1530) measured the intracellular Ca^{2+} concentration of hamster spermatozoa using a Ca^{2+}-sensitive fluorescent dye, Indo-1. They found that Ca_i^{2+} concentration in hyperactivated hamster spermatozoa with large flagellar beat amplitude is considerably higher than that in nonhyperactivated spermatozoa with much smaller flagellar beat amplitude (compare Fig. 36A and B). Interestingly, Ca_i^{2+} in hyperactivated spermatozoa is higher not only in the flagellar midpiece, but also in the head (acrosomal and postacrosomal) region (Table 5). In the flagellar region, Ca_i^{2+} oscillation is more or less synchronous with flagellar beating in a low viscosity medium (Fig. 36A,B). These facts seems to indicate that there is a close correlation between Ca_i^{2+} level and beat amplitude/frequency of the flagellum.

TABLE 4. *The possible relationship between intracellular condition and the mode of sperm motility, based on experiments using demembranated spermatozoa*

Motile state	Intracellular Ca^{2+}	Intracellular pH	Intracellular cAMP
Quiescent	High (>10 μM)[a]	Low (<6.8)	Low (<1 μM)
Activated	Low (<1 μM)[a]	High (6.6–7.8)	High (>10 μM)
Hyperactivated	High (>1 μM)[a]	High (>7.0)	High (>10 μM)

From refs. 1172 and 1173.

[a] According to the studies using fluorescent pH indicators fura-2 and quin-2 (698, 1586, 1627), the intracellular Ca^{2+} concentrations of membrane-intact hamster and bull spermatozoa are in the order of 100–200 nM, or 0.1–0.2 μM. It is possible that under the experimental conditions used, the naked (treated) axoneme was less sensitive to Ca^{2+} changes than the axoneme within membrane-intact spermatozoa. However, the trend in the Ca^{2+} effect on axonema probably remains unchanged.

Under optimal *in vitro* capacitation conditions, spermatozoa must be able to maintain (or attain) a cAMP level high enough for hyperactivation. There are close relationships between loss of sperm motility and a drop in cAMP level and dephosphorylation of a 55-kDa sperm protein (784). The failure of spermatozoa to exhibit hyperactivated motility, if it happens, could be due to the inability of the spermatozoa to generate a high level of cAMP essential for the initiation of hyperactivated motility. In such cases, addition of membrane-permeable dibutyryl cAMP or a phosphodiesterase inhibitor such as caffeine or pentoxifylline to the medium would allow the spermatozoa to exhibit hyperactivated motility (167,767,1340,1621) to facilitate fertilization (717,952).

Like the acrosome reaction, there may be true and false hyperactivation. *True* (physiological) hyperactivation occurs in live, motile spermatozoa, whereas the *false* occurs in moribund spermatozoa. As the plasma membrane of dying spermatozoa begins to lose its semiper-

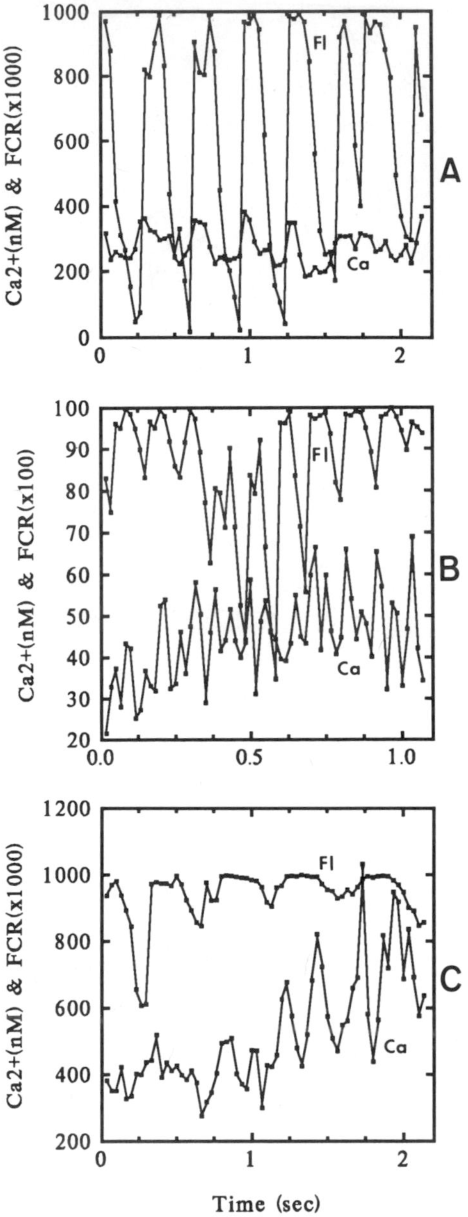

FIG. 36. $[Ca^{2+}]_i$ oscillations (Ca) and flagellar-bend oscillations (Fl) of the golden hamster sperm tail. (**A**) A hyperactivated spermatozoon. (**B**) A fresh, nonhyperactivated spermatozoon. (**C**), A hyperactivated spermatozoon placed in a viscous, 1.5% methyl cellulose-containing medium; the spermatozoon is prevented from displaying high amplitude flagellar beatings, but Ca^{2+} oscillations are not prevented. (From ref. 1530.)

meability, extracellular Ca^{2+} may enter the cell. It may cause a temporary increase in the tail beating frequency and amplitude. Spermatozoa may exhibit hyperactivatedlike movements that some investigators have witnessed in semen or among dying spermatozoa in culture.

For more details on the biochemical bases of activation and hyperactivation, readers are referred to refs. 475,734,974,1048,1049,1172,1275,1563 and 1668.

SPERM INTERACTION WITH CUMULUS OOPHORUS

The eggs of eutherian mammals are surrounded by vestments through which spermatozoa must pass before fusing with the egg plasma membrane. The zona pellucida, which lies immediately next to the egg proper, is a relatively thick, elastic coat composed of several glycoproteins. In most eutherian mammals, the zona is further surrounded at ovulation by the cumulus oophorus (Fig. 37). In some ungulates (e.g., sheep and cows), monotremes, and marsupials, the cumulus is shed either before or shortly after ovulation (63,414). In such cases, the zona is the only egg vestment the spermatozoa must pass through before effecting fertilization.

Some Properties of the Cumulus Oophorus

The cumulus is composed of cells and their matrix. The major component of the matrix is a polymerized hyaluronic acid (2500 kDa) (396) that is conjugated with proteins (1629). The matrix is secreted by cumulus cells during resumption of meiosis, causing a rapid expansion of the cumulus prior to ovulation (Fig. 38) (705, 921,922,1573,1581). In electron micrographs, the matrix of the fully expanded cumulus appears as a fibrous network among cumulus cells (1366,1558,1719). The matrix extends into pores in the outer region of the zona (1555,1573).

During oogenesis, the follicular cells immediately above the growing oocytes, called the corona radiata, extend slender processes through the zona to the surface of the oocyte. In many species, these processes are withdrawn from the zona during resumption of meiosis, but in some species (e.g., the rabbit), the withdrawal of the

TABLE 5. *Intracellular Ca^{2+} concentration (nM) in various regions of activated and hyperactivated hamster spermatozoa*

Sperm	Acrosomal region	Postacrosomal region	Proximal midpiece	Distal midpiece
Activated	38.5 ± 9.1	35.7 ± 11.6	7.7 ± 5.5	12.5 ± 6.7
Hyperactivated	124.6 ± 49.7	229.2 ± 80.7	161.2 ± 52.3	190.9 ± 51.5

From Ref. 1530.

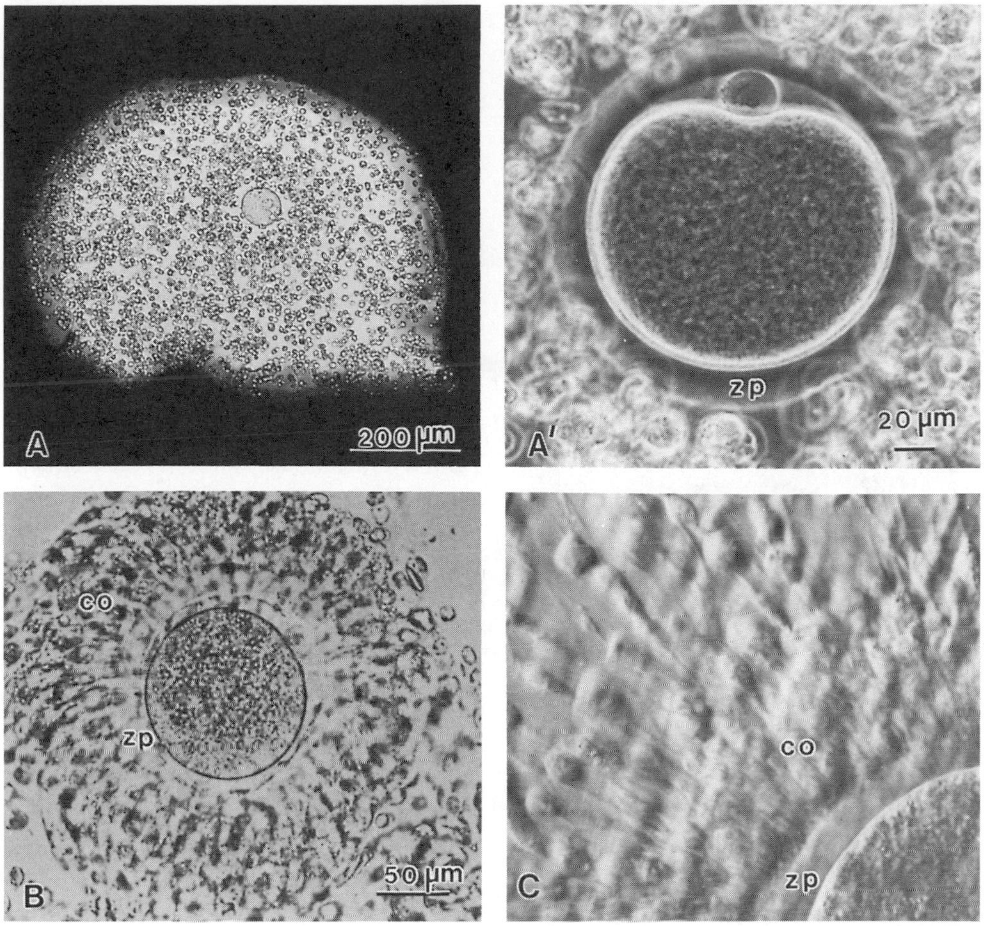

FIG. 37. Egg-cumulus complexes. (**A**) Golden hamster egg (*center*) in the cumulus oophorus; the cumulus is placed in India ink-containing medium to show the boundary of the cumulus clearly. (**A′**) A recently ovulated hamster egg under a higher magnification, slightly compressed between a slide and coverslip; corona and cumulus cells are indistinguishable from each other. (**B**) A recently ovulated rabbit egg surrounded by several layers of tightly packed corona cells; outer cumulus cells, more loosely packed, had been removed with hyaluronidase before photograph. (**C**) An ovarian cattle egg with radially arranged corona and cumulus cells. (B from ref. 877.)

processes is incomplete even after ovulation. In these species, the corona cells that surround the zona are readily distinguishable from the loosely packed outer cumulus cells (Fig. 37B) (877). In species where the withdrawal of the cytoplasmic processes from the zona is complete by the time of ovulation (e.g., mice and hamsters), corona and cumulus cells are morphologically indistinguishable from each other (Fig. 37A′). Cumulus cells may continue to synthesize and secrete progesterone and prostaglandins even after ovulation (1465).

The cumulus cells surrounding the growing oocyte are arranged radially (Fig. 37C). This radial arrangement of the cumulus cells is not evident in the fully expanded cumulus oophorus. But in the undisturbed (nondistorted) cumulus, there may be invisible radial acellular "channels" along which the spermatozoa swim.

Sperm Entry into the Cumulus

It was once thought that many spermatozoa surround each egg, loosening or dispersing the cumulus, so that one could penetrate the egg. This happens when eggs are inseminated *in vitro,* but not *in vivo,* with a large number of spermatozoa. Under natural *in vivo* conditions, very few spermatozoa are present near the egg at fertilization. During the course of fertilization, the sperm to egg ratio can be 1:1 or even less (120,533,1477,1500). Perhaps in most mammals, the cumulus oophorus disperses after, not before, fertilization (16,63).

Austin (19) was the first to report that spermatozoa must be capacitated in order to penetrate into the cumulus. Uncapacitated spermatozoa may attach to the surface of the cumulus, but fail to penetrate it. Capacitated

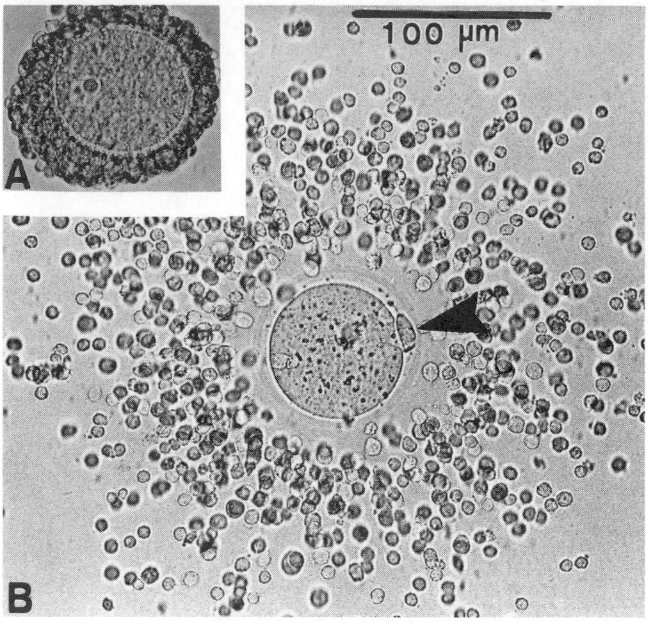

FIG. 38. Mouse cumulus oophorus before and after expansion. **(A)** A mouse egg isolated from a preovulatory antral follicle, with compact cumulus; **(B)** a recently ovulated mouse egg in an expanded cumulus. An *arrowhead* indicates the 2nd polar body. (From ref. 922a.)

spermatozoa, on the other hand, readily penetrate the cumulus (19,121,462,467,468,819,839). Interestingly, spermatozoa that have completed their acrosome reactions before encountering the cumulus stick to the surface of the cumulus and do not penetrate it (121, 462,468). Only capacitated spermatozoa with "intact" acrosomes are able to enter the cumulus. According to White et al. (1656), human spermatozoa do not seem to need to undergo a formal capacitation period after ejaculation in order to penetrate the cumulus. However, these investigators admitted the possibility that a small percentage of the spermatozoa they used could have been capacitated prior to insemination. In fact, some human spermatozoa may be capacitated *in vitro* very quickly (i.e., within 2 hr) (1230). Whether or not human spermatozoa require capacitation for cumulus penetration remains to be determined.

How do the capacitated spermatozoa pass through the cumulus to reach the surface of the zona pellucida? Are the acrosome reaction and acrosomal enzymes involved in this process? According to Talbot (467,1556) and Cherr et al. (103), most capacitated hamster spermatozoa penetrate through the cumulus and reach the zona without undergoing the acrosome reaction. Sea urchin and frog spermatozoa, which do not possess hyaluronidase, can penetrate the hamster cumulus with great ease (472). I have observed that rooster spermatozoa, which are lacking in hyaluronidase (cf. ref. 311) can penetrate the hamster cumulus without any difficulty (1735).

Do these observations mean that spermatozoa may pass through the cumulus without any aid from acrosomal enzymes or is the cumulus penetration by spermatozoa purely mechanical? What about hyaluronidase, which has been thought to be the cumulus lysin for many years? Is cumulus penetration by spermatozoa purely mechanical? Talbot and her associates (468,472) are of the opinion that hyaluronidase, although not essential, facilitates cumulus penetration. They (468,554) speculate that the plasma membrane of hamster spermatozoa carries hyaluronidase, and this surface hyaluronidase (not the hyaluronidase within the acrosome) aids in sperm passage through the cumulus. The notion that hyaluronidase on the sperm surface assists cumulus penetration by spermatozoa is not new (13,260,294,295,323), and hyaluronidase is not the only enzyme believed to be on the sperm surface. Other surface enzymes implicated for cumulus penetration include acrosin (1572), beta-galactosidase, and arylsulfatase (148,1294).

Where do these surface enzymes come from? Zao et al. (554) surmise that the sperm surface adsorbs these enzymes during spermatogenesis, epididymal transit, and/ or capacitation. The possibility that some acrosomal content escapes through the "intact" outer acrosomal and plasma membranes prior to the acrosome reaction has been considered (348,465,554), but unequivocal evidence to support this intriguing notion is yet to be presented.

Once spermatozoa enter the cumulus, not surprisingly, the pattern of their movement changes, perhaps because of high viscoelasticity of the cumulus matrix. Spermatozoa appear to require considerable thrust to advance through the cumulus matrix. Hamster spermatozoa within the cumulus matrix display a hatchetlike movement (Fig. 31) (889,1115). Apparently, the viscoelasticity of the cumulus matrix prevents spermatozoa from displaying high-amplitude flagellar movement. In fact, when the spermatozoa within the cumulus leave it, they immediately resume hyperactivated movement with a higher flagellar beat frequency and curvature (1114). Distortion, tearing, and compaction of the cumulus fibrous network, as revealed by electron microscopy (1719), reflect the physical resistance spermatozoa face when they swim in the cumulus matrix. High viscoelasticity may not be the only factor that alters the swimming pattern within the cumulus. According to Tesarik et al. (1580), human spermatozoa displaying nonprogressive, whiplash (hyperactivated) movement in the medium initiate a more progressive, linear movement within 5 min of exposure to the solubilized (hyaluronidase-digested) cumulus matrix material, which binds to the sperm surface (1576).

Inhibition of Sperm Penetration into the Cumulus

Since uncapacitated spermatozoa are unable to penetrate the cumulus, the sperm surface may appear very sticky to the matrix of the outer cumulus. At least something on the surface seems to be removed or altered during capacitation so that the sperm head becomes less sticky and is then able to slide through the cumulus. Cummins and Yanagimachi (121) reported that myocrisin and sodium heparin (hyaluronidase inhibitors) prevent capacitated hamster spermatozoa from entering the cumulus. Although this was interpreted as an indication of hyaluronidase involvement in sperm entry in the cumulus, one cannot rule out the possibility that these reagents make the sperm surface very sticky by altering its surface charge.

In some cases of infertility where spermatozoa cannot enter the cumulus efficiently, removal of the cumulus by hyaluronidase may improve *in vitro* fertilization (1156,1619). Although the presence of antiacrosomal enzyme antibodies within the cumulus was suspected (1156), inefficient sperm entry in the cumulus could be due in part to (i) the presence of anticumulus antibodies or (ii) an abnormality in the chemical characteristics of the cumulus matrix such that even capacitated spermatozoa are trapped on or in the cumulus.

Tesarik (1570) attempted to prevent *in vitro* human fertilization using anticumulus antibodies, with unexpected results. The antiserum, raised against solubilized (hyaluronidase digested) human cumulus matrix, failed to prevent cumulus disintegration by human spermatozoa, whereas it did prevent both the acrosome reaction and sperm–zona binding. The reason for this is unclear. In other studies, Tesarik (1582,1583) raised antibodies against the mouse cumulus–egg complex. When tested *in vitro*, the antibody reacted with both mouse cumulus and zona. Sperm binding to the zona was blocked by these antibodies (679). When female mice were injected with the antibody three times at 2-week intervals and then mated either on the day of the third injection or 3 weeks after the last injection, none became pregnant. When the same animals were mated 5 weeks after the last antibody injection, all animals became pregnant and delivered offspring of normal litter size. This transient contraceptive action of the antibody was not straightforward. The antibody, at high doses, disturbed egg maturation and ovulation for some unknown reason (1570).

Role of the Cumulus

Since the eggs of some eutherian species do not have a cumulus or have only remnants of the cumulus oophorus at the time of fertilization and the eggs of most species can be fertilized *in vitro* without an intact cumulus or cumulus components (530,843,1200), some investigators consider that the cumulus is unnecessary junk. However, in various species, including the mouse (1078,1377), Chinese hamster (359), pig (1121), and cattle (1717), the presence of cumulus oophorus or cumulus cells around the eggs is beneficial for *in vitro* fertilization. The beneficial effect is particularly evident when the sperm concentration (1487) or the concentration of albumin in the medium is low (171).

Figure 39 summarizes the results of experiments in which mouse eggs were inseminated *in vitro* with or without the cumulus oophorus (1078,1601). Spermatozoa from ten different males of the same strain were used. When inseminated at the same sperm concentration (2–3.5 × 10^5/mL), all or nearly all of the cumulus-intact eggs were fertilized, whereas cumulus-free eggs were fertilized erratically. Apparently, the cumulus reduces or minimizes individual variations of male fertility. Not all the males of a species are superfertile. For *in vitro* experiments, we tend to pick males that give high fertilization rates, eliminating the low-fertility males even if we know these males are completely fertile when they mate naturally.

The cumulus may be one of nature's efforts to reduce individual variations in male fertility. The cumulus factors beneficial to fertilization could be soluble components of the cumulus (715,850). Some cumulus factors are known to stimulate sperm motility (783), while others promote the acrosome reaction (1233,1489, 1568,1569,1581). Although cumulus components may indeed have the ability to induce the acrosome reaction, a more likely function of these components is the sensitization of spermatozoa to the zona pellucida, which carries acrosome reaction-inducing ligands. Observations by Cherr et al. (819) support this view. It is conceivable that spermatozoa "rub off" some of their surface coat while passing through the fibrous network of the cumulus. Other proposed functions of the cumulus include facilitation of fertilization by offering a larger target for spermatozoa to encounter (20,735), prolonging the fertile life of eggs (396), slowing down the process of zona hardening after ovulation (922,979), preventing acro-

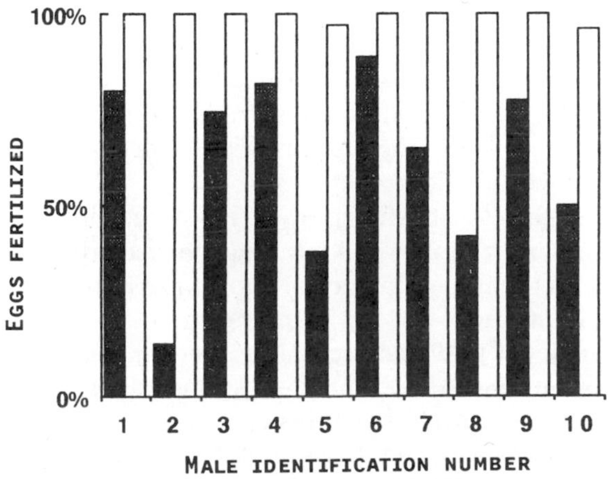

FIG. 39. *In vitro* fertilization of cumulus-intact (*white column*) and cumulus-free mouse eggs (*black column*), showing that the presence of the cumulus reduces individual variations of male fertility. (Drawn based on the data in refs. 1078 and 1601.)

some reacted spermatozoa from swimming away from the zona surface (758), filtering and admitting only a subpopulation of spermatozoa that are capable of interacting with the egg (938), and weeding out spermatozoa that are unable to swim strongly.

Another possible function is to aid sperm penetration into the zona. As already stated, the fibrous network of the cumulus is anchored to the zona (1719). This would prevent the zona (egg) from rotating within the cumulus when spermatozoa are moving on or in the zona. Zonae (eggs) in an immobilized state may allow the spermatozoa to push their heads against the zona strongly with less effort. When cumulus-free zona-intact eggs are inseminated *in vitro,* many spermatozoa attach to the zona surface. As the spermatozoa beat their tails, the eggs are rotated continuously. It is amazing that some spermatozoa are able to enter and pass through the zona under such seemingly hopeless circumstances where the zona (egg) keeps rotating.

Function of Acrosomal Hyaluronidase

The exact function of hyaluronidase in fertilization still remains unclear, although it was the first acrosomal enzyme identified and characterized almost 50 years ago (cf. 311). Lorton and First (302) maintain that bovine sperm hyaluronidase has no biological function because (i) hyaluronidase is unable to disperse the bovine cumulus oophorus surrounding ovarian eggs, and (ii) oviductal eggs shed the cumulus spontaneously within a few hours after ovulation. These investigators inferred that "this acrosomal enzyme is not functional in this species, but is a remnant of evolutional changes." However, there is room for argument. First of all, the inability of hyaluronidase to disperse the cumuli around ovarian eggs is not unique to this species. The cumuli of ovarian eggs of many other species are resistant to hyaluronidase. As mentioned earlier, synthesis and polymerization of hyaluronic acid is not complete until shortly before ovulation. Since bovine eggs recovered from the oviduct immediately after ovulation are surrounded by the cumulus oophorus (73), the conclusions of Lorton and First require reevaluation.

Nevertheless, the function of acrosomal hyaluronidase in fertilization is still puzzling, particularly in view of the fact that spermatozoa are able to pass through the cumulus without the acrosome reaction. According to Drobnis et al. (889), acrosomal contents (including hyaluronidase) released on the zona surface digests the cumulus matrix locally, and this enables the proximal region of the sperm tail to move more freely (Fig. 40). The sperm head confronting the zona will then be able to exhibit stronger and more efficient thrust and torque. Talbot (468) speculated that part of the hyaluronidase released on the zona surface following the acrosome reaction diffuses through the zona into the perivitelline space. This hyaluronidase, as well as the hyaluronidase bound to the sperm's inner acrosomal membrane, may digest hyaluronic acid in the zona and perivitelline space before the spermatozoon fuses with the egg plasma membrane (486).

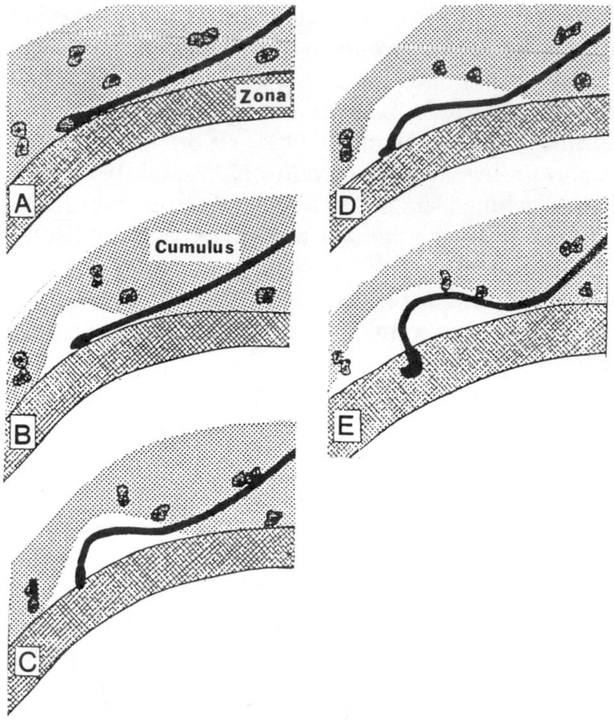

FIG. 40. Diagrams showing that hyaluronidase released from the acrosome at the zona surface depolymerizes the cumulus matrix locally to enable the proximal region of the sperm tail to move more freely. (From ref. 890.)

Recently Gmachil and Kreil (980a) suggested that hyaluronidase may be involved at the point of the sperm–zona interaction. According to them, the amino acid sequence of bee venom hyaluronidase has a considerable homology with the guinea pig PH-20, a protein that is believed to participate in sperm–zona binding (841, 1381). Although it is possible that hyaluronidase and PH-20 have similar protein characteristics, it has not been established that PH-20 has biochemical and biological characteristics similar to those of hyaluronidase. Thus the role of this enzyme in fertilization still remains uncertain.

SPERM INTERACTION WITH ZONA PELLUCIDA

Function of the Zona

The zona pellucida is a glycoprotein coat that protects the fragile eggs and embryos from physical damage (1291). Although normal fertilization and preimplantation development are possible *in vitro* in the absence of zona pellucida (1284,1561,1584,1602), its presence is essential for the development of the preimplantation embryo *in vivo*. Without the zona, the blastomeres of an embryo may dissociate from each other (909) or adhere to blastomeres of other embryos, thus losing the individuality of the embryos. Furthermore, the embryo may adhere to the oviductal epithelium and perish (787, 854,1256,1560). Suggested roles of the zona as a protection from invasive bacteria and leucocytes (1291) or from immunological attack (925a) are unlikely, because macromolecules like immunoglobulins (1329,1471) and even virus particles (1003), yeast (1131), and follicle cells (1724) pass easily through the zona. Incidentally, the oviductal luminal fluid in which preimplantation embryos develop is usually free of leucocytes and microorganisms. The oviduct may thus possess some mechanisms that inhibit invasion and/or survival of such invasive cells and organisms.

For the spermatozoa deposited in the female tract, the zona is the last physical barrier that they must pass before fertilizing the egg. The egg itself has an intrinsic mechanism to block the multiple entry of spermatozoa, but in most species part of this mechanism is shared with the zona (see the section on "Cortical Reaction and Polyspermy Block" of this review). In most animals, the perivitelline space of the fertilized egg contains macromolecules secreted by the egg before and after fertilization. In some mammals, macromolecules of oviductal origin are added to the perivitelline space (771,1111). Thus the zona also helps to provide a specialized microenvironment for the developing embryo.

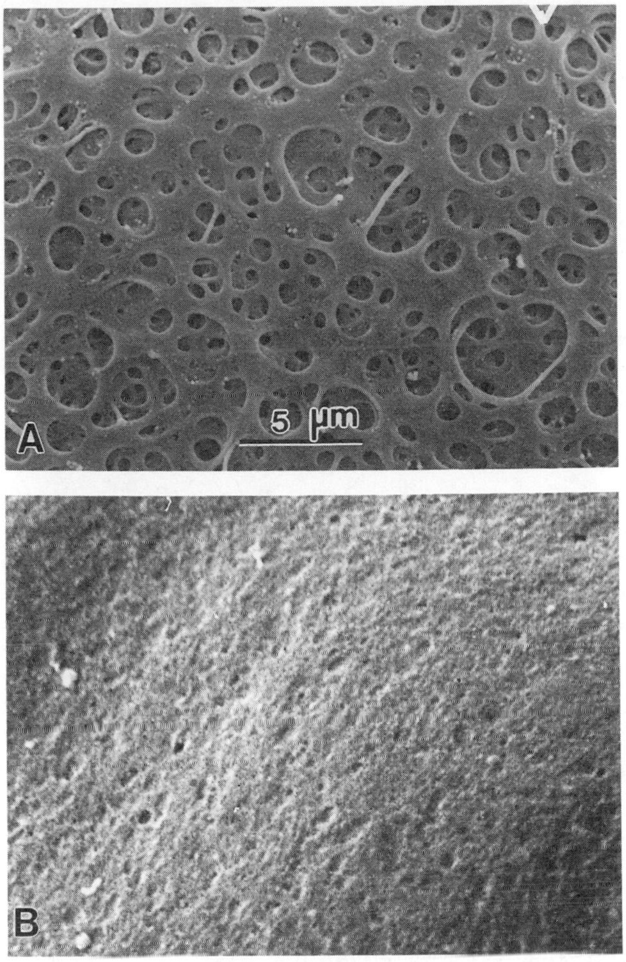

FIG. 41. Scanning electron micrographs of the outer (**A**) and inner (**B**) surfaces of the zona pellucida of the golden hamster egg. (From ref. 392.)

Properties of the Zona

Zona Morphology

The size (20) and rigidity (1115) of the zona pellucida varies greatly from one species to another, as does the thickness. It is very thin in some species (e.g., 1–2 μm in marsupials) and very thick in some others (e.g., 16 μm in pig) (898). In general, the material constituting the zona of a fully mature egg is more densely packed in the inner half than in the outer half. The outer zona surface has a fenestrated spongelike structure (Fig. 41A), perhaps the result of follicle cells' processes extending through the zona to the oocyte surface during oocyte growth. In contrast, the inner surface shows a fine granular appearance (Fig. 41B) (1364) or a fine microtubular appearance (927). The spongy appearance of the outer zona may reflect the maturity of zona (egg) and sperm penetrability, since human zonae with a smooth outer surface are less penetrable by spermatozoa than those with a spongy appearance (926).

The zona in some species has an almost even optical density throughout its thickness (e.g., the rat and mouse), whereas in others it has two or more zones or layers with different optical densities (898). In the golden hamster, the zona appears optically homogeneous before the egg enters the oviduct. Soon after entry of the egg into the oviduct, however, the outer region of the zona becomes much more light-refractory than the inner layer. This can be recognized easily by phase-contrast microscopy (1710). This zona alteration is due to the binding of an oviductal glycoprotein to the zona (see below). In some species (e.g., rabbit and pig), the zonae of oviductal eggs have two or more distinct layers with different optical densities (878,904). Whether this is due to the intrinsic nature of the zona or the addition of oviductal glycoproteins to the zona is not clear.

Zona Chemistry

The zona pellucida consists of several components. For example, pig zona includes 71% protein, 19% neutral hexose, 2.7% sialic acid, and 2.4% sulfate (140). The glycoprotein components of the zona have a polypeptide backbone that is deferentially glycosylated, yielding extensive charge heterogeneity. Three families of acidic

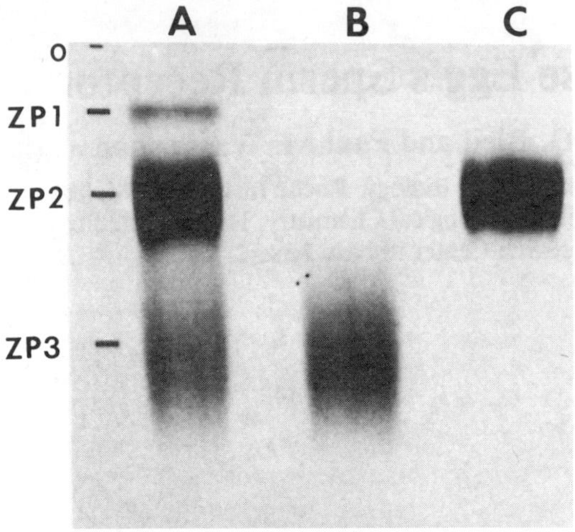

FIG. 42. SDS-PAGE analysis of purified mouse zona pellucida glycoproteins. (**A**) Three zona components; (**B**) purified ZP3; (**C**) purified ZP2. (From ref. 69.)

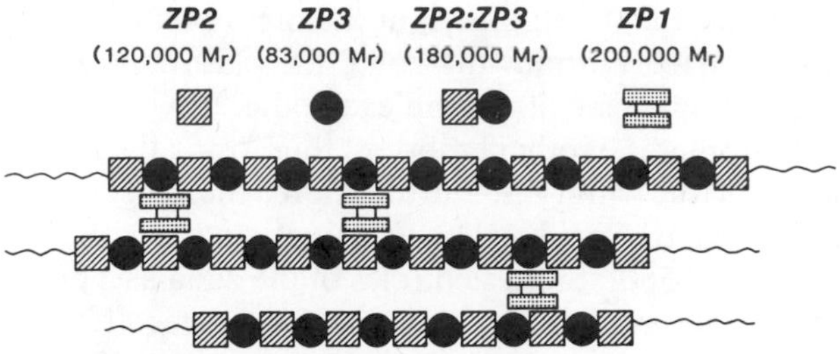

FIG. 43. Schematic representation of the arrangement of glycoproteins in mouse zona filaments, based on electron microscopy, immunological, and chemical cross-linking experiments. (From ref. 1639.)

glycoproteins and five components have been identified in the pig: (a) the 90-kDa family, which gives rise to the 65-kDa and 25-kDa components as a consequence of limited proteolysis and reduction of intermolecular —S—S— bonds; (b) the 55-kDa alpha family; and (c) the 55-kDa beta family (221,222,422,1028). When deglycosylated, average apparent molecular weights reduce to the following: the 90-kDa family (65–70 kDa), 65-kDa components (50–55 kDa), the 55-kDa alpha and beta families (36–40 kDa), and 25-kDa components (15 kDa). The 55-kDa alpha and beta families constitute 70% to 80% of total pig zona glycoproteins (1028), with the sperm receptor activity for zona located in the 55-kDa alpha family (1721). The structure of acidic N-linked saccharide chains of the 55-kDa glycoprotein has been determined (1295).

The mouse zona has three components: ZP1 (185–200 kDa), ZP2 (120–140 kDa), and ZP3 (83 kDa) (67,198,1484) (Fig. 42). The hamster zona also has three components: ZP1 (200–240 kDa), ZP2 (150 kDa), and ZP3 (56–80 kDa) (8,1262,1640). Likewise, the zonae of humans, rabbits, rats, and horses are each composed of three families of glycoproteins (684,1206,1240,1473), whereas the zona of the cat has only two families (1206). The chemistry and molecular biology of the zona pellucida and the molecular mechanism of zona-related phenomena have been intensively studied during the past several years. The considerable progress made in this area of research is due to the endeavors of many investigators, in particular the groups led by Wassarman and Dean who have used the laboratory mouse as a model. Table 6 shows some of the biochemical characteristics of the mouse zona glycoproteins. Figure 43 is a schematic representation of the arrangement of mouse ZP1, ZP2, and ZP3.

TABLE 6. *Characteristics of mouse zona pellucida glycoproteins*

Characteristics	Zona pellucida glycoproteins		
	ZP1	ZP2	ZP3
Relative amount in ZP	~44	~44	~11
Glycoprotein *Mr*			
a	200 kDa	120 kDa	83 kDa
b	185 kDa	140 kDa	83 kDa
Polypeptides			
No. per molecule	2	1	1
Subunit *Mr*	75 kDa	77 kDa	44 kDa
No. of amino acids		713	424
Intermolecular —S—S—	+	−	−
Intramolecular —S—S—	−	+	+
N-linked oligosacc.	+	+	+
(No.)	(?)	(6)	(3–4)
O-linked oligosacc.	+	+	+
(No.)	(?)	(?)	(?)
Sialylation	+	+	+
Sulfation	+	+	+

From refs. 1639 and 1643.

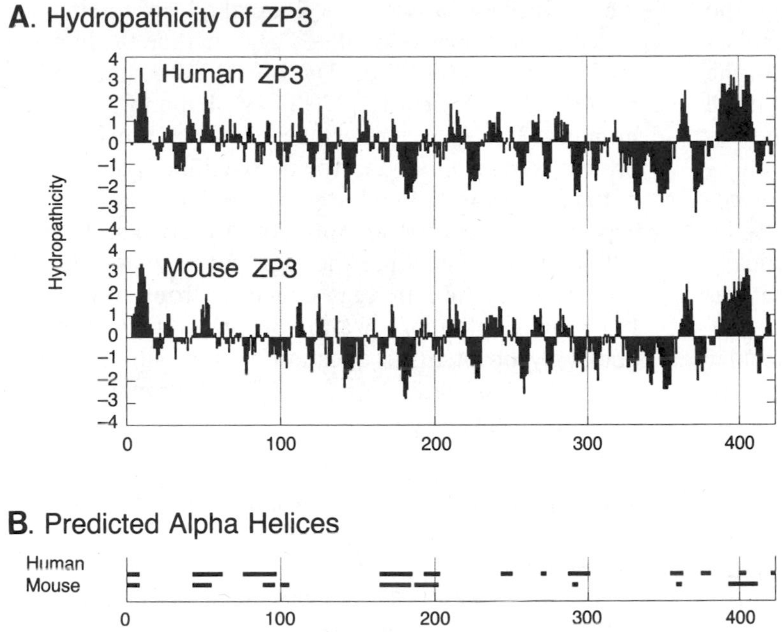

FIG. 44. Comparison of the secondary structure of human and mouse ZP3 proteins. (**A**) Hydropathicity of human and mouse ZP3, indicating the degree of conservation between the two proteins. (**B**) Alpha-helical structure of human and mouse ZP3. (From ref. 809.)

The nucleotide sequences of ZP3 mRNAs and the deduced amino acid sequence of ZP3 have been determined for the mouse (1124,1409), hamster (1125), rabbit (1467), and human (809). The mouse, human, and hamster ZP3 genes contain eight exons each. The encoding sequences of the mouse and human genes are 74% identical, and they encode proteins of 424 amino acids that are 67% identical. As evidenced by the similarity of their predicted secondary structure, many substitutions are conservative (Fig. 44) (809). The hamster gene encodes a 422 amino acid protein that is 81% identical to mouse ZP3 (1125). The overall structure of ZP3 mRNA is conserved among mammals (1409). The mouse ZP3 gene is on chromosome 5, approximately 9 cM distal to the GUS locus; the ZP2 gene is on chromosome 7, approximately 11 cM distal to the c locus (1191) (Fig. 45).

Origin and Biosynthesis of the Zona

The question of whether the zona material is synthesized and secreted by follicle cells or by the oocyte was controversial for many years (e.g., 821,1002,1010), but it is now clear from studies on the mouse that in this species, and perhaps in many others, the zona is produced exclusively by the oocyte. The evidence to support this view includes the following: (i) Growing oocytes freed from zonae are able to synthesize the mass of all glycoproteins found in the zona; and (ii) *in situ* hybridization assays of ovaries using ZP2 and ZP3 molecular probes (cDNAs and oligonucleotides) indicate that ZP glycoproteins are synthesized in the oocytes, but not in follicles or other cell types.

The synthesis and secretion (exocytosis) of zona glycoproteins begin as soon as the oocyte is surrounded by follicle cells and starts to grow. The synthesis and secretion continue until close to the time of ovulation, with a peak activity about the time when the oocytes attain full size (762,1169,1369,1420,1640). In the mouse, ZP2 and ZP3 (and perhaps ZP1) are synthesized and secreted si-

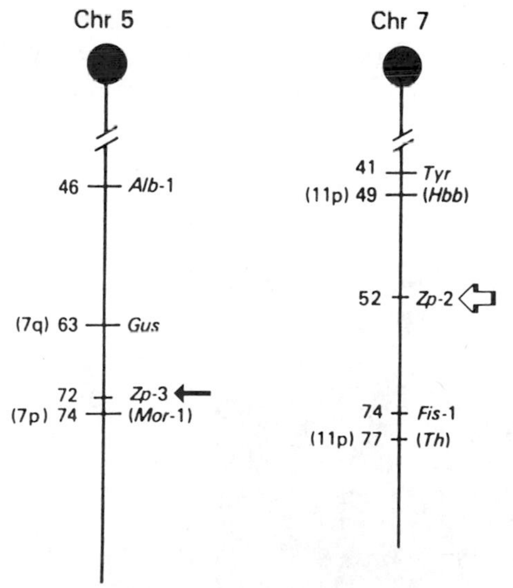

FIG. 45. Loci of mouse ZP2 and ZP3 genes on chromosomes 5 and 7. Numbers on the left indicate the approximate map distance of selected loci in centimeteres from the centromere (*black filled circles* at top of lines). The numbers in parentheses represent the chromosomal location of genes that have been mapped in the human. Relevant loci are listed on the *right*. (From ref. 1191.)

multaneously (Fig. 46), but, in other species (e.g., the pig), different glycoproteins may be synthesized and secreted at different stages of oocyte growth (1551). In the mouse, ZP3 is first synthesized as a 44-kDa polypeptide that is first core-glycosylated, giving rise to 53- and 56-kDa intermediates, and then processed to complex oligosaccharides prior to secretion as a mature 80-kDa glycoprotein (1440). Synthesis of ZP2 occurs similarly (997). The question of whether the zona is modified chemically and physically during the final stage of oocyte maturation remains controversial (cf. 856,1429 for references). For more details of zona biochemistry and molecular biology, readers are referred to reviews by Wassarman (1639,1640,1643) and Dean (866,867).

Other Zona Components

When examined by scanning electron microscopy, the outer surface of the zona has a spongy appearance, whereas the inner surface has an irregular particulate appearance (392). Hyaluronic acid, the major component of the cumulus oophorus, extends into the outer spongy region of the zona (470,1573), and therefore can be considered a part of the native zona.

It is generally believed that the chemical composition of the zona does not change drastically during the growth and maturation of the oocyte or even after ovulation. According to Fowler and Grainge (164), however, the mouse zona loses glycosaminoglycans several hours before ovulation. There is convincing evidence that glycoproteins of oviductal origin bind firmly to zonae as the eggs are transported from the ovary to the oviduct. In the case of the hamster, this glycoprotein has been identified as a 150–250-kDa molecule secreted by nonciliated epithelial cells of both the ampulla and isthmus of oviduct (667). Species in which oviductal glycoproteins are added to the zonae of ovulated eggs include the hamster (165,666,683,1109,1110,1310,1424,1710), sheep (973), pig (87,222,505), cattle (770,1648), baboon (771) and human (1399). In the mouse, a 214-kDa oviductal glycoprotein is incorporated in the perivitelline space instead of the zona (947,1111). In the baboon, an oviductal glycoprotein is incorporated into both the zona and perivitelline space (771). Since the eggs that have not seen the oviduct (e.g., human eggs collected from ovaries for IVF) can develop into healthy offspring, the role of oviductal glycoproteins in question must be supplemental, rather than essential, for normal fertilization and/or development of the eggs.

Sperm Binding to and Penetration through the Zona

Time Course

When eggs are collected from the oviducts of naturally mated females while fertilization is in progress, spermatozoa are seldom observed within the zona pellucida, suggesting that sperm passage through the zona is very rapid (17,64). Austin (17) estimated that the rat spermatozoon *in vivo* probably takes no more than a few minutes to pass through the zona. According to Sato and Blandau (432), who continuously observed sperm penetration through the zona pellucida of mouse eggs inseminated *in vitro,* spermatozoa took an average of 20 min (ranging from 15 min to 26 min) to cross the zona. This cannot be considered fast. If spermatozoa take more than 15 min to pass through the zona *in vitro,* one would expect to see spermatozoa within zonae rather frequently when eggs are collected and examined around the time of fertilization. Since this is not the case, it is

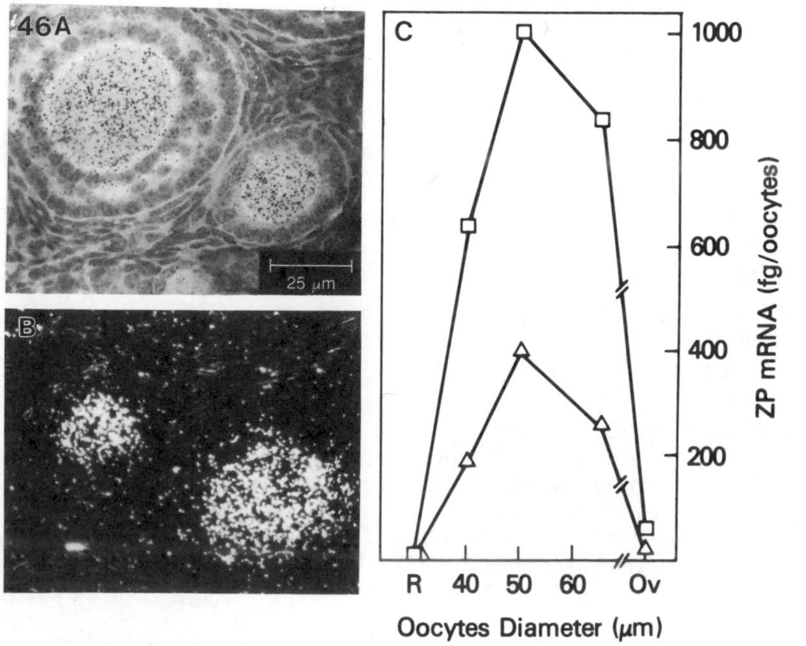

FIG. 46. Synthesis of ZP2 and ZP3 in the mouse. **(A)** *In situ* hybridization of ovarian tissue hybridized with ^{35}S-labelled ZP3 antisense RNA transcripts; grains represent endogenous ZP3 transcripts in the cytoplasm of growing eggs. **(B)** Same as A but viewed with dark field optics. **(C)** The amount of ZP2 and ZP3 produced during egg growth from resting stage (*R*) to ovulation (*OV*). (From ref. 867.)

possible that the conditions Sato and Blandau employed *in vitro* were not directly comparable to the situation *in vivo*.

The time when spermatozoa begin to penetrate eggs *in vitro* seems to be influenced greatly by the physiological state of spermatozoa. For instance, when golden hamster spermatozoa are collected from the cauda epididymidis and mixed immediately with eggs in a capacitation medium, many acrosome-intact spermatozoa attach to the zona surface almost immediately after insemination. These spermatozoa begin to undergo the acrosome reaction sometime thereafter and actual penetration of spermatozoa into the eggs occurs commonly 3 to 4 hr later (542). When hamster spermatozoa are capacitated prior to mixing with the eggs, sperm penetration of the zona can be seen as early as 10 min after insemination (524). Fully capacitated hamster spermatozoa can fertilize 100% of the eggs within 30 min of insemination *in vitro* (1516). Storey et al. (460) reported that *in vitro* "capacitated" mouse spermatozoa mixed with cumulus-intact eggs seldom penetrated zonae in less than 2 hr after insemination. According to Motomura and Toyoda (335), however, capacitated mouse spermatozoa penetrated the zona much faster. Heads of some spermatozoa were already within the zona by 5 min after insemination, and the zonae of 15% of the eggs were completely penetrated by sperm heads 11 min after insemination. By 20 min after insemination, the zonae of 80% of the eggs had been penetrated completely. Thus, the time spermatozoa spend on and in the zona seems to be influenced greatly by how well the spermatozoa are capacitated. At least in the hamster and mouse, fully capacitated spermatozoa in the most favorable environment do not seem to spend much time on and in the zona.

Biochemistry of Sperm–Zona Binding

Zona Ligands

Capacitated spermatozoa bind firmly to the surface of the zona pellucida before penetrating it. Sperm–zona binding is mediated by the interaction between the zona and sperm surface molecules. This was demonstrated first by Gwatkin and Williams (202), who found in the hamster that solubilized zonae pellucidae prevented capacitated spermatozoa from binding to the surface of intact zonae *in vitro*. The solubilized zonae apparently did not affect the motility of spermatozoa. Why were the spermatozoa unable to bind to the zona in the presence of solubilized zonae? It is reasonable to assume that the surface of spermatozoa carries receptors for zona molecules and that saturation of these receptors with solubilized zona molecules renders the spermatozoa incapable of binding to (or recognizing) native intact zonae. There is no doubt that the sperm membrane carries a molecule or molecules with strong affinity to the zona pellucida (372,463,1357).

The chemical nature of the zona molecules responsible for sperm–zona binding has been studied most extensively in the mouse. According to Wassarman and his associates (506,507,1638–1640,1643), two zona components, ZP2 and ZP3, have sperm-binding activities. In the mouse and perhaps many other species, ZP3 is the primary ligand that specifically binds to the plasma membrane over the acrosomal cap of acrosome-intact spermatozoa; ZP2 is the secondary ligand which preferentially binds to the inner acrosomal membrane of acrosome-reacted spermatozoa (Fig. 47) (69,760,1276).

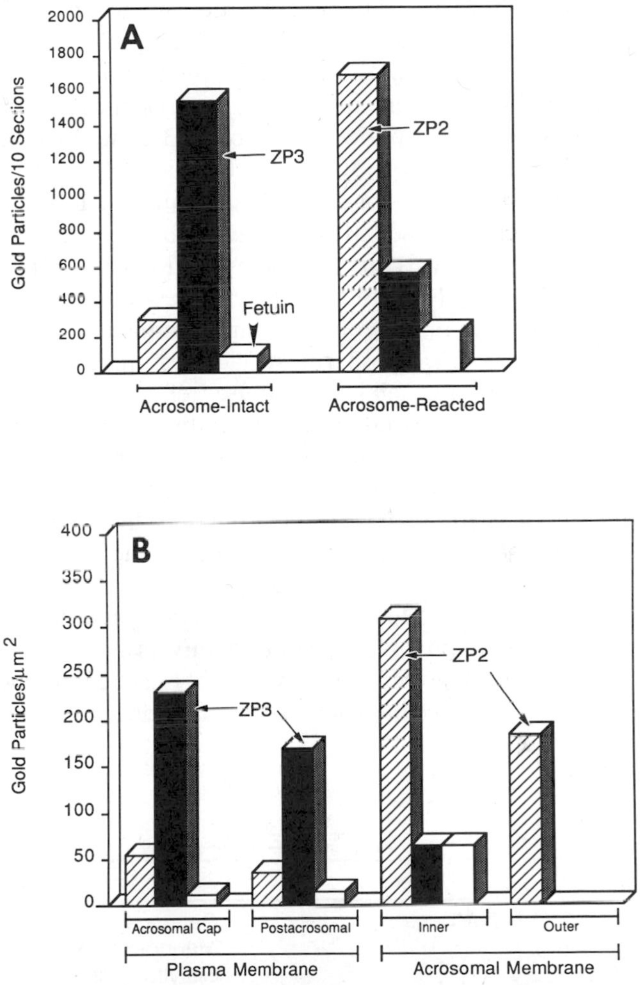

FIG. 47. Binding specificity of purified mouse ZP2 and ZP3. Acrosome-intact and acrosome-reacted mouse spermatozoa were exposed to purified ZP2 or ZP3 coupled with colloidal gold particles. The average number of particles on each 1 μm^2 of the plasma membrane and of the acrosomal membrane was determined. Fetuin, a plasma glycoprotein, was used as the control. (**A**) ZP3 and ZP2 each has preferential affinity to the acrosome-intact and acrosome-reacted spermatozoa, respectively. (**B**) ZP3 preferentially binds to the sperm plasma membrane, whereas ZP2 binds to the acrosomal membrane which is exposed after the acrosome reaction. (From ref. 1276: note that the acrosomal cap region defined in this report includes the equatorial segment which is exceptionally large in the mouse as shown in Fig. 15 of this review.)

Mouse ZP3 has both sperm-binding and acrosome reaction-triggering activities. Its O-linked carbohydrate moiety is responsible for binding of the acrosome-intact spermatozoa to the zona (163). The sperm-binding activity seems to reside within the carboxyl-terminal half of the ZP3 glycopolypeptide (1422). Although the importance of the carbohydrate moiety of the zona glycoprotein in the sperm–zona binding has been demonstrated in various species (670,763,1271,1475,1552,1603), the precise oligosaccharide sequence of the zona glycoprotein may not be critical for the sperm-binding activity. According to Beebe et al. (736), recombinant mouse ZP3, obtained from cells other than oocytes, has both sperm-binding and acrosome reaction-inducing activities equivalent to those of native ZP3, despite apparent differences in glycosylation between the two molecules.

The induction of the mouse sperm acrosome reaction requires the polypeptide moiety of ZP3 as well as the carbohydrate moiety (506,939). The possible mechanism by which ZP3 triggers the acrosome reaction has already been discussed. It is interesting to note that solubilized zona induces the acrosome reaction faster (162), more efficiently (68), and in a less species-specific manner (1263) than native zona. Perhaps, a larger number of ZP receptors on the sperm surface (estimated to be 10,000–50,000 per cell in the mouse [ref. 69]) bind ZP3 molecules when the latter are in solution compared to when the spermatozoon interacts with an intact zona. Zonae, after fixation with aldehydes, cannot be penetrated by spermatozoa, but they do retain the ability to bind spermatozoa (1457,1505) and induce the acrosome reaction (1615). As stated already, glycoproteins secreted by the oviduct bind to zonae as soon as the eggs enter the oviduct. Although this may not be a universal phenomenon, oviductal glycoprotein, when it is added to the zona, may enhance the zona's ability to induce the acrosome reaction (1710).

Zona Receptor of Spermatozoa

Freshly ejaculated spermatozoa, or spermatozoa collected from the epididymis are able to attach to the zonae of homologous or heterologous species (218,1545). Apparently, uncapacitated spermatozoa and, in some cases, even immature spermatozoa from the epididymis are able to attach to the zonae. Such attachment is weak, easily disturbed by repeated pipetting, and generally not species-specific. On the other hand, attachment between capacitated spermatozoa and the zona is not readily disturbed by physical manipulation (724,1072,1439), and it is thus considered to be the stronger chemical binding rather than a weak physical attachment. During the past several years, a variety of candidates for the sperm's zona receptor have been proposed (Table 7) (cf. 938,1099, 1138,1434). Sperm–zona interaction is a complex phenomenon. It consists of at least three steps: (i) binding of acrosome-intact spermatozoa with the zona, (ii) binding of acrosome-reacting and acrosome-reacted spermatozoa with the zona, and (iii) penetration of acrosome-reacted spermatozoa into and through the zona. The first two are designated as the primary and secondary zona binding, respectively (763,1276). Unfortunately, most studies in the past were carried out without differentiating between these first two steps, so it is not clear from these studies whether the molecules proposed are for the primary or secondary binding.

One of the candidates for the sperm's zona receptor is proacrosin/acrosin. Both Urch and Petel (1612) and Jones (1100) believe that proacrosin binds to the zona nonenzymatically and serves as a ligand for both primary and secondary sperm binding. If proacrosin/acrosin is involved in the primary binding of the acrosome-intact spermatozoa to the zona, then these enzymes must be on the outer surface of the sperm plasma membrane over the acrosome. Although acrosin on the

TABLE 7. *Some of proposed candidates for the sperm's zona receptor*

Species	Proposed zona receptor	Ref.
Mouse	Galactosyltransferase (60 kDa)	1190, 1486
	Mannosidase	1606
	Sialyltransferase	902
	95-kDa protein	1167, 1168
	56-kDa protein	764
	15-kDa protein	1410
Hamster	26-kDa protein	1532
	Acrosin	709
Guinea pig	60–64-kDa protein	1155, 1380
	Acrosin	709
Rabbit	87-kDa protein	1331
Pig	15-kDa protein	1097
	Proacrosin (53–55 kDa)	1100–1102, 1597, 1598, 1611
	Nonproacrosin protein (55 kDa)	1355
	18-kDa protein	1442, 1443
Horse and bull	Galactosyltransferase	929
Human	Lectinlike protein (54 kDa)	665
	Acrosin	1572

plasma membrane of pig and human spermatozoa has been reported by many investigators (1571,1572,1594, 1596), immunocytochemical electron-microscopic evidence has not been convincing in support of their conclusion. All of the acrosomal enzymes are believed to be packed within the acrosome during spermiogenesis. How then is it possible for the proacrosin within the acrosome to reach the outer surface of living spermatozoa prior to the acrosome reaction? It is difficult to conceive that macromolecules like proacrosin/acrosin can pass freely through both the outer acrosomal and the overlaying plasma membrane to reach the outer surface of the plasma membrane. However, there may be an unknown mechanism that allows large molecules like proacrosin/acrosin to pass through "intact" membranes. As there is no evidence that either the male or the female tracts secrete proacrosin/acrosin, one may surmise that proacrosin/acrosin is released from dead spermatozoa in the male or female tract (or in medium) and is picked up by the surface of living spermatozoa. It is very unlikely that spermatozoa rely solely on such an unreliable source of proacrosin/acrosin to carry out their important functions. Richardson et al. (1405) were unable to demonstrate sperm-surface acrosin in rabbit spermatozoa until after the acrosome reaction. Unless or until it can be proven unequivocally that proacrosin/acrosin can pass through intrasperm membranes and these enzymes persist on the outer surface of the sperm plasma membrane during capacitation, it should be considered that the sperm's primary zona receptors are molecules other than proacrosin/acrosin.

Kopf and Gerton (1138) have surmised that the putative primary zona receptor of mouse spermatozoa has two binding sites, one for ZP3's sperm binding ligand and the other for ZP3's acrosome reaction-triggering ligand (Fig. 48). A 95-kDa mouse sperm protein with tyrosine kinase activity (804,901,1165,1168) may be this molecule. At present, we cannot rule out the possibility that the putative primary zona receptors are the decapacitation-factor-like macromolecules originating from the epididymis and/or seminal plasma (1410,1442,1443) that are not removed completely from the sperm surface during capacitation.

The strongest candidate for the sperm's secondary zona receptor is, thus far, proacrosin/acrosin. A probable site of these enzymes is the inner acrosomal membrane (IAM), which recognizes the zona (249,530) and binds to ZP2 (760,1276). The reports by Barros and his associate (709,801) on the localization of acrosin on the IAM are very interesting. These investigators incubated hamster and guinea pig spermatozoa *in vitro,* allowing them to undergo spontaneous acrosome reactions. At various times before, during, and after the acrosome reaction, spermatozoa were examined for their binding ability to antihuman and antibovine acrosin antibodies, which cross-react with hamster, guinea pig, and mouse spermatozoa. These investigators detected acrosin on

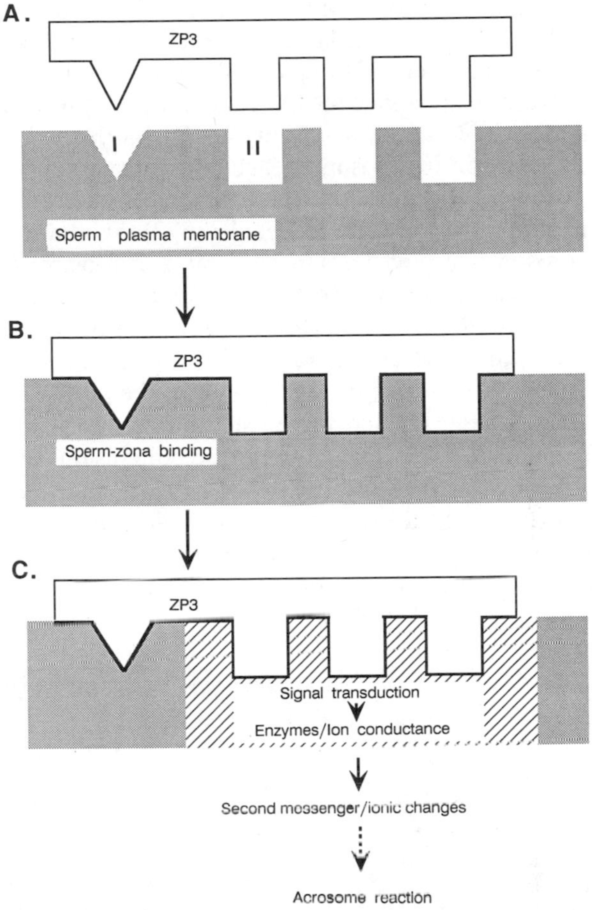

FIG. 48. Model for the interaction between zona glycoprotein ligand and the sperm plasma membrane receptor. **(A)** Sperm plasma membrane over the acrosome has at least two types of receptors, one for ZP3's sperm-binding ligand (*I*) and the other for ZP3's acrosome reaction-inducing ligand (*II*). **(B)** Successful sperm-zona binding is followed by sperm interaction with other ligands. **(C)** Once the interaction of ZP3 with sperm receptors is completed, signal transduction and second messenger/ion conductance change occurs culminating in the acrosome reaction. (Adapted from ref. 1138.)

the IAM of recently acrosome-reacted spermatozoa. Interestingly, the acrosin activity on the IAM of hamster spermatozoa disappeared rather quickly after the acrosome reaction, whereas that of the guinea pig spermatozoa did not. A fucoidin-binding substance demonstrated by Huang and Yanagimachi (240) on the IAM and on or in the equatorial segment of acrosome-reacted guinea pig spermatozoa could be proacrosin/acrosin because the fucoidin (fucose) -binding protein in boar spermatozoa has been identified as acrosin (1596).

When spermatozoa undergo the acrosome reaction on the zona, a part of the acrosomal contents is dispersed into the surrounding medium, while the less diffusible portion of the contents (together with vesiculated membranes, in some species) sticks firmly to the zona. This remnant or acrosomal ghost (545), has strong acrosin activity (709,801,1294,1571,1572,1707) and may assist sperm binding to and penetration of the zona (545,887,1362). A 64-kDa PH20 protein, believed to be the guinea pig sperm's zona receptor, migrates from the postacrosomal region to the IAM after the acrosome reaction (841,842,1383). According to Richardson et al. (1405), acrosin in acrosome-reacted rabbit spermatozoa is located in the anterior region of the postacrosomal area, not on the IAM. Tesarik et al. (1572) maintain that in acrosome-reacted human spermatozoa most of the acrosin is located in the equatorial segment and a small amount on the IAM. Arylsulfatase and galactosidase, which Nikolajczyk and O'Rand (1294) believe to be rabbit sperm's zona receptors, are found in the postacrosomal region after the acrosome reaction.

The considerable variations in the conclusions as to the chemical nature and site of the sperm's zona receptors seem to reflect the infantile stage of our research in this area. Common use of immunofluorescence technique at the light microscopic level could be the major cause of this apparent discrepancy. Unlike somatic cells, spermatozoa have complicated membrane systems. Membranes may be torn away or partly disintegrate after death of spermatozoa or chemical fixation. This results in the exposure of intracellular components (including acrosomal contents) to confuse localization experiments. Since no one using light microscopy can be sure of the degree of membrane integrity, living spermatozoa should be used for immunocytochemistry. Alternatively, specimens should be examined by electron microscopy (TEM, not SEM) at magnifications high enough to detect the structural integrity of the membranes. By doing so, we should be able to eliminate or at least reduce the confusion in the results of immunocytochemical studies.

Manner of Sperm Binding to, and Penetration into, the Zona

Uncapacitated mouse epididymal spermatozoa can bind to both the outer and inner surfaces of mouse zona (673,1545). Capacitated hamster spermatozoa bind

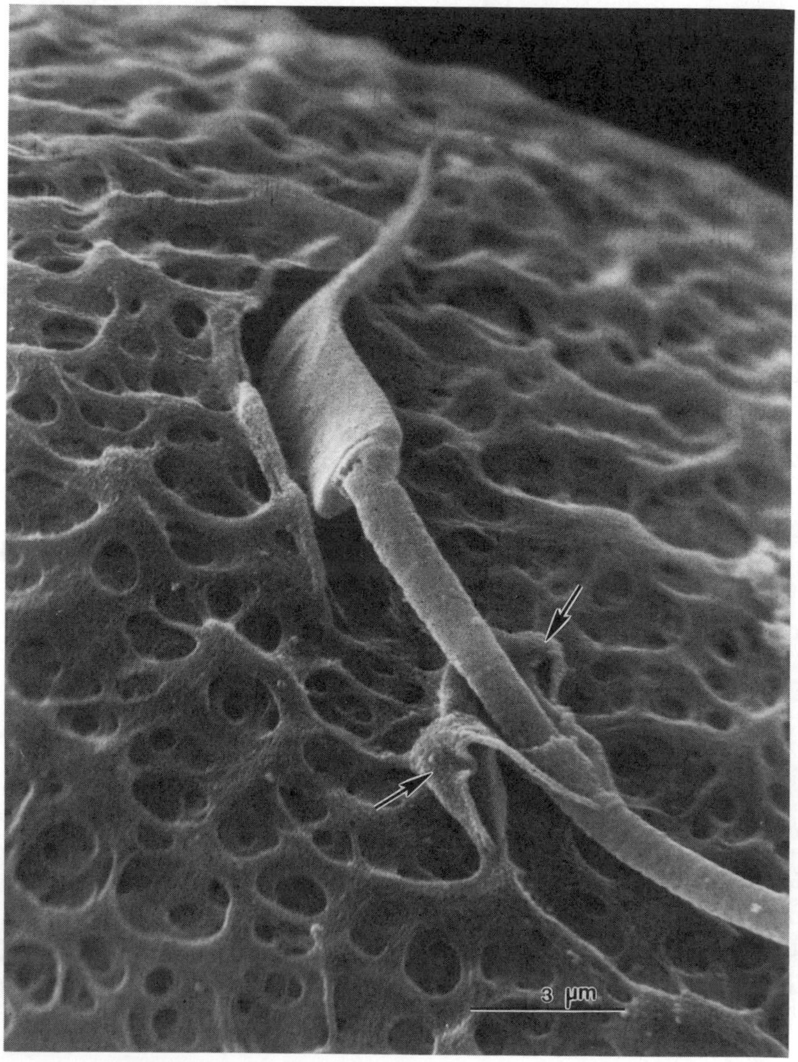

FIG. 49. Scanning electron micrograph of a golden hamster spermatozoon about to enter the zona pellucida. The acrosomal ghost (*arrow*) is seen encircling the midpiece of the spermatozoon. (From ref. 545.)

firmly to the outer surface, but may (202) or may not (392) bind to the inner surface of the zona. I found that the hamster spermatozoa, both capacitated and uncapacitated, are able to attach to the outer and inner surfaces of the zona, but the inner surface binding is considerably weaker. Spermatozoa on the inner surface of the zona do not stay there persistently (1735). Ng et al. (1290), who performed subzona insertion of human spermatozoa for infertile couples, found one human spermatozoon that appeared to have entered the zona from its inner surface. I have never observed such zona penetration by spermatozoa, at least in the hamster. ZP2 and ZP3 glycoproteins, which are responsible for sperm binding and the acrosome reaction, seem to be present throughout the zona as judged by the even distribution of the binding sites for anti-ZP monoclonal antibody (143a) and lectins (1424). It could be the physical state of the inner surface of the zona (e.g., the lack of a porous surface) or the lack of ligands that makes sperm binding and entry into the zona from the inside more difficult.

When eggs are collected from oviducts during the progression of fertilization and examined immediately, acrosome-reacted spermatozoa that are about to enter the zona or in the act of passing through the zona may be seen. Such spermatozoa almost always have acrosomal ghosts around their heads or have left the ghosts behind on the outer zona surface (Figs. 49 and 50) (115, 116,543). All prospective fertilizing spermatozoa on the zona oscillate their heads with the center of oscillation at either the inner acrosomal membrane or the equatorial segment (545). The spermatozoon passing through the zona beats its tail vigorously (Fig. 51) (175,432, 523,530,890,971,1696). The sperm head advances a little at a time and appears as though its narrowing front end cuts open the zona by an oscillatory, forward movement of the head (523,731,890). The peak force generated by the vigorous tail movement at this time is approximately 3000 μdyns, considered sufficient to break covalent bonds (887). The fertilizing spermatozoon always leaves a thin, sharply defined penetration slit in the zona. Spermatozoa of many species take curved paths through the zona (25,131,132), but vertical penetration has also been recorded (178,432,539). According to Yang et al. (548), hamster spermatozoa take an average of 7 min 3 sec (range from 4 min 20 sec to 10 min 53 sec) from the attachment to the zona until entry into the perivitelline space. Drobnis et al. (890) witnessed two hamster spermatozoa that passed through the zona in 11 min. Mouse spermatozoa take an average of 20 min (ranging from 15 to 26 min) to cross the zona (432). The

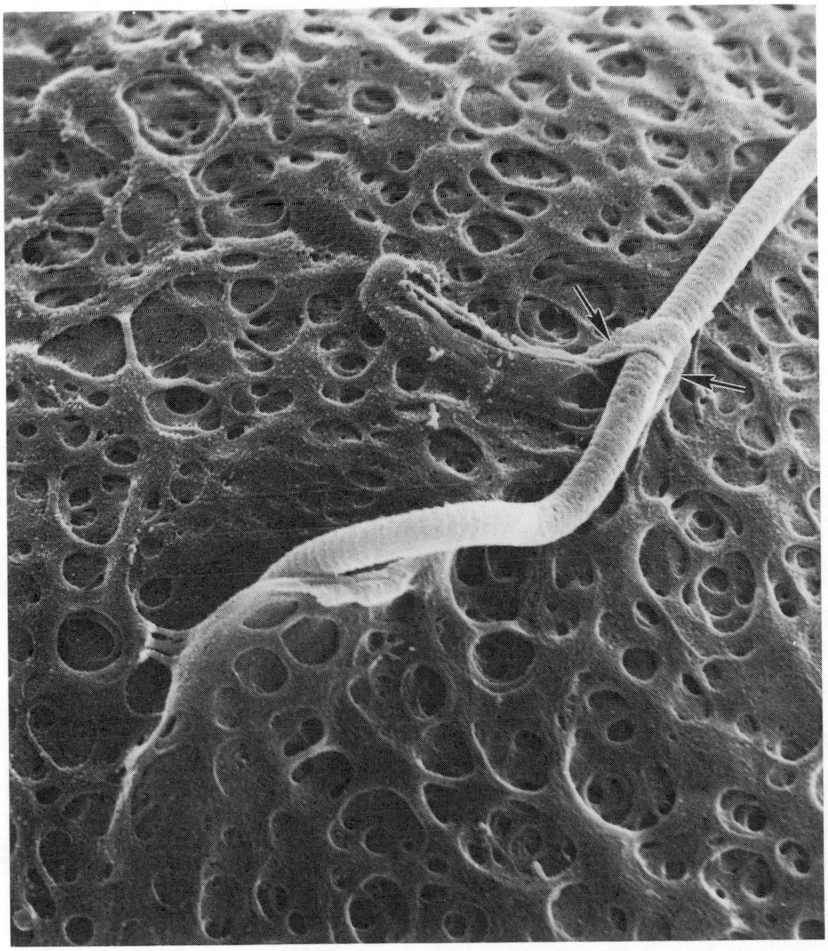

FIG. 50. Same as Fig. 49, but this spermatozoon head is deep inside the zona. (From ref. 545.)

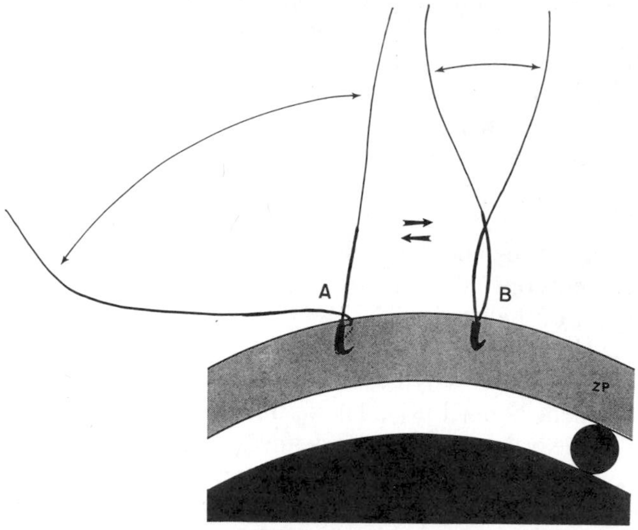

FIG. 51. Schematic representation of the tail beat shape of golden hamster spermatozoa during penetration through the zona pellucida (ZP). In all penetrating spermatozoa, motility is bimodal, having (**A**) a high-amplitude, low-frequency lever mode alternated with (**B**) a low-amplitude, high-frequency sinusoidal mode. When the zona is surrounded by intact cumulus matrix, penetration motility is also bimodal, but the distal portion of the tail is constrained by the matrix material. (Adapted from ref. 890.)

reason for large variations in time reported by these investigators is not clear, but it could be due to the differences in (i) the method of observation, (ii) the type of medium used, and, particularly, (iii) the capacitation status of spermatozoa at the time of insemination.

Mechanisms of Sperm Entry and Penetration through the Zona

In birds and the opossum, spermatozoa undergo the acrosome reaction upon contact with a very thin zona. Acrosomal enzymes released during the acrosome reaction make a hole in the zona, through which a spermatozoon swims (358,414). The major zona-hydrolyzing enzymes in these species are trypsinlike enzymes (281, 414,471a). The mechanism by which eutherian spermatozoa enter and pass through a thick zona is still not clear. For the sake of discussion, two scenarios are presented here.

Mechanical Hypothesis

In this hypothesis, sperm penetration through zona is purely mechanical. Acrosomal enzymes play no role in zona penetration by spermatozoa. The sole function of the acrosome reaction is to expose the *perforatorium,* which is the inner acrosomal membrane reinforced by underlining disulfide-rich material. The sharply pointed perforatorium cuts open the zona as the spermatozoon beats its tail vigorously. Strong sperm motility is the only requirement for sperm penetration through the zona. There is some support for this hypothesis as follows:

(i) The force generated by spermatozoon in the zona can be as great as 3000 μdyns, sufficient to break covalent bonds (887,890).

(ii) A fertilizing spermatozoon leaves a penetration slit in the zona with very sharply defined borders (25,39,43). It looks as though the spermatozoon

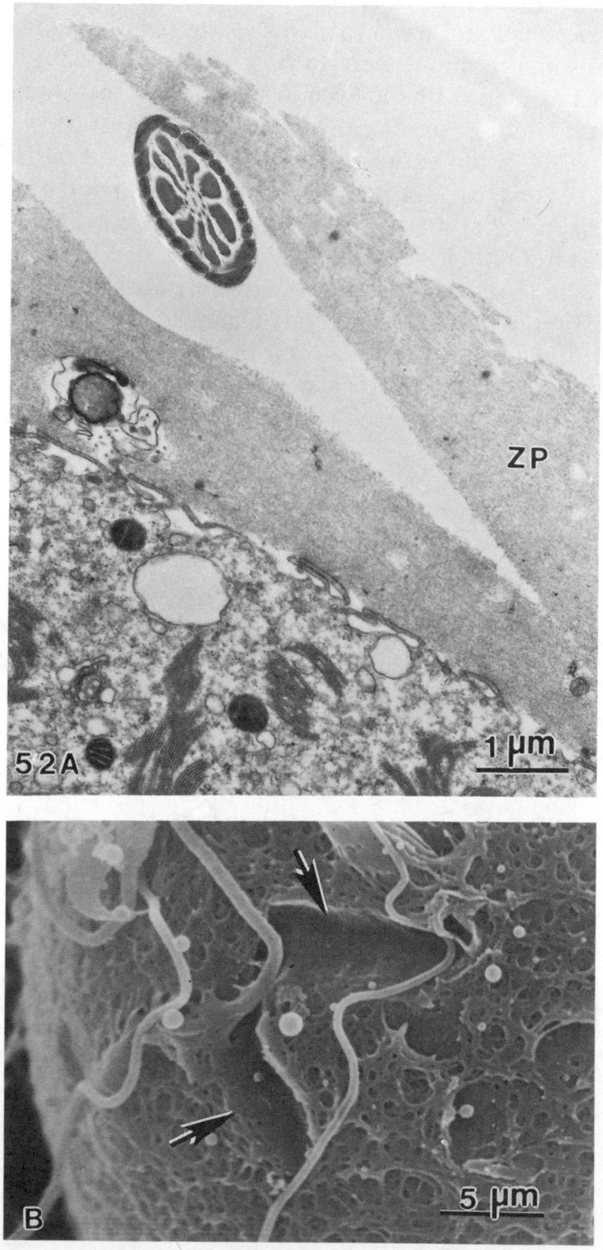

FIG. 52. (**A**) Sperm penetration slit in the zona pellucida (ZP) of Chinese hamster egg: note the sharply defined borders of the slit. (**B**) Sperm "tracks" (*arrows*) possibly made by two golden hamster spermatozoa on zona surface: eggs were inseminated *in vitro,* then washed to remove most spermatozoa. (cf. ref. 1090.) (B provided by Dr. Claudio Barros.)

physically cuts the zona rather than chemically dissolves it (Fig. 52A). Electron micrographs that show distortion and displacement of the zona's fibrous structure around the head of a penetrating spermatozoon (Fig. 53) (1361,1696) favor this view.

(iii) Proteinase inhibitors block the binding of spermatozoa to the zona surface, but once the binding is established, they can no longer prevent spermatozoa from passing through the zona (220,423).

(iv) No significant amount of acrosin is present on the inner acrosomal membrane after the acrosome reaction (1020,1057,1480,1707).

Enzymatic Hypothesis

In contrast to the above mechanical hypothesis, every step of sperm–zona interaction is enzyme-dependent. Sperm motility is of secondary importance. Enzymes (e.g., acrosin and galactosyltransferase) on the sperm plasma membrane (1196,1242,1572) serve as the sperm's primary zona receptor. The following acrosin hypothesis of sperm zona penetration is based on the findings by various investigators combined with my own perception. Acrosin, released from spermatozoa during the acrosome reaction, has unique properties. It hydrolyzes zona glycoproteins extensively in the same manner as trypsin, yet, unlike trypsin, it neither alters the gross macroscopic structure of the zona (138,788,900) nor destroys the zona's sperm-binding sites. In fact, it even enhances the zona's sperm-binding ability (1102).

Acrosin is first in its enzymatically inactive form, the proacrosin (Fig. 54A). This has a strong zona-binding ability (1611). Part of the proacrosin released from the spermatozoon during the acrosome reaction binds to the outer surface of the zona (1137,1571). Another part remains on the IAM of the spermatozoon (455,1031,1571, 1572). Proacrosin on both the zona and the IAM assists in maintaining acrosome-reacted spermatozoa on the zona. Autolytic conversion of proacrosin to an enzymatically active alpha-acrosin (Fig. 54B) is accelerated by low concentrations of zona glycoprotein, and is slowed down by high concentrations of the zona glycoprotein (1593). Therefore, on and in the native zona, where the concentration of zona molecules is very high, proacrosin may be progressively converted to alpha-acrosin a little at a time. Enzymatically active alpha-acrosin hydrolyzes and "softens" the zona (1613,1614), allowing an acrosome-reacted spermatozoon to insert its head into the substance of the zona. In the immediate vicinity of the sperm head, the zona surface appears eroded, forming a hole or sperm track (Fig. 52B) (1071,1090). This must reflect local hydrolysis of the zona surface. Further autolysis of alpha-acrosin results in the formation of beta-acrosin which still has zona-hydrolyzing ability, but no

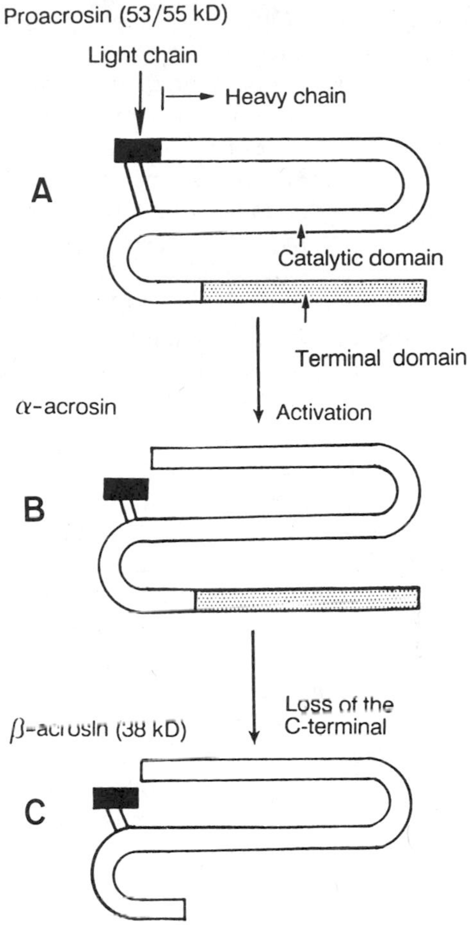

FIG. 54. Scheme of proacrosin activation pathway. Proacrosin (**A**) is activated by N-terminal cleavage of the Arg–Val bonds giving rise to the alpha-acrosin (**B**). Further processing by C-terminal cleavage results in the formation of the low molecular mass beta-acrosin (**C**). (From refs. 808, 1593a.)

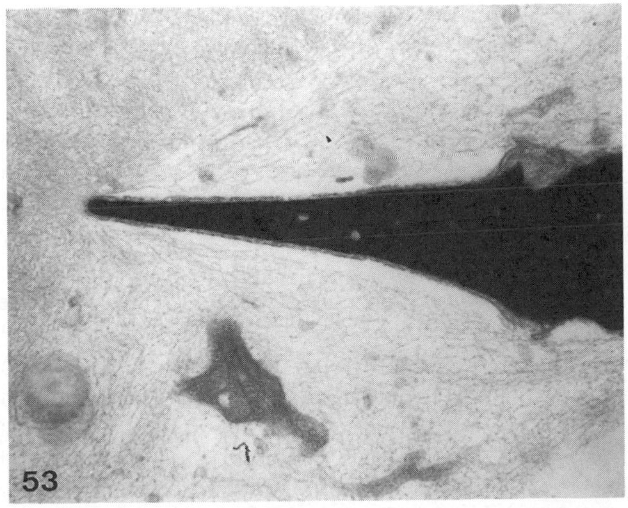

FIG. 53. A human spermatozoon in the human zona pellucida, showing displacement of zona fibers. (From ref. 1361.)

zona-binding activity (907,1611). Autodegradation of beta-acrosin is accelerated by the zona (907). Initially, when acrosome-reacted spermatozoon are on the zona surface, there are more proacrosin molecules on IAM than acrosin. As proacrosin autolysis proceeds, active acrosin hydrolyzes the zona allowing the spermatozoon to penetrate the zona. As long as the supply of proacrosin lasts, the binding of IAM proacrosin to the zona, the hydrolysis of the zona by alpha- and beta-acrosin, and the subsequent detachment of the IAM from the zona continue. This allows a spermatozoon to advance through the zona a little at a time. This is the principle of the so-called *binding-releasing* hypothesis (373,907, 1027,1596,1597,1611). In this hypothesis, sperm motility is considered necessary, but the degree of motility is not very important. As long as the spermatozoon is moderately motile, it can pass through the zona with the aid of acrosin.

For this hypothesis to be considered physiologically relevant, acrosin must be localized on the surface of acrosome-reacted spermatozoa. The time frame of proacrosin autolysis should be long enough and the concentration of acrosin present in all of its forms would be sufficient for the process of zona binding, zona hydrolysis, and penetration. If either time or concentration are not sufficient, acrosin will be exhausted before the sperm heads pass through the zona.

Considerations

If sperm penetration through the zona is purely mechanical, why then are the acrosomes of mammalian spermatozoa loaded with powerful zona-hydrolyzing enzymes? If the acrosome and acrosomal enzymes are relics of evolution, why do we not encounter a few mammals whose spermatozoa totally lack acrosomes and/or acrosomal enzymes? Since we have yet to find such species, acrosomal enzymes must have some very important function in fertilization. According to Overstreet et al. (379,1334), human spermatozoa enter the cervical mucus more efficiently when they are in the protease-rich seminal plasma than when they are in artificial salt solution without enzymes. Modification of the semen–mucus interface by seminal plasma proteases seems to facilitate sperm entry into the mucus. Similarly, acrosomal enzymes released by a spermatozoon on the zona surface may locally alter the physical properties of the zona. This may facilitate the binding and insertion of the sperm head into the zona matrix. Once the sperm head is within the zona, spermatozoa may no longer require acrosomal enzymes (including acrosin). The mechanical force generated by the tail only may be sufficient for the continuing advance of a spermatozoon through the zona. The disulfide-induced rigidity of the sperm head, an evolutionary development in eutherian mammals, seems to permit the tail's thrust to be translated along the axis of the head to the zona quite directly (731). Until convincing evidence is presented that acrosomal enzymes (including acrosin) on either the IAM or the equatorial or postacrosomal regions of acrosome-reacted spermatozoa play crucial roles in zona penetration by spermatozoa, we may assume that the acrosomal enzymes are important only during sperm binding and initial entry into the zona.

Species Specificity of the Sperm–Zona Interaction

It is puzzling that acrosome-reacted spermatozoa of some species (e.g., mouse and hamster) do not bind to and penetrate the zona (427; also 824, Fig. 2), whereas those of some other species (e.g., the guinea pig) are able to do so even when they have undergone the acrosome reaction hours before meeting the eggs (159,238). These apparent species differences could be due to differences in the stability of the proacrosin on the IAM. According to Barros and his associates (709,801), acrosin activity on the hamster sperm IAM is lost rather quickly after the acrosome reaction, whereas acrosin on guinea pig sperm IAM retains its activity for a much longer time. The ability of guinea pig sperm IAM to retain proacrosin/acrosin after the acrosome reaction has been reported previously (1104). Perhaps, successful zona penetration by hamster and mouse spermatozoa requires not only the IAM-bound proacrosin/acrosin, but also a large quantity of proacrosin/acrosin released from the acrosome to alter chemical characteristics of the zona surface. For guinea pig spermatozoa, proacrosin/acrosin on the IAM alone may be enough for sperm entry into the zona. According to Kusan et al. (274), acrosome-reacted rabbit spermatozoa collected from the perivitelline space of fertilized eggs are able to penetrate the zonae of other unfertilized eggs. If this observation is confirmed by others, we may infer that rabbit spermatozoa behave similarly to guinea pig spermatozoa with respect to the characteristics of the membrane-bound proacrosin and acrosin.

In general, fertilization or sperm–zona interaction is assumed to be quite species-specific. However, this is not the case in a strict sense (1330) as evidenced by the presence of many mammalian hybrids between closely related species (728,995). Deer mouse eggs, for example, can be fertilized by spermatozoa of various species of the same and even different genera (Table 8) (1197). Sperm binding and penetration into the zona is possible even between distantly related species, for example, golden hamster sperm × Chinese hamster egg (1419), ram sperm × bovine egg (1498), goat sperm × bovine and sheep eggs (1497), cheetah sperm × domestic cat egg (881), human sperm × gibbon egg (727), human sperm × gorilla egg (1151), and hamster sperm × human egg

TABLE 8. *Fertility of female deer mice (*Peromyscus maniculatus*) artificially inseminated with spermatozoa from other rodents*

Sperm donor species	*P. manuculatus* eggs fertilized (%)	Development up to
P. maniculatus (deer mouse)	62	Adult
P. polionotus (oldfield mouse)	58	Adult
P. leucopus (wood mouse)	15	Term
P. gossypinus (cotton mouse)	87	Term
P. truei (pinyon mouse)	52	4-cell
P. floridanus (Florida mouse)	13	4-cell
Oryzomys palustris (rice rat)	15	2-cell
Mesocricetus auratus (golden hamster)	9	2-cell
Sigmodon hispidus (cotton rat)	3	2-cell
Reithrodontomys humulis (harvest mouse)	8	Fert.
Ochrotomys nuttalli (golden mouse)	0	
Meriones unguiculatus (Mongolian gerbil)	0	
Mus musculus (laboratory house mouse)	0	
Ratus norvegicus (laboratory Norway rat)	0	

From ref. 1197.

(1615,1714). Reverse crosses of the above often do not work at all or are very inefficient.

Strong sperm binding is necessary but not a sufficient requirement for successful zona penetration by spermatozoa. Jedlicki and Barros (1090) examined the behavior of hamster and mouse spermatozoa on zonae of unfertilized and fertilized eggs of homologous and heterologous species. They found that successful sperm penetration of the zona is always preceded by strong sperm binding to the zona and the production of a "hole" into which the sperm head was inserted. This hole (Jedlicki and Barros called it the *sperm track*) was apparently produced by the lytic action of acrosomal enzymes. Thus, the success or failure of sperm entry into the zona may depend on the sperm's ability to bind to and hydrolyze at least the outer surface of zona.

Interference with the Sperm–Zona Interaction

As described previously, the spermatozoon and the zona pellucida each have complementary molecules for their interactions. In the spermatozoon, these are the primary and secondary zona receptors. Zona pellucida glycoproteins are ligands for these sperm receptors. Although not required for binding interaction, sperm motility must also be considered essential for zona penetration. It is expected that any conditions or reagents that affect these interacting molecules would interfere with sperm–zona binding; those affecting sperm motility should also interrupt sperm penetration.

In human IVF, it is common that some eggs are not fertilized in a group where a significant number are fertilized normally. Such failure is apparently due to the anomalies of the egg proper and/or the egg vestments. In some instances, none of the inseminated eggs are fertilized despite apparently normal egg morphology and normal sperm morphology and motility. Bedford and his associates (736,747) classified such total fertilization failure into four categories: (i) total failure of sperm binding to the zona, (ii) tangential sperm binding to the zona, with no sperm entry into the substance of the zona, (iii) frequent sperm binding to the surface of and occasional penetration into the substance of the zona, and (iv) frequent sperm binding to the surface, with several sperm penetrating as far as the inner region of the zona. The failure of sperm-zona binding in category (i) may be due to some inherent defects in sperm plasma membrane components (including zona receptors) and zona ligands, incomplete sperm maturation within the epididymis, and/or immunological block of sperm–zona interactions by antisperm or antizona antibodies. Category (ii) could be due to the failure of spermatozoa to undergo the acrosome reaction because of defective zona ligands and/or the sperm's zona receptors. In categories (iii) and (iv), at least some spermatozoa must have undergone the acrosome reaction on the zona surface. Their inability to cross the zona seem to be due to either the physical or chemical anomalies of the zona, in particular its inner half, or the lack of strong motility needed for complete zona penetration.

Nonimmunological Block

A variety of nonimmunological reagents and conditions are known to interfere with sperm–zona interactions. These include the following:

1. *Lectins* mask terminal oligosaccharides of zona glycoproteins (1308).

2. *Glycosidases* cleave oligosaccharide chains of zona glycoproteins (191,992,1509,1687,1688).
3. *Low concentrations of trypsin and pronase* cleave zona's peptide chains and the zona's sperm-binding sites, without dissolving the zona (202,1309,1388).
4. Solubilized zona or its components saturate sperm's zona receptors (202,745,761,897,1006).
5. *Protease inhibitors* (423) and *fucoidin* (146,1054, 1302,1356) bind to the sperm's ZP receptor proacrosin/acrosin.
6. *Mannose* or *mannoside* (1272,1605) and *uridine diphosphate* (445) saturate or inhibit sperm's zona receptor.
7. *Dithiothreitol* (537) probably changes tertiary and quaternary structures of both the zona and the sperm's zona receptor proteins by reducing —S—S— bonds.

Immunological Block

The use of antibodies to block sperm–zona interactions and subsequent fertilization has attracted the keen interest of both basic and clinical scientists, and considerable progress in this area has been made during the past 10 years. Extensive coverage of this topic is beyond the scope of this review, and readers are referred to recent reviews (804,867,1030,1345,1432,1496) as well as a book edited by Alexander et al. (677).

Shivers et al. (1485) were the first to report possible inhibition of mammalian fertilization by antizona antibodies (anti-ZP). Their pioneering *in vitro* experiment was followed by *in vivo* experiments in which crude anti-ZP antibodies were injected into female mice (1092) and hamsters (1311). In both cases, *in vivo* fertilization was blocked; reversibility of the block was shown in the hamster. Subsequent studies of active immunization using isolated zonae pellucidae yielded variable results with respect to the degree of undesirable side effects such as ovarian dysfunctions (1201,1495). No apparent side effects were observed when Swiss mice were immunized with synthetic ZP3 peptides (amino acids 328–343) (1239). These mice remained infertile as long as 9 months. However, a closely situated and partially overlapping ZP3 peptide (amino acids 328–342) caused a T-cell-mediated autoimmune oophoritis in some (e.g., B6AF$_1$, BALB/cBy, and A/J) but not all strains of mice (1402). Although deglycosylated zona proteins (DGZP) were suggested as safer antigens than native zona proteins (1098), even DGZP may produce undesirable side effects (e.g., depletion of primordial follicles) after long-term immunization (1346). The epitopes responsible for the induction of infertility and the undesirable side effects must be identified and segregated before zona molecules are used as a contraceptive vaccine (1346). Dean et al. (867) have suggested that in order to avoid cytotoxicity, ZP B-cell epitopes should be coupled with foreign T-cell epitopes, rather than using ZP T-cell epitopes.

The use of spermatozoa as immunogens to reduce male and female fertility has a long history (60,734). An interesting example of sperm-induced infertility occurs in both sexes of the guinea pig (60). In guinea pig males injected with guinea pig spermatozoa or testis homogenate, testicular lesions characterized by loss of germinal epithelium and decrease in testis weight and volume become evident in 1 to 2 months after injection. Neither Sertoli cells nor interstitial cells are affected. In guinea pig females treated similarly, fertilization occurs, but fertility drops significantly due to the high rate of fetal loss and resorption.

The use of sperm zona receptors as immunogens has been recently examined. According to Saling and Lakowski (1437), a monoclonal antibody against 220 to 240-kDa molecules in or on the plasma membrane over the acrosome blocks the acrosome reaction but not sperm attachment to or penetration of the zona. Antiacrosin antibody prevents *in vivo* fertilization of the rabbit (896) and hamster (870). An antibody against rabbit inner acrosomal membrane (that may carry acrosin) prevents rabbit spermatozoa from binding to the zona (1508). Intraacrosomal proteins (that again may include acrosin) as potential immunogens have also been investigated (961,1265).

An interesting series of studies has been published by Primakoff and his associates using the guinea pig. Guinea pig spermatozoa have a 64-kDa protein (PH-20) that is originally distributed over the entire surface of the sperm head. PH-20 migrates to the postacrosomal region during epididymal sperm maturation (1155,1359). After the acrosome reaction it migrates to the plasma membrane over the equatorial segment and the IAM (841). PH-20 is believed to mediate the binding of acrosome-reacted spermatozoa to the zona because this process is inhibited strongly *in vitro* by a monoclonal antibody against PH-20 (1381). When 10 to 50 μg of anti-PH-20 protein was injected into each male and female twice, at 1 month intervals, and the females were mated with normal males approximately 1 month after the last injection, none of PH-20-treated animals became pregnant. All the males similarly treated became infertile as well. The fertility of PH-20-treated females was gradually restored. After 6 months, 17% of the females were fertile. By 15 months after injection, all the females became fertile (1383). The PH-20 gene was cloned and the amino acid sequence of the PH-20 protein was determined (1155). Although the PH-20 gene seems to be conserved in mammals (at least in the mouse, rat, hamster, bovine, monkey, and human) (1155), it is unknown whether anti-PH-20 causes temporary or permanent infertility in other animals.

Storage of the Zonae and Preparation of Artificial Zonae

The zona is one of the toughest physical barriers the spermatozoa must negotiate before effecting fertilization. Therefore, spermatozoa capable of penetrating the zonae without difficulty are most likely fertile. Although the final tests for sperm fertility must be done using normal, living eggs surrounded by zonae, preliminary assessment of sperm fertility can be done using zonae of nonliving, frozen eggs (1336) or those of the eggs stored in high concentrations of neutral salts (1703). Burkman et al. (793) developed a hemizona assay to evaluate the fertility of human spermatozoa. This technique has been applied to the monkey (1303). The principle of this assay is simple. A frozen or salt-stored human egg is cut into halves of approximately equal size, washed to remove egg contents, half of the zona is inseminated with spermatozoa from a man of proven fertility (control) and the other half with spermatozoa from a man of unknown fertility (test subject). At a specified time (e.g., 4 hr) after insemination with approximately the same number and density of spermatozoa, the number of spermatozoa bound to the zona surfaces between control and test halves are compared (949,950).

Since strong sperm-zona binding is a necessary preliminary to successful fertilization, the degree of sperm-zona binding is believed to be closely related to the degree of sperm fertility. Clinical data support this view (1301). Vazquez et al. (1620) prepared silica gel beads covalently linked with mouse ZP3. When mouse spermatozoa were added to these beads, 10% to 25% of the beads had one or a few spermatozoa attached. The number of beads with bound spermatozoa reached a maximum 15 min after insemination, and then decreased. This is a potentially useful technique, but it requires improvement to increase the numbers bound and the rate of sperm-bead binding. Covalently linking ZP2 to beads together with ZP3 may allow the spermatozoa to stay on the beads for a longer period of time.

Since fertilization requires more than sperm-zona binding, these assays would not predict sperm fertility with 100% accuracy. The ability of spermatozoa to cross the zona must be assessed simultaneously to increase the physiological relevance of the assay. For any sperm fertil-

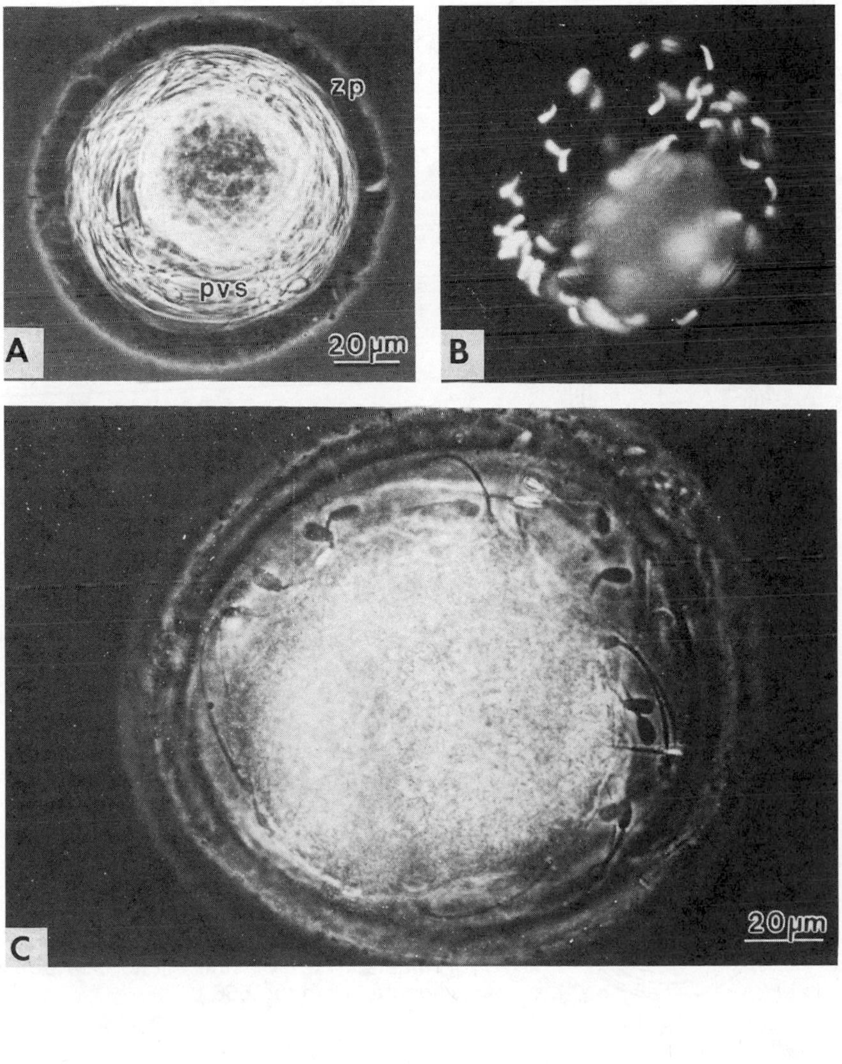

FIG. 55. Multiple sperm penetration into the perivitelline space of salt-stored unfertilized eggs. (**A**) A phase-contrast micrograph of a salt-stored golden hamster egg with numerous spermatozoa in the perivitelline space (pvs); this egg was washed thoroughly to remove spermatozoa from the zona surface. (**B**) The same as A, but examined with a fluorescence microscope after Hoechst 33324 staining to show sperm heads clearly. (**C**) A phase-contrast micrograph of salt-stored cattle egg with many spermatozoa in the perivitelline space; this salt-stored egg was heat-treated (75°C, 12 min) prior to insemination to restore the zona's penetrability by spermatozoa. (From ref. 1701.).

ity test, the use of fully matured, normal unfertilized eggs with intact zonae, either fresh or frozen, is recommended. If such eggs are not readily available for technical or ethical reasons, then nonliving frozen eggs (1336) or salt-stored eggs (1703) can be substituted. With salt-stored eggs, the vitellus is shrunken, creating a large perivitelline space. Since salt-stored eggs are dead and lack the mechanism to block polyspermy, many spermatozoa can cross the zona and enter the perivitelline space (Fig. 55A,B). The number of spermatozoa in the perivitelline space is considered proportional to the degree of sperm capacitation (766) and to the fertilizing ability of the spermatozoa under investigation. This method works nicely for the hamster and human but not for cattle (820,1221). Bull spermatozoa are barely capable of penetrating salt-stored bovine zona. Even hamster and human zonae tend to become less penetrable after long-term storage in salt solutions. Perhaps these effects are due to "salting-out" of certain zona glycoproteins. Precipitation of stable protein-salt mixtures may prevent sperm passage through the zona, which could be purely or partly mechanical (see above). A mild heat treatment is effective in increasing or restoring zona penetrability of salt-stored eggs in the hamster and bovine (1701) (Fig. 55C).

Recently, recombinant mouse ZP3 and rabbit ZP proteins (55 and 75 kDa) were produced by inserting ZP-cDNA in bacterial and viral promoters (739,1468). Since

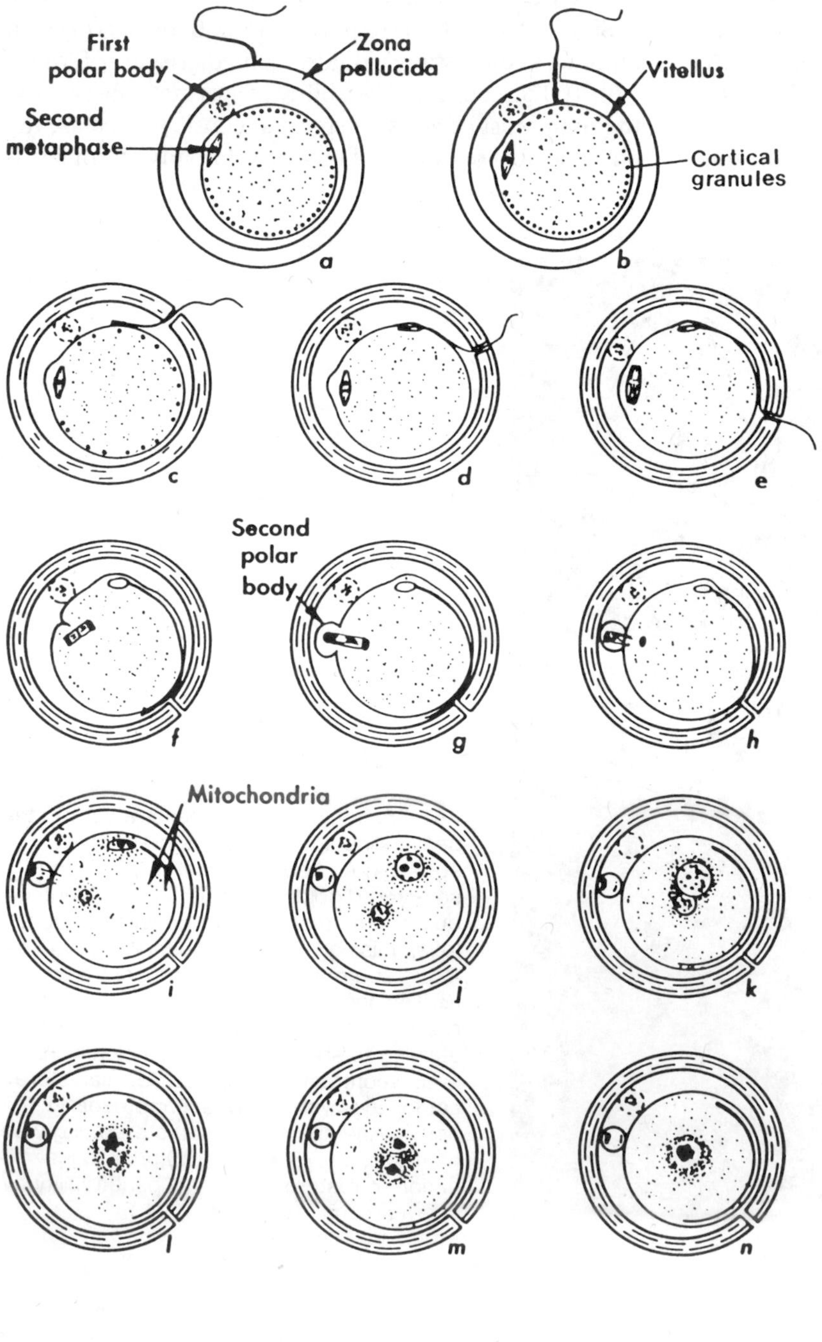

FIG. 56. Diagram of egg activation and pronuclei development in the rat. (*a–d*) Sperm–egg fusion and cortical granule exocytosis. Shading of the zona pellucida denotes the occurrence of the cortical granule mediated zona reaction. (*d–h*) Completion of the second meiosis. (*i–k*) Pronuclei development. (*l–m*) Reappearance of sperm and egg chromosomes. (*n*) Prometaphase of the first cleavage. (Adapted from ref. 556.)

recombinant mouse ZP3 was proven to be biologically active, mass production of such recombinant ZP molecules will make it possible to prepare a thin protein film containing both species-specific synthetic ZP molecules. With its thickness and hardness similar to native zona, this film could provide a zona substitute. If we can insert human ZP genes (1617) into animal genomes, transgenic human ZP products within animal zonae may make the latter penetrable by human spermatozoa. Animal eggs with such zonae would be very useful in assessing human sperm fertility in clinical laboratories (866). Insertion of transgenic hamster ZP3 into mouse zonae has been successful (1123).

SPERM–EGG FUSION

Manner of Sperm–Egg Fusion

Having passed through the zona pellucida, the fertilizing spermatozoon crosses the perivitelline space quickly. The sperm head then binds to the egg plasma membrane (oolemma) and soon the entire body of the spermatozoon is incorporated in the egg cytoplasm (ooplasm) (Fig. 56). This dynamic process can be observed continuously under carefully controlled *in vitro* conditions (178). Scanning electron micrographs give us an eye-catching three-dimensional view of this process (Fig. 57) (393,438,1478).

In all animals except eutherian mammals, the inner acrosomal membrane of acrosome-reacted spermatozoa fuses first with the oolemma (659). Eutherian mammals are unusual in this respect. It is the plasma membrane over the equatorial segment of the acrosome that fuses first with the oolemma, (Fig. 58) (50,329). The posterior region of the sperm head and the tail are subsequently incorporated by the egg via membrane fusion, whereas the anterior region of the head, where the inner acrosomal membrane is exposed, is engulfed by the egg in a phagocytic manner. The notion that the sperm plasma membrane of the postacrosomal region is the first to fuse with the oolemma was abandoned (660,1696), but it has been revived by Vigil (1626) who maintains that hamster spermatozoa that have lost their equatorial segments completely remain capable of fusing with the oolemma. It is important to note here that in common laboratory rodents, including the hamster, the equatorial segment extends from the main body of this segment to the rostral end of the sperm head (cf. Fig. 25 of ref. 951). Even if the main body of the equatorial segment is absent in cross sections of the sperm head, the rostral portion of the equatorial segment may still exist. Since Virgil's claim deserves attention and confirmation, further experiments should be performed using spermatozoa with simpler equatorial segments (e.g., those of the guinea pig, rabbit, cattle, or human). Unless it is proven unequivocally that spermatozoa are able to fuse with oolemma even after complete loss of the equatorial segment, we should hold to the currently accepted view that sperm–egg fusion begins between the oolemma and the plasma membrane over the sperm's equatorial segment.

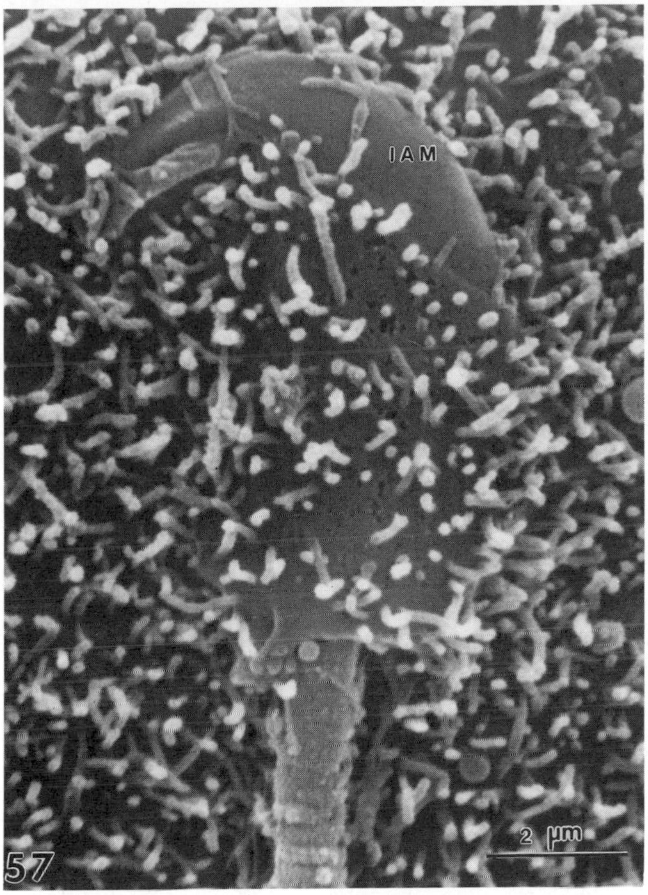

FIG. 57. A scanning electron micrograph of a golden hamster spermatozoon fusing with an egg. IAM, the inner acrosomal membrane to be incorporated in the egg later by "phagocytosis." (From ref. 530.)

Under ordinary conditions, the sperm membrane that makes the initial contact with the oolemma appears to be the inner acrosomal membrane followed by the plasma membrane of the equatorial segment/postacrosomal region. Scanning electron micrographs of spermatozoa that have landed on the oolemma (393,438,1365) give us the impression that head plasma membrane, including the inner acrosomal membrane, sticks to the egg microvilli. The oolemma has numerous microvilli except for the area immediately overlying the meiotic spindle, where the oolemma is either smooth or provides a large cytoplasmic protrusion (906). Sperm–egg fusion seldom occurs in this region (256,906). Although spermatozoa normally land on a field of microvilli, it is not clear whether the microvilli are essential for sperm–egg fusion (50). When zona-free hamster eggs were inseminated with acrosome-reacted spermatozoa in an acidic

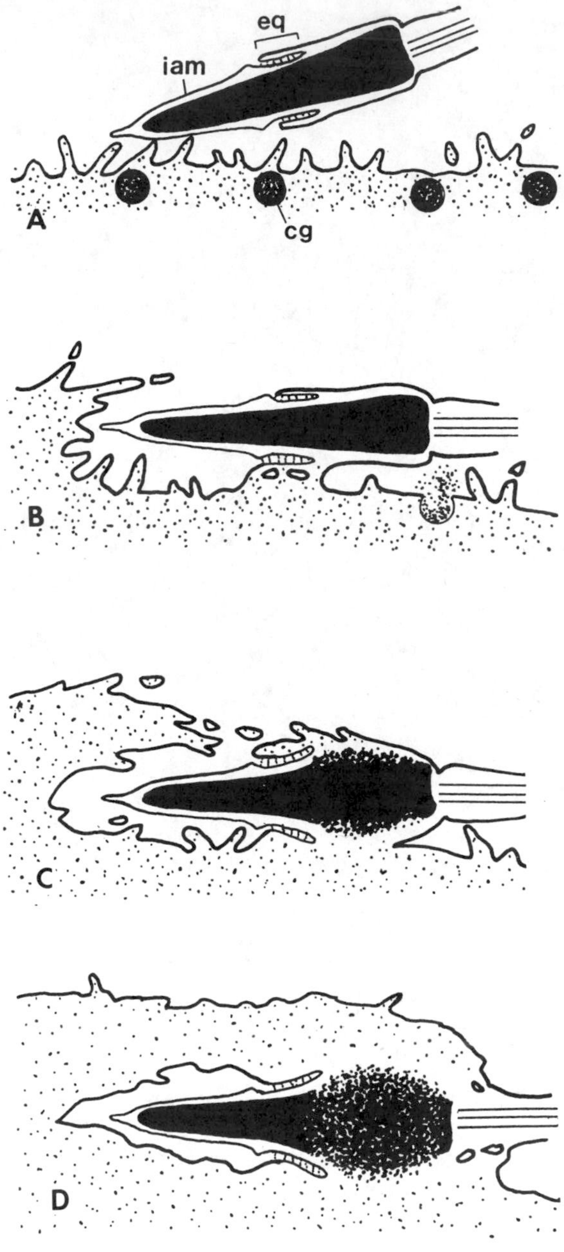

FIG. 58. Diagrams of the early stages of sperm–egg fusion. (*cg*) Cortical granule; (*eq*) equatorial segment; (*iam*) inner acrosomal membrane. (Adapted from ref. 50.)

(pH 6.0) medium, the spermatozoa became firmly attached to the oolemma, but fusion did not take place. Examination of these spermatozoa revealed that the plasma membrane over the equatorial segment was in close contact with a flat, microvillus-free oolemma (1704). Since these spermatozoa were capable of immediate fusion upon transfer of the gametes into normal medium (pH > 7.0), spermatozoa must be able to fuse with this microvillus-free oolemma. The inability or difficulty of the microvillus-free area above the meiotic spindle to fuse with spermatozoa could be due to a deficiency of sperm receptors rather than to absence of microvilli. This particular area of oolemma is known to be as fluid as the rest of the oolemma (514,1672).

One of the visible indications of sperm–egg fusion is the sudden reduction of sperm tail movement (659). This occurs not only in mammals (970,1676), but also in invertebrates such as the sea urchin (1194,1447). In the sea urchin (1033,1194) and perhaps in mammals, this tail immobilization occurs seconds after the onset of sperm–egg fusion.

As a rule, the entire sperm tail is incorporated into the egg (1035,1362,1364). Gaunt (977) clearly demonstrated the mingling of sperm and egg plasma membrane using immunofluorescence technique (Fig. 59). Sperm mitochondria, when they enter the egg, are transcriptionally

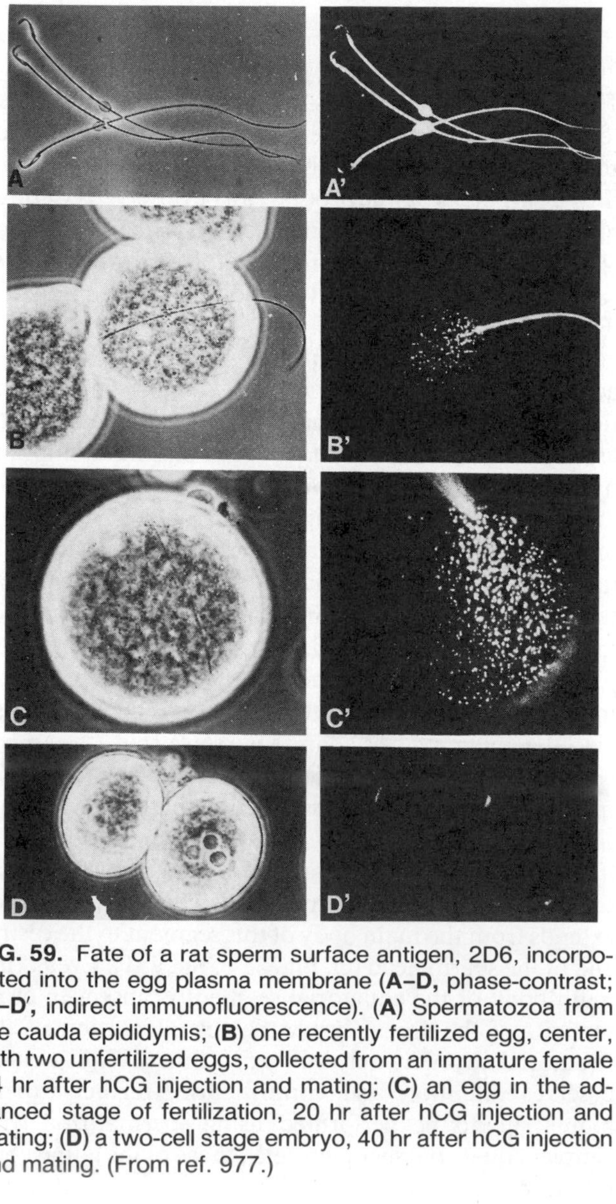

FIG. 59. Fate of a rat sperm surface antigen, 2D6, incorporated into the egg plasma membrane (**A–D,** phase-contrast; **A′–D′**, indirect immunofluorescence). (**A**) Spermatozoa from the cauda epididymis; (**B**) one recently fertilized egg, center, with two unfertilized eggs, collected from an immature female 14 hr after hCG injection and mating; (**C**) an egg in the advanced stage of fertilization, 20 hr after hCG injection and mating; (**D**) a two-cell stage embryo, 40 hr after hCG injection and mating. (From ref. 977.)

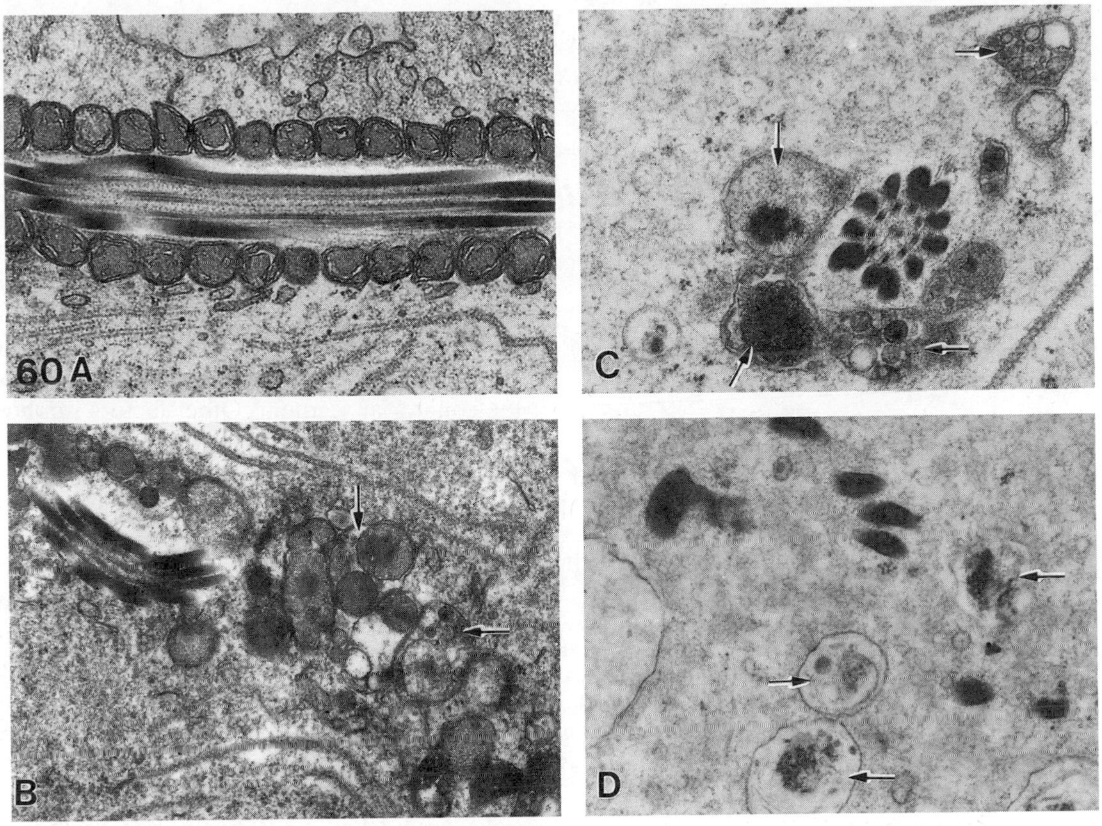

FIG. 60. Fate of sperm tail components in a golden hamster egg. (**A**) Midpiece in a recently fertilized egg. (**B**) Midpiece mitochondria engulfed by multivesicular bodies (*arrows*), in a two-cell stage embryo. (**C** and **D**) Multivesicular bodies (*arrows*) surrounding still intact [C] or dissociated [D] outer dense fibers, in late two-cell stage embryo. (A and B from ref. 1038.)

competent (676) but degenerate quickly (1038,1546) (Fig. 60A,B). However, some sperm mitochondrial DNA may survive. According to a calculation by Gyllensten et al. (1008), an order of 10^{-5} sperm mitochondrial DNA of the mouse persists and is transmitted to the next generation, the biological significance of which is not clear at present. Other structural components of the tail, such as the outer dense fibers and axoneme, are also destined to disintegrate (1038) (Fig. 60C,D). In a few species such as the field vole (26) and Chinese hamster (26,539), the tail components are "pushed out" of the eggs rather commonly after fertilization.

Under physiological conditions, only one spermatozoon fuses with the oolemma. *In vitro,* particularly when eggs are freed from zonae and inseminated with a high concentration of spermatozoa, multiple sperm entry into an egg as well as sperm-mediated egg-to-egg fusion may result (1347). In the hamster and pig, as many as 60 or more than 80 spermatozoa can fuse with one egg, respectively (587,1059), but fusion with an excessively large number of spermatozoa may result in cytolysis of the egg (587).

How Spermatozoa Become Capable of Fusing with the Eggs

The Acrosome Reaction as a Prerequisite to Sperm–Egg Fusion

The acrosome reaction is an absolute prerequisite for sperm–egg fusion. Acrosome-intact spermatozoa are unable to fuse with the oolemma, regardless of their capacitation status (530,660). When zona-free eggs are inseminated *in vitro* with acrosome-intact spermatozoa, the spermatozoa attach firmly to the oolemma (1365). With the pivotal center at the tip of their heads, all regions of the sperm head, including the equatorial segment, have ample chance to make contact with the oolemma, yet fusion never takes place (1735). Acrosome-reacted spermatozoa, on the other hand, are able to bind and fuse with the oolemma almost instantaneously (543a,1365). These observations suggest that, as the result of or concomitantly with the acrosome reaction, the plasma membrane over the equatorial segment undergoes a major physiological change that renders the spermatozoon competent to fuse (530,543b,660). I should point out here that the title of my original paper (ref. 5436) was misleading—it should have been: "Physiological changes in the *equatorial segment* region of mammalian spermatozoa: a necessary preliminary to the membrane fusion between sperm and egg cells." At that time, I thought that sperm–egg fusion begins in the postacrosomal region (or postnuclear cap region) rather than in the equatorial segment.

Mechanism by which the Plasma Membrane over the Equatorial Segment Becomes Fusogenic

When capacitated acrosome-intact mouse spermatozoa are stained with chlortetracycline (CTC) and examined with a fluorescence microscope, the equatorial segment area shows bright fluorescence. This region loses CTC fluorescence after the acrosome reaction (Fig. 21) (427,1522,1523,1634), indicating that something happens within the plasma membrane of the equatorial segment during or after the acrosome reaction. Although the mechanism by which the equatorial segment becomes fusogenic is not yet clear (530,660,1696), it seems natural to assume that the acrosomal contents released during the acrosome reaction alter the plasma membrane over the equatorial segment.

Dravland and Meizel (884) were the first to propose the possible involvement of acrosin in this process. This hypothesis was supported by Takano et al. (1554), who found that acrosin inhibitors prevented acrosome-reacting spermatozoa from becoming fusogenic. Interestingly, the inhibitors could not prevent fusion of acrosome-reacted spermatozoa once the spermatozoa had undergone their acrosome reactions in normal inhibitor-free medium. Acrosin may activate latent fusion proteins in the equatorial segment region or remove steric and/or charge barriers to the membrane apposition (1554). It is important to emphasize here that neither Dravland and Meizel (884) nor Takano et al. (1554) could inhibit sperm–egg fusion completely with acrosin inhibitors. Only the incidence of sperm–egg fusion was reduced, indicating that acrosin is perhaps not the sole enzyme or factor involved in the membrane change in the equatorial segment. Other factors implicated in the development of sperm's fusion competence include metalloendoprotease (875,876), calpain II (435,749), and plasminogen activator/plasmin (1056). F-actin appears in the equatorial segment and postacrosomal region of pig spermatozoa after the acrosome reaction (806), but its involvement in the development of fusion competence of spermatozoa remains to be investigated.

At present, no one is able to make acrosome-intact spermatozoa fusion competent. All attempts to make them fusible have failed (530,660,1554,1696). Fusion competence of spermatozoa may develop stepwise as shown in Fig. 61. The plasma membrane over the equatorial segment has a putative fusion protein (A). Sperm surface coat is removed or modified during capacitation (B). Immediately before the acrosome reaction, the plasma membrane over the acrosomal cap undergoes drastic changes either by zona or spontaneously (C). These changes permit the plasma membrane to fuse with

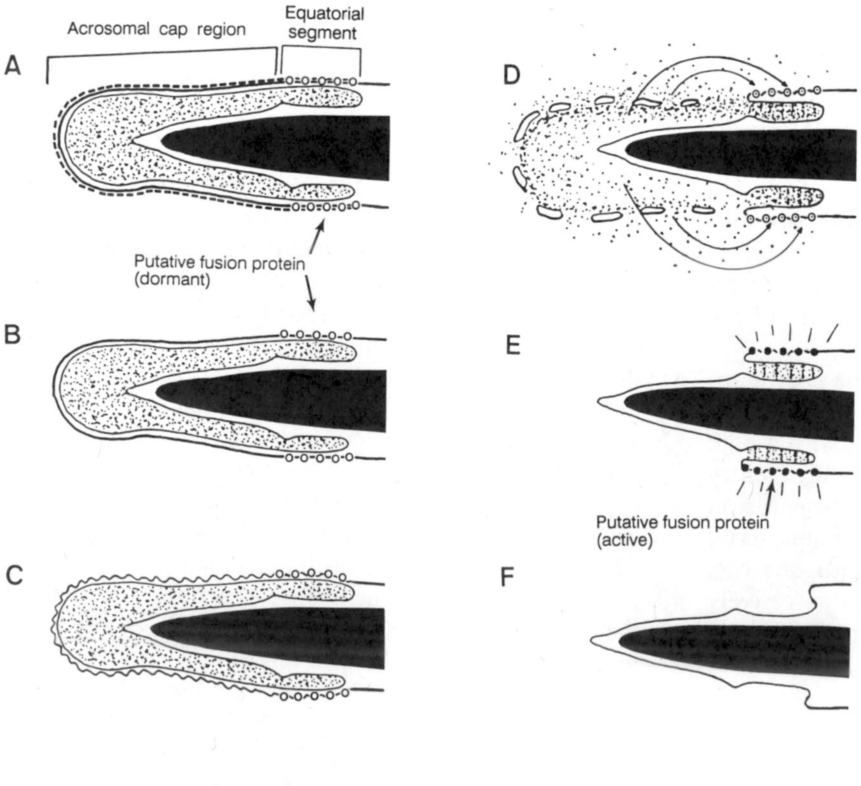

FIG. 61. Hypothetical pathways through which the spermatozoon becomes fusion competent. For explanation, see the text.

the underlying outer acrosomal membrane (see the section of acrosome reaction). Similar changes occur in the plasma membrane over the equatorial segment, but its fusion with the underlying outer acrosomal membrane is prevented because of the presence of intermembrane bridges stabilizing the outer acrosomal membrane in the equatorial segment (1431). The putative fusion proteins in altered plasma membrane are activated by acrosomal enzymes released during the acrosome reaction (D). Sperm membrane with active fusion proteins is now ready to fuse with the oolemma (E). With time, the equatorial segment may vesiculate and be lost (F), resulting in the loss of fusion competence of the spermatozoa. How quickly the spermatozoa become fusion competent is not known, but in the guinea pig the first fusion-competent spermatozoa appear approximately 2 min after the onset of acrosome membrane vesiculation (1735).

Fusion-Mediating Substances and Fusion Proteins in Spermatozoa

Lopez and Shur (1190) maintain that galactosyltransferase on the plasma membrane over the equatorial segment mediates sperm–egg fusion in the mouse. According to them, this surface galactosyltransferase is originally present on the plasma membrane over the acrosomal cap before the onset of the acrosome reaction. During the acrosome reaction, it is redistributed to the plasma membrane over the equatorial segment to mediate sperm attachment to the oolemma.

A 40-kDa protein, localized in the equatorial segment of mouse spermatozoa, has been proposed as a fusion mediator. The antibody to this protein (i) cross-reacts with the equatorial segment of both hamster and human spermatozoa (1438) (Fig. 62), and (ii) inhibits sperm–egg fusion in the mouse (1436). A 37-kDa protein of the caput epididymis origin, which is located in the equatorial segment of acrosome-reacted rat spermatozoa (1412), has been implicated for sperm–egg fusion (1411). It is unclear at present whether acrosin adsorbed on the plasma membrane of the equatorial segment and the postacrosomal region of acrosome-reacted rabbit (1405) and human (1572) spermatozoa is directly involved in sperm–egg fusion.

Okabe et al. (1312) believe that a 43-kDa protein on the surface of acrosome-reacted human spermatozoa mediates sperm–egg fusion. Its terminal amino acid sequence matches the protein CD46, which is known as a membrane adhesion molecule. Other membrane adhesion molecules on the human sperm surface implicated for sperm–egg fusion include fibronectin (967,1246) and the complement component Clq (968).

In the guinea pig, a protein called PH-30 is believed to be the fusion protein (1382). It consists of two subunits (60-kDa and 44-kDa). Its antibody inhibits sperm–egg

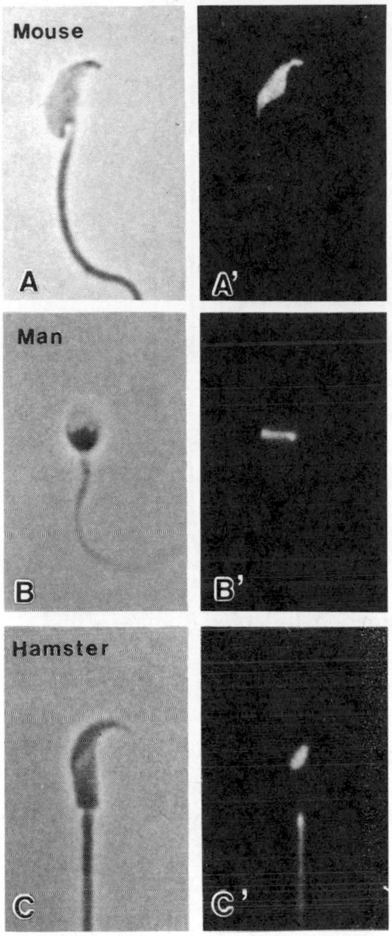

FIG. 62. Immunolocalization of the monoclonal antibody M29 on spermatozoa from the mouse, human, and golden hamster. The paired phase-contrast (**A,B,C**) and fluorescence micrographs (**A′,B′,C′**) demonstrate the specific localization of M29 to the equatorial segment in all of the species. Unlike mouse and human spermatozoa, hamster spermatozoa display nonspecific fluorescence in the midpiece. (From ref. 1438.)

fusion. The 60-kDa subunit contains a oolemma-binding site and the 44-kD subunit has a fusion peptide (Fig. 63) (765). The only question I have about PH-30 concerns its location on the spermatozoon. As stated already, the plasma membrane over the equatorial segment is believed to be the membrane that first fuses with the oolemma. Why then is PH-30 located in the postacrosomal region and not in the equatorial segment? It may be that the plasma membrane of the equatorial segment has another fusion protein, which has not yet been identified. PH-30 in the postacrosomal region may aid in the membrane fusion first initiated at the equatorial segment.

Sperm fusion proteins and viral fusion proteins may share biochemical characteristics. In viruses, the functions of binding to the target (host) cell surface and fusion with the membrane are carried out by either a single

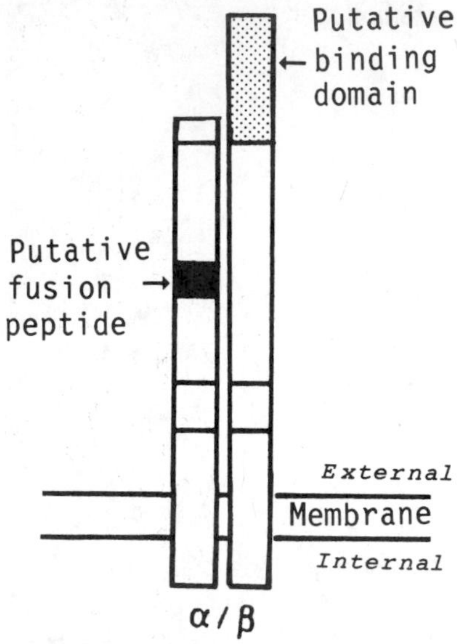

FIG. 63. A schematic model of mature PH-30 of the guinea pig spermatozoon. (Adapted from ref. 765.)

glycoprotein or separate glycoproteins (Table 9). Figure 64 is a diagrammatic representation of the HA glycoprotein of the influenza virus with two functional peptides in one molecule. Readers are referred to refs. 774a, 1305a, and 1658a for the possible mechanisms by which viral fusion proteins trigger membrane fusion.

Fusion of Subnormal and Abnormal Spermatozoa with Oolemma

Since Gordon and Talansky (987a) first reported that the incidence of mouse fertilization can be increased by drilling a hole in the zona pellucida, physical cutting of the zona prior to insemination or subzonal injection of spermatozoa have become a useful adjunct in dealing with certain types of human male infertility (cf. 829,830). Such microsurgical techniques are used when spermatozoa cannot penetrate zona normally or when the zona is too rigid for sperm penetration. As previously stated, spermatozoa must be acrosome-reacted before fusing with the oolemma. Thus, ideally, a single or a few recently acrosome-reacted spermatozoa should be placed in the perivitelline space so that sperm–egg fusion can occur immediately or at least without much delay. However, in practice, injecting spermatozoa of unknown acrosomal status sometimes serves the purpose. Some spermatozoa will undergo spontaneous acrosome reaction while swimming in the perivitelline space, then fuse with the oolemma. Others may undergo the acrosome reaction either on the inner surface of the zona or on the oolemma sometime after subzonal injection. As long as spermatozoa become acrosome-reacted before the eggs age excessively, normal fertilization will result. Subzonal injection of spermatozoa produced a baby for the first time in 1988 (1289).

Strong sperm motility is not essential for sperm–egg fusion (660). As long as spermatozoa (i) are acrosome-reacted and alive, (ii) retain a functional equatorial segment, and (iii) are given chances to contact the oolemma, they will fertilize eggs. Spermatozoa of infertile men with Kartagener's syndrome are motionless because of the lack of dynein arms (669). However, these motionless spermatozoa are capable of undergoing the acrosome reaction and fusing with the oolemma (674). Wolf et al. (1681,1682) reported the birth of a healthy girl after subzonal injection of spermatozoa from an infertile man whose spermatozoa swim slowly and abnormally due to the lack of outer dynein arms. Certain strains of bull produce tailless spermatozoa. These spermatozoa (heads only) are also able to undergo the acrosome reaction and fuse with the oolemma (1050). Boar spermatozoa collected from the rete testis are barely motile, yet they have the potential to undergo the acrosome reaction and fuse with the oolemma (1016).

Round-headed human spermatozoa, which apparently occur due to a recessive gene on the Y chromosome (1143a), have no acrosomes (1455) and are unable to bind to the zona and oolemma (744,1091,1148,1630a). Direct injection of these spermatozoa into ooplasm may be the only way to overcome the infertility of men with such spermatozoa (1152).

TABLE 9. *Viral fusion proteins*

Virus	Glycoprotein	Molecular weight (kDa)	Function
Sendai virus neuraminidase	HN	67	Binding and fusion
	F2 + F1	52, 11	Binding and fusion
Influenza virus	HA1 + HA2	44, 30	Binding and fusion
	NA	48–63	Neuraminidase
Vesicular stomatitis virus	G	61	Binding and fusion
Mouse mammalian tumor virus	gp 52	52	Fusion
Mouse hepatitis (90A) virus	90A + 90B	90, 90	Binding and fusion

From ref. 935.

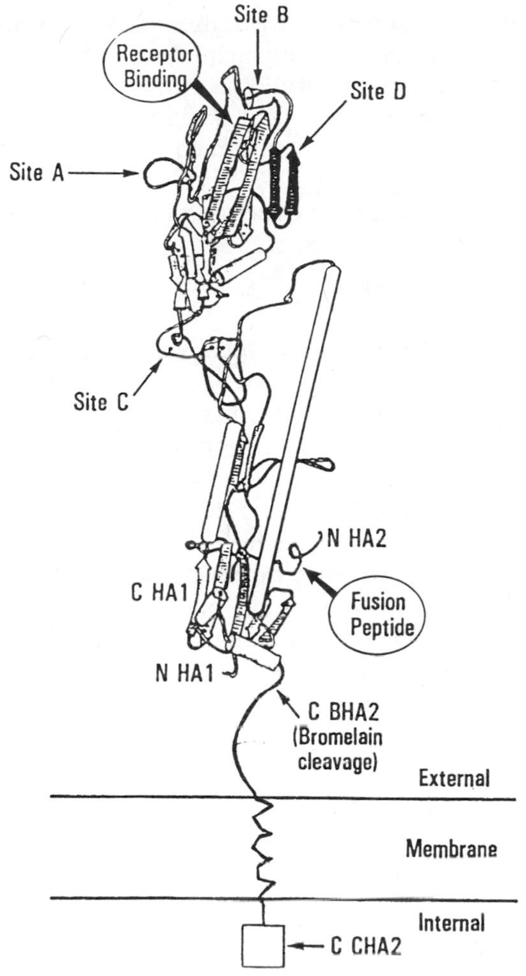

FIG. 64. A three-dimensional structure of influenza virus glycoprotein HA, showing the receptor binding site and the putative fusogenic hydrophobic segment, N HA2 amino terminus. (From refs. 1305,1664a.)

Fusion Competence of the Oolemma

Unlike sperm plasma membrane, the oolemma acquires its fusibility long before fertilization. In the golden hamster, the oolemma becomes fusible as soon as the primary oocyte is surrounded by follicle cells and starts to grow (1734). The fusibility, assessed by the number of spermatozoa fused with a zona-free oocyte, increases as the oocyte grows and reaches its maximum at maturity. Since the first acquisition of oocyte's fusibility and the beginning of zona pellucida formation are synchronous, Zuccotti et al. (1734) thought that part of the zona molecules might be inserted in the oolemma during the growth phase of oocyte development. However, at least in the mouse, there is no indication of the presence of a detectable amount of ZP2 and ZP3 molecules on or in the oolemma of fully mature eggs (143a,774) although the zona and oolemma share many common saccharides and antigens (797a,1218,1292).

In the mouse, the oolemma fusibility is reduced after the treatment of eggs with proteases such as trypsin, chymotrypsin, and pronase (775,777,1678). Of several surface proteins removed or modified by protease treatment, 94-kDa protein appears to be the one involved in the sperm–oolemma interaction (776). Interestingly, protease-treated eggs are capable of regenerating this protein in 3 to 6 hr when cultured *in vitro* (1045,1119). Concanavalin-affinity molecules on the oolemma appear and disappear in close association with the development and loss of oolemma's fusibility (1734). Therefore, it may be possible to isolate fusion-mediating molecules (778) by using this or similar lectins as molecular probes.

The situation in the golden hamster is quite different from that in the mouse. The hamster oolemma, unlike that of the mouse, is extremely resistant to proteolytic digestion. Even after treatments of 30 min with very high concentrations of relatively nonspecific proteases such as pronase, proteinase K, and thermolysin, the hamster oolemma remains fully capable of fusing with spermatozoa (1037,1378). Other proteases and various glycosidases are also unable to destroy the fusibility of the hamster oolemma. At present, the basis of such a conspicuous species difference between mouse and hamster is unclear. It is possible that the initial binding of spermatozoa with oolemma is mediated by general adhesion molecules such as those belonging to the integrin superfamily (786,967,969,1562a), Ig superfamily (1274), CD 46, a regulator of complement activation (1315), and cadhedrin family (1378).

As stated earlier, the equatorial segment of acrosome-reacted rat spermatozoa carries a 37-kDa protein, called DE, of epididymis origin (1412). Rat oolemma carries a molecule(s) that is complementary to the DE (1411). This oolemma molecule seems to participate in the fusion process rather than the prior sperm–oolemma binding. The nature of this molecule remains to be determined.

Detection of Sperm–Egg Fusion

Light Microscopy

Before the phase-contrast microscope, paraffin sectioning was the only way to ascertain the presence of spermatozoa within eggs. Phase-contrast microscopy enabled investigators to examine the presence or absence of sperm components within eggs without sectioning (20). The whole mount, fix, and stain method (726,812) made it possible to examine spermatozoa within opaque eggs loaded with nontransparent cytoplasmic inclusions. Bedford (726) lists the following as criteria for fertilization (successful sperm–egg fusion) in a single-cell egg, although not all are necessarily appropriate for every species:

1. Presence of a fertilizing sperm tail.
2. Swelling sperm head in ooplasm.
3. Male and female pronuclei.
4. Definitive first and second polar bodies.
5. Presence of sperm in the zona pellucida or the perivitelline space.
6. Appearance of the ooplasm.
7. Activation of the egg involving loss of cortica granules and rotation of meiotic spindle.

The presence of a swelling sperm head or a pronucleus with associated sperm tail in the ooplasm is an unequivocal evidence of successful sperm–egg fusion, but its absence does not necessarily imply that sperm–egg fusion did not occur. For example, sperm nuclei entering immature oocytes at the germinal vesicle stage (or those entering fertilized eggs at the pronuclear stage) remain condensed for hours until the metaphase-promoting factor becomes available (see below). Unfused spermatozoa on oolemmae in general can be removed by strong pipetting. If the spermatozoa are not removed even after repeated vigorous pipettings, then other methods (see below) must be used to ascertain the presence or absence of sperm nuclei within the ooplasm.

When zona-free mature eggs are inseminated *in vitro,* sperm–egg fusion may be detected by watching the response of spermatozoa to the egg surface. A spermatozoon that suddenly stops or almost stops its tail movement several seconds after its attachment to the oolemma is most likely fusing with the oolemma (Fig. 65) (659). The temporal relationship between the onset of membrane fusion and the cessation of tail movement has not been determined for mammals, but in sea urchins the sperm immobilization occurs about 6 sec after the onset of fusion (1033,1186). The reason for the sudden cessation of sperm tail movement is not clear, but it could be due to an influx of Ca^{2+} into the spermatozoon (1086) or depolarization of sperm tail membrane.

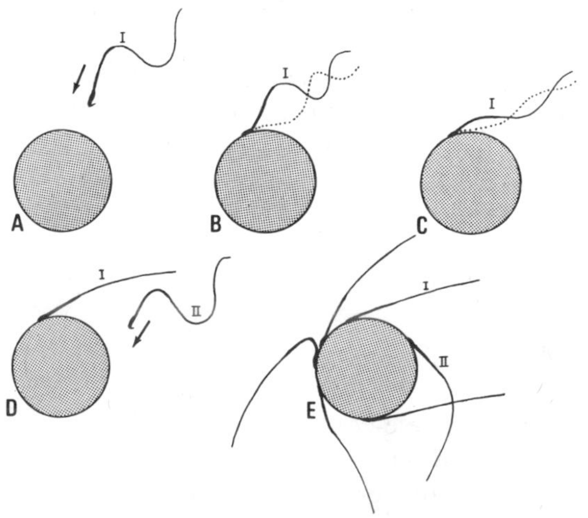

FIG. 65. Diagram showing that acrosome-reacted spermatozoa lose their motility rather abruptly soon after contact (fusion) with the oolemma: observations on zona-free golden hamster eggs inseminated *in vitro* with acrosome-reacted spermatozoa. Spermatozoa freely swimming (**A**) and those immediately after attachment (**B**) beat their tails vigorously. Between 5 and 15 sec after contact, tail beating slows down suddenly (**C**) and stops by the next 10 sec (**D**). By 5 min after insemination, each egg has many motionless spermatozoa stuck on its surface (**D**). (From ref. 659.)

Electron Microscopy

Transmission electron microscopy is straightforward. Although it is tedious and considerable time must be spent in searching for the site of sperm–egg interaction, transmission electron microscopy provides sufficient resolution to determine unequivocally whether or not the sperm and egg have fused. It is still one of the best and most reliable methods available (1187). Scanning electron microscopy provides excellent three-dimensional images of sperm–egg interaction, but its low resolution is not suitable for the study of initial phases of membrane fusion.

Dye Transfer Technique

This technique, developed by Hinkley et al. (1032,1033) for the study of membrane fusion of sea urchin gametes, has been applied successfully to mammals (834,1004,1517,1734). The procedure of the technique is simple: preload unfertilized eggs with the DNA-specific fluorochrome Hoechst 33743, rinse eggs thoroughly, and then inseminate. When fusion occurs, the fluorochrome enters the sperm and stains its DNA, resulting in a bright fluorescence of the sperm nucleus at the egg surface. Fixation of inseminated eggs at intervals is recommended to determine the time of fusion. Without fixation and permeabilization of the sperm nuclear envelope, the fluorochrome cannot reach the nuclei instantly. It is important to note that the fluorochrome loaded in the eggs will eventually diffuse out of the eggs. The speed of this varies from species to species. In the species whose eggs lose fluorochrome relatively quickly (e.g., hamster, 834), only a few eggs should be handled at one time. If too many fluorochrome-loaded eggs are placed in a small aliquot of the medium, fluorochrome diffusing out of the eggs will stain the nuclei of spermatozoa outside of the eggs. Green (996) suggested the use of membrane-impermeable fluorochromes, such as propidium iodide in order to overcome the problem of dye diffusion. Of course this dye must be injected microsurgically into eggs prior to experiments.

Differential Staining Technique

When sperm nuclei are incorporated in the ooplasm of mature eggs, —S—S— bonds in the sperm protamines are quickly reduced to —SH (1353) and the protamines are replaced by histones (865) even before nuclear decondensation begins. The same changes occur when spermatozoa enter immature oocytes (1735). According to Krzanowska (1141) and Miller and Masui (1243), mouse sperm nuclei are darkly stained with toluidine blue and Giemsa when they are in the ooplasm. The technique is simple. Fix inseminated eggs with acetic alcohol, air-dry on a slide, then stain with either toluidine blue or Giemsa. Sperm nuclei outside of the egg are unstained, whereas those within the ooplasm stain darkly. Polge (cited from ref. 1220) found that sperm nuclei within the ooplasm are stained more darkly with lacmoid than those outside the eggs. Differential staining of sperm nuclei inside and outside of the egg seems to depend on the SS–SH and protamine–histone status of the nucleus. Although these techniques can be used to estimate the location of unswollen sperm nuclei, one may encounter sperm nuclei with various degrees of stain reaction. This makes judgment as to the fertilization status difficult. No single method is perfect. The combined use of two or more different techniques is recommended when the location of unswollen sperm nuclei is questionable. For more details of the detection of sperm–egg fusion, readers are referred to Longo and Yanagimachi (1187).

Control of Sperm–Egg Fusion

Species Specificity of Sperm–Egg Fusion

Sperm interaction with the oolemma is much less species specific than the sperm–zona interaction (529). For example, mouse spermatozoa unable to penetrate the zona can readily fuse with the hamster oolemma. Similarly, mouse spermatozoa will fuse with the oolemmae (eggs) of the rat, guinea pig, and rabbit (660). The hamster oolemma can fuse with acrosome-reacted spermatozoa of a wide variety of mammalian species including monkey and human (660). However, it should be noted that, in general, membrane fusion occurs much more readily between gametes of homologous species than those of heterologous species.

Medium Components and Conditions Affecting Sperm–Egg Fusion

In experiments that aim to analyze the process and mechanism of sperm–egg fusion, it is advisable to free the eggs from both the cumulus cells and zonae pellucidae and inseminate them with recently acrosome-reacted spermatozoa. Under optimum conditions, sperm–egg fusion begins instantaneously and synchronously. Such systems allow us to study sperm–egg fusion directly.

Sperm–egg fusion is temperature dependent (1037). At an acidic pH (<6.0) sperm–egg fusion is reversibly blocked (1704). Mammalian spermatozoa, unlike sea urchin spermatozoa (1460,1553), require a millimolar concentration of extracellular Ca^{2+} to fuse with the oolemma (953,1694,1695).

Guinea pig spermatozoa can undergo the acrosome reaction in K^+-free medium but are unable to fuse with the oolemma in this medium (1414). This is because the spermatozoa require extracellular K^+ to become fusion competent during the acrosome reaction. Once the spermatozoa have undergone the acrosome reaction in a K^+-containing normal medium, they do not require extracellular K^+ to fuse with the oolemma (1698). The situation is different in the mouse whose spermatozoa require K^+ for sperm–oolemma fusion (773). The reason for such a species difference is unclear.

As already stated, spermatozoa require an intricate balance of ions, energy substrates, and macromolecules in the medium for their capacitation, acrosome reaction and interactions with egg vestments. In contrast, medium requirements are minimal for sperm–oolemma fusion. For example, one of the simplest media that support fusion of acrosome-reacted guinea pig spermatozoa with the oolemma (zona-free eggs) constitutes: 138 mM NaCl + 2 mM $CaCl_2$ + 12 mM $NaHCO_3$ + 4 mM glucose + 3 mg/mL serum albumin (1709). If necessary, NaCl in the medium can be replaced with 138 mM choline chloride, $NaHCO_3$ by 12 mM KH_2PO_4, and glucose by either 1 mM pyruvate or 9 mM lactate. An energy source and albumin are not essential for fusion per se, but their inclusion is recommended to keep eggs alive and prevent adhesion to the container and pipette. Polyvinyl alcohol or polyvinyl pyrrolidone (1 mg/mL) can be used instead of albumin. An organic buffer (e.g., HEPES and MOPS) can be used as substitutes for bicarbonate as long as the medium is maintained at a pH between 7.0 and 8.0.

Inhibition of Sperm–Egg Fusion

Table 10 lists some of the antisperm and antiegg antibodies that inhibit sperm–egg fusion *in vitro*. The mechanism by which these antibodies prevent fusion is not clear, but most of them appear to inhibit the binding of acrosome-reacted spermatozoa to the oolemma.

Only a few nonimmunological reagents that prevent sperm–egg fusion will be discussed here. High concentrations of monosaccharides may reduce the incidence of sperm–oolemma fusion. Inclusion of 40 to 60 mM N-acetylglucosamine, galactose, or L-fucose in insemination medium reduces the incidence of mouse sperm–egg fusion to 40% to 55% of control level (774). Okabe et al. (1313) tested 10 different oligosaccharides including the three saccharides mentioned above and found that D-

TABLE 10. *Antisperm and antiegg antibodies which inhibit in vitro sperm–egg fusion in homologous species*[a]

Antibody/ species	P, polycl. M, monocl. (name, if any)	Antigen site, if known	Ref.
Antisperm			
Mouse	M (OBF13)	Entire head surface	1314
	M (M29 mAb)	Equatorial segment	1436
Hamster	P (3.10)	Head	1267
	P, Fab	Head	1609
Guinea pig	P, dival.		1055
	P. dival.		1706
	M (PH30 mAb)	Postacr. region	1382
Rabbit	P, Fab	Inner acr. memb	1508
Antiegg			
Hamster	M (GHO 4/8)	Oolemma	1218

[a] Several reports that antihuman sperm antibodies inhibit sperm–egg fusion are not included in this table, because it is not clear from the descriptions in the reports whether the inhibition is due to inhibition of sperm–egg fusion per se or due to inhibition of the acrosome reaction.

glucosamine was most potent in inhibiting sperm–egg fusion in the mouse. This was confirmed for the hamster (1735). However, none of the oligosaccharides tested so far is as effective as fucoidan and ascophyllin (sulfated fucose polymers) in inhibiting sperm–egg fusion in both mouse and hamster (774,885,1735). In the presence of fucoidan or dextran sulfate (500 kDa), acrosome-reacted hamster spermatozoa are unable to attach firmly to the oolemma (1735). This may be due to binding of fucoidan to the equatorial segment and the inner acrosomal membrane of acrosome-reacted spermatozoa (240). Putative fusion-mediating molecules in these areas of the spermatozoon may be masked by fucoidan. The prevention of sperm–egg fusion by polyamines (936) may operate through the same or a similar mechanism.

Hirao and Yanagimachi (1036) have reported that of the many enzymes tested, only phospholipase C reduces the fusibility of the hamster oolemma. However, a highly purified preparation of this enzyme is without effect (823). Thus the effect reported by Hirao and Yanagimachi was likely due to the action of contaminants in the enzyme preparation they used. Isolation and identification of the contaminants would be interesting, but this has not yet been done.

Cytochalasin has been reported to reduce sperm penetration into ooplasm (1413). However, it seems to be postfusion events that are disturbed by cytochalasin, not the sperm–egg fusion per se (530,1163,1179,1735).

For more information about sperm–egg fusion in mammals, readers are referred to the refs. 660 and 1709. Important information is available about electrophysiological events that occur immediately before and during sperm–egg fusion in sea urchins (1222,1655).

EGG ACTIVATION

Upon fusion with the spermatozoon, the dormant egg awakens to initiate a series of morphological and biochemical events that lead to cell division/differentiation and the formation of a new individual. This arousal of the egg is referred to as activation. This does not mean that all cellular activities of the unfertilized egg are in a static state. The molecules comprising metaphase spindle, for example, are turning over very rapidly (986). Some other cellular components may well be very active in terms of molecular turnover and metabolism. Therefore, metaphorically speaking, an unfertilized egg may be like a racing car on the start line with its engine running, ready to go but waiting for the wheels to engage with the engine.

The most easily recognizable visible indications of egg activation in mammals are the exocytosis of cortical granules (Fig. 56 *a–d*) and the resumption of meiosis. The egg arrested at metaphase of the second meiosis before fertilization completes the meiosis after sperm–egg fusion (*d–h*). The resulting haploid complement of chromosomes then transforms into an egg pronucleus (*i–j*). Meanwhile, the sperm nucleus decondenses and transforms into a sperm pronucleus (*f–j*). DNA synthesis (chromosome duplication) begins in both the egg and sperm pronuclei several hours after sperm–egg fusion (282,283,1140,1192,1328). The fully developed sperm and egg pronuclei come into close approximation at the center of the egg (*k*), their nuclear envelopes disintegrate, and their chromosomes mingle prior to the first mitotic division (cleavage) (*l–n*) (1176). The mingling of chromosomes (syngamy) can be considered as the end of fertilization and the beginning of embryonic development.

The interval between sperm–egg fusion and the initiation of the first cleavage is a few hours or less in many invertebrates and nonmammalian vertebrates, but in mammals it usually takes 12 hr or more despite the high temperature (30–40°C) of the female's body in which fertilization takes place. The reason for this is not clear, but it could be related partly to differences in the nature of the maternal messenger RNA (mmRNA) stored in the egg cytoplasm during oogenesis. For example, sea urchins may already have transcribed mmRNA important for the cleavage program (648); this may include cyclin (580), which are postulated to be involved in control of embryonic mitosis. Although mammals also have mmRNAs (563), cleavage and early development appear to be relatively more sensitive to transcription inhibitors such as α-amanatin (581). Thus, in mammals, *de novo* mRNA transcription, in addition to mRNA translation, may be rate limiting to cleavage division.

Egg Activation in the Sea Urchin—A Model

The physiology and biochemistry of egg activation have been studied extensively in nonmammalian vertebrates (e.g., amphibians) and invertebrates, particularly the sea urchin (for review, see refs. 578,579,594,595, 618,652,653,916,917,1181,1544,1607). The large number of gametes readily available has facilitated biochemical study of egg activation in these species.

Figure 66 is the timetable of the major events that occur in the sea urchin egg within 80 min of insemination. Immediately after sperm–egg binding, ionic channels of the sperm membrane are incorporated into the egg plasma membrane, and the electrical continuity of two gametes is established (1222). This causes a transient opening of Na^+ channels and activation of voltage-dependent Ca^{2+} channels in the oolemma, resulting in a transient depolarization of the oolemma. This membrane depolarization prevents further spermatozoa from fusing with the oolemma (1084). Sperm–egg interaction then stimulates the breakdown of membrane phosphatidylinositol diphosphate (PIP_2), via the G-protein/phospholipase C cascade, with the resultant production of inositol triphosphate (IP_3) and diacylglycerol (DAG). IP_3 stimulates the release of Ca^{2+} from intracellular stores

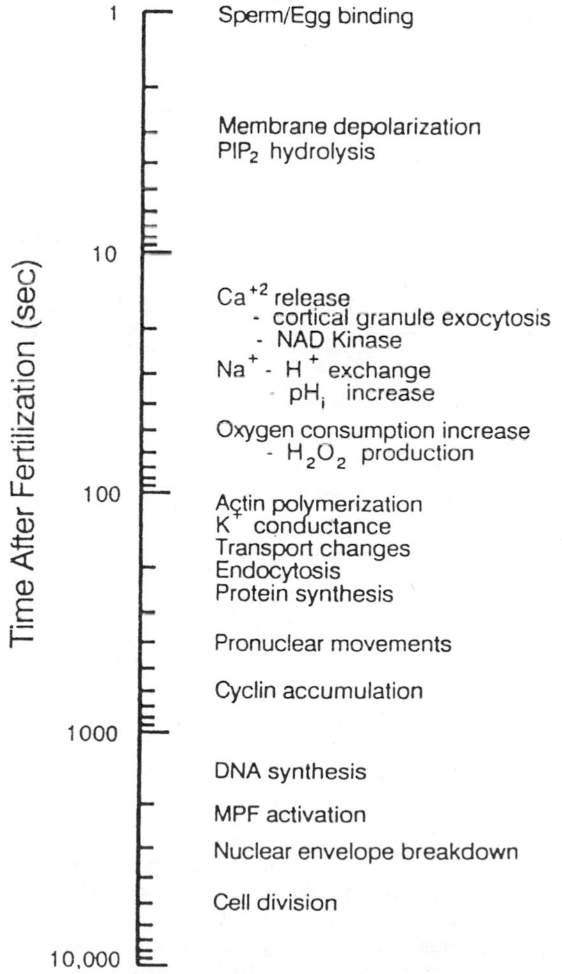

FIG. 66. The sequence of changes initiated by fertilization in the sea urchin, *Strongylocentrotus purpuratus*. (From ref. 917.)

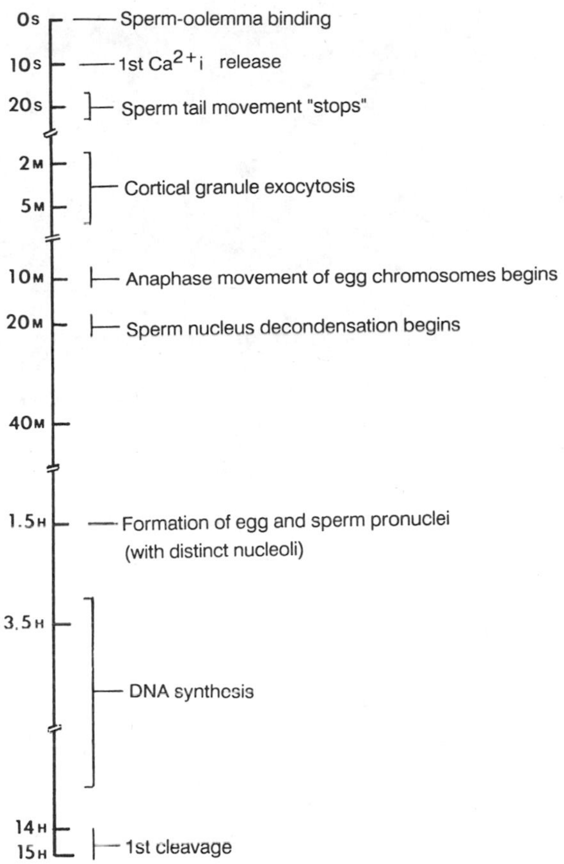

FIG. 67. The sequence of events in fertilization of the golden hamster. S, seconds; M, minutes; H, hours.

(594,1544,1607), which induces the exocytosis of cortical granules (916,1463,1652,1653) leading to the elevation and hardening of the egg envelope. Diacylglycerol stimulates H^+Na^+ exchange (1544), resulting in a rise of intracellular pH (6.9 to 7.3). Acclimations of the ooplasm apparently removes or masks inhibitory proteins in the egg cytoplasm, resulting in activation of the egg's oxidative pathways, lipid metabolism, nicotinamide nucleotide reduction, and protein and DNA syntheses (578,653,916,917,1544).

Transient Ca_i^{2+} Rises during Egg Activation in Mammals

The timetable of the events that occur following sperm–egg binding in the hamster is shown in Figure 67. As will be seen from this figure, all of the postfusion events take place much more slowly than in the sea urchin.

Analysis of egg activation in mammals began in 1981 when Miyazaki et al. (1251) and Cutherbertson et al. (861) reported that hamster and mouse eggs display a series of periodic membrane hyperpolarizations and $[Ca^{2+}]_i$ rises after sperm fusion. Since hyperpolarization of the egg plasma membrane (oolemma) is the result of an increased K^+ conductance of the oolemma due to

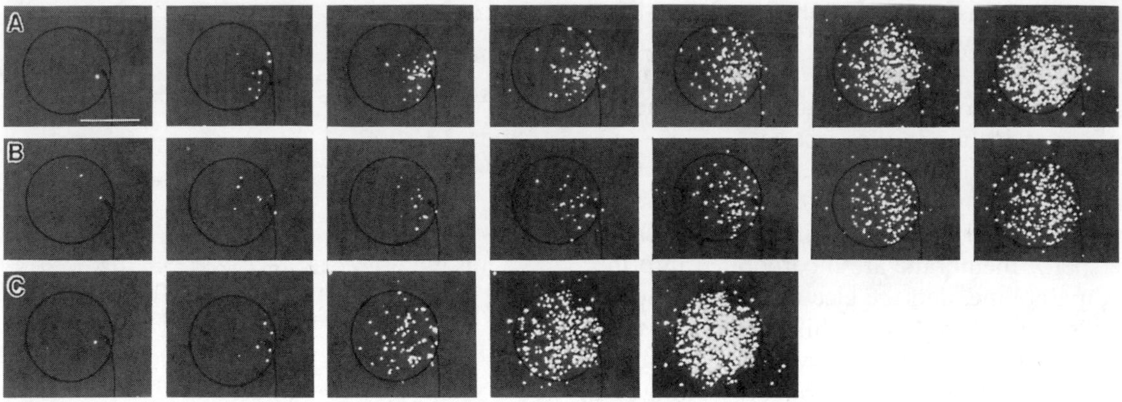

FIG. 68. Continuous accumulation of aequorin luminescent light spots during successive Ca_i^{2+} releases from a monospermic golden hamster egg. The first (A), second (B), and third (C) responses are shown. Each response shows the spread of Ca^{2+} rise from the vicinity of the sperm attachment site. In each row, photographs were taken (from *right to left*) at 0, 0.5, 1, 1.5, 2, 2.5 and 3 seconds (up to 2 sec in C). From ref. 617.

elevated $[Ca^{2+}]_i$ (1068,1252), these three phenomena occur simultaneously (1069). The level of Ca_i^{2+} can be monitored by using either a Ca^{2+}-sensitive microelectrode or a Ca^{2+}-binding photoprotein, aequorin. In the latter, luminescence generated by the Ca_i^{2+} is recorded using the phototon counting imaging apparatus with a supersensitive video camera. In the hamster, the first Ca_i^{2+} release occurs 10 to 30 sec after attachment of the fertilizing spermatozoon to the oolemma (617). The Ca_i^{2+} rise begins near the sperm attachment site, spreads throughout the egg within 4 to 7 sec (Ca^{2+} wave), and ends 15 to 20 sec later (Fig. 68). Transient Ca_i^{2+} rise occurs repeatedly (Ca^{2+} oscillations) at more or less regular intervals for 60 min or more (Fig. 69). A single injection of IP_3 causes a single transient Ca_i^{2+} increase without measurable delay (Fig. 70A) and multiple or continuous injections produce multiple Ca_i^{2+} releases (1250) (Fig. 70B). Injection of GTP$_r$S (a nonhydrolyzable analog of GTP which activates G protein continuously) induces repetitive Ca_i^{2+} increases that decline in amplitude with time (1248,1543) (Fig. 70C). A recent study using a function-blocking monoclonal antibody against the IP_3 receptor protein revealed that IP_3-induced Ca^{2+} release (IICR) from IP_3-sensitive stores is the cause of the initiation of a Ca_i^{2+} rise at the site of sperm attachment. Furthermore, IICR is the essential mechanism for the generation of Ca^{2+} wave and Ca^{2+} oscillations in fertilized eggs (1254,1255). These facts indicate unequivocally that the PIP_2 hydrolysis cascade is responsible for transient Ca_i^{2+} elevations in the fertilized egg (1249,1250).

Figure 71 illustrates possible mechanisms of sperm-induced Ca_i^{2+} release during activation of mature eggs (1253). Two possibilities are shown here. In the first, chain reactions leading to Ca_i^{2+} release are triggered by the binding of putative sperm ligand (X) with the oolemma's receptor (R). Phospholipase C (PLC) is activated by either G protein (G) or protein tyrosine kinase (PTK). In the second, the reactions are initiated by a soluble factor (Y) that is introduced by the spermatozoon into the egg during sperm–egg fusion (863,1281, 1519,1541,1542,1544).

The mechanism of Ca_i^{2+} oscillations has been analyzed

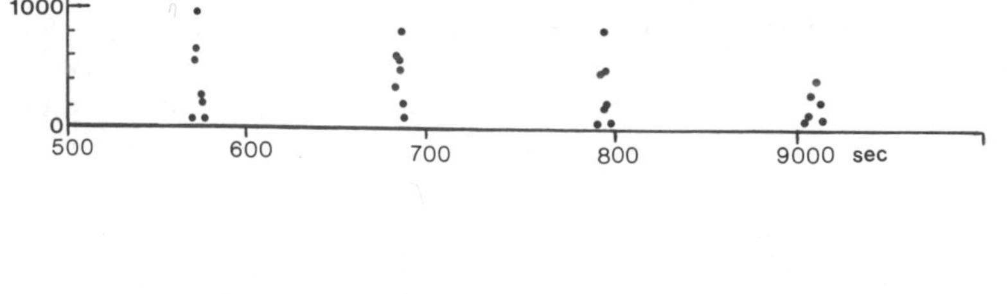

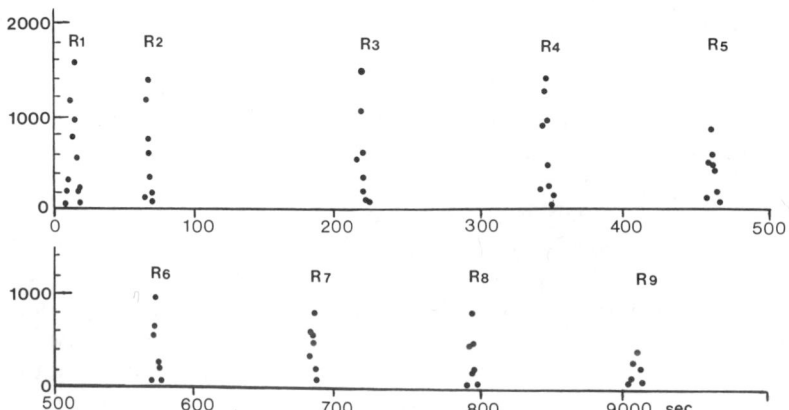

FIG. 69. Periodic Ca_i^{2+} elevations in the golden hamster egg. *Ordinate:* arbitrary unit of aequorin luminescence intensity in a central 21 × 21 μm region of the egg. *Abscissa:* time (sec) after sperm attachment to the oolemma. *One black dot* indicates the value in a 1-sec period. R_1, the first response; R_2, the second response, and so on. (From ref. 617.)

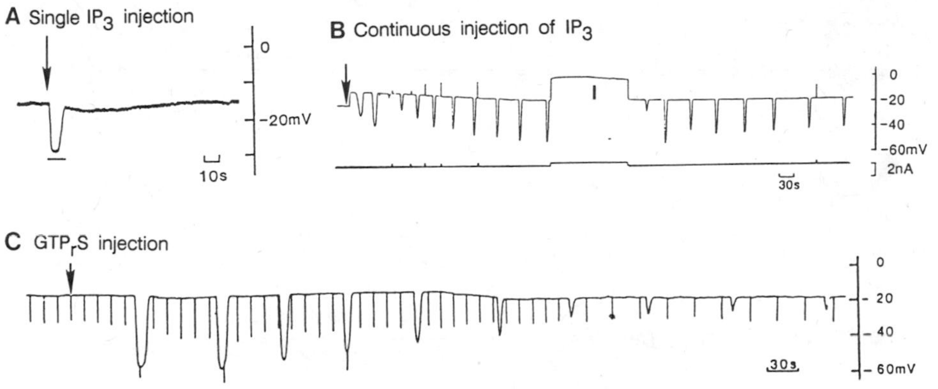

FIG. 70. Transient Ca_i^{2+} elevations by injection of IP_3 and GTP[S] into golden hamster egg; measured by their associated membrane potential hyperpolarization. (**A**) After a single IP_3 injection. (**B**) After continuous injection of IP_3; I, interrupted by sustained positive "backing" current applied to injection pipette. (**C**) After injection of GTP[S]. (From ref. 1248 [A and C]; ref. 1543 [B].)

by Miyazaki and his associates (1068,1248–1250, 1254,1255). Each transient Ca_i^{2+} elevation is due to IP_3-induced Ca_i^{2+} release from internal stores, but continuation of repetitive transient Ca_i^{2+} rises require external Ca^{2+}. Miyazaki et al. postulate that sperm–egg fusion causes a continuous increase in the permeability of the oolemma to Ca_e^{2+} as well as a persistent IP_3 production. Ca^{2+} entering the egg from the outside refills the previously emptied stores and sensitizes IP_3 receptors, leading to the next IP_3-induced Ca^{2+} release when the luminal $[Ca^{2+}]$ reaches a certain level (1253). These investigators propose a linkage between Ca^{2+} influx and Ca^{2+} release. The pathway of Ca^{2+} influx may be Ca^{2+} channels which are activated by IP_3 and or IP_4 (1075) or emptied Ca^{2+} stores (1385).

Figure 72 illustrates hypothetical pathways through which released Ca_i^{2+} triggers CG exocytosis and the resumption of meiosis. The early Ca_i^{2+} rises are undoubtedly important for the exocytosis of cortical granules (1128). Protein kinase C activated by DAG and free Ca_i^{2+} (743,832,833,1664) may break the balance of protein phosphorylation/dephosphorylation, leading to the modulation of membrane ionic channels and inactivation of metaphase promoting factor (MPF) and cytostatic factor (CSF). There is evidence that inactivation of MPF and CSF (1175,1288,1433,1482,1645,1728) and pH_i elevation allow the eggs to escape from the metaphase II arrest. Repetitive Ca_i^{2+} rises may also be important in inducing/controlling ooplasmic streaming and contraction of the fertilized egg (1715).

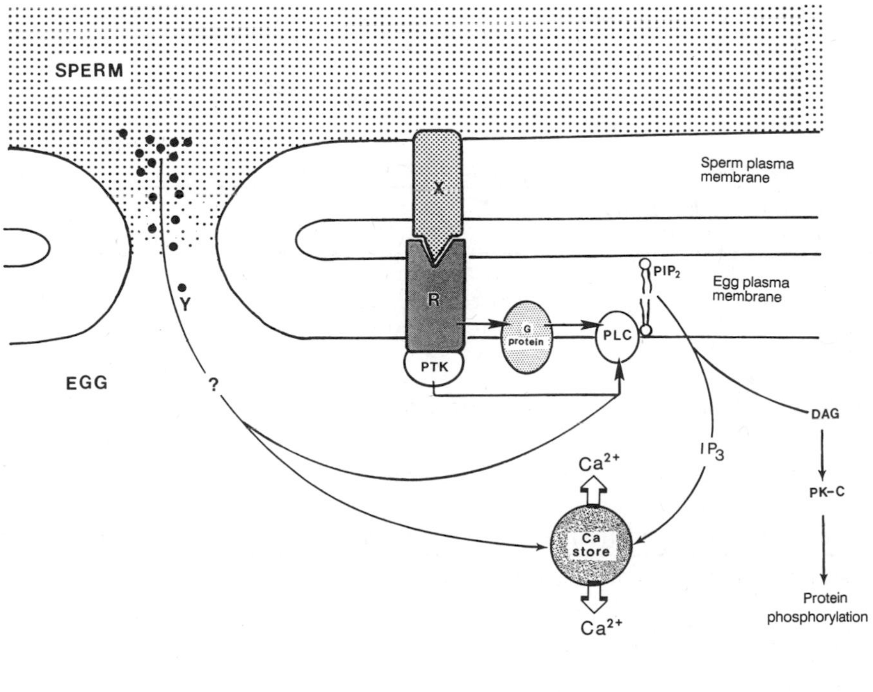

FIG. 71. Possible mechanisms of sperm-induced Ca_i^{2+} release during egg activation (modified from ref. 1253). For explanation, see the text; for full details refer to ref. 1253.

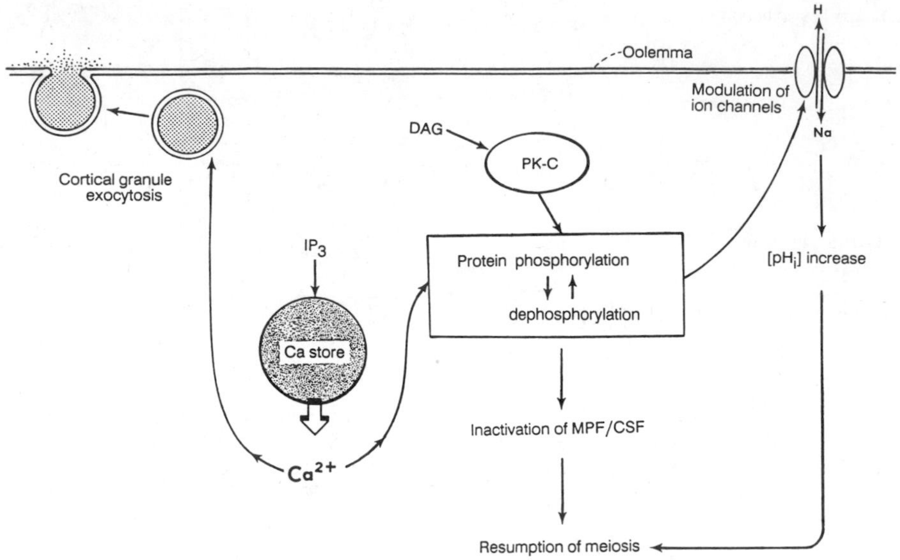

FIG. 72. Hypothetical pathways through which released Ca_i^{2+} triggers cortical granule exocytosis and the resumption of meiosis. For explanation, see the text.

Consequences of Mammalian Egg Activation

A raise in intracellular pH is one of the most important consequences of egg activation in the sea urchin, which is believed to trigger protein and DNA syntheses. According to Shibata et al. (1481), pH_i values of unfertilized and fertilized (pronuclear) hamster eggs are 6.80 ± 0.10 and 7.15 ± 0.08, respectively, which are about the same as those in the sea urchin. Table 11 lists several physical and biochemical parameters of mammalian eggs before and after fertilization. It is important to note that most investigators have not examined eggs continuously (or at short intervals) from the moment of fertilization or egg activation. By only comparing unfertilized eggs with fertilized eggs at the advanced pronuclear stage, they may have overlooked some temporal, yet very important changes that occur immediately or soon after egg activation.

When and How the Egg Becomes Activation Competent

Ovarian oocytes at the germinal vesicle (GV) can fuse with acrosome-reacted spermatozoa (646), but are unable to undergo cortical granule exocytosis (748, 893,1266). Activation competence, as determined by calcium ionophore-induced membrane depolarization (924) and cortical granule exocytosis (893), develops gradually after GV breakdown and reaches a maximum at the metaphase of the second meiosis. According to

TABLE 11. *Change in characteristics of mammalian eggs after fertilization*[a]

Parameters	Difference between unfertilized and fertilized (pronuclear) eggs[b]	Notes	Ref.
Intracellular Po_2	Not significant	ca. 50 mm Hg	1472
ATP/ADP ratio in ooplasm	Significant reduction after fertilization	Increase in cellular respiration?	604
Amino acid uptake	Not significant		588
Water permeability	Not significant		605
Glycerol permeability	Significant increase after fertilization	Within 3 hr after fertilization	592
Membrane lipid diffusibility	Not significant		656
	Significant reduction after fertilization		1095
Membrane capacitance	Significant increase after fertilization	Increase in microvilli?	685, 1689

[a] For the changes in protein and RNA syntheses and in metabolic activities unfertilized through blastocyst stages, see Wolf (1674).
[b] Time of fertilization (sperm–egg fusion) is not described specifically in all but one study (592).

Tombes et al. (1591), the intracellular store of Ca^{2+} increases fourfold during this period. Perhaps, the development (reassembly) of the endoplasmic reticulum in the egg cortex, which functions as calcium sequestered (cf. 895,1193), is closely related to the development of the egg's activation competence (818,891,892).

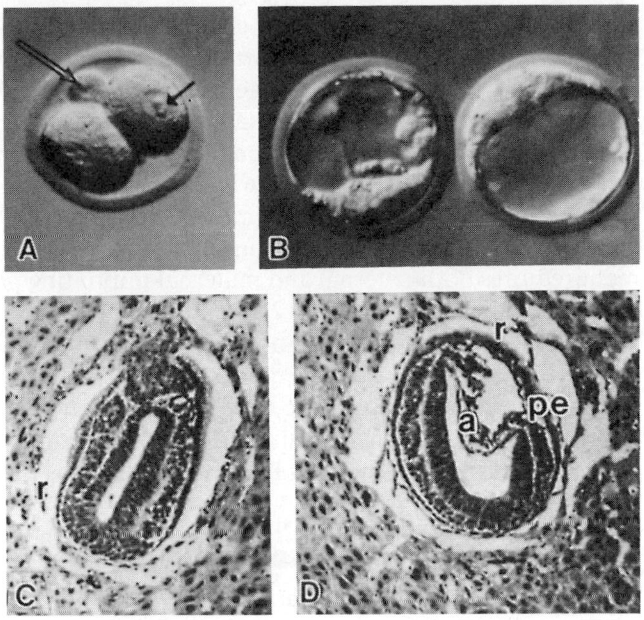

FIG. 73. Parthenogenetically developing mouse (LT/Sv) eggs. Eggs were collected from ovaries 48 hr after PMSG injection and cultured in Whitten's medium. Eggs cleaved (**A**) and developed into blastocysts (**B**) after spontaneous meiotic maturation. Some parthenogenetic blastocysts implanted and developed into 6-day stage (**C** and **D**). *a,* Amnion; *pe,* proximal endoderm; *r,* Reichert's membrane. (From ref. 919 [A, B] and ref. 1512 [C, D].)

Spontaneous Egg Activation

In most species, unfertilized eggs aging *in vivo* or *in vitro* do not activate spontaneously. The metaphase spindle disintegrates gradually and chromosomes scatter throughout the ooplasm, and in some cases individual chromosomes and/or groups of chromosomes may form multiple micropronuclei (1177,1180,1237). In some species, aging eggs activate spontaneously. Rat eggs, for example, commonly emit the second polar body after 4 to 5 hr of culture *in vitro,* but without formation of a pronucleus (1118). Golden hamster eggs are unusual in that a large proportion of them activate spontaneously during aging both *in vivo* and *in vitro.* They form pronuclei with or without emission of the second polar body. A few may reach the two-cell stage, but they do not develop further (694,1699). Although activated eggs may be morphologically similar to fertilized eggs, degenerative changes in various organelles are evident. Moreover, most of the cortical granules remain in the egg cortex (1178). In many species, oocytes in atretic follicles may activate and undergo pseudocleavage before degeneration. In hybrid mice (C57B/6J × AJL/J)F_1, for example, many ovarian oocytes activate when the females are injected with inhibitors of ovarian purine metabolism (882). Eggs develop within follicles up to the three-cell stage, but they do not develop further.

A rare example of true spontaneous egg activation occurs in an inbred LT/Sv strain of the mouse (681,919,920,1512,1514). Approximately 10% to 20% of oocytes activate parthenogenetically, either in the ovary or in the oviduct. Many of these activated eggs are diploid due to either the suppression of the second polar body formation or the fusion of the second polar body with the egg (923). They develop for 5 to 6 days as if they were fertilized normally (Fig. 73A,B). In the uterus, they become disorganized and die shortly after reaching the egg cylinder or primitive streak stage (Fig. 73C,D). In the ovary, the embryos may transform into teratomas.

TABLE 12. *Physical and chemical stimuli that can induce oocyte activation in mammals*[a]

Physical	Chemical
1. Mechanical	1. Enzymatic (e.g., trypsin, hyaluronidase)
(a) Pricking	2. Osmotic
(b) Manipulation of oocytes *in vitro*	(a) Hypertonicity
2. Thermal	(b) Hypotonicity
(a) Cooling	3. Ionic
(b) Heating	(a) Divalent cations
3. Electric	(b) Calcium ionophore
	4. Anesthetics
	(a) General (e.g., ethanol, chloral hydrate)
	(b) Local (e.g., procaine)
	5. Tranquilizers (e.g., phenothiazine)
	6. Protein synthesis inhibitors (e.g., puromycin, cycloheximide)
	7. Products in phosphoinoside cycle (e.g., IP_3, oleoyl-acetyl-glycerol)

[a] 1–5: See refs. 660, 654, 1406; 4: ethanol, ref. 860; 6: refs. 826, 1122, 1494, 1727; 7: ref. 1145.

When two parthenogenetic eight-cell embryos were aggregated with one normally fertilized eight-cell embryo and allowed to develop, chimeric offspring contained cells derived from parthenogenetic embryos, indicating that parthenogenetic cells are capable of differentiating into normal cells (1513,1515). The inability of parthenogenetic embryos to survive to term *in utero* is probably due to the fact that normal postimplantation development requires both paternal and maternal imprinting of the genomes (712,1040,1228,1264,1536).

Another interesting example of spontaneous parthenogenesis is the human ovarian teratoma, which is believed to result from parthenogenetic development of ovarian oocytes (1174). Whether parthenogenetic eggs exhibit Ca_i^{2+} and pH_i rises before they begin to develop has not been determined.

Induced (Artificial) Egg Activation

Mammalian eggs can be activated by a wide variety of physical and chemical stimuli (Table 12). Most of these activating stimuli seem to cause a rise in the intracellular Ca^{2+} concentration (1591,1659). Some stimuli (e.g., protein synthesis inhibitors) may activate eggs by inhibiting protein phosphorylation (1494), perhaps without causing a Ca_i^{2+} rise as in *Xenopus* (1728). Human eggs can be activated by continuous exposure to 10 μg/mL puromycin, but activation starts only after many hours of treatment (873).

Ethanol (860) is very effective in activating the eggs of mice and several other species. However, it cannot activate recently ovulated eggs very efficiently, and works more effectively as the eggs age in the oviduct (1143). This is true for egg activation by a Ca^{2+}-free medium (1537,1660). Despite such seemingly subphysiological situation, mouse eggs activated by a Ca^{2+}-free medium, for example, are able to develop into 25 somite embryos (1117). Similarly, Surani et al. (1535) obtained parthenogenetic diploid mouse blastocysts after activating mouse eggs by a 5- to 6-hr treatment with a Ca^{2+} and Mg^{2+}-free medium. When isolated cells of the inner cell mass were introduced into normal blastocysts, these blastocysts had developed chimeric embryos in 15 to 17 days. As noted earlier, cells from parthenogenetic embryos apparently can survive and differentiate in ectopic sites and contribute to the production of normal embryos. This was confirmed by Jagerbauer et al. (1088) who examined various tissue cells in chimeras produced by aggregation of a four- to eight-cell parthenogenetic mouse embryo with a normally fertilized two-cell embryo. Incidentally, ethanol can induce a long-lasting Ca_i^{2+} rise in mouse eggs, but not the repetitive, transient Ca_i^{2+} releases (1407,1483). It is a poor activating agent for human eggs (668,1666).

Electric shock as a mammalian egg activator was first used to activate mouse eggs by Tarkowski et al. (1562) and then by Gwatkin et al. (1007) in the hamster. Since then, many investigators have used electric shock not only to activate eggs, but also to fuse with anucleate eggs with blastomeres or other cells (779,1136,1229,1499, 1663,1712). Electric shock is believed to cause a reversible membrane lipid breakdown, allowing a temporary increase in membrane permeability to ions, including Ca^{2+} (1731). Ordinary fertilization media can be used during electric stimulation, but media with low electric conductivity (e.g., 300 mM mannitol supplemented with 0.05–0.1 mM $CaCl_2$ and $MgCl_2$) are preferable to avoid excessive ion influx. When a single shock or multiple shocks (e.g., 1.5 kV/cm, 50 μsec) is/are given, 50% to

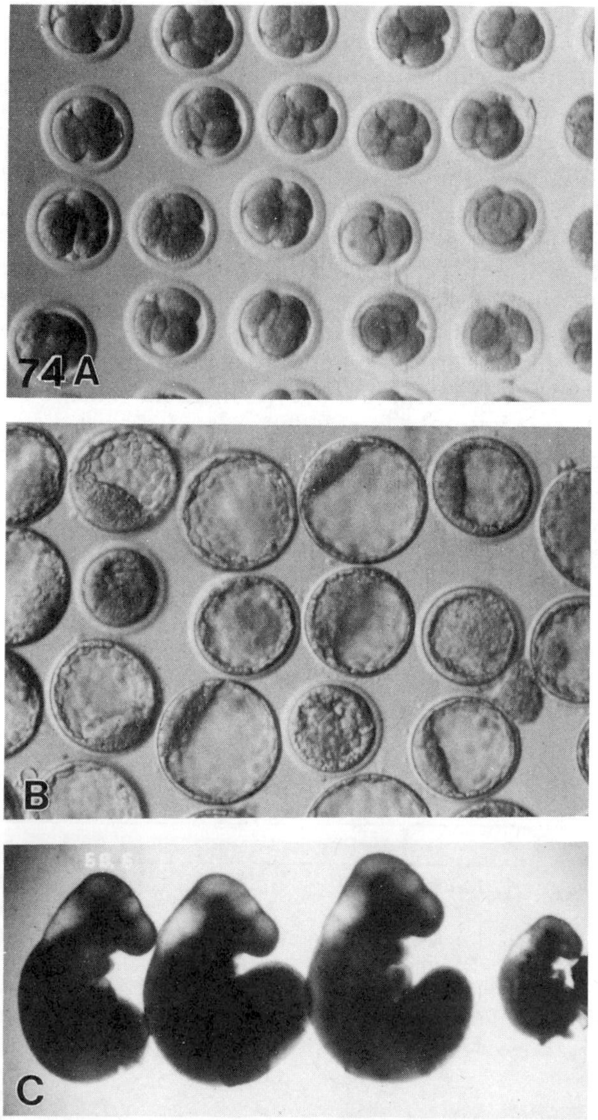

FIG. 74. Parthenogenetically developing rabbit embryos. Unfertilized eggs were repeatedly electrostimulated (e.g., 1.8 kV cm^{-1}, 22 pulses). (**A**) Eggs at the four- to eight-cell stage, 24 hr poststimulation; (**B**) blastocysts, 5 days poststimulation; (**C**) parthenogenetic fetuses on day 10 of pregnancy. (From ref. 1337.)

100% of the eggs are activated (extrusion of the second polar body and formation of pronucleus) (see 1384 and 1406 for refs). In the mouse, Ca^{2+} and Mg^{2+} in the stimulation medium is not essential, but their presence facilitates activation (1327,1406). In the pig, Ca^{2+} is needed in the medium (1534). In regard to hamster eggs, I have found that both calcium ionophore (1511) and electric stimulation (1304a) induce nuclear activation (resumption of meiosis) of hamster eggs very well, but the latter provokes cortical granule exocytosis better than the former (1735). Since a single electric stimulus is able to induce only a single Ca^{2+} transient (933,1534), multiple stimuli may be necessary to mimic the repetitive Ca_i^{2+} releases that occur during normal fertilization. Excellent egg activation and development of parthenogenetic embryos were obtained by Ozil (1337) who electrostimulated rabbit eggs repeatedly (Fig. 74). Here again, the inability of parthenogenetic embryos to develop to term was perhaps due to the lack of paternally imprinted genomes. By contrast, some insects and reptiles reproduce parthenogenetically from generation to generation (616,650). Fertile adult fish and amphibians also have been produced from artificially activated eggs without participation of male genomes (719,1247,1386). We may be able to produce viable parthenogenetic offspring in mammals when we learn more about the nature and mechanisms of genomic imprinting.

CORTICAL REACTION AND POLYSPERMY BLOCK

Sea Urchin—A Model

The sea urchin is the classical experimental animal for the studies of cortical granule exocytosis and block to polyspermy (1082,1084,1181,1463,1464). Although we must be cautious in extrapolating from the sea urchin to mammals, it may be useful to summarize the situation in this model.

Cortical granules (CGs) approximately 1 μm in diameter are assembled by the Golgi-apparatus and move to the periphery of the egg during maturation. Mature CGs contain sulfated mucopolysaccharides, a protein called hyaline, serine protease, and peroxidase among others. The thin vitelline envelope, which can be seen only by electron microscopy, is homologous to the mammalian zona pellucida. When eggs are inseminated, spermatozoa arrive at the vitelline envelope in less than a few seconds. The acrosome reaction occurs either on the vitelline envelope or within a jelly coat surrounding it. Upon insertion of ionic channels of the acrosomal membrane into the oolemma, the latter undergoes a depolarization (from −70 mV to + 10 mV) in 0.1 to 1 sec. This membrane depolarization is maintained and prevents additional sperm fusion until CG exocytosis is completed. This is called rapid (primary) block to polyspermy.

Exocytosis of CGs begins several microns away from the point of sperm–egg fusion (918), rapidly spreads over the entire surface of the egg, and is completed within 1 min. Part of the CG protein remains on the oolemma to form a hyaline layer, but other CG components contribute to the elevation of the vitelline coat. In addition, proteases in CGs are believed to facilitate swelling of the CG contents, elevation of the vitelline envelope, and removal of sperm-binding receptors from the vitelline envelope. CG peroxidase hardens the elevated vitelline envelope by cross-linking tyrosine residues of the vitelline coat protein using H_2O_2 generated by the egg as a burst during the first 15 min after sperm–egg fusion. Such alterations in the vitelline envelope constitute the slow (secondary) block to polyspermy. H_2O_2 is toxic to spermatozoa and in addition it hardens the elevated vitelline coat. This may provide an additional block to polyspermy. Although not functional during normal fertilization, the hyaline layer on the oolemma of the fertilized egg has the ability to prevent sperm–egg fusion. If fertilized eggs are deprived of both the vitelline envelope and the hyaline layer and reinseminated, eggs are penetrated again at all stages as far as blastula (1113,1531).

Cortical Granules and Cortical Reaction in Mammals

Cortical granules (CGs) in mammalian eggs were first observed in the hamster by Austin using the phase-contrast microscope (555). He observed many small granules in the egg cortex which disappeared after fertilization. Austin and Braden (23,555) inferred that these granules are homologous to the sea urchin CGs (577,619) that play a central role in the modification of the egg envelope during fertilization. Figure 75 shows the cortex of hamster egg before and after CG exocytosis: CGs within the cortex appear as small dark granules (0.1–0.5 μm in diameter; ref. 555) under the phase-contrast microscope (Fig. 57A). Since eggs of most other species have coarser granular cytoplasm with abundant inclusions, CGs can be seen clearly only by transmission electron microscopy (1547) or after labeling eggs with specific lectins (e.g., *Lens culinaris* agglutinin or LCA) with selective affinity for CGs (817,892) (Fig. 76C). They exist in the cortex of mature unfertilized eggs of all mammalian species including the human studied so far (699,1188,1445). Unlike sea urchin CGs (1279), CGs in the hamster egg cortex can be shifted by strong centrifugal force (1711).

Origin and Chemistry of Cortical Granules

Cortical granules are manufactured by the Golgi-complex and migrate to the periphery of the egg. Their

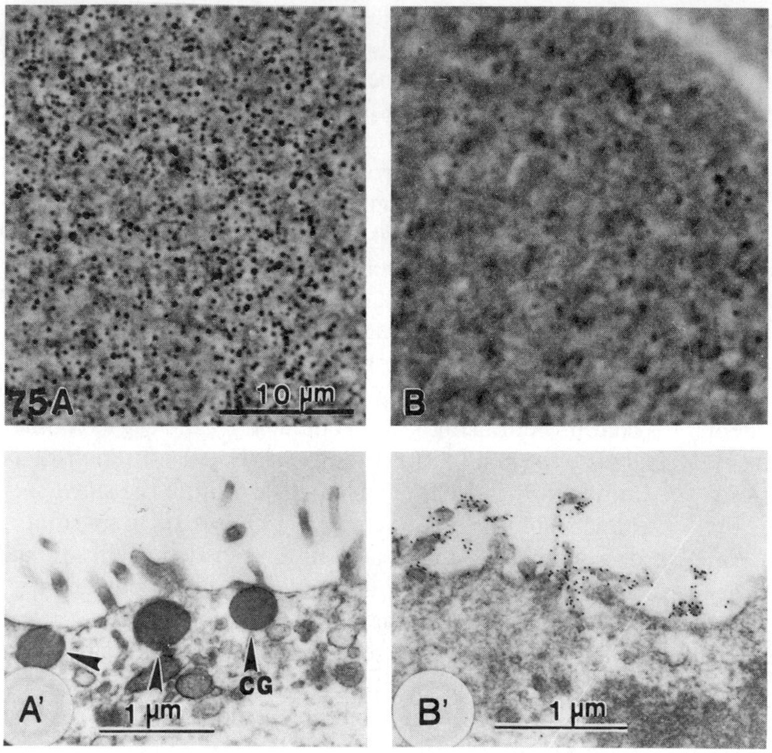

FIG. 75. Cortex of golden hamster eggs: phase-contrast micrographs of unactivated (**A**) and activated (**B**) eggs. Cortical granules are visible as small dark granules in the cortex of the unactivated egg. Sections through the cortex of unactivated (**A'**) and activated (**B'**) eggs. Materials extruded from cortical granules (CG) were labeled with gold-conjugated *Lens culnaris* agglutinin (**B'**). (Figures A' and B', from ref. 817.)

production and migration occur during oogenesis as well as meiotic maturation (583,630,844,1547). Unlike those of the sea urchin, mammalian CGs have a simple internal structure (Fig. 77). They contain mucopolysaccharides (934,1699), protease (203,1263), tissue-type plasminogen activator with serine protease activity (1730), acid phosphatase (1510) and peroxidase (1000).

Behavior of Cortical Granules before fertilization

The behavior of CGs during oocyte maturation was examined carefully by Ducibella and his associates who stained CGs in fixed mouse eggs using biotin-conjugated lectin LCA (892,894). In fully grown oocytes at the germinal vesicle stage, CGs are distributed evenly in the entire egg cortex. As oocytes approach metaphase I, a fairly large CG-free domain appears in the cortex above the meiotic spindle. Since this CG-free cortex is incorporated in the first polar body, the CG-free domain becomes temporarily small, but it becomes larger again as the oocytes approach the metaphase II. CG-free domain enlarges even after ovulation, occupying up to 40% of the entire cortex of an unfertilized mouse egg. The hamster egg cortex also develops a CG-free domain above the meiotic spindle, but it occupies only about 5% of the cortex in a mature unfertilized egg (625) (Fig. 76A,B). The development of the CG-free domain in the mouse and hamster is believed to reflect a local exocytosis and redistribution (lateral migration) of CGs (625,892). No distinct CG-free domain appears in the cat during oocyte maturation, indicating that premature CG exocytosis may not occur in this species (795).

The CG exocytosis prior to fertilization, either in the ovary or oviduct, has been called "premature" or "precocious" (622). This may be induced by a temporal $[Ca^{2+}]_i$ increase around the anaphase spindle, as it occurs in somatic cells (818,1391). Although premature CG exocytosis occurs very prominently above the meiotic spindle, it may occur to a limited extent in the rest of the egg cortex. We can see two populations of CG in transmission electron micrographs, one being more electrodense than the other. The so-called light CG seems to be preferentially involved in the premature CG exocytosis (113,622,630). The biological significance of premature CG exocytosis is not clear. Of many hypothesis proposed (795), I incline to support the view that it contributes to the separation of corona cell processes from the oolemma (1722) and the formation of the perivitelline space, which would facilitate sperm incorporation into the egg (625). However, it is possible that the premature CG exocytosis is a nonfunctional event induced by the transient $[Ca^{2+}]_i$ increase during meiotic maturation.

Cortical Granule Exocytosis at Fertilization

When zona-free hamster eggs are inseminated *in vitro* with acrosome-reacted spermatozoa, the first Ca_i^{2+} release takes place approximately 10 sec after sperm attachment to the egg, the second approximately 1 min later, and successive ones at intervals of 2 min (617).

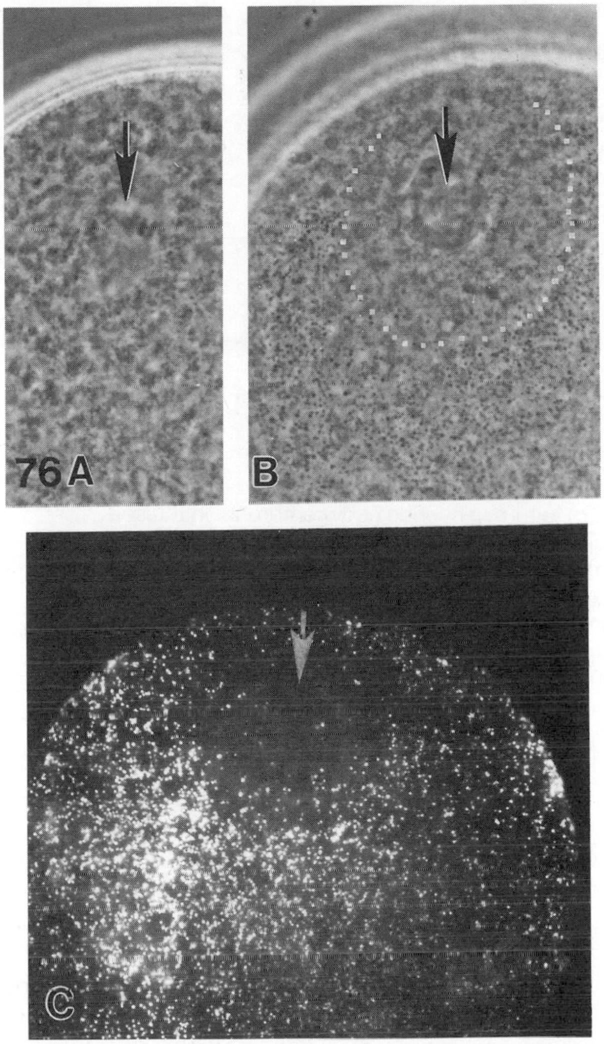

FIG. 76. **(A,B)** Phase-contrast micrographs of the cortex of unactivated golden hamster eggs, showing a cortical granule-free area (*circles with white dotted line*) above the metaphase spindle (*arrow*) of the second meiotic division; photographs A and B were taken at different focal planes. **(C)** Cortex of an unfertilized egg stained with FITC-conjugated *Lens culnaris* agglutinin after fixation and detergent treatment of the egg; numerous bright *dots* represent cortical granules. A *white arrow* in C indicates the cortical-granule-free area of the cortex. (From ref. 625 [A, B]; micrograph C was provided by Dr. Gary N. Cherr.)

Cortical granule exocytosis begins in less than 2 min after sperm–egg binding (see Fig. 67) and the majority (more than 95%) of CGs are exocytosed within the next 5 min (1735). Although Ca_i^{2+} release begins near the point of sperm–egg attachment and spreads to the opposite pole (617), the wavelike propagation of CG exocytosis that occurs in sea urchin and fish eggs, has not been witnessed in mammalian eggs. Perhaps, the first Ca^{2+} release triggers the exocytosis of most CGs, but the subsequent releases may induce the exocytosis of the remaining CGs as well. Part of exocytosed CG materials remain on the egg surface. In the mouse, they aggregate gradually to form large clumps. The clumps are aggregated further into a larger mass at the cleavage furrow and then disappear completely by the late two-cell stage (1161).

Virtually nothing is known about the molecular mechanism of mammalian CG exocytosis. Experiments using isolated sea urchin egg cortex with firmly attached CGs have demonstrated that micromollar Ca^{2+} triggers CG exocytosis, which is energy dependent. Ca^{2+} may induce conformational changes in the CG and plasma membranes necessary for membrane fusion. Ca^{2+} may also activate membrane-bound phospholipases A_2 and C, which hydrolyze membrane phospholipids to produce fusogenic lysophospholipids and diacyl glycerol (1082, 1463). Necessity of Ca^{2+} for mammalian egg CG exocytosis has been demonstrated in the mouse; mouse eggs preloaded with Ca^{2+} chelater BAPTA/AM fail to exhibit CG exocytosis in response to the parthenogenetic agent, ethanol (1591).

Immature eggs at the GV stage lack the ability to undergo CG exocytosis in response to spermatozoa or parthenogenetic agents. In the mouse, this ability begins to appear at metaphase I and reaches a normal level by metaphase II (818,981). Ducibella (818,891,892) attributed this to the development of the endoplasmic reticulum in the egg cortex during meiotic maturation. In other words, Ducibella considered that the CG exocytosis incompetence of immature GV eggs is due to the absence of the cortical membrane system, which stores and releases intracellular Ca^{2+}. Immature GV eggs of the hamster, like those of the mouse, are unable to undergo CG exocytosis (1266), but they are able to exhibit repetitive Ca_i^{2+} elevations in response to spermatozoa and IP_3 injection (964). Since the peak of each Ca^{2+} oscillation is about half of that in mature eggs (964), the CG exocytosis incompetence of immature hamster eggs could be due to a low level of released Ca_i^{2+}. Alternatively, it could be due to an incomplete assembly of CG and CG exocytosis mechanisms.

Egg Development without Cortical Granule Exocytosis

When healthy mature eggs are fertilized by normal spermatozoa, the vast majority of CG erupt quickly. Their exocytosis tends to be less complete in parthenogenetically activated eggs (994,999,1679). Nevertheless, mouse eggs parthenogenetically activated by a $Ca^{2+}Mg^{2+}$-free medium or ethanol are able to develop into forelimb bud embryos (1117,1536) or differentiate into normal somatic cells or germ cells (1535). Initiation of embryonic development without cortical reaction is certainly possible in the sea urchin (640) and fish (597). Although it is an exciting event in the fertilization process, CG exocytosis can be considered as a terminal event. Its prime function is to modify the egg vestment

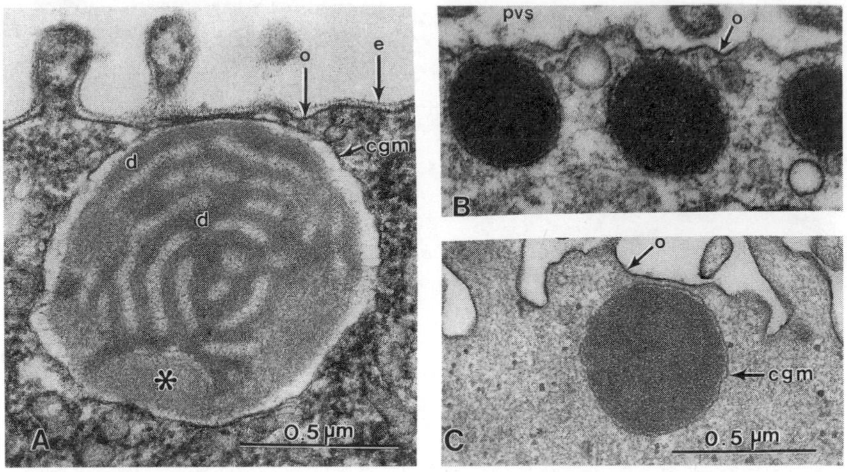

FIG. 77. Cortical granules of the sea urchin (**A**), human (**B**), and golden hamster (**C**). During exocytosis, cortical granule membrane (*cgm*) fuses with the oolemma (*o*) to form a hybride egg membrane. In the sea urchin *Hemicentrotus pulcherrimus* (see A), each cortical granule contains electron-dense lamellar (*d*) and electron-lucent semispherical (*) structures. The former are discharged into the perivitelline space (*pvs*) and join the overlying vitelline envelope (*e*) so that a delicate vitelline envelope transforms into an elevated and hardened fertilization envelope. The latter remains on the oolemma surface to become a component of the hyaline layer. In mammals the contents of individual cortical granules appear homogenous (see B and C), but part of the contents remains on the oolemma (*o*), while another part diffuses into the perivitelline space (*pus*) and alters the physical and chemical characteristics of the relatively thick zona pellucida. (Provided by Dr. Noriko Usui [A] and Dr. A. Henry Sathananthan [B].)

(and the oolemma?) to prevent polyspermic fertilization (see below).

Block to Polyspermy

The block to polyspermy in the sea urchin occurs in two steps (1084,1181,1186,1463). Within a few seconds after sperm attachment to it, the negatively charged oolemma is depolarized (from −70 mV to +10 mV), preventing additional sperm fusion until the cortical reaction is completed. Sperm–egg fusion begins approximately 5 sec after the onset of membrane depolarization. About 3 sec later CG exocytosis begins and is completed in the next 20 to 30 sec. Cortical-granule-mediated elevation and modification of the vitelline coat serve as the permanent block to polyspermy to replace the temporal electric block to polyspermy. The hyaline layer formed on the oolemma by CG also possesses the ability to block polyspermy.

The electric polyspermy block does not seem to occur in the mouse (1085), the only mammal investigated. Cortical-granule-mediated modification of the zona pellucida (zona reaction) and CG-independent change in the oolemma (plasma membrane block) are the major polyspermy-blocking mechanisms in mammals (20, 515,891). According to Yu and Wolf (1718), mouse eggs are capable of extruding the nuclei of supernumerary spermatozoa during or shortly after extrusion of the second polar body. Stewart-Savage and Bavister (1517) have suggested the possibility that supernumerary hamster spermatozoa may fuse with the oolemma, but are prevented from entering the vitellus. Whether these forms of polyspermy block occur in animals other than the mouse and hamster is not known. Eggs of salamanders and birds have no cortical granules. Numerous spermatozoa enter an egg and form pronuclei during normal fertilization (physiological polyspermy). However, only one of them unites with the female pronucleus; the rest become pycnotic and degenerate by some unknown mechanism (1081,1084). Such a polyspermy-blocking mechanism does not exist in mammals.

Relative Importance of Zona Reaction and Plasma Membrane Polyspermy Block

The mechanism by which eggs of a species prevent polyspermy can be inferred by examining the location and frequency distribution of supplemental spermatozoa within the perivitelline space of the eggs collected from oviducts after natural mating. If the eggs of a species seldom contain supplementary spermatozoa in the perivitelline space, this species must depend heavily on the zona reaction for polyspermy prevention. On the contrary, if monospermic eggs contain numerous supplementary spermatozoa in the perivitelline space, the plasma membrane block must be the primary mechanism for polyspermy prevention in this species. Thus, Austin (20) divided mammals into three groups: Group I depends primarily on the zona reaction, group II depends primarily on the plasma membrane block, and

TABLE 13. *Classification of animals based on the mechanisms of polyspermy block they use*

	Group I	Group II	Group III
Species	Golden hamster Dog Sheep Field vole Ferret Human[a]	Rat Mouse Guinea pig Cat	Rabbit Pika Mole Bat[b]
Characteristics of supplemental sperm in monospermic eggs	Supplemental sperm in PVS is rare if ever found	Often 1 (or less commonly few) in PVS	Regularly have supplemental sperm in PVS
Polyspermy block in normal fertilization depends primarily on	ZR	Both ZR and PMB	PMB

From ref. 12. PVS, perivitelline space; ZR, zona reaction; PMB, plasma membrane block.
[a] Ref. 632, 747.
[b] Ref. 1273.

group III depends on both (Table 13). Humans seem to belong to group I (632,747).

It is important to note that in all mammals the zona pellucida and egg plasma membrane (oolemma) work synergistically to reduce the chance of polyspermy. For example, rabbit zona, which do not exhibit a distinct zona reaction restricts the number of spermatozoa reaching the oolemma; without zonae many rabbit eggs become polyspermic *in vitro* (1223). The hamster oolemma seldom meets supernumerary spermatozoa under ordinary *in vivo* conditions, yet its ability to fuse with spermatozoa is reduced drastically upon fertilization (747,1517). In other words, eggs of all species have at least two safeguards against polyspermy.

Mechanism of the Zona Reaction

The involvement of CGs in the zona reaction was first inferred by Austin and Braden (23) and proven experimentally by Barros and Yanagimachi (31). Gwatkin and his associates (203,1005) first suggested the involvement of CG protease in the zona reaction. Subsequently, partial hydrolysis of zona proteins following fertilization was reported in various animals including the rat (1398), mouse (791), pig (1024,1029) and human (1473). In the mouse, a zona glycoprotein ZP2 (120 kD) is partially hydrolyzed upon fertilization or parthenogenetic activation (759) by a cortical granule-derived nontrypsinlike protease (1263). It becomes a 90-kD glycoprotein, $ZP2_f$ (Fig. 78), which remains as part of the zona due to persisting —S—S— bonds (1263). Another major ZP glycoprotein, ZP3, is altered simultaneously, but its change is undetectable in protein molecular weight or isoelectric point; perhaps CG glycosidase rather than protease modifies saccharide moiety of ZP3 (1638). A sudden increase in PAS-reactivity of mouse zona after fertilization (948) may be due to saccharide modification of ZP molecules. Not all the ZP2 and ZP3 molecules are

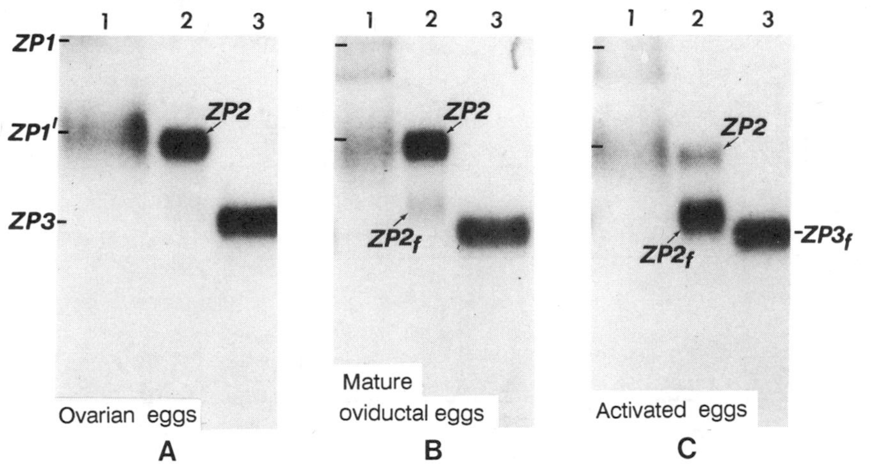

FIG. 78. Evidence that ZP2 is hydrolyzed upon egg activation: Discontinues SDS-PAGE of purified mouse zona pellucida glycoproteins from **(A)** mature ovarian eggs, **(B)** mature unfertilized oviductal eggs, and **(C)** eggs artificially activated by calcium ionophore. Note that after egg activation most of ZP2 are converted to ZP_{2f} with a lower molecular weight. The presence of a small amount of $ZP2_f$ in mature ovidicutal egg (B) is perhaps due to the premature cortical granule exocytosis that occurs in unfertilized mouse eggs in the oviduct. (From ref. 66.)

converted to $ZP2_f$ and $ZP3_f$. Yet it is enough to render the zona impenetrable by spermatozoa (759,761,939, 1638,1639,1642). The presence of residual ZP2 and ZP3 in the zonae of fertilized eggs accounts for the binding and the acrosome reaction of spermatozoa on the zonae of fertilized eggs that may occur after reinsemination of fertilized eggs with very high concentrations of spermatozoa (1642).

As already stated, mouse ovarian eggs exhibit an extensive precocious CG exocytosis during meiotic maturation while they are in the ovary, yet the zonae remain penetrable by spermatozoa (893). Perhaps fluid components surrounding ovarian eggs inactivate CG enzymes (see below). Eggs of some strains of mouse are known to reduce their fertilizability rather quickly after ovulation. In part, this could be due to the spontaneous CG exocytosis within oviducts (1107,1632) which do not carry CG enzyme inhibitors.

It is well known that zonae of many species become resistant to various reagents after fertilization (Table 14). The reason for this is not very clear. Although some investigators maintain that this zona hardening is due to cross-linking of tyrosine residues in the zona by the catalytic action of CG peroxidase (1000,1456), others cast doubt on this hypothesis. Conformational changes in ZP proteins by CG protease (1638) or an alternation of ZP saccharides by CG glycosidase (758,1189,1638) or lectinlike molecules (879) may be responsible for the zona hardening. In the hamster, hardening of the zona cannot be detected by chemical means (Table 14), but it can be demonstrated by sucking eggs (zonae) into a glass capillary (886). Postfertilization hardening of the zona does not appear directly related to the polyspermy block. For example, rabbit zonae exhibit a very distinct postfertilization hardening (993), yet they remain penetrable by spermatozoa for many hours after fertilization (Fig. 79A,B). The rabbit zona needs the oviductal mucin coat to block sperm penetration. The significance of the zona hardening, if any, is probably in the preimplantation development of zygotes, rather than polyspermy prevention.

Kinetics and Efficiency of the Zona Reaction

Since the zona reaction is the result of chemical interactions between zona molecules and CG materials, any reagents or conditions that interfere with CG exocytosis and zona-CG interaction would affect the zona reaction. The chronology of CG exocytosis and zona reaction may vary according to species. In the mouse and hamster, CG exocytosis seems to begin within a few minutes after sperm–egg fusion and is completed by 5 to 10 min after the fusion. Functional zona reaction could be established within a few minutes after sperm–egg fusion, but in most eggs the zona reaction seems to be completed when CG exocytosis is about to finish (711,1263, 1446,1518).

When CG exocytosis is slowed down by a local anesthetic, procaine, polyspermy results from multiple sperm penetration through the zona (671). An almost unlimited number of spermatozoa pass through the zona when the vitelli (and perhaps CGs too) are destroyed by concentrated solutions of neutral salts (766,1703). The high incidence of polyspermy in immature oocytes and aging eggs must be due, at least in part, to the immaturity or deterioration of the machinery involved in CG exocytosis, respectively (for details, see 891). Human eggs, which normally exhibit a rather strong zona reaction in the inner region of the zona, can be polyspermic. One possible cause of polyspermy in human IVF, according to Sathananthan and Trounson (632), is the delayed CG exocytosis and consequent delay in the zona reaction. Immaturity of the egg at the time of sperm penetration, excessive aging of eggs in culture, and/or an inherent zona defect could all result in polyspermy.

In some animals with relatively thin zonae (e.g., laboratory rodents), all or most of the supernumerary spermatozoa fail to insert their heads deep into the zonae of fertilized eggs. Apparently the soluble components of CGs spread out quickly and alter the entire thickness of the zona rather promptly. In some other species with relatively thick zonae (e.g., cats, pigs, and humans) many spermatozoa keep entering the zona even after fertiliza-

TABLE 14. *Block to multiple sperm penetration of the zona pellucida and the development of resistance to solublization by protease and mercaptoethanol*

Species	Block to multiple sperm penetration of zona	Increased resistance of zona pellucida to solubilization in		
		Trypsin	Pronase	Mercaptoethanol
Mouse	+	+	+	+
Rat	+	+		
Hamster	++	–	–	–
Rabbit	–	++	++	++
Sheep	++		–	

From ref. 199.

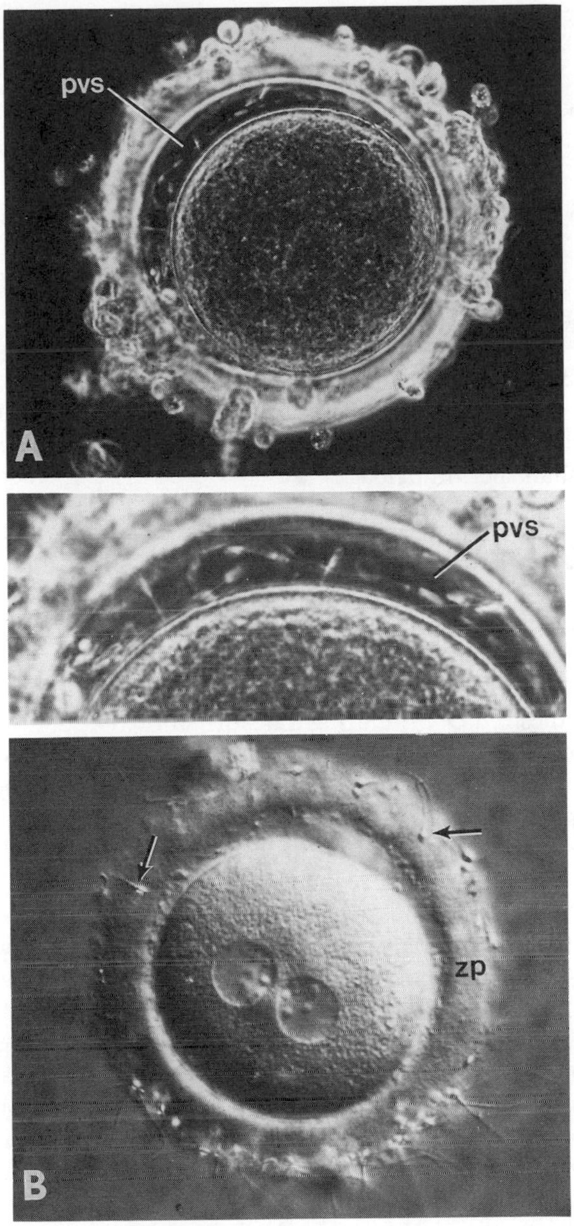

FIG. 79. Fertilized eggs of the rabbit (**A**) and human (**B**). In the rabbit, many surplus spermatozoa are seen in the perivitelline space (pvs) of a monospermically fertilized egg. In the human, surplus spermatozoa are seldom seen in the perivitelline space of normally fertilized eggs. Micrograph B shows that at least two spermatozoa (*arrows*) have entered deep inside the zona pellucida (*zp*) but failed to pass through it. (Provided by Dr. L. Michael Bedford [A] and Dr. Phillip Matson [B].)

tion. They advance half way through the zona, then stop (Fig. 79C) (132,747,1662), suggesting that zona modifications by CG material is prominent in the inner half of the zona where zona molecules are more tightly packed than the outer half. In the human, CG material may not mask or destroy the sperm receptor activity of the outer region of the zona, since eggs normally fertilized *in vitro* have as many spermatozoa bound to and intruding into the zona as sibling eggs unfertilized because of an impenetrable zona (736).

Spontaneous Zona Hardening In Vitro

As stated previously, preovulatory CG exocytosis in the mouse is very prominent. It involves 20% to 40% of the egg cortex around the meiotic spindle (891,1293). Obviously, this preovulatory CG exocytosis does not induce a zona reaction (892,894,1679), or all ovulated eggs would be infertile. When immature mouse oocytes are cultured in simple culture media such as Whittingham's medium with 0.4% bovine serum albumin, the oocytes undergo nuclear maturation normally, but the zonae of many oocytes are impenetrable by spermatozoa; zonae show resistance to various zona-dissolving reagents (883). This spontaneous zona hardening *in vitro* (869,879) can be prevented by incorporating serum or follicular fluid in egg culture media (868,883). Protease inhibitors (e.g., fetuin) in the follicular fluid (1462) seem to inactivate proteases released from the CG during meiotic maturation of the egg. Zhang et al. (1729) could prevent zona hardening of *in vitro* matured rat oocytes by including soybean trypsin inhibitor or mercaptoethanol in oocyte culture media. The spontaneous zona hardening *in vitro* does not occur in the cat whose oocytes exhibit insignificant or no preovulatory CG exocytosis (795).

Plasma Membrane Polyspermy Block

The egg plasma membrane (oolemma) is an important site of polyspermy block. Even in species whose eggs depend almost exclusively on the zona pellucida to prevent polyspermy (e.g., hamsters and humans), the oolemma drastically reduces its ability to fuse with spermatozoa after fertilization or parthenogenetic activation (817,1235,1290,1517,1734). In the case of the hamster, the oolemma does not lose its fusibility completely and remains capable of fusing with few spermatozoa until the two- to four-cell stage of embryonic development (646,1734).

Speed

Sato (1446) inseminated mouse eggs *in vitro* (between a slide and coverslip) and continuously examined the behavior of the fertilizing and supernumerary spermatozoa toward the oolemma. He found that none of the supernumerary spermatozoa fused with oolemma when they entered the perivitelline space later than 1 min after fusion of the fertilizing spermatozoon. In other words, polyspermy block of the oolemma appears to be established by 1 min after sperm–egg fusion. Although Sato did not examine CG exocytosis, it is most probable that the majority of CG were still in the egg cortex at that time. Stewart-Savage and Bavister (1518) considered the speed of the plasma membrane block in the hamster based on statistical analysis of the temporal relationship between sperm–egg fusion and CG exocytosis. They estimated that the plasma membrane polyspermy block is established by 6 min after sperm–egg fusion while CG exocytosis is still in progress, and that CG exocytosis is completed 9 min after sperm–egg fusion. These estimated time intervals between sperm–egg fusion and plasma membrane polyspermy block are considerably shorter and probably more accurate than those estimated by earlier researchers (711,1673).

Mechanism

Since CG membranes are integrated in the oolemma upon CG exocytosis (817,1161), it is tempting to speculate that both CG membrane and CG contents contribute to the establishment of plasma membrane polyspermy block. In fact, Wolf and Hamada (1677) reported that the mouse CG contents, collected from 200 fertilized eggs in 50 μl medium, could render approximately 30% of zona-free unfertilized mouse eggs incapable of fusing with spermatozoa. However, there is evidence suggesting that CG exocytosis is not directly related to the plasma membrane polyspermy block. For instance, when mouse eggs are activated by either calcium ionophore or mechanical stimulation, at least or more than 50% of CG undergo exocytosis, yet all the eggs remain capable of fusing (1679). Similarly, mouse eggs activated by ethanol undergo CG exocytosis (1001), yet the oolemmae remain fusible even at the late pronuclear stage (1204). In the hamster, the oolemma of the fertilized egg does not become *totally* rejective to excessive spermatozoa until the four to eight-cell stage (646,1734).

In the sea urchin, depolarization of the oolemma constitutes the fast (temporal) block to polyspermy, which is followed by the slower (permanent) CG-mediated block at the level of egg vestment (1084,1464). In the mouse, there is no indication of membrane potential change following fertilization (1085). The only prominent electrical change in the mouse and hamster is the transient membrane hyperpolarization which begins several seconds after sperm–egg fusion (126,861). This cannot be considered representing the permanent polyspermy block of the oolemma. Inseminated rabbit eggs exhibit membrane depolarization followed by a slow repolarization which may occur up to 36 times over a period of 90 ± 11 min (615). However, it is unlikely that such transient membrane changes block polyspermy permanently. It remains to be determined whether changes in membrane surface negative charge (836), membrane capacitance (685) and concanavalin-A-binding ability (988) contribute directly to the polyspermy block of the rabbit oolemma. The nature and mechanisms of the plasma membrane block to polyspermy in mammals must be the subject of further investigations.

DECONDENSATION OF THE SPERM NUCLEUS IN OOPLASM

Sperm Nucleus

Before discussing the process and mechanism of sperm nucleus decondensation, it is necessary to describe some of the features that characterize the mammalian sperm nucleus.

Histone and Protamine in the Nucleus

In somatic cells as well as spermatogonia and spermatocytes, histones are synthesized in the nucleus during interphase of the cell cycle and then bind to newly synthesized DNA. During transformation of round spermatids to spermatozoa, all or almost all of their histones are replaced by transitional proteins and then by more basic protamines, which are rich in arginine, serine, and cysteine (560,566,702,1126,1232,1374). This sequential protein replacement coincides with compaction of the chromatin and the repression of transcriptional activity in the nucleus (560,741,1025). In human and mouse spermatozoa, small amounts of histones remain bound to the DNA (e.g., 976,1300,1559). The persistence of transitional proteins in human sperm nuclei has been reported also (1210). In man, ejaculates commonly contain a variable proportion of spermatozoa with immature nuclei (733), and this may contribute to the presence of such proteins (657). In fact, the proportions of histones and transitional proteins are considerably higher in the spermatozoa of infertile men than in those of fertile men (703,757).

An unusual event within the sperm nucleus in eutherian mammals is the extensive conversion of protamine —SH to —S—S— during sperm passage (maturation) through the epididymis (47,49,94,566,1211, 1348,1470). This makes the nuclei of mature eutherian spermatozoa resistant to physical and chemical disruption (1112,1231,1257,1691,1702) (Fig. 80). The rigidity of the nucleus that the keratoid quality confers is believed to be beneficial for the mechanical passage of the sperm head through the thick, rather tough, zona pellucida (559,731; also see the section on "Sperm Interaction with Zona Pellucida").

Acridine orange (AO) can be used in assessing the SH/SS status of the sperm nuclei (1139). When the nuclei are treated with acid (e.g., acetic alcohol) while their DNA-associated protamines are not cross-linked by

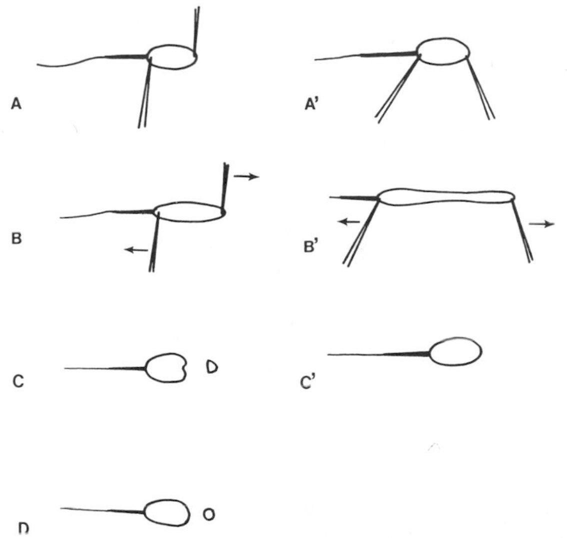

FIG. 80. Experiments showing the rigidity and elasticity of human sperm head (nucleus). When the head of a normal motile spermatozoon was grasped with two needles (*A*) and stretched with full tension of the needles (*B*), a small piece was broken off at the anterior end of the head. The head snapped back to its original shape except for the torn anterior head end (*C–D*). When the head of a 3-day-old, nonmotile, normal looking spermatozoon was similarly manipulated, the head was stretched markedly (*A′–B′*). Normal shape of the head was restored upon release of the head from the needles (*C′*). (Redrawn from ref. 1257.)

—S—S—, the DNA is denatured (becomes single-stranded). Acridine orange bound to denatured DNA aggregates to emit a "red" fluorescence. In contrast, when highly —S—S— cross-linked nuclei are treated with acid, the associated DNA is resistant to denaturation. In that case, AO binds to native (double-stranded) DNA as a monomer and emits a "green" fluorescence. As might be expected, the nuclei of all testicular spermatozoa typically exhibit a red fluorescence and all cauda epididymal spermatozoa show a green fluorescence. In other words, AO can differentiate immature sperm nuclei from mature ones, and vice versa. Although the principles are less clear, toluidine blue (1141), Giemsa or methylene blue (1243), and aniline blue (1567) can differentiate maturity and immaturity of spermatozoa by the staining reactions. Use of AO and aniline blue has become popular for the assessment of the maturity and fertility potential of human spermatozoa (690,831,925, 944,1565).

DNA Packing in the Sperm Nucleus

DNA is packed in a unique way within the sperm nucleus. In somatic cell nuclei, DNA is first packed into nucleosomes, in which approximately 140 base pairs of DNA are wrapped slightly less than twice around an octomer of histones; adjacent nucleosomes are then further coiled into a solenoid (Fig. 81A). According to one model (701,1636,1637), protamines in the sperm nucleus bind to DNA by lying lengthwise inside the minor groove, with DNA strands packed side by side in a linear array (Fig. 81B). Chromatins are arranged in an orderly way (1129,1132,1634a,1635,1636) within a nuclear matrix (741,742).

Figure 82 shows the intact nucleus of a human spermatozoon (arrow) and 22 chromosomes derived from the nucleus of another human spermatozoon penetrated into a golden hamster egg. Obviously sperm chromosomes are packed very tightly within a very small space. Despite such extreme compaction, sperm chromatins are not dehydrated. Water may contribute as much as one third of the volume of each nucleus of mature rat spermatozoa (864). Since the sperm nucleus apparently contains a DNA polymerase (1404), theoretically at least it might be activated during the pronuclear stage of fertilization to repair DNA damages inflicted on spermatozoa before fertilization (562,978,1219). The sperm nucleus also contains some RNA (794,1354), a DNA-dependent RNA polymerase (1026), and circular DNA (1227). Whether these minor components have specific functions during early embryogenesis or are just residues trapped during nuclear condensation is not known.

Under ordinary light and transmission electron microscopes, the mature sperm nucleus appears as a homogeneous structure of highly compacted chromatin. Individual chromosomes cannot be identified. However, it is now possible to determine the presence or absence of specific chromosomes (e.g., X and Y chromosomes, chromosomes 1, 17, and so on) in the sperm nucleus by *in situ* hybridization using specific molecular probes (Fig. 83) (835,1012,1013,1077,1105). Kinetochores (centromeres) can be visualized in sperm nuclei using specific antibodies (1009,1339,1450,1533).

The size and shape of the sperm head are determined by the size and shape of the nucleus and rostrally the acrosome. The mechanism by which the species-specific characteristics of these organelles are determined remains unknown (928,1375).

Sperm Nucleus Decondensation

The first visible change to occur in the sperm nucleus after its incorporation into the egg is the breakdown of the nuclear envelope, which, unlike that of somatic cells, has no pores overall except in its posterior region. The breakdown of the membrane begins at the level of the equatorial segment and proceeds anteriorly and posteriorly. The perinuclear material (theca) (742,1185,1326) begins to mingle with the ooplasm before decondensation of the sperm nucleus becomes distinct (Fig. 84). The speed of nucleus decondensation varies among species. In the golden hamster, for example, decondensation becomes distinct first in the middle of the sperm nucleus

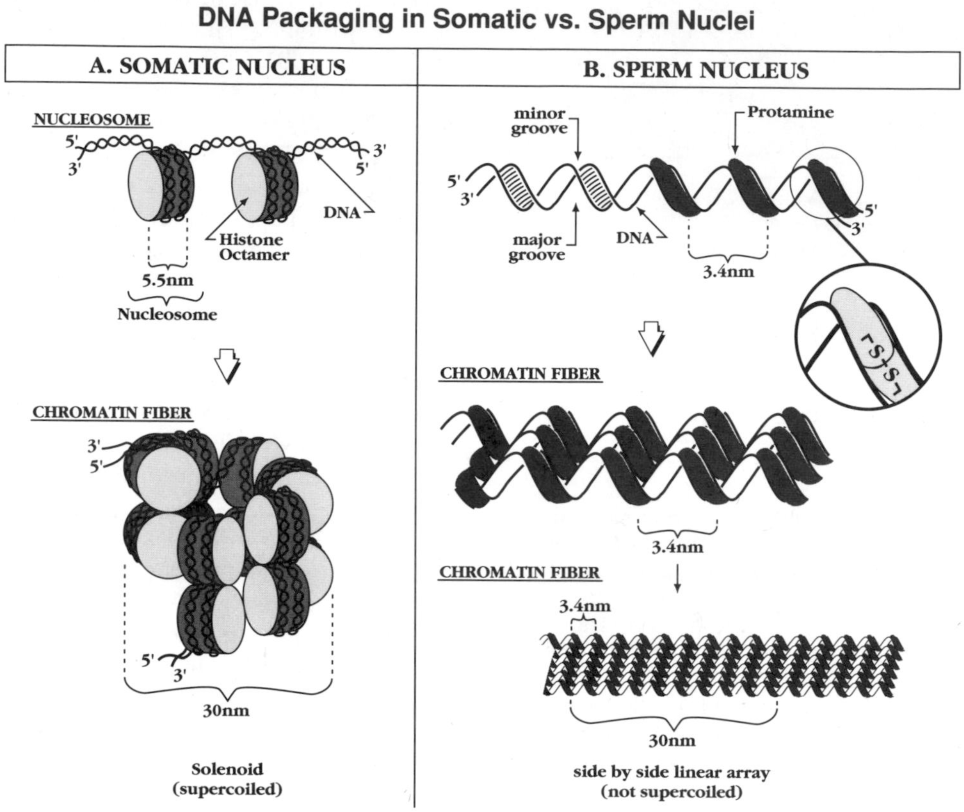

FIG. 81. Diagrams of DNA packaging in somatic (**A**) and sperm nuclei (**B**). For explanation, see the text. (From ref. 1636.)

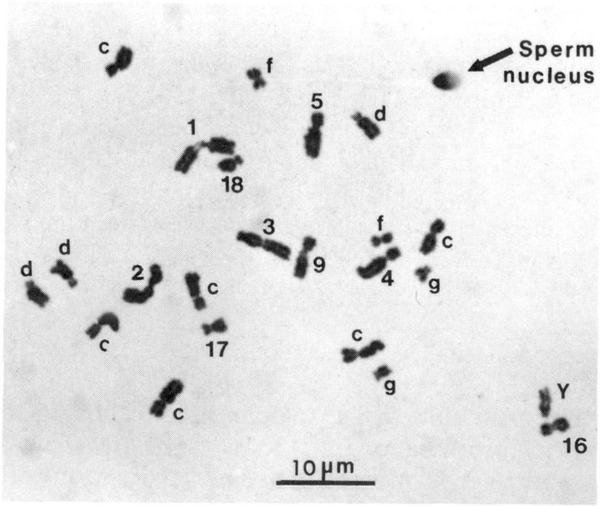

FIG. 82. A human sperm nucleus (*arrow*) and 22 chromosomes originated from another human sperm nucleus. This micrograph was a by-product of the human sperm chromosome analyses using zona-free hamster eggs. Chromosomes were from a spermatozoon penetrated into an egg. The intact nucleus is perhaps the nucleus of another spermatozoon that failed to fuse with the egg. The number or letter next to each chromosome is the chromosome identification number or denotes the chromosome group. (Provided by Dr. Yujiro Kamiguchi.)

approximately 20 min after sperm–egg fusion (Fig. 67) and is completed in the next 40 min (543a,711). The ooplasmic conditions that cause sperm nuclear decondensation and pronuclear development are apparently not species specific. Human sperm nuclei, for example, can decondense and develop into normal-looking pronuclei in hamster eggs (534,660,1708), frog eggs (623), and frog egg extracts (788a,1307). Although very inefficiently, the cytoplasm of some somatic cells may induce decondensation (1096,1203,1618) and DNA synthesis of sperm nuclei (1618).

Mechanism of Nuclear Envelope Breakdown

The nature of the factor responsible for the rapid disintegration of the sperm nuclear envelope is not known. It is tempting to speculate that sperm-born phospholipases (1403,1649) play a role, but concrete evidence for or against this notion is absent. According to Berrios and Bedford (748) and Szollosi et al. (1548), rabbit and mouse spermatozoa that have fused with immature oocytes at the GV stage retain their nuclear envelopes intact, inferring that the ooplasm of immature eggs lacks the ability to break down the nuclear envelope. The ob-

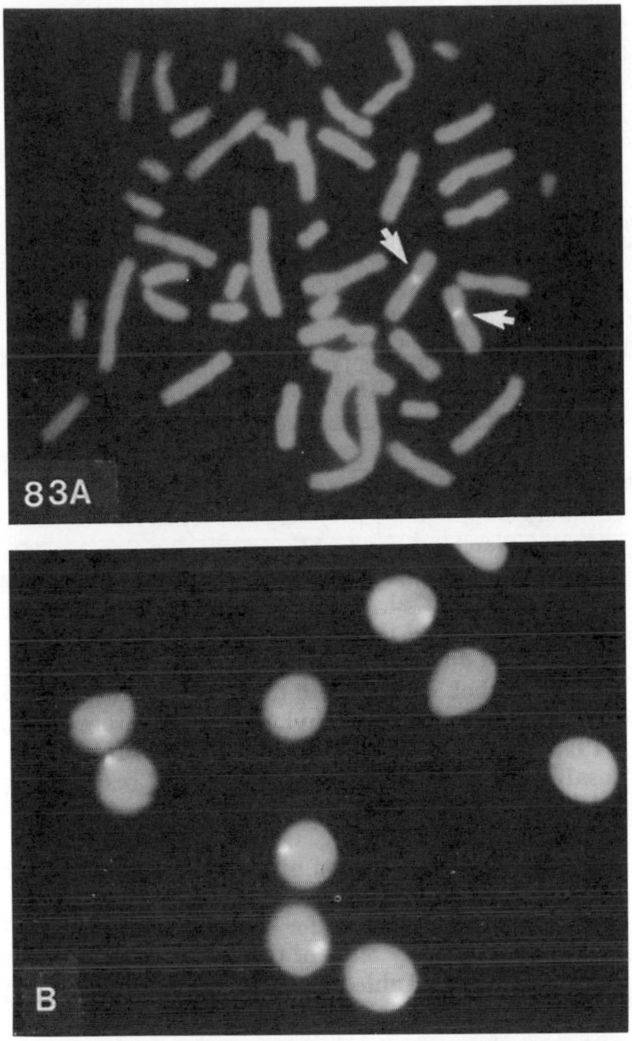

FIG. 83. Detection of specific chromosome(s) in nuclei using *in situ* hybridization. (**A**) Mitotic chromosomes from a lymphocyte of a human female; (**B**) human sperm nuclei partially decondensed with dithiothreitol. Each bright spot is the hybridization signal of an X chromosome-specific (TRX) probe. TRX is 400 base pairs long and recognizes 5,000 copies located in the centromeric region of the X chromosome. (From ref. 1013.)

servations by Usui and Yanagimachi (646,1735) contradict this. At least in the hamster, the intrinsic nuclear envelope disappears quickly; then a new envelope (without pores and resembling the intrinsic nuclear envelope) surrounds each nucleus. The same sequence of events occurs when spermatozoa fuse with fertilized eggs at the pronuclear or two-cell stage (646,1735). The disappearance of the nuclear envelopes from cattle sperm nuclei in GV oocytes has been reported by Crozet and Dumont (116). The discrepancy between the results from the mouse and rabbit with others could be due to the species difference. The breakdown of the intrinsic nuclear envelope during the interphase of cell cycle may be puzzling (1548), but one should remember that the sperm chromatin is highly condensed and the sperm nuclear envelope lacks a lamin lining (1185,1448). Although the breakdown of the nuclear envelope appears to be a necessary preliminary to the decondensation of the sperm nucleus and subsequent development into a large pronucleus (1690), the breakdown of the nuclear envelope does not necessarily lead to nuclear decondensation (646).

Mechanism of Sperm Nucleus Decondensation

A clue to the mechanism of sperm nucleus decondensation was obtained in 1971 when Calvin and Bedford (94) reported that mammalian sperm nuclei decondense readily in a simple medium containing dithiothreitol (DTT), an —S—S— reducing agent, and sodium dodecyl sulfate (SDS), an anionic detergent, but not in SDS or DTT alone. About the same time, other investigators (576,602) demonstrated that sperm nuclei lose protamines soon after their entry in the ooplasm. These and subsequent studies have led us to believe that reduction of —S—S— bonds in nuclear protamines and the replacement of protamines by histones are directly involved in the sperm nucleus decondensation in the ooplasm (for reviews, see 1350,1733).

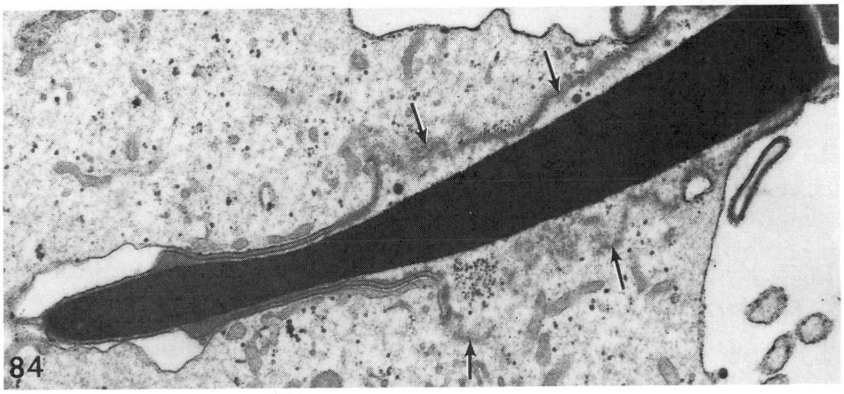

FIG. 84. Perinuclear material (*arrows*) dispersing into the ooplasm of a recently fertilized hamster egg, approximately 15 min after sperm-egg fusion. (From ref. 543a.)

Protamine Replacement by Histone

Nuclear proteins of frog spermatozoa are not cross-linked by —S—S— bonds (48), as are most vertebrate spermatozoa. When a spermatozoon enters an egg, protamines are replaced by histones within 5 min (1306). This replacement is accomplished by intermolecular competitions between DNA and nucleoplasmin towards protamines. Nucleoplasmin is the most abundant protein in the nuclear matrix (sap). Its large quantity is released from the GV into the ooplasm during breakdown of the GV envelope. Before spermatozoa enter mature eggs, sperm DNA is tightly bound to protamine. When a sperm nucleus enters nucleoplasmin-rich ooplasm, protamines leave DNA because of their stronger affinity to nucleoplasmin. Freed DNA then binds to histones, which are abundant in the ooplasm (1306,1368,1367). According to Ito et al. (1080), DTT-treated human sperm nuclei lose protamines and decondense within 30 min after being exposed to toad nucleoplasmin *in vitro.* Apparently nucleoplasmin–protamine binding is not species-specific.

Eutherian mammals differ from other species such as the frog in that protamine —S—S— must be reduced before protamines can be replaced by histones. There seems no doubt that this —S—S— reduction is accomplished by reduced glutathione (GSH) which is abundant in the ooplasm of mature eggs (567,799,1352). The fact that the ooplasm of the immature GV eggs is unable to decondense sperm nuclei (627,646,1135,1204) is most likely due to a lack of or deficiency in such substances as nucleoplasmin (1204) rather than a deficiency in GSH (627), because GSH concentration in GV oocytes is high (4–6 mM) although it is slightly lower than that in mature ovulated eggs (8–10 mM) (1352). In fact, within GV oocytes sperm protamine —S—S— is reduced within 30 min (1735).

How quickly does the reduction of sperm nuclear —S—S— take place within the ooplasm? Judging from the nuclear stainability with toluidine blue (1141), Giemsa (1243), and AO (1735), which enables differentiation of the —S—S—/—SH status of sperm protamines (1139), the reduction seems to begin before nuclear decondensation is detected by light microscopy. A drastic change in the staining reaction of the hamster sperm nucleus to ammoniacal $AgCl_2$ occurs within 5 min after sperm–egg fusion (573). This may be another indication of a rapid —S—S— reduction of sperm nuclear protamines within the ooplasm. In the mouse protamines are eliminated from the sperm nucleus during its decondensation (576). However, histone replacement is not completed until some time later (1297). In other words, there may be a transition period when part of sperm DNA is devoid of both protamines and histones. If this is true, it represents a most unusual situation, since, even in rapidly dividing somatic cells, histones are deposited almost immediately onto newly synthesized DNA (657). This point must be reinvestigated (1080). Figure 85 shows the probable sequence of events in sperm nucleus decondensation in the ooplasm.

Sperm Nucleus Decondensation and Egg Activation

Sperm nucleus decondenses during egg activation in normal fertilization. However, this does not imply that activation is a *sine qua non* for the nucleus decondensation. For example, when sperm nuclei are injected gently into mature unfertilized hamster eggs by microsurgery, the eggs remain unactivated, yet sperm nuclei decondense (1610). The same thing happens when the eggs are inseminated in the presence of colcemid (781, 1454a,1684), which apparently maintains the concentration of the metaphase-promoting factor (MPF) high (781,1023,1207) via its action on the metaphase spindle/chromosomes. As long as MPF concentration is high,

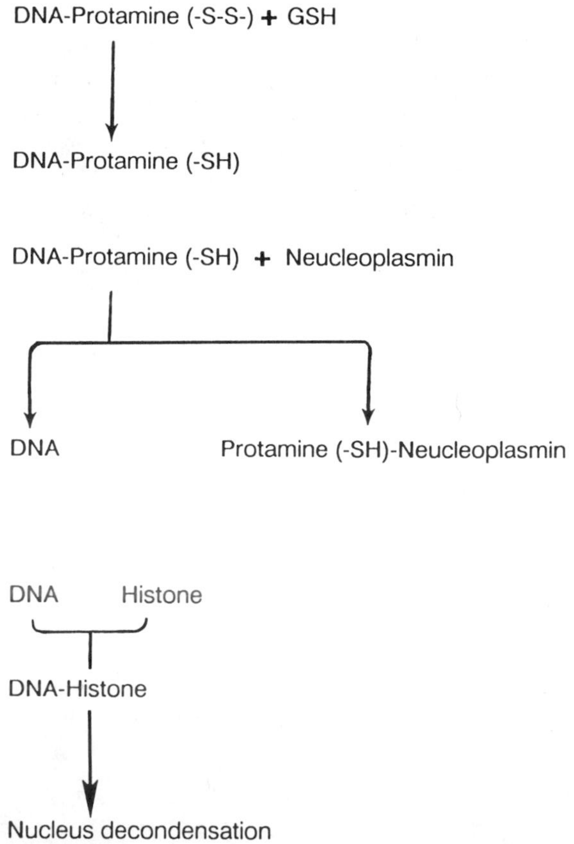

FIG. 85. Probable mechanism by which sperm protamines are replaced by histones during normal fertilization. In the ooplasm, sperm protamine —S—S— is quickly reduced to —SH by agent(s) such as reduced glutathione. Protamine then leaves DNA because of its stronger affinity to nucleoplasmin. Freed DNA immediately binds to histone.

decondensed sperm nuclei are unable to develop into pronuclei (see the next section).

Sperm Nucleus Decondensation In Vitro

Induction of sperm nuclear decondensation is possible without ooplasm. A simple medium containing anionic detergent and DTT (or mercaptoethanol), for example, can induce nuclear decondensation very efficiently (47,610,657). According to Jagar et al. (1087), heparin and several other polyanions (e.g., chondroitin sulfate) can decondense human sperm nuclei slowly. Heparin plus DTT decondense human sperm nuclei very rapidly. Even mouse and bull sperm nuclei, which do not respond to heparin alone, decondense in heparin plus DTT. Jager et al. inferred that heparin removes protamines from sperm chromatin. Thus heparin (and some polyanions) may mimic nucleoprotamine in freeing sperm DNA from protamines. Although Reyes et al. (1400) maintain that heparin and reduced glutathione are native sperm nucleus-decondensing factors, it must be nucleoplasmin, not heparin per se, that contributes to the sperm nuclear decondensation within the ooplasm. Several investigators have suggested the possible involvement of sperm nucleus-associated proteases in the sperm nucleus decondensation based on their observations that media containing both DTT (or mercaptoethanol) and protease can cause extensive decondensation of sperm nuclei (1070,1212,1213). Whether sperm nuclei really carry endogenous proteases and whether these proteases are directly involved in sperm nucleus decondensation during normal fertilization are still open questions.

COMPLETION OF OOCYTE MEIOSIS, PRONUCLEUS DEVELOPMENT, AND SYNGAMY

Completion of Oocyte Meiosis

In all eukaryotic cells, the cell division cycle is programmed by two cell-cycle-regulating proteins, cdc2 protein kinase and cyclin (Fig. 86) (1083,1144,1299). The former (34 kDa) is present in the cytoplasm all the time, whereas the latter (45–65 kDa, depending on species) changes its concentration during the cell cycle. During the G_1 phase, cyclin is synthesized and binds to cdc2 to form cdc2-cyclin complex or metaphase-prompting factor (MPF). Metaphase-prompting factor is activated when Tyrosin 15 residues (Y15) of cdc2 are dephospholylated and threonine 161 residues (T161) are phospholylated (1144,1245a). Activated MPF triggers a breakdown of the nuclear envelope and allows the cell to advance to the M-phase. Cyclin is then destroyed and the resultant loss of MPF activity leads the cell to the G_1 phase of the next cell cycle.

In mammals, the MPF concentration within ovarian eggs increases after breakdown of the germinal vesicle (1023). It disappears temporarily during the first meiotic division, then increases again as oocytes enter the second meiotic division (1023). The reason for mature unfertilized eggs being arrested at metaphase II for many hours is unknown. The speculation at the time was that (i) a cytostatic factor (CSF or c-mos protooncogen product, p^{39mos}) stabilizes MPF, directly or indirectly through its action on microtubules, to maintain a high MPF con-

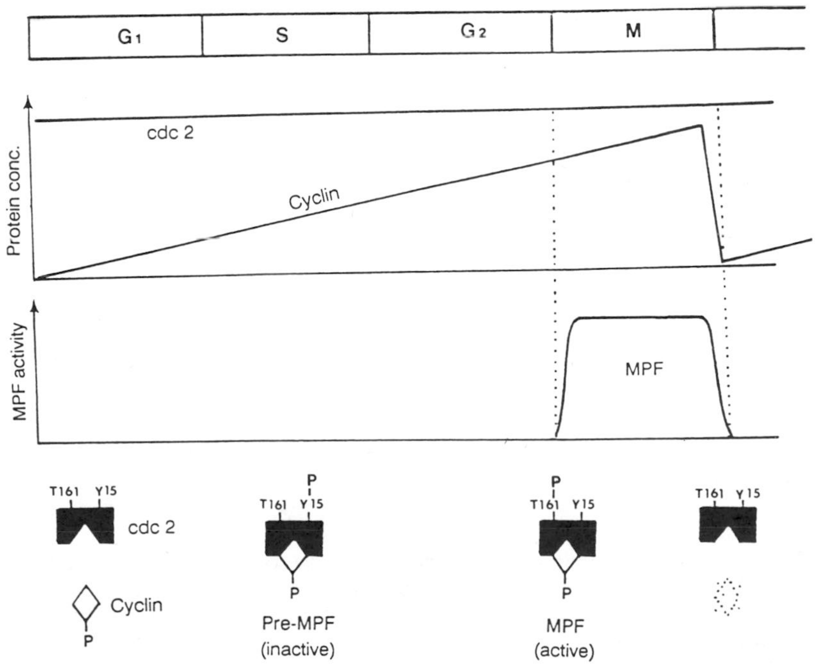

FIG. 86. Molecular changes in metaphase promoting factor (MPF) during cell cycle. For explanation, see the text.

centration (1214) and (ii) inactivation of CSF causes degradation of MPF, allowing the egg to escape from the metaphase arrest (1214). However, since MPF disappears from activated eggs before CSF does (1644,1646), the disappearance of MPF and of CSF from fertilized eggs appears to be independent phenomena. The lowering of CSF could prepare the egg for the next cell cycle rather than for degradation of MPF (1646). The sustained arrest of mammalian oocytes at metaphase II may be dependent on the synthesis of short-lived proteins (824,1494,1646). In the mouse, both MPF and CSF disappear after fertilization (965,1644). Transient Ca_i^{2+} elevation upon fertilization may trigger the degradation of these proteins (Fig. 87) (1214,1644). The importance of Ca_i^{2+} rising for the advancement of cell cycle from one to the next has been recognized (1654).

Polar Body Formation

Scanning electron micrographs of hamster oocytes at the metaphase of the first and second meiotic divisions revealed that the egg cortex above the metaphase spindle has prominent cytoplasmic protrusions (Fig. 88) (906,1035). According to Ebensburger and Barros (906), these protrusions disappear quickly when the eggs are removed from the oviduct into the culture media. The functional significance of the cytoplasmic protrusions is not clear. Okada et al. (625) have speculated that the membrane covering the protrusions becomes part of the membrane covering the first or second polar body. It is conceivable that the cortical region above the meiotic spindle actively synthesizes and stockpiles the plasma membrane necessary for the polar body formation. Perhaps substances emanating from metaphase chromosomes/spindle (1184) play a role in the cortical modifications and the synthesis of plasma membrane. Prevention of polar body formation by cytochalasin (1163,1179) is expected because this specialized cell division, as other cell divisions, requires actin for the formation of cleavage furrow.

Pronuclei Development

Egg Activation Is Required for Pronuclei Development

As noted earlier, egg activation is not required for decondensation of the sperm nucleus in the ooplasm. However, it is required for transformation of the decondensed sperm nucleus into a pronucleus. When immature mouse oocytes at metaphase I are inseminated and cultured, they progress to metaphase II, but they do not advance further. Meanwhile, the sperm nucleus within the ooplasm swells, then condenses to form a small mass of chromatin or chromosomelike structures (570,825). The same sequence of events occurs when immature human oocytes at metaphase I are inseminated *in vitro* (798,1458,1459,1574). Such a direct transformation, bypassing the pronuclear stage, is called *premature chromosome condensation* (PCC). Sperm PCC also occurs when mature eggs are inseminated in a medium containing microtubule inhibitors (e.g., colcemid). Sperm nuclei decondense, then recondense, and, unless the eggs are freed from the inhibitor, neither sperm nuclei nor egg chromosomes develop into pronuclei (Fig. 89) (781). The microtubule inhibitor seems to prevent pronuclear development by maintaining a high level of MPF (1023) via its action on the metaphase spindle. When the metaphase spindle is removed from an egg (or egg fragment), the sperm nucleus within ooplasm transforms into a pronucleus despite continuous presence of the inhibitor (781). This can be interpreted as indicating that removal of the metaphase spindle causes a rapid degradation of the MPF.

Other Factors Controlling Pronuclei Development

According to Mattiolo et al. (1220), pig ovarian eggs, when matured *in vitro* in the presence of follicle (granulosa) cells, are fertilized normally and sperm nuclei transform into well-developed pronuclei. In contrast, the eggs seldom support the development of pronuclei when

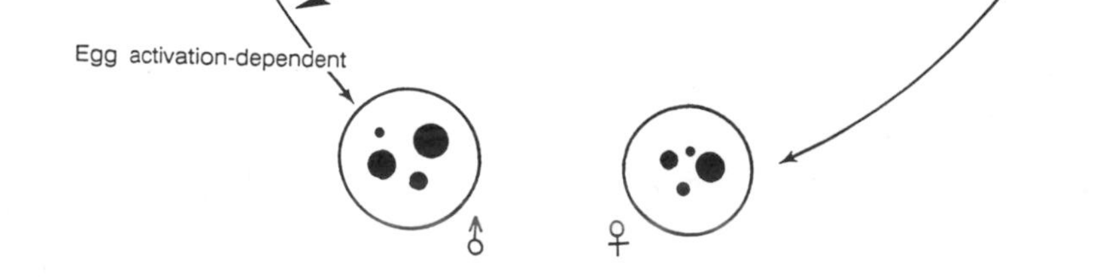

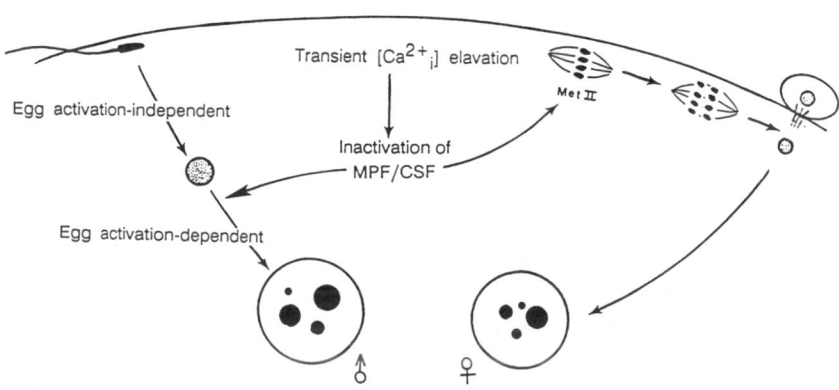

FIG. 87. A diagram illustrating that sperm nucleus decondensation is independent of egg activation, whereas the transformation of a decondensed sperm nucleus to a pronucleus is dependent on egg activation. Inactivation of MPF/CSF by transient $[Ca_i^{2+}]$ elevation seems to be of critical importance for egg activation.

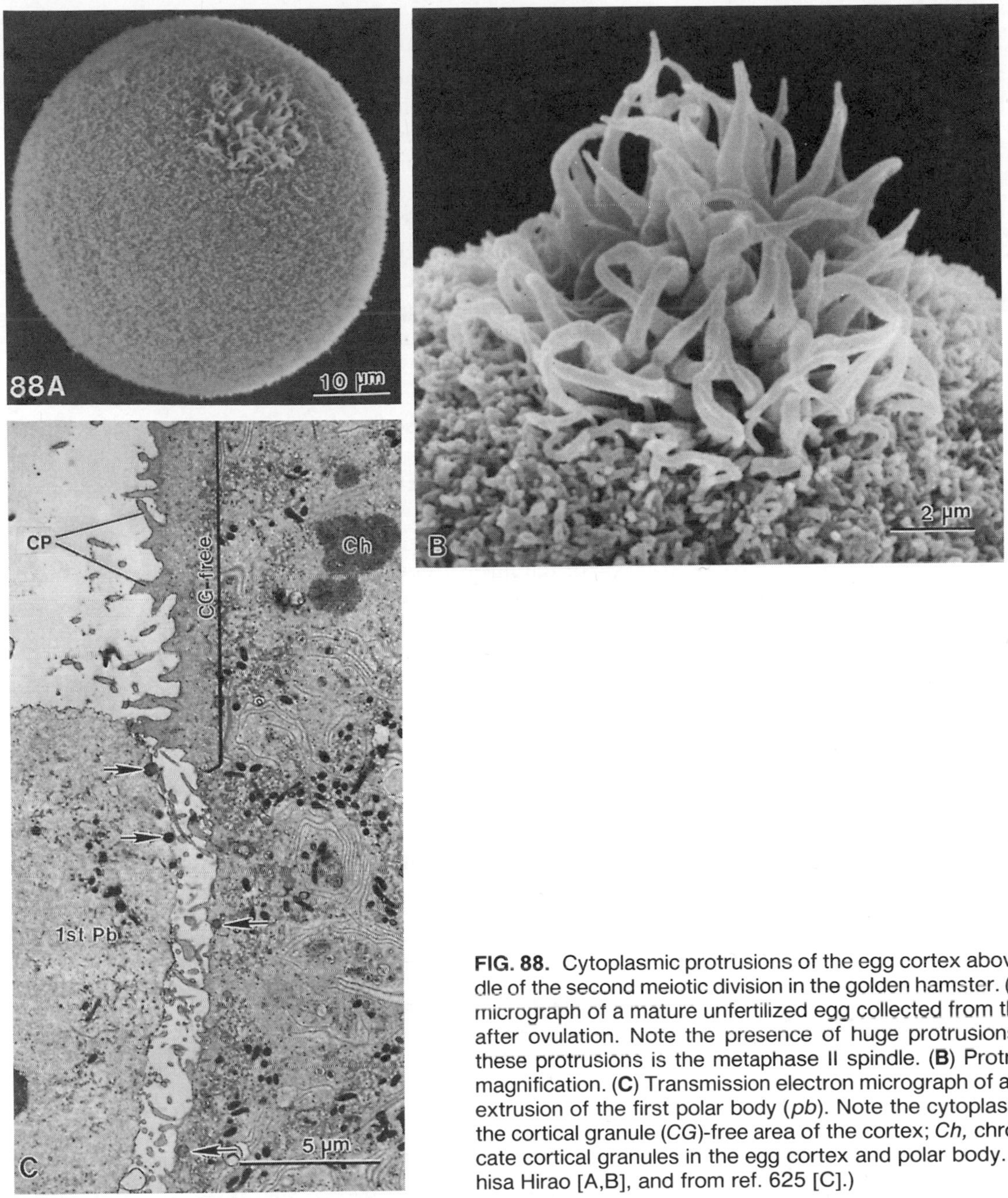

FIG. 88. Cytoplasmic protrusions of the egg cortex above the metaphase spindle of the second meiotic division in the golden hamster. (**A**) A scanning electron micrograph of a mature unfertilized egg collected from the oviduct a few hours after ovulation. Note the presence of huge protrusions in the cortex; under these protrusions is the metaphase II spindle. (**B**) Protrusions under a higher magnification. (**C**) Transmission electron micrograph of an ovarian egg after the extrusion of the first polar body (*pb*). Note the cytoplasmic protrusions (*CP*) in the cortical granule (*CG*)-free area of the cortex; *Ch,* chromosome. *Arrows* indicate cortical granules in the egg cortex and polar body. (Provided by Dr. Yukihisa Hirao [A,B], and from ref. 625 [C].)

they mature *in vitro* in the absence of granulosa cells. In these eggs, most sperm nuclei remain condensed in close approximation to the large egg pronuclei. Apparently, the so-called *male pronucleus growth factor* (MPGF) (645,1585) is not produced in the ooplasm of eggs matured in the absence of granulosa cells. Whether the ooplasmic factors controlling the development of sperm pronuclei and those for egg pronuclei are identical (1684) or different (530,587) is a question. The MPGF could be substances such as nucleoplasmin essential for sperm nucleus decondensation.

The amount of ooplasmic material necessary to support sperm and egg pronuclei formation seems to be limited (26). When one spermatozoon enters the egg, sperm and egg nuclei compete for this *pronucleus formative material* (PFM) (26). In the case of the rat and mouse, the sperm (male) pronucleus has a much greater affinity for PFM than the egg pronucleus, with the result that the sperm pronucleus is larger than the egg pronucleus (26,692,693,697). In dispermic rat eggs at the stage of maximum pronuclear size, the sum of the volumes of the egg pronucleus and the two sperm pronuclei does not

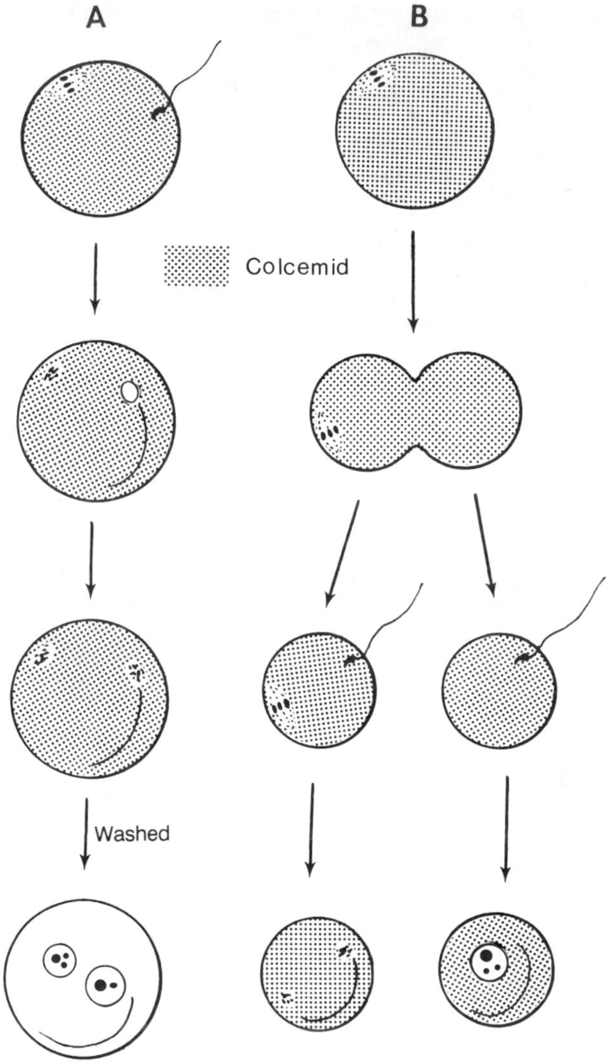

FIG. 89. Behavior of sperm and egg nuclei in mouse eggs inseminated in the presence of colcemid. *Dotted* eggs denote the eggs placed in a colcemid-containing medium. For explanation, see the text. (Drawn based on data in ref. 781.)

exceed the sum of the volume of normal pronuclei (26). When an excessive number of spermatozoa enter an egg, sperm nuclei compete for the material and only a few or none successfully develop into sperm pronuclei (587).

The PFMs are apparently not species specific. Transformation of sperm nuclei into normal-looking pronuclei is possible in the eggs of remote species (659, 1283,1351) (Fig. 90). The nuclei of some somatic cells (e.g., hepatocyte and thymocyte) (1283,1549) and even protein-free bacteriophage lambda DNA (740,943, 1287) also can produce pronucleuslike structures when incorporated into mature eggs.

As already stated, the sperm pronucleus is larger than the egg pronucleus throughout the pronuclear stage in the mouse and rat. This is not the case in some other species, such as golden hamsters (695) and humans (Fig. 79B). In humans, microsurgical removal of excess sperm pronuclei from polyspermic eggs after IVF has potential clinical significance. For example, dispermic eggs, which would not develop normally, can be rescued if one sperm pronucleus is successfully removed. In this case, the egg pronucleus should not be removed because normal embryonic development requires both male and female genomes, which are apparently imprinted differently (686,712,1040,1264). Unfortunately, thus far, there is no simple method to distinguish a sperm pronucleus from an egg pronucleus (987,1205,1661). The egg pronucleus is usually located closer to the second polar body than the sperm pronucleus, but not always. Someday, it may be possible to differentiate the sperm and egg pronuclei because in the mouse, for example, these pronuclei may not be identical in their chromatin organization and/or lamin composition of the nuclear envelope (822).

The endoplasmic reticulum (ER) is the major source of the nuclear envelope (NE). However, a recent study by Wilson and Newport (1665) has revealed that normal NE can be formed in "ER-depleted" frog egg homogenate. Two types of nuclear NE precursors, NEP-A and NEP-B, have been recognized (1625). NEP-B binds to chromatin, then NEP-A fuses with the chromatin-bound NEP-B (Fig. 91). Nuclear lamins contribute to the formation of the inner layer of NE (1379,1448), but its relationship to sperm chromatin and NEPs remains unclear. The NEPs in mammals have not been identified, but vesicular components in the ooplasm appear to be essential for pronuclear development. When hamster eggs are

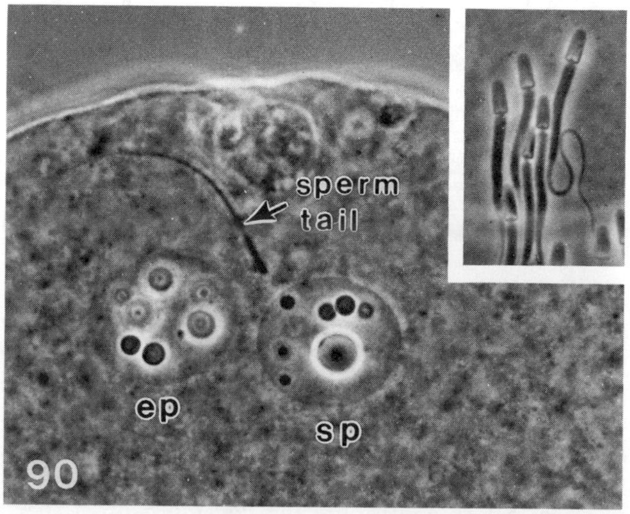

FIG. 90. A golden hamster egg injected microsurgically with a bat (*Myotis velifer*) spermatozoon, examined 5 hr later. The sperm pronucleus was indistinguishable from the egg pronucleus. Labels *sp* (sperm nucleus) and *ep* (egg pronucleus) were placed arbitrarily from the position of bat sperm tail (*arrow*). (From ref. 1735, with permission.)

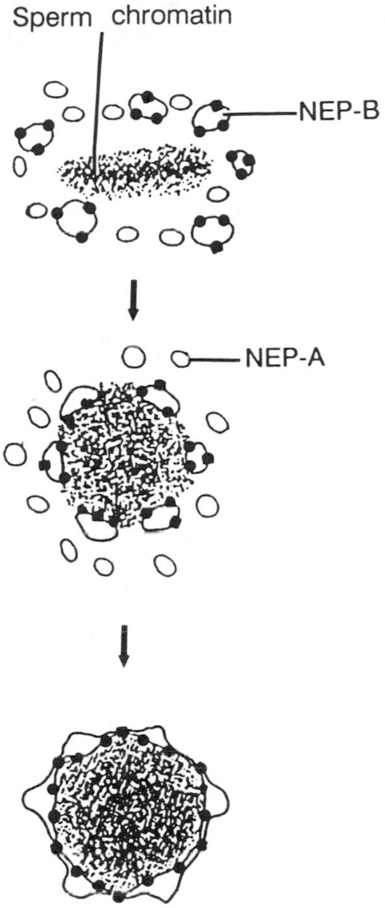

FIG. 91. A model for nuclear envelope assembly. A nuclear envelope precursor NEP-B binds to sperm chromatin in an ATP-independent manner. Another precursor NEP-A then fuses with chromatin-bound NEP-B; this step requires ATP. (From ref. 1625.)

freed from their zonae and centrifuged strongly, the contents of each egg are stratified, and each egg then divides into two, then into four or more fragments, depending on the intensity and duration of centrifugation. The "lightest" clear fragments receiving no vesicular materials can be penetrated by spermatozoa. In these fragments sperm nuclei decondense but never develop into pronuclei (Fig. 92A,B). Other fragments receiving vesicular materials support both sperm nucleus decondensation and normal pronucleus development (Fig. 92C) (1711).

DNA and Protein Synthesis During Pronuclei Development

During normal fertilization, DNA synthesis begins almost synchronously in the sperm and egg pronuclei. In the mouse, it begins about 8 hr after fertilization when pronuclei have distinct nucleoli, and is completed within the next 8 hr (Fig. 93) (880,1052,1140). This is one of the most radiosensitive stages in embryonic development (880,1686).

The timing of DNA synthesis seems to be determined largely by ooplasmic factors (1282). For example, hamster sperm nuclei within hamster ooplasm undergo DNA synthesis (and chromosome duplication) between 3 hr and 8 hr after fertilization (1283). Human sperm nuclei within hamster ooplasm also synthesize DNA about the

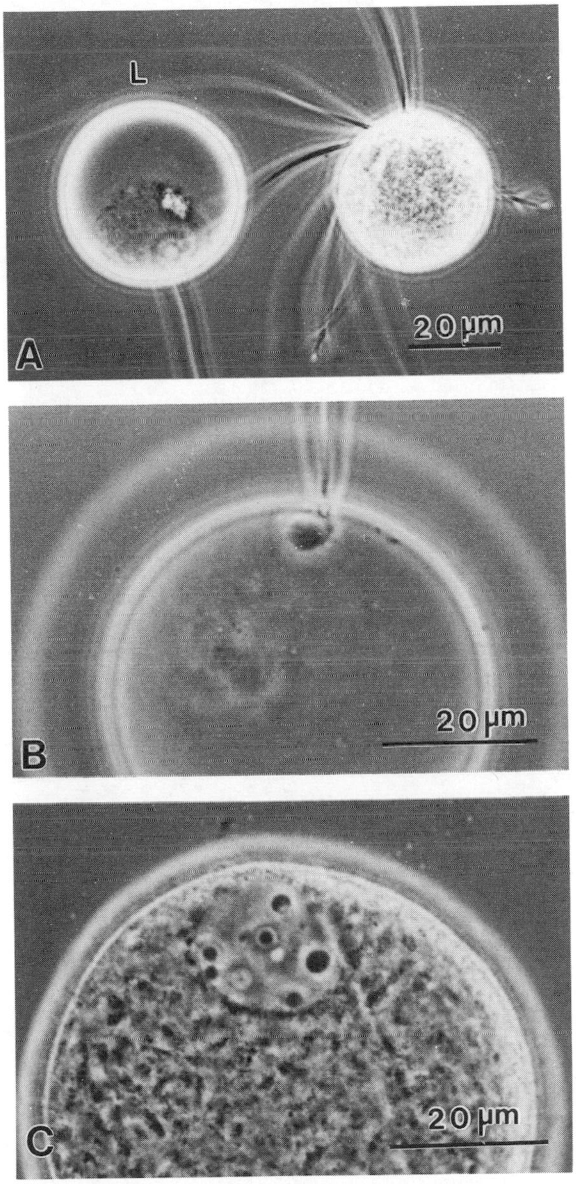

FIG. 92. Behavior of sperm nuclei incorporated in egg fragments. Mature unfertilized hamster eggs were freed from the zonae pellucidae and centrifuged strongly, in Percoll gradient, to divide each egg into four fragments or quarters. (A) shows the lightest quarter (*L*) and the next to the lightest quarter. Only the lightest quarters had virtually no vesicular materials. When inseminated, sperm–egg fusion occurred much less frequently in the lightest quarters than in other fragments. Within the lightest quarters sperm nuclei decondensed, but they never developed into pronuclei (B). Well-developed pronuclei appeared in other quarters (C). (From ref. 1711.)

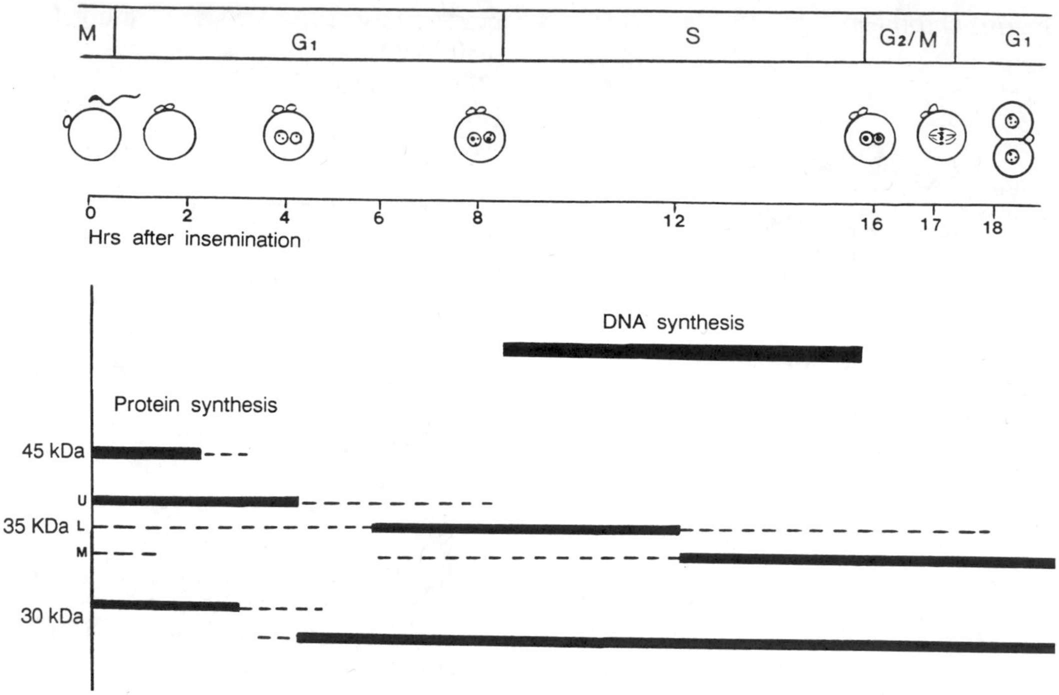

FIG. 93. Timing of DNA replication and protein synthesis during the first cell cycle of mouse development. For explanation, see the text. (Adapted from ref. 1052.)

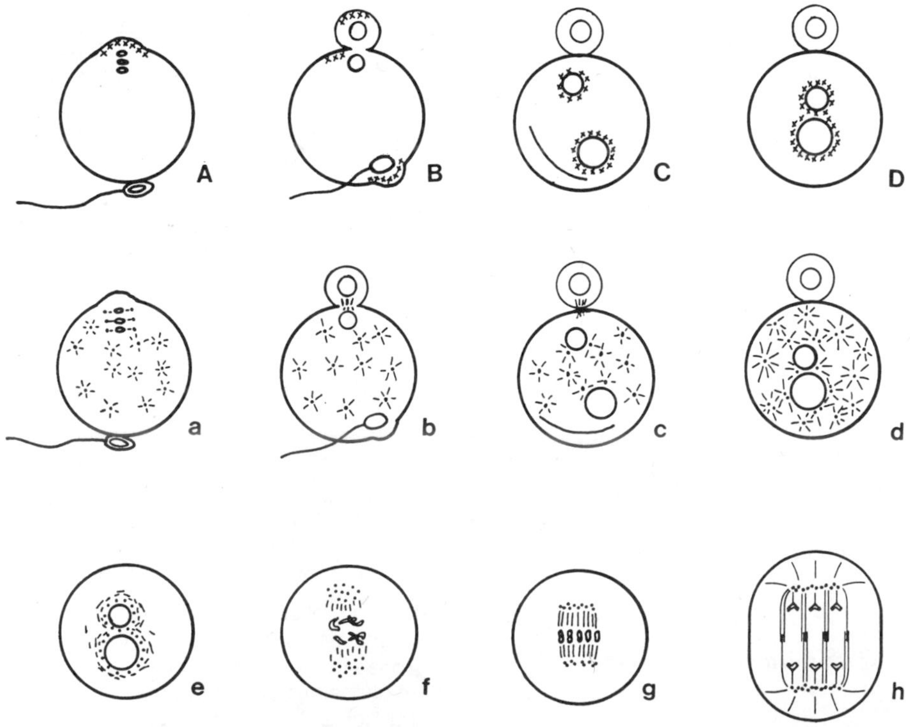

FIG. 94. Behavior of microfilaments (**A–D**) and microtubules (*a–h*) during fertilization and the first cleavage in the mouse. For explanation, see the text. (*x*) Microfilaments; (*dots*) centrosomal foci; (*lines*) microtubules. (Drawn based on information from refs. 611 and 637.)

same time (704), whereas those within native (human) ooplasm do not initiate DNA synthesis until approximately 12 hr after fertilization (1575). Hamster ooplasm can support DNA synthesis of foreign sperm nuclei (754,1108,1209,1564), but its DNA synthesis machinery seems to work most efficiently for sperm nuclei of its own species (1283).

Established for many years pronuclear eggs have translation activity and synthesize new proteins (785,815,827,857) perhaps using stored maternal mRNA. According to Howlett and Bolton (1052), at least five new proteins are synthesized during the pronucleus stage (Fig. 93). Some (e.g., one 45-kDa and one 35-kDa protein) are transiently synthesized within a few hours after sperm–egg fusion and then disappear. Some others appear several hours after sperm–egg fusion. The nature and functions of these proteins are not clear, but some could be mitosis-triggering proteins (1051), which are stockpiled during the long pronucleus stage for subsequent cleavages. A great change in the rate of protein synthesis occurs during the late pronucleus and mid two-cell stages (1154). In the mouse, transition from maternal control to zygotic control of transcription activity begins during the early and mid two-cell stage (1052,1199). Transition time varies among different species (1566).

Syngamy

The sequence of the migration of sperm and egg pronuclei to the center of the fertilized egg and their union (syngamy) have been studied extensively by both light- (20,26) and electron microscopy (607–609). The cytoskeletal system is believed to play important roles in these processes. Our knowledge of the behavior of cytoskeletal systems during mammalian fertilization has been expanded greatly due to the availability of many specific molecular probes for different cytoskeletal components (611–613,634–637,1163,1370,1397,1449).

The behavior of microfilaments (actins) and microtubules during normal fertilization in the mouse is summarized diagrammatically in Fig. 21. Actins exist throughout the cortex of the unfertilized egg (1182), but they are most conspicuous in the region above the meiotic spindle (Fig. 94A–D) (599). Actins and fodrin (a spectrinlike protein), which act together during fertilization, are not involved in sperm–egg fusion. They seem to be important in (i) anchoring the meiotic spindle to the egg cortex, (ii) determining the axis of cell division (extrusion of the polar-body and cleavages) (299,1452) and (iii) drawing the sperm nucleus deep into the egg (1647). Microtubules in the egg are essential for cell division (including polar-body extrusion) and the formation and migration of pronuclei (1207). Interestingly, in addition to the spindle microtubules, there are 16 cytoplasmic microtubule organizing centers or foci in an unfertilized mouse egg (Fig. 94a). Each centrosomal focus organizes an aster; after sperm incorporation, some foci, along with their asters, begin to associate with the developing pronuclei (Fig. 94b,c). When two pronuclei are closely apposed at the egg center, several foci are found in contact with the pronuclei and typically a pair reside between the adjacent pronuclei (Fig. 94d). Shortly before the envelopes of sperm and egg pronuclei disintegrate, all foci condense on the pronuclear surface; also, sheaths of microtubules circumscribe the adjacent pronuclei (Fig. 94e). At the prophase of the first mitosis (cleavage), the centrosomes detach from the nuclear region, appearing as two broad clusters (Fig. 94f) that aggregate into irregular bands at metaphase (Fig. 94g). At anaphase and telophase the centrosomes widen somewhat (Fig. 94h).

Microtubular organizing centers in fertilized mouse eggs are exclusively of maternal origin (637,1451). The ability of rabbit ooplasm to organize centrioles is evident from the observation by Szollosi and Ozil (1550) that, although not detectable in unfertilized eggs, centrioles

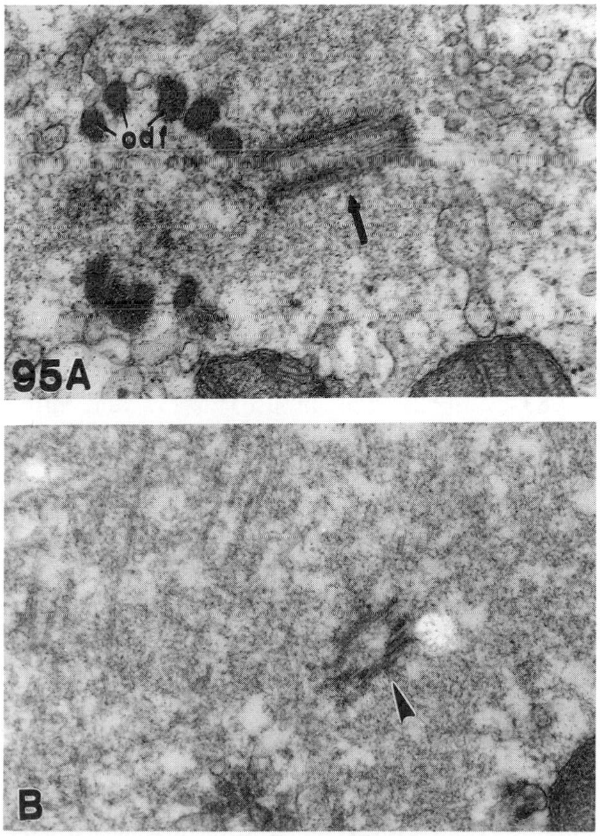

FIG. 95. Two centrioles (a single arrow and an arrowhead) in a fertilized sheep egg at the metaphase of the first cleavage. Somewhat dispersed outer dense fibers (*odf*) of the fertilizing spermatozoon are seen in **A.** (From ref. 852.)

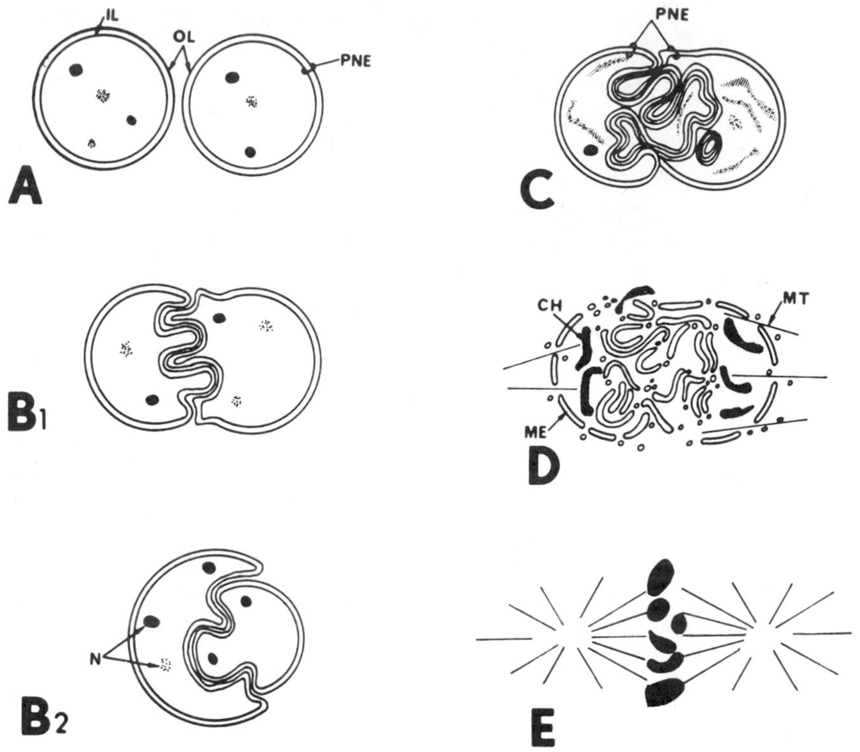

FIG. 96. Diagrams of the association of the sperm and egg pronuclei in the rabbit. (**A**) Apposition of the pronuclei. (**B$_1$**, **B$_2$**) Interdigitation of the proximal surfaces of the pronuclei. (**C**) Complex infolding of the proximal surface of the pronuclei. (**D**) Vesiculation of pronuclear envelopes and formation of mitotic spindle. (**E**) First metaphase mitotic apparatus. *CH,* chromatin; *IL,* inner lamina of pronuclear envelope; *ME,* membranous elements formed as a result of vesiculation of pronuclear envelope; *MT,* microtubules; *N,* nucleoli; *OL,* outer lamina of pronuclear envelope; *PNE,* pronuclear envelope. (From ref. 607.)

begin to appear in the blastomeres of parthenogenetically developing embryos. In the sheep (852), human (1444), and cow (Sathananthan, personal communication), a centriole is carried into the egg by the fertilizing spermatozoon. It duplicates and migrates to one pole of the mitotic spindle during the first cleavage (Fig. 95).

When egg and sperm pronuclei are in close proximity to one another, the proximal surfaces of the pronuclei become highly convoluted (Fig. 96). In the rabbit, convoluted NEs interlock (Fig. 96B,C) and fuse at several places before the entire NE breaks down (Fig. 96D) (607,983,1193). In the mouse (1723) and human (1445a), NEs of sperm and egg pronuclei breakdown separately without interlocking. A transient Ca_i^{2+} increase can be detected sometimes (not always) within 5 min before NE breakdown (1591). In the hamster, extracellular Ca^{2+} is not essential for the pronuclear development, but without it pronuclear eggs perish before reaching the two-cell stage (532).

When Does the Sperm Nucleus Become Competent to Take Part in Syngamy?

The egg nucleus is apparently ready for syngamy upon completion of meiosis. Is this true for the sperm nucleus? Recent studies in the hamster (1304,1304a) have shown the nuclei of round spermatids, when incorporated into mature eggs, are capable of duplicating their DNAs (chromosomes) and mingling with egg chromosomes. Although a definitive conclusion should be deferred until viable normal offspring are born after such manipulation, the results of these preliminary studies seem to suggest that the sperm nucleus, like the egg nucleus, is syngamy competent upon completion of meiosis. If this proves to be the case, all the postmeiotic modifications of the male germ cells can be considered as processes solely dedicated for the delivery of their nuclei into the eggs.

ACKNOWLEDGMENTS

The following colleagues provided valuable information, and I am grateful for their advice: Drs. J. Dean, D. Epel, J. Eppig, N.B. Hecht, D.D. Hoskins, C. Katagiri, C.D. Lindeman, Y. Masui, S. Miyazaki, P. Olds-Clarke, J.W. Overstreet, S.S. Suarez, U.A. Urch and P. Wassarman. I am indebted to Drs. H. Matsumoto, T.T.F. Huang, and T.T. Smith, and Mrs. C. Oser and Mrs. H. Yanagimachi for their help in the preparation of the manuscript.

My special thanks go to Drs. J.M. Bedford and C.L. Markert who were kind enough to read the original manuscript and supported me with invaluable advice and helpful suggestions.

REFERENCES

1. Abrescia P, Lombarli G, DeRosa M, Quagliozzi L, Guardiola L, Metafora S. Identification and preliminary characterization of a sperm-binding protein in normal human semen. *J Reprod Fertil* 1985;73:71–77.

2. Acott TS, Hoskins DD. Bovine sperm forward motility protein: binding to epididymal spermatozoa. *Biol Reprod* 1981;24:234–240.
3. Acott TS, Katz DF, Hoskins DD. Movement characteristics of bovine epididymal spermatozoa: effects of forward motility protein and epididymal maturation. *Biol Reprod* 1983;29:389–399.
4. Adams CE, Chang MC. Capacitation of rabbit spermatozoa in the fallopian tube and in the uterus. *J Exp Zool* 1962; 151:159–165.
5. Aguas AP, Pinto da Silva P. The acrosomal membrane of boar sperm: a Golgi-derived membrane poor in glycoconjugates. *J Cell Biol* 1985;100:528–534.
6. Ahuja KK. Fertilization studies in the hamster: the role of cell surface carbohydrates. *Exp Cell Res* 1982;140:353–362.
7. Ahuja KK. Carbohydrate determinants involved in mammalian fertilization. *Am J Anat* 1985;174:207–223.
8. Ahuja KK, Bolwell CP. Probable asymmetry in the organization of components of the hamster zona pellucida. *J Reprod Fertil* 1983;69:49–55.
9. Ahuja KK, Giebert DJ. Involvement of sperm sulphatase in early sperm-zona interactions in the hamster. *J Cell Sci* 1985;78:247–261.
10. Aketa K, Ohta T. When do sperm of the sea urchin, Pseudocentrotus depressus, undergo the acrosome reaction at fertilization? *Dev Biol* 1977;61:366–372.
11. Allison AC, Hartree EF. Lysosomal enzymes in the acrosome and their possible role in fertilization. *J Reprod Fertil* 1970;21:501–515.
12. Alvarez AC, Slorey BT. Taurine, hypotaurine, epinephrine and albumin inhibit lipid peroxidation in rabbit spermatozoa and protect against loss of motility. *Biol Reprod* 1983;29:548–555.
13. Anand SR, Kaur SP, Chaudhry PS. Distribution of β-N-acetylglucosamindiase, hyaluronoglucosaminidase and acrosin in buffalo and goat spermatozoa. *Hoppe-Seyler's Z Physiol Chem* 1977;358:685–688.
14. Aonuma S, Okabe M, Kawaguchi M, Kishi Y. Studies on sperm capacitation IX. Movement characteristics of spermatozoa in relation to capacitation. *Chem Pharm Bull (Tokyo)* 1980; 28:1497–1502.
15. Ashraf M, Peterson RN, Russell LD. Activity and location of cation-dependent ATPase on the plasma membrane of boar spermatozoa. *Biochem Biophys Res Commun* 1982;107: 1273–1278.
16. Austin CR. Function of hyaluronidase in fertilization. *Nature* 1948;162:63.
17. Austin CR. Observations on the penetration of the sperm into the mammalian egg. *Aust J Sci Res* [B] 1951;4:581–596.
18. Austin CR. The "capacitation" of the mammalian sperm. *Nature* 1952;170:326.
19. Austin CR. Capacitation and the release of hyaluronidase from spermatozoa. *J Reprod Fertil* 1960;3:310–311.
20. Austin CR. *The Mammalian Egg.* Springfield, Illinois: Charles C Thomas; 1961.
21. Austin CR. Capacitation of spermatozoa. *Int J Fertil* 1967;12:25–31.
22. Austin CR. Sperm maturation in the male and female genital tracts. In: Metz CB, Monroy A, eds. *Biology of Fertilization,* Vol. 2. New York: Academic Press; 1985:121–155.
23. Austin CR, Braden AWH. Early reaction of the rodent egg to spermatozoa penetration. *J Exp Biol* 1956;33:358–365.
24. Austin CR, Bishop MWH. Some features of the acrosome and perforatorium in mammalian spermatozoa. *Proc R Soc Lond [Biol]* 1958;149:234–240.
25. Austin CR, Bishop MWH. Role of the rodent acrosome and perforatorium in fertilization. *Proc R Soc Lond [Biol]* 1958;149:241–248.
26. Austin CR, Walton A. Fertilisation. In: Parkes AS ed. *Marshall's Physiology of Reproduction,* Vol. 1, Part 2. London: Longmans, Green; 1960:310–416.
27. Babcock DF. Examination of the intracellular ionic environment and of ionophore action by null point measurements employing the fluorescein chromophore. *J Biol Chem* 1983; 258:6380–6389.
28. Ball GD, Leibfried ML, Lenz RW, Ax RL, Bavister BD, First NL. Factors affecting successful in vitro fertilization of bovine follicular oocytes. *Biol Reprod* 1983;28:717–725.
29. Barros C, Bedford JM, Franklin LE, Austin CR. Membrane vesiculation as a feature of the mammalian acrosome reaction. *J Cell Biol* 1967;34:C1–C5.
30. Barros C, Jedliki A, Bize I, Aguirre E. Relationship between the length of sperm preincubation and zona penetration in the golden hamster: a scanning electron microscopy study. *Gamete Res* 1984;9:31–43.
31. Barros C, Yanagimachi R. Induction of the zona reaction in Golden hamster eggs by conical granule material. *Nature* 1971;233:268–269.
32. Bavister BD. Substitution of synthetic polymer for protein in a mammalian gamete culture system. *J Exp Zool* 1981;217: 45–51.
33. Bavister BD. Evidence for a role of post-ovulatory cumulus components in supporting fertilizing ability of hamster spermatozoa. *J Androl* 1982;3:365–372.
34. Bavister BD, Yanagimachi R. The effects of sperm extracts and energy sources on the motility and acrosome reaction of hamster spermatozoa *in vitro. Biol Reprod* 1977;16:228–237.
35. Bavister BD, Yanagimachi R, Teichman RJ. Capacitation of hamster spermatozoa with adrenal gland extracts. *Biol Reprod* 1976;14:219–221.
36. Bearer EL, Friend DS. Modifications of anionic lipid domains preceding membrane fusion in guinea pig sperm. *J Cell Biol* 1982;92:604–615.
37. Bedford JM. Changes in the electrophoretic properties of rabbit spermatozoa during passage through the epididymis. *Nature* 1963;200:1178–1180.
38. Bedford JM. Fine structure of the sperm head in ejaculate and uterine spermatozoa of the rabbit. *J Reprod Fertil* 1964;7:221–228.
39. Bedford JM. Ultrastructural changes in the sperm head during fertilization in the rabbit. *Am J Anat* 1968;123:329–358.
40. Bedford JM. Limitation of the uterus in the development of the fertility (capacitation) of spermatozoa. *J Reprod Fertil* 1969;8(Suppl):19–26.
41. Bedford JM. Sperm capacitation and fertilization in mammals. *Biol Reprod* 1970;2(Suppl):128–158.
42. Bedford JM. The saga of mammalian sperm from ejaculation to syngamy. In: Gibian H, Plotz EJ, eds. *Mammalian Reproduction.* New York: Springer-Verlag; 1970:124–182.
43. Bedford JM. An electron microscopic study of sperm penetration into rabbit egg after natural mating. *Am J Anat* 1972;133:213–254.
44a. Bedford JM. Biology of primate spermatozoa. In: Lucken WP, ed. *Contributions to Primatology,* Vol. 3. Basel: Karger; 1974:97–140.
44b. Bedford JM. Mechanisms involved in penetration of spermatozoa through the vestments of the mammalian egg. In: edited by Coutinho EM, Fuchs F, eds. *Physiology and Genetics of Reproduction.* Part B. New York: Plenum Press; 1974:55–68.
45. Bedford JM. Fertilization. In: Austin CR, Shon RV, eds. *Reproduction in Mammals I: Germ Cells and Fertilization.* London: Cambridge University Press; 1982:128–163.
46. Bedford JM. Significance of the need for sperm capacitation before fertilization in eutherian mammals. *Biol Reprod* 1983;28:108–120.
47. Bedford JM, Calvin HI. The occurrence and possible functional significance of —S—S— crosslinks in sperm heads, with particular reference to eutherian mammals. *J Exp Zool* 1974; 188:137–156.
48. Bedford JM, Calvin HI. Changes in —S—S— linked structures of the sperm tail during epididymal maturation, with comparative observation in sub-mammalian species. *J Exp Zool* 1974;187:181–204.
49. Bedford JM, Calvin HI, Cooper GW. The maturation of spermatozoa in the human epididymis. *J Reprod Fertil* 1973;18(Suppl):199–213.
50. Bedford JM, Cooper GW. Membrane fusion events in fertilization of vertebrate eggs. In: Poste G, Nicolson GL, eds. *Membrane Surface Reviews (Membrane Fusion),* Vol. 5. Amsterdam: North-Holland; 1978:65–125.

51. Bedford JM, Cross NL. Normal penetration of rabbit spermatozoa through a trypsin and acrosin resistant zona pellucida. *J Reprod Fertil* 1978;54:385–392.
52. Bedford JM, Moore HDM, Franklin LE. Significance of the equatorial segment of the acrosome of the spermatozoa in eutherian mammals. *Exp Cell Res* 1979;119:119–126.
53. Bellve AR, O Brien DA. The mammalian spermatozoa: structure and temporal assembly. In: Hanman JF, ed. *Mechanism and Control of Animal Fertilization.* New York: Academic Press; 1983:55–137.
54. Benau DA, Storey BT. Zona-binding site sensitive to trypsin inhibitors. *Biol Reprod* 1987;32:282–292.
55. Berger T, Clegg ED. Adenylate cyclase activity in porcine sperm in response to female reproductive tract secretions. *Gamete Res* 1983;7:169–177.
56. Bemal A, Torres J, Reyes A, Rosado A. Presence and regional distribution of sialyl transferase in the epididymis of the rat. *Biol Reprod* 1980;23:290–293.
57. Berruti G, Franchi E, Camatini M. Ca^{2+} localization in boar spermatozoa by the pyroantimonate technique and X-ray microanalysis. *J Exp Zool* 1986;237:257–262.
58. Bhattacharyya A, Roldan ERS, Yanagimachi R. Requirement of monovalent cations in the acrosome reaction of guinea pig spermatozoa. *Gamete Res* 1986;15:285–294.
59. Bhattacharyya AK, Zancveld LJD. Release of acrosin and acrosin inhibitor from human spermatozoa. *Fertil Steril* 1978; 30:70–78.
60. Bishop DW. Biology of spermatozoa. In: Young WC, ed. *Sex and Internal Secretions,* Vol. 2. Baltimore: Williams & Wilkins; 1961:707–796.
61. Bishop MWH, Smiles J. Induced fluorescence in mammalian gametes with acridine orange. *Nature* 1957;176:307–308.
62. Bize I, Santander G. Epinephrine decreases the potassium requirement of hamster sperm capacitation: furosemide blocks the effect of epinephrine. *J Exp Zool* 1985;235:261–267.
63. Blandau RJ. Biology of eggs and implantation. In: Young WC, ed. *Sex and Internal Secretions,* Vol. 2. Baltimore: Williams & Wilkins; 1961:797–882.
64. Blandau RJ, Odor DL. Observations on sperm penetration into the ooplasm and changes in the cytoplasmic components of the fertilizing spermatozoa in the rat ova. *Fertil Steril* 1952;3: 13–26.
65. Blazak WF, Overstreet JW. Instability of nuclear chromatin in the ejaculated spermatozoa of fertile men. *J Reprod Fertil* 1982;65:331–339.
66. Bleil JD, Beall CF, Wassarman PM. Mammalian sperm-egg interaction: fertilization of mouse eggs triggers modification of the major zona pellucida glycoprotein, ZP2. *Dev Biol* 1981; 86:189–197.
67. Bleil JD, Wassarman PM. Structure and function of the zona pellucida: identification and characterization of the proteins of the mouse ooeyte's zona pellucida. *Dev Biol* 1980;76:185–202.
68. Bleil JD, Wassarman PM. Sperm-egg interactions in the mouse: sequence of events and induction of the acrosome reaction by a zona pellucida glycoprotein. *Dev Biol* 1983;95:317–324.
69. Bleil JD, Wassarman PM. Autoradiographic visualization of the mouse egg's sperm receptor bound to sperm. *J Cell Biol* 1986;102:1363–1371.
70. Boatman DE, Bavister BD. Regulation of hamster sperm capacitation by bicarbonate ion-carbon dioxide. *J Cell Biol* 1983;97(5):40 (abst).
71. Boatman DE, Bavister BD. Stimulation of rhesus monkey sperm capacitation by cyclic nucleotide mediators. *J Reprod Fertil* 1984;71:357–366.
72. Boell EJ. Oxygen consumption of mouse sperm and its relationship to capacitation. *J Exp Zool* 1985;234:105–116.
73. Brackett BG, Bousquet D, Boice ML, Donawiek WJ, Evans JF, Dressel MA. Normal development following *in vitro* fertilization in the cow. *Biol Reprod* 1982;27:147–208.
74. Braden AW. Properties of the membranes of rat and rabbit eggs. *Aust J Sci Res* 1952;5:460–471.
75. Bradley MP, Forrester IT. A $[Ca^{2+} + Mg^{2+}]$-ATPase and active Ca^{2+} transport in the plasma membranes isolated from ram sperm flagella. *Cell Calcium* 1980;1:381–390.
76. Bradley MP, Forrester IT. A sodium-calcium exchange mechanism in plasma membrane vesicles isolated from ram sperm flagella. *FEBS Lett* 1980;121:15–18.
77. Bradley MP, Forrester IT. Sperm calcium homeostasis during maturation. In: Lobl TJ, Hafez ESE, eds. *Male Fertility and Its Regulation,* Boston: MIT Press; 1985:437–449.
78. Breitbart H, Darshan R, Rubinstein S. Evidence for the presence of ATPase-dependent calcium pump and ATPase activities in bull sperm head membranes. *Biochem Biophys Res Commun* 1984;122:479–489.
79. Breitbart H, Rubinstein S, Nass-Arden L. The role of calcium and Ca^{2+}-ATPase in maintaining motility in ram spermatozoa. *J Biol Chem* 1985;260:11548–11553.
80. Breitbart H, Stern B, Rubinstein S. Calcium transport and Ca^{2+}-ATPase activity in ram sperm plasma membrane vesicles. *Biochim Biophys Acta* 1983;728:349–355.
81. Brooks DE. Biochemical environment of sperm maturation. In: Fawcett DW, Bedford JM, eds. *The Spermatozoa.* Baltimore: Urban and Schwarzenberg; 1979:23–34.
82. Brooks DE. Purification of rat epididymal proteins 'D' and 'E', demonstration of shared immunological determinant, and identification of regional synthesis and secretion. *Int J Androl* 1982;5:513–524.
83. Brooks DE. Characterization of a 22 KDa protein with widespread tissue distribution but which is uniquely present in secretions of the testis and epididymis and on the surface of spermatozoa. *Biochim Biophys Acta* 1985;841:59–70.
84. Brooks DE, Means AR, Wright EJ, Singh SP, Tiver KK. Molecular cloning of the cDNA for two major androgen-dependent secretory proteins of 18.5 kilodaltons synthesized by the rat epididymis. *J Biol Chem* 1986;261:4956–4961.
85. Brooks DE, Tiver KK. Localization of epididymal secretory proteins on rat spermatozoa. *J Reprod Fertil* 1983;69:651–657.
86. Brown CR. Distribution of hyaluronidase in the ram spermatozoa. *J Reprod Fertil* 1975;45:537–539.
87. Brown CR, Cheng WKT. Changes in composition of the porcine zona pellucida during development of the oocyte to the 2- to 4-cell embryo. *J Embryol Exp Morphol* 1986;92:183–191.
88. Brown CR, von Glos KI, Jones R. Changes in plasma membrane glycoproteins of rat spermatozoa during maturation in the epididymis. *J Cell Biol* 1983;96:256–264.
89. Brown CR, Hartree EF. Distribution of a trypsin-like proteinase in the ram spermatozoa. *J Reprod Fertil* 1974;36:195–198.
90. Bryan JHD. Capacitation in the mouse: the response of murine acrosomes to the environment of the female genital tract. *Biol Reprod* 1974;10:414–421.
91. Bryan JHD, Akruk SR. A naphthol-yellow-S and erythrosin B staining procedure for use in studies of the acrosome reaction of rabbit spermatozoa. *Stain Technol* 1977;52:47–50.
92. Burkman LJ. Characterization of hyperactivated motility by human spermatozoa during capacitation: comparison of fertile and oligospermic sperm populations. *Arch Androl* 1984; 13:153–165.
93. Burkman LJ, Overstreet JW, Katz DF. A possible role for potassium and pyruvate in the modulation of sperm motility in the rabbit oviductal isthmus. *J Reprod Fertil* 1984;71:367–376.
94. Calvin HI, Bedford JM. Formation of disulfide bonds in the nucleus and accessory structures of mammalian spermatozoa during maturation in the epididymis. *J Reprod Fertil* 1971;13(Suppl):65–75.
95. Casillas ER. Accumulation of carnitin by bovine spermatozoa during maturation in the epididymis. *J Biol Chem* 1973; 248:8227–8232.
96. Casillas ER, Chaipayungpan S. Carnitin content of rabbit epididymal spermatozoa in organ culture. *J Reprod Fertil* 1982;65:247–251.
97. Castellani-Ceresa L, Berruiti G, Colombo R. Immunocytochemical localization of acrosin in boar spermatozoa. *J Exp Zool* 1983;227:297–304.
98. Chang MC. Fertilizing capacity of spermatozoa deposited in Fallopian tubes. *Nature* 1951;168:997–998.
99. Chang MC. Some aspects of mammalian fertilization. In: Tyler A, Van Bostel BC, Metz CB, eds. *The Beginning of Embryonic*

Development. Washington, DC: American Association for the Advancement of Science; 1957:109–134.
100. Chang MC. The meaning of sperm capacitation. *J Androl* 1984;5:45–50.
101. Chang MC, Hunter RHF. Capacitation of mammalian sperm: biological and experimental aspects. In: Greep RO, ed. *Handbook of Physiology,* Section 7, Vol. 5. Washington, DC: American Physiological Society, 1977:339–351.
102. Cheng WTK, Moor RM, Polge C. *In vitro* fertilization of pig and sheep oocytes matured *in vivo* and *in vitro. Theriogenology* 1986;25:146a.
103. Cherr GN, Lamben H, Meizel S, Kau DF. *In vitro* studies of the golden hamster sperm acrosome reaction: completion on the zona pellucida and induction by homologous solubilized zonae pellucidae. *Dev Biol* 1986;114:119–131.
104. Clegg EG. Mechanisms of mammalian sperm capacitation. In: Hartmann JF, ed. *Mechanism and Control of Animal Fertilization.* New York: Academic Press, 1983:177–212.
105. Collado ML, Castro G, Hicks JJ. Effect of spermatozoa upon carbonyl anhydrase activity of rabbit endometrium. *Biol Reprod* 1979;20:747–750.
106. Colwin LH, Colwin AL. Membrane fusion in relation to sperm–egg association. In: edited by Metz CB, Monroy A, eds. *Fertilization, Vol. 1.* New York: Academic Press; 1967:295–367.
107. Cooper GW, Bedford JM. Asymmetry of spermiation and sperm surface change patterns over the giant acrosome in the musk shrew Suncus murinus. *J Cell Biol* 1976;69:415–428.
108. Cooper GW, Overstreet JW, Katz DF. The motility of rabbit spermatozoa recovered from the female genital tract. *Gamete Res* 1979;2:35–42.
109. Cooper TG. The onset and maintenance of hyperactivated motility of spermatozoa from the mouse. *Gamete Res* 1984; 9:55–74.
110. Cornen LE, Meizel S. Stimulation of *in vitro* activation and the acrosome reaction of hamster spermatozoa by catecholamines. *Proc Natl Acad Sci USA* 1978;10:4954–4958.
111. Courot M. Transport and maturation of spermatozoa. *Prog Reprod Biol* 1981;8:67–79.
112. Courtens JL, Rozinek J, Fournier-Delpech S. Binding of epididymal proteins to the spermatozoa of the ram. *Andrologia* 1982;14:509–514.
113. Cran DG, Cheng WTK. The cortical reaction in pig oocytes during *in vivo* and *in vitro* fertilization. *Gamete Res* 1986;13:241–251.
114. Cross NL, Morales P, Overstreet JW. Two simple methods for detecting human sperm acrosome reactions. *J Androl* 1986;7:28a.
115. Crozet N. Ultrastructural aspects of *in vivo* fertilization in the cow. *Gamete Res* 1984;10:241–251.
116. Crozet N, Dumont M. The site of the acrosome reaction during *in vivo* penetration of the sheep oocyte. *Gamete Res* 1984;10:97–105.
117. Cuasnicu PS, Echeverria FG, Piazza A, Blaquier JA. Addition of androgens to cultured hamster epididymis increases zona recognition by immature spermatozoa. *J Reprod Fertil* 1984; 70:541–547.
118. Cummins JM. Hyperactivated motility patterns of ram spermatozoa recovered from the oviducts of mated ewes. *Gamete Res* 1982;6:53–63.
119. Cummins JM, Fleming AD, Crozel N, Kuehl TJ, Kosower NS, Yanagimachi R. Labeling of live mammalian spermatozoa with the fluorescent thio alkylating agent, monobromobimane (MB): immobilization upon exposure to ultraviolet light and analysis of acrosomal status. *J Exp Zool* 1986;237:375–382.
120. Cummins JM, Yanagimachi R. Sperm–egg ratios and the site of the acrosome reaction during *in vivo* fertilization in the hamster. *Gamete Res* 1982;5:239–256.
121. Cummins JM, Yanagimachi R. Development of ability to penetrate the cumulus oophorus by hamster spermatozoa capacitated *in vitro* in relation to the timing of the acrosome reaction. *Gamete Res.* 1986;15:187–212.
122. Dacheux JL, Paquignon M. Relations between the fertilizing ability, motility and metabolism of epididymal spermatozoa. *Reprod Nutr Dev* 1980;20:1085–1099.
123. D'Addario DA, Turner TT, Howards SS. Effect of vasectomy on the osmolarity of hamster testicular and epididymal intraluminal fluid. *J Androl* 1980;1:167–170.
124. Dan JC. Studies on the acrosome reaction. 1. Reaction to egg–water and other stimuli. *Biol Bull* 1952;103:54–66.
125. Dan JC. The acrosome reaction. *Int Rev Cytol* 1956;5:365–393.
126. Dan JC, Hashimoto S, Kubo M. The fine structure of the acrosome trigger. In: Afzelins BJ, ed. *The Functional Anatomy of the Spermatozoa,* New York: Pergamon Press; 1975:39–45.
127. Davis BK. Inhibitory effect of synthetic phospholipid vesicles containing cholesterol on the fertilizing capacity of rabbit spermatozoa. *Proc Soc Exp Biol Med* 1976;152:257–261.
128. Davis BK. Timing of fertilization in mammals: sperm cholesterol/phospholipid ratio as a determinant of the capacitation interval. *Proc Natl Acad Sci USA* 1981;78:7560–7564.
129. Davis BK, Byrne R, Hangund B. Studies on the mechanism of capacitation II. Evidence for lipid transfer between plasma membrane of rat sperm and serum albumin during capacitation *in vitro. Biochim Biophys Acta* 1979;558:257–266.
130. DeMayo FJ, Mizoguchi H, Dukelow WR. Fertilization of squirrel monkey and hamster ova in the rabbit oviduct. *Science* 1980;208:1468–1469.
131. Dickmann Z. The passage of spermatozoa through and into the zona pellucida of the rabbit egg. *J Exp Biol* 1964;41:177–182.
132. Dickmann Z, Dziuk PJ. Sperm penetration of the zona pellucida of the pig egg. *J Exp Biol* 1964;41:603–608.
133. Dravland JE, Llanus MN, Munn RJ, Meizel S. Evidence for the involvement of a sperm trypsin-like enzyme in the membrane events of the hamster acrosome reaction. *J Exp Zool* 1984;232:117–128.
134. Dravland JE, Meizel S. Stimulation of sperm capacitation and acrosome reaction *in vitro* by glucose and lactate and the inhibition by glycolytic inhibitor alpha-chlorohydrin. *Gamete Res* 1981;4:515–523.
135. Dudenhausen E, Talbot P. Detection and kinetics of the normal acrosome reaction of mouse sperm. *Gamete Res* 1982;6: 257–265.
136. Dudkiewicz AB, Garrison GA. Substrate preference of boar acrosin in zona pellucida lysis. *J Cell Biol* 1982;95:164.
137. Dunbar BS. Morphological, biochemical and immunochemical characterization of the mammalian zona pellucida. In: Hartmann JF, ed. *Mechanism and Control of Animal Fertilization.* New York: Academic Press; 1983:139–157.
138. Dunbar BS, Budkiewicz AB, Bundman DS. Proteolysis of specific porcine zona pellucida glycoproteins by boar acrosin. *Biol Reprod* 1985;32:619–630.
139. Dunbar BS, Munoz MG, Cordle CT, Metz CB. Inhibition of fertilization *in vitro* by treatment of rabbit spermatozoa with univalent isoantibodies to rabbit sperm hyaluronidase. *J Reprod Fertil* 1976;47:381–384.
140. Dunbar BS, Wardrip NJ, Hedrick JK. Isolation, physicochemical properties and macromolecular composition of the zona pellucida from porcine oocytes. *Biochemistry* 1980;19:356–365.
141. Dunbar BS, Wolgemuth DJ. Structure and function of the mammalian zona pellucida, a unique extracellular matrix. In: Satier BH, ed. *Modern Cell Biology,* Vol. 3. New York: Alan R. Liss; 1984:77–111.
142. Durr R, Shur B, Roth S. Sperm-associated sialyltransferase activity. *Nature* 1977;265:547–548.
143a. East IJ, Dean J. Monoclonal antibodies as probes of the distribution of ZP-2, the major sulfated glycoprotein of the mouse zona pellucida. *J Cell Biol* 1984;98:795–800.
143b. Echeverria FMG, Cuasnicu PS, Blaquier JA. Identification of androgen-dependent glycoproteins in the hamster epididymis and their association with spermatozoa. *J Reprod Fertil* 1982;64:1–7.
144. Eddy EM, Vernon RB, Muller CH, Hahnel AC, Fenderson BA. Immunodissection of sperm surface modifications during epididymal maturation. *Am J Anat* 1985;174:225–237.
145. Enders GC, Friend DS. Detection of anionic sites on the cytoplasmic surface of the guinea pig acrosomal membrane. *Am J Anat* 1985;173:241–256.
146. Eppig JJ. The relationship between cumulus cell-oocyte cou-

pling, oocyte meiotic maturation, and cumulus expansion. *Dev Biol* 1982;89:268–272.
147. Fain-Maurel ME, Danoune JP, Reger JF. A cytochemical study on surface charges and lectin-binding sites in epididymal and ejaculated spermatozoa of Macaca fasciculris. *Anat Rec* 1984;208:375–382.
148. Farooqui AA, Srivastava PN. Isolation, characterization and the role of rabbit testicular arylsulfatase A in fertilization. *Biochem J* 1979;181:331–337.
149. Farooqui A, Srivastava PN. Isolation of p-N-acetylhexosaminidase from rabbit semen and its role in fertilization. *Biochem J* 1980;191:827–834.
150. Fawcett DW. The mammalian spermatozoon. *Dev Biol* 1975;44:394–436.
151. Fawcett DW, Hollenberg RD. Changes in the acrosome of guinea pig spermatozoa during passage through the epididymis. *Zeit Zellforsch* 1963;60:276–292.
152. Flechon JE. Sperm glycoproteins of the boar, bull, rabbit, and ram: acrosomal glycoproteins. *Gamete Res* 1979;2:43–51.
153. Flechon JE. Ultrastructural and cytochemical analysis of the mammalian sperm plasma membrane during epididymal maturation. *Prog Reprod Biol* 1981;8:90–99.
154. Flechon JE. Sperm surface changes during the acrosome reaction as observed by freeze-fracture. *Am J Anat* 1985; 174:239–248.
155. Flechon JE, Harrison RAP, Flechon B, Escaig J. Membrane fusion events in the Ca^{2+}/ionophore-induced acrosome reaction of ram spermatozoa. *J Cell Sci* 1986;81:43–63.
156. Flemming AD, Kosower NS, and Yanagimachi R. Alteration of sperm thiol-disulfide status and capacitation in guinea pig. *Gamete Res* 1986;13:93–102.
157. Flemming AD, Kuehl TJ. Effects of temperature upon capacitation of guinea pig spermatozoa. *J Exp Zool* 1985;233:405–411.
158. Flemming AD, Yanagimachi R. Effects of various lipids on the acrosome reaction and fertilizing capacity of guinea pig spermatozoa, with special reference to the possible involvement of lysophospholipid in the acrosome reaction. *Gamete Res* 1981; 4:253–273.
159. Flemming AD, Yanagimachi R. Fertile life of acrosome-reacted guinea pig spermatozoa. *J Exp Zool* 1982;220:109–115.
160. Flemming AD, Yanagimachi R. Evidence suggesting the importance of fatty acids and fatty acid moieties of sperm membrane phospholipids in the acrosome reaction of guinea pig spermatozoa. *J Exp Zool* 1984;229:485–489.
161. Flemming AD, Yanagimachi R, Yanagimachi H. Spermatozoa of the atlantic bottlenosed dolphin, *Tursiops truncatus*. *J Reprod Fertil* 1981;63:509–514.
162. Florman HM, Storey BT. Mouse gamete interactions: the zona pellucida is the site of the acrosome reaction leading to fertilization *in vitro*. *Dev Biol* 1982;91:121–130.
163. Florman HM, Wassarman PM. O-linked oligosaccharides of mouse egg ZP-3 account for its sperm receptor activity. *Cell* 1985;4:313–324.
164. Fowler RE, Grainge C. A histochemical study of the changes occurring in the protein-carbohydrate composition of the cumulus-oocyte complex and zona pellucida in immature mice in response to gonadotropin stimulation. *Histochem J* 1985; 17:1235–1249.
165. Fox LL, Shivers CA. Immunologic evidence for addition of oviductal components to the hamster zona pellucida. *Fertil Steril* 1975;26:599–608.
166. Fraser LR. Motility patterns in mouse spermatozoa before and after capacitation. *J Exp Zool* 1977;202:439–444.
167. Fraser LR. Dibutyryl cyclic AMP decreases capacitation time *in vitro* in mouse spermatozoa. *J Reprod Fertil* 1981;62:63–72.
168. Fraser LR. Ca^2 is required for mouse sperm capacitation and fertilization *in vitro*. *J Androl* 1982;3:412–419.
169. Fraser LR. Potassium ions modulate expression of mouse sperm fertilizing ability, acrosome reaction and hyperactivated motility *in vitro*. *J Reprod Fertil* 1983;69:539–553.
170. Fraser LR. Mechanisms controlling mammalian fertilization. In: Finn CA, ed. *Oxford Review of Reproductive Biology,* Vol. 6. Oxford: Clarendon Press; 1984:174–225.
171. Fraser LR. Albumin is required to support the acrosome reaction but not capacitation in mouse spermatozoa *in vitro*. *J Reprod Fertil* 1985;74:185–196.
172. Fraser LR, Quinn PJ. A glycolytic product is obligatory for initiation of sperm acrosome reaction and whiplash motility required for fertilization in the mouse. *J Reprod Fertil* 1981;61:25–35.
173. Friend DS. The organization of the sperm membrane. In: Edidin M, Johnson MH, eds. *Immunobiology of Gametes*. Cambridge: Cambridge University Press; 1977:5–30.
174. Friend DS. Freeze-fracture alterations in guinea pig sperm membranes preceding gamete fusion. In: edited by Gilula NB, ed. *Membrane-Membrane Interactions*. New York: Raven Press; 1980:153–165.
175. Friend DS. Plasma-membrane diversity in a highly polarized cell. *J Cell Biol* 1982;93:243–249.
176. Friend DS, Orci L, Perrelet A, Yanagimachi R. Membrane particle changes attending the acrosome reaction in guinea pig spermatozoa. *J Cell Biol* 1977;74:561–577.
177. Funaki Y, Fukushima M, Ono H. Fertilization and cleavage of bovine follicular oocytes in rabbit reproductive tracts after maturation *in vitro*. *J Exp Zool* 1983;226:137–142.
178. Gaddum-Rosse P. Mammalian gamete interactions: What can be gained from observations on living eggs? *Am J Anat* 1985;173:347–356.
179. Gaddum-Rosse P, Blandau RJ. Comparative studies on the proteolysis of fixed gelatin membranes by mammalian sperm acrosomes. *Am J Anat* 1972;134:133–144.
180. Garbers DL. The elevation of cyclic AMP concentrations in flagella-less sea urchin sperm heads. *J Biol Chem* 1981; 256:620–624.
181. Gaunt SJ. Spreading of the sperm surface antigen within the plasma membrane of the egg after fertilization in the rat. *J Embryol Exp Morphol* 1983;75:257–270.
182. Go KJ, Wolf DP. The role of sterols in sperm capacitation. *Adv Lipid Res* 1983;20:317–330.
183. Go KJ, Wolf DP. Albumin-mediated changes in the sperm sterol contents during capacitation. *Biol Reprod* 1985;32: 145–153.
184. Goodpasture JC, Polakoski KL, Zaneveld LJD. Acrosin, proacrosin and acrosin inhibitor of human spermatozoa: extraction, quantitation and stability. *J Androl* 1980;1:16–27.
185. Goodpasture JC, Reddy JM, Zaneveld LJD. Acrosin, proacrosin, and acrosin inhibitor of guinea pig spermatozoa capacitated and acrosome-reacted *in vitro*. *Biol Reprod* 1981;25:44–55.
186. Gordon LM, Mobley PW. Membrane lipids, membrane fluidity, and enzyme activity. In: Aloia RC, Boggs JM, eds. *Membrane Fluidity in Biology,* Vol. 4. Orlando, Florida: Academic Press; 1985:1–49.
187. Gordon M. Localization of phosphatase activity on membranes of the mammalian sperm head. *J Exp Zool* 1973;185:111–120.
188. Gordon M, Dandekar PV, Bartoszewicz W. The surface coat of epididymal, ejaculated, and capacitated sperm. *J Ultrastruct Res* 1975;50:199–207.
189. Gordon M, Dandekar PV, Eager PR. Identification of phosphatases on the membranes of guinea pig sperm. *Anat Rec* 1978;191:123–133.
190. Gould JE, Overstreet JW, Hanson FW. Interaction of human spermatozoa with the human zona pellucida and zona-free hamster oocyte following capacitation by exposure to human cervical mucus. *Gamete Res* 1985;12:47–54.
191. Gould K, Zaneveld LJD, Srivastava PN, Williams WL. Biochemical changes in the zona pellucida of rabbit ova induced by fertilization and sperm enzymes. *Proc Soc Exp Biol Med* 1971;136:6–10.
192. Gould SF, Bernstein MH. The localization of bovine sperm hyaluronidase. *Differentiation* 1975;3:123–132.
193. Green DPL. Induction of the acrosome reaction in guinea pig spermatozoa *in vitro* by Ca ionophore A23187. *J Physiol* 1976;260:18–19.
194. Green DPL. The mechanism of the acrosome reaction. In: Johnson MH, ed. *Development in Mammals,* Vol. 3, New York: North-Holland; 1978:65–81.
195. Green DPL. The activation of proteolysis in the acrosome reaction of guinea pig spermatozoa. *J Cell Sci* 1978;32:153–164.
196. Green DPL, Hockaday AR. The histochemical localization of

acrosin in guinea pig sperm after the acrosome reaction. *J Cell Sci* 1978;32:177–184.
197. Green DPL, Purves TD. Mechanical hypothesis of sperm penetration. *Biophys J* 1984;45:659–662.
198. Greve JM, Wassarman PM. Mouse egg extracellular coat is a mixture of interconnected filaments possessing a structural repeat. *J Mol Biol* 1985;181:253–264.
199. Gwatkin RBL. *Fertilization Mechanisms in Man and Mammals.* New York: Plenum Press; 1977.
200. Gwatkin RBL, Andersen OF, Hulchison CF. Capacitation of hamster spermatozoa *in vitro:* the role of cumulus components. *J Reprod Fertil* 1972;30:389–394.
201. Gwatkin RBL, Klein D. Binding of solubilized zona by porcine sperm as they undergo the acrosome reaction. *J Androl* 1985;6:28a.
202. Gwatkin RBL, Williams DT. Receptor activity of the hamster and mouse solubilized zona pellucida before and after the zona reaction. *J Reprod Fertil* 1977;49:55–59.
203. Gwatkin RBL, Williams DT, Hartmann JF, Kniazuk M. The zona reaction of hamster and mouse eggs. Production *in vitro* of a trypsin-like protease from cortical granules. *J Reprod Fertil* 1973;32:259–265.
204. Haino K. Studies on the egg membrane lysin of *Tegula pfeifferi:* purification and properties of the egg–membrane lysin. *Biochim Biophys Acta* 1971;229:459–470.
205. Haino-Fukushima K. Studies on the egg membrane lysin of *Tegula pfeifferi:* the reaction mechanism of the egg membrane lysin. *Biochim Biophys Acta* 1974;352:459–470.
206. Hamilton DW. Steroid function in the mammalian epididymis. *J Reprod Fertil* 1971,13(Suppl):89–97.
207. Hamilton DW. UDP-galactose: N-acetylglucosamine galactosyltransferase in fluids from rat testis and epididymis. *Biol Reprod* 1980;23:377–385.
208. Hamilton DW. Evidence for alpha-lactoalbumin-like activity in reproductive tract fluids of the male rat. *Biol Reprod* 1981;25:385–392.
209. Hamilton DW, Fawcett DW. *In vitro* synthesis of cholesterol and testosterone from acetate by rat epididymis and vas deferens. *Proc Soc Exp Biol Med* 1970;133:693–695.
210. Hamilton DW, Gould RP. Galactosyltransferase activity associated with rat epididymis. *Anat Rec* 1980;196:71a.
211. Hammerstedt RH, Hay SR, Amann RP. Modification of ram sperm membranes during epididymal transit. *Biol Reprod* 1982;27:745–754.
212. Hammer CE, Fox SB. Biochemistry of oviductal secretions. In: Hafez ESE, Blandau RJ, eds. *The Mammalian Oviduct.* Chicago: University of Chicago Press; 1969:333–355.
213. Hammer CE, Jennings LL, Sojka NJ. Cat (*Feris catus* L.) spermatozoa require capacitation. *J Reprod Fertil* 1970; 23:477–480.
214. Handrow RR, Boehm SK, Lenz RW, Robinson JA, Aux RL. Specific binding of glycosaminoglycan 3H-heparine to bull, monkey and rabbit spermatozoa *in vitro. J Androl* 1984; 5:51–63.
215. Handrow RR, Lenz RW, Aux RL. Structural comparisons among glycosaminoglycans to promote an acrosome reaction in bovine spermatozoa. *Biochem Biophys Res Commun* 1982; 107:1326–1332.
216. Harrison RAP. The metabolism of mammalian spermatozoa. In: Greep RO, Koblinsky MA, eds. *Frontiers in Reproduction and Fertility Control.* Cambridge: MIT Press; 1975:379–401.
217. Harrison RAP. The acrosome, its hydrolase, and egg penetration. In: Andre J, ed. *The Sperm Cell.* The Hague: Martinus Nijhoff; 1983:259–273.
218. Hartmann JF. Mammalian fertilization: Gamete surface interactions *in vitro.* In: Hartman JF, ed. *Mechanism and Control of Animal Fertilization.* New York: Academic Press; 1985: 325–364.
219. Hartmann JF, Hutchison CF. Nature of the prepenetration contact interactions between hamster gametes *in vitro. J Reprod Fertil* 1974;36:49–57.
220. Hartmann JF, Hutchison CF. Is acrosin the lysin of the zona pellucida during fertilization? Proceedings of the 9th Annual Society of the Study of Reproduction Meeting, Philadelphia (abst. 2).
221. Hedrick JL, Wardrip NJ. Topographical radio-labeling of zona pellucida glycoproteins. *J Cell Biol* 1982;95:162a.
222. Hedrick JL, Wardrip NJ, Berger T. Difference in the macromolecular composition of the zona pellucida isolated from pig oocytes, eggs and zygotes. *J Exp Zool* 1986;241:257–262.
223. Helm G, Owman CH, Rosengren E, Sjoberg NO. Regional and cyclic variations in catecholamine concentrations of the human fallopian tube. *Biol Reprod* 1982;26:553–558.
224. Herz Z, Northey D, Lawyer M, First NL. Acrosome reaction of bovine spermatozoa *in vitro:* sites and effects of the stages of the estrous cycle. *Biol Reprod* 1985;32:1163–1168.
225. Hinkley RE, Wright BD, Greenberg CA. Induction of the acrosome reaction in sea urchin spermatozoa by the volatile anesthetic halothane. *Biol Reprod* 1986;34:119–125.
226. Hinrichsen AC, Topfer-Petersen E, Dietl T, Schmoeckel C, Schill WB. Immunological approach to the characterization of the acrosomal membrane of boar spermatozoa. *Gamete Res* 1985;11:143–155.
227. Hinrichsen-Kohane AC, Hinrichsen MJ, Schill WS. Molecular events leading to fertilization. *Andrologia* 1984;16:321–341.
228. Hirata F, Axelrod J. Phospholipid methylation and biological signal transmission. *Science* 1980;209:1082–1090.
229. Hirst PJ, DeMayo FJ, Dukelow WR. Xenogenous fertilization of laboratory and domestic animals in the oviduct of the pseudopregnant rabbit. *Theriogenology* 1981;15:67–75.
230. Hoffer AP, Shalev M, Frisch DH. Ultrastructure and maturational changes in spermatozoa in the epididymis of the pigtail monkey, *Macaca nemestrina. J Androl* 1981;2:140–146.
231. Holt WV. Development and maturation of the mammalian acrosome: a cytochemical study using phosphotungstic acid staining. *J Ultrastruct Res* 1979;68:58–71.
232. Holt WV. Surface-bound sialic acid on ram and bull spermatozoa: deposition during epididymal transit and stability during washing. *Biol Reprod* 1980;23:847–851.
233. Holt WV. Functional development of the mammalian sperm plasma membrane. In: Finn CA, ed. *Oxford Review of Reproductive Biology,* Vol. 4. Oxford: Clarendon Press; 1982: 195–240.
234. Holt WV. Membrane heterogeneity in the mammalian spermatozoa. *Int Rev Cytol* 1984;81:159–194.
235. Hoppe PC. Genetic influences on mouse sperm capacitation *in vivo* and *in vitro. Gamete Res* 1980;3:343–349.
236. Howards S, Lechene C, Vigetsky R. The fluid environment of the maturing spermatozoa. In: Fawcett DW, Bedford JM, eds. *The Spermatozoa.* Baltimore: Urban and Schwarzenberg; 1979:35–41.
237. Huacuja L, Delgado NM, Merchant H, Pancardo RM, Rosado A. Cyclic AMP induced incorporation of 33Pi into human sperm membrane components. *Biol Reprod* 1977;17:89–96.
238. Huang TTF, Flemming AD, Yanagimachi R. Only acrosome-reacted spermatozoa can bind and penetrate into zona pellucida: a study using guinea pig. *J Exp Zool* 1981;217:286–290.
239. Huang TTF, Hardy D, Yanagimachi H, Teuscher C, Tung K, Wild G, Yanagimachi R. pH and proteinase control of acrosomal content stasis and release during the guinea pig acrosome reaction. *Biol Reprod* 1985;32:451–462.
240. Huang TTF, Yanagimachi R. Fucoidin inhibits attachment of guinea pig spermatozoa to the zona pellucida through binding to the inner acrosomal membrane and equatorial domains. *Exp Cell Res* 1984;153:363–373.
241. Huang TTF, Yanagimachi R. Inner acrosomal membrane of mammalian spermatozoa: its properties and possible functions in fertilization. *Am J Anat* 1985;174:249–268.
242. Huneau D, Harrison RAP, Flechon JE. Ultrastructural localization of proacrosin and acrosin in ram spermatozoa. *Gamete Res* 1984;9:425–440.
243. Hunter AG, Nornes HO. Characterization and isolation of a sperm-coating antigen from rabbit seminal plasm with capacity to block fertilization. *J Reprod Fertil* 1969;20:419–427.
244. Hunter RHF. Pre-ovulatory arrest and periovulatory redistribution of competent spermatozoa in the isthmus of the pig oviduct. *J Reprod Fertil* 1984;72:203–211.

245. Hyne RV. Bicarbonate and calcium dependent induction of rapid guinea pig acrosome reaction by monovalent ionophore. *Biol Reprod* 1984;31:312–323.
246. Hyne RV, Edwards KP. Influence of 2-deoxyl-D-glucose and energy substrates on guinea-pig sperm capacitation and acrosome reaction. *J Reprod Fertil* 1985;73:59–69.
247. Hyne RV, Edwards KP, Smith JD. Changes in guinea pig sperm intracellular sodium and potassium content during capacitation and treatment with monovalent ionophore. *Gamete Res* 1985;12:65–73.
248. Hyne RV, Garbers DL. Calcium-dependent increase in adenosin 3′,5′-monophosphate and induction of the acrosome reaction in guinea pig spermatozoa. *Proc Natl Acad Sci USA* 1979;76:5699–5703.
249. Hyne RV, Higginson R, Kohlman D, Lopata A. Sodium requirement for capacitation membrane fusion during the guinea pig acrosome reaction. *J Reprod Fertil* 1984;70:83–94.
250. Infante JP, Huszagh VA. Synthesis of highly unsaturated phosphatidylcholine in the development of sperm motility: a role for epididymal glycerol-3-phosphorylcholine. *Mol Cell Biochem* 1985;69:3–9.
251. Inoue M, Wolf DP. Fertilization-associated changes in the murine zona pellucida: a time sequence study. *Biol Reprod* 1975;13:546–551.
252. Ishijima S, McCracken JA, Witman GB. Flagellar movement of intact and demembranated ram spermatozoa. *J Cell Biol* 1985;101:364a.
253. Johnson LA, Garner DL, Truitt-Gilbert AJ, Lessley A. Immunocytochemical acrosin on both acrosomal membranes and in the acrosomal matrix of porcine spermatozoa. *J Androl* 1983;4:222–229.
254. Johnson LL, Katz DF, Overstreet JW. The movement characteristics of rabbit spermatozoa before and after activation. *Gamete Res* 1981;4:275–282.
255. Johnson MH. The macromolecular organization of membranes and its bearing on events leading up to fertilization. *J Reprod Fertil* 1975;44:167–184.
256. Johnson MH, Eager D, Muggleton-Harris A. Mosaicism in organization of concanavalin A receptors on the surface membrane of mouse eggs. *Nature* 1975;257:321–322.
257. Jones HP, Lenz RW, Palevitz BA, Cormier MJ. Calmodulin localization in mammalian spermatozoa. *Proc Natl Acad Sci USA* 1980;77:2772–2776.
258. Jones R, Brown CR. Association of epididymal secretory proteins showing α-lactoalbumin-like activity with plasma membrane of rat spermatozoa. *Biochem J* 1982;206:161–164.
259. Joyce C. The antifertility activity of sperm hyaluronidase inhibitors. *Biol Reprod* 1982;26:117a.
260. Joyce C, Jeyendran RS, Zaneveld LJD. Release, extraction and stability of hyaluronidase associated with human spermatozoa: comparison with rabbit. *J Androl* 1985;6:152–161.
261. Katz DF, Yanagimachi R. Movement characteristics of hamster spermatozoa within the oviduct. *Biol Reprod* 1980;22:759–764.
262. Katz DF, Yanagimachi R. Movement characteristics of hamster and guinea pig spermatozoa upon attachment to the zona pellucida. *Biol Reprod* 1981;25:785–791.
263. Kinsey WH, Koehler JK. Cell surface charges associated with *in vitro* capacitation of hamster sperm. *J Ultrastruct Res* 1978;64:1–13.
264. Koehler JK. Fine structure of spermatozoa of the Asiatic musk shrew, Suncus murinus. *Am J Anat* 1977;149:135–152.
265. Koehler JK. The mammalian sperm surface: studies with specific labeling techniques. *Int Rev Cytol* 1978;54:73–108.
266. Koehler JK. Lectins as probes of the spermatozoa surface. *Arch Androl* 1981;6:197–217.
267. Koehler JK. Surface alterations during the capacitation of mammalian spermatozoa. *Am J Primatol* 1981;1:131–141.
268. Koehler JK, Gaddum-Rosse P. Media induced alterations of the membrane associated particles of the guinea pig sperm tail. *J Ultrastruct Res* 1975;51:106–118.
269. Koehler JK, Nudelman ED, Hakomori S. A collagen-binding protein of the surface of ejaculated rabbit spermatozoa. *J Cell Biol* 1980;86:529–536.
270. Kopecny V, Flechon JE. Fate of acrosomal glycoproteins during the acrosome reaction and fertilization: a light and electron microscope autoradiographic study. *Biol Reprod* 1981;24:201–216.
271. Kopecny V, Flechon JE, Pivko J. Binding of secreted glycoproteins to spermatozoa in the mammalian epididymis: a fine-structure autoradiographic study. *Anat Rec* 1984;208:197–206.
272. Koyama K, Hasegawa A, Isojima S. Effect of antisperm antibody on the *in vitro* development of rat embryos. *Gamete Res* 1984;10:143–152.
273. Krzanowska H. Toluidine blue staining reveals changes in chromatin stabilization of mouse spermatozoa during epididymal maturation and penetration of ova. *J Reprod Fertil* 1982;64:97–101.
274. Kusan F, Flemming AD, Seidel G. Successful fertilization *in vitro* of fresh intact oocytes by perivitelline (acrosome reacted) spermatozoa in the rabbit. *Fertil Steril* 1984;41:766–770.
275. Kvist U, Bjorndahl L. Zinc preserves and inherent capacity for human sperm chromatin decondensation. *Acta Physiol Scand* 1985;124:195–200.
276. Kvist U, Bjorndahl L, Roomans C, Lindholmer C. Nuclear zinc in human epididymal and ejaculated spermatozoa. *Acta Physiol Scand* 1985;125:297–303.
277. Lambert H. Temperature dependence of capacitation in bat sperm monitored by zona-free hamster ova. *Gamete Res* 1981;4:525–533.
278. Lambert H. Role of sperm-surface glycoproteins in gamete recognition in two mouse species. *J Reprod Fertil* 1984; 70:281–284.
279. Lambert H, Overstreet JW, Morales P, Hanson FW, Yanagimachi R. Sperm capacitation in the female reproductive tract. *Fertil Steril* 1985;43:325–327.
280. Lambert H, Van Le A. Possible involvement of a sialyated component of the sperm plasma membrane in sperm–zona interaction in mouse. *Gamete Res* 1984;10:153–163.
281. Langford BB, Howarth B. A trypsin-like enzyme in acrosomal extracts of chicken, turkey, and quail spermatozoa. *Poult Sci* 1974;53:834–837.
282. Langlais J, Plante L, Bleau G, Chapdelaine A, Roberts KD. Metabolism of lysophosphatidylcholine in relation to sperm capacitation. *Fertil Steril* 1982;38:135–136.
283. Langlais J, Roberts KD. A molecular membrane model of sperm capacitation and the acrosome reaction of mammalian spermatozoa. *Gamete Res* 1985;12:183–224.
284. Langlais J, Zollinger M, Plante L, Chapedelaine A, Bleau G, Roberts KD. Localization of cholesterol sulfate in human spermatozoa in support of a hypothesis of the mechanism of capacitation. *Proc Natl Acad Sci USA* 1981;78:7266–7270.
285. Leblond CP, Clemmont Y. Spermatogenesis of rat, mouse, hamster, and guinea pig as revealed by the periodic acid-fuchsin sulfurous acid technique. *Am J Anat* 1952;90:167–215.
286. Lechene C. Elemental and biochemical microanalysis of the male reproductive tract. *Ann NY Acad Sci* 1982;383:513–526.
287. Lee MA, Storey BT. Evidence for plasma membrane impermeability to small ions in acrosome intact mouse spermatozoa bound to mouse zonae pellucidae, using aminoacridine fluorescent pH probe. *Biol Reprod* 1985;33:235–246.
288. Lee MA, Storey BT. Bicarbonate is essential for fertilization of mouse eggs: mouse sperm require it to undergo the acrosome reaction. *Biol Reprod* 1986;34:349–356.
289. Legault Y, Bleau G, Chapdelaine A, Roberts KD. Steroid sulfatase activity of hamster reproductive tract during the estrous cycle. *Biol Reprod* 1980;23:720–725.
290. Legault Y, Bouthiller M, Bleau G, Chapedelaine A, Roberts KD. The sterol and sterol sulfate content of the male hamster reproductive tract. *Biol Reprod* 1979;20:1213–1219.
291. Leibfried ML, Bavisler BD. Effects of epinephrine and hypotaurine in *in vitro* fertilization in the golden hamster. *J Reprod Fertil* 1982;66:87–93.
292. LeLannou D, Colleu D, Boujard D, Segalin J. Stabilization of nuclear chromatin in human spermatozoa during capacitation *in vitro*. In: Testan J, Frydman R, eds. *Human In Vitro Fertilization*. Amsterdam: Elsevier; 1985:149–152.
293. Lenz RW, Bellin ME, Aux RL. Rabbit spermatozoa undergo an

acrosome reaction in the presence of glycoaminoglycans. *Gamete Res* 1983;8:11–19.
294. Lewin LM, Nevo Z, Gabsu A, Weissenberg R. The role of sperm bound hyaluronidase in the dispersal of the cumulus oophrus surrounding the rat ova. *Int J Androl* 1982;5:37–44.
295. Lewin LM, Nevo Z, Weissenberg R. The role of bound hyaluronidase in rat sperm–cumulus oophorus interaction. *Ann NY Acad Sci* 1981;383:473–474.
296. Lewis CA, Talbot CF, Vacquier VD. A protein from abalone sperm dissolves the egg vitelline layer by a nonenzymatic mechanism. *Dev Biol* 1982;92:227–239.
297. Llanos MN, Lui CW, Meizel S. Studies of phospholipase A2 related to the hamster sperm acrosome reaction. *J Exp Zool* 1982;221:107–117.
298. Llanos MN, Meizel S. Phospholipid methylation increases during capacitation of golden hamster sperm *in vitro*. *Biol Reprod* 1983;28:1043–1051.
299. Longo FJ, Chen DY. Development of cortical polarity in mouse eggs: involvement of the meiotic apparatus. *Dev Biol* 1985;107:382–394.
300. Lopez LC, Bayna EM, Litoff D, Shaper NL, Shaper JH, Shur BD. Receptor function of mouse sperm surface galactosyltransferase during fertilization. *J Cell Biol* 1985;101:1501–1510.
301. Lopo AC. Sperm-egg interactions in invertebrates. In: Hartmann JF, ed. *Mechanism and Control of Animal Fertilization,* New York: Academic Press; 1983:269–324.
302. Lonon SP, First NL. Hyaluronidase does not disperse the cumulus oophotus surrounding bovine ova. *Biol Reprod* 1979;21:301–308.
303. Lui CW, Cornett LE, Meizel S. Identification of the bovine follicular fluid protein involved in the *in vitro* induction of the hamster sperm acrosome reaction. *Biol Reprod* 1977;17:34–41.
304. Lui CW, Meizel S. Biochemical studies of the *in vitro* acrosome reaction inducing activity of bovine serum albumin. *Differentiation* 1977;9:59–66.
305. Lui CW, Meizel S. Further evidence in support of a role for hamster sperm hydrolytic enzymes in the acrosome reaction. *J Exp Zool* 1979;207:173–186.
306. Lui CW, Mrsny RJ, Meizel S. Procedure for obtaining high percentages of viable *in vitro* capacitated hamster sperm. *Gamete Res* 1979;2:207–211.
307. Mahadevan MM, Traunson AO. Removal of the cumulus oophorus from the human oocyte for *in vitro* fertilization. *Fertil Steril* 1985;43:263–267.
308. Mahanes MS, Ochs DL, Eng LA. Cell calcium of ejaculated rabbit spermatozoa before and following *in vitro* capacitation. *Biochem Biophys Res Commun* 1986;134:664–670.
309. Mahi CA, Yanagimachi R. The effect of temperature, osmolality and hydrogen ion concentration on the activation and acrosome reaction of golden hamster spermatozoa. *J Reprod Fertil* 1973;35:55–66.
310. Mahi CA, Yanagimachi R. Maturation and sperm penetration of canine ovarian oocytes *in vitro*. *J Exp Zool* 1976; 196:189–196.
311. Mann T. *The Biochemistry of Semen and of the Male Reproductive Tract.* New York: Methuen; 1964.
312. Mann T, Lutwak-Mann C. *Male Reproductive Function and Semen.* New York: Springer-Verlag; 1981.
313. Maro B, Johnson MH, Pickering SJ, Flach G. Changes in actin distribution during fertilization in the mouse egg. *J Embryol Exp Morphol* 1984;81:211–237.
314. Meizel S. The mammalian sperm acrosome reaction. A biochemical approach. In: Johnson MH, ed. *Development in Mammals.* New York: North-Holland; 1978:1–64.
315. Meizel S. The importance of hydrolytic enzymes to an exocytotic event, the mammalian sperm acrosome reaction. *Biol Rev* 1984;59:125–157.
316. Meizel S. Molecules that initiate or help stimulate the acrosome reaction by their interaction with the mammalian sperm surface. *Am J Anat* 1985;174:285–302.
317. Meizel S, Deamer DW. The pH of the hamster sperm acrosome. *J Histochem Cytochem* 1978;26:98–105.
318. Meizel S, Lui CW. Evidence for a role of a trypsinlike enzyme in the hamster sperm acrosome reaction. *J Exp Zool* 1976; 195:137–144.
319. Meizel S, Lui CW, Working PK, Mrsny RJ. Taurine and hypotaurine: their effects on motility, capacitation and the acrosome reaction of hamster sperm *in vitro* and their presence in sperm and reproductive tract fluids of several mammals. *Dev Growth Diff* 1980;22:483–494.
320. Meizel S, Turner KO. Stimulation of an exocytotic event, the hamster sperm acrosome reaction, by cis-unsaturated fatty acids. *FEBS Lett* 1983;161:315–318.
321. Meizel S, Turner KO. The effects of products and inhibitors of arachidonic acid metabolism on the hamster sperm acrosome reaction. *J Exp Zool* 1984;231:283–288.
322. Meizel S, Turner KO. Glycosaminoglycans stimulate the acrosome reaction of previously capacitated hamster sperm. *J Exp Zool* 1986;237:137–139.
323. Metz CB, Seiguer AC, Castro AE. Inhibition of the cumulus dispersing and hyaluronidase activities of sperm by heterologous and isologous antisperm antibodies. *Proc Soc Exp Biol Med* 1972;140:776–781.
324. Miller MA, Masui Y. Changes in the stainability and sulfhydryl level in the sperm nucleus during sperm–oocyte interaction in mice. *Gamete Res* 1982;5:167–179.
325. Miyamoto H, Chang MC. The importance of serum albumin and metabolic intermediates for capacitation of spermatozoa and fertilization of mouse eggs *in vitro*. *J Reprod Fertil* 1973;32:193–205.
326. Mohri H, Yanagimachi R. Characteristics of motor apparatus in testicular, epididymal and ejaculated spermatozoa: a study using demembranated sperm model. *Exp Cell Res* 1980; 127:191–196.
327. Monks NJ, Stein DM, Fraser LR. Mouse sperm adenylate cyclase is stimulated by calcium. *Proceedings of the 13th Annu Meeting of the Society for the Study of Fertility, London,* 1985 (abst. 10).
328. Moore HDM. The net surface charge of mammalian spermatozoa as determined by isoelectric focusing: changes following sperm maturation, ejaculation, incubation in the female tract, and after enzyme treatment. *Int J Androl* 1979;2:449–462.
329. Moore HDM, Bedford JM. The interaction of mammalian gametes in the female. In: Hartmann JF, ed. *Mechanism and Control of Animal Fertilization.* New York: Academic Press; 1983:453–497.
330. Moore HDM, Hibbitt KG. The binding of labelled basic proteins by boar spermatozoa. *J Reprod Fertil* 1976;46:71–76.
331. Moore DJ, Clegg ED, Lunstra DD, Mollenhauer HH. An electron-dense stain for isolated fragments of plasma and acrosomal membrane from porcine sperm. *Proc Soc Exp Biol Med* 1974;145:1–6.
332. Mortimer D, Courtol AM, Giovangrandi Y, Jeulin C, David G. Human sperm motility after migration into, and incubation in, synthetic media. *Gamete Res* 1984;9:131–144.
333. Morton B, Albagli L. Modification of hamster sperm adenyl cyclase by capacitation *in vitro*. *Biochem Biophys Res Commun* 1973;50:695–703.
334. Morton DB. Acrosomal enzymes: immunological localization of acrosin and hyaluronidase in ram spermatozoa. *J Reprod Fertil* 1975;45:375–378.
335. Motomura M, Toyoda Y. Scanning electron microscopic observations on the sperm penetration through the zona pellucida of mouse oocytes fertilized *in vitro*. *Jpn J Zootech Sci* 1980;51:595–601.
336. Mo GW, Vacquier VD. Immunoperoxidase localization of binding during the adhesion of sperm to sea urchin eggs. *Curr Top Dev Biol* 1979;13:31–44.
337. Mrsny RJ, Meizel S. Evidence suggesting a role for cyclic nucleotides in acrosome reactions of hamster sperm *in vitro*. *J Exp Zool* 1980;211:153–158.
338. Mrsny RJ, Meizel S. Potassium ion influx and Na^+, K^+-ATPase activity are required for the hamster sperm acrosome reaction. *J Cell Biol* 1981;91:77–82.
339. Mrsny RJ, Meizel S. Initial evidence for the modification of hamster sperm Na^+, K^+-ATPase activity by cyclic nucleotide

mediated processes. *Biochem Biophys Res Commun* 1983; 112:132–138.
340. Mrsny RJ, Meizel S. Inhibition of hamster sperm Na^+, K^+-ATPase activity by taurine and hypotaurine. *Life Sci* 1985; 36:271–275.
341. Mrsny RJ, Siiteri JE, Meizel S. Hamster sperm Na^+, K^+-adenosine triphosphatase: increased activity during capacitation *in vitro* and its relationship to cyclic nucleotides. *Biol Reprod* 1984;30:573–584.
342. Mrsny RJ, Waxman L, Meizel S. Taurine maintains and stimulates motility of hamster sperm during capacitation *in vitro. J Exp Zool* 1979;210:123–128.
343. Mujica A, Ruiz MAV. On the role of glucose in capacitation and acrosome reaction of guinea pig sperm. *Gamete Res* 1983;8:335–344.
344. Multamaki S, Pelliniemi LJ, Suominen J. Ultrastructural study of separated cell and acrosomal membranes of bull spermatozoa. *Fertil Steril* 1975;26:932–938.
345. Murphy SJ, Roldan ERS, Yanagimachi R. Effects of extracellular cations and energy substrates on the acrosome reaction of precapacitated guinea pig spermatozoa. *Gamete Res* 1986; 14:1–10.
346. Murphy SJ, Yanagimachi R. The pH-dependence of motility and the acrosome reaction of guinea pig spermatozoa. *Gamete Res* 1984;10:1–8.
347. Nakano M, Otsuka M, Akama K, Tobita T. Predominance of beta-structure in solubilized zona pellucida from porcine ova. *Biochem Int* 1984;9:39–43.
348. Nagai T, Yanagimachi R, Srivastava PN, Yanagimachi H. Acrosome reaction in human spermatozoa. *Fertil Steril* 1986;45:701–707.
349. Nagai T, Niwa K, Iritani A. Effect of sperm concentration during preincubation in a defined medium on fertilization *in vitro* of pig follicular oocytes. *J Reprod Fertil* 1984;70:271–275.
350. Nicander L, Sjoden I. An electron microscopical study of the acrosomal complex and its role in fertilization in the river lamprey, *Lampetra fluriatilis. J Submicrosc Cytol* 1971;3:309–317.
351. Nicolson GL, Usui N, Yanagimachi R, Yanagimachi H, Smith JR. Lectin-binding site on the plasma membranes of rabbit spermatozoa changes in surface receptors during epididymal maturation and after ejaculation. *J Cell Biol* 1977;74:950–962.
352. Nikolopoulou M, Soucek DA, Vary JC. Changes in the lipid content of boar sperm plasma membranes during epididymal maturation. *Biochem Biophys Acta* 1985;815:486–498.
353. Niwa K, Ohara K, Hoshi Y, Iritani A. Early events of *in-vitro* fertilization of cat eggs by epididymal spermatozoa. *J Reprod Fertil* 1985;74:657–660.
354. Ohzu E, Yanagimachi R. Acceleration of acrosome reaction in hamster spermatozoa by lysolecithin. *J Exp Zool* 1982; 224:259–263.
355. Oikawa T, Kurata S, Sendai Y. Discovery of a novel zona pellucida glycoprotein (ZP-0) having a sperm binding activity. *J Reprod Immunol* 1986;(Suppl):81.
356. Okabe M, Takada K, Adachi T, Kohama Y, Miura T, Aonuma S. Studies on sperm capacitation using monoclonal antibody—disappearance of an antigen from the anterior part of mouse sperm head. *J Pharmacol Dyn* 1986;9:55–60.
357. Okabe M, Takada K, Adachi T, Kohama Y, Miura T. Inconsistent reactivity of an anti-sperm monoclonal antibody and its relationship to sperm capacitation. *J Reprod Immunol* 1986;9:67–70.
358. Okamura F, Nishiyama H. The passage of spermatozoa through the vitelline membrane in the domestic fowl, *Gallus gallus. Cell Tissue Res* 1978;188:497–508.
359. Oliphant G, Reynolds AB, Thomas TS. Sperm surface components involved in the control of the acrosome reaction. *Am J Anat* 1985;174:269–283.
360. Olson GE. Changes in intramembranous particle distribution in the plasma membrane of *Didelphis virginiana* spermatozoa during maturation in the epididymis. *Anat Rec* 1980;197:471–488.
361. Olson GE, Danzo BJ. Surface changes in rat spermatozoa during epididymal transit. *Biol Reprod* 1981;24:431–443.
362. Olson GE, Orgebin-Crist MC. Sperm surface changes during epididymal maturation. *Ann NY Acad Sci* 1982;383:372–391.
363. Olson GE, Lifsics MR, Winfrey VP, Rifkin JM. Association of a 26KD polypeptide with the flagellar plasma membrane of rat spermatozoa during maturation in the epididymis. *J Androl* 1986;7:13a.
364. Olson GE, Winfrey VP. Substructure of a cytoskeletal complex associated with the hamster sperm acrosome. *J Ultrastruct Res* 1985;92:167–179.
365. Olson GE, Winfrey VP, Garbers DL, Noland TD. Isolation and characterization of macromolecular complex associated with the outer acrosomal membrane of bovine spermatozoa. *Biol Reprod* 1985;13:761–779.
366. Ono K, Yanagimachi R, Huang TTF. Phospholipase A of guinea pig spermatozoa: its preliminary characterization and possible involvement in the acrosome reaction. *Dev Growth Diff* 1982;24:305–310.
367. O'Rand MG. Restriction of a sperm surface antigen's mobility during capacitation. *Dev Biol* 1977;55:260–270.
368. O'Rand MG. Changes in sperm surface properties correlated with capacitation. In: Fawcett DW, Bedford JM, eds. *The Spermatozoa.* Baltimore: Urban and Schwarzenberg; 1979:195–204.
369. O'Rand MG. Modification of the sperm membrane during capacitation. *Ann NY Acad Sci* 1982;383:392–404.
370. O'Rand MG. Differentiation of mammalian sperm antigens. In: Metz CB, Monroy A, eds. *Biology of Fertilization,* Vol. 2. New York: Academic Press; 1985:103–119.
371. O'Rand MG, Fisher SJ. Localization of zona pellucida binding sites on rabbit spermatozoa and induction of the acrosome reaction by solubilized zonae. *Dev Biol* 1987;119:551–559.
372. O'Rand MG, Matthews JE, Welch JE, Fisher SJ. Identification of zona binding proteins of rabbit, pig, human and mouse spermatozoa on nitrocellulose blots. *J Exp Zool* 1985;235:423–428.
373. O'Rand MG, Welch JE, Fisher SJ. Sperm membrane and zona pellucida interactions during fertilization. In: Dhindsa DS, Bahl OP, eds. *Molecular and Cellular Aspects of Reproduction.* New York: Plenum Press; 1986:131–144.
374. Orgebin-Crist MC. Epididymal physiology and sperm maturation. *Prog Reprod Biol* 1981;8:80–89.
375. Orgebin-Crist MC, Fournier-Delpech S. Sperm–egg interaction: evidence for maturational changes during epididymal transit. *J Androl* 1982;3:429–433.
376. Orgebin-Crist MC, Olson GE, Danzo BJ. Factors influencing maturation of spermatozoa in the epididymis. In: Franchimont P, Channing CP, eds. *Intragonadal Regulation of Reproduction.* New York: Academic Press; 1981:393–417.
377. Oshio S, Kaneko S, Mohri H. Impurities in commercial preparations of bovine serum albumin inhibits the acrosome reaction of hamster spermatozoa. *Zool Sci* 1986;3:295–299.
378. Overstreet JW, Bedford JM. Transport, capacitation and fertilizing ability of epididymal spermatozoa. *J Exp Zool* 1974;189:203–214.
379. Overstreet JW, Coats C, Katz DK, Hanson FW. The importance of seminal plasma for sperm penetration of human cervical mucus. *Fertil Steril* 1980;34:569–572.
380. Overstreet JW, Cooper GW. Reduced sperm motility in the isthmus of the rabbit oviduct. *Nature* 1975;258:718–719.
381. Overstreet JW, Cooper GW, Katz DF. Sperm transport in the reproductive tract of the female rabbit II. The sustained phase of transport. *Biol Reprod* 1978;19:115–132.
382. Overstreet JW, Cooper GW. The time and location of the acrosome during sperm transport in the female rabbit. *J Exp Zool* 1979;209:97–104.
383. Overstreet JW, Cooper GW. Effect of ovulation and sperm motility on the migration of rabbit spermatozoa to the site of fertilization. *J Reprod Fertil* 1979;55:53–59.
384. Parks JE, Hammerstedt RH. Developmental changes occurring in the lipid of ram epididymal sperm plasma membranes. *Biol Reprod* 1985;32:653–668.
385. Parrish RF, Wincek TJ, Polakoski KL. Glycosaminoglycon stimulation of the *in vitro* conversion of boar proacrosin into acrosin. *J Androl* 1980;1:89–95.
386. Pellicciari C, Hosokawa Y, Fukuda M, Romanini MGM. Cytofluorometic study of nuclear sulphydryl and disulphide groups during sperm maturation in the mouse. *J Reprod Fertil* 1983;68:371–376.

387. Perreault S, Zaneveld LJD, Rogers BJ. Inhibition of fertilization in the hamster by sodium aurothiomalate, a hydronidase inhibitor. *J Reprod Fertil* 1980;60:461–467.
388. Perreault SD, Zirkin BR, Rogers BJ. Effect of trypsin inhibitors on acrosome reaction of guinea pig spermatozoa. *Biol Reprod* 1982;26:343–351.
389. Peterson RN, Henry L, Saxena W, Russell LD. Further characterization of boar sperm plasma membrane proteins with affinity for the porcine zona pellucida. *Gamete Res* 1985;12:91–100.
390. Peterson RN, Hunt WP, Henry LH. Interaction of boar spermatozoa with porcine oocytes: increase in proteins with high affinity for the zona pellucida during epididymal transit. *Gamete Res* 1986;14:57–64.
391. Peterson RN, Russell LD. The mammalian spermatozoon: a model for the study of regional specificity in the plasma membrane organization and function. *Tissue Cell* 1985;17:769–791.
392. Phillips DM, Shalgi RM. Surface properties of the zona pellucida. *J Exp Zool* 1980;213:1–8.
393. Phillips DM, Shalgi RM. Sperm penetration into rat ova fertilized *in vivo*. *J Exp Zool* 1982;221:373–378.
394. Picheral B, Charbonneau M. Anural fertilization: a morphological reinvestigation of some early events. *J Ultrastruct Res* 1982;81:306–321.
395. Piko L. Immunological phenomena in the reproductive process. *Int J Fertil* 1967;12:377–383.
396. Piko L. Gamete structure and sperm entry in mammals. In: Melz CB, Monroy A, eds. *Fertilization,* Vol. 2. New York: Academic Press; 1979:325–403.
397. Piko L, Tyler A. Fine structural studies of sperm penetration in the rat. *Proceedings of the 5th International Congress on Animal Reproduction,* Trento, Italy, Vol. 2. 1964:372–374.
398. Plummer JM, Watson PF. Ultrastructural localization of calcium ions in ram spermatozoa before and after cold shock is demonstrated by a pyroantimonate technique. *J Reprod Fertil* 1985;75:255–263.
399. Presti FT. The role of cholesterol in regulating membrane fluidity. In: Aloia RC, Boggs JM, eds. *Membrane Fluidity in Biology, Vol. 4: Cellular Aspects.* Orlando, Florida: Academic Press; 1985:97–146.
400. Quian Z, Tsai Y, Steinberg A, Lu M, Greenfield ARL, Haddox MK. Localization of ornithin decarboxylase in rat testicular cells and epididymal spermatozoa. *Biol Reprod* 1985;33: 1189–1195.
401. Quinn PJ, White IG. Active cation transport in dog spermatozoa. *Biochem J* 1967;104:328–340.
402. Quinn PJ, White IG. Distribution of adenosintriphosphatase activity in ram and bull spermatozoa. *J Reprod Fertil* 1968;15:449–452.
403. Rahi H, Srivastava PN. Hormonal regulation of lysosomal hydrolases in the reproductive tract of the rabbit. *J Reprod Fertil* 1983;67:447–455.
404. Rahi H, Srivastava PN. Lysosomal hydrolases in reproductive organs during estrous cycle of the hamster. *Gamete Res* 1984;10:57–66.
405. Rao VII, Sarmah BC, Bhattacharyya NK. Xenogenous fertilization of goat ova in the rabbit oviduct. *J Reprod Fertil* 1984;71:377–379.
406. Reddy JM, Joyce C, Zaneveld LJD. Role of hyaluronidase in fertilization: the antifertility activity of myocrisin, a nontoxic hyaluronidase inhibitor. *J Androl* 1980;1:28–32.
407. Reger JF, Fain-Maurel MA, Dadoune JP. A freeze-fracture study on epididymal and ejaculate spermatozoa of the monkey (*Macaca fascicularis*). *J Submicrosc Cytol* 1985;17:49–56.
408. Restall BJ, Wales RG. The fallopian tube of the sheep. III. The chemical composition of the fluid from the fallopian tube. *Aust J Biol Sci* 1966;19:687–698.
409. Restall BJ, Wales RG. The fallopian tube of the sheep. V. Secretion from the ampulla and isthmus. *Aust J Biol Sci* 1968;21:491–498.
410. Reyes A, Chavarria ME, Rosado A. Interference with spermatozoa capacitation. In: Cunningham GR, Schill WS, Hafez ESE, eds. *Regulation of Male Fertility.* The Hague: Martinus Nijhoff; 1980:135–149.
411. Reyes A, Magdaleno VM, Hernandez O, Rosado A, Delgado NM. Effect of zinc on decondensation of human spermatozoa nuclei by heparine. *Arch Androl* 1983;10:155–160.
412. Rifkin JM, Olson GE. Characterization of maturation-dependent extrinsic proteins of the rat sperm surface. *J Cell Biol* 1984;100:1582–1591.
413. Rikmenspoel R, Orris SE, Isles CA. Effect of vandate, Mg^{2+} and electric current injection on the stiffness of impaled bull spermatozoa. *J Cell Sci* 1981;51:53–61.
414. Rodger JC, Bedford JM. Separation of sperm pairs and sperm–egg interaction in the opossum *Didelphis virginiana. J Reprod Fertil* 1982;64:171–179.
415. Rogers BJ. Mammalian sperm capacitation and fertilization *in vitro:* a critique of methodology. *Gamete Res* 1978;1:165–223.
416. Rogers BJ, Garcia L. Effect of cAMP on acrosome reaction and fertilization. *Biol Reprod.,* 1979;21:365–372.
417. Roldan ERS, Shibata S, Yanagimachi R. Effect of Ca^{2+} channel antagonists on the acrosome reaction of guinea pig and golden hamster spermatozoa. *Gamete Res* 1986;13:281–292.
418. Romrell LJ, O'Rand MG, Sandow PS, Porter JP. Identification of surface autoantigens which appear during spermatogenesis. *Gamete Res* 1982;5:35–48.
419. Roomans GM. Calcium binding to the acrosomal membrane of human spermatozoa. *Exp Cell Res* 1975;96:23–30.
420. Russell LD, Kramper B, Hunt W, Peterson RN. Selective solubilization of major boar sperm plasma membrane (PM) polypeptides (PS) by detergents and buffer of various ionic strength. *Biol Reprod* 1984;30(Suppl. 1):111a.
421. Russell LD, Peterson NR, Hunt W, Strack LE. Posttesticular surface modifications and contributions of reproductive fluids to the surface polypeptide composition of boar spermatozoa. *Biol Reprod* 1984;30:959–978.
422. Sacco AG, Yurewicz EG, Subramanian MG. Carbohydrate influences the immunogenic and antigenic characteristics of the ZP3 macromolecule (Mr 55000) of the pig zona pellucida. *J Reprod Fertil* 1986;76:575–586.
423. Saling PM. Involvement of trypsin-like activity in binding of mouse spermatozoa to zona pellucida. *Proc Natl Acad Sci USA* 1981;78:6231–6235.
424. Saling PM. Development of the ability to bind zonae pellucidae during epididymal maturation. *Biol Reprod* 1982;26:429–436.
425. Saling PM, Bedford JM. Absence of species specificity for mammalian sperm capacitation *in vivo. J Reprod Fertil* 1981;63: 119–123.
426. Saling PM, Sowinski J, Storey BT. An ultrastructural study of epididymal mouse spermatozoa binding to zonae pellucidae *in vitro:* sequential relationship to the acrosome reaction. *J Exp Zool* 1979;209:229–238.
427. Saling PM, Storey BT. Mouse gamete interaction during fertilization *in vitro:* chlorfelracycline as a fluorescent probe for the mouse sperm acrosome reactions. *J Cell Biol* 1979;83:544–555.
428. Sano K. Acrosome reaction of echinoderm sperm. In: Hidaka H, Hartshorne DJ, eds. *Calmodulin Antagonists and Cellular Physiology.* New York: Academic Press; 1985:117–127.
429. Santos-Sacchi J, Gordon M. Induction of the acrosome reaction in guinea pig spermatozoa by cGMP analogues. *J Cell Biol* 1980;5:798–803.
430. Santos-Sacchi J, Gordon M. The effect of ATP depletion upon the acrosome reaction in guinea pig sperm. *J Androl* 1982;3:108–112.
431. Santos-Sacchi J, Gordon M, Williams WL. Potentiation of the cGMP-induced guinea pig acrosome reaction by zinc. *J Exp Zool* 1980;213:289–291.
432. Sato K, Blandau RJ. Time and process of sperm penetration into cumulus-free mouse eggs fertilized *in vitro. Gamete Res* 1979;2:295–304.
433. Saxena NK, Russell LD, Saxena N, Peterson RN. Immunofluorescence antigen localization on boar sperm plasma membrane: monoclonal antibodies reveal apparent new redistribution of surface antigens during sperm maturation and at ejaculation. *Anat Rec* 1986;214:238–252.
434. Schlegel RA, Hammerstedt R, Cofer GP, Kozarsky K. Changes in the organization of the lipid bilayer of the plasma membrane during spermatogenesis and epididymal maturation. *Biol Reprod* 1986;34:379–391.

435. Schollmeyer JE. Identification of calpain II in porcine sperm. *Biol Reprod* 1986;34:721–731.
436. Shalgi R, Kaplan R, Nebel L, Kraicer PF. The male factor in fertilization of rat eggs *in vitro*. *J Exp Zool* 1981;217:399–402.
437. Shalgi R, Phillips DM. Mechanics of *in vitro* fertilization in the hamster. *Biol Reprod* 1980;23:433–448.
438. Shalgi R, Phillips D. Mechanics of sperm entry in cycling hamsters. *J Ultrastruct Res* 1980;71:154–161.
439. Shams-Borham G, Harrison RAP. Production, characterization, and use of ionophore-induced, calcium-dependent acrosome reaction in ram spermatozoa. *Gamete Res* 1981;4: 407–432.
440. Shams-Borham G, Huneau D, Fleehon JE. Acrosin does not appear to be bound to the inner acrosomal membrane of bull spermatozoa. *J Exp Zool* 1979;209:143–149.
441. Shapiro BM, Schackmann RW, Tombes RM, Kazazoglan T. Coupled ionic and enzymatic regulation of sperm behavior. *Curr Top Cell Regul* 1985;26:97–113.
442. Sheikhnejad RG, Srivastava PN. Isolation and properties of a phospholidylcholine-specific phospholipase C from bull seminal plasma. *J Biol Chem* 1986;261:7544–7549.
443. Shimizu S, Tsuji M, Dean J. *In vitro* synthesis of three sulfated glycoproteins of murine zonae pellucidae by oocytes grown in follicle culture. *J Biol Chem* 1983;258:5858–5863.
444. Shinohara H, Yanagimachi R, Srivastava PN. Enhancement of the acrosome reaction of hamster spermatozoa by proteolytic enzymes, kallikrein, trypsin and chymotrypsin. *Gamete Res* 1985;11:19–28.
445. Shur BD, Hall NG. A role for mouse sperm surface galactosyltransferase in sperm binding to the egg zona pellucida. *J Cell Biol* 1982;95:574–579.
446. Siddiquey AKS, Cohen J. *In vitro* fertilization in the mouse and the relevance of difference sperm/egg concentrations and volumes. *J Reprod Fertil* 1982;66:237–242.
447. Singer SJ, Nicolson GL. The fluid mosaic model of the structure of the cell membrane. *Science* 1972;175:720–731.
448. Singh JP, Babcock DF, Lardy HA. Increased calcium ion influx is a component of capacitation of spermatozoa. *Biochem J* 1978;172:549–556.
449. Singh JP, Babcock DF, Lardy HA. Motility activation, respiratory stimulation, and alteration of Ca^{2+} transport in bovine sperm treated with amine local anesthetic and calcium transport antagonists. *Arch Biochem Biophys* 1983;221:291–303.
450. Snider DR, Clegg ED. Alteration of phospholipids in porcine spermatozoa during *in vivo* uterus and oviduct incubation. *J Anim Sci* 1978;40:269–274.
451. Soucek DA, Nikolopoulou M, Vary JC, Zirkin B. Fluidity measurements of sperm membranes from *in vitro* capacitated and acrosome reacted boar sperm. *J Cell Biol* 1985;101:263a.
452. Srivastava PN, Akruk SR, Williams WL. Dissolution of rabbit zona by sperm acrosome extract: effect of calcium. *J Exp Zool* 1979;207:521–529.
453. Srivastava PN, Brewer JM, White RA. Hydrolysis of p-nitrophenylphosphorylcholine by alkaline phosphatase and phospholipase C from rabbit sperm acrosome. *Biochem Biophys Res Commun* 1982;108:1120–1125.
454. Srivastava PN, Farooqui AA, Gould KG. Studies on hydrolytic enzymes of chimpanzee sperm. *Biol Reprod* 1981;25:363–369.
455. Srivastava PN, Munnell JF, Yang CH, Foley CW. Sequential release of acrosomal membrane and acrosomal enzymes of ram spermatozoa. *J Reprod Fertil* 1974;36:363–372.
456. Srivastava PN, Ninjour V. Isolation of rabbit testicular cathepsin D and its role in the activation of proacrosin. *Biochem Biophys Res Commun* 1982;109:63–69.
457. Stein DM, Fraser LR. Cyclic nucleotide metabolism in mouse epididymal spermatozoa during capacitation *in vitro*. *Gamete Res* 1984;10:283–299.
458. Stein DM, Fraser LR, Monks NJ. Adenosine and Gpp(NH)p modulate mouse sperm adenylate cyclase. *Gamete Res* 1986;13:151–158.
459. St. Jacques S, Forget A, Roberts KD. Monoclonal antibodies specific for an oviduct component associated with the zona pellucida. *J Reprod Immunol* 1986;(Suppl.):52.
460. Storey BT, Lee MA, Muller C, Ward CR, Wirtshafter DG. Binding of mouse spermatozoa to the zona pellucida of mouse eggs in cumulus: evidence that the acrosomes remain substantially intact. *Biol Reprod* 1984;3:1119–1128.
461. Suarez SS, Katz DF, Overstreet JW. Movement characteristics and acrosomal status of rabbit spermatozoa recovered at the site and time of fertilization. *Biol Reprod* 1983;29:1277–1287.
462. Suarez SS, Katz DF, Meizel S. Changes in motility that accompany the acrosome reaction in hyperactivated hamster spermatozoa. *Gamete Res* 1984;10:253–265.
463. Sullivan R, Bleau G. Interaction of isolated components from mammalian sperm and egg. *Gamete Res* 1985;12:101–116.
464. Suzuki F. Changes in intramembranous particle distribution in epididymal spermatozoa of the boar. *Anat Ree* 1981;199: 361–376.
465. Szollosi D, Hunter RHF. The nature and occurrence of the acrosome reaction in spermatozoa of the domestic pig, *Sus scrofa*. *J Anat* 1978;127:33–41.
466. Takahashi N, Yamagata T. Involvement of sialic acids in fertilization of the mouse. *Dev Growth Diff* 1982;24:407.
467. Talbot P. Events leading to fertilization in mammals. In: Harrison RF, Thompson JBW, eds. *Fertility and Sterility: Proceedings of the 11th World Congress on Fertilization and Sterilization.* Boston: MTP Press; 1984:121–131.
468. Talbot P. Sperm penetration through oocyte investments in mammals. *Am J Anat* 1985;174:331–346.
469. Talbot P, Chacon RS. A triple stain technique for scoring acrosome reaction of human sperm. *J Exp Zool* 1980;215:201–208.
470. Talbot P, DiCarlantonio G. The oocyte–cumulus complex: ultrastructure of the extracellular components in hamster and mice. *Gamete Res* 1984;10:127–142.
471a. Talbot P, DiCarlantonio G. Ultrastructure of opossum oocyte investing coats and their sensitivity to trypsin and hyaluronidase. *Dev Biol* 1984;103:159–167.
471b. Talbot P, DiCarlantonio G. Cytochemical localization of dipeptidyl peptidase II (DPP-II) in mature guinea pig sperm. *J Histochem Cytochem* 1985;33:1169–1172.
472. Talbot P, DiCarlantonio G, Zao P, Penkala J, Haimo LT. Motile cells lacking hyaluronidase can penetrate the hamster oocyte cumulus complex. *Dev Biol* 1985;108:387–398.
473. Talbot P, Kleve MG. Hamster sperm cross react with antiactin. *J Exp Zool* 1978;204:131–136.
474. Talbot P, Summers RG, Hylander BL, Keough EM, Franklin LE. The role of calcium in the acrosome reaction: an analysis using ionophore A23187. *J Exp Zool* 1976;198:383–392.
475. Tash JS, Means AR. Cyclic adenosin 3′, 5′ monophosphate, calcium and protein phosphorylation in flagella motility. *Biol Reprod* 1983;28:75–104.
476. Tesarik J. Topographic relations of intramembranal particle distribution patterns in human sperm membranes. *J Ultrastruct Res* 1984;89:42–55.
477. Tesarik J. Comparison of acrosome reaction-inducing activities of human cumulus oophorus, follicular fluid and ionophore A23187 in human sperm populations of proven fertilizing ability *in vitro*. *J Reprod Fertil* 1985;74:383–388.
478. Tezon JG, Ramella E, Cameo MS, Vazquez MH, Blacquier JA. Immunochemical localization of secretory antigens in the human epididymis and their association with spermatozoa. *Biol Reprod* 1985;32:591–597.
479. Thakkart JK, East J, Franson R. Modulation of phospholipase A2 activity associated with human sperm membranes by divalent cations and calcium. *Biol Reprod* 1984;30:679–689.
480. Thakkart JK, East J, Seyle D, Franson RC. Surface-active phospholipase A2 in mouse spermatozoa. *Biochim Biophys Acta* 1983;754:44–50.
481. Thompson RS, Smith DM, Zamboni L. Fertilization of mouse ova *in vitro:* an electron microscopic study. *Fertil Steril* 1974;25:222–249.
482. Topfer-Peterson E, Friess AE, Nguyen H, Schill WS. Evidence for a fucose-binding protein in boar spermatozoa. *Histochemistry* 1985;83:139.
483. Topfer-Peterson E, Friess AE, Sinowalz F, Bielz S, Schill WS. Immunocytological characterization of the outer acrosomal membrane (OAM) during acrosome reaction in boar. *Histochemistry* 1985;82:113–120.

484. Topfer-Peterson E, Schill WB. A new separation method of subcellular fraction of boar spermatozoa. *Andrology* 1981;13:174–176.
485. Topfer-Peterson E, Schill WS. Characterization of lectin receptors isolated from the outer acrosome membrane of boar spermatozoa. *Int J Androl* 1983;6:375–392.
486. Toyoda Y, Yokoyama M, Hoshi T. Studies on the fertilization of mouse eggs *in vitro. Jpn J Anim Reprod* 1971;16:147–157.
487. Tsunoda Y, Chang MC. *In vitro* fertilization of hamster eggs by ejaculated or epididymal spermatozoa in the presence of male accessory secretions. *J Exp Zool* 1977;201:445–450.
488. Uesugi S, Yamazoe S. Presence of sodium-potassium-stimulated ATPase in boar epididymal spermatozoa. *Nature* 1966;209:403.
489. Urch UA, Hedrick JL. Acrosin derived peptides bind the zona pellucida. *J Cell Biol* 1985;101:378a.
490. Urch UA, Wardrip NJ, Hedrick JL. Proteolysis of the zona pellucida by acrosin: the nature of the hydrolysis product. *J Exp Zool* 1985;236:239–243.
491. Urch UA, Wardrip NJ, Hedrick JL. Limited and specific proteolysis of the zona pellucida by acrosin. *J Exp Zool* 1985;233:479–483.
492. Usui N, Yanagimachi R. Cytochemical localization of membrane-bound Mg^{2+}-dependent ATPase activity in guinea pig sperm head before and during the acrosome reaction. *Gamete Res* 1986;13:271–280.
493. Vacquier VD, Moy GW. Isolation of binding: the protein responsible for adhesion of sperm to sea urchin eggs. *Proc Natl Acad Sci USA* 1977;74:2456–2460.
494. Velazquez A, Delgado ND, Rosado A. Taurine content and amino acid composition on human acrosome. *Life Sci* 1986;38:991–995.
495. Vernon RB, Hamilton MS, Eddy EM. Effects of *in vivo* and *in vitro* fertilization environments on the expression of a surface antigen of the mouse sperm tail. *Biol Reprod* 1985;32:669–680.
496. Vernon RB, Muller CH, Herr JC, Feuchter FA, Eddy EM. Epididymal secretion of a mouse sperm surface component recognized by a monoclonal antibody. *Biol Reprod* 1982;26:523–535.
497. Vijayasarathy S, Balarm P. Regional differentiation in bull sperm plasma membranes. *Biochem Biophys Res Commun* 1982;108:760–769.
498. Vijayasarthy S, Shivaji S. Bull sperm plasma and acrosomal membrane: fluorescence studies of lipid phase fluidity. *Biochem Biophys Res Commun* 1982;108:585–591.
499. Viriyapanich P, Bedford JM. Sperm capacitation in the fallopian tube of the hamster and its suppression by endocrine factors. *J Exp Zool* 1981;217:403–407.
500. Viriyapanich P, Bedford JM. The fertilization performance *in vivo* of rabbit spermatozoa capacitated *in vitro. J Exp Zool* 1981;216:169–174.
501. Virtanen I, Bradley RA, Paaivuo R, Lehto VP. Distinct cytoskeletal domains revealed in sperm cells. *J Cell Biol* 1984;99:1083–1091.
502. Volglmayr JK, Fairbanks G, Lewis RG. Surface glycoprotein changes in ram spermatozoa during epididymal maturation. *Biol Reprod* 1983;29:767–775.
503. Volglmayr JK, Sawyer FR. Surface transformation of ram spermatozoa in uterus, oviduct and cauda epididymal fluids *in vitro. J Reprod Fertil* 1986;78:315–325.
504. De Vries JWA, Willemsen R, Geuze HJ. Immunocytochemical localization of acrosin and hyaluronidase in epididymal and ejaculated porcine spermatozoa. *Eur J Cell Biol* 1985;37:81–88.
505. Wardrip NJ, Hedrick JL, Berger T. Comparison of pig zona pellucida from oocytes, eggs and zygotes. *Fed Proc* 1985;44:1778a.
506. Wassarman PM, Bleil JD, Florman HM, Greve JM, Roller RJ, Salizman GS, Samuels FG. The mouse eggs receptor for sperm: What is it and how does it work? *Cold Spring Harb Symp Quant Biol* 1985;50:11–19.
507. Wassarman PM, Florman HM, Greve JM. Receptor-mediated sperm–egg interactions in mammals. In: Metz CB, Monroy A, eds. *Fertilization,* Vol. 2. New York: Academic Press; 1985:341–360.
508. Watson PF, Plummer JM. Relationship between calcium binding sites and membrane fusion during the acrosome reaction induced by ionophore in ram spermatozoa. *J Exp Zool* 1986;238:113–118.
509. Weil AJ. The spermatozoa-coating antigen (SCA) of the seminal vesicle. *Ann NY Acad Sci* 1965;124:267–269.
510. Weinman DE, Williams WL. Mechanism of capacitation of rabbit spermatozoa. *Nature* 1961;203:423–424.
511. Westrick JC, Boatman DE, Bavister BD. Characteristics of acrosome reaction-inducing factor from hamster cumulus and follicular fluid. *Biol Reprod* 1985;37:351a.
512. White IG, Volglmayr JK. ATP-induced reactivation of ram testicular, caudal epididymal, and ejaculated spermatozoa extracts with Triton X-100. *Biol Reprod* 1986;34:183–193.
513. Wincek TJ, Parrish RF, Polakoski KL. Fertilization: a uterine glycosaminoglycan stimulates the conversion of sperm proacrosin to acrosin. *Science* 1979;203:553–554.
514. Wolf DE, Hagopian SS, Isojima S. Changes in sperm plasma membrane lipid diffusibility after hyperactivation during *in vitro* capacitation in the mouse. *J Cell Biol* 1986;102:1372–1377.
515. Wolf DP. The mammalian egg's block to polyspermy. In: Mastroianni L, Biggers BJ, eds. *Fertilization and Embryonic Development In Vitro.* New York: Plenum Press; 1981:183–197.
516. Wolf DP, Boldt J, Byrd W, Bechtol KB. Acrosomal status evaluation in human ejaculate sperm with monoclonal antibodies. *Biol Reprod* 1985;32:1157–1162.
517. Wong PYD, Tang AYE. Studies on the binding of a 32K rat epididymal protein to rat epididymal spermatozoa. *Biol Reprod* 1987;27:1239–1246.
518. Working PK, Meizel S. Preliminary characterization of a Mg^{2+}-ATPase in hamster sperm head membranes. *Biochem Biophys Res Commun* 1982;104:1060–1065.
519. Working PK, Meizel S. Correlation of increased intraacrosomal pH with the hamster sperm acrosome reaction. *J Exp Zool* 1983;227:97–107.
520. Yamasata T, Ito M, Takahashi K. The involvement of a saccharide-mediated recognition mechanism in the interaction between sperm and the zona pellucida of the egg cells of the mouse. In: Chester MA, Heingard D, Lundblad A, Sevenssen S, eds. *Glycoconjugates.* Lund: Rahmis i Lund; 1983:623–624.
521. Yamamoto N. Immunoelectron microscopic localization of calmodulin in guinea pig testis and spermatozoa. *Acta Histochem Cytochem* 1985;18:199–211.
522. Yanagimachi R. Sperm penetration into hamster egg *in vitro. Proceedings of the 3rd International Congress Animal Reproduction* Trento, 1964:321–324.
523. Yanagimachi R. Time and process of sperm penetration into hamster ova *in vivo* and *in vitro. J Reprod Fertil* 1966;11:359–370.
524. Yanagimachi R. *In vitro* capacitation of hamster spermatozoa by follicular fluid. *J Reprod Fertil* 1969;18:275–286.
525. Yanagimachi R. *In vitro* acrosome reaction and capacitation of golden hamster spermatozoa by bovine follicular fluid and its fractions. *J Exp Zool* 1969;170:269–280.
526. Yanagimachi R. *In vitro* capacitation of golden hamster spermatozoa by homologous and heterologous blood sera. *Biol Reprod* 1970;3:147–153.
527. Yanagimachi R. The movement of golden hamster spermatozoa before and after capacitation. *J Reprod Fertil* 1970;23:193–196.
528. Yanagimachi R. Fertilization of guinea pig eggs *in vitro. Anat Rec* 1977;174:9–20.
529. Yanagimachi R. Specificity of sperm-egg interaction. In: Edidin M, Johnson MH, eds. *Immunobiology of Gametes.* London: Cambridge University Press; 1977:255–295.
530. Yanagimachi R. Mechanisms of fertilization in mammals. In: Mastroianni L, Biggers JD, eds. *Fertilization and Embryonic Development In Vitro.* New York: Plenum Press, 1981:81–187.
531. Yanagimachi R. *In vitro* sperm capacitation and fertilization of golden hamster eggs in a chemically defined media. In: *In Vitro Fertilization and Embryo Transfer,* edited by Hafez ESE, Semm K, Lancaster: MTP Press; 1982:65–76.
532. Yanagimachi R. Requirement of extracellular calcium ions for various stages of fertilization and fertilization related phenomena in the hamster. *Gamete Res* 1982;5:323–344.

533. Yanagimachi R. Fertilization. In: Crosignani PG, Rubin BL, eds. *In Vitro Fertilization and Embryo Transfer,* London: Academic Press; 1983:65–100.
534. Yanagimachi R. Zona-free hamster eggs: their use in assessing fertilizing capacity and examining chromosomes of human spermatozoa. *Gamete Res* 1984;10:178–232.
535. Yanagimachi R, Chang MC. Fertilization of hamster eggs *in vitro. Nature* 1963;200:281–282.
536. Yanagimachi R, Cummins JM. Optical changes in the acrosomal caps of golden hamster spermatozoa prior to the acrosome reaction. *Proceedings of the Annual Conference of the Society for the Study of Reproduction,* Aberdeen; 1985:(abst. 20).
537. Yanagimachi R, Huang TTF, Flemming AD, Kosower NS, Nicolson GL. Dithiorestal, a disulfide-reducing agent, inhibits capacitation, acrosome reaction and interaction with eggs by guinea pig spermatozoa. *Gamete Res* 1983;7:145–154.
538. Yanagimachi R, Kamiguchi K, Mikamo K, Suzuki F, Yanagimachi H. Maturation of spermatozoa in the epididymis of the chinese hamster. *Am J Anat* 1985;172:317–330.
539. Yanagimachi R, Kamiguchi K, Sugawara S, Mikamo K. Gametes and fertilization in the chinese hamster. *Gamete Res* 1983;8:97–117.
540. Yanagimachi R, Mahi CA. The sperm acrosome reaction and fertilization in the guinea pig: a study *in vivo. J Reprod Fertil* 1976;16:49–54.
541. Yanagimachi R, Noda YD. Fine structure of the hamster sperm head. *Am J Anat* 1970;128:367–388.
542. Yanagimachi R, Noda YD. Ultrastructural changes in the hamster sperm head during fertilization. *J Ultrastruct Res* 1970;31:465–485.
543a. Yanagimachi R, Noda YD. Electron microscope studies of sperm incorporation into the hamster egg. *Am J Anat* 1970;128:429–462.
543b. Yanagimachi R, Noda YD. Physiological changes in the postnuclear cap region of mammalian spermatozoa: a necessary preliminary to the membrane fusion between sperm and egg cells. *J Ultrastruct Res* 1970;31:486–493.
544. Yanagimachi R, Noda YD, Fujimoto M, Nicolson GL. The distribution of negative surface charge of mammalian spermatozoa. *Am J Anat* 1972;135:497–520.
545. Yanagimachi R, Phillips DM. The status of acrosomal caps of hamster spermatozoa immediately before fertilization *in vitro. Gamete Res* 1984;9:1–19.
546. Yanagimachi R, Suzuki F. A further study of lysolecithin-mediated acrosome reaction of guinea pig spermatozoa. *Gamete Res* 1985;11:29–40.
547. Yanagimachi R, Usui N. Calcium dependence of the acrosome reaction and activation of guinea pig spermatozoa. *Exp Cell Res* 1974;89:161–174.
548. Yang WH, Lin LL, Wang JR, Chang MC. Sperm penetration through zona pellucida and perivitelline space in hamster. *J Exp Zool* 1972;179:191–206.
549. Yoshigaki N, Katagiri C. Acrosome reaction of sperm of the toad, *Bufo bufo japonicus. Gamete Res* 1982;6:343–352.
550. Young LG, Hinton BT, Gould FG. Surface changes in chimpanzee sperm during epididymal transit. *Biol Reprod* 1985;32:399–412.
551. Zahler WL, Doak GA. Isolation of the outer acrosomal membrane from bull sperm. *Biochim Biophys Acta* 1975;406: 479–488.
552. Zamboni L. Fertilization in the mouse. In: Moghissi KS, Hafez ESE, eds. *Biology of Mammalian Fertilization and Implantation.* Springfield, Illinois: Charles C. Thomas; 1972:213–262.
553. Zaneveld LJD, Polakoski KL, Williams WL. A proteinase and proteinase inhibitor of mammalian sperm acrosomes. *Biol Reprod* 1973;9:219–225.
554. Zao PZR, Meizel S, Talbot P. Release of hyaluronidase and beta-acetylhexosaminidase during *in vitro* incubation of hamster sperm. *J Exp Zool* 1985;134:63–71.
555. Austin CR. Cortical granules in hamster eggs. *Exp Cell Res* 1956;10:533–540.
556. Austin CR. *Fertilization.* Englewood Cliffs, New Jersey: Prentice-Hall; 1965.
557. Austin CR, Braden AWH. Observations on nuclear size and form in living rat and mouse eggs. *Exp Cell Res* 1955;8:163–172.
558. Balakier H, Tarkowski AK. The role of germinal vesicle karyoplasm in the development of male pronucleus in the mouse. *Exp Cell Res* 1980;128:79–86.
559. Bedford JM. Oocyte structure and the design and function of the sperm head in eutherian mammals. In: Andre J, ed. *The Sperm Cell.* London: Academic Press; 1983:75–89.
560. Bellve AR. The molecular biology of mammalian spermatogenesis. In: Finn CA, ed. *Oxford Reviews of Reproductive Biology,* Vol. 1. Oxford: Clarendon Press; 1979:159–261.
561. Bjorndahl L, Kjellberg S, Roomans GM, Kvist U. The human sperm nucleus takes up zinc at ejaculation. *Int J Androl* 1986;9:77–80.
562. Brandriff B, Pedersen RA. Repair of the ultraviolet-irradiated male genome in fertilized mouse eggs. *Science* 1981;211: 1431–1433.
563. Braude PR, Pelham HRB, Flach G, Lobatto R. Post transcriptional control in the early mouse embryo. *Nature* 1979;282: 102–105.
564. Brinster RL, Chen HY, Trumbauer ME, Payton BV. Secretion of proteins by the fertilized mouse ovum. *Exp Cell Res* 1981;134:291–296.
565. Calvin HI. Keratinoid proteins in the heads and tails of mammalian spermatozoa. In: Duckett JG, Racey PA, eds. *The Biology of the Male Gamete.* London: Academic Press; 1975:257–273.
566. Calvin HI. Comparative analysis of the nuclear basic proteins in rat, human, guinea pig, mouse and rabbit spermatozoa. *Biochim Biophys Acta* 1976;134:377–389.
567. Calvin HI, Grosshans K, Blake EJ. Estimation and manipulation of glutathion levels in prepuberal mouse ovaries and ova: relevance to sperm nucleus transformation in the fertilized egg. *Gamete Res* 1986;14:265–275.
568. Cavanagh A, Morton H, Roefe BA, Gidley-Baird AL. Ovum factor: a first signal of pregnancy? *Am J Reprod Immunol* 1982;2:97–101.
569. Chen HY, Brinster RL, Merz EA. Changes in protein synthesis following fertilization of the mouse ovum. *J Exp Zool* 1980;212:355–360.
570. Clarke HJ, Masui Y. Dose-dependent relationship between oocyte cytoplasmic volume and transformation of sperm nuclei to metaphase chromosomes. *J Cell Biol* 1987;104:831–840.
571. Clegg KB, Piko L. RNA synthesis and cytoplasmic polyadenylation in the one-cell mouse embryo. *Nature* 1982;295:342–345.
572. Dale B, DeFelice J, Ehrenstein G. Injection of soluble sperm fraction into sea urchin eggs triggers the cortical reaction. *Experientia* 1985;41:1068–1070.
573. Da-Yuan C, Longo FJ. A cytochemical study of nuclear changes in fertilized hamster eggs. *Anat Rec* 1983;207:327–334.
574. Delgado NM, Reyes R, Huacuja L, Carranco A, Merchant H, Rosado A. Decondensation of human sperm nuclei by glycosaminoglycan sulfate from sea urchin egg. *J Exp Zool* 1982;224:457–460.
575. Dube F, Dufresne-Duke L, Guerrier P. Sperm nuclear decondensation in *Barnea candida* (mollusca, pelecypoda) oocytes does not require germinal vesicle breakdown. *J Exp Zool* 1982;221:383–387.
576. Ecklund PS, Levine L. Mouse sperm basic nuclear protein: electrophoretic characterization and fate after fertilization. *J Cell Biol* 1975;66:251–262.
577. Endo Y. The role of the cortical granules in the formation of the fertilization membrane in eggs from Japanese sea urchins. *Exp Cell Res* 1952;3:106–118.
578. Epel D. The triggering of development at fertilization. In: Ebert J, Okada T, eds. *Mechanisms of Cell Change.* New York: John Wiley & Sons; 1979:17–31.
579. Epel D. The physiology and chemistry of calcium during the fertilization of eggs. In: Cheung WY, ed. *Calcium and Cell Function,* Vol. 2. New York: Academic Press; 1982:355–385.
580. Evans T, Rosenthal E, Youngblom J, Distel D, Hunt T. Cyclin: a protein specified by maternal mRNA in sea urchin eggs that is destroyed at each cleavage division. *Cell* 1983;33:389–396.
581. Flach G, Johnson MH, Braude PR, Taylor RAS, Holton VN.

The transition from maternal to embryonic control in the 2-cell mouse embryo. *EMBO J* 1982;1:681–686.
582. Fulton BP, Whittingham DG. Activation of mammalian oocytes by intercellular injection of calcium. *Nature* 1978;273: 149–151.
583. Gordon K, Brown DB, Ruddle FH. *In vitro* activation of human sperm induced by amphibian egg extract. *Exp Cell Res* 1985;157:409–418.
584. Graham CF. The production of parthenogenetic mammalian embryos and their use in biological research. *Biol Rev* 1974;49:399–422.
585. Gulyas BJ. Cortical granules of mammalian eggs. *Int Rev Cytol* 1980;63:357–392.
586. Hamaguchi Y, Hiramoto Y. Activation of sea urchin eggs by microinjection of calcium buffers. *Exp Cell Res* 1981;131: 171–179.
587. Hirao Y, Yanagimachi R. Development of pronuclei in polyspermic eggs of the golden hamster: is there any limit to the number of sperm heads that are capable of developing into male pronuclei? *Zool Mag* [*Tokyo*] 1979;88:24–33.
588. Holmberg SRM, Johnson MH. Amino acid transport in the unfertilized and fertilized mouse eggs. *J Reprod Fertil* 1979;36:223–231.
589. Hunter RHF. Polyspermic fertilization in pig during the luteal phase of the estrous cycle. *J Exp Zool* 1967;165:451–460.
590. Huret JL. Nuclear chromatin decondensation of human sperm. *Arch Androl* 1986;16:97–109.
591. Iwamatsu T, Ohta T. The changes in sperm nuclei after penetrating fish oocytes matured without germinal vesicle material in their cytoplasm. *Gamete Res* 1980;3:121–132.
592. Jackowski S, Leibo SP, Mazur P. Glycerol permeability of fertilized and unfertilized mouse ova. *J Exp Zool* 1988;212: 329–341.
593. Jaffe LA, Gould M. Polyspermy-preventing mechanisms. In: Metz CB, Monroy A, eds. *Biology of Fertilization*, Vol. 3. Orlando, Florida: Academic Press; 1985:223–250.
594. Jaffe LF. Sources of calcium in egg activation: a review and hypothesis. *Dev Biol* 1983;99:265–276.
595. Jaffe LF. The role of calcium explosions, waves and pulses in activating eggs. In: Metz CB, Monroy A, eds. *Biology of Fertilization*, Vol. 3. Orlando, Florida: Academic Press; 1985: 127–165.
596. Kamiguchi Y, Mikamo K. An improved, efficient method for analyzing human sperm chromosomes using zona-free hamster ova. *Am J Human Genet* 1986;38:724–740.
597. Kanoh Y, Yanagimachi R. Ueber den japanischen Hering (Clupea pallasii C. et V.) II. Der Beginn der Entwicklung ohne Zerfallen der Kortikalaveoli. *J Fac Sci Hokkaido Univ Ser VI* [*Zool*] 1956;12:264–272.
598. Katagiri C, Moiya M. Spermatozoan response to the toad egg matured after removal of germinal vesicle. *Dev Biol* 1976;50:235–241.
599. Karasiewicz J, Soltynska MS. Ultrastructural evidence for the presence of actin filaments in mouse eggs at fertilization. *Roux's Arch Dev Biol* 1985;194:369–372.
600. Kaufman MH. *Early Mammalian Development: Parthenogenesis Studies*. Cambridge: Cambridge University Press. 1983.
601. Kay ES, Shapiro BM. The formation of the fertilization membrane of the sea urchin egg. In: Metz CB, Monroy A, eds. *Biology of Fertilization*, Vol. 3. Orlando, Florida: Academic Press; 1985:45–80.
602. Kopecny V, Pavlok A. Autoradiographic study of mouse spermatozoan arginine-rich nuclear protein in fertilization. *J Exp Zool* 1975;191:85–96.
603. Kvist U. Spermatozoal thiol-disulphide interaction: a possible event underlying physiological sperm nuclear chromatin decondensation. *Acta Physiol Scand* 1980;115:503–505.
604. Leese HJ, Biggers JD, Mroz EA, Lechene C. Nucleotides in a single mammalian ovum or preimplantation embryo. *Anal Biochem* 1984;140:443–448.
605. Leibo SP. Water permeability and its activation energy of fertilized and unfertilized mouse ova. *J Membr Biol* 1980;53: 179–188.
606. Lohka MJ, Masui Y. The germinal vesicle material required for sperm pronuclear formation is located in the soluble fraction of egg cytoplasm. *Exp Cell Res* 1983;148:481–491.
607. Longo FJ. Fertilization: a comparative ultrastructural review. *Biol Reprod* 1973;9:149–215.
608. Longo FJ. Regulation of pronuclear development. In: Jagiello G, Vogel C, eds. *Regulators of Reproduction*. New York: Academic Press; 1981:529–557.
609. Longo FJ. Pronuclear events during fertilization. In: Metz CB, Monroy A, eds. *Biology of Fertilization*, Vol. 3. Orlando, Florida: Academic Press; 1985:251–298.
610. Mahi CA, Yanagimachi R. Induction of nuclear decondensation of mammalian spermatozoa *in vitro*. *J Reprod Fertil* 1975;44:293–296.
611. Maro B. Fertilization and the cytoskeleton in the mouse. *Bioessays* 1986;3:18–21.
612. Maro B, Howlett SH, Webb M. Non-spindle microtubule organization centers in metaphase II-arrested mouse oocytes. *J Cell Biol* 1985;101:1665–1672.
613. Maro B, Johnson MH, Pickering SJ, Flach G. Changes in actin distribution during fertilization of the mouse egg. *J Embryol Exp Morphol* 1984;81:211–237.
614. Masui Y, Clarke HJ. Oocyte maturation. *Int Rev Cytol* 1979;57:185–282.
615. McCulloh DH, Rexroad CE, Levitan H. Insemination of rabbit egg is associated with slow depolarization and repetitive diphasic membrane potentials. *Dev Biol* 1983;95:372–377.
616. Mittwoch U. Parthenogenesis. *J Med Genet* 1978;15:165–181.
617. Miyazaki S, Hashimoto N, Yoshimoto Y, Kishimoto T, Igusa Y, Hiramoto Y. Temporal and spatial dynamics of the periodic increase in intracellular free calcium at fertilization of golden hamster eggs. *Dev Biol* 1986;118:259–267.
618. Monroy A. *Chemistry and Physiology of Fertilization*. New York: Holt, Rinehart and Winston; 1965.
619. Moser F. Studies on cortical layer response to stimulating agents in the Arbacia eggs. I. Response to insemination. *J Exp Zool* 1939;80:423–446.
620. Mumford RA, Hartmann JF, Ashe BM, Zimmerman M. Proteinase activities of the golden hamster eggs and cells of the cumulus oophorus. *Dev Biol* 1981;81:332–335.
621. Naish SJ, Perreault SD, Foehner AL, Zirkin BR. DNA synthesis in the fertilizing hamster sperm nucleus: sperm template availability and egg cytoplasmic control. *Biol Reprod* 1987;36: 245–253.
622. Nicosia SV, Wolf DP, Inoue M. Cortical granule distribution and cell surface characteristics in mouse eggs. *Dev Biol* 1977;57:56–74.
623. Ohsumi K, Katagiri C, Yanagimachi R. Development of pronuclei from human spermatozoa injected microsurgically into frog (Xenopus) eggs. *J Exp Zool* 1986;237:319–325.
624. Oikawa T, Maruyama Y. Detection of differences in surface carbohydrates of unfertilized and fertilized golden hamster eggs using potato agglutinin. *J Exp Zool* 1983;227:139–143.
625. Okada A, Yanagimachi R, Yanagimachi H. Development of a cortical granule-free area of cortex and the perivitelline space in the hamster oocyte during maturation and following fertilization. *J Submicrosc Cytol* 1986;18:233–247.
626. Perreault SD, Barbee RR. Sperm nucleus decondensation depends on glutathione synthesis in maturing hamster oocytes. *Dev Growth Diff* 1986;28(Suppl):53(abst. 7).
627. Perreault SD, Wolff RA, Zirkin BR. The role of disulfide bond reduction during mammalian sperm nuclear decondensation *in vivo*. *Dev Biol* 1981;101:160–167.
628. Perreault SD, Zirkin BR. Sperm nuclear decondensation in mammals: role of sperm-associated proteinase *in vivo*. *J Exp Zool* 1982;224:253–257.
629. Rodman TC, Pruslin FH, Hoffmann HP, Alfrey VG. Turnover of basic chromosomal protein in fertilized eggs: a cytoimmunochemical study of events *in vivo*. *J Cell Biol* 1981;90:351–361.
630. Rousseau P, Meda P, Lecart C, Haumont S, Ferin J. Cortical granule release in human follicular oocytes. *Biol Reprod* 1977;16:104–111.
631. Sampson MM. Sperm filtrates and dialyzates: their action on ova of the same species. *Biol Bull* 1926;50:301–338.
632. Sathananthan AH, Trounson AO. The human pronuclear

ovum: fine structure of monospermic and polyspermic fertilization *in vitro*. *Gamete Res* 1985;12:385–398.
633. Schatten G, Maul GG, Schatten H, Chaly N, Simery C, Balczon R, Brown DL. Nuclear lamins and peripheral nuclear antigens during fertilization and embryogenesis in mice and sea urchins. *Proc Natl Acad Sci USA* 1985;82:4727–4731.
634. Schatten G, Simerly C, Cline H, Maul G. Cytoskeleton and nuclear lamin organization during mammalian fertilization and early development. *J Embryol Exp Morphol* 1984;(Suppl):74.
635. Schatten G, Simerly C, Schatten H. Microtubule configurations during fertilization, mitosis, and early development in the mouse and the requirement for egg microtubule-mediated motility during mammalian fertilization. *Proc Natl Acad Sci USA* 1985;82:4152–4156.
636. Schatten H, Schatten G. Motility and centrosomal organization during sea urchin and mouse fertilization. *Cell Motil Cytoskel* 1986;6:163–175.
637. Schatten H, Schatten G, Mazia D, Balczon R, Simerly C. Behavior of centrosomes during fertilization and cell division in mouse oocytes and in sea urchin eggs. *Proc Natl Acad Sci USA* 1986;83:105–109.
638. Schmell ED, Gulyas BJ, Hedrick JL. Egg surface changes during fertilization and the molecular mechanism of the block to polyspermy. In: Hartmann JF, ed. *Mechanism and Control of Animal Fertilization.* New York: Academic Press; 1986:365–413.
639. Schuel H. Secretory function of egg cortical granules in fertilization and development. *Gamete Res* 1978;1:299–382.
640. Schuel H. Functions of egg cortical granules. In: Metz CB, Monroy A, eds. *Biology of Fertilization,* Vol. 3. Orlando, Florida: Academic Press; 1985:1–43.
641a. Skoblina MN. Role of karyoplasm in the emergency of capacity of egg cytoplasm to induce DNA synthesis in transplanted sperm nuclei. *J Embryol Exp Morphol* 1976;36:67–72.
641b. Slack BE, Bell JE, Benos DJ. Inositol-1,4,5-trisphosphate injection mimics fertilization potentials in sea urchin eggs. *Am J Physiol* 1986;250:C340–C344.
642. Szollosi D. Time and duration of DNA synthesis in rabbit eggs after sperm penetration. *Anat Rec* 1965;159:209–212.
643. Takeuchi IK, Takeuchi YK. Changes in stainability of cortical granule materials with tannic acid before and after fertilization of ova. *Zool Sci* 1985;2:415–418.
644. Tarkowski AK. Induced parthenogenesis in the mouse. In: Markert CL, Papaconstantinon, J, eds. *Developmental Biology of Reproduction.* New York: Academic Press; 1975:107–129.
645. Thibault C, Gerard M. Cytoplasmic and nuclear maturation of rabbit oocytes *in vitro. Ann Biol Anim Biochim Biophys* 1973;13:145–156.
646. Usui N, Yanagimachi R. Behavior of hamster sperm nuclei incorporated into eggs at various stages of maturation, fertilization and early development. *J Ultrastruc Res* 1976;57:276–288.
647. Vacquier VD. The isolation of intact cortical granules from sea urchin eggs: calcium ions trigger granule discharge. *Dev Biol* 1975;43:62–74.
648. Wagenaar EB, Mazia D. The effect of emetine on the first cleavage division of the sea urchin, *Stronglyocentrotus purpuratus.* In: Dirksen ER, Prescott DM, Fox LF, eds. *Cell Reproduction.* New York: Academic Press; 1978:539–545.
649. Wassarman PM. The biology and chemistry of fertilization. *Science* 1987;235:553–554.
650. Went DF. Egg activation and parthenogenetic reproduction in insect. *Biol Reprod* 1982;57:319–344.
651. Whitaker MJ, Irvine RF. Inositol 1,4,5-triphosphate microinjection activates sea urchin eggs. *Nature* 1984;312:636–639.
652. Whitaker MJ, Steinhardt RA. Ionic regulation of egg activation. *Q Rev Biophys* 1982;15:593–666.
653. Whitaker MJ, Steinhardt RA. Ionic signaling in the sea urchin egg at fertilization. In: Metz CB, Monroy A, eds. *Biology of Fertilization,* Vol. 3. Orlando, Florida: Academic Press; 1985:167–221.
654. Whittingham DC. Parthenogenesis in mammals. In: Finn CA, ed. *Oxford Reviews of Reproductive Biology,* Vol. 2. Oxford: Clarendon Press; 1980:205–231.
655. Wiesel S, Schultz GA. Factors which may affect removal of protamine from sperm DNA during fertilization in rabbit. *Gamete Res* 1981;4:25–34.
656. Wolf DE, Edidin M, Handyside AH. Changes in the organization of the mouse egg plasma membrane upon fertilization and first cleavage: indications from the lateral diffusion rates of fluorescent lipid analogs. *Dev Biol* 1981;85:191–198.
657. Wolgemuth DJ. Synthetic activities of the mammalian early embryos: molecular and genetic alterations following fertilization. In: Hartmann JF, ed. *Mechanism and Control of Animal Fertilization.* New York: Academic Press; 1983:415–452.
658. Yamashita N. Enhancement of ionic currents through voltage-gated channels in the mouse oocyte after fertilization. *J Physiol* 1982;329:263–280.
659. Yanagimachi R. Sperm-egg association in mammals. In: Moscona AA, Monroy A, eds. *Current Topics in Developmental Biology,* Vol. 12. New York: Academic Press; 1978:83–105.
660. Yanagimachi R. Sperm-egg fusion. In: Duzgunes N, Bronner F, eds. *Current Topics in Membranes and Transport,* Vol. 32. San Diego: Academic Press; 1988:3–43.
661. Zamboni L. Fine morphology the follicle wall and follicle cell-oocyte association. *Biol Reprod* 1974;10:125–149.
662. Zirkin BR, Soucek DA, Chang TSK, Perreault SD. *In vitro* and *in vivo* studies of mammalian sperm nuclear decondensation. *Gamete Res* 1985;11:349–365.
663. Hedrick JL, ed. *The Molecular and Cellular Biology of Fertilization.* New York: Plenum Press; 1984.
664. Aarons D, Boettger-Tong H, Holt G, Poirier GR. Acrosome reaction induced by immunoaggregation of a proteinase inhibitor bound to the murine sperm. *Mol Reprod Dev* 1991;30: 258–264.
665. Abdullah M, Widgren EE, O'Rand MG. A mammalian sperm lectin related to rat hepatocyte lectin-2/3. *Molec Cell Biochem* 1991;103:155–161.
666. Abe H, Oikawa T. Ultrastructural evidence for an association between an oviductal glycoprotein and the zona pellucida of the golden hamster egg. *J Exp Zool* 1990;256:210–221.
667. Abe H, Oikawa T. Immunocytochemical localization of an oviductal zona pellucida glycoprotein in the oviductal epithelium of the golden hamster. *Anat Rec* 1991;229:305–314.
668. Abramczuk JW, Lopata A. Resistance of human follicular oocytes to parthenogenetic activation: DNA distribution and content in oocytes maintained *in vitro. Hum Reprod* 1990;5: 578–581.
669. Afzelius BA, Eliasson R, Johnson O, Lindholmer C. Lack of dynein arms in immotile human spermatozoa. *J Cell Biol* 1975;66:225–232.
670. Ahuja KK. Fertilization studies in the hamster: The role of cell-surface carbohydrates. *Exp Cell Res* 1982;140:353–362.
671. Ahuja KK. *In-vitro* inhibition of the block to polyspermy of hamster eggs by tertiary amine local anaesthetics. *J Reprod Fertil* 1982;65:15–22.
672. Ahuja KK. Lectin-coated agarose beads in the investigation of sperm capacitation in the hamster. *Dev Biol* 1984;104:131–142.
673. Aitken RJ, Richardson DW. Mechanism of sperm-binding inhibition by anti-zona antisera. *Gamete Res* 1981;4:41–47.
674. Aitken RJ, Ross A, Lees MM. Analysis of sperm function in Kartagener's syndrome. *Fertil Steril* 1983;40:696–698.
675. Albert M, Gallo JM, Escalier D, Parseghian N, Jouannet P, Schrevel J, David G. Unexplained *in-vitro* fertilization failure: implication of acrosomes with a small reacting region, as revealed by a monoclonal antibody. *Hum Reprod* 1992;7: 1249–1256.
676. Alcivar AA, Hake LE, Millette CF, Trasler JM, Hecht NB. Mitochondrial gene expression in male germ cells of the mouse. *Dev Biol* 1989;135:263–271.
677. Alexander NJ, Griffin D, Spieler JM, Waites GMH, eds. *Gamete Interaction: Prospects for Immunocontraception.* New York: Wiley and Sons; 1990.
678. Alvarez JG, Lee MA, Iozzo RV, Lopez I, Touchstone JC, Storey BT. Ethanol accelerates acrosome loss in human spermatozoa. *J Androl* 1988;9:357–366.
679. Amiel ML, Moos J, Tesarik J, Testart J. Evidence of new antigens in the mouse cumulus oophorus during preovulatory cumulus expansion. *Mol Reprod Dev* 1993;34:81–86.
680. Anakwe OO, Gerton GL. Acrosome biogenesis begins during meiosis: evidence from the synthesis and distribution of an acro-

somal glycoprotein, acrogranin, during guinea pig spermatogenesis. *Biol Reprod* 1990;42:317–328.
681. Anderson E, Hoppe PC, Lee GS. The karyotype and ultrastructural characteristics of spontaneous preimplantation mouse parthenotes. *Gamete Res* 1984;9:451–467.
682. Andrew JC, Bavister BD. Capacitation of hamster spermatozoa with the divalent cation chelators D-penicillamine, L-histidine, and L-cysteine in a protein-free medicine. *Gamete Res* 1989;23:159–170.
683. Araki Y, Kurata S, Oikawa T, Yamashita T, Hiroi M, Naiki M, Sendo F. A monoclonal antibody reacting with the zona pellucida of the oviductal egg but not with that of the ovarian egg of the golden hamster. *J Reprod Immunol* 1987;11:193–208.
684. Araki Y, Orgebin-Crist M-C, Tulsiani DRP. Qualitative characterization of oligosaccharide chains present on the rat zona pellucida glycoconjugates. *Biol Reprod* 1992;46:912–919.
685. Arnold WM, Schmutzler RK, Al-Hasani S, Krebs D, Zimmermann U. Differences in membrane properties between unfertilised and fertilised single rabbit oocytes demonstrated by electro-rotation. Comparison with cells from early embryos. *Biochim Biophys Acta* 1989;979:142–146.
686. Aronson J, Solter D. Developmental potency of gametic and embryonic genomes revealed by nuclear transfer. In: McLarene A, Siracusa G, eds. *Current Topics in Developmental Biology,* Vol. 23. San Diego: Academic Press; 1987:55–71.
687. Aruoma OI, Halliwell B, Hoey B, Butler J. The antioxidant action of taurine, hypotaurine and their metabolic precursor. *Biochem J* 1988;256:251–255.
688. Asch RH, Balmaceda JP, Johnston I, eds. *Gamete Physiology.* Norwell, Massachusetts: Serono Symposia USA; 1990.
689. Ashizawa K, Tokudome Y, Okauchi K, Nishiyama H. Effects of HeLa and BHK-21 cells on the survival of fowl, bull, ram and boar spermatozoa *in vitro. J Reprod Fertil* 1982;66:663–666.
690. Auger J, Mesbah M, Huber C, Dadoune JP. Aniline blue staining as a marker of sperm chromatin defects associated with different semen characteristics discriminates between proven fertile and suspected infertile men. *Int J Androl* 1990;13:452–462.
691. Austin CR. Observations on the penetration of the sperm into the mammalian egg. *Aust J Sci Res (Ser B)* 1951;4:581–596.
692. Austin CR. XIV—The formation, growth, and conjugation of the pronuclei in the rat egg. *J R Microscop Soc* 1951;71: 295–306.
693. Austin CR. The development of pronuclei in the rat egg, with particular reference to quantitative relations. *Aust J Sci Res* 1952;5:354–365.
694. Austin CR. Activation of eggs by hypothermia in rats and hamster. *J Exp Biol* 1956;33:338–347.
695. Austin CR. Ovulation, fertilization, and early cleavage in the hamster. *J R Microscop Soc* 1956;75:141–154.
696. Austin CR. *The Mammalian Egg.* Springfield, Illinois: Charles C. Thomas; 1961.
697. Austin CR, Braden AWH. Observation on nuclear size and form in living rat and mouse eggs. *Exp Cell Res* 1955;8: 163–172.
698. Babcock DF, Pfeiffer DR. Independent elevation of cytosolic [Ca^{2+}] and pH of mammalian sperm by voltage-dependent and pH-sensitive mechanisms. *J Biol Chem* 1987;262:15041–15047.
699. Baca M, Zamboni L. The fine structure of human follicular oocytes. *J Ultrastruc Res* 1967;19:354–381.
700. Baldi E, Casano R, Falsetti C, Krausz C, Maggi M, Forti G. Intracellular calcium accumulation and responsiveness to progesterone in capacitating human spermatozoa. *J Androl* 1991;12:323–330.
701. Balhorn R. A model for the structure of chromatin in mammalian sperm. *J Cell Biol* 1982;93:298–305.
702. Balhorn R, Gledhill BL, Wyrobek AJ. Mouse sperm chromatin proteins: quantitative isolation and partial characterization. *Biochemistry* 1977;16:4074–4080.
703. Balhorn R, Reed S, Tanphaichitr N. Aberrant protamine 1/protamine 2 ratios in sperm of infertile human males. *Experimentia* 1988;44:52–55.
704. Balkan W, Martin RH. Timing of human sperm chromosome replication following fertilization of hamster eggs *in vitro. Gamete Res* 1982;6:115–119.
705. Ball GD, Wieben ED, Bayers AP. DNA, RNA, and protein synthesis by porcine oocyte–cumulus complexes during expansion. *Biol Reprod* 1980;33:739–744.
706. Bamba K, Cran DG. Effect of rapid warming of boar semen on sperm morphology and physiology. *J Reprod Fertil* 1985;75: 133–138.
707. Barros C. Capacitation of mammalian spermatozoa. In: Coutinho EM, Fuchs F, eds. *Physiology and Genetics of Reproduction,* Vol. 2. New York: Plenum Press; 1974:3–24.
708. Barros C, Berrios M, Herrera A. Capacitation in vitro of guinea-pig spermatozoa in a saline solution. *J Reprod Fertil* 1973;34:547–549.
709. Barros C, Capote C, Perez C, Crosby JA, Becker M, De Ioannes A. Immunodetection of acrosin during the acrosome reaction of hamster, guinea-pig and human spermatozoa. *Biol Res (Chile)* 1992;25:31–40.
710. Barros C, Fujimoto M, Yanagimachi R. Failure of zona penetration of hamster spermatozoa after prolonged preincubation in a blood serum fraction. *J Reprod Fertil* 1973;35:89–95.
711. Barros C, Yanagimachi R. Polyspermy-preventing mechanisms in the golden hamster egg. *J Exp Zool* 1972;180:251–266.
712. Barton SC, Ferguson-Smith AC, Fundele R, Surani A. Influence of paternally imprinted genes on development. *Development* 1991;113:679–688.
713. Battalia DE, Yanagimachi R. Enhanced and co-ordinated movement of hamster oviduct during periovulatory period. *J Reprod Fertil* 1979;56:515–520.
714. Battalia DE, Yanagimachi R. The changes in oestrogen and progesterone levels triggers adovarian propulsive movement of the hamster oviduct. *J Reprod Fertil* 1980;59:243–247.
715. Bavister BD. Evidence for a role of post-ovulatory cumulus components in supporting fertilizing ability of hamster spermatozoa. *J Androl* 1982;3:365–372.
716. Bavister BD, Boatman DE, Liebfried L, Loose M, Vernon MW. Fertilization and cleavage of Rhesus monkey oocytes *in vitro. Biol Reprod* 1983;28:983–999.
717. Bavister BD, Boatmen DE, Morgan PM, Warikoo PK. Fertilization in Rhesus monkey. In: Dunbar BS, O'Rand GO, eds. *Overview of Mammalian Fertilization.* New York: Plenum Press; 1991:363–383.
718. Bavister BD, Cummins JM, Roldan ERS, eds. *Fertilization in Mammals.* Norwell, Massachusetts: Serono Symposia USA; 1990.
719. Beatty RA. Parthenogenesis in vertebrates. In: Metz CB, Monroy A, eds. *Fertilization,* Vol. I. New York: Academic Press; 1967:413–440.
720. Beaver FL, Friend DS. Morphology of mammalian sperm membranes during differentiation, maturation, and capacitation. *J Electr Microscop Tech* 1990;16:281–297.
721. Bedford JM. Development of the fertilizing ability of spermatozoa in the epididymis of the rabbit. *J Exp Zool* 1966;163: 319–330.
722. Bedford JM. Effects of duct ligation on the fertilizing ability of spermatozoa from different regions of the rabbit epididymis. *J Exp Zool* 1967;166:271–282.
723. Bedford JM. The importance of capacitation for establishing contact between eggs and sperm in the rabbit. *J Reprod Fertil* 1967;13:365–367.
724. Bedford JM. Experimental requirement for capacitation and observations on ultra-structural changes in rabbit spermatozoa during fertilization. *J Reprod Fertil* 1967;(Suppl. 2):35–48.
725. Bedford JM. Limitation of the uterus in the development of the fertilizing ability (capacitation) of spermatozoa. *J Reprod Fertil* 1969;(Suppl. 8):19–26.
726. Bedford JM. Techniques and criteria used in the study of fertilization. In: Daniel JC, ed. *Methods in Mammalian Embryology.* San Francisco: W. H. Freeman; 1971:37–63.
727. Bedford JM. Sperm/egg interaction: The specificity of human spermatozoa. *Anat Rec* 1977;188:477–488.
728. Bedford JM. Why mammalian gametes don't mix. *Nature* 1981;291:286–288.
729. Bedford JM. The bearing of epididymal function in strategies for *in vitro* fertilization and gamete intrafollopian transfer. *Ann NY Acad Sci* 1988;541:284–291.

730. Bedford JM. Effects of elevated temperature on the epididymis and testis. In: Zorgniotti AW, ed. *Temperature and Environmental Effects on the Testis.* New York: Plenum Press; 1991:19–32.
731. Bedford JM. The coevolution of mammalian gametes. In: Dunbar BS, O'Rand MG, eds. *A Comparative Overview of Mammalian Fertilization.* New York: Plenum Press; 1991:3–35.
732. Bedford JM, Bent MJ, Calvin H. Variations in the structural character and stability of the nuclear chromatin in morphologically normal human spermatozoa. *J Reprod Fertil* 1973;33: 19–29.
733. Bedford JM, Calvin H, Cooper GW. The maturation of spermatozoa in the human epididymis. *J Reprod Fertil* 1973;(Suppl. 18):199–213.
734. Bedford JM, Hoskins DD. The mammalian spermatozoa: morphology, biochemistry and physiology, In: Lamming GE, ed. *Marshall's Physiology of Reproduction,* Vol. 2. Edinburgh: Churchill Livingston; 1990:379–568.
735. Bedford JM. Kim HH. Cumulus oophorus as a sperm sequestering device, *in vivo. J Exp Zool* 1993;265:321–328.
736. Bedford JM, Kim HH. Sperm/egg binding patterns and oocyte cytology in retrospective analysis of fertilization failure *in vitro. Hum Reprod* 1993;8:453–463.
737. Bedford JM, Yanagimachi R. Epididymal storage at abdomal temperature reduces the time required for capacitation of hamster spermatozoa. *J Reprod Fertil* 1991;91:403–410.
738. Bedford JM, Yanagimachi R. Initiation of sperm motility after mating in the rat and hamster. *J Androl* 1992;13:444–449.
739. Beebe S, Leyton L, Burks D, Ishikawa M, Fuerst T, Dean J, Saling P. Recombinant mouse ZP3 inhibits sperm binding and induces the acrosome reaction. *Dev Biol* 1992;151:48–54.
740. Bell P, Dabauvalle MC, Scheer U. *In vitro* assembly of prenucleolar bodies in Xenopus egg extract. *J Cell Biol* 1992;118: 1297–1304.
741. Bellve AR. Biogenesis of the mammalian spermatozoon. In: Amann AP, Seidel GE, eds. *Prospects for Sexing Mammalian Sperm.* Boulder: Colorado Associated University Press; 1982:69–102.
742. Bellve AR, Chandrika R, Martinova YS, Barth AH. The perinuclear matrix as a structural element of the mouse sperm nucleus. *Biol Reprod* 1992;47:451–465.
743. Bement W. Signal transduction of calcium and protein kinase C during egg activation. *J Exp Zool* 1992;263:382–397.
744. Von Bemhardi R, De Ioannes AE, Blanco LP, Herrera E, Bustos-Obregon E, Vigil P. Round-headed spermatozoa: a model to study the role of the acrosome in early events of gamete interaction. *Andrologia* 1990;22:12–20.
744a. Bentz J, Ellens H, Alford D. An architecture for the fusion site of influenza hemagglutinin. *FEBS Lett* 1990;276:1–5.
745. Berger T, Davis A, Wardrip NJ, Hedrick JL. Sperm binding to the pig zona pellucida and inhibition of binding by solubilized components of the zona pellucida. *J Reprod Fertil* 1989;86: 559–565.
746. Berger T, Turner KO, Meizel S, Hedrick JL. Zona pellucida-induced acrosome reaction in boar spermatozoa. *Biol Reprod* 1989;40:525–530.
747. Berkeley AS, Bedford JM, Rosenwaks Z. Clinical aspects of human *in vitro* fertilization. In: Wassarman PM, ed. *Elements of Mammalian Fertilization,* Vol. II. Boca Raton, Florida: CRC Press; 1991:33–61.
748. Berrios M, Bedford JM. Oocyte maturation: aberrant post-fusion responses of the rabbit primary oocyte to penetrating spermatozoa. *J Cell Sci* 1976;39:1–12.
749. Berruti G. Evidence for Ca^{2+}-mediated F-actin-phospholipid binding of human sperm capacitation II. *Cell Biol Int Rep* 1991;15:917–927.
750. Berruti G, Franchi E. Calcium and polyphosphoinositides: their distribution in relation to the membrane changes occurring in the head of boar spermatozoa. *Eur J Cell Biol* 1986;41:238–245.
751. Beyler SA, Zaneveld LJD. The role of acrosin in sperm penetration through human cervical mucus. *Fertil Steril* 1979;32: 671–675.
752. Bhattacharyya A, Pakrash A. Requirement of an extracellular energy substrate for the guinea pig sperm acrosome reaction induced by calcium ionophore. *Mol Reprod Dev* 1991;28: 286–291.
753. Bhattacharyya A, Yanagimachi R. Synthetic organic pH buffers can support fertilization of guinea pig eggs, but not as efficiently as bicarbonate buffer. *Gamete Res* 1988;19:123–129.
754. Bird JM, Houghton JA. Cytogenetics of porcine sperm chromosomes following IVF of zona-free hamster oocytyes. *Arch Androl* 1990;25:45–57.
755. Bishop DW. Biology of spermatozoa. In: Young WC, ed. *Sex and Internal Secretions,* Vol. 1. Baltimore: Williams and Wilkins; 1961:707–796.
756. Blackmore PF. Thapsigargin elevates and potentiates the ability of progesterone to increase intracellular free calcium in human sperm: possible role of perinuclear calcium. *Cell Calcium* 1993;14:53–60.
757. Blanchard Y, Lescoat D, Le Lannou D. Anomalous distribution of nuclear basic proteins in round-headed human spermatozoa. *Andrologia* 1990;22:549–555.
758. Bleil JD. Sperm receptors of mammalian eggs. In: Wassarman PM, ed. *Elements of Mammalian Fertilization,* Vol. 1. Boca Raton, Florida: CRC Press; 1991:133–151.
759. Bleil JD, Beall CF, Wassarman PM. Mammalian sperm-egg interaction: fertilization of mouse eggs triggers modification of the major zona pellucida glycoprotein, ZP2. *Dev Biol* 1981;86: 189–197.
760. Bleil JD, Greve JM, Wassarman PM. Identification of a secondary sperm receptor in the mouse egg zona pellucida: role in maintenance of binding of acrosome-reacted sperm to eggs. *Dev Biol* 1988;128:376–385.
761. Bleil JD, Wasserman PM. Mammalian sperm–egg interaction: identification of a glycoprotein in mouse egg zonae pellucidae possessing receptor activity for sperm. *Cell* 1980;20:873–882.
762. Bleil JD, Wassarman PM. Synthesis of zona pellucida proteins by denuded and follicle-enclosed mouse oocytes during culture *in vitro. Proc Natl Acad Sci USA* 1980;77:1029–1033.
763. Bleil JD, Wassarman PM. Galactose at the nonreducing terminus of O-linked oligosaccharides of mouse egg zona pellucida glycoprotein ZP3 is essential for the glycoprotein's sperm receptor activity. *Proc Natl Acad Sci USA* 1988;85:6778–6782.
764. Bleil JD, Wassarman PM. Identification of a ZP3-binding protein on acrosome-intact mouse sperm by photoaffinity crosslinking. *Proc Natl Acad Sci USA* 1990;87:5563–5567.
765. Blobel CP, Wolfsberg TG, Turck CW, Myles DG, Primakoff P, White JM. A potential fusion peptide and an integrin ligand domain in a protein active in sperm–egg fusion. *Nature* 1992;356:248–252.
766. Boatman DE, Andrews JC, Bavister BD. A quantitative assay for capacitation: evaluation of multiple sperm penetration through the zona pellucida of salt-stored hamster eggs. *Gamete Res* 1988;19:19–29.
767. Boatman DE, Bavister BD. Stimulation of Rhesus monkey sperm capacitation by cyclic nucleotide mediators. *J Reprod Fertil* 1984;71:357–366.
768. Boatman DE, Robbins RT. Bicarbonate: carbon-dioxide regulation of sperm capacitation, hyperactivated motility, and the acrosome reaction. *Biol Reprod* 1991;44:806–813.
769. Boettger-Tong H, Aarons D, Biegler B, Lee T, Poirier GR. Competition between zonae pellucidae and a proteinase inhibitor for sperm binding. *Biol Reprod* 1992;47:716–722.
770. Boice ML, Mavrogianis PA, Murphy CN, Prather RS, Day BN. Immunocytochemical analysis of the association of bovine oviduct-specific glycoproteins with early embryo. *J Exp Zool* 1992;263:225–229.
771. Boice ML, McCarthy TJ, Mavrogianis PA, Fazleabas AT, Verhage HG. Localization of oviductal glycoproteins within the zona pellucida and perivitelline space of ovulated ova and early embryos in baboons (papio anubis). *Biol Reprod* 1990;43: 340–346.
772. Boitano S, Omoto CK. Trout sperm swimming patterns and role of intercellular Ca^{++}. *Cell Motil Cytoskel* 1992;21:74–82.
773. Boldt J, Casas A, Whaley E, Creazzo T, Lewis JB. Potassium dependence for sperm–egg fusion in mice. *J Exp Zool* 1991;257:245–251.
774. Boldt J, Howe AM, Parkerson JB, Gunter LE, Kuehn E. Carbohydrate involvement in sperm–egg fusion in mice. *Biol Reprod* 1989;40:887–896.
775. Boldt J, Howe AM, Preble J. Enzymatic alteration of the ability

of mouse egg plasma membrane to interact with sperm. *Biol Reprod* 1988;39:19–27.
776. Boldt J, Gunter LE, Howe AM. Characterization of cell surface polypeptides of unfertilized, fertilized, and protease-treated zona-free mouse eggs. *Gamete Res* 1989;23:91–101.
777. Boldt J, Wolf DP. An improved method for isolation of fertile zona-free mouse eggs. *Gamete Res* 1986;13:213–222.
778. Boldt J, Wolf DP. Isolation of ^{125}I-concanavalin A-labeled plasma membrane from unfertilized mouse eggs. *Gamete Res* 1987;16:303–310.
779. Bondioli KR, Westhusin ME, Looney CR. Production of identical bovine offspring by nuclear transfer. *Theriogenology* 1990;33:165–174.
780. Borrero C, Ord T, Balmaceda JP, Rojas FJ, Asch RH. The GIFT experiences: an evaluation of the outcome of 115 cases. *Hum Reprod* 1988;3:227–230.
781. Borsuk E, Manka R. Behavior of sperm nuclei in intact and bisected metaphase II mouse oocytes fertilized in the presence of colcemid. *Gamete Res* 1988;20:365–376.
782. Brackett BG, Server JB. Capacitation of rabbit spermatozoa in the uterus. *Fertil Steril* 1970;21:687–695.
783. Bradley MP, Garbers DL. The stimulation of bovine caudal epididymal sperm forward motility by bovine cumulus-egg complexes *in vitro*. *Biochem Biophys Res Commun* 1983;115:777–787.
784. Brandt H, Hoskins DD. A cAMP-dependent phospholylated motility protein in bovine epididymal sperm. *J Biol Chem* 1980;255:982–987.
785. Brinster RL, Chen HY, Trumbauer ME, Paynton BV. Secretion of proteins by the fertilized mouse ovum. *Exp Cell Res* 1981;134:291–296.
786. Bronson RA, Fusi F. Evidence that Arg–Gly–Asp adhesion sequence plays a role in mammalian fertilization. *Biol Reprod* 1990;43:1019–1025.
787. Bronson RA, McLaren A. Transfer to the mouse oviduct of eggs with and without the zona pellucida. *J Reprod Fertil* 1970;22:129–137.
788. Brown CR, Cheng WTK. Limited proteolysis of the porcine zona pellucida by homologous sperm acrosin. *J Reprod Fertil* 1985;74:257–260.
788a. Brown DB, Blake EJ, Wolgemuth DJ, Gordon K, Ruddle FH. Chromatin decondensation and DNA synthesis in human sperm activated *in vitro* by using *Xenopus laevis* egg extracts. *J Exp Zool* 1987;242:215–231.
789. Brown DB, Nagamani M. Use of *Xenopus laevis* frog egg extract in diagnosing human male unexplained infertility. *Yale J Biol Med* 1992;65:29–38.
790. Brucker C, Sandow BA, Blackmore PF, Lipford GB, Hodgen GD. Monoclonal antibody AG7 inhibits fertilization post sperm–zona binding. *Mol Reprod Dev* 1992;33:451–462.
791. Brunner S, Brinster RL. Radioiodination of unfertilized and fertilized mouse ova. *J Cell Biol* 1977;75(Suppl):61a (abst CJ530).
792. Burkman LJ. Hyperactivated motility of human spermatozoa during *in vitro* capacitation and implications for fertility. In: Gagnon G, ed. *Controls of Sperm Motility: Biological and Clinical Aspects.* Boca Raton, Florida: CRC Press; 1991:303–329.
793. Burkman LJ, Kruger TF, Coddington CC, Rosenwaks Z, Franken DR, Hodgen GD. The hemizona assay (HZA): development of a diagnostic test for the binding of human spermatozoa to the human hemizona pellucida to predict fertilization potential. *Fertil Steril* 1988;49:688–697.
794. Burzio LO, Yanez A, Pessot C, Urzua U, Brito M, Concha II, Zarrage AM. Characteristics of the RNA present in rat sperm. In: Baccetti B, ed. *Comparative Spermatology 20 Years After.* New York: Raven Press; 1991:13–17.
795. Byers AP, Barone MA, Donoghue AM, Wildt DE. Mature domestic cat oocyte does not express a cortical granule-free domain. *Biol Reprod* 1992;47:709–715.
796. Byrd W, Tsu J, Wolf DP. Kinetics of spontaneous and induced loss in human sperm incubated under capacitating and noncapacitating conditions. *Gamete Res* 1989;22:109–122.
797. Byrd W, Wolf DP. Acrosomal status in fresh and capacitated human ejaculated sperm. *Biol Reprod* 1986;34:859–869.
797a. Cahova M, Draber P. Inhibition of fertilization by a monoclonal antibody recognizing the oligosaccharide sequence GalNAcB1-4GalB1-4 on the mouse zona pellucida. *J Reprod Immunol* 1992;21:241–256.
798. Calafell JM, Badenas J, Catala V, Egozcue J, Santalo J. Premature chromosome condensation (PCC) as a sign of oocyte immaturity. *Hum Reprod* 1990;5(Suppl):78(abst 251).
799. Calvin HI, Grosshans K, Blake EJ. Estimation and manipulation of glutathione levels in prepuberal mouse ovaries and ova: relevance to sperm nucleus transformation in the fertilized egg. *Gamete Res* 1986;14:265–275.
800. Camatini M, Anelli G, Casale A. Immunochemical localization of calmoduline in intact and acrosome-reacted boar sperm. *Eur J Cell Biol* 1986;41:89–96.
801. Capote C, Perez C, Crosby J, Becker MI, De Ioannes A, Barros C. Acrosome reaction, acrosin and sperm penetration. In: Baccetti B, ed. *Comparative Spermatology, 20 Years After.* New York: Raven Press; 1991:113–117.
802. Cardullo RA, Baltz JM. Metabolic regulation in mammalian sperm: mitochondrial volume determines sperm length and flagellar beat frequency. *Cell Motil Cytoskel* 1991;19:180–188.
803. Carron CP, Mathias A, Saling PM. Antiidiotype antibodies prevent antibody binding to mouse sperm and antibody-mediated inhibition of fertilization. *Biol Reprod* 1989;40:153–162.
804. Carron CP, Saling PM. Sperm antigens and immunological interference of fertilization. In: Wassarman PM, ed. *Elements of Mammalian Fertilization.* Vol. II. Boca Raton, Florida: CRC Press; 1991:147–176.
805. Castellani-Ceresa L, Brivio MF, Radaelli G. Electron microscopic localization of F-actin in acrosome reacted boar spermatozoa by means of a phalloidin-FITC complex. *J Submicrosc Cytol Pathol* 1991;23:347–349.
806. Castellani-Ceresa L, Brivio MF, Radaelli G. F-actin in acrosome-reacted boar spermatozoa. *Mol Reprod Dev* 1992;33:99–107.
807. Castellani-Ceresa L, Mattioli M, Radaelli G, Barboni B, Brivio MF. Actin polymerization in boar spermatozoa: fertilization is reduced by the use of cytochalasin D. *Mol Reprod Dev* [in press].
808. Cechova D, Topfer-Petersen E, Zucker A, Jonakova V. Isolation, purification, and partial characterization of low molecular-mass boar proacrosin. *Biol Chem Hoppe-Seyler* 1990;371:317–323.
809. Chamberlin ME, Dean J. Human homology of the mouse sperm receptor. *Proc Natl Acad Sci USA* 1990;87:6014–6018.
810. Chan PJ, Hutz RJ, Dukelow WR. Nonhuman primate *in vitro* fertilization: seasonability cumulus cells, cyclic nucleotides, ribonucleic acid and viability assays. *Fertil Steril* 1982;38:609–615.
811. Chang MC. Fertilizing capacity of spermatozoa deposited into the fallopian tubes. *Nature* 1951;168:697–698.
812. Chang MC. Fertilization of rabbit ova and the effects of temperature *in vitro* on their subsequent fertilization and activation *in vivo*. *J Exp Zool* 1952;121:351–382.
813. Chang MC. Fertilization of rabbit ova *in vitro*. *Nature* 1959;184:466–467.
814. Chang MC. Development of fertilizing capacity of rabbit spermatozoa in the uterus. *Nature* 1955;175:1036–1037.
815. Chen HY, Brinster RL, Merz EA. Changes in protein synthesis following fertilization of the mouse ovum. *J Exp Zool* 1980;212:355–360.
816. Cheng WTK, Polge C, Moor RM. *In vitro* fertilization and development of farm animal oocytes matured *in vivo* and *in vitro*. *Proc Symp Dev Appl Biotech Agr* 1986;49:711–718.
817. Cherr GN, Drobnis EZ, Katz DF. Localization of cortical granule constituents before and after exocytosis in the hamster egg. *J Exp Zool* 1988;246:81–93.
818. Cherr GN, Ducibella T. Activation of the mammalian egg: cortical granule distribution, exocytosis, and the block to polyspermy. In: Bavister BD, Commins J, Roldan ERS, eds. *Fertilization in Mammals.* Norwell, Massachusetts: Serono Symposia USA; 1990:309–330.
819. Cherr GN, Lambert H, Meizel S, Katz DF. *In vitro* studies of the golden hamster sperm acrosome reaction: completion on the zona pellucida and induction by homologous soluble zonae pellucidae. *Dev Biol* 1986;114:119–131.
820. Chian RC, Niwa K, Okuda K. *In vitro* penetration of zona pellu-

cida of salt-stored bovine oocytes before and after maturation by frozen-thawed spermatozoa. *Theriogenologia* 1991;36:209–219.
821. Chiquoine AD. The development of the zona pellucida of the mammalian ovum. *Am J Anat* 1960;106:149–196.
822. Ciemerych MA, Czolowska R. Differential chromatin condensation of female and male pronuclei in mouse zygotes. *Mol Reprod Dev* 1993;34:73–80.
823. Clark JM, Koehler JK. Does phospholipase C inhibit fusion between sperm and zona-free eggs? *Gamete Res* 1988;19:339–348.
824. Clarke HJ, Masui Y. The induction of reversible and irreversible chromosome decondensation by protein synthesis inhibition during meiotic maturation of mouse oocytes. *Dev Biol* 1983;97:291–301.
825. Clarke HJ, Masui Y. Transformation of sperm nuclei to metaphase chromosomes in the cytoplasm of maturing oocyte of the mouse. *J Cell Biol* 1986;102:1039–1046.
826. Clarke HJ, Rossant J, Masui Y. Suppression of chromosome condensation during meiotic maturation induces parthenogenetic development of mouse oocytes. *Development* 1988;104:97–103.
827. Clegg KB, Piko L. RNA synthesis and cytoplasmic polyadenylation in the one-cell mouse embryo. *Nature* 1982;295:342–345.
828. Coddington C, Fulgham DL, Alexander NJ, Johnson DJ, Herr JC, Hodgen GD. Sperm bound to zona pellucida in hemizonal assay demonstrate acrosome reaction when stained with T-6 antibody. *Fertil Steril* 1990;54:504–508.
829. Cohen J, Alikani M, Adler A, et al. Microsurgical fertilization procedures: the absence of stringent criteria for patient selection. *J Assoc Reprod Genet* 1992;9:197–206.
830. Cohen J, Malter HE, Talansky BE, Grifo J., eds. *Micromanipulation of Human Gametes and Embryos.* New York: Raven Press; 1992.
831. Colleu D, Lescoat D, Boujard D, Le Lannou D. Human spermatozoal nuclear maturity in normozoospermia and asthenozoospermia. *Arch Androl* 1988;21:155–162.
832. Colonna R, Tatone C. Protein kinase C-dependent and independent events in mouse egg activation. *Mol Reprod Dev* [in press].
833. Colonna R, Tatone C, Malgaroli A, Eusebi F, Mangia F. Effects of protein kinase C stimulation and free Ca^{2+} rise in mammalian egg activation. *Gamete Res* 1989;24:171–183.
834. Conover JC, Gwatkin RBL. Pre-loading of mouse oocytes with DNA-specific fluorochrome (Hoechst 33342) permits rapid detection of sperm-oocyte fusion. *J Reprod Fertil* 1988;82:681–690.
835. Coonen E, Pieters MHEC, Dumoulin JCM, Meyer H, Evers JLH, Ramaekers FCS, Geraedts JPM. Nonisotopic *in situ* hybridization as a method for nondisjunction studies in human spermatozoa. *Mol Reprod Dev* 1991;28:18–22.
836. Cooper GW, Bedford JM. Charge density change in the vitelline surface following fertilization of the rabbit egg. *J Reprod Fertil* 1971;25:431–436.
837. Cooper TG. In defense of a function for the human epididymis. *Fertil Steril* 1990;54:965–975.
837a. Cooper TG. *The Epididymis, Sperm Maturation and Fertilization.* Berlin/New York: Springer-Verlag; 1986.
837b. Cooper TG. Epididymal proteins and sperm maturation. In: Nieschlag E, Habenicht UF, eds. *Spermatogenesis-Fertilization-Contraception.* Berlin/New York: Springer-Verlag; 1992:285–318.
838. Coronel CE, Lardy HA. Functional properties of caltrin proteins from seminal vesicle of the guinea pig. *Mol Reprod Fertil* 1992;33:74–80.
839. Corselli J, Talbot P. *In vitro* penetration of hamster oocyte-cumulus complexes using physiological numbers of sperm. *Dev Biol* 1987;122:227–242.
840. Cosson MP, Billard R, Letellier L. Rise of internal Ca^{2+} accompanies the initiation of trout sperm motility. *Cell Motil Cytoskel* 1989;14:424–434.
841. Cowan AE, Myles DG, Koppel DE. Migration of the guinea pig sperm membrane protein pH-20 from one localized surface domain to another does not occur by a simple diffusion-trapping mechanism. *Dev Biol* 1991;144:189–198.
842. Cowan AE, Primakoff P, Myles DG. Sperm exocytosis increases the amount of pH-20 antigen on the surface of guinea pig sperm. *J Cell Biol* 1986;103:1289–1297.
843. Cox JF. Effect of the cumulus on *in vitro* fertilization of *in vitro* matured cow and sheep oocytes. *Theriogenologia* 1991;35:191.
844. Cran DG, Cheng WTK. The cortical reaction in pig oocytes during *in vivo* and *in vitro* fertilization. *Gamete Res* 1986;13:241–251.
845. Cross NL, Meizel S. Methods for evaluating the acrosomal status of mammalian sperm. *Biol Reprod* 1989;41:635–641.
846. Cross NL, Morales P, Fukuda M, Benboodi E. Determinating acrosomal status of the cynomolgus monkey sperm by fluorescence microscopy. *Am J Primatol* 1989;17:157–163.
847. Cross NL, Morales P, Overstreet JM, Hanson FW. Two simple methods for detecting acrosome-reacted human sperm. *Gamete Res* 1986;15:213–226.
848. Cross NL, Morales P, Overstreet JW, Hanson FW. Induction of acrosome reactions by human zona pellucida. *Biol Reprod* 1988;38:235–244.
849. Cross NL, Overstreet JW. Glycoconjugates of the human sperm surface. *Gamete Res* 1987;16:23–35.
850. Cross PC, Brinster RL. *In vitro* development of mouse oocytes. *Biol Reprod* 1970;3:298–307.
851. Crozet N. Ultrastructural aspects of *in vitro* fertilization in the cow. *Gamete Res* 1984;10:241–251.
852. Crozet N. Behavior of the sperm centriole during sheep oocyte fertilization. *Eur J Cell Biol* 1990;53:326–332.
853. Crozet N, Dumont M. The site of the acrosome reaction during *in vivo* penetration of the sheep oocyte. *Gamete Res* 1984;10:97–105.
854. Cuasnicu PS, Bedford JM. Sperm entry into zona-free oocytes in the hamster oviduct: implications for the mechanisms of acrosome reaction induction. *Gamete Res* 1988;21:85–91.
855. Cuasnicu PS, Bedford JM. The effect of moderate epididymal aging on the kinetics of the acrosome reaction and fertilizing ability of hamster spermatozoa. *Biol Reprod* 1989;40:1067–1073.
856. Cuasnicu PS, Bedford JM. Hamster oocyte penetrability during preovulatory maturation. *Mol Reprod Dev* 1991;29:72–76.
857. Cullen B, Emigholz K, Monahan J. The transient appearance of specific proteins in one-cell mouse embryos. *Dev Biol* 1980;76:215–221.
858. Cummins JM, Robson SK, Rouse GW. The acrosome reaction in spermatozoa of the grey-headed flying fox (*Pteropus poliocephalus:* Chiroptera) exposes barded subacrosomal material. *Gamete Res* 1988;21:11–22.
859. Cummins JM, Woodall PE. On mammalian sperm dimensions. *J Reprod Fertil* 1985;75:153–175.
860. Cuthbertson KSR. Parthenogenetic activation of mouse oocytes *in vitro* with ethanol and benzyl alcohol. *J Exp Zool* 1983;226:311–314.
861. Cuthbertson KSR, Whittingham DG, Cobbold PH. Free Ca^{2+} increases in exponential phases during mouse oocyte activation. *Nature* 1981;294:754–757.
862. Dacheux JL, Dacheux F, Paquignon M. Changes in sperm surface membrane and luminal protein fluid content during epididymal transit in the boar. *Biol Reprod* 1989;40:633–651.
863. Dale B, DeFelice LJ. Soluble sperm factors, electrical events and egg activation. In: Dale B, ed. *Mechanism of Fertilization.* Berlin: Springer-Verlag; 1990:475–487.
864. Da Silva LB, Trebes JE, Balhorn R, et al. X-ray laser microscopy of rat sperm nuclei. *Science* 1992;258:269–271.
865. Da-Yuang C, Chen CY, Longo FJ. A cytochemical study of nuclear changes in fertilized hamster eggs. *Anat Rec* 1983;207:325–334.
866. Dean J. Biology of mammalian fertilization: role of the zona pellucida. *J Clin Invest* 1992;89:1055–1059.
867. Dean J, Millar SE, Liang L, Chamberlin ME, Lunsford RD. Molecular genetics of the mouse zona pellucida: implications for immunologic perturbations of fertilization. In: Wassarman PM, ed. *Elements of Mammalian Fertilization,* Vol. II. Boca Raton, Florida: CRC Press; 1991:133–146.
868. De Felici M, Salustri A, Siracusa G. "Spontaneous" hardening of the zona pellucida of mouse oocytes during *in vitro* culture. II. The effect of follicular fluid and glycosaminoglycans. *Gamete Res* 1985;12:227–235.
869. De Felici M, Siracusa G. "Spontaneous" hardening of the zona

pellucida of mouse oocytes during *in vitro* culture. *Gamete Res* 1982;6:107–113.
870. De Ioannes AE, Becker MI, Perez C, Capote C, Barros C. Role of acrosin and antibodies to acrosin in gamete interaction. In: Alexander NJ, et al., ed. *Gamete Interaction: Prospects of Immunocontraception.* New York: Wiley; 1990:185–195.
871. De Leeuw AW, Deh Daas JHG, Woelders H. The fix vital stain method simultaneous determination of viability and acrosomal status of bovine spermatozoa. *J Androl* 1991;12:112–118.
872. Demott RP, Suarez SS. Hyperactivated sperm progress in the mouse oviduct. *Biol Reprod* 1992;46:779–785.
873. De Sutter P, Dozortsev D, Cieslak J, Wolf G, Verlinsky Y, Dyban A. Parthenogenetic activation of human oocytes by puromycin. *J Assisted Reprod Genet* 1992;9:328–337.
874. Deutch DS, Katz DF, Overstreet JW. Increase in human sperm oxygen consumption at low cell concentrations. *Biol Reprod* 1985;32:865–871.
874a. De Vries JWA, Willemsen R, Geuze HJ. Immunocytochemical localization of acrosin and hyaluronidase in epididymal and ejaculated porcine spermatozoa. *Eur J Cell Biol* 1985;37:81–88.
875. Diaz-Perez E, Meizel S. Importance of mammalian sperm metalloendoprotease activity during the acrosome reaction to subsequent sperm–egg fusion: inhibitor studies with human sperm and zona-free hamster eggs. *Mol Reprod Dev* 1992;31:122–130.
876. Diaz-Perez E, Thomas P, Meizel S. Evidence suggesting a role for sperm metalloendoprotease activity in penetration of zona-free hamster eggs by human sperm. *J Exp Zool* 1988;248: 213–221.
877. Dickmann Z. Denudation of the rabbit egg: time-sequence and mechanism. *Am J Anat* 1963;113:303–335.
878. Dickmann Z, Dzuik PJ. Sperm penetration of the zona pellucida of the pig egg. *J Exp Biol* 1964;41:603–608.
879. Dolci S, Bertolani MV, Canipari R, De Felici M. Involvement of carbohydrates in the hardening of the zona pellucida of mouse oocytes. *Cell Biol Int Rep* 1991;15:571–579.
880. Domon M. Radiosensitivity variation during the cell cycle in pronuclear mouse embryos *in vitro. Cell Tissue Kinet* 1982;15:89–98.
881. Donoghue AM, Howard JG, Byers AP, et al. Correlation of sperm viability with gamete interaction and fertilization *in vitro* in the cheetah (*Acinonyx jubatus*). *Biol Reprod* 1992;46: 1047–1056.
882. Downs SM. Stimulation of parthenogenesis in mouse ovarian follicles by inhibitors of inosine monophosphate dehydrogenase. *Biol Reprod* 1990;43:427–436.
883. Downs SM, Schroeder AC, Eppig JJ. Serum maintains the fertilizability of mouse oocytes matured *in vitro* by preventing hardening of the zona pellucida. *Gamete Res* 1986;15:115–122.
884. Dravland JE, Meizel S. The effect of inhibitors of trypsin and phospholipase A_2 on the penetration of zona pellucida-free hamster eggs by acrosome-reacted hamster sperm. *Andrologia* 1982;3:388–395.
885. Dravland JE, Mortimer D. Role for fucose-sulfate-rich carbohydrates in the penetration of zona-pellucida-free hamster eggs by hamster spermatozoa. *Gamete Res* 1988;21:353–358.
886. Drobnis EZ, Andrew JB, Katz DF. Biophysical properties of the zona pellucida measured by capillary suction: Is zona hardening a mechanical phenomenon? *J Exp Zool* 1988;245:206–219.
887. Drobnis EZ, Katz DF. Videomicroscopy of mammalian fertilization. In: Wassarman PM, ed. *Elements of Mammalian Fertilization,* Vol. I. Boca Raton, Florida: CRC Press; 1991:269–300.
888. Drobnis EZ, Overstreet JW. 1. Natural history of mammalian spermatozoa in the female reproductive tract. In: Milligan SR, ed. *Oxford Review of Reprodive Biology,* Vol. 14. New York: Oxford University Press; 1992:1–45.
889. Drobnis EZ, Yudin AI, Cherr GN, Katz DF. Kinematics of hamster sperm during penetration of the cumulus cell matrix. *Gamete Res* 1988;21:367–383.
890. Drobnis EZ, Yudin AI, Cherr GN, Katz DF. Hamster sperm penetration of the zona pellucida: kinematic analysis and mechanical implications. *Dev Biol* 1988;130:311–323.
891. Ducibella T. Mammalian egg cortical granules and the cortical reaction. In: Wassarman PM, ed. *Elements of Mammalian Fertilization,* Vol. I. Boca Raton, Florida: CRC Press; 1991:205–231.
892. Ducibella T, Anderson E, Albertini DF, Aalberg J, Rangarajan S. Quantitative studies of changes in cortical granule number and distribution in the mouse oocyte during meiotic maturation. *Dev Biol* 1988;130:184–197.
893. Ducibella T, Duffy P, Reindollar R, Su B. Changes in the distribution of mouse oocyte cortical granules and ability to undergo the cortical reaction during gonadotropin-stimulated meiotic maturation and aging *in vivo. Biol Reprod* 1990;43:870–876.
894. Ducibella T, Kurasawa S, Rangarajan S, Kopf GS, Schultz RM. Precocious loss of cortical granules during mouse oocyte meiotic maturation and correlation with an egg-induced modification of the zona pellucida. *Dev Biol* 1990;137:46–55.
895. Ducibella T, Rangarajan S, Anderson E. The development of mouse oocyte cortical reaction competence is accompanied by major changes in cortical vesicles and not cortical granule depth. *Dev Biol* 1988;130:789–792.
896. Dudkiewicz AB. Inhibition of fertilization in the rabbit by anti-acrosin antibodies. *Gamete Res* 1983;8:183–197.
897. Dumont M, Crozet N. Inhibitory effect of homologous solubilized zona pellucida on rabbit *in vitro* fertilization. *Reprod Nutr Develop* 1988;28:1531–1540.
898. Dunbar BS. Morphological, biochemical, and immunochemical characterization of the mammalian zona pellucida. In: Hartmann JF, ed. *Mechanism and Control of Animal Fertilization.* New York: Academic Press; 1983:139–175.
899. Dunbar BS, O'Rand MG, eds. *A Comparative Overview of Mammalian Fertilization.* New York: Plenum Press; 1991.
900. Dunbar BS, Prasad SV, Timmons TM. Comparative structure and function of mammalian zonae pellucidae. In: Dunbar BS, O'Rand MG, eds. *A Comparative Overview of Mammalian Fertilization.* New York: Plenum Press; 1991:97–114.
901. Duncan AE, Fraser LR. Cyclic AMP-dependent phosphorylation of epididymal mouse sperm proteins during capacitation *in vitro:* identification of a M_r 95000 phosphpotyrosine-containing protein. *J Reprod Fertil* 1993;97:287–299.
902. Durr R, Shur B, Roth S. Sperm-associated sialtransferase activity. *Nature* 1977;265:547–548.
903. Dyson ALM, Orgebin-Crist MC. Effect of hypophysectomy, castration and androgen replacement upon the fertilizing ability of rat epididymal spermatozoa. *Endocrinology* 1973;93:391–402.
904. Dzuik PJ, Dickmann Z. Sperm penetration through the zona pellucida of the sheep egg. *J Exp Zool* 1965;158:237–240.
905. East IJ, Gulyas BJ, Dean J. Monoclonal antibodies to the murine zona pellucida protein with sperm receptor activity: effects on fertilization and early development. *Dev Biol* 1985;109: 268–273.
906. Ebensperger C, Barros C. Changes at the hamster oocyte surface from the germinal vesicle stage to ovulation. *Gamete Res* 1984;9:387–397.
907. Eberspaecher U, Gerwien J, Habenicht UF, Scheuning WD, Donner P. Activation and subsequent degradation of proacrosin is mediated by zona pellucida glycoproteins, negatively charged polysaccharides and DNA. *Mol Reprod Dev* 1991;30:164–170.
908. Eddy EM. The spermatozoa. In: Knobil E, Neil J, eds. *The Physiology of Reproduction.* New York: Raven Press; 1988:27–68.
909. Edwards RG. Cleavage of one- and two-celled rabbit eggs *in vitro* after removal of zona pellucida. *J Reprod Fertil* 1964;7:413–415.
910. Ehrenwald E, Foote RH, Parks JE. Bovine oviductal fluid components and their potential role in sperm cholesterol efflux. *Mol Reprod Dev* 1990;25:195–204.
911. Ehrenwald E, Parks JE, Foote RH. Cholesterol efflux from bovine sperm. I. *Gamete Res* 1988;20:145–157.
912. Eisenbach M, Ralt D. Precontact mammalian Sperm-egg communication and role in fertilization. *Am J Physiol* 1992;262:C1095–C1101.
913. Elliott M, Higgins JA. Capacitation and the acrosome reaction in guinea pig spermatozoa increase the availability of surface aminophospholipids for labelling by trinitrobenzene sulphonate. *Cell Biol Int Rep* 1983;7:1091–1096.
914. Elstein M. The role of cervical mucus in the physiology of sperm transport and its clinical assessment. In: Cohen J, Hendry F, eds. *Spermatozoa, Antibodies and Infertility.* Oxford: Blackwell; 1978:55–65.

915. Endo Y, Schultz RM, Kopf GS. Effects of phorbol esters and a diacylglycerol on mouse egg: inhibition of fertilization and modification of the zona pellucida. *Dev Biol* 1987;119:199–209.
916. Epel D. Arousal of activity in sea urchin egg at fertilization. In: Schatten H, Schatten G, eds. *The Cell Biology of Fertilization.* San Diego: Academic Press; 1989:361–385.
917. Epel D. The initiation of development at fertilization. *Cell Diff Dev* 1990;29:1–12.
918. Epel D, Patton C. Cortical granules of sea urchin eggs do not undergo exocytosis at the site of sperm–egg fusion. *Dev Growth Diff* 1985;27:361–369.
919. Eppig JJ. Developmental pottential of LT/Sv parthenotes derived from oocytes matured *in vivo* and *in vitro. Dev Biol* 1978;65:244–249.
920. Eppig JJ. Preimplantation embryonic development of spontaneous mouse parthenotes after oocyte meiotic maturation *in vitro. Gamete Res* 1981;4:3–13.
921. Eppig JJ. The relationship between cumulus cell–oocyte coupling, oocyte meiotic maturation, and cumulus expansion. *Dev Biol* 1982;89:268–272.
922. Eppig JJ. Mammalian oocyte development *in vivo* and *in vitro.* In: Wassarman PM, ed. *Elements of Mammalian Fertilization,* Vol. I. Boca Raton: CRC Press; 1991:57–76.
922a. Eppig JJ. Intercommunication between mammalian oocytes and companion somatic cells. *BioEssays* 1991;13:569–674.
923. Eppig JJ, Kozak LP, Eicher EM, Stevens LC. Ovarian teratomas in mice are derived from oocytes that have completed the first meiotic division. *Nature* 1977;269:517–518.
924. Eusebi F, Salustri A. Development of membrane sensitivity to the parthenogenetic agent calcium ionophore A23187 during meiotic maturation in the hamster oocyte. *Gamete Res* 1985;12:131–137.
925. Evenson DP, Darzynkiewicz Z, Melamed MR. Relation of mammalian sperm chromatin heterogenety to fertility. *Science* 1980;210:1131–1133.
925a. Ewoldsen MA, Ostlie NS, Warner CM. Killing of mouse blastocyst stage embryos by cytotoxic T lymphocytes directed to major histocompatibility complex antigens. *J Immunol* 1987;138:2764–2770.
926. Familiari G, Nottola SA, Micara G, Aragona C, Motta PM. Is the sperm-binding capacity of the zona pellucida linked to its surface structure? *J IVF-ET* 1988;5:134–143.
927. Familiari G, Nottola SA, Macchiarelli G, Micara G, Aragona C, Motta PM. Human zona pellucida during *in vitro* fertilization. *Mol Reprod Dev* 1992;32:51–61.
928. Fawcett DW, Anderson WA, Philips DM. Morphogenetic factors influencing the shape of the sperm head. *Dev Biol* 1971;26:220–251.
929. Fayrer-Hosken RA, Caudle AB, Shur BD. Galactosyltransferase activity is restricted to the plasma membranes of equine and bovine sperm. *Mol Reprod Dev* 1991;28:74–78.
930. Feinberg J, Weinman J, Weinman S, Walsh MP, Harricane MC, Gabrion J, Demaille JB. Immunocytochemical and biochemical evidence for the presence of calmodulin in bull sperm flagellum. *Biochim Biophys Acta* 1981;673:303–311.
931. Fenichel P, Hsi BL, Farahifar D, Donzeau M, Barrier-Delpech D, Yeh CJG. Evaluation of the human sperm acrosome reaction using a monoclonal antibody, GB24, and fluorescence-activated cell sorter. *J Reprod Fertil* 1989;87:699–706.
932. Feuchter FA, Tabet AJ, Green MF. Maturation antigen of the mouse sperm flagellum. I. Analysis of its secretion, association with sperm, and function. *Am J Anat* 1988;181:65–76.
933. Fissore RA, Robl JM. Intracellular Ca^{2+} response of rabbit oocytes to electrical stimulation. *Mol Reprod Dev* 1992;32:9–16.
934. Flechon JE. Nature glycoproteique des granules corticaux de l'oeuf de lapine. *J Microsc* 1970;9:221–242.
935. Flechon JE, Hunter RHF. Distribution of spermatozoa in the utero–tubal junction and isthmus of pigs, and their relationship with the luminal epithelium after mating. *Tissue Cell* 1981;13:127–139.
936. Fleming AD, Armstrong DT. Effects of polyamines upon capacitation and fertilization in the guinea pig. *J Exp Zool* 1985;233:93–100.
937. Flaherty SP, Olson GE. Membrane domains in guinea pig sperm and their role in the membrane fusion events of the acrosome reaction. *Anat Rec* 1988;220:267–280.
938. Florman HM, Babcock DF. Progress toward understanding the molecular basis of capacitation. In: Wassarman PM, ed. *Elements of Mammalian Fertilization,* Vol. 1. Boca Raton, Florida: CRC Press; 1991:105–132.
939. Florman HM, Bechtol KB, Wassarman PM. Enzymatic dissection of the functions of the mouse egg's receptor for sperm. *Dev Biol* 1984;106:243–255.
940. Florman HM, Corron ME, Kim TDH, Babcock DF. Activation of voltage-dependent calcium channels of mammalian sperm is required for zona pellucida-induced acrosomal exocytosis. *Dev Biol* 1992;152:304–314.
941. Florman HM, First NL. The regulation of acrosomal exocytosis I. Sperm capacitation is required for the induction of acrosome reactions by bovine zona pellucida *in vitro. Dev Biol* 1988;128:453–463.
942. Florman HM, Tombers RM, First NL, Babcock DF. An adhesion-associated agonist from the zona pellucida activates G protein-promoted elevation of internal calcium and pH that mediate mammalian sperm acrosomal exocytosis. *Dev Biol* 1989;135:133–136.
943. Forbes DJ, Kirschner MW, Newport JW. Spontaneous formation of nucleus-like structures around bacteriophage DNA microinjected into Xenopus eggs. *Cell* 1983;34:13–23.
944. Foresta C, Zorzi M, Rossato M, Varotto A. Sperm nuclear instability and staining with anilin blue: abnormal persistence of histones in spermatozoa in infertile men. *Int J Androl* 1992;15:330–337.
945. Forrler A, Dellenbach P, Nisand I, Moreau L, Cranz C, Clavert A, Rumpler Y. Direct intraperitoneal insemimation in unexplained and cervical infertility. *Lancet* 1986;1:916–907.
946. Fouquet JP, Fraile B, Kann ML. Sperm actin and calmodulin during fertilization in the hamster: an immune electron microscopic study. *Anat Rec* 1991;231:316–323.
947. Fowler RE, Barratt E. The uptake of [^{3}H] glucosamine-labeled glycoconjugates into the perivitelline space of preimplantation mouse embryo. *Hum Reprod* 1989;4:821–825.
948. Fowler RE, Kaufman MH, Grainge C. The secretions of the cumulus-oocyte complex in relation to fertilization and early mouse embryonic development: A histochemical study. *Histochem J* 1986;18:541–550.
949. Franken DR, Burkman LJ, Oehninger SC, Coddington, CC, Rosenwaks Z, Hodgen GD. Hemizona assay using salt-stored human oocytes: Evaluation of zona pellucida capacity for binding human spermatozoa. *Gamete Res* 1989;22:15–26.
950. Franken DR, Oehninger S, Burkman LJ, Coddington CC, Kruger TF, Rosenwaks Z, Acosta AA, Hodgen GD. The hemizona assay (HZA): a predictor of human sperm fertilizing potential in *in vitro* fertilization (IVF) treatment. *J In Vitro Fert Embryo Transf* 1989;6:44–50.
951. Franklin LE, Barros C, Fussell EN. The acrosomal region and the acrosome reaction in sperm of the golden hamster. *Biol Reprod* 1970;3:180–200.
952. Fraser LR. Accelerated mouse sperm penetration in vitro in the presence of caffeine. *J Reprod Fertil* 1979;57:377–384.
953. Fraser LR. Minimum and maximum extracellular Ca^{2+} requirements during mouse sperm capacitation and fertilization in vitro. *J Reprod Fertil* 1987;81:77–89.
954. Fraser LR. Sperm capacitation and its modulation. In: Bavister BD, et al., ed. *Mammalian Fertilization.* Norwell, Massachusetts: Serono Symposia USA; 1990:141–153.
955. Fraser LR. Requirements for successful mammalian sperm capacitation and fertilization. *Arch Path Lab Med* 1992;116:345–350.
956. Fraser LR, Ahuja KK. Metabolic and surface events in fertilization. *Gamete Res* 1988;20:491–519.
957. Fraser LR, Harrison RAP, Herod JE. Characterization of a decapacitation factor associated with epididymal mouse spermatozoa. *J Reprod Fertil* 1990;89:135–148.
958. Fraser LR, Herod JE. Expression of capacitation-dependent changes in chlorotetracycline fluorescence patterns in mouse spermatozoa requires a suitable glycolysable substrate. *J Reprod Fertil* 1990;88:611–621.

959. Fraser LR, Lane MR. Capacitation- and fertilization-related alterations in mouse oxygen consumption. *J Reprod Fertil* 1987;81:385–393.
960. Fraser LR, McDermott CA. Ca^{2+}-related changes in the mouse sperm capacitation state: a possible role for Ca^{2+}-ATPase. *J Reprod Fertil* 1992;96:363–377.
960a. Fraser LR, Umar G, Sayed S. Na^{+}-requiring mechanisms modulate capacitation and acrosomal exocytosis in mouse spermatozoa. *J Reprod Fert* 1993;97:539–549.
961. Freemerman AJ, Wright RM, Flickinger CJ, Herr JC. Coloning and sequencing of baboon and cynomolgus monkey intraacrosomal protein SP-10: Homology with human SP-10 and a mouse sperm antigen (MSA-63). *Mol Reprod Dev* 1993;34: 140–148.
962. Friend DS. Plasma-membrane diversity in a highly polarized cell. *J Cell Biol* 1982;93:243–249.
963. Friend DS, Rudolf I. Acrosomal disruption in sperm. *J Cell Biol* 1974;63:466–478.
964. Fujiwara T, Nakada K, Shirakawa H, Miyazaki S. Development of inositol triphosphate-induced calcium release mechanism during maturation of hamster oocytes. *Dev Biol* 1993;156: 69–79.
965. Fulka J Jr, Jung T, Moor RM. The fall of biological maturation promoting factor (MPF) and histone H1 kinase activity during anaphase and telophase in mouse oocytes. *Mol Reprod Dev* 1992;32:378–382.
966. Furuya S, Endo Y, Oba M, Nozawa S, Suzuki S. Effects of modulators of protein kinases and phosphatases on mouse sperm capacitation. *J Assisted Reprod Genet* 1992;9:391–399.
967. Fusi FM, Bronson RA. Sperm surface fibronectin expression following capacitation. *J Androl* 1992;13:28–35.
968. Fusi F, Bronson RA, Hong Y, Ghebrehiwei B. Complement component Clq and its receptor are involved in the interaction of human sperm with zona-free hamster eggs. *Mol Reprod Dev* 1991;29:180–188.
969. Fusi FM, Vignali M, Busacca M, Bronson RA. Evidence for the presence of an integrin cell adhesion receptor on the oolemma of unfertilized human oocytes. *Mol Reprod Dev* 1992;31: 215–222.
970. Gaddum-Rosse P, Blandau RJ, Langley LB, Sato K. Sperm tail entry into the mouse egg *in vitro*. *Gamete Res* 1982;6:215–223.
971. Gaddum-Rosse P, Blandau RJ, Langley LB, Battaglia DE. *In vitro* fertilization in the rat: observations on living eggs. *Fertil Steril* 1984;42:285–292.
972. Gall WE, Ohsumi Y. Decondensation of sperm nuclei *in vitro*. *Exp Cell Res* 1976;102:349–358.
973. Gandolfi F, Modina S, Brivini TAL, Galli C, Moor RM, Lauria A. Oviduct ampullary epithelium contributes a glycoprotein to the zona pellucida, perivitelline space and blastomeres membrane of sheep embryos. *Eur J Bas Appl Histochem* 1991; 35:383–392.
974. Garbers DL, Kopf GS. The regulation of spermatozoa by calcium and cyclic nucleotides. In: Greengard P, Robinson GA, ed. *Advances in Cyclic Nucleotide Research,* Vol. 13. New York: Raven Press; 1980:251–306.
975. Garty NB, Galiani D, Aharonhem A, Ho YK, Phillips DM, Dekel N, Salomon Y. G-proteins in mammalian gametes: an immunocytochemical study. *J Cell Sci* 1988;91:21–31.
976. Gatewood JM, Cook GR, Balhorn R, Schmid CW, Bradbury EM. Isolation of four core histones from human sperm chromatin representing a minor subset of somatic histones. *J Biol Chem* 1990;265:20662–20666.
977. Gaunt SJ. Spreading of a sperm surface antigen within the plasma membrane of the egg after fertilization in the rat. *J Embryol Exp Morphol* 1983;75:259–270.
978. Genesca A, Caballin MR, Miro R, Benet J, Germa JR, Egozcue J. Repair of human sperm chromosome aberrations in the hamster egg. *Hum Genet* 1992;89:181–186.
979. Gianfortoni JG, Gulyas BJ. The effect of short-term incubation (aging) of mouse oocytes on *in vitro* fertilization, zona solubility, and embryonic development. *Gamete Res* 1985;11:59–68.
980. Glassner M, Jones J, Kligman I, Woolkalis MJ, Gerton GL, Kopf GS. Immunocytochemical and biochemical characterization of guanine nucleotide-binding regulatory proteins in mammalian spermatozoa. *Dev Biol* 1991;146:438–450.
980a. Gmachl M, Gunther K. Bee venom hyaluronidase is homologous to a membrane protein of mammalian sperm. *Proc Natl Acad Sci USA* 1993;90:3569–3573.
981. Gnessie L, Ruff MR, Fraioli F, Pert CB. Demonstration of receptor-mediated chemotoxis by human spermatozoa. *Exp Cell Res* 1985;161:219–230.
982. Goltz JS, Gardner TK, Kanous KS, Lindemann CB. Interaction of pH and cyclic adenosin 3,5-monophosphate on activation of motility in Triton X-100 extracted bull sperm. *Biol Reprod* 1988;39:1129–1136.
983. Gondos B, Bhiraleus P, Conner LA. Pronuclear membrane alterations during approximation of pronuclei and initiation of cleavage in the rabbit. *J Cell Sci* 1972;10:61–78.
984. Goodpaster JC, Reddy JM, Zaneveld JD. Acrosin, proacrosin, and acrosin inhibitor of guinea pig spermatozoa capacitated and acrosome-reacted *in vitro*. *Biol Reprod* 1987;25:44–55.
985. Goodrowe KL, Miller AM, Wildt DE. Capacitation of domestic cat spermatozoa as determined by homologous zona pellucida penetration. *Proceedings of the 11th International Congress on Animal Reproduction and Artificial Insemination* 1988;3: 245–247.
986. Gorbsky GJ, Simerly C, Schatten G, Borisy GG. Microtubules in the metaphase-arrested mouse oocyte turn over rapidly. *Proc Natl Acad Sci USA* 1990;87:6049–6053.
987. Gordon JW, Navot D, Grunfeld L, Laufer N, Garrisi GJ. Successful microsurgical removal of a pronucleus from tripronuclear human zygotes. *Fertil Steril* 1989;52:367–372.
987a. Gordon JW, Talansky BE. Assisted fertilization by zona drilling: a mouse model for correction of oligospermia. *J Exp Zool* 1986;239:347–354.
988. Gordon M, Dandekar PV. Electron microscope assessment of fertilization of rabbit ova treated with concanaval in A and wheat germ agglutinin. *J Exp Zool* 1976;198:437–442.
989. Gottlieb W, Meizel S. Biochemical studies of metalloendoprotease activity in the spermatozoa of three mammalian species. *J Androl* 1987;8:14–24.
990. Gould JE, Overstreet JW, Hanson FW. Interaction of human spermatozoa with the human zona pellucida and zona-free hamster oocyte following capacitation by exposure to human cervical mucus. *Gamete Res* 1985;12:47–54.
991. Gould JE, Overstreet JW, Yanagimachi H, Yanagimachi R, Katz DF, Hanson FW. What functions of the sperm cells are measured by *in vitro* fertilization of zona-free hamster eggs. *Fertil Steril* 1983;40:344–352.
992. Gould KG, Srivastava PN, Cline EM, Williams WL. Inhibition of *in vitro* fertilization of rabbit ova with naturally occurring antifertility agents. *Contraception* 1971;3:261–267.
993. Gould K, Zaneveld LJD, Srivastava PN, Williams WL. Biochemical changes in the zona pellucida of rabbit ova induced by fertilization and sperm enzymes (35180). *Proc Soc Exp Biol Med* 1971;136:6–10.
994. Graham CF. The production of parthenogenetic mammalian embryos and their use in biological research. *Biol Rev* 1974;49:399–422.
995. Gray AP. *Mammalian Hybrids.* Farnham Royal Bucks, Commonwealth Agriculture Bureau, England; 1954.
996. Green DPL. Comparison of H 33342 and propidium iodide as fluorescent markers for sperm fusion with hamster oocytes. *J Reprod Fertil* 1993;96:581–591.
997. Greve JM, Salzmann GS, Roller RJ, Wassarman PM. Biosynthesis of the major zona pellucida glycoprotein secreted by oocytes during mammalian oogenesis. *Cell* 1982;31:749–759.
998. Greve JM, Wassarman PM. Mouse egg extracellular coat is a matrix of interconnected filaments possessing a structural repeat. *J Mol Biol* 1985;81:253–264.
999. Gulyas BJ. Cortical granules of mammalian eggs. *Int Rev Cytol* 1980;63:357–392.
1000. Gulyas BJ, Schmell ED. Ovoperoxidase activity in ionophore treated mouse eggs. I. Electron microscopic localization. *Gamete Res* 1980;3:267–277.
1001. Gulyas BJ, Yuan LC. Cortical reaction and zona hardening in

mouse oocytes following exposure to ethanol. *J Exp Zool* 1985;233:269–276.
1002. Guraya SS. Morphology, histochemistry and biochemistry of human oogenesis and ovulation. *Int Rev Cytol* 1974;37: 121–151.
1003. Gwatkin RBL. Effect of viruses on early mammalian development, I. Action of mengo encephalitis virus on mouse ova cultivated in vitro. *Proc Natl Acad Sci* 1963;50:576–581.
1004. Gwatkin RBL, Conover JC, Collins RL, Quigley MM. Failed fertilization in human *in vitro* fertilization analyzed with the deoxyribonucleic acid-specific fluorochrome Hoechst 33342. *Am J Obstet Gynecol* 1989;160:31–35.
1005. Gwatkin RBL, Williams DT. Heat sensitivity of the cortical granule protease from hamster eggs. *J Reprod Fertil* 1974;39: 153–155.
1006. Gwatkin RBL, Williams DT. Bovine and hamster zona solutions exhibit receptor activity for capacitated but not for noncapacitated sperm. *Gamete Res* 1978;1:259–263.
1007. Gwatkin RBL, Williams DT, Hartmann JF, Kniazuk M. The zona reaction of hamster and mouse eggs: prodaction *in vitro* by a trypsin-like protease from cortical granules. *J Reprod Fertil* 1973;32:259–265.
1008. Gyllensten U, Wharton D, Josefsson A, Wilson AC. Paternal inheritance of mitochondrial DNA in mice. *Nature* 1991; 352:255–257.
1009. Haaf T, Grunenberg H, Schmid M. Paired arrangement of nonhomologous centromeres during vertebrate spermiogenesis. *Exp Cell Res* 1990;187:157–167.
1010. Haddad A, Nagai MET. Radioautographic study of glycoprotein biosynthesis and renewal in the ovarian follicles of mice and the origin of the zona pellucida. *Cell Tissue Res* 1977; 177:347–369.
1011. Hamilton DW, Wenstrom JC, Baker JB. Membrane glycoproteins from spermatozoa: partial characterization of an integral Mr = ca. 24,000 molecule from the rat spermatozoa that is glycosylated during epididymal maturation. *Biol Reprod* 1986;34:925–936.
1012. Han TL, Ford JH, Webb GC, Flaherty SP, Correll A, Matthews CD. Simultaneous detection of X- and Y-bearing human sperm by double fluorescence *in situ* hybridization. *Mol Reprod Dev* 1993;34:308–313.
1013. Han TL, Webb GC, Flaherty SP, Correll A, Matthews CD, Ford JH. Detection of chromosome 17- and X-bearing human spermatozoa using fluorescence in situ hybridization. *Mol Reprod Dev* 1992;33:189–194.
1014. Handrow RR, First NL, Parrish JJ. Calcium requirement and increased association with bovine sperm during capacitation by heparin. *J Exp Zool* 1989;252:174–182.
1015. Hanson FW, Overstreet JW. The interaction of human spermatozoa with cervical mucus *in vivo. Am J Obstet Gynecol* 1981;140:173–178.
1016. Hirayama H, Kusunoki H, Kato S. Capacity of rete testicular and cauda epididymal boar spermatozoa to undergo the acrosome reaction and subsequent fusion with egg plasma membrane. *Mol Reprod Dev* 35:62–68.
1017. Harper MJK. Stimulation of sperm movement from the isthmus to the site of fertilization in the rabbit oviduct. *Biol Reprod* 1973;8:369–377.
1018. Harrison RAP. Hyaluronidase in ram semen. *Biochem J* 1988;252:865–874.
1019. Harrison RAP. Preliminary characterization of the multiple forms of ram sperm hyaluronidase. *Biochem J* 1988;252: 875–882.
1020. Harrison RAP, Flechon J-E, Brown CR. The location of acrosin and proacrosin in ram spermatozoa. *J Reprod Fertil* 1982;66:349–358.
1021. Harrison RAP, Roldan ERS. Phosphonositides and their products in the mammalian sperm acrosome reaction. *J Reprod Fertil* 1990;(Suppl. 42):51–67.
1021a. Hartman CG. Ovulation, fertilization and the transport and viability of eggs and spermatozoa. In: Allen E, Danforth CH, Doisy ED, eds. *Sex an Internal Secretion,* 2nd edition. Baltimore; Williams & Wilkins; 1939:630–719.
1022. Hartmann JF, ed. *Mechanism and Control of Animal Fertilization.* New York: Academic Press; 1983.
1023. Hashimoto N, Kishimoto T. Regulation of meiotic metaphase by a cytoplasmic maturation-promoting factor during mouse oocyte maturation. *Dev Biol* 1988;126:242–252.
1024. Hatanaka Y, Nagai T, Tobita T, Nakano M. Changes in the properties and composition of zona pellucida of pigs during fertilization *in vitro. J Reprod Fertil* 1992;95:431–440.
1025. Hecht NB. Mammalian protamines and their expression. In: Hnilica LS, Stern GS, Stern JL, eds. *Histones and Other Basic Proteins.* Boca Raton, Florida: CRC Press; 1989:347–372.
1026. Hecht NB, Williams JL. Nuclear and mitochondrial DNA-dependent RNA polymerases in bovine spermatozoa. *J Reprod Fertil* 1979;57:157–165.
1027. Hedrick JL, Urch UA, Hardy DM. Structure-function properties of the sperm enzyme acrosin. In: Witaker JR, Sonnett PE, eds. *Biocatalysis in Agricultural Biotechnology.* Washington, DC: American Chemical Society; 1989:212–229.
1028. Hedrick JL, Wardrip NJ. On the macromolecular composition of the zona pellucida from porcine oocytes. *Dev Biol* 1987;121:478–488.
1029. Hedrick JL, Wardrip NJ, Berger T. Differences in the macromolecular composition of the zona pellucida isolated from pig oocytes, eggs, and zygotes. *J Exp Zool* 1987;241:257–262.
1030. Henderson CJ, Hulme MJ, Aiken RJ. Contraceptive potential of antibodies to the zona pellucida. *J Reprod Fertil* 1988;83: 325–343.
1031. Herr JC, Flickinger CJ, Homyk M, Klotz K, John E. Biochemical and morphological characterization of the intra-acrosomal antigen SP-10 from human sperm. *Biol Reprod* 1990;42: 181–193.
1032. Hinkley RE, Edelstein RN, Ivonnet PI. Selective identification of sperm fused with the surface of echinoderm eggs by DNA-specific bisbenzimide (Hoechst) fluorochromes. *Dev Growth Diff* 1987;29:211–220.
1033. Hinkley RE, Wright BD, Lynn JW. Rapid visual detection of sperm-egg fusion using the DNA-specific fluorochrome Hoechst 33342. *Dev Biol* 1986;118:148–154.
1034. Hinsch KD, Hinsch E, Aumuller G, Tychowiecka I, Schultz G, Schill WB. Immunoligical identification of G protein alpha- and beta-subunits in tail membranes of bovine spermatozoa. *Biol Reprod* 1992;47:337–346.
1035. Hirao Y, Hiraoka J. Surface architecture of sperm tail entry into the hamster oocyte. *Dev Growth Diff* 1987;29:123–132.
1036. Hirao Y, Yanagimachi R. Effects of various enzymes on the ability of hamster egg plasma membranes to fuse with spermatozoa. *Gamete Res* 1978;1:3–12.
1037. Hirao Y, Yanagimachi R. Temperature dependence of sperm-egg fusion and post-fusion events in hamster fertilization. *J Exp Zool* 1978;205:433–438.
1038. Hiraoka J, Hirao Y. Fate of sperm tail components after incorporation into hamster egg. *Gamete Res* 1988;19:369–380.
1039. Hirayama T, Quinn P, Marrs R. Fertilizing ability of mouse spermatozoa from different regions of the epididymis microsurgically injected into the perivitelline space of oocytes. *Fertil Steril* 1991;(Suppl):S-11(abst. 0-025).
1040. Holliday R. A different kind inheritance. *Sci Amer* 1989; 260:60–74.
1041. Holt WV, North RD. Thermotropic phase transitions in the plasma membrane of spermatozoa. *J Reprod Fertil* 1986;78: 447–457.
1042. Hoos PC, Olson GE. Characterization of a 23 KDa sperm-binding polypeptide of the golden hamster epididymis. *Biol Reprod* 1988;39:131–140.
1043. Hoppe PC. Fertilizing ability of mouse sperm from different epididymal regions and after washing and centrifugation. *J Exp Zool* 1975;192:219–222.
1044. Horan AH, Bedford JM. Development of the fertilizing ability of spermatozoa in the epididymis of the syrian hamster. *J Reprod Fert* 1972;30:417–423.
1045. Horvath P, Kellom T, Caulfield J, Boldt J. Mechanistic studies of the plasma membrane block to polyspermy in mouse eggs. *Mol Reprod Dev* 1992;34:65–72.
1046. Hoshi K, Aita T, Yanagida K, Yoshimatsu N, Sato A. Variation in the cholesterol/phospholipid ratio in human spermatozoa and its relation with capacitation. *Hum Reprod* 1990;5:71–74.

1047. Hoshi M. Lysins. In: Metz CB, Monroy A, eds. *Biology of Fertilization,* Vol. 2. Orlando: Academic Press; 1985:431–462.
1048. Hoskins DD, Brandt H, Acott TS. Initiation of sperm motility in the mammalian epididymis. *Fed Proc* 1978;37:2534–2542.
1049. Hoskins DD, Vijayaraghavan S. A new view on the epididymal development of sperm motility: interrelationships among adenosine, calcium and cyclic AMP. In: Baccetti B, ed. *Comparative Spermatology 20 Years After.* New York: Raven Press; 1991:479–483.
1050. Hough SH, Foote RH. Usefulness of bull sperm with stump tail defect in studying fertilization. *Biol Reprod* 1986;34(Suppl 1):95(abst. 91).
1051. Howlett SK. A set of proteins showing cell cycle dependent modification in the early mouse embryo. *Cell* 1986;45:387–396.
1052. Howlett SK, Bolton VN. Sequence and regulation of morphological and molecular events during the first cell cycle of mouse embryogenesis. *J Embryol Exp Morphol* 1985;87:175–206.
1053. Huang TTF, Hardy D, Yanagimachi H, Teuscher C, Tung K, Wild G, Yanagimachi R. pH and protease control of acrosome content stasis and release during the guinea pig acrosome reaction. *Biol Reprod* 1985;32:451–462.
1054. Huang TTF, Ohzu E, Yanagimachi R. Evidence suggesting that L-fucose is part of a recognition signal for sperm-zona pellucida attachment in mammals. *Gamete Res* 1982;5:355–361.
1055. Huang TTF, Tung KSK, Yanagimachi R. Autoantibodies from vasectomized guinea pigs inhibit fertilization *in vitro. Science* 1981;213:1267–1269.
1056. Huarte J, Belin D, Bosco D, Sappino AP, Vassalli JD. Plasminogen activator and mouse spermatozoa: urokinase synthesis in the male genital tract and binding of the enzyme to the sperm cell surface. *J Cell Biol* 1987;104:1281–1289.
1057. Huneau D, Harrison RAP, Flechon J-E. Ultrastructural localization of proacrosin and acrosin in ram spermatozoa. *Gamete Res* 1984;9:425–440.
1058. Hunter AG, Polge C. *In vitro* fertilizability of spermatozoa from various regions of the boa epididymis. *Biol Reprod* 1986; 34(Suppl):99(abst. 100).
1059. Hunter RHF. Sperm-egg interactions in the pig: monospermy, extensive polyspermy, and the formation of chromatin aggregates. *J Anat* 1976;122:43–59.
1060. Hunter RHF. *Physiology and Technology of Reproduction in Female Domestic Animals.* New York: Academic Press; 1980.
1061. Hunter RHF. Sperm transport and reservoirs in the pig oviduct in relation to the time of ovulation. *J Reprod Fertil* 1981;63:109–117.
1062. Hunter RHF. *The Fallopian Tubes.* Berlin: Springer-Verlag; 1988.
1063. Hunter RHF. Fertilization in the pig and horse. In: Dunbar BS, O'Rand MG, eds. *Overview of Mammalian Fertilization.* New York: Plenum Press; 1991:329–349.
1064. Hunter RHF, Cook B, Poyser NL. Regulation of oviduct function in pigs by local transfer of ovarian steroids and prostoglandins. *Eur J Obstet Gynecol* 1983;14:225–232.
1065. Hunter RHF, Flechon B, Flechon JE. Pre- and peri-ovulatory distribution of viable spermatozoa in the pig oviduct. *Tissue Cell* 1987;19:423–436.
1066. Hunter RHF, Flechon B, Flechon JE. Distribution, morphology and epithelial interactions of bovine spermatozoa in the oviduct before and after ovulation. *Tissue Cell* 1991;23:641–656.
1067. Huret JL, Courtot AM. Effect of migration and capacitation on the nuclear stability of human sperm. *Arch Androl* 1984; 13:147–152.
1068. Igusa Y, Miyazaki S. Effects of altered extracellular and intracellular calcium concentration on hyperpolarizing responses of the hamster egg. *J Physiol* 1983;340:611–632.
1069. Igusa Y, Miyazaki S. Periodic increase of cytoplasmic free calcium in fertilized hamster eggs measured with calcium-sensitive electrodes. *J Physiol* 1986;377:193–205.
1070. Incharoensakdi A, Panyim S. *In vitro* decondensation of human sperm chromatin. *Andrologia* 1981;13:64–73.
1071. Inoue M, Kobayashi Y, Kaneko M, Fujii A. Sperm-zona interaction in the mouse-special reference to the time of acrosome reaction. *J Mamm Ova Res* (Japan) 1984;1:77–80.
1072. Inoue M, Wolf DP. Sperm binding characteristics of the murine zona pellucida. *Biol Reprod* 1975;13:340–346.
1073. Iqbal M, Shivaji S, Vijayasarathy S, Balaram. Synthetic peptides as chemoattractants for bull spermatozoa. *Biochem Biophys Res Commun* 1980;96:235–242.
1074. Irvine DS, Aitken RJ. Measurement of intracellular calcium in human spermatozoa. *Gamete Res* 1986;15:57–71.
1075. Irvine RF. Inositol tetrakisphosphate as a second messenger: confusions, contradictions, and a potential resolution. *BioEssay* 1991;13:419–429.
1076. Ishijima S, Mohri H. A quantitative description of flagellar movement in golden hamster spermatozoa. *J Exp Biol* 1985;114:463–475.
1077. Ishijima SA, Okuno M, Nakahori Y, Seki S, Nagafuchi S, Kaneko S, Mohri H. Identification of X- and Y-chromosome-bearing human sperm separated by free-flow electrophoresis using Y-chromosome-specific polymerase chain reaction. *Biochem Res* 1992;13:221–224.
1078. Itagaki Y, Toyoda Y. Effects of prolonged sperm preincubation and elevated calcium concentration on fertilization of cumulus-free mouse eggs *in vitro. J Reprod Dev (Japan)* 1992;38: 219–224.
1079. Ito M, Smith TT, Yanagimachi R. Effect of ovulation on sperm transport in the hamster oviduct. *J Reprod Fertil* 1991;93: 157–163.
1080. Itoh T, Ohsumi K, Katagiri C. Remodeling of human sperm chromatin mediated by nucleoplasmin from amphibian eggs. *Dev Growth Diff* 1993;35:59–66.
1081. Iwao Y, Elinson RP. Control of sperm nuclea behavior in physiologically polyspermic newt eggs: possible involvement of MPF. *Dev Biol* 1990;142:301–312.
1082. Jackson RC, Crabb JH. Cortical exocytosis in the sea urchin egg. In: Duzgunes N, Bronner F, eds. *Current Topics in Membranes and Transport,* Vol. 32. San Diego: Academic Press; 1988: 45–85.
1083. Jacobs T. Control of the cell cycle. *Dev Biol* 1992;153:1–15.
1084. Jaffe LA, Gould M. Polyspermy-preventing mechanisms. In: Metz CB, Monroy A, eds. *Biology of Fertilization,* Vol. 3. Orlando: Academic Press; 1985:223–250.
1085. Jaffe LA, Sharp AP, Wolf DP. Absence of an electrical polyspermy block in the mouse. *Dev Biol* 1983;96:317–323.
1086. Jaffe LF. The roles of intermembrane calcium in polarizing and activating eggs. In: Dale B, ed. *Mechanism of Fertilization: Plants to Humans,* Berlin: Springer-Verlag; 1990:389–417.
1087. Jager S, Wijchman J, Kremer J. Studies on the decondensation of human, mouse, and bull sperm nuclei by heparin and other polyanions. *J Exp Zool* 1990;256:315–322.
1088. Jagerbauer EM, Fraser A, Herbst EW, Kothary R, Fundele R. Parthenogenetic stem cells in postnatal mouse chimeras. *Development* 1992;116:95–102.
1089. Jasen RPS. Fallopian tube isthmus and ovum transport. *Science* 1978;201:349–351.
1090. Jedlicki A, Barros C. Scanning electron microscope study of *in vitro* prepenetration gamete interactions. *Gamete Res* 1985; 11:121–131.
1091. Jeyendran RS, Van Der Ven HH, Kennedy WP, Heath E, Perez-Pelaez M, Sobrero AJ, Zaneveld LJD. Acrosomeless sperm. A cause of primary male infertility. *Androgia* 1984; 17:31–36.
1092. Jilek F, Pavlok A. Antibodies against mouse ovaries and their effect on fertilization *in vitro* and *in vivo* in the mouse. *J Reprod Fertil* 1975;42:377–380.
1093. Jinno M, Burkman LJ, Coddington CC. Human sperm hyperactivated motility and egg penetration. *Biol Reprod* 1987; 36(Suppl 1):53(abst. 20).
1094. Johnson L, Varner DD. Effect of daily spermatozoan production but not age on transit time of spermatozoa through the human epididymis. *Biol Reprod* 1988;39:812–817.
1095. Johnson M, Ediddin M. Lateral diffusion in plasma membrane of mouse egg is restricted after fertilization. *Nature* 1978; 272:448–450.
1096. Johnson RT, Rao PN, Hughes S. Mammalian cell fusion III. A hela cell inducer of premature chromosome condensation active in cells from a variety of animal species. *J Cell Physiol* 1970;76:151–157.
1097. Jonakova V, Sanz L, Calvete JJ, Henschen A, Cechova D, Topfer-Petersen E. Isolation and biochemical characterization

of a zona pellucida-binding glycoprotein of boar spermatozoa. *FEBS* 1991;280:183–186.
1098. Jones GR, Sacco AG, Subramanian MG, Kruger M, Zhang S, Yurewicz EC, Moghissi KS. Histology of ovaries of female rabbits immunized with deglycosylated zona pellucida macromolecules of pigs. *J Reprod Fertil* 1992;95:513–525.
1099. Jones R. Identification and functions of mammalian sperm-egg recognition molecules during fertilization. *J Reprod Fertil* 1990;42(Suppl):89–105.
1100. Jones R. Interaction of zona pellucida glycoproteins, sulphated carbohydrates and synthetic polymers with proacrosin, the putative egg-binding protein from mammalian spermatozoa. *Development* 1991;111:1155–1163.
1101. Jones R, Brown CR. Identification of a zona-binding protein from boar spermatozoa as proacrosin. *Exp Cell Res* 1987; 171:503–508.
1102. Jones R, Brown CR, Lancaster RT. Carbohydrate-binding properties of boar sperm proacrosin and assessment of its role in sperm–egg recognition and adhesion during fertilization. *Development* 1988;102:781–792.
1103. Jones R, Shalgi R, Hoyland J, Phillips DM. Topographical rearrangement of a plasma membrane antigen during capacitation of rat spermatozoa *in vitro*. *Dev Biol* 1990;139:349–362.
1104. Jones R, Williams RM. Identification of zona- and fucoidan-binding proteins in guinea-pig spermatozoa and mechanism of recognition. *Development* 1990;109:41–50.
1105. Joseph AM, Gosden JR, Chandley AC. Estimation of aneuploidy levels in human spermatozoa using chromosome specific probes and *in situ* hybridisation. *Hum Genetics* 1984;66: 234–238.
1106. Joyce CL, Nuzzo NA, Wilson JRL, Zaneveld LJD. Evidence for a role of cyclooxygenase (prostaglandin synthetase) and prostaglandins in the sperm acrosome reaction and fertilization. *J Androl* 1987;8:74–82.
1107. Kaleta E. Sperm penetration *in vitro* into ovarian and tubal oocytes from mice of the inbred KE and C57 strains. *Gamete Res* 1979;2:99–104.
1108. Kamiguchi Y, Mikamo K. An improved, efficient method for analyzing human sperm chromosomes using zona-free hamster ova. *Am J Hum Genet* 1986;38:724–740.
1109. Kan FWK, Roux E, St-Jacques S, Bleau G. Demonstration by lectin-gold cytochemistry of transfer of glycoconjugates of oviductal origin to the zona pellucida of oocytes after ovulation in hamsters. *Anat Rec* 1990;226:37–47.
1110. Kan FWK, St-Jacques S, Bleau G. Immunocytochemical evidence for the transfer of an oviductal antigen to the zona pellucida of hamster ova after ovulation. *Biol Reprod* 1989;40: 585–598.
1111. Kapur RP, Johnson LV. Ultrastructural evidence that specialized regions of the murine oviduct contribute a glycoprotein to the extracellular matrix of mouse oocytes. *Anat Rec* 1988; 221:720–729.
1112. Katayose H, Matsuda J, Yanagimachi R. The ability of dehydrated hamster and human sperm nuclei to develop into pronuclei. *Biol Reprod* 1992;47:277–284.
1113. Kato KH, Iwaikawa Y, Sugiyama M. Fusion of spermatozoa with embryonic cells and somatic cells in the sea urchin. *Dev Growth Diff* 1983;25:571–583.
1114. Katz DF, Cherr GN, Lambert H. The evolution of hamster sperm motility during capacitation and interaction with the ovum vestments *in vitro*. *Gamete Res* 1986;14:333–346.
1115. Katz DF, Drobnis EZ, Overstreet JW. Factors regulating mammalian sperm migration through the female reproductive tract and oocyte vestments. *Gamete Res* 1989;22:443–469.
1116. Kaufman MH. *Early Mammalian Development: Parthenogenetic Studies*. London: Cambridge University Press; 1983.
1117. Kaufman MH, Barton SC, Surani MAH. Normal postimplantation development of mouse parthenogenic embryos to the forelimb bud stage. *Nature* 1977;265:53–55.
1118. Keefer C, Schuetz AW. Spontaneous activation of ovulated rat oocytes during *in vitro* culture. *J Exp Zool* 1982;224:371–377.
1119. Kellom T, Vick AA, Boldt J. Recovery of penetration ability in protease-treated zona-free mouse eggs occurs coincident with recovery of a cell surface 94 kD protein. *Mol Reprod Dev* 1992;33:46–52.
1120. Kholkute SD, Lian Y, Roudebush WE, Dukelow WR. Capacitation and the acrosome reaction of squirrel monkey spermatozoa evaluated by the chlortetracyclin fluorescent assay. *Am J Primatol* 1990;20:115–125.
1121. Kikuchi K, Nagai T, Motlik J. Effect of follicle cells on *in-vitro* fertilization of pig follicular oocytes. *Theriogenology* 1991; 35:225.
1122. Kim H, Schuetz AW. Regulation of parthenogenetic activation of metaphase II mouse oocytes by pyruvate. *J Exp Zool* 1991;257:375–385.
1123. Kinloch RA, Mortillo S, Wassarman PM. Transgenic mouse eggs with functional hamster sperm receptors in their zona pellucida. *Development* 1992;115:937–946.
1124. Kinloch RA, Roller RJ, Fimiani CM, Wassarman DA, Wassarman PM. Primary structure of the mouse sperm receptor polypeptide determined by genomic cloning. *Proc Natl Acad Sci USA* 1988;85:6409–6413.
1125. Kinloch RA, Ruiz-Seiler B, Wassarman PM. Genomic organization and polypeptide primary structure of zona pellucida glycoprotein hZP3, the hamster sperm receptor. *Dev Biol* 1990;142:414–421.
1126. Kistler WS, Geroch ME, Williams-Ashman HG. Specific basic proteins from mammalian testes: isolation and properties of small basic proteins from rat testes and epididymal spermatozoa. *J Biol Chem* 1973;248:4532–4543.
1127. Klemm U, Muller-Esterl W, Engel W. Acrosin, the peculiar sperm-specific serine protease. *Hum Genet* 1991;87:635–641.
1128. Kline D, Kline JT. Repetitive calcium transients and the role of calcium in exocytosis and cell cycle activation in the mouse egg. *Dev Biol* 1992;149:80–89.
1129. Koehler JK. A freeze-etching study of rabbit spermatozoa with particular reference to head structure. *J Ultrast Res* 1970;33: 598–614.
1130. Koehler JK, ed. *Gamete Surface and Their Interactions*. New York: Alan R. Liss; 1985.
1131. Koehler JK, Smith WD, Ravnik S. Phagocytosis of yeast by human oocytes: fine structural observations. *Gamete Res* 1987;17:237–244.
1132. Koehler JK, Wurschmidt U, Larsen MP. Nuclear and chromatin structure in rat spermatozoa. *Gamete Res* 1983;8:357–370.
1133. Kohane AC, Cameo MS, Pineiro L, Garberi JC, Blaquier JA. Distribution and site of production of specific proteins in the rat epididymis. *Biol Reprod* 1980;23:181–187.
1134. Kohane AC, Gonzalez Echeverria FMC, Pineiro L, Blaquier JA. Interaction of proteins of epididymal origin with spermatozoa. *Biol Reprod* 1980;23:737–742.
1135. Komar A. Fertilization of parthenogenetically activated mouse eggs. *Exp Cell Res* 1982;139:361–367.
1136. Kono T, Kwon OY, Nakahara T. Development of enucleated mouse oocytes reconstituted with embryonic nuclei. *J Reprod Fertil* 1991;93:165–172.
1137. Kopecny V, Flechon JE. Ultrastructural localization of labeled acrosomal glycoproteins during *in vivo* fertilization in the rabbit. *Gamete Res* 1987;17:35–42.
1138. Kopf GS, Gerton GL. The mammalian sperm acrosome and the acrosome reaction. In: Wassarman PM, ed. *Elements of Mammalian Fertilization,* Vol. 1. Boca Raton, Florida: CRC Press; 1991:153–203.
1139. Kosower NS, Katayose H, Yanagimachi R. Thiol-disulfide status and acridine orange fluorescence of mammalian sperm nuclei. *J Androl* 1992;13:342–348.
1140. Krishna M, Generoso WM. Timing of sperm penetration, pronuclear formation, pronuclear DNA synthesis, and first cleavage in naturally ovulated mouse eggs. *J Exp Zool* 1977;202: 245–252.
1141. Krzanowska H. Toluidine blue staining reveals changes in chromatin stabilization of mouse spermatozoa during epididymal maturation and penetration of ova. *J Reprod Fertil* 1982;64: 97–101.
1142. Krzanowska H. Interstrain competition amongst mouse spermatozoa inseminated in various proportiona, as affected by the genotype of the Y chromosome. *J Reprod Fertil* 1986;77: 265–270.
1143. Kubiak JZ. Mouse oocytes gradually develop the capacity for activation during the metaphase II arrest. *Dev Biol* 1989;136: 537–545.

1143a. Kullander S, Rausing A. On round-headed human spermatozoa. *Int J Fertil* 1975;20:33–40.
1144. Kumagai A, Dunphy WG. The cdc 25 protein controls tyrosine dephosphorylation of the cdc 2 protein in a cell-free system. *Cell* 1991;64:903–914.
1145. Kurasawa S, Schultz RM, Kopf GS. Egg-induced modifications of the zona pellucida of mouse eggs: effects of microinjected inositol 1,4,5-trisphosphate. *Dev Biol* 1989;133:295–304.
1146. Lakoski KA, Carron CP, Cabot CL, Saling PM. Epididymal maturation and the acrosomal reaction in mouse sperm: response to zona pellucida develops coincident with modification of M42 antigen. *Biol Reprod* 1988;38:221–233.
1147. Lakoski KA, William C, Saling P. Proteins of the acrosomal region in mouse sperm: immunological probes reveal posttesticular modifications. *Gamete Res* 1989;23:21–37.
1148. Lalonde L, Chapdelaine A, Langlais J, Roberts KD, Antaki P, Bleau G. Male infertility associated with round-headed acrosomeless spermatozoa. *Fertil Steril* 1988;49:316–321.
1149. Lambert H, Overstreet JW, Morales P, Hanson FW, Yanagimachi R. Sperm capacitation in the human female reproductive tract. *Fertil Steril* 1985;43:325–327.
1150. Lansford B, Haas GG, Debault LE, Wolf DP. Effect of sperm-associated antibodies on the acrosomal status of human sperm. *J Androl* 1990;11:532–538.
1151. Lanzendorf SE, Holmgren WJ, Johnson DE, Scobey MJ, Jeyndran RS. Hemizona assay for measuring zona binding in the lowland gorilla. *Mol Reprod Dev* 1992;31:264–267.
1152. Lanzendorf S, Maloney M, Ackerman S, Acosta A, Hodgen G. Fertilizing potential of acrosome-defective sperm following microsurgical injection into eggs. *Gamete Res* 1988;19:329–337.
1153. Lardy H, San Augustin J. Caltrin and calcium regulation of sperm activity. In: Schatten H, Schatten G, eds. *The Cell Biology of Fertilization.* San Diego: Academic Press; 1989:29–39.
1154. Lathan KE, Garrels JI, Chan C, Solter D. Quantitative analysis of protein synthesis in mouse embryos. I. Extensive reprogramming at the one-and two-cell stages. *Development* 1991;112: 921–932.
1155. Lathrop WF, Carmichael EP, Myles DG, Primakoff P. cDNA cloning reveals the molecular structure of a sperm surface protein, pH-20, involved in sperm–egg adhesion and the wide distribution of its gene among mammals. *J Cell Biol* 1990; 111:2939–2949.
1156. Lavy G, Boyers SP, DeCherney AH. Hyaluronidase removal of the cumulus oophorus increases *in vitro* fertilization. *J In Vitro Fertil Embryo Transf* 1988;5:257–260.
1157. Lee MA, Check JH, Kopf GS. A guanine nucleotide-binding regulatory protein in human sperm mediates acrosomal exocytosis induced by the human zona pellucida. *Mol Reprod Dev* 1992;31:78–86.
1158. Lee MA, Storey BT. Evidence for plasma membrane permeability to small ions in acrosome-intact mouse spermatozoa bound to mouse zona pellucidae, using an aminoacridine fluorescence probe. *Biol Reprod* 1985;33:235–246.
1159. Lee MA, Storey BT. Endpoint of first stage of zona pellucida-induced acrosome reaction in mouse spermatozoa characterized by acrosomal H^+ and Ca^{2+} permeability: population and single cell kinetics. *Gamete Res* 1989;24:303–326.
1160. Lee MA, Trucco GS, Bechtol KB, Wummer N, Kopf GS, Blasco L, Storey BT. Capacitation and acrosome reaction in human spermatozoa monitored by chlortetracycline fluorescence assay. *Fertil Steril* 1987;48:649–658.
1161. Lee SH, Ahuja KK, Gilburt DJ, Whittingham DG. The appearance of glycoconjugates associated with cortical granule release during mouse fertilization. *Development* 1988;102:595–604.
1162. Leeton J, Healy D, Rogers P, Yates C, Caro C. A controlled study between the use of gamete intrafallopian tube transfer (GIFT) and *in vitro* fertilization and embryo transfer in the management of idiopathetic and male infertility. *Fertil Steril* 1987;48:605–607.
1163. Le Guen P, Crozet N, Huneau D, Gall L. Distribution and role of microfilaments during early events of sheep fertilization. *Gamete Res* 1989;22:411–425.
1164. Lesec G, Manhes H, Hardy RI, et al. *In-vivo* transperitoneal fertilization. *Hum Reprod* 1989;4:521–526.
1165. Leyton L, LeGuen P, Bunch D, Saling PM. Regulation of mouse gamete interaction by a sperm tyrosine kinase. *Proc Natl Acad Sci USA* 1992;89:11692–11695.
1166. Leyton L, Robinson A, Saling P. Relationship between the M42 antigen of mouse sperm and the acrosome reaction induced by ZP3. *Dev Biol* 1989;132:174–178.
1167. Leyton L, Saling P. Evidence that aggregation of mouse sperm receptors by Zp3 triggers the acrosome reaction. *J Cell Biol* 1989;108:2163–2168.
1168. Leyton L, Saling P. 95KDa sperm proteins binds ZP3 and serve as tyrosine kinase substrates in response to zona binding. *Cell* 1989;57:1123–1130.
1169. Liang LF, Chamow SM, Dean J. Oocyte-specific expression of mouse ZP-2: developmental regulation of the zona pellucida gene. *Mol Cell Biol* 1990;10:1507–1515.
1170. Lindemann CB, Goltz JS, Kanous KS. Regulation of activation state and flagellar wave from in epididymal rat sperm: evidence for the involvement of both Ca^{2+} and cAMP. *Cell Motil Cytoskel* 1987;8:324–332.
1171. Lindemann CB, Goltz JS, Kanous KS, Gardner TK, Olds-Clarke P. Evidence for an increased sensitivity to Ca^{2+} in the flagella of sperm from $t^{w32}/+$ mice. *Mol Reprod Dev* 1990;26:69–77.
1172. Lindemann CB, Kanous KS. Regulation of mammalian sperm motility. *Arch Androl* 1989;23:1–22.
1173. Lindemann CB, Kanous KS, Gardner TK. The interrelationship of calcium and cAMP mediated effects on reactivated mammalian sperm models. In: Baccetti B, ed. *Comparative Spermatology 20 Years After.* New York: Raven Press; 1991:491–502.
1174. Linder D, McGaw BK, Hecht F. Parthenogenic origin of benign ovarian teratomas. *New Engl J Med* 1975;292:63–66.
1174a. Llanos M, Vigil P, Salgado AM, Morales P. Inhibition of the acrosome reaction by trypsin inhibitors and prevention of penetration of spermatozoa through the human zona pellucida. *J Reprod Fert* 1993, 97:173–178.
1175. Lohka MJ, Masui Y. Roles of cytosol and cytoplasmic particles in pronuclear formation in cell-free preparations from amphibian eggs. *J Cell Biol* 1984;98:1222–1230.
1176. Longo FJ. Fertilization: a comparative ultrastructural review. *Biol Reprod* 1973;9:149–215.
1177. Longo FJ. Ultrastructural changes in rabbit eggs aged *in vivo.* *Biol Reprod* 1974;11:22–39.
1178. Longo FJ. An ultrastructural analysis of spontaneous activation of hamster eggs aged *in vivo.* *Anat Rec* 1974;179:27–55.
1179. Longo FJ. Effects of cytochalasin B on sperm-egg interactions. *Dev Biol* 1978;67:249–265.
1180. Longo FJ. Aging of mouse eggs *in vivo* and *in vitro.* *Gamete Res* 1980;3:379–393.
1181. Longo FJ. *Fertilization.* New York: Chapman & Hall; 1987.
1182. Longo FJ. Actin-plasma membrane associations in mouse eggs and oocytes. *J Exp Zool* 1987;243:299–309.
1183. Longo FJ, Anderson E. Cytological events leading to the formation of the two-cell stage in the rabbit: association of the maternally and paternally derived genomes. *J Ultrastruc Res* 1969;29:86–118.
1184. Longo FJ, Chen DY. Development of cortical polarity in mouse egg: involvement of the meiotic apparatus. *Dev Biol* 1985; 107:382–394.
1185. Longo FJ, Krohne G, Franke WW. Basic proteins of the perinuclear theca of mammalian spermatozoa and spermatids: a novel class of cytoskeletal elements. *J Cell Biol* 1987;105:1105–1120.
1186. Longo FJ, Lynn JW, McCulloh DH, Chambers EL. Correlative ultrastructural and electrophysiological studies of sperm–egg interactions of the sea urchin, *Lytechinus variegatus.* *Dev Biol* 1986;118:155–166.
1187. Longo FJ, Yanagimachi R. Detection of sperm–egg fusion. In: Duzgunes N, ed. *Methods of Enzymology, Vol. 221: Membrane Fusion Techniques,* Part B. San Diego: Academic Press; pp. 249–260.
1188. Lopata A, Sathanathan AH, McBain JC, Johnston WIH, Speirs AL. The ultrastructure of the preovulatory human egg fertilized *in vitro.* *Fertil Steril* 1980;33:12–20.
1189. Lopez LC, Bayna EM, Litoff D, Shaper NL, Shaper JH, Shur BD. Receptor function of mouse sperm surface galactosyltransferase during fertilization. *J Cell Biol* 1985;101:1501–1510.

1190. Lopez LC, Shur BD. Redistribution of mouse sperm surface galactosyltransferase after the acrosome reaction. *J Cell Biol* 1987;105:1663–1670.

1191. Lunsford RD, Jenkins N, Kozak C, Silan C, Liang CF, Copeland NG, Dean J. Genomic mapping of mouse ZP-2 and ZP-3; two oocyte-specific genes encoding zona pellucida proteins. *Genomics* 1990;6:184–187.

1192. Luthardt FW, Donahue RP. Pronuclear DNA synthesis in mouse eggs. *Exp Cell Res* 1973;82:143–151.

1193. Luttmer S, Longo FJ. Ultrastructural and morphometric observations of cortical endoplasmic reticulum in *Arbacia, Spisula* and mouse eggs. *Dev Growth Diff* 1985;27:349–359.

1194. Lynn JW, Chambers EL. Voltage clamp studies of fertilization in sea urchin eggs. *Dev Biol* 1984;102:98–109.

1195. Macek MB, Lopez LC, Shur BD. Aggregation of beta-1,4-galacto-syltransferase on mouse sperm induces the acrosme reaction. *Dev Biol* 1991;147:440–441.

1196. Macek MB, Shur BD. Protein-carbohydrate complementarity in mammalian gamete recognition. *Gamete Res* 1988;20: 93–109.

1197. Maddock MB, Dawson WD. Artificial insemination of deermice (*Peromyscus maniculatus*) with sperm from other rodent species. *J Embryol Exp Morphol* 1974;31:621–634.

1198. Magargee SF, Kunze E, Hammerstedt RH. Changes in lectin-binding features of ram sperm surfaces associated with epididymal maturation and ejaculation. *Biol Reprod* 1988;38:667–685.

1199. Magnuson T, Epsteih CJ. Genetic expression during early mouse development. In: Bavister BD, ed. *The Mammalian Preimplantation Embryo.* New York: Plenum Press; 1987: 133–150.

1200. Mahadevan MM, Trounson AO. Removal of the cumulus oophorus from the human oocyte for *in vitro* fertilization. *Fertil Steril* 1985;43:263–267.

1201. Mahi-Brown CA, Yanagimachi R, Nelson ML, Yanagimachi H, Palumbo N. Ovarian histopathology of bitches immunized with porcine zonae pellucidae. *Am J Reprod Immunol Microbiol* 1988;18:94–103.

1202. Makler A, Reichler A, Stoller J, Feigin PD. A new model for investigating in real-time the existence of chemotaxis in human spermatozoa. *Fertil Steril* 1992;57:1066–1074.

1203. Maleszewski M. Decondensation of mouse sperm chromatin in cell-free extracts: a micromethod. *Mol Reprod Dev* 1990; 27:244–248.

1204. Maleszewski M. Behavior of sperm nuclei incorporated into parthenogenetic mouse eggs prior to the first cleavage division. *Mol Reprod Dev* 1992;33:215–221.

1205. Malter HE, Cohen J. Embryonic development after microsurgical repair of polyspermic human zygotes. *Fertil Steril* 1989;52:373–380.

1206. Maresh GA, Dunbar BS. Antigenic comparison of five species of mammalian zonae pellucidae. *J Exp Zool* 1987;244:299–307.

1207. Maro B, Johnson MH, Webb M, Flach G. Mechanism of polar body formation in the mouse oocyte: an interaction between the chromosomes, the cytoskeleton and the plasma membrane. *J Embryol Exp Morphol* 1986;92:11–32.

1208. Marquant-Le Guienne B, De Almeida M. Role of guinea-pig sperm autoantigens in capacitation and the acrosome reaction. *J Reprod Fertil* 1986;77:337–345.

1209. Martin RH. Human sperm karyotyping: a tool for the study of aneuploidy. In: Vig BK, Sandberg AA, eds. *Progress and Topics in Cytogenetics,* Vol. 7, Part B. New York: Alan R. Liss 1988;297–316.

1210. Martinage A, Arkhis A, Alimi E, Sautiere P, Chevaillier P. Molecular characterization of nuclear basic protein HPI1, a putative precursor of human sperm protamines HP2 and HP3. *Eur J Biochem* 1990;191:449–451.

1211. Marushige Y, Marushige K. Properties of chromatin isolated from bull spermatozoa. *Biochim Biophys Acta* 1974;340: 498–508.

1212. Marushige Y, Marushige K. Enzymatic unpacking of bull sperm chromatin. *Biochim Biophys Acta* 1975;403:180–191.

1213. Marushige Y, Marushige K. Dispersion of mammalian sperm chromatin during fertilization: an *in vitro* study. *Biochim. Biophys Acta* 1978;519:1–22.

1214. Masui Y. The role of "cytostatic factor (CSF)" in the control of oocyte cell cycles: a summary of 20 years of study. *Dev Growth Diff* 1991;33:543–551.

1215. Matano Y. Comparative mammalian spermatology with scanning electron microscopes V. Chiropters and Cetaceans. *Proceedings of the 10th International Congress on Anatomy,* Tokyo, 1975.

1216. Mate KE, Rodger JC. Stability of the acrosome of the bush-tailed possum and tammar wallaby *in vitro* and after exposure to conditions and agents known to cause capacitation or acrosome reaction of eutherian spermatozoa. *J Reprod Fertil* 1991;91: 41–48.

1217. Mathieu C, Guerin J, Cognat M, Lejeune H, Pinatel M, Lornage J. Motility and fertilizing capacity of epididymal human spermatozoa in normal and pathological cases. *Fertil Steril* 1992;57:871–876.

1218. Matsuda T. Production of monoclonal antibodies against hamster oocyte and their inhibitory effects on fertilization. *Adv. Obstet. Gynecol. (Japan)* 1986;38:373–381.

1219. Matsuda Y, Tobari I. Repair capacity of fertilized mouse eggs for X-ray damage induced in sperm and mature oocytes. *Mutat Res* 1989;210:35–47.

1220. Mattioli M, Galeati G, Seren E. Effect of folicule somatic cells during pig oocyte maturation on egg penetrability and male pronucleus formation. *Gamete Res* 1988;20:177–183.

1221. McBride CE, Fayrer-Hosken RA, Younis A, Brackett BG. Comparison of rabbit and bovine salt-stored zonae for sperm penetration. *J Androl* 1988;9(Suppl):34(abst 61).

1222. McCulloh DH, Chambers EL. Fusion of membranes during fertilization. *J Gen Physiol* 1992;99:137–175.

1223. McCulloh DH, Wall RJ, Levitan H. Fertilization of rabbit ova and the role of ovum investments in the block to polyspermy. *Dev Biol* 1989;120:385–391.

1224. McDonald JK, Kadhodayan S. A latent proteinase in guinea pig sperm. *Biochem Biophys Res Commun* 1988;151:827–835.

1225. McDonald LE, Sampson J. Intraperitoneal insemination of the heifer. *Proc Soc Exp Biol* 1957;95:815–816.

1226. McGaughey RW, Nemiro JS. Correlation of estrogen levels with oocytes aspirated and with pregnancy in a program of clinical tubal transfer. *Fertil Steril* 1987;48:98–106.

1227. McGrath JP, Evenson DP. Circular DNA in human and boar spermatozoa. *Gamete Res* 1982;5:379–393.

1228. McGrath J, Solter D. Completion of mouse embryogenesis requires both the maternal and paternal genomes. *Cell* 1984;37:179–189.

1229. McLaughlin KJ, Davies L, Seamark RF. *In vitro* embryo culture in the production of identical merino lambs by nuclear transplantation. *Reprod Fertil Dev* 1990;2:619–622.

1230. McMaster R, Yanagimachi R, Lopata A. Penetration of human eggs by human spermatozoa *in vitro. Biol Reprod* 1978;19: 212–216.

1231. Meistrich ML, Reid BO, Barcellona WJ. Changes in sperm nuclei during spermatogenesis and epididymal maturation. *Exp Cell Res* 1976;99:72–78.

1232. Meistrich ML, Trostle PK, Brock WA. Association of nucleoprotein transition with chromatin changes during rat spermatogenesis. In: Jagiello G, Vogel HJ, eds. *Bioregulations of Reproduction,* New York: Academic Press; 1981:151–166.

1233. Meizel S, Turner KT. Progesterone acts at the plasma membrane of human sperm. *Mol Cell Endocrinol* 1991;11:R1–R5.

1234. Mendoza C, Carreras A, Moos J, Tesarik J. Distinction between true acrosome reaction and degenerative acrosome loss by a one-step staining method using *Pisum sativum* agglutinin. *J Reprod Fertil* 1992;95:755–763.

1235. Menezes J, Peter J. Role of the vitellus in the block to polyspermy in golden hamster eggs. *Gamete Res* 1985;11:305–309.

1236. Metz CB, Monroy A, eds. *Biology of Fertilization,* Vols. I–III. New York: Academic Press; 1985.

1237. Meyer NL, Longo FJ. Cytological events associated with *in vitro* aged and fertilized rabbit eggs. *Anat Rec* 1979;195:357–374.

1238. Michod RE, Levin BR, eds. *The Evolution of Sex.* Saunderland, Massachusetts: Sinauer Associates; 1987.

1239. Millar SE, Chamow SM, Baur AW, Oliver C, Robey F, Dean J. Vaccination with a synthetic zona pellucida peptide produces long-term contraception in female mice. *Science* 1989;246: 935–938.

1240. Miller CC, Fayrer-Hosken RA, Timmons TM, Lee VH, Caudle AB, Dunbar BS. Characterization of equine zona pellucida glycoproteins by polyacrylamide gel electrophoresis and immunological techniques. *J Reprod Fertil* 1992;96:815–825.

1241. Miller DJ, Ax RL. Carbohydrates and fertilization in animals. *Mol Reprod Dev* 1990;26:184–198.

1242. Miller DJ, Macek MB, Shur BD. Complementarity between sperm surface B-1,4-galactosyltransferase and egg-coat ZP3 mediates sperm–egg binding. *Nature* 1992;357:589–593.

1243. Miller MA, Masui Y. Changes in the stainability and sulfhydryl level in the sperm nucleus during sperm–oocyte interaction in mice. *Gamete Res* 1982;5:167–179.

1244. Miller RL. Sperm chemo-orientation in the metazoa. In: Metz CB, Monroy A, eds. *Biology of Fertilization,* Vol. 2. Orlando: Academic Press; 1985:275–337.

1245. Miller RL. Synthetic peptides are not chemoattractants for bull sperm. *Gamete Res* 1985;5:395–401.

1245a. Minshull J. Cyclin synthesis: who needs it? *BioEssay* 1993;15: 149–155.

1246. Miranda PV, Tezon JG. Characterization of fibronectin as a marker for human epididymal sperm maturation. *Mol Reprod Dev* 1992;33:443–450.

1247. Mirza JA, Shelton WL. Induction of gynogenesis and sex reversal in silver carp. *Aquaculture* 1988;68:1–14.

1248. Miyazaki S. Inositol 1,4,5-trisphosphate-induced calcium release and guanine nucleotide-binding protein-mediated periodic calcium rises in golden hamster eggs. *J Cell Biol* 1988;106:345–353.

1249. Miyazaki S. Signal transduction of sperm-egg interaction causing periodic calcium transients in hamster eggs. In: Naccitelli R, Cherr GN, Clark WH, eds. *Mechanisms of Egg Activation.* New York: Plenum Press; 1989:231–246.

1250. Miyazaki S. Repetitive calcium transients in hamster oocytes. *Cell Calcium* 1991;12:205–216.

1251. Miyazaki S, Igusa Y. Fertilization potential in golden hamster eggs consists of recurring hyperpolarizations. *Nature* 1981;290: 702–704.

1252. Miyazaki S, Igusa Y. Ca-mediated activation of a K current at fertilization of golden hamster eggs. *Proc Natl Acad Sci USA* 1982;79:931–935.

1253. Miyazaki S, Shirakawa H, Nakada K, Honda Y. Essential role of the inositol 1,4,5-triphosphate receptor/Ca^{2+} release channel in Ca^{2+} waves and Ca^{2+} oscillations at fertilization of mammalian eggs. *Dev Biol* 1993;158: [in press].

1254. Miyazaki S, Shirakawa H, Nakada K, Honda Y, Yuzaki M, Nakada S, Mikoshiba K. Antibody to the inositol trisphosphate receptor blocks trimerosal-enhanced Ca^{2+}-induced Ca^{2+} release and Ca^{2+} oscillations in hamster eggs. *FEBS* 1992;309:180–184.

1255. Miyazaki S, Yuzaki M, Nakada K, Shirakawa H, Nakanishi S, Nakada S, Mikoshiba K. Block of Ca^{2+} wave and Ca^{2+} oscillation by antibody to the inositol 1,4,5-trisphosphate receptor in fertilized hamster eggs. *Science* 1992;257:251–255.

1256. Modlinski JA. The role of the zona pellucida in the development of mouse egg *in vivo. J Embryol Exp Morphol* 1970;23:539–547.

1257. Moench GL, Holt H. Microdissection studies on human spermatozoa. *Biol Bull* 1929;56:267–273.

1258. Moghissi KS. Composition and functions of cervical secretion. In: Greep RO, ed. *Handbook of Physiology, Sec. 7, Endocrinology,* Vol. 2. Washington DC: American Physiology Society; 1973:25–48.

1259. Mohri H, Awano M, Ishijima S. Maturation and capacitation of mammalian spermatozoa. In: Yoshinaga K, Mori T, eds. *Development of Preimplantation Embryos and Their Environment.* New York: Alan R. Liss; 1989:53–62.

1260. Mohri H, Ishijima S. Epididymal maturation and motility of mammalian spermatozoa. In: Serio M, ed. *Prospects in Andrology,* New York: Raven Press; 1989:291–298.

1261. Molenaar A, Forrester IT, Bradley MP. The localization of cyclic AMP-dependent protein kinase activity in ram spermatozoa. *Proc. Univ. Otago Med. School,* 1981;59:50–51.

1262. Moller CC, Bleil JD, Kinloch RA, Wassarman PM. Structural and functional relationships between mouse and hamster zona pellucida glycoproteins. *Dev Biol* 1990;137:276–286.

1263. Moller CC, Wassarman PM. Characterization of a proteinase that cleaves zona pellucida glycoprotein ZP2 following activation of mouse eggs. *Dev Biol* 1989;132:103–112.

1264. Monk M. Genomic imprinting. *Genes Dev* 1988;2:921–925.

1265. Moore A, Penfold LM, Johnson JL, Latchman DS, Moore HDM. Human sperm–egg binding is inhibited by peptides corresponding to core region of an acrosomal serine protease inhibitor. *Mol Reprod Dev* 1993;34:280–291.

1266. Moore HDM, Bedford JM. Ultrustructure of the equatorial segment of hamster spermatozoa during penetration of oocytes. *J Ultrastr Res* 1978;62:110–117.

1267. Moore HDM, Hartman TD. Localization by monoclonal antibodies of various surface antigens of hamster spermatozoa and the effect of antibody on fertilization *in vitro. J Reprod Fertil* 1984;70:175–183.

1268. Moore HDM, Smith CA, Hartman TD, Bye AP. Visualization and characterization of the acrosome reaction of human spermatozoa by immunolocalization with monoclonal antibody. *Gamete Res* 1987;17:245–259.

1269. Moore PB, Dedham JR. Calmodulin, a calmodulin acceptor protein, and calcimedins: unique antibody localization in hamster sperm. *J Cell Biol* 1984;25:99–107.

1270. Morales P, Cross NL. A new procedure for determining acrosomal status of very small numbers of human sperm. *J Histochem Cytochem* 1989;129:1291–1292.

1271. Morales P, Overstreet JW, Katz DF. Changes in human sperm motion during capacitation *in vitro. J Reprod Fertil* 1988;83: 119–128.

1272. Mori K, Daitoh T, Irahara M, Kamada M, Aono T. Significance of D-mannose as a sperm receptor site on the zona pellucida in human fertilization. *Am J Obstet Gynecol* 1989;161:207–211.

1273. Mori T, Uchida TA. Ultrastructural observations of fertilization in the Japanese long-fingered bat, *Miniopterus schreibersii fuliginosus. J Reprod Fertil* 1981;63:231–235.

1274. Mori T, Wu GM, Mori E. Expression of CD4-like structure on murine egg vitelline membrane and its signal transductive roles through $p56^{lck}$ in fertilization. *Am J Reprod Immunol* 1991;26:97–103.

1275. Morisawa M, Inoda T, Oda S. Regulation of sperm motility by osmotic pressure. In: Dale B, ed. *Mechanism of Fertilization.* Berlin: Springer-Verlag; 1990:143–154.

1276. Mortillo S, Wassarman PM. Differential binding of gold-labeled zona pellucida glycoproteins mZP2 and mZP3 to mouse sperm membrane compartments. *Development* 1991;113:141–149.

1277. Mortimer D. Sperm transport in the human female reproductive tract. In: Finn CA, ed. *Oxford Review of Reproductive Biology* Vol. 5. Oxford: Oxford University Press; 1983:30–61.

1278. Mortimer D, Leslie EE, Kelly RW, Templeton AA. Morphological selection of human spermatozoa *in vivo* and *in vitro. J Reprod Fertil* 1982;64:391–399.

1279. Moser F. Studies on cortical layer response to stimulating agents in the *Arbacia* eggs. I. Response to insemination. *J Exp Zool* 1939;80:423–446.

1280. Mullins KJ, Seake RG. Study of the functional anatomy of bovine cervical mucosa with special reference to mucus secretion and sperm transport. *Am J Anat* 1989;225:106–117.

1281. Naccitelli R. How do sperm activate eggs? In: Bode HR, eds. *Current Topics in Development Biology,* Vol. 25. Orlando: Academic Press, 1991:1–16.

1282. Naish SJ, Perreault SD, Foehner AL, Zirkin BR. DNA synthesis in the fertilizing hamster sperm nucleus: sperm template availability and egg cytoplasmic control. *Biol Reprod* 1987;36: 245–253.

1283. Naish SJ, Perreault SD, Zirkin BR. DNA synthesis following microinjection of heterologous sperm and somatic cell nuclei into hamster oocytes. *Gamete Res* 1987;18:109–120.

1284. Naito N, Toyoda Y, Yanagimachi R. Production of normal mice from oocytes fertilized and developed without zonae pellucidae. *Hum Reprod* 1992;7:281–285.

1285. Neill JM, Olds-Clark P. A computer-assisted assay for mouse sperm hyperactivation demonstrates that bicarbonate but not bovine serum albumin is required. *Gamete Res* 1987;18: 121–140.

1286. Nestor A, Handel MA. The transport of morphologically abnormal sperm in the female reproductive tract of mice. *Gamete Res* 1984;10:119–125.
1287. Newport J. Nuclear reconstruction *in vitro:* stages of assembly around protein-free DNA. *Cell* 1987;48:205–217.
1288. Newpot JW, Kirschner MW. Regulation of the cell cycle during early Xenopus development. *Cell* 1984;37:731–742.
1289. Ng SC, Bongso A, Ratnam SS, et al. Pregnancy after transfer of sperm under zona. *Lancet* 1988;2:790.
1290. Ng SC, Sathananthan AH, Bongso TA, Ratnam SS, Tok VCM, Ho JKC. Subzonal transfer of multiple sperm (MIST) into early human embryos. *Mol Reprod Dev* 1990;26:253–260.
1291. Nichols J, Gardner RL. Effect of damage to the zona pellucida on development of preimplantation embryos in the mouse. *Hum Reprod* 1989;4:180–187.
1292. Nicolson GN, Yanagimachi R, Yanagimachi H. Ultrastructural localization of lectin-binding sites of the zonae pellucidae and plasma membranes of mammalian eggs. *J Cell Biol* 1975;66: 263–274.
1293. Nicosia SV, Wolf DP, Inoue M. Cortical granule distribution and cell surface characteristics in mouse eggs. *Dev Biol* 1977;57:56–74.
1294. Nikolajczyk BS, O'Rand MG. Characterization of rabbit testis B-galactosidase and arylsulfatase A: purification and localization in spermatozoa during the acrosome reaction. *Biol Reprod* 1992;46:366–378.
1295. Noguchi S, Nakano M. Structure of the acidic N-linked carbohydrate chains of the 55-kDa glycoprotein family (PZP3) from porcine zona pellucida. *Eur J Biochem* 1992;209:883–894.
1296. Noland TD, Van Eldik LJ, Garbers DL, Burgess WH. Distribution of calmodulin and calmodulin-binding proteins in membranes from bovine spermatozoa. *Gamete Res* 1985;11: 297–303.
1297. Nonchev S, Tsanev R. Protamine-histone replacement and DNA replication in the male mouse pronucleus. *Mol Reprod Dev* 1990;25:72–76.
1298. Noyes RW. Fertilizing capacity of spermatozoa. *Western J Surg Obstet Gynecol* 1953;61:342–349.
1299. Nurse P. Universal control mechanism regulating onset of M-phase. *Nature* 1990;344:503–507.
1300. O'Brien DA, Bellve AR. Protein constituents of the mouse spermatozoon. *Dev Biol* 1980;75:386–404.
1301. Oehninger S, Burkman LJ, Coddington CC, Acosta AA, Scott R, Hodgen GD, Franken DA. Hemizona assay: assessment of sperm dysfunction and prediction of *in vitro* fertilization outcome. *Fertil Steril* 1989;51:665–670.
1302. Oehninger S, Clark GF, Fulgham D, Blackmore PF, Mahony MC, Acosta AA, and Hodgen GD. Effect of fucoidin on human sperm–zona pellucida interaction. *J Androl* 1992;13:519–525.
1303. Oehninger S, Franken DR, Scott RT, Acosta AA, Coddington CC, Hodgen GD. Validation of the hemizona assay in a monkey model: influence of oocyte maturational stages. *Fertil Steril* 1989;51:881–885.
1304. Ogura A, Yanagimachi R. Round spermatid nuclei injected into hamster oocytes form pronuclei and participate in syngamy. *Biol Reprod* 1993;48:219–225.
1304a. Ogura A, Yanagimachi R, Usui N. Behaviour of hamster and mouse round spermatid nuclei incorporated into mature oocytes by electrofusion. *Zygote* 1993;1:1–8.
1305. Ohnishi S. Fusion of viral envelopes with cellular membranes. In: Bronner F, ed. *Current Topics in Membrane and Transport,* Vol. 32. San Diego: Academic Press; 1988:257–296.
1306. Ohsumi K, Katagiri C. Characterization of the ooplasmic factor inducing decondensation of and protamine removal from toad sperm nuclei: involvement of nucleoplasmin. *Dev Biol* 1991;148:295–305.
1307. Ohsumi K, Katagiri C, Yanagimachi R. Human sperm nuclei can transform into condensed chromosomes in Xenopus egg extracts. *Gamete Res* 1988;20:1–9.
1308. Oikawa T, Nicolson GL, Yanagimachi R. Inhibition of hamster fertilization by phytoagglutinins. *Exp Cell Res* 1974;83: 239–246.
1309. Oikawa T, Nicolson GL, Yanagimachi R. Trypsin-mediated modification of the zona pellucida glycopeptide structure of hamster eggs. *J Reprod Fertil* 1974;43:133–136.
1310. Oikawa T, Sendai Y, Kurata S, Yanagimachi R. A glycoprotein of oviductal origin alters biochemical properties of the zona pellucida of hamster egg. *Gamete Res* 1988;19:113–122.
1311. Oikawa T, Yanagimachi R. Block of hamster fertilization by anti-ovary antibody. *J Reprod Fertil* 1975;45:487–494.
1312. Okabe M, Matzno S, Nagira M, Mimura T, Kawai Y, Mayumi T. A human sperm antigen possibly involved in binding and/or fusion with zona-free hamster eggs. *Fertil Steril* 1990;54: 1121–1126.
1313. Okabe M, Yagasaki M, Matzno S, Nagira M, Kohama Y, Mimura T. Glucosamine enhanced sperm–egg binding but inhibited sperm–egg fusion in mouse. *Experientia* 1989;45:193–194.
1314. Okabe M, Yagasaki M, Oda H, Matzno S, Kohama Y, Mimura T. Effect of a monoclonal anti-mouse sperm antibody (OBF 13) on the interaction of mouse sperm with zona-free mouse and hamster eggs. *J Reprod Immunol* 1988;13:211–219.
1315. Okabe M, Ying X, Nagira M, Ikawa M, Kohama Y, Mimura T, Tanaka K. Homology of an acrosome-reacted sperm-specific antigen to CD46. *J Pharmacobio-Dyn.,* 1992;15:455–459.
1316. Okamura N, Tanba M, Fukuda A, Sugita Y, Nagai T. Forskolin stimulates porcine sperm capacitation by increasing calcium uptake. *FEBS* 1993;316:283–286.
1317. Olds-Clarke P. Sperm from $t^{w32}/+$ mice: capacitation is normal, but hyperactivation is premature and nonhyperactivated sperm are slow. *Dev Biol* 1989;131:475–482.
1318. Olds-Clarke P. Variation in the quality of sperm motility and its relationship to capacitation. In: Bavister B, Cummins J, Roldan E, eds. *Fertilization in Mammals.* Norwell, Massachusetts: Serono Symposia USA; 1990:91–99.
1319. Olds-Clarke P. The genetics of sperm function in fertilization. *Ann NY Acad Sci* 1991;637:474–485.
1320. Olds-Clarke P, Johnson LR. t Haplotypes in the mouse compromise sperm flagellar function. *Dev Biol* 1993;155:14–25.
1321. Olds-Clarke P, Sego R. Calcium alters capacitation and progressive motility of uterine spermatozoa from +/+ and congenic $t^{w32}/+$ mice. *Biol Reprod* 1992;47:629–635.
1322. Oliphant G. Removal of sperm-bound seminal plasma components as a prerequisite to induction of the rabbit acrosome reaction. *Fertil Steril* 1976;27:28–38.
1323. Oliphant G, Brackett BG. Immunological assessment of surface changes of rabbit sperm undergoing capacitation. *Biol Reprod* 1973;9:404–414.
1324. Oliphant G, Reynolds AB, Thomas TS. Sperm surface components involved in the control of the acrosome reaction. *Am J Anat* 1985;174:269–289.
1325. Olson GE, Lifsics MR, Winfrey VP, Rifkin JM. Modification of the rat sperm flagellar plasma membrane during maturation in the epididymis. *J Androl* 1987;8:129–147.
1326. Olson GE, Winfrey VP. Characterization of postacrosomal sheath of bovine spermatozoa. *Gamete Res* 1988;20:329–342.
1327. Onodera M, Tsunoda Y. Parthenogenetic activation of mouse and rabbit eggs by electric stimulation *in vitro. Gamete Res* 1989;22:277–283.
1328. Oprescu S, Thibault C. Duplication de l'and dans les oeufs de lapine apres la fecondation. *Ann Biol Anim Biochem Biophys* 1965;5:151–156.
1329. O'Rand MG. The presence of sperm-specific surface isoantigens on the egg following fertilization. *J Exp Zool* 1977;202: 267–273.
1330. O'Rand MG. Sperm–egg recognition and barriers to interspecies fertilization. *Gamete Res* 1988;19:315–328.
1331. O'Rand MG, Widgren EE, Fisher SJ. Characterization of the rabbit sperm membrane autoantigen, RSA, as lectin-like zona binding protein. *Dev Biol* 1988;129:231–240.
1332. Oshio S, Kanako S, Mohri H. Impurities in commercial preparations of bovine serum albumin inhibits the acrosome reaction of hamster spermatozoa. *Zool Sci* 1986;3:295–299.
1333. Osman RA, Andria M, Jones D, Meizel S. Steroid induced exocytosis: the human sperm acrosome reaction. *Biochem Biophys Res Commun* 1989;160:828–833.
1334. Overstreet JW. Transport of gametes in the reproductive tract of the female mammal. In: Hartmann JF, ed. *Mechanism Controlling Animal Fertilization.* New York: Academic Press; 1983:499–543.
1335. Overstreet JW, Cooper GW. The time and location of the acro-

some reaction during sperm transport in the female rabbit. *J Exp Zool* 1979;209:97–102.

1336. Overstreet JW, Hembree WC. Penetration of the zona pellucida of nonliving human oocytes by human spermatozoa *in vitro. Fertil Steril* 1976;27:815–831.

1337. Ozil JP. The parthenogenetic development of rabbit oocytes after repetitive pulsatile electrical stimulation. *Development* 1990;109:117–127.

1338. Palermo G, Van Steirteghem A. Enhancement of acrosome reaction and subzonal insemination of a single spermatozoon in mouse eggs. *Mol Reprod Dev* 1991;30:339–345.

1339. Palmer DK, O'Day K, Margolis RL. The centromere specific histone CENP-A is selectively retained in discrete foci in mammalian sperm nuclei. *Chromosoma* 1990;100:32–36.

1340. Pang SC, Williams DB, Huang T, Wang C. Effects of pentoxifylline on sperm motility and hyperactivated motility *in vitro:* a preliminary report. *Fertil Steril* 1993;59:465–467.

1341. Parisel CC, Weinman JS, Escaig FT, Guyot MY, Iftode FC, Weinmam SJ, Damaille JG. Analytical subcellular distribution of cAMP-dependent protein kinase activity in bull spermatozoa. *Gamete Res* 1984;10:433–444.

1342. Parks JE, Ehrenwald E. Cholesterol efflux from mammalian sperm and its potential role in capacitation. In: Bavister BD, ed. *Fertilization in Mammals.* Norwell, Massachusetts: Serono Symposia USA; 1990:155–167.

1343. Parrish JJ, Susko-Parrish J, Winer MA, First NL. Capacitation of bovine sperm by heparin. *Biol Reprod* 1988;38:1171–1188.

1344. Parry RV, Baker PJ, Jones R. Characterization of low Mr zona pellucida binding proteins from boar spermatozoa and seminal plasma. *Mol Reprod Dev* 1992;33:108–115.

1345. Paterson M, Aitken RJ. Development of vaccines targeting the zona pellucida. *Current Opin Immunol* 1990;2:743–747.

1346. Paterson M, Koothan PT, Morris KD, O'Byrne KT, Braude P, Williams A, Aitken RJ. Analysis of the contraceptive potential of antibodies against native and deglycosylated procine ZP3 *in vivo* and *in vitro. Biol Reprod* 1992;46:523–534.

1347. Pavlok A, Travnik P, Kopecny V, Stastna J. Fusion of hamster and pig zona-free eggs stimulated by boar and guinea pig sperm at fertilization *in vitro. Gamete Res* 1982;6:189–197.

1348. Pellicciari C, Hosokawa Y, Fukuda M, Manfredi Romanini MG. Cytofluorometric study of nuclear sulphydryl and disulphide goups during sperm maturation in the mouse. *J Reprod Fertil* 1983;68:371–376.

1349. Pellicciari C, Redi CA, Garagna S, Fukuda M, Romanini GM. Cytochemical patterns of mouse sperm chromatin during the passage along the female genital tract. *Acta Histochem Cytochem* 1984;17:51–58.

1350. Perreault SD. Regulation of sperm nuclear reactivation during fertilization. In: Bavister BD, Cummins J, Roldan ERS, eds. *Fertilization in Mammals,* Norwell, Massachusetts: Serono Sympsia USA; 1990:285–296.

1351. Perreault SD, Barbee RR, Elstein K, Zucker RM, Keefer CL. Interspecies differences in the stability of mammalian sperm nuclei assessed *in vivo* by sperm microinjection and *in vitro* by flow cytometry. *Biol Reprod* 1988;39:157–167.

1352. Perreault SD, Barbee RR, Slott VL. Importance of glutathione in the acquisition and maintenance of sperm nuclear decondensing activity in maturing hamster oocytes. *Dev Biol* 1988;125:181–186.

1353. Perreault SD, Naish ST, Zirkin BR. The timing of hamster sperm nuclear decondensation and male pronucleus formation is related to sperm nuclear disulfide bond content. *Biol Reprod* 1987;36:239–244.

1354. Pessot CA, Brito M, Figueroa J, Concha II, Yanez A, Burzio LO. Presence of RNA in the sperm nucleus. *Biochem Biophys Res Commun* 1989;158:272–278.

1355. Peterson RN, Hunt WP. Identification, isolation, and properties of a plasma membrane protein involved in the adhesion of boar sperm to the procine zona pellucida. *Gamete Res* 1989;23:103–118.

1356. Peterson RN, Russel LD, Hunt WP. Evidence for specific binding of uncapacitated boar spermatozoa to porcine zonae pellucidae *in vitro. J Exp Zool* 1984;231:137–147.

1357. Peterson RN, Russell LD, Spaulding G, Bundman D, Buchanan J, Freund M. Electrophoretic and chromatographic properties of boar sperm plasma membranes: antigen and polypeptides with affinity for isolated zonae pellucidae. *J Androl* 1981;2:300–311.

1358. Phelps BM, Koppel DE, Primakoff P, Myles DG. Evidence that proteolysis of the surface is an initial step in the mechanism of formation of sperm cell surface domains. *J Cell Biol* 1990;111:1839–1847.

1359. Phelps BM, Myles DG. The guinea pig sperm plasma membrane protein, pH-20, reaches the surface via two transport pathways and becomes localized to a domain after an initial uniform distribution. *Dev Biol* 1987;123:63–72.

1360. Phillips DM. Comparative analysis of mammalian sperm motility. *J Cell Biol* 1972;53:561–573.

1361. Phillips DM. Structure and function of zona pellucida. In: Familiari G, Makabe S, Motta PM, eds. *Ultrastructure of the Ovary,* The Hague: Kluwer Academic Publisher; 1991:63–72.

1362. Phillips DM. Electron microscopy of mammalian fertilization. In: Wassarman PM, ed. *Elements of Mammalian Fertilization,* Vol. 1. Boca Raton, Florida: CRC Press; 1991:249–267.

1363. Phillips DM, Jones R, Shalgi R. Alterations in distribution of surface and intracellular antigens during epididymal maturation in rat spermatozoa. *Mol Reprod Dev* 1991;29:347–356.

1364. Phillips DM, Shalgi R. Surface architecture of the mouse and hamster zona pellucida and oocyte. *J Ultrast Res* 1980;72:1–12.

1365. Phillips DM, Yanagimachi R. Difference in the manner of association of acrosome-intact and acrosome-reacted hamster spermatozoa with egg microvilli as revealed by scanning electron microscopy. *Dev Growth Diff* 1982;24:543–551.

1366. Phillips DM, Zacharopoulos VR, Perotti ME. Structure of the cumulus oophorus at the time of fertilization. *Cell Tissue Res* 1990;261:249–259.

1367. Philpott A, Leno GH. Nucleoplasmin remodels sperm chromatin in Xenopus egg extracts. *Cell* 1992;69:759–767.

1368. Philpott A, Leno GH, Laskey RA. Sperm decondensation in Xenopus egg cytoplasm is mediated by neucleo-plasmin. *Cell* 1991;65:569–578.

1369. Philpott CC, Ringuette MJ, Dean J. Oocyte-specific expression and developmental regulation of ZP3, the sperm receptor of the mouse zona pellucida. *Dev Biol* 1987;121:568–575.

1370. Pickering SJ, Johnson MH, Braude PR, Houliston E. Cytoskeletal organization in fresh, aged and spontaneously activated human oocytes. *Hum Reprod* 1988;3:978–989.

1371. Piko L. Gamete structure and sperm entry in mammals. In: Metz CB, Monroy A, eds. *Fertilization* Vol. 2. New York: Academic Press; 1969:325–403.

1372. Pillai MC, Meizel S. Trypsin inhibitors prevent the progesterone-initiated increase in intracellular calcium required for the human sperm acrosome reaction. *J Exp Zool* 1991;258:384–393.

1373. Plachot M, Junca A, Mandelbaum J, Cohen J, Salat-Baroux J, Da Lage C. Timing of *in vitro* fertilization of cumulus-free and cumulus-enclosed human oocytes. *Hum Reprod* 1986;1:237–242.

1374. Poccia D. Remodeling of nucleoproteins during gametogenesis, fertilization, and early development. *Int Rev Cytol* 1986;105:1–65.

1375. Pogany GC, Balhorn R. Quantitative fluorometry of abnormal mouse sperm nuclei. *J Reprod Fertil* 1992;96:25–34.

1376. Pollard JW, Plante C, King WA, Hansen PJ, Betteridge KJ, Suarez SS. Fertilizing capacity of bovine sperm may be maintained by binding to the oviductal epithelial cells. *Biol Reprod* 1991;44:102–107.

1377. Pomeroy KO, Dodds JF, Seidel GE. Caffeine promotes *in vitro* fertilization of mouse ova within 15 minutes. *J Exp Zool* 1988;248:207–212.

1378. Ponce RH, Yanagimachi R, Urch UA, Yamagata T, Ito M. Retention of hamster oolemma fusibility with spermatozoa after various enzyme treatments: a search for the molecules involved in sperm–egg fusion. *Zygotes* 1993; in press.

1379. Prather RS, Schatten G. Construction of the nuclear matrix at the transition from maternal to zygotic control of development in the mouse: an immunocytochemical study. *Mol Reprod Dev* 1992;32:203–208.

1380. Primakoff P, Cowan A, Hyatt H, Tredick-Kline J, Myles DG. Purification of the guinea pig sperm pH-20 antigen and detec-

tion of a site-specific endoproteolytic activity in sperm preparations that cleaves pH-20 into two disulfide-linked fragments. *Biol Reprod* 1988;38:921–934.
1381. Primakoff P, Hyatt H, Myles DG. A role for the migrating sperm surface antigen pH-20 in guinea pig sperm binding to the egg zona pellucida. *J Cell Biol* 1985;101:2239–2244.
1382. Primakoff P, Hyatt H, Tredick-Kline J. Identification and purification of a sperm surface protein with a potential role in sperm–egg membrane fusion. *J Cell Biol* 1987;104:141–149.
1383. Primakoff P, Lathrop W, Woolman L, Cowan A, Myles D. Fully effective contraception in male and female guinea pig immunized with the sperm protein pH-20. *Nature* 1988;335:543–546.
1384. Prochazka R, Kanka J, Sutovsky P, Fulka J, Motlik J. Development of pronuclei in pig oocytes activation by a single electric pulse. *J Reprod Fertil* 1992;96:725–734.
1385. Putney RW. Inositol phosphates and calcium entry. In: Putney PW Jr, ed. *Inositol Phosphate and Calcium Signalling,* New York: Raven Press; 1992:143–160.
1386. Quillet E, Garcia P, Guyomard R. Analysis of the production of all homozygous lines of rainbow trout by gynogenesis. *J Exp Zool* 1991;257:367–374.
1387. Quinn P, Kerin JF, Warnes GM. Improved pregnancy rate in human *in vitro* fertilization with the use of a medium based on the composition of human tubal fluid. *Fertil Steril* 1985;44: 493–498.
1388. Quinn P, Stanger JD. Fertilization of pronase-treated mouse ova *in vitro. Aust J Biol Sci* 1981;34:245–248.
1389. Ralt D, Goldenberg M, Petterolf P, et al. Sperm attraction to a follicular factor(s) correlates with human egg fertilizability. *Proc Natl Acad Sci USA* 1991;88:2840–2844.
1390. Rankin TL, Tsuruta KJ, Holland MK, Griswold MD, Orgebin-Crist MC. Isolation, immunolocalization, and sperm-association of three proteins of 18, 25, and 29 killodaltons secreted by the mouse epididymis. *Biol Reprod* 1992;46:747–766.
1391. Ratan RR, Shelanski ML, Maxfield FR. Transition from metaphase to anaphase is accompanied by local changes in cytoplasmic free calcium in ptK2 kidney epithalial cells. *Proc Natl Acad Sci USA* 1986;83:5136–5140.
1392. Ravnik SE, Albers JJ, Muller CH. A novel view of albumin-supported sperm capacitation: role of lipid transfer protein-I. *Fertil Steril* 1993;59:629–638.
1393. Ravnik SE, Muller CH. Relationship between support of human sperm capacitation and lipid transfer activity among different albumin preparations. *J Androl* 1989;10:21a(abst 11).
1394. Ravnik SE, Zarutskie PW, Muller CH. Lipid transfer activity in human follicular fluid: relation to human sperm capacitation. *J Androl* 1990;11:216–226.
1395. Ravnik SE, Zarutskie PW, Muller CH. Purification and characterization of a human follicular fluid lipid transfer protein that stimulates human sperm capacitation. *Biol Reprod* 1992;47: 1126–1133.
1396. Redi CA, Garagna S, Pellicciari C, Romanini MGM, Capanna E, Winking H, Gropp A. Spermatozoa of chromosomally heterozygous mice and their fate in male and female genital tracts. *Gamete Res* 1984;9:273–286.
1397. Reima I, Lehtonen E. Localization of nonerythroid spectrin and actin in mouse oocytes and preimplantation embryos. *Differentiation* 1985;30:68–75.
1398. Repin VS, Akimova IM. The microelectrophoretic analysis of protein patterns of mammalian oocytes and zygotes zona pellucide. *Biokimia (USSR)* 1976;41:50–57.
1399. Reuter LM, O'Day-Bowman MB, Mavrogianis PA, Verhage HG. Association of a human oviduct-specific glycoprotein (HOGP) with hamster and human ovarian oocytes, but not with human sperm during *in vitro* incubation. *Biol Reprod* 1992:46(Suppl 1):78.
1400. Reyes R, Rosado A, Hernandez O, Delgado NM. Heparin and glutathion: physiological decondensing agentes of human sperm nuclei. *Gamete Res* 1989;23:39–47.
1401. Reynolds AB, Thomas TS, Wilson WL, Oliphant G. Concentration of acrosome stabilizing factor (ASF) in rabbit epididymal fluid and species-specificity of anti-ASF antibodies. *Biol Reprod* 1989;40:673–680.
1402. Rhim SH, Millar SE, Robey F, et al. Autoimmune disease of the ovary induced by a Zp3 peptide from the mouse zona pellucida. *J Clin Invest* 1992;89:28–35.
1403. Ribbes H, Plantavid M, Bennet PJ, Chap H, Douste-Blazy L. Phospholipase C from human sperm specific phosphoinositides. *Biochim Biophys Acta* 1987;919:245–254.
1404. Richards JM, Witkin SS. A nuclear DNA polymerase in bull spermatozoa. *J Reprod Fertil* 1978;54:43–47.
1405. Richardson RT, Nikolajcyzk BS, Abdullah LH, Beavers JC, O'Rand MG. Localization of rabbit sperm acrosin during the acrosome reaction induced by immobilized zona matrix. *Biol Reprod* 1991;45:20–26.
1406. Rickords LF, White KL. Electrofusion-induced intracellular Ca^{2+} flux and its effect on murine oocyte activation. *Mol Reprod Dev* 1992;31:152–159.
1407. Rickords LF, White KL. Electroporation of inositol 1,4,5-triphosphate induces repetitive calcium oscillations in murine oocytes. *J Exp Zool* 1993;265:178–184.
1408. Rigoni F, Dell'Antone P, Deana R. Evidence for a pH-driven Ca^{2+} uptake in EGTA-treated bovine spermatozoa. *Eur J Biochem* 1987;169:417–422.
1409. Ringuette MJ, Chamberlin ME, Baur AW, Sobieski DA, Dean J. Molecular analysis of cDNA coding for ZP3, a sperm binding protein of the mouse zona pellucida. *Dev Biol* 1988;127: 287–295.
1410. Robinson R, Richardson R, Hinds K, Clayton D, Poirier GR. Features of a seminal proteinase inhibitor—zona pellucida—binding component on murine spermatozoa. *Gamete Res* 1987;16:217–228.
1411. Rochwerger L, Cohen DJ, Cuasnicu PS. Mammalian sperm–egg fusion: The rat egg has complementary sites for a sperm protein that mediates gamete fusion. *Dev Biol* 1992;153:83–90.
1412. Rochwerger L, Cuasnicu P. Redistribution of a rat epididymal glycoprotein after *in vitro* and *in vivo* capacitation. *Mol Reprod Dev* 1992;31:34–41.
1413. Rogers BJ, Bastias C, Coulson RL, Russell L. Cytochalasin D inhibits penetration of hamster eggs by guinea pig and human spermatozoa. *J Androl* 1989;10:275–282.
1414. Rogers BJ, Ueno M, Yanagimachi R. Fertilization by guinea pig spermatozoa requires potassium ions. *Biol Reprod* 1981;25: 639–648.
1415. Roldan ERS, Fleming AD. Is a Ca^{2+}-ATPase involved in Ca^{2+} regulation during capacitation and the acrosome reaction of guinea-pig spermatozoa? *J Reprod Fertil* 1989;85:297–308.
1416. Roldan ERS, Harrison RAP. The absence of active protein kinase C in ram spermatozoa. *Biochem Biophys Res Commun* 1988;155:901–906.
1417. Roldan ERS, Harrison RAP. Molecular mechanisms leading to exocytosis during the sperm acrosome reaction. In: Bavister BD, Cummins J, Roldan ERS, eds. *Fertilization in Mammals.* Norwell, Massachusetts: Serono Symposia USA; 1990:179–196.
1418. Roldan ERS, Mollinedo F. Diacylglycerol stimulates the C^{2+}-dependent phospholipase A_2 of ram spermatozoa. *Biochem Biophys Res Commun* 1991;176:294–300.
1419. Roldan ERS, Yanagimachi R. Cross-fertilization between syrian and chinese hamster. *J Exp Zool* 1989;250:321–328.
1420. Roller RJ, Kinloch RA, Hiraoka BY, Li SS-L, Wassarman PM. Gene expression during mammalian oogenesis and early embryogenesis: quantification of three messenger RNAs abundant in fully grown mouse. *Development* 1989;106:251–261.
1421. Roomans GM, Afzelius BA. Acrosome reaction in human sperm. *J Submicrosc Cytol* 1975;7:61–69.
1422. Rosiere TK, Wassarman PM. Identification of a region mouse zona pellucida glycoprotein mZP3 that possesses sperm receptor activity. *Dev Biol* 1992;154:309–317.
1423. Rotem R, Paz GF, Homonnai ZT, Kalina M, Naor Z. Protein kinase C is present in human sperm: possible role in flagellar motility. *Proc Natl Acad Sci* 1990;87:7305–7308.
1423a. Rotem R, Paz GF, Homonnai ZT, Kalina M, Lax J, Breitbart H, Naor Z. Ca^{2+}-independent induction of acrosome reaction by protein kinase C in human sperm. *Endocrinology* 1992;131:2235–2243.
1424. Roux M, Kan FWK. Changes in glycoconjugate contents of the zona pellucida during growth and development in the golden

hamster: a quantitative cytochemical study. *Anat Rec* 1991;203:347–360.
1425. Rowland IW. Insemination of the guinea-pig by intraperitoneal injection. *J Endocrinol* 1957;16:98–106.
1426. Roy AC, Ratnam SS. Biosynthesis of prostaglandins by human spermatozoa *in vitro* and their role in acrosome reaction and fertilization. *Mol Reprod Dev* 1992;33:303–306.
1427. Royere D, Hamamah S, Nicolle JC, Lansac J. Etude de l'etat de la chromattine des spermatocoides humains de la capacitation *in vitro*. *Contracep Fertil Sex* 1988;16:559–561.
1428. Rubinstein S, Breitbart H. Role of spermine in mammalian sperm capacitation and acrosome reaction. *Biochem J* 1991;278:25–28.
1429. Rufas O, Shalgi R. Maturation-associated changes in the rat zona pellucida. *Mol Reprod Dev* 1990;26:324–330.
1430. Ruknudin A, Silver IA. Ca^{2+} uptake during capacitation of mouse spermatozoa and the effect of an anion transport inhibitor on Ca^{2+} uptake. *Mol Reprod Dev* 1990;26:63–68.
1431. Russell L, Peterson RN, Freund M. On the presence of bridges linking the inner and outer acrosomal membranes of boar spermatozoa. *Anat Rec* 1980;198:449–459.
1432. Sacco AG. Zona pellucida: current status as a candidate antigen for contraceptive vaccine development. *Am J Reprod Immunol Microbiol* 1987;15:122–130.
1433. Sagata N, Watanabe N, Van de Woude GF, Ikawa Y. The c-mos proto-oncogen product is a cytostatic factor responsible for meiotic arrest in vertebrate eggs. *Nature* 1989;342:512–518.
1434. Saling PM. Mammalian sperm interaction with extracellular matrices of the egg. In: Milligan SR, ed. *Oxford Review of Reproductive Biology,* Vol. II. Oxford: Oxford University Press; 1989:339–388.
1435. Saling PM. How the egg regulates sperm function during gamete interaction: facts and fantasies. *Biol Reprod* 1991;44:246–251.
1436. Saling PM, Irons G, Waibel R. Mouse sperm antigens that participate in fertilization. I. Inhibition of sperm fusion with the egg plasma membrane using monoclonal antibodies. *Biol Reprod* 1985;33:515–526.
1437. Saling PM, Lakoski KA. Mouse sperm antigens that participate in fertilization. II. Inhibition of sperm penetration through the zona pellucida using monoclonal antibodies. *Biol Reprod* 1985;33:527–536.
1438. Saling PM, Raines LM, O'Rand MG. Monoclonal antibody against mouse sperm blocks a specific event in the fertilization process. *J Exp Zool* 1983;227:481–486.
1439. Saling PM, Storey BT, Wolf DP. Calcium-dependent binding of mouse epididymal spermatozoa to the zona pellucida. *Dev Biol* 1978;65:515–525.
1440. Salzmann GS, Greve JM, Roller R, Wassarman PM. Biosynthesis of the sperm receptor during oogenesis in the mouse. *EMBO J* 1983;2:1451–1456.
1441. Sanchez R, Topfer-Petersen E, Aitken RJ, Schill WB. A new method for evaluation of the acrosome reaction in viable human spermatozoa. *Andrologia* 1991;23:197–203.
1442. Sanz L, Calvete JJ, Mann K, et al. The complete primary structure of the spermadhesion AWN, a zona pellucida-binding protein isolated from boar spermatozoa. *FEBS* 1992;300:213–219.
1443. Sanz L, Calvete JJ, Schafer W, Mann K, Topfer-Petersen E. Isolation and biochemical characterization of two isoforms of a boar sperm zona pellucida-binding protein. *Biochim Biophys Acta* 1992;1119:127–132.
1444. Sathananthan AH, Kola I, Osborne J, Trounson A, Bongso A, Ratnam SS. Centrioles in the beginning of human development. *Proc Natl Acad Sci USA* 1991;88:4806–4810.
1445. Sathananthan AH, Trounson AO. Ultrastructure of cortical granule release and zona interaction in monospermic and polyspermic human ova fertilized *in vitro*. *Gamete Res* 1982;6: 225–234.
1445a. Sathananthan AH, Trounson AO. The human pronuclear ovum: fine structure of monospermic and polyspermic fertilization *in vitro*. *Gamete Res* 1985;12:385–398.
1446. Sato K. Polyspermy-preventing mechanisms in mouse eggs fertilized *in vitro* (1). *J Exp Zool* 1979;210:353–359.
1447. Schatten G, Hulser D. Timing the early events during sea urchin fertilization. *Dev Biol* 1983;100:244–248.
1448. Schatten G, Maul GG, Schatten H, Chaly N, Simerly C, Balczon R, Brown DL. Nuclear lamins and peripheral nuclear antigens during fertilization and embryogenesis in mice and sea urchins. *Proc Natl Acad Sci USA* 1985;82:4727–4731.
1449. Schatten G, Schatten H. Cytoskeletal alterations and nuclear architectural changes during mammalian fertilization. In: McLaren A, Siracusa G, eds. *Current Topics in Developmental Biology,* Vol. 23. San Diego: Academic Press; 1987:23–53.
1450. Schatten G, Simerly C, Palmer DK, Margolis RL, Maul G, Andrews BS, Schatten H. Kinetochore appearance during meiosis, fertilization and meitosis in mouse oocytes and zygotes. *Chromosoma* 1988;96:341–352.
1451. Schatten G, Simerly C, Schatten H. Maternal inheritance of centrosomes in mammals? Studies on parthenogenesis and polyspermy in mice. *Proc Natl Acad Sci USA* 1991;88:6785–6789.
1452. Schatten H, Cheney R, Balczon R, Willard M, Cline C, Simerly C, Schatten G. Localization of fodrin during fertilization and early development of sea-urchins and mice. *Dev Biol* 1986;118:457–466.
1453. Schatten H, Schatten G, eds. *The Cellular Biology of Fertilization.* New York: Academic Press; 1989.
1454. Schatten H, Schatten G, eds. *The Molecular Biology of Fertilization.* New York: Academic Press; 1989.
1454a. Schatten H, Simerly C, Maul G, Schatten G. Microtubule assembly is required for the formation of the pronuclei, nuclear lamin acquisition, and DNA synthesis during mouse, but not sea urchin, fertilization. *Gamete Res* 1989;23:309–322.
1455. Schirren CG, Holstein AF, Schirren C. Ueber die morphgense rund koepfiger spermatozoen des menschen. *Andrologia* 1971;3:117–125.
1456. Schmell ED, Gulyas BJ. Ovoperoxidase activity in ionophore treated mouse eggs. II. Evidence for the enzyme's role in hardening the zona pellucida. *Gamete Res* 1980;3:279–290.
1457. Schmell ED, Gulyas BJ. Mammalian sperm–egg recognition and binding *in vitro*. I. *Biol Reprod* 1980;23:1075–1085.
1458. Schmiady H, Kentenich H. Premature chromosome condensation after *in vitro* fertilization. *Hum Reprod* 1989;4:689–695.
1459. Schmiady H, Sperling K, Kentenich SH, Stauber M. Prematurely condensed human sperm chromosomes after *in vitro* fertilization (IVF). *Hum Genet* 1986;74:441–443.
1460. Schmidt T, Patten C, Epel D. Is there a role for the calcium influx during fertilization of the sea urchin egg? *Dev Biol* 1982;90:284–290.
1461. Schoysman RJ, Bedford JM. The role of the human epididymis in sperm maturation and sperm storage as reflected in the consequences of epididymovasectomy. *Fertil Steril* 1986;46:293–299.
1462. Schroeder AC, Schultz RM, Kopf GS, Taylor FR, Becker RB, Eppig JJ. Fetuin inhibits zona pellucida hardening and conversion of ZP2 to $ZP2_f$ during spontaneous mouse oocyte maturation *in vitro* in the absence of serum. *Biol Reprod* 1990;43: 891–897.
1463. Schuel H. Secretory functions of egg cortical granules in fertilization and development: a critical review. *Gamete Res* 1978;1:299–382.
1464. Schuel H. Functions of egg cortical granules. In: Metz CB, Monroy A, eds. *Biology of Fertilization,* Vol. 3. Orlando: Academic Press; 1985:1–43.
1465. Schuetz AW, Dubin NH. Progesterone and prostaglandin secretion by ovulated rat cumulus cell–oocyte complexes. *Endocrinology* 1981;108:457–463.
1466. Schwartz R, Brooks W, Zinsser HH. Evidence for chemotaxis as a factor in sperm motility. *Fertil Steril* 1958;9:300–308.
1467. Schwoebel E, Prasad S, Timmons TM. Isolation and characterization of a full-length cDNA encoding the 55-kDa rabbit zona pellucida protein. *J Biol Chem* 1991;266:7214–7219.
1468. Schwoebel ED, Vandevoort CA, Lee VH, Lo YK, Dunbar BS. Molecular analysis of the antigenicity and immunogenicity of recombinant zona pellucida antigens in a primate model. *Biol Reprod* 1992;47:857–865.
1469. Seki N, Toyama Y, Nagano T. Changes in the distribution of filipin-sterol complexes in the boar sperm head plasma membrane during epididymal maturation and in the uterus. *Anat Rec* 1992;232:221–230.
1470. Seligman J, Shalgi R, Oschry Y, Kosower NS. Sperm analysis by

flow cytometry using the fluorescent thiol labeling agent monobromobimane. *Mol Reprod Dev* 1991;29:276–281.
1471. Sellens MH, Jenkinson EJ. Premeability of the mouse zona pellucida to immunoglobulin. *J Reprod Fertil* 1975;42:153–157.
1472. Sengoku K, Ishikawa M, Shibata S, Shimizu T. Oxygen tension of preimplantation hamster embryos. *Acta Obstet Gynecol (Japan)* 1986;38:1727–1732.
1473. Shabanowitz RB, O'Rand MG. Characterization of the human zona pellucida from fertilized and unfertilized eggs. *J Reprod Fertil* 1988;82:151–161.
1474. Shalgi R, Matityahn A, Gaunt SJ, Jones R. Antigens on rat spermatozoa with a potential role in fertilization. *Mol Reprod Dev* 1990;25:286–296.
1475. Shalgi R, Matityahn A, Nobel L. The role of carbohydrates in sperm-egg interaction in rats. *Biol Reprod* 1986;34:446–452.
1476. Shalgi R, Phillips DM. Sperm penetration into rat ova fertilized *in vitro*. *J Androl* 1982;3:382–387.
1477. Shalgi R, Phillips DM. Motility of rat spermatozoa at the site of fertilization. *Biol Reprod* 1988;39:1207–1213.
1478. Shalgi R, Phillips DM, Jones R. Status of the rat acrosome during sperm-zona pellucida interactions. *Gamete Res* 1989;22:1–13.
1479. Shalgi R, Smith TT, Yanagimachi R. A quantitative comparison of the passage of capacitated and uncapacitated hamster spermatozoa through the uterotubal junction. *Biol Reprod* 1992;46:419–424.
1480. Shams-Borham G, Huneau D, Flechon JE. Acrosin does not appear to be bound to the inner acrosomal membrane of bull spermatozoa. *J Exp Zool* 1979;209:143–149.
1481. Shibata S, Mizukami A, Takada H, Sengoku K, Ishikawa M, Shimizu T. Intercellular pH in fertilization of hamster eggs analyzed by microelectrode method. *Acta Obstet Gynecol* (Japan) 1988;40(Suppl):201(abst 215).
1482. Shibuya EK, Masui Y. Stabilization and enhancement of primary cytostatic (CSF) by ATP and NaF in amphibian egg cytosols. *Dev Biol* 1988;129:253–264.
1483. Shiina Y, Kaneda M, Matsuyama K, Tanaka K, Hiroi M, Doi K. Role of the extracellular Ca^{2+} on the intracellular Ca^{2+} changes in fertilized and activated mouse oocytes. *J Reprod Fertil* 1993;97:143–150.
1484. Shimizu S, Tsuji M, Dean J. *In vitro* biosynthesis of three sulfated glycoproteins of murine zona pellucida by oocytes grown in follicle culture. *J Biol Chem* 1983;258:5858–5863.
1485. Shivers CA, Dudkiewicz AB, Franklin LE, Fussell EN. Inhibition of sperm-egg interaction by specific antibody. *Science* 1972;178:1211–1213.
1486. Shur BD, Hall NG. Sperm surface galactosyltransferase activities during *in vitro* capacitation. *J Cell Biol* 1982;95:567–573.
1487. Siddiquey AKS, Cohen J. *In-vitro* fertilization in the mouse and the relevance of different sperm/egg concentrations and volumes. *J Reprod Fertil* 1982;66:237–242.
1488. Sidhu KS, Guraya SS. Cellular and molecular biology of capacitation and acrosome reaction in mammalian spermatozoa. *Int Rev Cytol* 1989;118:231–280.
1489. Siiteri JF, Dandekar P, Meizel S. Human sperm acrosome reaction-initiating activity associated with the human cumulus oophorus and mural granulosa cells. *J. Exp Zool* 1988;246:71–80.
1490. Silber SJ. Pregnancy caused by sperm from vasa efferentia. *Fertil Steril* 1988;49:373–375.
1491. Silber SJ. Apparent fertility of human spermatozoa from the caput epididymis. *J Androl* 1989;10:263–274.
1492. Silber SJ, Ord T, Borrero C, Balmaceda J, Asch R. New treatment for infertility due to congenital absence of vas deferens. *Lancet* 1987;2:850–851.
1493. Singer SL, Lambert H, Cross NL, Overstreet JW. Alteration of the human sperm surface during *in vitro* capacitation as assessed by lectin-induced agglutination. *Gamete Res* 1985;12:291–299.
1494. Siracusa G, Whittingham DG, Molinaro M, Vivarelli E. Parthenogenetic activation of mouse oocytes induced by inhibitors of protein synthesis. *J Embryol Exp Morphol* 1978;43:157–166.
1495. Skinner SM, Mills T, Kirchick HJ, Dunbar BS. Immunization with zona pellucida proteins results in abnormal ovarian follicular differentiation and inhibition of gonadotropin-induced steroid secretion. *Endocrinology* 1984;115:2428–2432.
1496. Skinner SM, Timmons TM, Schwoebel ED, Dunbar BS. The role of zona pellucida antigens in fertility and infertility. *Immun Allerg Clin North Am* 1990;10:185–197.
1497. Slavik T, Fulka J. *In vitro* fertilization of intact sheep and cattle oocytes with goat spermatozoa. *Theriogenology* 1992;38:721–726.
1498. Slavik T, Pavlok A, Fulka J. Penetration of intact bovine ova with ram sperm *in vitro*. *Mol Reprod Dev* 1990;25:345–347.
1499. Smith LC, Wilmut I. Factors affecting the viability of nuclear transplanted embryos. *Theriogenology* 1990;33:152–164.
1500. Smith TT, Koyanagi F, Yanagimachi R. Distribution and number of spermatozoa in the oviduct of the golden hamster after natural mating and artificial insemination. *Biol Reprod* 1987;37:225–234.
1501. Smith TT, Yanagimachi R. Capacitation status of hamster spermatozoa in the oviduct at various times after mating. *J Reprod Fert* 1989;86:255–261.
1502. Smith TT, Yanagimachi R. The viability of hamster spermatozoa stored in the isthmus of the oviduct: the importance of sperm-epithelium contact for sperm survival. *Biol Reprod* 1990;42:450–457.
1503. Smith TT, Yanagimachi R. Attachment and release of spermatozoa from the caudal isthmus of the hamster oviduct. *J Reprod Fertil* 1991;91:567–573.
1504. Smokovitis A, Kokolis N, Taitzoglou I, Rekkas C. Plasminogen activator: the identification of an additional proteinase at the outer acrosomal membrane of human and boar spermatozoa. *Int J Fertil* 1992;37:308–314.
1505. Soldani P, Rosati F. Sperm-egg interaction in the mouse using live and glutaraldehyde-fixed eggs. *Gamete Res* 1987;18:225–235.
1506. Spira B, Breitbart H. The role of anion channels in the mechanism of acrosome reaction in bull spermatozoa. *Biochim Biophys Acta* 1992;1109:65–73.
1507. Srivastava PN, Kumar VM, Arbtan KD. Neuraminidase induces capacitation and acrosome reaction in mammalian spermatozoa. *J Exp Zool* 1988;245:106–110.
1508. Srivastava PN, Sheikhnejad RG, Fryer-Hosken R, Malter H, Brackett BG. Inhibition of fertilization of the rabbit ova *in vitro* by the antibody to the inner acrosomal membrane of rabbit spermatozoa. *J Exp Zool* 1986;238:99–102.
1509. Srivastava PN, Zaneveld LJD, Williams WL. Mammalian sperm acrosomal neuraminidases. *Biochem Biophys Res Commun* 1970;39:575–582.
1510. Stastna J. Relationship of cortical granules to lysosomes in the rat ovum. *Folia Morphologica* 1974;22:234–236.
1511. Steinhardt RA, Epel D, Carroll EJ, Yanagimachi R. Is calcium ionophore a universal activator for unfertilised eggs? *Nature* 1974;252:41–43.
1512. Stevens LC. Teratocarcinogenesis and spontaneous parthenogenesis in mice. In: Markert CL, Papaconstantinou J, eds. *The Developmental Biology of Reproduction,* New York: Academic Press; 1975:93–106.
1513. Stevens LC. Totipotent cells of parthenogenetic origin in a chimaeric mouse. *Nature* 1978;276:266–267.
1514. Stevens LC, Varnum DS. The development of teratomas from parthenogenetically activated ovarian mouse eggs. *Dev Biol* 1974;37:369–380.
1515. Stevens LC, Varnum DS, Eicher EM. Viable chimaera produced from normal and parthenogenetic mouse embryos. *Nature* 1977;269:515–517.
1516. Stewart-Savage J. Effect of bovine serum albumin concentration and source on sperm capacitation in the golden hamster. *Biol Reprod* 1993;49:74–81.
1517. Stewart-Savage J, Bavister BD. A cell surface block to polyspermy occurs in golden hamster eggs. *Dev Biol* 1988;128:150–157.
1518. Stewart-Savage J, Bavister BD. Time course and pattern of cortical granule breakdown in hamster eggs after sperm fusion. *Mol Reprod Dev* 1991;30:390–395.
1519. Stice SL, Robl JM. Activation of mammalian oocytes by a factor obtained from rabbit sperm. *Mol Reprod Dev* 1990;25:272–280.

1520. Stock CE, Fraser LR. The acrosome reaction in human sperm from men of proven fertility. *Hum Reprod* 1987;2:109–119.
1521. Stock CE, Fraser LR. Divalent cations, capacitation and the acrosome reaction in human spermatozoa. *J Reprod Fertil* 1989;87:463–478.
1522. Storey BT. Sperm capacitation and the acrosome reaction. *Ann NY Acad Sci* 1991;637:457–473.
1523. Storey BT. Zona pellucida-induced acrosome reaction in mouse sperm: Sequence of acts and players. In: Baccetti B, ed. *Comparative Spermatology 20 Years After.* New York: Raven Press; 1991.
1524. Storey BT, Kopt GS. Fertilization in the mouse, II. Spermatozoa. In: Dunbar SB, O'Rand MG, eds. *A Comparative Overview of Mammalian Fertilization,* New York: Plenum Press; 1991:167–216.
1525. Suarez SS. Sperm transport and motility in mouse oviduct: observation *in situ. Biol Reprod* 1987;36:203–210.
1526. Suarez SS, Dai X. Hyperactivation enhances mouse sperm capacity for penetrating viscoelastic media. *Biol Reprod* 1992;46:686–691.
1527. Suarez SS, Dai X, DeMott RP, Redfern K, Mirando MA. Movement characteristics of boar sperm obtained from the oviduct or hyperactivated *in vitro. J Androl* 1992;13:75–80.
1528. Suarez SS, Katz DF, Owen DH, Andrew JB, Powell RL. Evidence for the function of hyperactivated motility in sperm. *Biol Reprod* 1991;44:375–381.
1529. Suarez SS, Osman RA. Initiation of hyperactivated flagellar bending in mouse sperm within the female reproductive tract. *Biol Reprod* 1987;36:1191–1198.
1530. Suarez SS, Varosi SM, Dai X. Intracellular calcium increases with hyperactivation in intact moving hamster sperm and oscillates with the flagellar beat cycle. *Proc Natl Acad Sci USA* 1993;90:4660–4664.
1531. Sugiyama M. Refertilization of the fertilized eggs of the sea urchin. *Biol. Bull* 1951;101:335–344.
1532. Sullivan R, Bleau G. Interaction of isolated components from mammalian sperm and egg. *Gamete Res* 1985;12:101–116.
1533. Sumner AT. Immunocytochemical demonstration of kinetochores in human sperm head. *Exp Cell Res* 1987;171:250–253.
1534. Sun FZ, Hoyland J, Huang X, Mason W, Moor RM. A comparison of intracellular changes in porcine eggs after fertilization and electroactivation. *Development* 1992;115:947–956.
1535. Surani MAH, Barton SC, Kaufman MH. Development to term of chimaeras between diploid parthenogenetic and fertilised embryos. *Nature* 1977;270:601–603.
1536. Surani MAH, Barton SC, Norris ML. Development of reconstituted mouse eggs suggests imprinting of the genome during gametogenesis. *Nature* 1984;308:548–550.
1537. Surani MAH, Kaufman MH. The influence of extracellular calcium and magnesium ions on the second meiotic division of mouse oocytes. *Dev Biol* 1977;59:86–90.
1538. Suzuki F. Changes in the distribution of intramembranous particles and Filipin-sterol complexes during epididymal maturation of golden hamster spermatozoa. *J Ultrast Mol Struct Res* 1988;100:39–54.
1539. Suzuki F. Morphological aspects of sperm maturation. In: Bavister BD, Cummins J, Roldan ERS, eds. *Fertilization in Mammals.* Norwell, Massachusetts: Serono Symposia USA; 1990: 65–75.
1540. Suzuki F, Yanagimachi R. Changes in the distribution of intra membranous particles and Filipin-reactive membrane sterols during *in vitro* capacitation of golden hamster spermatozoa. *Gamete Res* 1989;23:335–347.
1541. Swann K. A cytosolic sperm factor stimulates repetitive calcium increases and mimics fertilization in hamster eggs. *Development* 1990;110:1295–1302.
1542. Swann K. Different triggers for calcium oscillations in mouse eggs involve a ryanodine-sensitive calcium store. *Biochem J* 1992;287:79–84.
1543. Swann K, Igusa Y, Miyazaki S. Evidence for an inhibitory effect of protein kinase C on G-protein-mediated repetitive calcium transients in hamster eggs. *EMBO J* 1989;8:3711–3718.
1544. Swann K, Whitaker MJ. Second messengers at fertilization in sea-urchin eggs. *J Reprod Fertil* 1990;42(Suppl):141–153.
1545. Swenson CE, Dunbar BS. Specificity of sperm–zona interaction. *J Exp Zool* 1982;219:97–104.
1546. Szollosi D. The fate of sperm middle-piece mitochondria in the rat egg. *J Exp Zool* 1965;159:367–378.
1547. Szollosi D. Development of cortical granules and the cortical reaction in rat and hamster eggs. *Anat Rec* 1967;159:431–446.
1548. Szollosi D, Szollosi MS, Czolowska R, Tarkowski AK. Sperm penetration into immature mouse oocytes and nuclear changes during maturation: an EM study. *Biol Cell* 1990;69:53–64.
1549. Szollosi D, Czolowska R, Soltynska MS, Tarkowski AK. Remodelling of thymocyte nuclei in activated mouse oocytes: an ultrastructural study. *Eur J Cell Biol* 1986;42:140–151.
1550. Szollosi D, Ozil JP. *De novo* formation of centrioles in parthenogenetically activated, diploidized rabbit embryos. *Biol Cell* 1991;72:61–66.
1551. Takagi J, Araki Y, Dobashi M, Imai T, Hiroi M, Tonosaki A, Sendo F. The development of porcine zona pellucida using monoclonal antibodies. I. Immunocytochemistry and light microscopy. *Biol Reprod* 1989;40:1095–1102.
1552. Takahashi K, Yamagata T. Involvement of sialic acids in fertilization of the mouse. *Dev Growth Diff* 1982;24:407 (abst)
1553. Takahashi YM, Sugiyama M. Relation between the acrosome reaction and fertilization in the sea urchin. I. Fertilization in Ca-free seawater with egg-water treated spermatozoa. *Dev Growth Diff* 1973;15:261–267.
1554. Takano H, Yanagimachi R, Urch U. Evidence that acrosin activity is important for the development of fusibility of mammalian spermatozoa with oolemma: inhibitor studies using the golden hamster. *Zygotes* 1993;1:79–91.
1555. Talbot P. Hyaluronidase dissolves a component in the hamster zona pellucida. *J Exp Zool* 1984;229:309–316.
1556. Talbot P. Sperm penetration through oocyte investments in mammals. *Am J Anat* 1985;174:331–346.
1557. Talbot P, Chacon R. Detection of modifications in the tail of capacitated guinea pig sperm using lectins. *J Exp Zool* 1981;216:435–444.
1558. Talbot P, DiCarlantonio G. Architecture of the hamster oocyte-cumulus complex. *Gamete Res* 1984;9:261–272.
1559. Tanphaichitr N, Sobhon P, Talupphet N, Chalermisarachai M. Basic nuclear proteins in testicular cells and ejaculated spermatozoa in man. *Exp Cell Res* 1978;117:347–356.
1560. Tarkowski AK. Experiments on the transplantation of ova in mice. *Acta Theriogenol* 1959;2:251–267.
1561. Tarkowski AK. Mouse chimeras developed from fused eggs. *Nature* 1961;190:857–860.
1562. Tarkowski AK, Witkowska A, Nowicka J. Experimental parthenogenesis in the mouse. *Nature* 1970;226:162–165.
1562a. Tarone G, Russo MA, Hirsch E, et al. Expression of beta 1 integin complexes on the surface of unfertilized mouse oocyte. *Development* 1993;117:1369–1375.
1563. Tash JS. Protein phospholylation: the second messenger signal transducer of flagellar motility. *Cell Motil Cytoskel* 1989;14: 332–339.
1564. Tateno H, Mikamo K. A chromosomal method to distinguish between X- and Y-bearing spermatozoa of the bull in zona-free hamster ova. *J Reprod Fertil* 1987;81:119–125.
1565. Tejada RI, Mitchell JC, Norman A, Marik JJ, Friedman S. A test for the practical evaluation of male fertility by acridine orange (AO) fluorescence. *Fertil Steril* 1984;42:87–91.
1566. Telford NA, Watson AJ, Schultz GA. Transition from maternal to embryonic in early mammalian development: a comparison of several species. *Mol Reprod Dev* 1990;26:90–100.
1567. Terquem A, Dadoune JP. Aniline blue staining of human spermatozoon chromatin. Evaluation of nuclear maturation. In: Andre J, ed. *The Sperm Cell.* Hague: Martinus Nijhoff; 1983:249–252.
1568. Tesarik J. Comparison of acrosome reaction-inducing activities of human cumulus oophorus, follicular fluid and ionophore A23187 in human sperm populations of proven fertilizing ability *in vitro. J Reprod Fertil* 1985;74:383–388.
1569. Tesarik J. Appropriate timing of the acrosome reaction is a major requirement for the fertilizing spermatozoon. *Hum Reprod* 1989;4:957–961.
1570. Tesarik J. Immunoinhibition of human fertilization in vitro by

antibodies to the cumulus oophorus intercellular matrix. *J Reprod Fertil* 1989;87:193–198.
1571. Tesarik J, Drahorad J, Peknicova J. Subcellular immunochemical localization of acrosin in human spermatozoa during the acrosome reaction and zona pellucida penetration. *Fertil Steril* 1988;50:133–141.
1572. Tesarik J, Drahorad J, Testart J, Mendoza C. Acrosin activation follows its surface exposure and precedes membrane fusion in human sperm acrosome reaction. *Development* 1990;110:391–400.
1573. Tesarik J, Kopecny V. Late preovulatory synthesis of proteoglycans by the human oocyte and cumulus cells and their secretion into the oocyte-cumulus-complex extracellular matrices. *Histochemistry* 1986;85:523–528.
1574. Tesarik J, Kopecny V. Developmental control of the human male pronucleus by ooplasmic factors. *Hum Reprod* 1989;4:962–968.
1575. Tesarik J, Kopecny V. Nucleic acid synthesis and development of human male pronucleus. *J Reprod Fertil* 1989;86:549–558.
1576. Tesarik J, Kopecny V, Dverak M. Selective binding of human cumulus cell-secreted glycoproteins to human spermatozoa during capacitation in vitro. *Fertil Steril* 1984;41:919–925.
1577. Tesarik J, Mendoza C. Insights into the function of a sperm-surface progesterone receptor: evidence of ligand-induced receptor aggregation and the implication of proteolysis. *Exp Cell Res* 1993;205:111–117.
1578. Tesarik J, Mendoza C, Carreras A. Fast acrosome reaction measure: a highly sensitive method for evaluating stimulus-induced acrosome reaction. *Fertil Steril* 1993;59:424–430.
1579. Tesarik J, Mendoza C, Moos J, Fenichel P, Fehlmann M. Progesterone action through agglutination of receptor on sperm plasma membrane. *FEBS* 1992;308:116–120.
1580. Tesarik J, Oltras CM, Testart J. Effect of the human cumulus oophorus on movement characteristics of human capacitated spermatozoa. *J Reprod Fertil* 1990;88:665–675.
1581. Tesarik J, Pilka L, Drahorad J, Cechova D, Veselsky L. The role of cumulus cell-secreted proteins in the development of human sperm fertilizing ability: implication in IVF. *Hum Reprod* 1988;3:129–132.
1582. Tesarik J, Testart J, Leca G, Nome F. Reversible inhibition of fertility in mice by passive immunization with anticumulus oophorus antibodies. *Biol Reprod* 1990;43:385–391.
1583. Tesarik J, Testart J, Nome F. Effects of prolonged administration of anti-cumulus oophorus antibody on reproduction in mice. *J Reprod Fertil* 1990;90:605–610.
1584. Thadani VM. Mice produced from eggs fertilized *in vitro* at a very low concentration. *J Exp Zool* 1982;219:277–283.
1584a. Thibault C, Dauzier L, Wintenberger S. Etude cytologique de la fecondation in vitro de l'oeuf de la lapin. *C R Soc Sci Biol* 1954;148:789.
1585. Thibault C, Gerard M, Menezo Y. Acquisition par tion du noyau du spermatozoide fecondant (MPGF). *Ann. Biol Anim Biochem Biophys* 1975;15:705–714.
1586. Thomas P, Meizel S. An influx of extracellular calcium is required for initiation of the human sperm acrosome reaction induced by human follicular fluid. *Gamete Res* 1988;20:397–411.
1587. Thomas P, Meizel S. Effects of metalloendoprotease substrates on the human sperm acrosome reaction. *J Reprod Fertil* 1989;85:241–249.
1588. Thomas P, Meizel S. Phosphatidylinositol 4, 5-bis-phosphate hydrolysis in human sperm stimulated with follicular fluid or progestrone is dependent on calcium influx. *Biochem J* 1989;264:539–546.
1589. Thomas TS, Reynolds AL, Oliphant G. Evaluation of the site of synthesis of rabbit sperm acrosome stabilizing factor using immunocytochemical and metabolic labeling techniques. *Biol Reprod* 1984;30:693–705.
1590. Thorgaard GH. Chromosome set manipulation and sex control in fish. In: Hoar WS, Randall DJ, Donaldson EM, ed. *Fish Physiology*, Vol. 9B. New York: Academic Press; 1983:405–434.
1591. Tombes RM, Simerly C, Borisy GG, Schatten G. Meiosis, egg activation, and nuclear envelope breakdown are differentially reliant on Ca^{2+}, whereas germinal vesicle breakdown is Ca^{2+} independent in the mouse oocyte. *J Cell Biol* 1992;117:799–811.
1592. Tonkins PT, Hongton JA. The rapid induction of the acrosome reaction of human spermatozoa by electropermeabilization. *Fertil Steril* 1988;50:329–336.
1593. Topfer-Petersen E, Cechova D. Zona pellucida induces conversion of proacrosin to acrosin. *Int J Androl* 1990;13:190–196.
1593a. Topfer-Petersen E, Cechova D, Henschen A, Steinberger M, Friess AE, Zucker A. Cell biology of acrosomal proteins. *Andrologia* 1990;22(Suppl 1):110–121.
1594. Topfer-Petersen E, Friess AE, Nguyen H, Schill W-B. Evidence for a fucose-binding protein in boar spermatozoa. *Histochemistry* 1985;83:139–145.
1595. Topfer-Peterson E, Friess A, Sinowatz F, Biltz S, Schill WB. Immunological characterization of the outer acrosomal membrane during acrosome reaction in boar. *Histochemistry* 1985;82:113–120.
1596. Topfer-Petersen E, Henschen A. Acrosin shows zona and fucose binding, novel properties for a serine proteinase. *FEBS* 1987;226:38–42.
1597. Topfer-Petersen E, Henschen A. Zona pellucida-binding and fucose-binding of boar sperm acrosin is not correlated with proteolytic activity. *Biol Chem Hoppe-Seyler* 1988;369:69–76.
1598. Topfer-Petersen E, Steinberger M, Ebner Von Eschenbach C, Zucker A. Zona pellucida-binding of boar sperm acrosin is associated with the N-terminal peptide of the acrosin B-chain (heavy chain). *FEBS* 1990;265:51–54.
1599. Toshimori K, Tanii I, Araki S, Oura C. A rat sperm flagellar surface antigen that originates in the testis and is expressed on the flagellar surface during epididymal transit. *Mol Reprod Dev* 1992;32:399–408.
1600. Toyoda Y, Naito K. IVF in domestic animals. In: Bavister BD, et al., eds. *Fertilization in Mammals.* Norwell, Massachusetts: Serono Symposia USA; 1990:335–347.
1601. Toyoda Y, Sato E, Naito K. Role of the cumulus oophorus in mammalian fertilization. In: Mohri H, Takahashi M, Tachi C, eds. *Biology of the Germ Line in Animal and Man,* Tokyo: Japan Science Society Press/Basel: Karger; 1993:111–124.
1602. Trounson AO, Moore NW. The survival and development of sheep eggs following complete or partial removal of the zona pellucida. *J Reprod Fertil* 1974;41:97–105.
1603. Tulsiani DRP, Nagdas SK, Cornwall GA, Orgebin-Crist M-C. Evidence for the presence of high-mannose/hybrid oligosaccharide chain(s) on the mouse ZP2 and ZP3. *Biol Reprod* 1992;46:93–100.
1604. Tulsiani DRP, Skudlarek MD, Holland MK, Orgebin-Crist MC. Glycosylation of rat sperm plasma membrane during epididymal maturation. *Biol Reprod* 1993;48:417–428.
1605. Tulsiani DRP, Skudlarek MD, Orgebin-Crist M-C. Novel alpha-D-manosidase of rat sperm plasma membranes: characterization and potential role in sperm–egg inter-actions. *J Cell Biol* 1989;109:1257–1267.
1606. Tulsiani DRP, Skudlarek MD, Orgebin-Crist M-C. Human sperm plasma membranes possess alpha-D-mannosidase activity but no galactosyltransferase activity. *Biol Reprod* 1990;42:843–858.
1607. Turner PR, Jaffe LA. G-proteins and the regulation of oocyte maturation and fertilization. In: Schatten H, Schatten G, eds. *The Cell Biology of Fertilization.* San Diego: Academic Press; 1989:297–318.
1608. Turner TT. Spermatozoa are exposed to a complex microenvironment as they traverse the epididymis. *Ann NY Acad Sci* 1991;637:364–383.
1609. Tzartos SJ. Inhibition of *in-vitro* fertilization of intact and denuded hamster eggs by univalent anti-sperm antibodies. *J Reprod Fertil* 1979;55:447–455.
1610. Uehara T, Yanagimachi R. Behavior of nuclei of testicular, caput and cauda epididymal spermatozoa injected into hamster eggs. *Biol Reprod* 1977;16:315–321.
1611. Urch UA. Biochemistry and function of acrosin. In: Wassarman PM, ed. *Elements of Mammalian Fertilization.* Boca Raton, Florida: CRC Press; 1991:233–248.
1612. Urch UA, Patel H. The interaction of boar sperm proacrosin

with its natural substrate, the zona pellucida, and with polysulfated polysaccharides. *Development* 1991;111:1165–1172.
1613. Urch UA, Wardrip NJ, Hedrick JL. Limited and specific proteolysis of the zona pellucida by acrosin. *J Exp Zool* 1985; 233:479–483.
1614. Urch UA, Wardrip NJ, Hedrick JL. Proteolysis of the zona pellucida by acrosin: the nature of the hydrolysis products. *J Exp Zool* 1985;236:239–243.
1615. Uto N, Yoshimatsu N, Lopata A, Yanagimachi R. The zona-induced acrosome reaction of hamster spermatozoa. *J Exp Zool* 1988;248:113–120.
1616. Vandevoort CA, Tollner TL, Overstreet JW. Sperm-zona pellucida interaction in cynomolgus and rhesus macaques. *J Androl* 1992;13:428–432.
1617. Van Duin M, Polman JEM, Verkoelen CCEH, Bunschoten VH, Meyerink JH, Olijve W, Aitken RJ. Cloning and characterization of the human sperm receptor ligand ZP3: evidence for a second polymorphic allele with a different frequency in the Caucasian and Japanese populations. *Genomics* 1992;14: 1064–1070.
1618. Van Meel FCM, Pearson PL. Do human spermatozoa reactivate in the cytoplasm of somatic cells? *J Cell Sci* 1979;35:105–122.
1619. Vaught LK, Vaught WG, Huen N, Quinones R, Sher G, Maassarani G. Fertilization of human oocytes after cumulus oophorus removal by hyaluronidase. *Fertil Steril* 1991;(Suppl Ann Meet Fertil Soc):186 (abst).
1620. Vazquez MH, Phillips DM, Wassarman PM. Interaction of mouse sperm with purified sperm receptors covalently linked to silica beads. *J Cell Sci* 1989;92:713–722.
1621. Venessa JK, Coutts JRT, Robertson L. Pentoxifylline stimulates hyperactivation in human sperm. *J Reprod Fertil* 1992;9:48(abst 82).
1622. Verkuyl DAA. Oral conception. Impregnation via the proximal gastrointestinal tract in a patient with an aplastic distal vagina. Case report. *Br J Obstet Gynecol* 1988;95:933–934.
1623. Vernon RB, Muller CH, Eddy EM. Further characterization of a secreted epididymal glycoprotein in mice that binds to sperm tails. *J Androl* 1987;8:123–128.
1624. Veselsky L, Jonakova V, Sanz ML, Topfer-Peterson E, Cechova D. Binding of a 15kDa glycoprotein from spermatozoa of boars to surface of zona pellucida and cumulus oophorus cells. *J Reprod Fertil* 1992;96:593–602.
1625. Vigers GPA, Lohka MJ. A distinct vesicle population targets membranes and pore complexes to the nuclear envelope in Xenopus eggs. *J. Cell Biol* 1991;112:545–556.
1626. Vigil P. Gamete membrane fusion in hamster with reacted equatorial segment. *Gamete Res* 1989;23:203–213.
1627. Vijayaraghavan S, Hoskins D. Quantitation of bovine sperm cytoplasmic calcium with Quin-2 and Fura-2: evidence that external calcium does not have direct access to the sperm cytoplasm. *Cell Calcium* 1989;10:241–253.
1628. Vijayaraghvan S, Hoskins DD. Changes in the mitochondrial calcium influx and efflux properties are responsible for the decline in sperm calcium during epididymal maturation. *Mol Reprod Dev* 1990;25:186–194.
1629. Virji N, Phillips DM, Dunbar BS. Identification of extracellular proteins in the rat cumulus oophorus. *Mol Reprod Dev* 1990;25:339–344.
1630. Visconti P, Tezon JG. Phorbol esters stimulate cyclic adenosine 3′,5′-monophosphate accumulation in hamster spermatozoa during *in vitro* capacitation. *Biol Reprod* 1989;40:223–231.
1630a. Von Bernhardi R, De Ioannes AE, Blanco LP, Herrera E, Bustos-Obregon E, Vigil P. Round-headed spermatozoa: A model to study the role of the acrosome in early events of gamete interaction. *Andrology* 1990;22:12–20.
1631. Vreeburg JTM, Holland MK, Orgebin-Crist MC. Binding of epididymal proteins to rat spermatozoa *in vivo*. *Biol Reprod* 1992;47:588–597.
1632. Wabik-Sliz B. Number of cortical granules in mouse oocytes from inbred stains differing in efficiency of fertilization. *Biol Reprod* 1979;21:89–97.
1633. Waibel R, Granet R, Ficsor G, Ginsberg L. Caproyl esterase from rat testis: purification and action on cumulus cells. *Gamete Res* 1985;12:75–84.
1634. Ward CR, Storey BT. Determination of time course of capacitation in mouse spermatozoa using a chlortetracycline fluorescence assay. *Dev Biol* 1984;104:287–296.
1634a. Ward WS. Deoxyribonucleic acid loop domain tertiary structure in mammalian spermatozoa. *Biol Reprod* 1993;48: 1193–1201.
1635. Ward WS, Coffey DS. Identification of a sperm nuclear annulus: a sperm DNA anchor. *Biol Reprod* 1989;41:361–370.
1636. Ward WS, Coffey DS. DNA packaging and organization in mammalian spermatozoa: comparison with somatic cells. *Biol Reprod* 1991;44:569–574.
1637. Ward WS, Partin AW, Coffey DS. DNA loop domains in mammalian spermatozoa. *Chromosoma* 1989;98:153–159.
1638. Wassarman PM. The biology and chemistry of fertilization. *Science* 1987;235:553–560.
1639. Wassarman PM. Zona pellucida glycoproteins. *Annu Rev Biochem* 1988;57:415–442.
1640. Wassarman PM. Profile of a mammalian sperm receptor. *Development* 1990;108:1–17.
1641. Wassarman PM, ed. (1991): *Elements of Mammalian Fertilization,* Vols. I and II. Boca Raton, Florida: CRC Press.
1642. Wassarman PM, Bleil JD, Florman HM, Greve JM, Roller RJ, Salzmann GS, Samuels FG. The mouse egg's receptor for sperm: What is it and how does it work? *Cold Spring Harb Symp Quant Biol* 1985;50:11–19.
1643. Wassarman PM, Mortillo S. Structure of the mouse egg extracellular coat, the zona pellucida. *Int Rev Cytol* 1991;130: 85–110.
1644. Watanabe N, Hunt T, Ikawa Y, Sagata N. Independent inactivation of MPF and cytostatic factor (MOS) upon fertilization of Xenopus eggs. *Nature* 1991;352:247–248.
1645. Watanabe N, Van de Woude GF, Ikawa Y, Sagata N. Specific proteolysis of the C-mos-proto-oncogen by calpain on fertilization of *Xenopus* eggs. *Nature* 1989;324:505–511.
1646. Weber M, Kubiak JZ, Arlinghaus RB, Pines J, Maro B. C-mos proto-oncogene product is partly degraded after release from meiotic arrest and persists during interphase in mouse zygotes. *Dev Biol* 1991;148:393–397.
1647. Webster SD, McGaughey RW. The cortical cytoskeleton and its role in sperm penetration of the mammalian egg. *Dev Biol* 1990;142:61–74.
1648. Wegner CC, Killian GJ. *In vitro* and *in vivo* association of an oviduct estrus-associated protein with bovine zona pellucida. *Mol Reprod Dev* 1991;29:77–84.
1649. Weiman S, Ores-Carton F, Rainteau D, Puszkin S. Immunoelecton microscopic localization of calmodulin and phospholipase A_2 in spermatozoa. *J Histochem Cytochem* 1986;34: 1171–1179.
1650. Wendy TS, Wilson L, Reynold AB, Oliphant G. Chemical and physical characterization of rabbit sperm acrosome stabilizing factor. *Biol Reprod* 1986;35:691–703.
1651. Wenstrom JC, Hamilton DW. Dolichol concentration and biosynthesis in rat testis and epididymis *Biol Reprod* 1980;23: 1054–1059.
1652. Whitaker M. How calcium may cause exocytosis in sea urchin eggs. *Biosci. Rep* 1987;7:383–397.
1653. Whitaker MJ, Baker PE. Calcium-dependent exocytosis in an *in vitro* secretory granule plasma membrane preparation from sea urchin eggs and the effects of some inhibitors of cytoskeletal function. *Proc R Soc Lond* [Biol] 1983;218:397–413.
1654. Whitaker M, Patel R. Calcium and cell cycle control. *Development* 1990;108:525–542.
1655. Whitaker M, Swann K, Crossley I. What happens during the latent period at fertilization. In: Nuccitelli R, Cherr GN, Clark WH, eds. *Mechanisms of Egg Activation.* New York: Plenum Press; 1989:157–171.
1656. White DR, Phillips DM, Bedford JM. Factors affecting the acrosome reaction in human spermatozoa. *J Reprod Fertil* 1990; 90:71–80.
1657. White IG, Belanger L, Hough S, Ellington J, Foote RH. Biochemical changes in bull spermatozoa during capacitation *in vitro*. *Theriogenology* 1992;37:571–578.

1658. White IG, Kar A. Aspects of the physiology of sperm in the female genital tract. *Contraception* 1973;3:183–194.
1658a. White JM. Viral and cellular membrane fusion proteins. *Annu Rev Physiol* 1990;52:675–697.
1659. Whittingham DG. Parthenogenesis in mammals. In: *Oxford Reviews of Reproductive Biology,* Vol. 2. Oxford: Clarendon Press; 1980:205–231.
1660. Whittingham DG, Siracusa G. The involvement of calcium in the activation of mammalian oocytes. *Exp Cell Res* 1978;113: 311–317.
1661. Wiker S, Malter H, Wright G, Cohen J. Recognition of paternal pronuclei in human zygotes. *J In Vitro Fertil Embryo Transf* 1990;7:33–37.
1662. Wildt DE. Fertilization in cat. In: Dunbar BS, O'Rand GO, eds. *Overview of Mammalian Fertilization,* New York: Plenum Press; 1991:299–328.
1663. Willadsen SM. Nuclear transplantation in sheep embryos. *Nature* 1986;320:63–65.
1664. Williams CJ, Schultz RM, Kopf GS. Role of G proteins in mouse egg activation: stimulatory effects of acetylcholine on the ZP2 to $ZP2_f$ conversion and pronuclear formation in eggs expressing a functional ml muscarinic receptor. *Dev Biol* 1992;151:288–296.
1664a. Wilson IA, Skehel JJ, Wiley DC. Structure of the haemagglutinin membrane glyco protein of influenza virus at 3 A resolution. *Nature* 1981;280:366–373.
1665. Wilson KL, Newport J. A trypsin-sensitive receptor on membrane vesicles is required for nuclear envelope formation *in vitro. J Cell Biol* 1988;107:57–68.
1666. Winston N, Johnson M, Pickering S, Braude P. Parthenogenetic activation and development of fresh and aged human oocytes. *Fertil Steril* 1991;56:904–912.
1667. Wistrom CA, Meizel S. Evidence that progesterone-initiated human sperm acrosome reaction involves a putative GABA receptor/Cl^- channel complex and Cl^- influx. *Biol Reprod* 1992;46(Suppl 1):64a.
1667a. Winstrom CA, Meizel S. Evidence suggesting involvement of a unique human steroid receptor/Cl^- channel complex in the progesterone-induced acrosome reaction. *Dev Biol* 1993, in press.
1668. Witman GB. Introduction to cilia and flagella. In: Bloodgood RA, eds. *Ciliary and Flagella Membranes.* New York: Plenum Press; 1990:1–28.
1669. Wolf DE, Gadullo RA. Physical properties of the mammalian sperm plasma membrane, In: Baccetti B, ed. *Comparative Spermatology 20 Years After.* New York: Raven Press; 1991: 599–604.
1670. Wolf DE, Lipscomb AC, Maynard VM. Causes of nondiffusing lipid in the plasma membrane of mammalian spermatozoa. *Biochemistry* 1988;27:860–865.
1671. Wolf DE, Voglmayr JK. Diffusion and regionalization in membranes of maturing ram spermatozoa. *J Cell Biol* 1984;98: 1678–1684.
1672. Wolf DE, Ziomek CA. Regionalization and lateral diffusion of membrane proteins in unfertilized and fertilized mouse eggs. *J Cell Biol* 1983;96:1786–1790.
1673. Wolf DP. The block to sperm penetration in zona-free mouse eggs. *Dev Biol* 1978;64:1–10.
1674. Wolf DP. The ovum before and after fertilization. In: Zaueveld LD, Chatterton RT, eds. *Biochemistry of Mammalian Reproduction,* New York: Wiley & Sons; 1982:231–259.
1675. Wolf DP. Acrosomal status quantitation in human sperm. *Am J Reprod Immunol* 1989;20:106–113.
1676. Wolf DP, Armstrong PB. Penetration of the zona-free mouse egg by capacitated epididymal sperm: cinemicrographic observations. *Gamete Res* 1978;1:39–46.
1677. Wolf DP, Hamada M. Induction of zonal and egg plasma membrane blocks to sperm penetration in mouse eggs with cortical granule exudate. *Biol Reprod* 1977;17:350–354.
1678. Wolf DP, Inoue M, Stark RA. Penetration of zona-free mouse ova. *Biol Reprod* 1976;15:213–221.
1679. Wolf DP, Nicosia SV, Hamada M. Premature cortical granule loss does not prevent sperm penetration of mouse eggs. *Dev Biol* 1979;71:22–32.
1680. Wolf DP, Vanderoort CA, Meyer-Haas GR, Zelinski-Wooten MB, Hesse DL, Baugham WL, Stouffer RL. *In vitro* fertilization and embryo transfer in the Rhesus monkey. *Biol Reprod* 1989;41:335–346.
1681. Wolf JP, Feneux D, Escalier D, Paintrand I, Rodrigues D, Frydman R, Jouannet P. Pregnancy after subzonal insemination with human spermatozoa packing outer dynein arms. *Focus Reprod* 1992;2:12–13.
1682. Wolf JP, Feneux D, Escalier D, Rodrigues D, Frydman R. Pregnancy after subzonal insemination with spermatozoa lacking outer dynein arms. *J Reprod Fertil* 1993;97:487–492.
1682a. Wong PYD, Huang SJ, Leong AYH et al. Physiology and pathology of electrolyte transport in the epididymis. In: Nieschlag ES, Habenicht UF, eds. *Spermatogenesis-Fertilization-Contraception.* Berlin/New York: Springer-Verlag;1992:318–344.
1683. Wooten MW, Voglmayr JK, Wrenn RW. Characterization of cAMP-dependent protein kinase and its endogenous substrate proteins in ram testicular, cauda epididymal, and ejaculated spermatozoa. *Gamete Res* 1987;16:57–68.
1684. Wright SJ, Longo FJ. Sperm nuclear enlargement in fertilized hamster eggs is related to meiotic maturation of the maternal chromatin. *J Exp Zool* 1988;247:155–165.
1685. Xian M, Azuma S, Naito K, Kunieda T, Moriwaki K, Toyoda Y. Effect of a partial deletion of Y chromosome on *in vitro* fertilizing ability of mouse spermatozoa. *Biol Reprod* 1992; 47:549–553.
1686. Yamada T, Yukawa O, Matsuda Y, Ohkawa A. Changes in radiosensitivity of the *in vitro* fertilized mouse ova during zygotic stage from fertilization to first cleavage. *J Radiat Res* 1982;23:450–456.
1687. Yamagata T. The role of saccharides in fertilization of the mouse. *Dev Growth Diff* 1985;27:176–177.
1688. Yamagata T, Ito M, Takahashi N. Involvement of an asparagine-linked oligosaccaride located in the zona pellucida in mouse fertilization *in vitro. Zool Sci* 1985;1:933(abst).
1689. Yamashita N. Enhancement of ionic currents through voltage-gated channels in the mouse oocyte after fertilization. *J Physiol* 1982;329:263–280.
1690. Yamashita M, Onozato H, Nakanishi T, Nagahara Y. Breakdown of the sperm nuclear envelope is a prerequisite for male pronucleus formation: Direct evidence from the gynogenetic crucian carp *Carassius auratus langsdorfii. Dev Biol* 1990; 137:155–160.
1691. Yanagida K, Yanagimachi R, Perreault SD, Kleinfeld RG. Thermostability of sperm nuclei assessed by microinjection into hamster oocytes. *Biol Reprod* 1991;44:440–447.
1692. Yanagimachi R. Penetration of guinea-pig spermatozoa into hamster eggs *in vitro. J Reprod Fertil* 1972;28:477–480.
1693. Yanagimachi R. Acceleration of the acrosome reaction and activation of guinea pig spermatozoa by detergents and other reagents. *Biol Reprod* 1975;13:513–526.
1694. Yanagimachi R. Calcium requirement for sperm–egg fusion in mammals. *Biol Reprod* 1978;19:949–958.
1695. Yanagimachi R. Requirement of extracellular calcium ions for various stages of fertilization and fertilization-related phenomena in the hamster. *Gamete Res* 1982;5:323–344.
1696. Yanagimachi R. Mammalian fertilization. In: Knobil E, et al. *The Physiology of Reproduction,* Vol. 1, New York: Raven Press; 1988:135–185.
1697. Yanagimachi R. Sperm capacitation and gamete interaction. *J Reprod Fertil* 1989;38(Suppl):27–33.
1698. Yanagimachi R, Bhattacharyya A. Acrosome-reacted guinea pig spermatozoa become fusion competent in the presence of extracellular potassium ions. *J Exp Zool* 1988;248:354–360.
1699. Yanagimachi R, Chang MC. Fertilizable life of golden hamster ova and their morphological changes at the time of losing fertilizability. *J Exp Zool* 1961;148:185–203.
1700. Yanagimachi R, Chang MC. Sperm ascent through the oviduct of the hamster and rabbit in relation to the time of ovulation. *J Reprod Fertil* 1963;6:413–420.
1701. Yanagimachi R, Katayose H, Killian G, Lee CN, Carrel DT, Huang TTF. Moderate heat treatment increases the penetrability of zonae pellucidae of salt-stored oocytes by spermatozoa. *Zygote* 1993;[in press].
1702. Yanagimachi R, Katayose H, Matsuda J, Yanagida K. Stability

of mammalian sperm nuclei. In: Spera G, Fabbrini A, Gnessi L, Bardin CW, eds. *Molecular and Cellular Biology of Reproduction.* New York: Raven Press; 1992:157–176.
1703. Yanagimachi R, Lopata A, Odom CB, Bronson RA, Mahi CA, Nicolson GL. Retention of biologic characteristics of zona pellucida in highly concentrated salt solution: the use of salt-stored eggs for assessing the fertilizing capacity of spermatozoa. *Fertil Steril* 1979;31:562–574.
1704. Yanagimachi R, Miyashiro LH, Yanagimachi H. Reversible inhibition of sperm–egg fusion in the hamster by low pH. *Dev Growth Diff* 1980;22:281–288.
1705. Yanagimachi R, Nicolson GL. Lectin-binding properties of hamster egg zona pellucida and plasma membrane during maturation and preimplantation development. *Exp Cell Res* 1976;100:249–257.
1706. Yanagimachi R, Okada A, Tung KSK. Sperm autoantigens and fertilization: II. Effects of anti-guinea pig sperm autoantibodies on sperm–ovum interactions. *Biol Reprod* 1981;24:512–518.
1707. Yanagimachi R, Teichman RJ. Cytochemical demonstration of acrosomal proteinase in mammalian and avian spermatozoa by a silver proteinate method. *Biol Reprod* 1972;6:87–97.
1708. Yanagimachi R, Yanagimachi H, Rogers BJ. The use of zona-free animal ova as a test-system for the assessment of the fertilizing capacity of human spermatozoa. *Biol Reprod* 1976;15: 471–476.
1709. Yanagimachi R, Zuccotti M, Weems YS. Fusibilities of plasma membranes of mammalian gametes. In: Baccetti B, ed. *Comparative Spermatology 20 Years After,* Vol. 75, New York: Raven Press; 1991:271–276.
1710. Yang CH, Yanagimachi R. Differences between mature ovarian and oviductal oocytes: a study using the golden hamster. *Hum Reprod* 1989;4:63–71.
1711. Yang CH, Yanagimachi R, Yanagimachi H. Morphology and fertilizability of zona free hamster eggs separated into halves and quarters by centrifugation. *Biol Reprod* 1989;41:741–752.
1712. Yang X, Jiang SE, Kovacs A, Foote RH. Nuclear totipotency of cultured rabbit morulae to support full-term development following nuclear transfer. *Biol Reprod* 1992;47:636–643.
1713. Yoshimatsu N, Yanagimachi R. Effects of cations and other medium components on the zona-induced acrosome reaction of hamster spermatozoa. *Dev Growth Diff* 1988;30:651–659.
1714. Yoshimatsu N, Yanagimachi R, Lopata A. Zonae pellucidae of salt-stored hamster and human eggs: their penetrability by homologous and heterologous spermatozoa. *Gamete Res* 1988; 21:115–126.
1715. Yoshimoto Y, Hiramoto Y. Observation of intracellular Ca^{2+} with aequorine luminescence. *Int Rev Cytol* 1991;129:45–73.
1716. Young LG, Gould KG, Hinston BT. Lectin binding sites on the plasma membrane of epididymal and ejaculated chimpanzee sperm. *Gamete Res* 1986;14:75–87.
1717. Younis AI, Brackett BG. Importance of cumulus cells and insemination intervals for development of bovine oocytes into morulae and blastocysts *in vitro. Theriogenology* 1991;36: 11–21.
1718. Yu SF, Wolf DP. Polyspermic mouse eggs can dispose of supernumerary sperm. *Dev Biol* 1981;82:203–210.
1719. Yudin AI, Cherr GM, Katz DF. Structure of the cumulus matrix and zona pellucida in the golden hamster: a new view of sperm interaction with oocyte-associated extracellular matrices. *Cell Tissue Res* 1988;251:555–564.
1720. Yudin AI, Gottlieb W, Meizel S. Ultrastructural studies of the early events of the human sperm acrosome reaction as initiated by human follicular fluid. *Gamete Res* 1988;20:11–24.
1721. Yurewicz EC, Pack BA, Sacco AG. Isolation, composition, and biological activity of sugar chains of porcine oocyte zona pellucida 55K glycoproteins. *Mol Reprod Dev* 1991;30:126–134.
1722. Zamboni L. Fine morphology of the follicle wall and follicle cell-oocyte association. *Biol Reprod* 1974;10:125–149.
1723. Zamboni L, Chakraborty J, Smith DM. First cleavage division of the mouse zygote. an ultrastructural study. *Biol Reprod* 1972;7:170–193.
1724. Zamboni L, Smith DM, Thompson RS. Migration of follicle cells through the zona pellucida and their sequestration by human oocytes *in vitro. J Exp Zool* 1972;181:319–340.
1725. Zaneveld LJD, De Jonge CJ. Mammalian sperm acrosomal enzymes and the acrosome reaction. In: Dunbar BS, O'Rand MG, eds. *A Comparative Overview of Mammalian Fertilization,* New York: Plenum Press; 1991:63–79.
1726. Zaneveld LJD, De Jonge CJ, Anderson RA, Mack SR. Human sperm capacitation and the acrosome reaction. *Hum Reprod* 1991;6:1265–1274.
1727. Zernika-Goetz M. Spontaneous and induced activation of rat oocytes. *Mol Reprod Dev* 1991;28:169–176.
1728. Zhang SC, Masui Y. Activation of Xenopus laevis eggs in the absence of intracellular Ca activity by the protein phosphorylation inhibitor, 6-dimethylaminopurine (6-DMAP). *J Exp Zool* 1992;262:317–329.
1729. Zhang X, Rutledge J, Armstrong DT. Studies on zona hardening in rat oocytes that are matured *in vitro* in a serum-free medium. *Mol Reprod Dev* 1991;28:292–296.
1730. Zhang X, Rutledge J, Khamsi F, Armstrong DT. Release of tissue-type plasminogen activator by activated rat eggs and its possible role in the zona reaction. *Mol Reprod Dev* 1992; 32:28–32.
1731. Zimmermann U. Electric field-mediated fusion and related electrical phenomena. *Biochim Biophys Acta* 1982;694: 227–277.
1732. Zinaman M, Drobnis EZ, Morales P, et al. The physiology of sperm recovered from the human cervix: acrosomal status and response to inducers of the acrosome reaction. *Biol Reprod* 1989;41:790–797.
1733. Zirkin BR, Perreault SD, Naish SJ. Formation and function of the male pronucleus during mammalian fertilization. In: Schatten H, Schatten G, eds. *The Molecular Biology of Fertilization,* San Diego: Academic Press; 1989:91–114.
1734. Zuccotti M, Yanagimachi R, Yanagimachi H. The ability of hamster oolemma to fuse with spermatozoa: its acquisition during oogenesis and loss after fertilization. *Development* 1991; 112:143–152.
1735. Yanagimachi R, et al. Unpublished data.

The Physiology of Reproduction, Second Edition,
edited by E. Knobil and J.D. Neill,
Raven Press, Ltd., New York © 1994.

CHAPTER 6

Mammalian Embryogenesis

Roger A. Pedersen and Carol A. Burdsal

INTRODUCTION

This chapter is devoted to advances in the field of mammalian development. During the past two decades, we have witnessed revolutionary progress in our understanding of preimplantation and early postimplantation differentiation of mammalian embryos. Although much of this work has been carried out in laboratory animals, particularly rodents, embryo biotechnology has been increasingly extended to livestock species and to humans, with major economic and clinical benefits. These successes in the areas of embryo transfer in agricultural animals (see 1,2,3 for review) and human *in vitro* fertilization (see 4,5,6,7 for review) have commanded widespread attention to the potential for further application of our knowledge of mammalian embryos. Because these successful applications are extensively reviewed elsewhere, we focus here on advancements in basic understanding of early mammalian embryogenesis, which provide the technical and conceptual foundation for future insights and applications. This review addresses morphological, genetic, and molecular aspects of mammalian embryogenesis; gametogenesis and fertilization, although closely related to embryogenesis, are not treated here because they are the subjects of other chapters in this volume.

Laboratory of Radiobiology and Environmental Health; Departments of Radiology, Anatomy and Obstetrics, Gynecology and Reproductive Sciences; University of California, San Francisco, California 94143

Historical Overview of Mammalian Embryology

Since the time of Aristotle, the origin of mammalian embryos has attracted the attention of scholars and healers. This ultimately led to the seventeenth and eighteenth century discoveries of the sperm and egg as the cellular components of animal reproduction. Von Baer extended this observation to the mammal with his description of the dog's egg in 1828. The nineteenth century was characterized by intense activity in descriptive embryology, facilitated by development of histological techniques and culminating in intense philosophical debates over Haeckel's germ layer theory and Wolff's epigenetic theory of development (8,9). The advent of experimental embryology in the late nineteenth century in the work of Boveri and his contemporaries was largely confined to invertebrates and amphibians, which yielded abundant embryos for experimental analysis. However, there were early successes with mammalian embryos during this period, including the first embryo transfers by Heape (10) and light microscopic morphological descriptions of rodent embryos that are still unsurpassed in their detail (see 11 for review and references).

Our modern era of experimental mammalian embryology had its origins in the culture of mouse embryos by Whitten (12,14; see 15–17, for review) and the successful transfer of cultured embryos to foster mothers by McLaren and Biggers with development into live-born young (18). Another important contribution was development of methods for increasing the number and controlling the stage of mammalian embryos by superovulation using gonadotropins (19). Together, these innovations led to an outburst of research on the fate and potency of blastomeres, developmental genetics, and physiological and molecular properties of the mammalian embryo between the time of fertilization and completion of organogenesis. This rapid development of the field has been sustained by a wider perception of the need to gain control over human reproduction and to assess the risks of prenatal exposure to environmental pollutants. Moreover, advancements in this field will ultimately lead to an understanding of the causes of developmental abnormalities.

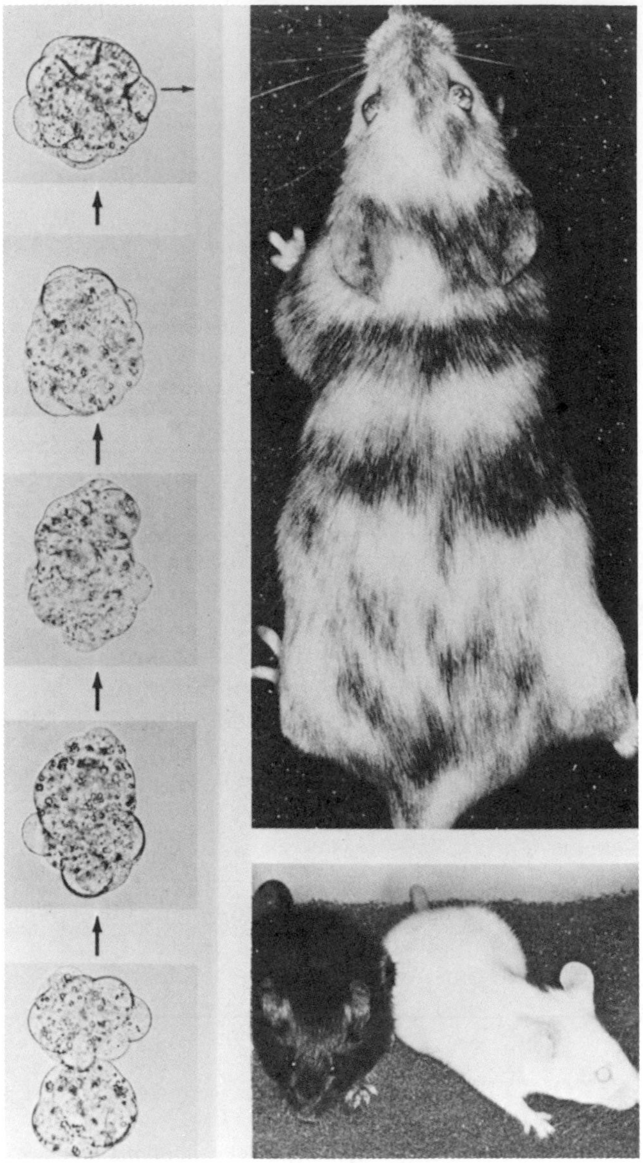

FIG. 1. Two cleavage-stage embryos (*lower left*) of pigmented and albino genotypes, respectively, aggregated after zonae pellucidae removal. Successive views show formation of one chimeric embryo from all the blastomeres of both. A chimeric mouse from one such chimera (*upper right*): note transverse clones of black and white in the coat and radiating clones in the eyes. Mating this mouse with a white male produced both pigmented and albino offspring (*lower right*). From Mintz (901).

Methods Used in Mammalian Embryology

Although some investigators have used traditional embryological approaches such as disaggregation or extirpation of blastomeres, the small and fragile mammalian embryo has required novel approaches. The most elegant of these have taken advantage of the accumulated genetic information about mammals. The first experimental approach unique to mammals was production of aggregation chimeras, pioneered by Tarkowski (20) and Mintz (21) (Fig. 1) (see 22 for a review of the early work using chimeras). These chimeras were formed by aggregating two 8- to 16-cell-stage mouse embryos after removing their zonae pellucidae. For analytical purposes, the embryos were obtained from strains which differed in coat or eye color, chromosomal morphology, or biochemical traits. The most commonly used biochemical markers were the isozymes of glucose phosphate isomerase (23), which could be readily resolved on gels prepared from even small amounts of embryonic tissue. As a marker for analyzing chimeras, glucose phosphate isomerase was advantageous because it was present in virtually all tissues of the embryo and the adult, whereas pigmented or rapidly dividing cells were not ubiquitous. This marker's disadvantage was that the resulting animal's three-dimensional structure was lost in preparing tissue extracts for analysis (see 22 for review).

These limitations spurred a quest for better markers. The criteria for an ideal marker include cell autonomy (i.e., the marker must not require other cells for its expression), ubiquity, heritability, and ease of detection

(24,25). Gardner (27) used the combination of cells mutant or wild type for malic enzyme to study postimplantation fate of extraembryonic endoderm cells. Also, Rossant and coworkers studied chimeras between closely related mouse species, using *in situ* hybridization with recombinant DNA probes to distinguish donor and host descendants (28,29). The bacterial gene for beta-galactosidase (*lacZ*) also fulfills the above criteria and has been used in numerous studies to identify the site of transcription of tissue-specific genes; its use as a lineage marker is discussed in a later section dealing with potency and fate in early embryogenesis. The methods, concepts, and applications involved in mammalian chimeras have recently been reviewed (30).

Micromanipulation of mammalian embryos, pioneered by Lin (31), has led to dramatic insights. Gardner's development of techniques for introducing individual cells into blastocysts (26) led to a new generation of chimera studies which assessed the fate and potency of cells at later stages and with greater resolution than was possible with aggregation chimeras (Fig. 2). In these studies, Gardner and coworkers generally used the biochemical markers developed for aggregation chimeras and analyzed the progeny either at midgestation or after birth.

Microinjection of cell lineage tracers into cells provides an alternative method for marking progenitor cells in lineage studies. Initially, oil droplets were used to mark cells, but this suffered from a propensity to segregate to a single blastomere (32,33). Pedersen and coworkers used horseradish peroxidase, initially used for lineage studies in amphibian and annelid embryos (34–36) to trace the lineages of marked progenitor cells during early stages of development of the mouse embryo (37, see 36 for review) (Fig. 3). Although such passively distributed markers are limited to short-term studies, because they become diluted during embryonic growth, they have provided for analysis of the fate of single cells while avoiding disturbance of the embryonic architecture.

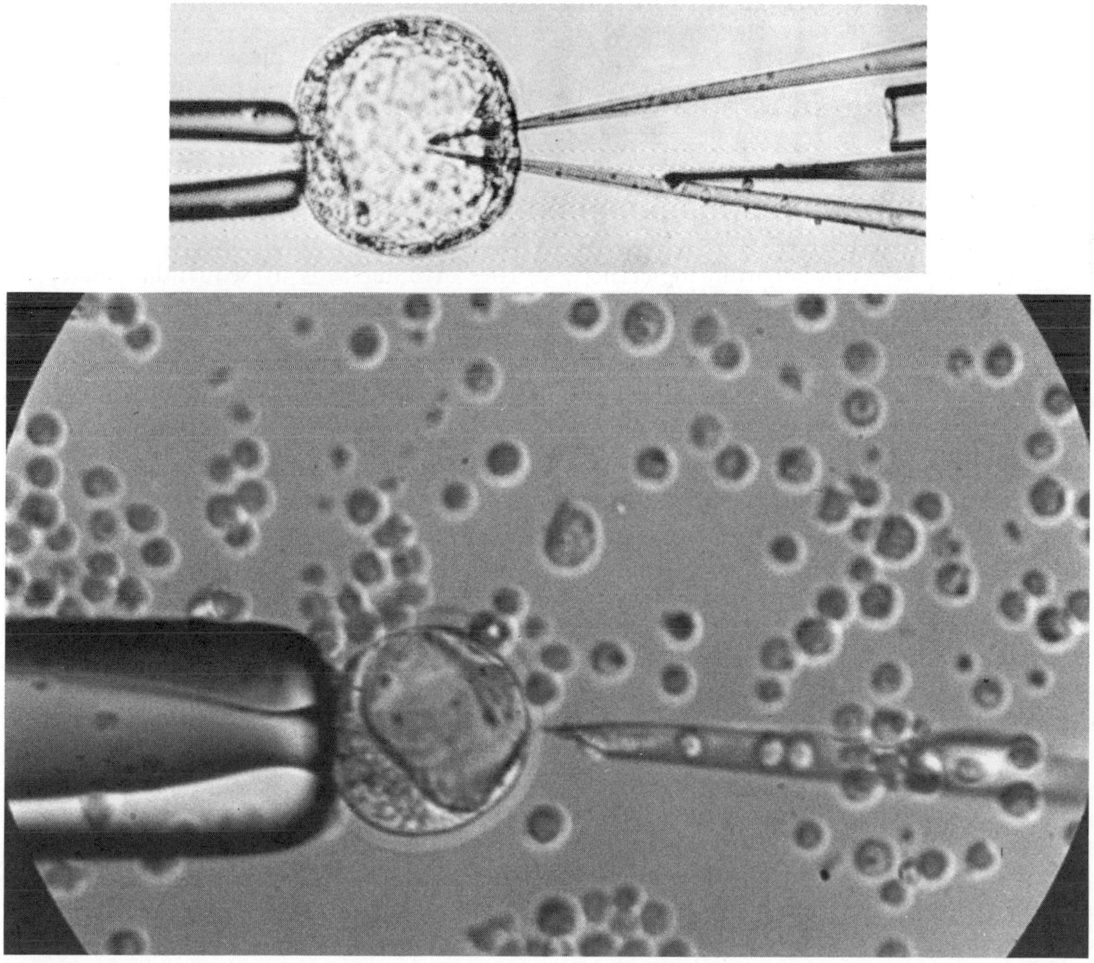

FIG. 2. Injection into the mouse blastocyst cavity through a triangular opening to generate chimeras at the blastocyst stage (*top*). From Gardner (442). Injection of embryonic stem cells into a mouse blastocyst using a beveled needle (*bottom*).

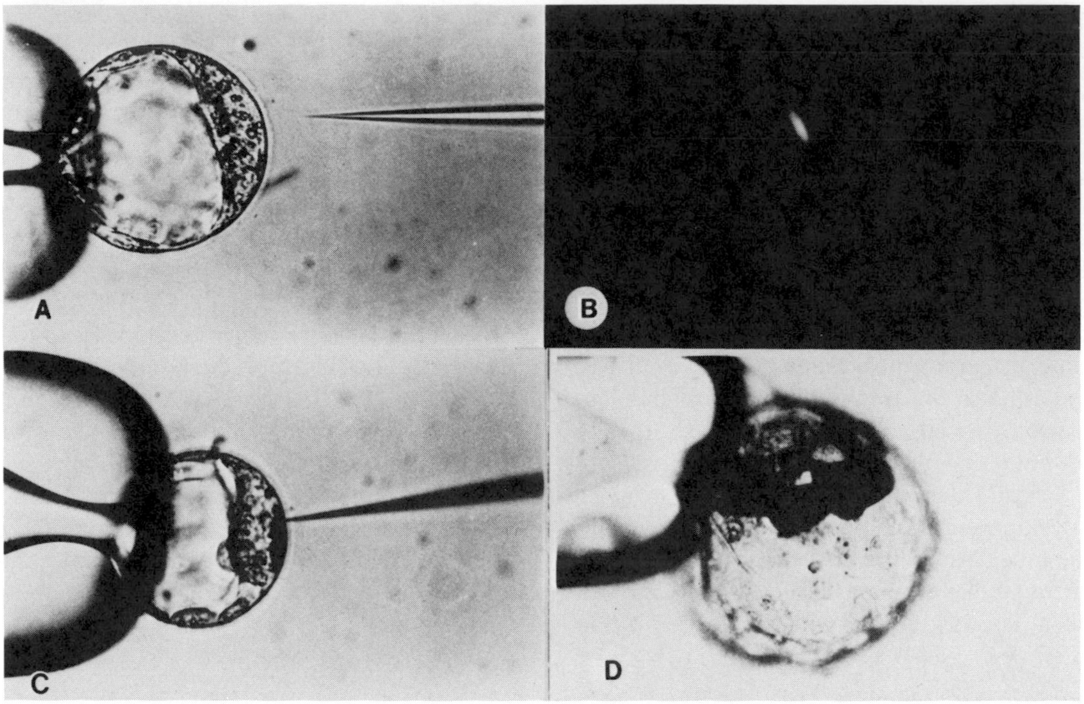

FIG. 3. Injection of horseradish peroxidase plus rhodamine-conjugated dextran into polar trophectoderm cells to analyze their fate during blastocyst growth. **A:** Midstage blastocyst prepared for microinjection into central polar trophectoderm cell. **B:** Fluorescence of rhodamine-conjugated dextran immediately after injection. **C:** Staining of injected cell with horseradish peroxidase immediately after injection. **D:** Staining of descendant cells with horseradish peroxidase after 48-hour culture, showing predominantly mural localization of stained trophectoderm cells. From Cruz and Pedersen (169).

The importance of nuclear transfer studies for understanding nuclear potency was evident from the earlier work on amphibian embryos by Briggs and King (38), who demonstrated the totipotency of blastula nuclei, and by Gurdon (39), who extended these observations to tadpole nuclei. The nuclear transfer method devised by McGrath and Solter (40) is based on fusion of microsurgically transferred karyoplast fragments at the zygote stage. Experiments using appropriate genetic markers for donor and host components have revealed unique roles for maternal and paternal pronuclei in early mouse embryogenesis, as discussed in a later section.

Production of transgenic animals by microinjecting exogenous DNA into the zygote pronucleus (41) has become a powerful method for studying mammalian embryogenesis. This method produces genetically novel animals which carry one or more copies of the exogenous DNA integrated into their genome. These integrated genes are inherited as Mendelian traits in subsequent generations and may be expressed in tissue-specific and temporally correct patterns (see 42 for review). Transgenic mice provide access to the mammalian genome for a wide variety of genetic, biochemical, and physiological studies, as subsequently described.

The demands of mammalian embryos have fostered other methodological innovations in addition to micromanipulation. Immunosurgery, the cytotoxic immune lysis of outer cells by sequential treatment with heat-inactivated antiserum and active complement (43), has been used to obtain pure populations of inner cells for molecular analysis and for making chimeras. Because of the small amount of material mammalian embryos provide, miniaturization is a universally applied method for studying them. Many investigators have ingeniously reduced the amounts of tissue required for their studies. They have also tended to treat the individual embryo as the experimental unit and to rely on small population sizes (44). This trend is epitomized in the physiological analysis of individual preimplantation embryos using techniques developed for single cells (46,47; see 45 for review). Another approach was to increase the sensitivity of an existing analytical technique so it could be used with embryos. Two-dimensional gel electrophoresis was used to identify polypeptide differences between inner cell mass and trophectoderm tissues of mouse embryos (48). This method has recently been extended to construct high-resolution protein databases for preimplantation-stage mouse embryos (49). Similarly, by refining the procedures for generating cDNA libraries, it has been possible to generate stage-specific libraries of cleavage- and blastocyst-stage mouse embryos (50). Exquisite sensitivities for detecting messenger RNA (mRNA) have been achieved by using reverse transcriptase and the polymerase chain reaction (RT-PCR) to amplify cDNA products of specific genes at various preimplantation stages (51,52). Similarly, *in situ* hybridization brings analysis of mRNA transcripts to the single embryo level of sensitivity, particularly when used as a whole-mount method (53,54). The ultimate combination of resolving power and sensitivity in analyzing embryonic transcription may be attained by combining RT-PCR with cDNA cloning to generate amplified libraries from single embryos (55). It is perhaps a reflection of the revolutionary state of the field of mammalian embryology that such technological innovations have often found their earliest applications with early mouse embryos.

An alternative strategy for analysis of mammalian development is to exploit pluripotent stem cells derived from germ-cell tumors or from embryos as cell culture systems for studying the differentiative events that occur in early embryos. Initial studies of such pluripotent cells by Stevens and by Pierce focused on the stem cells of teratomas, or embryonal carcinoma (EC) cells (56). Because of their pluripotency and their tendency to develop into clusters of cells (embryoid bodies) resembling the tissues of a normal embryo, EC cells have been widely studied as models for the early stages of mouse development (57). The observation (58,59) that EC cells could contribute to chimeras when they were injected into blastocysts led to extensive studies that characterized their limited capacity for germline contribution (60). The search for alternative systems led to the discovery that pluripotent stem cells could be grown directly from preimplantation-stage embryos (61,62). These cells, known as embryonic stem (ES) cells, have not been studied as extensively as models for embryonic differentiation as EC cells; however, they have become widely used as vehicles for introducing genes into mice, because of their capacity for contribution to the germline (Fig. 4) (reviewed in 63–65). Exploitation of ES cells for gene targeting in mice ranks as one of the major developments in mammalian genetics. This is discussed in a later section and is noted throughout this review where there are relevant results from ablating the functions of particular genes.

In sum, despite its small initial size and relative inaccessibility in the maternal reproductive tract, the mammalian embryo has yielded to numerous ingenious approaches. As a result, mammalian embryos are now being examined over a wide range of cellular, morphological, genetic, and molecular aspects. The success of the many investigators who have devoted themselves to mammalian embryology has thereby established the embryos of mammalian species, mice in particular, as uniquely valuable models for studies of vertebrate devel-

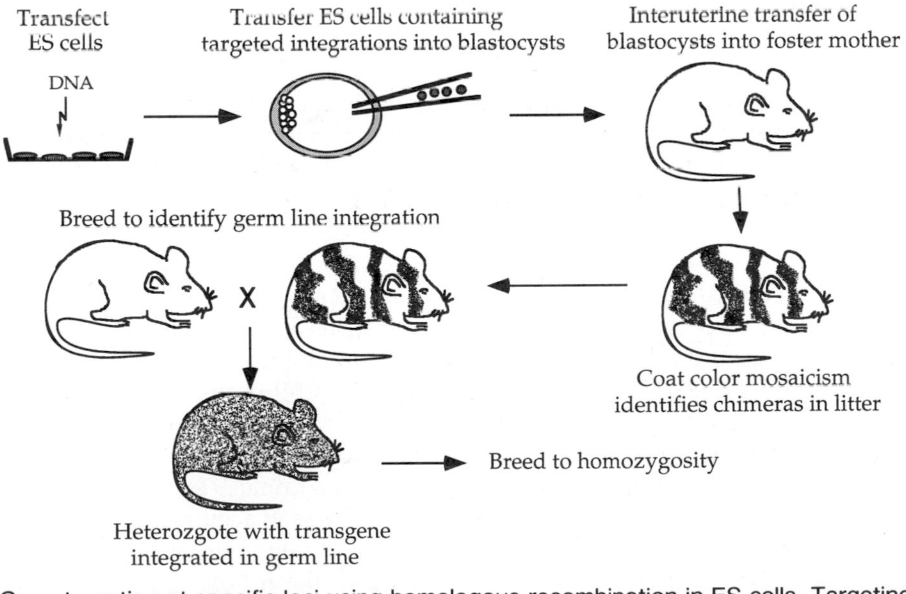

FIG. 4. Gene targeting at specific loci using homologous recombination in ES cells. Targeting vectors are constructed that will alter or replace specific genes by homologous recombination. After screening and selecting transformants, ES cells containing targeted integrations are injected into host blastocysts that are then transferred to the uteri of pseudopregnant foster mothers. By using ES cells and host blastocysts from strains of mice with different coat colors, chimeras generated from these manipulations can be identified by coat color mosaicism. The chimeras are then bred with mice having the host blastocyst genotype; if the ES cells have contributed to a chimera's germ line, the coat color of the ES line is passed on, and one copy of the targeted gene is present in the offspring. Interbreeding of these heterozygous mice will produce transgenic animals, one quarter of which will be homozygous at the targeted locus.

opment. Although the field has expanded to the extent that it is no longer possible to review it in its entirety, we present some of the major issues and findings and provide an indication about promising future research directions.

MORPHOLOGICAL ASPECTS

Timing of Early Morphogenesis

The events of fertilization occur relatively slowly in mammals compared to most other organisms. The time required for sperm-egg fusion and second polar body emission is 1–2 hours after insemination in the mouse (66,67) and 2–5 hours in the hamster (68). Pronuclei form about 6 hours after insemination, and DNA synthesis begins 2–4 hours later in most strains of mice studied (67,69). In the hamster, the time from insemination to pronuclear formation is about 4 hours; time to the beginning of DNA synthesis is about 8 hours (70). The time from insemination to sperm penetration varies in other species depending on the duration of capacitation (see the chapter by Yanagimachi, this volume, for details of capacitation). Given that ovulation occurs in mice at the midpoint of the dark period, by the middle of the day on which the copulatory plug is found [0.5 days of gestation (d.g.)], the embryos have progressed only to the pronuclear stage. By comparison, *Drosophila* embryos undergo cleavage at 10-minute intervals, and amphibian embryos cleave at approximately 30-minute intervals. Mouse embryos undergo their first and second cleavages at intervals of 20–26 hours *in vivo* in most strains studied (69). There is a marked effect of genetic background on cleavage time in the first two cycles; later cleavages occur at approximately 10-hour intervals in most strains of mice (71–73). However, there is an association between certain haplotypes at the H-2 locus and slow-versus-fast development (74). When mouse embryos are placed in culture, their development is retarded, with cleavage progressing 2 or more hours slower each cycle than *in vivo,* so that the time for development to the blastocyst stage *in vitro* may be an entire day longer than *in vivo* (75,76).

There is now considerable information about the cell cycle dynamics at various cleavage stages in the mouse embryo. Figure 5 details representative stages. In the first cell cycle, S phase lasts 4–8 hours and G2 + M ranges from 3 to 8 hours; in the second cycle, S takes 4–7 hours, and G2 + M ranges from 12 to 15 hours (67,69,77; see 78 for review). The comparable values for the third and fourth cycles are 7 hours for S and from 1 to 5 hours for G2 + M (79); for the fifth cycle, 8–9 hours; and G2 + M lasts 2 hours (80). The G1 phase of the cycle is brief at all cleavage stages (1–2 hours). These estimates are valuable when attempting to infer at what point important events in cell determination and differentiation occur. Human embryos also develop as slowly *in vitro* as do mouse embryos, dividing at intervals of 16–24 hours during early cleavages (81,82); in their first cell cycle, human embryos have an S phase of 3–5 hours, G2 phase of 3–6 hours, and M phase of 3.0–3.5 hours (83).

Cleavage is invariably asynchronous in mammalian embryos. Asynchronous division from the 2-cell stage creates a 3-cell embryo. The earlier dividing blastomere of the 2-cell mouse embryo in turn has descendants that divide earlier than descendants of the later dividing blastomere (73,84). The range from the earliest to latest division at late cleavage stages can reach several hours in culture, with longer times at the later cleavages (73).

During mid- to late cleavage stages of placental mammals, the blastomeres begin a process of compaction, during which individual blastomeres seem to lose their identity and merge into a single coherent mass of cells (85). This early morphogenetic event is marked by junctional differentiation in which gap junctions and incipient tight junctions form between outer blastomeres and initiate the process of epithelial differentiation, culminating in the formation of trophectoderm at the blastocyst stage (86–90; for review see 91–94). It is interesting that compaction does not occur in marsupial embryos; instead, the blastomeres accumulated by midcleavage stages adhere to the zona pellucida, eventually forming a single outer cell layer (unilaminar) at the blastocyst stage (95–97). In addition to the importance of compaction in eutherian embryos as one of the first visible signs of embryonic differentiation, it also reflects the onset of their cell-cell adhesion and junctional development, as discussed in a later section.

The next morphogenetic event in mammalian development is the formation of the blastocyst cavity, also known as the blastocoel, although it is not homologous to the amphibian blastocoel. Blastocyst formation manifests the beginning of fluid transport by the trophectoderm cells, as well as physical partitioning of cells between an inner compartment (the inner cell mass) and an outer epithelium (the trophectoderm), which envelops the inner cells and retains the blastocoel fluid. The mural trophectoderm surrounds the blastocoel, and the polar trophectoderm overlies the inner cell mass (see Fig. 5). The cell number at the time of blastocyst formation varies considerably among various species of placental mammals (85; see 95,98 for review). Generally, fluid begins to accumulate in late cleavage: after division to the 16-cell stage in the hamster and pig, the 32-cell stage in the mouse, the 64-cell stage in the sheep and human, and the 128-cell stage in the rabbit. Some rare species accumulate fluid at earlier stages; for example, the *Elephantulus* embryo begins accumulating its blastocoel fluid at the four-cell stage (95,98).

During blastocyst expansion, asynchrony between cell divisions increases and cell division slows in the mouse embryo (99–101). In the mural trophectoderm, this tendency culminates in giant cell transformation, a process

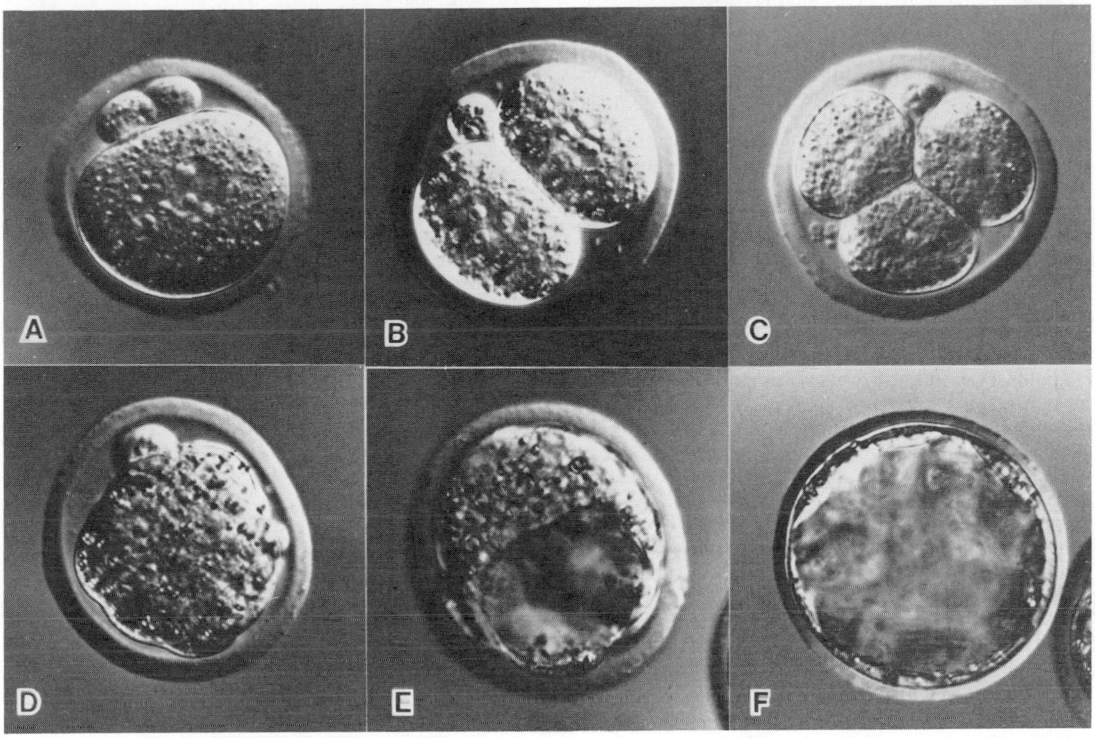

G
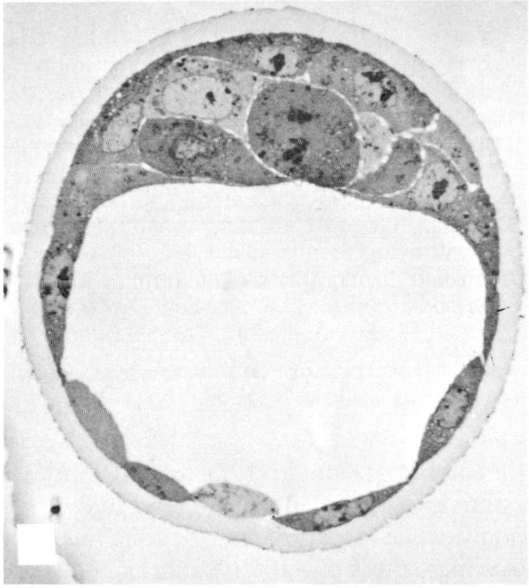

FIG. 5. Preimplantation stages of mouse embryo development. **A:** Zygote, 0.5 d.g.; **B:** 2-cell stage, 1.5 d.g.; **C:** 4-cell stage, 2.0 d.g.; **D:** Compacting morula, (8- to 16-cell stage), 2.5–3.0 d.g.; **E:** Early blastocyst stage, (32 cells), 3.5 d.g.; **F:** Expanded blastocyst stage (~64 cells); inner cell mass is out of focal plane. ×340. From Pedersen (78). **G:** Thick-section scanning electron micrograph of 3.5 d.g. mouse blastocyst showing large, rounded cells of inner cell mass and flattened cells of trophectoderm. ×595. From Pierce (902).

of endoreduplication (DNA synthesis without cell division), which begins in the abembryonic mural trophectoderm—opposite to the inner cell mass—at 4.5–6.5 d.g., depending on the species (102; reviewed in 95). The proportion of inner cell mass cells to total blastocyst cells decreases in both mouse and pig embryos during the late blastocyst stage despite maintaining similar mitotic indices as the trophectoderm, perhaps reflecting cell death in the inner cell mass (101,103). Approximately 10% of blastocyst cells are indeed necrotic during blastocyst expansion, suggesting that programmed cell death may occur at this stage (101).

At 4.0–4.5 d.g. in the mouse, hatching commences and the blastocyst escapes from the zona pellucida. By this time, the inner cell mass has differentiated into an outer layer of primitive endoderm surrounding an inner core of primitive ectoderm. Then the embryo begins to implant in the uterine wall, where the inner cell mass and polar trophectoderm-derived cells grow rapidly, transforming the rodent embryo into a cylindrical structure by 5.5 d.g. (Fig. 6). The inner core of this "egg cylinder" has two components, embryonic ectoderm and extraembryonic ectoderm, while the single outer component is primitive (or visceral) endoderm. An estimated

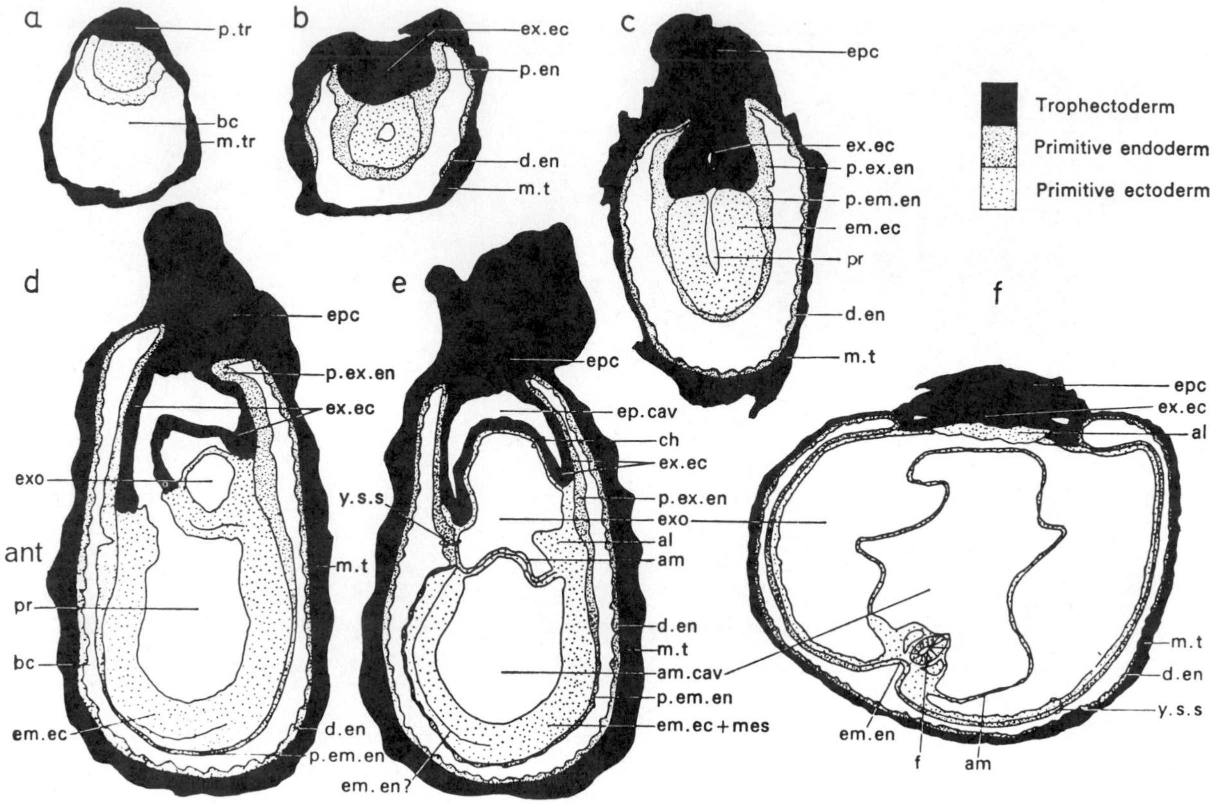

FIG. 6. Fate map of the trophectoderm (*solid*), primitive endoderm (*fine stippling*), and primitive ectoderm (*coarse stippling*) of the mouse late blastocyst projected onto successive developmental stages. **A:** 4.5 d.g. implanting late blastocyst. **B:** 5.0 d.g. proamniotic cavity stage early egg cylinder. **C:** 5.5 d.g. early pre-streak stage egg cylinder. **D:** 7.0 d.g. early gastrula stage egg cylinder. **E:** 7.5 d.g. mid-gastrula stage egg cylinder. **F:** 8.5 d.g. early somite stage embryo, in transverse section. The parts of the embryos are drawn to scale. al, allantois; am, amnion; am. cav, amniotic cavity; ant, anterior; bc, blastocoel; ch, chorion; d. en, distal (parietal) endoderm; em. ec, embryonic ectoderm (epiblast); em. en, definitive embryonic (gut) endoderm; epc, ectoplacental cone; ep. cav, extoplacental cavity; ex. ec, extraembryonic ectoderm; exo, exocoelom; f, fetus; mes, mesoderm; m. tr, mural trophectoderm; p. tr, polar trophectoderm; p. em. en, proximal (visceral) embryonic endoderm; p. ex. en, proximal (visceral) extraembryonic endoderm; pr, proamniotic cavity; y. s. s., yolk sac splanchnopluеure. From Gardner and Papaioannou (178).

cell cycle time for visceral endoderm of 10.7 hours was obtained for mouse embryos using the labeled mitoses method (104); an estimate of 6.6 hours was obtained from colcemid-blocked mitoses (105); and an estimate of population doubling times of 10.5 hours (anterior visceral endoderm) or 8.4 hours (posterior visceral endoderm) was obtained from single-cell HRP injections into axial endoderm at 6.7 d.g. (228). HRP injections into axial visceral endoderm cells one day later gave a population doubling time of 24 hours and revealed a substantial level of cell death; the surviving endoderm cells had a cell cycle time of 11.5 hours or less (227). The differences in results between studies may be a combination of method, stage, and tissue differences. Estimates of the cell cycle times in embryonic ectoderm (or epiblast) based on cell counts and mitotic indices led Snow (106) to postulate the existence of a proliferative zone anterior to the primitive streak, with a cell cycle time of 3 hours; labeled mitoses provided an estimate of cell cycle time for epiblast of 8 hours (107); and HRP injection gave an estimate of 7.5 hours (229). The latter two studies found no evidence for a proliferative zone but did not seek to eliminate this possibility. A thorough assessment of the epiblast population dynamics using various approaches in rat embryos revealed a cell cycle time for the luminal cells of the primitive streak of 3.0–3.5 hours and for the remainder of epiblast and mesoderm of 7.0–7.5 hours. The short cell cycle time in epiblast cells of the rat primitive streak resulted from reductions in all phases of the cell cycle (107a). This observation of an epiblast proliferative zone differs from that of Snow (106), not only in location but also in nature: it is located within the primitive streak rather than anterior to it, and it is a transitory phenomenon in the rat embryo, with cells resuming a more typical cell cycle once they emerge from the primitive streak as mesoderm rather than persisting within the epiblast as a stem cell population (904).

The differences in cell cycle times between stages and

tissues raise the question of what kind of clock regulates cell division and morphogenesis in the early embryo. This question has been approached experimentally using aggregation chimeras and other techniques. Neither increasing the number of cells in the mouse embryo by aggregating two or more embryos together nor decreasing the cell number by inducing tetraploidy appreciably changes the time of cavitation, but simply changes the number of cells in the embryo at the time the cavity forms (108). This observation led to the proposal that mouse embryos count time by nuclear divisions. Contrary to this idea, however, are the results of treating mouse embryos with phorbol esters, aphidicolin (an inhibitor of DNA polymerase alpha), or inhibitors of polyamine biosynthesis. These treatments cause cavitation with fewer cells and at earlier times than in the normal embryo (109 113). Thus, there may be a cytoplasmic component to timekeeping in the mammal as there is in the amphibian embryo (114), rather than a strictly nuclear clock as in the ascidian (115).

The mechanism of cell cycle control is an active topic in many embryonic and cell culture systems, including the early mouse embryo. In 1971, Masui and Markert discovered that cytoplasmic factors regulate the progression of meiosis in amphibian embryos (116). Maturation promoting factor (MPF), which is abundant in the mature amphibian oocyte, mouse oocyte, and in embryonic and somatic cells at the time of mitosis, induces nuclear breakdown and chromosomal condensation of meiotic as well as mitotic nuclei (117–122; see 123 for review). Complementary studies in yeast and *Xenopus* recently led to molecular identification of the components of MPF, $p34^{cdc2}$ and cyclin, and subsequent studies have revealed the alternating patterns of $p34^{cdc2}$ phosphorylation/dephosphorylation and cylin synthesis/degradation which are responsible for its cyclic M-phase-inducing activity (reviewed in 124). Antibodies against cdc2 protein have been used to detect this component of MPF in fertilized mouse embryos (125), and transcripts for cyclins B1 and B2 were also found in eggs and zygotes and in both inner cell mass and trophectoderm at the blastocyst stage (896). Thus, the molecular components of this universal cell cycle-regulating system are present also in mammalian embryos. Sorting out the mechanistic relationships between cell cycle events and morphogenesis is an even more complex problem that needs to be resolved before we can understand how early development is coordinated.

Potency of Isolated Blastomeres

Developmental biologists have long been interested in determining the potency of early cell types. Prospective potency is defined as the full range of developmental capabilities of an embryonic cell or tissue (126), and as such can only be characterized by experimental perturbation of the intact embryo. Restriction of potency—that is, determination—indicates that decisive events have limited the future capabilities of the cell or tissue. Understanding the molecular mechanisms which underlie this aspect of developmental decision-making is a fundamental problem of developmental biology, and assessing the potency of cells during mammalian development is of major importance. Not only are individual 2-cell blastomeres of mouse (127) and rabbit (128) embryos totipotent, the offspring that develop from single mouse two-cell blastomeres are normal in every detectable aspect (129,131). Tarkowski and Wroblewska (132) found, however, that most individual blastomeres isolated at the 4- and 8-cell stages developed into trophoblast vesicles devoid of inner cells. They proposed that the differentiation into trophectoderm and inner cell mass was determined by the outer or inner position of blastomeres at the morula stage (16 to 32 cells). This "inside-outside" hypothesis predicted that blastomeres would remain totipotent at least until they assume their positions at the morula stage. A substantial body of work confirms this prediction, showing that mouse embryo blastomeres maintain their potency at the 2- to 16-cell stages (127,133–136). A similar degree of totipotency seems to exist in cleavage-stage rabbit, horse, cow, and sheep embryos (see 98,137 for review). Beyond the morula stage, the increasing junctional differentiation of the outer cells that accompanies their incipient differentiation into trophectoderm makes it difficult to disaggregate the embryo and assess their potency (138). Nonetheless, outer cells of the late morula (~30 cell stage) have been shown to be totipotent in mouse embryos, as are the inner cells at this stage (135).

Furthermore, cells in the inner cell mass of the early mouse blastocyst are also totipotent because they can form trophectoderm when isolated by immunosurgery and grown in culture, and they can even differentiate into invasive giant cells when transferred to the uteri of foster mothers (139–142). Immunosurgery has also been used to isolate inner cells at later stages of blastocyst development. These studies show that the inner cells lose their totipotency during blastocyst expansion at approximately the time of the division from 32 to 64 cells (139–141). Inner cells isolated from expanded blastocysts either by immunosurgery or by microdissection form an outer layer of primitive endoderm cells, rather than of trophectoderm (143). It is difficult, however, to define the precise stage at which this important developmental transition occurs. Cells differentiating from individual inner cell masses isolated at the 32- to 64-cell stages often contain a mixture of trophectoderm and primitive endoderm cells (100,144). This heterogeneity could arise from asynchrony within the inner cell mass, with cells at their sixth cycle forming trophectoderm and cells at their seventh cycle forming primitive endoderm. Thus, restriction in the potency of inner cell occurs relatively late in preimplantation development.

Cell Allocation in Preimplantation Embryos

The totipotency of preimplantation mammalian embryo cells focuses our attention on the timing and mechanisms that allocate some of the blastomeres to the inner cell mass and others to the trophectoderm lineage. Several studies have made it clear that the position of a blastomere in the early embryo is crucial to its subsequent fate. When totipotent blastomeres of cleavage-stage embryos which had been experimentally marked with [^{3}H]-thymidine or differing in their glucose phosphate isomerase isozyme were placed on the outside of aggregation chimeras, they generally developed into trophectoderm. Conversely, cells on the inside generally developed into inner cell mass (133,134). These results fulfill a major prediction of the inside-outside hypothesis and raise the question of when and how cells acquire their positions in the intact embryo.

The early cleavage stages of mouse embryos have only outer cells, presumably because packing of equal-sized, round objects requires a minimum number to completely enclose one or more of them. This number ranges from 10 to 17 in modeling studies, depending on the deformability assumed for the objects (145,146). Inside cells are first observed in mouse embryos at the 10- to 16-cell stage, when 1–6 cells are enclosed, as determined by time lapse cinemicrography (146) or by paraffin serial sectioning, immunosurgery, or labeling intact embryos on their outer surface with fluorescent antibodies, then disaggregating them (147). The mean number of enclosed cells increases to 10–13 at the early blastocyst-stage (32-cell) mouse embryo (see Fig. 5), with some variation depending on the method used (100). The ratio of inner cells to total blastocyst cell number decreases from 0.40 in the early mouse blastocyst to 0.25 in the late blastocyst (128–256-cell stage) (99; see also 148).

The distribution of cleavage products into inner cell mass and trophectoderm is not random. First, mixing between regions of cleavage-stage mouse embryos is limited, as shown by aggregating [3H]thymidine-labeled and unlabeled 8-cell embryos and sectioning them for autoradiography at the blastocyst stage. The descendants of the labeled blastomeres tend to remain together in the same quadrant of the resulting chimera rather than mixing thoroughly (149,150). Likewise, when chimeras are made between the 4-cell descendants of earlier- and later-dividing 2-cell blastomeres, the earlier-dividing blastomere contributes slightly more cells to the inner cell mass than the later-dividing cell, also indicative of nonrandom contribution (84,151). This attribute of earlier-dividing blastomeres in aggregation chimeras is even more dramatic when 4- and 8-cell mouse embryos are combined, in which case the inner cell mass of the chimera is composed almost entirely of cells from the more advanced component (152). However, time-lapse analysis of intact embryos found no significant relationship between division order at the second and third cleavages and the division plane at the fourth cleavage, which appears to determine whether cells are allocated to the inner cell mass or trophectoderm lineages (73). These authors conclude that the disparity in division times between the blastomeres used in the chimera studies far exceed the differences in intact embryos, thus generating an artifact in chimeras. Nevertheless, the phenomenon of disproportionate contribution to the inner cell mass of chimeras by the more advanced blastomeres has been exploited to manufacture sheep-goat chimeras in which the primary fetal component is derived from the goat, but the sheep trophoblast constitution is compatible with development to term in a sheep foster mother (153). The mechanism for this differential contribution may involve the size or cell surface characteristics of the blastomeres, since smaller, advanced blastomeres tend to be engulfed by larger, earlier-stage blastomeres when they are combined in pairs (154,155). Even in the intact embryo, earlier-dividing blastomeres at the fourth cleavage division have a slightly greater tendency to divide into inner and outer cell pairs than the later-dividing blastomeres, which have a greater tendency to produce outer/outer pairs (73). Thus, intercellular interactions in the fourth cleavage division may influence the division plane and allocation of cells to yield greater contributions to the inner cell mass from the earlier-dividing blastomeres at this stage, which are also likely to be the earlier-flattening ones during recompaction of the embryo after cleavage (156).

Further evidence for an orderly partitioning of cleavage products into the inner cell mass and tophectoderm has been obtained by reaggregating outer and inner blastomeres of 16-cell mouse embryos. At this stage, the outer blastomeres of mouse embryos are slightly larger than the inner ones and are polarized, having a higher density of microvilli on their free surface than on portions of their membranes apposed to other blastomeres. In contrast to this polarized phenotype of the outer cells, inner cells are apolar (157,158). When labeled outer cells are combined in either inner or outer locations with various proportions of unlabeled inner or outer cells, the polarized outer cell invariably contributes at least one descendant to the trophectoderm of the resulting blastocyst. The developmental contributions of the apolar (inner) cells are not as constrained; they give rise to either inner cell mass or trophectoderm, depending primarily on their initial position in the aggregates (159,160). The polarization of rabbit embryo blastomeres occurs at a later stage of development (after the 32-cell stage, and thus after compaction), suggesting that the phenomenon of blastomere polarization before blastocyst formation may be a general property of eutherian mammals (161).

Unfortunately, this information does not allow us to make a conclusive statement about what controls differentiation into either trophectoderm or inner cell mass.

The predictions of the inside-outside hypothesis about totipotency and the role of position in cell fate are supported by available evidence, but this does not indicate what kind of signals might cause the differentiation of enclosed cells into inner cell mass and outer cells into trophectoderm. It is unlikely that diffusible substances in the blastocoel cavity cause or sustain inner cell mass differentiation because embryos at totipotent stages inserted with intact zonae pellucidae into the blastocoel of giant chimeras develop into morphologically normal blastocysts, rather than into inner cell masslike structures (162). The polarization hypothesis also accounts for many of the events leading to trophectoderm differentiation (163). In this hypothesis, the separation of cleaving blastomeres into two lineages is thought to be the result of the propensity of outer cells to polarize, owing to their asymmetric cell contacts (see 164 for review). When combined with the constraints of polarization discussed previously, this presumably leads to the allocation of polarized descendants to the trophectoderm at the blastocyst stage and of apolar descendants to the inner cell mass. The polarization hypothesis predicts that polarized blastomeres will maintain the capacity to generate apolar cells, and that apolar cells will maintain the capacity to polarize, until the two tissue lineages of the blastocyst become clonally distinct populations. It does not exclude the possibility that inner cell mass cells will have outer descendants. The inside-outside hypothesis predicts, however, that cells located on the inside at the morula or blastocyst stage will remain stably located in the inner cell mass lineage during subsequent postimplantation development.

The microinjection of horseradish peroxidase into individual blastomeres also demonstrates that developmental constraints appear during early development of the intact mouse embryo. Labeled descendants of 2-cell blastomeres almost always occupy both inner cell mass and trophectoderm. Single 8-cell blastomeres often have descendants in both inner cell mass and trophectoderm, but may have exclusively trophectoderm descendants (37). Outer, 16-cell blastomeres have principally trophectoderm descendants but may have inner cell mass descendants as well (167). Interestingly, the number of internal cells generated at the fourth and fifth cleavages varies between embryos, with an inverse proportion in the contributions by dividing 8-cell and outer 16-cell blastomeres to the inner cell population of an individual embryo (168). Ultimately, however, descendants of outer cells are exclusively located in the trophoblast lineage, with those marked at the 32- to 64-cell stages (early and expanding blastocysts) contributing only to polar or mural trophectoderm (169). Thus, an outer position at late cleavage stages constrains a mouse blastomere to produce at least one outer descendant in subsequent cleavages. This constraint appears to arise together with the polarized phenotype at the time of compaction, and the extent of contribution to trophectoderm coincides with the degree of epithelial differentiation that has occurred at each stage, so that by the early blastocyst stage outer cells are both allocated to and differentiated into trophectoderm.

Does the inner cell mass cell population of the early blastocyst constitute a similarly allocated population with descendants only in primitive endoderm and primitive ectoderm? In their study of reconstituted blastocysts using the *M. musculus-M. caroli* marker system, Rossant and Croy (170) found a small but highly significant incidence of inner cell mass descendants in the midgestation trophectoderm lineage of the placenta when early blastocyst inner cell masses were used as donors in the reconstitutions. These trophectoderm cells could have arisen from a systematic contribution of inner cells to the trophectoderm population, or from adventitious trapping or escape of injected inner cells into the outer layer of the host embryo. Analysis of inner cell fate in intact mouse blastocysts by injecting horseradish peroxidase into single inner cell mass cells and culturing the labeled embryos for 24 hours revealed labeled cells in the polar and mural trophectoderm, leading to the hypothesis that the inner cell mass contributes descendants to the polar trophectoderm (171). The companion study in which polar trophectoderm cells were injected with horseradish peroxidase (169) had led to the proposal that definitive polar trophectoderm is formed only during the later stages of blastocyst growth after such a contribution from inner cells was completed. Subsequent studies used different methods to test this hypothesis. Using fluorescent latex microparticles to label all trophectoderm in intact nascent blastocysts, Dyce et al. (172) found a low frequency of inner cell contribution to trophectoderm, but in these cases, only a few (unlabeled) inner cell mass-derived trophectoderm cells were present. Gardner and Nichols (173) transplanted microsurgically isolated inner cells or outer cells orthotopically to genetically distinct, synchronous late morula or blastocyst-stage embryos and found a low frequency of inner cell contributions to trophoblastic tissues in the resulting chimeras. They attributed these cases to tissue contamination rather than genuine chimerism. These studies thus do not support the above hypothesis (169,171), suggesting rather that inner cells are also allocated by the blastocyst stage so that trophectoderm and inner cell mass populations become mutually exclusive lineages as soon as trophectoderm differentiates, even though inner cell mass cells remain pluripotent at that stage (see 187 for review).

Trophectoderm and Primitive Endoderm Fates

The prospective fate of embryonic cells is defined as their normal contribution to tissues or organs that arise in subsequent development. It is to be distinguished from prospective potency, which is the full range of developmental capabilities of a cell under any experimental circumstances (126). The prospective fate of blastocyst cells during postimplantation development of the mouse embryo has been studied with injection chimeras and reconstituted blastocysts. These studies have generally been performed by injecting expanded, (3.5 d.g.) blastocysts containing approximately 64 cells. Using these approaches, it has been possible to assess the fate of inner cell mass and trophectoderm cells by combining genetically marked cells at the same stages and assessing their contributions to the conceptus at midgestation or at term. Similarly, it has been possible to determine the fate of the more advanced cells, particularly primitive endoderm and ectoderm obtained from the 4.5-d.g. embryo. Primitive endoderm from later stage embryos (6.5 and 7.5 d.g.) has also been used as a source of cells for blastocyst injection chimeras, but cells identified as primitive ectoderm from these stages have not produced descendants in chimeric blastocysts (174; see 175 for discussion).

These studies (reviewed in 176–178; summarized in Fig. 6) show that the mutual trophectoderm gives rise to the primary trophoblast giant cells (involved in implantation) and that polar trophectoderm gives rise to the ectoplacental cone and extraembryonic ectoderm, as well as to secondary giant cells which develop during postimplantation stages (170,179,180). These later trophectoderm descendants are confined to the chorioallantoic placenta. Trophectoderm is thus allocated to an extraembryonic fate during the earliest morphogenetic events of embryogenesis and makes no subsequent contribution to the fetus or to amnion or yolk sac. There is nonetheless some flexibility within the trophectoderm lineage because diploid trophectoderm cells of the blastocyst can be induced to proliferate by juxtaposing a donor inner cell mass. Moreover, diploid cells of the midgestation extraembryonic ectoderm and ectoplacental cone remain capable of producing trophoblast giant cells either *in vitro* or when transplanted to ectopic sites, with more rapid giant cell differentiation from the ectoplacental cone than from extraembryonic ectoderm (142,179,181). Also, extraembryonic ectoderm cells of 5.5- or 6.5-d.g. mouse embryos contribute to ectoplacental cone and trophoblast giant cells after injection into blastocysts (182). These observations lead to the conclusion that polar trophectoderm (in preimplantation embryos) and extraembryonic ectoderm (in postimplantation embryos) serve as the stem cell populations for the entire trophectoderm lineage (142,183,184).

The fate of primitive endoderm cells from 4.5-d.g. blastocysts has been studied by injecting them into 3.5-d.g. hosts. Synchronous hosts have not been used, owing to the lower rate of development after transfer to foster mothers at the late blastocyst stage. These studies have shown that primitive endoderm cells of the mouse embryo produce detectable descendants only in the visceral and parietal yolk sac endoderm during postimplantation development and do not contribute to the fetal gut (185,186; see 187 for further discussion). Interestingly, visceral yolk sac endoderm from later-stage embryos (6.5 and 7.5 d.g.) produced a similar pattern of descent, whereas parietal endoderm descendants of any donor age were invariably limited to the parietal endoderm population (188). These results suggest that primitive endoderm serves as a stem cell population for visceral and parietal endoderm at the late blastocyst stage, and visceral endoderm or a morphologically indistinguishable cell type serves as the stem cell for both types of extraembryonic endoderm at postimplantation stages (186). This model is supported by observations that visceral endoderm cells of the 7.5-d.g. mouse embryo are able to differentiate into parietal endoderm in culture (189), that peroxidase-labeled visceral embryonic endoderm cells overlying the anteriormost region of the mouse egg cylinder at 7.5 d.g. move into extraembryonic positions during 24 hours of culture (190), and that cells in the junction between visceral and parietal endoderm have a migratory phenotype (191).

A comparison of these models for trophectoderm and extraembryonic endoderm fate reveals a similar morphogenetic theme. Both lineages appear to be set aside early in development, before implantation and the period of dramatic growth begin. Once allocated, both lineages seem to emerge from relatively small stem cell populations of 20–30 cells. Both yield a pluripotent cell type (extraembryonic ectoderm in the trophectoderm lineage and visceral endoderm in the extraembryonic endoderm lineage). Both have terminally differentiated cell types that accumulate distally after a period of morphogenetic movement or translocation (trophoblast giant cells and parietal cells, respectively). Indeed, these latter two cell types form an intimate association with each other, constituting the parietal yolk sac (see Fig. 6). Thus, the pattern of growth of the major extraembryonic tissues of the mouse embryo during the periimplantation period can be visualized as the coordinated expansion of terminally differentiated cells by distal accretion of cells that move away from actively proliferating stem-cell populations. This does not, however, exclude the possibility of continued cell proliferation in the terminally differentiated cells, particularly parietal endoderm. Implicit in this interpretation is a series of binary decisions associated with the successive partitioning of lineages, totipotent cleavage-stage blastomeres forming either trophectoderm or inner cell mass; the former forming either polar or mural trophectoderm and the latter forming either primitive endoderm or ectoderm. Without similar studies in other species, it will never be known with certainty how generally this understanding applies. However, their morphological similarities during preimplantation stages suggest that such lineage partitions are a common feature of embryogenesis, at least in eutherian embryos (reviewed in 95) (Fig. 7). A similar argument can be made for postimplantation development of primitive ectoderm into the embryo proper where there is less morphological and topographical diversity than in the extraembryonic structures (95).

Primitive Ectoderm (Epiblast) Fate

Information about epiblast potency, allocation, and fate provides insight into the complex series of decisions whereby primitive ectoderm (also known as epiblast because of its overt homology with the avian embryo) differentiates into fetal mesoderm, endoderm, and ecto-

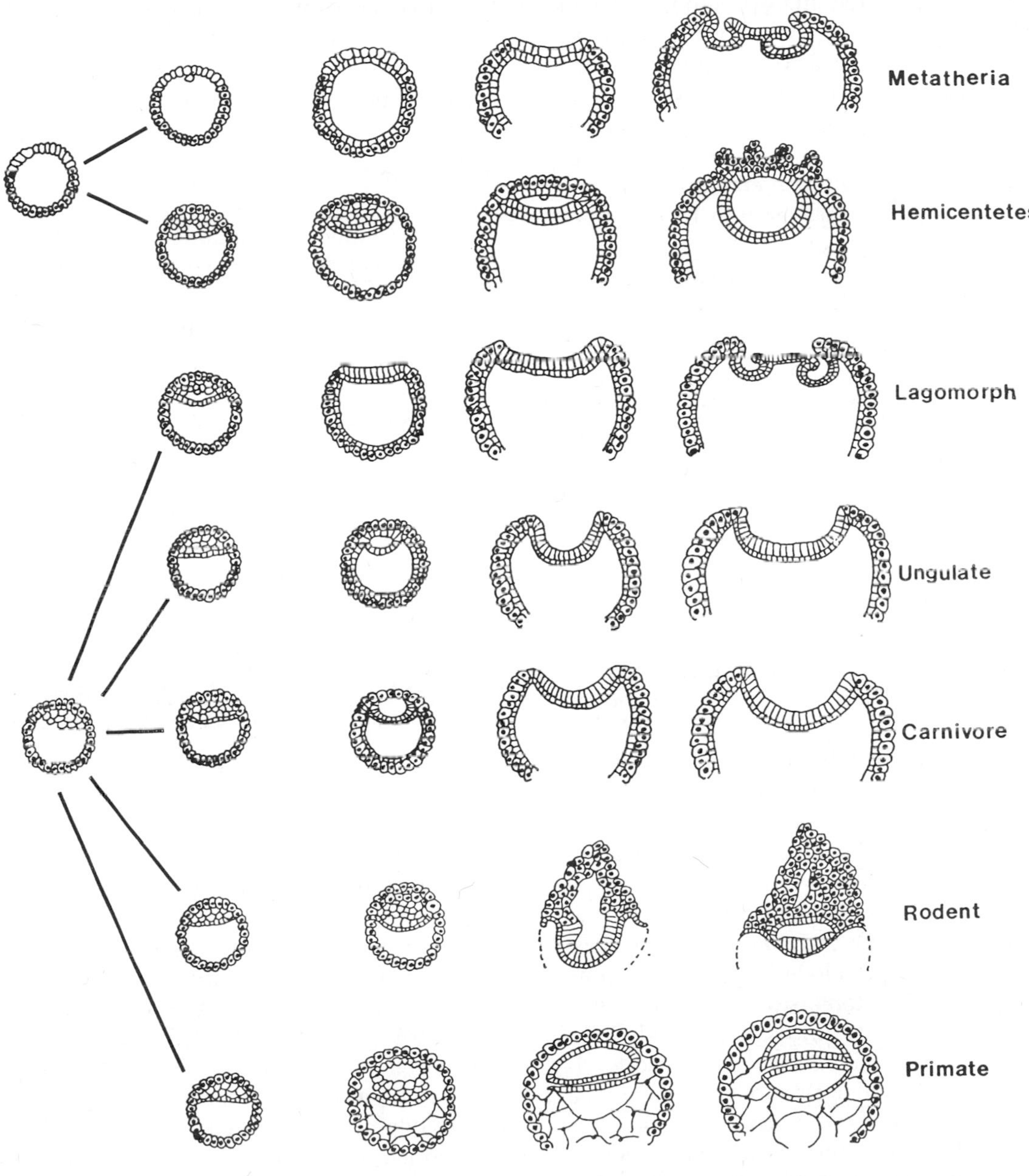

FIG. 7. Schematic comparison of embryonic and extraembryonic lineages in different mammals. Shown are cells of trophoblast lineage (*solid nuclei*); primitive ectoderm (epiblast) lineage (*tall, columnar cells*); primitive endoderm and its derivatives (visceral embryonic and extraembryonic endoderm and parietal endoderm) (*cuboidal cells*). In marsupials (metatheria) and in the primitive insectivore, *Hemicentites* (*top*) a unilaminar protoderm forms first, and the epiblast and primitive endoderm lineages are derived from it. In eutherians (*bottom*) the inner cell mass originates from blastomeres enclosed during cleavage and compaction, then gives rise to epiblast and primitive endoderm after blastocyst formation. From Cruz and Pedersen (95).

derm (192). In injection chimeras, primitive ectoderm cells from late blastocysts (4.5 d.g.) contribute descendants to all tissues of the fetus, including the gut. Primitive ectoderm also has descendants in the extraembryonic mesoderm of the visceral yolk sac, the amnionic ectoderm, and the mesoderm of the chorion (185; see 194 for review). There is evidence from the pattern of X-chromosome inactivation of primitive ectoderm descendants in mouse chimeras that primordial germ cells are also derived from this tissue (195,451). Primitive ectoderm has descendants neither in trophectoderm nor in extraembryonic endoderm, demonstrating that primitive ectoderm is a committed cell population by the time of implantation. Gardner (196) demonstrated that pure populations of primitive ectoderm isolated by enzymatic treatment and microdissection do not subsequently generate any cells resembling primitive endoderm, despite earlier reports of endoderm regeneration by immunosurgically isolated ectodermal cores from 4.5-d.g. mouse blastocysts (197–199). This result is consistent with the behavior of primitive endoderm and ectoderm as clonally distinct populations in blastocyst injection chimeras. Analysis of epiblast fate in postimplantation embryos has been carried out by four separate approaches: transferring tissues to ectopic sites in adult animals; culturing isolated tissues; generating postimplantation chimeras; and marking cells in intact embryos.

Analysis in Ectopic Sites

Tissue fragments of primitive-streak-stage rodent embryos develop into mature tissue in several ectopic sites, specifically, the anterior chamber of the eye, the kidney capsule, and the testis capsule (see 175,200 for review). The pioneering studies of Grobstein (201,202) demonstrated that epiblast forms a wide range of differentiated tissues, including derivatives of all three germ layers. This finding, which is incompatible with the notion of epiblast as definitive ectoderm, was later confirmed by other investigators who transferred tissues of rat (203,204) or mouse embryos (205,206) to ectopic sites. When visceral embryonic endoderm from the same stages was transferred to ectopic sites, it was resorbed (203,207) or developed only into parietal endoderm (205). Visceral extraembryonic endoderm likewise developed into tissue with a parietal endoderm phenotype (208). The broad developmental potential of epiblast is even more striking in the demonstration that all regions (anterior, distal, and posterior) of the epiblast (see Fig. 6) have the capacity to form derivatives of the three definitive germ layers in ectopic sites (206,209–211). It can be inferred from these results that the epiblast of the primitive-streak-stage rodent embryo contains cells that can differentiate into the three primary germ layers: ectoderm, mesoderm, and endoderm. However, these studies do not demonstrate that all three layers descend from single progenitor cells within the epiblast. Demonstration of the latter degree of totipotency requires a clonal analysis.

A restriction in the potency of epiblast in rodent embryos can be detected at the headfold stage, when isolated epiblast no longer differentiates into endoderm derivatives but still forms mesodermal tissues (207). Endoderm isolated from this stage does not survive, but combined with mesoderm, develops into both gut and mesoderm derivatives (207). The anterior and posterior fractions of these combined tissues produce complementary derivatives of the gut, suggesting that some regionalization of potential has occurred by the headfold stage.

Analysis In Vitro

A single analysis of explanted embryo fragments indicates that there is regionalization in the embryo before the headfold stage. In his study, Snow (212) dissected fragments of the intact primitive-streak-stage mouse embryo containing all three germ layers and cultured these for 24 hours. These multilayered fragments produced only a portion of the tissue repertoire of the embryo. Most notably, a region at the posterior end of the primitive streak was the only fragment capable of producing germ cells. This same region is the site where germ cells are first visible by alkaline phosphatase staining in the intact embryo (213). These results, together with the pluripotency of the isolated tissue layers at comparable stages, imply that regionalized restrictions in the fate of the rodent epiblast occur as the result of tissue interactions at or after the primitive-streak stage, but are not attributable to limited potency of the epiblast.

Analysis in Postimplantation Chimeras

Using an approach developed for the chick embryo (214), Beddington carried out an analysis of donor tissues in chimeric mouse embryos using [^{3}H]-thymidine as a marker (215,216). Groups of approximately 20 labeled epiblast cells were grafted into the same or a different site of the primitive-streak-stage embryo, and the tissue contributions of the labeled cells 36 hours later were scored by autoradiography (see Fig. 6). Transplanted anterior epiblast formed mainly neuroectoderm and surface ectoderm when placed in anterior and distal sites, and formed surface ectoderm and loose mesoderm even when placed in a posterior location. Transplanted posterior epiblast formed mainly surface ectoderm when placed in an anterior site and formed only mesoderm when placed into distal or posterior sites. Transplanted distal epiblast formed surface and neuroectoderm and mesoderm when placed in an anterior site, formed only mesoderm when placed in a posterior site, but formed mainly mesoderm and gut endoderm when placed in a distal site. These patterns of contribution indicate that there are regional differences in the fate of donor epiblast cells in the epiblast of postimplantation chimeras, despite the apparent totipotency of the isolated tissue (215,216; see 175 for review).

Using a similar approach, Copp (217) transferred [^{3}H]-thymidine-labeled grafts of embryonic epiblast with mesoderm obtained from the posterior part of the primitive streak to the same site at the base of the allantois, where they formed somatic cells and germ cells (as identified by alkaline phosphatase staining). Grafts of epiblast with mesoderm from lateral regions into the base of the allantois produced somatic descendants, but failed to produce germ cells. These results confirm that germ cells are epiblast-derived and reinforce the conclusion that donor epiblast cells in postimplantation chimeras show greater regionalization than is demonstrated by their pluripotency in ectopic sites (218,219; see 220 for review). A similar transplantation strategy using gold-conjugated wheat germ agglutinin as the label revealed the fate of 7.5 d.g. mouse epiblast in the neuroectoderm and in somitic and lateral mesoderm (221,222). When combined with the previous postimplantation chimera studies, these results indicate that cells in the anterior region give rise to fore- and midbrain neuroectoderm; distal-lateral epiblast cells give rise to hindbrain; and epiblast in the node region (anterior tip of the primitive streak) and lateral to the anterior portion of the streak gives rise to spinal cord. Cells in proximal region give rise to surface ectoderm of the head and oral regions, as well as ectodermal placodes and neural crest. Cells in distal-lateral regions and epiblast adjacent to the primitive streak gave rise to paraxial mesoderm, while primitive streak cells produce a diversity of tissues, including paraxial, lateral plate, and caudal mesoderm from its anterior and middle regions and extraembryonic mesoderm and primordial germ cells from its posterior region. These studies show that the segments of the central nervous system are already organized in the correct craniocaudal pattern and have their proper dorsoventral organization at the time of gastrulation. Moreover, the spatial array of brain segments is remarkably similar to the chick embryo at similar stages (222; see also 223,224). However, this evidence for regionalization of the epiblast should not be taken as reflecting the potency or fate of individual cells, which requires a clonal analysis.

Analysis in Intact Embryos

Analysis of cell fate in intact embryos has the advantage that it does not alter the normal tissue relationships within the embryo, thus revealing the fate of descendants of single marked progenitor cells in their undisturbed environment without invoking a test of their potency under altered circumstances (other than the marking procedure itself). Although studying radiation-induced somatic mosaicism has provided enormous insight into *Drosophila* cell lineages, the extreme radiation-sensitivity of the mammalian embryo precludes such an approach except for relatively late in gestation (225). Direct visual observation has been used in *C. elegans* embryos to determine their complete lineage, but this approach cannot be used in the intact early mammalian embryo, which lacks the polarity and cytoplasmic localizations that could serve as landmarks to identify blastomeres reproducibly. It has been possible to circumvent these limitations and achieve a clonal analysis of cell lineage in the mouse embryo by using the microinjected lineage tracer horseradish peroxidase in postimplantation embryos. The initial analysis (227) indicated that embryonic endoderm at the mid- to late primitive-streak stage of the mouse embryo is a mixed population consisting of cells that have descendants either in extraembryonic endoderm or in the embryonic gut, but not in both tissues. Further analysis of pre- and early primitive-streak stages indicated that progenitors of embryonic foregut endoderm appear in the midline of the endoderm layer near the anterior tip of the primitive streak early in gastrulation (228). The cells that appear a day later in this location are progenitors of midgut endoderm and notochord and constitute the head process (190). It can be inferred from these results that the progenitors of the embryonic gut arise progressively (anterior to posterior) from epiblast during gastrulation, replacing primitive endoderm cells, which move into the yolk sac where they form strictly extraembryonic descendants.

The analysis of mouse epiblast fate confirms this conclusion, showing that cells labeled by intracellular microinjection with a mixture of horseradish peroxidase and rhodamine-conjugated dextran can produce descendants in the embryonic gut endoderm, as well as the other primary germ layers (embryonic ectoderm and mesoderm), amniotic ectoderm and extraembryonic mesoderm (229) (Fig. 8A). The cuplike embryonic portion of the mouse egg cylinder (containing the epiblast) was divided into 11 arbitrary zones (Fig. 8B). The first tier of zones passes from the anterior of the epiblast to its posterior and is adjacent to the boundary of extraembryonic and embryonic ectoderm. Zone I is the anterior axial portion, and zone V is the posterior axial portion containing the base of the primitive streak; the second tier consists of zones VI–X, again passing from anterior to posterior, with zone VI at the anterior of the embryo and zone X at the posterior, including the tip of the primitive streak at the early streak stage. The rounded base of the cup forms zone XI, and it consists of the tip of the egg cylinder. Embryos labeled at 6.7 d.g. in epiblast at or near the anterior end of the primitive streak (zones V, IX, and X) and cultured one day had descendants in the head process and embryonic endoderm; those labeled in

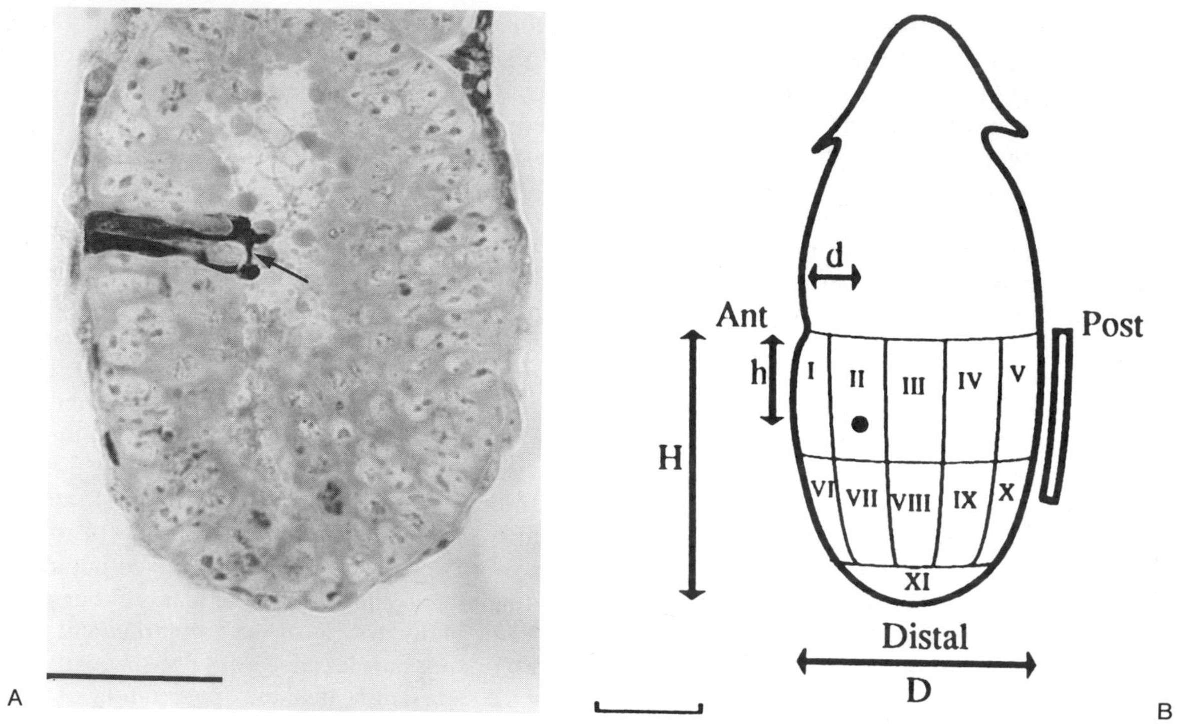

FIG. 8. Clonal analysis of mouse epiblast fate using microinjected lineage tracers and comparison of the mouse gastrula fate map to other vertebrate systems. **A:** Longitudinal section of the embryonic region of a 6.7-d.g. egg cylinder after injection of a single epiblast cell with horseradish peroxidase and rhodamine-conjugated dextran, stained and fixed without culture. An HRP-injected epiblast cell is connected to its sister cell by an apical (luminal) cytoplasmic bridge (*arrow*). Scale bar: 50 μm. **B:** Diagram of early gastrula stage (6.7 d.g.) mouse egg cylinder identifying zones I–XI marked by lineage tracer microinjection. ant, the anterior of the prospective craniocaudal axis (*left*); post, posterior (*right*); the typical extent of the primitive streak (*vertical rectangle, right*). The position of the injected epiblast was estimated along the H and D axes as distance h from the embryonic/extraembryonic border and distance d from the anterior margion of the embryo. Scale bar, 0.1 mm. From Lawson et al. (229).

the embryonic axis anterior to the primitive streak (zones I, VI, IX, and X) had descendants in ectoderm (surface and neuroectoderm); those labeled in lateral epiblast and primitive streak (zones II–V and VIII–X) had descendants in embryonic mesoderm; those labeled in anterior proximal epiblast (zones I and II) had descendants in amniotic ectoderm; and those labeled in posterolateral epiblast and the posterior portion of the primitive streak (zones IV and V) had descendants in extraembryonic mesoderm. Notably, labeled epiblast cells often had descendants in more than one germ layer, particularly after labeling in zone X, showing that single mouse epiblast cells are indeed pluripotent (229).

In an extension of these studies of epiblast cell fate, mouse embryos labeled at 6.7 d.g. were cultured for 36 hours and examined for the location of descendants in organ rudiments composed of embryonic ectoderm and embryonic or extraembryonic mesoderm (230,231). The pattern of descendants in the neural plate shows that this region, which develops primarily into the brain, is derived from more anterior and lateral regions (zones I and VII). In contrast to the origin of the majority of neural plate cells, midline cells of the hindbrain arise from more posterior areas (zones IX and X), near the primitive streak. Unlike other neural plate clones, which were generally pure neuroectoderm, these hindbrain descendants were often mixed clones, consisting of neuroectoderm, mesoderm, and notochord (the mesodermal descendants were located adjacent to the notochord). The origin of these hindbrain midline cells from pluripotent progenitors is particularly interesting because they are viewed as critical for the normal morphogenesis of the neural tube in other vertebrate systems, leading to elongation of the hindbrain and spinal cord. The pattern of descent in the spinal cord was not studied here because the embryos do not yet possess a spinal cord at the termination of the cultures (8 d.g.). The origin of embryonic and extraembryonic mesoderm was studied in embryos with one to five somites and concomitant development of heart, foregut, notochordal plate, neural folds, allantois, and blood islands in the yolk sac. Mesoderm is derived from most of the epiblast except for an axial strip anterior to the primitive streak, which generates only ectoderm. The proximal half of the epiblast is the source of the extraembryonic mesoderm (i.e., blood islands, yolk sac mesoderm, amnion mesoderm, and allantois) and also contributes to the extreme posterior portion of the primitive streak. The basal part of the allantois and the posterior portion of the streak are derived from the more anterior, paraxial region of epiblast (zone II). The absence of labeled descendants in embryonic mesoderm from precursors from zone V indicates that this region is incorporated into extraembryonic mesoderm, probably the mesoderm lining the exocoelom. Precursors from a slightly more caudal paraxial region in zones II and VII have descendants in the posterior portion of the streak and in posterior embryonic mesoderm. The blood islands are derived from the most posterior part of this region (zones IV and V), presumably from some of the first epiblast cells to enter the streak. The blood islands and adjacent extraembryonic mesoderm of the yolk sac share a common progenitor, since both cell types are commonly labeled after injection into zones IV and V. The remaining epiblast (zones VIII, IX and X) produces mesoderm in axial, paraxial, and lateral mesoderm; heart; and the anterior portion of the primitive streak. Thus, the bulk of the embryonic mesoderm at the early somite stage is derived from a relatively small region of the early-streak stage epiblast anterior and lateral to the anterior end of the primitive streak. The region at or nearest the streak makes the most extensive contribution to the axial mesoderm, and the region farthest away makes the smallest contribution. Lateral mesoderm is derived mainly from zone VIII, which occupies the middle portion of the streak at the late streak stage. Clones that contribute to the heart originate in the border of the regions overlapping presumptive extraembryonic and embryonic mesoderm (zones IV and VIII). These observations show that the early primitive streak extends partly by proliferation of a resident population already in the anterior portion of the streak by the early streak stage, and mainly through expansion of its posterior half by incorporating descendants from lateral and anterior epiblast. Thus, mesoderm formation and primitive streak elongation are concurrent processes, the posterior half of the streak being formed by the cells traveling through it into extraembryonic and lateral mesoderm, which is accomplished by the late streak stage. The anterior portion of the streak remains responsible for generating the axial and paraxial mesoderm.

The question remains of what mechanism is responsible for establishing the anterioposterior axis and thus the bilateral symmetry of the mammalian embryo. The results of morphological analysis of mouse blastocysts and early postimplantation conceptuses led Smith (232,233) to propose that a characteristic tilt of the inner cell mass/polar trophectoderm complex predicts the eventual anterioposterior axis and its orientation. Gardner and coworkers (234) examined this hypothesis by marking the direction of tilt of the ectoplacental cone with respect to the embryonic region of the early egg cylinder, using horseradish peroxidase microinjection and serial section reconstruction. They found that where a tilt was recognizable, it predicted the orientation of the anterioposterior axis but not its polarity, since the tilt was in the direction of the anterior of the embryo proper as often as to its posterior. Interestingly, the posterior of the conceptus lay slightly to the left of the site predicted from the tilt in either case. The mechanism(s) responsible for left-right assymetry are equally mysterious but may become accessible to analysis with the recent discovery of an experimentally-induced mutation that, when homozygous, reverses the handedness of mouse embryos (235). Evidence for the role of specific gene products in development of the embryonic axis is discussed in a later section.

In sum, the set of fate maps of the mouse epiblast derived from analysis of tissue fragments *in vitro* (212), postimplantation chimeras (222), and intact postimplantation embryos (229–231) reveals a reproducible pattern of regionization that strikingly resembles that of the chick embryo, in that the entire embryo proper is derived from epiblast (223,224). However, there is no evidence for restriction of mouse epiblast cells to particular germ layer fates before gastrulation, as has been reported for the chick embryo by Stern and Canning (237a); clonal analysis shows that the descendants of most labeled epiblast cells are not confined to a single germ layer or to extraembryonic mesoderm. The similarities of the mouse gastrula fate map to that of other vertebrates studied in similar detail (avian and amphibian; Fig. 9) imply that fundamental mechanisms such as axis and organ rudiment formation are highly conserved. These similarities provide compelling evidence for continuing to study the mouse embryos as a model system for understanding basic mechanisms of human development. Clonal analysis of tissue fate in later organ formation has also been fruitfully approached using similar labeling strategies (236), and with long-term markers such as retroviruses (220,226; reviewed in 237). Together, these studies provide a morphological basis for the studies on molecular aspects of cell allocation and differentiation.

Relationship Between Potency, Allocation, and Fate

The reduction of potency and the allocation of cells to mutually exclusive lineages in the extraembryonic lineages clearly implies a binary mode of decision making. These decisions occur late in the preimplantation period, coinciding with gradual morphological changes of undifferentiated cells into the trophectodermal and primitive endodermal phenotypes during blastocyst development. Epiblast cells appear to remain pluripotent until gastrulation, when they diverge into one or more of the primary germ layers or regions; it is not known whether epiblast differentiates into embryonic ectoderm, endoderm, and mesoderm and into amniotic ectoderm and

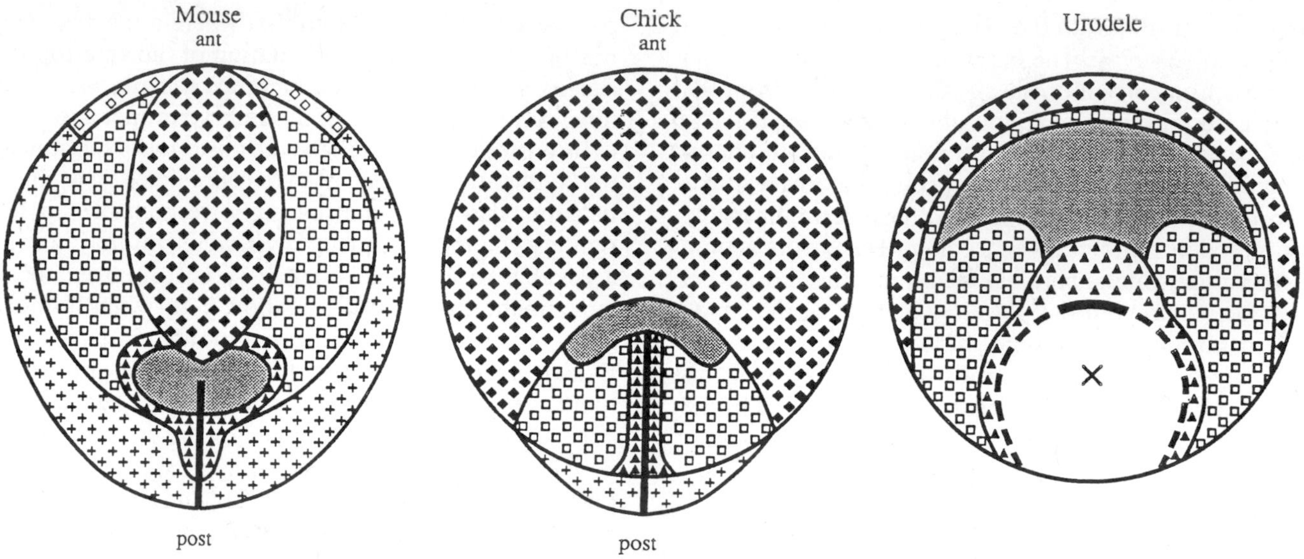

FIG. 9. Gastrula fate maps of the early gastrula stages of mouse, chick, and urodele embryos. The mouse epiblast at the early primitive streak stage has been flattened and the data has been interpolated to fill the gaps created by this projection; overlaps between the prospective germ layer fates have been removed for clarity. The map of the chick epiblast area pellucida is shown at stage 3 according to Vakaet (in 25). The urodele gastrula is viewed from its vegetal side, so that much of its prospective ectoderm and some prospective mesoderm is not visible. X, vegetal pole. Shown are the primitive streak of the mouse and chick embryos and the dorsal lip of the blastopore of the urodele embryo (*thickened bar*), embryonic ectoderm (*filled diamonds*); amnion ectoderm (*open diamonds*); embryonic mesoderm (*open squares*); embryonic endoderm (*filled triangles*); notochord (*stippled*); extraembryonic mesoderm (+). From Lawson et al. (229).

extraembryonic mesoderm by a series of binary decisions or simply on the basis epigenetic information contained in their immediate cellular environment. Clearly, the concept of determination does not apply to early mammalian embryonic development in the traditional sense of an event that precedes morphological differentiation (238). Rather, commitment appears to emerge during differentiation and may not be separable from morphological and biochemical aspects of phenotypic divergence of cells. Indeed, the earliest evidence that progenitors of a lineage have acquired a distinct fate is the allocation of cells to that lineage rather than a restriction in their potency, e.g., inner cell mass cells at the early blastocyst stage and epiblast cells during gastrulation. These examples of cell allocation during cleavage, blastocyst formation, and postimplantation growth indicate an active interaction between cells and their environment (reviewed in 573). This, in turn, implies a capacity for gene regulation even at early stages. As we shall see in the following section, there is substantial evidence for this conclusion.

GENETIC ASPECTS

Early Gene Expression

Although mammalian preimplantation development is sometimes compared to the morphologically similar processes of cleavage and blastulation in other vertebrate classes and in invertebrates, these similarities can be misleading because mammals use a fundamentally different reproductive strategy. Cleavage in nonmammals produces the cells of the blastula, which imminently begins gastrulation. By contrast, the events following cleavage in placental mammals establish the extraembryonic lineages necessary for viviparous survival. Another difference inherent in the mammalian strategy is the reduction of yolk. Only vestiges persist of the large stores of yolk seen in the eggs of amphibians, reptiles, birds, and egg-laying mammals (monotremes). Marsupial embryos have small but recognizable yolk deposits which they expel from their cytoplasm during early cleavage (reviewed in 96). For their nutrition, the early embryos of eutherians initially rely on protein and glycogen stores in the egg and diffusion of simple sugars and amino acids within the fluids of the maternal reproductive tract (reviewed in 239). Following implantation and gastrulation, they rely on maternal nutrient sources obtained through the visceral yolk sac and chorioallantoic placenta. Accordingly, unlike amphibians and several invertebrate systems, embryos of placental mammals show an early onset of embryonic gene expression, which is necessary for the differentiation of the specialized cells required for intrauterine growth. Because this mammalian reproductive strategy has perhaps resulted in the minimal egg mass for a vertebrate organism, the period from fertilization to implantation is genetically a critical transition from a program of gametogenesis to one of rapid proliferation and diversification. Detailed reviews (240,241) have discussed the evidence for preimplantation transcription of nuclear factors, cytoskeletal elements, membrane and secreted proteins (including growth factors and their receptors), as well as the metabolic machinery of mammalian embryos. Only the general properties of gene expression that accompany preimplantation development are discussed in this section (see also 242–245 for review). In a later section, we will discuss expression of specific genes during postimplantation development, when the embryo proper of various mammals and other vertebrate species more closely resemble one another.

Maternal mRNA

The newly ovulated mouse egg contains approximately 350 pg of "maternal" RNA, mostly ribosomal and transfer RNA (246). Judging by the quantity of poly A tracts in the egg, approximately 20 pg is poly A+ mRNA, assuming average poly A tract lengths of 63 nucleotides and mRNA lengths of 1700 nucleotides (246,247). The quantity of specific mRNA has been measured, showing 431 fg of actin mRNA and 167 fg of histone mRNA per ovulated oocyte (248,249), as well as measurable amounts of individual cloned transcripts (250). This maternal mRNA is capable of serving as a template for protein synthesis, as shown by *in vitro* translation (251). Although some of the changes in protein synthetic pattern following fertilization (1-cell to 2-cell stage) appear to result from posttranslational modifications (252–254), other changes seem to utilize the stored maternal mRNA (255). In contrast to the situation in *Xenopus* and sea urchin oocytes, cytoplasmic mRNA of mouse oocytes does not contain any excess of the repetitive sequences that indicate unprocessed mRNA (256). Furthermore, growing and fully grown mouse oocytes contain normal amounts of U1 RNA, an essential component of the mRNA splicing machinery. This also contrasts with the fully grown *Xenopus* oocyte and early sea urchin embryo, which are deficient in this regard (257,258).

Despite the apparent normality of the maternal mRNA in mouse eggs, translational efficiencies for actin and histone mRNAs are quite low—less than one-tenth of what occurs in blastocysts (244). Furthermore, the mouse egg has little spare translational capacity, as shown by the injection of mRNA (259) and the fact that the net rate of protein synthesis does not increase within the first 24 hours after fertilization (260,261). A possible explanation for these results is a deficiency in oocyte ribosomes (262). Increases in ribosome content and loading of ribosomes by mRNA accompany subsequent increases in the rate and efficiency of protein synthesis (246,263; see 244 for review).

Activation of Zygotic Genes

During early cleavage mammalian embryos begin to rely on products of the zygotic genome. During this transition, the total amount of mRNA and of specific transcripts decreases to only a fraction of that present in the oocyte (248,249). Whether this represents an active degradative process or normal rates of mRNA turnover is unclear. When exogenous globin mRNA is injected into embryos, it is available for translation for 15–17 hours, but is no longer functional as a template for protein synthesis after 48 hours (264).

Whereas protein synthesis before the 2-cell stage of mouse embryos is transcription independent (251,265), development beyond the 2-cell stage requires mRNA synthesis (268). At the 2-cell stage, poly A+ mRNA is synthesized at the rate of 0.2 pg/embryo/hour and ribosomal RNA at the rate of 0.4 pg/embryo/hour (269). The total amount of mRNA accumulated by the 8-cell stage approaches that present in the ovulated egg, but amounts of histone and actin mRNA are still only one-fourth to one-half that of the egg (248,249).

The use of genetic markers for zygote-specific products has made it possible to determine when the zygotic genome is activated. In mouse embryos the paternal isozyme of beta-glucuronidase is detected at the late 2-cell to early 4-cell stage (270). Similarly, the paternal isoforms of beta-2 microglobulin and hypoxanthine-guanine phosphoribosyl transferase first appears in 2-cell embryos (271,272). The transition to embryonic transcription occurs at the 2-cell stage in hamster embryos; between 2-cell and 16-cell stages in rabbit embryos; at the 4- to 8-cell stage in human embryos; at the 8- to 10-cell stage in pig embryos; and at the 8- to 16-cell stage in sheep and cow embryos (240,273–275).

Given the substantial time elapsed between fertilization and 2-cell stage of mouse embryos, it remains interesting to question whether any embryonic gene expression occurs at the earlier stages. There is evidence for considerable turnover of poly A tracts of mRNA and 3′ terminal AMP of transfer RNA (tRNA) in both 1- and 2-cell mouse embryos (247,269,276). Also, the mRNAs of both unfertilized and fertilized eggs show normal levels of cap structures (277,278). In addition to labeling of these terminal structures by $[^3H]$-adenosine and $[^3H]$-guanosine (279), $[^3H]$-adenosine labels internal sites in tRNA and in both poly A− and poly A+ heterogeneous RNA (presumed mRNA) of 1-cell and early 2-cell embryos, but at very low rates; ribosomal RNA synthesis is undetectable before the 2-cell stage (269). Therefore, a modest amount of mRNA synthesis (about one-fifth the 2-cell rate) probably occurs in 1-cell embryos, but its functional significance is unclear. Interestingly, this early transcription appears to be derived preferentially from the paternal pronucleus (280).

The morphogenetic events of compaction and blastocyst development require prior embryonic gene expression, as shown by stage-specific sensitivity to alpha amanitin (281–283). One consequence of this gene activity is the synthesis of lineage-specific polypeptides in trophectoderm and inner cell mass (284–286).

In sum, the pattern of gene expression in the preimplantation embryo changes from predominantly posttranscriptional and posttranslational control during early-cleavage stages to predominantly transcriptional control in successive stages, transcription being required for completion of preimplantation morphogenesis (240,241,283).

Mutations Affecting Early Development

Before direct measurements of gene expression were made on mammalian embryos, the only indication of early involvement of the embryonic genome was homozygous lethal mutations. Of approximately 700 known mutations in the mouse, about 20 adversely affect early development (287). None of these early-acting mutations will be described in depth here because they have been the subject of detailed reviews (212,288–292) (see also reviews of specific genetically complex regions *A*-locus: 293; *C*-locus: 294,295; and *T*-locus: 296–298]). Rather, this and the following section evaluate the results of studying these mutations and the prospects for producing additional mutations affecting specific genes or processes during preimplantation and early postimplantation development. Virtually all this work has been accomplished in the mouse because few genes affecting periimplantation development have been described in other species.

Mutations affecting early embryogenesis can be grouped into those visible at (a) cleavage stages, (b) blastocyst formation, (c) implantation stages, (d) early egg cylinder stages, and (e) late egg cylinder/gastrula stages (reviewed in 291–293). Those affecting cleavage stages are C^{25H}, a deletion at the albino locus, and *t*12 at the *t* locus. Mutations affecting blastocyst formation are ovum mutant, Tail short and T hairpin. Those affecting periimplantation stages are the a locus mutants, lethal nonagouti (a^x), lethal yellow (a^Y); oligosyndactyly; and three *t* complex mutants, t^{w73}, $t^{wPa\text{-}1}$ and T^{orl}. Mutations affecting early egg cylinder stages include two at the *t* locus, T^{orl} and t^{w5}, the albino locus mutant, C^{6H}, and deletions in the *c* complex affecting a gene (*exed*) necessary for development of extraembryonic ectoderm. Mutations affecting gastrulation are t^9, short ear, another *c* complex gene affecting mesoderm differentiation (*msd*) and fused (kinky). Most of these mutants have been known for years, owing largely to the pioneering work of L. C. Dunn, D. Bennett, S. Waelsch, W. and L. Russell, and their associates. The availability of the mutants consistently captures the imagination of developmental geneticists because they hold the promise of genetic inroads to developmental mechanisms. By comparison, saturation mutagenesis for processes involved in early developmental decisions has proved enormously useful in understanding *Drosophila* and *C. elegans* (315,316).

A limitation of existing, recessive mutations lethal during mammalian embryogenesis is that the homozygotes are generally first recognized as they become retarded and moribund. This complicates attempts to determine the primary causes of developmental arrest. In principle, this problem can be circumvented by using linked genetic markers. One such example is the *t* locus, in which mutant alleles can be recognized by a closely-linked polypeptide (340). Another is the A^Y allele, which is closely linked with an integrated proviral sequence (337). Mutant embryos can be identified by separating blastomeres at the 2-cell stage (440), then pooled for biochemical determinations at later stages. By using linked mutations, developmental geneticists have succeeded in isolating such genes, as described in a later section (338,339); however, the "reverse genetics" approach is laborious and is confined to those genes for which there are closely linked genes that can be used as entry points. Given the apparent existence of genes whose function is critical for early development on every autosome that has been examined in detail, it should be possible to isolate additional mutants using saturation mutagenesis as previously done with invertebrate species (315,316). The difficulty in this approach is that most autosomal defects will have to be established in homozygous form by multigenerational crosses before their effects are apparent. Although this complicates the analysis, it does not preclude collecting additional mutants for easily assayed phenotypes. This has been done for the t-region of mouse chromosome 17 (317). In order to apply this approach to the early stages of development, it would be necessary to devise screening criteria for developmentally interesting defects such as failure to differentiate into inner cell mass and trophectoderm, rather than death, owing to metabolic deficiencies. Another complication is that these new mutants would provide no more molecular accessibility to the affected genes than currently available mutants do. These limitations have provoked developmental geneticists to devise transgenic approaches for interfering with gene expression in mammalian embryos.

Transgenic Approaches

Pronuclear DNA Injection and Embryonic Virus Infection

Probably no single genetic approach has generated more excitement for developmental geneticists than the introduction of exogenous genes into the early embryo. This approach has flourished with the availability of recombinant DNA techniques for producing and analyzing DNA sequences. Furthermore, the use of cloned

DNA sequences to transform cultured cells (318) was a compelling incentive for studying the fate of these genes throughout the whole of development, when they could potentially be regulated during the growth and differentiation of the intact organism. However, the first attempt at genetically altering mammalian embryos by the introduction of foreign DNA used virus as the DNA source. Jaenisch microinjected SV40 DNA into the blastocoel cavity of mouse embryos and detected the sequences in the adult mice (319,320). Subsequent studies performed with cloned DNA focused on the pronuclear-stage mouse embryo (41) and on the early *Drosophila* embryo. When the injected DNA integrates into the host embryo genome, it is subsequently transmitted as a Mendelian trait, and the offspring of these novel individuals become unique strains. The first such mammals were termed *transgenic mice* (41,321–324). Subsequent similar studies have resulted in transgenic rabbits, sheep, goats, and pigs (325). This approach has been strikingly successful in generating informative integration events (see 326–330).

Although the earliest transgenic mice produced by pronuclear DNA injection did not express the exogenous genes, Wagner and associates (323) eventually obtained activity using the herpes simplex virus (HSV) thymidine kinase gene, while Brinster and associates (321) also obtained expression with a mouse metallothionein-HSV thymidine kinase fusion gene. These results stimulated numerous subsequent studies. The primary objectives of such studies have been to determine the requirements for efficient, tissue-specific expression and to localize the genetic determinants of this specificity. Successful studies of exogenous gene expression have provided numerous insights into the biochemical and physiological aspects of hematopoiesis, immune system development, tumorigenesis, and other subjects. As a consequence of recent results that show a high incidence of efficient expression, gene therapy involving hematopoietic stem cells in humans and gene augmentation in livestock are realistic goals (331,331a,359).

An important byproduct of transgenic approaches is insertional mutagenesis in molecular accessibility to the gene(s) at the site of integration (332). Endogenous retroviruses are responsible for two known mutations in mice, the *dilute* locus (333–335) and the *hairless* locus (336). Another mutation that is closely linked to a retrovirus is A^y (337). In this case, however, a translocation stock led to the discovery and cloning of the mutant *a* locus (338,339). Experimental retrovirus infection of embryos (341) also leads to insertional mutations and has been identified as the cause of the homozygous lethality of *Mov-13* mice at 12–13 d.g. (342). The insertional event took place in the first intron of the alpha 1 (I) collagen gene, completely blocking transcription of this gene, which is essential for development of blood vessels *in vivo* but not for epithelial branching of organ rudiments *in vitro* (343–347). Most notably, the unique DNA sequence of the exogenous retrovirus facilitated molecular cloning and identification of the flanking regions surrounding the integration site. This approach has been further refined by incorporating a bacterial tRNA suppressor gene into the retrovirus which simplifies the cloning process (348). The practical limitation of insertional mutagenesis by retroviruses is the relative rarity of mutations. Although retroviral infection and integration are efficient, there is a relatively low incidence of mutagenesis with this approach (342; reviewed in 349).

By contrast, the incidence of insertional mutagenesis resulting from pronuclear DNA injection appears to be relatively high. An unexpected discovery in zygote DNA injection transgenesis studies was that the injected DNA can act as a mutagen, producing developmental mutants at a frequency on the order of 10 percent (350). In the study by Wagner et al. (350), two out of six transgenic lines carried recessive lethal mutations as a result of integration of human growth hormone sequences. In the study by Palmiter et al. (351), one of seven transgenic lines produced by injecting a metallothionein/thymidine kinase fusion gene was unable to transmit the inserted DNA through males, even though these were fertile. This result suggests that the integration event disrupted a function essential during haploid stages of spermatogenesis, thus accounting for the pattern of its transmission. There is also a transgenic line containing a Rous sarcoma virus/chloramphenicol acetyl transferase fusion gene that shows transmission distortion and dominant lethality owing to an induced translocation (352). Another line produced by microinjection of a mammary tumor virus/myc fusion gene is characterized by a recessive limb abnormality (353). This latter mutant appears to be allelic to the known spontaneous mutation, limb deformity. A junction fragment has been cloned from the integration site, showing that this approach may yet fulfill the objective of identifying the molecular basis of certain developmentally significant genes. In the transgenic line studied by Woychik et al. (353), however, the integration event caused a deletion of approximately 1 kb of DNA, showing that injected DNA may cause rearrangements in the process of integration. These structural changes could significantly complicate the task of identifying the developmentally significant sequences from the cloned junction fragments. Nevertheless, insertional mutagenesis is a source of molecularly identifiable mutants, many of which are alleles of existing mutations, despite the apparent improbability of such events. Thus, the production and analysis of these mutants serve two purposes: addition of new mutants and insight into the known ones. In addition to more than 20 insertional mutations affecting posnatal or fetal development, several have been generated with effects on periimplantation development, including decompaction (354), arrest on day 5 (355), embryonic disorganization on day 7

(356), and egg cylinder inviability (357; reviewed in 332).

To date, hundreds of cloned gene sequences have been introduced into pronuclear-stage mouse embryos, with at least some degree of expression. Many such studies have demonstrated that tissue- and stage-specific expression of the transgene can be obtained. Interestingly, the mice varied widely in the level of specific synthesis, despite similar copy numbers of the exogenous genes. In studies by Brinster, Palmiter, and associates, the metallothionein promoter was used to obtain gene expression predominantly in the liver of transgenic mice. However, the correlation between levels of expression and number of integrated copies was poor (321,358). The major conclusions arising from these and other related studies (reviewed in 359) are that genomic sequences located adjacent (generally 5′) to the structural genes studied are indeed necessary and sufficient in many cases for tissue-specific gene expression. Recent studies have demonstrated the effectiveness of using reporter or indicator genes encoding distinctive products to study tissue-specific expression. Fusion genes containing *lacZ* and other fluorometrically or histochemically detectable reporter genes have been particularly useful because of the ease of visualization of the gene product. The expression of metallothionein promoter, regulated E. coli beta-galactosidase, was detected in single preimplantation embryos after microinjection and similar approaches have been used to detect expression of transgenes at later stages (360,362; see 365 for review). A particularly interesting finding using this approach was that enhancers are not necessary for transcription at the early zygote stage but only as cleavage progresses (363,364). Combining a minimal promoter with the DNA response element for retinoic acid has made it possible to visualize the sites and stages of retinoic acid release in mouse embryos (365,366).

Another innovation resulting from pronuclear DNA injection transgenic studies is the ablation of particular tissues by cell lineage-specific expression of a toxin encoded by the transgene, such as the diphtheria A subunit (367,368; reviewed in 369). However, owing to the immense number of DNA constructions and issues addressed by pronuclear DNA injection, a comprehensive review of the information gained through pronuclear DNA injection is beyond the scope of this chapter, and the reader is referred to existing reviews for further information obtained using this approach (328–332).

Homologous Recombination in Embryonic Stem Cells

Another means for introducing exogenous genes into the mouse germ line is genetic transformation of ES cells, followed by selection to identify clones that have undergone homologous recombination; these are propagated and used to generate chimeras that possess the modified allele (63,64) (see Fig. 4). The main advantage in using ES cells over previously studied EC cells for this purpose is their euploidy and the attendant high frequency with which they colonize the germ line in chimeras produced by blastocyst injection (370). Stewart and associates (371) used a retrovirus to introduce genes conferring neomycin resistance into mice, and subsequent studies showed the possibility of obtaining germ line integration by means of embryonic stem cell transformation, selection, and transfer to host blastocysts (372,373). Capecchi and other workers focused on the HPRT gene, using homologous recombination between an exogenous gene targeting vector and the native gene to knock out or correct the function of one allele in ES cells (374–377). A key development was the use of positive drug selection, followed by the use of a combination of positive and negative selection to identify and recover the rare homologous clonal events (378). These efforts have culminated in a generalizable method for gene targeting, with initial successes in targeting the *Hox 1.1* gene (379), the *engrailed-2* gene (380). The importance of this approach is that it incisively tests the role of the targeted gene in all the tissues of an otherwise intact organism, and unlike zygotic DNA injection, it does not alter the genetic context of the modified target gene. Ensuing studies have generated an outburst of information about the roles of specific genes in mouse development so extensive that it is no longer realistic to tabulate the more than 100 genes being studied. Because other reviews have addressed the development of this approach (63,381–385,426) and provided detailed methods (64,65,386,388), this chapter concentrates instead on describing gene targeting events that affect mouse embryogenesis. These results will be discussed in the appropriate sections.

Other developments involving ES cells, however, are also particularly noteworthy. By combining a weak promoter with a *lacZ* reporter gene, Gossler et al., (389) were able to "trap" enhancers on the basis of expression of the reporter gene in the resulting ES cell lines. Another "gene trap" or "promoter trap" construct containing a splice-acceptor site fused to the *lacZ* reporter gene has also been used to identify developmentally interesting endogenous genes by stage- and tissue-specific expression patterns (389–391). In the latter approach, the trapping vector was introduced either by electroporation or by retroviral infection, leading to characteristic patterns of gene expression when ES cells were injected into blastocysts and stained for beta-galactosidase expression in midgestation embryos; chimeras derived from these lines were mated to generate homozygosity, which led to embryonic lethality in 9 of 24 lines (390). This is anticipated from the fact that the integration of the gene- or promoter-trapping vector invariably disrupts the trapped gene by creating a fusion product with the *lacZ* reporter sequence. Further analysis of ES cell lines generated with this approach should reveal numerous additional mutations in developmentally-expressed genes. The major advantage of this approach over other methods of mutagenesis is that it facilitates identification and isolation of genes in redundant pathways solely on the basis of reporter gene expression, whereas other approaches would not detect visible consequences of disrupting just one component of the pathway (reviewed in 392).

Recently, Strauss et al. (393) and Gearhart, J. D., and coworkers (898) have succeeded in introducing large vectors consisting of physically intact yeast artificial chromosomes into ES cells by lipofection. These studies facilitate the introduction of entire genes with their intact promoter and enhancer sequences into mice for evaluation of the effects on the whole organism. Thus, it is now possible to circumvent the vector size limitations of DNA microinjection or electroporation and introduce even large genes in the several hundred kilobase to megabase range (for example, clotting factor VIII), thereby substantially expanding the nature of genetic alterations accessible through this technology.

Finally, recent studies show that it is possible to culture pluripotent ES-like cells not only from blastocysts, but also from primordial germ cells (395–397). These successes appear due to inclusion of particular growth factors, including steel factor, leukemia inhibitory factor, and basic fibroblast growth factor, in the culture medium (other roles of these factors are discussed in a later section). These findings may have important implications for understanding the embryonic origins of ES cells and for maintaining their pluripotent phenotype.

Interference with Development Using Antisense RNA

One additional novel strategy for specific genetic interference is based on blocking translation of mRNA by introducing an excess of the complementary, antisense strand. Tissue culture cells expressing antisense genes show reduced thymidine kinase activity (398). Similarly, microinjection of antisense mRNA directly into the cytoplasm blocks the translation of co-injected globin mRNA in Xenopus oocytes (399), although microinjection into fertilized eggs was less successful because the embryonic cytoplasm contained an enzyme activity that dissociated the antisense RNA from its complementary target (see 400 for review). Mouse embryos did not appear to have such RNA-duplex "melting" activity, however, although RNAs injected into the mouse zygote were rapidly degraded, as are endogenous maternal mRNAs (401). Injecting the antisense RNA into 2- and 4-cell stage embryos largely bypassed this problem, leading to a 75-percent inhibition in activity of the targeted beta-glucuronidase gene product. An alternative to microinjecting antisense RNAs is use of DNA oligonucleotides that can penetrate the membrane. This approach reduced the rate of progression to the blastocyst stage and decreased blastocyst cell number when cleavage-stage embryos were exposed to antisense oligonucleotides for insulinlike growth factor (IGF) II (403). Similarly, microinjection of antisense RNA or exposure to antisense deoxyoligonucleotides for epidermal growth factor receptor delayed blastocyst cavity formation in mouse embryos (402). In both of these cases, treatment with sense strand reagents or with antisense reagents to irrelevant gene products had no developmental consequences, so the effects observed can be regarded as indicating a required function of the gene product in preimplantation embryogenesis.

Effects of Aneuploidy and Other Chromosomal Abnormalities

The lethality of haploid and monosomic mouse embryos illustrates the importance of a balanced chromosome constitution for normal early development. Haploid embryos can be produced by parthenogenesis or by mechanically altering the number of pronuclei in the zygote (404–408). These genetically altered individuals die during cleavage and peri-implantation stages. Parthenogenesis often produces diploid embryos as a result of second polar body suppression, in which case development can continue to midgestation stages, as subsequently discussed. Therefore, it is the loss of an entire chromosome set in haploids, rather than some trauma associated with the experimental procedures, that is responsible for their early death.

The peri-implantation lethality of all mammalian monosomies also supports the argument that the intact diploid set of chromosomes must be present for normal embryonic development. Mouse embryos nullisomic for the X-chromosome begin to die at early cleavage stages (407,409,410). Mouse embryos monosomic for specific autosomes have been produced using the Robertsonian translocation stocks developed by Gropp (see 291,411 for review). These begin to die during late cleavage or early blastocyst stages (monosomies for chromosome 1, 2, 5, and 15) or at later stages in blastocyst development (monosomies 4, 10, 12, 14, 17, 18, and 19). Almost none of these embryos survive beyond implantation (412,413; see 291 for review). Although cells of monosomic embryos can be sustained in chimeras for a time, there appears to be a progressive reduction in the monosomic component, so that few of the resulting fetuses are chimeric at term (413–416; see 291 for review). The absence of monosomies in recognized human conceptions argues for a similar early stage of death, since they should be produced by nondisjunction at meiosis in equal frequencies as trisomies, which are frequent among spontaneous abortions during the first trimester of pregnancy (417,418). Trisomies in mice, as in humans, are generally capable of development to relatively advanced stages, but rarely to term (411). These results indicate that both diploid chromosome sets must be present for normal mammalian development. They do not rule out a deleterious effect of lethal genes in monosomies, although this seems unlikely in inbred strains of mice. Thus, the detrimental effects of monosomy may be due to the dosage-dependent decrease in gene products from the affected chromosome (419). Differences in stage of death among monosomies indicate that the genes present on different autosomes have distinct roles during early development.

A coherent explanation for some of these observations arose from studies of Robertsonian and reciprocal translocations in which maternal or paternal duplication of part or all of an autosome (with respective paternal/maternal deficiencies of the same regions) led to gestational or neonatal lethalities (420–423; reviewed in 424). This approach detected four autosomes that are lethal when they are maternally duplicated (2, 6, 7, and 11) and four that are lethal when they are paternally duplicated (2, 7, 11, and 17) (Fig. 10). Duplication of five autosomes led to differential recovery of offspring as compared with biparental inheritance (1, 5, 9, 14, and 17) while the remaining 10 autosomes had regions that remained untested (8, 10, 12, and 18) or showed completely normal complementation (3, 4, 13, 15, 16, and 19) (424). Because there is abnormal complementation when both autosomal regions are inherited from the same parental source in such cases, they fulfill the definition (425) of a chromosomally imprinted region whose behavior differs depending on its parent of origin. This discovery, and the complementary embryological observations, have had a major impact on concepts of gene regulation during mammalian embryogenesis, and are discussed in the following two related sections dealing with X-chromosome activity and imprinting of autosomal genes.

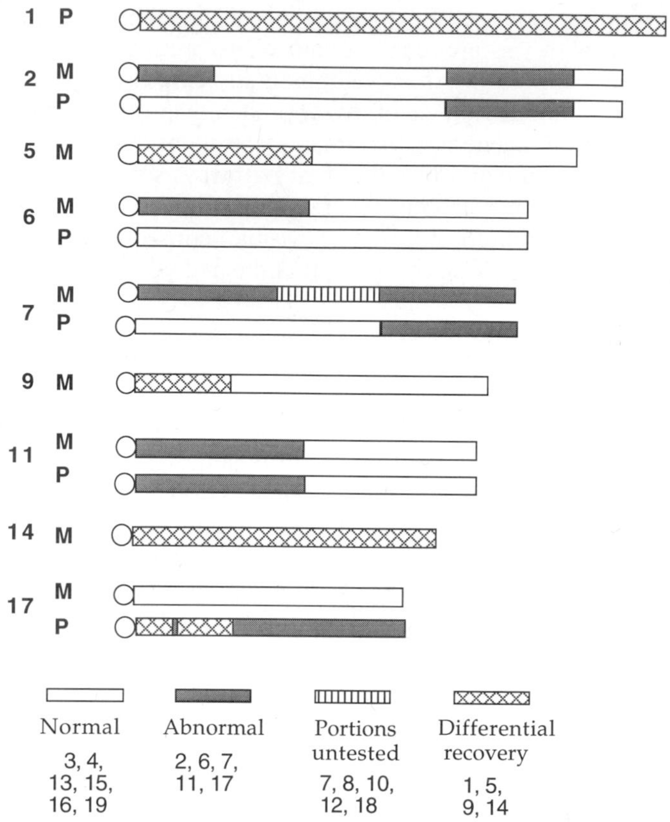

FIG. 10. Mouse autosomes showing developmental abnormalities when they are inherited as maternal duplications/paternal deficiencies or paternal duplications/maternal deficiencies. Regions are indicated where there is defective complementation when both autosomes (or indicated segments) are derived from the same parent. Abnormal phenotypes include prenatal and neonatal deaths. In some cases, the indicated duplication/deficiency condition is not lethal, but leads to differential recovery of offspring, as compared with normal (biparental) inheritance. Autosomes that do not cause abnormalities when inherited as duplications/deficiencies and other autosomes with untested portions are also indicated. M, maternal duplication/paternal deficiency; P, paternal duplication/maternal deficiency. Adapted from Cattanach and Beechey (424) and Pedersen et al. (474).

X Chromosome Activity During Development

One X chromosome of female placental mammals is inactivated during development, leading to dosage compensation of X-linked genes (426; see 427,428,428a for review). The process of X-inactivation is a paradigm for gene regulation because changes in X chromosome chromatin are correlated with changes in the expression of genes on this chromosome. Furthermore, the activity of the second X chromosome in females changes in a regular, well-documented sequence throughout the life cycle. Finally, the pattern of X chromosome inactivation in extraembryonic tissues confirms the existence of imprinting, because X-inactivation is nonrandom in extraembryonic lineages.

The status of X chromosome activity has been studied by cytogenetic techniques, ratios of autosomal and X-linked enzymes, and isozymic patterns of polymorphic X-linked genes. Cytogenetic approaches rely on the differential staining of the inactive X chromosome in interphase nuclei or metaphase chromosomes or on its asynchronous replication. The dosage of X-linked gene products is generally deduced from the absolute amounts of one or more gene products [including glucose-6-phosphate dehydrogenase (G6PD), hypoxanthine-guanine phosphoribosyl transferase (HPRT), and phosphoglycerate kinase (PGK)] or from the ratio of these activities to autosomal gene products. Isozymic variants in human and mouse G6PD and mouse HPRT and PGK have been used as qualitative indications of X chromosome activity. By combining the information from these approaches, we now have a detailed picture of the temporal and spatial aspects of X chromosome activity.

The activity ratios of X-linked enzymes in XX and XO mice indicate that both X chromosomes of normal females are active in the oocyte (429). This is confirmed by the isozyme patterns of G6PD in human ovaries early in gestation (430) and by the patterns of G6PD and HPRT in mice (431). Similar studies of germ cells isolated from various stages of M. caroli embryos indicate that onset of activity in the previously inactive X chromosome coincides with meiosis (431). By contrast, the X chromosome of spermatogenic cells appears to be expressed at a low level or not at all (432,433). Thus, X chromosome reactivation occurs during early stages of meiosis in the female, and this activity persists throughout oocyte growth until the time of ovulation, when transcription ceases (244).

Because of the relative inactivity of the X chromosome during spermatogenesis, it was important to determine whether both X chromosomes are expressed in the early embryo or only that inherited from the egg. Cytogenetic observations made at various stages of embryogenesis first revealed asynchronous X chromosome replication at the blastocyst stage; before this stage, both chromosomes have the appearance of active chromatin (434,435). Quantitative assays of X-linked gene products demonstrated a bimodal distribution when single embryos were assayed (436–439), presumably indicating the presence of embryos with one active X (males) and two active Xs (females). Epstein and associates accomplished a direct comparison of male and female embryos by separating blastomeres at the 2-cell stage, characterizing the sex of one-half of the embryo cytogenetically and assaying small groups of the other half of embryos for HPRT levels (440,441). Female embryos had 2-fold higher levels of HPRT on the average than males. Together, these results demonstrated that the female preimplantation mouse embryo has two active X chromosomes. This has been confirmed in studies of feral mice heterozygous for HPRT isozymes, showing that both X chromosomes are expressed at least from the 8-cell stage (see 428,428a for review). Therefore, the preimplantation embryo, like the egg, is characterized by activation of both X chromosomes.

When does X-inactivation occur? The cytogenetic observations suggest that inactivation begins at the late morula to early blastocyst stage (435) or the late blastocyst stage (434). However, evidence from injection chimera experiments using single inner cell mass cells from genetically marked mouse blastocysts (3.5–4.5 d.g.) reveals that both X chromosomes are active in the inner cell mass at these donor stages (442). This implies that the cytogenetic results on blastocysts are derived only from the trophectoderm cells. In addition, biochemical evidence indicates that there are two active X chromosomes in the embryonic ectoderm until day 6 of gestation (438,439,443). However, not all inner cell mass derivatives remain active until this time. Cytogenetic observations by Takagi and associates (444) showed that there is an early replicating X chromosome in the visceral endoderm as early as 5.3 d.g. and that this pattern changes to late replication in the visceral endoderm between 6.0 and 6.5 d.g. and in the extraembryonic ectoderm and ectoplacental cone. Although the significance of the shift from early to late replication is unknown, both stages reflect inactivity of the allocyclic X (445). Thus, X-chromosome inactivation accompanies cellular differentiation, occurring first in trophectoderm and its derivatives, then in primitive endoderm and its derivatives, and finally in the primitive ectoderm and its derivatives, including the germ cells (446). Only in early embryos and oocytes are both X chromosomes of a female individual active (Fig. 11).

Perhaps the most intriguing observation about the pattern of X-inactivation in early mouse embryos is that inactivation in the extraembryonic tissue lineages is nonrandom, the paternal X chromosome (Xp) being preferentially inactivated. This was first seen at the cytogenetic level (444) and was confirmed by analyzing PGK isozyme patterns in heterozygous female embryos (444,447–451). These studies demonstrate conclusively that the Xp is preferentially inactivated, while the Xm is

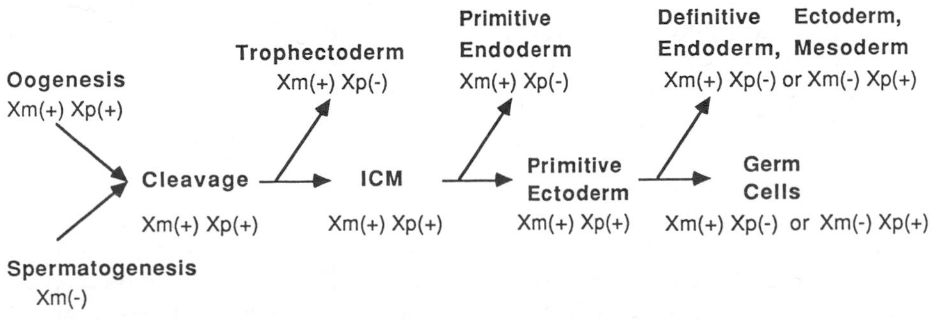

FIG. 11. Model linking X-chromosome inactivation to cellular differentiation in various cell lineages. Trophectoderm and primitive endoderm lineages show preferential inactivation of the paternally-inherited X-chromosome in female embryos, suggesting an imprinting mechanism that distinguishes the two chromosomes. This mechanism is nullified by gastrulation, when inactivation is random. m, maternal; p, paternal; +, active; −, inactive. Adapted from Monk and Harper (193).

active in the visceral and parietal endoderm, the ectoplacental cone, and the extraembryonic ectoderm. Of the extraembryonic tissues examined, only visceral yolk sac mesoderm had a mosaic pattern of random X-inactivation. This is another manifestation of heritable imprinting of maternal and paternal X chromosomes, presumably acquired during gametogenesis (see 428,428a for review). In marsupials, the paternal X chromosome is preferentially inactivated in somatic tissues (452). The similarity between the extraembryonic pattern of paternal X-inactivation and the extraembryonic developmental retardation in digynics and parthenotes implies a mechanistic relationship at the level of imprinting.

What information serves as the basis for nonrandom inactivation? The extraembryonic tissue lineages are notably all derived from cells that occupy external positions in the late preimplantation embryo, when inactivation of their X chromosome occurs. The pattern of preferential paternal X-inactivation in somatic tissues of the marsupial (452) reinforces this correlation because the unilaminar structure of its blastocyst results in all cells having an external position (96,97). X-inactivation in primitive ectoderm may also coincide with epithelial differentiation and formation of the proamniotic cavity. The correlation between embryonic position, epithelial differentiation, and precocious inactivation of the paternal X chromosome indicates there is an epigenetic source of critical information common to these processes, but it does not provide any hint about its content.

The alternating periods of X-chromosome activity and inactivity throughout the life cycle (see Fig. 11) imply that there is a mechanism for controlling X chromosome function. This process can be viewed either as inhibitory inactivation (453) or as stimulatory activation (428,428a,454). Although these models differ in their implications, both involve stage-specific synthesis of chromatin-modifying gene products and their subsequent dilution or degradation. The X-inactivation center (*Xce*) modifies X chromosome expression by governing the probability of inactivation, depending on the *Xce* allele present in somatic cells (see 536 for review). Recent studies have revealed the existence of a gene (located in a central syntenic region of mouse and human X chromosomes where mouse *Xce* resides) whose expression correlates completely with inactivation of the X chromosome: Human *XIST* and mouse *Xist* are both expressed exclusively from the inactive X chromosome (455–457). In the mouse, the mature inactive-X-specific Xist transcript is 15 kb long, and contains no open reading frame, suggesting that it may function as an RNA or as a chromatin organizing region of the DNA. The *Xist* gene is expressed in male germ cells during spermatogenesis, when the maternal X chromosome is inactive, but not in male somatic tissues (458–460). Moreover, the onset of specific paternal *Xist* expression in morula- and blastocyst-stage mouse embryos precedes inactivation of the paternal X chromosome in trophectoderm or primitive endoderm cells (899). Therefore, a currently viable hypothesis for the regulation of X chromosome activity is that expression of an *Xist* allele prevents the expression of the X chromosome on which it is located. Further information is needed to determine how the expression of *Xist* itself is regulated and how it exerts its effects on the X chromosome.

In summary, X chromosome inactivation during early development first occurs in extraembryonic tissue lineages as they differentiate (447). The pattern of inactivation in these tissues is nonrandom, resulting in preferential X inactivation, in contrast to the random inactivation occurring slightly later in the primitive ectoderm lineage. Finally, a transcript from a gene (*Xist*) that is tightly linked to the X-inactivation center, and may be identical to it, appears to be involved in the X-inactivation process. Because of similarities in the pattern of preferential Xp inactivation in the extraembryonic lineages and the developmental consequences genomic imprinting, X-inactivation could be useful as a model for understanding the mechanism(s) of imprinting of autosomal genes (reviewed in 424).

Genomic Imprinting

The importance of chromosome (or genomic) imprinting in mammalian developmental genetics was first recognized by Lyon and Glenister (463), who invoked differential expression of the maternal and paternal chromosomes as an explanation for the differential recovery of duplications/deficiencies, depending on whether they are inherited from the mother or father. As described earlier, the combined data of such studies constitute "an imprinting map which has defined regions of autosomes in which one or more genes appear to be modified as they pass through the germ lines of one, or other, or both parents, with the result that the maternal and paternal copies become functionally different in the zygote" (424). Evidence for differential roles of maternal and paternal genomes arose independently in developmental studies of isoparental mouse embryos (that is, diploid individuals with only maternal or paternal chromosomes) produced by experimental activation of oocytes (parthenogenones) or by nuclear transfer at the zygote stage (gynogenones and androgenones) (reviewed in 464,465).

Molecular analyses of mice with allelic markers has confirmed the basic premise that there is parent-allele-specific expression of certain (imprinted) genes, and recent studies have extended this conclusion to the human counterparts of some of these genes. Finally, attempts to account for the stable, parental-gender-specific patterns of gene expression have led to further studies on the role of DNA methylation in embryos and to speculation on the biological significance of this non-Mendelian genetic phenomenon.

Parthenogenesis

The phenomenon of virgin birth, or parthenogenesis, occurs in at least one species of every vertebrate class except mammals. There are parthenogenetic birds, reptiles, fish, and amphibians (466–469; 419 for review). Although the predominant strategy for reproduction in each of these vertebrate classes involves sexual recombination and mating, the existence of parthenogenetic species is conclusive evidence that development can occur in the absence of a paternal contribution to the genome: in other words, maternal and paternal genomes can be functionally equivalent in every significant way in those species (419). Despite earlier claims of successful development of mice both from normal and from parthenogenetic nuclei transferred to normally fertilized egg cytoplasm (471,472), it is now clear that the parthenogenetic mouse genome is incapable of supporting development to term, and anecdotal observations of isolated females of many species lead to the conclusion that this is true for mammals in general (see 469,473,474 for review).

Developmental failure of parthenogenones does not generally occur at preimplantation stages. Experimental parthenogenesis can be induced with a variety of treatments, all of which yield apparently normal activation, cleavage, and blastocyst formation in the diploid individuals that occur as a result of suppression of second polar body formation (see 468 for review). Some spontaneous diploidization of haploids also occurs. These diploid parthenogenetic individuals develop until postimplantation stages, with a rare few developing into small 25-somite embryos by day 10 of gestation (476,477). Spontaneous parthenogenesis occurs in ovarian oocytes of the LT/Sv strain of mice (478), leading to morphologically normal preimplantation embryos; these ultimately develop into ovarian teratomas, which often contain trophoblastic elements (479). Spontaneous parthenogenetic development of ovarian oocytes has also been observed in humans, resulting in disorganized structures which often include teeth, hair, and bone tissues, known as mature teratomas or dermoid cysts (480).

Despite their midgestation death, parthenogenones can contribute viable cells to chimeras made by aggregation or by injection of the parthenogenetic ICM into a normal blastocyst. Cells at the parthenogenones have been contributed to the germ line of fertile chimeras (481,482). The capacity of the parthenogenones to reach advanced developmental stages but not beyond day 10 indicates that functions not previously required become necessary for development at that stage. Because homozygous blastocysts could be produced by diploidizing a single pronucleus after removal of the other pronucleus from normally fertilized zygotes (483), it initially appeared possible that the failure of parthenogenetic mammalian development was due to a deficiency of some nonnuclear contribution normally made by the sperm during the process of fertilization. However, despite an early claim of success (484), several attempts to demonstrate the development to term of homozygous diploid maternal (digynic) or paternal (diandric) pronuclei have failed (419,470,473,485). However, homozygous cells of diploid, digynic uniparental mouse embryos can contribute to chimeras when aggregated with normal blastomeres at the 8- to 16-cell stage and have even produced viable gametes in a fertile female mouse derived in this way (486). Nonetheless, the low incidence of such contributions indicates that the digynic constitution is detrimental to development.

The development of an efficient method for nuclear transfer in mouse embryos using microsurgery and virus-mediated cell fusion (487) has stimulated rapid progress in defining the developmental potential of mouse pronuclei and determining the reasons for developmental arrest of parthenogenones. Transferring a normal pronuclear pair to parthenogenetic egg cytoplasm and carrying out the reciprocal transfer shows unequivocally that the failure of parthenogenones is determined by their nuclear rather than their cytoplasmic condition (488). Furthermore, gynogenones containing two maternal pronuclei, even from different strains of mice, manifest a pattern of developmental arrest essentially indistinguishable from that of parthenogenones (489,490). These embryos never develop to term but arrest at early postimplantation stages, sometimes reaching day 10 as a retarded embryo with sparse extraembryonic tissues (Fig. 12), leading Surani and co-workers (490) to hypothesize that paternal genes are uniquely necessary for extraembryonic lineages, particularly for trophoblast proliferation. It is clear that the developmental arrest of gynogenones and parthenogenones is a duplication/deficiency disorder that can be complemented only by substituting one of the two haploid egg nuclei with a sperm-derived nucleus.

Further studies of mouse parthenogenones document their phenotype in greater detail and show their fate in chimeras with normal, fertilized embryos. Parthenogenones that reach postimplantation stages have perturbed differentiation of their trophoblast and primitive endoderm lineages. Their ectoplacental cones consist primarily of trophoblast giant cells (491,900; reviewed in 474). In addition, there is abnormal differentiation of visceral extraembryonic endoderm cells, which lack the polarized organization of normal yolk sac endoderm, and in the more severely disturbed parthenogenones, the primitive endoderm lineage consists entirely of parietal endoderm cells. Therefore, the poor extraembryonic development of parthenogenetic embryos cannot be attributed to an inability to differentiate into the terminal cells of

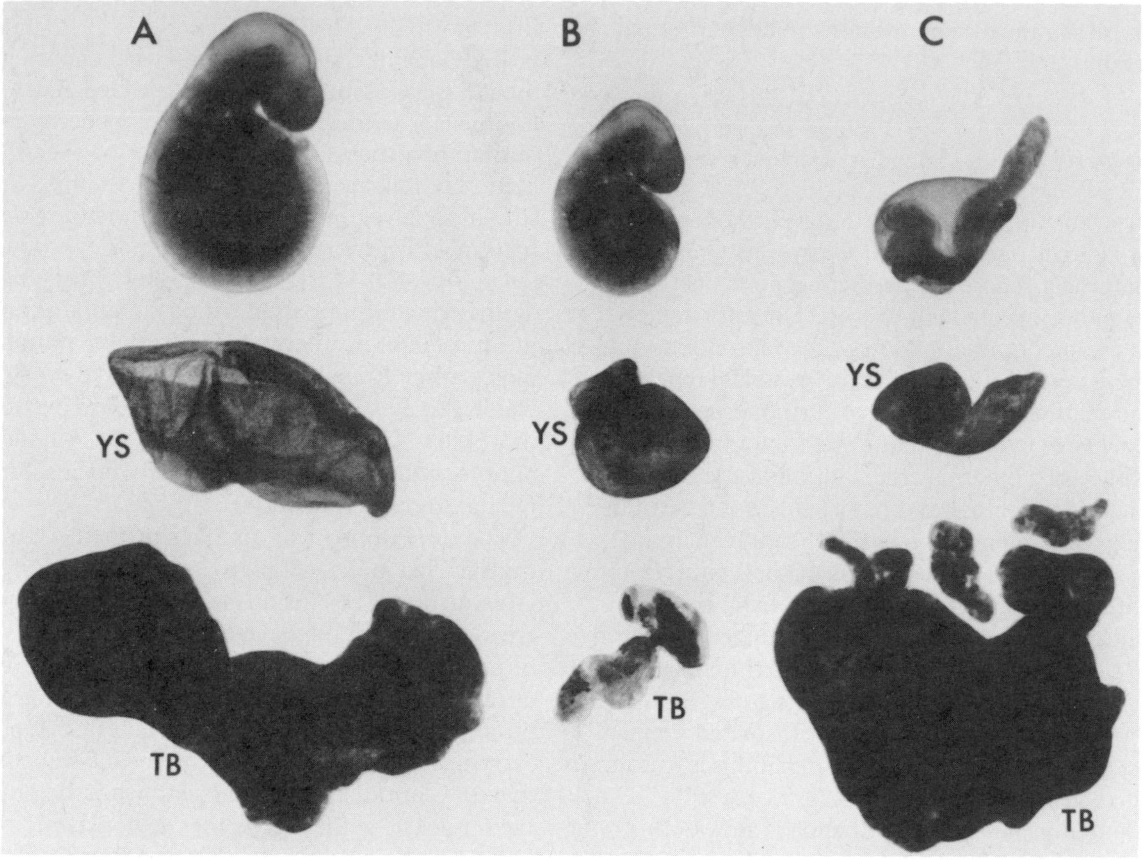

FIG. 12. Dissected components (embryo proper, yolk sac, and trophoblast) of normal (fertilized) mouse embryo (**A**), a gynogenone (**B**), and an androgenone (**C**). Note differences in the extent of embryonic and extraembryonic tissue development in the three different circumstances. YS, yolk sac; TB, trophoblast. From Surani et al. (535).

the extraembryonic lineages, but may rather be the result of a propensity for terminal differentiation without proliferation of sufficient stem cells to maintain a self-renewing population (reviewed in 474). This may account for the tendency of parthenogenetically-derived ovarian tumors to contain trophoblast cells, despite the apparent failure of trophoblast development in parthenogenones transferred to the uterus.

In chimeras made by aggregating cleavage-stage embryos with markers to distinguish between parthenogenetic and normal, fertilized embryos, clear differences in their tissue distribution and fate emerged. Despite allocation of parthenogenetic cells to both the trophectoderm and inner cell mass at the blastocyst stage (3.5 d.g.), they were eliminated from the trophoblast lineage by 6.5 d.g., and from primitive endoderm by midgestation stages (9.5–11.5 d.g.), despite their persistence in most lineages in the embryo proper (492–494). At later stages of fetal development and after birth, parthenogenetic cells did not contribute to skeletal muscle, and contributions to other tissues gradually declined, as if the parthenogenetic contribution underwent negative selection (except in the germ line of fertile adult females, where the parthenogenetic component persisted throughout fertile life) (481,482,495,496). Those fetuses and postnatal individuals with extensive parthenogenetic contribution, however, were smaller and grew slower than normal offspring. Embryonic stem cells generated from diploid parthenogenetic blastocysts can also contribute extensively to the embryonic tissues of chimeras (63,497), including female germ cells (Sturm, K. S. and Pedersen, R. A., 1993, *unpublished observations*). Although parthenogenetic ES cells have not been examined for their contribution to extraembryonic lineages, it seems unlikely they would do so because normal, fertilized embryo-derived ES cells make relatively little contribution to trophoblast and primitive endoderm of chimeras (498).

Androgenesis

Diandric mouse embryos can be produced by nuclear transfer, developing to early postimplantation stages when transferred to the uteri of foster mothers, but never reaching term (489,490). The postimplantation diandric embryos analyzed on day 10 of gestation have extremely rudimentary embryonic development, but the extent of trophoblast development is near (or in excess of) normal, and yolk sac development is intermediate (499) (see Fig. 12). The pattern of developmental arrest in experimentally-produced diploid diandric embryos is thus strikingly different from that of parthenogenones and digynic embryos, which have retarded extraembryonic growth (500). The differential phenotypes between parthenogenones and androgenones led Surani and co-workers to hypothesize a complementary relationship between the two parental genetic contributions, with the maternal component playing a unique role in development of the embryo proper (490). Because of the difficulty of the nuclear transfer procedures in generating androgenones and their low incidence of development to postimplantation stages, only a few have been described. However, recent studies have described the phenotypes of late gestation and neonatal chimeras made by aggregating androgenones with normal, fertilized embryos or injecting androgenetic cells into blastocysts (501,502). While most of these chimeras died at early postimplantation stages, those surviving into later gestation were larger than normal stage-matched embryos, and those surviving to birth had pronounced skeletal abnormalities, including hypertrophied rib structures. Interestingly, when ES cells were derived from androgenetic blastocysts and used to generate chimeras, an apparently identical phenotype emerged; moreover, when androgenetic ES cells were injected into mice, they formed teratomas with abundant muscle tissue (503). These results underscore the complementary phenotypes of pure parthenogenetic and androgenetic embryos and reaffirm the suggestion (504) that the genes affected by imprinting affect embryonic growth and differentiation.

Another case of androgenesis is the development of hydatidiform mole in the human, the result of fertilization by two spermatozoa (505; see 506 for review). These embryos become androgenetic, owing to failure of the maternal genome to participate in development, generally producing a 46 XY conceptus in which all of the chromosomes are from sperm. The trophoblastic hyperplasia and embryonic dysgenesis of moles is strongly reminiscent of the development of diandric mouse embryos. This observation is consistent with Surani's hypothesis, showing that as a result of imprinting, the paternal genome preferentially supports development of the extraembryonic tissues and fails to support development of the fetus (490).

Genes Affected by Imprinting in Mice

As discussed earlier, Robertsonian translocations have been used to generate chromosomally balanced young that had either maternal or paternal duplications with the corresponding paternal or maternal deficiencies for specific mouse chromosomes (424). These studies have identified three classes of imprinting effects. In the most severe class, embryos with the noncomplementing duplication die very early in development, as in the case of maternal duplication of proximal chromosome 2, maternal duplication of proximal chromosome 6, and paternal duplication of distal chromosome 7. A class with intermediate severity causes midfetal to early neonatal death, as in maternal duplication for distal chromosome 7 or proximal chromosome 7, and maternal deletion of proximal chromosome 17 (the *Tme* locus). The class of recognized imprinting effects with least severity causes phenotypic or behavioral abnormalities accompanying postnatal lethality/reduced viability, as in maternal or paternal duplication for distal chromosome 2 or proximal chromosome 11, maternal duplication of central chromosome 7, paternal duplication of proximal chromosome 7, or paternal duplication of distal chromosome 17 (424,514). It was not clear from the genetic studies whether the imprinting phenomenon is restricted to a few specific genes within these chromosomal regions, or if imprinting affects most or all of the genes in each region. Minimally, one gene in each region could account for the imprinting effect (two in those cases where there are both maternal and paternal duplication/deficiency effects) leading to a minimal estimate of nine or thirteen imprinted genes, and a maximal estimate of perhaps 10 percent of the genome.

To date, three mouse genes with differential parental allele-specific expression have been discovered on chromosome 7: insulinlike growth factor (IGF)-II, *H19,* and small nuclear ribonuclear protein N (*Snrpn*). The first of these to be recognized was the *Igf2* gene, which was inactivated by homologous recombination in male ES cells. Offspring resulting from male chimeras carrying the targeted *Igf2* gene were only 60 percent of normal weight; however, when they received the mutant gene from their mothers, they were normal size (507), leading to the discovery that the maternal allele was not transcribed, except in the choroid plexus and leptomeninges of the brain (508). Imprinting of this gene was confirmed in studies of mouse fetuses disomic for distal chromosome 7, where *Igf2* maps (509). A closely linked gene, *H19,* was identified as being imprinted using interspecific crosses between *Mus musculus domesticus* and *M. spretus* to generate allele-specific markers for the maternal and paternal mRNAs, and was found to be expressed only from the maternal allele (510). This gene, which is closely linked to *Igf2,* lacks a conserved open reading frame and has no known function but is widely transcribed in early extraembryonic tissues and is subsequently repressed in most tissues (511). Overexpression of *H19* in transgenic mice leads to late gestational death, suggesting that transcriptional dosage of this gene may have to be regulated carefully (512). The most recently discovered imprinted gene, *Snrpn,* is located in the central region of chromosome 7, in a region with homology to human chromosome 15 in the critical region for the Prader-Willi syndrome, as discussed below. The *Snrpn* gene appears to function as part of the mRNA splicing machinery and could be involved in processing the calcitonin gene-related peptide mRNA, a hypothalamic gene product; it is expressed abundantly in brain, but only from the paternal allele (513). Mice with maternal duplications in the region containing this gene show postnatal lethality with failure to thrive and could be considered a model for Prader-Willi syndrome (514).

Additional studies provide evidence for imprinting of two genes located on mouse chromosome 17. One of these is the T maternal effect gene (*Tme*), which is deleted in the T hairpin mutation (T^{hp}). This mutation, which is lethal when inherited maternally, is a nuclear rather than cytoplasmic effect (515–519). A molecular examination of the mutation revealed that the *Igf2r* gene is also located within the deletion, and is expressed only when inherited maternally; therefore, it was proposed that *Igf2r* is closely linked or identical to *Tme* (520). However, further genetic analysis of this locus revealed that *Tme* could be distinguished from *Igf2r,* depending on the allele of an unlinked gene designated as the *Imprintor-1* locus, upon which the imprinted state of *Tme* depends. By combining *Tme* with an *Imprintor-1* allele that does not induce maternal allele-specific expression of *Tme,* mice carrying the T^{hp} deletion survived without an active *Igf2r* gene (521). These mice were larger than their normal littermates, but this difference disappeared as they grew to adulthood. Three other genes examined for parental allele-specific expression within the T^{hp} deletion showed expression from both maternal and paternal alleles, showing that imprinting did not affect the entire region in which the imprinted genes reside. Similar findings emerged from studies of mouse chromosome 7, showing that genes adjacent to *Igf2* and *H19* are not imprinted (514,897). Therefore, based on minimal estimates for the number of imprinted genes, at least 4–8 imprinted genes remain to be discovered.

Extent of Imprinting in Other Species

If such a fundamental process as genomic imprinting occurs during mouse gametogenesis and is the inherent cause of parthenogenetic and androgenetic arrest in this species, then there should be evidence among other mammalian species for a similar phenomenon. The phenotype of ovarian cysts and hydatidiform moles in humans argues that a similar process limits development of these isoparental conceptions as in mouse (473). Moreover, there are several human diseases in which the onset, prevalence, or phenotype depends on the parental origin, including Prader-Willi syndrome/Angelman syndrome, Beckwith-Wiedeman syndrome, Wilms' tumor, and other cancers (reviewed in 522,523). Moreover, recent studies have documented parental allele-specific transcription of the human *Igf2* gene (paternally expressed), the *H19* gene (maternally expressed) and the *Snrpn* gene (maternally expressed) (524–529). Interestingly, the *Igf2* gene, which maps to the critical region for Beckwith-Wiedemann syndrome, is expressed from both parental alleles in the Wilms' tumors characteristic of this disease (526,527), leading to the proposal that overexpression of this gene is responsible for the symptoms of Beckwith-Wiedemann syndrome and that relaxation of imprinting of this gene leads to a predisposition to Wilms' tumor.

The conservation of the identity of these imprinted genes between rodents and humans argues that imprinting is widespread among eutherian mammals. In addition, the preferential paternal X chromosome inactivation in somatic tissues of marsupials suggests that imprinting phenomena exist there also.

Mechanism of Imprinting

In searching for molecular mechanism(s) for genomic imprinting, we should bear in mind the following prerequisites: (a) the mechanism(s) should be stable throughout the range of development that imprinting endures; (b) it should be capable of altering the function of the parental alleles without changing their primary sequence; (c) it should be erased and reset to the state of the opposite gamete at each subsequent life cycle; and (d) it should be capable of influencing transcription. While the previous studies established late cleavage or blastocyst stage (inner cell mass) as time limits for nuclear totipotency in mouse embryos (470,485,531; see 532 for review), they did not formally address the issue of whether genomic imprinting is stable throughout cleavage because the inability of more advanced nuclei to support early development could be due to asynchrony between donor nucleus and host cytoplasm. The study by Surani et al. (535), however, addressed this point by experimentally producing haploid gynogenetic or androgenetic embryos as a source of donor nuclei between the 2- and 16-cell stages. These were then transferred to haploid gynogenetic or androgenetic zygotes. Reconstituted diploids developed normally to term if they contained both maternal and paternal genetic contributions but not if they were digynic or diandric. The results indicate that genomic imprinting acquired during gametogenesis is stable at least through early cleavage. In addition, the observations of the expression patterns of imprinted genes show that they are stably expressed from one parental allele throughout development (with the exception of *Igf2,* which is expressed from both alleles in certain brain tissues). Therefore, the mechanism(s) by which the embryonic imprint is maintained must be extraordinarily stable.

Secondary modification of DNA structure, particularly by methylation of cytosines at CpG sequences, may provide a mechanism for stable differentiation of the maternal and paternal genetic contributions and has been considered in X chromosome inactivation during embryogenesis as well as in transcriptional regulation of known imprinted genes. The methylation of cytosine in CpG sequences often correlates with decreased expression in the affected or adjacent genes (reviewed in 539–540).

DNA methylation levels change dramatically during the mouse life cycle: Global levels of methylation are low in fetal and neonatal oocytes and high in sperm; methylation decreases during preimplantation development to a nadir at the blastocyst stage, then increases by the time of gastrulation in the primitive ectoderm lineage but remains at low levels in the trophoblast and primitive endoderm lineages (541–546). Methylation of specific DNA sequences (e.g., L1 repeats, mouse urinary protein genes) in mature sperm and eggs, however, is not as distinctive as in the immature gametes, suggesting that substantial methylation occurs during oocyte growth or maturation (546). Both maternal and paternal components become hypomethylated during early cleavage, despite the presence of high levels of DNA methyl transferase (547), and there is little evidence from these studies of global or specific sequence methylation that could serve to distinguish the parental alleles by the blastocyst stage. Therefore, a role of DNA methylation in the primary imprinting phenomenon has not been established by the general patterns of DNA methylation.

Studies of DNA methylation in X-linked genes have led to insights into the role of methylation in the initial events of X-inactivation (reviewed in 548). Paradoxically, there is global hypomethylation of DNA in the first tissues to show X-inactivation (trophectoderm and primitive endoderm) which are extensively hypomethylated (549–553). Moreover, methylation of strategic CpG sites on the inactive HPRT allele occurs after, rather than before, X-inactivation (554). On the other hand, examination of a specific methylation site in the 5′ region of the X-linked *PGK-1* gene shows that it is not methylated in sperm or eggs, so it cannot serve as the primary imprint for inactivation of this gene, but that it becomes methylated about the time of X-inactivation, by 6.5 d.g. (544,555). Results with cultured cells may indicate a role for DNA methylation in stabilizing X-inactivation. DNA from the inactive X-chromosome of adult tissues functions poorly in DNA-mediated transformation experiments with cultured HPRT-deficient cells (556). By contrast, DNA from the inactive X chromosome of extraembryonic tissues functions as well as DNA from the active X chromosome (557). Similar results were obtained with a transgenic mouse line containing an alpha-fetoprotein minigene integrated into the X chromosome. Unlike the endogenous X-linked genes, the exogenous alpha-fetoprotein gene was expressed in visceral endoderm even when it was paternally inherited, but it was not expressed on the inactive X chromosome in the fetal liver (558).

Studies of certain transgenes have shown a relationship between parental inheritance and DNA methylation (reviewed in 464). In the best example of this phenomenon, the maternal allele of the *RSV-Ig-mycA* transgene was highly methylated and repressed, whereas the paternal allele was only partially methylated and was expressed in the heart (559). Detailed examination of the history of methylation of this transgene showed that the methylation pattern was erased early in both male and female gametogenesis, primordial germ cell DNA being hypomethylated at all transgene CpG sites; the highly methylated maternal pattern was established during later stages of oogenesis, and was present in the mature (metaphase II) oocyte, which was maintained throughout later stages of development (560). By contrast, the paternal allele was inherited from the sperm in a partially methylated state, became completely demethylated during preimplantation stages, then reacquired the partially methylated adult pattern before gastrulation (by 6.5 d.g.). The methylation pattern of this transgene thus reflects the changing patterns of DNA methylation during early development, and is consistent with, but does not prove, a role for methylation in the imprinted regulation of this gene. The role of DNA methylation in transgene imprinting is complicated by the observation that hypermethylation in such cases depends not only on the transgene locus, but also on other genetic factors that act in *trans* to modify the methylation patterns (561). Furthermore, the high frequency of imprinted patterns of transgene methylation can also be interpreted as a consequence of embryonic defense mechanisms against exogenous genetic intrusions (562,563).

Therefore, studies of DNA methylation of endogenous imprinted genes have been carried out to address the relationship between patterns of gene expression and the state of methylation at sites of imprinted genes. Careful examination of the promoter regions of the mouse *Igf2* gene revealed no parental allele-specific methylation differences, and both alleles were in an open chromatin configuration. However, multiple CpG sequences located 3 kb upstream of the start site for this gene were more methylated in normal, fertilized embryos than in their maternal disomy 7 embryos, suggesting that the paternal chromosome, which is active, has the more highly methylated allele (564). Similar studies of the mouse *H19* gene show that there are specific CpG sites in the promoter region that are methylated only on the (nonexpressed) paternal gene, but these sites become methylated only sometime after fertilization, since they are not methylated in sperm (565,566). Finally, an extensive examination of the *Igf2r* gene detected two regions of parent-specific methylation, one near the transcription start site that becomes increasingly methylated on the (repressed) paternal allele during late gestation but is not methylated in sperm, and another that is 27 kb downstream from the start site and is methylated at morula, blastocyst, and later stages of development, but only on the (expressed) maternal allele (567). In sum, these recent findings provide new insights into the role of DNA methylation in regulating the expression of imprinted endogenous genes. First, the paternal allele-specific methylation patterns of the *H19* and *Igf2r* genes cannot be the primary imprint, because they are not present during gametogenesis; second, the *Igf2* and *Igf2r* genes have allele-specific methylation patterns in which methylation of the allele correlates with its expression rather than its repression. A similar correlation between DNA methylation and expression has recently been observed for the imprinted expression of a keratin 18/*lacZ* transgene. Such a role for DNA methylation in sustaining transcription of some genes could be explained by its effect on the binding of negative transcriptional regulators (568). Finally, these observations raise the possibility that the primary imprint consists of DNA-RNA or DNA-protein interactions that are maintained through the preimplantation period and ultimately stabilized by DNA methylation. DNA methylation is nevertheless critical to the manifestation of imprinting during development, as indicated by the midgestation lethality of mice homozygous for deletions in the predominant DNA methyltransferase gene (569) and the perturbations of imprinted patterns of gene expression in such individuals (Jaenisch, R., 1993, *unpublished observations*).

Biological Role of Imprinting

The combined observations in this section invite speculation about the evolutionary origin and biological role of the genomic imprinting of specific genes and its developmental consequences seen in mammals. Specializations of the parental genomes are not unique to mammals because they are also found in plants, insects, and other species (reviewed in 464). However, the unique functional consequences of genomic imprinting in preventing viable parthenogenesis in mammals suggests that imprinting may have arisen independently several times during plant and animal evolution. The evolutionary benefits of precluding parthenogenesis consist primarily of maintaining heterosis by diminishing the probability of inbreeding. If this were the basis of genomic imprinting, it should be found widespread at least among vertebrates. Another category of benefits in preventing parthenogenesis may apply specifically to placental mammals, which have an invasive chorioallantoic placenta that could diminish maternal fitness if its differentiation and growth were independent of the paternal genome, given the probability of spontaneous ovarian egg activation (see 522). A third category of explanation for the absence of parthenogenesis in mammals is conflicting interests between maternal and paternal organisms when one gender is responsible for the nutritional resources provided to the offspring, as is particularly true of viviparous mammals (570,571). This latter explanation provides the best accounting for the observed information about genomic imprinting, since there are unique functional consequences that seem restricted to mammals; this hypothesis also accounts for the existence of imprinting phenomena in marsupials. A definitive test of this hypothesis would require examining the extent of imprinting of specific genes in eutheria and marsupials, where it should be widespread, and among birds, reptiles, or other oviparous vertebrates, where it should be absent.

MOLECULAR ASPECTS

Transcriptional Control, Differentiation, and Pattern Formation

In the search for genes in the mouse embryo that control morphogenesis and pattern formation, a profitable approach has been the application of reverse genetics and molecular techniques combined with classical genetics. Using these strategies, a number of putative mammalian developmental control genes have been characterized whose function has been inferred from homologies to genes in other systems, or whose function has been assayed directly in transgenic mice, produced either by zygotic DNA injection or by homologous recombination in ES cells (reviewed in 572,573). We will focus on genes affecting the period from gastrulation through organogenesis in the mouse embryo.

Brachyury, Goosecoid, Motch

Brachyury mutant mice display a shortened tail as heterozygotes and homozygous embryos die around 10.0 d.g. with defects in tissues of mesodermal origin, including a greatly reduced allantois (574). In a landmark paper, Hermann et al. (575) described the cloning of the *Brachyury* (*T*) gene in the mouse embryo. Previously, genetic analyses had localized the *T* locus to chromosome 17 and subsequently, pieces of this chromosome were microdissected and cloned, which greatly facilitated the cloning of *Brachyury* (*T*). Chromosome walking along these fragments and the availability of independently-derived deletions and duplications over the entire *T* locus allowed the identification of a 110-kb region that contained the *T* gene. Within this region a single transcription unit was identified and sequenced. Confirmation that the *T* gene had been cloned was derived from an additional spontaneous *T* locus mutant, T^{Wis}. In this mutant, the presence of a retroviral-like element that disrupted the coding region of the newly identified gene was discovered (575; reviewed in 576). The *T* gene was expressed strongly in 8.5–9.5 d.g. embryos by Northern analysis and by *in situ* hybridization, and transcripts were localized to the embryonic ectoderm and mesoderm of the primitive streak (577). Expression was found to be restricted solely to the notochord in later development. Thus, the expression pattern correlated with tissues known to be affected in homozygous mutant embryos. The mouse *Brachyury* (*T*) gene does not encode a signal peptide or a potential transmembrane domain. Therefore, *Brachyury* (*T*) gene may encode a transcription factor that is first expressed at the primitive streak and that plays a role in the patterning of mesodermal tissues (575,578).

Embryonic stem cell lines from *Brachyury* (*T*) mutants were generated and they were combined with wild type cells in chimeras (579). *T*/+ ES cells formed normal chimeras when combined with +/+ ES cells, whereas *T*/*T* ↔ +/+ chimeras mimicked the *T*/*T* phenotype. Because wild type cells could not rescue the mutant phenotype, the *T* gene appears to act autonomously in the cells of the primitive streak and notochord. The presence of wild-type cells also did not rescue defects in the allantois, which was affected in *T* mutants but does not express the *T* gene. Therefore, the *T* gene may also act upstream in a signaling pathway that controls the formation of this tissue. Lastly, the tail defect in *Brachyury* (*T*) mice has been rescued in transgenic mice (578). Insertion of a single copy of the *T* gene was able to rescue the *T*-associated tail phenotype in heterozygous mice. Stott et al. (578) also reported that increased gene dosage of the *T* gene in mice heterozygous for the *T Curtailed* (T^C) allele caused an increased extension of the tail (i.e., the body axis). Therefore, the level of the *T* gene product correlated with the extension of the anteroposterior axis in this study. These data suggest that *Brachyury* (*T*) may act as a transcription factor and be involved in the process of anteroposterior axis formation during embryogenesis.

Two other genes have recently been characterized which are expressed at the primitive streak of the mouse embryo, *Goosecoid* and *Motch* (580–582). *Goosecoid* resembles *gooseberry* and *bicoid* in *Drosophila,* whereas *Motch* is the mouse homolog of the *Drosophila Notch* gene, a gene involved in cell-cell interactions and cell fate decisions in the fly embryo. *Goosecoid* accumulated as a patch in the embryonic ectoderm at the site where the primitive streak forms and later at 6.8–7.0 d.g. marked the anterior end of the streak. After that period, *goosecoid* expression ceased temporarily and was not detected again until the period of organogenesis around 10.0 d.g. (583). Treatment of mouse embryos with activin A, a molecule known to induce mesodermal tissue in *Xenopus* embryos, resulted in the accumulation of *goosecoid* over the entire epiblast. These results suggest that *goosecoid* acts early during primitive streak formation and that a localized signal in the posterior of the embryo may induce *goosecoid* expression. In contrast to *goosecoid, Motch* expression begins in the primitive streak and continues in the 9.5 day neuroepithelium, in mesodermally-derived tissues such as the somites, and in neural crest-derived tissues (581,582). In whole mount *in situ* hybridizations, *Motch* expression became concentrated around the midline of the embryo where future axial mesoderm will develop (581). Just prior to the condensation of the first somite, a dense band of *Motch* expression marked the site. *Motch* expression continued in a band one somite wide, at the anterior end of the presomitic mesoderm as successive somites formed. *Motch* expression was down-regulated in the newly generated somites, suggesting that it plays a role in somite formation. Thus, the expression pattern of *Motch* in the mouse embryo suggests it may function similarly as in *Drosophila,* that is, to mediate cell-cell interactions or cell fate decisions during axis formation.

Homeobox *Genes*

The *Hox* family of homeobox-containing genes were cloned in mammals based on their homology to genes in the *Drosophila* Antennapedia and Bithorax complexes (the HOM-C complex) which control pattern formation in fly embryos (reviewed in 584). There are 38 mouse (and human) *Hox* genes arranged in four clusters on separate chromosomes in the vertebrate homeotic complex (Hox-C). Note that throughout this review we are adhering to the newly adopted nomenclature for vertebrate *Hox* genes (585). Most mouse *Hox* genes are first expressed in broad regions of embryonic ectoderm and mesoderm of the late primitive streak at approximately 8.0 days of development (reviewed by 584,586). Along the developing embryonic axis the expression of different *Hox* genes becomes more restricted, with each gene exhibiting a distinct anterior border of expression, while in more posterior regions the expression domains of many *Hox* genes overlap. In addition, within the mouse Hox-C and in the *Drosophila* HOM-C, a striking correlation exists between the order of a gene within a cluster and its anterior boundary of expression: while transcription proceeds 5′ to 3′ through the complex, the more 3′ a gene lies in a cluster, the more anterior the border of its expression in the embryo (587,588). As development proceeds, the expression of most mouse *Hox* genes becomes restricted to smaller region-specific and still overlapping domains along the anteroposterior axis in the presomitic, somitic, or lateral mesoderm, and the neuroectoderm. While *Hox* gene expression at this stage of development generally exhibits a distinct anterior border within the ectoderm and mesoderm, posterior boundaries of expression are less distinct (584,586). Between 8.5 and 10.5 days of development domains of *Hox* expression in the ectoderm and the mesoderm begin to diverge, with expression in the ectodermally-derived neural tube (the developing central nervous system [CNS]) extending more anteriorly than the expression in the underlying mesoderm. In general, these region-specific domains of expression of individual *Hox* genes persist throughout subsequent organogenesis. Through 12.5–13.5 days of development the expression of *Hox* genes is also observed within limb buds and neural crest-derived structures such as the spinal ganglia and other components of the peripheral nervous system (PNS) (586,588). The expression of several genes in the mouse Hox-A and -B clusters, such as *HoxA6, HoxA7, HoxB5,* and *HoxB9,* extends to spinal ganglia and cranial nerves and expression in the PNS correlates with their anterior expression border within the CNS (586).

Because of their restricted expression pattern during embryogenesis and by analogy to *Drosophila* homeotic gene function, vertebrate *Hox* genes are proposed to encode transcription factors whose region-specific expression controls anteroposterior patterning in the ectoderm and mesoderm during development (586,587). Indeed, ectopic expression of both human and mouse *Hox* gene products induced homeotic transformations in *Drosophila* embryos (589,591). Additionally, in "gene swap" experiments, cis-regulatory elements of the *Drosophila deformed* (*dfd*) gene and cis-regulatory elements of the human homolog of *dfd, HOXB4,* directed the expression of *lacZ* reporter proteins to appropriate positions along the anteroposterior axis of the mouse and fly embryo, respectively (592,593). These data indicate that not only are the structure of mouse and *Drosophila* homeotic genes conserved, but also the overall mechanism for establishing region-specific gene expression along the anteroposterior axis of the embryo is conserved between arthropods and chordates.

In the mouse embryo, the hypothesis that *Hox* genes control anteroposterior patterning has been tested by creating null mutations at specific *Hox* loci using homologous recombination in ES cells (584). Null mutants of *HoxA1* and *HoxA3* have both been created; these mutants died just after birth with mutant embryos displaying structural deficiencies and a wide array of cranial and cardiac defects (594–596). Null mutants of *HoxA3* were athymic, aparathyroid, and displayed cardiac and craniofacial abnormalities that are comparable to DiGeorge syndrome in humans (594). This pattern of abnormalities is consistent with an effect on organs derived from multiple cell lineages including the mesoderm, pharyngeal endoderm, and neural crest. Null mutants of *HoxA1* displayed defects in the anatomy of the inner ear and loss of connections between cranial ganglia and the brainstem (595,596). These authors also reported that characteristic bulges or rhombomeres in the 9.5- to 11.5-day hindbrain are missing in the *HoxA1* null mutants. Comparison of the mutant phenotypes between *HoxA1*⁻ and *HoxA3*⁻ mutant embryos revealed no defects in common, showed that there was a limited region along the anteroposterior axis in which the defects of each were manifested, and showed that defective structures in both mutants were restricted to their anterior border of expression (595). Null mutants of *HoxC8* and *HoxB4* have also been generated by homologous recombination and these mutants died neonatally. In contrast to mutants that have lost the more anteriorly expressed *HoxA1* and *HoxA3,* null mutants of *HoxC8* and *HoxB4* showed distinct homeotic transformations in the identity of some axial structures, specifically the vertebrae (597–599). In *HoxC8*⁻ mutants, transformations occurred in which skeletal elements resembled their most anterior neighbor. For example, the 1st lumbar vertebra was transformed into a rib-bearing vertebra (resembling its neighboring, anterior thoracic vertebra) and in *HoxB4*⁻ mutants the 2nd cervical vertebra, the axis, was transformed so that it resembled the 1st cervical vertebra, the atlas. Defects in the morphogenesis of the sternum were also observed in *HoxB4*⁻ mutants. The phenotypic changes observed in the *HoxB4*⁻ mutants corresponded to the most anterior border of its expression in the vertebral column. Although the anterior limits of the skeletal transformations in the *HoxC8*⁻ mutants were more difficult to define, the anterior transformations produced by targeting the expression of these two *Hox* genes are consistent with the phenotypes of loss of function mutations in *Drosophila* homeotic genes in which anterior transformations are produced.

Apart from the *Hox* clusters, several homeobox genes with more divergent homeobox sequences including *Engrailed-1* (*En-1*) and *En-2* have been isolated in mice and humans (600,601). Mouse *En-1* and *En-2* are located on chromosome 5 and 1, respectively, and during development the expression of *En* transcripts becomes restricted to a band of cells spanning the junction of the mid- and hindbrain (587,602,603). The expression of *En-1* transcripts, but not of *En-2,* continues in spinal cord. Immunohistological techniques have also localized En-1 and -2 protein to presumptive myoblasts within the first branchial arch (604). Homozygous *En-2*⁻ mutants were generated via homologous recombination (603). These mice showed no overt phenotype; however, careful examination of the cerebellar anatomy revealed subtle alterations in the anatomy of folds in the cerebellum in null mutants. Joyner et al. (603) hypothesized that a further role for *En-2* in embryogenesis may be masked by a redundancy of expression with *En-1.* This may also be the case for *Hox* null mutants, including the *HoxB4*⁻ mutants described above, that show effects in axial structures of mesodermal origin but do not display gross or overt defects in the CNS or PNS, despite prominent gene expression in those regions in normal embryos.

The role of *Hox* gene products in development has also been tested in gain-of-function mutants by generating transgenic mice that overexpress or ectopically express certain *Hox* genes along the anteroposterior axis of the embryo (584). Transgenic mice which overexpress *HoxA4* displayed functional stenosis of the colon or megacolon (605). This lethal condition is thought to arise due to a deficiency in the innervation of the colon from neural crest-derived myenteric ganglion cells and suggests that the defect in the transgenic animals may lie in the neural crest lineage. In other experiments, when *HoxD4* was placed under the control of promoter sequences of the more anteriorly expressed *HoxA1,* the expression domain of the *HoxD4* in the mesoderm of transgenic animals was more rostral than its normal anterior boundary of expression (606). The effect of the ectopic transgene expression was the posterior transformation of occipital bones into cervical vertebrae in regions that normally do not express *HoxD4.* These transgenic mice displayed no altered phenotype in regions that normally express *HoxD4.* In contrast to the posterior transformations observed in the *HoxD4* transgenics, the anterior ectopic expression of three additional *Hox* genes, *HoxA7, HoxC8,* and *HOXC6* results in anterior transformations of axial structures (607–610). The ectopic anterior expression of *HoxC8* and *HOXC6* resulted in the appearance of an additional pair of ribs on a lumbar vertebra as was also observed in null mutations at the *HoxC8* locus (598). These studies suggest that over- or underexpression of *Hox* genes produces similar phenotypes in axial structures. These studies also support the hypothesis that *Hox* genes, acting in a complex combinatorial code, specify skeletal identity in vertebrates.

Transgenic mice have also been used to examine the cis-regulatory elements of various *Hox* genes. Numerous studies have identified specific positive elements that are necessary for the correct anterior border of *Hox* gene expression (611–616) and for the correct expression of *En-2* in neural tissues or in mandibular myoblasts (601). Furthermore, additional negative regulatory elements have been identified that are necessary for the downregulation of *Hox* gene expression in posterior embryonic regions and for the restriction of expression of *Hox* genes to certain subsets of cells: for example, the restriction of *HoxB4* expression to the neuroectoderm (615) or the restriction of *HoxA7* to prevertebrae (613). These data indicate that separate cis-regulatory regions play a role in setting up the initial pattern of *Hox* gene expression and that as development proceeds, additional elements control further *Hox* gene expression in different subsets of cells.

Despite the evidence from loss-of-function mutants and transgenic gain-of-function mutants which indicate that *Hox* genes acting as transcription factors determine axial identity, few if any downstream targets of *Hox* genes have been positively identified in mice. Experiments in tissue culture cells have shown that cotransfection of *Xenopus Hox* gene constructs modulates the activity of the mouse neural-cell adhesion molecule (NCAM) promoter and the chicken tenascin promoter (reviewed in 617). In similar experiments, mouse *Evx-1* also stimulated tenascin promoter activity (618). NCAM has also been proposed as a downstream target of *Pax-3* (619) (Pax genes are discussed below). These *in vitro* studies suggest that the region-specific expression of morphoregulatory molecules such as cell adhesion proteins may depend on local cues provided by homeobox genes and their encoded proteins during embryological development. The slow progress in identifying target genes for *Hox* gene activity in the mouse suggests that it may be fruitful to return to paradigms provided by the study of *Drosophila* development and search for genes in the mouse which are homologous to those known to act up- or downstream of the *Drosophila* HOM-C gene products.

Pax *Genes*

Murine paired-box, or Pax, genes constitute another class of homeobox genes that display region-specific expression during development and that are proposed to function in axial specification. *Pax* genes contain the classical homeobox domain plus a second motif, the paired box, found in their *Drosophila* homolog, the *paired* gene (reviewed in 620,621). There are currently nine *Pax* genes, and in contrast to the *Hox* genes, they do not display a clustered organization, but rather have been mapped to five different chromosomes. No *Pax* gene is expressed before 8.0 days of development in the mouse, but between 8.0 and 9.5 days, *Pax* expression is found in axial structures of both the ectoderm (the CNS) and the paraxial mesoderm (except for *Pax-1,* which is expressed only in the mesodermal derivatives such as the intervertebral disks and the sternum) (620,622). Again, in contrast to *Hox* genes that display distinct anterior boundaries of expression in the CNS, *Pax* genes are expressed the length of the neural tube; however, expression is restricted to discrete regions within the transverse plane of the neural tube. For example, *Pax-3* is expressed in the dorsal regions of the neural tube, including the roof plate and the neural crest, while *Pax-6* is expressed only in ventral regions of the neural tube.

Transgenic mice which lack *Pax* expression or express *Pax* genes ectopically have not been generated, but a role for *Pax* genes in development has been surmised from mouse and human mutants at various *Pax* loci. The first mutant examined was *undulated* (*un*), which exhibits distortions along the entire vertebral column including a "kinky" tail (623,624). *Pax-1* was mapped close to the *un* locus on chromosome 2. *Pax-1* is normally expressed in the intervertebral disk and sternum, and Balling et al. (625) determined that *un* mutants have a single nucleotide change in the conserved part of the *Pax-1* paired box. Thus, *Pax-1* has been implicated in the generation of the vertebral column. At another locus, *Splotch* (*Sp*) mutant mice exhibit abnormal development of the CNS, including exencephalus and spina bifida and dysgenesis of the heart and pigmentation (621,626,627). Three alleles of *Sp* (Sp^{2H}, Sp^{r}, and *Sp*) show alterations in the *Pax-3* gene and the phenotypes of these mutants are consistent with the pattern of *Pax-3* expression. Because of the observed defects in the neural tube and in neural crest-derived structures in *Sp* mutants, Moase and Trasler (619) used immunobiochemical techniques to examine the distribution of NCAM which is prominently expressed in these tissues. An altered form of NCAM was observed in the developing CNS in *Sp* mutants, suggesting that the posttranslational modification of NCAM is a downstream consequence of *Pax-3* expression.

Pax-9 was mapped to chromosome 12 while *Pax-6* mapped close to *small eye* (*Sey*) on chromosome 2 (621,628). In addition, *Pax-6* was found to be mutated in several *Sey* alleles (621). Homozygous *Sey* mutants do not develop eyes and lack nasal structures; therefore, *Pax-6* expression has been implicated in the normal development of these structures. In addition, mutations in the human homolog of *Pax-6* have been implicated in causing aniridia, the partial or complete absence of the iris (629). Lastly, the human homolog of *Pax-3, HuP2,* was found to be mutated in persons affected with Waardenburg syndromes I and III, which include pigmentary disturbances, eye defects, occasional deafness, and mental retardation (621,630). Therefore, counterparts of the mouse mutants *Sp* and *Sey* have been identified in humans, attesting to the evolutionary conservation of development of axial structures controlled by *Pax* genes.

POU *Genes*

POU-domain transcription factors contain a homeodomain distantly related to the classical *Antennapedia* homeodomain plus a second motif termed the *POU-specific domain.* This class of transcription factors was initially defined through the characterization of four different transcription factors: the mammalian Pit-1, Oct-1, and Oct-2 factors; and the nematode developmental regulator Unc-86 (631,632). POU transcription factors share the property of binding to a well-characterized octomer motif in target genes, and a number of genes for POU-domain transcription factors have been described in mammals, including *Brn-1* and *Brn-2* which probably encode rat homologs of mouse Oct proteins, the mouse Tst-1 factor, and the human *RDC-1* gene product (631,633–635).

The majority of POU factors were detected selectively or primarily in the CNS although they displayed no organized pattern of expression with respect to embryonic axes. The function of the CNS-specific POU factors may be similar to the function of the Oct-6 homolog in nematodes, Unc-86 (632). The *unc-86* locus is required for the commitment of several neuroblast lineages and the specification of various neurons (636,637). Mutant *unc-86* neuroblast cells reiterate the lineage of their mother cell rather than differentiating into daughter cells with novel identities, and this leads to the overproduction of certain cell types and the absence of others in the developing nematode. This evidence suggests that the Unc-86 transcription factor exerts its control over cell lineage by altering the pattern of gene expression, and mammalian POU-domain transcription factors are proposed to function similarly. Support for this hypothesis comes from the analysis of *dwarf* mouse mutants (638). Two *dwarf* alleles (*dw* and dw^J) encode disrupted *Pit-1* genes, and in *dwarf* mice three of five successive cell types that are supposed to differentiate in the anterior pituitary gland fail to do so.

In contrast to the CNS-specific POU factors, Oct3/4 was detected only in undifferentiated cells of the early embryo and in undifferentiated ES and embryonal carcinoma (EC) cells (631). After 9.0 days of mouse development, the expression of Oct3/4 became completely restricted to migrating primordial germ cells, and in adults expression continued only in germ cells. Therefore, in contrast to other Oct proteins, Oct3/4 expression correlated with cells that maintain a high degree of pluripotency. Oct3/4 expression is controlled by a retinoic acid repressible element in P19 EC cells, while possible downstream targets include *HoxA5* and *kFGF* (631,639). In conclusion, the analysis of *unc-86* and *dw* mutants supports the hypothesis that the POU-domain class of proteins play a role in specifying neuronal phenotypes and that they have a role in cell proliferation during differentiation events. To date, no transgenics have been constructed to test the role of specific POU-domain transcription factors in developmental processes.

Zinc Finger Genes

Mouse zinc finger genes encode a class of proteins homologous to the *Kruppel, snail,* and *twist* genes in *Drosophila* which bind DNA through the zinc finger motif and act as transcription factors with roles in pattern formation (reviewed in 640). Mouse *Krox-20* is a member of the zinc finger class of transcription factors and its expression pattern in the developing hindbrain provides one of the first molecular indications of hindbrain segmentation (641). The restricted domains of expression of *Krox-20* became apparent starting at 7.75–8.5 d.g., when two stripes of *Krox-20* expressing cells were observed in the hindbrain before the overt morphological appearance of rhombomeres. The expression boundaries of *Krox-20* came to delineate rhombomere (r)3 and r5 after their overt differentiation. Following the formation of rhombomeres, *Krox-20* expression was downregulated, suggesting that it could be part of the mechanism that generates hindbrain segmentation (642).

In the developing hindbrain, the homeobox gene, *HoxB2,* shows a restricted domain of expression in r3 and r5 when it is first expressed similar to that of *Krox-20* (643). For this reason, it was hypothesized that *Krox-20* may play a role in regulating *HoxB2* expression in the hindbrain. DNase footprinting revealed three *Krox-20* binding sites within an enhancer element of *HoxB2,* and Sham et al. (643) demonstrated that the *HoxB2* enhancer imposed r3/r5 expression of a *lacZ* fusion protein in transgenic mice. Sham et al. (643) constructed a second transgenic line in which the expression of *Krox-20* was directed to more posterior rhombomeres bordering on r6/r7 and used this line to examine *Krox-20* control of *HoxB2* expression. When a reporter construct containing the r3/r5 enhancer was integrated in the transgenic line that ectopically expressed *Krox-20, lacZ* expression was observed in r3 and r5, as normal, and expression also was observed in the more posterior r6/r7 domain. Thus, the ectopically expressed *Krox-20* was able to transactivate the reporter gene so that expression was also observed in the more posterior domain. These complex genetic manipulations indicate that *Krox-20* is part of the normal upstream regulatory cascade that governs segmental expression of *HoxB2* in the hindbrain *in vivo* and therefore may play a role in setting up hindbrain segmental identity.

A mouse homolog of the *Drosophila snail* gene, termed *Sna,* encodes a protein containing four zinc fingers (644). This protein was detected in gastrulating embryos throughout the primitive streak and in the entire mesodermal layer. By 10.5 d.g., *Sna* was expressed in most mesenchymal cells whether of neural crest or mesodermal origin. This pattern suggests that the *Sna* protein may play multiple roles in postimplantation development. Other zinc finger genes described in the mouse include *Evi-1* and *Ntfin12* (645,646). *Evi-1* was detected at a number of embryonic sites including the limb buds where expression peaked from 9.5–12.5 d.g. while *Ntfin12* expression was detected only in the neuroectoderm and later CNS and PNS derivatives. To date, no functional genetic analyses of *Sna, Evi-1,* or *Ntfin12* have been reported, and their precise role in mammalian embryogenesis remains to be determined.

Helix-Loop-Helix Genes

The family of basic helix-loop-helix (bHLH or HLH) proteins includes the structurally related proteins Myo-D, myogenin, E12, Myf-5 and Myf-6 (reviewed in 647). Transfection of these bHLH genes into a wide range of cultured cells induced a program of skeletal muscle differentiation indicating that these proteins act as cell-type specific transcription factors that activate muscle-specific genes. Different myogenic HLH genes can substitute for each other in the *in vitro* differentiation assays, and individual myogenic HLH proteins influence their own expression as well as that of other HLH factors in most cell lines; therefore, it has been difficult to ascribe functions to specific members of this family. In the developing mouse embryo, *Myf-5* was detected before any known muscle-specific protein and before other bHLH proteins in the dermamyotome of cranial somites at 8.0 d.g. in the mouse (648). Myogenin was subsequently expressed in early myotomes and then *Mfy-6* mRNA appeared. As Myf-5 levels dropped, Myo-D and other muscle-specific proteins, such as contractile proteins, were detected around 10.5 d.g. in differentiated myotomal cells (649). To assess the role of separate bHLH factors in muscle differentiation in the embryo, *Myf-5* and *Myo-D* were inactivated via homologous recombination in ES cells (650,651). Null mutants at the *Myo-D* locus were viable, fertile, and did not display any skeletal muscle abnormalities. *Myf-5* levels were elevated in postnatal mutant mice suggesting that, in accordance with the cell culture studies, genes inducing skeletal differentiation function redundantly during embryonic development. The appearance of muscle-specific markers was delayed approximately two days in *Myf-5* null mutants, suggesting that the early expression of *Myf-5* may be required for initiating myogenesis *in vivo;* however, these mutants displayed no abnormalities in skeletal muscles, indicating that the myogenic lineage is extremely plastic. Other bHLH family members were expressed at normal levels in *Myf-5*$^{-}$ mice. Null mutations at *Myf-5* were neonatally lethal; mutant mice were unable to breathe owing to the absence of the major distal part of the ribs. These results corroborate the findings when *Myo-D* was targeted, that is, that single members of the bHLH family are dispensable for the development of skeletal muscle, and suggest that *Myf-5* plays an additional role in the formation of lateral sclerotome derivatives such as the ribs.

Another member of this class of transcription factors is the Id protein. This factor contains the HLH structural motif but is missing the basic region adjacent to the HLH domain in Myo-D and other family members (652). Id can specifically associate with other members of the HLH family and when dimerized prevents their binding to DNA, thereby suppressing myogenic differentiation. *In situ* hybridization studies revealed that upon gastrulation, Id was expressed at high levels in almost all regions of the embryo, and that expression declined with further development (653). A human homolog of *Id, Id-2,* was detected in several fetal tissues including the developing nervous system (654). In addition, the retinoic acid-induced differentiation of neuroblastoma cell lines was accompanied by a decrease in *Id-2* mRNA. These results suggest that decreased *Id-2* expression may be required for neuronal and glial differentiation much the same as decreased *Id* expression allows myogenic differentiation. They also suggest that positive bHLH factors are present and play a role in neuronal differentiation. Genes encoding bHLH proteins that are currently known to be expressed in the nervous system include *c-myb, c-myc,* and *N-myc,* and *MASH1* (654–656). The elucidation of the interaction of bHLH proteins in muscle cell differentiation provides a model for the action of these proteins in other tissues and should aid in unraveling the role this family of proteins plays in the differentiation of neuronal and other tissues in the developing embryo.

Retinoic Acid

The teratogenic effects of exogenous retinoic acid (RA) on vertebrate embryos include severe craniofacial abnormalities and defects in limb anatomy and abnormal axial development. Accordingly, current hypotheses suggest that RA plays a role the normal limb development and anteroposterior axial morphogenesis. In the developing limb, when a region termed the *zone of proliferative activity* (ZPA) was transplanted, it induced a mirror image of the digits in the recipient limb bud (reviewed in 657). Further evidence for the role of RA in limb development came with the demonstration that RA-soaked beads, acting as a local source of RA, caused the duplication of normal anteroposterior pattern of digits, thus mimicking ZPA activity (658,659). In addition, in the chick limb bud, a shallow gradient of RA was detected consistent with the hypothesis that RA acts as (or induces) a morphogen that controls anteroposterior patterning in this system. Hensen's node from the chick primitive streak and the floor plate of the rat neural tube also mimicked ZPA activity when transplanted to the developing chick limb (660,661). In summary, RA has become a strong candidate molecule for a vertebrate morphogen, and recent investigations have focused on its role in anteroposterior patterning along the body axis.

A number of RA receptors (RARs) have been characterized in mammals and these receptors are classified into three families: α, β, and γ, all of which are steroid receptorlike transcription factors composed of separate domains for steroid and ligand binding and for DNA binding (reviewed in 657,662). RARs were detected at numerous sites, including a diffuse overall expression of RARα at 7.5–8.0 d.g., stronger expression of RARα in the neural crest at 9.0 d.g., RARβ expression in 7.5- to 8.5-day mesoderm and in proximal mesoderm of the limb bud at 9.0 d.g., and RARγ expression beginning at 8.0 d.g. in the posterior half of the embryo in all germ layers. RARα expression was ubiquitous (though lower in the brain than other RARs) and RARβ and RARγ, in general, appeared to be mutually exclusive in the developing neural tube. Multiple isoforms of each receptor have been characterized. The expression of some isoforms of RARβ were restricted to the CNS, while one isoform of RARγ was restricted to the skin. These complex expression patterns suggest that RARs play multiple roles during development; however, no RAR has yet been specifically targeted by homologous recombination in ES cells to test its role in embryonic development. In addition to the RARs, cellular retinoic acid binding proteins and cellular retinol binding proteins also exist. These proteins have been hypothesized to modify the concentration and distribution of RA in embryonic and adult tissues; however, their role in early embryogenesis remains to be determined. The embryonic expression of these proteins has been reviewed by Maden (663).

The clearest evidence for an affect of RA on anteroposterior patterning was provided by the detailed analysis of skeletal structures in embryos exposed to teratogenic levels of RA in utero (664). Embryos exposed to RA at 6.5 d.g. showed no effect, but embryos exposed at 7.3 days of development displayed severe deformations of the head, nonclosure of the neural tube in the cranial region, in addition to seven specific posterior transformations of vertebrae along the length of the vertebral column. In contrast, embryos exposed at approximately 8.0 d.g. displayed severe malformations in the posterior half of the body and four distinct, exclusively anterior transformations in the posterior half of the vertebral column (Fig. 13). Because segmental identity is proposed to be encoded by *Hox* genes, the expression of several *Hox* genes was examined in the RA-treated embryos. The boundary of *HoxA7* and *HoxC8* shifted to the anterior in treated embryos which correlated in general with the observed morphological posterior transformations in the thoracic regions of these embryos. Thus, the effect of the RA treatment was the same as ectopically expressing a posterior *Hox* gene in a more anterior segment (as discussed earlier). Those studies showed that such ectopic *Hox* gene expression resulted in an anterior segment assuming the identity apparently encoded by the normally more posteriorly expressed *Hox* gene.

Studies on whole embryos have been complemented with those in both human and mouse EC cells (665). No expression of 38 *HOX* genes was observed in undifferentiated NT2/D1 cells, a human EC cell line; however, 24 of these were activated after 1 week of culture in the presence of RA. Specifically, genes positioned in 3′ locations of *HOX* clusters activated. Within the HOX B cluster it was further determined that 3′ genes were induced by 10^{-8} M RA, whereas 10^{-5} M RA was required to activate 5′ genes fully. Additionally, in all HOX clusters, genes responding to RA were sequentially activated by 10^{-5} M RA in a 3′ to 5′ order. Similar results were obtained with mouse EC cells of the F9 line. Finally, *HOX* genes have been identified that are down-regulated in response to RA. It can be concluded from these *in vitro* studies in EC cells that *HOX* genes are differentially activated by RA according to their location within the four clusters, in a time- and concentration-dependent manner (665). Because this pattern correlates with the known expression patterns of *Hox* genes along the anteroposterior axis of humans and mice, it reaffirms the evolutionary conservation of the strict temporal and spatial relationships between the sequence of *Hox* gene expression, transcript location, and chromosomal position. This, in turn, implies that a temporally and spatially localized source of RA could activate *Hox* genes during vertebrate development.

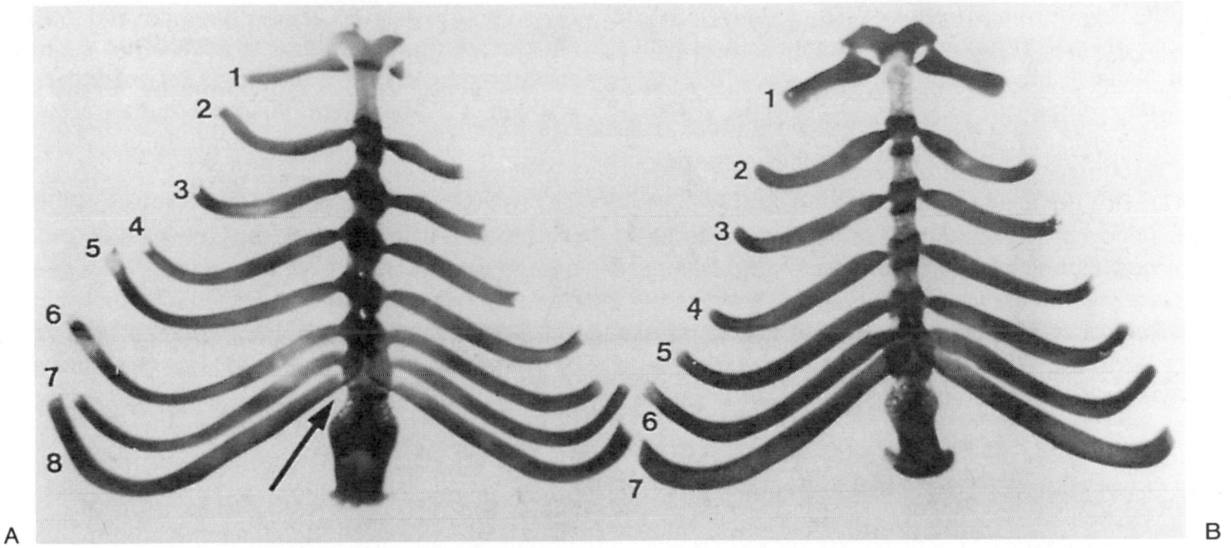

FIG. 13. Anterior transformation of vertebrae after treatment with RA. **A:** Sternum displaying eight ribs from an embryo exposed to retinoic acid. **B:** Sternum from control animal with seven ribs. The vertebral pattern in the retinoic-acid-treated sternum reflects an anterior transformation of the eighth thoracic vertebra (non-rib-bearing) so that it now resembles seventh thoracic (rib-bearing) vertebra. From Kessel and Gruss (664).

Two methodologies have been used to identify RA sources in the embryo: the construction of transgenic animals with reporter constructs sensitive to RA (666–668,901) and further transplantation studies utilizing portions of the developing mouse embryo (669). Hogan et al. (669) determined that 6.5-day egg cylinders could not mimic ZPA activity when transplanted to the developing chick wing bud. But, as development proceeds, the node region (the equivalent of Henson's node of chick embryos) of the primitive streak in headfold or neural-plate stage embryos (0–3 somites) when transplanted produced the highest rate of altered patterns of digits. In addition, the node region was also better at synthesizing RA from its biosynthetic precursor, all transretinol, than other embryonic regions tested. This result suggests an attractive model for activation of *Hox* gene expression. The node of the mammalian primitive streak would provide a source of RA; as mesoderm cells exit through the streak, exposure to RA could first activate transcription of 3′ genes; longer exposures, at higher concentrations (as gastrulation continues) could turn on more 5′ genes (669).

To provide an indication of RA production during normal development, several transgenic lines of mice have been constructed with *lacZ* under the control of the RARβ2 promoter (667,668;892) or under the more specific control of the RA response element (RARE) present in the RARβ gene (666). In these latter animals, *lacZ* expression was not observed until the time of neural plate formation. Expression of *lacZ* defined the posterior domain of RA production in the embryo with expression observed in all three germ layers. The anterior border of transgene expression coincided with the mouse node. The expression boundary of the transgene became more posterior and more restricted during organogenesis and mimicked the reported expression of the RARβ gene. Teratogenic doses of RA resulted in *lacZ* expression across the entire transgenic embryo: the posterior restriction in transgene expression was obliterated.

Because increased RA concentration in treated embryos alters the anteroposterior boundaries of these model RA target genes, these studies support the hypothesis of a role for RA in anteroposterior patterning along the body axis. Another observation that supports the hypothesis is that the anterior boundary of the RA indicator transgene at the headfold stage was found to correspond to the most anterior expression boundary of Hox C genes (670). Treatment of embryos with teratogenic doses of RA also altered portions of Hox C gene expression within the transgene expression domain at the time of exposure. These data support the concept that an RA signaling pathway is involved in specifying boundaries of gene expression along the anteroposterior axis of the embryo. Because the RA target gene is not activated until well after gastrulation and early mesoderm migration, this study does not indicate that RA plays a role in these processes.

If RA plays a role in anteroposterior patterning, target genes that function in embryogenesis and that are induced by RA remain to be identified. A RARE has been identified in one *Hox* gene, and one *Pax* gene (*Pax-3*) was shown to be RA-inducible *in vitro* (671,672). Other genes whose expression may be sensitive to RA *in vivo* have to date been characterized only in EC cell lines. For example, the rate of transcription of *HoxA5* changed in RA-induced EC cells (673) while the expression of two *Oct* genes, *Oct3/4* and *Oct-6*, was repressed with RA-induced differentiation of EC cells. Other genes whose expression changed in RA-treated EC cells include *MK1*, *REX-1* (a zinc-finger gene), and the transcription factor, *AP-2* (657). In conclusion, while significant advances have been achieved through the use of genetic constructs to determine the role of RA in mammalian development, there remains a large gap between the known teratogenic effects of RA, characterization of endogenous sources of RA, and the elucidation of molecular pathways by which RA may control pattern in the mouse embryo.

Induction and Growth

Cytokines: DIA/LIF and Steel Factor

Differentiation inhibiting activity or leukemia inhibitory factor (DIA/LIF) is a cytokine of 45–56 kD that displays pleiotropic effects on cells. Its activities include: (*a*) the induction or suppression of differentiation in different myeloid leukemia cell lines; (*b*) anabolic and catabolic effects on bone; (*c*) the induction of differentiation in neurons *in vitro;* and (*d*) the suppression of differentiation in totipotent ES cells (reviewed in 674–676). DIA/LIF has been cloned in the human, mouse, rat, sheep, and pig (677,678). The DIA/LIF gene is highly conserved (84 percent) between species in coding regions and in a 5′ region that encodes four TATA boxes, two transcriptional start sites, and the minimal region required for promoter function. In addition, analysis of protein sequences revealed that protein similarity ranged from 74 percent between mouse and sheep to 92 percent between rat and mouse. The evolutionary conservation of the coding regions of this gene and of portions of potential cis-acting control elements indicates the importance of the control of DIA/LIF expression and function in mammals.

The discovery that DIA/LIF inhibited the differentiation of ES cells *in vitro* greatly advanced ES cell technology and the generation of transgenics at specific genetic loci by homologous recombination in ES cells. It also spurred the search for sources of DIA/LIF during embryogenesis. During periimplantation stages of development in the uterus, DIA/LIF expression was observed in the uterine endometrial glands on the fourth day of pregnancy (679). Uterine expression coincided with blastocyst formation and always preceded implantation; the same results were observed in pseudopregnant mice and females undergoing delayed implantation, indicating that this expression was under maternal control. When the embryonic expression of DIA/LIF was examined by *in situ* hybridization, it was detected in extraembryonic tissues beginning at 7.5 d.g., and expression continued in extraembryonic tissues of 9.5- through 12.5-day embryos (680). DIA/LIF transcripts were also detected by PCR in preimplantation blastocysts (3.5 d.g.) and in extraembryonic tissues of the 7.5-day egg cylinder by PCR. Rathjen et al. (681) demonstrated that alternative splicing of the DIA/LIF transcript produced two products, LIF D, which encodes a diffusible form of the protein; and LIF M, which encodes a matrix-associated form of the protein. The expression of these two transcripts in the mouse embryo was examined by RNase protection; transcripts of LIF M were detected in embryonic regions of 6.5-day egg cylinders but not in the embryonic regions of 7.5-day egg cylinders (682). In agreement with the previous *in situ* hybridization analysis, LIF M and LIF D were found highly expressed in the extraembryonic regions of 6.5-day embryos and were expressed to a lesser extent in the extraembryonic regions of 7.5-day embryos. The demonstration that DIA/LIF inhibited ES cell differentiation *in vitro* and that DIA/LIF was expressed in the preimplantation embryo and in the embryonic region of the 6.5-day egg cylinder suggests that DIA/LIF may function to regulate stem cells, that is, maintain tissues in an undifferentiated state during development.

The DIA/LIF receptor has been cloned by the expression screening of a human placental library (683). It is an integral membrane protein whose transmembrane and cytoplasmic domains are most closely related to the gp-130 "signal-transducing" subunit of the human interleukin 6 (IL-6) receptor. This structural similarity places the LIF receptor in a family that includes the receptors for growth hormone, IL-2, -3, -4, -5, -6, and -7, granulocyte-macrophage colony stimulating factor (GM-CSF), and erythropoetin receptors (675). The expression pattern of the DIA/LIF receptor in the embryo has yet to be examined.

To determine the function of DIA/LIF during mouse development, Stewart et al. (684) used homologous recombination to mutate DIA/LIF in transgenic animals. Blastocysts produced by these mutants failed to implant and did not develop in homozygous mutant females. Mutant DIA/LIF blastocysts developed normally when transferred to pseudopregnant wild-type recipients, thus, DIA/LIF was shown to be unnecessary for prenatal development or early postnatal life. The failure of these blastocysts to implant in mutant females indicates that the uterine expression of DIA/LIF is essential for implantation; extension and application of these studies in humans may improve the establishment of successful pregnancies produced by *in vitro* fertilization (684).

The *Steel* locus encodes a cytokine important for the survival of a number of cell types (reviewed in 685). Mutants at the *Steel* (*Sl*) locus have defects in PGCs, pigment cells, and hematopoietic cells. Heterozygotes at the *Dominant Spotting* (*W*) locus display a white forehead blaze and areas of depigmentation on the ventral body wall while homozygous mutants at this locus display defects in coat color, PGC development, and hematopoetic development similar to *Sl* mutants. The *W* gene encodes the *c-kit* proto-oncogene, a transmembrane tyrosine kinase receptor, while the *Sl* locus encodes a cytokine given a number of names including the kit ligand, stem cell factor, mast cell factor, and the steel factor (685,686). Like the *DIA/LIF* gene, *Sl* encodes a gene that produces two polypeptides by alternative splicing, a membrane-bound form and a soluble form, and the expression of these forms of the steel factor was regulated in a tissue-specific manner. Another similarity between the steel factor and DIA/LIF is that both stimulated the proliferation of or acted as a survival factor for PGCs *in vitro* (687–691).

The *W* (*c-kit*) gene product and the steel factor were detected in complementary patterns during mouse development (692–694). The *c-kit* receptor protein was found on germ cells and hematopoetic and melanocyte stem cell populations while the steel factor was expressed by cells in the microenvironment of the affected stem cells (685). For example, *c-kit* was first expressed on neural crest cells approximately 12–24 hours after the neural crest emerged from the neural tube and later in presumptive melanoblasts. Eventually these cells were detected in the dermis and epidermis. In contrast, the steel factor was expressed within the dermis through which the melanocytes migrated.

Lastly, individuals affected by the human dominant genetic disorder, piebaldism, display alterations in pigment matching those observed in heterozygous *W* mice. In one individual, piebaldism was shown to result from a defect in the *W* (*c-kit*) gene (695,696). Because of the complementary actions of c-kit and steel factor in the mouse, these results suggest that other individuals with this disorder may have defects in the gene encoding steel factor.

Epidermal Growth Factor and Transforming Growth Factor-α

Epidermal growth factor (EGF) and transforming growth factor-α (TGF-α) are homologous polypeptides that share 35 percent sequence identity and induce growth-promoting responses in a number of cell types (reviewed in 697,698). In addition, these two growth factors bind to the same receptor, the epidermal growth factor receptor (EGFR) and both effect early development in mouse and human embryos (reviewed in 699,700). EGF and TGF-α have also been implicated in the formation of various organs including the tooth, the lung, and the kidney where epithelial-mesenchymal interactions are important for morphogenesis (698).

EGF has been cloned in humans and rodents and TGF-α has been cloned in humans and in the mouse, rat, and hamster (697,698,701–703). TGF-α was expressed in both pre- and postimplantation mouse embryos and in postimplantation rat embryos (699, 702,704–706). Maternal decidua in rats and rat syncytial trophoblast cells have also been reported to express transcripts for TGF-α (707,708). In contrast to the expression of TGF-α in preimplantation stages, EGF transcripts were not detected in preimplantation mouse embryos but were detected by 9 days of development.

Physiological effects of EGF and TGF-α were demonstrated when their addition to embryo cultures stimulated the development of 2-cell stage embryos to blastocysts and increased protein synthesis as measured by the incorporation of ^{35}S-methionine (700,709,710). At the morula-to-blastocyst transition, EGF stimulated protein synthesis but did produce a mitogenic effect (710). In addition, Dardik and Schultz (711) demonstrated that EGF and TGF-α stimulated the rate of blastocyst expansion, suggesting that at this stage of development, the function of the first embryonic epithelium, the trophectoderm, is sensitive to growth factor modulation.

The expression of EGF and TGF-α has been examined in a number of mammalian species (712–714). In cultured pig embryos, embryonic transcripts of TGF-α were expressed earlier than those of EGF which were detectable after the postelongation blastocyst stage of development, suggesting that EGF may also play a role in trophectoderm differentiation in this species (713,714). In bovine embryos, TGF-α was detectable by RT-PCR in all stages of preimplantation development and in agreement with findings in the mouse, EGF was not detectable in the preimplantation bovine embryo (714). Human embryos produced TGF-α, but not EGF, after 5–8 days of culture (712). The production of TGF-α correlated with the morula-to-blastocyst transition in the human embryos, and these results suggest that EGF may play a role in this process in the human.

To assess the role of TGF-α mediated signals in development, transgenic animals which were null at the TGF-α locus were constructed using homologous recombination (715,716). Homozygous null mutants were both viable and fertile. TGF-α null homozygotes displayed eye abnormalities and pronounced waviness of whiskers and fur. Thus, although TGF-α is expressed during preimplantation development it is not absolutely required for successful development. At later stages, when TGF-α and EGF are both expressed, EGF may have compensated for the lack of TGF-α; however, TGF-α does seem to be required for normal eye and follicle development. The phenotype of the TGF-α null homozygotes was similar to that of the mouse mutant *waved-1* (*wa-1*). Upon molecular and genetic examination of these animals it was determined that the *wa-1* phenotype was a mutation in the TGF-α gene. Of interest will be future studies targeting the *EGFR* gene; thereby creating null mice for both EGF and TGF-α trophic effects.

The EGFR has tyrosine kinase activity and undergoes autophosphorylation when transducing a mitogenic signal; this receptor has been cloned in the mouse and human (698,699). Consistent with the ability of early stage mouse embryos to respond to EGF and TGF-α, the EGFR was detected from the 2-cell through the blastocyst stage of development (697,699,706,717). These studies have localized EGFR expression to both the trophectoderm and the ICM in blastocysts. Therefore, an autocrine stimulation by TGF-α in the ICM and a paracrine stimulation of the polar trophectoderm by the ICM are both possible. Because TGF-α mRNAs were detected in the maternal decidua, it is suggested that embryos may also respond to maternal products at this time (708). EGFR has also been localized on human trophoblast cells (718).

In an elegant study, Brice et al. (719) used antibodies, antisense RNAs, and antisense deoxynucleotides to perturb EGFR function. Treatment of embryos with antibodies specific for the EGFR significantly accelerated the onset of cavitation. Antibody binding appeared to mimic ligand-receptor binding and initiate the cascade of responses typically induced by the EGFR's activity. In contrast, treatment of embryos with antisense nucleotides significantly delayed the onset of cavitation, presumably due to interference with EGFR production. Because the onset of cavitation (a late endpoint of trophectoderm differentiation) was scored in these experiments, antibodies and antisense nucleotides presumably interfered with earlier events which lead to cavitation; Brice et al. (719) therefore suggested that EGFR could function in the induction of trophectoderm differentiation.

Paria et al. (720) investigated the intracellular mechanisms by which EGFR transduces ligand binding. In this study, treatment of early embryos with EGF induced a twofold increase in tyrosine kinase activity in 3.5-day blastocysts, and tryphostin (a compound that specifically inhibits EGFR tyrosine kinase activity) diminished the autophosphorylation of the EGFR and abolished tyrosine kinase activity in tryphostin-treated blastocysts. EGF binding was unaffected in the treated embryos and in further experiments, tryphostin inhibited the development of 2-cells to blastocysts. These results suggest that the ligand activated-EGFR tyrosine kinase activity and the ensuing signaling cascade are important for mouse preimplantation development.

The Transforming Growth Factor-β Superfamily

Transforming growth factor-β1, -β2, and -β3 (TGF-β1, -β2, and -β3) are related polypeptides that have been characterized in mammals and that induce a wide variety of responses including: (a) the stimulation of cartilage growth; (b) angiogenesis; (c) the production of ECM proteins, adhesive receptors for ECM proteins, and proteases that degrade the ECM; and (d) cell migration (721). The mature form of TGF-β1 is identical in human, porcine, simian, and bovine cells except for one amino acid in the murine protein (721,722). A number of other proteins and genes including inhibin, activin, Müllerian inhibitory substance, the bone morphogenetic proteins (BMPs), the *decapentaplegic* gene that regulates dorsal-ventral patterning in *Drosophila* embryogenesis, and the *Vg-1* gene product in *Xenopus* embryos are members of the TGF-β superfamily of growth factors (721).

Interest in the role of TGF-β's role in development was heightened when it was demonstrated that mammalian TGF-β1, in conjunction with fibroblast growth factor (FGF) induced the *in vitro* differentiation of mesoderm in isolated tissues of the amphibian embryo (reviewed in 721,723,724). TGF-β2 acting alone was also an inducer of mesodermal tissue in *Xenopus* animal caps in that *in vitro* system. Lastly, the endogenous *Xenopus* protein, XTC-MIF, a potent mesodermal inducer, was determined to be activin. These results have spurred further investigations into the role of TGF-β family members in mesoderm differentiation and developmental processes in general, and in the mammalian embryo (reviewed in 725).

TGF-β1 transcripts were detected from fertilization through the blastocyst stage of development in the mouse embryo by RT-PCR and TGF-β1 protein was also detected by immunocytochemistry in blastocysts (51,705). TGF-β2 transcripts have also been detected by RT-PCR in preimplantation embryos (726). TGF-β2 protein has been detected from the 4-cell stage of development onward, and this expression was regulated as tissues differentiated. In blastocysts, trophectoderm cells expressed TGF-β2 but ICM cells did not (722). In the egg cylinder, both embryonic and extraembryonic visceral endoderm expressed TGF-β2; the embryonic ectoderm did not.

TGF-β expression in postimplantation mouse embryos has been examined by Northern analysis, *in situ* hybridization, and immunocytochemistry (727–735). The expression of TGF-β1, -β2, and -β3 was observed in a variety of tissues and organs, and the three isoforms displayed overlapping but distinct patterns of expression during later mouse development. TGF-β1 is expressed in blood islands of the visceral yolk sac and in hematopoietic precursor cells in the fetal liver. Interestingly, TGF-β1 was prominently expressed in epithelial regions undergoing morphogenic interactions with the underlying mesenchyme; for example, during the formation of the fetal heart, whiskers, and the secondary palate (721,736). In a number of instances where TGF-β1 protein is found in a mesenchyme, TGF-β1 mRNA is expressed in the adjacent epithelium (727,728).

An example of the adjacent expression of TGF-β1 mRNA and protein is provided by the developing fetal heart (731,736). During cardiac cushion formation in the embryonic heart (the morphogenesis of the region that will give rise to the valves and septae), TGF-β1 mRNA was localized to the endothelium overlying the cushion while TGF-β1 protein was localized in the mesenchyme of the cardiac cushion. The role that TGF-β1 may play in tissue remodeling during cushion (and later septae and valve) formation may be mediated by this growth factor's ability to regulate genes encoding ECM proteins, receptors for ECM proteins, and proteases capable of digesting the ECM (reviewed in 721,737).

In the localization studies, TGF-β2 expression correlated with growth and/or the differentiation of embryonic epithelia while TGF-β3 expression was observed in a number of specific tissues including bone, lung, amnion, and tissues of the CNS. The expression of TGF-β3 was also highest during periods of active morphogenesis in these tissues. TGF-β3 expression in the spinal cord became restricted to the intervertebral mesenchyme as it condensed to form the intervertebral discs. Interestingly, *Pax-1* shows the same expression pattern and while this coexpression does not establish a causal relationship, it suggests that the *TGF-β3* and *Pax*-1 genes may interact during formation of the vertebral column (732).

In human embryos, the distribution of TGF-β1, -β2, and -β3 was found to be broadly similar to that seen in mouse (738). For example, TGF-β1 was detected in human hematopoietic precursors and cardiac valve endothelia; the expression of TGF-β2 and -β3 was observed the developing human lung. In other mammals, TGF-β (and FGF) promoted the development of bovine embryos through the normally observed 8-cell block, and TGF-β2 was detected as a maternal transcript and throughout subsequent preimplantation development in bovine embryos (714,739).

In an attempt to delineate specific developmental roles of TGF-β1, this gene was disrupted by homologous recombination and transgenic mice null at this locus were generated (740,741). Considerable interuterine lethality was observed during these two studies, with only one-half to one-third of the expected number of homozygotes detected in litters produced from matings of TGF-$\beta 1^-$ heterozygotes. The remaining homozygotes died within approximately 3 weeks of birth and displayed an acute wasting syndrome and inflammation in a number of organs including the heart, lung, and stomach. No analysis of the embryonic lethality of the TGF-β1 null mutation was attempted in either study; therefore, the necessity of TGF-β1 in embryonic development remains uncharacterized.

The *nodal* gene, a novel member of the TGF-β superfamily has recently been described (742). *Nodal* mutant embryos failed during gastrulation when the embryonic epithelium overproliferated and then degenerated rather than giving rise to mesoderm. Transcripts of *nodal* were detected in prestreak and very early streak embryos by RT-PCR. By *in situ* hybridization, nodal transcripts were detected in a ring around the node of the primitive streak just as the node formed. This localization persisted to the headfold stage when transcripts were no longer detected concurrent with the disappearance of the node as a distinct structure. Zhou et al. (742) hypothesized that the *nodal* gene encodes a signaling molecule essential for mesoderm formation and subsequent development in the mouse.

The final group of TGF-β related proteins that will be discussed here is the inhibins and activins. Inhibins and activins are produced by the gonads and were first identified by their ability to regulate the release of follicle-stimulating hormone (FSH) from the pituitary (reviewed in 743). Inhibin is a heterodimer composed of an α and one of two β subunits, βA or βB. Activins are dimers of β subunits of which the βA/βB heterodimer (activin AB) and the βA/βA homodimer (activin A) have been best characterized, although a βB/βB homodimer (activin B) may also have biological activity. The discovery of *Xenopus* activin's *in vitro* ability to induce dorsal mesoderm in amphibian animal cap assays has led researchers to ask if mammalian activin might play the same role in the mouse. Indeed, a factor purified from the WEH3-3 mammalian cell line, activin A, functioned as a mesoderm inducer in the *Xenopus* system, indicating that certain pathways of induction are conserved evolutionarily between the two species (744).

The expression of the inhibin α and β subunits in mouse embryos was examined by RT-PCR and immunocytochemistry, and subunit expression was developmentally regulated during mouse embryogenesis (735, 745,746). The α, βA, and βB subunits were all detectable as maternal transcripts (746). Reports conflict on the presence or absence of α subunit mRNA in blastocysts, while the expression of βA subunit mRNA was consistently absent in blastocysts (745,746). In contrast, βB subunit transcripts were consistently detected in blastocysts and by immunocytochemistry β chain protein was detected specifically in the trophectoderm in 3.5-day on the presence or absence of α subunit mRNA in blastocysts, while the expression of βA subunit mRNA was consistently absent in blastocysts (745,746). In contrast, βB subunit transcripts were consistently detected in blastocysts and by immunocytochemistry β chain protein was detected specifically in the trophectoderm in 3.5-day blastocysts. By 4.5 d.g. the expression of the β subunit protein switched from the trophectoderm to the ICM (746). In 7.5- to 10.5-day embryos, βB transcripts were reduced, and βA subunit transcripts were now prominently expressed (745). Thus, activin subunits were sequentially expressed during mouse development with βA expression beginning after implantation at the time βB expression was reduced. In contrast to the changes observed in inhibin subunit expression, the transcripts for the activin receptor type II were present through all developmental stages. Thus, activins appear developmentally regulated during mouse development and transcripts for the βA subunit are present during primitive streak mesoderm differentiation and migration. The localization of activin proteins in postimplantation embryos remains to be determined; to date, no effect of activins on mesoderm differentiation in mammals has been demonstrated.

The *decapentaplegic-Vg*-related (*DVR*) proteins include the mammalian *Vgr-1* gene which is related to the *Xenopus Vg-1* gene (747), and the BMPs have been implicated in developmental processes in the mouse. These proteins have been reviewed by Lyons et al. (748), Wozney (749) and Rosen and Thies (750) and will not be discussed further.

The Fibroblast Growth Factor Family

Presently, seven distinct *fibroblast growth factor* genes (*FGF1-7*) (751) have been characterized in mammals and this family of growth factors is known to influence the proliferative and differentiative process in a number of cell types, mostly of mesodermal or neuroectodermal origin (reviewed in 752,753). *In vitro,* the activity of both FGF-1 (aFGF) and FGF-2 (bFGF) can be positively or negatively regulated by TGF-β depending on the cell type, suggesting that such interactions may also be important *in vivo.* Of the seven *FGF* gene products, four induce mesoderm in *Xenopus* animal caps and in contrast to the TGF-β-related activin, FGFs specifically induce posterior and ventral mesoderm. Searching for parallels in the mammalian embryo, the expression of members of the FGF family have been extensively characterized in peri- and postimplantation mouse embryos (755–761).

FGF-1 and FGF-2 are closely related polypeptides that share 55 percent homology (753). FGF-2 is highly conserved with bovine and human peptides, sharing 98.7 percent overall amino acid sequence identity, while FGF-1 is somewhat less conserved. The expression of these two FGF family members was examined in rat embryos and they displayed similar patterns of expression with both polypeptides expressed in cells of the CNS (neuroectodermal origin) and in most cells of mesodermal origin (756,757). Neither protein was expressed in endoderm-derived cells (757).

Fu et al. (757) examined FGF protein expression at a stage of rat embryonic development beyond the point where FGF might play a role in mesoderm induction or differentiation; however, in the mouse, genes encoding a number of FGF family members have been cloned (759) and the expression of these FGF family members before and during gastrulation has been examined by *in situ* hybridization (754,755,758,760,761).

By *in situ* hybridization, FGF-5 transcripts were present at a uniformly high level throughout the embryonic ectoderm in 5.0- to 7.5-day embryos (758,760). In contrast to the embryonic ectoderm, little to no *FGF-5* expression was detected in primitive streak mesoderm. The visceral endoderm in embryonic regions also expressed *FGF-5* but a sharp boundary of expression was observed with no extraembryonic tissue (extraembryonic ectoderm nor extraembryonic visceral endoderm) expressing this transcript. At later stages in the head process the splanchnic and lateral somatic mesoderm expressed FGF-5 mRNA (758,760).

FGF-3 (*int-2*) shows a strikingly different pattern of expression compared to *FGF-5* (754,755). Parietal but not visceral endoderm cells expressed *FGF-3,* and in embryonic regions of the egg cylinder only the newly forming mesodermal tissue expressed *FGF-3* (754). At 8.5 d.g. regions of the neuroepithelium adjacent to the developing otocyst prominently expressed transcripts of *FGF-3* and its later expression in sensory epithelia of the inner ear suggests *FGF-3* may play a role in development of the inner ear. The localization of FGF-3 mRNAs to the primitive streak mesoderm and parietal endoderm correlates with the migratory behavior of these cells and suggests expression of the *FGF-3* gene may be important for this phenotype.

The pattern of expression of *FGF-4* was overlapping but distinct from *FGF-5* and *FGF-3* (761). *FGF-4* was detected in the ICM of the late blastocyst and in the embryonic ectoderm through gastrulation, when *FGF-4* expression became restricted to the primitive streak region of the embryo. Both embryonic ectoderm and primitive streak mesoderm in the region of the primitive streak expressed *FGF-4.* As gastrulation continued and the streak elongated, *FGF-4* expression became restricted to the distal two-thirds of the streak. *FGF-4* was also transiently detected in branchial arches, the somitic myotome, the apical ectodermal ridge, and the tooth bud.

FGF-6 mRNA levels were also developmentally regulated in the mouse embryo (762). Peak expression was observed at 15.5 days of development with continued *FGF-6* expression detected in the adult testis, heart, and skeletal muscle.

What roles for the various FGF family members can be hypothesized from these data? Based on the expression of *FGF-4* in the pluripotent embryonic ectoderm until just prior to gastrulation and the expression of *FGF-5* in the embryonic ectoderm and loss of expression in differentiating mesoderm, it seems they may play a role in the maintenance of the undifferentiated state in the embryonic ectoderm. The restricted expression of *FGF-4* to tissues just entering or within the primitive streak and of *FGF-3* to mesoderm exiting the streak suggests that the sequential expression of these two genes may progressively influence mesoderm differentiation during mouse gastrulation (761). While these descriptive studies have localized mRNAs and not the secreted FGF proteins, it is possible that these factors act locally due to interactions with cell surface and ECM proteins (reviewed in 753,763). In addition, the restriction of *FGF-4* expression to the rostral two-thirds of the primitive streak in cells fated to form axial, paraxial, or lateral (but not extraembryonic) mesoderm suggests that it may play a role in mesoderm specification during gastrulation.

The expression pattern of *FGF-4* in mesoderm at the midstreak stage contrasts with that of syndecan-1 which is expressed in posterior (proximal) and lateral mesoderm (764). As discussed in a later section, syndecan-1 binds FGF-2 (bFGF) and modulates its activity; it is intriguing to suppose that syndecan-1 may also modulate the activity of secreted FGF-4 within the primitive streak mesoderm. The role of FGF family members in mesoderm induction in the mouse can be tested by eliminating specific FGF gene expression although the overlap in expression of these molecules may cloud interpretation.

In experiments in amphibian embryos, dominant negative mutation of the FGF receptor (FGFR-1) disrupted gastrulation and mesoderm formation (765) implicating this signaling pathway in the process of mesoderm induction. In the human and the mouse, four FGFRs have been identified and these receptors are highly homologous receptor tyrosine kinases (reviewed in 766,767). The expression of *FGFR-1* (the *flg* gene) has been examined and its pattern of expression correlates with mesoderm formation in the developing mouse embryo (766,768). The highest levels of FGFR-1 transcripts were detected in mesoderm adjacent to the primitive streak and by the late streak stage, expression was detected throughout the embryonic ectoderm and mesoderm. With further development, ectodermal expression of *FGFR-1* became restricted to the neuroectoderm and mesodermal expression became concentrated in the paraxial mesoderm and eventually in the rostral half of newly formed somites. These results suggest that *FGFR-1* may play a role in formation of the neuroectoderm and in specification of mesoderm within compartments in developing somites.

By *in situ* hybridization, *FGFR-2* was expressed predominantly in epithelia, in a pattern that overlaps that of *FGFR-1,* and *FGFR-3* (the *bek* gene product) was expressed in the neuroepithelium and the developing CNS (767,769,770). In contrast to *FGFR-1* which was not expressed in endodermal derivatives, *FGFR-4* expression was detected in the definitive endoderm of the embryonic gut and the extraembryonic endoderm of the yolk sac in 8.5- to 9.5-day embryos (771). FGFR-4 transcripts were also detected in the myotome of somites and later in skeletal muscle.

Currently *FGFR-1* is the best candidate for mediating FGF signaling during mesoderm differentiation. Complicating this interpretation was the observation that two forms of alternatively spliced FGFR-1 mRNA exist in mouse and humans (768,772) and that the probe used by Yamaguchi et al. (766) did not distinguish between the two. In addition, the two FGFR-1 isoforms in mouse and human display multiple and overlapping ligand specificities (772,775). A detailed analysis of the expression of FGF proteins, rather than transcripts, in specific embryonic tissues is necessary and may aid in unraveling the role of FGFR-mediated signaling during gastrulation in the mouse (766).

Platelet-Derived Growth Factor

Platelet-derived growth factor (PDGF) is a dimer composed of two closely related polypeptides, PDGFA and PDGFB (reviewed in 776). PDGFA and B are encoded by separate genes and in humans, with the A and B subunits sharing 56 percent amino acid identity. PDGF exists as an AA or BB homodimer or as an AB heterodimer. In general, PDGFs stimulate proliferation in a number of cultured cells and have been hypothesized to play a role in wound healing, atherosclerosis, and neoplastic transformation. The receptor for PDGF is also dimeric, existing as an α/α homodimer (PDGFRα), a β/β homodimer (PDGFβ), or an α/β heterodimer (PDGF$\alpha\beta$). Receptors containing the α subunit can bind PDGFA and B while the PDGFβ receptor can bind only PDGFB.

Transcripts for PDGFA, B and the PDGFRs have been characterized in the mouse embryo and may also play several roles during mammalian development (776). Transcripts of *PDGFA* were detected as maternal message and as zygotic transcripts from the 8-cell stage embryo through the blastocyst stage (51). *In situ* hybridization analyses demonstrated that all cells in the preimplantation embryo expressed transcripts of PDGFA and PDGFRα, and immunocytochemistry demonstrated that PDGFA protein was also present in all cells of blastocysts (51,777).

Mercola and coworkers cloned the mouse homologs of PDGFA, B, and the PDGFRα subunit and examined their expression in postimplantation embryos by RNAse protection, *in situ* hybridization, and immunohistochemistry (777,778). Prior to implantation *PDGFA* and *PDGFRα* were coexpressed, but after implantation, *PDGFA* and *PDGFRα* were no longer expressed in the same tissues. The embryonic ectoderm of the 7.5-day embryo prominently expressed transcripts of *PGDFA* whereas the mesoderm prominently expressed *PDGFRα* (777,779–781). PDGFA and PDGFRα transcripts were also observed in the visceral endoderm (780–782). Tyrosine kinase assays demonstrated that in both pre- and postimplantation embryos the PDGFRs were functional (777). By 8.0 d.g., the mesodermal expression of *PDGFRα* was observed in loose mesenchyme, developing somites, and neural crest-derived mesenchyme while *PDGFA* was observed in the surface ectoderm (777,779,780). Thus the embryonic ectoderm appears to produce PDGFA, while the primitive streak mesoderm expresses the PDGFRα, and this interaction may promote proliferation of mesoderm or even guide mesoderm migration during gastrulation similar to the effects observed during inflammation and wound healing (777). The expression *PDGFRα* then continues in mesodermal derivatives throughout organogenesis. Morrison-Graham et al. (782) also detected PDGFRα transcripts in nonneuronal derivatives of the neural crest in various organs including the thymus and the heart.

The necessity of a PDGFRα-mediated interaction in development was shown when the *Patch* (*Ph*) mutation was mapped to chromosome 5, next to the *W* (*c-kit*) gene, and was shown to be a deletion that includes the *PDGFRα* gene (783). *Ph* homozygous mutants die prenatally and display growth deficiencies in many mesodermally-derived structures, including the schlerotome of the 9.5-day embryo and connective tissues arising later in development. In addition, *Ph* homozygotes display abnormal development of craniofacial structures and organs to which neural crest mesenchyme contribute. These abnormal structures include a reduced thymus, a reduced thyroid, and incomplete septation of the outflow tract of the heart (776,781,782). The pattern of defects observed in *Patch* mutants is consistent with the expression of *PDGFRα* in normal embryos. Therefore, PDGFRα does not seem necessary for the formation of the mesoderm at the primitive streak but may act as a proliferation or survival factor that is necessary for subsequent normal development. The *Patch* deletion includes, but extends beyond, the *PDGFRα* gene; however, the expression of *W* or *c-kit,* the nearest gene for which probes are available, is normal in *Patch* mutants (776). Therefore, the phenotype observed in *Patch* mutants is probably the result of the deletion of the *PDGFRα* gene, but defects caused by the combined deletion of the *PDGFRα* and an uncharacterized adjacent gene cannot be ruled out (776). Lastly, the defects seen in *Patch* mutants are phenotypically similar to Waardenburg syndromes II and III in humans (reviewed in 784).

Other Selected Proto-Oncogenes

The transcription of the proto-oncogene, c-*fos,* is a component of the transcription complex termed *activating complex*-1 (AP-1), and is a member of the family of early response genes whose own transcription increases rapidly in response to growth factors (reviewed in 785–787). Expression of c-*fos* was low in embryonic tissues and high in extraembryonic tissues of mouse, human, and pig embryos (787,790–792). In RT-PCR assays, Neilsen et al. (793) demonstrated that TGF-α, EGF, human PDGF, recombinant PDGFAA homodimer, and FGF-2 (bFGF) induced the expression of c-*fos* mRNA in 7.5 mouse embryos. Thus, the induction of c-*fos* transcription indicated that the receptors for these ligands were functional at this stage of development. In contrast, PDGFRβ was not determined to be functional in 7.5-day embryos in these assays because PDGFBB did not induce increased transcription of c-*fos.*

The role of c-*fos* in the developing mouse embryo was also tested in transgenic mice that overexpress c-*fos* and in transgenic animals null at this locus (794,795). Both types of transgenic animal displayed bone and hematopoietic abnormalities including osteopetrosis in the c-*fos* null mutants.

The *myc* family of proto-oncogenes are proposed to play roles in cellular differentiation and proliferation (796). By *in situ* hybridization, N-*myc* expression was observed in the primitive streak and the embryonic mesoderm of postimplantation embryos (797). During and after organogenesis, N-*myc* was expressed in a number of tissues that include the epithelia of the CNS, structures of neural crest origin, the myocardium of the cardiac ventricles, lung, kidney, and gut (798). The N-*myc* gene has been targeted by homologous recombination, and transgenic mice null at this locus have been generated (799–801). N-*myc* null homozygotes displayed growth retardation and died between 10.5 and 12.5 d.g., displaying multiple defects in tissues and organs that normally express N-*myc.* Affected organs included the cranial and spinal ganglia which were reduced in size, lung, gut, and mutant hearts which failed to undergo normal morphogenesis. These studies demonstrate that N-*myc* plays a number of essential roles during mouse embryogenesis. An additional transgenic line was generated in which mutant and normal transcripts of N-*myc* were produced (800). These homozygous mutants died at birth and displayed a marked underdevelopment of the lung airway epithelium which resulted in insufficient oxygenation of their blood. This defect again correlated with a normal site of N-*myc* expression and these results suggest that N-*myc* is required for the proliferation of lung epithelium.

Wnt-1 was first characterized in mammary tumors and has since been identified as the mammalian homolog of the *Drosophila wingless* gene (reviewed in 802). The *Wnt-1* gene encodes a secreted glycoprotein that is proposed to function in intercellular signaling. In the developing mouse embryo, *Wnt-1* expression was localized to a circular band of cells just anterior to the mid-hindbrain junction and to dorsal regions of the diencephalon, mesencephalon, and spinal cord. Transgenic mice that lack *Wnt-1* have been generated by homologous recombination (803,804). The most severe phenotype of *Wnt-1* null homozygotes was neonatal death in embryos that were missing a substantial portion of the midbrain and cerebellum (Fig. 14). A viable adult mouse was also obtained that displayed more limited midbrain and anterior cerebellar deficiencies. The phenotype of these mice resembled that of the naturally occurring mutant, *swaying* (*sw*). Thomas et al. (805) demonstrated that the deletion of a single base pair from the *Wnt-1* proto-oncogene occurred in *Sw* mutants. Thus, *Wnt-1* expression is necessary for the early regional development of the midbrain and cerebellum. Development of other *Wnt-1* expression domains such as in the spinal cord were not affected in the *Wnt-1* null mutants; a possible explanation is that functional redundancy between Wnt family members may compensate for the lack of *Wnt-1* expression in these areas (802).

Finally, a transgenic line that ectopically expresses *Wnt-1* displayed congenital limb malformations (806).

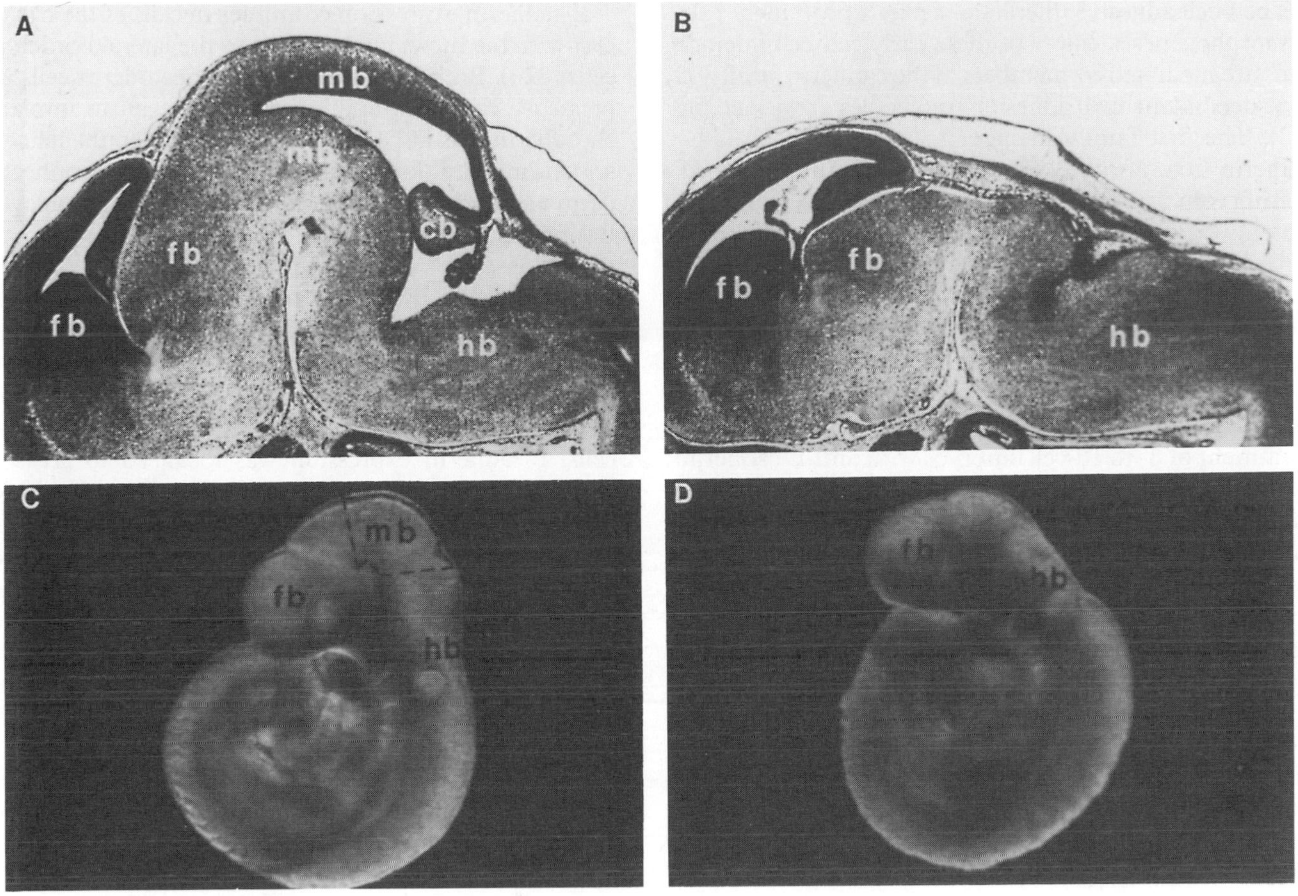

FIG. 14. Phenotype of mice homozygous for a disrupted *wnt-1* allele. Sagittal sections (*top*) through-14.5-day fetuses heterozygous (**A**) and homozygous (**B**) for the mutated *wnt-1* allele. Both the midbrain region and cerebellum are missing in the homozygous mouse, whereas forebrain and hindbrain appear normal. Whole embryo view (*bottom*) of 9.5-day embryos heterozygous (**C**) and homozygous (**D**) for the disrupted *wnt-1* allele. The midbrain region boxed in (C) is missing in the homozygous embryos. Other areas appear normal. mb, midbrain region; cb, cerebellum; fb, forebrain; hb, hindbrain. From McMahon and Bradley (803).

Although *Wnt-1* is not normally expressed in the limb bud, other Wnt family members are expressed there (807). The interaction of the ectopically expressed *Wnt-1* with endogenous Wnt receptor molecules was presumed to produce the aberrant phenotype in these transgenics.

Cell Adhesion and Migration

Both cell-cell and cell-extracellular matrix (ECM) interactions play vital roles in mammalian embryonic development and both have been investigated in extensive *in vitro* studies detailed below. Adhesive interactions during mammalian embryogenesis, implantation, and placentation have been recently reviewed by Damsky et al. (808).

Cell-Cell Adhesion

The event that triggers all mammalian developmental processes is the adhesion and subsequent fusion of two dissimilar cells, the sperm and egg, during fertilization. The mammalian oocyte is surrounded by the zona pellucida at the time of fertilization and the role of the ZP3, a zona glycoprotein, in sperm attachment to the zona pellucida has been described (reviewed in 809). Recently, PH-30, a molecule that may mediate the membrane interactions of the sperm and oocyte has been characterized (810,811). PH-30 is a sperm surface membrane protein composed of two integral membrane glycoprotein subunits, the a subunit containing a putative fusion protein typical of viral fusion proteins, and the b subunit containing a domain related to disintegrins, the family of soluble integrin-binding peptides first described from snake venom. The PH-30 molecule is therefore proposed to bind to an integrin on the oocyte membrane. Integrins have been localized to the surface of the oocyte (812,902), although the oocyte receptor for PH-30 remains as yet unknown (811). Further integrin-mediated interactions during mouse development will be discussed in a later section.

As mouse development proceeds through early cleavage, cell-cell adhesive interactions play a prominent role in morphogenesis. Many of these early cell-cell interactions are mediated by members of the cadherin family of Ca^{2+}-dependent cell adhesion molecules (reviewed in 813). The first family member to be synthesized is E-cadherin (uvomorulin) which is prominently expressed in embryonic and adult epithelia (813–816). E-cadherin protein was detected at the 1- to 2-cell stage of development with zygotic transcription of the molecule commencing at the 2-cell stage coincident with the activation of the embryonic genome (817,818). E-cadherin was distributed uniformly over the surface of blastomeres until compaction (8-cell stage), when its expression became restricted to cell membranes between adjacent cells. Treatment of 8- to 16-cell embryos with anti-E-cadherin antibodies blocked compaction and prevented subsequent embryogenesis, thus demonstrating the indispensable role of E-cadherin in this early morphogenetic process (814–816). This antibody-induced inhibition was reversible and embryos compacted and developed normally upon removal of the anti-E-cadherin antibodies.

In addition to the morphological changes during compaction, other physiological changes have been shown to accompany compaction, including changes in the pattern of phosphorylated proteins examined by two-dimensional gel electrophoresis (819). Several unique phosphoproteins were detectable only in compacting embryos, suggesting that specific metabolic pathways were functioning during compaction. Furthermore, E-cadherin present at the 4-cell stage and 8-cell stage could be distinguished by its phosphorylation status (820). Little phosphorylated E-cadherin was detectable by immunoprecipitation from early and late 4-cell embryos. In contrast, significant levels of phosphorylated E-cadherin were detected at the 8-cell stage just prior to compaction.

The ability of E-cadherin to mediate cell adhesion is dependent on a functional cytoplasmic domain, the location of the phosphorylation sites; therefore, changes in phosphorylation on E-cadherin could be a potent modulator of E-cadherin function during development. Treatment of 4- to 8-cell embryos with agents that activate protein kinase C (such as phorbol ester) had dramatic effects on compaction: Low concentrations induced premature compaction and caused a redistribution of E-cadherin to cell borders, as was observed in untreated, normally compacting embryos (821,822). These data suggest that protein kinase C plays a role in the initiation of compaction either directly through its effect on E-cadherin or indirectly through its effect on cytoskeletal elements associated with E-cadherin during the process of compaction (822). While E-cadherin and protein kinase C have been implicated in the initiation of compaction, β-1,4 galactosyltransferase has been implicated in maintaining the compacted state at the late morula stage (823).

E-cadherin expression continues in cells of the blastocyst with the molecule localized to the lateral borders of cells (824). Both ICM cells and trophectoderm cells expressed E-cadherin, and as embryos began to implant, E-cadherin was also detected on uterine epithelial cells and at implantation sites between the mural trophectoderm and uterine epithelium (824,825). In human cytotrophoblast cells, E-cadherin expression was high as cytotrophoblast cells aggregated, and it was lost with the fusion of cells during their differentiation into syncytial trophoblasts (826). P-cadherin, a cadherin first identified in mice placenta, was expressed on mural trophectoderm cells and on uterine decidual cells on day 5 of pregnancy (825). After degeneration of uterine epithelial cells, P-cadherin expression was localized to areas of contact between trophoblast giant cells and uterine decidual cells, thus suggesting that P-cadherin plays a role in the connection of embryonal tissues to maternal decidual cells. The human analogue of P-cadherin has been cloned and found to share 87 percent homology with mouse P-cadherin; however, P-cadherin does not seem to play a role in cell-cell binding in human placenta because both cytotrophoblast cells and maternal decidual cells express E-cadherin rather than P-cadherin (827).

E-cadherin has also been shown to play a role in the formation of the primitive endoderm at 3.5 d.g. (828). Isolated ICMs failed to develop an outer endodermal layer upon *in vitro* culture in the presence of antibodies against E-cadherin. These data imply that E-cadherin-mediated cell contacts are necessary for the segregation of the primitive endoderm from the ICM during normal development.

Through 6.5 d.g., E-cadherin expression remains strong in the embryonic ectoderm (epiblast) and in the visceral endoderm (hypoblast) (824). Perhaps the most important morphogenetic movements of cells during embryonic development occur next during gastrulation when the future body plan of the embryo is laid down. At approximately 7.0 d.g., cells in the posterior epiblast lose cell-cell contacts, ingress, and form the primitive streak. In contrast to the embryonic ectoderm, mesoderm cells, which have passed through the streak, did not express E-cadherin. Burdsal et al. (829) demonstrated that treatment of explants of embryonic ectoderm *in vitro* with function-perturbing antibodies against E-cadherin caused cells within the explant to lose cell-to-cell contacts, to assume a mesenchymal morphology, and to migrate on a fibronectin substratum (Fig. 15). In addition to the morphological changes, cells in anti-E-cadherin-treated epiblast explants began to express vimentin, an intermediate filament protein characteristic of mesoderm at this stage of development, and ceased to express SSEA-1 and E-cadherin itself, two markers characteristic of the embryonic ectoderm (824,830). These data suggest that loss of E-cadherin-mediated cell contacts in cells of the posterior embryonic ectoderm *in vitro* is sufficient to induce a phenotypic change that is characteristic of mesoderm differentiation at the primitive streak in the intact embryo.

Cell-Substratum Adhesion

Cell-substratum interactions during mouse development have been examined in a number of *in vitro* systems. For example, the outgrowth of trophectoderm cells from blastocysts cultured on various ECM components *in vitro* has provided a model system for implantation (831). At 10–15 hours after embryos hatch from the zonae pellucidae, blastocysts become adhesive, attach, and spread on fibronectin, laminin (and the E8 proteolytic fragment of laminin), and various collagens *in vitro* (832–835). Attachment to these proteins was blocked by the addition of function-perturbing antibodies (anti-extracellular matrix receptor, anti-ECMR antibodies) which recognize the $\beta 1$ and $\beta 3$ subfamilies of integrins, the superfamily of receptors known to mediate interactions with ECM glycoproteins, suggesting that integrin expression is important for outgrowth *in vitro* and implantation *in vivo* (834,836).

To determine whether changes in integrin expression might play a role during implantation, Sutherland et al. (893) examined the expression of integrins in periimplantation embryos by RT-PCR and immunoprecipitation. A set of receptors including those for fibronectin ($\alpha 5\beta 1$), laminin ($\alpha 6\beta 1$), and vitronectin ($\alpha v\beta 3$) were expressed continuously throughout early development. In contrast, three receptors, $\alpha 2$, $\alpha 6$A, and $\alpha 7$, (subunits of receptors capable of binding laminin and collagen) were first expressed coincident with endoderm differentiation and development of attachment competence in blastocysts. By 7.5 d.g.; $\alpha 2$, $\alpha 6$A, and $\alpha 7$ were detected only in the ectoplacental cone (the differentiating trophoblast) which is the region of the embryo that interacts with the maternal decidua, suggesting that these receptors may play specific roles in trophoblast adhesion. Trophoblast cells adhered to the E8 proteolytic fragment of laminin and studies using function-perturbing antibodies demonstrated that anti-$\alpha 6\beta 1$ antibodies did not block this interaction, suggesting that other laminin receptors mediate trophoblast interactions with the laminin in the maternal decidua (893).

Farach et al. (837) have reported that soluble heparin also inhibited blastocyst attachment and trophectoderm outgrowth on both fibronectin and laminin. These results demonstrate that multiple interactions occur during trophoblast attachment and outgrowth and that both

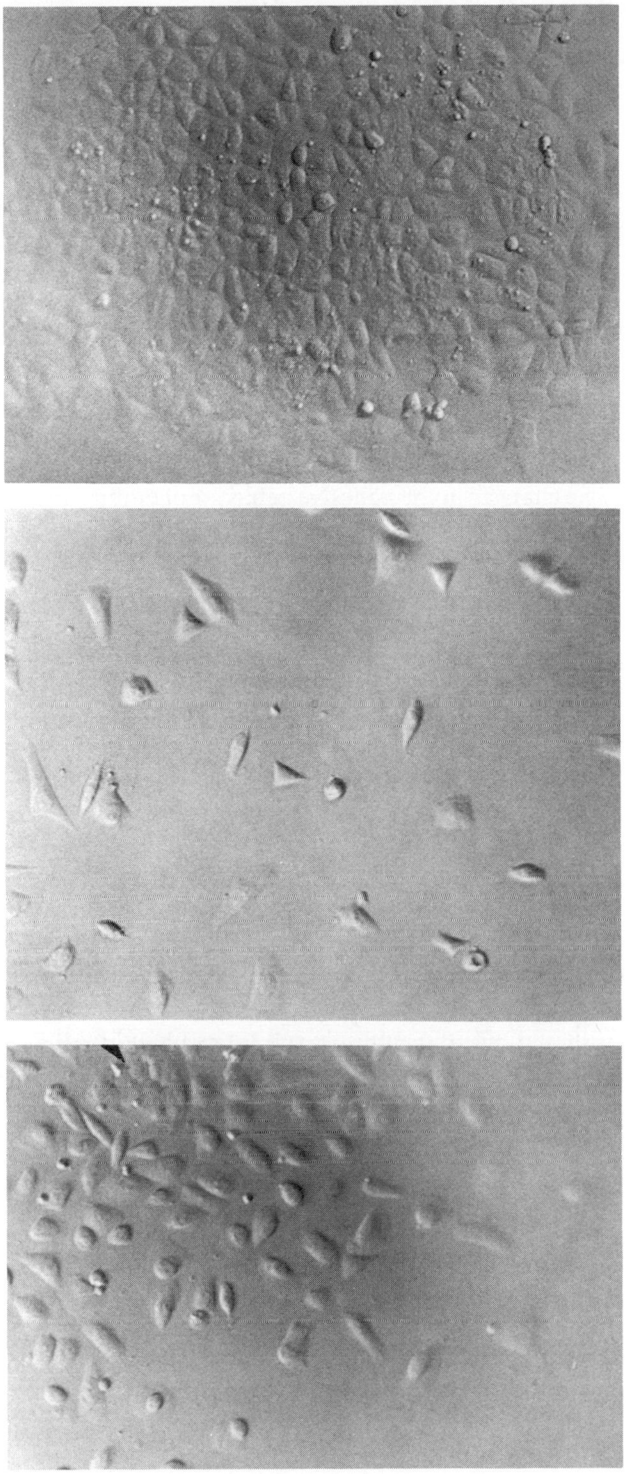

A

B

C

FIG. 15. Effect of function-perturbing anti-E-cadherin antibodies on explants of embryonic ectoderm (epiblast) from the primitive streak of the 7.5-day mouse embryo. **A:** Control epiblast explant: cells display the typical morphology of epithelial cells in culture; no cells have migrated away from the explant, which maintains a coherent border. **B:** Primitive streak mesoderm explant: cells display a fibroblastic morphology and have migrated away from the center of the explant and from each other. **C:** Anti-E-cadherin-treated epiblast explant: cells have undergone a mesenchymal transition, are more elongated and flattened compared to the control epiblast explant, and have migrated away from the explant, just as in mesoderm explants. Original center of the explant is shown (*arrowhead*). Altered from Burdsal et al. (829).

non-integrin-mediated and integrin-mediated events may play a role in both the attachment of blastocysts and in the establishment of the placenta during implantation.

During the invasion process trophoblast cells penetrate the uterine epithelium and then invade the uterine decidual stroma; in human embryos the expression of $\beta 1$ integrin, laminin, and the 72 kD type IV collagenase correlated with the timing of implantation, and this stage of development in the mouse was accompanied by the increased accumulation of transcripts for the metalloproteinases, stromelysin and collagenase (838,839; reviewed in 840). Glass et al. (831) and Behrendtsen et al. (841) have examined the role of metalloproteinases in mouse blastocyst outgrowths and demonstrated that trophoblast cells locally degraded the matrix upon which they were plated and that numerous proteinases, including type IV collagenase (92 kD M_r), were secreted into the culture medium. In addition, tissue inhibitor of metalloproteinases (TIMP) inhibited the proteinase activity secreted by blastocyst outgrowths, indicating that these were metalloproteinases. Addition of TIMP or of a blocking antibody to the 92 kD gelatinase abolished matrix degradation by the trophoblast cells. The invasion of early gestation human cytotrophoblast cells was also blocked by addition of function-perturbing antibodies against the 92 kD collagenase (842). The *Timp-1* gene has been disrupted via homologous recombination in ES cells, and when these cells were induced to differentiate by RA, they were more invasive than their undifferentiated counterparts (843). Work is in progress to use these cells to generate null mutant mice at this locus (C. A. Alexander and Z. Werb, 1993, *personal communication*). These results indicate that attachment to and degradation of the ECM both play an important role during the implantation of the mouse and human embryo (reviewed in 844).

Parietal endoderm cells migrate onto the trophoblast at the late blastocyst stage of development where they secrete Reichert's membrane and where they will later form the parietal yolk sac. Following 5.0–7.0 days of blastocyst outgrowth *in vitro,* parietal endodermlike cells migrate out onto the culture dish (893). These parietal endoderm cells migrated on fibronectin, laminin, and the E8 proteolytic fragment of laminin. In contrast to trophoblast, anti-$\alpha 6$ integrin antibodies did block parietal endoderm outgrowth on laminin, indicating that $\alpha 6\beta 1$ is a major laminin receptor for these cells.

At approximately 7.0 d.g. in the mouse, mesoderm cells ingress from the primitive streak and migrate to positions within the embryo where they will contribute to subsequent organogenesis. Primitive streak-stage mesoderm cells migrate in the extracellular space between the embryonic ectoderm and the visceral endoderm. Fibronectin, laminin, and type IV collagen have all been localized to this region immunohistologically (845–848). Nakatsuji et al. (849) have examined the migration of primitive streak mesoderm cells in cinemicrographic studies. In a similar *in vitro* system, Burdsal et al., (829) examined the adhesive behavior of primitive streak tissues. In attachment assays, epiblast explants adhered well to fibronectin, more poorly to laminin and collagen type IV, and not at all to vitronectin. In contrast, mesoderm explants attached well to all these proteins, correlating with the increased interaction of this tissue with these matrix components during migration. Adhesion of primitive streak mesoderm to fibronectin, vitronectin, laminin, and type IV collagen was completely blocked by anti-ECMR antibodies. In addition, antibodies specific for $\alpha 6\beta 1$ integrin selectively blocked attachment of mesoderm to laminin but not to fibronectin, indicating that $\alpha 6\beta 1$ is also a major laminin receptor for these cells. The changes in the adhesive behavior of embryonic ectoderm compared with the primitive streak mesoderm imply that integrins are developmentally regulated during gastrulation. However, there is still no *in vivo* evidence to suggest that these changes play a causal role in mesoderm migration at gastrulation. The *$\beta 1$ integrin* gene has been targeted in F9 and ES cells and the generation of null mutant mice at this locus is in progress (850; Stephens and C. Damsky, 1993, *personal communication*).

Other Embryonic Cell Migrations: Neural Crest and Primordial Germ Cells

Neural crest cells delaminate from the neural tube and migrate to numerous sites within the embryo where they differentiate into multiple cell types including the neurons and glia of the PNS, melanocytes, and chondrocytes (851). The role of integrins in neural crest migration has been demonstrated in the chick embryo where anti-integrin antibodies perturbed cranial neural crest migration (reviewed in 852); however, due to the inaccessibility of this cell population in the mammals, similar data are not available. In technically demanding experiments, Chan and Tam (853) and Serbedzija et al. (236) have followed the migration of the neural crest in the rat and mouse embryo, respectively. In these studies, cell tracers were injected into the amniotic cavity and these markers labeled the ectoderm (and neuroectoderm) at a stage prior to closure of neural tube. Premigratory neural crest cells were thus labeled and the migratory neural crest cells were studied histologically after their delamination from the closed neural tube. Distinct differences were observed in the migration pathway of the cranial neural crest between the chick, rat, and mouse; therefore, the cell-substratum interactions of the mammalian neural crest may also differ from the chick. In a landmark study, Stemple and Anderson (854) purified rat neural crest cells and propagated neural crest clones *in vitro.* The isolated neural crest cells were multipotent, generating both neurons and schwann cells in clonal cultures.

Upon serial propagation the neural crest clones also generated multipotent progeny. These data indicate that the mammalian neural crest are capable of self-renewal and are, therefore, a true stem cell population. Lastly, the composition of the substratum on which the neural crest clones were maintained was found to influence the overt differentiation of the multipotent cells. These results imply that such a mechanism may be operating *in vivo.*

Primordial germ cells (PGCs) can first be detected at the base of the allantois in the mouse embryo at approximately 7.5 d.g. (855). From this position the PCGs become incorporated into the wall of the hindgut by 8.5 d.g. and by 9.5 d.g. they begin to migrate. By 12.5 d.g., PGCs have migrated through the dorsal mesentery to their final destination, the genital ridge (856,857). The migration, potency, and proliferation of PGCs have been reviewed recently (691,894). In a recent study, the role of fibronectin in PCG migration was examined (859). Embryonic regions containing premigratory, migratory, and postmigratory PGCs were dissected, dissociated, and the adhesion of cells to fibronectin was quantified (in the cell mixtures, PCGs were identified by their cell-surface alkaline phosphatase activity). These *in vitro* assays demonstrated that a decrease in adhesion to fibronectin correlated with the initiation of migration in the PGC population between 8.5 and 9.5 d.g., and these data suggest that a developmentally regulated decrease in adhesion to fibronectin in the hindgut may allow PGCs to leave the area by active migration (859). De Felici and coworkers (691) have demonstrated that anti-integrin antibodies (anti-ECMR antibodies) and RGD-containing peptides block PGC adhesion to fibronectin *in vitro,* implicating these receptors in PGC migration. Changes in cell-cell adhesion may also play a role in the initiation of PGC migration; as PGCs exit the hindgut, they may down-regulate cell-cell adhesion molecules such as E-cadherin, but as of yet it is not known if PGCs express this molecule (894). Also, alkaline phosphatase has been implicated in PGC migration in the salamander, suggesting that it may act similarly in mammalian PCG migration, though this has not been investigated (860).

Other Adhesion Molecules

Thrombospondin is an ECM glycoprotein that serves as an attachment factor for a variety of cells. Thrombospondin binds both extracellular glycoproteins (including fibronectin and collagens) and the proteases, plasminogen and plasminogen activator. Thrombospondin has been hypothesized to play a role in morphogenesis because it may organize the ECM and locally direct protease activity in the ECM (861). In the mouse embryo, immunohistochemical studies utilizing a polyclonal antisera demonstrated that thrombospondin was deposited at cell-cell borders by the 8-cell stage of development, while in the blastocyst the molecule was enriched in the ICM and on the surface of the trophectoderm. Thrombospondin also supported the outgrowth of trophoblast *in vitro* (862). In the egg cylinder, thrombospondin was found enriched in the basement membrane separating the embryonic ectoderm and the visceral endoderm. During neurulation, thrombospondin was localized in the basement membrane of the surface ectoderm and the neuroectoderm and along the pathway of neural crest migration (862,863). Two thrombospondin genes have been identified in the mouse (864). Therefore, it is not clear if the immunolocalization pattern reported by O'Shea et al. (862) reflects one or both genes. In conclusion, a specific role for thrombospondin in postimplantation development remains to be demonstrated.

Another ECM glycoprotein that shows a unique tissue distribution during development is tenascin (865–867). A distinct characteristic of tenascin expression is its expression in mesenchyme at the sites of epithelial-mesenchymal interactions during morphogenetic processes (868–870). Such sites include the developing tooth bud, vibrissae, developing kidney, and the mammary gland. In contrast to its restricted distribution in epithelial-mesenchymal interactions, tenascin is more widely distributed in the central nervous system and may play a role in neuronal development (871,872). Because of tenascin's proposed role in important developmental events, Saga et al. (867) addressed the hypothesis that tenascin was necessary for normal development by creating mice with a null mutation at the tenascin locus using homologous recombination. Surprisingly, homozygous null mutant mice were born live with no anatomical abnormalities. In addition, mutant mice showed no signs of cerebellar defects or behavioral abnormalities that would correlate with abnormal development of the central nervous system due to the loss of tenascin expression. These results do not support the above hypothesis; however, in the complex environment of the developing embryo the possibility that other molecules substitute for tenascin's function cannot be dismissed. Aukhil and Erickson (873) have adopted the strategy of overexpressing tenascin in transgenic mice to assess its function. To date, mice overexpressing tenascin in ectopic sites within the central nervous system also show no defects (H. P. Erickson, 1993, *personal communication*).

A different type of molecule that associates with the ECM is the heparan sulfate proteioglycan, syndecan. The syndecans are a family of integral membrane proteoglycans prominently expressed in epithelia (reviewed in 874). Syndecan-1, the first family member to be described, binds ECM molecules extracellularly, and associates with the actin-containing cytoskeleton, intracellularly (874,875). In addition, syndecan-1 binds FGF-2 (bFGF) and acts as a low-affinity receptor to regulate its effects (876,877). During mouse embryogenesis, syndecan-1 expression undergoes striking spatial and temporal changes (764). Syndecan-1 protein was first detected at the 4-cell stage, and by the hatched blastocyst stage of development syndecan-1 expression was enriched in the basement membrane between the primitive ectoderm and the primitive endoderm. At 7.5 d.g., syndecan-1 continued to be expressed on the basolateral surfaces of two epithelia, the embryonic ectoderm and the visceral endoderm. These sites are consistent with syndecan-1's proposed role in matrix attachment (and epithelial organization). Interestingly, syndecan-1 was also expressed in the primitive streak mesoderm. The molecule was expressed strongly on posterior and lateral mesoderm cells and was barely detectable on anterior mesoderm. As discovered subsequently, FGF family members have been implicated in specifying mesodermal fate in amphibian embryos (723,724,764); Sutherland et al. (764) propose that the asymmetric expression of syndecan-1 on mouse primitive streak mesoderm cells is consistent with its reported role as a receptor for FGF and imply that syndecan-1 may play a role in establishing pattern in the mouse embryo.

CONCLUSIONS

The Mammalian Embryo *In Vitro:* Advantages and Limitations

The success of experimental approaches to early mammalian embryogenesis is largely attributable to work with cultured embryos. Since the 1950s, most investigators have used *in vitro* methods for part or all of their analysis. The enormous advantage conferred by this approach is the accessibility of the embryo itself for treatment and intervention. During preimplantation stages, the embryo is normally free in the oviduct or uterine lumen anyway, so the task of maintaining the embryo in a normal state is one of approximating the fluid and gas conditions of the native environment. Maintaining normal development *in vitro* throughout the preimplantation period has been accomplished with only a few species, including the mouse, rabbit, and human. In these cases, the successful culture was largely a result of empirically altering the growth conditions to optimize development, rather than mimicking reproductive tract conditions *in vivo:* these latter parameters are unknown except for a few species, and where such information has been applied to generate culture media, these have not substantially improved development. Rather, a novel approach involving simplex optimization appears to be the most efficient method yet devised for discovering media that support preimplantation development *in vitro* (905).

The ultimate test of the adequacy of preimplantation culture conditions for any species remains transfer of preimplantation stage embryos to the natural or a surrogate mother, with development to term as the endpoint (1). The alternative approach of culturing blastocysts to postimplantation stages as outgrowths, while a useful endpoint for evaluating blastocyst viability, yields a low incidence of successful development beyond gastrulation, and certain features are abnormal, including the two-dimensional growth of trophoblast derivatives as a monolayer on the substrate used for culture, and the retardation of the embryo proper. These phenomena may be related, in the sense that failure to maintain three-dimensionality *in vitro* may prevent normal cell-cell interactions necessary for placental morphogenesis and therefore embryonic nutrition; alternatively, autocrine factors produced by either placenta or embyro may become diluted by culture medium, thus depriving the embryo of essential growth-promoting substances.

The extent of normal growth rate and morphology for embryos explanted and cultured at postimplantation stages is limited to 2–3 days for rodents, which have been the subject of most experimental work (reviewed in 906). Returning cultured postimplantation embryos to the uterus has been only marginally successful, without development to term after transfer (907). Thus, despite the advantages of accessibility provided by culture, postimplantation embryos cannot be restored to their normal intrauterine potential for growth. However, dissecting midgestation embryos free of the uterus and decidua for *exo utero* development provides access for microsurgical intervention, including lineage tracing at late stages of embryogenesis and fetal development (852). Clearly, defining the nature of epigenetic interactions within the embryo and between embryonic and maternal tissues through membrane contacts, extracellular matrix, and humoral factors remains one of the major tasks in early mammalian embryology (573). At stake is an understanding not only of the requirements for successful *in vitro* development, but also of the molecular mechanisms for induction of the embryonic axes and the anteroposterior succession of axial structures that characterize vertebrates as bilaterally symmetrical quadripeds.

Mammalian Embryos as Models for Vertebrate Development

It should be apparent that the cumulative experimental approaches to the embryos of laboratory mammals have made them superb systems for many aspects of developmental biology. Sensitive techniques make it possible to study gene expression in the small tissue samples available from mammalian embryos; analysis of embryonic cell potency, allocation, and fate has provided insight into the architectural rules for construction of the mammalian embryo. The knowledge about regulation of tissue-specific gene expression and developmental mechanisms gained from transgenics and other genetic studies attests to the power of these approaches.

The compelling reason for studying mammals as model systems that has emerged from the current body of knowledge about their embryos is that development during and after gastrulation appears to be highly conserved. This conclusion is supported by the extensive similarity of the gastrula fate map of the mouse to that of the chick and urodele embryo (175,190,211,224,229) and the apparent conservation of the pattern of homeobox and PAX gene expression during the formation of segmental axial structures (584,620,621). Accordingly, it appears that the basic way of establishing the vertebrate body plan has remained essentially unchanged for the past 250–500 million years. Although this argument can also be used to justify using birds, frogs, fish, or even *Drosophila* as models for vertebrate development, mammals nonetheless have some features that justify their use. These pertain mainly, but not exclusively, to extraembryonic tissues and structures: their precocious differentiation and cell allocation; preferential paternal X chromosome inactivation in placental and yolk sac tissues; and the dramatic effects of genomic imprinting. Thus, mammals are deeply generalized in some aspects of their embryogenesis, yet uniquely specialized in others. This combination makes a compelling case for studying the developmental mechanisms of mammalian embryos. Analysis of these mechanisms in mammals should be informative of developmental phenomena among vertebrates in general, and should provide immediate opportunities for beneficial applications to problems of human health.

Transgenic Animals as Models for Human Disorders

The body of knowledge obtained from transgenic mice attests to the power of these novel approaches. The genetic transformation of mouse embryos and ES cells provide a technological advances and insights that are valuable for improving gene therapy. Specific benefits of transgenic approaches include elucidating the mechanisms of tissue specific gene regulation, optimizing procedures for introducing exogenous genes into cells, and determining which promoters are effective in a wide variety of target tissues. This information is the necessary background for clinically effective gene therapy to correct biochemical defects in human somatic cells.

The more than 20 preexisting (nontransgenic) mouse models for human genetic disorders that have already been identified by their phenotypic similarities and by comparative mapping include albinism, alpha- and beta-thalassemia, testicular feminization, X-linked muscular dystrophy, and others (reviewed in 784). The cumulative resolving power of recombinant inbred strains (899) and interspecific crosses (900) in mouse gene mapping studies provides a counterpart to the human genome effort for identifying syntenic regions and evaluating linkages. If both the human and mouse genes have been mapped, it is straightforward to evaluate the relevance of phenotypic similarities that a potential mouse model might have for a human disorder. No other laboratory or domestic species currently approaches the number of identified genes as the mouse system, which will therefore continue to increase in usefulness as a genetic and developmental model.

The high frequency of insertional mutagenesis from mouse zygotic DNA injection has led to numerous additional mutations, many of them allelic with existing mutations, including limb deformity, pigmy, Steel, *situs inversus viscerum,* and others (reviewed in 332). The relatively small number of the genes responsible for these phenotypes that has been cloned may indicate an inherent limitation of this approach. Nonetheless, all of these mutants can potentially provide additional models for specific human genetic disorders. In a few cases, the transgene itself creates a model for human disease by introducing a gene that is not present in mice (Table 1, part A). Although it is limited to genes that have already been cloned, homologous recombination in embryonic stem cells is potentially the largest source of mouse mutants as models, alreading leading to several phenotypes that are the counterparts of human disorders (Table 1,

TABLE 1. *Transgenic mouse models of human disease*

A. Transgenic lines generated by pronuclear injection

Transgene	Disease model (phenotype)	reference
Human poliovirus receptor	Poliovirus-sensitive mouse	878
Human collagenase	Pulmonary emphysema	879
Human neurofilament (heavy)	Amyotrophic lateral sclerosis (ALS)	880

B. Specific Loci targeted by homologous recombination in ES cells

Transgenic locus	Disease model (phenotype)	reference
Retinoblastoma-1 (Rb-1)	Embryonic lethal; abnormal neural and hematopoietic development	881,882,883
Cystic fibrosis transmembrane regulator (CFTR)	Abnormal choloride transport in epithelia	884
Apolipoprotein E	Hypercholesterolemia and atherosclerosis	885,886
c-fos	Osteopetrosis, growth retardation, and altered hematopoiesis	795
HoxA3	DiGeorge' Syndrome	594

part B). Finally, continued use of promoter-trap strategies will reveal additional mutations for specific developmental processes, stages, and tissues (392). Together, these and any additional novel approaches will accelerate the already geometric expansion in the utility of the mouse as a model for human disorders. The eventual extension of embryo and ES cell biotechnology to other species (386), especially the rat and bovine systems, will have equally profound implications for understanding the genetic basis of development and disease.

ACKNOWLEDGMENTS

Work in this laboratory was supported by the U.S. Department of Energy Office of Health and Environmental Research, Contract DE-AC03-76-SF01012 and by National Institute of Child Health and Human Development Program Project Grant HD26732. C.A.B. was a beneficiary of National Research Service Award ES07102 from the National Institute of Environmental Health Sciences. We thank Drs. Jean Latimer, Stephen Grout, and Clement Markert for their comments, and our numerous colleagues who responded to our request for and allowed us to cite their unpublished work. We are grateful to Ms. Liana Hartanto for her assistance with the manuscript.

REFERENCES

1. Adams CE. *Mammalian egg transfer.* Boca Raton, Florida: CRC Press; 1982.
2. Brackett BG, Seidel GE, Seidel SM, eds. *New technologies in animal breeding.* New York: Academic Press; 1981.
3. Hafez ESE, Semm K, eds. *In vitro fertilization and embryo transfer.* New York: Alan R. Liss; 1982:393.
4. Beier HM, Lindner HR, eds. *Fertilization of the human egg in vitro: biological basis and clinical application.* Berlin: Springer Verlog; 1983.
5. Jones HW Jr, Jones GS, Hodgen GD, Rosenwaks Z, eds. *In vitro fertilization.* Baltimore: Williams and Wilkins; 1986.
6. Seppala M, Edwards RG, eds. Volume 442: in vitro fertilization and embryo transfer. In: *Annals New York Acadamy of Sciences.* New York: New York Academy of Sciences; 1985.
7. Trounson A, Woods C, eds. *In vitro fertilization and embryo transfer.* Edinburgh: Churchill Livingstone; 1984.
8. Bodemer CW. The biology of the blastocyst in historical perspective. In: Blandau RJ, ed. *Biology of the blastocyst.* Chicago: University of Chicago Press; 1971:1–25.
9. Horder TJ, Witkowski JA, Wilie CC, eds. A history of embryology. In: *Proceedings of the eighth symposium of the British Society for Developmental Biology.* Cambridge, England: Cambridge University Press; 1986.
10. Heape W. Preliminary note on the transplantation and growth of mammalian ova within a uterine foster mother. *Proc Roy Soc Lond* 1891:48:457.
11. Rossant J, Papaioannou VE. The biology of embryogenesis. In: Sherman MI, ed. *Concepts in mammalian embryogenesis.* Cambridge, Massachusetts: MIT Press; 1977:1–36.
12. Whitten WK. Culture of tubal mouse ova. *Nature* 1956;177:96.
13. Brinster RL. Studies on the development of mouse embryos in vitro: II. the effect of energy source. *J Exp Zool* 1965;158:59–68.
14. Biggers JD. Whitten WK, Whittingham DG. The culture of mouse embryos in vitro. In: Daniel JC Jr, ed. *Methods in mammalian embryology.* San Francisco: WH Freeman; 1971:86–116.
15. Hogan B, Costantini F, Lacy E. *Manipulating the mouse embryo: a laboratory manual.* Cold Spring Harbor, New York: Cold Spring Harbor Laboratory; 1986:12–15.
16. Biggers JD. In vitro fertilization and embryo transfer in historical perspective. In: Trounson A, Wood C, eds. In vitro fertilization and embryo transfer. London: Churchill Livingstone; 1984:3–15.
17. Biggers JD. Pioneering mammalian embryo culture. In: Bavister BD, ed. *Mammalian preimplantation embryo: regulation of growth and different in vitro.* New York: Plenum Press; 1987:1–22.
18. McLaren A, Biggers JD. Successful development and birth of mice cultivated *in vitro* as early embryos. *Nature* 1958; 182:877–878.
19. Edwards RG, Gates AH. Timing of the stages of the maturation, divisions, ovulation, fertilization and the first cleavage of eggs of adult mice treated with gonadotrophins. *J Endocrinol* 1959; 18:292–304.
20. Tarkowski AK. Mouse chimeras developed from fused eggs. *Nature* 1961;190:857–860.
21. Mintz B. Formation of genetically mosaic mouse embryos, and early development of "lethal (t12/t12) normal" mosaics. *J Exp Zool* 1964;157:273–292.
22. McLaren A. *Mammalian chimeras.* London: Cambridge University Press; 1976.
23. Chapman VM, Ansell JD, McLaren A. Trophoblast giant cell differentiation in the mouse: expression of glucose phosphate isomerase (GPI-1) electrophoretic variants in transferred and chimeric embryos. *Dev Biol* 1972;29:48–54.
24. West JD. Volume 3: analysis of clonal growth using chimeras and mosaics. In: Johnson MH, ed. *Development in mammals.* North Holland, Amsterdam. 1978:413–460.
25. LeDourin N, McLaren A, eds. *Chimeras in developmental biology.* New York: Academic Press; 1984.
26. Gardner RL. Mouse chimeras obtained by the injection of cells into the blastocyst. *Nature* 1968;220:596–597.
27. Gardner RL. An in situ cell marker for clonal analysis of development of the extraembryonic endoderm in the mouse. *J Embryol Exp Morphol* 1984;80:251–288.
28. Rossant J, Vijh M, Siracusa LD, Chapman VM. Identification of embryonic cell lineages in histological sections of M. Musculus ↔ M. caroli chimaeras. *J Embryol Exp Morphol* 1983; 73:179–191.
29. Lo C. Localization of low abundance DNA sequences in tissue sections by in situ hybridization. *J Cell Sci* 1986;81:143–162.
30. Ng YK, Iannaccone PM. Experimental chimeras: current concepts and controversies in normal development and pathogenesis. *Curr Top Dev Biol* 1992;27:235–274.
31. Lin TP. Egg micromanipulation. In: Daniels JC Jr, ed. *Methods in mammalian embryology.* San Francisco: WH Freeman; 1971:157–185.
32. Wilson IB, Bolton E, Cutler RH. Preimplantation differentiation in the mouse egg as revealed by microinjection of vital markers. *J Embryol Exp Morphol* 1972;27:467–479.
33. Graham CF, Deussen ZA. Features of cell lineage in preimplantation mouse development. *J Embryol Exp Morphol* 1978; 48:53–72.
34. Jacobson M, Hirose G. Origin of the retina from both sides of the embryonic brain: a contribution to the problem of crossing at the optic chiasma. *Science* 1978;202:637–639.
35. Weisblat DA, Sawyer RT, Stent GS. Cell lineage analysis by intracellular injection of a tracer enzyme. *Science* 1978; 202:1295–1298.
36. Gimlich RL, Braun J. New fluorescent cell lineage tracers. *Dev Biol* 1985;115:340–352.
37. Balakier H, Pedersen RA. Allocation of cells to inner mass and trophectoderm lineages in preimplantation mouse embryos. *Dev Biol* 1982;90:352–362.
38. Briggs R, King TJ. Transplantation of living nuclei from blastula cells into enucleated frogs' eggs. *Proc Natl Acad Sci USA* 1952;38:455–463.
39. Gurdon JB. The developmental capacity of nuclei taken from intestinal epithelium cells of feeding tadpoles. *J Embryol Exp Morphol* 1962;10:622.
40. McGrath J, Solter D. Nuclear transplantation in the mouse embryo by microsurgery and cell fusion. *Science* 1983;220: 1300–1303.

41. Gordon JW, Scangos GA, Plotkin DJ, Barbosa JA, Ruddle FH. Genetic transformation of mouse embryos by microinjection of purified DNA. In: *Proc Nat Acad Sci, USA* 1980;77:7380–7384.
42. Brinster RL, Palmiter RD. Introduction of genes into the germ line of animals. In: *The Harvey Lectures,* New York: Alan R. Liss; 1986:1–38.
43. Solter D, Knowles B. Immunosurgery of mouse blastocyst. *Proc Natl Acad Sci USA* 1975;72:5099–5102.
44. Biggers JD, Brinster RL. Biometrical problems in the study of early mammalian embryos in vitro. *J Exp Zool* 1965;158:39–48.
45. Kaye PL. Metabolic aspects of the physiology of the preimplantation embryo. In: Rossant J, Pedersen RA, eds. *Experimental approaches to mammalian embryonic development.* New York: Cambridge University Press; 1986:267–292.
46. Clarke RN, Baltz JM, Lechene CP, Biggers JD. Use of ultramicrofluorometric methods for the study of single preimplantation embryos. *Poultry Science* 1989;68:972–978.
47. Gosden JR, West JD. Prospects for preimplantation diagnosis of genetic diseases. In: Gwatkin RBL, ed. *Genes in mammalian reproduction.* Wiley-Liss Inc; 1993:73–130.
48. van Blerkom J, Barton SC, Johnson MH. Molecular differentiation in the preimplantation mouse embryo. *Nature* 1976; 259:319–321.
49. Latham KE, Garrels JI, Chang C, Solter D. Analysis of embryonic mouse development: construction of a high-resolution, two-dimensional gel protein database. *App Theor Electrophoresis* 1992;2:163–170.
50. Rothstein JL, Johnson D, DeLoia JA, Skowronski J, Solter D, Knowles B. Gene expression during preimplantation mouse development. *Genes Dev* 1992;6:1190–1201.
51. Rappolee DA, Brenner CA, Schultz R, Mark D, Werb Z. Developmental expression of PDGF, TGF-a, and TGF-b genes in preimplantation mouse embryos. *Science* 1988;241:1823–1825.
52. Rappolee DA, Wang A, Mark D, Werb Z. Novel method for studying mRNA phenotypes in single or small numbers of cells. *J Cell Biochem* 1989;39:1–11.
53. Wilkinson DG, Green J. *In situ* hybridization and the three-dimensional reconstruction of serial sections. In: Copp AJ, Cockroft DL, eds. *Postimplantation mammalian embryos: a practical approach.* Oxford University Press; 1990:155–171.
54. Coulou RA, Herman BG. Detection of mRNA by *in situ* hybridization to postimplantation mouse embryo whole mounts. In: Wassarman PM, ed. *Guide to Techniques in Mouse Development. Methods Enzymol* 1993;225:373–383.
55. Varmuza S, Tate P. Isolation of epiblast-specific cDNA clones by differential hybridization with polymerase chain reaction-amplified probes derived from single embryos. *Mol Reprod Dev* 1992;32:339–348.
56. Martin GR. Teratocarcinomas and mammalian embryogenesis. *Science* 1980;209:768–776.
57. Hogan BLM, Barlow DP, Tilly R. F9 teratocarcinoma cells as a model for the differentiation of parietal and visceral endoderm in the mouse embryo. In: Gardner RL, ed. *Embryonic and germ cell tumours in humans and animals.* London: Imperial Cancer Research Fund; 1983:115–140.
58. Brinster RL. The effect of cells transferred into the mouse blastocyst on subsequent development. *J Exp Med* 1974;140:1049.
59. Mintz B, Illmensee K. Normally genetically mosaic mice produced from malignant teratocarcinoma cells. In: *Proc Natl Acad Sci USA* 1975;72:3585–3589.
60. Papaioannou VE, Rossant J. Effects of the embryonic environment on proliferation and differentiation of embryonal carcinoma cells. *Cancer Surv* 1983;2:165–183.
61. Martin GR. Isolation of a pluripotent cell line from early mouse embryos cultured in medium conditioned by teratocarcinoma stem cells. *Proc Natl Acad Sci USA* 1981;78:7634–7638.
62. Evans MI, Kaufman MH. Establishment in culture of pluripotential cells from mouse embryos. *Nature* 1981;292:154–156.
63. Robertson EJ, Bradley A. Production of permanent cell lines from early embryos and their use in studying developmental problems: In: *Experimental approaches to mammalian embryonic development.* New York: Cambridge University Press; 1986:475–508.
64. Robertson EJ. Embryo-derived stem cell lines. In: Robertson EJ, ed. *Teratocarcinoma and embryonic stem cells: a practical approach.* Oxford: Oxford University Press; 1987:71–112.
65. Joyner AL. *Gene targetting.* Oxford: Oxford University Press; 1983; [in press].
66. Gaddum-Rosse P, Bladau RJ, Langley LB, Sato K. Sperm tail entry into the mouse egg *in vitro. Gamete Res* 1982;6:215–223.
67. Howlett SK, Bolton VN. Sequence and regulation of morphological and molecular events during the first cell cycle of mouse embryogenesis. *J Embryol Exp Morph* 1985;87:175–206.
68. Yanagimachi R. Time and process of sperm penetration into hamster and ova *in vivo* and *in vitro. J Reprod Fertil* 1966; 11:359–370.
69. Molls M, Zamboglou N. Streffer C. A comparison of the cell kinetics of pre-implantation mouse embryos from two different mouse strains. *Cell Tissue Kinet* 1983;16:277–283.
70. Naish SJ, Perreault SD, Foehner AL, Zirkin A. DNA synthesis in the fertilizing hamster sperm nucleus: sperm template availability and egg cytoplasmic control. *Biol Reprod* [in press].
71. Shire JGM, Whitten WK. Genetic variation in the timing of first cleavage in mice: effect of paternal genotype. *Biol Reprod* 1980;23:363–368.
72. Shire JGM, Whitten WK. Genetic variation in the timing of first cleavage in mice: effect of maternal genotype. *Biol Reprod* 1980;23:369–376.
73. Sutherland AE, Speed TP, Calarco PG. Inner cell allocation in the mouse morula: the role of oriented division during fourth cleavage. *Dev Biol* 1990;137:13–25.
74. Goldbard SB, Warner CM. Genes affect the timing of early mouse embryo development. *Biol Reprod* 1982;27:419–424.
75. Harlow GM, Quinn P. Development of preimplantation mouse embryos *in vivo* and *in vitro. Aust J Biol Sci* 1982;35:187–193.
76. Streffer C, van Beuningen D, Molls M, Zamboglu N, Schultz S. Kinetics of cell proliferation in the preimplanted mouse embryo *in vivo* and *in vitro. Cell Tissue Kinet* 1980;13:135–143.
77. Sawicki W, Abramczuk J, Blaton O. DNA cycles in the second and third cell cycles of mouse preimplantation development. *Exp Cell Res* 1978;112:199–205.
78. Pedersen RA. Potency, lineage and allocation in preimplantation mouse embryos. In: Rossant J, Pedersen RA, eds. *Experimental approaches to mammalian embryonic development.* New York: Cambridge University Press; 1986:3–33.
79. Smith RKW, Johnson MH. Analysis of the third and fourth cell cycles of mouse early development. *J Reprod Fertil* 1986; 76:393–399.
80. Chisholm JC. Analysis of the fifth cell cycle of mouse development. *J Reprod Fertil* 1988;84:29–36.
81. Sundstrom P, Nilsson O, Liedholm P. Cleavage rate and morphology of early human embryos obtained after artificial fertilization and culture. *Actra Obstet Gynecol Scand* 1981;60:109–120.
82. Trouson AO, Mohr LR, Wood C, Leeton JF. Effect of delayed insemination on in-vitro fertilization, culture and transfer of human embryos. *J Reprod Fertil* 1982;64:285–294.
83. Balakier H, MacLusky NJ, Casper RF. Characterization of the first cell cycle in human zygotes: implications for cryopreservation. *Fertil Steril* 1993;59:359–365.
84. Kelly SJ, Mulnard JG, Graham CF. Cell division and cell allocation in early mouse development. *J Embryol Exp Morphol* 1978;48:37–51.
85. Lewis WH, Wright ES. On the early development of the mouse egg. *Carnegie Instit Contrib Embryol* 1935;25:113–143.
86. Ducibella T, Albertini DF, Anderson E, Biggers J. The preimplantation mammalian embryo: characterization of intracellular junctions and their appearance during development. *Dev Biol* 1975;45:231–250.
87. Magnuson T, Dempsey A, Stackpole CW. Characterization of intercellular junctions in the preimplantation mouse embryo by freeze-fracture and thin-section electron microscopy. *Dev Biol* 1977;61:252–261.
88. Magnuson T, Jacobson JB, Stackpole CW. Relationship between intercellular permeability and junctional organization in the preimplantation mouse embryo. *Dev Biol* 1978;67:214–224.
89. McLachlin JR, Caveney S, Kidder GM. Control of gap junction formation in early mouse embryos. *Dev Biol* 1983;98:155–164.
90. Goodall H, Johnson MH. The nature of intercellular coupling within the preimplantation mouse embryo. *J Embryol Exp Morphol* 1984;79:53–76.
91. Biggers JD, Bell JE, Benos DJ. Mammalian blastocyst: transport

functions in a developing epithelium: invited review. *Am J Physiol* 1988:255:419–432.
92. Wiley LM, Kidder GM, Watson AJ. Cell polarity and development of the first epithelium. *Bioessays* 1990;12:67–73.
93. Gueth-Hallonet C, Maro B. Cell polarity and cell diversification during early mouse embryogenesis. *Trends Genet,* 1992;8: 274–279.
94. Sobel JS. Membrane-cytoskeletal interactions in the early mouse embryo. *Cell Biol* 1990;1:341–348.
95. Cruz YP, Pedersen RA. Origin of embryonic and extraembryonic cell lineages in mammalian embryos. In: *Animal applications of research in mammalian development, current communications in cell and molecular biology series.* Cold Spring Harbor, NY: Cold Spring Harbor Laboratory Press; 1991:147–204.
96. Selwood L. Mechanisms underlying the development of pattern of marsupial embryos. *Curr Top Dev Biol* 1992;27:175–233.
97. Wimsatt WA. Some comparative aspects of implantation. *Biol Reprod* 1975;12:1–40.
98. Papaioannou VE, Ebert KM. Comparative aspects of embryo manipulation in mammals. In: Rossant I, Pedersen RA, eds. *Experimental approaches to mammalian embryonic development.* New York: Cambridge University Press; 1986:67–96.
99. Barlow P, Owen DAJ, Graham C. DNA synthesis in the preimplantation mouse embryo. *J Embryol Exp Morphol* 1972; 27:431–455.
100. Chisholm JC, Johnson MH, Warren PD, Fleming TP, Pickering SJ. Developmental variability within and between mouse expanding blastocysts and their ICMs. *J Embryol Exp Morphol* 1985;86:311–336.
101. Handyside AH, Hunter S. Cell division and death in the mouse blastocyst before implantation. *Roud's Arch Dev Biol* 1986; 195:519–526.
102. Dickson AD. The form of the mouse blastocyst. *J Anat* 1966;100:335–348.
103. Papaioannou VE, Ebert KM. The preimplantation pig embryo: cell number and allocation to trophectoderm and inner cell mass of the blastocyst *in vivo* and *in vitro. Development* 1988; 102:793–803.
104. Solter D, Skreb N. La durée des phases du cycle mitotique dans différentes régions du cylindreoeuf de la souris. *CR hebd Séanc Acad Sci (Paris)* 1968;267:659–661.
105. Lewis NE, Rossant J. Mechanism of size regulation in mouse embryo aggregates. *J Embryol Exp Morphol* 1982;72:169–181.
106. Snow MHL. Gastrulation in the mouse: growth and regionalization of the epiblast. *J Embryol Exp Morphol* 1977;42:293–303.
107. Poelmann RE. Differential mitosis and degeneration patterns in relation to the alteratins in the shape of the embryonic ectoderm of early post-implantation mouse embryos. *J Exp Morph* 1980;55:33–51.
107a. MacAuley A, Werb Z, Mirkes PE. Characterization of the unusually rapid cell cycles during rat gastrulation. *Development* 1993;117:873–883.
108. Smith R, McLaren A. Factors affecting the time of formation of the mouse blastocoel. *J Embryol Exp Morphol* 1977;41:79–92.
109. Sawicki W, Mystkowska ET. Phorbol estermediated modulation of cell proliferation and primary differentiation of mouse preimplantation embryos. *Exp Cell Res* 1981;136:455–458.
110. Alexandre H. The utilization of an inhibitor of spermidine and spermine synthesis as a tool for the study of determination of cavitation in the preimplantation mouse embryo. *J Embryol Exp Morphol* 1979;53:145–162.
111. Alexandre H. Effet de l'inhibition specifique de la replication de l'ADN par l'aphidicoline sur la differentiation primarie de l'oeuf de souris en preimplantation. *CR Acad Sci (Paris) III,* 1982;294:1001–1006.
112. Dean WL, Rossant J. Effect of delaying DNA replication on blastocyst formation in the mouse. *Differentiation* 1984;26:134–137.
113. Spindle AI, Nagano H, Pedersen RA. Inhibition of DNA replication in preimplantation mouse embryos by aphidicolin. *J Exp Zool* 1985;235:289–295.
114. Newport J, Kirschner M. A major developmental transition in early Xenopus embryos: II. control of the onset of transcription. *Cell* 1982;30:687–696.
115. Mita-Miyazawa I, Ikegami S, Satoh N. Histospecific acetylcholinesterase development in the presumptive muscle cells isolated from 16-cell-stage ascidian embryos with respect to the number of DNA replications. *J Embryol Exp Morphol* 1985;87:1–12.
116. Masui Y, Markert CL. Cytoplasmic control of nuclear behavior during meiotic maturation of frog oocytes. *J Exp Zool* 1971;117:129–146.
117. Newport J, Kirschner M. Regulation of the cell cycle during early Xenopus development. *Cell* 1984;37:731–742.
118. Kishimoto T, Yamazaki K, Kato Y, Koide SS, Kanatani H. Induction of starfish oocyte maturation by maturation-promoting factor of mouse and surf clam oocytes. *J Exp Zool* 1984;231:293–295.
119. Sorensen RA, Cyert MS, Pedersen RA. Active maturation promoting factor is present in mature mouse oocytes. *J Cell Biol* 1985;100:1637–1640.
120. Balakier H, Czolowska R. Cytoplasmic control of nuclear maturation in mouse oocytes. *Exp Cell Res* 1977;110:466–469.
121. Balakier H. Induction of maturation in small oocytes from sexually immature mice by fusion with meiotic or mitotic cells. *Exp Cell Res* 1978;112:137–141.
122. Balakier H, Masui Y. Chromosome condensation activity in the cytoplasm of anucleate and nucleate fragments of mouse oocytes. *Dev Biol* 1986;113:155–159.
123. Masui Y, Clarke JH. Oocyte maturation. *Int Rev Cytol* 1979;57:185–283.
124. Wickramasinghe D, Albertini DF. Cell cycle control during mammalian oogenesis. *Curr Topics Dev Biol* 1993;27:125–153.
125. McConnell J, Lee M. Presence of $cdc2^{+}$-like proteins in the preimplantation mouse embryo. *Development* 1989;107:481–487.
126. Weiss P. *Principles of development.* New York: Holt; 1939.
127. Tarkowski AK. Experiments on the development of isolated blastomeres of mouse eggs. *Nature* 1959;184:1286–1287.
128. Seidel F. Die Entwicklungspotenzen einer isolierten Blastomere des Zweizellenstadiums im Saugetierei. *Naturwissenschaften* 1952;39:355–356.
129. Papaioannou VE, Mkandawire J, Biggers JD. Development and phenotypic variability of genetically identical half mouse embryos. *Development* 1989;106:817–827.
130. Biggers JD, Papaioannou VE. Water-escape time in adult mice derived from manipulated preimplantation embryos. *In Vitro Fertil Embryo Trans* 1991;8:352–360.
131. Biggers JD, Papaioannou VE. Postnatal compensatory growth of manipulated mouse embryos. *Hum Reprod* 1991;6:36–44.
132. Tarkowski AK, Wroblewska J. Development of blastomeres of mouse eggs isolated at the 4- and 8-cell stage. *J Embryol Exp Morphol* 1967;18:155–180.
133. Kelly SJ. Studies of the developmental potential of 4- and 8-cell stage mouse blastomeres. *J Exp Zool* 1977;200:365–376.
134. Hillman N, Sherman MI, Graham CF. The effect of spatial arrangement on cell determination during mouse development. *J Embryol Exp Morphol* 1972;28:263–278.
135. Rossant J, Vijh KM. Ability of outside cells from preimplantation mouse embryos to form inner cell mass derivatives. *Dev Biol* 1980;76:475–482.
136. Ziomek CA, Johnson MH, Handyside AH. The developmental potential of mouse 16-cell blastomeres. *J Exp Zool* 1982;221:345–355.
137. Prather RS, Robl JM. Cloning by nuclear transfer and embryo splitting in laboratory and domestic animals. In: Pedersen RA, McLaren A, First N, eds. *Animal applications of research in mammalian development.* New York: Cold Spring Harbor Laboratory Press; 1991:205–232.
138. Stern MS. Experimental studies on the organization of the preimplantation mouse embryo: II. reaggregation of disaggregated embryos. *J Embryol Exp Morphol* 1992;28:255–261.
139. Handyside AH. Time of commitment of inside cells isolated from preimplantation mouse embryos. *J Embryol Exp Morphol* 1978;45:37–53.
140. Hogan B, Tilly R. In vitro development of inner cell masses isolated immunosurgically from mouse blastocysts: II. inner cell masses from 3.5- to 4.0-day p.c. blastocysts. *J Embryol Exp Morphol* 1978;45:107–121.
141. Spindle AI. Trophoblast regeneration by inner cell masses isolated from cultured mouse embryos. *J Exp Zool* 1978; 203:483–489.

142. Rossant J, Lis WT. Potential of isolated mouse inner cell masses to form trophectoderm derivatives *in vivo*. *Dev Biol* 1979; 70:255–261.
143. Rossant J. Investigation of the determinative state of the mouse inner cell mass: II. the fate of isolated inner cell masses transferred to the oviduct. *J Embryol Exp Morphol* 1975;33:991–1001.
144. Nichols J, Gardner RL. Heterogeneous differentiation of external cells in individual isolated early mouse inner cell masses in culture. *J Embryol Exp Morphol* 1984;80:225–240.
145. Izquierdo L, Ortiz ME. Differentiation in the mouse morulae. *Roux' Arch* 1975;177:67–74.
146. Daniel JC Jr. The first potential I.C.M. cell during cleavage of the rabbit ovum. *Roux's Arch* 1976;179:249–250.
147. Handyside AH. Immunofluorescence techniques for determining the numbers of inner and outer blastomeres in mouse morulae. *J Reprod Immunol* 1981;2:339–350.
148. Copp AJ. Interaction between inner cell mass and trophectoderm of the mouse blastocyst: I. a study of cellular proliferation. *J Embryol Exp Morphol* 1978;48:109–125.
149. Garner W, McLaren A. Cell distribution in chimaeric mouse embryos before implantation. *J Embryol Exp Morphol* 1974; 32:495–503.
150. Kelly SJ. Investigations into the degree of cell mixing that occurs between the 8-cell and the blastocyst stage of mouse development. *J Exp Zool* 1979;207:121–130.
151. Surani MAH, Barton SC. Spatial distribution of blastomeres is dependent on cell division order and interactions in mouse morulae. *Dev Biol* 1984;102:335–343.
152. Spindle AI. Cell allocation in preimplantation mouse chimeras. *J Exp Zool* 1982;219:361–367.
153. Meinecke-Tillmann S, Meinecke B. Experimental chimaeras—removal of reproductive barrier between sheep and goat. *Nature* 1984;307:637–638.
154. Surani MAH, Kimbers SJ, Barton SC. Differential adhesiveness as a mechanism of cell allocation to inner cell mass and trophectoderm in the mouse blastocyst. In: Neubert D, Merker HJ, eds. *Culture techniques: applicability for studies on prenatal differentiation and toxicity.* Berlin: W de Gruyter; 1981:397–412.
155. Kimber SJ, Surani MAH, Barton SC. Interactions of blastomeres suggest changes in cell surface adhesiveness during the formation of inner cell mass and trophectoderm in the preimplantation mouse embryo. *J Embryol Exp Morphol* 1982;58:231–249.
156. Garbutt CL, Johnson MH, George MA. When and how does cell division order influence cell allocation to the inner cell mass of the mouse blastocyst? *Development* 100:325–332.
157. Handyside AH. Distribution of antibody- and lectin-binding sites on dissociated blastomeres from mouse morulae: evidence of polarization at compaction. *J Embryol Exp Morphol* 1980; 60:99–116.
158. Ziomek CA, Johnson MH. Cell surface interaction induces polarization of mouse 8-cell blastomeres at compaction. *Cell* 1980;21:935–942.
159. Ziomek CA, Johnson MH. The roles of phenotype and position in guiding the fate of 16-cell mouse blastomeres. *Dev Biol* 1982;91:440–447.
160. Johnson MH, Ziomek CA. Cell interactions influence the fate of mouse blastomeres undergoing the transition from the 16- to the 32-cell stage. *Dev Biol* 1983;95:211–218.
161. Ziomek CA, Chatot CL, Manes C. Polarization of blastomeres in the cleaving rabbit embryo. *J Exp Zool* 1990;256:84–91.
162. Pedersen RA, Spindle AI. Role of the blastocoel microenvironment in early mouse embryo differentiation. *Nature* 1980; 284:550–552.
163. Johnson MH, Pratt HMP, Handyside AH. The generation and recognition of positional information in the preimplantation mouse embryo. In: Glasserand SR, Bullock DW, eds. *Cellular and molecular aspects of implantation.* New York: Plenum Publishing Co; 1981:55–74.
164. Johnson MH, Maro B. Time and space in the mouse early embryo: a cell biological approach to cell diversification. In: Rossant J, Pedersen RA, eds. *Experimental approaches to mammalian embryonic development.* New York: Cambridge University Press; 1986:35–65.
165. Fleming TP, Johnson MH. From egg to epithelium. *Ann Rev Cell Biol* 1988;4:459–485.
166. Pratt HPM. Marking time and making space: chronology and topography in the early mouse embryo. *Int Rev Cytol* 1989;117:99–130.
167. Pedersen RA, Wu K, Balakier H. Origin of the inner cell mass in mouse embryos: cell lineage analysis by microinjection. *Dev Biol* 1986;117:581–595.
168. Fleming TP. A quantitative analysis of cell allocation to trophectoderm and inner cell mass in the mouse blastocyst. *Dev Biol* 1987;119:520–531.
169. Cruz YP, Pedersen RA. Cell fate in the polar trophectoderm of mouse blastocysts as studied by microinjection of cell lineage tracers. *Dev Biol* 1985;112:73–83.
170. Rossant J, Croy BA. Genetic identification of tissue of origin of cellular populations within the mouse placenta. *J Embryol Exp Morphol* 1985;86:177–189.
171. Winkel GK, Pedersen RA. Fate of the inner cell mass in mouse embryos as studied by microinjection of lineage tracers. *Dev Biol* 1988;127:143–156.
172. Dyce J, George M, Goodall H, Fleming TP. Do trophectoderm and inner cell mass cells in the mouse blastocyst maintain discrete lineages? *Development* 1987;100:685–698.
173. Gardner RL, Nichols J. An investigation of the fate of cells transplanted orthotopically between morulae/nascent blastocysts in the mouse. *Hum Reprod* 1991;6:25–35.
174. Rossant J. Cell commitment in early rodent development. In: Johnson MH, ed. *Development in mammals,* Volume 2: Amsterdam: North Holland; 1977:119–150.
175. Beddington R. Analysis of tissue fate and prospective potency in the egg cylinder. In: Rossant J, Pedersen RA, eds. *Experimental approaches to mammalian embryonic development.* New York: Cambridge University Press; 1986:121–147.
176. Gardner RL. In vivo and in vitro studies on cell lineage and determination in the early mouse embryo. In: Lloyd CW, Rees DA, eds. *Cellular controls in differentiation,* London: Academic Press; 1981:257–278.
177. Gardner RL. Volume 24: origin and differentiation of extraembryonic tissues in the mouse. In: Richter GW, Epstein MA, eds. *International review of experimental pathology.* New York: Academic Press; 1983:63–133.
178. Gardner RL, Papaioannou VE. Differentiation in the trophectoderm and inner cell mass. In: Balls M, Wild AE, eds. *The early development of mammals, British society for developmental biology.* Symposium 2. Cambridge: Cambridge University Press; 1975:107–132.
179. Gardner RL, Papaioannou VE, Barton SC. Origin of the ectoplacental cone and secondary giant cells in mouse blastocysts reconstituted from isolated trophoblast and inner cell mass. *J Embryol Exp Morphol* 1973;30:561–572.
180. Papaioannou VE. Lineage analysis of inner cell mass and trophectoderm using microsurgically reconstituted mouse blastocysts. *J Embryol Exp Morphol* 1982;68:199–209.
181. Johnson MH. Molecular differentiation of inside cells and inner cell masses isolated from the preimplantation mouse embryo. *J Embryol Exp Morphol* 1979;53:335–344.
182. Rossant J, Gardner RL, Alexandre HL. Investigation of the potency of cells from the postimplantation mouse embryo by blastocyst injections: a preliminary report. *J Embryol Exp Morphol* 1978;48:239–247.
183. Copp AJ. Interaction between inner cell mass and trophectoderm of the mouse blastocyst: II. fate of the polar trophectoderm. *J Embryol Exp Morphol* 1979;51:109–120.
184. Rossant J, Tamura-Lis W. Effect of culture conditions on diploid to giant-cell transformation in postimplantation mouse trophoblast. *J Embryol Exp Morphol* 1981;62:217–227.
185. Gardner RL, Rossant J. Investigation of the fate of 4.5 day post-coitum mouse inner cell mass cells by blastocyst injection. *J Embryol Exp Morphol* 1979;52:141–152.
186. Gardner RL. Investigation of cell lineage and differentiation in the extraembryonic endoderm of the mouse embryo. *J Embryol Exp Morphol* 1982;68:175–198.
187. Rossant J. Development of extraembryonic cell lineages in the mouse embryo. In: Rossant J, Pedersen RA, eds. *Experimental approaches to mammalian embryonic development.* New York: Cambridge University Press; 1986:97–120.
188. Cockroft DL, Gardner RL. Clonal analysis of the developmental

potential of 6th and 7th day visceral endoderm cells in the mouse. *Development* 1987;101:143–155.
189. Hogan BLM, Tilly R. Cell interactions and endoderm differentiation in cultured mouse embryos. *J Embryol Exp Morphol* 1981;62:379–394.
190. Lawson KA, Meneses JJ, Pedersen RA. Cell fate and cell lineage in the endoderm of the presomite mouse embryo, studied with an intracellular tracer. *Dev Biol* 1986;115:325–339.
191. Hogan BLM, Newman R. A scanning electron microscope study of the extraembryonic endoderm of the 8th-day mouse embryo. *Differentiation* 1984;26:138–143.
192. Hashimoto K, Nakatsuji N. Formation of the primitive streak and mesoderm cells in mouse embryos—detailed scanning electron microscopial study. *Dev Growth Diff* 1989;31:209–218.
193. Monk M, Harper MI. Sequential X chromosome inactivation coupled with cellular differentiation in early mouse embryos. *Nature* 1979;281:311–313.
194. Rossant J. Somatic cell lineages in mammalian chimeras. In: LeDouarin N, McLaren A, eds. *Chimeras in developmental biology.* Orlando, Florida: Academic Press; 1984:89–109.
195. Gardner RL, Lyon MF, Evans EP, Burtenshaw MD. Clonal analysis of X-chromosome inactivation and the origin of the germ line in the mouse embryo. *J Embryol Exp Morphol* 1985;88:349–363.
196. Gardner RL. Regeneration of endoderm from primitive ectoderm in the mouse embryo: fact or artifact? *J Embryol Exp Morphol* 1985;88:303–326.
197. Pedersen RA, Spindle AI, Wiley LM. Regeneration of endoderm by ectoderm isolated from mouse blastocysts. *Nature* 1977; 270:435–437.
198. Dziadek M. Cell differentiation in isolated inner cell masses of mouse blastocysts in vitro: onset of specific gene expression. *J Embryol Exp Morphol* 1979;53:367–379.
199. Atienza-Samols SB, Sherman MI. In vitro development of core cells of the inner cell mass of the mouse blastocyst: effects of conditioned medium. *J Exp Zool* 1979;208:67–71.
200. Svajger A, Levak-Svajger B, Skreb N. Rat Embryonic ectoderm as renal isograft. *J Embryol Exp Morphol* 1986;94:1–27.
201. Grobstein C. Intraocular growth and differentiation of the mouse embryonic shield implanted directly and following in vitro cultivation. *J Exp Zool* 1951;116:501–525.
202. Grobstein C. Intraocular growth and differentiation of clusters of mouse embryonic shields cultured with and without primitive endoderm and in the presence of possible inductors. *J Exp Zool* 119:355–380.
203. Levak-Svajger B, Svajger A. Differentiation of endodermal tissues in homografts of primitive ectoderm from two-layered rat embryonic shields. *Experientia* 1971;27:683–684.
204. Skreb N, Svajger A. Experimental teratomas in rats. In: Solter D, ed. *Teratomas and differentiation.* London: Academic Press; 1975:83–97.
205. Diwan SB, Stevens LC. Development of teratomas from ectoderm of mouse egg cylinders. *J Natl Cancer Inst* 1976; 57:937–942.
206. Beddington RSP. Histogenic and neoplastic potential of different regions of the mouse embryonic egg cylinder. *J Embryol Exp Morphol* 1983;75:189–204.
207. Levak-Svajger B, Svajger A. Investigation of the origin of definitive endoderm in the rat embryo. *J Embryol Exp Morphol* 1974;32:445–459.
208. Solter D, Damjanov I. Explanation of extraembryonic parts of 7d mouse egg cylinders. *Experientia* 1973;29:701–703.
209. Skreb N, Svajger A, Levak-Svajger A. Developmental potentialities of the germ layers. In: *Embryogenesis in mammals. Ciba Found Symp* 1976;40:27–39.
210. Svajger A, Levak-Svajger B, Kostovic-Knezevic L, Bradamante Z. Morphogenetic behaviour of the rat embryonic ectoderm as a renal homograft. *J Embryol Exp Morphol* [Suppl] 1981;65: 243–267.
211. Tam PPL. The histogenetic capacity of tissues in the caudal end of the embryonic axis of the mouse. *J Embryol Exp Morphol* 1984;82:253–266.
212. Snow MHL. Autonomous development of parts isolated from primitive-streak-stage mouse embryos: is development clonal? *J Embryol Exp Morphol* [Suppl] 1981;65:269–287.
213. Ozdzenski W. Observations on the origin of the primordial germ cells in the mouse. *Zool Pol* 1967;17:367–379.
214. Rosenquist. A radioautographic study of labeled grafts in the chick blastoderm: development from primitive-streak stages to stage 12. *Carnegie Inst Wash Contrib Embryol* 1966;38:71–110.
215. Beddington RSP. An autoradiographic analysis of the potency of embryonic ectoderm in the 8th day postimplantation mouse embryo. *J Embryol Exp Morphol* 1981;64:87–104.
216. Beddington RSP. An autoradiographic analysis of tissue potency in different regions of the embryonic ectoderm during gastrulation in the mouse. *J Embryol Exp Morphol* 1982;69:265–285.
217. Copp AJ, Roberts HM, Polani PE. Chimaerism of primordial germ cells in the early postimplantation mouse embryo following microsurgical grafting of posterior primitive streak cells in vitro. *J Embryol Exp Morphol* 1986;15:95–115.
218. Soriano P, Jaenisch R. Retroviruses as probes for mammalian development: allocation of cells to the somatic and germ cell lineages. *Cell* 1986;46:19–29.
219. Wilkie TM, Brinster RL, Palmiter RD. Germline and somatic mosaicism in transgenic mice. *Dev Biol* 1986;118:9–18.
220. Rossant J. Cell lineage analysis in mammalian embryogenesis. *Curr Top Dev Biol* 1987;23:115–146.
221. Tam PPL, Beddington RSP. The formation of mesodermal tissues in the mouse embryo during gastrulation and early organogenesis. *Development* 1987;99:109–126.
222. Tam PPL. Regionalisation of the mouse embryonic ectoderm: allocation of prospective ectodermal tissues during gastrulation. *Development* 1989;107:55–67.
223. Gardner RL. The relation between cell lineage and differentiation in the early mouse embryo. In: Gehring WJ, ed. *Genetic mosaics and cell differentiation,* Heidelberg: Springer Verlog; 1978:205–241.
224. Beddington RSP. The origin of the foetal tissues during gastrulation in the rodent. In: Johnson MH, ed. *Development in mammals.* Volume 5. Amsterdam: Elsevier; 1983:1–32.
225. Russell LB, Russell WL. Analysis of the changing radiation response of the developing mouse embryo. *J Cell Comp Physiol* [Suppl 1]: 1954;43:103–147.
226. Sanes JR, Rubenstein JLR, Nicolas JF. Use of a recombinant retrovirus to study post-implantation cell lineage in mouse embryos. *EMBO J* 1986;5:3133–3142.
227. Lawson KA, Meneses JJ, Pedersen RA. Cell fate and cell lineage in the endoderm of the presomite mouse embryo, studied with an intracellular tracer. *Dev Biol* 1986;115:325–339.
228. Lawson KA, Pedersen RA. Cell fate, morphogenetic movement and population kinetics of embryonic endoderm at the time of germ layer formation in the mouse. *Development* 1987;101: 627–652.
229. Lawson KA, Meneses JJ, Pedersen RA. Clonal analysis of epiblast fate during germ layer formation in the mouse embryo. *Development* 1991;113:891–911.
230. Lawson KA, Pedersen RA. Clonal analysis of cell fate during gastrulation and early neurulation in the mouse. In: *postimplantation development in the mouse. Ciba Found Symp* 1992; 165:3–26.
231. Lawson KA, Pedersen RA. Early mesoderm formation in the mouse embryo. In: Bellairs et al., eds. *Formation and differentiation of early embryonic mesoderm.* New York: Plenum Press; 1992:33–46.
232. Smith LJ. Embryonic axis orientation in the mouse and its correlation with blastocyst relationships to the uterus: I. relationship between 82 hours and $4\frac{1}{4}$ days. *J Embryol Exp Morphol* 1980;55:257–277.
233. Smith LJ. Embryonic axis orientation in the mouse and its correlation with blastocyst relationships to the uterus: II. relationships from $4\frac{1}{4}$ to $9\frac{1}{2}$ days. *J Embryol Exp Morphol* 1985;89:15–35.
234. Gardner RL, Meredith MR, Altman DG. Is the anterior-posterior axis of the fetus specified before implantation in the mouse? *J Exp Zool* 1992;264:437–443.
235. Yokoyama T, Copland NG, Jenkins NA, Montgomery CA, Elder FFB, Overbeek PA. Reversal of left-right asymmetry: a situs inversus mutation. *Science* 1993;260:679–682.
236. Serbedzija GN, Bronner-Fraser M, Fraser SE. Vital dye analysis of cranial neural crest cell migration in the mouse embryo. *Development* 1992;116:297–307.

237. Beddington RSP, Lawson KA. Clonal analysis of cell lineages. In: Copp AJ, Cockroft DL, eds. *Postimplantation mammalian embryos: a practical approach.* Oxford: Oxford University Press; 1990:267–292.
237a. Stern CD, Canning DR. Origin of cells giving rise to mesoderm and endoderm in chick embryo. *Nature* 1990;343:273–275.
238. Johnson MH, Handyside AH, Braude PR. Volume 2: control mechanisms in early mammalian development. In: Johnson MH ed. *Development in mammals.* Amsterdam: North-Holland; 1977:67–97.
239. Kaye PL. Metabolic aspects of the physiology of the preimplantation embryo. In: Rossant J, Pedersen RA, eds. *Experimental approaches to mammalian embryonic development.* Cambridge: Cambridge University Press; 1986:267–292.
240. Telford NA, Watson AJ, Schultz GA. Transition from maternal to embryonic control in early mammalian development: a comparison of several species. *Mol Reprod Dev* 1990;26:90–100.
241. Kidder GM. Genes involved in cleavage, compaction, and blastocyst formation. In: Gwatkin RBL, ed. *Genes in mammalian reproduction.* Wiley-Liss Inc; 1993:45–71.
242. Johnson MH. The molecular and cellular basis of preimplantation mouse development. *Biol Rev* 1981;56:463–498.
243. Schultz GA, Clough JR, Braude PR, Pelham HRB, Johnson MH. A reexamination of messenger RNA populations in the preimplantation mouse embryo. In: Glasser SR, Bullock DW, eds. *Cellular and molecular aspects of implantation.* New York: Plenum Publishing Co; 1981:137–154.
244. Schultz GA. Utilization of genetic information in the preimplantation mouse embryo. In: Rossant J, Pedersen RA, eds. *Experimental approaches to mammalian embryonic development.* New York: Cambridge University Press; 1986:239–265.
245. Kidder GM. The genetic program for preimplantation development. *Dev Genet* 1992;13:319–325.
246. Piko L, Clegg KB. Quantitative changes in total RNA, total poly(A), and ribosomes in early mouse embryos. *Dev Biol* 1982;89:362–378.
247. Clegg KB, Piko L. Poly(A) length, cytoplasmic adenylation, and synthesis of poly A+ RNA in early mouse embryos. *Dev Biol* 1983;95:331–341.
248. Giebelhaus DH, Weitlauf HM, Schultz GA. Actin mRNA content in normal and delayed implanting mouse embryos. *Dev Biol* 1985;107:407–413.
249. Graves RA, Marzluff WF, Giebelhaus DH, Schultz GA. Quantitative and qualitative changes in histone gene expression during early mouse development. In: *Proc Nat Acad Sci, USA.* 1985;82:5685–5689.
250. Taylor KD, Piko L. Patterns of mRNA prevalence and expression of B1 and B2 transcripts in early mouse embryos. *Development* 1987;101:877–892.
251. Braude PR, Pelham H, Flach G, Lobatto R. Posttranscriptional control in the early mouse embryo. *Nature* 1979;282:102–105.
252. van Blerkom J. The structural relation and posttranslational modification of stage-specific proteins synthesized during early preimplantation development in the mouse. In: *Proc Natl Acad Sci USA* 1981;78:7629–7633.
253. van Blerkom J. Post-translational regulation of early development in the mammal. In: Venizale C, ed. *Differentiation and proliferations.* New York: Van Nostrand Reinhold; 1985:67–86.
254. van Blerkom J, Runner MN. Mitochondrial reorganization during resumption of arrested meiosis in the mouse oocyte. *Am J Anat* 1984;171:335–355.
255. Howlett SK, Bolton VN. Sequence and regulation of morphological and molecular events during the first cell cycle of mouse embryogenesis. *J Embryol Exp Morphol* 1985;87:175–206.
256. Kaplan G, Jelinek WR, Bachvarova R. Repetitive sequence transcripts and U1 RNA in mouse oocytes and eggs. *Dev Biol* 1985;109:15–24.
257. Forbes DJ, Kornberg TB, Kirschner MW. Small nuclear RNA transcription and ribonucleoprotein assembly in early Xenopus development. *J Cell Biol* 1983;97:62–72.
258. Zeller R, Nyffenegger T, DeRobertis EM. Nucleocytoplasmic distribution of snRNPs and stockpiled snRNA-binding proteins during oogenesis and early development in Xenopus laevis. *Cell* 1983;32:425–434.
259. Ebert KM, Brinster RL. Rabbit alpha-globin messenger RNA translation by the mouse ovum. *J Embryol Exp Morphol* 1983;74:159–168.
260. Brinster RL, Wiebold JL, Brunner S. Protein metabolism in preimplanted mouse ova. *Dev Biol* 1976;51:215–224.
261. Merz EA, Brinster RL, Brunner S, Chen HY. Protein degradation during preimplantation development of the mouse. *J Reprod Fertil* 1981;61:415–418.
262. Bachvarova R, De Leon V. Stored and polysomal ribosomes of mouse ova. *Dev Biol* 1977;58:248–254.
263. Kidder GM, Conlon RA. Utilization of cytoplasmic poly(A)+ RNA for protein synthesis in preimplantation mouse embryos. *J Embryol Exp Morphol* 1985;89:223–234.
264. Brinster RL, Chen HY, Trumbauer ME, Avarbock MR. Translation of rabbit globin messenger RNA by the mouse ovum. *Nature* 1980;283:499–501.
265. Petzoldt U, Hoppe PC, Illmensee K. Protein synthesis in enucleated fertilized and unfertilized mouse eggs. *Roux's Arch Dev Biol* 1980;189:215–219.
266. Flach G, Johnson MH, Braude PR, Taylor RAS, Bolton VN. The transition from maternal to embryonic control in the 2-cell mouse embryo. *EMBO J* 1982;1:681–686.
267. Bolton VN, Oades PJ, Johnson MH. The relationship between cleavage, DNA replication, and gene expression in the mouse 2-cell embryo. *J Embryol Exp Morphol* 1984;79:139–163.
268. Bensaude O, Babinet C, Morange M, Jacob F. Heat shock proteins, first major products of zygotic gene activity in the mouse embryo. *Nature* 1983;305:331–333.
269. Clegg KB, Piko L. Quantitive aspects of RNA synthesis and polyadenylation in 1-cell and 2-cell mouse embryos. *J Embryol Exp Morphol* 1983;74:169–182.
270. Wudl L, Chapman V. The expression of beta glucuronidase during preimplantation development of mouse embryos. *Dev Biol* 1976;48:104–109.
271. Sawicki JA, Magnuson T, Epstein CJ. Evidence for expression of the paternal genome in the two-cell mouse embryo. *Nature* 1982:294:450–451.
272. Moore TF, Whittingham DG. Imprinting of phosphoribosyltransferases during preimplantation development of the mouse mutant, Hprtb-m3. *Development* 1992;115:1011–1016.
273. Braude PR, Bolton V, Moore S. Human gene expression first occurs between the four- and eight-cell stages of preimplantation development. *Nature* 1988;332:459–461.
274. Seshagiri PB, Bavister BD, Williamson JL, Aiken JM. Qualitative comparison of protein production at different stages of hamster preimplantation embryo development. *Cell Differ Dev* 1990;31:161–168.
275. Jarrell VL, Day BN, Prather RS. The transition from maternal to zygotic control of development occurs during the 4-cell stage in the domestic pig, *Sus scrofa:* quantitative and qualitative aspects of protein synthesis. *Biol Reprod* 1991;44:62–68.
276. Young RJ, Sweeney K. Adenylation and ADPribosylation in the mouse 1-cell embryo. *J Embryol Exp Morphol* 1979;49:139–152.
277. Young RJ. Appearance of 7-methylguanosine-5′ phosphate in the RNA of 1-cell embryos three hours after fertilization. *Biochem Biophys Res Commun* 1977;76:32–39.
278. Schultz GA, Clough JR, Johnson MH. Presence of cap structures in messenger RNA of mouse eggs. *J Embryol Exp Morphol* 1980;56:139–156.
279. Young RJ, Sweeny K, Bedford JM. Uridine and guanosine incorporation by the mouse one-cell embryo. *J Embryol Exp Morphol* 1978;44:133–148.
280. Ram PT, Schultz RM. Reporter gene expression in G2 of the one cell mouse embryo. *Devel Biol* 1993;156:552–556.
281. Braude PR. Control of protein synthesis during blastocyst formation in the mouse. *Dev Biol* 1979;68:440–452.
282. Braude PR. Time-dependent effects of alpha-amanitin on blastocyst formation in the mouse. *J Embryo Exp Morphol* 1979;52:193–202.
283. Kidder GM, McLachlin JR. Timing of transcription and protein synthesis underlying morphogenesis in preimplantation mouse embryos. *Dev Biol* 1985;112:265–275.
284. van Blerkom J, Barton SC, Johnson MH. Molecular differentiation in the preimplantation mouse embryo. *Nature* 1976; 259:319–321.

285. Handyside AH, Johnson MH. Temporal and spatial patterns of the synthesis of tissue-specific polypeptides in the preimplantation mouse embryo. *J Embryol Exp Morphol* 1978;44:191–199.
286. Howe CC, Gmur R, Solter D. Cytoplasmic and nuclear protein synthesis during in vitro differentiation of murine ICM and embryonal carcinoma cells. *Dev Biol* 1980;74:351–363.
287. Green MC. *Genetic variants and strains of the laboratory mouse.* Stuttgart: Gustav Fischer; 1981:8–278.
288. McLaren A. Genetics of the early mouse embryo. *Ann Rev Genet* 1976;10:361–388.
289. Magnuson T, Epstein CJ. Genetic control of very early mammalian development. *Biol Rev* 1981;56:369–408.
290. Magnuson T. Genetic abnormalities and early mammalian development. In: Johnson MH, ed. *Development in mammals.* Volume 5 Amsterdam: Elsevier; 1983:209–249.
291. Magnuson T. Mutations and chromosomal abnormalities: how are they useful for studying genetic control of early mammalian development? In: Rossant J, Pedersen RA, eds. *Experimental approaches to mammalian embryonic development.* New York: Cambridge University Press; 1986:437–474.
292. Magnuson T, Epstein CJ. 1987.
293. Pedersen RA, Spindle AI. Cellular and genetic analysis of mouse blastocyst development. In: Glasser SR, Bullock DW, eds. *Cellular and molecular aspects of implantation.* New York: Plenum Press; 1981:91–108.
294. Gluecksohn-Waelsch S. Genetic control of morphogenetic and biochemical differentiation: lethal albino deletions in the mouse. *Cell* 1979;16:225–237.
295. Magnuson T, Sharan SK, Holdener-Kenny B. Mutations affecting early development in the mouse. In: Bavister BD, ed. *Preimplantation embryo development.* New York: Springer-Verlag; 1993:131–143.
296. Bennett D. The T locus of the mouse. *Cell* 1975;6:441–454.
297. Bennett D. The T-complex in the mouse: an assessment after 50 years of study. *Harvey Lect* 1980;74:1–21.
298. Silvers LM. Mouse t haplotypes. *Ann Rev Genet* 1985;19: 179–208.
299. Lewis SE. Developmental analysis of lethal effects of homozygosity for the c25H deletion in the mouse. *Dev Biol* 1978;65: 553–557.
300. Nadijcka MD, Hillman N, Gluecksohn-Waelsch S. Ultrastructural studies of lethal c25H/c25H mouse embryos. *J Embryol Exp Morphol* 1979;52:1–11.
301. Hillman N, Hillman R. Ultrastructural studies of tw32/tw32 mouse embryos. *J Embryol Exp Morphol* 1975;33:685–695.
302. Wakasugi N. Studies on fertility of DDK mice: reciprocal crosses between DDK and C57BL/6J strains and experimental transplantation of the ovary. *J Reprod Fertil* 1973;33:283–291.
303. Paterson HF. In vivo and in vitro studies on the early embryonic lethal tail-short (Ts) in the mouse. *J Exp Zool* 1980;211:247–256.
304. Babiarz B. Deletion mapping of the T/t complex: evidence for a second region of critical embryonic genes. *Dev Biol* 1983; 95:342–351.
305. Papaiannou VE, Mardon H. Lethal nonagouti (ax): description of a second embryonic lethal at the agouti locus. *Dev Genet* 1983;4:21–29.
306. Papaioannou VE, Gardner RL. Investigation of the lethal yellow Ay/Ay embryo using mouse chimaeras. *J Embryol Exp Morphol* 1979;52:153–163.
307. Paterson HF. In vivo and in vitro studies on the early embryonic lethal oligosyndactylism (Os) in the mouse. *J Embryol Exp Morphol* 1979;52:115–125.
308. Magnuson T, Epstein CJ. Oligosyndactyly: a lethal mutation in the mouse that results in mitotic arrest very early in development. *Cell* 1984;38:823–833.
309. Spiegelman M, Artzt K, Bennett D. Embryological study of a T/t locus mutation (tw73) affecting trophectoderm development. *J Embryol Exp Morphol* 1976;36:373–381.
310. Babiarz B, Garrisi GJ, Bennett D. Genetic analysis of the tw73 haplotype of the mouse using deletion mutations: evidence for a parasitic lethal mutation. *Genet Res* 1982;39:111–120.
311. Guenet J, Condamine H, Gaillard J, Jacob F. twPa-1, twPa-2, twPa-3: three new t-haplotypes in the mouse. *Genet Res* 1980;36:211–217.
312. Lewis SE, Turchin HA, Gluecksohn-Waelsch S. The developmental analysis of an embryonic lethal (c6H) in the mouse. *J Embryol Exp Morphol* 1976;36:363–371.
313. Nadijcka MD, Hillman N. Autoradiographic studies of tn/tn mouse embryo. *J Embryol Exp Morphol* 1975;33:725–730.
314. Gluecksohn-Schoenheimer S. The effect of an early lethal (t0) in the house mouse. *Genetics* 1940;25:391–400.
315. Nusslein-Volhard C, Wieschaus E, Kluding H. Mutations affecting the pattern of the larval cuticle of Drosophila melanogaster, I. Zygotic loci on the second chromosome. *Roux's Arch Dev Biol* 1984;193:267–282.
316. Sternberg PW, Horvitz HR. The genetic control of cell lineage during nematode development. *Ann Rev Genet* 1984;18: 489–524.
317. Bode VC. Ethylnitrosourea mutagenesis and the isolation of mutant alleles for specific genes located in the *t*-region of mouse chromosome 17. *Genetics* 1984;108:457.
318. Pellicer A, Robins D, Wold B, Sweet R, Jackson J, Lowy I, Roberts JM, Sim GK, Silverstein S, Axel R. Altering genotype and phenotype by DNA mediated gene transfer. *Science* 1980;29: 1414–1422.
319. Jaenisch R. Infection of mouse blastocysts with SV40 DNA: normal development of the infected embryos and persistence of SV40 specific DNA sequences in the adult animals. *Cold Spring Harbor Symp Quant Biol* 1974;39:375–380.
320. Jaenisch R, Mintz B. Simian virus 40 DNA sequences in DNA of healthy adult mice derived from preimplantation blastocysts injected with viral DNA. In: *Proceedings of the National Academy of Science, USA* 1974;71:1250–1254.
321. Brinster RL, Chen HY, Trumbauer ME, Denear AW, Warren R, Palmiter RD. Somatic expression of herpes thymidine kinase in mice following injection of a fusion gene into eggs. *Cell* 1981;27:223–231.
322. Costantini F, Lacy E. Introduction of a rabbit beta-globin gene into the mouse germ line. *Nature* 1981;294:92–94.
323. Wagner EF, Stewart TA, Mintz B. The human beta-globin gene and a functional viral thymidine kinase gene in developing mice. In: *Proc Natl Acad Sci USA* 1981;78:5016–6020.
324. Wagner TE, Hoppe PC, Jollick JD, Scholl DR, Hodinka RL, Gault JB. Microinjection of a rabbit beta-globin gene into zygotes and its subsequent expression in adult mice and their offspring. *Proc Natl Acad Sci USA* 1981;78:6376–6380.
325. Hammer R, Pursel VG, Rexroad Jr CE, Wall RJ, Bolt DJ, Ebert KM, Palmiter RD, Brinster RL. Production of transgenic rabbits, sheep, and pigs by microinjection. *Nature* 1985;315:680–683.
326. Gordon JW, Ruddle FH. DNA mediated genetic transformation of mouse embryos and bone marrow—a review. *Gene* 1985;33:121–136.
327. Palmiter RD, Brinster RL. Transgenic mice. *Cell* 1985; 14:343–345.
328. Brinster RL, Chen HY, Trumbauer M, Yagle MK, Palmiter RD. Factors affecting the efficiency of introducing foreign DNA into mice by microinjecting eggs. *Proc Natl Acad Sci USA* 1985;82:4438–4442.
329. Wagner EF, Stewart CL. Integration and expression of genes introduced into mouse embryos. In: Rossant J, Pedersen RA, eds. *Experimental approaches to mammalian embryonic development.* Cambridge University Press; 1986:509–549.
330. Brinster RL, Palmiter RD. Introduction of genes into the germ line of animals. *Harvey Lect* 1985;80:1–38.
331. Pedersen RA, McLaren A, First NL, eds. *Animal applications of research in mammalian development.* Cold Spring Harbor, NY: Cold Spring Harbor Laboratory Press; 1991.
331a. Pinkert CA, ed. *Methods in transgenic animal technology.* San Diego, CA: Academic Press Inc; 1993.
332. Meisler MH. Insertional mutation of 'classical' and novel genes in transgenic mice. *Trends Genet* 1992;8:341–344.
333. Jenkins NA, Copeland NG, Taylor BA, Lee BK. Dilute (d) coat colour mutation of DBA/2J mice is associated with the site of integration of an ecotropic MuLV genome. *Nature* 1981;293:370–374.
334. Copeland NG, Hutchison KW, Jenkins NA. Excision of the DBA ecotropic provirus in dilute coatcolor revertants of mice occurs by homologous recombination involving the viral LTRs. *Cell* 1983;33:379–387.
335. Mercer JA, et al. Novel myosin heavy chain encoded by murine dilute coat colour locus. *Nature* 1991;349:709–713.

336. Stoye JP, et al. Role of endogenous retroviruses as mutagens: The hairless mutation of mice. *Cell* 1988;54:383–391.
337. Copeland NG, Jenkins NA, Lee BK. Association of the lethal yellow (AY) coat-color mutation with an ecotropic murine leukemia virus genome. In: *Proc Natl Acad Sci, USA* 1983;80: 247–249.
338. Bultman SJ, Michaud EJ, Woychik RP. Molecular characterization of the mouse agouti locus. *Cell* 1992;71:1195–2204.
339. Miller MW, Duhl DM, Vrieling H, Cordes SP, Ollman MM, Winkes BM, Barsh GS. Cloning of the mouse agouti gene predicts a secreted protein ubiquitously expressed in mice carrying the lethal yellow mutation. *Genes and Development* 1993;7: 454–467.
340. Silvers LM, Uman J, Danska J, Garrels JI. A diversified set of testicular cell proteins specified by genes within the mouse t complex. *Cell* 1983;35:35–45.
341. Soriano P, Cone RD, Mulligan RC, Jaenisch R. Tissue-specific and ecotopic expression of genes introduced into transgenic mice by retroviruses. *Science* 1986;234:1409–1413.
342. Jaenisch R, Harbers K, Schnieke A, Lohler J, Chumakov I, Jahner D, Grotkopp D, Hoffman E. Germline integration of Moloney murine leukemia virus at the Mov 13 locus leads to recessive lethal mutation and early embryonic death. *Cell* 1983;32:209–216.
343. Schnieke A, Harbers K, Jaenisch R. Embryonic lethal mutation in mice induced by retrovirus insertion into the alphal(I) collagen gene. *Nature* 1983;304:315–320.
344. Harbers K, Kuehn M, Delius H, Jaenisch R. Insertion of retrovirus into the first intron of alpha1(I) collagen gene leads to embryonic lethal mutation in mice. In: *Proceedings of the National Academy of Science, USA* 1984;81:1504–1508.
345. Breindle M, Harbers K, Jaenisch R. Retrovirus-induced lethal mutation in collagen 1 gene is associated with altered chromatin structure. *Cell* 1984;38:916.
346. Lohler J, Timpl R, Jaenisch R. Embryonic lethal mutation in mouse collagen 1 gene causes repture of blood vessels and is associated with erythropoietic and mesenchymal cell death. *Cell* 1984;38:597–607.
347. Kratochwil K, Dziadek M, Lohler J, Harbers K, Jaenisch R. Normal epithelial branching morphogenesis in the absence of collagen 1. *Dev Biol* 1986;117:596–606.
348. Reik W, Weiher H, Jaenisch R. Replication competent Moloney leukemia virus carrying a bacterial suppressor tRNA gene: selective cloning of proviral and flanking host sequences. *Proc Natl Acad Sci USA* 1985;82:1141–1145.
349. Gridley T, Gray DA, Orr-weaver T, Soriano P, Barton DE, Franke U, Jaenisch R. Molecular analysis of the *mov*34 mutation: transcript disrupted by proviral integration in mice is conserved in *Drosophila*. *Development* 1990;109:235–242.
350. Wagner EF, Covarrubias L, Stewart TA, Mintz B. Prenatal lethalities in mice homozygous for human growth hormone gene sequences integrated in the germ line. *Cell* 1983;35:647–655.
351. Palmiter RD, Wilkie TM, Chen HY, Brinster RL. Transmission distortion and mosaicism in an unusual transgenic mouse pedigree. *Cell* 1984;36:869–877.
352. Mahon KA, Overbeek PA, Westphal H. Dominant prenatal lethality in a transgenic mouse line is associated with a chromosomal translocation. *J Cell Biol* 1986;103:146a.
353. Woychik RP, Stewart TA, Davis LG, D'Eustachio P, Leder P. An inherited limb deformity created by insertional mutagenesis in a transgenic mouse. *Nature* 1985;318:36–40.
354. Cheng SS, Constantini F. Morula decompaction (mdn), a preimplantation recessive lethal defect in a transgenic mouse line. *Dev Biol* 1993;156:265–277.
355. Mark WH, Signorelli K, Lacy E. An insertional mutation in a transgenic mouse line results in developmental arrest at day 5 of gestation. *Cold Spring Harbor Symposium Quantitative Biology* 1985;50:453–463.
356. Robertson EJ. Using embryonic stem cells to introduce mutations into mouse germ line. *Biol Reprod* 1991;44:238–245.
357. Tan SS. Liver-specific and position-specific expression of a retinol-binding protein-lacZ fusion gene (RBP-lacZ) in transgenic mice. *Dev Biol* 1991;146:24–37.
358. Palmiter RD, Chen HY, Brinster RL. Differential regulation of metallothionein-thymidine kinase fusion gene in transgenic mice and their offspring. *Cell* 1982;29:701–710.
359. Pursel VG, Pinkert CA, Miller KF, Bolt DJ, Campbell RG, Palmiter RD, Brinster RL, Hammer RE. Genetic engineering of livestock. *Science* 1989;244:1281–1288.
360. Stevens ME, Meneses JJ, Pedersen RA. Expression of a mouse metallothionein-*Escherichia coli* β-galactosidase fusion gene (MT-βgal) in early mouse embryos. *Exp Cell Res* 1989; 183:319–325.
360a. Nielsen LL, Pedersen RA. *Drosophila* alcohol dehydrogenase: a novel reporter gene for use in mammalian embryos. *J Exp Zool* 1991;257:128–133.
361. Kothary R, Clapoff S, Darling S, Perry MD, Moran LA, Rossant J. Inducible expression of an hsp68-lacZ hybrid gene in transgenic mice. *Development* 1989;105:707–714.
362. Overbeek P. Factors affecting transgenic animal production efficiencies. In: Pinkert CA, ed. *Methods in transgenic animal technology*. San Diego: Academic Press (in press). 1993.
363. Martinez-Salas E, Linney E, Hassell J, DePamphilis ML. The need for enhancers in gene expression first appears during mouse development with formation of the zygotic nucleus. *Genes Dev* 1989;10:1493–1506.
364. Bonnerot C, Vernet M, Grimber G, Briand P, Nicolas JF. Transcriptional selectivity in early mouse embryos: a qualitative study. *Nucl Acids Res* 1991;25:7251–7257.
365. Rossant J, Zirngibl R, Cado D, Shago M, Giguere V. Expression of a retinoic acid response element-hsp lacZ transgene defines specific domains of transcriptional activity during mouse embryogenesis. *Genes Dev* 1991;5:1333–1344.
366. Balkan W, Colbert M, Bock C, Linney E. Transgenic indicator mice for studying activated retinoic acid receptors during development. *Proc Natl Acad Sci USA*. 1992;89:3347–3351.
367. Breitman ML, Bryce DM, Giddens E, Clapoff S, Goring D, Tsui LC, Klintworth GK, Bernstein A. Analysis of lens cell fate and eye morphogenesis in transgenic mice ablated for cells of the lens lineage. *Development* 1989;106:457–463.
368. Palmiter RL, Behringer RR, Quaife CJ, Maxwell F, Maxwell IH, Brinster RL. Cell lineage ablation in transgenic mice by cell-specific expression of a toxin gene. *Cell* 1987;50:435–443.
369. Bernstein A, Breitman M. Genetic ablation in transgenic mice. *Mol Biol Med* 1989;6:523–530.
370. Bradley A, Evans M, Kaufman MH, Robertson E. Formation of germ line chimaeras from embryo derived teratocarcinoma cell lines. *Nature* 1984;309:255–256.
371. Stewart CL, Vanek M, Wagner EF. Expression of foreign genes from retroviral vectors in mouse teratocarcinoma chimaeras. *EMBO J* 1985;4:3701–3709.
372. Gossler A, Doetschman T, Korn R, Serfling E, Kemler R. Transgenesis via blastocyst-derived embryonic stem cell lines. *Proc Natl Acad Sci USA*. 1986;83:9065–9069.
373. Robertson E, Bradley A, Kuehn M, Evans M. Germ-line transmission of genes introduced into cultured pluripotential cells by retroviral vector. *Nature* 1986;323:445–448.
374. Thomas KR, Capecchi MR. Site-directed mutagenesis by gene targeting in mouse embryo-derived stem cells. *Cell* 1987;51: 503–512.
375. Doetschman T, Gregg RG, Maeda N, Hooper ML, Melton DW, Thompson S, Smithies O. Targeted correction of mutant HPRT gene in mouse embryonic stem cells. *Nature* 1987;330:576–578.
376. Doetschman T, Williams P, Maeda N. Establishment of hamster blastocyst-derived embryonic stem (ES) cells. *Dev Biol* 1988;127: 224–227.
377. Doetschman T, Maeda N, Smithies O. Targeted mutation of the HprT hene in mouse embryonic stem cells. *Proc Natl Acad Sci USA*. 1988;85:8583–8587.
378. Mansour SL, Thomas KR, Capecchi MR. Disruption of the proto-oncogene int-2 in mouse embryo-derived stem cells: a general strategy for targeting mutations to non-selectable genes. *Nature* 1988;336:348–352.
379. Zimmer A, Gruss P. Production of chimaeric mice containing embryonic stem (ES) cells carrying a homeobox Hox 1.1 allele mutated homologous recombination. *Nature* 1989;338:150–153.
380. Joyner AL, Skarnes WC, Rossant J. Production of a mutation in mouse En-2 gene by homologous recombination in embryonic stem cells. *Nature* 1989;338:153–156.

381. Baribault H, Kemler R. Embryonic stem cell culture and gene targeting in transgenic mice. *Mol Biol Med* 1989;6:481–492.
382. Mansour SL. Gene targeting in murine embryonic stem cells: introduction of specific alterations into the mammalian genome. *GATA* 1990;7:219–227.
383. Rossant J, Joyner AL. Towards molecular-genetic analysis of mammalian development. *Trends Genet* 1989;5:277–283.
384. Yamamura K, Wakasugi S. Manipulating the mouse genome: new approaches for the dissection of mouse development. *Dev Growth Diff* 1991;32:93–100.
385. Rossant J, Hopkins N. Of fin and fur: mutational analysis of vertebrate embryonic development. *Genes Dev* 1992;6:1–13.
386. Stewart CL. Prospects for the establishment of embryonic stem cells and genetic manipulation of domestic animals. In: Pedersen RA, McLaren A, First NL, eds. *Animal Applications of Research in Mammalian Development.* Cold Spring Harbor, NY: Cold Spring Harbor Laboratory Press, 1991;267–283.
387. Beddington R, Constantini F, Lacy E. *Manipulating the mouse embryo.* 2nd ed. New York: Cold Spring Harbor Laboratory Press; 1993.
388. Methods in Enzymology Volume, 1993.
389. Gossler A, Joyner AL, Rossant J, Skarnes WC. Mouse embryonic stem cells and reporter constructs to detect developmentally regulated genes. *Science* 1989;244:463–465.
390. Friedrich G, Soriano P. Promoter traps in embryonic stem cells: a genetic screen to identify and mutate developmental genes in mice. *Genes Dev* 1991;5:1513–1523.
391. Skarnes WC, Auerbach BA, Joyner AL. A gene trap approach in embryonic stem cells: the *lac*Z reporter is activated by splicing, reflects endogenous gene expression, and is mutagenic in mice. *Genes Dev* 1992;6:903–918.
392. Hill DP, Wurst W. Gene and enhancer trapping: mutagenic strategies for developmental studies. *Curr Top Dev Biol* 1993;28: 181–206.
393. Strauss WM, Dausman J, Johnson C, Lawrence J, Jaenisch R. Germline transmission of a yeast artificial chromosome spanning the murine COL1A1 (α_1(I) Collagen) locus. *Science* 1993; [in press].
394. Lamb BT, Sisodia SS, Lawler AM, Slunt HH, Kitt CA, Kearns WG, Pearson PL, Price DL, Gearhart JD. The introduction and expression of the 400 kb human genomic sequence of the amyloid precursor protein gene in embryonic stem cells and transgenic mice. *Nature Genet* 1993; [in press].
395. Dolci S, Williams DE, Ernst MK, Resnick JL, Brannan CI, Lock LF, Lyman SD, Boswell HS, Donovan PJ. Requirement for mast cell growth factor for primordial germ cell survival in culture. *Nature* 1991;352:809–811.
396. Godin I, Deed R, Cooke J, Zsebo K, Dexter M, Wylie CC. Effects of the steel gene product on mouse primordial germ cells in culture. *Nature* 1991;352:807–809.
397. Matsui Y, Zsebo K, Hogan BLM. Derivation of pluripotential embryonic stem cells from murine primordial germ cells in culture. *Cell* 1992;70:841–847.
398. Izant JG, Weintraub H. Inhibition of thymidine kinase gene expression by anti-sense RNA: a molecular approach to genetic analysis. *Cell* 1984;36:1007–1015.
399. Melton D. Injected anti-sense RNAs specifically block messenger-RNA translation in vivo. *Proc Natl Acad Sci USA* 1985;82: 144–148.
400. Melton DA, Rebogliati MR. Anti-sense RNA injections in fertilized eggs as a test for the function of localized mRNAs. *J Embryol Exp Morphol* [Suppl] 1986;97:211–221.
401. Bevilacqua A, Erickson RP, Heiber V. Antisense RNA inhibits endogenous gene expression in mouse preimplantation embryos: lack of double-stranded RNA "melting" activity. *Proc Natl Acad Sci USA* 1988;85:831–835.
402. Brice EC, Wu JW, Muraro R, Adamson ED, Wiley LM. Modulation of mouse preimplantation development by epidermal growth factor receptor antibodies, antisense RNA and deoxyoligonucleotides. *Dev Genet* 1993;[in press].
403. Rappolee DA, Sturm KS, Behrendtsen O, Schultz GA, Pedersen RA, Werb Z. Insulin-like growth factor II acts through an endogenous growth pathway regulated by imprinting in early mouse embryos. *Genes Dev* 1992;6:939–952.
404. Kaufman MH, Gardner RL. Diploid and haploid mouse parthenogenetic development following in vitro activation and embryo transfer. *J Embryol Exp Morphol* 1974;31:635–642.
405. Kaufman MH, Sachs L. The early development of haploid and aneuploid parthenogenetic embryos. *J Embryol Exp Morphol* 1975;34:645–655.
406. Modlinski JA. Haploid mouse embryos obtained by microsurgical removal of one pronucleus. *J Embryol Exp Morphol* 1975;33:897–905.
407. Tarkowski AK. In vitro development of haploid mouse embryos produced by bisection of one-cell fertilized eggs. *J Embryol Exp Morphol* 1977;38:187–202.
408. Tarkowski AK, Rossant J. Haploid mouse blastocysts developed from bissected zygotes. *Nature* 1976;259:663–665.
409. Luthardt FW. Cytogenetic analysis of oocytes and early preimplantation embryos from XO mice. *Dev Biol* 1976;54:73–81.
410. Burgoyne PS, Biggers JD. The consequences of X-dosage deficiency in the germ line: impared development in vitro of preimplantation embryos from XO mice. *Dev Biol* 1976;51:109–117.
411. Epstein CJ. *The consequences of chromosome imbalance: principles, mechanisms, models.* New York: Cambridge University Press; 1986.
412. Baranov VS. Chromosomal control of early embryonic development in mice: I. experiments on embryos with autosomal monosomy. *Genetica* 1983;61:165–177.
413. Magnuson T, Debrot S, Dimpfl J, Zweig A, Zamora T, Epstein CJ. The early lethality of autosomal monosomy in the mouse. *J Exp Zool* 1985;236:353–360.
414. Epstein CJ, Smith SA, Zamora T, Sawicki JA, Magnuson TR, Cox DR. Production of viable adult trisomy 17 ↔ diploid mouse chimeras. *Proc Natl Acad Sci USA* 1982;79:4376–4380.
415. Cox DR, Smith SA, Epstein LB, Epstein CJ. Mouse trisomy 16 as an animal model of human trisomy 21 (Down syndrome): production of viable trisomy 16 ↔ diploid mouse chimeras. *Dev Biol* 1984;101:416–424.
416. Epstein CJ, Smith SA, Cox DR. Production and properties of mouse trisomy 15 ↔ diploid chimeras. *Dev Genet* 1984;4: 159–165.
417. Boue J, Boue A, Lazar P. Retrospective and prospective epidemiological studies of 1500 karyotyped spontaneous human abortions. *Teratology* 1975;12:11–26.
418. Hassold TJ, Matsuyama A, Newlands JM, Matsuura JS, Jacobs PA, Manuel B, Tsuei J. A cytogenetic study of spontaneous abortions in Hawaii. *Ann Hum Genet* 1978;41:443–454.
419. Markert CL. Parthenogenesis, homozygosity, and cloning in mammals. *J Hered* 1982;73:390–397.
420. Cattanach BM, Kirk M. Differential activity of maternally and paternally derived chromosome regions in mice. *Nature* 1985;315:496–498.
421. Cattanach BM. Parental origin effects in mice. *J Embryol Exp Morphol* [Suppl] 1986;97:137–150.
422. Searle AG, Beechey CV. Complementation studies with mouse translocations. *Cytogenet Cell Genet* 1978;20:282–303.
423. Searle AG, Beechey CV. Non-complementation phenomena and their bearing on non-disjunctional effects. In: Dellarco VL, Voytek PE, Hollaender A, eds. *Aneuploidy, aetiology and mechanisms.* New York: Plenum Press; 1985:363–376.
424. Cattanach BM, Beechey CV. Autosomal and X-chromosome imprinting. *Development* [Suppl] 1990:63–72.
425. Crouse HV. The controlling element in sex chromosome behaviour in *Sciara. Genetics* 1960;45:1429–1443.
426. Lyon MF. Gene action in the X-chromosome of the mouse (*Mus musculus L.*). *Nature* 1961;190:372–373.
427. West JD. X-chromosome expression during mouse embryogenesis. In: Crosignani PG, Rubin BW, eds. *Genetic control of gamete production and function.* New York: Academic Press; 1982:49–91.
428. Chapman VM. X-chromosome regulation in oogenesis and early mammalian development. In: Rossant J, Pedersen RA, eds. *Experimental approaches to mammalian embryonic development.* New York: Cambridge University Press; 1986:365–398.
428a. Grant SG, Chapman VM. Mechanisms of X-chromosome regulation. *Ann Rev Genet* 1988;22:199–233.
429. Epstein CJ. Expression of the mammalian X chromosome before and after fertilization. *Science* 1972;175:1467–1468.
430. Migeon BR, Jelalian K. Evidence for two active X chromosomes

in germ cells of female before meiotic entry. *Nature* 1977;269: 242–243.
431. Kratzer PG, Chapman VM. X chromosome reactivation in oocytes of Mus caroli. *Proc Natl Acad Sci USA* 1981;78:3093–3097.
432. Lifschytz E, Lindsley DL. Sex chromosome activation during spermatogenesis. *Genetics* 1974;78:323–331.
433. Kramer JM, Erickson RP. Developmental program of PGK-1 and PGK-2 isozymes in spermatogenic cells of the mouse: specific activities and rates of synthesis. *Dev Biol* 1981;87:37–45.
434. Mukherjee AB. Cell cycle analysis and X-chromosome inactivation in the developing mouse. In: *Proc Natl Acad Sci USA* 1976;73:1608–1611.
435. Takagi N. Differentiation of X-chromosomes in early female mouse embryos. *Exp Cell Res* 1974;86:127–135.
436. Adler DA, West JD, Chapman VM. Expression of alpha-galactosidase in preimplantation mouse embryos: implications for X-chromosome inactivation. *Nature* 1977;267:838–839.
437. Monk M, Kathuria H. Dosage compensation for an X-linked gene in pre-implantation mouse embryos. *Nature* 1977;270: 599–601.
438. Monk M, Harper M. X-chromosome activity in preimplantation mouse embryos from XX and XO mothers. *J Embryo Exp Morphol* 1978;46:53–64.
439. Kratzer PG, Gartler SM. HGPRT activity changes in preimplantation mouse embryos. *Nature* 1978;274:503–504.
440. Epstein CJ, Smith S, Travis B, Tucker G. Both X-chromosomes function before visible X-chromosome inactivation in female mouse embryos. *Nature* 1978;274:500–502.
441. Epstein CJ, Travis B, Tucker G, Smith S. The direct demonstration of an X-chromosome dosage effect prior to inactivation. In: Russell LB, ed. *Genetic mosaics and chimeras in mammals.* New York: Plenum Press; 1978;261–267.
442. Gardner RL, Lyon MF. X-chromosome inactivation studies by injection of a single cell into the mouse blastocyst. *Nature* 1971;231:385–386.
443. Kratzer PG, Gartler SM. Hypoxanthine guanine phosphoribosyl transferase expression in early mouse development. In: Russell LB, ed. *Genetic mosaics and chimeras in mammals.* New York: Plenum Press; 1978:247–260.
444. Takagi N, Sugawara O, Sasaki M. Regional and temporal changes in the pattern of X-chromosome replication during the early post-implantation development of the female mouse. *Chromosoma* (Berl) 1982;85:275–286.
445. Sugawara O, Takagi N, Sasaki M. Allocyclic early replicating X chromosome in mice: genetic inactivity and shift into a later replication in early embryogenesis. *Chromosoma* (Berl) 1983;88: 133–138.
446. Monk M, Harper MI. Sequential X-chromosome inactivation coupled with cellular differentiation in early mouse embryos. *Nature* 1979;281:311–313.
447. West JD, Frels WI, Chapman VM, Papaioannou VE. Preferential expression of the maternally derived X-chromosome in the mouse yolk sac. *Cell* 1977;12:873–882.
448. Frels WI, Rossant J, Chapman VM. Maternal X chromosome expression in mouse chorionic ectoderm. *Dev Genet* 1979;1: 123–132.
449. Frels WI, Chapman V. Expression of the maternally derived X chromosome in the mural trophoblast of the mouse. *J Embryol Exp Morphol* 1980;56:179–190.
450. Papaioannou VE, West DD, Bucher T, Linke IM. Non-random X-chromosome expression early in mouse development. *Dev Genet* 1981;2:305–315.
451. McMahon A, Monk M. X-chromosome activity in female mouse embryos heterozygous for Pgk-1 and Searle's translocation, T (X;16)16H. *Genet Res* (Camb) 1983;41:69–83.
452. Van de Berg JL, Johnston PG, Cooper DW, Robinson ES. X-chromosome inactivation and evolution in marsupials and other mammals. In: Rattazzi MC, Scandalios JG, eds. *Isozymes: current topics in biological and medical research.* New York: Alan R Liss. 1983:201–218. (*Gene expression and development;* vol 9).
453. Gartler SM, Riggs AD. Mammalian X chromosome inactivation. *Ann Rev Genet* 1983;17:155–190.
454. Lyon MF. Mechanisms and evolutionary origins of variable X-chromosome activity in mammals. *Proc R Soc Lond* 1974;187B: 243–268.
455. Brown CJ, Ballabio A, Rupert JL, Lafreniere RG, Grompe M, Tonlorenzi R, Willard HF. A gene from the region of the human X inactivation centre is expressed exclusively from the inactive X chromosome. *Nature* 1991;349:38–44.
456. Borsani G, Tonlorenzi R, Simmler MC, Dandolo L, Arnau D, Capra V, Grompe M, Pizzuti A, Munzy D, Lawrence C, Willard HF, Avner P, Ballabio A. Characterization of a murine gene expressed from the inactive X-chromosome. *Nature* 1991; 351:325–329.
457. Brookdorff N, Ashworth A, Kay GF, Cooper P, Smith S, McCabe VM, Norris DP, Penny GD, Patel D, Rastan S. Conservation of position and exclusive expression of mouse *Xist* from the inactive X-chromosome. *Nature* 1991;351:329–331.
458. Salido EC, Yen PH, Mohandas TK, Shapiro LJ. Expression of the X-inactive associated gene *XIST* during spermatogenesis. *Nature Genet* 1992;2:196–199.
459. McCarrey JR, Dilworth DD. Expression of *Xist* in mouse germ cells correlates with X-chromosome inactivation. *Nature Genet* 1992;2:200.
460. Richler C, Soreq H, Wahrman J. X-inactivation in mammalian testis is correlated with inactive X-specific transcription. *Nature Genet* 1992;2:192–195.
461. Kay GF, Penny GD, Patel D, Ashworth A, Brockdorff N, Rastan S. Expression of *Xist* during mouse development suggests a role in the initiation of X-chromosome inactivation. *Cell* 1993; 72:171–182.
462. Brookdorff N, Ashworth A, Kay GF, McCabe VM, Norris DP, Cooper P, Swift S, Rastan S. The product of the mouse *Xist* gene is a 15 kb inactive X-specific transcript containing no conserved ORF and located in the nucleus. *Cell* 1992;71:515–526.
463. Lyon MF, Glenister PH. Factors affecting the observed number of young resulting from adjacent-2 disjunction in mice carrying a translocation. *Genet Res* 1977;29:83–92.
464. Solter D. Differential imprinting and expression of maternal and paternal genomes. *Ann Rev Genet* 1988;22:127–146.
465. Surani MA. Genomic imprinting: developmental significance and molecular mechanism. *Curr Opin Genet Dev* 1991;2: 241–246.
466. Beatty RA. Parthenogenesis in vertebrates. In: Metz RB, Monroy A, eds. *Fertilization,* Volume 1. New York: Academic Press; 1967.
467. Mittwoch U. Parthenogenesis. *J Med Genet* 1978;15:165–181.
468. Kaufman MH. *Early mammalian development: parthenogenetic studies.* London: Cambridge University Press; 1983.
469. Markert CL, Seidel GE Jr. Parthenogenesis, identical twins and cloning in mammals. In: Brackett BG, Seidel GE Jr, Seidel SM, eds. *New technologies in animal breeding.* New York: Academic Press; 1981:181–200.
470. Modlinski JA. The fate of inner cell mass and trophectoderm nuclei transplanted to fertilized mouse eggs. *Nature* 1981;292: 342–343.
471. Illmensee K, Hoppe PC. Nuclear transplantation in Mus musculus: developmental potential of nuclei from preimplantation embryos. *Cell* 1981;23:9–18.
472. Hoppe PC, Illmensee K. Full term development after transplantation of parthenogenetic embryonic nuclei into fertilized mouse eggs. In: *Proceedings of the National Academy of Science, USA.* 1982;79:1912–1916.
473. Surani MAH. Evidences and consequences of differences between maternal and paternal genomes during embryogenesis in the mouse. In: Rossant J, Pedersen RA, eds. *Experimental approaches to mammalian embryonic development.* New York: Cambridge University Press; 1986:401–435.
474. Pedersen RA, Sturm KS, Rappolee DA, Werb Z. Effects of imprinting on early development of mouse embryos. In: Bavister BD, ed. *Proceedings of the Serono Symposium on Preimplantation Embryo Development, August 15–18.* Boston, Massachusetts, 1993:212–226.
475. Surani MAH, Reik W, Norris ML, Barton SC. Influence of germline modifications of homologous chromosomes on mouse development. *J Embryol Exp Morphol* [Suppl] 1986;97:123–136.
476. Graham CF. The production of parthenogenetic mammalian

embryos and their use in biological research. *Biol Rev* 1974;49: 399–422.
477. Kaufman MH, Barton SC, Surani MAH. Normal post-implantation development of mouse parthenogenetic embryos to the forelimb bud stage. *Nature* (Lond) 1977;265:53–55.
478. Stevens LC. Teratocarcinogenesis and spontaneous parthenogenesis in mice. In: Markert CL, Papaconstantinou J, eds. *Developmental biology of reproduction.* New York: Academic Press; 1975:13–106.
479. Varmuza SL. Teratogenic effects of parthenogenetic cells from LTXBO mice, a strain which develops ovarian teratomas at high frequency. *Roux's Arch Dev Biol* 1992;201:142–148.
480. Stevens L. The origin and development of testicular, ovarian and embryo-derived teratomas. In: Silver L, Martin G, Strickland S, eds. *Teratocarcinoma stem cells.* Cold Spring Harbor, NY: Cold Spring Harbor Laboratory; 1983:23–36.
481. Stevens LC, Varnum DS, Eicher EM. Viable chimaeras produced from normal and parthenogenetic mouse embryos. *Nature* (Lond) 1977;269:515.
482. Surani MAH, Barton SC, Kaufman MH. Development to term of chimaeras between diploid parthenogenetic and fertilized embryos. *Nature* (Lond) 1977;270:601–602.
483. Markert CL, Petters RM. Homozygous mouse embryos produced by microsurgery. *J Exp Zool* 1977;201:295–302.
484. Hoppe PC, Illmensee K. Microsurgically produced homozygous-diploid uniparental mice. *Proc Natl Acad Sci USA* 1977;74: 5657–5661.
485. Modlinski JA. Preimplantation development of microsurgically obtained haploid and homozygous diploid mouse embryos and effects of pretreatment with cytochalasin B on enucleated eggs. *J Exp Embryol Morphol* 1980;60:153–161.
486. Anderegg C, Markert CL. Successful rescue of microsurgically produced homozygous, uniparental mouse embryos via production of aggregation chimeras. *Proc Natl Acad Sci USA* 1986;83: 6509–6513.
487. McGrath J, Solter D. Nuclear transplantation in the mouse embryo by microsurgery and cell fusion. *Science* 1983;220: 1300–1303.
488. Mann JR, Lovell-Badge RH. Inviability of parthenogenones determined by pronuclei, not egg cytoplasm. *Nature* (Lond) 1984;310:66–67.
489. McGrath J, Solter D. Completion of mouse embryogenesis requires both maternal and paternal genomes. *Cell* 1984;37: 179–183.
490. Surani MAH, Barton SC, Norris ML. Development of reconstituted mouse eggs suggests imprinting of the genome during gametogenesis. *Nature* (Lond) 1984;308:548–550.
491. Varmuza S, Mann M, Rogers I. Site of action of imprinted genes revealed by phenotypic analysis of parthenogenetic embryos. *Dev Genet* 1992;[in press].
492. Clarke HJ, Varmuza S, Prideaux VR, Rossant J. The developmental potential of parthenogenetically derived cells in chimeric mouse embryos: implications for action of imprinted genes. *Development* 1988;104:175–182.
493. Thomson J, Solter D. The developmental fate of androgenetic, parthenogenetic, and gynogenetic cells in chimeric gastrulating mouse embryos. *Genes Dev* 1988;2:1344–1351.
494. Thomson J, Solter D. Chimeras between parthenogenetic or androgenetic blastomeres and normal embryos: allocation to the inner cell mass and trophectoderm. *Dev Biol* 1988;131:580–583.
495. Nagy A, Sars M, Markulla M. Systematic non uniform distribution of parthenogenetic cells in adult mouse chimeras. *Development* 1989;106:321–324.
496. Fundele R, Norris M, Barton S, Fehlau M, Howlett S, Mills W, Surani MA. Temporal and spatial selection against parthenogenetic cells during development of fetal chimeras. *Development* 1990;108:203–211.
497. Evans M, Bradley A, Robertson EJ. EK contribution to chimeric mice: from tissue culture to sperm. In: Jaenisch R, Costantini F, eds. *Banbury Report 20. Genetic manipulation of the early mammalian embryo.* A Cold Spring Harbor, NY: Cold Spring Harbor Laboratory Press, 1985;93.
498. Beddington RS, Robertson EJ. An assessment of the developmental potential of embryonic stem cells in the midgestation mouse embryo. *Development* 1989;105:733–737.
499. Barton SC, Surani MAH, Norris ML. Role of paternal and maternal genomes in mouse development. *Nature* (Lond) 1984;311: 374–376.
500. Barton SC, Adams CA, Norris ML, Surani MAH. Development of gynogenetic and parthenogenetic inner cell mass and trophectoderm tissues in reconstituted blastocysts in the mouse. *J Embryol Exp Morphol* 1985;90:267–285.
501. Barton S, Ferguson-Smith A, Fundele R, Surani MA. Influence of paternally imprinted genes on development. *Development* 1991;113:679–687.
502. Mann J, Stewart C. Development to term of mouse androgenetic aggregation chimeras. *Development* 1991;113:1325–1333.
503. Mann J, Gadi I, Harbison M, Abbondanzo S, Stewart C. Androgenetic mouse embryonic stem cells are pluripotent and cause skeketal defects in chimeras: implications for genetic imprinting. *Cell* 1990;62:251–260.
504. Surani MA, Barton S, Howlett S, Norris M. Influence of chromosomal determinants on development of androgenetic and parthenogenetic cells. *Development* 1988;103:171–178.
505. Jacobs PA, Wilson C, Sprenkle JA, Rosenshein NB, Migeon BR. Mechanism of origin of complete hydatidiform moles. *Nature* (Lond) 1980;286:714–716.
506. Szulman AE, Surti V. Complete and partial hydatidiform moles: cytogenetic and morphological aspects. In: Patillo RA, Hussa RO, eds. *Human trophoblast and neoplasms.* New York: Plenum; 1984:135–146.
507. DeChiara TM, Efstratiadis A, Robertson EJ. A growth-deficiency phenotype in heterozygous mice carrying an insulin-like growth factor II gene disrupted by targeting. *Nature* 1990;345:78–80.
508. DeChiara TM, Robertson EJ, Efstratiadis A. Parental imprinting of the mouse insulin-like growth factor II gene. *Cell* 1991;64: 849–859.
509. Ferguson-Smith AC, Cattanach BM, Barton SC, Beechey CV, Surani MA. Embryological and molecular investigations of parental imprinting on mouse chromosome 7. *Nature* 1991;251: 667–670.
510. Bartolomei MS, Zemel S, Tilghman SM. Parental imprinting of the mouse H19 gene. *Nature* 1991;351:153–155.
511. Zemel S, Bartolomei MS, Tilghman SM. Physical linkage of two mammalian imprinted genes, *H19* and insulin-like growth factor 2. *Nature Genet* 1992;2:61–65.
512. Brunkow ME, Tilghman SM. Ectopic expression of the H19 gene in mice causes prenatal lethality. *Genes Dev* 1991;5:1092–1101.
513. Leff SE, Brannan CI, Reed ML, Ozçelik T, Francke U, Copeland NG, Jenkins NA. Maternal imprinting of the mouse *Snrpn* gene and conserved linkage homology with the human Prader-Willi syndrome region. *Nature Genet* 1992;2:259–264.
514. Cattanach BM, Barr JA, Evans EP, Burtenshaw M, Beechey CV, Leff SE, Brannan CI, Copeland NG, Jenkins NA, Jones J. A candidate mouse model for Prader-Willi syndrome which shows an absence of *Snrpn* expression. *Nature Genet* 1992;2:270–274.
515. McGrath J, Solter D. Maternal (T^{hp}) lethality in the mouse is a nuclear, non-cytoplasmic defect. *Nature* (Lond) 1984;308: 550–551.
516. Johnson DR. Hairpin-tail: a case of postreductional gene action in the mouse egg. *Genetics* 1974;76:795–805.
517. Johnson DR. Further observations on the hairpin tail (Thp) mutation in the mouse. *Genet Res* 1975;24:207–213.
518. McLaren A. The impact of pre-fertilization events on post-fertilization development in mammals. In: Newth DR, Balls M, eds. *Maternal effects in development.* London: Cambridge University Press; 1979:287–320.
519. Winking H, Silver LM. Characterization of a recombinant mouse t haplotype that expresses a dominant lethal maternal effect. *Genetics* 1984;108:1013–1020.
520. Barlow DP, Stoger R, Herrmann BG, Saito K, Schweifer N. The mouse insulin-like growth factor type-2 receptor is imprinted and closely linked to the *Tme* locus. *Nature* 1991;349:84–87.
521. Forejt J, Gregorova S. Genetic analysis of genomic imprinting: an *Imprintor-1* gene controls inactivation of the paternal copy of the mouse *Tme* locus. *Cell* 1992;70:443–450.
522. Hall JG. Genomic imprinting: review and relevance to human diseases. *Am J Hum Genet* 1990;46:857–873.
523. Ferguson-Smith AC, Reik W, Surani MA. Genomic imprinting and cancer. *Cancer Surv* 1990;9:487–503.

524. Zhang Y, Tycko B. Monoallelic expression of the human *H19* gene. *Nature Genet* 1992;1:40–44.
525. Ozçelik T, Leff S, Robinson W, Donlon T, Lalande M, Sanjines E, Schinzel A, Francke U. Small nuclear ribonucleoprotein polypeptide N (*SNRPN*), and expressed gene in the Prader-Willi syndrome critical region. *Nature Genet* 1992;2:265–269.
526. Ogawa O, Eccles MR, Szeto J, McNoe LZ, Yun K, Maw MA, Smith PJ, Reeve AE. Relaxation of insulin-like growth factor II gene imprinting implicated in Wilms' tumour. *Nature* 1993; 362:749–751.
527. Ranier S, Johnson LA, Dobry CJ, Ping AJ, Grundy PE, Feinberg AP. Relaxation of imprinted genes in human cancer. *Nature* 1993;362:747–749.
528. Giannoukakis N, Deal C, Paquette J, Goodyer CG, Polychronakos C. Parental genomic imprinting of the human IGF2 gene. *Nature Genet* 1993;4:98–101.
529. Ohlsson R, Nystrom A, Pfeifer-Ohlsson S, Tohonen V, Hedborg F, Schofield P, Flam F, Ekstrom TJ. *IGF2* is parentally imprinted during human embryogeneisis and in the Beckwith-Wiedemann syndrome. *Nature Genet* 1993;4:94–97.
530. Modlinski JA. Haploid mouse embryos obtained by microsurgical removal of one pronucleus. *J Exp Embryol Morphol* 1975;33:897–905.
531. McGrath J, Solter D. Inability of mouse blastomere nuclei transferred to enucleated zygotes to support development in vitro. *Science* 1984;226:1317–1319.
532. McGrath J, Solter D. Nucleocytoplasmic interactions in the mouse embryo. *J Embryol Exp Morphol* [Suppl] 1986;97: 277–289.
533. Robl JM, Gilligan B, Critser ES, First NL. Nuclear transplantation in mouse embryos: assessment of recipient cell stage. *Biol Reprod* 1986;34:733–739.
534. Willadson SM. Nuclear transplantation in sheep embryos. *Nature* 1986;320:63–65.
535. Surani MAH, Barton SC, Norris ML. Nuclear transplantation in the mouse: heritable differences between parental genomes after activation of the embryonic genome. *Cell* 1986;45:127–136.
536. Cattanach BM. Control of chromosome inactivation. *Ann Rev Genet* 1975;9:1–18.
537. Razin A, Cedar H, Riggs A, eds. *DNA methylation.* New York: Springer-Verlag; 1984.
538. Doerfler W. DNA methylation and gene activity. *Ann Rev Biochem* 1983;52:93–124.
539. Razin A, Cedar H. DNA methylation and gene expression. *Microbiol Rev* 1991;55:451–458.
540. Jost JP, Saluz HP, eds. *DNA methylation: molecular biology and biological significance.* Birkhauser Basel: 1993:572.
541. Sanford JP, Clark HJ, Chapman VM, Rossant J. Differences in DNA methylation during oogenesis and spermatogenesis and their persistence during early embryogenesis in the mouse. *Genes Dev* 1987;1:1039–1046.
542. Monk M, Boubelik M, Lehnert S. Temporal and regional changes in DNA methylation in the embryonic, extraembryonic and germ cell lineages during mouse embryo development. *Development* 1987;99:371–382.
543. Monk M. Changes in DNA methylation during mouse embryonic development in relation to X-chromosome activity and imprinting. Series B: biological sciences. *Philosophical Transactions of the Royal Society of London:* 1990;326:299–312.
544. Monk M, Grant M. Preferential X-chromosome inactivation, DNA methylation and imprinting. *Development* 1990;55:62–73.
545. Monk M. Changes in DNA methylation during mouse embryonic development in relation to X-chromosome activity and imprinting. *Phil Trans Roy Soc (Lond)* 1990;B326:179–187.
546. Howlett SK, Reik W. Methylation levels of maternal and paternal genomes during preimplantation development. *Development* 1991;113:119–127.
547. Carlson LL, Page AW, Bestor TH. Properties and localization of DNA methyltransferase in preimplantation mouse embryos: implications for genomic imprinting. *Genes Dev* 1992;6:2536–2541.
548. Riggs AD, Pfeiffer GD. X-chromosome inactivation and cell memory. *Trends Genet* 1992;8:169–173.
549. Manes C, Menzel P. Demethylation of CpG sites in DNA of early rabbit trophoblast. *Nature* 1981;293:589–590.
550. Chapman V, Forrester L, Sanford J, Hastie N, Rossant J. Cell lineage-specific undermethylation of mouse repetitive DNA. *Nature* 1984;307:284–286.
551. Razin A, Webb C, Szyf M, Ysraeli J, Rosenthal A, Naveh-Many T, Sciaky-Gallili N, Cedar H. Variations in DNA methylation during mouse cell differentiation in vivo and in vitro. *Proc Natl Acad Sci USA* 1984;81:2275–2279.
552. Young PR, Tilghman SM. Induction of alphafetoprotein synthesis by differentiation of teratocarcinoma cells is accompanied by a genome-wide loss of DNA methylation. *Mol Cell Biol* 1984;4:898–907.
553. Rossant J, Sanford JP, Chapman VM, Andrews GK. Undermethylation of structural gene sequences in extraembryonic lineages of the mouse. *Dev Biol* 1986;117:567–573.
554. Lock LF, Takagi N, Martin GR. Methylation of the *Hprt* gene on the inactive X occurs after chromosome inactivation. *Cell* 1987;48:39–46.
555. Singer-Sam J, Grant M, LeBon JM, Okuyama K, Chapman V, Monk M, Riggs AD. Use of a HpaII-polymerase chain reaction assay to study DNA methylation in the Pgk-1 CpG island of mouse embryos at the time of X-chromosome inactivation. *Mol Cell Biol* 1990;10:4987–4989.
556. Chapman V, Kartzer PG, Siracusa LD, Quarantillo BA, Evans R, Liskay RM. Evidence from DNA modification in the maintenance of X-chromosome inactivation of adult mouse tissues. *Proc Natl Acad Sci USA* 1982;79:5357–5361.
557. Kratzer PG, Chapaman VM, Lambert H, Evans RE, Liskay RM. Differences in the DNA of the inactive X-chromosomes of fetal and extraembryonic tissues of mice. *Cell* 1983;33:37–42.
558. Krumlauf R, Hammer RE, Brinster R, Chapman VM, Tilghman SM. Regulated expression of alphafetoprotein genes in transgenic mice. *Cold Spring Harbor Symp Quant Biol* 1985;50:371–378.
559. Swain JL, Stewart TA, Leder P. Parental legacy determines methylation and expression of an autosomal transgene: a molecular mechanism for parental imprinting. *Cell* 1987;50:719–727.
560. Chaillet JR, Vogt TF, Beier DR, Leder P. Parental-specific methylation of an imprinted transgene is established during gametogenesis and progressively changes during embryogenesis. *Cell* 1991;66:77–83.
561. Sapienza C, Paquette J, Tran TH, Peterson A. Epigenetic and genetic factors affect transgene methylation imprinting. *Development* 1989;107:165–168.
562. Bestor TH. DNA methylation: evolution of a bacterial immune function into a regulator of gene expression and genome structure in higher eukaryotes. *Phil Trans Roy Soc* (Lond) 1990; B326:179–187.
563. Doerfler W. Patterns of DNA methylation: evolutionary vestiges of foreign DNA inactivation as a host defence mechanism. *Biol Chem Hoppe Seiler* 1991;372:557–564.
564. Sasaki H, Jones PA, Chaillet JR, Ferguson-Smith AC, Barton SC, Reik W, Surani MA. Parental imprinting: potentially active chromatin of the repressed maternal allele of the mouse insulin-like growth factor II (*Igf2*) gene. *Genes Dev* 1992;6:1843–1856.
565. Ferguson-Smith AC, Sasaki H, Cattanach BM, Surani MA. Parental-origin-specific epigenetic modification of the mouse *H19* gene. *Nature* 1993;362:751–755.
566. Bartolomei MS, Webber AL, Brunkow ME. Thighman SM. Epigenetic mechanisms underlying the imprinting of the mouse *H19* gene. *Genes Devel* 1993 (in press).
567. Stoger R, Kubicka P, Liu CG, Kafri T, Razin A, Cedar H, Barlow DP. Maternal-specific methylation of the imprinted mouse *Igf2r* locus identifies the expressed locus as carrying the imprinting signal. *Cell* 1993;73:61–71.
568. Thorey IS, Pedersen RA, Linney E, Oshima RG. Parent-specific expression of a human keratin 18/b-galactosidase fusion gene in transgenic mice. *Dev Dynam* 1992;195:100–112.
569. Li E, Bestor TH, Jaenisch R. Targeted mutation of the DNA methyltransferase gene results in embryonic lethality. *Cell* 1992;69:915–926.
570. Haig D, Graham C. Genomic imprinting and the strange case of the insulin-like growth factor II receptor. *Cell* 1991;64: 1045–1046.
571. Moore T, Haig D. Genomic imprinting in mammalian development: a parental tug-of-war. *Trends Genet* 1991;7:45–49.
572. Lobe CG. Transcription factors and mammalian development. *Curr Topics Dev Biol* 1992;27:351–383.

573. Latimer JJ, Pedersen RA. Epigenetic interactions and gene expression in peri-implantation mouse embryo development. In: Gwatkin RBL, ed. *Genes in mammalian reproduction.* New York:Wiley-Liss Inc; 1993:131–171.
574. Gluecksohn-Schoenheimer S. The development of normal and homozygous brachy (T/T) mouse embryos in the extraembryonic coelom of the chick. *Proc Natl Acad Sci USA* 1944;134–140.
575. Herrmann BG, Labeit S, Poustka A, King TR, Lehrach H. Cloning of the T gene required in mesoderm formation in the mouse. *Nature* 1990;343:617–622.
576. Silver LM. At the crossroads of developmental genetics: the cloning of the classical mouse *T* locus. *Bioessays* 1990;12:377–380.
577. Wilkinson DG, Bhatt S, Herrmann BG. Expression pattern of the mouse *T* gene and its role in mesoderm formation. *Nature* 1990;343:657–659.
578. Stott D, Kispert A, Herrmann BG. Rescue of the tail defect of *Brachyury* mice. *Genes Dev* 1993;7:197–203.
579. Rashbass P, Cooke LA, Herrmann BG, Beddington RSP. A cell autonomous function of *Brachyury* in *T/T* embryonic stem cell chimaeras. *Nature* 1991;353:348–351.
580. Blum M, Gaunt SJ, Cho KWY, Steinbeisser H, Blumberg B, Bittner D, De Robertis EM. Gastrulation in the mouse: the role of the homeobox gene *goosecoid. Cell* 1992;69:1097–1106.
581. Reaume AG, Conlon RA, Zirngibl R, Yamaguchi TP, Rossant J. Expression analysis of a *Notch* homologue in the mouse embryo. *Dev Biol* 1992;154:377–387.
582. Del Amo FF, Smith DE, Swiatek PJ, Gendron-Maguire M, Greenspan RJ, McMahon AP, Gridley T. Expression pattern of *Motch,* a mouse homolog of *Drosophila Notch,* suggests an important role in early postimplantation mouse development. *Development* 1992;115:737–744.
583. Gaunt SJ, Blum M, De Robertis EM. Expression of the mouse *goosecoid* gene during mid-embryogenesis may mark mesenchymal cell lineages in the developing head, limbs, and body wall. *Development* 1993;117:769–778.
584. McGinnis W, Krumlauf R. Homeobox genes and axial patterning. *Cell* 1992;68:283–302.
585. Scott MP. Vertebrate homeobox gene nomenclature. [Letter]. *Cell* 1992;71:551–553.
586. Shashikant CS, Utset MF, Violette SM, Wise TL, Einat P, Pendleton JW, Schughart K, Ruddle FH. Homeobox genes in mouse development. *Eukar Gene Express* 1991;1:207–245.
587. Kessel M, Gruss P. Murine developmental control genes. *Science* 1990;249:374–379.
588. Gaunt SJ. Expression patterns of mouse hox genes: clues to understanding of developmental and evolutionary strategies. *Bioessays* 1991;13:505–512.
589. Malicki J, Schughart K, McGinnis W. Mouse *Hox-2.2* specifies thoracic segmental identity in Drosophila embryos and larvae. *Cell* 1990;63:961–967.
590. McGinnis N, Kuziora MA, McGinnis W. Human *Hox-4.2* and drosophila *deformed* encode similar regulatory specificities in Drosophila embryos and larvae. *Cell* 1990;63:969–976.
591. Zhao JJ, Lazzarini RA, Pick L. The mouse *Hox-1.3* gene is functionally equivalent to the *Drosophila Sex combs reduced* gene. *Genes Dev* 1993;7:343–354.
592. Awgulewitsch A, Jacobs D. *Deformed* autoregulatory element from *Drosophila* functions in a conserved manner in transgenic mice. *Nature* 1992;358:341–344.
593. Malicki J, Cianetti LC, Peschle C, McGinnis W. A human *HoxB4* regulatory element provides head-specific expression in *Drosophila* embryos. *Nature* 1992;358:345–346.
594. Chisaka O, Capecchi MR. Regionally restricted developmental defects resulting from targeted disruption of the mouse homeobox gene *Hox-1.5. Nature* 1991;350:473–479.
595. Chisaka O, Musci TS, Capecchi MR. Developmental defects of the ear, cranial nerves and hindbrain resulting from targeted disruption of the mouse homeobox gene Hox-1.6. *Nature* 1992;355:516–520.
596. Lufkin T, Dierich A, Lemeur M, Mark M, Chambon P. Disruption of the Hox-1.6 homeobox gene results in defects in a region corresponding to its rostral domain of expression. *Cell* 1991;66:1105–1119.
597. Le Mouellic H, Lallemand Y, Brûlet P. Targeted replacement of the homeobox gene *Hox-3.1* by the *Escherichia coli LacZ* in mouse chimeric embryos. *Proc Natl Acad Sci USA* 1990;87:4712–4716.
598. Le Mouellic H, Lallemand Y, Brûlet P. Homeosis in the mouse induced by a null mutation in the *Hox-3.1* gene. *Cell* 1992;69:251–264.
599. Ramirez-Solis R, Zheng H, Whiting J, Krumlauf R, Bradley A. *Hoxb-4* (*Hox-2.6*) mutant mice show homeotic transformation of cervical vertebra and defective closure of the sternal rudiments. *Cell* 1993;73:279–294.
600. Joyner A, Martin GR. *En-1* and *En-2,* two mouse genes with sequence homology to the *Drosophila engrailed* gene: expression during embryogenesis. *Genes Dev* 1987;1:29–38.
601. Logan C, Khoo WK, Cado D, Joyner AL. Two enhancer regions in the mouse *En-2* locus direct expression to the mid/hindbrain region and mandibular myoblasts. *Development* 1993;117:905–916.
602. Joyner AL, Skarnes WC, Rossant J. Production of a mutation in mouse *En-2* gene by homologous recombination in embryonic stem cells. *Nature* 1989;339:153–156.
603. Joyner AL, Herrup K, Auerbach A, Davis CA, Rossant J. Subtle cerebellar phenotype in mice homozygous for a targeted deletion of the *En-2* homeobox. *Science* 1991;251:1239–1243.
604. Davis CA, Holmyard DP, Millen KJ, Joyner AL. Examining pattern formation in mouse, chicken and frog embryos with an *En*-specific antiserum. *Development* 1991;111:287–298.
605. Wolgemuth DJ, Behringer RR, Mostoller MP, Brinster RL, Palmiter RD. Transgenic mice overexpressing the mouse homoeobox-containing gene *Hox-1.4* exhibit abnormal gut development. *Nature* 1989;337:464–467.
606. Lufkin T, Mark M, Hart CP, Dollé P, LeMeur M, Chambon P. Homeotic transformation of the occipital bones of the skull by ectopic expression of a homeobox gene. *Nature* 1992;359:835–842.
607. Balling R, Mutter G, Gruss P, Kessel M. Craniofacial abnormalities induced by ectopic expression of the homeobox gene *Hox-1.1* in transgenic mice. *Cell* 1989;58:337–347.
608. Kessel M, Balling R, Gruss P. Variations of cervical vertebrae after expression of a *Hox-1.1* transgene in mice. *Cell* 1990;61:301–308.
609. Pollock RA, Jay G, Bieberich CJ. Altering the boundaries of *Hox3.1* expression: Evidence for antipodal gene regulation. *Cell* 1992;71:911–923.
610. Jegalian BG, De Robertis EM. Homeotic transformations in the mouse induced by overexpression of a human *Hox3.3* transgene. *Cell* 1992;71:901–910.
611. Kress C, Vogels R, De Graaff W, Bonnerot C, Meijlink F, Nicolas JF, Deschamps J. Hox-2.3 upstream sequences mediate lacZ expression in intermediate mesoderm derivatives of transgenic mice. *Development* 1990;109:775–786.
612. Püschel AW, Balling R, Gruss P. Position-specific activity of the Hox1.1 promoter in transgenic mice. *Development* 1990;108:435–442.
613. Püschel AW, Balling R, Gruss P. Separate elements cause lineage restriction and specify boundaries of *Hox-1.1* expression. *Development* 1991;112:279–287.
614. Bieberich CJ, Utset MF, Awgulewitsch A, Ruddle FH. Evidence for positive and negative regulation of the *Hox-3.1* gene. *Proc Nat Acad Sci, USA.* 1990;87:8462–8466.
615. Whiting J, Marshall H, Cook M, Krumlauf R, Rigby PWJ, Stott D, Allemann RK. Multiple spatially specific enhancers are required to reconstruct the pattern of *Hox-2.6* gene expression. *Genes Dev* 1991;5:2048–2059.
616. Behringer RR, Crotty DA, Tennyson VM, Brinster RL, Palmiter RD, Wolgemuth J. Sequences 5′ of the homeobox of the *Hox-1.4* gene direct tissue-specific expression of *lacZ* during mouse development. *Development* 1993;117:823–833.
617. Edelman GM, Jones FS. Cytotactin: a morphoregulatory molecule and a target for regulation by homeobox gene products. *Trends Biochem* 1992;17:228–232.
618. Jones FS, Chalepakis G, Gruss P, Edelman GM. Activation of the cytotactin promoter by the homeobox-containing gene *Evx-1. Proc Natl Acad Sci USA* 1992;89:2091–2095.
619. Moase CE, Trasler DG. N-CAM alterations in splotch neural tube defect mouse embryos. *Development* 1991;113:1049–1058.
620. Deutsch U, Gruss P. Murine paired domain proteins as regula-

tory factors of embryonic development. *Dev Biol* 1991;2: 413–424.
621. Gruss P, Walther C. Pax in development. *Cell* 1992;69:719–722.
622. Deutsch U, Dressler GR, Gruss P. *Pax 1,* a member of a paired box homologous murine gene family, is expressed in segmented structures during development. *Cell* 1988;53:617–625.
623. Wright ME. *Undulated:* a new genetic factor in Mus musculus affecting the spine and tail. *Heredity* 1947;1:147–141.
624. Grüneberg H. Genetical studies on the skeleton of the mouse XII. The development of *undulated. J Genet* 1954;52:441–455.
625. Balling R, Deutsch U, Gruss P. *Undulated,* a mutation affecting the development of the mouse skeleton, has a point mutation in the paired box of *Pax 1. Cell* 1988;55:531–535.
626. Epstein DJ, Vekemans M, Gros P. *Splotch* (Sp^{2H}), a mutation affecting development of the mouse neural tube, shows a deletion within the paired homeodomain of Pax-3. *Cell* 1991;67:767–774.
627. Epstein DJ, Vogan KJ, Trasler DG, Gros P. A mutation within intron 3 of the *Pax-3* gene produces aberrantly spliced mRNA transcripts in the splotch (*Sp*) mouse mutant. *Proc Natl Acad Sci USA* 1993;90:532–536.
628. Wallin J, Mizutani Y, Imai K, Miyashita N, Moriwaki K, Taniguchi M, Kosek H, Balling R. A new Pax gene, *Pax-9* maps to mouse chromosome 12. *Mammal Genome* 1993;4:354–358.
629. Jordan T, Hanson I, Zaletayev D, Hodgson S, Prosser J, Seawright A, Hastie N, van Heyningen V. The human PAX6 gene is mutated in two patients with aniridia. *Nature Genet* 1992;1:328–332.
630. Hoth CF, Milunsky A, Lipsky N, Seffer R, Clarren SK, Baldwin CT. Mutations in the paired domain of the human Pax3 gene cause Kelin-Waardenburg syndrome (WS-III) as well as Waardenburg syndrome type I (WS-I). *Am J Hum Genet* 1993;52:455–462.
631. Schöler HR. Octamania: the POU factors in murine development. *Trends Genet* 1991;7:323–329.
632. Li S, Rosenfeld MG. POU-domain transcription factors in development and embryonic cell lineage determination. *Dev Biol* 1992;3:203–213.
633. He X, Treacy MN, Simmons DM, Ingraham HA, Swanson LW, Rosenfeld MG. Expression of a large family of POU-domain regulatory genes in mammalian brain development. *Nature* 1989;340:35–42.
634. Zimmerman EC, Jones CM, Fet V, Hogan BLM, Magnuson MA. Nucleotide sequence of mouse SCIP, cDNA, a POU-domain transcription factor. *Nuc Acids Res* 1991;19:956.
635. Collum RG, Fisher PE, Datta M, Mellis S, Thiele C, Huebner K, Croce CM, Israel MA, Theil T, Moroy T, DePinho R, Alt FW. A novel POU homeodomain gene specifically expressed in cells of the developing mammalian nervous system. *Nuc Acids Res* 1992;20:4919–4925.
636. Chalfie M, Horvitz HR, Sulston JE. Mutations that lead to reiterations in the cell lineages of *C. elegans. Cell* 1981;24:59–69.
637. Finney, Ruvkun G. The *unc-86* gene product couples cell lineage and cell identity in *C. elegans. Cell* 1990;63:895–905.
638. Li S, Crenshaw BE III, Rawson EJ, Simmons DM, Swanson LW, Rosenfeld MG. Dwarf locus mutants lacking three pituitary cell types result from mutations in the POU-domain gene *pit-1. Nature* 1990;347:528–533.
639. Ma YG, Rosfjord E, Huebert C, Wilder P, Tiesman J, Kelly D, Rizzino A. Transcriptional regulation of the murine k-FGF gene in embryonic cell lines. *Dev Biol* 1992;154:45–54.
640. Ashworth A, Denny P. Zinc finger protein genes in the mouse genome. *Mammal Genome* 1991;1:196–200.
641. Krumlauf R, Hunt P, Graham A, Wilkinson D. Patterning regional identity: spatially-restricted and dynamic expression patterns of *Krox-20* and *Hox* genes in the developing nervous system. *Dev Biol* 1991;2:375–384.
642. Wilkinson DG, Bhatt S, Chavrier P, Bravo R, Charnay P. Segment-specific expression of a zinc-finger gene in the developing nervous system of the mouse. *Nature* 1989;337:461–464.
643. Sham MH, Vesque C, Nonchev S, Marshall H, Frain M, Das Gupta R, Whiting J, Wilkinson D, Charnay P, Krumlauf R. The zinc finger gene *Krox20* regulates *HoxB2* (*Hox2.8*) during hindbrain segmentation. *Cell* 1993;72:1–20.
644. Smith DE, Del Amo FF, Gridley T. Isolation of Sna, a mouse gene homologous to the *Drosophila* genes *snail* and *escargot:* its expression pattern suggests multiple roles during postimplantation development. *Development* 1992;116:1033–1039.
645. Perkins AS, Mercer JA, Jenkins NA, Copeland NG. Patterns of *Evi-1* expression in embryonic an adult tissues suggest that *Evi-1* plays an important regulatory role in mouse development. *Development* 1991;111:479–487.
646. Noce T, Fujiwara Y, Ito M, Takeuchi T, Hashimoto N, Yamanouchi M, Higashinakawa T, and Fujimoto H. A novel murine zinc finger gene mapped within the t^{w18} deletion region expresses in germ cells and embryonic nervous system. *Dev Biol* 1992;155:409–422.
647. Weintraub H, Davis R, Tapscott S, Thayer M, Krause M, Benezra R, Blackwell TK, Turner D, Rupp R, Hollenberg S, Zhuang Y, Lassar A. The *myoD* gene family: nodal point during specification of the muscle cell lineage. *Science* 1991;251: 761–766.
648. Ott MO, Bober E, Lyons G, Arnold H, Buckingham M. Early expression of the myogenic regulatory gene, *myf-5,* in precursor cells of skeletal muscle in the mouse embryo. *Development* 1991;111:1097–1107.
649. Sassoon D, Lyons G, Wright WE, Lin, Lassar A, Wientraub H, Buckingham M. Expression of two myogenic regulatory factors myogenin and MyoD1 during mouse embryogenesis. *Nature* 1989;341:303–307.
650. Braun T, Rudnicki MA, Arnold HH, Jaenisch R. Targeted inactivation of the muscle regulatory gene *Myf-5* results in abnormal rib development and perinatal death. *Cell* 1992;71:369–382.
651. Rudnicki MA, Braun T, Hinuma S, Jaenisch R. Inactivation of *MyoD* in mice leads to up-regulation of the myogenic HLH gene *Myf-5* and results in apparently normal muscle development. *Cell* 1992;71:383–390.
652. Benezra R, Davis RL, Lockshon D, Turner DL, Weintraub H. The protein Id: a negative regulator of helix-loop-helix DNA binding proteins. *Cell* 1990;61:49–59.
653. Wang Y, Benezra R, Sassoon DA. Id expression during mouse development: A role in morphogenesis. *Dev Biol* 1992;194: 222–230.
654. Biggs J, Murphy FV, Israel MA. A human Id-like helix-loop-helix protein expressed during early development. *Proc Natl Acad Sci USA* 1992;89:1512–1516.
655. Lo LC, Johnson JE, Wuenschell CW, Saito T, Anderson DJ. Mammalian *achaete-scute* homolog 1 is transiently expressed by spatially restricted subsets of early neuroepithelial and neural crest cells. *Genes Dev* 1991;5:1524–1537.
656. Ellmeier W, Aguzzi A, Kleiner E, Kurzbauer R, Weith A. Mutually exclusive expression of a helix-loop-helix gene and N-*myc* in human neuroblastomas and in normal development. *EMBO J* 1992;11:2563–2571.
657. Linney E. Retinoic acid receptors: transcription factors modulating gene regulation, development, and differentiation. *Curr Trends Dev Biol* 1992;27:309–350.
658. Tickle C, Alberts B, Wolpert L, Lee J. Local application of retinoic acid to the limb bond mimics the action of the polarizing region. *Nature* 1982;296:564–565.
659. Summerbell D. The effect of local application of retinoic acid to the anterior margin of the developing chick limb. *J Embryol Exp Morphol* 1983;78:269–289.
660. Waddington CH. *The epigenetics of birds.* New York: Cambridge University Press; 1952.
661. Wagner M, Thaller C, Jessel T, Eichele G. Polarizing activity and retinoic synthesis in the floor plate of the neural tube. *Nature* 1990;345:819–823.
662. Ruberte E, Kastner P, Dollé P, Krust P, Leroy P, Mendelsohn C, Zelent A, Chambon P. Retinoic acid receptors in the embryo. *Dev Biol* 1991;2:153–159.
663. Maden M. Retinoid-binding proteins in the embryo. *Dev Biol* 1991;2:161–170.
664. Kessel M, Gruss P. Homeotic transformations of murine vertebrae and concomitant alteration of *Hox* codes induced by retinoic acid. *Cell* 1991;67:89–104.
665. Boncinelli E, Simeone A, Acampora D, Mavilio F. *HOX* gene activation by retinoic acid. *Trends Genet* 1991;7:329–334.
666. Rossant J, Zirngibl R, Cado D, Shago M, Giguere V. Expression of a retinoic acid response element-*hsplacZ* transgene defines specific domains of transcriptional activity during mouse embryogenesis. *Genes Dev* 1991;5:1333–1344.

667. Mendelsohn C, Ruberte E, LeMeur M, Morriss-Kay G, Chambon P. Developmental analysis of the retinoic acid-inducible RAR-$\beta 2$ promoter in transgenic animals. *Development* 1991;113: 723–734.
668. Balkan W, Colbert M, Bock C, Linney E. Transgenic indicator mice for studying activated retinoic acid receptors during development. *Proc Natl Acad Sci USA* 1992;89:3347–3351.
669. Hogan BLM, Thaller C, Eichele G. Evidence that Hensen's node is a site of retinoic acid synthesis. *Nature* 1992;359:237–241.
670. Conlon RA, Rossant J. Domains of retinoic acid action in post-implantation mouse embryos. *Mol Biol Cell* 1992;3:98a.
671. Goulding MD, Chalepakis G, Deutsch U, Erselius JR, Gruss P. Pax-3, a novel murine DNA binding protein expressed during early neurogenesis. *EMBO J* 1991;10:1135–1147.
672. Langston AW, Gudas LJ. Identification of a retinoic acid responsive enhancer 3′ of the murine homeobox gene Hox-1.6. *Mech Devel* 1992;38:217–227.
673. Murphy SP, Garbern J, Odenwald WF, Lazzarini RA, Linney E. Differential expression of the homeobox gene Hox-1.3 in F9 embryonal carcinoma cells. *Proc Natl Acad Sci USA* 1988;85: 5587–5591.
674. Kurzrock R, Estrov Z, Wetzler M, Gutterman JU, Talpaz M. LIF: not just a leukemia inhibitory factor. *Endocrine Rev* 1991;12:208–217.
675. Hilton DJ. LIF: lots of interesting functions. *Trends Biochem* 1992;17:72–76.
676. Smith AG, Nichols J, Robertson M, Rathjen PD. Differentiation inhibiting activity (DIA/LIF) and mouse development. *Dev Biol* 1992;151:339–351.
677. Stahl J, Gearing DP, Willson TA, Brown MB, King JA, Gough NM. Structural organization of the genes for murine and human leukemia inhibitory factor. *J Biol Chem* 1990;265:8833–8841.
678. Willson TA, Metcalf D, Gough NM. Cross-species comparison of the sequence of the leukemia inhibitory factor gene and its protein. *Eur J Biochem* 1992;204:21–30.
679. Bhatt H, Brunet LJ, Stewart CL. Uterine expression of leukemia inhibitory factor coincides with the onset of blastocyst implantation. *Proc Natl Acad Sci USA* 1991;88:11408–11412.
680. Conquet F, Brûlet P. Developmental expression of myleloid leukemia inhibitory factor gene in preimplantation blastocysts and in extraembryonic tissues of mouse embryos. *Mol Cell Biol* 1990;10:3801–3805.
681. Rathjen PD, Toth S, Willis A, Heath JK, Smith SG. Differentiation inhibiting activity is produced in matrix-associated and diffusible forms that are generated by alternate promoter usage. *Cell* 1990;62:1105–1114.
682. Rathjen PD, Nichols J, Toth S, Edwards DR, Heath JK, Smith AG. Developmentally programmed induction of differentiation inhibiting activity and the control of stem cell populations. *Genes Dev* 1990;4:2308–2318.
683. Gearing DP, Thut CJ, VandenBos T, Gimpel SD, Delaney B, King J, Price V, Cosman D, Beckmann MP. Leukemia inhibitory factor is structurally related to the IL-6 signal transducer, gp130. *EMBO J* 1991;10:2839–2848.
684. Stewart CL, Kasper P, Brunet LJ, Bhatt H, Gadi I, Köntgen F, Abbondanzo SJ. Blastocyst implantation depends on maternal expression of leukemia inhibitory factor. *Nature* 1992;359: 76–79.
685. Morrison-Graham K, Takahashi Y. Steel factor and *c*-Kit receptor: from mutants to a growth factor system. *Bioessays* 1993;15:77–83.
686. Williams DE, De Vries P, Namen AE, Widmer MB, Lyman SD. The *Steel* factor. *Dev Biol* 1992;151:368–376.
687. De Felici M, Dolci S. Leukemia inhibitory factor sustains the survival of mouse primordial germ cells cultured on TM_4 feeder layers. *Dev Biol* 1991;147:281–284.
688. Dolci S, Williams DE, Ernst MK, Resnick JL, Brannan CI, Lock LF, Lyman SD, Boswell HS, Donovan PJ. Requirement for mast cell growth factor for primordial germ cell survival in culture. *Nature* 1991;352:809–811.
689. Matsui Y, Toksoz D, Nishikawa S, Nishikawa SI, Williams D, Zsebo K, Hogan BLM. Effect of *Steel* factor and leukemia inhibitory factor on murine primordial germ cells in culture. *Nature* 1992;353:760–752.
690. Godin I, Deed R, Cooke J, Zsebo K, Dexter M, Wylie CC. Effects of the *steel* gene product on mouse primordial germ cells in culture. *Nature* 1991;352:807–809.
691. De Felici M, Dolci S, Pesce M. Cellular and molecular aspects of mouse primordial germ cell migration and proliferation in culture. *Int J Dev Biol* 1992;36:205–213.
692. Matsui Y, Zsebo KM, Hogan BLM. Embryonic expression of a haematopoietic growth factor encoded by the *Sl* locus and the ligand for *c-kit*. *Nature* 1990;347:667–669.
693. Keshet E, Lyman SD, Williams DE, Anderson DM, Jenkins NA, Copeland NG, Parada LF. Embryonic RNA expression patterns of the *c-kit* receptor and its cognate ligand suggest multiple functional roles in mouse development. *EMBO J* 1991;10: 2425–2435.
694. Motro B, Van der Kooy D, Rossant J, Reith A, Bernstein A. Contiguous patterns of *c-kit* and *steel* expression: analysis of mutations at the *W* and *Sl* loci. *Development* 1991;113:1207–1221.
695. Geibel LB, Spritz RA. Mutation of the *KIT* (mast/stem cell growth factor receptor) protooncogene in human piebaldism. *Proc Natl Acad Sci USA* 1991;88:8696–8699.
696. Fleischman RA, Saltman DL, Stastny V, Zneimer S. Deletion of the *c-kit* protooncogene in the human developmental defect piebald trait. *Proc Natl Acad Sci USA* 1991;88:10885–10889.
697. Adamson ED. Developmental activities of the epidermal growth factor receptor. In: Nilsen-Hamilton N, ed. *Growth factors and development.* New York: Academic Press Inc; 1990:1–29.
698. Partanen AM. Epidermal growth factor and transforming growth factor-α in the development of epithelial-mesenchymal organs of the mouse. In: Nilsen-Hamilton, ed. *Growth factors and development.* New York: Academic Press Inc; 1990:31–55.
699. Adamson ED. EGF receptor activities in mammalian development. *Mol Reprod Dev* 1990;27:16–22.
700. Werb Z. Expression of EGF and TGF-α in early mammalian development. *Mol Reprod Dev* 1990;27:10–15.
701. Derynck R, Roberts AB, Winkler ME, Chen EY, Goeddel DV. Human transforming growth factor-alpha: precursor structure and expression in *E. coli*. *Cell* 1984;38:287–297.
702. Lee DC, Rose TM, Webb NR, Todaro GJ. Cloning and sequence analysis of a cDNA for rat transforming growth factor-alpha. *Nature* 1985;313:489–491.
703. Chiang T, McBride J, Chou MY, Nishimura I, Wong DT. Molecular cloning of the complementary DNA encoding for the hamster TGF-alpha mature peptide. *Carcinogenesis* 1991;12: 529–532.
704. Twardzik DR. Differential expression of transforming growth factor-α during prenatal development of the mouse. *Cancer Res* 1985;45:5413–5416.
705. Rappolee DA, Sturm KS, Schultz GA, Pedersen RA, Werb Z. The expression of growth factor ligands and receptors in preimplantation mouse embryos. Heyner S, Wiley L, eds. *Early embryo development and paracrine relationships.* New York: Alan R Liss Inc. 1990:11–25.
706. Dardik A, Smith RM, Schultz RM. Colocalization of transforming growth factor-α and a functional epidermal growth factor receptor (EGFR) to the inner cell mass and preferential localization of the EGFR on the basolateral surface of the trophectoderm in the mouse embryo. *Dev Biol* 1992;154:396–409.
707. Han VKM, Hunter III, ES, Pratt RM, Zendegui JG, Lee DC. Expression of rat transforming growth factor alpha mRNA during development occurs predominantly in the maternal decidua. *Mol Cell Biol* 1987;7:2335–2343.
708. Wilcox JN, Derynck R. Developmental expression of transforming growth factors alpha and beta in mouse fetus. *Mol Cell Biol* 1988;8:3415–3422.
709. Wood SA, Kaye PL. Effects of epidermal growth factor on preimplantation mouse embryos. *J Reprod Fertil* 1989;85:575–582.
710. Paria BC, Dey SK. Preimplantation embryo development *in vitro:* cooperative interactions among embryos and role of growth factors. *Proc Natl Acad Sci USA* 1990;87:4756–4760.
711. Dardik A, Schultz RM. Blastocoel expansion in the preimplantation mouse embryo: stimulatory effect of TGF-α and EGF. *Development* 1991;113:919–930.
712. Hemmings R, Langlais J, Falcone T, Granger L, Miron P, Guyda H. Human embryos produce transforming growth factors α activity and insulin-like growth factors II. *Fertil Steril* 1992;58: 101–104.

713. Vaughan TJ, James PS, Pascall JC, Brown KD. Expression of the genes for TGFα, EGF, and the EGF receptor during early pig development. *Development* 1992;116:663–669.
714. Watson AJ, Hogan A, Hahnel A, Weimer KE, Schultz GA. Expression of growth factor ligand and receptor genes in the preimplantation bovine embryo. *Mol Reprod Dev* 1992;31:87–95.
715. Luetteke NC, Qui TH, Peiffer RL, Oliver P, Smithies O, Lee DC. TGF-α deficiency results in hair follicle and eye abnormalities in targeted and waved-1 mice. *Cell* 1993;73:263–278.
716. Mann BG, Fowler KJ, Gabriel A, Nice EC, Williams L, Dunn AR. Mice with a null mutation of the TGF-α gene have abnormal skin architecture, wavy hair, and curly whiskers and often develop corneal inflammation. *Cell* 1993;73:249–261.
717. Wiley LM, Wu JX, Harari I, Adamson ED. Epidermal growth factor receptor mRNA and protein increase after the four-cell preimplantation stage in murine development. *Dev Biol* 1992;149:247–260.
718. Kawagoe K, Akiyama J, Kawamoto T, Morishita Y, Mori S. Immunohistochemical demonstration of epidermal growth factor (EGF) receptors in normal human placental villi. *Placenta* 1990;11:7–15.
719. Brice EC, Wu JX, Muraro R, Adamson ED, Wiley LM. Modulation of mouse preimplantation development by epidermal growth factor receptor antibodies and by antisense RNA and deoxynucleotides. *Dev Genet* 1993;14:174–184.
720. Paria BC, Tsukamura H, Dey SK. Epidermal growth factor-specific protein tyrosine phosphorylation in preimplantation embryo development. *Biol Reprod* 1991;45:711–718.
721. Nilsen-Hamilton M. Transforming growth factor-β and its actions on cellular growth and differentiation. In: Nilsen-Hamilton, ed. *Growth factors and development.* New York: Academic Press Inc. 1990:95–136.
722. Slager HG, Lawson KA, van den Eijnden-van Raaij AJM, de Laat SW, Mummery CL. Differential localization of TGF-β2 in mouse preimplantation and early postimplantation development. *Dev Biol* 1991;145:205–218.
723. Slack JM. Growth factors as inducing agents in early *Xenopus* development. *J Cell Sci* [Suppl] 1990;13:119–130.
724. Jesell TM, Melton DA. Diffusible factors in vertebrate embryonic induction. *Cell* 1992;68:257–270.
725. Mummery CL, van den Eijnden-van Raaij AJM. Type β transforming growth factors and activins in differentiating embryonal carcinoma cells, embryonic stem cells and early embryonic development. *Int J Dev Biol* 1993;37:169–182.
726. Kelly D, Campbell J, Tiesman I, Rizzino A. Regulation and expression of transforming growth factor type β during early mammalian development. *Cytotechnology* 1990;4:227–242.
727. Heine UI, Munoz EF, Flanders KC, Ellingsworth LR, Lam HYP, Thompson NL, Roberts AB, Sporn MB. Role of transforming growth factor-β in the development of the mouse embryo. *J Cell Biol* 1987;105:2861–2876.
728. Lehnert SA, Arkhurst RJ. Embryonic expression pattern of TGF beta type-1 RNA suggests both paracrine and autocrine mechanisms of action. *Development* 1988;104:263–273.
729. Miller DA, Lee A, Chen EY, Moses HL, Derynck R. cDNA cloning of the murine TGF-β3 precursor and the comparative expression the TGF-β3 and TGF-β1 mRNA in murine embryos and adult tissues. *Mol Endocrinol* 1989;7:1926–1934.
730. Miller DA, Lee A, Pelton RW, Chen EY, Moses HL, Derynck R. Murine transforming growth factor beta 2 cDNA sequence and expression in adult tissues and embryos. *Mol Endocrinol* 1989b;3:1108–1114.
731. Arkhurst RJ, Lehnert SA, Faissner A, Duffie E. TGF beta in murine morphogenetic processes: the early embryo and cardiogenesis. *Development* 1990;108:645–656.
732. Pelton RW, Dickinson ME, Moses HL, Hogan BLM. *In situ* hybridization analysis of TGFβ3 RNA expression during mouse development: comparative studies with TGFβ1 and β2. *Development* 1990;110:609–620.
733. Pelton RW, Saxena B, Jones M, Moses HL, Gold LI. Immunohistochemical localization TGFβ1, TGFβ2, and TGFβ3 in the mouse embryo: expression patterns suggest multiple roles during embryonic development. *J Cell Biol* 1991;115:1091–1105.
734. Schmid P, Cox D, Bilbe G, Maier R, McMaster GK. Differential expression of TGFβ1, β2 and β3 genes during mouse embryogenesis. *Development* 1991;111:117–130.
735. Manova K, Paynton BV, Bachvarova RF. Expression of activins and TGFβ1 and β2 RNAs in early postimplantation mouse embryos and uterine decidua. *Mech Dev* 1992;36:141–152.
736. Arkhurst RJ, Fitzpatrick DR, Fowlis DJ, Gatherer D, Millan FA, Slager H. The role of TGF-βs in mammalian development. *Mol Reprod Dev* 1992;32:127–135.
737. Matrisian LM, Hogan BLM. Growth factor regulated proteases and extracellular matrix remodelling during mammalian development. In: Nilsen-Hamilton M, ed. *Growth factors and development.* New York: Academic Press Inc; 1990:219–259.
738. Gatherer D, Ten Dijke P, Baird DT, Arkhurst RJ. Expression of TGF-β isoforms during first trimester human embryogenesis. *Development* 1990;110:445–460.
739. Larson RC, Ignotz GG, Currie WB. Defined medium containing TGF-β and bFGF permits development of bovine embryos beyond the "8-cell block." *J Reprod Fertil* 1990;4:(abst).
740. Shull MM, Ormsby I, Kier AB, Pawlowski S, Diebold RJ, Yin M, Allen R, Sidman C, Proetzel G, Calvin D, Annunziata N, Doetschman T. Targeted disruption of the mouse transforming growth factor-β1 gene results in multifocal inflammatory disease. *Nature* 1992;359:693–699.
741. Kulkarni AB, Huh CG, Becker D, Geiser A, Lyght M, Flanders KC, Roberts AB, Sporn MB, Ward JM, Karlsson S. Transforming growth factor β1 null mutation in mice causes excessive inflammatory response and early death. *Proc Natl Acad Sci USA* 1993;90:770–774.
742. Zhou X, Sasaki H, Lowe L, Hogan BLM, Kuehn MR. Nodal is a novel TGF-β-like gene expressed in the mouse node during gastrulation. *Nature* 1993;361:543–547.
743. Ying S. Inhibins, activins and follistatins: gonadal proteins modulating the secretion of follicle-stimulating hormone. *Endocr Rev* 1988;9:267–293.
744. Albano RM, Godsave SF, Huylebroeck D, Van Nimmen K, Isaacs HV, Slack JMW, Smith JC. A mesoderm-inducing factor produced by WEHI-3 murine myelomonocytic leukemia cells is activin A. *Development* 1990;110:435–443.
745. van den Eijnden-van Raaij AJM, Feijen A, Lawson KA, Mummery CL. Differential expression of inhibin subunits and follistatin, but not of activin receptor type II, during early murine embryonic development. *Dev Biol* 1992;154:356–365.
746. Albano RM, Groome N, Smith JC. Activins are expressed in preimplantation mouse embryos and in ES and EC cells and are regulated on their differentiation. *Development* 1993;117:711–723.
747. Lyons K, Graycar JL, Lee A, Hashmi S, Lindquist PB, Chen EY, Hogan BLM, Derynck R. *Vgr-1,* a mammalian gene related to Xenopus *Vg-1,* is a member of the transforming growth factor β gene superfamily. *Proc Natl Acad Sci USA* 1989;86:4554–4558.
748. Lyons KM, Jones M, Hogan BLM. The DVR gene family in embryonic development. *Trends Genet* 1991;7:408–412.
749. Wozney JM. The bone morphogenetic protein family and osteogenesis. *Mol Reprod Dev* 1992;32:160–167.
750. Rosen V, Thies RS. The BMP proteins in bone formation and repair. *Trends Genet* 1992;8:97–102.
751. Baird A, Klagsburn M. Nomenclature meeting: report and recommendations: fibroblast growth factors family. *Ann NY Acad Sci* 1991;638:13–16.
752. Goldfarb M. The fibroblast growth factor family. *Cell Growth Differ* 1990;1:439–445.
753. Gospodarowicz D. Fibroblast growth factor and its involvement in developmental processes. In: Nilsen-Hamilton, M, ed. *Growth Factors and Development.* New York: Academic Press Inc; 1990:57–93.
754. Wilkinson DG, Peters G, Dickson C, McMahon AP. Expression of the FGF-related proto-oncogene *int-2* during gastrulation and neurulation in the mouse. *EMBO J* 1988;7:691–695.
755. Wilkinson DG, Bhatt S, McMahon AP. Expression pattern of the FGF-related proto-oncogene *int-2* suggests multiple roles in fetal development. *Development* 1989;105:131–136.
756. Gonzalez A, Buscalia M, Ong M, Baird A. Distribution of basic fibroblast growth factor in the 18-d rat fetus: localization in the basement membranes of diverse tissues. *J Cell Biol* 1990;110:753–765.
757. Fu YM, Spirito P, Yu ZY, Biro S, Sasse J, Lei J, Ferrans VJ, Epstein SE, Casscells W. Acidic fibroblast growth factor in the developing rat embryo. *J Cell Biol* 1991;114:1261–1273.

758. Haub O, Goldfarb M. Expression of the fibroblast growth factor-5 gene in the mouse embryo. *Development* 1991;112:397–406.
759. Hébert JM, Basilico C, Goldfarb M, Haub O, Martin GR. Isolations of cDNAs encoding four mouse FGF family members and characterization of their expression patterns during embryogenesis. *Dev Biol* 1990;138:454–463.
760. Hébert JM, Bole MB, Martin GR. mRNA localization studies suggest that murine FGF-5 plays a role in gastrulation. *Development* 1991;112:407–415.
761. Niswander L, Martin, GR. *Fgf-4* expression during gastrulation, myogenesis, limb and tooth development in the mouse. *Development* 1992;114:755–768.
762. de Lapeyriere O, Rosnet O, Benharroch D, Raybaud F, Marchetto S, Planche J, Galland F, Mattei MG, Copeland NG, Jenkins NA. Structure, chromosome mapping and expression of the murine Fgf-6 gene. *Oncogene* 1990;5:823–831.
763. Ruoslahti E, Yamaguchi Y. Proteoglycans as modulators of growth factor activities. *Cell* 1991;64:867–869.
764. Sutherland AE, Sanderson RD, Mayes M, Siebert M, Calarco PG, Bernfield M, Damsky CH. Expression of syndecan, a putative low affinity fibroblast growth factor receptor, in the early mouse embryo. *Development* 1991;113:39–351.
765. Amaya E, Musci TJ, Kirschner MW. Expression of a dominant negative mutant of the FGF receptor disrupts mesoderm formation in *Xenopus* embryos. *Cell* 1991;66:257–270.
766. Yamaguchi TP, Conlon RA, Rossant J. Expression of the fibroblast growth factor receptor FGFR-1/flg during gastrulation and segmentation in the mouse embryo. *Dev Biol* 1992;152:75–88.
767. Peters K, Ornitz D, Werner S, Williams L. Unique expression pattern of the FGF receptor 3 gene during mouse organogenesis. *Dev Biol* 1993;155:423–430.
768. Bernard O, Li M, Reid HH. Expression of two different forms of fibroblast growth factor receptor 1 in different mouse tissues and cell lines. *Proc Natl Acad Sci USA* 1991;88:7625–7629.
769. Orr-Urtreger A, Givol D, Yayon A, Yarden Y, Lonai P. Developmental expression of two murine fibroblast growth factor receptors, *flg* and *bek*. *Development* 1991;113:1419–1434.
770. Peters KGS, Werner G, Chen G, Williams T. Two FGF receptor genes are differentially expressed in epithelial and mesenchymal tissues during limb formation and organogenesis in the mouse. *Development* 1992;114:233–243.
771. Stark KL, McMahon JA, McMahon AP. FGFR-4, a new member of the fibroblast growth factor receptor family, expressed in the definitive endoderm and skeletal muscle lineages of the mouse. *Development* 1991;113:641–651.
772. Johnson DE, Lee PL, Lu J, Williams LT. Diverse forms of a receptor for acidic and basic fibroblast growth factors. *Mol Cell Biol* 1990;10:4728–4736.
773. Dionne CA, Crumley G, Bellor F, Kaplow JM, Searfoss GRM, Burgess WH, Jaye M, Schlessinger J. Cloning and expression of two distinct high-affinity receptors cross-reacting with acidic and basic fibroblast growth factors. *EMBO J* 1990:2685–2692.
774. Mansukhani A, Moscatelli D, Talarico D, Levytska V, Basilico C. A murine fibroblast growth factor (FGF) receptor expressed in CHO cells is activated by basic FGF and Kaposi FGF. *Proc Natl Acad Sci USA* 1990;87:4378–4382.
775. Safran A, Avivi A, Orr-Urtreger A, Neufeld G, Lonai P, Givol D, Yarden Y. The murine *flg* gene encodes a receptor for fibroblast growth factor. *Oncogene* 1990;5:635–643.
776. Bowen-Pope DF, van Koppen A, Schatteman G. Is PDGF really important? testing the hypotheses. *Trends Genet* 1991;7:413–418.
777. Palmieri SL, Payne J, Stiles CD, Biggers JD, Mercola M. Expression of mouse PDGF-A and PDGF α-receptor genes during pre- and post-implantation development: evidence for a developmental shift from an autocrine to a paracrine mode of action. *Mech Dev* 1992;39:181–191.
778. Mercola M, Wang C, Kelly J, Brownlee C, Jackson-Grusby L, Stiles CD, Bowen-Pope D. Selective expression of PDGF A and its receptor during early mouse embryogenesis. *Dev Biol* 1990;138:14–122.
779. Orr-Urtreger A, Lonai P. Platelet-derived growth factor-A and its receptor are expressed in separate, but adjacent cell layers of the mouse embryo. *Development* 1992;115:1045–1058.
780. Schatteman GC, Morrison-Graham K, van Koppen A, Weston JA, Bowen-Pope DF. Regulation and role of PDGF receptor α-subunit expression during embryogenesis. *Development* 1992;115:123–131.
781. Orr-Urtreger A, Bedford MT, Do MS, Eisenbach L, Lonai P. Developmental expression of the α receptor for platelet-derived growth factor, which is deleted in the embryonic lethal *Patch* mutation. *Development* 1992;115:289–303.
782. Morrison-Graham K, Schatteman GC, Bork T, Bowen-Pope DF, Weston JA. A PDGF receptor mutation in the mouse (*Patch*) perturbs the development of a non-neuronal subset of neural crest-derived cells. *Development* 1992;115:133–142.
783. Stephenson DA, Mercola M, Anderson E, Wang C, Stiles CD, Bowen-Pope DF, Chapman V. Platelet-derived growth factor receptor α-subunit gene (*Pdgfrα*) is deleted in the mouse patch (*Ph*) mutation. *Proc Natl Acad Sci USA* 1991;88:6–10.
784. Darling SM, Abbott CM. Mouse models of human single gene disorders I: non-transgenic mice. *Bioessays* 1992;14:359–366.
785. Pavelic K, Slaus NP, Spaventi R. Growth factors and proto-oncogenes in early mouse embryogenesis and tumorigenesis. *Int J Dev Biol* 1992;35:209–214.
786. Zelenka PS. Proto-oncogenes in cell differentiation. *Bioessays* 1990;12:22–26.
787. Adamson ED. Two proto-oncogenes that play dual roles in embryonal cell growth and differentiation. *Int J Dev Biol* 1993;37:11–116.
788. Adamson ED, Müller R, Verma I. Expression of *c-onc* genes, *c-fos* and *c-fms* in developing mouse tissues. *Cell Biol Int Rep* 1983;7:557–558.
789. Adamson ED, Meek J, Edwards SA. Product of the cellular oncogene, *c-fos,* observed in mouse and human tissues using an antibody to a synthetic peptide. *EMBO J* 1985;4:941–947.
790. Müller R, Tremblay JM, Adamson ED, Verma IM. Tissue and cell-type specific expression of *c-fos* expression of two human *c-onc* genes. *Nature* 1983a;304:454–456.
791. Müller R, Verma IM, Adamson ED. Expression of *c-onc* genes: *c-fos* and *c-fms* transcripts accumulate to high levels during development of mouse placenta, yolk sac, and amnion. *EMBO J* 1983b;2:679–684.
792. Whyte A, Stewart HJ. Expression of the proto-oncogene *fos* (*c-fos*) by preimplantation blastocysts of the pig. *Development* 1989;105:651–656.
793. Neilsen LL, Werb Z, Pedersen RA. Induction of *c-fos* transcripts in early postimplantation mouse embryos by TGF-α, EGF, PDGF, and FGF. *Mol Reprod Dev* 1991;29:227–237.
794. Ruther U, Wagner EF. The specific consequences of *c-fos* expression in transgenic mice. *Prog Nuc Acids Res Mol Biol* 1989;36:235–245.
795. Wang ZQ, Ovitt C, Grigoriadis AE, Möhle-Steinlein U, Rüther U, Wagner EF. Bone and haematiopoietic defected in mice lacking *c-fos. Nature* 1992;360:741–745.
796. Cole MD. The *myc* oncogene: Its role in transformation and differentiation. *Ann Rev Genet* 1986;20:361–384.
797. Downs KM, Martin GR, Bishop JM. Contrasting patterns of *myc* and N-*myc* expression during gastrulation of the mouse embryo. *Genes Dev* 1989;3:860–869.
798. Kato K, Kanamori A, Wakamatsu Y, Sawai S, Kondos H. Tissue distribution of N-myc expression in the early organogenesis period of the mouse embryo. *Dev Growth Differ* 1991;33:29–36.
799. Charron J, Malynn BA, Fisher P, Stewart V, Jeannotte L, Goff SP, Robertson EJ, Alt FW. Embryonic lethality in mice homozygous for a targeted disruption of the N-*myc* gene. *Genes Dev* 1992;6:2248–2257.
800. Moens CB, Auerbach AB, Conlon RA, Joyner AL, Rossant J. A targeted mutation reveals a role for N-*myc* in branching morphogenesis in the embryonic mouse lung. *Genes Dev* 1992;6:691–704.
801. Stanton BR, Perkins AS, Tessarollo L, Sassoon DA, Parada LF. Loss of N-*myc* function results in embryonic lethality and failure of the epithelial component of the embryo to develop. *Genes Dev* 1992;6:2235–2247.
802. McMahon AP. Pattern regulation in the vertebrate embryo: the role of the *wnt*-family of putative signalling molecules. *Sem Dev Biol* 1991:425–433.
803. McMahon AP, Bradley A. The *Wnt-1 (int-1)* proto-oncogene is required for development of a large region of the mouse brain. *Cell* 1990;62:1073–1085.
804. Thomas KR, Capecchi MR. Targeted disruption of the murine

int-1 proto-oncogene resulting in severe abnormalities in midbrain and cerebellar development. *Nature* 1990;346:847–850.
805. Thomas KR, Musci TS, Neumann PE, Capecchi MR. *Swaying* is a mutant allele of the proto-oncogene *Wnt-1*. *Cell* 1991;67: 969–976.
806. Zákány J, Duboule D. Correlation of expression of *Wnt-1* in developing limbs with abnormalities in growth and skeletal patterning. *Nature* 1993;362:546–549.
807. Gavin BJ, McMahon JA, McMahon AP. Expression of multiple novel *Wnt-1/int-1*-related genes during fetal and adult mouse development. *Genes Dev* 1990;4:2319–2332.
808. Damsky CH, Sutherland A, Fisher S. Adhesive interactions in early mammalian embryogenesis, implantation and placentation. *FASEB J* 1993; [in press].
809. Wasserman PM. Mouse gametic adhesion molecules. *Biol Reprod* 1992;46:186–191.
810. Blobel CP, White JM. Structure, function and evolutionary relationship of proteins containing a disintegrin domain. *Curr Op Cell Biol* 1992;4:760–765.
811. Blobel CP, Wolfsberg TG, Turck CW, Myles DG, Primakoff P, White JM. A potential fusion peptide and an integrin ligand domain in a protein active in sperm-egg fusion. *Nature* 1992;356: 248–252.
812. Fusi FM, Vignali M, Busacca M, Bronson RA. Evidence for the presence of an integrin cell adhesion receptor on the oolemma of unfertilized human oocytes. *Mol Reprod Dev* 1992;31:215–222.
813. Takeichi M. The cadherins: cell-cell adhesion molecules controlling animal morphogenesis. *Development* 1988;102:639–655.
814. Hyafil F, Morello D, Babinet C, Jacob F. A cell surface glycoprotein involved in the compaction of embryonic carcinoma cells and cleavage stage embryos. *Cell* 1980;21:927–934.
815. Damsky CH, Richa J, Solter D, Kundsen K, Buck CA. Identification and purification of a cell surface glycoprotein mediating intercellular adhesion in embryonic and adult tissue. *Cell* 1983;34: 455–466.
816. Vestweber D, Kemler R. Rabbit antiserum against a purified surface glycoprotein decompacts mouse preimplantation embryos and reacts with specific adult tissue. *Expl Cell Res* 1984;152: 169–178.
817. Ogous S, Okada TS, Takeichi M. Cleavage stage embryos share a common cell adhesion system with teratocarcinoma cells. *Dev Biol* 1982;92:521–528.
818. Vestweber D, Gossler A, Boller K, Kemler R. Expression and distribution of cell adhesion molecule uvomorulin in mouse preimplantation embryos. *Dev Biol* 1987;124:451–456.
819. Bloom T, McConnell J. Changes in protein phosphorylation associated with compaction of the mouse preimplantation embryo. *Mol Reprod Dev* 1990;26:199–210.
820. Sefton M, Johnson MH, Clayton L. Synthesis and phosphorylation of uvomorulin during mouse early development. *Development* 1992;155:313–318.
821. Bloom TL. The effects of phorbol ester on mouse blastomeres: a role for protein kinase C in compaction? *Development* 1989;106: 159–171.
822. Winkel GK, Ferguson JE, Takeichi M, Nuccitelli R. Activation of protein kinase C triggers premature compaction in the four-cell stage mouse embryo. *Dev Biol* 1990;138:1–15.
823. Bayna EM, Shaper JH, Shur BD. Temporally specific involvement of cell surface β-1,4, galactosyltransferase during mouse embryo morula compaction. *Cell* 1988;53:145–157.
824. Damjanov I, Damjanov A, Damsky CH. Developmentally regulated expression of the cell-cell adhesion glycoprotein cell-CAM 120/80 in peri-implantation mouse embryos and extraembryonic membranes. *Dev Biol* 1986;116:194–202.
825. Kadokawa Y, Fuketa I, Nose A, Takeichi M, Nakatsuji N. Expression pattern of E- and P-cadherin in mouse embryos and uteri during the periimplantation period. *Dev Growth Differ* 1989;31:23–30.
826. Coutifaris C, Kao LC, Sehdev HM, Chin U, Babalola GO, Blaschuk OW, Strauss III JF. E-cadherin expression during the differentiation of human trophoblasts. *Development* 1991;113: 767–777.
827. Shimoyama Y, Yoshida T, Terada M, Shimosato Y, Abe O, Hirohashi S. Molecular cloning of a human Ca^{2+}-dependent cell-cell adhesion molecule homologous to mouse placental cadherin: its low expression in human placental tissues. *J Cell Biol* 1989; 109:1787–1794.
828. Richa J, Damsky CH, Buck CA, Knowles BB, Solter D. Cell surface glycoproteins mediate compaction, trophoblast attachment, and endoderm formation during early mouse development. *Dev Biol* 1985;108:513–521.
829. Burdsal CA, Damsky CH, Pedersen RA. The role of E-cadherin and integrins in mesoderm differentiation and migration at the mammalian primitive streak. *Development* 1993;118:829–844.
830. Solter D, Knowles BB. Monoclonal antibody defining a stage specific mouse embryonic antigen (SSEA-1). *Proc Natl Acad Sci USA* 1978;75:5565–5569.
831. Glass RH, Aggeler J, Spindle A, Pedersen RA, Werb Z. Degradation of extracellular matrix by mouse trophoblast outgrowths: a model for implantation. *J Cell Biol* 1983;96:1108–1116.
832. Armant DR, Kaplan HA, Lennarz WI. Fibronectin and laminin promote in vitro attachment and outgrowth of mouse blastocysts. *Dev Biol* 1986;116:519–523.
833. Armant DR, Kaplan HA, Mover H, Lennarz WI. The effect of hexapeptides and attachment and outgrowth of mouse blastocysts cultured in vitro: evidence for the involvement of the cell recognition tripeptide Arg-Gly-Asp. *Proc Natl Acad Sci USA* 1986;83:6751–6755.
834. Sutherland AE, Calarco P, Damsky CH. Expression and function of cell surface extracellular matrix receptors in mouse blastocyst attachment and outgrowth. *J Cell Biol* 1988;106:1331–1348.
835. Carson DD, Tang JP, Gay S. Collagens support embryo attachment and outgrowth *in vitro:* effects of the Arg-Gly-Asp sequence. *Dev Biol* 1988;127:368–375.
836. Hynes RO, Lander AD. Contact and adhesive specificities in the associations, migrations, and targeting of cells and axons. *Cell* 1992;68:303–322.
837. Farach MC, Tang JP, Decker GL, Carson DD. Heparin/heparan sulfate is involved in attachment and spreading of mouse embryos in vitro. *Dev Biol* 1987;123:401–410.
838. Turpeenniemi-Hujanen T, Rönnberg L, Kauppila A, Puistola U. Laminin in the human embryo implantation: analogy to the invasion by malignant cells. *Fertil Steril* 1992;88:105–113.
839. Brenner CA, Adler RR, Rappolee DA, Pedersen RA, Werb Z. Genes for extracellular matrix-degrading metalloproteinases and their inhibitor, TIMP, are expressed during early mammalian development. *Genes Dev* 1989;3:848–859.
840. Werb Z, Alexander CM. Proteinases and matrix degradation. In: Kelly WN, Harris Jr ED, Ruddy S, Sledge CB, eds. *Textbook of rheumatology.* 4th ed. Philadelphia: WB Saunders Co. 1992: 248–268.
841. Behrendtsen O, Alexander CM, Werb Z. Metalloproteinases mediate extracellular matrix degradation by cells from mouse blastocyst growths. *Development* 1992;114:447–456.
842. Librach CL, Werb Z, Fitzgerald ML, Chiu K, Corwin NM, Esteves RA, Grobelny D, Galardy R, Damsky CH, Fisher SJ. 92-kD type IV collagenase mediates invasion of human cytotrophoblasts. *J Cell Biol* 1991;113:437–449.
843. Alexander CM, Werb Z. Targeted disruption of the tissue inhibitor of metalloproteinases gene increases the invasive behaviour of primitive mesenchymal cells derived from embryonic stem cells in vitro. *J Cell Biol* 1992;118:727–739.
844. Strickland S, Richards WG. Invasion of the trophoblasts. *Cell* 1992;71:355–357.
845. Wartiovaara I, Leivo I, Vaheri A. Expression of the cell surface-associated glycoprotein fibronectin in the early mouse embryo. *Dev Biol* 1979;69:247–257.
846. Adamson ED, Ayers SE. The localization and synthesis of some collagen types in developing mouse embryos. *Cell* 1979;69: 953–965.
847. Leivo I, Vaheri A, Timpl R, Wartiovaara J. Appearance and distribution of collagens and laminin in the early mouse embryo. *Dev Biol* 1980;76:100–114.
848. Leivo I. Structure and composition of early basement membranes: studies with early embryos and teratocarcinoma cells. *Med Biol* 1983;61:1–30.
849. Nakatsuji N, Snow MHL, Wylie CC. Cinemicrographic study of the cell movement in primitive-streak stage mouse embryo. *J Embryol Exp Morph* 1986;96:99–109.
850. Stephens L, Fitzgerald M, Damsky C. Targeted mutagenesis of β1

integrins in embryonal carcinoma and embryonic stem cells. *Mol Biol Cell* 1992;3:130a.
851. Le Douarin N. *The neural crest.* New York: Oxford University Press; 1982.
852. Bronner-Fraser M. Mechanisms of neural crest cell migration. *Bioessays* 1993;15:221–230.
853. Chan WY, Tam PPL. A morphological and experimental study of the mesencephalic neural crest cells in the mouse embryo using wheat germ agglutinin-gold conjugates as the cell marker. *Development* 1988;102:427–442.
854. Stemple DL, Anderson DJ. Isolation of a stem cell for neurons and glia from the mammalian neural crest. *Cell* 1992;71: 973–985.
855. Ginsberg M, Snow MHL, McLaren A. Primordial germ cells in the mouse embryos during gastrulation. *Development* 1990;110: 521–528.
856. Clark JM, Eddy EM. Fine structural observations on the origin and associations of primordial germ cells of the mouse. *Dev Biol* 1975;47:136–155.
857. Tam PPL, Snow MHL. Proliferation and migration of primordial germ cells during compensatory growth in mouse embryos. *J Embryol Exp Morphol* 1981;64:133–147.
858. Wylie CC, Heasman J. Migration, proliferation, and potency of primordial germ cells. *Sem Dev Biol* 1993; [*Submitted*].
859. Ffrench-Constant C, Hollingsworth A, Heasman J, Wylie CC. Response to fibronectin of mouse primordial germ cells before, during and after migration. *Development* 1991;113:1365–1373.
860. Zackson SL, Steinberg MS. A molecular marker for cell guidance information in the axolotl embryo. *Dev Biol* 1988;127:435–442.
861. Silverstein RL, Nachman RL. Thrombospondin-plasminogen interactions: modulation of plasmin generation. *Sem Thromb Hemostasis* 1987;13:335–342.
862. O'Shea KS, Liu LHJ, Kinnunen LH, Dixit VM. Role of the extracellular matrix protein thrombospondin in the early development of the mouse embryo. *J Cell Biol* 1990;111:2713–1723.
863. O'Shea KS, Dixit VM. Unique distribution of the extracellular matrix component thrombospondin in the developing mouse embryo. *J Cell Biol* 1988:2737–2748.
864. Bornstein P, O'Rourke K, Wikstrom K, Wolf FW, Katz R, Li P, Dixit VM. A second expressed thrombospondin gene (Thbs2) exists in the mouse genome. *J Biol Chem* 1991;266:12821–12824.
865. Crossin KL, Hoffman S, Grummet M, Thiery JP, Edelman GM. Site-restricted expression of cytotactin during development of the chicken embryo. *J Cell Biol* 1986;102:1917–1930.
866. Ekblom P, Aufderheide E. Stimulation of tenascin expression in mesenchyme by epithelial-mesenchymal interactions. *Int J Dev Biol* 1989;33:71–79.
867. Saga Y, Yagi T, Ikawa Y, Sakakura T, Aizawa S. Mice develop normally without tenascin. *Genes Dev* 1992;6:1821–1831.
868. Chiquet-Ehrismann R, Mackie EJ, Pearson CA, Sakakura T. Tenascin: an extracellular matrix protein involved in tissue interactions during fetal development and oncogenesis. *Cell* 1986;47: 131–139.
869. Thesloff LE, Mackie E, Vanio S, Chiquet-Ehrismann R. Changes in the distribution of tenascin during tooth development. *Development* 1987;101:289–296.
870. Aufderheide ER, Chiquet-Ehrismann R, Ekblom P. Epithelial-mesenchymal interactions in the developing kidney lead to the expression of tenascin in the mesenchyme. *J Cell Biol* 1987; 105:599–608.
871. Husmann K, Faissner A, Schachner M. Tenascin promotes cerebellar granule cell migration and neurite outgrowth by different domains in the fibronectin type III repeats. *J Cell Biol* 1992;116:1475–1486.
872. Mege RM, Nicolet M, Pincon-Raymond M, Murawsky M, Reiger F. Cytotactin is involved in synaptogenesis during regeneration of the frog neuromuscular system. *Dev Biol* 1992;149: 381–394.
873. Aukhil I, Erickson HP. Transfected BHK cells and transgenic mice expressing specific splice variants of tenascin. *Mol Biol Cell* 1992;3:128a.
874. Bernfield M, Kokenyesi R, Kato M, Hinkes MT, Spring J, Gallo RL, Lose EJ. Biology of the syndecans: a family of transmembrane heparan sulfate proteoglycans. *Ann Rev Cell Biol* 1992;8:365–393.
875. Bernfield M, Sanderson RD. Syndecan, a developmentally regulated cell surface proteoglycan that binds extracellular matrix and growth factors. *Phils Trans R Soc London* 1990;B327:171–186.
876. Yayon A, Klagsbrun M, Esko JD, Leder P, Ornitz DM. Cell surface, heparin-like molecules are required for binding of basic fibroblast growth factor to its high affinity receptor. *Cell* 1991;64:841–848.
877. Bernfield M, Hooper KC. Possible regulation of FGF activity by syndecan, an integral membrane heparan sulfate proteoglycan. *Ann NY Acad Sci* 1991;638:182–194.
878. Koike S, Taya C, Kurata T, Abe S, Ise I, Yonekawa H, Nomoto A. Transgenic mice susceptible to poliovirus. *Proc Natl Acad Sci USA* 1991;88:951–955.
879. D'Armiento J, Dalal SS, Okada Y, Berg RA, Chada K. Collagenase expression in the lungs of transgenic mice causes pulmonary emphysema. *Cell* 1992;71:955–961.
880. Côté F, Collard JF, Julien JP. Progressive neuronopathy in transgenic mice expressing the human neurofilament heavy gene: a mouse model of amyotrophic lateral sclerosis. *Cell* 1993;73: 35–46.
881. Clarke AR, Maandag ER, van Roon M, van der Lugt NM, vad der Valk M, Hooper ML, Berns A, te Riele H. Requirement for a functional *Rb-1* gene in murine development. *Nature* 1992;359: 328–330.
882. Jacks T, Fazeli A, Schmitt EM, Bronson RT, Goodell MA, Weinberg RA. Effects of an Rb mutation in the mouse. *Nature* 1992:295–300.
883. Lee EYHP, Chang CY, Hu N, Wang YCJ, Lai CC, Herrup K, Lee WH, Bradley A. Mice deficient for Rb are nonviable and show defects in neurogenesis and hametopoiesis. *Nature* 1992;359: 288–294.
884. Clarke LL, Grubb BR, Gabriel SE, Smithies O, Koller BH, Boucher RC. Defective epithelial choloride transport in a gene-targeted mouse model of cystic fibrosis. *Science* 1992;257: 1125–1128.
885. Plump AS, Smith JD, Hayek T, Aalto-Setälä K, Walsh A, Verstuyft JG, Rubin EM, Breslow JL. Severe hypercholesterolemia and atherosclerosis in apolipoprotein E-deficient mice created by homologous recombination in ES cells. *Cell* 1992;71:343–353.
886. Zhang SH, Reddick RL, Piedrahita JA, Maeda N. Spontaneous hypercholesterolemia and arterial lesions in mice lacking apolipoprotein E. *Science* 1992;258:468–471.
887. Chapman and Wolgemuth [*Submitted*].
888. Villar A and Pedersen RA [*Submitted*].
889. Gearhart JD et al. [*Submitted*].
890. Rastan S [*Submitted*].
891. Sturm KS et al. [*Submitted*].
892. Colbert MC, Linney E, LaMantia A-S. Local sources of retinoic acid coincide with retinoid-mediated transgene activity during embryonic development. *Proc Natl Acad Sci USA* 1993; 90:6572–6576.
893. Sutherland et al. [*Submitted*].
894. Wylie and Heasman [*Submitted*].
895. Perry JS. The mammalian fetal membranes. *J Reprod Fert* 1981;62:321–335.
896. Lawitts JA, Biggers JD. Optimization of mouse embryo culture media using simplex methods. *J Reprod Fert* 1991;91:543–556.
897. Copp AJ, Cockroft DL (eds). *Postimplantation mammalian embryos: A practical approach.* Oxford: Oxford University Press, 1990.
898. Beddington RSP. The development of 12th day fetuses following reimplantation of pre- and early- primitive streak-stage mouse embryos. *J Embryol Exp Morphol* 1985;88:281–291.
899. Taylor BA. Recombinant inbred strains. In: Lyon MF, Searle AG, eds. *Genetic Variants and Strains of the Laboratory Mouse, 2nd Ed.* Oxford: Oxford University Press, 1989;773–796.
900. Auner P, Amar L, Dandolo L. Guenet JL. Genetic analysis of the mouse using interspecific crosses. *Trends Genet* 1988;4:18–23.
901. Mintz B. Allophenic mice of multi-embryo origin. In: Daniel JC, Jr. *Methods in mammalian embryology.* San Francisco: WH Freeman 1971;186–214.
902. Pierce GB. The cancer cell and its control by the embryo. *Am J Pathol* 1983;113:117–124.
903. Wylie CC, Heasman J. Migration, proliferation and potency of primordial germ cells. *Sem Dev Biol* 1993;4:161–170.

The Physiology of Reproduction, Second Edition,
edited by E. Knobil and J.D. Neill,
Raven Press, Ltd., New York © 1994.

CHAPTER 7

Biology of Implantation

H. M. Weitlauf

Implantation of embryos in the wall of the uterus is a basic feature of mammalian reproduction. It is the result of a complex series of interactive steps beginning with fixation of the blastocyst in the uterus and ending with formation of a definitive placenta. Details of the intervening steps vary in different species, but the fundamental elements of embryo attachment and penetration of the epithelium with invasion into the endometrium, as well as formation of decidual tissue by the uterus, are features common to many animals. Furthermore, in the species studied so far, it appears the embryos and the uterus must be "synchronized"; typically, this means that the embryos have reached the expanded blastocyst stage and that the endometrium has undergone certain hormone-dependent changes that cause it to become "receptive" to the embryo.

Because of its complexity, the process of implantation is difficult to study *in toto,* and most research has been carried out on those component steps that can be dissected out for description or definition. This approach has been quite successful, and a vast literature has grown up over the past 50 years in which detailed accounts have been compiled describing the processes of embryo attachment, and penetration of the epithelium, the endocrine basis for uterine receptivity, and cytologic and biochemical changes associated with initiation of the decidual reaction and differentiation of decidual tissue. However, because they have focused on selected facets of the process, often in only one species, investigators have sometimes been tempted to look for and champion single mechanisms as the "cause" of implantation. But implantation is not an isolated event established at a moment in time, or even necessarily involving the same mechanisms in different species, and thus, there is no single cause or mechanism that can be singled out; the resulting controversies have tended to dominate the literature. Because it is difficult to develop an overview of implantation from the perspective of the conflicts, those findings that are most consistent and that seem to reflect common elements in various species are emphasized in this chapter. Several extensive reviews dealing with specific aspects of implantation should be consulted for further details regarding the controversial issues (1–14).

Texas Tech University Health Sciences Center, Department of Cell Biology and Anatomy, Lubbock, Texas 79430

CELLULAR ASPECTS OF IMPLANTATION

Details of implantation vary in different species. However, in all animals it ultimately involves a direct interaction of the trophoblast with the luminal epithelium of the uterus. This basic step has been described in detail from a morphologic perspective and provides a framework on which physiologic and biochemical observations can be organized.

Attachment

For descriptive purposes, it has been useful to consider that the attachment of embryos to the uterine epithelium occurs in two phases, apposition and adhesion (8); the processes involved are quite distinct. The term *apposition* denotes the progressively increasing intimacy of contact between the trophoblast and the uterine epithelium. In mice and rats, the uterine lumen closes down around the embryos in the earliest phase of implantation, and thus the uterus has the appearance of "clasping" the blastocysts (15). However, in animals such as the rabbit, the blastocyst enlarges to fill the uterine lumen and hence brings the trophoblast into apposition with the epithelium without general obliteration of the lumen (8,16). In either case, investment of embryos with maternal epithelium seems to provide the initial mechanism for their immobilization within the uterus. At this stage, the blastocyst can be dislodged without damage by gentle perfusion of the uterus, and hence the earliest fixation of the embryo is functional rather than involving structural connections between the two individuals. During this phase, there is a progressive interdigitation of microvilli and an increasingly intimate association between the membranes of the blastocyst and endometrium. The microvilli become shorter, more blunted, and irregular (17–22), and there is the appearance of large bulbous cytoplasmic projections, particularly on the antimesometrial surface (2,23). The obliteration of the uterine lumen with progressively closer apposition of the apical ends of the endometrial epithelial cells and the trophoblast has been referred to as the *attachment reaction* (18).

The mechanisms responsible for development of apposition, clasping, and the attachment reaction have not been worked out in detail, although in mice, rats, hamsters, and guinea pigs the changes appear to be associated with a more generalized closure of the uterine lumen that is dependent on the endocrine status of the mother (16,19–21,24–30). For instance, the uterine lumen remains relatively open in ovariectomized mice given no replacement hormones and becomes obliterated only after the animals are injected with progesterone (31,32). After treatment with progesterone alone, the process of closure tends to be arrested at the stage characterized by simple interdigitation of microvilli and does not show the progressively closer apposition characteristic of normal pregnancy. This "first stage" of closure can be maintained with progesterone for prolonged periods in castrated animals and is induced to progress to the "second stage" only by adding estrogen to the regimen (33). As might be expected, then, some degree of closure and clasping has been reported to occur in mice with lactational or experimentally induced delayed implantation (27,34). In those situations, the interaction between uterine epithelium and trophoblast is characterized by simple interdigitation of the microvilli as long as the animals are nursing or are maintained with progesterone. However, after the addition of estrogen, the association between the embryo and the uterus becomes more intimate, with a reduction in microvilli and progression to the typical attachment reaction (32). With the development of more intimate apposition in response to estrogen, there is apparently increased pressure on the blastocysts as their surfaces become marked and distorted by corresponding irregularities in the uterine epithelium (35). There is some degree of clasping of delayed-implanting rats embryos (26), but the preponderance of evidence indicates that, in that species also, estrogen must be added for a typical attachment reaction (36,37).

It is now generally assumed that uterine closure and clasping of embryos or other objects (38,39) involves both endocrine-dependent resorption of fluid from the lumen, presumably by way of the irregular cytoplasmic projections referred to as *pinopods* (40–42), and a mild generalized edema that occurs throughout the endometrium in response to estrogen (43,44). However, associated changes in the apical membranes of the uterine epithelial cells (45) and the occurrence of increased membrane turnover (46) indicate that processes associated with uterine closure are not limited to the removal of luminal fluid. Furthermore, although closure and clasping appear to be primarily hormone-dependent uterine functions, it has been reported that the presence of blastocysts (or oil droplets) in the lumen hastens the second stage of closure and appearance of the attachment reaction (47), and presumably such objects in the lumen provide an additional stimulus to the epithelium.

The significance of closure and the attachment reaction in mice and rats may be that a period of stability is provided during which adhesion between the embryo and uterus can develop. However, in animals such as the rabbit, the mink, or the rhesus monkey, there does not appear to be a typical closure of the uterine lumen or clasping of the embryos (16,48), and it seems to be the expansion of the blastocyst that is primarily responsible for establishing the initial apposition between trophoblast and epithelium. It is interesting in this regard that there is no evidence for pinopod-mediated uptake of fluid from the lumen of the rabbit uterus (49). In large domestic species also, with their superficial epitheliochorial-type implantation, the interdigitation of microvilli is particularly extensive, and embryos appear to be firmly fixed in the uterus even though a typical attachment reaction with progressive loss of microvilli is not observed (50–52).

Adhesion of trophoblast cells to the apical end of uterine epithelial cells develops as the apposition phase progresses. Cytologic evidence most often cited as demonstrating the development of adhesiveness is twofold. First, with tissue taken from progressively later stages in the early phase of implantation, there is an increase in the amount and frequency of distortion of one or both surfaces. This is thought to occur as a normal part of the attachment process and to be exaggerated as a differential shrinkage artifact when the tissues are fixed for microscopy. Second, not only are there extensive areas where closely apposed membranes of trophoblast and apical ends of the uterine cells are parallel and separated by less than 150 to 200 Å, but primitive junctional complexes are established (8,9). Although some descriptions of these regions have indicated the existence of mature septate-type desmosomal junctions and areas of cytoplasmic confluence (21,26), the usual observation is of more primitive and less specialized types of junctional complexes in the absence of cytoplasmic confluence (8,9,15,27,53). Once the epithelium is penetrated, however, typical mature junctional complexes are often observed to be shared between uterine epithelium and the invading trophoblast (53).

The molecular basis for initial adhesion of trophoblast and uterine epithelium at implantation has not yet been determined with certainty. However, because of the widespread involvement of various cell surface glycoproteins and extracellular matrix molecules as cell-adhesion/substrate-adhesion molecules, and the fundamental role of cell surface glycoconjugates in cell-recognition/adhesion phenomena during embryogenesis and tumor metastasis (54–57), attention has been focused on the search for such molecules on the surface of peri-implantation blastocysts and uterine epithelium: In as much as the initial interaction between the embryo and the uterus involves the outer surface of the blastocyst (i.e., trophectoderm) and the luminal surface of the epithelial cells, it is presumed that complementary factors relevant to embryo attachment will be expressed at the apical ends of those highly polarized cell types. Furthermore, because the maternal hormones impose a relatively short "window of receptivity" on the uterus, and it is only during that time that implantation can occur, those glycoconjugates on the apical surface of trophectoderm or uterine epithelium that are hormone responsive are the most likely candidates for a role in embryo attachment.

In some of the earliest studies, it was shown that there are striking hormone-dependent changes in the glycocalyx on the apical surface of uterine epithelial cells in the peri-implantation period. The changes are qualitative as well as quantitative (e.g., the thickness and morphologic appearance of the glycocalyx change at the time of expected implantation and the amount of negative charge associated with the surface is reduced due to removal of sialic acid residues). Thus, Enders and Schlafke (58), using a combination of colloidal thorium, ruthenium red, and concanavalin A-peroxidase, demonstrated the extensive distribution of negative charges and acidic glycoproteins on the surface of mouse uterus during the fourth and fifth days of normal pregnancy and on the seventh day of lactation-delayed implantation. Although those workers were the first to suggest that there is a reduction in the thickness of the glycocalyx at implantation, the methods used were not considered to be quantitative. Others, however, have confirmed that there is both a generalized loss of anionic sites and a reduction in thickness of the uterine glycocalyx at about the time of implantation; rabbit (59), rat (60,61), mouse (62,63), and primate (64). And there are reports of corresponding changes in the ability of uterine epithelium to bind certain lectins indicating qualitative changes in carbohydrate residues of specific cell surface glycoconjugates occur as well, especially marked is the appearance of galactose residues (62–69). Interestingly, these changes are apparently not dependent on the presence of embryos, because they occur in pseudopregnant as well as pregnant animals. In the ferret, however, the uterine glycocalyx does appear to be reduced in thickness initially at the specific points of contact between the embryo and uterus, indicating that the embryo plays a role in the process of modifying the uterine surface (70). A reduction in thickness of the glycocalyx could be associated with the removal of masking residues and thus be responsible for opening a variety of specific binding sites. Indeed, the report by Chavez and Anderson (62) indicating that binding sites for the *Ricinus communis* lectin (i.e., binds D-galactose) appear at both implantation and interimplantation areas in mouse uterus during the peri-implantation phase of pregnancy has been used to support the suggestion that lectinlike receptors for galactose, appearing on the embryos, could bind to those sites and act as part of the adhesion mechanism at implantation.

More recently, the results of extensive biochemical analyses have provided hard evidence for hormone-dependent changes in specific cell surface glycoconjugates on the uterine epithelium as well. Dutt et al. (71) provided the first systematic description of steroid hormone effects on overall assembly of uterine glycoproteins in mice. Other reports describe changes in uterine production of specific classes of glycoconjugates including hyaluronate (72); lactosaminoglycans and galactosyltransferases (63,73–79); and heparin/heparan sulfate proteoglycans and their binding proteins (80–84). These molecules are all known to be components of different cell-adhesion systems and are localized at the apical surface of the uterine epithelial cells where they would have the potential to be involved in the cell recognition/adhesion necessary for initial embryo attachment. By contrast, some other extracellular matrix molecules with the potential for involvement in cell-adhesion mechanisms (i.e., laminin, collagen, and fibronectin) and which are abundant in the endometrium are conspicuously absent from the apical surface of the uterine epithelium. Thus, although these glycoproteins are presumably available for later steps in implantation, including penetration of the basement membrane and invasion of the endometrial stroma, they are not likely to have a role in the initial attachment phase of implantation (85–87).

Surface molecules have also been observed to change on embryos at the time of attachment. For instance, histocompatibility antigens (H-2) on dormant delayed-implanting mouse blastocysts decrease during reactivation (88,89), suggesting that these glycoprotein factors are either removed or masked, and there is a reduction in the thickness of the glycocalyx and in binding of positively charged colloidal iron, as well as indicating a decrease in the density of negative surface charges (90–92). This histochemical finding was confirmed by the results of experiments using free-zone electrophoresis (93,94). Such changes in the embryos are compatible with removal of terminal sialic acid residues or larger moieties of the oligosaccharide components of surface glycoproteins at the time of attachment and at the initiation of implantation.

In related experiments, lectins have been used to probe the glycocalyx of the embryo for changes in the "accessibility" of specific sugars at the time of implantation. Because it appears, in many species, that the initial attachment of embryos occurs on specific limited regions of their surfaces (58,70,95,96), it might be anticipated that those regions would acquire adhesiveness earlier than other areas on the embryos and, therefore, that changes in lectin binding that are relevant to implantation would have corresponding temporal and regional patterns. Although binding of different lectins has been observed by several investigators, in most cases the anticipated temporal and regional changes have not been found. Thus, it was shown with the electron microscope that concanavalin A-peroxidase binds to the surfaces of both embryos and the uterus of mice, but there was no evidence of a change with implantation or of regional distribution on the blastocysts (58,97). Chavez and Enders (98,99), using ferritin-conjugated lectins on days 5 and 6 of normal pregnancy as well as during delayed implantation, found stage-specific changes in the binding of peanut agglutinin and the agglutinin from *Ricinus communis* to the surface of blastocysts as they prepared to implant (these lectins bind preferentially to *N*-acetylgalactosamine and D-galactose, respectively), but neither change could be implicated as a factor in the acquisition of adhesiveness because the binding pattern was not different in nonadhesive delayed-implanting embryos. However, those same workers (100) reported that the lectin from *Dolichos biflorus* (specific for *N*-acetylglucosamine) did bind to delayed-implanting embryos but did not bind to embryos that were reactivated. Although regional differences were not seen, they suggested that the loss of binding sites is associated with the acquisition of adhesiveness. With concanavalin A bound to red blood cells, Sobel and Nebel (101,102) observed increased agglutination over the abembryonic pole of mouse blastocysts, and similarly, concanavalin A attached to latex beads was shown to bind preferentially to the abembryonic end of delayed-implanting blastocysts (103). However, again, there was no change in this regional pattern of binding on reactivation and subsequent implantation. From such observations, it cannot be determined whether changes in the glycocalyx that lead to changes in lectin binding are simply not related to the acquisition of regional adhesiveness or whether the methods used are too insensitive to demonstrate subtle differences in binding. By contrast, the observation that binding of molecular [^{3}H]concanavalin A to delayed-implanting embryos decreases in the abembryonic region during reactivation prompted the suggestion that there is a regional change in availability of mannoselike sugars or membrane fluidity that is related to the development of adhesiveness (104,105). A similar temporal and regional change in the glycocalyx during reactivation of delayed-implanting mouse embryos was inferred from increased staining of the abembryonic pole with Alcian blue (103). Although the precise nature of changes in the glycocalyx cannot be deduced from such information, the observation of such temporal and regional patterns is compatible with the interpretation that they are related to the acquisition of localized adhesiveness on the embryo at the time of implantation.

Pinsker and Mintz (106) are often credited with the first attempts to establish qualitative differences in composition of surface glycoproteins in preimplantation mouse embryos. Those workers labeled two- to four-cell embryos or morula-early blastocysts differentially with [^{3}H]- and [^{14}C]glucosamine, combined them, and removed the glycocalyx with trypsin; the trypsinate was treated with pronase, and the digest was subjected to gel filtration. They found more label and generally larger fragments in the material from blastocysts but were unable to determine whether the change was due to synthesis of qualitatively new glycoproteins or due to differentially regulated expression of those present in the earlier stages. In either case, they did not examine blastocysts at the time they acquire adhesiveness, and therefore, their results do not provide information strictly about changes associated with implantation. Similarly, the observation by Surani (107) that tunicamycin reduces synthesis of glycoconjugates by mouse embryos did not particularly advance our understanding of the role of changes on the embryonic surface at implantation.

Immunocytochemical methods have also provided direct evidence for the expression of several basement membrane molecules and components of known cell-adhesion systems on blastomeres of early embryos (see ref. 108 for a caveat). Thus, laminin appears to be present as early as the two-cell stage (109) and is found in areas of contact between cells at the eight- to 16-cell stage; nidogen appears at this stage also (109–111). Entactin is first observed at the hatched blastocyst stage (111). Immunoreactive basement membrane collagens may be expressed as early as the two- to four-cell stage, with type III collagen becoming localized to the intercellular areas at the blastocyst stage (112). With expansion of the blastocysts and formation of endoderm, the laminin nidogen and entactin tend to colocalize to areas of developing extracellular matrix (109,111). Type IV collagen and fibronectin are expressed in the inner cell mass (ICM) of late blastocyst stage embryos and thus also correspond to formation of early basement membrane (110,113–116).

Immunohistochemical methods have been used to demonstrate expression of the closely related cell-adhesion molecules CAM 120/80 (117,118), uvomorulin (119,120), and cadhedrin (121) in mouse embryos as early as the two-cell stage. Antibodies to these cell-adhesion molecules typically disrupt compaction and cell–cell adhesion within the embryo. There are several other reports of less well-defined antigenic determinants on the surfaces of cells at the eight-cell-morula stage, and in some cases, the antibodies were also able to block compaction (e.g., see refs. 122–124). And at least one report has appeared of the expression of a receptor for fucosylated oligosaccharides on eight-cell embryos that is essential for compaction (i.e., as demonstrated by disruption of compaction with the putative ligand) (125). The spatiotemporal distribution of most of these cell–adhesion molecules and the fact that in many cases antibodies against them cause decompaction of late morula stage embryos and disrupt blastulation make it seem likely that they are involved in cell–cell interactions within the embryo rather than with attachment to the uterus. By contrast, at least one cell-adhesion molecule (i.e., CAM 105 originally described in rat liver) is expressed only on the surface of early blastocysts and appears to be down-regulated on mural trophectoderm at about the time of attachment; thus, CAM 105 may play a role in embryo–uterine interactions at implantation (126).

Interactions between galactosyltransferase and multivalent lactosaminoglycans are recognized as being important for cell–cell adhesion (127) and components of a potential galactosyltransferase/lactosaminoglycan cell-adhesion system have been reported on mouse embryos as early as the four- to eight-cell stage. Matricorena et al. (128), Babiarz and Hathaway (129), and Hathaway and Babiarz (130) used a monoclonal antibody to the II3C determinant on F9 cells to demonstrate the presence of that specific lactosaminoglycan on compacted morula and attaching blastocysts. Bayna et al. (131) found that an antibody to β-1,4 galactosyltransferase (from milk) recognized a determinant between cells of the late morula and reported that the antigen disrupted compaction. Sato et al. (132) also presented immunologic evidence for the presence of a galactosyltransferase on mouse embryos from the eight-cell through early blastocyst stages of development; Hjortberg and Nilsson (133) and Svalander et al. (134) reported that a galactose-containing determinant is expressed on the surface of the blastocyst at about the time of implantation. Thus, a cell-adhesion system using lactosaminoglycans and galactosyltransferase is a potential candidate for a role in the process of embryo attachment and the initiation of implantation. It is interesting in this regard that Chavez (63) reported being able to inhibit implantation *in vivo* by intrauterine instillation of compounds that interfere with galactosyltransferase.

Heparin/heparan sulfate proteoglycans represent still another group of glycoconjugates with the potential to function in cell adhesion mechanisms. And it has been reported that an antibody against heparan sulfate basement membrane proteoglycans recognized determinants on preimplantation mouse embryos from the two-cell through blastocyst stage (135); it appears to colocalize with laminin and nidogen as the embryos begin to produce early basement membrane. More recently, a specific heparan sulfate/chondroitin sulfate containing membrane proteoglycan (designated syndecan) has also been detected on the surface of embryos from the four-cell-early blastocyst stage; as endoderm is formed, it becomes localized to cell–cell boundaries and is ultimately restricted to the site of first matrix deposition. Because of the spatiotemporal pattern, syndecan is thought to be an unlikely participant in the implantation process *per se* (86,136).

In other work with immunologic probes, the expression of certain soluble lectins with specificity for lactosamine-based structures has been observed on the surface of trophectoderm of hatched blastocysts [i.e., Mac-2, L14 (137), and L14 (138)]. This finding, along with the appearance of appropriate glycoconjugate ligands on the apical surface of the uterine epithelium at about the time of implantation (62,63,68,79), raises the possibility that highly specific ligand-receptor recognition mechanisms using soluble lectins on the embryo and lactosaminoglycan-based structures on the uterus are available at the appropriate time and, thus, might be involved in the initial attachment of embryos to the uterus.

The mere demonstration of components of putative adhesion systems does not prove that they function at the time of implantation. And an extensive body of work in which the attachment and outgrowth of mouse embryos on defined substrata *in vitro* has been blocked with specific molecules provides additional information implicating some of these factors (in a functional way) to the mechanism(s) responsible for embryo adhesion to the uterine lining. For simplicity, the work is grouped as follows: Farach et al. (139) reported that disruption of overall glycoconjugate assembly in the blastocyst (with *p*-nitrophenyl-D-xylosides) prevented (reversibly) attachment and outgrowth of embryos *in vitro;* it was concluded that production of glycoconjugates is critical for normal attachment. Lindenberg et al. (140) reported that the milk oligosaccharide lacto-*N*-fucopentaose I inhibits attachment of mouse blastocysts on uterine epithelial monolayers and proposed that a surface receptor on the trophectoderm normally interacts with similar determinants on the uterine epithelium to affect embryo attachment; there is evidence for hormonal regulation of such a carbohydrate epitope in the uterus of mice (78,79). Richa et al. (117) reported that antibodies (i.e., GP 140 and SMF I) against a group of cell-substratum-adhesion glycoproteins prevented attachment and outgrowth of mouse blastocysts cultured in medium containing serum. However, no epithelial ligand has been identified, and because the molecules defined by those antibodies are similar to the CAM 120/80 and have essentially the same distribution in the embryo (118,141), it has been considered probable that they are involved in attachment of the cells to the embryonic extracellular matrix rather than to the uterus. Nevertheless, these molecules are expressed early on the surface of trophectoderm, and the possibility that they are involved in attachment and invasion of embryos *in vivo* must be considered. An interesting series of experiments have been reported that deals with integrin receptors on embryos that recognize peptides containing the sequence RGD (see ref. 86). First, it was established that mouse blastocysts will attach to and spread out on a defined substrate consisting of laminin, fibronectin, vitronectin, or collagen (types II, IV, and VI). Subsequently, it was found that the outgrowth on (but not the attachment to) fibronectin and collagen types II and IV was blocked by peptides containing the RGD sequence (142–146). Because peptides with the RGD sequence have differential effects on attachment and outgrowth with different substrates, it was concluded that there must be several mechanisms responsible for embryo attachment to the basement membrane and extracellular matrix molecules. That there were temporal differences in gaining competence to attach to different substrates (as well as for different domains on the same substrate) suggested that the several mechanisms with different specificities were developmentally regulated (85). Farach et al. (144) investigated the role of heparin/heparan sulfate proteoglycans in attachment and outgrowth of mouse blastocysts on defined extracellular matrix components as well as uterine epithelial cell monolayers. Results of that work provided several lines of evidence to implicate heparin/heparan sulfate proteoglycans in the mechanisms responsible for attachment to and outgrowth on a variety of matrices: (a) soluble heparin inhibited attachment and outgrowth on platelet factor IV and decreased the rate of attachment and outgrowth on laminin and fibronectin as well as on monolayers of uterine epithelium; (b) digestion of the surface components of embryos with heperinase slowed the rate of outgrowth; (c) selective staining for sulfated proteoglycans and labeling surface components with I^{125} demonstrated that heparin/heparan sulfate proteoglycans are a major component of the blastocyst surface; and (d) the additional findings that binding proteins for heparin/heparan sulfate proteoglycans exist on the apical surface of uterine epithelial cells (84) and that heparan sulfate is a potent inducer of the decidual reaction (12) makes this cell-adhesion system particularly interesting as a potential mechanism for embryo attachment or signal transduction at the time of implantation. The emerging concept that mechanisms responsible for initial attachment of the embryos are separate from those involved in penetration of the basement membrane and endometrial stroma is an important one and will lead to more focused experiments in the future.

Because there are changes in the appearance and chemical composition of the glycocalyx on both the uterine and the embryonic sides, it now seems probable that specific complementary molecules will eventually be shown to be responsible for attachment of mammalian embryos to the uterine wall. However, it remains to be determined precisely which molecules are involved and how they are regulated.

Penetration of the Epithelium

It is clear that, with the exception of those species having a superficial (i.e., epitheliochorial) type of placentation, all mammalian embryos penetrate the uterine epithelium and its associated basal lamina to establish a definitive vascular relationship with the mother. However, the process varies considerably from species to species in terms of both timing and precise cytologic features, and the early literature was replete with what appeared to be conflicting observations. Some conceptual order was brought to this complex problem when Schlafke and Enders (9) pointed out that there are really three general strategies for penetrating the uterine epithelium and that different animals have adopted one or another of these approaches. Many of the apparent inconsistencies disappear when comparisons are confined to a single type of penetration. A brief description of the essential cytologic details in each of the three categories is useful to demonstrate the different ways in which different species have solved the problem of breaching the epithelial barrier.

Intrusive Penetration

In species that have adopted the intrusive approach to penetration of the epithelium, the embryos are generally considered to be highly "invasive"; the ferret provides an excellent example (70,147). Attachment initially occurs at specialized regions (i.e., ectoplasmic pads) of developing syncytial trophoblast. Whereas the broader regions of syncytial plaque generally follow the contour of the apical end of the epithelial cells, the ectoplasmic pads tend to indent them and appear to provide the initial points of attachment. The first penetration of epithelium is seen as the projection of a thin fold of syncytial trophoblast between adjacent epithelial cells. Initially, the processes are ectoplasmic, but as they enlarge and progress to the basal lamina, the cytoplasm is found to contain the usual array of organelles. The trophoblastic membrane is observed to share both apical junctional complexes and punctate desmosomes with the lateral membrane of adjacent epithelial cells. It is not known how the original epithelial apical junctional complexes are breached, but the process typically occurs at many sites that are separated by only a few cells. Although the trophoblast eventually surrounds large numbers of epithelial cells and there is evidence of cell death and phagocytosis, the overwhelming impression is of apparently undisturbed epithelial cells adjacent to the trophoblast. Indeed, it has been suggested that healthy epithelium is necessary for anchoring the trophoblast as it penetrates deeper into the endometrium (70). The trophoblastic processes pause at the basal lamina and are disposed along it for a brief time and then proceed to invade the stroma where they surround but do not penetrate the basal lamina of the capillaries. Other species having the intrusive type of penetration include the guinea pig (53,148,149) and the rhesus monkey (48). There are subtle but potentially important differences in detail in these animals. For example, the syncytial trophoblastic processes of both the monkey and the ferret typically pause at the epithelial basal lamina; in the monkey, they then go on to invade the basal lamina of endometrial blood vessels, something not seen in the ferret.

The intrusion of the cellular trophoblast to form the isolated endometrial cups responsible for secretion of gonadotropin in the horse provides an interesting variation in this form of epithelial penetration that appears to be unrelated to the process of implantation *per se* (150).

Displacement Penetration

The rat and the mouse provide typical examples of displacement penetration (15,151). As the apposition phase proceeds and the first signs of decidualization appear in the subjacent stroma, there is typically evidence of cell death in the epithelial layer and of detachment of cells either singly or in groups. With the light microscope, these cells occasionally appear as dark masses (W-bodies) between the embryo and the endometrium and were originally thought to reflect the passage of some material from the embryo to the uterus (152). However, it was subsequently shown with the electron microscope that these masses are really dead epithelial cells that are being phagocytized by the trophoblast (151). As the trophoblast comes into contact with the basal lamina, it pauses and sends out processes that undermine adjacent cells and thus extends the epithelial defect and increases the area available for contact with the embryo. The basal lamina is then breached, apparently not by the trophoblast but rather by ectoplasmic processes of underlying decidual cells (153).

The mechanism responsible for death and detachment of epithelium in this type of implantation is not known. However, it does appear to be intrinsic to the uterus because it occurs in the "implantation chambers" associated with an oil-induced decidual reaction in pseudopregnant mice (154–157) and is blocked by administration of actinomycin D (158). Considerable histochemical evidence has been presented that indicates that the activity of different lysosomal enzymes decreases in the epithelial cells adjacent to an implanting embryo but not in interimplantation areas or in pseudopregnant animals (159–164), and it has been argued on this basis that the cells are undergoing autolysis in response to an embryonic signal (165). When the sloughing of epithelium was prevented by actinomycin D, mouse blastocysts became attached to the epithelium but were unable to penetrate to the basal lamina or stroma and thus could not truly implant (158). Hence, mouse blastocysts seem to be only weakly invasive, and an intact uterine epithelium may be an effective barrier to implantation. Therefore, autolytic destruction of the epithelium seems to be an important precondition for implantation in that species at least, and the finding that mouse blastocysts transferred to the uteri of cyclic females implant only if the epithelium is disrupted (166) supports this suggestion.

Fusion Penetration

The rabbit provides an example of fusion penetration (53,95,167,168). First attachment occurs between syncytial knobs of the abembryonic trophoblast and individual epithelial cells. The apical membrane of the epithelial cell fuses with that of the trophoblastic knob, resulting in cytoplasmic confluency. As the epithelial cell is converted to syncytium, it becomes cytologically distinct from its neighbors and appears, using the light or electron microscope, as a "peg" of trophoblast extending to the basal lamina. The original nucleus is present for some time, and the lateral plasma membrane retains the original junctional complexes with its apparently normal neighboring cells. There may be more than one peg per trophoblastic knob, and after some delay, the basal lamina is penetrated at the locations of these pegs and the trophoblastic processes proceed to penetrate the endometrial blood vessels. Subsequently, there is widespread formation of epithelial symplasma, and fusion occurs in areas between the trophoblastic knobs (169).

Localized Changes in the Stroma

In rats and mice, the endometrial stroma eventually undergoes dramatic cytologic changes to form a decidua in response to the implanting embryo. This process is discussed in detail later, but it should be noted here that subtle changes occur locally in the endometrium as an early part of the decidual response. The most obvious of these are the increases in alkaline phosphatase activity (155) and vascular permeability (170–172), which occur in the stroma immediately adjacent to the embryos even before they have penetrated the epithelium.

It is clear, even from these strictly morphologic accounts of early pregnancy, that at least two different sorts of changes occur in the peri-implantation uterus. First, there are certain hormone-dependent changes in the endometrium that make subsequent steps possible. These "enabling" changes, such as closure of the lumen and the acquisition by epithelium of the potential for self-destruction, occur throughout the endometrium, apparently without regard to the presence of an embryo. By contrast, there are other changes in the endometrium that must be provoked by a stimulus, from either an embryo or a suitable experimental substitute. These "evoked" responses, such as autolysis of epithelial cells or decidual transformation of stromal cells, are typically localized to the endometrium adjacent to the embryo or the site of experimental stimulation. Although the actual roles of many of these changes have not been established with certainty, it is presumed that they are important for the implantation process; a great deal of work has been directed at defining their molecular and cellular basis. The process of decidual transformation and the associated enabling changes leading to acquisition of sensitivity by the endometrium may be of the most thoroughly studied of all.

Decidualization

Decidual transformation of the endometrium in response to an implanting embryo results in grossly observable increases in the size and weight of the uterus. This growth is due not only to proliferation and differentiation of the endometrial stromal cells but also to infiltration of the endometrium by a variety of cells derived from the bone marrow and swelling of the tissue caused by localized increases in vascular permeability and the development of tissue edema. Thus, after attachment, the embryo typically becomes embedded in an enlarging mass of decidual tissue, each so-called nidus being separated from the others by intervening areas of nontransformed endometrium. Formation of the decidua is a conspicuous part of the process of implantation, and although the function of this specialized tissue has not been determined with certainty, it is generally believed to be a critical component of the mother's response to the embryo.

The discovery by Loeb (173–175) nearly 80 years ago that a similar transformation of the endometrium could be induced by indifferent stimuli in the uteri of animals that were suitable prepared with ovarian steroid hormones has led to the development of an experimental model for this maternal response to the implanting embryo. Several investigators have pointed to subtle differences between the "deciduomata" of the experimental model and naturally occurring decidua, particularly with respect to the timing of development and minor morphologic details (176–178). However, the basic processes responsible for decidual transformation in response to the embryo appear to be the same as those leading to formation of experimental decidoumata, and the model has come to be widely accepted (179).

One of the most important observations made with the experimental model has been that the decidual response can be obtained only during a limited time in pregnancy or pseudopregnancy (180–181) and that this period varies with the nature of the experimental stimulus. Thus, a grossly traumatic stimulus such as crushing or cutting the uterus was found to be effective during a period of 3 or 4 days early in pseudopregnancy, whereas less traumatic stimuli such as intraperitoneal injection of pyrathiazine or the intraluminal instillation of different chemical substances can elicit a response only during a period of a few hours (154,182–188). Furthermore, this period of maximum sensitivity to the so-called nontraumatic stimuli was found to correspond to the period of uterine receptivity for blastocysts as established by asynchronous embryo transfer experiments (189–196).

With this information in hand, it then became possible to determine the endocrine basis for developing uterine sensitivity. In an extensive series of experiments with mice and rats, it was eventually shown that although progesterone alone would support the development of a deciduoma in response to traumatic stimuli, it is estrogen acting on the endometrium after preconditioning with progesterone for at least 2 days that is responsible for entraining the pattern of sensitivity and subsequent refractoriness characteristic of the peri-implantation period (1–3,179,188). As might be anticipated, this endocrine regimen is essentially the same as that necessary to obtain implantation of blastocysts in ovariectomized rats and mice (170,197,198).

Once it was established that formation of this new "decidual organ" (199) was dependent on appropriate hormonal conditioning and the application of a suitable stimulus during a limited time, the emphasis of investigators shifted to defining those chemical and cytologic changes within the endometrium that are associated with establishing receptivity and the differentiation of decidual tissue (1–7).

Preparation of the Endometrium

Hormone-dependent changes in cell proliferation and differentiation occur in all compartments of the endometrium, and although it has not been possible to determine how the changes are related to the acquisition of receptivity or to the development of the decidual reaction, it is generally thought that they are essential.

Cell Proliferation

Changes in the rates of proliferation of endometrial components have been examined in intact animals during the estrous cycle and early pregnancy and pseudopregnancy: mice (200–202), rats (203–206), guinea pig (207–209), and hamster (210).

Luminal Epithelium

Mitotic activity in luminal epithelium of mice varies during the ovarian cycle, with a peak at about the time of ovulation and a smaller secondary peak 3 days later. The secondary peak falls on the third day of pregnancy if mating has occurred, and there is little or no mitotic activity in the luminal epithelium thereafter (200,201). A similar pattern appears in the rat, with the first peak at about the time of ovulation and a second one 2 days later on the second day of pregnancy or pseudopregnancy (203–205). It has been reported similarly that in guinea pigs, there is mitotic activity at about the time of ovulation and a secondary peak 2 to 3 days later (207–209). With hamsters also, mitotic activity is found in the epithelium at the time of ovulation, with a marked increase 2 days later (210).

Synthesis of DNA, as demonstrated by incorporation of [^{3}H]thymidine and autoradiographic or scintillation counting techniques, follows the same pattern. Incorporation of [^{3}H]thymidine increases in luminal epithelium of the mouse on the second day of pseudopregnancy and decreases thereafter (201,211). In rats also, the epithelium is labeled with [^{3}H]thymidine on the second and third days of pseudopregnancy (212).

Glandular Epithelium

Proliferation of endometrial glands tends to be low in mice at and before ovulation but shows a marked increase 3 days later, coincident with the second peak of epithelial mitosis (200,202). The pattern appears to be similar in the rat, with a peak on the second day of pregnancy (204,205,213); a corresponding incorporation of [^{3}H]thymidine has been observed on the second day of pregnancy (214). Mitotic activity in the glands of the guinea pig is of relatively greater extent than that in the mouse and the rat and appears somewhat later, with a peak on the fourth day of the estrous cycle (207–209).

Stroma

A small amount of mitotic activity is observed in the stroma of the mouse just before ovulation and is minimal thereafter until a marked increase occurs on the fourth day of pseudopregnancy or pregnancy; the high levels of mitotic activity carry over into the fifth day, when implantation occurs (200,201). There appears to be some preferential distribution of the active cells near the luminal epithelium, although mitosis occurs throughout the endometrium. A similar pattern is observed in the rat, with stromal mitosis appearing late on the third day and peaking on the fourth day, and the active cells appear to be concentrated in the subepithelial antimesometrial stroma (204–206). The pattern in the guinea pig seems to peak between the sixth and seventh days of the cycle (207–209).

Incorporation of [^{3}H]thymidine into DNA is observed in the stroma of mice and rats after epithelial mitosis has ceased. It is maximal on the fourth and fifth days of pseudopregnancy (201,211,212) in the subepithelial cells of the antimesometrial region (215) and appears to be a consequence of estrogen action after preparation by progesterone (216).

The endocrine regulation of cell division in the different tissue compartments of the endometrium has been examined critically using ovariectomized animals given replacement therapy: mice (217–222); rats (206,216, 223); guinea pig (207,208); and rabbit (224,225). The relationships between changes in the endocrine milieu and mitotic activity in the luminal epithelium, the glands, and the stroma have been most completely established for mouse endometrium. A description of these relationships in the mouse therefore seems useful as a basis for comparison. The observations on intact mice fit well with what has been discovered about endocrine regulation of these tissues in replacement experiments with ovariectomized animals; the observations also fit well with what is known about the changing levels of ovarian steroid hormones in the estrous cycle and early pregnancy (3,4).

Luminal Epithelium

Mitotic activity is nil in the luminal epithelium of ovariectomized mice given no hormone replacement. However, after a single injection of estrogen, there is an increase in mitotic activity; the response is biphasic with peaks at about 24 and 36 h (217–220,222,226–230). If estrogen is administered continuously, the effect on mitotic activity in epithelial cells is maintained for 2 days and then drops off (221). Progesterone administered by itself has no stimulatory effect on luminal epithelium but markedly reduces the effect on estrogen if the two hormones are administered simultaneously; typically, the first peak of mitotic activity is reduced and the second peak is blocked completely. The effect of progesterone can be obtained up to about 17 h after estrogen (231,232). However, if progesterone is given for 3 days, a subsequent injection of estrogen has no effect on mitotic activity in the epithelium (233). The rat is apparently similar to the mouse in that estrogen stimulates mitotic activity in luminal epithelial cells within 24 h and pretreatment with progesterone suppresses that effect (206,223). The rabbit seems to respond differently in that estrogen stimulates epithelium only mildly whereas progesterone alone (in sufficiently high doses) is the more effective stimulus; it has been reported, however, that priming with estrogen reduces the amount of progesterone needed for the mitogenic effect (224,225). In the ovariectomized guinea pig, estrogen stimulates epithelial mitosis (207,208) and pretreatment with progesterone prevents this effect (207).

Glandular Epithelium

A single injection of estrogen has no effect on mitosis in uterine glands of mice (220). However, with continuous administration of estrogen, a wave of mitosis is seen in the glands at 72 h; this is followed by a second wave of mitotic activity 72 h after terminating treatment (221). Progesterone given beforehand suppresses both waves of activity, whereas progesterone given with the estrogen, or after estrogen treatment, blocks only the second wave. In the rat, estrogen causes an increase in mitosis in the glands within 24 h and causes a further increase at 48 h; again, pretreatment with progesterone suppresses that effect (206,223). In rabbits, there is reported to be some mitotic activity in the glands after treatment with estrogen alone, but the response is much greater with progesterone (225). There is a question regarding control of mitosis in uterine glands of the guinea pig because some investigators have achieved proliferation with estrogen alone and suggest that the guinea pigs are like mice and rats (207); whereas others have reported that mitotic activity is stimulated by progesterone after estrogen priming and suggest, therefore, that guinea pigs are similar to rabbits (208).

Stroma

Neither estrogen nor progesterone alone appears to have an effect on mitotic activity in stroma in mice. However, progesterone is able to induce stromal mitosis if a priming dose of estrogen has been given previously (234). Furthermore, if progesterone is given for 3 days, the stroma undergoes marked hypertrophy in response to a subsequent injection of estrogen regardless of whether priming estrogen was given (220,233). Priming with estrogen appears to compress the progesterone-induced changes into just 2 days (235). Interestingly, a second injection of estrogen given to progesterone-treated animals at 48 h will cause a second increase in mitotic activity, but if it is given between 12 and 36 h after the first injection, the endometrium is refractory and the estrogen is redirected to affect the epithelium (236). In the rat also, estrogen has no effect on stromal mitosis unless there has been pretreatment with progesterone (206,223). Also, it appears the mitotic activity in the rat is concentrated in the antimesometrial stroma adjacent to the luminal epithelium (223). With the rabbit, estrogen alone causes a modest increase in stromal mitosis (225). Again, there is a question in the cased guinea pigs because some investigators find that progesterone alone stimulates little mitotic activity in the stroma, which increases dramatically when estrogen is added as it does in the mouse (207), whereas others report that progesterone after estrogen priming causes massive increases in stromal mitosis and suggest that the guinea pig is like the rabbit (208).

Associated with changes in proliferation during the peri-implantation period, there are marked changes in the levels of steroid receptors (237–241). However, it has been difficult to evaluate the significance of the changes with respect to development of endometrial receptivity and mitotic activity, not only because of the heterogeneity within the receptor populations (242,243) but also because in many cases the measurements were made on whole uterus rather than in the different tissue compartments or cell populations of the endometrium. It must be remembered that the myometrium accounts for as much as 90% of the mass of the uterus and that measurements of the whole organ tend to reflect changes in that compartment rather than in the endometrium. The significance of this distinction was demonstrated by Glasser and McCormack (7), who observed that, as measured in whole uterus, the concentrations of both nuclear and cytosol estrogen receptor decrease from the second or third day of pregnancy onward, whereas in stroma the content actually increases. Martel and Psychoyos (244) likewise found differential changes in cytosol estrogen receptor levels in the different uterine compartments in response to progesterone, with increases occurring in stroma after 48 h accompanied by simultaneous decreases in the epithelium. Although the concentration of estrogen receptor is correlated with the mitogenic effect of estrogen in the peri-implantation period, levels of receptor do not appear to be the limiting factor (244) and the acquisition of sensitivity to estrogen after 48 h of progesterone appears to involve other regulatory factors.

In general, then, estrogen stimulates proliferation of both luminal and glandular epithelium, whereas progesterone inhibits the mitogenic effect of estrogen on epithelium. Furthermore, estrogen given after several days of progesterone treatment causes stroma, rather than epithelium, to proliferate. Pretreatment of the uterus with estrogen reduces the time necessary for this effect of progesterone to become manifest. The changes in mitotic activity are reflected, as would be expected, by parallel changes in the incorporation of [^{3}H]thymidine into DNA. In the light of these findings, the patterns of mitotic activity in cyclic and pregnant mice and rats have led to the hypothesis that it is the estrogen released at about the time of ovulation that initiates the first wave of epithelial proliferation, its withdrawal being responsible for a wave of activity in the glands on the third day of pregnancy. According to this hypothesis, progesterone from the corpus luteum then conditions the stroma, and the nidatory estrogen induces proliferation of the stroma on the fourth and fifth days in preparation for implantation. Thus, the hormone regimen necessary to establish a typical peri-implantation pattern of mitotic activity in the endometrium of ovariectomized mice appears to be the same as that required to develop maximum uterine sensitivity to a nontraumatic intraluminal stimulus for decidualization (188). It is not known whether this pattern of proliferative activity enables the endometrium to respond to a decidual stimulus or merely accompanies the acquisition of sensitivity.

Cell Differentiation

Morphologic Changes

Results of morphologic examination of the endometrium in cyclic and pregnant animals or castrated animals given different hormone replacements demonstrate clearly again that changes occur in all compartments of the endometrium in response to ovarian steroid hormones. The cytologic changes indicate that there are significant differences in overall synthetic activity in the stromal cells as the endometrium moves from presensitivity through the sensitive phase and becomes refractory.

Luminal Epithelium

Uterine luminal epithelium becomes atrophic after removal of the ovaries. The typical high columnar cells quickly change to a more cuboidal shape, with the nucleus located in a middle position. The cytoplasm becomes weakly basophilic, with meager amounts of endoplasmic reticulum, and the Golgi complex is small. Numerous lipid droplets accumulate in the basal regions of the cells, and the apical microvilli become short, with little evidence of surface coat material. After the injection of estrogen, the cells increase in height, the cytoplasm becomes intensely basophilic, and there is an increase in the amount and prominence of the endoplasmic reticulum. The nuclei come to occupy a more basal position, the Golgi complex increases markedly and may occupy the lateral as well as the supranuclear area of the cells, and the apical microvilli increase in length. It is estimated that the apical surface area of the cells increases by as much as 50% and becomes covered with a "fuzz" (226–228,245). It is generally presumed that this extracellular material is a typical glycocalyx composed of negatively charged acidic glycoproteins (26,27,58, 246). Other consistent findings after administration of estrogen are the rapid dissipation of basal lipid droplets (247–251) and increases in several enzymatic activities, including alkaline phosphatase and nonspecific esterase (252–255).

Progesterone, given by itself to ovariectomized animals, also leads to an increase in cell height. However, the cytoplasm remains pale-staining, and there is increased accumulation of lipid in the basal area of the cells (31). Although cathepsin D activity increases in the luminal epithelium on stimulation with progesterone (256), there is no increase in alkaline phosphatase activity (254). Probably the most dramatic cytologic change in epithelium treated for several days with progesterone is the development of extensive interdigitation of the apical microvilli on the apposed luminal surfaces (31–33) and the formation of pinopods (23,96,257,258). It will be recalled that these features are characteristic of the first phase of uterine closure and are, therefore, associated with "presensitive" endometrium.

The addition of estrogen in this situation leads to loss of the lipid droplets, increased prominence of the rough endoplasmic reticulum, and a reduction in the number and size of the microvilli. Subsequently, the apical membranes are more closely apposed and the surface becomes irregular, with attainment of the second stage of uterine closure characteristic of postsensitive or refractory endometrium (33). Although the transition from first to second stage of closure appears to be dependent on ovarian steroid hormones, the fact that it occurs more rapidly in the presence of an embryo or oil droplet in the lumen indicated that some additional factors are involved (47). The luminal epithelium of intact cyclic, or pregnant, animals shows corresponding changes in lipid and in the activity of several enzymes, presumably in response to changing levels of ovarian steroid hormones (256,259–263).

Uterine Glands

There is relatively little information about endocrine-dependent cytodifferentiation of the glandular epithelium in ovariectomized animals, and most attention has been directed at the hormonal basis for secretory activity. It is reported that continuous treatment of ovariectomized mice with progesterone (with or without estrogen priming) leads to increased glandular secretion after 8 days; simultaneous injection of progesterone and estrogen leads to more massive secretory activity in just 5 days, whereas injection of estrogen after 3 days of progesterone leads to maximum secretion 48 h later (264). Cells of the uterine glands in mice are typically more cuboidal in the shape than luminal epithelium; they also have less lipid and appear to respond more slowly to ovarian steroid hormones (265). By the fourth day of pregnancy, the gland cells are found to have large lucent apical vesicles that disappear on the fifth and sixth day, as the lumen becomes distended (266). With cytochemical methods, it has been shown that this material contains carbohydrate and appears first in multivesicular bodies and on the concave, but not the convex, surface of the Golgi complex. The lumen is narrowed during the progesterone domination characteristic of delayed implantation; the Golgi complex is typically located lateral to the nucleus, although there is abundant smooth and rough endoplasmic reticulum (267). The addition of estrogen after several days of progesterone domination leads to the second stage of uterine closure within 24 h, and the glands start to become distended, although there are no significant ultrastructural changes in the cells. However, by 48 h the grandular lumen becomes filled with carbohydrate-rich material, and electron-dense granules are found at the apical border of the cells; the Golgi complex is located apical to the nucleus, and rough endoplasmic reticulum is present in increased amounts. That the glands are normally active on the sixth to seventh day of pregnancy or pseudopregnancy (i.e., 48 h after nidatory estrogen is imposed on progesterone domination) correlates well with the observed changes in endocrine replacement studies.

Stroma

The stromal cells also show hormone-dependent changes, particularly in the nucleoli (268). Tachi et al. (269) demonstrated, with the electron microscope, that after ovariectomy (a) the nucleoli in stromal cells are small and the fibrous component predominates, (b) there is a reduction in the amount of cytoplasm, and (c) the rough endoplasmic reticulum is less prominent. After treatment with estrogen alone, there is only a slight increase in the granular component of the nucleoli and no significant change in cytoplasmic features. By contrast, after treatment with progesterone, there is a marked enlargement of the nucleoli, with augmentation of the granular component. There are also increases in the rough endoplasmic reticulum, which becomes distended, and the cytoplasm has many polyribosomes. If estrogen is added after progesterone pretreatment, all aspects of these changes are accentuated. Another prominent hormone-dependent feature in presensitive stroma is the development of a generalized edema that leads, in part, to the first phase of uterine closure (43,44,197,270).

Metabolic Changes

The results of extensive studies of uterine metabolism demonstrate that there are hormone-dependent changes at the molecular level in the peri-implantation period that correlate with the changes in proliferation and cytodifferentiation.

The metabolism of uterine RNA has been examined in some detail. Incorporation of [^{3}H]uridine into RNA increases between the second and third day of pregnancy or pseudopregnancy in mice and rats (271–273). In rats, the rate of incorporation is biphasic, with a small peak on the third day and a more sustained increase on the fifth day; it then decreases unless decidualization occurs (274,275). This change appears to be largely in the nuclear fraction, is thought to be associated with increased processing of ribosomal RNA (276,277), and is correlated temporally with increased numbers of polyribosomes in stroma on the fifth day (276). Measurements of DNA template activity with bacterial RNA polymerase *in vitro* generally confirm the biphasic nature of the pattern of RNA synthesis, with the greatest activity in chromatin prepared from uteri on the third and fifth day (6,278). Furthermore, it has been inferred from DNA/RNA competitive hybridization studies that there are species of RNA synthesized on the fifth day of pregnancy that are not present on the second or the seventh day (278). Although increases in the synthesis of RNA were found in all compartments of the endometrium, the greatest increase was in the stroma (279). It is of particular interest that the activity was found to be greater in pregnant horns than in pseudopregnant horns even before attachment of the embryo.

Ornithine decarboxylase activity increases within 4 h of estrogen administration, and this change is prevented by cycloheximide (280). There is a biphasic peak in ornithine decarboxylase activity, with increases on the third and fifth day; this persists in implantation sites but not in interimplantation areas (281,282).

Synthesis of uterine proteins, as inferred from the incorporation of labeled amino acids, also has a biphasic pattern in the peri-implantation period. Thus, incorporation of label increases on the third day of pregnancy, decreases on the fourth day, and increases again on the fifth (283,284). The increased rates of synthesis are maintained beyond the fifth day in implantation sites but not in interimplantation areas. With estrogen alone, the increases are greatest in epithelium; with progesterone alone, the increase is more dramatic in stroma (285). Along with the increase in overall protein synthesis, specific and apparently new proteins appear. These migrate in the post-transferrin region during electrophoresis on polyacrylamide gels (286,287). Interestingly, the pattern in pseudopregnant animals is different in that there is no increase in protein synthesis on the fifth day, again suggesting that the embryos provide some stimulus to the uterus even before attachment (284).

Chemical analysis of endometrium for lipid throughout the peri-implantation period confirms the cytologic observations. There are changes in both total lipid and the relative proportions of neutral triglycerides (288). The studies have been undertaken with both intact cyclic, or pregnant, animals as well as with ovariectomized animals given replacement ovarian steroid hormone therapy. Although there are some species differences, it appears in general that estrogen reduced total lipid, primarily by influencing neutral triglycerides, whereas progesterone causes an increase; progesterone is particularly effective in this regard when it has been preceded by estrogen (289–293). Neutral triglycerides tend to accumulate in the endometrium, both epithelium and stroma, in the first 4 days of pregnancy, presumably because of the effect of luteal progesterone. Interestingly, lipids decrease in the implantation sites, but not interimplantation areas, on days 6 and 7 as decidualization proceeds (294). Although different investigators have suggested that neutral lipids provide an energy source for the developing embryo and that phospholipids may be important for synthesis of such components as cell membrane and prostaglandins during decidualization, it has not been possible to directly relate changes in lipids to regulation of proliferation or differentiation of the endometrium.

Endocrine-dependent changes have also been observed in the intermediary metabolism of the endometrium during the estrous cycle and in the early progestational period in the rat. Attempts have been made to relate differing patterns of intrauterine oxygen tension, activity of glycolytic enzymes, uterine respiration, and glucose use to the shift in stromal cells away from mitotic activity and toward cytodifferentiation and the development of progestational sensitivity (5,259,295–303). Although it is clear that hormone-dependent changes in cell proliferation, in cytodifferentiation, and in the different metabolic and synthetic patterns must ultimately be responsible for the development of uterine receptivity, none of the observations has provided a clear understanding of the process at the molecular level.

However, some observations have been made that provide clues to the mechanisms involved. Thus, Yochim and colleagues have shown that the ovarian steroid hormones regulate availability of the pyridine nucleotide cofactor nicotinamide adenine dinucleotide phosphate and hence ultimately control pentose shunt activity in the endometrium (303–306). And Glasser and McCormack (307) reported that treatment of ovariectomized rats with progesterone leads to an increase of more than 500% in the number of RNA initiation sites available in the endometrium, whereas template activity is markedly restricted after the injection of estrogen. It may be then that progestational sensitivity develops in the endometrium because increased levels of cofactor lead to increased pentose shunt activity and provide endometrial cells with increased capacity for reductive biosynthesis and sugars for nucleic acid synthesis, which, in conjunction with increased template activity, would facilitate cytodifferentiation, whereas the consequent reduced flux in the nicotinamide adenine dinucleotide salvage path would limit production of ADP-ribose and impair DNA synthesis and cell division. Receptivity, which develops after an injection of estrogen superimposed on progesterone, then, may be the result of restricting template activity and increasing salvage pathway activity, which favors DNA synthesis and cell division (308–310).

Transformation of the Endometrium

Sensitization of the endometrium by the ovarian steroid hormones appears to be a universal requirement for decidualization, but there are significant species differences in the reaction itself. Thus, for example, the reaction is quite robust in rats and mice and more modest in rabbits. Or again, although predecidual changes occur spontaneously in human endometrium during the late secretory phase of the menstrual cycle (311), a signal from the embryo is normally involved in eliciting the reaction in laboratory rodents. Hence, care must be taken in interpreting results of experiments on decidualization, and in what follows, an attempt has been made to focus on those features that appear to be most consistent.

Fibroblast-like Stromal Cells

Although uterine stroma comprises several cell types that presumably have distinct roles in decidualization (312), results of most morphologic and autoradiographic studies support the concept that it is the fibroblastlike stromal elements that give rise to the definitive decidual cells (212,215,313–317). And despite differences in details of timing, the need for a stimulus and the extent of endometrial involvement among different species, the basic cytologic changes associated with decidualization of stromal cells appear to be similar in different animals (270,313,314,318,319). Among the earliest changes to be observed are the development of edema (29,171,193, 194,320) and an increase in alkaline phosphatase activity in the fibroblastlike precursor cells (155). Subsequently, these cells become slightly enlarged, the nuclei become rounded, and there is typically an increase in the prominence of the nucleoli. The cells tend to align themselves into a continuous layer beneath the epithelium (15,21); and while mitotic activity in the central area declines and finally ceases, there is continued proliferation of cells in the areas adjacent to the developing nidus (200,206,321–323). As the process continues, the cells assume an epithelioid appearance (i.e., a characteristically rounded shape) and typically contain two or more polyploid nuclei (323). At the ultrastructural level, differentiation of decidual cells is characterized by the accumulation of glycogen, often in association with lipid droplets, and by progressively increasing amounts of fibrillar material organized into parallel arrays and appearing as bundles in the cytoplasm. There is an increase in the number of polyribosomes, as well as in the amount and distention of rough endoplasmic reticulum;

the nucleoli become enlarged with an increase in the granular component (15,29,178,324–328). It has recently been reported that the amount of fibronectin on the surface of these cells decreases as they undergo differentiation and that this change may be important in the development of their characteristic rounded shape (329). A consistent finding in the different electron microscopic studies of decidualization is that the cells are crowded closely together, with fingerlike projections and many junctions of the adherens and gap types (15,315,330,331). The temporal aspect of the development of these junctions has been described in detail (324,332). Essentially the same cytologic transformation occurs when presensitized endometrial stromal cells are placed *in vitro* and cultured in the presence of progesterone: rat (333–336), mouse (337), and human (311).

Cell proliferation and the cytologic differentiation associated with decidualization in rats typically starts in compact areas of the subepithelial antimesometrial stroma adjacent to the site of embryo attachment and is associated with destruction of the uterine luminal epithelial cells surrounding the blastocyst by a process resembling apoptosis or programmed cell death (see ref. 338). It begins in response to a signal that has not yet been defined and spreads ventrally and laterally before finally involving the mesometrial endometrium (223,316,317, 326,339). Welsh and Enders (340–342) were able to observe in the mesometrial region that processes from the decidual cells penetrate the basal lamina of the luminal epithelium and undermine the cells before their destruction. The decidual processes appear to spread out on the denuded luminal surface and deposit an extensive extracellular matrix rich in cross-banded collagen fibers; similar processes become insinuated between endothelial cells of the maternal blood sinuses. Those decidual cells in close proximity to trophoblast die (apparently also due to a form of programmed cell death) and are replaced with proliferating endothelium or trophoblast. Simultaneously with these changes, there is migration of endothelial cells onto the luminal surface, which establishes continuity between the maternal sinusoids and the mesometrial chamber and leads to the flow of maternal blood into trophoblastic sinusoids and the mesometrial portion of the uterine lumen before development of the chorioallantoic placenta. In the mouse, similar changes are observed in the epithelium in response to the embryo (157,338) although the initial changes in stroma can be found throughout the antimesometrial region (343).

Localized changes in vascular permeability is one of the earliest responses of the sensitive endometrium to any kind of deciduogenic stimulus and is most easily demonstrated by the extravascular accumulation of intravenously injected macromolecular dye (170,171). The development of fenestrations and gaps in the endothelium of endometrial blood vessels at implantation sites but not between implantations has been described and provides an explanation at the ultrastructural level for the so-called Pontamine Blue reaction in those areas (326,344). Although Lundkvist and Ljungkvist (324) argued that some cytologic changes precede the appearance of overt edema and the Pontamine Blue reaction, it has subsequently been shown, in the rat, that labeled albumin leaks from the vessels within 15 min of a decidualizing stimulus (345). Thus, the development of edema is still one of the earliest changes known to be associated with the endometrial response to a decidualizing stimulus. These changes can occur while blastocysts are still enclosed in the zona pellucida, and thus the signal does not require direct contact between trophoblast and uterine epithelium (172,346).

Leukocytes

Besides the fibroblastlike stromal cells that are transformed during decidualization, the endometrium contains a variety of other cells that may be important for implantation and pregnancy. Most nonfibroblast stromal cells are infiltrating leukocytes of two types, macrophages and granulated large lymphocytelike cells. These cells are of bone marrow origin and hence express the common leukocyte antigen (CLA). They are found in the uteri of humans as well as laboratory animals, where they accumulate in the endometrium apparently in response to estrogen and progesterone. The patterns of leukocyte distribution in naturally occurring decidua and experimentally induced deciduomata are indistinguishable, and hence, the accumulation of these cells is apparently not driven by immunologic (or other) signals from the embryo (see refs. 312,347–368).

A significant proportion of $CLA^{[+]}$ cells in the endometrium of both humans and laboratory animals are macrophages. The numbers of these cells appear to fluctuate during the estrous cycle and to increase dramatically with decidualization. Because changes in numbers of uterine macrophages occur during the cycle, and their accumulation and distribution are similar in pregnant and pseudopregnant animals, it is generally believed that they are regulated by ovarian steroid hormones and do not require a specific signal from the conceptus. Many of the cells in the placenta have been identified as macrophages as well, and these cells are of fetal origin (see refs. 351,352,354,355,362,364,369–382). Morphology of macrophages in the uteroplacental tissues tends to be quite variable, and they have been most successfully identified by means of monoclonal antibodies to a variety of typical macrophage antigens. In humans, the cells are found to express CD 14, CD11c and class II proteins of the major histocompatibility complex (HLA-DR; some express HLA-DP and HLA-DQ as well) but are CD11b (Mac-1) negative. Interestingly, some cells in the endometrium that are most strongly $HLA\text{-}DR^{[+]}$ are not macrophages (371,372,374,375,377,381,383). In rodents, the CLA$^{[+]}$, F4/80$^{[+]}$, Fcγ receptor$^{[+]}$, I-A$^{k[+]}$, and cells in endometrium (i.e., the macrophages) not only fluctuate during the estrous cycle but have been shown to decrease markedly after ovariectomy and to be restored with injections of estrogen and progesterone (379,380). The increase in the number of endometrial macrophages during the first half of pregnancy (376) follows a biphasic pattern that may be related to changes in the amount of intact luminal epithelium and associated CSF-1 (384). There are relatively few macrophages in the primary decidual zone, but they are more numerous in the secondary decidual zone; this appears to be true in normal implantation sites as well as in the artificially induced deciduomata of pseudopregnant animals (385,386).

The roles played by uterine macrophages in implantation and pregnancy are not known, but it has been suggested that they are important as phagocytes and producers of extracellular enzymes for tissue remodeling (see ref. 312); involved in antigen presentation (387); and local modulators of the immune response via secretion of different cytokines and PGE_2 (388,389).

In humans, the granulated endometrial stromal cells (also referred to as Kornchenzellen [K cells]) are the second most numerous CLA-positive cell type. They have excentric round or oval hyperchromatic nuclei and are characterized by varying numbers of cytoplasmic granules that stain with pholoxine-tartrazine (350,390–392). These cells are found in the stroma surrounding blood vessels and glands in late secretory phase endometrium, and their numbers increase up to the time of implantation and are maintained through the first trimester after which they decrease in number; in nonpregnant cycles they disappear 1 to 2 days before menstruation (349,367,392,393). Although these granulated stromal cells have been observed to undergo mitosis *in situ,* it is not known to what extent infiltration versus proliferation contribute to their accumulation in the endometrium (392). Besides expressing CLA, granulated endometrial cells display the T-lineage differentiation markers CD2 (OKT 11), CD7, and CD38 (OKT 10) and the natural killer antigen CD56 (Leu-19; NKH-1); they apparently do not express the classic mature T-cell antigens CD3 (OKT3; Leu-4), CD4 (Leu-3a), CD5, CD8 (OKT 8), the IL-2 receptor (CD25), or the natural killer cell antigens CD16 (Leu-11) and Leu-7 (349,350,366, 392,394–396). However, the granulated endometrial cells do produce perforin, have at least some natural killer activity against K562 cells, and apparently proliferate in response to IL-2 (366,397–399, but see refs. 392 and 400). At least some of these cells also express TCR$\gamma\delta$ (401) and may be derived from the unique subpopulation of peripheral lymphocytes (i.e., CD3$^{[-]}$, CD16$^{[-]}$, CD56$^{[+]}$) described by Lanier et al. (402). Similar cells have been widely reported to exist in the uteri of rodents, where they are designated granulated metrial gland (GMG) cells (see refs. 347,348,350,360,361,403–406), and they have been identified in sheep as well (365).

The roles of these granular endometrial leukocytes in pregnancy have not yet been established, but as more monoclonal antibodies are developed and used to probe the endometrium and better methods are devised for isolating the cells without destroying their surface characteristics, the dynamics of different subpopulations and their precise functions should become clear.

Molecular Changes

Development of mature decidual tissue involves both proliferation and differentiation of cells in the endometrial stroma. It is not surprising, therefore, that significant changes in both the total content and rates of synthesis of DNA, RNA, and protein have been observed (see ref. 6). As indicated earlier, the synthesis of DNA can be demonstrated in endometrial stromal cells on the fourth and fifth days of pseudopregnancy or pregnancy by incorporation of [^{3}H]thymidine (201,212,216,316). This increase in synthetic activity in the stroma follows the decline in proliferation of the epithelium. It occurs in response to the nidatory estrogen and accompanies the progression through the receptive phase and into the refractory phase (211). The synthesis of DNA continues on the sixth day in areas undergoing decidualization, but not in those areas between implantations (214). And it appears that once the decidual cells have become differentiated they no longer synthesize DNA; rather it is those cells peripheral to the forming nidus that continue to incorporate the labeled thymidine (215). It has been observed in mice that there are two populations of cells that begin DNA synthesis at about 11 to 15 h after the decidualizing stimulus; one differentiates into mature decidual cells without dividing, the other goes on to divide before differentiating (407). The peak in DNA synthesis occurs about 30 h after application of the decidual stimulus (408); chemical measurements of total DNA content revealed that changes are substantial, with increases of up to 70% per day in the second and third day after the experimentally applied stimulus (409). As might be expected, this increase in DNA content did not occur when decidualization was prevented by the antiestrogen MER-25 (410).

The decidual cells typically become binucleate and polyploid (321,322). Production of these nuclei, some containing as much as 32n DNA in rats and 64n DNA in mice, involves endoreplication rather than fusion (323) and reaches a maximum at about 96 h after application of the decidualizing stimulus (317). With rats, it has been possible to separate decidual cells on the basis of ploidy by means of differential sedimentation velocity on serum albumin gradients (411). It appears that those cells destined to develop the highest ploidy will synthesize DNA on the fourth day of pseudopregnancy, whereas those engaged in synthesis of DNA on the fifth day will typically develop lower ploidy (412,413). However, it appears that it is those cells that are synthesizing DNA early in the process of transformation that remain in the 2n to 4n population, whereas those synthesizing DNA later tend to end up in the 6n to 8n range. Thus, Moulton (412) found evidence to support the concept that there are two populations of stromal cells in rats as well: one that differentiates without dividing, and a second that divides before undergoing differentiation. It appears, then, that the rat is similar to the mouse (407) in this regard. The continued synthesis of DNA (and RNA) by decidual cells in ovariectomized animals is dependent on progesterone replacement, apparently more so in the cells at 4n to 8n DNA than in smaller cells. In contrast, synthesis of proteins is more progesterone-dependent in smaller cells than it is in the 4n to 8n population (412).

Although synthesis of RNA occurs in the uterine stroma of pregnant and pseudopregnant mice and rats before the acquisition of sensitivity, further increases are observed with decidual transformation. Synthesis and accumulation of uterine RNA change dramatically on formation of mature decidual tissue, with increases in content being observed as little as 5 h after the systemic injection of pyrathiazine as the decidualizing stimulus (318). This early change in RNA was localized, by histochemical means, to the superficial cells of the antimesometrial stroma in rat (319). The increase is limited to decidualizing tissue and is not observed in those areas that fail to become transformed (273,275); it can be detected within 8 h of the intraluminal application of the decidualizing stimulus (414). The overall increase in RNA content of decidual tissue has been estimated at 95% to 110% on the first day after stimulation (409,414). A corresponding increase in uridine incorporation is observed and thought to reflect largely increased processing of ribosomal RNA (277,278); however, increases in activity of both RNA polymerase types I and III have been reported in the mouse (415), and template activity is significantly increased in decidualizing tissue on the sixth day of pregnancy, suggesting that there are substantial changes in the synthesis of all classes of RNA (6,279). Ornithine decarboxylase increases in a biphasic manner early in decidual transformation, presumably to support nucleic acid synthesis; the increases are blocked by cycloheximide, actinomycin D (416), and indomethacin (417).

Overall protein content in the rat deciduoma increases by as much as 70% per day in the second and third days after stimulation (409). In the mouse, there is a biphasic increase in protein: a two- to threefold increase in the first 24 h, and a secondary and more sustained increase of four- or fivefold on the third and fourth days (408). Rates of protein synthesis, as measured by incorporation of single radiolabeled amino acids, increase on the third and fourth days and then fall. A larger and more sustained increase that is localized in implantation sites occurs on the fifth day (284,418). Increases in protein synthesis are dependent on appropriate hormonal preparation of the endometrium as well as on the decidualizing stimulus and can be blocked with antiestrogens (MER-25) (410), tamoxifen (285), and cycloheximide (418); these treatments also block the decidual transformation. Progesterone appears to be necessary for continued high levels of protein synthesis by decidual tissue and may be acting primarily on the smaller stromal cells (i.e., those with 2 to 4n DNA) (412). Because decidual transformation is associated with significant increases in tissue mass, it is not surprising that there are marked increases in synthesis of DNA, RNA, and protein. However, because cytodifferentiation associated with the decidual reaction evolves over time and is regionalized within the endometrium, such measurements of overall changes in macromolecular synthesis in the uterus have not provided insights into either the nature of this unique process or the potential functional significance of the new tissue (419).

As it became clear that increases in general protein synthesis accompanied the decidual transformation, efforts were made to determine whether decidual cell-specific proteins could be identified that might provide a clue to the function of this developing organ. Yoshinaga (420) prepared rabbit antiserum to crude extracts of rat deciduomata and found that it would prevent decidualization in both the rat and mouse (420,421); he suggested that some proteins in decidual tissue of these species have similar immunologic characteristics. Similarly, Joshi et al. (422) reported the existence of a decidua-specific antigen in the baboon, and Sacco and Mintz (423) reported a uterine-specific antigen on the fourth day of pregnancy in mice. Although none of these antigens has been characterized further, their existence demonstrates the potential for unique proteins in this tissue to subserve specific functions.

Several investigators have demonstrated the existence of unique decidual proteins by resolving dual radiolabeled proteins on polyacrylamide gels (424–430). Again, however, none of these proteins has been described in sufficient detail to determine if they are the same between species. Denari et al. (426) observed a unique protein within 1 h of the stimulus for decidualization in the rat. In terms of electrophoretic mobility, this protein (protein A) was similar to estrogen-induced uterine protein (i.e., IP) (431–433). However, it (i.e., protein A) was not increased in animals treated with estrogen alone and was not observed in nonstimulated uteri; it seems unlikely that this protein is the IP. Another protein with characteristics similar to those of IP was found to be synthesized maximally on the fourth and sixth days of pregnancy and depressed on the fifth day; the investigators suggested that it is associated with regulation of cell division (430). Although this protein was presumed to be IP because of its electrophoretic mobility, it was found to be greatly increased in deciduomata when there were no concomitant increases in estrogen, and because it was shown that IP is induced by estrogen in all cell layers (434), it seems unlikely that this protein is the IP. Also, a pregnancy-associated protein was found in the post-transferrin region of the same gels. Its synthesis increased from the fourth through the sixth day of pregnancy and remained elevated in implantation sites but not in inter-implantation areas (288,427,428).

With the increased resolution provided by two-dimensional polyacrylamide gel electrophoresis, it has recently been possible to demonstrate in the rat that at least four new peptides appear with decidualization and that several others decrease (435). Furthermore, in the hamsters, several decidua-specific nuclear and cytoplasmic proteins are modulated both positively and negatively by progesterone (436), and more significantly, decidual cells continue to produce these distinctive proteins *in vitro* (437). In a most important paper, Glasser and Julian (438) reported that production of intermediate filament proteins is markedly increased in decidual cells. Those workers were able to show by means of a variety of techniques, including two-dimensional polyacrylamide electrophoresis, Western blots, and indirect immunocytochemistry, that while production of vimentin increases in proportion to the overall change in protein synthesis with decidualization, production of desmin is increased inordinately. And it appears from that work that desmin is the decidual protein 4 reported by Lejeune et al. (435) and the decidual protein 8 reported by Leavitt et al. (437). This finding is particularly important because it ties a change in a specific protein to the differentiation of decidual cells.

The hormone-dependent nature of these different changes led some investigators to examine differences in steroid receptors in the endometrium. Martel and Psychoyos (439) reported that the amount of estrogen receptor in implantation sites decreases relative to DNA and protein and that there is little evidence of receptor in the nucleus. This seems to be compatible with the observation of decreased uptake of [^{3}H]estradiol by implantation versus interimplantation sites (440,441). The conflicting report by Logeat et al. (239) that estrogen receptor increases markedly in implantation sites identified by Trypan Blue dye appears to be based on the artifactual binding of steroids by the dye (439,442). However, Moulton and Koenig (442) reported that the number of estrogen receptors in cells with high ploidy increases relative to DNA, whereas McConnell et al. (443) reported that progesterone receptors in the same cells decrease relative to DNA; Sartor (444) claimed that uptake of progesterone is high in implantation sites and low in the nondecidualized regions between implantation sites. These several observations exemplify the problem of examining an organ with distinct anatomic compartments and marked cellular heterogeneity. The work of Glasser and McCormack (7), which points out that nuclear and cytoplasmic receptors for estrogen increase in stromal cells at the same time they are decreasing in epithelial cells, clearly demonstrates the futility of attempting to understand uterine function by examining changes in overall receptor content. Thus, although it is clear that differences in steroid receptors are related to specialized functions of decidual tissue and different aspects of the process of implantation, the significance of much of that work remains obscure.

Remodeling of Endometrial Extracellular Matrix

During the proliferative phase of the reproductive cycle, uterine interstitial matrix is characterized by a dense network of cross-linked fibrillar collagens including types I, III, IV, V, and VI, as well as fibronectin. Type VI collagen, which is particularly abundant during the proliferative phase and is typically responsible for cross-connecting large fibrils of the major collagens, decreases dramatically with decidualization and ultimately is found only in association with blood vessels. It has been suggested that removal of type VI collagen, by specific proteases released from differentiated decidual cells, could reduce cross-linking between major interstitial collagen types without destroying them and, thus, lead to loosening of the stroma without compromising its overall strength (13,391,419,445–454). Similarly, it has been suggested that the progressive unmasking of type V collagen because of a reduction in the amount of its binding to fibronectin or type I collagen also results in relaxation of the matrix (329,419,453). These possibilities are not mutually exclusive, and a bewildering array of hormone-responsive proteolytic activities and naturally occurring inhibitors that might subserve such functions have been associated with implanting trophoblast as well as with normal and decidualized endometrial stroma (455–468). Also, differentiated decidual cells produce a nonfibrillar matrix composed of type IV collagen, laminin, entactin, fibronectin, heparan sulfate proteoglycan, and a family of glycoproteins recognized by the monoclonal antibody [G71] (13,329,445,446,453,469–475). This material becomes organized into a characteristic bilaminar basal lamina ("aura") surrounding the mature decidual cells. It is penetrated by cellular processes containing matrix material that is being exported to the extracellular compartment (445). This pericellular basement membrane material may serve to stabilize the surrounding interstitial matrix and immobilize the decidual cells (447,448). With loosening of the matrix and development of edema, the hydrated glycosaminoglycans and proteoglycans of the endometrial ground substance act as space-filling molecules and presumably facilitate cell movement and provide anchoring sites for migration. It is interesting in this regard that Carson et al. (72) observed a several fold increase in production of hyaluronate by mouse uteri at about the time of implantation. Thus, remodeling of the uterine extracellular matrix during the peri-implantation phase of pregnancy appears to involve selective and controlled degradation of some filamentous elements coupled with a switch to production of more nonfibrillar basal laminal and ground substance molecules.

Changes in Secreted Proteins

Leuteotrophic activity associated with late secretory phase (and decidualized) human endometrium has been shown to be authentic prolactin (476–487). It is localized to decidual cells and glandular epithelium and its production requires progesterone *in vitro* as well as *in vivo* (311,478). Prolactin is not stored as secretory granules in the endometrium as it is in the pituitary, and the mechanism responsible for regulating its production and release is not the same as that involved in the pituitary (488–490). It has been suggested that endometrial prolactin acts, in humans at least, primarily as a paracrine factor, possibly to facilitate electrolyte exchange across the chorioamnion where the existence of appropriate receptors has been demonstrated (13,491). A similar polypeptide with luteotrophic activity is synthesized and secreted by decidual cells of the rat as early as day 6 of pregnancy. It apparently has electrophoretic properties similar to those for prolactin and competes for authentic receptors (see refs. 492,493) but is immunologically distinct from prolactin (492–495).

Another major secretory product of late secretory phase human endometrium and decidua in the first and second trimester is a protein of approximately 29 kDa designated as pregnancy-associated endometrial α-1 globulin (α_1-PEG). It is localized to predecidual cells and, after implantation, to decidual cells and becomes the main somatomedin/insulinlike growth factor-I (IGF-I) binding protein in amniotic fluid (496–500). α_1-PEG has physicochemical and immunochemical characteristics similar to the soluble placental protein 12 (PP 12), and they both bind IGF-I. However, there appear to be slight differences in their amino acid sequences, and it has been suggested that although both are produced by the endometrium, they function in different compartments of the conceptus (501–504; and see ref. 505).

A second pregnancy-associated endometrial protein designated α_2-PEG by Bell and co-workers is a dimeric glycoprotein (subunit molecular weight, 28,000) with significant amino acid homology to β-lactoglobulin. It is produced by the glandular epithelium and can be detected in culture supernatants as well as in uterine flushings (496,497,503,506–508); it may not be particularly important for implantation but rather acts as a retinol binding/transporting protein during placentation and embryogenesis (13,505). There are reports by other groups of independent observations of uterine-secreted proteins designated α-uterine protein (AUP), progestagen-associated endometrial protein (PEP), and the soluble PP14, which are in reality synonyms for α_2-PEG (503, 509–518).

Lactotransferrin has been described in glandular epithelium from secretory phase human endometrium (519) and is a major secretory product of mouse (but apparently not rat) endometrium; its production is markedly increased in response to estrogen (520). Uteroferrin is a progesterone-induced iron binding glycoprotein produced by pig endometrium; it can be detected at about the time of embryo elongation and is a main secretory product after implantation (521).

Uteroglobin is a main uterine-secreted protein (15.7 kDa) of rabbit endometrium during pregnancy (522–525); it is composed of two identical chains of 70 amino acids connected by disulfide bonds (526,527), and its production by noncilliated epithelium is markedly stimulated by progesterone both *in vivo* and *in vitro* (522,524,528–533). The function of uteroglobin is unclear, but it is known to be capable of binding progesterone (534,535), inhibiting trypsin activity (523), and blocking antigenicity of blastocysts and sperm *in vitro* (536,537).

Low levels of the enzyme diamine oxidase have been detected in human proliferative and secretory phase endometrium; activity increases dramatically during the first trimester of pregnancy and can be recovered from medium used to culture decidualized endometrium (538). Diamine oxidase is also reported in the uteri of pregnant hamsters and rats several days after implantation (539–542). Interest in the enzyme was stimulated by the marked changes in accumulation, synthesis, and degradation of the polyamines putrescine, spermidine, and spermine in the early placenta, and it is presumed that its importance is related primarily to postimplantation events (see ref. 505).

Endometrial Cytokines

The localized changes in cell proliferation and differentiation, reorganization of the extracellular matrix, and recruitment of cells from the bone marrow that are associated with decidualization and embryo implantation are similar in many ways to those in inflammatory reactions and wound healing. And as might have been anticipated, cytokines known for their roles in inflammation are being found in the uterus. Indeed, it is becoming clear that a network of cytokines interacting with the ovarian hormones and a variety of cell types in the uterus will ultimately be shown to be important for local mediation of the events that support implantation. Although a bewildering number of papers have already appeared in which uterine production of many of these factors is described and the existence of the appropriate receptors is documented, as yet little is known with certainty about the mechanisms that regulate them or their specific roles in implantation (see refs. 543–547).

Human endometrium has been shown to produce bioactive interleukin-1 (IL-1) in response to bacterial endotoxin (548), and immunoreactive IL-1_β and its mRNA are present in human decidua (549). Interleukin-1_α and IL-1_β mRNAs have been localized to macrophagelike cells in the subepithelial uterine stroma of mice, and IL-1 protein and mRNA appear to increase in response to estrogen (550–552). High-affinity receptors for IL-1 are present on human endometrial epithelial cells, and recombinant IL-1_α has been shown to stimulate production of prostaglandin E_2, IL-6, and the expression of class II proteins of the major histocompatibility complex (HLA-DR) by those cells; addition of estrogen significantly reduces the IL-1-induced expression of HLA-DR (545,553–555). Interleukin-1 apparently promotes development of preimplantation embryos resulting from certain genetic crosses (556), and although it remains to be determined how production of this cytokine is regulated and precisely which cells in the endometrium are involved, it is clear that the IL-1 gene and its products are present in the uterus and have the potential to influence events in the peri-implantation phase of pregnancy.

Interleukin-2 (IL-2) mRNA has been demonstrated in syncytiotrophoblast of human placenta (557), and the protein can be detected in human placenta and amnion (558). Interleukin-2 has not been detected in the uteroplacental units of rats or mice, and indeed, when injected intraperitoneally before the time of implantation, IL-2 appears to be detrimental to the establishment of pregnancy in mice (559).

The presence of interleukin-3 (IL-3) has not been confirmed in the uterus, but it is presumed that uterine T cells produce it; Athanassakis et al. (560) have shown that recombinant IL-3 is stimulatory to placental cells in culture and suggested that it plays a role in maintaining the uteroplacental unit in mice.

Interleukin-6 (IL-6) protein and mRNA have been detected in mouse uterus during pregnancy as well as during the cycle, and it can be markedly increased in ovariectomized animals by treatment with estrogen combined with progesterone (551,552). Immunoreactive IL-6 has been localized in scattered stromal and epithelial cells in human endometrium (561). Also, several isoforms of IL-6 have been shown to be produced by human endometrial stromal cells *in vitro* in response to the inflammatory cytokines IL-1_α, IL-1_β, tumor necrosis factor-α (TNF_α), and interferon-γ (INF_γ); of these, IL-1_α is most potent inducer (554). This effect of IL-1 is reduced in the presence of estrogen, and because IL-6 is known to strongly inhibit proliferation of human epithelial cells, it has been proposed that hormone-dependent changes in proliferative activity of endometrial epithelium during the cycle reflect a local interaction between ovarian steroids and IL-6 from the subjacent stroma (554). Furthermore, human trophoblast cells apparently have receptors for IL-6 and will release human chorionic gonadotropin (hCG) in response to it as well as to gonadotropin-releasing hormone (GnRH); the IL-6 system and the GnRH system regulate hCG release by the trophoblast cells independently (562). Thus, possible roles for IL-6 as a component of the endocrine/paracrine system responsible for regulating local changes within the uterus at the time of implantation are beginning to emerge.

Interferon-γ has been shown to induce differential expression of class II proteins of the main histocompatibility complex by human endometrial epithelial cells (HLA-DR > HLA-DP and HLA-DQ) and to inhibit their proliferation *in vitro* (563–566). Furthermore, it has been observed that although expression of HLA-DR molecules by mammary as well as uterine epithelium is influenced by ovarian steroids, it is markedly enhanced and constant in those basal epithelial elements of uterine glands that are adjacent to lymphoid aggregates containing large numbers of activated T cells (i.e., secretors of INF_γ) (564,567,568). By contrast, in both the human and rhesus monkey, proliferation of those cells appears to be reduced relative to epithelium in other areas of the uterus (563,565,566,568–577). Because the epithelial receptors for INF_γ remain relatively constant throughout the cycle (571), it has been suggested that localized variations in hormone-dependent expression of HLA-DR molecules by epithelium, as well as focal differences in proliferative activity during the menstrual cycle, are due in part to paracrine effects of INF_γ produced by activated T cells within the endometrium (546); those T cells apparently do have estrogen receptors and thus presumably are targets for ovarian hormones (578).

Biologically active TNF_α has been identified in supernatants of human decidual and placental cell cultures, and receptors for TNF_α are present in human placenta (579–581). Recombinant TNF_α causes increased production of a host of bioactive factors by human placental cells *in vitro* (e.g., matrix metalloproteinase, tissue collagenase, stromeolysin, urokinase type-plasminogen activator, and prostaglandin E_2) (582). Bioactive TNF_α and its mRNA have been demonstrated in the mouse uterus in pregnancy as well as during the cycle (551,552). Tumor necrosis factor alpha has been shown to promote development of preimplantation mouse embryos of certain genetic crosses (556), and although it is not yet known which uterine cells are responsible for its production, it has been presumed that it has a role in implantation, remodeling of the endometrium, and early development of the placenta.

Epidermal growth factor (EGF) and its receptor have been demonstrated in the uteri of a variety of animals both as proteins and the mRNA transcripts (583–592). Immunocytologic and *in situ* hybridization studies of EGF in mouse uterus show localization, particularly in luminal and glandular epithelium (592). Estrogen causes an increase in the amount of EGF protein in immature uteri (583), but its effect in the mature uterus is not clear. Huet-Hudson et al. (592) concluded from results of their studies *in vivo* that estrogen increases *de novo* synthesis of EGF in the uteri of ovariectomized adult mice, whereas DiAugustine et al. (586) reported that estrogen does not stimulate synthesis of the EGF precursor *in vitro.*

It has been reported that the binding affinity of EGF to uterine membranes increases during the preimplantation phase of pregnancy (593) and that estrogen causes an increase in the overall uterine content of EGF receptor in mature as well as immature animals (584,585, 587,594). However, there is no evidence of differences in binding of EGF to human endometrium removed at different times of the menstrual cycle (589); similarly, there is little indication from immunohistochemical studies of variation in amounts of EGF receptor during the menstrual cycle (595,596). It does appear that there are increases in amounts and distribution of the EGF receptor during human pregnancy (597), and there is a localized increase in binding to the uterus at the implantation site in mice even before the attachment of embryos (598). Epidermal growth factor has been shown to stimulate proliferation of endometrial cells from immature uteri (599–601) as well as to increase the production of progesterone receptors in cells from the uteri of fetal guinea pigs (600). Epidermal growth factor is able to substitute for estrogen and induces uterine growth and production of lactoferrin in ovariectomized adult mice (602), and receptors have been detected in the placenta (603). Thus, it seems probable that EGF will be shown to play a major role in the endocrine/paracrine mechanism responsible for regulating localized changes within the uterus at the time of implantation.

Multiple fibroblast growth factor (FGF)-like activities have been detected in the uterus of the pregnant pig; these factors have been shown to have molecular characteristics similar to acidic FGF and basic FGF (see ref. 543).

Platelet-derived growth factor (PDGF) is expressed in preimplantation mouse embryos (604), and the mRNA for the β chain as well as for the PDGF receptor have been detected in human placenta (605).

The spatiotemporal expression of transforming growth factor-alpha (TGF_{α}) protein and its mRNA has been described in the uterus of mice during the peri-implantation period of pregnancy; it is initially localized in glandular and luminal epithelium and then, after implantation, is found in decidual cells at the fetomaternal interface in both mice and rats (606–608). Expression of TGF_{α} has also been demonstrated in preimplantation mouse embryos (604). Although it has been suggested that TGF_{α}, working through EGF receptors, is involved in estrogen-dependent proliferation in rodent uterus or has an effect on development of the placenta, its specific function at implantation has not been determined.

Expression of transforming growth factor-beta (TGF-β) has been demonstrated in preimplantation mouse embryos (604). Immunoreactive TGF-β and its mRNA have been described in first trimester human decidua, where it was localized to cells at the fetomaternal interface, placenta, and extraembryonic membranes (549, 609). The spatiotemporal pattern of TGF-β_1 expression, as determined by immunocytochemistry and *in situ* hybridization, has been described in the peri-implantation mouse uterus (610). Transforming growth factor-β_1 mRNA was concentrated primarily in epithelium before implantation and was found throughout the decidua afterward; the protein was also localized to the epithelium before implantation and was associated with extracellular matrix afterward. Transforming growth factor-β_2 bioactivity and mRNA have been identified in pregnant mouse uterus and found to peak at about midpregnancy (611,612). Transforming growth factor-beta is released into the extracellular compartment as an inactive precursor and must be modified by esterases or INF_{γ} to become active (613–615). Because the antibodies used for immunocytochemical localization of TGF-β typically recognize the mature rather than the inactive form, localization of the protein in immunohistochemical studies has not always been in good agreement with results of *in situ* hybridization to identify the cells containing the TGF-β mRNA, and caution has been urged when interpreting such data (546,616). Receptors for TGF-β have not been described in endometrium, but from their widespread distribution in other tissues, it is presumed that types I, II, and III will be found (546). A TGF-β-like immunosuppressive factor (i.e., promotes anchorage independent cell growth) has been described in the pregnant mouse uterus; because it is neutralized by antibodies to TGF-β_2 but not by those to TGF-β_1, it has been presumed to be similar to (or the same as) TGF-β_2 (611,617).

Macrophage colony stimulating factor (M-CSF) is present in large amounts in the uteri of pregnant mice and humans (618–622). The M-CSF mRNA has been localized exclusively to the epithelial compartment in the endometrium and is present as early as day 3 of pregnancy in mice (621). The uterine concentrations of M-CSF mRNA and protein increase dramatically during pregnancy, apparently in response to estrogen and progesterone (621,623,624). The receptor for M-CSF is the product of the c-*fms* proto-oncogene, and its mRNA is expressed in the placenta of mice (621,624–626) and humans (627). The coordinated spatiotemporal expression of M-CSF and its receptor has led to the speculation that it is important for growth and development of the placenta (see ref. 544). Thus, the finding that osteopetrotic mice (op/op) that lack M-CSF are infertile was of particular interest (628). However, the additional findings that heterozygous males can breed successfully with such females and that the large amounts of M-CSF normally present in the uterus during pregnancy are apparently not critical in those animals remain to be explained. Indeed, Tartakovsky et al (629) reported that the injection of small amounts of M-CSF during the preimplantation period totally blocks pregnancies resulting from certain genetic crosses. Thus, although M-CSF will undoubtedly be shown to play a critical role in the cytokine network responsible for local regulation within the developing implantation site, its peculiar function is still obscure.

Granulocyte/macrophage colony stimulating factor (GM-CSF) promotes development of preimplantation embryos resulting from specific genetic crosses (556), and GM-CSF bioactivity is found in supernatants of day 12 decidual cell cultures (630). Granulocyte/macrophage colony stimulating factor stimulates proliferation of mouse placental cells (560) and, thus, may also be involved in the cytokine network responsible for development of the uteroplacental unit.

The insulinlike growth factor–I (IGF-I) and its mRNA have been reported in the rat uterus (631–634), and in the presence of estrogen, exogenous IGF-I stimulates DNA synthesis by endometrial cells (635). The protein and its mRNA have been detected in human placenta as well (636–638), and the protein has been identified in uterine fluid of pigs (639). Kapur et al. (640) described its spatiotemporal expression in the peri-implantation phase of pregnancy in mice by means of immunocytochemistry and *in situ* hybridization; it was found that early in the preimplantation period, IGF-I is expressed principally in luminal and glandular epithelium, and that about the time of implantation, it is also expressed in stroma and the decidual cells. Insulinlike growth factor 1 protein and its mRNA are stimulated and increase in the uteri of immature rats (631,632,641), pigs (642), and ovariectomized mice (640) after the injection of estrogen. In ovariectomized adult mice, it has been shown that estrogen stimulates expression of IGF-I primarily in the epithelial compartment of the uterus, whereas progesterone induces its production primarily in stroma (640). Insulinlike growth factor II mRNA and protein have been detected in human trophoblast after the time of implantation (637,638,643) as well as in the endometrium (644). And IGF-II mRNA has been reported in adult rat uterus, where it is expressed at a low level and apparently cannot be stimulated with estrogen (632,633).

Receptors for IGF-I are reported to exist in the uterus of rats and humans and are found to respond to ovarian hormones; they are localized principally in the myometrium (645–647). Binding of IGF-II to trophoblast outgrowths has been reported (648), and IGF-I causes increases in activity of 3β-hydroxysteroid dehydrogenase activity in human cytotrophoblast cells (649).

The IGFs are transported bound to a family of high-affinity binding proteins (IGFBPs). Insulinlike growth factor binding protein-I is identical to PP 12 (502) and similar to α_1-PEG (503; but see ref. 504). The protein and its mRNA are localized to luminal and glandular epithelium and expressed in predecidual stroma as well as decidual cells (503,634,650,651). Insulinlike growth factor binding protein-1 is a major endometrial secretory product (651,652) and is down-regulated by estrogen (647). Although the function of the IGFBPs in the uterus is unclear, it has been suggested that these proteins modulate IGF activity (634,653,654), and hence, their being regulated in turn by ovarian hormones provides the potential for another control mechanism in the endocrine/paracrine system responsible for local changes within the uterus at the time of implantation.

Leukemia inhibitory factor (LIF) is expressed in mouse uterine glands and is essential for development of stem cells from the inner cell mass (655). Expression of this cytokine increases at about the time of implantation, is under maternal control, and apparently is essential for embryo implantation (656); the specific role played by LIF remains unknown.

Proenkephalin A mRNA has been detected in mouse endometrial glands, and the amounts increase markedly in cells near the feto–maternal interface with decidualization (657); again, beyond demonstrating the potential for this cytokine to play a role as a link in the endocrine/paracrine system responsible for local regulation in the uterus, nothing is known about its function at implantation.

The above outline attempts only to provide an overview of what is appearing currently with respect to the detection of different cytokines and their receptors in the endometrium and is by no means exhaustive; this literature is growing so rapidly that it is difficult to put the findings in proper perspective. And although it seems probable that the paracrine and autocrine factors outlined above will prove to be important in regulating cell proliferation, differentiation, and function in the uterus at implantation, as they do in typical inflammatory reactions, it must be emphasized that it is still too early to assign them specific roles or attempt to define the controlling mechanisms. What is clear is that the existence of a variety of paracrine factors in the different cellular compartments of the endometrium, some of which appear to interact with ovarian steroid hormones, provides the uterus with the potential for translating systemic endocrine signals into the localized changes in the endometrium that are characteristic of developing implantation sites.

Initiation of Decidualization

That transformation of sensitized endometrium can be initiated by a variety of stimuli and will proceed in the absence of an embryo implies not only that elements necessary for decidualization are intrinsic to the uterus but also that events entrained by the different stimuli converge at a common physiologic point. It has been proposed that histamine and prostaglandins, released locally in the uterus in response to the different stimuli, provide the common locus and that these factors initiate the vascular and cellular changes of decidualization.

Histamine

The hypothesis that it is histamine released from uterine mast cells by the nidatory surge of estrogen that is responsible for initiating the decidual reaction was formulated over a period of several years by Shelesnyak and colleagues, based on the following observations: (a) Histamine antagonists instilled into the uterine lumen prevent the formation of deciduomata and reduce the number of implantations in rats (658,659); (b) histamine injected intraluminally, as well as histamine releasers administered systemically, induced decidual reactions in pseudopregnant rats (658–660); and (c) histamine content of rat uteri is reduced at the time of implantation (661), as well as in the uteri of ovariectomized rats after the injection of estrogen (662,663). Several investigators have disputed this hypothesis (179,664) and raise the following objections: (a) Intraluminal stimulators of the decidual response may be nonspecific (184,185,665); (b) systemic antihistamines are not particularly effective in blocking the decidual response (666,667); (c) in the hands of other investigators, instillation of histamine in the uterine lumen has not elicited greater responses than the vehicle alone, nor can a dose-response relationship be demonstrated (664,668,669); (d) depletion of histamine in mast cells with 48/80 does not prevent the decidual reaction (179); and (e) the decidual reaction normally occurs only in the vicinity of the embryo or as discrete foci after administration of a systemic stimulus, and it would be expected that a generalized release of mast cell histamine in response to nidatory estrogen would result in a response throughout the uterus (179).

Although many of the objections can be argued away, the failure of systemic antihistamines to block decidualization was seen as damaging; thus, the hypothesis was not universally accepted. The subsequent finding that there are two types of histamine receptors (H_1 and H_2) and that both may have to be blocked for a complete antihistamine effect suggested that the early failures (i.e., typically with blockers of H_2 receptors) did not constitute evidence against a role for histamine in implantation. Thus, interest was renewed when Brandon and Wallis (670) reported that implantation and decidualization were reduced in rats treated with a combination of blockers of H_1 and H_2 receptors (pyrilamine and burimamide, respectively). This finding seemed even more significant when coupled with the demonstration that rabbit blastocysts have H_2 receptors, whereas endometrium has the H_1 type (671). However, more recently, Brandon and Raval (672) were unable to block the attachment of embryos with another specific and more potent blocker of the H_2 receptor (i.e., metiamide), and it has now been questioned whether the earlier effect with burimamide (670) was actually mediated through an effect on H_2 receptors (673).

Although the question of histamine receptors is still open, other evidence seems to support the hypothesis that histamine from mast cells is important in the uterine response. Thus, Ferrando and Nalbandov (674) depleted areas of the endometrium of mast cells by localized freezing and found that although this prevented implantation and decidualization, the effect could be overcome by instillation of histamine into the uterine lumen. Furthermore, Dey et al. (675) found that inhibition of histamine release from mast cells by means of intraluminal instillation of disodium cromoglycate prevented implantation and the decidual reaction in the rabbit and concluded that mast cell histamine plays a critical role in decidualization and, thus, in implantation.

From these observations, as well as those of Shelesnyak and colleagues, it seems probable that histamine has something to do with decidual transformation and implantation. However, many of the objections raised by DeFeo (179) are still relevant, and a role for uterine histamine remains to be clearly defined.

Prostaglandins

The proposition that uterine prostaglandins have an obligatory role in the development of endometrial vascular permeability and subsequent decidual transformation is based on several lines of evidence (676,677). First, it has been shown that blocking the synthesis of prostaglandins with indomethacin during the first few days of pregnancy inhibits or delays implantation in mice (678,679), rats (680–682), hamsters (683), and rabbits (684). It was generally observed in those experiments that, after treatment with indomethacin, the implantation sites appeared later and were smaller than in control animals and that embryonic development was retarded. Furthermore, the expected localized increases in vascular permeability associated with implantation are blocked or delayed by indomethacin in rats (681,685) and rabbits (686,687). In some cases, exogenous prostaglandins partially overcame the effects of indomethacin (679,684,688). That this effect is on the uterus rather than on the embryos or on the production of steroid hormones by the ovary was shown by experiments with spayed animals given progesterone and estrogen replacement to achieve uteri with maximum sensitivity to decidualizing stimuli. Again, it was found that indomethacin blocked or greatly attenuated the artificially stimulated decidual response (689–694).

Second, the concentration of prostaglandins is observed to increase in decidualizing tissue in both normal pregnant animals and those with artificially stimulated deciduoma; again, this increase is blocked by indomethacin (681,685,692,695–699). Furthermore, exogenous prostaglandins placed in the lumen of sensitized uteri are able to stimulate an increase in vascular permeability, even when endogenous prostaglandin synthesis is inhibited. There has been some disagreement about which of the prostaglandins is most effective. For example, Kennedy (685) found that prostaglandin E-2 (PGE-2) instilled into the lumen was effective in increasing vascular permeability, whereas prostaglandin F-2α (PGF-2α) was not. However, constant infusion of PGF-2α was as effective as PGE-2 (694). Complete decidual transformation can be elicited by intraluminal application of prostaglandins, with or without suppressing endogenous synthesis with indomethacin; PGF-2α instilled into the lumen is reported to be effective (700), and implants of PGE-2 and PGF-2α are both effective (701). More recently, it has been shown that there are specific receptors for PGE-2 in the stroma of rat endometrium (702) and that their concentration increases with progesterone, reaching a maximum on the fifth and sixth days of pseudopregnancy. There are no receptors for PGF-2α in the rat endometrium (703). It is suggested, therefore, that any effect of PGF-2α on decidual tissues is a result of its conversion to PGE-2 or because PGF-2α cross-reacts with PGE-2 receptors. This could provide an explanation for the effect of PGF-2α after constant infusion, when instillation as a bolus was less effective (685,694). However, the uterus is in a neutral state after several days of progesterone, and there was no change of PGE-2 receptor concentration on addition of estrogen to develop the sensitive or receptive state (704). It has been reported that progesterone translocation to the nucleus is mediated by prostaglandins (705). Furthermore, production of prostaglandins increases in uterine tissue on the fifth day of pregnancy or pseudopregnancy (682) did not find such differences in ovariectomized animals treated with ovarian steroid hormones, even though the expected increase in vascular permeability in response to intraluminal PGE-2 (or saline) was present. Thus, the acquisition of endometrial sensitivity does not appear to be directly correlated to the ability of the uterus to produce prostaglandins, and it appears that no simple relationship exists between the condition of endometrial receptivity and the level of prostaglandin production of receptors.

Several observations have been made that suggest that changes in cyclic AMP mediate the decidualizing effects of prostaglandin at the cellular level. Thus, there is a rapid and dramatic increase in cyclic AMP after artificial stimulation of the decidual response (692,706–708), and this is inhibited by indomethacin (692,708). Furthermore, the instillation of cholera toxin causes increases in both vascular permeability and decidualization (707). Although the process of decidualization after cholera toxin may not be identical with that associated with PGE-2 (709), there are at least the typical changes in permeability and steroid receptors (710). However, intrauterine instillation of cyclic AMP or dibutyryl cyclic AMP does not induce decidualization (701,706,707,711) but will induce implantation if embryos are present (712,713). Thus, it is clear that prostaglandins have some obligatory role in implantation, presumable involving the increase in vascular permeability associated with decidualization, but the importance of their role in the overall decidual transformation and the process of implantation remains unclear.

Embryonic Signals

It has long been suspected that some form of embryonic signaling is necessary for the process of implantation and the "maternal recognition of pregnancy" (714,715). However, the nature of the putative signals and how they function remain very controversial. There are several problems: First, the localized nature of the uterine response during the apposition phase of implantation implies that some type of embryonic signal acts at short range, whereas systemic changes associated with the maternal recognition of pregnancy, such as maintenance of the corpus luteum and modulation of the immune response, indicate that some are effective at longer range. Therefore, it seems probable that in many cases there are more than one embryonic signal. Second, even when the purpose of embryonic signaling is the same in two species, the mode of action may be quite different. For example, in women and nonhuman primates, it is the production of a chorionic gonadotropin that is responsible for "rescuing" the corpus luteum (716), and although there is controversy about whether that embryonic signal is actually synthesized by preimplantation blastocysts, it is clear that it operates as a luteotrophic factor (11). By contrast, in domestic animals such as the sheep, pig, and cow, it is the production of an antiluteolysin by the embryo that is essential to neutralize the effect of uterine PGF-2α and thus prevent destruction of the corpus luteum.

Many reports have appeared during the past 25 years

that deal with the attempts to demonstrate that different potential signal substances are synthesized and released by preimplantation embryos. At one time or another, carbon dioxide, steroids, histamine, prostaglandins, and proteins of embryonic origin have all been proposed as signals. Besides diffusible chemical factors, it has even been suggested that physical contact between the embryo and the endometrium provides a signaling mechanism. In reviewing the evidence for these different factors, it should be kept in mind that it is unlikely that any one factor will be identified that could be considered as "the" signal for implantation in all animals; furthermore, in most cases, there is no reason to suggest that any of the proposed factors are mutually exclusive.

Physical Stimuli

Two observations have been used to support the hypothesis that it is physical contact between the embryo and the epithelium that is responsible for signaling at implantation. The first is the finding that embryo-sized beads of glass, paraffin, or agar produce decidual reactions in pseudopregnant rats (717,718). Although it is interesting, this hypothesis has not been supported by results of other experiments with different kinds of artificial or surrogate embryos. For example, unfertilized rat eggs, two-cell embryos, or mouse or sea urchin eggs apparently had little or no ability to elicit reaction in rats (718); McLaren (719) found that beads made of glass or an acrylic polymer did not produce deciduomas in pseudopregnant mice, and Blandau (717) was unable to obtain the reaction in pseudopregnant guinea pigs by using beads made of glass or paraffin. The second proposal is that because microvilli of the trophoblast interdigitate with those of the epithelium, pulsations of the blastocyst at this stage (720,721) might lead to distortion of the epithelium (676,722) and augment a physical signal. However, the finding that localized edema will occur when embryos are still in the zona pellucida (172,407) makes the significance of this mechanism questionable. Although it may eventually be possible to demonstrate that such physical contact results in epithelial distortion and that it is important, the findings to date have not been convincing, and none of the observations is clear-cut enough to assign a specific role to contact-mediated signals at implantation.

Carbon Dioxide

The possibility that carbon dioxide (produced as a metabolic by-product of developmentally active blastocysts) is important as a signal for implantation was originally proposed by Boving (723,724). It was hypothesized that carbon dioxide removed from the rabbit embryo as bicarbonate ion is converted to carbonic acid and an alkaline carbonate salt in the uterine epithelium, with the carbonic acid subsequently being converted to carbon dioxide by carbonic anhydrase. It was envisioned that a resulting increase in pH could have local effects on the uterus. Hetherington (186,725) also suggested that embryonic carbon dioxide might be involved in eliciting the decidual reaction, because small bubbles of that gas or air were more effective in inducing a decidual response in pseudopregnant mice than was N_2 or O_2. Although there is no direct evidence to support this hypothesis, the observation that ethoxzolamide (an inhibitor of carbonic anhydrase) reduces the number of implantations in pregnant rabbits (724) is difficult to discount, and the question of a role for embryonic carbon dioxide as a unique embryonic signal at implantation remains unresolved.

Steroids

The concept that the embryos synthesize steroid hormones, which then play a role in implantation, has evolved from the original observation by Huff and Eik-Nes (726) that 6-day-old rabbit blastocysts were not only capable of forming pregnenolone from [^{14}C]acetate but that they "biotransformed" pregnenolone, 17α-hydroxypregnenolone, progesterone, and androstenedione to other phenolic compounds. The question of synthesis of estrogen by blastocysts and the putative involvement of such "embryonic estrogen" in implantation (727) has been controversial. However, steroid metabolism by preimplantation embryonic tissue has been found in many of the animals that have been studied in detail (714,715,728,729). The observations in different species are summarized as follows.

Pig

It has been known for more than 10 years that 12- to 14-day-old pig trophoblast is capable of synthesizing estrogens from labeled androstenedione, dehydroepiandrosterone, and testosterone and thus that the embryos have aromatase activity (728,730–732). The finding that pig blastocysts convert labeled progesterone and pregnenolone to estrogen, in the presence of a system for generating cofactors, demonstrates functional Δ^5-3β- and 17β-hydroxysteroid dehydrogenase activities as well as those of the steroid C-17-20 lyase (733). Similar results have recently been reported by Fischer et al. (734), who demonstrated that estrogen can be produced from labeled progesterone by pig embryos. Estradiol production was first observed at the large spherical blastocyst stage: Estrone and estradiol were synthesized by tubular embryos, with amounts decreasing at the filamentous stage and increasing again between days 16 and 25. The enzymatic activity was demonstrated definitively in these studies by conversion of labeled substrates *in vitro,* as well as recovery and recrystallization (to constant specific activity) of the products. The results confirmed earlier histochemical findings on changing levels of Δ^5-3β- and 17β-hydroxysteroid dehydrogenase in the embryos between days 12 and 16 (735). Furthermore, the blastocysts have relatively high concentrations of estrogen and progesterone *in utero,* and the gradients between mother and embryo make it appear likely that the steroids are of embryonic rather than maternal origin (733,736).

The maternal recognition of pregnancy in the pig occurs between day 10 and 12 (737), and involves an antiluteolytic effect. Bazer and Thatcher (738) have argued that estrogen of embryonic origin is involved as follows: (a) PGF-2α from the uterus is the luteolysin in the pig and is reduced in utero-ovarian blood between days 12 and 20 of gestation (739,740), but its concentration in the uterine lumen is increased at that time (741); (b) systemic estrogen duplicates this pattern of changes in PGF-2α (739,740); and (c) it is estrogen from the embryo that is responsible for redirecting the secretion of endometrial prostaglandin from the bloodstream to the uterine lumen and thus spares the corpus luteum. Pig endometrium incubated with an embryo also has the capacity to convert progesterone to estrogen. There is no evidence for endometrial conversion of progesterone to estrogen by pseudopregnant animals, and therefore, the embryo must be responsible for altering the endometrial cells (734). A second possibility has been raised, namely, that estrogen from the embryo is sulfated in the endometrium (714,731,742) and, in the conjugated form, goes to the ovary, where it is luteotrophic (715). A third possibility has recently been raised with the report that pig blastocysts have the capacity for synthesis of catechol estrogens from estradiol (743). Because catechol estrogens have been implicated in regulation of prostaglandin synthesis and because the transient increase in estrogen 2,4-dioxylase activity occurs at the time of maternal recognition of pregnancy, Mondschein et al. (743) suggested that estrogen synthesized by the embryo as a result of increased aromatase activity, between days 10 and 14 of pregnancy, is used in the formation of catechol estrogen, which acts as a signal in implantation. It is of interest in this regard that catechol estrogens have been reported to cause implantation in delayed-implanting mice (744) and to stimulate production of prostaglandins by preimplantation rabbit embryos and endometrium (745). The endometrium of pigs also appears to be responsible for concentrating steroids in the lumen that may act as substrates for embryos (746).

Rabbit

The hypothesis that steroids of embryonic origin are important not only for development of the blastocyst but also locally to induce implantation (747,748) has been controversial. As applied to rabbits, this concept has been attacked on several grounds, including lack of specificity of the histochemical assay (749); the supposition that high concentrations of steroids in rabbit blastocysts (750,751) are of maternal origin rather than from the embryo (752–754); and the argument that the presence of enzymatic capacity does not necessarily mean that it functions *in vivo* (755). Nevertheless, definitive measurements were eventually made of the conversion of dehydroepiandrosterone to androstenedione by 5-day-old rabbit embryos and of conversion of testosterone to estradiol by 7-day-old embryos (756). Coupled with demonstrations of aromatase activity in cell-free lysates of embryos in the presence of an NADPH-generating system (757) and in whole blastocysts *in vitro* (758), these observations appear to establish that the enzymatic capacity for synthesis of estrogen exists in preimplantation rabbit blastocysts.

The question of a function for steroids associated with embryos, whether of maternal or embryonic origin, is unresolved. The several observations that implicate estradiol as a factor in preimplantation development and implantation in the rabbit are (a) incubation of blastocysts with the antiestrogen CI-628 reduces their ability to implant when transferred to pseudopregnant recipients, and the effect is reversible (759); (b) instillation of CI-628 into the uterine lumen reduces the number of implantations (760) and prevents the increases in acid phosphatase that are expected in luminal epithelium adjacent to the embryos (761); and (c) estradiol binds to a soluble cytosolic protein in rabbit blastocysts, and this binding is blocked by CI-628 (759). Although these findings implicate estradiol in development and implantation in the rabbit, they do not prove that it is of embryonic origin. Indeed, the finding that an inhibitor of aramatase (4-hydroxy-4-androstene-3,17-dione) reduces blastocyst production of estradiol from testosterone *in vitro* but does not interfere with either embryo development or implantation (758) is difficult to reconcile with that premise. The further finding that rabbit endometrium can synthesize labeled estrogen from [^{3}H]progesterone and [^{3}H]androstenedione and that the presence of the embryo influences this metabolic activity complicates this problem further (762).

Rat, Mouse, and Hamster

Enzymatic capacity for steroid metabolism in preimplantation embryos of small laboratory rodents has also been inferred from the histochemical demonstration of Δ^5-3β- and 17β-hydroxysteroid dehydrogenase activities in rats (763–766), and hamsters (767). Dickmann and colleagues published an extensive series of articles in which it has been proposed that estrogen of embryonic origin is important for the development of preimplantation stage rat, mouse, and hamster embryos as well as for the initiation of implantation (748,768). The hypothesis is supported largely by the histochemical evidence for changes in enzyme activity at the morula and blastocyst stages and the observation that CI-628 blocks embryo development at the morula stage (769) and interferes with implantation (161,770). Although this concept has not generally been accepted with respect to embryos of pigs and rabbits, largely because it has been possible to demonstrate enzymatic conversion of precursors to estrogen with biochemical techniques in addition to the histochemistry, that has not been the case with the embryos of the small laboratory rodents. Indeed, attempts by several investigators to identify transformed products of pregnenolone, progesterone, androstenedione, and dehydroepiandrosterone with preimplantation embryos of mouse and rat by radioimmunoassay (771–773) or chromatographic methods have been unsuccessful (771–774). Although the different studies with CI-628 seem to point to estrogen of embryonic origin (161,761,769, 770), a question has been raised as to whether the effects are due to nonspecific toxicity (769); these effects may be difficult to reconcile in the light of the conflicting observations that there is little estrogen receptor in the nucleus at implantation sites (439). Levels of enzymatic activity in hamsters do not change with development (775), and inhibitors of aromatase (776) and steroidogenesis (777) do not block implantation, at least in hamsters.

Other Species

Estrogen production by horse blastocysts *in vitro* has been reported (778), and in a comparative study with tissue from sheep, cows, roe deer, ferrets, cats, a plains viscacha, rabbits, and pigs, Gadsby et al. (732) reported observing significant aromatase activity and estrogen synthesis in pig trophoblast, whereas it was appreciably lower in all other species. In that study, labeled estrogens were recovered only from incubations of allantochorionic tissue of roe deer recovered shortly after implantation, as well as from pooled samples of tissue from early bovine embryos.

Histamine

It has been reported that preimplantation embryos of rabbits (779) and mice (780) have the enzymatic capacity to synthesize histamine from histidine *in vitro* (i.e., histidine decarboxylase). In rabbits, the activity peaks on the sixth day of pregnancy and intraluminal instillation of low doses of an inhibitor of histidine decarboxylase (α-methylhistidine dihydrochloride) on the fifth day of pregnancy delayed implantation and, at higher doses, interrupted implantation; simultaneous administration of histidine counteracted the inhibitor (781). Blastocyst formation of mice was also inhibited with α-methylhistidine, and again this effect was overcome with histidine (780). These findings, along with the observation that histamine reduces the requirement for estrogen in inducing implantation in hypophysectomized progesterone-treated rats (782), prompted the suggestion that histamine synthesized by the embryo is important for development of the blastocyst and acts as a local signal to the endometrium at the time of implantation. Although the hypothesis that histamine produced by the embryo is involved in causing localized changes in the endometrium at implantation is appealing, it has not been substantiated and is difficult to reconcile with the report that histamine-releasing implants did not induce a significant decidual reaction in pseudopregnant rabbits (686). Furthermore, it is clear that localized decidual reactions will occur without an embryo being present.

Prostaglandins

Several approaches have been taken in evaluating the ability of preimplantation embryos of different species to synthesize prostaglandins and in assessing their role in the process of implantation (783). Thus, it has been possible to demonstrate that some biologic processes are suppressed in blastocysts *in vitro* by inhibitors of prostaglandin synthesis; it has been shown *in vitro* that the quantity of prostaglandin within the embryo or released into the medium increases with time; and in some cases, it has been possible to demonstrate the synthesis of labeled prostaglandins from radioactive arachidonic acid supplied either exogenously or from endogenous pools. The reported observations made with these different approaches can be summarized as follows.

Rabbit

The presence of prostaglandins in preimplantation blastocysts was first reported by Dickmann and Spilman (784). Prostaglandin of the F and E series was detected by radioimmunoassay in freshly recovered blastocysts on the sixth day of development. An increase in the content of PGF was also observed in rabbit blastocysts incubated *in vitro* for 24 h (785), demonstrating that they do have the capacity for prostaglandin synthesis. Dey et al. (785) did not observe the release of prostaglandins into the medium during incubation of rabbit blastocysts. However, more recent studies have demonstrated both synthesis and release of PGE and PGF by 6- and 7-day-old rabbit embryos (786). Although it has not been possible to demonstrate the synthesis of labeled prostaglandins by rabbit blastocysts from exogenous arachidonic acid, it has been shown that when the endogenous phospholipid pools were prelabeled *in vitro* with $[^3H]$-

arachidonic acid and released by a calcium-specific ionophore, labeled prostaglandins were synthesized and released into the medium (783). From these observations, it seems clear that rabbit blastocysts have the ability to synthesize and release prostaglandins to influence the endometrium locally. Furthermore, it appears that treatment with indomethacin early in pregnancy reduces the number of implantation sites in rabbits (684) and, therefore, that prostaglandins are involved in the process of implantation in this species. However, it remains unproven as to whether the local changes in endometrium (786) and the increase in concentration of prostaglandins at implantation sites (787) are caused by embryonic prostaglandins.

Cow

Measurable amounts of immunoreactive prostaglandins of E and F series were observed in cow blastocysts recovered on the thirteenth through the sixteenth day of development and incubated for up to 48 h *in vitro;* the amounts increased in proportion to the ages of the embryos (788). Similarly, increasing amounts of radiolabeled prostaglandins were recovered after incubation of 16- and 19-day-old bovine embryos with radioactive precursors (789). Clearly, cow blastocysts have the capacity to synthesize prostaglandins, and again the suggestion that they (or other metabolites of arachidonic acid) might be important for embryonic development, act as local signals to the uterus, or be involved in maintenance of the corpus luteum (789) remains unproven.

Rat and Mouse

It has not been possible to detect the synthesis of prostaglandins by preimplantation embryos of rat using radioimmunoassay methods, even after incubation of up to 220 embryos for 24 h (677). Similarly, it has not been possible to demonstrate synthesis of labeled prostaglandins by mouse blastocysts from either exogenous or endogenous [^{3}H]arachidonic acid (783). However, in the case of the mouse at least, there is strong evidence that prostaglandins of embryonic origin are involved in expansion of the blastocyst, because several antagonists suppress the process of hatching *in vitro* (790–792). Although instillation of some of these prostaglandin antagonists into the uterine lumen also interfered with implantation, the degree of their effectiveness was not the same as that for suppression of hatching (793), and it is not clear if they act at the level of the embryo or the endometrium. Because prostaglandins of the E series are often involved in water transport across epithelia, Biggers and colleagues suggested that these prostaglandins are important for that function in the blastocyst as well and thus could be involved in implantation by virtue of maintaining the turgidity necessary for apposition and adhesion of the blastocyst and endometrium rather than as local signal factors (790,793). It must be recognized that these possibilities are not mutually exclusive.

Sheep

Sheep blastocysts (at days 12 and 15 of development) were found to synthesize prostaglandins of the E and F series when incubated with labeled arachidonic acid (794), and the total amounts released into the medium in $8\frac{1}{2}$ h was 28 times the amount contained in the embryos at the time of recovery (795). Although the concentrations of PGE and PGF were shown to be high in both 14- and 23-day-old blastocysts and synthesis of PGF in the endometrium increased after day 14, indomethacin had no effect on implantation in this species (796).

Taken together, these findings provide strong evidence for production of prostaglandins by preimplantation embryos of the rabbit, sheep, and cow. The evidence for the mouse is indirect and less compelling, and as pointed out by Racowsky and Biggers (783), alternative methods will have to be used before the question can be settled with respect to the rat. When embryonic prostaglandins function as local signals to the uterus or are important to the embryo simply for maintaining normal cell function is unclear.

Proteins

It has been known for almost 20 years that proteins of embryonic origin are important for the maternal recognition of pregnancy in sheep. Evidence is now beginning to accumulate that supports the suggestion that such embryonic protein factors are involved in establishing pregnancy in a number of other species as well.

Sheep

The concept that a protein signal of embryonic origin plays a role in maternal recognition of pregnancy in sheep dates back to the observations by Moor and Rowson (797–800) that luteolysis is prevented if a conceptus is present between days 12 and 13 or if homogenates of 14- to 15-day-old conceptuses are instilled into the uterine lumen. The active principal in the homogenates was heat labile and presumed, therefore, to be a protein. In similar experiments, Martal et al. (801) confirmed this observation and demonstrated that the active material (which they called *trophoblastin*) from 14- to 16-day-old embryos was not only heat labile but was ineffective after treatment with protease. That extracts from older embryos [i.e., 21 and 23 days old (801) or 25 days old (800)] were ineffective in prolonging the life of the corpus luteum led to the suggestion that the protein was synthesized by the embryos only during the period from day 13 to day 21. This protein factor is presumably of trophoblast origin because transfer of trophoblastic vesicles (from 11- to 13-day-old embryos) to the uteri of nonpregnant ewes (on day 12 of the cycle) prolonged luteal life (802).

Although the signal has not been definitively identified, it has recently been shown *in vitro* that stage-specific proteins are synthesized and secreted by preimplantation sheep blastocysts. Thus, Godkin et al. (803) demonstrated with two-dimensional polyacrylamide gel electrophoresis that the major labeled product of 13-day-old sheep embryos incubated *in vitro* with [^{3}H]leucine was a low-molecular-weight (17,000), acidic (PI 5.5) protein initially designed protein X). Although several other proteins were synthesized and secreted by embryos between days 14 and 21, protein X was predominant up to day 23, when it could no longer be detected. This protein is apparently synthesized in trophoblast, as shown by immunocytochemical methods (804), and has been redesignated "ovine trophoblast protein 1" (oTP-1). It binds to receptors in the endometrium with high affinity and apparently changes the pattern of protein synthesis in endometrium *in vitro* (804). This protein is the main translation product of trophoblastic mRNA, in a cell-free wheat-germ lysate system, and its production appears to peak in 13-day-old embryos (805). Also, instillation of oTP-1 into the uterine lumen of cyclic ewes prolongs the life of the corpus luteum (806). However, this protein does not compete for luteinizing-hormone receptors on the corpus luteum nor does it stimulate progesterone synthesis (804), and thus it is apparently not the luteotrophic factor in conceptus homogenates reported by Godkin et al. (807) and Ellinwood et al. (808). For these reasons, it has been suggested that oTP-1 is the embryonic protein factor involved in protecting against luteolysis (trophoblastin), presumably because its interaction with the uterine epithelium leads to altered release or metabolism of endometrial PGF-2α (805). Also, Masters et al. (809) reported that the major glucosamine-labeled product, purified by ion-exchange and gel-filtration chromatography of medium from 14- to 16-day-old embryos, is a large glycoprotein (600,000 Da), consisting of at least 50% carbohydrate (largely *N*-acetylglucosamine and galactose) and relatively resistant to proteolysis. A similar embryonic-secreted factor has been observed in the cow and pig, but no functional significance has been ascribed to this glycoprotein as yet.

Cow

The cow is similar to the sheep and pig in that the presence of conceptus tissues *in utero* (before day 17) results in the maintenance of the corpus luteum (810–812). Furthermore, the infusion of homogenates of 17- and 18-day-old embryos has been shown to delay luteal regression, although it is not known if the active principal is sensitive to heat or protease as it is in sheep (812). Preattachment bovine conceptuses have been shown to synthesize and secrete a complex array of stage-specific proteins between days 16 and 24 of development (813). The individual proteins were separated by two-dimensional polyacrylamide gel electrophoresis and ion-exchange and gel-filtration chromatography. The amount of radiolabel incorporated into secreted material increases from day 16 through day 22 and decreases by day 24. Several low-molecular-weight acidic proteins are secreted during this period that are similar to, but not identical with, those secreted by ovine trophyoblast. These factors are no longer evident by day 29 and thus are restricted to the period of maternal recognition of pregnancy in the cow. Also, a large glycoprotein labeled with [^{3}H]glucosamine was secreted by tissue from all stages including postimplantation (day 69) chorion. This may be the same factor isolated earlier by Masters et al. (809) using similar techniques.

Pig

The time of maternal recognition of pregnancy in the pig is day 10 to day 12, and as with the sheep and the cow, a conceptus must be present *in utero* (before day 13) if the corpus luteum is to survive (737,814). It has been known for some time that the preattachment pig blastocyst is active in synthesizing and releasing proteins (815–817). Stage-specific proteins have been demonstrated in the pig *in vitro* by incubation of preattachment-stage embryos with radiolabeled precursors and by analysis of the conditioned medium using two-dimensional polyacrylamide gel electrophoresis (818). The main labeled products between $10\frac{1}{2}$ and 12 days appear to be a group of low-molecular-weight acidic proteins similar to those reported for the sheep and the cow. However, between days 13 and 16, the main products are larger and more basic, and after day 18, the main secreted products are a group of serum proteins synthesized by the embryo rather than by the trophoblast. A large glycoprotein labeled with [^{3}H]glucosamine and similar to that observed in sheep and cows was isolated with ion-exchange and gel-filtration chromatography from all stages (809).

Mouse

The concept that proteins secreted by the preimplantation mouse embryo might be involved in signaling at implantation dates back to the observation by Fishel and Surani (819) that a labeled glycoprotein (approximately 87,000 Da) could be recovered from the medium after incubating blastocysts with [^{3}H]glucosamine. More recently, it has been demonstrated that a complex array of stage-specific proteins are synthesized and secreted when preimplantation mouse blastocysts are incubated with [^{35}S]methionine (820). The proteins were isolated from conditioned medium and separated with two-dimensional polyacrylamide gel electrophoresis. It was found that synthesis and secretion of labeled proteins increased between days 4 and 5 of pregnancy, and as with embryos of the sheep, pig, and cow, there were several low-molecular-weight acidic proteins released before implantation. Of special interest was the finding that some of the proteins secreted by the mouse embryos were decreased in amount as embryos entered the dormant phase associated with delayed implantation. Those proteins that decreased as embryos became dormant typically increased as the embryos were reactivated. Furthermore, the appearance of these secreted factors was correlated temporally with the appearance of the Pontamine Blue reaction in the uterus. Although these findings are highly suggestive of a signal role for secreted proteins in preimplantation mouse embryos, that function remains to be demonstrated.

Early Pregnancy Factor

Several observations have been reported that indicate that other systemic signals of embryonic origin are involved in the maternal recognition of pregnancy. Of these, the so-called early pregnancy factor (EPF) has received the most attention. The existence of EPF was hypothesized after the observation that lymphocytes from pregnant mice had less activity in the rosette inhibition test with a standard antilymphocyte serum than did those from nonpregnant animals (821). Subsequently, it was found that the activity was a serum factor that enhanced the ability of rabbit antimouse serum to prevent rosette formation with normal red blood cells and spleen cells in the presence of complement (822,823). The amount of activity appeared to vary with the number of fetuses and to drop quickly once the embryos were removed (824). The factor was reported to suppress "adoptive transfer" of contact sensitivity to trinitrochlorobenzene, and it was suggested that it regulates cellular immunity *in vivo* (825). There are at least two types of EPF activity that appear at characteristic times in pregnancy (i.e., pre- and postimplantation). The early form is a large molecule [mice, 180,000 Da by gel filtration (826); sheep, 250,000 Da (827)] that can be separated into a nonactive protein fraction and an active factor (50,000 Da) by ion-exchange chromatography; recombining these fractions returns activity. It appears, then, that the early form of EPF is associated with a normal serum protein carrier. The active principal in the early form of EPF consists of two components, EPF-A and EPF-B. These components can be separated by differential precipitation with 40% NH_4SO_4; neither component alone has any effect, but activity is restored when they are recombined (827–829). In the mouse, EPF-A is secreted by the oviduct in an inactive form and will not alter the rosette inhibition test until EPF-B is added; EPF-B is secreted by the ovary [in the presence of a pituitary factor shown to be prolactin (830)] in response to a factor secreted by the fertilized or parthenogenically stimulated ovum (831–833). The early form of mouse EPF has been purified by immunoabsorption, electrofocusing, and gel filtration (834); the monomeric form has a molecular weight of 21,000 and can be resolved into peptides of three sizes (at 10,501 Da is EPF-A; at 7,200 and at 3,400 Da combine to form EPF-B). In mice, the late form of EPF appears to be produced by the embryo as the oviduct and ovary lose the capacity to synthesize components of the early form by about day 7 of pregnancy, but EPF activity can still be detected in the serum and urine in those animals as well as in animals ovariectomized on day 4 of pregnancy (826). Similar activity has been reported in sheep (828,833,835,836), humans (823,837–841), rats (842), pigs (843), and cows (833). It appears that EPF from mice, sheep, pigs, and humans have similar characteristics with respect to the effect on the rosette inhibition test and the appearance of different forms in each stage of pregnancy. Furthermore, there appears to be no species specificity; for example, human and pig ova produce a factor that will work in the mouse after intraperitoneal injection and extracts of fertilized mouse ova (but not unfertilized ova) elicit EPF activity when injected into the sheep oviduct (833).

Whether EPF functions in regulation of the maternal immune system in pregnancy, or exists at all, has been questioned by some investigators (844,845). However, because it (a) has been detected early in pregnancy in all species studied, (b) requires the presence of a viable embryo (or fetus), and (c) appears to last through at least the first half of pregnancy, some investigators have proposed that it be used as a diagnostic test for pregnancy (846–851).

Other Signals

Several other putative signal-response mechanisms have been reported that may be related to early pregnancy factors. For example, two-cell hamster embryos are reported to release an octapeptide that inhibits ovulation (852–854); fertilized horse ova are transported into the uterus while unfertilized ova are retrained in the oviduct (855,856); lactate levels in the mouse oviduct remain elevated longer in animals with viable embryos than in pseudopregnant animals (857); and thrombocytopenia occurs in mice from the first day to the seventh day of pregnancy and does not occur in pseudopregnant mice (858). This latter response can be observed, however, within 3 h of the transfer of fertilized embryos to pseudopregnant mice and thus seems to be initiated by an embryonic signal. Although the importance of these different signal factors to the biology of implantation and the precise mechanism of their action in different animals remain obscure, the study of embryonic factors is of major importance and will be an important area for research in the next few years.

Influence of the Uterine Environment on Blastocyst Development

Besides observations that indicate that blastocysts can effect local and systemic changes in the mother during the peri-implantation period, it has become clear that development of the embryos is, in turn, influenced by the uterine environment. The uterine potential for regulating development of preimplantation embryos is dramatically illustrated by the phenomenon of delayed implantation. In that situation, development is arrested at the blastocyst stage for a period of several days, or even months, and resumes only in response to a change in the maternal endocrine status. During this phase of development quiescence, the blastocysts typically have reduced levels of metabolic and synthetic activity, and cell division actually stops. In some species, such a period of embryonic diapause occurs as an obligatory part of pregnancy; in others, it may or may not occur, depending on conditions in the maternal environment. In either case, after reactivation, the "dormant" blastocysts resume development, and the subsequent implantation and fetal development are normal (859,860). It is generally accepted that the uterus is responsible for the embryonic quiescence associated with delayed implantation, because removing blastocysts to extrauterine sites either *in vivo* or *in vitro* leads to their metabolic reactivation (861). The presumed mechanism, as proposed 50 years ago by Brambell (862), is that the uterus regulates development in delayed implantation by either (a) restricting a critical "growth factor" or (b) secreting an "inhibitory substance" into the lumen. Most studies directed at defining the mechanisms responsible for embryonic quiescence in delayed implantation have made use of the fact that the blastocysts become "reactivated" *in vitro* after being removed from the uterus and incubated for a few hours in different tissue culture media. In this case, reactivation is characterized by (a) increases in metabolic activity and macromolecular synthesis, as occurs with reactivation of embryos *in vivo* (861,863,864), and (b) the outgrowth of trophoblast cells, which has been likened to the initial changes associated with implantation *in utero* (865–870).

The observations most often cited to support the concept that restriction of essential factors is a mechanism for delayed implantation can be summarized as follows: Trophoblast outgrowth does not occur *in vitro* in the absence of certain amino acids (867–870), serum factors (867,868), or glucose (869,871,872). It has been suggested from such observations that the uterus might impose developmental quiescence on the embryos by restricting one or more of these factors or even restricting concentrations of different ions (872–878) during delayed implantation. However, the level of amino acids in uterine fluid from delayed-implanting mice appears to be the same as that in normal animals (879), and although deletion of amino acids or serum from the culture medium prevents outgrowth, it apparently does not prevent metabolic activation (880). The suggestion that embryos do not develop beyond the blastocyst stage *in vitro* in the absence of glucose because they are energy deficient and thus that developmental arrest *in vivo* is due to the same cause (881) has not proven tenable. Dormant embryos actually have a higher ATP/ADP ratio than reactivated embryos, and indeed, it appears that reduced use of glucose by dormant embryos (882,883) is due to allosteric inhibition of glycolysis because of the high-energy state of the cells (884). Furthermore, it has been impossible to maintain metabolic quiescence *in vitro* by restricting the concentrations of different ions in the medium, and it now seems unlikely that this is a mechanism by which the uterus renders the embryos quiescent *in vivo* (885). Several investigators have reported the results of experiments in which embryos were incubated in uterine fluid and examined for changes in metabolic activity or shedding of the zona pellucida (864,886–891). Results indicate that there is a factor present in flushings of uteri from cyclic or pseudopregnant animals that reduces RNA synthesis by blastocysts *in vitro*. The factor is heat stable and dialyzable and is neutralized in the uteri of pregnant but not pseudopregnant animals 6.5 h after the injection of estrogen (891). The nature of this putative inhibitory factor has not been determined. It is not known if the blastotoxic factor reported by Psychoyos and Casimiri (892) is the same one responsible for these changes, and although these results provide support for the interesting possibility that the uterus can inhibit embryonic growth, this proposal has not been proven conclusively and has not been universally accepted.

SUMMARY

It is obvious from the foregoing presentation that implantation of mammalian embryos is a complex phenomenon in which a variety of interactive processes occur between the conceptus and the mother. It should also be clear that although different facets of the process have been described in much detail, relatively little is known at the molecular or cellular level about the actual mechanisms responsible for implantation in any one species, let alone in a comparative sense. However, despite our failure to understand totally this critical aspect of mammalian reproduction, it is possible to develop a general overview of the process in the hope that it will allow the reader to focus on common and, thus, presumably important features.

1. The embryo and the uterus must be synchronized. From work in mice and rats, this seems to be related largely to the ability of the uterus to respond to an appropriate stimulus from a blastocyst, with changes in both the epithelium and stroma leading to attachment and the formation of a decidua. The period of uterine receptivity is limited, and the changes responsible for this condition are entrained by estrogen in progesterone-conditioned endometrium. The transition from nonsensitivity to receptivity and on to refractoriness is associated with many changes in the endometrium, including altered rates of synthesis of RNA and protein, cell proliferation, and different changes in cytologic characteristics. However, it is not clear, at the cellular or molecular level, what uterine receptivity is; at present, sensitivity is only an operational definition that describes an essential condition for implantation.
2. In response to a locally effective signal from the embryo, the sensitized endometrial stroma undergoes the process of decidual transformation. This reaction is similar to an inflammatory response and involves a variety of cytokines that may drive cellular proliferation and differentiation, as well as the development of localized increases in vascular permeability, polyploid nuclei, dramatic cytologic changes, and synthesis of unique species of RNA and protein. The so-called decidua that are formed typically provide a solid mass of cells into which the conceptus is embedded. The process responsible for formation of decidual tissue appears to require an intact epithelium to conduct the embryonic signal to the stroma and may use histamine and/or the local release of PGE-2 to initiate the reaction. Although formation of the decidua is a conspicuous part of the process of implantation in many species and it seems to represent the development of an entirely new organ at implantation, its actual function remains unknown.
3. The trophoblast of the embryo and the luminal epithelium of the uterus become adherent, with or without subsequent penetration of the endometrium. Adhesion of embryos to the uterine epithelium presumably involves changes in the glycoprotein molecules on one or both surfaces. Changes in lectin binding may reflect the expression of complementary surface glycoproteins and, thus, might be related to the acquisition of adhesiveness. However, it has not yet been shown which of these changes are causally related to attachment and implantation.
4. In response to a variety of signal factors from preimplantation embryos, there are local and systemic changes in the mother that can be considered to constitute the "maternal recognition of pregnancy." It is generally assumed that implantation and subsequent pregnancy will not be successful unless such recognition takes place.

REFERENCES

1. Psychoyos A. Hormonal control of ovoimplantation. In: Harris RS, Munson PL, Diczfalusy E, Grover J, eds. *Vitamins and Hormones: Advances in Research and Applications,* Vol 31. New York: Academic Press, 1973;201–256.
2. Psychoyos A. Endocrine control of egg implantation. In: Greep RO, Astwood EB, eds. *Handbook of Physiology, Section 7: Endocrinology,* Vol II, Part 2. Washington, DC: American Physiological Society, 1973;187–215.
3. Finn CA. The implantation reaction. In: Wynn R, ed. *Biology of the Uterus.* New York: Plenum Press, 1977;245–308.
4. O'Grady JE, Bell SC. The role of the endometrium in blastocyst implantation. In: Johnson MH, ed. *Development in Mammals,* Vol. 1. New York: North-Holland, 1977;165–243.
5. Yochim JM. Development of the progestational uterus: metabolic aspects. *Biol Reprod* 1975;12:106–133.
6. Glasser SR, Clark JH. A determinant role for progesterone in the development of uterine sensitivity to decidualization and ovo-implantation. In: Markert SL, Papaconstantinou J, eds. *The Developmental Biology of Reproduction.* New York: Academic Press, 1975;311–345.
7. Glasser SR, McCormack SA. Cellular and molecular aspects of decidualization and implantation. In: Beier HM, Karlson P, eds. *Proteins and Steroids in Early Pregnancy.* New York: Springer-Verlag, 1981;245–310.
8. Enders AC. Mechanisms of implantation of the blastocyst. In: Velardo JT, Kasprow BA, eds. *Biology of Reproduction: Basic and Clinical Studies.* Symposium on Reproductive Biology, Sponsored by Third Pan American Congress of Anatomy, 1972;313–333.
9. Schlafke S, Enders AC. Cellular basis of interaction between trophoblast and uterus at implantation. *Biol Reprod* 1975;12:41–65.
10. Wimsatt WA. Some comparative aspects of implantation. *Biol Reprod* 1975;12:1–40.
11. Heap RB, Flint APF, Gadsby JE. Role of embryonic signals in the establishment of pregnancy. *Br Med Bull* 1979;35:129–135.
12. Finn CA. Implantation, menstruation and inflammation. *Biol Rev* 1986;61:313–328.
13. Aplin JD. Cellular biochemistry of the endometrium. In: Wynn RM, Jollie WP, eds. *Biology of the Uterus.* New York: Plenum Medical Book Company, 1989;89–129.
14. Parr MB, Parr ER. The implantation reaction. In: Wynn RM, Jollie WP, eds. *Biology of the Uterus.* New York: Plenum, 1989;233–277.
15. Enders AC, Schlafke S. A morphological analysis of the early implantation stages in the rat. *Am J Anat* 1967;120:185–226.
16. Hedlund K, Nilsson O, Reinius S, Aman G. Attachment reaction of the uterine luminal epithelium at implantation: light and electron microscopy of the hamster, guinea-pig, rabbit and mink. *J Reprod Fertil* 1972;29:131–132.
17. Nilsson BO. Structural differentiation of luminal membrane in rat uterus during normal and experimental implantations. *Z Anat* 1966;125:152–159.
18. Nilsson BO. Some ultrastructural aspects of ovo-implantation. In: Hubinens PO, Lercy F, Robyn C, Leleux P, eds. *Ovo-Implantation. Human Gonadotropins and Prolactin.* New York: S Karger, 1970;52–72.
19. Young MP, Whicher JT, Potts DM. The ultrastructure of implantation in the golden hamster (*Cricetus auratus*). *J Embryol Exp Morphol* 1968;19:341–345.
20. Potts DM. The attachment phase of ovoimplantation. *Am J Obstet Gynecol* 1966;96:1122–1128.
21. Potts DM. The ultrastructure of implantation in the mouse. *J Anat* 1968;103:77–90.
22. Potts M. The ultrastructure of egg-implantation. In: McLaren A,

ed. *Advances in Reproductive Physiology.* London: Logos, 1969;241–267.
23. Psychoyos A, Mandon P. Scanning electron microscopy of the surface of the rat uterine epithelium during delayed implantation. *J Reprod Fertil* 1971;26:137–138.
24. Nilsson O. Attachment of rat and mouse blastocysts onto uterine epithelium. *Int J Fertil* 1967;12:5–13.
25. Reinius S. Ultrastructure of blastocyst attachment in mouse. *Z Zellforsch Mikrosk Anat* 1967;77:257–266.
26. Potts DM, Psychoyos A. Evolution de l'ultrastructure des relations ovoendometriales sous l'influence de l'oestrogene, chez la ratte en retard experimental de nidation. *C R Acad Sci Paris Ser D* 1967;264:370–373.
27. Potts DM, Psychoyos A. L'ultrastructure des relations ovoendometriales au cours du retard experimental de nidation chez la souris. *C R Acad Sci Paris Ser D* 1967;264:956–958.
28. Mayer G, Nilsson O, Reinius S. Cell membrane changes of uterine epithelium and trophoblast during blastocyst attachment in rat. *Z Anat Entwick* 1967;126:43–48.
29. Tachi S, Tachi C, Lindner HR. Ultrastructural features of blastocyst attachment and trophoblastic invasion in the rat. *J Reprod Fertil* 1970;21:37–56.
30. Parkening TA. Apposition of uterine luminal epithelium during implantation in senescent golden hamster. *J Gerontol* 1979;34: 335–344.
31. Martin L, Finn CA, Carter J. Effects of progesterone and oestradiol on the luminal epithelium of the mouse uterus. *J Reprod Fertil* 1970;21:461–469.
32. Hedlund K, Nilsson O. Hormonal requirements for the uterine attachment reaction and blastocyst implantation in the mouse, hamster and guinea-pig. *J Reprod Fertil* 1971;26:267–269.
33. Pollard RM, Finn CA. Ultrastructure of the uterine epithelium during the hormonal induction of sensitivity and insensitivity to a decidual stimulus in the mouse. *J Endocrinol* 1972;55:293–298.
34. McLaren A. A study of blastocysts during delay and subsequent implantation of lactating mice. *J Endocrinol* 1968;42:453–463.
35. Lundkvist O, Nilsson BO, Bergstrom S. Studies on the trophoblast-epithelial complex during decidual induction in rats. *Am J Anat* 1979;154:211–230.
36. Warren R, Enders AC. An electron microscope study of the rat endometrium during delayed implantation. *Anat Rec* 1964;148: 177–195.
37. Ljungkvist I. Attachment reaction of rat uterine luminal epithelium. IV. The cellular changes in the attachment reaction and its hormonal regulation. *Fertil Steril* 1972;23:847–865.
38. Tachi S, Tachi C. Ultrastructural studies on maternal-embryonic cell interactions during experimentally induced implantation of rat blastocysts to the endometrium of the mouse. *Dev Biol* 1979;68:203–223.
39. McLaren A, Nilsson O. Electron microscopy of luminal epithelium separated by beads in the pseudopregnant mouse uterus. *J Reprod Fertil* 1971;26:379–381.
40. Enders AC, Nelson DM. Pinocytotic activity of the uterus of the rat. *Am J Anat* 1973;138:277–300.
41. Leroy F, Van Hoeck J, Bogaert C. Hormonal control of pinocytosis in the uterine epithelium of the rat. *J Reprod Fertil* 1976;47:59–62.
42. Parr MR, Parr EL. Uterine luminal epithelium: protrusions mediate endocytosis, not apocrine secretion, in the rat. *Biol Reprod* 1974;11:220–233.
43. Lundkvist O. Morphometric estimation of stromal edema during delayed implantation in the rat. *Cell Tissue Res* 1979;199: 339–348.
44. Yochim JM, Saldarini RJ. Glucose utilization by the myometrium during early pseudopregnancy in the rat. *J Reprod Fertil* 1969;20:481–489.
45. Murphy CR, Swift JG, Mukherjee TM, Rogers AW. Changes in the fine structure of the apical plasma membrane of endometrial epithelial cells during implantation in the rat. *J Cell Sci* 1982;55:1–12.
46. Parr M. Apical vesicles in rat uterine epithelium during early pregnancy: a morphometric study. *Biol Reprod* 1982;26: 915–924.
47. Pollard RM, Finn CA. Influence of the trophoblast upon differentiation of the uterine epithelium during implantation in the mouse. *J Endocrinol* 1974;62:669–674.
48. Enders AC, Hendrickx AG, Schlafke S. Implantation in the rhesus monkey: initial penetration of endometrium. *Am J Anat* 1983;167:275–598.
49. Parr MB, Parr EL. Relationship of apical domes in the rabbit uterine epithelium during the peri-implantation period to endocytosis, apocrine secretion and fixation. *J Reprod Fertil* 1982;66:739–744.
50. Bjorkman N. Fine structure of the fetal-maternal area of exchange in the epitheliochorial and endotheliochorial types of placentation. *Acta Anat* 1973;61(suppl 86):1–22.
51. Boshier DP. A histological and histochemical examination of implantation and early placentome formation in sheep. *J Reprod Fertil* 1969;19:51–61.
52. Wathes DC, Wooding FBP. An electron microscopic study of implantation in the cow. *Am J Anat* 1980;159:285–306.
53. Enders AC, Schlafke S. Cytological aspects of trophoblast–uterine interaction in early implantation. *Am J Anat* 1969; 125:1–30.
54. Frazier W, Glaser L. Surface components and cell recognition. *Annu Rev Biochem* 1979;48:491–523.
55. Edelman GM. Cell adhesion molecules. *Science* 1983;219:450–457.
56. Edelman GM. Expression of cell adhesion molecules during embryogenesis and regeneration. *Exp Cell Res* 1984;161:1–16.
57. Trinkaus JP. Cell adhesion. III. Mechanisms. In: *Cells Into Organs: The Forces That Shape the Embryo.* Englewood Cliffs, NJ: Prentice-Hall, 1984;120–178.
58. Enders AC, Schlafke S. Surface coats of the mouse blastocyst and uterus during the implantation period. *Anat Rec* 1974;180: 31–46.
59. Anderson TL, Hoffman LH. Alterations in epithelial glycocalyx of rabbit uteri during early pseudopregnancy and pregnancy, and following ovariectomy. *Am J Anat* 1984;171:321–334.
60. Hewitt K, Beer AE, Grinnell F. Disappearance of anionic sites from the surface of the rat endometrial epithelium at the time of blastocyst implantation. *Biol Reprod* 1979;21:691–707.
61. Enders AC, Schlafke S, Welsh AO. Trophoblastic and uterine luminal epithelial surfaces at the time of blastocyst adhesion in the rat. *Am J Anat* 1980;159:59–72.
62. Chavez DJ, Anderson TL. The glycocalyx of the mouse uterine luminal epithelium during estrus, early pregnancy, the peri-implantation period and delayed implantation. I. Acquisition of *Ricinus communis* I binding sites during pregnancy. *Biol Reprod* 1985;32:1135–1142.
63. Chavez DJ. Possible involvement of D-galactose in the implantation process. In: Denker H, Aplin JD, eds. *Trophoblast Invasion and Endometrial Receptivity. Novel Aspects of the Cell Biology of Embryo Implantation. Trophoblast Res* 1990;4:259–272.
64. Anderson TL, Simon JA, Hodgen GD. Histochemical characteristics of the endometrial surface related temporally to implantation in the non-human primate (*Macaca fascicularis*). In: Kenker H, Aplin JD, eds. *Trophoblast Invasion and Endometrial Receptivity. Novel Aspects of the Cell Biology of Embryo Implantation. Trophoblast Res* 1990;4:273–284.
65. Lampelo SA, Ricketts AP, Bullock DW. Purification of rabbit endometrial plasma membranes from receptive and non-receptive uteri. *J Reprod Fertil* 1985;75:475–484.
66. Nalbach BP, Denker HW. Stage-dependent changes in lectins binding patterns of rabbit uterus and blastocysts during the preimplantation period and implantation. *Eur J Cell Biol* 1983;4(suppl):13.
67. Bukers A, Friedrich NJ, Nalbach BP, Denker HW. Changes in lectin binding patterns in rabbit endometrium during pseudopregnancy, early pregnancy and implantation. In: Denker H, Aplin JD, eds. *Trophoblast Invasion and Endometrial Receptivity. Novel Aspects of the Cell Biology of Embryo Implantation. Trophoblast Res* 1990;4:285–305.
68. Anderson TL, Olson GE, Hoffman LH. Stage-specific alterations in the apical membrane glycoproteins of endometrial epithelial cells related to implantation in rabbits. *Biol Reprod* 1986;34: 701–720.
69. Hoffman LH, Winfrey VP, Anderson TL, Olson GE. Uterine receptivity to implantation in the rabbit: evidence for a 42 kDa

glycoprotein as a marker of receptivity. In: Denker H, Aplin JD, eds. *Trophoblast Invasion and Endometrial Receptivity. Novel Aspects of the Cell Biology of Embryo Implantation. Trophoblast Res* 1990;4:243–258.

70. Enders AC, Schlafke S. Implantation in the ferret: epithelial penetration. *Am J Anat* 1972;133:291–316.
71. Dutt A, Tang J, Welply JK, Carson DD. Regulation of *N*-linked glycoprotein assembly in uteri by steroid hormones. *Endocrinology* 1986;118:661–673.
72. Carson DD, Dutt A, Tang JP. Glycoconjugate synthesis during early pregnancy: hyaluronate synthesis and function. *Dev Biol* 1987;120:228–235.
73. Nelson JD, Jato-Rodriguez JJ, Mookerjea S. Effect of ovarian hormones on glycosyltransferase activities in the endometrium of ovariectomized rats. *Arch Biochem Biophys* 1975;169:181–191.
74. Dutt A, Tang J, Carson DD. Lactosaminoglycans are involved in uterine epithelial cell adhesion *in vitro*. *Dev Biol* 1987;119:27–37.
75. Dutt A, Tang J, Carson DD. Estrogen preferentially stimulates lactosaminoglycan-containing oligosaccharide synthesis in mouse uteri. *J Biol Chem* 1988;263:2270–2279.
76. Dutt A, Carson DD. Lactosaminoglycan assembly, cell surface express, and release of mouse uterine epithelial cells. *J Biol Chem* 1990;265:430–438.
77. Barbiarz BS, Hathaway HJ. Hormonal control of the expression of antibody-defined lactosaminolglycans in the mouse uterus. *Biol Reprod* 1988;39:699–706.
78. Kimber SJ, Lindenberg S, Lundblad A. Distribution of some Galβ1-3(4) GlcNAc related carbohydrate antigens on the mouse uterine epithelium in relation to the peri-implantational period. *J Reprod Immunol* 1988;12:297–313.
79. Kimber SJ, Lindenberg S. Hormonal control of a carbohydrate epitope involved in implantation in mice. *J Reprod Fertil* 1990;89:13–21.
80. Munakata H, Isemura M, Yosizawa Z. Effects of female hormones on the activity of 3′-phosphoadenylylsulfate: desulphated heparan sulphate sulphotransferase in the endometrium of rabbit uterus. *Int J Biochem* 1985;17:1077–1083.
81. Tang J, Julian J, Glasser SR, Carson DD. Heparan sulfate proteoglycan synthesis and metabolism by mouse uterine epithelial cells cultured *in vitro*. *J Biol Chem* 1987;262:12832–12842.
82. Morris JE, Potter SW, Gaza-Bulseco G. Estradiol induces an accumulation of free heparan sulfate glycosaminoglycan chains in uterine epithelium. *Endocrinology* 1988;122:242–253.
83. Morris JE, Potter SW, Gaza-Bulseco G. Estradiol-stimulated turnover of heparan sulfate proteoglycan in mouse uterine epithelium. *J Biol Chem* 1988;263:4712–4718.
84. Wilson O, Jacobs AL, Stewart S, Carson DD. Expression of externally-disposed heparin/heparan sulfate binding sites by uterine epithelial cells. *J Cell Physiol* 1990;143:60–67.
85. Carson DD, Wilson OF, Dutt A. Glycoconjugate expression and interactions at the cell surface of mouse uterine epithelial cells and peri-implantation-stage embryos. In: Denker H, Aplin JD, eds. *Trophoblast Invasion and Endometrial Receptivity. Novel Aspects of the Cell Biology of Embryo Implantation. Trophoblast Res* 1990;4:211–241.
86. Fisher SJ, Sutherland A, Moss L, et al. Adhesive inveractions of murine and human trophoblast cells. In: Denker H, Aplin JD, eds. *Trophoblast Invasion and Endometrial Receptivity. Novel Aspects of the Cell Biology of Embryo Implantation. Trophoblast Res* 1990;4:115–137.
87. Denker HW. Trophoblast-endometrial interactions at embryo implantation: a cell biological paradox. In: Denker H, Aplin AJ, eds. *Trophoblast Invasion and Endometrial Receptivity. Novel Aspects of the Cell Biology of Embryo Implantation, Trophoblast Res* 1990;4:3–29.
88. Hakansson S, Sundkvist KG. Decreased antigenicity of mouse blastocysts after activation for implantation from experimental delay. *Transplantation* 1975;19:479–484.
89. Hakansson S, Heyner S, Sundkvist KG, Bergstrom S. The presence of paternal H-2 antigens on hybrid mouse blastocysts during experimental delay of implantation and the disappearance of these antigens after onset of implantation. *Int J Fertil* 1975;20:137–140.
90. Nilsson O, Lindqvist I, Ronquist G. Decreased surface charge of mouse blastocysts at implantation. *Exp Cell Res* 1973;83:421–423.
91. Nilsson O, Lindqvist I, Ronquist G. Blastocyst surface charge and implantation in the mouse. *Contraception* 1975;11:441–450.
92. Jenkinson EJ, Searle RF. Cell surface changes on the mouse blastocyst at implantation. *Exp Cell Res* 1977;106:386–390.
93. Clemetson CAB, Moshfeghi MM, Mallikarjuneswara VR. Electrophoretic mobility of the rat blastocyst. *Contraception* 1970;1:357–360.
94. Nilsson BO, Hjerten S. Electrophoretic quantification of the changes in the average net negative charge density of mouse blastocysts implanting *in vivo* and *in vitro*. *Biol Reprod* 1982;27:485–493.
95. Enders AC, Schlafke S. Penetration of the uterine epithelium during implantation in the rabbit. *Am J Anat* 1971;132:219–240.
96. Bergstrom S, Nilsson O. Blastocyst attachment and early invasion during oestradiol-induced implantation in the mouse. *Anat Embryol* 1976;149:149–154.
97. Konwinski M, Vorbrodt A, Solter D, Koprowski H. Ultrastructural study of concanavalin-A binding to the surface of preimplantation mouse embryos. *J Exp Zool* 1977;200:311–324.
98. Chavez DJ, Enders AC. Temporal changes in lectin binding of peri-implantation mouse blastocysts. *Dev Biol* 1981;87:267–276.
99. Chavez DJ. Cell surface of mouse blastocysts at the trophectoderm-utrine interface during the adhesive stage of implantation. *Am J Anat* 1986;176:153–158.
100. Chavez DJ, Enders AC. Lectin binding of mouse blastocysts: appearance of dolichos biflorus binding sites on the trophoblast during delayed implantation and their subsequent disappearance during implantation. *Biol Reprod* 1982;26:545–552.
101. Sobel JS, Nebel L. Concanavalin A agglutinability of the developing mouse trophoblast. *J Reprod Fertil* 1976;47:399–402.
102. Sobel JS, Nebel L. Changes in concanavalin A agglutinability during development of the inner cell mass and trophoblast of mouse blastocysts *in vitro*. *J Reprod Fertil* 1978;52:239–248.
103. Nilsson BO, Naeslund G, Curman B. Polar differences of delayed and implanting mouse blastocysts in binding of alcian blue and concanavalin A. *J Exp Zool* 1980;214:177–180.
104. Carollo JR, Weitlauf HM. Regional changes in the binding of [^{3}H] concanavalin A to mouse blastocysts at implantation: an autoradiographic study. *J Exp Zool* 1981;218:247–251.
105. Wu JT, Chang MC. Increase in concanavalin A binding sites in mouse blastocysts during implantation. *J Exp Zool* 1978;105:447–453.
106. Pinsker MC, Mintz B. Change in cell-surface glycoproteins of mouse embryos before implantation. *Proc Natl Acad Sci USA* 1973;70:1645–1648.
107. Surani MAH. Glycoprotein synthesis and inhibition of glycosylation by tunicamycin in pre-implantation mouse embryos: compaction and trophoblast adhesion. *Cell* 1979;18:217–227.
108. Leivo I. Structure and composition of early basement membranes: studies with early embryos and teratocarcinoma cells. *Med Biol* 1983;61:1–30.
109. Dziadek M, Timpl R. Expression of nidogen and laminin in basement membranes during mouse embryogenesis and teratocarcinoma cells. *Dev Biol* 1985;111:372–382.
110. Leivo I, Vaheri A, Timpl R, Wartiovaara J. Appearance and distribution of collagens and laminin in the early mouse embryo. *Dev Biol* 1980;76:100–114.
111. Wu T, Wan Y, Chung AE, Damjanov I. Immunohistochemical localization of entactin and laminin in mouse embryos and fetuses. *Dev Biol* 1983;100:496–505.
112. Sherman MI, Shalgi R, Rizzino A, Sellens MH, Gay S, Gay R. Changes in the surface of the mouse blastocyst at implantation. In: *Maternal Recognition of Pregnancy*. CIBA Foundation Symposium No. 64 (new series). New York: Excerpta Medica, 1979;33–52.
113. Wartiovaara J, Levivo L, Vaheri A. Expression of the cell surface-associated glycoprotein, fibronectin, in the early mouse embryo. *Dev Biol* 1979;69:247–257.
114. Adamson ED, Ayers SE. The localization and synthesis of some collagen types in developing mouse embryos. *Cell* 1979;16:953–965.
115. Sherman MI, Gay R, Gay S, Miller EJ. Association of collagen

with preimplantation and peri-implantation mouse embryos. *Dev Biol* 1980;74:470–478.
116. Zetter BR, Martin GR. Expression of a high molecular weight cell surface glycoprotein (LETS protein) by preimplantation mouse embryos and teratocarcinoma cells. *Proc Natl Acad Sci USA* 1978;75:2324–2328.
117. Richa J, Damsky CH, Buck CA, Knowles BB, Solter D. Cell surface glycoproteins mediate compaction, trophoblast attachment, and endoderm formation during early mouse development. *Dev Biol* 1985;108:513–321.
118. Damjanov I, Damjanov A, Damsky CH. Developmentally regulated expression of the cell–cell adhesion glycoprotein cell-CAM 120-80 in peri-implantation mouse embryos and extraembryonic membranes. *Dev Biol* 1986;116:194–202.
119. Vestweber D, Gossler A, Boller K, Kemler R. Expression and distribution of cell adhesion molecule uvomorulin in mouse preimplantation embryos. *Dev Biol* 1987;124:451–456.
120. Vestweber D, Kemler R. Rabbit antiserum against a purified surface glycoprotein decompacts mouse preimplantation embryos and reacts with specific adult tissues. *Exp Cell Res* 1984;152: 169–178.
121. Yoshida-Noro C, Suzuki N, Takeichi M. Molecular nature of the calcium-dependent cell–cell adhesion system in mouse teratorcarcinoma and embryonic cells studied with a monoclonal antibody. *Dev Biol* 1984;101:19–27.
122. Hyafil F, Morello D, Babinet C, Jacob F. A cell surface glycoprotein involved in the compaction of embryonal carcinoma cells and cleavage stage embryos. *Cell* 1980;21:927–934.
123. Ducibella T. Divalent antibodies to mouse embryonal carcinoma cells inhibit compaction in the mouse embryo. *Dev Biol* 1980;79:356–366.
124. Sato M, Muramatsu T. Oncodevelopment carbohydrate antigens: distribution of ECMA 2 and 3 antigens in embryonic and adult tissues of the mouse and in teratocarcinomas. *J Reprod Immunol* 1986;9:123–135.
125. Bird JM, Kimber SJ. Oligosaccharides containing fucose linked α(1-3) and α(1-4) to *N*-acetylglucosamine cause decompaction of mouse morulae. *Dev Biol* 1984;104:449–460.
126. Svalander PC, Odin P, Nilsson BO, Obrink B. Trophectoderm surface expression of the cell adhesion molecule cell-CAM 105 on rat blastocysts. *Development* 1987;100:653–660.
127. Shur BD. The receptor function of galactosyltransferase during cellular interactions. *Mol Cell Biochem* 1984;61:143–158.
128. Martricorena P, Hogan B, DiMeo A, Artzt K, Bennett D. Carbohydrate changes in pre- and peri-implantation mouse embryos as detected by a monoclonal antibody. *Cell Differentiation* 1983;12:1–10.
129. Babiarz BS, Hathaway HJ. Immunofluorescent localization of a monoclonally defined cell surface antigen, (IIC3) during mouse development. *Exp Cell Res* 1986;163:221–232.
130. Hathaway HJ, Babiarz BS. Developmental regulation of the monoclonally defined IIC3 antigen during primary and secondary trophoblast differentiation *in vitro*. *Cell Differentiation* 1988;24:55–66.
131. Bayna EM, Shaper JH, Shur BD. Temporally specific involvement of cell surface β-1,4 galactosyltransferase during mouse embryo morula compaction. *Cell* 1988;53:145–157.
132. Sato M, Muramatsu T, Berger EG. Immunological detection of cell surface galactosyltransferase in preimplantation mouse embryos. *Dev Biol* 1984;102:514–518.
133. Hjortberg M, Nilsson BO. Appearance, shedding and endocytosis of a blastocyst surface galactose-galacotsamine derivative detected with a monoclonal antibody. In: Denker H, Aplin JD, eds. *Trophoblast Invasion and Endometrial Receptivity. Novel Aspects of the Cell Biology of Embryo Implantation. Trophoblast Res* 1990;4:179–189.
134. Svalander PC, Hjortberg M, Gronvik K-O, Nilsson BO. Mouse blastocyst surface expression of galactose-containing epitopes coinciding with trophoblast differentiation. *Cell Differ Dev* 1989;21:191–200.
135. Dziadek M, Fujiwara S, Paulsson M, Timpl R. Immunological characterization of basement membrane types of heparan sulfate proteoglycan. *EMBO J* 1985;4:905–912.
136. Sutherland AE, Sanderson RD, Mayes M, et al. Expression of syndecan, a putative low affinity fibroblast growth factor receptor, in the early mouse embryo. *Development* 1991;113:339–351.
137. Weitlauf HM, Knisley KA. Changes in surface antigens on preimplantation mouse embryos. *Biol Reprod* 1992;46:811–816.
138. Poirier F, Timmons PM, Chan C-TJ, Guenet J-L, Rigby PWJ. Expression of the L14 lectin during mouse embryogenesis suggests multiple roles during pre- and post-implantation development. *Development* 1992;115:143–155.
139. Farach MC, Tang JP, Decker GL, Carson DD. Differential effects of *P*-nitrophenyl-D-xylosides on mouse blastocysts and uterine epithelial cells. *Biol Reprod* 1988;39:443–455.
140. Lindenberg S, Sundenberg K, Kimber SJ, Lundblad A. The milk oligosaccharide, lacto-*N*-fucopentaose I, inhibits attachment of mouse blastocysts on endometrial monolayers. *J Reprod Fertil* 1988;83:149–158.
141. Damsky CH, Richa J, Solter D, Knudsen K, Buck CA. Identification and purification of a cell surface glycoprotein mediating intercellular adhesion in embryonic and adult tissue. *Cell* 1983;34:455–466.
142. Armant DR, Kaplan HA, Lennarz WJ. Fibronectin and laminin promote *in vitro* attachment and outgrowth of mouse blastocysts. *Dev Biol* 1986;116:519–523.
143. Armant DR, Kaplan HA, Mover H, Lennarz WJ. The effect of hexapeptides on attachment and outgrowth of mouse blastocysts cultured *in vitro:* evidence for the involvement of the cell recognition tripeptide arg-gly-asp. *Proc Natl Acad Sci* 1986;83: 6751–6755.
144. Farach MC, Tang JP, Decker GL, Carson DD. Heparin/heparan sulfate is involved in attachment and spreading of mouse embryos *in vitro*. *Dev Biol* 1987;123:401–410.
145. Carson DD, Tang J, Gay S. Collagens support embryo attachment and outgrowth *in vitro:* effects of the arg-gly-asp sequence. *Dev Biol* 1988;127:368–375.
146. Sutherland AE, Calarco PG, Damsky CH. Expression and function of cell surface extracellular matrix receptors in mouse blastocyst attachment and outgrowth. *J Cell Biol* 1988;106:1331–1348.
147. Gulamhusein AP, Beck F. Light and electron microscopic observations at the pre- and early post-implantation stages in the ferret uterus. *J Anat* 1973;115:159–174.
148. Enders AC, Schlafke S. The fine structure of the blastocyst: some comparative studies. In: Wolstenholme GEW, O'Connor M, eds. *Preimplantation Stages of Pregnancy*. CIBA Foundation Symposium. Boston: Little, Brown, 1965;29–59.
149. Parr EL. Shedding of the zona pellucida by guinea pig blastocysts: an ultrastructural study. *Biol Reprod* 1973;8:531–544.
150. Allen WR, Hamilton DW, Moor RM. The origin of equine endometrial cups. II. Invasion of the endometrium by trophoblast. *Anat Rec* 1973;177:485–502.
151. Finn CA, Lawn AM. Transfer of cellular material between the uterine epithelium and trophoblast during the early stages of implantation. *J Reprod Fertil* 1968;15:333–336.
152. Wilson IB. A new factor associated with the implantation of the mouse egg. *J Reprod Fertil* 1963;5:281–282.
153. Enders AC, Schlafke S. Comparative aspects of blastocyst–endometrial interactions at implantation. In: Whelan J, ed. *Maternal Recognition of Pregnancy*. CIBA Foundation Symposium No. 64 (new series). New York: Excerpta Medica, 1979;3–32.
154. Finn CA, Hinchliffe JR. Histological and histochemical analysis of the formation of implantation chambers in the mouse uterus. *J Reprod Fertil* 1965;9:301–309.
155. Finn CA, Hinchliffe JR. Reaction of the mouse uterus during implantation and deciduoma formation as demonstrated by changes in the distribution of alkaline phosphatase. *J Reprod Fertil* 1964;8:331–338.
156. Hinchliffe JR, El-Shershaby AM. Epithelial cell death in the oil-induced decidual reaction of the pseudopregnant mouse: an ultrastructural study. *J Reprod Fertil* 1975;45:463–468.
157. El-Shershaby AM, Hinchliffe JR. Epithelial autolysis during implantation of the mouse blastocyst: an ultrastructural study. *J Embryol Exp Morphol* 1975;33:1067–1080.
158. Finn CA, Bredl JCS. Studies on the development of the implantation reaction in the mouse uterus: influence of actinomycin D. *J Reprod Fertil* 1973;34:247–253.
159. Moulton BC, Elangovan S. Lysosomal mechanisms in blastocyst

implantation and early decidualization. In: Glasser SR, Bullock DW, eds. *Cellular and Molecular Aspects of Implantation.* New York: Plenum Press, 1981;335–344.
160. Roy SK, Sengupta J, Manchanda SK. Histochemical study of β-glucuronidase in the rat uterus during implantation and pseudopregnancy. *J Reprod Fertil* 1983;68:161–164.
161. Sengupta J, Paria BC, Manchanda SK. Effect of an oestrogen antagonist on implantation and uterine leucylnaphthylamidase activity in the ovariectomized hamster. *J Reprod Fertil* 1981;62:437–440.
162. Van Hoorn G, Denker HW. Effect of the blastocyst on a uterine amino acide arylamidase in the rabbit. *J Reprod Fertil* 1975;45:359–362.
163. Boshier DP. Effects of the rat blastocyst on neutral lipids and nonspecific esterases in the uterine luminal epithelium at the implantation site. *J Reprod Fertil* 1976;46:245–247.
164. Moulton BC. Ovum implantation and uterine lysosomal enzyme activity. *Biol Reprod* 1974;10:543–548.
165. Finn CA. Cellular changes in the uterus during the establishment of pregnancy in rodents. *J Reprod Fertil* 1982;31(suppl): 105–111.
166. Cowell TP. Implantation and development of the mouse eggs transferred to the uteri of non-progestational mice. *J Reprod Fertil* 1969;19:239–245.
167. Steer HW. The trophoblastic knobs of the preimplanted rabbit blastocyst: a light and electron microscopic study. *J Anat* 1970;107:315–325.
168. Steer HW. Implantation of the rabbit blastocyst: the invasive phase. *J Anat* 1971;110:445–462.
169. Larsen JF. Electron microscopy of the implantation site in the rabbit. *Am J Anat* 1961;109:319–334.
170. Psychoyos A. La réaction déciduale est precédée de modifications précoces de la perméabilité capillarie de l'uterus. *C R Soc Biol* 1960;154:1384–1387.
171. Psychoyos A. Perméabilité capillarie et décidualisation utérine. *C R Acad Sci (Paris)* 1961;252:1515–1517.
172. McLaren A. Can mouse blastocysts stimulate a uterine response before losing the zona pellucida? *J Reprod Fertil* 1969;19: 199–201.
173. Loeb L. Wounds of the pregnant uterus. *Proc Soc Exp Biol Med* 1907;4:93–96.
174. Loeb L. The production of decidoumata and the relation between the ovaries and formation of the decidua. *JAMA* 1908;50: 1897–1901.
175. Loeb L. The experimental production of the maternal part of the placenta of the rabbit. *Proc Soc Exp Biol Med* 1908;5:102–105.
176. Deanesly R. The differentiation of the decidua at ovo-implantation in the guinea-pig contrasted with that of the traumatic deciduoma. *J Reprod Fertil* 1971;26:91–97.
177. Lundkvist O, Nilsson BO. Endometrial ultrastructure in the early uterine response to blastocysts and artificial deciduogenic stimuli in rats. *Cell Tissue Res* 1982;225:355–364.
178. Welch AO, Enders AC. Light and electron microscopic examination of the mature decidual cells of the rat with emphasis on the antimesometrial decidua and its degeneration. *Am J Anat* 1985;172:1–29.
179. DeFeo VJ. Decidualization. In: Wynn RM, ed. *Cellular Biology of the Uterus.* New York: Appleton-Century-Crofts, 1967;191–290.
180. Long JA, Evans HM. The oestrus cycle in the rat and its associated phenomena. *Mem Univ Calif* 1922;6:1–148.
181. Parkes AS. The functions of the corpus luteum. II. The experimental production of placentoma in the mouse. *Proc R Soc Lond (Biol)* 1929;104:183–188.
182. Kraicer PF, Shelesnyak MC. Détermination de la période de sensibilité maximale de l'endomètre a la décidualisation au moyen de déciduomes provoqués par un traitement empruntant la voie vasculaire. *C R Acad Sci (Paris)* 1959;248:3213–3215.
183. Shelesnyak MC, Kracier PF. Time-limits of uterine sensitivity to decidualization during progestation. *Proc 1st Int Congr Endocrinol (Copenh)* 1960.
184. DeFeo VJ. Determination of the sensitive period for the induction of deciduomata in the rat by different inducing procedures. *Endocrinology* 1963;73:488–497.
185. DeFeo VJ. Temporal aspect of uterine sensitivity in the pseudopregnant or pregnant rat. *Endocrinology* 1963;72:305–316.
186. Hetherington CM. The development of deciduomata induced by two nontraumatic methods in the mouse. *J Reprod Fertil* 1968;17:391–393.
187. Harper MJK. Deciduomal response of the golden hamster uterus. *Anat Rec* 1969;163:563–574.
188. Finn CA, Martin L. Endocrine control of the timing of endometrial sensitivity to a decidual stimulus. *Biol Reprod* 1972;7:82–96.
189. McLaren A, Michie D. Studies on the transfer of fertilized mouse eggs to uterine foster-mothers. I. Factors affecting the implantation and survival of native and transferred eggs. *J Exp Biol* 1956;33:394–416.
190. Psychoyos A. Control de la nidation chez les mammiferes. *Arch Anat Microsc Morphol Exp* 1965;54:85–104.
191. Psychoyos A. Etude des relations de l'oeuf et de l'endometre au cours du retard de la nidation ou des premieres phases du processes de la nidation chez la ratte. *C R Acad Sci Paris Ser D* 1966;263:1755–1758.
192. Psychoyos A. Recent researches of egg-implantation. In: Wolstenholme GEW, O'Connor M, eds. *Egg Implantation.* CIBA Foundation Study Group 23. London: Churchill, 1966;4–28.
193. Psychoyos A. Hormonal factors governing decidualization. *Excerpta Med Found Int Congr Serv* 1969;184:935–938.
194. Psychoyos A. Hormonal requirements for egg implantation. In: Raspe G, ed. *Advances in BioSciences. IV. Mechanisms Involved in Conception.* London: Pergamon Press, 1969;275–290.
195. Noyes RW, Dickmann Z. Relationship of ovular age to endometrial development. *J Reprod Fertil* 1960;1:186–196.
196. Dickmann Z, Noyes RW. The fate of ova transferred into the uterus of the rat. *J Reprod Fertil* 1960;1:197–212.
197. Psychoyos A. The hormonal interplay controlling egg-implantation in the rat. In: McLaren A, ed. *Advances in Reproductive Physiology.* London: Logos Press, 1967;257:277.
198. Humphrey KW. The induction of implantation in the mouse after ovariectomy. *Steroids* 1967;10:591–600.
199. Shelesnyak MC. Decidualization: the decidua and the deciduoma. *Perspect Biol Med* 1962;5:503–518.
200. Finn CA, Martin J. Patterns of cell division in the mouse uterus during early pregnancy. *J Endocrinol* 1967;39:593–597.
201. Zhinkin LN, Samoshkina NA. DNA synthesis and cell proliferation during formation of deciduomata in mice. *J Embryol Exp Morphol* 1967;17:593–605.
202. Hall K. Uterine mitosis, alkaline phosphatase and adenosine triphosphatase during development and regression of deciduomata in pseudopregnant mice. *J Endocrinol* 1969;44:91–100.
203. Leroy F, Galand P, Chretien J. The mitogenic action of ovarian hormones on the uterine and vaginal epithelium during the oestrus cycle in the rat: an autoradiographic study. *J Endocrinol* 1969;45:441–447.
204. Chaudhury RR, Sethi A. Effects of an intra-uterine contraceptive device on mitosis in the rat uterus on different days of pregnancy. *J Reprod Fertil* 1970;22:33–40.
205. Marcus GJ. Mitosis in the rat uterus during the estrous cycle, early pregnancy and early pseudopregnancy. *Biol Reprod* 1974;10:447–452.
206. Tachi C, Tachi S, Lindner HR. Modification by progesterone of oestradiol-induced cell proliferation, RNA synthesis and oestradiol distribution in the rat uterus. *J Reprod Fertil* 1972;31:59–76.
207. Mehrotra SN, Finn CA. Cell proliferation in the uterus of the guinea-pig. *J Reprod Fertil* 1974;37:405–409.
208. Marcus GJ. Hormonal control of proliferation in the guinea-pig uterus. *J Endocrinol* 1974;63:89–97.
209. Schmidt IG. Proliferation in the genital tract of the normal mature guinea pig treated with colchicine. *Am J Anat* 143;73:59–80.
210. Krueger WA, Maibenco HC. DNA replication and cell division in the hamster uterus. *Anat Rec* 1972;173:229–234.
211. Herken R. Cell kinetics of early gestation mouse uterus. *Cell Tissue Kinet* 1983;16:419–428.
212. Galassi L. Autoradiographic study of the decidual cell reaction in the rat. *Dev Biol* 1968;17:75–84.
213. Leroy F, Galand P. Radioautographic evaluation of mitotic parameters in the endometrium during the uterine sensitivity period in pseudopregnant rat. *Fertil Steril* 1969;20:980–922.

214. O'Grady JE, Heald PJ. Uterine nucleic acid and phospholipid metabolism in the early stages of rat pregnancy. *J Endocrinol* 1976;68:33P–34P.
215. Lobel BL, Levy E, Shelesnyak MC. Studies on the mechanism of nidation. XXXIV. Dynamics of cellular interactions during progestation and implantation in the rat. *Acta Endocrinol* 1967;123(suppl):7–109.
216. Clark BF. The effect of oestrogen and progesterone on uterine cell division and epithelial morphology in spayed-hypophysectomized rats. *J Endocrinol* 1973;56:341–342.
217. Allen E, Smith GM, Gardner WU. Accentuation of the growth effect of Theelin on genital tissues of the ovariectomized mouse by arrest of mitosis with colchicine. *Am J Anat* 1937;61:321–341.
218. Perrotta CA. Initiation of cell proliferation in the vaginal and uterine epithelia of the mouse. *Am J Anat* 1962;111:195–204.
219. Epifanova OI. Mitotic cycles in estrogen-treated mice: an autoradiographic study. *Exp Cell Res* 1966;42:562–577.
220. Martin L, Finn CA. Hormonal regulation of cell division in epithelial and connective tissues of the mouse uterus. *J Endocrinol* 1968;41:363–371.
221. Finn CA, Martin L. Endocrine control of gland proliferation in the mouse uterus. *Biol Reprod* 1973;8:585–588.
222. Martin L, Finn CA, Trinder G. Hypertrophy and hyperplasia in the mouse uterus after oestrogen treatment: an autoradiographic study. *J Endocrinol* 1973;56:133–144.
223. Clark BF. The effects of oestrogen and progesterone on uterine cell division and epithelial morphology in spayed adrenalectomized rats. *J Endocrinol* 1971;50:527–528.
224. Lee A, Dukelow WR. Synthesis of DNA and mitosis in rabbit uteri after oestrogen and progesterone injections and during early pregnancy. *J Reprod Fertil* 1972;31:473–476.
225. Koeski Y, Fujimoto GI. Progesterone effects contrasted with 17-β estradiol on DNA synthesis in epithelial nuclear proliferation in the castrate rabbit uterus. *Biol Reprod* 1974;10:596–604.
226. Nilsson O. Ultrastructure of mouse uterine surface epithelium under different estrogenic influences. 1. Spayed animals and oestrus animals. *J Ultrastruct Res* 1958;1:375–396.
227. Nilsson O. Ultrastructure of mouse uterine surface epithelium under different estrogenic influences. 3. Late effect of estrogen administered to spayed animals. *J Ultrastruct Res* 1958;2:185–199.
228. Nilsson O. Ultrastructure of mouse uterine surface epithelium under different estrogenic influences. 2. Early effect of estrogen administered to spayed animals. *J Ultrastruct Res* 1958;2:73–95.
229. Das RM. The effects of oestrogen on the cell cycle in epithelial and connective tissues of the mouse uterus. *J Endocrinol* 1972;55:21–30.
230. Das RM. The time-course of the mitotic response to oestrogen in the epithelium and stroma of the mouse uterus. *J Endocrinol* 1972;55:203–204.
231. Martin L, Das RM, Finn CA. The inhibition by progesterone of uterine epithelial proliferation in the mouse. *J Endocrinol* 1973;57:549–554.
232. Das RM, Martin L. Progesterone inhibition of mouse uterine epithelial proliferation. *J Endocrinol* 1973;59:205–206.
233. Martin L, Finn CA. Duration of progesterone treatment required for a stromal response to oestradiol-17β in the uterus of the mouse. *J Endocrinol* 1969;44:279–280.
234. Finn CA, Martin L. The role of the oestrogen secreted before oestrus in the preparation of the uterus for implantation in the mouse. *J Endocrinol* 1970;47:431–438.
235. Finn CA, Martin L. The control of implantation. *J Reprod Fertil* 1974;39:195–206.
236. Finn CA, Martin L, Carter J. A refractory period following oestrogenic stimulation of cell division in the mouse uterus. *J Endocrinol* 1969;44:121–126.
237. Talley DJ, Tobert JA, Armstrong EG Jr, Villee CA. Changes in estrogen receptor levels during deciduomata development in the pseudopregnant rat. *Endocrinology* 1977;101:1538–1544.
238. Armstrong EG Jr, Tobert JA, Talley DJ, Villee CA. Changes in progesterone receptor levels during deciduomata development in the pseudopregnant rat. *Endocrinology* 1977;101:1545–1551.
239. Logeat F, Sartor P, Vu Hai MT, Milgrom E. Local effect of the blastocyst on estrogen and progesterone receptors in the rat endometrium. *Science* 1980;207:1083–1085.
240. Vu Hai MT, Logeat F, Milgrom E. Progesterone receptors in the rat uterus: variations in cytosol and nuclei during the oestrous cycle and pregnancy. *J Endocrinol* 1978;76:43–48.
241. Martel D, Psychoyos A. Progesterone-induced oestrogen receptors in the rat uterus. *J Endocrinol* 1978;76:145–154.
242. Clark JH, Markaverich B, Upchurch S, Eriksson H, Hardin JW, Peck EJ. Heterogeneity of estrogen binding sites: relationship to estrogen receptors and estrogen response. *Recent Prog Horm Res* 1980;36:89–134.
243. Do YS, Leavitt WW. Characterization of a specific progesterone receptor in decidualized hamster uterus. *Endocrinology* 1978; 102:443–451.
244. Martel D, Psychoyos A. Behavior of uterine steroid receptors at implantation. In: Leroy F, Finn CA, Psychoyos A, Hubinont PO, eds. *Progress in Reproductive Biology,* Vol 7. New York: Karger, 1980;216–233.
245. Nilsson O. Ultrastructure of mouse uterine surface epithelium under different estrogenic influences. 4. Uterine secretion. *J Ultrastruct Res* 1959;2:331–341.
246. Nilsson BO. Changes of the luminal surface of the rat uterus at blastocyst implantation: scanning electron microscopy and ruthenium red staining. *Z Anat Entwick* 1974;144:337–342.
247. Alden RH. Implantation of the rat egg. II. Alterations in osmiophilic epithelial lipids of the rat uterus under normal and experimental conditions. *Anat Rec* 1947;97:1–19.
248. Elftman H. Estrogen control of the phospholipids of the uterus. *Endocrinology* 1958;62:410–415.
249. Elftman H. Estrogen induced changes in the Golgi apparatus and lipid of the uterine epithelium of the rat in the normal cycle. *Anat Rec* 1963;146:139–143.
250. Fuxe K, Nilsson O. The effect of oestrogen on the histology of the uterine epithelium of the mouse. *Exp Cell Res* 1963;32:109–117.
251. Boshier DP, Holloway H. Effects of ovarian steroid hormones on histochemically demonstrable lipids in the rat uterine epithelium. *J Endocrinol* 1973;65:59–67.
252. Hall K. Lactic dehydrogenase and other enzymes in the mouse uterus during the peri-implantation period of pregnancy. *J Reprod Fertil* 1973;34:79–91.
253. Hall K. Lipids in the mouse uterus during early pregnancy. *J Endocrinol* 1975;65:233–243.
254. Enders AC. Comparative studies on the endometrium of delayed implantation. *Anat Rec* 1961;139:483–497.
255. Smith MSR, Wilson IB. Histochemical observations on early implantation in the mouse. *J Embryol Exp Morphol* 1971;25: 165–174.
256. Wood C, Psychoyos A. Activité de certaines enzymes hydrolytiques dans l'endomètre au cours de la pseudogestation et de divers états de réceptivité utérine chez la ratte. *C R Acad Sci Paris Ser D* 1967;265:141–144.
257. Bergstrom S. Delay of blastocyst implantation in the mouse by ovariectomy or lactation. A scanning electron microscope study. *Fertil Steril* 1972;23:548–561.
258. Bergstrom S, Nilsson O. Ultrastructural response of blastocysts and uterine epithelium to progesterone deprivation during delayed implantation in mice. *J Endocrinol* 1972;55:217–218.
259. Christie GA. Implantation of the rat embryo: glycogen and alkaline phosphatases. *J Reprod Fertil* 1966;12:279–294.
260. Abraham R, Hendy R, Dougherty WJ, Fulfs JC, Golberg L. Participation of lysosomes in early implantation in the rabbit. *Exp Mol Pathol* 1970;13:329–345.
261. Elangovan S, Moulton BC. Blastocyst implantation in the rat and the immunohistochemical distribution and rate of synthesis of uterine lysosomal cathespin D. *Biol Reprod* 1980;23:663–668.
262. Moulton BC, Ingle CB. Uterine lysosomal cathespin D activity, rate of synthesis and immunohistochemical localization following initiation of decidualization in pseudopregnant rats. *Biol Reprod* 1981;25:393–398.
263. Moulton BC. Progesterone and estrogen control of the response of rat uterine lysosomal cathespin D activity to a deciduogenic stimulus. *Endocrinology* 1982;110:1197–1202.
264. Finn CA, Martin L. Endocrine control of the proliferation and

secretion of uterine glands in the mouse. *Acta Endocrinol* 1971;155(suppl):139.
265. Enders AC, Given RL. The endometrium of delayed and early implantation. In: Wynn RM, ed. *Biology of the Uterus.* New York: Plenum Press, 1977;203–243.
266. Given RL, Enders AC. Mouse uterine glands during the peri-implantation period: fine structure. *Am J Anat* 1980;157: 169–179.
267. Given RL, Enders AC. Mouse uterine glands during the delayed and induced implantation periods. *Anat Rec* 1978;190:271–284.
268. Hooker CW, Forbes TR. A bio-assay for minute amounts of progesterone. *Endocrinology* 1947;41:158–169.
269. Tachi C, Tachi S, Lindner HR. Effects of ovarian hormones upon nucleolar ultrastructure in endometrial stromal cells of the rat. *Am J Anat* 1974;10:404–413.
270. Fainstat T. Extracellular studies of uterus. I. Disappearance of the discrete collagen bundles in endometrial stroma during various reproductive states in the rat. *Am J Anat* 1963;112:337–370.
271. Miller BG, Emmens CW. The effects of oestradiol and progesterone on the incorporation of tritiated uridine into the genital tract of the mouse. *J Endocrinol* 1969;43:427–436.
272. Miller BG, Owen WH, Emmens CW. The incorporation of tritiated uridine in the uterus and vagina of the mouse during early pregnancy. *J Endocrinol* 1968;41:189–195.
273. Miller BG, Owen WH, Emmens CW. Uridine incorporation in the rat genital tract during early pregnancy. *J Endocrinol* 1968;42:351–352.
274. Heald PJ, O'Grady JE. The uptake of [^{3}H] uridine into the nucleic acids of the rat uterus during early pregnancy. *Biochem J* 1970;117:65–71.
275. O'Grady JE, Heald PJ, O'Hare A. Incorporation of [^{3}H] uridine into the ribonucleic acid of rat uterus during pseudopregnancy and in the present of I.C.I. 46474 [*trans*-1-(*p*-β-dimethylaminoethoxyphenyl)-1,2-diphenylbut-1-ene]. *Biochem J* 1970;119:609–613.
276. Heald PJ, O'Grady JE, O'Hare A, Vass M. Changes in uterine RNA during early pregnancy in the rat. *Biochim Biophys Acta* 1972;262:66–74.
277. Heald PJ, O'Grady JE, Moffat GE. The incorporation of [^{3}H] uridine into nuclear RNA in the uterus of the rat during early pregnancy. *Biochim Biophys Acta* 1972;281:347–352.
278. O'Grady JE, Moffat GE, McMinn L, Vass MA, O'Hare A, Heald PJ. Uterine chromatin template activity during the early stages of pregnancy in the rat. *Biochim Biophys Acta* 1975;407:125–132.
279. Heald PJ, O'Grady JE, O'Hare A, Vass M. Nucleic acid metabolism of cells of the luminal epithelium and stroma of the rat uterus during early pregnancy. *J Reprod Fertil* 1975;45:129–138.
280. Kaye AM, Icekson I, Lindner HR. Stimulation by estrogens of ornitinine and *S*-adenosylmethionine decarboxylases in the immature rat uterus. *Biochim Biophys Acta* 1971;252:150–159.
281. Saunderson R, Heald PJ. Ornithine decarboxylase activity in the uterus of the rat during early pregnancy. *J Reprod Fertil* 1974;39:141–143.
282. Heald PJ. Changes in ornithine decarboxylase during early implantation in the rat. *Biol Reprod* 1979;20:1195–1199.
283. Reid RJ, Heald PJ. Uptake of ^{3}H-leucine into proteins of rat uterus during early pregnancy. *Biochim Biophys Acta* 1970;204: 278–279.
284. Reid RJ, Heald PJ. Protein metabolism of the rat uterus during the oestrous cycle, pregnancy and pseudopregnancy and as affected by an anti-implantation compound, ICI 46,474. *J Reprod Fertil* 1971;27:73–82.
285. Smith JA, Martin L, King RJB, Vertes M. Effects of oestradiol-17β and progesterone on total and nuclear-protein synthesis in epithelial and stromal tissues of the mouse uterus and of progesterone on the ability of these tissues to bind oestradiol-17β. *Biochem J* 1970;119:773–784.
286. Bell SC, Reynolds S, Heald PJ. Presumptive induced protein synthesis in the rat uterus during early pregnancy. *J Endocrinol* 1976;68:34p–35p.
287. Bell SC, Reynolds S, Heald PJ. Uterine protein synthesis during the early stages of pregnancy in the rat. *J Reprod Fertil* 1977;49:177–181.
288. Beall JR. Uterine lipid metabolism—a review of the literature. *Comp Biochem Physiol* [B] 1972;42:175–195.
289. Goswami A, Kar AB, Chowdhury SR. Uterine lipid metabolism in mice during the oestrous cycle: effect of ovariectomy and replacement therapy. *J Reprod Fertil* 1963;6:287–295.
290. Aizawa Y, Mueller GC. The effect *in vivo* and *in vitro* of estrogens on lipid synthesis in the rat uterus. *J Biol Chem* 1961;236: 381–386.
291. Davis JS, Alden RH. Hormonal influence on lipid metabolism of rat uterus. *Anat Rec* 1959;134:725–737.
292. Ray SC, Morin RJ. Lipid composition of the non-gravid and gravid rabbit endometrium. *Proc Soc Exp Biol Med* 1965;120: 849–853.
293. Morin RJ, Carrion M. *In vitro* incorporation of acetate-1-^{4}C into the phospholipids of rabbit and human endometria. *Lipids* 1968;3:349–353.
294. Beall JR, Werthessen NT. Lipid metabolism of the rat uterus after mating. *J Endocrinol* 1971;51:637–644.
295. Yochim JM. Intrauterine oxygen tension during the preimplantation period. In: Blandau RJ, ed. *Biology of the Blastocyst.* Chicago: University of Chicago Press, 1971;363–382.
296. Battellino LJ, Sabulsky J, Blanco A. Lactate dehydrogenase isoenzymes in rat uterus: changes during pregnancy. *J Reprod Fertil* 1971;25:393–399.
297. Clark SW, Yochim JM. Effect of ovarian steroids on lactic dehydrogenase activity in endometrium and myometrium of the rat uterus. *Endocrinology* 1971;89:358–365.
298. Clark SW, Yochim JM. Lactic dehydrogenase in the rat uterus during progestation, its relation to intrauterine oxygen tension and the regulation of glycolysis. *Biol Reprod* 1971;5:152–160.
299. Saldarini RJ, Yochim JM. Metabolism of the uterus of the rat during early pseudopregnancy and its regulation by estrogen and progesterone. *Endocrinology* 1967;80:453–466.
300. Surani MAH, Heald PJ. The metabolism of glucose by rat uterus tissue in early pregnancy. *Acta Endocrinol* 1971;66:16–24.
301. Yochim JM, Clark SW. Lactic dehydrogenase activity in the uterus of the rat during the estrous cycle and its relation to intrauterine oxygen tension. *Biol Reprod* 1971;5:146–151.
302. Yochim JM, Mitchell JA. Intrauterine oxygen tension in the rat during progestation: its possible relation to carbohydrate metabolism and the regulation of nidation. *Endocrinology* 1968;82: 706–713.
303. Yochim JM, Pepe GJ. Effect of ovarian steroids on nucleic acids, protein, and glucose-6-phosphate dehydrogenase activity in endometrium of the rat: a metabolic role for progesterone in "progestational differentiation." *Biol Reprod* 1971;5:171–182.
304. Mallonee RC, Yochim JM. Uterus of the rat during progestation: pyridine nucleotide activity and its relation to preimplantation changes in pentose cycle activity. *Biol Reprod* 1980;23:588–594.
305. Yochim JM, Mallonee RC. Hormonal control of pyridine nucleotide activity in the uterus: a model for progestational differentiation. *Biol Reprod* 1980;23:595–605.
306. Pepe GJ, Yochim JM. Pentose cycle activity in endometrium of the rat during progestation: its regulation by intrauterine oxygen and its relation to the "progestational" action of progesterone. *Endocrinology* 1971;89:366–377.
307. Glasser SR, McCormack SA. Estrogen-modulated uterine gene transcription in relation to decidualization. *Endocrinology* 1979;104:1112–1118.
308. Cummings AM, Yochim JM. Nicotinamide adenine dinucleotide in rat uterus: role of progesterone in the regulation of preimplantation differentiation. *Endocrinology* 1983;112:1407–1422.
309. Cummings AM, Yochim JM. Nicotinamide adenine dinucleotide kinase in the rat uterus: regulation by progesterone and decidual induction. *Endocrinology* 1983;112:1412–1419.
310. Yochim JM. Modulation of uterine sensitivity to decidual induction in the rat by nicotinamide: challenge and extension of a model of progestational differentiation. *Biol Reprod* 1984;30: 637–645.
311. Daly DC, Maslar IA, Riddick DH. Prolactin production during *in vitro* decidualization of proliferative endometrium. *Am J Obstet Gynecol* 1983;145:672–678.
312. Padykula HA. Shifts in uterine stromal cell populations during

pregnancy and regression. In: Glasser SR, Bullock DW, eds. *Cellular and Molecular Aspects of Implantation.* New York: Plenum Press, 1981;197–216.
313. Krehbiel RH. Cytological studies of the decidual reaction in the rat during pregnancy and in the production of deciduomata. *Physiol Zool* 1937;10:212–238.
314. Velardo JT, Dawson AB, Olsen AG, Hisaw FL. Sequence of histological changes in the uterus and vagina of the rat during prolongation of pseudopregnancy associated with the presence of deciduomata. *Am J Anat* 1953;92:273–305.
315. Jollie W, Benscome SA. Electron microscopic observations on primary decidua formation in the rat. *Am J Anat* 1965;116: 217–236.
316. Kleinfeld RG, O'Shea JD. Spatial and temporal patterns of deoxyribonucleic acid synthesis and mitosis in the endometrial stroma during decidualization in the pseudopregnant rat. *Biol Reprod* 1983;28:691–702.
317. Leroy F, Bogaert C, Van Hoeck J, Delcroix C. Cytophotometric and autoradiographic evaluation of cell kinetics in decidual cell growth in rats. *J Reprod Fertil* 1974;38:441–449.
318. Lobel BL, Tic L, Shelesnyak MC. Studies on the mechanisms of nidation. XVII. Histochemical analysis of decidualization in the rat. Part 2. Induction. *Acta Endocrinol* 1965;50:469–485.
319. Lobel BL, Tic L, Shelesnyak MC. Studies on the mechanism of nidation. XVII. Histochemical analysis of decidualization in the rat. Part 3. Formation of the deciduomata. *Acta Endocrinol* 1965;50:517–536.
320. Finn CA, McLaren A. A study of the early stages of implantation in mice. *J Reprod Fertil* 1967;13:259–267.
321. Sachs L, Shelesnyak MC. The development and suppression of polyploidy in the developing and suppressed deciduoma in the rat. *J Endocrinol* 1955;12:146–151.
322. Dupont H, Duluc JA, Mayer G. Evolution cytologique et genese de la polyploidie dans le dèciduome expérimental chez la ratte en gestation unilatérale. *C R Acad Sci Paris Ser D* 1971;272: 2360.
323. Ansell JD, Barlow PW, McLaren A. Binucleate and polyploid cells in the decidua of the mouse. *J Embryol Exp Morphol* 1974;31:223–227.
324. Lundkvist O, Ljungkvist I. Morphology of the rat endometrial stroma at the appearance of the pontamine blue reaction during implantation after an experimental delay. *Cell Tissue Res* 1977;184:453–466.
325. Parkening TA. An ultrastructural study of implantation in the golden hamster. III. Initial formation and differentiation of decidual cells. *J Anat* 1976;122:485–498.
326. O'Shea JD, Kleinfeld RG, Morrow HA. Ultrastructure of decidualization in the pseudopregnant rat. *Am J Anat* 1983;166: 271–298.
327. Abrahamsohn P. Ultrastructural study of the mouse antimesometrial decidua. *Anat Embryol* 1983;166:263–274.
328. Enders AC, Welsh AO, Schlafke S. Implantation in the rhesus monkey: endometrial responses. *Am J Anat* 1985;173:147–169.
329. Grinnell F, Head IR, Hoffpauir J. Fibronectin and cell shape *in vivo:* studies on the endometrium during pregnancy. 1982;94: 597–606.
330. Finn CA, Lawn AM. Specialized junctions between decidual cells in the uterus of the pregnant mouse. *J Ultrastruct Res* 1967;20:321–327.
331. Lawn AM, Wilson EW, Finn CA. The ultrastructure of human decidual and predecidual cells. *J Reprod Fertil* 1971;26:85–90.
332. Kleinfeld R, Morrow HA, DeFeo VJ. Intercellular functions between decidual cells in the growing deciduoma of the pseudopregnant rat uterus. *Biol Reprod* 1976;15:593–603.
333. Vladimirsky F, Chen L, Amsterdam A, Zor U, Lindner HR. Differentiation of decidual cells in cultures of rat endometrium. *J Reprod Fertil* 1977;49:61–68.
334. Sananes N, Weiller S, Baulieu E-E, Goascogne CL. *In vitro* decidualization of rat endometrial cells. *Endocrinology* 1978;103: 86–95.
335. Sananes N, Weiller S, Baulieu E-E, Goascogne CL. Decidualization *in vitro:* effects of progesterone and indomethacin. *Prog Reprod Biol* 1980;7:125–134.
336. Peleg S, Lindner HR. Role of steroid hormones and prostaglandins in the regulation of DNA synthesis by decidual cells in culture. *Mol Cell Endocrinol* 1980;20:209–218.
337. Bell SC, Searle RF. Differentiation of decidual cells in mouse endometrial cell cultures. *J Reprod Fertil* 1981;61:425–433.
338. Parr EL, Tung HN, Parr MB. Apoptosis as the mode of uterine epithelial cell death during embryo implantation in mice and rats. *Biol Reprod* 1987;26:211–225.
339. Bell SC. Decidualization: regional differentiation and associated function. *Oxford Rev Reprod Biol* 1983;5:220–271.
340. Welsh AO, Enders AC. Trophoblast–decidual cell interaction and establishment of maternal blood circulation in the parietal yolk sac placenta of the rat. *Anat Rec* 1987;217:203–219.
341. Welsh AO, Enders AC. Chorioallantoic placenta formation in the rat: I. Luminal epithelial cell death and extracellular matrix modifications in the mesometrial region of implantation chambers. *Am J Anat* 1991;192:215–231.
342. Welsh AO, Enders AC. Chorioallantoic placenta formation in the rat: II. Angiogenesis and maternal blood circulation in the mesometrial region of the implantation chamber prior to placental formation. *Am J Anat* 1991;192:347–365.
343. Ledford BE, Rankin JC, Froble VL, Serra MJ, Markwald RR, Baggett B. The decidual cell reaction in the mouse uterus: DNA synthesis and autoradiographic analysis of response cells. *Biol Reprod* 1978;18:506–509.
344. Abrahamsohn P, Lundkvist O, Nilsson O. Ultrastructure of the endometrial blood vessels during implantation of the rat blastocyst. *Cell Tissue Res* 1983;229:269–280.
345. Milligan SR, Mirembe FM. Time course of the changes in uterine vascular permeability associated with the development of the decidual cell reaction in ovariectomized steroid-treated rats. *J Reprod Fertil* 1984;70:1–6.
346. Hoos PC, Hoffman LH. Temporal aspects of rabbit uterine vascular and decidual responses to blastocyst stimulation. *Biol Reprod* 1980;23:453–459.
347. Bulmer D, Peel S. The demonstration of immunoglobulin in the metrial gland cells of the rat placenta. *J Reprod Fertil* 1977;49:143–145.
348. Peel S, Bulmer D. The fine structure of the rat metrial gland in relation to the origin of the granulated cells. *J Anat* 1977; 123:687–696.
349. Bulmer N, Sunderland CA. Immunohistological characterization of lymphoid cell populations in the early human placental bed. *Immunology* 1984;52:349–357.
350. Bulmer JN, Hollings D, Ritson A. Immunocytochemical evidence that endometrial stroma granulocytes are granulated lymphocytes. *J Pathol* 1987;153:281–287.
351. Padykula HA. Cellular mechanisms involved in cyclic stromal renewal of the uterus. III. Cells of the immune response. *Anat Rec* 1976;184:49–72.
352. Padykula HA, Campbell AG. Cellular mechanisms involved in cyclic stromal renewal of the uterus. II. The albino rat. *Anat Rec* 1976;184:27–48.
353. Padykula HA, Taylor JM. Cellular mechanisms involved in cyclic stromal renewal of the uterus. I. The opossum, *Didelphis virginiana. Anat Rec* 1976;184:5–26.
354. Padykula HA, Driscoll SG, Cardasis CA. Decidual differentiation in the normal early gestational human uterus includes lymphoid infiltration. *Anat Rec* 1978;190:500–501 (abst).
355. Padykula HA, Tansey TR. The occurrence of uterine stromal and intra-epithelial monocytes and heterophils during normal late pregnancy in the rat. *Anat Rec* 1979;193:329–336.
356. Bernard O, Ripoche M-A, Bennett D. Distribution of maternal immunoglobulins in the mouse uterus and embryo in the days after implantation. *J Exp Med* 1977;145:58–75.
357. Bernard O, Scheid MP, Ripoche M-A, Bennett D. Immunological studies of mouse decidual cells. I. Membrane markers of decidual cells in the days after implantation. *J Exp Med* 1978;148:580–591.
358. Rachman F, Bernard O, Scheid MP, Bennett D. Immunological studies of mouse decidual cells. II. Studies of cells in artificially induced decidua. *J Reprod Immunol* 1981;3:41–48.
359. Kearns M, Lala PK. Bone marrow origin of decidual cell precursors in the pseudopregnant mouse uterus. *J Exp Med* 1982;155:1537–1554.

360. Peel S, Stewart IJ, Bulmer D. Experimental evidence for the bone marrow origin of granulated metrial gland cells of the mouse uterus. *Cell Tissue Res* 1983;233:647–656.
361. Mitchel BS, Peel S. Identification of cells bearing leucocyte surface antigens in metrial gland tissue from rats of different gestational ages, strains or parities. *Immunology* 1984;53:63–68.
362. Tachi C. Mechanisms underlying regulation of local immune responses in the uterus during early gestation of eutherian mammals. I. Distribution of immuno-competent cells which bind anti-IgG antibodies in the post-nidatory uterus of the mouse. *Zool Sci* 1985;2:341–348.
363. Johnson S, Lala PK. Bone marrow origin of decidual cell precursors in murine pregnancy. *J Reprod Immunol* 1986;122(suppl 1)(abst).
364. Tachi C, Tachi S. Macrophages and implantation. *Ann NY Acad Sci* 1986;476:158–182.
365. Lee CS, Gogolin-Ewens K, Brandon MR. Identification of a unique lymphocyte subpopulation in the sheep uterus. *Immunology* 1988;63:157–164.
366. King A, Birkby C, Loke YW. Early human decidual cells exhibit NK activity against the K562 cell line but not against first trimester trophoblast. *Cell Immunol* 1989;118:337–344.
367. King A, Loke YW. Uterine large granular lymphocytes: a possible role in embryonic implantation? *Am J Obstet Gynecol* 1990;162:308–310.
368. Kachkache M, Acker GM, Chaouat G, Noun A, Garabedian M. Hormonal and local factors control the immunohistochemical distribution of immunocytes in the rat uterus before conceptus implantation: effects of ovariectomy, fallopian tube secretion and injection. *Biol Reprod* 1991;45:860–868.
369. Moskalewski S, Ptak W, Strzyzewska J. Macrophages in mouse placenta: morphologic and functional identification. *J Reticuloendothelial Soc* 1974;16:9–14.
370. Nehemiah JL, Schnitzer JA, Schulman H, Novikoff AB. Human chorionic trophoblasts, decidual cells and macrophages: a histochemical and electron microscopic study. *Am J Obstet Gynecol* 1981;140:261–268.
371. Bulmer N, Johnson PM. Macrophage populations in the human placenta and amniochorion. *Clin Exp Immunol* 1984;57:393–403.
372. Sutton L, Mason DY, Redman CWG. HLA-DR positive cells in the human placenta. *Immunology* 1983;49:103–105.
373. Sutton L, Gadd M, Mason Y, Redman CWG. Cells bearing class II MHC antigens in the human placenta and amniochorion. *Immunology* 1986;58:23–29.
374. Kabawat SE, Mostoufi-Zadeh M, Driscoll SG, Bhan AK. Implantation site in normal pregnancy. A study with monoclonal antibodies. *Am J Pathol* 1985;118:76–84.
375. Kabawat SE, Mostoufi-Zadeh M, Berkowitz RS, Driscoll SG, Goldstein DP, Bhan AK. Implantation site in complete molar pregnancy: a study of immunologically competent cells with monoclonal antibodies. *Am J Obstet Gynecol* 1985;152:97–99.
376. Hunt JS, Manning LS, Mitchell D, Selanders JR, Wood GW. Localization and characterization of macrophages in murine uterus. *J Leukoc Biol* 1985;38:255–265.
377. Khong TY. Immunohistologic study of the leukocytic infiltrate in maternal tissues in normal and pre-eclamptic pregnancies at term. *Am J Reprod Immunol Microbiol* 1987;15:1–8.
378. Goldstein J, Braverman M, Salafia C, Buckley PB. The phenotype of human placental macrophages and its variation with gestational age. *Am J Pathol* 1988;133:648–659.
379. Zheng Y, Zhou Z-Z, Lyttle CR, Teuscher C. Immunohistochemical characterization of the estrogen-stimulated leukocyte influx in the immature rat uterus. *J Leukoc Biol* 1988;44:27–32.
380. De M, Wood GW. Influence of oestrogen and progesterone on macrophage distribution in the mouse uterus. *J Endocrinol* 1990;126:417–424.
381. Laguens G, Goni JM, Laguens M, Goni JM, Laguens R. Demonstration and characterization of HLA-DR positive cells in the stroma of human endometrium. *J Reprod Immunol* 1990;18:179–186.
382. Yagel S, Livni N, Zacut D, Gallily R. Characterization and localization of human placental mononuclear phagocytes by monoclonal antibodies and other cell markers. *Isr J Med Sci* 1990;26:243–249.
383. Bulmer JN, Morrison L, Smith JC. Expression of class II MHC gene products by macrophages in human uteroplacental tissue. *Immunology* 1988;63:707–714.
384. De M, Wood GW. Analysis of the number and distribution of macrophages, lymphocytes, and granulocytes in the mouse uterus from implantation through parturition. *J Leukoc Biol* 1991;50:381–392.
385. De M, Choudhuri R, Wood GW. Determination of the number and distribution of macrophages, lymphocytes, and granulocytes in the mouse uterus from mating through implantation. *J Leukoc Biol* 1991;50:252–262.
386. Choudhuri R, Wood GW. Leukocyte distribution in the pseudopregnant mouse uterus. *Am J Reprod Immunol* 1992;27:69–76.
387. Oksenberg JR, Yosef M, Schenker E, Mozes Y, Brautbar C. Antigen presenting cells in human decidual tissue. *Am J Reprod Immunol Microbiol* 1986;11:82–88.
388. Hunt JS, Manning LS, Wood GW. Macrophages in murine uterus are immunosuppressive. *Cell Immunol* 1984;85:499–510.
389. Tawkik OW, Hunt JS, Wood GW. Implication of prostaglandin E_2 in soluble factor-mediated immune suppression by murine decidual cells. *Am J Reprod Immunol Microbiol* 1986;12:111–117.
390. Hamperl H, Hellweg G. Granular endometrial stromal cells. *Obstet Gynecol* 1958;2:379–387.
391. Dallenbach-Hellweg G. *Histopathology of the Endometrium.* New York: Springer-Verlag, 1981.
392. Bulmer JN, Ritson A, Pace D. Endometrial leukocytes in human pregnancy. *Trophoblast Res* 1990;4:431–451.
393. King A, Wellings V, Gardner L, Loke YW. Immunocytochemical characterization of the unusual large granular lymphocytes in human endometrium throughout the menstrual cycle. *Hum Immunol* 1989;24:195–205.
394. Bulmer N, Johnson PM. Immunohistological characterization of the decidual leucocyte infiltrate related to endometrial gland epithelium in early human pregnancy. *Immunology* 1985;55:35–44.
395. Starkey POM, Sargent IL, Redman CWG. Cell populations in human early pregnancy decidua: characterization and isolation of large granular lymphocytes by flow cytometry. *Immunology* 1988;65:129–134.
396. Redline RW, Lu CY. Localization of fetal major histocompatibility complex antigens and maternal leukocytes in murine placenta. Implications for maternal–fetal immunological relationship. *Lab Invest* 1989;61:27–36.
397. Lin PY, Joag SV, Young JD, Change Y-S, Soong Y-K, Kuo T-T. Expression of perforin by natural killer cells within first trimester endometrium in humans. *Biol Reprod* 1991;45:698–703.
398. Manaseki S, Searle RF. Natural killer (NK) cell activity of first trimester human decidua. *Cell Immunol* 1989;121:166–173.
399. Ferry BL, Starkey PM, Sargent IL, Watt GMO, Jackson M, Redman CWG. Cell populations in the human early pregnancy decidua: natural killer activity and response to interleukin-2 of CD56-positive large granular lymphocytes. *Immunology* 1990;70:446–452.
400. Bulmer N, Johnson PM. The T-lymphocyte population in first-trimester human decidua does not express the interleukin-2 receptor. *Immunology* 1986;58:685–687.
401. Mincheva-Nilsson L, Hammarstrom S, Hammarstrom M-R. Human decidual leukocytes from early pregnancy contain high numbers of $\gamma\delta[+]$ cells and show selective down-regulation of alloreactivity. *J Immunol* 1992;149:2203–2211.
402. Lanier LL, Le AM, Civin CI, Loken MR, Phillips JH. The relationship of CD16 (Leu-11) and Leu-19 (NKH-1) antigen expression on human peripheral blood NK cells and cytotocix T lymphocytes. *J Immunol* 1986;136:4480–4486.
403. Stewart I. A morphological study of granulated metrial gland cells and trophoblast cells in the labrinthine placenta of the mouse. *J Anat* 1984;139:627–638.
404. Parr EL, Parr MB, Young JD-E. Localization of a pore-forming protein (perforin) in granulated metrial gland cells. *Biol Reprod* 1987;37:1327–1335.
405. Parr EL, Young LHY, Parr MB, Young D-E. Granulated metrial gland cells of pregnant mouse uterus are natural killer-like cells

that contain perforin and serine esterases. *J Immunol* 1990; 145:2365–2372.
406. Heyborne KD, Cranfill RL, Carding SR, Born WK, O'Brien RL. Characterization of $\delta\delta$ T lymphocytes at the maternal–fetal interface. *J Immunol* 1992;149:2872–2878.
407. Das RM, Martin L. Uterine DNA synthesis and cell proliferation during early decidualization induced by oil in mice. *J Reprod Fertil* 1978;53:125–128.
408. Ledford BE, Rankin JC, Markwald RR, Baggett B. Biochemical and morphological changes following artificially stimulated decidualization in the mouse uterus. *Biol Reprod* 1976;15:529–535.
409. Shelesnyak MC, Tic L. Studies on the mechanism of decidualization. IV. Synthetic processes in the decidualizing uterus. *Acta Endocrinol* 1963;42:465–472.
410. Shelesnyak MC, Tic L. Studies on the mechanism of decidualization. V. Suppression of synthetic processes of the uterus (DNA, RNA, and protein) following inhibition of decidualization by an antioestrogen, ethanoxytriphetol (MER-25). *Acta Endocrinol* 1963;43:462–463.
411. Moulton BC, Blaha GC. Separation of deciduomal cells by velocity sedimentation at unit gravity. *Biol Reprod* 1978;18:141–147.
412. Moulton BC. Effect of progesterone on DNA, RNA and protein synthesis of deciduoma cell fractions separated by velocity sedimentation. *Biol Reprod* 1979;21:667–672.
413. Moulton BC, Koenig BB. Uterine deoxyribonucleic acid synthesis during preimplantation in precursors of stromal cell differentiation during decidualization. *Endocrinology* 1984;115: 1302–1307.
414. Miller BG. Metabolism of RNA and pyrimidine nucleotides in the uterus during the early decidual cell reaction. *J Endocrinol* 1973;59:275–283.
415. Serra MJ, Ledford BE, Rankin JC, Baggett B. Changes in RNA polymerase activity in isolated mouse uterine nuclei during the decidual cell reaction. *Biochim Biophys Acta* 1978;521:267–273.
416. Barkai U, Kraicer PF. Definition of period of induction of deciduoma in the rat using ornithine decarboxylase as a marker of growth onset. *Int J Fertil* 1978;23:106–111.
417. Collawn SS, Rankin J, Ledford BE, Baggett B. Ornithine decarboxylase activity in the artificially stimulated decidual cell reaction in the mouse uterus. *Biol Reprod* 1981;24:528–533.
418. Tarachand U, Sivabalan R, Eapen J. Protein anabolism in endometrium and myometrium during the growth of induced deciduoma in rats. *Experientia* 1980;36:1154–1156.
419. Glasser SR. Biochemical and structural changes in uterine endometrial cell types following natural or artificial deciduogenic stimuli. In: Denker H, Aplin JD, eds. *Trophoblast Invasion and Endometrial Receptivity. Novel Aspects of the Cell Biology of Embryo Implantation. Trophoblast Res* 1990;4:377–416.
420. Yoshinaga K. Rabbit antiserum to rat deciduoma. *Biol Reprod* 1972;6:51–57.
421. Yoshinaga K. Interspecific cross-reactivity of deciduoma antiserum: interaction between mouse deciduoma and anti-serum to rat deciduoma. *Biol Reprod* 1974;11:50–55.
422. Joshi SG, Szarowski DH, Bank J. Decidua-associated antigens in the baboon. *Biol Reprod* 1981;25:591–598.
423. Sacco AG, Mintz B. Mouse uterine antigens in the implantation period of pregnancy. *Biol Reprod* 1975;12:498–503.
424. Denari JH, Rosner JM. Studies on biochemical characteristics of an early decidual protein. *Int J Fertil* 1978;23:123–127.
425. Umapathesivam K, Jones WR. An investigation of decidual specific proteins in the rat. *Int J Fertil* 1978;23:138–142.
426. Denari JH, Germino NI, Rosner JM. Early synthesis of uterine proteins after a decidual stimulus in the pseudopregnant rat. *Biol Reprod* 1976;15:1–8.
427. Bell SC. Synthesis of 'decidualization-associated protein' in tissues of the rat uterus and placenta during pregnancy. *J Reprod Fertil* 1979;56:255–262.
428. Bell SC. Protein synthesis during deciduoma morphogenesis in the rat. *Biol Reprod* 1979;20:811–821.
429. Bell SC. Immunochemical identify of decidualization-associated proteins and α_2 acute-phase macroglobulin in the pregnant rat. *J Reprod Immunol* 1979;1:193–206.
430. Bell SC, Hamer J, Heald PJ. Induced protein and deciduoma formation in rat uterus. *Biol Reprod* 1980;23:935–940.
431. Notides A, Gorski J. Estrogen-induced synthesis of a specific uterine protein. *Proc Natl Acad Sci USA* 1966;56:230–235.
432. Manak R, Wertz N, Slabaugh M, Denari H, Wang JT, Gorski J. Purification and characterization of the estrogen-induced protein (IP) of the rat uterus. *Mol Cell Endocrinol* 1980;17:119–132.
433. Katzenellenbogen BS. Synthesis and inducibility of the uterine estrogen-induced protein, IP, during the rat estrous cycle: clues to uterine estrogen sensitivity. *Endocrinology* 1975;96:289–297.
434. Dupont-Mairess N, Galand P. Estrogen action: induction of the synthesis of a specific protein (IP) in the myometrium, the stroma and the luminal epithelium of the rat uterus. *Endocrinology* 1975;96:1587–1591.
435. Lejeune B, Lecocq R, Lamy F, Leory F. Changes in the pattern of endometrial protein synthesis during decidualization in the rat. *J Reprod Fertil* 1982;66:519–523.
436. MacDonald RG, Morency KO, Leavitt WW. Progesterone modulation of specific protein synthesis in the decidualized hamster uterus. *Biol Reprod* 1983;2:753–766.
437. Leavitt WW, MacDonald RG, Shwaery GT. Characterization of deciduoma proteins in hamster uterus: detection in decidual cell cultures. *Biol Reprod* 1985;32:631–643.
438. Glasser SR, Julian J. Intermediate filament protein as a marker of uterine stromal cell decidualization. *Biol Reprod* 1986;35: 463–474.
439. Martel D, Psychoyos A. Estrogen receptors in the nidatory sites of the rat endometrium. *Science* 1981;211:1454–1455.
440. Ward WF, Frost AG, Orsini MW. Estrogen binding by embryonic and interembryonic segments of the rat uterus prior to implantation. *Biol Reprod* 1978;18:598–601.
441. Sartor P. Exogenous hormone uptake and retention in the rat uterus at the time of ova-implantation. *Acta Endocrinol* 1977;84:804–812.
442. Moulton BC, Koenig BB. Estrogen receptor in deciduoma cells separated by velocity sedimentation. *Endocrinology* 1981;108: 484–488.
443. McConnell KN, Sillar RG, Young BD, Green B. Ploidy and progesterone-receptor distribution in flow-sorted deciduomal nuclei. *Mol Cell Endocrinol* 1982;25:99–104.
444. Sartor P. Cell proliferation and decidual morphogenesis. *Prog Reprod Biol* 1980;7:115–124.
445. Kisalus LL, Herr JC, Little CD. Immunolocalization of extracellular matrix proteins and collagen synthesis in first-trimester human decidua. *Anat Rec* 1987;218:402–415.
446. Aplin JD, Charlton AK, Ayad S. An immunohistochemical study of human and endometrial extracellular matrix during the menstrual cycle and first trimester of pregnancy. *Cell Tissue Res* 1988;253:231–240.
447. Aplin JD, Charlton AK. The role of matrix macromolecules in the invasion of decidua by trophoblast: model studies using BeWo cells. In: Denker H, Aplin JD, eds. *Trophoblast Invasion and Endometrial Receptivity. Novel Aspects of the Cell Biology of Embryo Implantation. Trophoblast Res* 1990;4:139–158.
448. Foidart JM, Christiane Y, Emonard H. Interactions between the human trophoblast cells and the extracellular matrix of the endometrium. Specific expression of α-galactose residues by invasive human trophoblastic cells. In: Denker H, Aplin JD, eds. *Trophoblast Invasion and Endometrial Receptivity. Novel Aspects of the Cell Biology of Embryo Implantation. Trophoblast Res* 1990;4: 159–177.
449. Wienke EC, Filberto Calvazos S, Hall DS, Lucas LV. Ultrastructure of the endometrial stromal cell during the menstrual cycle. *Am J Obstet Gynecol* 1968;102:65–77.
450. More IAR, Armstrong EM, Carty M, McSeveney D. Cyclical changes in the ultrastructure of the normal endometrial stromal cell. *Br J Obstet Gynaecol* 1974;81:337–347.
451. Wynn RM. Ultrastructural development of the human decidua. *Am J Obstet Gynecol* 1974;118:652–670.
452. Cornille FJ, Lauweryns JM, Brosens IA. Normal human endometrium. An ultrastructural survey. *Gynecol Obstet Invest* 1985;20:113–129.
453. Glasser SR, Lampelo S, Munir MI, Julian JA. Expression of desmin, laminin and fibronectin during *in situ* differentiation (decidualization) of rat uterine stromal cells. *Differentiation* 1987;35: 132–142.

454. Mulholland J, Aplin JD, Ayad S, Hong L, Glasser SR. Loss of collagen type VI from rat endometrial stroma during decidualization. *Biol Reprod* 1992;46:1136–1143.
455. Denker HW. Implantation: the role of proteinases, the blockage of implantation by proteinase inhibitors. *Adv Anat Embryol Cell Biol* 1977;53:3–123.
456. Yagel S, Parhar RS, Jeffrey JJ, Lala PK. Normal nonmetastatic human trophoblast cells share *in vitro* invasive properties of malignant cells. *J Cell Physiol* 1988;136:455–462.
457. Owers NO, Blandau RJ. Proteolytic activity of the rat and guinea pig blastocysts *in vitro*. In: Blandau RJ, ed. *The Biology of the Blastocyst*. Chicago: University of Chicago Press, 1971;207–223.
458. Glass RH, Aggeler J, Spindle A, Pedersen RA, Werb Z. Degradation of extracellular matrix by mouse trophoblast outgrowths: a model for implantation. *J Cell Biol* 1983;96:1108–1116.
459. Strickland S, Reich E, Sherman MI. Plasminogen activator in early embryogenesis: enzyme production by trophoblast and parietal endoderm. *Cell* 1976;9:231–240.
460. Kubo H, Spindle A, Pedersen RA. Inhibitions of mouse blastocyst attachment and outgrowth by protease inhibitors. *J Exp Zool* 1981;216:445–451.
461. Tansey TR, Padykula HA. Cellular responses to experimental inhibition of collagen degradation in the postpartum rat uterus. *Anat Rec* 1978;191:287–296.
462. Edwards DR, Murphy G, Reynolds JJ, et al. Transforming growth factor beta modulates the expression of collagenase and metalloproteinase inhibitors. *EMBO J* 1987;6:1899–1904.
463. Brenner CA, Adler RR, Rappolee, DA, Pedersen RN, Werb Z. Genes for extracellular matrix-degrading metalloproteinases and their inhibitor, TIMP, are expressed during early mammalian development. *Genes Dev* 1989;3:848–859.
464. Fisher SJ, Leitch MS, Kantor MS, Basbaum CB, Kramer RH. Degradation of extracellular matrix by trophoblastic cells of first trimester human placentas. *J Cell Biochem* 1985;27:31–41.
465. Fisher SJ, Cui T, Zhang L, et al. Adhesive and degradative properties of human placental cytotrophoblast cells *in vitro*. *J Cell Biol* 1989;109:891–902.
466. Kliman HJ, Feinberg RF. Human trophoblast-extracellular matrix (ECM) interactions *in vitro*: ECM thickness modulates morpholoby and proteolytic activity. *Proc Natl Acad Sci USA* 1990;87:3057–3061.
467. Lala PK, Graham CH. Mechanisms of trophoblast invasiveness and their control: the role of proteases and protease inhibitors. *Cancer Metastasis Rev* 1990;9:369–379.
468. Pastore GN, Dicola LP, Dollahon NR, Gardner RM. Effect of estriol on the structure and organization of collagen in the lamina propria of the immature rat uterus. *Biol Reprod* 1992;47:83–91.
469. Aplin JD, Seif MW. Basally located epithelial cell surface component identified by a novel monoclonal antibody technique. *Exp Cell Res* 1985;160:550–555.
470. Aplin JD, Seif MW. A monoclonal antibody to a cell surface determinant in human endometrial epithelium: stage-specific expression in the menstrual cycle. *Am J Obstet Gynecol* 1987;156:250–255.
471. Faber M, Wewer UM, Berthelsen JG, Liotta LA, Albrechtsen R. Laminin production by human endometrial stromal cells relates to the cyclic and pathologic state of the endometrium. *Am J Pathol* 1986;124:384–398.
472. Wan Y-J, Wu T-C, Chung AE, Damjanov I. Monoclonal antibodies to laminin reveal the heterogeneity of basement membranes in the developing and adult mouse tissues. *J Cell Biol* 1984;98:971–979.
473. Charpin C, Kopp F, Pourreau-Schneider N, et al. Laminin distribution in human decidual and immature placenta. An immunoelectron microscopic study (avidin-biotin-peroxidase complex method). *Am J Obstet Gynecol* 1985;151:822–826.
474. Wewer UM, Faber M, Liotta LA, Albrechtsen R. Immunochemical and ultrastructural assessment of the nature of the pericellular basement membrane of human decidual cells. *Lab Invest* 1985;53:624–633.
475. Wewer UM, Damjanov A, Weiss J, Liotta LA, Damjanov I. Mouse endometrial stromal cells produce basement-membrane components. *Differentiation* 1986;32:49–58.
476. Riddick DH, Luciano AA, Kusmik WF, Maslar IA. *De novo* synthesis of prolactin by human decidua. *Life Sci* 1978;23:1913–1922.
477. Riddick DH, Daly DC, Walters CA. The uterus as an endocrine compartment. *Clin Perinatol* 1983;10:627–639.
478. Riddick DH, Daly DC. Decidual prolactin production in human gestation. *Semin Perinatol* 1982;6:229–237.
479. Golander A, Hurley T, Barrett J, Hizi A, Handwerger S. Prolactin synthesis by human chorion-decidual tissue: a possible source of prolactin in the amniotic fluid. *Science* 1978;202:311–313.
480. Maslar IA, Riddick RH. Prolactin production by human endometrium during the normal menstrual cycle. *Am J Obstet Gynecol* 1979;135:751–754.
481. Maslar IA, Kaplan BM, Luciano AA, Riddick DH. Prolactin production by the endometrium of early human pregnancy. *J Clin Endocrinol Metab* 1980;51:78–83.
482. Markoff E, Zeitler P, Peleg S, Handwerger S. Characterization of the synthesis and release of prolactin by an enriched fraction of human decidual cells. *J Clin Endocrinol Metab* 1983;56:962–968.
483. Braverman MB, Bagni A, deZiegler D, Den T, Gurpide E. Isolation of prolactin-producing cells from first and second trimester decidua. *J Clin Endocrinol Metab* 1984;58:521–525.
484. Heffner LJ, Iddenden DA, Lyttle CR. Electrophorectic analysis of secreted human endometrial proteins: identification and characterisation of luteal phase products. *J Clin Endocrinol Metab* 1986;62:1288–1295.
485. Kauma S, Shapiro SS. Immunoperoxidase localisation of prolactin in endometrium during normal menstrual, luteal phase defect and corrected luteal phase defect cycles. *Fertil Steril* 1986;46:37–41.
486. McRae MA, Newman GR, Walker SM, Jasani B. Immunohistochemical identification of prolactin and 24k protein in secretory phase endometrium. *Fertil Steril* 1986;45:643–648.
487. Tomita K, McCoshen JA, Fernandez CS, Tyson JE. Immunologic and biologic characteristics of human decidual prolactin. *Am J Obstet Gynecol* 1982;142:420–426.
488. Golander A, Barrett J, Hurley T, Barry S, Handwerger S. Failure of bromocriptine, dopamin, and thyrotropin-releasing hormone to affect prolactin secretion by human decidual tissue *in vitro*. *Endocrinology* 1979;49:787–789.
489. Handwerger S, Barry S, Conn PM. Different subcellular storage sites for decidual and pituitary-derived prolactin: possible explanation for differences in regulation. *Mol Cell Endocrinol* 1984;37:83–87.
490. Handwerger S, Hamman I, Costello A, Markoff E. cAMP inhibits the synthesis and release of prolactin from human decidual cells. *Mol Cell Endocrinol* 1987;50:99–106.
491. Herington AC, Graham J, Healy DL. The presence of lactogen receptors in human chorion laeve. *J Clin Endocrinol Metab* 1980;51:1466–1468.
492. Gibori G, Kalison B, Basuray R, Rao MC, Hunzicker-Dunn M. Endocrine role of the decidual tissue: decidual luteotropin regulation of luteal adenylyl cyclase activity, luteinizing hormone receptors, and steroidogenesis. *Endocrinology* 1984;115:1157–1163.
493. Jayatilak PG, Glaser LA, Warshaw ML, Herz Z, Gruber JR, Gibori G. Relationship between luteinizing hormone and decidual luteotropin in the maintenance of luteal steroidogenesis. *Biol Reprod* 1984;31:556–564.
494. Basuray R, Gibori G. Luteotropic action of decidual tissue in the pregnant rat. *Biol Reprod* 1980;23:507–512.
495. Basuray R, Jaffe RC, Gibori G. Role of decidual luteotropin and prolactin in the control of luteal cell receptors for estradiol. *Biol Reprod* 1983;28:551–556.
496. Bell SC, Patel S, Hales MW, Kirwan PH, Drife JO. Immunochemical detection and characterisation of pregnancy-associated endometrial α_1- and α_2-globulins secreted by human endometrium and decidua. *J Reprod Fertil* 1985;74:261–270.
497. Bell SC, Hales MW, Patel S, Kirwan PH, Drife JO. Protein synthesis and secretion by the human endometrium and decidua during early pregnancy. *Br J Obstet Gynaecol* 1985;92:793–803.
498. Bell SC, Patel S, Kirwan PH, Drife JO. Protein synthesis and secretion by the human endometrium during the menstrual cycle and the effect of progesterone *in vitro*. *J Reprod Fertil* 1986;77:221–231.

499. Bell SC, Hales MW, Patel S, Kirwan PH, Drife JO, Milford-Ward A. Amniotic fluid levels of secreted pregnancy-associated endometrial α_1- and α_2-globulins (α_1- and α_2-PEG). *Br J Obstet Gynaecol* 1986;93:909–915.
500. Waites GT, Walker RA, Bell SC. Immunohistological localization of endometrial somatomedin-IGF binding protein or α_1-PEG by using monoclonal antibodies. *J Reprod Fertil* 1988;36 (suppl):182.
501. Wahlstrom T, Teisner B, Folkersen J. Tissue localisation of pregnancy-associated plasma protein A (PAPP-A) in normal placenta. *Placenta* 1981;2:253–258.
502. Koistinen R, Kalkkinen N, Huhtala M-L, Seppala M, Bohn H, Rutanen E-M. Placental protein 12 is a decidual protein that binds somatomedin and has an identical N-terminal amino acid sequence with somatomedin-binding protein from human amniotic fluid. *Endocrinology* 1986;118:1375–1378.
503. Bell SC, Bohn H. Immunochemical and biochemical relationship between human pregnancy-associated secreted endometrial α_1- and α_2-globulins (α_1- and α_2-PEG) and soluble placental proteins 12 and 14 (PP12 and PP14). *Placenta* 1986;7:283–294.
504. Bell SC, Keyte JW. N-terminal amino acid sequence of human pregnancy-associated endometrial α_1-globulin, an endometrial insulin-like growth factor (IGF) binding protein—evidence for two small molecular weight IGF binding proteins. *Endocrinology* 1988;123:1202–1204.
505. Bell SC. Secretory endometrial/decidual proteins and their function in early pregnancy. *J Reprod Fertil* 1988;36(suppl):109–125.
506. Bell SC, Keyte JW, Waites GT. Pregnancy-associated endometrial α_2-globulin (α_2-PEG), the major secretory protein of the luteal phase and first trimester pregnancy endometrium, is not glycosylated prolactin but related to β-lactoglobulins. *J Clin Endocrinol Metab* 1987;65:1067–1071.
507. Bell SC, Dore-Green F. Detection and characterisation of human secretory, "pregnancy-associated" endometrial α_2-globulin (α_2-PEG) in uterine luminal fluid. *J Reprod Immunol* 1987;11: 13–29.
508. Bell SC, Smith S. The endometrium as a paracrine organ. In: Chamberlin GVP, ed. *Contemporary Obstetrics and Gynecology,* Vol 1, Part 2. London: Butterworths, 1988;273–299.
509. Sutcliffe RG, Brock DJH, Nicholson LVB, Dunn E. Fetal- and uterine-specific antigens in human amniotic fluid. *J Reprod Fertil* 1978;54:86–90.
510. Sutcliffe RG, Bolton AE, Sharp F, Nicholson LVB, Mackinnon R. Purification of human alpha uterine protein. *J Reprod Fertil* 1980;58:435–442.
511. Sutcliffe RG, Kukulska-Langlands BM, Coggins JR, Hunter JB, Gore CH. Studies on human pregnancy-associated plasma protein A. Purification by affinity chromatography and structural comparison with α_2-macroglobulin. *Biochem J* 1980;191: 799–809.
512. Sutcliffe RG, Joshi SG, Patterson WF, Bank JF. Serological identify between human alpha uterine protein and human progestagen-dependent endometrial protein. *J Reprod Fertil* 1982;65:207–209.
513. Joshi SG, Ebert KM, Swartz DP. Detection and synthesis of a progestagen-dependent protein in human endometrium. *J Reprod Fertil* 1980;59:273–285.
514. Joshi SG, Ebert KM, Smith RA. Properties of the progestagen-dependent protein of the human endometrium. *J Reprod Fertil* 1980;59:287–296.
515. Joshi SG, Bank JF, Szarowski DH. Radioimmunoassay for a progestagen-associated protein of the human endometrium. *J Clin Endocrinol Metab* 1981;52:1185–1192.
516. Joshi SG. A progestagen-associated protein of the human endometrium: basic studies and potential clinical applications. *J Steroid Biochem* 1983;19:751–757.
517. Julkunen M, Raikar RS, Joshi SG, Bohn H, Seppala M. Placental protein 14 and progestagen-dependent endometrial protein are immunologically indistinguishable. *Hum Reprod* 1986;1:7–8.
518. Huhtala M-L, Seppala M, Narvanen A, Palomaki P, Julkunen M, Bohn H. Amino acid sequence homology between human placental protein 14 and β-lactoglobulins from various species. *Endocrinology* 1987;120:2620–2622.
519. Tourville DR, Ogra SS, Lippes J, Tomasi TB. The human female reproductive tract: immunohistological localization of γA, γG, γM, secretory "pieces," and lactoferrin. *Am J Obstet Gynecol* 1970;108:1102–1108.
520. Pentecost BT, Teng CT. Lactotransferrin is the major estrogen inducible protein of mouse uterine secretions. *J Biol Chem* 1987;262:10134–10139.
521. Chen TT, Bazer FW, Cetorelli JJ, Pollard WE, Roberts RM. Purification and properties of a progesterone-induced basic glycoprotein from the uterine fluid of pigs. *J Biol Chem* 1973;248: 8560–8566.
522. Beier HM. Uteroglobin: a hormone sensitive endometrial protein involved in blastocyst development. *Biochim Biophys Acta* 1968;160:289–291.
523. Beier HM. Uteroglobin and related biochemical changes in the reproductive tract during early pregnancy in the rabbit. *J Reprod Fertil* 1976;25(suppl):53–69.
524. Bullock DW, Conell KM. Occurrence and molecular weight of rabbit uterine "blastokinin." *Biol Reprod* 1973;9:125–132.
525. Daniel JC. Blastokinin and analogous proteins. *J Reprod Fertil* 1976;25(suppl):71–83.
526. Nieto A, Ponstingel H, Beato M. Purification and quaternary structure of the hormonally induced protein uteroglobin. *Arch Biochem Biophys* 1977;180:82–92.
527. Morize I, Surcouf E, Vaney MC, et al. Refinement of the $L222_1$ crystal form of oxidised uteroglobin at 1.34 Å resolution. *J Mol Biol* 1987;194:725–741.
528. Rajkumar K, Bigsby R, Lieberman R, Gerschenson LE. Uteroglobulin production by cultured rabbit uterine epithelial cells. *Endocrinology* 1983;112:1490–1498.
529. Rajkumar K, Bigsby R, Lieberman R, Gerschenson LE. Effect of progesterone and 17β-estradiol on production of uteroglobulin by cultured rabbit uterine epithelial cells. *Endocrinology* 1983;112:1499–1505.
530. Aumuller G, Setiz J, Heyns W, Kirchner C. Ultrastructural localization of uteroglobin immunoreactivity in rabbit lung and endometrium, and rat ventral prostate. *Histochemistry* 1985;83: 413–417.
531. Loosfelt H, Fridlansky F, Savouret J-F, Atger M, Milgrom E. Mechanism of action of progesterone in the rabbit endometrium. Induction of uteroglobin and its mRNA. *J Biol Chem* 1981;256:3465–3470.
532. Tsai M-J, Bullock DW, Woo SLC. Hormonal regulation of rabbit uteroglobin gene transcription. *Endocrinology* 1983;112:871–876.
533. Kirchner C. Uteroglobin in the rabbit. I. Intracellular localization in the oviduct, uterus and preimplantation blastocyst. *Cell Tissue Res* 1976;170:415–424.
534. Beato M, Beier HM. Characteristics of the purified uteroglobin-like protein from rabbit lung. *J Reprod Fertil* 1978;53:305–314.
535. Tancredi T, Temussi PA, Beato M. Interaction of oxidized and reduced uteroglobin with progesterone. *Eur J Biochem* 1982;122: 101–104.
536. Mukherjee AB, Ulane RE, Agrawal AK. Role of uteroglobin and transglutaminase in masking antigenicity of implanting rabbit embryos. *Am J Reprod Immunol* 1982;2:135–141.
537. Mukerjee DC, Agrawal AK, Marjunath R, Mukherjee AB. Suppression of epididymal sperm antigenicity in the rabbit by uteroglobin and transglutaminase *in vitro. Science* 1983;219:989–991.
538. Holinka CF, Gurpide E. Diamine oxidase activity in human decidua and endometrium. *Am J Obstet Gynecol* 1984; 150:359–363.
539. Spilman CH, Bergstrom KK, Beuving DC. Effects of prostaglandins and peripheral progesterone and uterine diamine oxidase in the pregnant hamster. *Prostaglandins* 1980;20:1061–1074.
540. Guha SK, Janne J. The synthesis and accumulation of polyamines in reproductive organs of the rat during pregnancy. *Biochim Biophys Acta* 1976;437:244–252.
541. Maudsley DV, Kobayashi Y. Biosynthesis and metabolism of putrescine in the rat placenta. *Biochem Pharmacol* 1977;26: 121–124.
542. Bacus B, Kim KS. Subcellular distribution of diamine oxidase. *Comp Gen Pharmacol* 1970;1:196–200.
543. Brigstock DR, Heap RB, Brown KD. Polypeptide growth factors in uterine tissues, and secretions. *J Reprod Fertil* 1989;85: 747–758.

544. Pollard JW. Regulation of polypeptide growth factor synthesis and growth factor-related gene expression in the rat and mouse uterus before and after implantation. *J Reprod Fertil* 1990;88: 721–731.
545. Tabibzadeh SS. Cytokine regulation of human endometrial function. *Ann NY Acad Sci* 1991;622:89–98.
546. Tabibzadeh SS. Human endometrium: an active site of cytokine production and action. *Endoc Rev* 1991;12:272–290.
547. Simmen FA, Simmen RCM. Peptide growth factors and protooncogenes in mammalian conceptus development. *Biol Reprod* 1991;44:1–5.
548. Romero R, Wu YK, Brody DT, Oyarzun E, Duff GW, Durum SK. Human decidua: a source of interleukin-1. *Obstet Gynecol* 1989;73:31–34.
549. Kauma S, Matt D, Strom S, Eierman D, Turner T. Interleukin-1β, human leukocyte antigen HLA-DRα, and transforming growth factor-β expression in endometrium, placenta, and placental membranes. *Am J Obstet Gynecol* 1990;163:1430–1437.
550. Takacs L, Kovacs EJ, Smith MR, Young HA, Durum SK. Detection of IL-1α and IL-1β gene expression by *in situ* hybridization: tissue localization of IL-1 mRNA in the normal C57BL/6 mouse. *J Immunol* 1988;141:3081–3095.
551. De M, Sanford TH, Wood GW. Detection of interleukin 1, interleukin-6, and tumor necrosis factor-α in the uterus during the second half of pregnancy in the mouse. *Endocrinology* 1992;131:14–20.
552. De M, Sanfrod TH, Wood GW. Interleukin-1, interleukin-6, and tumor necrosis factor-α are produced in the mouse uterus during the estrous cycle and are induced by estrogen and progesterone. *Dev Biol* 1992;151:297–305.
553. Tabibzadeh SS, Kaffka KL, Satyaswaroop PG, Kilian PL. Interleukin-1 (IL-1) regulation of human endometrial function: present of IL-1 receptor correlates with IL-1-stimulated prostaglandin E_2 production. *J Clin Endocrinol Metab* 1990;70: 1000–1009.
554. Tabibzadeh SS, Santhanam U, Sehgal PB, May LT. Cytokine-induced production of IFN-β_2/IL-6 by freshly explanted human endometrial stromal cells. *J Immunol* 1989;142:3134–3139.
555. Tabibzadeh SS, Sivarajah A, Carpenter D, Ohlsson-Wilhelm O, Satyaswaroop PG. Modulation of HLA-DR expression in epithelial cells by interleukin 1 and estradiol-17β. *J Clin Endocrinol Metab* 1990;71:740–747.
556. Tartakovsky B, Ben-Yair E. Cytokines modulate preimplantation development and pregnancy. *Dev Biol* 1991;146:345–352.
557. Boehm KD, Kelley MF, Ilan J, Ilan J. The interleukin 2 gene is expressed in the syncytiotrophoblast of human placenta. *Proc Natl Acad Sci* 1989;86:656–660.
558. Soubiran PL, Zapitelli J-P, Schaffar L. IL-2-like material present in human placenta and amnion. *J Reprod Immunol* 1987;12: 225–234.
559. Tezabwala BU, Johnson PM, Rees RC. Inhibition of pregnancy viability in mice following IL-2 administration. *Immunology* 1989;67:115–119.
560. Athanassakis I, Bleackley C, Paetkan V, Guilbert L, Barr P, Wegmann TG. The immunostimulatory effect of T cells, and T cell lymphokines on murine fetally derived placental cells. *J Immunol* 1987;138:37–44.
561. Tabibzadeh SS, Poubouridis D, May LT, Sehgal PB. Interleukin-6 immunoreactivity in human tumors. *Am J Pathol* 1989;135: 427–433.
562. Nishino E, Matsuzaki N, Masuhiro K, et al. Trophoblast-derived interleukin-6 (IL-6) regulates human chorionic gonadotropin release through IL-6 receptor on human trophoblasts. *J Clin Endocrinol Metab* 1990;71:436–441.
563. Tabibzadeh SS, Gerber MA, Satyaswaroop PG. Induction of HLA-DR antigen expression in human endometrial epithelial cells *in vitro* by recombinant γ-interferon. *Am J Pathol* 1986;125:90–96.
564. Tabibzadeh SS, Pondichery G, Satyaswaroop PG, Rao PN. Antiproliferative effect of interferon-γ in human endometrial epithelial cells *in vitro:* potential local growth modulatory role in endometrium. *J Clin Endocrinol Metab* 1988;67:131–138.
565. Tabibzadeh SS, Kaffka KL, Kilian PL, Satyaswaroop PG. Human endometrial epithelial cell lines for studying steroid and cytokine actions *in vitro. Cell Dev Biol* 1990;26:1173–1179.
566. Tabibzadeh SS, Satyaswaroop PG. Differential expression of HLA-DR, HLA-DP, and HLA-DQ antigenic determinants of the major histocompatibility complex in human endometrium. *Am J Reprod Immunol Microbiol* 1988;18:124–130.
567. Klareskog L, Forsum U, Peterson PA. Hormonal regulation of the expression of Ia antigens on mammary gland epithelium. *Eur J Immunol* 1980;10:958–963.
568. Tabibzadeh SS, Bettica A, Gerber MA. Variable expression of Ia antigens in human endometrium and in chronic endometritis. *Am J Clin Pathol* 1986;86:153–160.
569. Tabibzadeh SS, Mortillo S, Gerber MA. Immunoultrastructural localization of Ia antigens in human endometrium. *Arch Pathol Lab Med* 1987;111:32–37.
570. Kamat BR, Isaacson PG. The immunocytochemical distribution of leukocytic subpopulations in human endometrium. *Am J Pathol* 1987;127:66–73.
571. Tabibzadeh SS. Evidence of T-cell activation and potential cytokine action in human endometrium. *J Clin Endocrinol Metab* 1990;71:645–649.
572. Tabibzadeh SS. Proliferative activity of lymphoid cells in human endometrium throughout the menstrual cycle. *J Clin Endocrinol Metab* 1990;70:437–443.
573. Morris H, Edwards J, Tiltman A, Emms M. Endometrial lymphoid tissue: an immunohistological study. *J Clin Pathol* 1985;38:644–652.
574. Padykula HA, Coles LG, McCracken JA, King NW Jr, Longcope C, Kaiserman-Abramof IR. A zonal pattern of cell proliferation and differentiation in the rhesus endometrium during the estrogen surge. *Biol Reprod* 1984;31:1103–1118.
575. Padykula HA, Coles LG, Okulicz WC, et al. The basalis of the primate endometrium: a bifunctional germinal compartment. *Biol Reprod* 1989;40:681–690.
576. Kaiserman-Abramof H, Padykula HA. Ultrastructural epithelial zonation of the primate endometrium (rhesus monkey). *Am J Anat* 1989;184:13–30.
577. Ferenczy A, Bertrand G, Gelfand MM. Proliferation kinetics of human endometrium during the normal menstrual cycle. *Am J Obstet Gynecol* 1979;133:859–866.
578. Tabibzadeh SS, Pondichery G, Satyaswaroop RG. Sex steroid receptors in lymphoid cells of human endometrium. *Am J Clin Pathol* 1989;91:656–663.
579. Casey ML, Cox SM, Beutler B, Milewich L, MacDonald PC. Cachectin/tumor necrosis factor-α formation in human decidual. Potential role of cytokines in infection-induced preterm labor. *J Clin Invest* 1989;83:430–436.
580. Jaattela M, Kuusela P, Saksela E. Demonstration of tumor necrosis factor in human amniotic fluids and supernatants of placental and decidual tissues. *Lab Invest* 1988;58:48–52.
581. Eades DK, Corneium P, Pekala PH. Characterization of tumor necrosis factor receptor in human placenta. *Placenta* 1988;9: 247–251.
582. So T, Ito A, Sato T, Mori Y, Hirakawa S. Tumor necrosis factor-α stimulates the biosynthesis of matrix metalloproteinases and plasminogen activator in cultured human chorionic cells. *Biol Reprod* 1992;46:772–778.
583. Gonzalez F, Lakshmanan J, Hoath S, Fisher DA. Effect of oestradiol-17β uterine epidermal growth factor concentration in immature mice. *Acta Endocrinol (Copenh)* 1984;105:425–428.
584. Mukku VR, Stancel GM. Receptors for epidermal growth factor in the rat uterus. *Endocrinology* 1985;117:149–154.
585. Mukku VR, Stancel GM. Regulation of epidermal growth factor receptor by estrogens. *J Biol Chem* 1985;260:9820–9824.
586. DiAugustine RP, Petrusz P, Bell GI, et al. Influence of estrogens on mouse uterine epidermal growth factor precursor protein and messenger ribonucleic acid. *Endocrinology* 1988;122:2355–2363.
587. Lingham RB, Stancel GM, Loose-Mitchell DS. Estrogen regulation of epidermal growth factor receptor messenger ribonucleic acid. *Mol Endocrinol* 1988;2:230–235.
588. Sheets EE, Tibris JCM, Cook NI, Virgin SD, Spellacy WN. *In vitro* binding of insulin and epidermal growth factor to human endometrium and endocervix. *Am J Obstet Gynecol* 1985;153: 60–65.

589. Hofmann GE, Rao CV, Barrow GH, Schultz GS, Sanfilippo JS. Binding sites for epidermal growth factor in human uterine tissues and leiomyomas. *J Clin Endocrinol Metab* 1984;58:880–884.
590. Sorrentino JM, Hendrix JC. EGF receptor binding studies in endometrial cell culture. *Life Sci* 1984;34:1769–1774.
591. Reynolds RK, Talavera F, Roberts JA, Hopkins MP, Menon KMJ. Characterization of epidermal growth factor receptor in normal and neoplastic human endometrium. *Cancer* 1990;66:1967–1974.
592. Huet-Hudson YM, Chakraborty C, De KS, Suzuki MY, Andrews GK, Dey SK. Estrogen regulates the synthesis of epidermal growth factor in mouse uterine epithelial cells. *Mol Endocrinol* 1990;4:510–523.
593. Chakraborty C, Tawfik OW, Dey SK. Epidermal growth factor binding in rat uterus during the peri-implantation period. *Biochem Biophys Res Commun* 1988;153:564–569.
594. Gardener RM, Verner G, Kirkland JL, Stancel GM. Regulation of uterine epidermal growth factor (EGF) receptors by estrogen in the mature rat and during the estrous cycle. *J Steroid Biochem* 1989;32:339–343.
595. Berchuck A, Soisson AP, Olt J, et al. Epidermal growth factor receptor expression in normal and malignant endometrium. *Am J Obstet Gynecol* 1989;161:1247–1252.
596. Chengini N, Rao CV, Wakin N, Sanfilippo J. Binding of ^{125}I-epidermal growth factor in human uterus. *Cell Tissue Res* 1986;246:543–548.
597. Damjanov I, Mildner B, Knowles BB. Immunohistochemical localization of the epidermal growth factor receptor in normal human tissues. *Lab Invest* 1986;55:588–592.
598. Brown MJ, Zogg JL, Schultz GS, Hilton FK. Increased binding of epidermal growth factor at preimplantation sites in mouse uteri. *Endocrinology* 1989;124:2882–2888.
599. Tomooka Y, DiAugustine RF, McLachlan JA. Proliferation of mouse uterine epithelial cells *in vitro*. *Endocrinology* 1986;118:1011–1018.
600. Sumida C, Lecerf F, Pasqualini J. Control of progesterone receptors in fetal uterine cells in culture: effects of estradiol, progestins, antiestrogens, and growth factors. *Endocrinology* 1988;122:3–11.
601. Gerschenson LE, Conner EA, Yang J, Anderson M. Hormonal regulation of proliferation in two populations of rabbit endometrial cells in culture. *Life Sci* 1979;24:1337–1343.
602. Nelson KG, Takahashi T, Bossert NL, Walmer DK, McLachlan JA. Epidermal growth factor replaces estrogen in the stimulation of female genital-tract growth and differentiation. *Proc Natl Acad Sci USA* 1991;88:21–25.
603. Smith WC, Talamantes F. Characterization of the mouse placental epidermal growth factor receptor: changes in receptor number with day of gestation. *Placenta* 1986;7:511–522.
604. Rapolee DA, Brenner CA, Schultz R, Mark D, Werb Z. Developmental expression of PDGF, TGF_α and TGF_β genes in preimplantation mouse embryos. *Science* 1988;241:1823–1825.
605. Goustin AS, Betsholtz C, Pfeifer-Ohlsson S, et al. Coexpression of the *sis* and *myc* protoncogenes in developing human placenta suggests autocrine control of trophoblast growth. *Cell* 1985;41:301–312.
606. Han VKM, Hunter S III, Pratt RM, Zendegui JG, Lee DC. Expression of rat transforming growth factor alpha mRNA during development occurs predominantly in the maternal decidua. *Mol Cell Biol* 1987;7:2335–2343.
607. Lee DC. TGF-alpha: expression and biological activities of the integral membrane precursor. *Mol Reprod Dev* 1990;27:37–45.
608. Tamada H, Das SK, Andrews GK, Dey SK. Cell-type-specific expression of transforming growth factor-α in the mouse uterus during the peri-implantation period. *Biol Reprod* 1991;45:365–372.
609. Frolik CA, Dart LL, Meyers CA, Smith DM, Sporn MB. Purification and initial characterization of a type β transforming growth factor from human placenta. *Proc Natl Acad Sci USA* 1983;80:3676–3680.
610. Tamada H, McMaster MT, Flanders KC, Andrew GK, Dey SK. Cell type-specific expression of transforming growth factor-β-1 in the mouse uterus during the peri-implantation period. *Mol Endocrinol* 1990;4:965–972.
611. Altman DJ, Schnieder SL, Thompson DA, Cheng H-L, Tomasi TB. A transforming growth factor β_2 (TGF-β_2)-like-immunosuppressive factor in amniotic fluid and localization of TGF-β_2 in the pregnant uterus. *J Exp Med* 1990;172:1391–1401.
612. Lea RG, Flanders KC, Harley CB, Manuel J, Banwatt D, Clark DA. Release of a transforming growth factor (TGF)-β_2-related suppressor factor from post-implantation murine decidual tissue can be correlated with the detection of a subpopulation of cells containing RNA for TGF-β_2. *J Immunol* 1992;148:778–787.
613. Miyazono K, Yuki K, Takaku F, et al. Latent forms of TGF-β: structure and biology. *Ann NY Acad Sci* 1990;593:51–58.
614. Roberts AB, Kim S-J, Kondiah P, et al. Transcriptional control of expression of the TGF-βs. *Ann NY Acad Sci* 1990;593:43–50.
615. Twardzik DR, Mikovits JA, Ranchalis JE, Purchio AF, Ellingworth L, Ruscetti FW. γ-Interferon-induced of latent transforming growth factor-β by human monocytes. *Ann NY Acad Sci* 1990;593:276–284.
616. Akhurst RJ, Lehnert SA, Gatherer D, Duffie E. The role of TGF-β in mouse development. *Ann NY Acad Sci* 1990;593:259–271.
617. Clark DA, Flanders KC, Banwatt D, et al. Murine pregnancy decidua produces a unique immunosuppressive molecule related to transforming growth factor β-2. *J Immunol* 1990;144:3008–3014.
618. Bradley TR, Stanley ER, Summer MA. Factors from mouse tissues stimulating colony growth of mouse bone marrow cells *in vitro*. *Aust J Exp Biol Med Sci* 1971;49:595–603.
619. Rosendaal M. Colony-stimulating factor (CSF) in the uterus of the pregnant mouse. *J Cell Sci* 1975;19:411–423.
620. Bartocci A, Pollard JW, Stanley ER. Regulation of colony stimulating factor-1 during pregnancy. *J Exp Med* 1986;164:956–961.
621. Arceci RJ, Shanhan F, Stanley ER, Pollard JW. Temporal expression and location of colony stimulating factor 1 (CSF-1) and its receptor in the female reproductive tract are consistent with CSF-1 regulated placental development. *Proc Natl Acad Sci USA* 1989;86:8818–8822.
622. Azuma C, Saji F, Kimura T, et al. Steroid hormones induce macrophage colony stimulation factor (Mcsf) and Mcsf receptor messenger RNAs in the human endometrium. *J Mol Endocrinol* 1990;5:103–110.
623. Pollard JW, Bartocci A, Areci R, Orlofsky A, Lander MB, Stanley ER. Apparent role of the macrophage factor, CSF-1 placental development. *Nature* 1987;330:484–486.
624. Regenstreif LJ, Rossant J. Expression of the c-*fms* proto-oncogene and of the cytokine, CSF-1 during mouse embryogenesis. *Dev Biol* 1989;133:284–294.
625. Muller R, Slamon DJ, Adamson ED, et al. Transcription of c-Onc genes c-*ras*^{ki} and c-*fms* during mouse development. *Mol Cell Biol* 1983;3:1062–1069.
626. Muller R, Verma IM, Adamson ED. Expression of c-Onc genes: c-*fos* transcripts accumulate to high levels during development of mouse placenta, yolk sac and amnion. *EMBO J* 1983;2:679–684.
627. Hosina M, Nishio A, Bo M, Boime I, Mochizuki M. The expression of the oncogene fms in human chorionic tissue. *Acta Obstet Gynecol Jpn* 1985;27:2791–2798.
628. Pollard JW, Hunt JS, Wiktor-Jedrzejczak W, Stanley ER. A pregnancy deficit in the osteopetrotic (op/op) mouse demonstrates the requirement for CSF-1 in female fertility. *Dev Biol* 1991;148:273–283.
629. Tartakovsky B, Goldstein O, Brosh N. [a] Colony-stimulating factor-1 blocks early pregnancy in mice. *Biol Reprod* 1991;44:906–912.
630. Wegman TG, Athanassakis I, Branch D, Dy M, Menu E, Chaouat G. The role of M-CSF and GM-CSF in fostering placental growth, fetal growth, and fetal survival. *Transplant Proc* 1988;21:566–568.
631. Murphy LJ, Murphy LC, Friesen HG. Estrogen induces insulin-like growth factor-I expression in the rat uterus. *Mol Endocrinol* 1988;1:445–450.
632. Norstedt G, Levinovitz A, Eriksson H. Regulation of uterine insulinlike growth factor I mRNA and insulinlike growth factor II mRNA by estrogen in the rat. *Act Endocrinol (Copenh)* 1989;120:466–472.
633. Murphy LJ, Bell GI, Friesen HG. Tissue distribution of insulin-

like growth factor I and II messenger ribonucleic acid in the adult rat. *Endocrinology* 1987;120:1279–1282.
634. Murphy LJ, Ghahary A. Uterine insulinlike growth factor-1: regulation of expression and its role in estrogen-induced uterine proliferation. *Endocr Rev* 1990;11:443–453.
635. Ghahary A, Chakrabarti S, Murphy LJ. Localization of the sites of synthesis and action of insulin-like growth factor-I in the rat uterus. *Mol Endocrinol* 1990;4:191–195.
636. Wang C-Y, Daimon M, Shen S-J, Engelmann GL, Ilan J. Insulinlike growth factor-I messenger ribonucleic acid in the developing human placenta and in term placenta of diabetics. *Mol Endocrinol* 1988;2:217–229.
637. Ohlsson R, Holmgren L, Glaser A, Szpecht A, Pfeifer-Ohlsson S. Insulinlike growth factor 2 and short-range stimulating loops in control of human placental growth. *EMBO J* 1989;8:1993–1999.
638. Fant M, Munro H, Moses AC. An autocrine/paracrine role for insulinlike growth factors in the regulation of human placental growth. *J Clin Endocrinol Metab* 1986;63:499–505.
639. Simmen RCM, Simmen FA, Ko Y, Bazer FW. Differential growth factor content of uterine luminal fluids from large white and prolific meishan pigs during the estrous cycle and early pregnancy. *J Anim Sci* 1989;67:1538–1545.
640. Kapur S, Tamada H, Dey SK, Andrews GK. Expression of insulinlike growth factor-I (IGF-I) and its receptor in the peri-implantation mouse uterus, and cell-specific regulation of IGF-I gene expression by estradiol and progesterone. *Biol Reprod* 1992;46:208–219.
641. Schoenle E, Zapf J, Humbel RE, Foresch ER. Insulinlike growth factor I stimulates growth in hypophysectomized rats. *Nature* 1982;296:252–253.
642. Simmen RCM, Simmen FA, Hofig A, Farmer SJ, Bazer FW. Hormonal regulation of insulinlike growth factor gene expression in the pig uterus. *Endocrinology* 1990;127:2166–2174.
643. Ohlsson R, Larsson E, Nilsson O, Wahlstrom T, Sundstrom P. Blastocyst implantation procedes induction of insulinlike growth factor II gene expression in human trophoblasts. *Development* 1989;106:555–559.
644. Letcher R, Simmen RCM, Bazer FW, Simmen FA. Insulinlike growth factor-I expression during early conceptus development in the pig. *Biol Reprod* 1989;41:1143–1151.
645. Tommala P, Pekonen F, Rutanen EM. Binding of epidermal growth factor and insulinlike growth factor I in human myometrium and leiomata. *Obstet Gynecol* 1989;74:658–662.
646. Chandrasekhar Y, Marayan S, Singh P, Nagamani M. Binding of insulinlike growth factor-I to rat uterus: variations during sensitization and decidualization. *Acta Endocrinol (Copenh)* 1990; 123:243–250.
647. Ghahary A, Murphy LJ. Regulation of uterine insulinlike growth factor receptors by estrogen and variation throughout the estrous cycle. *Endocrinology* 1989;125:597–604.
648. Mattson BA, Rosenblum IY, Smith KM, Heyner S. Autoradiographic evidence for insulin and insulinlike growth factor binding to early mouse embryos. *Diabetes* 1988;37:585–589.
649. Nestler JE. Insulin and insulinlike growth factor-I stimulate the 3β-hydroxysteroid dehydrogenase activity of human placental cytotrophoblasts. *Endocrinology* 1989;125:2127–2133.
650. Fazleabas AT, Jaffe RC, Verhage HG, Waites G, Bell SC. An insulinlike growth factor-binding protein in the baboon (*Popio anutuis*) endometrium: synthesis, immunocytochemical localization, and hormonal regulation. *Endocrinology* 1989;124: 2321–2329.
651. Waites GT, James RFL, Bells SC. Immunohistochemical localization of the human endometrial secretory protein pregnancy-associated endometrial a1-globulin, an insulinlike growth factor-binding protein, during the menstrual cycle. *J Clin Endocrinol Metab* 1988;67:1100–1104.
652. Bell SC, Patel SR, Jackson JA, Waites GT. Major secretory protein of human decidualized endometrium in pregnancy is an insulinlike growth factor-binding protein. *J Endocrinol* 1988; 118:317–328.
653. Elgin RG, Busby WH Jr, Clemmons DR. An insulinlike growth factor (IGF) binding protein enhances the biological response to IGF-1. *Proc Natl Acad Sci USA* 1987;84:3254–3258.
654. Rutanen E-M, Pekonen F, Makinen T. Soluble 34k binding protein inhibits the binding of insulingrowth factor I to its cell receptors in human secretory phase endometrium: evidence for autocrin/paracrine regulation of growth factor action. *J Clin Endocrinol Metab* 1988;66:173–180.
655. Bhatt H, Brunet LJ, Stewart CI. Uterine expression of leukemia inhibitory factor coincides with the onset of blastocyst implantation. *Proc Natl Acad Sci USA* 1991;88:11408–11412.
656. Stewart CL, Kaspar P, Brunet LJ, et al. Blastocyst implantation depends on maternal expression of leukemia inhibitory factor. *Nature* 1992;359:76–79.
657. Rosen H, Itin A, Schiff R, Keshet E. Local regulation within the female reproductive tract and upon embryonic implantation: identification of cells expressing proenkephalin A. *Mol Endocrinol* 1990;4:146–154.
658. Shelesnyak MC. Inhibition of decidual cell formation in the pseudopregnant rat by histamine antagonists. *Am J Physiol* 1952;170:522–527.
659. Shelesnyak MC. Some experimental studies on the mechanism of ovo-implantation in the rat. *Recent Prog Horm Res* 1957;13: 269–317.
660. Kraicer PF, Shelesnyak MC. The induction of deciduomata in the pseudopregnant rat by systemic administration of histamine and histamine releasers. *J Endocrinol* 1958;17:324–328.
661. Shelesnyak MC. Fall in uterine histamine associated with ovum implantation in pregnant rat. *Proc Soc Exp Biol Med* 1959;100:380–381.
662. Spaziani E, Szego CM. The influence of estradiol and cortisol on uterine histamine of the ovariectomized rat. *Endocrinology* 1958;63:669–678.
663. Spaziani E, Szego CM. Further evidence for mediation by histamine of estrogenic stimulation of the rat uterus. *Endocrinology* 1959;64:713–723.
664. Humphrey KW, Martin L. Attempted induction of deciduomata in mice with mast-cell, capillary permeability and tissue inflammatory factors. *J Endocrinol* 1968;42:129–141.
665. Wrenn TR, Bitman J, Cecil HC, Gilliam DR. Uterine deciduomata: role of histamine. *J Endocrinol* 1964;28:149–152.
666. Finn CA, Keen PM. Influence of systemic antihistamines on formation of deciduoma. *J Endocrinol* 1962;24:381–382.
667. Harper MJK. Failure of various antihistiminic drugs to prevent implantation in rats. *J Reprod Fertil* 1965;9:359–361.
668. Finn CA, Keen PM. Failure of histamine to induce deciduomata in the rat. *Nature* 1962;194:602–603.
669. Banik UK, Ketchel MM. Inability of histamine to induce deciduomata in pregnant rats and pseudopregnant rats. *J Reprod Fertil* 1964;7:259–261.
670. Brandon JM, Wallis RM. Effect of mepyramine, a histamine H_1-, and burinamide, a histamine H_2-receptor antagonist, on ovum implantation in the rat. *J Reprod Fertil* 1977;50:251–254.
671. Dey SK, Villanueva C, Abdou NI. Histamine receptors on rabbit blastocyst and endometrial cell membranes. *Nature* 1979;278: 648–649.
672. Brandon JM, Raval PJ. Interaction of estrogen and histamine during ovum implantation in the rat. *Eur J Pharmacol* 1979;57:171–177.
673. Brandon JM. Some recent work on the role of histamine in ovum implantation. In: Leroy F, Finn CA, Psychoyos A, Hubinont P, eds. *Blastocyst-Endometrium Relationships, Progress in Reproductive Biology,* Vol 7. New York: S Karger, 1980;244–252.
674. Ferrando G, Nalbandov AV. Relative importance of histamine and estrogen on implantation in rats. *Endocrinology* 1968;83: 933–937.
675. Dey SK, Villanueva C, Chien SM, Crist RD. The role of histamine in implantation in the rabbit. *J Reprod Fertil* 1978;53: 23–26.
676. Kennedy TG. Embryonic signals and initiation of blastocyst implantation. *Aust J Biol Sci* 1983;36:531–543.
677. Kennedy TG, Armstrong DT. The role of prostaglandins in endometrial vascular changes at implantation. In: Glasser SR, Bullock DW, eds. *Cellular and Molecular Aspects of Implantation.* New York: Plenum Press, 1981;349–363.
678. Lau IF, Saksena SK, Chang MC. Pregnancy blockade by indomethacin, an inhibitor of prostaglandin synthesis: its reversal by

prostaglandins and progesterone in mice. *Prostaglandins* 1973;4:795–803.
679. Holmes PV, Gordashko BJ. Evidence of prostaglandin involvement in blastocyst implantation. *J Embryol Exp Morphol* 1980;55:109–122.
680. Gavin MA, Dominguez Fernandez-Tejerina JC, Montanes de las Heras MF, Vijil Maeso E. Efectos de un inhibidor de la biosintesis de las prostglandinas (indometacina) sobre la implantacion en la rata. *Reproduccion* 1974;1:177–186.
681. Kennedy TG. Evidence for a role for prostaglandins in the initiation of blastocyst implantation in the rat. *Biol Reprod* 1977;16:286–291.
682. Phillips CA, Poyser NL. Studies on the involvement of prostaglandin in implantation in the rat. *J Reprod Fertil* 1981;62:73–81.
683. Evans CA, Kennedy TG. The importance of prostaglandin synthesis for the initiation of blastocyst implantation in the hamster. *J Reprod Fertil* 1978;54:255–261.
684. Hoffman LH. Antifertility effects of indomethacin during early pregnancy in the rabbit. *Biol Reprod* 1978;18:148–153.
685. Kennedy TG. Prostaglandins and increased endometrial vascular permeability resulting from the application of an artificial stimulus to the uterus of the rat sensitized for the decidual cell reaction. *Biol Reprod* 1979;20:560–566.
686. Hoffman LH, DiPietro DL, McKenna TJ. Effects of indomethacin on uterine capillary permeability and blastocyst development in rabbits. *Prostaglandins* 1978;15:823–829.
687. Hoos PC, Hoffman LH. The effect of histamine receptor antagonists and indomethacin on implantation in the rabbit. *Biol Reprod* 1983;29:833–840.
688. Saksena SK, Lau IF, Chang MC. Relationship between oestrogen, prostaglandin F_{2a} and histamine in delayed implantation in the mouse. *Acta Endocrinol* 1976;81:801–807.
689. Castracane VD, Saksena SK, Shaikh AA. Effect of IUDs, prostaglandins and indomethacin on decidual cell reaction in the rat. *Prostaglandins* 1974;6:397–404.
690. Sananes N, Baulieu EE, LeGoascogne C. Prostaglandin(s) as inductive factor of decidualization in the rat uterus. *Mol Cell Endocrinol* 1976;6:153–160.
691. Tobert JA. A study of the possible role for prostaglandins in decidualization using a nonsurgical method for the instillation of fluids into the rat uterine lumen. *J Reprod Fertil* 1976;47:391–393.
692. Rankin JC, Ledford BE, Jonsson HT, Baggett B. Prostaglandins, indomethacin and the decidual cell reaction in the mouse uterus. *Biol Reprod* 1979;20:399–404.
693. Miller MM, O'Morchoe CCC. Decidual cell reaction induced by prostaglandin F_{2a} in the mature oophorectomized rat. *Cell Tissue Res* 1982;225:189–199.
694. Kennedy TG, Lukash LA. Induction of decidualization in rats by the intrauterine infusion of prostaglandins. *Biol Reprod* 1982;27:253–260.
695. Kennedy TG. Timing of uterine sensitivity for the decidual cell reaction: role of prostaglandins. *Biol Reprod* 1980;22:519–525.
696. Jonsson HT, Rankin JC, Ledford BE, Baggett B. Uterine prostaglandin levels following stimulation of the decidual cell reaction: effects of indomethacin and tranylcypromine. *Prostaglandins* 1979;18:847–857.
697. Kennedy TG. Estrogen and uterine sensitization for the decidual cell reaction: role of prostaglandins. *Biol Reprod* 1980;23:955–962.
698. Kennedy TG, Zamecnik J. The concentration of 6-keto-prostaglandin F_{1a} is markedly elevated at the site of blastocyst implantation in the rat. *Prostaglandins* 1978;16:599–605.
699. Hoffmann LH, Davenport GR, Brash AR. Endometrial prostaglandins and phospholipase activity related to implantation in rabbits: effects of dexamethasone. *Biol Reprod* 1984;30:544–555.
700. Miller MM, O'Morchoe CCC. Inhibition of artificially induced decidual cell reaction by indomethacin in the mature oopherectomized rat. *Anat Rec* 1982;204:223–230.
701. Hoffman LH, Strong GB, Davenport GR, Frolich JC. Deciduogenic effect of prostaglandins in the pseudopregnant rabbit. *J Reprod Fertil* 1977;50:231–237.
702. Kennedy TG, Martel D, Psychoyos A. Endometrial prostaglandin E_2 binding: characterization in rats sensitized for decidual cell reaction and changes during pseudopregnancy. *Biol Reprod* 1983;29:556–564.
703. Martel D, Kennedy TG, Moneir MN, Psychoyos A. Failure to detect binding sites for prostaglandin F-2_a in membrane preparations from rat endometrium. *J Reprod Fertil* 1985;75:265–274.
704. Kennedy TG, Martel D, Psychoyos A. Endometrial prostaglandin E_2 binding during the estrous cycle and its hormonal control in ovariectomized rats. *Biol Reprod* 1983;29:565–571.
705. Peleg S, Lindner HR. The effect of prostaglandins on progestin receptor translocation and on decidual cell reaction *in vivo* and *in vitro*. *Endocrinology* 1982;110:1647–1652.
706. Leroy F, Vansande J, Shetgen G, Brasseur D. Cyclic AMP and triggering of the decidual reaction. *J Reprod Fertil* 1974;39:207–211.
707. Rankin JC, Ledford BE, Baggett B. Early involvement of cyclic nucleotides in the artificially stimulated decidual cell reaction in the mouse uterus. *Biol Reprod* 1977;17:549–554.
708. Kennedy TG. Prostaglandin E_2, adenosine 3′:5′-cyclic monophosphate and changes in endometrial vascular permeability in rat uterus sensitized for decidual cell reaction. *Biol Reprod* 1983;29:1069–1076.
709. Johnston MEA, Kennedy TG. Estrogen and uterine sensitization for the decidual cell reaction in the rat: role of prostaglandin E_2, and adenosine 3′:5-cyclic monophosphate. *Biol Reprod* 1984;31:959–966.
710. Alleua JJ, Kenimer JG, Jordan AW, Lamanna C. Induction of estrogen and progesterone receptors and decidualization in the hamster uterus of cholera toxin. *Endocrinology* 1983;11:2095–2106.
711. Webb FTG. The inability of dibutyryl adenosine 3′,-5′-monophosphate to induce the decidual reaction in intact pseudopregnant mice. *J Reprod Fertil* 1975;42:187–188.
712. Webb FTG. Implantation in ovariectomized mice treated with dibutyryl adenosine 3′,5′-monophosphate (dibutyryl cyclic AMP). *J Reprod Fertil* 1975;42:511–517.
713. Holmes PV, Bergstrom S. Induction of blastocyst implantation in mice by cyclic AMP. *J Reprod Fertil* 1975;43:329–332.
714. Heap RB, Flint APF, Gadsby JE, Rice C. Hormones, the early embryo and the uterine environment. *J Reprod Fertil* 1979;55:267–275.
715. Flint APF, Burton RD, Gadsby JE, Saunders PTK, Heap RB. Blastocyst estrogen synthesis and the maternal recognition of pregnancy. In: *Maternal Recognition of Pregnancy.* CIBA Foundation Symposium No. 64 (new series). New York: Excerpta Medica, 1979;209–238.
716. Atkinson LE, Hotchkiss J, Fritz GR, Surve AH, Neill JD, Knobil E. Circulating levels of steroids and chorionic gonadotropin during pregnancy in the rhesus monkey, with special attention to the rescue of the corpus luteum in early pregnancy. *Biol Reprod* 1975;12:335–345.
717. Blandau RJ. Embryo–endometrial interrelationship in the rat and guinea pig. *Anat Rec* 1949;104:331–360.
718. Alden RH, Smith MJ. Implantation of the rat egg. IV. Some effects of artificial ova on the uterus. *J Exp Zool* 1959;142:215–226.
719. McLaren A. Can beads stimulate a decidual response in the mouse uterus? *J Reprod Fertil* 1968;15:313–315.
720. Cole RJ. Cinemicrographic observations on the trophoblast and zona pellucida of the mouse blastocyst. *J Embryol Exp Morphol* 1967;17:481–490.
721. Bitton-Casimiri V, Brun J-L, Psychoyos A. Comportement *in vitro* des blastocysts du 5[e] jour de la gestation chez la ratte; etude microcinematographique. *C R Acad Sci Paris Ser D* 1970;270:2979–2982.
722. Lejeune B, Van Hoeck J, Leroy F. Transmitter role of the luminal uterine epithelium in the induction of decidualization in rats. *J Reprod Fertil* 1981;61:235–240.
723. Boving BG. Implantation. *Ann NY Acad Sci* 1959;75:700–725.
724. Boving BG. Implantation mechanisms. In: Hartman CG, ed. *Mechanisms Concerned with Conception.* New York: Pergamon Press, 1963;321–396.
725. Hetherington CM. Induction of deciduomata in the mouse by carbon dioxide. *Nature* 1968;219:863–864.
726. Huff RL, Eik-Nes KB. Metabolism *in vitro* of acetate and certain

steroids by six-day-old rabbit blastocysts. *J Reprod Fertil* 1966;11:57–63.

727. Dickmann Z, Dey SK. Two theories: the preimplantation embryo is a source of steroid hormones controlling (1) morula-blastocyst transformation, and (2) implantation. *J Reprod Fertil* 1973;35:615–617.
728. Heap RB, Flint APF, Gadsby JE. Embryonic signals and maternal recognition. In: Glasser SR, Bullock DW, eds. *Cellular and Molecular Aspects of Implantation.* New York: Plenum Press, 1981;311–325.
729. Sauer MJ. Hormone involvement in the establishment of pregnancy. *J Reprod Fertil* 1979;56:725–743.
730. Perry JS, Heap RB, Amoroso EC. Steroid hormone production by pig blastocysts. *Nature* 1973;245:45–47.
731. Perry JS, Heap RB, Burton RD, Gadsby JE. Endocrinology of the blastocyst and its role in the establishment of pregnancy. *J Reprod Fertil* 1976;25(suppl):85–104.
732. Gadsby JE, Heap RB, Burton RD. Oestrogen production by blastocyst and early embryonic tissue of various species. *J Reprod Fertil* 1980;60:409–417.
733. Gadsby JE, Burton RD, Heap RB, Perry JS. Steroid metabolism and synthesis in early embryonic tissue of pig, sheep, and cow. *J Endocrinol* 1976;71:45P–46P.
734. Fischer HE, Bazer FW, Fields MJ. Steroid metabolism of endometrial and conceptus tissues during early pregnancy and pseudopregnancy in gilts. *J Reprod Fertil* 1985;75:69–78.
735. Flood DF. Steroid-metabolizing enzymes in the early pig conceptus and in the related endometrium. *J Endocrinol* 1974;63: 413–414.
736. Heap RB, Flint APF, Hartmann PE, et al. Oestrogen production in early pregnancy. *J Endocrinol* 1981;89:77–94
737. Dhindsa DS, Dziuk PJ. Effect of pregnancy in the pig after filling embryos or fetuses in one uterine horn in early gestation. *J Anim Sci* 1968;27:122–126.
738. Bazer FW, Thatcher WW. Theory of maternal recognition of pregnancy in swine based on estrogen controlled endocrine versus exocrine secretion of prostaglandin F_{2a} by uterine endometrium. *Prostaglandins* 1977;14:397–401.
739. Frank M, Bazer FW, Thatcher WW, Wilcox CJ. A study of prostaglandin F_2 as the leuteolysin in swine. III. Effects of estradiol valerate on prostaglandin F, progestins, estrone, and estradiol concentrations in the utero-ovarian vein of nonpregnant gilts. *Prostaglandins* 1977;14:1183–1196.
740. Moeljono MPE, Thatcher WW, Bazer FW, Frank M, Owens LJ, Wilcox CJ. A study of prostaglandin F_{2a} as the leuteolysin in swine. II. Characterization and comparison of prostaglandin F, estrogens and progestin concentrations in utero-ovarian vein plasma of nonpregnant and pregnant gilts. *Prostaglandins* 1977;14:543–555.
741. Zavy MT, Bazer FW, Thatcher WW, Wilcox CJ. A study of prostaglandin $F_{2\text{-}a}$ as the leuteolysin in swine. V. Comparison of prostaglandin F, progestins, estrone and estradiol in uterine flushings from pregnant and nonpregnant gilts. *Prostaglandins* 1980;20: 837–851.
742. Heap RB, Perry JS, Gadsby JE, Burton KD. Endocrine activities of the blastocyst and early embryonic tissue in the pig. *Biochem Soc Trans* 1975;3:1183–1188.
743. Mondschein JS, Hersey RM, Dey SK, Davis DL, Weisz J. Catechol estrogen formation by pig blastocyst during the preimplantation period: biochemical characterization of estrogen-2/4-dioxylase and correlation with aromatase activity. *Endocrinology* 1985;117:2339–2346.
744. Hoeversland RC, Dey SK, Johnson DC. Catechol estradiol induced implantation in the mouse. *Life Sci* 1982;30:1801–1804.
745. Pakrasi PL, Dey SK. Catechol estrogens stimulate synthesis of prostaglandin in the preimplantation rabbit blastocyst and endometrium. *Biol Reprod* 1983;29:347–354.
746. Stone BA, Seamark RF. Steroid hormones in uterine washings and in plasma of gilts between days 9 and 15 after oestrus and between days 9 and 15 after coitus. *J Reprod Fertil* 1985;75: 209–221.
747. Dickmann Z, Dey SK, Sengupta J. Steroidogenesis in rabbit preimplantation embryos. *Proc Natl Acad Sci USA* 1975;72: 298–300.
748. Dickmann Z, Dey SK, Sengupta J. A new concept: control of early pregnancy by steroid hormones originating in the preimplantation embryo. *Vitam Horm* 1976;34:215–242.
749. Bleau G. Failure to detect Δ^5-3β-hydroxysteroid oxidoreductase activity in the preimplantation rabbit embryo. *Steroids* 1981;37: 121–132.
750. Seamark RF, Lutwak-Mann C. Progestins in rabbit blastocysts. *J Reprod Fertil* 1972;29:147–148.
751. Fuchs AR, Beling C. Evidence for early ovarian recognition of blastocysts in rabbits. *Endocrinology* 1974;95:1054–1058.
752. Borland RM, Erickson GF, Ducibella T. Accumulation of steroids in rabbit preimplantation blastocysts. *J Reprod Fertil* 1977;49:219–224.
753. Singh MM, Booth WD. Studies on the metabolism of neutral steroids by preimplantation rabbit blastocysts *in vitro* and the origin of blastocyst oestrogen. *J Reprod Fertil* 1978;53:297–304.
754. Fujimoto S, Sundaram K. The source of progesterone in rabbit blastocysts. *J Reprod Fertil* 1978;52:231–233.
755. Bullock DW. Steroids from the pre-implantation blastocyst. In: Johnson MH, ed. *Development in Mammals,* Vol 2. New York: North-Holland, 1977;199–208.
756. George FW, Wilson JD. Estrogen formation in the early rabbit embryo. *Science* 1978;199:200–201.
757. Hoversland RC, Dey SK, Johnson DC. Aromatase activity in the rabbit blastocyst. *J Reprod Fertil* 1982;66:259–263.
758. Wu J-T, Lin GM. Effect of aromatase inhibitor on oestrogen production in rabbit blastocysts. *J Reprod Fertil* 1982;66: 655–662.
759. Bhatt BM, Bullock DW. Binding of oestradiol to rabbit blastocysts and its possible role in implantation. *J Reprod Fertil* 1974;39:65–70.
760. Dey SK, Dickmann Z, Sengupta J. Evidence that the maintenance of early pregnancy in the rabbit requires "blastocyst estrogen." *Steroids* 1976;28:481–485.
761. Sengupta J, Roy SK, Manchanda SK. Hormonal control of implantation: a possible role of lysosomal function in the embryo–uterus interaction. *J Steroid Biochem* 1979;11:729–744.
762. Wise T, Heap RB. Effects of the embryo upon endometrial estrogen synthesis in the rabbit. *Biol Reprod* 1983;28:1097–1106.
763. Dey SK, Dickmann Z. Estradiol-17β-hydroxysteroid dehydrogenase activity in preimplantation rat embryos. *Steroids* 1974;24: 57–62.
764. Dey SK, Dickmann Z. Δ^5-3β-Hydroxysteroid dehydrogenase activity in rat embryos on days 1 through 7 of pregnancy. *Endocrinology* 1974;95:321–322.
765. Dickmann Z, Dey SK. Steroidogenesis in the preimplantation rat embryo and its possible influence on morula-blastocyst transformation and implantation. *J Reprod Fertil* 1974;37:91–93.
766. Dickmann Z, Dey SK. Evidence that Δ^5-3β-Hydroxysteroid dehydrogenase activity in rat blastocysts is autonomous. *J Endocrinol* 1974;61:513–514.
767. Dickmann Z, Sengupta J. Δ^5-3β-Hydroxysteroid dehydrogenase activity in preimplantation hamster embryos. *Dev Biol* 1974;40: 196–198.
768. Dickmann Z, Sengupta J, Dey SS. Does 'blastocyst estrogen' initiate implantation? *Science* 1977;195:687–688.
769. Sengupta J, Dey SK, Dickmann Z. Is mouse preimplantation embryogenesis controlled by estrogen originating in the preimplantation embryo? *Anat Rec* 1977;187:709 (abst).
770. Sengupta J, Roy SK, Manchanda SK. Effect of an anti-oestrogen on implantation of mouse blastocysts. *J Reprod Fertil* 1981;62: 433–436.
771. Chew NJ, Sherman MI. Biochemistry of differentiation of mouse trophoblast: Δ^5,3β-hydroxysteroid dehydrogenase. *Biol Reprod* 1975;12:351–359.
772. Sherman MI, Atienza SB. Production and metabolism of progesterone and androstenedione by cultured mouse blastocysts. *Biol Reprod* 1977;16:190–199.
773. Marcal JM, Chew NJ, Salomon DS, Sherman MI. Δ^5,β-Hydroxysteroid dehydrogenase activities in rat trophoblast and ovary during pregnancy. *Endocrinology* 1975;96:1270–1279.
774. Antila E, Koskinen J, Niemela P, Saure A. Steroid metabolism by mouse preimplantation embryos *in vitro*. *Experientia* 1977;33: 1374–1375.

775. Niimura S, Ishida K. Histochemical studies of Δ^5-3β-,20α- and 20β-hydroxysteroid dehydrogenases and possible progestagen production in hamster eggs. *J Reprod Fertil* 1976;48:275–278.
776. Brodie AMH, Wu JT, Marsh DA, Brodie HJ. Aromatase inhibitors. III. Studies on the antifertility effect of 4-acetoxy-4-androstene-3,17-dione. *Biol Reprod* 1978;18:365–370.
777. Evans CA, Kennedy TG. Blastocyst implantation in ovariectomized, adrenalectomized hamsters treated with inhibitors of steroidogenesis during the pre-implantation period. *Steroids* 1980;36:41–52.
778. Zavy MT, Mayer R, Vernon MW, Bazer FW, Sharp DC. An investigation of the uterine lumenal environment of non-pregnant and pregnant pony mares. *J Reprod Fertil* 1979;27 (suppl):403–411.
779. Dey SK, Johnson DC, Santos JG. Is histamine production by the blastocyst required for implantation in the rabbit? *Biol Reprod* 1979;21:1169–1173.
780. Dey SK, Johnson DC. Histamine formation by mouse preimplantation embryos. *J Reprod Fertil* 1980;60:457–460.
781. Dey SK. Role of histamine in implantation: inhibition of histidine decarboxylase induces delayed implantation in the rabbit. *Biol Reprod* 1981;24:867–869.
782. Johnson DC, Dey SK. Role of histamine in implantation: dexamethasone inhibits estradiol-induced implantation in the rat. *Biol Reprod* 1980;22:1136–1141.
783. Racowsky C, Biggers JD. Are blastocyst prostaglandins produced endogenously? *Biol Reprod* 1983;29:379–388.
784. Dickmann Z, Spilman CH. Prostaglandins in rabbit blastocysts. *Science* 1975;190:997–998.
785. Dey SK, Chien SM, Cox CL, Crist RD. Prostaglandin synthesis in the rabbit blastocyst. *Prostaglandins* 1980;19:449–453.
786. Harper MJ, Norris CJ, Rajkumar K. Prostaglandin release by zygotes and endometria of pregnant rabbits. *Biol Reprod* 1983;28:350–362.
787. Pakrasi PL, Dey SK. Blastocyst is the source of prostaglandins in the implantation site in the rabbit. *Prostaglandins* 1982;24:73–77.
788. Shemesh M, Milaguir F, Ayalon N, Hansel W. Steroidogenesis and prostaglandin synthesis by cultured bovine blastocysts. *J Reprod Fertil* 1979;56:181–185.
789. Lewis GS, Thatcher WW, Bazer FW, Curl JS. Metabolism of arachidonic acid *in vitro* by bovine blastocysts and endometrium. *Biol Reprod* 1982;27:431–439.
790. Biggers JD, Leonov BV, Baskar JF, Fried J. Inhibition of hatching of mouse blastocysts *in vitro* by prostaglandin antagonists. *Biol Reprod* 1978;19:519–533.
791. Baskar JF, Torchiana DF, Biggers JD, Corey EJ, Andersen NH, Subramanian N. Inhibition of hatching of mouse blastocysts *in vitro* by various prostaglandin antagonists. *J Reprod Fertil* 1981;63:359–363.
792. Hurst PR, MacFarlane DW. Further effects of nonsteroidal anti-inflammatory compounds on blastocyst hatching *in vitro* and implantation rates in the mouse. *Biol Reprod* 1981;25:777–784.
793. Biggers JD, Baskar JF, Torchiana DF. Reduction of fertility of mice by the intrauterine injection of prostaglandin antagonists. *J Reprod Fertil* 1981;63:365–372.
794. Marcus GJ. Prostaglandin formation by the sheep embryo and endometrium as indication of maternal recognition of pregnancy. *Biol Reprod* 1981;25:56–64.
795. Hyland JH, Manns JG, Humphrey WD. Prostaglandin production by ovine embryos and endometrium *in vitro*. *J Reprod Fertil* 1982;65:299–304.
796. Lacroix MC, Kann G. Comparative studies of prostaglandins F_{2a} and E_2 in late cyclic and early pregnant sheep: *in vitro* synthesis by endometrium and conceptuses. Effects of *in vivo* indomethacin treatment on establishment of pregnancy. *Prostaglandins* 1982;23:507–526.
797. Moor RM, Rowson LEA. Influence of the embryo and uterus on luteal function in the sheep. *Nature* 1964;201:522–523.
798. Moor RM, Rowson LEA. The corpus luteum of the sheep: functional relationship between the embryo and the corpus luteum. *J Endocrinol* 1966;34:233–239.
799. Moor RM, Rowson LEA. The corpus luteum of the sheep: effect of the removal of embryos on luteal function. *J Endocrinol* 1966;34:497–502.
800. Rowson LEA, Moor RM. The influence of embryonic tissue homogenate infused into the uterus, on the life span of the corpus luteum in the sheep. *J Reprod Fertil* 1967;13:511–516.
801. Martal J, Lacroix MC, Loudes C, Saunier M, Winterberger-Torres S. Trophobastin, an antiluteolytic protein present in early pregnancy in sheep. *J Reprod Fertil* 1979;56:63–73.
802. Heyman Y, Camous S, Fevre J, Meziou W, Martal J. Maintenance of the corpus luteum after uterine transfer of trophoblastic vesicles to cyclic cows and ewes. *J Reprod Fertil* 1984;70:533–540.
803. Godkin JD, Bazer FW, Moffatt J, Sessions F, Roberts RM. Purification and properties of a major, low molecular weight protein released by the trophoblast of sheep blastocysts at days 13–21. *J Reprod Fertil* 1982;65:141–150.
804. Godkin JD, Bazer FW, Roberts RM. Ovine trophoblast protein 1, an early secreted blastocyst protein, binds specifically to uterine endometrium and affects protein synthesis. *Endocrinology* 1984;114:120–130.
805. Hansen PJ, Anthony RV, Bazer FW, Baumbach GA, Roberts RM. *In vitro* synthesis and secretion of ovine trophoblastic protein-1 during the period of maternal recognition of pregnancy. *Endocrinology* 1985;117:1424–1430.
806. Godkin JD, Bazer FW, Thatcher WW, Roberts RM. Proteins released by cultured days 15–16 conceptuses prolong luteal maintenance when introduced into the uterine lumen of cyclic ewes. *J Reprod Fertil* 1984;71:57–64.
807. Godkin JD, Cote C, Duby RT. Embryonic stimulation of ovine and bovine corpora lutea. *J Reprod Fertil* 1978;54:375–378.
808. Ellinwood WE, Nett TM, Niswender GD. Maintenance of the corpus luteum of early pregnancy in the ewe. I. Luteotropic properties of embryonic homogenates. *Biol Reprod* 1979;21:281–288.
809. Masters RA, Roberts RM, Lewis GS, Thatcher WW, Blazer FW, Godkin JD. High molecular weight glycoproteins released by expanding, pre-attachment sheep, pig and cow blastocysts in culture. *J Reprod Fertil* 1982;66:571–583.
810. Betteridge KJ, Eaglesome MD, Randall GCB, Mitchell D, Sugden EA. Maternal progesterone levels as evidence of luteotrophic or antiluteolytic effects of embryos transferred to heifers 12–17 days after estrus. *Theriogenology* 1978;9:86.
811. Sreeran JM. Non-surgical embryo transfer in the cow. *Theriogenology* 1978;9:69–83.
812. Northey DL, French LR. Effect of embryo removal and intrauterine infusion of embryonic homogenates on the lifespan of the bovine corpus luteum. *J Anim Sci* 1980;50:298–302.
813. Bartol FF, Roberts RM, Bazer FW, Lewis GS, Godkin JD, Thatcher WW. Characterization of proteins produced *in vitro* by peri-attachment bovine conceptus. *Biol Reprod* 1984;32:681–693.
814. Bazer FW, Geisert RE, Thatcher WW, Roberts RM. The establishment and maintenance of pregnancy. In: Cole JA, Foxcroft GR, eds. *Control of Pig Reproduction.* London: Butterworths, 1982;227–252.
815. Wyatt C. Endometrial components involved in protein synthesis by 16-day pig blastocyst tissue in culture. *J Physiol (Lond)* 1976;260:73P–74P.
816. Saunders PTK, Ziecik AJ, Flint APF. Gonadotrophinlike substance in pig placenta and embryonic membranes. *J Endocrinol* 1980;85:25.
817. Rice C, Ackland N, Heap RB. Blastocyst–endometrial interaction and protein synthesis during preimplantation development in the pig studied *in vitro. Placenta* 1981;2:129–142.
818. Godkin JD, Bazer FW, Lewis GS, Geisert RD, Roberts RM. Synthesis and release of polypeptides by pig conceptuses during the period of blastocyst elongation and attachment. *Biol Reprod* 1982;27:977–987.
819. Fishel SB, Surani MAH. Evidence for the synthesis and release of a glycoprotein by mouse blastocysts. *J Reprod Fertil* 1980;59:181–185.
820. Nieder GL, Weitlauf HM, Hartman M. Synthesis and secretion of stage specific proteins by peri-implantation mouse embryos. *Biol Reprod* 1986;36:687–699.

821. Morton H, Hegh V, Clunie GJA. Immunosuppression detected in pregnant mice by rosette inhibition test. *Nature* 1974;249: 459–460.
822. Morton H, Hegh V, Clunie GJA. Studies of the rosette inhibition test in pregnant mice: evidence of immunosuppression? *Proc R Soc Lond (Biol)* 1976;193:413–419.
823. Morton H, Rolfe B, Clunie GJA, Anderson MJ, Morrison J. An early pregnancy factor detected in human serum by the rosette inhibition test. *Lancet* 1977;i:394–397.
824. Nancarrow CD, Evison BM, Scaramuzzi RJ, Turnbull KE. Detection of induced death of embryos in sheep by the rosette inhibition test. *J Reprod Fertil* 1979;57:385–389.
825. Noonan FP, Halliday WJ, Morton H, Clunie GJA. Early pregnancy factor is immunosuppressive. *Nature* 1979;278:649–650.
826. Clarke FM, Morton H, Clunie GJA. Detection and separation of two serum factors responsible for depression of lymphocyte activity in pregnancy. *Clin Exp Immunol* 1978;32:318–323.
827. Clarke FM, Morton H, Rolfe BE, Clunie GJA. Partial characterization of early pregnancy factor in the sheep. *J Reprod Immunol* 1980;2:151–162.
828. Wilson S, McCarthy R, Clarke F. In search of early pregnancy factor: isolation of active polypeptides from pregnant ewe's sera. *J Reprod Immunol* 1983;5:275–286.
829. Clarke FM, Wilson S. Biochemistry of early pregnancy factor. In: Grudzinskas, Teisner B, Seppala M, eds. *Pregnancy Proteins.* New York: Academic Press, 1982;407–412.
830. Morton H, Rolfe B, Cavanagh A. Early pregnancy factor: biology and clinical significance. In: Grudzinkas JG, Teisner B, Seppala M, eds. *Pregnancy Proteins.* New York: Academic Press, 1982;391–405.
831. Morton H, Rolfe BE, McNeill L, Clarke P, Clarke FM, Clunie GJA. Early pregnancy factor: tissues involved in its production in the mouse. *J Reprod Immunol* 1980;2:73–82.
832. Cavanagh AC, Morton H, Rolfe BE, Gidley-Baird A. Ovum factor: a first signal of pregnancy? *Am J Reprod Immunol* 1982;2:97–101.
833. Nancarrow CD, Wallace ALC, Grewal AS. The early pregnancy factor of sheep and cattle. *J Reprod Fertil* 1981;30(suppl): 191–199.
834. Cavanagh AC. Production *in vitro* of mouse early pregnancy factor and purification to homogeneity. *J Reprod Fertil* 1984;71: 581–592.
835. Morton H, Clunie GJA. A test for early pregnancy in sheep. *Res Vet Sci* 1979;26:261–262.
836. Morton H, Nancarrow CD, Scaramuzzi RJ, Evison BM, Clunie GJA. Detection of early pregnancy factor in sheep by rosette inhibition test. *J Reprod Fertil* 1979;56:75–80.
837. Morton H, Tinnenberg HR, Rolfe B, Wolf M, Mettler L. Rosette inhibition test: a multicentre investigation of early pregnancy factor in humans. *J Reprod Immunol* 1982;4:251–261.
838. Smart YC, Roberts TK, Clancy RL, Cripps AW. Early pregnancy factor: its role in mammalian reproduction research review. *Fertil Steril* 1981;35:397–402.
839. Koh LY, Jones WR. The rosette inhibition test in early pregnancy diagnosis. *Clin Reprod Fertil* 1982;1:229–233.
840. Tinnenberg HR, Staves RP, Semm K. Improvement of the rosette inhibition assay for the detection of early pregnancy factor in humans using the monoclonal antibody, anti-human-lyt-3. *Am J Reprod Immunol* 1984;5:151–156.
841. Rolfe BE, Morton H, Cavanagh AC, Gardiner RA. Detection of an early pregnancy factorlike substance in sera of patients with testicular germ cell tumors. *Am J Reprod Immunol* 1983;3: 97–100.
842. Koch E, Morton H, Ellendorff F. Early pregnancy factor: biology and practical application. *Br Vet J* 1983;139:52–58.
843. Morton H, Morton DJ, Ellendorff F. The appearance and characteristics of early pregnancy factor in the pig. *J Reprod Fertil* 1983;69:437–446.
844. Cooper DW, Aitken RJ. Failure to detect altered rosette inhibition titres in human pregnancy serum. *J Reprod Fertil* 1981;61: 241–245.
845. Whyte A, Heap RB. Early pregnancy factor. *Nature* 1983;304: 121–122.
846. Smart YC, Fraser IS, Clancy RL, Roberts TK, Crippis AW. Early pregnancy factor as a monitor for fertilization in women wearing intrauterine devices. *Fertil Steril* 1982;37:201–204.
847. Smart YC, Roberts TK, Fraser IS, Cripps AW, Clancy RL. Validation of rosette inhibition test for detection of early pregnancy in women. *Fertil Steril* 1982;37:779–785.
848. Shaw FD, Morton H. The immunological approach to pregnancy diagnosis: a review. *Vet Rec* 1980;106:268–270.
849. Rolfe B, Cavanagh A, Forde C, Bastin CC, Morton H. Modified rosette inhibition test with mouse lymphocytes for detection of early pregnancy factor in human pregnancy serum. *J Immunol Methods* 1984;70:1–11.
850. Rolfe BE, Morton H, Clarke FM. Early pregnancy factor is an immuno-suppressive contaminant of commercial preparations of human chorionic gonadotrophin. *Clin Exp Immunol* 1983;51: 45–52.
851. Rolfe BE. Detection of fetal wastage. *Fertil Steril* 1982;37: 655–660.
852. Kent HA Jr. A polypeptide from oviductal contents which influences ovarian function. *Biol Reprod* 1973;8:38–42.
853. Kent HA Jr. Contraceptive polypeptide from hamster embryos: sequence of amino acids in the compound. *Biol Reprod* 1975;12:504–507.
854. Kent HA Jr. The two to four-cell embryos as source tissue of the tetrapeptide preventing ovulations in the hamster. *Am J Anat* 1975;144:509–512.
855. Van Niekerk CH, Gerncke WH. Persistence and pathologic cleavage of tubal ova in the mare. *Onderstepoort J Vet Res* 1966;32:195–232.
856. Betteridge KJ, Mitchell D. Retention of ova by the fallopian tube in mares. *J Reprod Fertil* 1972;31:515.
857. Nieder GL, Corder C. Pyruvate and lactate levels in oviducts of cycling, pregnant, and pseudopregnant mice. *Biol Reprod* 1983;28:566–574.
858. O'Neill C. Thrombocytopenia is an initial maternal response to fertilization in mice. *J Reprod Fertil* 1985;73:559–566.
859. Renfree MB, Calaby JH. Background to delayed implantation and embryonic diapause. *J Reprod Fertil* 1981;29(suppl):1–9.
860. Aitken RJ. Embryonic diapause. In: Johnson MH, ed. *Development in Mammals,* Vol I. New York: North-Holland, 1977; 307–359.
861. McLaren A. Blastocyst activation. In: Segal SJ, Crozier R, Corman PA, Condliffe PG, eds. *The Regulation of Mammalian Reproduction.* Springfield, IL: Charles C Thomas, 1973;321–328.
862. Brambell FWR. The influence of lactation on implantation of the mammalian embryo. *Am J Obstet Gynecol* 1937;33:942–953.
863. Weitlauf HM. *In vitro* uptake and incorporation of amino acids by blastocysts from intact and ovariectomized mice. *J Exp Zool* 1973;183:303–308.
864. Psychoyos A, Bitton-Casimiri V, Brun JL. Repression and activation of the mammalian blastocyst. In: Talwar GP, ed. *Regulation and Differentiated Function in Eukaryote Cells.* New York: Raven Press, 1975;509–514.
865. Mintz B. Formation of genetically mosaic mouse embryos and early development of "lethal (t^{12}/t^{12})-normal" mosaics. *J Exp Zool* 1964;157:273–292.
866. Cole RJ, Paul J. Properties of cultured preimplantation mouse and rabbit embryos and cell strains derived from them. In: *Preimplantation Stages of Pregnancy.* CIBA Foundation Symposium. Boston: Little, Brown, 1965;82–111.
867. Gwatkin RBL. Defined media and development of mammalian eggs *in vitro. Ann NY Acad Sci* 1966;139:79–90.
868. Gwatkin RBL. Amino acid requirements for attachment and outgrowth of the mouse blastocyst *in vitro. J Cell Physiol* 1966;68:335–344.
869. Naeslund G. The effect of glucose-, arginine-, and leucine-deprivation on blastocyst outgrowth *in vitro. Upsala J Med Sci* 1979;84:9–20.
870. Naeslund G, Lundkvist O, Nilsson BO. Transmission electron microscopy of mouse blastocysts activated and growth arrested *in vivo* and *in vitro. Anat Embryol* 1980;159:33–48.
871. Wordinger RJ, Brinster RL. Influence of reduced glucose levels

on the *in vitro* hatching, attachment and trophoblast outgrowth of the mouse blastocyst. *Dev Biol* 1976;53:294–296.

872. Van Blerkom J, Chavez DJ, Bell H. Molecular and cellular aspects of facultative delayed implantation in the mouse. In: *Maternal Recognition of Pregnancy.* CIBA Foundation Symposium No. 64 (new series). New York: Excerpta Medica, 1979;141–172.
873. Aitken RJ. Delayed implantation in roe deer (*Capreolus capreolus*). *J Reprod Fertil* 1974;39:225–233.
874. Aitken RJ. Calcium and zinc in the endometrium and uterine flushings of the roe deer (*Carreoulus carreolus*) during delayed implantation. *J Reprod Fertil* 1974;40:333–340.
875. Van Winkle LJ. Low Na^+ concentration: a factor contributing to diminished uptake and incorporation of amino acids by diapausing mouse blastocysts? *J Exp Zool* 1977;202:275–281.
876. Van Winkle LJ. Activation of amino acid accumulation in delayed implantation mouse blastocysts. *J Exp Zool* 1981;218: 239–246.
877. Van Winkle LJ, Campione AL, Webster DI. Sodium ion concentrations in uterine flushings from "implanting" and "delayed implanting" mice. *J Exp Zool* 1983;226:321–324.
878. Surani MAH. Cellular and molecular approaches to blastocyst uterine interactions at implantation. In: Johnson MH, ed. *Development in Mammals,* Vol I. New York: North-Holland, 1977;245–305.
879. Gwatkin RBL. Nutritional requirements for post-blastocyst development in the mouse. *Int J Fertil* 1969;14:101–105.
880. Weitlauf HM, Kiessling AA. Activation of 'delayed implanting' mouse embryos *in vitro. J Reprod Fertil* 1981;29(suppl):191–202.
881. Nilsson BO, Magnusson C, Widehn S, Hillensjo T. Correlation between blastocyst oxygen consumption and trophoblast cytochrome oxidase reaction at initiation of implantation of delayed mouse blastocysts. *J Embryol Exp Morphol* 1982;71:75–82.
882. Torbit CA, Weitlauf HM. Production of carbon dioxide *in vitro* by blastocysts from intact and ovariectomized mice. *J Reprod Fertil* 1975;42:45–50.
883. Menke TM, McLaren A. Carbon dioxide production by mouse blastocysts during lactational delay of implantation or after ovariectomy. *J Endocrinol* 1970;47:287–294.
884. Nieder GL, Weitlauf HM. Regulation of glycolysis in the mouse blastocyst during delayed implantation. *J Exp Zool* 1984;231: 121–129.
885. Nieder GL, Weitlauf HM. Effects of metabolic substrates and ionic environment on *in-vitro* activation of delayed implanting mouse blastocysts. *J Reprod Fertil* 1985;73:151–157.
886. Weitlauf HM. Effect of uterine flushings on RNA synthesis by 'implanting' and 'delayed implanting' mouse embryos *in vitro. Biol Reprod* 1976;14:566–571.
887. Weitlauf HM. Factors in mouse uterine fluid that inhibit the incorporation of [3H] uridine by blastocysts *in vitro. J Reprod Fertil* 1978;52:321–325.
888. Psychoyos A, Bitton-Casimiri V. Captation *in vitro* d'un priecurseur d'acide ribonucleique (ARN)-(uridine 5-^{3}H) par le bastocyste de rat: differences entre blastocysts normaux et blastocysts en diapause. *C R Soc Biol (Paris)* 1969;268:188–190.
889. Aitken RJ. The culture of mouse blastocysts in the presence of uterine flushings collected during normal pregnancy, delayed implantation, and pro-oestrus. *J Embryol Exp Morphol* 1977;41: 295–300.
890. O'Neill C, Quinn P. Interaction of uterine flushings with mouse blastocysts *in vitro* as assessed by the incorporation of [^{3}H] uridine. *J Reprod Fertil* 1981;62:257–262.
891. O'Neill C, Quinn P. Inhibitory influence of uterine secretions on mouse blastocysts decreases at the time of blastocyst activation. *J Reprod Fertil* 1983;68:269–274.
892. Psychoyos A, Casimiri V. Uterine blastotoxic factors. In: Glasser SR, Bullock DW, eds. *Cellular and Molecular Aspects of Implantation.* New York: Plenum Press, 1981;327–334.

The Physiology of Reproduction, Second Edition,
edited by E. Knobil and J.D. Neill,
Raven Press, Ltd., New York © 1994.

CHAPTER 8

Anatomy and Genesis of the Placenta

Peter Kaufmann[1] and Graham Burton[2]

HISTORICAL SURVEY

By virtue of the scientific method, our understanding of any subject inevitably evolves with time. Often this is a painstakingly slow process, but on occasions, great leaps forward may be made either through the advent of new technology or the occurrence of a contemporary advance in a different but related field of study. This premise applies as well to our knowledge of the placenta as to that of any other organ system, and the purpose of this brief historical survey is to highlight the most significant stages in the development of our understanding of placental structure and function.

Although the placenta was venerated by the early Egyptians, DeWitt (1) credited the Greek physician Diogenes of Apollonia (ca 480 BC) with being the first to ascribe the function of fetal nutrition to the organ. Aristotle (384–322 BC) developed this idea further, realizing that the fetus is fully enclosed within membranes, which he termed the *chorion.* He thus challenged the previously held Hippocratic theories that the fetus is nourished by suckling from uterine paps or cotyledons. Instead, Aristotle believed that the vessels of the umbilical cord trans-

[1]Institut für Anatomie, RWTH Aachen, D 5100 AACHEN, Germany
[2]Department of Anatomy, University of Cambridge, Cambridge CB2 3DY, United Kingdom

mitted nutrients by communicating directly with those of the uterus, vein to vein and artery to artery.

Aristotle's teachings were further reinforced by the next notable contributor, Galen (AD 130–200). Galen synthesized both Hippocratic and Aristotelian ideas on reproduction into a series of theoretic constructs. Thus, he believed that the embryo is formed from the menstrual blood that is no longer shed after conception and that whereas the allantois forms from the female semen, the chorion forms from coagulation of the male sperm mass (1). Despite this rather teleologic approach, Galen was a great experimenter, accurately describing the anatomy of the fetal membranes of ruminants and correctly deducing that the fetus excretes urine into the allantoic sac. These animal studies most likely colored his appreciation of the human situation, however, for he too believed that the vessels of the umbilical cord communicate directly with their maternal counterparts, opening on the surface of the uterine caruncles. Indeed, Amoroso (2) held the view that both Aristotle and Galen probably never actually dissected the human body.

This state of affairs persisted throughout the Middle Ages. For example, during this period it was commonly held that the human uterus was a seven-chambered structure similar to that of the pig, and it was Leonardo da Vinci (1452–1519) who first illustrated it correctly as a *uterus simplex* (3). Leonardo's manuscripts are justly famed for their beautiful illustrations, but often the accompanying notes indicate meticulous observations. In these, he asserted that the veins of the fetus are not directly connected to those of the uterus, thus challenging one of the most basic precepts of the ancients' teachings.

Despite these major contributions, Leonardo continued to propagate through his illustrations the misconception that the human placenta is cotyledonary in nature. He was not alone in his confusion, however, and in his defense, it must be recognized that the common domestic animals display a bewildering array of placental types. The next great anatomist, Andreas Vesalius (1514–1564), depicted the human placenta as being of the zonary type characteristic of carnivores in the first edition of *De Humani Corporis Fabrica* (Fig. 1). This he corrected in the second edition, but the discoidal placenta then shown still bears many similarities to a single cotyledon from a ruminant, with large vessels running over the free chorion and the intimation of the presence of a large allantoic sac.

After nearly 1,300 years of stagnation since the time of Galen, scholastic activity suddenly blossomed during the Renaissance. Realdus Columbus (1516–1559) introduced the term *placenta* in 1559 (4), derived from the Latin root for a flat "cake." Julius Caesar Arantius (1530–1589) made great strides forward, not only in considering the placenta as a uterine liver involved in the "purification" of the fetal blood but also by establishing through many comparative dissections the independence of the maternal and fetal circulations. Despite Leonardo's earlier notes, which admittedly were not published as an anatomic text, Arantius is generally accredited with this fundamental discovery (5).

The idea was not readily accepted, however. Thus, Hieronymus Fabricius (1537–1619), a detailed observer of the placenta of a number of species, wavered for many years but was finally convinced by the weight of evidence in favor of the ancient teachings. His pupil Adrianus Spigelius (1578–1625) adopted a compromise position, believing that maternal blood flows from the uterine vessels into the open mouths of the umbilical veins but that the umbilical arteries end in the placenta and do not communicate with their uterine equivalents. It is arguable that neither of these men really furthered knowledge of placental function, but what cannot be denied is the exquisite beauty of their illustrations (6) (Fig. 2).

The next main advance in our understanding of the

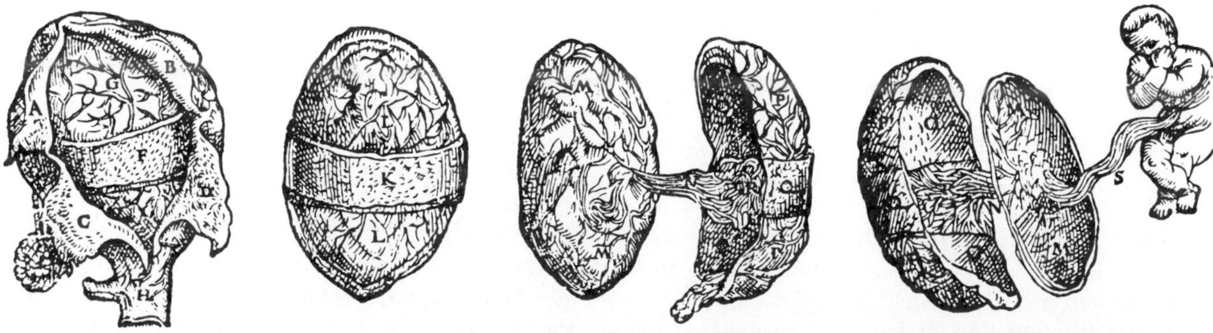

FIG. 1. When preparing first edition of De Humani Corporis Fabrica in 1543, Vesalius incorrectly extrapolated from the canine to the human situation. In this illustration, he depicts human placenta as being zonary in type. Furthermore, in right-hand figure, there is the suggestion that a flange of membrane is attached halfway along umbilical cord. This is typical of the arrangement in the dog, where the large allantoic sac results in intra-amnionic and intra-allantoic parts to the umbilical cord. Some commentators have interpreted such errors as indicating that classical anatomists had relatively few opportunities to dissect reproductive material.

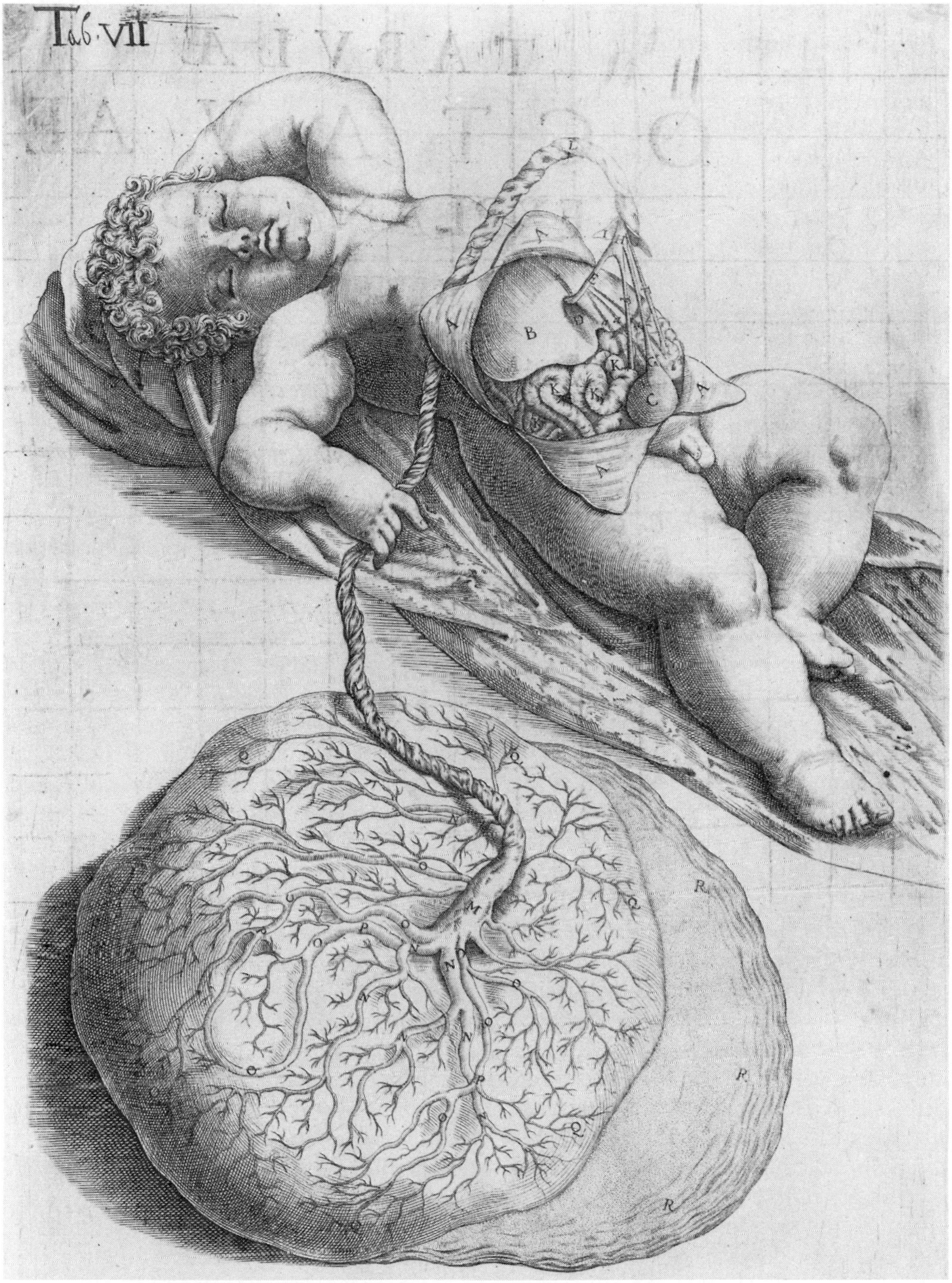

FIG. 2. One of the plates from De Formato Foetu of Spigelius (1626), demonstrating the exquisite beauty of illustrations from this period.

placenta was through the work of William Harvey (1578–1657) and his theories on the circulation of blood. He continued to see the main function of the organ as nutritive rather than respiratory and argued on the basis of his understanding of the circulation that the fetal and maternal blood streams must be separate. Nevertheless, Harvey could still not explain the vital step of how blood passed from arteries to veins, and it was not until after his death that Malpighi in 1660 provided the answer with his discovery of capillaries. It was also Malpighi who first suggested that the placenta is a substitute for the lungs while those of the fetus are at rest, and we come close to a correct appreciation of the organ's function when in 1668 John Mayow asserted that the maternal blood supplies the fetus with "nitro-aerial spirits" or oxygen. He proposed the replacement of Arantius' uterine liver concept with that of a uterine lung, but now at least two of the principal functions of the organ were clearly established.

No historical survey of the placenta, however brief, would be complete without due acknowledgment of the enormous contributions made by the brothers William (1718–1783) and John (1728–1792) Hunter. Through their renowned studies involving the injection of molten wax into the circulation of gravid uteri, graphically depicted by Corner (5), they succeeded in providing confirmatory experimental proof of the independence of the maternal and fetal circulations, first suggested by Leonardo almost 250 years earlier. Their writings suggested that the brothers had a clear appreciation of the way in which the uterine arteries open into what we now refer to as the intervillous space. For them, however, it was simply a large blood-filled space because the concept of placental villi was not realized until nearly halfway through the nineteenth century, when use of the microscope became more widespread.

Almost contemporaneously in the 1840s, Weber and Dalrymple (7) published virtually identical drawings of isolated villi, illustrating within their core the fetal capillary network uniting umbilical artery to vein. Although these drawings accurately reflect the gross morphology of the villi, ideas concerning their histologic nature were still confused. An epithelial covering to the villi was clearly depicted, but for many years, this was believed to be maternal in origin. The illustrations of Ercolani from 1877 (see Fig. 9 in ref. 8) reflect contemporary opinion of how this was achieved, for in these the uterine vessels are shown opening through the basal plate and expanding into thin-walled sac-like structures that envelop the fetal villi like a glove. Only 5 years later in 1882, Theodor Langhans (9) demonstrated that both layers of the epithelial covering, now referred to as the cytotrophoblast and the syncytiotrophoblast, are, in fact, fetal in origin, so establishing our current understanding of villous structure.

That such confusion should have existed is perhaps not surprising, for this was a time of intense debate on the issues of evolution and of the diversity of animals after the publication of Darwin's *The Origin of Species* in 1859. It saw the heyday of comparative anatomy, and the placental membranes certainly did not escape the attention of avid investigators intent on demonstrating phylogenetic links. Large collections of material were amassed by zoologists such as Hubrecht (10), and indeed it was he who first introduced the term *trophoblast* when describing the early development of the hedgehog in 1889. In recognition of its direct nutritive significance to the embryo, Hubrecht conferred the term on that part of the epiblast that forms the outer layer of the blastocyst and so is in immediate contact with the maternal tissues. As is seen later, when viewed in the context of the bewildering array of placental types demonstrated by even the more common domestic and laboratory mammals, the ideas and extrapolations of Ercolani and his contemporaries do not seem so outrageous.

Necessary order was imposed on the broader zoologic scene largely by Otto Grosser, who proposed a classification system based on the number of tissue layers that, under the light microscope, appear to separate the maternal and fetal blood streams (11,12). Hence the terms *epitheliochorial, syndesmochorial, endotheliochorial,* and *hemochorial* were coined, and although this system has had to be updated in the light of subsequent findings and has on occasions been misconstrued, in general it has provided a useful framework for subsequent comparative studies. These have advanced our understanding of placental function enormously and mention must be made of the major contributions provided by, for example, the works of Mossman (13) and Amoroso (14). Grosser did not restrict himself to animal material, however, and his descriptions of the histologic structure of the human placenta were also detailed and accurate.

Focusing on the human situation, it should now be apparent that the foundations of our present understanding of placental structure were in place by the start of the twentieth century. Shortly after in 1905, as a result of a series of astute observations, Halban (15) concluded that the organ must produce "active substances" and correctly pronounced that "during pregnancy the placenta usurps the protective function of the ovary and carries it to a higher degree." Although Halban obviously had no detailed knowledge of estrogen and progesterone, the third main function of the placenta, that of an endocrine organ, had clearly been recognized.

However, although an extensive body of knowledge concerning the structure of the mature placenta was beginning to be established at the beginning of the century, relatively little was known about earlier stages and, in particular, about implantation. The small amount of information available was based on very rare specimens recovered fortuitously during surgical or autopsy procedures, and many of these have since been interpreted as being pathologic. To rectify this situation, in the mid-1920s Streeter established a breeding colony of rhesus monkeys at the Carnegie Institute in Washington and so pioneered the systematic study of early embryologic development. In conjunction with collaborators such as Hartman, Heuser, and Wislocki, a series of detailed descriptions of macaque development resulted (16). These not only yielded unique information on that species but also provided a yardstick of development against which the more occasional human specimens could be compared. The success of these studies prompted attempts to recover early human embryos on a more systematic basis from hysterectomy material, and this led to the establishment of the renowned Hertig-Rock collection (17). The subsequent descriptions of human development based on this collection laid the foundations for much of modern embryology.

Although the Carnegie Institute played a pivotal role, others (e.g., Stieve [18]) also made notable contributions through their meticulous observations of early specimens. Stieve is perhaps more widely remembered for his papers describing the configuration of the mature villous tree, which at the time were highly controversial. As stated, the general architecture of a placental villus had been known quite accurately since the illustrations of Weber and Dalrymple, but how these were arranged within the organ was another matter. The prevailing view was that the villi resembled a tree, with its "roots" attached to the chorionic plate and ever-diminishing branches extending toward the basal plate. A few were believed to attach to the uterine wall as "anchoring villi," but most were thought to hang freely in the intervillous space as terminal villi. Stieve (19), however, considered that fusion between the tips of terminal villi was commonplace and that this converted the villous tree into a lattice-type network through which the fetal blood flows. However, Spanner (20) believed that the main trunk of the tree first extended to the basal plate and that the principal branches then recurved toward the chorionic plate before giving off terminal villi (see Figs. 171–173 in ref. 4). Subsequent studies and three-dimensional reconstructions have now irrefutably confirmed that the traditional view is the correct picture, although as will be seen later, some fusion between villi does occur.

These differences in arrangement might at first sight appear unimportant and the subject of esoteric debates between morphologists, but when considering placental exchange, it is critical to have an appreciation of the relative directions of the maternal and fetal blood flows. On the maternal side, one problem that had taxed investigators since the time of the Hunter brothers was how the direction of blood flow was regulated in the intervillous space. The problem they and their contemporaries rapidly perceived was why does the maternal blood, when delivered into a large space with no preformed channels, circulate to bathe all the villi rather than passing directly from the arterial to the nearest venous opening? One solution to the problem was offered by Bumm in 1893 (see Figs. 19 and 20 in ref. 21), who maintained that the openings of the arteries and veins are widely separated. Whereas the uterine veins open through the basal plate, he believed the mouths of the uterine arteries are to be found distributed over the surface of the placental septa. These Bumm mistakenly considered to be of maternal origin, and the basis of his theory was that maternal arterial blood is delivered from the septa to the lateral surface of the villous tree and that it then drains toward the basal plate.

Spanner (20) refuted these findings and instead proposed that although arterial openings are distributed at intervals over the basal plate, the venous openings are found exclusively at the margins of the placental disc. In his view, arterial blood flows toward a relatively villous-free area beneath the chorionic plate, the subchorial lake, and then disperses laterally into a marginal sinus before entering the uterine veins (see Fig. 21 in ref. 21). Spanner formulated his theory on the basis of injection studies, and although it was enthusiastically received at that time, it is likely that he was misled by artifacts arising from premature hardening of his injection medium, celloidin.

Resolution of the problem of arteriovenous shunting in the intervillous space was finally provided by the introduction of cineradiography. This was pioneered in the human by Borell and co-workers (22), but the problem of radiation dosage limited systematic study. Again, the macaque colony at the Carnegie Institute played a vital role, and it was largely through the elegant work of Ramsey and her collaborator Donner that the "physiologic concept" was confirmed. In this, it is proposed that arterial blood is delivered to the central region of a lobe through an opening in the basal plate and that the incoming force sends it in a fountainlike spurt toward the chorionic plate. These are often referred to eponymously as *Borell jets*. As the blood disperses laterally between the villi, it displaces the existing supply into the mouths of the uterine veins. Some refinement of this concept may prove to be necessary if the recent finding from direct visualization during chorionic villus sampling that blood flow through the intervillous space does not commence until the end of the first trimester (23) is confirmed by subsequent studies. Nonetheless, for the remainder of gestation the physiologic concept holds true and indeed has recently been confirmed by nuclear magnetic resonance imaging (24).

The midpart of the twentieth century saw other major advances in the correlation of structure and function, resultant again on the introduction of new technologies. During the 1940s, the elaboration and refinement of histochemical techniques, pioneered in their application to the placenta by workers such as Dempsey and Wislock (25), enabled enzymatic activity and hormone synthesis to be localized to specific sites and tissues. Furthermore, it became possible to explore how patterns of activity may vary at different stages of gestation and under different antenatal conditions. Shortly after, in the next decade, the cellular organelles involved could be visualized through the advent of the transmission electron microscope.

With the superior resolution offered by the instrument, the detailed nature of, for example, the microvillous border, the vacuolar transport systems, the synthetic and degradatory organelles, and the relationship between the syncytium and the cytotrophoblast at once became apparent (26,27). The images obtained provided powerful evidence that the trophoblast does not act as a simple homogeneous semipermeable membrane and influenced physiologists greatly in their thinking on the mechanisms of transplacental transport.

Since these early studies, advances in microscope technology and in allied preparative techniques have permitted evermore sophisticated structural studies to be performed. Membrane receptors, growth factors, extracellular matrix molecules, and other molecules regulating placental development can be localized and quantified by autoradiographic and immunolabeling procedures. Cytoskeletal proteins can be mapped in three dimensions using fluorescent probes and confocal microscopy. Models of how placental growth and differentiation are regulated can be proposed on the basis of these findings and corroborated or refuted by subsequent *in vitro* studies. *In situ* hybridization is now even allowing us to localize messenger ribonucleic acid (RNA), and so it is becoming possible to dissect placental structure, development, and function down to the molecular level.

In the light of these few findings, it is necessary to update and reappraise our theories on placental development constantly. The placenta is manifestly the result of materno–fetal interaction, however, and mention must be made of the enormous contribution that immunology has made during the second half of this century. For many years, it has been known that trophoblast extends beyond the placenta down the necks of the spiral arteries, in a process that destroys their media and is thought to be necessary to ensure an adequate uteroplacental supply. Trophoblast also migrates through the endometrium between the uterine glands, mingling with cells of the maternal immune system. Recent advances in our understanding of histocompatibility antigens and of the autocrine and paracrine effects of cytokines released through these cellular interactions are beginning to clarify how the disparate genetic tissues may successfully coexist and how the depth of placental invasion may be regulated.

COMPARATIVE PLACENTATION

When one reviews the wide array of placenta types demonstrated by even the domestic mammals, it is little wonder that they have been the source of such confusion over the centuries. Interspecies differences are marked, and it is essential that they continue to be borne in mind when extrapolating physiologic, endocrinologic, immunologic, or any other data from the animal to the human situation. This section highlights some of the more major differences, but for details on individual species, readers are directed to the specialist texts (14,28,29).

Placental types may be classified at several complementary levels, reflecting, for example, both gross and microscopic structure, the histologic nature of the materno–fetal interface, or the relative directions of the maternal and fetal blood flows.

The most fundamental level relates to the origin of the fetal vessels that vascularize the chorion. The chorion is intrinsically an avascular tissue, and so for it to take part in materno–fetal exchange, it must develop a functional circulation. This may be derived from vessels running in the extraembryonic mesodermal covering of either the yolk sac or the allantois. The former situation gives rise to a *choriovitelline* placenta, and this represents the main form of placentation in many marsupials. By contrast, among most mammals, the yolk sac is a very transient structure, functioning only for nutritive and respiratory exchange in the earliest stages of pregnancy.

Notable exceptions to this general rule are the rodents and lagomorphs in which the yolk sac often persists throughout gestation, although it does not actually vascularize the chorion. In some species, such as the mouse and rabbit, the yolk sac is highly elaborated into the complete inverted type. Breakdown of the overlying chorion and of the outer wall of the yolk sac exposes the endodermal lining to the secretions of the uterine glands. This represents an important pathway in the absorption of proteins and the transport of maternal immunoglobulins, which continues to function until term.

In these species, as in most mammals, the definitive placenta is vascularized by vessels associated with the allantois. The allantois is a diverticulum of the hindgut, whose initial embryonic development is slightly later than that of the yolk sac. It may expand into the extraembryonic coelom as a large fluid-filled sac in species such as the pig, cow, and horse or remain a rudimentary structure penetrating only the proximal end of the connecting stalk, as in the human. In either case, development of its vasculature is prolific, and on making contact with the chorion, it establishes the *chorioallantoic* placenta. Further description will be limited to this form of placentation, in view of its paramount importance in mammalian materno–fetal exchange.

Placental Shape

The second level of classification to be considered relates to the gross morphology of the placenta. Four main types are recognized in a scheme that dates back to the

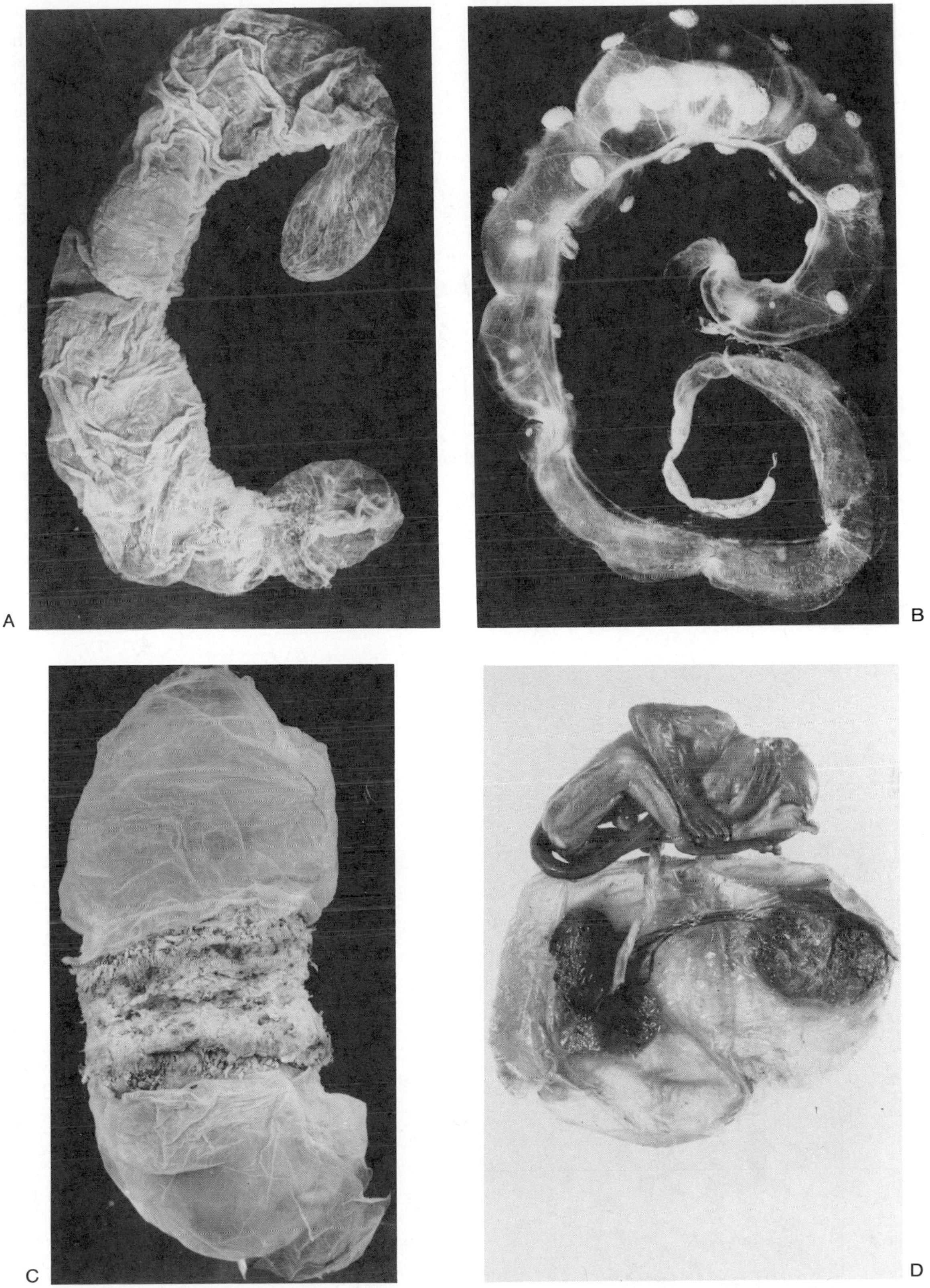

FIG. 3. Montage showing (**A**) diffuse placenta of domestic pig, (**B**) cotyledonary placenta of cow, (**C**) zonary placenta of dog, and (**D**) double discoid placenta of leaf-eating monkey.

time of Hieronymus Fabricius. The basis of the classification is whether physical interaction between the maternal and fetal tissues occurs over all the available surface of the chorionic sac or whether it is restricted to specialized regions. In the simplest situation, as in, for example, the pig, interaction takes place over virtually the entire sac, and so these placentas are described as *diffuse* (Fig. 3A). By contrast, interaction only occurs in ruminants opposite specialized nonglandular areas of the endometrium known as caruncles. The number, shape, and size of the caruncles is species-specific, ranging in number from 100 to 120 in the sheep to only four in some types of deer. Intervening areas of the chorion are smooth and relatively avascular, and so the resultant placentas are termed *cotyledonary* (Fig. 3B). Among several unrelated orders, including the carnivores, physical interaction is restricted to an equatorial belt encircling the chorionic sac, giving rise to a *zonary* placenta (Fig. 3C). In *discoi-*

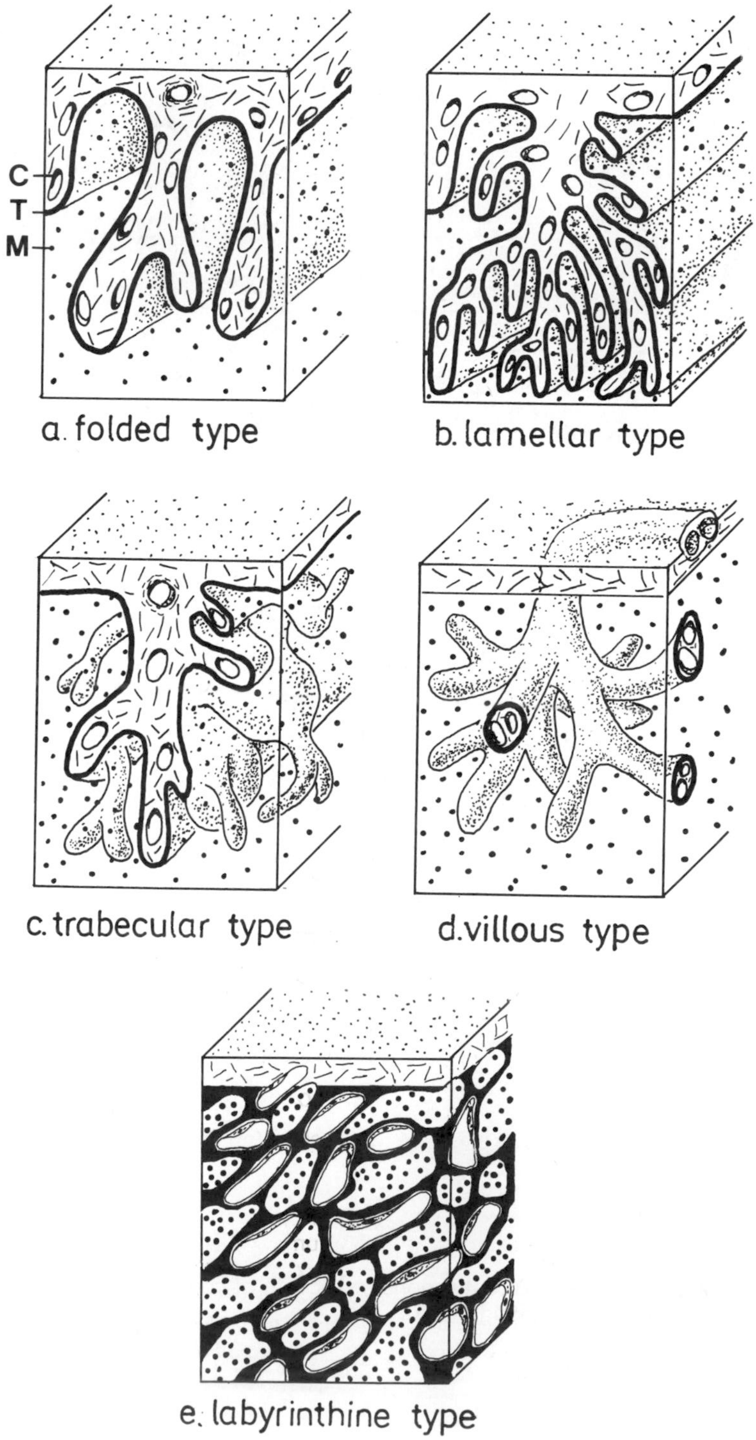

FIG. 4. Types of interdigitation between maternal and fetal tissues. *M,* maternal tissue or maternal blood (*larger dots*); *T,* fetal trophoblast (*black*); and *C,* fetal capillaries and fetal connective tissue. (Modified and extended after ref. 29, with permission.)

dal placentas, which may be single or double, interaction is confined to a roughly circular area. This situation is characteristic of the primates and many laboratory rodents (Fig. 3D).

Materno–Fetal Interdigitation

Within each of these gross forms, variations exist in the manner by which the maternal and fetal tissues interact. Again the simplest situation, *folded,* is typified by the pig. The uterine surface is thrown into a series of undulations, referred to as primary folds, and the fetal chorion is initially draped over these (Fig. 4A). As gestation advances, a series of smaller ripples, the secondary folds, develop at the interface, so increasing the surface area of mutual contact. A generally similar but more exaggerated type of folding is seen among the carnivores. Within the zonary placenta of the cat or dog, the maternal and fetal tissues interdigitate through an elaborate series of tall, slender, parallel folds or sheets. Because of their size and orientation, this arrangement is referred to as *lamellar* (Fig. 4B). In other species, for instance some of the higher primates, the parallel folds are not complete and so arrays of broad palmate branches are created (Fig. 4C). This pattern is described as *trabecular* and foreshadows the development of the *villous* configuration in which the fetal tissues form a three-dimensional tree-like structure, repeatedly branching into more slender units (Fig. 4D). Finally, the maternal and fetal tissues may each form a highly complex three-dimensional framework, which interlocks in a similar fashion to the substance and pores of a sponge (Fig. 4E). This *labyrinthine* arrangement is found in the placentas of rodents, lagomorphs, and insectivores.

Materno–Fetal Barrier

Allied to these gross morphologic and microscopic variants are differences in the fundamental relationship between the trophoblast and the uterine tissues. In most species, the trophoblast is simply apposed to the uterine epithelium, and there is no destruction or invasion of the maternal tissues. The conceptus therefore remains in the uterine lumen throughout gestation, and use of the term *implantation* is somewhat of a misnomer. Nonetheless, this situation is often referred to as "central implantation" and the histologic relationship between the fetal and maternal tissues is classified as *epitheliochorial* (Fig. 5A). Although individual species variations exist in the detailed nature of the placental barrier, this arrangement is found in the pig, ruminants, and horse. Thus, in the ruminant the fetal placental villi interdigitate with the crypts of the maternal caruncles, a configuration that may well have generated in the ancient's minds the im-

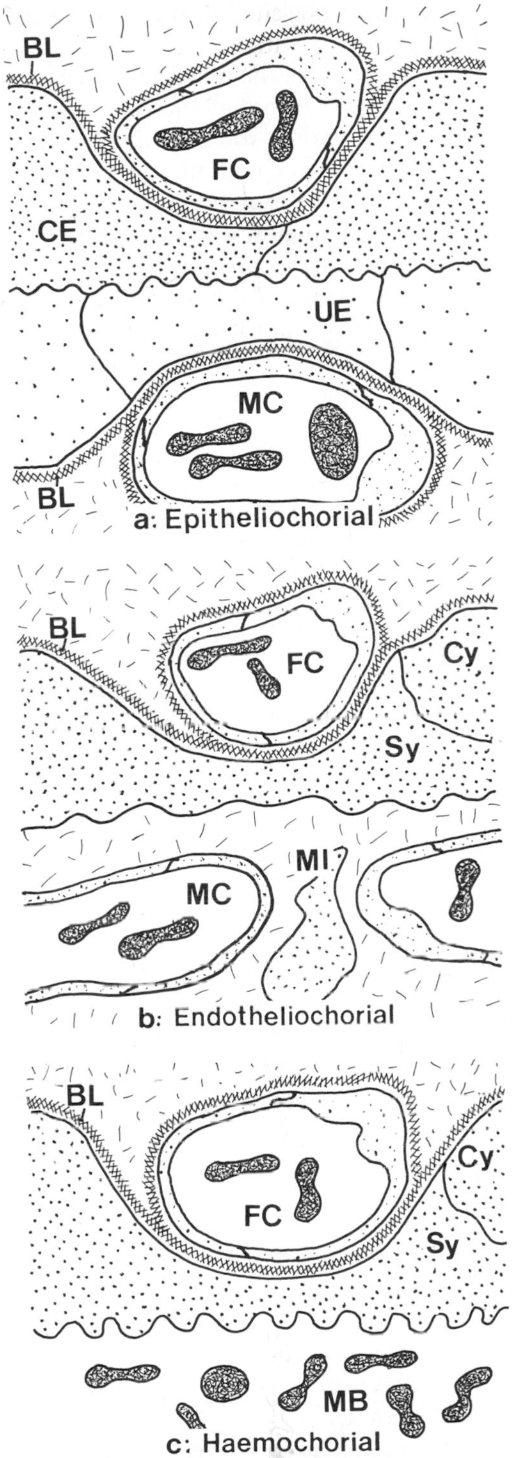

FIG. 5. Tissue layers of materno–fetal barrier according to Grosser classification. *MC,* maternal capillary; *MB,* maternal blood; *FC,* fetal capillary; *BL,* basal laminas; *CE,* chorionic epithelium (trophoblast); *Sy,* syncytiotrophoblast; *Cy,* cytotrophoblast; *UE,* uterine epithelium; and *MI,* maternal interstitium. Fetal components are comprised under the name *chorion.* Maternal components are reduced step by step until, in the hemochorial situation, chorion comes into direct contact with maternal blood. (Modified from ref. 283, with permission.)

pression of the fetal vessels "plugging into" their maternal counterparts.

By contrast, invasion of the maternal tissues is seen in five apparently unrelated orders of mammals, namely, the carnivores, insectivores, rodents, bats, and primates. Limited destruction of the endometrium occurs in the carnivores, in many species of insectivores and bats, and among some lower primates. The uterine epithelium is removed, and in the carnivores, this typically occurs opposite the equatorial zone of the chorionic sac. The trophoblast is now apposed to the maternal capillaries embedded in an acellular matrix of basal lamina-type material, a relationship classified as *endotheliochorial* (Fig. 5B).

Further invasion results in erosion into the maternal vessels, so that the trophoblast is bathed directly by the mother's blood. This is termed *hemochorial* placentation (Fig. 5C) and is typical of the rodents and primates. Even within this category, variations occur. Depending on whether the trophoblast is one, two, or three layers thick, the *hemomonochorial* placenta of, for example, the man and guinea pig, the *hemodichorial* placenta of the rabbit, and the *hemotrichorial* placenta of the rat and mouse are recognized (30). These layers may be a combination of cellular and syncytial elements, and so the detailed histologic nature of the placental membrane is of key importance when considering facilitated and active transport or vesicular transfer.

Despite this seemingly aggressive behavior of the trophoblast in most cases, the depth of invasion is still relatively superficial and limited, so that the bulk of the conceptus remains within the uterine lumen. This is known as *superficial implantation,* and it is only among the great apes that the blastocyst becomes completely embedded within the endometrium and *interstitial implantation* takes place.

Vascular Arrangement

A main danger of classification systems is that once proposed, the information contained within them may be wrongly extrapolated to support hypotheses in fields quite different from those for which the scheme was originally devised. The history of the Grosser classification exemplifies this point.

When first put forward, the histologic classification scheme provided a main advance by clarifying the different types of materno–fetal interface observed among mammals. Assumptions were soon made, however, that the permeability of the placental barrier was dictated by the numbers of layers separating the two circulations. The epitheliochorial placenta was thus considered to be of lower efficiency and more "primitive" than its hemochorial counterpart, a supposition that dogged placental physiology for many decades.

As mentioned previously, although the number of tissue layers present may influence the *mechanisms* by which active transport or vesicular transfer occurs, there is no evidence to suggest it has any bearing on the efficiency of these processes. Equally, for diffusional transport, it is now clear that the rate will be proportional to the area and the mean thickness of the placental barrier. With regard to the latter, it is a common phenomenon in many species possessing an epitheliochorial placenta for the fetal capillaries to invaginate deeply into the chorionic epithelium as gestation advances. As a result, the overall thickness of the interhemal barrier may be little different from that in the hemochorial situation, a fact that is lost when comparing placentas on their histologic basis alone.

Another important determinant of the rate of diffusional exchange is the relative directions of the maternal and fetal blood flows. Several different arrangements can be envisaged, as illustrated in Fig. 6, and these will all have contrasting exchange characteristics (31–33). The most inefficient system would be that of *concurrent* flow, in which both the maternal and fetal bloodstreams run in the same direction. Perhaps for this reason, it does not seem to form the basis of any placental circulation. At the opposite extreme is the *countercurrent* system, in which the two bloodstreams run in opposite directions. This is highly efficient, theoretically allowing arteriovenous equilibration, and is seen in the placentas of rodents, lagomorphs, and equids.

In many ruminant species, there seems to be a mixture of both concurrent and countercurrent flow at different points along the villous interdigitations. As a result, the net effect is considered to be *cross-current.* A more clearly defined cross-current flow is seen within the lamellar placenta of carnivores. Finally, in those higher primates possessing a villous hemochorial placenta, the highly three-dimensional branching of the villous tree ensures that there will be an unpredictable and varying combination of all three patterns of relative blood flow. The term *multivillous* flow has been used to describe this situation.

These differences in the geometric arrangements of the fetal and maternal vascular networks and their influence on diffusional exchange are reflected in the fetoplacental weight ratio at term (pig, cross-current 9:1; rodents, countercurrent up to 20:1) (33). Again, on the basis of the Grosser classification, one might suppose that the villous hemochorial placenta of the human, providing such intimate contact between the two circulations, would be highly efficient. However, a combination of arteriovenous shunting through the intervillous space and multivillous blood flow conspire to ensure that the fetoplacental weight ratio remains at a lowly 6:1. Maintaining the maternal circulation in a geometrically defined network clearly confers some advantages.

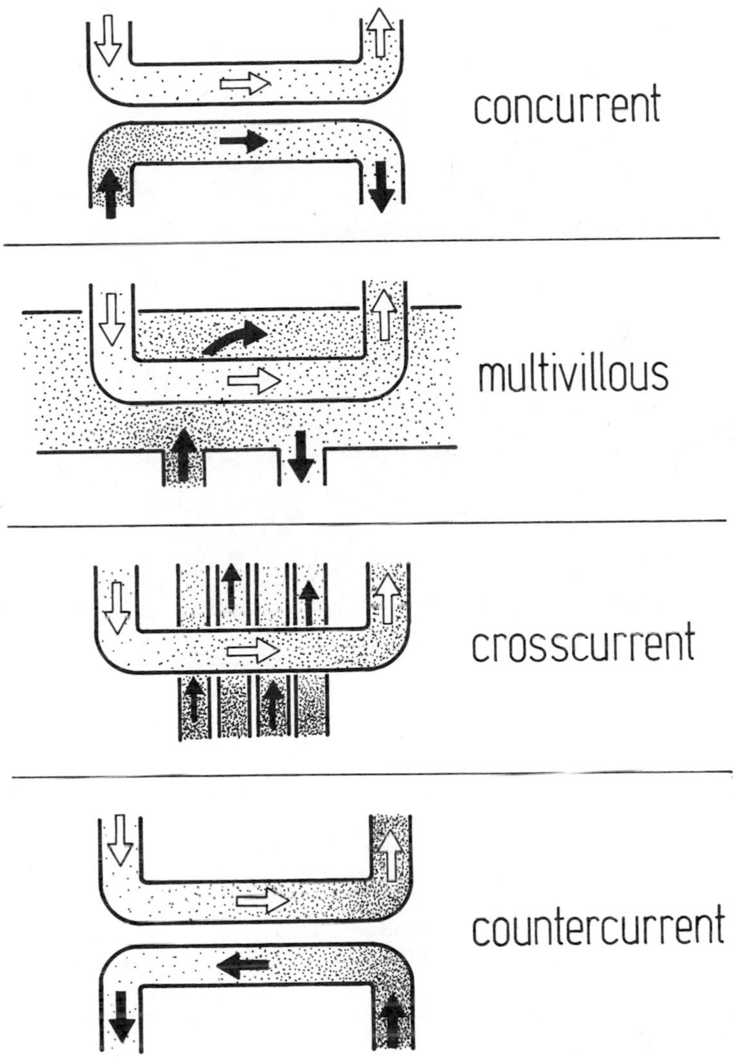

FIG. 6. Idealized arrangement of fetal (*white arrows*) and maternal (*black arrows*) bloodstreams of different placental exchange types. Density of dots in venous limbs of fetal vessel loops (*upper right vessel of each drawing*) illustrates efficiency of different exchangers. (From ref. 33, with permission.)

MACROSCOPY OF THE DELIVERED PLACENTA

The full-term human placenta is usually a circular disc-like organ, but in approximately 10% of cases, it displays abnormal shapes, such as bilobate placenta, placenta succenturiata, duplex placenta, bidiscoidal placenta, zonary placenta, or placenta membranacea (34). The latter three types are comparable with placental shapes of other species (cf. section on Comparative Placentation). At term, the delivered organ is, on average, 22 cm in diameter and 2.5 cm thick at the center and weighs 470 g. These data show considerable interindividual variation and, moreover, are strongly dependent on the mode of delivery. Factors such as the time of clamping of the umbilical cord and the time elapsed between delivery and fixation are critical because loss of fetal and/or maternal blood have a major impact on the dimensions of this highly vascularized organ.

On the fetal (chorionic or amnionic) surface, the umbilical cord most frequently inserts in a slightly eccentric position. The avascular and glossy amnion covers the chorionic plate, including the chorionic vessels (Fig. 7). The latter are continuous with those of the umbilical cord and branch in a starlike pattern. Their final branches supply the villous trees. Where arteries and veins cross, the arterial branches are usually closer to the amnion, and according to Wentworth (35), only about 3% of cases show the opposite relationship. White

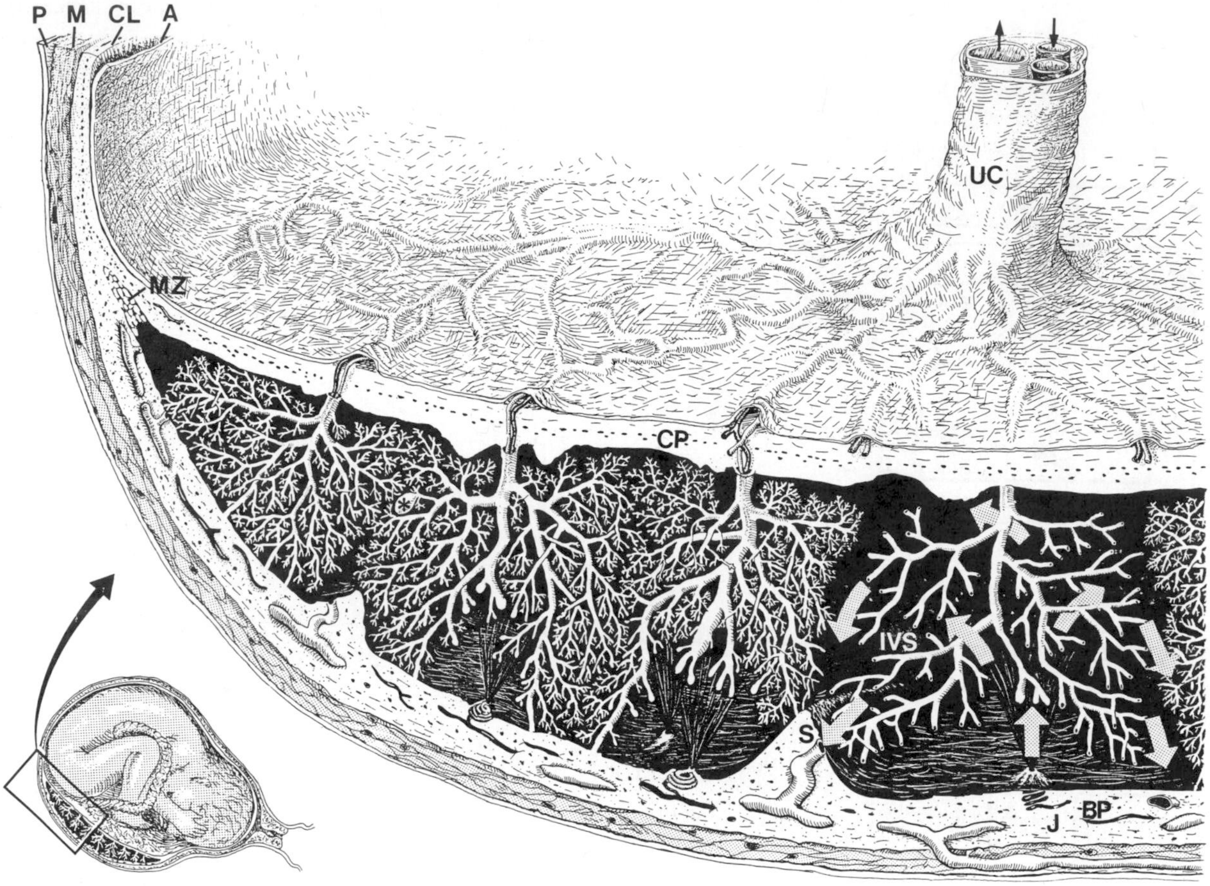

FIG. 7. Summarizing survey diagram of nearly mature human placenta *in situ.* Loose centers of villous trees, arranged around maternal arterial inflow area, are frequent features. *P,* perimetrium; *M,* myometrium; *CL,* chorion laeve; *A,* amnion; *MZ,* marginal zone between placenta and fetal membranes, with obliterated intervillous space and ghost villi; *, cell island; *S,* septum; *J,* junctional zone; *BP,* basal plate; *CP,* chorionic plate; *IVS,* intervillous space; and *UC,* umbilical cord. (From ref. 284, with permission.)

opaque stripes often accompanying the larger chorionic vessels are due to increased number of collagen fibers. Corresponding opaque spots located between the chorionic vessels (bosselations) usually point to larger subchorionic deposits of Langhans' fibrinoid.

Near the placental margin, where the chorionic plate and the basal plate form the chorion laeve (Fig. 7), the transparency of the chorionic plate decreases, thus forming a largely incomplete, opaque subchorial closing ring. It connects the placenta with the rest of the fetal membranes. If the closing ring is peripherally undergrown by villous trees, the specimen is called a placenta circumvallata. In such cases, the membranes are connected superficially to the fetal surface of the placenta.

The uterine (maternal) surface of the placenta is an artificial surface, originating from the separation of the organ from the uterine wall. It is composed of a heterogeneous mixture of trophoblastic and decidual cells, embedded in large amounts of extracellular debris, fibrinoid, and blood clot. An incomplete system of flat grooves or deeper clefts subdivides the basal surface of the placenta into ten to 40 slightly elevated areas called lobes. Inside the placenta, the grooves correspond to the septa (Fig. 7). The grooves are the postpartal results of tearing at sites of minor mechanical resistance, because the basal central parts of the septa are often characterized by necrotic zones and pseudocysts. The septa should not be misunderstood as true separating structures that subdivide the intervillous space into chambers. Rather, they are irregular pillars or short sails that only trace the lobular borders.

The lobes show a fairly good correspondence with the position of the villous trees. From the chorionic plate at term, 60 to 70 villous trees (or fetal lobules) arise. Thus, according to Boyd and Hamilton (4) and Kaufmann (36), each lobe is occupied by one to four villous trees (Fig. 7). Small marginal lobes are likely to be occupied only by one single villous tree and thus correspond to what Schuhmann (37) described to represent a placentone.

Terms such as *fetal placenta* for the chorionic plate including villous trees and intervillous space or *maternal placenta* for the basal plate should be strictly avoided because they are inappropriate, misleading, and often cause misinterpretation (e.g., as soon as morphologically inexperienced scientists isolate respective parts of the organ and trusting in their putative judgment designate material to be solely of maternal or fetal origin). Both plates usually represent a colorful mixture of fetal and maternal tissues. Macroscopic dissection of placental structures can never guarantee the entirely fetal or maternal composition of the isolated probes. A corresponding warning is necessary regarding the placental bed, which is often thought to represent the maternal remains after separation of the placenta. Trophoblastic streamers deeply invading the endometrium, even reaching the myometrium, remain *in utero* after delivery.

Structurally impressive parameters such as placental shape and site of cord insertion are usually regarded as functionally unimportant. However, as has been recently stressed by Becker (38), both are influenced by the intrauterine position of the placenta, the location of the cord insertion representing the epicenter of implantation (39). Eccentric or marginal cord insertion thus point to an eccentric implantation on the anterior or posterior uterine wall. This causes an asymmetric development of the organ for mechanical and nutritional reasons, and thus functional implications cannot be totally excluded.

EARLY DEVELOPMENT

Prelacunar Stage

Formation of the placenta begins as soon as the blastocyst has become attached to the endometrium, a process that is believed to occur at about day 6 to 7 postconception. At this stage, the blastocyst has hatched from the zona pellucida and consists of an outer wall, comprising a single layer of uninucleate trophoblast cells, surrounding the blastocoel and the inner cell mass (Fig. 8A). Cell lineage studies have now confirmed that the placenta and extraembryonic membranes are largely derived from the trophoblast, whereas the embryo and umbilical cord arise exclusively from the inner cell mass.

The inner cell mass confers an axis of symmetry on the blastocyst, for it is eccentrically placed in contact with the trophoblast wall. The overlying cells are referred to as polar trophoblast and are involved in making the first crucial attachments of the blastocyst with the endometrial epithelium. Variations in the orientation of the blastocyst at the time of implantation almost certainly account for abnormalities in the site of insertion of the umbilical cord into the placental disc (40).

Implantation normally takes place in the upper part of the body of the uterus near the midsagittal plane and with almost equal frequency on the anterior and posterior walls. A more lateral siting may lead to attachment occurring on both walls, resulting in a bilobed placenta or other variant. It is intriguing that a higher incidence of both abnormal placental shapes and eccentric insertions of the umbilical cord has been reported in pregnancies arising from *in vitro* fertilization techniques compared with controls (41). One conclusion might be that the normal pattern of materno–fetal interactions regulating implantation is disturbed in this group.

The earliest *in vivo* specimens available for study are those in the collection of Hertig et al. (42). Even the youngest of these, estimated to be at day 7 postconception, displays a blastocyst that is almost completely embedded within the endometrium (cf. Fig. 8B). Therefore, in an attempt to study the initial stages of attachment, Lindenberg and co-workers (43) cultured hatched blastocysts obtained after *in vitro* fertilization on monolayers of human endometrial epithelium. In this somewhat simplified system, all the blastocysts became adherent to the monolayer and three of four were considered to "implant," as evidenced by outgrowth of the trophoblastic cells. The polar trophoblast cells covering the inner cell mass produced long slender processes that penetrated the intercellular spaces between adjacent endometrial cells. There was no evidence of phagocytosis by the trophoblast, and the endometrial cells were displaced laterally where they formed a multilayer three to four cells thick. Having penetrated between the endometrial cells, the trophoblast cells in the center of the "implantation" site transformed into an early multinucleated syncytium or *syncytiotrophoblast*.

In the *in vivo* situation, the partially embedded specimens available all show a similar but more extensive syncytial transformation in those peripheral elements of the trophoblast abutting the maternal endometrium. The trophoblast cells that formed the original wall of the blastocyst remain unicellular and are now referred to as *cytotrophoblast* cells. These act as a stem cell population, and their rapid division and subsequent fusion with the syncytiotrophoblast leads to the continual expansion of this mantle.

Lacunar Stage

Toward the end of day 8 postconception, a series of fluid-filled spaces or vacuoles develop within the syncytiotrophoblastic mass (Fig. 8C). Although initially isolated, these vacuoles soon coalesce to form larger *lacunae,* which are separated by attenuated *trabeculae* of syncytiotrophoblast. This marks the start of the lacunar or trabecular stage of development, lasting from days 8 to 12 postconception.

At the end of this period, implantation may be considered to be complete. The blastocyst, or conceptus as it

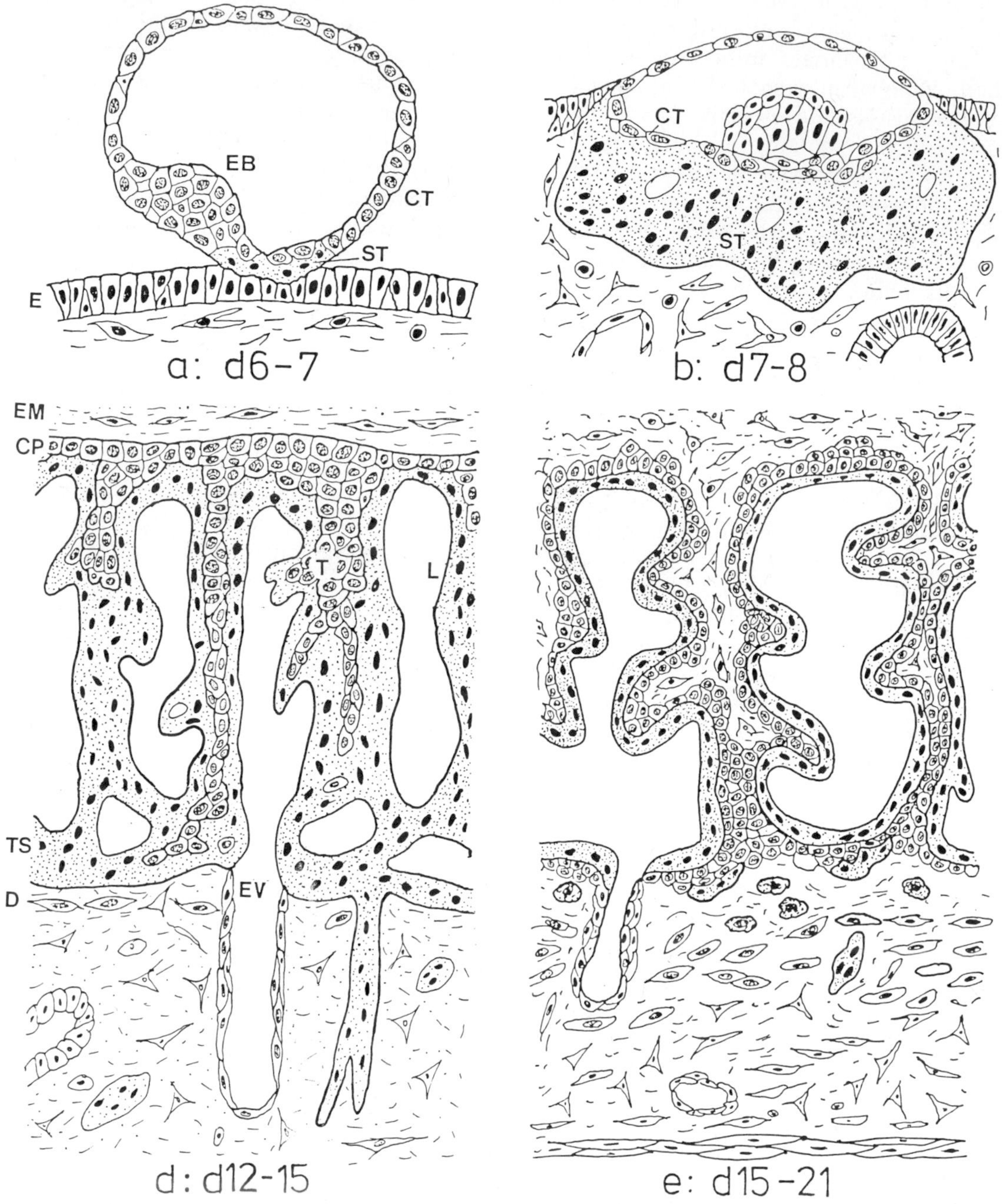

FIG. 8. Simplified drawings of typical stages of early placental development. (**A** and **B**) Prelacunar stages; (**C**) lacunar stage; (**D**) transition from lacunar to primary villous stage; (**E**) secondary villous stage; and (**F**) tertiary villous stage. *E,* endometrial epithelium; *EB,* embryoblast; *CT,* cytotrophoblast; *ST,* syncytiotrophoblast; *EM,* extraembryonic mesoderm; *CP,* chorionic plate; *T,* trabeculae and primary villi; *L,* maternal blood lacunae; *TS,* trophoblastic shell; *EV,* endometrial vessel; *D,* decidua; *RF,* Rohr's fibrinoid; *NF,* Nitabuch's fibrinoid; *G,* trophoblastic giant cell; *x,* X cells or extravillous cytotrophoblast; *BP,* basal plate; *PB,* placental bed; and *J,* junctional zone. (Altered from ref. 284, with permission.)

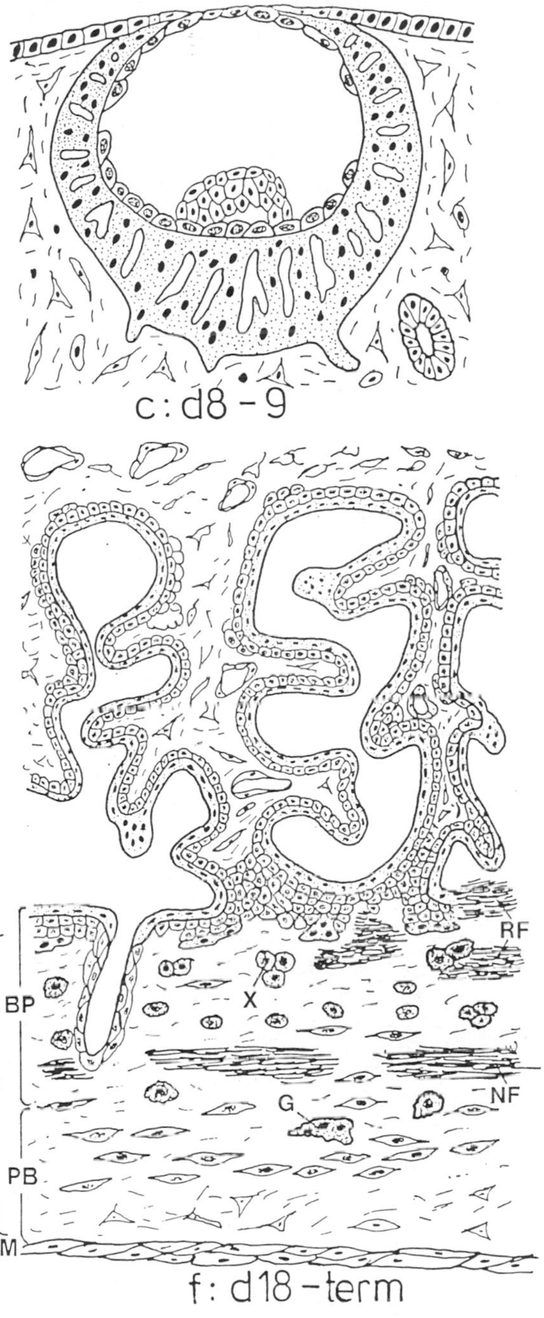

FIG. 8. *Continued.*

may now be better called, is totally embedded within the uterine wall, and the endometrial epithelium has regrown over the site. The syncytiotrophoblastic mantle surrounds the conceptus, but it is thicker and the lacunae are better developed beneath the embryonic pole. By this stage, the inner cell mass has transformed into the bilaminar germ disc, and extraembryonic mesoderm, derived from the most caudal end of the future primitive streak (44), has begun to spread over the inner aspect of the trophoblast wall (Fig. 8D). The new combination of trophoblast and extraembryonic mesoderm is termed the *chorion,* and so the original wall of the blastocyst may now be referred to as the chorionic sac.

Formation of the lacunae subdivides the trophoblastic mantle into three fundamental zones: the primary chorionic plate facing the embryo; the lacunar system together with the trabeculae; and the trophoblastic shell abutting the endometrium. The lacunae are clearly the forerunners of the intervillous space of the mature placenta, whereas the primary chorionic plate and the trophoblastic shell become the chorionic and basal plates, respectively. In the mature placenta, these are connected by anchoring villi, which represent the derivatives of the trabeculae as follows.

Commencing on day 12, cytotrophoblast cells originating from the primary chorionic plate penetrate into the trabeculae, extending as far as tips by day 14 (Fig. 8D). At this point, they extend laterally, establishing contacts with counterparts in adjacent trabeculae and so contribute to the trophoblastic shell. Indeed, many come to lie on the deepest side of the shell, in contact with the endometrial cells. From this position, many migrate into the endometrial stroma between the uterine glands and around the spiral arteries (45). Because of their location, these are referred to as extravillous cytotrophoblast, and as will be seen later, they represent a unique subset of trophoblast cells characterized by different cell markers. Suffice to say at present that one of their roles appears to be the transformation of the spiral arteries into dilated capacitance vessels, thus ensuring an adequate uteroplacental circulation later in gestation. This process involves the destruction of the arterial media and the replacement of the endothelial lining with trophoblast in a retrograde fashion.

Invasion into the tips of the maternal vessels is seen from day 12 onward, and initially the escaping maternal blood passes into the lacunae through communicating channels through the trophoblastic shell. The mouths of the spiral arteries soon become plugged with trophoblast, however, so that these communications are reduced to an interconnecting network of intercellular spaces (4,23). These plugs act as a filtering system, and there is evidence from direct vision of the intervillous space by hysteroscopy that for the first 12 weeks of pregnancy the space is free from maternal blood cells (46).

Doppler studies have indicated that turbulence within the intervillous space, suggesting an active maternal circulation, is likely only to be seen at the end of the first trimester, an event that coincides with morphologic evidence of loosening of the trophoblastic plugs. The implication of this would be that up until this stage of development, the conceptus is reliant on oxygen carried in solution by the maternal plasma filtrate that passes into the lacunar system. Hence, organogenesis is carried out under conditions of relatively low pO_2. It is notable that at the end of this period, there is a switch from the production of embryonic hemoglobins, which are able to combine with oxygen at the very low tension and pH of interstitial fluid, to fetal hemoglobins (47). Interestingly, in pathologic cases, maternal blood may be seen circulating within the early intervillous space, suggesting that trophoblastic invasion has been abnormal (46).

Early Villous Stage

Proliferation within the cytotrophoblastic core of the trabeculae results in a considerable increase in their length. Around day 13, the trabeculae begin to develop side branches composed entirely of trophoblast that protrude into the lacunae (Fig. 8D). These are termed *primary villi,* and the lacunae can now justifiably be referred to as the intervillous spaces.

Shortly after, extraembryonic mesoderm derived from the primary chorionic plate invades the trabeculae. It does not penetrate to their tips, and so the more distal parts of the trabeculae connecting with the trophoblastic shell remain composed of cytotrophoblast alone, often without a syncytiotrophoblastic covering. These segments are referred to as the cytotrophoblastic cell columns and are the actively proliferating source of the extravillous cytotrophoblast. The mesoderm does penetrate the primary villi, however, and in doing so, transforms them into *secondary villi* (Fig. 8D).

Within this villous mesoderm, hemangioblastic progenitor cells differentiate, and beginning between days 18 and 20, these give rise to the first fetal capillaries (48,49). Vascularization marks the formation of *tertiary villi* (Fig. 8E).

Hence, this form of villous classification reflects basic stages in the development of new villi, a process that continues throughout gestation. The first two categories represent transitory stages, and as tertiary villi accumulate, they soon come to form the bulk of the placental tissue.

Initially, villi develop over the entire surface of the chorionic sac, although as mentioned previously, they are more profuse over the deeper embryonic pole than over the abembryonic pole. The villi at the latter interact with the endometrium that has overgrown the implanting blastocyst, the decidua capsularis. As the conceptus enlarges, the decidua capsularis becomes progressively stretched and the placental villi in this region are compressed. By the end of the second month, the implantation site bulges into the cavity of the uterus, but the decidua capsularis has yet to fuse with the opposite wall of the uterus. As a result, the villi over the embryonic pole may receive a relatively poor supply of nutrients, which could account for the fact that beginning around the ninth week postconception they begin to degenerate. This regression extends in an equatorial direction and is accompanied by a disappearance of the associated intervillous space and by fusion of the primary chorionic plate with the trophoblastic shell. The chorionic sac becomes secondarily smooth in this region and is referred to as the chorion laeve. At the end of this process, villi only remain at the embryonic pole, where they constitute the definitive discoidal placenta.

Attention will now be turned to the tissue components within this organ.

BASIC VILLOUS STRUCTURE

Syncytiotrophoblast

The syncytiotrophoblast forms the outer covering of the villous tree (Fig. 9A and B) and the surface of the chorionic plate directed toward the intervillous space. It is a continuous multinucleated syncytial layer that contains a high concentration of organelles (Fig. 10).

Microvilli are found over the entire surface throughout gestation, although their density and morphology may vary according to the antenatal and fixation conditions (50). Receptors for many factors such as insulin, low-density lipoprotein, transferrin, and immunoglobulin (Ig) G have been detected on the microvillous surface. For reviews, see Benirschke and Kaufmann (51) and Jones and Fox (52). These receptors tend to cluster at the base of the microvilli where clathrin-coated pits are found (53). One proposed function of the microvilli is that they present a large surface area containing receptors to the maternal blood and that movement of receptor and bound ligand into the region of a coated pit with subsequent internalization provides a means for concentration. The microvillous surface is also rich in different enzymes, particularly in alkaline phosphatase, which may exist in several isoforms. Other enzymes include 5′-nucleotidase, hexokinase, α-amylase, protein kinases, and galactosyl and sialyl transferases. Actin filaments provide a supporting framework for the microvilli and link with a dense meshwork of both microtubules and microfilaments lying just beneath the syncytial surface (54).

Within the cytoplasm are many pinocytotic vesicles, free ribosomes, mitochondria, lipid droplets, and different multivesicular and dense bodies (52,55). Endoplasmic reticulum, Golgi apparatus, and secretory droplets are also plentiful, confirming the wide range of metabolic activities in which the syncytiotrophoblast is involved.

The nuclei within this layer show varying chromatin patterns, and as gestation advances, an increasing number display a dense aggregation of the chromatin beneath the nuclear membrane. Most of these appear to be sequestered into tightly packed clumps known as syncytial

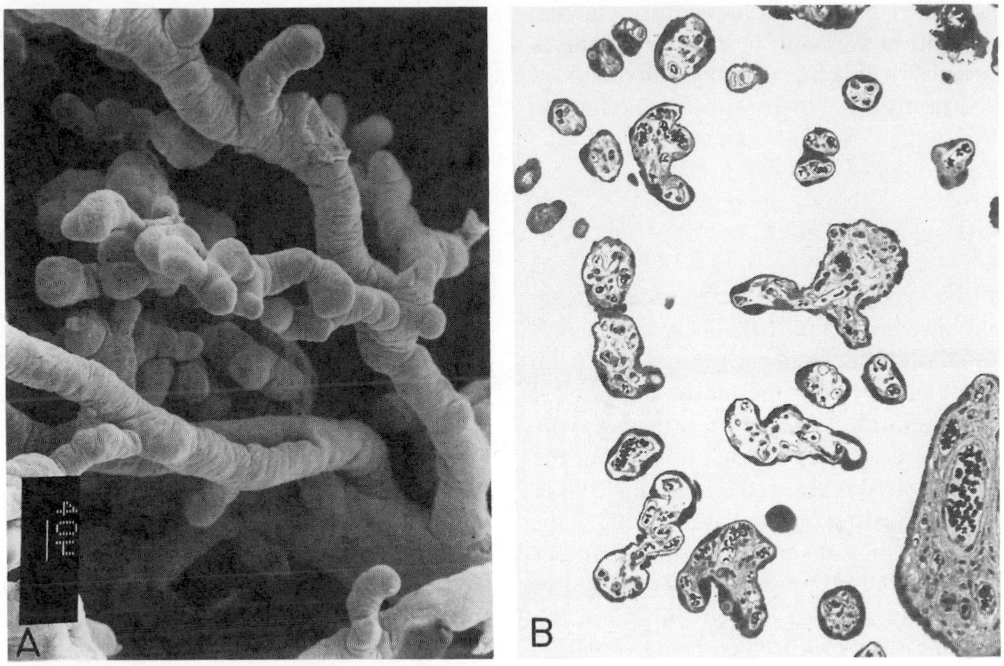

FIG. 9. Villi from normal, mature placenta, fortieth week of gestation. (**A**) In this scanning electron micrograph, long, slender, slightly curved mature intermediate villi with a moderate number of grapelike terminal villi are dominating features. All villi are covered by velvetlike, continuous layer of syncytiotrophoblast, separating villous interior from surrounding maternal blood (removed). (**B**) In corresponding histologic section, many oblique and cross sections of villi can be seen. Dark surface layer represents trophoblast. ×120. (From ref. 285, with permission.)

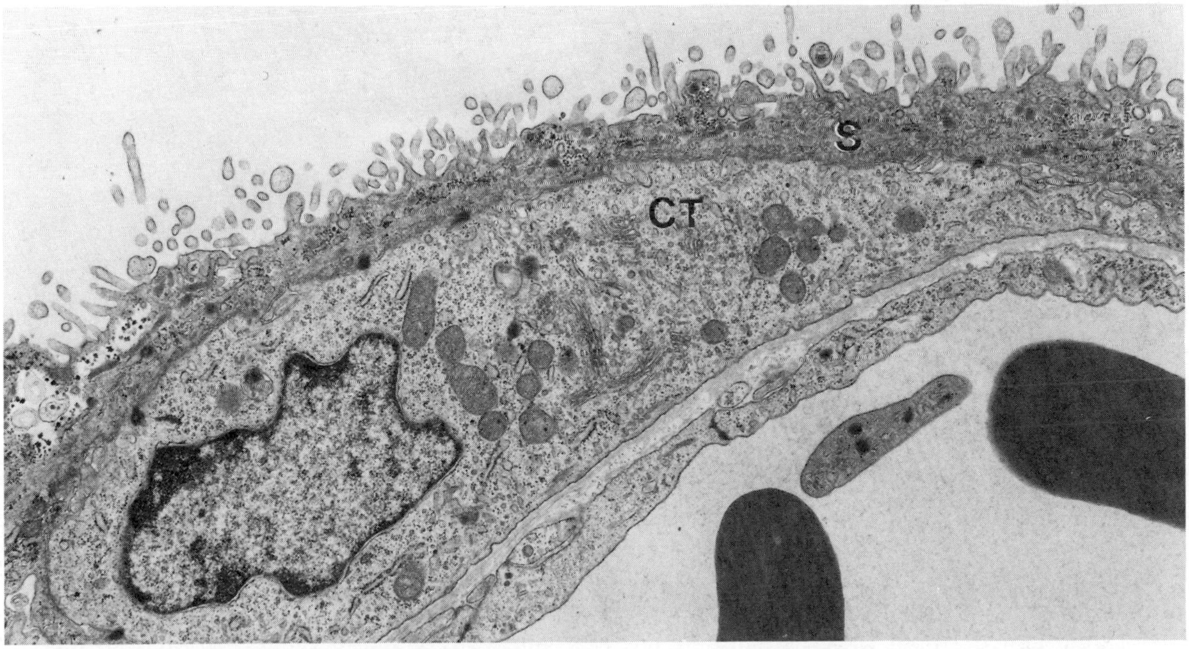

FIG. 10. Transmission electron micrograph of placental barrier separating intervillous space with maternal blood (*above*) and fetal blood in fetal capillaries (*lower right*). Barrier consists of syncytiotrophoblast (*S*), villous cytotrophoblast, Langhans' cells (*CT*), slender cleft with basal laminas, and fetal endothelium. ×9,800. (From ref. 286, with permission.)

knots. Mitosis has never been observed within syncytial nuclei, and transcription seems to be reduced. Generation and maintenance of this layer therefore depend on the continual incorporation of cytotrophoblast cells into it (56,57).

Cytotrophoblast (Langhans' Cells)

Lying deep to the syncytial layer are the uninucleate villous cytotrophoblast cells (Fig. 10). These appear frequently in sectioned material from early gestation, to the extent that for much of the first trimester the trophoblast is a two-layered epithelium. As gestation progresses, the cytotrophoblast cells are seen less often, and most of the villous surface (about 80%) is covered by the single layer of syncytiotrophoblast resting on the basal lamina. This has led to the common misconception that the number of cytotrophoblast cells falls as pregnancy advances. Recent stereologic studies have shown that this is not the case but that the total number of cells increases steadily until term (58). The real situation is that as the villous surface rapidly expands, the cytotrophoblast cells become widely separated and so *appear* less numerous in sectioned material. This has important consequences for materno–fetal immunoglobulin transfer, for unlike the syncytiotrophoblast and endothelial cells, cytotrophoblast cells do not express Fcg receptors (59). Transport of immunoglobulins may therefore only become possible in later pregnancy, when the cytotrophoblastic layer becomes incomplete.

The control of cytotrophoblastic proliferation is uncertain, although it does seem to be heavily influenced by the prevailing oxygen tension (60). Culture in hypoxic conditions (61) or pregnancy at high altitude (Reshetnikova, *unpublished observations*) leads to an increase in numbers. The volume of trophoblast associated with each cytotrophoblast nucleus appears to remain constant throughout gestation, indicating that trophoblastic growth is purely hyperplastic in nature (58).

Resting, or undifferentiated, cytotrophoblast cells are generally cuboidal in shape, and their cytoplasm displays a paucity of organelles. Secretory droplets are infrequent, and the overall appearance is of a cell type that is metabolically quiescent. Further development leads to the formation of fewer intermediate cells, which as their name implies are intermediate in morphologic appearance between the resting state and syncytiotrophoblast (52). These cells are more active, as evidenced by the display of enzymes for both aerobic and anaerobic glycolysis (51,62). The presence of messenger RNA for the human chorionic gonadotropin (hCG) α subunit has also been demonstrated in intermediate cells (63).

The cytoplasm of these cells finally comes to resemble that of the overlying syncytiotrophoblast, and fusion with the latter soon follows. Desmosomes normally attach the cytotrophoblast cells to the deep surface of the syncytium, and during recruitment, gap junctions form in the intervening areas. Their formation appears to initiate fusion, and soon isolated remnants of the cell membranes, some still carrying desmosomes, are all that remain (for review, see ref. 51). The circulation of these remnants within the syncytioplasm may result in the incorporation of redundant junctional complexes into the microvillous surface (64). It is intriguing that at the time of implantation in the marmoset, there is considerable retroviral expression at the interface between the syncytiotrophoblast layer and the cytotrophoblast cells, leading to speculation that retroviral proteins may be involved in the fusion process (65).

Throughout gestation, the trophoblast rests on a well-developed basal lamina, composed largely of type IV collagen, laminin, and fibronectin. The thickness of the lamina is very variable from point to point on the villous surface, but in general, it increases toward term. Excessive thickening has been reported in pregnancies associated with maternal diabetes, hypertension, and cigarette smoking.

Fixed Connective Tissue

One of the principal components of the stromal villous core is the fixed connective tissue cells. The appearance of these varies greatly, depending on the degree of maturity of the villi in question, and so they are described in relation with the development of the villous tree later.

Hofbauer Cells

Hofbauer cells are fetal macrophages that are found within the villous stroma at all stages of gestation. They possess a very characteristic morphology, for their surface is thrown into a complex system of lamellipodia and microplicae, and their cytoplasm contains many vacuoles and lysosomes (Figs. 11 and 12). The origin of these cells has been the topic of much debate, but it now appears that there may be different sources. In the first month of pregnancy, Hofbauer cells possibly originate from mesenchymal cells in the villous stroma (49), but this supply may be augmented by differentiation from fetal bone marrow–derived macrophages once the fetal circulation is established (66). Moreover, it has been shown that the macrophage population may increase through mitotic division (67).

Several diverse functions have been ascribed to Hofbauer cells including the regulation of stromal fluid balance, modulation of vasculogenesis and stromal cell growth, and the absorption of immune complexes. Comparison of class II major histocompatibility complex (MHC) antigen expression by the cells at different stages

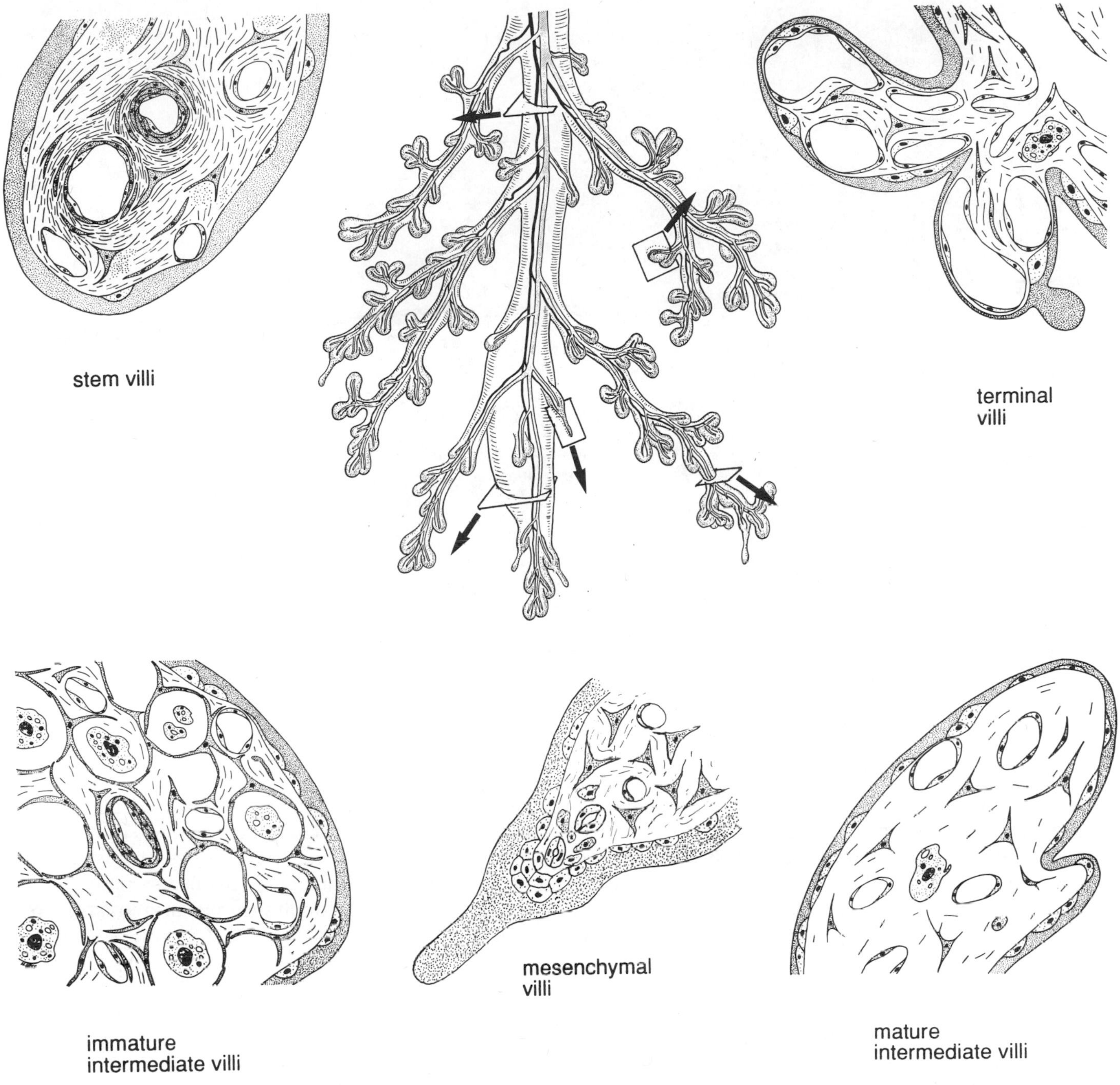

FIG. 11. Simplified representation of peripheral part of mature placental villous tree, together with typical cross sections of different villous types. (From ref. 284, with permission.)

of pregnancy has shown that they are progressively activated as gestation advances. They may thus also play an important role as antigen-presenting cells, acting as an active second line of defence to any infectious agent that has succeeded in beaching the trophoblastic layer. In this regard, it should be noted that a subpopulation of Hofbauer cells are CD4 positive and so may act as portals of entry to the fetus or reservoirs for the human immunodeficiency virus (for review, see ref. 66).

Fetal Vessels

The fetal vascular network is lined by a nonfenestrated endothelium throughout (Fig. 12). At least two populations of endothelial cells may be present, although the functional significance of this is not yet clear (68). One cell type is characterized by the presence of many microfilaments, which have been identified as predominantly vimentin and are therefore considered to have a struc-

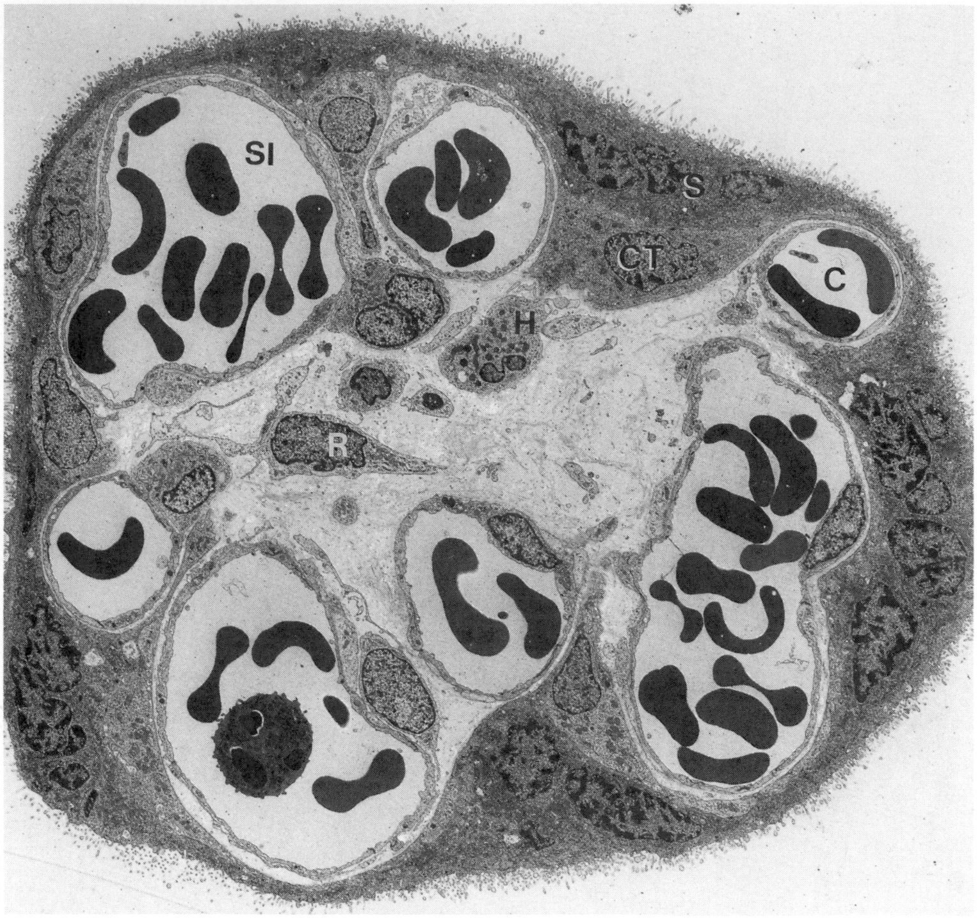

FIG. 12. Survey electron micrograph of typical, well-preserved terminal villus. It illustrates high degree of fetal capillarization, with some of the capillaries (*C*) narrow and others dilated, forming sinusoids (*SI*). Sparse connective tissue is composed of macrophages (*H*), different fixed connective tissue cells (*R*), and connective tissue fibers. Stroma is surrounded by a structurally highly variable layer of syncytiotrophoblast (*S*) below which few cytotrophoblastic cells (*CT*) can be seen. ×2,000. (From ref. 286, with permission.)

tural rather than a contractile role (54). The second type possesses a well-developed rough endoplasmic reticulum and contains many secretory granules. Both cell types may be represented within a single cross section of a capillary, but as yet it is not known whether there are regional variations in distribution throughout the villous tree.

Junctional complexes link adjacent cells and serve to both stabilize the endothelium and to limit the permeability of the paracellular transport route, particularly in respect to anionic molecules. Large molecules, including IgG, are transported across the epithelium by plasmalemmal vesicles, which are present within both of the cell types described above (69).

The capillaries within the terminal villi are only surrounded by a basement membrane during the last third of pregnancy (49) (Fig. 12), and this contains type IV collagen, laminin, and fibronectin (70). It is secreted by both the endothelial cells and their associated pericytes. The pericytes may also contribute to angiogenesis within the villi (49).

Further proximally in the villous tree, arteries and arterioles are found within the stem and intermediate villi (Fig. 11). These possess a smooth muscle coat, but elastic laminae are generally absent and the adventitia gradually blends with the fixed connective tissue of the stromal core. Because of the lack of neural innervation in the placenta, the caliber of the fetal vasculature must be controlled by paracrine and autocrine factors produced in response to physical stimuli such as transmural pressure or flow rate (71).

Integrity of the Placental Barrier

There is physiologic evidence for the existence of two different routes of transfer across the placental barrier, a transcellular and a paracellular route (72). The transcellular route involves transfer across the plasma membranes and the cytosol of the syncytiotrophoblast; the paracellular route is thought to be an extracellular, water-filled pathway. The existence of the latter pathway has been proven with physiologic *in vitro* and *in vivo* measurements. However, it is difficult to understand it morphologically because the villous syncytiotrophoblast has for a long time been thought to be a continuous uninterrupted layer, completely separating maternal and fetal circulations.

Three issues shall be addressed in this section, each of which might explain the paracellular pathway:

Is the syncytiotrophoblast really a syncytial continuum or is it composed of larger syncytial units separated by lateral intercellular clefts?

Areas of syncytial denudation closed by fibrin clot do exist. Do they provide a paracellular route?

Membrane-lined transtrophoblastic channels connecting apical and basal surfaces of the syncytiotrophoblast have been described as possible paracellular transfer routes.

The syncytiotrophoblast is a continuous, generally uninterrupted layer that extends over the surfaces of all villous trees (Fig. 9A), as well as over parts of the inner surfaces of the chorionic and basal plates. It thus lines the intervillous space. As a consequence, every substance passing from the maternal to the fetal circulation was thought to do so under the control of this trophoblastic layer. Recently, a few reports have pointed to the existence of vertical cell membranes that are said to subdivide the syncytium into "syncytial units" (for review, see ref. 51). After careful study, we were able to detect extremely few of such lateral intercellular clefts. In our opinion, these findings have an accidental rather than a real basis. They represent the results of a syncytiotrophoblastic repair mechanism (51) after syncytial rupture (cf. below). Therefore, terms such as *syncytial cells* and *syncytiotrophoblasts,* widely used in experimental disciplines, are inappropriate and should be avoided. Because of the paucity of these structures, they are very unlikely to provide effective transfer routes.

Recent research has shown that the integrity and completeness of the syncytiotrophoblastic barrier is not perfect. Where the syncytiotrophoblast is interrupted by degeneration or by mechanical forces, the gap is filled by fibrin (so-called perivillous fibrin) as a result of blood clotting. Corresponding fibrin spots replacing the syncytiotrophoblast are regular findings in every placenta throughout pregnancy. Such areas may serve as paratrophoblastic routes for materno–fetal macromolecule transfer bypassing the syncytiotrophoblast; horseradish peroxidase (48,000 D; 3.0-nm molecular radius) was shown to pass through the fibrin spots from the maternal circulation into the fetal villous stroma. According to Nelson and co-workers (73), perivillous fibrin accounts for about 7% of the villous surface of the normal human term placenta. This may offer a relevant paratrophoblastic transfer route for macromolecules.

Another paratrophoblastic transfer route for smaller molecules can be provided by the transtrophoblastic channels (74–76). Transport experiments by Stulc and co-workers (77) provided the first evidence for the existence of water-filled routes, so-called pores or channels, across the rabbit placenta. Their radius was calculated to be approximately 10 nm. This finding has been confirmed for the guinea pig placenta by Thornburg and Faber (78) and Hedley and Bradbury (79). Application of lanthanum hydroxide as an extracellular tracer through the maternal or fetal circulation by Kaufmann and co-workers (74) resulted in the demonstration of membrane-lined channels in the isolated guinea pig placenta and in the isolated human placental lobule (75). The channels have luminal diameters of 15 to 25 nm (80) and pass through the syncytiotrophoblast as winding and branching channels from the apical to basal surface. They are likely to be routes for membrane recycling from the basal to the apical syncytiotrophoblastic plasmalemma because there are morphologic hints for a respective baso-apical membrane flux (75,80).

These results are in agreement with experimental findings obtained in the guinea pig placenta (81) and in the *in vitro* perfused human placenta (75). In the fully isolated, artificially perfused organ, hydrostatic and colloid osmotic forces cause feto–maternal fluid shifts; an elevation in the fetal venous pressure of 5 to 17 mm Hg was sufficient to cause a shift 30% to 50% of the arterial perfusion volumes into the maternal circulation. Ultrastructurally, the channels identified are initially slender but later dilate into baglike structures (74). As soon as the fetal venous pressure was reduced to normal values, the fluid shift ceased and the baglike channels disappeared. The only possible explanation is the existence of preexisting transtrophoblastic channels, which can be dilated under conditions of elevated pressures. It is likely that the channels traced with lanthanum hydroxide are identical to those dilated experimentally under the conditions of fluid shift and those postulated in transfer experiments by the physiologists mentioned above.

Functionally, the transtrophoblastic channels are possible sites of transfer for water-soluble, lipid-insoluble molecules with an effective molecular diameter of about 1.5 nm (72,78). Under the conditions of feto–maternal fluid shift caused by fetal venous pressure increase or fetal decrease of osmotic pressure, they may dilate to such an extent that even larger molecules may pass (74,81). Moreover, pressure-dependent dilatation and closure of the channels may act as an important factor in fetal osmoregulation and water balance. Excessive fetal hydration will cause an increase of fetal venous pressure and a decrease of osmotic pressure. Both factors have been experimentally proven to dilate initially narrow channels, thus allowing feto–maternal fluid shift and equilibration of the surplus water.

VILLOUS TREES

Structure of Villous Types

The pattern of trabeculae seen during early development lays down the foundations of the arrangement of the villi in the mature organ. Hence, the villi are clustered together into a series of spherical units known as lobules or placentones (82). Each lobule arises from the chorionic plate by a thick villous trunk (Fig. 7), which is derived ultimately from a trabecula. The main trunk branches repeatedly, and although some subdivisions extend as far as the basal plate, the anchoring villi, most end freely in the intervillous space (Fig. 9A). Five types of villi have been distinguished on the basis of their caliber, stromal characteristics, and vessel structure, and these types largely reflect differing subdivisions of this villous tree (4,83–85) (Fig. 11).

1. **Stem villi** (4,83) (Fig. 11). These represent the first five to 30 generations of unequal dichotomous branchings and serve to give mechanical support to the villous tree. They are characterized by a compact fibrous stroma containing centrally located arteries or larger arterioles and veins or venules. Capillaries are relatively infrequent, and so these villi probably play little part in placental exchange. Their physiologic significance lies in the fact that the smaller branches are most likely the site of the fetal resistance vessels.
2. **Mature intermediate villi** (83) (Figs. 9A and 11). Repeated branching of stem villi results in the formation of long slender intermediate villi, ranging from 80 to 120 μm in diameter. These are often gently curving, and terminal villi arise at intervals from all aspects of their surface (Fig. 9A). Internally, they consist of a loose stromal core, with scant fibers and cells, and embedded within this are occasional arterioles. Fetal vessels occupy at least half the villous volume, and most are now in the form of capillaries. This increased degree of vascularization and the high level of enzyme activity within the syncytiotrophoblast indicate that this villous type may play a significant role in materno–fetal exchange and hormone synthesis.
3. **Terminal villi** (4,83) (Figs. 9A, 11, and 12). These are the final branches of the villous tree and are physiologically its most important component. They are short stubby protuberances up to 100 μm in length and 80 μm in diameter, although some possess a more narrow neck region. Most (95%) arise from the surface of mature intermediate villi, and one of their principal characterizing features is the high degree of capillarization (more than 50% of overall volume).

   When viewing sections of terminal villi, it is immediately apparent that the thickness of the syncytiotrophoblast, and indeed of the villous membrane in general, is not uniform over the villous surface. Instead, there are areas where the syncytium is extremely attenuated and is devoid of nuclei or other large organelles. Underlying such an area is a dilated segment of a fetal capillary, known as a sinusoid, and hence the thickness of the villous membrane separating the maternal and fetal circulations may be as little as 0.5 to 2.0 μm (Fig. 12). These sites have been referred to as α zones, epithelial plates, and nephro-pneumoid regions in the past, but now the term *vasculo-syncytial membrane* is most widely used. Their morphology suggests they play an important role in diffusional exchange, and their formation will be considered later in connection with the fetal angioarchitecture.

   At other points on the villous surface, the syncytiotrophoblastic layer is relatively thick (Fig. 12). Here are found the nuclei, sometimes clustered into syncytial knots, and other major organelles. The terms β *zones* or *enteroid regions* have been used to denote these areas, and as the latter suggests, they are the most important sites of metabolic and endocrine activities.

   Hence, different areas of the surface of terminal villi are responsible for different placental functions. Put in simple terms, this ensures that two of the placenta's main tasks, to act as a fetal lung and as a fetal liver, are arranged in parallel rather than in series. This is almost certainly to the benefit of diffusional exchange, for evidence from several biologic systems indicates that for maximum efficiency the intervening barrier should be as thin as possible.
4. **Immature intermediate villi** (83) (Fig. 11). As their title suggests, these represent peripheral continuations of stem villi that are in the process of development. Thus, although common in immature placentas, their distribution in the mature organ is generally limited to the central regions of the lobules (Fig. 7), which are considered the principal germinal zones.

   Externally, these villi are rather bulbous, whereas in section they display highly characteristic profiles. The fixed stromal cells possess large sail-like processes that link together to form a series of fiber-free intercommunicating channels oriented parallel to the long axis of the villus (Fig. 11). Hofbauer cells appear morphologically to be able to move along and cross between these channels. Embedded among the stromal cells are arterioles, confirming that these villi are the forerunners of stem villi. It is important that their presence is recognized and that they are not incorrectly interpreted as edematous villi.
5. **Mesenchymal villi** (86) (Fig. 11). These are again a transient population, seen predominantly in the earliest stages of pregnancy in which they are the precursors of immature intermediate villi. In the more mature placenta, they are inconspicuous and may differentiate directly into mature intermediate villi. Structurally, they possess a stromal core that is not yet organized into stromal channels. Fetal vessels are poorly developed, but Hofbauer cells may be visible.

Development of Villous Trees

As mentioned previously, the development of the villous tree starts by the formation of side branches on the trabeculae. The earliest of these are composed of syncytiotrophoblast alone and so are termed *syncytial* or *trophoblastic sprouts.* In early gestation, these are seen arising in an apparently random pattern from the surfaces of mesenchymal and immature intermediate villi (50,86) (Fig. 13). Similar structures are seen along the surfaces of all villous types. In later pregnancy, they are signs of syncytiotrophoblastic nuclear sequestration rather than of villous sprouting (87).

At all stages of gestation, it appears that a proportion of the sprouts break away, and the resulting syncytial globules are exported in the maternal blood, most becoming lodged in the pulmonary capillary bed. It has been estimated that up to 150,000 such globules enter the maternal circulation each day (88). The functional significance of this phenomenon is not known, but it may act as a mechanism by which excessive or unnecessary syncytial nuclei can be shed. Alternatively, it has been suggested that it plays a role in modifying the maternal immune system, although how this is achieved by tissue that is devoid of MHC antigens remains uncertain.

Mesenchymal invasion into the proximal end of the nonshed true sprout is soon followed by the formation of capillaries, so rendering conversion into a tertiary villus complete. Up until the fifth week postconception, mesenchymal villi formed in this way progress to become primitive stem villi. However, after this point mesenchymal villi differentiate into immature intermediate villi (86). The latter continue to produce many new syncytial sprouts until they themselves are transformed into stem villi. Hence, growth of the more structural elements of the villous tree is very rapid during the first trimester.

The situation changes considerably during the third trimester. Placental growth tends to slow, and differentiation of the remaining villous types is seen. Mesenchymal villi no longer transform into immature intermediate villi but form mature intermediate villi instead. The remaining immature intermediate villi gradually differentiate into stem villi and so become scarce at term, normally being restricted to the centers of the placentones. Throughout the third trimester, terminal villi, the more functional components of the placenta, are elaborated from the surfaces of mature intermediate villi.

This switch in differentiation pathways at the start of the third trimester is of key importance in placental development (85,86). If it takes place too early, the organ stops growing too soon and differentiates prematurely. Consequently, the terminal villi are very densely packed because of a deficit of later generations of stem villi. This may have an adverse effect on blood flow through the intervillous space. Alternatively, if the switch is delayed, the placenta is characterized by persisting immaturity and a relative lack of terminal villi.

Fetal Angioarchitecture

Close to the point of insertion of the cord into the chorionic plate, in most (96%) placentas, the umbilical

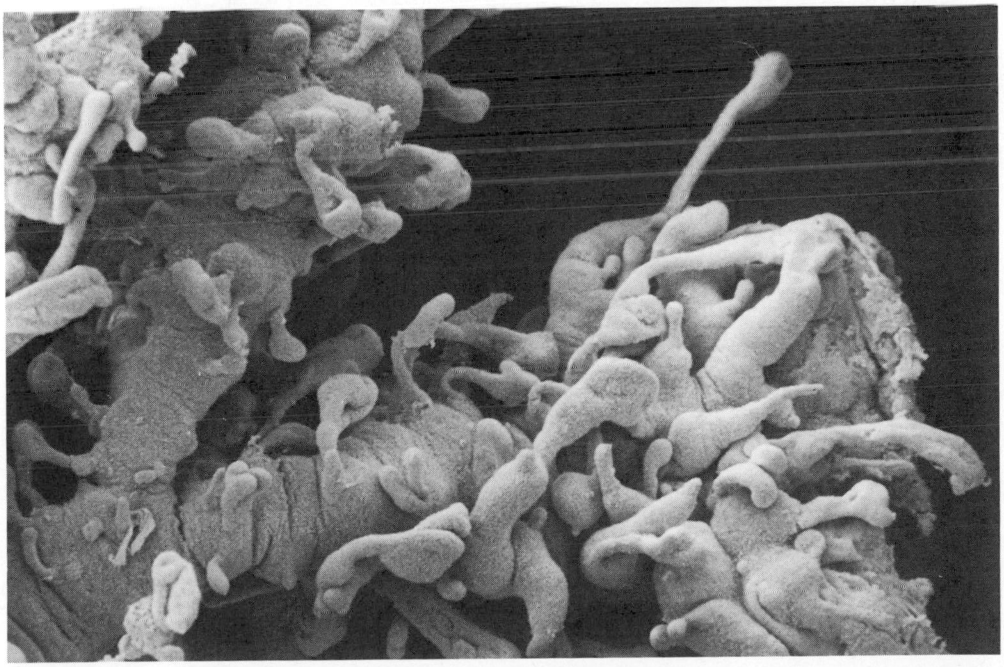

FIG. 13. Scanning electron micrograph of placental villi from eighth week of gestation. At this stage of pregnancy, central stems are covered with profusion of developing side branches. Early sprouts are slender and cylindical, but these later develop expanded distal ends. ×130. (From ref. 287, with permission.)

arteries are linked by Hyrtl's anastomosis. This most likely ensures even pressures in the chorionic arteries as they ramify over the chorionic plate. At intervals, branches of these arteries penetrate the plate and take up a central location within stem villi. Such vessels are surrounded by a few layers of smooth-muscle cells and by an adventitia, which is two to three times as thick as the media.

As the villous tree branches, so do the arteries. Within the smaller stem villi and both mature and immature intermediate villi, arterioles are found (89,90). They are surrounded by an intercommunicating system of long, slender capillaries, referred to as the paravascular network (90–92). This is orientated parallel to the longitudinal axis of the villi. Many functions have been ascribed to it in the past, the most popular of which has been the nutrition of deeper parts of the villous core for which diffusion from the intervillous space is arguably inadequate. Equally plausible, however, is the claim that the network represents a vestige of an earlier stage in development when the villi were better vascularized (4). What does seem clear as a result of exploring its connections through serial reconstructions is that there is no real basis for suggestions that it regulates fetal blood flow resistance by acting as an arteriovenous shunting system (51).

Within mature intermediate villi, the arterioles and venules give way to long coiled capillary loops. Elongation of this capillary plexus is rapid during the third trimester and exceeds that of the containing villi. As a result, capillary coils are formed, which protrude from the surface, raising a blister of trophoblast before them (89). In this way, new terminal villi are formed, and the same capillary may run through several terminal villi in series (Fig. 14) before communicating with a venule.

The caliber of the capillary is not uniform within a terminal villus, for dilated regions, known as sinusoids, occur at intervals along its length (Figs. 12 and 14). At these points, the lumen may reach 40 μm in diameter, and it has been proposed that they serve to reduce blood flow resistance, so ensuring an even distribution of flow through peripheral parts of the villous tree. Because the resistance of a vessel is inversely proportional to the fourth power of the radius, their presence could have a significant impact on blood flow. Sinusoids are only seen in the final stages of placental development, and their formation coincides with increasing length of the fetal capillaries (89,90). Moreover, within the otherwise iden-

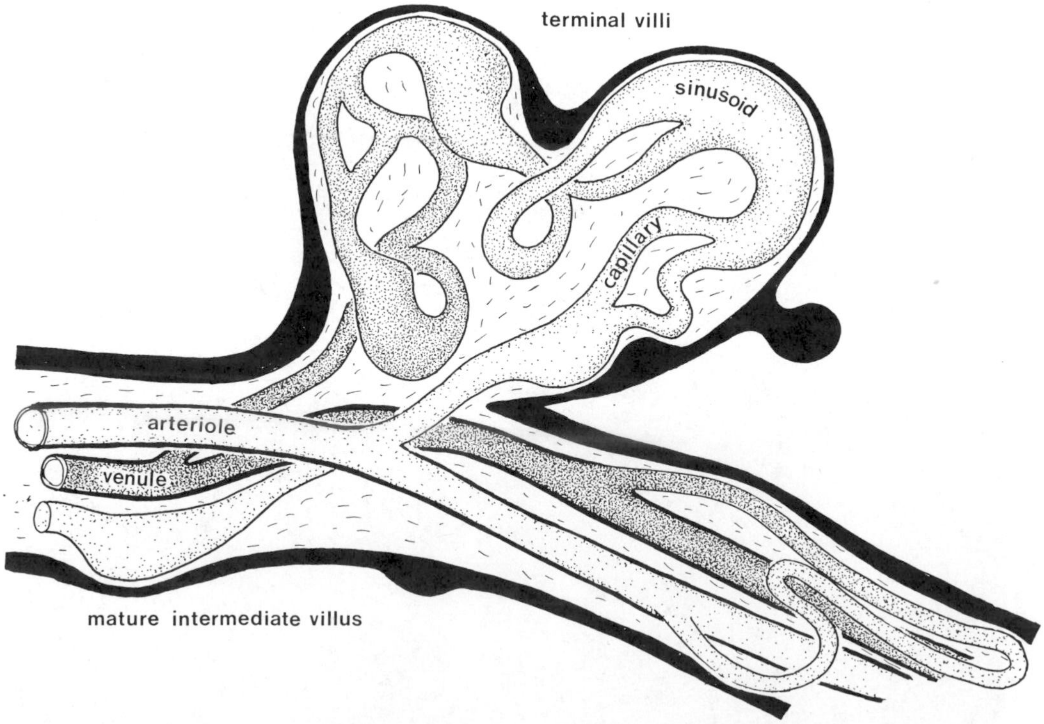

FIG. 14. Arrangement of fetal vessels in two terminal villi and one mature intermediate villus. Note highly complex loop formation of terminal fetal capillaries. Branching is usually followed shortly later by refusion of two capillary branches. Such a branching pattern avoids basal short-cuts. Thus, each erythrocyte has to pass terminal capillaries in full length. Local dilations, or sinusoids, reduce blood flow resistance. (From ref. 284, with permission.)

tical placentas of the capybara and guinea pig, sinusoids only occur in the capybara where the fetal capillaries are considerably longer (51).

In terms of their formation, it is notable that the sinusoids are almost invariably located on the outside wall of a tight capillary bend. Wall tension will be greatest at this point, and consequently this will be the site of dilatation under the influence of the high transmural pressure operating in later gestation. This dilatation will bring the outer wall of the capillary loop into close contact with the overlying syncytiotrophoblast, and constant pressure exerted on the latter may lead to remodeling, resulting in its local attenuation. As a result, a vasculo-syncytial membrane is formed (93,94).

Sinusoids are not totally ephemeral structures, however, reliant on a distending pressure for their existence. They may be seen, albeit to a reduced extent, after cessation of the fetal circulation in material that has been immersion fixed (50). The increased wall tension experienced by the endothelial cells may lead to their remodeling and an increase in surface area or may stimulate local angiogenesis. Incorporation of daughter cells into the vessel wall would result in a more permanent dilatation.

Recent experiments involving the perfusion of term placentas at different pressures have revealed that the walls of the sinusoids display elastic properties. As the pressure rises, the percentage of the overall villous volume represented by the sinusoids increases, as does the capillary surface area (95). This results in the further elaboration of vasculo-syncytial membranes, for the mean thickness of the villous membrane falls. Consequently, there is always a very close and precise relationship between the volume of the fetal capillaries and mean membrane thickness (96).

The physiologic significance of this mechanism may be considerable. For example, as the fetal blood pressure and hence capillary transmural pressure rises during the last trimester, thinning of the villous membrane will occur. In the acute situation, if the fetus becomes hypoxic, blood pressure will also increase (97,98). Not only will this lead to increased fetal blood flow, but the same changes will take place. In both cases, oxygen diffusion across the placenta will be facilitated. Restricting capillary dilatation to the sinusoids has the advantage to the fetus that maximal reduction in membrane thickness can be achieved with the minimal increase in extracorporeal blood volume.

The formation of terminal villi, sinusoids, and vasculo-syncytial membranes are therefore inextricably interlinked. Another benefit of sinusoids proposed in the past is that they serve to reduce the rate of blood flow opposite the attenuated regions of the trophoblast. This will only be of physiologic significance should the rate of diffusion across the membrane be a limiting factor. Alternatively, it could be argued that erythrocytes passing around the inner aspect of the capillary bend will be disadvantaged by their presence, for they will be further removed from the oxygen source. It seems likely, however, that given the marked changes in caliber, the pattern of blood flow through these regions will be complex, although not turbulent. This will be sufficient to ensure adequate mixing and more uniform oxygenation.

Intervillous Space

The directional relationship between the maternal and fetal blood flow is of considerable physiologic significance, as discussed previously in relation to comparative placental types. To understand the pattern of maternal blood flow in the human placenta, one needs a knowledge of the configuration of the intervillous space.

The fetal villi are arranged into 40 to 60 inverted cup-shaped lobules or placentones, each arising from the chorionic plate by a main stem villous. From the distribution of villous types and enzyme activity, it is clear that the central region of a lobule is the germinative zone (82). Here, the villi are loosely packed, and indeed as gestation advances, villous-free central cavities can be detected ultrasonographically (99). A series of radiographic and injection studies has confirmed that the arterial blood released from the openings of the maternal spiral arteries through the basal plate is delivered into these cavities (100,101) (Fig. 7). This constant relationship suggests that the pattern of maternal arterial inflow plays a key role, either hemodynamically or by differing oxygen tensions, in the formation and location of the lobules (102).

The openings of the uterine veins are positioned opposite the more peripheral parts of the lobule (Fig. 8). As a result, the maternal blood disperses radially through the lobule in a centrifugal fashion. This led Wigglesworth (101) to distinguish three zones in the lobule: an arterial zone consisting of the villous-free central area; a capillary zone comprising the dense meshwork of villi; and a venous zone situated peripherally and under the chorionic plate. Although accurate measurements are difficult to obtain *in vivo,* it is likely that the oxygen tension in the intervillous space varies correspondingly.

Because of the complex arrangement of villi described above, the interrelationship of the fetal and maternal blood flows cannot be assigned to one of the geometrically defined flow systems, such as concurrent, countercurrent, or crosscurrent. The situation in the human placenta comprises components of all these exchange systems (33) and corresponds to what Moll (32) defined as a multivillous flow system.

The rate of maternal blood flow through the lobule will be dictated principally by two factors. The first is the driving force, which is the pressure differential between the uterine arteries and veins, and the second is the resistance presented by the gaps between adjacent villi. As described in the historical introduction, our appreciation of the configuration of the intervillous space has changed over the years. Scanning electron microscopy has resolved many of the uncertainties, however, and it is now clear that within the bulk of the lobule, it comprises a series of irregular cleftlike spaces (50). These are generally of capillary dimensions only but are in free communication with one another. The width of the intervillous clefts is difficult to estimate, for not only are the walls very irregular but the spaces are influenced by several artificial phenomena. Using data for partum intervillous blood volume (23.3–37.9% of the placental volume) and the villous surface area at term (11–13.3 m^2), the mean width has been calculated as ranging from 16.4 to 32.0 μm (51). One must bear in mind that there is a considerable subchorial lake and large spaces in the centers of the lobules. Thus, the real "intervillous" volume is likely to be lower than that quoted above, and so the intervillous clefts are even narrower. Occasional fusion does occur between neighboring villi (87,103), although not to the extent claimed by Stieve (19). The main significance of these points of fusion is that they can be disrupted (103). The resulting syncytial injury may then provide a stimulus for fibrin deposition, as is discussed later.

Resin injection studies have demonstrated that the shape of the lobule, and the disposition of the villi within it, are heavily dependent on the perfusion pressure of the fetal vasculature (104). Equally, the volume of the intervillous space is approximately halved if clamping of the umbilical cord is delayed (105). It thus appears that the fetal vessels provide hydraulic support of the villous tree and, in doing so, may determine the shape and size of the intervillous clefts. Perfusion studies of delivered placenta at different pressure have confirmed that over the physiologic range as the pressure rises, the gaps between the villi increase (95). How these can be measured more precisely will be considered in the section on stereology. It is envisaged that increasing turgidity of the fetal vasculature leads to straightening of intermediate and smaller stem villi and their movement into the otherwise relatively villous-free interlobular and subchorionic regions. In this way, the pressures within the fetal circulation could influence the pattern of maternal blood flow. Larger gaps between neighboring villi will not only reduce the resistance to maternal blood flow, but they will also promote a more even perfusion throughout the lobule and reduce the risk of arteriovenous shunting through the basal region.

The converse situation has also been proposed, whereby the pressures in the intervillous space could control the fetal circulation. This concept was formulated into the sluice-flow principle put forward by Power and Longo (106), in which it was suggested that if pressure in the intervillous space exceeds umbilical venous pressure, the villous capillaries will be compressed. The experimental evidence for placental sluice-flow was soon challenged by Berman and co-workers (107) following studies conducted on sheep. However, more recent Doppler flow studies have demonstrated a rapidly reversible increase in the umbilical pulsatility index when women move from either the standing or the lateral position to the supine position (108,109). Because this increase in vascular resistance is independent of changes in the fetal heart rate, it is thought to be due to raised pressure in the intervillous space. This, in turn, results from impeded venous drainage, consequent on partial occlusion of the inferior vena cava by the gravid uterus (108,110). The delicate nature of vasculo-syncytial membranes and the elastic properties of the fetal capillaries (95) provide morphologic evidence that the peripheral elements of the fetal vasculature are vulnerable to compression.

The corollary of this may be that the size of the fetal capillaries and the thickness of the villous membrane varies throughout the lobule in relation to the local intervillous pressure. Although, like oxygen tension, this is almost impossible to measure accurately *in vivo,* it is probable that a central-peripheral pressure gradient exists. A higher pressure differential between the fetal capillary lumina and the intervillous space could explain the finding of increased vasculo-syncytial membranes in the more venous parts of the lobule (111,112).

A further factor that can potentially influence the relationship between maternal and fetal blood flows is the deposition of fibrin within the intervillous space (cf. section on Fibrinoid). This occurs to a limited extent during the course of all normal pregnancies, principally in the relatively villous-free area immediately beneath the chorionic plate. Maternal blood flow through this region is particularly sluggish, and the fibrin enmeshes the roots of the main stem villi. Because these are not involved in materno–fetal exchange, the deposition is of little physiologic significance. Only if it is particularly excessive will it compromise placental surface area, but it may serve to remodel the intervillous space and reduce the volume of "redundant" regions.

Oxygen as Regulator of Villous Development

Transplacental oxygen transfer is only one of many placental functions. However, its particular importance becomes evident from the fact that it is nearly the only placental function that on disturbance immediately may cause fetal death. Because of this, it is not surprising that the maternal oxygen supply to the placenta affects placental growth and differentiation to an higher extent than any other known parameter.

Respective pathohistologic reports unanimously describe that the amount of villous cytotrophoblast is increased in all those pathologic conditions that are thought to be related to intrauterine hypoxia (61,113–115). Arnholdt and co-workers (116) found evidence that this is not only due to an increased mitotic index but also to a reduction of the length of the cell cycle. These results are supported by the finding that unusually good oxygenation of villi reduces the amount of villous cytotrophoblast (51,115,117). Pathohistologic (118) and experimental (119,120) evidence has also shown that the villous syncytiotrophoblast is affected by hypoxia; it is reduced in thickness and produces increased numbers of syncytial knots. Tominaga and Page (119) interpreted this as a sign of adaptation by reducing diffusion distances. However, more stringent stereologic studies have suggested that the changes are more likely caused by degenerative processes (120).

All hypoxic *in vitro* studies have been performed on villous explants rather than on villous cytotrophoblast cultures. Because of this, it is still an open question whether cytotrophoblast responds directly to variations of the oxygen partial pressure or whether this response is mediated by factors released by other hypoxic tissue components such as syncytiotrophoblast or villous macrophages. There are several candidates for factors that might mediate hypoxic signals: epidermal growth factor (EGF) is produced by syncytiotrophoblast (for review, cf. ref. 121); its mitogenic action on trophoblast has been shown by Lysiak and co-workers (122); and its receptors have been detected in cytotrophoblast (123). Transforming growth factor α (TGF-α) (122) and tumor necrosis factor α (TNF-α), the latter produced by macrophages (124), and colony stimulating factor 1 (CSF-1) produced by mesenchymal cells (125,126) are other candidates. Finally, TGF-β1 and TGF-β2, both produced by macrophages (124) and by trophoblast (127), seem to be involved in the regulation of syncytial fusion of the postproliferative cytotrophoblast to regenerate the hypoxically damaged syncytiotrophoblast.

The villous connective tissue also responds to variations in the intrauterine oxygen supply. Chronic hypoxia results in poor fibrosis of the villi (51,128); in contrast, higher levels of intravillous po_2 increase villous fibrosis (117,128). Possible mediators are macrophage products such as TGF-β that stimulates collagen-I transcription (129) or interleukin-1 that, among other functions, regulates fibroblast proliferation (130).

Several studies have dealt with the reaction of fetal villous endothelium to hypoxia. Complicated pregnancies suffering from intrauterine hypoxia show villous hypercapillarization (131); the same is valid for placentas obtained from pregnancies from high altitude (132). However, using *in vitro* culture of villous explants, it is difficult to find clear experimental evidence for this correlation (61,119,120,133) because the isolated fragments of fetal endothelial tubes tend to disintegrate in culture.

Experimental chronic hypoxia in pregnant guinea pigs resulted in an increased fetal capillarization and in an elevated carbon monoxide diffusion capacity (134). More detailed studies revealed that this was due to stimulated sprouting and branching of capillaries: The mean capillary length and the mean capillary diameter were reduced, and the number of parallel capillary loops was considerably raised (135). Because the trophoblastic thickness also decreased, the mean materno–fetal diffusion distance was much shorter as compared with normoxic placentas (134).

Clear evidence for the respective cell biologic regulations was obtained from endothelial culture experiments (136–138). Surprisingly, endothelial cells showed reduced mitotic rates and reduced motility when cultured under hypoxic conditions (137,138). However, addition of conditioned medium obtained from hypoxic macrophages stimulated endothelial proliferation (137). The same authors have shown that increased production of basic fibroblast growth factor (bFGF) by the hypoxic macrophages and enhanced expression of bFGF receptor by the hypoxic endothelium were responsible for the enhanced endothelial proliferation. Other angiogenetic factors that must be considered to mediate hypoxic signals, comprise platelet-derived endothelial cell growth factor (PDECGF), which is probably of trophoblastic origin (139); the platelet-derived growth factor B (PDGF-B) produced by villous cytotrophoblast (140); and an amitogenic angiogenesis factor secreted by hypoxic macrophages (136).

There are only very few data concerning hypoxic influences on the maternal vascularization of the placenta. In the guinea pig under hypoxic conditions, volume and surface of maternal blood lacunae are reduced (134). In contrast, in human placentas from high altitude the intervillous space was described to be increased (132). For the cow placenta, Reynolds and co-workers (141) demonstrated maternal endothelial mitogens of endometrial origin. However, up to now these data do not give a clear concept how uteroplacental oxygenation modulates maternal vascularization of the placenta.

Summarizing the above data, we arrive at the following conclusions regarding villous reactions to hypoxia: Hypoxia damages villous syncytiotrophoblast, which in turn stimulates cytotrophoblastic proliferation and subsequent syncytial fusion. Despite these attempts to regenerate the damaged syncytiotrophoblast, the volume and the thickness of the latter are reduced, thus facilitating materno–fetal oxygen diffusion. Villous connective tissue, which is also reduced under these conditions, may add to the same effects. Fetal oxygen uptake is furthermore facilitated by expansion of the villous capillary bed by sprouting and nonsprouting angiogenesis, both processes probably being stimulated by growth factors derived from hypoxic macrophages and hypoxic trophoblast. Widening of the capillary bed with reduction of the length of the individual capillaries causes reduction of fetoplacental blood flow resistance and thus may be advantageous for the hypoxically maltreated fetal cardiovascular system.

Stereologic Data

In the past, many attempts have been made to quantify different aspects of placental structure, with the aim of producing a measure of the organ's functional capabilities. Some investigations have examined fresh villi under phase-contrast microscopy and used the number of syncytial sprouts observed as an index of trophoblastic growth (118,142). Most, however, have worked with sectioned material and have largely presented either planar morphometric data, such as profile areas and perimeter lengths, or stereologic ratios (e.g., component volume or surface area density per reference volume). These data have recently been exhaustively reviewed by Benirschke and Kaufmann (51).

Although such results are easily obtained and may be sufficient to draw comparisons between different regions or treatment groups, their physiologic significance can be difficult to interpret. For example, the number of vasculo-syncytial membranes per 100 villous profiles provides little indication of the overall diffusing capacity for several reasons. First, there are the problems of defining what actually constitutes a vasculo-syncytial membrane and how one accounts for the influence of the plane of sectioning on apparent membrane thickness. Second, such an index does not take into account the areal extent of these specializations. A few large vasculo-syncytial membranes may have the same impact on gaseous exchange as many small ones. What is required is a descriptor that takes all these factors into account and provides a measure of membrane thickness that can be substituted directly into physiologic diffusion equations. In this case, it is the harmonic mean thickness that is of key importance. Whenever possible, it is therefore advisable to convert all planar data into component densities and true thicknesses, and this is the domain of stereology. The component densities should, in turn, be converted into absolute values (e.g., total lengths, surface areas, and numbers) by relating them to the reference volume (i.e., the total volume of the placenta). Doing such conversions enables an absolute value for each placental parameter to be calculated. It is then easy to see whether changes in one compartment are mirrored or compensated for by alterations in another, so avoiding problems of misinterpretation.

When considering the results of a stereologic study, detailed attention must be given to the manner in which the placentas have been collected, sampled, and processed. Because the placenta is such a highly vascular organ, the timing of the clamping of the cord has a profound impact on the values of many parameters (105). The problem here is essentially the major, but unpredictable, shift of extracorporeal placental blood back to the body at the time of delivery, the placental transfusion. For this reason, placentas delivered by cesarean section are volumetrically different from those delivered vaginally (143). Furthermore, even material obtained after cesarean section differs considerably from that aspirated directly from the still maternally perfused placenta *in situ* (144).

After delivery, the picture is complicated by leakage of fetal blood occurring from villous tissue torn during delivery and the effects of postdelivery ischemia. Thus, even in cesarean-delivered placentas in which the cord is clamped immediately and remains clamped throughout, repeated sampling at intervals over a period of 20 min demonstrates major changes (20–30%) in the size of the fetal vessels and the thickness of the villous membrane (145,146). Most of these changes take place in the first 5 min postdelivery. To overcome this problem, perfusion fixation has been used (143,147), but in view of the elasticity of the fetal capillaries recently demonstrated, one might legitimately query what is the appropriate pressure and should it be the same for all placentas?

Clearly, for a study to be internally consistent, the collection of material must be uniform throughout, and if the data are to reflect the situation *in vivo,* it is essential the samples are taken immediately after delivery. From the description of the villous trees, it should now be apparent that the placenta is not a homogeneous organ, and so the site of sampling is also highly relevant. For comparative studies, sampling from defined areas, such as the central and peripheral parts of a lobule, is justified. However, if the aim is to acquire data that are representative of the entire organ, it is crucial that all areas have an equal and independent chance of being sampled. Strategies by which this can be achieved were outlined by Mayhew and Burton (148).

In the past, many samples have been fixed in formal saline and embedded in paraffin wax. This can result in linear shrinkages of 20% to 30%, representing volume shrinkage of 50% to 60%. It is therefore important when interpreting absolute values to check that shrinkage has been taken into consideration (149). This is not such a problem with glutaraldehyde fixation and resin embedding, when the linear shrinkage is only 2% (150). Resin embedding also confers the advantage that thinner sections (0.5–1.0 μm) can be cut, allowing easier identification of villous types (83). Stereologically, such sections reduce the problems caused by image overprojection (87,151), and the superior resolution they provide enables more accurate identification of tissue boundaries.

Having obtained histologic sections of placental material, the question then arises as to how and what to measure. During the past decade, there have been many advances in stereologic techniques, and these have been thoroughly reviewed by Gundersen and co-workers (152,153) and Mayhew (154). With regard to what can be measured, we shall restrict ourselves here to those parameters that are of the most direct physiologic relevance (Table 1).

Total placental volume is of key importance because it provides the means of converting component densities into absolute quantities. The total volume can then be broken down into the volumes of components of interest. For example, a knowledge of the volumes of the maternal and fetal circulations is necessary when considering the bulk flow of compounds or when assessing the rate of blood flow through the organ. Equally, the volume of trophoblast correlates strongly with assays of several placental synthetic products (155).

Many substances cross the placenta by passive diffusion, and so their rate of transfer will be governed by the Fick equation. In the human placenta, all diffusion must proceed across the trophoblast and then across the fetal capillary endothelium, or vice versa. It is therefore reasonable to use the mean of these two exchange surfaces as an estimate of the effective surface area of the tissue barrier. Studies on placentas from women living at altitudes, and thus exposed to hypobaric hypoxia, has led to conflicting results; reduced villous surface area being reported by Jackson and co-workers (132) and the converse by Kádar and Saldana (156). In the former study, it was considered that the reduction was part of the general pattern of diminished growth at altitude. In the latter, the increase was interpreted as a compensatory change in response to reduced oxygen supply. Placental hypertrophy has also been reported in cases of maternal anemia (157). Whether this translates into increased villous surface area is not yet known.

According to the Fick equation, the rate of diffusional exchange is inversely proportional to the membrane thickness. However, as previously discussed, the thickness of the villous membrane is not uniform throughout the villous tree or even over the surface of terminal villi. Therefore, what is required is the mean of the reciprocal local thicknesses, and this is the harmonic mean thickness. The use of this term rather than the arithmetic mean emphasizes the contribution made to diffusional exchange by the vasculo-syncytial membranes. Substituting values for the harmonic mean thickness and the effective exchange surface area into the Fick equation enables the gas conductance of the human placental membrane to be estimated, and values of 3 to 5 ml/min/mm Hg have been obtained (158,159). Recent studies have demonstrated that the thickness of the villous membrane may be reduced under conditions of low oxygen tension, again suggesting placental adaptation aimed at improving diffusional exchange (149,160). By contrast an increase in membrane thickness has been found in placentas from women who smoked cigarettes during pregnancy (161), and in both situations, the changes seem to be mediated through alterations in the fetal vasculature.

Hence, quantification of relatively straightforward structural parameters can provide a powerful insight into the diffusional capacity of the placenta under different conditions. It must be repeatedly stressed, however, that all these studies are based on delivered placentas, and the situation may be much more dynamic *in utero*. Even the few data obtained from biopsies out of the still maternally perfused placenta *in utero* (144) are difficult to interpret and should not be mistaken as "*in vivo*" data because biopsy was performed during cesarean section, after opening of the uterus and delivery of the baby. De-

TABLE 1. *Stereologic data for normal term placentas*

	Aherne and Dunhill (1966)	Laga et al. (1973)	Bouw et al. (1976)	Mayhew et al. (1984, 1986)	Feneley and Burton (1991)
Placental volume (cm^3)	488	448	540	408	—
Total villous membrane (cm^3)	224	204	239	—	—
Volume of intervillous space (cm^3)	144	110	210	173	—
Volume of fetal vessels (cm^3)	45.0	36.0	74.9	43.5	—
Volume of trophoblast (cm^3)	58.0	57.3	47.6	—	—
Villous surface area (m^2)	11.0	16.7	13.3	7.0	—
Capillary surface area (m^2)	12.2	12.4	15.8	5.4	—
Arithmetic mean thickness of villous membrane (μm)	3.5	—	—	—	4.5
Harmonic mean thickness of villous membrane (μm)	—	10.0	—	4.9	3.6

spite these limitations, these latter data are very likely to be the most trustable ones. As previously discussed, the pressure differential between the fetal and maternal circulations has a major impact on the thickness of the villous membrane. Regional and temporal variations in gas conductance may therefore be occurring throughout the organ.

Application of more recent stereologic techniques to the placenta is only just beginning. For example, mention has already been made to the counting of cytotrophoblast cells at different stages of gestation (58). This study took advantage of the "dissector" technique, which allows the numbers of particles to be estimated without assumptions about their size or shape (162). Our own work in progress suggests that the "star volume" (153) may provide a useful index of the size of the spaces between individual villi. In simplistic terms, this technique estimates the volume of an irregular space that can be "seen" in all directions from a random point falling within it and again is free from bias caused by plane of sectioning. It therefore has potential as a guide to maternal blood flow through the intervillous space.

With further research, more aspects of placental function may be quantified stereologically, yielding hard data with which to test hypotheses. These may concern placental growth and development, or adaptation and compensation, but the key will always be the quality of the placental material on which the measurements are based.

NONVILLOUS PARTS

Chorionic Plate, Umbilical Cord, and Membranes

The development of the chorionic plate, the umbilical cord, and the membranes are closely related to that of the amnion. At day 13 postconception, the blastocystic cavity is occupied by a loose meshwork of cells, the so-called extraembryonic mesoderm, which surrounds the embryoblast. The embryoblast is composed of two vesicles, the amnionic vesicle and the primary yolk sac. Where both vesicles are in contact with each other, they form the double-layered embryonic disc. From day 14 onward, the extraembryonic mesoderm cells are rearranged in such a way that they only line the inner surface of the trophoblastic vesicle (thus forming the chorion) and the surfaces of the two embryonic vesicles (making up the embryo). In between, the exocoelomic cavity forms. The exocoelom is bridged by a bundle of mesenchymal cells, which is referred to as the connecting stalk. It links the embryonic vesicles to the trophoblast and is the early forerunner of the umbilical cord. During the same period, a ductlike extension of the hindgut originating in the caudal region of the embryo, penetrates the proximal end of the connecting stalk. This structure is the allantois, the primitive extraembryonic urinary bladder.

In the course of the following weeks, one of the two embryonic vesicles, namely, the amnionic vesicle, enlarges considerably. It extends around the embryonic disc and the yolk sac and finally covers the connecting stalk. The latter is thus transformed into the umbilical cord. Further fluid accumulation within the amnionic cavity causes its continued expansion until it completely occupies the former blastocystic cavity surrounding the fetus. In the course of this process, the amnionic mesenchyme locally touches and finally fuses with the chorionic mesoderm lining the inner surface of the trophoblastic vesicle. This process starts in the vicinity of the insertion of the cord into the chorionic plate and continues until the middle of pregnancy, by which time the amnionic and chorionic mesenchyme are fused throughout. Unlike the situation in the cord in which the amnion fuses firmly with the underlying connective tissue, fusion of the amnion with chorionic plate or remaining membranes is never complete. Rather, amnion and chorion can always easily slide against each other. Histologically, they seem to be separated by a system of slender, fluid-filled clefts, the intermediate layer of the chorionic plate, and the membranes.

Already in the third week postconception, the allantois becomes supplied with fetal vessels. The human allantoic vessels, two allantoic arteries originating from the internal iliac arteries and one allantoic vein that enters into the hepatic vein, invade the placenta and become connected to the villous vessels. In recognition of the allantoic participation in vascularizing the organ, the human placenta falls in to the category of "chorioallantoic" placentas previously described. Fusion of the allantoic vessels with the intravillous vessel system establishes a complete fetoplacental circulation in the course of the fifth week postconception.

In the same period, the developing cord has a length of between 0.5 and 1.0 cm; by the fourth month, it has grown to between 16 and 18 cm; by the sixth month to between 33 and 35 cm; and at term, it reaches a final length of about 50 cm, with extreme values ranging from 18 to 122 cm (4).

Even in early pregnancy, the cord is characterized by a spiral twisting, the number of turns increasing up to a maximum of 300 as pregnancy advances. In most cases, the twist is sinistral, or anticlockwise. The twists have been interpreted as the result of rotary movements of the fetus, caused by asymmetric uterine contractions (51).

At day 14 postconception, the primary chorionic plate consists of three layers: syncytiotrophoblast, cytotrophoblast, and extraembryonic mesenchyme (Fig. 8D). They separate the intervillous space from the blastocystic cavity. Trophoblastic proliferation with subsequent degeneration and fibrinoid transformation (Langhans' fibrinoid) causes continuous growth of the primary chorionic plate. Around the fourth and fifth week of pregnancy, allantoic blood vessels reach the primary chorionic plate through the connecting stalk (cf. above) and start protruding into the stem villi, which branch off from the chorionic plate. As soon as the expanding amnionic sac comes into close contact with the mesenchymal surface of the chorionic plate (eighth to tenth week postconception), the definitive chorionic plate is formed. It is composed of the following layers: Langhans' fibrinoid lining the intervillous space and largely replacing the original syncytiotrophoblast; one or several layers of cytotrophoblast; chorionic mesenchyme; a spongy layer with many clefts, which indicate the border between chorion and amnion; amnionic mesoderm; and amnionic epithelium, which lines the amnionic cavity (for further details, cf. refs. 51,163, and 164).

To understand the development of the fetal membranes, it is necessary to recollect that the villous developmental steps described above are valid only for the implantation pole (i.e., that part of the blastocystic circumference that becomes attached to the endometrium and that implants first). The other parts of the blastocystic circumference implant a few days later and undergo corresponding, although delayed development (Fig. 8B). As early as the fourth week, they already show the first signs of regression; these parts are called the capsular chorion frondosum. The newly formed villi degenerate, and the surrounding intervillous space obliterates. Finally, the chorionic plate, the obliterated intervillous space, villous remnants, and the basal plate all fuse, forming a multilayered compact lamella termed the *smooth chorion* (*chorion laeve*). The first patches of the smooth chorion appear opposite to the implantation pole at the so-called abembryonic or antiimplantation pole. From there, they spread over about 70% of the surface of the chorionic sac until the fourth lunar month.

On the maternal surface, the smooth chorion is lined by capsular decidua. With complete implantation, the decidua closes again over the blastocyst, forming the capsular decidua. With the increasing diameter of the chorionic sac, the capsular decidua bulges into the uterine lumen and locally touches the parietal decidua of the opposing uterine wall. Between the fifteenth and twentieth week postconception, both decidual layers fuse with each other, thus obliterating the uterine cavity. From this point onward, the smooth chorion has contact over nearly its entire surface with the decidual surface of the uterine wall and may function as a paraplacental exchange organ. Because of the deficiency of a fetal vascularization of both the smooth chorion and the amnion, all paraplacental exchange between fetal membranes and fetus has to pass the amnionic fluid.

The mean thickness of the fetal membranes at term, after separation from the uterine wall, is about 200 to 300 μm. The membranes show some similarity with the structure of the chorionic plate (165). The innermost layer, the amnionic epithelium, encloses the amnionic fluid (Fig. 7). It is involved in the production of the latter and also in its resorption. Moreover, experimental results (166) indicate that the amnionic epithelium contains abundant carbonic anhydrase, an enzyme being involved in removal of carbon dioxide and in pH regulation. The epithelium rests on a thin layer of amnionic mesoderm.

The next layer is continuous with the connective tissue of the chorionic plate and is directly adherent to the outer cytotrophoblastic layer. The latter is of varying thickness. Near the placental margin, persisting ghost villi, embedded in fibrinoid, split the cytotrophoblast into two layers. These continue into the placenta and become confluent with the chorionic and basal plates, respectively. Attached to the outer surface of the cytotrophoblast is a decidual layer. The latter indicates that separation of the membranes, as in the placenta, does not take place along the materno–fetal interface but, instead, it cleaves somewhat deeper.

Basal Plate and Uteroplacental Vessels

The basal plate and its early forerunner, the trophoblastic shell, are formed at the base of the lacunar system at day 8 postconception (Fig. 8C and D). Initially, it is a purely trophoblastic layer. From day 13 postconception onward, detaching trophoblast cells penetrate into the surrounding endometrium, thus forming the junctional zone. A few invading trophoblast cells come into close contact with each other and fuse to form syncytial giant cells. Where they are separated from each other, they may undergo higher differentiation into so-called X cells (interstitial trophoblast or intermediate trophoblast) (Fig. 8F). Increasing numbers of endometrial stroma cells undergo considerable hypertrophy and become transformed into decidua cells.

Because of a combination of phagocytic, cytotoxic, and immunologic activities, varying amounts of degenerating trophoblast, decidua, extracellular matrix, and intermingled fibrinogen condense and form a homogeneous extracellular material called fibrinoid. Where the latter is in close contact with the intervillous space, it is called Rohr's fibrinoid (Fig. 8F). More deeply positioned layers of fibrinoid, which surround groups of trophoblastic and/or decidua cells, are named Nitabuch's fibrinoid. The entire materno–fetal "battlefield" stretches from the intervillous space down to the myometrium. It is described as the junctional zone (Fig. 8F). The superficial part of it, adhering to the placenta after placental separation, is the basal plate. It represents the bottom of the intervillous space and consists of trophoblastic and endometrial cells and much fibrinoid (167–169). Its intervillous surface may partly be lined by maternal endothelium derived from the maternal veins. Those parts of the junctional zone that remain in the uterus after delivery are called the placental bed. This consists mainly of intact and necrotic endometrial tissue, with trophoblastic cells intermingled (170).

By the invasive capacities of the penetrating trophoblast, endometrial arteries (spiral arteries) and veins become eroded and thus connected with the intervillous space. There is general agreement that the number of corresponding maternal vessels that supply the placenta, although originally high, is reduced considerably toward term by obliteration (4). The final number of spiral arteries given for the term placenta is about 100 and that for venous openings is 50 to 200.

As early as the second month of pregnancy, the walls of the arteries and veins exhibit regressive changes. Endothelial necrosis is followed by degeneration of the muscle cells of the media. In most places, inelastic tubes result, constructed only of amorphous extracellular material (171,172). This process is accompanied by dilation of the lumina, in particular of those segments near the intervillous space. Parallel to the above vessel changes, rounded trophoblast cells, so-called intra-arterial trophoblast, invade the arterial lumina from the intervillous space. In some places, these cells may completely occlude the arterial lumina, although this may be a temporary phenomenon restricted to the first trimester. In others, they replace the degenerative endothelium, thus forming a new internal cellular vessel lining (173). Uteroplacental veins undergo similar changes, but to a much lesser degree; they always remain free of intravascular trophoblast (4). However, their endothelial lining tends to proliferate toward the intervillous space and may partly line its basal surface.

Even though apparently degenerative, these pregnancy changes of the uteroplacental vessels are described as "physiologic processes" (174), necessary for normal placentation. Complete absence, or reduced physiologic vessel transformations, are regularly combined with pregnancy-associated hypertension complicated by fetal growth retardation (173,174).

Placental Septa

Placental septa are dome-shaped or sail-like extensions of the basal plate into the intervillous space, rather than real septa dividing the intervillous space into separately maternally perfused chambers (175) (Fig. 7). Their tissue composition is identical with that of the basal plate, namely, a fibrinoid matrix with interspersed trophoblastic and decidual cells. Even maternal vessels, mostly veins, may extend into the septa. The septa are interpreted as dislocations of basal plate tissue into the intervillous space, caused by lateral movement and folding of the uterine wall and basal plate over each other (51).

Cell Columns and Cell Islands

Cell columns are the trophoblastic connections of larger stem villi, the so-called anchoring villi, to the basal plate. These are segments of the villous trees that persist in the primary villus stage, because mesenchymal invasion during formation of secondary villi does not reach the most basal segments of the anchoring villi (Fig. 8E and F). Because of continuous cytotrophoblastic proliferation at the stromal–trophoblastic interface (123,176), the cell columns serve as segments of longitudinal growth of the anchoring villi. From their distal ends, cytotrophoblast may invade the basal plate, thus contributing to the growth of the latter. Because of this, cell columns serve as one of the richest sources for the so-called extravillous cytotrophoblast. Fibrinoid deposition at the surface of the cell columns slowly "buries" them into the basal plate. As soon as they are completely incorporated into the latter, the cytotrophoblastic proliferation slows down. After partial degeneration of the cells and complete disintegration of their structure, cell columns largely disappear in the course of the last trimester and can only rarely be observed in the term placenta.

Cell islands obviously are largely comparable structures (123,177,178). They, too, are formed from villous tips that have not been opened up by connective tissue during the transition from primary to tertiary villi. The only difference is that these villous tips were not connected to the basal plate, as are anchoring villi. Also, the cytotrophoblast of the cell islands proliferates and later becomes largely transformed into fibrinoid, which surrounds clusters and strings of surviving extravillous cytotrophoblast. Sometimes central degeneration and liquefaction causes the development of fluid-filled cysts inside the cell islands. Cell biologic studies concerning proliferative behavior of villous cytotrophoblast, the expression of growth factor receptors and of oncogene protein products, and the interactions with extracellular matrix did not reveal any differences between cell islands and cell columns (123,177,178).

Extravillous Trophoblast

Most cellular and syncytial trophoblast from the implanted blastocyst is consumed in the development of the placental villi. The remaining trophoblast, which is not used for villus formation, the extravillous trophoblast, is the basic material for the development of all other parts of the placenta (e.g., the smooth chorion, the chorionic plate, the basal plate including the cell columns, the septa, and the cell islands).

The nomenclature of the trophoblast residing outside of the villi is confusing. Because some doubt existed in the past regarding its derivation, the first name used was *X cells*. Later its trophoblastic origin was proven (179), and many authors proposed new designations: extravillous trophoblast, extravillous cytotrophoblast, nonvillous trophoblast, intermediate trophoblast, specialized trophoblast, interstitial trophoblast, intravascular trophoblast, intra-arterial trophoblast, trophoblastic giant cells, trophocytes, spongiotrophoblastlike cells, placental site giant cells, etc. Regrettably, everyone of these terms has a slightly different definition. We, therefore, propose the use of the term *extravillous trophoblast* as the most general heading for all types of trophoblast occurring outside of villi. When syncytial elements can be excluded, the name *extravillous cytotrophoblast* may be more appropriate. It is still an open question whether the two subpopulations (the intra-arterial trophoblast, lining the spiral artery lumina and partly occluding those, and the interstitial trophoblast, comprising all those extravillous trophoblast cells that are not located inside vessel lumina) are different only regarding their location or rather represent separate lines of differentiation (for literature, see ref. 51).

One of the crucial problems in histopathology and in experimental studies of the placenta for the unexperienced placentologist seems to be the discrimination between extravillous cytotrophoblast and decidua. Reliable markers for decidual cells as opposed to trophoblastic cells are antiprolactin (180) and antivimentin (181). However, extravillous trophoblast as opposed to decidual cells can be identified by binding anticytokeratin (181) and anti-human placental lactogen (182–185).

FIBRINOID

In paraffin sections of normal and pathologic placentas of all stages of development, one finds an acellular, homogeneous material that preferably binds acid stains. This material was first described by Langhans (186) as fibrin. Later, it was named *fibrinoid* by Hitschmann and Lindenthal (187) because there were some doubts as to the mere derivation from blood clotting.

Fibrinoid has been described in different localizations and under different names: as Langhans' stria or subchorial fibrinoid at the intervillous surface of the chorionic plate, as perivillous fibrin or perivillous fibrinoid encasing or partly covering placental villi, as intravillous fibrinoid or villous fibrinoid necrosis in the villous stroma, as Rohr's stria at the surface of the basal plate (Fig. 8F) facing the intervillous space, or as Nitabuch's stria or uteroplacental fibrinoid in the depth of the basal plate where maternal and fetal cells come in close contact to each other (Fig. 8F). Moreover, fibrinoid deposits can be found in placental septa and cell islands, in the walls of uteroplacental vessels replacing the usual constituents of vessels walls, and in the smooth chorion where it fills the former intervillous space.

Studying all these locations in detail, it is tempting to speculate that fibrinoid is formed in all those places where syncytiotrophoblast as materno–fetal barrier is disrupted or degenerated (e.g., perivillous fibrinoid) or where syncytiotrophoblast never did exist to separate maternal and fetal tissues (e.g., uteroplacental fibrinoid) (cf. below).

Composition

Fibrinoid has been shown to contain fibrinogen and fibrin (188–191). Kisalus and Herr (192) found immunocytochemical proof for a decidual secretion of heparan sulfate proteoglycan into the surrounding fibrinoid. Depending on the site of fibrinoid deposition, different amounts of other substances are added [e.g., hyaluronic acid and sialic acid (193,194), IgG, IgA, IgM, complement C3 (189,190), and albumins (188,195,196)]. Our own recent immunohistochemical studies (Malekzadeh et al., *unpublished data*) provided evidence that fibrinoid is a heterogeneous material. In most locations, it shows intense reaction with antifibrin and antifibrinogen antibodies (fibrin-type fibrinoid); this is particularly true for fibrinoid related to the intervillous space. However, in deeper layers of fibrinoid and in some special locations not in contact with the intervillous space, an immunohistochemically different composition has been observed. At these sites, oncofetal fibronectin and tenascin have been found, whereas fibrin is no longer detectable (non-fibrin fibrinoid). Histologically, this latter type of fibrinoid is always related to trophoblast cells. Such findings indicate that fibrinoid is partly derived from blood clot but that also cellular secretion and/or cellular degeneration may contribute to it. Both types may partly mix, but in most locations, they are clearly separate.

Functional Aspects

It is no longer justified to classify fibrinoid merely as being the result of degenerative processes, caused by placental aging or altered blood flow and nutrition (i.e., simply as an indicator for placental "degeneration"). Rather, most authors consider that fibrinoid is an unavoidable constituent of the normal placenta. Four different aspects are under discussion.

1. Hörmann (197) pointed to fibrinoid as "constructive principle" of the placenta, serving for mechanical stability of the organ.
2. Additional importance may be attributed to fibrinoid as regulator of the intervillous circulation (51). The intervillous space is an open, cleftlike communicating and continuously growing system. Problems in perfusion are to be expected. One possibility to adapt the shape of the intervillous space to the maternal

blood flow is to obstruct all poorly perfused areas by clotting of blood and fibrinoid deposits. Morphogenetically active extracellular matrix constituents such as tenascin (177) and oncofetal fibronectin (178) detected in such fibrinoid demonstrate high morphogenetic activities of the villous trees in those locations. Thus, fibrinoid may act as a limb in a complex process to adapt the shape of the villous trees to intervillous circulation.

3. The occurrence of fibrinoid at the materno–fetal junction correlates with invasive placentation (198). Because of this, it has been discussed as a barrier to limit the invasiveness of the trophoblast (199–201). However, the presence of oncofetal fibronectin and tenascin around just extravillous cytotrophoblast may locally facilitate migration and invasiveness.
4. Many authors discuss an immunologically protective function (190,202–207). An immunoprotective role of sialic acid as normal constituent of fibrinoid has been stressed by Currie and Bagshawe (204). This molecule may mask fetal antigens and thus prevent their recognition by maternal cells; moreover, sialic acid is thought to protect fetal cells from already sensitized maternal lymphocytes. Also, heparan sulfate proteoglycan, secreted by decidual cells into the surrounding uteroplacental fibrinoid (192), has been suggested as a molecule for immunoprotection.

Swinburne (208) proposed that the fibrinoid expresses target antigens that bind circulating maternal antibodies; the resulting immune complexes contribute to deposition of fibrinoid. The same concept was favored by Chaouat and co-workers (209) and by Hunziker and Wegmann (210). According to Raghupathy and co-workers (211), antibodies bound to fibrinoid are internalized and degraded within 4 to 6 h; the capacity of this antigen sponge is regenerated within 48 h.

In the noninvasive epitheliochorial placentation of artiodactyla and perissodactyla, which largely lack fibrinoid, the trophoblast is uninterrupted and serves with the trophoblastic glycocalix as a perfect immune barrier. In contrast, the trophoblast and its glycocalix are multiply interrupted in hemochorial placentation and may thus raise the demand for an additional focal immune barrier. Because fibrinoid is deposited in all sites where the trophoblast is discontinuous, the fibrinoid may serve as a substitute (51,73,177).

CELL BIOLOGIC TRENDS IN PLACENTAL RESEARCH[a]

The human placenta is a ready source for human hormones, proteins, and nucleic acids. This may be one of the main reasons that it became the target of a wide range of highly active cell biologic and molecular biologic studies. Because many of these may also serve as a basis for studies in other fields of placentology, the aim of this chapter is to act as a guide to the recent respective literature in some of these exciting fields of placental research.

Cell Isolation and Culture

An important approach to the understanding of cell biologic interactions in any organ is the possibility to isolate and to cultivate its cells for *in vitro* studies. A technique for isolating cytotrophoblast cells was established by Kliman and co-workers (213); some laboratories have added certain modifications (214,215). Several methods have been published to isolate the Hofbauer cells (macrophages) using proteolytic enzymes (216,217), a combination of enzymatic digestion and density gradient centrifugation (218), or mechanical action and density gradient centrifugation without the use of enzymes (219). The latter approach has the advantage of not damaging the surface antigen pattern of the macrophages. Drake and Loke (220) recently established a technique to isolate endothelial cells from uteroplacental vessels, and placental fibroblasts have been separated by Fant (221). Attempts to isolate and culture fetal villous endothelial cells have not been successful yet.

Growth Factors, Growth Factor Receptors, and Oncogenes

The placenta produces many polypeptide growth factors, possesses a complex array of respective receptors, and expresses several proto-oncogene protein products (for reviews, see refs. 222–224). EGF is detectable in amniotic fluid, umbilical vessels, and placental tissue (225). Morrish and co-workers (226) showed that this growth factor induces morphologic differentiation of the trophoblast together with increased production of hCG and HPL *in vitro*. Correspondingly, its receptor (EGF-R) was found in the syncytiotrophoblast as well as in the villous and extravillous cytotrophoblast (123,227,228).

Structurally related to EGF-R is the protein product of the proto-oncogene c-erbB-2, which encodes a receptor protein for a yet unknown ligand (229,230). In the human placenta, expression could be observed in the villous syncytiotrophoblast as well as in the differentiated and nonproliferating extravillous cytotrophoblast (123).

Insulinlike growth factors (IGF) 1 and 2 are expressed primarily in highly proliferative cytotrophoblast populations, as, for example, in cell islands and cell columns (231). Because many IGF receptors are expressed in villous cytotrophoblast, it has been suggested that IGF mediates autocrine and/or short-range paracrine growth control of trophoblast (231).

[a] The contents of this section are based on a contribution by P. Kaufmann and M. Castellucci to ref. 212.

Insulin receptor (I-R) has been described to be present mainly at the villous syncytiotrophoblastic surface in the first trimester, whereas in the second and in the third trimesters trophoblastic expression becomes weaker. By contrast, increasing I-R activities are seen in the fetal endothelium (232). According to these results, maternal insulin and its receptors may be involved in the regulation of villous growth throughout the first trimester, whereas villous growth regulating activities of fetal insulin seem to dominate in later pregnancy.

PDGF and its receptors (PDGF-R) are expressed in the human placenta (140,233). It has been shown that PDGF is coexpressed with the *myc* proto-oncogene in proliferative cytotrophoblast, and it has been suggested that PDGF influences the "pseudomalignant" phenotype of the early human placenta (233). Also, Holmgren and co-workers (140) proposed an important role for PDGF-B and its receptors in placental angiogenic processes.

Another growth factor detected in the human placenta and structurally related to PDGF is PDECGF. It stimulates endothelial cell growth and chemotaxis *in vitro* and angiogenesis *in vivo* (234); by immunohistochemistry, it is mainly detected in the stromal cells of the chorionic villi and in the villous trophoblast.

TGF-β and TGF-β messenger RNA have been isolated from human placenta (235). It has been suggested that it may play an important role in the inhibition of trophoblastic invasion of the uterine wall during placental development (236). It may also regulate the local immune response and prevent rejection of the fetus. Moreover, Morrish and co-workers (237) have shown that it acts as a major inhibitor of trophoblast differentiation and concomitant peptide secretion.

Proteases

Proteolytic enzymes and their inhibitors play an important role during migration and invasion of trophoblast cells and during remodeling of the villous stroma in the course of placental development. It has been shown that trophoblast expresses interstitial and type IV collagenolytic activities (238–240), and the former has been also detected in villous fibroblasts (239). Inhibitors of such proteases (e.g., tissue inhibitor of metalloproteases are involved in the regulation of trophoblast invasion, the latter inhibitor being probably produced by trophoblast and decidual cells (241).

Plasminogen activators (uPA and tPA) and their inhibitors have been shown to be present in amniotic fluid (242) and to be produced by the trophoblast (240–245) (for reviews, see refs. 241 and 246). Interestingly, plasminogen activator inhibitor type 1 (PAI-1) is mainly present in invading cytotrophoblast cells, whereas PAI-2 is prominent in the villous syncytiotrophoblast (244).

Extracellular Matrix Molecules

Recent research has strongly emphasized the role of extracellular matrix molecules in morphogenetic and invasive processes. Tenascin (177,247) has been shown to be expressed in fetal stroma related both to proliferative trophoblast and to trophoblastic defects covered by fibrinoid. It has been discussed to support postmitotic migration of the cytotrophoblast.

Fibronectins are well known to be expressed in the villous stroma (70,248,249). In particular, the oncofetal isoform, absent from the villous stroma, is specifically expressed in cell columns and neighboring parts of the basal plate (250). It has been speculated that this isoform could mediate implantation and placental–uterine attachment throughout gestation. Fibronectins are involved in attaching cells to extracellular matrix through integrins such as $\alpha 5/\beta 1$ (for a review, see ref. 247).

Different from most other organs, molecules such as laminin, collagen IV, and heparan sulfate are not only detectable in the basement membrane but also weakly expressed throughout the villous stroma in the human placenta (70,252,253). The universal presence of these molecules in the extracellular matrix may facilitate remodeling of basement membranes and thus may increase morphogenetic and functional flexibility of the various villous cell populations.

Moreover, collagen types I, III, V, and VI have been found by immunohistochemistry in the stroma of the chorionic villi (252–254). Also, decorin, a small leucine-rich proteoglycan that seems to have a primary function in the organization of the extracellular matrix has been detected in the villous stroma (255). Interestingly, the core protein of decorin (whose synthesis is induced by TGF-β) binds and neutralizes TGF-β (256).

There is an increasing use of extracellular matrix molecules for *in vitro* studies of the trophoblast. It has been demonstrated that such molecules influence trophoblast differentiation (73,257,258); they can play a pivotal role in repair mechanisms (73), may participate in modulating hormone and protein production (258), and can influence the morphology and proteolytic activity of the trophoblast (215,259).

MORPHOLOGIC ASPECTS OF DIAGNOSTIC METHODS

Ultrasound

Ultrasound was first introduced into clinical obstetric practice in the late 1950s and has subsequently proved to be a simple, safe, and accurate way of imaging the placenta *in vivo*. From the outset, one of the great benefits it conferred was the ability to localize the placenta, but as the technology improves, it has become possible to monitor the organ's growth and assess its consistency.

The development of the transvaginal probe has enabled the events taking place during even the first few weeks of pregnancy to be visualized, and these were recently reviewed by Schaaps (260). Only a few days after the expected menstrual period, it is possible to distinguish a gestational sac buried within the uterine mucosa. The center of the sac appears as a fluid-filled echo-free cavity and is surrounded by an echo-rich peripheral zone corresponding to the proliferating trophoblastic mantle. An amniotic cavity and secondary yolk sac become visible ultrasonographically during the third week postconception. By this time, it is therefore also possible to distinguish multiple pregnancies and to diagnose whether these are mono- or dichorial and mono- or diamniotic.

At the end of the third week, the peripheral zone is 3 to 4 mm thick, and this thickness triples over the next 2 weeks. Regression of chorionic villi and formation of the chorion laeve is indicated during weeks 7 to 11 of gestation by an increasing disparity in the thickness of the peripheral zone at the embryonic and abembryonic poles. There is no difference in echogenicity at these two sites, however. That part destined to become the definitive placenta continues to expand, and uterine vessels become more prominent in the adjacent endometrium. Although the echo patterns suggest circulatory activity in these vessels, recent evidence, as previously discussed, suggests the spiral arteries do not under normal conditions communicate with the intervillous space until the end of the first trimester (46).

In terms of ultrasonographic appearances, further placental development is best described by reference to the classification scheme proposed by Grannum and coworkers (99). Although based on static gray scale images rather than the current real-time scanning techniques, this pioneering work has largely stood the test of time. Within the scheme, four grades of placental appearances are recognized:

Grade 0: All placentas at the end of the first trimester start with this configuration. The chorionic plate is smooth, and in echogenic terms, the substance of the placenta is homogeneous. The basal area is devoid of echogenic densities.

Grade 1: The chorionic plate displays subtle undulations, and linear echogenic densities are randomly dispersed throughout the substance of the organ. These densities are orientated so that their long axis is parallel to the chorionic plate. The basal plate is still free of echogenic densities.

Grade 2: Commalike echogenic densities extend from the chorionic plate toward but not as far as the basal plate. The scattered echogenic densities become more numerous and increasingly dense. The hallmark of this grading is the appearance of similarly orientated echogenic densities within the basal plate, which at times may be so frequent as to become confluent.

Grade 3: The placenta is divided into compartments by the commalike echogenic densities that now appear to extend from chorionic to basal plate. Midway between the two plates spherical echolucent areas develop.

Although no direct attempts were made to correlate these ultrasonographic appearances with placental histology, it is generally believed that the commalike densities represent placental septa, and the echolucent areas correspond to the central villous-free parts of the lobules (cf. Fig. 7). The higher grades are therefore taken to indicate increasing maturity of the placenta, although it is not unusual for individual cases to display a mixture of features. Not all placentas will progress to a grade 3 configuration at term, however. The grade 1 configuration is generally seen at approximately 31 weeks of gestation, but in normal pregnancies, 40% of cases will remain grade 1 at term. Grade 2 placenta appears at approximately 36 weeks of gestation, and 45% of cases will retain this configuration until term. The grade 3 placenta appears at 38 weeks and accounts for the remaining 15% of cases at term.

The main aim of the classification scheme was not to describe placental development as such but rather to gain a noninvasive measure of fetal maturity. In general, the correlation between placental grading and fetal biparietal diameter is poor (99,261). By contrast, the correlation with fetal lung maturation is much stronger. In the original study of Grannum et al. (99) of normal patients, occurrence of grade 1 was associated with a 65% mature lecithin/sphingomyelin ratio in the amniotic fluid, grade 2 with 87.5%, and grade 3 with 100%. These findings were confirmed by Petrucha et al. (262) and Tabsh (263), but others have reported weaker correlations (264,265).

Ultrasonic examination of the placenta can therefore provide an indication of the degree of maturation of the organ and hence of the fetus. Much work has yet to be done to determine how the echogenic densities correspond to areas of placental calcification and infarction, and volumetric estimation of the placenta ultrasonographically still produces variable results. Until these aspects are better understood and preferably quantified in some way, it is unlikely that simple ultrasonic examination of the placenta can yield further information of physiologic importance. At present, its great strengths lie in the pathologic arena and in the diagnosis of complications such as placenta previa, abruptio placentas, and hydatidiform mole.

Doppler Ultrasound

The application of the Doppler principle to ultrasound has opened up new possibilities for imaging the fetoplacental unit by permitting blood flow velocities to be measured noninvasively. When an ultrasound acoustic wave is directed at a moving target, the energy backscattered undergoes a frequency change that is proportional to the relative velocity of the target and to the cosine of the angle of intersection between the target and the beam. Pulsed Doppler has the advantage of being range selective and so allows velocities at specific points to be measured. It can be combined with conventional ultrasound imaging, and so these points can be accurately located within the placenta or uterine wall. The refinement of color Doppler enables relative velocities to be more easily discriminated and blood flow to be determined in smaller vessels than is possible with traditional Doppler techniques.

The Doppler signals obtained represent the summation of multiple Doppler shift frequencies backscattered by erythrocytes traveling at different velocities. These velocities vary according to the phase of the cardiac cycle, and so in real-time imaging, a flow velocity waveform (FVW) is displayed. Analysis of this waveform can provide qualitative information such as the presence or direction of blood flow and also quantitative or semiquantitative data on velocity. The shape of the FVW also gives an indication of the degree of resistance to flow offered by the vessel in question and its subsequent ramifications. In low resistance networks, end-diastolic velocities indicate that some blood flow occurs during all phases of the cardiac cycle. By contrast in high-resistance vascular beds, flow is only observed during systole. In the most severe cases, reverse flow may even occur during diastole. Several indices, such as the resistance index and pulsatility index, have therefore been devised, and these are all based on a comparison of the peak systolic and end-diastolic velocities (266).

Doppler ultrasound can thus provide information on velocity and resistance, but of greater interest to physiologists is the volume of blood flow. This will be determined by a combination of the mean velocity and the vessel cross-sectional area. Measurements of the latter with ultrasound imaging have, for technical reasons, been less successful and so, in general quantitative measurements of blood flow, have proved to be unreliable and poorly reproducible (267).

Using color Doppler techniques, it is possible to visualize blood flow in the umbilical vessels at 7 weeks of gestation. During the first trimester, the FVW indicates a high vascular resistance in the placenta and no end-diastolic velocities (268). At the end of this period, between weeks 12 and 14 of gestation, end-diastolic velocities develop and are maintained throughout the remainder of pregnancy in normal cases. The factors underlying this change are not yet certain, but it is clear that alterations in the fetal cardiac output heart rate and blood pressure have no impact on the pulsatility index of the umbilical artery (269). It coincides with a progressive increase in the vascularity of the placental villi, as evidenced by an increase in the fractional volume represented by the capillaries and an increase in their length density (270). It also coincides with the establishment of continuous maternal blood flow within the intervillous space, and as discussed previously, alterations in the transmural pressure operating between the two circulations can have a major impact on the caliber of the fetal vessels. Changes in the concentration of oxygen or metabolites could also exert an effect on the umbilical circulation (270).

On the maternal side, a progressive reduction in resistance to blood flow in the uterine arteries is observed during the first trimester (271,272). This fall continues until approximately the twentieth week of gestation, from which point onward the resistance remains stable. A combination of hormonal changes and endovascular trophoblastic invasion is the most likely cause for this phenomenon.

Later in gestation, during the second and third trimesters, there is a progressive fall in the pulsatility index within the fetal placental circulation (273). To the term fetus, the organ therefore represents a low-resistance arteriovenous shunt.

The situation may be complicated in certain pathologic conditions, however. Different attempts have been made to correlate placental changes with abnormal FVW patterns (274–278). These studies have largely been qualitative or semiquantitative and have included mixed pathologies such as maternal hypertension, intrauterine growth retardation, cigarette smoking, diabetes mellitus, and chromosomal abnormalities. This large number of variables has led to a confused picture, but the most consistent finding is that raised placental resistance is often associated with a reduction in the number of fetal arteries within the stem villi. As stressed previously, it is likely that vascular resistance will be determined by absolute values of structural parameters, such as the total length or cross-sectional area of the stem villous arteries. To date, such data have not been correlated with FVW profiles.

Mathematical modeling of the placental circulation, incorporating morphologic information obtained from vascular casts, has also been attempted (279,280). Systematic alteration of the variables within such models may provide insight into which structural parameters exert the greatest influence on the FVW profile.

Nuclear Magnetic Resonance Imaging

Nuclear magnetic resonance imaging is another safe and noninvasive imaging technique that has potential for monitoring the placenta *in vivo*. Its use could enable the volumetric growth of the organ to be assessed sequentially during gestation in a more accurate way than is possible with ultrasound at present. Equally, the high resolution and texture details that it provides might allow areas of infarction or other pathology to be diagnosed antenatal and correlated more precisely with the clinical history.

Injection of a contrast medium into the circulation allows the blood to be visualized and its rate of flow determined in a manner that is independent of the angle between the vessel and the receiver. As yet, it has only been applied to the rhesus monkey and to the human placenta perfused *in vitro* (24). The results have been encouraging and have largely confirmed the patterns of fetal and maternal blood flow previously described. The ease and reproducibility of the technique indicates that it has considerable potential for monitoring the uteroplacental circulation *in vivo,* either sequentially to assess normal patterns of development or in cases of suspected pathology and growth retardation.

Chorionic Villus Sampling

Chorionic villus sampling is a technique by which a sample of villi can be removed from the chorion frondosum during the first, and sometimes even second, trimester. Because of the small size of the sample available and the rather imprecise localization of the sampling site, the opportunities for morphologic studies are limited. Recent quantitative studies on material from terminations of pregnancy have revealed, however, that even in the first trimester structural differences can be identified in the placentas of women smoking cigarettes (270). Further studies are required to determine whether other pathologic changes are established at a similarly early stage of pregnancy.

By contrast, much information on genetic and metabolic disorders can be obtained by chorionic villus sampling (281). For this reason, the technique has had greater impact on the clinical management of early pregnancies than on our understanding of fetoplacental physiology. The procedure does carry a risk of spontaneous miscarriage, and so other ways of retrieving fetal cells are being investigated. Possibilities for the future are trophoblast cells deported in the maternal circulation or nucleated fetal erythrocytes released by defects in the placental barrier (282).

REFERENCES

1. DeWitt F. An historical study on theories of the placenta to 1900. *J Hist Med* 1958;14:360–374.
2. Amoroso EC. Early theories of the placenta form: fancies to facts. The JY Simpson Oration. In: *Royal College of Obstetricians and Gynaecologists, 42 Annual Report.* 1971;76–91.
3. McMurrich JP. *Leonardo da Vinci the Anatomist (1452–1519).* London: Baillere, Tindall and Cox, 1930.
4. Boyd JD, Hamilton WJ. *The Human Placenta.* Cambridge: Heffers, 1970.
5. Corner GC. Exploring the placental maze. The development of our knowledge of the relation between the blood-streams of mother and infant *in utero. Am J Obstet Gynecol* 1963;86: 408–418.
6. Steven DH. Placenta depicta—illustrations and ideas. In: Steven DH, ed. *Comparative Placentation. Essays in Structure and Function.* London: Academic Press, 1975;1–24.
7. Dalrymple J. On the structure and functions of the human placenta. *Med Chir Trans Lond* 1842;25:21–29.
8. Steven DH. Historical introduction: concepts of the trophoblast and of its role in placentation. In: Loke YW, Whyte A, eds. *Biol Trophoblast.* Amsterdam: Elsevier, 1983;3–21.
9. Langhans T. Über die Zellschicht des menschlichen Chorion. *Anat Physiol Festschrift für Henle* 1882;69–79.
10. Hubrecht AAW. Studies in mammalian embryology. I. The placentation of *Erinaceus europaeus,* with remarks on the phylogeny of the placenta. *J Microsc Sci* 1889;30:283–404.
11. Grosser O. *Vergleichende Anatomie und Entwicklungsgeschichte der Eihäute und der Placenta.* Wien, Leipzig: W Braumüller, 1909.
12. Grosser O. *Frühentwicklung, Eihautbildung und Placentation des Menschen und der Säugetiere.* München: JF Bergmann, 1927.
13. Mossman HW. *Vertebrate Fetal Membranes: Comparative Ontogeny and Morphology; Evolution; Phylogenetic Significance; Basic Functions; Research Opportunities.* London: Macmillan, 1987.
14. Amoroso EC. Placentation. In: Parkes AS, ed. *Marshall's Physiology of Reproduction,* Ed 3, Vol 2. London: Longmans Green, 1952;127–311.
15. Halban J. Die innere Sekretion von Ovarium und Placenta und ihre Bedeutung für die Funktion der Milchdrüse. *Arch Gynäkol* 1905;75:353–441.
16. Wislocki GB, Streeter GL. On the placentation of the macaque (*Macaca mulatta*) from the time of implantation until formation of the definitive placenta. *Carnegie Contributions Embryol* 1938;27:1–65.
17. Hertig AT, Rock J. Two human ova of the pre-villous stage, having an ovulation age of about 11–12 days respectively. *Carnegie Contributions Embryol* 1941;29:127–156.
18. Stieve H. Ein 131/2 Tage altes, in der Gebärmutter erhaltenes und durch Eingriff gewonnenes menschliches Ei. *Arch Mikr Anat* 1926;7:295–402.
19. Stieve H. Die Entwicklung und der Bau der menschlichen Placenta. Teil 2. Zotten: Zottenraumgitter und Gefäße in der zweiten Hälfte der Schwangerschaft. *Z Mikrosk Anat Forsch* 1941;50:1–20.
20. Spanner R. Mütterlicher und kindlicher Kreislauf der menschlichen Placenta und seine Strombahnen. *Z Anat Entwicklungsgesch* 1935;105:163–242.
21. Ramsey EM. Circulation in the maternal placenta of the rhesus monkey and man, with observations on the marginal lakes. *Am J Anat* 1956;98:159–190.
22. Borell U, Fernström I, Westman A. Eine arteriographische Studie des Plazentarkreislaufs. *Geburtshilfe Frauenheitkd* 1958;18:1–9.
23. Hustin J, Schaaps JP, Lambotte R. Anatomical studies of the utero-placental vascularization in first time trimester of pregnancy. *Trophoblast Res* 1988;3:49–60.
24. Panigel M, Coulam C, Wolf G, Zeleznik A, Leone F, Podesta C. Magnetic resonance imaging (MRI) of the placental circulation using gadolinium—DTPA as a paramagnetic marker in the rhesus monkey *in vivo* and the perfused human placenta *in vitro. Trophoblast Res* 1988;3:271–282.
25. Dempsey EW, Wislocki GB. Observations on some histochemical reactions in the human placenta, with special reference to the significance to the glycogen and iron. *Endocrinology* 1944;35: 409–429.
26. Boyd JD, Hughes AFW. Observations on human chorionic villi using the electron microscope. *J Anat* 1954;88:356–362.
27. Wislocki GB, Dempsey EW. Electron microscopy of the human placenta. *Anat Rec* 1955;123:133–167.
28. Steven DH. Anatomy of the placental barrier. In: Steven DH, ed. *Comparative Placentation. Essays in Structure and Function.* London: Academic Press, 1975;25–57.

29. Kaufmann P. Functional anatomy of the non-primate placenta. *Placenta* 1981;(suppl I):13–28.
30. Enders AC. A comparative study of the fine structure in several hemochorial placentas. *Am J Anat* 1965;116:29–67.
31. Faber JJ. Application of the theory of heat exchangers to the transfer of inert materials in placentas. *Circ Res* 1969;24: 221–234.
32. Moll W. Gas exchange in concurrent, countercurrent and crosscurrent flow systems: the concept of the fetoplacental unit. In: Longo LD, Bartels H, eds. *Respiratory Gas Exchange and Blood Flow in the Placenta.* DHEW Publ. No. (NIH), Dept. Health, Education and Welfare, 1972;73–361.
33. Dantzer V, Leiser R, Kaufmann P, Luckhardt M. Comparative morphological aspects of placental vascularisation. *Trophoblast Res* 1988;3:235–260.
34. Torpin R. *The Human Placenta.* Springfield, Illinois: Thomas, 1969.
35. Wentworth P. Some anomalies of the foetal vessels of the human placenta. *J Anat* 1965;99:273–282.
36. Kaufmann P. Basic morphology of the fetal and maternal circuits in the human placenta. *Contrib Gynecol Obstet* 1985;13:5–17.
37. Schuhmann R. Plazenton: Begriff, Entstehung, funktionelle Anatomie. In: Becker V, Schiebler TH, Kubli F, eds. *Die Plazenta des Menschen.* Stuttgart, New York: Thieme Verlag, 1981; 199–207.
38. Becker V. Plazenta. In: Becker V, Roeckelein G, eds. *Pathologie der Plazenta und des Abortes.* Berlin, Heidelberg, New York: Springer-Verlag, 1989;1–155.
39. Schultze BS. Über velamentöse und placentale Insertion der Nabelschnur. *Arch Gynäkol* 1987;30:47–56.
40. McLennan JE. Implications of eccentricity of the human umbilical cord. *Am J Obstet Gynecol* 1968;101:1124–1130.
41. Jauniaux E, Englert Y, Vanesse M, Hidden M, Wilkin P. Pathologic features of placentas from singleton pregnancies obtained by *in vitro* fertilization and embryo transfer. *Obstet Gynecol* 1990;76:61–64.
42. Hertig AT, Rock J, Adams EC. A description of 34 human ova within the first 17 days of development. *Am J Anat* 1956;98:435–494.
43. Lindenberg S, Hyttel P, Lenz S, Holmes PV. Ultrastructure of the early human implantation *in vitro*. *Hum Reprod* 1986;1: 533–538.
44. Luckett WP. Origin and differentiation of the yolk sac and extraembryonic mesoderm in presomite human and rhesus monkey embryos. *Am J Anat* 1978;152:59–97.
45. Pijnenborg R. Trophoblast invasion and placentation in the human: morphological aspects. *Trophoblast Res* 1990;4:33–47.
46. Schaaps JP, Hustin J. *In vivo* aspect of the maternal-trophoblastic border during the first trimester of gestation. *Trophoblast Res* 1988;3:39–48.
47. Salvo G, Samoggia P, Petti S, et al. Haemoglobin switching in human embryos: asynchrony of z-a and e-g-globulin switches in primitive and definitive erythropoietic lineage. *Nature* 1985;313: 235–238.
48. Dempsey DE. The development of capillaries in the villi of early human placentas. *Am J Anat* 1972;134:221–238.
49. Demir R, Kaufmann P, Castellucci M, Erbengi T, Kotowski A. Fetal vasculogenesis and angiogenesis in human placental villi. *Acta Anat* 1989;136:190–203.
50. Burton GJ. The fine structure of the human placental villus as revealed by scanning electron microscopy. *Scanning Microsc* 1987;1:1811–1828.
51. Benirschke K, Kaufmann P, eds. *Pathology of the Human Placenta,* Ed 2. New York: Springer, 1990.
52. Jones CJP, Fox H. Ultrastructure of the normal human placenta. *Electron Microsc Rev* 1991;4:129–178.
53. Ockleford CD, Whyte A. Differentiated regions of human placental cell surface associated with exchange of material between maternal and fetal blood: coated vesicles. *J Cell Sci* 1977;25:293–312.
54. Ockleford CD, Wakely J. The skeleton of the placenta. In: Harrison RJ, Holmes RL, eds. *Progress in Anatomy.* Vol II. London: Cambridge University Press, 1981;19–48.
55. Dearden L, Ockleford CD. Structure of human trophoblast: correlation with function. In: Loke YW, Whyte A, eds. *Biology of Trophoblast.* Amsterdam: Elsevier, 1983;69–110.
56. Kim CK, Benirschke K. Autoradiographic study of the "X cells" in the human placenta. *Am J Obstet Gynecol* 1971;109:96–102.
57. Kaufmann P, Nagl W, Fuhrmann B. Die funktionelle Bedeutung der Langhanszellen der menschlichen Placenta. *Anat Anz* 1983;77:435–436.
58. Simpson RA, Mayhew TM, Barnes PR. From 13 weeks to term, the trophoblast of human placenta grows by the continuous recruitment of new proliferative units: a study of nuclear number using the disector. *Placenta* 1992;13:501–512.
59. Bright NA, Ockleford CD. Fcg receptor bearing cells in human term amniochorion. *J Anat* (*in press*).
60. Kaufmann P. Untersuchunger über die Langhanszellen in der menschlichen Placenta. *Z Zellforsch* 1972;128:283–302.
61. Fox H. Effect of hypoxia on trophoblast in organ culture. A morphologic and autoradiographic study. *Am J Obstet Gynecol* 1970;107:1058–1064.
62. Kaufmann P, Stark J. Enzymhistochemische Untersuchungen an reifen menschlichen Placentazotten. I. Reifungs- und Alterungsvorgänge am Trophoblasten. *Histochemistry* 1972;29:65–82.
63. Hoshina M, Boothby M, Hussa R, Pattillo R, Camel HM, Boime I. Linkage of human chorionic gonadotrophin and placental lactogen biosynthesis to trophoblast differentiation and tumorigenesis. *Placenta* 1985;6:163–172.
64. Reale E, Wang T, Zaccheo D, Maganza C, Pescetto G. Junctions on the maternal blood surface of the human placental syncytium. *Placenta* 1980;1:245–258.
65. Smith CA, Moore HDM. Expression of C-type viral particles at implantation in the marmoset monkey. *Hum Reprod* 1988;3: 395–398.
66. Castellucci M, Kaufmann P. Hofbauer cells. In: Benirschke K, Kaufmann P, eds. *Pathology of the Human Placenta.* New York: Springer, 1990;71–80.
67. Castellucci M, Celona A, Bartels H, Steininger B, Benedetto V, Kaufmann P. Mitosis of the Hofbauer cell: possible implications for a fetal macrophage. *Placenta* 1987;8:65–76.
68. Nikolov SD, Schiebler TH. Über das fetale Gefäßsystem der reifen menschlichen Placenta. *Z Zellforsch* 1973;139:309–350.
69. Leach L, Eaton BM, Firth JA, Contractor SF. Immunogold localisation of endogeneous immunoglobulin-G in ultrathin frozen sections of the human placenta. *Cell Tissue Res* 1989;257: 603–607.
70. Yamada T, Isemura M, Yamaguchi Y, Munakata H, Hayashi N, Kyogoku M. Immunohistochemical localization of fibronectin in the human placentas at their different stages of maturation. *Histochemistry* 1987;86:579–584.
71. Myatt L. Control of vascular resistance in the human placenta. *Placenta* 1992;13:329–341.
72. Stulc J. Extracellular transport pathways in the haemochorial placenta. *Placenta* 1989;10:113–119.
73. Nelson DM, Crouch EC, Curran EM, Farmer DR. Trophoblast interaction with fibrin matrix. Epithelialization of perivillous fibrin deposits as a mechanism for villous repair in the human placenta. *Am J Pathol* 1990;136:855–865.
74. Kaufmann P, Schröder H, Leichtweiss H-P. Fluid shift across the placenta: II. Feto-maternal transfer of horseradish peroxidase in the guinea pig. *Placenta* 1982;3:339–348.
75. Kertschanska S, Kaufmann P. Morphological evidence for the existence of transtrophoblastic channels in human placental villi. *Placenta* 1992;13:A33.
76. Kertschanska S, Kosanke G, Kaufmann P. Morphological evidence for the existence of transtrophoblastic channels in human placental villi. *Trophoblast Res* 7 (*in press*).
77. Stulc J, Friederich R, Jiricka Z. Estimation of the equivalent pore dimensions in the rabbit placenta. *Life Sci* 1969;8:167–180.
78. Thornburg K, Faber JJ. Transfer of hydrophilic molecules by placenta and yolk sac of the guinea pig. *Am J Physiol* 1977;233:C111–C124.
79. Hedley R, Bradbury MBW. Transport of polar non-electrolytes across the intact and perfused guinea-pig placenta. *Placenta* 1980;1:277–285.

80. Kaufmann P, Schröder H, Leichtweiss H-P, Winterhager E. Are there membrane-lined channels through the trophoblast? A study with lanthanum hydroxide. *Trophoblast Res* 1987;2:557–571.
81. Schröder H, Nelson P, Power B. Fluid shift across the placenta. I. The effect of dextran T40 in the isolated guinea pig placenta. *Placenta* 1982;3:327–338.
82. Schuhmann RA. Placentome structure of the human placenta. *Bib Anat* 1982;22:46–57.
83. Kaufmann P, Sen DK, Schweikhart G. Classification of human placental villi. 1. Histology. *Cell Tissue Res* 1979;200:409–423.
84. Sen DK, Kaufmann P, Schweikhart G. Classification of human placental villi. II. Morphometry. *Cell Tissue Res* 1979;200: 425–434.
85. Kaufmann P. Development and differentiation of the human placental villous tree. *Bib Anat* 1982;22:29–39.
86. Castellucci M, Scheper M, Scheffen I, Celona A, Kaufmann P. The development of the human placental villous tree. *Anat Embryol* 1989;181:117–128.
87. Cantle SJ, Kaufmann P, Luckhardt M, Schweikhart G. Interpretation of syncytial sprouts and bridges in the human placenta. *Placenta* 1987;8:221–234.
88. Iklé FA. Trophoblastzellen in strömenden Blut. *Schweiz Med Wochenschr* 1961;91:934–945.
89. Kaufmann P, Bruns U, Leiser R, Luckhardt M, Winterhager E. The fetal vascularization of term human placental villi. II. Intermediate and terminal villi. *Anat Embryol* 1985;173:203–214.
90. Kaufmann P, Luckhardt M, Leiser R. Three-dimensional representation of the fetal vessel system in the human placenta. *Trophoblast Res* 1988;3:113–137.
91. Boe F. Studies on the vascularization of the human placenta. *Acta Obstet Gynecol Scand* 1953;32(suppl 5):1–92.
92. Arts NF. Investigations on the vascular system of the placenta. Part I. General introduction and fetal vascular system. *Am J Obstet Gynecol* 1961;82:147–158.
93. Pisarski T, Topilko A. Comparative study of the vascular syncytial membranes of the human placenta in light and electron microscopy. *Pol Med J* 1966;5:630–638.
94. Burton GJ, Tham SW. Formation of vasculo-syncytial membranes in the human placenta. *J Dev Physiol* 1992;18:43–47.
95. Karimu AL, Burton GJ. Compliance of the human placental villous membrane at term: the concept of the fetoplacental unit as an autoregulating gas exchange system. *Trophoblast Res* 7 (*in press*).
96. Burton GJ, Feneley MR. Capillary volume fraction is the principal determinant of villous membrane thickness in the normal human placenta at term. *J Dev Physiol* 1992;17:39–45.
97. Mott JC, Walker DW. Neural and endocrine regulation of circulation in the fetus and newborn. In: Shepherd JT, Abboud FM, Geiger SR, eds. *Handbook of Physiology. Section 2. Circulation, Vol III. Peripheral Circulation and Organ Blood Flow, Part 2.* Bethesda, Maryland: American Physiological Society, 1983; 837–883.
98. Dawes GS. The fetoplacental circulation: anatomy, physiology, pathology and assessment of function by ultrasound. In: Redman CWG, Sargent IL, Starkey PM, eds. Oxford: Blackwell Scientific Publishers, 1993;579–587.
99. Grannum PAT, Berkowitz RL, Hobbins JC. The ultrasonic changes in the maturing placenta and their relation to fetal pulmonic maturity. *Am J Obstet Gynecol* 1979;133:915–922.
100. Nelson JH, Bernstein RL, Huston JW, Garcia NA, Gartenlaub C. Percutaneous retrograde femoral arteriography in obstetrics and gynaecology. *Obstet Gynecol Surv* 1961;16:1–19.
101. Wigglesworth J. Vascular anatomy of the human placenta and its significance for placental pathology. *J Obstet Gynaecol Br Cwlth* 1969;76:979–989.
102. Reynolds SRM. Formation of fetal cotyledons in the hemochorial placenta. A theoretical consideration of the functional implications of such an arrangement. *Am J Obstet Gynecol* 1966;94:425–439.
103. Burton GJ. Scanning electron microscopy of intervillous bridges in the human placenta. *J Anat* 1986;147:245–254.
104. Freese UE. The uteroplacental vascular relationship in the human. *Am J Obstet Gynecol* 1968;101:8–16.
105. Bouw GM, Stolte LAM, Baak JPA, Oort J. Quantitative morphology of the placenta. I. Standardization of sampling. *Eur J Obstet Gynecol Reprod Biol* 1976;6:325–331.
106. Power GG, Longo LD. Sluice flow in placenta: maternal vascular pressure effects on fetal circulation. *Am J Physiol* 1973;225: 1490–1496.
107. Berman W, Goodlin RC, Heymann MA, Rudolph AM. Relationships between pressure and flow in the umbilical and uterine circulations of the sheep. *Circ Res* 1976;38:262–266.
108. Marx GF, Patel S, Berman JA, Farmakides G, Schulman H. Umbilical blood flow velocity waveforms in different maternal positions and with epidural analgesia. *Obstet Gynecol* 1986;68:61–64.
109. van Katwijk C, Wladimiroff JW. Effect of maternal posture on the umbilical artery flow velocity waveform. *Ultrasound Med Biol* 1991;17:683–685.
110. Scott DB, Kerr MG. Inferior vena cava pressure in late pregnancy. *J Obstet Gynecol* 1963;70:1044–1049.
111. Teasdale F. Functional significance of the zonal morphologic differences in the normal human placenta. A morphometric study. *Am J Obstet Gynecol* 1978;130:773–781.
112. Critchley GR, Burton GJ. Intralobular variations in barrier thickness in the mature human placenta. *Placenta* 1987;8:185–194.
113. Fox H. The villous cytotrophoblast as an index of placental ischaemia. *J Obstet Gynaecol Br Cwlth* 1964;71:885–893.
114. Piotrowicz B, Niebroj TK, Sieron G. The morphology and histochemistry of the full term placenta in anaemic patients. *Folia Histochem Cytochem* 1969;7:435–444.
115. Kaufmann P, Gentzen DM, Davidoff M. Die Ultrastruktur von Langhanszellen in pathologischen menschlichen Placenten. *Arch Gynäkol* 1977;22:319–332.
116. Arnholdt H, Meisel F, Fandrey K, Löhrs U. Proliferation of villous trophoblast of the human placenta in normal and abnormal pregnancies. *Virchows Arch [B] Cell Biol* 1991;60:365–372.
117. Panigel M, Myers RE. Histological and ultrastructural changes in rhesus monkey placenta following interruption of fetal placental circulation by fetectomy or interplacental umbilical vessel ligation. *Acta Anat* 1972;81:481–506.
118. Alvarez H, Benedetti WL, Morel RL, Savarelli M. Trophoblast gradient and its relationship to placental hemodynamics. *Am J Obstet Gynecol* 1970;106:416–420.
119. Tominaga T, Page EW. Accommodation of the human placenta to hypoxia. *Am J Obstet Gynecol* 1966;94:679–685.
120. Ong PJL, Burton GJ. Thinning of the placental villous membrane during maintenance in hypoxic organ culture: structural adaptation or syncytial degeneration? *Eur J Obstet Gynecol Reprod Biol* 1991;39:103–110.
121. Prager D, Weber MM, Herman-Bonert V. Placental growth factors and releasing/inhibiting peptides. *Semin Reprod Endocrinol* 1992;2:83–94.
122. Lysiak J, Khoo N, Conelly I, Stettler-Stevenson W, Peeyush L. Role of transforming growth factor (TGF) and epidermal growth factor (EGF) on proliferation, invasion, and hCG production by normal and malignant trophoblast. *Placenta* 1992;A41.
123. Mühlhauser J, Crescimanno C, Kaufmann P, Höfler H, Zaccheo D, Castellucci M. Differentiation and proliferation patterns in human trophoblast revealed by c-erbB-2 oncogene product and EGF-R. *J Histochem Cytochem* (*in press*).
124. Hunt JS. Macrophages in human uteroplacental tissues: a review. *Am J Reprod Immunol* 1989;21:119–122.
125. Jokhi P, Chumbley G, King A, Gardner L, Loke W. Expression of the colony stimulating factor-1 receptor by cells at the uteroplacental interface. *Placenta* 1992;13:29(abst).
126. Shorter S, Clover L, Starkey P. Evidence for both an autocrine and paracrine role for the colony-stimulating factors in regulating placental growth and development. *Placenta* 1992;13:58(abst).
127. Graham CH, Lala PK. Mechanism of control of trophoblast invasion *in situ*. *J Cell Physiol* 1991;148:228–234.
128. Fox H. *Pathology of the Placenta.* London: WB Saunders, 1978.
129. Rossi P, Karsenty G, Roberts AB, Roche NS, Sporn MB, De Crombrugghe B. A nuclear factor 1 binding site mediates the transcriptional activation of a type I collagen promoter by transforming growth factor-β. *Cell* 1988;52:405–414.
130. Schmidt JA, Mizel SB, Cohen D, Green I. Interleukin 1: a potential regulator of fibroblast proliferation. *J Immunol* 1982;128: 2177–2182.

131. Hölzl M, Lüthje D, Seck-Ebersbach K. Placentaveränderungen bei EPH-Gestose. *Arch Gynäkol* 1974;217:315–334.
132. Jackson MR, Mayhew TM, Haas JD. Morphometric studies on villi in human term placentae and the effects of altitude, ethnic grouping and sex of newborn. *Placenta* 1987;8:487–495.
133. Amaladoss ASP, Burton GJ. Organ culture of human placental villi in hypoxic and hyperoxic conditions: a morphometric study. *J Dev Physiol* 1985;7:13–118.
134. Bacon BJ, Gilbert RD, Kaufmann P, Smith AD, Trevino FT, Longo LD. Placental anatomy and diffusing capacity in guinea pigs following long-term maternal hypoxia. *Placenta* 1984;5: 475–488.
135. Scheffen I, Kaufmann P, Philippens L, Leiser R, Geisen C, Mottaghy K. Alterations of the fetal capillary bed in the guinea pig placenta following long-term hypoxia. In: Piiper J, Goldstick TK, Meyer D, eds. *Oxygen Transfer to Tissue, XII.* New York: Plenum Press, 1990;779–790.
136. Werb Z. How the macrophage regulates its extracellular environment. *Am J Anat* 1983;166:237–256.
137. Ogawa S, Leavy J, Clauss M, et al. Modulation of endothelial cell (EC) function in hypoxia: alterations in cell growth and the response to monocyte-derived mitogenic factors. *J Cell Biochem* 1991;suppl 15F:213.
138. Shreeniwas R, Ogawa S, Cozzolino F, et al. Macrovascular and microvascular endothelium during long-term hypoxia: alterations in cell growth, monolayer permeability, and cell surface coagulant properties. *J Cell Physiol* 1991;146:8–17.
139. Jackson MR, Carney EW, Lye SJ, Ritchie JWK. Immunolocalisation of two angiogenic factors (PDECGF and VEGF) in human placental villi throughout gestation. *Placenta* 1992;13:27(abst).
140. Holmgren L, Glaser A, Pfeifer-Ohlsson S, Ohlsson R. Angiogenesis during human extraembryonic development involves the spatiotemporal control of PDGF ligand and receptor gene expression. *Development* 1991;113:749–754.
141. Reynolds LP, Killilea SD, Redmer DA. Angiogenesis in the female reproductive system. *FASEB J* 1992;6:886–892.
142. Aladjem S. The syncytial knot: a sign of active syncytial proliferation. *Am J Obstet Gynecol* 1967;99:350–358.
143. Burton GJ, Ingram SC, Palmer ME. The influence of the mode of fixation on morphometrical data derived from terminal villi in the human placenta at term: a comparison of immersion and perfusion fixation. *Placenta* 1987;8:37–51.
144. Schweikhart G, Kaufmann P. Zur Abgrenzung normaler, artefizieller und pathologischer Strukturen in reifen menschlichen Plazentazotten. I. Ultrastruktur des Syncytiotrophoblasten. *Arch Gynäkol* 1977;222:213–230.
145. Kaufmann P. Influence of ischemia and artificial perfusion on placental ultrastructure and morphometry. *Contrib Gynecol Obstet* 1985;13:18–26.
146. Feneley MR, Burton GJ. Villous composition and membrane thickness in the human placenta at term: a stereological study using unbiased estimators and optimal fixation techniques. *Placenta* 1991;12:131–142.
147. Jauniaux E, Moscoso JG, Vanesse M, Campbell S, Driver M. Perfusion fixation for placental morphologic investigation. *Hum Pathol* 1991;22:442–449.
148. Mayhew TM, Burton GJ. Methodological problems in placental morphometry: apologia for the use of stereology based on sound sampling practice. *Placenta* 1988;9:565–581.
149. Jackson MR, Joy CF, Mayhew TM, Haas JD. Stereological studies on the true thickness of the villous membrane in human term placentae: a study of placentae from high-altitude pregnancies. *Placenta* 1985;6:249–258.
150. Burton GJ, Palmer ME. Eradicating fetomaternal fluid shift during perfusion fixation of the human placenta. *Placenta* 1988;9:327–332.
151. Weibel ER. *Stereological Methods, Volume 1, Practical Methods for Biological Morphometry.* London: Academic Press, 1979.
152. Gundersen HJG, Bendtsen TF, Korbo L, et al. Some new simple and efficient stereological methods and their use in pathological research and diagnosis. *Acta Pathol Microbiol Immunol Scand* 1988;96:379–394.
153. Gundersen HJG, Bagger P, Bendtsen TF, et al. The new stereological tools: disector, fractionator and point-sampled intercepts and their use in pathological research. *Acta Pathol Microbiol Immunol Scand* 1988;96:857–881.
154. Mayhew TM. The new stereological methods for interpreting functional morphology from slices of cells and organs. *Exp Physiol* 1991;76:639–665.
155. Vermeulen RCW, Kurver PH, Arts NFT, van Kessel H, Wilson GR, Klopper A. The relationship between the surface area of the trophoblast and some placental products. *Placenta* 1982;3: 359–366.
156. Kádar L, Saldana M. La placenta de la altura. 1. Caracteristicas macroscópicas y morfometria. *Ginecol Obstet Lima* 1971;17: 2–23.
157. Beischer NA, Sivasamboo R, Vohra S, Silpisornkosal S, Reid S. Placental hypertrophy in severe pregnancy anaemia. *J Obstet Gynaecol Br Cwlth* 1970;77:398–409.
158. Laga EM, Driscoll SG, Munro HN. Quantitative studies of human placenta. 1. Morphometry. *Biol Neonate* 1973;23:231–259.
159. Mayhew TM, Jackson MR, Haas JD. Microscopical morphology of the human placenta and its effects on oxygen diffusion: a morphometric model. *Placenta* 1986;7:121–131.
160. Reshetnikova OS, Burton GJ, Milovanov AP. The effects of hypobaric hypoxia on the terminal villi of the human placenta. *J Physiol* 1993;459:308P.
161. Burton GJ, Palmer ME, Dalton KJ. Morphometric differences between the placental vasculature of non-smokers, smokers and ex-smokers. *Br J Obstet Gynaecol* 1989;96:907–915.
162. Sterio DC. The unbiased estimation of number and sizes of arbitrary particles using the disector. *J Microsc* 1984;134:127–136.
163. Wiese K-H. Licht- und elektronenmikroskopische Untersuchungen an der Chorionplatte der reifen menschlichen Placenta. *Arch Gynäkol* 1975;218:243–259.
164. Weser H, Kaufmann P. Lichtmikroskopische und histochemische Untersuchungen an der Chorionplatte der reifen menschlichen Placenta. *Arch Gynäkol* 1978;225:15–30.
165. Bourne GL. *The Human Amnion and Chorion.* London: Lloyd-Luke Ltd, 1962.
166. Mühlhauser J, Crescimanno C, Rajaniemi H, Castellucci M, Kaufmann P. Localization of carbonic anhydrase isoenzymes in amnion and human placenta by immunofluorescence techniques. *Anat Anz* 1992;174(suppl):128.
167. Hein K. Licht- und elektronenmikroskopische Untersuchungen an der Basalplatte der reifen menschlichen Plazenta. *Z Zellforsch* 1971;122:323–349.
168. Kaufmann P, Stark J. Die Basalplatte der reifen menschlichen Placenta. I. Semidünnschnitt-Histologie. *Z Anat Entwickl-Gesch* 1971;135:1–1971.
169. Stark J, Kaufmann P. Die Basalplatte der reifen menschlichen Placenta. II. Gefrierschnitthistochemie. *Z Anat Entwickl-Gesch* 1971;135:185–201.
170. Robertson WB, Warner B. The ultrastructure of the human placental bed. *J Pathol* 1974;112:203–211.
171. Brosens I, Robertson WB, Dixon HG. The physiological response of the vessels of the placental bed to normal pregnancy. *J Pathol Bacteriol* 1967;93:569–579.
172. De Wolf F, de Wolf-Peeters C, Brosens I. Ultrastructure of the spiral arteries in the human placental bed at the end of normal pregnancy. *Am J Obstet Gynecol* 1973;117:833–848.
173. Sheppard BL, Bonnar J. The maternal blood supply to the placenta in pregnancy complicated by intrauterine fetal growth retardation. *Trophoblast Res* 1988;3:69–82.
174. Brosens I. The utero-placental vessels at term—the distribution and extent of physiological changes. *Trophoblast Res* 1988;3: 61–68.
175. Becker V, Jipp P. Über die Trophoblastschale der menschlichen Plazenta. *Geburtshilfe Frauenheilkd* 1963;23:466–474.
176. Okudaira Y, Yoshiaki M, Kanoh H. Morphological variability of human trophoblasts in normal and neoplastic conditions. In: Soma H, ed. *Placenta: Basic Research for Clinical Application.* Basel: Karger, 1991;176–187.
177. Castellucci M, Classen-Linke I, Mühlhauser J, Kaufmann P, Zardi L, Chiquet-Ehrismann R. The human placenta: a model for tenascin expression. *Histochemistry* 1991;95:449–458.
178. Castellucci M, Crescimanno C, Arezio P, Mühlhauser J, Cinti S,

Kaufmann P. Extracellular matrix molecules in the morphogenesis of the human placenta. *Placenta* 1991;12:376.
179. Faller TH, Ferenci P. Der Aufbau der Placenta-Septen. Untersuchungen mit Hilfe der Quinacrinfluorescenzfärbung des Y-Chromatins. *Z Anat Entwickl-Gesch* 142:207–2177.
180. Rosenberg SM, Maslar IA, Riddick DH. Decidual production of prolactin in late gestation: further evidence for a decidual source of amniotic fluid prolactin. *Am J Obstet Gynecol* 1980;138: 681–685.
181. Beham A, Denk H, Desoye G. The distribution of intermediate filament proteins, actin and desmoplakins in human placental tissue as revealed by polyclonal and monoclonal antibodies. *Placenta* 1988;9:479–492.
182. Gosseye S, Fox H. An immunohistological comparison of the secretory capacity of villous and extravillous trophoblast in the human placenta. *Placenta* 1984;5:329–348.
183. Kurman RJ, Main CS, Chen H-C. Intermediate trophoblast: a distinctive form of trophoblast with specific morphological, biochemical and functional features. *Placenta* 1984;5:349–370.
184. Kurman RJ, Young RH, Norris HJ, Main CS, Lawrence WD, Sculley RE. Immunocytochemical localization of placental lactogen and chorionic gonadotropin in the normal placenta and trophoblastic tumors, with emphasis on intermediate trophoblast and the placental site trophoblastic tumor. *Int J Gynecol Pathol* 1984;3:101–121.
185. Beck T, Schweikhart G, Stolz E. Immunohistochemical location of HPL, SP1 and β-HCG in normal placentas of varying gestational age. *Arch Gynecol* 1986;239:63–74.
186. Langhans Y. Untersuchungen über die menschliche Plazenta. *Arch Anat Physiol Anat Abt* 1877;188–267.
187. Hitschmann J, Lindenthal OT. Der weisse Infarkt der Placenta. *Arch Gynäkol* 1903;69:587–628.
188. Moe N. Deposits of fibrin and plasma proteins in the normal human placenta. *Acta Pathol Microbiol Scand* 1969;76:74–88.
189. Gille J, Börner P, Reinecke J, Krause P-H, Deicher H. Über die Fibrinoidablagerungen in den Endzotten der menschlichen Placenta. *Arch Gynäkol* 1974;217:263–271.
190. Faulk P, Trenchev P, Dorling J, Holborow J. Antigens on postimplantation placentae. In: Edwards RG, Howe CWS, Johnson MH, eds. *Immunobiology of Trophoblast.* Cambridge: University Press, 1975.
191. Sutcliffe RG, Davies M, Hunter JB, Waters JJ, Parry JE. The protein composition of the fibrinoid material at the human uteroplacental interface. *Placenta* 1982;3:297–308.
192. Kisalus LL, Herr JC. Immunocytochemical localization of heparan sulfate proteoglycan in human decidual cell secretory bodies and placental fibrinoid. *Biol Reprod* 1988;39:419–430.
193. Bradbury S, Billington WD, Kirby DRS. A histochemical and electron microscopical study of the mouse placenta. *J R Microsc Soc* 1965;84:199–211.
194. Bagshawe K, Lawler S. The immunogenicity of the placenta and trophoblast. In: Edwards RG, Howe CWS, Johnson MH, eds. *Immunobiology of Trophoblast.* London: Cambridge University Press, 1975;171–182.
195. Brzosko W, Nowoslawski A, Pisarki T. Analiza immunohistochemiczna mas wloknikowatych w lozysku ludzkim. *Ginekol Pol* 1965;36:121–130.
196. Brzosko W, Nowoslawski A, Pisarski I. Immunohistochemical analysis of the fibrinoid masses in human placenta. *Pol Med J* 1965;5:114–123.
197. Hörmann G. Die Fibrinoidisierung des Chorionepithels als Konstruktionsprinzip der menschlichen Plazenta. *Z Geburtshilfe Gynäkol* 1965;164:263–269.
198. Pijnenborg R, Robertson WB, Brosens I, Dixon G. Trophoblast invasion and the establishment of haemochorial placentation in man and laboratory animals. *Placenta* 1981;2:71–92.
199. Badarau L, Gavrilita L. Intervillous fibrin deposition, the Rohr, Nitabuch and Langhans striae. *Am J Obstet Gynecol* 1967;98: 252–260.
200. Wynn RM. Fetomaternal cellular relations in the human basal plate: an ultrastructural study of the placenta. *Am J Obstet Gynecol* 1967;97:832–850.
201. Wynn RM. Cytotrophoblastic specializations: an ultrastructural study of the human placenta. *Am J Obstet Gynecol* 1972;114:339–353.
202. Bardawil WA, Toy BL. The natural history of choriocarcinoma: problems of immunity and spontaneous regression. *Ann NY Acad Sci* 1959;80:197–261.
203. Kirby DRS, Billington WD, Bradbury S, Goldstein DJ. Antigen barrier of mouse placenta. *Nature* 1964;204:548–549.
204. Currie CA, Bagshawe KD. The masking of antigens on trophoblast and cancer cells. *Lancet* 1967;i:708–710.
205. McCormick JN, Faulk WP, Fox H, Fuddenberg HH. Immunohistological and elution studies of the human placenta. *J Exp Med* 1971;91:1–13.
206. Azab I, Okamura H, Beer A. Decidual cell production of human placental fibrinoid. *Obstet Gynecol* 1972;40:186–193.
207. Wynn RM. Fine structure of the placenta. In: Gruenwald P, ed. *The Placenta and Its Maternal Supply Line.* Lancaster: Medical Technology Publications, 1975.
208. Swinburne LM. Leucocyte antigens and placental sponge. *Lancet* 1970;ii:592–593.
209. Chaouat G, Kolb JP, Wegmann TG. The murine placenta as an immunological barrier between the mother and the fetus. *Immunol Rev* 1983;75:31–60.
210. Hunziker RD, Wegmann TG. Placental Immunoregulation. *Crit Rev Immunol* 1987;613:245–285.
211. Raghupathy R, Singh B, Wegmann TG. Fate of antipaternal H-2 antibodies bound to the placenta *in vivo. Transplantation* 1984;37:296.
212. Kaufmann P, Castellucci M. Development and anatomy of the placenta. In Fox H, ed. *Haines and Taylor's Textbook of Obstetrical and Gynaecological Pathology.* London: Churchill Livingstone (*in press*).
213. Kliman HJ, Nestler JE, Sermasi E, Sanger JM, Strauss JF III. Purification, characterization and *in vitro* differentiation of cytotrophoblasts from human term placenta. *Endocrinology* 1986; 118:1567–1582.
214. Douglas GC, King BF. Isolation of pure villous cytotrophoblast from term human placenta using immunomagnetic microspheres. *J Immunol Methods* 1989;119:259–268.
215. Bischof P, Friedli E, Martelli M, Campana A. Expression of extracellular matrix degrading metalloproteinases by cultured human cytotrophoblast cells. Effects of cell adhesion and immunopurification. *Am J Obstet Gynecol* 1991;165:1791–1801.
216. Flynn A, Finke JH, Hilfiker ML. Placental mononuclear phagocytes as a source of interleukin-1. *Science* 1982;218:475–477.
217. Frauli M, Ludwig H. Immunocytochemical identification of mitotic Hofbauer cells in cultures of first trimester human placental villi. *Arch Gynecol Obstet* 1987;241:47–51.
218. Uren S, Boyle W. Isolation of macrophages from human placenta. *J Immunol Methods* 1985;78:25–34.
219. Zaccheo D, Pistoia V, Castellucci M, Martinoli C. Isolation and characterization of Hofbauer cells from human placental villi. *Arch Gynecol Obstet* 1989;246:189–200.
220. Drake BL, Loke YW. Isolation of endothelial cells from human first trimester decidua using immunomagnetic beads. *Hum Reprod* 1991;6:1156–1159.
221. Fant ME. *In vitro* growth rate of placental fibroblasts is developmentally regulated. *J Clin Invest* 1991;88:1697–1702.
222. Adamson ED. Review article: expression of proto-oncogenes in the placenta. *Placenta* 1987;8:449–466.
223. Blay J, Hollenberg MD. The nature and function of polypeptide growth factor receptors in the human placenta. *J Dev Physiol* 1989;12:237–248.
224. Ohlsson R. Growth factors, protooncogenes and human placental development. *Cell Differ Dev* 1989;28:1–16.
225. Scott SM, Buenaflor GG, Orth DN. Immunoreactive human epidermal growth factor concentrations in amniotic fluid, umbilical artery and vein serum, and placenta in full-term and preterm infants. *Biol Neonate* 1989;56:246–251.
226. Morrish DW, Bhardwaj D, Dabbagh LK, Marusyk H, Siy O. Epidermal growth factor induces differentiation and secretion of human chorionic gonadotropin and placental lactogen in normal human placenta. *J Clin Endocrinol Metab* 1987;65:1282–1290.
227. Bulmer JN, Thrower S, Wells M. Expression of epidermal growth

factor receptor and transferrin receptor by human trophoblast populations. *Am J Reprod Immunol* 1989;21:87–93.
228. Ladines-Llave CA, Maruo T, Manalo AS, Mochizuki M. Cytologic localization of epidermal growth factor and its receptor in developing human placenta varies over the course of pregnancy. *Am J Obstet Gynecol* 1991;165:1377–1382.
229. Lupu R, Colomer R, Kannan B, Lippman ME. Characterization of a growth factor that binds exclusively to the erbB-2 receptor and induces cellular responses. *Proc Natl Acad Sci USA* 1992;89:2287–2291.
230. Peles E, Bacus SS, Koski RA, et al. Isolation of the neu/HER-2 stimulatory ligand: a 44 kd glycoprotein that induces differentiation of mammary tumor cells. *Cell* 1992;69:205–216.
231. Ohlsson R, Holmgren L, Glaser A, Szpecht A, Pfeifer-Ohlsson S. Insulin-like growth factor 2 and short-range stimulatory loops in control of human placental growth. *EMBO J* 1989;8:1993–1999.
232. Desoye G, Hartmann M, Blaschitz A, Dohr G, Kohnen G, Kaufmann P. Insulin receptors in syncytiotrophoblast and fetal endothelium of human placenta. Immunohistochemical evidence for developmental changes in distribution patter. *J Clin Endocrinol Metab* (*submitted*).
233. Goustin AS, Betsholtz C, Pfeifer-Ohlsson S, et al. Coexpression of the *sis* and *myc* proto-oncogenes in developing human placenta suggests autocrine control of trophoblast growth. *Cell* 1985;41: 301–312.
234. Ishikawa F, Miyazono K, Hellman U, et al. Identification of angiogenic activity and the cloning and expression of platelet-derived endothelial cell growth factor. *Nature* 1989;338: 557–562.
235. Frolik CA, Dart LL, Meyers CA, Smith DM, Sporn MB. Purification and initial characterization of a type β transforming growth factor from human placenta. *Proc Natl Acad Sci USA* 1983;80:3676–3680.
236. Dungy LR, Siddiqi TA, Khan S. Transforming growth factor-β_1 expression during placental development. *Am J Obstet Gynecol* 1991;165:853–857.
237. Morrish DW, Bhardwaj D, Paras MT. Transforming growth factor β1 inhibits placental differentiation and human chorionic gonadotropin and placental lactogen secretion. *Endocrinology* 1991;129:22–26.
238. Emonard H, Christiane Y, Smet M, Grimaud JA, Foidart JM. Type IV and interstitial collagenolytic activities in normal and malignant trophoblast cells are specifically regulated by the extracellular matrix. *Invasion Metastasis* 1990;10:170–177.
239. Moll UM, Lane BL. Proteolytic activity of first trimester human placenta: localization of interstitial collagenase in villous and extravillous trophoblast. *Histochemistry* 1990;94:555–560.
240. Librach CL, Werb Z, Fitzgerald ML, et al. 92-kd type IV collagenase mediates invasion of human cytotrophoblasts. *J Cell Biol* 1991;113:437–449.
241. Lala PK, Graham CH. Mechanisms of trophoblast invasiveness and their control: the role of proteases and protease inhibitors. *Cancer Metastasis Rev* 1990;9:369–379.
242. Kjaeldgaard A, Pschera H, Larsson B, Gaffney P, Åstedt B. Plasminogen activators and inhibitors in amniotic fluid. *Fibrinolysis* 1989;3:203–206.
243. Åstedt B, Hägerstrand I, Lecander I. Cellular localisation in placenta of placental type plasminogen activator inhibitor. *Thromb Haemost* 1986;56:63–65.
244. Feinberg RF, Kao L-C, Haimowitz JE, et al. Plasminogen activator inhibitor types 1 and 2 in human trophoblasts. PAI-1 is an immunocytochemical marker of invading trophoblasts. *Lab Invest* 1989;61:20–26.
245. Radtke K-P, Wenz K-H, Heimburger N. Isolation of plasminogen activator inhibitor-2 (PAI-2) from human placenta. Evidence for vitronectin/PAI-2 complexes in human placenta extract. *Biol Chem Hoppe Seyler* 1990;371:1119–1127.
246. Bischof P, Martelli M. Proteolysis in the penetration phase of the implantation process. *Placenta* 1992;13:17–24.
247. Damsky CH, Fitzgerald ML, Fisher J. Distribution patterns of extracellular matrix components and adhesion receptors are intricately modulated during first trimester cytotrophoblast differentiation along the invasive pathway, *in vivo*. *J Clin Invest* 1992;89:210–222.
248. Virtanen I, Laitinen L, Vartio T. Differential expression of the extra domain-containing form of cellular fibronectin in human placentas at different stages of maturation. *Histochemistry* 1988;90:25–30.
249. Earl U, Estlin C, Bulmer JN. Fibronectin and laminin in the early human placenta. *Placenta* 1990;11:223–231.
250. Feinberg RF, Kliman HJ, Lockwood CJ. Is oncofetal fibronectin a trophoblast glue for human implantation? *Am J Pathol* 1991;138:537–543.
251. Akiyama SK, Nagata K, Yamada KM. Cell surface receptors for extracellular matrix components. *Biochim Biophys Acta* 1990;1031:91–110.
252. Nanaev AK, Rukosuev VS, Shirinsky VP, et al. Confocal and conventional immunofluorescent and immunogold electron microscopic localization of collagen types III and IV in human placenta. *Placenta* 1991;12:573–595.
253. Rukosuev VS. Immunofluorescent localization of collagen types I, III, IV, V, fibronectin, laminin, entactin, and heparan sulphate proteoglycan in human immature placenta. *Experientia* 1992;48:285–287.
254. Amenta PS, Gay S, Vaheri A, Martinez-Hernandez A. The extracellular matrix is an integrated unit: ultrastructural localization of collagen types I, III, IV, V, VI, fibronectin, and laminin in human term placenta. *Collagen Rel Res* 1986;6:125–152.
255. Bianco P, Fisher LW, Young MF, Termine JD, Robey PG. Expression and localization of the two small proteoglycans biglycan and decorin in developing human skeletal and non-skeletal tissues. *J Histochem Cytochem* 1990;38:1549–1563.
256. Yamaguchi Y, Mann DM, Ruoslahti E. Negative regulation of transforming growth factor-β by the proteoglycan decorin. *Nature* 1990;346:281–284.
257. Kao L-C, Caltabiano S, Wu S, Strauss JF III, Kliman HJ. The human villous cytotrophoblast: interaction with extracellular matrix proteins, endocrine function, and cytoplasmic differentiation in the absence of syncytium formation. *Dev Biol* 1988;130:693–702.
258. Castellucci M, Kaufmann P, Bischof P. Extracellular matrix influences hormone and protein production by human chorionic villi. *Cell Tissue Res* 1990;262:135–142.
259. Kliman HJ, Feinberg RF. Human trophoblast-extracellular matrix (ECM) interactions *in vitro*: ECM thickness modulates morphology and proteolytic activity. *Proc Natl Acad Sci* 1990;87: 3057–3061.
260. Schaaps J-P. Ultrasound features of the early gestational sac. In: Barnea ER, Hustin J, Jauniaux E, eds. *The First Twelve Weeks of Gestation*. Berlin: Springer Verlag, 1992;65–77.
261. Petrucha RA, Golde SH, Platt LD. Real-time ultrasound of the placenta in assessment of fetal pulmonic maturity. *Am J Obstet Gynecol* 1982;142:463–467.
262. Petrucha RA, Golde SH, Platt LD. The use of ultrasound in the prediction of fetal pulmonary maturity. *Am J Obstet Gynecol* 1982;144:931–934.
263. Tabsh KMA. Correlation of real-time ultrasonic placental grading with amniotic fluid lecithin/sphingomyelin ratio. *Am J Obstet Gynecol* 1983;145:504–508.
264. Harman CR, Manning FA, Stearns E, Morrison I. The correlation of ultrasonic placental grading and the fetal pulmonary maturation in five hundred sixty-three pregnancies. *Am J Obstet Gynecol* 1982;143:941–943.
265. Gast MJ, Ott W. Failure of ultrasonic placental grading to predict severe respiratory distress in a neonate. *Am J Obstet Gynecol* 1983;146:464–465.
266. Griffin D, Cohen-Overbeek T, Campbell S. Fetal and utero-placental blood flow. *Clin Obstet Gynecol* 1983;10:565–602.
267. Jurkovic D, Jauniaux E, Campbell S. Doppler ultrasound investigations of pelvic circulation during the menstrual cycle and early pregnancy. In: Barnea ER, Hustin J, Jauniaux E, eds. *The First Twelve Weeks of Gestation*. Berlin: Springer Verlag, 1992;78–96.
268. Fisk MN, MacLachlan N, Ellis C, Tannirandorn Y, Tonge HM, Rodeck CH. Absent end-diastolic flow in first trimester umbilical artery. *Lancet* 1988;2:1256–1257.

269. Wladimiroff JW, Huisman TWA, Stewart PA. Fetal and umbilical flow velocity waveforms between 10-16 weeks' gestation: a preliminary study. *Obstet Gynecol* 1991;78:812–814.
270. Jauniaux E, Burton GJ. The effect of smoking in pregnancy on early placental morphology. *Obstet Gynecol* 1992;79:645–648.
271. Stabile I, Bilardo C, Panella M, Campbell S, Grudzinskas JG. Doppler measurement of uterine blood flow in the first trimester of normal and complicated pregnancies. *Trophoblast Res* 1988;3:301–307.
272. Den Ouden M, Cohen-Overbeek TE, Wladimiroff JW. Uterine and fetal umbilical artery flow velocity waveforms in normal first trimester pregnancies. *Br J Obstet Gynaecol* 1990;97:716–719.
273. Maulik D, Yarlagadda P, Willoughby L. Doppler assessment of fetoplacental circulation. *Trophoblast Res* 1988;3:293–300.
274. Giles WB, Trudinger BJ, Baird PJ. Fetal umbilical artery flow velocity waveforms and placental resistance: pathological correlation. *Br J Obstet Gynaecol* 1985;92:31–38.
275. McCowan LM, Mullen BM, Ritchie K. Umbilical artery flow velocity waveforms and the placental vascular bed. *Am J Obstet Gynecol* 1987;157:900–902.
276. Nessmann C, Huten Y, Uzan M. Placental correlates of abnormal umbilical Doppler index. *Trophoblast Res* 1988;3:309–323.
277. Jimenez E, Vogel M, Arabin B, Wagner G, Mirsalim P. Correlation of ultrasonographic measurement of the utero-placental and fetal blood flow with the morphological diagnosis of placental function. *Trophoblast Res* 1988;3:325–334.
278. Rochelson B, Kaplan C, Guzman E, Arato M, Hansen K, Trunca C. A quantitative analysis of placental vasculature in the third-trimester fetus with autosomal trisomy. *Obstet Gynecol* 1990;75:59–63.
279. Guiot C, Piantà PG, Todros T. Modelling the feto-placental circulation: I. A distributed network predicting umbilical haemodynamics throughout pregnancy. *Ultrasound Med Biol* 1992;18:535–544.
280. Todros T, Guiot C, Piantà PG. Modelling the feto-placental circulation: 2. A continuous approach to explain normal and abnormal flow velocity waveforms in the umbilical arteries. *Ultrasound Med Biol* 1992;18:545–551.
281. Brambati B. Prenatal diagnosis and invasive techniques in the first trimester of pregnancy. In: Barnea ER, Hustin J, Jauniaux E, eds. *The First Twelve Weeks of Gestation.* Berlin: Springer Verlag, 1992;393–416.
282. Wachtel S, Elias S, Price J, et al. Fetal cells in the maternal circulation: isolation by multiparameter flow cytometry and confirmation by polymerase chain reaction. *Hum Reprod* 1991;6:1466–1469.
283. Burton GJ. Human and animal model: limitations and comparisons. In: Barnea ER, Hustin J, Jeauniaux E, eds. *The First Twelve Weeks of Gestation: A New Frontier for Investigation and Intervention.* Berlin: Springer, 1992;469–485.
284. Kaufmann P, Scheffen I. Placental development. In: Polin R, Fox W, eds. *Fetal and Neonatal Physiology, Vol 1.* Philadelphia: WB Saunders, 1992;47–56.
285. Kaufmann P, Luckhardt M, Schweikhart G, Cantle SJ. Cross-sectional features and three-dimensional structure of human placental villi. *Placenta* 1987;8:235–247.
286. Schiebler TH, Kaufmann P. Reife Plazenta. In: Becker V, Schiebler TH, Kubli F, eds. *Die Plazenta des Menschen.* Stuttgart: Thieme, 1981;51–111.
287. Burton GJ. The fine structure of the human placental villus as revealed by scanning electron microscopy. *Scanning Microsc* 1987;1:1811–1828.

The Reproductive Systems

The Female

The Physiology of Reproduction, Second Edition,
edited by E. Knobil and J.D. Neill,
Raven Press, Ltd., New York © 1994.

CHAPTER 9

Embryology of Mammalian Gonads and Ducts

Anne Grete Byskov[1] and Poul Erik Høyer[2]

Gonadal formation in mammals takes place early in fetal life. Although the genetic sex is determined at conception, the morphologic sexual differences between fetuses can first be recognized at the time when their gonads become sex-differentiated. The gonads evolve when germ cells and different somatic cells migrate and settle in the gonadal ridges to interact in a finely regulated manner. The following modeling of the embryonic gonads into an ovary or a testis depends on differentiation of the somatic cell lines supporting the germ cells. This differentiation is crucial for priming the fetus in the female or male direction. Inadequate sexual differentiation of the gonad may alter production of sex hormones and other substances necessary for growth and differentiation of the sex ducts, external genitalia, and other secondary sex characteristics, as well as sex priming of the brain.

EARLY GONADAL FORMATION

The gonads develop along the ventral cranial part of the mesonephros. Several simultaneously occurring events characterize the initial gonadal formation: migration of primordial germ cells (PGCs) into the coelomic epithelium and the underlying mesenchymal tissue covering the mesonephros; release and migration of mesonephric cells and other cell types into the same area; and establishment of the germ cells supporting cell lineages.

Primordial Germ Cells

The migratory pathway and, in particular, the precise origin of the PGC are difficult to establish because they are not easy to distinguish from surrounding cells. For decades, it was believed that the PGC originated in the

[1] Laboratory of Reproductive Biology, University Hospital of Copenhagen, Rigshospitalet Section 5821, DK-2100 Copenhagen, Denmark
[2] Institute of Medical Anatomy, The Panum Institute, University of Copenhagen, DK-2200 Copenhagen, Denmark

so-called germinal epithelium (i.e., the coelomic epithelium lining the gonad). However, as early as 1880, Nussbaum (1) proposed an extragonadal origin of the PGC in frog and trout. Subsequently, PGCs have also been identified in extragonadal sites in many mammalian species (rat [2,3], mouse [4–6], human [7,8], rabbit [9]). The PGCs were originally identified in the endoderm-derived yolk sac by the alkaline phosphatase technique (7). Different studies, however, suggest that the stem cells of the PGC are not of endodermal but of ectodermal origin (10–13). Grafting studies indicate that PGCs reside in the epiblast of the inner cell mass of the blastocyst (14,15) and that they are restricted to the derivatives of the epiblast in the posterior primitive streak (16). Studies of X chromosome inactivation during mouse embryogenesis suggest that somatic cell lines are allocated before the germ cell line (17). However, labeling of four- to 16-cell mouse embryos with retroviruses and analyzing the distribution of proviruses in the different tissues developing from such embryos suggests that a germ cell line is set aside very early, maybe in the four- to eight-cell stage, and before allocation of somatic tissues (18).

In summary, the migratory route taken by the PGC from the extra embryonic site is to the embryonic mesoderm of the primitive streak, then further to the visceral endoderm of the yolk sac, and to the developing hindgut from where the PGC migrates up through the dorsal mesentery and finally reaches the gonads.

The mechanisms by which the PGCs are translocated from extragonadal sites to the gonadal ridges are poorly understood. The mobility of PGCs suggests that these cells may migrate actively (for review, see ref. 19). The guidance of oriented migration toward the gonads is also uncertain. It appears that fibronectin is present along the migratory pathway (20), stimulating the migration of PGCs (21). The locomotion of PGCs *in vitro* is also enhanced by fibronectin in the substrate (22). Migrating rat PGCs possess a unique surface glycoconjugate with ter-

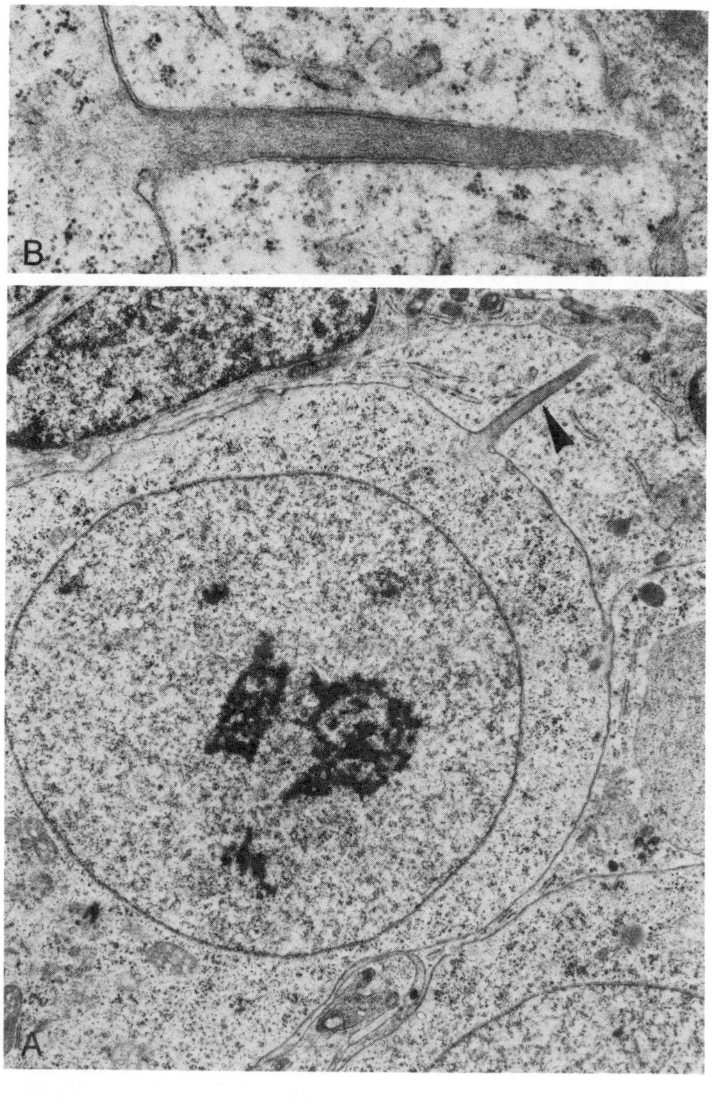

FIG. 1. Oogonium of 9-week-old fetal human ovary. Plasmalemma forms a fingerlike projection (*arrowhead*) with bundles of microfilaments. (**A**) ×5,800; (**B**) ×30,000.

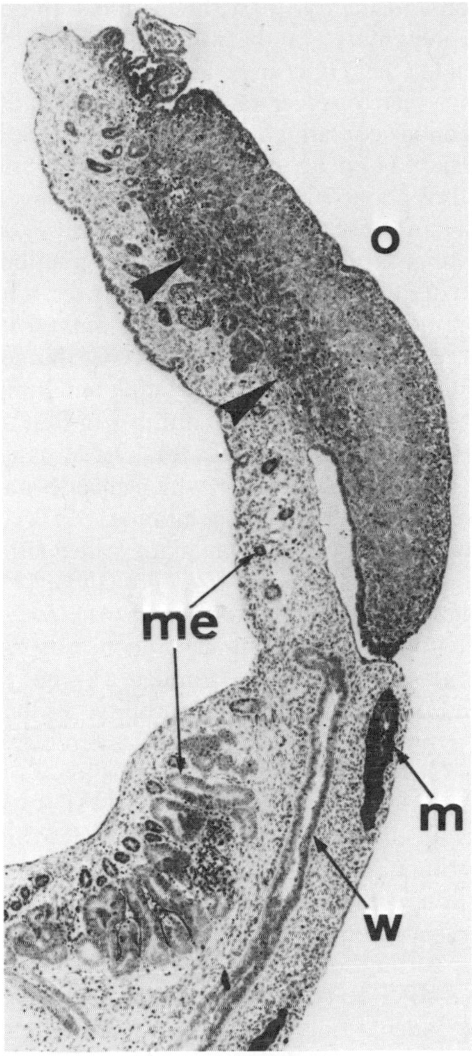

FIG. 2. Ovary–mesonephric complex of 11-week-old human fetus. The ovary (*o*) is attached to cranial part of mesonephros (*arrowheads*). Caudally, mesonephric tubules (*me*), wolffian duct (*w*), and müllerian duct (*m*) are seen. ×200.

minal α-*N*-acetylgalactosamine, which is lost by arrival to the gonads (23). In the mouse PGC, a slightly different glycoconjugate was detected, indicating differences between genera in the distinctive glycoconjugate coats of migrating PGCs (24). Such specific glycoconjugate coats of the PGC may be important for cell recognition and guidance of migration.

A more passive translocation of PGCs may occur during the morphogenic rearrangements of the developing tissues (e.g., during invagination of the hindgut) (15,25,26). Finally, it is possible that the PGCs are attracted by chemotactic substances produced by the gonad (7) as visualized by the time-lapse films of chick PGCs in culture (27). This attractant does not seem to be class-specific because mouse germ cells settle in chick gonads when mouse hindgut-containing germ cells are transplanted into the coelomic cavity of chick embryos (28). In culture, mouse gonadal ridges exerted a long-range attracting effect on PGCs (29). This seemed to be mediated by transforming growth factor (TGF-β_1), which also inhibits proliferation of PGCs (30).

As mentioned above, tracing and counting of PGCs are facilitated by the cytochemical demonstration of their relatively high activity of alkaline phosphatase (31). Ultrastructural studies have shown that the reaction products are mainly localized to the plasma membrane. It is believed that this enzyme is involved in the transfer of metabolites across the cell surface (4). The alkaline phosphatase-stained PGCs have been counted from the time they are seen in the primitive streak until they reach

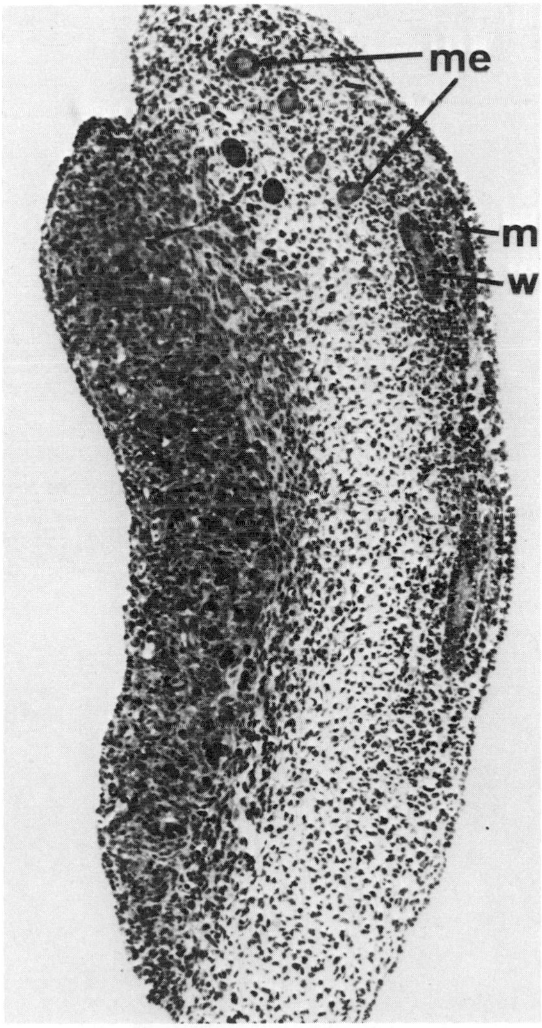

FIG. 3. Ovary–mesonephric complex of $12\frac{1}{2}$-day-old mouse fetus. The ovary appears as a rather dense homogeneous cell mass. *m,* müllerian duct; *me* mesonephric tubules; *w,* wolffian duct. ×400.

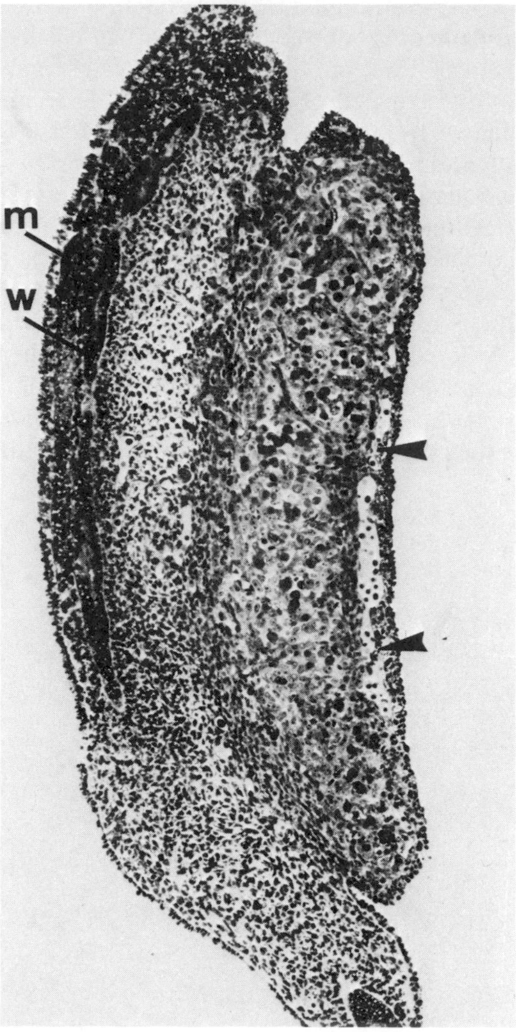

FIG. 4. Testis–mesonephric complex of $12\frac{1}{2}$-day-old mouse fetus. Beneath surface epithelium, tunica albuginea (*arrowheads*) is developing. Testicular cords have begun to form in cranial part of testis. *m,* müllerian duct; *w,* wolffian duct. ×425.

the gonad and then go past the allantois, the hindgut, and the mesentery. In the 8-day-old mouse embryo, about ten to 100 PGCs can be identified (5,6,32). During migration, their number rapidly increases, and by day 13, the gonads contain about 10,000 germ cells (33). In the 5-week-old human embryo, the number of migrating germ cells is about 700 to 1,300 (7), and by week 8, the germ cell number of the developing gonad is 600,000 (34).

Surprisingly little is known about the regulation of proliferation of PGCs. For many years, however, it has been clear that mutations in the mouse *dominant white spotting* (W) gene reduce the number of PGCs that reach the gonad (35). Later, it was discovered that mutations in the *Steel* (Sl) gene also reduce the number of PGCs during migration (for review, see ref. 36). The W is identical with the proto-oncogene c-*kit,* which encodes a tyrosine kinase receptor of the cell membrane (37,38). The Sl gene encodes a peptide growth factor, called either *stem cell factor* (SCF) (39) or *mast cell growth factor* (MGF) (40), which is a c-kit receptor ligand (41). *In vitro,* the c-kit receptor–ligand system acts in concert with *leukemia inhibitory factor* (LIF) to stimulate a limited proliferation and/or survival and/or motility of the PGCs (42,43). However, addition of *basic fibroblast growth factor* (bFGF) to such cultures of PGCs allows continued proliferation for at least 20 passages (44,45). Because the W exerts its effect within the cell, whereas Sl probably induces somatic cells to produce growth factors, a synergistic action at the local site is probably important for PGC survival/proliferation and stresses the importance of the supporting somatic cells.

When the PGCs arrive at the coelomic epithelium covering the gonadal ridges, they seem to be "trapped" by processes from the epithelial cells (46). Soon thereafter, PGCs are present in the underlying tissue as well. Morphologically, it is not possible to distinguish between PGCs that have just arrived to the gonadal tissue and those that are still migrating within extragonadal tissues.

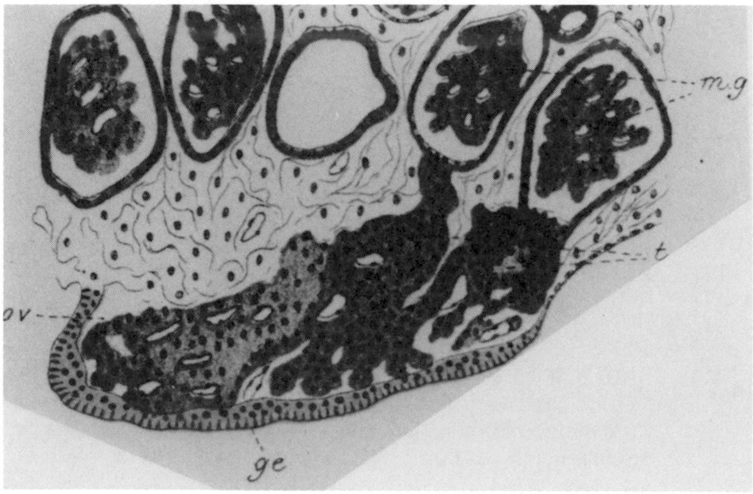

FIG. 5. Cell streams connect parietal layer of Bowman's capsule with somatic cells of developing gonad. This drawing, made by F. M. Balfour in 1878 (see ref. 69), is probably one of the first illustrations indicating that mesonephros contributes cells to the gonad. *ov,* ovary; *ge,* germinal epithelium; *t,* tubuliferous tissue, derived from Malpighian bodies; *mg,* Malpighian body.

The PGCs are transformed into oogonia or prespermatogonia from the time the gonadal sex is recognizable. The oogonia of early fetal human and pig ovaries occasionally exhibit unique straight fingerlike projections with closely packed parallel microfilaments (Fig. 1), the function of which is unknown.

X Chromosome Inactivation

The sex of migrating primordial germ cells may be recognized by their sex chromatin status. Generally, female cells contain a chromatin body, the Barr body, which represents the inactive X chromosome. Lyon (47) proposed that a dose compensation mechanism is achieved by X chromosome inactivation to avoid the aneuploidy effect by the presence of more than one X chromosome. In somatic cells, inactivation occurs during embryonic life (48–50). Gene mapping has confirmed that homology between the human and the monotreme X chromosome is conserved, whereas only a putative Y chromosome is present in these ancestral mammals (51) although still exerting male determination. In marsupials, the paternal X is preferentially inactivated although sometimes incomplete (52). In the female mouse, preferential inactivation of the paternal X chromosome is seen only in the extraembryonic membranes, whereas X chromosome activity in the embryonic tissues changes during embryonic development, resulting in switching on and off the paternal and maternal X chromosome activity (for review, see ref. 53). In female germ cells, one X chromosome is also inactivated during migration (54,55), but reactivation has been noticed by the time they reach the ovarian anlage (56–58). In oogonia of human and mouse, only one X chromosome is active (50,59), but reactivation occurs when germ cells enter leptonema of the first meiotic prophase (60,61). There is substantial evidence that deoxyribonucleic acid (DNA) methylation is correlated with the maintenance of inactivation of genes on the inactive X chromosome in adult female somatic tissues (62; for review, see ref. 63). In the female PGC, however, the inactive X chromosome escapes methylation, which may explain later activation at meiosis (64,65). The X chromosomes remain active during oocyte growth and maturation.

Mesonephros

The mesonephros is the second of the three consecutive nephric structures (pro-, meso-, and metanephros), which develop consecutively during fetal life of all mammals. All three kidneys arise in the nephrogenic cord, which forms from the segmented intermediate mesoderm early in embryonic life. The pronephros develops first from the most cranial segment, the mesonephros develops somewhat later from the intermediate segment, and finally the metanephros, the permanent kidney, arises from the most caudally placed one. The pronephros never functions in mammals, but the pronephric duct serves as an inducer for the formation of the mesonephros and the metanephros (66). The nephrons of mesonephros develop from the nephrogenic cord in a cranial caudal direction and successively form a connection with the pronephric duct, now called the *wolffian duct*.

In some species (e.g., pig, sheep, rabbit, and human), the mesonephros is a functioning kidney with well-developed glomeruli and tubuli (Fig. 2). However, in

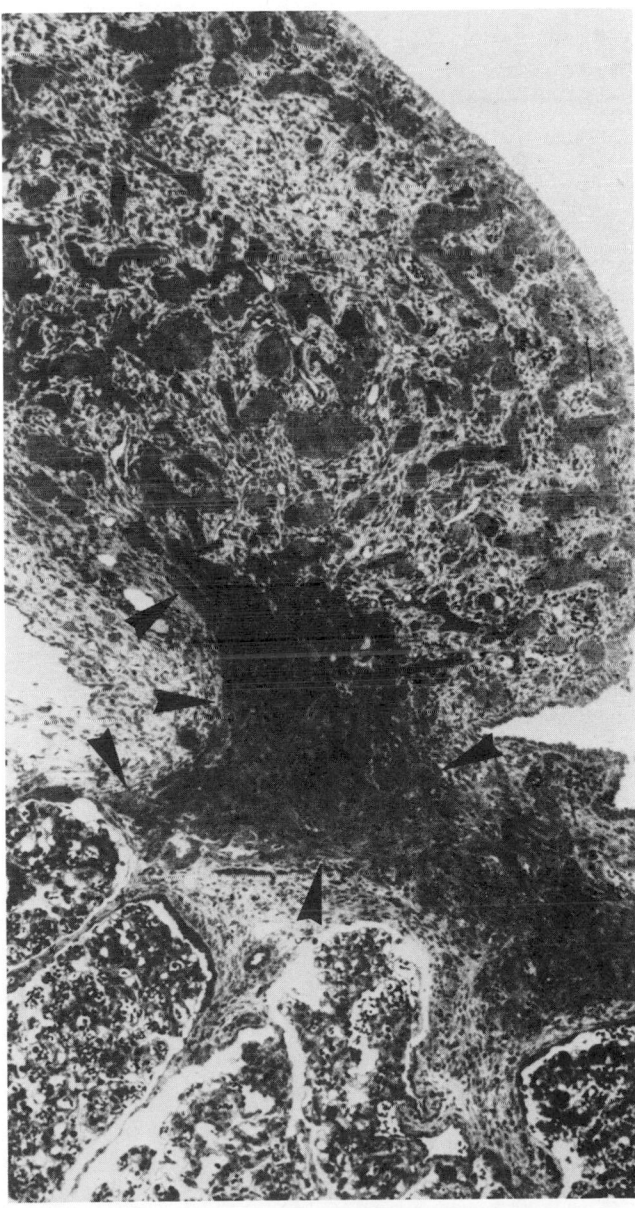

FIG. 6. Part of ovary and mesonephros of 42-day-old pig fetus. Dense cell masses (*arrowheads*) of mesonephric origin connect germ cell cords of ovary with parietal layers of Bowman's capsules. ×200.

other species (e.g., guinea pig and mouse), the mesonephric tissue consists only of tubuli, which in some cases may develop Bowman's capsules but without functional glomeruli (67) (Figs. 3 and 4).

Although Waldeyer (68) and Balfour (69) proposed more than a century ago that the central cell mass of the gonad originated in the mesonephros (Fig. 5), this idea was virtually neglected until Witschi came to the same conclusion while studying amphibian (70) and mammalian gonads (71). Subsequently, many studies have lent support to this idea. In the mouse, for example, the mesonephric connection is obvious from the time the gonads are formed (72–75). In the bovine fetus, a broad stream of cells exhibiting strong alkaline phosphatase activity was observed to connect the glomerular tuft and the developing gonad (76). Similar cell streams that connect the gonads with the mesonephric tissue have been described in other species, supporting the idea that the mesonephros and the gonads are closely interacting (human [77]; sheep [78,79]; rabbit [80,81]) (see Figs. 2, 6, and 7). The cell streams that connect the mesonephric tissue proper and the gonads are called the rete ovarii and the rete testis in female and male, respectively. In the fetal mouse, the mesonephric tubules and the rete of both sexes exhibit strong immunoreactivity for the nerve cell adhesion molecule (NCAM) (82).

Different experiments have shown that the mesonephros influences gonadal development and function and germ cell differentiation. When fetal undifferentiated mouse ovaries are stripped from mesonephric tissues, in this case the rete ovarii, ovarian differentiation and meiosis are prevented or inhibited when transplanted subcutaneously into mice (83). In mouse ovaries cultured with or without mesonephros, meiosis resumes as normal (84,85). The meiosis-inducing influence by mesonephric tissue is also seen *in vivo* in the fetal mouse testis: Germ cells left outside the testicular cords may enter meiosis if situated close to the mesonephric-derived epi-

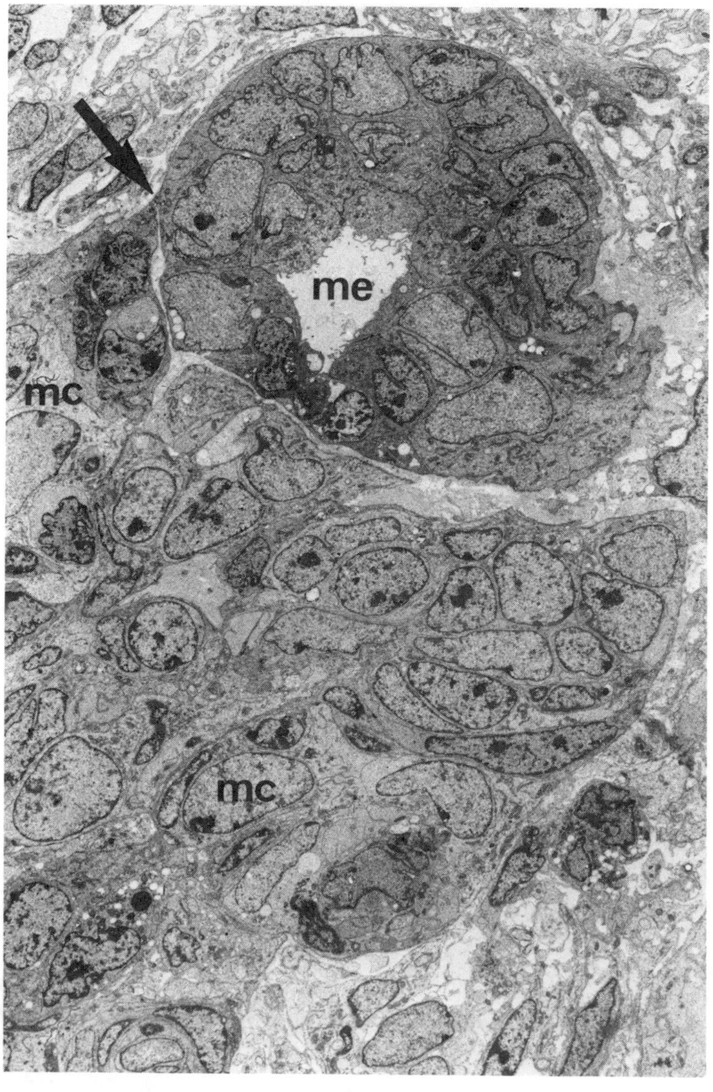

FIG. 7. Cranially placed mesonephric tubule (*me*) and mesonephric-derived cell mass (*mc*) of a 9-week-old female human fetus. An opening of the tubule is shown by an *arrow*. ×1,820.

didymis (86). Also, the steroid synthesis by cultured fetal rabbit gonads is influenced by the mesonephros (87,88) (see *Differentiation of the Testis* section).

The mesonephros seems to be crucial not only for gonadal development but also for the formation of the fetal adrenal cortex (71,89). Moreover, recent experiments indicate that the mesonephros may provide some signal for limb outgrowth in the chick embryo (90).

Coelomic Epithelium and Other Cell Types

The early, nondifferentiated gonad consists of a loose mesenchymal tissue covered by the coelomic epithelium and supported by the developing mesonephric tissue.

Mesenchymal cells can be recognized throughout gonadal development of both sexes. At very early stages, the developing gonad is invaded by capillaries (91). A limited amount of information is available on early innervation of the gonads. However, it is likely that an ingrowth of nerves follows the invasion of blood vessels.

The epithelium that covers the gonads has previously been termed the *germinal epithelium*. This term is very unfortunate because the germ cells do not derive from the epithelium but only pass through it (see *Primordial Germ Cells* section). Before gonadal sex differentiation takes place, no complete separation between the epithelium proper and the underlying tissue exists, because the basal lamina is not yet intact. The epithelial layer consists of pleomorphic proliferating cells, which at places have a cylindrical appearance (92,93). Primordial germ cells, probably in the process of migration, are often contained in the epithelium (94,95).

During gonadal sex differentiation, the coelomic epithelium covering the gonads develops differently in the two sexes. In the male, the epithelium is soon delineated by an intact basal lamina, whereby the developing testicular cords become separated from the epithelium. Simultaneously, the epithelium and the outermost testicular

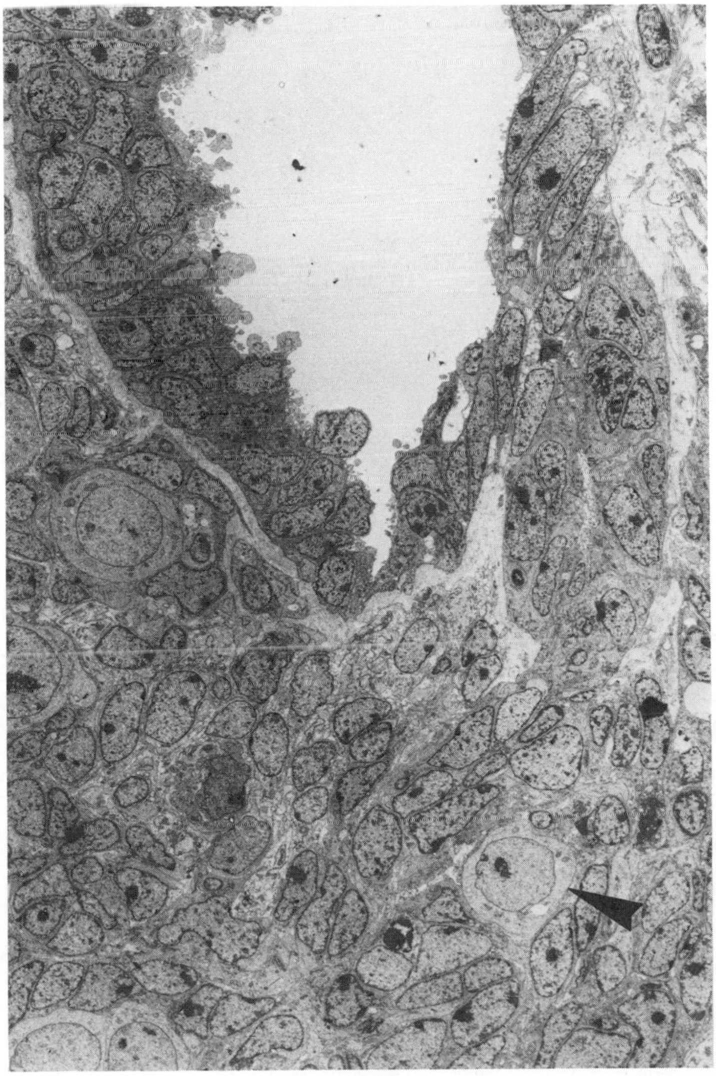

FIG. 8. Part of ovarian cortex of 9-week-old human fetus, showing connections between down-growing surface epithelium and oogonium (*arrowhead*). ×1,820.

cords become separated by a mesenchymal tissue, which differentiates into the developing tunica albuginea. The coelomic epithelium initially becomes cuboidal; then later when the testis rapidly increases its volume, it becomes flattened. In the female, the basal lamina of the coelomic epithelium becomes completed much later in development. As a consequence, the epithelium remains, at some locations, in contact with the underlying germ cells (Fig. 8). Germ cells may even be seen within the epithelium a long time after gonadal sex differentiation begins (96) (Fig. 9).

A conspicuous cell type with some resemblance to undifferentiated blood cells, particularly lymphocytes, has been found in differentiating gonads of both sexes from different species (H. Peters, A. G. Byskov, and P. E. Høyer, *unpublished observations:* human, rabbit, mouse). The cells are rounded and contain many ribosomes, sparse endoplasmic reticulum, and a relatively small, often spherical, nucleus with dense peripheral chromatin. They occur one by one or form aggregates situated close to the germ cells (Fig. 10). In the mouse, such cells disappear after the first week after birth. The function of these cells remains to be determined.

Dual Origin of the Supporting Cell Lineage?

The developing gonad often contains germ cells in cords or clumps that are not only connected to mesonephros at the basal part of the gonad (97) but also to the surface epithelium (guinea pig [98]; rat [99,100]; human [92,101,102]). These observations lend support to the idea that the surface epithelium proliferate downward and/or mesponephic cells move up in between the germ cells, giving rise to the germ cell supporting cell lineages, granulosa cells, and Sertoli cells (103). Byskov (72) and Wartenberg (77) proposed a dual origin of the granulosa cells/Sertoli cells, from mesonephros and from the surface epithelium.

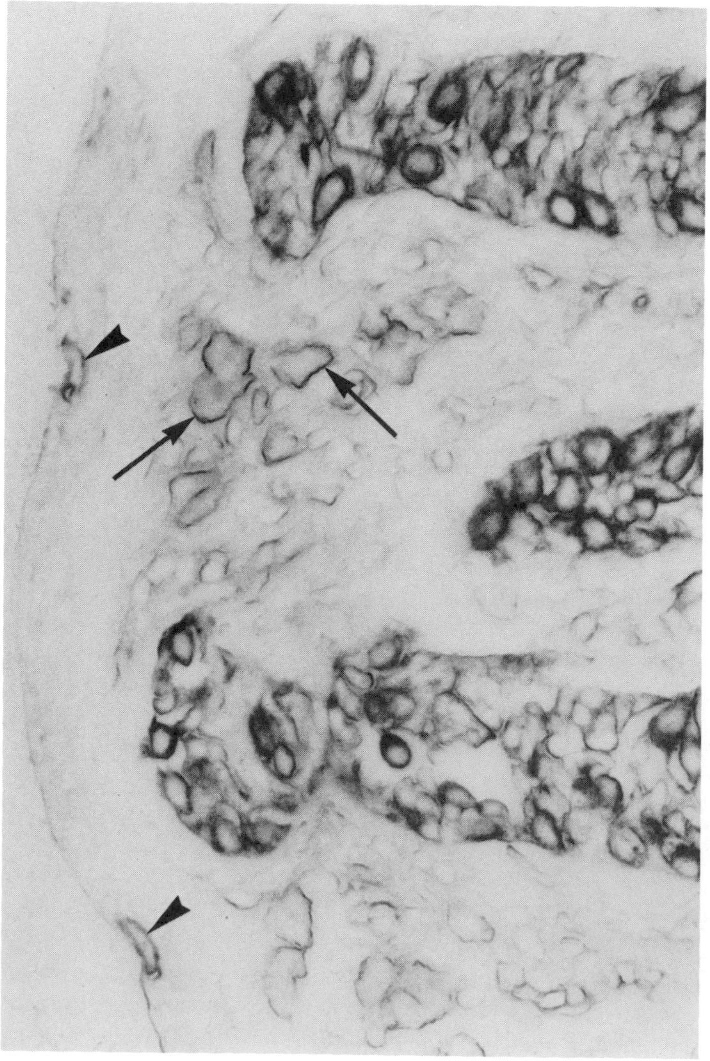

FIG. 9. Alkaline phosphatase activity in a cryosection of 12-week-old human fetal testis. Germ cells of testicular cords and of surface epithelium (*arrowheads*) as well as plasmalemma of Leydig cells (*arrows*) exhibit activity. ×311.

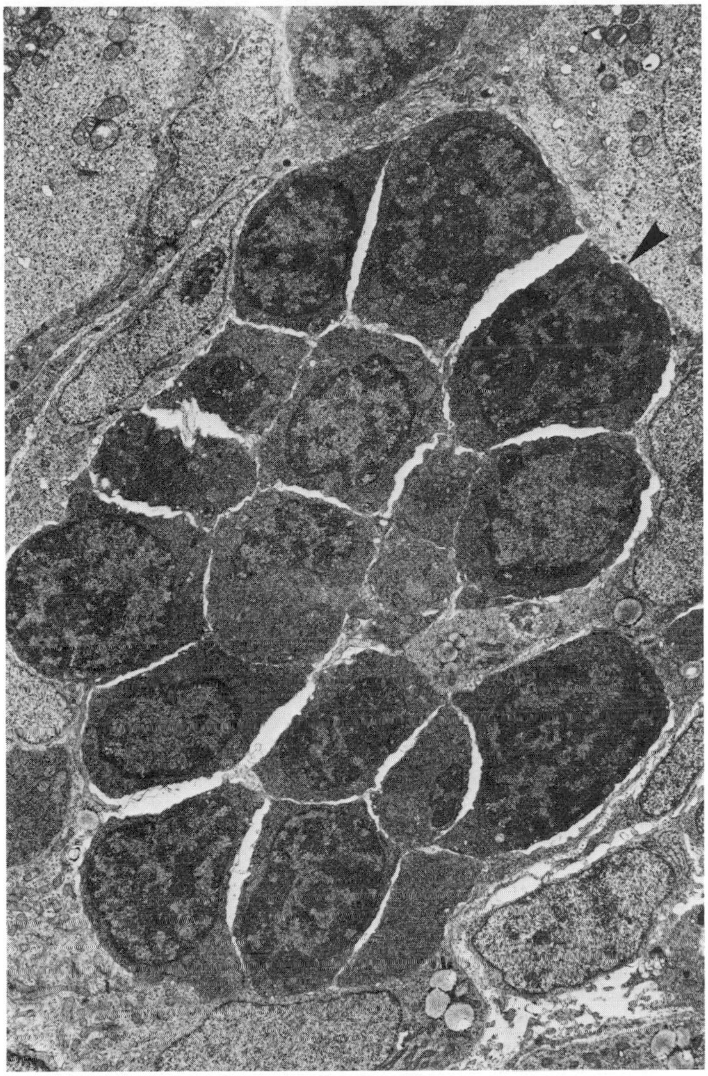

FIG. 10. Aggregate of lymphocytelike cells in newborn mouse ovary. At some places, such cells are in contact with oocytes (*arrowhead*). ×4,560.

Granulosa cells and Sertoli cells share many features of structural and functional characters that support their common origin. They are both epithelial cell types enclosed in a specific germ cell compartment. They are equipped for steroid production, possess receptors for the same stimulators (e.g., gonadotrophins and growth factors), and secrete inhibin in concert with follicle-stimulating hormone (FSH). They are both able to express antimüllerian hormone responsible for regression of the müllerian duct in the male, although in very different temporal patterns (104,105) (see *Sertoli Cells, Experimental Masculinization of the Ovary,* and *Male Differentiation of Genital Ducts* subsections). Neither Sertoli cells nor granulosa cells of small follicles show positive immunohistochemical reaction for NCAM, whereas granulosa cells of larger follicles react positively (82). During growth and differentiation of follicles, many features of the granulosa cells change, whereby cytologic markers of origin are easily blurred.

Whether Sertoli cells and granulosa cells originate in common or different cell lineage(s) has been studied in mouse chimeras (XX-XY) (for review, see ref. 106). Burgoyne et al. (107) found that in the adult testis, all Sertoli cells were XY but that granulosa cells might contain XY cells (108). Patek et al. (106) visualized that both XX and XY cells were present in all gonadal tissues of the XX-XY chimeras but that Sertoli cells were predominantly XY and granulosa cells mainly XX. Later, Palmer and Burgoyne (109) found that Sertoli cells of fetal chimeric testes had a higher proportion of XX cells than in Sertoli cells of adult chimeric testes. Thus, a selection against XX cells among Sertoli cells seems to be favored supporting the studies of Mullen and Whitten (110). The studies by Patek et al. (106) give some support to the idea that the coelomic epithelium, which was almost exclusively XX in the chimeric mice, contributes cells to both the Sertoli cell and the granulosa cell lineage but that other cell types also participate. An early selection against one or the other somatic cell lineage may play an important role in gonadal sex differentiation.

An elegant experiment of orthotopic transplantation of a quail mesonephric anlage to a chicken embryo showed a dual origin of the somatic cells of the gonad. The experiment is based on the nuclear marker of the quail cells, which is not present in the chicken cells. The coelomic epithelial cells were found to colonize the gonad very early, whereas mesonephric proliferation starts later, not until gonadal sex differentiation (111). These results support observations of a developing primate gonad that somatic cells derive from the coelomic epithelium during an early stage of gonadal formation and that mesonephric contribution takes place later (112).

The mesonephros is large, long-lived, and functional in both the quail and the monkey. In the mouse and other mammals, in which the mesonephros is small and nonfunctioning, mesonephric cells seem to participate in gonadal formation before gonadal sex differentiation (72,74). It is possible that the degree and timing of somatic cell migration into the developing gonad depend on the functional status of the mesonephros in that species. Whether the supporting cell lineage originates in the same or different cell types may be important for the understanding of gonadal sex differentiation.

DIFFERENTIATION OF THE GONADAL SEX

Genetic Control of Gonadal Sex

Gonadal sex in mammals is normally determined by the genetic sex (113). In the fruitfly, *Drosophila,* it was discovered in 1916 (114) that embryos with one X chromosome develop as males and embryos with two X chromosomes become females regardless of the presence of the Y chromosome. In mammals, however, it was not until 1959 that the presence of a Y chromosome was found to be associated with development of a testis (115–118). Individuals with sex chromosome constitutions XY, XXY, or even XXXXY develop as phenotypical males, and those with XO, XX, or XXX develop as females (119,120). Many studies have shown that the Y chromosome carries a testis-determining sequence(s), which has been designated testis-determining factor (TDF) or testis-determining gene on the Y in humans (TDY) and in mice (Tdy) (121,122). In 1966, TDY was localized to the short arm of the Y chromosome (123). Later, it was proposed that the testis-determining substance on the short arm might be identical with the male-specific H-Y antigen (124), also known as the classical *histocompatible Y antigen* (125). This hypothesis was attractive because, until recently, it was found that almost all mammals possessing a testis were H-Y-positive independent of their karyotype (126). The detection of H-Y antigen in these studies was based on serologic tests in which it was assumed that antisera raised against male cells would recognize H-Y antigen (serologically detectable male [SDM]) (127). McLaren (128) discovered, however, that certain male mice of variants of sex-reversed XX (Sxr XX mice) develop as phenotypical males with testes but lack H-Y antigenecity as determined by tests using T-lymphocyte-mediated histocompatibility response as the originally defined H-Y antigen. Previously, phenotypical males with testes, although sterile, have been found to be SDM antigen-negative (man [129]; mouse [130]). Although theoretical models apparently explained why H-Y negative males develop testes (131,132), it is now clear that H-Y antigen does not play a primary role in sex determination. Thus, the H-Y and TDY genes map to different portions of the Y chromosome (133,134).

In 1971, Cattanach et al. (135) proposed that a sex-reversing factor, Sxr, determines XX mouse embryos to develop as males. Although the Sxr XX mice do not have a Y chromosome, they develop as males because a small, sex-determining portion of the Y chromosome is attached to the paternally derived X chromosome (136–138). The Sxr is passed through XY Sxr carrier males with an abnormal Y chromosome carrying a duplication of the sex-determining region, one copy of which is often transferred to the X chromosomes during meiosis. Apart from the primary testis determinant Tdy, two other genetic functions have so far been localized within the Sxr region: Hya, a gene controlling the H-Y expression (139) and Spy, a factor involved in spermatogenesis (140,141).

Y-DNA hybridization assays have shown that many human XX males have TDY in one of the X chromosomes (142) and that some human XY females have a Y chromosome in which this factor is absent (143). By studying the sequences present in a human XX male and absent in a human XY female patient with a translocation between the Y chromosome and an autosome, X,t(Y;22), Page et al. (144) localized TDY to within a 140-kb segment of the short arm of the Y chromosome. All 140 kb of DNA in the 1A2 segment were isolated and cloned, and a new gene was identified. ZFY, as it was termed, contained DNA sequences that are highly conserved during mammalian evolution. For example, ZFY has two Y-linked homologues in mice (145,146), Zfy-1 and Zfy-2. The nucleotide sequence of this conserved DNA suggested that it coded for a protein with multiple cysteine- and histidine-rich "finger" domains. In these domains, paired cysteines and paired histidines were thought to be pulled into a tetrahedral coordination complex with a zinc cation, leaving the intervening residues to form a loop ideal for binding DNA. Consequently, it was proposed that this "zinc-finger" protein might bind to nucleic acids in a sequence-specific manner, which might regulate transcription (144,147). This feature made ZFY, Zfy-1, and Zfy-2 candidate genes for TDY/Tdy. However, several observations compromised this theory. For example, it was less consistent with ZFY being TDY that a ZFY homologue, ZFX, is present on the X chromosome in many species and that an additional autosomal homologue is present in mice (144,148). Also, a sequence related to ZFY is present on autosomes but not on sex chromosomes of marsupials (149).

Direct evidence that ZFY/Zfy is not the TDF came from two studies in 1989. First, Koopman et al. (150) showed that Zfy-1, but not Zfy-2, is expressed in differentiating embryonic testes of normal mice. However, neither Zfy-1 nor Zfy-2 was expressed in embryonic testes of W^e/W^e mutant mice, which are virtually devoid of germ cells (see *Primordial Germ Cells* subsection). This indicated that Zfy-1 is not expressed in the somatic supporting cell lineages that are believed to be crucial for gonadal sex determination (109,151,152) (see *Transformation of the Gonadal Sex* subsection). Koopman et al. (150) suggested that Zfy-1 may instead have a role in male germ cell development. Second, Palmer et al. (153) found three XX men and one XX intersex who all were indubitably male but lacked ZFY. In all four XX males, exchange of Y-specific sequences was found within a maximum of 60 kb next to the pseudoautosomal boundary. This indicated that the testis-determining gene is located in segment 1A1 of the short arm of the Y chromosome and not in segment 1A2 as found by Page et al. (144). This apparent contradiction was, however, resolved when Page et al. (154) discovered that their X,t(Y;22) female patient (144) had suffered a second deletion, removing just that testis-determining sequence in segment 1A1 that Palmer et al. (153) had detected in the XX males.

In 1990, the genetic switch on the Y chromosome that triggers the gonads to develop into testes rather than ovaries was finally discovered. It was named SRY in humans and Sry in mice, for the gene in the sex determining region of the *Y* (155,156). SRY was mapped to within 35 kb proximal to the pseudoautosomal boundary and was shown to be conserved and Y-specific among a wide range of mammals (155). Strong evidence that SRY is normally necessary for testis determination was provided by the detection of two sex-reversed women who had *de novo* mutations in SRY (157,158). The corresponding mouse gene, Sry, was deleted in a line of XY female mice—known to be mutant in Tdy (159,160)—and was expressed on day 11.5 post coitus in the male urogenital ridge but not in the female urogenital ridge (156). Further, Koopman et al. (161) detected Sry transcripts in the testis anlage of 11.5 day post coitus embryos but not in the adjacent mesonephros or any other tissue tested. One day later, after testis cord formation, Sry transcription ceased. This made Koopman et al. (161) suggest that "Sry initiates a cascade of gene expression, but is not required for the maintenance of gene activity in the developing testis." Moreover, unlike Zfy-1 and Zfy-2, Sry was normally expressed in the genital ridge of W^e/W^e mutant mice, indicating that Sry is expressed in somatic cell lineages of the developing testis (161). Also, the Zfy genes exhibit normal structure and expression in XY female mice mutant in Tdy (160). Finally, the predicted protein product of SRY/Sry includes a domain characterized by a region of homology with several known or putative DNA-binding proteins (156).

Final proof that Sry alone is able to initiate testis determination came from transgenic experiments by Koopman et al. in 1991 (162). They showed that Sry on a 14-kb genomic DNA fragment is sufficient to induce testis differentiation and subsequent male development when introduced into chromosomally female mouse embryos.

As indicated above, gonadal sex determination is dependent on the sex chromosome constitution. Chromosomal errors, particularly those affecting the X and Y, which can arise in germ cells during meiosis or in the early mitotic divisions during embryogenesis, may interfere with gonadal differentiation (for review, see ref. 106). However, several chromosomal errors (e.g., XO [Turner's syndrome], XXY [Klinefelter's syndrome], and Tfm [testicular feminization]) do not seem to affect the primary sex determination of the gonad but rather later stages of gonadal differentiation.

An individual in which the gonad develops with both ovarian and testicular tissues is a hermaphrodite, or sex mosaic, and has been described in many species (128), including humans (163). They could develop from fused XX and XY embryos (i.e., chimeras), which also have been made experimentally (164,165) or by injecting male embryonic stem cells into blastocysts (166), or as a result of Y chromosome nondisjunction (167). The sex of gonads of chimeras do not differentiate according to the relative proportion of male (XY) and female (XX) clones (106,168). Most XX/XY chimeras develop as male phenotypes in more than 40% of the cases if the XY cells comprise more than one-third of the cells in the gonads (169). However, most XX/XY chimeras possess ovotestes during fetal life, but subsequently the testicular part takes over (170,171). As a result, adult chimeric ovotestes are rare (for review, see ref. 128). A dominant influence of the male tissue over the female tissue is also demonstrated by the inhibition of growth of the müllerian duct in fetal mouse hermaphrodites, in which only 15% of testicular tissue caused normal male inhibition of müllerian duct growth (172).

Transformation of Gonadal Sex

The gonadal sex of mammals is highly stable and cannot be changed by altering environmental conditions (e.g., the temperature during differentiation as in certain reptiles) (173) or by oral administration of sex steroids as in some fish (174,175).

A complete gonadal sex transformation would imply changes in the form and function of the somatic elements that support the germ cells and that female germ cells developed into spermatozoa and male germ cells into oocytes, a phenomenon that seems not to occur in mammals. Masculinization of the mammalian ovary usually means lack of follicles and appearance of structures with resemblance to testicular cords. Feminization of the testis includes lack of testicular cords. It is widely accepted to consider the mammalian female development as a default pathway and the male development as a result of Y chromosome activity, diverting the female pathway into the male direction.

The time window during which the gonadal sex is determined is narrow in the nonmammalian vertebrates also. It seems that experimental modulation of the gonadal structure can only take place during or before this window when the supporting somatic cell lineage of the gonads has not yet differentiated. In cultures of fetal mouse gonads, Byskov and Grinsted (176) defined the time window during which the gonadal sex could be influenced *in vitro* to range from day 10 to day $12\frac{1}{2}$ of fetal life, a schedule also suggested by Palmer and Burgoyne (109). The genetic imprinting of the somatic cell line is apparently not an immediate event but needs time for synthesis of different promotors and receptors in the affected cell types. Lowell-Badge (177) stressed that the Sry gene "appears to act only for a very brief period just before testis cord formation" but that its expression must be regulated by other factors of the supporting cell lineage.

From experiments with castrated rabbit fetuses, Jost (178,179) concluded that the genital structures basically are "programmed" for femaleness and that development in the male direction opposes the female program. Therefore, the gonadal primordium is considered to develop into an ovary unless a male organizer counteracts this trend and imposes testicular differentiation (180). It is assumed that, in contrast to the gonadal sex determination, the secondary male or female sex characteristics are mainly, if not entirely, dependent on the hormone/substances produced by the differentiated testis, respectively

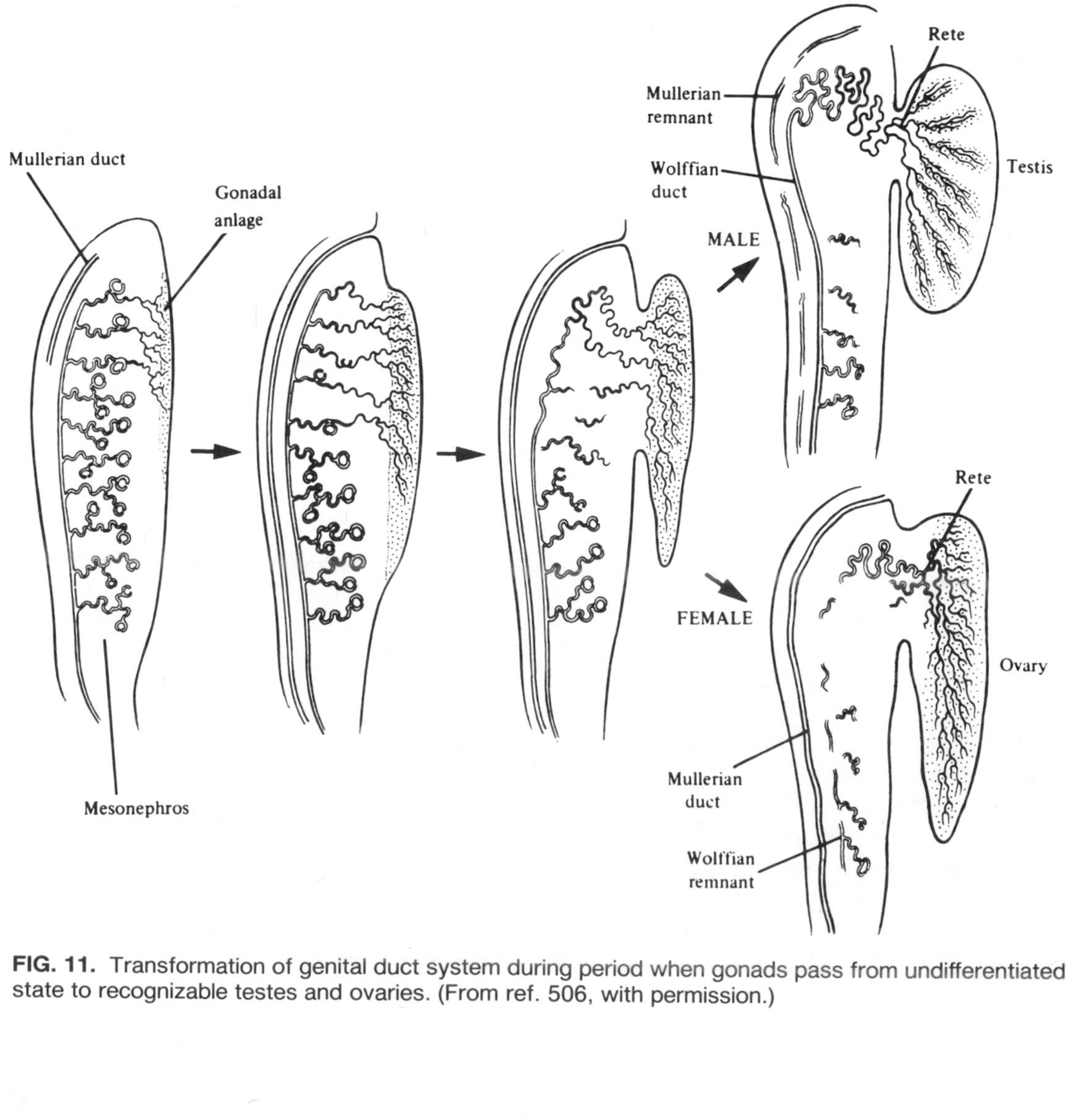

FIG. 11. Transformation of genital duct system during period when gonads pass from undifferentiated state to recognizable testes and ovaries. (From ref. 506, with permission.)

ovary. Many studies have shown that gonadal hormones have a direct effect on secondary sex characteristics. Mammalian gonadal sex differentiation can, however, not be changed by gonadal sex steroids. Only in the primitive young marsupials the gonadal sex has been experimentally influenced *in vivo* by sex steroids. In the newborn male opossum (103,181) and wallabies (182), the testicular anlage can develop into an ovotestis or an ovary by giving low doses of estradiol propionate. Such testicular changes could not be repeated by Moore and Thurstam (183), although the estradiol treatment resulted in inhibition of testicular formation and complete feminization of external and internal genitalia.

Differentiation of the gonads is, like most other organs, a result of a series of intervening events that among others includes cell–cell interaction, cell proliferation, growth inhibition, programmed cell death, and promotion of selected cell types. Specific influence on one of these important events may alter structure and function of the differentiating mammalian gonad but will probably not, as mentioned before, change a female or a male gonad into a functional gonad of the other sex. Chimeric gonads of mice, whether *natural* or *man*-made, have provided tools for the study of gonadal sex transformation (106). Transgenic mice represent another powerful model in which the function of structural genes involved in the differentiation of gonads can be studied (162,184).

DIFFERENTIATION OF THE OVARY

A functional ovary depends on three main events taking place during early stages of gonadogenesis: the initiation of meiosis, enclosure of germ cells into a specific compartment (the follicle), and the differentiation of other steroid-producing cells, the theca cells, and interstitial cells outside the follicle. These events depend on differentiation of the supporting cell lineage, the granulosa cells being enclosed in the follicle compartment with the oocyte.

Different Patterns of Early Ovarian Differentiation

Somatic cell lineages deriving from mesonephros, coelomic epithelium, or the "preexisting" mesenchyme populate the gonad together with invading germ cells before morphologic sex differentiation takes place. The

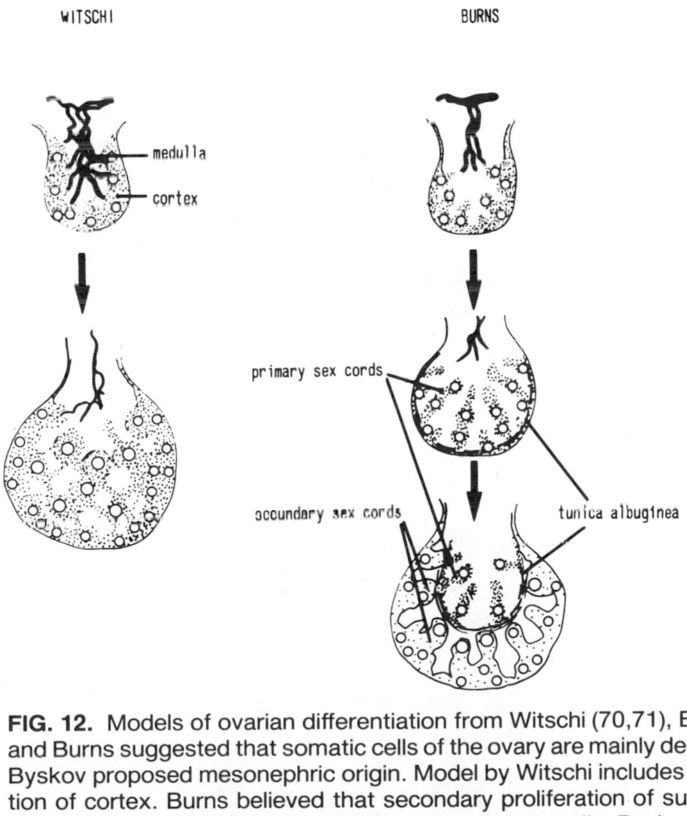

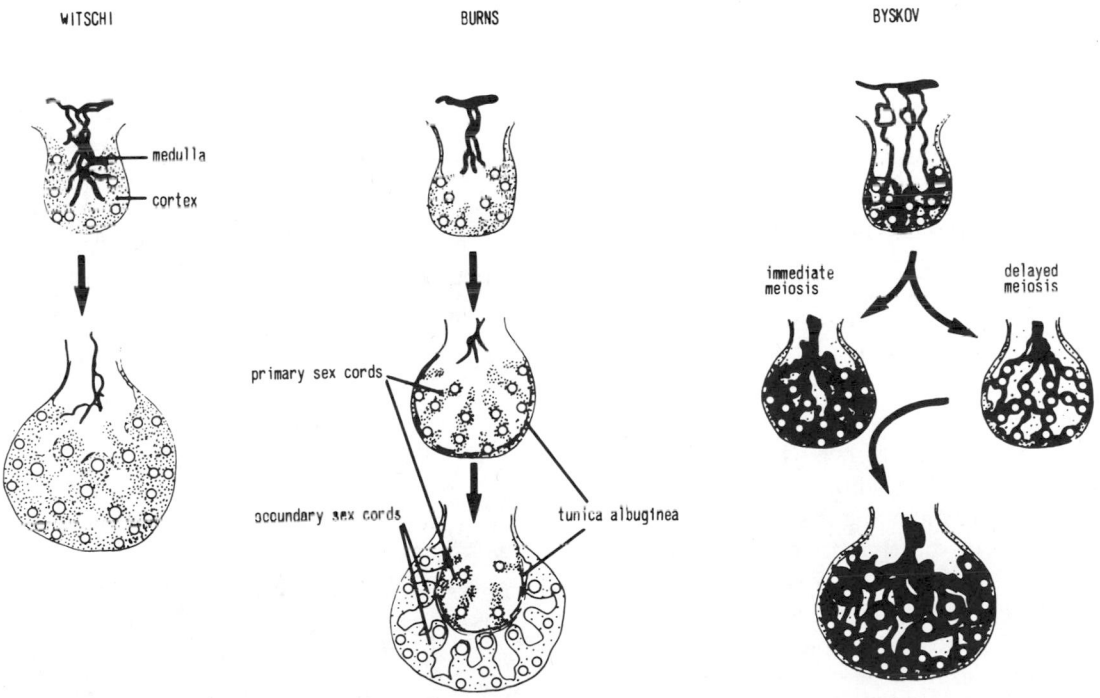

FIG. 12. Models of ovarian differentiation from Witschi (70,71), Burns (103), and Byskov (334). Witschi and Burns suggested that somatic cells of the ovary are mainly derived from surface epithelium, whereas Byskov proposed mesonephric origin. Model by Witschi includes degeneration of medulla and proliferation of cortex. Burns believed that secondary proliferation of surface epithelium forms secondary sex cords, which contribute the bulk of ovarian somatic cells. Byskov's model involves two types of transitory stages of ovarian differentiation, one in which meiosis starts almost simultaneously with gonadal sex differentiation (immediate meiosis) and another in which meiosis is more or less delayed with respect to sex differentiation (delayed meiosis). In both cases, mesonephric-derived cells are main contributors to ovarian cell mass. (From ref. 272, with permission.)

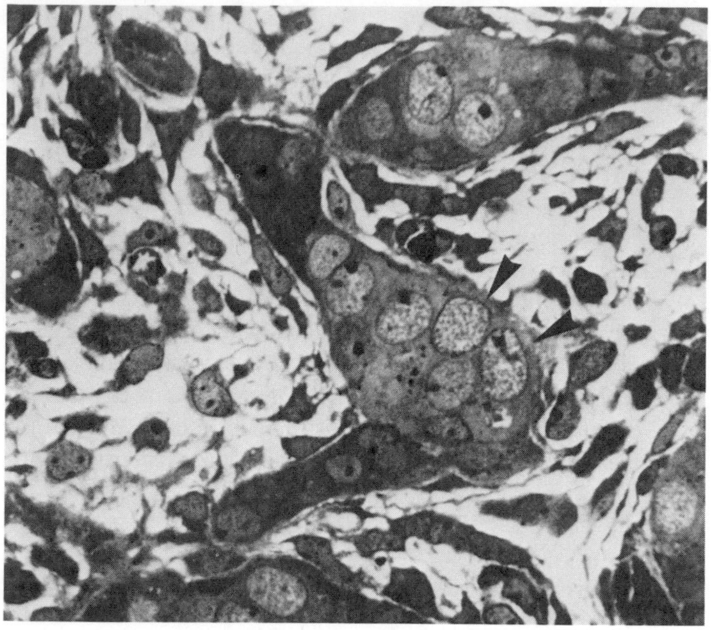

FIG. 13. Germ cell cords of 42-day-old pig ovary. Cords are tightly packed with somatic cells and germ cells (*arrowheads*). ×1,000.

ovarian–mesonephric connection is retained during ovarian differentiation, although the mesonephric tissue gradually regresses (Figs. 6 and 11). In fact, mesonephric function may affect formation of the ovary (67). In many species, the central part of the differentiating ovary becomes occupied by the invading mesonephric cells (i.e., the intraovarian rete), which push the germ cells toward the periphery (Fig. 2). An ovarian cortex richly populated with germ cells and a medulla consisting mainly of mesonephric cells are thereby formed. Cells of the surface epithelium are often in contact with—and seem to grow into—the underlaying tissue, thus contributing cells to the ovarian anlage (185) (see *Dual Origin of the Supporting Cell Lineage?* subsection).

Two main patterns of ovarian differentiation can be recognized depending on whether the germ cells of the ovary undergo "immediate" meiosis without previous steroid production or "delayed" meiosis (Fig. 12) with steroid secreted before meiosis begins (186). In species with immediate meiosis (e.g., mouse, rat, hamster), the germ cells of the ovary enter the first meiotic prophase simultaneously with or shortly after gonadal sex can be recognized morphologically. These ovaries produce little or no steroids *de novo* until follicles are formed. In species with "delayed" meiosis (e.g., pig, sheep, dog, cow), the beginning of meiosis in the female is delayed up to 45 days (cow) with respect to testicular differentiation (i.e., a delay period). In contrast to species with immediate meiosis, such ovaries produce different amounts of steroids during the delay period (see *Steroid Hormone Production in the Developing Gonads* section).

In species with immediate meiosis, the ovary appears compact when meiosis begins at an early stage of sex differentiation. The germ cells are distributed uniformly, often in clusters throughout the entire ovarian tissue (e.g., mouse, hamster), or in a basically well-defined cortical area (e.g., human).

In ovaries of species with delayed meiosis, the germ cells become enclosed in germ cell cords during the delay period. In some species (pig [187]; cat, mink, ferret [97];

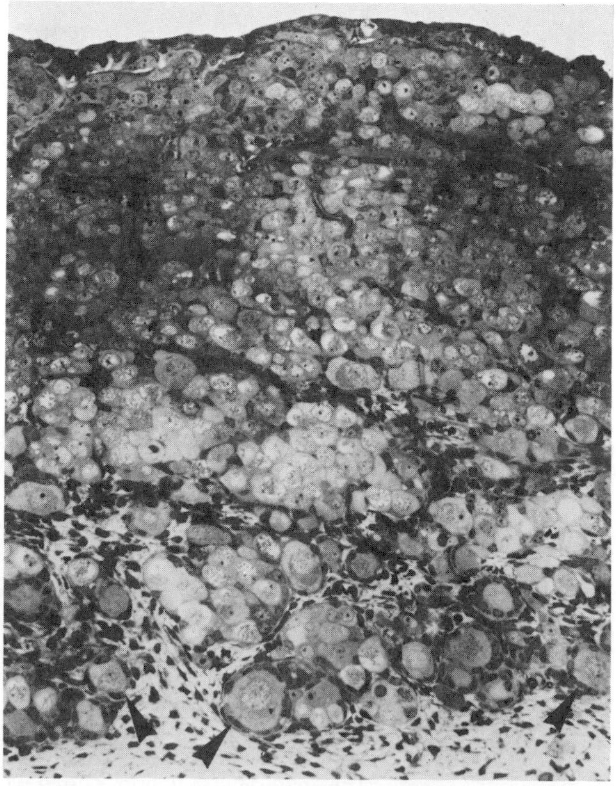

FIG. 14. Part of ovary from 21-week-old human fetus. Small follicles (*arrowheads*) are present in inner part of cortex. Middle part contains oocytes in different stages of meiosis, whereas peripheral layer still contains oogonia. ×360.

sheep [76]; cow [188]), the germ cell cords are lined with a basal lamina and clearly defined from the surrounding loose mesenchyme (Fig. 13). The cords are irregularly shaped and are tightly packed with somatic cells and germ cells. By the end of the delay period, the cell cords begin to break up in the central part of the ovary close to the intraovarian mesonephric cell cords (i.e., intraovarian rete). This process is related to the beginning of meiosis (see *Meiotic Prophase* subsection).

In other species (e.g., the rabbit), the germ cell cords are more closely packed in the ovarian cortex, and well-defined cords are only clearly recognizable in the inner part, where they connect with the intraovarian rete cords.

The development of the human fetal ovary represents a transitory example between immediate and delayed meiosis. Although there is a delay period of 2 to 3 weeks, no or very little steroids are produced *de novo*. Intraovarian mesonephric cell cords occupy the medulla before meiosis starts, and the cortically placed germ cells are not confined to cords but are rather gathered into large clusters (Fig. 14).

Meiotic Prophase

Although meiosis represents similar events in germ cells of the two sexes, the time schedule and the resulting number of haploid germ cells differ between ovary and testis.

In the female germ cells, meiosis is initiated at early stages of development, often during fetal life. The first germ cells to begin meiosis are always localized at the inner part of the cortex. However, meiosis is arrested in late prophase of the first meiotic phase, and the divisions are delayed and do not take place until much later in the mature animal (around ovulation time). In the male germ cells, meiosis begins at puberty and proceeds without significant delay (Fig. 15).

The two meiotic divisions are unique for germ cells. During the first meiotic division, maternal and paternal genes are exchanged before the pairs of chromosomes are divided into the two daughter cells, each containing 1n chromosomes and 2c DNA. The second meiotic division occurs without being preceded by DNA synthesis. This division results in formation of the haploid germ

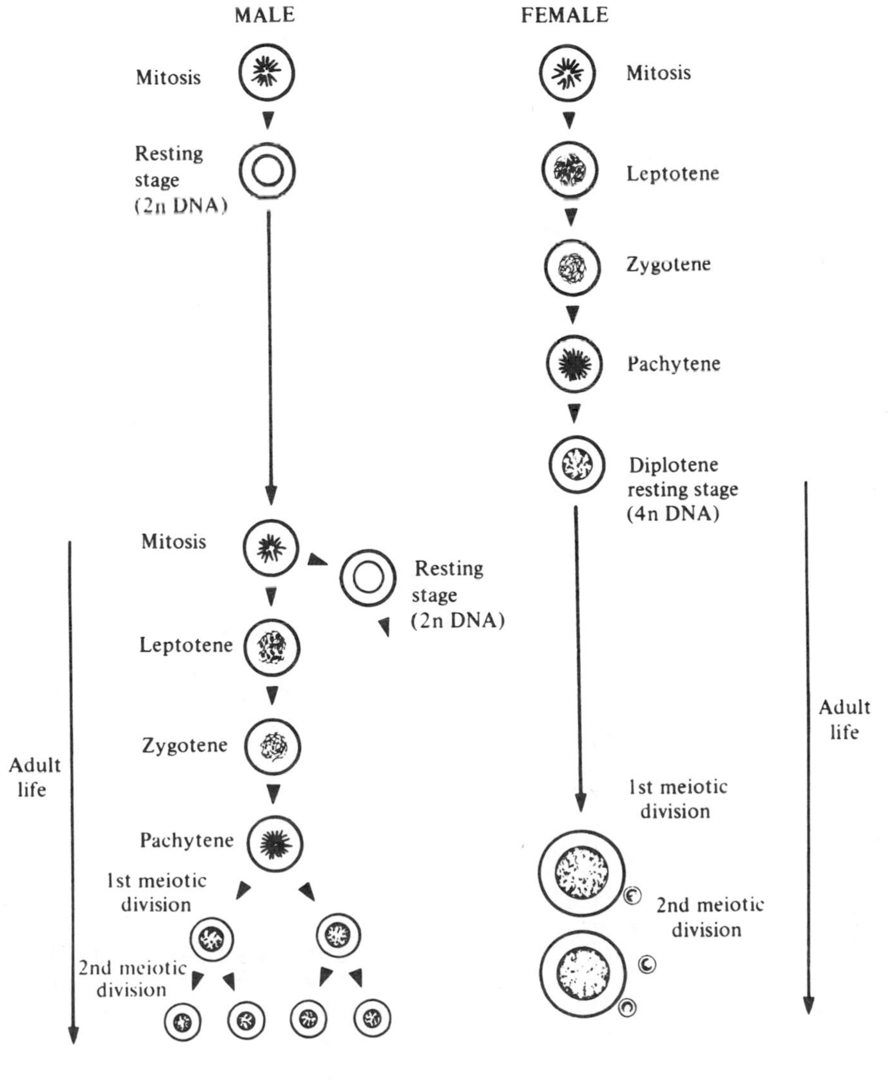

FIG. 15. Life cycles of male and female germ cells. Germ cells of both sexes divide mitotically until, or shortly after, gonadal sex differentiation. Female germ cells all enter meiosis at early stages of development, whereas male germ cells keep a resting stem cell population that can divide mitotically and from which meiotic cells continue to emerge throughout life. Male germ cells rest with 2c DNA (2c = 2n), whereas female germ cells rest in diplotene stage with 4c DNA (4c = 4n). (From ref. 506, with permission.)

cells with a 1n set of chromosomes and 1c DNA (for review, see ref. 189).

Meiosis in a female germ cell is not completed until after fertilization and results in a single egg and two abortive cells, the polar bodies, whereas four spermatozoa are produced by each male germ cell entering meiosis (Fig. 15), all possessing 1c DNA and 1n chromosomes.

Proliferation and Premeiotic DNA Synthesis of Oogonia

The oogonia continue to divide mitotically until they enter meiosis. Fluctuations in the total number of germ cells in fetal and neonatal ovaries of different mammalian species are seen in Fig. 16 (190). The rate of mitosis during the time preceding meiosis varies between species. In species with delayed meiosis, the mitotic activity is low during most of the delay period, but it increases rapidly shortly before meiosis starts (pig [191]). In species in which meiosis starts shortly after gonadal sex differentiation, the period with low mitotic activity in the oogonial population is nonexistent (mouse) or very short (rat), and meiosis is introduced by a series of mitotic divisions shortly after gonadal sex differentiation (192). Often groups of germ cells divide synchronously. When meiosis begins, similar groups exhibit synchrony while passing through transitory stages of meiosis (193,194). Germ cells of such groups are often connected by intercellular bridges (195). It has been proposed that a single-stem cell gives rise to such germ cell groups (196). The bridges may be used to transfer different substances (e.g., gene products) between germ cells (195,197).

The premeiotic DNA synthesis is an important event because this DNA persists throughout the lifetime of the oocyte, lasting until either fertilization or atresia. The premeiotic DNA synthesis has been studied by means of incorporated isotope-labeled thymidine followed by autoradiography (194,198–200). These studies have shown that no neoformation of oocytes takes place after they enter meiosis. Experiments in which germ cells of fetal ovaries have been eliminated by irradiation confirm these results (201–203). An exception from this concept

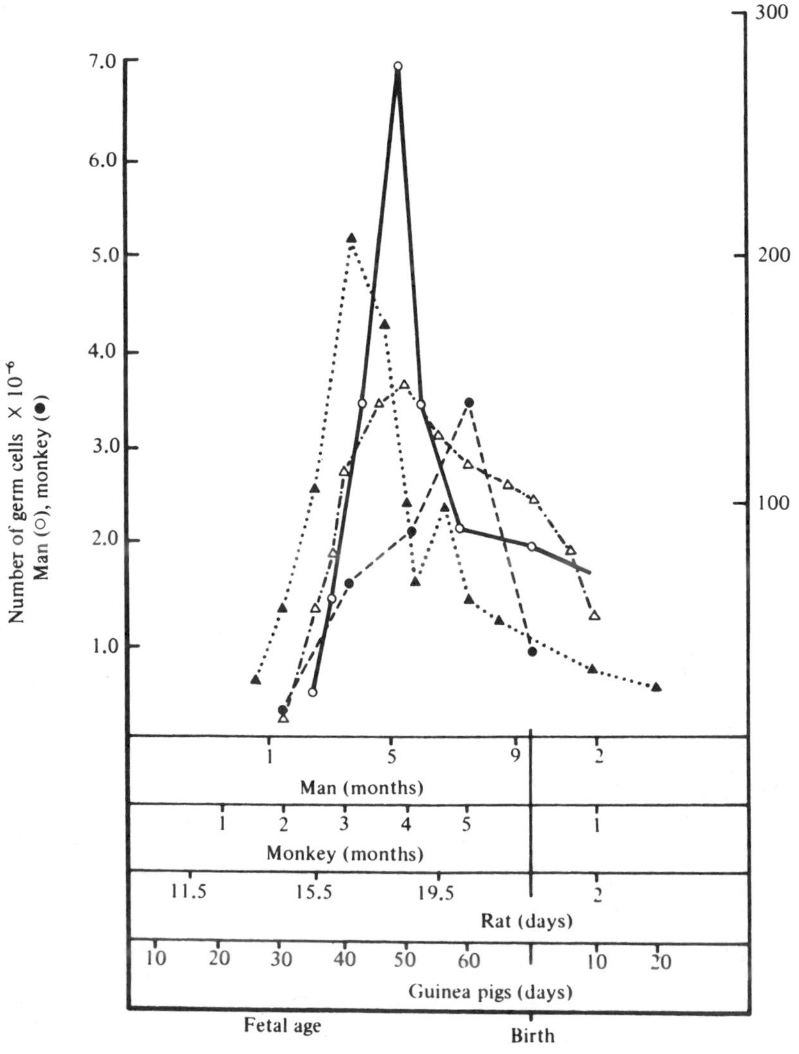

FIG. 16. Numbers of germ cells in ovaries of fetuses and neonates in humans, monkeys, rats, and guinea pigs. (From ref. 190, with permission.)

occurs in prosimians in which oogonialike cells of the adult ovary exhibit DNA synthesis (204,205). An additional low level of DNA synthesis also occurs during pachytene stages (see below).

Germ cells of the proliferative phases that precede meiosis are extremely sensitive to irradiation (for review, see ref. 206). It seems that the premeiotic division stage is the most sensitive and that sensitivity decreases as meiosis advances (207,208).

Transitory Stages of the Meiotic Prophase in Oocytes

The first meiotic prophase is subdivided into five consecutive stages, namely, leptonema, zygonema, pachynema, diplonema, and diakinesis. ("The adjectives corresponding to the first four stages are leptotene, zygotene, pachytene and diplotene and are often used as nouns" Goodenough and Levine [189].)

The leptotene stage is resumed by the end of the premeiotic DNA synthesis. In the immature rabbit, DNA synthesis still seems to take place in leptotene cells (209). In some species, a preleptotene condensation stage has been recognized (human [210]; mouse [86]; rabbit [211]; sheep [212]; horse [213]). During the preleptotene and leptotene stages, the chromosomes begin to condense; they appear in the light microscope as thin coiled threads with chromomeric periodicity (Fig. 17). Each thread consists of identical sister chromatids.

During the zygotene stage, the homologous sister chromatids pair and the synaptonemal complexes are formed (Fig. 18). The synaptonemal complexes are structures that hold the two homologous chromatids together. Detailed information about the synaptonemal complexes has been provided by three-dimensional reconstructions from serial thin sections of chromosomes (214,215). The process of pairing can also be studied in great detail by the surface spreading technique (216). The chromatids coil increasingly during zygonema (Fig. 17). In pachynema, synapsis is completed between homologous chromatids in which coiling and condensation is maximal (Fig. 17). The maternal and paternal chromatids are now in the position for gene exchange (i.e., crossing-over) between nonsister-chromatid bivalents (set of homologs) in the following stage (i.e., diplonema), allowing meiotic recombination to take place (for review, see refs. 217 and 218). In oocytes of late pachytene and early diplotene stage, chiasmata can be recognized even in the light microscope (219). Chiasmata represent the sites at the chromatids that break and reunite with the other nonsister chromatid, as shown by different labeling of the chromatids (218,220). The amount of chromosomal material that is exchanged between paternal and maternal chromatids can be evaluated by labeling premeiotic oogonia in S-phase with bromodeoxyuridine and studying the oocyte in the metaphase of the second meiotic division (221).

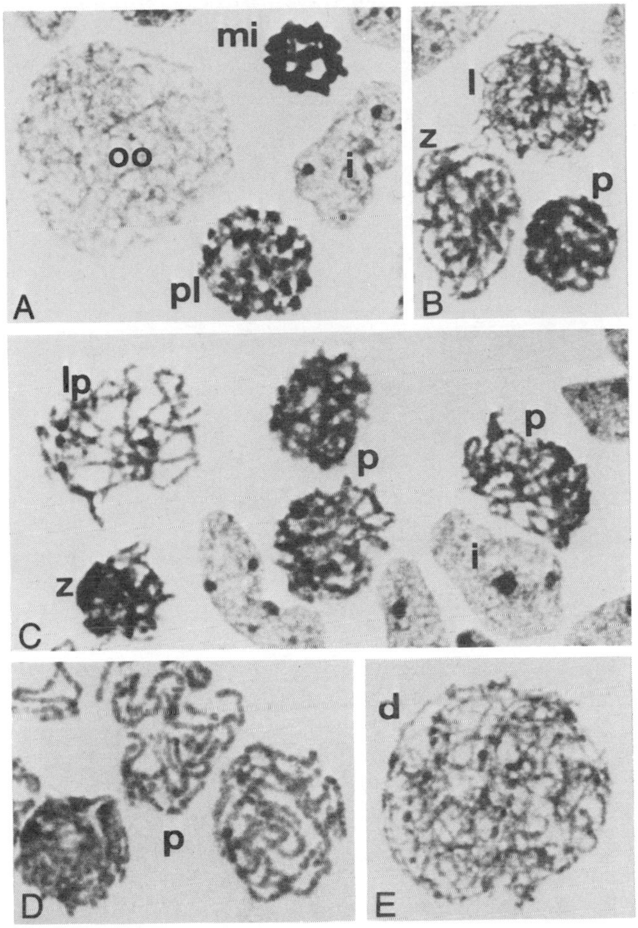

FIG. 17. Feulgen-stained squash preparations of fetal mouse ovaries, showing germ cells in different stages of meiosis. ×3,500. **(A)** A $13\frac{1}{2}$-day-old fetus showing an oogonium (*oo*), preleptotene cells (*pl*), somatic cells in interphase (*i*), and one cell in mitosis (*mi*). **(B, C)** A $16\frac{1}{2}$-day-old fetus. *l*, leptotene; *z*, zygotene; *p*, pachytene; and *lp*, late pachytene stage. **(D, E)** A $19\frac{1}{2}$-day-old fetus. *d*, diplotene stage.

Chiasmata and crossing-over have been considered a 1:1 relationship (222), with a higher frequency in female germ cells than in male germ cells (223). In the Turkish hamster, however, this pattern is reversed, with the oocytes having less recombinations than the spermatocytes (224). This observation led to the hypothesis that the hormonal environment might influence genetic recombination, as female hamster germ cells enter meiosis after birth remote from the intrauterine hormonal influences.

In the newborn mouse ovary, a low level of DNA synthesis takes place in a small fraction of oocytes in early diplotene stage when the synaptonemal complexes dissolve, which may be a result of DNA repair in these oocytes (225). In spermatocytes, low incorporation of ^{3}H-thymidine occurs in pachytene stage (226), which possibly could be related to the chromatid pairing (218).

In mammals, the diplotene stage (or diplonema) (Fig. 17) lasts for a long time and may (e.g., in the human)

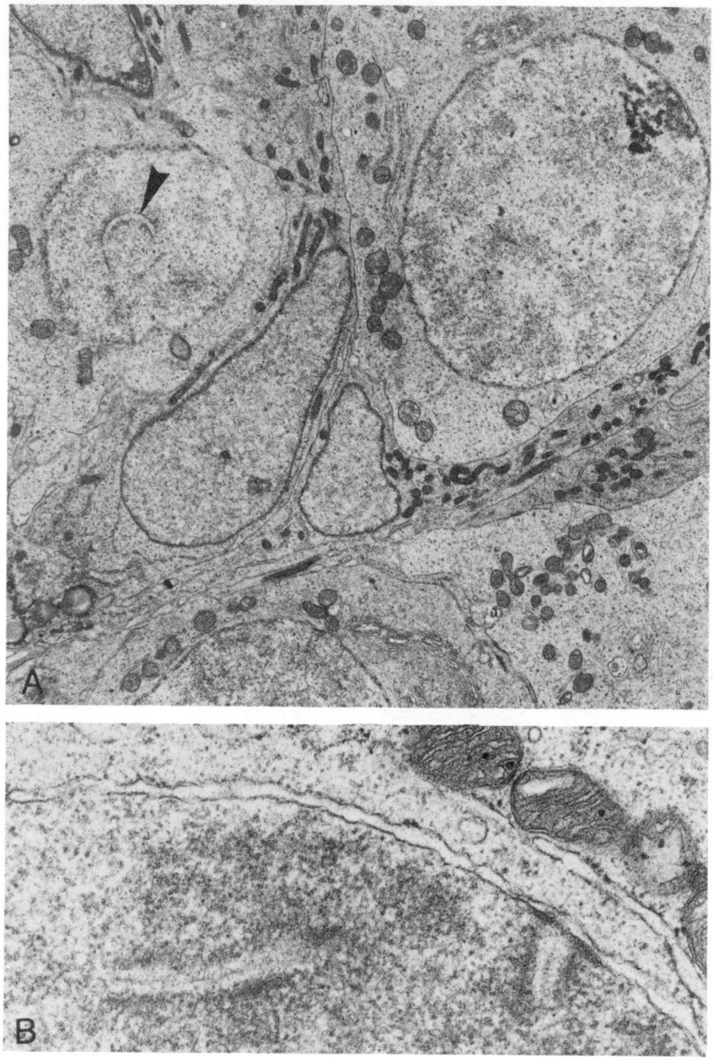

FIG. 18. (**A**) Part of ovary of 19-day-old fetal mouse, showing oocytes in meiosis (pachytene stage with synaptonemal complex, *arrowhead*). ×6,250. (**B**) Higher magnification of two synaptonemal complexes of an oocyte in pachytene stage. ×38,000.

take more than 50 years. In general, the chromosomal material becomes very diffuse and is therefore only hardly seen after DNA staining. In some species, the chromosomes form lampbrush structures in the diplotene stage, which has been referred to as the *dictyate stage* (227). This condition seems to be related to high radiosensitivity (206).

Germ cells passing through the transitory stages of the meiotic prophase appear to be extremely vulnerable. A large percentage of oocytes that enter meiosis will not reach the diplotene stage but will instead become pyknotic, particularly when entering the zygotene and pachytene stages (228). In the fetal human ovary, only about 5% of the peak number of germ cells reach the diplotene stage (34).

It seems that the presence of two active X chromosomes from the beginning of meiosis (see *Early Gonadal Formation* section) promotes the survival and function of oocytes. Germ cells of human XO (Turner's syndrome) ovaries begin to degenerate about the third month of fetal life (when meiosis starts), and often these women develop sterile ovaries (229,230). XO mice, however, are fertile, although many oocytes degenerate during meiosis (231). Oocyte loss in XO mice and women may be due to X dosage deficiency as both XX are active from onset of meiosis (232). Survival of XO germ cells in the mouse is possibly the result of a complete inactivation of critical X-linked genes and their absence or restricted expression from the Y chromosome, genes that in the human X escape inactivation (233). It was proposed that germ cells, which during the pachytene stage have unpaired or incompletely paired chromosomes, are selectively destroyed (234,235) or may result in meiotic nondisjunction. Such chromosomes would behave as univalents without normal disjoining from each other causing "unbalanced" oocytes after the first meiotic division (236). Henderson and Edwards (236) proposed that oocytes entering meiosis late in fetal life had more nondisjunctions (fewer chiasmata formations) than oocytes entering meiosis early. According to their "production line hypothesis," those oocytes that are first entering meiosis are also the first to be released by ovulation later in life (first in–first out, last in–last out). Thus, increasing nondisjunctions in oocytes toward the end of fetal life would explain the adult age-dependent increase in oocyte chromosome anomalies. Although the theory about nondisjunctions has been tested with various results, the first in—first out, last in—last out theory was only recently confirmed (237).

The synthesis of ribonucleic acid (RNA) has been studied during the transitory stages of meiosis by autoradiography after uptake of ^{3}H-uridine [rat (192); monkey (238)]. In the rat, it was shown that the incorporation of the radioactive tracer in oocytes in pachytene stage was ten times higher than in the previous stages of meiosis, indicating higher RNA synthesis in this stage (192).

Formation of Follicles

When the oocyte reaches diplonema, it must become enclosed in a follicle together with the supporting granulosa cells (Fig. 19). In most species, single oocytes are surrounded by presumptive granulosa cells, which are delineated by an intact basal lamina. In some species, more than one oocyte is enclosed within the same follicle (i.e., polyovular follicle) (e.g., primate [239]; dog [240]) (Fig. 20), a phenomenon also seen in other species during the immature period (241). If the oocyte in the diplotene stage fails to be enclosed into the follicle, it invariably degenerates. Ultrastructural analysis of cells involved in folliculogenesis has recently been reviewed (242).

Follicles begin to form in the inner part of the ovarian cortex where oocytes first reach diplonema (Figs. 14 and 21). In many species, the granulosa cells of these developing follicles are connected with the intraovarian mesonephric-derived rete cords (243) (Fig. 22). That the mesonephric-derived rete cells contribute to the granulosa cell layer has been supported by transplantation experiments by Byskov et al. (244), who showed that follicle formation depended on whether a sufficient number of mesonephric cells had invaded the developing ovary.

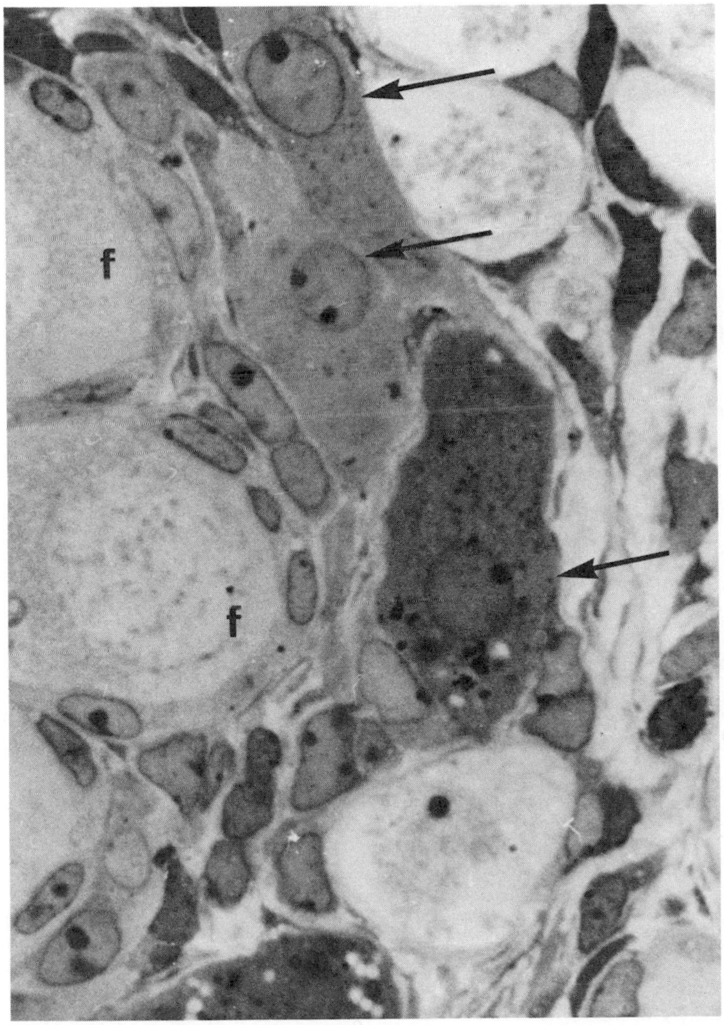

FIG. 19. Part of ovarian cortex of 23-week-old human fetus, showing three interstitial cells (*arrows*) with different content of osmiophilic granules (i.e., various degrees of differentiation), oocytes, and two small follicles (*f*). ×1,275.

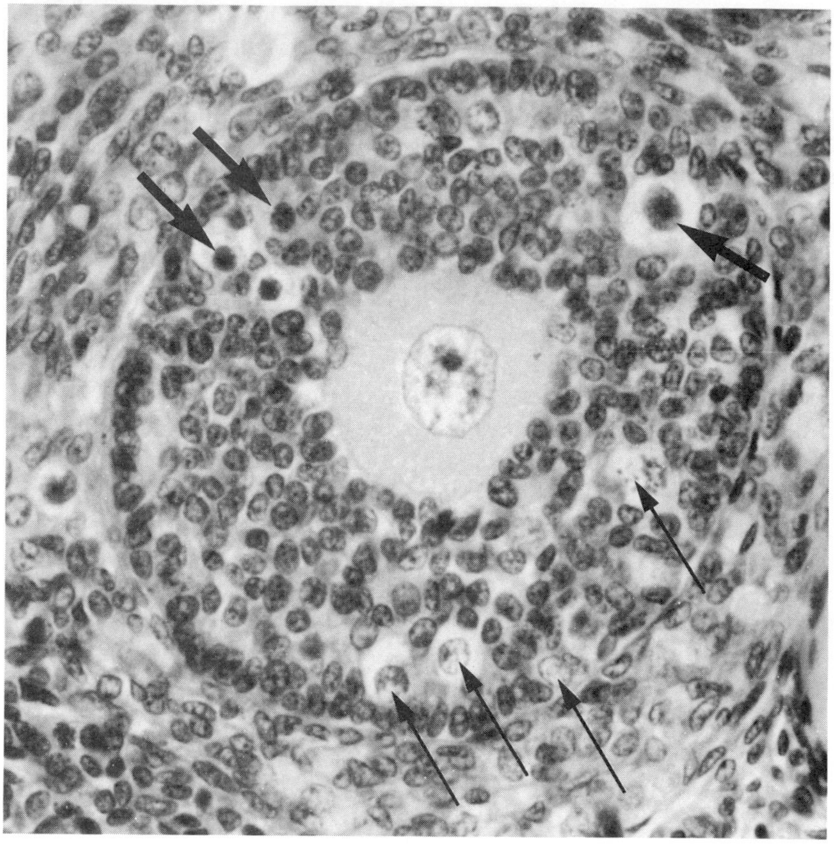

FIG. 20. Polyovular follicle from a 39-week-old human ovary. Small apparently healthy oocytes (*thin arrows*) and small oocytes with pyknotic nuclei (*thick arrows*) are seen in granulosa layer of a growing follicle. ×800.

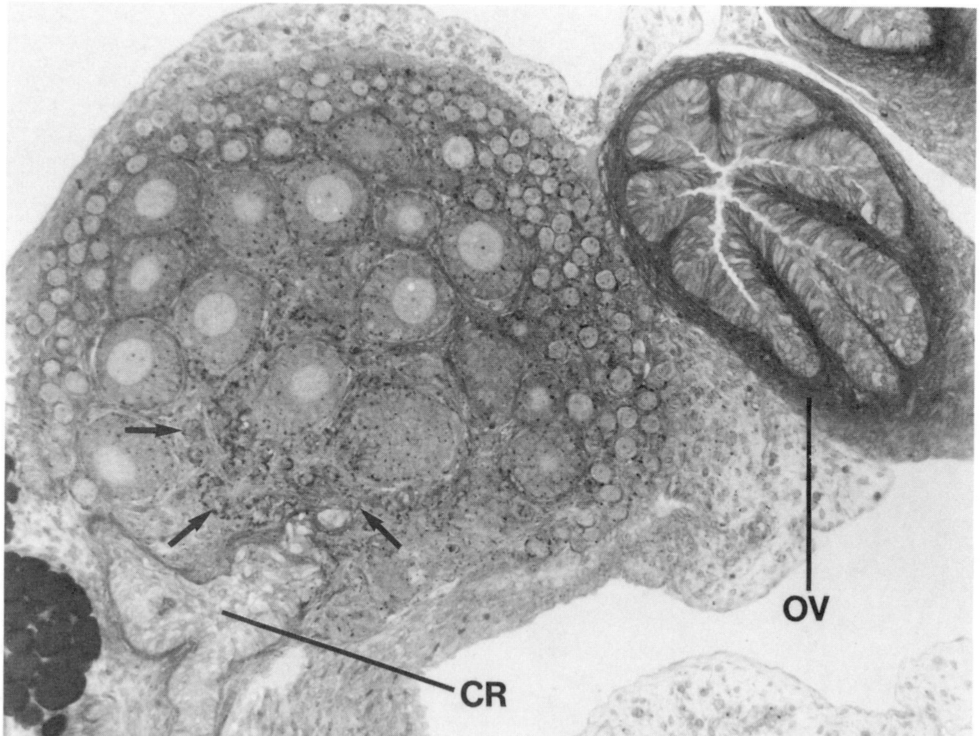

FIG. 21. Developing ovary and oviduct (*Ov*) from a 7-day-old immature mouse. Growing follicles are seen in inner part and small nongrowing follicles in outer part of the ovary. Lipid droplets are present in intraovarian rete cords in center of ovary (*arrows*). *CR,* connecting rete. ×400.

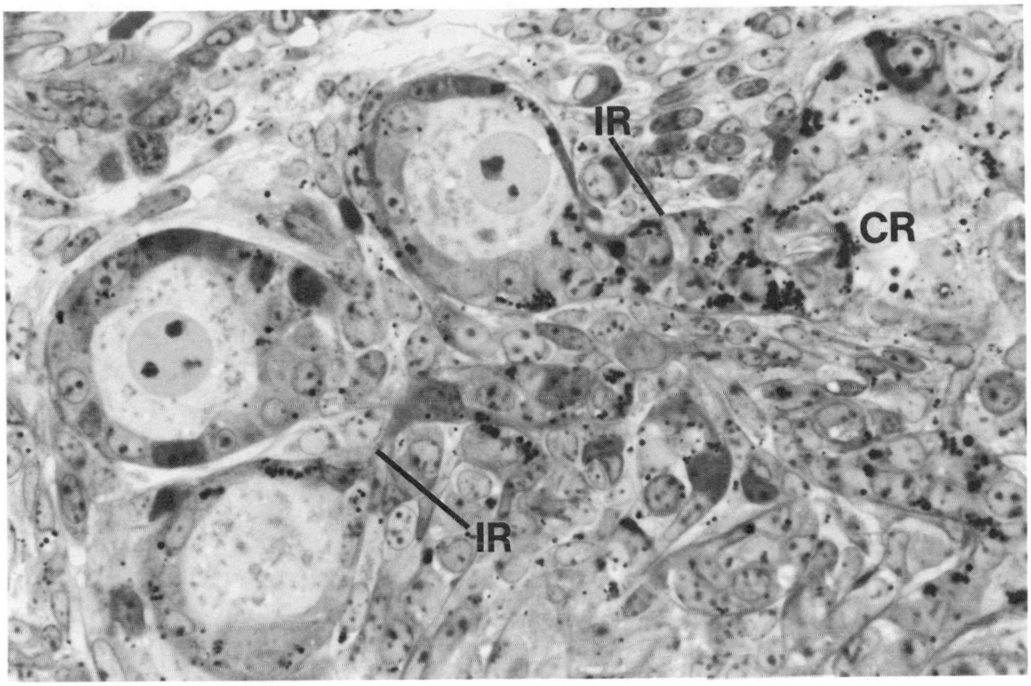

FIG. 22. Small, centrally placed follicles of 7-day-old immature ovary. Intraovarian rete cords (*IR*) with lipid droplets connect follicles and connecting rete (*CR*). ×1,000.

These experiments also indicated that the disappearance of the ovarian surface epithelium did not influence early folliculogenesis, making it unlikely that this epithelium is an important source of granulosa cells, at least during formation of these first follicles. Such observations do not exclude contribution of cells from the surface epithelium—or from mesenchymal cells—to the granulosa cell layer. It is possible that late-formed follicles at the periphery of the ovary contain fewer mesonephric cells than the early formed, centrally placed follicles.

Initiation of Oocyte and Follicle Growth

The first-formed follicles in the center of the fetal or neonatal ovary exhibit a different pattern of formation, growth, and differentiation compared with the follicles in the mature ovary (245). This may reflect that the granulosa cells change in respect to origin, sensitivity to hormones, and growth factors, depending on at which stage of development the follicles are formed. This is closely related to the geographically placement of the follicle within the ovary. Early folliculogenesis in the center of the ovary depends on migration of mitotically dividing extraovarian rete cells into the intraovarian rete surrounding the centrally placed oocytes (246). Some of these cells become granulosa cells, whereas other intraovarian rete cells appear to differentiate into the first interstitial cells (247) (Fig. 22). By arrival into the ovary, where the connecting rete cells contact the germ cells, they stop proliferation as reported in the rat (246). The accumulation of these early granulosa cells is therefore a result of migration and differentiation of rete cells rather than local proliferation. In contrast, in the *mature* ovary the recruitment of follicles for growth is a result of proliferation of preexisting granulosa cells of the small, resting follicle. Thus, the formation of the first growing follicles is fast compared with the time course of follicular growth in the adult animal (248–250). In other respects, early formed follicles appear to differ from those of the mature ovary. The theory has been advanced that those follicles that remain connected to the intraovarian rete contain an atretic oocyte and are in the process of degeneration (247). The elimination of the connection to the rete may depend on whether the oocyte is healthy and able to induce the surrounding granulosa cells to gather and enclose themselves into the follicular unit. Long-time cultures of fetal mouse gonads, with or without mesonephros, has also accentuated the role of this organ in survival and growth of oocytes, being stimulatory during early stages and inhibitory later in fetal life (251).

The mechanisms that trigger initial follicular growth are unknown. Exogenous gonadotrophins have been reported to stimulate the onset of follicular growth in the mouse (252), and gonadotrophins seem to support follicular growth in the fetal/infant monkey (253). Various studies of cultured preantral follicles have shown that successful follicular development depends on FSH (mouse [254–256]; hamster [257,258]). Follicular growth is retarded in hypophysectomized fetal monkeys (253) and rats (259), in anencephalic human fetuses (260), and in infant mice treated with antigonadotrophins (261). In juvenile monkeys treated with a gonadotropin-releasing hormone (GnRH)-antagonist, small follicles developed normally indicating that pulsatile release of gonadotrophins does not affect growth of small follicles; also, these small follicles were unaffected by diethylstilbestrol (DES), suggesting that initial stimulus of follicular growth may occur within the ovary itself (262).

The role of growth factors on follicular growth and development has been studied during the past few years. In the hamster, preantral follicular growth is stimulated by both epidermal growth factor (EGF) and TGFα, *in vitro* and *in vivo* (263). Moreover, preliminary results with cultured newborn mouse ovaries suggest a role of EGF in initiation of follicular growth (264). Other growth factors, in particular those that stimulate both growth and steroidogenesis (e.g., insulinlike growth factor I and II [265] and fibroblast growth factor (FGF) [266]) are likely candidates for initiation of follicular growth.

In cultures of fetal ovaries without added hormones, growth of oocytes as well as follicles will resume, but addition of FSH, luteinizing hormone (LH) will increase growth and promote the follicular structure (254), accentuating a role of these hormones in the very beginning of growth initiation. The modulators of FSH (inhibin and activin) have been localized by immunocytochemical methods in fetal human and monkey testes and ovaries (267). Weak immunoreactivity of β_B subunit was only detected in a few small follicles of the human fetal ovary. All three subunits (α, β_A, and β_B) were found in many small and growing follicles in the monkey ovary in late gestation, suggesting an intraovarian and endocrine role of these proteins.

In a simple organ culture of fetal mouse ovaries, it was shown that the characteristic geographically determined growth pattern of oocytes is being imprinted shortly after meiosis is initiated (i.e., even before the oocytes have reached diplotene stage [268]). When such ovarian cultures contain few oocytes, almost all of them are growing, whereas in ovaries with many oocytes, only a small fraction will be growing. This study also confirms the theory of Krarup et al. (269) that the number of growing follicles of the ovary is inversely correlated to the number of small nongrowing follicles. How small follicles escape the resting pool and begin to grow is not known. Small growing follicles are, in fact, neighbors to small nongrowing ones (Fig. 23).

In a morphologic study of the neonatal rat ovary, Rajah et al. (270) hypothesized that initial mesenchymal-presumptive granulosa cell association is crucial for folliculogenesis and that the rete ovarii may induce follicle assembly.

The time at which follicles form in different species depends on when the oocytes reach the diplotene stage. This may occur during fetal life (e.g., human, pig, guinea pig) or after birth (e.g., mouse, rat, rabbit, and ferret) (for reviews, see refs. 271 and 272).

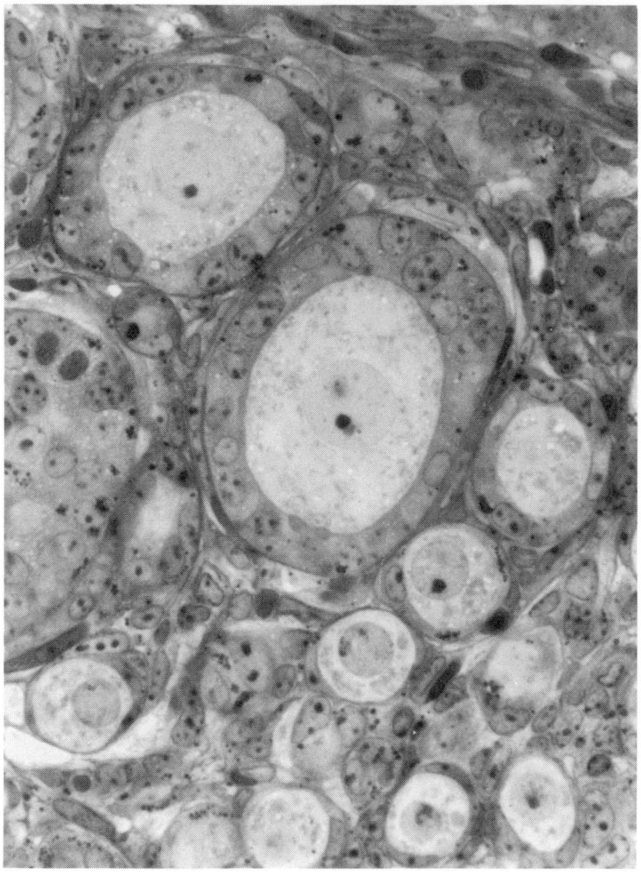

FIG. 23. Several small, nongrowing follicles in close apposition to two growing ones in cortex of 6-day-old immature mouse ovary. ×1,000.

Steroid-Producing Cells

In the adult ovary, the steroid-producing cells comprise mainly theca cells and granulosa cells of large follicles, corpora lutea cells, and interstitial cells. In the developing ovary, large follicles and corpora lutea are absent, but other cell types, possibly precursors of later steroid-producing cells, actively participate in steroid secretion.

A "typical" steroid-producing cell is traditionally characterized by many mitochondria with tubular cristae, abundant smooth endoplasmic reticulum, and many lipid droplets (273). However, steroid production by the mammalian ovary may occur at times when cells with such characteristics cannot be found (e.g., in the fetal rabbit ovary [274]). By day 19, the fetal rabbit ovary is able to convert testosterone to estrogen (275) and is also able to secrete steroids *de novo* in cultures (79). The cells that seem to be responsible for this steroidogenesis lack the typical ultrastructural characteristics of steroid-producing cells, except for their content of lipid droplets. However, these cells, which are localized in the mesonephric-derived medulla, do exhibit activity of 3β-hydroxy-Δ^5-steroid dehydrogenase as shown by quantitative cytochemistry (276).

In species with immediate meiosis, ovarian *de novo* steroidogenesis does not take place until follicles are formed (see *Steroid Hormone Production in the Developing Gonads* section). When follicles appear, cells containing mitochondria with tubular cristae, smooth endoplasmic reticulum, and lipid droplets (i.e., the interstitial cells) are recognized in the ovary (276). In the human, these cells are first seen after the twelfth week in the inner part of the cortex, close to the follicles (277,278) (Figs. 14 and 19). At the fourteenth week, high reduced nicotinamide adenine dinucleotide phosphate (NADH) diaphorase activity is present in some cells situated in the inner part of the cortex (Fig. 24), but not until the twentieth week do a few of these cells show activity of 3β-hydroxy-Δ^5-steroid dehydrogenase (278) and ultrastructural characteristics of steroid-producing cells (Fig. 25). In the 23-week-old fetus, most of these cells are situated in the inner part of the cortex, but some may also have a more peripheral location.

The origin of the early steroid-producing cells, in particular, theca cells, is not clear, and different hypotheses have been put forward. Their stem cells could be fibroblasts or "stroma" cells (279), revealing similar morphology as fibroblasts (280). Other studies support the concept that the early steroid-producing cells share a common ancestor, with the granulosa cells being derived from cells of mesonephric origin (276). This concept is supported by studies that show that the mesonephros itself is steroidogenic in the rabbit embryo (281). In the mouse, the ontogeny of the first interstitial, steroid-producing cells was studied by quantitative cytochemical detection of 3β-hydroxy-Δ^5-steroid dehydrogenase activity in the intraovarian rete cells of the immature mouse ovary (247). It was shown that, by day 7, only those rete cells that position themselves close to the oocytes develop this enzyme activity. During the next 2 weeks, the connection between the granulosa cells and the intraovarian rete cells becomes eliminated in some follicles. Only the peripherally situated granulosa cells of these isolated follicles retain some activity of 3β-hydroxy-Δ^5-steroid dehydrogenase, whereas the cells closer to the oocytes lose it. However, oocytes, possibly atretic ones,

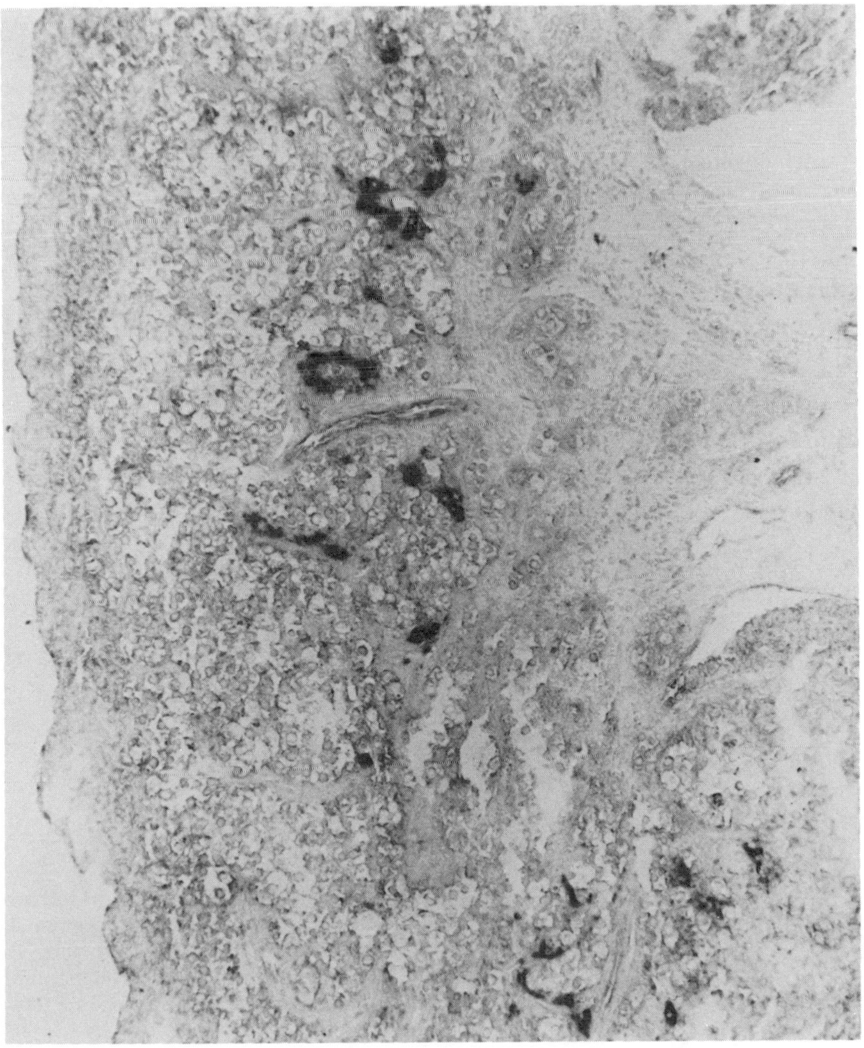

FIG. 24. Part of ovary of 20-week-old human fetus. Cells located in inner part of cortex exhibit strong NADH diaphorase activity. ×120.

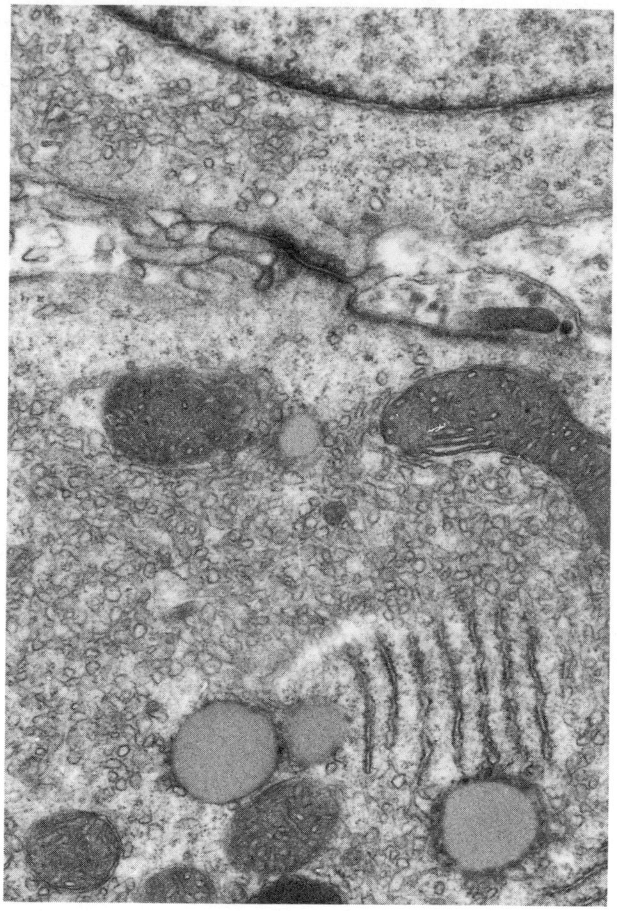

FIG. 25. Part of two early interstitial cells of 20-week-old human ovary. Note abundant agranular endoplasmic reticulum, stacks of granular endoplasmic reticulum and mitochondria with tubular cristae, and lipid droplets. ×22,000.

that remain connected to the intraovarian rete show a uniform enzyme activity in their surrounding granulosa cells (see *Formation of Follicles* subsections). The activity of these cells, as well as that in cells of the intraovarian rete cords proper, shows a steady increase during the third week of life (Fig. 26) and represents the first interstitial tissue (247).

In some species, a so-called hilar rete body, which is formed from the connecting rete (97,282), contains "interstitial hilar gland cells" that exhibit 3β-hydroxy-Δ^5-steroid dehydrogenase activity and have a hormone-dependent morphology. In the human fetus, ovarian hilar cells are present from the thirteenth week onward (282). However, high human chorionic gonadotropin (hCG) levels appear to have little effect on the formation of hilar cells because they are also present in anencephalic fetuses (283).

Experimental Masculinization of the Ovary

As mentioned above, the mammalian gonadal sex is very stabile and controlled by a battery of genes (see *Genetic Control of Gonadal Sex* subsection). It is, however, possible to affect the morphologic differentiation of both the ovarian and testicular anlage by means other than genetic manipulations. Such experiments provide information on the mechanisms controlling gonadal sex differentiation.

Although functional sex change of the mammalian ovary has not yet been achieved, certain characteristics of a testis can be induced. These structures are described as epithelial cords, as tubules with resemblance to seminiferous cords, or as "testicular cords" (for review, see ref. 284). The latter term is probably unfortunate because male germ cells are not present within them and also because well-defined cords and tubules containing oogonia/oocytes differentiate during normal ovarian formation in many species, in particular in species with delayed meiosis (186) (Figs. 6 and 13).

Many studies have been inspired by the old observation that testicular tissue secretes substances during development that virilize neighboring tissue, in particular sex ducts. Masculinizing influences of fetal testicular tissue (285–289) and of adult testis (290) on ovarian differentiation have been widely reported. Not only testicular tissue but also other adult male organs (e.g., the kidney)

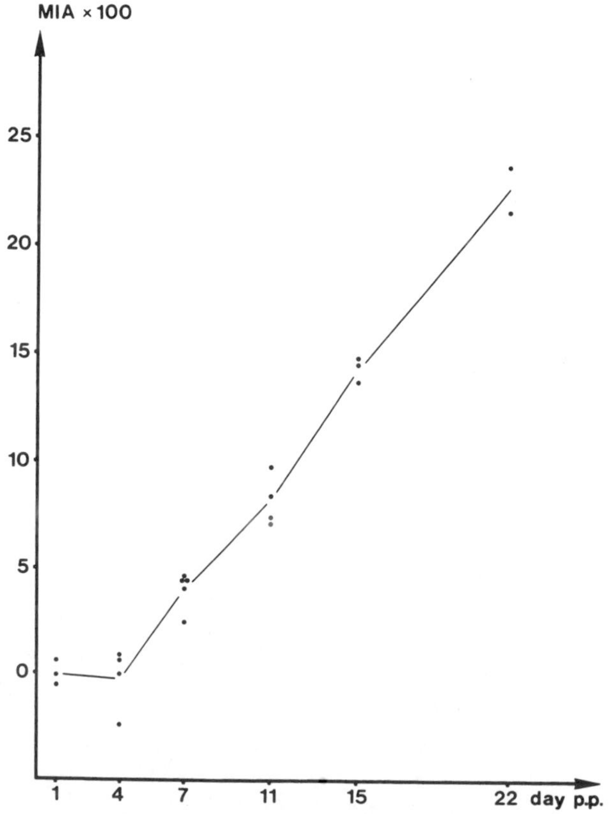

FIG. 26. Changes in activity (*MIA* ×*100:* mean integrated absorbance ×100) of 3β-hydroxy-Δ^5-steroid dehydrogenase in intraovarian rete cells of immature mouse ovary from day 1 to day 22 postpartum (*p.p.*). Each point represents the mean of measurements obtained from one animal of separate litters. (From ref. 247, with permission.)

seem to induce "testicular cords" in transplanted fetal ovaries (291,292).

However, these results could not be reproduced by Ozdzenski et al. (293), or by Burgoyne et al. (294), who suggest instead that the ovarian testicular cords might be structures of mesonephric origin. Neither in cocultures of embryonic mouse ovaries and testes (295) nor of fetal and neonatal rabbit testes and ovaries (186) did any testicular structures develop in the ovaries. It is possible that the length of culture/grafting explains the diversity of these results.

Testicular masculinization of female reproductive organs exists in *nature's* own experiment with freemartins of cattle in which a female and a male twin are connected through the blood circulation (296,297). It was believed that masculinization of the female twin gonads and sex ducts was caused by hormones produced by the male twin. Later, Jost (178) proposed that another substance, which was not testosterone, might be produced in the twin testes, being responsible for the female twin masculinization, in particular for the regression of the müllerian duct (298). This substance is the antimüllerian hormone (AMH), also known as müllerian-inhibiting substance (MIS) (see *Sertoli Cells* subsection). Vigier et al. (299) showed that also the ovaries of fetal rats become affected, like the freemartins after culture in purified bovine AMH. Not only does the number of germ cells decrease and "testislike cords" develop in the ovary, but the steroidogenic capacity also changes: Ovine fetal ovaries exposed to ovine AMH secrete testosterone rather than estradiol because of inhibition of aromatase activity (299). Moreover, fetal rat ovaries, which have been long-time cultured in conditioned media from cultures of fetal or young rat testes, develop cords with germ cells and produce AMH (284).

DIFFERENTIATION OF THE TESTIS

As in the ovary, testicular differentiation and function depend on the enclosure of germ cells into specific compartments (the testicular cords) (Fig. 27). The subsequent differentiation of the two characteristic cell lineages (Leydig cells and Sertoli cells) depends on testicular cord formation: the steroid-producing Leydig cells outside the compartment and the Sertoli cells secreting AMH inside. This compartmentalization appears to be a rather new evolutionary event. In primitive fish, only the secondary spermatocytes and Sertoli cells are separated by the formation of a basement membrane immediately before meiosis begins. Thus, the primary spermatogonia are left outside the compartment. In mammals (in fact, all amniotes), all germ cells and Sertoli cells are, however, confined into the common compartment of testicular cords (300).

Testicular Cords

The first event leading to testicular differentiation seems to be that germ cells gather closely together with

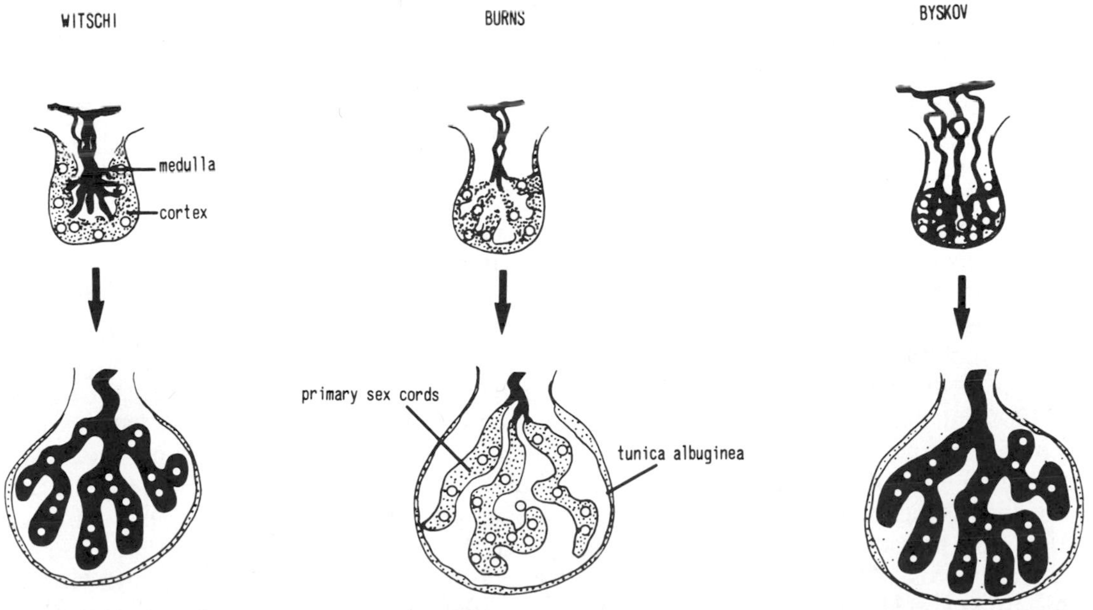

FIG. 27. Models of testicular differentiation from Witschi (70,71), Burns (103), and Byskov (334). Witschi and Byskov proposed that testicular somatic cells originate mainly in mesonephros. In Witschi's model, epithelial-derived cortex degenerates, whereas mesonephric-originated medulla proliferates. In Byskov's model, the epithelium never plays an important role. Burns suggested that surface epithelium proliferates to form primary sex cords, or medulla cords, which develop further into testicular cords. (From ref. 272, with permission.)

some somatic cells, the future Sertoli cells, thereby forming testicular cords. Because the first sign of male gonadal differentiation is noticed in the presumptive Sertoli cells, it is likely that this cell lineage is expressing Sry and initiating testicular formation. Different experiments indicate that germ cells may not be necessary for this process. Testicular cords form in mice in which very few germ cells are present (e.g., in certain mutations [301,302], after irradiation [186], or after treatment with busulphan [100]). The trigger mechanism for the gathering of somatic and germ cells remains uncertain. It has been proposed that the male-specific cell surface histocompatibility antigen (H-Y antigen) of the Sertoli cells may play a role (see *Differentiation of the Gonadal Sex* section). Clusterin, a glycoprotein (present in the rete testis fluid), which performs a cell-aggregating function and which is possibly secreted by the Sertoli cells, may play a role in the early gathering of germ cells (303). Testicular differentiation appears to be independent of the influence of gonadotrophins (304) and steroid hormones (180).

In the differentiating testis of the human embryo (14-mm crown–rump length), germ cells and presumptive Sertoli cells become tightly packed to form one single plate that, in the 30- to 35-mm embryo, is transformed into a network of anastomosing cords (305). Such a reticulum of testicular cord precursors has been reconstructed in the fetal rabbit testis (306). In the newly differentiated fetal rat testis of day 17, the testicular cords are simple arch-formed structures that are arranged more or less perpendicular to the long axis of the testis and connected to the rete testis. During testicular growth, the arches grow in length and become more and more convoluted to form a palisadelike structure without anastomosis (307). Serial sections of the differentiating fetal mouse testis of day 13 indicate that the first aggregations form a few plates or simple arches (Fig. 28) perpendicular to the long axis, thereby resembling the rat model.

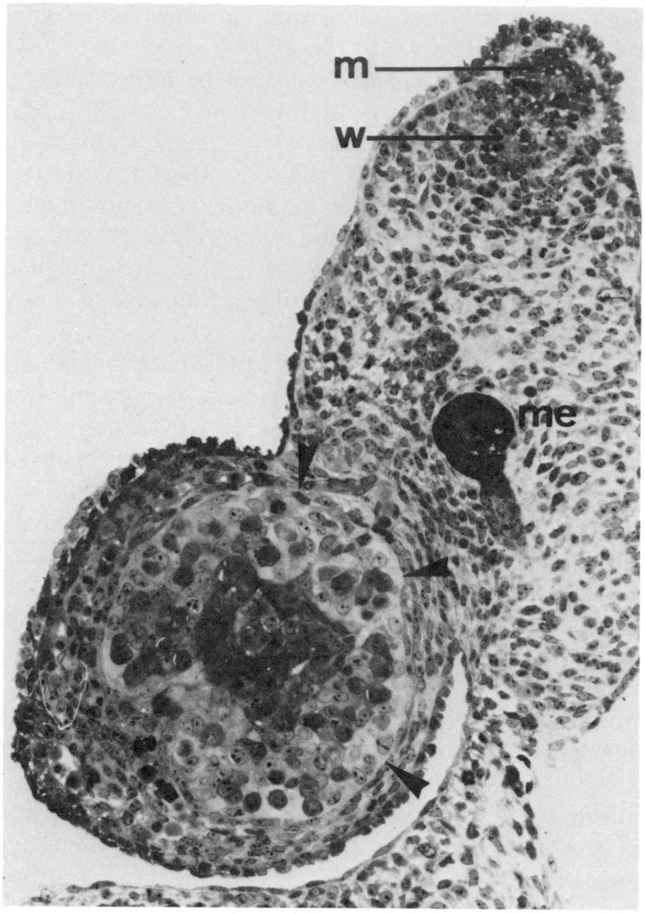

FIG. 28. Cross section of testicular–mesonephric complex of $12\frac{1}{2}$-day-old mouse fetus. A newly differentiated testicular cord forms a simple arch (*arrowheads*). *me,* mesonephric tubule; *m,* müllerian duct; *w,* wolffian duct. ×400.

The precise mechanisms involved in testicular cord formation are not known. However, ultrastructural studies indicate that the formation of an intact basal lamina surrounding the cords is an early and essential event (rat [308], pig [91,309], rabbit [306]). The process of the enclosure of testicular cords occurs fast. In the rat, it takes less than 24 h (308) and often results in cutting off cytoplasm that extends from the Sertoli cells (308,310) (Fig. 29). Simultaneously, a layer of microfilaments is seen in the Sertoli cells close to the basal surface of the cells. It was suggested that this filamentous layer participates in forming the testicular cords (311). In particular, the deposition of fibronectin in and along the site of the forming basal lamina (312), and the expression of types I and III collagens in the Sertoli cells, may play an important role in this morphogenesis (99). Cocultures of rat Sertoli cells and peritubular myoid cells indicated that the formation of the basal lamina requires cooperation between the two cell types (313). Another important morphogenic element in testicular cord formation is probably the intermediate filament proteins keratin and vimentin. While vimentin is constantly expressed during Sertoli cell differentiation, keratins are a transient and early feature of these cells (314,315).

Throughout testicular differentiation, the proximal ends of the testicular cords remain connected to the mesonephric-derived rete testis tissue, which in the human has been called the *rete blastema* (for review, see ref. 94) (Fig. 30). Thus, the mesonephric cells have "free access to the intratubular as well as the interstitial space contributing to the Sertoli cell and the Leydig cell precursor" (81). These cells exhibit high NADH diaphorase activity in the 9-week-old human male (Fig. 31).

During early stages of testicular differentiation, the coelomic epithelium is connected to the testicular cords for a short period while approximately the same cords basally in the gonads are connected to mesonephric rete strands (306). In the rat, the deposition of a continuous layer of fibronectin under the surface epithelium is seen simultaneously with retraction of the testicular cords from the coelomic epithelium (312). At the same time, an increase in the formation of basal lamina material and other extracellular components is seen beneath the surface epithelium (312). These events represent the formation of the tunica albuginea (Fig. 30).

As the testicular anlage grows, the vascularization becomes more prominent. In the fetal pig testis, it was proposed that the ingrowing capillaries could stimulate the differentiation of the testicular cords (91). It was described that testicular cords are first differentiated in the periphery; this area is also the first to become vascularized.

Factors Influencing Testicular Cord Formation

The success of testicular cord formation seems to be correlated to an almost complete separation of the testicular tissue from the mesonephric tissue (310). Almost simultaneously with the cord formation, the testis rounds up, whereby the connection to the mesonephros becomes thin. In the 14-day-old fetal mouse, the testis consists only of a few tiny cords that connect the testicular cords with the developing tubules of the epididymis. In cultures of fetal undifferentiated mouse testes, testicular cord formation can be more or less prevented by leaving the mesonephros together with the testis. In such cultures, the separation between the testis and the mesonephros is impaired; also, the testis does not become rounded, and it retains a broad connection to the mesonephros (310). The formation of testicular cords *in vitro* can also be prevented in the rat by adding serum from rat and other species (316). In contrast, horse serum in cultures of fetal mouse testis seems to be crucial for testicular cord formation (317). Analogs of adenosine cyclic monophosphate also have a preventive effect on testicular cord formation in cultures of fetal mouse testes (318). Forskolin virtually feminizes fetal mouse testis *in vitro* (264,319), an effect also seen in cultures of fetal rat testes (Byskov, *unpublished data*).

It is, in fact, much easier to obtain an immediate effect on testicular differentiation *in vitro* than an effect on the ovary, suggesting that activation/inactivation of genes

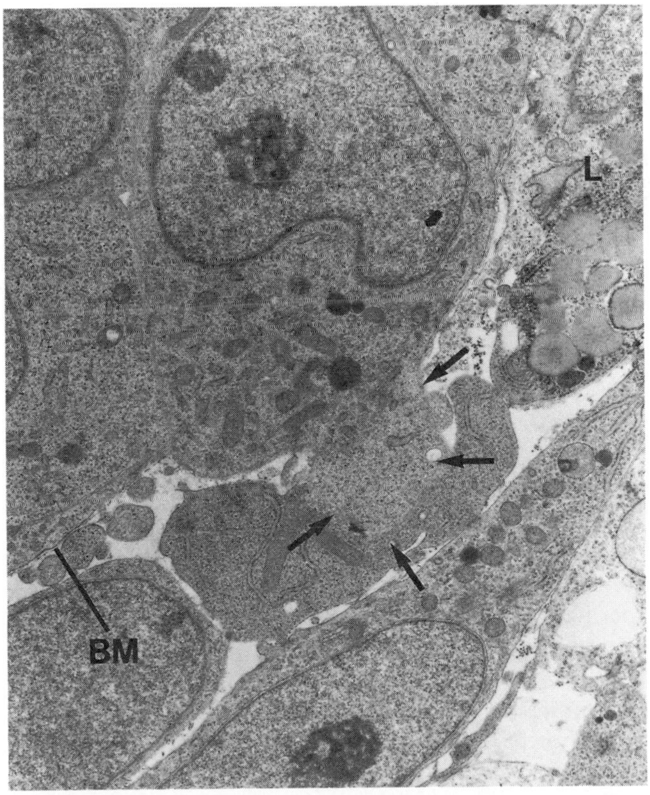

FIG. 29. Part of testicular cord of 14-day-old fetal mouse testis. Cytoplasm of a Sertoli cell (*arrows*) protrudes through basement membrane (*BM*). An early differentiated Leydig cell (*L*) with lipid droplets is seen. ×11,000.

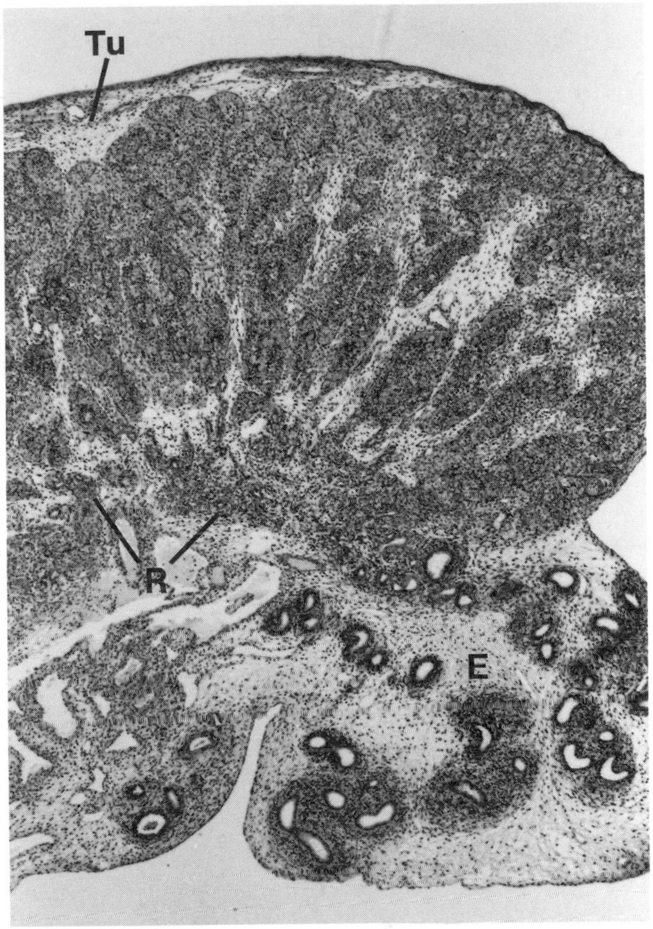

FIG. 30. Part of testis and epididymis (*E*) of a 21-week-old human fetus. The rete testis (*R*) connects testicular cords and epididymis. At places, the tunica albuginea is well demarcated (*Tu*). ×350.

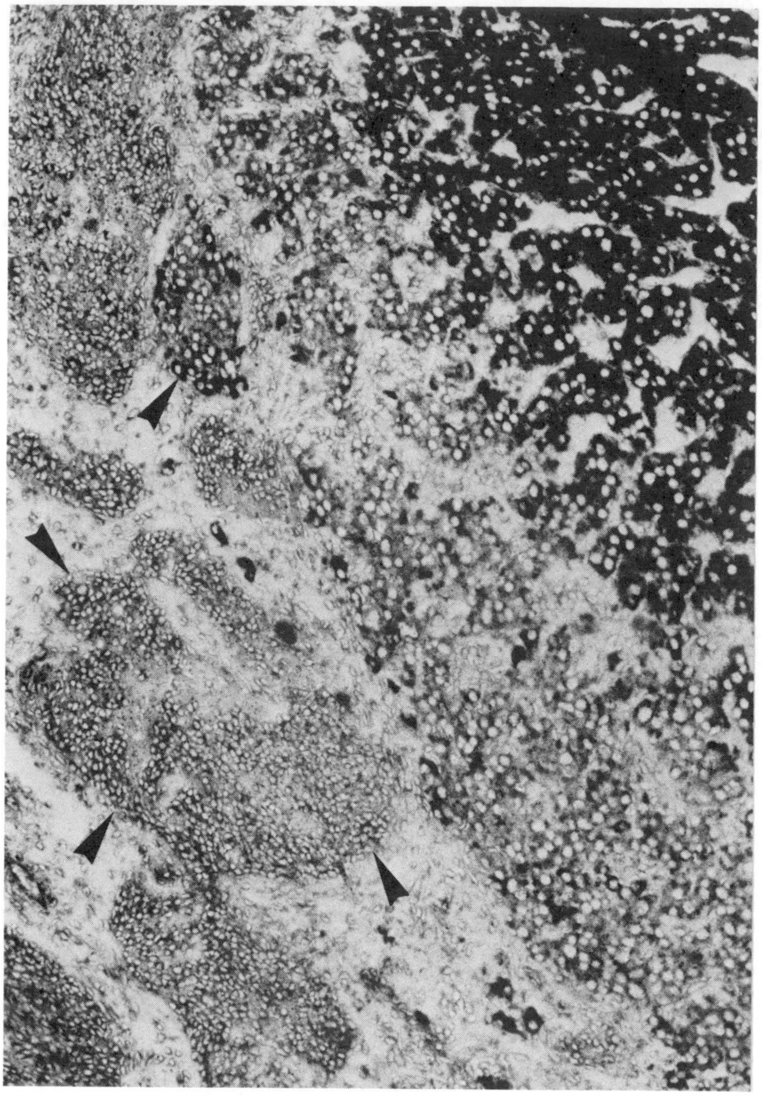

FIG. 31. Cryosection of 9-week-old human fetal testis, showing very strong NADH-diaphorase activity in cells of the testicular cords (*upper right corner*). Strong activity is also present in invading mesonephric cells (*arrowheads*). ×162.

that determine testicular formation are heavily influenced by the environment.

Prespermatogonia

When the male germ cells become enclosed in testicular cords, they are termed *prespermatogonia* (320) (Fig. 32). If the germ cells are not enclosed in testicular cords, they invariably degenerate. However, enclosure itself does not necessarily ensure normal differentiation. During early testicular development, the prespermatogonia enter waves of mitotic divisions, and simultaneously they undergo morphologic differentiation. These events are referred to as *prespermatogenesis* by Hilscher et al. (321), who studied this process in detail in the rat (see also ref. 322). In the fetal rodents (rat [322]; mouse [323,324]), many prespermatogonia divide mitotically shortly after testicular differentiation. They are often gathered in clusters in which the cells divide synchronously. Like oogonia, they are connected by intercellular bridges (197,325–327) (Fig. 33). About day 18 in the rat and day 50 in the pig, prespermatogonia enter the so-called cap phase (328), in which the nucleus becomes eccentric and other organelles agglomerate, forming a cap near the nucleus (Fig. 33). This phenomenon is also seen in the fetal pig prespermatogonia (187). The prespermatogonia in the cap phase of the rat is arrested in interphase (G1) containing 2c DNA (rat [322]; mouse [329,330]). In many species, virtually no mitoses are seen until the second proliferation wave of mitosis begins, shortly before puberty, but in the mouse, mitotic activity is resumed shortly after birth (331).

The pattern of proliferation of the prespermatogonia of other species (e.g., the rabbit and the pig) differs from that of the rat. In both these species, the wave of mitotic

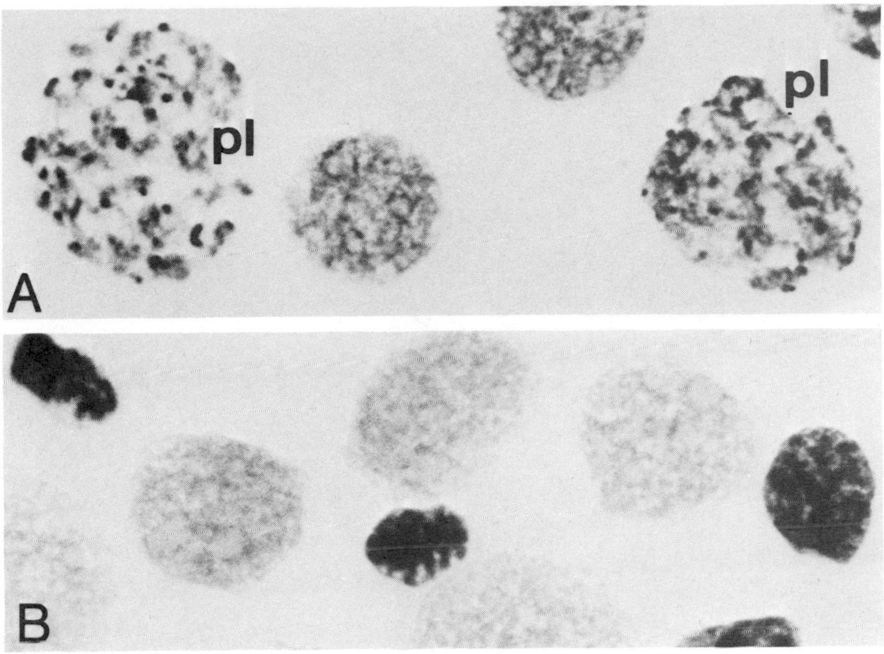

FIG. 32. Feulgen-stained squash preparations of fetal mouse testes showing prespermatogonia. ×5,000. (**A**) A $14\frac{1}{2}$-day-old fetus with two prespermatogonia and two other germ cells in early preleptotene (*pl*) stage. (**B**) A $19\frac{1}{2}$-day-old fetus with several lightly stained prespermatogonia and dark somatic cells.

divisions is delayed with respect to the time of testicular differentiation (rabbit [332]; pig [191]). This period corresponds to the delay period of the oocytes in these species. Thus, the wave of mitosis in prespermatogonia coincides in time with the onset of meiosis in the female (see *Control of Meiosis* section).

In a certain mouse strain (Hi line), it has been shown that in some mice an extended proliferation period of prespermatogonia is correlated to a high incidence of testicular teratomas (323). However, in another group of the same Hi line, about 12% of fetuses at 16 to 18 days of gestation had very few germ cells. All these had testicular teratomas. It appears that germ cell proliferation must be strictly controlled to ensure their normal differentiation. However, the rate of germ cell degeneration during and shortly after proliferation is normally high (rat [333]; rabbit [332]). The reason for this high rate of degeneration is not known, but it has been proposed that a certain ratio between germ cells and Sertoli cells is important for germ cell development (332).

The reaction for alkaline phosphatase remains positive in prespermatogonia, whereas it is lost in diplotene oocytes (see *Transitory Stages of the Meiotic Prophase in Oocytes* subsection). In contrast to oocytes in transitory stages of meiosis, the RNA synthesis remains low in prespermatogonia (192).

Sertoli Cells

Like the granulosa cells, the origin of the Sertoli cells is still uncertain. Various studies indicate that cells derived from the mesonephros contribute to the Sertoli cell population (mouse [75]; sheep [79]) and Witschi (71) and Byskov (334) proposed that testicular somatic cells, including the Sertoli cells, are, in fact, mainly derived from the mesonephros (for review, see ref. 272), although cells of the coelomic epithelium probably also contribute (272). Wartenberg proposed a dual origin of Sertoli cells in the human (77) and rabbit (335), in which a dense dark cell population (the MI cells) could be distinguished from a population of light cells (the MP cells). He proposed that the MI cells (the putative meiosis-inducing cells derived from mesonephros) and the MP cells might be meiosis-preventing cells with origin in the coelomic epithelium. However, in the rat, a cellular marker of the dark cells that could trace them as mesonephric cells could not be found (336). Instead, ultrastructural similarities between early Sertoli cells and mesenchymal cells support the concept that the Sertoli cells differentiate from a central gonadal blastema (337) as proposed by Gropp and Ohno (338). Finally, Sertoli cells have been proposed to originate in the coelomic epithelium (112,339).

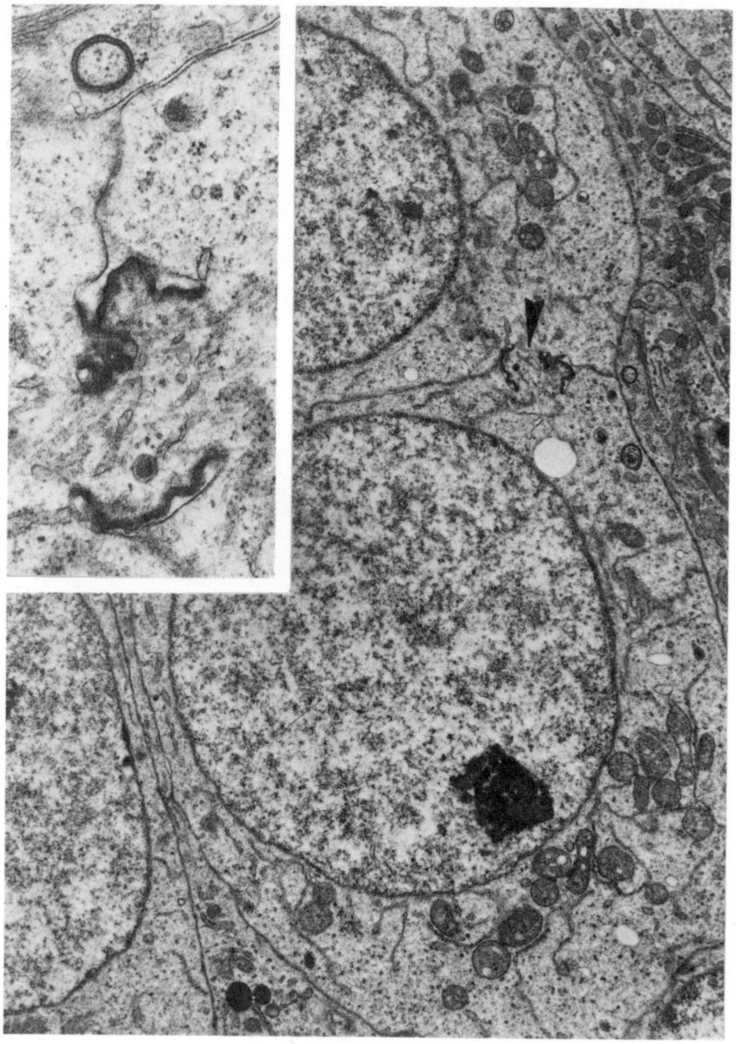

FIG. 33. Part of a testis of 50-day-old fetal pig, showing an intercellular bridge (*arrowhead*) between two prespermatogonia, the lower one having most organelles arranged at one side of its nucleus, thus forming a cap. ×7,640 (**Inset**) Higher magnification of intercellular bridge. ×30,000.

The Sertoli cells proliferate throughout fetal and neonatal development, but when spermatogenesis begins, mitosis in Sertoli cells ceases (340–343). The highest proliferative activity occurs on day 16 in the fetal rat (331).

The remodeling of the "indifferent" gonad into a morphologically recognizable testis has been carefully described in various species (rat [337]; rabbit [306]; pig [309]; mouse [74]; sheep [344]). At the initial stages of testicular differentiation, the Sertoli cells range from irregular to columnar in shape, with the germ cells embedded between them. Gradually, their shape becomes irregular, with cytoplasmic extensions protruding from the apical and lateral borders into neighboring Sertoli cells. This occurs simultaneously with the changed position of the prespermatogonia from a central to a peripheral location (345). Initially, the Sertoli cells are only involved in the formation of desmosomes (346), but gradually the development of incomplete tight junctions and small gap junctions occurs (347). The "tight" junctions lack the parallel and interlacing pattern characteristic of occlusive tight junctions of the fully differentiated Sertoli cells of the adult testis (347). Thus, the fetal Sertoli cells have not yet developed the complex junction attachments that later form the blood–testis barrier in the adult. It has been proposed that the rearrangement of germ cells from a central to a peripheral position may be caused by a series of formations and disruptions of Sertoli cell junctions (347).

Initially, the ultrastructure of the Sertoli cells resembles that of mesenchymal cells with a paucity of organelles (rabbit [348]; rat [205,349]; pig [91,187]). During later stages, the rough endoplasmic reticulum becomes more prominent, a peak in testosterone production is seen (350,351), and close approximations between the endoplasmic reticulum and the plasma membrane have been observed in the pig (187) (Fig. 34).

Little information is available concerning steroidogenic capacity of the fetal Sertoli cells. Androgen secretion was found in explanted fetal guinea pig testes at a stage when no Leydig cells were distinguishable (352). It was suggested that the androgens came from the prospective Leydig cells, although all cell types destined to form

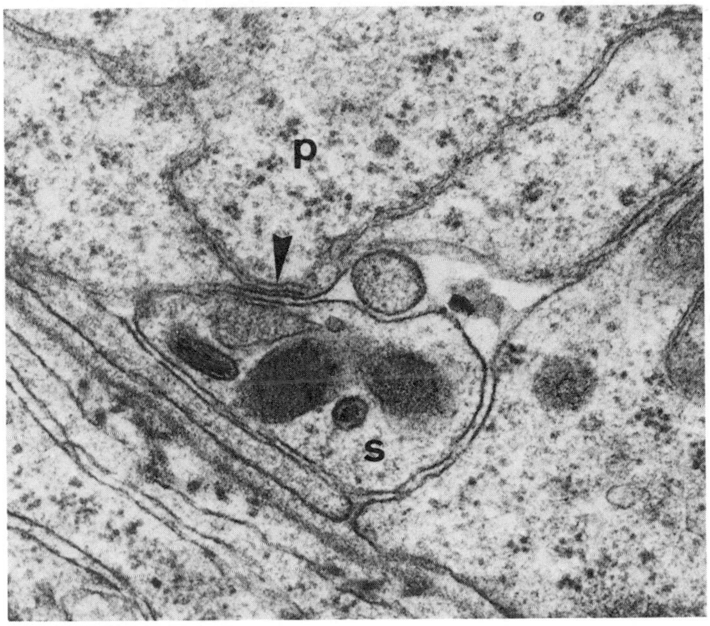

FIG. 34. Peripheral part of testicular cord from 50-day-old fetal pig testis. The endoplasmic reticulum of a Sertoli cell (*s*) and of a prespermatogonium (*p*) is in close proximity to plasma membranes (*arrowhead*). ×50,000.

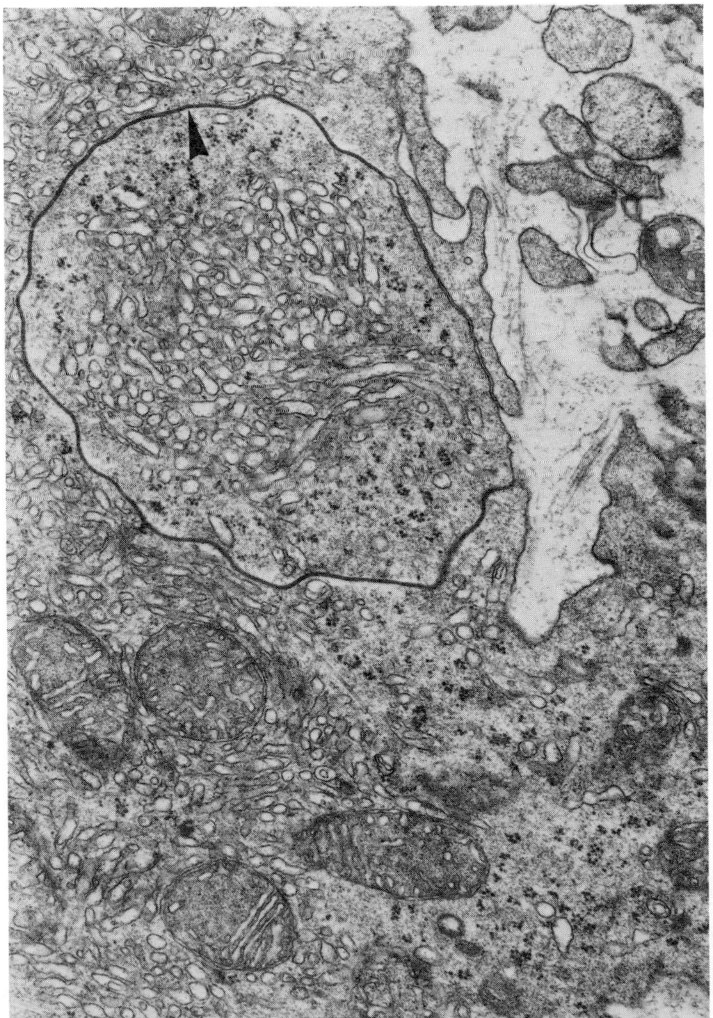

FIG. 35. Leydig cells of a 15-week-old human fetal testis, showing abundant agranular endoplasmic reticulum, mitochondria with tubular cristae, and a gap junction between two adjacent cells (*arrowhead*). ×18,400.

testicular cords, including pre-Sertoli cells, were also present. However, a transitory high activity of 3β-hydroxy-Δ^5-steroid dehydrogenase has been detected in the newly formed testicular cord of fetal pig testes before the early differentiation of Leydig cells takes place (353). Moreover, in the early fetal guinea pig, Black and Christensen (354) observed that some Sertoli cells resembled differentiating Leydig cells with regard to some structural features that may be related to steroidogenesis.

After Jost's discovery in 1947 (178) that the fetal testis induced regression of the müllian duct, it was shown that the Sertoli cells were responsible for the secretion of the AMH, also termed MIS (see *Male Differentiation of Genital Ducts* subsection). Anti-Müllerian hormone is a member of the TGF-β family and has been cloned in several species (for review, see 355). Anti-Müllerian hormone is the first known secretory product of the Sertoli cells. Its initial secretion may be regulated indirectly by Sry, the expression of which in the fetal mouse precedes AMH by 2 days (356). As described later, different physiologic roles besides its regressive activity on müllerian duct have been ascribed to AMH (e.g., inducing descent of the testis in the neonate) (357).

Leydig Cells

In contrast to the ovary, the steroid-producing cells of the testis, namely, the Leydig cells, develop shortly after gonadal sex differentiation has taken place, correlating with the onset of testosterone production. They can first be recognized between the testicular cords in the center of the testis as rounded cells with a dense cytoplasm that is stained by the periodic acid-Schiff (PAS) technique (358). The origin of the fetal Leydig precursor cells has not yet been clarified. They may arise from mesenchymal cells (mouse [331]; human [273,359]; pig [91]) or from mesonephric cells (human, rabbit [335]; mouse [72]; sheep [88]). The Leydig cells only proliferate at a

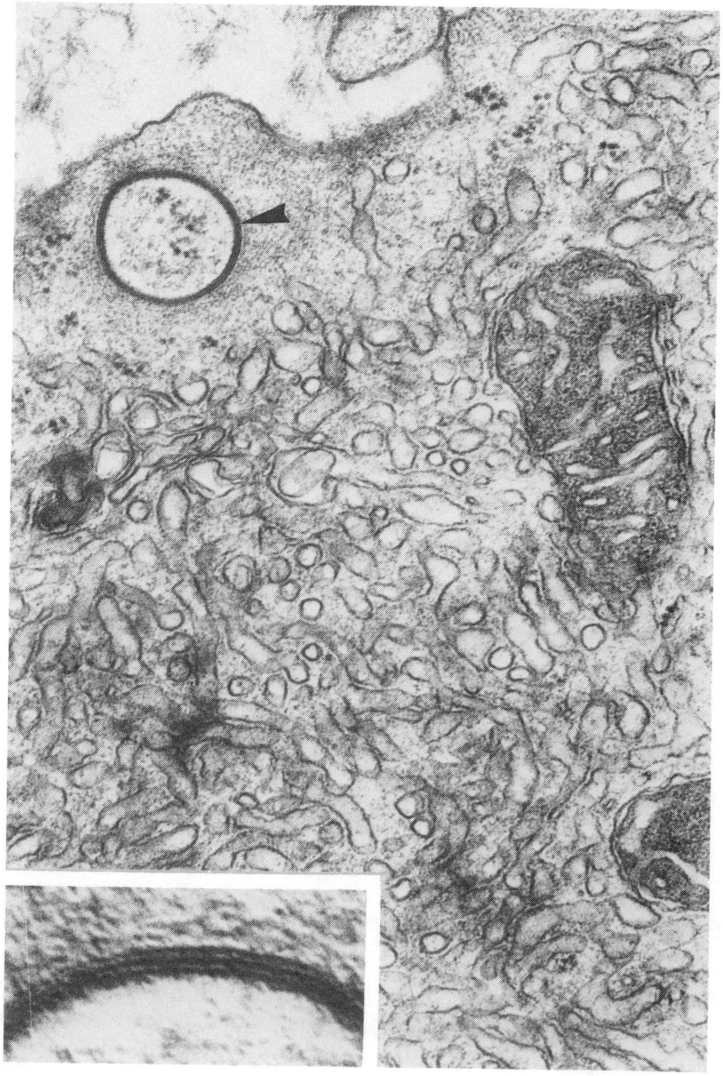

FIG. 36. Peripheral part of cytoplasm from a Leydig cell of 15-week-old human fetal testis, showing a gap junction between two adjacent cells, one of which forms a fingerlike protrusion into the other (*arrowhead*). ×45,600. (**Inset**) Higher magnification of part of the gap junction. ×182,400.

slow rate during early stages of differentiation (331). After birth, mitotic figures in Leydig cells are rarely seen (345). At pubertal life, the number of Leydig cells increases as does the proliferation rate, reaching a peak before maturity (331). This fluctuation in the number of Leydig cells has fostered ideas that these cells might, in fact, arise in fetal life, dedifferentiate around the time of birth, and redifferentiate at puberty (360). However, the response to hCG by fetal Leydig cells diverges from that of adult ones indicating that the fetal Leydig cell population is different from those present in the adult testis (361). The differentiating Leydig cells rapidly gain the typical morphological appearance of steroid-producing cells, with abundant agranular endoplasmic reticulum, mitochondria with tubular cristae, and lipid droplets (for review, see ref. 273) (Fig. 35). Small aggregates of particles as well as gap junctions have been detected on the plasma membrane of differentiating rabbit Leydig cells (195). Gap junctions are also present between differentiated fetal human Leydig cells around the fifteenth week of fetal life (Figs. 35 and 36). The rise in testosterone secretion by the testis is closely correlated with cytodifferentiation and increase in volume of the Leydig cells (320,358,362,363) as well as increase in their number (364). Similarly, testosterone secretion declines when the Leydig cells dedifferentiate during late fetal life (101,348). The well-differentiated Leydig cells also exhibit high activity of 3β-hydroxy-Δ^5-steroid dehydrogenase, NADPH and NADH diaphorases, and glucose-6-phosphate dehydrogenase (365,366) (Figs. 37 and 38). At the same time, high alkaline phosphatase activity is present in the plasma membrane of the Leydig cells (Fig. 9).

What triggers the differentiation of the Leydig cells is not known. However, testicular cord formation always precedes the morphologic differentiation of Leydig cells, and some experiments support the idea that compartmentalization of the testis by the formation of testicular cords is crucial for the formal differentiation and function of the Leydig cells. Cultures of minced fetal mouse

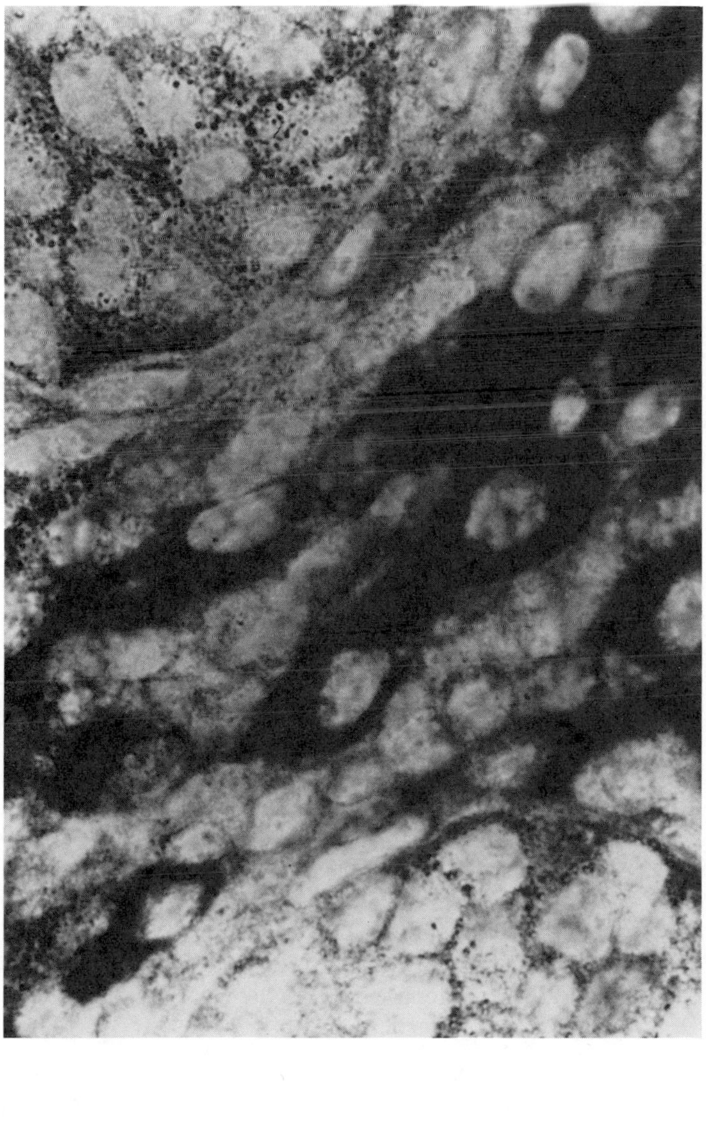

FIG. 37. Cryosection of a 12-week-old human fetal testis, showing very strong NADH-diaphorase activity in Leydig cells (*center*). Cells of testicular cords (*top, bottom*) also show activity. ×1,244.

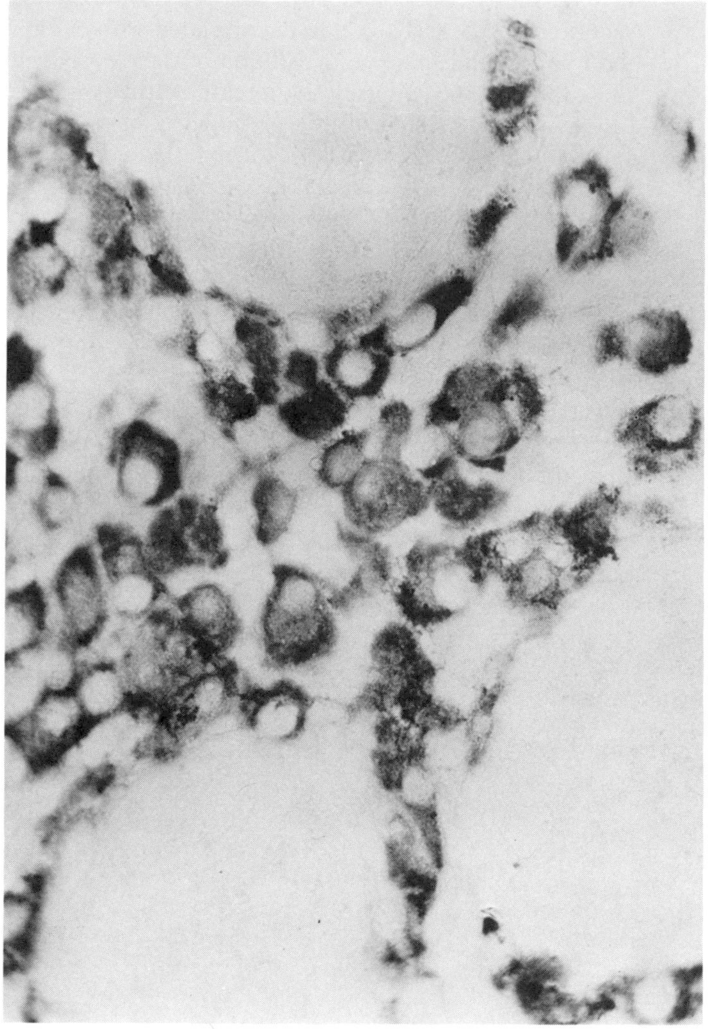

FIG. 38. Cryosection of a 12-week-old human fetal testis, showing NADPH-diaphorase activity in Leydig cells, whereas cells of testicular cords show no or very low activity. ×496.

testes, in which the structure of the testicular cords is disrupted, produce significantly less testosterone, but more progesterone, than do cultures of intact testes (310). The mitochondria of Leydig cells in the minced testes have laminar cristae, and the endoplasmic reticulum is mainly of the granular type, indicating that impaired testicular cord formation influences functional and morphologic differentiation of the Leydig cells.

In vitro, testicular cord formation of the fetal mouse testis is also impaired if a low dose of progesterone (2 μg/ml) is added to the culture medium (367), whereas higher doses do not interfere. Thus, with respect to testicular cord formation, it may be crucial that steroidogenesis by the fetal Leydig cells is delayed.

In the fetal rat testis *in vitro,* testicular cord formation can be prevented when the testicular anlage is cultured in a medium containing fetal calf serum (368,369), human serum, or an α-globulin fraction of human serum (318). In such cordless testes, cells exhibiting 3β-hydroxy-Δ^5-steroid dehydrogenase activity can be traced, but production of testosterone is considerably lower than in the control cultures (370). Despite that, it was concluded that cytodifferentiation of the Leydig cells does not depend on normal differentiation of testicular cords.

The influence of gonadotrophins on Leydig cell differentiation and maintenance has been studied in many species (272). The concentration of chorionic gonadotrophin peaks shortly before Leydig cells differentiate (371); by that time, gonadotrophin receptors are present in fetal testicular cells (372,373). Furthermore, *in vitro* studies of hormone production by fetal rabbit testes indicate that some extrinsic factors initiate steroid synthesis by the fetal testis (87,371). In anencephalic male fetuses, in which the concentration of gonadotrophins is low, few Leydig cells are present (283). Hypophysectomy of fetal monkeys (374) and decapitation of fetal rabbits (304) and fetal monkeys (375) result in depletion of Leydig cells, indicating that the pituitary gland of the fetus is needed for maintenance of Leydig cells. By contrast, in the syndrome of testicular feminization caused by lack

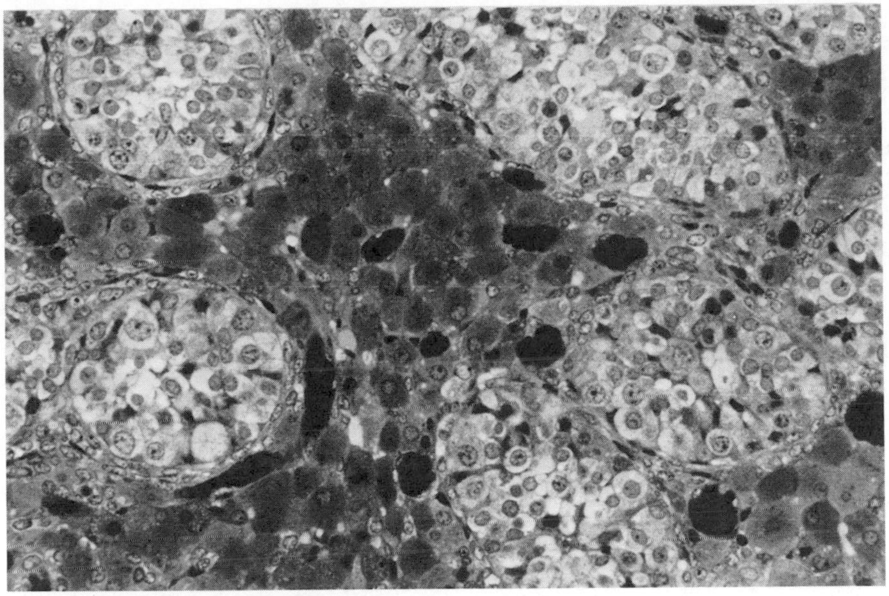

FIG. 39. Part of testis from 20-week-old human fetus with testicular feminization. Number and size of Leydig cells are greatly increased. ×500.

of androgen receptors, the number of Leydig cells is greatly increased (Fig. 39) and the concentration of gonadotrophins is higher than normal (119). These two conditions also suggest the importance of gonadotrophic stimulation of Leydig cell differentiation and maintenance.

CONTROL OF MEIOSIS

The time at which the germ cells enter meiosis differs not only between sexes but also between females of different species (see *Female Germ Cells* and *Male Germ Cells* subsections). Generally, meiosis begins early in life in the female, whereas in the male, meiosis does not start until puberty. This paradigm has led to the theory that an "internal clock" of male and female germ cells might regulate meiosis (14). However, the finding that ectopic mouse germ cells of both sexes, which are localized to the fetal adrenal gland, begin meiosis at the same time that female germ cells enter meiosis in the ovary (376) apparently substantiates the concept that a "meiotic clock" may operate autonomously. However, a meiosis-inducing substance has been detected in the fetal human adrenal glands of both sexes at the time when female meiosis starts (L. Westergaard et al., *unpublished results*). It is therefore uncertain whether the germ cells that enter meiosis in the fetal adrenal gland are triggered by a so-called internal clock or by substances produced by the somatic cells, as proposed by Byskov (186) and Tarkowski (377).

The factors that control the different timing of onset of meiosis in female and male germ cells may depend on their genetic constitution. In the female germ cells, it seems that both X chromosomes must be active before meiosis begins (47,59,378). However, *in vivo,* male germ cells are able to enter meiosis simultaneously with the female germ cells if they are situated in the vicinity of the mesonephric tissue, outside the testicular cords (379), or in the adrenal gland (186).

It is conceivable that initiation of meiosis is not controlled by a single parameter but that a series of factors are interacting, such as a "genetic clock," formation of a specific micromilieu around the germ cells, and local production of growth factors or hormones (e.g. steroids) (380). In cultures of late fetal rabbit ovaries, the pituitary gland promoted meiosis, indicating an important role of this gland, at least in this species (381). Specific meiosis-regulating substances are also suggested to play an important role. A meiosis-inducing substance is produced in cultures of ovaries or testes with germ cells undergoing meiosis (295) and a meiosis-preventing substance (MPS) is produced by fetal testes in which meiosis is held in abeyance (379). The activity of the two substances is evaluated by their ability to induce or prevent meiosis in cultured fetal mouse testes or ovaries, respectively (186). Although the nature of the two substances is not yet fully understood, different experiments indicate that meiosis-inducing substance is a small molecule (less than 2 kDa) with lipophilic and to some extent also hydrophilic characteristics and that MPS is a small peptide (367). Previous suggestions that meiosis-inducing substance might be a PAS-positive substance (97), possibly a glycoprotein incorporating ^{3}H-fucose (382), have not yet been confirmed. Meiosis-inducing substance and MPS are apparently not species-specific because media containing these substances (obtained from testes of bulls and humans) induce and prevent (respectively) meiosis in fetal mouse testes/ovaries (186). Recent *in vitro* studies of fetal mouse testes indicate that receptors for meiosis-inducing substance exist in germ cells and/or neighboring cells (319).

Regulatory Genes and Meiosis

Germ cells and somatic cells are subject to different genetic regulatory systems in particular because germ cells at a certain stage of development must switch from mitosis to meiosis and undergo the unique meiotic divisions. Although the list of genes for regulatory proteins expressed during meiosis in mammals is growing (383), little is still known about the role of these proteins early in meiosis, in particular in female germ cells. In the adult mouse testis, a new gene, *meg1,* has been identified, characterized, and localized with most abundance in pachytene spermatocytes (384). Whether this gene is also expressed in female meiotic germ cells is unknown. In the mouse, a zinc-finger protein gene is especially expressed after the pachytene stage in both male and female germ cells (385). A gene product responsible for initiation of meiosis has not yet been identified.

As mentioned earlier (see *Primordial Germ Cells* subsection), differential DNA methylation is correlated to activation–inactivation–reactivation of the X chromosome. In the human fetal ovary, the early meiotic oocytes appear to be unmethylated (65), whereas male germ cells become methylated postnatally in connection with the onset of meiosis and spermatogenesis (386).

Female Germ Cells

The first germ cells that enter meiosis in the fetal ovary are always seen in the central basal part of the ovary, close to the mesonephric connection (for review, see ref. 272). Gradually, more peripherally situated oogonia enter meiosis (Fig. 14). For instance, in the human fetal ovary, the first meiotic germ cells are seen around the third month, whereas peripherally situated germ cells are still entering meiosis during the eighth month (34). Therefore, if an "internal clock" does exist, it must obviously be influenced by factors of the local environment. The old observations that meiosis is initiated close to the mesonephric connection led to the hypothesis that mesonephric-derived cells induce meiosis (329). In support of this theory are the findings that meiosis in cultures of fetal ovaries is dependent on the presence of mesonephric tissue of the mouse (83) and hamster (387). However, in other species, meiosis appears not to be influenced by the mesonephros (rat [388]; rabbit [186]). This discrepancy may be related to the pattern of ovarian development in different species (e.g., between species with immediate and delayed meiosis) (see *Different Patterns of Early Ovarian Differentiation* subsection). In the rabbit ovary, which exhibits delayed meiosis, it has not been possible to induce meiosis during the delay period (186). This may be a result of the enclosure of germ cells in cordlike structures, which may create an unfavorable milieu comparable with the conditions in the fetal testicular cords. As mentioned in the *Different Patterns of Early Ovarian Differentiation* subsection, steroids are secreted by ovaries during the delay period. It is possible that onset of meiosis does not occur simultaneously with production of substantial amounts of steroids in the ovary.

That a meiosis-inducing substance is secreted by ovaries at the time when meiosis begins has been shown in cocultures between fetal mouse ovaries and testes. Ovaries containing germ cells in early stage of meiosis induce meiosis in the male germ cells of cocultured fetal testes (295). Meiosis-inducing substance is also present in follicular fluid of preovulatory follicles of human and cow in increasing concentration from 6 h after the preovulatory gonadotrophic peak until ovulation (389,390).

The hypothesis has been advanced that meiosis of female germ cells is triggered by meiosis-inducing substance and arrested in the diplotene stage by the action of MPS (186) or the so-called oocyte maturation inhibitor (OMI), produced by the granulosa cells (391; for review, see ref. 392). Thus, meiosis of female germ cells may be controlled by the relative concentration of meiosis-inducing substance and MPS (186). In oocytes of amphibians and other vertebrate classes, cytostatic factors, which stabilize maturation promoting factor (MPF), could also be responsible for oocyte arrest in the diplotene stage (for review, see ref. 393).

Male Germ Cells

In the adult testis, several genes have been cloned that are specifically expressed during different stages of spermatogenesis (383,394). Normally male germ cells do not enter meiosis until puberty. However, meiotic germ cells are seen in fetal testes of different species at the same time that meiosis begins in the ovary of the coeval female fetus (mouse [86]; cat [55]; human [395]). Such meiotic male germ cells are situated outside the testicular cords, in close apposition to the mesonephric tissue (86). As in the female, it seems likely that meiosis-inducing substance is produced by the mesonephric-derived tissue and that male germ cells are able to respond to the substance by entering meiosis. The reason that germ cells within testicular cords do not enter meiosis may be because of the presence of MPS within the testicular cords (379). The presence of MPS in testes has been demonstrated in fetal testes cocultured with fetal ovaries in which meiosis became inhibited (295) and in immature and adult testes that secrete MPS during short-time cultures (396). Because meiosis-inducing substance is also produced by the pubertal and adult testes, it is possible that also in the testis, meiosis may be regulated by the relative concentration of these two substances.

STEROID HORMONE PRODUCTION IN THE DEVELOPING GONADS

Ovary

For a long time, it has been assumed that the fetal ovary was incapable of *de novo* synthesis of steroids. The human fetal ovary, for instance, has been reported to secrete steroids only in the last part of fetal life (397). However, other species, namely, those with delayed meiosis, often produce large amounts of estrogen at early stages of ovarian differentiation during the delay period (sheep [398]; rabbit [88,275]; cow [399]; guinea pig [400]). Obviously, the time at which *de novo* steroid synthesis begins varies greatly between species. However, the enclosure of germ cells in specific compartments (either germ cell cords or follicles) seems to play a major role in differentiation of the steroid-producing cells. In primates in which specific germ cell cords are not formed and in which meiosis begins early, estradiol production *de novo* is not seen until follicles begin to grow late in fetal life (401–403), but the aromatizing system responsible for conversion of androgens to estrogens is already active at the eighth week of fetal life (404). In ovaries of other species, steroid production *de novo* is nil or very low during the period when meiosis occurs (mouse [405]; rat [2,406]).

Early *de novo* steroid production in species with delayed meiosis takes place only during the delay period, when germ cells are enclosed in cordlike structures. By the end of the delay period when meiosis begins, the steroid production decreases or ceases, but it rises again when follicles form (399).

It is not known how steroid synthesis is initiated in the ovary. Thus, it is unclear whether the high level of hCG

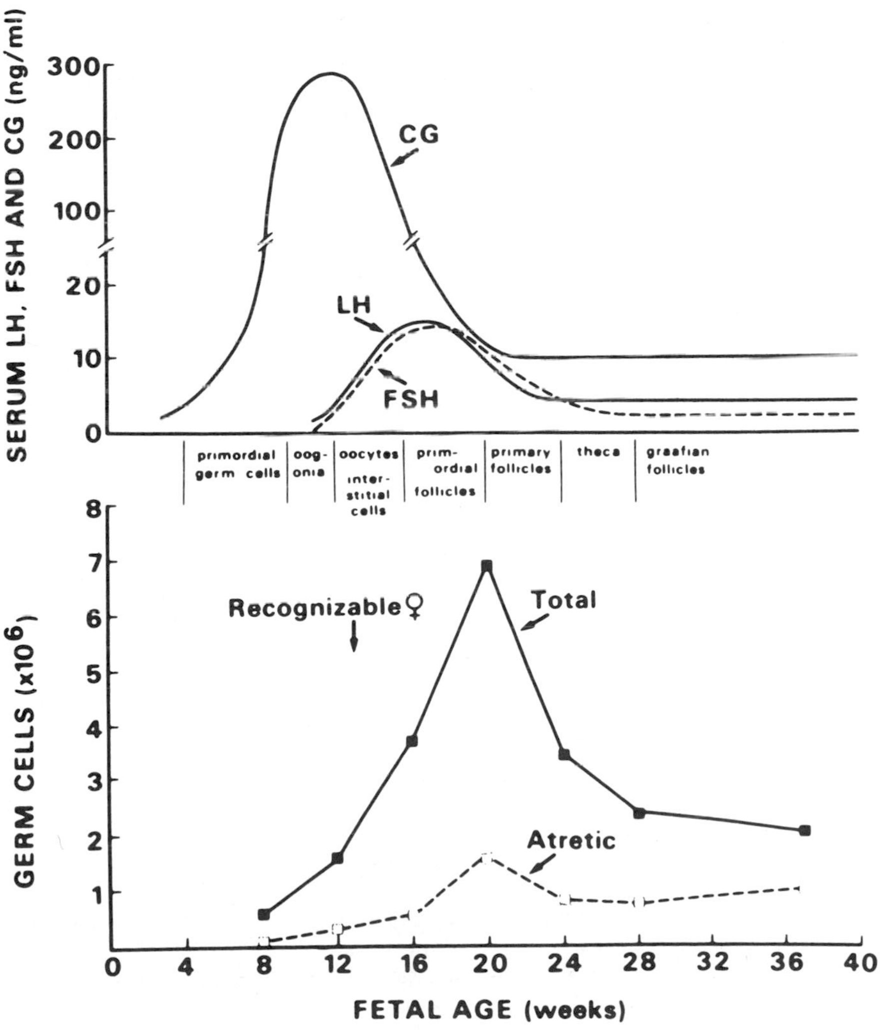

FIG. 40. Schematic summary of temporal relationship in female human fetus between mean serum concentrations of hCG (*CG*), LH, and FSH; ovarian morphology; and the ovarian content of germ cells. From ref. 424, with permission.

present before and during early differentiation of the fetal ovary initiates steroid production, but very early, enzymes necessary for conversion of androgens to estrogens are present (guinea pig [407]; rat [408]) (Fig. 40).

Fetal ovarian steroid synthesis by rabbit (350) and rat (406) seems independent of gonadotrophins, whereas gonadotrophins stimulate steroid synthesis by the fetal mouse ovary (405). However, estradiol production by the fetal bovine ovary is stimulated by LH during the delay period, but the ovary becomes refractory by the end of the delay period (399). Steroid synthesis by the fetal pig ovary *in vitro* is enhanced by exposure to hCG or LH (409) during the delay period.

It is not known to what extent fetal ovarian cells use other steroids (e.g., those that originate in the liver [410] or in the adrenal cortex [411]).

Testis

In all the mammalian species that have been studied, the newly sex-differentiated testis is able to synthesize testosterone *de novo* from acetate (for review, see ref. 412). Testicular steroids are responsible for maintenance of growth and differentiation of the internal and external genitalia (178–180,413). Moreover, fetal testicular androgens are generally believed to be necessary for priming the brain in the male direction at early developmental stages (414–417). Recent studies on cultured dopaminergic neurons from 14-day-old rat fetuses show, however, that sexual dimorphism developed *in vitro* (418). Because systemic differences in testosterone concentration do not occur until around day 18 in the fetal rat (419), it seems that factors other than androgens—possibly genetic sex?—are responsible for sexual differentiation of the brain (420). Also, hormones or substances of testicular origin, in particular AMH, may control testicular descent from the abdominal position into the scrotum (421,422).

As in the ovary, the mechanisms that cause initiation of the steroid synthesis in the fetal testis are not known. *In vitro* experiments have shown that steroid production by sex-differentiated testes can be stimulated by hCG and LH (for review, see ref. 423). In the human, it is possible that hCG stimulates fetal androgen production by the testis, because the rise, peak, and fall in hCG content are closely mirrored by testosterone secretion (human [424]) (Fig. 41). In cultures of hCG-treated human fetal testicular tissues, the secretion of testosterone is facilitated by low-density lipoprotein (LDL) cholesterol (425). Because the content of LDL receptors fluctuates with the level of hCG, it is possible that the concentration of LDL cholesterol is regulated by hCG (425). The content of gonadotrophin receptors in fetal testicular tissue rises concomitantly with increasing testosterone secretion. In the human, for example, the number of hCG

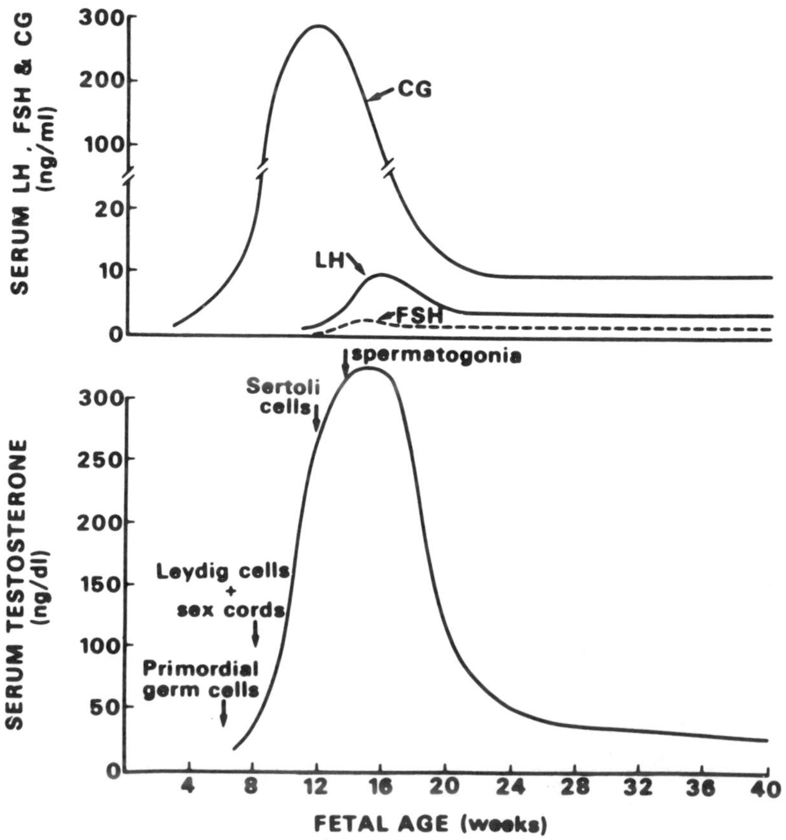

FIG. 41. Schematic summary of temporal relationship in the male human fetus between mean serum concentrations of hCG (*CG*), LH, and FSH and of mean serum concentration of testosterone and testicular morphology. (From ref. 424, with permission.)

receptors and the amount of testosterone both reach a peak between the fifteenth and the eighteenth week of gestation (426). In the fetal rat, the content of LH receptors rises simultaneously with increase in testosterone secretion, but the content of LH receptors continues to increase until after birth, whereas the levels of intratesticular testosterone and hCG decrease (427). The fall in placental hCG during the latter part of fetal life seems to be crucial for the decrease of testosterone production. This may be of particular importance because fetal Leydig cells, at least *in vitro,* remain sensitive to hCG stimulation. In contrast to the adult, cultured fetal Leydig cells of human, monkey, and rat are able to respond to sustained concentration of gonadotrophin by testosterone production without being desensitized (428).

The time at which the peak of testosterone occurs during fetal life also seems to be very important for maturation of the central nervous system. In rat fetuses of stressed mothers, in which the surge of testosterone appears earlier than normal, the male offspring achieves a feminized behavioral pattern (425). Other steroids (e.g., from fetal adrenal gland) may also interfere with testosterone production, because fetal rat testes secrete more testosterone after stimulation with adrenocorticotrophin (429).

FORMATION AND DIFFERENTIATION OF GENITAL DUCTS

In contrast to gonadal formation, the reproductive tracts of male and female (the wollfian duct and the müllerian duct, respectively) differ from the very beginning of their formation (Fig. 42). Their ability to differentiate into functional reproductive tracts depends completely on the gonadal sex. In the male, testicular secretion of testosterone is responsible for growth and differentiation of the wollfian duct to form epididymis, vas deferens, and seminal vesicle, whereas testicular secretion of AMH causes müllerian duct regression (Fig. 43). In the female, these two hormones are not present at this stage of development, allowing the müllerian duct to grow and give rise to the oviduct, uterus, and the upper part of vagina, whereas the wollfian duct degenerates in the absence of testosterone (Fig. 43). Apparently, devel-

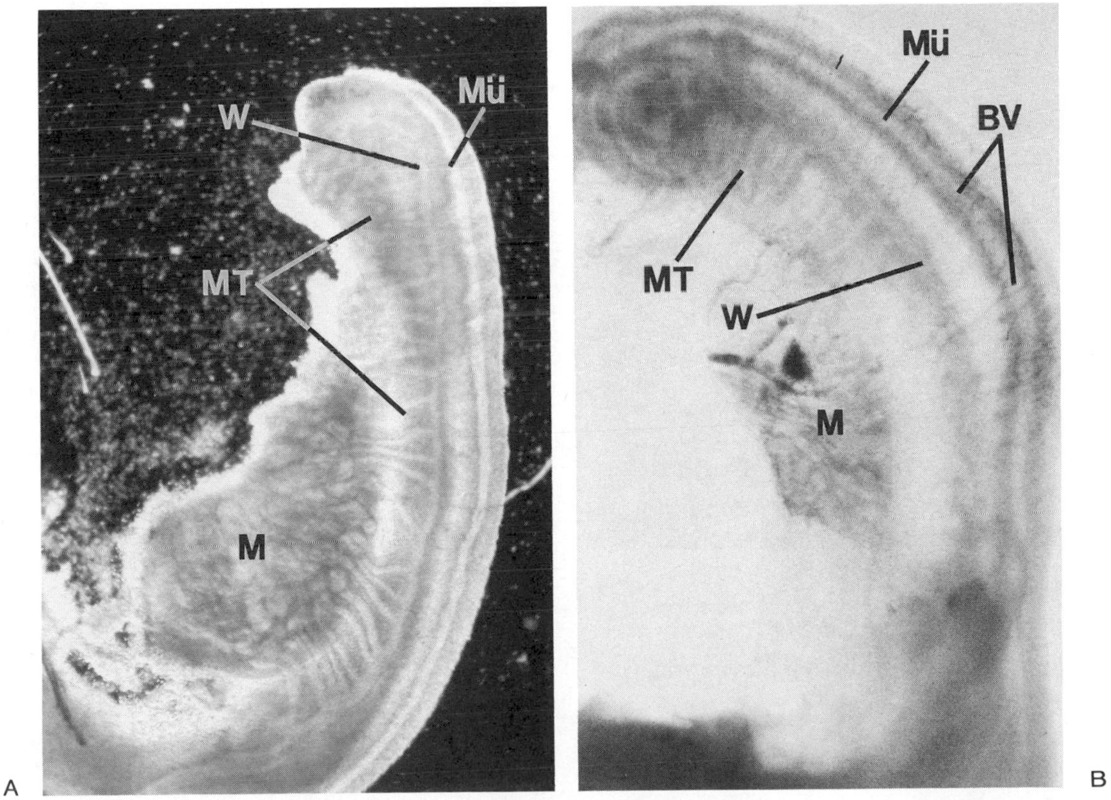

FIG. 42. Whole mount preparations of cranial and middle parts of urogenital ducts and mesonephros of two human female fetuses from which gonads have been removed. (**A**) 9 weeks old. Mesonephros (*M*) is still prominent, with many tubules connecting to wolffian duct (*W*). Müllerian duct (*Mü*) is still rather thin. (**B**) 12 weeks old. Mesonephros is regressing and only cranially placed tubules (*MT*) connect to the wolffian duct (*W*). Müllerian duct (*Mü*) is well developed, wrapped in a network of blood vessels (*Bv*), and with a distinct lumen.

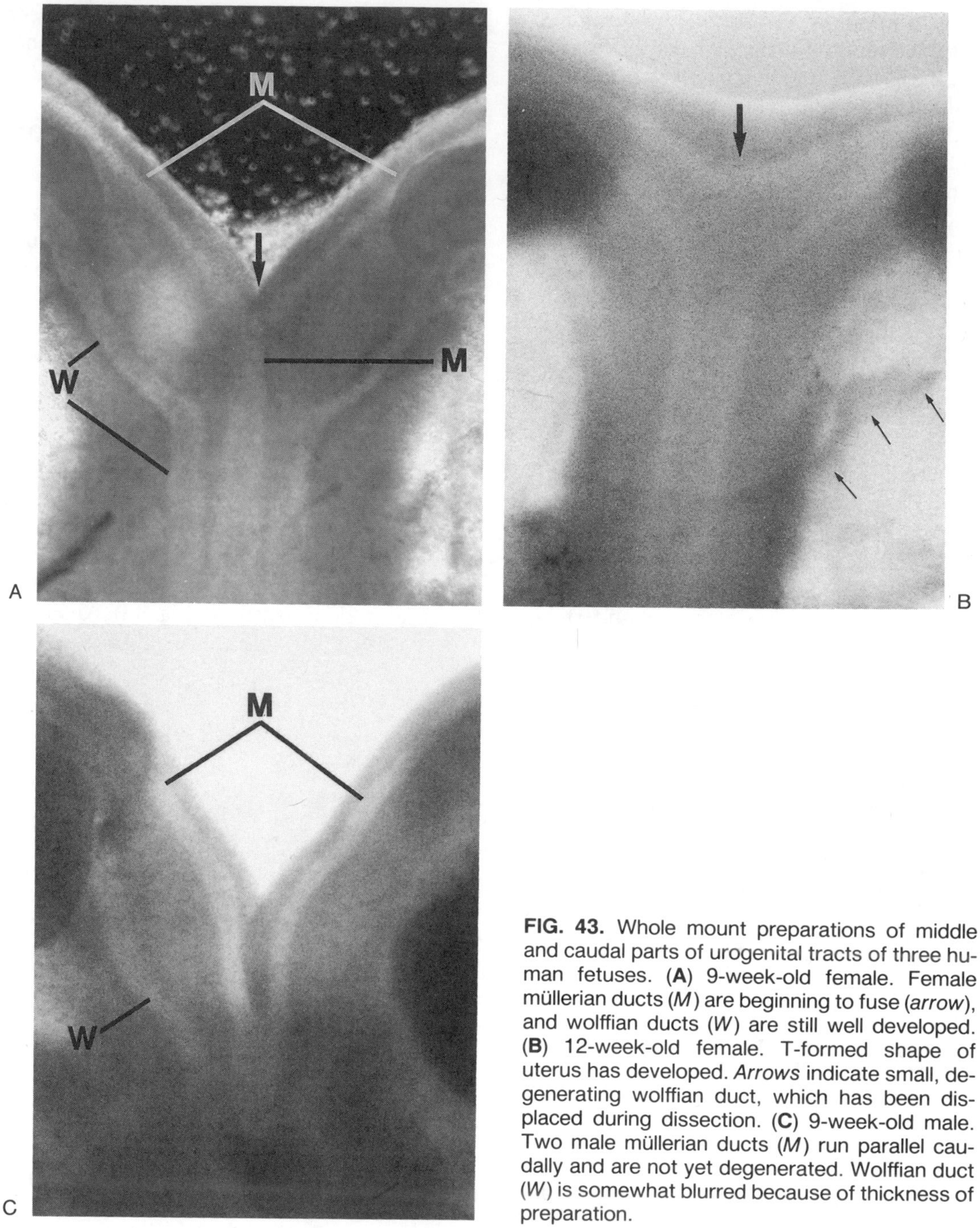

FIG. 43. Whole mount preparations of middle and caudal parts of urogenital tracts of three human fetuses. (**A**) 9-week-old female. Female müllerian ducts (*M*) are beginning to fuse (*arrow*), and wolffian ducts (*W*) are still well developed. (**B**) 12-week-old female. T-formed shape of uterus has developed. *Arrows* indicate small, degenerating wolffian duct, which has been displaced during dissection. (**C**) 9-week-old male. Two male müllerian ducts (*M*) run parallel caudally and are not yet degenerated. Wolffian duct (*W*) is somewhat blurred because of thickness of preparation.

opment/regression of ducts in the female are independent of ovarian secretions.

Undifferentiated Ducts

The Müllerian and Wolffian ducts do not arise simultaneously. The Wolffian duct is the excretory duct of the mesonephros (see *Mesonephros* subsection); it is recognizable well before the gonads form (Fig. 11). The müllerian duct (i.e., the paramesonephric duct) develops in a cranial–caudal direction along the wolffian duct around the time when the gonads form. The literature provides various conflicting hypotheses on the ontogeny of the paramesonephric duct. The wolffian duct may simply serve as guidance for the early growth of the müllerian duct (430,431). Other studies based on morphologic observations suggest, however, that the wolffian duct releases epithelial cells that contribute to the developing müllerian duct as it is growing caudally (432–434). Experiments with chick embryos provide evidence for autonomous growth of the müllerian duct, without excluding cellular contribution from the wolffian duct (435). Applying immunohistochemical methods in fetal hamster genital ducts, Viebahn et al. (436) provided results that do not support the concept of cellular contribution from the wolffian duct to the müllerian duct: The pattern of expression of intermediate filaments (vimentin and keratins) differed between the müllerian and the wolffian ducts but virtually not between sexes of the same duct. The initial formation of the müllerian duct appears to start by invagination of the coelomic epithelium lateral to the cranial end of the mesonephric duct. This invagination persists in the female and develops into the abdominal ostium (437). However, in the fetal rabbit, the anlage of the müllerian duct seems to arise from a cell cord that develops in close proximity to the cranial part of the wolffian duct (A. G. Byskov and P. E. Høyer, *unpublished results*). A similar pattern of development has been described in the chick (438). When the caudal blind tips of the müllerian ducts reach the pelvic area, they have crossed ventrally to the wolffian ducts to reach and fuse with each other in the midline dorsocranially to the urogenital sinus.

At early stages of differentiation, both mesonephric and paramesonephric ducts are simple straight tubules lined with a single-layered epithelium consisting of cells ranging from squamous to cylindrical. As they grow, the epithelium becomes taller, with the nuclei situated in the basal part. The epithelial cells of the early wolffian duct of rat and mouse are rich in glycogen, dense bodies, and lysosomes (439). The rat müllerian duct has a tiny lumen at the time of sex differentiation. The tightly packed columnar cells are rich in free ribosomes and contain a well-developed supranuclear Golgi apparatus (440). Parallel to the epithelial growth, mesenchymal cells are arranged in concentric layers around the ducts. Further differentiation of the genital ducts is dependent on mesenchymal–epithelial interaction, in which the mesenchyme probably is the target and mediator of morphogenic action by hormones and other substances (for review, see ref. 441).

Female Differentiation of Genital Ducts

Female Müllerian Duct

In the female, the cranial part of the müllerian duct develops into the oviduct, or the fallopian tubes, the middle part develops into the uterus, and the caudal part may contribute to the cranial part of the vagina (Figs. 2, 42, and 43). In some species, the müllerian tubes remain separated as paired uteri (e.g., mouse and rat), whereas in others they fuse to form a simplex type of uterus (442). The early differentiating oviduct can be distinguished from the uterus by its coiling and smaller diameter. A muscular layer develops around the oviductal tubules, the epithelium of which invaginates and folds. The epithelial cells may either develop cilia or later become secretory (443). Relatively early in development, the oviduct differentiates into three segments: the ampulla, the infundibulum, and the isthmus. In humans and the guinea pig, both of which have an extended gestational period, most of these developmental steps occur during the midgestational period. In species that have a shorter gestation (e.g., the hamster, the mouse, and the rat), differentiation of the oviduct takes place after birth (443).

Differentiation of the uterus starts simultaneously with that of the oviduct. The junction between uterus and oviduct early becomes clearly distinguishable by the abrupt increase in uterine diameter. Demarcation between uterus and vagina takes place later; in the human, this occurs in the latter part of the third month (444) when the vaginal fornices develop. In the human fetus at about $9\frac{1}{2}$ weeks, the uterus begins to differentiate into an upper part (the corpus) and a lower part (the cervix) (445). They are both initially the same length, but the cervix gradually reaches two-thirds of the total length at birth (442). During the second trimester, the main components, such as glands and muscular coat, develop. Glands are first seen in the cervical part at 17 weeks and then appear about 2 weeks later in the corpus. At midgestation, mesenchyme surrounding both wolffian and müllerian ducts condenses and forms the early muscular layer of the uterus (442). The growing muscular layer of the upper part of the corpus participates in formation of the convex-shaped fundus (445). During the third trimester, mucinous cells appear in the cervix, whereas secretory cells only occasionally are seen in the endometrium at birth. These cytologic characteristics may be induced by estrogens and/or progesterone (446). However, it is not certain how endometrial growth and differentiation are controlled during early stages of fetal life.

Early development and growth of the müllerian duct are generally considered to occur autonomously (447). Apparently, no stimulation is required for differentiation of the female genital tract. Neither decapitation nor castration of fetal female rabbit fetuses prevented growth of the müllerian duct (178,304). Normal development also takes place in genital tracts of fetal rats cultured in steroid-free culture medium (448). Therefore, neither gonadotrophins nor the ovary are necessary for differentiation of the female genital tract (449). Development of the müllerian duct also appears to be independent of bFGF in contrast to the male reproductive tract (450).

Although the development of the paramesonephric duct is not an estrogen-dependent process (178), estrogen receptors have been detected in müllerian ducts of fetal rats (447) and guinea pigs (451) during the last part of gestation. In the mouse, estrogen receptors were detected by immunocytochemical assays and immunoblots already from day 15 of fetal life (452). Exposure of DES, a synthetic estrogen, to the developing female reproductive tract caused deleterious and permanent alterations in human and mice (453,454) and even affected the ovary of the offspring (455). These studies suggest that exogenous estrogens can affect the development of the female reproductive tract, although the role—if any—of the endogenous estrogens is unclear. In a transfilter coculture between fetal mouse genital ridges and ovaries, Byskov and Hansen (456) showed that the ovary influences growth and differentiation of the oviduct when placed closely together: Newly differentiated fetal mouse ovaries stimulate growth of the stromal tissue of the female duct system; older fetal ovaries suppress growth of both müllerian duct epithelium and the surrounding stroma of younger fetuses, indicating ovarian secretion of duct-inhibitory substances. Secretion of AMH is, however, not detected in the ovary until postnatally, when it is first visualized in the mouse ovary on day 6 in the granulosa cells of growing follicles (356). Because the fetal female müllerian duct regresses when exposed to AMH, it is crucial that AMH expression is not induced in the ovary until later. That the fetal female müllerian duct can respond to AMH was shown in the classical experiments by Jost (178): Grafts of fetal rabbit testes into fetal rabbit females, close to the genital ducts, induced degeneration of the female müllerian duct, whereas implants of crystals of testosterone had no effect.

Female Wolffian Duct

During normal female development, the wolffian duct invariably degenerates because of the lack of androgens. Degeneration begins shortly after gonadal sex differentiation (Fig. 2). In the human, it is generally finished at the beginning of the third trimester (439). However, before degeneration is completed, the caudal part of the wolffian duct gives origin to the ureteric bud and contributes to the bladder and urethra (437). It may also be incorporated in the vaginal plate (457,458).

The wolffian duct of both sexes of rabbits castrated early in fetal life degenerates unless exposed to implants of testosterone (178). Moreover, in cultures of genital ridges of fetal rats (459,460) and mice, growth and differentiation of the wolffian duct only occur when cocultured with testicular tissue or by adding testosterone. Prenatal exposure to DES also seems to prevent the total regression of the wolffian duct, indicating presence of estrogen receptors also in this part of the duct system (461).

Male Differentiation of Genital Ducts

Male Wolffian Duct

In the male, the cranial part of the wolffian duct develops into the epididymis, the central portion becomes the vas deferens, and the caudal part forms the ejaculatory duct and the seminal vesicle (Figs. 30 and 43). Some of the cranial mesonephric tubules, which are connected to the rete testis, are retained as efferent ductules of the epididymis. During differentiation of the epididymis, the wolffian duct grows in length and becomes heavily convoluted. The epithelium of the duct is columnar and develops many microvilli and later develops cilia (rat [462]; sheep [463]). In the human, secretory activity is seen in the third trimester (464). The epididymal duct becomes surrounded by concentrically arranged mesenchymal cells, which differentiate into a thin layer of smooth muscle cells. The connection between epididymis and vas deferens becomes clearly marked by the formation of trilaminar smooth muscle layers of the latter duct (465).

The primitive seminal vesicle arises from a distention of the caudal portion of the wolffian duct, which in the human fetus occurs at the 60-mm stage (96). The seminal vesicle is covered by a tall nonsecretory columnar epithelium with a well-defined basement membrane (466). During differentiation, the lumen of the seminal vesicle gradually attains a complicated folded form.

In the human, the caudal part of the wolffian duct, which becomes the ejaculatory duct, is not clearly demarcated from the seminal vesicle until the third trimester (467). In contrast to the cranial part, no secretory granules are seen during fetal life (467).

Growth and differentiation of the wolffian duct are controlled by testosterone. This was shown in fetal rabbits (178) and rats (459,460) *in vitro* (see *Female Differentiation of Genital Ducts* subsection). It seems that testosterone itself rather than dihydrotestosterone (DHT) is responsible for differentiation of the wolffian duct (468–470), although DHT may be important for the development of the epididymis (471). All reproductive organs contain androgen receptors in the mesenchymal/stromal cells of the fetal mouse from day 13, whereas androgen receptors of the epithelial cells are only detected after day 16 of fetal life (472), indicating an inductive role of the mesenchymal tissue on the epithelium (for review, see ref. 473). Estrogen receptors have also been detected in the fetal male reproductive tract tissue of the mouse, although somewhat later than androgen receptors (474), but their role in the male fetus still remains unclear.

The mechanism by which testosterone induces differentiation of the male wolffian duct is not well understood. Gupta (475), using *in vitro* organ culture bioassays of genital tract differentiation, found that prostaglandin E_2 is able to masculinize the internal genital tract of the fetal mouse in the absence of testosterone. Later, Gupta and Bentlejewski (476) demonstrated that antibody against prostaglandin E_2 inhibited differentiation of the fetal mouse wolffian duct in a dose-dependent manner using embryonic male explants containing fetal testes. Moreover, both phospholipase A_2 inhibitors (cortisone and dexamethasone) and cyclooxygenase inhibitors (aspirin and indomethacin) blocked wolffian duct differentiation, and these effects could be reversed by prostaglandin E_2 supplementation (476). These results indicate that the testosterone-dependent wolffian duct differentiation requires ongoing prostaglandin synthesis within the reproductive tract.

Basic fibroblast growth factor also seems to play a role in the development of the male reproductive tract. Antiserum to bFGF infused into a mouse kidney, in which fetal male mouse ducts were transplanted, resulted in severe impairment of the wolffian duct development, in particular in the part developing into epididymis (450).

The wolffian duct becomes dependent on testosterone during the period immediately after sex differentiation, the "critical period," simultaneously with degeneration of the mesonephros (for review, see ref. 67). The enzyme that metabolizes testosterone to DHT, namely, 5α-reductase, only appears after "stabilization" of the wolffian duct (465), which occurs during the critical period.

Male Müllerian Duct and AMH

In normal males, the müllerian ducts begin regression shortly after testicular differentiation. The regression depends on Sertoli cell secretion of a specific müllerian inhibitor, which is not testosterone (178). This inhibitor is the glycoprotein mentioned in previous sections, namely, AMH, also termed MIS; it has a molecular mass of about 140 kDa (477). Josso and colleagues in Paris, Donahoe and colleagues in Boston, and others have purified the protein and cloned the genes for AMH (bovine [478,479]; human [479,480]; mouse [356]; rat [481]). There is 95% homology between the C termini of AMH from these four species, and AMH shares a striking similarity to proteins of the TGF-β family (for review, see ref. 482). Anti-Müllerian hormone is secreted by Sertoli cells from early stages of testicular differentiation (483–485). Anti-Müllerian hormone is interspecies-specific because AMH from one species can induce regression of the müllerian duct of other species (486,487). These activities of AMH have mainly been assayed *in vitro,* using $14\frac{1}{2}$-day-old fetal rat müllerian ducts and a bioassay developed by Picon (448) and others (484,488).

A receptor for AMH has not yet been cloned, but receptors are most likely present in the fetal müllerian duct, not only in the male but also in the female müllerian duct, which also regresses when exposed to AMH (299). The masculinizing effect of AMH on the fetal ovary (105,284), its interaction with epidermal growth factor (EGF) in cells from fetal rat lung (489), its synthesis in postnatal granulosa cells (105,298), and its antiproliferative effect on tumor cells (for review, see refs. 490 and 491) also indicates that receptors for AMH are present in a variety of cell types. These and other observations indicate that AMH has other physiologic roles than inducing müllerian duct regression.

The müllerian duct is sensitive to AMH only during a limited period after gonadal sex differentiation. Exposure before or after this critical period is ineffective (492,493). Studies on grafted human embryonic reproductive tracts indicate that the effect of AMH is permanent and irreversible (493).

In some species, however, AMH is produced for an extended period, even when there is no müllerian duct tissue left (494). It has been proposed that this delayed secretion of AMH might serve other purposes (e.g., inhibition of meiosis [495] and initiation of testicular descent [465,484]).

One of the first signs of regression of the müllerian duct is the formation of densely packed fibroblasts around the duct (496,497), indicating that the mesenchyme is an important target in the action of AMH (498). Concomitant with the periductal condensation of mesenchyme, a degradation of the extracellular matrix in this area takes place (499). Biochemical studies indicate that AMH may act by dephosphorylation of membrane proteins (500). Also, histochemical studies have shown that the membrane-bound enzyme nucleotide pyrophosphatase, which exhibits a broad hydrolytic activity, is localized over the regressing male müllerian duct of the rat but absent in the female müllerian duct (501).

The effect of AMH on the male müllerian duct can be prevented by exogenous estrogens (502). The müllerian ducts persist in males that have been exposed to DES during fetal life (503,504). Also in mice carrying the testicular feminization mutation gene (Tfm), prenatal exposure to DES inhibits regression of the müllerian duct (505). Thus, the regression of the müllerian ducts in males must occur during a critical period of development and depends on a proper hormonal balance.

ACKNOWLEDGMENTS

The authors thank Mr. Keld B. Ottosen for excellent preparation of the illustrations and Dr. Lars Kayser and Mrs. Kirsten Krogh for valuable help with typing the manuscript.

REFERENCES

1. Nussbaum M. Die Differenzierung des Geschlechts im Tierreich. *Arch Mikrosk Anat* 1880;18:1–121.
2. Rauh W. Ursprung des weiblichen Keimzellen und die chromatischen Vorgänge bis zur Entwicklung der Synapsisstadium. Beobachtet an des Ratte. (*Mus. decum alb.*). *Z Anat* 1929;78: 637–668.
3. Eddy EM, Clark JM. Electron microscopic study of migrating germ cells in the rat. In: Hess M, ed. *Electron Microscopic Concepts of Secretion. Ultrastructure of Endocrine and Reproductive Organs.* New York: Wiley & Sons, 1975;151–167.

4. Zamboni L, Merchant H. The fine morphology of mouse primordial germ cells in extragonadal locations. *Am J Anat* 1973;137:299–335.
5. Chiquoine AD. The identification, origin and migration of the primordial germ cells in the mouse embryo. *Anat Rec* 1954;118:135–145.
6. Mintz B, Russell ES. Gene induced embryological modification of primordial germ cells in the mouse. *J Exp Zool* 1957;134:207–230.
7. Witschi E. Migration of the germ cells of human embryos from the yolksac to the primitive gonadal fold. *Contrib Embryol* 1948;32:67–80.
8. McKay DC, Hertig AT, Adams EC, Danziger S. Histochemical observations on the germ cells of human embryos. *Anat Rec* 1953;117:201–219.
9. Chretien FC. Étude de l'origine, de la migration et de la multiplication des cellules germinales chez l'embryon de lapin. *J Embryol Exp Morphol* 1966;16:591–607.
10. Gardner RL, Rossant J. Investigation of the fate of 4.5 day post-coitum mouse inner cell mass cells by blastocyst injection. *J Embryol Exp Morphol* 1979;52:141–152.
11. McMahon A, Fosten M, Monk M. Random X-chromosome inactivation in female primordial germ cells in the mouse. *J Embryol Exp Morphol* 1981;64:251–258.
12. Noguchi M, Noguchi T, Watanabe M, Muramatsu T. Localization of receptors for Dolichos biflorus agglutinin in early postimplantation embryos in mice. *J Embryol Exp Morphol* 1982;72:39–52.
13. Hahnel AC, Eddy EM. Cell surface markers of mouse primordial germ cells defined by two monoclonal antibodies. *Gamete Res* 1986;15:25–34.
14. McLaren A. *Germ Cells and Soma: A New Look at an Old Problem.* New Haven, London: Yale University Press, 1981.
15. Snow MHL, Monk M. Emergence and migration of mouse primordial germ cells. In: McLaren A, Wylie CC, eds. *Current Problems in Germ Cell Differentiation.* Cambridge: Cambridge University Press, 1983;115–135.
16. Copp AJ, Robets HM, Polani PE. Chimaerism of primordial germ cells in the early postimplantation mouse embryo following microsurgical grafting of posterior primitive streak cells *in vitro. J Embryol Exp Morphol* 1986;95:94–115.
17. McMahon A, Fosten M, Monk M. Random X-chromosome inactivation in female primordial germ cells in the mouse. *J Embryol Exp Morphol* 1981;64:251–258.
18. Soriano P, Jaenisch R. Retroviruses as probes for mammalian development: allocation of cells to the somatic and germ cell lineages. *Cell* 1986;46:19–29.
19. Eddy EM, Clark JM, Gong D, Fenderson BA. Origin and migration of primordial germ cells in mammals. *Gamete Res* 1981;4:333–362.
20. Fujimoto T, Yoshinaga K, Kono I. Distribution of fibronectin on the migratory pathway of primordial germ cells in mice. *Anat Rec* 1985;211:271–278.
21. Ffrench-Constant C, Hollingsworth A, Heasman J, Wylie CC. Response to fibronectin of mouse primordial germ cells before, during and after migration. *Development* 1991;113:1365–1373.
22. Alvarez-Buylla A, Merchant-Larios H. Mouse primordial germ cells use fibronectin as a substrate for migration. *Exp Cell Res* 1986;165:362–368.
23. Fazel AR, Schulte BA, Thompson RP, Spicer SS. Presence of a unique glycoconjugate on the surface of rat primordial germ cells during migration. *Cell Differ* 1987;21:199–211.
24. Fazel AR, Schulte BA, Spicer SS. Glycoconjugate unique to migrating primordial germ cells differs with genera. *Anat Rec* 1990;228:177–184.
25. Snow MHL. Autonomous development of parts isolated from primitive streak stage mouse embryos. Is development clonal? *J Embryol Exp Morphol* 1981;65(suppl.):269–287.
26. Niewkoop PD, Sutasurya LA. *Primordial Germ Cells in the Chordates.* London: Cambridge University Press, 1979.
27. Kuwana T, Maeda-Suga H, Fujimoto T. Attraction of chick primordial germ cells by gonadal anlage *in vitro. Anat Rec* 1986;215:403–406.
28. Rogulska R, Ozdzenski W, Komar A. Behaviour of mouse primordial germ cells in the chick embryo. *J Embryol Exp Morphol* 1971;25:155–164.
29. Godin I, Wylie CC, Heasman J. Genital ridges exert long-range effects on mouse primordial germ cell numbers and direction of migration in culture. *Development* 1990;108:357–363.
30. Godin I, Wylie CC. TGFβ_1 inhibits proliferation and has a chemotropic effect on mouse primordial germ cells in culture. *Development* 1991;113:1451–1457.
31. Hardisty MW. Primordal germ cells and the vertebrate germ line. In: Jones RE, ed. *The Vertebrate Ovary.* New York: Plenum Press, 1978;1–45.
32. Ozdzenski W. Observations on the origin of primordial germ cells in the mouse. *Zool Pol* 1967;17:367–379.
33. Tam P, Snow MHL. Proliferation and migration of primordial germ cells during compensatory growth in the mouse embryo. *J Embryol Exp Morphol* 1981;64:133–147.
34. Baker TG. A quantitative and cytological study of germ cells in the human ovaries. *Proc R Soc Lond B* 1963;158:417–433.
35. Mintz B, Russel ES. Gene-induced embryological modification of primordial germ cells in the mouse. *J Exp Zool* 1957;134:207–237.
36. Russel ES. Hereditary anemias of the mouse: A review for geneticists. *Adv Genet* 1979;20:357–459.
37. Chabot B, Stephenson DA, Chapman VM, Besmer P, Bernstein A. The proto-oncogene c-kit encoding a transmembrane tyrosine kinase receptor match to the mouse W locus. *Nature* 1988;335:88–89.
38. Geissler EN, Ryan MA, Housman DE. The dominant white spotting (W) locus of the mouse encodes the c-kit protooncogene. *Cell* 1988;55:185–192.
39. Zsebo KM, Wypych J, McNiece IK, et al. Identification, purification and biological characterization of stem cell factor from Buffalo rat liver conditioned medium. *Cell* 1990;63:195–201.
40. Godin I, Deed R, Cooke J, Zsebo K, Dexter M, Wylie CC. Effect of the steel gene product on mouse primordial germ cells in culture. *Nature* 1991;352:807–809.
41. Zsebo KM, Williams DA, Geissler EN, et al. Stem cell factor is encoded at the Sl locus of the mouse and is the ligand for the c-kit tyrosine kinase receptor. *Cell* 1990;63:213–224.
42. Dolci S, Williams DE, Ernst MK, et al. Requirement for mast cell growth factor for primordial germ cell survival in culture. *Nature* 1991;352:809–811.
43. Matsui Y, Toksoz D, Niskikawa S, et al. Effect of steel factor and leukaemia inhibitory factor on murine primordial germ cells in culture. *Nature* 1991;353:750–752.
44. Matsui Y, Zsebo K, Hogan BLM. Derivation of pluripotential embryonic stem cells from murine primordial germ cells in culture. *Cell* 1992;70:841–847.
45. Resnick JL, Bixler LS, Cheng L, Donovan PJ. Long term proliferation of mouse primordial germ cells in culture. *Nature* 1992;359:550–551.
46. Merchant-Larios H, Alvarez-Buylla A. The role of extracellular matrix and tissue topographic arrangement in mouse and rat primordial germ cell migration. In: Eshkol A, Eckstein B, Dekel N, Peters H, Tsafriri A, eds. *Development and Function of the Reproductive Organs. Serono Symposia Review No. II.* New York: Raven Press, 1986;1–11.
47. Lyon MF. Gene action in the X-chromosome of the mouse (*Mus musculus*). *Nature* 1961;190:372–373.
48. Lyon MF. Sex chromosome activity in germ cells. In: Fuchs F, Coutinho EM, eds. *Physiology and Genetics of Reproduction.* New York: Plenum Press, 1974;63–71.
49. Cattanach BM. Control of chromosome inactivation. *Annu Rev Genet* 1975;9:1–17.
50. Gartler SM, Rivewst M, Cole RE. Cytological evidence for an inactive X chromosome in murine oogonia. *Cytogenet Cell Genet* 1980;28:203–207.
51. Watson JM, Riggs A, Graves JAM. Gene mapping studies confirm the homology between the platypus X and echidna X, chromosomes and identify a conserved ancestral monotreme X chromosome. *Chromosoma* 1992;101:596–601.
52. Marshall-Graves JA. The evolution of mammalian sex chromosomes and dosage compensation: clues from marsupials and monotremes. *Trends Genet* 1987;3:252–256.

53. Cattanach BM, Beechey CV. Autosomal and X-chromosome imprinting. *Development* 1990;(suppl.):63–72.
54. Monk M, Grant M. Preferential X-chromosome inactivation, DNA methylation and imprinting. *Development* 1990;(suppl.): 55–62.
55. Ohno S, Klinger HP, Atkin WB. Human oogenesis. *Cytogenetics* 1962;1:42–51.
56. Teplitz R, Ohno S. Postnatal induction of oogenesis in the rabbit (*Oryctolagus cuniculus*). *Exp Cell Res* 1963;31:183–189.
57. Ohno S. *Sex Chromosomes and Sex Linked Genes.* Berlin: Springer-Verlag, 1967.
58. Migeon BR, Jelalian K. Evidence for two active X chromosomes in germ cells of female before meiotic entry. *Nature* 1977;269:242–243.
59. Gartler SM, Andina R, Gant N. Ontogeny of X-chromosome inactivation in the female germ line. *Exp Cell Res* 1975;91:454–457.
60. Andina RJ. A study of X chromosome regulation during oogenesis in the mouse. *Exp Cell Res* 1978;111:211–218.
61. West J. X chromosome expression during mouse embryogenesis. In: Crosignani PG, Rubin BL, Fraccaro M, eds. *Genetic Control of Gamete Production and Function.* London: Academic Press, 1982;49–91.
62. Monk M. Methylation and the X chromosome. *Bioessays* 1986;4:204–208.
63. Pourcel C. Imprinting and Methylation. In: Gwatkin RBL, ed. *Genes in Mammalian Reproduction.* New York: Wiley-Liss, 1993;173–184.
64. Grant M, Zuccotti M, Monk M. Methylation of CpG sites of two X-linked genes coincides with X-inactivation in the female mouse embryo but not in the germ line. *Nature* 1992;2:161–166.
65. Singer-Sam J, Goldstein L, Dai A, Gartler SM, Riggs AJ. A potentially critical Hpa II site of the X chromosome linked PGK1 gene is unmethylated prior to the onset of meiosis of human oogenic cells. *Proc Natl Acad Sci* 1992;89:1413–1417.
66. Du Bois AM. The embryonic kidney. In: Rouiller C, Muller AF, eds. *The Kidney. Vol. 1.* New York: Academic Press, 1969;1–59.
67. Grinsted J, Aagesen L. Mesonephric excretory function related to its influence on differentiation of fetal gonads. *Anat Rec* 1984;210:551–556.
68. Waldeyer W. *Eierstock und Ei.* Leipzig: Engelman, 1870.
69. Balfour FM. On the structure and development of the vertebrate ovary. *Q J Microsc Sci* 1878;XVIII:383–445.
70. Witschi E. Studies on sex differentiation and sex determination in amphibians. V. Range of the cortex-medulla antagonism in parabiotic twins of Ranidae and Hylidae. *J Exp Zool* 1931;58:113–145.
71. Witschi E. Embryogenesis of the adrenal and the reproductive glands. *Recent Prog Horm Res* 1951;6:1–23.
72. Byskov AG. The anatomy and ultrastructure of the rete system in the fetal mouse ovary. *Biol Reprod* 1978;19:720–735.
73. Fraedrich J. Licht- und elektronmikroskopische Untersuchungen über den Zusammenhang der Mesonephros-und frühen Gonadenentwicklung der weissen Maus. *Dissertation.* Bonn: Med Fak, 1979;1–58.
74. Upadhyay S, Luciani JM, Zamboni L. The role of the mesonephros in the development of the indifferent gonads and ovaries of the mouse. *Ann Biol Anim Biochim Biophys* 1979;19(4b): 1179–1196.
75. Upadhyad S, Luciani JM, Zamboni L. The role of the mesonephros in the development of the mouse testis and its excurrent pathways. In: Byskov AG, Peters H, eds. *Development and Function of Reproductive Organs.* Amsterdam: Excerpta Medica, 1981;18–27.
76. Gropp A, Ohno S. Presence of a common embryonic blastema for ovarian and testicular parenchymal (follicular, interstitial and tubular) cells in cattle, Bos taurus. *Z Zellforsch Mikrosk Anat* 1966;74:505–528.
77. Wartenberg H. Human testicular development and the role of the mesonephros in the origin of a dual Sertoli cell system. *Andrologia* 1978;10:1–21.
78. Zamboni L, Bézard J, Mauléon P. The role of the mesonephros in the development of the sheep fetal ovary. *Ann Biol Anim Biochim Biophys* 1979;19(4B):1153–1178.
79. Zamboni L, Upadhyay S, Bezard J, Mauleon P. The role of the mesonephros in the development of the sheep testis and its excurrent pathways. In: Byskov AG, Peters H, eds. *Development and Function of Reproductive Organs.* Amsterdam: Excerpta Medica, 1981;31–40.
80. Kinsky I. Bildung des somatischen Gonadenblastems durch die degenerierende Urniereteile des Kaninchens. *Verh Anat Ges* 1979;73:403–406.
81. Wartenberg H. Der Mesonephros und die Gonadenentwicklung. *Verh Anat Ges* 1979;73:385–401.
82. Møller CJ, Byskov AG, Roth J, Celis JE, Bock E. NCAM in developing mouse gonads and ducts. *Anat Embryol* 1991;184: 541–548.
83. Byskov AG. Does the rete ovarii act as a trigger for the onset of meiosis? *Nature* 1974;252:396–397.
84. Byskov AG, Grinsted J. Feminizing effect of mesonephros on cultured differentiating mouse gonads and ducts. *Science* 1981;212:817–818.
85. McLaren A, Buehr M. Development of mouse germ cells in cultures of fetal gonads. *Cell Differ Dev* 1990;31:185–195.
86. Byskov AG. The meiosis inducing interaction between germ cells and rete cells in the fetal mouse gonad. *Ann Biol Anim Biochim Biophys* 1978;18:327–334.
87. Grinsted J, Byskov AG, Christensen IJ, Jensenius JC. Influence of the mesonephros on fetal and neonatal rabbit gonads. I. Sex-steroid release by the testis in vitro. *Acta Endocrinol* 1982;99:272–280.
88. Grinsted J. Influence of mesonephros on foetal and neonatal rabbit gonads. II. Sex-steroid release by the ovary *in vitro*. *Acta Endocrinol (Copenh)* 1982;99:281–287.
89. Crowder RE. The development of the adrenal gland in man, with special reference to origin and ultimate location of cell types and evidence in favor of the "cell migration" theory. *Contrib Embryol* 1957;251:194–221.
90. Geduspan JS, Solursh M. A growth-promoting influence from the mesonephros during limb outgrowth. *Dev Biol* 1992;151: 242–250.
91. Pelliniemi LJ. Ultrastructure of gonadal ridge in male and female pig embryos. *Anat Embryol* 1975;147:19–34.
92. Wartenberg H. Development of the early human ovary and role of the mesonephros in the differentiation of the cortex. *Anat Embryol* 1982;165:253–280.
93. Wagenen GV, Simpson ME. *Embryology of the Ovary and Testis. Homo Sapiens and Macaca mulatta.* New Haven: Yale University Press, 1965.
94. Wartenberg H. The influence of the mesonephric blastema on gonadal development and sexual differentiation. In: Byskov AG, Peters H, eds. *Development and Function of Reproductive Organs.* Amsterdam: Excerpta Medica, 1981;3–12.
95. Peters H, McNatty KP. *The Ovary. A Correlation of Structure and Function in Mammals.* London: Granada Publishing, 1980.
96. Jirasek JE. *Development of the Genital System and Male Pseudohermaphroditism.* Baltimore: Johns Hopkins Press, 1971.
97. Byskov AG. The role of the rete ovarii in meoisis and follicle formation in the cat, mink and ferret. *J Reprod Fertil* 1975;45:210–219.
98. Jeppesen T. Surface epithelium of the fetal guinea pig ovary. A light and electron microscopic study. *Anat Rec* 1975;183: 499–515.
99. Paranko J. Expression of type I and III collagen during morphogenesis of fetal rat testis and ovary. *Anat Rec* 1987;219:91–101.
100. Merchant H. Rat gonadal and ovarian organogenesis with and without germ cells. An ultrastructural study. *Dev Biol* 1975;44:1–21.
101. Pelliniemi LJ, Dym M. The fetal gonad and sexual differentiation. In: Tulchinsky D, Ryan KJ, eds. *Maternal–Fetal Endocrinology.* Philadelphia: WB Saunders, 1980;252–280.
102. Gelly JL, Richoux JP, Lehenp BP, Grignon G. Immunolocalization of type IV collagen and laminin during rat gonadal morphogenesis and postnatal development of the testis and epididymis. *Histochemistry* 1989;93:31–37.
103. Burns RK. Role of hormones in the differentiation of sex. In: Young WC, ed. *Sex and Internal Secretions.* Baltimore: Williams & Wilkins, 1961;76–160.

104. Vigier B, Picard JY, Tran D, Legeai L, Josso N. Production of anti-müllerian hormone: another homology between Sertoli and granulosa cells. *Endocrinology* 1984;114:1315–1320.
105. Takahashi M, Hayashi M, Manganaro TF, Donahoe PK. The ontogeny of müllerian inhibiting substance in granulosa cells of the bovine ovarian follicle. *Biol Reprod* 1986;35:447–453.
106. Patek CE, Kerr JB, Gosden RG, et al. Sex chimaerism, fertility and sex determination in the mouse. *Development* 1991;113: 311–325.
107. Burgoyne PS, Buehr M, Koopman P, Rossant T, McLaren A. Cell-autonomous action of the testis-determining gene: Sertoli cells are exclusively XY in XX-XY chimaeric mouse testes. *Development* 1988;102:443–450.
108. Burgoyne PS, Buehr M, McLaren A. XY follicle cells in ovaries of XX-XY female mouse chimaeras. *Development* 1988;104: 683–688.
109. Palmer S, Burgoyne PS. *In situ* analysis of fetal, prepubertal and adult XX-XY chimaeric mouse testes: Sertoli cells are predominantly but not exclusively XY. *Development* 1991;112:265–268.
110. Mullen RJ, Whitten WK. Relationship of genotype and degree of chimerism in coat color to sex ratios and gametogenesis in chimeric mice. *J Exp Zool* 1971;178:165–176.
111. Rodemer-Lenz E. On cell contribution to gonadal soma formation in quail-chick chimeras during the indifferent stage of gonadal development. *Anat Embryol* 1989;179:237–242.
112. Yoshinaga K, Hess DL, Hendrickx AG, Zamboni L. The development of the sexually indifferent gonad in the prosimian, Galago crassicaudatus crassicaudatus. *Am J Anat* 1988;181:89–105.
113. Polani PE. Pairing of X and Y chromosomes, non-inactivation of X-linked genes, and the maleness factor. *Hum Genet* 1982;60:207–211.
114. Bridges CB. Non-disjunction as proof of the chromosome theory of heredity. *Genetics* 1916;1:1–51, 107–163.
115. Jacobs PA, Strong JA. A case of human intersexuality having a possible XXY sex-determining mechanism. *Nature* 1959;183: 302–303.
116. Ford CE, Jones KW, Polani PE, de Almeida JC, Briggs JH. A sex-chromosome anomaly in a case of gonadal dysgenesis (Turner's Syndrome). *Lancet* 1959;1:711.
117. Welshons WJ, Russell LB. The Y chromosome as the bearer of male determining factors in the mouse. *Proc Natl Acad Sci* 1959;45:560–566.
118. Beatty RA. Genetic basis for the determination of sex. *Philos Trans R Soc Lond (Biol)* 1970;259:3–13.
119. Grumbach MM, Conte FA. Disorders of sexual differentiation. In: Wilson JD, Foster DW, eds. Philadelphia: WB Saunders, 1985;312–401.
120. Polani PE. Sex chromosome anomalities in man. In: Hamerton JL, ed. *Chromosomes in Medicine. Little Club Clinics in Developmental Medicine, No.* 5. London: National Spastic Society with William Heinemann Medical Books Ltd., 1962;74–133.
121. Eicher EM, Washburn LL. Genetic control of primary sex determination in mice. *Annu Rev Genet* 1986;20:327–360.
122. McLaren A. Sex determination in mammals. *Trends Genet* 1988;4:153–157.
123. Jacobs PA, Ross A. Structural abnormalities of the Y chromosome in man. *Nature* 1966;210:352–354.
124. Wachtel SS, Ohno S, Koo GL, Boyse EA. H-Y antigen and male development. In: Troen P, Nankin HR, eds. *Testis in Normal and Infertile Men.* New York: Raven Press, 1975;35–43.
125. Eichwald EJ, Silmer CR. Skin. Communication. *Transplant Bull* 1955;2:148–149.
126. Wachtel SS, Koo GC. H-Y antigen in gonadal differentiation. In: Austin CR, Edwards RG, eds. *Mechanisms of Sex Differentiation in Animals and Man.* London: Academic Press, 1981;255–299.
127. Silvers WK, Gasser DL, Eicker EM. H-Y antigen, serologically detectable male antigen and sex determination. *Cell* 1982;28:439–440.
128. McLaren A. Chimeras and sexual differentiation. In: LeDouarin N, McLaren A, eds. *Chimeras in Developmental Biology.* New York: Academic Press, 1984;381–399.
129. Teyssier JR, Amice-Chambon U, Bajolle F, Pigeon F. H-Y antigen negativity associated with a normal male phenotype. *Arch Androl* 1983;11:253–258.
130. Meldvold RW, Kohn HI, Yerganian G, Fawcett DW. Evidence suggesting the existence of two H-Y antigens in the mouse. *Immunogenetics* 1977;5:33–41.
131. Ohno S. The Y-linked testis determining gene and H-Y plasma membrane antigen gene: are they one and the same? *Endocr Rev* 1985;6:421–431.
132. Simpson E, McLaren A, Chandler P. Evidence for two male antigens in mice. *Immunogenetics* 1982;15:609–614.
133. McLaren A, Simpson E, Tomonari K, Chandler P, Hogg H. Male sexual differentiation in mice lacking H-Y antigen. *Nature* 1984;312:552–555.
134. Simpson E, Chandler P, Goulmy E, Disteche CM, Ferguson-Smith MA, Page DC. Separation of the genetic loci for the H-Y antigen and for testis determination on human Y chromosome. *Nature* 1987;326:876–878.
135. Cattanach BM, Pollard CE, Hawkes SG. Sex reversed mice: XX and XO males. *Cytogenetics* 1971;10:318–337.
136. Singh L, Jones KW. Sex reversal in the mouse (*Mus musculus*) is caused by a recurrent nonreciprocal crossover involving the X and an aberrant Y chromosome. *Cell* 1982;28:205–216.
137. Evans EP, Burtenshaw MD, Cattenach BM. Meiotic crossing-over between the X and Y chromosomes of male mice carrying the sex-reversing (Sxr) factor. *Nature* 1982;300:443–445.
138. Burgoyne PS. Genetic homology and crossing over in the X and Y chromosomes of mammals. *Hum Genet* 1982;61:85–90.
139. Simpson E, McLaren A, Chandler P, Tomomonari K. Expression of H-Y antigen by female mice carrying Sxr. *Transplantation* 1984;37:17–21.
140. Burgoyne PS, Levy ER, McLaren A. Spermatogenic failure in mice lacking H-Y antigen. *Nature* 1986;320:170–172.
141. Roberts C, Weith A, Passage E, Michot JL, Matei MG, Bishop CE. Molecular and cytogenetic evidence for the location of Tdy and Hya on the mouse Y chromosome short arm. *Proc Natl Acad Sci* 1988;85:6446–6449.
142. Guellaen G, Casanova M, Bishop C, et al. Human XX males with Y single-copy DNA fragments. *Nature* 1984;307:172–173.
143. Disteche CM, Casanova M, Sall H, et al. Small deletions of the short arm of the Y chromosome in 46, XY females. *Proc Natl Acad Sci* 1986;83:7841–7844.
144. Page DC, Mosher R, Simpson EM, et al. The sex-determining region of the human Y chromosome encodes a finger protein. *Cell* 1987;51:1091–1104.
145. Mardon G, Mosher R, Disteche CM, Nishioka Y, McLaren A, Page DC. Duplication, deletion, and polymorphism in the sex-determining region of the mouse Y chromosome. *Science* 1989;243:78–80.
146. Nagamine CM, Chan K, Kozak CA, Lau Y-F. Chromosome mapping and expression of a putative testis-determining gene in mouse. *Science* 1989;243:80–83.
147. Mitchell MJ, Bishop CE. A structural analysis of the Sxr region of the mouse Y chromosome. *Genomics* 1992;12:26–34.
148. Schneider-Gädicke A, Beer-Romero P, Brown LG, Nussbaum R, Page DC. ZFX has a gene structure similar to ZFY, the putative human sex determinant, and escapes X inactivation. *Cell* 1989;57:1247–1258.
149. Sinclair AH, Foster JW, Spencer JA, et al. Sequences homologous to ZFY, a candidate human sex-determining gene, are autosomal in marsupials. *Nature* 1988;336:780–783.
150. Koopman P, Gubbay J, Collignon J, Lovell-Badge R. Zfy gene expression patterns are not compatible with a primary role in mouse sex determination. *Nature* 1989;342:940–942.
151. Burgoyne PS, Buehr M, Koopman P, Rossant J, McLaren A. Cell-autonomous action of the testis-determining gene: Sertoli cells are exclusively XY in XX-XY chimaeric mouse testes. *Development* 1988;102:443–450.
152. McLaren A. Development of the mammalian gonad: the fate of the supporting cell lineage. *Bioessays* 1991;13:151–156.
153. Palmer MS, Sinclair AH, Berta P, et al. Genetic evidence that ZFY is not the testis-determining factor. *Nature* 1989;342: 937–939.
154. Page DC, Fisher EMC, McGillivray B, Brown LG. Additional deletion in sex-determining region of human Y chromosome resolves paradox of X,t(Y;22) female. *Nature* 1990;346:279–281.
155. Sinclair AH, Berta P, Palmer MS, et al. A gene from the human

sex-determining region encodes a protein with homology to a conserved DNA-binding motif. *Nature* 1990;346:240–244.
156. Gubbay J, Collignon J, Koopman P, et al. A gene mapping to the sex-determining region of the mouse Y chromosome is a member of a novel family of embryonically expressed genes. *Nature* 1990;346:245–250.
157. Berta P, Ross Hawkins J, Sinclair AH, Taylor A, Griffiths BL. Genetic evidence equating SRY and the testis-determining factor. *Nature* 1990;348:448–454.
158. Jäger RJ, Anvret M, Hall K, Scherer G. A human XY female with a frame shift mutation in the candidate testis-determining gene SRY. *Nature* 1990;348:452–454.
159. Lovell-Badge R, Robertson E. XY female mice resulting from a heritable mutation in the primary testis-determining gene, Tdy. *Development* 1990;109:635–646.
160. Gubbay J, Koopman P, Collignon J, Burgoyne P, Lovell-Badge R. Normal structure and expression of Zfy genes in XY female mice mutant in Tdy. *Development* 1990;109:647–653.
161. Koopman P, Münsterberg A, Capel B, Vivian N, Lovell-Badge R. Expression of a candidate sex-determining gene during mouse testis differentiation. *Nature* 1990;348:450–452.
162. Koopman P, Gubbay J, Vivian N, Goodfellow P, Lovell-Badge R. Male development of chromosomally female mice transgenic for Sry. *Nature* 1991;351:117–121.
163. Niekerk WAV, Retief AE. The gonads of human true hermaphrodites. *Hum Genet* 1981;58:117–122.
164. Tarkowski AK. Mouse chimeras developed from fused eggs. *Nature* 1961;190:857–860.
165. McLaren A. *Mammalian Chimeras.* Cambridge: Cambridge University Press, 1976.
166. Hooper ML, Hardy K, Handyside A, Hunter S, Monk M. HPRT deficient (Lesch-Nyhan) mouse embryos derived from germline colonisation by cultured cells. *Nature* 1987;326:292–295.
167. Eicher EM, Beamer WG, Washburn LL, Whitten WH. A cytogenetic investigation of inherited true hermaphroditism in BALBc/Wt mice. *Cytogenet Cell Genet* 1980;28:104–115.
168. Ford CE. Cytogenetics and sex determination in man and mammals. *J Biosoc Sci* 1970;(suppl):2:7–30.
169. Whitten WK, Beamer WG, Byskov AG. The morphology of fetal gonads of spontaneous mouse hermaphrodites. *J Embryol Exp Morphol* 1979;52:63–78.
170. Whitten WK. Chromosomal basis for hermaphroditism in mice. In: Markert CL and Papaconstantantinou J, eds. *The 33rd Symposium of the Society for Developmental Biology.* New York: Academic Press, 1975;189–205.
171. Bradbury MW. Testes of XX-XY chimeric mice develop from fetal ovotestes. *Dev Genet* 1987;8:207–218.
172. Yding Andersen C, Byskov AG, Grinsted J. Growth pattern of the sex ducts in foetal mouse hermaphrodites. *J Embryol Exp Morph* 1983;73:59–68.
173. Deeming DC, Ferguson MW. Environmental regulation of sex determination in reptiles. *Philos Trans R Soc B* 1988;322:19–39.
174. Gallien L. Development in sexual organogenesis. *Adv Morphog* 1967;6:259–317.
175. Goudie CA, Redner BD, Simco BA, Davis KB. Feminization of channel cat fish by oral administration of steroid sex hormones. *Trans Am Fish Soc* 1983;112:670–672.
176. Byskov AG, Grinsted J. Feminizing effect of mesonephros on cultured differentiating mouse gonads and ducts. *Science* 1981;212:817–818.
177. Lowell-Badge R. The role of Sry in mammalian sex determination. In: *Postimplantation Development in the Mouse. Ciba Foundation Symp. 165.* Chichester: Wiley, 1992;162–182.
178. Jost A. Recherches sur la différenciation sexuelle de l'embryon de lapin, III. Role des gonades foetales dans la différenciation sexuelle somatique. *Arch Anat Microsc Morphol* 1947;36: 271–315.
179. Jost A. Problemes in fetal endocrinology. The gonadal and hypophyseal hormones. *Recent Prog Horm Res* 1953;8:379–418.
180. Jost A. General outline about reproductive physiology and its developmental background. In: Gibian H, Plotz EJ, eds. *Mammalian Reproduction.* Berlin: Springer Verlag, 1970;4–32.
181. Burns RK. Sex transformation in the opossum: Some new results and a retrospect. *Arch Anat Microsc* 1950;39:467–483.
182. Alcorn GT. Ovarian development in the tammar wallaby *Macropus eugenii.* Ph.D. Thesis, MacQuarie University, Australia, 1975.
183. Moore HD, Thurstam SM. Sexual differentiation in the grey short-tailed opposum, *Monodelphis domestica,* and the effect of oestradiol benzoate on development in the male. *J Zool* 1990;221:639–658.
184. Behringer RR, Cate RL, Froelick GJ, Palmiter RD, Brinster RL. Abnormal sexual development in transgenic mice chronically expressing Müllerian inhibiting substance. *Nature* 1990;345: 167–170.
185. Wartenberg H. Ultrastructure of fetal ovary including oogenesis. In: von Blerkom J, Motta PM, eds. *Ultrastructure of Human Gametogenesis and Early Embryogenesis.* Boston: Kluwer Academic Publishers, 1989;61–85.
186. Byskov AG. Regulation of meiosis in mammals. *Ann Biol Anim Biochim Biophys* 1979;19:1251–1261.
187. Byskov AG, Høyer PE, Björkman N, Mørk AB, Olsen B, Grinsted J. Ultrastructure of germ cells and adjacent somatic cells correlated to initiation of meiosis in the fetal pig. *Anat Embryol* 1986;175:57–67.
188. Hashimoto Y, Eguchi Y. Histological observations on the gonads in the cattle and the horse fetus. I. The cattle fetus. *Jpn J Zootech* 1955;26:259–266.
189. Goodenough V, Levine RP. *Genetics.* London: Holt, Rinehart & Winston, 1974.
190. Baker TG. Oogenesis and ovarian development. In: Balin H, Glasser S, eds. *Reproductive Biology.* Amsterdam: Excerpta Medica, 1972;398–437.
191. Byskov AG, Grinsted J. Production of germ cells and regulation of meiosis. In: Jagiello G, Vogel HJ, eds. *Bioregulators of Reproduction.* New York: Academic Press, 1981;109–117.
192. Hilscher B, Hilscher W, Bulthoff-Ohnolz B, et al. Kinetics of gametogenesis. I. Comparative histological and autoradiographic studies of oocytes and transitional prespermatogona during oogenesis and prespermatogenesis. *Cell Tissue Res* 1974;154: 443–470.
193. Borum K. Oogenesis in the mouse. A study of meiotic prophase. *Exp Cell Res* 1961;24:495–507.
194. Peters H, Levy E, Crone M. Oogenesis in rabbits. *J Exp Zool* 1965;158:169–180.
195. Gondos B. Oogonia and oocytes in mammals. In: Jones RE, ed. *The Vertebrate Ovary.* New York: Plenum Press, 1978;83–120.
196. Rüsse I. Oogenesis in cattle and sheep. *Bibl Anat* 1983;24:77–92.
197. Gondos B. Intercellular bridges and mammalian germ cell differentiation. *Differentiation* 1973;1:177–182.
198. Kenelly JJ, Foote RH, Jones RC. Duration of premeiotic deoxyribonucleic acid synthesis and the stages of prophase in rabbit oocytes. *J Cell Biol* 1970;47:477–484.
199. Lima-Di-Faria A, Borum K. The period of DNA synthesis prior to meiosis in the mouse. *J Cell Biol* 1962;14:381–388.
200. Peters H, Crone M. DNA synthesis in oocytes of mammals. *Arch Microsc Morphol Exp* 1967;56(suppl. 3–4):160–170.
201. Mintz B. Continuity of the female germ cell line from embryo to adult. *Arch Anat Microsc Morphol Exp* 1959;48:155–172.
202. Beaumont HM. Radiosensitivity of oogonia and oocytes in the foetal rat. *Int J Radiat Biol* 1961;3:59–72.
203. Mandl AM. The radiosensitivity of germ cells. *Biol Rev* 1964;39:288–371.
204. Ioannou JM. Oogenesis in adult prosimians. *J Embryol Exp Morphol* 1967;17:139–145.
205. Anand Kumar TC. Oogenesis in the lorises. *Loris tardigradus lydekkerianus* and *Nucticebris coucang. Proc R Soc Lond (Biol)* 1968;169:167–176.
206. Baker TG. The effects of ionizing radiation on the mammalian ovary with particular reference to oogenesis. In: Hamilton DW, Greep RO, eds. *Handbook of Physiology. Endocrinology. Vol. V.* Washington, DC: American Physiology Society, 1973;349–361.
207. Beaumont HM. The short term effect of acute X-irradiation on oogonia and oocytes. *Proc R Soc Lond (Biol)* 1965;161:550–570.
208. Oakberg EF, Clark E. Species comparisons of radiation response of the gonads. In: Carlson WD, Gassner FY, eds. *Effects of Ionizing Radiation in the Reproductive System.* Oxford: Pergamon Press, 1963;11–24.
209. Larsen J, Byskov AG, Christensen IJ. Flow cytometry and sorting

of meiotic prophase cells of female rabbits. *J Reprod Fertil* 1986;76:587–596.
210. Stahl A, Luciani JM. Individualization d'un stade preleptotene de condensation chromosomique au debut meiose chez l'ovocyte foetal humain, *C R Acad Sci* 1971;272:2041–2044.
211. Devictor-Vuillet M, Luciani JM, Stahl A. Étude des stades de debut de la méiose chez l'ovocyte de lapin: comparaison avec l'ovocyte humain. *Ann Biol Anim Biochim Biophys* 1973; 13:73–78.
212. Mauléon P, Devictor-Vuillet M, Luciani JM. The preleptotene chromosome condensation and decondensation in the ovary of the sheep embryo. *Ann Biol Anim Biochim Biophys* 1976;16:293–296.
213. Deanesly R. Germ cell development and the meiotic prophase in the fetal horse ovary. *J Reprod Fertil (Suppl)* 1975;23:547–552.
214. Holm PB, Rasmussen SW. Human meiosis. I. The human pachytene karyotype analyzed by three dimensional reconstruction of the synaptonemal complex. *Carlsberg Res Commun* 1977;42: 283–323.
215. Bojko M. Human meiosis. IX. Crossing over and chiasma formation in oocytes. *Carlsberg Res Commun* 1985;50:43–72.
216. Speed RM. Meiosis in the foetal mouse ovary. 1. An analysis at the light microscope level using surface spreading. *Chromosoma* 1982;85:427–437.
217. Resnick MA. Investigating the genetic control of biochemical events in meiotic recombination. In: Moens PB, ed. *Meiosis.* New York: Academic Press, 1987;157–210.
218. Roeder GS. Chromosome synapsis and genetic recombination. *Trends Genet* 1990;6:385–389.
219. Fang JS, Jagiello GM. An analysis of the chromomere map and chiasmata characteristics of human diplotene oocytes. *Cytogenet Cell Genet* 1988;47:52–57.
220. Jones GH. Chiasmata. In: Moens PB, ed. *Meiosis.* London, New York: Academic Press, 1987;213–244.
221. Polani PE, Crolla JA, Seller MJ. An experimental approach to female mammalian meiosis: Differential chromosome labeling and an analysis of chiasmata in the female mouse. In: Jagiello G, Vogel H, eds. *Bioregulators of Reproduction.* New York: Academic Press, 1981;59–87.
222. Whitehouse HLK. *Towards an Understanding of the Mechanisms of Heredity.* New York: St. Martins Press, 1973.
223. Callan HG, Perry PE. Recombination in male and female meiocytes contrasted. *Philos Trans R Soc Lond B* 1977;277: 227–233.
224. Fang JS, Jagiello GM. Unique state of sexual dimorphism of crossing-over in diplotene spermatocytes and oocytes of *Mesocricetus brandti,* a species with neonatal oogenesis. *Biol Reprod* 1991;45:447–454.
225. Crone M, Peters H. Unusual incorporation of tritiated thymidine into early diplotene oocytes of mice. *Exp Cell Res* 1968;50:664–668.
226. Meistrich ML, Reid BO, Barcellona WJ. Meiotic DNA synthesis during mouse spermatogenesis. *J Cell Biol* 1975;64:211–222.
227. Baker TG, Franchi LL. The origin of cytoplasmatic inclusions from the nuclear envelope of mammalian oocytes. *Z Zellforsch Mikrosk Anat* 1967;93:45–55.
228. Beaumont HM, Mandl AH. A quantitative and cytological study of oogonia and oocytes in the foetal and neonatal rat. *Proc R Soc Lond (Biol)* 1962;155:557–579.
229. Singh RP, Carr DH. The anatomy and histology of XO human embryos and fetuses. *Anat Rec* 1966;155:369–384.
230. Ford CE, Jones KW, Polani PE, De Almeida JCC, Briggs JH. A sex-chromosome anomaly in a case of gonadal dysgenesis (Turners syndrome). *Lancet* 1959;1:711–713.
231. Burgoyne PS, Baker TG. Perinatal oocyte loss in XO mice and its implications for the aetiology of gonadal dysgenesis in XO women. *J Reprod Fertil* 1985;75:633–645.
232. Burgoyne PS. The genetics of sex in development. In: Hamilton D, Naftolin F, eds. *Basic Reproductive Medicine, Vol. 1: Basis and Development of Reproduction.* Cambridge: MIT Press, 1981;1–31.
233. Ashworth A, Rastan S, Lovell-Badge R, Kelly G. X-chromosome inactivation may explain the difference in viability of XO humans and mice. *Nature* 1991;351:406–408.
234. Miklos GLG. Sex-chromosome pairing and male fertility. *Cytogenet Cell Genet* 1974;13:558–577.
235. Burgoyne PS, Baker TG. Meiotic pairing and gametogenic failure. In: Evans CW, Dickinson HG, eds. *Controlling Events in Meiosis.* Cambridge: Company of Biologists, 1984;349–362.
236. Henderson SA, Edwards RG. Chiasma frequency and maternal age in mammals. *Nature* 1968;218:22–28.
237. Polani PE, Crolla JA. A test of the production line hypothesis of mammalian oogenesis. *Hum Genet* 1991;88:64–70.
238. Baker TG, Beaumont HM, Franchi LL. The uptake of tritiated uridine and phenylalanine by the ovaries of rats and monkeys. *J Cell Sci* 1969;4:655–675.
239. Wagenen GV, Simpson ME. *Postnatal Development of the Ovary in Homo sapiens and Macaca mulatta.* New Haven, CT: Yale University Press, 1973.
240. Andersen AC, Simpson ME. *The Ovary and the Reproductive Cycle of the Dog (Beagle).* Los Altos, CA: Geron-X, Inc, 1973.
241. Brambell FWR. Ovarian changes. In: Parkes AS, ed. *Marshall's Physiology of Reproduction.* London: Longmans Green, 1956;397–542.
242. Makabe S, Naguro T, Nottula SA, Pereda J, Motta PM. Migration of germ cells, development of the ovary, and folliculogenesis. In: Familiari G, Makabe S, Motta PM, eds. *Ultrastructure of the Ovary.* Boston, Dordrecht, London: Kluwer Academic Publishers, 1991;1–27.
243. Byskov AG, Lintern-Moore S. Follicle formation in the immature mouse ovary: the role of the rete ovarii. *J Anat* 1973;116:207–217.
244. Byskov AG, Skakkebæk NE, Stafanger G, Peters H. Influence of ovarian surface epithelium and rete ovarii on follicle formation. *J Anat* 1977;123:77–86.
245. Mossman HW, Duke KL. *Comparative Morphology of the Mammalian Ovary.* Madison: The University of Wisconsin Press, 1973.
246. Stein LE, Anderson EH. A qualitative and quantitative study of rete ovarii development in the fetal rat: correlation with the onset of meiosis and follicle cell appearance. *Anat Rec* 1979; 193:197–211.
247. Høyer PE, Byskov AG. A quantitative cytochemical study of 3β-hydroxysteroid dehydrogenase activity in the rete system of the immature mouse ovary. In: Byskov AG, Peters H, eds. *Development and Function of Reproductive Organs.* Amsterdam: Excerpta Medica, 1981;216–224.
248. Hirshfield AN. Development of follicles in the mammalian ovary. *Int Rev Cytol* 1991;124:43–101.
249. Pedersen T. Follicle growth in the mouse ovary. In: Biggers JD, Schuetz AW, eds. *Oogenesis.* London: Butterworths, 1972; 261–276.
250. Peters H. Folliculogenesis in mammals. In: Jones RE, ed. *The Vertebrate Ovary,* New York: Plenum Press, 1978;121–144.
251. Nikitin A, Byskov AG. Mesonephric influence on the survival of fetal mouse germ cells; preliminary results. In: Byskov AG, Peters H, eds. *Development and Function of Reproductive Organs.* Amsterdam: Excerpta Medica, 1981;51–57.
252. Lintern-Moore S. Initiation of follicular growth in the infant mouse ovary by exogenous gonadotrophin. *Biol Reprod* 1977;17:635–639.
253. Gulyas BJ, Hodgen GD, Tullner WW, Ross GT. Effects of fetal or maternal hypophysectomy on endocrine organs and body weight in infant rhesus monkeys (*Macaca mulatta*): with particular emphasis on oogenesis. *Biol Reprod* 1977;16:216–227.
254. Baker TG, Neal P. Initiation and control of meiosis and follicular growth in ovaries of the mouse. *Ann Biol Anim Biochim Biophys* 1973;13:137–144.
255. Nayudu PL, Osborn SM. Factors influencing the rate of preantral and antral growth of mouse ovarian follicles *in vitro. J Reprod Fertil* 1992;95:349–362.
256. Wang X, Roy SV, Greenwald GS. *In vitro* DNA synthesis by isolated preantral to preovulatory follicles from the cyclic mouse. *Biol Reprod* 1991;44:857–863.
257. Challoner S. Studies of oogenesis and follicular development in the golden hamster. 2. Initiation and control of meiosis in vitro. *J Anat* 1975;119:149–156.
258. Roy SK, Greenwald GS. Hormonal requirements for the growth

and differentiation of hamster preantral follicles in long-term culture. *J Reprod Fertil* 1989;87:103–114.
259. Hirshfield AN. Comparison of granulosa cell proliferation in small follicles of hypophysectomized, prepuberal, and mature rats. *Biol Reprod* 1985;32:979–987.
260. Baker TG, Scrimgeour JB. Development of the gonad in normal and anencephalic human fetuses. *J Reprod Fertil* 1980;60: 193–199.
261. Eshkol A, Lunenfeld B, Peters H. Ovarian development in infant mice. Dependence on gonadotrophic hormones. In: Butt WR, Crooke AC, Ryle M, eds. *Gonadotrophins and Ovarian Development.* Edinburgh: Livingstone, 1970;249–258.
262. Koering MJ, Danforth DR, Hodgen GD. Early folliculogenesis in primate ovaries: testing the role of estrogen. *Biol Reprod* 1991;45:890–897.
263. Roy SK, Greenwald GS. Mediation of follicle-stimulating hormone action on follicular desoxyribonucleic acid synthesis by epidermal growth factor. *Endocrinology* 1991;129:1903–1908.
264. Byskov AG, Bagger P, Andersen CY, Wilken-Jensen C, Westergaard L. Differentiation, growth and maturation of oocytes. In: Haseltine FP, Findlay JK, eds. *Growth Factors in Fertility Regulation.* New York: Cambridge University Press, 1991;3–11.
265. Voutilainen R, Miller WL. Developmental and hormonal regulation of mRNAs for insulin-like growth factor II and steroidogenic enzymes in human fetal adrenals and gonads. *DNA* 1988; 7:9–15.
266. Gospodarowicz D, Ferrara N. Fibroblast growth factor and the control of pituitary and gonad development and function. *J Steroid Biochem* 1989;32:183–191.
267. Rabinovici J, Goldsmith PC, Roberts VJ, Vaughan J, Vale W, Jaffe RB. Localization and secretion of inhibin/activin subunits in the human and subhuman primate fetal gonads. *J Clin Endocrinol Metab* 1991;73:1141–1149.
268. Guoliang X, Byskov AG, Høyer PE. Postnatal growth pattern of mouse oocytes is imprinted during embryonic life. *In preparation.* 1993.
269. Krarup T, Pedersen T, Faber M. Regulation of oocyte growth in the mouse ovary. *Nature* 1969;224:187–188.
270. Rajah R, Glaser EM, Hirshfield AN. The changing architecture of the neonatal rat ovary during histogenesis. *Dev Dynamics* 1992;194:177–192.
271. Mauleon P, Mariana JC. Oogenesis and folliculogenesis. In: Cole HH, Cupps PT, eds. *Reproduction in Domestic Animals.* New York: Academic Press, 1976;175–202.
272. Byskov AG. Differentiation of mammalian embryonic gonad. *Physiol Rev* 1986;66:71–117.
273. Christensen AK. Leydig cells. In: Greep RO, Astwood EB, eds. *Handbook of Physiology. Vol. V.* Baltimore: Williams & Wilkins, 1975;57–94.
274. Gondos B, George FW, Wilson JD. Granulosa cell differentiation and estrogen synthesis in the fetal rabbit ovary. *Biol Reprod* 1983;29:791–798.
275. Milewich L, George FW, Wilson JD. Estrogen formation by the ovary of the rabbit embryo. *Endocrinology* 1977;100:187–196.
276. Byskov AG, Høyer PE, Westergaard L. Origin and differentiation of the endocrine cells of the ovary. *J Reprod Fertil* 1985;75:299–306.
277. Gondos B, Hobel CJ. Interstitial cells in the human fetal ovary. *Endocrinology* 1973;93:736–739.
278. Høyer PE. Histoenzymology of the human ovary: dehydrogenases directly involved in steroidogenesis. In: Motta PM, Hafez ES, eds. *Biology of the Ovary.* The Hague: Nijhoff, 1980;52–67.
279. Erickson GF, Magoffin DA, Dyer CA, Hafeditz C. The ovarian androgen producing cells: a review of structure/function relationships. *Endocr Rev* 1985;6:371–399.
280. Quattropani SL. Morphogenesis of the ovarian interstitial tissue in the neonate mouse. *Anat Rec* 1973;177:569–584.
281. Grinsted J. Influence of mesonephros on foetal and neonatal rabbit gonads. II. Sex-steroid release by the ovary *in vitro. Acta Endocrinol* 1982;99:281–287.
282. Gougeon A. Aspects originaux de la glande interstitielle ovarienne chez la Hérisson: morphologie, histogenese, hyperplasie, enzymes de la steroidogenese. *Ann Biol Anim Biochim Biophys* 1974;14:53–66.
283. Zondek LH, Zondek T. Ovarian hilar cells and testicular Leydig cells in anencephaly. *Biol Neonate* 1983;43:211–219.
284. Prépin J, Hida N. Influence of age and medium on formation of epithelial cords in the rat fetal ovary *in vitro. J Reprod Fertil* 1989;87:375–382.
285. Buyse A. The differentiation of transplanted mammalian gonad primordia. *J Exp Zool* 1935;70:1–41.
286. Moore CR, Price D. Differentiation of embryonic reproductive tissues of the rat after transplantation into postnatal hosts. *J Exp Zool* 1942;90:229–265.
287. Holyoke EA. The differentiation of embryonic gonads transplanted to the adult omentum in the albino rat. *Anat Rec* 1949;103:675–699.
288. McIntyre MN. Effect of fetal testis on ovarian differentiation in heterosexual embryonic rat gonad transplant. *Anat Rec* 1956;124:27–46.
289. Turner CD, Asakawa H. Experimental reversal of germ cells in ovaries of fetal mice. *Science* 1964;143:1344–1345.
290. Turner CD. Experimental reversal of germ cells. *Embryologia* 1969;10:206–230.
291. Taketo T, Merchant-Larios H, Koide SS. Induction of testicular differentiation on the fetal mouse ovary by transplantation into adult male mice. *Proc Soc Exp Biol Med* 1984;176:148–153.
292. Taketo-Hosotani T. Factors involved in the testicular development from fetal mouse ovaries following transplantation. *J Exp Zool* 1987;241:95–100.
293. Ozdzenski W, Rogulska T, Batakier H, Brzozowska M, Rembiszewska A, Stepinska U. Influence of embryonic and adult testis on the differentiation of embryonic ovary in the mouse. *Arch Anat Microsc Morphol Exp* 1976;65:285–294.
294. Burgoyne PS, Ansell J-D, Tournay A. Can the indifferent mammalian XX gonad be sex reversed by interaction with testicular tissue? In: Eshkol A, Eckstein B, Dekel N, Peters H, Tsafriri A, eds. *Development and Function of the Reproductive Organs. Serono Symposia Review No. 11.* New York: Raven Press, 1986;23–39.
295. Byskov AG, Saxen L. Induction of meiosis in foetal mouse testis *in vitro. Dev Biol* 1976;52:193–200.
296. Lillie FR. The free-martin: A study of the action of sex hormones in the foetal life of cattle. *J Exp Zool* 1917;23:371–452.
297. Jost A, Virgier B, Prépin J. Freemartins in cattle: the first steps of sexual organogenesis. *J Reprod Fertil* 1972;29:349–379.
298. Virgier B, Tran D, Legai L, Bézard J, Josso N. Origin of anti-müllerian hormone in bovine freemartins fetuses. *J Reprod Fertil* 1984;70:473–479.
299. Vigier B, Forest NG, Eychenne B, et al. Anti-müllerian hormone produces endocrine sex reversal of fetal ovaries. *Proc Natl Acad Sci* 1989;86:3684–3688.
300. Grier HJ. Chordate testis: The extracellular matrix hypothesis. *J Exp Zool* 1992;261:151–160.
301. McCoshen JA. *In vivo* sex differentiation of congeneric germinal cell aplastic gonads. *Am J Obstet Gynecol* 1982;142:83–88.
302. Mintz B, Russell ES. Developmental modifications of primordial germ cells, induced by W-series genes in the mouse embryo. *Anat Rec* 1955;122:443–449.
303. Blaschuk O, Burdzy K, Fritz IB. Purification and characterization of a cell-aggregating factor (Clusterin), the major glycoprotein in ram rete testis fluid. *J Biol Chem* 1983;258:7714–7720.
304. Jost A. Recherches sur la differenciation sexuelle de l'embryon de lapin. IV. Organogenese sexuelle masculine apres decapitation du foetus. *Arch Anat Microsc Morphol Exp* 1951;40:247–281.
305. Elias H. Frühentwicklung der Samenkanälchen beim Menschen. *Verh Anat Ges Versamml* 1974;68:123–131.
306. Wartenberg H, Kinsky J, Viebahn C, Schmolke C. Fine structural characteristics of testicular cord formation in the developing rabbit gonad. *J Electron Microsc Tech* 1991;19:133–157.
307. Clermont Y, Huckins C. Microscopic anatomy of the sex cords and seminiferous tubules in growing and adult albino rats. *Am J Anat* 1961;180:79–97.
308. Magre S, Jost A. The initial phases of testicular organogenesis in the rat. An electron microscopy study. *Arch Anat Microsc Morphol* 1980;69:297–318.
309. Pelliniemi LJ. Ultrastructure of the indifferent gonad in male and female pig embryos. *Tissue Cell* 1976;8:163–174.

310. Byskov AG, Yding Andersen C, Westergaard L. Dependence of the onset of meiosis on the internal organization of the gonad. In: McLaren A, Wylie CC, eds. *Current Problems in Germ Cell Differentiation.* Cambridge: Cambridge University Press, 1983; 215–224.
311. Magre S, Jost A. Early stages of differentiation of the rat testis: regulations between Sertoli and germ cells. In: McLaren A, Wylie CC, eds. *Current Problems in Germ Cell Differentiation.* Cambridge: Cambridge University Press, 1983;201–214.
312. Paranko J, Pelliniemi LJ, Vaheri A, Foidart JM, Lakkala-Paranko T. Morphogenesis and fibronectin in sexual differentiation of rat embryonic gonads. *Differentiation* 1983;(suppl.)23: 72–81.
313. Fritz IB, Skinner MK, Tung PS. The nature of somatic cell interactions in the seminiferous tubule. In: Eshkol A, Eckstein B, Dekel N, Peters H, Tsafriri A, eds. *Development and Function of Reproductive Organs. Serono Symposia Review No. 11.* New York: Raven Press, 1986;85–91.
314. Parenko J, Kallajoki M, Pelliniemi LJ, Lehto VP, Virtanen L. Transient coexpression of cytokeratin and vimentin in differentiating rat Sertoli cells. *Dev Biol* 1986;117:35–44.
315. Stosiek P, Kasper M, Karsten U. Expression of cytokeratins 8 and 18 in human Sertoli cells of immature and atrophic seminiferous tubules. *Differentiation* 1990;43:66–70.
316. Chartrain I, Magre S, Maingurd M, Jost A. Effect of serum on organogenesis of the rat testis *in vitro. In Vitro Cell Dev Biol* 1984;20:912–922.
317. Taketo T, Seen CD, Koide SS. Requirement of serum components for the preservation of primordial germ cells in the testis cords during early stages of testicular differentiation *in vitro* in the mouse. *Biol Reprod* 1986;34:919–924.
318. Taketo T, Thau RB, Adeyemo O, Koide SS. Influence of adenosine 3′,5′-cyclic monophosphate analogues on testicular organization of fetal mouse gonads *in vitro. Biol Reprod* 1984;30:189–198.
319. Byskov AG, Fenger M, Westergaard L, Yding Andersen C. Forskolin and the meiosis inducing substance synergistically initiate meiosis in fetal male germ cells. *Mol Reprod Dev* 1993;34:47–52.
320. Gondos B. Development and differentiation of the testis and male reproductive tract. In: Steinberger A, Steinberger E, eds. *Testicular Development, Structure and Function.* New York: Raven Press, 1980;3–20.
321. Hilscher W, Hilscher B, Gauss G, Lippers P, Bülthoff B. Untersuchung zur Kinetik der Gonocyten und Stützzellen der Wistarratte. *Andrologie* 1972;4:311–325.
322. Hilscher W. T1-Prospermatogonia (Primordial Spermatogonia of Rauh): the "ameiotic" counter part of early oocytes. *Fortschr Androl* 1981;7:21–32.
323. Nogushi T, Stevens LC. Primordial germ cell proliferation in fetal testes in mouse strains with high and low incidences of congenital testicular teratomas. *J Natl Cancer Inst* 1982;69:907–913.
324. Peters H. Migration of gonocytes into the mammalian gonad and their differentiation. *Philos Trans R Soc Lond (Biol)* 1970;259:91–101.
325. Hilscher W. Kinetics of prespermatogenesis and spermatogenesis of the Wistar rat under normal and pathological conditions. *Fortschr Androl* 1970;1:17–20.
326. Huckins C, Clermont Y. Evolution of gonocytes in the rat testis during late embryonic and early post-natal life. *Arch Anat Histol Embryol* 1968;51:343–354.
327. Mauger A, Clermont Y. Ultrastructure des gonocytes et des spermatogonies de jeune rat. *Arch Anat Microsc Morphol Exp* 1974;63:133–146.
328. Rauh W. Das chondriom in der ersten Keimzellen der Ratte. Eine Keimbahnuntersuchung. *Z Ges Anat* 1929;89:271–309.
329. Larsen JK, Byskov AG, Grinsted J. Growth and differentiation of foetal mouse gonads in culture studied by flow cytometry on nuclear suspensions. *Acta Pathol Microbiol Immunol Scand (A)* 1981;(suppl.)274:178–182.
330. Kluin PM, Kramer MF, de Rooij DG. Proliferation of spermatogonia and Sertoli cells in maturing mice. *Anat Embryol* 1984;169:73–78.
331. Vergouwen RPFA, Jacobs SGPM, Huiskamp R, Davids JAG, de Rooij DG. Proliferative activity of gonocytes, Sertoli cells and interstitial cells during testicular development in mice. *J Reprod Fertil* 1991;93:233–243.
332. Gondos B, Byskov AG. Germ cell kinetics in the neonatal rabbit testis. *Cell Tissue Res* 1981;215:143–151.
333. Beaumont HM, Mandl AM. A quantitative study of primordial germ cells in the male rat. *J Embryol Exp Morphol* 1963;11:715–740.
334. Byskov AG. Primordial germ cells and regulation of meiosis. In: Austin CR, Short RV, eds. *Reproduction in Mammals. Book 1. Germ Cells and Fertilization.* Cambridge: Cambridge University Press, 1981;1–16.
335. Wartenberg H. Structural aspects of gonadal differentiation in mammals and birds. In: Müller U, Franke WW, eds. *Differentiation.* Berlin: Springer Verlag, 1983;64–71.
336. Jost A. Initial stages of gonadal development. *Arch Anat Microsc Morphol Exp* 1985;74:39–41.
337. Magre S, Jost A. Sertoli cells and testicular differentiation in the rat fetus. *J Electron Microsc Tech* 1991;19:172–188.
338. Gropp A, Ohno S. Presence of a common embryonic blastema for ovarian and testicular parenchymal (follicular, interstitial and tubular) cells in cattle, *Bos taurus. Z Zellforsch Mikrosk Anat* 1966;74:505–528.
339. Merchant-Larios H. The onset of testicular differentiation in the rat: an ultrastructural study. *Am J Anat* 1976;145:319–330.
340. Clermont Y, Perey B. Quantitative study of the cell population of the seminiferous tubules in immature rats. *Am J Anat* 1957;100:241–268.
341. Nagy F. Cell division kinetics and DNA synthesis in the immature Sertoli cells of the rat testis. *J Reprod Fertil* 1972;28:389–395.
342. Steinberger A, Steinberger E. The Sertoli cells. In: Johnson AD, Gomes WR, eds. *The Testis.* New York: Academic Press, 1977;371–399.
343. Sun EL, Gondos B. Proliferative activity in the rabbit testis during postnatal development. In: Byskov AG, Peters H, eds. *Development and Function of Reproductive Organs. International Congress Series No. 559.* Amsterdam: Excerpta Medica, 1981; 140–148.
344. Zamboni L, Upadhyay S. The contribution of the mesonephros to the development of the sheep fetal testis. *Am J Anat* 1982;165:339–356.
345. Gondos B. Testicular development. In: Johnson AD, Gomes WR, eds. *The Testis. Vol. IV.* New York: Academic Press, 1977;1–37.
346. Jost A, Magre S. Testicular development phases and dual hormonal control of sexual organogenesis. In: Serio M, Motta M, Zanisi M, Martini L, eds. *Sexual Differentiation: Basic and Clinical Aspects. Serono Symposa Publications. Vol. 11.* New York: Raven Press, 1984;1–15.
347. Gondos B, Sun EL. Cell membrane modifications during human fetal gonadal development. In: Byskov AG, Peters H, eds. *Development and Function of the Reproductive Organs.* Amsterdam: Excerpta Medica, 1981;31–40.
348. Gondos B, Conner LA. Ultrastructure of the developing germ cell in the fetal rabbit testis. *Am J Anat* 1973;136:23–42.
349. Magre S. Différenciation des cellules de Sertoli et morphogenese testiculaire chez le foetus de Rat. *Arch Anat Microsc Morphol Exp* 1985;74:64–68.
350. George FW, Wilson JD. The regulation of androgen and estrogen formation in fetal gonads. *Ann Biol Anim Biochim Biophys* 1979;19(4B):1297–1306.
351. Raeside JI, Sigman DM. Testosterone levels in early fetal testes of domestic pigs. *Biol Reprod* 1975;13:318–321.
352. Ortiz E, Price D, Zaaijer JJP. Organ culture studies of hormone secretion in endocrine glands of fetal guinea pigs. II. Secretion of androgenic hormone in adrenals and testes during early stages of development. *Koninkl Nederl Akademie van Wetenschappen* 1966;69:400–408.
353. Moon YS, Raeside JI. Histochemical studies on hydroxysteroid dehydrogenase activity of fetal pig testis. *Biol Reprod* 1972;7:278–287.
354. Black VH, Christensen AK. Differentiation of interstitial cells and Sertoli cells in fetal guinea pig testes. *Am J Anat* 1969;124:211–238.

355. Cate RL, Wilson CA. Müllerian inhibiting substance. In: Gwatkin RBL, ed. *Genes in Mammalian Reproduction*. New York: Wiley-Liss, 1993;185–205.
356. Münsterberg A, Lowell-Badge R. Expression of the mouse anti-müllerian hormone gene suggests a role in both male and female sexual differentiation. *Development* 1991;113:613–624.
357. Hudson J, Donahoe PK. The hormonal control of testicular descent. *Endocr Rev* 1986;7:270–283.
358. Roosen-Runge EC, Anderson D. The development of the interstitial cells in the testis of the albino rat. *Acta Anat* 1959;37:125–137.
359. Pelliniemi LJ, Niemi M. Fine structure of the human foetal testis. I. The interstitial tissue. *Z Zellforsch* 1969;99:507–522.
360. Kerr JB, Knell CM. The fate of fetal Leydig cells during the development of the fetal and postnatal rat testis. *Development* 1988;103:535–544.
361. Leinonen PJ, Jaffe RB. Leydig cell desensitization by human chorionic gonadotropin does not occur in the human fetal testis. *J Clin Endocrinol Metab* 1985;61:234–238.
362. Picon R. Testosterone secretion by foetal rat testis *in vitro*. *J Endocrinol* 1976;71:231–238.
363. Weisz J, Ward IL. Plasma testosterone and progesterone titers of pregnant rats, their male and female fetuses and neonatal offspring. *Endocrinology* 1980;106:306–316.
364. Tapanainen J, Kuopio T, Pelliniemi LJ, Huhtaniemi I. Rat testicular endogenous steroids and number of Leydig cells between the fetal period and sexual maturity. *Biol Reprod* 1984;31:1027–1035.
365. Niemi M, Ikonen M, Hervonen A. Histochemistry and fine structure of interstitial tissue in human foetal testis. In: Woltenholme GEW and O'Connor M, eds. *Endocrinology of the Testis. Ciba Foundation Colloquium on Endocrinology. Vol. 16*. London: J & A Churchill Ltd., 1967;31–55.
366. Orth J, Weisz J. Development of 3β-hydroxysteroid dehydrogenase and glucose-6-phosphatase activity in Leydig cells of the fetal rat testis: a quantitative cytochemical study. *Biol Reprod* 1980;22:1201–1209.
367. Yding Andersen C, Byskov AG, Grinsted J. Partial purification of the meiosis inducing substance (MIS). In: Byskov AG, Peters H, eds. *Development and Function of Reproductive Organs*. Amsterdam: Exerpta Medica, 1981;73–80.
368. Magre S, Agelopoulou R, Jost A. Action du serum de foetus de veau sur la differenciation in vitro on le mantien des cordons seminiferes du testicule du foetus du rat. *C R Acad Sci (Paris)* 1981;292:85–89.
369. Agelopoulou R, Magre S, Patsavoudi E, Jost A. Initial phases of the rat testis differentiation *in vitro*. *J Embryol Exp Morphol* 1984;83:15–31.
370. Patsavoudi E, Magre S, Castanier M, Scholler R, Jost A. Dissociation between testicular morphogenesis and functional differentiation of Leydig cells. *J Endocrinol* 1985;105:235–238.
371. Clements JA, Reyes FI, Winter JSD, Faiman C. Studies on human sexual development. III. Fetal pituitary and serum, and amniotic fluid concentrations of LH, CG and FSH. *J Clin Endocrinol Metab* 1976;42:9–19.
372. Catt KJ, Dufau ML, Neaves WB, Walsh PC, Wilson JD. LH-HCG receptors and testosterone content during differentiation of the testis in the rabbit embryo. *Endocrinology* 1975;97:1157–1165.
373. George FW, Simpson ER, Milewich L, Wilson JD. Studies on the regulation of the onset of steroid hormone biosynthesis in fetal rabbit gonads. *Endocrinology* 1979;105:1100–1106.
374. Gulyas BJ, Tullner WW, Hodgen GD. Fetal and maternal hypophysectomy in rhesus monkeys (*Macaca mulatta*): effects on the development of testes and other endocrine organs. *Biol Reprod* 1977;17:650–660.
375. Tseng MT, Alexander NJ, Kittinger GW. Effects of fetal decapitation on the structure and function of Leydig cells in rhesus monkeys (*Macaca mulatta*). *Am J Anat* 1975;143:349–362.
376. Zamboni L, Upadhyay S. Germ cell differentiation in mouse adrenal glands. *J Exp Zool* 1983;228:173–193.
377. Tarkowski AK. Are genetic factors controlling sexual differentiation of somatic and germinal tissues of a mammalian gonad stable or labile? In: Kretchmer N, Walcher DN, eds. *Environmental Influences on Genetic Expression*. Bethesda, MD: National Institutes of Health, 1969;49–68.
378. Kratzer PG, Chapman VM. X chromosome reactivation in oocytes of *Mus caroli*. *Proc Natl Acad Sci USA* 1981;78:3093–3097.
379. Byskov AG. Regulation of initiation of meiosis in fetal gonads. *J Androl (Suppl)* 1978;2:29–39.
380. Angelova P, Jordanov J. Meiosis-inducing and meiosis-preventing effects of sex steroid hormones on hamster fetal ovaries in organ culture. *Arch Anat Microsc* 1987;75:149–159.
381. Mazur M, Younglai EV. Role of the pituitary in controlling oogenesis in the rabbit. *Biol Reprod* 1986;35:191–197.
382. Jagiello GM, Dennis J, Hiura M, Ducayen MB. Incorporation of L-^{3}H-fucose in the rete and ovary of the fetal mouse. *Gamete Res* 1983;7:155–160.
383. Wolgemuth DJ, Watrin F. List of cloned mouse genes with unique expression pattern during spermatogenesis. *Mammal Genome* 1991;1:283–288.
384. Don J, Wolgemuth DJ. Identification and characterization of the regulated pattern of expression of a novel mouse gene, meg1, during the meiotic cell cycle. *Cell Growth Differ* 1992;3:495–505.
385. Noce T, Fujiwara Y, Sezaki M, Fujimoto H, Higashinakagawa T. Expression of a mouse zinc finger protein gene in both spermatocytes and oocytes during meiosis. *Dev Biol* 1992;153:356–367.
386. Driscoll DJ, Migeon BR. Sex difference in methylation of single-copy genes in human meiotic germ cells: implications for X chromosome inactivation, parental imprinting, and origin of CpG mutations. *Somat Cell Mol Genet* 1990;16:267–282.
387. Fajer AB, Schneider J, McCall D, Ances IG, Polakis SE. The induction of meiosis by ovaries of newborn hamsters and its relation to the action of the extra ovarian structures in the mesovarium (rete ovarii). *Ann Biol Anim Biochim Biophys* 1979;19(4B):1273–1278.
388. Stein LE, Anderson E. *In vitro* analysis of ovarian differentiation and the initiation of meiosis in the rat. *Acta Anat* 1981;10:189–205.
389. Westergaard L, Byskov AG, VanLook PFA, et al. Meiosis-inducing substances in human preovulatory follicular fluid related to time of follicle aspiration and to the potential of the oocyte to fertilize and cleave *in vitro*. *Fertil Steril* 1985;44:663–667.
390. Westergaard L, Callesen H, Hyttel P, Greve T, Byskov AG. Meiosis inducing substance (MIS) in bovine preovulatory follicles. *Zuchthygiene* 1985;20:217–221.
391. Tsafriri A, Channing CP. An inhibitory influence of granulosa cells and follicular fluid upon porcine oocyte meiosis *in vitro*. *Endocrinology* 1975;96:922–927.
392. Tsafriri A, Dekel N, Bar-Ami S. The role of oocyte maturation inhibitor in follicular regulation of oocyte maturation. *J Reprod Fertil* 1982;64:541–551.
393. Masui Y. The role of "cytostatic factor (CSF)" in the control of oocyte cell cycles: a summary of 20 years of study. *Dev Growth Differ* 1991;33:543–551.
394. Erickson RP. Molecular genetics of mammalian spermatogenesis. In: Gwatkin RBL, ed. *Genes in Mammalian Reproduction*. New York: Wiley-Liss, 1993;1–26.
395. Luciani JM, Devictor-Vuillet M, Stahl A. Preleptotene chromosome condensation stage in human foetal and neonatal testes. *J Embryol Exp Morphol* 1977;38:175–186.
396. Grinsted J, Byskov AG. Meiosis inducing and meiosis preventing substances in human male reproductive organs. *Fertil Steril* 1981;35:199–204.
397. Reyes FI, Winter JSD, Faiman C. Studies on human sexual development. I. Fetal gonadal and adrenal sex steroids. *J Clin Endocrinol Metab* 1973;37:74–78.
398. Mauléon P, Bezard J, Terqui M. Very early and transient secretion of oestradiol-17β by foetal sheep ovary *in vitro*. *Ann Biol Anim Biochim Biophys* 1977;17:399–401.
399. Shemesh M. Estradiol-17β biosynthesis by the early bovine fetal ovary during the active and refractory phases. *Biol Reprod* 1980;23:577–582.
400. Sholl SA, Goy RW. Androgen and estrogen synthesis in the fetal guinea pig gonad. *Biol Reprod* 1978;18:160–169.
401. Taylor T, Coutts JRT, Macnaughton MC. Human foetal synthe-

sis of testosterone from perfused progesterone. *J Endocrinol* 1974;60:321–326.
402. Payne AH, Jaffe RB. Androgen formation from pregnenolone sulfate by the human fetal ovary. *J Clin Endocrinol Metab* 1974;39:300–304.
403. Resko JA, Ploem JG, Stadelman HL. Estrogens in fetal and maternal plasma of the rhesus monkey. *Endocrinology* 1975; 97:425–430.
404. George FW, Wilson JD. Conversion of androgen to estrogen by the human fetal ovary. *J Clin Endocrinol Metab* 1978; 47:550–555.
405. Terada N, Kuroda H, Namiki M, Kitamura Y, Matsumoto K. Augmentation of aromatase activity by FSH in ovaries of fetal and neonatal mice in organ culture. *J Steroid Biochem* 1984;20:741–745.
406. Weniger JP, Chouraqui J, Zeis A. Steroid conversions by the 19-day old foetal rat ovary in organ culture. *Biol Chem* 1985;366:555–559.
407. Rigaudière N. Evolution des teneurs en testostérone et dihydrotestostérone dans le plasma le testicule et l'ovaire chez la cobaye au cours de la vie foetale. *C R Acad Sci (Paris)* 1977;285:989–992.
408. Picon R. Stades initiaux de la stéroidogenèse dans les gonade de mammifères. *Arch Anat Microsc Morphol Exp* 1986;74:81–86.
409. Raeside JI. Gonadotrophic stimulation of androgen secretion by the early fetal pig ovary in organ culture. *Biol Reprod* 1983;28:128–133.
410. Carr BR, Simpson ER. Cholesterol synthesis in human fetal tissues. *J Clin Endocrinol Metab* 1982;55:447–452.
411. Diczfalusy E, Manuso S. Oestrogen metabolism in pregnancy. In: Klopper A, Diczfalus E, eds. *Foetus and Placenta.* Oxford: Blackwell Scientific Publications, 1969;191–248.
412. Eik-Nes KB. Biosynthesis and secretion of testicular steroids. In: Greep RO, Astwood EB, eds. *Handbook of Physiology. Vol. V.* Baltimore: Williams & Wilkins, 1975;95–115.
413. Raynard A, Frilley M. Etat de développement des ébauches mammaires et du cordon vaginal chez les foetus males et femelles de souris, dont le ébauches génitales ont été détruites par une irradiation au moyen des rayons X, a l'age de treize jours. *C R Acad Sci (Paris)* 1947;225:1380–1382.
414. Forest MG. Role of androgens in fetal and pubertal development. *Horm Res* 1983;18:69–83.
415. McEwen BS. Gonadal steroids and brain development. *Biol Reprod* 1980;22:43–48.
416. Resko JA. Fetal hormones and development of the central nervous system in primates. *Adv Sex Horm Res* 1977;3:139–168.
417. Ward IL, Weisz J. Maternal stress alters plasma testosterone in fetal males. *Science* 1980;207:328–329.
418. Kolburger W, Trepel M, Beyer C, Pilgrim Ch, Reisert I. The influence of genetic sex on sexual differentiation of diencephalic dopaminergic neurons *in vitro* and *in vivo. Brain Res* 1991;544:349–352.
419. Baum ML, Woutersen PJA, Slob AK. Sex difference in whole-body androgen content in rat on fetal days 18 and 19 without evidence that androgen passes from males to females. *Biol Reprod* 1991;44:747–751.
420. Reisert I, Pilgrim Ch. Sexual differentiation of monoamninergic neurons—genetic or epigenetic? *Trends Neurosci* 1991;14: 468–473.
421. Habenicht U-F. Hormonal regulation of testicular descent. *Adv Anat Embryo Cell Biol* 1983;81:1–54.
422. Hutson JM, Donahoe PK. The hormonal control of testicular descent. *Endocr Rev* 1986;7:270–283.
423. Winter JSD, Faiman C, Reyes F. Sexual endocrinology of fetal and perinatal life. In: Austin CR, Edwards RG, eds. *Mechanisms of Sex Differentiation in Animals and Man.* London: Academic Press, 1981;205–253.
424. Winter JSD, Faiman C, Reyes FI. Sex steroid production by the human fetus: its role in morphogenesis and control by gonadotrophins. In: Blandau RJ, Bergma D, eds. *Morphogenesis and Malformation of the Genital System.* New York: Alan R. Liss, 1977;41–58.
425. Carr BR, Parker CR, Ohashi M, MacDonald PC, Simpson ER. Regulation of human fetal testicular secretion of testosterone: low-density lipoprotein-cholesterol and cholesterol synthesized *de novo* as steroid precursor. *Am J Obstet Gynecol* 1983;146:241–246.
426. Molsberry RL, Carr BR, Mendelson CR. Human chorionic gonadotropin binding to human fetal testes as a function of gestational age. *J Clin Endocrinol Metab* 1982;55:791–794.
427. Warren DW, Huhtaniemi IT, Tapanainen J, Dufau ML, Catt KJ. Ontogeny of gonadotropin receptors in the fetal and neonatal rat testis. *Endocrinology* 1984;114:470–476.
428. Leinonen PJ, Jaffe RB. Leydig cell desensitization by human chorionic gonadotropin does not occur in the human fetal testis. *J Clin Endocrinol Metab* 1985;61:234–238.
429. Warren DW, Schmitt CA, Franzino SJ. Adrenocorticotropin stimulates testosterone production by fetal rat testis. *Ann N Y Acad Sci* 1984;438:677–680.
430. Dohr G, Tarmann T. Contacts between wolffian and müllerian cells at the tip of the outgrowing müllerian duct in rat embryos. *Acta Anat* 1984;120:123–128.
431. Felix W. The development of the urogenital organs. In: Keibl F, Mall FP, eds. *Manual of Human Embryology.* Philadelphia: JB Lippincott, 1912;752–879.
432. Grünwald P. The relation of the growing müllerian duct to the wolffian duct and its importance for the genesis of malformations. *Anat Rec* 1941;81:1–19.
433. Burkl W, Pollitzer G. Über die genetischen Beziehungen des Müllerschen Ganges zum Wolffschen Gang beim Menschen. *Z Anat Entw Gesch* 1952;116:552–572.
434. Frutiger P. Zur Frühentwicklung der Ductus paramesonephrici und des Müllerschen Hügels beim Menschen. *Acta Anat* 1969;72:233–245.
435. Bishop-Calame S. Étude expérimentale de l'organogénèse du système uro-génitale de l'embryon de poulet. *Arch Anat Microsc Morphol Exp* 1966;55:215–309.
436. Viebahn C, Lane EB, Ramaekers CS. The mesonephric (wolffian) and paramesomephric (müllerian) ducts of golden hamsters express different intermediate-filament proteins during development. *Differentiation* 1987;34:175–188.
437. Hamilton WJ, Mossman HW. *Human Embryology.* Baltimore: Williams & Wilkins, 1972.
438. Didier E. Recherches sur la morphogénèse du canal de Müller chez les oiseaux. *Roux Arch Entw Mech Org* 1973;172:271–302.
439. Josso N. Differentiation of the genital tract: stimulators and inhibitors. In: Austin CR, Edwards RG, eds. *Mechanisms of Sex Differentiation in Animals and Man.* London: Academic Press, 1981;165–203.
440. Price JM, Donahoe PK, Ito Y, Hendren WH III. Programmed cell death in the müllerian duct induced by müllerian substance. *Am J Anat* 1977;149:353–376.
441. Cunha GR, Shannon JM, Neubauer BL, et al. Mesenchymal–epithelial interactions in sex differentiation. *Hum Genet* 1981;58:68–77.
442. O'Rahilly R. The embryology and anatomy of the uterus. In: Norris HJ, Hertig AT, Abell MR, eds. *The Uterus.* Baltimore: Williams & Wilkins, 1973;17–39.
443. Price D, Zaaijer JJP, Ortiz E. Hormonal influences on genetic expression as demonstrated in organ culture studies of reproductive ducts of fetal guinea pigs. *Konink Nederl Akademie van Wetenshappen Proc Ser C* 1969;72:370–384.
444. Patten BM. *Human Embryology.* New York: McGraw-Hill, 1953.
445. Hunter PH. Observations on the development of the human female genital tract. *Contrib Embryol Carnegie Inst* 1930; 22:91–108.
446. Davies J, Kusama H. Developmental aspects of the human cervix. *Ann N Y Acad Sci* 1962;97:534–550.
447. Jost A. Basic sexual trends in the development of vertebrates. In: *Sex, Hormones and Behaviour. Ciba Foundation Symposium, No. 62.* Amsterdam: Excerpta Medica, 1979;5–18.
448. Picon R. Action du testicule foetal sur le development in vitro des canaux de Müller chez le rat. *Arch Anat Microsc* 1969;58:1–9.
449. Somjen GJ, Kaye AM, Lindner H. Demonstration of 8-*S*-cytoplasmic oestrogen receptor in rat müllerian duct. *Biochim Biophys Acta* 1976;428:787–791.
450. Alarid ET, Cunha GR, Young P, Nicoll CS. Evidence for an

organ- and sex-specific role in basic fibroblast growth factor in the development of the fetal mammalian reproductive tract. *Endocrinology* 1991;129:2148–2154.

451. Pasqualini JR, Sumida C, Gelly C, Nguyen BL. Specific ^{3}H-estradiol binding in the fetal uterus and testis of guinea pig. Quantitative evolution of ^{3}H-estradiol receptors in the different fetal tissues (kidney, lung, uterus and testis) during fetal development. *J Steroid Biochem* 1976;7:1031–1038.
452. Greco TL, Furlow JD, Duello TM, Gorski J. Immunodetection of estrogen receptors in fetal and neonatal femal mouse reproductive tracts. *Endrocrinology* 1991;129:1326–1332.
453. Bibbo M, Gill WB, Freidoon A, et al. Follow-up study of male and female offspring of DES-exposed mother. *J Obstet Gynecol* 1977;49:1–7.
454. McLachlan JA, Newbold RR, Bullock BC. Long-term effects of the female mouse genital tract associated with prenatal exposure to diethylstilbestrol. *Cancer Res* 1980;40:3988–3999.
455. Newbold RR, Bullock BC, McLachlan JA. Exposure to diethylstilbestrol during pregnancy permanently alters the ovary and oviduct. *Biol Reprod* 1983;28:735–744.
456. Byskov AG, Hansen JL. Ovarian influence on the müllerian duct differentiation. In: Eshkol A, Eckstein B, Decke N, Peters H, Tsafriri A, eds. *Development and Function of Reproductive Organs. Serono Symposia Review, No. II.* New York: Raven Press, 1986;85–91.
457. Bok G, Drews U. The role of the wolffian ducts in the formation of the sinus vagina: an organ culture study. *J Embryol Exp Morphol* 1983;73:275–295.
458. Acién P. Embryological observations on the female genital tract. *Hum Reprod* 1992;7:437–445.
459. Price D, Pannabecker R. Comparative responsiveness of homologous sex ducts and accessory glands of fetal rats in culture. *Arch Anat Microsc* 1959;48:223–244.
460. Josso N. Action de la testostérone sur le canal de Wolff du foetus de rat en culture organotypique. *Arch Anat Microsc* 1970;59:37–50.
461. Haney AF, Newbold RR, Fetter BF, McLachlan JA. Paraovarian cysts associated with prenatal diethylstilbestrol exposure. *Am J Pathol* 1986;124:405–411.
462. Flickinger CJ. Fine structure of the wolffian duct and cytodifferentiation of the epididymis in fetal rats. *Z Zellforsch* 1969;96:344–360.
463. Tiedemann K. Die Ultrastruktur des Epithels des Wolffschen Ganges und des Ductus Deferens beim Schafembryo. *Z Zellforsch* 1971;113:230–248.
464. Zondek LH, Zondek T. The secretory activity of the maturing epididymis compared with maturational changes in other reproductive organs of the foetus, infant and child. *Acta Paediatr Scand* 1965;54:295–305.
465. Wilson JD, Griffin JE, George FW, Leshim M. The endocrine control of male phenotypic development. *Aust J Biol Sci* 1983;36:101–128.
466. Flickinger CJ. The fine structure and development of the seminal vesicles and prostate in the fetal rat. *Z Zellforsch* 1970;109:1–14.
467. Aumüller G. Prostate gland and seminal vesicles. In: Oksche A and Vollrath L, eds. *Handbook der Mikroskopischen Anatomie des Menschen, 7. Band. Harn-und Geschlechtapparat, 6. Teil.* Berlin: Springer Verlag, 1979.
468. Wilson JD, Siiteri K. Developmental pattern of testosterone synthesis in the fetal gonad of the rabbit. *Endocrinology* 1973;92:1182–1191.
469. Wilson JD, Lasnitski I. Dihydrotestosterone formation in fetal tissues of the rabbit and rat. *Endocrinology* 1971;89:659–668.
470. Siiteri PK, Wilson JD. Testosterone formation and metabolism during male sexual differentiation in the human embryo. *J Clin Endocrinol Metab* 1974;38:113–125.
471. Tsuji M, Shima H, Cunha GR. *In vitro* androgen-induced growth and morphogenesis of the wolffian duct within urogenital reach. *Endocrinology* 1991;128:1805–1811.
472. Cooke PS, Young P, Cunha GR. Androgen receptor expression in the developing reproductive organs. *Endocrinology* 1991; 128:2867–2873.
473. Cunha GR. Development of the urogenital tract. In: Timiris P, Meisami E, eds. *Handbook of Human Growth and Developmental Biology. Vol. II: Endocrines, Sexual Development, Growth, Nutrition and Metabolism. Part A: Endocrines and Sexual Development.* Boca Raton, FL: CRS Press, 1989;247–261.
474. Cooke PS, Young P, Hess RA, Cunha GR. Estrogen receptor expression in developing epididymis, efferent ducturus, and other male reproductive organs. *Endocrinology* 1991;128:2874–2879.
475. Gupta C. Prostaglandins masculinize the mouse genital tract. *Endrocrinology* 1989;124:1781–1787.
476. Gupta C, Bentlejewski CA. Role of prostaglandins in the testosterone-dependent wolffian duct differentiation of the fetal mouse. *Biol Reprod* 1992;47:1151–1160.
477. Picard JY, Tran D, Josso N. Biosynthesis of iodinated anti-müllerian hormone by fetal testes: evidence for the glycoprotein nature of the hormone and for its disulfide-bonded structure. *Mol Cell Endocrinol* 1978;12:17–30.
478. Picard JY, Benarous R, Guerrier D, Josso N, Kahn A. Cloning and expression of cDNA for anti-müllerian hormone. *Proc Natl Acad Sci* 1986;83:5464–5468.
479. Cate RL, Mattaliano RJ, Hession C, et al. Isolation of the bovine and human genes for müllerian inhibiting substance and expression of the human gene in animal cells. *Cell* 1986;45:685–698.
480. Guerrier D, Boussin L, Mader S, Josso N, Kahn A, Picard JY. Expression of the gene for anti-müllerian hormone. *J Reprod Fertil* 1990;88:695–706.
481. Haqq C, Lee MM, Tizard R, et al. Isolation of the rat gene for müllerian inhibiting substance. *Genomics* 1992;12:665–669.
482. Massague J. The transforming growth factor-beta family. *Annu Rev Cell Biol* 1990;6:597–641.
483. Blanchard MG, Josso N. Source of the anti-müllerian hormone synthesized by the fetal testis: müllerian-inhibiting activity of fetal bovine Sertoli cells in tissue culture. *Pediatr Res* 1974;8:968–971.
484. Donahoe PK, Ito Y, Price JM, Hendren WH III. Müllerian inhibiting substance activity in bovine fetal, newborn and prepuberal testes. *Biol Reprod* 1977;16:238–243.
485. Tran D, Josso N. Localization of anti müllerian hormone in the rough endoplasmic reticulum of the developing bovine Sertoli cell using immunocytochemistry with a monoclonal antibody. *Endocrinology* 1983;111:1562–1567.
486. Josso N. Evolution of the müllerian inhibiting activity of the human testis. Effect of fetal, peri-natal and post-natal human testicular tissue on the müllerian duct of the fetal rat in organ culture. *Biol Neona* 1972;20:368–379.
487. Tran D, Josso N. Relationship between ovarian and mammalian anti-müllerian hormones. *Biol Reprod* 1977;16:267–273.
488. Josso N, Picard J-Y, Tran D. The anti-müllerian hormone. *Recent Prog Horm Res* 1977;33:117–163.
489. Catlin EA, Uitvlugt ND, Donahoe PK, Powell DM, Hayashi M, MacLaughlin DT. Müllerian inhibiting substance blocks epidermal growth factor receptor phosphorylation in fetal rat lung membranes. *Metabolism* 1991;40:1178–1184.
490. Donahoe PK, Cate RL, MacLaughlin DT, et al. Müllerian inhibiting substance: gene structure and mechanism of action of a fetal regressor. *Recent Prog Horm Res* 1987;43:431–467.
491. Cate RL, Donahoe PK, MacLaughlin DT. Müllerian-inhibiting substance. In: Sporn MB, Roberts AB, eds. *Peptide Growth Factors and Their Receptors, II.* Berlin: Springer-Verlag, 1990;179–210.
492. Josso N, Picard J-Y. Anti-müllerian hormone. *Physiol Rev* 1986;66:1038–1090.
493. Taguchi O, Cunha GR, Lawrence WD, Robboy SJ. Timing and irreversibility of müllerian duct inhibition in the embryonic reproductive tract of the human male. *Dev Biol* 1984;106:394–398.
494. Picon R. Modifications chez le rat, au cours du developpement du testicule, de son action inhibitrice sur les canaux de Müller *in vitro. C R Acad Sci* 1970;271:2370–2372.
495. Jost A, Vigier B, Prépin J. Freemartins in cattle: the first steps of sexual organogenesis. *J Reprod Fertil* 1972;29:349–379.
496. Dyche WJ. A comparative study of the differentiation and involution of the müllerian duct and wolffian duct in the male and female mouse. *J Morphol* 1979;162:175–210.
497. Wartenberg H. Morphological studies on the role of the periductal stroma in the regression of the human male müllerian duct. *Anat Embryol* 1985;171:311–323.

498. Hayashi HH, Shima H, Hayashi K, Tvelstaadt RL, Donahoe PK. Immunocytochemical localization of müllerian inhibiting substance in the rough endoplasmic reticulum and Golgi apparatus in Sertoli cells of the neonatal calf testis using a monoclonal antibody. *J Histochem Cytochem* 1984;32:649–654.
499. Ikawa H, Trelstad RL, Hutson JM, Manganaro TF, Donahoe PK. Changing patterns of fibronectin, laminin, type IV collagen and a basement membrane proteoglycan during rat müllerian duct regression. *Dev Biol* 1984;102:260–263.
500. Hutson JM, Fallat ME, Kamagata S, Donahoe PK, Budzik GP. Phosphorylation events during müllerian duct regression. *Science* 1984;233:586–589.
501. Fallat ME, Hutson JM, Budzik GP, Donahoe PK. The role of nucleotide pyrophosphatase in müllerian duct regression. *Dev Biol* 1983;100:358–364.
502. Wolff E. L'action du diethylstilbestrol sur les organes genitaux de l'embryon de poulet. *C R Acad Sci* 1939;208:1532–1535.
503. McLachlan JA, Newbold RR, Bullock B. Reproductive tract lesions in male mice exposed prenatally to diethylstilbestrol. *Science* 1975;190:991–992.
504. Newbold RR, Suzuki Y, McLachlan JA. Müllerian duct maintenance in heterotypic organ culture after *in vivo* exposure to diethylstilbestrol. *Endocrinology* 1984;115:1863–1868.
505. Kobayashi S. Induction of müllerian duct derivatives in testicular feminized (Tfm) mice by prenatal exposure to diethylstilbestrol. *Anat Embryol* 1984;169:35–39.
506. Byskov AG. In: Austin CR, Short RV, eds. *Germ Cells and Fertilization.* Cambridge: Cambridge University Press, 1982.

The Physiology of Reproduction, Second Edition,
edited by E. Knobil and J.D. Neill,
Raven Press, Ltd., New York © 1994.

CHAPTER 10

Cyclic Changes in the Primate Oviduct and Endometrium

Robert M. Brenner and Ov Daniel Slayden

There are several reviews on the hormonal regulation of the primate endometrium (1) and oviduct (2), but none focus on the similarities and differences in the effects of estrogens and progestins in these two organs. In both tissues, estradiol (E_2) drives proliferation and cell differentiation and primes the tissue for progesterone (P) action by elevating the progesterone receptor (PR). But in the estrogen-primed oviduct, P acts solely as an estrogen antagonist. In the estrogen-primed endometrium, P antagonizes estrogen action but also stimulates cell differentiation, arterial growth, decidualization, and development of a progestational state. In this review, we explore these differences in steroid hormone action in these two compartments of the primate reproductive tract.

CYCLIC CHANGES IN CELL DIFFERENTIATION IN THE PRIMATE OVIDUCT

Several reviews of the biology and cellular ultrastructure of the mammalian oviduct have been published (2–9). The older literature on the comparative gross anatomy of the primate oviduct was summarized by Eckstein (10). Most recently, fairly comprehensive studies of the cyclic changes in the oviducts of cynomolgus (11) and pig-tailed macaques (12–14) have been completed. Also, some recent definitive studies (15,16) on the oviducts of women have been reported.

Human Oviduct

Novak and Everett (17) showed that in the postmenstrual period, the ciliated and secretory cells increased in height to a maximum near midcycle and then diminished in height to a minimum in the premenstrual and menstrual phases. The ciliated cells shrunk more rapidly than the secretory cells, and the apices of the latter projected well beyond the tips of the cilia during the latter part of the cycle. In the older literature (17), these protruding secretory cells were referred to as "peg" cells and erroneously assumed to be a third cell type of the oviductal epithelium. Verhage et al. (15) noted that although there was general agreement that secretory cells varied in cell height in cyclical fashion, there was considerable dis-

Division of Reproductive Sciences, Oregon Regional Primate Research Center, Beaverton, Oregon 97006

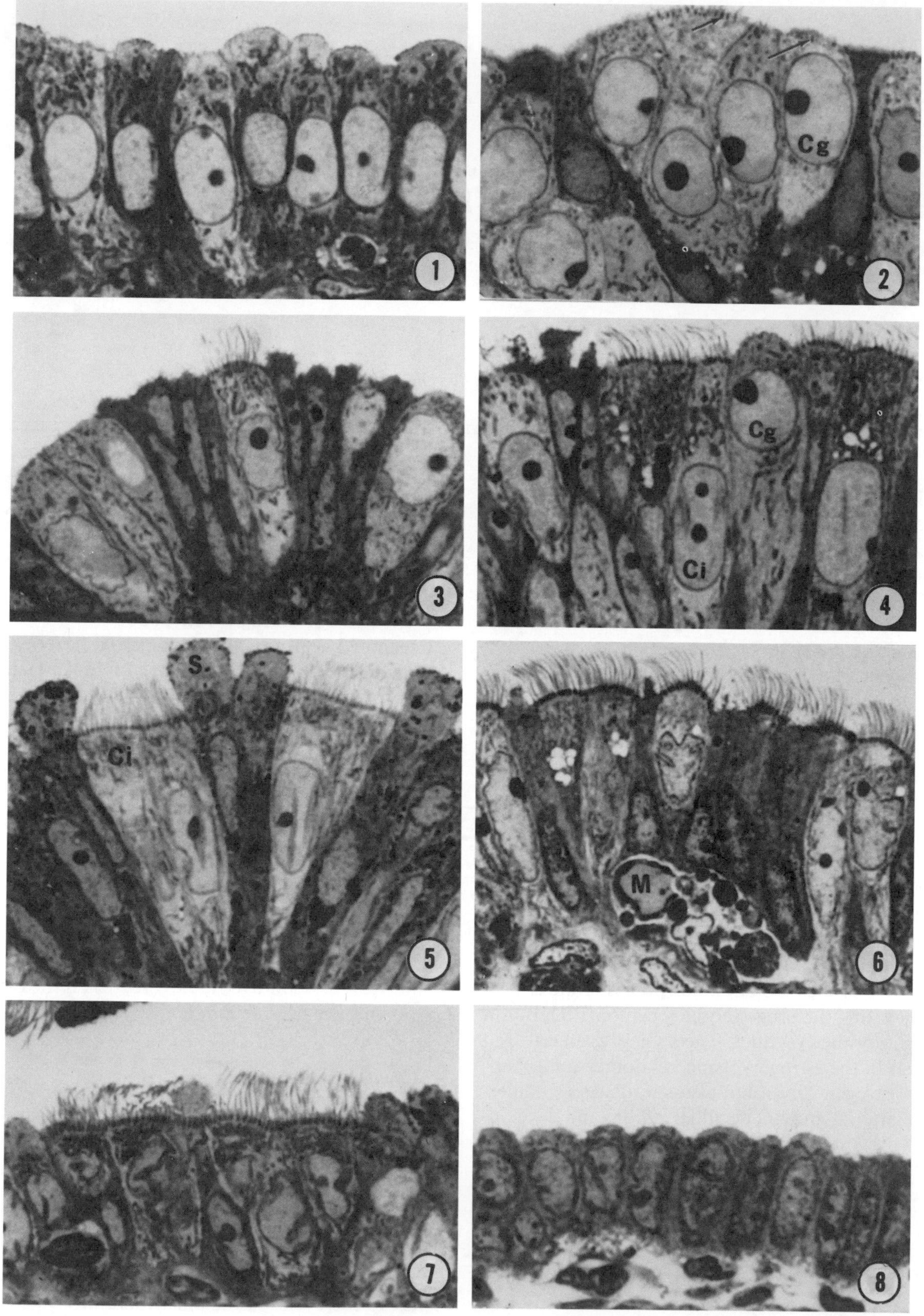
1
Cg
2
3
Cg
Ci
4
S.
Ci
5
M
6
7
8

agreement on the ciliated cells. Some authors (18–21) reported no change in percentage ciliation during the cycle, whereas others (22) observed ciliogenesis with the electron microscope. Verhage et al. (15) studied the oviducts of 24 normally cycling women, six each during the early follicular, late follicular, early luteal, and late luteal phases of the menstrual cycle. Six additional samples were obtained from pregnant women and six from women during the postpartum phase. The cytomorphometrics showed that the epithelial cells attained their maximum height and degree of ciliation during the late follicular phase in both the fimbriae and the ampulla. At the end of the luteal phase, some atrophy and deciliation had occurred, especially in the fimbriae. Hypertrophy and reciliation occurred during the early follicular phase. Approximately 10% to 12% of the cells formed new cilia in both the fimbriae and the ampulla during each menstrual cycle. During pregnancy and through the postpartum period, there was further atrophy and deciliation (from 57% ciliation and 30 μm cell height at midcycle to 24% ciliation and 20 μm at parturition). Atrophy and deciliation were associated with elevated serum P levels, hypertrophy and reciliation with low P and moderate E_2 levels. Ultrastructural studies of these tissues showed that the pattern of ciliogenesis was very similar to that described for the rhesus monkey (23). This definitive study indicated that although the ciliation–deciliation cycles that occur in the human oviduct are less extensive than in the oviducts of macaques, P antagonizes and E_2 stimulates epithelial cell hypertrophy, secretion, and ciliogenesis in both species.

The most recent study of the human oviduct (16) confirmed these conclusions and added that an increase in epithelial mitotic activity occurred during the follicular phase when P was essentially undetectable. Moreover, these workers agreed that deciliation, decrease of epithelial height, and a loss of mitotic activity coincided with elevated levels of P; continuous progestin therapy had the same antiestrogenic effect on the tubal epithelium that was exerted by endogenous P during the luteal phase. The same laboratory had shown previously (24) that estrogens could induce oviductal ciliogenesis in menopausal women. These findings confirm and extend the earlier observations by Andrews (25) that estrogens stimulate oviductal ciliogenesis in postparturient women and that progestins can inhibit this effect.

Jansen (8) described the hormonal regulation of oviductal secretions, especially of the human and nonhuman primate oviduct. He noted that around the time of ovulation, the secretions of the isthmic region become much more viscous than those of the ampulla. Indeed, the lumen of the isthmus fills with a viscous plug that renders the cilia invisible by scanning electron microscopy. This material was most abundant at midcycle when E_2 levels were highest; P suppressed this secretion. Jansen (8) suggested that this isthmic mucous layer may, like the analogous mucous column in the endocervix, play an important regulatory role in the transport of sperm through the isthmus toward the ampullary-isthmic junction where fertilization normally occurs.

Verhage's laboratory has shown that estrogens can stimulate secretion of specific glycoproteins by the baboon and human oviduct *in vivo* and *in vitro* and that this secretion was suppressed in oviducts of ovariectomized or E_2 + P-treated baboons (26,27).

Nonhuman Primate Oviduct

Oviductal cycles have been observed in pig-tailed macaques in a series of studies from Dr. Blandau's laboratory (12–14). The results showed that the fimbriae were extensively ciliated during midcycle and sparsely ciliated in the early follicular and late luteal phases. There was evidence of extensive ciliogenesis early in the cycle and signs of ciliary degeneration and shedding late in the cycle. Ovariectomy resulted in almost complete deciliation in the fimbriae and ampulla, but not in the isthmus. Treatment with estradiol benzoate restored the epithelium to its heavily ciliated, fully secretory, midcycle appearance.

In our own laboratory, we have focused primarily on cynomolgus and rhesus macaques. To evaluate changes during the natural menstrual cycle, we sampled the reproductive tracts of 27 cynomolgus macaques during the menstrual cycle and correlated the cytologic changes in

←

FIG. 1. *Preciliogenic.* Ampulla. All cells are hypertrophied, and their nuclei are swollen. No basal bodies can be seen by light microscopy. ×1050. **FIG. 2.** *Ciliogenic.* Fimbriae. Ciliogenic (*Cg*) cells are light, hypertrophied cells with swollen nuclei and enlarged nucleoli; basal bodies (*arrows*) are present in apical cytoplasm. Dark cells are future secretory cells. ×1050. **FIG. 3.** *Ciliogenic-ciliated.* Ampulla. Most of light cells are ciliogenic, but a few have become ciliated. Dark cells are future secretory cells. ×1050. **FIG. 4.** *Ciliated-ciliogenic.* Ampulla. Most of light cells have become ciliated (*Ci*), but some are still ciliogenic (*Cg*). Dark cells are secretory. ×1050. **FIG. 5.** *Ciliated-secretory.* Ampulla. Light cells are ciliated; dark cells are secretory. Note pronounced degree of secretory tip extension. ×1050. **FIG. 6.** *Early regression.* Fimbriae. Large numbers of macrophages (*M*) filled with nuclear and cellular fragments are present in epithelium. ×1050. **FIG. 7.** *Late regression.* Ampulla. Epithelium consists of atrophied ciliated and secretory cells with shriveled nuclei. Deciliation is more extensive in some regions than others during this phase. ×1050. **FIG. 8.** *Full regression.* Fimbriae. Epithelial cells are maximally atrophied and dedifferentiated, and their nuclei are maximally shriveled. ×1050.

the oviductal epithelium with changes in the serum levels of E_2 and P and with the histology of the ovaries and the endometria (11).

Ciliated cell height and percentage ciliation were measured in the fimbriae, ampulla, and isthmus, as previously described (28). We also found that "secretory tip extension," the distance that the tips of the secretory cells extend beyond the ciliated cells, was a useful morphometric index of secretory cell development. Additional cytologic features assessed included size and roundness of epithelial nuclei, degree of mitotic activity, extent of ciliogenesis as marked by basal body formation, content of glycogen and granules in secretory cells, and degree of pinching-off of ciliated cell tips (2). Two additional criteria were the presence of intraepithelial apoptotic bodies (29,30), an indicator of cell death by apoptosis, and the presence of macrophages filled with nuclear and cellular fragments in subepithelial and intraepithelial locations. In the monkey, oviductal apoptosis and macrophage invasion occur during the early luteal phase of the natural cycle or 2 to 5 days after the onset of P treatment in an artificial-cycle. In hamsters, apoptosis in the uterine luminal epithelium is induced by the sharp decline in E_2 combined with the rise in P that occurs during the proestrus-estrus transition (31). A similar rapid decline in E_2 after the preovulatory surge and a rise in serum P occurs in the periovulatory period in primates, and this hormonal shift is probably also responsible for the occurrence of apoptosis and macrophage invasion that occurs in the oviducts of cynomolgus and rhesus monkeys. Because of the large number of parameters we assessed, we were able to define eight specific stages through which the oviduct passes during the menstrual cycle. We have named these stages in order of their appearance as follows: preciliogenic, ciliogenic, ciliogenic-ciliated, ciliated-ciliogenic, ciliated-secretory, early regression, late regression, and full regression. A description of each stage is presented below, and the stages are illustrated in Figures 1 to 8. The descriptions were developed through study of the oviducts of cynomolgus macaques, but the same stages occur in rhesus macaques.

Preciliogenic (Fig. 1): This phase is marked by the onset of swelling of epithelial cell nuclei, smoothing of the nuclear contours, cellular hypertrophy, and mitotic activity. Light and dark cells are not apparent; generally, no basal bodies are evident.

Ciliogenic (Fig. 2): Mitosis and cellular hypertrophy continue; epithelial nuclei are round and smooth; light and dark cells can now be distinguished, and basal bodies may be apparent in the apical cytoplasm of the light, hypertrophied cells.

Ciliogenic-Ciliated (Fig. 3): All the features of the ciliogenic phase persist, but many ciliated cells have now developed. Secretory (dark) cells are present but not prominent. The word *ciliogenic* is placed first in the name of this phase to emphasize that ciliogenic cells predominate over ciliated ones.

Ciliated-Ciliogenic (Fig. 4): In this phase, most cells have become ciliated, but a few cells undergoing ciliogenesis can still be found scattered through the epithelium. Moreover, mitotic activity has not yet ceased. Secretory cells have become much more prominent and have developed bulbous tips filled with granules and glycogen. The word *ciliated* is placed first in the name of this phase to emphasize that ciliated cells predominate over ciliogenic ones.

Ciliated-Secretory (Fig. 5): In this phase, most epithelial cells are either ciliated or secretory, and ciliogenic phases are extremely rare. Secretory cells are fully developed, with bulbous tips rich in granules, glycogen, and some vacuoles. These tips extend well beyond the basal body row in the fimbriae and well past the cilia in the ampulla and isthmus. Epithelial cell nuclear contours are less smooth than during ciliogenesis.

Early regression (Fig. 6): In this phase, there are apoptotic epithelial cells scattered throughout the epithelium. Macrophages have invaded the epithelium and are phagocytosing dead cells. There are no other differences from the ciliated-secretory phase.

Late regression (Fig. 7): In this phase, the epithelium is atrophied, secretory activity has diminished, considerable deciliation has occurred, and many ciliated cells appear to be pinching off their tips. Dead cells and macrophages are still present. Epithelial cell nuclei now appear definitely shriveled.

Full regression (Fig. 8): In this phase, the epithelium is maximally atrophied and deciliated, epithelial cell nuclei are maximally shriveled, and secretory activity is at a minimum. There are very few dead cells left, and macrophages are less common.

All the cyclic changes, with one exception, are most evident in the fimbriae, less so in the ampulla, and least in the isthmus. The exception is secretory tip extension, which is least in the fimbriae, larger in the ampulla, and greatest in the isthmus (Fig. 9).

In Table 1, we list for each animal the predominant ovarian features, the levels of serum E_2 and P, the predominant endometrial features, the mean percentage ciliation in the fimbriae, the oviductal stage, and the days elapsed since the onset of the last menses (cycle day). The animals are presented from the top down in the order of their oviductal (not menstrual) cycles.

Table 1 also indicates that the oviductal stages are roughly equivalent to the typical ovarian stages of the primate menstrual cycle as follows: Preciliogenic and ciliogenic = early follicular; ciliogenic-ciliated = midfollicular; ciliated-ciliogenic = late follicular; ciliated-secretory = periovulatory; early regression = early luteal; late regression = midluteal; and full regression = late luteal.

Because the delimiters between these stages are not absolutely precise, we conclude that the rate of E_2-driven

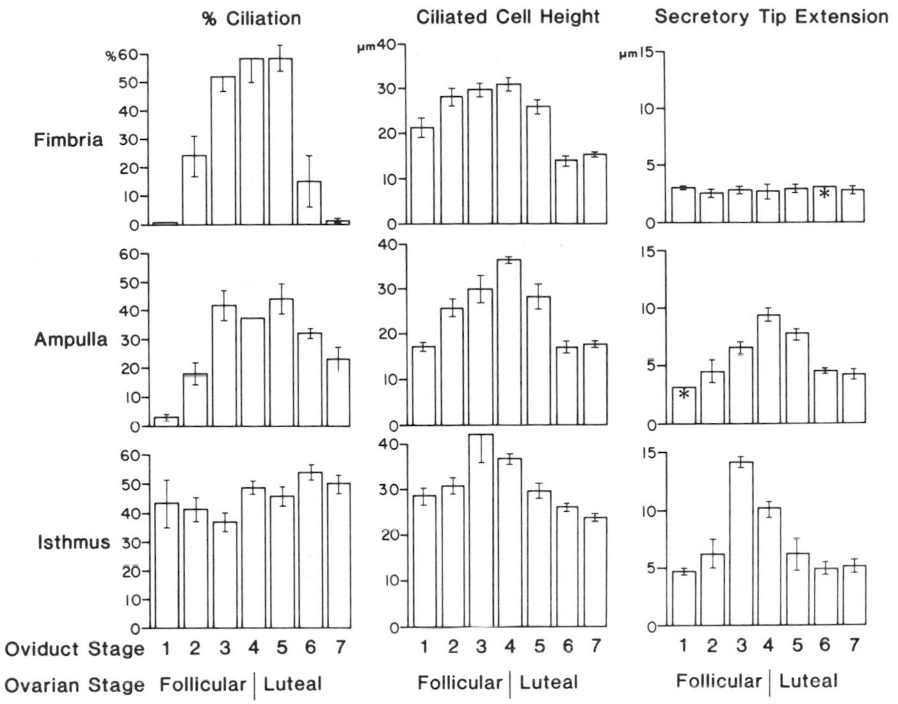

FIG. 9. Percentage ciliation, cell height, and secretory tip extension in fimbriae, ampulla, and isthmic regions of oviduct of cynomolgus macaques are compared at different times during menstrual cycle. Data were grouped according to oviductal staging sequence described in text. For convenience of presentation in graphic form, oviductal stages were given group numbers as follows: *Group 1:* preciliogenic-ciliogenic (n = 3); *Group 2:* ciliogenic-ciliated (n = 6); *Group 3:* ciliated-ciliogenic (n = 3); *Group 4:* ciliated-secretory (n = 2); *Group 5:* early regression (n = 4); *Group 6:* late regression (n = 2); and *Group 7:* full regression (n = 7). Data are presented as means with standard error bars where appropriate. *, sample of one.

ciliogenesis differs among individual ciliogenic cells. In the ciliogenic-ciliated stage, those few ciliated cells present were either the first to enter or the quickest to complete the ciliogenic process, and in the ciliated-ciliogenic phase, those few ciliogenic cells still present were either the last to enter or the slowest to complete ciliogenesis. Even in the ciliated-secretory state, when most cells were either ciliated or secretory, a few ciliogenic cells could still be found; presumably, the latter cells had lagged greatly behind most those cells destined to form cilia.

After ovulation, cell death occurs in some (but not all) of the epithelial cells. Those that die are apparently extremely sensitive to the combination of estrogen withdrawal and progestin increase characteristic of this period; most of the epithelial cells simply atrophy during this time. Differences in the rate of regression during the remainder of the luteal phase also exist. In the fimbriae, many cells lose their cilia quickly, most lose them eventually, but some never deciliate. Even in long-term ovariectomized animals, a few shrunken and shriveled but fully ciliated cells may persist in the fimbriae. The factors that make some cells so sensitive and others so insensitive to the same hormonal changes are unknown.

Fimbrial-Endometrial Relationships

To facilitate comparisons between the oviduct and endometrium, we present micrographs (Figs. 10–16) here of the histologic differences in these organs at key points in the menstrual cycle. During menstruation, when the endometrium is sloughing because of P withdrawal, the fimbrial epithelium is undergoing ciliogenesis (Figs. 10 and 11). When the endometrium is in the late proliferative stage because of elevated E_2, the fimbrial epithelium is in the ciliated-secretory state (Figs. 12 and 13). When the endometrium becomes hypertrophied and progestational because of elevated P, the fimbrial epithelium undergoes severe regression (Figs. 14–16).

CYCLIC CHANGES IN LOCALIZATION AND REGULATION OF ESTROGEN AND PROGESTIN RECEPTORS IN THE OVIDUCT

The above data suggest that estrogens stimulate growth of all the cellular components of the oviduct, and progestins inhibit these effects (Fig. 17). To understand

TABLE 1. *Oviductal, ovarian, and endometrial features in 27 cycling cynomolgus macaques*

Animal	Cycle day	Mean percentage ciliation in fimbriae	Oviduct stage	E_2 (pg/ml)	P (ng/ml)	Ovarian features	Endometrial stage
9414	1	0	Preciliogenic	93	0.30	Regressing CL[a]	Menses
9413	2	0	Ciliogenic	36	0.33	Regressing CL	Menses
9449	3	0	Ciliogenic	109	0.54	Regressing CL	Menses
9437	2	5.4	Ciliogenic-ciliated	35	0.85	Regressing CL	Menses-repair
9420	4	10.5	Ciliogenic-ciliated	76	0.18	Medium follicles	Menses-repair
8819	4	12.0	Ciliogenic-ciliated	152	0.90	Medium follicles	Early proliferative
9425	6	30.0	Ciliogenic-ciliated	88	0.10	Medium follicles	(Tissue lost)
9411	6	50.5	Ciliogenic-ciliated	124	0.10	Large follicle	Early proliferative
9421	6	34.0	Ciliogenic-ciliated	171	0.11	Medium follicle	Early proliferative
9439	13	56.5	Ciliated-ciliogenic	406	0.57	Preovulatory follicle	Midproliferative
9430	11	41.5	Ciliated-ciliogenic	583	0.50	Preovulatory follicle	Midproliferative
9417	10	56.5	Ciliated-ciliogenic	298	0.12	Preovulatory follicle	Midproliferative
8838	40	65.3	Ciliated-secretory	202	0.10	Preovulatory follicle	Late proliferative
8808	14	49.0	Ciliated-secretory	139	2.32	Fresh CL	Late proliferative
8817	13	57.0	Early regression	56	0.65	Fresh CL	Proliferative-progestational
9436	25	48.5	Early regression	56	2.28	Fresh CL	Proliferative-progestational
8833	13	66.8	Early regression	49	2.41	Fresh CL	Proliferative-progestational
8821	18	61.0	Early regression	63	4.13	Fresh CL	Proliferative-progestational
8828	25	23.5	Late regression	131	5.69	Functional CL	Midprogestational
9442	28	5.5	Late regression	62	0.81	Regressing CL	Late progestational
8837	25	2.0	Full regression	62	2.90	Functional CL	Midprogestational
9416	28	1.0	Full regression	56	0.74	Regressing CL	Midprogestational
8815	22	1.0	Full regression	119	12.15	Functional CL	Late progestational
8810	32	1.0	Full regression	19	0.20	Regressing CL	Late progestational
8825	27	2.0	Full regression	75	7.11	Functional CL	Late progestational
8818	30	1.0	Full regression	45	2.66	Functional CL	Late progestational
8836	2	2.0	Full regression	60	0.10	Regressing CL	Menses

From ref. 11, with permission.
[a] CL, corpus luteum.

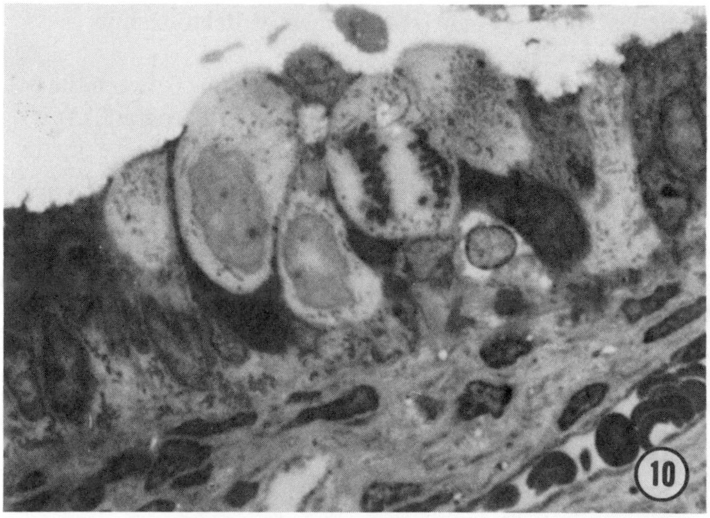

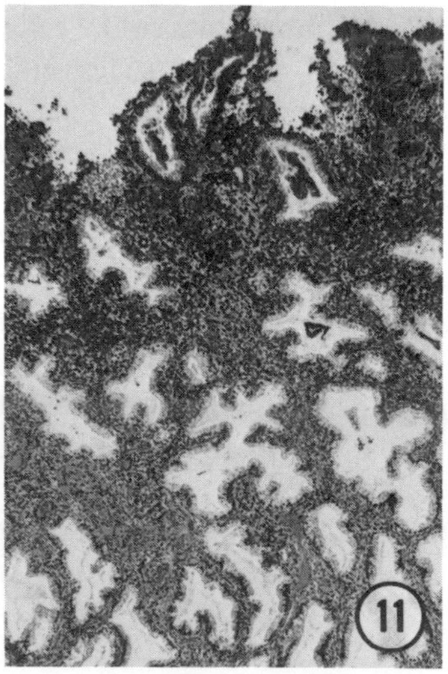

FIG. 10. *Fimbriae.* Ciliogenic state. A mitotic figure is evident, and there are several light, hypertrophied ciliogenic cells. Darker epithelial cells are future secretory cells. ×788.
FIG. 11. *Endometrium.* Menses. Typical sloughing of upper zones is evident. ×20.

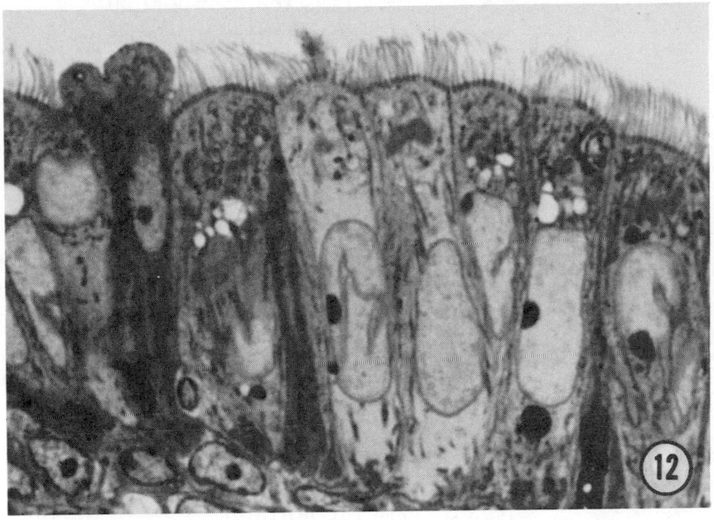

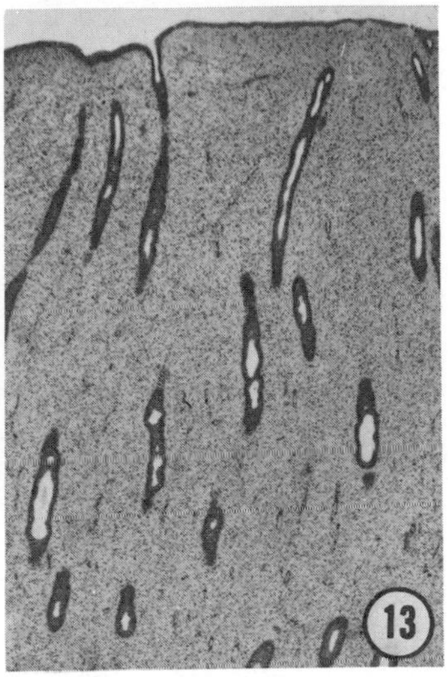

FIG. 12. *Fimbriae.* Ciliated-secretory stage. ×1575.
FIG. 13. *Endometrium.* Late proliferative stage. ×20.

further the mechanisms underlying these processes, we measured estrogen receptor (ER) and PR levels in the oviduct through binding and immunoassays during the natural cycle and under different hormonal conditions and localized these receptors to specific cell types by immunocytochemical (ICC) techniques with monoclonal antireceptor antibodies.

In our earliest study (28), two consecutive artificial menstrual cycles were produced in spayed monkeys by daily injection of a sequential E_2-P regimen. One oviduct was removed from each of nine animals during Cycle I, and the remaining oviduct was removed from each during Cycle II. Also, other animals were treated to produce two cycles and were sampled at three critical times: after 14 days of E_2 alone, after 21 days of E_2 plus P, and after 14 more days of E_2 alone. The results showed that ciliogenesis and the development of secretory activity occurred when E_2 acted alone at levels of 100 to 200 pg/ml, and atrophy, deciliation, and cessation of secretion took place when P levels were elevated above 1 ng/ml, even though E_2 levels remained constant at approximately 200 pg/ml.

Sucrose gradient assays were used to quantify the amount of cytosolic ER at these different time points. Estrogen receptor levels increased with E_2 treatment, decreased during sequential P administration, and recov-

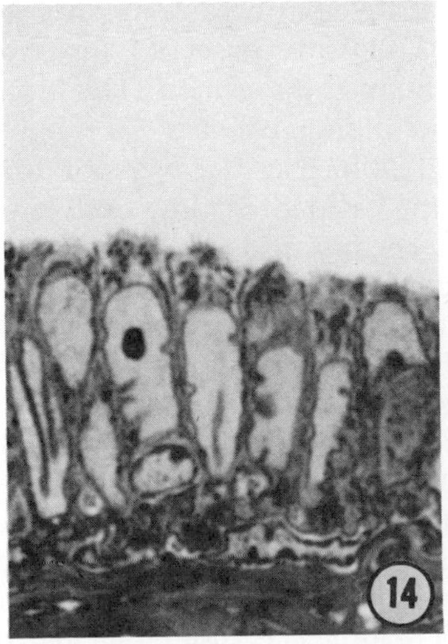

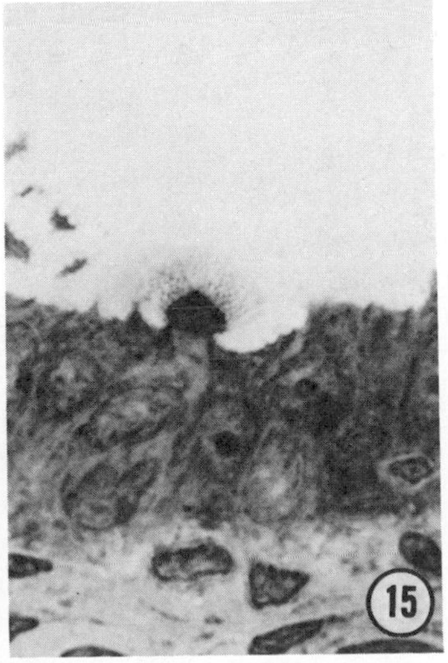

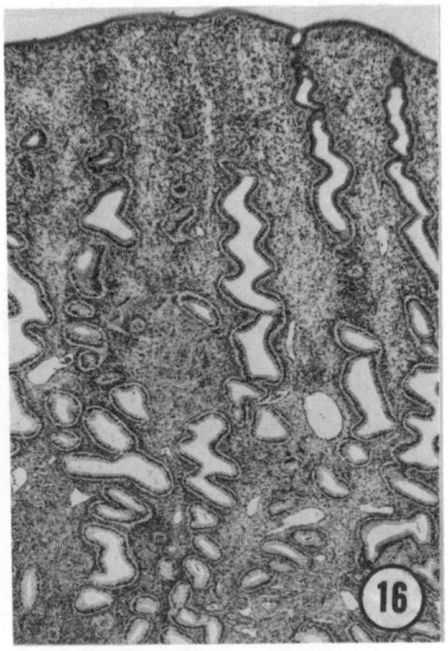

FIG. 14. *Fimbriae.* Full regression stage. ×1575.
FIG. 15. *Fimbriae.* Another region of the epithelium shown in Fig. 14. An example of apocrinelike process by which tips of ciliated cells are pinched off is shown. ×1575.
FIG. 16. *Endometrium.* Late progestational stage. Endometrial glands are highly sacculated. ×20.

17

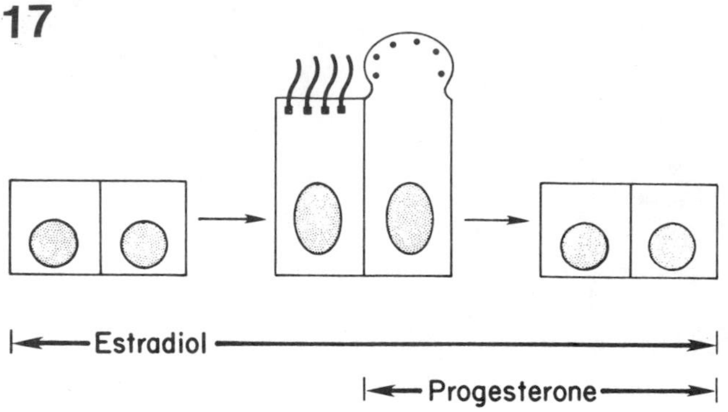

FIG. 17. Effects of E_2 and P on the oviductal epithelium. E_2 stimulates differentiation to a ciliated-secretory state; P suppresses that effect of E_2.

ered when P treatment ceased. Overall, the waxing and waning of epithelial cell height and percentage ciliation was accompanied by parallel increases and decreases in the level of cytosolic ER. Measurements of the tissue concentrations of E_2 showed that there was significantly less E_2 bound to the oviductal tissues when P was administered, even though serum E_2 levels remained constant (28,32).

We have also used binding and exchange assays to measure both cytosolic and nuclear ER per milligram DNA. Total ER was the sum of the nuclear and cytosolic values. These assays (see the tabular data attached to Fig. 19A, B, and C) showed that ER levels (total, cytosolic, and nuclear) were elevated by 14 days of E_2 treatment and suppressed by 14 days of E_2 plus P treatment. We have also measured cyclic changes in oviductal ER during the course of the natural menstrual cycle (33), and data from the same animals that were described in Table 1 are presented in the lower portion of Figure 18. When the cytosolic and nuclear ER levels from ciliogenic oviducts were compared with oviducts in late and full regression, it was clear that P could suppress ER in the presence of elevated levels of serum E_2 (Table 2). Consequently, we concluded that in both the natural cycle and in hormonally treated animals, P could antagonize the effects of E_2 on oviductal differentiation by suppressing ER levels below the threshold required to facilitate E_2 action. Similar observations of the effects of E_2 versus P on ER have been made in several species by several workers (34–36).

Immunocytochemical Findings

Development of ICC methods to visualize ER and PR with monoclonal antibodies made it possible to localize ER and PR in discrete cell populations (37–40). In the spayed oviduct, where binding assays showed most of the receptor was cytosolic, ICC indicated that all the specific staining was in the nuclei of stromal and epithelial cells (Fig. 19A). E_2 treatment increased the number of positively stained cells (Fig. 19B), and sequential P treatment greatly suppressed ER staining (Fig. 19C). Total, nuclear, and cytosolic ER levels are shown in the lower part of Figure 19. These findings support the view that the ER is a nuclear protein that is synthesized in the cytoplasm and spontaneously enters the nucleus in the absence of ligand, as in spayed animals. Some receptor molecules may "shuttle" back and forth between nucleus and cytoplasm (41), but at any time, most of the receptor population is in the nucleus. Estrogen receptor is always detected in cell nuclei in frozen sections by ICC regardless of the hormonal state of the animal because the protein is trapped there by the freezing technique. The reason there is so much receptor in the cytosol is probably that homogenization dislocates weakly bound receptor protein into the cytosolic fraction. Similar conclusions concerning the ligand-independent nuclear localization of ER as well as PR have been reached by many laboratories that have used ICC and biochemical techniques to study intact tissues and organs under physiologic conditions (37,42,43).

In all our studies, ICC showed that ER was only present in stromal cells, smooth-muscle cells, and secretory cells. Ciliated cells were *not* stained for ER (Figs. 20 and 21). After P treatment, the stromal and secretory cells lost all detectable staining for ER in parallel with the suppression in total ER measured by binding and exchange assays (Fig. 19C). This suppressive effect of P on stromal and secretory cell ER occurred within 24 h of P treatment. Figure 22 shows a series of ICC preparations of oviducts from animals treated for 14 days with E_2 (Fig. 22A) and then sampled 1 h (Fig. 22B), 3 h (Fig. 22C), and 12 to 24 h (Fig. 22D) after onset of P treatment, with E_2 treatment maintained throughout. The first clearly detectable evidence of suppression of ER staining occurred between 12 and 24 h. Thus, 1 day after P treatment began, ER was suppressed to very low levels in stromal and secretory cells. The first evidence of deciliation and suppression of secretion was usually evident within 48 to 72 h of the onset of P treatment; thus, the decline in ER preceded the biologic effects of P. This supports the role of this decline as a causal factor in P antagonism of E_2 action, but the absence of ER in ciliated cells suggests that this antagonism is indirect.

Immunocytochemistry of PR showed that staining was present in stromal, smooth-muscle, and secretory epithelial cells but *was also absent* from ciliated cells, which suggests that the effects of P on ciliated cells may *also* be indirect. The intensity of PR staining, which was minimal in spayed animals, was increased after E_2 treat-

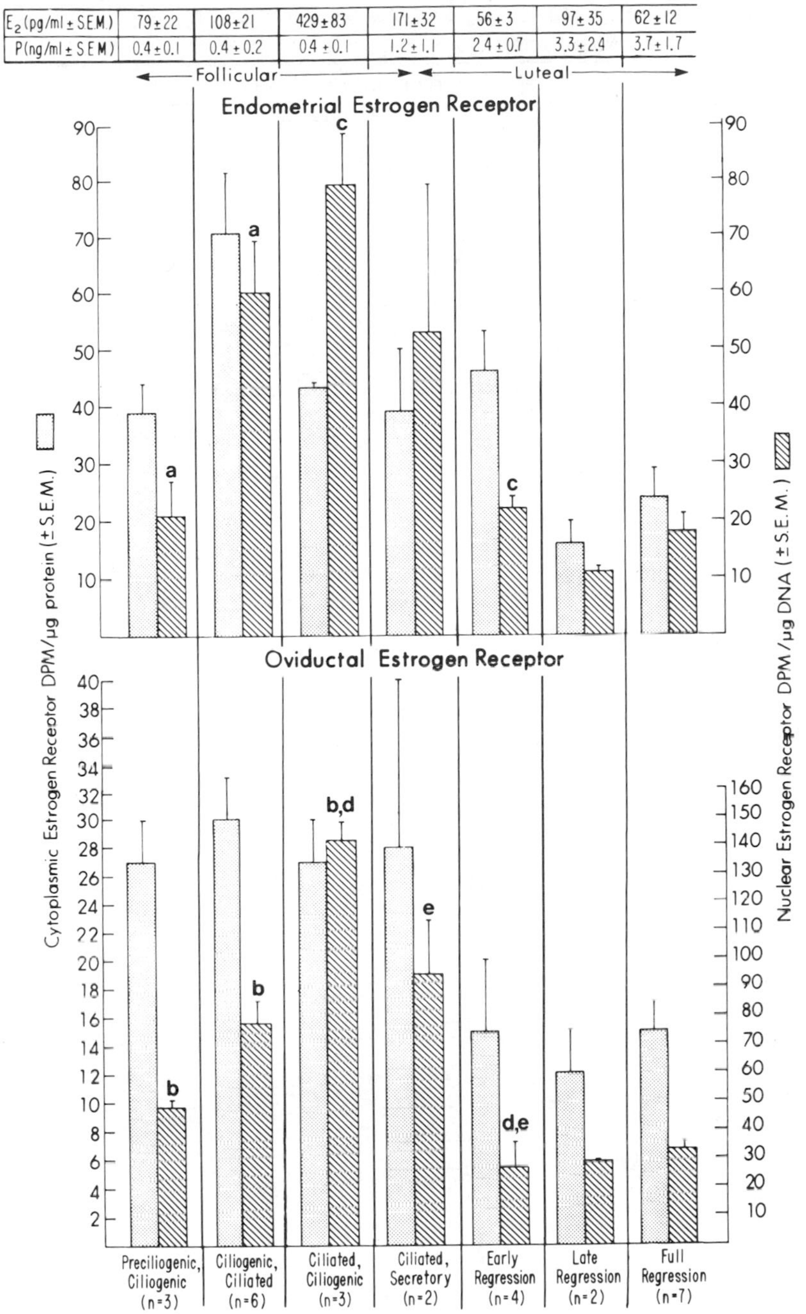

FIG. 18. Nuclear and cytoplasmic estradiol (E_2) receptors in oviducts and endometrium of cynomolgus macaques during menstrual cycle. Abscissa is a time scale of the cycle from early follicular (*left*) to late luteal (*right*). Data are grouped according to number of animals in each of oviductal stages. Mean serum levels of E_2 and P in each of these stages are presented in tabular form at top of figure. Nuclear receptor levels in groups with same *lowercase letter* are significantly different from one another (Student's *t*-test, $P < .05$). (From ref. 33, with permission.)

ment in the stromal, smooth-muscle, and secretory cells, the only cell types that contain ER (Fig. 23). In the animals treated with a sequential E_2 + P regimen, staining for PR was suppressed in the secretory cells (so that the entire epithelium was negative for PR) but remained readily detectable in the stroma (Fig. 24). This surprising finding strongly suggested that the effects of P on the epithelium were mediated by the stroma. To check the sensitivity of the ICC technique, we prepared thick frozen sections (30 μm, in contrast to the usual thickness of 5 μm) to increase the concentration of PR antigen in the sections. Immunocytochemistry of these thicker sections showed that the epithelium remained negative for PR, whereas the stromal cells stained excessively dark for PR (Fig. 25). We concluded that the absence of PR in the oviductal epithelium of P-suppressed oviducts was real and not due to insensitivity of the ICC technique.

Measurements of PR by binding assays confirmed that sequential P treatment down-regulated total PR (44). In six E_2-treated animals, the levels of total PR were 14.8 ± 2.6 pmol/mg DNA. In eight sequential E_2 + P-treated animals, PR levels were significantly reduced

TABLE 2. *Comparison of serum steroids with oviduct ER in the early follicular and late luteal phases of the natural menstrual cycle*[a]

	Stage of the menstrual cycle		
	Late luteal (n = 9)	Early follicular (n = 9)	P
Serum steroids			
E_2 (pg/ml ± SEM)	70 ± 12	98 ± 16	NS
P (ng/ml ± SEM)	3.6 ± 1.4	0.38 ± 0.11	<.05
Estrogen receptor levels			
Cytosol (dpm/μg protein ± SEM)	15 ± 1	29 ± 2	<.001
Nuclear (dpm/μg DNA ± SEM)	32 ± 3	68 ± 7	<.001
Morphologic stage	Late and full regression	Preciliogenic-ciliogenic Ciliogenic-ciliated	

[a] In this tabulation, data on nine animals in the late luteal phase (last two oviductal stages) are specifically compared with data on nine animals in the early follicular phase (first three oviductal stages). The table is based on data in ref. 33. The two main columns in the table under the heading "Stage of the menstrual cycle" compare different data from the late luteal and early follicular phases. These data are serum estradiol (E_2), serum progesterone (P), nuclear and cytosolic estrogen receptor, and morphologic stage. For each parameter, a Student's t-test was used to determine whether the differences between the follicular and luteal phases were significant. The P values for each comparison are presented in the last column on the right side of the table.

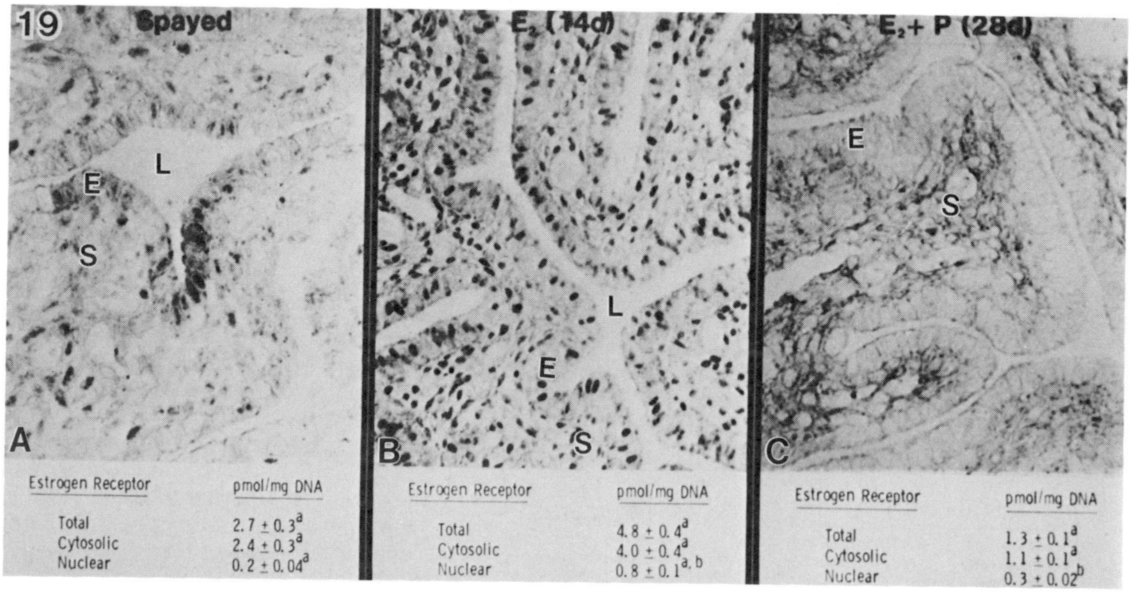

FIG. 19. Effects of three treatments on oviductal ER. **A:** Spayed, untreated; **B:** Spayed, treated with E_2 for 14 days; **C:** Spayed, treated with E_2 for 14 days and E_2 plus P for additional 14 days. Top part of each is a photomicrograph of oviductal epithelium (ampulla) stained for ER. Bottom part of each is a tabulation of amount of ER measured by binding assays in oviducts from the same treatment groups. Values with the same superscript letter are significantly different between groups (P < .01). Note that in spayed animals, a few stromal and epithelial cells are positive for ER. After E_2 treatment, this number goes up in both stromal and epithelial cells, and after P treatment, the number of ER-positive cells in stroma and epithelium is reduced to less than in spayed animals. Total receptor levels follow the same pattern. Note that all positive staining is confined to cell nuclei. Original magnification: A, ×630; B, ×400; C, ×630. E, epithelium; L, lumen; S, stroma.

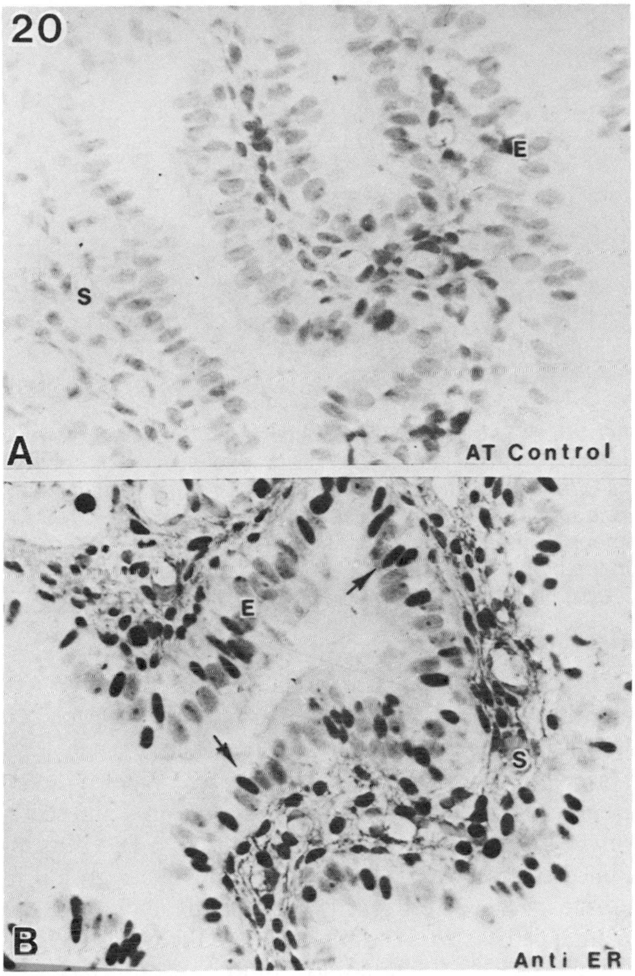

FIG. 20. ER staining in oviductal epithelium (ampulla) in fully ciliated-secretory state. **A:** Stained with AT, a control antibody and hematoxylin to show nuclei. **B:** Stained with H222 for ER, and hematoxylin for nuclei. Comparison of A and B shows that not all nuclei in the epithelium are positive for ER. This heterogeneity is highly consistent, and careful examination shows that ER-positive nuclei are stromal and secretory cells. This heterogeneity can also be seen in Fig. 19B. E, epithelium; S, stroma. Original magnification: ×400.

($P < .001$) to 1.03 ± 0.31. This suppression by P of its own receptor has been found in different P target organs in different species (45). Our ICC results suggest, however, that this suppression is cell type-specific, with complete suppression in the epithelium and much less suppression in the stromal and the smooth-muscle compartments.

These data raise several questions concerning the mode of action of E_2 and P at the genomic level. First, ER and PR are both lacking from ciliated cells, yet E_2 stimulates ciliogenesis and P inhibits it. How can the dramatic effects of both E_2 and P on the ciliated cells occur when the ciliated cells lack receptors for both steroids?

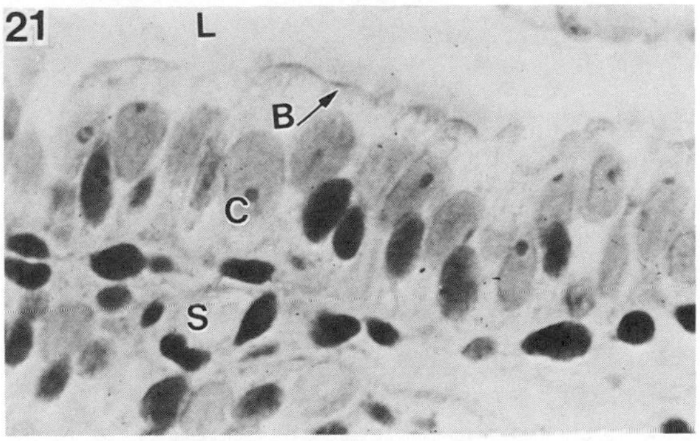

FIG. 21. ER staining in oviductal epithelium (fimbriae) in ciliated-secretory state. The epithelial heterogeneity is because ciliated cells are ER-negative and stromal and secretory cells are ER-positive. Cilia are difficult to discern in photomicrographs of frozen sections, but the basal bodies of the cilia are readily apparent. *B*, basal bodies; *C*, ciliated cell; L, lumen; *S*, stroma. Original magnification: ×900.

Second, P suppresses its own receptor, yet as long as P treatment is continued it will continue to act as an estrogen-antagonist even though the levels of PR are greatly reduced. How does P maintain its effects while suppressing its own receptor?

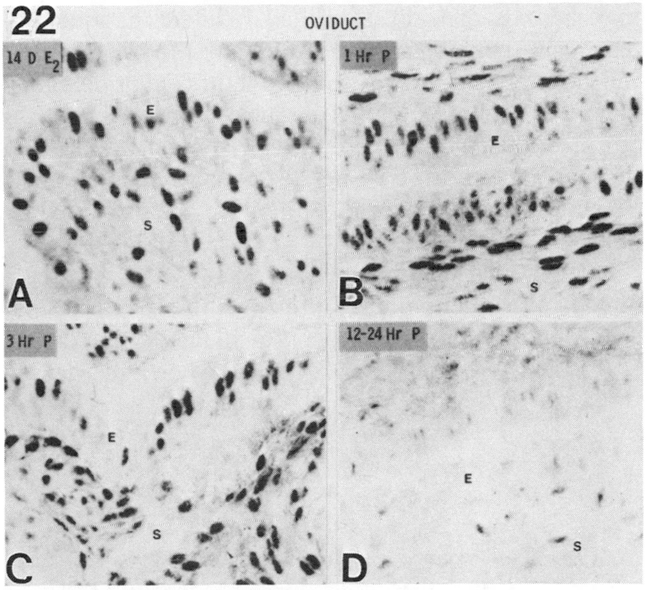

FIG. 22. Effect of P on oviductal (fimbriae) ER at **(A)** 0 h, **(B)** 1 h, **(C)** 3 h, and **(D)** 12 to 24 h after implantation of a P capsule into animals that had been treated with an E_2 implant for the previous 14 days. Staining for ER was not clearly reduced until 12 to 24 h after P treatment, and it was suppressed in stromal and secretory cells at approximately same rate. Binding assays for cytosolic and nuclear ER were also performed at same time intervals (117). Nuclear ER was significantly lowered within 1 to 3 h, but cytosolic and total ER were not significantly lowered until 12 to 24 h. Nuclear staining did not decrease until total ER was significantly lowered. E, epithelium; S, stroma.

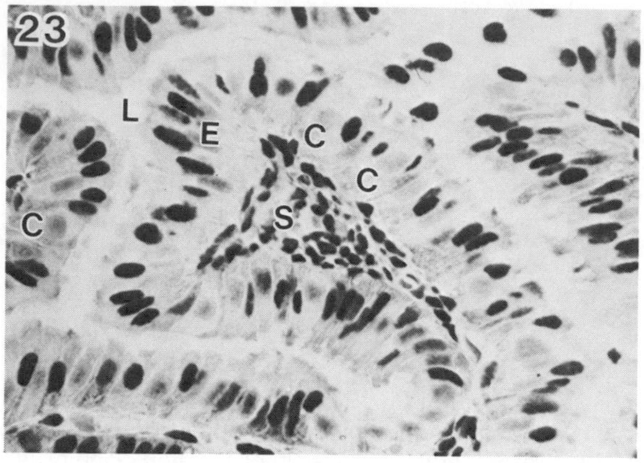

FIG. 23. Distribution of PR in the oviductal epithelium (ampulla) in the ciliated-secretory state. As with ER, only stromal and secretory cells are PR-positive. C, ciliated cell; E, epithelium; L, lumen; S, stroma. Original magnification: ×630.

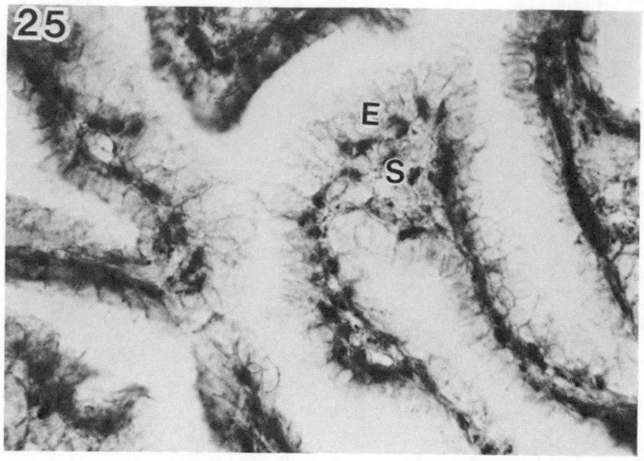

FIG. 25. PR staining in thick section (30 μm) of oviductal epithelium (fimbriae) in fully regressed state induced by sequential E_2 plus P treatment. In such a thick section, antigen concentration would be increased five- to sixfold over the amount normally present in a 5-μm section. Yet PR remains undetectable in epithelium, while it is overstained in stroma. E, epithelium; S, stroma. Original magnification: ×630.

New Model of Hormone Action in the Oviductal Epithelium

We suggest that many of the effects of E_2 and P on the state of differentiation of the oviductal epithelium are mediated indirectly through soluble growth factors (or other currently unknown mediators) secreted by stromal cells. There is extensive evidence from other laboratories that steroids can affect epithelial differentiation indirectly via the subjacent mesenchyme (46,47). Stromal cells are separated from the epithelium by a definitive basement membrane, so it is unlikely that such effects are mediated by direct junctional contact. In electron microscopic studies, we never observed such contacts (2), and to our knowledge, none have been reported by others.

In this paracrine model (Figs. 26 and 27), E_2 would act directly at the genomic level through the ER in stromal cells to induce the secretion of growth factors that diffuse across the basement membrane and stimulate growth and differentiation in the ER-negative ciliogenic cells. In the epithelium, E_2 could act directly at the genomic level in secretory cells as these cells have ER. When P levels rise, P can act directly in PR-positive stromal and secretory cells to suppress ER in both cell types and thus inhibit the secretion of E_2-dependent oviductal glycoproteins from the secretory cells and growth factors from the stromal cells. Also, P might stimulate the release of specific growth or differentiation inhibitors from stromal cells.

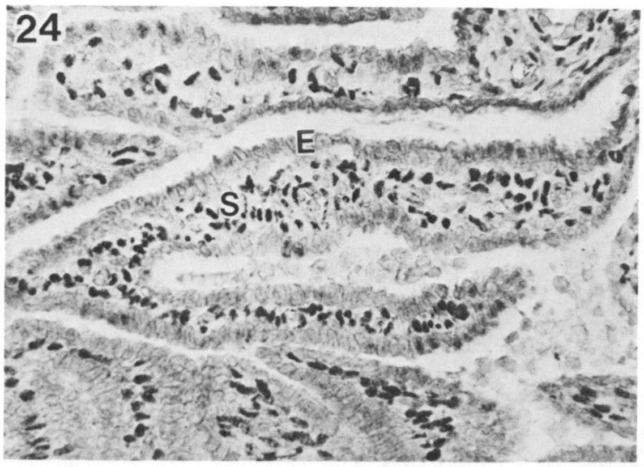

FIG. 24. Distribution of PR in oviductal epithelium in fully regressed state induced by sequential E_2 plus P treatment. PR remains easily detectable in the stroma but is undetectable in most epithelial cells. E, epithelium; S, stroma. Original magnification: ×630.

26

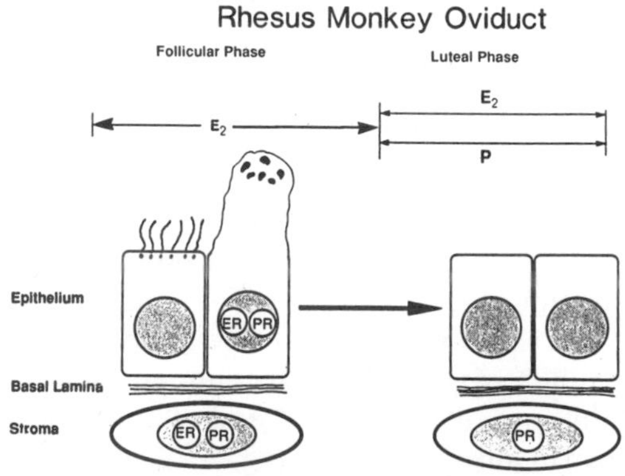

FIG. 26. Although E_2 induces ciliated-secretory state, ER is only present in stromal and secretory cells. Estradiol also induces PR but only in stromal and secretory cells. When P acts, it suppresses effects of E_2 on ciliated and secretory cells, even though PR is only present in stromal and secretory cells when P action begins. After P has acted for 2 weeks, only stromal cells maintain PR, so these cells must be responsible for maintenance of P effect that persists as long as P treatment is maintained.

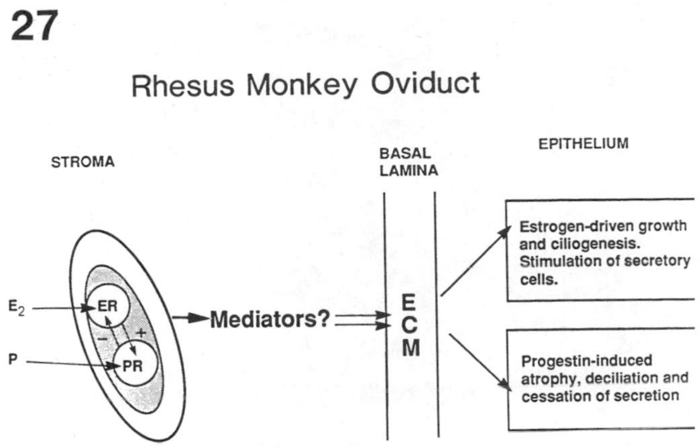

FIG. 27. New model of steroid hormone action in oviductal epithelium. Estradiol and P act through their respective receptors in stromal cells to regulate secretion of mediators, probably growth factors. It is these mediators that directly influence state of differentiation of oviductal epithelium. Progesterone acts through PR in stromal cells to lower stromal ER, and this leads to lowered secretion of E_2-dependent mediators. Withdrawal of these mediators leads to oviductal dedifferentiation, as if E_2 itself had been withdrawn.

As P continues to act, it eventually down-regulates PR greatly in the secretory cells but only partially in the stromal cells. Because the suppressive effects of P on E_2 action in the epithelium continue indefinitely until P treatment is stopped and because only stromal cells retain detectable levels of PR during sustained P action, we suggest that the sustained antagonism of the entire epithelium by P is mediated by the stroma. Specifically, we suggest it is the suppression by P of ER in stromal cells that is responsible for the inability of E_2 to act in the presence of E_2 and P. Once P treatment is stopped, ER can recover spontaneously (as it does in spayed animals) to levels adequate to mediate E_2 actions in stromal and secretory cells. These cells can then increase their ER and PR levels in response to E_2, the stromal cells can secrete their specific mediators that drive ciliogenesis, and the cycle of differentiation of the oviductal epithelium can begin anew.

What are these presumed stromal mediators? Are they well known growth factors or unknown, oviduct-specific molecules? Novel ICC data recently presented by Wang et al. (48) showed that reactivity for the epidermal growth factor receptor (EGFR) in the human oviduct was most intense in the stromal cells and undetectable in the epithelium. Wang et al. (48) also examined the localization of the C-*erb*B-2 protein and found it only in the epithelium, *not* the stroma. The C-*erb*B-2 gene is the human homologue of the rat *neu* oncogene and highly homologous to the human EGFR gene (C-*erb*B-1). It codes for an 185-kDa transmembrane glycoprotein, which is believed to be a growth factor receptor with a yet unidentified ligand (49). Epidermal growth factor may therefore directly affect the stroma but not the epithelium, and a currently unknown ligand for the C-*erb*B-2 protein may directly affect the epithelium but not the stroma.

There also have been recent reports that all the members of the insulinlike growth factor family (peptides, receptors, and binding proteins) are present in human oviductal tissues (50,51). Research into the role of these different growth factors in the control of oviductal differentiation should be highly rewarding.

ENDOMETRIUM OF HIGHER PRIMATES

Anatomy and Histology

On the basis of gross anatomy, the uterus can be divided into three parts: the fundus (dome-shaped top), the corpus (body), and the isthmus (neck), which leads into the cervix. The mucosa that lines the uterine cavity, the endometrium, is surrounded by a muscular wall, the myometrium. The endometrial surface consists of a simple columnar epithelium, ciliated in women (52–54), that is continuous with many simple tubular or branched glands that extend to the base of the endometrial-myometrial border. Its lamina propria or stroma is a highly cellular connective tissue with an amorphous extracellular matrix containing relatively few connective tissue fibers. The border between the endometrium and the myometrium is irregular and indistinct.

Bartelmez described four zones or layers in rhesus (55) and human (56) endometrium (Fig. 28D). Zone I consists of the surface epithelium and an underlying band of stromal cells. Zone II contains the straight necks of the glands that run perpendicular to the surface surrounded by a relatively dense cellular stroma. Zone III contains the bodies of the glands, which are frequently branched (55) and surrounded by a looser stroma. Zone IV is the basal layer adjacent to the myometrium, in which the blind ends of the glands terminate. An alternate classification, more commonly applied to the human endometrium, describes three zones. A superficial layer, the compacta, consists of densely packed stromal cells around the straight necks of the glands. This is equivalent to Bartelmez's zones I and II. Beneath this is the spongiosa, a thick, spongy layer containing the tortuous bodies of the glands, comparable with zone III, and then the basalis, a basal layer equivalent to zone IV. The compacta and upper spongiosa are also referred to as the functionalis (as opposed to the basalis) because they appear to be more dramatically affected by fluctuations in circulating levels of steroid hormones, derive their blood supply from specialized spiral arteries rather than the basal arteries that supply the basal endometrium, and are either partially lost or extensively remodeled after menstruation.

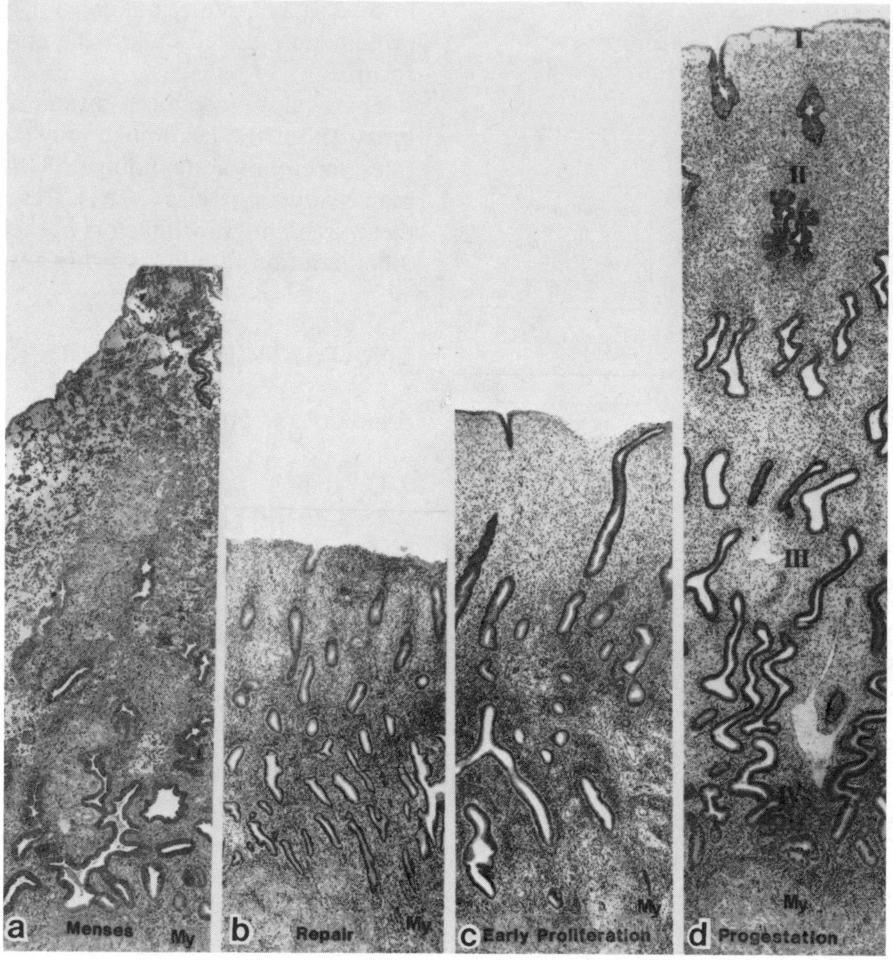

FIG. 28. Endometrium throughout cycle showing zones. **A:** Menses; **B:** Repair; **C:** Early proliferation; **D:** Progestation. *My,* Myometrium. ×20.

Cyclic Changes

The only ovarian factors required to elicit complete maturational and functional responses of the primate endometrium are the ovarian steroids E_2 and P. This concept, last reviewed in 1961 (1), has stood the test of time. Hodgen (57) reported that pregnancy could be established in spayed monkeys treated with Silastic implants of E_2 and P in sequential fashion to recreate the pattern of serum E_2 and P that occurs during the fertile menstrual cycle. The pregnancy was initiated by transfer of an embryo into the fimbrial ostium, so both tubal transport and implantation were supported in these spayed animals. Estradiol and P may induce paracrine factors within the reproductive tract (58), but the evidence is convincing that no other ovarian factors are essential for normal tract function.

Noyes, Hertig, and Rock (59) described a scheme for classifying the histology of the endometrium relative to an ideal 28-day cycle in which the first day of menstruation is day 1. During days 4 to 7, the early proliferative period, the glands are straight, short, and narrow, and the stroma is compacted. During the mid-proliferative period, days 8 to 10, the surface epithelium is columnar, the glands are longer and very mitotically active, and the stroma is somewhat edematous. Stromal mitoses are numerous. During the late proliferative stage, days 11 to 14, the glands, which are growing rapidly, become tortuous. The glandular epithelium appears pseudostratified because of the accelerated proliferation of the elongated cells. The stroma is less edematous than during the mid-proliferative stage and is also actively growing.

When fertilization and implantation do not occur, the luteal phase of a normal cycle usually lasts for 12 to 14 days. The effects of P become evident on day 16, the second day after ovulation, when glycogen accumulates in the basal portion of the glandular epithelium, displacing the nuclei and producing a pseudostratified configuration. In formalin-fixed material, the glycogen is solubilized, leaving large vacuoles in the base of the cells. On day 17, the nuclei of the glandular epithelial cells form an orderly row with homogeneous cytoplasm above them and large vacuoles below (59). By day 18, the vacuoles in the glandular epithelium are smaller as the glycogen moves into the apex of the cells and then into the lumens of the glands. On day 19, very few vacuoles remain in the glandular epithelial cells, and most of the nuclei are once more basal in location.

During the final days of the cycle, the glands are dilated and the glandular epithelium has a saw-toothed appearance, with shrunken nuclei and jagged apical surfaces. This appearance, referred to as secretory exhaustion, is highly variable. Changes in the stroma are more reliable indicators of cycle stage. On cycle days 21 and 22, the endometrial stroma becomes highly edematous. At this stage, the stromal cells are small with dense nuclei and filamentous cytoplasm. On day 23, stromal cells surrounding the spiral arterioles begin to enlarge. This, along with stromal mitoses, constitute the earliest visible predecidual change (59). By day 24, predecidual cells are observed cuffing the spiral arterioles, and stromal mitoses are more numerous. By day 25, hypertrophied stromal cells are also present under the surface epithelium, and by day 27, the upper portion of the endometrial

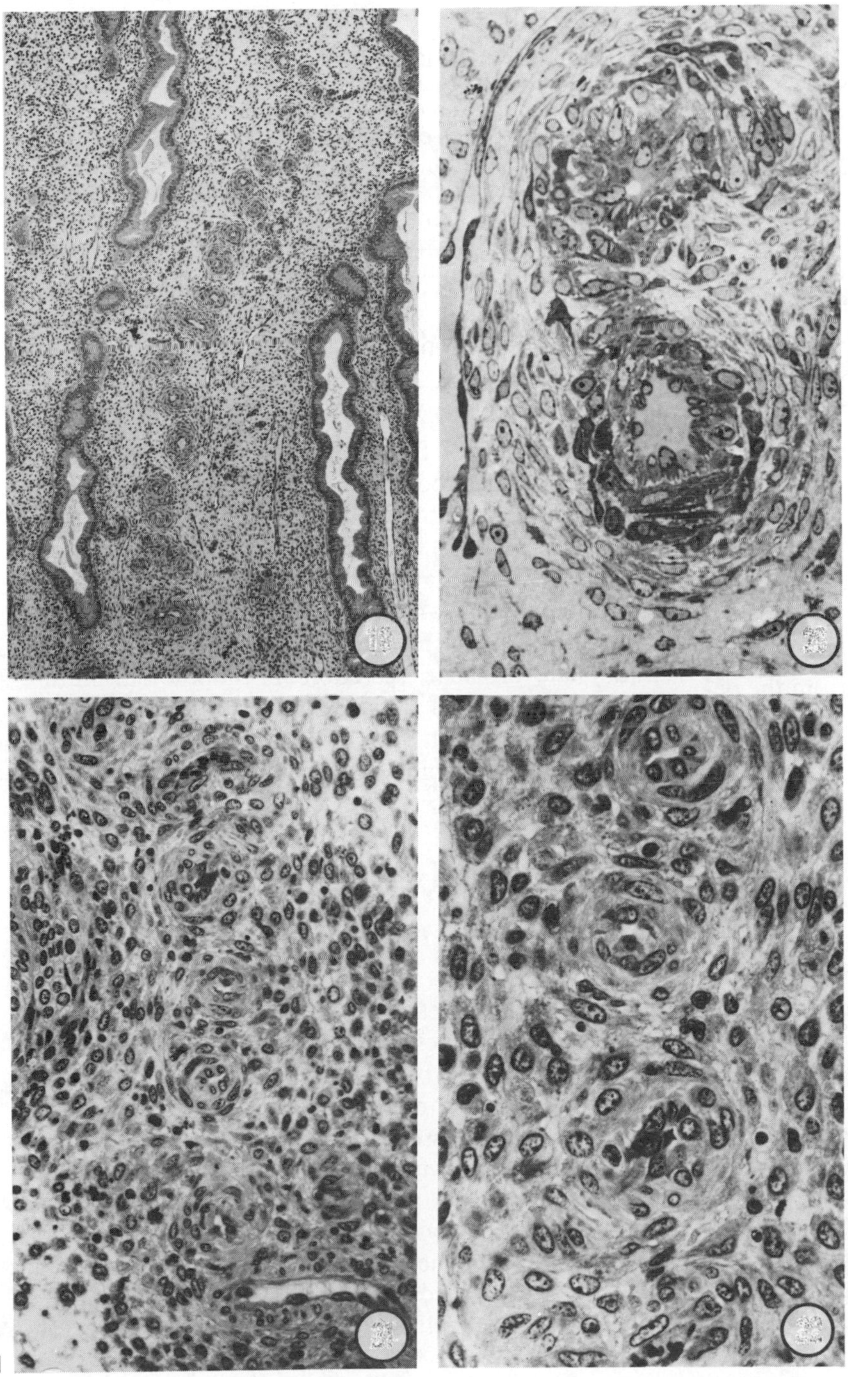

29 30 31 32

Figures 29 to 32 compare spiral arteries and periarteriolar stromal cells in macaque and human endometrium during luteal phase. Enlargement of periarteriolar stromal cells occurs in both species but is more extreme in human endometrium. **FIG. 29.** Macaque. ×140. (From ref. 11, with permission.) **FIG. 30.** Macaque. ×480. (From ref. 11, with permission.) **FIG. 31.** Human. ×250. **FIG. 32.** Human. ×500.

stroma consists of a sheet of well-developed decidual-like cells. Lymphocytes and polymorphonuclear leukocytes invade the upper regions on days 25 to 27 (59,60).

Similar cyclic changes have been described in the endometrium of nonhuman primates [e.g., baboons (60–62) and macaques]. The morphology of the macaque endometrium throughout the ovarian cycle (Fig. 28) (55,56) and early gestation (56,63) and during a variety of steroid hormone treatments (64–68) has been described in detail.

A significant difference in the cyclic changes observed in human and rhesus endometrium is the degree to which the periarteriolar stromal cells differentiate during the final week of the menstrual cycle. In women, the decidual reaction begins around the spiral arterioles and then spreads throughout the upper $\frac{2}{3}$ of the endometrium. In contrast, the changes that occur in the stroma of the late secretory macaque endometrium are minimal. Most stromal cells enlarge somewhat, but the only stromal cells that enlarge-substantially are those surrounding the spiral arterioles. Figures 29 and 30 illustrate spiral arteries in late luteal macaque endometrium, and Figures 31 and 32 illustrate them in late luteal human endometrium. Pregnancy, or extended P treatment, results in a more dramatic hypertrophy of most of the stromal cells in macaque endometrium and has been called a decidual reaction (55,63). Thus, the reaction of macaque stromal cells to P is similar in kind although not in degree to that of human stromal cells. A recent report indicates that a mechanical deciduogenic stimulus can be used to induce decidualization in nonpregnant rhesus monkeys just as in other species (69).

The endometrial stroma consists of several different cell types that are presumed to have different functions. Stromal cells may protect maternal tissues from the destructive invasion of the trophoblast (70) or contribute to the protection of the allogenic fetoplacental unit from rejection by the maternal immune system (71,72). Endometrial granulocytes or "Kornchenzellen" (73,74) may be a functionally distinct population of T cells in the decidua (73). These cells, along with the assortment of lymphocytes, lymphoblasts, and macrophages present in the endometrium, may represent a unique hormone-dependent component of the immune system (74,75). In the human endometrium, there is a population of lymphocytes concentrated in the basalis region that may be part of such a system (76).

Several laboratories have developed methods for isolation and culture of human endometrial stromal and epithelial cells (77–79). Progesterone treatment of stromal cell cultures increases expression of 17-β estradiol dehydrogenase (80), relaxin (81,82), prolactin (83–85) vitamin D (86), and insulinlike growth factor (IGF) binding protein (87,88). Explants of proliferative human endometrium exposed to 50 to 100 ng/ml of P released decidual prolactin (dPRL) by the third or fourth day in culture (89,90) and its production increased with time (Fig. 33). The precise role of these and other stromally derived molecules (91–95) in endometrial function is unknown. Recently, Zhu et al. (96) reported that prolactin secretion is maximal when stromal cells are treated with P and then relaxin in sequence. IGF-I is also reported to stimulate prolactin secretion in endometrial cultures. Relaxin and IGF-I are very similar proteins, sharing approximately 35% homology (96), and relaxin as well as the IGFs may be an important paracrine factor in the endometrium.

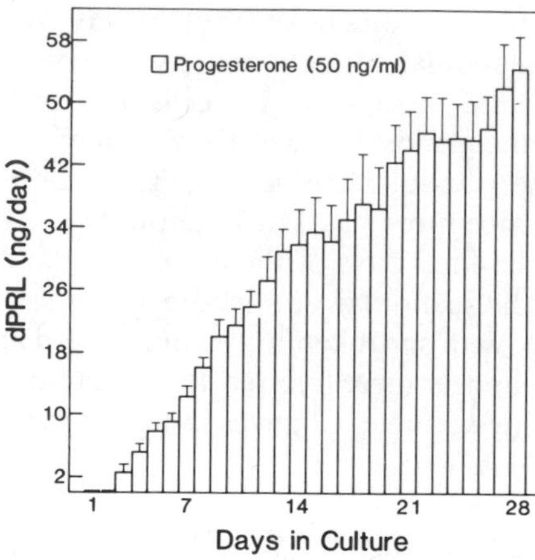

FIG. 33. Prolactin (*dPRL*) production by proliferative endometrium during organ culture in presence of P. Explants prepared from four samples of proliferative endometrium were cultured in medium containing 50 ng/ml P for 28 days (two or three cultures from each tissue). Culture medium was replaced daily, and spent medium was assayed for dPRL. The amounts of dPRL measured in the medium harvested from cultures prepared from the same tissue were averaged, and the values for the four tissues were combined. Each bar represents the mean SEM ($n = 4$) amount of dPRL measured in the medium on each day, expressed as nanograms per day per culture. (From ref 89, with permission)

MENSTRUAL AND REPAIR PHASE OF THE CYCLE

In the older literature, the concept was promulgated that the entire functionalis was lost during menstruation and that a new functionalis arose from proliferating stem cells located in the basalis (97). Hartman (98) had shown that an entire endometrium could regenerate from remnants left after dissecting out the endometrium with a scalpel and then wiping the uterine cavity clean with a cotton swab. In one animal so prepared, a pregnancy was established 22 days after hysterotomy. This provided convincing evidence that a functional endometrium *could* regenerate from the deepest portion of zone IV.

However, Bartelmez (55,56,99) and Markee (100)

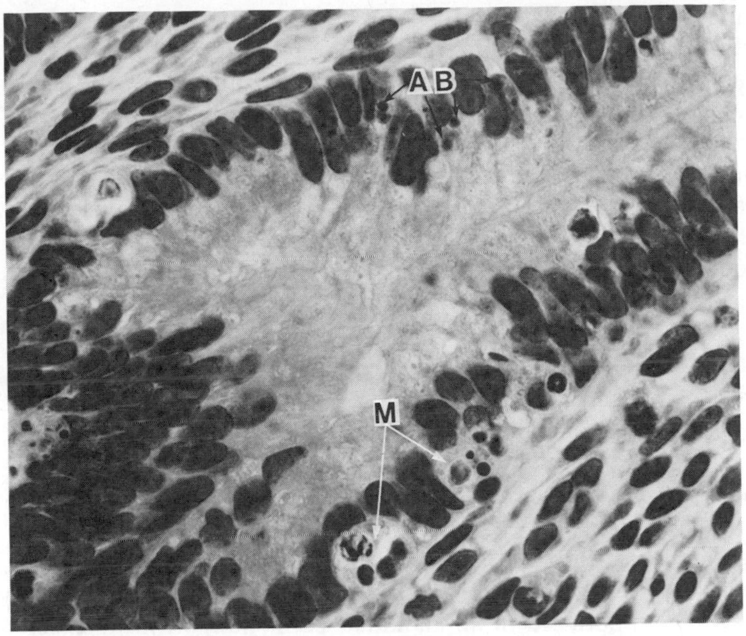

FIG. 34. Zone IV (basalis) from menstruating macaque. *White arrows* indicate macrophages (*M*) and *black arrows* point to apoptotic bodies (*AB*). ×750.

concluded that during natural menstruation very little tissue was shed and that the reduction in the thickness of the endometrium is primarily due to loss of fluid and the resulting shrinkage of the spongy layer. McLennan and Rydell (101) concluded, after an extensive survey, that regeneration of the new surface commonly occurs from a residuum of spongiosa rather than from the most basal elements of the endometrium. Bensley (102) found that mitotic activity was very low in the basal region until midcycle when it increased around the periovulatory period and then decreased. Ferenczy et al. (103) noted that during the early repair phase, DNA synthesis occurred primarily in the gland and surface epithelial cells, involved both cellular migration and replication, and was essentially a wound-healing reaction that was not dependent on E_2. Also, Ferenczy et al. (104) reported that the highest rates of proliferation were evident on days 8 to 10 in the upper third of the functionalis, not the basalis.

Padykula et al. (105) obtained endometrial biopsies 1 h after a single intravascular injection of ^{3}H-thymidine during the follicular phase. Again, epithelial labeling indexes were higher in the functionalis than in the basalis. In zone IV, the percentage of labeled cells increased from 1% at 2 days before the estrogen surge to 7% by 3 days after the estrogen surge (approximately 1 day postovulation). Subsequent analysis of two additional biopsies obtained 5 days after the estrogen surge indicated that the labeling index in zone IV continued to increase to reach 9% during the early luteal phase. These data and a report by Okulicz (106) strongly suggest that in macaques P can stimulate proliferation in the glands of zone IV but it inhibits glandular proliferation in the upper zones. Padykula et al. (107) suggested that the cells produced in zone IV of the basalis during the luteal phase were progenitors for the new endometrium that develops after menstruation, but the fate of the thymidine-labeled cells from zone IV in subsequent cycles has not been reported.

Other workers (108,109) suggested that cellular atrophy, apoptosis, and phagocytosis of dead cells play major roles in the remodeling of the endometrium. Flowers (110) concluded that the secretory spongiosa remains viable during the menstrual period and is converted by autophagocytosis and heterophagocytosis into a replicating endometrium. We have noted that during menstruation, extensive apoptosis occurs in the basalis (Fig. 34). This is probably a result of the withdrawal of P, which is trophic to this zone in macaques (106). Overall, it seems unlikely that the new cells produced during the luteal phase in the deep basalis contribute in a major way to endometrial regeneration after menstruation during natural cycles, although they retain the potential to reorganize and regenerate an entire functional endometrium after endometriectomy, as originally shown by Hartman (98).

REGULATION AND LOCALIZATION OF ESTROGEN AND PROGESTIN RECEPTORS IN THE ENDOMETRIUM

All reports on ER fluctuations during natural menstrual cycles in both human and monkey endometrium agree that nuclear and cytosolic ER levels are higher during the follicular than the luteal phase. Figure 18 (upper part) presents data from our laboratory on changes in endometrial ER (33) during the natural cycle. These data were obtained from the same 27 cynomolgus macaques presented in Table 1. Note that the decline in ER occurs at a time when the endometrium undergoes extensive progestational development in preparation for implantation. One might expect that P receptor levels would remain elevated during this period to sustain P action. However, cytosolic levels of the P receptor are lower during the luteal than the follicular phase, and nuclear P receptor levels are reported to be significantly higher only at midcycle or during the first few days of elevated P in the circulation (111–114). The progestational development of the primate endometrium requires continuous P action during the cycle, but as in the oviduct (115,116), the action of P tends to decrease the level of its own receptor. Because binding assays performed on homogenized tissues mask differences between cell types, we have used ICC to further explore receptor regulation in specific cell types in the endometrium. We have examined the uteri of rhesus (*Macaca mulatta*), cynomolgus (*Macaca fascicularis*), and pig-tail (*Macaca nemestrina*) monkeys either after hormonal treatments or during natural cycles and have found convincing evidence that stromal–epithelial interactions play important roles in regulating the growth and differentiation of the primate endometrium, just as in the oviduct.

We examined spayed macaques that were either untreated, treated with a 2-cm E_2 implant for 2 weeks, or treated first with E_2 for 2 weeks and then E_2 plus P for 2 additional weeks (117). The binding assays showed that in untreated spayed animals, most of the ER was cytosolic, but the ICC studies indicated that all specific staining was nuclear (Fig. 35A). After E_2 treatment, more ER was found in both the cytosolic and nuclear fractions, and there was an increase in the number of positively stained cells (Fig. 35B). Sequential P treatment lowered cytosolic and nuclear ER in the oviduct and endometrium significantly below the amount present in these tissues in E_2-treated animals, and lowered the cytosolic, but not the nuclear levels, significantly below the levels found in spayed animals. After such sequential P treatment, nuclear staining was undetectable, well below the amount seen in spayed animals (Fig. 35C). Thus, the nuclear staining for ER detected by ICC paralleled the total ER (cytosolic plus nuclear) measured by binding assays and was increased by treatment with E_2 and decreased by sequential P treatment. These findings are similar to those we described above for the oviduct.

Immunocytochemistry also showed that in the E_2-treated animals, there was an increase in the intensity of nuclear staining of the PR in the stromal fibroblasts and the glandular epithelium of all endometrial zones (Fig. 36) compared with spayed untreated animals. The induction of PR by E_2 treatment in rhesus monkey endometrium has also been noted by Okulicz et al. (118). After 14 days of E_2 plus P treatment, PR staining was suppressed in all glandular epithelium with the exception of zone IV (Fig. 37). However, stromal PR remained easily detectable in all zones (Fig. 38). Therefore, just as in the oviduct, the sustained effects of P on the glands of the functionalis in the late luteal phase may be mediated through the stroma, as the stromal cell population was the only one with detectable PR in the functionalis during most of the luteal phase. During sequential P treatment, ER became undetectable in most stromal cells in all regions, although it remained detectable in the glandular epithelium of zone IV. Also, ER remained detectable in the perivascular stroma and smooth-muscle walls of the spiral arteries in the functionalis. The great reduction of ER in the stroma and glandular epithelium throughout the functionalis argues against any significant direct role for estrogen on these cells during proges-

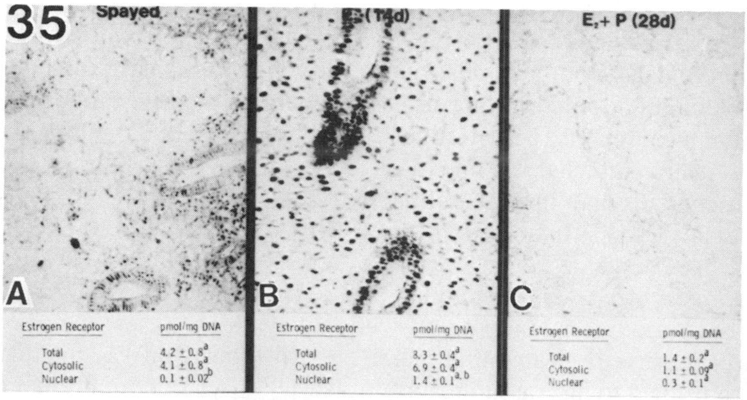

FIG. 35. Immunocytochemistry of ER in functionalis zone of endometrium is compared with a tabulation of binding assays of ER in whole endometrium from spayed animals that were either (**A**) untreated, (**B**) treated for 14 days with E_2, or (**C**) treated for 14 days with E_2 then 14 days with E_2 and P. Immunocytochemical shows that ER is low but detectable in nuclei of spayed untreated animals, that E_2 treatment increases the number of cells positive for ER, and that sequential P treatment suppresses ER below detectable levels in functionalis. In the tabulation, treatment groups with the same superscript letter were significantly different (student's *t*-test, $P < .01$). Original magnification, ×250.

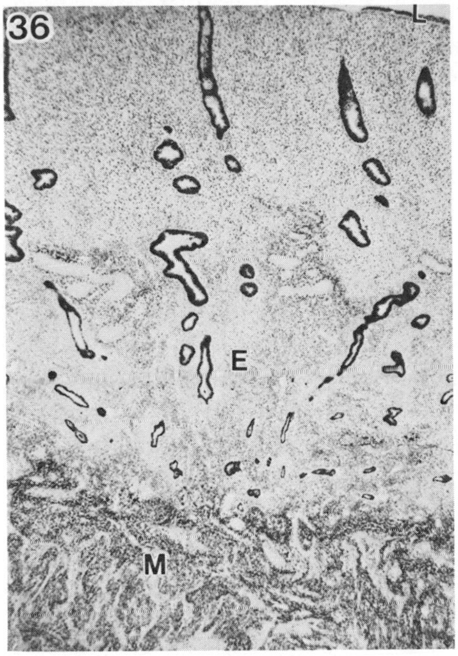

FIG. 36. Immunocytochemistry of PR in animals treated for 14 days with E_2. Positive staining is evident in stroma and glandular epithelium throughout entire thickness of endometrium. *L,* lumen; *E,* endometrium; *M,* myometrium. Original magnification, ×45.

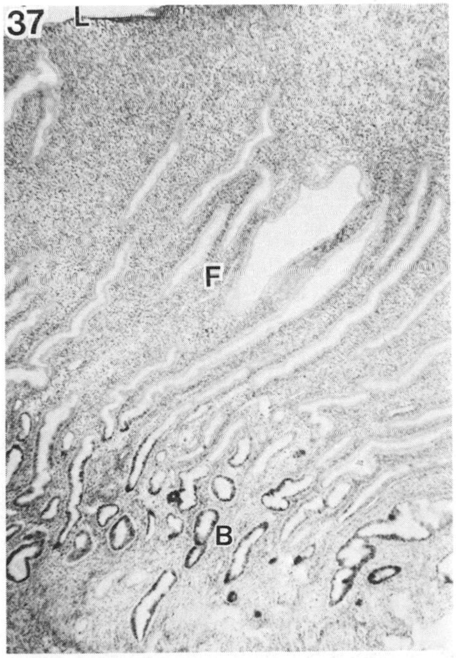

FIG. 37. Immunocytochemistry of PR in animals treated with 14 days of E_2 followed by 14 days of E_2 plus P. Progesterone receptor staining is greatly reduced in glandular epithelium of all zones except deeper portions of basalis. Stromal cells retain PR staining throughout all zones. This is more clearly seen in Fig. 4. *L,* lumen; *F,* functionalis; *B,* basalis. Original magnification, ×45.

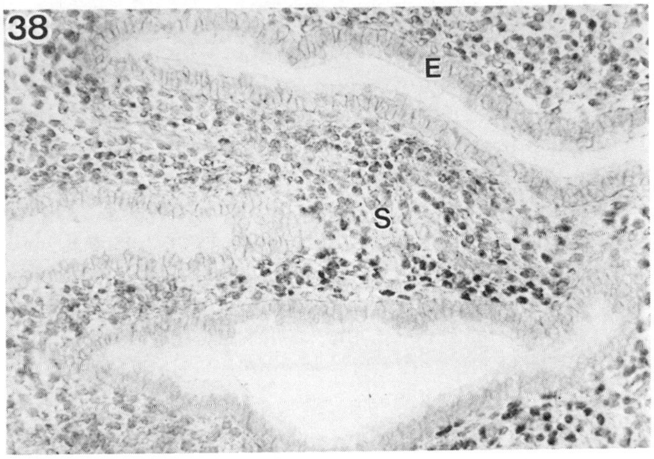

FIG. 38. Immunocytochemistry of PR in functionalis of E_2 and P-treated animals. After P treatment, PR staining becomes undetectable in glandular epithelium but remains detectable in stromal cells. *E,* glandular epithelium; *S,* stroma. Original magnification, ×400.

tational development of this endometrial zone, but the retention of ER in the vascular muscle regions of the spiral arteries indicates that E_2 could directly affect these blood vessels during the luteal phase. Progesterone receptor staining was also retained in the walls of the spiral arteries in the functionalis during sequential P treatment so P could also directly affect these vessels.

In naturally cycling macaques, we found that the pattern of ER and PR staining in the endometrium throughout the cycle was essentially as described above for the hormonally treated ones. Also, the results in cycling and pregnant baboons were essentially the same as in the rhesus monkey (119). In baboons during the luteal phase or after treatment with sequential P, there was a loss of ER from both stroma and glandular epithelium, except in the glandular epithelium in the basalis (zone IV), but PR was maintained in all the stroma as well as the glands of the deep basalis. During early pregnancy in the baboon, ER was absent from the endometrial glands and stroma but was present in the walls of spiral arteries and in the myometrium despite continual high levels of circulating P. The ER in the human endometrium behaved similarly (120,121). Significantly, in women as in nonhuman primates, stromal cells retained PR staining throughout the entire endometrium during the luteal phase. Clearly, receptor regulation in the primate endometrium is cell type-specific.

LUTEAL-FOLLICULAR TRANSITION

The period between menstrual cycles is known as the luteal-follicular transition (LFT) and is marked by a dramatic decline in serum P while serum E_2 remains constant or increases slightly. Consequently, P antagonism of ER is diminished and ER levels rise (33). We considered this an important time period in which to study cell type-specific receptor regulation. To do this, we created artificial menstrual cycles through the use of E_2 and P-filled Silastic capsules in spayed monkeys and sampled the endometrium during the LFT between the end of one cycle and the first few days of the next (122,123). We measured ER levels with binding assays and used ICC to evaluate changes in the distribution of ER and PR among the different uterine cell types. In these studies, after one artificial cycle, the P (but not the E_2) implants were withdrawn, and uteri were removed 0, 0.5, 1, 2, 3, 4, 5, 7, and 14 days later.

Morphologic Reorganization in the LFT

On day 0 of the LFT, the endometria were similar to those taken from monkeys in the late luteal phase of the natural cycle (122). After 12 hours of P withdrawal, there was a variable increase in stromal edema and a consistent, dramatic increase in cell death by apoptosis, especially in the basalis. Between days 0 and 3, mitotic activity was nil. By 1 or 2 days of P withdrawal, there was considerable compaction of the stroma and a great increase in close associations between the basal lamina of the endometrial glands and the subepithelial stromal cells. In zones III and IV of the basalis, there were many dead and dying glandular epithelial cells undergoing apoptosis and an increased number of macrophages filled with cellular debris and nuclear fragments. By the third and fourth days of P withdrawal, typical surface hemorrhage and sloughing of surface tissue had occurred and the stroma had become further compacted. On day 4, the mitotic index was only 0.2%, but on day 5, the mitotic activity rose tenfold to 2%. By day 5, epithelial cells had migrated from the mouths of the glands and formed a new luminal surface. Epithelial mitoses were abundant except in the basalis. In all animals, the surface had healed by day 7 of P withdrawal, and distinct zones I and II were apparent. In all endometria from day-7 and -14 animals, the mitotic indices were approximately 2%. Mitoses were not found in the lower basalis except in the 14-day group.

The histologic changes in the artificial LFT were similar to those previously described for the natural LFT by Bartelmez in his classic study of the endometrium of the rhesus monkey (55). He used the terms *premenstrual regression* and *regressive phase* to describe the stromal compaction that occurs in the endometrium at the beginning of this period, and he mentioned widespread cell death in the glands without specifying the basalis. However, in his study of the menstruating human uterus (99), he presented drawings of dying cells in the basalis (see his figures 35, 36, and 37 in Plate 15) that are excellent illustrations of apoptosis. The withdrawal of P that occurs with the demise of the corpus luteum is likely responsible for apoptosis during the natural cycle in the endometrial basalis in macaques and women.

ER and PR during the LFT

Binding assays showed that endometrial ER concentrations increased linearly during the LFT (122). However, ICC revealed that up to and including the time when epithelial mitotic activity began, most of the ER (Fig. 39A–D) and PR (Figs. 40 and 41) were specifically localized in the stromal fibroblasts, not in the epithelial cells that were mitotically active. These results suggested that estrogen-dependent mitotic renewal began in ER/PR-negative glandular epithelial cells under the influence of the stroma.

In a further test of this hypothesis, we combined ICC with ^{3}H-thymidine autoradiography to determine whether the specific cells making DNA during the LFT contained ER or PR (123). Also, we retreated animals with P during the LFT to determine whether P could antagonize the effects of E_2 on epithelial mitosis when

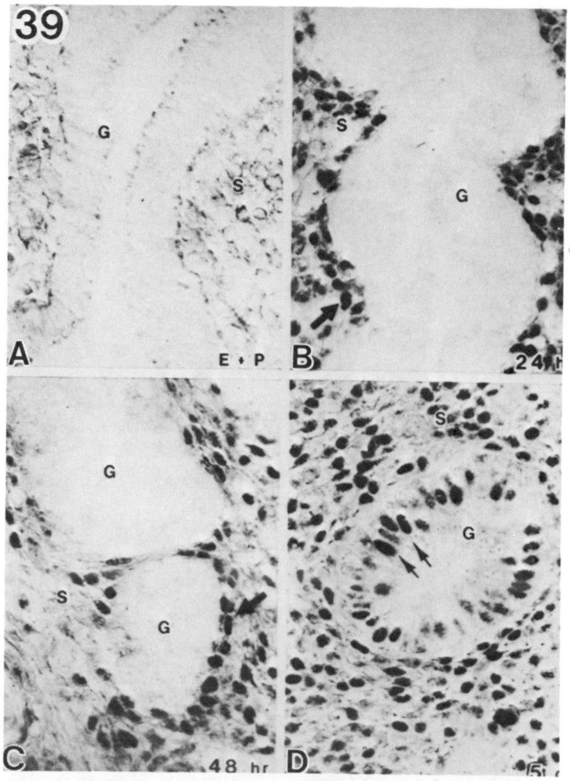

FIG. 39. Immunocytochemistry of ER in the functionalis during LFT. Estrogen receptor staining is (**A**) negative in stroma and glands after 28 days of sequential E_2 plus P administration and is positive only in the stroma (**B**) 24 and (**C**) 48 h after P withdrawal and does not become positive in large numbers of glandular epithelial cells until (**D**) 5 days after P withdrawal. *G*, glands, *S*, stroma. Original magnification, ×400. (From ref. 122, with permission.)

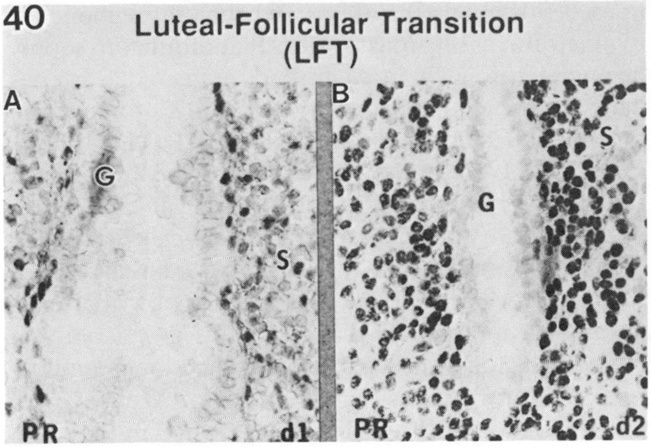

FIG. 40. Immunocytochemistry of PR in the functionalis during days 1 and 2 of LFT. Progesterone receptor staining is only detectable in stroma, not glandular epithelium on (**A**) days 1 and (**B**) 2 of P withdrawal. G, gland; S, stroma. Original magnification, ×400. (From ref. 122, with permission.)

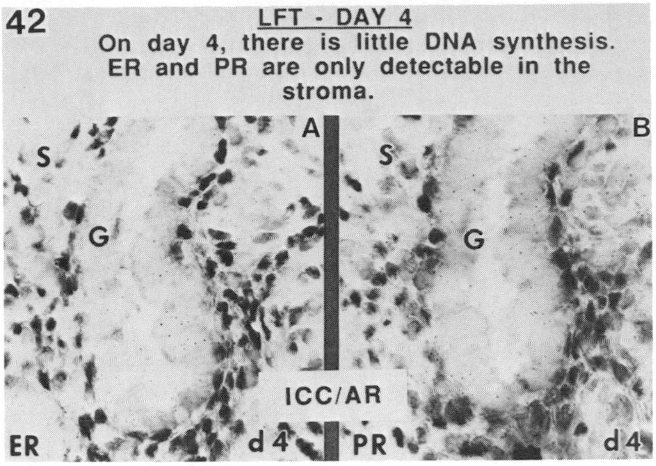

FIG. 42. Day 4 of LFT. Combined immunocytochemical/-autoradiographic (*ICC/AR*) preparations showing (**A**) ER on left and (**B**) PR on right in sections labeled with ^{3}H-thymidine. Estrogen receptor and PR are only detectable in stroma, and there are no cells making DNA. G, gland; S, stroma. Original magnification, ×400. (From ref. 122, with permission.)

PR was only present in stromal cells. To simplify the analysis, we confined our studies to that region of the functionalis (zone II/III) that remains after menstrual sloughing, because this is the region that undergoes estrogen-dependent proliferation after serum P declines. At 4 days after P withdrawal, there was little ^{3}H-thymidine uptake (Fig. 42). At 4.5 days after P withdrawal, there was a burst of DNA synthesis in the epithelium, but most epithelial cells that were autoradiographically positive for ^{3}H-thymidine uptake were immunocytochemically negative for both ER and PR (Fig. 43). By day 5 of P withdrawal, most of the ^{3}H-thymidine positive cells were still PR-negative and many were still ER-negative, although ER had become detectable in many ^{3}H-thymidine positive cells (Fig. 44). Retreatment with P on days 3 and 4 of the LFT (when PR was only present in the stroma) significantly inhibited DNA synthesis in epithelial cells, as measured by a decrease in the number of ^{3}H-thymidine-labeled cells (Fig. 45). Progesterone retreatment also significantly lowered the amount of total endometrial ER measured biochemically, but ICC showed that this suppressive effect of P on ER occurred only in the stroma (123). Taken together, these data indicated that E_2 treatment could stimulate

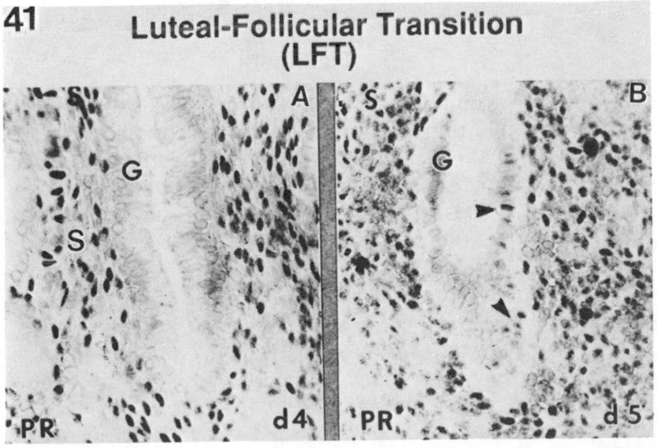

FIG. 41. Immunocytochemistry of PR in functionalis during days (**A**) 4 and (**B**) 5 of LFT. Progesterone receptor is detectable in stroma throughout this period but does not appear in glandular epithelium until day 5. *Arrowheads* point to PR-positive nuclei in glandular epithelium on day 5. G, gland; S, stroma. Original magnification, ×400. (From ref. 122, with permission.)

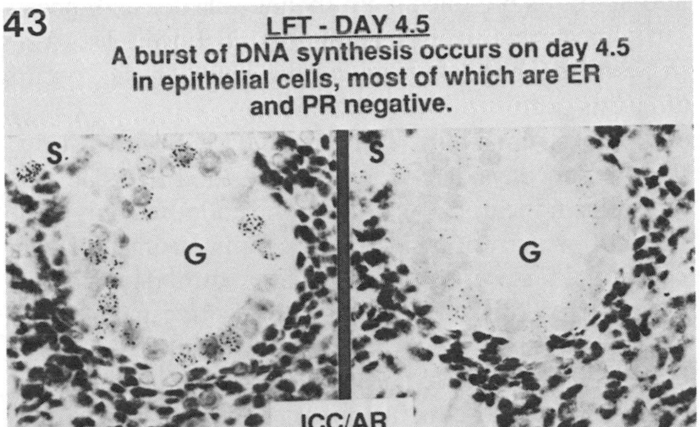

FIG. 43. Day 4.5 of LFT. Combined immunocytochemical/autoradiographic (*ICC/AR*) preparations showing (A) ER on left and (B) PR on right in sections labeled with ^{3}H-thymidine. On day 4.5, DNA synthesis is evident in many glandular epithelial cells, most of which are negative for (A) ER and (B) PR. In both A and B, slight nuclear staining evident is due to hematoxylin staining of chromatin. Only stroma contains detectable levels of ER and PR. G, gland; S, stroma. Original magnification, ×400. (From ref. 122, with permission.)

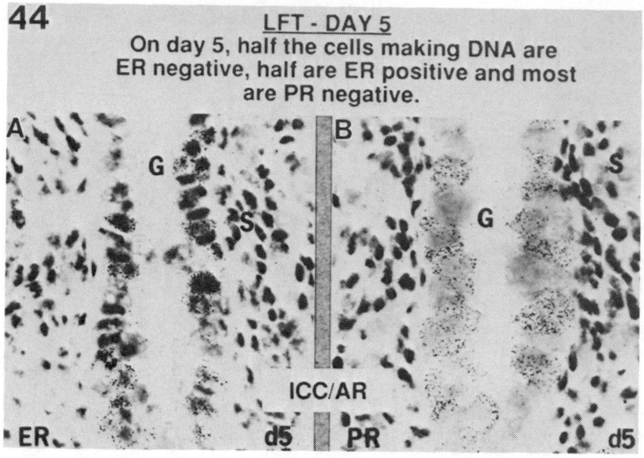

FIG. 44. Day 5 of LFT. Combined immunocytochemical/autoradiographic (*ICC/AR*) preparations. As above, (**A**) ER is on left and (**B**) PR is on right in sections labeled with ^{3}H-thymidine. About half the cells making DNA have become (A) ER-positive by day 5, but almost none are PR-positive. G, gland; S, stroma. Original magnification, ×400. (From ref. 122, with permission.)

DNA synthesis in epithelial cells that lacked ER, and P treatment could suppress DNA synthesis in epithelial cells that lacked PR. These findings (Fig. 46) suggest that the effects of E_2 on epithelial DNA synthesis in endometrial zone II/III during the very early proliferative phase of the menstrual cycle in nonhuman primates may be mediated indirectly through factors released from the stroma. Whether stromal cells continue to mediate the effects of E_2 on epithelial mitosis as the cycle progresses remains to be determined. Estrogen receptor is present in both stromal and glandular epithelial cells after days 5 and 6, but its presence in epithelial cells does not necessarily mean that stromal mediators no longer play a role in the E_2-dependent epithelial proliferation that occurs after this time.

Not all stromal fibroblasts became ER-positive during the first few days of P withdrawal in the LFT. The stromal cells in the upper regions of the endometrium [zone I and upper part of zone II (55,56)] that reorganize after menstrual loss were also ER-negative until days 4 and 5. Estrogen receptor staining was also negative in the epithelial cells that migrated from the mouths of the glands to form the new luminal epithelial surface (Fig. 47). These data confirm the conclusions of Ferenczy that surface repair is essentially a wound healing process and does not require direct estrogen stimulation (103,124).

RECEPTOR LOCALIZATION IN ENDOMETRIAL ARTERIES

In the rhesus macaque, the pattern of uterine circulation has been described in a series of classic papers (125–127) and reviewed by Ramsey (128). The uterine artery on each side enters the uterus and runs throughout the myometrium as an arcuate artery that ramifies to supply the myometrium. The arcuate sends many radial arteries that enter the endometrium, where they continue as the so-called coiled or spiral arteries that Daron (125) classified as Type I arteries. These vascularize the functionalis [zones I, II, and upper part of III; (55)]. The radials also give off much smaller branches, the so-called basal or Type II arteries that only vascularize the basalis [zones IV and lower part of zone III; (55)]. The basal arteries produce a capillary bed that maintains the viability of the lower regions when the upper layers slough and degenerate during menstrual breakdown. We have reported (122) that ER was detectable by ICC in the spiral arteries but had not previously commented on zonal differences or on the basal arteries. We have recently observed that in zone IV, the basal arteries and the spiral arteries in zone IV were negative for ER. Others have noted that ER was present in the walls of spiral arteries in

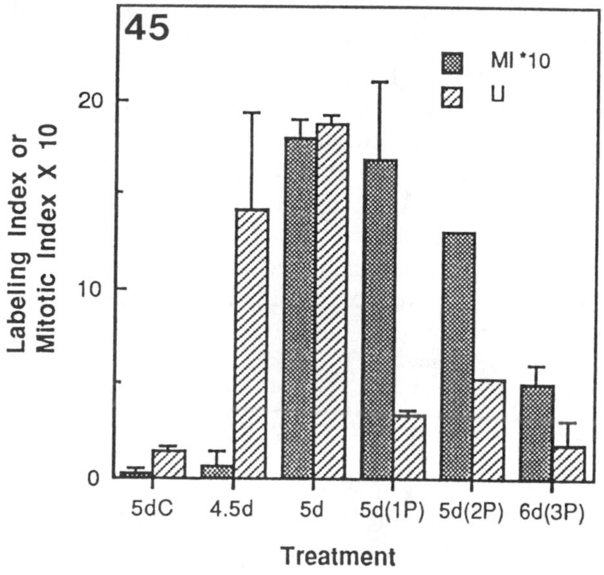

FIG. 45. Labeling index (*LI*) and mitotic index (*MI*) in endometrial zone II/III under different hormonal conditions associated with LFT. In each case, animals had been treated with sequential P regimen for 28 days before procedures below were initiated. The treatments indicated by the code under each pair of bars are as follows:

Code	Treatment
5dC	Controls, sampled on day 5 after withdrawal of both E_2 and P capsules
4.5d	Samples on day 4.5 of LFT
5d	Sampled on day 5 of LFT
5d(1P)	Sampled on day 5 of LFT but with P reinserted 1 day previously
5d(2P)	Sampled on day 5 of LFT but with P reinserted 2 days previously
6d(3P)	Sampled on day 6 of LFT but with P reinserted 3 days previously

$n = 3$ except for group 5d(2P), where $n = 2$.

(From ref. 122, with permission.)

the baboon (119) and the human (129) endometrium, but these authors also did not comment on zonal differences or on the basal arteries. Recently (130), we have shown a positive signal for ER mRNA by *in situ* hybridization in the walls of the spiral arteries in zones II and III and a lack of signal in the spiral arteries in zone IV closest to the myometrium. Also, many of the radial and arcuate arteries in the myometrium were negative for both ER protein and ER mRNA. The basal (Type II) arteries, which can be recognized in sections because of their small diameter and location close to the myometrial border, were also consistently negative for ER mRNA. We have recently observed that the PR of the vascular wall is also present in the spiral arteries of the functionalis but not the basalis. Consequently, we suggest that the genomic actions of estrogens and progestins on some uterine vascular elements are likely to be indirect. Only in the functionalis, where ER and PR are both present in the vascular wall, could the actions of these steroids be direct.

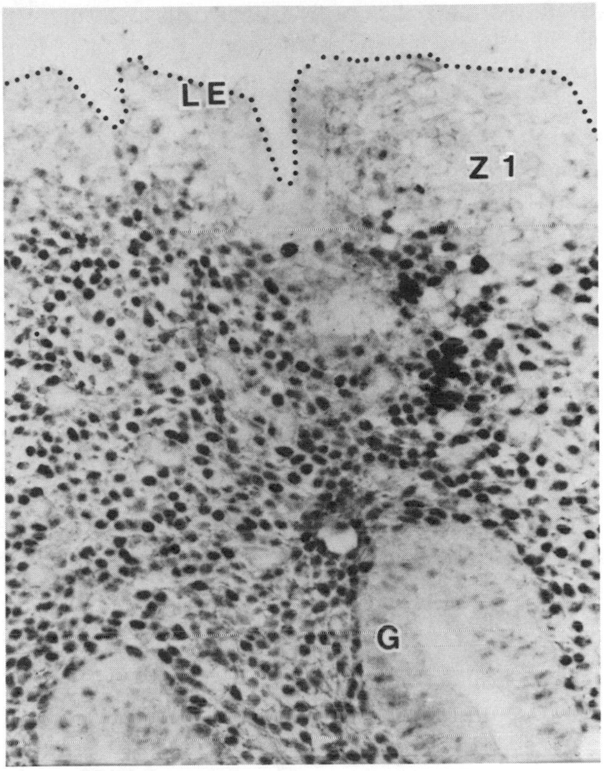

FIG. 47. Frozen section of upper endometrial functionalis (zone I and upper part of II) on day 5 of P withdrawal. Luminal epithelium (*LE*) and stromal nuclei of zone I (*Z1*) were ER-negative throughout day 5, which included the period of surface healing. Surface is outlined with a *dotted line* for clarity. ×150. (From ref. 122, with permission.)

POTENTIAL MEDIATORS: ENDOMETRIAL GROWTH FACTORS

The above studies and others in primate (119,122, 123,129) and nonprimate species (46,131–133) indicate that estrogens can stimulate epithelial mitosis in the endometrium when ER is only detectable in the endometrial stroma and that P can influence the epithelium when PR is only present in the stroma. Moreover, there is growing recognition that ovarian steroids stimulate synthesis of specific peptides (134), growth factors, and/or growth factor binding proteins (135), which have the potential to regulate cell proliferation in target tissues. Steroid stimulation of several growth factors has been reported (134), but none has been *unequivocally* identified as a physiological mediator of steroid action in the primate uterus. Among the likely contenders are IGF and EGF families.

46

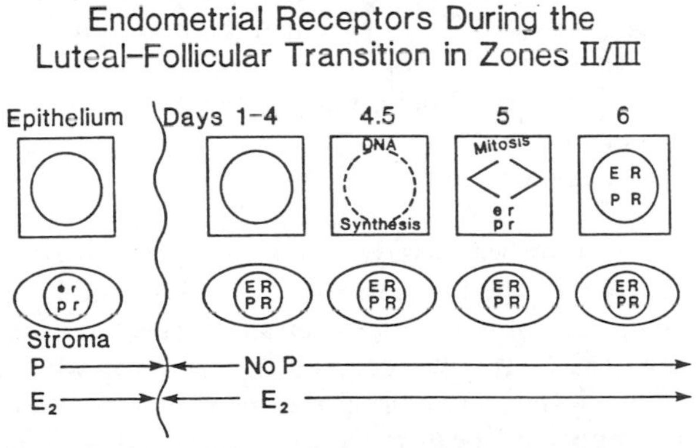

FIG. 46. Cellular localization of endometrial ER and PR during LFT. *Wavy vertical line* indicates end of one artificial menstrual cycle and beginning of the next. Estrogen receptor and PR increase in stromal cells immediately but do not appear in epithelial cells until day 5. Estradiol-dependent DNA synthesis begins in ER-negative epithelium on day 4.5. Retreatment with P during days 3 and 4 prevents E_2-dependent DNA synthesis even though PR is absent from the epithelium (see text and ref. 123). These data suggest that during LFT, E_2 can act through stroma to drive epithelial proliferation. If administered on days 2 to 4, P can block this effect of E_2 on epithelium even though PR is only in stroma.

Insulinlike Growth Factor System

Insulinlike growth factor I and II (IGF-I, IGF-II) are two homologous polypeptides that stimulate mitosis in a wide variety of tissues (136). Regulation of IGFs in the uterus has been studied extensively in rats, in which the predominant stimulator of IGF-I secretion is estrogen (137). Within 6 h after a single injection of E_2, IGF-I mRNA increased 14- to 22-fold (138,139) over that of untreated control animals, whereas E_2 treatment had no effect on hepatic synthesis of IGF-I (140). Ghahary et al. (139) showed by *in situ* hybridization that estrogen-stimulated expression of IGF-I mRNA is detectable in all uterine compartments, but expression is most abundant in myometrial smooth-muscle cells and outer stromal cells. In pseudopregnant rats, expression of IGF-I mRNA occurs in periglandular and periepithelial stroma (141).

Cell membrane receptors for IGF-I and IGF-II have been identified in the uterus of the rat (142) and in human endometrium during both the proliferative and secretory phases (143). Like IGF-I, expression of IGF-I receptors in the rat uterus appears to be stimulated by estrogen (137). Localization by autoradiography has indicated that IGF-I receptors in the rat occur in all uterine layers but are most abundant in the myometrium (142).

In biologic fluids, IGFs are found bound to specific IGF binding proteins (IGFBPs). These IGFBPs bind IGFs with affinity comparable with that of the IGF-I and II receptors, and it is believed that these binding proteins function as carrier proteins in transport of IGFs and as modulators of IGF action within target tissues (87,135,144). To date, six IGFBPs have been sequenced and expression of IGFBP-1, -2, and -3 has been reported in reproductive tract tissues of women (41,135) and the baboon (144).

Human uterine IGFBP-1 is an approximately 25-kDa nonglycosylated protein (145). This protein is structurally and genetically similar to the endometrial/placental proteins previously called placental protein 12 (PP12) and α_1-PEG (87,145,146). In women, IGFBP-1 has been localized immunocytochemically in decidualized stromal cells during both the luteal phase of the cycle and during pregnancy (146). Insulinlike growth factor binding proteins-1 mRNA is reported to be expressed by the secretory but not proliferative human endometrium (145), and IGFBP-1 has been detected by radioimmunoassay in explant cultures of proliferative and secretory endometrium treated with P (147,148). Fazleabas et al. (149) have identified by affinity cross-linking and Western blot analysis, an IGFBP in the baboon that is immunologically and biochemically similar to the IGFBP-1 reported in humans. This IGFBP can be detected immunocytochemically in the endometrium of baboons during the late luteal phase of the cycle, pregnancy, and after E_2 plus P treatment but not during follicular phase or after E_2 treatment alone (144,150). However, the histologic distribution of IGFBP-1 in baboon appears to be different from that observed in women. In the nonpregnant baboon, IGFBP-1 synthesis is confined to the epithelial cells of the deep basal glands during the late luteal phase (150) and shifts to the decidualized stromal cells during pregnancy (144). This pattern of IGFBP localization closely parallels ICC staining of PR during the luteal phase of the cycle and during pregnancy as reviewed above, which supports the hypothesis that P induces both IGFBP-1 secretion and decidualization in humans and nonhuman primates.

Two other IGFBPs, IGFBP-2 and IGFBP-3, have been examined in the human (87,135) and baboon (144) endometrium. Insulinlike growth factor binding proteins-2 is a 31-kDa nonglycosylated protein and is the main IGFBP reported in human and rat nervous system (151,152). Insulinlike growth factor binding protein-3 is a glycoprotein with a 29-kDa core protein and circulates as the main serum IGFBP (153,154). Giudice et al. (87,135) have shown that IGFBP-2 mRNA and IGFBP-3 mRNA are present in the proliferative and secretory endometrium of women. Western blot analysis showed that both IGFBP-2 and IGFBP-3 are synthesized *in vitro* by endometrial stromal cell cultures. In these cultures, E_2 plus P treatment increased IGFBP-2, but not IGFBP-3, levels significantly (200-fold) compared with untreated controls. Insulinlike growth factor binding protein-2 and IGFBP-3 are expressed by cultured explants of baboon endometrium collected during early pregnancy and are presumably up-regulated by P, but their precise regulation in baboons has not been studied (144).

The role of the IGFBPs in the reproductive tract is only poorly understood. If IGFs in the proliferative endometrium of primates are up-regulated by estrogen, as is reported for rat IGF-I, then P induction of IGFBPs may result in modulation of IGF action during the transition to a secretory endometrium. Insulinlike growth factor binding proteins may also modulate IGF-stimulated events during implantation, perhaps limiting the extent of trophoblast invasion (87). Additional research on the interactions among these different elements is needed to clarify their roles in the primate endometrium.

Epidermal Growth Factor

Estrogens are reported to induce EGF mRNA and EGF peptide (155) in rodent uteri, and EGF has been shown to have estrogenlike effects on uterine growth (156) in rodents. Epidermal growth factor mRNA is present in human endometrium (157), and the EGF peptide has been detected by ICC (158–160).

Receptors for EGF (EGFR) in the human endometrium have been assayed by several laboratories using different methodologies. Specific binding of radiolabeled EGF to human endometrial tissues is reported (161,162), but these reports do not agree on whether receptor levels vary during the menstrual cycle. Several attempts have been made to localize EGFR by ICC in the human uterus (159,160,163). Wang et al. (48) recently showed that reactivity for EGFR was most intense in the stromal cells and only minimally detectable in the glandular epithelium during the follicular phase and that stromal reactivity increased during the luteal phase. Wang et al. (48) also examined the localization of the C-*erb*B-2 protein and found it in the glandular epithelium, *not* the stroma, where its expression was also increased during the luteal phase. These results raise the intriguing possibility that EGF could affect the stroma directly and another ligand affect the epithelium directly, just as we noted above for the oviduct. Several questions remain concerning the possible role of stromal EGFR and epithelial C-*erb*B-2 as important components of a steroid-regulated paracrine system in the primate endometrium.

FINAL OVERVIEW

At the end of the menstrual cycle, the oviduct and endometrium are in two entirely different states. The oviduct is atrophied and regressed, but the endometrium is hypertrophied and progestational. In both tissues, luteal P has suppressed ER dramatically in the epithelium and the stroma, so that the effects of E_2 during the luteal phase are suppressed in both organs. Progesterone receptor has remained easily detectable in the stroma but usually undetectable in the epithelium in both tissues. Notable exceptions include the spiral arteries in the functionalis and the glands of the basalis, where ER and PR both persist. Thus, at the end of the cycle in both organs, the genomic actions of P must be primarily mediated through the stroma. When the functional corpus luteum finally regresses and serum P declines, the endometrium responds within a few days by menstruating, and the oviduct responds by entering into the ciliogenic process. Consequently, menstruation must also be considered a stromal function, as the only cells in the functionalis with PR that could "sense" P withdrawal are in the stroma and the walls of the spiral arteries.

After menstruation, as the next cycle begins, the endometrial surface repairs itself and E_2-dependent glandular proliferation begins. But ER reappears first in the underlying stroma and does not reappear in the glandular epithelium until after DNA synthesis begins. Thus, the stroma probably plays a key role in the first wave of E_2-dependent proliferation in the glandular epithelium, although later in the follicular phase, after ER has developed in the glands, E_2 could directly stimulate epithelial proliferation.

During menstruation, in the oviduct, the decline in P leads to elevations in ER, and E_2 then acts to drive oviductal differentiation. The lack of ER in fully ciliated cells and its presence in the stroma further implies that the effects of estrogen on ciliogenesis may be indirectly mediated by the stroma. However, E_2 may act directly on the ER-positive secretory cells.

At midcycle, serum P rises again and serum E_2 returns to early follicular phase levels. The endometrium steadily responds by stromal cell enlargement, gland cell enlargement in all zones, increased glandular sacculation, spiral artery development, increased stromal edema, and (in macaques) increased mitotic activity in zone IV of the basalis (102,105). Progesterone acts to induce the expression of an array of steroid-regulated genes in both stromal and epithelial cells, but epithelial cells lack PR during much of the time they are responding to P. Thus, the stroma may generate P-dependent mediators that affect epithelial cell response during the late luteal phase. The oviduct, however, atrophies and dedifferentiates as serum P levels increase, and the fully regressed oviduct presents a stark contrast to the fully stimulated, hypertrophied endometrium. Progesterone receptor is retained in the stroma, so the ability of P to keep the epithelium suppressed may be a function of PR-positive stromal cells. In sum, the stroma of both organs is probably involved to a much greater degree than previously realized in the cyclic changes in the entire tract.

Our emphasis on the role of the stroma is not meant to imply that all E_2-dependent epithelial events occur in ER-negative cells or that all P-dependent epithelial events occur in PR-negative cells. The glands of the basalis, which maintain PR throughout the luteal phase, enter mitosis when P levels rise and undergo apoptosis when P levels fall. These events could all be directly receptor-mediated, as PR is easily detectable within the affected cells. Oviductal secretory cells have ER and PR, so E_2 and P could also have direct genomic actions in these cells.

However, the role of the stroma in the adult cycling primate reproductive tract has been relatively neglected, and our goal in this review has been to stimulate research into the still unknown processes that underlie the familiar waxing and waning of the female tract. Through such research, reproductive scientists can lay the groundwork for improved, rational therapies for endometrial adenocarcinoma, fibromyoma, endometriosis, and other diseases of the tract and hopefully make an important contribution to the reproductive health of womankind.

ACKNOWLEDGMENTS

This review, Publication No. 1880 of the Oregon Regional Primate Research Center, was supported by grants HD-19182, P30 HD-18185, HD-19917, and RR-00163 from the National Institutes of Health. We thank Drs. Maryanne McClellan, Neal West, and Ila Maslar for their help and for graciously permitting us to use their findings in this review, Kunie Mah for technical assistance and help in assembling the figures, and Angela Adler for word processing assistance. Thanks also to Mr. Ron Severson, science teacher, Lakeridge High School, Lake Oswego, Oregon, for the photomicrograph in Fig. 34, taken during his tenure as a Science Teacher Intern at the Oregon Regional Primate Research Center, Summer 1985.

REFERENCES

1. Hisaw FL, Hisaw FL Jr. Action of estrogen and progesterone on the reproductive tract of lower primates. In: Young WC, ed. *Sex and Internal Secretions.* Baltimore: Williams & Wilkins 1961;556–589.
2. Brenner RM, Anderson RGW. Endocrine control of ciliogenesis

in the primate oviduct. In: Greep RO, Astwood EB, eds. *Handbook of Physiology, Section 7: Endocrinology, Vol. II, The Female Reproductive System, Part 2.* Baltimore: Williams and Wilkins, 1973;123–140.
3. Hafez ESE, Blandau RJ. *The Mammalian Oviduct.* Chicago: The University of Chicago Press, 1969.
4. Blandau RJ. Gamete transport in the female mammal. In: Greep RO, Astwood EB, eds. *Handbook of Physiology, Section 7: Endocrinology, Vol. II, The Female Reproductive System, Part 2.* Baltimore: Williams and Wilkins, 1973;53–163.
5. Hafez ESE. Endocrine control of the structure and function of the mammalian oviduct. In: Greep RO, Astwood EB, eds. *Handbook of Physiology, Section 7: Endocrinology, Vol. II, The Female Reproductive System, Part 2.* Baltimore: Williams and Wilkins, 1973;97–122.
6. Hafez ESE. Anatomy and physiology of the mammalian uterotubal junction. In: Greep RO, Astwood EB, eds. *Handbook of Physiology, Section 7: Endocrinology, Vol. II, The Female Reproductive System, Part 2.* Baltimore: Williams and Wilkins, 1973;87–95.
7. Johnson AD, Foley CW. *The Oviduct and Its Functions.* New York: Academic Press, 1974.
8. Jansen RPS. Endocrine response in the fallopian tube. *Endocr Rev* 1984;5:525–551.
9. Croxatto HB, Villalon M, eds. International Symposium on the Biology of the Oviduct. *Arch Biol Med Exp (Santiago)* 1991;24:213–422.
10. Eckstein P. Internal reproductive organs. In: Hofer H, Schultz AH, Starck D, eds. *Primatologia.* Vol. 3, Part 1. Basel: Karger, 1958;542–629.
11. Brenner RM, Carlisle KS, Hess DL, Sandow BA, West NB. Morphology of the oviducts and endometria of cynomolgus macaques during the menstrual cycle. *Biol Reprod* 1983;29:1289–1302.
12. Rumery RE, Gaddum-Rosse P, Blandau RJ, Odor DL. Cyclic changes in ciliation of the oviductal epithelium in the pig-tailed macaque (*Macaca nemestrina*). *Am J Anat* 1978;153:345–365.
13. Odor DL, Gaddum-Rosse P, Rumery RE, Blandau RJ. Cyclic variations in the oviductal ciliated cells during the menstrual cycle and after estrogen treatment in the pig-tailed monkey, *Macaca nemestrina.* Anat Rec 1980;198:35–57.
14. Odor DL, Gaddum-Rosse P, Rumery RE. Secretory cells of the oviduct of the pig-tailed monkey *Macaca nemestrina,* during the menstrual cycle and after estrogen treatment. *Am J Anat* 1983;166:149–172.
15. Verhage HG, Bareither ML, Jaffe RC, Akbar M. Cyclic changes in ciliation, secretion and cell height of the oviductal epithelium in women. *Am J Anat* 1979;156:505–521.
16. Donnez J, Casanas-Roux F, Caprasse J, Ferin J, Thomas K. Cyclic changes in ciliation, cell height, and mitotic activity in human tubal epithelium during reproductive life. *Fertil Steril* 1985;43:554–559.
17. Novak E, Everett HS. Cyclical and other variations in the tubal epithelium. *Am J Obstet Gynecol* 1928;16:499–530.
18. Patek E. The epithelium of the human fallopian tube. A surface ultrastructural and cytochemical study. *Acta Obstet Gynecol Scand* 1974;53(suppl):31.
19. Clyman MJ. Electron microscopy of the human fallopian tube. *Fertil Steril* 1966;17:281–301.
20. Brosens IA, Vasquez G. Fimbrial microbiopsy. *J Reprod Med* 1976;16:171–178.
21. Critoph FN, Dennis KJ. The cellular composition of the human oviduct epithelium. *Br J Obstet Gynaecol* 1977;84:219–221.
22. Oberti C, Gomez-Rogers C. "De novo" ciliogenesis in the human oviduct during the menstrual cycle. In: Velardo JT, Kasprow BA, eds. *Symposium on Biology of Reproduction,* Vol. 3. New Orleans: Pan American Congress of Anatomy, 1972;241–248.
23. Anderson RGW, Brenner RM. The formation of basal bodies (centrioles) in the rhesus monkey oviduct. *J Cell Biol* 1971;50:10–34.
24. Donnez J, Casanas-Rouss F, Ferin J, Thomas K. Changes in ciliation and cell height in human tubal epithelium in the fertile and post-fertile years. *Maturitas* 1983;5:39–45.
25. Andrews MC. Epithelial changes in the puerperal fallopian tube. *Am J Obstet Gynecol* 1951;62:28–37.
26. Verhage HG, Boice ML, Mavrogianis P, Donnelly K, Fazleabas A. Immunological characterization and immunocytochemical localization of oviduct-specific glycoproteins in the baboon (*Papio anubis*). *Endocrinology* 1989;124:2464–2472.
27. Verhage HG, Mavrogianis PA, Boice ML, Li W, Fazleabas AT. Oviductal epithelium of the baboon: hormonal control and the immuno-gold localization of oviduct-specific glycoproteins. *Am J Anat* 1990;187:81–90.
28. Brenner RM, Resko JA, West NB. Cyclic changes in oviductal morphology and residual cytoplasmic estradiol binding capacity induced by sequential estradiol-progesterone treatment of spayed rhesus monkeys. *Endocrinology* 1974;95:1094–1104.
29. Kerr JFR, Wyllie AH, Currie AR. Apoptosis: a basic biological phenomenon with wide ranging implications in tissue kinetics. *Br J Cancer* 1972;26:239–257.
30. Wyllie AH, Kerr JFR, Currie AR. Cell death: the significance of apoptosis. *Int Rev Cytol* 1980;68:251–306.
31. Sandow BA, West NB, Norman RL, Brenner RM. Hormonal control of apoptosis in hamster uterine luminal epithelium. *Am J Anat* 1979;156:15–36.
32. Resko JA, Boling JL, Brenner RM, Blandau RJ. Sex steroids in reproductive tract tissues: regulation of estradiol concentrations by progesterone. *Biol Reprod* 1976;15:153–157.
33. West NB, Brenner RM. Estrogen receptor levels in the oviducts and endometria of cynomolgus macaques during the menstrual cycle. *Biol Reprod* 1983;29:1303–1312.
34. Jänne O, Isomaa V, Isotalo H, Kokko E, Vierikko P. Uterine estrogen and progestin receptors and their regulation. *Ups J Med Sci Suppl* 1978;22:62–70.
35. Clark JH, Hsueh AJW, Peck EJ Jr. Regulation of estrogen receptor replenishment by progesterone. *Ann NY Acad Sci USA* 1977;286:161–179.
36. Leavitt WW, MacDonald RG, Okulicz WC. Hormonal regulation of estrogen and progesterone receptor systems. In: Litwack G, ed. *Biochemical Actions of Hormones, Vol X.* New York: Academic Press, 1983;323–356.
37. King WJ, Greene GL. Monoclonal antibodies localize oestrogen receptor in the nuclei of target cells. *Nature* 1984;307:745–747.
38. McClellan MC, West NB, Tacha DE, Greene GL, Brenner RM. Immunocytochemical localization of estrogen receptors in the macaque reproductive tract with monoclonal antiestrophilins. *Endocrinology* 1984;114:2002–2014.
39. Press MP, Nousek-Goebl N, King WJ, Herbst AL, Greene GJ. Immunohistochemical assessment of estrogen receptor distribution in the human endometrium throughout the menstrual cycle. *Lab Invest* 1984;51:495–503.
40. Perrot-Applanat M, Groyer-Picard M-T, Lorenzo F, et al. Immunocytochemical study with monoclonal antibodies to progesterone receptor in human breast tumors. *Cancer Res* 1987;47:2652–2661.
41. Guiochon-Mantel A, Lescop P, Christin-Maitre S, Loosfelt H, Perrot-Applanat M, Milgrom E. Nucleocytoplasmic shuttling of the progesterone receptor. *EMBO J* 1991;10:3851–3859.
42. Gasc J-M, Baulieu E-E. Steroid hormone receptors: intracellular distribution. *Biol Cell* 1986;56:1–6.
43. Press MF, Xu S, Wang J, Greene GL. Subcellular distribution of estrogen receptor and progesterone receptor with and without specific ligand. *Am J Pathol* 1989;135:857–864.
44. West NB, Hess DL, Brenner RM. Differential suppression of progesterone receptor by progesterone in the reproductive tract of primate macaques. *J Steroid Biochem* 1986;25:497–503.
45. Clarke CL, Sutherland RL. Progestin regulation of cellular proliferation. *Endocr Rev* 1990;11:266–301.
46. Cunha GR, Bigsby RM, Cooke PS, Sugimura Y. Stromal-epithelial interactions in adult organs. *Cell Differ* 1985;17:137–148.
47. Boutin EL, Sanderson RD, Bernfield M, Cunha GR. Epithelial-mesenchymal interactions in uterus and vagina alter the expression of the cell surface proteoglycan, syndecan. *Dev Biol* 1991;148:63–74.
48. Wang D, Fujii S, Konishi I, et al. Expression of c-*erb*B-2 protein and epidermal growth factor receptor in normal tissues of the female genital tract and in the placenta. *Virchows Archiv A Pathol Anat* 1992;420:385–393.
49. Schimmelpenning H, Eriksson ET, Falkmer UG, Azavedo E, Svane G, Auer GU. Expression of the c-*erb*B-2 proto-oncogene product and nuclear DNA content in benign and malignant hu-

man breast parenchyma. *Virchows Archiv A Pathol Anat* 1992;420:433–440.

50. Giudice LC, Dsupin BA, Irwin JC, Eckert RL. Identification of insulinlike growth factor binding proteins in human oviduct. *Fertil Steril* 1992;57:294–301.
51. Giudice LC, Dsupin BA, Vu TH, Jin IH, Hoffman AR. Differential expression of insulinlike growth factor-I (IGF-I), IGF-II and Type I and Type II IGF receptor messenger RNAs in human oviduct. Abstract #P-002. *Abstracts of 40th Ann Mtg Pacific Coast Fert Soc* 1992;A11–A12.
52. White AJ, Buchsbaum HJ. Scanning electron microscopy of the human endometrium. *Gynecol Oncol* 1973;1:330–339.
53. Ferenczy A, Richart RM. Scanning and transmission electron microscopy of the human endometrial surface epithelium. *J Clin Endocrinol Metab* 1973;36:999–1008.
54. Ferenczy A. Surface ultrastructural response of the human uterine lining epithelium to hormonal environment. A scanning electron microscopic study. *Acta Cytol* 1977;21:566–572.
55. Bartelmez GW. Cyclic changes in the endometrium of the rhesus monkey (*Macaca mulatta*). *Contrib Embryol* 1951;34:99–144.
56. Bartelmez GW. The phases of the menstrual cycle and their interpretation in terms of the pregnancy cycle. *Am J Obstet Gynecol* 1957;74:931–955.
57. Hodgen GD. Surrogate embryo transfer combined with estrogen-progesterone therapy in monkeys. *JAMA* 1983;250:2167–2171.
58. Cunha GR, Chung LWK, Shannon JM, Taguchi O, Fujii H. Hormone-induced morphogenesis and growth: role of mesenchymal–epithelial interactions. *Recent Prog Horm Res* 1983;39:559–598.
59. Noyes RW, Hertig AT, Rock J. Dating the endometrial biopsy. *Fertil Steril* 1950;1:3–25.
60. Kraemer DC, Maqueo M, Hendrickx AG, Vera Cruz NC. Histology of the baboon endometrium during the menstrual cycle and pregnancy. *Fertil Steril* 1977;28:482–487.
61. MacLennan AH, Wynn RM. Menstrual cycle of the baboon. *Obstet Gynecol* 1971;38:350–358.
62. Dollar JR, Hand GS, Beck LR, Boots LR. The baboon as a primate model for the study of endometrium. *Am J Obstet Gynecol* 1979;134:305–309.
63. Enders AC, Welsh AO, Schlafke S. Implantation in the rhesus monkey: endometrial responses. *Am J Anat* 1985;173:147–169.
64. Hisaw FL, Meyer K, Fevold HL. Production of a premenstrual endometrium in castrated monkeys by ovarian hormones. *Proc Soc Exp Biol* 1930;27:400–403.
65. Cleveland R. Cytologic and histologic observations on the epithelial, connective and vascular tissues of the endometrium of macaques under various experimental conditions. *Endocrinology* 1941;28:388–405.
66. Rossman I. The deciduomal reaction in the rhesus monkey (*Macaca mulatta*). *Am J Anat* 1940;66:277–365.
67. Dallenbach-Hellweg G, Dawson AB, Hisaw FL. The effect of relaxin on the endometrium of monkeys: histological and histochemical studies. *Am J Anat* 1966;119:61–78.
68. Kelly WA, Marston JH, Eckstein P. Effect of an intra-uterine device on endometrial morphology and the deciduomal reaction in the rhesus monkey. *J Reprod Fertil* 1969;19:331–340.
69. Ghosh D, Sengupta J. Endometrial responses to a deciduogenic stimulus in ovariectomized rhesus monkeys treated with oestrogen and progesterone. *J Endocrinol* 1989;120:51–58.
70. Mossman HW. Comparative morphogenesis of the fetal membranes and accessory uterine structures. *Contrib Embryol* 1937;158:133–247.
71. Golander G, Zakuth V, Schechter Y, Spirer Z. Suppression of lymphocyte reactivity *in vitro* by a soluble factor secreted by explants of human decidua. *Eur J Immunol* 1981;11:849–851.
72. Bischof P, DuBerg S, Sizonenko MT, et al. *In vitro* production of pregnancy-associated plasma protein A by human decidua and trophoblast. *Am J Obstet Gynecol* 1984;148:13–18.
73. Bulmer JN, Sunderland CA. Immunohistological characterization of lymphoid cell populations in the early human placental bed. *Immunology* 1984;52:349–357.
74. Bulmer JN, Sunderland CA. Bone-marrow origin of endometrial granulocytes in the early human placental bed. *J Reprod Immunol* 1983;5:383–387.
75. Laguens RM, Laguens RP. Isolation and characteristics of a macrophage population of human uterine mucosa. *Gynecol Obstet Invest* 1983;16:136–141.
76. Tabibzadeh S. Proliferative activity of lymphoid cells in human endometrium throughout the menstrual cycle. *J Clin Endocrinol Metab* 1990;70:437–443.
77. Kleinman D, Sharon Y, Sarov I, Insler V. Human endometrium in cell culture: a new method for culturing human endometrium as separate epithelial and stromal components. *Arch Gynecol* 1983;234:103–112.
78. Rinehart CA Jr, Lyn-Cook BD, Kaufman DG. Gland formation from human endometrial epithelial cells *in vitro*. *In Vitro Cell Dev Biol* 1988;24:1037–1041.
79. Osteen KG, Hill GA, Hargrove JT, Gorstein F. Development of a method to isolate and culture highly purified populations of stromal and epithelial cells from human endometrial biopsy specimens. *Fertil Steril* 1989;52:965–972.
80. Markiewicz L, Gurpide E. *In vitro* evaluation of estrogenic, estrogen antagonistic and progestagenic effects of a steroidal drug (Org OD-14) and its metabolites on human endometrium. *J Steroid Biochem* 1990;35:535–541.
81. Bigazzi M, Nardi E, Bruni P, Petrucci F. Relaxin in human decidua. *J Clin Endocrinol Metab* 1980;51:939–941.
82. Koay ESC, Bagnell CA, Bryant-Greenwood GD, Lord SB, Cruz AC, Larkin LH. Immunocytochemical localization of relaxin in human decidua and placenta. *J Clin Endocrinol Metab* 1985;60:859–863.
83. Chen G, Huang JR, Mazella J, Tseng L. Long-term effects of progestin and RU 486 on prolactin production and synthesis in human endometrial stromal cells. *Hum Reprod* 1989;4:355–358.
84. Braverman MB, Bagni A, deZiegler D, Den T, Gurpide E. Isolation of prolactin-producing cells from first and second trimester decidua. *J Clin Endocrinol Metab* 1984;58:521–525.
85. Hochner-Celnikier D, Ron M, Eldor A, et al. Growth characteristics of human first trimester decidual cells cultured in serum-free medium: production of prolactin, prostaglandins and fibronectin. *Biol Reprod* 1984;31:827–836.
86. Weisman Y, Harell A, Edelstein S, David M, Spirer Z, Golander A. 1α,25-dihydroxyvitamin D_3 and 24,25-dihydroxyvitamin D_3 *in vitro* synthesis by human decidua and placenta. *Nature* 1979;281:317–319.
87. Giudice LC, Milkowski DA, Lamson G, Rosenfeld RG, Irwin JC. Insulinlike growth factor binding proteins in human endometrium: steroid-dependent messenger ribonucleic acid expression and protein synthesis. *J Clin Endocrinol Metab* 1991;72: 779–787.
88. Tabanelli S, Tang B, Gurpide E. *In vitro* decidualization of human endometrial stromal cells. *J Steroid Biochem Molec Biol* 1992;42:337–344.
89. Maslar IA, Ansbacher R. Effects of progesterone on decidual prolactin production by organ cultures of human endometrium. *Endocrinology* 1986;118:2102–2108.
90. Maslar IA, Powers-Craddock P, Ansbacher R. Decidual prolactin production by organ cultures of human endometrium: effects of continuous and intermittent progesterone treatment. *Biol Reprod* 1986;34:741–750.
91. MacLaughlin DT, Richardson GS, Sylvan PE. Analysis of human endometrial protein secretions *in vivo* and *in vitro:* effects of estrogens and progesterone. In: Jasonni VM et al., eds. *Steroids and Endometrial Cancer.* New York: Raven Press, 1983;93–104.
92. Bell SC, Patel S, Hales MW, Kirwan PH, Drife JO. Immunochemical detection and characterization of pregnancy-associated endometrial alpha$_1$ and alpha$_2$-globulins secreted by human endometrium and decidua. *J Reprod Fertil* 1985;74:261–270.
93. Iacobelli S, Marchetti P, Bartoccioni E, Natoli V, Scambia G, Kaye AM. Steroid-induced proteins in human endometrium. *Mol Cell Endocrinol* 1981;23:321–331.
94. Strinden ST, Shapiro SS. Progesterone-altered secretory proteins from cultured human endometrium. *Endocrinology* 1983;112: 862–870.
95. Heffner LJ, Iddenden DA, Lyttle CR. Electrophorectic analyses of secreted human endometrial proteins: identification and characterization of luteal phase prolactin. *J Clin Endocrinol Metab* 1986;62:1288–1295.
96. Zhu HH, Huang JR, Mazella J, Rosenberg M, Tseng L. Differential effects of progestin and relaxin on the synthesis and secretion of immunoreactive prolactin in long term culture of human en-

dometrial stromal cells. *J Clin Endocrinol Metab* 1990;71: 889–899.
97. Schroder R. Anatomische Studien zur normalen und pathologischen Physiologie des Menstruationszyklus. *Arch Gynakol* 1915;104:27–102.
98. Hartman CG. Regeneration of the monkey uterus after surgical removal of the endometrium and accidental endometriosis. *West J Surg Obstet Gynecol* 1944;52:87–102.
99. Bartelmez GW. Histological studies on the menstruating mucous membrane of the human uterus. *Contrib Embryol* 1933;142: 142–186.
100. Markee JE. Menstruation in intraocular endometrial transplants in the rhesus monkey. *Contrib Embryol* 1940;28:219–308.
101. McLennan CE, Rydell AH. Extent of endometrial shedding during normal menstruation. *J Obstet Gynecol* 1965;26:605–621.
102. Bensley CM. Cyclic fluctuations in the rate of epithelial mitosis in the endometrium of the rhesus monkey. *Contrib Embryol* 1951;34:87–98.
103. Ferenczy A, Bertrand G, Gelfand MM. Studies on the cytodynamics of human endometrial regeneration III. *In vitro* short-term incubation historadioautography. *Am J Obstet Gynecol* 1979; 134:297–304.
104. Ferenczy A, Bertrand G, Gelfand MM. Proliferation kinetics of human endometrium during the normal menstrual cycle. *Am J Obstet Gynecol* 1979;133:859–867.
105. Padykula HA, Coles LG, McCracken JA, King NW Jr, Longcope C, Kaiserman-Abramof IR. A zonal pattern of cell proliferation and differentiation in the rhesus endometrium during the estrogen surge. *Biol Reprod* 1984;31:1103–1118.
106. Okulicz WC, Tast J, Balsamo M. Progesterone regulation of endometrial proliferation during the secretory phase in artificial menstrual cycles of the rhesus monkey (Abstract). *J Cell Biol* 1991;115:10a (#51).
107. Padykula HA, Coles LG, Okulicz WC, et al. The basalis of the primate endometrium: a bifunctional germinal compartment. *Biol Reprod* 1989;40:681–690.
108. Hopwood D, Levison DA. Atrophy and apoptosis in the cyclical human endometrium. *J Pathol* 1976;119:159–166.
109. Davie R, Hopwood D, Levison DA. Intercellular spaces and cell junctions in endometrial glands: their possible role in menstruation. *Br J Obstet Gynaecol* 1977; 84:467–476.
110. Flowers CE Jr. New observations on the physiology of menstruation. *Obstet Gynecol* 1978;51:16–24.
111. Levy C, Robel P, Gautray JP, et al. Estradiol and progesterone receptors in human endometrium: normal and abnormal menstrual cycles and early pregnancy. *Am J Obstet Gynecol* 1980;136:646–651.
112. Bayard F, Damilano S, Robel P, Baulieu E-E. Cytoplasmic and nuclear estradiol and progesterone receptors in human endometrium. *J Clin Endocrinol Metab* 1978;46:635–648.
113. Ochiai K. Cyclic variation and distribution in the concentration of cytosol estrogen and progesterone receptors in the normal human uterus and myoma. *Acta Obstet Gynecol Jpn* 1980;32: 945–952.
114. Lukola A, Punnonen R. Estrogen and progesterone receptors in human uterus and oviduct. *J Endocrinol Invest* 1983;6:179–183.
115. Pollow K, Inthraphuvasak J, Manz B, Grill H-J, Pollow B. A comparison of cytoplasmic and nuclear estradiol and progesterone receptors in human fallopian tube and endometrial tissue. *Fertil Steril* 1981;36:615–622.
116. Pino AM, Devoto L, Davila M, Soto E. Changes during the menstrual cycle in cytosolic and nuclear concentrations of progestagen receptor in the human fallopian tube. *J Reprod Fertil* 1984;70:481–485.
117. West NB, McClellan MC, Sternfeld MD, Brenner RM. Immunocytochemistry versus binding assays of the estrogen receptor in the reproductive tract of spayed and hormone treated macaques. *Endocrinology* 1987;121:1789–1800.
118. Okulicz WC, Savasta AM, Hoberg LM, Longcope C. Immunofluorescent analysis of estrogen induction of progesterone receptor in the rhesus uterus. *Endocrinology* 1989;125:930–934.
119. Hild-Petito S, Verhage HG, Fazleabas AT. Immunocytochemical localization of estrogen and progestin receptors in the baboon (*Papio anubis*) uterus during implantation and pregnancy. *Endocrinology* 1992;130:2343–2353.
120. Garcia E, Bouchard P, De Brux J, et al. Use of immunocytochemistry of progesterone and estrogen receptors for endometrial dating. *J Clin Endocrinol Metab* 1988;67:80–87.
121. Bergeron C, Ferenczy A, Toft DO, Schneider W, Shyamala G. Immunocytochemical study of progesterone receptors in the human endometrium during the menstrual cycle. *Lab Invest* 1988;59:862–869.
122. McClellan M, West NB, Brenner RM. Immunocytochemical localization of estrogen receptors in the macaque endometrium during the luteal-follicular transition. *Endocrinology* 1986;119: 2467–2475.
123. McClellan MC, Rankin S, West NB, Brenner RM. Estrogen receptors, progestin receptors and DNA synthesis in the macaque endometrium during the luteal-follicular transition. *J Steroid Biochem Molec Biol* 1990;37:631–641.
124. Ferenczy A. Studies on the cytodynamics of experimental endometrial regeneration in the rabbit. Historadioautography and ultrastructure. *Am J Obstet Gynecol* 1977;128:536–545.
125. Daron GH. The arterial pattern of the tunica mucosa of the uterus in macacus rhesus. *Am J Anat* 1936;58:349–419.
126. Bartelmez GW. Premenstrual and menstrual ischemia and the myth of endometrial arteriovenous anastomoses. *Am J Anat* 1956;98:69–95.
127. Bartelmez GW. The form and the functions of the uterine blood vessels in the rhesus monkey. *Contrib Embryol* 1957;36:153–182.
128. Ramsey EM. Placental vasculature and circulation. In: Greep RO, ed. *Handbook of Physiology. Section 7: Endocrinology, Vol. II. Female Reproductive System, Part 2,* Ed 2. Washington, DC: American Physiological Society, 1973;323–337.
129. Perrot-Applanat M, Groyer-Picard MT, Garcia E, Lorenzo F, Milgrom E. Immunocytochemical demonstration of estrogen and progesterone receptors in muscle cells of uterine arteries in rabbits and humans. *Endocrinology* 1988;123:1511–1519.
130. Koji T, Brenner RM. Localization of estrogen receptor messenger RNA in rhesus monkey uterus by nonradioactive in situ hybridization with digoxigenin labeled oligodeoxynucleotides. *Endocrinology* 1993; 132:382–392.
131. Cunha GR, Shannon JM, Vanderslice KD, McCormick K, Bigsby RM. Autoradiographic demonstration of high affinity nuclear binding and finite binding capacity of ^{3}H-estradiol in mouse vaginal cells. *Endocrinology* 1983;113:1427–1430.
132. Bigsby RM, Aixin L, Luo K, Cunha GR. Strain differences in the ontogeny of estrogen receptors in murine uterine epithelium. *Endocrinology* 1990;126:2592–2596.
133. Bigsby RM. Progesterone inhibition of estrogen-induced epithelial proliferation in the rodent uterus requires stromal factors. In: *Program and Abstracts of 72nd Annual Meeting of The Endocrine Society* (held in Atlanta, GA, June 20–23, 1990). 1990;199.
134. Fay TN, Grudzinskas JG. Human endometrial peptides: a review of their potential role in implantation and placentation. *Hum Reprod* 1991;6:1311–1326.
135. Giudice LC, Lamson G, Rosenfeld RG, Irwin JC. Insulinlike growth factor-II (IGF-II) and IGF binding proteins in human endometrium. *Ann NY Acad Sci* 1991;626:295–307.
136. Rechler MM, Nissley SP. Insulinlike growth factors. In: Sporn MB, Roberts AB, eds. *Peptide Growth Factors and Their Receptors I.* New York: Springer-Verlag, 1991;263–367.
137. Murphy LJ, Ghahary A. Uterine insulinlike growth factor-1: regulation of expression and its role in estrogen-induced uterine proliferation. *Endocr Rev* 1990;11:443–453.
138. Murphy LJ, Murphy LC, Friesen HG. Estrogen induces insulinlike growth factor-I expression in the rat uterus. *Mol Endocrinol* 1987;1:445–450.
139. Ghahary A, Chakrabarti S, Murphy LJ. Localization of the sites of synthesis and action of insulinlike growth factor-I in the rat uterus. *Mol Endocrinol* 1990;4:191–195.
140. Murphy LJ, Friesen HG. Differential effects of estrogen and growth hormone on uterine and hepatic insulinlike growth factor I gene expression in the ovariectomized hypophysectomized rat. *Endocrinology* 1988;122:325–332.
141. Croze F, Kennedy TG, Schroedter IC, Friesen HG, Murphy LJ. Expression of insulinlike growth factor-I and insulinlike growth factor-binding protein-1 in the rat uterus during decidualization. *Endocrinology* 1990;127:1995–2000.
142. Ghahary A, Murphy LJ. Uterine insulinlike growth factor-I re-

ceptors: regulation by estrogen and variation throughout the estrous cycle. *Endocrinology* 1989;125:597–604.
143. Talavera F, Reynolds RK, Roberts JA, Menon KMJ. Insulinlike growth factor I receptors in normal and neoplastic human endometrium. *Cancer Res* 1990;50:3019–3024.
144. Tarantino S, Verhage HG, Fazleabas AT. Regulation of insulinlike growth factor-binding proteins in the baboon (*Papio anubis*) uterus during early pregnancy. *Endocrinology* 1992;130: 2354–2362.
145. Julkunen M, Koistinen R, Aalto-Setälä K, Seppälä M, Jänne OA, Kontula K. Primary structure of human insulinlike growth factor-binding protein/placental protein 12 and tissue-specific expression of its mRNA. *FEB* 1988;236:295–302.
146. Waites GT, James RFL, Bell SC. Immunohistological localization of the human endometrial secretory protein pregnancy-associated endometrial a_1-globulin, an insulinlike growth factor-binding protein, during the menstrual cycle. *J Clin Endocrinol Metab* 1988;67:1100–1104.
147. Rutanen E-M, Koistinen R, Wahlstrom T, Bohn H, Ranta T, Seppälä M. Synthesis of placental protein 12 by human decidua. *Endocrinology* 1985;116:1304–1309.
148. Rutanen E-M, Koistinen R, Sjöberg J, et al. Synthesis of placental protein 12 by human endometrium. *Endocrinology* 1986;118: 1067–1071.
149. Fazleabas AT, Verhage HG, Waites G, Bell SC. Characterization of an insulinlike growth factor binding protein, analogous to human pregnancy-associated secreted endometrial α_1-globulin, in decidua of the baboon (*Papio anubis*) placenta. *Biol Reprod* 1989;40:873–885.
150. Fazleabas AT, Jaffe RC, Verhage HG, Waites G, Bell SC. An insulinlike growth factor-binding protein in the baboon (*Papio anubis*) endometrium: synthesis, immunocytochemical localization, and hormonal regulation. *Endocrinology* 1989;124: 2321–2329.
151. Lamson G, Pham H, Oh Y, Ocrant I, Schwander J, Rosenfeld RG. Expression of the BRL-3A insulinlike growth factor binding protein (rBP-30) in the rat central nervous system. *Endocrinology* 1989;123:1100–1102.
152. Rosenfeld RG, Pham H, Conover CA, Hintz RL, Baxter RC. Structural and immunological comparison of insulinlike growth factor binding proteins of cerebrospinal and amniotic fluids. *J Clin Endocrinol Metab* 1989;68:638–646.
153. Hintz RL, Liu F. Demonstration of specific plasma protein binding sites for somatomedin. *J Clin Endocrinol Metab* 1977;45:988–995.
154. Baxter RC, Martin JL, Tyler MI, Howden MEH. Growth hormone-dependent insulinlike growth factor (IGF) binding protein from human plasma differs from other human IGF binding proteins. *Biochem Biophys Res Commun* 1986;139:1256–1261.
155. DiAugustine RP, Petrusz P, Bell GI, et al. Influence of estrogens on mouse uterine epidermal growth factor precursor protein and messenger ribonucleic acid. *Endocrinology* 1988;122:2355–2363.
156. Nelson KG, Takahashi T, Bossert NL, Walmer DK, McLachlan JA. Epidermal growth factor replaces estrogen in the stimulation of female genital-tract growth and differentiation. *Proc Natl Acad Sci USA* 1991;88:21–25.
157. Haining REB, Schofield JP, Jones DSC, Rajput-Williams J, Smith SK. Identification of mRNA for epidermal growth factor and transforming growth factor-α present in low copy number in human endometrium and decidua using reverse transcriptase-polymerase chain reaction. *J Mol Endocrinol* 1991;6:207–214.
158. Haining REB, Cameron IT, van Papendorp C, et al. Epidermal growth factor in human endometrium: proliferative effects in culture and immunocytochemical localization in normal and endometriotic tissues. *Hum Reprod* 1991;6:1200–1205.
159. Chegini N, Rossi MJ, Masterson BJ. Platelet-derived growth factor (PDGF), epidermal growth factor (EGF), and EGF and PDGF β-receptors in human endometrial tissue: localization and *in vitro* action. *Endocrinology* 1992;130:2373–2385.
160. Hofmann GE, Scott RT Jr, Bergh PA, Deligdisch L. Immunohistochemical localization of epidermal growth factor in human endometrium, decidua, and placenta. *J Clin Endocrinol Metab* 1991;73:882–887.
161. Smith K, LeJeune S, Harris AH, Rees MCP. Epidermal growth factor receptor in human uterine tissues. *Hum Reprod* 1991;6:619–622.
162. Troche V, O'Connor DM, Schaudies RP. Measurement of human epidermal growth factor receptor in the endometrium during the menstrual cycle. *Am J Obstet Gynecol* 1991;165: 1499–1503.
163. Berchuck A, Soisson AP, Olt GJ, et al. Epidermal growth factor receptor expression in normal and malignant endometrium. *Am J Obstet Gynecol* 1989;161:1247–1252.

The Physiology of Reproduction, Second Edition,
edited by E. Knobil and J.D. Neill,
Raven Press, Ltd., New York © 1994.

CHAPTER 11

Follicular Steroidogenesis and Its Control[1]

Robert E. Gore-Langton and David T. Armstrong

The follicles are the principal functional units of the mammalian ovary. The function of each follicle is to provide the support system necessary for the female germ cell (oocyte) to attain its maximum potential—that of uniting with a male germ cell (spermatozoan) to produce an embryo capable of development leading to the birth of a normal viable offspring.

The somatic cells of the follicle contribute in several ways to accomplish this function, essential for the reproduction and survival of the species. First, they provide the nutritive requirements of the growing oocyte and, perhaps, the stimulus that initiates its growth. Later they control both the nuclear and cytoplasmic maturation of the oocyte contained in those follicles that are selected for ovulation and contribute to the atresia and oocyte destruction in those that are not. These direct effects of the follicle cells on the development and fate of the enclosed oocyte are mediated via changes they bring about in the microenvironment within the follicle, wrought in large part by products they secrete into the follicular fluid bathing the oocyte. In addition, specialized granulosa cells (cumulus cells) in the innermost layer surrounding the oocyte are coupled, metabolically, to the oocyte by gap junctions through which nutrient substances and regulatory molecules are delivered directly to the ooplasm.

The best-known and best-characterized secretory products of the follicle are the steroid hormones. The follicular steroids fulfill a number of important functions related to reproduction. They function as hormones, in the classical sense, being transported via the circulation to act on a wide variety of "target" tissues and organs comprising not only the reproductive system, but also several other organs and systems, including the central nervous system, musculoskeletal system, cardiovascular system, immune system, liver, and adipose and cutaneous tissues. Steroid actions at many levels contribute to the success of the reproductive process. For example, by action on brain centers that control sexual behavior, they ensure that females are willing and able to mate at the time that mature oocytes are released from the follicle. Actions on the musculature and cilia of the oviduct per-

Department of Physiology and Obstetrics and Gynecology, The University of Western Ontario, London, Ontario N6A 5A5, Canada

[1] Reprinted from *The Physiology of Reproduction,* edited by Ernst Knobil and Jimmy D. Neill, et al. Raven Press, Ltd., New York © 1988, pp. 331–385.

mit the cumulus–oocyte complex to be picked up by the oviductal fimbria and retained at the site of fertilization, while at the same time assisting with the transport of spermatozoa to that site. Oviductal and uterine smooth muscles, under the influence of steroid hormones, determine the time of entry of the fertilized egg into the uterus, and steroids bring about endometrial changes required for implantation of the developing embryo to occur, for maintenance of pregnancy once it is established, and for delivery of the full-term fetus.

In addition to acting as hormones on structures remote from the ovary, the steroids produced by follicle cells also act locally within the follicles in which they are produced, both as "paracrine" agents, acting on adjacent cells, and as "autocrine" agents, acting on or within the cells in which they are produced. As will be discussed later in this chapter, as well as elsewhere in this volume, steroids produced by the granulosa cells can influence the secretory pattern of the theca cells and the meiotic maturation of the oocyte. They also act on the granulosa cells themselves, influencing both their mitotic rate and their differentiation.

CLASSES OF FOLLICULAR STEROIDS

Chemical Classification

The steroid hormones may be classified on the basis either of their chemical structure or of their principal physiological actions. The hormones of main concern in this chapter are the sex steroids belonging to three major classes: progestins (gestagens, progestagens), androgens, and estrogens. Steroids belonging to all three classes are produced by the ovarian follicles at one or more stage(s) of development.

The chemical classification system relates all steroids to one of several parent, or stem, compounds, all of which comprise a ring complex, made up of three cyclohexane rings (A,B,C) and a cyclopentane ring (D), as illustrated in Fig. 1. To this fully saturated ring complex, referred to as the perhydrocyclopentanophenanthrene nucleus (or, more simply, the steroid nucleus), are attached additional components that vary according to steroid class. The ovarian steroids are all related to, and can be considered as chemical derivatives of, one of the four parent compounds illustrated in Fig. 1.

Cholestane, which comprises the steroid nucleus with methyl groups at the junctions between the A and B rings (at C-10) and the C and D rings (at C-13), and an eight-membered side chain attached to C-17, is the parent compound of cholesterol and other sterols, the biosynthetic precursors of all the steroids to be considered in this chapter. Fission of the side chain between C-20 and C-22 leads to the formation of the C_{21}-steroids (pregnane series), the chemical class to which the progestins belong. Further cleavage of the side chain between C-17 and C-20 produces the C_{19}-steroids (androstane series) to which the androgens belong. Finally, removal of the angular methyl group at C-10 leads to the formation of C_{18}-steroids (estrane series), the class to which the estrogens and related C_{18}-compounds belong.

A systematic method of nomenclature is used to identify each steroid according to which of the above series it belongs, as well as the nature and location of various modifications and chemical substitutions on the parent structure. Modifications of the parent structure include (a) introduction of double bonds between adjacent car-

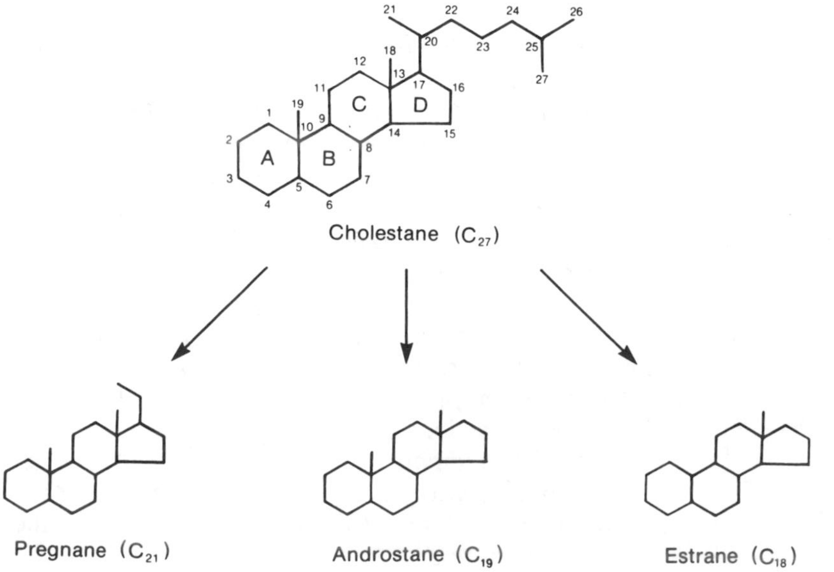

FIG. 1. Chemical classification for the parent structures from which the three main categories of ovarian steroids are derived. All steroid structures are derivatives of cholestane, the parent compound of cholesterol. Decreasing numbers of carbons occur as cholesterol is metabolized to progestins (pregnane series), androgens (androstane series), and estrogens (estrane series).

bon atoms, either in the ring structure or the side chain; (b) hydroxyl (OH) substituents; and (c) carbonyl groups resulting from oxidation of the hydroxyl substituents. Since the steroid nucleus has a well-defined structure with three-dimensional conformation, the stereochemistry of substitutions must be considered, in order to distinguish between the stereoisomers resulting from substitutions at asymmetric carbons.

Stereoisomers resulting from substituents on the steroid nucleus are distinguished from each other by nomenclature that signifies the side of the plane of the molecule on which the substituent is located. By convention, substituents on the same side of the plane as the angular methyl group at C-10 are considered as having the β-configuration and are signified by a solid valency line (–); those with substituents on the opposite side of the plane have the α-configuration, signified by a broken line (- - -). For the steroids dealt with here, isomerization at C-3 and C-17 is of particular importance.

The other position of asymmetry of special interest in this chapter is that which occurs at C-5 as a result of orientation of the hydrogen atom there, which can occur on either the α- or β-side of the molecule. This results in *cis–trans* isomerism about the A-B ring junction, the *trans*-isomer resulting when the C-5-hydrogen atom is on the α-side of the molecule, i.e., *trans* to the orientation of the angular methyl group at C-10, and the *cis*-isomer resulting when this hydrogen is in the 5β-configuration. The conformation of the steroid nucleus differs markedly, depending on the orientation of the hydrogen at C-5, the A and B rings of 5α-reduced steroids lying in essentially the same plane, whereas those of 5β-reduced steroids are approximately at right angles to each other.

For a more detailed description of steroid structure, including stereochemistry and nomenclature, the reader is referred to the recent concise review by Kellie (1).

Biological Classification

Ovarian steroids are also classified on the basis of their principal biological function into one of the three major classes: progestins, androgens, and estrogens, which for the most part are represented by compounds belonging to the C_{21} (pregnane), C_{19} (androstane), and C_{18} (estrane) series, respectively.

Estrogens

Physiologically, the estrogens, estrone and estradiol-17β, are the most important of the follicular steroids. Their trivial names are reflections of their roles in induction of sexual receptivity (estrus) in female mammals, but they play key roles in many other aspects of female reproductive physiology, as will be considered later. Estrone (3-hydroxy-estra-1,3,5[10]-trien-17-one) was the first sex steroid to be isolated and identified. Doisy et al. (2) crystallized this steroid from human pregnancy urine in 1929, and later from follicular fluid of sows (3). Estradiol-17β (estra-1,3,5[10]-triene-3,17β-diol) is approximately 10 times as potent as estrone in most biological assays and, on a molar basis, is the most active of all steroids produced by the ovary. Several hydroxylated derivatives of these C_{18}-steroids, all of which possess an aromatic A-ring, have been identified recently in follicular fluids and tissues and are therefore assumed to be of follicular origin. These include 2-hydroxyestrone (2,3-dihydroxy-estra-1,3,5[10]-trien-17-one), 2-hydroxy-estradiol, and their 2-methylated derivatives, as well as 4-OH-, 6-OH-, and 16-OH-derivatives of estrone and estradiol-17β (4–6).

In addition to the aromatic C_{18}-steroids, other compounds of the estrane series, 19-norandrostenedione (estra-4-ene-3,17-dione) and 19-nortestosterone (17β-hydroxy-estra-4-en-3-one) have been identified in the follicular fluid of the mare (4,7) and sow (8). The physiological function of these nonaromatic C_{18}-steroids remains to be determined.

Androgens

Biological evidence that the ovary produces androgens dates back to observations that ovaries grafted to the ears of male mice were able to reverse castration-induced atrophy of their seminal vesicles and prostate glands (9). The identification of androstenedione and testosterone in follicular fluid (10) followed by the demonstration of formation of these compounds from radiolabeled precursors by follicle cells (11) established the follicle as a significant source of ovarian androgens. As will be considered below, androstenedione and testosterone are the immediate biosynthetic precursors of the estrogenic steroids, estrone and estradiol-17β, respectively, because they are amenable to aromatization.

A number of nonaromatizable C_{19}-steroids, produced by saturation of the A-ring of the steroid nucleus, have also been identified as ovarian androgens of considerable importance (12–14). Ovarian 5α-reduced androgens that have been identified in several species include 5α-dihydrotestosterone (17β-hydroxy-5α-androstan-3-one) (DHT), 5α-androstane-3,17-dione, androsterone and epiandrosterone, and 5α-androstane-3α,17β-diol and its 3β-epimer. There is also recent evidence for ovarian production of 5β-reduced androgens in at least one species, the hamster (15).

Several 16-unsaturated steroids (androsta-4,16-dien-3-one, 5α-androst-16-en-3-one, and 3α-OH-5α-androst-16-ene) have been identified in ovarian tissue following incubation with radiolabeled precursors (16).

Progestins

Pregnenolone (3β-OH-pregn-5-en-20-one) is the most important progestin produced by the follicle because of its key position as the precursor of all the steroid hormones. Its most abundant C_{21} product in the follicle is progesterone (pregn-4-ene-3,20-dione), produced as a biosynthetic intermediate by follicles at all growing stages of development and as a secretory end product in the peri- and postovulatory periods. Other C_{21}-steroids of follicular origin include 17α-OH-progesterone (the immediate precursor of the aromatizable androgens), 20α-dihydroprogesterone (20α-hydroxy-pregn-4-en-3-one) and its 20β-epimer, and 17α,20α- and 17α,20β-pregnenediols. In addition, ring-A-reduced metabolites of each of these pregn-4-ene compounds have been shown to be produced by ovarian tissues of several species (particularly rodents) under certain physiological conditions (13,14,17).

PATHWAYS OF BIOSYNTHESIS AND KEY ENZYMES

Much of our knowledge of steroid biosynthetic processes has been gleaned from investigations on tissues other than the ovary. In particular, studies with adrenal cortex, testis, and human placenta have contributed to most of our current understanding of the steroidogenic enzymes, including their subcellular organization and control mechanisms. The available evidence indicates a high degree of similarity between the processes that are common to the different steroidogenic tissues, including the follicle. We have not attempted to present an exhaustive review of the extensive literature that has led to the present state of knowledge of the subject. The reader is referred to a number of excellent textbooks and reviews (18–20). Our aim in this section, rather, is to provide a summary of the biosynthetic pathways, identifying those individual enzymatic steps and processes that have been shown to be subject to physiological regulation. This brief review will provide a background for the remainder of the chapter, which deals with the control mechanisms as they apply specifically to the steroids of follicular origin. Other chapters will deal with aspects of steroidogenesis that pertain to the corpus luteum and the testis.

Steroid Precursors

The follicular steroids are produced from cholesterol derived from one of three possible sources: (a) preformed cholesterol taken up from the blood, primarily in the form of circulating lipoproteins; (b) preformed cholesterol stored within the ovarian cell, either as free cholesterol, a constituent of cell membranes, or liberated from cholesterol esters stored within cytoplasmic lipid droplets; and (c) cholesterol synthesized *de novo* in the ovarian cell from 2-carbon components derived from metabolism of carbohydrate, fat, or protein within the cell. The extent to which one or another of these sources of cholesterol is utilized for ovarian steroidogenesis varies with animal species and with cell type involved. Utilization of each may be subject to regulation with the quantitative importance of one source or another varying with the physiological state (21).

Most studies of the role of cholesterol from different sources as ovarian steroidogenic precursors have utilized extrafollicular tissues, e.g., corpus luteum (21), interstitial tissue (22), or luteinized granulosa cells in culture (23–25). In these tissues, cholesterol in circulating lipoproteins appears to be the most important source of steroidogenic cholesterol. Considerable evidence has been accumulated supporting a mechanism of uptake that involves binding of extracellular lipoproteins via their apoprotein component to specific receptors located on the cell membrane, followed by internalization of the lipoprotein-receptor complex, uptake of the complexes by lysosomes, degradation of lipoproteins by lysosomal esterases, and release of free cholesterol, which is then able to gain access to the steroidogenic enzymes. Cholesterol from both low-density lipoproteins (LDL) and high-density lipoproteins (HDL) has been implicated as steroidogenic precursor in these tissues (23). Species differences occur in the relative importance of the two classes of lipoproteins; HDL appears to be of greater quantitative importance in rodents, whereas cholesterol associated with LDL is the major circulating form of steroidogenic cholesterol in other species, including humans.

Differences in the vascular anatomy of the various cellular components of the ovary influence the degree to which circulating lipoproteins may serve as steroidogenic precursors. Thus, the corpus luteum, like the adrenal cortex, has an abundant blood supply and a highly permeable capillary endothelium, enabling the large lipoprotein molecules to gain access to lipoprotein receptors on luteal cells *in vivo.* The theca interna of the follicle receives blood from a similarly rich vascular supply and may therefore also be in a position to utilize lipoprotein cholesterol. On the other hand, the granulosa layers of the follicle are isolated from direct contact with the blood supply by a relatively impermeable basement membrane that provides a barrier to large molecules such as LDL (26–28). Only after luteinization has been initiated by the preovulatory luteinizing hormone (LH) surge *in vivo* does penetration of the capillary network occur through the basement membrane, allowing more ready access of lipoproteins to the granulosa cell component of the follicles. Predictions based on these anatomical considerations have been supported by recent experiments with cultured follicles (29) in which steroidogenesis in theca cells was influenced considerably more by the presence or absence of lipoprotein in the culture media than was that in granulosa cells.

Ovarian cells, particularly those in a position to take up extracellular cholesterol from circulating lipoproteins, store substantial amounts of cholesterol in intracellular lipid droplets, primarily as esters of long-chain fatty acids. An equilibrium between the cholesterol–fatty acyl esters in these intracellular depots and free cholesterol is maintained by a balance between two enzymes, acyl coenzyme A:cholesterolacyl transferase (ACAT) (commonly called cholesterol ester synthetase) and sterol ester hydrolase (cholesterol esterase), the former favoring storage of excess cholesterol in esterified form and the latter catalyzing release of the stored cholesterol. The activities of both these enzymes, as well as of 3-hydroxy-3-methylglutaryl coenzyme A-reductase (HMG CoA reductase), the rate-limiting enzyme in cholesterol biosynthesis (Fig. 2), are under hormonal control, in addition to being regulated by intracellular levels of cholesterol (21). The state of equilibrium between cholesterol esters and free cholesterol and the relative contributions to steroidogenesis of extracellular cholesterol, intracellularly stored cholesterol, and cholesterol synthesized *de novo* from smaller molecular precursors may differ considerably under different prevailing physiological conditions.

Cholesterol (C_{27}-Sterol) Side-Chain Cleavage

The first step in the conversion of cholesterol to steroids, and the step generally believed to be rate limiting in steroidogenesis under most conditions, is the cleavage of the C-20,22 bond resulting in the C_{21} compound, pregnenolone, and a 6-carbon fragment, isocaproic aldehyde. The enzyme system that catalyzes this reaction is located on the matrix side of the inner mitochondrial membranes (30). It is a multienzyme complex comprising three components: cytochrome P-450 side-chain cleavage (SCC), which is the terminal (electron-acceptor) oxygenase, a flavin adenine dinucleotide (FAD)-containing flavoprotein, and the sulfur-containing heme protein luteodoxin or adrenodoxin (in luteal and adrenal cells, respectively), which serves to shuttle an electron between the other two components (21). The reaction utilizes nicotinamide adenine dinucleotide phosphate (NADPH) generated within the mitochondria by oxidation of Krebs cycle intermediates or fatty acids. Three moles each of NADPH and of oxygen are utilized per mole of cholesterol undergoing side-chain cleavage.

The generally accepted pathway for biosynthesis of pregnenolone from cholesterol is illustrated in Fig. 2. Evidence summarized by Lieberman et al. (31) suggests that the overall reaction *in vivo* probably does not involve stable, free hydroxylated intermediates as shown here. Instead, it has been proposed that the substrate cholesterol and subsequent transient hydroxylated intermediates remain bound to the $P\text{-}450_{SCC}$ until the ultimate product, pregnenolone, is formed and released. The free hydroxylated intermediates that have been isolated from disrupted cell preparations may merely be "inadvertent by-products of the processes which are formed when the cytochrome $P\text{-}450_{SCC}$-substrate complex is denatured" (31).

Metabolism of Pregnenolone

Pregnenolone is the key steroidogenic intermediate common to all classes of steroid hormones produced by the follicles, as well as by other steroidogenic tissues. It is converted to progesterone by a microsomal enzyme, or enzyme complex, Δ^5-3β-hydroxysteroid dehydrogenase:$\Delta^{5\text{-}4}$-isomerase. Although separation of the dehydrogenase from the isomerase activities has been achieved for a bacterial enzyme system, the two enzyme activities in mammalian steroidogenic tissues, including the ovary, have not been separated and appear to function physiologically as a single entity (32). The enzyme utilizes NAD+ as an electron acceptor, and the reaction is essentially irreversible under physiological conditions. Similar, but perhaps not identical enzymes, bring about the conversion of 17α-OH-pregnenolone and dehydroepiandrosterone (DHEA) to 17α-OH-progesterone and androstenedione, respectively (Fig. 2).

C_{21}-Steroid Side-Chain Cleavage

The rate-limiting step in the biosynthesis of androgens in the follicle, as in other androgen-secreting organs, is the 17α-hydroxylase:C-17,20-lyase enzyme complex. A component of the membranes of the agranular endoplasmic reticulum (microsomes), this enzyme system is a cytochrome P-450-containing mixed-function oxidase, requiring NADPH and molecular oxygen. As with the cholesterol side-chain cleavage system, the two reactions (17α-hydroxylation and cleavage of the C-17,20 bond) occur in a concerted fashion in which the 17α-hydroxy intermediate probably remains bound to the enzyme complex without appearing in free form. The reaction can utilize either pregnenolone or progesterone as substrate, resulting in formation of the respective products, DHEA or androstenedione. These two alternative pathways are referred to as the 5-ene-3β-hydroxy (or Δ^5) pathway and the 4-en-3-oxo (or Δ^4) pathway, respectively, although it is uncertain whether the same or separate enzymes are involved (Fig. 2) (33).

This enzymic step is subject to hormonal and feedback regulation, and is one of the key points at which

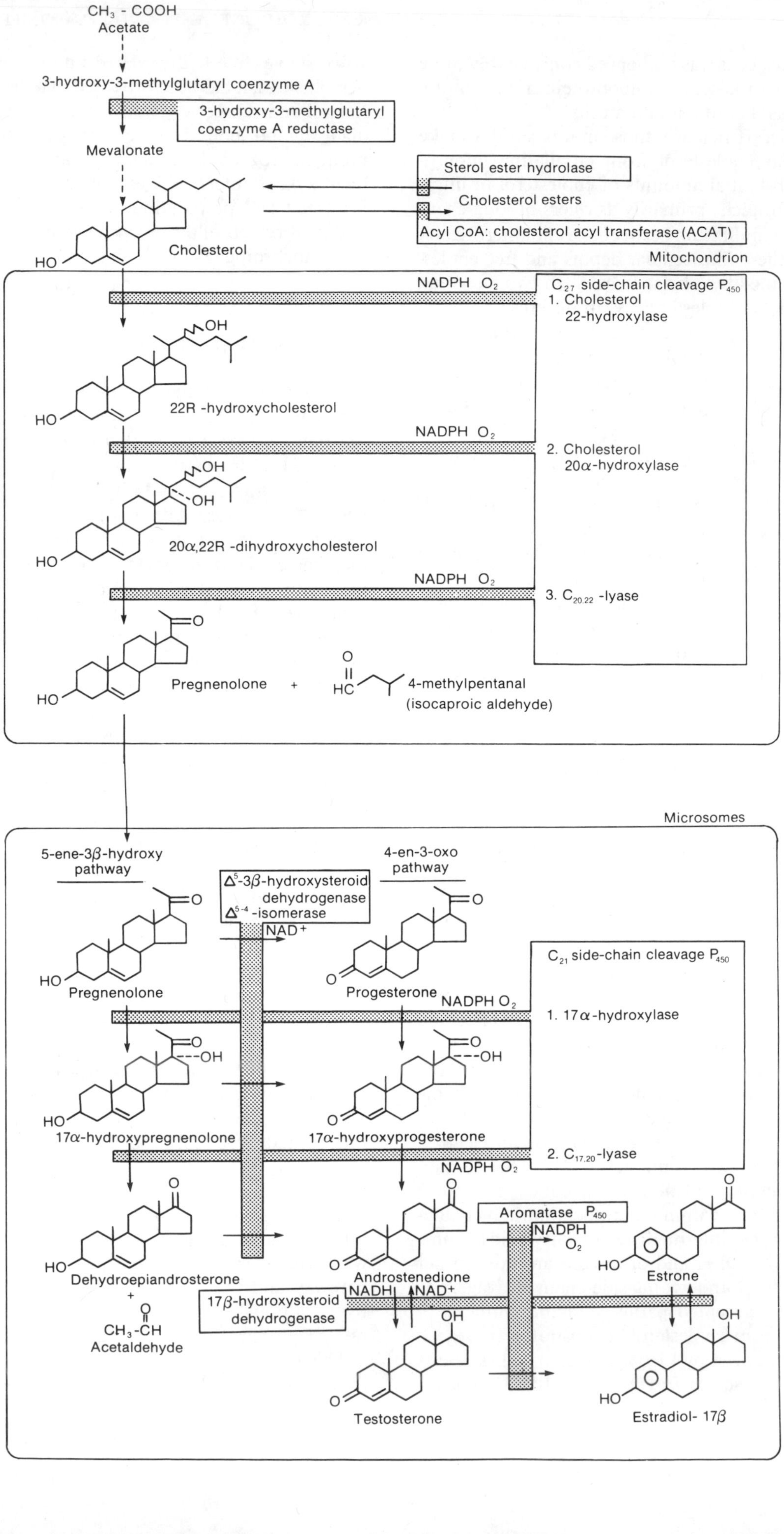

CH3 - COOH
Acetate
3-hydroxy-3-methylglutaryl coenzyme A
3-hydroxy-3-methylglutaryl coenzyme A reductase
Mevalonate
Sterol ester hydrolase
Cholesterol esters
Acyl CoA: cholesterol acyl transferase (ACAT)
HO
Cholesterol
Mitochondrion
NADPH O2
C27 side-chain cleavage P450
1. Cholesterol 22-hydroxylase
OH
22R -hydroxycholesterol
2. Cholesterol 20α-hydroxylase
20α,22R -dihydroxycholesterol
3. C20,22 -lyase
O
Pregnenolone
+
HC
4-methylpentanal
(isocaproic aldehyde)
Microsomes
5-ene-3β-hydroxy pathway
4-en-3-oxo pathway
Δ5-3β-hydroxysteroid dehydrogenase
Δ5-4 -isomerase
NAD+
C21 side-chain cleavage P450
Pregnenolone
Progesterone
1. 17α-hydroxylase
17α-hydroxypregnenolone
17α-hydroxyprogesterone
2. C17,20-lyase
Aromatase P450
NADPH
O2
Dehydroepiandrosterone
+
CH3-CH
Acetaldehyde
Androstenedione
Estrone
17β-hydroxysteroid dehydrogenase
NADH
NAD+
Testosterone
Estradiol- 17β

physiological control of follicular steroid secretion occurs.

An alternative mechanism for formation of C_{19}-steroids, involving side-chain cleavage of pregnenolone and progesterone without prior 17-hydroxylation, has been demonstrated in boar testis. The products of the reaction, androst-5,16-dien-3β-ol and androst-4,16-dien-3-one, respectively, have also been identified in porcine and human follicular fluid, suggesting that this minor pathway may function in follicular steroidogenesis under certain conditions (33).

Aromatization of C_{19}-Steroids

The 4-ene-C_{19}-steroids, androstenedione and testosterone, are converted to the estrogens, estrone and estradiol-17β, respectively, by an enzyme complex located in the membranes of the agranular endoplasmic reticulum of several ovarian cell types (to be considered in detail below). This enzyme complex, referred to as "aromatase" because of the aromatic structure of the products, is a cytochrome P-450-containing mixed-function oxidase that catalyzes a multiple-step reaction leading to removal of the methyl group at C-10 as formic acid, followed by rearrangement of ring A to the aromatic structure.

The reaction requires NADPH, and 3 moles of O_2 are consumed. Two of these are involved in two consecutive hydroxylations at C-19, and the overall reaction involves a third hydroxylation, but the exact site of this has not been established with certainty. The overall reaction, illustrating three proposed alternative mechanisms to account for the third mole of oxygen consumed, is depicted as a sequence of steps (Fig. 3). Most evidence supports a concept of enzyme-bound intermediates that do not exist as free compounds, but rather as transition states in which the substrate remains bound to the enzyme complex and undergoes the entire series of reactions before release of the product from the enzyme (31). The final step resulting in the formation of the aromatic A-ring with the loss of the angular methyl group as formic acid may be nonenzymatic and could occur after release from the enzyme complex. Although the mechanisms of the various steps in the overall reaction have been determined largely from studies of human placental microsome preparations, the available evidence suggests that the reaction in follicle cells proceeds along similar lines (34,35).

Reductive Metabolism of Ovarian Steroids

5α-Reduced Pathways of Progestin and Androgen Metabolism

Enzymatic reduction of 4-en-3-oxo-steroids of both C_{21} and C_{19} classes occurs in ovarian tissues of a variety of species. The enzyme(s) that catalyze this reduction are stereospecific 5α- or 5β-reductase(s) located in the agranular endoplasmic reticulum and utilize(s) NADPH as the source of the reducing protons. In most ovarian systems studied, the reductase is specific for the 5α-configuration (36–38), although 5β-reduced products have been identified from preparations of hamster ovaries (15,39).

In many of the systems studied, 5α-reduction is followed directly by stereospecific reduction of the 3-oxo-group by 3α-hydroxysteroid dehydrogenase leading to formation of 3α-OH-derivatives of the 5α-reduced metabolites. Both the 5α- and 3α-reductions can occur either before or after cleavage of the C-17,20 bond (40), with the result that ring A reduction products of both progestins and androgens are formed by ovarian preparations. Whether these are products of separate enzymes specific for the two classes of steroids or of the same enzymes that do not discriminate between C_{19} and C_{21} steroid substrates has not been established with certainty (see Fig. 4).

3β-Hydroxy derivatives of 5α-reduced progestins and androgens have also been reported following incubation of ovarian homogenates (41,42), suggesting the presence of a 3β-hydroxysteroid dehydrogenase capable of using 5α-reduced steroids as substrates. Because 3β-hydroxy metabolites could not be identified in ovarian vein blood (43) or following incubation of intact ovarian preparations with radiolabeled progesterone (17), the possibility has been raised that 3β-hydroxy products represent artifacts when cell disruption enables the 5α-reduced compounds to gain access to the membrane-bound Δ^5-3β-hydroxysteroid dehydrogenase whose function in conjunction with the $\Delta^{5\text{-}4}$-isomerase in the intact cell is

FIG. 2. The principal biosynthetic pathways in the ovary for production of the progestins, androgens, and estrogens. Cholesterol may be synthesized *de novo* from acetate or derived from preformed sources. The metabolism of cholesterol to the sex steroids is carried out sequentially by several enzyme systems, each with several catalytic functions. Thus, the conversion of cholesterol to androgens involves three enzyme systems: cholesterol (C_{27}-sterol) side-chain cleavage P-450, C_{21}-steroid side-chain cleavage P-450, and Δ^5-3β-hydroxysteroid dehydrogenase: $\Delta^{5\text{-}4}$-isomerase. Subsequent conversion of C_{19}-steroids to estrogens is carried out by aromatase P-450 enzyme(s). The enzyme systems are distributed in different subcellular sites as indicated.

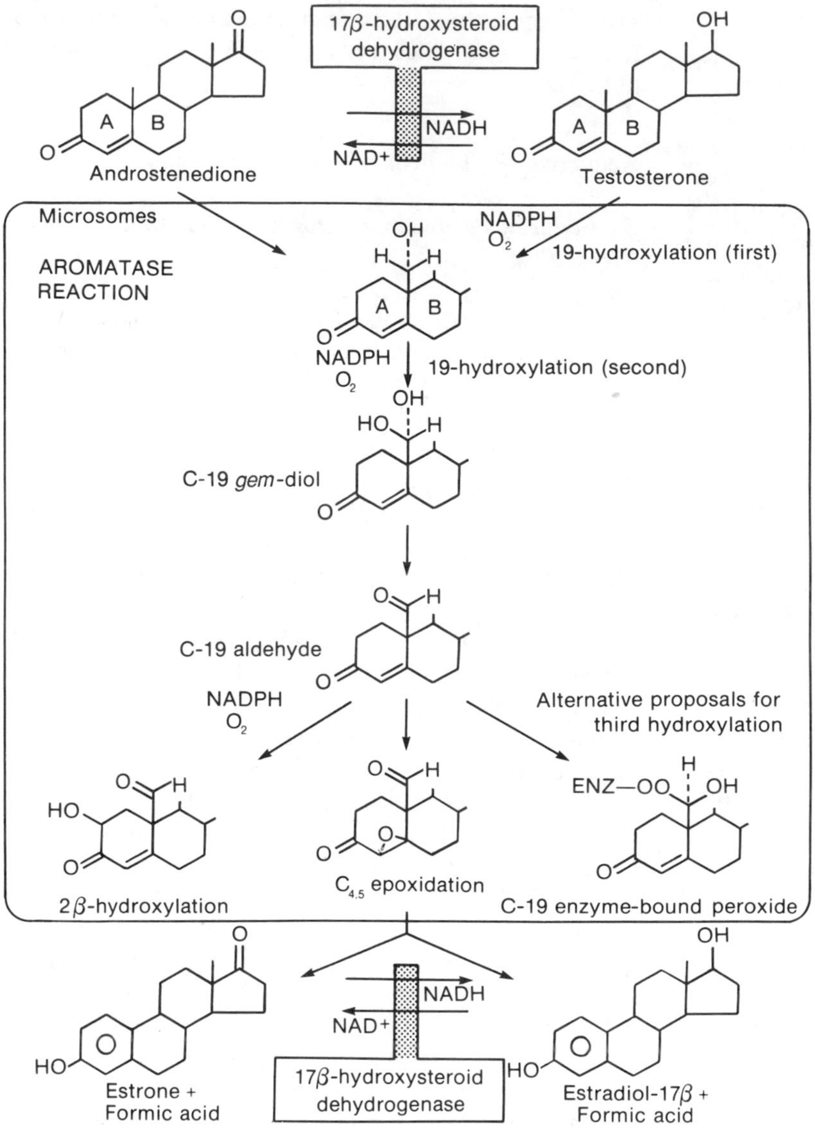

FIG. 3. Proposed sequence of reactions in the aromatization of androstenedione and testosterone. The aromatase enzyme system catalyzes a concerted reaction of enzyme-bound transition states involving three hydroxylations, the first two occurring at C-19, while the site of the third remains controversial: Hydroxylation at C-2β is considered most probable, but alternative mechanisms involving epoxidation or an enzyme-bound peroxide have also been proposed. Note that the C-19 aldehyde form of the enzyme-bound intermediate is more stable than the C-19 *gem* diol and forms spontaneously. Also, the final step resulting in C-10,19 cleavage and rearrangement to the aromatic ring-A may occur by a nonenzymatic mechanism.

conversion of pregnenolone to progesterone (17). On the other hand, high circulating levels of 5α-androstane-3β,17β-diol have been reported in prepubertal rats; these have been found to drop considerably following ovariectomy (44), suggesting that at least a portion of this 3β-reduced androstanediol is of ovarian origin and attesting to the possible physiological significance of the 3β-epimer (45).

20-Hydroxysteroid Dehydrogenases

The C-20-carbonyl group of C_{21} steroids, including progesterone, 17α-hydroxyprogesterone, and ring A-saturated progestins, can undergo enzymic reduction to the corresponding 20-hydroxy derivative(s). The stereospecificity of the 20-hydroxysteroid dehydrogenase enzyme in ovarian cells (corpus luteum, follicles, intersti-

FIG. 4. Reductive pathways of progestin and androgen metabolism in the ovary. *Notes:* 1. The 20α-hydroxysteroid dehydrogenase occurs in ovaries of most species (shown), while in bovines a different enzyme has 20β stereospecificity (not shown). 2. 5α-Reduction occurs similarly for C_{21}- and C_{19}-steroids, but it is not known whether it is the same 4-ene-5α-reductase enzyme acting in each instance. 5β-Reduction, an important reaction in the peripheral metabolism of C_{21}- and C_{19}-steroids, is an additional pathway present in the hamster ovary. 3. Conversion of 5α-reduced steroids via the 3α-hydroxysteroid dehydrogenase (shown) is well documented. An alternative pathway involving a 3β-hydroxysteroid dehydrogenase (not shown) has been demonstrated under limited conditions. The expected 3β-hydroxy products are similar to those shown. The 3β-epimer of androsterone is epiandrosterone.

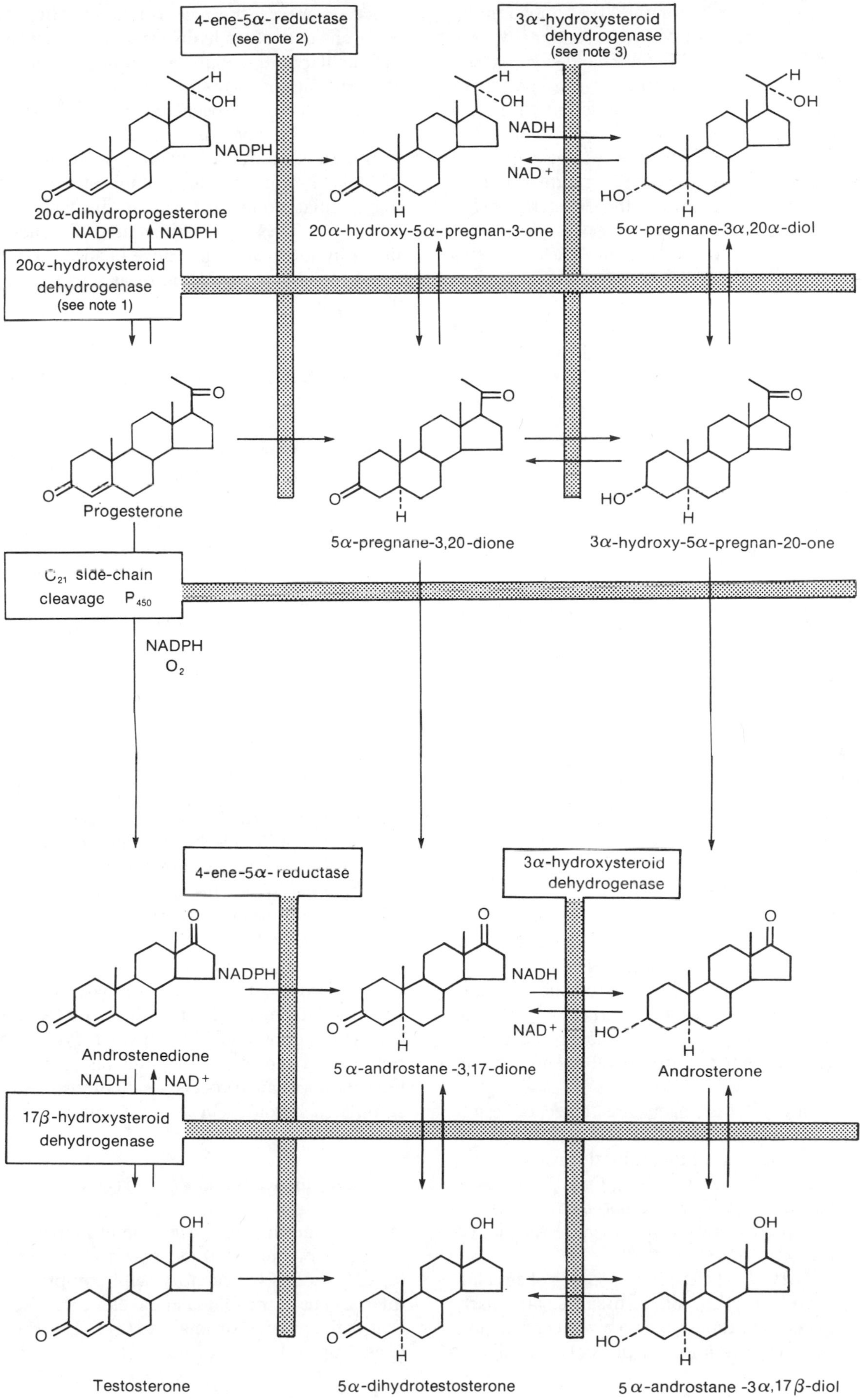
4-ene-5α-reductase (see note 2)
3α-hydroxysteroid dehydrogenase (see note 3)
NADPH
NADH
NAD+
20α-dihydroprogesterone
20α-hydroxy-5α-pregnan-3-one
5α-pregnane-3α,20α-diol
NADP
NADPH
20α-hydroxysteroid dehydrogenase (see note 1)
Progesterone
5α-pregnane-3,20-dione
3α-hydroxy-5α-pregnan-20-one
C21 side-chain cleavage P450
NADPH
O2
4-ene-5α-reductase
3α-hydroxysteroid dehydrogenase
NADPH
NADH
NAD+
Androstenedione
5 α-androstane -3,17-dione
Androsterone
NADH
NAD+
17β-hydroxysteroid dehydrogenase
Testosterone
5α-dihydrotestosterone
5 α-androstane -3α,17β-diol

tial cells) of most species is for the 20α configuration, although the bovine corpus luteum, exceptionally, produces the 20β-hydroxy metabolite. The 20-hydroxysteroid dehydrogenases are located in the cytosol portion of those ovarian cells studied, and they preferentially utilize NADPH as the hydrogen donor. The 20α-hydroxysteroid dehydrogenase of rodent corpora lutea undergoes hormonal regulation, thereby providing a means of influencing the biological potency of the C_{21}-steroid product secreted by this organ since the product 20α-hydroxy-pregn-4-en-3-one is considerably less active as a progestational agent than is its precursor, progesterone (46).

Since 20α-reduced steroids are poor substrates for C-17,20-lyase, the activity of the 20α-hydroxysteroid dehydrogenase may play a significant role in determining the amount of C_{21}-substrate available for conversion to androgens in follicular cells (47).

17β-Hydroxysteroid Dehydrogenase

17-Hydroxy- and 17-oxo-steroids are readily interconvertible by a reversible 17β-hydroxysteroid dehydrogenase present in microsomes of several steroidogenic tissues, including the follicle. Enzymes with cofactor requirements for both NAD+ and NADP+ have been described (33). Although both androgens and estrogens serve as substrates for this reaction (Figs. 2,3), it is uncertain whether this is because of a lack of rigorous substrate specificity of the ovarian 17β-hydroxysteroid dehydrogenase or because there are separate enzymes for the C_{18}-steroids and for the C_{19}-steroids, either of the 4-en-3-oxo-, 5-en-3β-hydroxy-, or ring-A-reduced variety.

Hydroxylation of Estrogens

Several hydroxylated estrogens have been reported in follicular fluid of a number of species and are therefore assumed to be of follicular cell origin. These include 2-OH-, 4-OH-, 6-OH-, and 16-OH-estrone and estradiol. Like all hydroxylase reactions, the ovarian enzymes that catalyze these hydroxylations are cytochrome P-450-containing enzymes that require NADPH and molecular oxygen.

The 2-OH- and 4-OH-estrogens are "catechol" estrogens, with 2-OH-estrone and 2-OH-estradiol being of particular interest because of their putative roles in regulation of gonadotropin secretion (48). Once formed, the catechol estrogens are rapidly metabolized to their O-methylated derivatives by the enzyme, catechol-*O*-methyl transferase.

The liver is believed to be the major source of circulating catechol estrogens, but other tissues, particularly various regions of the brain, have received considerable attention as sites of formation of physiological significance. However, the recent demonstration of catechol estrogens and other hydroxylated estrogen metabolites in follicular fluid and tissue (5,6) suggests the follicle may also be a site of formation of this class of compounds. The presence of estrogen-2- and 4-hydroxylase activity in porcine follicular tissues, particularly in membrana granulosa of preovulatory follicles, provides support for follicular production of catechol estrogens and further suggests that production increases during follicular maturation (49). These findings raise questions about the possible physiological significance of these compounds either in follicular regulation or as secretory products of the follicle (50).

STEROIDOGENESIS AND ITS CONTROL BY CELL TYPE

Our intention in this section is to review the individual contributions of the follicular and interstitial cell types to steroidogenesis, with particular regard to the cellular sites of the steroidogenic enzymes and their regulation by gonadotropins, intraovarian steroidal actions, and other known or putative regulatory factors, and to consider the importance of cooperation of the different cell types in the overall steroidogenic process in the follicle. We will not consider the molecular mechanisms of gonadotropin action, which are beyond the scope of this chapter, nor will we review the extensive literature that has developed to support the concept that gonadotropins —follicle-stimulating hormone (FSH) and luteinizing hormone (LH)—regulate steroidogenesis and other aspects of follicular maturation by stimulating the production of cyclic AMP (cAMP), the so-called second messenger. These topics have been previously reviewed (51,52). Suffice it to say, cAMP is now well established as the principal, if not the only intracellular mediator of FSH and LH/human chorionic gonadotropin (hCG) actions on the follicular cell types. FSH and LH satisfy virtually all of the criteria originally set out by Sutherland and colleagues (53) and subsequently extended by Kuo and Greengard (54) to indicate that a hormone mediates its actions via cAMP and cAMP-dependent phosphorylation of proteins. Calcium has a permissive role in the steroidogenic process, as demonstrated for FSH-stimulated steroidogenesis in rat granulosa cells (55).

Steroidogenic Cells and Their Origins

In all mammalian species the principal cell types involved in follicular steroidogenesis are of two basic types: (a) LH-responsive secretory cells, comprising the theca interna cells of the follicular envelope and the interstitial cells of the ovarian stroma, and (b) FSH-responsive cells, consisting exclusively of granulosa cells, which only later in follicular maturation also acquire the ability to respond to LH. These two basic cell types fulfill distinct roles in the steroidogenic process by virtue of their different regulatory hormones and their dissimilar expression of steroidogenic enzymes.

Granulosa and theca/interstitial cells have distinct embryological origins. Granulosa cells appear to be derived mainly, although perhaps not exclusively, from certain cells within the intraovarian rete ovarii which closely resemble granulosa cells in terms of their organelles (56) and microfilaments (57–60). The intraovarian rete ovarii in the prefollicular ovary consists of cell cords and tubules and of mesenchymal cells in the ovarian medulla. Early follicular development occurs centrally in the innermost part of the cortex within the rete cords as rete cells move between and attach to oocytes, differentiate into granulosa cells, and then organize follicles (56,61).

Once follicles form and the granulosa cells become fully enclosed by the follicular basement membrane, it is clear that these cells alone proliferate to produce the membrana granulosa layer. However, this population of granulosa cells does not remain uniform, but as the antral follicle develops, these cells become organized into morphologically distinguishable regions with specialized functions. The granulosa cells in the layer immediately adjacent to the oocyte (i.e., corona radiata cells) establish intimate contact with the oocyte up until the preovulatory stage by means of cellular processes traversing the zona pellucida and forming gap junctional complexes with the oolema. These cells serve as "nurse" cells, providing nutrients for oocyte growth and also presumably exchanging regulatory factors with the oocyte, thereby relaying signals required for the coordinated maturation of the follicle and the oocyte. The cumulus granulosa cells comprise the cellular mass that surrounds the oocyte (i.e., the cumulus oophorus) and attaches the oocyte to the follicle wall. The cumulus cells physically support the oocyte within the follicle and may contribute to its nutritional and regulatory needs. Following ovulation the oocyte–cumulus complex facilitates pick-up by the oviduct and may contribute to the final maturation of the oocyte, as well as the capacitation of spermatozoa that must penetrate through the extracellular material formed by the cumulus cells. The majority of granulosa cells form the so-called mural or parietal granulosa cells lining the follicular cavity. Those mural cells adjacent to the follicular basement membrane are the first to differentiate steroidogenic responsiveness to LH based on the acquisition of LH binding sites (62,63), the expression of Δ^5-3β-hydroxysteroid dehydrogenase activity (64), and the level of cytochrome P-450 (65). In addition, mural granulosa cells at this stage lose the differentiation antigen that is uniformly present on granulosa cells of earlier follicular stages (66). Other *in vitro* evidence suggests that subpopulations of granulosa cells may exist with respect to differential sensitivity to FSH and vasoactive intestinal peptide (VIP) (67).

The theca cells appear to differentiate from mesenchymal cells in the ovarian stroma (68,69). Since the theca layer is not present in primary follicles but differentiates as follicles grow and mature, it is evident that theca cells arise continually throughout reproductive life; the mesenchymal progenitor cells are perhaps pluripotent stem cells that also contribute to cells of loose connective tissue. It has been suggested that in the immature mouse the theca layer might also be formed from certain intraovarian rete cells that are initially contiguous with cells forming the follicular granulosa cells but become separated from association with the oocyte as the follicle is enclosed (70,71). There is similar evidence in the rabbit (72). However, these cells in the mouse appear to give rise principally to the primary interstitial cells (70). Primary interstitial cells in fetal ovaries of the human appear to have distinct steroidogenic activities (see section on the prefollicular ovary, below).

Secondary interstitial cells found in the adult ovary are derived from theca cells of atretic follicles (73–77). Whereas the oocyte and surrounding granulosa cells of an atretic follicle degenerate and are eliminated from the ovary, the theca cells in the follicular envelope survive as small islands of steroidogenic cells in the ovarian stroma. On this basis, certain similarities in function of theca and secondary interstitial cells of adult ovaries might reasonably be expected. However, theca and interstitial cells probably do not have identical biosynthetic properties since the interstitial cells, in contrast with the theca cells, are less likely to be influenced by paracrine regulatory substances secreted by the membrana granulosa; instead, they may receive direct sympathetic innervation. Secondary interstitial cells also differ from theca cells in that their androgen biosynthetic activity not only persists throughout reproductive life (78–80) but continues in aged ovaries (81,82).

In later sections of this chapter we consider the evidence for steroidogenic functions of interstitial cells, theca cells, and granulosa cells in the early stages of ovarian organogenesis and at various stages of follicular development in the adult ovary. However, the characteristic steroidogenic functions of theca and secondary interstitial and granulosa cells in adult ovaries and mature follicles, typical of the follicular phase, are now described.

Pathways and Their Control by Gonadotropins (FSH and LH)

Theca and Interstitial Cells

The most abundant steroid products of mature theca cells of all species are C_{19}-compounds, including the 4-ene-3β-hydroxysteroids and 5α-reduced androgens, which are produced from the catabolism of cholesterol by pathways previously described. As discussed earlier, since the theca interna becomes highly vascularized as the follicle matures, it is reasonable that the internalization of blood-borne lipoprotein provides the major source of cholesterol for steroidogenesis by theca cells *in vivo*. Steroidogenesis in the absence of lipoprotein cholesterol *in vitro* is limited (83).

The preferred enzymatic route for the conversion of cholesterol to androgens in the theca of human (84) and bovine (85) ovary is via the 5-ene-3β-hydroxysteroid pathway. DHEA produced via this pathway is then metabolized to androstenedione. It is apparent that rat ovarian interstitial cell cultures (i.e., consisting of interstitial cells and follicular cell types) produce both 5-ene-3β-hydroxy and 4-en-3-oxo intermediates (86).

LH action via specific receptors present on the theca cells at all follicular stages (87–93), and consequent production of cAMP (81,94–96), provides the principal stimulus for these steroidogenic activities. Studies with cultured ovarian interstitial cells isolated from hypophysectomized rats indicate that the cells constitutively express Δ^5-3β-hydroxysteroid dehydrogenase and have functional LH receptors but are not steroidogenically active unless induced to differentiate with either LH or prostaglandin E_2 (PGE_2) (97). These results with ovarian interstitial cell cultures might reflect similar control mechanisms occurring in thecal tissue, which also responds to LH or PGE_2 with increased androgen secretion (96,98,99).

The steroidogenic action of LH on theca cells apparently increases the activities of 17α-hydroxylase:C-17,20-lyase in ovaries or follicles of rat (100,101,102) and hamster (103). These enzyme activities are rate-limiting and appear to be the site at which LH stimulates C_{19}-steroid production by theca cells, as follicles progress from small antral stages to early preovulatory follicles in the rat (102), and where ovarian androgen production is substantially restricted in late preovulatory follicles (104) (also see the section on preovulatory follicles, below). Recent studies have employed immunoblot analysis to measure the specific contents (i.e., amount of enzyme protein per microgram of tissue protein) of this and other steroidogenic enzymes and their electron donors in follicles dissected from bovine ovaries of mature animals (105). These studies have demonstrated that 17α-hydroxylase P-450 in follicles increased fivefold between medium-sized (9–11 mm) and large (14–18 mm) follicles, indicating that an increase in enzyme protein occurs in the follicular cells (granulosa and theca) as follicles mature. Significantly, this enzyme protein was undetectable in bovine corpora lutea throughout the luteal phase, consistent with the loss of the enzyme activity as follicles luteinize in response to the LH surge. (This aspect is discussed later with respect to late preovulatory follicles after the LH surge.) These changes showed specificity for the 17α-hydroxylase P-450 since its electron donor, NADPH-cytochrome P-450 reductase, has a similar specific content during follicle development and in corpora lutea.

Although progesterone is apparently not limiting as an intermediate for thecal androgen production in small antral follicles, progesterone accumulation in isolated small antral and preovulatory rat follicles is stimulated *in vitro* by hCG, indicating that activation of the LH receptor also stimulates a step in the conversion of cholesterol to progesterone (102). Further studies tended to rule out the possibility that this action was due to decreased progesterone metabolism. Isolated theca cells from small antral and preovulatory rat follicles also produced increased progesterone when stimulated with cAMP, this stimulation being much greater with theca from preovulatory follicles (102). Therefore, it is evident from these studies that progesterone production by theca cells is also hormonally regulated and varies with the stage of follicular development. This effect of LH is probably the result of increased activity of C_{27} side-chain cleavage and is consistent with increased pregnenolone production in LH-stimulated rat ovarian interstitial cell cultures (86). Ultrastructural immunocytochemical visualization of P-450_{SCC} in ovaries of immature rats indicates that this mitochondrial enzyme is initially found in only a few theca cells, but the number of theca cells containing this enzyme increases after pregnant mare serum gonadotropin (PMSG) treatment (30). Significantly, these studies showed a strong reaction for P-450_{SCC} in interstitial cells even before PMSG treatment, with no apparent change as a result of hormonal stimulation.

Androstenedione is the principal aromatizable C_{19}-steroid produced by isolated theca interna tissue or cells, with lesser amounts of testosterone occurring, as described in the rat (94), hamster (103,106), pig (107), sheep (194), cow (85,108,109), and human (110,111). The greater abundance of androstenedione than testosterone is due to a deficiency in 17β-hydroxysteroid dehydrogenase, a fact that has significance in the steroidogenic cooperation of theca and granulosa cells, as discussed later. Rat ovarian interstitial preparations in culture are also active in 5α-reduction of C_{19}-steroids; the major LH-stimulated product is androsterone (86), which may be produced by sequential action of 5α-reductase and 3α-hydroxysteroid dehydrogenase (Fig. 4). The next most abundant 5α-reduced metabolite is 5α-androstane-3α,17β-diol, which can be derived from testosterone according to the same reactions described above for androstenedione or, alternatively, might result from conversion of androsterone to 5α-androstane-3α,17β-diol in a reversible reaction catalyzed by the apparently weak thecal activity of 17β-hydroxysteroid dehydrogenase. It has been demonstrated that 3α-hydroxy-5α-pregnan-20-one is converted to 5α-androstane-3α,17β-diol by supernatants of ovarian homogenates from immature rats, suggesting that this pregnane may be an earlier intermediate in a pathway to the androstanediol (112). Activity of 5α-reductase in thecal tissue from hamster preovulatory follicles may not be regulated by LH (103) but is subject to LH control in thecal/interstitial cells in prepubertal rat ovaries (100,101). There is no change in thecal 5α-reductase activity in the adult rat during pregnancy as follicles develop from small antral to preovulatory stages (113). Activity of ovarian 5α-reductase, which is greatest before the onset of puberty (14,40,45), is greatly decreased in ovaries of adult rats (114–116) and in immature rats in which puberty has been advanced with PMSG (42). The physiological significance of 5α-reduced androgens in the immature rat is indicated by the effect of exogenous 5α-androstane-3β,17β-diol, but not its 3α-epimer, to advance the onset of puberty (117) and by there being sufficient concentrations of the 3β-epimer in blood to account for these changes at puberty (37). FSH has also been shown to induce an epimerization reaction in the immature rat ovary that converts 5α-androstane-3α,17β-diol to the biologically active 3β-epimer (118).

Alternate routes of progesterone catabolism, in addition to those involved in the production of androgens, also occur in theca cells. Transiently increased production of 17α-hydroxyprogesterone in the human at midcycle (119,120) may primarily arise in the theca cells before similar pathways are fully active in the granulosa cells. The corpus luteum becomes the principal source of this steroid in the luteal phase of the human (121). In rat interstitial cells, the principal C_{21} metabolite is 20α-dihydroprogesterone (86). The production of this metabolite is increased by LH treatment, but the amount produced is still less than that of intermediates and products of the 4-en-3-oxosteroid pathway.

Theca cells may also aromatize androgens and contribute directly to ovarian estrogen secretion in varying degrees depending on species and follicular stage, e.g., in human (122–124), monkey (125), mare (126,127), cow (85), hamster (106), sheep (128), and pig (107). However, results of most studies indicate that aromatase activity (i.e., conversion of C_{19}-steroids to estrogens) in the theca cells either is not significantly greater than that in the granulosa cells (e.g., as in pig and sheep) or is considerably less than in the granulosa cells. In studies with cultures of follicular tissue from immature pigs, theca initially has considerably less aromatase activity than granulosa cells expressed on a per follicle basis, but when follicular growth and maturation was induced with PMSG treatment, aromatase activity in theca cells increased substantially while that in granulosa cells declined slightly (107). Studies with sheep follicle cell types also indicate substantially increased estrogen production by theca cells as follicles mature (128). Therefore, in mature follicles of pig and sheep, both theca and granulosa cells appear to have similar abilities *in vitro* to produce estrogens, either from endogenous androgen (theca cells) or supplied substrate (granulosa cells).

Most studies with human theca cells in culture agree that the quantity of estrogen secretion is significant but small (129), regardless of whether the theca is obtained from small or large follicles or at various stages of the menstrual cycle (110). For the preovulatory human follicle it was estimated that 99.9% of the aromatase activity resides in the membrana granulosa (130,131), and there is an excellent positive correlation between granulosa aromatase activity and the concentration of estradiol in follicular fluid (130). These results strongly indicate that thecal cell production of estrogen in the human is relatively minor in comparison to the aromatizing capabilities of granulosa cells from large antral follicles. Results of other studies with human follicle cells in culture (111,124) are difficult to interpret in terms of relative theca and granulosa cell aromatase activities since data are often expressed as estradiol production per culture without corrections for cell number.

There is little direct information to distinguish the steroidogenic functions of secondary interstitial cells from those of the theca interna cells, and the biosynthetic pathways are generally assumed to be similar. However, as already noted, the immunocytochemical staining for P-450$_{SCC}$ in interstitial cells of immature rat ovary is greater than in theca cells; also, it does not depend on exogenous gonadotropin treatment (30). Whether this difference reflects similar differences in enzymic activity is not known. *In vitro* studies using dispersed ovarian preparations from hypophysectomized rats (designated as ovarian interstitial cells but containing all ovarian cell types) have investigated the regulation of the LH-responsive cell types (86,97). The biosynthetic activities of these mixed cell cultures are similar to those already described for theca cells. Specific isolation of secondary interstitial cells from rat ovarian stroma has not been feasible without significant contamination by theca and follicle cell types but is more readily accomplished in humans and in larger animals. Nevertheless, true interstitial cells (i.e., glandular cells) in the ovarian stroma of the human constitute only about 1% of the ovarian volume during the menstrual cycle, with this value increasing to 4–6% in late pregnancy (132). Human stromal cells obtained on cycle day 18 were incubated with [^{3}H]pregnenolone and [^{14}C]progesterone and were shown to use both 4-en-3-oxo and 5-ene-3β-hydroxy pathways, with the products being androstenedione (the major product), testosterone, progesterone, 17α-hydroxyprogesterone (133), and, under some circumstances, estrone and estradiol (134). Production of these steroids was increased by treatment with hCG. In other studies, cultures of human stromal cells synthesized, androstenedione, 17α-hydroxyprogesterone, progesterone, and estradiol but in lesser amounts than by theca cells (123,135).

Granulosa Cells

Whereas the steroidogenic pathways in the theca and interstitial cells function primarily in the *de novo* production of androgens, the pathways in the granulosa cells are organized principally for the metabolism of C_{19}-steroids (i.e., androgens) to estrogens and for the *de novo* synthesis of progesterone and its C_{21} metabolites. As will be discussed in following sections, cooperation of the theca and granulosa cell compartments appears to be crucial to the control by gonadotropins of follicular steroid hormone secretion in all species studied. This cooperation takes the form of exchange of steroid pathway intermediates, direct steroidal effects on enzyme activities, and paracrine regulation.

Evidence from both *in vivo* and *in vitro* studies indicates that the granulosa cells of large antral and preovulatory follicles are the principal, although not exclusive, site in all species of ovarian aromatase activity and estrogen biosynthesis. Regulation of androgen aromatization in the granulosa cells of all species studied appears to be by the action of FSH (136), which in rat granulosa cell cultures stimulates aromatase enzyme activity as measured in a cell-free assay (137) and requires RNA and protein synthesis for expression of this action (138). Recent studies with rat granulosa cells suggest that aromatase cytochrome P-450, as detected in radiolabeled immunoisolates, is induced by FSH or dibutyryl cAMP (139). In addition, FSH or dibutyryl cAMP has been reported to stimulate two to three times the amount of the NADPH-cytochrome P-450 reductase detected in cultured rat granulosa cells (in immunoisolates and by immunoblot analysis), but this component is apparently in excess of the specific aromatase cytochrome P-450 (140). In addition to this action of FSH to induce aromatase enzyme in granulosa cells, estrogen biosynthesis requires the cooperation of the theca cells in supplying the androgen substrates for the aromatization reaction. This important aspect is discussed in detail in a following section.

The production of progesterone and its metabolites (i.e., progestins) is one of the major biosynthetic activities of granulosa cells in large antral and preovulatory follicles. Progesterone biosynthesis occurs in granulosa cells initially in response to FSH stimulation, but this action is later augmented by LH after its receptors have differentiated. In culture, FSH stimulates progesterone biosynthesis in undifferentiated granulosa cells from immature rats (141–145) and in granulosa cells from various other species, including human (124,129,146), simian (147), porcine (24), and avian (148). A similar effect of FSH on progesterone production has also been shown for cumulus granulosa cells of rat (149). In contrast, LH alone does not stimulate progesterone biosynthesis in cultured granulosa cells from hypophysectomized, estrogen-treated rats but is an effective stimulus *in vitro* following either a 24-hr *in vivo* treatment with FSH to induce LH receptors (142) or after 2 days of FSH priming *in vitro* (150). Many studies in various species substantiate the stimulation of progesterone production by LH in mature granulosa cells from antral follicles. In all species studied the greatest stimulation of progesterone biosynthesis *in vivo* follows the LH surge, often after a transient decrease in production, as granulosa cells undergo differentiation (i.e., luteinization) to form granulosa-lutein cells.

The progesterone biosynthetic pathway (see Fig. 2 and the first three sections on biosynthetic pathways, above) in granulosa cells is typical of all steroidogenic cells, involving conversion of cholesterol to pregnenolone and then to progesterone. In antral and preovulatory follicular stages, intracellular cholesterol is probably almost entirely derived from *de novo* synthesis and perhaps to a small extent from endogenous lipid stores, since cholesterol associated with lipoproteins in blood (28,151) cannot penetrate the avascular granulosa cell layer. Only after ovulation is extracellular lipoprotein likely to be a major source of cholesterol as a precursor for biosynthesis in granulosa-lutein cells (23,152).

The apparent rate-limiting reaction for progesterone biosynthesis, regulated by FSH action on granulosa cells, is cholesterol side-chain cleavage (144,153,154). The effects of hormonal stimulation on this enzyme activity have been suggested to involve an increase in the association of cholesterol with the P-450_{SCC} via a low-molecular-weight activator peptide and to increase the supply of intramitochondrial cholesterol by a cytoskeleton-mediated process, as appears to be the situation in the adrenal cortex (32). There is similar evidence in the ovary for stimulatory effects of LH/hCG on cholesterol transport and activation of the cholesterol side-chain cleavage enzyme (155–157). In rat granulosa cells, FSH stimulates pregnenolone production in the presence of cyanoketone, which inhibits metabolism to progesterone; 25-hydroxycholesterol, which readily enters the mitochondria, further enhances this effect of FSH, suggesting that FSH may also increase cholesterol side-chain cleavage activity in this cell type (153). Concomitant increases in mitochondrial activity of side-chain cleavage enzyme in ovaries of rat (158) and pig (154) further suggest that synthesis of this enzyme may be increased. However, immunoblot analysis of C_{27} side-chain cleavage cytochrome P-450 and its electron donor, adrenodoxin, in dissected bovine follicles has not shown increases in specific contents of either of these enzyme proteins as follicles mature from medium to large sizes (105). These studies report that both P-450_{SCC} and adrenodoxin increase only in corpora lutea at the early-mid luteal phase, which suggests that induction at this stage is primarily the result of earlier LH stimulation.

Additional actions of LH, in luteal tissue of various species, include enhancement of cholesterol availability by (a) stimulating 3-hydroxy-3-methylglutaryl coenzyme A reductase, which is rate-limiting for cholesterol biosynthesis (159); (b) acutely stimulating cholesterol esterase, thereby increasing the availability of free cholesterol from intracellular stores of fatty acid esters (160–162); and (c) increasing the number of lipoprotein receptors (163), thereby enhancing uptake of cholesterol in the form of lipoprotein.

FSH (87), and subsequently LH (164–167), greatly stimulate rat granulosa cell activity of Δ^5-3β-hydroxysteroid dehydrogenase:$\Delta^{5\text{-}4}$-isomerase. It has been suggested that $\Delta^{5\text{-}4}$-isomerase activity may be present in excess in adrenal and testis tissue (168,169), but the issue of whether this enzyme activity and the Δ^5-3β-hydroxysteroid dehydrogenase are separate entities or a single enzyme remains unresolved. Following gonadotropin stimulation, activity of Δ^5-3β-hydroxysteroid dehydrogenase is apparently not limiting for progesterone synthesis in cultured granulosa cells from immature rats, which do not substantially accumulate pregnenolone during FSH-stimulated synthesis of progesterone and 20α-dihydroprogesterone (170). This may not be true in the pig, in which cultured granulosa cells accumulate greater quantities of pregnenolone than progesterone (171).

The metabolism of progesterone to 20α-dihydroprogesterone in granulosa cells (see section on 20-hydroxysteroid dehydrogenase, above) is influenced by FSH stimulation of the 20α-hydroxysteroid dehydrogenase enzyme, as demonstrated by *in vivo* experiments with hypophysectomized, estrogen-treated rats (172) and with cultured rat granulosa cells (173). In contrast, LH is apparently not required for maximal activity of this enzyme in ovaries of proestrous rats (174), and hCG is not an effective stimulus in FSH-primed rat granulosa cells in culture (164). However, various studies in the rat have reported inhibitory or stimulatory actions of LH/hCG on 20α-hydroxysteroid dehydrogenase, concomitant with luteotropic or luteolytic actions, respectively (46,175–177). The conversion of progesterone to 20α-dihydroprogesterone in the rat corpus luteum (178,179) is important in regulating progestational activity during pregnancy (180) and parturition (181,182). The same pathway to 20α-dihydroprogesterone occurs in mouse (183) and human (184); however, in bovine corpus luteum, the principal metabolite is 20β-dihydroprogesterone (184).

Other C_{21} metabolites of progesterone result from the sequential action of 5α-reductase and 3α-hydroxysteroid dehydrogenase, the products being 5α-pregnane-3,20-dione and 3α-hydroxy-5α-pregnan-20-one, respectively (Fig. 4). The extent of formation of these products depends on the 5α-reductase activity, which is greatest in immature rats (115,185). Similar sequential catabolism of 20α-dihydroprogesterone to 20α-hydroxy-5α-pregnan-3-one and then 5α-pregnane-3α,20α-diol is expected (Fig. 4); the latter metabolite has been found to be a significant product in long-term cultures of rat granulosa cells (186). A fully reversible conversion of 5α-pregnane-3,20-dione to 3β-hydroxy-5α-pregnan-20-one is also expected to be catalyzed by the 3β-hydroxysteroid dehydrogenase (see section on 5α-reduced pathways, above), but little is known about the regulation involved.

In contrast with theca cells, granulosa cells of all species studied, with the apparent exception of the bovine (85), do not have significant activities of C_{21} side-chain cleavage enzymes and synthesize little or no C_{19}-steroids from either pregnenolone or progesterone (85,94,99, 187–192).

Granulosa cells possess considerable activity of the 17β-hydroxysteroid dehydrogenase enzyme (103,193–196), which acts on both C_{19}-steroids, androstenedione and testosterone, as well as aromatization products, estrone and estradiol (Fig. 2). Although androstenedione is the major ovarian androgen in most species, the 17β-hydroxysteroid dehydrogenase reaction favors the production of estradiol as the major ovarian estrogen. The presence of 5α-reductase and 3α-hydroxysteroid dehydrogenase in granulosa cells also permits theca-derived androgens to be converted to several ring A-reduced metabolites (Fig. 4) according to the same reactions occurring for progesterone metabolism described above. FSH does not influence the production of 5α-reduced metabolites of testosterone (i.e., androsterone and 5α-androstane-3α,17β-diol) in rat granulosa cell cultures (141). Furthermore, FSH was ineffective in maintaining elevated 5α-reductase activity in prepubertal rats after hypophysectomy (197).

From a physiological viewpoint, aromatization of theca-derived androgens is perhaps the most important pathway of androgen metabolism in the granulosa cell. This key concept of cooperation of the follicle cell types in the regulation of estrogen biosynthesis is considered next. Other important actions of theca-derived androgens on estrogen biosynthesis via paracrine mechanisms are considered later (see section on estrogens, below).

Cooperation of Theca and Granulosa Cells

The functional basis of the modern concept of cellular cooperation in follicular estrogen biosynthesis has already been described: Theca cells are stimulated by LH to produce aromatizable androgens, and granulosa cells respond to FSH with increased aromatase activity but without *de novo* production of C_{19}-steroid substrates. We will briefly discuss the historical development of the current "two-cell-type, two-gonadotropin" theory of steroidogenic regulation and then consider the direct *in vitro* experimental evidence in animals and humans that supports this concept and other aspects of cooperation in follicular steroid metabolism.

The early literature implicated the follicle in estrogen biosynthesis (198), with some authors favoring the theca interna cells as the principal site of synthesis (199–201) and others suggesting the follicular epithelium (i.e., membrana granulosa) as the primary source (202). The first substantial evidence of the cooperation of ovarian cell types in estrogen biosynthesis was provided by Falck in 1959 (203) in now-classic experiments in which ovarian cell types in the rat were transplanted either alone or in combination into the anterior eye chamber together with estrogen-sensitive vaginal epithelium as a biological indicator of estrogen production. These studies established that estrogen biosynthesis required the cooperation of granulosa or lutein cells with theca or interstitial cells. Falck mistakenly interpreted these findings as indicating a permissive influence of granulosa or lutein cells (perhaps mediated by progesterone) on estrogen secretion by theca or interstitial cells in the rat. Although this proposal was incorrect for the rat, where thecal biosynthesis does not contribute significantly to estrogen production, in at least certain species C_{21}-steroids from the granulosa cells may indeed be utilized by theca cells for androgen production, thereby contributing to estrogen production by both cell types.

A two-cell theory of the sort suggested by Falck was subsequently proposed for the mare (187), with the additional proposal that granulosa cells have only weak 17α-hydroxylase and little C-17,20-lyase activities. Further studies with isolated ovarian cell types in the pig demonstrated that granulosa cells converted pregnenolone to progestins, but not to androgens, while readily interconverting exogenous testosterone and androstenedione (i.e., by the 17β-hydroxysteroid dehydrogenase) and aromatizing these androgens (193). It was later proposed that C_{19}-steroid precursors in the pig are produced by the theca and are then transferred to the granulosa for conversion to testosterone (188). In this way, estrogen was presumed to be synthesized by granulosa as well as theca cells, although aromatase activity in pig theca was believed to be higher (193).

The next major step in the development of the modern concept of regulation of estrogen biosynthesis was the determination of the cellular sites of FSH and LH action. Much earlier work by Greep and coworkers (204) in hypophysectomized immature rats provided the first hints that FSH and LH act upon different cell types to promote estrogen formation. Subsequently, Hollander and Hollander (205) demonstrated that FSH action *in vivo* or *in vitro* stimulated [^{14}C]testosterone conversion to estradiol by canine ovarian slices. However, up until the 1970s, LH was still considered to be the key, if not the only, steroidogenic hormone in the follicle for a variety of reasons. The action of LH via cAMP was becoming established as an important control mechanism, LH was known to stimulate both androgen and estrogen production by luteal and stromal ovarian preparations (184), and it was later shown to stimulate acute estrogen production by the isolated rabbit follicle (206). Furthermore, use of relatively impure FSH cast doubts on the active hormone in earlier studies. The crucial role of FSH in controlling follicular estrogen biosynthesis in the rat was then established with the findings that explanted ovaries from hypophysectomized immature rats produced estrogen in response to FSH but not to LH and that they required the addition of testosterone as substrate (207). Similar findings with isolated rat granulosa cells in culture determined that FSH acted directly on the granulosa cells to stimulate aromatization (136), thereby extending earlier work demonstrating a similar action of FSH on testicular Sertoli cells (208).

The results of these *in vitro* studies led to the formulation of a modern two cell-type, two gonadotropin theory in which theca interna cells (and perhaps also interstitial cells) are stimulated by LH to produce androgens, which in turn traverse the follicular basement membrane to be utilized for estrogen biosynthesis in an FSH-stimulated reaction within the granulosa cells. Current evidence indicates that this concept is valid for antral and preovulatory follicles in the rat and most other species, despite additional and sometimes significant production of estrogens by theca cells in certain species. Evidence in various species of the exclusive localization of FSH binding sites on granulosa cells and of LH binding sites initially on theca/interstitial and only later on granulosa cells supports the two-cell-type, two-gonadotropin concept described above. The *in vitro* evidence directly supporting the concept of metabolic cooperation in estrogen biosynthesis by the two cell types is of three kinds. First, there is evidence that androgens produced in the theca layer exit from these cells in order to participate in estrogen biosynthesis, the inference being that extracellular androgens diffuse into the granulosa cell layer. Second, the evidence indicates that addition of aromatizable androgens to granulosa cells is essential for significant estrogen production, and addition of pregnenolone or other C_{21} precursors to thecal cells tends to increase androgen production. Third, recombination of isolated theca tissue and granulosa cells by coincubation demonstrates synergism in estrogen synthesis, provided that the two cell types either are stimulated with the appropriate gonadotropins *in vitro* or are derived from mature steroidogenically active follicles. This supporting evidence is discussed below.

First, *in vivo* evidence that FSH and LH act at separate sites and by separate mechanisms in stimulating estrogen secretion has been obtained in studies with hypophysectomized rats. Treatment of hypophysectomized rats with LH has been demonstrated to enhance ovarian androgen (testosterone and dihydrotestosterone) content; however, concomitant administration of FSH was required to elevate estradiol levels. Substitution of LH with aromatizable androgen (testosterone or androstenedione) led to similar increases in estradiol production, provided that the rats had also been treated with FSH (209). Thus, these findings are consistent with a stimulatory action of LH on production of androgens that were then used as substrate for conversion to estradiol in the presence of FSH, thus providing *in vivo* support for the two-cell, two-gonadotrophin mechanism for control of estrogen biosynthesis in the rat.

This cell-cooperation hypothesis requires that androgens of thecal origin must diffuse across the basement membrane separating the granulosa and thecal layers of the follicle in order for androgens to gain access to the aromatase enzyme in the granulosa cells. There is ample evidence that such diffusion does, in fact, occur. Concentrations of aromatizable androgens (i.e., androstenedione and testosterone) in follicular fluid are consistent with their serving as efficient substrates for aromatization by the granulosa cells. Furthermore, even higher concentrations of androgens might be achieved at the level of mural granulosa cells as the result of an androgen gradient, presumed to exist from the theca cells across the follicular basement membrane to the mural cells and finally to the follicular fluid. One study, using an experimental ovarian model in sheep, has provided indirect evidence that extracellular androgen produced in the theca layer must cross into the follicle to allow estrogen biosynthesis by the granulosa cells. In this study, ovaries of ewes were autotransplanted to the carotid–jugular circulation, and endogenous LH pulses were observed to result in episodic secretion of estradiol into the jugular vein (210). Following infusion into the ovarian artery of a high-titer antiserum against androgen, the normally episodic secretion of estradiol was inhibited, suggesting that passage of androgen across the follicular membrane was prevented by binding to antibodies. There is also indirect evidence in the pig that suggests thecal androgen transference to the granulosa cells (107).

Various studies in pig (107), sheep (128), and human (99,124,135,191,211) provide the evidence that granulosa cells must be supplied with an extracellular source of aromatizable androgen substrate in order to synthesize estrogens.

Evidence of substantial theca-granulosa cell synergism in estrogen production *in vitro* has been obtained in coculture studies with follicle cells of sheep (194), hamster (103), and human (122,124,135). Also, evidence of stromagranulosa synergism in estrogen production in the human was found in one study (124) but not in another (135). Similar studies in sheep have shown that follicle wall preparations (theca and granulosa) were far more effective in the production of estrogen than either cell type alone (128). In the rat, evidence of exclusive production of androgens by theca cells (212) and of aromatization in granulosa cells (141), combined with information that preovulatory estrogen production by the follicle is regulated by LH-stimulated thecal androgen production (102), provides convincing support for the original concept.

Apart from estrogen biosynthesis, there are other forms of follicle cell cooperation in steroid production and metabolism. Theca-granulosa cell synergism has been found for the production of thecal androgen in the sheep (128) and human (124,135). Other studies in the mare (189,213), hamster (103), rat (214), and pig (215) provide evidence that C_{21}-steroid precursors, which may be produced in the granulosa layer, can be metabolized to androgens by the theca cells. In other studies in the rat, comparisons of production of immunoreactive androgen (perhaps DHT) by intact preovulatory follicles or isolated cell types suggest that coordinated activities of both granulosa and theca cells are required for this biosynthetic function (102). Furthermore, theca-granulosa (124,135), as well as stroma–granulosa (135), synergism is also involved in progesterone synthesis in the human.

Intraovarian Regulation by Follicular Steroids

Estrogens

Early experiments demonstrated that estrogens had a stimulatory effect on the ovary (216–223). In experiments in which estrogen was administered to hypophysectomized immature rats, ovarian weight was maintained and ovaries became more responsive to gonadotropic stimulation. Furthermore, the ovarian weight response to gonadotropins was inhibited by antiserum to estradiol (224). Treatment of hypophysectomized rats with gonadotropins increased the number of atretic follicles per ovary, and administration of estrogen partially reversed this effect (225).

Specific uptake and retention of [^{3}H]estradiol *in vivo* by ovaries of immature rats (226,227), incorporation of estradiol into granulosa cells (228), and binding of estradiol to nuclear fractions of rat granulosa (229) and luteal cells (230) indicate the presence of estrogen binding sites in the ovary. Saidudduin and Zassenhaus (231) have characterized estrogen binding components from ovaries of immature rats. Their results suggested that ovarian estrogen binding sites are similar to specific, high-affinity estrogen receptors in uterine tissue.

There is evidence suggesting that estrogen acts within the ovary to inhibit androgen production, the estrogen presumably originating from granulosa cells and androgen from theca. Treatment of intact immature rats with estradiol suppressed ovarian testosterone and 5α-dihydrotestosterone production. Concomitant administration of gonadotropins failed to overcome the inhibition by estrogen, indicating that the effect was not mediated by decreased circulating gonadotropin (232). To provide further evidence for a direct intraovarian action of estrogen, Silastic implants of estradiol were embedded under the ovarian bursa unilaterally. Under these conditions, LH-stimulated androgen content of the ipsilateral ovary was considerably lower than that of the contralateral ovary (232). An inhibitory effect of estradiol on LH-induced androgen content of ovaries from immature hypophysectomized rats was reported as further evidence that a pituitary factor was not involved (232).

Results of *in vitro* experiments have demonstrated similar effects of estrogen on ovarian androgen synthesis. Whole ovaries from estrogen-treated immature, intact, or hypophysectomized rats responded to LH-stimulation *in vitro* with decreased androgen production when compared to that of ovaries obtained from rats that were not treated with estrogen. Dibutyryl cAMP did not increase testosterone production by cultured ovaries of estrogen-pretreated rats (233). Estradiol treatment of immature rats *in vivo* also suppressed androgen secretion by isolated thecal tissue *in vitro* (234). In culture experiments with isolated porcine thecal tissue (234) or dispersed theca cell preparations (235), addition of estrogens directly to the culture medium inhibited LH-stimulated androgen production in a dose-dependent manner, establishing that the inhibitory action of estrogens is directly on theca cells.

All indications are that estrogen inhibits ovarian androgen synthesis at a site distal to cAMP production, probably at an enzymatic step(s) in the steroidogenic pathway between androgens and their C_{21} precursors. In accordance with this hypothesis, estrogen pretreatment of ovaries from intact immature rats *in vivo* has been shown to inhibit conversion of radioactively labeled progesterone to androgens (testosterone, androstenedione, and androsterone) *in vitro*. On the other hand, incorporation into 3α-hydroxy-5α-pregnan-20-one is enhanced, suggesting that estrogen may act by inhibiting the 17α-hydroxylase:C-17,20-lyase enzyme system or by diverting C_{21} substrates into a pathway resulting in the formation of 5α-reduced pregnane compounds (233). In another study, treatment of immature rats with estradiol suppressed the stimulation by hCG of androstenedione, testosterone, 17α-hydroxyprogesterone, and 17α-hydroxy-pregnenolone production by dispersed ovarian cells in culture. Pregnenolone production was unchanged, while progesterone production was markedly enhanced. Estradiol had no effect on hCG binding capacity, hCG-stimulated cAMP synthesis, or the viability of ovarian steroidogenic cells. It was concluded that exogenous estradiol blocked ovarian androgen formation by reducing the activity of the 17α-hydroxylase enzyme (236). Further *in vitro* evidence with rat ovarian interstitial cell cultures indicates that estradiol directly causes rapid inhibition of 17α-hydroxylase and C-17,20-lyase enzyme activities (237).

There is evidence that estrogens are capable of regulating metabolism of androgens by a direct action on 5α-reductase. Eckstein and Nimrod (238) have shown an inhibitory effect of estradiol on 5α-reductase activity in microsomal preparations from immature rat ovaries. Since the minimal effective concentration of estradiol required to inhibit enzyme activity was in the range measurable in follicular fluid, the authors suggested that estradiol may be physiologically significant in the regulation of androgen metabolism.

Administration of LH to intact immature rats has been shown to affect ovarian progesterone metabolism in a manner identical to that of estrogen. Measured *in vitro,* ovarian androgen production was reduced and 3α-hydroxy-5α-pregnan-20-one secretion stimulated (233). Exposure of ovaries isolated from prepubertal rats to LH alters progesterone metabolism, favoring formation of 5α-reduced pregnane compounds while decreasing androgen and 5α-reduced androgen biosynthesis (239). In cultured preovulatory follicles from PMSG-treated immature rats, LH inhibited C-17,20-lyase activity. Addition of inhibitors of steroid synthesis prevented the inhibitory action of LH on the conversion of 17α-hydroxy-progesterone to androgens but did not affect basal lyase activity. These experiments suggested that the inhibitory action of LH on androgen synthesis may be mediated by the action of another ovarian steroid. That this steroid is estrogen is supported by experiments showing that the aromatase inhibitor, 4-acetoxy-androstane-3,17-dione, blocks the negative effect of LH on androgen synthesis by rat preovulatory follicles *in vitro* (240).

After the ovulatory surge of LH, androgen levels in ovarian tissue, follicular fluid, and ovarian venous blood and serum initially rise and then fall precipitously several hours later (241–243). This apparent inhibitory effect of LH on androgen production raises the possibility that this inhibition represents a physiological role of estrogens in the intrafollicular control of androgen biosynthesis. In support of this possibility, Smith et al. (244) and Kalra and Kalra (245) have measured serum hormone concentrations during the rat estrous cycle and have shown that, shortly after the LH surge on the day of proestrus, estradiol peaks and then rapidly declines. That the rise is dependent on the LH surge has been demonstrated in proestrous hamsters by blocking LH secretion with injections of phenobarbital (246). It may be that the surge of LH initially stimulates theca cells to produce androgens, which are aromatized to estrogens by granulosa cells. The estrogens then inhibit the thecal 17α-hydroxylase:C-17,20-lyase enzyme system, thereby limiting further synthesis of androgens and their subsequent use as substrates for aromatization. The ability of low doses of estradiol to enhance progesterone production by isolated bovine theca cells (247) may be a reflection of precursor accumulation following the inhibitory action of estrogens. This action may contribute to the transition of the follicle from primarily an estrogen-secreting to a progesterone-secreting structure, initiated by the LH surge. The role of estrogens in regulation of the corpus luteum is beyond the scope of this chapter and will be discussed elsewhere in the volume.

Another intrafollicular regulatory action of estrogens that has been clearly established is their ability to enhance ovarian estrogen production through direct actions on granulosa cells. Clomiphene citrate, a weak estrogen, increased estradiol and estrone synthesis from radiolabeled androstenedione by superfused canine ovaries *in vivo* (248). Clomiphene citrate (249), estradiol, estrone, hexestrol, moxestrol, ethinyl estradiol, chlorotrianisene, mestranol (250), and triphenylethylene antiestrogens (251) have also been reported to have similar effects on FSH-induced estrogen synthesis by cultured granulosa cells isolated from ovaries of immature hypophysectomized, DES-primed rats. FSH-induced aromatase activity in rat granulosa cells was enhanced by *in vitro* addition of DES (252). Good correlation was found between receptor binding affinity and biological potency of both natural and synthetic estrogens or antiestrogens, and the stimulatory effect could not be accounted for by increased granulosa cell viability or protein mass (250).

In support of the hypothesis that estrogens are physiological regulators of granulosa cell aromatase activity, the minimal effective dose of estradiol required to elicit a response (3.7×10^{-10} M) is well within the range of estradiol in antral fluid of preovulatory follicles (250). Thus, estrogens may function within the ovary or in individual follicles as end-product amplifiers to enhance FSH-induced aromatase.

Estrogens have been shown to decrease progesterone secretion by porcine (253–256), bovine (247), rat (257), and human (258,259) granulosa cells and by large follicles from bovine ovaries (260). The inhibitory action of estrogens on porcine granulosa cells was both time- and dose-dependent and was demonstrable in short-term, but not long-term, cultures at estradiol concentrations similar to those found *in vivo* (261). Estrogen-inhibition of progesterone production was not dependent on cell density in culture or due to a cytotoxic effect, degree of follicular maturation, or accelerated metabolism of 20α-dihydroprogesterone. Instead, the action of estrogen appeared to limit the conversion of pregnenolone to progesterone, resulting in enhanced pregnenolone accumulation in culture. Increased pregnenolone production in the presence of estrogen was also the result of enhanced cholesterol side-chain cleavage activity (154,261) and mitochondrial content of P-450 (154).

The inhibitory action of estrogen on progesterone production has been corroborated *in vivo*. Administration of estradiol for 3 days decreased LH-induced ovarian progesterone content in hypophysectomized immature rats but not in intact animals. Also, in ovaries of estradiol-treated hypophysectomized rats, dibutyryl cAMP, but not LH, restored *in vitro* progesterone production to values comparable to those of ovaries from control animals. This result suggests that estrogen inhibits progesterone synthesis by acting at a step early in the stimulative cascade, possibly prior to cAMP generation (262).

There are also reports of stimulatory effects of estrogen on progesterone secretion in porcine (24,263) and rat (257,264,265) granulosa cells. Unlike the inhibitory action of estrogen, the stimulatory effect on porcine granulosa cells in culture was only demonstrable in longer-term incubations and was found to be dependent on the density of granulosa cells in culture and the maturational status of the follicle from which cells were isolated (261). Granulosa cells from small, but not larger, follicles responded to estrogen with increased progesterone secretion, an effect that was found to be due to increased activity of Δ^5-3β-hydroxysteroid dehydrogenase:$\Delta^{5\text{-}4}$-isomerase. In addition, with estrogen treatment, pregnenolone accumulation was increased, as were cholesterol side-chain cleavage activity and hydrolysis of endogenous cholesterol esters.

Catechol estrogens, which may be synthesized within the follicle (49), have also been shown to stimulate steroidogenesis in rat granulosa cells *in vitro* (266) and corpora lutea (267).

Androgens

With the establishment of the obligatory role of androgens as substrates for estrogen biosynthesis, other possible roles of androgens in follicular function at first received little attention or were dismissed. The antiandrogen, hydroxyflutamide had little or no effect on FSH-induction of enzyme activity or LH receptors in diethylstilbestrol (DES)-primed, hypophysectomized immature rats, suggesting that androgens are not essential for FSH to initiate development of antral follicles (268). In support of this hypothesis, Neumann et al. (269) demonstrated that cyproterone acetate, another antiandrogen, did not disrupt estrous cycles or interfere with ovulation in adult rats. In addition, Lyon and Glenister (270) have reported that Tfm/O mice, a strain in which females carry a gene conferring androgen resistance, have normal reproductive cycles; follicular maturation, conception, and pregnancy occur.

More recently, however, evidence of several sorts has appeared providing convincing evidence of other regulatory functions of androgens in the follicle. Specific androgen binding sites have been identified in ovaries from estrogen-primed, hypophysectomized immature rats (271) and later localized to the granulosa cell compartment (272). Similar androgen-binding proteins are found in sheep granulosa cells (273) and human ovarian cytosol (274).

In healthy, rather than atretic, follicles there is an inverse relationship between intrafollicular concentrations of androgens and estrogens. High ratios of androgens to estrogens in follicular fluid have been associated with nonovular and atretic follicles (229,275,276). However, from these data it is difficult to determine whether the predominance of androgen over estrogen is the cause of atresia or merely a result of the process. Both androgens (221,277) and hCG (278), which stimulate ovarian androgen synthesis, have been shown to promote atresia in rats. Coadministration of antiandrogens or antiserum raised against androgen (278) alleviated this effect of hCG. Further, treatment of immature, hypophysectomized, PMSG-treated rats with DHT induced atresia (279). This latter effect could be at least partially overcome by estradiol. Recently, Opavsky and Armstrong (280) showed an inhibitory effect of LH on the superovulatory response of immature rats to FSH. Although there is considerable circumstantial evidence to implicate androgens in the process of follicular atresia, the mechanisms of this process and the specific role of androgens in controlling the process are poorly understood.

In view of the rather substantial evidence in favoring a negative role for androgens in follicular maturation, it is perhaps surprising to find that androgens have positive effects on follicular growth. Ovarian degeneration occurred in androgen-resistant Tfm/O mice (281), and an antiandrogen accelerated atresia in preovulatory rat follicles (282). Somewhat similarly, treatment of diestrous rats with flutamide resulted in decreased growth and maturation of ovarian follicles (283). Also, an inhibitory action of androgen antisera on hCG-induced ovulation has been reported in hypophysectomized rats (284).

In trying to reconcile the apparent discrepancies between androgen effects within the ovarian follicles, it is worth noting that the antagonistic action of androgen on follicular events, as has been implicated in atresia, is believed to affect only those follicles at the preantral and early antral stages of development. The facilitory effect of androgen may be reserved for those large follicles that have already entered the final stages of development (285).

In culture, androgens have been shown to stimulate progesterone biosynthesis by intact follicles dissected from ovaries of cycling ewes (286) and cows (260) and by granulosa cells isolated from pig (255,256), rat (257,287) and mouse (288) ovaries. In addition, administration of androgens to intact immature rats increased subsequent progesterone accumulation by their isolated ovarian cells *in vitro* (289). Since both aromatizable and nonaromatizable androgens were effective, the response appears to be androgenic rather than dependent on aromatization of androgens to estrogens. This hypothesis is supported by data for the pig, in which implants of antiandrogens (flutamide or hydroxyflutamide) placed in the ovarian interstitium decreased progesterone secretion by isolated granulosa cells *in vitro* (290). Hydroxyflutamide and cyproterone acetate suppressed the stimulatory effect of testosterone on progesterone production by rat granulosa cell incubations (257).

Androgens, in addition to having their own stimulatory effects, enhance FSH-stimulated progestin synthesis (143–145,291). This action was blocked by hydroxyflutamide (292), and the potency of various androgens appeared to be correlated with the extent to which they were converted to testosterone or DHT (195).

Depending on the animal model used, androgens have been shown to act at both pre- and post-cAMP sites. Using granulosa cells isolated from ovaries of immature hypophysectomized, estrogen-treated rats, androstenedione enhanced stimulation of progestin production by the cAMP analog dibutyryl cAMP but had no effect on [^{125}I]FSH binding to the cells, FSH-stimulated cAMP production, or conversion of cAMP to AMP by the phosphodiesterase enzyme (144). On the other hand, in granulosa cells isolated from ovaries of intact immature rats, androgens enhance FSH-responsiveness, as measured by the FSH stimulation of cAMP production (292–294) and [^{125}I]FSH binding (294,295), and suppress cAMP metabolism (292).

Increased C_{21}-steroid production in the presence of androgen is not a reflection of decreased catabolism by 5α-reductase (144), although androgens have been reported to regulate catabolism of progesterone (296,297) through inhibition of 20α-hydroxysteroid dehydrogenase (298). Androgens alone or in combination with FSH have no effect on levels of free or esterified cholesterol in cultured rat granulosa cells (299). However, in these cells, androgen and FSH act synergistically to enhance lipoprotein utilization (300). Both FSH and testosterone independently enhance conversion of cholesterol to pregnenolone, indicating a stimulatory action on cholesterol side-chain cleavage. Combined treatment results in synergism (153,291,299). Transport of cholesterol into mitochondria is unaffected by FSH or androgen (299). Effects of androgens on 3β-hydroxysteroid dehydrogenase are equivocal. Some data suggest that androgens act synergistically with FSH to increase conversion of pregnenolone to progesterone (291), while other data indicate that androgens are ineffective at this site (141).

In contrast to the work using rat tissue, aromatizable androgens have a negative influence on progesterone production by human granulosa cells (124) and on FSH-stimulated progesterone accumulation by granulosa cells isolated from porcine ovaries (171,301). Although estradiol had a similar inhibitory action and nonaromatizable androgens were ineffective, the effect of aromatizable androgens could not be accounted for by conversion to estrogens since 4-acetoxy-4-androstene-3,17-dione, an inhibitor of aromatase, failed to prevent the testosterone-induced decrease in progesterone production (301).

Similar to the action of FSH, dibutyryl cAMP stimulated progesterone production by porcine granulosa cells. Addition of testosterone to cultures suppressed the stimulatory effect of dibutyryl cAMP, indicating that testosterone acts at a site distal to cAMP generation (171). Further studies revealed that androgens had no effect on progesterone metabolism (301); however, they did enhance pregnenolone synthesis in FSH-treated granulosa cell cultures (171). Thus, decreased progesterone production in the presence of androgen appears to be due to restricted conversion of pregnenolone to progesterone through inhibition of Δ^5-3β-hydroxysteroid dehydrogenase:$\Delta^{5\text{-}4}$-isomerase activity. A direct inhibitory action of testosterone on this enzyme has recently been demonstrated (302).

Very little work has been done to investigate intraovarian effects of androgens on thecal steroidogenesis. Androgen has been shown to enhance progesterone secretion by human thecal tissue in culture. The effect on granulosa cell progesterone synthesis was negative, and in combined incubations of theca or stroma plus granulosa cells, no effect of androgen could be discerned (124).

As discussed above, FSH has a regulatory role in ovarian estrogen secretion through induction of aromatase activity in rat granulosa cells. Studies using cultured rat granulosa cells from intact immature rats have demonstrated that, in addition to acting as substrates for FSH-stimulated aromatase, androgens also enhance FSH-induction of enzyme activity (303). Both aromatizable and nonaromatizable androgens were effective, although nonaromatizable androgens (5α-dihydrotestosterone and androsterone) were only 50% as potent as aromatizable androgens (testosterone and androstenedione). Thus, it is clear that this action of androgens is not dependent on their conversion to estrogens. This contention is supported by experiments showing that androgen enhancement of FSH-induced aromatase activity is suppressed by hydroxyflutamide (an androgen receptor blocker) (304,305) and is not affected by 4-acetoxy-4-androstene-3,17-dione (an inhibitor of aromatase) (252) or nafoxidine (an estrogen receptor blocker) (252).

There is evidence to suggest that, in the intact immature rat model, androgens influence granulosa cell aromatase activity by action at a site before cAMP production. Although testosterone enhances FSH-induced aromatase activity, it has no effect on cAMP-induced estrogen synthesis. Androgens enhance the responsiveness of cultured granulosa cells to FSH in the production of cAMP, as well as in stimulating cellular [^{125}I]FSH binding (294).

Aromatization of testosterone to estradiol by granulosa cells, isolated from the largest follicles in ovaries of rats showing diestrous II and proestrous vaginal smears, has been shown to be competitively inhibited by 5α-reduced androgens (306). The same phenomenon was described using human follicles excised at all stages of maturity (307). Apart from alterations in aromatase enzyme activity itself, follicular estrogen biosynthesis may be influenced by the amount of C_{19} substrate available and variation in the ratio of aromatizable to nonaromatizable androgens as the result of changes in 5α-reductase activity. Rat (40) and human (110,308) ovaries have been shown to convert aromatizable androgens actively to 5α-reduced androgens. Since high concentrations of estrogen in follicular fluid have been associated with healthy antral follicles and low estrogen with apparently degenerating follicles (275), alterations in the capacity of granulosa cells to convert androgens to estrogens may be a physiologically important mechanism for regulating concentrations of intrafollicular steroid hormones and development of individual follicles.

Siiteri and Thompson (309) have reported a 2.5-fold increase in 5α-reductase activity and a 5-fold decrease in aromatase activity within a few hours of exposure of ovaries of PMSG-treated rats to hCG. Katz and Armstrong (310) observed a similar decline in aromatase activity following LH treatment. The increased activity of 5α-reductase could contribute to the decreased estradiol secretion, which occurs dramatically following the LH surge, in two ways: (a) by decreasing the intrafollicular levels of aromatizable androgens through increased 5α-reductase activity and (b) by increasing intrafollicular levels of 5α-reduced androgens, which serve as competitive inhibitors of the aromatase enzyme system.

Progestins

It is uncertain whether progestins have any direct role in the intraovarian regulation of ovarian function, and reports are often contradictory. Some investigators have found that administration of exogenous progesterone to estrogen-primed, hypophysectomized immature rats had no effect on ovarian morphology (229,311,312), while others have presented evidence that progesterone has an inhibitory effect on follicular development when given to intact animals (313–316). That the effect of progesterone in these latter experiments might be mediated indirectly by depression of pituitary secretion of gonadotropins, rather than direct inhibition at the follicular level, is suggested by the observation that retardation of follicular growth by progesterone occurs only when plasma concentrations of both FSH and LH are significantly reduced (316). Goodman and Hodgen (317) attempted to avoid this problem by placing progesterone directly in the monkey ovary and suggested that their results supported a direct inhibitory action of progesterone on follicular development.

In prepubertal rats, progesterone implants decrease serum LH concentrations and reduce estradiol accumulation by the isolated follicles but, surprisingly, facilitate the stimulatory effects of low-dose hCG treatment on the growth of small antral follicles and on estrogen synthesis (318). It was suggested that progesterone may facilitate LH action under physiological circumstances when basal LH is low. On the other hand, even in the presence of elevated serum progesterone, preovulatory follicular maturation at the end of pregnancy (i.e., follicles functionally indistinguishable from those at proestrus) is supported by small sustained increases in serum LH, suggesting that progesterone may have no direct inhibitory effect on follicle cell maturation (319).

In support of a direct action of progesterone on ovarian regulation, specific progesterone receptors have been identified in rat ovary (320,321) and subsequently in rat granulosa cells (322,323). Similarly, ovarian progestin binding sites have been reported in rabbit (324), guinea pig (325), cow (326), and human (274,327).

Progesterone has been shown to enhance the ability of cultured rat granulosa cells to respond to FSH in the production of cAMP (293). In another study, synthetic progestin (R5020) increased FSH-stimulation of progesterone and 20α-dihydroprogesterone synthesis in granulosa cells isolated from immature hypophysectomized, estrogen-treated rats. Similarly, R5020 enhanced LH-stimulated progestin production by cells that had previously been primed with FSH to induce LH-receptor formation. Furthermore, in the presence of cyanoketone, an inhibitor of Δ^5-3β-hydroxysteroid dehydrogenase, progesterone augmented the ability of FSH to stimulate pregnenolone synthesis (328). The major criticism of this latter work is that the concentration (1×10^{-6} M) of synthetic progestin required to elicit a response is at the extreme upper limit of physiological progestin concentrations. The possibility that the action of progestin was mediated by nonspecific binding to androgen receptors was considered; however, the apparent autoregulatory actions of progestins were not altered by treatment with antiandrogens, indicating that the effect was not due to binding of progestin to androgen receptors (329).

The effects of several progestins on FSH-stimulated estrogen production by cultured rat granulosa cells isolated from ovaries of immature hypophysectomized, DES-treated rats have been examined (330). FSH-enhanced estrogen secretion was reduced following treatment with progesterone, 20α-dihydroprogesterone, or R5020, a potent synthetic progestin. A study of the relative potencies of the progestins revealed that R5020 was the most effective compound, followed by progesterone and 20α-dihydroprogesterone. This pattern was found to reflect the relative abilities of the progestins to bind to ovarian progestin receptors. Later experiments investigated the mechanism by which R5020 inhibits FSH-induction of aromatase activity. It was concluded that the synthetic progestin acts at a site distal to cAMP production and that it is not a competitive inhibitor of aromatase (331).

In another study of the effect of progesterone on FSH-stimulated estradiol synthesis by cultured rat granulosa cells, it was questioned whether progesterone has the same effect on aromatase activity once activity has been induced *in vivo* (332). In granulosa cells isolated on the morning of proestrus from follicles of immature rats previously treated with PMSG (4 IU), progesterone had a slight suppressive effect on estradiol synthesis. However, it was evident that once aromatizing activity had been induced estradiol synthesis was much less sensitive to inhibition by progesterone.

Likewise, an inhibitory effect of progesterone on estrogen secretion has been demonstrated *in vivo* (246). Progesterone administered to hamsters on the morning of the day of proestrus resulted in a fall in serum estradiol concentration without a concomitant change in blood levels of gonadotropins. The fact that concomitant administration of testosterone did not reverse the effect of progesterone indicated that progesterone acted at the level of the aromatase enzyme system. This study led the authors to speculate that the inhibitory effect of progesterone is one factor in the sharp decline in the serum concentration of estrogen that occurs after the LH surge in normally cycling hamsters (333).

Regulation of androgen production in the ovary by progestins has not been reported; however, both progesterone (334) and 5α-pregnane-3,20-dione (335) are effective inhibitors of the C-17,20-lyase, indicating their potential in intraovarian regulation of androgen biosynthesis.

Other Regulatory Factors and Hormones

Prolactin

Prolactin has long been known as a "luteotrophic" hormone, particularly in rodents but also in several other species. As such, it is involved in initiating luteinization of granulosa cells, in maintaining their level of progesterone synthesis as luteal cells, and in inhibiting the activity of the progesterone catabolizing enzyme, 20α-hydroxysteroid dehydrogenase, the latter particularly in rodents (336). The appearance of specific prolactin receptors in granulosa cells late in follicular development and their induction by FSH in culture (249) indicate the likelihood that prolactin may exert a physiological action on granulosa cells at the stage of terminal differentiation, when they are transformed into luteal cells. In support of this, prolactin has been demonstrated to enhance progesterone production in cultured granulosa cells obtained from preovulatory rat follicles (337) and porcine follicles (338). Striking morphological changes, characteristic of luteinization, were also induced by prolactin in cultured rat granulosa cells (337).

Stimulatory effects of prolactin on steroidogenesis in prepubertal (i.e., nonluteinized) ovaries have also been reported. Thus, prolactin injections (339) or hyperprolactinemia induced by *in vivo* administration of dopaminergic receptor blockers (339,340) have been found to induce precocious puberty, as well as to increase ovarian responsiveness to LH in immature rats. The latter effect appeared to be mediated, in part, by an increase in ovarian LH receptors (339). There is also evidence for a role of prolactin in induction and maintenance of LH receptors on luteal cells at late gestational stages in the rat (341).

In contrast to the stimulatory action of prolactin on progesterone secretion by granulosa cells at a late stage of differentiation, progesterone production by granulosa cells from small immature porcine follicles was markedly inhibited by physiological concentrations of prolactin (338). Exposure of the latter granulosa cells to estradiol reversed this inhibitory effect (342).

Another inhibitory effect of prolactin, on estrogen secretion, was reported for cultured rat granulosa cells obtained from follicles at both preantral and preovulatory stages (343,344). Decreased estrogen secretion *in vitro* appears to be due, at least in part, to an inhibitory action of prolactin on FSH induction of aromatase activity (345,346). The site of this action of prolactin appears to be distal to adenylate cyclase, as prolactin also inhibited the stimulatory action of dibutyryl cAMP. The inhibitory effect of prolactin on rat follicle aromatase activity has also been demonstrated by *in vivo* exposure of intact rats to the hormone (347). In addition, prolactin has been reported to suppress basal and gonadotropin-stimulated estradiol secretion by human ovaries perfused *in vitro* (348).

Evidence for an inhibitory influence of prolactin on androgen secretion, presumably by action on the theca and/or interstitial cells, of rat ovaries has also been reported. Levels of androstenedione in preovulatory follicles of adult rats were significantly decreased by prolactin (347), whereas hypoprolactinemia, induced *in vivo* by bromoergocryptine, was accompanied by markedly increased secretion of 5α-androstane-3α,17β-diol, the major androgen secreted by the prepubertal rat ovary in response to hCG stimulation (349). Addition of prolactin to cultured rat theca–interstitial cell preparations at concentrations within the physiological range for the female rat, and consistent with the binding affinity observed for the specific binding sites (receptors) that have been found on rat theca–interstitial cells, caused a dose-dependent inhibition of LH-stimulated androgen formation (androsterone, 5α-androstandiol) (350). As with granulosa cells, the inhibitory action of prolactin on theca–interstitial cells appears to be exerted at a step after adenylate cyclase, since the stimulatory action of 8-bromo-cAMP, as well as of other activators of adenylate cyclase (PGE_2, choleratoxin), was similarly inhibited by prolactin.

Gonadotropin-releasing Hormonelike Peptides

Evidence that systemic administration of gonadotropin-releasing hormone (GnRH) or its agonists paradoxically inhibit reproductive functions (351) was first attributed exclusively to indirect effects on the hypothalamic–pituitary–gonadal axis. There is indeed evidence showing that continuous or intermittent administration of GnRH or its agonists can cause the pituitary to become refractory to the releasing hormone (352–355) and, through the release of gonadotropins, can induce ovarian receptor loss and desensitization to these hormones (356–359). However, numerous other studies, particularly in the rat, have since established that GnRH binding sites are present in various extrapituitary tissues, including the gonads, and that direct actions of GnRH on somatic cells of ovary and testis occur (329,360). Furthermore, products with biological activities similar to those of hypothalamic GnRH have been reported in the ovary, testis, placenta, pancreas, other central nervous system (CNS) structures, and in some tumor types (360). We will review only those studies pertinent to possible intraovarian actions of GnRH-like peptides.

Ovarian cell types in the rat that have been demonstrated to have specific high-affinity binding sites for GnRH are granulosa (361,362), luteal (362,363), and theca (364) cells, at all stages of differentiation (364). These binding sites, presumed to be receptors by virtue of the various biological effects reported, are localized in the plasma membrane (365). In granulosa cells, GnRH receptors have been shown to be regulated by GnRH itself (inhibitory and stimulatory effects) and maintained by FSH (362,366). Two binding components have been identified in granulosa cells, of which one is similar to the pituitary GnRH receptor (367,368). Only binding sites of low affinity (369,370) or moderate affinity (371) have been found in human corpus luteum (369,370), consistent with the prolonged treatment required to observe inhibitory effects on progesterone biosynthesis by human granulosa cells *in vitro* (372). One study reports the absence of inhibitory effects of GnRH on progesterone biosynthesis by human granulosa cells (373). Biological effects of GnRH on ovarian cells in rabbit (374), pig (375), and chicken (376,377) also suggest the presence of GnRH-sensitive mechanisms. Lack of ovarian inhibition by GnRH in mice (378) and rhesus monkeys (379) and the absence of specific binding sites in ovine, bovine, and porcine ovaries (380) and in monkey corpora lutea (381) suggest that these species may not share the same GnRH sensitivity found in the rat.

The first evidence for a direct extrapituitary effect of a

GnRH agonist on the rat ovary was provided by the study of Rippel and Johnson (382), which showed inhibition of the hCG-stimulated ovarian and uterine weight gains in immature hypophysectomized animals. These findings were substantiated by extrapituitary inhibitory effects of GnRH and its agonists on FSH-stimulated ovarian weight gain and aromatase activity in immature hypophysectomized, estrogen-treated rats and on FSH-stimulated estrogen and progesterone production in cultured rat granulosa cells (383,384). GnRH inhibition of ^3H_2O release from [1β-^{3}H]testosterone, as a measure of aromatase activity, has also been demonstrated in cells from immature estrogen-primed rats (385,386). Other studies in hypophysectomized, PMSG-treated female rats demonstrated that a potent GnRH agonist also inhibited follicular maturation and steroidogenesis (387).

The effect of GnRH in decreasing FSH-stimulated progesterone production appears to be due to actions at several sites, causing inhibition of pregnenolone production (presumed to be an effect on the cholesterol side-chain cleavage enzyme), inhibition of Δ^5-3β-hydroxysteroid dehydrogenase activity (153,386,388), and stimulation of 20α-hydroxysteroid dehydrogenase activity (389), thereby reducing progesterone production and increasing its conversion to 20α-dihydroprogesterone. Inhibitory influences of GnRH on LH/hCG-stimulated estrogen and progesterone production were also demonstrated in cultured rat granulosa cells previously primed with FSH (164,390). Differences in the mechanisms of inhibition of progesterone production were seen with different stimulatory agents. Thus, the inhibitory action on LH/hCG-stimulated progesterone production appeared to involve decreased pregnenolone production (164), whereas the inhibition of prolactin and β-adrenergic agonist-stimulated progesterone production appeared to be the result of an action of GnRH to increase the activity of 20α-hydroxysteroid dehydrogenase, without influencing pregnenolone production (390,391).

Direct effects of GnRH on steroidogenesis in granulosa cells are not limited to inhibition. In the absence of other stimulatory agents, GnRH and its agonists act on granulosa cells from normal or immature hypophysectomized, estrogen-primed rats to increase aromatase activity (386) and the production of pregnenolone, progesterone, and 20α-dihydroprogesterone (153,170,386, 388,392). These and other studies indicate that GnRH stimulates the cholesterol side-chain cleavage enzyme (153,170), the Δ^5-3β-hydroxysteroid dehydrogenase (386,388), and 20α-hydroxysteroid dehydrogenase (173). However, GnRH and GnRH agonists do not activate steroidogenesis nearly as well as FSH does. The direct effects of GnRH, either inhibitory or stimulatory, on follicular steroidogenesis *in vivo* appear to depend on the duration of exposure and on the stage of follicular maturation (393,394).

GnRH also has diverse effects on other aspects of granulosa cell cytodifferentiation that may be responsible for some or all of the observed influences on steroidogenesis. FSH-induced formation of LH and prolactin receptors (384,395) and stimulation of receptors for epidermal growth factor (EGF) on rat granulosa cells is inhibited by GnRH and its agonists (396). GnRH also inhibits FSH-stimulated cAMP production in rat (397–399) and porcine (375) granulosa cells. This effect in rat granulosa cells is apparently due to two actions: (a) inhibition of adenylate cyclase (399), which has been attributed to a decrease in the FSH receptor content and to an inhibition of the FSH-regulated increase in its own receptor (400); and (b) stimulation of extracellular phosphodiesterase activity (399), although there are indications that intracellular and total phosphodiesterase activity is decreased by GnRH (401). The inhibition of adenylate cyclase by GnRH is dependent on the type of activating stimulus, since stimulation by isoproterenol or prostaglandin E is not inhibited (400). In contrast, following FSH-stimulation the subsequent increase in cAMP production induced by LH, isoproterenol, or PGE_2 is inhibited by GnRH, in a process requiring calcium (402). Since the inhibitory effects of GnRH can be seen when steroidogenesis is stimulated by cAMP analogs (or by various agents that stimulate cAMP production), it is probable that GnRH causes these effects by actions at site(s) distal to cAMP production. A GnRH agonist partially inhibits dibutyryl cAMP-stimulated aromatase activity in rat granulosa cells in the presence of an inhibitor of phosphodiesterase, indicating that cAMP catabolism is unlikely to fully explain the inhibitory actions (385). Inhibition of the FSH-stimulated increase in cAMP binding sites in rat granulosa cells (170) might be one additional factor in the direct inhibitory effects of GnRH.

Other FSH-stimulated responses that are augmented by GnRH include cellular protein production (403) and prostaglandin synthesis (397). GnRH alone also stimulates cellular protein content (404) and production of lactate (405), plasminogen activator (406), prostaglandins (392), and fibronectin (407). Additional effects of GnRH on phospholipid labeling from ^{32}P and phosphatidylinositol metabolism (408–412) and on arachidonic acid release (413) suggest that pathways involving phosphoinositide metabolism, perhaps related to calcium mobilization and calcium-activated enzymes (414,415), may mediate some of the actions of GnRH at sites distal to cAMP. Neither prostaglandins nor cAMP appears to mediate stimulatory effects of GnRH on progesterone production by granulosa cells from preovulatory rat follicles (416), although a GnRH agonist in the presence of a phosphodiesterase inhibitor has been found to cause very low levels of cAMP to accumulate in the culture medium of granulosa cells from immature estrogen-treated rats (386).

The independent stimulatory actions of GnRH on granulosa cells may activate certain physiological mechanisms since GnRH agonists cause meiotic maturation of follicle-enclosed oocytes *in vitro* (417) and *in vivo* in estrogen- or PMSG-primed, hypophysectomized rats (418,419), as well as ovulation in hypophysectomized rats (420,421). Tertiary atretic follicles seem to be most susceptible to the meiosis-inducing action of GnRH (418). Degenerative changes in oocytes and premature luteinization of granulosa cells, occurring without ovulation (384,400), have been reported as a result of GnRH agonist treatment, suggesting that GnRH both stimulates and disturbs normal regulatory mechanisms. A more recent study indicates that GnRH agonist-induced oocyte maturation in the rat is not abnormal (418), in contrast to earlier reports.

GnRH also has inhibitory effects on ovarian interstitial cells prepared from hypophysectomized immature rats (422). LH-induced differentiation of interstitial cells is blocked by GNRH, and inhibition of androgen production is by selective inhibition of the 17α-hydroxylase:C-17,20-lyase enzyme (423).

The presence of specific receptors for GnRH in ovarian cell types in the rat is reason enough to suspect a physiological role involving locally produced GnRH factors. Yet it is apparent that GnRH decapeptide produced by the hypothalamus is unlikely to have a peripheral action on the ovary by virtue of its extremely low concentrations; the highest concentration in human plasma, collected during the periovulatory period, is on the order of 8×10^{-12} M (424). The first suggestion of a local source of GnRH-like factor(s), so-called gonadocrinins, was the report of an acid-extractable factor in rat follicular fluid and in rat granulosa cell conditioned-medium that was capable of releasing FSH and LH from rat pituitary cells *in vitro* but that was immunologically and chromatographically distinct from GnRH (425). However, the investigators who first reported this factor have been unable to reproduce their findings (426). Other investigators have since found two components in extracts from luteinized rat ovaries that resemble GnRH in a radio-receptor assay using ovarian plasma membranes but that show little immunoassayable activity (427). These ovarian GnRH-like factors are protease sensitive and have molecular weights between 1,000 and 10,000 daltons. They differ from hypothalamic GnRH in that they are more sensitive to heat (inactivated at 50 or 60°C for 5 min), and they are distinct by reverse-phase high-performance liquid chromatography. Since significant quantities of this receptor-active material have also been found in liver and kidney, it would appear that the factors may not be specific ovarian products.

The physiological function(s) of ovarian GnRH-like peptides are unknown. It is conceivable that they are natural GnRH agonists that mediate paracrine or autocrine regulation within the ovary, the biological actions perhaps being similar to those already outlined for GnRH and its synthetic agonists. From this perspective, the direct antigonadotropic actions of GnRH shown in the rat might suggest a role in follicular atresia, perhaps related to selection of the dominant follicle. Alternatively, GnRH-like peptides might be GnRH antagonists. However, evidence obtained in estrogen-primed, hypophysectomized rats indicates that the action of FSH on follicle development is potentiated by a synthetic GnRH antagonist but is inhibited by exogenous GnRH (428). This result suggests that the antagonist was competitive to a GnRH-like factor, presumably of ovarian origin, that inhibits the action of FSH on follicle recruitment to the preovulatory stage.

Glucocorticoids

The influence of the adrenal glands and glucocorticoid treatments on ovarian function has long been recognized from various studies in mice (429) and rats (430–433) and in women (434,435). Although many of the effects of glucocorticoids may be mediated by actions on the hypothalamus and/or pituitary gland (431–433,436), a direct action of these steroids on the ovary cannot be discounted.

Glucocorticoid receptors have been characterized in rat ovaries (437) and localized to granulosa cells (438). Cortisol or dexamethasone have been shown to inhibit FSH-stimulated aromatase activity (439,440) but to enhance FSH-stimulated progesterone production in cultured rat granulosa cells (439,441). The action of glucocorticoids on progesterone production is associated with increased Δ^5-3β-hydroxysteroid dehydrogenase and reduced 20α-hydroxysteroid dehydrogenase activities, resulting in enhanced synthesis and concomitant suppression of metabolism. In porcine granulosa cell incubations, cortisol has no effect on basal progesterone production but is stimulatory in the presence of insulin (442). The physiological significance of these observations is obscure. Concentrations of glucocorticoids required to elicit responses *in vitro* were considered pharmacological. Nevertheless, these observations are interesting from a pathological point of view, and the presence of an ovarian glucocorticoid receptor, as well as of cortisol-binding globulin concentrated in follicular fluid (443,444), suggests that glucocorticoids may be of some physiological significance in the regulation of follicular function.

Growth Factors and Insulin

It is now quite clear that several well-characterized "growth factors" have *in vitro* modulatory effects on granulosa cell differentiation, including effects on steroidogenesis in several species. However, it is uncertain what the concentrations of these factors are within the follicles at different stages, what the cellular sources are either within the ovary or in extraovarian tissues, and what the regulatory or permissive actions are *in vivo*. These factors most likely influence cytodifferentiation in its many facets, rather than specifically affecting the steroidogenic mechanisms. A complete review of this expanding area of investigation is beyond the scope of this chapter, and readers are referred to the reviews available (329,445). We outline below the principal actions of growth factors on steroidogenesis by ovarian cell cultures.

EGF has been shown to bind to high-affinity, low-capacity receptors (446) and to have different influences on the steroidogenic pathways for estrogen and progesterone production in rat granulosa cells. EGF inhibits FSH-stimulated estrogen biosynthesis (i.e., aromatase activity) in granulosa cells from immature hypophysectomized, estrogen-treated rats (446,447), while it augments FSH-stimulated progestin biosynthesis and independently stimulates production of pregnenolone, progesterone, and 20α-dihydroprogesterone (446). EGF has also been reported to impair FSH-stimulated progesterone production in rat granulosa cells by increasing catabolism to 20α-dihydroprogesterone (448). The stimulatory actions of EGF (and perhaps its inhibitory actions as well) may involve sites distal to cAMP production since EGF has been reported to decrease FSH-stimulated cAMP production and to increase cAMP catabolism (448). In studies with pig granulosa cells, EGF inhibited FSH-stimulated estrogen biosynthesis but consistently inhibited FSH or hCG-stimulated progesterone production only after longer periods of treatment in culture (449). In contrast with these actions on rat and pig cells, EGF acts on cultured hen granulosa cells to inhibit LH-stimulated progesterone biosynthesis, apparently by inhibitory actions at the levels of cAMP production, as well as distal to this step but before C_{27} side-chain cleavage (450). Other studies in the rat have shown that the EGF receptor content of granulosa cells is regulated by LH and FSH and is maximum at proestrus of the cycle (396,446), indicating that EGF action may be coordinated with other hormonally regulated events. EGF has also been shown to inhibit androgen production by rat ovarian theca–interstitial cells (451). The only *in vivo* effect of EGF on the follicle so far demonstrated is the retardation of development of early stage follicles when administered to neonatal mice (452). However, there is no evidence to relate this effect to inhibition of estrogen biosynthesis, and it could be due to inhibitory effects on the pituitary.

The source of EGF would appear to be extraovarian, and it has been found in several tissues, as well as in mouse plasma and milk (453). EGF has been purified from submaxillary glands of mice and rats (454,455) and from human urine (456); the structures of the material isolated from these sources are similar but not identical. The fact that androgens greatly stimulate EGF levels in submaxillary glands and plasma (453,457) suggests a possible mechanism for self-regulation of androgen production via EGF action on the theca-interstitial cells. The possibility that EGF-like peptides might be produced locally and have autocrine actions affecting follicular function must also be considered. The EGF-like growth factor, α transforming growth factor (TGF-α), is known to interact with EGF receptors and has been found in several normal tissues (458–460). Also, normal bovine pituitary cells in culture have been reported to produce EGF, EGF-like, and TGF-α-like peptides (461).

Platelet-derived growth factor (PDGF) also increases FSH-stimulated progestin production, which may involve increased sensitivity to FSH and cAMP (448). This *in vitro* action suggests that PDGF release from platelets during follicular rupture may act to stimulate luteal cell production of progesterone.

Several modulatory actions on steroidogenesis have also been shown for insulin and the insulinlike growth factors (IGFs); these latter factors, classically thought to be of hepatic origin, are known as IGF-I (or somatomedin C [Sm-C]) and IGF-II in humans (or rIGF-II/MSA [multiplication stimulating activity] in the rat). Receptors for SM-C/IGF-I have been reported in granulosa cells of immature pigs (462,463) and of rat (445). Insulin receptors have also been reported on granulosa or luteal cells of rat, pig, and human (464–468). It is not clear whether the effects of insulin on granulosa cells are mediated through insulin receptors or type I IGF receptors (which preferentially bind IGF-I but also bind IGF-II and insulin). However, IGF-I does not appear to interact with insulin receptors.

There is evidence in the rat (445) and pig (469,470) for IGF-I production by granulosa cells in culture and for measurable quantities of IGF-I in follicular fluid from porcine (471,472) and human ovaries (445). Moreover, immunoreactive IGF-I in ovarian extracts increases following treatment of hypophysectomized, estrogen-treated rats with growth hormone (GH) (473), suggesting regulation of ovarian IGF production. Insulin has also been measured in fluid from porcine (472) and human (474) follicles.

The effects of IGF-I on rat granulosa cells cultured under serum-free conditions are to augment the stimulation by FSH of progesterone and 20α-dihydroprogesterone production (475,476) and of aromatase activity (477). In porcine granulosa cells, IGF-I alone or synergistically with FSH increases progesterone production (462) and also appears to stimulate pregnenolone, progesterone, and 20α-dihydroprogesterone independently, without synergism with FSH (463). Independent stimulatory effects of rIGF-II/MSA have been shown on progesterone production by porcine granulosa cells when cultured in the absence of serum (478), although another study has shown only a synergism with FSH (462). Insulin has also been shown to act synergistically amplifying the stimulatory effect of LDL on progesterone biosynthesis by porcine granulosa cells, the mechanisms involving increased binding, internalization, and degradation of LDL (479).

GH has been shown to augment FSH-stimulated progesterone and 20α-dihydroprogesterone production by cultured granulosa cells from hypophysectomized, estrogen-treated rats by mechanisms involving increased cAMP, as well as stimulation at a site distal to cAMP (480). It has not yet been determined whether this is a direct effect of GH or whether GH-stimulated production of IGF is responsible.

Insulin has steroidogenic effects similar to those of IGF-I, and since effects of insulin and IGF-I are not additive, it is likely that they employ the same mechanism. Progesterone production by rat (464,481) and pig (442,466,467,478,482,483) granulosa cells is stimulated by insulin, as is FSH-stimulated aromatase activity in rat (481) and human (484) granulosa cells. In contrast, insulin inhibits or is without effect on aromatase activity in porcine granulosa cells (478,485).

Neuroregulatory Substances and Ovarian Innervation

The innervation of the mammalian ovary has been well documented. Although considerable variation exists among species, sympathetic nerves, to a large extent accompanying blood vessels, innervate the ovarian interstitial tissue and perifollicular regions in several species, with follicles at all stages of development having adrenergic nerve terminals in close proximity to the blood vessels of the theca externa. Neither blood vessels nor nerves penetrate the basement membrane to reach the granulosa layers of follicles at any stage of development (486).

Although the physiological significance of the ovarian nerves remains to be established, considerable research has centered around the possible role of adrenergic neurotransmitters in controlling follicular function. Studies by Bahr and Ben-Jonathan (487) have shown that stimulation of the rat ovary with gonadotropin depletes the ovary of the catecholamine. A 40% reduction of ovarian concentrations of noradrenaline occurred 12 hr after PMSG administration to prepubertal rats; this was followed by a further 40% reduction 4 hr after the preovulatory LH surge. FSH, rather than LH or PRL, was found to be the pituitary hormone primarily involved in depletion of noradrenaline from Graafian follicles (488). Noradrenaline levels in porcine follicular fluid have been reported to vary with the stage of the estrous cycle, the highest levels being observed during the follicular phase (days 16–20) (489).

In vivo evidence for possible involvement of ovarian nerves in regulation of steroid secretion has come from ovarian denervation and ovarian nerve stimulation experiments. Decreased activity of Δ^5-3β-hydroxysteroid dehydrogenase was seen in both the interstitial gland cells and corpus luteum of the pregnant rat following ovarian denervation (490). Subsequently, Capps et al. (491) showed that electrical stimulation of the nerves in the ovarian plexus of hypophysectomized rats caused the interstitial cells to hypertrophy and develop ultrastructural features typical of active steroid-secreting cells.

The possible role of catecholamines in the direct regulation of steroid biosynthesis by follicle cells has been examined both *in vivo* and *in vitro*. *In vivo* experiments involved intrafollicular injection of adrenergic agonists and antagonists in rabbits. Beta-adrenergic, but not α-adrenergic, agonists resulted in increased progesterone output by the ovary, without influencing estrogen secretion (492). *In vitro* studies have shown catecholamine stimulation of progesterone production by dispersed luteal or granulosa cells in culture (492–496). These effects could be blocked by the β-adrenergic antagonist propranolol. The steroidogenic response (progesterone synthesis) of cultured rat granulosa cells to noradrenaline and isoproterenol was markedly enhanced by pretreatment of the cells with FSH *in vivo* or *in vitro* (496). Perhaps related to this is the observation of increased levels of high-affinity β_2-adrenergic receptors on granulosa cells during the proestrus associated with puberty in the rat (497). Catecholamine responsiveness of granulosa cells in preovulatory follicles of the rat apparently develops only after the preovulatory LH surge (498).

The interstitial tissue, the most richly innervated component of the ovaries, also contains β_2-adrenergic receptors (497), and addition of the β_2-agonist zinterol to cultured rat interstitial tissue ("residual" tissue, after removal of most granulosa cells) increased output of testosterone and androstenedione from this tissue on the day of proestrus, the peripubertal stage in which the greatest concentration of β_2-receptors were present (497). Addition of epinephrine, norepinephrine and isoproterenol to cultured theca-interstitial cells from hypophysectomized rats also markedly enhanced the secretion of certain androgens in the presence of hCG stimulation. The catecholamines were ineffective in stimulating basal (i.e., in the absence of hCG stimulation) secretion of steroids by the theca-interstitial tissue (despite the fact that they are effective, by themselves, in stimulating cAMP output) (499). Other neurotransmitters that have been detected in the ovary include acetylcholine (based on demonstration of acetylcholinesterase activity) (500), dopamine (487,501), substance P (502,503), VIP (504), and γ-aminobutyric acid (GABA) (329). Although high-affinity binding sites in ovarian tissue have been reported for some of these compounds and certain *in vitro* effects on steroidogenesis occur (505), suggesting possible regulatory roles, information is lacking about the specific effects of these neurotransmitters on steroid biosynthesis in the follicle.

STEROIDOGENESIS AND ITS CONTROL BY FOLLICLE TYPE

Introductory Description of Follicle Types

In the foregoing sections we have described the characteristic steroidogenic functions and control of the separate cell types of the mature ovarian follicle. The purpose of this section is to reexamine the evidence from the perspective of follicular development stage, drawing on related examples from human and animal studies to illustrate principles. It is intended to place the previous discussion of cellular details of steroid formation and regulation into the context of the follicle as a developing biosynthetic structure. We shall consider the dynamic processes of steroid synthesis and secretion occurring within the follicles as follicular maturation proceeds under the control of the pituitary gonadotropic hormones. Although the follicular contribution to ovarian steroid production is at any time the composite secretion of steroids by follicles at various functionally different stages, the most important contribution eventually comes from one or several dominant follicles forming a cohort destined to ovulate.

The stages of follicular development have been described by several classifications that distinguish follicles in terms of oocyte morphology and size, and the number of supporting granulosa cells and their organization. Similar schemes for mouse (506) and human (507) ovaries have defined eight principal types of follicle. The general categories of follicle types are the following: small nongrowing follicles (i.e., primordial follicles classified as types 1–2 in human and 1–3a in mouse); preantral follicles (i.e., single-layered primary and multilaminar secondary follicles classified as types 3–5 in the human and types 3b–5b in the mouse), which are characterized mainly by increases in oocyte size and number of granulosa cells; and antral follicles (i.e., tertiary or Graafian follicles classified as types 6–8 in human and mouse), which feature formation of a fluid-filled antrum and further increases in granulosa cell number. In addition, antral follicles of several species have been referred to previously as either small or large to indicate the extent of their expansion, so this description is also used here. Moreover, large antral follicles are described as either nonovulatory or preovulatory to indicate their maturity according to accepted functional criteria. We shall discuss the differing steroidogenic functions of follicles according to several of these morphological categories.

Initially, a prefollicular phase will be considered. This phase does not represent a follicular stage but, rather, a brief period in ovarian organogenesis before the onset of folliculogenesis, the process whereby germ cells associate with the follicular cells to form primordial follicles. This prefollicular phase can occur in embryonic life, in the neonate, or even in later prepubertal stages depending on the species.

The Prefollicular Ovary

The prefollicular phase of ovarian development would appear to be largely devoid of steroidogenic function in some, but not all, species. However, this view may reflect the great difficulty in assessing steroid production at early stages in certain smaller animals.

Steroid synthesis in rodent ovaries is undetectable or very limited before follicles form (70,508). The rat ovary, which begins forming follicles on postnatal day 1 (509,510), was shown to be unresponsive to gonadotropic stimulation of estrogen production during the fetal period (511). Histochemical activity of Δ^5-3β-hydroxysteroid dehydrogenase has been demonstrated in prefollicular ovaries of rat (512) but only in the interstitial cells, with no activity apparent in granulosa cells. In neonatal mouse ovaries, in which folliculogenesis begins on postpartum day 2 (513–515), significant histochemical activity for Δ^5-3β-hydroxysteroid dehydrogenase first appears in the intraovarian rete cells at 7 days of age (70). However, in all these studies, the presence of histochemical enzyme activity does not establish that the enzyme is functioning as part of a biosynthetic pathway.

In contrast to studies in rodents, prefollicular ovaries of rabbit (516), sheep (517), and cow (518) apparently synthesize or have certain functional enzymes required to synthesize steroids even before initiation of meiosis in the oocytes, which precedes follicle formation. Studies in the rabbit demonstrated conversion of testosterone to estradiol by ovaries at day 18 of gestation, but the presence of endogenous androgen substrate was not determined (516). Other studies showed that gonadotropins were able to stimulate progesterone production by cultured rabbit granulosa cells, isolated from ovaries at the early postnatal period, but only after follicles had formed (519); folliculogenesis begins in this species at 14 days of age (520–522). In bovine ovaries, in which folliculogenesis begins about day 95 of fetal life (523), estradiol production has been detected as early as 45 ± 3 days of fetal age but was biphasic and subsequently declined (518,524). The onset of ovarian estradiol production occurred when the sex of the embryonic gonad was first distinguishable. *De novo* synthesis is believed to occur at this early fetal age since both testosterone and estradiol have been shown to be present in the ovaries. Furthermore, estradiol production *in vitro* is stimulated by LH. Progesterone and prostaglandins are produced even earlier, at day 30 of gestation (518). At much later gestational stages in the bovine, at least a month before term, ovaries *in vitro* convert [^{14}C]progesterone to several hydroxylated metabolites of C_{21}-steroids and to C_{19}-steroids, as well as convert [^{14}C]androstenedione to testosterone and estradiol (525). These conversions most probably involve enzymes present in both follicular and interstitial cells.

Steroidogenic function in prefollicular human ovaries has not been adequately investigated, but histochemical enzyme activity for Δ^5-3β-hydroxysteroid dehydrogenase has been demonstrated at this stage in the interstitial cells (526–528). Evidence for early steroidogenic function in human fetal ovaries following folliculogenesis is considered later (see section on preantral and early antral follicles, below).

Morphological evidence suggests biosynthetic and secretory activity in granulosa cells in prefollicular ovaries of various species. In general, these cells have numerous ribosomes and branching mitochondria and well-developed Golgi complexes, and they often contain lipid droplets. However, these features are not specific indicators of steroid-synthesizing cells, and they may reflect other biosynthetic functions associated with granulosa cell-oocyte cooperation. In the prefollicular ovary, oocytes and granulosa cells exist together within the irregular cords and nests of the ovarian cortex. The arrangement of oocytes and granulosa cells is closely packed, with extremely close apposition of plasma membranes, since at this time there is no zona pellucida to separate the granulosa cells from the oocyte. At this stage, therefore, granulosa cells may serve primarily to provide nutrients to the oocyte, a function that is certainly continued, in the developing follicles of adults, by the specialized granulosa cells of the corona radiata (60). Granulosa cells in prefollicular ovaries also appear to be active in the phagocytosis of degenerating germ cells.

Oocytes and granulosa cells are entirely interdependent in the formation of follicles, without which neither substantial steroidogenesis nor oocyte growth can occur. Therefore, a most important aspect of the prefollicular phase is the establishment of granulosa cell and oocyte associations leading to folliculogenesis. When the number of oocytes in the fetal ovary is greatly decreased by a genetic defect or destructive treatments, follicles rarely form, and the ovary is deficient in normal steroid production. An example is Turner's syndrome in humans, where the 45,X chromosome constitution results in a failure to differentiate oocytes and follicle organization is disrupted (529–531). The XO condition in mice is far less severe, and females are fertile and appear normal with the exceptions of reduced numbers of oocytes, a shorter reproductive life span (532), and developmental retardation (533). Destruction of oocytes in ovaries of fetal rats by treatment with the antimitotic drug busulphan (534,535) or irradiation (536) leads to a similar conclusion: Without oocytes, follicles do not form, and the resultant ovary consists mainly of stroma containing networks of cords and tubules resembling the intraovarian rete ovarii. Such ovaries lack steroidogenic functions and fail to develop responsiveness to gonadotropins (537).

In summary, the cells of the prefollicular phase in some, but not all, species appear to be steroidogenically inactive and to be unresponsive to gonadotropins in terms of steroid production. However, it is necessary to interpret the significance of these findings cautiously since apparent inactivity may reflect inadequate sensitivity of the assay procedures, while apparent activity of certain enzyme steps need not necessarily indicate biologically important *de novo* production of steroid hormones. Early differentiation of granulosa cells and their organization into follicles would appear to be influenced largely by interactions of these cells with oocytes and gonadotropins, but little is known about other local factors controlling early ovarian differentiation and folliculogenesis, including steroidogenesis.

Preantral and Early Antral Follicles

Preantral follicles develop from primary follicles by enlargement of the oocyte and proliferation of the supporting granulosa cells. The factors responsible for initiation of growth of follicles from the nongrowing pool are unknown but have previously been discussed in terms of regulation by the oocyte or granulosa cells (538). Subsequent development of preantral follicles is not dependent on gonadotropins and continues after hypophysectomy (539). As the follicle enlarges, theca cells differentiate from cells within the ovarian stroma, thereby forming a sheath of flattened cells around the follicular basement membrane. Formation of the theca layer is quite variable among individual follicles in the mouse but becomes distinct at the multilaminar stage. In the hamster, theca appears to differentiate in follicles with seven or eight layers of granulosa cells (540). In the mouse, only later, when the antrum forms, does the theca differentiate further into theca interna and externa (541,542).

Evidence of various types, largely indirect, suggests that in several species limited steroidogenic activity is probably acquired at the preantral stage of follicle development, although it is weakly expressed until the antral stage. FSH receptors are found on rat granulosa cells at all follicular stages, including early preantral follicles

(543,544). However, the precise contributions of preantral follicles to ovarian steroid production are not well understood, primarily because of difficulties in studying the relatively low secretory activities of these follicles *in vivo* and because methodology for isolating preantral follicles is not well developed. Only recently has an improved enzymatic and mechanical method been developed for the isolation of various stages of intact preantral follicles in the hamster (540). Research on early follicles has also been neglected in favor of the functionally more important Graafian follicle. Several different approaches for deducing the steroidogenic function of preantral follicles are discussed below.

The formation of preantral follicles in the neonatal period of the rat provides an opportunity to examine gonadotropin responsiveness and steroidogenesis in ovaries containing only small follicles, early preantral follicles, and interstitial cells. Since theca cells from the immature rat produce negligible amounts of estrogens (190) and rat ovarian interstitial cell preparations in culture produce only small quantities of estrogens (86), neonatal ovarian synthesis of estrogens *in vitro* may be an indicator of aromatase activity in the granulosa cells. However, it is also possible that neonatal thecal and interstitial cells at this age differ from those in older rats and are capable of significant estrogen biosynthesis.

Follicle growth in the neonatal rat begins by postpartum day 2, with multilaminar follicles forming by day 6, but it is not until about day 10 that the first follicles containing antra appear in significant numbers. The available data suggest that preantral follicles of the neonatal period may respond to gonadotropins and produce steroids. Quattropani and Weisz (545) have shown that Δ^5-3β-hydroxysteroid dehydrogenase activity is present histochemically in interstitial cells of day 4 rat ovaries and that as early as day 5, ovaries are capable of converting [^{3}H]progesterone to estrogens. These investigators suggested that the interstitial cells were solely responsible for these steroidogenic activities in the neonatal rat. However, FSH binding sites, which are thought to be specific for granulosa cells, have also been demonstrated in the ovary as early as day 5 (546), and FSH has been found to stimulate both cAMP and steroid production by ovaries of 4-day-old rats (547).

Other studies with cultured ovaries from 4-day-old rats have shown that progesterone production is stimulated by $(Bu)_2$cAMP and conversion of testosterone to estradiol is stimulated by $(Bu)_2$cAMP or FSH (548). Furthermore, estrogen production in these studies was not substantially stimulated by FSH alone, but was greatly augmented by FSH in combination with LH (548), which is consistent with a "two-cell type, two-gonadotropin" form of regulation at this early developmental stage.

Recent studies involving similar *in vitro* incubations of rat ovaries have established that purified FSH, LH, or PGE_2 will each stimulate, to a different extent, the production of progesterone, androstenedione, and estradiol by ovaries at day 6 but not earlier (547). In these studies, secondary preantral follicles were the most advanced stages present at this time, suggesting that gonadotropin-regulated *de novo* synthesis of the three major classes of steroids might be produced by the developing preantral follicles in cooperation with the interstitial cells. In these studies, LH was by far the most potent stimulus for androstenedione and estradiol production, but addition of the phosphodiesterase inhibitor 3-isobutyl-1-methylxanthine (MIX) resulted in enhanced responsiveness to both FSH and LH, with FSH then having a potency equal to that of LH. The contention that phosphodiesterase activity limits steroidogenic responsiveness to gonadotropins in early ovaries was confirmed in incubations of 4-day-old ovaries, which only in the presence of MIX allowed increases in androstenedione secretion in response to PGE_2, LH, and FSH and increases in estradiol in response to PGE_2 alone (547). These results indicate that steroidogenic capabilities differentiate in neonatal rat ovaries even before acquisition of full responsiveness to gonadotropins, and certainly well before formation of antral follicles. The responsiveness to LH might also be regulated by local steroid action since other investigators have shown that estrogen treatment of neonatal rats advances the age at which LH-stimulated cAMP can be demonstrated *in vitro* (549).

The extent to which steroidogenic activities seen in neonatal rat ovaries might be influenced by the high circulating levels of FSH (550,551) and other pituitary hormones (552) present during this period is uncertain. It can only be speculated that the steroidogenic pathways seen in neonatal rat ovaries might be similarly expressed as a result of the cooperation of preantral follicles and interstitial cells present in ovaries at later developmental ages, including adults. Steroids secreted by preantral follicles at all developmental ages might influence local concentrations within the ovary, thereby affecting follicular function or maturation. However, the studies described above with whole neonatal ovary incubations do not provide conclusive evidence that significant steroidogenesis occurs within the follicular compartment, as opposed to the interstitial cells.

Similarly, there is no direct information on the steroidogenic function of preantral follicles in the adult human ovary. However, studies have investigated steroidogenic activity of fetal ovarian tissue *in vitro*. Most of the studies have obtained ovarian tissue at fetal ages later than the beginning of folliculogenesis, which occurs at about 8 weeks of gestation in the human (553). Therefore, steroidogenic activities reported might partly reflect functions of early follicles. However, another potentially important steroidogenic cell population is found in the interstitium of ovaries from human fetuses at 12 to 20 weeks gestation (554). These interstitial cells of the embryonic ovary, also called primary interstitial cells (97), are located in the medullary region beneath the cortical cords and are often adjacent to blood vessels. Their fine structure is typical of steroidogenic cells, and they are relatively large (>30 μm greatest diameter).

The evidence for steroidogenesis in human fetal ovaries is based on experiments in which fetal ovarian tissues were incubated in the presence of radioactive steroid precursors. The ability to convert [^{3}H]testosterone or androstenedione into estradiol and estrone was not apparent in undifferentiated gonads of human fetuses at approximately 6 to 8 weeks gestation but was acquired at about 8 to 10 weeks and continued to be present until at least midgestation (555). However, George and Wilson cautioned that their results alone do not give evidence of *de novo* estrogen synthesis from endogenous substrates. Earlier studies with ovaries from more advanced fetuses (16–22 weeks gestation) did not find evidence of C_{19}-steroid synthesis from [^{14}C]progesterone (556) or from [1-^{14}C]acetate (557), but in the latter study acetate was converted to lanosterol, cholesterol, and smaller quantities of pregnenolone and progesterone. A further study in which fetal ovarian tissue was incubated with [^{14}C]-pregnenolone found progesterone to be the main product, but products of the 5-ene-3β-hydroxy-steroid pathway, 17α-hydroxypregnenolone and dehydroepiandrosterone, were also identified (558). An earlier study demonstrated the active conversion of [^{14}C]progesterone to 20α-dihydroprogesterone in fetal ovaries at 19 weeks but not at 12 to 15 weeks of gestation (559). More recently, in organ cultures of ovaries from three fetuses (12, 20, and 22 weeks gestation), release of progesterone, dehydroepiandrosterone, androstenedione, estrone, and estradiol (560) was reported. It was also found that progesterone production *in vitro* was stimulated by $(Bu)_2$cAMP and, to a lesser extent, by LH/FSH.

A most interesting finding is the substantial conversion by fetal human ovaries (at approximately 12.5–17.5 weeks gestation) of [^{3}H]pregnenolone sulfate into pregnenolone, 17α-hydroxypregnenolone, dehydroepiandrosterone, and androstenedione but without formation of progesterone, testosterone, or estrogens (561). This indicates the presence of steroid sulfatase activity in the fetal ovary and the ability to convert C_{21}-steroids to C_{19}-steroids via the 5-ene-3β-hydroxysteroid pathway, similar to the preferred pathway to androstenedione in the adult ovary (84). The presence of a high concentration of pregnenolone sulfate in fetal blood (562) suggests there is a natural substrate available. These studies indicate that the human fetal ovary is steroidogenically active at developmental stages after initiation of folliculogenesis but when embryonic interstitial cells are also present. It is possible that both early follicular cells and interstitial cells contribute to the conversions observed. However, the presence of the interstitial cells precludes deductions regarding the steroidogenic functions of early stages of human follicles. As mentioned previously, interstitial cells in the human ovary are histochemically reactive for Δ^5-3β-hydroxysteroid dehydrogenase even in prefollicular stages.

One study with fetal ovaries of rhesus monkeys indicates that the capacity for *de novo* production of estradiol is acquired only in late gestation, when multilayered and antral follicles have already developed (563); this suggests that preantral follicles may not contribute significantly to estrogen production in this species, at least during fetal life.

A more direct, but little used approach to assess steroidogenesis in preantral follicles at various stages of development has been to obtain dispersed follicles by enzymatic and/or mechanical procedures. In one study, dispersed ovarian tissues from immature mice were cultured *in vivo* as transplants, either implanted subcutaneously in gelfoam sponges or diffusion chambers or as cells implanted into intraocular sites (564). Intraocular transplants were accompanied by a fragment of vaginal epithelium as a biological indicator of estrogen production. These studies demonstrated that subcutaneous transplants into ovariectomized mice caused vaginal opening and onset of estrous cycles similar to that seen in nonovariectomized controls, and intraocular transplants promoted cornification of the vaginal fragment. In the latter situation, follicles transplanted together with dispersed ovarian cells, presumably containing androgen-secreting interstitial cells, were far more effective in causing vaginal cornification. Most importantly, it was noted that vaginal cornification, taken as a measure of estrogen production, was apparent only when growth of follicles and concomitant maturation of antra were observed. Therefore, while preantral follicles might have contributed to estrogen production by transplants of dispersed ovarian tissues, these studies suggest that substantial secretion of estrogens requires antral follicles.

Enzymatic dispersion of the ovarian compartments has also been used successfully to harvest all but the most mature antral follicles from rabbit ovaries (565). Measurements of follicular steroid content, which undoubtedly reflect steroid uptake from other compartments and follicles at different stages, as well as biosynthesis, suggest a progressive increase in levels of progesterone and estrogen as follicles develop from small primary to large antral stages. However, since *de novo* synthesis was not conclusively demonstrated, these results do not necessarily establish the steroidogenic abilities of early rabbit follicles.

Preantral follicles have been isolated from ovaries of cyclic hamsters and incubated *in vitro* to assess LH-stimulated steroid production (566). These studies indicate that isolated preantral follicles show a shift in LH-stimulated steroid products, depending on the time of follicle isolation relative to the endogenous LH surge. Before the LH surge during proestrus, androstenedione production predominated; immediately following the endogenous LH surge, the isolated preantral follicles produced only progesterone. The ability to produce androstenedione, and additionally estradiol, reappeared in follicles isolated on the afternoon of estrus. Subsequently, isolated small antral follicles, which had developed from preantral follicles present at estrus, produced mainly estradiol and androstenedione, with only smaller amounts of progesterone. It is apparent that steroidogenesis can occur in isolated preantral hamster follicles and that *in vivo* the LH surge may act to synchronize steroidogenesis by these follicles (566).

Many *in vivo* studies with immature normal or hypophysectomized rats indicate that ovaries consisting primarily of larger preantral follicles are steroidogenically responsive to gonadotropins (FSH and/or LH). However, these animal models do not allow the action of FSH in inducing steroidogenic activity to be distinguished from the concurrent effect of FSH on formation of follicular antra. Large preantral follicles that form in hypophysectomized rats do not show autonomous synthesis of estrogens but require stimulation with FSH and either LH or aromatizable androgen (209). It would appear that significant aromatase activity occurs only as antral follicles form in response to FSH stimulation.

Several models exist for the culture of granulosa cells from ovaries containing primarily small and preantral follicles. Granulosa cells can be obtained either from normal immature rats before large antral follicles have formed or from immature hypophysectomized rats, in which very few small tertiary follicles will form in the absence of gonadotropin stimulation. In both models, treatment with estrogen is often used to stimulate the numbers of relatively uniform preantral follicles; in addition, this treatment greatly increases the responsiveness of the cells to FSH. Regardless of the model employed, granulosa cells isolated from ovaries of these animals show minimal production of progestins or estrogens when cultured without gonadotropins, even in the presence of aromatizable substrates. Other features of granulosa cytodifferentiation, such as LH receptor formation, are also absent in cells cultured without gonadotropins, indicating that these cells are minimally differentiated. Therefore, it is apparent that key steroidogenic enzymes are lacking or weakly expressed in granulosa cells of preantral follicles in hypophysectomized or normal immature rats. Since preantral follicles can, and probably do, develop without gonadotropin support, it is likely that the granulosa cells of at least early preantral stages are not very active steroid producers. However, it is probably that cyclical increases in circulating gonadotropins act in a coordinate fashion to stimulate cytodifferentiation and steroidogenesis in granulosa cells of late preantral follicles. Granulosa cells from preantral follicles of rats respond in culture to FSH with increased secretion of C_{21}-steroids and increased aromatase activity. These steroidogenic effects *in vitro* usually appear after a delay of about 24 hr, suggesting the need for induction of steroidogenic enzymes.

Certain steroidogenic enzymes are present (although perhaps not maximally expressed) in preantral follicles that have not been stimulated with gonadotropins. Granulosa cells isolated from immature rats and placed in culture are able to convert exogenous pregnenolone to progesterone, 20α-dihydroprogesterone, and, probably in lesser amounts, 5α-reduced C_{21}-steroid metabolites (47). They also convert testosterone rapidly to its 5α-reduced metabolites, including 5α-androstane-$3\alpha,17\beta$-diol and androsterone (141). Histochemical demonstration of Δ^5-3β-hydroxysteroid dehydrogenase activity in the rat ovary indicates that this enzyme is strongly expressed in granulosa cells of preovulatory follicles but is only weakly expressed in earlier antral stages (567). This is consistent with the biochemical evidence that induction of this enzyme requires FSH stimulation of the granulosa cells (141).

A variety of factors might be responsible for limiting the steroidogenic competency of preantral follicles. Although the granulosa cells have FSH receptors that, at least in late preantral follicles, are functionally coupled to adenylate cyclase, these receptors do not function optimally since estrogen is required to augment FSH-stimulated cAMP production. This increased cAMP response in turn allows FSH to increase aromatase activity and estrogen synthesis and to increase the number of gonadotropin receptors and cAMP binding sites (568). These changes are associated with development of the antral follicle. Further, although it is generally assumed that circulating FSH and LH are similarly available to the granulosa cells of preantral and later-stage follicles by diffusion from capillaries of the theca layer through the follicular wall and into the granulosa cell layers, this assumption has not been critically tested. However, molecular size per se is not a limiting factor for gonadotropin penetration of the follicular membrane (569). The ability of healthy and steroidogenically active follicles to concentrate gonadotropins in follicular fluid suggests the probable importance of the availability of FSH to steroid production. Thus, while it is clear that follicle cells isolated from large preantral follicles respond to gonadotropins and require them for steroid production, it is uncertain to what extent preantral follicles from various species secrete steroids *in vivo* in response to normal cyclical fluctuations in circulating gonadotropin levels.

Antral to Early Preovulatory Follicles

There is general agreement that the antral stages of follicular development, and especially the early preovulatory follicles, are by far the most important source of ovarian steroids during the female cycle. This changing pattern of steroid secretion is associated with increased follicle cell growth and cytodifferentiation and considerable expansion of the antrum, which occur in response to changing levels of FSH and LH. The ability to secrete significant quantities of estrogens, a function acquired as antral follicles form, is of key importance in increasing the responsiveness of the granulosa cells to FSH and subsequently to LH (570–572). The direct action of estrogen at the follicular level and the additional indirect effect of feedback inhibition of gonadotropin secretion are important contributing factors in follicular selection.

The formation of the fluid-filled antrum provides a convenient morphological marker of the stage in follicle development when gonadotropin-dependent growth of the follicle approximately begins and steroid secretion greatly increases. Antrum formation is induced by the action of FSH, but not LH alone, and presumably reflects changes in the FSH-dependent secretory function of the granulosa cells, as well as influx of interstitial fluid (569,573). Increased follicular vascularization and steroidal effects on follicular vascular permeability could also be factors in antral fluid accumulation (569). However, antrum formation is apparently not a necessary feature of preovulatory follicular maturation in all species, since in several exceptional families (i.e., *Tenrecidae* and *Erinaceidae*), ovaries do not form antral follicles (574).

Granulosa cells of early antral follicles do not generally have ultrastructural features characteristic of steroid-secreting cells. This was originally taken as evidence of their nonsteroidogenic function until later histochemical and biochemical evidence changed that view. Only after the LH surge are substantial ultrastructural changes seen in organelles associated with steroidogenesis in the granulosa cells. These changes, which are considered the earliest signs of morphological luteinization and may occur prior to ovulation in certain species (575), are discussed in the next section.

We have already reviewed the evidence for steroid pathways present in mature granulosa and theca cells of antral follicles and considered the types of cellular cooperation involved in regulating steroid production at this stage. In this section, we consider only the additional evidence indicating that the major sources of ovarian estrogens and progesterone during the follicular phase are the large antral and preovulatory follicles, and that both small and large antral follicles are significant sources of androgens prior to the LH surge. This evidence comes mainly from measurements comparing steroid levels in ovarian venous plasma or in follicular fluid with those in peripheral plasma.

Steroid measurements in ovarian venous plasma reflect rates of ovarian secretion into the circulation. For example, a close relationship between follicular production of certain steroids and secretion into blood is apparent, since pulsatile release of LH in sheep is followed rapidly by steroid secretion into the ovarian vein, with peak levels of estradiol and androstenedione occurring 30 min after each pulse (576). In comparison, steroid measurements in follicular fluid provide a static profile of the pool of steroids secreted primarily by the granulosa and theca cells of one follicle. However, the concentrations of steroids in follicular fluid reflect not only secretion into the fluid, but also changes due to metabolism and dilution as fluid accumulates. Transfer of steroids from follicular fluid to venous plasma occurs only slowly. As demonstrated in the mare, the hourly transfer of radiolabeled pregnenolone and androstenedione from follicular fluid to ovarian vein was approximately 3% to 9% (189). The export of free and conjugated steroids from follicular fluid might also be impaired by binding globulins in the fluid (577,578). In this regard, species differences occur since sex hormone-binding globulin is present in blood plasma and follicular fluid of the cow and sheep but not the pig (579).

Estrogens

Estrogen secretion in women is highest during the late follicular phase of the menstrual cycle (580). At this time, estrogen levels are significantly higher in ovarian venous plasma from ovaries containing a large antral follicle (>8 mm diameter) compared with contralateral ovaries containing small antral follicles (<8 mm diameter) (581). This difference is about 15-fold for estradiol and 7-fold for estrone. Furthermore, venous plasma levels of estrogens from ovaries containing small follicles are only about 1.6-fold greater than levels in peripheral plasma, indicating the relatively low rate of estrogen secretion by small antral follicles. At other times in the cycle, from menstruation to the early follicular phase, when peripheral estrogen levels are low, there are no differences in venous plasma levels between right and left ovaries (581).

Follicular fluid levels of estrogens measured in small and large antral follicles (according to the sizes described above) throughout the human menstrual cycle provide additional evidence that it is the large antral follicles of the middle and late follicular phase that secrete the greatest quantities of estrogens (581,582). In several different studies, fluids from large follicles at late follicular phase have been reported to have mean estradiol concentrations in the range of 1,500 to 2,400 ng/ml (581–585). In contrast with these types of follicles, fluid obtained from large antral follicles at early follicular or luteal phases of the cycle had low estrogen concentrations that did not differ from those in small antral follicles (581). Furthermore, small antral follicles (<8 mm diameter) showed only small fluctuations in concentrations of estrogens throughout the follicular and luteal phases. However, a more recent study in the human indicates that relatively high intrafollicular concentrations of estradiol (>200 ng/

ml) are also found in certain small antral follicles (4–7 mm in diameter) from follicular and luteal phases of the cycle (586), when these follicles are judged to be healthy. In this study, a healthy follicle was defined as having a nondegenerative oocyte and at least 50% of the maximum number of granulosa cells present for a given follicular diameter. Therefore, estrogen concentrations in human follicular fluid are substantially elevated only in healthy antral follicles and are greatest in healthy large antral follicles that have developed at the appropriate stage of the cycle, i.e., preovulatory follicles.

Consistent with the observations on follicular fluid levels of estrogens, much higher levels of aromatase activity, determined *in vitro,* are present in large preovulatory follicles compared with nonovulatory antral follicles taken during the late follicular phase in women (131,587). Furthermore, aromatase activity in granulosa cells of the dominant follicle in humans becomes maximal during the midfollicular phase and cannot be further stimulated by FSH *in vitro* (131,586). In comparison, when FSH and LH levels are suppressed by steroid negative feedback from the corpus luteum during the human luteal phase, follicles are not recruited for preovulatory estrogen biosynthesis; hence, follicular fluid concentrations of estrogens remain low.

Estrogenic follicles in the human are distinguished by two other important features. First, elevated estradiol concentrations in these follicles occur only when intrafollicular FSH is also elevated (>1.3 mU/ml), indicating the key regulatory role of FSH (582). Second, the importance of granulosa cells in estrogen production is further indicated by the positive relation between the number of granulosa cells and the intrafollicular estradiol concentration for a given size of antral follicle (588). Thus, it appears that preovulatory follicles prior to the midcycle LH surge are characterized by much higher estrogen biosynthetic activity and estrogen content, higher FSH concentrations, and more granulosa cells than in nonovulatory or atretic follicles (131,584,589,590).

Studies of numerous other species—including sheep (591), cows (109), pigs (592), rabbits (593), and rats (594)—report similarly high levels of estrogens in follicular fluid from large antral follicles, with maximal concentrations occurring in the preovulatory period, before or immediately after the LH surge. On the other hand, fluid from atretic follicles of various species, like the human, characteristically exhibits substantially lower estradiol concentrations (109,276,588,595,596).

Over 90% of the circulating estradiol secreted during the late follicular phase of monotocous species originates from the dominant follicle (597,598). In women, normally only one antral follicle matures to preovulatory eminence. Estradiol levels in the fluid of the dominant follicle before the midcycle LH surge is on the order of 1 to 2 μg/ml (131,569,597), and similar estrogen levels have been found in fluids from ovaries of cyclic (597,599–602) and gonadotropin-stimulated (603,604) women. Results from various other monotocous species are comparable (187,213,603,605–607). Therefore, this evidence indicates that the dominant follicle is the principal source of the preovulatory estrogen surge that appears in plasma. This conclusion has been directly supported by studies in women that measured the large decrease in ovarian venous plasma levels of estradiol and estrone following surgical enucleation (i.e., intact removal) of the largest follicle (608). This preovulatory estrogen production is apparently regulated by LH-stimulated production of aromatizable androgens in the theca cells (discussed below; see also the section on post-LH surge preovulatory follicles), in agreement with evidence that granulosa aromatase activity is already maximally stimulated in early preovulatory follicles and cannot be further stimulated by FSH in cells from follicles >12 mm in diameter at midfollicular phase (586).

Some insight into the physiological factors regulating follicular estrogen biosynthesis during the preovulatory period has been provided from *in vitro* incubations of follicles at different stages of the estrous cycle. In the rat, regulation of estradiol production by isolated preovulatory follicles appears to be principally at the level of production of aromatizable androgens. When follicles from ovaries of 5-day cycling rats were incubated individually, accumulation of estradiol in the culture medium increased from low levels at diestrus I to high levels at proestrus (609). Estradiol accumulation by follicles obtained at either diestrus or proestrus was increased by addition of androstenedione or testosterone (indicating the presence of aromatase activity) or by addition of 17α-hydroxyprogesterone or progesterone (indicating the presence of 17α-hydroxylase:C-17,20-lyase enzyme required for conversion of progesterone to androgens). In these studies measurements of follicular enzyme activities at diestrus and proestrus demonstrated little change in lyase activity and a small increase in aromatase activity at proestrus. Since C-17,20-lyase activity was always more limiting than aromatase activity, it was concluded that increased estradiol production at proestrus might be due to an increase in endogenous production of progesterone, with greater conversion to androgens. This was supported by the finding that pregnenolone accumulation in medium from follicle incubations, carried out in the presence of cyanoketone to inhibit metabolism to progesterone, increased between diestrus and proestrus (609). Other studies (as already discussed in the section on the theca) have indicated that increased thecal cell activities of 17α-hydroxylase:C-17,20-lyase are principally responsible for the increases in androgen production that occur as small antral follicles become preovulatory (102). Therefore, together, these results are consistent with the idea that LH-stimulated production of thecal androgens (via affects on C_{21} and C_{27} side-chain cleavage) is the controlling factor in estrogen secretion at proestrus in the rat. In this respect, the regulation of preovulatory estrogen secretion in the rat and human appears to be similar.

The regulation of follicular estrogen biosynthesis in developing follicles might in part be accomplished by secreted regulatory protein(s) that have been identified in fluids of preovulatory follicles in the human (610,611) and pig (612) and that have been shown to inhibit granulosa cell aromatase activity and reduce responsiveness to gonadotropins (611–613). The regulatory protein(s) might be one means by which the "selected" or dominant follicle in monotocous species causes neighboring follicles to become atretic. The positive relationship in preovulatory follicles between estrogen concentrations in follicular fluid and levels of aromatase-inhibiting activity suggests that the dominant follicle is insensitive to this inhibitor (613). Evidence in women that this factor is secreted into the venous blood of ovaries containing a preovulatory follicle but not of contralateral ovaries suggests that interovarian, as well as intraovarian, regulation may be involved (614).

Androgens

Follicular fluid measurements demonstrate that antral follicles at all stages of the menstrual cycle in women are significant sources of C_{19}-steroids including androstenedione, testosterone, and their 5α-reduced metabolites. Since androstenedione and testosterone are not synthesized *de novo* in significant quantities by granulosa cells, they must be secreted into the follicular fluid by the theca cells of the follicle and perhaps also by the interstitial cells. However, granulosa and theca cells are capable of 5α-reduction of testosterone to 5α-dihydrotestosterone and further metabolism to 5α-androstane-3α,17β-diol and androsterone, so these metabolites might arise partly by conversion in the granulosa cells. Follicular fluid of women (275,615) and pigs (616) and extracts of rat ovary (79) contain 5α-dihydrotestosterone. The relative levels of androstenedione and testosterone in follicular fluid are probably also influenced by interconversion via 17β-hydroxysteroid dehydrogenase in the granulosa cells, as discussed earlier.

In women, the dominant androgen, androstenedione, has been measured in small and large antral follicles throughout the menstrual cycle (581). Concentrations of androstenedione in follicular fluid are between 100 and 500 times that in peripheral plasma (569). The highest concentrations of androstenedione in follicular fluid are found at midfollicular phase (745 ng/ml), with a substantial decrease occurring by the late follicular phase (120 ng/ml) (584). At the late follicular phase there is a significantly greater concentration of androstenedione in small antral follicles (726 ng/ml) than in large antral follicles (266 ng/ml) (581). At all other phases of the menstrual cycle, the differences between androgen concentrations in large and small antral follicles are not significant. Concentrations of testosterone, although considerably lower than androstenedione, show a similar pattern of change, with the highest levels occurring in small antral follicles at midcycle (104 ng/ml) but with lower concentrations in large antral follicles throughout the follicular phase (25–38 ng/ml) (581).

Androgen concentrations might be less in large antral follicles at the late follicular phase partly because of substantially greater conversion to estrogens and partly because of greater secretion into the blood due to the increased vascularization of the theca (581,617). Another contributing factor in the declining level of androgens observed in follicular fluid during the later stages of preovulatory follicle growth may be the inhibitory influence of the increasing estradiol concentrations on androgen biosynthesis in the theca cells (618,619). This possibility is supported by observations that the decline in androstenedione concentration occurring between the middle and late follicular phases is seen only in normal healthy follicles characterized by detectable levels of FSH in follicular fluid, while increased androstenedione concentrations are observed in follicles with undetectable FSH (584). Therefore, the role of FSH in inducing aromatase activity in granulosa cells appears to be an important factor in regulating follicular androgen concentrations. Estradiol, produced as a result of FSH-induced aromatase activity in granulosa cells, may feed back on the theca cells to inhibit production of its precursors, the aromatizable androgens. Such an intrafollicular negative-feedback system could be significant in limiting the rate of increase of estrogen secretion during the final stages of follicular growth; this would provide adequate time for completion of the process of cytoplasmic maturation of the oocyte before ovulation. An intrafollicular negative-feedback mechanism such as this could be particularly significant in polytocous species as a means of holding in check the most mature follicles in the selected ovulatory population: The less mature of the selected follicles could thereby continue to develop, thus resulting in a synchronous population by the time of the LH surge.

In bovine antral follicles, as in the human, changes in androgen and estrogen concentrations in follicular fluid are inversely related as follicles mature. Estradiol concentrations increase greatly as bovine follicles progress from small to large sizes, while androstenedione and testosterone concentrations decrease (620). A sharper decline in testosterone than androstenedione suggests that, as previously demonstrated (621,622), testosterone is the preferred substrate for aromatization in bovines, in contrast to the situation in the human. Another apparent difference from humans is that the concentration of FSH in bovine follicular fluid is not related to the high ratio of estradiol to androgen found in large follicles (620). This suggests that intrafollicular FSH is less likely to be a limiting factor for aromatization in bovine follicles than in human follicles. The bovine follicle may be exceptional also in another respect, since granulosa cells in this species have been reported to convert pregnenolone to 17α-hydroxprogesterone, and 17α-hydroxypregnenolone to androstenedione, indicating a possible role for these cells in C_{19}-steroid formation (85).

In the hamster, a different relationship of whole follicular concentrations of androgens and estrogens was seen in antral follicles stimulated with PMSG (623). After treatment with PMSG, testosterone and estrogen levels initially increased, the greatest concentrations occurring in middle-sized follicles; at longer intervals, however, testosterone concentrations decreased sharply in medium and large follicles, while estradiol and estrone concentrations declined less abruptly. Therefore, according to this model system in the hamster, a possible difference from other species is that androgen availability might become limiting to estrogen biosynthesis even before large antral follicles have formed.

Nonaromatic C_{18}-steroids are present in the follicular fluid of the mare and sow and are presumed to be products of follicular steroidogenesis. Equine follicular fluid was first shown to contain high levels of 19-norandrostenedione, with concentrations of this steroid at estrus being 30 to 160 ng/ml (4). More recently, 19-nortestosterone was also identified as a minor component in equine follicular fluid (6). Equine granulosa cells convert testosterone primarily to estrogens but also produce 19-nortestosterone and, apparently, lower amounts of 19-norandrostenedione (126), indicating an intrafollicular site of 19-norsteroid biosynthesis. Limited studies on follicular stages in the mare report that the highest concentrations of 19-norandrostenedione are present in fluids from large and preovulatory follicles, with lower levels present in less mature and atretic follicles (7). Porcine follicular fluid from preovulatory follicles obtained on days 19 and 20 of the estrous cycle also contains high concentrations of 19-norandrostenedione (21–25 μmol/liter, 5720–6810 ng/ml), with 19-nortestosterone being tentatively identified as a minor component (8). Follicular fluid concentrations of 19-norandrostenedione were increased after treatment of immature pigs with PMSG and decreased following subsequent hCG treatment (624). The physiological significance of 19-norsteroids in the follicle is not known, but they have been proposed as possible intermediates in estrogen biosynthesis in the mare (7) and as competitive inhibitors of aromatization in the pig (8). Furthermore, 19-norandrostenedione (0.5 μmol/liter) acts synergistically with cAMP to inhibit porcine oocyte maturation *in vitro,* suggesting another possible regulatory role in this species (625). Human ovarian tissue *in vitro* has been reported to convert testosterone to 19-norsteroids (626), but it has not been established that these steroids are present in human ovaries.

Progestins

Progesterone concentrations in follicular fluid of human follicles are much lower than in tissue of corpora lutea (627), but they vary substantially during the menstrual cycle and in small and large antral follicles. During the late follicular phase, concentrations are significantly higher in large antral follicles ($\sim$1300 ng/ml) than in small ones ($\sim$270 ng/ml) (582). Furthermore, the increase in follicular fluid progesterone concentration in large antral follicles occurs during the transition from midfollicular (760 ng/ml) to late follicular phases (1720 ng/ml), and this increase is associated with the presence of detectable levels of LH in the fluid (582). These increases in progesterone in the late follicular phase presumably reflect the increased secretion by granulosa cells; increased granulosa stimulation by LH would be expected as LH levels progressively rise in the second half of the follicular phase, at a time when FSH levels decline (628). LH has been shown to stimulate progesterone secretion by human granulosa cells from large antral follicles treated with FSH and estrogen (629). This effect of LH on human granulosa cells is presumably as a consequence of LH receptor induction, similar to that demonstrated in rat granulosa cells *in vivo* (87) and in culture (329). Luteinization of human granulosa cells appears to begin before ovulation since cells isolated in the preovulatory period produce large amounts of progesterone (630).

Pregnenolone, the immediate precursor of progesterone, is also substantially increased in fluid from large antral follicles at middle and late follicular phases in women (582). Levels on the order of 10 μg/ml are reported. Pregnenolone concentrations are also elevated in fluid from human preovulatory follicles aspirated 32 to 33 hr after treatment with hCG at midcycle, before the LH surge (631). Pregnenolone has been measured in bovine follicular fluid, with concentrations exceeding those of progesterone in the large preovulatory follicles present at proestrus (109).

Although the cellular origin of follicular fluid pregnenolone is uncertain, the likelihood that the granulosa cells are the source is supported by observations of high rates of pregnenolone secretion by cultured porcine granulosa cells (215). Evidence has been presented to suggest that pregnenolone in follicular fluid, secreted by granulosa cells, may undergo metabolism to progesterone by bovine theca cells (632) and to aromatizable androgens by porcine theca cells (215).

Preovulatory Follicles After the LH Surge

The ovulation-inducing LH surge causes concomitant changes in follicle cell structure, proliferative activity, and steroidogenesis of the preovulatory follicles. These changes occur in the interval between the LH peak and ovulation, this interval being relatively constant for each species; for example, 12 to 15 hr in mouse or rat and approximately 28 to 36 hr in human (633).

Ultrastructural changes occurring in granulosa cells of women prior to ovulation include a continuous change from granular to smooth endoplasmic reticulum (634,635) and a change to a more homogeneous chromatin structure (636). Typical characteristics of luteinization, such as an increase in smooth endoplasmic reticulum and the appearance of mitochondria with tubular cristae, begin to appear even before ovulation in many species (575). The ovulatory stimulus is also associated with changes in the quantities and types of gap junctions present between granulosa cells, as in the rabbit (637,638).

Mitoses are abundant in granulosa cells of large preovulatory follicles of certain species, including human (639), hamster (640), and guinea pig (641), but mitotic activity declines sharply between the LH surge and ovulation. In women the high mitotic index and nucleocytoplasmic ratio of granulosa cells in preovulatory follicles are apparently lowered even before the beginning of the LH surge (639). In the estrous rabbit, mitotic activity is greatest in cells of nonvesicular follicles but similarly declines following the mating-induced LH surge (642). These observations suggest that either the LH surge or perhaps related events preceding it are involved in suppressing granulosa cell proliferative activity as cells begin to luteinize. It is unknown whether these proliferative and steroidogenic changes are causally related. However, *in vivo* studies of PMSG/hCG superovulated rats indicate that increased steroidogenic activity develops only after DNA synthesis arrests (158,643), and recent *in vitro* studies with rat granulosa cells suggest that cell proliferation in culture and steroidogenic expression are inversely related (186).

Histochemical evidence of increased steroidogenic activity is also apparent as ovulation approaches. Activity of Δ^5-3β-hydroxysteroid dehydrogenase is weak in granulosa cells of developing antral follicles but increases about the time of the estrogen surge (644,645). Similarly in the hamster, activity of this enzyme increases towards the time of ovulation (640,646,647), when follicular progesterone synthesis increases (648). This enzyme is also active in granulosa cells of preovulatory human follicles, whereas it is limited to thecal cells in smaller antral follicles (585,649). In contrast with these changes in the granulosa cells, theca interna cells show high activity of Δ^5-3β-hydroxysteroid dehydrogenase throughout the maturation of the follicle.

Steroid production is substantially altered in the preovulatory period following the LH surge. Within minutes of the LH surge there is a transient increase in progesterone and estrogen secretion in several animal species, including rat, monkey, and rabbit, followed by a marked decline to basal levels within several hours (241, 310,593,650–653). This inhibitory phase following the LH surge or after hCG treatment is marked by decreased concentrations of aromatizable androgens and estrogens in follicular fluid or ovaries of all species studied, including rat (243), hamster (654), sheep (655), bovine (656), and human (657,658).

In the rat, a large preovulatory peak of progesterone and 20α-dihydroprogesterone occurs close to the time of the LH peak. These extremely high levels of progestins (i.e., greater than in the short luteal phase at diestrus) are probably derived from the granulosa cells as they begin the process of luteinization, although the extent of contributions from theca-interstitial cells is uncertain. LH stimulates progesterone secretion *in vitro* by mature granulosa cells of the rat (293,571), and *in vivo* pretreatment with testosterone significantly enhances this secretion (289). Measurements of steroids in follicular fluid of preovulatory follicles have been made in rats first given low-dose PMSG treatment to induce follicle maturation and then LH to induce ovulation (243). In these studies, the progesterone concentration in follicular fluid increased sevenfold within 1 hr of LH treatment and remained elevated throughout the 10-hr study. Androstenedione and estradiol concentrations in fluid were elevated before LH treatment, increased slightly 1 to 2 hr after LH, and then fell to extremely low levels by 6 hr. In other studies, inhibition of steroidogenesis, and in particular of estradiol production, occurs during the latter half of the preovulatory period in rat (104,310,650,653), sheep (659), and pig (660). In the rabbit, where the LH surge is a reflex response induced by mating, follicles isolated at 2 and 12 hours after mating showed, respectively, a rapid rise then a fall in progesterone and estradiol synthesis from [^{14}C]acetate (651).

A similar type of steroidogenic regulation occurs in the human ovary following the LH surge. Human ovarian slices initially showed increased conversion of [^{14}C]-acetate into pregnenolone, progesterone, 17α-hydroxyprogesterone, androstenedione (principal androgen), and estrogens (661). Subsequently, there was substantial reduction in the synthesis of pregnenolone and 17α-hydroxyprogesterone and, at the same time, almost complete inhibition of androgen and estrogen production (661). Fluid from human follicles after the LH surge also shows a progressive decrease over 38 hr in concentrations of estradiol and androstenedione, testosterone, and dehydroepiandrosterone (657). Similar results have been obtained in other studies (588,615,631). Despite the decrease in estradiol concentrations in human follicular fluid following the LH surge, preovulatory follicles still have the ability to aromatize androgens *in vivo* (583) and *in vitro* (662). Progesterone production decreases only slightly in the preovulatory period and then rises steadily toward ovulation (630,663), while estradiol synthesis remains low (651). Luteinization is well advanced

15 to 20 hr after the beginning of the LH surge, as indicated by high progesterone concentrations in follicular fluid (~13 μg/ml), with a further increase occurring (~18 μg/ml) after more than 27 hr (662). Progesterone concentrations in follicular fluid have been observed to peak between 5 and 25 hr after the onset of the LH surge, while the concentrations of 17α-hydroxyprogesterone change little (657). Measurements of steroids in blood during the preovulatory period in women provide similar evidence of changes in ovarian steroid secretion (630).

Regulation of the transient inhibition of steroid production in the preovulatory period of all species probably occurs at several levels. Evidence from luteal cells (356,357,664) and granulosa cells (358,359) indicates that relatively high concentrations of LH cause a transient desensitization at the gonadotropin receptor level such that target cells become refractory to gonadotropin stimulation of adenylate cyclase and steroid production. Desensitization in granulosa cells is followed by a down-regulation of receptors for LH, FSH, and estrogen (665,666). Normally during the luteal phase new receptors form and cells regain their sensitivity to LH at a time when progesterone production greatly increases. Pulsatile release of tonic levels of LH during the follicular phase may be important in preventing desensitization and down-regulation, which naturally occur in response to high concentrations and prolonged exposure to LH at midcycle.

Inhibition of estradiol production following the preovulatory LH surge is primarily the result of decreased androgen production in theca and interstitial cells. In an *in vitro* study with rat Graafian follicles in culture, inhibition of androgen secretion appeared to result from reduced 17α-hydroxylase and/or C-17,20-lyase activity since there was a concomitant inhibition of estradiol, androstenedione, and testosterone accumulation 4 to 6 hr after LH treatment (104). The authors of this study suggested that an LH-stimulated protein factor might inhibit enzymes required for cleavage of the C-17 side chain of progesterone. A subsequent study with PMSG-primed immature rats showed that a maximal ovulatory dose of LH *in vivo* caused an initial increase in ovarian androgen after 2 hr and then a reduction in androgens and estradiol 4 to 8 hr after LH injection, with serum concentrations declining after 6 hr (310). Aromatase activity in the ovarian microsomal fraction was also inhibited in a noncompetitive manner between 4 and 8 hr after LH treatment *in vivo,* consistent with either inactivation of the aromatase complex or reduced biosynthesis and rapid turnover of this enzyme. These results led to the suggestion that LH-induced inhibition of estrogen production in the rat occurred mainly at the level of 17α-hydroxylase:C-17,20-lyase, followed by a secondary decrease in aromatase activity (310). Other *in vivo* and *in vitro* studies in rats provide clear evidence that the major cause of the rapid decline in estrogen secretion after the LH surge is limited availability of aromatizable androgens, due to the decreased rate of C_{21} side-chain cleavage. The decreased ovarian content of estradiol following injection of hCG could be completely prevented by *in vivo* administration of testosterone (667) or by *in vitro* incubation of isolated follicles with aromatizable substrate (668). The decreased levels of 17α-hydroxylase:C-17,20-lyase responsible for the declining androgen production have been found to be associated with a marked reduction in the microsomal cytochrome P-450 levels in the preovulatory ovary. These experiments involving inhibitors of RNA and protein synthesis provided evidence that the LH-induced decline in activity of these rate-limiting enzymes was dependent on continuing synthesis of RNA and protein (669).

Recent studies indicate that the inhibition of the C_{21} side-chain cleavage reaction following treatment of proestrous rats with an ovulatory dose of hCG is at the levels of NADPH- and NADH-linked lyase reactions and selectively at the NADH-linked 17α-hydroxylase (670). It is possible that these apparently distinct lyase and hydroxylase activities detected after cell disruption do not reflect the true nature of the C_{21} side-chain cleavage system. As mentioned previously, direct immunoblot measurements of cytochrome P-450 for this enzyme in bovine follicles established that the enzyme protein decreases to undetectable levels at the earliest stage of corpora lutea formation (105). Inhibition of aromatase cannot be ruled out as a minor regulatory mechanism following LH treatment. Preovulatory estrogen secretion, which peaks slightly before the LH surge, has been suggested to mediate the inhibitory action on androgen production by a direct intraovarian action on the ovary (233). Support for this idea has been provided by results of *in vitro* studies indicating that estradiol inhibits androgen production by rat ovarian interstitial cell preparations (86). Evidence for a similar inhibitory effect of estradiol on androgen production by isolated porcine theca cells has also been reported (619) and recently confirmed (235).

Morphological signs of theca cell regression suggest that the activity of this cell type is reduced in the late preovulatory period in sheep (671) and human (672). Other studies of advanced human preovulatory follicles show that there are fewer theca cells and that they are associated with hemorrhagic lesions when androgen synthesis is minimal (661). However, in the rat, estrogen-priming *in vivo* actually increases the *in vitro* LH-stimulated progesterone response of theca cell preparations, suggesting that viability of theca cells is maintained despite reduced androgen production (234).

Prostaglandins may also be involved in steroidogenic regulation during the preovulatory period. High levels of prostaglandins (F and E series) are found in follicular fluid of the late preovulatory follicles of many species, including the rabbit (673,674), rat (675–677), pig

(678,679), and human (680). Prostaglandin synthesis is presumably stimulated via the action of LH in increasing cAMP. PGF is undetectable in human follicular fluid prior to the LH peak but is high in ovulatory follicles and at ovulation (569,678). Prostaglandins may be involved in desensitization to gonadotropins. However, PGE_2, which stimulates progesterone production by human granulosa cells *in vitro* (681), may also maintain or increase progesterone secretion in the late preovulatory period. Furthermore, PGE_2 stimulates androgen production by thecal cells (99,682). Adenylate cyclase is desensitized to LH and FSH at this time, but granulosa cells remain responsive to PGE_2 (665). Prostaglandins might also mediate effects of LH on increased blood flow and intraovarian distribution of blood (683), thereby influencing steroid secretion into the circulation. A further important role of prostaglandins at ovulation is probably in follicular rupture since this process is blocked by inhibitors of prostaglandin synthetase (684,685) and by systemic (686) or intrafollicular injection of antiserum against prostaglandins (675).

SUMMARY AND CONCLUDING COMMENTS

As reviewed in this chapter, the follicle is the principal steroidogenic unit of the ovary. Its biosynthetic activities, and the factors that regulate them, change greatly as it emerges from the pool of resting follicles and undergoes progressive stages of differentiation. This progression leads ultimately to ovulation and luteinization of a small minority of those follicles that leave the resting pool, with the vast majority being aborted in atresia.

The steroidogenic output of the follicle at essentially all stages is a function of the concerted actions of its two types of somatic cells, the theca and granulosa cells, whose steroidogenic profiles differ in some significant ways. These differences are the result of differences in hormone receptors on their cell membranes, in specific steroidogenic enzyme activities, and in compartmentalization within the follicle, which restricts vascularization to the thecal layers and thus creates substantially different microenvironments for the two cell types.

The steroidogenic cells of the follicle are under primary control by the pituitary gonadotropic hormones, FSH and LH, with many of the actions of these hormones being influenced or modulated by a number of intraovarian factors, principally the steroid products of these cells. The gonadotropins initiate the chain of responses in their respective target cells through interaction with specific high-affinity binding sites (receptors) on the cell surfaces. Variation in the cellular concentrations of these receptors appears to dictate the fate of a given follicle, including its level of steroid output at a given stage of development.

The actions of FSH are restricted to the granulosa cells, as all other ovarian cell types appear to lack FSH receptors. In contrast, LH actions are exerted on both follicle cell types, as well as on cells of the interstitial gland and corpus luteum. Granulosa cells at all stages of follicular development appear to possess FSH receptors, whereas they acquire LH receptors and responsiveness only at later developmental stages. Theca cells acquire LH receptors and responsiveness at considerably earlier stages of follicular development than do granulosa cells.

FSH and LH exert major effects on steroidogenesis in their respective follicle target cells at least in part through activation of membrane-bound adenylate cyclase, thereby increasing the rate of synthesis of cAMP from ATP. The resulting increased intracellular cAMP levels bring about a variety of physiological responses of the cells through coupling mechanisms that generally involve phosphorylation and activation of protein kinases. Steroidogenic responses depend upon the identity and levels of rate-limiting enzymes that the particular target cells possess at the time of stimulation or acquire subsequently.

The earliest steroidogenic response of undifferentiated granulosa cells (those present at early preantral stages of follicle development) to FSH is increased activity of the aromatase enzyme complex. Given an adequate supply of aromatizable androgens (testosterone or androstenedione), the granulosa cells, thus stimulated, are able to increase their rate of synthesis and secretion of estrogens. However, because of an essential absence of the androgen biosynthetic enzymes (17α-hydroxylase:C-17,20-lyase complex) in granulosa cells, estrogen secretion following FSH stimulation depends on an exogenous supply of androgen, and substrate supply becomes the rate-limiting factor *in vivo* and *in vitro* for estrogen biosynthesis by granulosa cells at early developmental stages.

FSH also increases the ability of the granulosa cells to secrete progestins through induction of two other rate-limiting steps in the steroidogenic pathway, cholesterol side-chain cleavage P-450_{SCC} and the Δ^5-3β-hydroxysteroid dehydrogenase: $\Delta^{5\text{-}4}$-isomerase enzyme complex. The cholesterol substrate required by the granulosa cells for progestin production *in vivo* (over and above that provided by low rates of constitutive synthesis in the granulosa cells themselves) is provided in the form of lipoprotein-bound cholesterol reaching the follicle via the blood supply. Lack of vascularization of the granulosa cell layer and essential impermeability of the basement membrane surrounding the granulosa layer to the large lipoprotein molecules limit progesterone production by granulosa cells until later preovulatory stages.

As the follicle matures, plasma membrane receptors for LH and prolactin are acquired by the granulosa cells. FSH appears to be the primary inducer of these receptors, but the induction is enhanced by autocrine and/or paracrine actions of the estrogen produced intracellu-

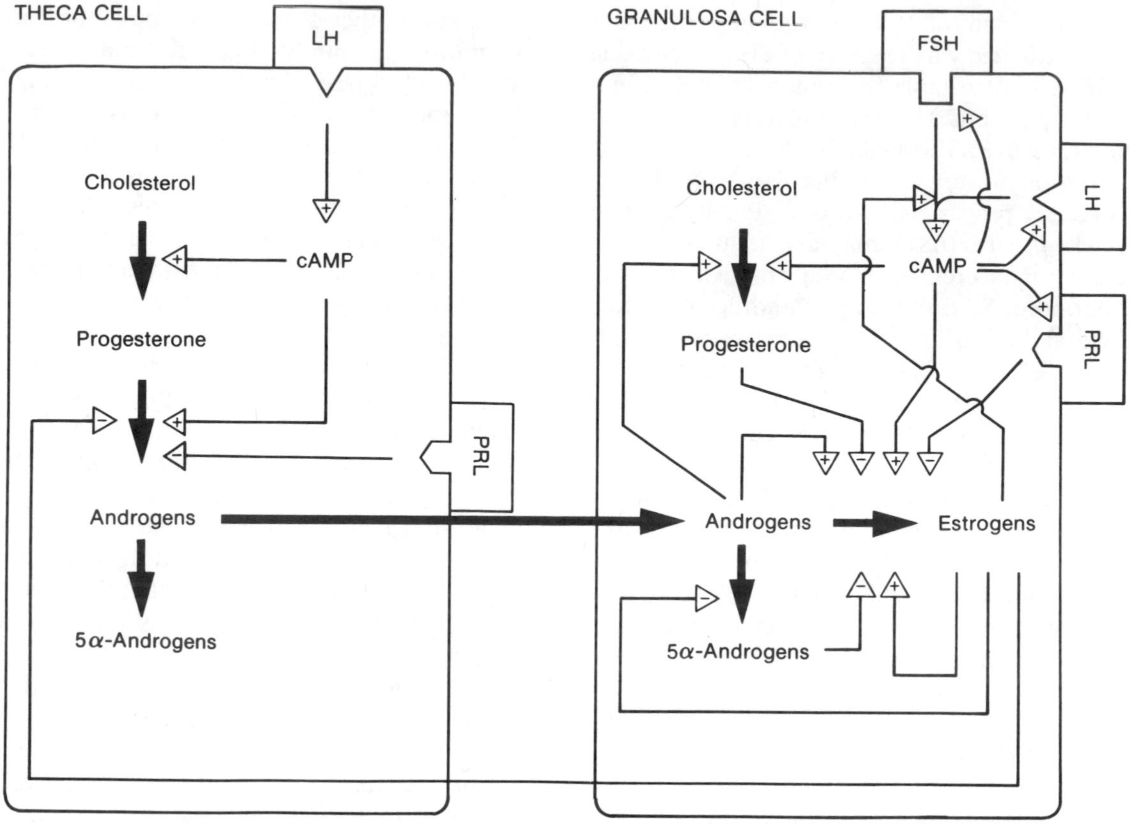

FIG. 5. Principal sites of regulation of follicular steroidogenesis in the rat. The scheme compresses into one diagram the principal regulatory sites of action of gonadotropins and steroids that have been demonstrated either at various stages of follicular maturation *in vivo* or with isolated cell types. (See section on steroidogenesis and its control by cell type for details.) The proposed sequence of events is as follows. Undifferentiated granulosa cells initially respond exclusively to FSH, by a cAMP-dependent mechanism, thereby stimulating activities of enzymes required for the metabolism of cholesterol to progesterone and for the conversion of theca-derived androgens to estrogens. Steroid biosynthesis in the theca cells is stimulated exclusively by LH. As the follicle matures, plasma membrane receptors for LH and prolactin (PRL) are acquired by the granulosa cells as a result of both FSH action and stimulation by estrogen on this process. LH may initially contribute to granulosa cell differentiation by augmenting the various cAMP-dependent processes. A variety of steroidal influences on the activities of steroidogenic enzymes may come into play as the follicles become more biosynthetically active. These effects may occur as the result of receptor-mediated actions of estrogens, androgens, and progesterone, thereby influencing responsiveness to FSH and LH, or steroids may directly alter enzymatic activities; these different actions of steroids are not distinguished in the above scheme. The apparent induction of aromatase activity is augmented by androgenic and estrogenic actions but is inhibited by progestins under certain circumstances. 5α-Reduced metabolites of androgens may competitively inhibit the aromatase enzyme, and estrogens may inhibit 5α-reductase. Prolactin has been shown to inhibit the induction of aromatase activity *in vitro* and also does so *in vivo* under certain physiological conditions, but its role in regulating estrogen synthesis during the ovarian cycle is still uncertain. Androgens may also facilitate the synthesis of progesterone. Following the LH surge, steroid production is briefly stimulated and then suppressed as granulosa and theca cells become desensitized to gonadotropin stimulation. Transiently increased estrogen secretion by granulosa cells causes inhibition of follicular estrogen biosynthesis by inhibiting androgen biosynthesis in the theca cells. Progesterone biosynthetic activity is restored subsequently and increases greatly as follicle cells luteinize.

larly in response to FSH stimulation and acting synergistically with FSH. Once the granulosa cells acquire receptors for LH, this gonadotropin becomes an additional stimulus to cAMP-regulated processes, particularly the further stimulation of the progesterone-synthesizing enzymes.

Androgen production appears to be the principal steroidogenic function of the theca cells. These cells therefore play a major role in enabling production of estrogen by the follicle, as they supply the substrate that is the rate-limiting factor in estrogen biosynthesis by the aromatase enzyme complex in granulosa cells. Since LH is required for significant rates of androgen production by the theca cells, this gonadotropin may be regarded as the primary regulatory factor in controlling estrogen secretion by all but the most immature of follicles. It is this action of LH on theca cells, together with the action of FSH in induction of aromatase activity in granulosa cells, that forms the basis of the "two-cell, two-gonadotropin" theory for control of estrogen secretion in the follicle.

The increased androgen secretion by theca cells, under LH stimulation, appears to be the result of increased activities of two sets of steroidogenic enzymes—the cholesterol side-chain cleavage system and the 17α-hydroxylase:C-17,20-lyase complex. Under certain physiological conditions, when the latter enzyme complex is rate-limiting, the products of the former may accumulate with the result that the theca cells become a significant source of C_{21}-steroid (progestin) secretion. Under other conditions, C_{21}-steroid synthesis may not keep pace with the activity of the 17α-hydroxylase:C-17,20-lyase complex, in which case exogenous progestin of granulosa cell origin may provide significant amounts of the C_{21}-substrate for theca cell androgen output. This, then, forms the basis of a second two-cell theory, for follicular steroidogenesis, in which granulosa and theca cells cooperate in the production of androgens by the follicle.

Under certain conditions, in some species more than others, the theca cells appear to possess a sufficient aromatase enzyme system to become a significant source of estrogen secretion as well.

Various steroidal influences on the activities of the steroidogenic enzymes in both granulosa and theca cells come into play as the follicles become more steroidogenically active under the influence of FSH and LH, as summarized in Fig. 5. At least some of the modulating effects of steroids appear to be mediated via intracellular steroid receptor, i.e., the demonstrated existence of estrogen receptors in granulosa cells, and the intraovarian actions of estrogens mentioned above. Other steroid effects appear to occur through direct action on steroidogenic enzymes.

In granulosa cells, the action of FSH in induction of aromatase is enhanced by androgens, as well as by estrogens, and inhibited, under certain circumstances, by 5α-reduced androgens and perhaps by progesterone. The 5α-reduced androgens also act as competitive inhibitors of the aromatase system. Both stimulatory and inhibitory actions of androgens have been reported on FSH-induced progesterone biosynthesis in granulosa cells. The stimulatory action, studied extensively in rat granulosa cells, appears to involve enhancement of FSH induction of the cytochrome P-450_{SCC} and the Δ^5-3β-hydroxysteroid dehydrogenase: $\Delta^{5\text{-}4}$-isomerase enzymes. The inhibitory action, demonstrated with porcine granulosa cells, appears to be primarily at the level of the Δ^5-3β-hydroxysteroid dehydrogenase:$\Delta^{5\text{-}4}$-isomerase complex.

Estrogens have been shown to influence androgen biosynthesis by theca cells, through inhibition at the level of the 17α-hydroxylase:C-17,20-lyase system. This paracrine action of estrogen may function as an intrafollicular negative-feedback system to limit its own production in granulosa cells through regulation of substrate availability.

Prolactin appears to exert inhibitory influences on estrogen biosynthesis, by inhibiting both FSH-induced aromatase activity in granulosa cells and LH-induced androgen production by theca/interstitial cells. A further well-established action of prolactin is its role in stimulating progesterone production by granulosa cells undergoing luteinization during the periovulatory period. The resulting high levels of progesterone may further contribute to the inhibition of estrogen synthesis in the follicle by prolactin.

The cyclic changes in follicular steroid biosynthesis during the estrous or menstrual cycle—as well as the more basal secretion rates of follicular activity during other physiological states such as pregnancy, seasonal and lactational anestrus (or amenorrhea), and prepuberty—can probably be explained on the bases of the coordinated actions of those cellular mechanisms and regulatory agents discussed in this chapter. The physiological importance of the pituitary gonadotropins and prolactin, as well as of the steroidal products of the follicular cells, is widely accepted. There are a number of other regulatory molecules whose specific roles in ovarian regulation are less well established but for which there is mounting evidence, largely from *in vitro* studies with isolated ovarian cells, of at least a supporting or permissive role in follicular regulation. Those we have included in this review are GnRH-like peptides, corticosteroids, insulin and other growth factors, and various neurotransmitters. We have undoubtedly overlooked others of emerging importance. Whether the demonstrated effects of these substances represent physiologically important actions or merely modulations peculiar to the *in vitro* systems remains uncertain. Nevertheless, it is abundantly clear that the follicular microenvironment, as embodied in the fluid of antral follicles, contains a wide array of varied substances (including steroids, eicosanoids, peptides, proteins, glycoproteins, and proteoglycans), some of which have hormonal or other biological activities *in vitro* and which could have significant regulatory effects on gonadotropin action and/or follicular steroidogenesis.

ACKNOWLEDGMENTS

We wish to thank Dr. S. A. J. Daniel for expert assistance in preparing material for portions of this chapter and Dr. M. W. Khalil for valuable discussions. We are also indebted to Mr. G. Barbe, Mrs. H. E. Ross, and Ms.

U. Williams for diligent assistance in the preparation of the manuscript. The authors' research is supported by a group grant from the Medical Research Council (MRC) of Canada; D.T.A. is a Career Investigator of the MRC, and R.E.G.-L. is the recipient of a Career Scientist Award from the Ontario Ministry of Health, Health Research Personnel Development Program.

REFERENCES

1. Kellie AE. Structure and nomenclature. In: Makin HLJ, ed. *Biochemistry of Steroid Hormones.* Oxford, UK: Blackwell Scientific; 1984:1–19.
2. Doisy EA, Veler CD, Thayer S. Folliculin from urine of pregnant women. *Am. J. Physiol.* 1929;90:329–330.
3. MacCorquodale DW, Thayer SA, Doisy EA. The isolation of the principal estrogenic substance of liquor folliculi. *J. Biol. Chem.* 1936;115:435–448.
4. Short RV. Steroid concentrations in the follicular fluid of mares at various stages of the reproductive cycle. *J. Endocrinol.* 1961;22:153–163.
5. Dehennin L, Blacker C, Reiffsteck A, Scholler R. Estrogen 2-, 4-, 6- or 16-hydroxylation by human follicles shown by gas chromatography-mass spectrometry associated with stable isotope dilution. *J. Steroid Biochem.* 1984;20:465–471.
6. Silberzahn P, Almahbobi G, Dehennin L, Merouane A. Estrogen metabolite in equine ovarian follicles; gas chromatographic-mass spectrometric determinations in relation to follicular ultrastructure and progestin content. *J. Steroid Biochem.* 1985;22: 501–505.
7. Silberzahn P, Dehennin L, Zwain I, Reiffsteck A. Gas chromatography-mass spectrometry of androgens in equine ovarian follicles at ultrastructurally defined stages of development. Identification of 19-nortestosterone in follicular fluid. *Endocrinology* 1985;117:2176–2181.
8. Khalil MW, Walton JS. Identification and measurement of 4-oestren-3,17-dione (19-norandrostenedione) in porcine ovarian follicular fluid using high performance liquid chromatography and capillary gas chromatography-mass spectrometry. *J. Endocrinol.* 1985;107:375–381.
9. Hill RT. Ovaries secrete male hormone. I. Restoration of the castrate type of seminal vesicle and prostate glands to normal by grafts of ovaries in mice. *Endocrinology* 1937;21:495–502.
10. Short RV. Steroids present in the follicular fluid of the mare. *J. Endocrinol.* 1960;20:147–156.
11. Ryan KJ, Petro Z. Steroid biosynthesis by human ovarian granulosa and thecal cells. *J. Clin. Endocrinol. Metab.* 1966;26:46–52.
12. Springer C, Eckstein B. Regulation of production in vitro of 5α-androstane-3α,17β-diol in the immature rat ovary. *J. Endocrinol.* 1971;50:431–439.
13. Zmigrod A, Lindner HR, Lamprecht SA. Reductase pathways of progesterone metabolism in the rat ovary. *Acta Endocrinol. (Copenh.)* 1972;69:141–152.
14. Karakawa T, Karachi K, Aono T, Matsumoto K. Formation of 5α-reduced C_{19}-steroids from progesterone in vitro by a pathway through 5α-reduced C_{21}-steroids in ovaries of late prepubertal rats. *Endocrinology* 1976;98:571–579.
15. Tsuji M, Terada N, Sato B, Matsumoto K. 5β- and 5α-reductases for 4-ene-3-ketosteroids in golden hamster ovaries at different stages of development. *J. Steroid Biochem.* 1982;16:207–213.
16. Gower DB. 16-Unsaturated C_{19}-steroids. A review of their chemistry, biochemistry and possible physiological role. *J. Steroid Biochem.* 1972;3:45–103.
17. Armstrong DT. Alterations of progesterone metabolism in immature rat ovaries by luteinizing hormone. *Biol. Reprod.* 1979;21:1025–1033.
18. Fieser LF, Fieser M.(1959): *Steroids* Reinhold, New York.
19. Dorfman RT, Ungar F. (1965): *Metabolism of Steroid Hormones.* Academic, New York.
20. Makin HLJ. (ed.) (1984): *Biochemistry of Steroid Hormones.* Blackwell, Oxford, UK.
21. Strauss III, JF, Schuler LA, Rosenblum MF, Tanaka T. Cholesterol metabolism by ovarian tissue. *Adv. Lipid Res.* 1981;18: 99–157.
22. Solod EA, Armstrong DT, Greep RO. Action of luteinizing hormone on conversion of ovarian cholesterol stores to steroid secreted in vivo and synthesized in vitro by the pseudopregnant rabbit ovary. *Steroids* 1966;7:607–620.
23. Gwynne JT, Strauss III, JF. The role of lipoproteins in steroidogenesis and cholesterol metabolism in steroidogenic glands. *Endocr. Rev.* 1982;3:299–329.
24. Veldhuis JD, Klase PA, Strauss III, JF, Hammond JM. Facilitative interactions between estradiol and luteinizing hormone in the regulation of progesterone production by cultured swine granulosa cells: relation to cholesterol metabolics. *Endocrinology* 1982;111:441–447.
25. Rajendran KC, Hwang J, Menoir KMJ. Binding, degradation and utilization of plasma high density and low density lipoproteins for progesterone production in cultured rat luteal cells. *Endocrinology* 1983;112:1746–1753.
26. Shalgi R, Kraicer P, Renoir A, Pinto M, Soferman N. Proteins of human follicular fluid: the blood-follicle barrier. *Fertil. Steril* 1973;24:429–434.
27. Chang SCS, Jones JD, Ellefson RD, Ryan RJ. The porcine ovarian follicle: I. Selected chemical analysis of follicular fluid at different developmental stages. *Biol. Reprod.* 1976;15:321–328.
28. Simpson ER, Rochelle DB, Carr BR, MacDonald PC. Plasma lipoproteins in follicular fluid of human ovaries. *J. Clin. Endocrinol. Metab.* 1980;51:1469–1471.
29. Wang SC, Greenwald GS. Effect of lipoproteins, 25-hydroxycholesterol and luteinizing hormone on in vitro follicular steroidogenesis in the hamster and rat. *Biol. Reprod.* 1984;31:271–279.
30. Farkash Y, Timberg R, Orly J. Preparation of antiserum to rat cytochrome P-450 cholesterol side chain cleavage, and its use for ultrastructural localization of the immunoreactive enzyme by protein A-gold technique. *Endocrinology* 1986;118:1353–1365.
31. Lieberman S, Greenfield NJ, Wolfson A. A heuristic proposal for understanding steroidogeneic processes. *Endocr. Rev.* 1984;5: 128–148.
32. Hall PF. Cellular organization for steroidogenesis. *Int. Rev. Cytol.* 1984;86:53–95.
33. Gower DB. The role of cytochrome P-450 in steroidogenesis and properties of some of the steroid-transforming enzymes. Makin HLJ, ed. In: *Biochemistry of Steroid Hormones.* Oxford, UK: Blackwell Scientific, 1984: 230–292.
34. Kautsky MP, Hagerman DD. Kinetic properties of steroid 19-hydroxylase and estrogen synthetase from porcine ovary microsomes. *J. Steroid Biochem.* 1980;13:1283–1290.
35. Brodie AM, Schwarzel WC, Brodie HJ. Studies on the mechanism of estrogen biosynthesis in the rat ovary. *J. Steroid Biochem.* 1976;7:787–793.
36. Mason NR. Steroid A-ring reduction by rat ovaries. *Endocrinology* 1970;87:350–355.
37. Eckstein B, Ravid R. On the mechanism of the onset of puberty: identification and pattern of 5α-androstane-3β,17β-diol and its 3α-epimer in peripheral blood of immature female rats. *Endocrinology* 1974;94:224–229.
38. Mizutani S, Akashi S, Terada N, Matsumoto K. A comparison of metabolism of progesterone to 5α-steroids in monkey, mouse and rat ovaries. *J. Steroid Biochem.* 1979;10:549–552.
39. Furubayashi Y, Terada N, Sato B, Matsumoto K. Localization of Δ^4-5β- and 5α-reductases and 17β-ol-dehydrogenase in immature golden hamster testis. *Endocrinology* 1982;111:269–272.
40. Inaba T, Imori T, Matsumoto K. Formation of 5α-reduced C_{19}-steroids from progesterone in vivo by 5α-reduced pathway in immature rat ovaries. *J. Steroid Biochem.* 1978;9:1105–1110.
41. Zmigrod A, Lindner HR. Metabolism of progesterone by the rat ovary: formation of 3β-hydroxy-5α-pregnan-20-one by ovarian microsomes. *Acta Endocrinol. (Copenh.)* 1969;61:618–628.
42. Armstrong DT, Kraemer MA, Hixon JE. Metabolism of progesterone by rat ovarian tissue: influence of pregnant mare serum gonadotrophin and prolactin. *Biol. Reprod.* 1975;12:599–608.

43. Ichikawa S, Morioka H, Sawada T. Identification of the neutral steroids in the ovarian venous plasma of LH-stimulated rats. *Endocrinology* 1971;88:372–383.
44. Eckstein B. The origin of 5α-androstane-3α,17β-diol and its 3β epimer in peripheral blood of immature female rats. *J. Steroid Biochem.* 1974;5:577–580.
45. Eckstein B. Blood concentrations and biological effects of androstanediols at the onset of puberty in the female rat. *J. Steroid Biochem.* 1983;19:883–886.
46. Hashimoto I, Wiest WG. Luteotrophic and luteolytic mechanisms in rat corpora lutea. *Endocrinology* 1969;80:886–892.
47. Goldring NB, Orly J. Concerted metabolism of steroid hormones produced by cocultured ovarian cell types. *J. Biol. Chem.* 1985;260:913–920.
48. MacLusky NJ, Naftolin F, Krey LC, Franks S. The catechol estrogens. *J. Steroid Biochem.* 1981;15:111–124.
49. Hammond JM, Hershey RM, Walega MA, Weisz J. Catecholestrogen production by porcine ovarian cells. *Endocrinology* 1986;118:2292–2299.
50. Ball R, Knuppen R. Catechol oestrogens (2- and 4-hydroxyoestrogen): chemistry, biogenesis, metabolism, occurrence and physiological significance. *Acta Endocrinol. (Copenh.)* 1980;93(Suppl. 232):1–27.
51. Richards JS. Hormonal control of ovarian follicular development. *Rec. Prog. Horm. Res.* 1979;35:343–368.
52. Richards JS. Maturation of ovarian follicles: actions and interactions of pituitary and ovarian hormones on follicular cell differentiation. *Physiol. Rev.* 1980;60:51–89.
53. Robison GA, Butcher RW, Sutherland EW. *Cyclic AMP.* Academic, New York.
54. Kuo JF, Greengard P. Cyclic nucleotide-dependent protein kinases. IV, Widespread occurrence of adenosine 3′,5′-monophosphate-dependent protein kinase in various tissues and phyla of the animal kingdom. *Proc. Natl. Acad. Sci. USA* 1969;64:1349–1355.
55. Carnegie J, Tsang BK. Follicle-stimulating hormone-regulated granulosa cell steroidogenesis: involvement of the calcium-calmodulin system. *Am. J. Obstet. Gynecol.* 1983;145:223–228.
56. Byskov AG. The anatomy and ultrastructure of the rete system in the fetal mouse ovary. *Biol. Reprod.* 1978;19:720–735.
57. Byskov AG, Rasmussen G. Ultrastructural studies of the developing follicle. In: Peters H, ed. *The Development and Maturation of the Ovary and Its Function, International Congress Series No. 267.* Excerpta Medica; Amsterdam: 1973:55–62.
58. Bjersing L. On the ultrastructure of follicles and isolated follicular granulosa cells of porcine ovary. *Z. Zellforsch. Mikrosk. Anat.* 1967;82:173–186.
59. Motta P, Didio LJA. Microfilaments in granulosa cells during the follicular development and transformation in corpus luteum in the rabbit ovary. *J. Submicrosc. Cytol.* 1974;6:15–27.
60. Zamboni L. Fine morphology of the follicle wall and follicle cell-oocyte association. *Biol. Reprod.* 1974;10:125–149.
61. Byskov AG. The role of rete ovarii in meiosis and follicle formation in the cat, mink and ferret. *J. Reprod. Fertil.* 1975;45:201–289.
62. Amsterdam A, Koch Y, Lieberman ME, Lindner HR. Distribution of binding sites for human chorionic gonadotropin in the preovulatory follicle of the rat. *J. Cell Biol.* 1975;67:894–900.
63. Midgley Jr, AR. Gonadotropin binding to frozen sections of ovarian tissue. In: Saxena BB, Beling CG, and Gandy HM, eds. *Gonadotropins,* Wiley-Interscience, New York: 1972:248–260.
64. Zoller LC, Weisz J. A quantitative cytochemical study of glucose-6-phosphate dehydrogenase and Δ^5-3β-hydroxy-steroid dehydrogenase activity in membrana granulosa of the ovulable type of follicle of the rat. *Histochemistry* 1979;62:125–135.
65. Zoller LC, Weisz J. Identification of cytochrome P-450 and its distribution in the membrana granulosa of the preovulatory follicle using quantitative cytochemistry. *Endocrinology* 1978;103:310–313.
66. Erickson GF, Hofeditz C, Unger M, Allen WR, Dulbecco R. A monoclonal antibody to a mammary cell line recognizes two distinct subtypes of ovarian granulosa cells. *Endocrinology* 1985;117:1490–1499.
67. Kasson BG, Median R, Davoren JB, Hsueh AJW. Identification of subpopulations of rat granulosa cells: sedimentation properties and hormonal responsiveness. *Endocrinology* 1985;117:1027–1034.
68. Weakly BS. Electron microscopy of the oocyte and granulosa cells in thedeveloping ovarian follicles of the golden hamster. *J. Anat.* 1966;100:503–534.
69. Hoage TR, Cameron IL. Folliculogenesis in the ovary of the mature mouse: an autoradiographic study. *Anat. Rec.* 1976;184:699–710.
70. Høyer PE, Byskov AG. (1981): A quantitative cytochemical study of Δ^5, 3β-hydroxysteroid dehydrogenase activity in the rete system of the immature mouse ovary. In: *Development and Function of Reproductive Organs,* edited by AG Byskov and H Peters, pp. 216–224. Excerpta Medica, Amsterdam.
71. Quattropani SL. Morphogenesis of the ovarian interstitial tissue in the neonatal mouse. *Anat. Rec.* 1973;177:569–584.
72. Mori H, Matsumoto K. On the histogenesis of the ovarian interstitial gland in rabbits. I. Primary interstitial gland. *Am. J. Anat.* 1970;129:289–306.
73. Kingsbury BF. Atresia and the interstitial cells of the ovary. *Am. J. Anat.* 1939;65:309–331.
74. Dawson AB, McCabe M. The interstitial tissue of the ovary in infantile and juvenile rat. *J. Morphol.* 1951;88:543–571.
75. Rennels EG. Influence of hormones on the histochemistry of ovarian interstitial tissue in the immature rat. *Am. J. Anat.* 1951;88:63–108.
76. Deanesly R. Origins and development of interstitial tissue in ovaries in rabbit and guinea-pig. *J. Anat.* 1972;113:251–260.
77. Guraya SS, Greenwald GS. A comparative histochemical study of interstitial tissue and follicular atresia in the mammalian ovary. *Anat. Rec.* 1968;149:411–434.
78. McNatty KP. Hormonal correlates of follicular development in the human ovary. *Aust. J. Biol. Sci.* 1981;34:249–268.
79. Bélanger A, Cusan L, Caron S, Barden N, Dupont A. Ovarian progestins, androgens and estrogen throughout the 4-day estrous cycle in the rat. *Biol. Reprod.* 1981;24:591–596.
80. Sridaran R, Gibori G. Intraovarian localization of luteinizing hormone/human chorionic gonadotropin stimulation of testosterone and estradiol synthesis in the pregnant rat. *Endocrinology* 1983;112:1770–1776.
81. Dennefors BL, Janson P, Knutson F, Hamberger L. Steroid production and responsiveness to gonadotrophin in isolated stromal tissue of human menopausal ovaries. *Am. J. Obstet. Gynecol.* 1980;136:997–1002.
82. Longcope C, Hunter R, Franz C. Steroid secretion by the postmenopausal ovary. *Am. J. Obstet. Gynecol.* 1980;138:564–568.
83. Dyer CA, Erickson GF, Curtiss LK. Functional heterogeneity in the ability of high density lipoproteins to enhance gonadotropin-induced androgen production in cultured rat theca-interstitial cells. In: Strauss III JF and Menon KMJ, eds. *Lipoprotein and Cholesterol Metabolism in Steroidogenic Tissues.* Strickley, Philadelphia: 1985:141–146.
84. Aakvaag A. Pathways in the biosynthesis of androstenedione in the human ovary in vitro. *Acta Endocrinol. (Copenh.)* 1969;60:517–526.
85. Lacroix E, Eechaute W, Leusen I. The biosynthesis of oestrogens by cow follicles. *Steroids* 1974;23:337–356.
86. Magoffin DA, Erickson GF. Primary culture of differentiating ovarian androgen-producing cells in defined medium. *J. Biol. Chem.* 1982;257:4507–4513.
87. Zeleznik AJ, Midgley Jr, AR, Reichert Jr, LE. Granulosa cell maturation in the rat: increased binding of human chorionic gonadotropin following treatment with follicle-stimulating hormone in vivo. *Endocrinology* 1974;95:818–825.
88. Lindner HR, Amsterdam A, Salomon Y, Tsafriri A, Nimrod A, Lamprecht SA, Zor U, Koch Y. Intraovarian factors in ovulation: determinants of follicular response to gonadotropins. *J. Reprod. Fertil.* 1977;51:215–235.
89. Zeleznik AJ, Schuler HM, Reichert Jr, LE. Gonadotropin-binding sites in the rhesus monkey ovary: role of the vasculature in the selective distribution of human chorionic gonadotropin in the preovulatory follicle. *Endocrinology* 1981;109:356–362.

90. Oxberry BA, Greenwald GS. An autoradiographic study of the binding of ^{125}I-labelled follicle-stimulating hormone, human chorionic gonadotrophin and prolactin to the hamster ovary throughout the estrous cycle. *Biol. Reprod.* 1982;27:505–516.
91. Shaha C, Greenwald GS. Development of steroidogenic activity in the ovary of the prepubertal hamster. I. Response to in vivo or in vitro exposure to gonadotropins. *Biol. Reprod.* 1983;28: 1231–1241.
92. Uilenbroek JTJ, van der Linden R. Changes in gonadotrophin binding to rat ovaries during sexual maturation. *Acta Endocrinol. (Copenh.)* 1983;104:413–419.
93. Henderson KM, Kieboom LE, McNatty KP, Lun S, Heath DA. ^{125}I-HCG binding to bovine thecal tissue from healthy and atretic antral follicles. *Mol. Cell. Endocrinol.* 1984;34:91–98.
94. Hamberger L, Hillensjö T, Ahren K. Steroidogenesis in isolated cells of preovulatory rat follicles. *Endocrinology* 1978;103: 771–777.
95. Weiss TJ, Armstrong DT, McIntosh JEA, Seamark RF. Maturational changes in sheep ovarian follicles: gonadotrophic stimulation of cyclic AMP production by isolated theca and granulosa cells. *Acta Endocrinol. (Copenh.)* 1978;89:158–165.
96. Tsang BK, Moon YS, Simpson CW, Armstrong DT. Androgen biosynthesis in human ovarian follicles: cellular source, gonadotropic control, and andenosine 3′,5′-monophosphate mediation. *J. Clin. Endocrinol. Metab.* 1979;48:153–158.
97. Erickson GF, Magoffin DA, Dyer CA, Hofeditz C. The ovarian androgen producing cells: a review of structure/function relationships. *Endocr. Rev.* 1985;6:371–399.
98. Erickson GF, Ryan KJ. Stimulation of testosterone production in isolated rabbit thecal tissue by LH/FSH, dibutyryl cyclic AMP, $PGF_{2\alpha}$, and PGE_2. *Endocrinology* 1976;99:452–458.
99. Tsang BK, Armstrong DT, Whitfield JF. Steroid biosynthesis by isolated human ovarian follicular cells in vitro. *J. Clin. Endocrinol. Metab.* 1980;51:1407–1411.
100. Fukuda S, Terakawa N, Sato B, Imori T, Matsumoto K. Hormonal regulation of activities of 17β-ol-dehydrogenases, aromatase and 4-ene-5α-reductase in immature ovaries. *J. Steroid Biochem.* 1979;11:1421–1427.
101. Aono T, Kitamura Y, Fukuda S, Matsumoto K. Localization of 4-ene-5α-reductase, 17β-ol-dehydrogenase and aromatase in immature rat ovary. *J. Steroid Biochem.* 1981;14:1369–1377.
102. Bogovich K, Richards JS. Androgen biosynthesis in developing ovarian follicles: evidence that luteinizing hormone regulates thecal 17α-hydroxylase and $C_{17\text{-}20}$-lyase activities. *Endocrinology* 1982;111:1201–1208.
103. Makris A, Ryan KJ. The source of follicular androgen in the hamster follicle. *Steroids* 1980;35:53–64.
104. Lieberman ME, Barnea A, Bauminger S, Tsafriri A, Collins WP, Lindner HR. LH effect on the pattern of steroidogenesis in cultured Graafian follicles of the rat: dependence on macromolecular synthesis. *Endocrinology* 1975;96:1533–1542.
105. Rodgers RJ, Waterman MR, Simpson ER. Cytochromes $P\text{-}450_{scc}$, $P\text{-}450_{17\alpha}$, adrenodoxin, and reduced nicotin-amide adenine dinucleotide phosphate-cytochrome P-450 reductase in bovine follicles and corpora lutea. Changes in specific contents during the ovarian cycle. *Endocrinology* 1986;118:1366–1374.
106. Makris A, Ryan KJ. Progesterone, androstenedione, testosterone, estrone, and estradiol synthesis in hamster ovarian follicle cells. *Endocrinology* 1975;96:694–701.
107. Evans G, Dobias M, King GJ, Armstrong DT. Estrogen, androgen, and progesterone biosynthesis by theca and granulosa of preovulatory follicles in the pig. *Biol. Reprod.* 1981;25:673–682.
108. McNatty KP, Heath DA, Lun S, Fanin JM, McDiarmid JM, Henderson KM. Steroidogenesis by bovine theca interna in an in vitro perfusion system. *Biol. Reprod.* 1984;30:159–170.
109. Fortune JE, Hansel W. Concentrations of steroids and gonadotropins in follicular fluid from normal heifers and heifers primed for superovulation. *Biol. Reprod.* 1985;32:1069–1079.
110. McNatty KP, Makris A, Reinhold VN, DeGrazia C, Osathanondh R, Ryan KJ. Metabolism of androstenedione by human ovarian tissues in vitro with particular references to reductase and aromatase activity. *Steroids* 1979;34:429–443.
111. McNatty KP, Makris A, Osathanondh R, Ryan KJ. Effects of luteinizing hormone on steroidogenesis by thecal tissue from human ovarian follicles in vitro. *Steroids* 1980;36:53–63.
112. Lerner N, Eckstein B. Identification of two 5α-reduced pregnanes as major metabolites of progesterone in immature rat ovaries (1000 × g supernatant) in vitro. *Endocrinology* 1976;98:179–188.
113. Bogovich K, Scales LM, Higginbottom E, Ewing LL, Richards JS. Short term androgen production by rat ovarian follicles and long term steroidogenesis by thecal explants in culture. *Endocrinology* 1986;118:1379–1386.
114. Eckstein B, Mechoulam R, Burstein SH. The identification of 5α-androstane-3α,17β-diol as a principal metabolite of pregnenolone in rat ovary at the onset of puberty. *Nature* 1970;228: 866–868.
115. Suzuki K, Kawakura K, Tamaoki BI. Effect of pregnant mare's serum gonadotrophin on the activities of 5α-reductase, aromatase, and other enzymes in the ovaries of immature rats. *Endocrinology* 1978;102:1595–1605.
116. Eckstein B, Ravid R. Changes in pathways of steroid production taking place in the rat ovary around the time of the first ovulation. *J. Steroid Biochem.* 1979;11:593–597.
117. Eckstein B, Golan R, Mishinsky JS. Onset of puberty in the immature female rat induced by 5α-androstane-3β,17β-diol. *Endocrinology* 1973;92:941–945.
118. Eckstein B, Springer C. Induction of an ovarian epimerase system catalyzing the transformation of 5α-androstane-3α,17β-diol to 5α-androstane-3β,17β-diol after treatment of immature rats with gonadotropins exhibiting FSH-like activity. *Endocrinology* 1971;89:347–352.
119. Florensa E, Sommerville IF, Harrison RF, Johnson MW, Youssefnejadian E. Plasma 20α-dihydroprogesterone, progesterone and 17-hydroxyprogesterone: daily and four-hourly variations during the menstrual cycle. *J. Steroid Biochem.* 1976;7:769–777.
120. Holmdahl TH, Johansson EDB. Peripheral plasma levels of 17α-hydroxyprogesterone, progesterone and oestradiol during normal menstrual cycles in women. *Acta Endocrinol. (Copenh.)* 1972; 71:743–754.
121. Aedo AR, Langren BM, Cekan Z, Diczfalusy E. Studies on the pattern of circulating steroids in the normal menstrual cycle. *Acta Endocrinol. (Copenh.)* 1976;82:600–616.
122. Ryan KJ, Petro Z, Kaiser J. Steroid formation by isolated and recombined ovarian granulosa and theca cells. *J. Clin. Endocrinol. Metab.* 1968;28:355–358.
123. Channing CP. Steroidogenesis and morphology of human ovarian cell types in tissue culture. *J. Endocrinol.* 1969;45:297–308.
124. Batta SK, Wentz AC, Channing CP. Steroidogenesis by human ovarian cell types in culture: influence of mixing of cell types and effect of added testosterone. *J. Clin. Endocrinol. Metab.* 1980;50:274–279.
125. Channing CP, Wentz AC, Jones G. Steroid secretion by monkey and human ovarian cell types in vivo and in vitro. In: Scholler R, ed. *Symposium on the Ovary held in Fresnes, France.* Editions Sepe, Paris: 1978:71–86.
126. Ryan KJ, Short RV. Formation of estradiol by granulosa and thecal cells of the equine ovarian follicle. *Endocrinology* 1965;76:108–114.
127. Channing CP, Grieves SA. Studies on tissue culture of equine ovarian cell types: steroidogenesis. *J. Endocrinol.* 1969;43: 391–402.
128. Armstrong DT, Weiss TJ, Selstam G, Seamark RF. Hormonal and cellular interactions in follicular steroid biosynthesis by the sheep ovary. *J. Reprod. Fertil. (Suppl. 30),* 1981;30:143–154.
129. Moon YS, Tsang BK, Simpson C, Armstrong DT. 17β-Estradiol biosynthesis in cultured granulosa and thecal cells of human ovarian follicles: stimulation by follicle-stimulating hormone. *J. Clin. Endocrinol. Metab.* 1978;47:263–267.
130. Hillier SG. Regulation of follicular oestrogen biosynthesis: a survey of current concepts. *J. Endocrinol.* 1981;89:3P–18P.
131. Hillier SG, van den Boogaard AJM, Reichert Jr, LE, van Hall EV. Control of preovulatory follicular estrogen biosynthesis in the human ovary. *J. Clin. Endocrinol. Metab.* 1981;52:847–856.
132. Mossman HW, Koering MJ, Ferry Jr, D. Cyclic changes of interstitial gland tissue of the human ovary. *Am. J. Anat.* 1964;115:235–256.

133. Leymarie P, Savard K. Steroid hormone formation in the human ovary. VI. Evidence for two pathways of synthesis of androgens in the stromal compartment. *J. Clin. Endocrinol. Metab.* 1968;28: 1547–1554.
134. Marsh JM, Savard K, LeMaire WJ. Steroidogenic capacities of the different compartments of the human ovary. In: James VHT, Serio M, and Giusti G, eds. *The Endocrine Function of The Human Ovary.* Academic; London: 1976:37–45.
135. McNatty KP, Makris A, De Grazia C, Osathanondh R, Ryan KJ. Steroidogenesis by recombined follicular cells from the human ovary in vitro. *J. Clin. Endocrinol. Metab.* 1980;51:1286–1292.
136. Dorrington JH, Moon YS, Armstrong DT. Estradiol-17β biosynthesis in cultured granulosa cells from hypophysectomized immature rats; stimulation by follicle-stimulating hormone. *Endocrinology* 1975;97:1328–1331.
137. Gore-Langton RE, Dorrington JH. FSH induction of aromatase in cultured rat granulosa cells measured by a radiometric assay. *Mol. Cell. Endocrinol.* 1981;22:135–151.
138. Wang C, Hsueh AJW, Erickson GF. The role of cyclic AMP in the induction of estrogen and progestin synthesis in cultured granulosa cells. *Mol. Cell. Endocrinol.* 1982;25:73–83.
139. Mendelson CR, Durham C, Evans C, Simpson ER. The induction of aromatase activity in estrogen-producing cells is mediated by the increased synthesis of aromatase cytochrome P-450. *67th Annual Meeting of The Endocrine Society,* (Abstr. 307) 1985:77.
140. Durham CR, Zhu H, Masters BSS, Simpson ER, Mendelson CR. Regulation of aromatase activity of rat granulosa cells: induction of synthesis of NADPH-cytochrome P-450 reductase by FSH and dibutyryl cyclic AMP. *Mol. Cell. Endocrinol.* 1985;40:211–219.
141. Dorrington JH, Armstrong DT. Effect of FSH on gonadal functions. *Rec. Prog. Horm. Res.* 1979;35:301–342.
142. Hillier SG, Zeleznik AJ, Ross GT. Independence of steroidogenic capacity and luteinizing hormone receptor induction in developing granulosa cells. *Endocrinology,* 1978;102:937–946.
143. Armstrong DT, Dorrington JH. Androgens augment FSH-induced progesterone secretion by cultured rat granulosa cells. *Endocrinology,* 1976;99:1411–1414.
144. Nimrod A. Studies on the synergistic effect of androgen on the stimulation of progestin secretion by FSH in cultured rat granulosa cells: a search for the mechanism of action. *Mol. Cell. Endocrinol.* 1977;8:201–211.
145. Nimrod A, Lindner HR. A synergistic effect of androgen on the stimulation of progesterone secretion by FSH in cultured rat granulosa cells. *Mol. Cell. Endocrinol.* 1976;5:315–320.
146. McNatty KP, Makris A, De Grazia C, Osathanondh R, Ryan KJ. The production of progesterone, androgens and oestrogens by human granulosa cells in vitro and in vivo. *J. Steroid Biochem.* 1979;11:775–779.
147. Channing CP. Temporal effects of LH, hCG, FSH and dibutyryl cyclic 3′,5′-AMP upon luteinization of rhesus monkey granulosa cells in culture. *Endocrinology* 1974;94:1215–1223.
148. Hammond RW, Burke WH, Hertelendy F. Influence of follicular maturation of progesterone release in chicken granulosa cells in response to turkey and ovine gonadotropins. *Biol. Reprod.* 1981;24:1048–1055.
149. Hillensjö T, Magnusson C, Svensson U, Thelander H. Effects of luteinizing hormone and follicle-stimulating hormone on progesterone synthesis by cultured rat cumulus cells. *Endocrinology* 1981;108:1920–1924.
150. Wang C, Hsueh AJW, Erickson GF. LH stimulation of estrogen secretion in cultured granulosa cells. *Mol. Cell. Endocrinol.* 1981;24:17–28.
151. Chang SCS, Jones JD, Ellefson RD, Ryan RJ. The porcine ovarian follicle. I. Selected chemical analysis of follicular fluid at different developmental stages. *Biol. Reprod.* 1976;15:321–328.
152. Carr BR, MacDonald PC, Simpson ER. The role of lipoproteins in the regulation of progesterone secretion by the human corpus luteum. *Fertil. Steril.* 1982;38:303–311.
153. Jones PBC, Hsueh AJW. Pregnenolone biosynthesis by cultured granulosa cells: modulation by follicle-stimulating hormone and gonadotropin-releasing hormone. *Endocrinology* 1982;111: 713–721.
154. Toaff ME, Strauss III, JF, Hammond JM. Regulation of cytochrome P-450_{SCC} in immature porcine granulosa cells by FSH and estradiol. *Endocrinology* 1983;112:1156–1158.
155. Boyd GS, Arthur JR, Beckett GJ, Mason JI, Trzeciak WH. The role of cholesterol and cytochrome P-450 in the cholesterol side-chain cleavage reaction in adrenal cortex and corpora lutea. *J. Steroid Biochem.* 1975;6:427–436.
156. Robinson J, Stevenson PM, Boyd GS, Armstrong DT. Acute in vivo effects of hCG and LH on ovarian mitochondrial cholesterol utilization. *Mol. Cell. Endocrinol.* 1975;2:149–155.
157. Mori M, Marsh JM. The site of luteinizing hormone stimulation of steroidogenesis in mitochondria of the rat corpus luteum. *J. Biol. Chem.* 1982;257:6178–6183.
158. Naumoff PA, Stevenson PM. The differential development of mitochondrial cytochrome P-450 and the respiratory cytochromes in rat ovary. *Biochim. Biophys. Acta.* 1981;673: 359–365.
159. Schuler LA, Toaff ME, Strauss III, JF. Regulation of ovarian cholesterol metabolism: control of 3-hydroxy-3-methylglutaryl coenzyme A reductase and acyl coenzyme A:cholesterol acyltransferase. *Endocrinology* 1981;108:1476–1486.
160. Behrman HR, Armstrong DT. Cholesterol esterase stimulation by luteinizing hormone in luteinized rat ovaries. *Endocrinology* 1969;85:474–480.
161. Caffrey JL, Fletcher PW, Diekman MA, O'Callaghan PL, Niswender GD. The activity of ovine luteal cholesterol esterase during several experimental conditions. *Biol. Reprod.* 1979;21: 601–608.
162. Henderson KM, Gorban AMS, Boyd GS. Effect of LH factors regulating ovarian cholesterol metabolism and progesterone synthesis in PMSG-primed immature rats. *J. Reprod. Fertil.* 1981;61.373–380.
163. Hwang J, Menon JMJ. Characterization of low density and high density lipoprotein receptors in the rat corpus luteum and regulation by gonadotropin. *J. Biol. Chem.* 1983;258:8020–8027.
164. Jones PBC, Valk CA, Hsueh AJW. Regulation of progestin biosynthetic enzymes in cultured rat granulosa cells: Effects of prolactin, β_2-adrenergic agonist, human chorionic gonadotropin and gonadotropin-releasing hormone. *Biol. Reprod.* 1983;29: 572–585.
165. Rubin BL, Deane HW, Hamilton JA, Driks EC. Changes in Δ^5-3β-hydroxysteroid dehydrogenase activity in the ovaries of maturing rats. *Endocrinology* 1963;72:924–930.
166. Koritz SB. (1967): On the regulation of pregnenolone synthesis. In: *Functions of the Adrenal Cortex,* edited by K. McKerns, pp. 27–48. Appleton-Century-Crofts, New York.
167. Madej E. Effect of exogenous hormones on the activity of Δ^5-3β-hydroxysteroid dehydrogenase in cultured granulosa cells from proestrous and preovulatory rat ovarian follicles. *Acta Histochem.* 1980;67:253–260.
168. Neville AM, Engel LL. Steroid Δ-isomerase of the bovine adrenal gland: kinetics, activation by NAD and attempted solubilization. *Endocrinology* 1968;83:864–872.
169. Philpott JE, Peron FG. A microassay procedure for Δ^5-3β-hydroxysteroid dehydrogenase based on substrate depletion. *Endocrinology* 1971;88:1082–1085.
170. Dorrington JH, McKeracher HL, Chan A, Gore-Langton RE. Luteinizing hormone-releasing hormone independently stimulates cytodifferentiation of granulosa cells. In: McKerns KW, and Naor Z, eds. *Hormonal Control of The Hypothalamo-pituitary-gonadal Axis. Biochemical Endocrinology Series,* Plenum; New York:1984:467–478.
171. Lischinsky A, Evans G, Armstrong DT. Site of androgen inhibition of FSH-stimulated progesterone production in porcine granulosa cells. *Endocrinology* 1983;113:1999–2003.
172. Eckstein B, Nimrod A. Effect of human chorionic gonadotropin and prolactin on 20α-hydroxysteroid dehydrogenase activity in granulosa cells of immature rat ovary. *Endocrinology* 1979;104:711–714.
173. Jones PBC, Hsueh AJW. Direct stimulation of ovarian progesterone metabolizing enzyme by gonadotropin-releasing hormone in cultured granulosa cells. *J. Biol. Chem.* 1981;256:1248–1254.
174. Eckstein B, Raanan M, Lerner N, Cohen S, Nimrod A. The appearance of 20α-hydroxysteroid dehydrogenase activity in preov-

ulatory follicles of immature rats treated with pregnant mare serum gonadotropin. *J. Steroid Biochem.* 1977;8:213–216.
175. Hickman-Smith D, Kuhn NJ. A proposed sequence of hormones controlling the induction of luteal 20α-hydroxysteroid dehydrogenase and progesterone withdrawal in the late-pregnant rat. *Biochem. J.* 1976;160:663–670.
176. Loewit K, Zambelis N. Progesterone and 20α-hydroxysteroid dehydrogenase regulation in the corpus luteum of the pregnant rat. *Acta Endocrinol. (Copenh.)* 1979;90:176–184.
177. Suzuki K, Tamaoki BI. Enzymological studies of rat luteinized ovaries in relation to acute reduction of aromatizable androgen formation and stimulated production of progestins. *Endocrinology* 1979;104:1317–1323.
178. Wiest WG. Conversion of progesterone to 4-pregn-20α-ol-3-one by rat ovarian tissue in vitro. *J. Biol. Chem.* 1959;234: 3115–3121.
179. Wiest WG, Kidwell WR, Kirschbaum TH. Induction of rat ovarian 20α-hydroxysteroid dehydrogenase activity by gonadotrophic hormone administration. *Steroids* 1963;2:617–630.
180. Csapo AI, Wiest WG. An examination of the quantitative relationship between progesterone and the maintenance of pregnancy. *Endocrinology* 1969;85:735–746.
181. Wiest WG. On the function of 20α-hydroxypregn-4-en-3-one during parturition in the rat. *Endocrinology* 1968;83:1181–1184.
182. Diaz-Zagoya JC, Wiest WG, Arias F. 20α-Hydroxysteroid oxidoreductase activity and 20α-dihydroprogesterone concentration in human placenta before and after parturition. *Am. J. Obstet. Gynecol.* 1979;133:673–676.
183. Loutfi G, Peron F, Dorfman RI. Formation of 20α-hydroxy-Δ^4-pregnen-3-one and Δ^4-androsten-3,17-dione in rodent ovaries. *Endocrinology* 1962;71:983–985.
184. Savard K, Marsh JM, Rice BF. Gonadotropins and ovarian steroidogenesis. *Rec. Prog. Horm. Res.* 1965;21:285–356.
185. Eckstein B, Lerner N. Changes in ovarian 5α-steroid reductase and 20α-hydroxysteroid dehydrogenase activity produced by induction of first ovulation with gonadotropin. *Biochim. Biophys. Acta* 1977;489:143–149.
186. Epstein-Almog R, Orly J. Inhibition of hormone-induced steroidogenesis during cell proliferation in serum-free cultures of rat granulosa cells. *Endocrinology* 1985;116:2103–2112.
187. Short RV. Steroids in the follicular fluid and the corpus luteum of the mare: A "two-cell type" theory of ovarian steroid synthesis. *J. Endocrinol.* 1962;24:59–63.
188. Bjersing L, Carstensen H. Biosynthesis of steroids by granulosa cells of the porcine ovary in vitro. *J. Reprod. Fertil.* 1967;14:101–111.
189. Younglai EV, Short RV. Pathways of steroid biosynthesis in the intact Graafian follicle of mares in oestrus. *J. Endocrinol.* 1970;47:321–331.
190. Fortune JE, Armstrong DT. Hormonal control of 17β-estradiol biosynthesis in proestrous rat follicles: estradiol production by isolated theca versus granulosa cells. *Endocrinology* 1978;102: 227–235.
191. Fowler RE, Fox NL, Edwards RG, Walters DE, Steptoe PC. Steroidogenesis by cultured granulosa cells aspirated from human follicles using pregnenolone and androgen as precursors. *J. Endocrinol.* 1978;77:171–183.
192. Johnson DC, Hoversland RC. Oestradiol synthesis by granulosa cells from immature rats treated with pregnant mare's serum gonadotrophin. *Acta Endocrinol. (Copenh.)* 1983;104:74–79.
193. Bjersing L, Carstensen H. The role of the granulosa in the biosynthesis of ovarian steroids. *Biochim. Biophys. Acta* 1964;86: 637–639.
194. Moor RM. Sites of steroid production in ovine Graafian follicles in culture. *J. Endocrinol.* 1977;73:143–150.
195. Nimrod A, Rosenfield RL, Otto P. Relationship of androgen action to androgen metabolism in isolated rat granulosa cells. *J. Steroid Biochem.* 1980;13:1015–1019.
196. Moon YS, Duleba AJ. Comparative studies of androgen metabolism in theca and granulosa cells of human follicles in vitro. *Steroids* 1982;39:419–430.
197. Terakawa N, Kondo K, Aono T, Kurachi K, Matsumoto K. Hormonal regulation of 4-ene-5α-reductase activity in prepubertal rat ovaries. *J. Steroid Biochem.* 1978;9:307–311.
198. Allen E, Doisy EA. Ovarian and placental hormones. *Physiol. Rev.* 1927;7:600–650.
199. Mossman HW. The thecal gland and its relation to the reproductive cycle. A study of the cyclic changes in the ovary of the pocket gopher, *Geomys Bursarius* (Shaw). *Am. J. Anat.* 1937;61: 289–319.
200. Corner GW. The sites of formation of estrogenic substances in the animal body. *Physiol. Rev.* 1983;18:154–172.
201. Hisaw FL. Development of the Graafian follicle and ovulation. *Physiol. Rev.* 1947;27:95–119.
202. Allen E. Glandular physiology and therapy. *JAMA* 1941;116: 405–413.
203. Falck B. Site of production of oestrogen in rat ovary as studied in micro-transplants. *Acta Physiol. Scand. Suppl. 47* 1959;163: 1–101.
204. Greep RO, van Dyke HB, Chow BF. Gonadotropins of the swine pituitary. I. Various biological effects of purified thylakentrin (FSH) and pure metakentrin (ICSH). *Endocrinology* 1942;30: 635–649.
205. Hollander N, Hollander V. The effect of follicle-stimulating hormone on the biosynthesis in vitro of estradiol-17β from acetate-1-C^{14}. *J. Biol. Chem.* 1958;233:1097–1099.
206. Mills TM, Davies PJA, Savard K. Stimulation of estrogen synthesis in rabbit follicles by luteinizing hormone. *Endocrinology* 1971;88:857–862.
207. Moon YS, Dorrington JH, Armstrong DT. Stimulatory action of follicle-stimulating hormone on estradiol-17β secretion by hypophysectomized rat ovaries in organ culture. *Endocrinology* 1975;97:244–247.
208. Dorrington JH, Armstrong DT. Follicle-stimulating hormone stimulates estradiol-17β synthesis in cultured Sertoli cells. *Proc. Natl. Acad. Sci. USA* 1975;72:2677–2681.
209. Armstrong DT, Papkoff H. Stimulation of aromatization of exogenous and endogenous androgens in ovaries of hypophysectomized rats in vivo by follicle-stimulating hormone. *Endocrinology* 1976;99:1144–1151.
210. Baird DT. Evidence in vivo for the two-cell hypothesis of ovarian estrogen synthesis by the sheep Graafian follicle. *J. Reprod. Fertil.* 1977;50:183–185.
211. Fowler RE, Fox NL, Edwards RG, Steptoe PC. Steroid production from 17α-hydroxypregnenolone and dehydroepiandrosterone by human granulosa cells in vitro. *J. Reprod. Fertil.* 1978;54:109–117.
212. Fortune JE, Armstrong DT. Androgen production by theca and granulosa isolated from proestrous rat follicles. *Endocrinology* 1977;100:1341–1347.
213. Short RV. Steroids present in the follicular fluid of the cow. *J. Endocrinol.* 1962;23:401–411.
214. Fortune JE. Bovine theca and granulosa cells interact to promote androgen and progestin production. *Biol. Reprod. (Suppl. 1)* 1981;24:39A (abstr. 33).
215. Lischinsky A, Armstrong DT. Granulosa cell stimulation of thecal androgen synthesis. *Can. J. Physiol. Pharmacol.* 1983;61: 472–477.
216. Pencharz RI. Effect of estrogens and androgens alone and in combination with chorionic gonadotropin on the ovary of the hypophysectomized rat. *Science* 1940;91:554–555.
217. Williams PC. Effect of stilbestrol on the ovaries of hypophysectomized rats. *Nature* 1940;145:388–389.
218. Simpson ME, Evans HM, Fraenkel-Conrat HL, Li CH. Synergism of estrogens with pituitary gonadotropins in hypophysectomized rats. *Endocrinology* 1941;28:37–41.
219. Williams PC. Ovarian stimulation by oestrogens: effects in immature hypophysectomized rats. *Proc. R. Soc. London [Biol.]* 1944;132:189–199.
220. Payne RW, Hellbaum AA. The effect of estrogens on the ovary of the hypophysectomized rat. *Endocrinology* 1955;57:193–199.
221. Payne RW, Runser RH. The influence of estrogen and androgen on the ovarian response of hypophysectomized immature rats to gonadotropins. *Endocrinology* 1958;62:313–321.
222. Bradbury JT. Direct action of estrogen on the ovary of the immature rat. *Endocrinology* 1961;68:112–120.
223. Smith BD. The effect of diethylstilbestrol on the immature rat ovary. *Endocrinology* 1961;69:238–245.

224. Reiter EO, Goldenberg RL, Vaitukaitis JL, Ross GT. Evidence for a role of estrogen in ovarian augmentation reaction. *Endocrinology* 1972;91:1518–1522.
225. Harman SM, Louvet JP, Ross GT. Interaction of estrogen and gonadotrophins on follicular atresia. *Endocrinology* 1975;96:1145–1152.
226. Saiduddui S. ^{3}H-estradiol uptake by the rat ovary. *Proc. Soc. Exp. Biol. Med.* 1971;138:651–660.
227. Saiduddui S, Milo Jr, GE. Effect of hypophysectomy and pretreatment on uptake and retention of estradiol by the ovary. *Proc. Soc. Exp. Biol. Med.* 1974;146:513–517.
228. Stumpf WE. Nuclear concentration of ^{3}H-estradiol in target issues. Dry-mount autoradiography of vagina, oviduct, ovary, testis, mammary tumor, liver and adrenal. *Endocrinology* 1969;85:31–37.
229. Richards JS. Estradiol receptor content of rat granulosa cells during follicular development: modification by estradiol and gonadotropins. *Endocrinology* 1975;97:1174–1184.
230. Richards JS. Estradiol binding to rat corpora lutea during pregnancy. *Endocrinology* 1974;95:1046–1053.
231. Saiduddin S, Zassenhaus HP. Estradiol-17β receptors in the immature rat ovary. *Steroids* 1977;29:197–213.
232. Leung PCK, Goff AK, Kennedy TG, Armstrong DT. An intraovarian inhibitory action of estrogen and androgen production in vivo. *Biol. Reprod.* 1978;19:641–647.
233. Leung PCK, Armstrong DT. Estrogen treatment of immature rats inhibits ovarian androgen production in vitro. *Endocrinology* 1979;104:1411–1417.
234. Leung PCK, Armstrong DT. Further evidence in support of a short-loop feedback action of estrogen on ovarian androgen production. *Life Sci.* 1980;27:415–420.
235. Hunter MG, Armstrong DT. Estrogens inhibit steroid production by dispersed porcine thecal cells. *Biol. Reprod. (Suppl. 1)* 1986;34:196 (abstr. 293).
236. Magoffin DA, Erickson GF. Mechanism by which 17β-estradiol inhibits ovarian androgen production in the rat. *Endocrinology* 1981;108:962–969.
237. Magoffin DA, Erickson GF. Direct inhibitory effects of estrogen on LH-stimulated androgen synthesis by ovarian cells cultured in defined medium. *Mol. Cell. Endocrinol.* 1982;28:81–89.
238. Eckstein B, Nimrod A. Properties of microsomal Δ^4-3-ketosteroid 5α-reductase in immature rat ovary. *Biochim. Biophys. Acta* 1977;499:1–9.
239. Armstrong DT. Alterations of progesterone metabolism in immature rat ovaries by luteinizing hormone. *Biol. Reprod.* 1979;21:1025–1033.
240. Evans G, Leung PCK, Brodie AMH, Armstrong DT. Effect of an aromatase inhibitor (4-acetoxy-4-androstene-3,17-dione) on the stimulatory action of luteinizing hormone on estradiol-17β synthesis by rat preovulatory follicles in vitro. *Biol. Reprod.* 1981;25:290–294.
241. Armstrong DT, Dorrington JH, Robinson J. Effects of indomethacin and aminoglutethimide phosphate in vivo on luteinizing-hormone-induced alterations on cyclic adenosine monophosphate, prostaglandin F, and steroid levels in preovulatory rat ovaries. *Can. J. Biochem.* 1976;54:796–802.
242. Bahr JM. Simultaneous measurement of steroids in follicular fluid and ovarian venous blood in the rabbit. *Biol. Reprod.* 1978;18:193–197.
243. Goff AK, Henderson KM. Changes in follicular fluid and serum concentrations of steroids in PMS-treated immature rats following LH administration. *Biol. Reprod.* 1979;20:1153–1157.
244. Smith MS, Freeman ME, Neill JD. The control of progesterone secretion during the estrous cycle and early pseudo-pregnancy in the rat: prolactin gonadotropin and steroid levels associated with rescue of the corpus luteum of pseudopregnancy. *Endocrinology* 1975;96:219–226.
245. Kalra SP, Kalra PS. Temporal interrelationships among circulating levels of estradiol, progesterone and LH during the rat estrous cycle: effects of exogenous progesterone. *Endocrinology* 1974;95:1711–1718.
246. Saidapur SK, Greenwald GS. Regulation of 17β-estradiol synthesis in the proestrous hamster: role of progesterone and luteinizing hormone. *Endocrinology* 1979;105:1432–1439.
247. Fortune JE, Hansel W. The effects of 17β-estradiol on progesterone secretion by bovine theca and granulosa cells. *Endocrinology* 1979;104:1834–1838.
248. Engels JA, Friedlander RL, Eik-Nes KB. An effect in vivo of clomiphene on the rate of conversion of androstenedione-C^{14} to estrone-C^{14} and estradiol-C^{14} by the canine ovary. *Metabolism* 1968;17:189–198.
249. Zhuang L-Z, Adashi EY, Hsueh AJW. Direct enhancement of gonadotropin-stimulated ovarian estrogen biosynthesis by estrogen and clomiphene citrate. *Endocrinology* 1982;110:2219–2221.
250. Adashi EY, Hsueh AJW. Estrogens augment the stimulation of ovarian aromatase activity by follicle-stimulating hormone in cultured rat granulosa cells. *J. Biol. Chem.* 1982;257:6077–6083.
251. Welsh Jr, TH, Jia X-C, Jones PBC, Zhuang L-Z, Hsueh AJW. Disparate effects of triphenylethylene antiestrogens on estrogen and progestin biosyntheses by cultured rat granulosa cells. *Endocrinology* 1984;115:1275–1282.
252. Daniel SAJ, Armstrong DT. Involvement of estrogens in the regulation of granulosa cell aromatase activity. *Can. J. Physiol. Pharmacol.* 1983;61:507–511.
253. Thanki KH, Channing CP. Influence of serum, estrogen, and gonadotropins upon growth and progesterone secretion by cultures of granulosa cells from small porcine follicles. *Endocr. Res. Commun.* 1976;3:319–333.
254. Thanki KH, Channing CP. Effects of follicle-stimulating hormone and estradiol upon progesterone secretion by porcine granulosa cells in tissue culture. *Endocrinology* 1978;103:74–80.
255. Schomberg DW, Stouffer RL, Tyrey L. Modulation of progestin secretion in ovarian cells by 17β-hydroxy-5-androstan-3-one (dihydrotestosterone): a direct demonstration in monolayer culture. *Biochem. Biophys. Res. Commun.* 1976;68:77–81.
256. Hancy AF, Schomberg DW. Steroidal modulation of progesterone secretion by granulosa cells from large porcine follicles: a role for androgens and estrogens in controlling steroidogenesis. *Biol. Reprod.* 1978;19:242–248.
257. Hillier SG, Knazek RA, Ross GT. Androgenic stimulation of progesterone production by granulosa cells from preantral ovarian follicles: further in vitro studies using replicate cell cultures. *Endocrinology* 1977;100:1539–1549.
258. Bieszczad RR, McClintock JS, Pepe GJ, Dimino MJ. Progesterone secretion by granulosa cells from different sized follicles of human ovaries after short term incubation. *J. Clin. Endocrinol. Metab.* 1982;55:181–184.
259. Veldhuis JD, Klase PA, Sandon BA, Kolp LA. Progesterone secretion by highly differentiated human granulosa cells isolated from preovulatory Graafian follicles, induced by endogenous gonadotropins and human chorionic gonadotropin. *J. Clin. Endocrinol. Metab.* 1983;57:287–291.
260. Shemesh M, Ailenberg M. The effect of androstenedione on progesterone accumulation in cultures of bovine ovarian follicles. *Biol. Reprod.* 1977;17:499–505.
261. Veldhuis JD. Bipotential actions of estrogens on progesterone biosynthesis by ovarian cells. II. Relation of estradiol's stimulatory actions to cholesterol and progestin metabolism in cultured swine granulosa cells. *Endocrinology* 1985;117:1076–1083.
262. Leung PCK, Armstrong DT. A mechanism for the intraovarian inhibitory action of estrogen on androgen production. *Biol. Reprod.* 1979;21:1035–1042.
263. Goldenberg RL, Bridson WE, Kohler PO. Estrogen stimulation of progesterone synthesis by porcine granulosa cells in culture. *Biochem. Biophys. Res. Commun.* 1972;48:101–107.
264. Bernard J. Effect of follicular fluid and oestradiol on the luteinization of rat granulosa cells in vitro. *J. Reprod. Fertil.* 1975;45:453–460.
265. Welsh Jr, TH, Zhuang L-Z, Hsueh AJW. Estrogen augmentation of gonadotropin-stimulated progestin biosynthesis in cultured rat granulosa cells. *Endocrinology* 1983;112:1916–1924.
266. Hudson KE, Hillier SG. Catechol estradiol control of FSH-stimulated granulosa cell steroidogenesis. *J. Endocrinol.* 1985;106:R1–R4.
267. Khan MI, Gibori G. Catechol estrogens and their role in luteal steroidogenesis. *Biol. Reprod.* 1984;30(Suppl. 1):127 (abstr. 194).
268. Zeleznik AJ, Hillier SG, Ross GT. Follicle-stimulating hormone-

induced follicular development: an examination of the role of androgens. *Biol. Reprod.* 1979;21:673–681.
269. Neumann F, von Berswordt-Wallrabe R, Elger W, Steinbeck K, Hann JD, Kramer M. Aspects of androgen-dependent events as studied by antiandrogens. *Recent Prog. Horm. Res.* 1970;26: 337–410.
270. Lyon MF, Glenister PH. Evidence from Tfm/O that androgen is inessential for reproduction in female mice. *Nature* 1974;247: 366–367.
271. Schreiber JR, Reid R, Ross GT. A receptor-like testosterone binding protein in ovaries from estrogen-stimulated hypophysectomized immature female rats. *Endocrinology* 1976;98:1206–1213.
272. Schreiber JR, Ross GT. Further characterization of rat ovarian testosterone receptor with evidence for nuclear translocation. *Endocrinology* 1976;99:590–596.
273. Campo SM, Carson RS, Findlay JK. (1984): Distribution and characterisation of specific androgen-binding sites within the ovine follicle. *15th Annual Conference of the Australian Society for Reproductive Biology, Canberra,* p. 27 (abstr.).
274. Milwidsky A, Younes MA, Besch NF, Besch PK, Kaufman RH. Receptor-like binding proteins for testosterone and progesterone in the human ovary. *Am. J. Obstet. Gynecol.* 1980;138:93–98.
275. McNatty KP, Moore Smith D, Makris A, Osathanondh R, Ryan KJ. The microenvironment of the human antral follicle: interrelationships among the steroid levels in antral fluid, the population of granulosa cells, and the status of the oocyte in vivo and in vitro. *J. Clin. Endocrinol. Metab.* 1979;49:851–860.
276. Carson RS, Findlay JK, Clarke IJ, Burger HG. Estradiol, testosterone, and androstenedione in ovine follicular fluid during growth and atresia of ovarian follicles. *Biol. Reprod.* 1981;24: 105–113.
277. Hillier SG, Ross GT. Effects of exogenous testosterone on ovarian weight, follicular morphology and intraovarian progesterone concentration in estrogen-primed hypophysectomized immature female rats. *Biol. Reprod.* 1979;20:261–268.
278. Louvet JP, Harman SM, Schreiber JR, Ross GT. Evidence for a role of androgens in follicular maturation. *Endocrinology* 1975;97:366–372.
279. Bagnell CA, Mills TM, Costoff A, Mahesh VB. A model for the study of androgen effects of follicular atresia and ovulation. *Biol. Reprod.* 1982;27:903–914.
280. Opavsky MA, Armstrong DT. The effectiveness of FSH in inducing superovulation is influenced by LH. *Biol. Reprod.* 1985;32 (Suppl. 1):71 (abstr. 67).
281. Ohno S, Christian L, Attardi B. Role of testosterone in normal female function. *Nature* 1973;243:119–120.
282. Peluso JJ, Brown I, Steger RW. Effects of cyproterone acetate, a potent antiandrogen, on the preovulatory follicle. *Biol. Reprod.* 1979;21:929–936.
283. Kumari GL, Datta JK, Das RP, Roy S. Evidence for a role of androgens in the growth and maturation of ovarian follicles in rats. *Horm. Res.* 1978;9:112–120.
284. Mori T, Suzuki A, Nishimura T, Kambegawa A. Evidence for androgen participation in induced ovulation in immature rats. *Endocrinology* 1977;101:623–626.
285. Tsafriri A, Braw RH. Experimental approaches to atresia in mammals. In: Clarke RE, ed. *Oxford Reviews of Reproductive Biology* Vol. 6, Oxford: Clarendon Press; 1984:226–265.
286. Moor RM, Hay MF, Seamark RF. The sheep ovary: regulation of steoidogenic, haemodynamic and structural changes in the largest follicle and adjacent tissue before ovulation. *J. Reprod. Fertil.* 1975;45:595–604.
287. Lucky AW, Schreiber JR, Hillier SG, Schulman JD, Ross GT. Progesterone production by cultured preantral rat granulosa cells: stimulation by androgens. *Endocrinology* 1977;100: 128–133.
288. Corredor A, Flickinger GL. Hormonal regulation of progesterone secretion by cultured mouse granulosa cells. *Biol. Reprod.* 1983;29:1142–1146.
289. Leung PCK, Goff AK, Armstrong DT. Stimulatory action of androgen administration in vivo on ovarian responsiveness to gonadotropins. *Endocrinology* 1979;104:1119–1123.
290. Schomberg DW, Williams RF, Tyrey L, Ulberg LC. Reduction of granulosa cell progesterone secretion in vitro by intraovarian implants of antiandrogen. *Endocrinology* 1978;102:984–987.
291. Welsh Jr, JH, Jones PBC, Ruiz de Galaretta CM, Fanjul LF, Hsueh AJW. Androgen regulation of progestin biosynthetic enzymes in FSH-treated rat granulosa cells in vitro. *Steroids* 1982;40:691–700.
292. Hillier SG, deZwart FA. Androgen/antiandrogen modulation of cyclic AMP-induced steroidogenesis during granulosa cell differentiation in tissue culture. *Mol. Cell. Endocrinol.* 1982;28: 347–361.
293. Goff AK, Leung PCK, Armstrong DT. Stimulatory action of follicle-stimulating hormone and androgens on the responsiveness of rat granulosa cells to gonadotropins in vitro. *Endocrinology* 1979;104:1124–1129.
294. Daniel SAJ, Armstrong DT. Site of action of androgens on follicle-stimulating hormone-induced aromatase activity in cultured rat granulosa cells. *Endocrinology* 1984;114:1975–1982.
295. Knecht M, Darbon JM, Ranta T, Baukal AJ, Catt KJ. Estrogens enhance the adenosine 3′,5′-monophosphate-mediated induction of follicle-stimulating hormone and luteinizing hormone receptors in rat granulosa cells. *Endocrinology* 1984;115:41–49.
296. Duleba AJ, Takahashi H, Moon YS. Androgenic modulation of progesterone metabolism by rat granulosa cells in culture. *Steroids* 1983;42:321–330.
297. Moon YS, Duleba AJ, Takahashi H. Differential actions of LH and androgens on progesterone catabolism by rat granulosa cells. *Biochem. Biophys. Res. Commun.* 1984;119:694–699.
298. Moon YS, Duleba AJ, Kuir KS, Yuen BH. Alterations of 20α-hydroxysteroid dehydrogenase activity in cultured rat granulosa cells by follicle-stimulating hormone and testosterone. *Biol. Reprod.* 1985;32:998–1009.
299. Nimrod A. On the synergistic action of androgen and FSH on progestin secretion by cultured rat granulosa cells. Cellular and mitochondrial cholesterol metabolism. *Mol. Cell. Endocrinol.* 1981;21:51–62.
300. Schrieber JR, Nakamura K, Weinstein DB. Androgen and FSH synergistically stimulate rat ovary granulosa cell utilization of rat and human lipoproteins. In: G Greenwald and PF Terranova, eds. *Factors Regulating Ovarian Function,* New York: Raven Press; 1983:311–315.
301. Evans G, Lischinsky A, Daniel SAJ, Armstrong DT. Androgen-inhibition of FSH-stimulated progesterone production by granulosa cells of pre-pubertal pig. *Can. J. Physiol. Pharmacol.* 1984;62:840–845.
302. Tan CH, Armstrong DT. FSH-stimulated 3β-HSD activity of porcine granulosa cells: inhibition by androgens. *Proceedings of the 3rd Joint Meeting of the British Endocrine Societies, Edinburgh,* Abstr. 12. 1984.
303. Daniel SAJ, Armstrong DT. Enhancement of follicle-stimulating hormone-induced aromatase by androgens in cultured rat granulosa cells. *Endocrinology* 1980;107:1027–1033.
304. Armstrong DT, Daniel SAJ, Salhanick AR, Sheela Rani CS. Hormonal interactions in regulation of steroid biosynthesis by the ovarian follicle. In: Makesh VB, Muldoon TG, Saxena BB, and Sadler WA, eds. *Functional Correlates of Hormone Receptors in Reproduction.* North-Holland, New York: Elsevier; 1980: 245–260.
305. Hillier SG, deZwart FA. Evidence that granulosa cell induction/activation by follicle-stimulating hormone is an androgen receptor-regulated process in vitro. *Endocrinology* 1981;109: 1303–1305.
306. Hillier SG, van den Boogaard AMJ, Reichert Jr, LE, van Hall EV. Alterations in granulosa cell aromatase activity accompanying preovulatory follicular development in the rat ovary with evidence that 5α-reduced C_{19} steroids inhibit the aromatase reaction in vitro. *J. Endocrinol.* 1980;84:409–419.
307. Hillier SG, van den Boogaard AMJ, Reichert Jr, LE, van Hall EV. Intraovarian sex steroid hormone interactions and the regulation of follicular maturation: aromatization of androgens by human granulosa cells in vitro. *J. Clin. Endocrinol. Metab.* 1980;50: 640–647.
308. Smith OW, Ofner P, Vena RL. In vitro conversion of testoster-

one-4-^{14}C to androgens of the 5α-androstane series by normal human ovary. *Steroids* 1974;24:311–315.

309. Siiteri PK, Thompson EA. Studies of human placental aromatase. *J. Steroid Biochem.* 1975;6:317–322.
310. Katz Y, Armstrong DT. Inhibition of ovarian estradiol-17β secretion by luteinizing hormone in prepubertal, pregnant mare serum-treated rats. *Endocrinology* 1976;99:1442–1447.
311. Saidudduin S, Zassenhaus HP. Effect of testosterone and progesterone on the estradiol receptor in the immature rat ovary. *Endocrinology* 1978;102:1069–1076.
312. Smith BD, Bradbury JT. Influence of progestins on ovarian responses to estrogen and gonadotrophins in immature rats. *Endocrinology* 1966;78:297–301.
313. Jesel L. Données nouvelles sur le contrôle exercé par le corps jaune sur la croissance folliculaire au début du cycle oestral chez le Cobaye. *C. R. Acad. Sci., Ser D* 1970;271:1693–1696.
314. Hori T, Kato G, Miyake T. Acute effects of ovarian steroids upon follicular growth in the cycling rat. *Endocrinol. Jpn.* 1973;20: 475–482.
315. Buffler G, Roser S. New data concerning the role played by progesterone in the control of follicular growth in the rat. *Acta Endocrinol.* 1974;75:569–578.
316. Beattie CW, Corbin A. The differential effects of diestrous progesterone administration on proestrous gonadotrophin levels. *Endocrinology* 1975;97:885–890.
317. Goodman AL, Hodgen GD. Systemic versus intraovarian progesterone replacement after luteectomy in rhesus monkeys: differential patterns of gonadotropins and follicle growth. *J. Clin. Endocrinol. Metab.* 1977;45:837–840.
318. Richards JS, Bogovich K. Effect of human chorionic gonadotropin and progesterone on follicular development in the immature rat. *Endocrinology* 1982;111:1429–1438.
319. Bogovich K, Richards JS, Reichert Jr, LE. Obligatory role of LH in the initiation of preovulatory follicular growth in the pregnant rat: specific effects of human chorionic gonadotropin and follicle-stimulating hormone on LH receptors and steroidogenesis in theca, granulosa and luteal cells. *Endocrinology* 1981;109: 860–867.
320. Schrieber JR, Hsueh AJW. Progesterone "receptor" in rat ovary. *Endocrinology* 1979;105:915–919.
321. Schreiber JR, Hsueh AJW, Baulieu EE. Binding of the anti-progestin RU-486 to rat ovary steroid receptors. *Contraception* 1983;28:77–85.
322. Schreiber JR, Erickson GF. Progesterone receptor in the rat ovary: further characterization and localization in the granulosa cell. *Steroids* 1979;34:459–469.
323. Naess O. Characterization of cytoplasmic progesterone receptors in rat granulosa cells: evidence for nuclear translocation. *Acta Endocrinol.* 1981;98:288–294.
324. Philibert D, Ojasoo T, Raynaud JP. Properties of the cytoplasmic progestin-binding protein in the rabbit uterus. *Endocrinology* 1977;101:1850–1861.
325. Pasqualini JR, Nguyen BJ. Progesterone receptors in fetal uterus and ovary of the guinea pig. Evolution during fetal development and induction and stimulation in estradiol-primed animals. *Endocrinology* 1980;106:1160–1165.
326. Jacobs BR, Smith RG. Evidence for a receptor-like protein for progesterone in bovine ovarian cytosol. *Endocrinology* 1980;106: 1276–1282.
327. Jacobs BR, Suchocki S, Smith RG. Evidence for human ovarian progesterone receptor. *Am. J. Obstet. Gynecol.* 1980;138: 332–336.
328. Fanjul LF, de Galarreta R, Hsueh AJW. Progestin augmentation of gonadotrophin-stimulated progesterone production by cultured rat granulosa cells. *Endocrinology* 1983;112:405–407.
329. Hsueh AJW, Adashi EY, Jones PBC, Welsh TH. Hormonal regulation of the differentiation of cultured ovarian granulosa cells. *Endocr. Rev.* 1984;5:76–127.
330. Schreiber JR, Nakamura K, Erickson GF. Progestins inhibit FSH-stimulated steroidogenesis in cultured rat granulosa cells. *Mol. Cell. Endocrinol.* 1980;19:165–173.
331. Schreiber JR, Nakamura K, Erickson GF. Progestins inhibit FSH-stimulated granulosa estrogen production at a post-cAMP site. *Mol. Cell. Endocrinol.* 1981;21:161–170.
332. Fortune JE, Vincent SE. Progesterone inhibits the induction of aromatase activity in rat granulosa cells in vitro. *Biol. Reprod.* 1983;28:1078–1089.
333. Greenwald GS. Gonadotropin regulation of follicular development. In: Mondgal NR, ed. *Gonadotropins and Gonadal Function.* New York: Academic; 1974:205–212.
334. Mahajan DK, Samuels LT. Inhibition of 17,20(17-hydroxyprogesterone)-lyase by progesterone. *Steroids* 1975;25:217–228.
335. Brophy PJ, Gower DB. Studies on the inhibition by 5α-pregnane-3.20-dione of the biosynthesis of 16-androstenes and dehydroepiandrosterone in boar testis preparations. *Biochim. Biophys. Acta* 1974;360:252–259.
336. Rothchild I. The regulation of the mammalian corpus luteum. *Rec. Prog. Horm. Res.* 1981;37:183–298.
337. Crisp TM. Hormone requirements for early maintenance of rat granulosa cell cultures. *Endocrinology* 1977;101:1286–1297.
338. Veldhuis JD, Klase P, Hammond JM. Divergent effects of prolactin upon steroidogenesis by porcine granulosa cells in vitro: influence of cytodifferentiation. *Endocrinology* 1980;107:42–46.
339. Advis JP, Richards JS, Ojeda SR. Hyperprolactinemia-induced precocious puberty: studies on the mechanism(s) by which prolactin enhances ovarian progesterone responsiveness to gonadotropins in prepubertal rats. *Endocrinology* 1981;108:1333–1342.
340. Advis JP, Ojeda SR. Hyperprolactinemia-induced precocious puberty in the female rat: ovarian site of action. *Endocrinology* 1978;103:924–935.
341. Gibori G, Richards JS. Dissociation of two distinct luteotropic effects of prolactin: regulation of luteinizing hormone-receptor content and progesterone secretion during pregnancy. *Endocrinology* 1978;102:767–774.
342. Veldhuis JD, Hammond JM. Oestrogens regulate divergent effects of prolactin in the ovary. *Nature* 1980;284:262–264.
343. Wang C, Hsueh AJW, Erickson GF. Prolactin inhibition of estrogen production by cultured rat granulosa cells. *Mol. Cell. Endocrinol.* 1980;20:135–144.
344. Wang C, Chan V. Divergent effects of prolactin on estrogen and progesterone production by granulosa cells of rat Graafian follicles. *Endocrinology* 1982;110:1085–1093.
345. Dorrington J, Gore-Langton RE. Prolactin inhibits oestrogen synthesis in the ovary. *Nature* 1981;290:600–602.
346. Dorrington JH, Gore-Langton RE. Antigonadal action of prolactin: further studies on the mechanism of inhibition of follicle-stimulatory hormone-induced aromatase activity in rat granulosa cell cultures. *Endocrinology* 1982;110:1701–1707.
347. Tsai-Morris CH, Ghosh M, Hirshfield AN, Wise PM, Brodie AMH. Inhibition of ovarian aromatase by prolactin in vivo. *Biol. Reprod.* 1983;29:342–346.
348. Demura R, Ono M, Demura H, Shizume K, Oouchi H. Prolactin directly inhibits basal as well as gonadotropin-stimulated secretion of progesterone and 17β-estradiol in the human ovary. *J. Clin. Endocrinol. Metab.* 1982;54:1246–1250.
349. Advis JP, Wiener SL, Ojeda SR. Changes in ovarian 3α-androstanediol response to human chorionic gonadotropin during puberty in the rat: modulatory role of prolactin. *Endocrinology* 1981;109:223–228.
350. Magoffin DA, Erickson GP. Prolactin inhibition of luteinizing hormone-stimulated androgen synthesis in ovarian interstitial cells cultured in defined medium: mechanism of actions. *Endocrinology* 1982;111:2001–2007.
351. Fraser HM. Antifertility effects of GnRH. *J. Reprod. Fertil.* 1982;64:503–515.
352. de Koning J, van Dieten JAMJ, van Rees GP. Refractoriness of the pituitary gland after continuous exposure to luteinizing hormone releasing hormone. *J. Endocrinol.* 1978;79:311–318.
353. Rippel RH, Johnson ES, White WF. Effect of consecutive injections of synthetic gonadotropin-releasing hormone on LH release in anestrous and ovariectomized ewes. *J. Anim. Sci.* 1974;39: 907–914.
354. Sandow J, van Rechenberg W, Kuhl H, Baumann R, Krauss B, Jerzabek G, Killie S. Inhibitory control of the pituitary LH secretion by LHRH in male rats. *Horm. Res.* 1979;11:303–317.

355. Fraser HM, Laird NC, Blakeley DM. Decreased pituitary responsiveness and inhibition of the luteinizing hormone surge and ovulation in the stump-tailed monkey (*Macaca arctoides*) by chronic treatment with an agonist of luteinizing hormone-releasing hormone. *Endocrinology* 1980;106:452–457.
356. Conti M, Harwood JP, Hsueh AJW, Dufau ML, Catt KJ. Gonadotropin-induced loss of hormone receptors and desensitization of luteal adenylate cyclase in the ovary. *J. Biol. Chem.* 1976;251: 7729–7731.
357. Hunzicker-Dunn M, Birnbaumer L. Adenylate cyclase activities in ovarian tissues. IV. Gonadotropin-induced desensitization of luteal adenylyl cyclase throughout pregnancy and pseudopregnancy in the rabbit and rat. *Endocrinology* 1976;99:211–222.
358. Jonassen JA, Richards JS. Granulosa cell desensitization: effects of gonadotropins on antral and preantral follicles. *Endocrinology* 1980;106:1786–1794.
359. Jonassen JA, Bose K, Richards JS. Enhancement and desensitization of hormone-responsive adenylate cyclase in granulosa cells of preantral and antral ovarian follicles: effects of estradiol and follicle-stimulating hormone. *Endocrinology* 1982;111:74–79.
360. Hseuh AJW, Jones PBC. Extrapituitary actions of gonadotropin-releasing hormone. *Endocr. Rev.* 1981;2:437–461.
361. Jones PBC, Conn PM, Marian J, Hsueh AJW. Binding of gonadotropin-releasing hormone agonist to rat ovarian granulosa cells. *Life Sci.* 1980;27:2125–2132.
362. Pieper DR, Richards JS, Marshall JC. Ovarian gonadotropin-releasing hormone (GnRH) receptors: characterization, distribution, and induction by GnRH. *Endocrinology* 1981;108: 1148–1155.
363. Clayton RN, Harwood JP, Catt KJ. Gonadotropin-releasing hormone analogue binds to luteal cells and inhibits progesterone production. *Nature* 1979;282:90–92.
364. Pelletier G, Sequin C, Dube D, St.-Arnaud R. Distribution of LHRH receptors in the rat ovary. *Biol. Reprod.* 1982;26(Suppl. 1):151 (abstr. 230).
365. Marian J, Conn PM. Subcellular localization of the receptor for gonadotropin-releasing hormone in pituitary and ovarian tissue. *Endocrinology* 1983;112:104–112.
366. Ranta T, Knecht M, Kody M, Catt KJ. GnRH receptors in cultured rat granulosa cells: mediation of the inhibitory and stimulatory actions of GnRH. *Mol. Cell. Endocrinol.* 1983;27:233–240.
367. Hazum E, Nimrod A. Photoaffinity-labeling and fluorescence-distribution studies of gonadotropin-releasing hormone receptors in ovarian granulosa cells. *Proc. Natl. Acad. Sci. USA* 1982;79: 1747–1750.
368. Hazum E. Photoaffinity labeling of luteinizing hormone releasing hormone receptor of rat pituitary membrane preparations. *Endocrinology* 1981;109:1281–1283.
369. Clayton RN, Huhtaniemi IT. Absence of gonadotropin-releasing hormone receptors in human gonadal tissue. *Nature* 1982; 299:56–59.
370. Popkin R, Bramley TA, Currie A, Shaw RW, Baird DT, Fraser HM. Specific binding of luteinizing-hormone releasing hormone to human luteal tissue. *Biochem. Biophys. Res. Commun.* 1983;114:750–756.
371. Bramley TA, Menzies GS, Baird DT. Specific binding of gonadotropin-releasing hormone and an agonist to human corpus-luteum homogenates—characterization, properties, and luteal phase levels. *J. Clin. Endocrinol. Metab.* 1985;61:834–841.
372. Tureck RW, Mastroianni Jr, L, Blasco L, Strauss III, JF. Inhibition of human granulosa cell progesterone secretion by a gonadotropin-releasing hormone agonist. *J. Clin. Endocrinol. Metab.* 1982;54:1078–1080.
373. Casper RF, Erickson GF, Rebar RW, Yen SSC. The effect of luteinizing hormone releasing factor and its agonist on cultured human granulosa cells. *Fertil. Steril.* 1982;37:406–409.
374. Koos RD, Ahren KEB, Janson PO, LeMaire WJ. (1982): Effect of a GnRH agonist on the rabbit ovary perfused in vitro. *64th Annual Meeting of the Endocrine Society,* p. 178 (abstr. 395).
375. Massicotte J, Veilleux R, Lavoie M, Labrie F. An LHRH agonist inhibits FSH-induced cyclic AMP accumulation and steroidogenesis in porcine granulosa cells in culture. *Biochem. Biophys. Res. Commun.* 1980;94:1362–1366.
376. Takats A, Hertelendy F. Adenylate cyclase activity of avian granulosa: effect of gonadotropin-releasing hormone. *Gen. Comp. Endocrinol.* 1982;48:515–524.
377. Hertelendy F, Linker F, Asem EK, Raab B. Synergistic effect of gonadotropin releasing hormone on LH-stimulated progesterone production in granulosa cells of the domestic fowl (*Gallus domesticus*). *Gen. Comp. Endocrinol.* 1982;48:117–122.
378. Bex FJ, Corbin A, France E. Resistance of the mouse to the antifertility effects of LHRH agonists. *Life Sci.* 1982;30:1263–1269.
379. Asch RH, Eddy CA, Schally AV. Lack of luteolytic effect of D-Trp-6-LH-RH in hypophysectomized rhesus monkeys (*Macaca mulatta*). *Biol. Reprod.* 1981;25:963–968.
380. Brown JL, Reeves JJ. Absence of specific luteinizing hormone releasing hormone receptors in ovine, bovine and porcine ovaries. *Biol. Reprod.* 1983;29:1179–1182.
381. Asch RH, VanSickle M, Rettori V, Balmaceda JP, Eddy CA, Coy DH, Schally AV. Absence of LHRH binding sites in corpora lutea from rhesus monkeys (*Macacca mulatta*). *J. Clin. Endocrinol. Metab.* 1981;53:215–217.
382. Rippel RH, Johnson ES. Inhibition of hCG-induced ovarian and uterine weight augmentation in the immature rat by analogs of GnRH. *Proc. Soc. Exp. Biol. Med.* 1976;152:432–436.
383. Hsueh AJW, Erickson GF. Extrapituitary action of gonadotropin-releasing hormone: direct inhibition of ovarian steroidogenesis. *Science* 1979;204:845–855.
384. Hsueh AJW, Wang C, Erickson GF. Direct inhibitory effect of gonadotropin-releasing hormone upon follicle-stimulating hormone induction of luteinizing hormone receptor and aromatase activity in rat granulosa cells. *Endocrinology* 1980;106: 1697–1705.
385. Gore-Langton RE, Lacroix M, Dorrington JH. Differential effects of luteinizing hormone-releasing hormone on follicle-stimulating hormone-dependent responses in rat granulosa cells and Sertoli cells in vitro. *Endocrinology* 1981;108:812–819.
386. Dorrington JH, McKeracher HL, Chan AK, Gore-Langton RE. Hormonal interactions in the control of granulosa cell differentiation. *J. Steroid Biochem.* 1983;19:17–32.
387. Ying S-Y, Guilleman R. (DTrp^6-Pro^9-NEt)-luteinising hormone-releasing factor inhibits follicular development in hypophysectomised rats. *Nature* 1979;280:593–595.
388. Jones PBC, Hsueh AJW. Regulation of 3β-hydroxysteroid dehydrogenase by gonadotropin-releasing hormone and follicle-stimulating hormone in cultured rat granulosa cells. *Endocrinology* 1982;110:1663–1671.
389. Jones PBC, Hsueh AJW. Regulation of ovarian 20α-hydroxysteroid dehydrogenase by gonadotropin-releasing hormone and its antagonist in vitro and in vivo. *J. Steroid Biochem.* 1981;14: 1169–1175.
390. Jones PBC, Hsueh AJW. Direct effects of gonadotropin-releasing hormone and its antagonist upon ovarian functions stimulated by FSH, prolactin and LH. *Biol. Reprod.* 1981;24:747–759.
391. Jones PBC, Hsueh AJW. Regulation of progesterone metabolizing enzyme by adrenergic agents, prolactin and prostaglandins in cultured rat ovarian granulosa cells. *Endocrinology* 1981;109: 1347–1354.
392. Clark MR. Stimulation of progesterone and prostaglandin E accumulation by luteinizing hormone-releasing hormone (LHRH) and LHRH analogs in rat granulosa cells. *Endocrinology* 1982;110:146–152.
393. Sheela Rani CS, Ekholm C, Billig H, Magnusson C, Hillensjö T. Biphasic effect of gonadotropin releasing hormone on progestin secretion by rat granulosa cells. *Biol. Reprod.* 1983;28:591–597.
394. Popkin R, Fraser HM, Jonassen J. Stimulation of androstenedione and progesterone release by LHRH and LHRH agonist from isolated rat preovulatory follicles. *Mol. Cell. Endocrinol.* 1983;29: 169–179.
395. Hsueh AJW, Ling NC. Effect of an antagonistic analog of gonadotropin-releasing hormone upon ovarian granulosa cell function. *Life Sci.* 1979;25:1223–1230.
396. St.-Arnaud R, Walker P, Kelly PA, Labrie F. Rat ovarian epidermal growth factor receptors: characterization and hormonal regulation. *Mol. Cell. Endocrinol.* 1983;31:43–52.
397. Clark MR, Thibier C, Marsh JM, LeMaire WJ. Stimulation of

prostaglandin accumulation by luteinizing hormone-releasing hormone (LHRH) and LHRH analogs in rat granulosa cells in vitro. *Endocrinology* 1980;107:17–23.

398. Knecht M, Katz MS, Catt KJ. Gonadotropin-releasing hormone inhibits cyclic nucleotide accumulation in cultured rat granulosa cells. *J. Biol. Chem.* 1981;256:34–36.
399. Knecht M, Catt KJ. Gonadotropin-releasing hormone: regulation of adenosine 3′,5′-monophosphate in ovarian granulosa cells. *Science* 1981;214:1346–1348.
400. Ranta T, Baukal A, Knecht M, Korhonen M, Catt KJ. Inhibitory actions of a gonadotropin-releasing hormone agonist on ovarian follicle-stimulating hormone receptors and adenylate cyclase in vitro. *Endocrinology* 1983;112:956–964.
401. Jones PBC, Hsueh AJW. Modulation of steroidogenic enzymes by gonadotropin-releasing hormone in cultured granulosa cells. In: Greenwald GS and Terranova PF, eds. *Factors Regulating Ovarian Function.* New York: Raven Press; 1983:275–279.
402. Ranta T, Knecht M, Darbon J-M, Baukal AJ, Catt KJ. Calcium dependence of the inhibitory effect of gonadotropin-releasing hormone on luteinizing hormone-induced cyclic AMP production in rat granulosa cells. *Endocrinology* 1983;113:427–429.
403. Hsueh AJW, Jones PBC. Direct hormonal modulation of ovarian granulosa cell maturation: effects of gonadotropin-releasing hormone. In: Rolland R, Van Hall EV, Hillier SG, McNatty KP, and Schoemaker J, eds. *Proceedings IVth Regnier de Graaf Symposium: Follicular Maturation and Ovulation.* Amsterdam: Excerpta Medica; 1982:9–13.
404. Hsueh AJW, Jones PBC. Regulation of ovarian granulosa and luteal cell functions by gonadotropin-releasing hormone and its antagonist. *Adv. Exp. Med. Biol.* 1982;147:223–262.
405. Billig H, Magnusson C, Ekholm C, Hillensjö T. Biphasic effect of a GnRH agonist on glycolysis in cultured rat granulosa cells. *Biol. Reprod.* 1982;26(Suppl. 1):152A (abstr. 231).
406. Wang C. Luteinizing hormone-releasing ·hormone stimulates plasminogen activator production by rat granulosa cells. *Endocrinology* 1983;112:1130–1132.
407. Dorrington JH, Skinner MK. Cytodifferentiation of granulosa cells induced by gonadotropin-releasing hormone promotes fibronectin secretion. *Endocrinology* 1986;118:2065–2071.
408. Naor Z, Yavin E. Gonadotropin releasing hormone stimulates phospholipid labeling in cultured granulosa cells. *Endocrinology* 1982;111:1615–1619.
409. Leung PCK, Raymond V, Labrie F. Stimulation of phosphatidic acid and phosphatidylinositol labeling in luteal cells by luteinizing hormone-releasing hormone. *Endocrinology* 1983;112: 1138–1140.
410. Davis JS, Farese RV, Clark MR. Gonadotropin-releasing hormone (GnRH) stimulates phosphatidylinositol metabolism in rat granulosa cells: mechanism of action of GnRH. *Proc. Natl. Acad. Sci. USA* 1983;80:2049–2053.
411. Davis JS, West LA, Farese RV. Gonadotropin-releasing hormone (GnRH) rapidly stimulates the formation of inositol phosphates and diacylglycerol in rat granulosa cells: further evidence for the involvement of Ca^{2+} and protein kinase C in the action of GnRH. *Endocrinology* 1986;118:2561–2571.
412. Minegishi T, Leung PCK. Effects of prostaglandins and luteinizing hormone-releasing hormone on phosphatidic acid-phosphatidylinositol labelling in rat granulosa cells. *Can. J. Physiol. Pharmacol.* 1985;63:320–324.
413. Minegishi T, Leung PCK. Luteinizing hormone-releasing hormone stimulates arachidonic acid release in rat granulosa cells. *Endocrinology* 1985;117:2001–2007.
414. Berridge MJ. Phosphatidylinositol hydrolysis: a multifunctioned transducing mechanism. *Mol. Cell. Endocrinol.* 1981;24: 115–140.
415. Nishizuka Y. The role of protein kinase C in cell surface signal transduction and tumour promotion. *Nature* 1984;308:693–698.
416. Zilberstein M, Sakut H, Eli Y, Naor Z. Regulation of prostaglandin E, progesterone, and cyclic adenosine monophosphate production in ovarian granulosa cells by luteinizing hormone and gonadotropin-releasing hormone and gonadotropin-releasing hormone agonist: comparative studies. *Endocrinology* 1984;114: 2374–2381.
417. Hillensjö T, LeMaire WJ. Gonadotropin-releasing hormone agonists stimulate meiotic maturation of follicle-enclosed rat oocytes in vitro. *Nature* 1980;287:145–146.
418. Banka CL, Erickson GF. Gonadotropin-releasing hormone induces classical meiotic maturation in subpopulations of atretic preantral follicles. *Endocrinology* 1985;117:1500–1507.
419. Dekel N, Sherizly I, Phillips DM, Nimrod A, Zilberstein M, Naor Z. Characterization of the maturational changes induced by a GnRH analogue in the rat ovarian follicle. *J. Reprod. Fertil.* 1985;75:461–466.
420. Corbin A, Bex FJ. Luteinizing hormone releasing hormone agonists induce ovulation in hypophysectomized proestrous rats: direct ovarian effect. *Life Sci.* 1981;29:185–192.
421. Ekholm C, Hillensjö T, Isaksson O. Gonadotropin-releasing hormone agonists stimulate oocyte meiosis and ovulation in hypophysectomized rats. *Endocrinology* 1981;108:2022–2024.
422. Magoffin DA, Reynolds DS, Erickson GF. Direct inhibitory effect of GnRH on androgen secretion by ovarian interstitial cells. *Endocrinology* 1981;109:661–663.
423. Magoffin DA, Erickson GF. Mechanism by which GnRH inhibits androgen synthesis directly in ovarian interstitial cells. *Mol. Cell. Endocrinol.* 1982;27:191–198.
424. Elkind-Hirsch K, Ravnikar V, Schift I, Tulchinsky D, Ryan KJ. Determinations of endogenous immunoreactive luteinizing hormone-releasing hormone in human plasma. *J. Clin. Endocrinol. Metab.* 1982;54:602–607.
425. Ying S-Y, Ling N, Bohlen P, Guillemin R. Gonadocrinins: peptides in ovarian follicular fluid stimulating the secretion of pituitary gonadotropins. *Endocrinology* 1981;108:1206–1215.
426. Esch F, Ling N, Ying S-Y, Guillemin R. Peptides of gonadal origin involved in reproductive biology. In: McCann SM, and Dhindsa DS, eds. *Role of Peptides and Proteins in Control of Reproduction.* Bethesda, MD: Proceedings of National Institute of Health Workshop; 1982.
427. Aten RF, Williams T, Behrman HR. Ovarian gonadotropin-releasing hormone-like protein(s): demonstration and characterization. *Endocrinology* 1986;118:961–967.
428. Birnbaumer L, Shahabi N, River J, Vale W. Evidence for a physiological role of gonadotropin-releasing hormone (GnRH) or GnRH-like material in the ovary. *Endocrinology* 1985;116: 1367–1370.
429. Jarrett RJ. Effect and mode of action of adrenocortico-trophic hormone upon the reproductive tract of the female mouse. *Endocrinology* 1965;76:434–440.
430. Ramaley JA. Role of the adrenal in PMSG-induced ovulation before puberty: effect of adrenalectomy. *Endocrinology* 1973;92: 881–887.
431. Baldwin DM, Sawyer CH. Effect of dexamethasone on LH release and ovulation in the cyclic rat. *Endocrinology* 1974;94: 1397–1403.
432. Yaginuma T, Kobayashi T. Effect of stress, metyrapone and adrenalectomy on compensatory ovarian hypertrophy. *Endocrinol. Jpn.* 1977;24:403–407.
433. Baldwin DM. The effect of glucocorticoids on estrogen-dependent luteinizing hormone release in the ovariectomized rat and on gonadotropin secretion in the intact female. *Endocrinology* 1979;105:120–128.
434. Cortes-Gallegos V, Gallegos AJ, Bedolla Tovar N, Cervantes C, Parra A. Effect of paramethasone acetate on ovarian steroids and gonadotropins. I. Normal menstrual cycle. *J. Clin. Endocrinol. Metab.* 1975;41:215–220.
435. Cunningham GR, Goldzieher JW, de la Pena A, Oliver M. The mechanism of ovulation inhibition by triamcinolone acetonide. *J. Clin. Endocrinol. Metab.* 1978;46:8–14.
436. Hagino N, Watanabe M, Goldzieher JW. Inhibition by adrenocorticotrophin of gonadotrophin-induced ovulation in immature female rats. *Endocrinology* 1969;84:308–314.
437. Schreiber JR, Nakamura K, Erickson GF. Rat ovary glucocorticoid receptor: identification and characterization. *Steroids* 1982;39:569–584.
438. Louvet JP, Baislic M, Bayard F, Boulard C. Glucocorticoid receptors in rat ovarian granulosa cell cytosol. *59th Annual Meeting of the Endocrine Society,* (abstr. 601). 1977:363.

439. Hsueh AJW, Erickson GF. Glucocorticoid inhibition of FSH-induced estrogen production in cultured rat granulosa cells. *Steroids* 1978;32:639–648.
440. Schoonmaker JN, Erickson GF. Glucocorticoid modulation of follicle-stimulating hormone-mediated granulosa cell differentiation. *Endocrinology* 1983;113:1356–1363.
441. Adashi EY, Jones PBC, Hsueh AJW. Synergistic effect of glucocorticoids on the stimulation of progesterone production by follicle-stimulating hormone in cultured rat granulosa cells. *Endocrinology* 1981;109:1888–1894.
442. Channing CP, Tsai V, Sachs D. Role of insulin, thyroxin and cortisol in luteinization of porcine granulosa cells grown in chemically defined media. *Biol. Reprod.* 1976;15:235–247.
443. Mahajan DK, Little AB. Specific cortisol binding protein in porcine follicular fluid. *Biol. Reprod.* 1978;17:834–842.
444. Mahajan DK, Billiar RB, Little AB. Isolation of cortisol binding globulin (CBG) from porcine follicular fluid by affinity chromatography. *J. Steroid Biochem.* 1980;13:67–71.
445. Adashi EY, Resnick CE, D'ercole AJ, Svoboda ME, Van Wyk JJ. Insulin-like growth factors as intraovarian regulators of granulosa cell growth and function. *Endocr. Rev.* 1985;6:400–420.
446. Jones PBC, Welsh Jr, TH, Hsueh AJW. Regulation of ovarian progestin production by epidermal growth factor in cultured rat granulosa cells. *J. Biol. Chem.* 1982;257:11268–11273.
447. Hsueh AJW, Welsh Jr, TH, Jones PBC. Inhibition of ovarian and testicular steroidogenesis by epidermal growth factor. *Endocrinology* 1981;108:2002–2004.
448. Knecht M, Catt KJ. Modulation of cAMP-mediated differentiation in ovarian granulosa cells by epidermal growth factor and platelet-derived growth factor. *J. Biol. Chem.* 1983;258: 2789–2794.
449. Schomberg DW, May JV, Mondschein JS. Interactions between hormones and growth factors in the regulation of granulosa cell differentiation in vitro. *J. Steroid Biochem.* 1983;19:291–295.
450. Pulley DD, Marrone BL. Inhibitory action of epidermal growth factor on progesterone biosynthesis in hen granulosa cells during short term culture: two sites of action. *Endocrinology* 1986;118: 2284–2291.
451. Erickson GF, Case E. Epidermal growth factor antagonizes ovarian theca-interstitial cytodifferentiation. *Mol. Cell. Endocrinol.* 1983;31:71–76.
452. Lintern-Moore S, Moore GPM, Panaretto BA, Robertson D. Follicular development in the neonatal mouse ovary; effect of epidermal growth factor. *Acta Endocrinol. (Copenh.)* 1981;96: 123–126.
453. Byyny RL, Orth DN, Cohen S, Doyne ES. Epidermal growth factor: effects of androgens and adrenergic agents. *Endocrinology* 1974;95:776–782.
454. Savage CR, Cohen S. Epidermal growth factor and a new derivative: rapid isolation procedures and biological and chemical characterization. *J. Biol. Chem.* 1972;247:7609–7611.
455. Moore Jr, JB. Purification and partial characterization of epidermal growth factor isolated from the male rat submaxillary gland. *Arch. Biochem. Biophys.* 1978;189:1–7.
456. Cohen S, Carpenter G. Human epidermal growth factor: isolation and chemical and biological properties. *Proc. Natl. Acad. Sci. USA* 1975;72:1317–1321.
457. Byyny RL, Orth DN, Cohen S, Island DP. Epidermal growth factor radioimmunoassay: effects of age, androgen and adrenergic agents on EGF storage and release. *53rd Annual Meeting of the Endocrine Society,* (abstr. 6) 1971:A45.
458. Nexo E, Hollenberg MD, Figueroa A, Pratt RM. Detection of epidermal growth factor-urogastrone and its receptor during fetal mouse development. *Proc. Natl. Acad. Sci. USA* 1980;77: 2782–2785.
459. Sporn MB, Roberts AB, Shull JH, Smith JM, Ward JM, Sodek J. Polypeptide transforming growth factors isolated from bovine sources and used for wound healing in vivo. *Science* 1983;219: 1329–1331.
460. Twardzik DR, Ranchalis JE, Todaro GJ. Mouse embryonic transforming growth factors related to those isolated from tumour cells. *Cancer Res.* 1982;42:590–593.
461. Kudlow JE, Korbin MS. Secretion of epidermal growth factor-like mitogens by cultured cells from bovine anterior pituitary glands. *Endocrinology* 1984;115:911–917.
462. Baranao JLS, Hammond JM. Comparative effects of insulin and insulin-like growth factors on DNA synthesis and differentiation of porcine granulosa cells. *Biochem. Biophys. Res. Commun.* 1984;124:484–490.
463. Veldhuis JD, Furlanetto RW. Trophic actions of human somatomedin C/insulin-like growth factor I on ovarian cells: in vitro studies with swine granulosa cells. *Endocrinology* 1985;116: 1235–1242.
464. Ladenheim RG, Tesone M, Charreau EH. Insulin action and characterization of insulin receptors in rat luteal cells. *Endocrinology* 1984;115:752–756.
465. Rein MS, Schomberg DW. Characterization of insulin receptors on porcine granulosa cells. *Biol. Reprod.* 1982;26(Suppl. 1):113A (abstr. 154).
466. Otani T, Mauro T, Yukimur N, Mochizuki M. Effect of insulin on porcine granulosa cells: implications of a possible receptor mediated action. *Acta Endocrinol. (Copenh.)* 1985;108:104–110.
467. Veldhuis JD, Tamura S, Kolp L, Furlanetto RW, Larner J. Mechanisms subserving insulin action in the gonad: evidence that insulin induces specific phosphorylation of its immunoprecipitable receptor on ovarian cells. *Biochem. Biophys. Res. Commun.* 1984;120:144–149.
468. Poretsky L, Grigorescu F, Flier JS. Insulin but not IGF-I receptors are widely distributed in normal human ovary. *67th Annual Meeting of the Endocrine Society,* (abstr. 814) 1985:204.
469. Hammond JM, Knight AP, Rechler MM. Somatomedin secretion by porcine granulosa cells: a potential mechanism for regulating ovarian follicular growth. *Clin. Res.* 1984;32:485A (abstr.) 1985:204.
470. Hammond JM, Baranao JLF, Skaleris DA, Rechler MM, Knight AP. Somatomedin (Sm) production by cultured porcine granulosa cells (GC). *J. Steroid Biochem.* 1984;20:1597 (abstr. 128).
471. Hammond JM. Peptide regulators in the ovarian follicle. *Aust. J. Biol. Sci.* 1981;34:491–504.
472. Hammond JM, Yoshida K, Veldhuis JD, Rechler MM, Knight AP. Intrafollicular role of somatomedins: comparison with effect of insulin. In: Greenwald GS, and Terranova PF, eds. *Factors Regulating Ovarian Function.* New York: Raven Press; 1983:197–201.
473. Davoren JB, Hsueh AJW. Growth hormone increases ovarian levels of immunoreactive somatomedin C/insulin-like growth factor I in vivo. *Endocrinology* 1986;118:888–898.
474. Diamond MP, Webster BW, Carr RK, Wentz AC, Osteen KG. Human follicular-fluid insulin concentrations. *J. Clin. Endocrinol. Metab.* 1985;61:990–992.
475. Adashi EY, Resnick CE, Svoboda ME, Van Wyk JJ. A novel role for somatomedin-C in the cytodifferentiation of the ovarian granulosa cell. *Endocrinology* 1984;115:1227–1229.
476. Adashi EY, Resnick CE, Svoboda ME, Van Wyk JJ. Somatomedin-C synergizes with follicle-stimulating hormone in the acquisition of progesterone biosynthetic capacity by cultured rat granulosa cells. *Endocrinology* 1985;116:2135–2142.
477. Adashi EY, Resnick CE, Brodie AMH, Svoboda ME, Van Wyk JJ. Somatomedin-C-mediated potentiation of follicle-stimulating hormone-induced aromatase activity of cultured rat granulosa cells. *Endocrinology* 1985;117:2313–2320.
478. Veldhuis JD, Kolp LA, Toaff ME, Strauss III, JF, Demers LM. Mechanisms subserving the trophic actions of insulin on ovarian cells: in vitro studies using swine granulosa cells. *J. Clin. Invest.* 1983;72:1046–1057.
479. Veldhuis JD, Nestler JE, Strauss III, JF, Gwynne JT. Insulin regulates low density lipoprotein metabolism by swine granulosa cells. *Endocrinology* 1986;118:2242–2253.
480. Jia X-C, Kalmijn J, Hsueh AJW. Growth hormone enhances follicle-stimulating hormone-induced differentiation of cultured rat granulosa cells. *Endocrinology* 1986;118:1401–1409.
481. Davoren JB, Hsueh AJW. Insulin enhances FSH-stimulated steroidogenesis by cultured rat granulosa cells. *Mol. Cell. Endocrinol.* 1984;35:97–105.
482. Veldhuis JD, Kolp LA. Mechanisms subserving insulin's differentiating actions on progestin biosynthesis by ovarian cells: stud-

ies with cultured swine granulosa cells. *Endocrinology* 1985;116: 651–659.

483. Ciancio MJ, LaBarbera AR. Insulin stimulates granulosa cells: increased progesterone and cAMP production in vitro. *Am. J. Physiol.* 1984;10:E468–E474.
484. Garzo VG, Dorrington JH. Aromatase activity in human granulosa cells during follicular development and the modulation by follicle-stimulating hormone and insulin. *Am. J. Obstet. Gynecol.* 1984;148:657–662.
485. May JV, Schomberg DW. Granulosa cell differentiation in vitro: effect of insulin on growth and functional integrity. *Biol. Reprod.* 1981;25:421–431.
486. Burden HW. Adrenergic innervation in ovaries of the rat and guinea pig. *Am. J. Anat.* 1972;133:455–462.
487. Bahr JM, Ben-Jonathan N. Preovulatory depletion of ovarian catecholamine. *Endocrinology* 1981;108:1815–1820.
488. Ben-Jonathan N, Brown RH, Laufer N, Reich R, Bahr JM. Norepinephrine in Graafian follicles is depleted by follicle-stimulating hormone. *Endocrinology* 1982;110:457–461.
489. Bahr JM, Ben-Jonathan N. Elevated catecholamine in porcine follicular fluid before ovulation. *Endocrinology* 1985;117: 620–623.
490. Burden HW, Lawrence IE. The effects of denervation on the localization of Δ^5-3β-hydroxysteroid dehydrogenase activity in the rat ovary during pregnancy. *Acta Anat.* 1977;97:286–290.
491. Capps ML, Lawrence IE, Burden HW. Ultrastructure of the cells of the ovarian interstitial gland in hypophysectomized rats. The effects of stimulation of the ovarian plexus and of denervation. *Cell Tissue Res.* 1978;193:433–442.
492. Bahr J, Kao L, Nalbandov AV. The role of catecholamine and nerves in ovulation. *Biol. Reprod.* 1974;10:273–290.
493. Condon WA, Black DL. Catecholamine-induced stimulation of progesterone by the bovine corpus luteum in vitro. *Biol. Reprod.* 1976;15:573–578.
494. Jordan III, AW, Caffrey JL, Niswender GD. Catecholamine-induced stimulation of progesterone and adenosine 3′,5′-monophosphate production by dispersed ovine luteal cells. *Endocrinology* 1978;103:385–392.
495. Kliachko S, Zor U. Increase in catecholamine-stimulated cyclic AMP and progesterone synthesis in rat granulosa cells during culture. *Mol. Cell. Endocrinol.* 1981;23:23–32.
496. Adashi EY, Hsueh AJW. Stimulation of β-adrenergic responsiveness by follicle-stimulating hormone in rat granulosa cells in vitro and in vivo. *Endocrinology* 1981;108:2170–2178.
497. Aguado LI, Petrovic SL, Ojeda SR. Ovarian β-adrenergic receptors during the onset of puberty: characterization, distribution and coupling to steroidogenic responses. *Endocrinology* 1982; 110:1124–1132.
498. Sheela Rani CS, Nordenstrom K, Norjavaara E, Ahren K. Development of catecholamine responsiveness in granulosa cells from preovulatory rat follicles—dependence on preovulatory luteinizing hormone surge. *Biol. Reprod.* 1983;28:1021–1031.
499. Dyer CA, Erickson GF. Norepinephrine amplifies human chorionic gonadotropin-stimulated androgen biosynthesis by ovarian theca-interstitial cells. *Endocrinology* 1985;116:1645–1652.
500. Burden HW, Lawrence Jr, IE. Experimental studies on the acetylcholinesterase-positive nerves in the ovary of the rat. *Anat. Rec.* 1978;190:233–242.
501. Farrar JA, Handeberg GM, Hartley ML, Pennefather JN. Catecholamine levels in the guinea pig ovary, myometrium and costouterine muscle during the estrous cycle and in the ovary remaining after unilateral ovariectomy. *Biol. Reprod.* 1980;22:473–479.
502. Ojeda SR, Costa ME, Katz KH, Hersh LB. Evidence for the existence of substance P in the prepubertal rat ovary. I. Biochemical and physiological studies. *Biol. Reprod.* 1985;33:286–295.
503. Dees WL, Kozlowski GP, Dey R, Ojeda SR. Evidence for the existence of substance P in the prepubertal rat ovary. II. Immunocytochemical localization. *Biol. Reprod.* 1985;33:471–476.
504. Larson LI, Fahrenkrug J, Schaffalitsky de Misckadell OB. Vasoactive intestinal polypeptide occurs in nerves of the female genitourinary tract. *Science* 1977;197:1374–1375.
505. Davoren JB, Hsueh AJW. Vasoactive intestinal peptide: a novel stimulator of steroidogenesis by cultured rat granulosa cells. *Biol. Reprod.* 1985;33:37–52.
506. Pedersen T, Peters H. Proposal for a classification of oocytes and follicles in the mouse ovary. *J. Reprod. Fertil.* 1968;17:555–557.
507. Peters H, Byskov AG, Grinsted J. Follicular growth in fetal and prepubertal ovaries in humans and other primates. In: Ross GT, and Lipsett MB, eds. *Clinics in Endocrinology and Metabolism. Reproductive Endocrinology.* London: Saunders; 1978:469–485.
508. Noumura T, Weisz J, Lloyd CW. In vitro conversion of 7-H^3 progesterone to androgens by the rat testis during the second half of fetal life. *Endocrinology* 1966;78:245–253.
509. Arai H. On the postnatal development of the ovary (albino rat) with special reference to the number of ova. *Am. J. Anat.* 1920;27:405–462.
510. Beaumont H, Mandl AM. A quantitative and cytological study of oogonia and oocytes in the foetal and neonatal rat. *Proc. R. Soc. London [Biol.]* 1962;155:557–579.
511. Levina SE, Gyevai A, Horvath E. Responsiveness of the ovary to gonadotrophins in pre- and perinatal life: estrogen secretion in tissue and organ cultures. *J. Endocrinol.* 1975;65:219–223.
512. Schlegel RJ, Farias E, Russo NC, Moore JR, Gardner LI. Structural changes in the fetal gonads and gonaducts during maturation of an enzyme, steroid 3β-ol-dehydrogenase, in the gonads, adrenal cortex and placenta of fetal rats. *Endocrinology* 1967;81:565–572.
513. Brambell FWR. The development and morphology of the gonads of the mouse. I. The morphogenesis of the indifferent gonad and of the ovary. *Proc. R. Soc. London [Biol.]* 1927;101:391–408.
514. Borum K. Oogenesis in the mouse. A study of the meiotic prophase. *Exp. Cell Res.* 1961;24:495–507.
515. Peters H. The development of the mouse ovary from birth to maturity. *Acta Endocrinol. (Copenh.)* 1969;62:98–116.
516. Milewich L, George FW, Wilson JD. Estrogen formation by the ovary of the rabbit embryo. *Endocrinology* 1977;100:187–196.
517. Mauléon P, Bezard J, Terqui M. Very early and transient 17β-estradiol secretion by fetal sheep ovary—in vitro study. *Ann. Biol. Anim. Biochim. Biophys.* 1977;17:339–401.
518. Shemesh M, Ailenberg M, Milaguir F, Ayalon N, Hansel W. Hormone secretion by cultured bovine pre- and postimplantation gonads. *Biol. Reprod.* 1978;19:761–767.
519. Erickson GF, Challis JRG, Ryan KJ. A developmental study on the capacity of rabbit granulosa cells to respond to trophic hormones and secrete progesterone in vitro. *Dev. Biol.* 1974;40: 208–224.
520. Mauléon P. Utilization de la colchicine dans l'étude des divisions goniales de l'ovaire d'embryons de brebis et analyse de quelques résultats. *Ann. Biol. Anim. Biochem. Biophys.* 1961;1:70–73.
521. Teplitz R, Ohno S. Postnatal induction of ovogenesis in the rabbit (*Oryctolagus cuniculus*). *Exp. Cell Res.* 1963;31:183–189.
522. Peters H, Levy E, Crone M. Oogenesis in rabbits. *J. Exp. Zool.* 1965;158:169–180.
523. Mauléon P. Cinétique de l'ovogenèse chez les mammifères. *Arch. Anat. Microsc. Morphol. Exp.* (Suppl).3/4:1967:125–150.
524. Shemesh M. Estradiol-17β biosynthesis by the early bovine fetal ovary during the active and refractory phases. *Biol. Reprod.* 1980;23:577–582.
525. Roberts JD, Warren JC. Steroid biosynthesis in the fetal ovary. *Endocrinology* 1964;74:846–852.
526. Goldman AA, Yakovac WC, Bongiovanni AM. Development of activity of 3β-hydroxysteroid dehydrogenase in human fetal tissues and in two anencephalic newborns. *J. Clin. Endocrinol. Metab.* 1966;26:14–22.
527. Cavallero C, Magrini U. Histochemical studies on 3β-hydroxysteroid dehydrogenase and other enzymes in the steroid-secreting structures of human foetus. In: Martini L, Fraschini F, and Motta M, eds. *Second International Congress on Hormonal Steroids, International Congress Ser. 132.* Amsterdam: Excerpta Medica; 1966:667–674.
528. Brandau H, Lehmann V. Histoenzymatische untersuchungen an menschlichen gonaden wahrend der intrauterinen entwicklung. *Z. Geburtshilfe Gynaekol.* 1970;173:233–249.

529. Singh RF, Carr DH. The anatomy and histology of XO human embryos and fetuses. *Anat. Rec.* 1966;155:369–383.
530. Morishima A, Grumbach MM. The interrelationship of sex chromosome constitution and phenotype in the syndrome of gonadal dysgenesis and its variants. *Ann NY Acad. Sci.* 1968;155: 695–715.
531. Weiss L. Additional evidence of gradual loss of germ cells in the pathogenesis of streak ovaries in Turner's syndrome. *J. Med. Genet.* 1971;8:540–544.
532. Lyon MF, Hawker SG. Reproductive lifespan in irradiated and unirradiated chromosomally XO mice. *Genet. Res.* 1973;21: 185–194.
533. Burgoyne PS, Baker TG. The XO ovary—development and function. In: Byskov AG, and Peters H, eds. *Development and Function of Reproductive Organs, International Congress Series No. 559.* Amsterdam: Excerpta Medica; 1981:122–128.
534. Vanhems E, Bousquet J. Influence du misulban sur le développement de l'ovaire du rat. *Ann. Endocrinol. (Paris)* 1971;33:119–128.
535. Merchant Larios H. The role of germ cells in the morphogenesis and cytodifferentiation of the rat ovary. In: Müller-Bérat N, ed. *Progress in Differentiation Research.* Amsterdam: North-Holland; 1976:453–462.
536. Beaumont HM. Radiosensitivity of oogonia and oocytes in the foetal rat. *Int. J. Rad. Biol.* 1961;3:59–72.
537. Reddoch RB, Pelletier RM, Barbe GJ, Armstrong DT. Lack of ovarian responsiveness to gonadotropic hormones in infantile rats sterilized with Busulfan. *Endocrinology* 1986;119:879–886.
538. Edwards RG, Fowler RE, Gore-Langton RE, et al. Normal and abnormal follicular growth in mouse, rat and human ovaries. *J. Reprod. Fertil.* 1977;51:237–263.
539. Nakano R, Mizuno T, Katayama K, Tojo S. Growth of ovarian follicles in the absence of gonadotrophins. *J. Reprod. Fertil.* 1975;45:545–546.
540. Roy SK, Greenwald GS. An enzymatic method for dissociation of intact follicles from the hamster ovary: histological and quantitative aspects. *Biol. Reprod.* 1985;32:203–215.
541. Brambell FWR. The development and morphology of the gonads of the mouse. 3. The growth of the follicles. *Proc. R. Soc. London [Biol.]* 1928;102:258–272.
542. Harrison RJ, Weir BJ. (1977): Structure of the mammalian ovary. In: Zuckerman S, and Weir BJ, eds. *The Ovary,* Vol. 1. New York: Academic; 1977:113–217.
543. Presl J, Pospisil J, Figarova V, Krabec Z. Stage dependent changes in binding of iodinated FSH during ovarian follicle maturation in rats. *Endocrinol. Exp. (Bratisl.)* 1974;8:291–298.
544. Nimrod A, Erickson GF, Ryan KJ. A specific FSH receptor in rat granulosa cells: properties of binding in vitro. *Endocrinology* 1976;98:56–64.
545. Quattropani SL, Weisz J. Conversion of progesterone to estrone and estradiol in vitro by the ovary of the infantile rat in relation to the development of its interstitial tissue. *Endocrinology* 1973;53:1269–1276.
546. Peluso JJ, Steger RW, Hafez ESE. Development of gonadotropin-binding sites in the immature rat ovary. *J. Reprod. Fertil.* 1976;47:55–58.
547. Reddoch RB, Armstrong DT. Interactions of a phosphodiesterase inhibitor, 3-isobutyl-1-methyl xanthine, with prostaglandin E_2, follicle-stimulating hormone, luteinizing hormone, and dibutyryl cyclic 3′,5′-adenosine monophosphate (cAMP) in cAMP and steroid production by neonatal rat ovaries in vitro. *Endocrinology* 1984;115:11–18.
548. Funkenstein B, Nimrod A, Lindner HR. The development of steroidogenic capability and responsiveness to gonadotropins in cultured neonatal rat ovaries. *Endocrinology* 1980;106:98–106.
549. Kolena J. Reversal of the unresponsiveness of neonatal rat ovary to LH in cAMP synthesis by estrogen. *Horm. Res.* 1976;7: 152–157.
550. Dohler KD, Wuttke W. Changes with age in levels of serum gonadotropins, prolactin and gonadal steroids in prepubertal male and female rats. *Endocrinology* 1975;97:898–907.
551. Meijs-Roelofs HMA, deGreef WJ, Uilenbroek JTJ. Plasma progesterone and its relationship to serum gonadotropins in immature female rats. *J. Endocrinol.* 1975;64:329–334.
552. Ramaley JA. Development of gonadotropin regulation in the prepubertal mammal. *Biol. Reprod.* 1979;20:1–31.
553. van Wagenen G, Simpson ME. *Embryology of The Ovary and Testis. Homo Sapiens and Macaca Mulatta.* New Haven, CT: Yale University Press; 1965.
554. Gondos B, Hobel CJ. Interstitial cells in the human fetal ovary. *Endocrinology* 1973;93:736–739.
555. George FW, Wilson JD. Conversion of androgen to estrogen by the human fetal ovary. *J. Clin. Endocrinol. Metab.* 1978;47: 550–555.
556. Taylor T, Coutles JRT, MacNaughton MC. Human foetal synthesis of testosterone from perfused progesterone. *J. Endocrinol.* 1974;60:321–326.
557. Jungmann RA, Schweppe JS. Biosynthesis of sterols and steroids from acetate ^{14}C by human fetal ovaries. *J. Clin. Endocrinol. Metab.* 1968;28:1599–1604.
558. Schindler AE, Friedrich E. Steroid metabolism of foetal tissues. I. Metabolism of pregnenolone-4-^{14}C by human foetal ovaries. *Endokrinologie* 1975;65:72–79.
559. Bloch E. Metabolism of [4-^{14}C]-progesterone by human fetal testis and ovaries. *Endocrinology* 1964;74:833–845.
560. Wilson EA, Jawad MJ. The effects of trophic agents on fetal ovarian steroidogenesis in organ culture. *Fertil. Steril.* 1979;32:73–79.
561. Payne AH, Jaffe RB. Androgen formation from pregnenolone sulfate by the human fetal ovary. *J. Clin. Endocrinol. Metab.* 1974;39:300–304.
562. Huhtaniemi I, Vihko R. Determination of unconjugated and sulfated neutral steroids in fetal blood of early and midpregnancy. *Steroids* 1970;16:197–206.
563. Ellinwood WM, McClellan MC, Brenner RM, Resko JA. Estradiol synthesis by fetal monkey ovaries correlates with antral follicle formation. *Biol. Reprod.* 1983;28:505–516.
564. Grob HS. Growth and endocrine function of isolated ovarian follicles cultivated in vivo. *Biol. Reprod.* 1969;1:320–323.
565. Nicosia SV, Evangelista I, Batta SK. Rabbit ovarian follicles. I. Isolation technique and characterization at different stages of development. *Biol. Reprod.* 1975;13:423–447.
566. Terranova PF, Garza F. Relationship between the preovulatory luteinizing hormone (LH) surge and androstenedione synthesis of preantral follicles in the cyclic hamster: Detection by in vitro responses to LH. *Biol. Reprod.* 1983;29:630–636.
567. Høyer PE, Anderson H. Histochemistry of 3β-hydroxysteroid dehydrogenase in rat ovary. *Histochemistry* 1977;51:167–193.
568. Richards JS. Maturation of ovarian follicles: actions and interactions of pituitary and ovarian hormones on follicular cell differentiation. *Physiol. Rev.* 1980;60:51–89.
569. McNatty KP. Follicular fluid. In: Jones RE, ed. *The Vertebrate Ovary.* New York: Plenum Press; 1978:215–259.
570. Richards JS, Jonasson JA, Rolfes AI, Kersey K, Reichert Jr, LE. Adenosine 3′,5′-monophosphate, luteinizing hormone receptor, and progesterone during granulosa cell differentiation: effects of estradiol and follicle-stimulating hormone. *Endocrinology* 1979; 104:765–773.
571. Sheela Rani CS, Salhanick AR, Armstrong DT. Follicle-stimulating hormone induction of luteinizing hormone receptor in cultured rat granulosa cells: an examination of the need for steroids in the induction process. *Endocrinology* 1981;108:1379–1385.
572. Wang C, Hsueh AJW, Erickson GF. Induction of functional prolactin receptors by follicle-stimulating hormone in rat granulosa cells in vivo and in vitro. *J. Biol. Chem.* 1979;254:11330–11336.
573. Edwards RG. Follicular fluid. *J. Reprod. Fertil.* 1974;37: 189–219.
574. Mossman HW, Duke KL. *Comparative Morphology of the Mammalian Ovary.* Madison: University of Wisconsin Press; 1973.
575. Bjersing L. Maturation, morphology, and endocrine function of the follicular wall in mammals. In: Jones RE, ed. *The Vertebrate Ovary.* New York: Plenum; 1978:181–214.
576. Baird DT, Swanston I, Scaramuzzi RJ. Pulsatile release of LH and secretion of ovarian steroids in sheep during the luteal phase of the estrous cycle. *Endocrinology* 1976;98:1490–1496.
577. Giorgi EP, Addis M, Columbo G. The fate of free and conjugated oestrogens injected into the Graafian follicles of equines. *J. Endocrinol.* 1969;43:37–50.
578. Martin B, Rotten D, Jolivet A, Gautray JP. Binding of steroids by

proteins in follicular fluid of the human ovary. *J. Clin. Endocrinol. Metab.* 1981;53:443–447.
579. Cook B, Hunter RHF, Kelly ASL. Steroid-binding proteins in follicular fluid and peripheral plasma from pigs, cows and sheep. *J. Reprod. Fertil.* 1977;51:65–71.
580. Baird DT. Ovarian steroid secretion and metabolism in women. In: James VHT, Seiro M, and Giusti G, eds. *The Endocrine Function of the Human Ovary.* London: Academic; 1976:125–133.
581. McNatty KP, Baird DT, Bolton A, Chambers P, Corker CS, McLean H. Concentration of oestrogens and androgens in human ovarian venous plasma and follicular fluid throughout the menstrual cycle. *J. Endocrinol.* 1976;71:77–85.
582. McNatty KP, Hunter WM, McNeilly AS, Sawers RS. Changes in the concentration of pituitary and steroid hormones in the follicular fluid of human Graafian follicles throughout the menstrual cycle. *J. Endocrinol.* 1975;64:555–571.
583. Kemeter P, Salzer H, Breitenecker G, Friedrich F. Progesterone, oestradiol-17β, and testosterone levels in the follicular fluid of tertiary follicles and Graafian follicles of human ovaries. *Acta Endocrinol. (Copenh.)* 1975;80:686–704.
584. McNatty KP, Baird DT. Relationship between follicle-stimulating hormone, androstenedione and oestradiol in human follicular fluid. *J. Endocrinol.* 1978;76:527–531.
585. Breitenecker G, Friedrich F, Kemeter P. Further investigations on the maturation and degeneration of human ovarian follicles and their oocytes. *Fertil. Steril.* 1978;29:336–341.
586. McNatty KP. (1982): Ovarian follicular development from the onset of luteal regression in humans and sheep. In: Rolland R, van Hall EV, Hillier SG, McNatty KP, and Schoemaker J, eds. *Proceedings IVth Regnier de Graaf Symposium: Follicular Maturation and Ovulation.* Excerpta Medica; Amsterdam. 1982.1–18.
587. Hillier SG, van Hall EV, van den Boogaard AJM, de Zwart FA, Keyzer R. Activation and modulation of the granulosa cell aromatase system: experimental studies with rat and human ovaries. In: Rolland R, van Hall EV, Hillier SG, McNatty KP, and Schoemaker J, eds. *Proceedings IVth Regnier de Graaf Symposium: Follicular Maturation and Ovulation.* Amsterdam: Excerpta Medica; 1982:51–70.
588. Bomsel-Helmreich O, Gougeon A, Thebault A, et al. Healthy and atretic human follicles in the preovulatory phase: differences in evolution of follicular morphology and steroid content of follicular fluid. *J. Clin. Endocrinol. Metab.* 1979;48:686–694.
589. Westergaard L, McNatty KP, Christensen I, Larsen JK, Byskov AG. Flow cytometric deoxyribonucleic acid analysis of granulosa cells aspirated from human ovarian follicles. A new method to distinguish healthy and atretic ovarian follicles. *J. Clin. Endocrinol. Metab.* 1982;55:693–698.
590. McNatty KP, Hillier SG, van den Boogaard AMJ, Trimbos-Kemper TCM, Reichert Jr, LE, van Hall EV. Follicular development during the luteal phase of the human menstrual cycle. *J. Clin. Endocrinol. Metab.* 1983;56:1022–1031.
591. McNatty KM, Gibb M, Dobson C, Thurley DC, Findlay JK. Changes in the concentration of gonadotrophic and steroidal hormones in the antral fluid of ovarian follicles throughout the estrous cycle of the sheep. *Aust. J. Biol. Sci.* 1981;34:67–80.
592. Eiler H, Nalbandov AV. Sex steroids in follicular fluid and blood plasma during the estrous cycle of pigs. *Endocrinology* 1977;100:331–338.
593. Patwardhan VV, Lanthier A. Effect of an ovulatory dose of luteinizing hormone on the concentration of oestrone, oestradiol and progesterone in the rabbit ovarian follicles. *Acta Endocrinol. (Copenh.)* 1976;82:792–800.
594. Fujii T, Hoover DJ, Channing CP. Changes in inhibin activity, and progesterone, oestrogen and androstenedione concentrations in rat follicular fluid throughout the oestrous cycle. *J. Reprod. Fertil.* 1983;69:307–314.
595. Moor RM, Hay MF, Dott HM, Cran DG. Macroscopic identification and steroidogenic function of atretic follicles in sheep. *J. Endocrinol.* 1978;77:309–318.
596. Tsuji K, Sowa M, Nakano R. Relationship among the status of the human oocyte, the 17β-estradiol concentration in the antral fluid and the follicular size. *Endocrinol. Jpn.* 1983;30:251–254.
597. Baird DT, Fraser IS. Concentration of oestrone and oestradiol-17β in follicular fluid and ovarian venous blood of women. *Clin. Endocrinol.* 1975;4:259–266.
598. Baird DT. Factors regulating the growth of the preovulatory follicle in the sheep and human. *J. Reprod. Fertil.* 1983;69:343–352.
599. Smith OW. Estrogens in the ovarian fluids of normally menstruating women. *Endocrinology* 1960;67:698–707.
600. Short RV, London DR. Defective biosynthesis of ovarian steroids in the Stein-Leventhal syndrome. *Br. Med. J.* 1961;1:1764–1727.
601. deJong FH, Baird DT, van der Molen HJ. Ovarian secretion rates of oestrogens, androgens and progesterone in normal women and in women with persistent ovarian follicles. *Acta Endocrinol. (Copenh.)* 1974;77:575–587.
602. Sanyal MK, Berger MJ, Thompson IE, Taymor ML, Horne Jr, HW. Development of Graafian follicles in adult human ovary. I. Correlation of estrogen and progesterone concentration in antral fluid with growth of follicles. *J. Clin. Endocrinol. Metab.* 1974;38:828–835.
603. Short RV. Steroid concentrations in the fluid from normal and polycystic (Stein-Leventhal) ovaries. In: *Proceedings of the Second International Congress of Endocrinology. International Congress Ser. No. 83,* pp. 940–943. Amsterdam: Excerpta Medica; 1964:940–943.
604. Edwards RG, Steptoe PC, Abraham GE, Walters E, Purdy JM, Fotherby K. Steroid assays and preovulatory follicular development in human ovarics primed with gonadotrophins. *Lancet* 1972;2:611–615.
605. Knudsen O, Velle W. Ovarian oestrogen levels in the nonpregnant mare: relationship to histological appearance of the uterus and to clinical status. *J. Reprod. Fertil.* 1961;2:130–137.
606. Short RV. Steroid concentrations in normal follicular fluid and ovarian cyst fluid from cows. *J. Reprod. Fertil.* 1962;4:27–45.
607. Channing CP, Coudert SP. Contribution of granulosa cells and follicular fluid to ovarian estrogen secretion in the rhesus monkey in vivo. *Endocrinology* 1976;98:590–597.
608. Aedo AR, Pedersen PH, Pedersen SC, Diczfalusy E. Ovarian steroid secretion in normally menstruating women. I. The contribution of the developing follicle. *Acta Endocrinol. (Copenh.)* 1980;95:212–221.
609. Uilenbroek JTJ, van der Schoot P, den Besten D, Woutersen PJA. Control of steroidogenesis during growth and early atresia of preovulatory rat follicles. In: Rolland R, van Hall EV, Hillier SG, McNatty KP, and Schoemaker J, eds. *Proceedings of the IVth Regnier De Graaf Symposium. Follicular Maturation and Ovulation.* Amsterdam: Excerpta Medica; 1982:71–82.
610. diZerega GS, Marrs RP, Roche PC, Campeau JD, Kling OR. Identification of proteins in pooled human follicular fluid which suppress follicular response to gonadotropins. *J. Clin. Endocrinol. Metab.* 1983;56:35–41.
611. diZerega GS, Marrs RP, Campeau JD, Kling OR. Human granulosa cell secretion of protein(s) which suppress follicular response to gonadotropins. *J. Clin. Endocrinol. Metab.* 1983;56:147–155.
612. Kling OR, Roche PC, Campeau JD, Nishimura K, Nakamura RM, diZerega GS. Identification of protein(s) in porcine follicular fluid which suppress follicular response to gonadotropins. *Biol. Reprod.* 1984;30:564–572.
613. diZerega GS, Campeau JD, Nakamura RM, Ujita EL, Lobo R, Marrs RP. Activity of a human follicular fluid protein(s) from spontaneous and induced ovarian cycles. *J. Clin. Endocrinol. Metab.* 1983;57:838–846.
614. diZerega GS, Goebelsman U, Nakamura RM. Identification of protein(s) secreted by the preovulatory ovary which suppresses the follicle response to gonadotropins. *J. Clin. Endocrinol. Metab.* 1982;54:1091–1096.
615. Brailly D, Gougeon A, Milgrom E, Bomsel-Helmreich O, Papiernik E. Androgen and progestins in the human ovarian follicle: differences in the evolution of preovulatory, healthy nonovulatory and atretic follicles. *J. Clin. Endocrinol. Metab.* 1981;53:128–134.
616. Veldhuis JD, Klase PA, Hammond JM. Sex steroids modulate prolactin action in spontaneously luteinizing porcine granulosa cells in vitro. *Endocrinology* 1981;108:1463–1468.
617. Schaar H. Funktionelle morphologie der theca interna im blas-

chenfollikel des menschlichen ovars. *Acta Anat.* 1976;94: 283–298.
618. Leung PCK, Armstrong DT. Interactions of steroids and gonadotropins in the control of steroidogenesis in the ovarian follicle. *Annu. Rev. Physiol.* 1980;42:71–82.
619. Tsang BK, Leung PCK, Armstrong DT. Inhibition by estradiol-17β of porcine thecal androgen production in vitro. *Mol. Cell. Endocrinol.* 1979;14:131–139.
620. Henderson KM, McNeilly AS, Swanston IA. Gonadotrophin and steroid concentrations in bovine follicular fluid and their relationship to follicle size. *J. Reprod. Fertil.* 1982;65:467–473.
621. Henderson KM, Swanston IA. Androgen aromatization by luteinized bovine granulosa cells in tissue culture. *J. Reprod. Fertil.* 1978;52:131–134.
622. Henderson KM, Moon YS. Luteinization of bovine granulosa cells and corpus luteum formation associated with loss of androgen aromatizing ability. *J. Reprod. Fertil.* 1979;56:89–97.
623. Matson PL, Tyler JPP, Collins WP. Follicular steroid content and oocyte meiotic status after PMSG stimulation of immature hamsters. *J. Reprod. Fertil.* 1981;61:443–452.
624. Khalil MW, Snow K. 19-norandrostenedione (4-estren-3,17-dione) levels in follicular fluid during ovarian follicular development in gilts. *Biol. Reprod.* 1985;32(Suppl. 1):122 (abstr. 170).
625. Daniel SAJ, Khalil MW, Armstrong DT. 19-Norandrostenedione (4-estrene-3,17-dione) inhibits porcine oocyte maturation in vitro. *Gamete Res.* 1986;13:173–184.
626. Axelrod LR, Goldzieher JW. The effect of cofactors on steroid biosynthesis in normal ovarian tissue. *Biochim. Biophys. Acta* 1970;202:349–353.
627. Swanston I, McNatty KP, Baird DT. The concentration of prostaglandin $F_{2\alpha}$ and steroids in the human corpus luteum. *J. Endocrinol.* 1977;73:115–122.
628. Yen SSC. The human menstrual cycle (integrative function of the hypothalamic-pituitary-ovarian-endometrial axis). In: Yen SSC, and Jaffe RB, eds. *Reproductive Endocrinology.* Philadelphia: Saunders; 1978:126–151.
629. McNatty KP, Sawers RS. Relationship between the endocrine environment within the Graafian follicle and the subsequent rate of progesterone secretion by human granulosa cells in vitro. *J. Endocrinol.* 1975;66:391–400.
630. Laborde N, Carril M, Cheviakoff S, Croxatto HD, Pedroza E, Rosner JM. The secretion of progesterone during the periovulatory period in women with certified ovulation. *J. Clin. Endocrinol. Metab.* 1976;43:1157–1163.
631. Fowler RE, Chan STH, Walters DE, Edwards RG, Steptoe PC. Steroidogenesis in human follicles approaching ovulation as judged from assays of follicular fluid. *J. Endocrinol.* 1977;72: 259–271.
632. Fortune JE. Bovine theca and granulosa cells interact to promote androgen and progestin production. *Biol. Reprod.* 1981;24 (Suppl. 1):39A (abstr.).
633. Peters H, McNatty KP. (1980): *The Ovary.* Granada, London.
634. Mestwerdt W. Die follikel-granulosazellen in beziehung zur steroid-biosynthese in der periovulationsphase. *Fortschr. Med.* 1977;95:361–365.
635. Mestwerdt W, Müller O, Brandau H. Die differenzierte struktur und funktion der granulsa und theka in verschiedenen follikelstadien menschlicher ovarien. 2. Mittleilung: der reifende, reife, sprungreife und frisch geplatzte follikel. *Arch. Gynaekol.* 1977;222:115–136.
636. Mestwerdt W, Müller O, Brandau H. Die differenzierte struktur und funktion der granulosa und theka in verschiedenen follikelstadien menschlicher ovarien. 1. mitteilung: der primordial-, primar-, sekundar- und ruhende tertiarfollikel. *Arch. Gynakol.* 1977;222:45–71.
637. Albertini DF, Anderson E. The appearance and structure of intercellular connections during the ontogeny of the rabbit ovarian follicle with particular reference to gap junctions. *J. Cell Biol.* 1974;63:234–250.
638. Bjersing L, Cajander S. Ovulation and the mechanism of follicle rupture. VI. Ultrastructure of theca interna and the inner vascular network surrounding rabbit Graafian follicles prior to induced ovulation. *Cell Tissue Res.* 1974;153:31–44.
639. Delforge JP, Thomas K, Roux F, Carneiro de Siqueira J, Ferin J. Time relationships between granulosa cell growth and luteinization, and plasma luteinizing hormone discharge in human. I. A morphometric analysis. *Fertil. Steril.* 1972;23:1–11.
640. Norman RL, Greenwald GS. Follicular histology and physiological correlates in the preovulatory hamster. *Anat. Rec.* 1972;173:95–108.
641. Hermreck AS, Greenwald GS. The effects of unilateral ovariectomy on follicular maturation in the guinea pig. *Anat. Rec.* 1964;148:171–176.
642. Boucek RJ, Telegdy G, Savard K. Influence of gonadotropin on histochemical properties of the rabbit ovary. *Acta Endocrinol. (Copenh.)* 1967;54:295–310.
643. Klinken SP, Stevenson PM. Changes in enzymatic activities during the artificially stimulated transition from follicular to luteal cell types in rat ovary. *Eur. J. Biochem.* 1977;81:327–332.
644. Pupkin M, Bratt H, Weisz J, Lloyd CW, Balogh Jr, K. Dehydrogenases in the rat ovary. I. A histochemical study of Δ^5-3β- and 20α-hydroxysteroid dehydrogenases and enzymes of carbohydrate oxidation during the estrous cycle. *Endocrinology* 1966;79:316–327.
645. Bjersing L. Ovarian histochemistry. In: Zuckerman S, and Wier BJ, eds. *The Ovary,* Vol. 1. New York: Academic; 1977:303–391.
646. Wingate AL. A histochemical study of the hamster ovary. *Anat. Rec.* 1970;166:399 (abstr.).
647. Blaha GC, Leavitt WW. The distribution of Δ^5-3β-hydroxysteroid activity in the golden hamster during the estrous cycle, pregnancy, and lactation. *Biol. Reprod.* 1970;3:362–368.
648. Norman RL, Greenwald GS. Effect of phenobarbital, hypophysectomy, and X-irradiation on preovulatory progesterone levels in the cyclic hamster. *Endocrinology* 1971;89:598–605.
649. Friedrich F, Breitenecker G, Salzer H, Holzner JH. The progesterone content of the fluid and the activity of the steroid-3β-ol-dehydrogenase within the wall of the ovarian follicles. *Acta Endocrinol. (Copenh.)* 1974;76:343–352.
650. Hillensjö T, Bauminger S, Ahrén K. Effect of luteinizing hormone on the pattern of steroid production by preovulatory follicles of pregnant mare's serum gonadotropin-injected immature rats. *Endocrinology* 1976;99:996–1002.
651. LeMaire WJ, Marsh JM. Interrelationships between prostaglandins, cyclic AMP and steroids in ovulation. *J. Reprod. Fertil.* 1975;22(Suppl.):53–74.
652. Younglai EV. Steroid production by isolated rabbit ovarian follicles: effects of luteinizing hormone from mating to implantation. *J. Endocrinol.* 1977;73:59–65.
653. Hori T, Ide M, Miyake T. Pituitary regulation of preovulatory oestrogen secretion in the rat. *Endocrinol. Jpn.* 1969;16:351–360.
654. Hubbard CJ, Greenwald GS. Cyclic nucleotides, DNA, and steroid levels in ovarian follicles and corpora lutea of the cyclic hamster. *Biol. Reprod.* 1982;26:230–240.
655. Murdoch WJ, Dunn TG. Alterations in follicular steroid hormones during the preovulatory period in the ewe. *Biol. Reprod.* 1982;24:1171–1181.
656. Dieleman SJ, Bevers MM, Poortman J, van Tol HTM. Steroid and pituitary hormone concentrations in the fluid of preovulatory bovine follicles relative to the peak of LH in the peripheral blood. *J. Reprod. Fertil.* 1983;69:641–649.
657. Testart J, Castanier M, Feinstein M-C, Frydman R. Pituitary and steroid hormones in the preovulatory follicle during spontaneous or stimulated cycles. In: Rolland R, van Hall EV, Hillier SG, McNatty KP, and Schoemaker, eds. *Follicular Maturation and Ovulation.* Amsterdam: Excerpta Medica; 1982:193–201.
658. Van Look PFA, Templeton AA, Swantson IA, et al. The effect of hCG on steroid levels in human Graafian follicles. *Proceedings of the 3rd Joint Meeting of the British Endocrine Societies, Edinburgh,* Abstract. 1984.
659. Moor RM. The ovarian follicle of the sheep: inhibition of oestrogen secretion by luteinizing hormone. *J. Endocrinol.* 1974;61: 455–463.
660. Bockaert J, Hunzicker-Dunn M, Birnbaumer L. Hormone-stimulated desensitization of hormone-dependent adenylyl cyclase: dual action of luteinizing hormone on pig Graafian follicle membranes. *J. Biol. Chem.* 1976;251:2653–2663.
661. Mori T, Fujita Y, Suzuki A, Kinoshita Y, Nishimura T, Kambegawa A. Functional and structural relationships in steroidogene-

sis in vitro by human ovarian follicles during maturation and ovulation. *J. Clin. Endocrinol. Metab.* 1978;47:955–966.
662. Edwards RG, Steptoe PC, Fowler RE, Baille J. Observations on preovulatory human ovarian follicles and their aspirates. *Br. J. Obstet. Gynaecol.* 1980;87:769–779.
663. Landgren B-M, Aedo A-R, Nunez M, Cekan SZ, Diczfalusy E. Studies on the pattern of circulating steroids in the normal menstrual cycle. *Acta Endocrinol. (Copenh.)* 1977;84:620–632.
664. Kirchick HJ, Birnbaumer L. Luteal adenylyl cyclase does not develop sensitivity to desensitization by human chorionic gonadotropin in the absence of nonluteal ovarian tissue. *Endocrinology* 1983;113:2052–2058.
665. Richards JS, Ireland JJ, Rao MC, Bernath GA, Midgley Jr, AR, Reichert Jr, LE. Ovarian follicular development in the rat: hormone receptor regulation by estradiol, follicle-stimulating hormone and luteinizing hormone. *Endocrinology* 1976;99: 1562–1570.
666. Rao MC, Richards JS, Midgley Jr, AR, Reichert Jr, LE. Regulation of gonadotropin receptors by luteinizing hormone in granulosa cells. *Endocrinology* 1977;101:512–523.
667. Suzuki K, Tamaoki BI. Postovulatory decrease in estrogen production is caused by the diminished supply of aromatizable androgen to ovarian aromatase. *Endocrinology* 1980;107: 2115–2116.
668. Hillensjö T, Hamberger L, Ahrén K. Effect of androgens on the biosynthesis of estradiol-17β by isolated preovulatory follicles. *Mol. Cell. Endocrinol.* 1977;9:183–193.
669. Suzuki K, Tamaoki BI. Acute decrease by human chorionic gonadotropin of the activity of preovulatory ovarian 17α-hydroxylase and C-17-20-lyase is due to decrease of microsomal cytochrome P-450 through de novo synthesis of ribonucleic acid and protein. *Endocrinology* 1983;113:1985–1991.
670. Eckstein B, Tsafriri A. The steroid C-17,20-lyase complex in isolated Graafian follicles: effects of human chorionic gonadotropin. *Endocrinology* 1986;118:1266–1270.
671. Bjersing L, Hay MF, Kann G, et al. Changes in gonadotrophins, ovarian steroids and follicular morphology in sheep at oestrus. *J. Endocrinol.* 1972;52:465–479.
672. Watzka M. Weibliche genitalorgane. Das ovarium. In: Mollendorf MV, and Bargmann W, eds. *Handbuch der Mikroskopischen Anatomies des Menschen,* Vol. 7. Berlin: Springer;1957:1–178.
673. LeMaire WJ, Yang NST, Behrman HH, Marsh JM. Preovulatory changes in the concentration of prostaglandins in rabbit Graafian follicles. *Prostaglandins* 1973;3:367–376.
674. Yang NST, Marsh JM, LeMaire WJ. Postovulatory changes in the concentrations of prostaglandins in rabbit Graafian follicles. *Prostaglandins* 1974;6:37–44.
675. Armstrong DT, Moon YS, Zamecnik J. Evidence for a role of prostaglandins in ovulation. In: Moudgal NR, ed. *Gonadotropins and Gonadal Function.* New York: Academic; 1974:341–356.
676. Armstrong DT, Zamecnik J. Pre-ovulatory elevation of rat ovarian prostaglandin F, and its blockade by indomethacin. *Mol. Cell. Endocrinol.* 1975;2:125–131.
677. Bauminger S, Lindner HR. Periovulatory changes in ovarian prostaglandin formation and their hormonal control in the rat. *Prostaglandins* 1975;9:737–751.
678. Ainsworth L, Baker RD, Armstrong DT. Pre-ovulatory changes in follicular fluid prostaglandin F levels in swine. *Prostaglandins* 1975;9:915–925.
679. Tsang BK, Ainsworth L, Downey BR, Armstrong DT. Preovulatory changes in cyclic AMP and prostaglandin concentrations in follicular fluid of gilts. *Prostaglandins* 1979;17:141–148.
680. Plunkett ER, Moon YS, Zamecnik J, Armstrong DT. Preliminary evidence of a role for prostaglandin F in human follicular function. *Am. J. Obstet. Gynecol.* 1975;123:391–397.
681. Henderson KM, McNatty KP. A biochemical hypothesis to explain the mechanism of luteal regression. *Prostaglandins* 1975;9:779–798.
682. Armstrong DT. Prostaglandins and follicular functions. *J. Reprod. Fertil.* 1981;62:283–291.
683. Janson PO. Effects of luteinizing hormone on blood flow in the follicular rabbit ovary as measured by radioactive microspheres. *Acta Endocrinol. (Copenh.)* 1975;79:122–133.
684. Armstrong DT, Grinwich DL. Blockade of spontaneous and LH-induced ovulation in rats by indomethacin, an inhibitor of prostaglandin biosynthesis. *Prostaglandins* 1972;1:21–28.
685. Grinwich DL, Kennedy TG, Armstrong DT. Dissociation of ovulatory and steroidogenic actions of luteinizing hormone in rabbits with indomethacin, an inhibitor of prostaglandin synthesis. *Prostaglandins* 1972;1:89–95.
686. Lau IF, Saksena SK, Chang MC. Prostaglandins F and ovulation in mice. *J. Reprod. Fertil.* 1974;40:467–469.

The Physiology of Reproduction, Second Edition,
edited by E. Knobil and J.D. Neill,
Raven Press, Ltd., New York © 1994.

CHAPTER 12

Follicular Development and Its Control[3]

Gilbert S. Greenwald[1] and Shyamal K. Roy[2]

"One of the most intriguing mysteries in ovarian physiology is what factors determine whether one follicle remains quiescent, another begins to develop but later becomes atretic, while still a third matures and ovulates" (1).

The above description of the fate of three primordial follicles sets the theme for this chapter. In view of the paucity of information about primordial follicles, emphasis is upon follicles once they have entered into the growing pool. We hope to provide a balanced account of follicular development in the cyclic, pregnant, and lactating animal. A comparative approach is stressed, which will point out significant species similarities and differences. Moreover, an attempt will be made to cover all aspects of folliculogenesis.

Folliculogenesis has attracted a great deal of attention, and, where feasible, this chapter focuses on recent findings. Table 1 lists a series of relevant reviews and chapters—which is by no means complete. Further entree to the literature on follicular development can be gained by consulting the volumes published during the past 15 years (Table 2).

[1]Department of Physiology, University of Kansas Medical Center, Kansas City, Kansas 66160
[2]Departments of Obstetrics and Gynecology and Physiology and Biophysics, University of Nebraska Medical Center, Omaha, Nebraska 68198

[3]For additional discussion of follicular development and its control in primates, see Chapter 49.

EARLY STAGES OF FOLLICULAR DEVELOPMENT

About 50 years ago, investigators established that primordial germ cells (PGCs) in the mouse first appear by 8 days post coitum in the yolk sac endoderm where they are readily visualized by their high content of alkaline phosphatase (for references, see ref. 49). A recent study

TABLE 1. *Reviews and chapters relevant to follicular development*

Year	Author
1947	Hisaw (2)
1956	Brambell (3)
1959	Falck (4)
1974	Greenwald (5)
1977	Channing and Tsafriri (6)
1977	Lindner et al. (7)
1977	Armstrong and Dorrington (8)
1980	Richards (9)
1981	diZerega and Hodgen (10)
1983	Erickson (11)
1984	Hsueh et al. (12)
1984	Tsafriri and Braw (13)
1985	Hillier (14)
1985	Adashi et al. (15)
1986	Erickson (16)
1987	Amsterdam and Rotmensch (17)
1987	Ireland (18)
1988	Richards and Hedin (19)
1988	Greenwald and Terranova (20)
1989	Tonetta and diZerega (21)
1989	Familiari et al. (22)
1990	Adashi (23)
1990	Buccione et al. (24)
1991	Hirshfield (25)
1992	Ackland et al. (26)
1992	Giudice (27)
1993	Findlay (28)
1993	Roy (29)

(49) employing whole mounts has demonstrated a cluster of PGCs at an even earlier time—day 7 post coitum—in extraembryonic mesoderm posterior to the primitive streak. The mean number of PGCs is 8 at the earliest detectable stage on day 7 and rises to 124 cells by early day 8. Excision of the cluster area on day 7 results 48 h later in embryos lacking PGCs. The PGCs normally migrate to the gonad by 12 days post coitum. Both rat and mouse PGCs have specific surface glycoconjugates, which disappear once they have entered the gonad (50). An *in vitro* comparison of the behavior of migratory and postmigratory PGCs reveals that the former cells (at 10 days post coitum) are very motile and will spread and actually displace cells of a feeder layer of inactivated STO cells, whereas postmigratory PGCs (day 12 post coitum) will not (51). Moreover, the postmigratory PGCs will continue to proliferate and divide in culture. It is estimated that the number of PGCs increases from 100 to about 4,000 entering the genital ridges (cited in ref. 52). Although the nature of the ovarian chemoattractants for PGC is not yet fully clear, it has been suggested that TGF-β_1 (transforming growth factor-β_1) produced by the gonad is one of the factors responsible for the chemotropic attraction of PGCs. However, *in vitro* TGF-β_1 inhibits the proliferation of 8.5-day PGCs; this effect is reversed by anti-TGF-β_1 (52). Evidently, other factors are responsible for the proliferation of PGCs as they migrate through the dorsal mesentery. One of the factors interfering with germ cell development is associated with the W locus, which differs from the normal WW phenotype in that it interferes with hematopoiesis and germ cell development. The cause of the sterility was established by Mintz and Russell in 1957 (53). The number of germ cells is normal at day 8, and the PGCs are in their normal tissue site. However, beginning at day 9 and thereafter, a disparity develops between W genotypes and control ww embryos with the number of PGCs lagging further and further behind in the former group. A related independent allele, steel, also affects PGCs, coat color and hematopoiesis and mast cells. It has recently been shown that W encodes a protooncogene *c-kit* receptor tyrosine kinase, located in the germ cell, while steel encodes a ligand expressed in the cells surrounding the

TABLE 2. *Relevant books on the ovarian follicle: 1977–1985*

Year	Title	Author(s)
1977	*The Ovary.* 2nd ed.	Zuckerman and Weir (30)
1978	*The Vertebrate Ovary*	Jones (31)
1978	*Control of Ovulation*	Crighton et al. (32)
1979	*Ovarian Follicular Development and Function*	Midgley and Sadler (33)
1979	*Ovarian Follicular and Corpus Luteum Function*	Channing, Marsh and Sadler (34)
1980	*Conception in the Human Female*	Edwards (35)
1980	*Biology of the Ovary*	Motta and Hafez (36)
1980	*The Ovary*	Peters and McNatty (37)
1981	*Dynamics of Ovarian Function*	Schwartz and Hunzicker-Dunn (38)
1982	*Intraovarian Control Mechanisms*	Channing and Segal (39)
1983	*Factors Regulating Ovarian Function*	Greenwald and Terranova (40)
1982–84	*Reproduction in Mammals.* 2nd ed.	Austin and Short (41)
1984	*Marshall's Physiology of Reproduction.* 4th ed.	Lamming (42)
1985	*Biology of Ovarian Follicles in Mammals*	Guraya (43)
1985	*Proceedings of the Fifth Ovarian Workshop*	Toft and Ryan (44)
1987	*The Primate Ovary*	Stouffer (45)
1988	*Nonsteroidal Gonadal Factors*	Hodgen et al. (46)
1989	*Growth Factors and the Ovary*	Hirshfield (47)
1991	*Signaling Mechanisms and Gene Expression in the Ovary*	Gibori (48)

germ cell (for references, see ref. 54). Mast cell growth factor is encoded by the steel locus (55), and its essentiality for primordial germ cells is demonstrated by culturing PGCs (8.5–10.5 days) on feeder cells. PGCs survive for less than 24 h *in vitro* in the absence of feeder cells but survive for 24 h in the presence of STO or NIH-3T3 cells but not CV-1 cells (55). Transfecting STO cells with a mast cell growth factor construct or adding mast cell growth factor directly to the cultures prolongs the survival time but not the proliferation of PGCs. *In situ* hybridization reveals in adult female mice that oocytes at all stages of development express c-*kit* and surrounding cells express the steel factor (54). A similar distribution is observed in 9- to 12.5-day embryos. Presumably, cell-cell interactions bind the steel factor to the germ cell *kit* receptor and thus initiates tyrosine autophosphorylation and transduction of second messenger systems.

According to Hilscher (56), the female germ cells undergo only one proliferative wave of oogonial divisions, whereas male gametogenesis involves two waves, the first one an exponential multiplication (prespermatogenic) corresponding to oogonial proliferation and a second spermatogenic wave culminating in the enormous number of sperm in the mature testis. The first differences between male and female germ cells are evident at the end of the first wave by differences in metaphase labeling (57).

Several experimental manipulations influence the number of oogonia. Rat ovaries explanted on day 13.5 post coitum and cultured for 4 to 6 days in the presence of thymulin or cocultured with fetal thymus contain significantly more oogonia than in their absence (58). Coculture of the explant with thymus and corticosterone (which prevents secretion of thymulin) reversed the effects of the thymus. However, it is not clear whether the thymus protects the oogonia from undergoing degeneration or leads to an actual increase in germ cell numbers. These results are especially intriguing in light of experiments involving rabbit fetuses hypophysectomized at 19 days of age and maintained in utero until day 28 (59). This procedure obviously deprives the fetus of growth hormone and tropic hormones but leads to thymic hypertrophy. Following hypophysectomy, the number of oogonia is significantly increased at day 28, suggesting an interesting interaction of the pituitary-thymic-ovarian axis.

The conversion of oogonia into primary oocytes depends on contact with cells derived from the rete ovarii, which is of mesonephric origin (60). The first germ cells to enter meiosis are located at the inner border of the ovary, where germ cell-somatic cell interactions first occur. It is postulated that the cells produce a meiosis-inducing substance. This can be demonstrated using grafted fetal mouse ovaries with or without the mesonephros attached. If the separation is performed early enough, the ovary lacks follicles and meiosis is blocked (60). The nature of meiosis-inducing substance is unknown, but it evidently involves second messenger systems, since incubation of gonadal ridges from 11.5-days post coitum fetal mice with forskolin or lithium induces meiosis in the treated testes (the contralateral gonad served as a control and was also incubated for 3 to 6 days [61]). Germ cells isolated from mouse gonads (12.5–13.5 days post coitum) labeled with a fluorescent dye and seeded on granulosa cells (from prepubertal mice) establish contact and transfer the dye within 2 to 3 h of culture, but not when fibroblasts are substituted as the feeder layer. Therefore, two-way traffic between germ and somatic cells is established at very early stages of development.

The majority of mammals restrict oogonial proliferation to prenatal development or to shortly after birth (62); the rare exceptions are lemurs where mitotic activity of germ cells is demonstrable even in the adult (63). Thus, in most mammals before or soon after birth, oogonia are transformed into primary oocytes characterized by a prolonged meiotic prophase and surrounded by a squamous layer of pregranulosa cells. These *primordial follicles* constitute the resting stockpile of nongrowing follicles, which are progressively depleted during the reproductive life span. Primordial follicles continuously (presumably) leave the nongrowing pool by being converted into *primary follicles* in which the oocyte is surrounded by a unilaminar layer of cuboidal granulosa cells—the descendents of the pregranulosa cells. The follicle is then launched on its career as a growing or developing follicle, culminating in either ovulation or the more likely fate of atresia at some stage in its subsequent development. According to Peters and colleagues (64) the initiation of follicle growth is not dependent on gonadotropins, since unilateral ovariectomy of 2-day-old mice does not change the number of normal developing follicles present 12 days later. On the other hand, continuous daily injection from birth of an antiserum to gonadotropins leads to signs of altered follicular development by 5 days of age and definite effects from 7 days onward (65). Follicular development in gonadotropin-deprived mice rarely progresses beyond the 40-cell stage, corresponding to a type 3b follicle: the smallest medium-sized follicle with an oocyte slightly larger than 20 μm in diameter (66). Transplantation of ovaries of 1-day-old rats to ovariectomized or ovariectomized-hypophysectomized adult female rats results 15 days later in the same number of small and medium follicles (up to two layers of granulosa cells), but the transplants in the gonadotropin-rich environment contain many more secondary follicles (multilaminar granulosa layers) and large follicles with incipient formation of an antral cavity. The oocytes are also considerably larger in the transplants in the ovariectomized hosts (67). The conclusion is that gonadotropins, especially follicle-stimulating hormones (FSH), enhance early follicle cell development and early oocyte growth. In the immature mouse (66) and rat (68), more follicles start to grow per day in young animals

(7-day-old mice, 16-day-old rats) than in older ones. This perhaps can be explained on the basis of high levels of gonadotropins in the prepubertal rodent (rat [69]; hamster [70]). The reduced number of growing follicles recruited per day in 3-week-old mice has been attributed to a factor produced by atretic follicles, which reduces growth initiation (64). The fact that large follicles have already differentiated by 21 days of age (66) raises the possibility that production of steroids and/or inhibin by the enlarging follicles can act via the hypothalamic-pituitary axis to account for fewer follicles entering into the growing pool. Several recent papers emphasize the role of high levels of FSH in the prepubertal rat. Serum FSH can be reduced during the first 10 days of life by injection of sodium glutamate (71), nonaromatizable androgens (72), and an antagonist of luteinizing hormone-releasing hormone (73). All three treatments drastically lower serum FSH and, to various degrees, serum luteinizing hormone (LH), and lead to retardation in follicular growth and a gradual loss of growing follicles.

With age, the number of primordial follicles declines in parallel with the number of growing follicles (mouse [74,75]; rat [76]; human [77,78]). A number of studies have revealed an interesting phenomenon: the migration and loss of primordial oocytes through the ovarian surface epithelium. This is especially clear-cut in the newborn mouse where the loss of oocytes into the periovarian sac reaches a peak in the first week of life and continues until about day 28 (79). The pregranulosa cells are left behind while the healthy oocyte penetrates between the epithelial cells and herniates, presumably by amoeboid movements, and exits the ovary.

Henderson and Edwards (80) showed a decline in chiasma frequency with increasing age of female mice. They attributed this to a "production line" gradient, with the earliest oocytes formed at meiosis being the first to be released from puberty and on. Oocytes developing later in the fetal ovary would show a decreased frequency of chiasmata and therefore a greater likelihood of producing univalents frequently producing unbalanced ova and zygotes. The hypothesis has been validated by a combined *in vitro-in vivo* approach in which fetal mouse ovaries were labeled *in vitro* with [^{3}H]thymidine on day 14 or days 16 and 17 and prepared for either air-dry spreading or transplanted to the kidney capsule of spayed young adult female mice (81). The ovaries labeled on day 14 had a very high proportion of labeled pachytene-diplotene stages compared to the labeling index at late gestation. On transfer to the spayed recipients, approximately twice as many follicles in the former group were labeled consistent with the belief that ova do not mature at random but are formed and released according to the time of entry into meiosis. The size of the pool of primordial follicles determines the fraction that is stimulated to grow. A reduction in the size of the pool reduces the number recruited into the growing pool. In the mouse, this relationship holds true whether the nongrowing pool is reduced by age or artificially by injection of dimethylbenzanthracene (74) or by early androgenization (64). There is considerable individual variation in the number of primordial follicles in man (41) and rhesus (82). The number of primordial follicles shows significant differences among three strains of rats (83). Interestingly, the strain with the greatest number of primordial follicles also has the greatest number of growing follicles and is most responsive to exogenous FSH. It is disconcerting, however, that this strain is the less fecund, judged by a higher incidence of sterile matings and smaller litter sizes; whether there are differences in ovulation rate between the strains is unknown (84).

A recent paper (85) has described a simple enzymatic method for isolating primordial follicles from the porcine ovary, but tremendous contamination with somatic cells makes it difficult to obtain a pure sample of primordials for biochemical analysis. The use of late fetal ovaries might alleviate this problem, but for routine purposes logistics dictate the use of ovaries of prepubertal animals. The porcine primordial follicles show several polypeptide bands differing or in common with oocytes from mature follicles but with considerable differences from somatic cells. The best sources of primordial follicles are by far the porcine, ovine, or bovine ovaries, based on the large numbers situated in the peripheral cortex, directly underlying the surface epithelium (86). At present, rapid separation of primordial follicles from somatic cells is the limiting factor in answering a number of unsolved questions about the nongrowing pool.

One of the most critical steps in folliculogenesis is the transformation of primordial into primary follicles. Intuitively, it seems likely that the conversion of the flattened pregranulosa cells into a cuboidal epithelium depends on cues provided by the oocytes, but the nature of the signal is unclear. Several lines of evidence indicate that the pregranulosa cells are unable to form follicles in the absence of the oocyte. Injection of busulfan (an alkylating agent) into pregnant rats destroys all primordial germ cells, and consequently a sterile gonad devoid of steroidogenic tissue is formed (87). Similarly, a mutant mouse strain may have 2 to 20 oocytes at birth, but their disappearance by 3 months prevents any further follicular development (88). Thymectomy of mice on day 3 also drastically decreases the total number of follicles as early as day 8 and especially affects the population of primordial follicles (89).

By a series of mitotic divisions, the unilaminar primary follicle is converted into a multilaminated preantral stage designated a *secondary follicle;* at various times in its life history the secondary follicle becomes invested with thecal cells. An elegant study deals with a mutant allele at the steel locus, which produces infertility but by a different route than depletion of germ cells (90). The mice have normal numbers of primordial follicles at birth and thereafter, but possess greater numbers of unilaminar and bilaminar follicles and virtually no growing follicles with three or more layers of granulosa cells (90). The block at the early secondary follicle stage can be overcome by fusing mutant steel ova with wild-type ova, and the resulting chimerids are fertile. A series of experiments points to a defect in ovarian stromal cells rather than the granulosa cells as the cause of the infertility; this most likely reflects failure of thecal differentiation, which is evident in normal mice when the follicle has three or more layers of granulosa cells (91). Daily injection of mice with epidermal growth factor from days 1 to 5 increases the number of small-growing follicles and decreases the number of primordial follicles (92). Whether deficiency of epidermal growth factor or other growth factors accounts for the block in follicular development (90) remains to be tested.

With the appearance of an antral cavity, the secondary follicle is converted into a *tertiary follicle.* The granulosa population of a large tertiary follicle in the mouse consists of about 50,000 cells (91). An intriguing question is what is the original number of precursor cells from which the final follicle is derived. This has been addressed by a very clever approach (93). An X-linked glycolytic enzyme, phosphoglycerate kinase-1, with two isoforms has been used to analyze tissue mosaicism in granulosa cells. The frequency distributions show that most follicles contain various proportions of the two phenotypes. Binomial statistics indicate that about five precursor cells give rise to the total population. Moreover, when cumulus cell activity is plotted against mural granulosa phosphoglycerate kinase-1, a linear relationship exists with a correlation coefficient of $r = .899$, implying that both compartments had the same precursors. The multiclonal nature of the granulosa cells correlates with the finding that most primordial follicles have three to six pregranulosa cells.

The morphologic and biochemical changes associated with these changes will be discussed later. At this point, we are concerned with a very basic issue: Is the growth and differentiation of primary and secondary follicles under the influence of gonadotropins, or is it only with the development of an antral cavity that the tertiary follicle becomes dependent on FSH and LH?

The relatively constant number of preantral follicles throughout the estrous cycle has often been cited as evidence that they are unaffected—or at most slightly affected—by changes in gonadotropins. Thus, throughout the cycle of the mouse no cyclic changes in numbers exist for follicles of types 3a to 6 (type 6: incipient formation of antral cavity [94]). However, incorporation of $[^3H]$thymidine into preantral mouse follicles begins to increase on the afternoon of proestrus and peaks on the morning of estrus, correlating with periovulatory changes in gonadotropins (91). Based on large sample sizes (11–18 rats per day of cycle) at least 21 follicles per ovary are recruited from smaller than 260 μm into larger than 260 μm between proestrus and estrus (95). Moreover, the number of smaller follicles (70–110 μm) significantly increases at diestrus; a definite antrum (i.e., a tertiary follicle) is present in follicles 120 to 130 μm in diameter. Hence preantral follicles *do* change in numbers during the estrous cycle of the rat. It is noteworthy that rat follicles less than 70 μm in diameter are never atretic (95). Similarly, in the periovulatory period of the rhesus monkey, there is a significant increase in the percentage of small preantral follicles ranging from 100 to 200 μm in diameter; the transition to an antral follicle occurs between 200 and 250 μm (82). Based on the terminology of Pedersen and Peters (96), there are significantly more types 3b and 4 follicles in the rat ovary at estrus and metestrus than on other days of the cycle (97). Of perhaps greater significance, the duration of the DNA-synthesis phase is shorter for all primary and secondary follicles at estrus than at other stages of the cycle (97), and this is also true for the cyclic mouse (94). The number of preantral follicles with two to five layers of granulosa cells does not vary during the hamster cycle (98). However, preantral hamster follicles, with one to five layers of granulosa cells show significant increases in $[^3H]$thymidine incorporation on proestrus and estrus as evaluated by autoradiography (99) or after *in vitro* incubation with $[^3H]$thymidine (100). Thus, the dogma of the unchanging number and responsiveness of preantral follicles is refuted in a number of species.

Still another way of demonstrating that preantral follicles *can* be stimulated in intact animals by gonadotropins is by evaluating the effects of superovulation induced by pregnant mare serum (PMS). For example, 26- to 28-day-old mice ovulate 60 ova in response to 10 IU PMS, followed 56 h later by 5 IU human chorionic gonadotropin (hCG): rats 24–30 days old ovulate 50 eggs after 30 IU PMS and an ovulating dose of 10 IU hCG (101). Adult rats injected with 50 IU PMS and a subsequent injection of 15 IU hCG 3 days later ovulate 43 ova per animal (102). The number of ova ovulated hardly makes it feasible that reduced atresia of tertiary follicles can solely account for these results; rather, recruitment of preantral follicles seems to be an essential component. Unequivocal evidence that preantral follicles are recruited by PMS treatment is provided by the cyclic hamster. Injection of 30 IU PMS on estrus (day 1 of cycle) results in the ovulation of 54 ova by the next cycle, and this is associated by day 2 with a doubling in the number of follicles greater than 267 μm in diameter (103). Within 4 h after the injection of 30 IU PMS on estrus, hamster follicles with four to five layers of granulosa cells respond by a significant reduction in their numbers and a concomitant increase in follicles with incipient formation of an antral cavity (104). Collectively, these results point to significant effects of gonadotropins on secondary (and even primary) follicles in intact animals.

It is frequently stated that gonadotropic hormones are unessential for early growth of follicles and that FSH and LH become indispensable for further development only at the transformation of the secondary to a tertiary follicle. Although species differences may exist, a careful perusal of the literature indicates that early follicular development *is* influenced by gonadotropins, but the picture is confusing because of the frequent subjective, anecdotal evaluations and the way even quantitative data have been presented. What follows, then, is a species by species account of the effects of hypophysectomy on follicular development which attempts to provide a balanced view of this important subject.

Rat

Rats hypophysectomized at 28 days of age were killed at various postoperative intervals, and healthy follicles were classified as primary or vesicular; the former category includes preantral follicles with two or more layers of granulosa cells (105). By 10 and 38 days after hypophysectomy, the average number of primary follicles was 102 and 20, respectively, compared to 213 on the day after operation; similarly, the number of vesicular follicles at the same time intervals were 99 and 3 compared to 160 on day 1. The maximal diameter of follicles maintained posthypophysectomy was 250 μm, but the number obviously falls sharply with time. An often-cited, but somewhat confusing, study of Paesi (106) dealt with hypophysectomy of young rats weighing 61–72 g. One week later, there was a 71% increase in the smallest follicles (23–32 μm in diameter). Since primordial follicles were not counted, presumably these were primary follicles with one layer of cuboidal granulosa cells. Approximately 20% of the small follicles showed signs of beginning atresia. One week after hypophysectomy, the largest follicles present were 360 μm compared preoperatively to 576 μm. The accumulation of small follicles might represent a decrease in the number of follicles developing into larger stages per unit of time (106). An excellent, thorough study by de Reviers (107) dealt with follicular development in the immature rat with follicles classified by the volume of granulosa cells. Volume ranged from 1,259 μm^2 for primary follicles to 25,200 μm^2 for large tertiary follicles. Following hypophsectomy at 27 days of age, 10 days later there is a 43% reduction in the number of smallest follicles (types 3b and 4) and a 37% reduction in intermediate follicles (types 5a and 6) and no larger stages (types 6–8) present compared to intact 28-day-old rats. In hypophysectomized rats killed 105 or 135 days later, the total number of small follicles varied from 8 to 48 and only sporadic numbers of intermediate follicles were present. De Reviers pointed out that long-term hypophysectomy of male rats leads to the development of gonadotropinlike cells in the pars tuberalis as evidenced by immunocytology (107). Even the long-term hypophysectomized rat may therefore not be completely devoid of some gonadotropin reserve. Ovine FSH is capable of stimulating follicular growth in rats hypophysectomized for as long as 25 days, and this effect is manifested in all stages of folliculogenesis. The action of FSH—depending on dose—involves diminished atresia but also increased recruitment. The recruitment may even affect primordial follicles as demonstrated by injecting [^{3}H]-thymidine 1 h before hypophysectomy, with the rats killed 72 h later. There was approximately a threefold greater labeling index in type 3b follicles after FSH treatment (107).

An unpublished study has considered follicular development in adult hypophysectomized rats with the endpoint—21 days later—expressed as numerical density of follicles based on their diameter (cited in ref. 108). Follicles smaller than 60 μm were not measured. The results indicate a significant decline in follicles larger than 175 μm by 3 weeks after hypophysectomy. A single injection of Armour FSH (4 mg) resulted 24 h later in a significant increase in the number of follicles 75 to 125 μm in diameter. A recent study reconfirms a number of the above findings: Rats hypophysectomized at 26 days of age, 3 days later show significant declines in secondary and tertiary follicles; for example, the number of follicles with two to three layers of granulosa cells is reduced to 107 ± 12 per ovary from the normal value of 175 ± 22 (109). The number of healthy tertiary follicles is even more affected by 3 days: 4.5 ± 1.2 versus 39 ± 3 in intact controls. In another study, hypophysectomy was the only treatment that decreased the loss of primordial follicles (intact: 4,688 ± 263 per ovary) with serum FSH and LH reduced to negligible levels (110). Intact rats on a restricted food diet (50% of intake of controls) had elevated FSH levels, but the number of primordial follicles was comparable to the controls, whereas the number of follicles that are 280 μm or smaller was significantly reduced. Long-term injection of a gonadotropin-releasing factor (GnRH) agonist greatly increases the percentage of follicles smaller than 35 μm, while decreasing the percentage of follicles larger than 35 μm from 14% in controls to 1% in the treated group (111). Bokser and colleagues (111) define follicles smaller than 35 μm as follicles with "little or no proliferative activity"; follicles larger than 35 μm are "unequivocally proliferating." Similarly, treatment of adult female rats for 7 weeks with a GnRH antagonist altered the ratio of small follicles (<30 μm) to large follicles (>30 μm) from the normal ratio of 3:1 to 11:1 (112).

The above results are so striking that one wonders why there is any question about the dependency of preantral rat follicles on gonadotropin support. In part, this is because some investigators have been more impressed by the ability of at least *some* follicles in the hypophysectomized rat to maintain some semblance of normal function. Thus, rats hypophysectomized on day 22 and injected 10 days later with [^{3}H]thymidine show a similar degree of labeling of granulosa cells in small follicles to intact animals (113). Nakano and colleagues (113) state "although many follicles were atretic, a few follicles with more than one layer of granulosa cells persisted." In another study, hypophysectomized rats were implanted 5 days postsurgery with pumps containing [^{3}H]thymidine and killed 8 days later (114). Follicles were heavily labeled over the granulosa cells: "some of the labeled follicles were healthy" but "many labeled follicles were atretic." Again, Hirshfield (114) is more impressed with the qualitative aspects—not quantitative—of follicular growth after hypophysectomy.

Mouse

Hypophysectomy of postpubertal mice results in few follicles developing beyond the two-layered granulosa stage, but Faddy and colleagues (115) recognized the tentativeness of the conclusion because of the heterogeneous ages of the mice and different times before they were killed. It is interesting, however, in intact cyclic mice that follicles are committed to either normal development or atresia by the time the third layer of granulosa cells has differentiated; a clearly established thecal layer is evident at this stage (116).

In adult mice hypophysectomized at random stages of the estrous cycle, by 4 days after hypophysectomy the number of preantral and antral follicles is reduced by 40% to 60% and large preovulatory follicles have vanished (117). The decline in antral follicles is not associated with any change in the rate of atresia. At 12 days following hypophysectomy, daily injections of FSH and LH for 4 days increases the number of healthy follicles for all stages and restores DNA synthesis to normal levels (118).

The dwarf Snell mouse shows a significantly lowered labeling index of small preantral follicles compared to littermate controls (119). Within 3 h after administering 1 μg rat FSH, the labeling index of primary follicles (one layer of granulosa cells) begins to increase, and by 24 hours, unilaminar and bilaminar follicles show major increases in the labeling index, especially in the dwarf mice. The hypogonadal mouse is deficient in GnRH, and consequently the ovaries lack antral follicles and the number of preantral follicles is reduced (120). Treatment with 1 μg of a highly purified FSH increases the number of primary follicles, presumably by increasing the rate at which primordial follicles enter the growing pool. Incubation of preantral mouse follicles with two to three layers of granulosa cells with FSH enables them to grow to normal large antral size in 6 to 7 days (121).

Hamster

In hamsters hypophysectomized on estrus, 1 to 28 days postsurgery, 99% of the follicles have five or fewer layers of granulosa cells, which is considerably below the size of the largest preantral follicle (122). With time, a greater percentage of follicles than normal accumulate in the group with two to three layers of granulosa cells. After a hiatus of 1 week, daily injection of 200 μg ovine FSH (NIH-S7) for 4 days, followed by hCG, resulted in the ovulation of an average of 32 ova. Interestingly, 200 μg FSH on the first day of treatment followed by 50 μg per day thereafter led to ovulation of 9 ova—a regimen and number of ovulations simulating the pattern in the intact cyclic hamster. Three days after immature hamsters were hypophysectomized, the number of healthy secondary and tertiary follicles was reduced from 405 to 251 per ovary and there was already a significant reduction in follicles with two to eight layers of granulosa cells and larger follicles had vanished (109). Similar results have also been observed in the adult hypophysectomized hamster (123). Four days after hypophysectomy of adult hamsters, considerable amounts of FSH can still be eluted from the nonluteal ovary and with significantly greater FSH receptor affinity than from follicles of intact hamsters (124). This finding has two important implications: Small preantral follicles have a greater affinity for FSH than large ones (there is no appreciable FSH binding by the interstitium), and it may take considerable time, depending on the species, before FSH completely disappears from the ovary of the hypophysectomized animal and a truly anhormonal environment is established.

A recent series of papers dealing with the hamster establish without doubt the importance of FSH for growth of preantral follicles. Thus, preantral follicles respond to the primary and secondary FSH surge on estrus and proestrus by increasing incorporation of [^{3}H]thymidine (100). Preantral follicles with one to four layers of granulosa cells and lacking theca have FSH and prolactin receptors but no human chorionic gonadotropin receptors (125). Small preantral follicles respond *in vitro* to FSH—but not to LH—by increasing DNA synthesis within 2 h (126), and this is associated with the synthesis of progesterone (127). Finally, long-term incubation (4 days) of preantral follicles in a serum-free medium with FSH doubles the DNA content per follicle and transforms large solid preantral follicles into small antral stages (128).

Guinea Pig

An often-cited paper (129) reported on three hypophysectomized animals which were killed 12 days later: "There was no reduction in the number of nonvesicular follicles." This is strictly an anecdotal account. Subsequently, 3- to 4-week-old guinea pigs were hypophysectomized, and groups of three or four animals were killed over the next 4 days (130). Follicles in the range of 140 to 800 μm in diameter were counted. The percentage of normal follicles from 140 to 356 μm did not appreciably differ between controls and hypophysectomized guinea pigs over the next 14 days. Only one of three animals killed on day 4 had any normal vesicular follicles, and in the other animals all follicles beyond the primordial stage were atretic. Paradoxically, by 6 and 14 days all ovaries contained vesicular follicles and a greater percentage were healthy: 63% versus 14% on day 4. No explanation was offered for these unusual results. Is it a matter of small sample size, or, with time, does another source of gonadotropins develop in the hypophysectomized guinea pig (pars tuberalis)?

Sheep

Ewes were hypophysectomized at estrus, with one ovary removed 4 days later and the other removed 70 days after treatment (131). All follicles with three or more layers of granulosa cells were counted. Four days after hypophysectomy the number of preantral follicles (<0.06 to 0.2 mm) did not differ from controls, but by 70 days posthypophysectomy there were fewer follicles from 0.06 to 0.2 mm compared to the day 4 control group (approximately 50% less in each size range). In hypophysectomized ewes—even in the short-term group —all follicles larger than 2.0 mm were atretic. The long-term hypophysectomized ewes had about 30 healthy small vesicular follicles. Thus, the ewe seems to be relatively impervious to a lack of gonadotropic hormones in developing small tertiary follicles. One wonders how *soon* after hypophysectomy of the ewe changes become apparent in the follicular population.

After long-term hypophysectomy (about 70 days) follicles in Boorola ewes were always less than 2 to 3 mm in diameter and were small antral follicles, despite the fact that plasma FSH and LH were nondetectable (132). It is especially significant that when the follicles from the hypophysectomized ewes were incubated with FSH and LH for 1 h, tissue cAMP did not differ from control follicles, nor were there any differences between the two sets of follicles at 0 h. Does this mean that the ewe (and possibly other barnyard species) differs from the rodent in the latter's dependency on FSH for preantral and early antral development?

Pituitary stalk-sectioned ewes on day 6 of the cycle and consequently treated with bovine follicular fluid had suppressed FSH levels through day 11 of the cycle (133). This resulted in restricted numbers of visible follicles (≥2 mm) to about one per animal. Stalk sectioning and saline injections resulted in about 2.5 visible follicles per pair of ovaries, and stalk sectioning plus FSH restored the number of visible follicles to the normal number of 15 per animal.

A hypogonadotropic model was produced in ewes by administering a GnRH agonist by osmotic minipumps for 5 weeks (134). Plasma FSH concentration fell to 10.2 μg/L compared to 25.9 μg/L in control ewes on day 8 of the cycle, and no LH pulses were recorded. The largest follicles were less than 2 mm. Intravenous infusion of a high dose of FSH (which simulated normal blood levels) restored the full range of follicular diameters to the distribution of luteal phase controls and also restored follicular estradiol production to control values. However, FSH infusion plus pulsatile LH infusion prevented follicular growth beyond 2.5 mm by doubling the number of small follicles. Evidently the critical point in follicular development in the ewe involves follicles between 2.0 and 3.0 mm in diameter (135).

Human

The effects of hypophysectomy on follicular development in the ovary have not been considered. However, two interesting clinical syndromes are pertinent. Follicular development past the primordial stage is rarely observed in women with hypogonadotropic hypogonadism and anosmia (olfactogenital dysplasia) (136). Total urinary gonadotropins are below the limits of detection in a mouse uterine bioassay, but exogenous gonadotropins can induce ovulation. In contrast, in the gonadotropin-resistant ovary syndrome, serum FSH and LH levels are elevated and can be further increased by LHRH (137), and the ovaries are not responsive to human menopausal gonadotropin (138). Follicular development is limited to primordial and a few primary follicles. It is assumed that there is a deficiency in gonadotropin receptors or a postreceptor defect. Hence long-term follicular development is severely impaired in the human ovary in the absence of physiologically effective actions of gonadotropins.

From the above account, it seems that a strong case can be made for several species that folliculogenesis—even early stages—is influenced by gonadotropins; following hypophysectomy some follicles can progress to the secondary stage, but, quantitatively, follicular growth is severely curtailed. Obviously, more research involving quantitative evaluation of follicular development in a number of species is required to definitely establish the precise effects of gonadotropins on early stages of folliculogenesis.

STRUCTURE AND FUNCTION OF THE ANTRAL FOLLICLE: THE GRANULOSAL COMPARTMENT

A biphasic pattern of oocyte and follicle growth in eutherian mammals was clearly established in studies performed 50 to 60 years ago (3). During the first phase, oocyte and follicle growth are linearly and positively correlated. Once the oocyte is close to its maximal size, shortly before formation of the antral cavity, a second phase ensues where follicle growth, consisting of mitotic activity of the granulosa and thecal cells and accumulation of follicular fluid, becomes the dominant element. This same relationship exists in monotremes and marsupials (139).

A very intimate relationship exists between the oocyte and surrounding granulosa cells. Oocytes of the nongrowing pool in the mouse ovary are surrounded by two to eight squamous follicle cells but are active in RNA synthesis and have low but significant levels of RNA polymerase (140). When nine follicle cells surround the oocyte, 96% of the follicular epithelium is cuboidal and oocyte growth is initiated, detected by an increase in nucleolar RNA polymerase. Of the total oocyte population in 30-day-old mouse ovaries, 81% were in the nongrowing pool, and only 2% of the total population were surrounded by nine or more granulosa cells. It is well established that RNA synthesis in mammalian oocytes increases during follicle growth and reaches a peak before an antral cavity is formed (for references, see ref. 141). Thereafter, uptake of [^{3}H]uridine declines rapidly and is low in the oocytes of mature follicles. Protein synthesis by mouse oocytes increases linearly and is greatest in medium (60–70 μm vitellus diameter) and large (75–90 μm vitellus diameter) oocytes; the large oocyte was collected from large antral follicles (142). That the oocyte in turn influences granulosa development is illustrated in several experiments. An oocyte-specific antigen from Lewis rats was collected and an antiserum raised in male rats; only oocytes reacted with the antiserum (143). When dissociated ovarian cells were incubated in the presence of normal rat serum, 40–50% reaggregated in a folliclelike structure, whereas when anti-oocyte serum was used, the percentage of granulosa cells forming "follicles" was reduced to 20–30%. A specific oocyte antigen, which is trypsin-labile, may therefore induce follicular differentiation.

The oocyte obviously has a very intimate relationship with the surrounding granulosa cells. Metabolic cooperativity is especially evident in the mouse in that denuded oocytes barely grow when dissociated from cumulus cells because of the lack of gap junctions to transport various compounds, which are first picked up by granulosa cells and then conveyed to the oocyte (144). Conversely, evidence is accumulating that the egg in turn influences the granulosa cells, and potentially thecal development, by the presence of various peptides in the oocyte. Thus, mature oocytes (from large preovulatory follicles) of rat, mouse, and hamster possess FSH binding sites and human chorionic gonadotropin receptors are present in the mouse and hamster but not in the rat or rabbit (145). Using specific antisera to FSH or LH, immunocytochemistry reveals immunodetectable FSH in primordial follicles and both FSH and LH in the oocytes of primary and secondary follicles in prepubertal rats (146). Similarly, epidermal growth factor is localized in the oocytes of hamster primordial follicles on day 2 of the cycle (147). Tumor necrosis factor-α (TNF-α) is present in rat primordial follicles (cited in ref. 148), and incubation of theca-interstitial cells with TNF-α causes the cells to migrate and form clusters after 4 days of treatment (148).

As previously mentioned, the sequence of the c-*kit* protooncogene predicts receptor tyrosine kinase activity, and *in situ* hybridization reveals its presence in oocytes from primordial to preovulatory stages in the adult mouse ovary (149). These findings suggest a link—albeit a tenuous one—to how the egg can influence early and late growth and differentiation of granulosa cells. When cumulus-oocyte complexes isolated from antral follicles of prepubertal mice are cultured for 4 h and [^{3}H]-thymidine added for an additional 3 h, the labeling index of the granulosa cells is significantly reduced by surgically removing the oocyte at the time of incubation (150). Moreover, oocyte-conditioned medium doubled the labeling index of preantral follicles.

In preantral rat follicles with oocyte diameter greater than 80 μm, the granulosa cells nearest the oocyte have a much higher labeling index than more distant cells, and after antral formation, the labeling and mitotic indices in cumulus cells are three times as great as in the mural granulosa (151). A gradient in labeling index also is demonstrable in the mural granulosa, with the layer adjacent to the antrum having a much higher labeling index than the deeper layers. Similarly, proestrous rats exposed to continuous infusion of [^{3}H]thymidine for 24 h show a centripetal labeling pattern with intensive marking of granulosa cells bordering on the antral cavity and in the cumulus oophorus (152). In contrast, in 27-day-old rats similar-sized follicles do not show this regional distribution.

Morphometric analysis of sheep oocytes reveals that in the smallest follicles (0.2–0.4 mm in diameter), the Golgi apparatus is located at the periphery and the cell membrane is folded and consists of numerous slender villi so that the surface area is about fivefold greater than a sphere of similar dimensions (153). As the follicle grows to about 2 mm, the mitochondria align along the periphery of the oocyte and the microvilli now only increase the surface area of the oocyte by a factor of 2.

The most intimate relationship of the oocyte and cumulus cells obviously involves the granulosa cells that ultimately form the corona radiata, and this relationship is established by the primary follicle (for references, see ref. 154). A series of follicular villi abut as gap junctions on the plasmalemma of the oocyte, before the zona pellucida develops, and greater than 85% of the nutrients are first taken up by the neighboring granulosa cells before being transferred to the oocyte (for references, see ref. 155). However, nonpolar amino acids such as leucine and valine may be able to bypass granulosa cells and interact directly with the mouse oocyte, whereas most amino acids cooperatively enter mouse oocytes (156). The origin of the zona pellucida has long been controversial, and species differences may very well account for the uncertainty whether it is derived from the oocyte, follicle cells, or both (154). Recent biochemical evidence indicates that denuded mouse oocytes synthesize and secrete zona pellucida proteins (157,158). Similarly, zona immunoreactive activity is demonstrable in hamster oocytes from primordial and primary follicles up through antral stages, whereas the granulosa cells are unstained (159). In the rabbit, using immunocytochemistry, the zona pellucida proteins are first observed in the oocyte when it is still surrounded by squamous follicle cells. The extracellular assemblage of the glycoproteins forming the zona pellucida intensifies when two or more layers of follicular cells have formed and the antigens are then apparent not only in the oocyte but in the inner layer of granulosa cells as well (160). This suggests a joint derivation of the zona pellucida. Granulosa cells from primary and early secondary follicles of immature rabbits express zona pellucida proteins *in vitro* in the absence of oocytes (161). However, posttranslational modifications of these proteins is inefficient in the absence of oocytes. Rabbits immunized with porcine zonae pellucidae ultimately show impeded follicular growth with no normal follicles with two or more layers of granulosa cells differentiating (162). The stage of follicular development affected by the increasing titer of zona pellucida antibodies is when the extracellular matrix first appears between the oocyte and follicle cells. There is a reduction in the number of primordial and primary follicles. It is interesting that deglycosylated zonae pellucidae raise high antibody titers in rabbits but without disrupting folliculogenesis (163). In this connection, it is intriguing that neonatal thymectomy or in naturally occurring athymic nude mice, a similar type of ovarian dysgenesis develops with age (see ref. 164). One wonders whether a common thread runs through both situations, involving disruption of the formation of a normal zona pellucida.

With the onset of formation of the antral cavity, follicular growth is accelerated, due to increased mitotic activity and accumulation of follicular fluid. Throughout the estrous cycle of the rat, 90% of the follicles are less than 300 μm, and the volume of follicular fluid first increases in amount when a diameter of 300 μm is reached (165). Mitotic activity in granulosa and theca is maximal in follicles from 200 to 300 μm in diameter and approximately threefold higher in granulosa cells (165). The mitotic index then falls in a linear fashion with the nadir for both compartments reached in follicles from 600 to 700 μm in diameter. There is a metestrous peak in mitotic activity in both granulosa and theca in follicles 401 to 500 μm, which presumably results in their ovulation at the next estrus. The volume of the antral cavity in the rat shows three distinct growth phases: a low plateau in follicles 200 to 300 μm, accelerated growth between 300 to 600 μm, and a final preovulatory spurt in follicles 700 μm. In follicles 600 μm in diameter the volume of granulosa, theca, and antrum are about 6:2:1, respectively. Primary follicular fluid is produced by the antral follicle until shortly before ovulation and to a great extent represents a plasma transudate plus granulosal secretions (for references, see ref. 166). It is interesting that the oxygen tension of follicular fluid falls as the human follicle matures; the fall in Po_2 correlates with a decrease in pH and a rise in Pco_2 as follicular size increases from 12 mm to 20 mm (167).

Three peaks of mucopolysaccharides are present in porcine follicular fluid: chondroitinlike material, heparin sulfate, and an unidentified peak; expressed as micrograms per follicle, all three fractions are maximal in follicles 6–12 mm in diameter (168). A more detailed biochemical analysis of proteoglycans in porcine follicular fluid is provided in Yanagishita and colleagues (169). Porcine FSH stimulates the incorporation of [^{3}H]-glucosamine into mucopolysaccharides by granulosa cells from small porcine follicles (<2 mm) and the stimulating effects are mimicked by dibutyryl cAMP and prostaglandin E_2 (170). The function of proteoglycans in follicular fluid is still unknown but conceivably may provide the microenvironment necessary for granulosal viability and proliferation.

Both the granulosa and thecal compartments act as functional syncitia through the presence of homocellular gap junctions, which persist in rat preantral follicles even after 90 days of hypophysectomy (171). However, within 48 h of injection of estradiol the gap junction surface area is increased in granulosa cells (fivefold greater than control values in intact rats); hCG has a similar effect on theca. Neither hormone is effective on the other compartment. A quantitative ultrastructural study of granulosa cell gap junctions in rat and rabbit follicles confirmed previous observations that an ovulatory dose of human chorionic gonadotropin within 5 to 12 h leads to rapid loss of gap junctions; in the rabbit, granulosa cells of ruptured follicles have only 15% of the amount of junctional membrane found in unstimulated large follicles (172). The importance of granulosa gap junctions in cell-to-cell communication is reinforced by a recent study (173). Granulosa cells were aspirated from preovulatory follicles of mature sows at days 18–20 of the cycle (when they have already been exposed to increasing levels of LH). Only 20% to 35% of the granulosa cells bound FSH or human chorionic gonadotropin and yet at 70% to 80% confluency nearly all granulosa cells contained dissociated cAMP-dependent protein kinase; at less than 20% confluency only one-third or fewer cells had dissociated protein kinase. Hence the importance of gap junctions in spreading a hormonal signal among granulosa cells.

There are considerable species differences in the ability of granulosa cells to convert pregnenolone to progesterone. In most species, it is not until shortly before the onset of the preovulatory surge in gonadotropins that significant 3β-hydroxysteroid dehydrogenase (3β-HSD) activity is evident in granulosa cells. For example, in the sheep the dominant follicle shows significant 3β-HSD activity in the theca (histochemically detectable), whereas the enzyme is not present in the membrana granulosa until a few hours before ovulation (174). The ultrastructural characteristics of the granulosa from large preovulatory follicles from sheep show few of the features associated with steroidogenesis, and even in the immediate period prior to ovulation there is no evidence of structural changes indicative of luteinization (175). In the human, the granulosa cells show ultrastructural characteristics of protein synthesis until the periovulatory increase in LH when morphometric analysis reveals a striking increase in smooth endoplasmic reticulum and other features indicative of increased steroidogenesis (176). Histochemical detection of 3β-HSD is also low in the preovulatory human follicle compared to the thecal reaction (177). Similarly, the ultrastructural organization of granulosa cells from preovulatory rhesus follicles shows features not associated with steroidogenesis, whereas atretic follicles have extensive smooth endoplasmic reticulum and large mitochondria with tubular cristae (178). These electron microscopic features are more indicative of 3β-HSD than other enzymes, since in both species granulosal cells can convert androgens to estrogens. Does the buildup of progesterone in follicular fluid in the immediate preovulatory period in humans represent a granulosa or thecal derivative? An enlightening histochemical comparison showed a much more intense reaction for 3β-HSD in the granulosa and theca of preovulatory follicles of the rat than hamster—both qualitatively and quantitatively (179). The activity in both species was much greater in the peripheral granulosa cells bordering on the basal lamina. Could this difference, in part, account for the premature histologic and biochemical signs of luteinization of granulosa cells observed in the preovulatory rat follicle compared to most other species? In summary, 3β-HSD activity is sparse in granulosa cells of most species until rising titers of LH enhance its ability to synthesize progesterone (see ref. 180). In the cow follicle, the major steroid product of the granulosa cells is pregnenolone, which is apparently then exported to the thecal layer for ultimate conversion to androgens (181). Hence there is traffic in both directions between theca and granulosa. In the proestrous hamster follicle neither pregnenolone nor progesterone are synthesized by granulosa cells incubated for 2 h with or without LH, whereas isolated theca produces considerable amounts of pregnenolone in response to LH (182).

One of the key steps in follicular steroidogenesis is the conversion of cholesterol to pregnenolone. In incubated rat granulosa cells (from preantral follicles), progestins preferentially use newly synthesized cholesterol rather than intracellular cholesterol (183). Addition of FSH and androstenedione leads to a marked increase in progesterone secretion but does not affect the percentage of unesterified cholesterol in the plasma membrane. The enzyme involved in this reaction is cytochrome P-450 side-chain cleavage (P-450_{SCC}), and immunofluorescence localization has been used to analyze the temporal sequence of follicular changes following administration of PMS to immature rats (184). Before treatment, the P-450_{SCC} is restricted to the interstitium. This is followed 24 h later by the appearance of the enzyme in the theca interna. By 48 h, P-450_{SCC} appears in the mural granulosa cells of preovulatory follicles, but there is no labeling in smaller follicles. Finally, at the early onset of the endogenous LH surge, P-450_{SCC} is detected for the first time in cumulus cells. When cumulus-oocyte complexes are isolated and cultured 48 h after PMS treatment in the presence of FSH or LH, about 85% of the complexes are positive 10 h later for P-450_{SCC} (185).

It has become evident in recent years that granulosa cells do not constitute a homogeneous tissue but rather show interesting regional specializations. This has been especially well demonstrated by quantitative cytochemistry. In the rat, there are distinctive differences between the peripheral portion of the membrana granulosa, the periantral granulosa cells, and the cumulus region. At proestrus, cells of the peripheral one-half to two-thirds of the membrana granulosa are pseudostratified, with cell processes extending to the basal lamina; these follicles are the ones destined to ovulate (186). In contrast, the rest of the membrana granulosa consists of stratified, rounded cells with rounded nuclei. On proestrus, growing follicles with a diameter of 400 μm first show signs of pseudostratification, and there are about three times as many showing this reaction as the number expected to ovulate. Elimination of the excess number of pseudostratified follicles proceeds rapidly after diestrus 1 and is completed by the evening of diestrus 2. Thus, the ovulable type of follicle is distinguished on the basis of the organization of the peripheral granulosa cells. On estrus and diestrus 1, there is little appreciable difference in 3β-HSD activity between peripheral, antral, and cumulus granulosa cells (187). However, by diestrus 2 and proestrus, 3β-HSD is two- to three-fold higher in peripheral granulosa. A similar regional difference is demonstrable for glucose 6-phosphate dehydrogenase of the type associated with hydroxylation reactions involved in steroid biosynthesis (187). Other evidence of granulosa heterogeneity is provided by a difference in lysosomal membrane permeability, which is greatest in peripheral granulosa cells, followed by periantral and then cumulus cells (188); presumably the former is the most active steroidogenic region of the granulosa.

Flow cytometry of human follicular aspirates (189) or granulosa cells from rats treated with diethylstilbestrol or PMS (190) demonstrate two populations of granulosa cells. Whether this heterogeneity reflects regional differences between mural and cumulus cells is unknown. In the case of the diethylstilbestrol model, light and electron microscopy shows two distinct sizes of granulosa cells, which also differ in their steroidogenic activity when the cells are incubated with FSH and androstenedione (191). Lipid droplets are also concentrated in the peripheral granulosa cells but much less than in the theca interna (179). The one characteristic feature of the cumulus cells of ovulable rat follicles is that PAS-positive granules are restricted to this region. A morphometric ultrastructural study of rat preovulatory follicles also confirms regional differences in the granulosa (179). The peripheral region contains the greatest volume of mitochondria, smooth endoplasmic reticulum, and lipid droplets. In contrast, the cumulus oophorus has the highest volume of rough endoplasmic reticulum—indicative of protein synthesis—and no lipid droplets. The oocyte-cumulus complex of rats collected before the LH surge secretes low amounts of progesterone throughout 2 days of culture (<10 pg/cumulus/day), whereas cumulus cells harvested after the LH surge accumulate 300 to 400 pg progesterone per day (192).

A mouse monoclonal antibody generated against a mammary tumor cell line recognizes a surface antigen in rat granulosa cells (193). Throughout the development of the preantral follicle, the plasma membrane of all granulosa cells gives a strong positive response for the antibody. However, once the antral cavity appears, 75% of the granulosa cells in the mural granulosa lack the antibody and its disappearance is initiated by FSH treatment within 12 h. A dramatic demonstration of the symbiosis between cumulus cells and oocyte is provided by culturing denuded, corona enclosed, and cumulus enclosed ovine oocytes for 24 h before transferring them to suitable inseminated recipients (194). For the three classes, the percentage of transferred ova developing into blastocysts was 1.9%, 1.8%, and 42.6%, respectively. However, when corona oocytes were supplemented with 5×10^6 granulosa cells (presumably mural cells), 37.2% developed into blastocysts.

Regional differences in FSH, hCG, and prolactin receptors have also been demonstrated in granulosa cells. In the preantral follicle, FSH binding sites are limited to granulosa cells and LH (hCG) binding sites are restricted to the theca. With time, LH binding sites appear in granulosa cells and the mature ovulable follicle therefore can be distinguished by LH and FSH binding sites in granulosa and LH binding in theca (for references see refs. 7, 9, 11, 12). A monoclonal anti-LH receptor shows distinct differences in its localization in the sow ovary (195). Immunoreactivity first appears on the theca of preantral follicles (100–200 μm); in large preovulatory follicles, the inner layer of theca bordering on the basement membrane is unlabeled. The granulosa cells were also now labeled but with a distinct gradient with very heavy labeling of the mural granulosa cells bordering on the basement membrane. The oocyte was not labeled. *In situ* hybridization of the rat antral follicle for LH receptor mRNA showed the most intensive reaction in the cells adjacent to the basement membrane (196). The oocyte and cumulus cells were negative.

Hypogonadal mice, injected intravenously with labeled hormones, bind hCG only to thecal and interstitial cells and FSH to granulosa cells. When treated with LH-RH for 5 days, mature follicles differentiate with some showing hCG binding now encompassing both theca and granulosa (197). In small sheep follicles (1–3 mm in diameter) cAMP production by granulosa cells is stimulated by FSH but not hCG (198), and similar observations have been made for porcine granulosa cells (see ref. 199). Topical autoradiography using slices of porcine ovaries reveals that granulosa cells from small follicles (1–2 mm) bind much more FSH than medium (3–5 mm) or large (6–10 mm) follicles, and hCG binding is slight in granulosa cells until large follicles are developed (200). When the largest antral follicles are collected on each day of the rat estrous cycle, the binding of FSH to granulosa cells is constant throughout the cycle at about 3,000 cpm/μg DNA, whereas hCG binding does not begin to increase until diestrus 2 with maximal values obtained on proestrus, increasing dramatically even before the preovulatory surges of gonadotropins (201). Maximal hCG binding to theca also occurs on proestrus. Intravenous injection of rats with labeled hCG, followed by autoradiography, showed that mural granulosa cells adjacent to the basement membrane demonstrated maximal grain counts, tenfold greater than the periantral layer (202). It is noteworthy that hCG binding to cumulus and oocyte is no greater than background (202). A quantitative study showed no binding of hCG to the rat oocyte; the affinity to cumulus and mural granulosa cells was the same, but the number of binding sites was very different: 223 sites per cumulus cell versus 2,000 sites per mural cell (203). Using topical autoradiography, and determining grain densities, there is no hCG binding to granulosa cells of rat follicles 400 to 500 μm in diameter, which are small antral follicles (204). The first noticeable binding to hCG was in the outermost granulosa layers of 500- to 600-μm follicles, and with increased size hCG binding spread to finally encompass the entire mural granulosa in follicles greater than 600 μm. Throughout the estrous cycle, hCG binding to cumulus and oocyte was no greater than background.

An autoradiographic study of the hamster ovary revealed that FSH binding to granulosa cells was present in the smallest preantral to large antral follicle and also the *oocyte* with increasing intensity as the oocyte enlarged; hCG or prolactin (PRL) did not bind to the granulosa of preantral follicles, but newly formed antral follicles on day 2 showed light activity in peripheral granulosa cells, which gradually spread to engulf all of the mural granulosa (205).

The presence of FSH binding sites on the granulosa cells of hamster preantral follicles have been demonstrated by topical autoradiography. The results of quantitative radioreceptor assays of FSH, hCG, and prolactin receptors agree with the autoradiographic finding and suggest further that granulosa cells of preantral follicles express a higher number of prolactin binding sites; however, hCG receptors do not appear until follicles have five to six layers of granulosa cells and a developing theca layer (125).

Normal functioning and viability of granulosa cells depend very much on functional FSH receptors on the cell surface. Although much evidence has been put forward to suggest that FSH and cAMP and its analogues can induce FSH receptors in ovarian granulosa cells (206,207), and epidermal growth factor and activin can modulate FSH binding sites (208,209), a clear-cut understanding of the control mechanism of FSH receptor induction in granulosa cells is warranted. Two follicular peptides have been implicated as possible local regulators of follicular FSH receptor expression: (1) activin, a member of the TGF-β gene family, and (2) follistatin. Both of these proteins are present in follicular fluid (210–212). Follistatin is produced by rat (213) and bovine (214) granulosa cells and is regulated by FSH (213,214). Follistatin message has been detected exclusively in granulosa cells (215). Activin receptors are present in rat granulosa cells (216). Exposure of cultured rat granulosa cells (diethylstilbestrol-primed, immature rats) to activin (3–100 ng/ml) significantly and dose-dependently increases FSH receptor levels by inducing more receptors; however, follistatin drastically reduces, in a dose-dependent manner, the activin-induced increase in FSH receptors. Although FSH alone causes a downregulation of granulosa cell FSH receptors, concurrent treatment with high doses of activin reverses the negative effects of FSH (217). Moreover, pretreatment of rat granulosa cells with activin markedly enhances aromatase activity, progesterone, and inhibin production (217). Contradictory results on the role of activin in folliculogenesis have been reported in an *in vivo* study involving 25-day-old rats (218). The experimental design consisted of unilateral intrabursal injection of activin with the other ovary serving as an *uninjected* control. When the animals were killed 24 h later, follicles greater than 500 μm were missing from the treated ovary, and 6% of antral follicles contained pyknotic nuclei compared to the control ovary. Several differences in experimental design could explain the disparate results, but it is disconcerting that only one set of ovaries were used in the latter study for the statistical analysis. Although more critical studies are needed to address the cellular and molecular mechanisms of FSH receptor induction in granulosa cells and the relation between these two follicular peptides and follicular atresia, all these lines of evidence point to a promising new area of research on the regulation of folliculogenesis.

Neither hCG nor PRL binding was detected on the mural granulosa or oocyte of preantral follicles. Hamster oocytes from which the zona pellucida has been removed still show specific FSH binding sites (145). Hydroxysteroid dehydrogenases have been demonstrated histochemically in the oocytes of several species (219), and one wonders whether mammalian oocytes are capable of producing steroids in response to gonadotropins, a well-established phenomenon in amphibians. An interesting observation is that in the guinea pig follicle 3β-HSD is restricted to the theca; the granulosal compartment is negative except for one layer of cumulus cells adjacent to the oocyte (220). Thus, regional differences in receptor distribution in mural and cumulus granulosa cells parallel morphologic and biochemical localizations.

It has been recognized for over 50 years that estrogen acts directly on the ovary of the hypophysectomized rat and synergizes with FSH to produce massive development of antral follicles (for references, see ref. 221). Although this is true for some species, others do not fit this model, as will be apparent from this section. A direct effect of estrogen on folliculogenesis in the rabbit has been demonstrated by the insertion of Silastic implants containing estradiol to one ovary of mature rabbits (222). This resulted in increased percentages of active follicles (i.e., preantral and antral follicles) in *both* ovaries. This is consistent with results, which revealed that 3 days treatment with FSH resulted in estrogen receptors—but not progesterone receptors—in granulosa cells of large preovulatory rabbit follicles but not in thecal cells (223). Injection of hCG resulted 6 h later in the disappearance of granulosal estrogen receptors and the appearance of progesterone receptors, as a prelude to luteinization. When all follicles larger than 1 mm in diameter were ruptured in rabbit ovaries, insertion of implants containing estradiol raised circulating estradiol by approximately 50 pg/ml; this resulted in the same number of follicles developing 3 days later (224). However, where estradiol concentration was further increased by addition of more implants, follicular recruitment was not affected, but there were no follicles larger than 2 mm.

The ovary of the hypophysectomized mouse, like the rat, responds to exogenous estrogen by increasing the number of preantral and small antral follicles by preventing atresia (225). Moreover, estrogen synergizes with FSH to restore all parameters of folliculogenesis to normal levels, including [^{3}H]thymidine incorporation to all stages of follicles from preantral to large preovulatory (225). Injecting an esterified estrogen or diethylstilbestrol (DES) into intact immature mice significantly increases ovarian weight and increases the number of preantral follicles (226). In untreated immature mice, ovarian estrogen binding sites are five- to seven-fold higher than in rabbit or guinea pig ovaries, respectively (226).

A series of recent *in vivo* and *in vitro* studies have reaffirmed the importance of the direct trophic effects of estrogen on folliculogenesis in the rat. Injection of intact immature rats with DES resulted 12 h later in increased DNA synthesis only in small follicles (<200 μm) but by 48 h medium (200–400 μm) and large follicles (>400 μm) showed increased incorporation of [^{3}H]thymidine

(227). After DES, the number of granulosa cells expressed from medium and large follicles increased at 36 to 48 h and 48 h, respectively. Contrary to the stimulating effects of one or two injections of DES (227) with three or four injections (every 24 h), [^{3}H]thymidine incorporation was significantly reduced in medium-sized follicles as well as aromatase activity and protein content (228). Also, the number of granulosa cells in medium-sized follicles declined after three or four injections. Since serum gonadotropin levels were not monitored, it is possible that DES may be acting via the hypothalamic-axis as well as directly, although the relative normality of small and large follicles favors the latter possibility. Chakravorty and associates (228) hypothesize that prolonged DES exposure induces an inhibitory peptide factor in medium-sized follicles, which acts in an autocrine or paracrine manner to inhibit follicular growth. Treatment of immature rats for 4 days with DES implants led to a fourfold increase in viable granulosa cells (229). Granulosa cells obtained from control rats showed very low levels of incorporation of [^{3}H]thymidine—in the presence or absence of insulin. In contrast, granulosa cells from DES-implanted rats showed higher incorporation rates but only after longer incorporation periods of 24 to 36 h. However, when granulosa cells were incubated with conditioned medium of thecal cells—exposed to estrogen—there was a 12-fold increase in [^{3}H]thymidine incorporation. These results are consistent with previously cited research, which has shown that the theca produces mitogenic factors (transforming growth factor-β) that enhance granulosal cell proliferation (see below). *In vivo,* DES stimulates a sevenfold expression of TGF-β_2 mRNA in rat granulosa cells but not in thecal cells (230).

In vitro evidence indicating that estrogen directly affects rat granulosa cell function is shown by the fact that estradiol increases GnRH turnover of phosphoinositide metabolism to produce diacylglycerol and inositol triphosphate (231). Since GnRH inhibits FSH-stimulable steroidogenesis, it is possible that under these circumstances, estrogen acts as a negative feedback controller of its own production. When cell-to-cell connections are disrupted in rat granulosa cells by EGTA, FSH fails to induce LH receptor, contrary to cells where gap junctions are intact (232). However, when estradiol plus FSH is added, LH receptors are induced, indicating a role for estrogen in promoting cellular interactions.

When immature rat ovaries are perifused continuously with FSH, [^{3}H]thymidine incorporation is lost after 24 h of perifusion while estrogen secretion by granulosa cells is unabated (233). The uncoupling of FSH-induced mitogenesis and steroidogenesis after 24 h can be reversed by perifusion with insulin, which turns on DNA synthesis and concurrently suppresses estradiol secretion.

Although in several species estrogen exerts direct stimulatory effects on folliculogenesis, in others the picture is cloudier. As pointed out elsewhere in this chapter, several lines of evidence suggest that estrogen is not directly involved in follicular growth in the macaque ovary, although other reports are positive. Unlike the rat, injection of hypophysectomized hamsters with estrogen fails to initiate growth of antral follicles, although it does significantly increase the number of small preantral follicles with up to five layers of granulosa cells (109). Whereas in the rat estrogen augments the stimulation of granulosal aromatase by FSH, in the hamster incubation with 10 ng estradiol depressed aromatase activity by 71% (234). In the same vein, incubation of preantral hamster follicles for 24 h with 1 or 10 μg estradiol induces follicular atresia (128). Long-term culture of isolated large preovulatory hamster follicles with estradiol has minimal effects on follicular structure and only transiently increases progesterone accumulation for the first 24 h (235). Again, this contrasts with the hyperresponsiveness of rat follicles to estrogen. Similarly, intrafollicular injection of estrogen antagonists or estradiol antiserum into explanted hamster follicles fails to affect the proportion of immature oocytes (i.e., intact germinal vesicles), suggesting that estradiol plays a minimal role in arresting meiosis (236).

Scatchard analysis has been used to compare estrogen receptors in the ovaries of immature hamsters and rats (237). The K_d for cytosolic receptors was greater in the rat (K_d = 0.52 nmol for the rat vs 1.41 nmol for the hamster) and the number of cytosolic binding sites was approximately twofold greater in the rat. Thus, the hamster does appear to have estrogen binding sites. A subsequent study has extended this approach by comparing estrogen receptors in large preovulatory follicles (221). The cytosolic and nuclear K_d's for the rat follicle are approximately twice as great as the hamster, but this difference is most likely not of biologic consequence. An intriguing species difference is that the total amount of estrogen receptors (sum of the number of cytosolic and nuclear binding sites) was approximately tenfold higher in the hamster than the rat. Thus, the failure of large hamster follicles to respond to estrogen cannot be explained by a lack of estrogen receptors. The estrogen resistance of the hamster follicle could result from a subtle change in the amino acid sequence of the receptor or perturbations in the postligand receptor interaction. These results suggest that the immunohistochemical localization of follicular estrogen receptors may not necessarily correlate with the functional ability of ligand-receptor interactions.

THECAL STRUCTURE AND FUNCTION

Primordial follicles in the mouse ovary 4 to 6 days after birth are surrounded by a unilaminar layer of connective tissue; on the transformation of primordial to primary follicles (i.e., a single layer of cuboidal granulosa cells) a theca folliculi begins to differentiate, consisting of fibroblasts and epithelial cells and possibly transitional cells (238). Even after the administration of PMS and hCG, the same cell types are present in the differentiated theca of graafian follicles (238). In the rat, a theca externa is first apparent around small antral follicles, 0.1–0.25 mm in diameter, consisting of fibroblasts, smooth muscle cells, and an intermediate variety (239). Some of the cells definitely show the ultrastructural characteristics of smooth muscle cells, and this is reinforced by the immunofluorescent demonstration of actin and myosin in several cell layers of the theca externa surrounding large graafian follicles (240). In "smaller" rat follicles, the fluorescent band is only one to four layers thick and often incomplete; follicles surrounded by one or two layers of granulosa cells already show a weak but definite fluorescence indicative of actin and myosin. Homocellular gap junctions link thecal cells in multilaminar follicles in the hypophysectomized rat, and hCG treatment increases the size and frequency of gap junctions and leads to thecal hypertrophy (171). Based on the definite presence of smooth muscles in the theca externa, the possibility has been raised for a number of species of a contractile component involved in ovulation (see references in refs. 241 and 242). This is consistent with the distribution of cholinergic and adrenergic nerves in the theca externa of numerous species and the ability to stimulate contractility of the bovine follicle *in vitro* and induce ovulation in the *in vitro* perfused rabbit ovary (243,244). Using a monoclonal antibody to actin, immunocytochemistry and immunoblots identify the theca externa of preantral and antral hamster follicles (245). A digestive fraction rich in thecal cells (identified by the antibody) was grown for 4 days in culture before [^{3}H]-thymidine was added; most of the theca externa cells had initiated DNA synthesis. When cultured cells were exposed to a Ca^{2+} ionophore, contractions were observed.

Several recent studies have considered the distribution of cholinergic and adrenergic fibers (246) and regulatory peptides (247) in the ovaries of various species. The former paper confirms that in the rat, adrenergic nerves are present in blood vessels in the theca interna, fibromuscular cells in theca externa and branches running through the stroma (246). Cholinergic activity is exhibited by a dense zone in the theca externa, which reaches its maximal intensity in the preovulatory follicle. It is intriguing that nerve fibers containing substance P course close to primordial follicles in the cortical stroma of rats (247). A number of the regulatory peptides, demonstrated by immunocytochemistry, are found in blood vessels as well as the theca externa and vary in abundance. For example, immunoreactivity for vasoactive intestinal peptide is present in small numbers of fibers in the ovaries of rat, cow, and pig and in moderate numbers of fibers in the human ovary. The most abundant regulatory peptide was neuropeptide Y, which formed an "almost single-layered network" of varicosities in the theca externa. A precursor of neuropeptide is present in follicular fluid obtained from patients undergoing *in vitro* fertilization (248); neuropeptide colocalizes with norepinephrine (cited in ref. 248). Vasoactive intestinal peptide acting in its physiologic dose range induces cytochrome P-450_{SCC} synthesis in granulosa cells from immature estrogen-primed rats (249). When ovarian denervation is performed by freezing the ovarian pedicle (thus eliminating ovarian sympathetic innervation for 10 days), normal ovulation rates continue (250). Nerve growth factor (NGF) is synthesized in ovarian sympathetic nerves of the juvenile rat as evidenced by the presence of NGF mRNA and NGF protein (251). Denervation of the ovary leads to increased ovarian NGF concentration. NGF mRNA in the denervated ovary is unaffected by injecting hypophysectomized rats with prolactin, FSH, or hCG. Administration of an antibody to NGF for the first 3 postnatal days blocks the development of ovarian sympathetic innervation (252). This is associated, at 29 to 30 days of age, with a greater percentage of small antral follicles from 250 to 300 μm in diameter and a concomitant reduction in follicles greater that 451 μm. In turn, this is reflected in a delay in the time of first ovulation and impaired release of testosterone and dihydrotestosterone from ovaries incubated for 3 h in the presence or absence of hCG. However, NGF antibody-treated females caged with fertile males results in 50% successful pregnancies. The reasons for the recovery of normal ovarian function in some animals is unknown. Autotransplantation of ovaries of 23-day-old rats next to the jugular vein results in the reinnervation of the ovaries by sensory (substance P-positive) and sympathetic (tyrosine hydroxylase-positive) nerve fibers 7 days after the transplantation and return of serum levels of gonadotropins to normal values (253). Moreover, ovulation occurs in these animals 21 days posttransplantation. However, when innervation to the transplanted ovaries is prevented with antibodies to NGF, serum gonadotropins fail to return to normal levels, suggesting the importance of innervation in maintaining the functional competence of the ovary. Immunocytochemical and *in situ* hybridization studies have revealed that follicular theca cells express both NGF receptor mRNA and proteins, and their expression disappears following ovulation (254). The interaction of the nervous system and folliculogenesis is obviously an area of increasing research interest.

The aggregation and ultimate differentiation of the theca folliculi is assumed to occur under the influence of growth factors emanating from the oocyte-granulosa complex, but there is no direct evidence to substantiate a causal relationship. In combined cultures of porcine thecal and granulosa cells, the reaggregated "follicle" tends to have the thecal cells arranged as the peripheral tissue (255). A causal relationship between the number of granulosa cell gap junctions and thecal development has been suggested for growing rat follicles (256). After the induction of ovulation by hCG in the rabbit, the temporal sequence in growing follicles is an increase in the labeling index of granulosa cells by 20–28 h and a lag until 40 h for an increase in the labeling index of endothelial thecal cells (257). On the other hand, a cytosol thecal extract (porcine) enhances the *in vitro* proliferation of granulosa cells and BALB/3T3 cells (258). Reciprocal interactions undoubtedly exist between theca and granulosa, which must be constantly kept in mind when the morphologic, biochemical, and steroidogenic properties of the isolated compartments are considered. For example, when bovine theca or follicle wall (theca plus granulosa) are incubated for 3 days with or without LH, the follicle wall secretes about four times as much androstenedione as an equal amount of theca (181). Follicle wall and granulosa cells secrete considerably more pregnenolone than theca, and addition of estradiol leads to a 12-fold increase in pregnenolone production by granulosa cells. In turn, culture of theca plus pregnenolone enhances the synthesis of androstenedione. Hence a positive feedback loop exists between the thecal and granulosal compartments. Further evidence of a feedback loop is provided by culturing bovine thecal cells with estradiol: This enhances the secretion of androstenedione and testosterone over a 6-day culture period with about ten-fold more androstenedione produced than testosterone (259).

A series of interesting studies has shown how growth factor production by the theca can influence the granulosa by paracrine pathways (260). Rat thecal/interstitial cells secrete transforming growth factor-β (261). Thecal-conditioned medium, alone or plus FSH, increases DNA synthesis in granulosa cells (262). Similar results are obtained by coculture of bovine theca and granulosa cells (263). Paracrine interactions on theca can also be inhibitory. Culture of human thecal cells for 4 days with LH and insulinlike growth factor-I causes about a 15-fold increase in androstenedione accumulation. Addition of 1 or 10 ng/ml of activin dose-dependently decreases androgen production with 50% inhibition at the higher dose (264).

The theca interna of sheep follicles, less than 3.0 mm in diameter, already consists of 8 to 12 layers of flattened cells and capillaries; 20% of the cells have the ultrastructural features of steroidogenically active cells; others are fibroblasts, and the majority are undifferentiated (265). In follicles 3–5.9 mm, approximately 40% of the theca interna cells possess tubular endoplasmic reticulum and the largest follicle on day 15 contained about 50% steroidogenically active cells. In all species, the theca interna is separated from the granulosa cells by a distinct PAS-positive band (e.g., in the cow [266])—the basal lamina. In the mouse, the basal layer consists of laminin, a noncollagenous glycoprotein (267) believed to be synthesized by basal epithelial or endothelial cells rather than fibroblasts. Several studies have revealed that granulosa cells in culture secrete fibronectin, a very important component of the extracellular matrix and therefore of consequence in the formation of the basement membrane in early folliculogenesis (268). The basal lamina is intact until shortly before ovulation. The time of appearance of a well-differentiated theca interna relative to the development of granulosa cells varies from species to species: mouse: three layers of granulosa cells (116); hamster: six layers of granulosa cells (269); sheep: follicles 2–3 mm (265); rhesus: three layers of granulosa cells; 100–125 μm in diameter (M. Koering, personal communication); human: preantral 180–240 μm in diameter (78). It is intriguing for the first three species that following hypophysectomy normal development of granulosa cells can proceed to the stage before a differentiated theca interna is found, albeit with a greatly reduced number of healthy follicles.

In the sheep follicle, maximal differentiation of the theca interna occurs in late estrus, but even then not all cells contain smooth endoplasmic reticulum (265). It is not until late estrus that numerous lipid droplets accumulate in the ovine theca interna—a usual sign of reduction in steroidogenesis; the first signs of discontinuity in the basal lamina also then appear (265). Bovine thecal cells separated from small (<5 mm), medium (5–10 mm), and large (>10 mm) antral follicles were cultured for 6 to 8 days in a serum-free medium in the presence or absence of hCG and insulin (270). In the first 3 days of culture, all preparations produce androstenedione in response to hCG and again about ten-fold more androstenedione than testosterone. After 3 days, steroidogenesis shifted from androstenedione to progesterone. It is noteworthy that there was a decline in proteins greater than 100 kDa secreted by thecal cells removed from small versus larger follicles. In the bovine theca interna, 3 to 4 days before ovulation, two cell populations emerge, consisting of large epithelial cells with round nuclei increasing in area and another group of fibroblastlike cells in which nuclear area does not increase; ultimately, the fibroblastic thecal cells contribute to the small luteal cells at the periphery of the corpus luteum and the epithelial variety disperse into the stroma (266).

It is possible with large porcine follicles (1.0–1.2 cm in diameter) to separate the theca interna as a discrete layer, mince it with scissors, and then with gentle trypsinization disperse the thecal cells (271). The thecal cells from these large preovulatory follicles differ in several respects from porcine granulosa cells in that the former contain many more lipid droplets; histochemically they show very intense 3β-hydroxysteroid dehydrogenase activity and in the first 2 days of culture produce 13 times more estrogen than granulosa cells. Similar substantial thecal production of estrogens has been observed in mature pig follicles obtained after injection of PMSG and hCG (272). Cultured porcine thecal cells—from follicles greater than 10 mm in diameter—show increased aromatase activity (using a radiometric assay) in response to hCG (273); thecal progesterone secretion is also stimulated by hCG. The theca was maintained in a serum-free medium. When theca was separated from 4 to 6 mm porcine follicles, optimal *in vitro* steroidogenesis resulted from a combination of LH, 1% fetal bovine serum and insulinlike growth factor-I (274), with androstenedione production declining after 1 day as progesterone accumulation increased over the next 3 days. Since porcine granulosa cells increase their production of insulinlike growth factor-I in response to epidermal growth factor or transforming growth factor-α (275), another route of communication exists between granulosa and thecal cells. Factors regulating thecal cell function are reviewed in a recent article (276). Cultured human thecal cells produce *in vitro* high levels of androstenedione for 2 days (30 ng $\times$ 10^5 cells), moderate levels of estradiol (2 ng $\times$ 10^5 cells), and, beyond day 4, nondetectable levels of these steroids. On the other hand, progesterone is produced at high levels (20 ng $\times$ 10^5 cell) throughout the 10 days of culture (277).

An abundant literature on rodents and many other species points to the theca as the major source of androgen precursors, which are then transported to the granulosa compartment for conversion to estrogens (see ref. 276 for references). In the rat, theca from small antral follicles do not accumulate testosterone, dihydrotestosterone, or androstenedione in response to 8-bromo-cAMP in contrast to large preovulatory follicles (278). Similarly, thecal cells from rat follicles increase progesterone synthesis in response to dibutyryl cAMP or hCG with comparable values in interstitial gland cells (279). Stromal cells (theca and interstitium) have considerably more 5α reductase activity than granulosa cells from both small and large rat follicles, consistent with a much greater production of 5α-pregnane-3,20-dione and 5α-androstene-3,17-dione. These findings agree with a topical autoradiographic study of the rat ovary, which showed that hCG binding to theca interna was detectable in follicles 100–200 μm in diameter and grain density doubled once again in follicles larger than 600 μm (204).

It seems quite likely that LH receptors must develop in the theca folliculi before it can differentiate into theca externa and interna, but so far this critical stage has not been studied. A fluorescein-hCG conjugate, injected intravenously, is localized in scattered patches of interstitial cells during the early follicular phase of cynomolgus monkeys; although at this stage numerous antral follicles are present, no concentrated band of hCG is evident and none is demonstrable on preantral follicles (280). On day 7, a single follicle in both ovaries was surrounded by a fluorescent ring of hCG, although there were as many as 4 to 8 follicles 1–3 mm in diameter per ovary. The fluorescent follicle—the putative dominant follicle—was not the largest. However, on day 9 the dominant follicle was surrounded by 8 to 14 layers of thecal cells, was more intensively fluorescent than on day 7, and was the largest follicle present.

In addition to its differentiation as a steroidogenic tissue, the theca interna pari passu develops a vascular supply and the two events may very well be related. Primordial rat follicles do not have an independent blood supply; it is not until a multilaminar granulosa and theca have formed (follicular diameter: 80–160 μm) that a vascular wreath develops in the inner portion of the theca interna adjacent to the membrana granulosa (281). The theca interna vasculature, in turn, is linked to an outer series of arterioles and venules in the theca externa. This pattern is unchanged throughout development except for expansion of blood vessels to keep pace with follicular growth. The pattern described for the vasculature of the rat follicle is essentially duplicated in all mammals. In ovaries removed from rhesus monkeys on day 9 or 10 of the cycle, morphometric analysis of the dominant follicle showed that 48% of the theca was vascularized compared to 25% vascularity in smaller antral follicles (282). When iodinated hCG was injected intravenously, the theca of the dominant follicle was heavily labeled, whereas smaller follicles showed little if any activity. Thus, selective vascularization of one follicle was associated with its greater ability to extract and concentrate hCG from the peripheral circulation. The steroidogenic output of androstenedione by perfused bovine theca correlates with the flow rate of the medium in the presence or absence of LH; the theca were from large preovulatory follicles, less than 10 mm in diameter (283).

The blood supply of the ovary can be increased by several mechanisms: (1) intraovarian growth of new blood vessels (angiogenesis); (2) growth of larger blood vessels; (3) vasodilation of existing capillaries; (4) an increase in the delivery of blood to the ovary. We will concentrate on angiogenesis. Based on earlier studies (281,282) it is possible that follicular growth is angiogenic-dependent, that is, the increase in granulosal and thecal cells must be accompanied and/or preceded by an increase in new capillaries that grow toward and within the theca of growing follicles. Ovaries excised from PMS-treated rats exhibit considerable vascularity 3 days after being placed on the chorioallantoic membrane of chicken eggs (284). Ovaries from non-PMS-treated rats showed moderate to no vascularization. In the PMS-treated rat, vascularity was most intense around follicles, and the theca was filled with nucleated chicken erythrocytes; however, these vessels did not penetrate the basal lamina. It is hypothesized that the granulosa cells may be the likely source of angiogenic factor because the new capillaries grow into the theca toward the granulosa cells (284).

Several lines of evidence support this hypothesis. Conditioned medium from granulosa cells obtained from preovulatory rat follicles has mitogenic activity on cultured endothelial cells resulting in a seven- to eight-fold

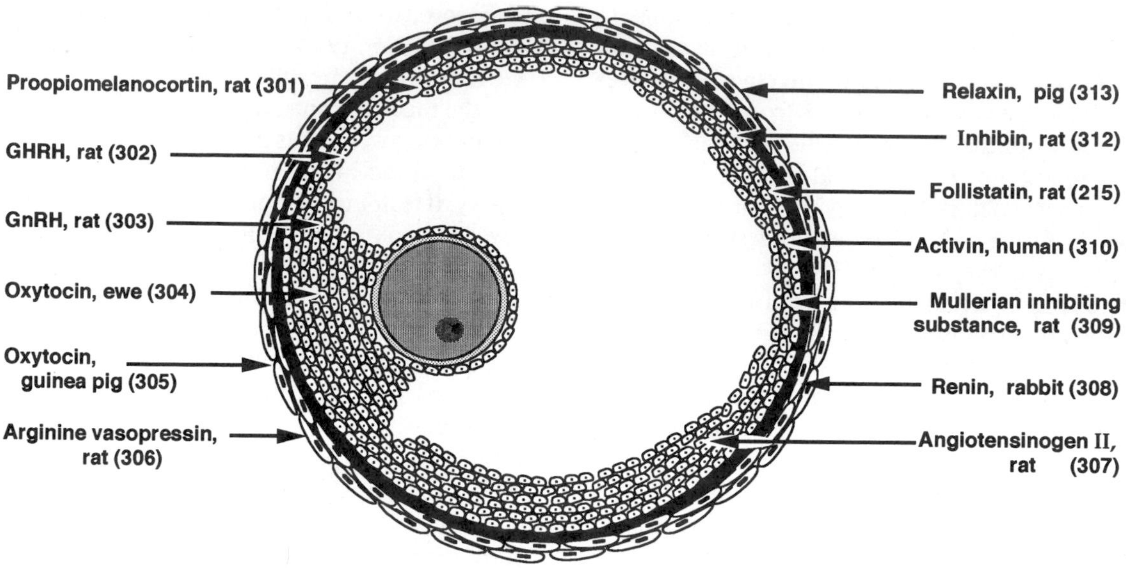

FIG. 1. Peptide hormones localized in granulosa and thecal compartments of mammalian antral follicles.

increase in proliferation (285). Preliminary characterization shows that the mitogenic activity is heat-resistant, partially destroyed by trypsin, and represents a high molecular weight fraction greater than 30,000. Spent medium from rat granulosa cells possesses chemotactic activity in addition to mitogenic activity with bovine aortic endothelium as the test tissue (286). Both activities are present in the same fraction (<10,000 Da) and it appears to be a lipoprotein by thin layer chromatography. A bewildering number of factors possess angiogenic activity, but one of the more likely candidates in the ovary is fibroblastic growth factor (FGF) that has a high affinity for heparin and heparin sulfate (287–289). Basic FGF is a potent angiogenic factor inducing endothelial cell migration, invasion, and production of plasminogen activator (290). FGF is secreted by endothelial cells and modulates a host of mitogenic and nonmitogenic functions of these cells (291,292). Basic FGF has been localized in theca cells of the fetal rat ovary (293), and the expression of the FGF gene has been detected in rat theca by reverse transcription and polymerase chain reaction amplification of thecal messenger RNA (294). The caveat is that the thecal layer is highly vascularized and therefore mRNA, used for reverse transcription and polymerase chain reaction, would invariably contain RNA from endothelial cells, which also express the FGF gene. Nevertheless, these results indicate a potential role of FGF in thecal angiogenesis. Crude glycosaminoglycans extracted from mouse ovaries potentiate the angiogenic activity of EGF, which is active in its own right in inducing capillary proliferation (295). Vascular endothelial growth factor, another member of the heparin-binding family, also has angiogenic properties. *In situ* hybridization of its mRNA in the primate ovary reveals a weak signal in granulosa cells and a stronger signal close to the basement membrane (296). It is not clear whether this zone corresponds to the peripheral mural granulosa cells or theca, but in the late follicular phase cynomolgus ovary (n = 1 ovary!) the largest follicle was most reactive.

Consistent with this concept, follicular fluid from porcine and human ovaries contains an angiogenic product (297,298), and the corpus luteum is also a source of an angiogenic factor (299). Using gel filtration with ammonium sulfate precipitation, two fractions of angiogenic activity were found in follicular fluid using as an endpoint aortic endothelial cell movement and proliferation *in vitro* and corneal angiogenesis *in vivo* (298). One factor with a molecular weight of 45,000 to 65,000 and another fraction of less than 1,500 exhibited angiogenic activity. On the other hand, proliferation of cultured bovine capillary endothelial cells is enhanced by extracts of porcine luteal and thecal cells but *not* by granulosa cells or follicular fluid (300). Hence the normally vascularized follicular compartment may have intrinsic ability to increase local angiogenesis. It is unknown whether the bovine thecal cells per se or the contained endothelial component is the source of the angiogenic factor(s).

Figure 1 summarizes the localization of various peptides in the antral follicle based on immunohistochemistry, *in situ* hybridization, or receptor studies. Most of these orphan peptides were first isolated from other endocrine glands—except for the inhibin family—and reasonable explanations for their functions exist; the same cannot be said for the roles of most of them in follicular function. At least a few generalizations can be made, but it obviously will be several years before the picture is clarified. Species differences exist in the abundance or absence of the peptides. The best example is GnRH-like activity in rat granulosa cells, whereas in other species it is either absent or binding sites with only low affinity are present. Several of the peptides do not reach peak levels until shortly before ovulation, suggesting that their presence is related more to luteal than follicular function. Conversely, some peptides disappear late on proestrus and are missing from the corpus luteum or atretic follicles so that a role in normal folliculogenesis is more likely. The same peptide may be identified in thecal or granulosal compartments of different species, which could affect their autocrine or paracrine activities. Even within the granulosal compartment, regional differences in distribution can occur, for example, more intense activity in cumulus cells than in membrana granulosa. In this instance, this implies a greater role on oocyte maturation than other follicular components.

FOLLICULAR ATRESIA

Follicular atresia is a universal phenomenon, characteristic of both mammalian and nonmammalian vertebrates (314). In the latter group, follicles are obliterated by massive phagocytic activity by granulosa cells, which in turn degenerate; morphologic changes are usually more subtle in the case of atresia in the mammalian ovary. It is estimated that greater than 99% of follicles become atretic in the human ovary and about 77% in the mouse (315). The number of follicles developing to the preovulatory stage are thus far fewer than the number undergoing atresia. Follicles can become atretic at any stage of development. Once a follicle enters the growing pool it either goes on to ovulate or becomes atretic; the chances are that it will become atretic, since more follicles are recruited during a cycle than usually ovulate. However, follicles in the nongrowing pool may also degenerate (316). The factors initiating atresia have intrigued scientists for many years and the factors regulating such a finely controlled mechanism are obviously worthy of investigation. Another intriguing question is: Can one predict when a follicle will become atretic—that is, what biochemical markers indicate that a follicle is destined for atresia (assessed morphologically)? In the search for these markers several models of atresia have been developed and they will be discussed later. First, a description of the process of natural atresia will be provided.

The Normal Process of Atresia: Membrana Granulosa

Two patterns of atresia are discernible in canine follicles. Type A involves prominent necrotic changes in oocyte and zona pellucida, whereas alterations of the granulosa cells are secondary; type B atresia is typified by distinctive degenerative changes in the granulosa with an almost unchanged oocyte and zona pellucida (317). Type A atresia predominates in secondary follicles (i.e., preantral), with type B atresia the only variety encountered in tertiary follicles.

It is difficult to discern when follicular atresia begins. Some investigators have used as the major criterion the presence of one or two pyknotic granulosa nuclei in the largest cross section of the follicle. This definition seems somewhat arbitrary, since even in the rodent tertiary follicle there are thousands of cells. A much more reliable number for early atresia was set up by Byskov (318), who used 5% pyknotic granulosa cells (in the largest cross section) as a sign of definite but early atresia. Healthy nonovulatory human follicles have a low pyknotic index (mean $\pm$ SE = 1.2%) and a high mitotic index (11.5%), whereas atretic follicles contain 10.9% pyknotic nuclei (319). Correlating flow cytometry of granulosa cells and follicular fluid estradiol in human follicles reveals that a DNA-S phase of 16% or more correlates with follicular health (86%), whereas an S-fraction of less than 16% includes 95% atretic follicles (320). Morphologic analysis of the largest follicle in ovaries from eight monkeys revealed that pyknosis normally occurs to some degree even in the dominant viable follicle. Moreover, the pyknotic index may vary considerably from one histologic section to another (321). This reinforces the difficulty of assessing the onset of spontaneous follicular atresia.

The degeneration of granulosa cells as atresia advances has all the characteristics of apoptotic cell death (322). Immature rats injected with PMS show definite histologic signs of follicular atresia on day 4 postinjection, which is paralleled by the appearance of an apoptotic pattern of DNA fragmentation (323). Similarly, granulosa cells recovered from diethylstilbestrol-treated rats are undifferentiated and do not express endonuclease activity, whereas 48 h after pregnant mare serum granulosa cell DNA has undergone about 30% degradation (324). Granulosa cells obtained from PMS-treated rats cultured in serum-free medium first begin to show significant spontaneous apoptosis by 16 h of incubation (325). Cellular death was partially suppressed by epidermal growth factor, transforming growth factor-α, or basic fibroblast growth factor but not by insulinlike growth factor-I, insulin, transforming growth factor-β or tumor necrosis factor-α. The combined effects of several growth factors was not tested. Since FSH induces EGF activity in hamster granulosa cells (147) and prolonged incubation of preantral hamster follicles with FSH prevents atresia (128), the modus operandi of FSH is obviously linked to growth factors. Advanced follicular atresia in the chicken and pig is easily recognized by the gross appearance of the follicles. Total DNA prepared for ethidium bromide staining or 3′ end labeling of internucleosomal DNA cleavage also distinguishes normal from atretic follicles (326). Whether DNA laddering is recognizable before or after histologic changes is unknown. Porcine follicles (3–6 mm) have been identified as healthy or atretic based on follicular opacity, and the latter category was confirmed by reduced follicular fluid estrogen (327). The decline in follicular estrogen was paralleled by decreases in aromatase in RNA, and, not unexpectedly, decreased FSH and LH receptor mRNA. Whereas there were no changes in 28S and 18S ribosomal RNA between healthy and atretic follicles, internucleosomal DNA fragmentation was evident in the latter group.

It has been proposed by Byskov (318) that atresia in the granulosa cell layer in the mouse occurs in three progressive phases:

Stage I: Up to 20% of the granulosa cells of the earliest atretic follicles exhibit pyknosis and fragmentation and these cells usually are adjacent to the antral cavity. This coincides with a reduction in [^{3}H]thymidine incorporation by the granulosa cells (expressed as labeling index, the number of labeled cells expressed as a percent of the total granulosa cells counted). Others have also reported a decreased uptake of [^{3}H]thymidine in atretic mouse (94) and dog (317) follicles as well as decreased ^{32}P uptake in rabbit follicles (328), both of which relate to the reduction in mitosis. An early study by Deane (329) revealed the presence of Feulgen-positive globules that were probably the fragmented nuclei of pyknotic cells observed by Byskov (318). In Stage I atresia and in normal follicles the basement membrane is intact. Two days after pulse labeling, mouse follicles in Stage I atresia show a marked increase in labeling index compared to the index at time zero presumably because of a reutilization of DNA released from dying cells by granulosa cells that are still viable (318). In addition, normal follicles exhibit essentially no pyknotic granulosa cells.

Stage II: A step further into atresia; the granulosa cells incorporate little, if any, [^{3}H]thymidine, and pyknotic granulosa cells are abundant (5–20%). Leukocytes begin to invade the membrana granulosa, correlating with a breakdown of the basement membrane. Lymphoid cells migrate into rat follicles on the evening of late diestrus as an antecedent to irreversible atresia (330). Subsequent studies involving immunoperoxidase staining have shown that Stage II atretic rat follicles are occasionally invaded by cytotoxic T lymphocytes, suggesting a role of the immune system in follicular differentiation and degeneration (331).

Stage III: The follicles are shrunken. Most of the parameters are similar to Stage II atresia except that the percentage of pyknotic cells was only 5%, probably due to a clearing of pyknotic granulosa cells from the follicles by macrophages and other scavenger-type cells. Markers of late stages of atresia include the appearance of angiotensin II receptors in rat granulosa cells (332) and high prorenin level in follicular fluid of bovine atretic follicles (333). These are most likely a consequence of atresia rather than causal antecedents.

In adult cyclic rats, the number of midsized follicles (350–550 μm) increases from estrus to diestrus. When the percentage of viable granulosa cells is measured by trypan blue exclusion and compared with the viability of the oocyte—as judged by fluorescence on exposure to fluorescin diacetate, a positive correlation is apparent (334). At diestrus and proestrus, follicles >550 mm with >60% granulosa viability were associated with healthy oocytes; for example, at proestrus, of 7.3 large antral follicles per ovary only 4 were normal. As rat follicles become atretic, ultrastructurally, intercellular spaces between granulosa cells increase (335), most likely representing a loss of gap junctions, which are reduced in atretic follicles (256). In medium-sized preantral follicles in the rat, incipient atretic changes in granulosa cells have a patchy distribution in that some cells show nuclear condensation (pyknosis) and marked dilatation of cytoplasmic organelles with cytoplasm and microvilli of the oocyte were still well preserved (336). Adjacent normal granulosa cells were undergoing mitosis. The granulosa cells also become flattened and lose cytoplasmic evaginations during atresia, whereas normal granulosa cells are spherical and have irregular cytoplasmic projections. These cytoplasmic projections normally correlate with the development of LH binding to granulosa cells (337). Thus, the loss of microvilli corresponds to loss of LH binding and the onset of atresia (338). With the loss of gap junctions and the loss of LH binding to granulosa cells, it is highly probable that the intercellular communication and trophic actions of LH needed to maintain an intact, well-structured membrane granulosa are lost. A monoclonal antibody (anti-OA-2) that recognizes a protein expressed only in granulosa cells of atretic follicles has been described (339) and used with models of atresia including hypophysectomized immature rats, diethylstilbestrol-primed, from which the diethylstilbestrol capsules were removed or 3 days of daily injections of hCG or testosterone. Indirect fluorescence of atretic *preantral* follicles revealed strong anti-OA-2 binding in a zone of granulosa cells adjacent to the basal lamina. Moreover, this distribution of reactive cells coincided with the localization observed with classical markers of atresia such as lipid droplets, acid phosphatase, and lysosomal nonspecific esterase. It is interesting that there was a distinct zonation of atresia; while the peripheral granulosa cells were degenerating, those closest to the egg were still normal.

An unusual variant of granulosa degeneration is present in the sheep follicle (340). The process again begins in granulosa cells bordering on the antral cavity. Phagocytic cells representing transformed granulosa cells increase in number as atresia progresses (akin to the process in nonmammalian vertebrates [314]). During secondary atresia, atretic bodies develop from the fusion of many nuclei and these multinucleated structures vary in diameter from 15 to 400 μm. Atretic sheep follicles (2–6 mm in diameter) have been reported to "regenerate" *in vitro* within 3 days by increased thickness of the granulosa layer by a factor of two- to four-fold (341). However, no mitotic figures are observed, and histologically the cells are definitely not normal granulosa cells.

It is possible to grossly identify atretic and healthy follicles in sheep (342), pig (343), and cow (344), based primarily on the vascularization of the theca, integrity of the membrana granulosa, and the translucency of the follicle. In fact, in the ewe normal and advanced atretic follicles, judged by their gross appearance, agreed with histologic criteria in over 95% of the cases (342).

During atresia the granulosa cells from atretic follicles of the rabbit take up less ^{35}S (345), suggesting a decrease in the synthesis of mucopolysaccharides containing sulfate. In contrast, atretic bovine follicles have low amounts of estrogen but high amounts of progesterone and chondroitin sulfate in follicular fluid (346). This relationship is significant when chondroitin sulfate concentration is plotted against estrogen or the estrogen:progesterone ratio but not when histology is used as the variable.

Histochemical and biochemical alterations in granulosa cells often precede definite morphologic changes in atretic granulosa cells (for references, see ref. 347). These include an increase in lysosomal enzymes such as acid phosphatase and aminopeptidase (348), and their role in the induction of atresia has been recently evaluated (349). In atretic follicles of a number of species, the histochemical appearance of 3β-hydroxysteroid dehydrogenase and lipid droplets in granulosa cells are characteristic markers of atresia, for example, in the human (350). The ovary of the 21- to 22-day-old rat consists mainly of primary and medium-sized preantral follicles. A single injection of DHT results 12–18 h later in drastic reductions of serum FSH and LH, and this is associated 48 h postinjection with a significant increase in cathepsin-D activity (a lysosomal enzyme) in aspirated granulosa cells (351). The deleterious effects of DHT are reversed by concurrent administration of FSH.

Granulosa cells from healthy human follicles maintained *in vitro* for 48 h produce large amounts of estradiol, progesterone, and small amounts of androstenedione without added steroid precursors (352). The follicles were judged to be normal, based on their possessing at least 75% of the maximal number of granulosa cells for their diameters. Follicles with less than 50% of optimal cell numbers of granulosa cells were judged atretic, and they frequently had a degenerating oocyte, low levels of estradiol, and undetectable levels of FSH in follicular fluid. Incubation of these granulosa cells produced elevated levels of androstenedione, testosterone, and dihydrotestosterone but negligible amounts of progesterone and estradiol. Thus, atresia of human follicles was associated with differentiation of granulosa cells into androgen-producing cells.

Oocyte

The common characteristic of atresia in the oocyte from the large follicles of many species is the meiosislike alterations called "pseudomaturation or pseudocleavage." This includes breakdown of the germinal vesicle, alignment of the chromosomes in metaphase and possibly expulsion of a polar body (353). One of the first signs of atresia in some follicles is the shrinkage of the oocyte (316,354). This is then either accompanied or followed by pseudomaturation. An increase in argyrophilic substances is observed in the oocytes of atretic rat follicles prior to the degenerative changes in the granulosa cells (355). This correlates ultrastructurally with an increase in granules in oocytes from atretic rat follicles (356). In nonpregnant women, synchronous degeneration of oocyte and granulosa cells occurs even in small antral follicles (357). Previous studies have shown that the organelles of the oocyte from atretic follicles tend to aggregate (356,358). The nuclear envelope loses its bilaminar appearance, increases its width, becomes uneven (356), or ruptures (359); thus, the plasmalemma of the oocyte becomes less distinct compared to that of healthy follicles.

A change in the histochemical staining properties of the porcine zona pellucida of atretic follicles is quite striking. In healthy follicles the zona pellucida stains uniformly green with Shorr's S3 and hematoxylin (360). In obviously atretic follicles the zona pellucida stains a bright orange. In some follicles (presumably healthy and with no morphologic signs of atresia), the zona pellucida was partially stained orange and green. These results indicate that Shorr's S3 stain may reveal a very early sign of atresia prior to observable changes in the follicular wall. Apparently, there are biochemical alterations in the mucopolysaccharides that reflect these changes in staining of the zona pellucida (360). Based on the altered staining properties of the atretic zona pellucida, it was estimated that 56% of preantral pig follicles were atretic compared to 73% and 84%, respectively, of medium sized (3–5 mm) and large follicles (6–12 mm). Shorr's stain is frequently used in exfoliative cytology to identify cornified vaginal cells, which biochemically represent a stage involving the formation of disulfide bonds in the epithelium. It is possible that physicochemical changes in the mucoproteins of the porcine zona pellucida may lead to similar changes during atresia. The strongest staining intensity of periodic acid-Schiff (PAS) occurs in the zona pellucida of atretic hamster follicles (361). PAS splits one or two glycol groups of glycoprotein complexes. Transmission and scanning electron microscopic examinations of atretic mouse follicles show that even the earliest stages of atresia are associated with structural changes of the zona pellucida: a compact reticulum of packed globular units connected to short interconnected filaments (362). These changes are associated with the loss of gap junctions in the corona radiata cells, thus isolating the ovum from its normal microenvironment and presumably leading to its ultimate death.

Follicles of most species in late stages of atresia exhibit germinal vesicle breakdown. When the oocytes from atretic rat follicles are cultured, germinal vesicle breakdown increased; however, 23% of the oocytes fragmented (356). Addition of pyruvate, which facilitates germinal vesicle breakdown (363), did not increase germinal vesicle breakdown in atretic follicles (356). During atresia the cumulus cells lose contact with the rat oocyte (316). Ultrastructurally, small gap junctions exist between the oocyte and the cumulus and these are reduced in atretic follicles (364).

In atretic rat follicles, the degeneration of the entire granulosa wall, until induced changes are observed in the oocyte, is estimated to take 24 h, and another 24 h elapse before the oocyte is completely denuded of cumulus cells (365). The ultimate death of the oocyte is typical of most mammals. However, the oocyte of the atretic sheep follicle (3–5 mm) is extremely resistant to degenerative changes: Oocytes cultured in atretic follicles for 24 h with FSH, LH, and estradiol and then transferred to the oviducts of inseminated ewes developed into blastocysts in 46% of the transfers (366).

Theca

In a number of species, including rodents (367) and primates (368), thecal hypertrophy is characteristic of follicles undergoing atresia. Ultrastructural examination of the thecal cells in atretic rat follicles reveals lipid droplets, an agranular endoplasmic reticulum, and mitochondria with tubular cristae typical of steroid secreting cells (369). The thecal cells of atretic follicles are cuboidal with a large nucleus to cytoplasm ratio and excessively folded plasma membranes. This transformation of rat thecal cells during atresia is similar to the morphology of the secondary interstitium, and thus in many species the theca cells of atretic follicles are progenitors of the secondary interstitium. The fact that these cells are functionally similar to interstitial cells is shown by the large amounts of progesterone secreted *in vitro* in response to hCG (369) and the presence of 3β-hydroxysteroid dehydrogenase activity (367,369). In hamster models of atresia, isolated theca respond to LH *in vitro* with an increase in progesterone, whereas theca from healthy antral follicles produce only small amounts of progesterone (370,371).

In several species, the ultimate fate of the theca is complete regression without any contribution to the interstitium. This is exemplified by the pig (360), cow (266), and sheep (372). This has been especially well studied in sheep (372) where during secondary atresia, thecal cells undergo condensation, fragmentation, and ultimate phagocytosis by still healthy thecal cells. Thecal regression in sheep therefore arises from the phenomenon of apoptosis (372), a basic process in kinetics of normal and abnormal tissue growth.

Degenerating cellular material accumulates and blocks the thecal capillaries of the atretic ovine follicle. This is an occasional finding in primary atresia, which becomes more marked as atresia progresses (372). Similarly, in tertiary atresia, the number of red blood cells per unit area and capillary area is significantly reduced in the ovine follicle (340). Estimates of follicular blood flow by radiolabeled microspheres fail to show any difference between normal and early atretic ovine follicles (373). The results may be confounded by the use of halothane to induce anesthesia. However, a similar study with conscious sheep also failed to distinguish between normal and early atretic follicles by thecal capillary blood flow. It was only in more advanced stages of atresia that thecal blood flow was reduced compared to normal follicles (cited in ref. 374). Thus, the evidence accumulated so far indicates that altered blood flow is a secondary rather than controlling factor in the onset of atresia. However, subtle changes in redistribution of blood between the inner and outer capillary wreaths of the theca would be difficult to evaluate with present methodology.

The basement membrane forms a semipermeable barrier between the theca interna and adjacent granulosa and consists of laminin, type IV collagen with fibronectin localized in the peripheral granulosa cells of small and medium follicles. As atresia progresses, the basal lamina in rat follicles thickens and fragments, and there is intense accumulation of fibronectin in the thecal-granulosa boundary (375). This phenomenon has been observed in rat, cow, and pig follicles.

One of the last steps in atresia is complete collapse of the follicle. Shortening of smooth muscle cells in the theca externa of atretic follicles has been reported in mice (376), and this may be causal to the final shrinkage.

After considering atretic changes in granulosa and theca, it is appropriate to review altered steroidogenesis during spontaneous follicular atresia. Slices of human antral follicles, classified into stages of atresia by histology, were incubated with [^{14}C]acetate (377). Stage I atresia was defined as crumbling regressing granulosa cells, and Stage II as virtual complete disappearance of granulosa cells and hypertrophy and hyperplasia of thecal cells; Stage III represents regression of the theca. In all three stages, androstenedione was the principal steroid product without any incorporation of acetate into progesterone. During the third stage of atresia, 17-hydroxyprogesterone was the only other steroid formed. As previously mentioned, granulosa cells from atretic human follicles lose their capacity to produce estradiol, estrone, and progesterone correlated with the absence of FSH in follicular fluid (378). Theca from human healthy and atretic follicles incubated for 15 h, show significantly greater production of progesterone and testosterone by the atretic theca (379). Addition of 5 or 10 ng LH/ml enhanced the production of androstenedione, testosterone, and dihydrotestosterone to the same extent, whereas the theca of atretic follicles showed no increases in estrone or estradiol but a greatly enhanced ability to accumulate progesterone (with 10 ng of LH).

Incubation of healthy and atretic porcine follicles for 24 h has shown that atretic follicles produce less estradiol but considerably more androstenedione, testosterone, and dihydrotestosterone (343). Progesterone secretion by atretic follicles is not increased in response to hCG. Follicular fluid concentrations of estrogen, testosterone and androstenedione are significantly less in atretic porcine follicles (380). Estrogen production by pig granulosa cells in the presence or absence of equimolar amounts of testosterone or androstenedione was highly elevated in granulosa from healthy follicles, and this is also true for progesterone production after the addition of FSH. Conversely, production of estradiol was much less by the theca of atretic follicles, but the production rates of testosterone and androstenedione were virtually identical between normal and healthy theca. The conclusion is that the loss of aromatase activity by porcine granulosa cells is the first step affected by atresia, in agreement with a similar sequence in the human follicle (378).

Steroid concentrations in pools of ovine antral fluid show that in normal follicles the molar ratio of estrogen:testosterone plus androstenedione is always greater than 1 (381). As atresia progresses the ratio shifts in favor of androgen dominance, primarily due to a fall in estradiol. In large (>3.5 mm) atretic follicles—judged by morphologic criteria—follicles with signs of early degeneration have reduced aromatase activity, consistent with the idea that in the ewe, lack of androgen substrate is not the limiting factor (382). In atretic ovine follicles (>4 mm), binding of [^{125}I]FSH and LH do not differ from healthy follicles until the most advanced stage of atresia (383). However, for intermediate-sized antral follicles (2–4 mm) the loss of FSH binding by granulosa cells precedes the decline in hCG binding. The authors conclude that the decreased binding of the labeled gonadotropins as atresia progresses is more likely a consequence than a cause of follicular regression. In PMSG/hCG-treated rats, atretic tertiary follicles do not express any LH receptor mRNA (384).

Bovine follicles from days 3 to 13 of the estrous cycle were assigned to healthy or atretic status based on follicular concentration of estradiol (estrogen-active or inactive) and histology (385). From days 3 to 7, a single large estrogen-active follicle is present. During this time span the estrogen inactive follicles have significantly less binding of hCG to theca and granulosa and reduced FSH binding to granulosa. The analysis of the data is complicated by the few estrogen-inactive follicles, their significantly fewer granulosa cells on days 5 and 7, and a lack of agreement between histologic classification and follicular fluid ratios of estrogen to progesterone. There is no difference in [^{125}I]hCG binding to bovine theca interna from healthy and atretic antral follicles (344). When perifused *in vitro,* the output of androstenedione by theca interna of normal bovine follicles is considerably enhanced by equimolar concentrations of LH or hCG, but the theca of atretic follicles is not responsive. Lack of available receptors, therefore, does not seem to account for the failure of androgen production by large atretic bovine follicles. Rather, distal events seem to be affected. A subsequent study (386) classified the theca of large bovine follicles (>8 mm) into three types based on the numbers and steroidogenic capacities of the associated granulosa cells. Type I theca (normal follicles) when perfused *in vitro* with LH responded by secreting increased cAMP, androstenedione, and testosterone. Type II theca (from possibly early atretic follicles) secreted increased cAMP and progesterone—but not androgens. Type III theca (definitely atretic), in response to LH, did not increase cAMP or steroids. The theca of all three types contained LH receptors. These results are strikingly similar to findings with some of the rodent models (see below).

Experimental Induction of Follicular Atresia

During the past 15 years several models involving rodents have been developed to study atresia with a number of the experimental designs based on previously described procedures (Table 3). Despite disparity in species

TABLE 3. *Rodent models of follicular atresia*

Model	Reference(s)
1. Hypophysectomy of proestrous rat	Braw et al., 1981 (387)
2. Hypophysectomy + PMS followed by anti-PMS (hamster)	Bill and Greenwald, 1981 (388)
3. Pentobarbital delay of ovulation in rat	Braw and Tsafriri, 1980 (389) Uilenbroek et al., 1980 (390)
4. Phenobarbital delay of ovulation in hamster	Terranova, 1980 (391)
5. PMS to immature mouse	Peters et al., 1975 (392)
6. PMS to immature rat	Peluso and Steger, 1978 (393) Braw and Tsafriri, 1980 (394)
7. PMS to immature hamster	Matson et al., 1984 (395)
8. Hypophysectomy of prepubertal rat Treatment with E_2 or DES, then hormone withdrawal	Schwall and Erickson, 1981 (369)
9. Androgen treatment of hypophysectomized rat	Bagnell et al., 1982 (396)

PMS, pregnant mare serum; E_2, estradiol; DES, diethylstilbestrol.

and experimental design, the models are remarkably similar in the conclusions reached and differ in key aspects from spontaneous atresia in sheep and human (see above). With one exception (369), the models focus on tertiary follicles, but they could just as well be utilized to study atresia of preantral follicles. As to be expected, the models using hypophysectomized animals show more rapid onset of morphologic and steroidogenic changes indicative of atresia than the use of intact animals. Thus, following hypophysectomy of proestrous rats, within 12 h *in vitro* accumulation of progesterone is significantly increased by explanted follicles, and, conversely, estradiol is approximately halved (387). Morphologic signs of early atresia are evident by 24 h with about 10% of the granulosa cells pyknotic, although mitotic figures are still present. By 2 days after hypophysectomy, germinal vesicle breakdown and polar body exclusion had occurred in most oocytes and the resumption of meiosis was associated with a 95% increase in oxygen consumption by the oocyte (397).

The onset of atresia is even more dramatic when pregnant mare serum (PMS) is neutralized by anti-PMS in the hypophysectomized hamster: Within 1 h, serum estradiol is reduced 55% (388) and the earliest histologic signs of atresia are discernible within 4 h by a significant increase in pyknotic cells in the cumulus oophorus, from 0.3% to 23.4% (398). At 2 h after anti-PMS, cAMP increased 108% above control levels, while cGMP rose 117% at 4 h; beginning at 12 h cAMP steadily declined (399). Pyknotic cells begin to appear in the mural granulosa by 8 h when there are still 65 mitotic figures in the largest cross section of the follicle. By 48 h, the number of pyknotic granulosa nuclei is maximal, and mitoses are now lacking. By 72 h, the granulosa layer is virtually eliminated and DNA values indicate that only 20% of the original number of cells are left in the follicle (399). The thickness of the theca showed a transitory increase at 12 h (398), which did not persist, unlike the situation observed during spontaneous atresia in the hamster. Steroid production by isolated hamster granulosa and theca paralleled the structural demise of the follicle. Necrotic changes in the granulosa cells were too widespread beyond 24 h to warrant steroid determinations beyond that point (371). The salient observations were that thecal shells exposed to LH produced large amounts of androstenedione and 17-hydroxyprogesterone for the first 24 h after anti-PMS but continued to produce appreciable quantities of progesterone for at least 72 h. This confirms previous observations with this model when intact follicles were incubated with 200 ng LH; cAMP was also increased for up to 72 h by this dose of LH, presumably a response of the theca (400). Thus, the loss of *C*-17,20-lyase in theca of the atretic hamster follicle is a critical event in atresia, an observation consistent with several other rodent models (see below). In 24 hours after administration of anti-PMS, grain counts of ^{125}I-labeled FSH and LH on granulosa cells are reduced by 69% and 53%, respectively, of control values and receptor binding declines to 5% and 24%, respectively, at 72 h (401). It is noteworthy that hCG binding to thecal cells and the interstitium was maintained at the same levels throughout the 72 h after the induction of atresia, which points to the extreme resistance of these tissues to hormone withdrawal. Using the same model, it has recently been shown that the earliest stage of atresia occurs 4 h after anti-PMS by the appearance of pyknotic cells in the cumulus oophorus, when thecal vasculature is still normal (402). The most drastic regressive changes occurred between 12 and 18 h, associated with germinal vesicle breakdown and a marked reduction in DNA synthesis in the mural granulosa. Despite all of the regressive changes in the follicle, the ovum is viable for at least 48 h as judged by maximal fluorescence after addition of fluorescein diacetate. DNA labeling of thecal endothelial cells also dropped sharply by 18 h, coinciding with a fall in thecal vascularity. However, the theca never contained pyknotic nuclei.

Another series of models deals with the administration of barbiturates at proestrus to block preovulatory surges of LH and FSH and hence extend the life span of antral follicles beyond their normal 2 to 3 days duration (Table 3, models 4–6). With these models, atresia unfolds at a slower pace. In the cyclic hamster after 3 days of ovulatory delay by repeated injections of phenobarbital, early signs of atresia are manifested by pyknotic nuclei in the membrana granulosa cells bordering on the antral cavity and in granulosa cells of the cumulus oophorus plus oocyte changes (391). During the period of ovulatory delay the tertiary follicles continue to enlarge, expanding from 561 μm in diameter at proestrus to 680 μm on the next day. A new set of follicles is recruited by 3 days of ovulatory delay, possibly in response to elevated serum levels of FSH. After 2 days of phenobarbital treatment, spontaneous ovulation results in about 18 ova being shed, most likely representing a composite of both delayed and new follicles. On days 2 and 3 of delay, follicles incubated in the presence of LH produce more progesterone and less androstenedione and estradiol than proestrous follicles (403). However, when explanted follicles were provided with androstenedione as a precursor, estrogen accumulation was maintained at high levels, indicating that impaired estrogen secretion by the follicle is not attributable to loss of aromatase activity but rather to a deficiency of androgen precursor. The *in vitro* ability of the hamster theca to respond to LH by producing androstenedione decreased as ovulatory delay was lengthened but with a concomitant increase in progesterone accumulation (370). Determination of FSH and LH (hCG) receptors in delayed follicles revealed that LH binding increased slightly or remained essentially unchanged during 3 days of delay (404); FSH binding decreased steadily throughout delay. Binding favored LH, and therefore increased receptors may account for the increase in progesterone secretion in delayed follicles.

Similar results are obtained in the proestrous rat injected with pentobarbitone (model 3). After 3 or 4 days of pentobarbital (Nembutal) treatment, most of the oocytes were in the dictyate stage but pyknotic nuclei, as well as mitotic figures, characterize the membrana granulosa. Meiosislike changes in the oocyte were observed by 4 days of ovulatory delay (389). Stage I atresia existed by day 3 and Stages I and II by day 4. By day 4 of treatment, injection of hCG resulted in the ovulation of 3.4 ova per animal compared to 11.0 on proestrus. A more drastic regimen consists of nembutal injected at proestrus (day 0) along with 4 mg progesterone (405). Preovulatory follicles regressed 2 days later and were being replaced by a new set of follicles, capable of a full ovulatory response to hCG (10.8 ova) by the next day. The reason for the rapidity of replacement of the preovulatory follicles was a drastic curtailment in LH secretion and a second surge of FSH on day 2.

Before morphologic signs of atresia are apparent in the pentobarbital-treated rat, steroid secretion is modified within 1 day as evidenced by estradiol and androgen accumulations of about 20–25% of proestrous values (389,390). On the other hand, progesterone accumulation over a 4-h period is unaffected (390). One day after ovulation is blocked, specific binding of hCG to follicles is significantly increased and FSH binding is comparable to proestrous values. Changes in receptor numbers therefore occur as a secondary event in this model of atresia as well as in others. *In vitro* steroidogenic activity of the delayed ovulating rat follicles duplicates the pattern in the hamster: Accumulation of androgen and estradiol is drastically decreased by 1 day of pentobarbital treatment and addition of testosterone to the medium leads to a fivefold increase in estradiol (390). Measurement of steroidogenic enzymes by ^{3}H exchange assays showed that 1 day of pentobarbital treatment significantly reduced *C*-17,20-lyase and 17α-hydroxylase, with a fall in aromatase activity by day 2 (406). Again the unavailability of androgen substrate, presumably thecal in origin, was one of the first biochemical markers of atresia. When bromocryptine—a dopaminergic agonist—is injected daily along with pentobarbital, the ability to ovulate in response to hCG is prolonged for as long as 3 days, associated with the maintenance of normal follicular structure and the *in vitro* ability to secrete high levels of estrogen (407). It is presumed that bromocryptine acts by decreasing prolactin secretion, which may have direct inhibitory effects on follicular secretion of estrogen. As enumerated several times in this chapter, the secretion of high levels of estrogen is sine qua non for normal tertiary follicles. The pattern of atresia in rat follicles after pentobarbitone administration parallels the sequence observed in spontaneous atresia with a delay of about 2 days in all events (408). During the cycle the life span of antral follicles in the rat can only be extended to a total of 5 to 6 days before regressive changes become evident.

Another group of models of induced follicular atresia involves the injection of immature animals with PMS, which leads to the waxing and waning of preovulatory antral follicles (Table 3, models 5–7). For example, injection of 22-day-old mice with 5 IU PMS results 24 h later in no change in the total number of "large" follicles, but the balance between healthy and atretic follicles is shifted so that only 33% of the population is atretic compared to 76% in controls (392). Similarly, administration of 15 IU PMS to 26-day-old rats does not alter the total number of preantral and antral follicles present 24 h later but decreases the proportion between nonatretic and atretic follicles (394). Both of these studies emphasize that PMS "rescues" follicles from atresia in mice and rats, but species differences and the dose of PMS administered suggest recruitment of follicles as another important role for the hormone in inducing superovulation (see below).

In 26-day-old rats, follicles capable of ovulating to hCG are present 48 h after IP injection of 5 IU PMS and they then rapidly degenerate by 60–72 h (409). The follicles can no longer ovulate by 72 h in response to a challenging dose of hCG; by 60 h acid phosphatase begins to build up in the membrana granulosa. By 60 h after PMS, LH binding was reduced by 46% (409), whereas FSH binding was unaffected until 56 h (393). Incorporation of [^{3}H]thymidine into the total ovary did not vary between 48 and 96 h after PMS, but the labeling index of antral follicles fell significantly at 96 h; this marked the onset of early atresia, as judged by the appearance of pyknotic granulosa cells (393). The critical role of FSH in maintaining an optimal environment for the granulosa cells is evident. Ultrastructurally, the earliest signs of atresia are apparent by 72 h; 28% of tertiary follicles are atretic as evidenced by focal areas of degeneration in granulosa cells, while others are normal (335). By 96 h all antral follicles contained at least two pyknotic nuclei and microvilli were diminishing. Thus, cell-to-cell communication is disrupted. Ovarian concentrations of testosterone and estradiol are significantly lowered by 72 and 96 h compared to 48 post-PMS (335).

Immature hamsters (25 days old) injected with 40 IU PMS—a superovulatory dose—show at 72–78 h normal *in vitro* follicular outputs of progesterone, 17β-hydroxyprogesterone and estradiol in response to LH (395). After 96–102 h, advanced atresia (established histologically) had affected antral follicles in some ovaries and this correlated *in vitro* with significantly higher accumulations of progesterone and greatly elevated plasma levels of the hormone. An estrogen-progesterone shift is thus demonstrably comparable to the changes observed in healthy tertiary follicles on proestrus after the preovulatory release of gonadotropins.

The above models concentrated on atresia induced in

antral follicles. It is noteworthy that hypophysectomized diethylstilbestrol (DES)-treated rats (immature animals) begin to show signs of atresia—judged by pyknotic granulosa cells—as early as 4 days postoperatively: About 55% of follicles greater than 200 μm are affected (410). This casts some doubt on the physiologic validity of this model, which is so extensively utilized. Another model deals with preantral follicles and emphasizes thecal changes: The protocol consists of hypophysectomized 21-day-old rats with Silastic implants of DES, which are removed from half the animals on day 24 and with subsequent necropsy 2 and 4 days later (369). In the animals with maintained estrogen levels numerous preantral follicles with fibroblastic thecal cells are present. In contrast, after DES withdrawal the thecal cells hypertrophy and develop the ultrastructural features of steroidogenic tissues. It is fascinating that these thecal changes occur in a presumably anhormonal environment. After DES withdrawal, hCG binding and the number of 3β-hydroxysteroid reactive cells increases, presumably reflecting thecal and interstial cells. At 4 days after estrogen withdrawal, when follicular activity is maximal, *in vitro* steroidogenesis in the presence of hCG is greatly enhanced for progesterone, 20-dihydroprogesterone, and androstenedione. In both control and estrogen-withdrawn cells, testosterone, dihydrotestosterone, and estrogen were undetectable. The increase in androgen production by the theca-interstitium therefore occurred apparently as a secondary event in atresia of preantral follicles.

Considerable attention has been devoted to a possible atretogenic role of androgens as opposed to anti-atretic effects of estrogens (411–413). For example, in PMS-hCG-treated immature rats, pretreatment with the antiandrogens cyproterone acetate or flutamide reduces the ovulation rate to hCG by 50% (414). Ovarian concentrations of estradiol, testosterone, and progesterone were, however, unaffected by flutamide; a better endpoint would have been *in vitro* accumulation of steroids by the antral follicles. In control rats, 48 h after PMS, 76% of the follicles greater than 500 μm were healthy; injection of either flutamide or CI 628 (an antiestrogen) decreased the number of nonatretic follicles to 14% and 9%, respectively (414). Granulosa cell viability, assessed by trypan blue exclusion, was reduced and 20 times more sensitive to the antiestrogen than the antiandrogen.

Since granulosa cells have specific androgen receptors (415,416) it is likely that the atretrogenic actions of androgens are exerted directly on these cells. Interestingly, testosterone reduces the availability of estrogen receptors (417). A role for dihydrotestosterone (DHT) in inducing atresia has been the subject of several studies. Thus, DHT administered to hypophysectomized PMS-treated rats causes a significant reduction in primary, secondary, and tertiary follicles and coadministration of estrogen reverses this effect (396). However, using the same animal model and the same protocol a recent study has failed to demonstrate a direct atretogenic effect of DHT (418). In the immature rat, DHT reduces the formation of LH receptors induced by FSH (419,420). Since DHT did not alter FSH stimulable adenylate cyclase and estradiol production, it is postulated that it acted as an antiestrogen by blocking the action of estradiol on the estradiol receptor and thus promoted atresia. Estradiol is required for FSH action in rat granulosa cells (421). Another possible mechanism of action of DHT is to block aromatase activity in rat granulosa cells (422). It has been suggested that if androgen production exceeds the ability of granulosa cells to aromatize it to estrogen, then DHT will be formed and might lead to atresia (8). Excessive LH stimulation of the theca of small rat follicles increases DHT significantly, whereas in large follicles, the granulosa cell population is large enough to convert most of the androgen to estrogen (422). At least for the rat, a proper balance between LH stimulation, androgen production, and aromatization is necessary to promote estrogen formation and the prevention of atresia. In other species, such as human and sheep, the presence of high levels of androgens in follicular fluid of atretic follicles may not be causative but merely represent the accumulation of large amounts of precursors because of insufficient aromatase activity.

Collectively, the rodent models of atresia show a consistent pattern. The morphologic changes duplicate those observed during spontaneous atresia. The steroid profiles demonstrate a fall in estrogen as the primary steroidogenic effect, attributable to a shutdown in thecal androgen secretion. The same changes prevail in the normal preovulatory period of rat and hamster (for references, see ref. 423). In contrast, comparable to the changes during atresia, in the proestrous ewe the abrupt fall in serum levels of estradiol are not associated with concomitant declines in androgens (424). Species differences may therefore exist in the hormonal basis of estrogen withdrawal.

A charge frequently leveled against models of atresia is that they may not accurately reflect events in normal, spontaneous atresia. However, excellent agreement exists between the morphologic and hormonal changes encountered during induced and spontaneous atresia. In a recent study, the experimental design consisted of dissecting the ten largest follicles from one ovary of intact cyclic hamsters for each day of the cycle (425). The follicles were incubated for a baseline 1 hour period followed by the addition of LH for another hour. The media were saved for determinations of steroids and the follicles then prepared for histology to assess whether they were healthy or atretic. Follicles with the earliest histologic signs of atresia have steroid profiles comparable to healthy follicles and normal vascularity, judged by the number of red blood cells present in thecal capillaries. When approximately one-third to one-half of the membrana granulosa cells are pyknotic and degenerating, a concurrent fall in *both* androstenedione and estradiol accumulation is apparent in the baseline and LH-stimulated incubations. Thecal vascularity is then also drastically reduced.

All of the aforementioned models of atresia have dealt with polytocous species. A model for inducing atresia in rhesus monkeys is based on exposure to elevated levels of estradiol-17β in Silastic implants for 24 h (426). After treatment at day 5, the contents of the single dominant follicle are aspirated on day 10. Follicular fluid concentrations of estrogen and progesterone were reduced three- and seven-fold, respectively, from control follicles. In light of the previous discussion on spontaneous atresia in the human, it would have been worthwhile to also measure androgens. The viability of granulosa cells has already diminished in the estrogen-treated follicles, but treatment with human FSH restored progesterone to control levels. At the end of 3 days of culture, the percentage of granulosa cells binding [^{125}I]hFSH did not differ between control and treated animals. Atresia was also induced in the dominant day 6 follicle of rhesus monkeys by subcutaneous administration of estradiol for 24 h (426). This resulted on day 10 in reduced viability of granulosa cells in the treated follicle and a sevenfold fall in follicular fluid estrogen and a concomitant threefold fall in progesterone. These findings obviously did not rule out a central site of estrogen to decrease FSH secretion. To rule out this possibility, 100 μg of estradiol was injected into the ovary (again on day 6) in the vicinity of the dominant follicle (427). There was a transitory increase in serum estradiol 6 h later but no changes in FSH or LH levels. A subsequent study in which estradiol was again administered subcutaneously for 24 h revealed that follicular fluid concentration of both estrogen and progesterone were drastically reduced within 24 h (428). Another protocol involved subcutaneous injection of estradiol plus various gonadotropin preparations rich in FSH for 2 to 4 days (429). In most instances, the combined treatment failed to reverse the atretogenic effects of exogenous estrogen. These studies suggest a direct effect of estrogen on the ovary. On the other hand, elevating normal serum estradiol from 60 to 90 ng/ml (with Silastic implants containing estradiol) is sufficient to lower FSH and lengthen the follicular phase of rhesus monkeys by about 5 days (430). Evidently, this treatment only temporarily affected the dominant follicle but did not induce atresia as evidenced by the short delay to ovulation. A mathematical model has been proposed to account for follicular selection in the mammalian ovary (431) and has been applied to the primate ovary, based on the studies of Zeleznik and Dierschke (432).

FOLLICULAR DEVELOPMENT AND SUPEROVULATION

An experimental increase in ovulation rate is an important procedure in analyzing follicular regulation in laboratory species, farm animals, and humans for *in vitro* fertilization programs. For our purposes, superovulation is defined as an approximate doubling in the normal ovulation rate (see ref. 433 for a recent review). Table 4 lists the various methods that have been used, all of which act by affecting either exogenous or endogenous levels of gonadotropins. Three mechanisms of actions have been suggested for the effects of gonadotropins on follicular development: (1) follicles already undergoing early atresia are "rescued," presumably as a result of vigorous mitotic activity in granulosa and/or thecal compartments; (2) smaller healthy follicles are recruited into a more active growth phase; (3) the rate of follicular atresia is reduced. The last two mechanisms are not mutually exclusive and indeed are the most likely combination accounting for superovulation.

Pregnant mare serum (PMS), since its isolation some 50 years ago, has been the most extensively utilized gonadotropin for inducing superovulation in laboratory and large domestic species (434). This unique molecule is structurally akin to hCG (435) and functions almost exclusively as an LH-like hormone in the mare and stallion (436,437). In other species, however, PMS serves in a dual capacity as an FSH and LH molecule (436–439). In one study using radioreceptor assays for FSH and LH the molar ratio of FSH:LH was 0.20 in the pig, 0.25 in rat tissue, and 0.0 in the horse (439). Rat, cow, and pig gonadal tissues bind as much labeled PMS as LH on a molar basis, whereas equine tissues bind only under 4% as much PMS as LH (436). For this reason, several authors have substituted "equine chorionic gonadotropin" for PMS.

The FSH:LH bioactivity ratio of PMS is almost impossible to evaluate because of the various endpoints that have been used in various studies. Equine pituitary LH also has significant FSH activity in rats and pigs (437,439). Two other features of PMS contribute to its efficacy in stimulating follicular growth: its long half-life, attributable to its high sialic acid content (435), and its ability to increase P-450$_{SCC}$, cholesterol esterase activity, and "cytochrome P-450" when injected into immature rats (440), and therefore overall increased steroidogenesis in rabbits (441), hamsters (442) and in other species.

TABLE 4. *Methods of inducing superovulation*

1. Administration of pregnant mare serum (domestic species; laboratory rodents)
2. Effects of follicle-stimulating hormone and luteinizing hormone
3. Active immunization with steroids (sheep)
4. Passive immunization with steroid antisera (sheep)
5. Bovine follicular fluid (sheep)
6. Pulsatile administration of gonadotropin-releasing hormone
7. Clomiphene citrate, human menopausal gonadotropin (human)
8. Effects of anti-luteinizing hormone

At the same time, in large domestic species increased steroid levels in response to PMS can be detrimental by disturbing the hypothalamic-pituitary axis.

The effects of PMS on follicular development have been established for several species. Administration of PMS on days 2 or 3 of the ovine cycle results in the formation of numerous large follicular cysts (>20 mm), which ultimately become luteinized without ovulating (443). If, however, PMS is injected on days 5–7, an average of 7.3 luteinized follicles with stigmata (indicative of ovulation) are present 9 to 10 days later and concomitantly the number of cystic follicles is reduced. For a number of species, including sheep, the follicular population of the two ovaries of one animal show considerably less variation than between animal variations (sheep: 444; hamsters: 445; heifers: 446), and a number of studies have taken advantage of this feature in their experimental design. In one investigation, sheep were either ovariectomized on day 12 of the cycle (controls) or injected with PMS and the other ovary removed 24 or 40 h later (447). In the control group, 74% of the follicles were between 2 and 2.9 mm in diameter and 7% were between 3 and 3.9 mm. At 24 h after PMS, only 50% of the follicles were in the smallest size category and 24% were now in the 2–2.9 mm range. Moreover, between 24 and 48 h after PMS, the number of healthy follicles >2 mm was substantially increased but with no change in the number of atretic follicles. The conclusion was that either recruitment and/or reduced atresia account for the greater number of large follicles after PMS. A recent study synchronized the cycles of Merino ewes by insertion of progesterone-impregnated vaginal sponges, which were removed 14 days after insertion (448). A day before sponge removal, laparotomies were performed, the three largest follicles in each ovary marked and PMS injected. At a second laparotomy, 24 h after PMS treatment, follicles that were less than 3 mm at the first laparotomy were recruited into the PMS group and by a third laparotomy (49–38 h after sponge removal), still more smaller "new" follicles were additionally recruited, especially among animals treated with 1,500 versus 750 IU PMS. Thus, recruitment of small follicles and sustained growth of larger follicles accounts for superovulation.

Similar conclusions were reached for heifers that were unilaterally ovariectomized on day 7, immediately injected with PMS and the remaining ovary removed 148 ± 23 h later—after the onset of the preovulatory surge of LH (446). Follicles larger than 70 μm were counted and assessed for normality or early to late atresia. An antral cavity began to form between 115 and 280 μm. Unilateral ovariectomy alone did not affect the number of normal preantral or antral follicles or the number of atretic follicles. After PMS, the remaining ovary significantly increased the number of preantral follicles and follicles with incipient formation of an antral cavity; the number of antral follicles was not affected. For the first two categories of follicles, PMS approximately doubled the mitotic index without changing that for normal or early atretic antral follicles. PMS treatment delayed the formation of an antrum for follicles less than 0.5 mm. After PMS, follicles larger than 5 mm contained significantly lower numbers of granulosa cells than control ovaries, suggesting that the antrum was correspondingly larger in the former group. The authors believe that some follicles were "rescued" from early atresia because abundant pyknotic cells were sometimes present in fresh corpora lutea and especially in luteinized follicles. The above findings on increased numbers of preantral and early antral follicles after PMS lends more credence to recruitment and reduced atresia as the factors responsible for increased numbers of healthy follicles. Similar conclusions were reached in another study where four cows were injected with PMS, and 48 h later, the entire antral population of follicles (>3 mm) was analyzed (449). In the PMS-treated animals, 70% of the follicles were healthy or very early atretic compared to 35% in the untreated controls. For the category of healthy follicles, the percentages were 38.4% and 16.2%, respectively. Repeated superovulations in cows induced by PMS did not affect the ovulation rate or viable embryos recovered (449), and similar results have been obtained in the hamster (450). Hence antibody formation to repeated exposure to PMS is not a problem. The ovulatory response in PMS-treated cows is enhanced by injection of PMS antiserum on the day of standing heat (451). The number of corpora lutea increased to 15.7 compared to 9.4 in PMS-treated controls and the number of large unruptured follicles decreased from 6.5 to 2.8.

Human menopausal gonadotropin (hMG) is frequently administered to increase ovulation rate in the human female (452). A single injection of hMG was administered at different days of the menstrual cycle and 4 to 5 days later ovaries were removed or wedge resections performed. Follicular histology was evaluated by examining all follicles ≥2 mm. The results indicate that injection of hMG in the early follicular stage led to an almost threefold increase in mitotic index, whereas treatment at later times, such as late follicular, did not alter granulosal cell mitotic index. We believe that hMG in the early follicular phase does not significantly increase the percentage of healthy follicles even though there were about 12% more healthy follicles in the stimulated cycle. It is postulated that hMG acts by accelerating follicular development so that the normal 15 days required for maturation is shortened to 10 days.

The hamster is the rodent species par excellence for evaluating the effects of PMS on ovulation and follicular development (453). This stems from the precision of the 4-day cycle and the ease with which spontaneous superovulation can be induced, contrary to the rat (see below). On day 1 of the cycle (estrus), each ovary of the hamster has normally recruited 10 *developing follicles,* which are large preantral stages. In the ensuing days, the preantral follicles mature into antral stages and the number is reduced to approximately 5 per ovary between days 3 and 4 (morning of proestrus), thus accounting for the normal ovulation of about 10 ova. When a small dose of PMS (5 IU) is injected on day 1, the hamsters ovulate 20 eggs by preventing atresia of the developing follicles, normally eliminated between days 3 and 4. In the light of recent findings on the dual FSH and LH actions of PMS on the rodent ovary, one wonders whether one or both of these gonadotropin activities save the developing follicles. As higher doses of PMS are administered on day 1, a plateau of 70 ovulations is reached with 30 or 60 IU PMS resulting from the recruitment of smaller *reserve follicles*, which normally would have taken several cycles before they were large preovulatory stages. Within 24 h of the injection of 30 IU PMS, the hamster ovary contains 27 ± 4 follicles larger than 267 μm compared to 14 ± 3 follicles in controls, and the combined developing and reserve follicles are maintained for the rest of the cycle (103). In the hamster clear-cut recruitment and subsequent reduced atresia represent the follicular responses to PMS. This is further substantiated in a later investigation: as early as 4 h after PMS, preantral follicles with four to eight or more layers of granulosa cells are mobilized (these are the reserve follicles) and begin to develop antral cavities (104). This also illustrates the rapidity with which follicles in the rodent ovary can be recruited by various perturbations contrary to the large domestic species where follicular kinetics operate at a much different pace. The combined effect of the developing and reserve follicles ultimately results in a three- to four-fold increase in the number of antral follicles, and this results in enormous increases in estrogen. For example, after 30 IU PMS on day 1 of the hamster cycle, serum estradiol on the afternoon of day 3 is 929 pg/ml, which, however, does not interfere with the normal operation of the hypothalamic-pituitary axis and ovulation of an average of 63 ova at the end of a normal 4-day cycle (454).

The effects of PMS administration to the cyclic rat are quite different. After the injection of 5 IU PMS during estrus, follicular development is accelerated, and there is a prompt appearance on the same day of approximately three times as many follicles larger than 55×10^6 μm^3 than in untreated animals, but only the normal number of ova are spontaneously ovulated (102). Higher doses of PMS (10–50 IU) recruit an even greater number of healthy follicles, but there is no spontaneous ovulation, although hCG treatment on day 3 causes the ovulation of 29 to 43 ova. It is presumed that rising and excessive titers of estrogens impair the proestrous release of LH and consequently ovulation is prevented. The salient point from this study (102) is that higher doses of PMS *can* increase the rate of recruitment of follicles and reduce atresia in the cyclic rat. Injection of 7.5 IU PMS on day 24 to immature rats results 24 h later in high mitotic indices in granulosa cells of all sizes of follicles, and this is already manifested in the smallest follicles studied, which have 90 cells in the largest cross section (114). This corresponds to follicles that are about 120 μm in diameter (455), and they are therefore very small preantral stages.

In addition to PMS, ovulation and superovulation have been induced in several species with "purified" preparations of FSH. One of the earliest studies removed LH contamination from ovine FSH by immunoabsorption with an antiserum to the β subunit of ovine LH (456). Proestrous rats were injected with nembutal to block the normal gonadotropic surge and therefore prevent ovulation. The effects of pentobarbital (Nembutal) were reversed by the purified FSH preparation and the animals ovulated 12 eggs the next morning. Hypophysectomized immature rats injected with 15 IU PMS ovulate in response to either hCG or recombinant FSH (recFSH) (457). Another experiment, in the same study, substituted recFSH for PMS; following a bolus injection of hCG or recFSH, superovulation of equal magnitude occurred. In the same vein, recFSH injected for 4 days into hypophysectomized immature rats increases ovarian weight and aromatase activity but without increasing serum estradiol (458). We have used a different model: adult mice hypophysectomized for 12 days, followed by daily injection of 4 μg ovine FSH for 4 days (118). The 12-day hiatus before treatment is initiated reduces ovarian function to baseline levels such that the largest follicles present are small antral stages lacking FSH and LH/hCG receptors (117). The injection of FSH stimulated the reappearance of large preovulatory follicles in 2 days, but at the end of 4 days, estradiol in *in vitro* incubations and serum were no different than hypophysectomized controls (118). Superovulation can be induced in these animals with hCG (FH) or recFSH (FF), but *in vivo* only 5% of fertilized FH ova advance to the four-celled stage and none in the FF group (459). After *in vitro* culture for 4 days 22% of two-celled FH embryos are converted to blastocysts compared to 80% of "normal" ova (459). Thus, inadequacy of the oocyte developing in an abnormal steroidal environment in the follicle and oviduct militates against the sole use of FSH to induce antral follicle development.

A similar situation may prevail in the human female. After long-term suppression of ACTH and gonadotropins by prednisone and GnRH, a woman with a deficiency of 17α-hydroxylase was treated with "purified FSH" for 14 days, at which time three follicles greater than 15 mm were detected (460). Following administration of hCG, the follicles were aspirated. Incubation of granulosa-luteal cells revealed elevated production of progestins but a marked reduction in androgens, 17-hydroxyprogesterone, and basal estradiol. When the cells were cultured with testosterone or androstenedione, estradiol production increased but was still only one-sixth of control values. The same deficiency in androgens and estradiol existed in aspirated follicular fluid. A subsequent study with the same patient shed additional light and showed that plasma FSH and LH (before FSH treatment was initiated) were both somewhat elevated compared to normal early follicular phase levels (461). Once treatment with FSH was begun, there was about a threefold increase in plasma FSH, whereas LH was unchanged. Throughout this period, plasma estradiol was undetectable. One day after the addition of sperm to the cumulus-oocyte complexes, two pronuclei were observed in two of the ova and both reached the seven-cell stage before degenerating. In the above patient, there were still measurable levels of endogenous gonadotropins.

In women with isolated gonadotropin deficiency, a regimen of purified FSH (with less than 1% LH contamination) for 10 days sharply increased plasma FSH, whereas LH was unaffected (462). Plasma estradiol showed a delayed rise to normal preovulatory levels, but the levels were only one-third of those obtained when hMG (with combined FSH and LH activity) was administered. On the other hand, androstenedione did not change over the 10-day period. Ultrasonography revealed obvious follicular growth and injection of hCG induced ovulation in seven women treated with FSH. A similar study utilized recFSH in a patient with extremely low serum levels of FSH and LH (463). After 12 days of treatment, serum estradiol was low, comparable to early follicular phase levels. Similarly, follicular fluid concentrations of estradiol and androstenedione were miniscule compared to controls. Comparable to the rat and mouse models (see above), the lack of even baseline levels of LH leads to inadequate androstenedione production, which in turn accounts for the estrogen deficiency, but this is not incompatible with follicles attaining preovulatory size.

One of the most provocative findings is the ability of LH to induce superovulation in cyclic hamsters and guinea pigs (123). High tonic levels of the hormone are maintained in hamsters by implanting an osmotic minipump on day 1 of the cycle. When 400 μg of ovine LH was infused, approximately 32 ova were shed at the next estrus. Several experiments eliminated the possibility that FSH contamination accounted for these results. It is even more striking that hamsters hypophysectomized on day 1 and implanted with LH maintained large antral follicles through day 4. Infusion of LH into guinea pigs doubled the ovulation rate whereas similar treatment of cyclic mice and rats was ineffective. Possibly excessive levels of estrogen may be acting as a negative feedback influence in the mouse and rat. The failure of spontaneous ovulation in the PMS-treated adult rat is distinctly different from the cyclic PMS-treated hamster in which serum levels of 1,000 pg/ml on proestrus do not interfere with the hypothalamic-pituitary axis.

Daily doses of 25 IU PMS for 4 days to intact, cyclic, or hypophysectomized adult rats increase the number of preantral and antral follicles, but, interestingly, concurrent treatment with prolactin blocks the development of antral follicles (464). The latter group indicates that prolactin can interfere with folliculogenesis directly at the ovarian level as well as at the hypothalamic-pituitary axis. Hyperprolactinemia can be induced in adult rats by transplantation of two donor pituitaries to the kidney capsule of adult pseudopregnant rats (465). Incubation of small antral follicles, with or without hCG, revealed significantly less accumulation of estradiol compared to diestrous control follicles. However, in the presence of testosterone, estradiol accumulation was restored to normal levels in the hyperprolactinemic follicles, suggesting that the inhibitory effects of prolactin were exerted at the theca.

In contrast to the cyclic rat, extensive use has been made of the immature rat to explore the superovulatory effects of PMS. For example, it was shown 30 years ago that immature rats injected with 30 IU PMS and 56 h later with 10 IU hCG showed temporal changes in the number of eggs ovulated (101). A maximum of 55 ova were ovulated at 23 to 32 days of age falling to 18 ova at 39 or 40 days of age. A greater rate of recruitment and reduced atresia most likely account for these results. As pointed out in the section on atresia, the immature rat not injected with hCG begins to show signs of atresia as early as 72 h after PMS.

The PMS-immature rat model has been utilized extensively to produce fully differentiated antral follicles capable of responding to hCG. For example, ovarian aromatase activity increases 12-fold after a single injection of 20 IU PMS (466). After injecting 10 IU PMS, maximal levels of FSH receptor mRNA and FSH binding are found at 52 h (467). Immature rats injected with 8 IU PMS spontaneously ovulate 12 eggs at 72 h (468), but concurrent treatment with DHT halves the number of ovulations and increases the number of atretic follicles. It is interesting that the deleterious effects of DHT are reversible by simultaneous injection of estradiol. DHT treatment reduces follicular content of estradiol in follicles larger than 200 μm, and this is associated with reduced aromatase activity in harvested granulosa cells.

Continuous infusion of LH increases blood flow to the hamster ovary on day 3 and induces a depletion of ovarian histamine (469). Injection of an antihistamine reduces the number of ova shed in LH implanted hamsters but not in controls. It is possible that increased ovarian blood flow may enhance delivery of FSH to the ovary, which seems necessary as a synergist for LH induced superovulation. In the hamster, thousands of mast cells are located in the hilum of the ovary surrounding blood vessels that enter and exit from the ovary (470). Since the LH surge on proestrus causes mast cell degranulation in the hamster (470) and LH causes ovarian histamine discharge (469,471,472), it seems plausible that mast cells and histamine are mediators in part of LH-induced superovulation in the hamster. Indeed, antihistamines block ovulation in several species by preventing follicular rupture (473–475). Several questions arise from this section: What factors are involved in LH-induced increase in ovarian blood flow? Do PMS and FSH induce ovulation by the same mechanism(s)? Are mast cells essential for LH-induced superovulation?

Other methods to induce superovulation rely upon the experimental manipulation of endogenous gonadotropin levels (Table 4). Active immunization of female sheep against estrogens increases basal levels of LH and FSH and increases pulsatile LH release to levels encountered in ovariectomized animals (see references in ref. 476). The ovulation rate is increased to 3 versus 1.5 by this treatment. Active immunization against androstenedione increases ovulation rate from 1.50 ± .25 to 2.00 ± 0 and the number of surface follicles larger than 3 mm in diameter is 1 and 3, respectively (477). It is proposed that active immunization against steroids increases the ovulation rate by disrupting the normal negative feedback effects of estradiol and/or by a reduction in follicular atresia. A variation on this technique is by passive immunization with antisera to steroids given as a single intravenous injection on the first day of estrus (478). Controls ovulate 1.3 ova compared to 2.1 ova after administration of the estradiol antisera, and the mean number of lambs born alive was 1.3 versus 1; this was attributable to a higher incidence of twinning in the group treated with the antisera. A mixture of antisera to estradiol, estrone, androstenedione, and testosterone was the most efficacious, increasing the ovulation rate to 2.1 and the lambing rate to 1.5.

The intravenous injection of bovine follicular fluid to ewes from days 1–11 of the cycle increased the ovulation rate to 3.4 ± 0.3 from 2.3 ± 0.3 in controls (479). The treatment significantly lowered FSH levels over the first 7 days and thereafter FSH returned to control values. Throughout the luteal phase, daily LH concentrations and pulse frequency and amplitude were significantly increased in the treated group. With the onset of induced luteolysis, the ewes injected with follicular fluid showed fourfold greater levels of FSH and about a twofold increase in LH compared to controls. The authors point out that the treatment prevented the postestrous surge of FSH and that the hypersecretion of FSH at the onset of the follicular phase therefore presumably accounts for the increased ovulation rate. However, since the onset of estrus was significantly delayed (89 vs 41 h), the return to control levels of FSH on day 8 and thereafter may constitute the time when "privileged follicles" may have been exposed to amounts of FSH required for their ultimate selection after luteal regression.

Another approach is to immunize sheep with a purified α subunit of inhibin with the expectation that the antisera generated would neutralize inhibin and thus increase circulating FSH (480). The immunized animals ovulated threefold more ova than controls. Injecting prepubertal rats with an antiserum to inhibin increases serum FSH concentrations within 8 h and doubles the ovulation rate at first estrus (481). A single injection of inhibin antiserum to 5-day cyclic rats on diestrus 1 results 8 h later in an increase in FSH, which is sustained for 48 h (482). This is associated at 48 h with a significant increase in the number of follicles larger than 260 μm and a less impressive (albeit significant) decrease in atretic follicles. Deferring the treatment to diestrus 2 almost doubles the ovulation rate. Again, the critical importance of FSH in follicular recruitment is evident. Indeed, exogenous FSH has been used extensively to induce superovulation in a variety of species.

The pulsatile infusion of GnRH using Alza osmotic minipumps has been used to increase ovulation rate and estrus in zoo maintained animals (483). The advantages are that synthetic GnRH seems to be universally capable of stimulating the species' own FSH and LH; consequently, physiologic stimulation of the ovaries is simulated and "natural" mating behavior is elicited.

Various regimens have been used to induce superovulation in the human (484), including clomiphene citrate followed by hCG, clomiphene plus human menopausal gonadotropin followed by hCG, and human menopausal gonadotropin followed by hCG. There is still room for improvement in the methodology. A new approach has been the intravenous infusion of pulsatile LH-RH or FSH with a controlled LH surge, similar to the system described for zoo-maintained species. A detailed consideration of superovulation in the human is beyond the scope of this chapter.

A chance discovery led to the surprising finding that a potent equine antiserum to bovine LH (anti-LH) is able to induce superovulation in several species. A single injection of anti-LH interrupted pregnancy in the hamster or rat and at subsequent estrus, the hamster superovulated 29 ova, whereas the rat ovulated the normal number of 13 eggs (485). Cyclic hamsters injected SC with 100 μl anti-LH at estrus (day 1) spontaneously ovulated 31.5 eggs after a cycle lengthened to 5 days from the normal 4-day duration (486). The major effect of the anti-LH was to induce atresia of the larger preantral follicles by day 2 followed by a rebound in follicular recruitment by the next day so that a greater than normal number of antral and intermediate follicles repopulated the ovaries. Quite distinct from the superovulatory effects of PMS, with anti-LH, serum levels of estradiol throughout the cycle are within the normal limits of control animals; hence aromatase activity is not increased. The anti-LH was only effective in inducing superovulation in the cyclic hamster when it was administered on estrus or proestrus; that is, at times when serum levels of FSH are normally elevated. After removal of the interfering LH antibodies from serum by Sephadex G-200 chromatography, radioimmunoassays for FSH and LH revealed normal levels of FSH throughout the cycle but LH levels were undetectable on day 2 and in most hamsters on day 3 (487). We had anticipated that anti-LH treatment would elicit a castration response and consequent hypersecretion of FSH and LH; indeed, the possibility cannot be discounted that more frequent samples between days 2 and 3 might detect a rebound release of elevated levels of FSH and/or LH. However, if the results are taken at face value, the sustained secretion of progesterone for 2 days by the autonomous corpora lutea might act as a sufficient negative feedback influence to prevent hypersecretion of gonadotropins. Our hypothesis on the mechanism of anti-LH's ability to induce superovulation in the hamster is that by temporarily eliminating LH action on the ovary, a "pure" FSH effect is manifested, thus increasing its mitogenic properties on granulosa cells (see ref. 487 for pertinent references on FSH:LH ratios). Several recent papers also point to altered FSH:LH ratios affecting follicular development, with higher amounts of LH reducing the mitogenic action of FSH. Thus, administration to immature rats of PMS with different FSH:LH ratios, followed by an ovulating dose of hCG, shows reduced ovulation rates at lower ratios (438). Similarly, immature rats with miniosmotic pumps delivering 240 μg porcine FSH/day ovulated 69 ± 10 eggs. When FSH was held constant and increasing amounts of LH concurrently infused, ovulation rate progressively declined (488). On the other hand, *hypophysectomized* proestrous hamsters injected daily with 5 μg/day ovine FSH plus 5, 10, or 20 μg LH did not reduce the number of follicles maturing or ovulating in response to hCG (489).

The ability of anti-LH to induce superovulation in the cyclic hamster is restricted to its first administration; a second injection—even 3 months later—results in the ovulation of only six ova at the end of a 4-day cycle (450). Injection of normal horse serum at estrus followed 14 days later by anti-LH results in the ovulation of only 18 ova. Evidently, after the initial exposure, the hamster rapidly forms antibodies to equine immunoglobulins. Injection of guinea pigs on day 12 of the cycle with 0.8 ml anti-LH prolonged the estrous cycle by 3 days and increased the ovulation rate from 2.9 to 5.6 ova (490). To our knowledge this treatment is the only one that has increased ovulation rate in the guinea pig other than the continuous infusion of LH (123). Equine anti-bovine LH injected on day 10 of the cycle also increases the number of ova shed in cyclic ewes from 2.1 ± 0.1 in control animals to 2.7 ± 0.2 and with estrus delayed by 0.6 days (491). It has likewise been successful in increasing the ovulation rate in pregnant mice injected with anti-LH on day 4; on day 8 the animals (from a control line) ovulated 16 eggs compared to a normal ovulation rate of 8.8 at estrus. A high-ovulating strain, which normally ovulates 16 eggs, ovulated 30 eggs when similarly treated (M. Barkley and G. Greenwald, unpublished observations). However, anti-LH does not increase the ovulation rate of pregnant (485) or cyclic rats (P. Terranova and G. Greenwald, unpublished observations). This intriguing model deserves further study.

Still another way to increase the ovulation rate is by selective breeding for large litter size in mice which increases the ovulation rate from 10.3 eggs (c strain) to 17.4 ova (SI strain) (492). A kinetic analysis of follicular development between the two strains shows some interesting differences. The SI strain decreased the incidence of atresia in large preovulatory follicles; there was a highly significant increase at proestrus in almost all classes of follicles and a faster transit time from one stage to another. It was estimated that the time required from primordial follicle recruitment to graafian follicle formation was reduced from 39.1 days in the c strain to 33.4 in the SI strain (492). Highly inbred mouse strains were injected at day 28 with 5 IU PMS and 5 IU hCG 48 h later (493). There was an enormous spread of ovulation rates varying from 8.8 to 53.5. Analysis of parental and F_1 and F_2 generations showed that the variation was attributable to three or four loci. A subsequent study (494) showed that the genetic differences in hormone-induced ovulation is not due to differences in the time of puberty and persists in adult mice. FSH is as effective as PMS and, significantly, injection of hCG—without PMS priming—did not show strain differences in ovulation rate. This suggests that differences in endogenous gonadotropins in the prepubertal mice are most likely not involved. A summary of these interesting studies is now available (495) and links the strain differences in ovulation to the H2 locus on chromosome 17 as well as two or three loci independent of H2. To our knowledge, steroid and peptide hormones (as well as growth factors) have not been measured in any of the mouse studies.

The homozygous Booroola Merino sheep (FF) ovulates more than five ova; the F+ (heterozygous) ovulates 2.8 eggs and noncarrier ewes (++) ovulate 1.2 ova (496). The only consistent correlation is that the FF ewes have significantly higher levels of FSH and LH compared to noncarriers with F+ having intermediate values. On the other hand, ovarian secretion rates of progesterone, androstenedione, and estradiol do not differ among the three genotypes. Consistent with chronic exposure to higher levels of gonadotropins, follicles in FF and F+ animals mature at smaller diameters than noncarrier ewes: approximately 3 mm, 4 mm, and 5 mm, respectively.

EFFECTS OF UNILATERAL OVARIECTOMY ON FOLLICULAR DEVELOPMENT

Unilateral ovariectomy (ULO) is a time honored procedure which has been useful in elucidating follicular kinetics in species as disparate as pigs, chickens, *Drosophila* (for references, see ref. 497), geckos (498), and the California leaf-nosed bat (499). The latter species normally always ovulates from the right ovary, but following its removal the left ovary takes over.

The effects of ULO in mammals can be analyzed in terms of compensatory hypertrophy of the contralateral ovary (i.e., increased weight) representing persistence of increased numbers of corpora lutea (e.g., the rat) as well as enhanced follicular activity. For our purposes, the effects of ULO on follicular development within the cycle in which the procedure was performed is a more meaningful endpoint, providing information on how late in the cycle successful follicular recruitment and hence increased ovulation rate can be elicited. This can be contrasted with the long term effects of ULO on follicular compensation, which involve different adjustments in pituitary-ovarian function.

The first experiment involving ULO dates back to an often-quoted study of John Hunter (500), who followed the farrowing records of two sows, one of which had been semispayed. Over the first 8 litters, the intact sow produced 87 young compared to 76 for the semispayed sow, but thereafter the control animal delivered 5 more litters consisting of 75 young. A pioneering study of Arai (501) established ovarian compensation in the rat after ULO and demonstrated that the surviving ovary had about twice as many corpora lutea and a greater number of mature follicles than in the intact animal. Working with the rabbit, Lipschutz (502) proposed that ovarian hypertrophy, following ULO, was caused by increased follicular development dependent on some "general body factor." He proposed one of the basic tenets of follicular selection, the law of follicular constancy: "The number of ova entering into follicular development, the rhythm of follicular development, and the degree attained by follicular development are constant and are controlled by somatic factors outside the ovary. Ovarian hypertrophy means those integrative processes that take place in the ovarian fragment after partial castration, which are not to be characterized by the increase in weight but only by those processes dictated by the "law of follicular constancy" (502).

Short-Term Effects of Unilateral Ovariectomy

The first species in which the immediate effects of unilateral ovariectomy (ULO) on compensatory ovulation were established was the hamster (445). Removal of one ovary at 9 A.M. for the first 3 days of the 4-day estrous cycle was followed by doubling in the number of ovulations from the remaining ovary. It was initially believed that a reduction in atresia of larger follicles between days 3 and 4 spared follicles and therefore resulted in compensatory ovulation (445). Recently, however, it was shown that ULO on day 3 within 4 h mobilizes preantral follicles with 6 or 7 layers of granulosa cells and converts them into small antral follicles (503). This puts the hamster in line with other species (see below) and also points to the rapidity with which follicles can respond in species with short estrous cycles.

Compensatory ovulation in cyclic rats, after ULO, depends on the length of the estrous cycle: In rats with 4-day cycles, ULO as late as day 3 results in doubling the number of ovulations from the remaining ovary. Slightly more leeway exists in rats with 5-day cycles where removal of one ovary as late as 2 A.M. of diestrus 2 results in follicular compensation (504). Increased proliferation of smaller follicles results in doubling the number of large follicles following ULO and consequently maintains the normal ovulation rate characteristic of the rat (505). After ULO of 4-day cyclic rats at 5 P.M. or 8 P.M. of diestrus, compensatory ovulation does not occur, although a surge in FSH begins 6 h later (506). However, if a day is added to the cycle by treatment with pentobarbital on proestrus, the animals *do* compensate by reduced follicular atresia as well as recruitment of smaller follicles.

A very detailed analysis of the effects of ULO on diestrus 1 on temporal changes in hormone levels in the cyclic rat is now available (507). Within 12 h, plasma FSH dramatically increases with no change observed in LH. By 24 h after ULO, injection of hCG almost doubles the ovulation rate of the remaining ovary. Ovarian venous plasma at 2 h showed a twofold increase in inhibin activity and abrupt increases in estradiol, testosterone, and progesterone.

Mice unilaterally ovariectomized at random times during the cycle, invariably double the number of ova shed within 3 days after the procedure (508). As an induced ovulator, the rabbit's response to ULO is of interest. Within 48 h of ULO, the number of approximately 1-mm follicles increase two- to three-fold in the remaining ovary, and injection of hCG 4 days later results in ovulation of 11.4 ova (509). Rabbits were unilaterally ovariectomized and on day 11 the remaining ovary and blood supply were removed *en bloc* and *in vitro* steroidogenesis measured (510). After ULO, compared to control animals estradiol and progesterone secretion increased, luteal weight increased, but there was no increase in luteal cell numbers. However, there was a significant increase in vessel space and endothelial cell volume in the ULO group. In contrast, following unilateral luteectomy (with the treated ovary left *in situ*) progesterone but not estradiol production was increased in the contralateral ovary and the number of luteal cells increased significantly.

What are the effects of ULO in species with long estrous cycles? The guinea pig can compensate as late as day 10 of the cycle by doubling the ovulation rate from the remaining ovary, and an increased rate of transformation of smaller sized follicles into larger ones accounts for the results (511). In contrast, ULO of Finn-Dorset sheep on day 2, 8, or 14 does not affect the number of ova shed (measured by number of corpora lutea) at the very next estrus (512). On the other hand, unilateral ovariectomy of Leicester-Merino ewes at day 14 results by the next cycle in compensatory ovulation (ULO: 2 corpora lutea; intact: 1.70) but is only partially effective when hemicastration is deferred to day 16 (513). In a breed of sheep with high ovulation rate (2.4 corpora lutea), ULO on day 10 of the cycle results in an overall ovulation of 2.2 from the remaining ovary (131). Four days after ULO, there is no significant increase in any size range of preantral follicles and antral follicles (131).

Unilateral ovariectomy on day 2 of the porcine estrous cycle results by day 13 in a compensatory increase in the number of large follicles (5–12.9 mm in diameter) (514). Sows unilaterally ovariectomized on day 2 of the estrous cycle ovulate as many ova at the next estrus as intact animals: 18.1 and 16.0 corpora lutea, respectively (515). There are obvious species differences between the sow and the ewe. The ewe after ULO ultimately does increase its ovulation rate per ovary, but the 2-year lamb production is significantly lower than that of intact ewe: 1.35 versus 1.61 (516). Evidently, follicles cannot be recruited as readily in the ewe as in other species. In contrast, within 6 h after ULO on day 3 of the hamster cycle, there is already a depletion of 66% of Stage 4 follicles (with 4 layers of granulosa cells) into Stage 5 (5-layered follicles) (269). Moreover, by 6 h after ULO, incubation of follicles with [^{3}H]thymidine shows a significantly lower rate of incorporation than comparable follicles from intact animals (517).

What are the effects of ULO on species which are normally monovular? In the cow, ULO on day 8 of the cycle results by the next estrus in a redistribution of follicular size with greater representation in the 9- to 16-mm class than in controls. However, in the one ovary group, the largest follicle is smaller than in the control, but the next largest follicle in the ULO group is consistently larger (518). Saidudden and colleagues (518) raise the interesting question of whether the potential for twin ovulation is enhanced in the ULO group, but to our knowledge this possibility has never been tested. Unilateral ovariectomy of the heifer results 7 days later in a significant increase in the number of follicles 5 or 6 mm and >9 mm in diameter; this increase can be blocked by daily injection of bovine follicular fluid (519).

Rhesus monkeys hemicastrated for 3 months show ovarian hypertrophy of the remaining ovary and histologically numerous "large follicles and corpora lutea in various stages of development" (520). Hemiovariectomized cynomolgus monkeys have more ovulatory cycles per 13 months than the intact group: 9.8 versus 5.8 and in 49% of cycles serum progesterone was greater than 9 ng/ml, whereas these levels were reached in only 26% of the intact group (521). Ovulation was verified by laparoscopy on days 11 and 21 of each cycle and evidently there was no increase in ovulation rate, which would surely have been noted. The ability of the primate ovary to restore normal function after massive extirpation is remarkable. For example, removal of one ovary and 90% of the other ovary from cynomolgus monkeys on days 2 to 4 leads to elevated levels of FSH and LH over the next 11 days, culminating in a preovulatory gonadotropin surge on 20 ± 3 days (522). This is followed by normal serum progesterone levels indicative of ovulation. Another group of animals were subjected to the same procedures and the majority of animals maintained 28 day cycles for 5 months to a year. These results are different from the effects of equally heroic surgery of the cyclic rat where after removal of $1\frac{1}{2}$ ovaries, there is no short-term or long-term compensatory ovulation (523).

As expected, there is even more of a dearth of information about the effects of ULO in the human female. The only concrete evidence, albeit incomplete, is provided in a study by Speert and colleagues (524), consisting of a series of 16 patients who required a second laparotomy within 2 years after removal of one ovary for complications of tubal pregnancy. In six patients the ovary was enlarged because of luteal or follicular cysts, but the remaining ovary appeared normal in the other patients. A long-term unilaterally ovariectomized woman had only one corpus luteum in the remaining ovary (525). The availability of sonographic techniques to visualize temporal changes in large follicles now makes it feasible to explore the long-term effects of ULO in primates.

It is apparent from the literature discussed so far, that compensatory follicular development (and therefore, ultimately, maintenance of the number of ovulations characteristic of the species) depends on rapid recruitment of small follicles as an acute response to ULO. What hormonal changes account for such a prompt response? Before the advent of radioimmunoassays, one proposal was that ULO resulted in no increase in pituitary gonadotropins but rather a "sparing effect" so that the amount normally available to two ovaries now exerted its actions on the remaining ovary. What is now established beyond doubt is that the acute effect of ULO or ablation of the dominant follicle is manifested in a sharp transient increase in serum levels of FSH with variable and less striking changes in LH. This has now been observed in the hamster (526), rat (for references, see ref. 527), rabbit (509), gilt (528), cow (519), ewe (513), and human (529). The increase in FSH, after ULO, is analogous to the periovulatory increase, which occurs in most mammals and is believed to recruit the next cohort of follicles. In the immediate period following ULO there is no change in serum levels of estradiol in the hamster (530) or rat (527). Hence removal of negative steroid feedback does not seem to be the major factor accounting for the transient increase in FSH. In rats, hemicastrated on diestrus

2—when antral follicles are present—the effects of ULO are reversed by administration of inhibin, suggesting that this may be the key ingredient removed by semispaying (527). Similarly, compensatory ovarian hypertrophy is prevented in unilaterally ovariectomized gilts by daily treatment with porcine follicular fluid (528). Redmer and coworkers (528) caution that their results do not rule out a direct inhibitory effect on follicular growth, although serum FSH was significantly increased in semispayed gilts injected with porcine serum.

At various times, it has been suggested that ovarian nerves play a role in compensatory follicular development, but ovarian sympathectomy by injecting 6-hydroxydopamine into an artifically closed ovarian bursa fails to prevent increased follicular numbers after ULO of the contralateral ovary (reviewed in ref. 531).

Long-Term Effects of Unilateral Ovariectomy

Following ULO of the cyclic hamster, compensatory ovulation occurs in the next 14 cycles without deviating from the normally rigid 4-day cycle (532). The hemicastrated rat, on the other hand, compensates completely for only 10 cycles and thereafter ovulates seven to nine ova from the remaining ovary. Comparable results for the rat were obtained by Peppler (533), who observed that rats hemiovariectomized for 3 months shed 10.9 ova from the remaining ovary, whereas by 6 months only 4.9 ova were ovulated. In long-term hemicastrated rats (3 months), the remaining ovary when examined at metestrus contained a similar number of follicles (>357 μm) than in intact animals (533), which suggests that follicular selection took place later in the cycle. In rats hemicastrated for 20 to 30 days, by metestrus, the total number of large antral follicles (>400 μm) was the same in ULO and intact rats, and it appears that this was accomplished by a significant reduction in atresia of follicles in the 350 to 399 μm category (534). A subsequent paper by Hirshfield (535) explored the problem in greater detail. In semispayed rats, follicles >450 μm are twice as numerous on proestrus than in intact rats, thus accounting for compensatory ovulation. By metestrus and diestrus there are already twice as many follicles in the semispayed group and this was associated with decreased atresia. Compensatory growth in the regenerating liver is associated with increased expression of several protooncogenes, such as c-*myc* and c-*fos* (536). However, in ULO rats, 3 and 14 days later—although compensatory ovarian weight occurs—there is no change in protooncogene expression. Alvarez and coworkers (536) suggest that compensatory ovarian hypertrophy involves a pathway different from the hyperplastic changes in regenerating liver.

At 70 days after unilateral ovariectomy of sheep, there is a significant increase in the number of small preantral follicles (<0.06 to 0.07 mm in diameter) and antral follicles, especially in the range of 2.0 to 3.6 mm (131). Again, this indicates the sluggish responsiveness of sheep follicles to ULO, but it must be realized that the increase in number of follicles may occur considerably earlier than the third or fourth cycle.

What hormonal patterns can account for follicular compensation in the long-term hemicastrate? For both the rat (537) and hamster (526) the second surge of FSH, which is normally restricted to estrus, is extended into the second day of the cycle, and this appears to be the signal that recruits additional follicles (300–450 μm in the rat) into the ovulatory range.

It is beyond the scope of this chapter to consider the effects of ULO on truly long-term reproductive performance. The primary studies were carried out by Zuckerman and his associates in rats (reviewed in ref. 538). When retired breeder rats (>1 year of age) were unilaterally ovariectomized for 90 days, the number of primordial follicles was about halved from the number present in one ovary of sham-operated controls (539). The ULO rats had increased plasma FSH and decreased LH compared to sham-operated animals. In ULO rats (surgery on day 50), the first time that reduced numbers of primordial follicles were found was at 250 days of age, and this again correlated with elevated levels of FSH. It appears likely that the greater concentration of FSH may accelerate the rate of entry of primordial follicles into the growing phase, although this cannot be proven by the distribution of healthy follicles. At 250 days there were significantly fewer unilaminar follicles in the ULO animals. A recent study shows that Stage I follicles (one layer of flattened granulosa cells) which constitute the "follicular pool" are significantly reduced by 4 weeks in hemicastrated mice, but the number of growing follicles is maintained or even increased (538). There is no difference in the percentage of oocytes undergoing atresia between semispayed and control mice for any stage of follicular development, but the stage of the estrous cycle when the animals were killed was not taken into account.

Proestrous mice were unilaterally ovariectomized or sham operated at 41–45 days old and killed 40–50 days later and the number of preantral follicles determined (540). The analysis revealed that many more small unilaminar and bilaminar follicles were dying than normal, whereas the number of the largest preantral follicles were similar to animals with two ovaries. Most atresia was observed in antral follicles in the controls and the incidence was halved by ULO, accounting for the greater ovulation rate.

Long-term effects of ULO have also been evaluated in gilts (541). Over four consecutive cycles, estrous cycle length was unaltered from controls and laparoscopy revealed approximate doubling of the ovulation rate. The most significant evidence of compensation was a doubling of follicles larger than 3.5 mm, associated with increased estrogen in ovarian venous effluent and greater concentrations of progesterone and estrogen in follicular fluid. Removal of one ovary from prepubertal gilts leads to a rapid increase in serum FSH but not LH—during the first 24 h compared to sham-operated animals (542). There is a transient increase in inhibin in ovarian venous serum on days 2 and 4 following ULO with levels returning to baseline on day 8 (543). The increased inhibin may act to inhibit sustained levels of serum FSH.

The overall impression from both the short-term and long-term effects of ULO is that FSH is essential for either increased follicular recruitment and/or reduced atresia. Whether FSH is acting through the now classical cyclic nucleotide pathways has not been established for any of the experimental models for ULO. The one dissenting paper to the critical role of transient increments in FSH involves hypophysectomizing intact or ULO ewes, treated with PMS for 56 h before injecting hCG (544). Under these circumstances the ULO group had the same number of ovulations as the animals with both ovaries.

FOLLICULAR DEVELOPMENT DURING THE ESTROUS CYCLE OF RAT AND HAMSTER

The rat and hamster have been selected as representative rodent species with short cycles in which follicular events occur at a much different rate than in mammals with long cycles such as sheep and humans. Schwartz and colleagues (545) were among the first to propose that the secondary surge of FSH on estrus initiates recruitment of growing follicles in the rat and these follicles are ovulated at the next estrus (4 or 5 days later). However, other factors preceding the (secondary) FSH surge of the immediate cycle are apparently also involved in the regulation of follicle development. Kinetic studies using the mouse, hamster, and rat have shown that the large preovulatory follicles ovulating in response to the LH surge actually enter the growing pool of follicles around 20 days earlier. These follicles may have been recruited by a gonadotropin surge and were then exposed to three or four consecutive surges of gonadotropins until ovulation.

It appears that primordial follicles enter the growing pool at a constant rate regardless of the day of the mouse estrous cycle as evidenced by a similar rate of incorporation of tritiated thymidine by granulosa cells of small follicles on each day of the cycle (94). Follicles entering the growing pool on day 1 (estrus) when FSH levels are elevated may be stimulated by the gonadotropic stimulus to move into more advanced stages of development. For example, in the hamster, Stage I follicles (2–3 layers of granulosa cells) that are present on estrus progress to Stage II (4–5 layers of granulosa cells) after 8 days (546). At the next estrus (when FSH levels are elevated) these follicles migrate after an additional 8 days to the next stage of development (Stage III, 6–7 layers of granulosa cells). However, Stages III and IV follicles (8 or more layers of granulosa cells but no antrum) present on estrus may either move into the preovulatory stages within 4 days or become atretic. Thus, from Stage I to the preovulatory phase takes approximately 20 days. It is unknown how long it takes for primary follicles to be transformed into Stage I follicles in the hamster. Based on [^{3}H]-thymidine studies in the cyclic rat, follicles with one or two layers of granulosa cells (type 3b) take approximately 22 days to develop to Stage 6 (antral follicle: 200 μm in diameter) (97). If 4 days is included for the transit time through types 7 and 8 (547,548), then a total of approximately 27 days elapses from types 3b to 8.

During the 20 to 30 days of growth the follicles are exposed to four to five consecutive LH/FSH surges at recurring intervals. These surges have been shown to affect small developing follicles in the rat and hamster (549,550). In the hypophysectomized estradiol-treated immature rat, treatment with 5 IU hCG followed by 2 μg human FSH resulted in a 15-fold increase in granulosal cell LH receptors by 36 h; FSH receptor increased threefold by 48 h and antral follicular development was markedly enhanced (549). Neither FSH nor hCG alone increased the FSH and LH receptors to maximal levels. In fact, FSH followed by hCG 12 h later was unable to increase the granulosa cell FSH and LH receptors to the same magnitude as hCG followed by FSH. The major point is that hCG (in synergy with FSH) increased its own receptor in the developing antral follicles. This action of hCG is similar to that of FSH on small antral follicles. The mechanism by which hCG increases the action of FSH is unknown. Very low levels of hCG binding sites are present in the theca and granulosa cells of estradiol primed rats (206,551,552) and hCG can stimulate theca cell hypertrophy. Therefore, hCG may synergize with FSH, using a thecal cell intermediary product (549). Neither testosterone nor estradiol mimicked the concerted effect of hCG and FSH to increase hCG receptor sites (549).

The LH surge in the hamster enhances progesterone production and inhibits androstenedione production in theca of preantral follicles (550). Large preantral follicles (Stages III and IV) isolated immediately before, during, and after the LH surge on proestrus were incubated *in vitro* with LH to stimulate steroidogenesis. Before the LH surge, follicles produced 2.4 ± 0.3 ng androstenedione per follicle and very low amounts of progesterone (<250 pg) and estradiol (<100 pg). During the peak of the LH surge preantral follicles produced 1.8 ± 0.2 ng progesterone, 1.9 ± 0.1 ng androstenedione, and less than 100 pg estradiol. Immediately after the LH surge preantral follicles were unable to produce androstenedione and estradiol, but the follicles produced 8.1 ± 3.1 ng progesterone at 3 P.M. on estrus and androstenedione secretion was also restored. Thereafter, steroid secretion returned to levels similar to that observed prior to the surge. These results have their exact counterpart in the altered steroidogenic profile of large preovulatory follicles after exposure to the ovulatory surges of gonadotropins. The LH surge may therefore synchronize the onset of androstenedione and estradiol synthesis during follicular development. LH appears to inhibit FSH action on steroidogenesis immediately after the surge but synergizes with FSH at later stages of development. FSH then acts on steroidogenically synchronized follicles after recruitment into the growing population.

For most species, the steroidogenic potential of small preantral follicles during the estrous cycle is still an enigma. However, recent studies using isolated, intact preantral follicles from adult hamsters (ranging from 55 to 330 μm) have revealed that preantral follicles, including small primary follicles with a single layer of granulosa cells and no theca, are capable of producing progesterone and androstenedione *in vitro* when challenged with FSH (127). However, de novo estrogen production is only evident for follicles with five or six layers of granulosa cells and a developing thecal layer. Steroidogenesis of preantral follicles shows a typical "estrogen-progesterone shift" following the periovulatory gonadotropin surges (127). Similarly, isolated intact human preantral follicles that are 90 to 150 μm in diameter are also capable of synthesizing steroids *in vitro* when stimulated by FSH (553).

Clear-cut evidence that small growing follicles are influenced by periovulatory changes in gonodotropins is provided in a series of recent studies based on the ability to dissect intact follicles from the hamster ovary by an enzymatic method (269). Small preantral follicles with one to five layers of granulosa cells lack any thecal investment. When such follicles are incubated with [^{3}H]-thymidine for 4 h a significant increase in incorporation occurs between the morning of proestrus and 3 P.M.—when the preovulatory surges of FSH and LH are in progress (100). A second increase in DNA synthesis is evident on the morning of estrus, which not only involves the smallest preantral follicles but now includes all larger healthy stages as well. These results are consistent with a previous autoradiographic study (99). Phenobarbital injected at 1 P.M. proestrus blocks the normal rise in FSH and LH and prevents the increase in [^{3}H]thymidine incorporation in all follicular stages; however, the effects can be reversed in the small preantral follicles by injection of FSH but not LH (517). The ability of FSH to enhance DNA synthesis of small preantral follicles can also be demonstrated *in vitro* where it is associated with increased cAMP activity (126). A similar situation probably exists in the cyclic rat. When the proestrous surge of FSH is blocked for several consecutive cycles by pentobarbital, by the fourth or fifth cycle no follicles larger than 0.4 mm are present (554). Addition of exogenous hCG failed to restore normal follicular growth, whereas FSH was effective. Insler and colleagues (554) suggest that in the third cycle before the ovulatory one, the periovulatory FSH surge determines the follicles selected for the next three cycles.

Estrus

In the hamster on the first day of the cycle (estrus), serum FSH is elevated and two- to six-fold higher than on day 2 (555–557). There is a biphasic pattern on day 4 (proestrus) with peak FSH levels attained at 4 P.M. on day 4, a decline to low levels by 9 P.M., and then a steady increase to the high levels observed on day 1. The secondary FSH surge in the rat is not as discrete as in the hamster (558,559). A single increase of serum FSH in the rat lasts for about 24 hours (afternoon of proestrus until just before noon estrus). The reason for the increase in estrous levels of FSH in the rat is the decline late on proestrus and early on estrus in ovarian venous blood levels of inhibinlike activity (560), coinciding with a decrease in follicular fluid levels of inhibin (561) and a decline in secretion of inhibin by granulosa cells in culture (562). A negative correlation also exists between the decrease in the number of antral follicles (due to ovulation) and rising FSH levels (563). In the hamster, charcoal-treated extracts of ovaries collected on proestrus reduce the serum levels of FSH but not ovaries gathered on other days of the cycle (564). It thus appears that the proestrous follicles produce substantial amounts of inhibin with granulosa cells as the principal source (565). Immunocytochemical and *in situ* hybridization studies with the rat ovary show that the granulosa cells of primary follicles and the theca cells of tertiary follicles express inhibin-α mRNA, while inhibin-β mRNA is expressed only in the granulosa cells of tertiary follicles (312). Moreover, inhibin-α message and protein are present in rat primordial follicles (312). The periovulatory gonadotropin surges decrease inhibin-β and increase inhibin-α gene expression in the granulosa cells (312).

A strong inverse relationship exists between peripheral serum levels of FSH and inhibin levels in ovarian venous plasma in the rat (560). Inhibin activity was determined by its ability to reduce the 24 h secretion of FSH in a dispersed rat pituitary cell culture system. On proestrus, in association with the LH surge, ovarian venous inhibin levels decreased, indicating that early luteinization altered the ability of the granulosa cells from mature follicles to produce inhibin (560,566). Thus, the pituitary was released of its FSH feedback regulation by a decrease in inhibin levels, and the subsequent secondary FSH surge ensued (567). A factor structurally related to inhibin is mullerian-inhibiting substance. In the prepubertal rat, mullerian-inhibiting substance mRNA is expressed in preantral and small antral follicles, especially in granulosa cells adjacent to the oocyte, but the message is missing from primordial follicles or large preovulatory follicles (568).

In the hamster, the major targets of FSH on estrus are large preantral follicles (with eight or more layers of granulosa cells) (98,569) and in the rat, antral follicles 350–550 μm in diameter (334,505,548). Histologic methods used to assess these changes in follicle development include quantitative analysis of the number and size of follicles on each day of the cycle and quantitative autoradiography of the extent of incorporation of [^{3}H]-thymidine into granulosa cells of the various sized follicles. Using autoradiography, these classes of follicles possess FSH and LH receptors in both species (201,205). In rats and hamsters, FSH receptors are located on granulosa cells (205,570). LH receptors are located on the theca of large preantral follicles and on the granulosa of antral follicles.

Although topical autoradiography using ^{125}I-labeled FSH and hCG has demonstrated the cellular distribution of gonadotropin binding sites in the ovaries of a variety of species (see ref. 29), recent molecular approaches with FSH and LH receptor cDNAs have elegantly demonstrated the dynamics of gonadotropin receptor expression in ovarian cell types. FSH receptor message is expressed only in the granulosa cells of preantral and antral rat follicles while LH receptor gene is expressed only in the theca and interstitial cells (571). *In vitro* exposure to PMS markedly increases FSH receptor message in granulosa cells. On the other hand, hCG sharply reduces FSH receptor mRNA within 6 to 12 h (571). These results provide important information concerning the dynamics of FSH receptors during follicular development, that is, a decrease in functional receptors may be due to a combination of internalization, degradation, and inhibition of receptor gene expression. The intraovarian factors regulating gonadotropin receptor gene expression will be a worthwhile area for future research.

Evidently, FSH induces granulosa cell steroidogenesis and increased numbers of LH receptors associated with preovulatory follicular development. In the immature rat (either intact or hypophysectomized) local ovarian effects of exogenous estrogen enhance the responsiveness of the ovary to FSH (572–574). Two types of estrogen receptors have been characterized in rat granulosa cells: One species is present only in the cytosol and does not appear to be involved in genomic responses; the other has the K_a and steroid specificity typical of estrogen-binding systems (575). In the intact and hypophysectomized immature hamster, however, estrogens do not increase the number of large preantral follicles (109). Either 1 or 2 mg of estradiol cyclopentylpropionate or diethylstilbestrol given daily on days 23 to 25 to intact or hypophysectomized immature hamsters and rats led to drastic differences in ovarian follicular development (hamster: reduced; rat: enhanced), whereas increases in uterine weights are similar in the two species.

Several lines of evidence indicate that *both* FSH and LH control follicular development in the hamster and rat. The release of FSH on estrus after (or coincidental with) the decline in inhibin secretion stimulates follicular development. In the hamster, injection of estradiol cyclopentylpropionate, a long-acting estrogen, on estrus prevents the secondary FSH surge at the next cycle and thus mature follicles fail to develop (576). When FSH secretion on estrus is reduced by injections of bovine follicular fluid, the number of ovulations in hamsters is proportional to the release of FSH during estrus (577). Complete inhibition of estradiol secretion and ovulation in the next cycle occurs only after abolishment of the preceding proestrous and estrous surges of FSH (577), whereas another study reported complete inhibition of the secondary FSH surge and of ovulation with estradiol cyclopentylpropionate given as a single injection on estrus (576). The differences in the two studies may be due to the degree of suppression of FSH secretion.

A significant correlation exists between the estrous release of FSH and the recruitment of large preantral follicles (Stage IV)—the pool from which the ovulatory follicles are selected 4 days later (578). The preovulatory secretion of FSH on proestrus may also be important in recruiting follicles because neutralization of circulating FSH with appropriate antisera decreased the secretion of estradiol and the number of ova shed at the next cycle in the hamster (579). Immature hamsters injected with PMS show maximal *in vitro* incorporation of [^{3}H]-thymidine by 18 h; intraperitoneal injection of FSH antiserum in the initial 8 h—but not later—inhibits the response (579). Hence the continued presence of PMS is not necessary. The same methodology nicely demonstrates the synergistic interaction of estrogens alone or with FSH in the immature rat. Unfortunately, the effects of estrogen were not tested in the hamster model.

As previously mentioned, hamster follicles that will ovulate at the subsequent cycle can be identified on the morning of estrus (day 1) as preantral follicles with 8 to 12 layers of granulosa cells (98). In chronically hypophysectomized hamsters follicles do not grow beyond Stages 2 or 3 (122). In order to stimulate growth of preovulatory follicles either a single large dose of FSH (200 μg) is required initially or the normal endogenous secondary surge of FSH is required (123,489). This must be followed by LH (123,489) or LH and FSH (489). A normal or exogenous surge of FSH is therefore essential to initiate development of preantral follicles that will ovulate 4 days later.

There are many actions of FSH that ensure proper development of the follicle to the preovulatory stage (see Table 5). FSH-stimulated secretion of estradiol by rat granulosa cells has a lag period of about 1 day *in vitro* (565), coinciding with antrum formation (in the hamster) and the onset of estradiol secretion (in the hamster and rat) on diestrus 1 or 2 (day 2 or 3) of the cycle

TABLE 5. *Some actions of FSH on follicular steroids and receptors during the early stages of development*

Action	Citation
Increase in 3β-hydroxysteroid dehydrogenase	Zeleznik et al., 1974 (570)
Induction of LH (hCG) receptors	
Stimulates estradiol secretion by granulosa cells when incubated with testosterone	Dorrington et al., 1975 (580)
Adenyl cyclase stimulation and progesterone secretion	Hillier et al., 1978, 1980 (581, 582)
Stimulates aromatase activity	Erickson and Hsueh, 1978 (565)
Stimulates prolactin receptor formation	Wang et al., 1979 (583)
Stimulates EGF and FSH receptor formation	Jones et al., 1982 (EGF) (584) Richards et al., 1976 (FSH) (206) Ireland and Richards, 1978 (FSH) (585)
Induces EGF activity in preantral follicles	Roy and Greenwald, 1990 (147)
Increases DNA polymerase-α	Roy and Greenwald, 1989 (586)
Induces TGF-β_2 activity in granulosa cells	Roy et al., 1992 (587)
Inhibits granulosa cell 5α-reductase	Payne et al., 1992 (588)
Stimulates bFGF receptors in granulosa cells	Shikone et al., 1992 (589)
Enhances IGF-I stimulable DNA synthesis by granulosa cells	Bley et al., 1992 (590)

FSH, follicle-stimulating hormone; LH, luteinizing hormone; hCG, human chorionic gonadotropin; EGF, epidermal growth factor; TGF, transforming growth factor; bFGF, basic fibroblast growth factor; IGF-I, insulinlike growth factor, stage I.

(98,559,591). It has long been known that both FSH and LH are necessary to maintain the secretion of estradiol by growing follicles (592–594). Even though FSH is capable of stimulating estradiol and aromatase, *in vitro* studies with FSH-primed rat granulosa cells have shown that LH also maintains estrogen production (595,596). Supporting *in vivo* evidence of this concept comes from the hamster hypophysectomized on estrus (when FSH levels *in sera* are elevated) and given constant infusion of LH using osmotic minipumps (123) or daily injections of hCG (489). Treatment with LH induces the development of normal estrogen-secreting preovulatory follicles 3 days later. The ability of LH alone to maintain follicle development depends on the time of prior FSH priming, that is, LH pumps inserted immediately and 6 h (but not 12 h) after FSH priming induced normal follicular growth (597).

Does this mean that after estrus, only LH or hCG is required for normal follicular development? In hypophysectomized hamsters treated with 5 μg ovine FSH on days 1 and 20 μg LH in polyvinylpyrrolodinone from days 1 to 4, serum levels of FSH are undetectable beyond day 2, but on day 4 the number of occupied FSH receptors in large antral follicles is two-thirds the value in follicles from intact hamsters (124). This is consistent with the observation that the hamster anterior pituitary on estrus (when the second serum peak of FSH is in progress) contains greater than 80% of FSH, which migrates after electrofocusing at PI values of 4.5 or less (598). The high glycoprotein content of FSH on estrus, therefore, may affect its plasma half-life and postreceptor biologic activity. In the intact hamster, a potent FSH antiserum blocks ovulation when injected on every day of the cycle except for the morning of proestrus (599). Hence the antral follicle is dependent for FSH throughout most of its existence. The point is that both FSH and LH are needed for normal follicular maturation, but their ratios and importance may vary at different stages of the cycle. This is most impressively demonstrated in studies involving perifusion of rat ovaries for 4 days with changing FSH:LH ratios comparable to the *in vivo* profiles found during the normal 4-day estrous cycle (600). Follicular growth culminates 4 days later in ovulation of an average of 4.3 oocytes per ovary.

Although FSH and LH are the primary gonadotropins for follicular development, a host of information is now available for the critical modulatory roles of multiple intraovarian factors, especially the growth factors (21,29,601). Among the growth factors, epidermal growth factor (EGF), transforming growth factor-α (TGF-α), insulinlike growth factors I and II, and basic fibroblast growth factor have received considerable attention. In the rat, immunohistochemical studies have revealed that TGF-α protein is present only in the theca-interstitial cells. Moreover, TGF-α mRNA is detected in the theca-interstitial cells by Northern blot analysis (602). Kudlow and associates (602) have also shown that treatment of immature rats with FSH increases TGF-α message level without changing the protein. It has not been explained, however, how FSH can influence theca-interstitial cells that are devoid of FSH receptors. Skinner and colleagues (603) have also identified an EGF-like substance in rat theca-interstitial cells, which later was identified as TGF-α. Contrary to the rat ovary, critical immunohistochemical studies using polyclonal EGF antibody have shown that in the hamster ovary, EGF activity is present only in the granulosa cells of preantral and small antral follicles (147). Moreover, hypophysectomy results in a drastic attenuation of follicular development with an associated drop in follicular EGF activity.

FSH, but not LH, however, restores folliculogenesis and EGF activity (147). EGF stimulated proliferation of rat granulosa cells *in vitro* (604) and significantly enhanced [^{3}H]thymidine incorporation by hamster preantral follicles (605). Moreover, EGF appears to mediate FSH action on hamster granulosa cell proliferation (606). The role of cAMP as an intermediary in FSH and EGF regulation of follicular DNA synthesis should not be overlooked. Although cAMP is a long-established second messenger for FSH, its functions have so far been considered in relation to follicular steroidogenesis. A low dose of cAMP induces *in vitro* follicular DNA synthesis in the hamster (126). Later it was shown that both FSH- and cAMP-induced follicular DNA syntheses are blocked by EGF-specific antibody (606), suggesting that cAMP does participate in the cascade of events leading to DNA synthesis. cAMP also stimulates *in vitro* granulosa cell proliferation and oocyte growth in mouse primary ovarian follicles cultured in collagen gels (607). EGF increases *in vitro* progesterone production by hamster preantral follicles (605) and inhibits aromatase activity in rat granulosa cells (608). Using topical autoradiography with [^{125}I]-EGF, EGF binding sites in the rat ovary are localized both in the theca and granulosa cell of secondary and tertiary follicles (609).

Similar to EGF/TGF-α, insulinlike growth factor-I (IGF-I) also modulates ovarian cell function in many species (15). IGF-I protein has been localized in the oocyte, granulosa cells, and theca-interstitial cells of developing rat follicles (610,611). Both IGF-I and IGF-II genes are expressed in theca and granulosa cells (612). Consistent with EGF activity in the hamster ovary, hypophysectomy in the rat also causes a marked depletion of follicular IGF-I immunoreactivity (610), suggesting possible regulation of ovarian IGF-I activity by pituitary gonadotropins. The expression of IGF-I gene has been detected in rat ovary by both Northern and *in situ* hybridization techniques (613). Treatment with diethylstilbestrol causes a significant increase in ovarian IGF-I message. Moreover, IGF-I mRNA is detected in the granulosa cells of both developing preantral and antral follicles but not in atretic follicles or luteal cells, suggesting that IGF-I expression is turned off when granulosa cells terminally differentiate into lutein cells. In fact, in preovulatory follicles, IGF-I message is localized only in the antral and mural granulosa cells (613). IGF-I stimulates DNA synthesis and progesterone production by hamster preantral follicles *in vitro* (605). It has been suggested that IGF-I has no clear-cut effect on the proliferation of rat granulosa cells (601); however, a recent study (614) has shown that rat granulosa cells, when plated at 3–5 $\times$ 10^5 cells/cm^2 on collagen-coated culture surface, respond to low doses of FSH (2–20 ng/ml) and 8-bromo-3′,5′-cAMP to synthesize DNA. Both insulin and IGF-I (100 ng/ml) significantly stimulate granulosa cell [^{3}H]-thymidine incorporation. Moreover, the DNA synthetic action of IGF-I is markedly augmented in the presence of 8-bromo-cAMP (590). These results corroborate the results of IGF-I on DNA synthetic activity of hamster granulosa cells in culture (605). IGF-I selectively stimulates P-450$_{SCC}$ gene expression in rat theca-interstitial cells and potentiates LH effects on theca-interstitial androgen biosynthesis (615). IGF-I also potentiates FSH-induced progesterone biosynthesis by rat granulosa cells in culture (601). All these lines of evidence suggest that IGF-I plays a crucial role in modulating gonadotropin effects on rat and hamster follicular cells. Although the role of IGF-II in follicular development remains to be investigated, the expression of IGF-II gene in rat theca cells has been reported (612).

The emerging role of IGF binding proteins (BP) in ovarian cell functions needs to be addressed. IGFBPs represent a family of related proteins, which bind and modulate IGF action (611,616). IGFBP inhibits FSH-induced [^{3}H]thymidine uptake and progesterone and estradiol production by rat granulosa cells in culture (616). Most interestingly, intrabursal injection of IGFBP-3 results in a 55% attenuation of equine chorionic gonadotropin-hCG–induced ovulation in immature rats (617). Recently, an antigonadotropic role has been ascribed to IGFBP-3 in the rat (618). Solution hybridization-RNase protection assay of total RNA from immature rat ovary has revealed that IGFBP-3 mRNA and protein are expressed exclusively in theca-interstitial cells. Hypophysectomy results in a significant reduction in IGFBP-3 mRNA expression, which is further augmented by either FSH or diethylstilbestrol. However, growth hormone replacement causes a marked elevation of IGFBP-3 message expression in the ovary. Although these results suggest that an attenuation of IGFBP-3 production is one of the mechanisms through which FSH or estrogen stimulates rat ovarian functions, the studies remain incomplete without testing LH, the primary target of which is theca-interstitial cells due to the presence of LH receptors. These results, however, are in contrast to those found in the pig and in the human where IGFBP-3 is localized in granulosa cells (see later sections).

In contrast to EGF or IGF-I, basic fibroblast growth factor (bFGF) significantly attenuates FSH-induced LH receptor synthesis and aromatase activity in rat granulosa cells (619,620). However, for hamster preantral follicles, bFGF stimulates [^{3}H]thymidine incorporation, albeit to a lesser extent, than either EGF or IGF-I (605). Basic FGF, on the other hand, is mitogenic to bovine granulosa cells (see later section). Both bFGF protein and message have been detected in rat theca cells (293,294). In cultured rat theca-interstitial cells, basic FGF strongly attenuates hCG-induced androstenedione production (621). Basic FGF is also a potent inhibitor of P-450$_{17\alpha}$ activity in the rat theca (621). Basic FGF appears to attenuate FSH-induced increase in the regulatory subunit (RIIβ) of the cAMP-dependent protein kinase via a protein kinase C-dependent mechanism in cultured diethylstilbestrol-treated immature rat granulosa cells and thus prevents FSH-induced cytodifferentiation (622). Recently, a role of bFGF in rat oocyte maturation has been proposed (623). Basic FGF stimulates cAMP production by rat granulosa cells and induces message expression for tissue-plasminogen activator in the rat ovary (623). Basic FGF also induces 10–80% germinal vesicle breakdown over a dose range of 0.6 to 333 nmol in follicle-enclosed oocytes and induces prostaglandin production in the same follicles. These findings clearly indicate that bFGF can mimic certain important functions of LH. Whether bFGF is part of the LH-regulation of follicular function is a subject for further research.

For normal follicular development, cell proliferation should be offset at some point by cell differentiation. Because of the fast rate of granulosa cell multiplication, it is logical to assume that certain factor(s) in the ovary should counteract the proliferative action of the above mentioned mitogens, and harmonize follicular development. One such factor is transforming growth factor-β (TGF β). TGF-β is a 25-kDa, multifunctional, heterodimeric protein, which exists in three isoforms in mammals (624). The detailed biochemistry and physiology of TGF-β will be discussed in another chapter, but some of its roles in follicular development are worth mentioning here. TGF-β_1 was first localized in mouse theca cells (625). Later, it was localized in rat theca (626–629). In a systematic study using hamster ovaries, it has been shown that TGF-β_1 is expressed in theca and interstitial cells, while intense TGF-β_2 immunoreactivity is localized in the granulosa cells of all follicles (587). Moreover, FSH selectively upregulates granulosa cell TGF-β_2 activity, while LH influences TGF-β_1 (587). The latter study is the first one to establish a relationship between gonadotropins and ovarian TGF-β activities. Besides TGF-β_2 proteins, TGF-β_2 message has been detected by reverse transcription polymerase chain reaction in diethylstilbestrol-treated immature rat granulosa cells (630); however, unlike the hamster ovary, Mulheron and Schomberg (630) have found that FSH downregulates granulosa cell TGF-β_2 message expression (630). In the presence of FSH, TGF-β stimulates the proliferation of immature rat granulosa cells in culture, and the effect of TGF-β can be interrupted by a TGF-β antibody, suggesting the specificity of TGF-β action on rat granulosa cells (631). From these results, Dorrington and colleagues (631) have suggested that FSH action on rat granulosa cells is mediated by TGF-β. However, FSH-induced *in vitro* [^{3}H]thymidine incorporation in the hamster preantral follicle cannot be inhibited by either anti-TGF-β_1 or anti-TGF-β_2 antibody (632), indicating that TGF-β may not be a mediator of FSH action on follicular DNA synthesis (627). The mode of action of TGF-β on granulosa cells is quite different from other mitogens, such as EGF/TGF-α or IGF-I or FSH (628). For example, TGF-β lengthens the G1 phase of the cell cycle rather than moving cells into the S phase (633); longer G1 may allow more cells to enter the G1 phase from the G0 and also to reach the G1-S boundary with a resultant increase in net [^{3}H]thymidine incorporation when TGF-β action is dissipated (632,634).

Besides DNA synthesis, TGF-β also enhances granulosa cell differentiation. TGF-β stimulates FSH-induced aromatase activity, LH receptor and EGF receptor induction, and progesterone production by rat granulosa cells (631,635,636). TGF-β_1 inhibits androgen biosynthesis in the rat ovary, perhaps by blocking the activity of P-$450_{17\alpha}$ (628). In contrast to these results, TGF-β augments FSH-stimulated aromatase activity (311) and cAMP accumulation (637) by hypophysectomized diethylstilbestrol-treated immature rat granulosa cells in culture. All these lines of evidence suggest that TGF-β in conjunction with other proliferative growth factors critically regulates follicle developmental process. Moreover, the activities of the positive and negative growth factors depend very much on pituitary gonadotropins.

Besides the typical gonadal cell types, the mammalian ovary contains numerous macrophages within the interstitium (638). Macrophages synthesize a multitude of cytokines, such as interleukins (IL) and tumor necrosis factor-α (TNF-α) and also noncytokine growth factors, such as bFGF, TGF-α, and TGF-β (see ref. 23). In diethylstilbestrol-primed rat granulosa cell cultures, IL-1, but not IL-2, significantly inhibits FSH-induced 3′,5′-cAMP formation and associated reduction of progesterone and LH-receptor induction; however, IL-1 alone has no significant effect on the process of granulosa cell differentiation (639). Moreover, IL-1β is more potent than IL-1α in suppressing FSH action on rat granulosa cells in culture. In the pig, IL-1 also stimulates granulosa cell growth but reduces progesterone (640) and 3′,5′-cAMP accumulation (641). Similarly, IL-1 significantly downregulates, in a dose-dependent manner, hCG-induced androgen production by rat granulosa cells *in vitro* (642). Moreover, a four- to five-fold increase in ovarian IL-1β transcripts has been reported in the PMS-primed rat ovary 6 h following a single injection of hCG (643); IL-1β mRNA is expressed exclusively in theca-interstitial cells (643). Most interestingly, treatment of ovarian cells in culture with recombinant IL-1β (10 ng/ml) results within 4 to 12 h in a marked increase in IL-1β message expression (643) suggesting the presence of an IL-1 autoregulatory system in ovarian cells. IL-1 activity has been detected in porcine (644) and human (645) follicular fluid. Contrary to the effects of IL-1 on progesterone production, IL-6 significantly stimulates progesterone accumulation by diethylstilbestrol-exposed rat granulosa cells *in vitro* (646). These cells also secrete bioassayable IL-6 in culture, which is further augmented by FSH exposure. In addition to their localization in stroma, macrophages are also present in the granulosa cells of rat follicles, albeit in small numbers (647). The macrophages were identified by specific monoclonal antibodies. Granulosa cells labeled with [^{3}H]thymidine in the presence of peritoneal macrophages show an increased labeling index and thus may play a role in normal proliferation and not just as scavenging cells.

Similar to interleukins, TNF-α has a profound effect on granulosa cell functions (23,648). TNF-α inhibits FSH-induced aromatase activity in rat granulosa cells in culture, but does not influence steroidogenesis when present alone (649). This inhibition of aromatase activity is, however, not due to interference with FSH binding, receptor activity, or cAMP generation (648). Although the ovarian source of TNF-α is still controversial, TNF-α inhibits *in vitro* estrogen production and stimulates progesterone by hamster preovulatory follicles (650). Therefore, it is again very clear that granulosa and theca cell proliferation and differentiation, the underlying events in folliculogenesis, are critically regulated by a variety of intraovarian signals. A thorough appreciation of this complex regulatory process is essential for better understanding the mechanisms of folliculogenesis. Some of these factors are directly regulated by gonadotropins, while others are modulated either by intraovarian growth factors or by autoregulatory mechanisms. What determines the spatiotemporal interactions of these growth factors during follicular development from primordial to antral stages? How do follicular cells and oocytes select the required factors from this vast library? Do gonadotropins induce such qualities in follicular cells during development? Time will provide answers to these queries. Figure 2 summarizes the localization of these factors in the mammalian preovulatory follicle.

A major factor in follicular development is the proliferation of granulosa cells. Although hormones such as FSH and estradiol-17β and growth factors such as EGF, IGF-I and TGF-α induce the proliferation of follicular granulosa cells, a host of intracellular events is intimately associated with the progression of granulosa cells in the S phase of the cell cycle and mitosis. The rapid induction of protooncogenes—c-*fos*, c-*myc* and members of the *jun* family—is a hallmark of almost all proliferating cells (651–654). Treatment of immature rats with equine chorionic gonadotropin results in a rapid induction of c-*fos* and c-*myc* message expression in ovarian cells (655). The FSH-induction of c-*fos* gene expression appears to be mediated by a C-kinase-dependent mechanism (656). In perfused immature rat ovaries, granulosa cells, when exposed to FSH and insulin, show a rapid increase in DNA synthesis with associated induction of c-*fos*, c-*myc*, and c-*jun* protooncogenes, suggesting their involvement during gonadotropin-induced follicular growth (657). However, the critical question is whether this protooncogene expression represents a typical characteristic of proliferating granulosa cells or do these protooncogene products actually mediate the mitogenic effects on follicular DNA synthesis.

Diestrus

During early diestrus, serum levels of progesterone are elevated in the hamster and rat (559,591,658), coinciding with luteal secretion of progesterone (659–662). Fol-

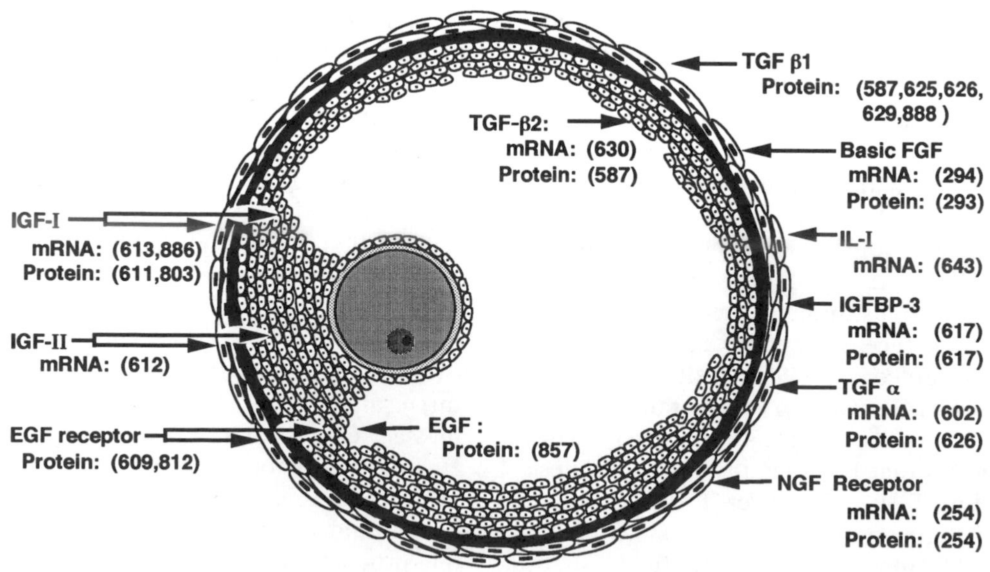

FIG. 2. Location of various growth factors and cytokines in granulosa and thecal compartments of antral follicles.

licles continue to grow during diestrus in the rat and LH levels begin to increase (663,664). When the largest follicles were excised from 4-day cyclic rats and steroid content determined, follicular estrogen first increased significantly on diestrus (e.g., at 11 A.M. to 78 pg/follicle); in contrast, measurable levels of progestogens were first detected at 11 A.M. of proestrus—about 1 ng/follicle (665). In granulosa cells from small to medium-sized rat follicles, 1 μg/ml FSH but not LH (10–100 μg/ml) stimulated cAMP formation, whereas both gonadotropins enhanced cAMP synthesis by granulosa cells from preovulatory follicles (666). These results are similar to experiments on isolated granulosa cells from porcine follicles of different sizes. The elevated LH is presumably causal in enhancing follicular development in the rat. On diestrus 1, circulating levels of LH are highest compared with other days of the cycle except for the afternoon of proestrus. The elevation in peripheral LH is due to an increase in LH pulse amplitude and a shortening of the LH pulse interval (663). This confirms previous reports that LH levels are elevated on diestrus 1 in the rat (664,667–669) but importantly establishes that LH levels are then pulsatile. Although it is not definitely known why LH levels increase on diestrus 1, it has been hypothesized that the low serum levels of progesterone and estradiol are causal factors (663,670). Injection of an LH-RH antagonist on diestrus 1 reduces mean LH by changing amplitude but not frequency and leads within 8 h to an increased percentage of early atretic follicles from 351 to 450 μm in diameter (671). In rats, pentobarbital administered on diestrus 1 delays vaginal cornification and uterine ballooning, presumably by decreasing circulating LH levels and, therefore, estradiol secretion (672,673); hCG given concurrently with pentobarbital restores vaginal cornification and uterine ballooning to normal levels. It has also been shown that injection of LH antisera on various days of the cycle in the hamster and rat prolong the cycle by 1 or 2 days (486,674,675) indicating that LH during this phase of the cycle is crucial in follicular development.

Additional evidence for the necessity of LH in follicle development in the hamster and rat comes from studies using subcutaneous injection of progesterone on various days of the cycle. Injection of progesterone (2.5–5 mg given on day 1 of the cycle) delays ovulation 1–5 days in the hamster (676,677). If the day of progesterone administration is shifted to day 3 of the hamster cycle, then 25–50 μg progesterone consistently reduces serum LH and delays ovulation by one day (678), whereas in the rat 250 μg progesterone on diestrus 2 postpones ovulation (679). In the hamster, progesterone injected on day 3 reduces serum levels of LH, estradiol, and thecal androstenedione production by antral follicles *in vitro;* follicular aromatizing ability is unaffected (680). Exogenous LH (combined with progesterone) restored estradiol secretion on day 3 by the antral follicles. Thus, exogenous progesterone induces a decline in LH causing reduced thecal secretion of androstenedione by antral follicles; in turn, this reduces the amount of precursor available for aromatization to estradiol. Ovulation is delayed by 1 day presumably because of the lack of positive feedback action of estradiol at the hypothalamic-pituitary axis, thus postponing the surge of gonadotropins until estradiol levels return to normal. It is also possible that at this phase of the cycle progesterone has a direct inhibitory action on the secretion of GnRH. Paradoxically, in the adult rat the LH pulse height and the mean serum LH are lower on diestrus 2 (day 3) than on day 2 when progesterone levels in the sera are basal (664). Thus, the decline in progesterone associated with luteal regression is accompanied by a decline in LH levels, even though follicular development and estradiol secretion are increasing. Within 1 hour of a single subcutaneous injection of 800 μg progesterone at 9 A.M. on diestrus 2 of the rat cycle, a precipitous decline in serum estradiol occurs associated with a fall in LH lasting for 48 h, a temporary decline in FSH but no change in serum testosterone (681). Follicular LH (hCG) receptors increase during the early antral phase of development, (9) and therefore the sensitivity of the follicle to LH may increase dramatically. In hamsters and rats with 4-day cycles, functional luteolysis on day 3 is not associated with any increase in ovarian venous blood flow (682,683), although this may not necessarily reflect the picture at the level of thecal blood supply. A long-term increase in exogenous progesterone (via Silastic implants) in adult cyclic mice affects the growth and death rate of follicles at all stages of development (684). Surprisingly, the number of small preantral follicles moving from stage to stage was accelerated, but the greater number did not transform into antral stages but rather became atretic as large solid follicles. It is possible that an altered FSH:LH ratio may account for these results.

Hourly LH pulses *in vitro* plus tonic FSH or tonic LH alone induce follicular growth within 3 h in ovaries of diestrous (diestrus 1) adult rats (685). It was estimated that in the larger size classes of follicles, tonic LH increased the number of cells by 5×10^4, attesting to the rapidity of response of the rodent ovary. During early diestrus, small antral follicles arising from the large preantral follicles present the day before have differentiated in the hamster (99,686). In the rat, the range in size of small antral follicles observed on estrus (352–517 μm in diameter) decreases on diestrus to 448–517 μm and thereafter they grow about 50–60 μm per day until proestrus (505). Immature 26-day-old rats primed with 10 IU PMS and killed at intervals corresponding to mid-diestrus and later show a striking *in vitro* increase in testosterone accumulation by granulosa cells at late diestrus, with levels then reverting to low values (687).

Follicles at late diestrus were small and medium-sized stages. A caveat to this study and others is that priming with PMS may alter the steroidogenic pathways and may not represent the status of adult cyclic animals.

It is postulated for the cyclic rat that the largest follicles on day 1 (estrus) may become atretic the next day and that the follicles destined to ovulate 4 days later are derived from a smaller group of follicles present on day 1 (455). This hypothesis is based on the observation that the number of granulosa cells (in the largest cross section) of the largest healthy follicles on day 2 have 1,200 cells rather than the expected 1,700 cells. Proliferation rates of granulosa cells determined on day 1 indicate that the follicles with 1,200 cells on day 2 would have been derived from follicles with 750 cells in the largest cross section. The largest healthy follicles on day 1 may therefore not necessarily give rise to the follicles ovulating 3 to 4 days later, although there are conflicting observations in the literature.

On days 3 and 4 of the cycle, follicles in both species continue to grow presumably (and primarily) under the influence of LH. During this period, subtle pulses of LH continue (663,664). In progesterone delayed ovulation of immature rats, slight but sustained increases in circulating LH occur after removal of the progesterone implants (688). The small increases in LH are presumably required for continued follicular maturation, production of estradiol, and increased LH binding to the follicle. The synchrony in the timing of ovulation following removal of the progesterone implants was similar to the effects of the normal decline in serum progesterone associated with luteal regression. Studies of Schwartz (661) and Greenwald (686) suggested that the decline in luteal production of progesterone regulated the time of onset of the next ovulation. For example, 5-day cyclic rats exhibit an extra day of luteal progesterone secretion (689–691). Conversely, injection of rats with bromocryptine, which decreases prolactin secretion, shortens the estrous cycle from 5 to 4 days by prematurely withdrawing luteal support (692,693).

Interestingly, no significant differences in the number and size of the larger (preovulatory) follicles on diestrus 2 are observed between bromocryptine-treated (4-day cycle) and 5-day cyclic rats (692). The failure of bromocryptine to affect follicular diameter was later reconfirmed, although follicular size was significantly larger in 4-day than in 5-day cyclic rats irrespective of whether they received bromocryptine (693). Shortening of the cycle to 4 days with bromocryptine did not alter the ovulation rate (approximately 10 ova/rat) as assessed by the number of fresh corpora lutea at the end of the next cycle. Follicular estradiol accumulation *in vitro* (4-h incubation) by large antral follicles taken on diestrus 2 is greater from rats treated with bromocryptine than control animals (9.0 ± 0.8 and 7.0 ± 0.4 pmol/follicle/4 h, respectively) (692), indicating that prolactin and/or progesterone may suppress follicular production of estradiol.

The change after luteolysis has been termed the "luteal-follicular" shift because of the coincident demise of the corpus luteum and the rise of follicular dominance (686). In 4-day cyclic rats, follicular progesterone, testosterone, and estrogen significantly increase at diestrus when serum progesterone declines (561). Steroid levels in the serum, corpora lutea, and nonluteal portion of the ovary of the cyclic hamster during this period reveal an inverse relationship between progesterone and estradiol (660) and the ratio of FSH to LH changes in favor of LH, which agrees with the hypothesis that LH is a major factor regulating follicular secretion of estrogen (688).

It has been proposed that during the luteal phase of the cycle, progesterone might be inhibitory by either a direct or indirect action on the follicle, since secretion of estrogen is impaired. However, for intact animals there is no evidence supporting a direct inhibitory action of progesterone on the ovary; in fact, progesterone stimulates ovarian responsiveness to hCG in the immature rat (694). A long-term inhibitory effect of progesterone on production of estradiol by proestrous rat follicles has been demonstrated, but the amounts of progesterone required are probably pharmacologic (695).

Evidence for an inhibitory action of prolactin on follicular estradiol synthesis is derived from a model using prolactin treated cyclic rats (696). Injection of 100 μg prolactin at 3 P.M. diestrus 1 and 9 A.M. and 5 P.M. of diestrus 2 reduces follicular estradiol production compared to controls. Of 7 animals injected with prolactin, 3 exhibited activated corpora lutea as evidenced by elevated serum levels of progesterone; this group also had lower serum levels of LH and estradiol (this mechanism of inhibition of follicular estradiol has been described earlier as a result of progesterone's ability to suppress LH secretion). In the remaining prolactin-treated animals, serum progesterone, LH, and estradiol levels were the same as saline injected rats; however, follicular estradiol production was suppressed *in vitro*. The mechanism by which prolactin inhibits follicular estradiol production may involve effects on the aromatase or P-$450_{17\alpha}$ enzyme systems. Since prolactin receptors are present on the granulosa cells of graafian follicles (551) and on theca-interstitial cells (552), both of these sites may be potential targets for prolactin induced suppression of estradiol secretion.

Prolactin also has been shown to inhibit estradiol synthesis *in vitro*. Granulosa cells taken from diethylstilbestrol-FSH–treated immature hypophysectomized rats were cultured for 2 to 4 days in the presence of 10^{-7} M androstenedione and 100 ng/ml of either FSH or LH (596). Addition of increasing quantities of prolactin to the culture media suppressed, in a dose-response manner, the secretion of estradiol but not progesterone. These results indicate that prolactin may have a specific inhibitory effect on granulosal cell aromatase. However, long-term culture of ovarian (theca-interstitial) cells from hypophysectomized immature rats reveals that prolactin inhibits LH-induced androgen synthesis (697). Progesterone was not produced in large quantities, even when androgen secretion was maximal.

FOLLICULAR DEVELOPMENT DURING THE ESTROUS CYCLES OF SHEEP, COW, AND SOW

These species are singled out for consideration because of the considerable research attention they have received and their different mode(s) of coping with the problem of follicular selection compared to species with short cycles. Strain differences exist, especially in sheep, but for the sake of convenience the generic designations will be used when feasible. The length of the estrous cycle is usually about 17 days in the sheep, 21 days in the cow, and 21 days in the sow. The first day of estrus is designated as day 0 of the cycle.

Ewe

Before turning to follicular kinetics in the ewe, it is worthwhile describing peripheral levels of gonadotropins and steroids throughout the estrous cycle. Following the proestrous surge of FSH, a second elevation in FSH occurs 1 or 2 days later (424,698), although this has not been observed consistently in all studies even with blood samples taken at frequent intervals (699,700). Occasional sporadic peaks of FSH are detectable during the luteal phase but with no definite rhythms recurring at intervals of several days. Pulses of FSH occur about every 2 h during the luteal and follicular phases of the cycle (424). In contrast, episodic pulses of LH recur about every 2.5 h during the luteal phase, accelerating to about 1 per h during the follicular phase. Peripheral serum levels of estradiol are at peak levels (10–25 pg/ml) on days 4–6 of the cycle (700,701) with a second increase apparent at the onset of luteolysis. The first peak in estradiol occurs when circulating levels of both FSH and LH are high. Pulsatile release of estradiol is linked to LH and the relationship is especially apparent when estradiol is measured in ovarian venous blood (for references, see ref. 424). The secretion of androstenedione and testosterone are correlated with that of estradiol. The corpus luteum has a life span of 14 or 15 days, and at its peak of progesterone secretion in the midluteal phase, serum LH and FSH are at their nadir. During the luteal phase, the peripheral concentration and secretion rate of progesterone are not influenced by the pulsatile release of LH (702). With the demise of the corpus luteum, a progressive fivefold increase in serum LH is elicited; there seems little doubt that negative feedback action of progesterone is the major regulatory steroid affecting LH secretion (701) and hence the selection of the ovulable follicle(s). In ovariectomized ewes, Silastic implants of estradiol plus progesterone, which duplicate the hormone profiles of intact animals, restore tonic LH levels to normal values but are unable to depress the postcastrational hypersecretion of FSH (699). Inhibin is the most likely choice for the putative hormone.

Several recent studies reaffirm the primacy of inhibin in regulating FSH levels in the ewe. Thus, across the estrous cycle there is an inverse relationship between peripheral plasma levels of FSH and inhibin (703). When all visible follicles are ablated by electrocautery, within 10 minutes ovarian venous blood concentration of estrogen is reduced by 81%, whereas inhibin is reduced by only 35%. It is noteworthy that the fall in peripheral inhibin levels during the first 3 days of the cycle coincides with the second rise in FSH. Confirming the above results on the effects of extirpating follicles, large estrogenic follicles (>3 mm) account for 90% of the total of *in vitro* estradiol secreted but only 55% of total inhibin production (704). A good correlation exists between inhibin secretion *in vitro* and the diameter of the follicle. Treatment with a GnRH agonist for 5 weeks suppresses plasma FSH and LH to about half control values and in most animals restricts follicular growth to less than 2.5 mm (705). Infusion of FSH for 72 h restores follicular growth beyond 2.5 mm, and the size distribution of follicles is not appreciably altered by ovine follicular fluid or an inhibin antiserum. The conclusion is that the latter two treatments are not exerted directly on the ovary but by altering plasma FSH levels. In contrast, after all visible follicles are extirpated on day 12, the stimulatory effects of PMS (58% of the follicles larger than 4 mm on day 15) are reversed by a charcoal extracted ovine fluid follicular preparation so that new follicles smaller than 2 mm are present (706). In this connection, injections of bovine follicular fluid for 3 days after luteolysis is induced on day 10 reduce plasma FSH for 4 days followed by a rebound to threefold-high levels and consequently almost doubles the ovulation rate (707).

In cyclic Texel ewes, an antral cavity begins to form in follicles about 0.5 mm in diameter and a pair of ovaries contains on average about 32% healthy tertiary follicles (708). Of the normal tertiary follicles, 83% are less than 2 mm in diameter, and for follicles larger than 2 mm, there is an average of 3.6 normal and 8.7 atretic. Based on follicular volumes, two "waves" of follicular development were discerned: The first, from days 1 to 12, culminates in a large tertiary follicle on days 7 to 9, which ultimately becomes atretic, and a second wave from days 12 to 0 usually recruits two large follicles, which grow rapidly in size on day 15 following luteolysis on day 14. Although Brand and deJong (708) referred to waves of follicular development, they were well aware of the constant presence of small follicles (up to 2 mm in diameter) throughout the cycle and they emphasized "that during the oestrous cycle the tertiary follicle population is constant and that an equilibrium exists between the production of follicles in a certain size class and their disappearance from that class, either by passing to a higher size class or by atresia." The fate of the two largest follicles (F_1 and F_2) on day 10 or 14 has been monitored by marking them with india ink, followed within 1 h by intravenous injection of gonadotropins (709). In uninjected ewes, the marked follicles on day 10 never ovulated, while on day 14, the F_1 as well as some unmarked follicles ovulated but none of the F_2 group. In the absence of the corpus luteum, cauterization of the largest follicle on day 0, 3.5, or 7 is followed by a surge of FSH and ovulation occurs approximately 4 days later (ref. 708). After luteolysis induced by a prostaglandin analogue (cloprostenol), follicles 2–4 mm or larger than 4 mm in diameter have the ability to trigger an LH surge within the normal time span: 55–60 h (710). If, however, the largest follicles are 2 mm (after cauterization of the larger ones), the LH surge is delayed by 24 h. Thus, considerable flexibility exists in the size range of follicles in the final selection process. The corpus luteum exerts a local effect on follicular development in the ewe; during the luteal phase there are more follicles 4 mm or larger on the ovary bearing the corpus luteum than on the contralateral ovary (711). A very thorough paper (712) documents changes in follicular dynamics in Merino ewes by estimating the doubling time of granulosa cells utilizing mitotic index and an estimate of 0.43 h for mitotic time (obtained by using colchicine). The growth rate of follicles up to 0.7 mm was slow (estimated times in classes 1 to 6 = 37 days) and accelerated in larger stages: approximately 8 days to reach a size of 5 mm. An important point is that a follicle ovulating at the end of any cycle would have been about 0.5 mm in diameter on day 6 or 7 of the cycle. Early atresia was rare in follicles less than 1 mm in diameter. Following the subcutaneous injection of PMS, 48 h later there were twice as many follicles (>0.5 mm) as in untreated ewes, with the greatest increase in follicles larger than 2.5 mm. This was associated with significantly higher mitotic indices and a concomitant reduction in atresia for the larger classes of follicles. A recent study confirms and extends these findings (713). Small antral follicles can be classified according to the percentage of atresia into two classes: Class I with a mean size less than 0.82 mm have an atretic rate of 5.2%; class II follicles are larger than 0.82 mm with 52% of the follicles atretic. There thus appears to be an inflection in the growth of the granulosa layers in follicles >0.82 mm, possibly accounting for the high rate of atresia.

A similar study compared follicular kinetics for two stains of ewes with different ovulation rates: Romano (average ovulation: 3.0) and Ile-de-France (1.6 ovulations) (714). Only follicles with three or more layers of granulosa cells were counted and antrum formation began at a follicular diameter of 0.2 mm for both strains. There was no difference between breeds in follicular growth rates, although there are 1.5 to 2.0 times more follicles (greater than 0.09 mm) in the Romanov versus Ile-de-France ewes (444). After pooling the data from the two breeds, it was estimated that the mean time for a follicle to pass from three layers of granulosa cells (200 cells) to the start of antrum formation (5,000 cells) was 130 days and to the preovulatory stage another 45 days for a total of about 6 months. Small follicles, less than 0.07 mm diameter, were compared between the two breeds by morphologic features: follicular diameter, number of cells per section, and oocyte diameter (715). Based on these criteria, it is postulated that growth of these small follicles can be classified into three stages: dormant, transitory (independent of gonadotropins), and growth phase (dependent on gonadotropins). The dormant phase follicles have a low incidence of cuboidal cells and are clustered in "nests" and, therefore, fit the definition of primordial follicles. Follicles in the growth phase have three to four layers of granulosa cells. The ovaries of the Ile-de-France ewes (low ovulation rate) differed from the Romanov breed in that the small follicles were significantly larger and contained more granulosa cells per section than in the latter group. The Romanov ewes have fewer follicles in the dormant and transitory categories but more in the growth phase, suggesting a greater rate of recruitment in response to gonadotropins.

Another study compared follicular growth in a high ovulating breed, D'Man (mean ovulation rate = 2.9), and a low ovulating breed, Timahite (1.1 Cl) (716). The major differences between the two breeds were that the D'Man ewes have a greater number of follicles larger than 1,285 μm (large follicles with an antrum) and a lower rate of atresia (54.9 vs 66.7%) for follicles 1,084–2,141 μm in diameter. In addition, there are significantly more follicles 118–462 μm (follicles beginning to develop an antrum)—a critical phase in follicular growth—in the D'Man ewe.

A breed that has attracted considerable and justifiable attention is the Booroola ewe; some animals ovulate as many as 10 to 11 eggs. There is a genetic basis for this high spontaneous ovulation rate (see references in ref. 717). One possible factor accounting for the prolificacy of the breed is that on day 3 of the cycle, pituitary content of FSH is approximately doubled in the Booroola compared to control ewes; however, there is no qualitative difference in FSH as determined by electrofocusing (718). There are obvious problems in extrapolating pituitary content to peripheral levels of FSH. However, the inhibin content of ovaries of Booroola ewes—collected at the midluteal phase—is only one-third the value of control animals (717), which is consistent with the possibility of higher circulating levels of FSH. Alternatively, the increased ovulation rate may be attributable to increased sensitivity to normal levels of gonadotropins. This possibility has been explored by comparing Booroola × Romney ewes ovulating 3.3 ova (F+) to animals ovulating 1.1 (++) (719). The animals were injected with cloprostenol on day 10, and from 0 to 48 h later, blood samples were collected and all follicles 2 mm and larger in diameter were dissected. The main finding was that in F+ ewes, follicles mature at a smaller diameter (3.5 mm compared to 5 mm) as evidenced by their ability to synthesize estradiol. The fact that there is no difference in androstenedione output in response to LH between the two strains points to differences in aromatase activity by the granulosa cells as the controlling factor. Two interesting correlations were evident: Nonatretic follicles from F+ ewes have about one-third as many granulosa cells as the + + ewes; the corpus luteum of the F+ ewes weigh 0.39 times the weight of the + + corpus luteum. From this observation, the logical conclusion is reached that a granulosa mass from 3F+ follicles equals the estrogen production rate of one follicle from the + + group. In comparing highly fecund F+ and Boorola ewes to control flocks with ovulation rates of 1.4, the Booroolas ovulate significantly earlier (7.5 h) but with usually no differences in peak LH concentrations or the interval between the onset of estrus and LH discharge (720). This again points to differences in follicular responsiveness established in the late luteal phase as the principal factors leading to increased ovulation rate in the Booroola.

These conclusions have been confirmed by destroying all visible follicles in both ovaries after inducing luteolysis on day 14 (721). The higher ovulation rate in Boorola-crossed ewes does not involve recruiting more follicles 3 or 4 mm in diameter but by late follicular selection of smaller preovulatory sized follicles. When all follicles were destroyed except for the dominant follicle (F_1), the ovaries were replenished with follicles 4 days later, indicating that the F_1 follicle did not inhibit growth of smaller stages. Further evidence that dominance does not exist in ewes is that injection of PMS during the luteal or follicular phase does not influence the subsequent ovulation rate (722). Moreover, coculturing of follicles larger than 5 mm with follicles 1.5–2.5 mm did not reduce the mitotic index of the smaller follicles.

Three methods for evaluating follicular dynamics, namely, ink labeling, histologic measurement of follicular size and granulosa cell number, and *in vitro* production of estradiol and estrone were used to compare large antral follicles in breeds with different ovulation rates (723). Excellent agreement exists between the three techniques. Between the late luteal and early follicular phase, the number of growing follicles did not differ between the low- and high-ovulating breeds. However, by the next day the number of estrogen-active follicles was reduced to the number that ultimately ovulated, with the remaining follicles becoming atretic.

On day 13 of the cycle, the corpus luteum is still functional in Welsh mountain sheep and the concentration of progesterone in ovarian venous plasma is about 1,000-fold higher than peripheral levels (724). Even at this stage, however, the largest nonatretic follicle secretes appreciable quantities of estrogen: from 145 to 390 pg/ml in ovarian venous plasma. This trend is accentuated on day 15 when, in most instances, the corpus luteum is regressing.

It is evident that demise of the ovine corpus luteum triggers the final stages of follicular development. This is especially well illustrated in experiments in Merino ewes where antibodies against progesterone were raised by injecting them with a progesterone-protein conjugate (725). Whereas control animals ovulated every 17 or 18 days, the ewes that actively developed progesterone antibodies ovulated at 6- to 10-day intervals, usually showed an increased ovulation rate, and at the end of several cycles the ovaries contained as many as five corpora lutea, representing their persistence over several shortened cycles.

From days 2 to 5, the largest follicle secreting estrogen has the enzyme 3β-hydroxysteroid dehydrogenase restricted to the theca interna, and after a hiatus on days 8 to 11, beginning on day 13 to day 0, a presumably new set of follicles shows enzymatic activity limited to the theca (174). Within 24 to 48 h after the injection of PMS on day 13, the number of 5-mm follicles increases, and, concomitantly, strong 3β-hydroxysteroid dehydrogenase activity is demonstrable in the theca—but not in the granulosa—of all these follicles.

A subsequent investigation revealed that an *in vivo* exposure to PMS for only 5 min enables about 25% of the follicles greater than 2 mm in diameter to secrete estrogen *in vitro* (726). Lengthening the time of exposure to PMS to 12 h fails to increase the proportion of estrogen-secreting follicles, consistent with the finding that for any follicular class about one-third of the follicles are nonatretic (e.g., ref. 708). Thus, the concept for the ewe of estrogen "activated" versus "nonactivated" follicles is extremely important with only one or two of the largest follicles falling into the former category. The one notable exception is between days 2 and 4 of the cycle when *many* of the explanted follicles are steroidogenically active (726) at a time approximating the second surge of FSH. Secretion rates of androstenedione and estradiol are increased (but not significantly) on day 3 of the cycle (727). The concentration of FSH in follicular fluid is about threefold higher in follicles in which the estradiol:androstenedione ratio is greater than 1, and the FSH values are comparable to peripheral levels (727). In experiments involving ewes with ovary and adnexa autotransplanted to the neck, between days 12 and 15, the secretion rate of estradiol—but not progesterone—increased within 5 min of each pulse of LH; everything points to a causal relationship between the two events (702). Addition of 0.25 to 10.0 μg of LH to explanted follicles of PMS-treated ewes, results at 48 h in drastic curtailment of estrogen production, whereas progesterone production increases dramatically by 24 h (728). However, within 4 h of the addition of LH, a transitory increase in estrogen accumulation occurs and this is followed by inhibition. It must be kept in mind that the amounts of LH added *in vitro* were comparable to estrous surge levels and not to the pulsatile pattern encountered on days 12–14.

An interesting approach combined topical autoradiography of [^{125}I]hCG binding sites with determinations of follicular fluid concentrations of steroids (729). During the luteal phase of the ewe, all follicles larger than 2 mm were dissected, antral fluid aspirated, and the follicle prepared for autoradiography. Follicles fell into three categories of hCG binding: to theca and granulosa (type I); LH receptors restricted to theca (type II); no LH receptors in either cell type (type III). During the luteal phase, the type I follicles contained the highest values of progesterone in follicular fluid (ca. 120 ng/ml), which were 10-fold higher than the concentrations of testosterone and estradiol. During the follicular phase, these follicles had the highest concentration of estradiol (120 ng/ml). During the follicular phase, the type II follicles contained high levels of testosterone (55 ng/ml) and very low levels of estradiol (2.5 ng/ml). LH was detectable (>2.5 ng/ml) in 86% of follicles examined without significant differences between small (<5 mm) and large follicles (>5 mm), except during behavioral estrus (727).

As is already evident, the follicles destined to ovulate in the ewe do not differentiate until about the time of luteolysis (730). This has been demonstrated during the normal estrous cycle (e.g., ref. 724) and following induced luteolysis and other experimental manipulations. Utilizing ovarian or uteroovarian autotransplants, with luteolysis induced on day 10, there is an abrupt two- to three-fold increase in the episodic rate of release of LH with no change in pulse amplitude; concomitantly the pulse rate of plasma FSH was unchanged with the pulse amplitude reduced by 60% (424). The episodic release of LH was mirrored within a few minutes by a rise in estradiol and androgens. As luteolysis progressed, plasma FSH dropped because of the reduced amplitude of the pulses. A surge of FSH accompanied the LH peak, followed by a second FSH peak about 22 h later. Very similar results are obtained in ewes with ovaries *in situ* and with luteolysis induced by prostaglandins (with or without PMS) on days 9 and 10 (731). The ewes were ovariectomized from 0 to 48 h after the onset of luteolysis and all follicles larger than 1.0 mm diameter were dissected and the follicles classified as healthy or atretic based on whether they contained more or less than 50% of the maximal number of granulosa cells for a given follicular diameter. It was not until 10 h after the induction of luteolysis that a large estrogen-activated follicle (>5 mm in diameter) was consistently present. Analysis of the percentage of healthy follicles by diameters suggests that the dominant follicle is capable of doubling the number of granulosa cells in 6–10 h. As the dominant follicles rise to prominence, there is a steady fall in the number of healthy follicles (>1 mm) from 50% at time zero to less than 20% by 24 h, possibly related to the decrease in FSH levels. Injection of PMS temporarily delays at 10 h the fall in follicular numbers apparently by recruiting smaller stages, but by 24 h the percentage of healthy follicles reverts to control levels. Another approach to identifying the ovulatory follicle is to synchronize estrus by using progesterone implants; removal of the implants sets in motion the same set of changes already described following spontaneous or induced regression of the corpus luteum (732). As the preovulatory period progressed, the dominant follicles compared to the nonovulatory follicles were larger, had greater concentrations of estradiol in follicular fluid and increased numbers of LH-hCG receptors in theca and granulosa cells. Suffolk sheep have an ovulation rate of 1.3, whereas Finnish Landrace ovulate 2.7 ova. Correlated with these rates, Suffolk ewes have 1.2 follicles with hCG binding to both theca and granulosa cells compared with 2.9 follicles in Finnish Landrace (732). Chronic administration for 6 weeks of a GnRH agonist reduces gonadotropin levels and follicular growth to baseline levels (733). When the ewes were then infused for 3 days with FSH, equivalent to the mean luteal phase, no follicles >2.5 developed nor was *in vitro* production of estradiol increased. In contrast, when FSH in doses simulating peak luteal phase amounts was infused, preovulatory estrogen active follicles matured.

It is apparent from these studies that the differentiation of the dominant follicles is associated with increased LH levels but with FSH unaffected and, if anything, reduced. In support of this contention, intravenous administration of LH-RH (luteinizing hormone-releasing hormone) antiserum in the preovulatory period promptly eliminates the pulsatile release of LH without affecting basal levels; the pulsatile release of estradiol is abolished with no change in secretion rate of testosterone or plasma levels of FSH (734).

Anestrous ewes have 35 follicles larger than 1 mm diameter, whereas on days 9–10 of the estrous cycle, there are 24 follicles (735). The anestrous pattern is associated with elevated levels of FSH and progesterone and, conversely, a reduction in the number of high amplitude LH peaks (2.4/9 h vs. 5.3/9 h on day 10 of the cycle). Continuous infusion of low doses of GnRH in anestrous ewes results in 23/24 ovulating with estrus detected an average of 37 h after the start of infusion (736). Serum LH concentration significantly increased; FSH values were not reported. The corpus luteum induced by GnRH were functional for at least 9 days. Intravenous pulse administration of LH (10 μg every 1 or 2 h for 29 to 91 days) to anestrous ewes simulates pulse rates comparable to luteal and follicular phases (735). This regimen is sufficient to induce normal cyclic progestational activity for at most two cycles; the period of subsequent acyclicity is associated with reduced FSH concentrations. Injection of anestrous ewes with bovine follicular fluid lowered plasma FSH concentrations by 70% and reduced the number of healthy follicles larger than 2 mm in diameter. Hourly intravenous injections of 50 μg FSH plus follicular fluid reverses the effects and significantly increases the number of large non-atretic follicles (>3 mm) (737). The mean number of ovulations during the breeding season is approximately 3.4 in Finnish Landrace and approximately 1.4 in Scottish Blackface (cited in ref. 738). During seasonal anestrus, an ovulatory dose of hCG induced the mean number of ovulations characteristic of the breed (738). The ovaries also contained the same number of estrogen active follicles typical of the breeding season, and these follicles were larger and with greater LH receptor binding than the inactive follicles. To turn to the other extreme, these differences in ovulation rate exist even in prepubertal ewes: Injection of hCG at 3.5 or 4 months resulted in ovulation rates comparable to natural ovulation rates, making this a useful technique to identify lambs carrying the Booroola gene (739).

Collectively, these results suggest that following the onset of luteolysis, pulsatile release of LH is the controlling factor in emergence of the dominant follicles with FSH in a strictly subordinate role. This does not rule out a possible primary role of FSH at earlier critical stages of follicular maturation. Indeed, injection of 500 IU PMS, along with prostaglandins, increases the ovulation rate in Romney ewes (731). Moreover, infusion of FSH from 24 h before until 60 h after induced luteolysis results in a mean ovulation rate of eight compared with three for ewes in which infusion was started concurrent with the induction of luteolysis (Baird and Webb, personal communication cited in ref. 730). Similarly, after prostaglandin-induced luteal regression, intravenous injection of bovine follicular fluid significantly decreases FSH levels without affecting the number of ovulations (740). Infusion of ovine FSH for 48 h plus injection of follicular fluid resulted in an ovulation rate of 14.6 ova.

In sheep, as in most other species, FSH and basal levels of LH are the major signals for follicular recruitment and selection (741), but it has become increasingly obvious that their effects on the ovary are modulated by numerous growth factors (742). For example, FSH increases insulinlike growth factor-I stimulation of progesterone secretion by granulosa cells from small ovine follicles (1–3 mm) and insulinlike growth factor-I increases DNA synthesis and proliferation to a greater extent in small follicles than large follicles (5–7 mm) (742).

Cow

Following the estrous surge there is a very definite second peak of circulating FSH, lasting for 2 or 3 days (385,743). The levels of FSH have been reported to show peaks on days 4, 8, 12 or 13, 17, and 18, but these are based on relative percentage changes (743). Schams and colleagues (743) believe these peaks are temporally related to periods of enhanced follicular growth. During the early luteal phase (day 4), 8.5 pulses of FSH are recorded per 12 h compared to 6.3 on day 11 and pulse amplitude is also unchanged (18.5 ng/ml versus 16.6) (744). Separate FSH pulses (with minimal LH increases) are encountered about 41% of the time in the midluteal phase; these are concomitant with or soon followed by pulses of progesterone (744). With the onset of luteolysis, no change in plasma FSH is observed up to 12 h later (745,746) with the levels falling significantly by 24 to 36 h (745). The second postestrous peak in FSH on day 4 is not associated with an increase in LH. On day 4, eight peaks of LH occur per 12 h with the number falling to 3.6 on day 11 when progesterone levels are maximal (744). About 96 percent of all LH-FSH pulses are followed within 60 min by a peak in estradiol (744). With the onset of induced luteolysis, a significant increase of mean plasma LH occurs within 1 to 3 h, related to a fourfold increase in pulse frequency and amplitude (744,746). During the luteal phase, plasma estradiol rises to a peak of 6 pg/ml on day 6 (747) and there are seven pulses of estradiol per 12 h; by the midluteal phase this value is halved in conjunction with the change in frequency of LH pulses (744). Following induced luteolysis, the pulse frequency for estradiol increases within 4 to 6 h but without changes in pulse amplitude (745). In healthy preantral follicles, the principal thecal androgen produced *in vitro* is androstenedione, with about one-fifth as much testosterone accumulated (283). During the early follicular phase, the average width of the theca interna is considerably thinner than in the preovulatory follicle (72.8 vs 237 μm) (748). Presumably, before the LH surge, 3β-hydroxysteroid dehydrogenase is deficient in granulosa cells from cows as is the case in sheep and numerous other species. A slow increase in peripheral levels of estradiol begins before progesterone falls (747).

Progesterone levels in the cyclic cow begin to increase from about day 4, reach a plateau around day 10 and decline to basal levels by day 17 or 18 (743). Luteal phase levels of progesterone average about 4 ng/ml (744,746) with pulse amplitude and mean concentrations peaking at about day 11. Progesterone drops very rapidly after induced luteolysis, falling 67% by 20 min (745). An inverse relationship exists between progesterone and LH levels in the cow (749) as in the ewe. Insertion of vaginal coils loaded with progesterone into cattle during the luteal or follicular phase usually lowers serum LH, but

FSH is unaffected. On removal of the coils and injection of $PGF_{2\alpha}$, serum LH increases but not FSH. Hence a case can be made for FSH being controlled by a separate releasing hormone, or, more likely, by the secretion of inhibin (749).

How do these cyclic changes in hormone levels relate to follicular development in the cow? When the largest follicle was marked between days 9 and 17, none of them ovulated; the likelihood of the largest follicle ovulating increased abruptly at day 18, and in five of six animals, the largest or next to largest follicle was selected by day 18 (750). When the largest follicle (F_1) and second largest follicle (F_2) are marked on different days of the cycle and examined 5 days later, the follicles are still present on days 8 and 13 but have regressed considerably by day 18 (751). Thus, between days 13 and 18, there is an increase in the rate of replacement and turnover of large follicles. This is further accentuated by day 18 in that the F_1 follicle only ovulated when ovulation occurred within 3 days. The greatest number of small follicles (1–3 mm) is observed on day 3, presumably in response to the second FSH surge (751). Medium-sized follicles (3–6 mm) are most numerous on day 13. In contrast, the number of large follicles (>6 mm) does not vary throughout the cycle. When all follicles larger than 5 mm in diameter are destroyed on day 13, it takes 5 days for F_1 and F_2 follicles to emerge from the medium-sized group. Similarly, if the ovary bearing the F_1 follicle is removed between days 4 and 12, the remaining ovary compensates within 4 days, but if the ovary contralateral to the F_1 follicle is removed, follicular development is unchanged (752). The dominant follicle may therefore inhibit smaller follicles by an intraovarian mechanism. When all grossly visible follicles are eliminated from both ovaries on day 10 by electrocautery and x-irradiation of the ovaries, luteal life span is significantly extended (753). This indicates that the normal presence of follicles during mid- to late diestrus is essential for luteolysis in the bovine. The above results are consistent with earlier histologic studies, which showed that 23.7% normal and 76.3% atretic follicles were present per pair of ovaries during the cycle (754). Follicles undergoing early atresia (defined in ref. 754) constituted 20.3% of the atretic population. Normal follicles larger than 5 mm were not found during the luteal phase, whereas 8- to 18-mm follicles developed during the follicular phase. Based on the mitotic time of sheep granulosa cells, the time required for bovine follicles to pass from one class to another has been analyzed (755). The time required for graafian follicles to grow from 0.4 to 10 mm is about 22 days—the approximate length of the estrous cycle. It is therefore tempting to speculate that the postestrous FSH surge stimulates the follicles that will ultimately ovulate 20–22 days later. Histologic signs of atresia were first observed in follicles at least 1.7 mm in diameter (755). The maximum growth rate of granulosa cells in cow follicles is reached in larger follicles (1.5 mm diameter) than in the sheep (0.10 mm diameter), suggesting for the cow that graafian follicles need to persist longer and grow to a greater size before they can respond to an ovulatory amount of luteinizing hormone. There is an excellent correlation between macroscopic and histologic criteria for follicular normality (93.3%) and atresia (95.5%) in bovine follicles ranging from 2 to 22 mm in diameter (756). As to be expected, for follicles from 2 to 5 mm in diameter, there is a progressive decline in follicular fluid estradiol as atresia proceeds from early to advanced stages (756).

The number of large follicles (>8 mm) increases from day 6 (1.3) to day 12 (1.8) and day 18 (2.1), and healthy follicles with FSH binding to granulosa cells and hCG binding to granulosa and thecal cells are already present at day 6 (757). Thus, even at day 6, follicles that could be thought of as preovulatory have differentiated, since removal of the corpus luteum or treatment with prostaglandins results in ovulation 2 or 3 days later. However, the ultimate normal fate of these follicles is atresia. On day 18, two large follicles are invariably present, one with considerably more estradiol content than the other, the latter evidently destined to degenerate (757).

Knowledge of follicular dynamics in cattle has been vastly extended by the application of ultrasonography, which yields information by nonsurgical intervention available by no other technique (758). During the bovine estrous cycle, two or three waves of follicular development are usually discernible (759). Cycles with three waves are invariably longer. In two-wave cycles, the first dominant follicle (F_1) is first detected on the day of estrus; the growth phase ends on day 6 although regression is not evident until day 13. The ovulatory follicle is detected on day 10, reaches a maximal diameter of 16.5 mm; 11 days elapse between first detection and ovulation. The growth of the F_1 follicle from wave 1 can be delayed by daily injections of follicular fluid beginning shortly after the onset of estrus (760). This is associated with depressed plasma FSH and estradiol, but LH is unaffected. A rebound in FSH then occurs and the F_1 follicle is first detected at 4.5 days. In most of the treated heifers there were only two waves of follicular development, whereas in the control group there were usually three waves. The secondary FSH surge is therefore important in initiating recruitment of the first F_1 follicle. Previous studies have shown significant differences in follicular development and ovulation between the right and left ovaries (see ref. 761 for references). Daily ultrasound examination confirmed this finding: There are significantly more 4- to 6-mm follicles in the right ovary, regardless of the presence or absence of a corpus luteum. During the first half of the cycle, there is a tendency for more follicles (>13 mm) on the ovary bearing the corpus luteum, but as luteolysis progresses, the right ovary becomes dominant. However, there is no evidence for alternation of ovulation. A key but hitherto unresolved question in the cow has always been whether a surge of FSH precedes the recruitment of the F_1 follicle of each wave. A statistical analysis, correlating the mean day of emergence of the dominant follicle with the day of maximum FSH shows that two-wave heifers have two FSH surges and three-wave animals have three FSH surges during the interovulatory period. The surges usually begin 2 to 4 days before follicles of 4 and 5 mm developed (762).

The dominant follicle of the first wave never reaches maturity presumably because of high concentrations of progesterone secreted by the corpus luteum. As previously mentioned, injection of a prostaglandin analogue on day 7 destroys the corpus luteum, and this results in the F_1 follicle continuing to develop. In 80% of animals ovulating 48 to 120 h post-PGF, the F_1 follicle was the ovulating follicle (763).

In the cow, unlike the ewe, the dominant follicle inhibits the development of smaller follicles. This observation has now been confirmed by ultrasonography. The experimental design consists of cauterizing the F_1 follicle on day 3 or 5 or sham surgery (764). When the F_1 follicle was ablated, the regression of the subordinate follicle was delayed and the F_1 follicle of the next wave prematurely emerged.

As already noted, the demise of the corpus luteum triggers the follicular phase in which the ovulatory follicle is selected. In spontaneous luteal-follicular shifts, hormone levels and follicular diameters were normalized to the LH surge (765). The mean diameter of the ovulating dominant follicle was 6 mm on day 4 (day 0 = LH surge) and reached maximal size (14 mm) before the LH surge. A definite increase in estradiol was noted at day 2, when progesterone levels were approaching their nadir. Plasma FSH gradually declined from late luteal phase values to the lowest point 6 h before the LH surge. By 24 h after the LH surge a small increase in FSH was observed in three of five animals. An inverse relationship exists between FSH and estradiol suggesting that estrogen and inhibin may act to suppress FSH, as in the case of the ewe.

Selection of the follicle destined to ovulate occurred between days 16 and 17 (day 4 to day 3 before ovulation). This was the time when growth of the F_1 and F_2 follicles began to diverge (766). Injection of PMS on day 14 or 16 (i.e., before or on the day of follicular selection) resulted in superovulation of 9 ova, whereas deferring the injection until day 18 gave mixed results, with some animals lacking corpora lutea and others with multiple corpora lutea. The effects of PMS treatment, therefore, corroborate days 16 and 17 as the turning point; beyond this time follicles larger than 7 mm—not including the F_1 follicle—have become atretic (766).

What are the effects on follicular dominance if progesterone levels are artificially prolonged by intravaginal insertion of Silastic devices containing progesterone from days 14 to 28 (767)? Cycle length is prolonged by 9 and 10 days, respectively, with one or two of the devices (groups 2 and 3) correlated with greater levels of progesterone in group 3. There were 3.8 waves in progesterone-treated animals of group 2 and 2.7 in group 2 controls. One of the most interesting observations is that insertion of one device almost doubled the life span of the F_1 follicle and this was associated with basal levels of LH (comparable to the normal luteal phase) and gradually increasing plasma estradiol. The prolonged persistence of the dominant follicle in group two suppresses recruitment of smaller follicles.

Ovaries collected from cows (with no information available about their reproductive history) had follicular fluid aspirated from all surface follicles and the follicles classified into three size classes based on the volume of antral fluid (768). As follicle size increased, FSH concentration in follicular fluid was unchanged, LH decreased significantly by 27%, and prolactin increased twofold. These changes were associated with a shift in the estradiol:androgen ratio such that 83% of the large follicles were predominantly estrogenic compared to only 7% of the small follicles. From days 3 to 7 of the cycle, the number of estrogen-active follicles (based on steroid determinations from follicular fluid) decreased from two to one per heifer with a gradual increase to day 7 in follicular diameter (14 mm) and number of granulosa cells (12×10^6) (385). Through day 7, an average of one large estrogen-inactive follicle was present per heifer, which was usually judged to be atretic on histologic grounds. On day 9, all follicles were estrogen-inactive; by day 13, however, small active follicles (10 mm) reappeared. The estrogen active follicle is distinguishable by specific hCG binding to both theca and granulosa cells and FSH binding to granulosa cells; this was especially evident on day 17 when receptor levels were about twice as high in both compartments compared to the inactive follicle (385). Dominant follicles during the follicular phase were superfused for 10 h (769). An excellent correlation existed between follicle size and estradiol secretion but not with testosterone or progesterone. The correlation with estradiol most likely represents an increase in granulosa cell numbers. It is interesting that dominant follicles obtained 48–60 h after prostaglandin injection have high intrafollicular concentrations of estradiol but very low levels of inhibin (770). In contrast, dominant nonovulatory follicles on day 6 of the estrous cycle have about one-third the concentration of estradiol as their counterparts during the follicular phase, but inhibin levels are approximately threefold higher in the nonovulatory follicle.

The proestrous follicle (24 h after progesterone declined to <1 ng/ml) average 16 mm in diameter with follicular fluid concentrations of LH and FSH of 1.48 ng/ml and 0.42 ng/ml, respectively. Estrogen concentration in the follicle (estradiol plus estrone, with the latter about 20-fold less) was 39 times the combined concentration of testosterone and androstenedione (771). This correlates with increased serum levels of LH but unchanged FSH levels (746). The estrogen-activated follicle has significantly greater FSH binding to granulosa cells and hCG binding to granulosa and thecal cells than the large estrogen-inactive follicles which are usually atretic by histologic criteria. Large atretic follicles have estradiol concentrations 150-fold lower than normal preovulatory follicles (771). Thus, in the cow as in the ewe, regression of the corpus luteum leads to the final selection of the ovulatory follicle, principally as a result of increased LH activity, after FSH and LH priming actions.

Ovaries were removed from cows 2 h after behavioral estrus and the nine largest follicles from each pair were dissected; the dominant follicle was 15 mm in diameter, others were as small as 2 or 3 mm (772). Estradiol secretion by the largest follicle *in vitro* was at a rate of 2 to 3 orders of magnitude greater than the smaller follicles, but small follicles ipsilateral to the dominant follicle secreted three times as much estradiol than the population on the contralateral ovary. Injection of porcine FSH for 4 days beginning on day 9 of the bovine cycle results, after induced luteolysis, in superovulation of 11 eggs per animal (773). At 12 h after the onset of estrus, estrogen concentrations in follicular fluid were similar to those observed in normal preovulatory follicles except for much lower amounts of estradiol.

Oxytocin has recently been found in the corpora lutea of numerous species, including cattle. As might be anticipated, oxytocin is secreted in increasing amounts by cultured granulosa cells as follicular development progresses (774). The highest secretion rate by granulosa cells was after the onset of estrus; the theca produced only small and variable amounts of oxytocin. Cultured bovine granulosa cells changed the pattern of hormone production as the cells shifted from follicular to luteal status, that is, secretion of inhibin and estradiol fell to basal levels after 3 days of culture, whereas oxytocin and progesterone significantly increased after 4 days of culture (775). These temporal changes were reflected in corresponding changes in mRNAs for inhibin and oxytocin. The increase in oxytocin and progesterone are not linked events, since addition of aminoglutethimide to cultured granulosa cells suppresses progesterone secretion by 95%, but oxytocin production is unaffected (776).

Undoubtedly, autocrine and paracrine factors transduce the effect of FSH and LH on the bovine follicle. For example, insulin plus FSH synergize to enhance viability of fully differentiated granulosa cells and also to increase progesterone secretion (777). Similar results have been obtained with follicles perifused for 4 or 21 h (778). Insulin or insulin plus FSH and LH stimulated DNA synthesis throughout the culture period with insulin acting as the principal mitogen. Insulinlike growth factor-I (IGF-I) appears to be the local growth factor involved in proliferation and differentiation of granulosa cells. Very small concentrations of IGF-I (1 ng/ml) effectively stimulate mitosis in granulosa cells collected from 4- to 6-mm bovine follicles (779). Higher doses of IGF-I (20 ng/ml) stimulates bovine granulosa cell proliferation *in vitro;* however, the effect cannot be further increased by supplementing with high-density lipoprotein and/or insulin in the medium, suggesting that IGF-I action may be independent of other factors that can induce granulosa cell proliferation (779).

Similar to rodents, folliculogenesis in the cow is also influenced by gonadal peptides. Because granulosa cell function is a key event in follicular development, studies have been conducted on cultured bovine granulosa cells to understand the roles of different growth factors on cell functions (780). Basic fibroblast growth factor (b-FGF) has been immunohistochemically localized in the granulosa cells of growing and mature bovine follicles; however, no staining is detectable for stromal cells (781). These results are diametrically opposed to what has been reported for rat granulosa cells (164). Bovine granulosa cells express 7- and 3.5-kb mRNA transcripts of bFGF gene and these messages are translated into a 16-kDa bFGF-like protein (782). Moreover, the synthesized factor induces proliferation of bovine granulosa cells. Bovine theca cells synthesize TGF-β-like protein (626). These findings clearly indicate that folliculogenesis in the bovine ovary may also be locally regulated by various growth factors made by follicular cells.

Pig

A recent study has shed considerable light on follicular kinetics in the gilt, utilizing colchicine treatment of five prepubertal sows (783). Thecal investment was a late event, not consistently observed until the preantral follicles were 206–287 μm in diameter, when there was an average of 11 layers of granulosa cells. It is estimated that a primary follicle (one to two layers of granulosa cells) grew to small antral size (400 μm) in 84 days, and further growth to a 3-mm follicle required 14 days. To reach a preovulatory size of about 8 mm, the follicle requires another 5 days. It is therefore postulated that at the beginning of the 19-day estrous cycle, small antral follicles ($\sim$400 μm) are the pool from which the ovulatory follicles are derived.

Serum FSH shows a minor rise, concomitant with the proestrous LH surge and a second rise in FSH about 27 h later, paralleling an increase in progesterone (784). Mean values of FSH are maximal on day 3 when estradiol is minimal. Contrary to the ewe and cow, the gilt shows greater pulsatile activity for FSH and LH during the luteal than follicular phase of the cycle. On day 12 of the cycle, pulsatile release of LH was usually followed within about an hour by pulses of estradiol. Two separate surges of prolactin are observed during the cycle, one during the proestrous increase of estradiol and one during estrus. Maximal values of serum progesterone are reached between days 9 and 14 of the cycle before drastically falling on day 15 (784,785). The hormonal pattern in the pig has not been studied as closely as other domestic species, but the available evidence indicates that the demise of luteal function does not increase basal or pulsatile levels of LH (784). This has now been substantiated, in part, in gilts given PGF on day 12 to facilitate luteolysis; plasma was collected from the jugular vein and ovarian venous effluent from days 11 to 16 (786). On day 14, LH pulse amplitude is halved and LH concentration is unchanged from days 11–16. On the other hand, LH pulse frequency is doubled on days 14–16 compared to days 11–13. For FSH, pulse frequency and concentration were relatively stable throughout the sampling period and there was a steady downward drift in pulse amplitude. Estradiol secretion increased concomitantly with the fall in progesterone but before any increase in pulsatile secretion of LH. Plasma concentrations of estrone and estradiol do not begin to increase during proestrus until plasma progesterone falls between days 15 and 18, and other than the proestrous surge, levels range between 8 and 12 pg/ml throughout the rest of the cycle (785).

The use of microdialysis systems to sample hormone levels in freely moving animals is a very promising technique, applicable to numerous organs and tissues. A microdialysis system was implanted into the wall of large tertiary follicles of miniature pigs on day 19 or 20 with the effluent collected every 30 minutes over the next 7 days (787). The follicles released estradiol, progesterone, oxytocin, and angiotensin II in a pulsatile pattern. Application of the latter two compounds directly to preovulatory follicles did not affect steroidogenesis. While androstenedione infusion greatly increased estradiol secretion, hCG had no effect on follicular estradiol or progesterone release.

Heterogeneity of porcine granulosa cells has been demonstrated by separating cells with strong attachments to each other or cells lacking such connections (788). The aggregates of tightly bound cells are frequently associated with a sharp profile on one edge so that they most likely represent mural granulosa cells. These cells are about twice as large as the weakly associated cells which may correspond to cumulus cells. The two subpopulations differ in that the tightly bound cells spontaneously secrete estradiol and progesterone during 40 h of culture and accumulation of both steroids is enhanced by FSH or LH much more so than the weakly associated cells.

LH receptor RNA drops to baseline levels in porcine granulosa cells (from <3 mm follicles) by 72 h of culture (789). Specific binding of labeled hCG is significantly increased to about the same extent, by either FSH, insulin or estradiol. When the three compounds are combined ("stimulating medium") hCG receptor increases after 48 h of exposure. Goxe and coworkers (789) conclude that both transcriptional and translational events are involved in the regulation of the LH receptor.

The pig is one of the few species in which thecal cells, from large follicles (>8 mm) have an active aromatase system (790). A follicle regulatory protein (FRP) is secreted by porcine granulosa cells but not theca (791) and is especially secreted by medium-sized follicles (3–6 mm). Immunoreactivity of FRP in spent medium is considerably enhanced in granulosa cells of small follicles by FSH plus dihydrotestosterone. It is hypothesized that FRP is an atretogenic local factor which can override low estradiol production of subordinate follicles (see below). In cultured thecal cells from medium-sized follicle, FRP does not affect aromatase activity over the first 48 h, and then enhances activity. This is paralleled by estradiol secretion (790). On the other hand, FRP does not affect secretion of testosterone and androstenedione. The reader is referred to a recent review article for more details on FRP (21).

The selection of follicles for ovulation occurs some time before day 17 of the porcine estrous cycle, as evidenced by the lack of compensatory ovulation when unilateral ovariectomy is performed on day 15 or 17 (792). On day 3 of the cycle no follicles larger than 4 mm are present in the ovaries, but by day 9 follicles between 4 and 8 mm begin to repopulate the ovary (793). On day 13, the largest follicles are 3 to 6 mm, with an average diameter of 4 mm (794). By day 16, average diameter is 4.8 mm, and only one of six gilts possessed large follicles (6–9 mm). Injection of 1,000 IU hCG on day 12 results in the presence on day 16 of both medium and large follicles in all animals with follicular estrogen and progesterone concentrations 2- and 40-fold greater, respectively, than the levels in control follicles. In randomly selected gilts, the right ovary on day 13 contained 48 follicles from 1 to 6 mm; by day 19, 29 follicles were in this size range and there was an average of only 1.5 large follicles (7–10 mm) per ovary (792). Follicular selection is evidently completed by day 17, since 91% of 5- to 6-mm follicles marked between days 17 and 21 are represented 6 days later by corpora lutea (795).

When all grossly visible follicles (>1 mm) are destroyed by electrosurgical cauterization on day 14 (late luteal phase), 6 days later the largest clear follicles present were 8 mm in diameter for Poland China gilts (796). Thus, the follicles grew 7 mm or 0.4515 log mm^3/day. Based on this figure, it is estimated that the ultimate ovulatory follicles, which are 7–11 mm at estrus, begin to develop around day 5 or 6 and are estimated to require 15.6 days to complete their development. Again, the second postestrous FSH increase may be an important selective factor. A very clear-cut surge of FSH occurs 2 to 4 days after the LH peak, with peak values 2 or 3 times greater than preovulatory concentrations (797). The secondary FSH surge correlates with a decline in inhibin which precedes the FSH peak (798).

As in the case of the other barnyard species, the largest follicles present at metestrus (>8 mm) have significantly greater follicular fluid levels of estrogens than androgens, and this relationship persists through diestrus and proestrus (799). Similarly, prepubertal gilts treated with PMS, show a daily follicular increase of 1–2 mm in diameter, associated with increasing concentration of estrone, estradiol, and progesterone in follicular fluid, comparable to the concentrations in the cyclic sow before and at the onset of estrus (800).

In cyclic or PMS-stimulated gilts, considerable follicular heterogeneity exists as evidenced by a range of follicular diameters of around 2 mm; follicles of the same size may show considerable differences in follicular steroid concentration (801). Similarly, the number of granulosa cells per follicle is also quite variable. This suggests that biochemical and histologic differences lead to follicles responding to the LH surge in different ways, presumably reflecting different stages of maturation. This has consequences for luteal function and embryonic development. Although fertilization rates in swine are approximately 95%, embryonic mortality in the first 30 days of pregnancy may be as high as 30% (802). Within a litter, blastocyst differentiation varies on day 12 with large blastocysts possibly representing "the leading edge" of mature follicles (802). As the more advanced blastocysts begin secreting estrogen this may directly or indirectly affect adversely the growth of smaller blastocysts which consequently die.

Because of the ready availability of large amounts of ovarian tissue, numerous studies on growth factor regulation of follicular activities have been carried out in the pig (see ref. 15). Porcine granulosa cells in culture produce measurable amounts of insulinlike growth factor (IGF-I) (803), and IGF-I stimulates porcine granulosa cell DNA synthesis (804,805). Moreover, FSH, estrogen, and cAMP enhance secretion of immunoreactive IGF-I by cultured porcine granulosa cells (806), suggesting the possible involvement of an important autocrine mechanism in gonadotropin-regulated follicular growth and differentiation. A systematic study on follicular IGF-I concentration and IGFBP-2 and -3 (binding proteins) has shown that fluid from small porcine follicles contains a maximum concentration of IGF-I and IGFBP-2; however, IGFBP-3 shows no particular relationship with IGF-I (807). Moreover, follicular fluid contains significantly more IGF-I at the late follicular phase compared to other phases of the cycle. Howard and Ford (807) have shown that, although PMS enhances follicular IGF-I concentration, hCG significantly decreases follicular IGF-I content within 10 h. Using multiple combinations of epidermal growth factor (EGF), IGF-I, and transforming growth factor-β (TGF-β), and with cell proliferation as the end point, it has been convincingly demonstrated that both EGF and IGF-I, either separately or combined, enhance the proliferation of porcine granulosa cells cultured in a platelet-poor defined medium (808). However, TGF-β either enhances or attenuates EGF-induced cell proliferation, depending on the concentration of platelet-poor plasma derived serum in the medium. IGF-I stimulates, in a dose-dependent manner, progesterone and 20α-hydroxypregn-4-ene-3-one production by cultured porcine granulosa cells (809). Contrary to these findings, IGF-I cannot stimulate progesterone production by cultured porcine granulosa cells unless accompanied by FSH (804). Using [^{125}I]IGF-I and topical autoradiography in the ewe, high-affinity IGF-I receptors have been localized only in the granulosa cells; however, IGFBPs have been detected in the entire ovary (810).

Besides IGF-I, EGF/TGF-α also stimulates DNA synthesis in cultured porcine granulosa cells; however, the culture medium must be fortified with platelet-poor plasma-derived serum (808). TGF-α, which evokes EGF-like response in target cells, stimulates basal estrogen production by the granulosa cells of prepubertal pigs, and TGF-α is much more potent than FSH in inducing follicular aromatase activity (811). Interestingly, genistein, a specific tyrosine kinase blocker, inhibits TGF-α-induced estrogen production, suggesting the involvement of a tyrosine kinase in the activation process. On the contrary, EGF significantly attenuates hCG-induced estrogen production by adult porcine theca cells. In the pig, specific EGF receptors are present only in the granulosa cells of growing preantral follicles and no specific binding is present in the thecal cells (812). EGF receptors in the granulosa cells appear to be upregulated by FSH (812). These reports clearly indicate that follicular cells undergo marked maturation with the onset of cyclic gonadotropins during the postpubertal period, and, consequently, their responses to different intraovarian factors differ. These studies also indicate that careful interpretation of experimental results is essential when extrapolating information across and within species.

While experiments utilizing granulosa cells predominate in the research on follicular development and regulation, studies using pure thecal cells are scanty. Because it is feasible to separate theca interna from porcine follicles, the issue of growth factor regulation of theca cell functions by culturing pure porcine theca cells in plasma-derived serum has been addressed (813). In this culture, cells proliferate after the addition of platelet-derived growth factor but not in response to EGF; a modest increase occurs in response to IGF-I. However, platelet-derived growth factor and EGF synergistically interact to enhance the proliferative activity of the former growth factor (813). These results, along with the findings that IGF-I is present in and stimulates porcine granulosa cells, are beginning to establish a possible cell-to-cell interaction through cell-specific growth factor response as local regulators of folliculogenesis.

Although TGF-β has long been used in porcine granulosa cell cultures, its presence in the porcine ovary has not been demonstrated until recently. Using porcine granulosa and theca cell-conditioned media and a sensitive granulosa cell bioassay, a high concentration of latent TGF-β_1 activity is detectable in porcine theca cell-conditioned medium (814). However, no TGF-β_1-like activity has been detected in granulosa cell cultures (814). Interestingly, TGF-β activity is present in porcine luteal cells, reinforcing the involvement of theca cells in forming the corpora lutea. These results, taken together with that of hamster ovarian TGF-β activity (587), strongly suggest a clear-cut partitioning of growth factors and their isoforms within follicular cell compartments. Similar to the results of May and colleagues (808), both TGF-β_1 and TGF-β_2 have been found to inhibit porcine granulosa cell proliferation in short- and long-term cultures (815). Moreover, in the latter studies, TGF-β, at low doses (10 pg/ml) potentiates and at high doses (1–10 ng/ml) inhibits epidermal growth factor-stimulated IGF-I production. TGF-β also inhibits FSH-induced progesterone production in both long- and short-term cultures of porcine granulosa cells (815). Therefore, a critical local interaction of growth factors may fine-tune gonadotropin-mediated folliculogenesis.

FOLLICULAR DEVELOPMENT DURING THE MENSTRUAL CYCLE OF SUBHUMAN PRIMATES AND HUMAN

Subhuman Primates

Follicles from *Macaca mullata* pass from preantral to antral stages between 200 and 250 μm (82). A significant increase in the mean percentage of follicles 100–200 μm is evident in the periovulatory period, evidently influenced by the midcycle increases in steroids (estrogens?) and gonadotropins (FSH?). Atresia is very limited in preantral follicles from 40 to 159 μm in diameter varying from less than 1% to a maximum of about 3%. Primordial follicles constitute 80–95% of the preantral follicles and range from 26,000 to 242,000 per pair of ovaries. In general, the mean number of preantral follicles varies directly with the size of the primordial follicle pool; similar numbers of primordial and preantral follicles are present in the right and left ovaries (82). As already noted, the interaction of ovarian innervation and follicular development is a field of increasing interest. In the rhesus ovary, primordial follicles are occasionally encountered almost completely surrounded with vasoactive intestinal polypeptide-positive fibers (816). It is suggested that these follicles are being selected for recruitment. The number of sympathetic and sensory fibers reaches a peak at the time of puberty, associated with theca interna and externa. In contrast, ovaries from senescent monkeys (20–27 years) show reduced numbers of vasoactive intestinal polypeptide fibers but no change in sympathetic or sensory nerves.

Small follicles (<100 μm) in cynomolgus monkeys can be classified into four categories: primordial, intermediary, primary, and secondary (817). The first two classes represent nongrowing follicles and constitute the majority of small follicles—approximately 90% in control ovaries. The range of primordial follicles from different animals is considerable (21,200-230,300), but the number in right and left ovaries from the same animal is similar. Administration of human menopausal gonadotropin and FSH for 7 days did not change the distribution of small follicles, but exogenous gonadotropins plus implants of a GnRH agonist significantly increased the number of intermediary follicles. Analysis of correlation between numbers of intermediary and secondary follicles revealed that in the unstimulated or gonadotropin-treated animals there is a positive correlation between the two classes but not in the GnRH-treated group. The results suggest that GnRH partially inhibits follicular growth by blocking the conversion of nongrowing to growing follicles.

Very few antral follicles larger than 1 mm are present during the luteal phase of rhesus until the corpus luteum shows histologic signs of regression in the premenstrual period (818). This coincides with a significant increase in serum FSH without a change in LH levels (e.g., refs. 819,820). The greatest number of atretic follicles throughout the cycle are 0.5–1.0 mm in diameter—medium-sized follicles (818). During the midluteal phase, preantral follicles (<257 μm in diameter) incorporate [^{3}H]thymidine with labeling frequency from 10% in follicles with one layer of granulosa cells to 60% in follicles with six or more layers (821). Hence the failure of advanced follicular development during the luteal phase is not attributable to a deficiency in growing preantral follicles. The limited follicular development during the luteal phase is most likely due to changes in pulse frequency and amplitude of gonadotropins as GnRH pulses are modulated. Thus, in measuring bioactive LH during the early luteal phase, an average of about 1 pulse per 90 min occurs, which changes to 1 pulse per 7–8 h during the late luteal phase (822). During the early follicular phase (days 2–5) the largest healthy follicles are 2 mm or less and there are usually two follicles about the same size. However, by days 7–9 in 3 of 4 sets of ovaries, one follicle was considerably larger than the other and this was further accentuated by days 11–13 (preovulatory stage) when the largest follicle was usually about 6 mm. Based on *in vivo* observations, the largest follicle grows from 1.7 mm to 9.4 mm during the 11 days before the LH surge, and the dominant follicle, destined to ovulate, can be confidently identified 7 days before the peak in 75% of repeated laparoscopies and in 100% of cases by 5 days before the LH peak (823). As the day of the LH peak approaches, the follicle grows at about 1 mm per day compared to 0.5 mm daily 10 days before the LH peak. Peripheral levels of estradiol increase rapidly from days 3 to 0 (the day of the LH surge), presumably reflecting the activity of the dominant follicle.

As follicle diameter increases from 1 to 7 mm, serum FSH decreases, but thereafter increased diameter correlates with rising levels of FSH. Ovulation occurs with equal frequency in each ovary, regardless of the location of the previous corpus luteum (824). By day 8 of the cycle, the ovarian venous effluent on the side of the dominant follicle already contains significantly more estradiol than the contralateral drainage (819). Even on day 8 or 12 of the cycle the dominant follicle may contain as many as 1.2% pyknotic granulosa cells and still be normal. Thus, the presence of 1 or 2 pyknotic nuclei is hardly grounds for classifying any follicle as atretic.

As already mentioned, a technique which has yielded a great deal of useful information about follicular development in large domestic species is extirpation of follicles and corpora lutea and it has been equally successful in primates. Cautery of the largest follicle present on day 10–12 of the rhesus cycle blocks ovulation, and surges of LH and FSH occur 12.4 days later (825). Hence the follicle destined to ovulate was already selected and no others were able to immediately substitute for its loss. Following follicle cautery, basal levels of LH and FSH (measured daily in ketamine-injected monkeys) were relatively stable, although a few monkeys showed slightly elevated levels the next day. Similarly, aspiration of the contents of the dominant follicle on day 10 lengthens the rhesus cycle to 39 days compared to the normal 30 days (826). About 65% of the animals did not have an LH surge on day 10, and it is this group that experienced a lengthened cycle. Following luteectomy, 4–6 days after the LH surge, preoperative levels of LH and FSH were maintained until 12.8 days later when typical midcycle surges of the gonadotropins were observed (825). Ovulation invariably occurred in the contralateral ovary (for references, see ref. 827) and in monkeys with both ovaries present; within 4 days after luteectomy, the contralateral ovary already had more medium-sized (0.5–1.0 mm) and large (1.1–1.5 mm) follicles (819). Another study revealed that after luteectomy on days 17–19 of the cycle, the new dominant follicle always originated on the side opposite the ovarian vein that had the highest concentration of progesterone (828).

The fact that ovulation in about 90% of cases occurred in the contralateral ovary raised the possibility that trauma following follicular ablation or luteectomy might have temporarily affected the ipsilateral ovary. Therefore, the above experiments were repeated in hemiovariectomized rhesus monkeys (827). Under these circumstances, after luteal extirpation a sustained and large increase in serum FSH was always observed, suggesting that in animals with two ovaries the contralateral ovary was responsible for the negative feedback on tonic FSH release—presumably now thought to be due to its production of inhibin. Collectively, these experiments led to the concept of recruitment of follicles at the end of the luteal phase and selection of the dominant follicle by days 5–7 of the follicular phase (for references, see ref. 829).

Presumably the higher levels of FSH in the early follicular phase aid in the selection of the dominant follicle. When charcoal-treated porcine follicular fluid was injected intraperitoneally every 8 h from days 1–4, serum FSH decreased 50 to 80% with no change in LH (830). Following this treatment, on days 10–14, the dominant follicle was much smaller than usual and contained very few granulosa cells; *in vitro* these cells secreted negligible amounts of progesterone and did not luteinize. Moreover, within 4 days the cells became necrotic. When porcine follicular fluid was administered daily from days 1–3, serum FSH was depressed from days 2 to 4, followed by a rebound to elevated levels on day 6 (820). Nevertheless, the animals ovulated with a follicular phase comparable in duration to control cycles. The resultant corpus luteum, secreted significantly less progesterone during the first half of the luteal phase.

Porcine follicular fluid administered from days 1 to 5 or days 6 to 12 significantly reduced serum FSH concentrations and estradiol without affecting LH (831). After cessation of porcine follicular fluid there was a rebound in FSH levels. Treatment during menses led to a delay in midcycle FSH and LH peaks until day 17 with formation of a normal, functional corpus luteum. On the other hand, when porcine follicular fluid was deferred until days 6–12, midcycle gonadotropin surges were delayed until day 26. It appears that the early treatment deferred appearance of the dominant follicle, whereas later treatment resulted in atresia. The dominant follicle, therefore, requires the continued presence of FSH throughout its development.

Cynomolgus monkeys injected daily with a GnRH antagonist to suppress gonadotropin secretion were then infused with FSH and LH delivered as 1 pulse/h (832). When plasma estradiol began to increase, the dose of FSH infused was reduced 12.5% per day and estradiol levels rose similar to the profile observed during the normal follicular phase. The conclusion is that the developing follicle continues to develop and secrete estrogen in the face of falling titers of FSH. It is proposed that exquisite sensitivity of negative feedback control of FSH release by estradiol therefore blocks smaller subordinate follicles from developing and consequently they become atretic. Furthermore, multiple follicles mature if the duration of pulsatile FSH treatment is prolonged. This argues against the dominant follicle inhibiting the growth of smaller follicles by decreasing their responsiveness to FSH and LH. The hypothesis is contrary to speculation that follicular regulatory protein production or other paracrine factors act locally to inhibit growth of other members of the follicular cohort.

Cynomolgus monkeys were infused with GnRH (1 pulse/h) with continuous infusion of an ovine antiestradiol superimposed for 20 days (833). This led to a sustained rise in serum FSH and LH and this was reflected in increased follicular development: 28 follicles larger than 2 mm compared to nine follicles in control animals. This reinforces the suppressive effects of estrogen on both FSH and LH in primates.

At least in the marmoset, granulosa cells from large follicles (>2.0 mm) secrete high concentrations of inhibin, which are responsive to LH *in vitro* (834). Granulosa cells from small follicles produce low amounts of inhibin, but FSH stimulates higher levels and FSH + testosterone or FSH + estradiol synergize to produce maximal amounts of inhibin.

The clear opposite of reducing serum FSH levels by porcine follicular fluid is to increase circulating levels by treatment with human menopausal gonadotropin (831). When human menopausal gonadotropin was administered from days 1 to 3 or 4 to 6, estradiol secretion increased immediately as more follicles were recruited. However, when human menopausal gonadotropin was administered after day 7 (when the dominant follicle has emerged) the other follicles were now unable to respond with increased estradiol secretion; presumably most of them were now atretic. Thus, after the selection of the dominant follicle, the other follicles, members of the same cohort, are unresponsive. Evidence has been presented that a follicular regulatory protein produced by the dominant follicle supresses estrogen production by other developing antral follicles without affecting FSH levels; it is therefore distinct from inhibin (reviewed in ref. 829). The maturing follicle in cynomolgus monkeys is the source of increasing titers of estradiol. When estradiol antibodies are infused from days 5 to 10, after unilateral ovariectomy on day 0, serum FSH and LH increases, and 10 days after hemispaying the remaining ovary of three animals contained two, two, and four large follicles (835). According to this interpretation, the dominant follicle's production of estrogen acts as the principal modulator of development of other follicles by its ability to suppress gonadotropin levels. This again is contrary to the notion that a follicular regulatory protein produced by the dominant follicle accounts for its outstripping the other members of the cohort.

Another approach to analyzing follicular development in the rhesus is to induce follicular atresia by Silastic implants of estradiol on days 5 to 7 of the cycle (see references in ref. 836). The resultant serum concentrations of estradiol of 100–400 pg/ml for 24 h, led to transient declines in FSH and LH, followed by a rebound and unusually high levels of both hormones on day 8. Dierschke and colleagues (836) believe that exogenous estrogen acts directly at the ovary or indirectly by the transitory depression of FSH to induce follicular atresia. It seems equally plausible that the rebound in LH is responsible for atresia: injection of hCG (1,000 IU) on day 9 or 11, prior to the spontaneous midcycle surges of LH and FSH, leads to apparent atresia of the dominant follicle as evidenced by the absence of midcycle increases in peripheral estrogen and gonadotropins (837). Progesterone administration by injection or Silastic implants on day 6 of the rhesus cycle similarly affects the dominant follicle resulting in very low levels of serum estradiol (30–50 pg/ml) maintained throughout the course of treatment (for references, see ref. 838).

During the follicular phase of the rhesus cycle, as follicles increase in size from 3 to 6 mm to 6 to 8 mm, follicular fluid estrogen increases from 100 ng/ml to 2,200 ng/ml (839) in agreement with the estrogen-activated follicles already described for other species. *In vitro* progesterone secretion and morphologic luteinization of granulosa cells are minimal for cells cultured for 2–8 days, from follicles smaller or larger than 6 mm (839). On the other hand, follicles removed during the early LH surge (when they are 6–8 mm) or mid-LH surge (10–11 mm) show *in vitro* morphologic luteinization of granulosa cells and significant progesterone secretion by granulosa and thecal cells. Moreover, the theca (without the addition of an androgen precursor) produces considerable amounts of estrogen, whereas the granulosa cells are inactive.

These results have been confirmed in short-term (3-h) incubations of granulosa and thecal cells from dominant follicles removed on day 12 of the rhesus cycle—2 days before the normal LH surge (840). The follicles were 5.2 mm in diameter and contained 3.32×10^6 granulosa cells. A tritiated exchange assay with [^{3}H]1,2-androstenedione (a measure of aromatase activity) showed that granulosa cells produced 341 fmol of ^3H_2O compared to 89 fmol by thecal cells. In this connection, when peripheral estradiol was greater than 150 pg/ml, aspiration of as many granulosa cells as possible from the dominant follicle results 15 min later in a fall of about 70% in the concentrations of progesterone, estradiol, and androstenedione from preaspiration levels (841).

A paper that has aroused considerable interest involves indirect immunocytochemical localization of estrogen and progesterone receptors in ovaries of cynomolgus throughout the menstrual cycle (842). Estrogen receptors were never detected in any ovarian component, whereas progesterone receptors were conspicuous in theca interna and externa. The important point is that the granulosa cells never displayed either receptor except in the follicle after the LH surge when the cells undergoing luteinization began to show progesterone receptors. However, these conclusions have been challenged in a recent study in which the presence of estrogen receptor in the rhesus ovary was documented by immunocytochemistry and steroid autoradiography (843). The receptor, by both procedures, was localized in antral follicles in granulosa and theca cells, interstitium, germinal epithelium, and very intensively in the corpus luteum. The estrogen binding was specific, competitive, and saturable. The reasons for the discrepancy between the two papers is unknown and especially difficult to determine, since the same monoclonal antibody (H222) to the estrogen receptor was used in both studies. In the baboon ovary, estrogen receptors are present in 30–40% of the granulosa cells of healthy antral follicles but the theca "were largely unlabeled" (844). Only a few preantral follicles were positive. This immunocytochemical study also used the H222 antibody. The results of the latter two studies with rhesus and baboon are consistent with results in the human ovary (see below).

In the immature cynomolgus (12–22 months) the hypothalamic-pituitary axis is immature, but exogenous GnRH can stimulate the ovary (cited in ref. 845). When juvenile monkeys were injected for 14 days with diethylstilbestrol or diethylstilbestrol plus a GnRH antagonist (to further eliminate endogenous gonadotropins as factors) the number of preantral and medium-sized follicles was reduced (845). The reduction was not associated with an increase in early atretic follicles. It is thus concluded that exogenous estrogen rather than stimulating antral follicular growth actually inhibits development. A recent review (846) sums up the literature, which shows that the well-established direct role of estrogen on follicular development in the rat may not apply to all species. The area is obviously in a state of flux.

Several features in folliculogenesis in the marmoset also differ from the rat. For example, GnRH binding sites are lacking in granulosa cells, as well as in other primates (847). A GnRH agonist did not inhibit FSH action on steroidogenesis or cAMP production. A GnRH agonist analogue partially suppressed estradiol and progesterone and cAMP. In rat granulosa cells, the same dose of GnRH reduced steroid and cAMP to 10–20% of control levels. Granulosa cells from small marmoset follicles also do not show any synergistic interactions of estradiol and FSH on progesterone accumulation or aromatase activity (848), again contrary to the rat. However, if the cells are exposed to estradiol for 48 h and then to FSH, there is a greater increase in steroidogenesis than to FSH alone.

The issue of effects of estrogen on the primate follicle is far from resolved, since the application of other tests for estrogen binding and combined theca and granulosa cell incubations may very well yield contradictory results.

Human

Until recently, quantitative histologic analyses of the human ovary were extremely limited—for obvious reasons. It is well established that the number of primordial and growing (>100 μm) follicles diminish with age: *primordial* ages 6 to 9: 484,000 compared to 8,236 at ages 40 to 44; *growing* ages 6 to 9: 15,220 compared to 6,190 at ages 40 to 44 (77). The number of graafian follicles (>1 mm) averaged 63 per pair of ovaries over the same time span, with only three of seven women having follicles in this size range at ages 40 to 44. Another frequently cited study dealt with follicular development during the menstrual cycle, with histologic evaluation of the endometrium used to date the ovaries (849). The heart of the paper is Table 21, based on 17 ovaries from women aged 18 to 33 y. The table shows the gradual emergence during the late follicular phase (days 11–14) of a large viable follicle, 10–13 mm in diameter, whereas on day 1 of the cycle the largest follicles are 3–4 mm. There are more small antral follicles from 1 to 2 mm in diameter present from days 12 to 14 (15.2 per ovary) than in the earlier follicular phase; the number of healthy small follicles declines in the earlier luteal phase (days 16–18) to an average of 8.5 per ovary with the maximal number present from days 20 to 27 (28 per ovary). Although a heroic amount of effort went into Block's studies (849), the knowledge gained was rather limited.

The situation has dramatically changed by a series of interesting and provocative findings by Alain Gougeon (78,850). The studies are based on histologic analyses of ovaries of 33 women with regular menstrual cycles (28 ± 2 days) and ovariectomized for extraovarian pathology. Days of the cycle were judged on plasma levels of estradiol, progesterone, LH, FSH, and, in some instances, by endometrial biopsy. Serial sections (10 μm) were cut for each ovary; both ovaries were available for sectioning from 22 patients.

Some of the salient findings are outlined in Table 6. The follicles are classified in 8 stages, based primarily on diameter and number of granulosa cells. Estimates of the doubling time of granulosa cells is calculated from *in vitro* determinations of the mitotic time (which turned out to be similar to the ewe [712]) and the mitotic index (851). Based on these estimates, the times spent in each class of follicular development are listed in Table 6. The mean time for a preantral follicle (Stage 1) to ovulate is about 85 to 90 days, thus entailing development over 3-1/2 cycles. Note in Table 6 that the most active stages in granulosa proliferation occur in classes 4–7. The overall rates of atresia are also shown in Table 6. Atresia of follicles 1 to 2 mm, classes 1–4, is relatively constant throughout the menstrual cycle and unaffected by cyclic hormone changes (852). In contrast, for classes 5 and 6, the atretic rate is higher and inversely proportional to circulating gonadotropin levels and highest during the

TABLE 6. *Follicular development in the human ovary*

Class of follicle	Description and time of entry into class	Diameter and number of granulosa cells	Mitotic index of granulosa cells	Time in each class (days)	Atretic follicles[a] (%)
1	Preantral with theca: Cycle 1 Luteal	190–240 μm 3–5 × 10^3	3.8	25	23.6
2	Beginning antrum: Cycle 2 End follicular phase	400 μm 15 × 10^3	4.1	20	35.4
3	Antral: Cycle 3 Follicular phase	1 mm 75 × 10^3	5.3	15	15.3
4	Antrum: Cycle 3 Midcycle phase	2 mm 375 × 10^3	8.5	10	24.2
5	Antrum: Cycle 3 Late luteal phase	5 mm 1.9 × 10^6	10.1	5	58.0
6	Antrum: Cycle 4 Early follicular phase	10 mm 9.4 × 10^6	10.6	5	76.8
7	Antrum: Cycle 4 Midfollicular phase	16 mm 47 × 10^6	10.7	5	50.0
8	Preovulatory: Cycle 4 Late follicular phase	20 mm 60 × 10^6	5.2[b] 0.5[c]	5	0

From Gougeon, refs. 78 and 850.
[a] Throughout cycle.
[b] Before LH surge.
[c] After LH surge.

early and midluteal phase, when almost all class 8 follicles are atretic. Table 6 lists the overall mitotic indices throughout the cycle (851). These rates, however, are not constant, and there is an especially brisk increase for classes 5 and 6 follicles at the end of the cycle (day 28) (852). Analysis of the largest healthy and atretic follicles throughout the cycle revealed that the dominant follicle could be identified by size during the early follicular phase—days 1 to 5—although morphologically it did not differ in vascularization, thecal, or granulosa development from other healthy follicles. By days 6 and 10, the dominant follicle (now 13.3 mm) did differ in these features from other healthy follicles (525). Excluding the dominant follicle, the next healthiest follicle never exceeded 6 mm in the follicular phase and 4 mm in the luteal phase. Based on the mitotic index, follicles 2–5 mm in diameter (classes 4 and 5 in Table 6) are very active in the late luteal phase and represent the population from which the dominant follicle may be already selected. It is interesting that the largest healthy follicle was invariably located on the ovary contralateral to the previous ovulation (525). A subsequent study showed that ovulation occurred in 87.6% of cases on the ovary opposite to the previous ovulation (853). This conclusion was based on the ability to histologically identify the age of the corpus luteum over 5 cycles. If the histologic criteria are valid, this would be quite contrary to previous assertions that ovulation in the human is a random event, uninfluenced by the side of the last corpus luteum. The pattern of alternating ovulations is explained on the basis of differences in the intraovarian hormonal milieu, such that a 5-day asynchrony exists in the population of follicles developing in the "ovulating" ovary or the contralateral one (854). It is proposed that this local effect comes into play when the follicles begin to develop an antral cavity (class 2). The follicles on the side of the corpus luteum, that is, the ovulating ovary, have a significantly higher mitotic index but are smaller in size than in the contralateral side; in the next cycle classes 3 and 4 follicles now develop earlier in the ipsilateral nonovulating ovary. Alternation of ovulation is an interesting and unsettling phenomenon if true; ultrasonography should be able to show whether, in fact, it is occurring. Unfortunately, such evidence from normal, spontaneously cyclic women is still unavailable. Table 6 shows when follicles pass from one stage to another during the menstrual cycle, illustrating how a class 1 follicle that will ovulate approximately 3 months later is selected. It is postulated that follicles move continuously out of the resting pool into class 1 and that the growth of follicles less than 2 mm requires only small amounts of gonadotropins, whereas larger sizes are influenced by cyclic changes in gonadotropin levels (855). The critical step for class 1 follicles is whether their development is initiated in the periovulatory period. These "privileged" follicles develop a theca under the influence of high levels of LH at the midcycle surge; consequently, these follicles may have greater ability to produce androgens which transported to the granulosa compartment enhance estrogen secretion (the last speculation is by G.S.G.). Class 1 follicles developing at other times during the cycle are destined to become atretic at some stage of their subsequent history. Thus, a class 1 follicle fortuitously emerging in the proper hormonal milieu is the one selected to ovulate. This scheme proposes a very early stage for follicular selection and is probably too rigid. There is more leeway in the system as evidenced by the effects of administering human menopausal gonadotropin, which acts on much more advanced classes of follicles (see below).

Additional insight in the hormonal regulation of the human follicle is provided in studies using a potent GnRH antagonist (Nal-Glu) to disrupt gonadotropin release (856). When the antagonist is injected subcutaneously for 3 days in the midfollicular phase, LH falls by 75% by 2 days of treatment and FSH declines by 21 ± 10% (not significant). Estradiol was reduced to the limits of detection of the radioimmunoassay and returned to pretreatment values 6 days after the last injection of Nal-Glu. Cycle length was prolonged to 37 vs 26 days and ultrasound examination revealed that the largest follicle at the onset of treatment regressed and was replaced by a new dominant follicle. Similar treatment at the late follicular phase—when the follicle was 16 mm—caused a now significant decrease in FSH (47%) and a 65% decrease in LH. Ultrasonography revealed that follicular growth was retarded, but ultimately the initial dominant follicle recovered and the follicular phase was lengthened from 12.6 to 19.2 days.

Another study used the same GnRH antagonist, administered for 3 or 4 consecutive days, with treatment initiated when the lead follicle (by ultrasonography) was 16–18 mm (857). A nice feature of the experimental design was that the women were monitored through two consecutive menstrual cycles: a control and treatment cycle. Serum LH and FSH reached their nadirs on the fourth day of treatment—approximately 10% of baseline levels. Similar to the previous study, the dominant follicle ovulated in 8 of 10 cycles. The gonadotropin surge occurred 4 days later. Thus, as the dominant follicle approaches the time of ovulation it becomes more and more independent of circulating levels of FSH and LH, presumably because of its greater numbers of FSH and LH receptors.

The point remains that the overwhelming number of follicles leaving the resting pool undergo atresia. It must be kept in mind, however, that even large preovulatory follicles (12–27 mm in diameter) contain pyknotic nuclei (1 ± 0.2%), but this is balanced by a moderate mitotic index (4.6 ± 0.8%) (319). In contrast, frankly atretic large follicles (>6 mm) have a high pyknotic index (10.9 ± 2.1%) 2 days before the LH surge. Healthy dominant human follicles show a strong reaction for 3β-hydroxysteroid dehydrogenase in the theca and limited activity in the granulosa; it is not until after the LH surge that an intense reaction develops in the granulosa cells. Follicles in advanced atresia show low or moderate 3β-hydroxysteroid dehydrogenase activity in the theca and almost none in the granulosa.

Criteria proposed for determining whether a follicle has the potential for further development are whether it contains (a) more than 50% of the maximal complement of granulosa cells for its size and (b) a normal oocyte (378). Thus, a 4-mm follicle has about 1×10^6 granulosa cells and a 12-mm normal follicle has 10×10^6 granulosa cells. Based on these criteria and concentration of steroids in follicular fluid, 90% of follicles larger than 1 mm in diameter were undergoing degenerative changes. After reaching a diameter of 4 mm only one or at most two follicles per follicular phase of the cycle are capable of continued mitotic activity to reach the 50–100 million granulosa cells characteristic of the preovulatory follicle. According to the aforementioned histologic studies of Gougeon and hormonal correlates from antral fluid (858), it is evident that the follicle destined to ovulate has normally emerged by days 1 to 5 as a healthy 4-mm follicle. On day 1 of the cycle, although the dominant follicle can not be grossly identified, ovarian venous plasma collected from both ovaries of a few patients already shows unilateral higher concentrations of progesterone, estradiol, and estrone and this is even more apparent by days 4–9 and thereafter when a large follicle can be identified (859–861). Moreover, by the midfollicular phase, high unilateral concentrations of the above steroids in ovarian effluent are also associated with asymmetry in levels of androstenedione and testosterone.

Granulosa cells harvested from 6- to 9 mm follicles on day 9, produce small amounts of estradiol (2 ng/10^6 cells) for 3 h with 10^{-7} M testosterone or androstenedione but show an eightfold increase when FSH is combined with either of the androgens (422). In contrast, granulosa cells collected from a large dominant follicle (20 mm), accumulate 60 ng estradiol/10^6 cells/3 h in the presence of testosterone and FSH has no synergistic action. Thus, the early developing follicle depends on FSH for regulation of aromatase enzymes in granulosa cells. It is interesting that 5α reduced androgens, at physiologic concentrations, can inhibit aromatization of testosterone in FSH-stimulated granulosa cells of small follicles (5–9 mm) (422).

For follicles less than 8 mm in diameter, the follicular fluid concentration of FSH is maximal at the early follicular, early luteal, and late luteal phases, during or just after peak levels of FSH in peripheral plasma (862). Large follicles appear during the midfollicular phase with 38% having detectable levels of FSH in follicular fluid; 11% of these follicles contain measurable amounts of LH. By the late follicular phase, 83% of large follicles have detectable FSH in follicular fluid and 70% of these follicles similarly have LH present. Follicles with high concentrations of FSH in follicular fluid also have a high ratio of estradiol to androstenedione in antral fluid (863). Judged by ultrasound scanning, the volume and diameter of the dominant follicle averaged 9.8 mm (range: 6–13 mm) 5 days before ovulation and thereafter an exponential growth phase ensued, culminating in a maximal diameter of 21 ± 3.5 mm (SD) with a range from 14 to 28 mm (864). During the 9 days post-LH peak, all follicles from 4 to 10 mm are usually atretic, based on histologic criteria (177). Such follicles invariably have an androstenedione:estradiol ratio greater than unity (865). Progesterone concentrations in follicular fluid are maximal in the late follicular phase, which correlates with detectable antral fluid levels of LH and FSH (865). Progesterone secretion by granulosa cells increases from 6 to 30 μg/24 h/10^6 cells as follicles enlarge from 5 to 25 mm (866).

Transvaginal ultrasound examination of normal cycling women provides a method for visualizing all follicles larger than 2 mm (867). During the early and late follicular phases and luteal phase, the mean number of follicles did not differ between the dominant and nondominant ovaries: 5.9 and 7.4 for the dominant ovary versus 5.8 to 7.5 for the nondominant ovary. The dominant follicle was first detectable on average 1.4 days before the LH surge, at a mean diameter of approximately 10 mm. At this time, the next largest follicle was on average 6 mm in diameter. The dominant follicle measured approximately 21 mm at the LH surge, whereas the nondominant follicles never exceeded 11 mm.

Addition of LH to granulosa cells from follicles of 5–15 mm diameter enhances progesterone secretion by 2.5-fold but does not stimulate further increases in larger follicles. For 5- to 18-mm follicles, 5 μg estradiol/ml significantly decreases progesterone secretion, with almost 60% inhibition of progesterone by granulosa cells from 18-mm follicles (866). Luteinizing hormone receptors in one or two of the largest follicles for various days of the follicular phase have now been determined (868). Baseline binding capacity is minimal on days 0 and 1 of the cycle and by days 7–14 a threefold increase occurs. As to be expected, atretic follicles on days 18 and 22 have reduced binding. These results are consistent with an earlier study based on granulosa cells, utilizing labeled hCG (869). The number of hCG binding sites increased from 0.82 ± 5 (fmol/mg protein) on days 5–6 compared to 1.36 ± 0 on day 13. These results agree with findings in every species that has been investigated, that is, follicular maturation is associated with increased LH (hCG) binding in the granulosal compartment.

Prolactin in follicular fluid is maximal in the early follicular phase and falls to lowest levels during the late follicular phase for all sized follicles with a second peak in the midluteal stage (862). In situations where peripheral levels of prolactin are greater than 100 ng/ml, 96% of the follicles lack detectable amounts of FSH and antral fluid concentration of estradiol is depressed (865). In addition, accompanying hyperprolactinemia, follicles greater than 4 mm were apparently undergoing atresia, based on the reduced number of granulosa cells for their diameter.

In large preovulatory follicles, both diced theca and granulosa cells appear capable of producing progesterone, androstenedione, and estradiol with progesterone the dominant steroid secreted by granulosa cells and androstenedione the major thecal product (for references, see ref. 870). When expressed as ng steroid/mg protein × 2 h, thecal and granulosa cells release estradiol at approximately the same rate in the absence or presence of hCG (870). In contrast, collagenase dispersed thecal and granulosa cells, incubated with a fixed amount of testosterone, show that granulosa cells have at least 700 times the aromatase activity of the theca when expressed as steroid/10^5 cells/24 h (422). Considerable differences in experimental design make it difficult to compare the two studies.

Based on these findings and others, McNatty (858,865) proposes that a preantral follicle destined for further development is transformed to an antral stage concurrent with high levels of FSH in plasma and its antral fluid. The latter minimizes atresia by increasing mitotic activity of granulosa cells and increasing aromatase activity in the cells, thus enhancing estrogen secretion. The combined interactions of FSH and estrogen act as a positive feedback to further enhance granulosa cell mitosis and estrogen accumulation in the follicle. The action of LH on the theca stimulates androstenedione, which in the favored follicle is converted to estrogens, thus further shifting the estrogen:androgen ratio. Preantral follicles not emerging when the concentration of follicular fluid FSH can be increased are therefore much more likely to be androgenic follicles and hence prone to atresia.

The potential to recruit follicles for ovulation obviously encompasses larger follicles—presumably around 4 mm at the onset of the follicular phase—as demonstrated by the ability of human menopausal gonadotropin or FSH administered on days 3 and 4 to increase the number of oocytes induced by hCG administered on day 8 (see ref. 871 for further references). Injection of human menopausal gonadotropin at the late luteal phase instead of the early follicular phase is even more successful in increasing the mitotic index of granulosa cells and increasing the induced ovulation rate to 3.7 ova (872). As previously mentioned, the secondary FSH surge, at the transition between the luteal and follicular phase, is believed to be the trigger for the next cohort of follicles to mature during the next follicular phase. A clear-cut increase in FSH is evident beginning about 15 days after the LH surge, at a time when LH remains at baseline levels (873). Frequent blood samples were taken over a 48-hour period at different times during the luteal-follicular shift. An increase in serum FSH occurred 11 days after the LH surge. This correlates with a dramatic increase in LH pulse frequency: from approximately 3 pulses/24 hours to 13.5 pulses and is inversely related to the log of serum progesterone. Pulsatile FSH secretion is rarely seen during the menstrual cycle but is observed during the transitional period with 80% of the FSH pulses concomitant with LH pulses. The most logical interpretation of these findings is that, as progesterone reaches its nadir, GnRH pulse frequency increases with serum FSH rising "3.5-fold compared to a 2-fold increase in mean LH" (873).

The human—like the rhesus—responds to removal of the dominant follicle or corpus luteum by ovulating 12.7 and 14.6 days later, respectively (874). Following either procedure, ovulation invariably occurs in the ipsilateral ovary, contrary to the situation in the rhesus. Unlike the rhesus, there is a clear-cut, transient increase in FSH and LH after follicular ablation in the human (529,875). Whether a true species difference exists or whether effects of anesthesia are responsible remains to be established. It would indeed be unusual if recruitment of the next follicle in the rhesus is not associated with transient increases in gonadotropins. The restraining influence of the human corpus luteum on gonadotropin levels is evident.

Contrary to the conflicting findings in the cynomolgus monkey (842), estrogen receptors are present in the human preovulatory follicle, as demonstrated by immunohistochemistry (876). Estrogen receptors are undetectable in primordial or preantral follicles and reach their peak in granulosa cells before the LH surge and thereafter decline rapidly. Progesterone receptors are present in theca interna and first appear in granulosa cells after the LH surge. Granulosa cells obtained from follicles aspirated 36 h after hCG administration cultured for several days—and therefore really granulosa-lutein cells—increase $P\text{-}450_{SSC}$ and progesterone secretion in response to either FSH, hCG, or cAMP (877). On the other hand, $P\text{-}450_{17\alpha}$ mRNA was not demonstrable after any of the treatments. A very interesting and thorough study involved harvesting immature granulosa cells during the late luteal phase or the first part of the follicular phase compared to mature cells from follicles during the second half of the follicular phase, before the LH surge (878). For the immature cells the ratio of [^{3}H]thymidine uptake to progesterone secretion was tenfold greater than for granulosa-lutein cells in basal incubations. FSH, but not LH, in two of four cases increased DNA synthesis in immature granulosa cells, whereas the reverse was true for mature granulosa. Regardless of the maturity of the granulosa cells, insulinlike growth factor-I (IGF-I) stimulated DNA synthesis as well as steroidogenesis. These results suggest an inverse relationship between proliferation and steroid synthesis of granulosa cells as they differentiate consistent with observations in other species. Somewhat divergent results were found in another study; FSH greatly enhanced basal production of progesterone by granulosa cells from normal and stimulated follicles, ranging from 5 to 20 mm in diameter (879). By itself, IGF-I was ineffective in stimulating progesterone production, but when combined with physiologic amounts of FSH or hCG there was a marked amplification in responsiveness. In a previous study, the estrogen responsiveness of the same granulosa preparations was evaluated with the cells cultured with androstenedione, hCG, FSH, or IGF-I (880). Estradiol production was stimulated to the same extent by FSH or IGF-I, but IGF-I acted synergistically with either FSH or hCG to produce about a fourfold increase in estradiol secretion. Whereas IGF-I stimulates and sustains *in vitro* $P\text{-}450_{arom}$ activity by granulosa cells, epidermal growth factor inhibits FSH-stimulated estradiol production of granulosa cells aspirated from normal follicles under 10 mm in diameter (881). The essentiality of IGF-I for follicular granulosal proliferation and differentiation is questioned in a study involving a Laron-type dwarf, where IGF-I deficiency exists secondary to growth hormone receptor abnormalities (882). During two courses of IVF treatment, serum estradiol was elevated despite barely measurable IGF-I and very high levels of IGFBP-I (binding protein). Aspirated follicular fluid showed the same profiles of IGF-I and IGFBP-1 but normal levels of estradiol and progesterone. Thus, the role of IGF-I in normal follicular development requires critical evaluation. Of course, the possibility exists that other growth factors could be acting in lieu of IGF.

As mentioned earlier, studies on fresh human ovarian materials are limited, and very few studies are documented using unstimulated, premenopausal human follicular tissues. Using an enzymatic dissociation procedure, preantral human follicles were isolated from ovaries of premenopausal women and cultured for 5 days in a serum-free defined medium (553). Class 1 and 2 follicles have 2 and 5 or 6 layers of granulosa cells, respectively, but no theca. In these studies the follicles showed significant increases in DNA content and [^{3}H]-thymidine incorporation when stimulated by human FSH. Moreover, class 2 preantral follicles developed into antral follicles within 5 days in response to FSH, while follicles in control cultures became atretic. Follicular steroidogenesis (progesterone, androstenedione, estradiol) also showed a significant rise following FSH exposure. These results corroborate the findings on hamster preantral follicles and provide strong and direct evidence that, like the hamster, the growth of human preantral follicles depends on FSH.

Among all the growth factors already described, IGF-I has been studied relatively extensively in relation to human follicular activities. Granulosa cells obtained from premenopausal women possess insulin and insulin receptors but not IGF-I binding sites (883). Contrary to these findings, granulosa cells obtained from follicles stimulated by clomiphene and human menopausal gonadotropins (as a part of IVF programs) respond *in vitro* to IGF-I to produce significantly higher amounts of $P\text{-}450_{arom}$ message and enzyme than control cells; however, epidermal growth factor attenuates FSH-induced aromatase activity in these cells (884), suggesting that human granulosa cells do have IGF-I receptors. The caveat, of course, is that the latter cells are exposed to high levels of exogenous hormones. When human granulosa cells from single follicles from spontaneous and hMG-hCG-stimulated cycles are exposed to a physiologic concentration of IGF-I (ED_{50} = 8 ng/ml), a significant increase in estradiol-17β production is observed. Moreover, IGF-I shows a synergistic effect with FSH in stimulating granulosa cell estradiol production (880), thus further attesting to the presence of IGF-I receptors in human granulosa cells and suggesting the possible role of IGF-I in human follicular activity. Granulosa cells from cystic follicles also respond to IGF-I in producing estradiol-17β (885). Recently, using 3′- and 5′-specific antisense probes for IGF-I and RNase protection assays, IGF-I message has been detected in whole premenopausal and menopausal ovaries but not in the granulosa cell compartment (886). The molecular data have been substantiated by immunocytochemical findings. On the contrary, mRNA for IGF-II has been localized in luteinized granulosa cells as well. The genes for IGF-I and IGF-II receptors, on the other hand, do not show any cellular specificity (886). These lines of evidence suggest that IGF-I and possibly IGF-II play significant local regulatory roles in human folliculogenesis. Fluid from cystic follicles of polycystic ovary syndrome contains significantly higher concentration of IGFBP than healthy follicles, thus establishing a reciprocal relationship between IGFBP expression and follicular health (887).

Transforming growth factor (TGF)-βs are members of a superfamily of related polypeptides including mullerian inhibiting substance inhibin and activin. Recent immunohistochemical studies on premenopausal human ovary have also shown that TGF-β_1 immunoreactivity is present in all cell types, while TGF-β_2 is present only in theca and small cells of the corpus luteum (888). No significant changes in TGF-β activities during the menstrual cycle have been noted. Obviously, more physiologic studies on human granulosa and theca cells are needed to reveal whether the activities of human granulosa cells, hence folliculogenesis, are indeed influenced by TGF-βs.

The distribution of the related peptide, mullerian inhibiting substance, has been established by *in situ* hybridization (889). The mRNA is present in highest levels in the cytoplasm of oocytes of primordial follicles with diminished levels as the oocytes mature. Positive staining, but to a lesser extent, was also apparent in the granulosa cells of primordial, preantral, and antral follicles. A point worth reiterating is the presence in the mammalian oocyte of a variety of growth factors and gonadotropin binding sites. Inhibin has been demonstrated in the granulosa cells of several species and in human follicular fluid (for references, see ref. 890). Measurement of plasma inhibin, estradiol, and progesterone during the menstrual cycle shows an excellent correlation between inhibin and estradiol during the follicular phase and inhibin and progesterone during the luteal phase, suggesting that both follicles and corpus luteum are the sources of inhibin.

FOLLICULAR DEVELOPMENT DURING PREGNANCY

This topic is of interest for several reasons:

1. Is there any "wavelike" development of follicles during pregnancy comparable to the length of the estrous cycle and, therefore, recurring every *n* days?
2. How does the negative feedback effect of high steroid levels affect the hypothalamic-pituitary axis and hence follicular growth?
3. In species in which corpora lutea are essential throughout pregnancy and produce progesterone as the main hormone, the follicles obviously are the principal source of ovarian estrogens.
4. Are follicles developing during pregnancy "mature" enough to ovulate in response to hCG?

Follicular development in the pregnant mouse can be divided into three stages:

1. From days 1 to 8 (day 1 = morning after mating) the largest follicles present are up to 473 μm in diameter and atresia of large follicles is minimal.
2. From days 10 to 14, follicular atresia is maximal and the largest follicles are usually 373 μm or less.
3. From days 16 to 19, follicular atresia is again minimal, and from day 18 on, large follicles reappear in preparation for postpartum ovulation (891).

This profile correlates with the ability to induce ovulation with 5 IU hCG. Thus, between days 12 and 14 only 37% of the injected animals ovulate, reaching the nadir at day 12 when the mean number of ovulations is 5.2—only half the normal number. The subcutaneous injection of 5 IU PMS on day 10 followed by hCG on day 12 results in 91% of the mice ovulating an average of 11.2 ova (891).

When pregnant mice were pulse-labeled by injecting [^{3}H]thymidine, small to large follicles were labeled on every day, which shows that there is continuous growth of follicles (96). At any time during pregnancy about 14 small follicles began to grow compared to 19 per day during the estrous cycle, but there is no difference in the transit time. It is interesting that the labeling index of types 6 and 7 follicles (incipient formation of antral cavity and coalesced cavity, respectively) tend to decrease during midpregnancy (cf. above results on induced ovulation with hCG). It was estimated that type 3b follicles (with 21–60 granulosa cells) moving out of the resting pool on day 1 of pregnancy are the ones that ultimately ovulate at postpartum estrus.

These morphologic findings show interesting correlations with the gonadotropin pattern during mouse pregnancy. Using 50 μl of plasma, there are peaks in LH on days 4 and 11 of gestation with no significant changes in FSH throughout this period (892). However, from days 12 to 15, LH is frequently undetectable in the amount of plasma assayed, whereas plasma FSH does not differ from earlier values. On the day of parturition, there is a sharp increase in both FSH and LH (892) coincident with follicular kinetics being restored to the pattern characteristic of the estrous cycle (96).

Follicular growth and gonadotropin profiles are quite different between the pregnant mouse and rat. Until day 14 of pregnancy in the rat, healthy follicles up to 600 μm are present, but this is followed by a hiatus on days 16 and 18 when the largest antral follicles are only 400 to 500 μm. Differentiation of larger follicles begins on day 20 culminating in follicles larger than 600 μm on day 22 and at delivery on day 23 (893). Follicles 300–400 μm in diameter are always present on every day of pregnancy and are especially abundant on the first 4 days of gestation. Ovulation with 20 IU hCG (sc) could not be induced before day 21, but priming with 25 IU PMS on day 15, 72 h before hCG treatment, resulted in ovulation. It was concluded that, even though medium and large antral follicles are present throughout most of gestation, the follicles were "physiologically immature." Subsequently, several other investigators injected pregnant rats with hCG and the results differed, depending possibly on differences in strain, colony, and route of administration (894). However, the consensus was that days 15 and 16 represented the nadir in follicular responsiveness to hCG.

In this connection, it is interesting that serum levels of FSH and LH are at their lowest values on day 16 with serum LH abruptly increasing on days 20 and 22 and with FSH recovering on day 18 (895). Furthermore, on day 16 the corpora lutea of pregnancy have the highest concentration of estradiol with the lowest levels in the nonluteal ovary, suggesting that between days 14 and 18, secretion of testosterone and estradiol represents proportionately more luteal than follicular activity. Ovarian venous plasma on day 15 of pregnancy also does not contain detectable amounts of inhibin, a further indication of the nonfunctional status of the follicles (896).

Richards and colleagues (897–900) have explored this problem in depth, focusing on follicular development on day 16 of pregnancy. Between days 14 and 19, FSH and hCG binding reach their nadir in granulosa cells and hCG receptors in thecal shells are also minimal (897). This was associated with minimal accumulation of estradiol *in vitro,* although providing testosterone as a substrate increased estrogen levels to values observed on days 4–12. Hence on day 15 the aromatizing system is still intact in the granulosa compartment. Follicular morphology on day 16 revealed that the follicles lacked the features typical of steroidogenically active tissue (898). Following daily injection on days 14 and 15 of 1.5 IU hCG, however, the theca hypertrophied and the orientation of granulosa cells was altered with extensive lipid deposition in both tissues. The most salient finding was that isolated thecal shells produced considerable testosterone *in vitro* after exposure to hCG: from 17 pg per theca per 5 h to 175 pg per theca per 5 h (898). The action of hCG is specific in that twice daily injections of FSH on days 14 and 15 fail to increase thecal LH receptor content or intrinsic ability of follicles to accumulate estradiol (899). The small antral follicles normally present on day 16, when incubated with [^{3}H]progesterone fail to convert it appreciably to labeled 17α-OH progesterone or androgens compared to normal preovulatory follicles on day 23 (900). Collectively, these experiments demonstrate that the relative paucity of serum LH on day 16, accounts for inadequate biochemical development of the theca with a consequent deficit in 17α-hydroxylase and C17-20 lyase. This condition is then reversed by rising titers of LH commencing on day 20 of gestation.

Ovariectomy of pregnant rats on day 7 results 24 h later in highly significant increases in peripheral LH and increased pulse amplitude and frequency of LH (901). When rats were implanted after ovariectomy with estradiol and progesterone capsules all parameters were restored to control levels, but either steroid alone was ineffective, that is both were necessary for the normal negative feedback control of LH. The pregnant rat exhibits postpartum estrus and ovulation and, as previously mentioned, this is associated with renewed follicular growth and abrupt increases in serum FSH (on day 16) and LH (on days 20–22). In intact control pregnant rats, between days 21 and 22 there are significant increases in peripheral LH and the amplitude and pulse frequency; this correlates with unchanged plasma estradiol but with a 60% reduction in progesterone (902). When animals were ovariectomized at day 21 the only major change was increased blood LH; however, replacement with physiologic levels of estradiol and progesterone did not restore all LH parameters to normal values. However, a combination of both steroids and porcine follicular fluid was successful, suggesting a possible role of inhibin. This is consistent with a significant increase in inhibin in ovarian venous plasma at the end of gestation in the rat (896).

Functional luteolysis in the pregnant rat occurs between days 18 and 21 (895) correlating with increased responsiveness to GnRH infusion on day 22 compared to day 18 (903). Rats delivering in the morning have an LH surge in the afternoon and ovulate that night (reference cited in ref. 903). Therefore, an ovulatory cycle is initiated as the luteal activity wanes so that the animals deliver on the equivalent of proestrus (903).

Follicular development in the pregnant hamster is diametrically opposed to the pattern described for the rat. Large healthy antral follicles greater than 415 μm in diameter are always present in the hamster ovary with about 10 per pair of ovaries from days 4 to 10, increasing to a peak of 35 to 40 on day 12 (904). This is paralleled by the ability of hCG to induce ovulation at any time during gestation with a mean number of 10 to 13 ovulations from days 4 to 8, culminating in a peak of 35 ovulations per animal on day 12 (904). Hence at midpregnancy, the hamster matures sufficient follicles to result in superovulation. Healthy follicles 277–322 μm in diameter (the smallest ones measured) were continuously present throughout gestation, indicating constant recruitment of preantral stages. The concentration of FSH on day 1 of the 16-day pregnancy was about fivefold greater than the levels on subsequent days (905). When sampled at 9 A.M. at 2-day intervals throughout pregnancy, serum FSH was approximately twice as great as 9 A.M. proestrous values (180 ng/ml vs 93 ng/ml) and serum LH was 20 ng/ml, which was comparable to 9 A.M. proestrous values (906). In contrast, in the pregnant rat, serum FSH is comparable to proestrous values, but LH ranges from 4 to 8 ng/ml from day 4 to 18, whereas on the morning of proestrus, serum LH is approximately 30 ng (681). Thus, the relative deficiency of LH may account for the differences in follicular development between the pregnant rat and hamster. Hamster follicles *in vitro* can be stimulated by 10 ng LH at any time during gestation to accumulate estradiol, although the response is drastically curtailed by day 16—the day of delivery (906), again a striking difference from the rat.

Follicular development in the pregnancy rabbit resembles the pattern found in the hamster. The intravenous injection of 25 IU hCG up to 12 days of pregnancy results in the ovulation of 11 ova, but similar treatment on day 21 leads to the ovulation of an average of 21 eggs (907). The enhanced ovulatory response to hCG is associated with increasing numbers of antral follicles 1 mm or greater in diameter: on days 8–11 a mean number of 14 follicles compared to day 17 when the ovaries average 23 follicles (907). Serum levels of FSH and LH measured at 3-day intervals throughout rabbit pregnancy do not correlate with the midgestational change in follicular numbers (908), but the sampling intervals tested in the hamster and other species are also not frequent enough for any valid comparisons. In estrous does, approximately half the follicles are less than 1.6 mm or greater in diameter (909). Some of these large follicles contain elevated levels of testosterone and progesterone but low estradiol; presumably these follicles are atretic. After inducing ovulation with hCG, only 15% of the remaining follicles are large, but by day 6 of pseudopregnancy, there is a redistribution with 75% of the follicles now classified as large. Correlated with the recruitment of large follicles, on day 6, the follicles now contain high levels of estradiol, testosterone, and progesterone. Rabbit corpora lutea first become dependent on estrogen on day 6 and the large follicles recruited by the periovulatory surge of FSH on days 1 and 2—with tonic levels of LH—(908) evidently fulfill this need.

The pregnant guinea pig resembles the hamster and rabbit in that large preovulatory follicles (500–700 μm) are present throughout gestation with the peak number attained on day 66 in preparation for postpartum estrus (910,911). Ovulation can be induced at any time in pregnant guinea pigs by the intravenous injection of 50 IU of hCG (912); the follicles on days 8–20 are less sensitive than from days 41 to 62 and the average ovulation rate is about twice as great in the last trimester (2.0 vs 3.9, respectively).

There is very little information available about follicular development during pregnancy in large domestic species. In cross-bred pigs, the total number of follicles up to 8 mm in diameter is greater up to 40 days of gestation, and by 110 days (shortly before delivery) there are no 7- to 8-mm follicles and few in the 4- to 6-mm class (913). Small follicles (1–2 mm) were relatively constant from days 23 to 63 in three breeds of sow, and over the same time span medium follicles (3–5 mm) were also fairly constant with large follicles (6–10 mm) averaging 4.8 per pregnant sow (914).

The number of normal and atretic follicles in the pregnant cow are 32.6% and 67.4%, respectively (754). Follicles larger than 5 mm in diameter are absent throughout pregnancy and in late pregnancy (243 days) the largest follicles are only 2 mm. Small follicles less than 1 mm in diameter are present throughout pregnancy and in fact constitute the dominant group. Despite the paucity of follicular development, plasma estradiol and estrone rise progressively throughout gestation with peak levels reached in the last trimester (915). At term, estrone levels are eight times as high as estradiol; evidently, an extraovarian source of estrogens exists. During bovine gestation, FSH pulses/12 h average 5 or 6 throughout pregnancy, whereas LH pulses average between 1 and 2 in the first and third trimesters and are almost wholly abolished in midgestation (915). The relationship between these peripheral hormone values and follicular quiescence during pregnancy is most likely related to differences from the bovine estrous cycle in which basal levels of progesterone, estradiol, and FSH are considerably less than during gestation and LH pulses per 12 h are 3- to 7-fold greater during the cycle (916). Hence reduced steroid feedback characterizes the estrous cycle with resultant modifications in pulsatile FSH and LH patterns.

Ultrasonography has shed considerable light on follicular dynamics in pregnant heifers. From days 0 to 70 of pregnancy, waves emerge approximately every 9 days (917). During pregnancy, from the second wave on the dominant follicle is invariably smaller compared to the first wave of nonbred and pregnant heifers. In contrast, the largest subordinate follicle (~8 mm in diameter) did not vary from wave to wave. Usually, the subordinate follicle grows for 3 days before further growth is impaired. Interestingly, during pregnancy from wave three and on the corpus luteum and dominant follicle were usually located in opposite ovaries in 75% of all cases (918). During early pregnancy (days 24–36) the largest follicle and total number of follicles were significantly greater in the ovary contralateral to the corpus luteum (919). This inequality in follicular development is abolished by hysterectomy, suggesting that the conceptus or uterus itself is responsible for the local inhibition of follicular development. Determination of follicular aromatase on day 17 of pregnancy showed that contrary to day 17 of the estrous cycle, the subordinate follicle possessed greater aromatase activity and higher follicular fluid concentration of estrogen than the dominant follicle.

Gestation in the ewe lasts 150 days. The total ovarian follicular population was compared between ewes killed at 140 days of pregnancy and day 5 postpartum in nonsuckling ewes (920). Plasma LH and FSH are very low in late gestation (see references in ref. 920), and this is reflected in the paucity of healthy antral follicles greater than 1 mm: 97% of follicles 1 mm or larger were atretic on day 140. At late pregnancy, preantral follicles constituted 76.1% of the total population and 94% were nonatretic. At 5 days postpartum, the number of preantral follicles—even the smallest stage—was significantly increased, suggesting an increased rate of recruitment of primordial follicles possibly in response to increasing gonadotropin levels. As reported for other species, the number of primordial follicles varied considerably from animal to animal ranging from 7,670 to 76,221 in the pregnant ewes.

There are no quantitative accounts available for the human ovary during pregnancy. Up to 10 weeks the ovary is populated by large graafian follicles (averaging 10 mm in diameter) that are atretic based on the usual degenerative status of the ovum, a granulosa layer only three cells thick, and an undeveloped thecal layer (921). This is very similar to the condition of the ovary shortly after ovulation. After 10 weeks, many new graafian follicles differentiate but rarely grow much larger than 4 mm and ultimately all show signs of atresia; degeneration of the granulosa cells is accompanied by excessive development of the theca. A later paper of Govan (922) dealt with ovarian activity from 26 to 40 weeks. During the first 7 weeks, there was little follicular activity, but beginning from 33 weeks until term, graafian follicles up to 2–4 mm reappear with considerable mitotic activity in the granulosa cells. Usually, however, most of these follicles were atretic. When the follicles were approximately 3 mm, mitoses appear in the theca layer and the theca persists after the complete disappearance of granulosa cells, but lacks 3β-ol dehydrogenase. A characteristic finding during pregnancy is the proliferation and luteinization of thecal cells surrounding both normal and atretic follicles (923) presumably in response to the elevated levels of hCG. In another study, involving samples collected at cesarean section, 298 follicles were available for analysis (924). The average diameter (extrapolated from follicular fluid measurements) was 2.75 mm, and degenerative changes were apparent in the failure to recover oocytes from 50% of the follicles; from the remaining follicles, 79% of the recovered oocytes were undergoing lysis. At term no follicles larger than 6 mm were present. After 2 hours of incubation, the predominant steroid released was androstenedione, about eightfold more than progesterone and estradiol (925). High concentrations of prostaglandin E_2 or F_2 (10 μg/ml) significantly increased cAMP formation by the follicles, whereas hCG was ineffective. The still functioning theca was presumably the source of the androgen and also was the tissue responsive to the prostaglandins. During the third trimester of human pregnancy, follicles normally develop to about 6 mm in diameter, and based on flow cytometry, only 7% are judged to be healthy (926). The steroid profiles in follicular fluid differed from aspirates from cycling women by having higher concentrations of progesterone and lower levels of androstenedione in the samples from pregnant women.

These scattered observations indicate that the human ovary is not quiescent during pregnancy but follicles grow only to about 4–6 mm before degenerative changes intervene. The puzzling question is what gonadotropins account for even this limited proliferation of follicles in view of the very low and frequently undetectable levels of FSH during human gestation (927,928). Human chorionic gonadotropin is obviously the principal circulating gonadotropin, and at various times it has been proposed that hCG has intrinsic but variable FSH activity. It is interesting that deglycosylated hCG acts as a partial agonist at the FSH receptor in rat granulosa cells, whereas native hCG shows only negligible cross-reactivity (929). Moreover, the relative binding affinity of deglycosylated hCG for LH receptors is twofold higher than native hCG. It is therefore possible that modified hCG may be able to substitute in part for FSH in stimulating follicular recruitment, but only to a limited extent.

An alternative explanation is that growth of small antral follicles (1–6 mm) may be more dependent on autocrine factors than gonadotropins. In the third trimester of pregnancy, follicular fluid was aspirated (930). The diameter of each follicle was estimated from the volume of fluid collected. The fluid contained very high levels of epidermal growth factor in concentrations severalfold higher than in serum. There was an inverse correlation between follicular diameter and epidermal growth factor concentration. However, follicular concentrations of progesterone and estradiol were unchanged over the range of follicular diameters: an average of 448 nmol/L for progesterone and 156 nmol/L for estradiol.

Very few reports are available on follicular development in pregnant monkeys (for references, see ref. 931). In the pigtailed macaque, serum FSH shows only minor fluctuations throughout pregnancy, and the levels are comparable to those found during the follicular phase of the menstrual cycle. This is distinctly different from the situation in the human. Serum estradiol and estrone begin to increase between days 100 and 120 and peak levels are reached at parturition. Following bilateral ovariectomy at day 35, estrogen profiles are similar to intact animals, indicating that the placenta is the primary source of the hormone. At 150 days, the ovary resembles a polycystic ovary with numerous atretic antral follicles of different sizes ranging from follicles with pyknotic granulosa cells to large cystic structures totally devoid of granulosa cells. However, some of the medium-sized follicles are histologically normal.

EFFECTS OF LACTATION ON FOLLICULAR DEVELOPMENT

In all mammals that have been studied, lactation impairs follicular development. Among laboratory species, this has been most clearly demonstrated in the rat where the suckling stimulus of small versus large litters influences the degree of follicular inhibition (reviewed in ref. 932). Thus, mothers nursing eight pups show a decrease in follicular numbers with the nadir reached at day 8 of lactation; between days 4 and 12, follicles larger than 400 μm are absent, whereas a few in this range are always present in dams nursing two pups (932). Follicular immaturity in rats with eight pups was reflected in very low levels of estradiol—*in vivo* and *in vitro.* On removal of the litter on day 3 of lactation, a significant increase is evident by 30 h in the number of follicles 201–600 μm in diameter and the animals ovulate by 96 h (933). The hormone profiles found in rats nursing eight pups exemplify a rather universal pattern during lactation: normal cyclic serum levels of FSH, elevated prolactin, and extremely reduced LH. Daily injection of 0.5–1.0 IU of hCG or 50 μg ovine LH from days 2 to 5, followed by an ovulatory injection of hCG results by the next morning in ovulation of the normal complement of ova (932). After the removal of the litter on day 3 of lactation at 11 A.M., 24 h later significant increases occur in serum LH and FSH with a concurrent fall in prolactin (933). The missing ingredient during intense suckling stimulus therefore appears to be LH. *In vitro* production rates of testosterone and estradiol by the nonluteal ovary are drastically reduced in rats nursing two or eight pups on day 2 of lactation but with a positive staircase increase for the former group over the next 8 days. It thus appears likely that the deficiency in LH leads to decreased androgen production by the theca and presumably reduced estrogen production by the granulosa compartment. Reduced estrogen secretion may also reflect less aromatase activity. When rats nursing eight pups are injected from days 2 to 4 of lactation with LH, ovulation of the normal number of ova ensues following an injection of hCG (934). Within 24 h of the first injection of LH, the concentration of estradiol in ovarian venous plasma increases dramatically, and this is paralleled by increased inhibin activity. This does not negate the role of high levels of prolactin during lactation, which may act directly or indirectly on the ovary. For example, high levels of prolactin inhibit follicular estrogen production in the rat (696,935). The respective roles of LH and prolactin in affecting follicular function during lactation is a theme recurring throughout this section. In addition to the high baseline levels of prolactin during lactation, the suckling induced response must also be considered. In rats suckling eight pups, the magnitude of prolactin release in 20-day postpartum mothers is considerably reduced and the return to baseline levels is also accelerated (936). Substituting 10-day-old pups with the 20-day postpartum mother does not enhance prolactin release, indicating that the intensity of suckling stimulus is not a factor. As will be seen later with other species, the hypothalamic-pituitary mechanism mediating suckling release of prolactin becomes refractory with time. Rats with prolonged lactation for 72 to 105 days (produced by substituting litters at approximately 2-week intervals) and then mated, usually deliver at 22 days (937). This suggests that FSH and LH—especially the latter—are of greater significance in the rat than suckling release of prolactin in regulating follicular development.

Bromocryptine treatment of suckling rats mated at postpartum estrus suppresses serum prolactin and progesterone levels and the uterus contains unimplanted embryos, even if progesterone is injected concurrently with bromocryptine (938). Removal of prolactin evidently fails to increase secretion of follicular estrogen, which is the key to triggering ovulation in the rat. This also suggests that the primary role of prolactin is at the hypothalamic-pituitary axis, not at the follicular level. In postpartum rats nursing seven pups, diestrus lasts for 3 weeks and is associated with reduced LH secretion, hyperprolactinemia, and increased serum progesterone (939). Daily administration of bromocryptine to lactating rats shortens the duration of diestrus to 11 days by depressing the secretion of both prolactin and progesterone to baseline levels.

It is well established that lactation prevents the postcastration rise in gonadotropins in the rat (reviewed by ref. 940), and with the increase in understanding of neuroendocrine mechanisms it was logical to implicate the hypothalamic-pituitary axis as a controlling factor. Indeed, there is a significant fall during lactation in pituitary GnRH receptor concentration (941). There is no change in pituitary affinity for GnRH receptors, but there are about 50% fewer binding sites than at estrus (942). Moreover, removal of an eight-pup litter from ovariectomized mothers results 24 h later in a brisk increase in GnRH pituitary receptors. Rats ovariectomized on day 10 show a significant increase in LH secretion by the next day, which can be blocked by exogenous prolactin without, however, affecting the LH response to GnRH (940). The action of prolactin is therefore presumably exerted in part at the hypothalamic level. On the other hand, pituitaries of lactating rats nursing eight pups exposed *in vitro* to pulsatile GnRH release as much FSH but considerably less LH than pituitaries from animals nursing two pups (943). This points to an action of the suckling stimulus (prolactin?) directly modifying pituitary response to GnRH. When rats nursing eight pups are ovariectomized on day 2, plasma LH does not increase until day 20, whereas in ovariectomized dams with two pups a gradual rise in LH occurs throughout lactation (944). Thus, the suckling stimulus rather than ovarian factors is mainly responsible for the suppression of FSH and LH in the first half of lactation. As will become apparent, changes in the frequency and magnitude of GnRH release most likely account for the low serum levels of LH during lactation.

Swiss mice nursing six young show a pattern very similar to the rat. During the first 11 days postpartum the largest vesicular follicles are 350 μm in diameter; thereafter the follicles enlarge to 450 μm, the corpora lutea of pregnancy regress and the vagina becomes mucified: indicative of estrogen-progesterone interaction (945).

The most extreme effect of lactation on follicular development has been observed in the hamster. Unlike the rat and mouse, there is no postpartum ovulation in the hamster; instead, the large number of vesicular follicles developed during pregnancy quickly regress, and consequently the thecal cells are incorporated into the interstitium (946). The net result is an ovary characterized by interstitial hypertrophy and with follicular development limited to preantral follicles with 7 to 8 layers of granulosa cells. This unusual ovary is maintained by as few as one to two suckling young. Removal of all young on days 2 or 14 of lactation results in ovulation exactly 4 days later (946). The hormonal basis for the acyclic ovary is a daily massive release at 4 P.M. of FSH and LH (947) evidently in a ratio incompatible with the differentiation of antral follicles. Concomitant with the daily gonadotropin surge, there is an increase in serum progesterone with increasing levels as lactation progresses. The progesterone is secreted by the interstitium, and several lines of evidence indicate its release is in response to the surge of LH (947).

Because of its economic importance, considerable attention has been devoted to follicular development in the postpartum cow. The degree of follicular inhibition is influenced by two factors: Suckling and its intensity delays the return to estrus, for example, beef cows that were nonsuckled, suckled once daily for 30 min or suckled ad libitum by two calves ovulated, respectively, an average of 31, 41, and 76 days postpartum, respectively (948). Another factor complicating follicular development in the bovine is the well-documented inhibitory effect of the corpus luteum of pregnancy or the ipsilateral uterine horn (949). In nonsuckling dairy cows, nonatretic follicles begin to form an antral cavity at 0.16 mm in diameter (950). On day 15 postpartum, 77% of the largest healthy antral follicles present are 0.16 to 1.6 mm and by day 35 only 1.5% of the smallest class are represented. Thus, during the early postpartum period, there is no constant replenishment of small antral follicles by preantral stages. On day 15 the percentage of follicles from 0.29 to 1.6 mm increased, presumably at the expense of the smallest antral follicles. At all times the ovary containing the corpora lutea had more nonatretic follicles than the contralateral ovary. In another study, follicles >3 mm were removed from ovaries of beef cows on day 5 postpartum from suckling and nonsuckling animals (949). Based on estrogen content in follicular fluid and histology, the number of healthy and atretic follicles was estimated. Follicles from the nonsuckled cows were already considerably larger: 50% were greater than 6 mm compared to 33% for follicles from suckled cows. Moreover, individual follicles from suckled cows had half the concentration of estrogen compared to follicles from the nonsuckled group. The "carryover" effect of the corpus luteum was also evident in that the percentage of follicles containing estrogen in the ovary with the corpus luteum was about one-third the value of the contralateral ovary (949). Another study evaluated follicular parameters in beef cows that were suckled or weaned on day 21 postpartum with the endpoint on day 25 (951). For combined follicles from 1 to larger than 6 mm in the weaned group, there was a 68% increase in LH receptors but no difference in FSH binding sites. The only hormone that differed in follicular fluid concentration was prolactin, which was 53% higher in follicles from the weaned cows. Subsequently, Walters and colleagues (952) measured changes at 24-h intervals after weaning on day 21 postpartum. Utilizing the largest follicle in the ovary, an increase in FSH receptors was observed 48 h after weaning, whereas the increase in hCG receptors did not occur until 96 h.

In the suckling cow, serum levels of FSH and LH are depressed compared to weaned animals (953), and this is associated with an altered pattern of gonadotropin release. In cows nursing two young ad libitum, the LH pulse is about 1 per 6 h contrasted to 3 per 6 h in weaned animals (948). After weaning on day 21, the number of LH pulses is approximately threefold greater in the weaned animals (951). In milked cows, FSH is secreted in the early postpartum period in discrete pulses comparable in frequency and magnitude to the profiles during pregnancy; there is a gradual increase in pulsatile release of LH in the first 1 or 2 weeks postpartum (see 954). Again, LH levels are more affected by lactation in the cow than FSH. When pituitary explants of weaned and suckled cows are exposed to GnRH, LH secretion is doubled in the former group (952). Following weaning, over the next 4 days, basal levels of serum LH increase in linear fashion, whereas FSH is unaffected (952). It has frequently been noted that the first cycle after parturition in the cow is significantly shorter than subsequent ones judged both by serum progesterone levels and behavioral estrus. This inadequate luteal phase is similar to a disorder of the human female and in both cases inadequate gonadotropin priming of follicles may be responsible. On day 7 postpartum, comparing suckled and nonsuckled beef cows, lower serum concentrations and pulse frequencies of LH and FSH are observed in the suckled group (953). The FSH was measured by a homologous radioimmunoassay, but in another study where a heterologous FSH radioimmunoassay was used, serum levels of FSH were within the normal estrous range (955). A recent review article (956) summarizes the effects of suckling in beef cows on steroid and gonadotropin levels.

In summary, suckling stimulus in the bovine alters the frequency of LH (and FSH?) pulses and, consequently, follicular development is impaired. As one might anticipate, pulsatile injection of GnRH has been used to reverse this situation and to induce ovulation within 4 days of treatment of suckling cows (957). The dominant follicle, as revealed by ultrasound, first appears 10 days after calving in suckling beef cows (958). However, only 11% of the dominant follicles ovulate, and in the others the follicle regresses to be replaced by a new one. Thus, prolonged anestrus is attributable to lack of ovulation rather than delayed development of follicles. In lactating dairy cattle the dominant follicle (>10 mm; again judged by ultrasound) appears on day 7 followed by a second wave on day 12 with ovulation occurring on day 20 (959). Most animals (81%) have two waves of follicular growth with the remaining cows showing three waves of growth. It should be stressed that the cattle were milked twice daily and not naturally suckling.

In ewes, as in cows, the first postpartum ovulation occurs more often (62.5%) in the ovary contralateral to the one bearing the corpus luteum (960). The time to postpartum ovulation was also shortened by 8 days when the ovulating ovary did not contain the corpus luteum of pregnancy.

Lactational anestrus in the sow usually lasts 6 weeks or longer and is—as usual—associated with altered follicular development (for a review article, see ref. 961). During the first 4 weeks of lactation only 47% of the follicles larger than 1 mm in diameter are normal and the largest healthy follicles are less than 4 mm (962). Beginning at the 6th week normal follicles comprise 64% of the population and a few follicles begin to emerge that are approximately 4 mm. On the day after weaning, there are numerous follicles less than 5 mm in diameter and by 4.8 days, the ovaries contain an average of seven follicles larger than 10 mm and 15 follicles 5 to 10 mm in diameter (1963). Follicular development in the sow is therefore held in abeyance until the suckling stimulus is removed. Before weaning, serum FSH values are similar to those observed during the estrous cycle, whereas LH values are depressed (964). Unilateral ovariectomy on day 20 of lactation is followed 24 h later by a significant increase in plasma FSH without any change in LH levels (965). By 48 h post-unilateral ovariectomy, ovarian venous plasma concentration of estradiol is twice as great as in sham-suckled sows and follicular fluid weight is already significantly elevated. Evidently, the responsiveness of the hypothalamic-pituitary axis is not blunted in the suckling sow. Serum prolactin is elevated compared to cyclic values. Pigs ovariectomized 2 to 4 days after farrowing show a prompt increase in FSH throughout a 30-day period of lactation, while serum LH did not differ over this period between ovariectomized and intact animals (966). The divergent profiles evidently result from two different control mechanisms, with FSH being normally restrained in the intact sow by inhibin produced by the numerous 1- to 5-mm follicles present throughout the postpartum period. After weaning, significant increases in serum FSH and LH presumably are responsible for the rapid maturation of follicles (963). Weaning to estrous intervals ranges from 3 to 10 days, and prolactin levels decline to basal concentration 1 or 2 h after weaning (967). Both LH and FSH concentrations rose in the 12 h postweaning period and an increase in pulse frequency per 12 h was especially pronounced for LH. As a corollary to these results, pulsatile administration of GnRH to lactating sows 25 days postpartum, is as effective as weaning in leading to fertile estrus within 4 days (968). Ablation of follicles larger than 3 mm, 36 h before weaning does not prolong the duration of postweaning estrus (969). At 24 h later, a significant increase in FSH —but not LH—is evident, and presumably the transitory exposure to higher levels of FSH accelerates the growth of smaller follicles so that the time to estrus and ovulation rate is not altered.

Although there is no morphologic evidence on follicular growth during lactation in the primate, indirect monitoring of gonadotropins and steroid hormones indicates that suckling inhibits follicular development. For example, in lactating rhesus monkeys, weaning normally occurs 9 to 12 months postpartum. Under these circumstances, serum LH is low during the first 9 months postpartum, and values typical of the follicular phase of the cycle are not attained until about 1 year (970). In the absence of a suckling stimulus, basal LH levels begin to rise after the first month. Serum FSH is also reduced during the first 6 months postpartum in lactating rhesus and normal follicular levels are not attained until 10 months. LH surges cannot be consistently elicited by injection of estradiol benzoate until 10 months in lactating monkeys, whereas in nonsuckling females they can be elicited within the first month postpartum. This included a group of cycling monkeys who served as foster mothers after being primed twice daily with thyrotropin-releasing hormone to become hyperprolactinemic. They responded to estradiol benzoate exactly like the normal postpartum suckling monkeys, which rules out pregnancy per se as the factor responsible for ovarian refractoriness in lactating animals.

In suckling or nonsuckling rhesus monkeys ovariectomized on days 24–25 postpartum, serum LH—and FSH—are suppressed by lactation (971) (compare with results in the sow). It is also noteworthy that pituitaries of lactating females contain only about 8% as much LH compared to a pool of pituitaries from cycling rhesus; FSH concentrations were similar between the two groups.

Basal serum prolactin gradually falls in lactating rhesus but from 60 to 180 days still runs at about 150 ng/ml, whereas it drastically declines within 48 h in nonsuckled monkeys (970). The diurnal rhythm of prolactin secretion, which is absent during pregnancy, is resumed within the first week postpartum (972). These altered patterns of gonadotropin secretion associated with lactation are also reflected in low serum levels of estradiol and progesterone (970,972). In the former study, serum progesterone averaged 0.4 ± 0.1 ng/ml for up to 80 days postpartum, which is confirmatory that suckling can partially "rejuvenate" the corpus luteum of pregnancy and restore some modicum of secretory activity—albeit at a low level. This is consistent with recent observations that bromocryptine administered to suckling monkeys curtails serum prolactin and progesterone (973). Suckling and nonsuckling Japanese macaque were monitored during the breeding season for resumption of ovulation by weekly venipuncture and measurement of progesterone (974). The nonsuckling monkeys showed cyclic changes in progesterone and menstruation, while only sporadic fluctuations and infrequent menstruation were observed in the suckling animals over a 6-month period.

In women, lactation delays the onset until first ovulation but the duration and patterns of suckling stimulus are variables that confound the results (reviewed in refs. 975 and 976). No morphologic studies are available, so that the extent to which follicular maturation is impaired is unknown. By 3 weeks after delivery, FSH levels are within the range of normal follicular values (977,978) and LH is reported to be within the normal range by 4 or 5 weeks (977). However, the pulsatile secretion of LH appears to be too low to induce estradiol secretion (978). Urinary estrogen is low in breast-feeding women until 40 weeks after delivery (976). The first ovulation in nonlactating women occurred between 43 and 87 days from delivery and was associated with increases in urinary pregnanediol or plasma progesterone (978). In the lactating group, there was no evidence of ovarian cyclicity until after weaning or after at least 150 days of lactation. After injection of 1 mg estradiol benzoate, a positive feedback increase in LH was still missing from seven lactating women at 100 days postpartum. For the first 2 weeks after delivery of nonnursing mothers, the response to GnRH is negative, followed by gradual increasing responsiveness with FSH responding before LH (979). Similar results have been reported for lactating and nonlactating women with both showing similar normal profiles of FSH and LH in response to GnRH by 4 or 5 weeks postpartum (977).

Prolactin levels decline rapidly after delivery but are maintained by suckling in lactating women for long periods of time (see ref. 980). The question then is: With fairly early resumption of basal levels of FSH and LH and response to GnRH, why is follicular maturation delayed so long in lactating women? More data are needed before the question can be resolved whether in women prolactin—directly or indirectly—plays a role or whether changes in GnRH pulsatile release is the controlling factor in lactational amennorhea (see ref. 981).

Still another factor involved in decreased LH secretion in the suckling animal is the proopiomelanocortin gene. For example, in suckled anestrous beef cows intravenous injection of naloxone increases the release of LH (982). Intracerebral infusion of naloxone in the vicinity of GnRH neurons stimulated LH release in suckling ewes within 20 minutes, but serum prolactin was not significantly lowered (983). Intracerebral infusion of an antibody to β-endorphin disinhibited GnRH-LH release when infused into the rostral preoptic area nucleus, whereas an antibody to metenkephalin was effective in anterior or mediobasal hypothalamus (984). In the bovine brain, immunocytochemically, GnRH and proopiomelanocortin neurons overlap extensively in the median eminence (985). Presumably, the same interactions of GnRH and proopiomelanocortin exist in the suckling rodent, since in the cyclic rat proopiomelanocortin mRNA is low on the afternoon of proestrus—when GnRH triggers the LH surge, and, conversely, proopiomelanocortin mRNA is elevated on estrus correlating with low tonic levels of LH (986).

CONCLUSIONS AND SPECULATIONS

Knowledge of primordial germ cells has progressed rapidly in recent years, primarily involving the mouse as a model. The ability to recover primordial germ cells at 10 days post coitum and observing their behavior and growth on a feeder layer of cells is a very important advance as well as the analysis of various mutants which lead to sterility. One can confidently predict the *in situ* hybridization, immunocytochemistry, and *in vitro* manipulations will unravel the paracrine and autocrine factors involved in their migration to the gonadal ridge and subsequent postmigratory proliferation. An especially intriguing observation is that rat and mouse primordial germ cells acquire specific surface glycoconjugates, which disappear once they have reached the gonad. For the first time, experimental evidence is available to support the Henderson-Edwards hypothesis that the earliest oocytes formed at meiosis are the first to exit from the ovary at puberty. Strategically timed injections of [^{3}H]-thymidine or bromodeoxyuridine (BrDu) directly into the early amniotic cavity might be a way of testing the theory by a strictly *in vivo* approach.

Knowledge of the nongrowing pool of follicles—the primordial stages—is still woefully lacking. At present, rapid separation of primordial follicles from somatic cells is the limiting factor in answering a number of unsolved questions about the nongrowing pool. The critical question is whether their conversion into primary follicles is strictly by chance or influenced by hormones, growth factors, or proximity to neurotransmitters. The latter possibility is suggested by several studies reviewed in this chapter, and there are some hints in the literature that primordial follicles in the rat *can* be influenced by gonadotropins.

It has become increasingly clear for a number of species that primary and secondary follicles, that is, preantral stages, *are* dependent on gonadotropins. We have now shown for the hamster, mouse, and human that *in vivo* or *in vitro* development requires FSH, and this is especially well established in the hamster where a variety of studies have shown the essentiality of FSH for steroidogenesis and DNA synthesis. Despite evidence to the contrary, a number of investigators still cling to the belief that rat preantral follicles are independent of gonadotropin support based on the qualitative ability of some follicles to develop following hypophysectomy, although the number is drastically reduced from intact animals. Careful qualitative studies are needed for the rat focusing on follicular development (healthy and atretic) in the post-hypophysectomy period and recrudescence in response to FSH and other hormones. However, there may very well be species differences in how far follicular development proceeds in the absence of gonadotropins. For example, 70 days after hypophysectomy, follicles in the ewe progress to small antral stages, usually less than 2 mm in diameter. Moreover, follicles of this size from hypophysectomized ewes respond to FSH or LH by significantly increasing tissue cAMP to levels comparable to control follicles. It is noteworthy that suppression of growth of follicles to a maximum of 2 mm can also be obtained in pituitary stalk-sectioned ewes treated with follicular fluid or by chronic administration of a GnRH agonist.

One of the critical steps in folliculogenesis is the emergence into the growing pool of primary follicles, that is, an oocyte surrounded by a unilaminar investiture of granulosa cells. Ultimately this will develop into a multilayered granulosa surrounded by thecal cells. From the earliest stage, communication is established between the oocyte and granulosa cells. One of the best examples is provided by the ovary of adult mice in which all oocytes express a protooncogene c-*kit* receptor tyrosine kinase, while the surrounding granulosa cells express a ligand. It is now known that oocytes of some species contain insulinlike growth factor, epidermal growth factor, tumor necrosis factor-α, or mullerian inhibiting substance. Moreover, in several species, receptors for FSH and LH-hCG are present in the oocyte, and immunodetectable FSH and LH are localized in the oocyte of primary and secondary rat follicles. A number of procedures destroy primordial germ cells, and, consequently, a sterile gonad lacking steroidogenic tissue is formed. Finally, addition of an oocyte to *in vitro* cells significantly increases DNA synthesis. Collectively, all of these observations point to the fact that symbiosis between granulosa cells and oocyte is obligatory, but at the earliest stages the oocyte may be the controlling factor in preantral follicular differentiation.

We and others have now shown that intact preantral follicles can be isolated from hamster, human, mouse, and rat ovaries by enzymatic dissociation. Under these circumstances, the geometry of the follicle is maintained with the normal relationships between oocyte, granulosa, and thecal compartments affording communication and transfer of signals from one compartment to the other. We believe that this method has significant advantages over previous techniques in studying the functions of preantral follicles.

An interesting finding of the past decade is the observation that regional differences exist in the granulosal compartment of antral follicles. This is reflected in distinct localization of peptide receptors, enzymes, steroidogenic potential, and presumably metabolic processes as well between the membrana granulosa and the cumulus oophorus. These structural and functional distinctions originate from the intimate relationship between the oocyte and its surrounding investment of granulosa cells. One wonders how early in the history of the preantral follicle can the future differences between cumulus and membrana granulosa be discerned. The different roles of the membrana granulosa and the cumulus-oocyte complex in the postovulatory period are obviously related to their different topographic and functional organizations in the maturing follicle.

A variety of observations point to the critical role of FSH in follicular recruitment. For example, in rodents:

1. The increased FSH levels at estrus correlate with changes in number of large preantral or antral follicles.
2. Unilateral ovariectomy results in transient increases in FSH and mobilization of additional follicles.

3. Injection of increasing amounts of inhibin during the periovulatory period leads to progressive decrease in the number of ova ovulated.
4. Injection of FSH induces superovulation.
5. *In vitro* addition of FSH increases DNA synthesis.

Numerous examples can be cited for other species as well. The extreme example of the efficacy of FSH is provided in human and rodent models by the ability of purified preparations of the hormone (without evident LH activity) to produce full-blown antral follicles, not secreting estrogen but capable of ovulating in response to exogenous gonadotropins. The effects of FSH are undoubtedly magnified by various growth factors such as epidermal growth factor in the case of the cyclic hamster. The primacy of FSH in follicular recruitment does not negate the importance of simultaneous low tonic levels of LH. Thus, administration at estrus of anti-LH to neutralize LH leads to follicular atresia in the face of normal serum levels of FSH. During estrus, the significance of the secondary surge of FSH for follicular recruitment has long been recognized in cyclic rodents, but clear-cut evidence of its importance in human and cattle folliculogenesis is now established as the factor launching the cohort of follicles that will next ovulate. Moreover, it seems likely that the periovulatory changes in gonadotropins are responsible for increasing the growth rate of even the smallest preantral follicles, which therefore receive a boost at several successive cycles.

While high titers of FSH are responsible for granulosal proliferation, aromatase activity, and antrum formation, LH becomes increasingly important in the final phase of maturation of the follicle. To a great extent, its actions are directed toward the theca by inducing its own receptors, increasing the production of androgens and increasing vascularity. The appearance of LH receptors in granulosa cells (induced by FSH and possibly LH as well) is invariably found in large preovulatory follicles of all species. The demise of luteal function accelerates follicular development and estrogen secretion. Thus, the main variable in determining the duration of the estrous cycle in the rat is whether the corpora lutea secrete progesterone for 2 or 3 days. The precision of the 4-day cycle of the hamster correlates with the rigid 2-day life span of the corpus luteum. In the sheep and cow, the follicular phase is clearly demarcated by the spontaneous or induced regression of the corpus luteum. One of the most striking examples of the significance of luteolysis on follicular development is provided by ewes injected with a progesterone-protein complex, which produces antibodies to progesterone. Under these circumstances, the normally lengthened estrous cycle is converted into a series of short cycles with corpora lutea accumulating similar to the cyclic rat. The luteal-follicular shift, therefore, is of paramount importance in the final selection of the ovulatory follicle(s) and is associated with withdrawal of progesterone. In most cases, after luteolysis, baseline levels of FSH are maintained but LH increases as a consequence of an increased pulsatile release pattern. In most species, the prolonged activity of the corpus luteum during pregnancy invariably blunts follicular growth and similar results ensue after prolonged administration of progesterone.

Pencharz and Williams (987,988) established in 1940 that diethylstilbestrol directly affected ovarian weight in hypophysectomized rats and subsequently it was shown that estrogens synergize with FSH to cause a dramatic increase in the number of antral follicles. Since then, the direct effects of estrogen in folliculogenesis have been extrapolated to all species, and a good case can be made for the mouse and possibly the rabbit. As pointed out in this review, estrogen receptors are demonstrable by immunocytochemistry in the human follicle, but the results are still contradictory in cynomolgus. The one glaring exception is the hamster, but other species need to be investigated before the generalization can be universally applied.

Recent years have witnessed renewed interest in follicular degeneration based on models to induce atresia or investigations of the spontaneous event. Species seem to be divided into two categories in terms of the hormonal withdrawal pattern by antral follicles: In rodents, the loss of thecal androgen seems to precede the loss of granulosal aromatase activity, whereas in the ewe and human the reverse sequence exists. In both groups, the ultimate loss of estrogen secretion by the atretic follicle is the common denominator. The deficit in estrogen secretion in a young antral follicle presumably curtails mitosis in the granulosa cells, and the follicle therefore lags further and further behind. The question remains, however, whether the loss of estrogen (or androgen) production is a primary or secondary event in atresia of tertiary follicles. It is virtually impossible to answer this question by examining follicles undergoing spontaneous atresia because of the difficulty in pinpointing the moment when degeneration begins and determining the criteria for this early step. The histologic presence of a few pyknotic nuclei may be normal and of no consequence to a granulosa population of several thousand to million cells (depending on the species). By the time the follicle can definitely be classified as atretic, it is too late to establish causal relationships. Hence it is our prejudice that experimental models in which atresia occurs as a timed, predictable event will be the only way to determine the prime mover. Although emphasis on atresia has focused on tertiary follicles, certainly the process is even more widespread in younger follicles, and entirely different mechanisms may be involved in their regression. A few studies have looked at FSH and LH receptors at the onset of atresia and found no differences in total numbers from normal follicles. A more meaningful endpoint may be the number of occupied receptors that are coupled to adenylate cyclase. We believe that a change distal to the peptide receptor may be the earliest signal of atresia.

The most dramatic histologic signs of atresia occur in the granulosa cells, and, consequently, this compartment has received the most attention. O'Shea (265) was the first to recognize the role of apoptosis in the atretic ovine follicle, although it had long been known that the appearance of pyknotic nuclei was the earliest sign of degeneration. Recently, several papers have appeared using DNA laddering as a biochemical sign of atresia. Whether this occurs concurrent with histologic evidence of regression or slightly precedes it is as yet unknown. However, in all likelihood, the histologic and biochemical changes in granulosa cells are secondary events rather than causative. Perhaps the vulnerability of granulosa cells in large antral follicles stems from their dependency for viability on being constantly bathed by the liquor folliculi. It will be interesting to determine whether significant changes occur in the proteoglycan and glycosaminoglycan constituents of follicular fluid in early stages of atresia. The theca is the most resistant portion of the atretic follicle, and morphologic alterations may not occur until several days after granulosa cells are affected. It is possible though—at least for rodents—that the theca may be the key to antral follicular development and atresia. Hisaw (2) originally postulated that an "undeveloped" theca might be responsible for atresia. Although the morphologic development of the theca in rodents may be normal, we suggest that biochemical "immaturity" may lead to atresia by impaired production of androgens, which in turn deprives the granulosa cells of substrate for conversion to estrogens. We base this belief on the pattern of steroidogenesis in induced and spontaneous atresia and the ability of exogenous LH or hCG to salvage the developing follicles that normally become atretic between days 3 and 4 of the hamster estrous cycle. This does not exclude an additional role for LH in recruiting more than the normal number of 20 developing follicles in the hamster. The critical factor in the final maturation of developing follicles may be the LH receptor level in theca interna cells. This may determine the ability of the cells to produce androstenedione and the vascularity of the theca. These two properties of the theca are so inextricably bound that it may be impossible to dissociate them. At present, however, it appears that the inception of atresia is not associated with decreases in vascularity, which may be a secondary event comparable to the sequence in luteolysis. Although the theca may be the pivotal tissue in rodent atresia, in other species the receptor deficiency may reside in the granulosa compartment involving LH and/or FSH receptors. Reasons for this possibility have been cited. It is noteworthy that in several species: pig, sheep, and possibly human, the theca of atretic follicles undergoes rapid regression so that there is little in the way of secondary interstitium in these species.

In this account, the follicle has largely been considered as an isolated component, uninfluenced by other ovarian compartments. The interrelationships between follicles and corpora lutea, follicles, and interstitium have been barely touched. Moreover, do tertiary follicles affect preantral stages if they share a common vascular supply? Coculture of these various tissues might be a rewarding approach.

A wide variety of stimuli induce superovulation, including pituitary and placental gonadotropins, antisera to sex steroids, antisera to inhibin, and clomiphene—an estrogen antagonist. It appears that highly pure FSH-like compounds (with high FSH:LH ratios) stimulate development of supernumerary follicles better than gonadotropins containing low FSH:LH ratios. However, in the hamster and guinea pig, continuous LH stimulation can induce spontaneous superovulation. Superovulation may result from a combination of recruitment of new follicles into the population and prevention of atresia of larger follicles; this may depend on the stage of the cycle that gonadotropic stimulus is provided. We do not believe that follicles already in early stages of atresia can be rescued. The mechanisms of superovulation may also involve an increase in ovarian blood flow, and thus the delivery rate of essential nutrients for the sudden increase in follicular growth. The temporal changes in ovarian blood flow after a superovulatory stimulus are largely unknown. It is tempting to speculate that increases in ovarian blood flow parallel (or precede) increases in the number of follicles.

The estrous cycles of hamster, rat, and mouse usually recur at 4- to 5-day intervals, as compared with 18 to 22 days for sheep, pigs, and cows. One would intuitively assume that folliculogenesis proceeds at different rates depending on cycle length and indeed this is the case. For the laboratory rodents, it is estimated that about 3 to 4 weeks are required between the time a follicle enters the growing pool and ovulates. In contrast, similar estimates are 6 months for the ewe, 103 days for the pig, and 85 days for the human. Consequently, perturbations are quickly sensed and promptly responded to by rodent follicular populations, as exemplified by their rapid mobilization after unilateral ovariectomy or administration of pregnant mare serum and their possible rapid onset of regression after hypophysectomy.

As anticipated, ultrasonography has shed considerable light on temporal changes in follicular dynamics. Based on histologic criteria, Gougeon (78) postulated that alternation of ovulation occurred with high frequency in the human ovary. This unexpected and somewhat unsettling notion could be resolved by ultrasound, but to our knowledge the technique has not yet been used with normal cyclic women. Ultrasound has been especially valuable in analyzing follicular growth in cyclic and pregnant cattle and mares. Although the waxing and waning of large follicles is referred to as a "wave," it must be kept in

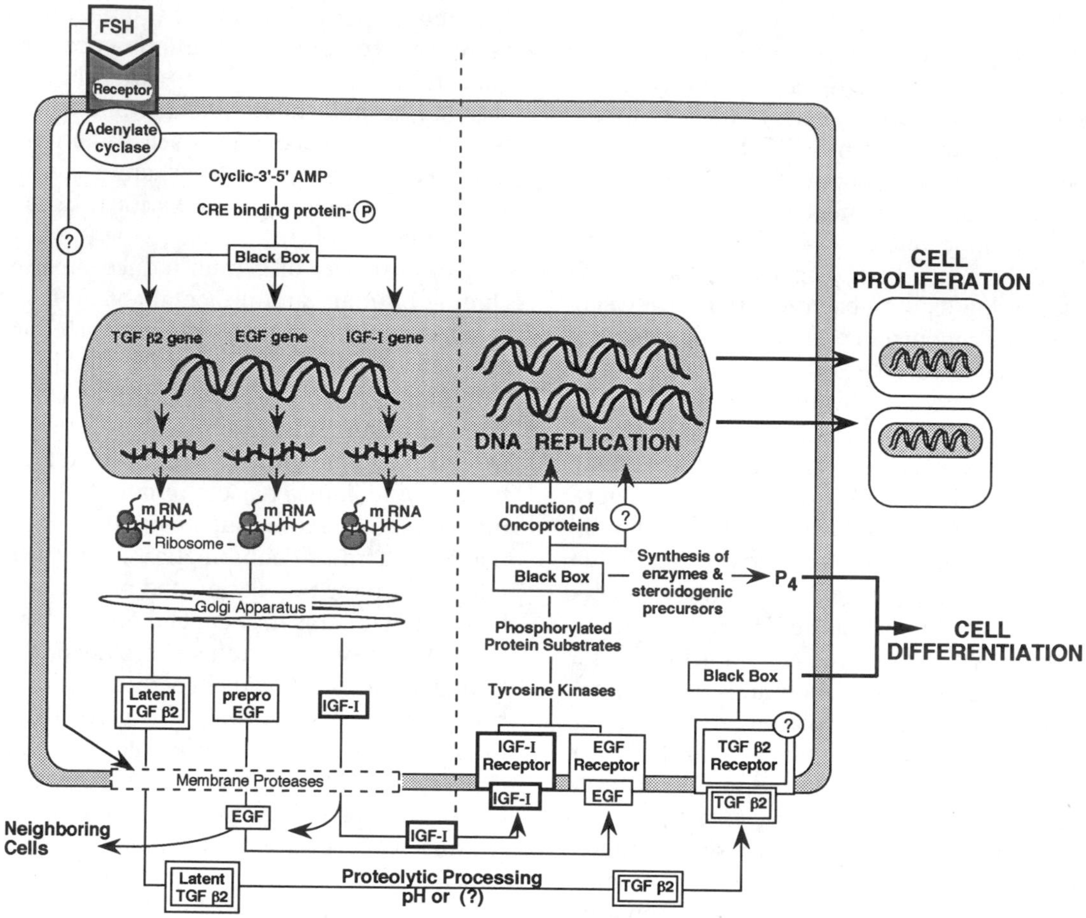

FIG. 3. A model of interactions of FSH with growth factors on granulosa cells. *CRE,* cAMP responsive element.

mind that recruitment of small preantral follicles probably occurs as a continuous daily event. Fluctuations in hormones and/or growth factors may be superimposed to produce follicles large enough to be visualized. In this connection, a statistical correlation exists during the bovine estrous cycle between a surge of FSH and the emergence of the dominant follicle of each wave.

Follicular development during lactation is impaired because of altered pulsatile release of LH and elevated levels of prolactin. The problem of hormonal control during lactation is also complicated by species differences. What remains to be established are the relative roles of gonadotropin-releasing hormone, prolactin, and proopiomelanocortin and their interactions and how much of the effects of prolactin are exerted indirectly or directly at the follicular level by impairing thecal production of androgens or granulosal production of estrogens.

The past decade has witnessed an explosion of information about ovarian growth factors and cytokines, but in most instances, it is premature to evaluate their functional significance. The area is complicated by species differences in localization of the factors, possibly changing roles as folliculogenesis progresses, a bewildering variety of inhibitory and stimulatory factors so that the ultimate outcome may depend on the algebraic summation of negative and positive signals. Based on our research and others', we propose a simplified working hypothesis for interactions of FSH and growth factors in modulating granulosa cell function (Fig. 3). To duplicate the effects of FSH, combined administration of several growth factors may be needed. These problems will be solved with time, but it is important not to lose sight of the fact that these are secondary factors transducing the prime movers: steroid and peptide hormones.

ACKNOWLEDGMENTS

The original work of the authors in this chapter was supported by NIH grants HD-00596 (GSG) and HD-02528 (SKR).

We thank Darlene Limback for her help in assembling the bibliography and computer drawing of the diagrams and Joella Judd for valiantly straightening our scribbled pages and typing the manuscript. We also thank Dr. Paul F. Terranova for his contributions to the first edition version of this chapter.

REFERENCES

1. Greenwald GS. Of eggs and follicles [Editorial]. *Am J Anat* 1972;135:1–4.
2. Hisaw FL. Development of the graafian follicle and ovulation. *Physiol Rev* 1947;27:95–119.
3. Brambell FWR. Ovarian changes. In: Parkes AS, ed. *Marshall's physiology of reproduction.* New York: Longmans, Green; 1956:397–542.
4. Falck B. Site of production of oestrogen in rat ovary as studied in micro-transplants. *Acta Physiol Scand* 1959;47[Suppl 163]:5–101.
5. Greenwald GS. Role of follicle-stimulating hormone and luteinizing hormone in follicular development and ovulation. In: Knobil E, Sawyer WH, eds. *Handbook of physiology/endocrinology.* Vol 4: Part 2. Washington D. C.: American Physiological Society; 1974:293–323.
6. Channing CP, Tsafriri A. Mechanism of action of luteinizing hormone and follicle-stimulating hormone on the ovary in vitro. *Metabolism* 1977;26:413–468.
7. Lindner HR, Amsterdam A, Salomon Y, et al. Intraovarian factors in ovulation: determinants of follicular response to gonadotrophins. *J Reprod Fertil* 1977;51:215–235.
8. Armstrong DT, Dorrington JH. Estrogen biosynthesis in the ovaries and testes. In: Thomas JA, Singhal RH, eds. *Regulatory mechanisms affecting gonadal hormone action.* Baltimore: University Park Press; 1977:215–258.
9. Richards JS. Maturation of ovarian follicles: actions and interactions of pituitary and ovarian hormones on follicular cell differentiation. *Physiol Rev* 1980;60:51–89.
10. diZerega GS, Hodgen GD. Folliculogenesis in the primate ovarian cycle. *Endocrine Rev* 1981;2:27–49.
11. Erickson GF. Primary cultures of ovarian cells in serum-free medium as models of hormone-dependent differentiation. *Mol Cell Endocrinol* 1983;29:21–49.
12. Hsueh AJW, Adashi EY, Jones PBC, Welsh TH Jr. Hormonal regulation of the differentiation of cultured ovarian granulosa cells. *Endocrine Rev* 1984;5:76–127.
13. Tsafriri A, Braw RH. Experimental approaches to atresia in mammals. *Oxford Rev Reprod Biol* 1984;6:226–265.
14. Hillier SG. Sex steroid metabolism and follicular development in the ovary. *Oxford Rev Reprod Biol* 1985;7:168–222.
15. Adashi EY, Resnick CE, D'Ercole AJ, Svoboda ME, VanWyk JJ. Insulin-like growth factors as intraovarian regulators of granulosa cell growth and function. *Endocrine Rev* 1985;6:400–420.
16. Erickson GF. An analysis of follicle development and ovum maturation. *Semin Reprod Endocrinol* 1986;4:233–254.
17. Amsterdam A, Rotmensch S. Structure-function relationships during granulosa cell differentiation. *Endocrine Rev* 1987;8: 309–337.
18. Ireland JJ. Control of follicular growth and development. *J Reprod Fertil* 1987;34[Suppl]:39–54.
19. Richards JS, Hedin L. Molecular aspects of hormone action in ovarian follicular development, ovulation, and luteinization. *Annu Rev Physiol* 1988;50:441–463.
20. Greenwald GS, Terranova PF. Follicular selection and its control. In: Knobil E, Neill J, eds. *The physiology of reproduction.* New York: Raven Press; 1988:387–445.
21. Tonetta SA, diZerega GS. Intragonadal regulation of follicular maturation. *Endocrine Rev* 1989;10:205–229.
22. Familiari G, Makabe S, Motta PM. The ovary and ovulation: a three-dimensional ultrastructural study. In: Van Blerkom J, Motta PM, eds. *Ultrastructure of human gametogenesis and early embryogenesis.* Norwell, MA: Kluwer Academic Publishers; 1989:85–124.
23. Adashi EY. The potential relevance of cytokines to ovarian physiology: the emerging role of resident ovarian cells of the white blood cell series. *Endocrine Rev* 1990;11:454–464.
24. Buccione R, Schroeder AC, Eppig JJ. Interactions between somatic cells and germ cells throughout mammalian oogenesis. *Biol Reprod* 1990;43:543–547.
25. Hirshfield AN. Development of follicles in the mammalian ovary. *Int Rev Cytol* 1991;124:43–101.
26. Ackland JF, Schwartz NB, Mayo KE, Dodson RE. Nonsteroidal signals originating in the gonads. *Physiol Rev* 1992;72:731–787.
27. Giudice LC. Insulin-like growth factors and ovarian follicular development. *Endocrine Rev* 1992;13:641–669.
28. Findlay JK. An update on the roles of inhibin, acturin, and follistation as local regulators of folliculogenesis. *Biol Reprod* 1993;48:15–23.
29. Roy SK. Regulation of ovarian follicular development: a review of microscopic studies. *J Electron Microsc* 1993;In press.
30. Zuckerman SS, Weir BJ, eds. *The ovary.* 2nd ed. New York: Academic Press; 1977.
31. Jones RE, ed. *The vertebrate ovary: comparative biology and evolution.* New York: Plenum Press; 1978.
32. Crighton DB, Foxcroft GR, Haynes NB, Lamming GE. *Control of ovulation.* Boston: Butterworth; 1978.
33. Midgley AR Jr., Sadler WA, eds. *Ovarian follicular development and function.* New York: Raven Press; 1979.
34. Channing CP, Marsh JM, Sadler WA, eds. *Ovarian follicular and corpus luteum function.* New York: Plenum Press; 1979.
35. Edwards RG. *Conception in the human female.* New York: Academic Press; 1980.
36. Motta PM, Hafez ESE, eds. *Biology of the ovary.* The Hague: Martinus Nijhoff; 1980.
37. Peters H, McNatty KP. *The ovary: a correlation of structure and function in mammals.* Los Angeles: University of California Press; 1980.
38. Schwartz NB, Hunzicker-Dunn M, eds. *Dynamics of ovarian function.* New York: Raven Press; 1981.
39. Channing CP, Segal SJ, eds. *Intraovarian control mechanisms.* New York: Plenum; 1982.
40. Greenwald GS, Terranova PF, eds. *Factors regulating ovarian function.* New York: Raven Press; 1983.
41. Austin CR, Short RV, eds. *Reproduction in mammals.* 2nd ed. New York: Cambridge University Press; 1982–84.
42. Lamming GE, ed. *Marshall's physiology of reproduction.* 4th ed. Vol 1: *Reproductive cycles of vertebrates.* New York: Churchill Livingstone; 1984.
43. Guraya SS. *Biology of ovarian follicles in mammals.* New York: Springer-Verlag; 1985.
44. Toft DO, Ryan RJ, eds. *Proceedings of the fifth Ovarian Work Shop.* Champaign, IL: Ovarian Work Shops; 1985.
45. Stouffer RL, ed. *The primate ovary.* New York: Plenum Press; 1987.
46. Hodgen GD, Rosenwaks Z, Spieler JM, eds. *Nonsteroidal gonadal factors: physiological roles and possibilities in contraceptive development.* Norfolk, VA: Jones Institute Press; 1988.
47. Hirshfield AN, ed. *Growth factors and the ovary.* New York: Plenum Press; 1989.
48. Gibori G, ed. *Signaling mechanisms and gene expression in the ovary.* New York: Springer-Verlag; 1991.
49. Ginsburg M, Snow MHL, McLaren A. Primordial germ cells in the mouse embryo during gastrulation. *Development* 1990; 110:521–528.
50. Fazel AR, Schulte BA, Spicer SS. Glycoconjugate unique to migrating primordial germ cells differs with genera. *Anat Rec* 1990;228:177–184.
51. Donovan PJ, Stott D, Cairns LA, Heasman J, Wylie CC. Migratory and postmigratory mouse primordial germ cells behave differently in culture. *Cell* 1986;44:831–838.
52. Godin I, Wylie CC. TGF β_1 inhibits proliferation and has a chemotropic effect on mouse primordial germ cells in culture. *Development* 1991;113:1451–1457.
53. Mintz B, Russell ES. Gene-induced embryological modifications of primordial germ cells in the mouse. *J Exp Zool* 1957;134: 207–237.
54. Motro B, Van Der Kooy D, Rossant J, Reith A, Bernstein A. Contiguous patterns of c-kit and steel expression: analysis of mutations at the W and Sl loci. *Development* 1991;113:1207–1221.
55. Dolci S, Williams DE, Ernst MK, et al. Requirement for mast cell growth factor for primordial germ cell survival in culture. *Nature* 1991;352:809–811.
56. Hilscher W. The genetic control and germ cell kinetics of the female and male germ line in mammals including man. *Hum Reprod* 1991;6:1416–1425.

57. Hilscher W, Hilscher B. Details of the female and male pathway of the Keimbahn determined by enzyme histochemical and autoradiographic studies. *Basic Appl Histochem* 1990;34:21–34.
58. Prepin J. Le thymus foetal et la thymuline stimulent la proliferation des ovogonies dans l'ovaire foetal de rat in vitro. *C R Acad Sci Paris* 1991;313:407–411.
59. Prepin J, Jost A. Augmentation du nombre des ovogonies dans l'ovaire de foetus de lapin hypophysectomisé par décapitation: rôle probable du thymus. *C R Acad Sci Paris* 1991;313:81–85.
60. Byskov AG. Regulation of meiosis in mammals. *Ann Biol Anim Biochem Biophys* 1979;19:1251–1261.
61. Byskov AG, Tinggaard H, Andersen CY. Role of second messengers in early differentiation of gonads and sex ducts. In: Hirshfield AN, ed. *Growth factors and the ovary.* New York: Plenum Press; 1989:23–32.
62. Mauleon P. Cinétique de l'ovogenèse chez les mammifères. *Arch Anat Microsc Morphol Exp* 1967;56:125–150.
63. Gerard P, Herlant M. Sur la persistance de phenomènes d'oogenèse chez les lemuriens adultes. *Arch Biol* 1953;64:97–111.
64. Peters H, Byskov AG, Faber M. Intraovarian regulation of follicle growth in the immature mouse. In: Peters H, ed. *The development and maturation of the ovary and its functions.* Amsterdam: Excerpta Medica; 1973:20–23.
65. Lunenfeld B, Kraiem Z, Eshkol A. The function of the growing follicle. *J Reprod Fertil* 1975;45:567–574.
66. Peters H. The development of the mouse ovary from birth to maturity. *Acta Endocrinol* 1969;62:98–116.
67. de Wolff-Exalto EA. Influence of gonadotrophins on early follicle cell development and early oocyte growth in the immature rat. *J Reprod Fertil* 1982;66:537–542.
68. Hage AJ, Groen-Klevant AC, Welschen R. Follicle growth in the immature rat ovary. *Acta Endocrinol* 1978;88:375–382.
69. Uilenbroek JTJ, de Wolff-Exalto EA, Blankenstein MA. Serum gonadotrophins and follicular development in immature rats after early androgen administration. *J Endocrinol* 1976;68: 461–468.
70. Vomachka AJ, Greenwald GS. The development of gonadotropin and steroid hormone patterns in male and female hamsters from birth to puberty. *Endocrinology* 1979;105:960–966.
71. Fagbohun CF, Dada MO, Metcalf JP, Ashiru OA, Blake CA. Blockade of the selective increase in serum follicle-stimulating hormone concentration in immature female rats and its effects on ovarian follicular development. *Biol Reprod* 1990;42: 625–632.
72. Smith SS, Ojeda SR. Neonatal release of gonadotropins is essential for development of ovarian follicle-stimulating hormone receptors. *Biol Reprod* 1986;34:219–227.
73. Van Cappellen WA, Meijs-Roelofs HMA, Kramer P, Van Den Dungen HM. Ovarian follicle dynamics in immature rats treated with a luteinizing hormone-releasing hormone antagonist (Org. 30276). *Biol Reprod* 1989;40:1247–1256.
74. Krarup T, Pedersen T, Faber M. Regulation of oocyte growth in the mouse ovary. *Nature* 1969;224:187–188.
75. Gosden RG, Laing SC, Felicio LS, Nelson JF, Finch CE. Imminent oocyte exhaustion and reduced follicular recruitment mark the transition to acyclicity in aging C57BL/6J mice. *Biol Reprod* 1983;28:255–260.
76. Mandl AM, Shelton M. A quantitative study of oocytes in young and old nulliparous laboratory rats. *J Endocrinol* 1959;18: 444–450.
77. Block E. Quantitative morphological investigations of the follicular system in women: variations at different ages. *Acta Anat* 1952;14:108–123.
78. Gougeon A. *Cinetique de la croissance et de l'involution des follicules ovariens pendant le cycle menstruel chez la femme* [Dissertation]. Paris: University of Pierre and Marie Curie, 1981.
79. Wordinger R, Sutton J, Brun-Zinkernagel A-M. Ultrastructure of oocyte migration through the mouse ovarian surface epithelium during neonatal development. *Anat Rec* 1990;227:187–198.
80. Henderson SA, Edwards RG. Chiasma frequency and maternal age in mammals. *Nature* 1968;218:22–28.
81. Polani PE, Crolla JA. A test of the production line hypothesis of mammalian oognesis. *Hum Genet* 1991;88:64–70.
82. Koering MJ. Preantral follicle development during the menstrual cycle in the *Macaca mulatta* ovary. *Am J Anat* 1983;166: 429–433.
83. Mauleon P, Rao KH. Variations génétiques des populations foliculaires dans les ovaires de rates impubères. *Ann Biol Anim Biochem Biophys* 1963;3:21–31.
84. Mauleon P, Pelletier J. Variations génétiques du fonctionnement hypophysaire de trois souches de rattes immatures, rélations avec la fertilité. *Ann Biol Anim Biochem Biophys* 1964;4:105–112.
85. Greenwald GS, Moor RM. Isolation and preliminary characterization of pig primordial follicles. *J Reprod Fertil* 1989;87: 561–571.
86. Gosden RG, Telfer E. Numbers of follicles and oocytes in mammalian ovaries and their allometric relationships. *J Zool [Lond]* 1987;211:169–175.
87. Merchant H. Rat gonadal and ovarian organogenesis with and without germ cells: an ultrastructural study. *Dev Biol* 1975;44: 1–21.
88. Merchant-Larios H, Centeno B. Morphogenesis of the ovary from the sterile W/Wv mouse. In: *Eleventh International Congress of Anatomy: advances in the morphology of cells and tissues.* New York: Liss; 1981:383–392.
89. Kosiewicz MM, Michael SD. Neonatal thymectomy affects follicle populations before the onset of autoimmune oophoritis in B6A mice. *J Reprod Fertil* 1990;88:427–440.
90. Kuroda H, Terada N, Nakayama H, Matsumoto K, Kitamura Y. Infertility due to growth arrest of ovarian follicles in Sl/Sl^t mice. *Dev Biol* 1988;126:71–79.
91. Wang X, Roy SK, Greenwald GS. In vitro DNA synthesis by isolated preantral to preovulatory follicles from the cyclic mouse. *Biol Reprod* 1991;44:857–863.
92. Byskov AG, Bagger P, Andersen CY, Wilken-Jensen C, Westergaard L. Differentiation, growth and maturation of oocytes. In: Haseltine FP, Findlay JK, eds. *Growth factors in fertility regulation.* New York: Cambridge University Press; 1988:3–11.
93. Telfer E, Ansell JD, Taylor H, Gosden RG. The number of clonal precursors of the follicular epithelium in the mouse ovary. *J Reprod Fertil* 1988;84:105–110.
94. Pedersen T. Follicle kinetics in the ovary of the cyclic mouse. *Acta Endocrinol* 1970;64:304–323.
95. Butcher RL, Kirkpatrick-Keller D. Patterns of follicular growth during the four-day estrous cycle of the rat. *Biol Reprod* 1984;31:280–286.
96. Pedersen T, Peters H. Follicle growth and cell dynamics in the mouse ovary during pregnancy. *Fertil Steril* 1971;22:42–52.
97. Groen-Klevant AC. An autoradiographic study of follicle growth in the ovaries of cyclic rats. *Acta Endocrinol* 1981;96:377–381.
98. Greenwald GS. Quantitative aspects of follicular development in the untreated and PMS-treated cyclic hamster. *Anat Rec* 1974;178:139–143.
99. Chiras DD, Greenwald GS. Analysis of ovarian follicular development and thymidine incorporation in the cyclic golden hamster. *Am J Anat* 1980;157:309–317.
100. Roy SK, Greenwald GS. Quantitative analysis of in vitro incorporation of [^{3}H]thymidine into hamster follicles during the oestrous cycle. *J Reprod Fertil* 1986;77:143–152.
101. Zarrow MX, Wilson ED. The influence of age on superovulation in the immature rat and mouse. *Endocrinology* 1961;69: 851–855.
102. Welschen R, Rutte M. Ovulation in adult rats after treatment with pregnant mare serum gonadotrophin during oestrus. *Acta Endocrinol* 1971;68:41–49.
103. Greenwald GS. Analysis of superovulation in the adult hamster. *Endocrinology* 1962;71:378–389.
104. Chiras DD, Greenwald GS. Ovarian follicular development in cyclic hamsters treated with a superovulatory dose of pregnant mare's serum. *Biol Reprod* 1978;19:895–901.
105. Lane CE, Greep RO. The follicular apparatus of the ovary of the hypophysectomized immature rat and the effects of hypophyseal gonadotropic hormones on it. *Anat Rec* 1935;63:139–146.
106. Paesi FJA. The influence of hypophysectomy and of subsequent treatment with chorionic gonadotrophin on follicles of different size in the ovary of the rat. *Acta Endocrinol* 1949;3:89–104.
107. de Reviers MM. *Etude quantitative de l'action des hormones gonadotropes hypophysaires sur la population folliculaire de l'ovaire*

de ratte immature: signification biologique du dosage de l'hormone folliculo-stimulante par le test de Steelman et Pohley [Dissertation]. L'Université de Tours, 1974.
108. Edwards RG, Fowler RE, Gore-Langton RE, et al. Normal and abnormal follicular growth in mouse, rat and human ovaries. *J Reprod Fertil* 1977;51:237–263.
109. Kim I, Shaha C, Greenwald GS. A species difference between hamster and rat in the effect of oestrogens on growth of large preantral follicles. *J Reprod Fertil* 1984;72:179–185.
110. Meredith S, Kirkpatrick-Keller D, Butcher RL. The effects of food restriction and hypophysectomy on numbers of primordial follicles and concentrations of hormones in rats. *Biol Reprod* 1986;35:68–73.
111. Bokser L, Srkalovic G, Szepeshazi K, Schally AV. Recovery of pituitary-gonadal function in male and female rats after prolonged administration of a potent antagonist of luteinizing hormone-releasing hormone (SB-75). *Neuroendocrinology* 1991; 54:136–145.
112. Ataya K, Tadros M, Ramahi A. Gonadotropin-releasing hormone agonist inhibits physiologic ovarian follicular loss in rats. *Acta Endocrinol (Copenh)* 1989;121:55–60.
113. Nakano R, Mizuno T, Katayama K, Tojo S. Growth of ovarian follicles in rats in the absence of gonadotrophins. *J Reprod Fertil* 1975;45:545–546.
114. Hirshfield AN. Comparison of granulosa cell proliferation in small follicles of hypophysectomized, prepubertal, and mature rats. *Biol Reprod* 1985;32:979–987.
115. Faddy MJ, Jones EC, Edwards RG. An analytical model for ovarian follicle dynamics. *J Exp Zool* 1976;197:173–186.
116. Oakberg EF. Follicular growth and atresia in the mouse. *In Vitro* 1979;15:41–49.
117. Wang X-N, Greenwald GS. Hypophysectomy of the cyclic mouse. I. Effects on folliculogenesis, oocyte growth and follicle-stimulating hormone and human chorionic gonadotropin receptors. *Biol Reprod* 1993;48:585–594.
118. Wang X-N, Greenwald GS. Hypophysectomy of the cyclic mouse. II. Effects of follicle-stimulating hormone (FSH) and luteinizing hormone (LH) on folliculogenesis, FSH and human chorionic gonadotropin receptors, and steroidogenesis. *Biol Reprod* 1993;48:595–605.
119. de Reviers MM. Sequential effects of FSH on the first stages of ovarian follicular development in normal and dwarf Snell mice. *Acta Endocrinol* 1988;117:26–32.
120. Halpin DMG, Charlton HM. Effects of short-term injection of gonadotrophins on ovarian follicle development in hypogonadal (hpg) mice. *J Reprod Fertil* 1988;82:393–400.
121. Nayudu PL, Osborn SM. Factors influencing the rate of preantral and antral growth of mouse ovarian follicles in vitro. *J Reprod Fertil* 1992;95:349–362.
122. Moore PJ, Greenwald GS. Effect of hypophysectomy and gonadotropin treatment on follicular development and ovulation in the hamster. *Am J Anat* 1974;139:37–48.
123. Garza F, Shaban MA, Terranova PF. Luteinizing hormone increases the number of ova shed in the cyclic hamster and guinea-pig. *J Endocrinol* 1984;101:289–298.
124. Kim I, Greenwald GS. Occupied and unoccupied FSH receptors in follicles of cyclic, hypophysectomized or hypophysectomized/gonadotropin-treated hamsters. *Mol Cell Endocrinol* 1986;44: 141–145.
125. Roy SK, Wang SC, Greenwald GS. Radioreceptor and autoradiographic analysis of FSH, hCG and prolactin binding sites in primary to antral hamster follicles during the periovulatory period. *J Reprod Fertil* 1987;79:307–313.
126. Roy SK, Greenwald GS. In vitro effects of follicle-stimulating hormone, luteinizing hormone, and prolactin on follicular deoxyribonucleic acid synthesis in the hamster. *Endocrinology* 1988;122:952–958.
127. Roy SK, Greenwald GS. In vitro steroidogenesis by primary to antral follicles in the hamster during the periovulatory period: effects of follicle-stimulating hormone, luteinizing hormone, and prolactin. *Biol Reprod* 1987;37:39–46.
128. Roy SK, Greenwald GS. Hormonal requirements for the growth and differentiation of hamster preantral follicles in long-term culture. *J Reprod Fertil* 1989;87:103–114.
129. Dempsey EW. Follicular growth rate and ovulation after various experimental procedures in the guinea pig. *Am J Physiol* 1937;120:126–132.
130. Perry JS, Rowlands IW. Hypophysectomy of the immature guinea-pig and the ovarian response to gonadotrophins. *J Reprod Fertil* 1963;6:393–404.
131. Dufour J, Cahill LP, Mauleon P. Short- and long-term effects of hypophysectomy and unilateral ovariectomy on ovarian follicular populations in sheep. *J Reprod Fertil* 1979;57:301–309.
132. McNatty KP, Heath DA, Hudson N, Clarke IJ. Effect of long-term hypophysectomy on ovarian follicle populations and gonadotrophin-induced adenosine cyclic 3′,5′-monophosphate output by follicles from Booroola ewes with or without the F gene. *J Reprod Fertil* 1990;90:515–522.
133. Larson GH, Mallory DS, Dailey RA, Lewis PE. Gonadotropin concentrations, follicular development, and luteal function in pituitary stalk-transected ewes treated with bovine follicular fluid. *J Anim Sci* 1991;69:4104–4111.
134. Picton HM, Tsonis CG, McNeilly AS. The antagonistic effect of exogenous LH pulses on FSH-stimulated preovulatory follicle growth in ewes chronically treated with a gonadotrophin-releasing hormone agonist. *J Endocrinol* 1990;127:273–283.
135. McNeilly AS. The ovarian follicle and fertility. *J Steroid Biochem Mol Biol* 1991;40:29–33.
136. Goldenberg RL, Powell RD, Rosen SW, Marshall JR, Ross GT. Ovarian morphology in women with anosmia and hypogonadotropic hypogonadism. *Am J Obstet Gynecol* 1976;126:91–94.
137. Lim HT, Meinders AE, deHaan LD, Bronkhorst FB. Anovulation presumably due to the gonadotrophin-resistant ovary syndrome. *Eur J Obstet Gynecol Reprod Biol* 1984;16:327–337.
138. Talbert LM, Raj MHG, Hammond MG, Greer T. Endocrine and immunologic studies in a patient with resistant ovary syndrome. *Fertil Steril* 1984;42:741–744.
139. Lintern-Moore S, Moore GPM. Comparative aspects of oocyte growth in mammals. In: Calaby JH, Tyndale-Biscoe CH, eds. *Reproduction and evolution. Proceedings of the fourth symposium on comparative biology of reproduction of the Australian Academy of Science.* Canberra City: Australian Academy of Science, 1977:215–219.
140. Lintern-Moore S, Moore GPM. The initiation of follicle and oocyte growth in the mouse ovary. *Biol Reprod* 1979;20:773–778.
141. Moore GPM, Lintern-Moore S, Peters H, Faber M. RNA synthesis in the mouse oocyte. *J Cell Biol* 1974;60:416–422.
142. Canipari R, Pietrolucci A, Mangia F. Increase of total protein synthesis during mouse oocyte growth. *J Reprod Fertil* 1979;57:405–413.
143. Muller U, Urban E. An oocyte-specific antigen and its possible role in the organization of the ovarian follicle of the rat. *Differentiation* 1981;20:274–277.
144. Heller DT, Cahill DM, Schultz RM. Biochemical studies of mammalian oogenesis: metabolic cooperativity between granulosa cells and growing mouse oocytes. *Dev Biol* 1981;84:455–464.
145. Roy SK, Greenwald GS. Evidence for binding sites for FSH and hCG in mammalian oocytes. In: Toft DO, Ryan RJ, eds. *Proceedings of the fifth Ovarian Workshop.* Champaign, IL: Ovarian Workshops, 1985:143–147.
146. Mulheron GW, Quattropani SL, Nolin JM. The ontogeny of immunoreactive, endogenous FSH and LH in the rat ovary during early folliculogenesis. *Proc Soc Exp Biol Med* 1989;190:91–97.
147. Roy SK, Greenwald GS. Immunohistochemical localization of epidermal growth factor-like activity in the hamster ovary with a polyclonal antibody. *Endocrinology* 1990;126:1309–1317.
148. Zachow RJ, Tash JS, Terranova PF. Tumor necrosis factor-α induces clustering in ovarian theca-interstitial cells in vitro. *Endocrinology* 1992;131:2503–2513.
149. Manova K, Nocka K, Besmer P, Bachvarova RF. Gonadal expression of c-kit encoded at the W locus of the mouse. *Development* 1990;110:1057–1069.
150. Vanderhyden BC, Telfer EE, Eppig JJ. Mouse oocytes promote proliferation of granulosa cells from preantral and antral follicles in vitro. *Biol Reprod* 1992;46:1196–1204.
151. Takaoka H, Satoh H, Makinoda S, Moriya S, Ichinoe K. Granulosa-cell growth factor in oocyte and its transport systems. *Acta Obstet Gynaecol Jpn* 1985;37:92–98.

152. Hirshfield AN. Patterns of [^{3}H]thymidine incorporation differ in immature rats and mature, cycling rats. *Biol Reprod* 1986;34: 229–235.
153. Cran DG, Moor RM, Hay MF. Fine structure of the sheep oocyte during antral follicle development. *J Reprod Fertil* 1980;59: 125–132.
154. Tesoriero JV. Comparative cytochemistry of the developing ovarian follicles of the dog, rabbit, and mouse: origin of the zona pellucida. *Gamete Res* 1984;10:301–318.
155. Shimizu S, Tsuji M, Dean J. In vitro biosynthesis of three sulfated glycoproteins of murine zonae pellucidae by oocytes grown in follicle culture. *J Biol Chem* 1983;258:5858–5863.
156. Colonna R, Mangia R. Mechanisms of amino acid uptake in cumulus-enclosed mouse oocytes. *Biol Reprod* 1983;28:797–803.
157. Wassarman PM, Bleil JD, Cascio SM, et al. Programming of gene expression during mammalian oogenesis. In: Jagiello G, Vogel HJ, eds. *Bioregulators of reproduction.* New York: Academic Press; 1981:119–150.
158. Dunbar BS. Morphological, biochemical, and immunochemical characterization of the mammalian zona pellucida. In: Hartmann JF, ed. *Mechanism and control of animal fertilization.* New York: Academic Press; 1983:139–175.
159. Léveilé MC, Roberts KD, Chevalier S, Chapdelaine A, Bleau G. Formation of the hamster zona pellucida in relation to ovarian differentiation and follicular growth. *J Reprod Fertil* 1987;79: 173–183.
160. Wolgemuth DJ, Celenza J, Bundman DS, Dunbar BS. Formation of the rabbit zona pellucida and its relationship to ovarian follicular development. *Dev Biol* 1984;106:1–14.
161. Maresh GA, Timmons TM, Dunbar BS. Effects of extracellular matrix on the expression of specific ovarian proteins. *Biol Reprod* 1990;43:965–976.
162. Skinner SM, Mills T, Kirchick HJ, Dunbar BS. Immunization with zona pellucida proteins results in abnormal ovarian follicular differentiation and inhibition of gonadotropin-induced steroid secretion. *Endocrinology* 1984;115:2418–2432.
163. Jones GR, Sacco AG, Subramanian MG, et al. Histology of ovaries of female rabbits immunized with deglycosylated zona pellucida macromolecules of pigs. *J Reprod Fertil* 1992;95:513–525.
164. Michael SD. Interactions of the thymus and the ovary. In: Greenwald GS, Terranova PF, eds. *Factors regulating ovarian function.* New York: Raven Press; 1983:445–464.
165. Lane CE, Davis FR. The ovary of the adult rat. I. Changes in growth of the follicle and in volume and mitotic activity of the granulosa and theca during the estrous cycle. *Anat Rec* 1939;73:429–442.
166. Gosden RG, Hunter RHF, Telfer E, Torrance C, Brown N. Physiological factors underlying the formation of ovarian follicular fluid. *J Reprod Fertil* 1988;82:813–825.
167. Fischer B, Kunzel W, Kleinstein J, Gips H. Oxygen tension in follicular fluid falls with follicle maturation. *Eur J Obstet Gynecol Reprod Biol* 1992;43:39–43.
168. Ax RL, Ryan RJ. The porcine ovarian follicle. IV. Mucopolysaccharides at different stages of development. *Biol Reprod* 1979;20:1123–1132.
169. Yanagishita M, Rodbard D, Hascall VC. Isolation and characterization of proteoglycans from porcine ovarian follicular fluid. *J Biol Chem* 1979;254:911–920.
170. Schweitzer M, Jackson JC, Ryan RJ. The porcine ovarian follicle. VII. FSH stimulation of in vitro [^{3}H]-glucosamine incorporation into mucopolysaccharides. *Biol Reprod* 1981;24:332–340.
171. Burghardt RC, Anderson E. Hormonal modulation of gap junctions in rat ovarian follicles. *Cell Tissue Res* 1981;214:181–193.
172. Larsen WJ, Tung HN, Polking C. Response of granulosa cell gap junctions to human chorionic gonadotropin (hCG) at ovulation. *Biol Reprod* 1981;25:1119–1134.
173. Fletcher WH, Greenan JRT. Receptor mediated action without receptor occupancy. *Endocrinology* 1985;116:1660–1662.
174. Hay MF, Moor RM. Distribution of Δ5-3β-hydroxysteroid dehydrogenase activity in the graafian follicle of the sheep. *J Reprod Fertil* 1975;43:313–322.
175. Cran DG, Hay MF, Moor RM. The fine structure of the cumulus oophorus during follicular development in sheep. *Cell Tissue Res* 1979;202:439–451.
176. Mestwerdt W, Muller O. Elektronenoptisch-morphometrische Untersuchungen zum Luteinisierungsprozess der Follikelgranulosazelle menschlicher Ovarien. *Arch Gynaekol* 1978;225:51–65.
177. Bomsel-Helmreich O, Gougeon A, Thebault A, et al. Healthy and atretic human follicles in the preovulatory phase: differences in evolution of follicular morphology and steroid content of follicular fluid. *J Clin Endocrinol Metab* 1979;48:686–694.
178. Amin H, Richart RM, Brinson AO. Preovulatory granulosa cells and steroidogenesis: an ultrastructural study in the rhesus monkey. *Obstet Gynecol* 1976;47:562–568.
179. Zoller LC. A comparison of rat and hamster preovulatory follicles: an examination of differences in morphology and enzyme activity using qualitative and quantitative analyses. *Anat Rec* 1984;210:279–291.
180. Bjersing L. Maturation, morphology, and endocrine function of the follicular wall in mammals. In: Jones RE, ed. *The vertebrate ovary: comparative biology and evolution.* New York: Plenum; 1978:181–214.
181. Fortune JE. Bovine theca and granulosa cells interact to promote androgen production. *Biol Reprod* 1986;35:292–299.
182. Makris A, Olsen D, Ryan KJ. Significance of the Δ5 and Δ4 steroidogenic pathways in the hamster preovulatory follicle. *Steroids* 1983;42:641–651.
183. Lange Y, Schmit VM, Schreiber JR. Localization and movement of newly synthesized cholesterol in rat ovarian granulosa cells. *Endocrinology* 1988;123:81–86.
184. Orly J. Orchestrated expression of steroidogenic side-chain cleavage cytochrome P-450 during follicular development in the rat ovary. *J Reprod Fertil* 1989;37[Suppl]:155–162.
185. Goldschmit D, Kraicer P, Orly J. Periovulatory expression of cholesterol side-chain cleavage cytochrome P-450 in cumulus cells. *Endocrinology* 1989;124:369–378.
186. Weisz J, Zoller LC. Quantitative cytochemistry in the study of regional specialization in the membrana granulosa of the ovulable type of follicle. In: Pattison JR, Bitensky L, Chayen J, eds. *Quantitative cytochemistry and its applications.* New York: Academic Press; 1979:269–283.
187. Zoller LC, Weisz J. A quantitative cytochemical study of glucose-6-phosphate dehydrogenase and Δ5-3β-hydroxysteroid dehydrogenase activity in the membrana granulosa of the ovulable type of follicle of the rat. *Histochemistry* 1979;62:125–135.
188. Zoller LC, Enelow R. A quantitative histochemical study of lactate dehydrogenase and succinate dehydrogenase activities in the membrana granulosa of the ovulatory follicle of the rat. *Histochem J* 1983;15:1055–1064.
189. Whitman GF, Boldt JP, Martinez JE, Pantazis CG. Flow cytometric analysis of induced human graafian follicles. I. Demonstration and sorting of two luteinized cell populations. *Fertil Steril* 1991;56:259–264.
190. Rao IM, Allsbrook WC Jr, Conway BA, et al. Flow cytometric analysis of granulosa cells from developing rat follicles. *J Reprod Fertil* 1991;91:521–530.
191. Rao IM, Mills TM, Anderson E, Mahesh VB. Heterogeneity in granulosa cells of developing rat follicles. *Anat Rec* 1991;229: 177–185.
192. Hillensjo T, Magnusson C, Svensson U, Thelander H. Effect of luteinizing hormone and follicle-stimulating hormone on progesterone synthesis by cultured rat cumulus cells. *Endocrinology* 1981;108:1920–1924.
193. Erickson GF, Hofeditz C, Unger M, Allen WR, Dulbecco R. A monoclonal antibody to a mammary cell line recognizes two distinct subtypes of ovarian granulosa cells. *Endocrinology* 1985;117:1490–1499.
194. Staigmiller RB, Moor RM. Effect of follicle cells on the maturation and developmental competence of ovine oocytes matured outside the follicle. *Gamete Res* 1984;9:221–229.
195. Meduri G, Vuhai-Luuthi MT, Jolivet A, Milgrom E. New functional zonation in the ovary as shown by immunohistochemistry of luteinizing hormone receptor. *Endocrinology* 1992;131: 366–373.
196. Peng X-R, Hsueh AJW, LaPolt PS, Bjersing L, Ny T. Localization of luteinizing hormone receptor messenger ribonucleic acid expression in ovarian cell types during follicle development and ovulation. *Endocrinology* 1991;129:3200–3207.

197. Charlton HM, Parry D, Halpin DMG, Webb R. Distribution of ^{125}I-labelled follicle-stimulating hormone and human chorionic gonadotrophin in the gonads of hypogonadal (hpg) mice. *J Endocrinol* 1982;93:247–252.
198. Armstrong DT, Weiss TJ, Selstam G, Seamark RF. Hormonal and cellular interactions in follicular steroid biosynthesis by the sheep ovary. *J Reprod Fertil* 1981;30[Suppl]:143–154.
199. Channing CP, Schaerf FW, Anderson LD, Tsafriri A. Ovarian follicular and luteal physiology. In: Greep RO, ed. *Reproductive physiology III. International review of physiology.* Baltimore: University Park Press; 1980:117–201.
200. Nakano R, Sasaki K, Shima K, Kitayama S. Follicle-stimulating hormone and luteinizing hormone receptors on porcine granulosa cells during follicular maturation: an autoradiographic study. *Exp Clin Endocrinol* 1983;81:17–23.
201. Uilenbroek JTJ, Richards JS. Ovarian follicular development during the rat estrous cycle: gonadotropin receptors and follicular responsiveness. *Biol Reprod* 1979;20:1159–1165.
202. Amsterdam A, Koch Y, Lieberman ME, Lindner HR. Distribution of binding sites for human chorionic gonadotropin in the preovulatory follicle of the rat. *J Cell Biol* 1975;67:894–900.
203. Lawrence TS, Dekel N, Beers WH. Binding of human chorionic gonadotropin by rat cumuli oophori and granulosa cells: a comparative study. *Endocrinology* 1980;106:1114–1118.
204. Bortolussi M, Marini G, Reolon ML. A histochemical study of the binding of ^{125}I-HCG to the rat ovary throughout the estrous cycle. *Cell Tissue Res* 1979;197:213–226.
205. Oxberry BA, Greenwald GS. An autoradiographic study of the binding of ^{125}I-labeled follicle-stimulating hormone, human chorionic gonadotropin and prolactin to the hamster ovary throughout the estrous cycle. *Biol Reprod* 1982;27:505–516.
206. Richards JS, Ireland JJ, Rao MC, Bernath GA, Midgley AR Jr, Reichert LE Jr. Ovarian follicular development in the rat: hormone receptor regulation by estradiol, follicle stimulating hormone and luteinizing hormone. *Endocrinology* 1976;99:1562–1570.
207. Knecht M, Darbon JM, Ranta T, Baukal AJ, Catt KJ. Estrogens enhance the adenosine 3′,5′-monophosphate-mediated induction of follicle-stimulating hormone and luteinizing hormone receptors in rat granulosa cells. *Endocrinology* 1984;115:41–49.
208. May JV, Buck PA, Schomberg DW. Epidermal growth factor enhances [^{125}I]iodo-follicle-stimulating hormone binding by cultured porcine granulosa cells. *Endocrinology* 1987;120:2413–2420.
209. Hasegawa Y, Miyamoto K, Abe Y, et al. Induction of follicle stimulating hormone receptor by erythroid differentiation factor on rat granulosa cell. *Biochem Biophys Res Commun* 1988;156:668–674.
210. Vale W, Rivier J, Vaughan J, et al. Purification and characterization of an FSH releasing protein from porcine ovarian follicular fluid. *Nature* 1986;321:776–779.
211. Robertson DM, Klein R, de Vos FL, et al. The isolation of polypeptides with FSH suppressing activity from bovine follicular fluid which are structurally different to inhibin. *Biochem Biophys Res Commun* 1987;149:744–749.
212. Ying SY, Becker A, Swanson G, et al. Follistatin specifically inhibits pituitary follicle stimulating hormone release in vitro. *Biochem Biophys Res Commun* 1987;149:133–139.
213. Saito S, Nakamura T, Titani K, Sugino H. Production of activin-binding protein by rat granulosa cells in vitro. *Biochem Biophys Res Commun* 1991;176:413–422.
214. Klein R, Robertson DM, Shukovski L, Findlay JK, de Kretser DM. The radioimmunoassay of follicle stimulating hormone (FSH)-suppressing protein (FSP): stimulation of bovine granulosa cell FSP secretion by FSH. *Endocrinology* 1991;128:1048–1056.
215. Nakatani A, Shimasaki S, Depaolo LV, Erickson GF, Ling N. Cyclic changes in follistatin messenger ribonucleic acid and its protein in the rat ovary during the estrous cycle. *Endocrinology* 1991;129:603–611.
216. LaPolt PS, Soto D, Su JG, et al. Activin stimulation of inhibin secretion and messenger RNA levels in cultured granulosa cells. *Mol Endocrinol* 1989;3:1666–1673.
217. Xiao S, Robertson DM, Findlay JK. Effects of activin and follicle-stimulating hormone (FSH)-suppressing protein/follistatin on FSH receptors and differentiation of cultured rat granulosa cells. *Endocrinology* 1992;131:1009–1016.
218. Woodruff TK, Lyon RJ, Hansen SE, Rice GC, Mather JP. Inhibin and activin locally regulate rat ovarian folliculogenesis. *Endocrinology* 1990;127:3196–3205.
219. Niimura S, Ishida K. Histochemical demonstration of hydroxysteroid dehydrogenases in the oocytes in antral follicles of pigs, cattle and horses. *Jpn J Anim Reprod* 1983;29:150–153.
220. Dupont E, Luu-The V, Labrie F, Pelletier G. Light microscopic immunocytochemical localization of 3β-hydroxy-5-ene-steroid dehydrogenase/Δ5-Δ4-isomerase in the gonads and adrenal glands of the guinea pig. *Endocrinology* 1990;126:2906–2909.
221. Kawashima M, Greenwald GS. Comparison of follicular estrogen receptors in rat, hamster and pig. *Biol Reprod* 1993;47:172–179.
222. Wallach EE, Noriega C. Effects of local steroids on follicular development and atresia in the rabbit. *Fertil Steril* 1970;21:253–267.
223. Iwai T, Fujii S, Nanbu Y, et al. Effect of human chorionic gonadotropin on the expression of progesterone receptors and estrogen receptors in rabbit ovarian granulosa cells and the uterus. *Endocrinology* 1991;129:1840–1848.
224. Erb Meuli L, Lacker HM, Thau RB. Experimental evidence supporting a mathematical theory of the physiological mechanism regulating follicle development and ovulation number. *Biol Reprod* 1987;37:589–594.
225. Wang X-N, Greenwald GS. Synergistic effects of steroids with FSH on folliculogenesis, steroidogenesis and FSH- and hCG-receptors in the hypophysectomized mouse. *J Reprod Fertil* 1993;In press.
226. Kim I, Greenwald GS. Effect of estrogens on follicular development and ovarian and uterine estrogen receptors in the immature rabbit, guinea pig and mouse. *Endocrinol Jpn* 1987;34:871–878.
227. Chakravorty A, Mahesh VB, Mills TM. Regulation of follicular development by diethylstilboestrol in ovaries of immature rats. *J Reprod Fertil* 1991;92:307–321.
228. Chakravorty A, Mahesh VB, Mills TM. Inhibition by diethylstilboestrol of proliferative potential of follicles of different sizes in immature rat ovaries. *J Reprod Fertil* 1991;92:323–332.
229. Bley MA, Simon JC, Saragueta PE, Baranao JL. Hormonal regulation of rat granulosa cell deoxyribonucleic acid synthesis: effects of estrogens. *Biol Reprod* 1991;44:880–888.
230. Mulheron GW, Schomberg DW. Effects of diethylstilbestrol on rat granulosa cell and thecal/interstitial cell transforming growth factor-β2 mRNA expression in vivo: analysis by reverse transcription-polymerase chain reaction. *Biol Reprod* 1992;46:546–550.
231. Iida K, Imai A, Tamaya T. Stimulatory effects of estrogen on gonadotropin-releasing hormone-induced phosphoinositide turnover in granulosa cells. *J Steroid Biochem Mol Biol* 1991;38:583–586.
232. Farookhi R, Desjardins J. Luteinizing hormone receptor induction in dispersed granulosa cells requires estrogen. *Mol Cell Endocrinol* 1986;47:13–24.
233. Peluso JJ, Delidow BC, Lynch J, White BA. Follicle-stimulating hormone and insulin regulation of 17β-estradiol secretion and granulosa cell proliferation within immature rat ovaries maintained in perifusion culture. *Endocrinology* 1991;128:191–196.
234. Hutz RJ, Krueger GS, Meller PA, Sholl SA, Dierschke DJ. FSH-induced aromatase activity in hamster granulosa cells: effect of estradiol-17β in vitro. *Cell Tissue Res* 1987;250:101–104.
235. Hutz RJ, Schaller M, Kitzman P, Bejvan SM. Oestradiol-17β affects differentially viability, progesterone secretion, and apical surface morphology of hamster ovarian follicles in vitro. *Zool Sci* 1991;8:81–88.
236. Racowsky C, Baldwin KV. Modulation of intrafollicular oestradiol in explanted hamster follicles does not affect oocyte meiotic status. *J Reprod Fertil* 1989;87:409–420.
237. Kim I, Greenwald GS. Estrogen receptors in ovary and uterus of immature hamster and rat: effects of estrogens. *Endocrinol Jpn* 1987;34:45–53.
238. Hiura M, Fujita H. Electron microscopy of the cytodifferentiation of the theca cell in the mouse ovary. *Arch Histol Jpn* 1977;40:95–105.
239. O'Shea JD. An ultrastructural study of smooth muscle-like cells

in the theca externa of ovarian follicles in the rat. *Anat Rec* 1970;167:127–140.
240. Amsterdam A, Lindner HR, Stewart UG. Localization of actin and myosin in the rat oocyte and follicular wall by immunofluorescence. *Anat Rec* 1977;187:311–328.
241. Capps ML, Lawrence IE Jr, Burden HW. Cellular junctions in perifollicular contractile tissue of the rat ovary during the preovulatory period. *Cell Tissue Res* 1981;219:133–141.
242. Muglia U, Vizza E, Familiari G, Motta PM. The smooth muscle cells in the ovary. In: Motta PM, ed. *Ultrastructure of smooth muscle.* Norwell, MA: Kluwer Academic Publishers; 1990: 221–235.
243. Walles B, Edvinsson L, Owman C, Sjoberg NO, Sporrong B. Cholinergic nerves and receptors mediating contraction of the graafian follicle. *Biol Reprod* 1976;15:565–572.
244. Kobayashi Y, Sjoberg NO, Walles B, et al. The effect of adrenergic agents on the ovulatory process in the in vitro perfused rabbit ovary. *Am J Obstet Gynecol* 1983;145:857–864.
245. Self DA, Schroeder PC, Gown AM. Hamster thecal cells express muscle characteristics. *Biol Reprod* 1988;39:119–130.
246. Ishwar S, Sankaranarayanan A, Bawa SR. Neurogenic involvement in follicular development and ovulation: a probability. *Int J Fertil* 1987;32:388–393.
247. Kannisto P, Ekblad E, Helm G, et al. Existence and coexistence of peptides in nerves of the mammalian ovary and oviduct demonstrated by immunocytochemistry. *Histochemistry* 1986; 86:25–34.
248. Jorgensen JC, O'Hare MMT, Andersen CY. Demonstration of neuropeptide Y and its precursor in plasma and follicular fluid. *Endocrinology* 1990;127:1682–1688.
249. Trzeciak WH, Ahmed CE, Simpson ER, Ojeda SR. Vasoactive intestinal peptide induces the synthesis of the cholesterol side-chain cleavage enzyme complex in cultured rat ovarian granulosa cells. *Proc Natl Acad Sci USA* 1986;83:7490–7494.
250. Wylie SN, Roche PJ, Gibson WR. Ovulation after sympathetic denervation of the rat ovary produced by freezing its nerve supply. *J Reprod Fertil* 1985;75:369–373.
251. Lara HE, McDonald JK, Ojeda SR. Involvement of nerve growth factor in female sexual development. *Endocrinology* 1990; 126:364–375.
252. Lara EL, Hill DF, Katz KH, Ojeda SR. The gene encoding nerve growth factor is expressed in the immature rat ovary: effect of denervation and hormonal treatment. *Endocrinology* 1990; 126:357–363.
253. Lara HE, Dees WL, Hiney JK, Dissen GA, Rivier C, Ojeda SR. Functional recovery of the developing rat ovary after transplantation: contribution of the extrinsic innervation. *Endocrinology* 1991;129:1849–1860.
254. Dissen GA, Hill DF, Costa ME, Ma YJ, Ojeda SR. Nerve growth factor receptors in the peripubertal rat ovary. *Mol Endocrinol* 1991;5:1642–1650.
255. Stoklosowa S, Gregoraszczuk E, Channing CP. Estrogen and progesterone secretion by isolated cultured porcine thecal and granulosa cells. *Biol Reprod* 1982;26:943–952.
256. Merk FB, Albright JT, Botticelli CR. The fine structure of granulosa cell nexuses in rat ovarian follicles. *Anat Rec* 1973;175: 107–126.
257. Kranzfelder D, Korr H, Mestwerdt W, Maurer-Schultze B. Follicle growth in the ovary of the rabbit after ovulation-inducing application of human chorionic gonadotropin. *Cell Tissue Res* 1984;238:611–620.
258. Makris A, Klagsbrun MA, Yasumizu T, Ryan KJ. An endogenous ovarian growth factor which stimulates BALB/3T3 and granulosa cell proliferation. *Biol Reprod* 1983;29:1135–1141.
259. Roberts AJ, Skinner MK. Estrogen regulation of thecal cell steroidogenesis and differentiation: thecal cell-granulosa cell interactions. *Endocrinology* 1990;127:2918–2929.
260. Knecht M, Feng P, Catt KJ. Transforming growth factor-beta: autocrine, paracrine, and endocrine effects in ovarian cells. *Semin Reprod Endocrinol* 1989;7:12–20.
261. Mulheron GW, Danielpour D, Schomberg DW. Rat thecal/interstitial cells express transforming growth factor-β type 1 and 2, but only type 2 is regulated by gonadotropin in vitro. *Endocrinology* 1991;129:368–374.
262. Bendell JJ, Dorrington J. Rat thecal/interstitial cells secrete a transforming growth factor-β-like factor that promotes growth and differentiation in rat granulosa cells. *Endocrinology* 1988;123:941–948.
263. Bendell JJ, Lobb DK, Chuma A, Gysler M, Dorrington JH. Bovine thecal cells secrete factor(s) that promote granulosa cell proliferation. *Biol Reprod* 1988;38:790–797.
264. Hillier SG, Yong EL, Illingworth PJ, Baird DT, Schwall RH, Mason AJ. Effect of recombinant activin on androgen synthesis in cultured human thecal cells. *J Clin Endocrinol Metab* 1991;72:1206–1211.
265. O'Shea JD, Cran DG, Hay MF, Moor RM. Ultrastructure of the theca interna of ovarian follicles in sheep. *Cell Tissue Res* 1978;187:457–472.
266. Priedkalns J, Weber AF, Zemjanis R. Qualitative and quantitative morphological studies of the cells of the membrana granulosa, theca interna and corpus luteum of the bovine ovary. *Z Zellforsch* 1968;85:501–520.
267. Wordinger RJ, Rudick VL, Rudick MJ. Immunohistochemical localization of laminin within the mouse ovary. *J Exp Zool* 1983;228:141–143.
268. Carnegie JA. Secretion of fibronectin by rat granulosa cells occurs primarily during early follicular development. *J Reprod Fertil* 1990;89:579–589.
269. Roy SK, Greenwald GS. An enzymatic method for dissociation of intact follicles from the hamster ovary: histological and quantitative aspects. *Biol Reprod* 1985;32:203–215.
270. Roberts AJ, Skinner MK. Hormonal regulation of thecal cell function during antral follicle development in bovine ovaries. *Endocrinology* 1990;127:2907–2917.
271. Stoklosowa S, Bahr J, Gregoraszczuk E. Some morphological and functional characteristics of cells of the porcine theca interna in tissue culture. *Biol Reprod* 1978;19:712–719.
272. Tsang BK, Ainsworth L, Downey BR, Marcus GJ. Differential production of steroids by dispersed granulosa and theca interna cells from developing preovulatory follicles of pigs. *J Reprod Fertil* 1985;74:459–471.
273. Tonetta SA, DeVinna RS, diZerega GS. Modulation of porcine thecal cell aromatase activity by human chorionic gonadotropin, progesterone, estradiol-17β, and dihydrotestosterone. *Biol Reprod* 1986;35:785–791.
274. Engelhardt H, Gore-Langton RE, Armstrong DT. Luteinization of porcine thecal cells in vitro. *Mol Cell Endocrinol* 1991;75: 237–245.
275. Mondschein JS, Hammond JM. Growth factors regulate immunoreactive insulin-like growth factor-I production by cultured porcine granulosa cells. *Endocrinology* 1988;123:463–468.
276. Magoffin DA. Regulation of differentiated functions in ovarian theca cells. *Semin Reprod Endocrinol* 1991;9:321–331.
277. Katayama E. Monolayer culture of human ovarian thecal cells: a study on morphological and functional characteristics. *Acta Obstet Gynaecol Jpn* 1984;36:927–936.
278. Bogovich K, Richards JS. Androgen synthesis during follicular development: evidence that rat granulosa cell 17-ketosteroid reductase is independent of hormonal regulation. *Biol Reprod* 1984;31:122–131.
279. Koninckx PR. *New aspects of ovarian function in man and in rat* (Dissertation). Belgium: Katholieke Universiteit Leuven, 1981.
280. diZerega GS, Hodgen GD. Fluorescence localization of luteinizing hormone/human chorionic gonadotropin uptake in the primate ovary. II. Changing distribution during selection of the dominant follicle. *J Clin Endocrinol Metab* 1980;51:903–907.
281. Bassett DL. The changes in the vascular pattern of the ovary of the albino rat during the estrous cycle. *Am J Anat* 1943;73: 251–291.
282. Zeleznik AJ, Schuler HM, Reichert LE Jr. Gonadotropin-binding sites in the rhesus monkey ovary: role of the vasculature in the selective distribution of human chorionic gonadotropin to the preovulatory follicle. *Endocrinology* 1981;109:356–362.
283. McNatty KP, Heath DA, Lun S, Fannin JM, McDiarmid JM, Henderson KM. Steroidogenesis by bovine theca interna in an in vitro perifusion system. *Biol Reprod* 1984;30:159–170.
284. Koos RD, LeMaire WJ. Factors that may regulate the growth and regression of blood vessels in the ovary. *Semin Reprod Endocrinol* 1983;1:295–307.
285. Koos RD. Stimulation of endothelial cell proliferation by rat

granulosa cell-conditioned medium. *Endocrinology* 1986;119: 481–489.

286. Lin MT, Wei SJ, Wing LYC. Chemotactic and mitogenic activities of granulosa cells in developing follicles. *Mol Cell Endocrinol* 1992;84:47–54.
287. Findlay JK. Angiogenesis in reproductive tissues. *J Endocrinol* 1986;111:357–366.
288. Koos RD. Potential relevance of angiogenic factors to ovarian physiology. *Semin Reprod Endocrinol* 1989;7:29–40.
289. Reynolds LP, Killilea SD, Redmer DA. Angiogenesis in the female reproductive system. *FASEB J* 1992;6:886–892.
290. Montesano R, Vassalli JD, Baird A, Guillemin R, Orci L. Basic fibroblast growth factor induces angiogenesis in vitro. *Proc Natl Acad Sci USA* 1986;83:7297–7301.
291. Platt T. Transcription termination and the regulation of gene expression. *Annu Rev Biochem* 1986;55:339–372.
292. Rosenberg M, Court D. Regulatory sequences involved in the promotion and termination of RNA transcription. *Annu Rev Genet* 1979;13:319–353.
293. Gonzalez AM, Buscaglia M, Ong M, Baird A. Distribution of basic fibroblast growth factor in the 18-day rat fetus: localization in the basement membrane of diverse tissues. *J Cell Biol* 1990;110:753–765.
294. Koos RD, Olson CE. Expression of basic fibroblast growth factor in the rat ovary: detection of mRNA using reverse transcription-polymerase chain reaction amplification. *Mol Endocrinol* 1989;3:2041–2048.
295. Sato E, Tanaka T, Takeya T, Miyamoto H, Koide S. Ovarian glycosaminoglycans potentiate angiogenic activity of epidermal growth factor in mice. *Endocrinology* 1991;128:2402–2406.
296. Ravindranath N, Little-Ihrig L, Phillips HS, Ferrara N, Zeleznik AJ. Vascular endothelial growth factor messenger ribonucleic acid expression in the primate ovary. *Endocrinology* 1992;131: 254–260.
297. Frederick JL, Shimanuki T, diZerega GS. Initiation of angiogenesis by human follicular fluid. *Science* 1984;224:389–390.
298. Frederick JL, Nuguyen H, Preston DS, et al. Initiation of angiogenesis by porcine follicular fluid. *Am J Obstet Gynecol* 1985;152:1073–1078.
299. Gospodarowicz D, Cheng J, Lui GM, Baird A, Esch F, Bohlen P. Corpus luteum angiogenic factor is related to fibroblast growth factor. *Endocrinology* 1985;117:2283–2391.
300. Makris A, Ryan KJ, Takehiko Y, Hill CL, Zetter BR. The nonluteal porcine ovary as a source of angiogenic activity. *Endocrinology* 1984;15:1672–1677.
301. Melner MH, Young SL, Czerwiec FS, et al. The regulation of granulosa cell proopiomelanocortin messenger ribonucleic acid by androgens and gonadotropins. *Endocrinology* 1986;119: 2082–2088.
302. Bagnato A, Moretti C, Ohnishi J, Frajese G, Catt KJ. Expression of the growth hormone-releasing hormone gene and its peptide product in the rat ovary. *Endocrinology* 1992;130:1097–1102.
303. Jones PBC, Conn PM, Marian J, Hsueh AJW. Binding of gonadotropin releasing hormone agonist to rat ovarian granulosa cells. *Life Sci* 1980;27:2125–2132.
304. Wathes DC, Kendall PAD, Perks C, Brown D. Effects of stage of the cycle and estradiol-17β on oxytocin synthesis by ovine granulosa and luteal cells. *Endocrinology* 1992;130:1009–1016.
305. Zhang L, Dreifuss JJ, Dubois-Dauphin M, Tribollet E. Autoradiographical localization of oxytocin-binding sites in the guinea-pig ovary at different stages of the oestrous cycle. *J Endocrinol* 1991;131:421–426.
306. Lolait SJ, Autelitano DJ, Markwick AJ, Toh BH, Funder JW. Co-expression of vasopressin with β-endorphin and dynorphin in individual cells from the ovaries of Brattleboro and Long-Evans rats: immunocytochemical studies. *Peptides* 1986;7:267–276.
307. Thomas WG, Sernia C. The immunocytochemical localization of angiotensinogen in the rat ovary. *Cell Tissue Res* 1990;261: 367–373.
308. Féral C, Reznik Y, Le Gall S, Mahoudeau J, Corvol P, Leymarie P. Stimulation by hCG of ovarian inactive renin synthesis in rabbit preovulatory theca cells. *J Reprod Fertil* 1990;89:407–414.
309. Ueno S, Kuroda T, Maclaughlin DT, Ragin RC, Manganaro TF, Donahoe PK. Mullerian inhibiting substance in the adult rat ovary during various stages of the estrous cycle. *Endocrinology* 1989;125:1060–1066.
310. Rabinovici J, Spencer SJ, Doldi N, Goldsmith PC, Schwall R, Jaffe RB. Activin-A as an intraovarian modulator: actions, localization, and regulation of the intact dimer in human ovarian cells. *J Clin Invest* 1992;89:1528–1536.
311. Ying SY, Becker A, Ling N, Ueno N, Guillemin R. Inhibin and beta type transforming growth factor (TGF-β) have opposite modulating effects on the follicle stimulating hormone (FSH)-induced aromatase activity of cultured rat granulosa cells. *Biochem Biophys Res Commun* 1986;136:969–975.
312. Meunier H, Cajander SB, Roberts VJ, et al. Rapid changes in the expression of inhibin α-, βA- and βB-subunits in ovarian cell types during the rat estrous cycle. *Mol Endocrinol* 1988;2: 1352–1363.
313. Bagnell CA. Production and biologic action of relaxin within the ovarian follicle: an overview. *Steroids* 1991;56:242–246.
314. Saidapur SK. Follicular atresia in the ovaries of nonmammalian vertebrates. *Int Rev Cytol* 1978;54:225–244.
315. Byskov AG. Follicular atresia. In: Jones RE, ed. *The vertebrate ovary: comparative biology and evolution.* New York: Plenum; 1978:533–562.
316. Ingram DL. Atresia. In: Zuckerman SS, Mandl AM, Eckstein P, eds. *The ovary.* New York: Academic Press; 1962:247–273.
317. Spanel-Borowski K. Morphological investigations on follicular atresia in canine ovaries. *Cell Tissue Res* 1981;214:155–168.
318. Byskov AGS. Cell kinetic studies of follicular atresia in the mouse ovary. *J Reprod Fertil* 1974;37:277–285.
319. Brailly S, Gougeon A, Milgrom E, Bomsel-Helmreich O, Papiernik E. Androgens and progestins in the human ovarian follicle: differences in the evolution of preovulatory, healthy nonovulatory, and atretic follicles. *J Clin Endocrinol Metab* 1981;53: 128–133.
320. Westergaard L, McNatty KP, Christensen I, Larsen JK, Byskov AG. Flow cytometric deoxyribonucleic acid analysis of granulosa cells aspirated from human ovarian follicles: a new method to distinguish healthy and atretic ovarian follicles. *J Clin Endocrinol Metab* 1982;55:693–698.
321. Koering MJ, Goodman AL, Williams RF, Hodgen GD. Granulosa cell pyknosis in the dominant follicle of monkeys. *Fertil Steril* 1982;37:837–844.
322. Gerschenson LE, Rotello RJ. Apoptosis: a different type of cell death. *FASEB J* 1992;6:2450–2455.
323. Hughes FM Jr, Gorospe WC. Biochemical identification of apoptosis (programmed cell death) in granulosa cells: evidence for a potential mechanism underlying follicular atresia. *Endocrinology* 1991;129:2415–2422.
324. Zeleznik AJ, Ihrig LL, Bassett SG. Developmental expression of Ca^{++}/Mg^{++}-dependent endonuclease activity in rat granulosa and luteal cells. *Endocrinology* 1989;125:2218–2220.
325. Tilly JL, Billig H, Kowalski KI, Hsueh AJ. Epidermal growth factor and basic fibroblast growth factor suppress the spontaneous onset of apoptosis in cultured rat ovarian granulosa cells and follicles by a tyrosine kinase-dependent mechanism. *Mol Endocrinol* 1992;6:1942–1950.
326. Tilly JL, Kowalski KI, Johnson AL, Hsueh AJW. Involvement of apoptosis in ovarian follicular atresia and postovulatory regression. *Endocrinology* 1991;129:2799–2801.
327. Tilly JL, Kowalski KI, Schomberg DW, Hsueh AJW. Apoptosis in atretic ovarian follicles is associated with selective decreases in messenger ribonucleic acid transcripts for gonadotropin receptors and cytochrome P450 aromatase. *Endocrinology* 1992;131: 1670–1676.
328. Odeblad E. Contributions to the theory and technique of quantitative autoradiography with ^{32}P with special reference to the granulosa tissue of the graafian follicles in the rabbit. *Acta Radiol (Stockh)* [*Suppl*] 1952;93:1–123.
329. Deane HW. Histochemical observations on the ovary and oviduct of the albino rat during the estrous cycle. *Am J Anat* 1952;91:363–414.
330. Bukovsky A, Presl J, Zidovsky J. Migration of lymphoid cells into the granulosa of rat ovarian follicles. *IRCS Med Sci* 1979;7: 603–604.
331. Bukovsky A, Presl J, Holub M. The ovarian follicle as a model for

the cell-mediated control of tissue growth. *Cell Tissue Res* 1984;236:717–724.
332. Daud AI, Bumpus FM, Husain A. Evidence for selective expression of angiotensin II receptors on atretic follicles in the rat ovary: an autoradiographic study. *Endocrinology* 1988;122:2727–2734.
333. Mukhopadhyay AK, Holstein K, Szkudlinski M, Brunswig-Spickenheier B, Leidenberger FA. The relationship between prorenin levels in follicular fluid and follicular atresia in bovine ovaries. *Endocrinology* 1991;129:2367–2375.
334. Peluso JJ, England-Charlesworth C. Development of preovulatory follicles and oocytes during the oestrous cycle of mature and aged rats. *Acta Endocrinol* 1982;100:434–443.
335. Peluso JJ, England-Charlesworth C, Bolender DL, Steger RW. Ultrastructural alterations associated with the initiation of follicular atresia. *Cell Tissue Res* 1980;211:105–115.
336. Gondos B. Ultrastructure of follicular atresia in the rat. *Gamete Res* 1982;5:199–206.
337. Ryan RJ, Lee CY. The role of membrane bound receptors. *Biol Reprod* 1976;14:16–29.
338. Peluso JJ, Steger RW, Hafez ESE. Surface ultrastructural changes in granulosa cells of atretic follicles. *Biol Reprod* 1977;16: 600–604.
339. Erickson GF, Magoffin DA, Unger M, Allen WR, Dulbecco R. A monoclonal antibody recognizes a 39 kDa protein expressed in atretic granulosa cells. *Mol Cell Endocrinol* 1988;60:177–187.
340. Hay MF, Cran DG, Moor RM. Structural changes occurring during atresia in sheep ovarian follicles. *Cell Tissue Res* 1976; 169:515–529.
341. Hay MF, Moor RM, Cran DG, Dott HM. Regeneration of atretic sheep ovarian follicles in vitro. *J Reprod Fertil* 1979;55:195–207.
342. Moor RM, Hay MF, Dott HM, Cran DG. Macroscopic identification and steroidogenic function of atretic follicles in sheep. *J Endocrinol* 1978;77:309–318.
343. Meinecke B, Meinecke-Tillmann S, Gips H. Experimentelle Untersuchungen zur Steroidsekretion intakter und atretischer Follikel in vitro. *Berl Munch Tierarztl Wochenschr* 1982;95:107–111.
344. Henderson KM, Kieboom LE, McNatty KP, Lun S, Heath DA. [^{125}I]hCG binding to bovine thecal tissue from healthy and atretic antral follicles. *Mol Cell Endocrinol* 1984;34:91–98.
345. Zachariae F. Studies in the mechanism of ovulation: autoradiographic investigations on the uptake of radioactive sulphate (^{35}S) into the ovarian follicular mucopolysaccharides. *Acta Endocrinol* 1957;26:215–224.
346. Bellin ME, Ax RL. Chondroitin sulfate: an indicator of atresia in bovine follicles. *Endocrinology* 1984;114:428–434.
347. Guraya SS. Follicular atresia. *Proc Indian Natl Sci Acad* 1973;39:311–332.
348. Lobel BL, Rosenbaum RM, Deane HW. Enzymic correlates of physiological regression of follicles and corpora lutea in ovaries of normal rats. *Endocrinology* 1961;68:232–247.
349. Ryan RJ. Follicular atresia: some speculations of biochemical markers and mechanisms. In: Schwartz NB, Hunzicker-Dunn M, eds. *Dynamics of ovarian function.* New York: Raven Press; 1981.
350. Breitenecker G, Friedrich F, Kemeter P. Further investigations on the maturation and degeneration of human ovarian follicles and their oocytes. *Fertil Steril* 1978;29:336–341.
351. Dhanasekaran N, Moudgal NR. Studies on follicular atresia: role of tropic hormone and steroids in regulating cathepsin-D activity of preantral follicles of the immature rat. *Mol Cell Endocrinol* 1986;44:77–84.
352. McNatty KP, Makris A, De Grazia C, Osathanondh R, Ryan KJ. Steroidogenesis in granulosa cells and corpus luteum: the production of progesterone, androgens and oestrogens by human granulosa cells in vitro and in vivo. *J Steroid Biochem* 1979;11: 775–779.
353. Austin CR. *The mammalian egg.* Oxford: Blackwell; 1961.
354. Byskov AG. Atresia. In: Midgley AR, Sadler WA, eds. *Ovarian follicular development and function.* New York: Raven Press; 1979:41–57.
355. Dawson AB. Argyrophilic inclusions in the cytoplasm of the ova of the rat in normal and atretic follicles. *Anat Rec* 1952;112: 37–59.
356. Peluso JJ, Bolender DL, Perri A. Temporal changes associated with the degeneration of the rat oocyte. *Biol Reprod* 1979;20: 423–430.
357. Westergaard L. Follicular atresia in relation to oocyte morphology in non-pregnant and pregnant women. *J Reprod Fertil* 1985;74:113–118.
358. Vasques-Nin GH, Sotelo JR. Electron microscope study of the atretic oocytes of the rat. *Z Zellforsch Abt Histochem* 1967;80:518–533.
359. Baker TG, Franchi LL. The fine structure of oogonia and oocytes in human ovaries. *J Cell Sci* 1967;2:213–234.
360. Centola GM. Light microscopic observations of alterations in staining of the zona pellucida of porcine follicular oocytes: possible early indications of atresia. *Gamete Res* 1982;6:293–304.
361. Delgado MV, Zoller LC. A quantitative and qualitative cytochemical analysis of glycosaminoglycan content in the zona pellucida of hamster ovarian follicles. *Histochemistry* 1987;87: 279–287.
362. Familiari G, Nottola SA, Familiari A, Motta PM. The three-dimensional structure of the zona pellucida in growing and atretic ovarian follicles of the mouse: scanning and transmission electron-microscopic observations using ruthenium red and detergents. *Cell Tissue Res* 1989;257:247–253.
363. Donahue RP, Stern S. Follicular cell support of oocyte maturation: production of pyruvate in vitro. *J Reprod Fertil* 1968;17: 395–398.
364. Albertini DF, Anderson E. The appearance and structure of intercellular connections during the ontogeny of the rabbit ovarian follicle with particular reference to gap junctions. *J Cell Biol* 1974;63:234–250.
365. Osman P. Rate and course of atresia during follicular development in the adult cyclic rat. *J Reprod Fertil* 1985;73:261–270.
366. Moor RM, Trounson AO. Hormonal and follicular factors affecting maturation of sheep oocytes in vitro and their subsequent developmental capacity. *J Reprod Fertil* 1977;49:101–109.
367. Guraya SS, Greenwald GS. A comparative histochemical study of interstitial tissue and follicular atresia in the mammalian ovary. *Anat Rec* 1964;149:411–434.
368. Mossman HW, Koering MJ, Ferry D Jr. Cyclic changes of interstitial gland tissue of the human ovary. *Am J Anat* 1964;115: 235–256.
369. Schwall R, Erickson GF. Functional and morphological changes in rat theca cells during atresia. In: Schwartz NB, Hunzicker-Dunn M, eds. *Dynamics of ovarian function.* New York: Raven Press; 1981:29–34.
370. Terranova PF, Martin NC, Chien S. Theca is the source of progesterone in experimentally induced atretic follicles of the hamster. *Biol Reprod* 1982;26:721–727.
371. Silavin SL, Greenwald GS. Steroid production by isolated theca and granulosa cells after initiation of atresia in the hamster. *J Reprod Fertil* 1984;71:387–392.
372. O'Shea JD, Hay MF, Cran DG. Ultrastructural changes in the theca interna during follicular atresia in sheep. *J Reprod Fertil* 1978;54:183–187.
373. Bruce NW, Moor RM. Capillary blood flow to ovarian follicles, stroma and corpora lutea of anaesthetized sheep. *J Reprod Fertil* 1976;46:299–304.
374. Findlay JK, Carson RS. Selective binding of gonadotrophins and the control of follicular growth and atresia. In: Flerko B, Setalo G, Tima L, eds. *Advances in physiological science.* Vol 15: *Reproduction and development.* Budapest: Pergamon; 1980:79–89.
375. Bortolussi M, Zanchetta R, Doliana R, Castellani I, Bressan GM, Lauria A. Changes in the organization of the extracellular matrix in ovarian follicles during the preovulatory phase and atresia: an immunofluorescence study. *Basic Appl Histochem* 1989;33: 31–38.
376. Motta PM, Familiari G. Occurrence of contractile tissue in the theca externa of atretic follicles in the mouse ovary. *Acta Anat* 1981;109:103–114.
377. Mori T, Fujita Y, Nihnobu K, Ezaki Y, Kubo K, Nishimura T. Steroidogenesis in vitro by human ovarian follicles during the process of atresia. *Clin Endocrinol* 1982;16:391–400.
378. McNatty KP, Smith DM, Makris A, Osathanondh R, Ryan KJ. The microenvironment of the human antral follicle: interrelationships among the steroid levels in antral fluid, the population of granulosa cells, and the status of the oocyte in vivo and in vitro. *J Clin Endocrinol Metab* 1979;49:851–860.
379. McNatty KP, Makris A, Osathanondh R, Ryan KJ. Effects of

luteinizing hormone on steroidogenesis by thecal tissue from human ovarian follicles in vitro. *Steroids* 1980;36:53–63.
380. Maxson WS, Haney AF, Schomberg DW. Steroidogenesis in porcine atretic follicles: loss of aromatase activity in isolated granulosa and theca. *Biol Reprod* 1985;33:495–501.
381. Carson RS, Findlay JK, Clarke IJ, Burger HG. Estradiol, testosterone and androstenedione in ovine follicular fluid during growth and atresia of ovarian follicles. *Biol Reprod* 1981;24: 105–113.
382. Tsonis CG, Carson RS, Findlay JK. Relationships between aromatase activity, follicular fluid oestradiol-17β and testosterone concentrations, and diameter and atresia of individual ovine follicles. *J Reprod Fertil* 1984;72:153–163.
383. Carson RS, Findlay JK, Burger HG, Trounson AO. Gonadotropin receptors of the ovine ovarian follicle during follicular growth and atresia. *Biol Reprod* 1979;21:75–87.
384. Peng X-R, Hsueh AJW, LaPolt PS, Bjersing L, Ny T. Localization of luteinizing hormone receptor messenger ribonucleic acid expression in ovarian cell types during follicle development and ovulation. *Endocrinology* 1991;129:3200–3207.
385. Ireland JJ, Roche JF. Development of nonovulatory antral follicles in heifers: changes in steroids in follicular fluid and receptors for gonadotropins. *Endocrinology* 1983;112:150–156.
386. McNatty KP, Lun S, Heath DA, Kieboom LE, Henderson KM. Influence of follicular atresia on LH-induced cAMP and steroid synthesis by bovine thecae interna. *Mol Cell Endocrinol* 1985;39:209–215.
387. Braw RH, Bar-Ami S, Tsafriri A. Effect of hypophysectomy on atresia of rat preovulatory follicles. *Biol Reprod* 1981;25: 989–996.
388. Bill CH II, Greenwald GS. Acute gonadotropin deprivation. I. A model for the study of follicular atresia. *Biol Reprod* 1981;24:913–921.
389. Braw RH, Tsafriri A. Follicles explanted from pentobarbitone-treated rats provide a model for atresia. *J Reprod Fertil* 1980;59:259–265.
390. Uilenbroek JTJ, Woutersen PJA, van der Schoot P. Atresia of preovulatory follicles: gonadotropin binding and steroidogenic activity. *Biol Reprod* 1980;23:219–229.
391. Terranova PF. Effects of phenobarbital-induced ovulatory delay on the follicular population and serum levels of steroids and gonadotropins in the hamster: a model for atresia. *Biol Reprod* 1980;23:92–99.
392. Peters H, Byskov AG, Himelstein-Braw R, Faber M. Follicular growth: the basic event in the mouse and human ovary. *J Reprod Fertil* 1975;45:559–566.
393. Peluso JJ, Steger RW. Role of FSH in regulating granulosa cell division and follicular atresia in rats. *J Reprod Fertil* 1978;54:275–278.
394. Braw RH, Tsafriri A. Effect of PMSG on follicular atresia in the immature rat ovary. *J Reprod Fertil* 1980;59:267–272.
395. Matson PL, Gledhill B, Collins WP. Effect of LH on steroidogenesis by hamster follicles isolated at defined stages of development. *J Reprod Fertil* 1984;70:675–681.
396. Bagnell CA, Mills TM, Costoff A, Mahesh VB. A model for the study of androgen effects on follicular atresia and ovulation. *Biol Reprod* 1982;27:903–914.
397. Magnusson C, Bar-Ami S, Braw R, Tsafriri A. Oxygen consumption by rat oocytes and cumulus cells during induced atresia. *J Reprod Fertil* 1983;68:97–103.
398. Hubbard CJ, Greenwald GS. Morphological changes in atretic graafian follicles during induced atresia in the hamster. *Anat Rec* 1985;212:353–357.
399. Hubbard CJ, Greenwald GS. Changes in DNA, cyclic nucleotides and steroids during induced follicular atresia in the hamster. *J Reprod Fertil* 1981;63:455–461.
400. Hubbard CJ, Greenwald GS. In vitro effects of luteinizing hormone on induced atretic graafian follicles in the hamster. *Biol Reprod* 1983;28:849–859.
401. Shaha C, Greenwald GS. Autoradiographic analysis of changes in ovarian binding of FSH and hCG during induced follicular atresia in the hamster. *J Reprod Fertil* 1982;66:197–201.
402. Greenwald GS. Temporal and topographic changes in DNA synthesis after induced follicular atresia. *Biol Reprod* 1989;40: 175–181.
403. Terranova PF. Steroidogenesis in experimentally induced atretic follicles of the hamster: a shift from estradiol to progesterone synthesis. *Endocrinology* 1981;108:1885–1890.
404. Na JY, Garza F, Terranova PF. Alterations in follicular fluid steroids and follicular hCG and FSH binding during atresia in hamster. *Proc Soc Exp Biol Med* 1985;179:123–127.
405. Mizuno O, Otani T, Shirota M, Sasamoto S. Maturation of ovarian follicles after inhibition of ovulation in rats. *J Endocrinol* 1983;97:113–119.
406. Uilenbroek JTJ, van der Linden R, Woutersen PJA. Changes in oestrogen biosynthesis in preovulatory rat follicles after blockage of ovulation with pentobarbitone sodium. *J Reprod Fertil* 1984;70:549–555.
407. van der Schoot P, den Besten D, Uilenbroek JTJ. Atresia of preovulatory follicles in rats treated with sodium pentobarbital: effects of bromocriptine. *Biol Reprod* 1982;27:189–199.
408. Freeman ME, Butcher RL, Fugo NW. Alteration of oocytes and follicles by delayed ovulation. *Biol Reprod* 1970;2:209–215.
409. Peluso JJ, Steger RW, Hafez ESE. Sequential changes associated with the degeneration of preovulatory rat follicles. *J Reprod Fertil* 1977;49:215–218.
410. Sadrkhanloo R, Hofeditz C, Erickson GF. Evidence for widespread atresia in the hypophysectomized estrogen-treated rat. *Endocrinology* 1987;120:146–155.
411. Louvet JP, Harman SM, Schreiber JR, Ross GT. Evidence for a role of androgens in follicular maturation. *Endocrinology* 1975;97:366–372.
412. Hillier SG, Ross GT. Effects of exogenous testosterone on ovarian weight, follicular morphology and intraovarian progesterone concentration in estrogen-primed hypophysectomized immature female rats. *Biol Reprod* 1979;20:261–268.
413. Harmon SM, Louvet JP, Ross GT. Interaction of estrogen and gonadotrophins on follicular atresia. *Endocrinology* 1975;96: 1145–1152.
414. Peluso JJ, Charlesworth J, England-Charlesworth C. Role of estrogen and androgen in maintaining the preovulatory follicle. *Cell Tissue Res* 1981;216:615–624.
415. Schreiber JR, Reid R, Ross GT. A receptor-like testosterone-binding protein in ovaries from estrogen-stimulated hypophysectomized immature female rats. *Endocrinology* 1976;98:1206–1213.
416. Schreiber JR, Ross GT. Further characterization of a rat ovarian testosterone receptor with evidence for nuclear translocation. *Endocrinology* 1976;99:590–596.
417. Saiduddin S, Zassenhaus HP. Effect of testosterone and progesterone on the estradiol receptor in the immature rat ovary. *Endocrinology* 1978;102:1069–1076.
418. Kohut JK, Jarrell JF, Younglai EV. Does dihydrotestosterone induce atresia in the hypophysectomized immature female rat treated with pregnant mare's serum gonadotropin? *Am J Obstet Gynecol* 1985;151:250–255.
419. Farookhi R. Effects of androgen on induction of gonadotropin receptors and gonadotropin-stimulated adenosine 3′-5′-monophosphate production in rat ovarian granulosa cells. *Endocrinology* 1980;106:1216–1223.
420. Farookhi R. Atresia: a hypothesis. In: Schwartz NB, Hunzicker-Dunn M, eds. *Dynamics of ovarian function*. New York: Raven Press; 1981:13–23.
421. Tonetta SA, Spicer LJ, Ireland JJ. CI628 inhibits follicle-stimulating hormone(FSH)-induced increases in FSH receptors of the rat ovary: requirement of estradiol for FSH action. *Endocrinology* 1985;116:715–722.
422. Hillier SG, van den Boogaard AMJ, Reichert LE Jr, van Hall EV. Intraovarian sex steroid hormone interactions and the regulation of follicular maturation: aromatization of androgens by human granulosa cells in vitro. *J Clin Endocrinol Metab* 1980;50: 640–647.
423. Greenwald GS, Limback D. Effects of treatment with cycloheximide at proestrus on subsequent in vitro follicular steroidogenesis in the hamster. *Biol Reprod* 1984;30:1105–1116.
424. Baird DT, Swanston IA, McNeilly AS. Relationship between LH, FSH, and prolactin concentration and the secretion of androgens and estrogens by the preovulatory follicle in the ewe. *Biol Reprod* 1981;24:1013–1025.
425. Greenwald GS. How does daily treatment with hCG induce su-

perovulation in the cyclic hamster. *Biol Reprod* 1993;48: 133–142.

426. Hutz RJ, Dierschke DJ, Wolf RC. Markers of atresia in ovarian follicular components from rhesus monkeys treated with estradiol-17β. *Biol Reprod* 1986;34:65–70.
427. Hutz RJ, Dierschke DJ, Wolf RC. Induction of atresia of the dominant follicle in rhesus monkeys (*Macaca mulatta*) by the local application of estradiol-17β. *Am J Primatol* 1988;15:69–77.
428. Hutz RJ, Krueger GS, Morgan PM, Dierschke DJ, Wolf RC. Atresia of the dominant ovarian follicle in rhesus monkeys is detected within 24 hours of estradiol treatment. *Am J Primatol* 1989;18:237–243.
429. Hutz RJ, Dierschke DJ, Wolf RC. Estradiol-induced follicular atresia in rhesus monkeys is not prevented by exogenous gonadotropins. *Am J Primatology* 1991;23:247–255.
430. Zeleznik AJ. Premature elevation of systemic estradiol reduces serum levels of follicle-stimulating hormone and lengthens the follicular phase of the menstrual cycle in rhesus monkeys. *Endocrinology* 1981;109:352–355.
431. Lacker HM, Beers WH, Erb Meuli L, Akin E. A theory of follicle selection. I. Hypotheses and examples. *Biol Reprod* 1987;37: 570–580.
432. Lacker HM, Beers WH, Erb Meuli L, Akin E. A theory of follicle selection. II. Computer simulation of estradiol administration in the primate. *Biol Reprod* 1987;37:581–588.
433. Thibault C. Croissance finale du follicule, ovulation, superovulation et qualité de l'ovocyte. *Contraception Fertil Sex* 1990;18: 691–698.
434. Cole HH. Studies on reproduction with emphasis on gonadotropins, antigonadotropins and progonadotropins. *Biol Reprod* 1975;12:194–211.
435. Moore WT Jr, Burleigh BD, Ward DN. Chorionic gonadotropins: comparative studies and comments on relationships to other glycoprotein hormones. In: Segal SJ, ed. *Chorionic gonadotropin.* New York: Plenum; 1980:89–126.
436. Stewart F, Allen WR. The binding of FSH, LH and PMSG to equine gonadal tissues. *J Reprod Fertil* 1979;27[Suppl]:431–440.
437. Licht P, Gallo AB, Aggarwal BB, Farmer SW, Castelino JB, Papkoff H. Biological and binding activities of equine pituitary gonadotrophins and pregnant mare serum gonadotrophin. *J Endocrinol* 1979;83:311–322.
438. Murphy BD, Mapletoft RJ, Manns J, Humphrey WD. Variability in gonadotrophin preparations as a factor in the superovulatory response. *Theriogenology* 1984;21:117–125.
439. Combarnous Y, Guillou F, Martinat N, Cahoreau C. Origine de la double activité FSH + LH de la choriogonadotropine equine (eCG/PMSG). *Ann Endocrinol (Paris)* 1984;45:261–268.
440. Leaver HA, Boyd GS. Action of gonadotrophic hormones on cholesterol side-chain cleavage and cholesterol ester hydrolase in the ovary of the immature rat. *J Reprod Fertil* 1981;63:101–108.
441. Younglai EV. Effects of pregnant mare's serum gonadotrophin administered in vivo on steroid accumulation by isolated rabbit ovarian follicles. *Acta Endocrinol* 1984;107:531–537.
442. Matson PL, Tyler JPP, Collins WP. Follicular steroid content and oocyte meiotic status after PMSG stimulation of immature hamsters. *J Reprod Fertil* 1981;61:443–452.
443. Cran DG. Follicular development in the sheep after priming with PMSG. *J Reprod Fertil* 1983;67:415–423.
444. Cahill LP, Mariana JC, Mauleon P. Total follicular populations in ewes of high and low ovulation rates. *J Reprod Fertil* 1979;55:27–36.
445. Greenwald GS. Quantitative study of follicular development in the ovary of the intact or unilaterally ovariectomized hamster. *J Reprod Fertil* 1961;2:351–361.
446. Monniaux D, Mariana JC, Gibson WR. Action of PMSG on follicular populations in the heifer. *J Reprod Fertil* 1984;70: 243–253.
447. Dott HM, Hay MF, Cran DG, Moor RM. Effect of exogenous gonadotrophin (PMSG) on the antral follicle population in the sheep. *J Reprod Fertil* 1979;56:683–689.
448. Driancourt MA, Fry RC. Effect of superovulation with pFSH or PMSG on growth and maturation of the ovulatory follicles in sheep. *Anim Reprod Sci* 1992;27:279–292.
449. Moor RM, Kruip TAM, Green D. Intraovarian control of folliculogenesis: limits to superovulation? *Theriogenology* 1984;21: 103–116.
450. Greenwald GS, Terranova PF. Development in the cyclic hamster of refractoriness to the superovulatory action of anti-LH serum. *J Reprod Fertil* 1983;69:297–301.
451. Dhondt D, Bouters R, Spincemaille J, Coryn M, Vandeplassche M. The control of superovulation in the bovine with a PMSG-antiserum. *Theriogenology* 1978;9:529–534.
452. Gougeon A, Testart J. Influence of human menopausal gonadotropin on the recruitment of human ovarian follicles. *Fertil Steril* 1990;54:848–852.
453. Greenwald GS. Analysis of superovulation in the hamster: 1962–1978. *Ann Biol Anim Biochem Biophys* 1979;19:1483–1487.
454. Greenwald GS. Effect of an anti-PMS serum on ovulation and estrogen secretion in the PMS-treated hamster. *Biol Reprod* 1973;9:437–446.
455. Hirshfield AN. Stathmokinetic analysis of granulosa cell proliferation in antral follicles of cyclic rats. *Biol Reprod* 1984;31:52–58.
456. Tsafriri A, Lieberman ME, Koch Y, et al. Capacity of immunologically purified FSH to stimulate cyclic AMP accumulation and steroidogenesis in graafian follicles and to induce ovum maturation and ovulation in the rat. *Endocrinology* 1976;98:655–661.
457. Galway AB, Lapolt PS, Tsafriri A, Dargan CM, Boime I, Hsueh AJW. Recombinant follicle-stimulating hormone induces ovulation and tissue plasminogen activator expression in hypophysectomized rats. *Endocrinology* 1990;127:3023–3028.
458. Mannaerts B, De Leeuw R, Geelen J, et al. Comparative in vitro and in vivo studies on the biological characteristics of recombinant human follicle-stimulating hormone. *Endocrinology* 1991; 129:2623–2630.
459. Wang X-N, Greemwald GS. hCG or human recombinant FSH induced ovulation and subsequent fertilization and preimplantation embryo development in hypophysectomized FSH-primed mice. *Endocrinology* 1993;132:2009–2016.
460. Pariente C, Rabinovici J, Lunenfeld B, et al. Steroid secretion by granulosa cells isolated from a woman with 17α-hydroxylase deficiency. *J Clin Endocrinol Metab* 1990;71:984–987.
461. Rabinovici J, Blankstein J, Goldman B, et al. In vitro fertilization and primary embryonic cleavage are possible in 17α-hydroxylase deficiency despite extremely low intrafollicular 17β-estradiol. *J Clin Endocrinol Metab* 1989;68:693–697.
462. Couzinet B, Lestrat N, Brailly S, Forest M, Schaison G. Stimulation of ovarian follicular maturation with pure follicle-stimulating hormone in women with gonadotropin deficiency. *J Clin Endocrinol Metab* 1988;66:552–556.
463. Schoot DC, Bennink HJTC, Mannaerts BMJL, Lamberts SWJ, Bouchard P, Fauser BCJM. Human recombinant follicle-stimulating hormone induces growth of preovulatory follicles without concomitant increase in androgen and estrogen biosynthesis in a woman with isolated gonadotropin deficiency. *J Clin Endocrinol Metab* 1992;74:1471–1473.
464. Larsen JL, Bhanu A, Odell WD. Prolactin inhibition of pregnant mare's serum stimulated follicle development in the rat ovary. *Endocr Res* 1990;16:449–459.
465. Jonassen JA, Baker SP, McNeilly AS. Long-term hyperprolactinaemia reduces basal but not androgen-stimulated oestradiol production in small antral follicles of the rat ovary. *J Endocrinol* 1991;129:357–362.
466. Brandt ME, Puett D, Covey DF, Zimniski SJ. Characterization of pregnant mare's serum gonadotropin-stimulated rat ovarian aromatase and its inhibition by 10-propargylestr-4-ene-3,17-dione. *J Steroid Biochem* 1988;31:317–324.
467. LaPolt PS, Tilly JL, Aihara T, Nishimori K, Hsueh AJW. Gonadotropin-induced up- and down-regulation of ovarian follicle-stimulating hormone (FSH) receptor gene expression in immature rats: effects of pregnant mare's serum gonadotropin, human chorionic gonadotropin, and recombinant FSH. *Endocrinology* 1992;130:1289–1295.
468. Conway BA, Mahesh VB, Mills TM. Effect of dihydrotestosterone on the growth and function of ovarian follicles in intact immature female rats primed with PMSG. *J Reprod Fertil* 1990;90:267–277.
469. Krishna A, Terranova PF, Matteri RL, Papkoff H. Histamine and increased ovarian blood flow mediate LH-induced superovulation in the cyclic hamster. *J Reprod Fertil* 1986;76:23–29.

470. Krishna A, Terranova PF. Alterations in mast cell degranulation and ovarian histamine in the proestrous hamster. *Biol Reprod* 1985;32:1211–1217.
471. Szego CM, Gitin ES. Ovarian histamine depletion during acute hyperaemic response to luteinizing hormone. *Nature* 1964; 201:682–684.
472. Lipner H. Ovulation from histamine depleted ovaries. *Proc Soc Exp Biol Med* 1971;136:111–114.
473. Wallach EE, Wright KH, Hamada Y. Investigation of mammalian ovulation with an in vitro perfused rabbit ovary preparation. *Am J Obstet Gynecol* 1978;132:728–738.
474. Knox E, Lowry S, Beck L. Prevention of ovulation in rabbits by antihistamine. In: Midgley AR, Sadler WA, eds. *Ovarian follicular development and function.* New York: Raven Press; 1979: 159–163.
475. Kobayashi Y, Wright KH, Santulli R, Kitai H, Wallach EE. Effect of histamine and histamine blockers on the ovulatory process in the in vitro perfused rabbit ovary. *Biol Reprod* 1983;28: 385–392.
476. Scaramuzzi RJ, Martensz ND, Van Look PFA. Ovarian morphology and the concentration of steroids, and of gonadotropin during the breeding season in ewes actively immunized against oestradiol 17β or oestrone. *J Reprod Fertil* 1980;59:303–310.
477. Scaramuzzi RJ, Baird DT, Clarke IJ, Martensz ND, Van Look PFA. Ovarian morphology and the concentration of steroids during the oestrous cycle of sheep actively immunized against androstenedione. *J Reprod Fertil* 1980;58:27–35.
478. Land RB, Morris BA, Baxter G, Fordyce M, Forster J. Improvement of sheep fecundity by treatment with antisera to gonadal steroids. *J Reprod Fertil* 1982;66:625–634.
479. Wallace JM, McNeilly AS. Increase in ovulation rate after treatment of ewes with bovine follicular fluid in the luteal phase of the oestrous cycle. *J Reprod Fertil* 1985;73:505–515.
480. Forage RG, Brown RW, Oliver KJ, et al. Immunization against an inhibin subunit produced by recombinant DNA techniques results in increased ovulation rate in sheep. *J Endocrinol* 1987;114:R1–R4.
481. Sander HJ, Meijs-Roelofs HMA, van Leeuwen ECM, Kramer P, van Cappellen WA. Initial ovulation rate and follicle population after injection of inhibin-neutralizing antiserum in the late-prepubertal rat. *J Endocrinol* 1991;130:289–296.
482. Sander HJ, Kramer P, van Leeuwen ECM, van Cappellen WA, Meijs-Roelofs HMA, DeJong FH. Ovulation rate, follicle population and FSH levels in cyclic rats after administration of an inhibin-neutralizing antiserum. *J Endocrinol* 1991;130:297–303.
483. Lasley BL. Treating infertility: CRES employs innovative method. *CRES Rep* 1984;2.
484. Jones GS. Update on in vitro fertilization. *Endocr Rev* 1984;5: 62–75.
485. Terranova PF, Greenwald GS. Antiluteinizing hormone: chronic influence on steroid and gonadotropin levels and superovulation in the pregnant hamster. *Endocrinology* 1979;104:1013–1019.
486. Greenwald GS, Terranova PF. Induction of superovulation in the cyclic hamster by a single injection of antiluteinizing hormone serum. *Endocrinology* 1981;108:1903–1908.
487. Terranova PF, Greenwald GS. Alteration of the serum follicle-stimulating hormone to luteinizing hormone ratio in the cyclic hamster treated with antiluteinizing hormone: relationship to serum estradiol, free antiluteinizing hormone and superovulation. *Endocrinology* 1981;108:1909–1914.
488. Opavsky MA, Armstrong DT. The effectiveness of FSH in inducing superovulation is influenced by LH. *Biol Reprod* 1985;32 [Suppl 1]:71.
489. Kim I, Greenwald GS. Hormonal requirements for maintenance of follicular and luteal function in the hypophysectomized cyclic hamster. *Biol Reprod* 1984;30:1063–1072.
490. Terranova PF, Greenwald GS. Increased ovulation rate in the cyclic guinea pig after a single injection of antiserum to LH. *J Reprod Fertil* 1981;61:37–42.
491. Fitzgerald JA, Ruggles AJ, Hansel W. Increased ovulation rate of adult ewes treated with anti-bovine LH antiserum during the normal breeding season. *J Anim Sci* 1985;60:749–754.
492. Spearow JL. Changes in the kinetics of follicular growth in response to selection for large litter size in mice. *Biol Reprod* 1986;35:1175–1186.
493. Spearow JL. Major genes control hormone-induced ovulation rate in mice. *J Reprod Fertil* 1988;82:787–797.
494. Spearow JL. Characterization of genetic differences in hormone-induced ovulation rate in mice. *J Reprod Fertil* 1988;82: 799–806.
495. Spearow JL, Erickson RP, Edwards T, Herbon L. The effect of H-2 region and genetic background on hormone-induced ovulation rate, puberty, and follicular number in mice. *Genet Res* 1991;57:41–49.
496. McNatty KP, Henderson KM. Gonadotrophins, fecundity genes and ovarian follicular function. *J Steroid Biochem* 1987;27: 365–373.
497. Peppler RD. *Method and mechanism of ovulatory compensation following unilateral ovariectomy in the rat* (Dissertation). Lawrence: University of Kansas, 1968.
498. Jones RE, Summers CH. Compensatory follicular hypertrophy during the ovarian cycle of the house gecko, *Hemidactylus frenatus. Anat Rec* 1984;209:59–65.
499. Bleier WJ, Ehteshami M. Ovulation following unilateral ovariectomy in the California leaf-nosed bat (*Macrotus californicus*). *J Reprod Fertil* 1981;63:181–183.
500. Hunter J. An experiment to determine the effect of extirpating one ovarium upon the number of young produced. *Phil Trans* 1787;17:233–239.
501. Arai H. On the cause of the hypertrophy of the surviving ovary after simispaying (albino rat) and on the number of ova in it. *Am J Anat* 1920;28:59–79.
502. Lipschutz A. New developments in ovarian dynamics and the law of follicular constancy. *Br J Exp Biol* 1928;5:283–291.
503. Chiras DD, Greenwald GS. Acute effects of unilateral ovariectomy on follicular development in the cyclic hamster. *J Reprod Fertil* 1978;52:221–225.
504. Peppler RD, Greenwald GS. Effects of unilateral ovariectomy on ovulation and cycle length in 4- and 5-day cycling rats. *Am J Anat* 1970;127:1–8.
505. Peppler RD, Greenwald GS. Influence of unilateral ovariectomy on follicular development in cycling rats. *Am J Anat* 1970;127: 9–14.
506. Otani T, Sasamoto S. Plasma and pituitary hormone changes and follicular development after unilateral ovariectomy in cyclic rats. *J Reprod Fertil* 1982;65:347–353.
507. Sasamoto S, Taya K, Arakawa H, Kishi H. Inhibin secretion and suppression of the FSH surge in superovulating animals. In: Burger HG, de Kretser DM, Findlay JK, Igarashi M, eds. *Inhibin-non-steroidal regulation of follicle stimulating hormone secretion.* New York: Raven Press; 1987:219–232.
508. McLaren A. Regulation of ovulation rate after removal of one ovary in mice. *Proc R Soc Lond* [*Biol*] 1966;166:316–340.
509. Fleming MW, Rhodes RC III, Dailey RA. Compensatory responses after unilateral ovariectomy in rabbits. *Biol Reprod* 1984;30:82–86.
510. Dharmarajan AM, Zanagnolo VL, Dasko LM, Hardy MP, Wallach EE. Changes in rabbit corpus luteum progesterone secretion and cellular morphology following unilateral luteectomy or ovariectomy. *Biol Reprod* 1992;46:251–255.
511. Hermreck AS, Greenwald GS. The effects of unilateral ovariectomy on follicular maturation in the guinea pig. *Anat Rec* 1964;148:171–176.
512. Land RB. Ovulation rate of Finn-Dorset sheep following unilateral ovariectomy or chlorpromazine treatment at different stages of the oestrous cycle. *J Reprod Fertil* 1973;33:99–105.
513. Findlay JK, Cumming IA. The effect of unilateral ovariectomy on plasma gonadotropin levels, estrus and ovulation rate in sheep. *Biol Reprod* 1977;17:178–183.
514. Brinkley HJ, Young EP. Effects of unilateral ovariectomy or the unilateral destruction of ovarian components on the follicles and corpora lutea of the nonpregnant pig. *Endocrinology* 1969;84: 1250–1256.
515. Brinkley HJ, Wickersham EW, First NL, Casida LE. Effect of unilateral ovariectomy on the structure and function of the corpora lutea of the pig. *Endocrinology* 1964;74:462–467.
516. Sundaram SK, Stob M. Effect of unilateral ovariectomy on reproduction and induced ovulation in ewes. *J Anim Sci* 1967;26: 374–376.
517. Roy SK, Greenwald GS. The effects of FSH and LH on incorpora-

tion of [^{3}H]thymidine into follicular DNA. *J Reprod Fertil* 1986;78:201–209.
518. Saiduddin S, Rowe RF, Casida LE. Ovarian follicular changes following unilateral ovariectomy in the cow. *Biol Reprod* 1970;2:408–412.
519. Johnson SK, Smith MF, Elmore RG. Effect of unilateral ovariectomy and injection of bovine follicular fluid on gonadotropin secretion and compensatory ovarian hypertrophy in prepuberal heifers. *J Anim Sci* 1985;60:1055–1060.
520. Cochrane RL, Holmes RL. Unilateral ovariectomy and hypophysectomy in the rhesus monkey. *J Endocrinol* 1966;35: 427–428.
521. Sopelak VM, Hodgen GD. Contralateral tubal-ovarian apposition and fertility in hemiovariectomized primates. *Fertil Steril* 1984;42:633–637.
522. Danforth DR, Chillik CF, Hertz R, Hodgen GD. Effects of ovarian tissue reduction on the menstrual cycle: persistent normalcy after near-total oophorectomy. *Biol Reprod* 1989;41:355–360.
523. Peppler RD. Effect of removing one ovary and a half on ovulation number in cycling rats. *Experentia* 1975;31:243–244.
524. Speert H, Na Sh W, Kaplan AL. Tubal pregnancy: some observations on external migration of the ovum and compensatory hypertrophy of the residual ovary. *Obstet Gynecol* 1956;7:322–324.
525. Gougeon A, Lefevre B. Evolution of the diameters of the largest healthy and atretic follicles during the human menstrual cycle. *J Reprod Fertil* 1983;69:497–502.
526. Bast JD, Greenwald GS. Acute and chronic elevations in serum levels of FSH after unilateral ovariectomy in the cyclic hamster. *Endocrinology* 1977;100:955–966.
527. Welschen R, Dullaart J, deJong FH. Interrelationships between circulating levels of estradiol-17β, progesterone, FSH and LH immediately after unilateral ovariectomy in the cyclic rat. *Biol Reprod* 1978;18:421–427.
528. Redmer DA, Christenson RK, Ford JJ, Day BN. Effect of follicular fluid treatment on follicle-stimulating hormone, luteinizing hormone and compensatory ovarian hypertrophy in prepuberal gilts. *Biol Reprod* 1985;32:111–119.
529. Baird DT, Backstrom T, McNeilly AS, Smith SK, Wathen CG. Effect of enucleation of the corpus luteum at different stages of the luteal phase of the human menstrual cycle on subsequent follicular development. *J Reprod Fertil* 1984;70:615–624.
530. Baranczuk R, Greenwald GS. Peripheral levels of estrogen in the cyclic hamster. *Endocrinology* 1973;92:805–812.
531. Curry TE Jr, Lawrence IE Jr, Burden HW. Effect of ovarian sympathectomy on follicular development during compensatory ovarian hypertrophy in the guinea-pig. *J Reprod Fertil* 1984;71:39–44.
532. Chatterjee A, Greenwald GS. The long-term effects of unilateral ovariectomy of the cycling hamster and rat. *Biol Reprod* 1972;7:238–246.
533. Peppler RD. Effects of unilateral ovariectomy on follicular development and ovulation in cycling, aged rats. *Am J Anat* 1971;132:423–428.
534. Hirshfield AN. Follicular recruitment in long-term hemicastrate rats. *Biol Reprod* 1982;27:48–53.
535. Hirshfield AN. Compensatory ovarian hypertrophy in the long-term hemicastrate rat: size distribution of growing and atretic follicles. *Biol Reprod* 1983;28:271–278.
536. Alvarez RD, Grizzle WE, Smith LJ, Miller DM. Compensatory ovarian hypertrophy occurs by a mechanism distinct from compensatory growth in the regenerating liver. *Am J Obstet Gynecol* 1989;161:1653–1657.
537. Butcher RL. Changes in gonadotropins and steroids associated with unilateral ovariectomy of the rat. *Endocrinology* 1977;101: 830–839.
538. Baker TG, Challoner S, Burgoyne PS. The number of oocytes and the rate of atresia in unilaterally ovariectomized mice up to 8 months after surgery. *J Reprod Fertil* 1980;60:449–456.
539. Meredith S, Dudenhoeffer G, Butcher RL, Lerner SP, Walls T. Unilateral ovariectomy increases loss of primordial follicles and is associated with increased metestrous concentration of follicle-stimulating hormone in old rats. *Biol Reprod* 1992;47:162–168.
540. Gosden RG, Telfer E, Faddy MJ, Brook DJ. Ovarian cyclicity and follicular recruitment in unilaterally ovariectomized mice. *J Reprod Fertil* 1989;87:257–264.
541. Kramer KK, Lamberson WR. Long-term effects of unilateral ovariectomy on ovarian function in gilts. *Anim Reprod Sci* 1991;26:137–149.
542. Redmer DA, Christenson RK, Ford JJ, Day BN. Effect of unilateral ovariectomy on compensatory ovarian hypertrophy, peripheral concentrations of follicle-stimulating hormone and luteinizing hormone, and ovarian venous concentrations of estradiol-17β in prepuberal gilts. *Biol Reprod* 1984;31:59–66.
543. Redmer DA, Christenson RK, Ford JJ, Day BN, Goodman AL. Inhibin-like activity in ovarian venous serum after unilateral ovariectomy in prepubertal gilts. *Biol Reprod* 1986;34:357–362.
544. Fry RC, Clarke IJ, Cahill LP. Changes in gonadotrophin concentrations are not necessarily involved in ovarian compensation after unilateral ovariectomy in sheep. *J Reprod Fertil* 1987;79: 45–48.
545. Schwartz NB, Cobbs SB, Ely CA. What is the function(s) of the proestrous FSH surge in the rat? In: *Endocrinology. Proceedings of the fourth International Congress of Endocrinology.* Amsterdam: Excerpta Medicus; 1972:897–902.
546. Chiras DD, Greenwald GS. An autoradiographic study of long-term follicular development in the cyclic hamster. *Anat Rec* 1977;188:331–337.
547. Welschen R. Amounts of gonadotropins required for normal follicular growth in hypophysectomized adult rats. *Acta Endocrinol (Copenh)* 1973;72:137–155.
548. Hirshfield AN, Midgley AR Jr. Morphometric analysis of follicular development in the rat. *Biol Reprod* 1978;19:597–605.
549. Ireland JJ, Richards JS. A previously undescribed role for luteinizing hormone (LH:hCG) on follicular cell differentiation. *Endocrinology* 1978;102:1458–1465.
550. Terranova PF, Garza F. Relationship between the preovulatory luteinizing hormone (LH) surge and androstenedione systhesis of preantral follicles in the cyclic hamster: detection by in vitro responses to LH. *Biol Reprod* 1983;29:630–636.
551. Richards JS, Midgley AR Jr. Protein hormone action: a key to understanding follicular and luteal cell development. *Biol Reprod* 1976;14:82–94.
552. Midgley AR Jr. Autoradiographic analysis of gonadotropin binding to rat ovarian tissue sections. *Adv Exp Med Biol* 1973;36:365–378.
553. Roy SK, Treacy BJ. Isolation and long-term culture of human preantral follicles. *Fertil Steril* 1993;59:783–790.
554. Insler V, Kleinman D, Sod-Moriah U. Role of midcycle FSH surge in follicular development. *Gynecol Obstet Invest* 1990;30: 228–233.
555. Bast JD, Greenwald GS. Serum profiles of follicle-stimulating hormone, luteinizing hormone and prolactin during the estrous cycle of the hamster. *Endocrinology* 1974;94:1295–1299.
556. Bex FJ, Goldman BD. Serum gonadotropins and follicular development in the Syrian hamster. *Endocrinology* 1975;96:928–933.
557. Siegel HI, Bast JD, Greenwald GS. The effects of phenobarbital and gonadal steroids on periovulatory serum levels of luteinizing hormone and follicle stimulating hormone in the hamster. *Endocrinology* 1976;98:48–55.
558. Gay VL, Midgley AR Jr, Niswender GD. Patterns of gonadotropin secretion associated with ovulation. *Fed Proc* 1970;29: 1880–1887.
559. Butcher RL, Collins WE, Fugo NW. Plasma concentrations of LH, FSH, prolactin, progesterone and estradiol-17β throughout the 4-day estrous cycle of the rat. *Endocrinology* 1974;94: 1704–1708.
560. DePaolo LU, Shander D, Wise PM, Barraclough CA, Channing CP. Identification of inhibin-like activity in ovarian venous plasma of rats during the estrous cycle. *Endocrinology* 1979;105: 647–654.
561. Fujii T, Hoover DJ, Channing CP. Changes in inhibin activity, and progesterone, oestrogen and androstenedione concentrations, in rat follicular fluid throughout the oestrous cycle. *J Reprod Fertil* 1983;69:307–314.
562. Sander HJ, van Leeuwen ECM, de Jong FH. Inhibin-like activity in media from cultured rat granulosa cells collected throughout the oestrous cycle. *J Endocrinol* 1984;103:77–84.
563. Welschen R, Hermans WP, deJong FH. Possible involvement of inhibin in the interrelationship between numbers of antral folli-

cles and peripheral FSH concentrations in female rats. *J Reprod Fertil* 1980;60:485–493.
564. Chappel SC. Cyclic fluctuations in ovarian FSH-inhibiting material in golden hamsters. *Biol Reprod* 1979;21:447–453.
565. Erickson GF, Hsueh AJW. Secretion of inhibin by rat granulosa cells in vitro. *Endocrinology* 1978;103:1960–1963.
566. Lee VWK. PMSG treated immature female rat: a model system for studying control of inhibin secretion. In: Greenwald GS, Terranova PF, eds. *Factors regulating ovarian function.* New York: Raven Press; 1983:157–161.
567. Schwartz NB, Channing CP. Evidence for ovarian "inhibin": suppression of the secondary rise in serum follicle stimulating hormone levels in proestrous rats by injection of porcine follicular fluid. *Proc Natl Acad Sci USA* 1977;74:5724.
568. Hirobe S, He W-W, Lee MM, Donahoe PK. Mullerian inhibiting substance messenger ribonucleic acid expression in granulosa and Sertoli cells coincides with their mitotic activity. *Endocrinology* 1992;131:854–862.
569. Chiras DD, Greenwald GS. Effects of steroids and gonadotropins on follicular development in the hypophysectomized hamster. *Am J Anat* 1978;152:307–320.
570. Zeleznik AJ, Midgley AR Jr, Reichert LE Jr. Granulosa cell maturation in the rat: increased binding of human chorionic gonadotropin following treatment with follicle stimulating hormone in vivo. *Endocrinology* 1974;95:818–825.
571. Camp TA, Rahal JO, Mayo KE. Cellular localization and hormonal regulation of follicle-stimulating hormone and luteinizing hormone receptor messenger RNAs in the rat ovary. *Mol Endocrinol* 1991;5:1405–1417.
572. Pencharz RI. Effect of estrogens and androgens alone and in combination with chorionic gonadotropin on the ovary of the hypophysectomized rat. *Science* 1940;91:554–555.
573. Williams PC. Effect of stilbestrol on the ovaries of hypophysectomized rats. *Nature* 1940;145:388–389.
574. Smith BD, Bradbury JT. Ovarian response to gonadotropins after pre-treatment with diethyl stilbestrol. *Am J Physiol* 1963;204: 1023–1027.
575. Kudolo GB, Elder MG, Myatt L. A novel oestrogen-binding species in rat granulosa cells. *J Endocrinol* 1984;102:83–91.
576. Greenwald GS. Proestrous hormone surges dissociated from ovulation in the estrogen treated hamster. *Endocrinology* 1975;97: 878–884.
577. Chappel SC, Selker F. Relation between the secretion of FSH during the periovulatory period and ovulation during the next cycle. *Biol Reprod* 1979;21:347–352.
578. Greenwald GS, Siegel HI. Is the first or second periovulatory surge of FSH responsible for follicular recruitment in the hamster? *Proc Soc Exp Biol Med* 1982;170:225–230.
579. Sheela Rani CS, Moudgal NR. Role of the proestrous surge of gonadotropins in the initiation of follicular maturation in the cyclic hamster: a study using antisera to follicle stimulating hormone and luteinizing hormone. *Endocrinology* 1977;101: 1484–1494.
580. Dorrington JH, Moon YS, Armstrong DT. Estradiol biosynthesis in cultured granulosa cells from hypophysectomized immature rats: stimulation by follicle stimulating hormone. *Endocrinology* 1975;97:1328–1331.
581. Hillier SG, Zeleznik AJ, Ross GT. Independence of steroidogenic capacity and luteinizing hormone receptor induction in developing granulosa cells. *Endocrinology* 1978;102:937–946.
582. Hillier SG, Zeleznik AJ, Knazek RA, Ross GT. Hormonal regulation of preovulatory follicle maturation in the rat. *J Reprod Fertil* 1980;60:219–229.
583. Wang C, Hsueh AJW, Erickson GF. Induction of functional prolactin receptors by follicle stimulating hormone in rat granulosa cells in vivo and in vitro. *J Biol Chem* 1979;254:11330–11336.
584. Jones PBC, Welsh TH Jr, Hsueh AJW. Regulation of ovarian progestin production by epidermal growth factor in cultured rat granulosa cells. *J Biol Chem* 1982;257:11268–11273.
585. Ireland JJ, Richards JS. Acute effects of estradiol and FSH on specific binding of human [I^{125}]iodo FSH to rat ovarian granulosa cells in vivo and in vitro. *Endocrinology* 1978;102:876–883.
586. Roy SK, Greenwald GS. Deoxyribonucleic acid polymerase-α activity in hamster follicles during the estrous cycle: roles of follicle stimulating hormone and luteinizing hormone. *Mol Cell Endocrinol* 1989;61:157–166.
587. Roy SK, Ogren CL, Roy C, Lu B. Cell-type-specific localization of transforming growth factor-β2 and transforming growth factor-β1 in the hamster ovary: differential regulation by follicle-stimulating hormone and luteinizing hormone. *Biol Reprod* 1992;46:595–606.
588. Payne DW, Packman JN, Adashi EY. Follicle-stimulating hormone inhibits granulosa cell 5α-reductase activity. *J Biol Chem* 1992;267:13348–13355.
589. Shikone T, Yamoto M, Nakano R. Follicle-stimulating hormone induces functional receptors for basic fibroblast growth factor in rat granulosa cells. *Endocrinology* 1992;131:1063–1068.
590. Bley MA, Simon JC, Estevez AG, Jimenez de Asua L, Baranao JL. Effect of follicle-stimulating hormone on insulin-like growth factor-I-stimulated rat granulosa cell deoxyribonucleic acid synthesis. *Endocrinology* 1992;131:1223–1229.
591. Page RD, Butcher RL. Follicular and plasma patterns of steroids in young and old rats during normal and prolonged estrous cycles. *Biol Reprod* 1982;27:383–392.
592. Fevold HL. Synergism of follicle stimulating hormone and luteinizing hormone in producing estrogen secretion. *Endocrinology* 1941;28:33–36.
593. Greep RO, Van Dyke HB, Chow BF. Gonadotropins of the swine pituitary. I. Various biological effects of purified thylakentrin (FSH) and pure metakentrin (ICSH). *Endocrinology* 1942;30: 635–639.
594. Lostroh A, Johnson RE. Amounts of interstitial cell stimulating hormone and follicle stimulating hormone required for development, uterine growth and ovulation in the hypophysectomized rat. *Endocrinology* 1966;79:991–996.
595. Erickson GF, Wang C, Hsueh AJW. FSH induction of functional LH receptors in granulosa cells cultured in a chemically defined medium. *Nature* 1979;279:336–337.
596. Wang C, Hsueh AJW, Erickson GF. LH stimulation of estrogen secretion in cultured granulosa cells. *Mol Cell Endocrinol* 1981;24:17–28.
597. Goodwin JA, Terranova PF. Relationship between LH dependency of preantral follicles and the secondary FSH surge: effects of hypophysectomy and correlation with hCG and FSH binding and follicular steroids. In: Toft DO, Ryan RJ, eds. *Proceedings of the fifth Ovarian Workshop.* New York: Raven Press; 1985: 243–248.
598. Cameron JL, Chappel SC. Follicle-stimulating hormone within and secreted from anterior pituitaries of female golden hamsters during the estrous cycle and after ovariectomy. *Biol Reprod* 1985;33:132–139.
599. Sheela Rani CS, Moudgal NR. Examination of the role of FSH in periovulatory events in the hamster. *J Reprod Fertil* 1977;50: 37–45.
600. Gruenberg ML, Steger RW, Peluso JJ. Follicular development, steroidogenesis and ovulation within ovaries exposed in vitro to hormone levels which mimic those of the rat estrous cycle. *Biol Reprod* 1983;29:1265–1275.
601. Adashi EY, Resnick CE, Svoboda ME, VanWyk JJ. Somatomedin-C synergizes with follicle-stimulating hormone in the acquisition of progestin biosynthetic capacity by cultured rat granulosa cells. *Endocrinology* 1985;116:2135–2142.
602. Kudlow JE, Kobrin MS, Purchio AF, et al. Ovarian transforming growth factor-α gene expression: immunohistochemical localization to the theca-interstitial cells. *Endocrinology* 1987;121: 1577–1579.
603. Skinner MK, Lobb D, Dorrington JH. Ovarian thecal/interstitial cells produce an epidermal growth factor-like substance. *Endocrinology* 1987;121:1892–1899.
604. Bendell JJ, Dorrington JH. Epidermal growth factor influences growth and differentiation of rat granulosa cells. *Endocrinology* 1990;127:533–540.
605. Roy SK, Greenwald GS. In vitro effects of epidermal growth factor, insulin-like growth factor-I, fibroblast growth factor, and follicle stimulating hormone on hamster follicular deoxyribonucleic acid synthesis and steroidogenesis. *Biol Reprod* 1991;44: 889–896.
606. Roy SK, Greenwald GS. Mediation of follicle-stimulating hor-

mone action on follicular deoxyribonucleic acid synthesis by epidermal growth factor. *Endocrinology* 1991;129:1903–1908.
607. Carrol J, Whittingham DG, Wood MJ. Effects of dibutyryl cyclic adenosine monophosphate on granulosa cell proliferation, oocyte growth and meiotic maturation in isolated mouse primary ovarian follicles cultured in collagen gels. *J Reprod Fertil* 1991;92:197–207.
608. Hsueh AJW, Welsh TH, Jones PBC. Inhibition of ovarian and testicular steroidogenesis by epidermal growth factor. *Endocrinology* 1981;108:2002–2004.
609. Chabot JG, St. Arnaud R, Walker P, Pelletier G. Distribution of epidermal growth factor receptors in the rat ovary. *Mol Cell Endocrinol* 1986;44:99–108.
610. Andersson I, Billig H, Fryklund L, et al. Localization of IGF-I in adult rats: immunohistochemical studies. *Acta Physiol Scand* 1986;126:311–312.
611. Hansson HA, Nilsson A, Isgaard J, et al. Immunohistochemical localization of insulin-like growth factor I in the adult rat. *Histochemistry* 1988;89:403–410.
612. Hernandez ER, Roberts CT Jr, Hurwitz A, LeRoith D, Adashi EY. Rat ovarian insulin-like growth factor II gene expression is theca-interstitial cell-exclusive: hormonal regulation and receptor distribution. *Endocrinology* 1990;127:3249–3251.
613. Oliver JE, Aitman TJ, Powell JF, Wilson CA, Clayton RN. Insulin-like growth factor I gene expression in the rat ovary is confined to the granulosa cells of developing follicles. *Endocrinology* 1989;124:2671–2679.
614. Bley MA, Simon JC, Estevez AG, Jimenez de Asua L, Baranao JL. Effect of follicle-stimulating hormone on insulin-like growth factor-I-stimulated rat granulosa cell deoxyribonucleic acid synthesis. *Endocrinology* 1992;131:1223–1229.
615. Magoffin DA, Kurtz KM, Erickson GF. Insulin-like growth factor-I selectively stimulates cholesterol side-chain cleavage expression in ovarian theca-interstitial cells. *Mol Endocrinol* 1990;4:489–496.
616. Drop SL. On the nomenclature of the insulin-like growth factor binding proteins. *Mol Cell Endocrinol* 1989;67:243–244.
617. Bicsak TA, Ling N, DePaolo LV. Ovarian intrabursal administration of insulin-like growth factor-binding protein inhibits follicle rupture in gonadotropin-treated immature female rats. *Biol Reprod* 1991;44:599–603.
618. Ricciarelli E, Hernandez ER, Tedeschi C, et al. Rat ovarian insulin-like growth factor binding protein-3: a growth hormone-dependent theca-interstitial cell-derived antigonadotropin. *Endocrinology* 1992;130:3092–3094.
619. Mondschein JS, Schomberg DW. Growth factors modulate gonadotropin receptor induction in granulosa cell cultures. *Science* 1981;211:1179–1180.
620. Baird A, Esch F, Mormede P, et al. Molecular characterization of fibroblast growth factor: distribution and biological activities in various tissues. *Recent Prog Horm Res* 1986;42:143–205.
621. Hurwitz A, Hernandez ER, Resnick CE, Packman JN, Payne DW, Adashi EY. Basic fibroblast growth factor inhibits gonadotropin-supported ovarian androgen biosynthesis: mechanism(s) and site(s) of action. *Endocrinology* 1990;126:3089–3095.
622. Oury F, Faucher C, Rives I, Bensaid M, Bouche G, Darbon J-M. Regulation of cyclic adenosine 3′,5′-monophosphate-dependent protein kinase activity and regulatory subunit RIIβ content by basic fibroblast growth factor (bFGF) during granulosa cell differentiation: possible implication of protein kinase C in bFGF action. *Biol Reprod* 1992;47:202–212.
623. LaPolt PS, Yamoto M, Veljkovic M, et al. Basic fibroblast growth factor induction of granulosa cell tissue-type plasminogen activator expression and oocyte maturation: potential role as a paracrine ovarian hormone. *Endocrinology* 1990;127:2357–2363.
624. Roberts AB, Sporn MB. Transforming growth factor-β. *Adv Cancer Res* 1988;51:107–145.
625. Thompson NL, Flanders KC, Smith JM, Ellingsworth LR, Roberts AB, Sporn MB. Expression of transforming growth factor-β1 in specific cells and tissues of adult and neonatal mice. *J Cell Biol* 1989;108:661–669.
626. Skinner MK, Keski-Oja J, Osteen KG, Moses HL. Ovarian thecal cells produce transforming growth factor-β which can regulate granulosa cell growth. *Endocrinology* 1987;121:786–792.
627. Bendell JJ, Dorrington J. Rat thecal/interstitial cells secrete a transforming growth factor-β-like factor that promotes growth and differentiation in rat granulosa cells. *Endocrinology* 1988;123:941–948.
628. Hernandez ER, Hurwitz A, Payne DW, Dharmarajan AM, Purchio AF, Adashi EY. Transforming growth factor-β1 inhibits ovarian androgen production: gene expression, cellular localization, mechanism(s) and site(s) of action. *Endocrinology* 1990; 127:2804–2811.
629. Teerds KJ, Dorrington JH. Immunohistochemical localization of transforming growth factor-β_1 and -β_2 during follicular development in the adult rat ovary. *Mol Cell Endocrinol* 1992;84:R7–13.
630. Mulheron GW, Schomberg DW. Rat granulosa cells express transforming growth factor-β type 2 messenger ribonucleic acid which is regulatable by follicle-stimulating hormone in vitro. *Endocrinology* 1990;126:1777–1779.
631. Dorrington JH, Chuma AV, Bendell JJ. Transforming growth factor β and follicle stimulating hormone promote rat granulosa cell proliferation. *Endocrinology* 1988;123:353–359.
632. Roy SK. Epidermal growth factor and transforming growth factor-β modulation of follicle-stimulating hormone-induced deoxyribonucleic acid synthesis in hamster preantral and early antral follicles. *Biol Reprod* 1993;48:552–557.
633. Lahio M, DeCaprio JA, Ludlow JW, Livingston DM, Massague J. Growth inhibition by TGF-β linked to suppression of retinoblastoma protein phosphorylation. *Cell* 1990;62:175–185.
634. Roy SK. Transforming growth factor-β potentiation of follicle-stimulating hormone-induced deoxyribonucleic acid synthesis in hamster preantral follicles is mediated by a latent induction of epidermal growth factor. *Biol Reprod* 1993;48:558–563.
635. Feng P, Catt KJ, Knecht M. Transforming growth factor-β regulates the inhibitory actions of epidermal growth factor during granulosa cell differentiation. *J Biol Chem* 1986;261:14167–14170.
636. Dodson WC, Schomberg DW. The effect of transforming growth factor-β on follicle-stimulating hormone-induced differentiation of cultured rat granulosa cells. *Endocrinology* 1987;120:512–516.
637. Knecht M, Feng P, Catt KJ. Bifunctional role of transforming growth factor-β during granulosa cell development. *Endocrinology* 1987;120:1243–1249.
638. Hume DA, Halpin D, Charlton H, Gordon S. The mononuclear phagocyte system of the mouse defined by immunohistochemical localization of antigen F4/80: macrophages of endocrine organs. *Proc Natl Acad Sci USA* 1984;81:4174–4177.
639. Gottschall PE, Katsura G, Dahl RR, Hoffman ST, Arimura A. Discordance in the effects of interleukin-1 on rat granulosa cell differentiation induced by follicle-stimulating hormone or activators of adenylate cyclase. *Biol Reprod* 1984;39:1074–1085.
640. Fukuoka M, Yasuda K, Taii S, Takakura K, Mori T. Interleukin-1 stimulates growth and inhibits progesterone secretion in cultures of porcine granulosa cells. *Endocrinology* 1989;124: 884–890.
641. Fukuoka M, Taii S, Yasuda K, Takakura K, Mori T. Inhibitory effects of interleukin-1 on luteinizing hormone-stimulated adenosine 3′,5′-monoophosphate accumulation by cultured porcine granulosa cells. *Endocrinology* 1989;125:136–143.
642. Hurwitz A, Payne DW, Packman JN, et al. Cytokine-mediated regulation of ovarian function: interleukin-1 inhibits gonadotropin-induced androgen biosynthesis. *Endocrinology* 1991;129:1250–1256.
643. Hurwitz A, Ricciarelli E, Botero L, Rohan RM, Hernandez ER, Adashi EY. Endocrine- and autocrine-mediated regulation of rat ovarian (theca-interstitial) interleukin-1β gene expression: gonadotropin-dependent preovulatory acquisition. *Endocrinology* 1991;129:3427–3429.
644. Takakura K, Taii S, Fukuoka M, et al. Interleukin-2 receptor/p55 (Tac)-inducing activity in porcine follicular fluid. *Endocrinology* 1989;125:618–623.
645. Khan SA, Schmidt K, Hallin P, Di Pauli R, De Geyter C, Nieschlag E. Human testis cytosol and ovarian follicular fluid contain high amounts of interleukin-1-like factor(s). *Mol Cell Endocrinol* 1988;58:221–230.
646. Gorospe WC, Hughes FM Jr, Spangelo BL. Interleukin-6: effects on and production by rat granulosa cells in vitro. *Endocrinology* 1992;130:1750–1752.

647. Fukumatsu Y, Katabuchi H, Naito M, Takeya M, Takahashi K, Okamura H. Effect of macrophages on proliferation of granulosa cells in the ovary in rats. *J Reprod Fertil* 1992;96:241–249.
648. Adashi EY, Resnick CE, Croft CS, Payne DW. Tumor necrosis factor-α inhibits gonadotropin hormonal action in nontransformed ovarian granulosa cells: a modulatory noncytotoxic property. *J Biol Chem* 1989;264:11591–11597.
649. Emoto N, Baird A. The effect of tumor-necrosis factor/cachectin on follicle-stimulating hormone-induced aromatase activity in cultured rat granulosa cells. *Biochem Biophys Res Commun* 1988;153:792–798.
650. Roby KF, Terranova PF. Tumor necrosis factor-α alters follicular steroidogenesis in vitro. *Endocrinology* 1988;123:2952–2954.
651. Armelin HA, Armelin MCS. The interactions of peptide growth factors and oncogenes. In: Guroff G, ed. *Oncogenes, genes, and growth factors.* New York: Wiley; 1987:331–373.
652. Lamph WW, Wamsley P, Sassone-Corsi P, Verma IM. Induction of proto-oncogene JUN/AP-1 by serum and TPA. *Nature* 1988;334:629–631.
653. Heikkila R, Schwab G, Wickstrom E, et al. A c-myc antisense oligodeoxynucleotide inhibits entry into S phase but not progress from G0 to G1. *Nature* 1987;328:445–449.
654. Studzinski GP, Brelvi ZS, Feldman SC, Watt RA. Participation of c-myc protein in DNA synthesis of human cells. *Science* 1986;234:467–470.
655. Delidow BC, White BA, Peluso JJ. Gonadotropin induction of c-fos and c-myc expression and deoxyribonucleic acid synthesis in rat granulosa cells. *Endocrinology* 1990;126:2302–2306.
656. Pennybacker M, Herman B. Follicle-stimulating hormone increases c-fos mRNA levels in rat granulosa cells via a protein kinase C dependent mechanism. *Mol Cell Endocrinol* 1991,80. 11–20.
657. Delidow BC, Lynch JP, White BA, Peluso JJ. Regulation of proto-oncogene expression and deoxyribonucleic acid synthesis in granulosa cells of perifused immature rat ovaries. *Biol Reprod* 1992;47:428–435.
658. Saidapur S, Greenwald GS. Peripheral blood and ovarian levels of sex steroids in the cyclic hamster. *Biol Reprod* 1978;18: 401–408.
659. Leavitt NN, Barcom CR, Bagwell JN, Blaha CC. Structure and function of the hamster corpus luteum during the estrous cycle. *Am J Anat* 1973;136:235–250.
660. Terranova PF, Greenwald GS. Steroid and gonadotropin levels during the luteal-follicular shift of the cyclic hamster. *Biol Reprod* 1978;18:170–175.
661. Schwartz NB. A model for the regulation of ovulation in the rat. *Rec Prog Horm Res* 1969;25:1–55.
662. Smith MS, Freeman ME, Neill JD. The control of progesterone secretion during the estrous cycle and early pseudopregnancy in the rat: prolactin, gonadotropin and steroid levels associated with rescue of the corpus luteum of pseudopregnancy. *Endocrinology* 1973;96:219–226.
663. Gallo RV. Pulsatile LH release during periods of low level LH secretion in the rat estrous cycle. *Biol Reprod* 1981;24:771–777.
664. Fox SR, Smith MS. Changes in the pulsatile pattern of luteinizing hormone secretion during the rat estrous cycle. *Endocrinology* 1985;116:1485–1492.
665. Szoltys M. Oestrogens and progestagens in rat ovarian follicles during the oestrous cycle. *J Reprod Fertil* 1981;63:221–224.
666. Hamberger L, Nordenstrom K, Rosberg S, Sjogren A. Acute influence of LH and FSH on cyclic AMP formation in isolated granulosa cells of the rat. *Acta Endocrinol* 1978;88:567–579.
667. Naftolin F, Brown-Grant K, Corker CS. Plasma and pituitary luteinizing hormone and peripheral plasma oestradiol concentrations in the normal oestrous cycle of the rat and after experimental manipulation of the cycle. *J Endocrinol* 1972;53:17–30.
668. Kalra SP, Kalra PS. Temporal interrelationships among circulating levels of estradiol, progesterone and LH during the rat estrous cycle. *Endocrinology* 1974;95:1711–1718.
669. Goodman RL. A quantitative analysis of the physiological role of estradiol and progesterone in the control of tonic and surge secretion of luteinizing hormone in the rat. *Endocrinology* 1978;102: 142–150.
670. Goodman RL, Daniel K. Modulation of pulsatile luteinizing hormone secretion by ovarian steroids in the rat. *Biol Reprod* 1985;32:217–225.
671. Devorshak-Harvey E, Peluso JJ, Bona-Gallo A, Gallo RV. Effect of alterations in pulsatile luteinizing hormone release on ovarian follicular atresia and steroid secretion on diestrus 1 in the rat estrous cycle. *Biol Reprod* 1985;33:103–111.
672. Okamoto MT, Nobunaga T, Suzuki Y. Delay in ovulation with pentobarbital anesthesia applied at various stages of the 4-day cyclic rat. *Endocrinol Jpn* 1972;19:11–17.
673. Dominquez R, Smith ER. Barbiturate blockade of ovulation on days other than proestrus in the rat. *Neuroendocrinology* 1974;14:212–223.
674. Schwartz NB, Gold JJ. Effect of a single dose of anti-LH serum at proestrus on the rat estrous cycle. *Anat Rec* 1967;157:137–150.
675. Laurence KA, Ichikawa S. Effects of antiserum to bovine LH on the estrous cycle and early pregnancy in the female rat. *Int J Fertil* 1969;14:8–15.
676. Greenwald GS. Effect of a single injection of diethylstilbestrol or progesterone on the hamster ovary. *J Endocrinol* 1965;33:13–23.
677. Greenwald GS. Exogenous progesterone: influence on ovulation and hormone levels in the cyclic hamster. *J Endocrinol* 1977;73:151–155.
678. Greenwald GS. Modification by exogenous progesterone of estrogen and gonadotropin secretion in the cyclic hamster. *Endocrinology* 1978;103:2315–2322.
679. Beattie CW, Corbin A. The differential effects of diestrus progestogen administration on proestrous gonadotropin levels. *Endocrinology* 1975;97:885–890.
680. Garza F, Terranova PF. Inhibition of thecal androstenedione production by exogenous progesterone in the cyclic hamster. *J Reprod Fertil* 1984;70:493–498.
681. Taya K, Terranova PF, Greenwald GS. Acute effects of exogenous progesterone on follicular steroidogenesis in the cyclic rat. *Endocrinology* 1981;108:2324–2330.
682. Varga B, Greenwald GS. Cyclic changes in utero-ovarian blood flow and ovarian hormone secretion in the hamster: effects of adrenocorticotropin, luteinizing hormone, and follicle-stimulating hormone. *Endocrinology* 1979;104:1525–1531.
683. Varga B, Horvath E, Folly G, Stark E. Study of the luteinizing hormone-induced increase of ovarian blood flow during the estrous cycle in the rat. *Biol Reprod* 1985;32:480–488.
684. Telfer E, Gosden RG, Faddy MJ. Impact of exogenous progesterone on ovarian follicular dynamics and function in mice. *J Reprod Fertil* 1991;93:263–269.
685. Peluso JJ, Luttmer S, Gruenberg ML. Modulatory action of FSH on LH-induced follicular growth in rats. *J Reprod Fertil* 1984;72:173–177.
686. Greenwald GS. Follicular activity in the mammalian ovary. In: Jones RE, ed. *The vertebrate ovary.* New York: Plenum; 1978:639–689.
687. Nordenstrom K, Johanson C. Steroidogenesis in isolated rat granulosa cells: changes during follicular maturation. *Acta Endocrinol* 1985;108:550–556.
688. Richards JS, Jonassen JA, Kersey KA. Evidence that changes in tonic luteinizing hormone secretion determine the growth of preovulatory follicles in the rat. *Endocrinology* 1980;107: 641–647.
689. Roser S, Bloch RB. Etude comparative des variations de la progesterone plasmalique ovarienne au cours de cycles de respectivement 4 et 5 jours, chez la ratte. *C R Soc Biol* 1971;165: 1995–1998.
690. van der Schoot P, de Greef WJ. Dioestrous progesterone and pro-oestrous luteinizing hormone in 4- and 5-day cycles of female rats. *J Endocrinol* 1976;70:61–68.
691. Nequin LG, Alvarez J, Schwartz NB. Measurement of serum steroid and gonadotropin levels and uterine and ovarian variables throughout 4-day and 5-day estrous cycles in the rat. *Biol Reprod* 1979;20:659–670.
692. van der Schoot P, Uilenbroek JTJ. Reduction of 5-day cycle length of female rats by treatment with bromocriptine. *J Endocrinol* 1983;97:83–89.
693. Boehm N, Plas-Roser S, Aron C. Prolactin and the control of cycle length in the female rat. *Acta Endocrinol* 1984;106: 188–192.

694. Richards JS, Bogovich K. Effects of human chorionic gonadotropin and progesterone on follicular development in the immature rat. *Endocrinology* 1982;111:1429–1438.
695. Fortune JE, Vincent SE. Progesterone inhibits the induction of aromatase activity in rat granulosa cells in vitro. *Biol Reprod* 1983;28:1078–1089.
696. Uilenbroek JTJ, van der Schoot P, den Besten D, Lankhorst RR. A possible direct effect of prolactin on follicular activity. *Biol Reprod* 1982;27:1119–1125.
697. Magoffin DA, Erickson GF. LH induction of androgen biosynthesis in cultured ovarian cells: inhibitory effect on prolactin. In: Schwartz NB, Hunzicker-Dunn M, eds. *Dynamics of ovarian function.* New York: Raven Press; 1981:55–60.
698. L'Hermite M, Niswender GD, Reichert LE Jr, Midgley AR Jr. Serum follicle-stimulating hormone in sheep as measured by radioimmunoassay. *Biol Reprod* 1972;6:325–332.
699. Goodman RL, Pickover SM, Karsch FJ. Ovarian feedback control of follicle-stimulating hormone in the ewe: evidence for selective suppression. *Endocrinology* 1981;108:772–777.
700. McNatty KP, Dobson C, Gibb M, Kieboom L, Thurley DC. Accumulation of luteinizing hormone, oestradiol and androstenedione by sheep ovarian follicles in vivo. *J Endocrinol* 1981;91: 99–109.
701. Hauger RL, Karsch FJ, Foster DL. A new concept for control of the estrous cycle of the ewe based on the temporal relationships between luteinizing hormone, estradiol and progesterone in peripheral serum and evidence that progesterone inhibits tonic LH secretion. *Endocrinology* 1977;101:807–817.
702. Baird DT, Swanston I, Scaramuzzi RJ. Pulsatile release of LH and secretion of ovarian steroids in sheep during the luteal phase of the estrous cycle. *Endocrinology* 1976;98:1490–1495.
703. Findlay JK, Clarke IJ, Robertson DM. Inhibin concentrations in ovarian and jugular venous plasma and the relationship of inhibin with follicle-stimulating hormone and luteinizing hormone during the ovine estrous cycle. *Endocrinology* 1990;126:528–535.
704. Mann GE, McNeilly AS, Baird DT. Hormone production in vivo and in vitro from follicles at different stages of the oestrous cycle in the sheep. *J Endocrinol* 1992;132:225–234.
705. McNeilly AS, Crow W, Campbell BK. Effect of follicular fluid and inhibin immunoneutralization on FSH-induced preovulatory follicle growth in the ewe. *J Endocrinol* 1991;131:401–409.
706. Cahill LP, Driancourt MA, Chamley WA, Findlay JK. Role of intrafollicular regulators and FSH in growth and development of large antral follicles in sheep. *J Reprod Fertil* 1985;75:599–607.
707. Henderson KM, Prisk MD, Hudson N, et al. Use of bovine follicular fluid to increase ovulation rate or prevent ovulation in sheep. *J Reprod Fertil* 1986;76:623–635.
708. Brand A, deJong WHR. Qualitative and quantitative micromorphological investigations of the tertiary follicle population during the oestrous cycle in sheep. *J Reprod Fertil* 1973;33:431–439.
709. Bherer J, Matton P, Dufour JJ. Fate of the two largest follicles in the ewe after injection of gonadotrophins at two stages of the estrus cycle. *Proc Soc Exp Biol Med* 1977;154:412–414.
710. Tsonis CG, Cahill LP, Carson RS, Findlay JK. Identification at the onset of luteolysis of follicles capable of ovulation in the ewe. *J Reprod Fertil* 1984;70:609–614.
711. Dailey RA, Fogwell RL, Thayne WV. Distribution of visible follicles on the ovarian surface in ewes. *J Anim Sci* 1982;54: 1196–1204.
712. Turnbull KE, Braden AWH, Mattner PE. The pattern of follicular growth and atresia in the ovine ovary. *Aust J Biol Sci* 1977;30:229–241.
713. Yenikoye A, Mariana JC, Celeux G. Follicular growth during the oestrous cycle in Peul sheep. *Anim Reprod Sci* 1989;21:201–211.
714. Cahill LP, Mauleon P. Influences of season, cycle and breed on follicular growth rates in sheep. *J Reprod Fertil* 1980;58:321–328.
715. Cahill LP, Mauleon P. A study of the population of primordial and small follicles in the sheep. *J Reprod Fertil* 1981;61:201–206.
716. Lahlou-Kassi A, Mariana JC. Ovarian follicular growth during the oestrous cycle in two breeds of ewes of different ovulation rate, the D'man and the Timahdite. *J Reprod Fertil* 1984;72: 301–310.
717. Cummins LJ, O'Shea T, Bindon BM, Lee VWK, Findlay JK. Ovarian inhibin content and sensitivity to inhibin in Booroola and control strain Merino ewes. *J Reprod Fertil* 1983;67:1–7.
718. Robertson DM, Ellis S, Foulds LM, Findlay JK, Bindon BM. Pituitary gonadotrophins in Booroola and control Merino sheep. *J Reprod Fertil* 1984;71:189–197.
719. McNatty KP, Henderson KM, Lun S, et al. Ovarian activity in Booroola × Romney ewes which have a major gene influencing their ovulation rate. *J Reprod Fertil* 1985;73:109–120.
720. Bindon BM, Piper LR, Thimonier J. Preovulatory LH characteristics and time of ovulation in the prolific Booroola Merino ewe. *J Reprod Fertil* 1984;71:519–523.
721. Castonguay F, Dufour JJ, Minvielle F, Estrada R. Follicular dynamics and dominance in Booroola × Finnish Landrace and Booroola × Suffolk ewes heterozygous for the F gene. *J Reprod Fertil* 1990;89:193–203.
722. Driancourt MA, Webb R, Fry RC. Does follicular dominance occur in ewes? *J Reprod Fertil* 1991;93:63–70.
723. Webb R, Gauld IK, Driancourt MA. Morphological and functional characterization of large antral follicles in three breeds of sheep with different ovulation rates. *J Reprod Fertil* 1989;87: 243–255.
724. Bjersing L, Hay MF, Kann G, et al. Changes in gonadotrophins, ovarian steroids and follicular morphology in sheep at oestrus. *J Endocrinol* 1972;52:465–479.
725. Thomas GB, Oldham CM, Hoskinson RM, Scaramuzzi RJ, Martin GB. Effect of immunization against progesterone on oestrus, cycle length, ovulation rate, luteal regression and LH secretion in the ewe. *Aust J Biol Sci* 1987;40:307–313.
726. Hay MF, Moor RM. Functional and structural relationships in the graafian follicle population of the sheep ovary. *J Reprod Fertil* 1975;45:583–593.
727. McNatty KP, Gibb M, Dobson C, Thurley DC, Findlay JK. Changes in the concentration of gonadotrophic and steroidal hormones in the antral fluid of ovarian follicles throughout the oestrous cycle of the sheep. Aust J Biol Sci 1981;34:67–80.
728. Moor RM. The ovarian follicle of the sheep: inhibition of oestrogen secretion by luteinizing hormone. *J Endocrinol* 1974;61: 455–463.
729. England BG, Webb R, Dahmer MK. Follicular steroidogenesis and gonadotropin binding to ovine follicles during the estrous cycle. *Endocrinology* 1981;109:881–887.
730. Driancourt MA, Gibson WR, Cahill LP. Follicular dynamics throughout the oestrous cycle in sheep: a review. *Reprod Nutr Dev* 1985;25:1–15.
731. McNatty KP, Gibb M, Dobson C, et al. Preovulatory follicular development in sheep treated with PMSG and/or prostaglandin. *J Reprod Fertil* 1982;65:111–123.
732. Webb R, England BG. Identification of the ovulatory follicle in the ewe: associated changes in follicular size, thecal and granulosa cell luteinizing hormone receptors, antral fluid steroids, and circulating hormones during the preovulatory period. *Endocrinology* 1982;110:873–881.
733. Picton HM, McNeilly AS. Evidence to support a follicle-stimulating hormone threshold theory for follicle selection in ewes chronically treated with gonadotrophin-releasing hormone agonist. *J Reprod Fertil* 1991;93:43–51.
734. McNeilly AS, Fraser HM, Baird DT. Effect of immunoneutralization of LH releasing hormone on LH, FSH and ovarian steroid secretion in the preovulatory phase of the oestrous cycle in the ewe. *J Endocrinol* 1984;101:213–219.
735. McNatty KP, Hudson NL, Henderson KM, et al. Changes in gonadotrophin secretion and ovarian antral follicular activity in seasonally breeding sheep throughout the year. *J Reprod Fertil* 1984;70:309–321.
736. McLeod BJ, Haresign W, Lamming GE. Induction of ovulation in seasonally anoestrous ewes by continuous infusion of low doses of Gn-RH. *J Reprod Fertil* 1983;68:489–495.
737. McNatty KP, Hudson N, Gibb M, et al. FSH influences follicle viability, oestradiol biosynthesis and ovulation rate in Romney ewes. *J Reprod Fertil* 1985;75:121–131.
738. Webb R, Baxter G, McBride D, Ritchie M, Springbett AJ. Mechanism controlling ovulation rate in ewes in relation to seasonal anoestrus. *J Reprod Fertil* 1992;94:143–151.
739. Driancourt MA, Bodin L, Boomaroy O, Thimonier J, Elsen JM. Number of mature follicles ovulating after a challenge of human chorionic gonadotropin in different breeds of sheep at different physiological stages. *J Anim Sci* 1990;68:719–724.

740. McNeilly AS. Effect of changes in FSH induced by bovine follicular fluid and FSH infusion in the preovulatory phase on subsequent ovulation rate and corpus luteum function in the ewe. *J Reprod Fertil* 1985;74:661–668.
741. Driancourt MA. Follicular dynamics in sheep and cattle. *Theriogenology* 1991;35:55–79.
742. Monniaux D, Pisselet C. Control of proliferation and differentiation of ovine granulosa cells by insulin-like growth factor-I and follicle-stimulating hormone in vitro. *Biol Reprod* 1992;46:109–119.
743. Schams D, Schallenberger E, Hoffman B, Karg H. The oestrous cycle of the cow: hormonal parameters and time relationships concerning oestrus, ovulation, and electrical resistance of the vaginal mucus. *Acta Endocrinol* 1977;86:180–182.
744. Walters DL, Schams D, Schallenberger E. Pulsatile secretion of gonadotrophins, ovarian steroids and ovarian oxytocin during the luteal phase of the oestrous cycle in the cow. *J Reprod Fertil* 1984;71:479–491.
745. Schallenberger E, Schams D, Bullermann B, Walters DL. Pulsatile secretion of gonadotrophins, ovarian steroids and ovarian oxytocin during prostaglandin-induced regression of the corpus luteum in the cow. *J Reprod Fertil* 1984;71:493–501.
746. Ireland JJ, Roche JF. Development of antral follicles in cattle after prostaglandin-induced luteolysis: changes in serum hormones, steroids in follicular fluid, and gonadotropin receptors. *Endocrinology* 1982;111:2077–2086.
747. Glencross RG, Munro IB, Senior BE, Pope GS. Concentrations of oestradiol-17β, oestrone and progesterone in jugular venous plasma of cows during the oestrous cycle and in early pregnancy. *Acta Endocrinol* 1973;73:374–384.
748. Dieleman SJ, Kruip TAM, Fontijne P, de Jong WHR, van der Weyden GC. Changes in oestradiol, progesterone and testosterone concentrations in follicular fluid and in the micromorphology of preovulatory bovine follicles relative to the peak of luteinizing hormone. *J Endocrinol* 1983;97:31–42.
749. Roche JF, Ireland JJ. The differential effect of progesterone on concentrations of luteinizing hormone and follicle-stimulating hormone in heifers. *Endocrinology* 1981;108:568–572.
750. Dufour J, Whitmore HL, Ginther OJ, Casida LE. Identification of the ovulating follicle by its size on different days of the estrous cycle in heifers. *J Anim Sci* 1972;34:85–87.
751. Matton P, Adelakoun V, Couture Y, Dufour JJ. Growth and replacement of the bovine ovarian follicles during the estrous cycle. *J Anim Sci* 1981;52:813–820.
752. Staigmiller RB, England BG. Folliculogenesis in the bovine. *Theriogenology* 1982;17:43–52.
753. Fogwell RL, Cowley JL, Wortman JA, Ames NK, Ireland JJ. Luteal function in cows following destruction of ovarian follicles at midcycle. *Theriogenology* 1985;23:389–398.
754. Choudary JB, Gier HT, Marion GB. Cyclic changes in bovine vesicular follicles. *J Anim Sci* 1968;27:468–471.
755. Scaramuzzi RJ, Turnbull KE, Nancarrow CD. Growth of graafian follicles in cows following luteolysis induced by the prostaglandin F2α' analogue, cloprostenol. *Aust J Biol Sci* 1980;33:63–69.
756. Kruip TAM, Dieleman SJ. Macroscopic classification of bovine follicles and its validation by micromorphological and steroid biochemical procedures. *Reprod Nutr Dev* 1982;22:465–473.
757. Merz EA, Hauser ER, England BG. Ovarian function in the cycling cow: relationship between gonadotropin binding to theca and granulosa and steroidogenesis in individual follicles. *J Anim Sci* 1981;52:1457–1468.
758. Fortune JE, Sirois J, Turzillo AM, Lavoir M. Follicle selection in domestic ruminants. *J Reprod Fertil* 1991;43(Suppl):187–198.
759. Ginther OJ, Knopf L, Kastelic JP. Temporal associations among ovarian events in cattle during oestrous cycles with two and three follicular waves. *J Reprod Fertil* 1989;87:223–230.
760. Turzillo AM, Fortune JE. Suppression of the secondary FSH surge with bovine follicular fluid is associated with delayed ovarian follicular development in heifers. *J Reprod Fertil* 1990;89:643–653.
761. Pierson RA, Ginther OJ. Follicular populations during the estrous cycle in heifers. II. Influence of right and left sides and intraovarian effect of the corpus luteum. *Anim Reprod Sci* 1987;14:177–186.
762. Adams GP, Matteri RL, Kastelic JP, Ko JCH, Ginther OJ. Association between surges of follicle-stimulating hormone and the emergence of follicular waves in heifers. *J Reprod Fertil* 1992;94:177–188.
763. Savio JD, Boland MP, Hynes N, Mattiacci MR, Roche JF. Will the first dominant follicle of the estrous cycle of heifers ovulate following luteolysis on day 7? *Theriogenology* 1990;33:677–687.
764. Ko JCH, Kastelic JP, Del Campo MR, Ginther OJ. Effects of a dominant follicle on ovarian follicular dynamics during the oestrous cycle in heifers. *J Reprod Fertil* 1991;91:511–519.
765. Kaneko H, Terada T, Taya K, et al. Ovarian follicular dynamics and concentrations of oestradiol-17β, progesterone, luteinizing hormone and follicle stimulating hormone during the periovulatory phase of the oestrous cycle in the cow. *Reprod Fertil Dev* 1991;3:529–535.
766. Pierson RA, Ginther OJ. Follicular populations during the estrous cycle in heifers. III. Time of selection of the ovulatory follicle. *Anim Reprod Sci* 1988;16:81–95.
767. Sirois J, Fortune JE. Lengthening the bovine estrous cycle with low levels of exogenous progesterone: a model for studying ovarian follicular dominance. *Endocrinology* 1990;127:916–925.
768. Henderson KM, McNeilly AS, Swanston IA. Gonadotrophin and steroid concentrations in bovine follicular fluid and their relationship to follicle size. *J Reprod Fertil* 1990;65:467–473.
769. Zimmermann RC, Westhof G, Thatcher S, Peukert-Adam I, Grunert E, Braendle W. Follicular size and steroid secretion of dominant bovine follicles. *Zentral bl Gynakol* 1990;112:1279–1283.
770. Martin TL, Fogwell RL, Ireland JJ. Concentrations of inhibins and steroids in follicular fluid during development of dominant follicles in heifers. *Biol Reprod* 1991;44:693–700.
771. Fortune JE, Hansel W. Concentrations of steroids and gonadotropins in follicular fluid from normal heifers and heifers primed for superovulation. *Biol Reprod* 1985;32:1069–1079.
772. Staigmiller RB, England BG, Webb R, Short RE, Bellows RA. Estrogen secretion and gonadotropin binding by individual bovine follicles during estrus. *J Anim Sci* 1982;55:1473–1482.
773. Thayer KM, Forrest DW, Welsh TH Jr. Real-time ultrasound evaluation of follicular development in superovulated cows. *Theriogenology* 1985;23:233.
774. Voss AK, Fortune JE. Oxytocin secretion by bovine granulosa cells: effects of stage of follicular development, gonadotropins, and coculture with theca interna. *Endocrinology* 1991;128:1991–1999.
775. Luck MR, Rodgers RJ, Findlay JK. Secretion and gene expressin of inhibin, oxytocin and steroid hormones during the in vitro differentiation of bovine granulosa cells. *Reprod Fertil Dev* 1990;2:11–25.
776. Luck MR. Ovarian oxytocin and progesterone are secreted independently of one another. *Mol Cell Endocrinol* 1988;56:149–155.
777. Saumande J. Culture of bovine granulosa cells in a chemically defined serum-free medium: the effect of insulin and fibronectin on the response to FSH. *J Steroid Biochem Mol Biol* 1991;38:189–196.
778. Peluso JJ, Hirschel MD. Role of gonadotropins and insulin in controlling steroidogenesis and growth of antral bovine follicles in perifusion culture. *Theriogenology* 1987;28:503–512.
779. Savion N, Lui GM, Laherty R, Gospodarowicz D. Factors controlling proliferation and progesterone production by bovine granulosa cells in serum-free medium. *Endocrinology* 1981;109:409–420.
780. Gospadarowicz D, Ferrara N, Schweigerer L, Neufeld G. Structural characterization and biological functions of fibroblast growth factor. *Endocrine Rev* 1987;8:95–114.
781. Grothe C, Unsicker K. Immunocytochemical localization of basic fibroblast growth factor in bovine adrenal gland, ovary and pituitary. *J Histochem Cytochem* 1989;37:1877–1883.
782. Neufeld G, Ferrara N, Schweigerer L, Mitchell R, Gospodarowicz D. Bovine granulosa cells produce basic fibroblast growth factor. *Endocrinology* 1987;121:597–603.
783. Morbeck DE, Esbenshade KL, Flowers WL, Britt JH. Kinetics of follicle growth in the prepubertal gilt. *Biol Reprod* 1992;47:485–491.
784. van de Wiel DFM, Erkens J, Koops W, Vos E, van Landeghem AAJ. Periestrous and midluteal time courses of circulating LH,

FSH, prolactin, estradiol-17β and progesterone in the domestic pig. *Biol Reprod* 1981;24:223–233.
785. Magness RR, Christenson RK, Ford SP. Ovarian blood flow throughout the estrous cycle and early pregnancy in sows. *Biol Reprod* 1983;28:1090–1096.
786. Flowers B, Cantley TC, Martin MJ, Day BN. Episodic secretion of gonadotrophins and ovarian steroids in jugular and utero-ovarian vein plasma during the follicular phase of the oestrous cycle in gilts. *J Reprod Fertil* 1991;91:101–112.
787. Einspanier A, Jarry H, Pitzel L, Holtz W, Wuttke W. Determination of secretion rates of estradiol, progesterone, oxytocin, and angiotensin II from tertiary follicles and freshly formed corpora lutea in freely moving sows. *Endocrinology* 1991;129:3403–3409.
788. Ford JJ, Lunstra DD. Differential production of estradiol by subpopulations of porcine granulosa cells. *J Reprod Dev* 1992;38: 91–98.
789. Goxe B, Salesse R, Remy JJ, Genty N, Garnier J. LH receptor RNA and protein levels after hormonal treatment of porcine granulosa cells in primary culture. *J Mol Endocrinol* 1992;8: 119–129.
790. Tonetta SA, DeVinna RS, diZerega GS. Effects of follicle regulatory protein on thecal aromatase and 3β-hydroxysteroid dehydrogenase activity in medium- and large-sized pig follicles. *J Reprod Fertil* 1988;82:163–171.
791. Tonetta SA, Yanagihara DL, DeVinna RS, diZerega GS. Secretion of follicle-regulatory protein by porcine granulosa cells. *Biol Reprod* 1988;38:1001–1005.
792. Clark JR, Brazier SG, Wiginton LM, Stevenson GR, Tribble LF. Time of ovarian follicle selection during the porcine estrous cycle. *Theriogenology* 1982;18:697–709.
793. Parlow AF, Anderson LL, Melampy RM. Pituitary follicle-stimulating hormone and luteinizing hormone concentrations in relation to reproductive stages of the pig. *Endocrinology* 1964;75:365–376.
794. Guthrie HD, Knudsen JF. Follicular growth and production of estrogen and progesterone after injection of gilts with human chorionic gonadotropin on day 12 of the estrous cycle. *J Anim Sci* 1984;59:1295–1302.
795. Hunter RHF, Baker TG. Development and fate of porcine graafian follicles identified at different stages of the oestrous cycle. *J Reprod Fertil* 1975;43:193–196.
796. Dailey RA, Clark JR, Staigmiller RB, First NL, Chapman AB, Casida LE. Growth of new follicles following electrocautery in four genetic groups of swine. *J Anim Sci* 1976;43:175–183.
797. Kelly CR, Socha TE, Zimmerman DR. Characterization of gonadotropic and ovarian steroid hormones during the periovulatory period in high ovulating select and control line gilts. *J Anim Sci* 1988;66:1462–1474.
798. Taya K, Kaneko H, Watanabe G, Sasamoto S. Inhibin and secretion of FSH in oestrous cycles of cows and pigs. *J Reprod Fertil* 1991;43(Suppl):151–162.
799. Bamberg E, Choi HS, Hassaan NK, Klaring WJ, Mostl E, Stockl W. Steroidhormongehalt in Blut und Ovarfollikeln des Rindes wahrend des Zyklus. *Zentralbl Vet Med* 1980;27:186–194.
800. Ainsworth L, Tsang BK, Downey BR, Marcus GJ, Armstrong DT. Interrelationships between follicular fluid steroid levels, gonadotropic stimuli, and oocyte maturation during preovulatory development of porcine follicles. *Biol Reprod* 1980;23:621–627.
801. Hunter MG, Wiesak T. Evidence for and implications of follicular heterogeneity in pigs. *J Reprod Fertil* 1990;40(Suppl):163–177.
802. Pope WF. Embryogenesis recapitulates oogenesis in swine. *Proc Soc Exp Biol Med* 1992;199:273–281.
803. Hammond JM, Baranao JL, Skaleris D, Knight AB, Romanus JA, Rechler MM. Production of insulin-like growth factors by ovarian granulosa cells. *Endocrinology* 1985;117:2553–2555.
804. Baranao JLS, Hammond JM. Comparative effects of insulin and insulin-like growth factors on DNA synthesis and differentiation of porcine granulosa cells. *Biochem Biophys Res Commun* 1984;124:484–490.
805. Hammond JM, English HF. Regulation of deoxyribonucleic acid synthesis in cultured porcine granulosa cells by growth factors and hormones. *Endocrinology* 1987;120:1039–1046.
806. Hsu CJ, Hammond JM. Gonadotropins and estradiol stimulate immunoreactive insulin-like growth factor-I production by porcine granulosa cells in vitro. *Endocrinology* 1987;120:198–207.
807. Howard HJ, Ford JJ. Relationships among concentrations of steroids, inhibin, insulin-like growth factor-I (IGF-I), and IGF-binding proteins during follicular development in weaned sows. *Biol Reprod* 1992;47:193–201.
808. May JV, Frost JP, Schomberg DW. Differential effects of epidermal growth factor, somatomedin-C/insulin-like growth factor-I, and transforming growth factor-β on porcine granulosa cell deoxyribonucleic acid synthesis and cell proliferation. *Endocrinology* 1988;123:168–179.
809. Veldhuis JD, Furlanetto RW, Juchter D, Garmey J, Veldhuis P. Trophic actions of human somatomedin C/insulin-like growth factor I on ovarian cells: in vitro studies with swine granulosa cells. *Endocrinology* 1985;116:1235–1242.
810. Monget P, Monniaux D, Durand P. Localization, characterization and quantification of insulin-like growth factor-I-binding sites in the ewe ovary. *Endocrinology* 1989;125:2486–2493.
811. Gangrade BK, Davis JS, May JV. A novel mechanism for the induction of aromatase in ovarian cells in vitro: role of transforming growth factor alpha-induced protein tyrosine kinase. *Endocrinology* 1991;129:2790–2792.
812. Fujinaga H, Yamoto M, Nakano R, Shima K. Epidermal growth factor binding sites in porcine granulosa cells and their regulation by follicle stimulating hormone. *Biol Reprod* 1992;46:705–709.
813. May JV, Bridge AJ, Gotcher ED, Gangrade BK. The regulation of porcine theca cell proliferation in vitro: synergistic actions of epidermal growth factor and platelet-derived growth factor. *Endocrinology* 1992;131:689–697.
814. Gangrade BK, May JV. The production of transforming growth factor-β in the porcine ovary and its secretion in vitro. *Endocrinology* 1990;127:2372–2380.
815. Mondschein JS, Canning SF, Hammond JM. Effects of transforming growth factor-β on the production of immunoreactive insulin-like growth factor I and progesterone and on [^{3}H]-thymidine incorporation in porcine granulosa cell cultures. *Endocrinology* 1988;123:1970–1976.
816. Schultea TD, Dees WL, Ojeda SR. Postnatal development of sympathetic and sensory innervation of the rhesus monkey ovary. *Biol Reprod* 1992;47:760–767.
817. Gougeon A, Lefevre B, Testart J. Influence of a gonadotrophin-releasing hormone agonist and gonadotrophins on morphometric characteristics of the population of small ovarian follicles in cynomolgus monkeys (*Macaca fascicularis*). *J Reprod Fertil* 1992;95:567–575.
818. Koering MJ. Cyclic changes in ovarian morphology during the menstrual cycle in *Macaca mulatta. Am J Anat* 1969;126: 73–101.
819. Koering MJ, Baehler EA, Goodman AL, Hodgen GD. Developing morphological asymmetry of ovarian follicular maturation in monkeys. *Biol Reprod* 1982;27:989–997.
820. Stouffer RL, Hodgen GD, Ottobre AC, Christian CD. Follicular fluid treatment during the follicular versus luteal phase of the menstrual cycle: effects on corpus luteum function. *J Clin Endocrinol Metab* 1984;58:1027–1033.
821. Zeleznik AJ, Wildt L, Schuler HM. Characterization of ovarian folliculogenesis during the luteal phase of the menstrual cycle in rhesus monkeys using [^{3}H]thymidine autoradiography. *Endocrinology* 1980;107:982–988.
822. Ellinwood WE, Norman RL, Spies HG. Changing frequency of pulsatile luteinizing hormone and progesterone secretion during the luteal phase of the menstrual cycle of rhesus monkeys. *Biol Reprod* 1984;31:714–722.
823. Clark JR, Dierschke DJ, Meller PA, Wolf RC. Hormonal regulation of ovarian folliculogenesis in rhesus monkeys. II. Serum concentrations of estradiol-17β and follicle stimulating hormone associated with growth and identification of the preovulatory follicle. *Biol Reprod* 1979;21:497–503.
824. Clark JR, Dierschke DJ, Wolf RC. Hormonal regulation of ovarian folliculogenesis in rhesus monkeys: I. Concentrations of serum luteinizing hormone and progesterone during laparoscopy and patterns of follicular development during successive menstrual cycles. *Biol Reprod* 1978;17:779–783.
825. Goodman AL, Nixon WE, Johnson DK, Hodgen GD. Regulation of folliculogenesis in the cycling rhesus monkey: selection of the dominant follicle. *Endocrinology* 1977;100:155–161.
826. Hutz RJ, Dierschke DJ, Wolf RC. Temporal and endocrine se-

quelae of aspirating follicular contents in rhesus monkeys. *Am J Primatology* 1987;13:195–202.

827. Goodman AL, Nixon WE, Hodgen GD. Between-ovary interaction in the regulation of follicle growth, corpus luteum function, and gonadotropin secretion in the primate ovarian cycle. III. Temporal and spatial dissociation of folliculogenesis and negative feedback regulation of tonic gonadotropin release after lutectomy in rhesus monkeys. *Endocrinology* 1979;105:69–73.
828. diZerega GS, Hodgen GD. The interovarian progesterone gradient: a spatial and temporal regulator of folliculogenesis in the primate ovarian cycle. *J Clin Endocrinol Metab* 1982;54: 495–499.
829. diZerega GS, Campeau JD, Ujita EL, et al. The possible role for a follicular protein in the intraovarian regulation of folliculogenesis. *Semin Reprod Endocrinol* 1983;1:309–320.
830. Channing CP, Anderson LD, Hoover DJ, Gagliano P, Hodgen G. Inhibitory effects of porcine follicular fluid on monkey serum FSH levels and follicular maturation. *Biol Reprod* 1981;25: 885–903.
831. diZerega GS, Turner CK, Stouffer RL, Anderson LD, Channing CP, Hodgen GD. Suppression of follicle-stimulating hormone-dependent folliculogenesis during the primate ovarian cycle. *J Clin Endocrinol Metab* 1981;52:451–456.
832. Zeleznik AJ, Kubik CJ. Ovarian responses in macaques to pulsatile infusion of follicle-stimulating hormone (FSH) and luteinizing hormone: increased sensitivity of the maturing follicle to FSH. *Endocrinology* 1986;119:2025–2032.
833. Zeleznik AJ, Hutchison JS, Schuler HM. Passive immunization with anti-oestradiol antibodies during the luteal phase of the menstrual cycle potentiates the perimenstrual rise in serum gonadotrophin concentrations and stimulates follicular growth in the cynomolgus monkey (*Macaca fascicularis*). *J Reprod Fertil* 1987; 80:403–410.
834. Hillier SG, Wickings EJ, Saunders PTK, et al. Control of inhibin production by primate granulosa cells. *J Endocrinol* 1989; 123:65–73.
835. Zeleznik AJ, Hutchison JS, Schuler HM. Interference with the gonadotropin-suppressing actions of estradiol in macaques overrides the selection of a single preovulatory follicle. *Endocrinology* 1985;117:991–999.
836. Dierschke DJ, Hutz RJ, Wolf RC. Induced follicular atresia in rhesus monkeys: strength-duration relationships of the estrogen stimulus. *Endocrinology* 1985;117:1397–1403.
837. Williams RF, Hodgen GD. Disparate effects of human chorionic gonadotropin during the late follicular phase in monkeys: normal ovulation, follicular atresia, ovarian acyclicity, and hypersecretion of follicle-stimulating hormone. *Fertil Steril* 1980;33:64–68.
838. Wilks JW, Spilman CH, Campbell JA. Arrest of folliculogenesis and inhibition of ovulation in the monkey following weekly administration of progestins. *Fertil Steril* 1983;40:688–692.
839. Channing CP. Progesterone and estrogen secretion by cultured monkey ovarian cell types: influences of follicular size, serum luteinizing hormone levels, and follicular fluid estrogen levels. *Endocrinology* 1980;107:342–352.
840. Vernon MW, Dierschke DJ, Sholl SA, Wolf RC. Ovarian aromatase activity in granulosa and theca cells of rhesus monkeys. *Biol Reprod* 1983;28:342–349.
841. Marut EL, Huang SC, Hodgen GD. Distinguishing the steroidogenic roles of granulosa and theca cells of the dominant ovarian follicle and corpus luteum. *J Clin Endocrinol Metab* 1983;57: 925–930.
842. Hild-Petito S, Stouffer RL, Brenner RM. Immunocytochemical localization of estradiol and progesterone receptors in the monkey ovary throughout the menstrual cycle. *Endocrinology* 1988;123:2896–2905.
843. Hutz RJ, Wagner N, Krause P, et al. Localization of estrogen receptors in rhesus monkey ovary. *Am J Primatol* 1993;In press.
844. Billiar RB, Loukides JA, Miller MM. Evidence for the presence of the estrogen receptor in the ovary of the baboon (*Papio anubis*). *J Clin Endocrinol Metab* 1992;75:1159–1165.
845. Koering MJ, Danforth DR, Hodgen GD. Early folliculogenesis in primate ovaries: testing the role of estrogen. *Biol Reprod* 1991;45:890–897.
846. Hutz RJ. Disparate effects of estrogens on in vitro steroidogenesis by mammalian and avian granulosa cells. *Biol Reprod* 1989; 40:709–713.
847. Wickings EJ, Eidne KA, Dixson AF, Hillier SG. Gonadotropin-releasing hormone analogs inhibit primate granulosa cell steroidogenesis via a mechanism distinct from that in the rat. *Biol Reprod* 1990;43:305–311.
848. Shaw HJ, Hodges JK. Effects of oestradiol-17β on FSH-stimulated steroidogenesis in cultured marmoset granulosa cells. *J Endocrinol* 1992;132:123–131.
849. Block E. Quantitative morphological investigations of the follicular system in women. Variations in the different phases of the sexual cycle. *Acta Endocrinol* 1951;8:33–54.
850. Gougeon A. Rate of follicular growth in the human ovary. In: Rolland R, van Hall EV, Hillier SG, McNatty KP, Schoemaker J, eds. *Follicular maturation and ovulation. Proceedings of the fourth Reinier de Graaf Symposium.* Princeton, NJ: Excerpta Medica; 1981:155–163.
851. Gougeon A. Vitesse de croissance des follicules dans l'ovaire humain. Contraception Fertil Sex 1984;12:839–845.
852. Gougeon A. Influence des variations hormonales cycliques (stéroides et gonadotropines) sur la croissance folliculaire dans l'ovaire humain. Contraception Fertil Sex 1984;12:615–620.
853. Gougeon A, Lefevre B. Histological evidence of alternating ovulation in women. *J Reprod Fertil* 1984;70:7–13.
854. Gougeon A. Croissance folliculaire dans l'ovaire humain pendant le cycle menstruel: mise en évidence de regulations intraovariennes. Contraception Fertil Sex 1984;12:733–738.
855. Gougeon A. Le follicule ovulatoire humain: à quel moment du cycle est-il selectionne et par quels mecanismes?—une tentative de reponse. Contraception Fertil Sex 1984;12:1397–1405.
856. Hall JE, Bhatta N, Adams JM, Rivier JE, Vale WW, Crowley WF Jr. Variable tolerance of the developing follicle and corpus luteum to gonadotropin-releasing hormone antagonist-induced gonadotropin withdrawal in the human. *J Clin Endocrinol Metab* 1991;72:993–1000.
857. Ditkoff EC, Cassidenti DL, Paulson RJ, et al. The gonadotropin-releasing hormone antagonist (Nal-Glu) acutely blocks the luteinizing hormone surge but allows for resumption of folliculogenesis in normal women. *Am J Obstet Gynecol* 1991;165: 1811–1817.
858. McNatty KP. Hormonal correlates of follicular development in the human ovary. *Aust J Biol Sci* 1981;34:249–268.
859. Lloyd CW, Lobotsky J, Baird DT, et al. Concentration of unconjugated estrogens, androgens and gestagens in ovarian and peripheral venous plasma of women: the normal menstrual cycle. *J Clin Endocrinol* 1971;32:155–166.
860. deJong FH, Baird DT, van der Molen HJ. Ovarian secretion rates of oestrogens, androgens and progesterone in normal women and in women with persistent ovarian follicles. *Acta Endocrinol* 1974;77:575–587.
861. Baird DT, Fraser IS. Blood production and ovarian secretion rates of estradiol-17β and estrone in women throughout the menstrual cycle. *J Clin Endocrinol Metab* 1974;38:1009–1017.
862. McNatty KP, Hunter WM, McNeilly AS, Sawers RS. Changes in the concentration of pituitary and steroid hormones in the follicular fluid of human graafian follicles throughout the menstrual cycle. *J Endocrinol* 1975;64:555–571.
863. McNatty KP, Baird DT. Relationship between follicle-stimulating hormone, androstenedione and oestradiol in human follicular fluid. *J Endocrinol* 1978;76:527–531.
864. Queenan JT, O'Brien KGD, Bains LM, Simpson J, Collins WP, Campbell S. Ultrasound scanning of ovaries to detect ovulation in women. *Fertil Steril* 1980;34:99–105.
865. McNatty KP. Cyclic changes in antral fluid hormone concentrations in humans. *Clin Endocrinol Metab* 1978;7:577–600.
866. Bieszczad RR, McClintock JS, Pepe GJ, Dimino MJ. Progesterone secretion by granulosa cells from different-sized follicles of human ovaries after short term incubation. *J Clin Endocrinol Metab* 1982;55:181–184.
867. Pache TD, Wladimiroff JW, deJong FH, Hop WC, Fauser BCJM. Growth patterns of nondominant ovarian follicles during the normal menstrual cycle. *Fertil Steril* 1990;54:638–642.
868. Yamoto M, Nakano R, Iwasaki M, Ikoma H, Furukawa K. Luteinizing hormone receptors in human ovarian follicles and cor-

pora lutea during the menstrual cycle. *Obstet Gynecol* 1986;68: 200–203.
869. Rajaniemi MJ, Ronnberg L, Kauppila A, et al. Luteinizing hormone receptors in human ovarian follicles and corpora lutea during menstrual cycle and pregnancy. *J Clin Endocrinol Metab* 1981;108:307–313.
870. Dennefors BL, Nilsson L, Hamberger L. Steroid and adenosine 3′,5′-monophosphate formation in granulosa and thecal cells from human preovulatory follicles in response to human chorionic gonadotropin. *J Clin Endocrinol Metab* 1982;54:436–441.
871. Bernardus RE, Jones GS, Acosta AA, et al. The significance of the ratio in follicle-stimulating hormone and luteinizing hormone in induction of multiple follicular growth. *Fertil Steril* 1985;43: 373–378.
872. Gougeon A, Lefevre B, Testart J. Recrutement et sélection du follicule dominant pendant le cycle menstruel spontane ou stimule chez la femme. In: *Periode peri-ovulatoire. Colloque de la societe francaise pour l'etude de la fertilite.* 1984;1–11.
873. Hall JE, Schoenfeld DA, Martin KA, Crowley WF Jr. Hypothalamic gonadotropin-releasing hormone secretion and follicle-stimulating hormone dynamics during the luteal-follicular transition. *J Clin Endocrinol Metab* 1992;74:600–607.
874. Nilsson L, Wikland M, Hamberger L. Recruitment of an ovulatory follicle in the human following follicle-ectomy and luteectomy. *Fertil Steril* 1982;37:30–34.
875. Araki S, Chikazawa K, Akabori A, Ijima K, Tamada T. Hormonal profile after removal of the dominant follicle and corpus luteum in women. *Endocrinol Jpn* 1983;30:55–70.
876. Iwai T, Nanbu Y, Iwai M, Taii S, Fujii S, Mori T. Immunohistochemical localization of oestrogen receptors and progesterone receptors in the human ovary throughout the menstrual cycle. *Virchows Arch Pathol Anat [A]* 1990;417:369–375.
877. Voutilainen R, Tapanainen J, Chung B-C, Matteson KJ, Miller WL. Hormonal regulation of P450scc (20,22-desmolase) and P450c17 (17α-hydroxylase/17,20-lyase) in cultured human granulosa cells. *J Clin Endocrinol Metab* 1986;63:202–207.
878. Yong EL, Baird DT, Yates R, Reichert LE Jr, Hillier SG. Hormonal regulation of the growth and steroidogenic function of human granulosa cells. *J Clin Endocrinol Metab* 1992;74: 842–849.
879. Erickson GF, Garzo VG, Magoffin DA. Progesterone production by human granulosa cells cultured in serum free medium: effects of gonadotrophins and insulin-like growth factor I (IGF-I). *Hum Reprod* 1991;6:1074–1081.
880. Erickson GF, Garzo VG, Magoffin DA. Insulin-like growth factor-I regulates aromatase activity in human granulosa and granulosa luteal cells. *J Clin Endocrinol Metab* 1989;69:716–724.
881. Mason HD, Margara R, Winston RML, Beard RW, Reed MJ, Franks S. Inhibition of oestradiol production by epidermal growth factor in human granulosa cells of normal and polycystic ovaries. *Clin Endocrinol* 1990;33:511–517.
882. Dor J, Ben-Shlomo I, Lunenfeld B, et al. Insulin-like growth factor-I (IGF-I) may not be essential for ovarian follicular development: evidence from IGF-I deficiency. *J Clin Endocrinol Metab* 1992;74:539–542.
883. Poretsky L, Grigorescu F, Seibel M, Moses AC, Flier JS. Distribution and characterization of insulin and insulin-like growth factor-I receptors in normal human ovary. *J Clin Endocrinol Metab* 1985;61:728–734.
884. Steinkampf MP, Mendelson CR, Simpson ER. Effects of epidermal growth factor and insulin-like growth factor I on the levels of mRNA encoding aromatase cytochrome P-450 of human ovarian granulosa cells. *Mol Cell Endocrinol* 1988;59:93–99.
885. Erickson GF, Magoffin DA, Cragun JR, Chang RJ. The effects of insulin and insulin-like growth factors-I and II on estradiol-17β production by granulosa cells of polycystic ovaries. *J Clin Endocrinol Metab* 1990;70:894–902.
886. Hernandez ER, Hurwitz A, Vera A, et al. Expression of the genes encoding the insulin-like growth factors and their receptors in the human ovary. *J Clin Endocrinol Metab* 1992;74:419–425.
887. Cataldo NA, Giudice LC. Follicular fluid insulin-like growth factor binding protein profiles in polycystic ovary syndrome. *J Clin Endocrinol Metab* 1992;74:695–697.
888. Chegini N, Flanders KC. Presence of transforming growth factor-β and their selective cellular localization in human ovarian tissue of various reproductive stages. *Endocrinology* 1992;130: 1707–1715.
889. Whitman GF, Pantazis CG. Cellular localization of mullerian inhibiting substance messenger ribonucleic acid during human ovarian follicular development. *Am J Obstet Gynecol* 1991;165: 1881–1886.
890. Tsonis CG, Messinis IE, Templeton AA, McNeilly AS, Baird DT. Gonadotropic stimulation of inhibin secretion by the human ovary during the follicular and early luteal phase of the cycle. *J Clin Endocrinol Metab* 1988;66:915–921.
891. Greenwald GS, Choudary JB. Follicular development and induction of ovulation in the pregnant mouse. *Endocrinology* 1969;84:1512–1516.
892. Murr SM, Bradford GE, Geschwind II. Plasma luteinizing hormone, follicle-stimulating hormone and prolactin during pregnancy in the mouse. *Endocrinology* 1974;94:112–116.
893. Greenwald GS. Ovarian follicular development and pituitary FSH and LH content in the pregnant rat. *Endocrinology* 1966;79:572–578.
894. Taya K, Sasamoto S. Induction of ovulation by exogenous gonadotrophin during pseudopregnancy, pregnancy or lactation in rats. *J Reprod Fertil* 1977;51:467–468.
895. Taya K, Greenwald GS. In vivo and in vitro ovarian steroidogenesis in the pregnant rat. *Biol Reprod* 1981;25:683–691.
896. Taya K, Kimura J, Sasamoto S. Inhibin activity in ovarian venous plasma during pregnancy, pseudopregnancy and lactation in the rat. *Endocrinol Jpn* 1984;31:427–433.
897. Richards JS, Kersey KA. Changes in theca and granulosa cell function in antral follicles developing during pregnancy in the rat: gonadotropin receptors, cyclic AMP and estradiol-17β. *Biol Reprod* 1979;21:1185–1201.
898. Carson RS, Richards JS, Kahn LE. Functional and morphological differentiation of theca and granulosa cells during pregnancy in the rat: dependence on increased basal luteinizing hormone activity. *Endocrinology* 1981;109:1433–1441.
899. Bogovich K, Richards JS, Reichert LE Jr. Obligatory role of luteinizing hormone (LH) in the initiation of preovulatory follicular growth in the pregnant rat: specific effects of human chorionic gonadotropin and follicle-stimulating hormone on LH receptors and steroidogenesis in theca, granulosa, and luteal cells. *Endocrinology* 1981;109:860–867.
900. Bogovich K, Richards JS. Androgen biosynthesis in developing ovarian follicles: evidence that luteinizing hormone regulates thecal 17α-hydroxylase and C17-20-lyase activities. *Endocrinology* 1982;111:1201–1208.
901. Gallo RV, Bona-Gallo A, O'Sullivan D. Ovarian steroid regulation of pulsatile luteinizing hormone release during early gestation in the rat. *J Neuroendocrinol* 1990;2:883–888.
902. Devorshak-Harvey E, Bona-Gallo A, Gallo RV. Ovarian regulation of pulsatile luteinizing hormone secretion during late gestation in the rat. *J Neuroendocrinol* 1989;1:257–264.
903. Koiter TR, van der schaaf-Verdonk GC, Schuiling GA. Effects of luteolysis during late pregnancy on pituitary responsiveness to gonadotrophin-releasing hormone in the rat. *J Endocrinol* 1991;128:411–418.
904. Greenwald GS. Induction of ovulation in the pregnant hamster. *Am J Anat* 1967;121:249–258.
905. Bast JD, Greenwald GS. Daily concentrations of gonadotrophins and prolactin in the serum of pregnant or lactating hamsters. *J Endocrinol* 1974;63:527–532.
906. Greenwald GS, Voogt JL, Limback D. In vitro follicular and luteal steroidogenesis in the pregnant hamster with preliminary studies in the rat. *Biol Reprod* 1984;30:93–104.
907. Adams CE. Ovarian response to human chorionic gonadotrophin and egg transport in the pregnant and post-parturient rabbit. *J Endocrinol* 1968;40:101–105.
908. Osteen KG, Mills TM. Serum LH and FSH levels in the pregnant rabbit. *Proc Soc Exp Biol Med* 1979;162:454–457.
909. Osteen KG, Mills TM. Changes in the size, distribution and steroid content of rabbit ovarian follicles during early pseudopregnancy. *Biol Reprod* 1980;22:1040–1046.
910. Labhsetwar AP, Diamond M. Ovarian changes in the guinea pig during various reproductive stages and steroid treatments. *Biol Reprod* 1970;2:53–57.
911. Bujard E. L'ovaire de cobaye (etudes statistiques des follicules

ovariques). I. L'ovaire gravide. *Rev Suisse Zool* 1953;60: 615–652.
912. Rowlands IW. The corpus luteum of the guinea pig. In: Wolstenholme G, Millar E, eds. *Ciba Foundation Colloquia on Ageing.* Boston: Little, Brown; 1956:69–85.
913. Melampy RM, Henricks DM, Anderson LL, Chen CL, Schultz JR. Pituitary follicle-stimulating hormone and luteinizing hormone concentrations in pregnant and lactating pigs. *Endocrinology* 1966;78:801–804.
914. Dufour JJ, Fahmy MH. Follicular and luteal changes during early pregnancy in three breeds of swine. *Can J Anim Sci* 1974;54:29–33.
915. Schallenberger E, Rampp J, Walters DL. Gonadotrophins and ovarian steroids in cattle. II. Pulsatile changes of concentrations in the jugular vein throughout pregnancy. *Acta Endocrinol* 1985;108:322–330.
916. Schallenberger E, Schondorfer AM, Walters DL. Gonadotrophins and ovarian steroids in cattle. I. Pulsatile changes of concentrations in the jugular vein throughout the oestrous cycle. *Acta Endocrinol* 1985;108:312–321.
917. Ginther OJ, Knopf L, Kastelic JP. Ovarian follicular dynamics in heifers during early pregnancy. *Biol Reprod* 1989;41:247–254.
918. Ginther OJ, Kastelic JP, Knopf L. Intraovarian relationships among dominant and subordinate follicles and the corpus luteum in heifers. *Theriogenology* 1989;32:787–795.
919. Thatcher WW, Driancourt MA, Terqui M, Badinga L. Dynamics of ovarian follicular development in cattle following hysterectomy and during early pregnancy. *Domestic Anim Endocrinol* 1991;8:223–234.
920. Al-Gubory KH, Martinet J. Comparison of the total ovarian follicular populations at day 140 of pregnancy and at day 5 postpartum in ewes. *Theriogenology* 1986;25:795–808.
921. Govan ADT. The human ovary in early pregnancy. *J Endocrinol* 1968;40:421–428.
922. Govan ADT. Ovarian follicular activity in late pregnancy. *J Endocrinol* 1970;48:235–241.
923. Starup J, Visfeldt J. Ovarian morphology in early and late human pregnancy. *Acta Obstet Gynecol Scand* 1974;53:211–218.
924. Dekel N, David MP, Yedwab GA, Kraicer PF. Follicular development during late human pregnancy. *Int J Fertil* 1977;22:24–29.
925. Dennefors BL, Nilsson L. Steroid production and responsiveness to gonadotropin and prostaglandins of human ovarian follicles at term pregnancy. *Fertil Steril* 1981;35:232–233.
926. Westergaard L, McNatty KP, Christensen IJ. Steroid concentrations in fluid from human ovarian antral follicles during pregnancy. *J Endocrinol* 1985;107:133–136.
927. Parlow AF, Daane TA, Dignam WJ. On the concentration of radioimmunoassayable FSH circulating in blood throughout human pregnancy. *J Clin Endocrinol* 1970;31:213–214.
928. Mishell DR Jr, Thorneycroft IH, Nagata Y, Nakamura RM. Steroid and gonadotropin levels in normal pregnancies and pregnancies following HMG therapy. In: Rosemberg E, ed. *Gonadotropin in Female Infertility.* Amsterdam: Excerpta Medica; 1973: 201–207.
929. Ranta T, Chen HC, Shimohigashi Y, Baukal AJ, Knecht M, Catt K. Enhanced follicle-stimulating hormone activity of deglycosylated human chorionic gonadotropin in ovarian granulosa cells. *Endocrinology* 1985;116:59–64.
930. Westergaard LG, Andersen CY, Byskov AG. Epidermal growth factor in small antral ovarian follicles of pregnant women. *J Endocrinol* 1990;127:363–367.
931. Chandrashekar V, Dierschke DJ, Wolf RC. Excessive ovarian follicular development in pregnant pigtailed macaques (*Macaca nemestrina*). *Am J Primatol* 1987;13:145–153.
932. Taya K, Greenwald GS. Mechanisms of suppression of ovarian follicular development during lactation in the rat. *Biol Reprod* 1982;27:1090–1101.
933. Taya K, Sasamoto S. Initiation of follicular maturation and ovulation after removal of the litter from the lactating rat. *J Endocrinol* 1980;87:393–400.
934. Taya K, Sasamoto S. Induced development of ovulatory follicles during the early stages of lactation by the administration of LH in the rat. *J Endocrinol* 1988;116:115–122.
935. Tsai-Morris CH, Ghosh M, Hirshfield AN, Wise PM, Brodie AMH. Inhibition of ovarian aromatase by prolactin in vivo. *Biol Reprod* 1983;29:342–346.
936. Selmanoff M, Selmanoff C. Role of pup age, estradiol 17-β and pituitary responsiveness in the differences in the suckling-induced prolactin response during early and late lactation. *Biol Reprod* 1983;29:400–411.
937. Bruce HM. Observations on the suckling stimulus and lactation in the rat. *J Reprod Fertil* 1961;2:17–34.
938. Gosden RG, Russell JA, Clarke J, Piper I. Effects of inhibiting prolactin secretion on the maintenance of embryonic diapause in the suckling rat. *J Endocrinol* 1981;88:197–203.
939. Hansen S, Sodersten P, Eneroth P. Mechanisms regulating hormone release and the duration of dioestrus in the lactating rat. *J Endocrinol* 1983;99:173–180.
940. Smith MS. Site of action of prolactin in the suppression of gonadotropin secretion during lactation in the rat: effect on pituitary responsiveness to LHRH. *Biol Reprod* 1981;24:967–976.
941. Reeves JJ, Tarnavsky GK, Platt T. Pituitary and ovarian luteinizing hormone releasing hormone receptors during the estrous cycle, pregnancy and lactation in the rat. *Biol Reprod* 1982; 27:316–319.
942. Smith MS. Effects of the intensity of the suckling stimulus and ovarian steroids on pituitary gonadotropin-releasing hormone receptors during lactation. *Biol Reprod* 1984;31:548–555.
943. Smith MS. Effect of pulsatile gonadotropin-releasing hormone on the release of luteinizing hormone and follicle-stimulating hormone in vitro by anterior pituitaries from lactating and cycling rats. *Endocrinology* 1982;110:882–890.
944. Taya K, Sasamoto S. Mechanisms responsible for suppression of FSH and LH during lactation in the rat. *J Endocrinol* 1991;129:119–130.
945. Greenwald GS. A histological study of the reproductive tract of the lactating mouse. *J Endocrinol* 1958;17:17–23.
946. Greenwald GS. Histologic transformation of the ovary of the lactating hamster. *Endocrinology* 1965;77:641–650.
947. Bridges RS, Goldman BD. Diurnal rhythms in gonadotropins and progesterone in lactating and photoperiod induced acyclic hamsters. *Biol Reprod* 1975;13:617–622.
948. Garcia-Winder M, Imakawa K, Day ML, Zalesky DD, Kittok RJ, Kinder JE. Effect of suckling and ovariectomy on the control of luteinizing hormone secretion during the postpartum period in beef cows. *Biol Reprod* 1984;31:771–778.
949. Bellin ME, Hinshelwood MM, Hauser ER, Ax RL. Influence of suckling and side of corpus luteum or pregnancy on folliculogenesis in postpartum cows. *Biol Reprod* 1984;31:849–855.
950. Dufour JJ, Roy GL. Distribution of ovarian follicular populations in the dairy cow within 35 days after parturition. *J Reprod Fertil* 1985;73:229–235.
951. Walters DL, Kaltenbach CC, Dunn TG, Short RE. Pituitary and ovarian function in postpartum beef cows. I. Effect of suckling on serum and follicular fluid hormones and follicular gonadotropin receptors. *Biol Reprod* 1982;26:640–646.
952. Walters DL, Short RE, Convey EM, Staigmiller RB, Dunn TG, Kaltenbach CC. Pituitary and ovarian function in postpartum beef cows. II. Endocrine changes prior to ovulation in suckled and nonsuckled postpartum cows compared to cycling cows. *Biol Reprod* 1982;26:647–654.
953. Williams GL, Talavera F, Petersen BJ, Kirsch JD, Tilton JE. Coincident secretion of follicle-stimulating hormone and luteinizing hormone in early postpartum beef cows: effects of suckling and low-level increases of systemic progesterone. *Biol Reprod* 1983;29:362–373.
954. Peters AR, Pimentel MG, Lamming GE. Hormone responses to exogenous GnRH pulses in post-partum dairy cows. *J Reprod Fertil* 1985;75:557–565.
955. Webb R, Lamming GE, Haynes NB, Foxcroft GR. Plasma progesterone and gonadotrophin concentrations and ovarian activity in post-partum dairy cows. *J Reprod Fertil* 1980;59:133–143.
956. Williams GL. Suckling as a regulator of postpartum rebreeding in cattle: a review. *J Anim Sci* 1990;68:831–852.
957. Walters DL, Short RE, Convey EM, Staigmiller RB, Dunn TG, Kaltenbach CC. Pituitary and ovarian function in postpartum beef cows. III. Induction of estrus, ovulation and luteal function with intermittent small-dose injections of GnRH. *Biol Reprod* 1982;26:655–662.

958. Murphy MG, Boland MP, Roche JF. Pattern of follicular growth and resumption of ovarian activity in post-partum beef suckler cows. *J Reprod Fertil* 1990;90:523–533.
959. Taylor C, Rajamahendran R. Follicular dynamics, corpus luteum growth and regression in lactating dairy cattle. *Can J Anim Sci* 1991;71:61–68.
960. Schirar A, Levasseur MC. Resumption of ovarian activity in post-partum ewes: carry-over effect of the corpus luteum of pregnancy. *Anim Reprod Sci* 1989;19:91–97.
961. Britt JH, Armstrong JD, Cox NM, Esbenshade KL. Control of follicular development during and after lactation in sows. *J Reprod Fertil* 1985;33(Suppl):37–54.
962. Kunavongkrit A, Einarsson S, Settergren I. Follicular development in primiparous lactating sows. *Anim Reprod Sci* 1982;5:47–56.
963. Cox NM, Britt JH. Relationships between endogenous gonadotropin-releasing hormone, gonadotropins, and follicular development after weaning in sows. *Biol Reprod* 1982;27:70–78.
964. Edwards S, Foxcroft GR. Endocrine changes in sows weaned at two stages of lactation. *J Reprod Fertil* 1983;67:161–172.
965. Martin MJ, Redmer DA, Ford JJ, Christenson RK, Day BN. Ovarian compensatory hypertrophy following unilateral ovariectomy in the suckled sow. *J Anim Sci* 1986;63:572–578.
966. Stevenson JS, Cox NM, Britt JH. Role of the ovary in controlling luteinizing hormone, follicle-stimulating hormone, and prolactin secretion during and after lactation in pigs. *Biol Reprod* 1981;24:341–353.
967. Shaw HJ, Foxcroft GR. Relationships between LH, FSH and prolactin secretion and reproductive activity in the weaned sow. *J Reprod Fertil* 1985;75:17–28.
968. Cox NM, Britt JH. Pulsatile administration of gonadotropin releasing hormone to lactating sows: endocrine changes associated with induction of fertile estrus. *Biol Reprod* 1982;27:1126–1137.
969. Cox NM, Armstrong JD, Britt JH. Influence of follicular ablation during lactation on postweaning interval to estrus, ovulation rate, and endocrine function in sows. *Domestic Anim Endocrinol* 1987;4:87–93.
970. Plant TM, Schallenberger E, Hess DL, McCormack JT, Dufy-Barbe L, Knobil E. Influence of suckling on gonadotropin secretion in the female rhesus monkey (*Macaca mulatta*). *Biol Reprod* 1980;23:760–766.
971. Weiss G, Butler WR, Dierschke DJ, Knobil E. Influence of suckling on gonadotropin secretion in the postpartum rhesus monkey. *Proc Soc Exp Biol Med* 1976;153:330–331.
972. Williams RF, Hodgen GD. Reinitiation of the diurnal rhythm of prolactin secretion in postpartum rhesus monkeys. *Biol Reprod* 1980;23:276–280.
973. Richardson DW, Goldsmith LT, Pohl CR, Schallenberger E, Knobil E. The role of prolactin in the regulation of the primate corpus luteum. *J Clin Endocrinol Metab* 1985;60:501–504.
974. Maeda K-I, Tsukamura H, Ohkura S, Kanaizuka T, Suzuki J. Suppression of ovarian activity during the breeding season in suckling Japanese monkey (*Macaca fuscata*). *J Reprod Fertil* 1991;92:371–375.
975. Thomson AM, Hytten FE, Black AE. Lactation and reproduction. *Bull WHO* 1975;52:337–349.
976. Howie PW, McNeilly AS. Effect of breast-feeding patterns on human birth intervals. *J Reprod Fertil* 1982;65:545–557.
977. Jeppsson S, Rannevik G, Thorell JI, Wide L. Influence of LH/FSH releasing hormone (LRH) on the basal secretion of gonadotrophins in relation to plasma levels of oestradiol, progesterone and prolactin during the post-partum period in lactating and in non-lactating women. *Acta Endocrinol* 1977;84:713–728.
978. Baird DT, McNeilly AS, Sawers RS, Sharpe RM. Failure of estrogen-induced discharge of luteinizing hormone in lactating women. *J Clin Endocrinol Metab* 1979;49:500–506.
979. Keye WR Jr, Jaffe RB. Changing patterns of FSH and LH response to gonadotropin-releasing hormone in the puerperium. *J Clin Endocrinol Metab* 1976;42:1133–1138.
980. McNeilly AS. Prolactin and the control of gonadotrophin secretion in the female. *J Reprod Fertil* 1980;58:537–549.
981. McNeilly AS, Glasier A, Jonassen J, Howie PW. Evidence for direct inhibition of ovarian function by prolactin. *J Reprod Fertil* 1982;65:559–569.
982. Whisnant CS, Kiser TE, Thompson FN, Barb CR. Opioid inhibition of luteinizing hormone secretion during the postpartum period in suckled beef cows. *J Anim Sci* 1986;63:1445–1448.
983. Malven PV, Stanisiewski EP, Haglof SA. Ovine brain areas sensitive to naloxone-induced stimulation of luteinizing hormone release. *Neuroendocrinology* 1990;52:373–381.
984. Weesner GD, Malven PV. Intracerebral immunoneutralization of beta-endorphin and met-enkephalin disinhibits release of pituitary luteinizing hormone in sheep. *Neuroendocrinology* 1990;52:382–388.
985. Leshin LS, Rund LA, Crim JW, Kiser TE. Immunocytochemical localization of luteinizing hormone-releasing hormone and proopiomelanocortin neurons within the preoptic area and hypothalamus of the bovine brain. *Biol Reprod* 1988;39:963–975.
986. Bohler HCL Jr, Tracer H, Merriam GR, Petersen SL. Changes in proopiomelanocortin messenger ribonucleic acid levels in the rostral periarcuate region of the female rat during the estrous cycle. *Endocrinology* 1991;128:1265–1269.
987. Pencharz RI. Effects of estrogens and androgens alone and in combination with chorionic gonadotropin on the ovary of the hypophysectomized rats. *Science* 1940;91:554–555.
988. Williams PC. Effects of stilbestrol on the ovaries of hypophysectomized rats. *Nature* 1940;145:388–389.

The Physiology of Reproduction, Second Edition,
edited by E. Knobil and J.D. Neill,
Raven Press, Ltd., New York © 1994.

CHAPTER 13

Ovulation

Lawrence L. Espey[1] and Harry Lipner[2]

Mammalian ovulation is a distinct biologic phenomenon that requires the rupture of healthy tissue at the surface of the ovary. In most mammals, the whole follicle protrudes markedly from the ovarian surface at the time of ovulation, and in many instances, a thin translucent stigma, the macula pellucida, forms at the apex of the follicle as the final sign of impending rupture. This unique morphologic change has left a striking impression on those who have actually observed it. Kelly (1) was so fascinated while observing a rabbit follicle near rupture that he stated, "As tension within the follicle increases, the transparent portion around the pole begins to bulge. . . . It now stands out like the nipple on a breast." The moment of rupture sometimes appears as an explosive event, leading observers to compare it to a "volcano erupting" (2) or a "blister that bursts" (3).

Some years ago, Walton and Hammond (4) provided a detailed account of the macroscopic changes that can be observed in a laboratory animal such as the rabbit. The changes that take place in the tissue at the site of rupture are pathophysiologic in that they involve a fracture in the dense layers of collagenous tissue that encapsulates the follicle, and there is invariable hemorrhage in the vicinity of this ovarian lesion. However, the structural modifications are not limited only to the apically protruding stigma of the follicle. There is ample evidence that the ovulatory surge in gonadotropic hormones transforms the entire ovarian follicle into a highly secretory corpus luteum. In fact, there is reason to believe that the primary action of the gonadotropins is luteinization and that rupture of the follicular surface is somewhat of a fortuitous event that is contingent on the local softening of tissues and proliferation of fibroblasts that occur during the early stages of remodeling of the ovarian follicle into a corpus luteum (5).

This chapter provides a chronologic account of the basic research on ovulation up to the 1970s, and then it concentrates on the information that has accumulated during the past several decades on the biochemical events of ovulation. The contents are not intended to be all-inclusive. For example, this chapter does not cover as many details about ovarian innervation and vascularity as the chapter on ovulation in the previous edition of these volumes (6).

Innumerable reviews on different aspects of ovulation have been written during the past 60 years. Some of these reviews are listed in this paragraph, whereas others are identified at more appropriate sites in this chapter. In 1932, Hartman (7) wrote the first comprehensive review of the work on ovulation, and his account provides many interesting insights into the early history of this

[1]Department of Biology, Trinity University, San Antonio, Texas 78212
[2]Department of Biological Sciences, Florida State University, Tallahassee, Florida 32306

subject. Also, there are several other reviews of the earlier work on ovulation (3,8–18). In more recent times, there has been an exponential growth in the number of studies on ovulation. Much of this more recent work has been described in detail in innumerable reviews that have appeared in the past 15 years. These include reviews of a comprehensive nature (19–26) on ovarian follicular development and ovulation (27,28) on the structure and morphology of follicles (29–32), on the biochemistry of ovulation (33–36), on ovarian smooth muscle (37), on applications of the ovarian perfusion model (38), on ovulation and the immune system (39,40), on the molecular aspects of ovulation (41–43), on signal transduction processes in ovulation (44), on ovulation as an inflammatory process (45,46), and on ovulation in relation to the menstrual cycle (47,48).

An initial note on terminology is also in order. It is common to use the expressions *preovulatory, ovulatory,* and *ovulation* all in reference to the entire gonadotropin-induced process. However, in this chapter, the adjective *ovulatory* will be applied to the entire process, whereas the term *preovulatory* will be used in reference to mature follicles that have not yet been stimulated to enter the ovulatory process. The term *ovulation* may indicate either the process or the moment of egg release, but in instances where clear delineation of the latter phenomenon is important, the term *follicular rupture* will be used for clarity.

HISTORICAL BACKGROUND

In the beginning, ovulation was studied mainly *in vivo,* simply with the naked eye. Observations of the follicular contents "oozing" or "bursting" from the ovary made a strong impression on the early investigators who managed to catch a glimpse of the phenomenon. The initial theories about the mechanism of ovulation keyed on the possible role of smooth muscle and the potential for such tissue to create intrafollicular pressures of sufficient magnitude to cause healthy follicular tissue to rupture. When light microscopy was first applied to studies of the microanatomy of visceral organs, the pioneering anatomists labeled much of the cellular component of the follicle as smooth-muscle tissue. However, it is now clear that most of this tissue in and around mature ovarian follicles is collagenous connective tissue, which has arisen from resident fibroblasts. Nevertheless, the first 100 years of investigation into the mechanism of ovulation centered on the smooth-muscle and the pressure theories. Therefore, the segments of this chapter that deal with the history of ovulation key on these two early theories and how they eventually gave way to the so-called enzyme theory of ovulation.

Early Years

Ovarian follicles were first identified in 1672, when de Graaf examined human ovaries and observed vesicles on their surface, which he mistakenly referred to as ova (49). More than a century later, Cruikshank (50) discovered ova in the fallopian tubes of rabbits, and eventually von Baer (28) realized that the mammalian oocyte was quite unlike the large avian and amphibian eggs but instead was a relatively small cell within the follicular mass (Figs. 1 and 2).

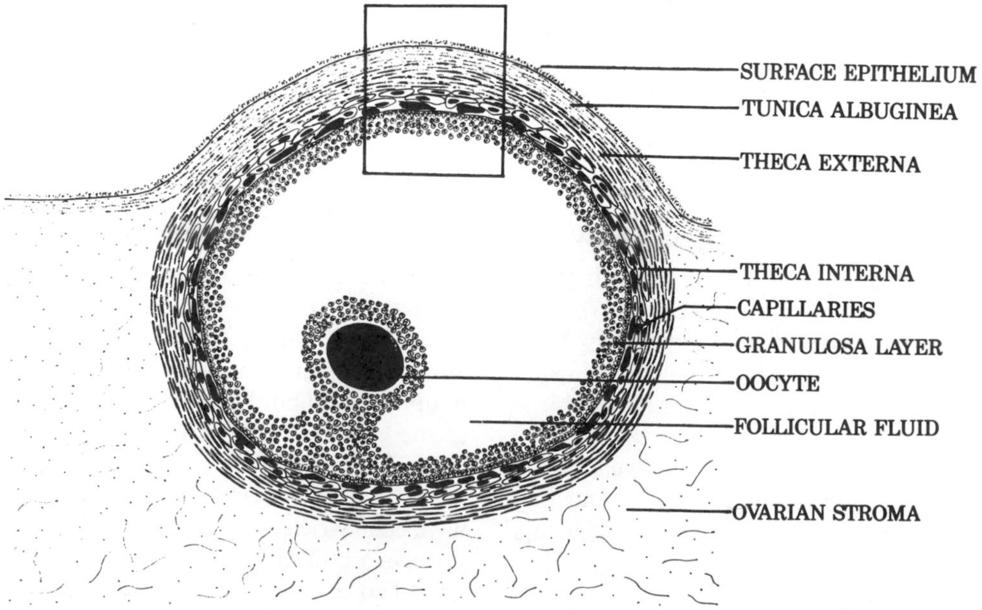

FIG. 1. Structural organization of a mature ovarian follicle from the rabbit. (From reference 5, with permission.)

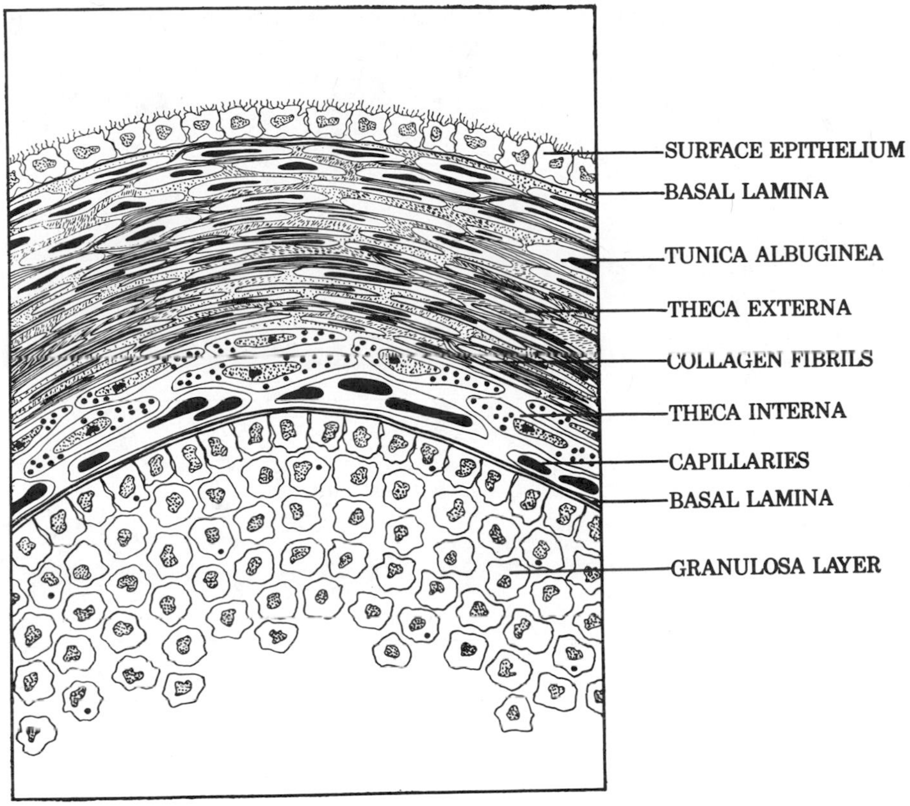

FIG. 2. Close-up view of the components of the follicle wall of a rabbit. (From reference 5, with permission.)

In the middle of the nineteenth century, von Kolliker (51) was the first to mention that smooth muscle was a structural constituent of the ovary. In 1858, Rouget (52) suggested that ovarian smooth-muscle activity impaired venous return and caused congestion and "erection" of ovulatory follicles in a manner that increased intrafollicular pressure and caused rupture. That same year, von Luschka (53) concluded that the follicular fluid was derived primarily from secretions of the granulosa cells and secondarily from fluids transported to them from the blood vessels of the theca interna. A year later, Pfluger (54) observed the motion of frog ovaries and concluded that the "peristalsis" that they exhibited was responsible for ovulation, but he was apparently unaware of the fact that the amphibian ovary is in a state of constant movement even out of the sexual season (11). Two years later, Aeby (55) used acetic and nitric acid staining techniques to identify what he considered to be smooth-muscle cells in the theca externa of avian and mammalian follicles, and he suggested that similar cells were responsible for the "peristaltic" contractions of the frog ovarian stroma. Several years later, Grohe (56) described the course of the muscle fibers in the ovary of the pig, and his observations led him to support the idea that congestion from impaired venous return caused rupture of mature follicles. In 1870, Waldeyer (57) agreed with Luschka's view of fluid formation, and he went on to hypothesize that a rapid hypertrophy of the theca interna increased intrafollicular pressure and caused rupture. There was little additional work on ovulation for the remainder of the nineteenth century, but the "smooth-muscle" and "pressure" theories of ovulation were already firmly established by that time.

Smooth-Muscle Theory

First Quarter of This Century

The smooth-muscle theory of ovulation has been one of the most controversial issues in the field of reproductive physiology. The controversy has been perpetuated mainly by persistent reports that the dominant cell type in the theca externa layer of the follicle wall is a typical smooth-muscle cell. At the beginning of the present century, von Winiwarter and Sainmont (58) demonstrated what they called smooth muscle in the wall of the cat and human follicle, even though they were unable to demonstrate that either electrical or chemical stimuli could cause the follicle to rupture. In 1919, Thomson (59) carried out extensive histological studies and concluded that muscular contractions on an engorged follicle naturally increases the intrafollicular pressure and causes the follicle to rupture. In contrast, Corner (60) reported that

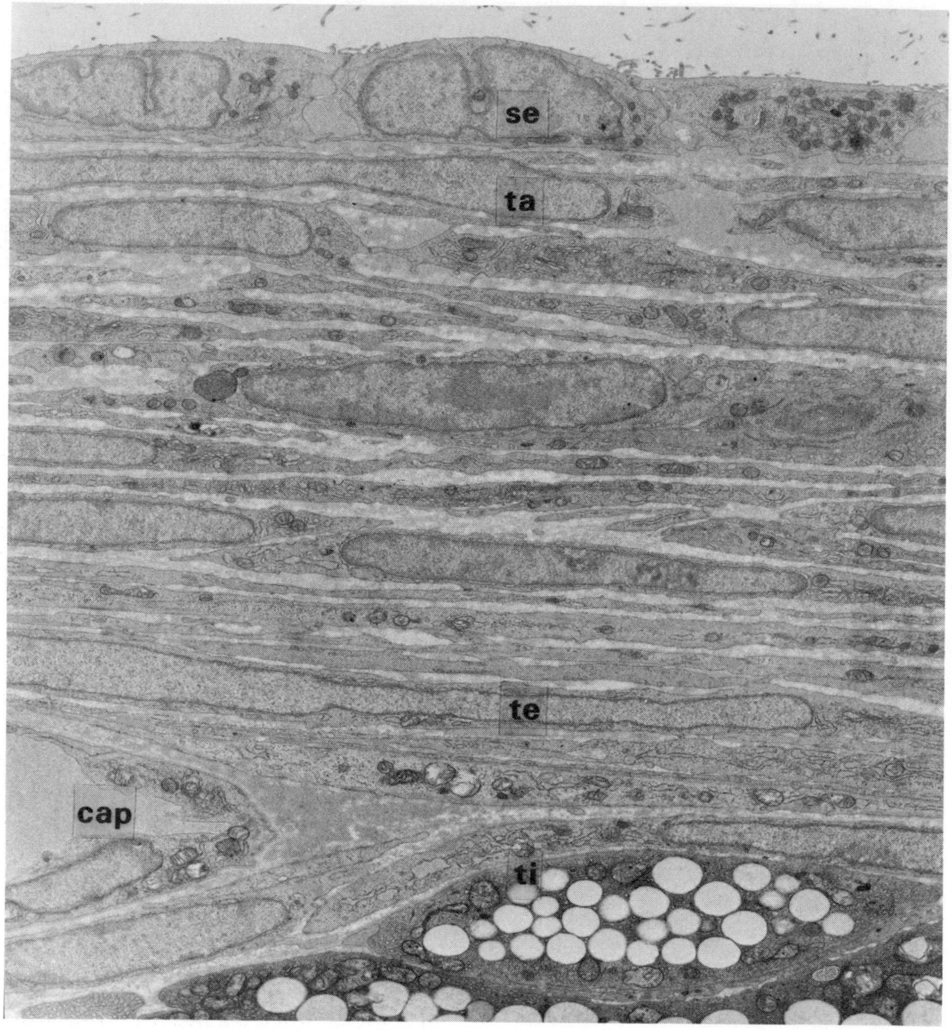

FIG. 3. A cross-sectional view of the thecal tissue between the surface epithelium (*se*) and theca interna (*ti*) at the apex of a mature rat follicle. Collagen fibers are relatively inconspicuous in the tunica albuginea (*ta*) and theca externa (*te*) of this section which has been fixed with glutaraldehyde and stained with Reynolds' lead citrate. A capillary (*cap*) is present in the region of the theca interna. (From reference 150, with permission.)

same year his findings from an extensive study of the histology of the granulosa and thecal layers, and he concluded that the theca externa consisted of collagenous fibrils and long spindle-shaped "fibroblasts" that became mitotic just before rupture (Fig. 3). Two years later, Guttmacher and Guttmacher (61) again reported histological evidence of thecal smooth muscle in the sow follicle, and they claimed that strips of these follicles contracted in response to solutions of HCl, barium chloride, and physostigmine sulfate. However, they also noted after 72 injections of ovarian and uterine arteries with saline that "even though one braced himself against a wall and pushed the piston of the injection syringe with all the physical strength available," rupture did not occur in a single instance, although one could see the follicular vessels wash out clearly. In the end, they admitted that their experiments were so inconsistent that they were unable to conclude that muscle tissue had a role in the rupture of a follicle.

Middle of This Century

More than a quarter of a century later, in 1947, Kraus (9) conducted an extensive study of ovulation in frogs, hens, and rabbits and found that attempts to induce contractility and ovulation with smooth-muscle stimulants or electrical impulses invariably failed. That same year, Claesson (62) attempted to resolve the smooth-muscle issue by examining cow, swine, rabbit, guinea pig, and rat ovaries under a polarization microscope. By this method, he failed to find the high intrinsic birefringence that is characteristic of muscle but instead found birefringence that is typical of connective tissue. The reliabil-

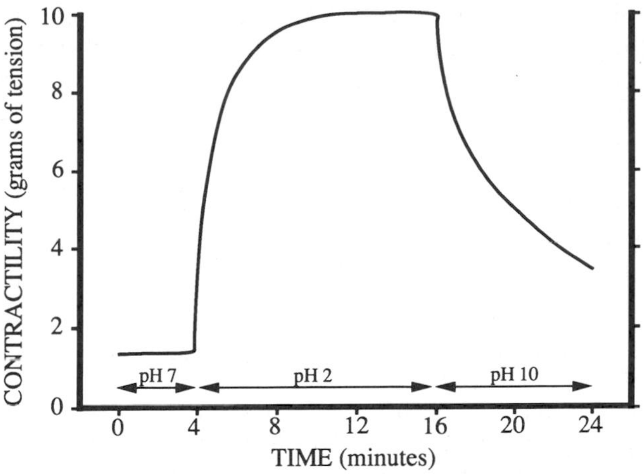

FIG. 4. Effect of pH on contractility of the follicle wall from a mature pig ovary. When the pH is lowered below pH 3.0, collagen fibers in the follicle wall undergo significant contraction. Increasing pH to the alkaline range promotes "relaxation" of the collagen fibers. (Adapted from reference 65.)

ity of the method negated virtually all previous histological evidence, including Claesson's own, of smooth muscle in the follicle wall and threw doubt on the reliability of any physiologic data. However, some years later, in 1960, Lipner and Maxwell (63) supported the smooth-muscle theory by demonstrating visible muscle-like contractions in the follicles of ovarian tissue autotransplanted into the anterior chamber of the rabbit's eye. However, several years later, Espey (12) attempted to duplicate the earlier experiments by the Guttmachers. He found that strips of sow follicles would contract only in response to HCl, that such contractions were tetanic in nature, that the tissue would relax only if it was exposed to alkaline solutions, and that such contractility could be attributed to collagen fibrils in the thecal layers of the follicle (Fig. 4). Three years later, Espey (64) used transmission electron microscopy to confirm the distribution of collagenous connective tissue and fibroblasts in the theca externa of the follicle, and he conducted further studies to verify that follicular collagen contracts when it is exposed to acidic solutions (65).

1970s Surge in Interest

The smooth-muscle controversy became more intense during the 1970s, when an avalanche of new reports claimed, on the basis of different kinds of evidence, that smooth-muscle activity is an integral part of the ovulatory process. The reader is referred to an earlier review for enumeration of these reports (37). In brief, this review concluded that typical smooth-muscle tissue is confined mainly to the hilar and medullary regions of the mammalian ovary. The many reports of myoid tissue in peri- and parafollicular areas are probably due to the overenthusiastic identification of "smooth-muscle" tissue primarily on the observation of cytoplasmic filaments in the cells of the theca interna, without realizing that such structures are also a normal component of thecal fibroblasts (66–68). At the time of ovulation and especially during luteinization, there may be some differentiation of these thecal fibroblasts into myofibroblasts to facilitate wound healing and the removal of granulation tissue during luteolysis, but there is no convincing evidence that such tissue has an essential role in the mechanism of ovulation (37).

After the Surge

Despite substantial evidence that ovarian contractions are not necessary for ovulation, there have been several more recent reports that continue to support the idea that smooth muscle is an important component in the mechanism of ovulation. Most of the effort to preserve the theory have come from Talbot, Martin, Schroeder, and collaborators (69–75), who continue to claim that there is a discrete layer of smooth-muscle cells at least in the basal hemisphere of the follicle and that such muscular tissue is necessary for extrusion of the oocyte. This lingering view is supported by further reports that myocytes are present in the follicles of many mammals (76), that such cells are syncytially linked by several types of surface junctions (77), that these cells contain actin fibrils characteristic of smooth-muscle cells (78), and that ovarian contractility and ovulation can be influenced by a wide range of agents that agonize and antagonize smooth-muscle contractions (71,79–82).

Also, Schroeder and Talbot (83) reported that intrafollicular pressure changes during preovulatory contractility in the follicle. However, two decades earlier, Espey and Lipner (84) pointed out that such rhythmic fluctuations in intrafollicular pressure are rare and are not essential for ovulation. More recently, Kobayashi et al. (85) have also shown that perfused rabbit ovaries can ovulate in the absence of ovarian smooth-muscle contractions, and Lofman et al. (86) have found that perfused rat ovaries can ovulate with no visible circumfollicular muscular activity.

Thus, there is still no convincing evidence that ovarian contractile activity is necessary for ovulation. Nevertheless, the existing data suggest that some kind of rhythmic motion is occasionally expressed by ovarian tissue near the time of ovulation, and the nature of this mechanical activity has not been adequately explained. Negligible attention has been given to the possibility that the rhythmic pulsations might be the consequence of vascular spasms in the blood vessels that enter the hilar region of the ovary (37). Also, it is possible that intraovarian pressure could fluctuate as a result of spasms in the tubo-uterine vasculature, because vessels of this origin anastomose with ovarian arteries (87). In considering this alternative explanation, it may be relevant to note that Markee (88) observed that the uterine vasculature sometimes undergoes rhythmic spasms at 15- to 20-sec intervals, depending on the "hormonal" conditions of the tissue. Therefore, it is possible that an agent like prostaglandin $F_{2\alpha}$, which is known to stimulate contraction of ovarian arterial smooth muscle (89) and which is known to increase markedly in the ovary during ovulation (33), may be promoting spasms in the ovarian vasculature near the time of ovulation.

Finally, it is worth mentioning that lutein follicles have been likened to granulation tissue (44,45). A granuloma is a firm nodular mass that forms in conjunction with angiogenesis and fibroplasia that develops during the wound healing process in injured and inflamed tissues (90–93). Such granulation tissue usually contains myofibroblasts that contract and relax in a similar way to smooth muscle cells (94). If this information is considered in conjunction with earlier ovarian studies that suggest that corpora lutea in particular may contain well-defined coats of smooth muscle (95), it is also possible that some of the reported ovarian contractility may be associated with myofibroblasts within luteinized, unruptured follicles. Thus, certain aspects of the smooth-muscle theory may deserve further investigation.

Summary

In summary, there are still differing opinions about the extent to which smooth-muscle cells are distributed in and around mammalian follicles. Some investigators continue to believe that the theca externa consists of typical smooth-muscle cells, whereas others report that the theca externa is predominantly a matrix of collagenous connective tissue with typical fibroblasts making up the cellular component. In any event, it is now rather clear that ovarian contractility is not a necessary feature of the ovulatory process. Still, there remains the possibility that some of the fibroblasts begin to differentiate into myofibroblasts as a ruptured follicle transforms into a corpus luteum, and the potential role of such myoid tissue in luteinization, or luteolysis, may deserve further investigation.

Pressure Theory

Superficial Observations

At the beginning of this century, additional attention was given to the hypothesis that an increase in intrafollicular pressure might be responsible for rupture of a mature ovarian follicle. Heape (96) stressed the role of increasing pressure as the cause of ovulation, and he believed that vasodilation and bursting blood vessels contributed to the ovulatory pressure. However, Schochet (97) did not think the follicular circulation could be responsible for intrafollicular pressure because he noted that follicle pressure probably was greater than the blood pressure within the capillaries because the capillaries appeared to be compressed by the antral pressure. However, Wester (98) suggested that some kind of pressure "necrosis" of the follicular wall was the final cause of rupture. However, the Guttmacher twins (61) subjected sow follicles to unusually high pressures of 300 to 350 mm Hg for hours without inducing ovulation, and the negative results of this test do not support a role for pressure in the mechanism of ovulation.

The impressive studies of rabbit ovulation in 1928 by Walton and Hammond (4) emphasized that the first sign of approaching ovulation is the gradual formation of the stigma (i.e., the macula pellucida) at the apex of a follicle. They reported that the whole follicle protrudes more markedly from the ovarian surface, and then the stigma suddenly "blows out as a pimple" in a manner that suggested an increase in internal pressure. The small blood vessels at the base of the stigma were seen to rupture before the stigma broke open, and they noted some extravasation of blood into the follicular antrum near the time of follicular rupture. They concluded that the process was comparable to "the formation and rupture of a boil" and that an increase in internal pressure was probably of primary importance in causing rupture. These observations were supported 3 years later by Kelly (1). Several years after that report, Hill et al. (2) made the first movies of ovulation, using the rabbit as their subject. These investigators emphasized that follicular rupture "is truly an explosive phenomenon." Likewise, in sheep, McKenzie and Terrill (99) reported that in some cases rupture occurred with "a decided spurt." They also noticed that the apical-most area of a follicle usually became very clear and transparent about an hour before rupture and that one or more small cones about 1 to 3 mm high ballooned out from this clear area a few minutes before rupture. In comparison, 10 years later, Kraus (9) reported that injections of pressurized saline into rabbit follicles could promote rupture but without stigma formation. Furthermore, she noticed that in such cases of artificial induction of ovulation the edge of the rupture site was fine and smooth, whereas in normal ovulation, the rupture point was circular and the edge of the follicle opening was blunt and rough. Also, unlike previous observers, Kraus (9) only saw the follicular fluid "ooze" from the rupture site instead of spurt out. In view of these characteristics, she concluded that the pressure theory was unable to explain the observable morphologic changes. Similarly, Hartman (7) pointed out that follicles of pigs, cattle, and sheep become flabby a few hours before ovulation, and this fact does not favor the idea of an increase in intrafollicular pressure.

Osmotic Pressure Hypothesis

Another version of the pressure theory was based on the idea that osmotic pressure might increase in ovarian follicles near the time of ovulation. While performing the Friedman pregnancy test on rabbits, Smith (100) became interested in what caused the tiny ovarian "blebs to swell up and burst within the course of a few hours." On measuring the total osmotic pressure of rabbit follicular fluid, he found a moderately higher osmolarity in ovulatory follicles when compared with unstimulated follicles. In a subsequent study, Smith and Ketteringham (101) speculated that so-called Call and Exner bodies of the granulosa layer of the follicle contained a glycogenlike substance that depolymerized near the time of ovulation and "contributed something to the follicle fluid which increases its osmotic tension so that it takes up fluid from the surrounding tissue and so increases the content of the follicle until it reaches the bursting point." Twenty years later, Zachariae and Jensen (102,103) advanced the osmosis hypothesis by reporting that preovulatory hyaluronidase activity depolymerized the acid mucopolysaccharides of the follicular fluid, "resulting in an increase in the intrafollicular colloid-osmotic pressure, increased volume, and follicular rupture." However, the presence of a follicular mucopolysaccharidase was never confirmed, and this theory of ovulation has faded.

Hydrostatic Pressure Measurements

Eventually, as technologies improved, Espey and Lipner (84) used an ultrasensitive Statham pressure transducer to measure the hydrostatic pressure within the follicular antrum during ovulation. Continuous

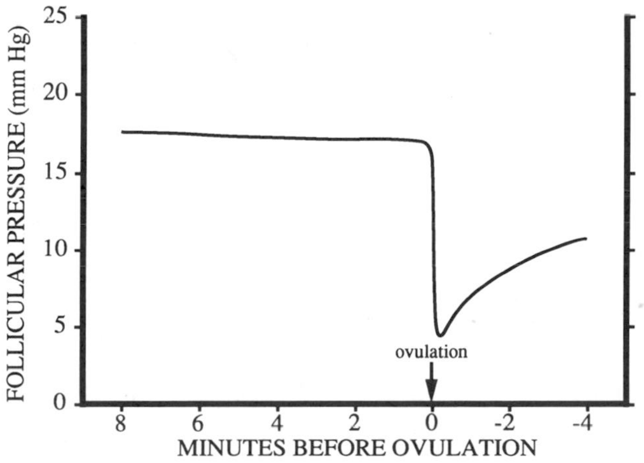

FIG. 5. Follicular pressure during ovulation in the rabbit. The moment of follicular rupture was confirmed by observation with a dissecting microscope. Intrafollicular hydrostatic pressure increases after rupture, as a blood clot forms at the apex of the follicle. (Adapted from reference 84.)

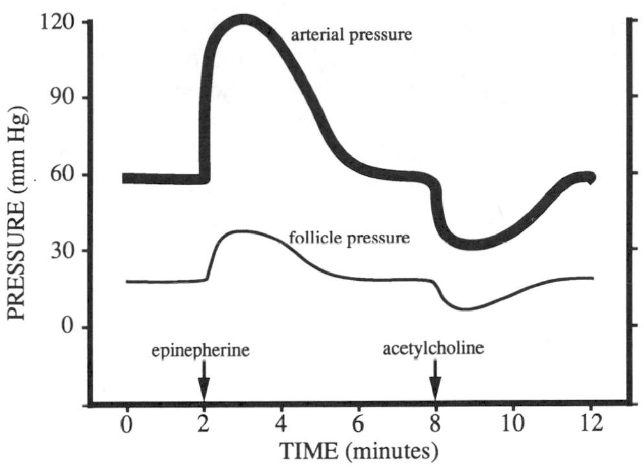

FIG. 6. Relationship of follicular pressure to systemic blood pressure. Alteration of carotid pressure by injections of epinephrine or acetylcholine resulted in a concomitant change in intrafollicular pressure. (Adapted from reference 84.)

monitoring clearly demonstrated that there is no increase in intrafollicular pressure during the hours preceding rupture and that the existing steady pressure of 15 to 20 mm Hg is directly dependent on the mean hydrostatic pressure of the ovarian arterial supply (Figs. 5 and 6). Concomitant with this study, Blandau and Rumery (104) adapted a water manometer to make static pressure measurements in the antra of rat follicles at different stages of development, and they found that the intrafollicular pressure remained within the range of capillary blood pressure during the ovulatory process. The results of these two experiments, which demonstrated a constant intrafollicular pressure, were confirmed a year later by a similar study conducted by Rondell (105). Some 15 years later, Bronson et al. (106) also could not detect any increase in pressure in pig follicles as the time of ovulation approached. Thus, it has been firmly established that follicular rupture is not caused by an increase in intrafollicular pressure.

Summary

In summary, intrafollicular pressure does not increase during ovulation but remains at a relatively constant 15 to 20 mm Hg that is dependent on the hydrostatic pressure in the extensive capillary network of the theca interna. This moderate pressure probably exerts a constant force on the follicle wall and may be an important factor in the ballooning of the stigma in a morphologically weaker area of the follicular apex. Also, the question of whether the moment of rupture is explosive or passive may have arisen from the fact that the superficial appearance of the phenomenon probably depends on the extent to which the arterial supply has been impaired during surgical exposure of the ovaries for visual observation during ovulation. If blood flow is reduced, intrafollicular pressure would be low and the contents of the follicle would ooze from the stigma area; whereas if the vascular supply is of normal patency, the moderate intrafollicular pressure may be of sufficient force to cause a weakening follicle wall to rupture under what appears to be a relatively strong head of pressure.

Proteolytic Enzyme Theory

Earlier Studies

As it gradually became apparent that neither the smooth-muscle theory nor the pressure theory adequately explained the mechanical events leading to ovulation, more and more attention was given to the possibility that the morphologic changes that occur at the apex of an ovulatory follicle might be the result of enzymic degradation of the thecal connective tissue. Descriptions of the disappearance of thecal tissue at the stigma and of the erosion of the rupture point by early investigators such as Long and Evans (107) made it clear that ovulation was not the consequence of any violent tearing of the follicular wall. In view of this kind of information, Irving Hardesty suggested to Schochet (97) that the liquor folliculi might "exert some special digestive action on the resisting tissues" of the follicle wall. With this idea in mind, Schochet collected follicular fluid randomly from large sow follicles and conducted several crude chemical tests that led him to conclude that the fluid was indeed the source of "a proteolytic ferment or enzyme" that contributes "to the digestion of the theca folliculi." Although his experiment has never been confirmed and although it is doubtful that the follicular fluid is the source of the proteases that degrade the follicle wall, Schochet is usually given credit for the proteolytic enzyme theory of ovulation.

In testing the enzyme hypothesis, Rugh (108) found that the external application of solutions of pepsin and hydrochloric acid initiated follicular rupture in frogs. A year later, Markee and Hinsey (109) noticed that ovulatory rabbit follicles develop an avascular area surrounded by dilated vessels, suggesting that local morphologic changes were a prerequisite for stigma formation. At about the same time, McKenzie and Terrill (99) reported similar morphologic changes in the sheep, noting a thinner, more transparent area at the apex of ovulatory follicles. A decade later, Moricard and Gothie (110) revived Schochet's hypothesis with tenuous evidence that gonadotropins cause the secretion of a "diastase" (a term that means any kind of enzyme in French) having proteolytic activity that digests the different layers of the follicle wall and results in rupture. A year later, Kraus (9) confirmed the earlier report of Rugh by showing that immersion of frog ovaries in an acidic solution of pepsin caused erosion of the follicle wall, but the amphibian ova were not fully extruded. Furthermore, all her attempts to identify a proteolytic enzyme in frog follicles failed, and her applications of proteolytic enzymes to the follicles of hens and rabbits were without effect. As a result of these negative findings, Kraus concluded that neither the pressure nor the enzyme theory fit the facts and that the immediate cause of ovulation remained a mystery.

Initial Enzyme Assays

As different assays for proteolytic enzymes became available around the middle of this century, some investigators began attempting to identify specific enzymes in follicular tissue. One of the first major efforts was by Jung and Held (111), who evaluated proteolytic enzymes and alkaline and acid phosphatases in small, intermediate, and large follicles of the pig. All three enzymes were found in significantly greater concentrations in the small follicles, compared with the larger ones, and most of the activity was at pH 2.5 to 3.5. That same year, Jung and Kides (112) reported that human follicular fluid contained a significant amount of cathepsinlike activity at acid pH but no trypsin activity at neutral pH. In a subsequent report (113), these same investigators assayed for endopeptidase, leucine-aminopeptidase, and glycyl-glycyl-dipeptidase and found that all these ovarian proteases were more abundant in small follicles compared with large ripe follicles. They concluded that such activity must be dependent on follicle-stimulating hormone (FSH) rather than luteinizing hormone (LH) and that the role of these enzymes in ovulation was uncertain. At about this same time, Reichert (114) roughly estimated ovarian proteinase activity in rats by homogenizing and extracting the ovaries and then measuring the optical absorbance of the extracts at 280 nm. He found that ovaries at diestrus and estrus contained significantly more "protease" activity than ovaries of pregnant and pseudopregnant animals. However, this crude method did not demonstrate any increase in acid or alkaline proteolytic activity on the morning of estrus, when the assays were conducted on tissue that was taken closest to the time of ovulation. Lee and Malvin (115) detected similar acid protease activity in follicular homogenates of sows. However, Espey (116) reported that the pH of sow follicular fluid remains in the alkaline range during ovulation, and therefore it is doubtful that the acid proteases reported in the above studies have any significant role in ovulation.

Intrafollicular Injections of Proteases

Further support for the enzyme theory came from experiments in which Espey and Lipner (13) injected small quantities of concentrated enzyme preparations directly into the antrum of rabbit follicles and showed that such injections rapidly induced morphologic changes similar to normal swelling, stigma formation, and rupture of the follicles. In the initial studies, clostridiopeptidase-A (a bacterial collagenase), nagarse, and pronase (also microbial enzymes) were the most effective in inducing rupture. Later experiments revealed that injections of mammalian collagenase or trypsin could also induce rupture of rabbit follicles (unpublished observations).

Change in Follicular Distensibility

In 1964, Rondell (105) studied the elasticity of rabbit follicles by simultaneously inserting two micropipettes into follicles. One pipette was for injecting set quantities of saline, and the other pipette was for pressure measurements. By measuring the pressure increase after injection of a unit quantity of saline, he was able to demonstrate a substantial increase in the distensibility of rabbit follicles that were near rupture. He concluded that such a change in the physical characteristics of the follicle wall were an essential part of the mechanism of ovulation. Several years later, Espey (65) also measured the tensile strength of the wall of sow follicles and found that follicles close to rupture are more *labile* when subjected to physical stress. He also showed that treatment of preovulatory follicles with a solution of collagenase caused the follicle walls to dissociate when they were subjected to only slight tension. Several years later, Espey (116) further demonstrated that elastase, trypsin, a general protease extract, α-chymotrypsin, and to a lesser extent, β-chymotrypsin could also significantly reduce the tensile strength of the sow follicle. Thus, it became evident that the follicle wall becomes progressively weaker as the time of rupture approaches and that treatment of strips of the follicle wall with different preparations of proteolytic enzymes can mimic this preovulatory degradation of the follicular connective tissue.

Efforts to Measure Collagenase

In view of much of the above information, Espey and Rondell (117,118) attempted to measure collagenolytic activity in sow and rabbit follicles by using a synthetic peptide substrate. However, the results revealed a decrease in enzyme activity rather than an increase as the time of rupture approached. In a further effort to assay collagenolytic activity, Espey and Coons (18) cultured sections of rabbit follicles on gels composed of reconstituted collagen. Although the follicular tissue digested the collagen gels when incubated in either acid or alkaline media, the results did not clearly demonstrate any increase in this activity during the ovulatory process. The following year, Morales et al. (119) used a more specific synthetic substrate to identify collagenase activity in rat follicles. Several years later, Morales et al. (120) applied an assay based on the digestion of endogenous collagen to measure "true" collagenase in rat ovaries, but they were unable to detect any significant change in such activity during ovulation. Thus, the measurement of an increase in ovarian collagenolytic activity has been a rather elusive goal. This difficulty is not particularly surprising because it is well known that mammalian collagenases are quite difficult to assay (16,18). Several more recent attempts to detect ovarian collagenolytic activity are discussed later in this chapter in the section on chemical events of the ovulatory process.

Summary

In summary, it is firmly established that the collagenous layers of the theca externa and tunica albuginea at the apex of a follicle must be degraded before a follicle can rupture. Furthermore, it is apparent that this follicular connective tissue becomes flaccid and distensible near the time of ovulation. Several *in vivo* and *in vitro* studies have shown that a number of metalloproteinases and serine proteases can decompose the follicle wall, but it has been difficult to measure collagenolytic activity in the ovary during normal ovulation. Part of the reason for the elusive nature of this activity may be because mammalian collagenases are highly destructive enzymes that must be inactivated rapidly to confine the damage to a localized area.

FUNCTIONAL ANATOMY OF THE OVARIAN FOLLICLE

General Morphology

Earlier reviews containing information on the anatomy of ovarian follicles include those by Hartman (7) and Harrison (121). The first report that dealt specifically with the ultrastructure of ovulatory follicles was in 1967 by Espey (64). Several years later, Bjersing and Cajander (122–127) published a series of papers that contain a much more complete analysis of the ultrastructure of the ovarian follicle of the rabbit, and Parr (128) published a vivid description of the ovarian follicle of the rat. Additional reviews on the morphology of ovarian follicles have been published by Lipner (15), Mossman and Duke (129), Bjersing (29), and Espey (19) and more recently by Balboni (30), Guraya (31), Lipner (6), and Espey (32).

Ovarian follicles begin as primordial spheres consisting of a single layer of flattened epithelial cells that surround individual oocytes (121) (Fig. 7). These primordial follicles persist for years in the outer cortical layers of the ovary until they eventually are selected to

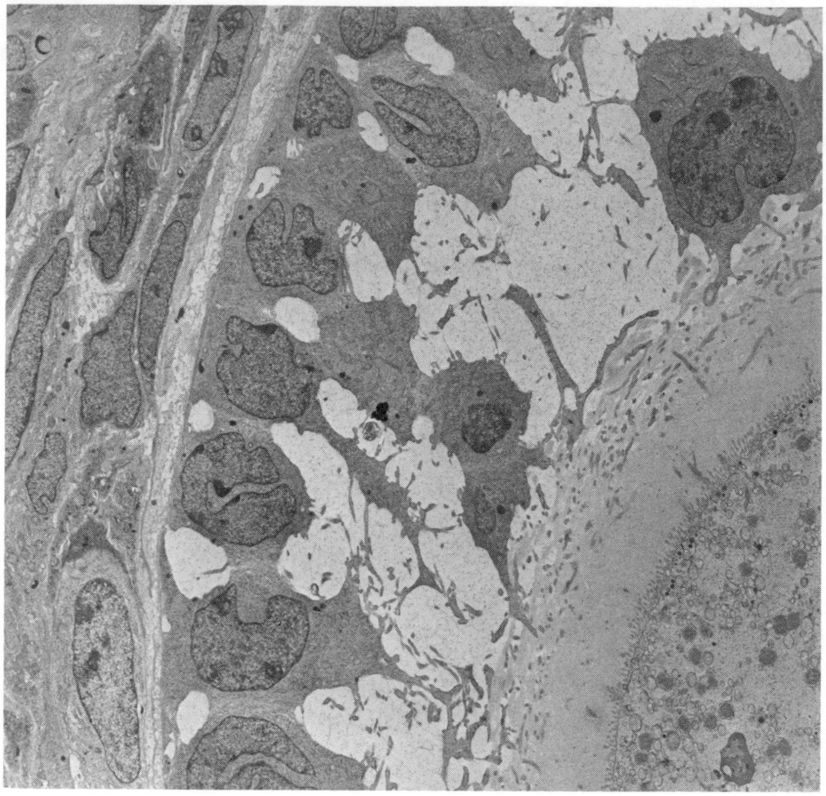

FIG. 7. A primordial follicle in a rabbit ovary. The oocyte and surrounding zona pellucida are located in the lower right corner of the photomicrograph. The layer of granulosa (follicular) cells is 1–2 cells deep. Fibroblasts in the loose connective tissue of the ovarian stroma have not yet differentiated into the secretory cells of the theca interna.

develop under the influence of gonadotropin stimulation. In the early stages of development, the granulosa cells increase in number and begin to form layers (130). Eventually, the granulosa cells promote the organization of a sheath of stromal fibroblasts that encapsulate the developing follicle and form the thecal layers around the follicle. As the follicle continues to grow, antral spaces begin to form within the sphere of granulosa cells, and these fluid-filled cavities eventually coalesce and expand into a single large cavity that makes the mature follicle appear like a blister on the surface of the ovary. In a given species of mammal, the size of a mature follicle is usually proportional to the body weight of the adult female.

The anatomy of rabbit follicles has been studied quite extensively, and most of the following description is based on the morphology of ovarian tissue in this species (Figs. 1 and 2). At the apex of a mature follicle, the outer portion of the follicle wall consists of a surface epithelium, which is a single layer of cuboidal or low columnar epithelial cells that adhere to the surface of a thin basal lamina. This epithelial covering around the ovary is probably a modified coelomic epithelium (i.e., a continuation of the peritoneum) (121). The tunica albuginea, which lies just inside the surface epithelium, is a layer of dense collagenous connective tissue that also surrounds the entire ovary. The theca externa is the distinct layer of collagenous connective tissue that delineates the follicle from the surrounding ovarian stroma. At the follicular apex where rupture normally occurs, these two connective tissue layers (i.e., the tunica albuginea and the theca externa) blend together in a fashion that makes it difficult to distinguish one from the other, except that the tunica layer has more extracellular collagen (64). The tensile strength of these two layers of collagenous connective tissue must be degraded for a follicle to rupture.

The theca interna is a thin layer of large oval cells that differentiate from thecal fibroblasts during follicular maturation (19). In some species, this layer is the principal site of estrogen synthesis during the final maturation of a follicle (131,132). One of the most prominent features of the theca interna is the extensive network of large capillaries that line the inner border of these steroid-secreting cells. These capillaries do not normally penetrate the basal lamina (i.e., the membrana propria) that separates the theca interna from the granulosa layer, which lines the inside of the follicle wall (19,29). The granulosa cells are relatively small polyhedral cells that are linked together by an elaborate system of gap junctions (133). The granulosa cells that lie closest to the theca interna are columnar in shape and appear to be firmly attached to the basal lamina, which separates these two layers of the follicle wall. The innermost granulosa cells are more cuboidal. At some point along the inner circumference of the follicle, clusters of granulosa cells project toward the center of the follicular antrum and form the cumulus oopherous, which contains the oocyte. This egg-bearing pedestal is surrounded by follicular fluid. The follicular fluid is a mixture of exudate from the granulosa tissue and transudate from the thecal blood supply (19,134). The same general morphology is characteristic of mature follicles in ovaries that have been perfused in an *in vitro* system (135).

Surface Epithelium

General Features

All mammalian ovaries are covered by a single layer of cuboidal cells that are loosely attached to a thin basal lamina at the surface of the connective tissue sheath (i.e., the tunica albuginea) that surrounds the ovary (19,32,136). In a cross-sectional view of the follicular apex, these cells contain large indented nuclei (64). Their cytoplasm has relatively small, yet conspicuous, mitochondria. However, the most striking feature of these cells is the dense cytoplasmic spheres of mucinlike material that often dominate the basal side of the cells (Fig. 8). A massive network of microvilli project from the peritoneal surface of this epithelial layer. The cells are held together at their lateral surfaces by zona occludens (64).

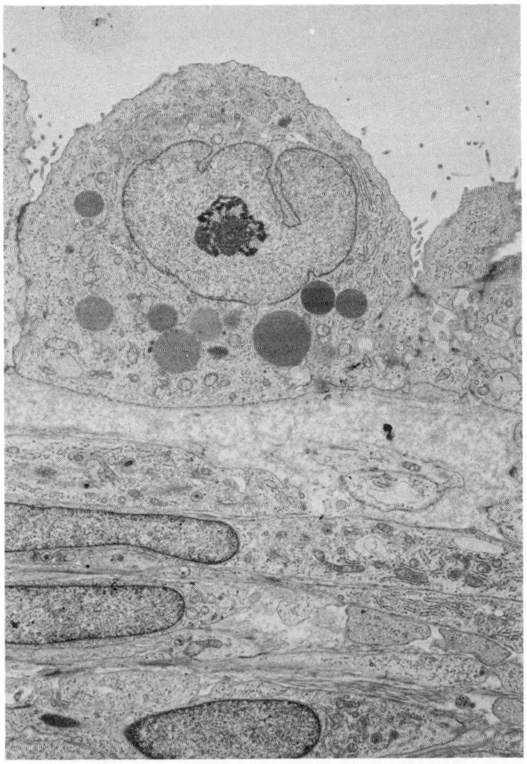

FIG. 8. Cross-sectional view of a surface epithelial cell at the apex of a mature rabbit follicle. Dense cytoplasmic granules are usually concentrated in the inner half of the cell. A prominent nucleolus is apparent in the nucleus of this cell. Note that fibroblasts are densely distributed within the underlying tunica albuginea. (From reference 152, with permission.)

Cytoplasmic Granules

In her studies on mice, Byskov (137) reported that the ovulatory degradation of the follicular apex starts at the outside and successively progresses to the interior of the follicle wall. Five years later, Bjersing and Cajander (122–124,138) reported a similar pattern of degradation in the ovulatory rabbit follicle and concluded that the surface epithelium is the source of hydrolytic enzymes that cause ovulation. In their series of papers on the surface epithelium, they described a rapid increase in the number and size of granules in the cells of the surface epithelium of rabbit follicles that had been induced to rupture. Furthermore, they concluded that many of these granules were lysosomes that released their enzymes toward the underlying tunica albuginea a few hours before follicular rupture. This hypothesis received indirect support from an earlier study by Rondell (14), who reported that collagenaselike activity exudes from the surface of follicles that are about to rupture.

This idea that cells of the surface epithelium contain massive lysosomes that extrude their proteolytic contents into the thecal layers of the follicle is intriguing, but the hypothesis has not been supported by other studies. Although the surface epithelium is intact in some follicles at the time of ovulation, more often this layer is no longer a constituent of the follicle wall at the site where rupture occurs (17,64,123,139,140). Also, if the surface epithelium is scraped from mature follicles, some of the follicles will still ovulate after stimulation by gonadotropin (141). Furthermore, contrary to the impression of Bjersing and Cajander (124), Rawson and Espey (141) carried out a quantitative study of the concentration of dense granules in the epithelial cells and found a twofold increase in these granules during the ovulatory process rather than a decrease. Also, Narimoto et al. (142) reported that the granules do not react like lysosomes when the follicular tissue is treated with Gomori's lead medium for acid phosphatase. Therefore, it is difficult to conclude that the surface epithelium has a significant role in the mechanism of ovulation. Nevertheless, future studies that might identify the chemical composition of the cytoplasmic granules in this layer could contribute significantly to the existing knowledge about the function of the surface epithelium.

Polymorphous Nuclei

As a matter of routine, almost every study of the ultrastructure of ovarian follicles has been conducted on tissues that have been oriented in a manner that shows a cross-sectional view of the follicle wall. Such orientation allows the investigator to see each of the follicle layers from the outer surface epithelium to the inner stratum granulosum. From such a "side" angle, the cells of the surface epithelium usually contain what appear to be large, somewhat notched, nuclei (19,64,124). However, if one orients the tissue so that *tangential* sections can be cut through the apex of ovulatory follicles, the nuclei of the epithelial cells appear to be multinucleate (32) (Fig. 9). In view of this characteristic, Espey (32) compared these cells to polymorphonuclear leukocytes and suggested that they might function as an outer defense mechanism to protect the vital procreative elements of the ovary from peritoneal microbes. Still, the precise function of the surface epithelium remains to be determined.

Scanning View of Follicular Apex

Transmission electron microscopy has revealed that the surface epithelial cells become grossly necrotic and tend to "slough off" when follicles are about to rupture (64) (Fig. 10). Later studies using scanning electron microscopy made it clear that the surface cells become detached from the stigma region of ovulatory follicles in the rabbit (123,140,143), rat (140,144), mouse (140,145), and hamster (145,146). Tsujimoto et al. (144) stated that the apical regions without surface epithelial cells display flattened and densely arranged fibroblasts of the tunica albuginea.

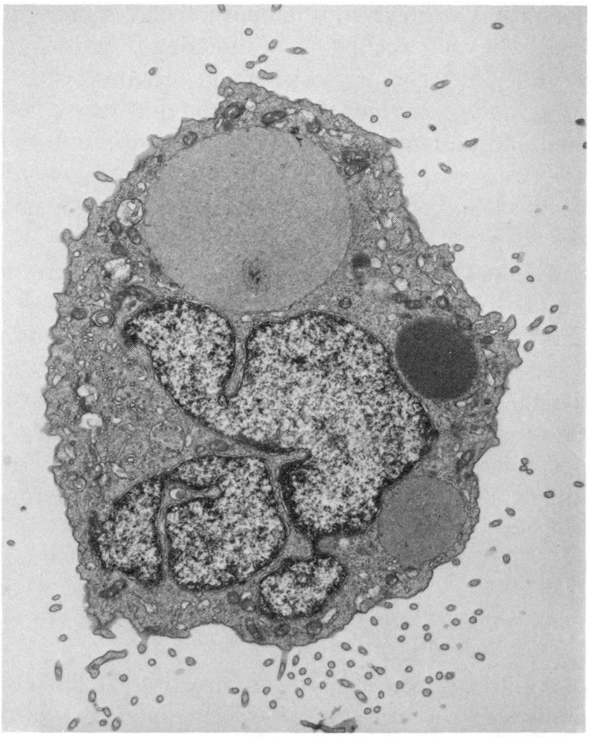

FIG. 9. Tangential view of a surface epithelial cell. When thin sections are made on a plane that is tangential to the apical surface of a follicle, the nuclei of the surface epithelial cells usually appear to be polymorphous.

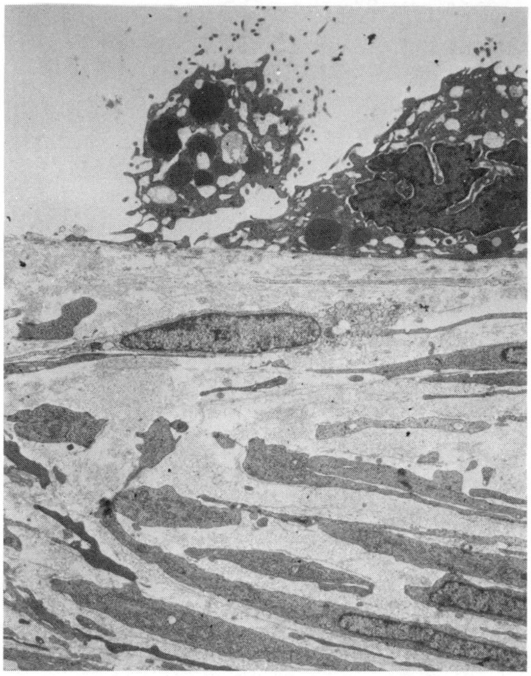

FIG. 10. Cross-sectional view of surface epithelial cells adjacent to a rabbit follicle that is within minutes of rupturing. Notice that the cells have become highly necrotic and are beginning to slough away from the follicular surface. The fibroblasts in the underlying tunica albuginea have dissociated and are now more sparsely distributed within this layer. (From reference 152, with permission.)

Tunica Albuginea

General Features

The tunica albuginea is a layer of dense collagenous connective tissue that surrounds the entire ovary (64,126). The outer border of this layer is delineated by the basal lamina that separates it from the cells of the surface epithelium. This layer consists almost exclusively of fibroblasts and an extracellular matrix of collagen fibers that are embedded in an amorphous matrix of ground substance (Fig. 8). In most mammals, the fibroblasts are about five to seven cells deep. These cells contain prominent oblong nuclei that have relatively smooth surfaces. Their cytoplasm is dominated by rough endoplasmic reticulum that is probably involved in the synthesis of tropocollagen. It appears that cytoplasmic processes are a common feature of the distal ends of these fibroblasts.

Collagen Matrix

At the site where rupture normally occurs at the apex of a follicle, the collagenous tissue of the tunica albuginea (and to a lesser extent, the theca externa) provides most of the strength of the follicle wall. Before hormonal stimulation of the ovulatory process, this dense connective tissue is quite tenacious. Such strength is to be expected, because individual collagen fibrils have a tensile strength estimated to be greater than that of cast iron (147). However, as Gross (148) pointed out three decades ago, the tenacity of a matrix of thecal connective tissue depends not only on the strength of the collagen fibrils but also on the mucopolysaccharide matrix that "cements" these fibrils into collagenous bundles. Therefore, it may not be necessary for the proteolytic enzymes that degrade the follicle wall to meet all the criteria of a "true collagenase" (i.e., they may not necessarily be enzymes that specifically hydrolyze the collagen fibrils). Instead, it is possible that less-specific serine proteases like plasminogen activator, kallikrein, or trypsinlike enzymes may digest the extracellular ground substance and allow the collagen fibrils to dissociate from one another under the force of a low, but constant, intrafollicular pressure (19,44).

In 1974, Parr (128) reported that rat follicles are exceptional in that they have no collagen at their apex where rupture normally occurs. This report implied that the term *thecal tissue* might be a misnomer in the rat follicle because, by definition, thecal tissue should contain fibrous collagen. Nevertheless, on the basis of his observations, Parr (17) concluded that collagenolytic activity may not be important in the mechanism of ovulation because collagen was not detectable in his electron micrographs. However, also in 1974, Rhodin (149) described collagen in the rat follicle. The discrepancy in these publications was clarified later by evidence that

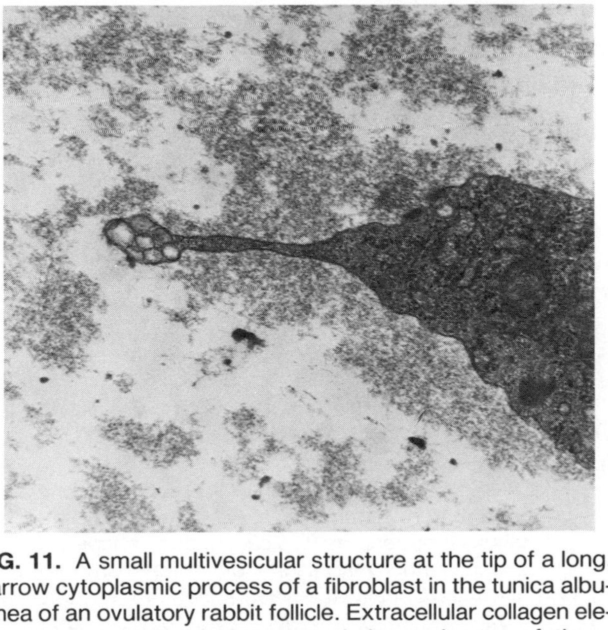

FIG. 11. A small multivesicular structure at the tip of a long, narrow cytoplasmic process of a fibroblast in the tunica albuginea of an ovulatory rabbit follicle. Extracellular collagen elements are usually absent around the perimeter of these structures. (From reference 153, with permission.)

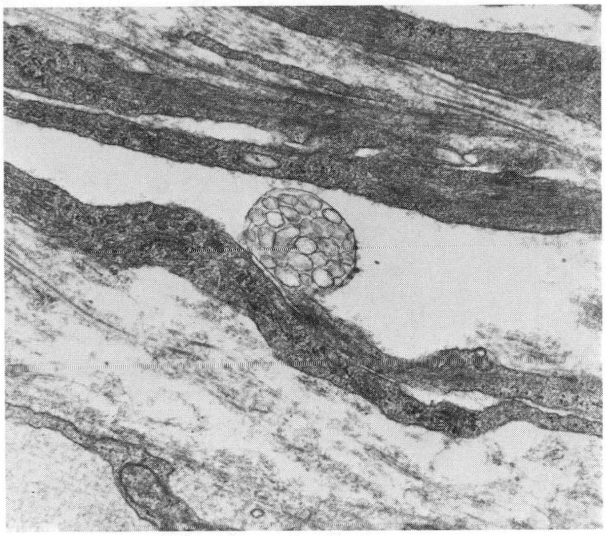

FIG. 12. Another multivesicular structure at the tip of a cytoplasmic process of a thecal fibroblast in a rabbit follicle. The cell body and nucleus) of the cell is to the right. Notice the absence of extracellular material around this multivesicular structure. (From reference 153, with permission.)

glutaraldehyde fixatives can cause collagen to lose its usual resistance to penetration by an electron beam (150). By staining thin sections of the follicle wall of the rat with a 1% solution of phosphotungstic acid, the collagen fibrils of the tunica albuginea and theca externa become much more visible in electron micrographs. Such staining reveals that the apex of a rat follicle has a substantial amount of extracellular collagen distributed evenly among the fibroblasts of the tunica albuginea and the theca externa.

Multivesicular Structures of Follicular Fibroblasts

One of the more interesting features of ovulatory follicles is the multivesicular structures that protrude from the surface of the plasma membranes of the fibroblasts in the collagen layers (19,32,151,152). These unusual structures are especially common at the leading edges of the pseudopodlike processes that extend from the cytoplasm of the proliferating fibroblasts in follicles that are about to rupture (Figs. 11 and 12). Espey (153) noted that the concentration of these structures increases approximately ninefold during the ovulatory process (Fig. 13). In some instances, it is evident that the extracellular matrix of collagen is decomposed in the vicinity of these multivesicular bodies (151,154). The general features of these structures strongly suggest that they may contribute in some important way to the opening of interstitial pathways for the movement of proliferating fibroblasts in ovulatory follicles. However, these unique entities are difficult to preserve for cytochemical analysis, and there

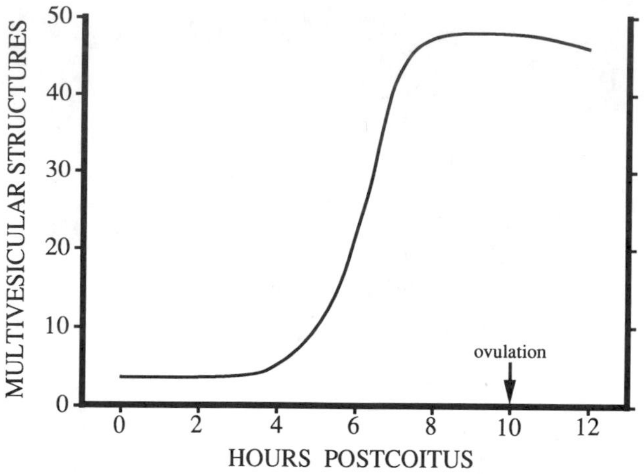

FIG. 13. Increase in the concentration of multivesicular structures associated with thecal fibroblasts of an ovulatory rabbit follicle. (Adapted from reference 151.)

is negligible information about their chemical composition (32). Therefore, their potential role in the mechanism of ovulation remains uncertain.

Theca Externa

General Features

The theca externa is an outer sphere of collagenous connective tissue that delineates a mature follicle from the surrounding ovarian stroma (19,32,64,152). Like the tunica albuginea, this layer of connective tissue appears to contain only one type of cell, namely, fibroblasts (Fig. 3). At the apex of a follicle, where the elements of the tunica albuginea and the theca externa are adjacent to one another, it is difficult to distinguish between these two layers in rabbit ovaries except for the fact that the theca externa contains fewer collagen fibers (32,64). In contrast, in the rat, the density of collagen fibers appears to be evenly distributed between the theca externa and the tunica albuginea (150).

Thecal Fibroblasts

As mentioned earlier, there continues to be some controversy over whether the cells of the theca externa are fibroblasts or smooth-muscle cells. The controversy has arisen in part from the fact that a significant portion of the cells appear to be spindle-shaped if the thin sections for transmission electron microscopy are cut perpendicular to the ovarian surface (64). However, if the thin sections are cut on a plane that is tangential to the ovarian surface, it becomes apparent that the cells of both the theca externa and the tunica albuginea are platter-shaped fibroblasts rather than spindle-shaped muscle cells (32) (Figs. 14 and 15). Besides the oval appearance of the fibroblasts, the tangential sections render the extracellular collagen more conspicuous, and it is more obvious that the collagenous fibrils are secretory products of these cells. Thus, fibroblasts are the dominant cell type in both the theca externa and the tunica albuginea.

Ovulatory Changes in the Thecal Connective Tissue

During the first several hours after initiation of the ovulatory process, there is very little change in the appearance of the theca externa and tunica albuginea (64,126,152). The first signs of change occur at about 4 h after stimulation in rabbit follicles, at which time edema begins to develop in the theca interna and the fibroblasts in this area begin to dissociate (126). As the ovulatory process progresses, there is surprisingly little change in

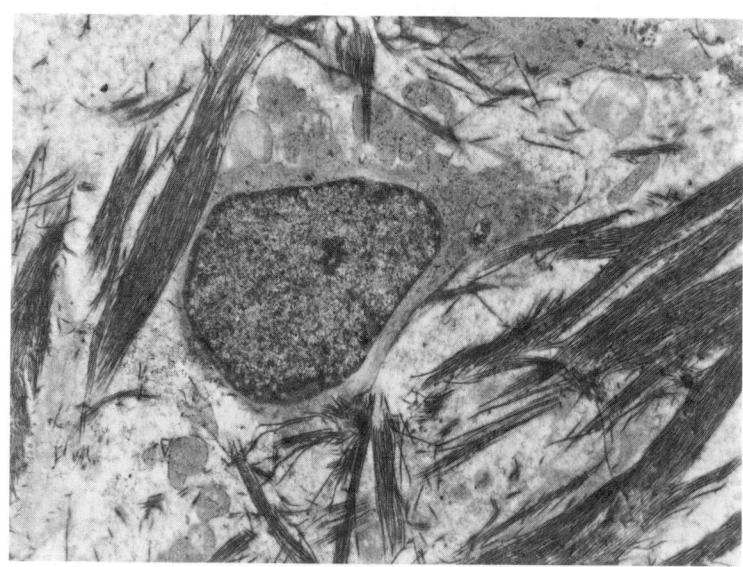

FIG. 14. Tangential view of a fibroblast at the apex of a mature rabbit follicle. From this angle, the cells always appear as typical ''platter-shaped'' fibroblasts, rather than as spindle-shaped smooth muscle cells. Usually, the plasma membrane is undiscernible, and the prominent extracellular collagen fibrils appear to be in direct contact with the cytoplasm that is rich in unpolymerized tropocollagen. (From reference 32, with permission.)

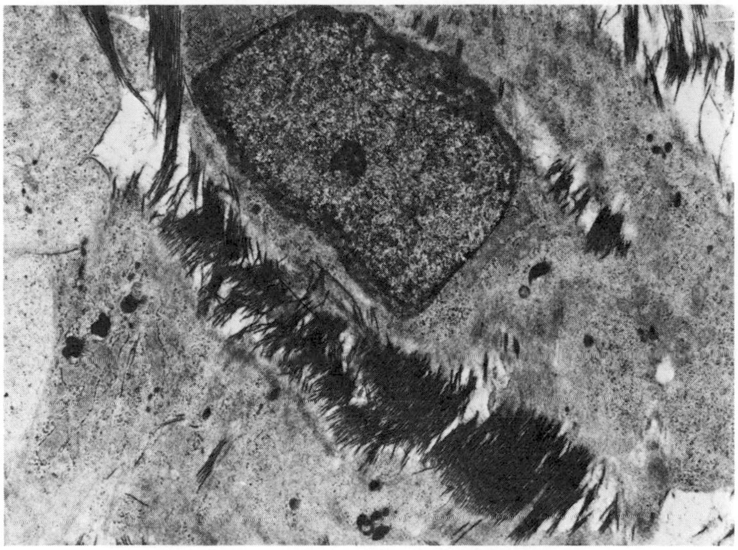

FIG. 15. Tangential view of another fibroblast at the apex of a mature rabbit follicle. Typically, the plasma membrane is undiscernible from this angle, and the prominent extracellular collagen fibrils appear to be in direct contact with the cytoplasm that is rich in unpolymerized tropocollagen. (From reference 32, with permission.)

the appearance of the follicle wall until the final hour before rupture. During this last hour, the fibroblasts and collagenous elements undergo marked dissociation in the apical region of the follicle wall (64,126,152) (Fig. 10). The concentration of collagen fibrils per square micron of cross-sectional area decreases to only about 28% of the value that was present before induction of the ovulatory process (64). Also, in the final minutes before rupture, the average depth of the collagenous tissue at the apex of a rabbit follicle decreases to only 27% of its original value (64) (Fig. 16). Thus, at the apex where rupture normally occurs, the follicle wall becomes thinner, and the connective tissue elements within the follicle wall become sparser. By this stage, extravasated blood cells are common within the extracellular spaces around the fibroblasts (152). This internal hemorrhaging is an indication that rupture is imminent. Espey (19,32,152) reported that the tenacious collagenous layers of the theca externa and tunica albuginea are usually the final tissue to break.

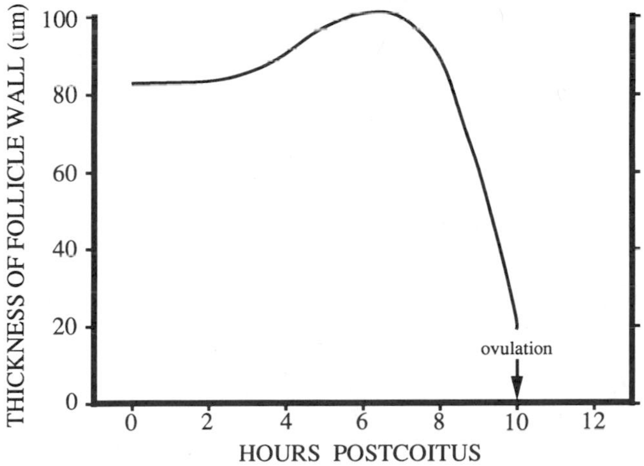

FIG. 16. Decline in thickness of collagenous layers of the follicle wall during final stages of the ovulatory process in the rabbit. Measurements were made from the outer surface of the tunica albuginea into the membrana propria at the inner surface of the theca interna. The modest increase in thickness of the follicle wall during the middle of the ovulatory process may reflect edematous swelling. (Adapted from reference 64.)

Theca Interna

General Features

The theca interna, which is approximately two cells thick, is bounded on the outer side by the fibroblasts of the theca externa and on the inner side by the basal lamina (membrana propria) that separates it from the granulosa layer (64,127). The embryologic origin of the cells of the theca interna has been debated for many years (121). Erickson et al. (155) reviewed most of the literature on the development and function of these cells and concluded that they are derived from ovarian stromal cells. These "interstitial" cells of the theca interna have large oval nuclei with very prominent nucleoli (Fig. 17). Their cytoplasm is dominated by lipid droplets, numerous mitochondria, some Golgi networks, and a few small lysosomal-like bodies. Such cytologic features are highly characteristic of active steroidogenic cells (156,157). The lipid droplets, which are a conspicuous feature of these cells, are filled with cholesterol to provide substrate for steroid biosynthesis.

Steroid Synthesis

It has been well established that a developing ovarian follicle produces more and more estrogen as it ap-

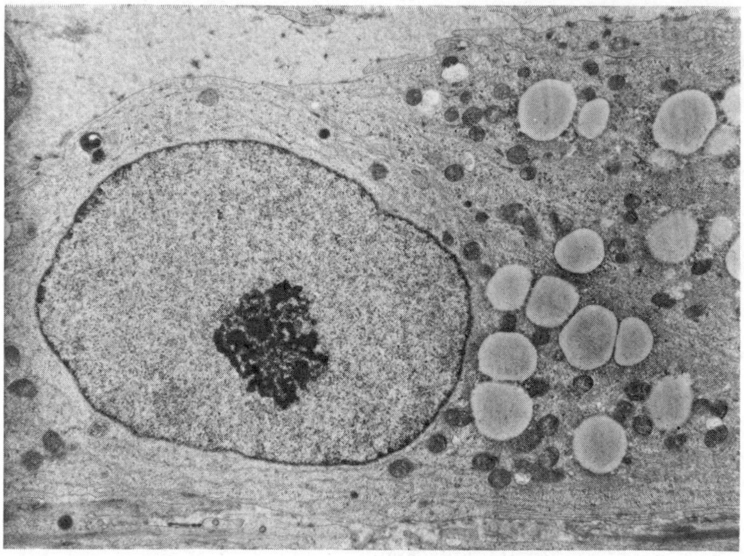

FIG. 17. Steroid secreting cell of the theca interna of a preovulatory rabbit follicle. Lipid droplets and mitochondria are characteristic of these cells, which may be active in 17β-estradiol production. Large, oval nuclei with prominent nucleoli are also characteristic of these cells. (From reference 32, with permission.)

proaches maturity (i.e., as it acquires the capacity to respond to an ovulatory surge in LH or exogenous chorionic gonadotropin (CG)) (158). Earlier studies on the histochemistry and cytochemistry of ovarian steroid synthesis have been reviewed by Guraya (159). Since that time, several investigators have reported that the estrogens, principally 17β-estradiol, are actively secreted by the cells of the theca interna, whereas the granulosa cells appear to be relatively inactive (132,136,160–163). However, in 1959, Falck (164) transplanted different combinations of granulosa and theca interna tissue into the anterior chamber of the rat eye and assessed subsequent estrogen secretion. He found that estrogen secretion occurred only when thecal interstitial cells and granulosa cells were transplanted together. Thus, on the basis of this synergisticlike action of the two follicular tissues, he concluded that two types of cells were necessary for estrogen synthesis in the ovarian follicle—with the theca interna carrying out the initial biosynthetic steps of androgen production and the granulosa cells converting the androgens to estrogens. Several years later, Bjersing (165) modified this "two-cell-type" theory by proposing that side-chain cleavage of cholesterol and 17α-hydroxylation are probably limited to the thecal interstitial cells, whereas aromatization to 17β-estradiol may take place in both theca and granulosa cells. However, the ultrastructure of the different layers of the follicle wall certainly make it appear as though the interstitial cells of the theca interna are the most active steroidogenic cells in preovulatory follicles (32,64,127). Therefore, further assessment of the steroid composition and relevant mRNA transcripts in the theca and granulosa cells may be required to confirm the two-cell theory of ovarian steroid secretion.

When a mature follicle has been stimulated by an ovulatory surge in gonadotropin, the local elevation in cyclic AMP mediates several changes in follicular steroidogenic activity. Within 1 h, estrogen and androgen secretion increases even further, but several hours later, the ovarian level of these two types of steroids declines sharply, while ovarian progesterone synthesis begins to rise significantly (161,163,166–177). By the time of ovulation, there are changes in the ultrastructure of the granulosa cells that reflect this increase in progesterone synthesis (32,159). The potential role of progesterone in the mechanism of ovulation is discussed later in this chapter in the section on ovarian steroids.

Vascular System

Most of the ovarian blood supply circulates to the mature ovarian follicles and to the wreath of large capillaries that lie along the inner border of the theca interna (19). This dense network of capillaries delivers nutrients to the steroidogenic cells of the theca interna, and it indirectly supplies the metabolic needs of the avascular granulosa layer, the cumulus oophorus, and the oocyte. The first detailed account of this elaborate blood supply was described at the turn of the century by Clark (178). The next half-century of work on the changes in this vascular pattern during the sexual cycles of mammals has been nicely summarized by Bassett (179) and by Burr and Davies (180). More recently, Ellinwood et al. (181) made a thorough review of the ovarian vasculature, and Lipner (6) updated this information.

The ovarian blood supply has been studied by several experimental methods. One approach has been to prepare corrosion casts for scanning electron microscopy of the follicle vasculature (182–185). Resin leakage during preparation of such casts has provided indirect evidence to support reports that the permeability of the thecal capillary network increases significantly during the ovulatory process (102,186,187).

Macroscopic observations of ovulatory follicles are all that are needed to detect the vascular blushing and hyperemia that are characteristic of ovulatory follicles. In their studies of rabbit ovulation in 1935, Hill et al. (2) noted that the capillary blood supply increases in ovulatory follicles. Also, in 1951, Burr and Davies (180) referred to the "hyperemia" that occurs in the rabbit ovary before ovulation. However, several attempts to measure this increase in ovarian blood flow have not provided a very consistent picture of the vascular changes that occur. By following the movement of radioactive microspheres into the ovarian vascular compartment, Murdoch et al. (188,189) concluded that the supply of ovarian blood to the follicle wall of the ewe initially increases after the LH surge, but then it declines during the 10 to 12 h preceding follicular rupture. However, Brown et al. (190) used the microsphere technique and found that capillary blood flow in the ewe ovary is significantly greater near ovulation. In the rabbit, studies with radioactive microspheres (191–193) have shown that ovarian blood flow increases significantly as early as 10 min after LH/hCG administration, reaches a maximum approximately 4 h later, and remains elevated throughout the ovulatory process. In contrast, in the gonadotropin-primed immature rat, Damber et al. (194) reported that the relative follicular blood flow did not increase during the ovulatory process. However, by using radioactive isotopes to estimate ovarian fractional blood flow, Wurtman (195) claimed that there was a rapid increase in ovarian hyperemia after the injection of LH into the rat. Similarly, Abisogun et al. (196) measured an increase in ovarian and follicular blood flow, with the most pronounced change occurring at 1.5 h after administering hCG into rats. Several other studies used either drop-flow counters (197), thermocouples (198), perfusion systems (199), ultrasonography with color-flow mapping (200), or transmission electron microscopy (201,202) to estimate ovarian hyperemia, but these methods have not clarified the changes in ovarian blood flow and blood volume during the ovulatory process.

Studies on the relationship between ovarian hyperemia and the well-known increase in prostaglandins during ovulation have been no more enlightening. Some reports have suggested that prostaglandins increase ovarian blood flow and/or blood volume (193,203); others have indicated that prostaglandins decrease ovarian blood flow (188,204); and yet another has concluded that eicosanoids have no effect on blood flow but may decrease permeability of the ovarian vasculature (196). In a recent study on the gonadotropin-primed immature rat, Tanaka et al. (205) used a spectrophotometric method to systematically measure hemoglobin in ovarian extracts during ovulation. This method showed that ovarian blood volume increases significantly beginning 4 h after hCG administration, and it reaches a peak that is approximately sevenfold greater than the control level at 10 h after hCG (i.e., at the time when follicles begin to rupture in the rat) (Fig. 18). In this model, indomethacin partially inhibited the increase in ovarian blood volume, suggesting that eicosanoids might function as mediators of ovarian hyperemia during the ovulatory process.

One of the more distinct changes in the vascular pattern of ovulatory follicles is the angiogenic activity that develops near the time of ovulation. One-half century ago, Bassett (179) reported that "shortly after rupture of a follicle, the granulosa is invaded at many points by vascular sprouts from the inner capillary wreath." This early observation has been confirmed by electron microscopy (185,202,206). Kranzfelder et al. (207) suggested that products from the granulosa cells regulate this angiogenic response, whereas Rose and Koos (208) suggested that a combination of factors in serum and in follicular fluid can govern the mitogenesis of new blood vessels in ovulatory follicles.

Granulosa Layer

General Features

The stratum granulosum is a multilayer of epithelial cells that extend inward from the membrana propria (basal lamina) that delineates the granulosa from the theca interna (32,64,125,137,209). There are several thorough reviews on the morphology of this innermost layer of the follicle (29,210). The granulosa is usually about five to ten cells deep, except for the cumulus mass, which protrudes randomly from any part of this stratum and suspends the oocyte more toward the center of the follicular antrum. More than a century ago, Sobotta (211) realized that the position of the cumulus in the follicle is entirely one of chance. The granulosa cells that are adjacent to the membrana propria are usually more

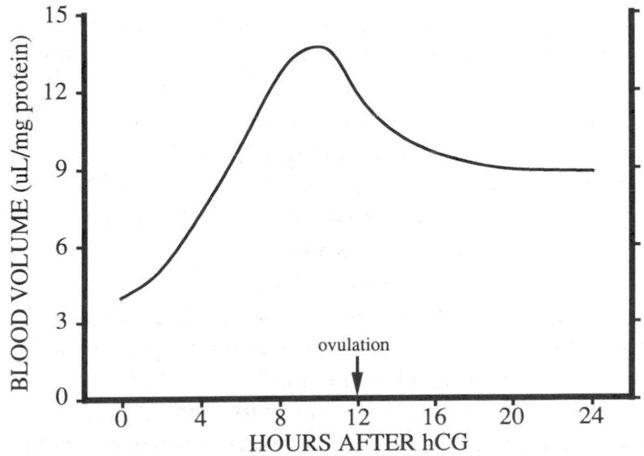

FIG. 18. Increase in ovarian blood volume during ovulation in the gonadotropin-primed immature rat. (Adapted from reference 205.)

columnar in shape, whereas the remainder of the cells in this layer are polyhedral or cuboidal (19,64). Granulosa cells of mature follicles contain some smooth endoplasmic reticulum, Golgi networks, granular mitochondria, and occasional lipid granules. Bjersing (29) reported that these cells undergo hypertrophy near the time of ovulation, and Espey (19) noted that they contain a greater number of lipid granules, which may reflect an increase in their steroid metabolism in response to gonadotropic stimulation. However, the most conspicuous morphologic changes in this layer occur shortly after ovulation, when large lipid droplets begin to dominate the cytoplasm of the cells of the lutein granulosa, when thecal fibroblasts begin to proliferate into the area to lay down new luteal connective tissue, and when the thecal blood vessels begin to penetrate this stratum for the first time.

In species such as the rabbit and sheep, which form ovulatory stigma, the granulosa layer is often absent from the apical-most area of follicles that are about to rupture (7,64,125,128). Apparently, as the follicle wall begins to balloon out during the final stages of the ovulatory process, the thin membrana propria between the granulosa layer and the theca interna dissociates and retracts in a circular pattern at the base of the developing stigma. In the process of this retraction, the apical granulosa cells and the thecal vascular tissue also disassociate and leave a thinner stigma lacking blood vessels. As the remaining collagenous tissue undergoes enzymatic decomposition during the final minutes before rupture, the stigma becomes translucent. At the base of the stigma, the broken blood vessels and extravasated blood may form a "rosette" around the pending site of rupture (4,7,99).

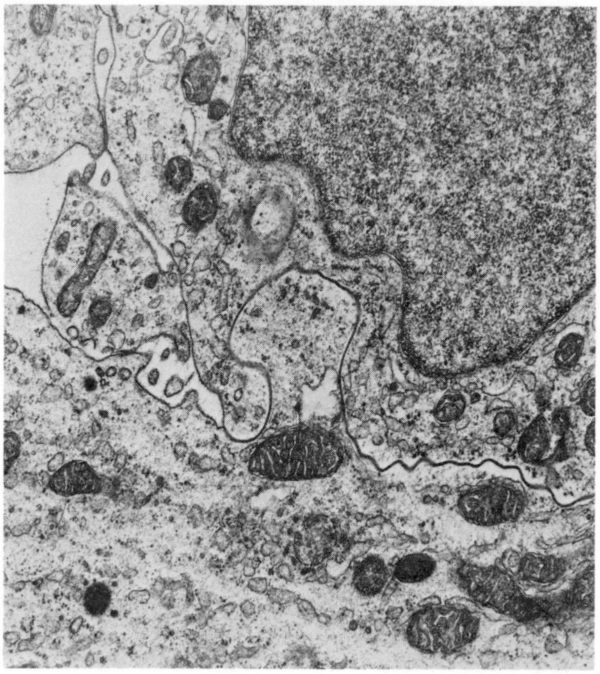

FIG. 19. Two adjacent granulosa cells in a rabbit follicle are fused together by a gap junction. The cytoplasmic process that extends from one cell into the other is characteristic of this cellular layer of the follicle. A conspicuous mitochondrion is present at the base of the cytoplasmic process. Such processes are commonly pinched-off i.e., phagocytosed) entirely into the cytoplasm of recipient granulosa cells. (From reference 133, with permission.)

Granulosa Gap Junctions

One of the more interesting features of the stratum granulosum is the elaborate network of gap junctions that link this layer of epithelial cells into a continuum (Fig. 19). These membrane junctions were originally described by Merk et al. (212,213) and by Espey and Stutts (133). As these investigators pointed out, besides providing intercellular cohesion, the tight junctions might (i) be necessary for the transport of ions and nutrients across the granulosa layer, (ii) be involved in routing the primary follicular fluid from the granulosa cells to the antrum, or (iii) be important in conducting fluctuations in membrane potentials throughout this stratum and perhaps even to the oocyte. Also, Espey and Stutts (133) noted that cytoplasmic invaginations commonly occur along the site where two cell membranes fuse into a gap junction (Fig. 19). Such invaginations can be pinched off or "phagocytozed" in a manner that can result in complete incorporation of a section of a gap junction into one of the two adjacent cells. This phagocytic activity results in the formation of a so-called annular gap junction completely within the cytoplasm of the recipient cell. This unusual phenomenon results in an exchange of cytoplasm between the two cells that shared a common gap junction. The physiologic value of this transfer of cytoplasm remains uncertain. It was initially thought that internalization of the gap junctions might increase during ovulation and that such a process might loosen the granulosa cells and the cumulus mass by the time of follicular rupture (133). In examining this hypothesis, Bjersing and Cajander (125) presented data from rabbits showing a decrease in the intercellular sharing of these gap junctions and a simultaneous increase in the internalized spherical gap junctions in the cytoplasm of individual granulosa cells as follicles progressed toward ovulation. Coons and Espey (214) conducted a more quantitative analysis of the distribution of these gap junctions during ovulation, and although they measured a significant decrease in the surface area of gap junctions situated between adjacent granulosa cells of follicles about to rupture, they also observed a decrease in the number of internalized gap junctions. These observations suggest that ovulation may be preceded by a separation of the gap junctions between cells, rather than by internalization of these junctions. Subsequent studies have further characterized the morphology of the granulosa gap junctions (162,215–221), but the specific function of these structures remains uncertain. They probably unify the granulosa cells into a syncytial layer during follicular growth and development, but it is not clear whether they have any important role in the chemical and/or electrical coupling of these cells during ovulation. Forty years ago, Zuckerman (222) stated that the oocyte is the dynamic center of follicular activity and that it maintains a constant influence on the membrana granulosa. Thus, it is possible that gap junctions couple the granulosa cells electrically into a syncytial network that influences the resumption of meiosis of the oocyte during ovulation, or conversely, it is possible that a meiotically rejuvenated oocyte might exert some ovulatory influence on the cumulus cells around it and this signal might be transmitted to the remainder of the granulosa layer through the gap junctions.

Other Anatomic Considerations

Follicular Fluid

Mature ovarian follicles in most mammalian species contain an antral cavity filled with follicular fluid. As early as 1918, Robinson (223) recognized different kinds of follicular fluid within developing follicles. He said that a "primary" viscous fluid is secreted from the granulosa cells during follicular growth and this liquid eventually coalesces to form the central antral cavity. A mature follicle contains a more serious "secondary" liquid that rapidly increases in volume shortly before ovulation. Some years later, Burr and Davies (180) recognized that the secondary liquid is probably a transudate from blood. The actual composition of the follicular fluid has been thoroughly reviewed by McNatty (134) and by Lipner (6). When a primordial follicle begins to grow, the hyperplastic granulosa cells secrete proteoglycans and related gelatinous materials that form the primary follicular fluid. The secondary fluid that transudes into the follicular antrum during ovulation is similar to blood plasma except that it contains much lower levels of fibrinogen, a slightly lower pH, and the protein, carbohydrate, and steroid profile of the fluid can fluctuate with the metabolic stage of the follicle (6,134).

The specific function of follicular fluid is unknown. As McNatty (134) pointed out, "The formation of a fluid-filled cavity within enlarging follicles provides a means by which intrafollicular cells of one follicle may be exposed to an environment that is different from that in adjacent follicles and from that in peripheral blood," and this may "provide an intraovarian mechanism to limit the number of follicles that can go on to ovulate." It is also feasible that the follicular fluid could serve to isolate the cumulus oophorus from blood-borne growth factors that might otherwise disturb the dormant meiotic state of the oocytes in preovulatory follicles. Yet, the more relevant question that remains unanswered is whether the follicular fluid contributes in some important way to the mechanism of ovulation. One possible function that has received negligible attention is that the follicular fluid, along with the zona pellucida and the corona radiata cells that surround the oocyte, may serve as defense mechanisms to protect the delicate egg from the acute onslaught of proteolytic activity that disrupts the collagenous layers of the follicle wall during ovulation. A second possibility is that the lubricative texture of the fluid may facilitate the smooth extrusion of the cumulus mass and oocyte out the rupture point. A more remote possibility is that the follicular fluid might contribute in some positive way to the postovulatory healing and luteinization processes that occur after ovulation. However, the precise functions of the fluid remain to be determined.

Innervation of Ovarian Follicles

Innervation of the mammalian ovary by sympathetic and parasympathetic fibers has been reviewed by several investigators (6,37,224,225). The sympathetic nerves originate from the lower thoracic region of the spinal cord and pass through the celiac plexus and ovarian ganglia before entering the hilar region of the ovary. The parasympathetic fibers, which are probably of vagal origin, also enter the hilus along with the ovarian blood vessels. These autonomic nerves converge, for the most part, on the ovarian vasculature (224), especially around vessels in the hilum and medulla (95,226,227). However, a portion of the nerves pass to the cortex of the ovary and form a plexus around the ovarian follicles. Walles et al. (228–230) reported that this follicular innervation is extensive, but McReynolds et al. (231) reported that it is essentially nonexistent. Within the follicle, nerves can be found in both the theca externa and the theca interna but not inside the granulosa (224). Besides making contact with the thecal vasculature, some of the nerves may terminate on myofibroblasts in this area of the follicle (232–234). Many investigators believe that the nerves regulate ovarian "contractility" and thereby contribute to the mechanism of ovulation. Espey (37) reviewed these different reports and noted that α-adrenergic agonists, β-adrenergic antagonists, and cholinergic antagonists all appear to promote some kind of contractile response in ovarian tissues. Since that review, there have been several additional reports that catecholamines and/or adrenergic receptors may participate in the process of ovulation (235–240). However, there is no convincing evidence that nerve excitation is a crucial event in the ovulatory process (37). In a series of studies almost two decades ago, Weiner et al. (87,241,242) showed that denervation of the rabbit ovary did not reduce the number of ovulations, pregnancies, or corpora lutea. Likewise, Wylie (243) froze the sympathetic nerve supply to the rat ovary and found that follicular rupture was not affected by the absence of this innervation. Furthermore, it has been demonstrated repeatedly that ovulation can occur in the *in vitro* perfusion system (38,244) and ovulatorylike changes can be induced within cultured ovaries (245), even though such experimental models totally lack innervation. Therefore, although one cannot completely rule out the possibility that adrenergic agents might have some modest influence on ovulation, it is, nevertheless, quite apparent that nervous activity is not an essential component of the ovulatory mechanism.

BIOCHEMICAL EVENTS IN OVULATION

Membrane Phenomena and Related Events

Gonadotropin Surge

The ovulatory process is initiated at the moment when follicular tissue is stimulated by a surge of pituitary gonadotropins. The pituitary surge in LH secretion can lead to as much as a 100-fold increase in the circulating level of the hormone (246). In the earlier years, it was generally presumed that LH was solely responsible for initiating the ovulatory process (8), but it is now apparent that other hormones can substitute for LH. Chorionic gonadotropin (CG), which has a peptide sequence that is highly homologous with LH, is commonly used as a substitute for LH (247). Likewise, FSH, which is named for its role in follicular development, can, by itself, induce ovulation (248,249). As early as 1973, Nalbandov et al. (250) concluded that "the ovulation-inducing hormones consist of a mixture of FSH and LH and that it is not LH alone." Subsequently, Greenwald and Papkoff (251) found that FSH preparations were more potent than LH in inducing ovulation in the hamster. More recently, Galway et al. (252) treated hypophysectomized rats with recombinant FSH and demonstrated that this pure hormone preparation can induce both follicular development and ovulation. Equally interesting is the growing evidence that gonadotropin-releasing hormone (GnRH) can induce ovulation in hypophysectomized animals (253–258). However, there is at least one contradictory report that claims that GnRH inhibits LH-induced ovulation in hypophysectomized rats (259). In any event, under normal conditions, LH and FSH probably act together to initiate the ovulatory process.

The concept that LH and FSH act in a complementary fashion to induce ovulation has been more readily accepted since there is now evidence that these two hormones are usually released in unison in response to GnRH, that they have relatively homologous peptide sequences, and that their respective receptors display considerable sequence similarity (247,260). LH and FSH, along with CG and thyroid-stimulating hormone (TSH), are members of a family of heterodimer glycoprotein hormones composed of a common α-subunit that is connected to a distinct β-subunit that confers receptor binding specificity (247).

Gonadotropin Receptors

Ovulation occurs only in mature ovarian follicles that have acquired an adequate concentration of LH receptors (42,247,260). Two decades ago, Midgley and coworkers (261,262) used ^{125}I-hCG to localize the site of LH binding in mature follicles. Their autoradiographs revealed that most of the binding occurred on the plasma membranes of the theca interna cells of the rat ovary, whereas the granulosa cells were generally free of the isotope-labeled gonadotropin. A subsequent study, which used fluorescence localization of hCG, supports this view (263). However, other investigations have shown that, although the highest density of labeled hormone *may be* in the theca interna, the layers of granulosa cells closest to the membrana propria also contain LH receptors (28,264–269). However, the cumulus cells and oocyte appear to be devoid of LH receptors (264,267). Acquisition of a sufficient concentration of LH receptors is dependent on the actions of estradiol, FSH, and probably some LH itself (28,266,268).

Several investigators have shown that the natural LH receptor has a molecular size of approximately 93 kDa (270–273). McFarland et al. (247) recently isolated and sequenced cDNA for the rat LH receptor. Decoding this cDNA has yielded a 674-residue polypeptide with a molecular size of 75 kDa and six unoccupied, *N*-linked glycosylation sites within its domain that account for the difference in its size when compared with the natural receptor. The receptor has a relatively large 341-residue extracellular domain and a 333-residue membrane-spanning region that is characteristic of the G-protein receptor family with seven transmembrane segments. Leung and Steele (260) recently reviewed the literature on the nature of this receptor, its relationship to the FSH receptor, and the intracellular signaling pathways by which it stimulates phospholipase activity in the gonads. The initial response to hormone/receptor coupling appears to be an elevation in intracellular cyclic AMP (42,260).

There is no clear evidence to indicate whether other membrane receptors are also involved in the ovulatory stimulus. With regard to prolactin (PRL), Piquette et al. (274) reported that this gonadotropin induces an increase in LH receptors in granulosa cells, and such an effect should increase the responsiveness of follicles to the ovulatory surge in gonadotropins. However, several other reports suggest that PRL interferes with ovulation (275–277). With regard to serotonin, this neurohumoral agent binds, like the gonadotropins, to a G-protein-coupled receptor (247). Although serotonin has been implicated in the mechanism of ovulation (278,279), there is at least one report that suggests that it does not increase significantly in human follicles at the time of ovulation (239), and its role remains uncertain. Other agents that might influence ovulation include vasoactive intestinal peptide (VIP) (260,280,281), neuropeptide Y (NPY) (240), oxytocin (282,283), and growth hormone-releasing factor (GRH) (260).

Cyclic AMP and Other Second Messengers

Two decades ago, Marsh et al. (284–287) demonstrated that rabbit follicles produce cyclic AMP, and these investigators suggested that this second messenger might be involved in the steroidogenic action of LH. Shortly thereafter, several other studies confirmed that LH action on ovarian steroidogenesis and luteinization is mediated by cyclic AMP (199,250,288–299). This second messenger increases within 10 min after exposure of a follicle to LH, and it reaches a peak within several hours (199,292,293,295). In contrast, there is a reciprocal decline in cyclic GMP (174,300). Cells of the theca interna are the principal source of cyclic AMP, but granulosa cells also respond in a similar manner to LH stimulation (293,294,296,301,302). Cyclic AMP acts through protein kinases to induce cholesterol side-chain cleavage cytochrome P450 ($P450_{scc}$) mRNA and to promote enzyme activity that catalyzes the first rate-limiting step in follicular progesterone synthesis (42,301,303–311). Besides its stimulatory effect on follicular progesterone synthesis, some reports suggest that cyclic AMP may also increase follicular prostaglandin synthesis (38,286, 312,313), but at least one study has come to the opposite conclusion (314). Equally confusing are reports that prostaglandins (particularly prostaglandin E_2) may (293,295, 314) or may not (312,315) promote the formation of cyclic AMP in ovulatory follicles.

Other second messengers may also be generated by the signal transduction processes in ovarian follicular cells that have been stimulated by an ovulatory surge in LH. Luteinizing hormone probably provokes a sustained increase in inositol triphosphate (IP_3) and diacylglycerol (DAG) (316,317), and Veldhuis (318,319) reported that the formation of these second messengers may be influenced by prostaglandin synthesis in granulosa cells. Also, the stimulation of progesterone synthesis by LH and cyclic AMP is probably affected by intracellular Ca^{2+} (307,320–322), but the precise role of this cation in ovarian steroidogenesis has not been established. Intracellular Ca^{2+} is considered to be a second messenger because it increases in cells shortly after ligand-receptor coupling and because it is required for activation of protein kinase C and for the subsequent phosphorylation of several metabolically active proteins (44).

Protein Kinases

When a hormone such as LH binds to membrane receptors on follicular cells, the events of signal transduction activate phosphorylation processes. The energy within phosphate bonds flows in an organized pattern through several effector enzymes and regulatory proteins that are sequentially energized to undergo conformational changes and mediate cellular responses (44,323). The kinds of protein kinases that are generated by gonadotropic hormone stimulation of ovarian follicles are only beginning to be deciphered. Hunzicker-Dunn and Jungmann (324,325) conducted several of the earliest studies on protein kinases in follicles. They reported that preovulatory (i.e., unstimulated) follicles contain only a single species of protein kinase and that the induction of ovulation and luteinization promotes the expression of two additional species of protein kinases. Richards and co-workers (298,326–330) conducted a detailed study of a regulatory subunit (RII_{51}) of cyclic AMP-dependent protein kinase type II. They found that this inhibitor of the catalytic subunit of cyclic AMP-dependent protein kinase increases in granulosa and theca cells in response to FSH and estradiol as a follicle matures. The LH/hCG surge causes a dramatic decrease in this regulatory subunit (298), but the significance of this change is uncertain, except that the decline coincides with the decrease in ovarian estrogen and androgen synthesis during ovulation.

Other studies have shown that protein kinase C activity, which usually increases after activation of phospholipase C and the formation of DAG, has an inhibitory effect on ovarian progesterone synthesis (307,331), and this action might be related to the stimulation of prostanoid synthesis (332–334). In contrast, other reports indicate that protein kinase C stimulates progesterone synthesis in differentiated granulosa cells, and this might be mediated by tumor necrosis factor-α (335–338). Thus, the actions of protein kinases in ovulation are uncertain. Nevertheless, it seems quite likely that protein phosphorylation plays an intermediary role in the ovulatory process (339).

Mobilization of Membrane Phospholipids

In the course of hormone binding to G-protein-coupled receptors such as the LH receptor, there is usually stimulation of adenylyl cyclase and a local increase in intracellular cyclic AMP (247). The phosphorylation of such receptors and their associated G proteins

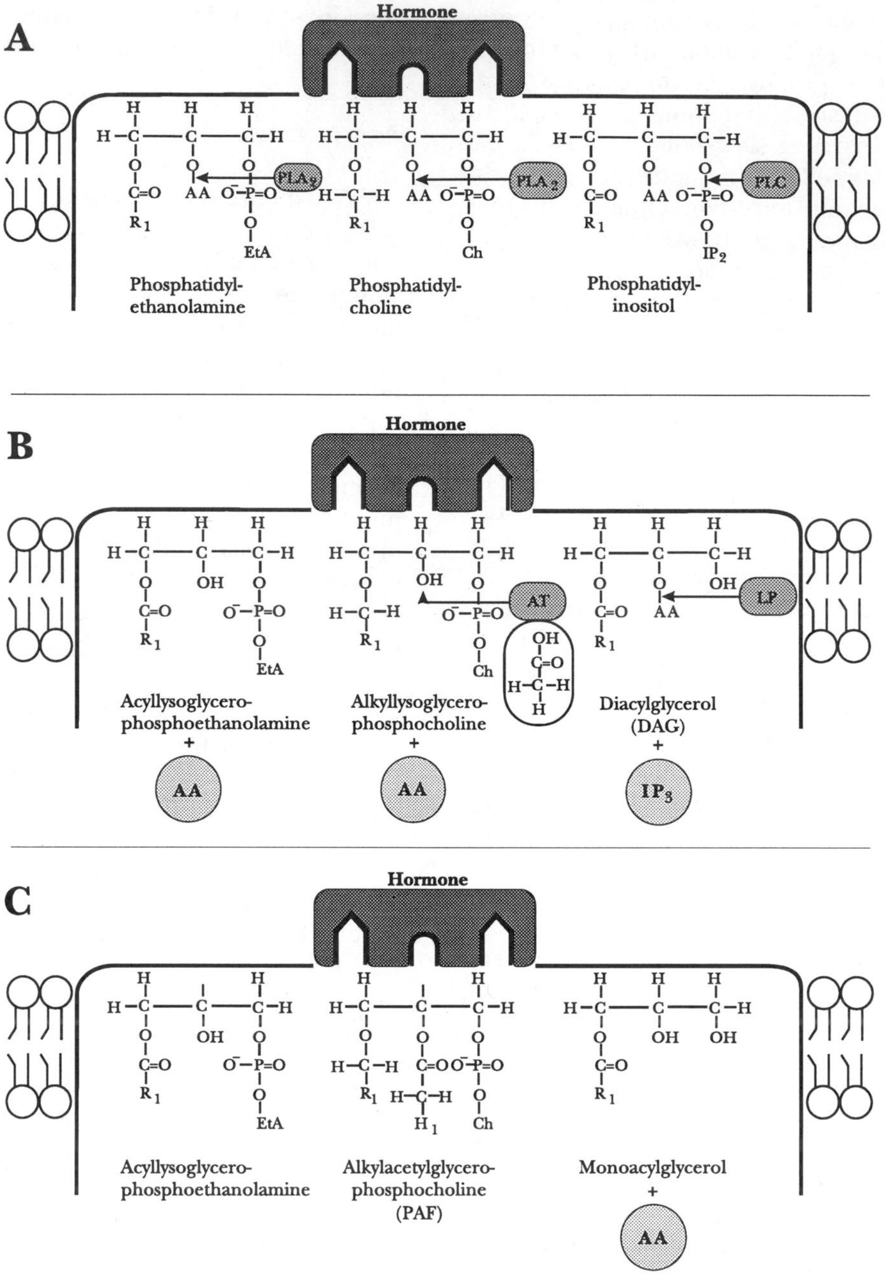

FIG. 20. Metabolism of common membrane phospholipids following hormone-receptor interaction. (A and B) Phosphatidylethanolamine and phosphatidylcholine are the two most common phospholipids in the membranes of most mammalian cells. Phosphatidylinositol is present in lesser, but significant, amounts. Phosphorylation of G-proteins leads to the activation of a number of phospholipases, including phospholipase A_2 (PLA_2) and phospholipase C (PLC). PLA_2 hydrolyzes the phosphatidylate molecule at the *sn*-2 position and releases a fatty acid such as arachidonic acid (AA). PLC hydrolyzes the phosphatidylate molecule at the *sn*-3 position. R_1 is an alkyl group. (B and C) After PLA_2 has released AA from the *sn*-2 position of phosphatidylcholine, an acetyl group can be added to this position by the action of acetyl transferase (AT) to form platelet-activating factor (PAF). Also, after PLC has acted on phosphatidylinositol to form diacylglycerol (DAG) and inositol 1,4,5-triphosphate (IP_3), the DAG molecule can be further hydrolyzed by lipases (LP) to yield even more AA. (From reference 44, with permission.)

also leads to the activation of phospholipases, which serve as signal amplifying enzymes by hydrolyzing common membrane phospholipids that serve as the substrates for second-messenger formation (44,340,341) (Fig. 20). Phospholipase C and phospholipase A_2 are two such amplifying enzymes that have been studied extensively in a variety of experimental models. There is now indirect evidence that these enzymes also contribute to the biochemical events of ovulation, and their potential roles have been reviewed recently by Espey (44) and by Leung and Steele (260).

Phospholipase C hydrolyzes phosphatidyl inositol-4,5-biphosphate, a complex lipid that comprises as much as 5% to 10% of the total membrane phospholipids in animal cells (44,342) (Fig. 20). The products of this enzyme action are IP_3 and DAG, two second messengers that release calcium ions from the endoplasmic reticulum and activate protein kinase C, respectively (44,260). Diacylglycerol can be further hydrolyzed by DAG lipase to yield arachidonic acid, the principal substrate for eicosanoid metabolism in ovarian follicles (44). In comparison, phospholipase A_2 can act directly on phosphatidylethanolamine and phosphatidylcholine, which together comprise about 75% of the phospholipids in the membranes of most mammalian cells, to generate arachidonic acid (44). Because this type of enzymatic activation of the arachidonate "cascade" occurs after almost any condition that stimulates the plasma membrane (343–346), similar de-esterification of membrane phospholipids is almost certain to occur in ovarian follicles that have been stimulated to ovulate. The liberated arachidonic acid is then available for the cyclooxygenase and lipoxygenase pathways of eicosanoid metabolism in ovulatory follicles, as discussed later in this chapter.

In closely related metabolic events, after phospholipase A_2 has hydrolyzed phosphatidylcholine into arachidonic acid and an alkyllysoglycerophosphocholine, this modified phosphocholine can then be acetylated at the *sn*-2 position to form platelet-activating factor (PAF) (44,347,348). Platelet-activating factor is actually a family of acetylated glycerophospholipids that usually form in acute inflammatory reactions and tissue injury (349–353). This family of phospholipids is formed by a wide variety of cells, including epithelial and endothelial cells, fibroblasts, mast cells, and leukocytes (352,354–357). In inflammatory processes, they are potent inducers of vascular permeability, and they elicit acute extravasation of plasma proteins and cause local accumulation of platelets and neutrophils (350,358,359). In rat ovaries, PAF is released (or labilized) during the first several hours after gonadotropic hormone stimulation of the ovulatory process (Fig. 21), and the changes in this bioactive phospholipid are characteristic of what happens to PAF in inflamed tissues (360). Also, there are reports that antagonists of PAF can suppress ovulation in a dose-dependent manner (361,362). Therefore, it is possible

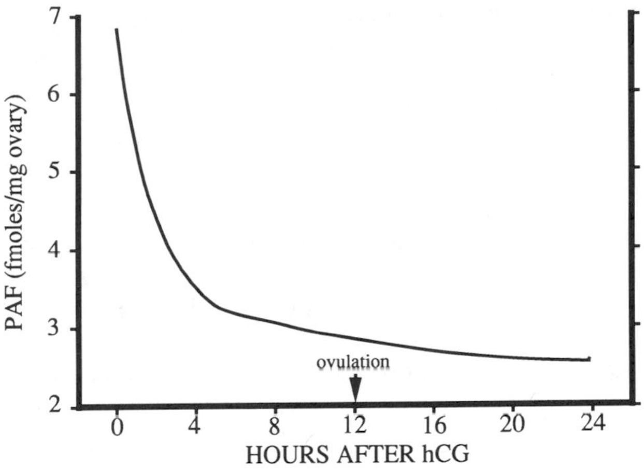

FIG. 21. Decrease in ovarian platelet-activating factor (PAF) during ovulatory process in the gonadotropin-primed immature rat. Figure based on (Adapted from reference 360.)

that PAF and related membrane phospholipids mediate some of the earlier events of the ovulatory process.

RNA and Protein Synthesis

It is natural to expect the signal transduction processes that are initiated by the gonadotropin surge to lead to transcription and translation activity in the theca and granulosa cells. The first indirect evidence of such activity was provided by Pool and Lipner (363,364), who found that actinomycin D (an inhibitor of mRNA synthesis) and cycloheximide (an inhibitor of protein synthesis) both block ovulation. These original observations were confirmed by several subsequent studies that demonstrated that protein synthesis is an essential part of the ovulatory process (365–370). The increase in protein synthesis is associated with an increase in mRNA formation that begins as early as 1 h after LH stimulation of mature follicles (365,366) and that persists until a few hours before the follicles rupture (371,372). The sites of synthesis of mRNA and protein appear to be mainly in the theca interna and the granulosa layer. The types of mRNA and protein are only beginning to be deciphered. Richards and co-workers conducted pioneering studies on the nature of the nucleic acids and enzymes responsible for ovarian steroid (42,302,310,311,373,374) and ovarian prostanoid (42,375–380) metabolism. Also, there is preliminary information about ovarian mRNA transcripts for kallikrein (381), plasminogen activator (PA) (252,382–384), collagenase (385), and metalloproteinase inhibitors (385–388), and these factors might be involved in the regulation of follicular proteolytic activity. Also, mRNA for a variety of growth factors has been identified in developing follicles, but it is not yet clear whether these cytokines contribute to the mechanism of ovulation (389–393).

Vasoactive Agents and Related Substances

Histamine

The first physical event that is known to occur in ovulatory follicles is the hyperemia that was described earlier in this chapter. Such an increase in blood flow and/or blood volume to a local area of irritation is usually associated with a release of histamine stores from mast cells and basophils (45). A main source of the ovarian histamine may be the mast cells in the walls of the large blood vessels in the ovarian hilum (394,395), and there is evidence that H_1 and H_2 receptors for histamine exist in these main ovarian vessels (396). Szego and Gitin (397,398) originally suggested that the release of histamine might be a physiologically significant event in ovulation. Their observations were supported by subsequent reports that antihistamines such as chlorpheniramine and pyrilamine (H_1-receptor antagonists) and cimetidine (an H_2-receptor antagonist), either separately or in combination, can inhibit ovulation *in vivo* and *in vitro* (395,399–402). Further support came from evidence that histamine, by itself, could induce ovulation *in vitro* in perfusion systems (395,401,403,404). This information, along with measurements that suggest there may be degranulation of mast cell histamine during ovulation, has led to speculation that this vasoactive agent might act as a paracrine mediator of the ovulatory process (405). However, the importance of histamine in ovulation has not been firmly established. More than 20 years ago, Lipner (406) used histamine-releasing drugs and antihistamines to show that this agent may not have a major role in ovulation. Furthermore, several other studies could not confirm the reported antiovulatory action of various H_1- and H_2-receptor antagonists (403,407–409). Also, several studies have revealed that histamine cannot induce the characteristic increase in prostanoid synthesis in follicular tissue (408,410), and this information casts further doubt on the idea that histamine by itself can mediate the ovulatory process. The question that remains unanswered is whether histamine is a causative agent in the mechanism of ovulation or whether this agent (and the associated hyperemia it generates) is merely an effect of (i.e., a response to) the degradative events of the ovulatory process.

Bradykinin

The nonapeptide bradykinin and other mammalian kinins are commonly generated at the site of tissue injury or inflammation (44–46). These kinins are produced by proteolytic cleavage of plasma kininogens by kallikrein (411,412). These vasoactive agents mediate a broad spectrum of biologic responses including vasodilation, increased vascular permeability, prostaglandin synthesis, cell proliferation, and inflammation (413–416). The first suggestions that bradykinin might be involved in ovulation came from a report by Smith and Perks (417) that plasma kininogen decreases in several mammals around the time of ovulation and from a review by Espey (45) that hypothesized that kinins might mediate the inflammatorylike events of the ovulatory process. Now, there is a variety of evidence that kinin-forming enzymes increase in the ovary at the time of ovulation (81,381,413,418–422) (Fig. 22). Also, there are reports that bradykinin can induce ovulation *in vitro* in perfused ovaries (423–425). Of particular interest are the reports that bradykinin can stimulate prostaglandin synthesis in mature ovarian follicles (423–425), although one study raises some question about this action of kinins on follicular prostanoid formation (410). Furthermore, there is evidence that bradykinin can promote the synthesis and release of eicosanoids in other experimental models (426–428), and this correlation suggests that kinins might be responsible, at least in part, for the well-known increase in eicosanoid metabolism in ovulatory follicles.

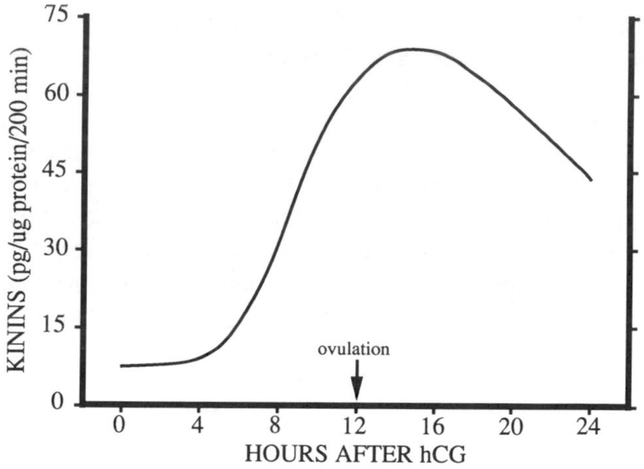

FIG. 22. Increase in ovarian kinin-generating capacity during ovulation in the gonadotropin-primed immature rat. (Adapted from reference 413.)

Angiotensin II

Angiotensin II is well known as a regulator of systemic blood pressure and fluid homeostasis. This vasoactive octapeptide is indirectly related to bradykinin in that the enzyme that converts angiotensin I into angiotensin II also acts as a kininase to degrade bradykinin (429). Angiotensin II has recently been implicated as a mediator of the ovulatory process because prorenin, which forms the enzyme to convert angiotensinogen into angiotensin I, increases in follicles in response to gonadotropic stimulation (430), angiotensin I-converting enzyme is detectable on the surface of granulosa cells (431), and receptors for angiotensin II are present in ovarian follicles (432–435) and especially because of reports that the angiotensin antagonist saralasin blocks ovulation (436–438). However, the importance of angiotensin II in ovulation has not been firmly established, because the converting enzyme responsible for formation of this agent does not increase during the periovulatory period (431), the converting enzyme inhibitor captopril does not affect ovulation (431), and several extensive efforts to confirm the reported antiovulatory action of saralasin have not been successful (439,440).

Prostaglandins

With the possible exception of ovarian steroids, no group of agents has been studied as extensively as the prostaglandins during the past two decades of work on ovulation. Prostaglandins are produced from arachidonic acid that is formed from membrane phospholipids in response to virtually any type of environmental condition that disturbs the plasma membrane (44,344,345). The prostanoids are commonly associated with inflammatory reactions, but they also form during immune reactions and hormonal responses. Although this group of eicosanoids are generally thought to mediate proinflammatory processes, there is also evidence that they might exert some anti-inflammatory action (441–447). Prostaglandin E_1, in particular, may be effective as an anti-inflammatory agent, and this prostanoid may act by inhibiting collagenase gene expression (446,448). These paradoxical pro- and anti-inflammatory theories of prostaglandin action may not be as contradictory as they seem at first; instead, the differences may reflect the complex nature of inflammatory reactions. Such reactions simultaneously involve degradative and reparative metabolic processes, and the prostanoids may be contributing to both of these processes in a temporal or biphasic pattern that has not yet been completely deciphered (45). It does appear that the E-type prostaglandins have an effect on the vascular supply to irritated and inflamed tissues. This subclass of prostanoids causes a variety of vascular responses, including the mediation of vasodilation and local hyperemia (45,46,442,445).

The first association of prostanoids to the mechanism of ovulation was two decades ago when Labhsetwar (449,450) reported that prostaglandin $F_{2\alpha}$ could induce ovulation in several different laboratory animals. However, his studies did not establish whether this prostanoid was acting directly on the ovary or indirectly via stimulation of LH secretion. Within a year of these first reports, a number of investigators demonstrated that indomethacin, a well-known inhibitor of prostaglandin synthesis, could prevent ovulation in several different laboratory animals (451–455), and this antiovulatory action of indomethacin has been confirmed many times (176,205, 407,413,456–473). Shortly thereafter, LeMaire and coworkers (474–477) reported a marked increase in prostaglandins E and F in rabbit follicles during the ovulatory process, and this association between prostanoid synthesis and the ovulatory process has also been confirmed many times (176,458,459,468,478–495) (Fig. 23). The early work on prostaglandins and ovulation has been reviewed by LeMaire and Marsh (496) and by Armstrong (497).

Even though prostaglandins have been studied extensively, their importance and functions in ovulation have not been fully established. Most investigators have keyed on prostaglandin $F_{2\alpha}$ as the more prominent prostanoid in the mechanism of rupture, whereas several studies (455,469,488,498,499) have suggested that prostaglandin E_2 may be more important. After Marsh and coworkers (284–286) first demonstrated that LH induces cyclic AMP synthesis in mature ovarian follicles, several studies suggested that prostaglandins (particularly prostaglandin E_2) might function to augment this action of LH on follicular cyclic AMP formation (295,500). However, other reports indicated that prostaglandins *do not* mediate the action of LH on cyclic AMP synthesis (314,315,460,462,501,502), and it now seems rather clear that the reverse is the case (i.e., that cyclic AMP mediates LH-induced prostaglandin synthesis in ovulatory follicles) (286,292,312,313,469,503). Also, there is indirect evidence to suggest that protein kinase C might augment the production of different prostaglandins in granulosa cells (332–334). Initial reports indicated that the LH-induced signal transduction process in ovulatory follicles results in an increase in prostaglandin synthesis mainly in granulosa cells (480,482,504), but other studies have suggested that cells of the theca interna are equally important as a source of prostanoids during ovulation (505–507). More recent studies that applied the techniques of molecular biology have shown that the

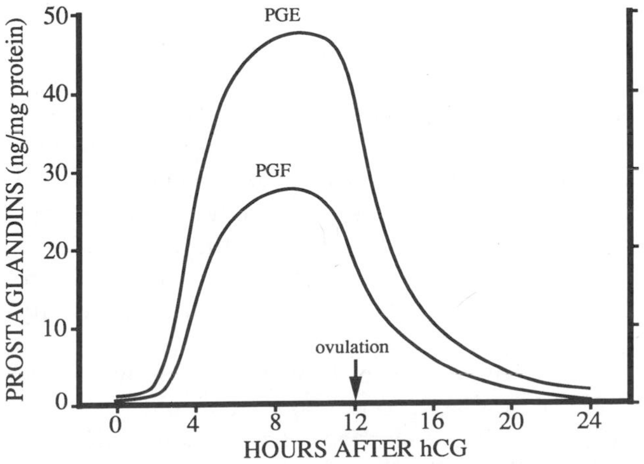

FIG. 23. Transient increase in prostaglandin E_2 (PGE) and prostaglandin $F_{2\alpha}$ (PGF) during ovulation in the gonadotropin-primed immature rat. (Adapted from references 176 and 494.)

granulosa, rather than the theca, is the principal follicular layer that responds to LH by forming mRNA for prostaglandin synthetase (375,377–379).

Considerable attention has been given to the relationship between follicular prostaglandin synthesis and steroid synthesis. The earliest studies indicated that prostaglandins do not mediate gonadotropin-induced steroidogenesis and luteinization of mature ovarian follicles (453,508), and this observation has been confirmed many times (193,292,404,458,460,463,472,473,492, 505,509–519). However, in contradiction, some investigators have reported that prostaglandins, especially of the E type, have at least a minor (520,521) and possibly a major (504,522–525) effect on ovarian progesterone synthesis during ovulation. Also, there are reports that prostaglandin E_2 stimulates progesterone synthesis in corpora lutea but that prostaglandin $F_{2\alpha}$ inhibits such steroid synthesis (526,527).

Several attempts have been made to determine whether ovarian prostaglandins are related either to the vasoactive agents that cause follicular hyperemia or to the proteolytic agents that have been implicated in the ovulatory process. However, most of these efforts have led to inconsistent or contradictory conclusions. Ovarian perfusion studies have shown that prostaglandin $F_{2\alpha}$ or histamine individually can induce ovulation (401,408), and these observations suggest a metabolic relationship between these two agents. Yet, perfusion studies have also shown that prostaglandin-induced ovulation is not blocked by antihistamines, and, conversely, histamine-induced ovulation is not blocked by inhibitors of prostaglandin synthesis. Therefore, prostaglandins and histamine do not appear to have an interdependent effect on ovulation (408). This conclusion is further corroborated by a report that histamine has no stimulatory effect on the synthesis of prostanoids (410). With regard to bradykinin, one report concludes that while this vasoactive agent can stimulate the production of F-type prostaglandins in perfused ovaries, such bradykinin-induced prostanoid synthesis is not essential for ovulation (423). Several other studies have found that bradykinin has little or no stimulatory effect on prostanoid synthesis (410,425). With regard to ovarian proteolytic activity, several experiments suggest that prostaglandins may be involved in the regulation of plasminogen activator production in the ovary (528,529), but other studies indicate that eicosanoids have a relatively insignificant effect on such proteolytic activity in the ovary (421,530–532), and this latter observation is consistent with the results from other experimental models (533). Similarly, some reports conclude that prostaglandins mediate follicular collagenolysis during ovulation (473,492,534), whereas other studies have arrived at the opposite conclusion (535,536). Also, there are studies that suggest that prostaglandins selectively inhibit collagen synthesis at the apex of developing follicles to facilitate rupture at this site (537) or that prostaglandins promote collagen synthesis and facilitate the healing process that sets in after ovulation (538,539).

Indomethacin has been very widely used in studies on ovulation because of its consistent inhibition of ovarian prostaglandin synthesis and follicular rupture (451–473). Such studies have also assessed the effect of indomethacin on changes in the ultrastructure of ovulatory follicles (152,465,529,540–542). Initial reports ignored the fact that this compound is a potent anti-inflammatory agent, but it is now clear that any strong nonsteroidal anti-inflammatory drug can inhibit ovulation (407,470). This group of drugs characteristically suppresses acute inflammatory reactions, whereas *steroidal* anti-inflammatory drugs (such as dexamethasone) have little effect on acute reactions, and they do not inhibit ovulation (407,543). Indomethacin is effective when administered either before or after initiation of the ovulatory process by gonadotropins, and it can be given almost up to the time of anticipated rupture (421,466,468). This wide "window" for its administration may be at least in part because the drug has a half-life of at least 5 h. Also, there is evidence that indomethacin has a very rapid effect on ovarian prostaglandin metabolism. When the drug is administered intravenously during the ovulatory process, the normally elevated levels of prostaglandins E_2 and $F_{2\alpha}$ decline significantly within 1 to 2 min (468). The inhibitory action of indomethacin on ovulation is dose-dependent rather than an all-or-none effect. One of the more peculiar features of indomethacin-induced blockage of ovulation is that the highest possible doses of the drug still permit the rupture of a limited number of follicles (468,543,544). Even more puzzling is the observation by Espey and coworkers (468,470,543,544) that relatively low doses of indomethacin that significantly inhibit the normal preovulatory rise in ovarian prostaglandins have no significant effect on the ovulation rate in rabbits and rats (Fig. 24). Conversely, cycloheximide can strongly inhibit ovulation while having minimal effect on follicular prostaglandin levels (370). This poor correlation between ovarian prostaglandin levels and ovulation rate has raised questions about the reliability of indomethacin as a "specific" inhibitor of prostanoid synthesis and about the importance of prostaglandins in the mechanism of ovulation.

As mentioned above, the implication of prostaglandins in the mechanism of ovulation has been based, in part, on the measurable increase in this group of compounds in follicular tissue during ovulation and on the capacity of indomethacinlike drugs to inhibit prostaglandin synthesis and ovulation. Also, there have been many efforts to confirm a role for prostaglandins by treating animals with prostanoids to either induce ovulation or to reverse the inhibitory action of agents such as indomethacin. However, the collective information from these ex-

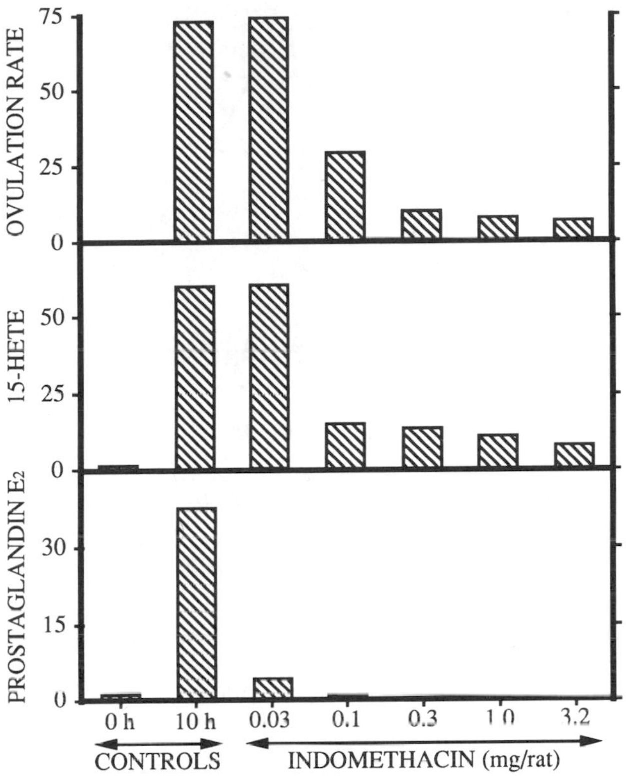

FIG. 24. Effect of graded doses of indomethacin on ovulation rate and ovarian 15-hydroxyeicosatetraenoic acid (15-HETE) and prostaglandin E_2 in the gonadotropin-primed immature rat. Ovulation rates are based on the number of ova in the oviducts at 24 hours after induction of the ovulatory process with hCG. The "controls" indicate the ovarian eicosanoid levels just before hCG and at 10 hours after hCG. The graded doses of indomethacin were administered at 1 hour after hCG. Note, in particular, that ovulation is not inhibited when prostaglandin E_2 is significantly reduced by 0.03 mg indomethacin/rat. (Adapted from references 472 and 544.)

periments has led to confusion rather than clarifying the role of these compounds in the mechanism of ovulation. Several earlier reports stated that mixtures of prostaglandins E_2 and $F_{2\alpha}$ can overcome the antiovulatory action of indomethacin (451,524), but a more recent study contradicts this observation (545). Other reports conclude that prostaglandin E_2 alone can promote follicular rupture (498,499) and can reverse the inhibitory effect of indomethacin (455,469,525,546,547), but these claims are neutralized by studies that show that prostaglandin E_2 cannot induce or restore ovulation that has been inhibited by indomethacin (404,517,541,548,549). Furthermore, several tests suggest that prostaglandin E_2 might actually inhibit ovulation (545,550). This same kind of confusion arises from studies with prostaglandin $F_{2\alpha}$ alone. There are reports that this prostanoid can induce ovulation in perfused ovaries (408,515,529) and can overcome the anti-ovulatory action of indomethacin (515,517,525,541,546,548,549,551–553) or ergocornine (554), yet several studies conclude that prostaglandin $F_{2\alpha}$ is relatively ineffective in restoring ovulation (498,547) and that ovulation can proceed unabated when production of this prostanoid is significantly inhibited by indomethacin (468,470,472,543,544) or prednisolone (555). Still, in support of a role for prostaglandin $F_{2\alpha}$, there are several claims that antisera to this prostanoid can inhibit ovulation (457,556). Other prostanoids, such as thromboxane (492) and prostacyclin (557), have also been implicated in ovulation, but their potential role(s) in ovulation remain even more uncertain than the E and F types of prostaglandins. In view of all this conflicting information, it may be important to keep in mind that the ovulatory process involves degradative events that lead to ovulation, yet a healing phase sets in shortly after the follicle ruptures (45,46). Therefore, it is possible that the prostanoids may contribute to either the damage, or the repair, or to both of these processes. In future studies, it might be worthwhile to examine the effects of prostaglandin E_1 on ovulation, because this agent is known to suppress collagenolytic activity and impair inflammatory-like processes (446,448).

Lipoxygenase Products

Arachidonic acid serves as a precursor not only for the prostaglandins but also for the biologically important leukotrienes and lipoxins that arise from different lipoxygenase-catalyzed reactions (346,558–560). The prostanoid products of arachidonic acid have been given the most attention in ovulation studies probably because of early development of radioimmunoassays for their measurement and because of the initial interest in the inhibition of prostaglandin synthesis and ovulation by indomethacin (545). However, in recent years, some attention has been given to the lipoxygenase products of arachidonate metabolism. Reich et al. (561,562) initially reported that nordihydroguaiaretic acid (NDGA) and 3 amino-1-(3-trifluro-methyphenyl)-2-pyrazoline hydrochloride (BW755c), two presumably specific inhibitors of lipoxygenase activity, can both block ovulation. The same laboratory has recently reported that esculetin and caffeic acid also inhibit the lipoxygenase pathway and ovulation (563). In support of these observations, Yoshimura et al. (564) found that NDGA blocks hCG-induced ovulation in a perfusion system. In contrast, Hellberg et al. (565) reported that NDGA and caffeic acid both actually increase, rather than decrease, the ovulation rate in the perfusion system. Also, several *in vivo* tests have failed to detect any antiovulatory action by NDGA (472,566). However, there is confirmation that BW755c can reduce the ovulation rate, but the specificity of this inhibitor is questionable (472). Likewise, there is now evidence that indomethacin, which has been commonly presumed to be a specific inhibitor of prostanoid synthesis, may also reduce the action of 12- and 15-

lipoxygenase activities (472,544,567,568). Therefore, the specificity of eicosanoid-inhibiting agents may not be as reliable as previously thought.

The family of enzymes that make up the lipoxygenases include 5-lipoxygenase for leukotriene formation and 15-lipoxygenase for lipoxin production (346, 472,494,543). These eicosanoids have been implicated in inflammatory reactions, where they may have diverse effects on blood vessels, leukocytes, glandular tissues, smooth muscles, and sensory neurons (346,560,569–571). Therefore, because the process of ovulation has been likened to an inflammatory reaction (45) and especially because it is not yet clear whether the prostaglandins contribute more to the degradative or to the reparative events in ovulatory follicles (545), it seems important to explore the potential role(s) of different lipoxygenase products in the ovulatory process. The significance of ovarian leukotrienes is presently the least understood. Several reports suggest that 5-lipoxygenase activity (which regulates leukotriene formation) increases only slightly during the first half of the ovulatory process and then declines long before follicles actually begin to rupture (494,543) (Fig. 25). Other reports claim a two- to fivefold increase in 5-lipoxygenase activity beginning midway through the process, with enzyme activity continuing to rise up to the time of ovulation (561, 562). Still, another study could not detect a significant rise in leukotrienes until after follicular rupture (566). More recent measurements of relatively stable metabolites of lipoxygenase enzymes have revealed a rather modest and transient increase in 5-hydroxyeicosatetraenoic acid (5-HETE) during the early stages of the ovulatory process, whereas 12- and 15-HETE increase over 12-fold by the time follicles begin to rupture (494,544) (Fig. 26). The ovulatory increase in 15-HETE can be inhibited in a dose-dependent manner by indomethacin (472,544) and

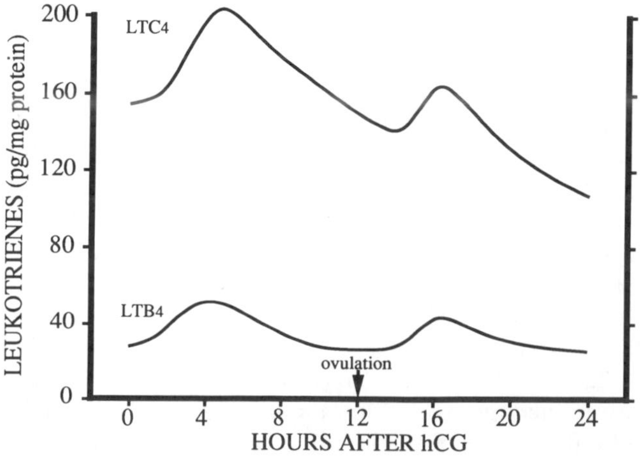

FIG. 25. Changes in ovarian leukotrienes B_4 (LTB_4) and C_4 (LTC_4) during ovulation in the gonadotropin-primed immature rat. (Adapted from reference 543.)

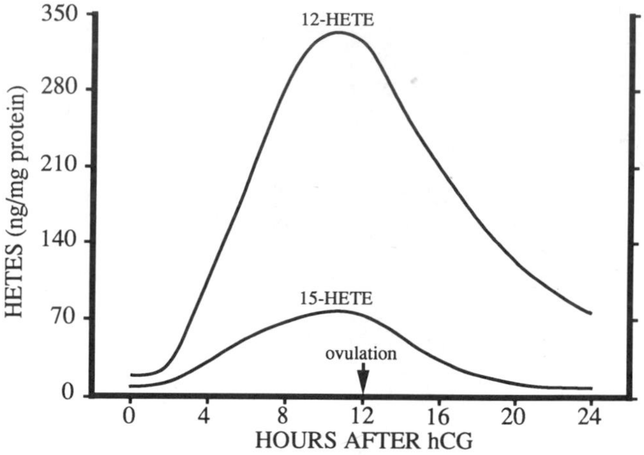

FIG. 26. Increase in 12-HETE and 15-HETE during ovulation in the gonadotropin-primed immature rat. (Adapted from references 494 and 544.)

by epostane (472). The optimum time to administer the latter agent to block ovulation is during the first one-third of the ovulatory process (494,572). Collectively, the present information indicates that the lipoxygenase products of arachidonate metabolism may contribute in some important way to the ovulatory process. There is preliminary evidence to suggest that they might stimulate progesterone and prostaglandin formation (260, 573) or promote collagenolysis in the follicle wall (534, 574,575), but their precise role(s) has not yet been established.

Ovarian Steroids

Early Studies

One of the first reviews of the role of steroids in mammalian ovulation was at a 1960 conference, "Control of Ovulation," which keyed on the ability of steroids to inhibit the gonadotropin surge that initiates ovulation (576). In the printed discussions following that report, Frederick Hisaw pointed out that a better understanding of steroid actions might provide answers to "the physiology of the follicle itself." The following year, at another conference, Hisaw (577) concluded his discussion by again stressing that the accumulation of progesterone over estrogen "might take a responsible part in the process of ovulation." He also noted that his thoughts were "supported by the observations of several workers who report the induction of experimental ovulation, *in vivo* and *in vitro,* in several species by the addition of progesterone—but not estrogen." A decade later, Lipner and co-workers (406,578), along with Ying and Greep (579), began confirming this hypothesis by demonstrating that agents such as aminoglutethimide and cyanoketone, which interfere with steroid synthesis, also inhibit ovulation. This earlier work has been reviewed by Lipner (15), Rondell (580), and LeMaire and Marsh (496). More recent reviews on the status of steroids in ovulation have been presented by Tsafriri et al. (35), Richards and Hedin (42), and Espey (36).

Response to the Gonadotropin Surge

It is common knowledge that mature ovarian follicles secrete a relatively large amount of estradiol, along with some androgens. It is also generally understood that synthesis of these steroids increases during the first several hours after the ovulatory process has been initiated by appropriate gonadotropic stimulation, but then it declines as ovarian progesterone synthesis begins to increase significantly (Fig. 27). As described earlier, this steroidogenic activity is probably mediated by cyclic AMP (284–299), and it may be influenced by the calcium/calmodulin system (320–322). Although this is the usual "textbook" account of ovarian steroid output during ovulation, the data in the literature reveal many variations in this basic pattern. The reported differences may be due, at least in part, to the fact that assorted studies have been conducted on different species of both immature and adult animals *in vivo* and *in vitro,* and the steroid assays have been performed either on whole ovaries, follicle walls, follicular fluids, ovarian perfusates, ovarian venous blood, or peripheral blood (36). Also, it is possible that some of the variability is related to the type and amount of gonadotropin(s) that were used to initiate the ovulatory process. For example, when relatively pure FSH has been given to induce ovulation in hypophysectomized hamsters (251) or in perfused rat ovaries (581), this hormone stimulated 17β-estradiol levels without initiating the usual ovulatory increase in progesterone. However, when LH or hCG is used in *in vivo* studies, the

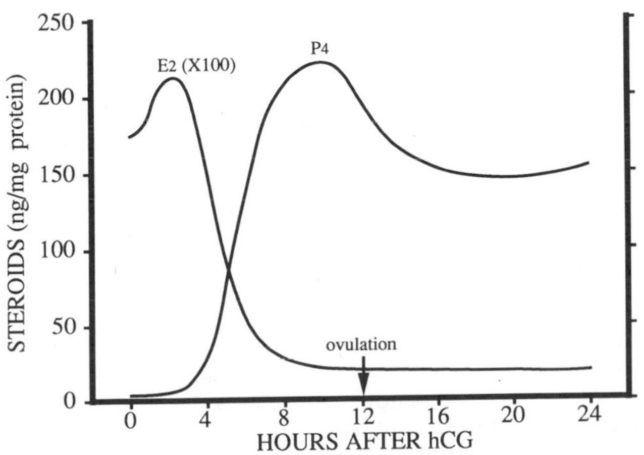

FIG. 27. Reciprocal relationship between ovarian 17β-estradiol (E_2) secretion and progesterone (P_4) during ovulation in the gonadotropin-primed immature rat. (Adapted from references 176 and 494.)

synthesis of 17β-estradiol, testosterone, androstenedione, and 17α-hydroxyprogesterone declines to negligible levels by the time of ovulation, while progesterone synthesis increases substantially within a few hours into the ovulatory process (169,171–176,494,572,582,583), although there may be some moderation in the output of this progestin near the time of follicular rupture (167, 170,192,492,494,523,573). Saidapur and Greenwald (173) reported that progesterone causes the decline in estrogen synthesis *in vivo,* whereas this progestin enhances 17β-estradiol production *in vitro* (173). This correlation seems to also hold true for *in vitro* perfusion studies, in which progesterone and 17β-estradiol are usually secreted in parallel (256,469,485,489,515,584–588). However, *in vitro* studies of "cultured" follicular tissue show a reciprocal relationship in the secretion of progesterone and 17β-estradiol (174,177,589–591). Higuchi and Espey (244) presented evidence that the differences in steroid secretion patterns of perfused ovaries versus nonperfused ovarian tissues may be related to adsorption properties of the perfusion system or to the large volume of the perfusion reservoir.

Sites of Steroid Synthesis

The sex steroids are synthesized along common pathways that originate with cholesterol (157). Cholesterol is converted into pregnenolone by cholesterol side-chain cleavage enzyme ($P450_{scc}$) and then into progesterone by 3β-hydroxysteroid dehydrogenase (3β-HSD). Subsequently, progesterone is converted into androgens, including testosterone, mainly by the actions of 17α-hydroxylase ($P450_{17\alpha}$) and C_{17-20}-lyase. Eventually, testosterone is converted into 17β-estradiol by the action of aromatase ($P450_{arom}$). Evidence of the cytochrome enzymes $P450_{scc}$, $P450_{17\alpha}$, and $P450_{arom}$ within experimental cells and tissues is commonly used to identify the sites of progesterone, androgen (especially androstenedione and testosterone), and estrogen (especially 17β-estradiol) synthesis. Such enzymes are frequently identified simply by the type(s) of steroids a given cell produces or, in recent years, by the detection of specific mRNA transcripts.

More than three decades ago, Falck (164) conducted histologic studies that led to the conclusion that both granulosa and theca interna cells might be required for estrogen formation. This hypothesis quickly lead to a number of modified versions of the so-called two-cell theory of granulosa-thecal cell steroidogenesis. Earlier accounts of the different forms of this theory have been summarized by Moor (592), Bjersing (29), and Ryan (593). Although it is difficult to establish a composite theory from these accounts, the preponderance of the earlier evidence seems to suggest that in mature ovarian follicles only thecal cells have the requisite enzymes for androgen synthesis, and therefore any estrogen synthesis by the granulosa is dependent on diffusion of precursor steroids from the theca interna. (However, this might be a "species variable" process [593,594]). The theory is supported by more recent evidence that the thecal cells of mature follicles produce substantially more androstenedione than granulosa cells (591,595–597), that granulosa cells lack $P450_{17\alpha}$ required for androgen formation (303,598), and that granulosa cells nevertheless generate 17β-estradiol (597). These observations do not rule out simultaneous estrogen synthesis by thecal cells, and, in fact, when aromatizable androgens are absent from the culture media, theca interna cells can produce substantially more estrogen than granulosa cells (591). Also, the "two-cell theory" is not supported by a report that granulosa cells have a potent $P450_{17\alpha}$ system (599). Furthermore, there are morphologic studies that describe the stratum granulosum as a steroidogenically inactive layer in mature follicles (32,132,600). In summary, the most relevant insight from these diverse studies is that a mature ovarian follicle is basically an androgen- and estrogen-secreting gland before its stimulation by an ovulatory surge in gonadotropin(s).

The pattern and sites of steroid synthesis during the ovulatory process have been established with greater certainty. There is a variety of physical (32,131,601,602) and chemical evidence (301–303,305,374,591,603,604) that ovulatory follicles lose their capacity to produce 17β-estradiol and that both the theca interna and the granulosa layers begin producing substantial amounts of progesterone. There is limited evidence to suggest that the granulosa might be the initial site of this progesterone synthesis, with thecal tissue contributing increasing amounts of this hormone as the follicle progresses toward luteinization (605). Also, there is evidence that interleukin-Iα might mediate this steroidogenic activity in the theca interna (606). In any event, once this cyclic AMP-dependent progesterone synthesis has been initiated, the $P450_{scc}$ gene no longer requires LH/hCG or cyclic AMP to sustain transcription of the enzymes for progesterone production (310,311,607). Also, as luteinization progresses, the granulosa cells develop the capacity to form $P450_{arom}$ mRNA and synthesize 17β-estradiol in a similar independent manner (608).

Importance of Steroids in Ovulation

The modest increase in synthesis of 17β-estradiol, androstenedione, and testosterone in follicles during the first hours of the ovulatory process raises the question of whether these steroids might contribute in some way to the ovulatory process. Ying and Greep (579) reported that when ovulation was blocked by aminoglutethimide, this inhibitory action could be overcome by the administration of exogenous 17β-estradiol or testosterone. However, several recent studies have concluded that 17β-estradiol is not essential for ovulation (588,609,610), and current opinion is that this steroid is not involved in the mechanism of ovulation. Presumably, androgens may not be important either, but there is negligible evidence to support this common assumption. It has also been suggested that the well-known decline in 17β-estradiol synthesis during the first one-half of the ovulatory process might be a prerequisite for follicular rupture (611). However, this idea is not supported by tests that show that the maintenance of artificially high 17β-estradiol levels throughout the ovulatory process does not impair normal ovulation rates (612).

Considerably more attention has been given to the role of progesterone in ovulation, because follicles produce substantial amounts of this steroid during the last one-half of the ovulatory process. A wide range of experimental approaches have provided evidence that progesterone has a significant role in ovulation (35,170, 275,370,406,472,492,523,524,572,578,580,613–617), but other studies appear to contradict this conclusion (586,588,618–623). Still, there is now little doubt that progesterone makes some important contribution to the events that lead to degradation of the follicle wall and rupture. One of the first experiments to firmly establish a role for this steroid was conducted by Snyder et al. (615), who clearly demonstrated that the inhibition of follicular steroidogenesis and ovulation by epostane could be overcome on treatment of the experimental animals with exogenous progesterone (Fig. 28). This observation was highly complementary to the less convincing evidence of Ying and Greep (579), who showed that progesterone could overcome the blockage of ovulation by aminoglutethimide. More recently, it has been established that the optimum time to administer epostane is during the hour preceding the ovulatory increase in progesterone synthesis, that this inhibitory agent severely impairs all steroidogenic activity in the ovary within a few minutes after its injection, that it causes only minor inhibition of follicular prostaglandin synthesis, that its antisteroidogenic effect is transient, and that ovarian progesterone synthesis approaches normal levels by the time inhibited follicles would have normally ruptured (472,494,572). Thus, these studies provide several potentially valuable bits of information about ovarian steroid metabolism during ovulation. First, they show that when ovarian steroid synthesis is blocked by a strong inhibitor like epostane (and probably by aminoglutethimide), the residual steroids rapidly dissipate from the ovarian tissue. This observation is significant because it indicates that exogenous steroids probably need to be administered in extraordinarily large quantities to mimic the locally high levels within the follicular cells where the specific hormones are normally produced. Second, the existing data reveal that there is a relatively narrow "temporal window" in the early stages of the

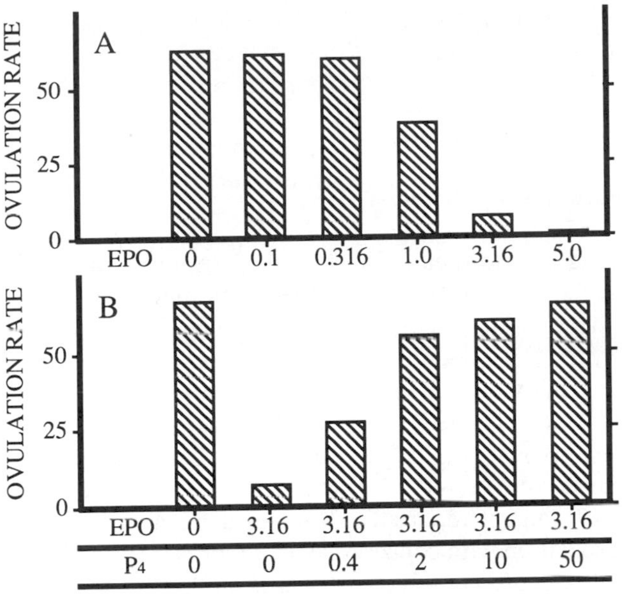

FIG. 28. Effects of epostane (EPO) and progesterone (P_4) on ovulation rate in gonadotropin-primed immature rats. Epostane inhibited ovulation in a dose-dependent manner when administered at 3 hours after hCG (frame A). The inhibitory action of epostane could be overcome by treating the animals with the designated amounts of P_4. (Adapted from reference 572.)

ovulatory process (i.e., at approximately the time when the progesterone levels begin to rise), during which it is vital for follicular steroidogenesis to proceed unabated. However, in contrast, it should be mentioned that when an animal such as the ewe is treated for an extended period of time with moderate amounts of epostane, this synthetic steroid increases the number of developing follicles and actually increases the ovulation rate (621,623,624).

Inhibitors of Steroidogenesis and Ovulation

As just indicated, it is now clear that epostane is an effective inhibitor of ovarian steroid synthesis and ovulation (35,472,494,572,615). Epostane is reportedly a competitive inhibitor of 3β-hydroxysteroid dehydrogenase (615,621,625), and therefore it probably exerts its antiovulatory action by blocking the conversion of pregnenolone into progesterone. In view of the effectiveness of this inhibitor, it is unfortunate that it is not readily available on the commercial market. A related synthetic steroid, trilostane, also inhibits 3β-hydroxysteroid dehydrogenase [–HSD] (626), and this compound can also inhibit ovulation (unpublished observation). However, trilostane is much weaker than epostane, and the quantities that are required to block ovulation make it less suitable as an experimental agent. Aminoglutethimide is probably a more practical antisteroidogenic and antiovulatory agent for experimental purposes. Since its original use by Lipner and Greep (578) and by Ying and Greep (579), at least one other laboratory has found it to be an effective agent for inhibiting ovulation *in vivo* (176), but it did not affect ovulation in an *in vitro* perfusion system (620). The inhibition of ovarian steroids by aminoglutethimide causes only a minor reduction in follicular prostaglandin synthesis (176,627).

Along with epostane and aminoglutethimide, the progesterone antagonist RU486 is in interesting antiovulatory agent. This agent has been used successfully in a number of instances to delay or block ovulation (35,628–634), and in only one known case did it fail to effect ovulation (622). Although RU486 has been assumed to act by blocking progesterone receptors in ovulatory follicles, one report has suggested that this agent may act at least in part by reducing the amount of LH release, but such an explanation cannot account for its antiovulatory effect in experimental animals in which the ovulatory process has been initiated by exogenous hCG (630,632). Another possibility is that RU486 may inhibit 3β-HSD, based on recent evidence that isolated follicles that have been treated with this agent lose some of their capacity to convert pregnenolone into progesterone (634). Finally, besides these inhibitory agents, a variety of other substances reportedly interfere with progesterone action and block ovulation (370,613,614,616, 635–637), and in at least two of these cases, the inhibitory effect was overcome by exogenous progesterone (616,636).

Luteinized Unruptured Follicles

There is ample evidence that gonadotropin-stimulated follicles that have been exposed to ovulation-inhibiting doses of indomethacin continue to produce normal amounts of progesterone (176,193,292, 312,460,472,473,492,516,519), and the unruptured follicles undergo luteinization (453,458,463,508,510,511, 514,517,518,542). There is also evidence that indomethacin treatment fails to affect established luteal function (513) or to shorten the normal length of pseudopregnancy (509), although progesterone secretion by luteal tissue might be somewhat less than normal after indomethacin (521). Occasionally, unruptured follicles spontaneously luteinize in the absence of indomethacin (638), and such anovulatory luteinization could be the consequence of an inadequate gonadotropin surge (639).

This phenomenon of luteinized unruptured follicles, which has been studied most extensively by Armstrong and co-workers (458,460,463,508,510), provides several valuable pieces of information about the mechanism of ovulation. First, the phenomenon makes it perfectly clear that the luteinization process that is normally initiated by a gonadotropin surge can proceed virtually unabated even when a stimulated follicle does not physically rupture. Second, the phenomenon makes it apparent that, although ovulation and luteinization are both normally initiated by the same gonadotropic stimulus, the two processes can be at least partially separated from one another. However, when this information is coupled with the fact that the ovulatory process is blocked by agents that inhibit follicular progesterone synthesis (i.e., that inhibit the central event of the luteinization process), the existing data strongly suggest that follicular rupture is fundamentally dependent on the steroidogenic activity that takes place during the early stages of luteinization.

Other Considerations

Several other features of steroid metabolism have received only limited attention but nevertheless may be worthy of further examination in future investigations. First, several reports suggest some kind of relationship between PRL and progesterone. It has been noted that progesterone stimulates PRL release (640). However, it has been reported that PRL inhibits ovarian progesterone synthesis and ovulation (275,641), yet some studies conclude that the antiovulatory action of PRL does not influence ovarian progesterone secretion (276,277). Second, although it is quite clear that prostanoids have negligible influence on follicular steroid metabolism, there are several reports that arachidonic acid (642) or lipoxygenase products of arachidonic acid (472,494,572,573) might influence ovarian steroid metabolism during ovulation. Now that more convenient methods exist for assaying these eicosanoids, the elucidation of their contribution(s) to the mechanism of ovulation should be forthcoming. Third, many years ago, Pincus and Merrill (576) pointed out that "one of the possibilities very much overlooked is that some of these (sex) steroids are mitosis-stimulating and others mitosis-inhibiting," and more recently, Clarke and Sutherland (643) reviewed the mechanisms by which progestins affect cell proliferation. Therefore, it might be worthwhile to examine in more detail the potential relationships between the ovulatory increase in progesterone synthesis and the common growth factors and cytokines. In this regard, progesterone might influence not only cellular proliferation within the luteinizing theca interna and granulosa, but it is also possible that this steroid might regulate the activation and proliferation of fibroblasts within the connective tissue layers of ovulatory follicles (32). Last, progesterone may play an *anti-inflammatory* role in arthritis (45,644) and in other models of inflammation (645,646). Therefore, although it is now quite apparent that progesterone contributes to the degradative events within the follicle during the early stages of the ovulatory process, it is still possible that this steroid might have some role in regulating the healing process that sets in shortly after ovulation (36,44).

Proteolytic Enzymes

Plasminogen Activator

As described earlier in this chapter, a mature ovarian follicle contains a tenacious collagen matrix at the apex where rupture occurs, and it is generally thought that proteolytic enzymes weaken this connective tissue at the time of ovulation. Plasminogen activator has been given considerable attention as a contributing agent in this process because this serine protease has been implicated in many types of tissue degradation and cellular movement (647), and it reportedly is secreted from fibroblasts in association with collagenase (648,649). In 1975, Beers et al. (650–652) conducted the first studies on the role of PA in ovulation. In initial experiments, it appeared as though FSH might be the principal gonadotropin that regulated ovarian PA activity, but now there is evidence that FSH (252,384,528,653–658), LH/hCG (276,421, 531,532,655,659–663), or GnRH (383,384,663) can promote follicular PA activity, whereas PRL reportedly inhibits the expression of this enzyme (276,277,664). The active gonadotropins mainly promote tissue-type PA activity rather than urokinase-type PA. The stimulatory effect of gonadotropins is probably mediated by cyclic AMP (651,652,655,657), although there is one study that suggests that the use of phosphodiesterase inhibitors to increase cyclic AMP levels may actually depress PA activity rather than increase it (665).

Most of the studies on ovarian PA activity have been conducted on granulosa cells (382–384,528,650–652, 655,657,658) or the closely related cumulus mass (656, 659). It has been reported that this enzyme is mainly in the granulosa layer (666), although molecular techniques have failed to find tPA mRNA in gonadotropin-stimulated granulosa (386). Other work indicates that the theca interna may also contain a significant amount of PA (660,663,667,668). In fact, some studies conclude that PA activity is distributed throughout most of the cells in the follicle wall and that it may be especially abundant in fibroblasts in the apical area where rupture normally occurs (661,667,669). In general, it appears that PA activity increases just before or very close to the expected time of ovulation (421,531,660,663,667,669–674) (Fig. 29), although there is one report that maximum activity is expressed during the first one-third of the ovulatory process and then declines (662).

Unfortunately, the highly relevant experiments that assess the effects of eicosanoids and steroids on ovarian PA activity have yielded conflicting results. In their original studies, Strickland and Beers (652) found that prostaglandins of the E type stimulated granulosa cells to pro-

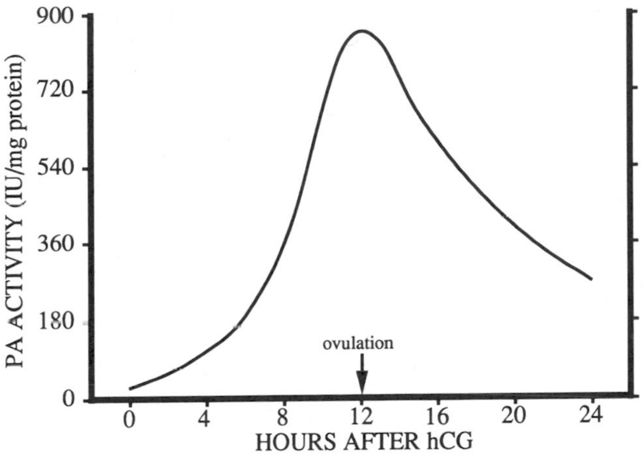

FIG. 29. Increase in ovarian plasminogen activator (PA) activity during ovulation in the gonadotropin-primed immature rat. (Adapted from reference 421.)

duce PA, whereas prostaglandins of the F type were without effect, yet Miyazaki et al. (529) recently reported that prostaglandin $F_{2\alpha}$ promotes PA activity in the follicle wall during ovulation. Similar contradiction is found on comparing one report that indomethacin suppresses PA secretion (528) with several other studies that claim that doses of indomethacin that significantly inhibit ovulation have no apparent effect on ovarian PA activity (421,530–532). The results from studies with steroids are equally confusing. Earlier experiments concluded that none of the principal ovarian steroids affected PA activity (652). More recent studies have suggested that 17β-estradiol may be especially important in inducing granulosa cell PA activity, whereas progesterone and testosterone appear to have only a minor role (35,532,658,666). Other reports suggest that testosterone (653) and progesterone (421,636) may be at least partially responsible for the expression of ovarian PA activity, whereas still another study suggests that ovarian prostaglandin synthesis may not be essential to the expression of this activity by granulosa cells (654). Experiments with a variety of agents that reportedly are specific inhibitors of PA activity have not clarified the above confusion about the role of this enzyme in ovulation (531,675–677). Thus, in summary, the nature of ovarian PA activity and its relationship to ovarian eicosanoids and steroids in the ovulatory process are not yet fully understood.

Kallikrein and Kinin-Generating Activity

Kallikreins are a family of serine proteases that are usually activated by tissues that have become irritated or inflamed (678–681). Besides their capacity to generate kinins, as discussed earlier in this chapter, kallikreins also convert procollagenase into its active form (682,683). In view of this action of kallikreins, 15 years ago Espey (684) suggested that such enzymes might be involved in the activation of procollagenase in ovulatory follicles. However, only a few experiments have been carried out on this potentially important protease. Espey et al. (420) used a relatively nonspecific chromogenic peptide substrate in studies that showed that follicular kallikrein activity may increase about sixfold in gonadotropin-primed immature rats (420) (Fig. 30). This ovulatory increase in activity is moderately (but, significantly) reduced by indomethacin treatment (413,420,421), which suggests that it might be related to eicosanoid metabolism in the follicle. Ovarian kallikrein activity is also suppressed by epostane treatment, and this inhibitory action can be reversed by treatment of the experimental animals with exogenous progesterone (421).

More precise information about the contribution of ovarian kallikrein activity to the ovulatory process may be forthcoming from new studies based on the methods of molecular biology. For example, Clements et al. (381) recently found that the granulosa cells of gonadotropin-treated rats express mRNA for several kallikrein gene family members, and further work should reveal which of these kallikreinlike enzymes are responsible for the ovarian kallikrein activity that peaks at about the same time as the onset of follicular rupture. Also, there is evidence that the subunits of nerve growth factor and epidermal growth factor (EGF) have peptide sequences that are similar to tissue kallikrein (428,685), and therefore it might be worthwhile in future studies to assess whether the internalization of proteolytic fragmentation of growth factor/receptor complexes might generate kallikrein activity during ovulation (44). Also, it might be worthwhile to examine whether several other novel proteases that have been implicated in the ovulatory process

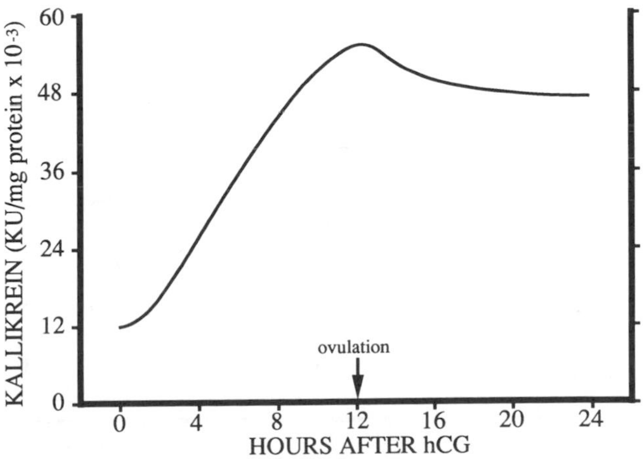

FIG. 30. Increase in ovarian kallikrein activity during ovulation in the gonadotropin-primed immature rat. (Adapted from references 420 and 421.)

(686,687) happen to belong to the kallikrein family of enzymes.

Collagenolytic Activity

The thecal layers of the follicle wall contain a substantial amount of collagenous connective tissue, and there can be little doubt that such tissue must be significantly weakened for a follicle to rupture under the force of a relatively modest intrafollicular pressure of approximately 20 mm Hg. The first evidence that collagenolytic enzymes might be involved in this process came about when Espey and Lipner (13) injected minute amounts of bacterial collagenase into rabbit follicles *in situ* and observed rupture of the follicles only a few minutes after the injections. At about this same time, there were several reports containing indirect (105) and direct (65) evidence that the tenacity of the follicle wall declines during the ovulatory process. Shortly thereafter, it became apparent that mammalian collagenase, elastase, trypsin, and chymotrypsin also can significantly reduce the tensile strength of the follicle wall (116). Morphologic studies also showed that the collagen and cellular elements of the follicle wall dissociate and that the wall becomes thinner at the apex as the time of ovulation approaches (64,126,688). However, initial attempts by Espey and Rondell (117,118) to measure an increase in ovarian collagenolytic activity were unsuccessful. Similarly, Parr (689) was unable to detect any neutral protease activity in ovulatory rat follicles, nor could he find any collagen fibers in the follicle wall (128). On the basis of this information, he concluded that rupture of the ovarian follicle was not mediated by collagenolytic enzymes. To the contrary, it is now clear that the thecal tissue in rat follicles *does* contain significant amounts of collagen (150), and several additional efforts have been made to identify the nature of enzymes that might degrade this connective tissue during ovulation. The earlier work on ovarian proteolytic and collagenolytic activity has been summarized in several reviews (16,18).

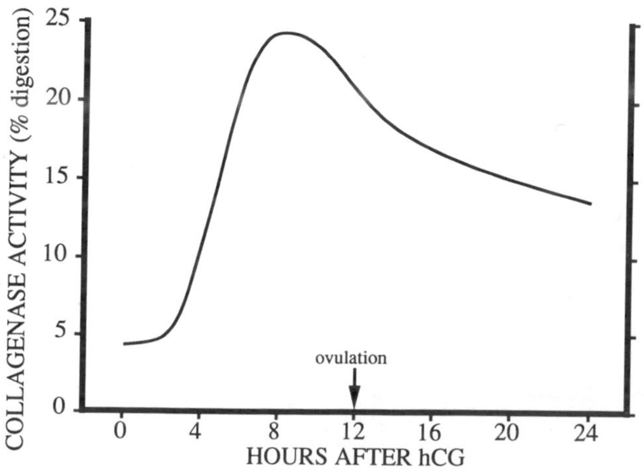

FIG. 31. Increase in ovarian collagenolytic activity during ovulation in the gonadotropin-primed immature rat. (Adapted from reference 690.)

More recent efforts to detect follicular collagenolytic activity have used assays based on the digestion of reconstituted collagen gels (18), ^{3}H-labeled collagen (120,534,676,690,691) (Fig. 31), synthetic peptide substrates (119,692,693), or substrates for gelatinase and proteoglycanase (694). Collectively, the results from these different studies indicate there is a substantial increase in ovarian collagenolytic enzymes during the ovulatory process. Complementary to these findings, Reich et al. (385) recently reported the detection of an ovarian mRNA for collagenase that increases 25-fold during ovulation. Curry and co-workers (387,388,695) reported that such activity might be locally regulated at least in part by tissue-derived inhibitors of metalloproteinases (TIMPs), which are produced by follicular cells in increasing amounts during the ovulatory process, and this observation has been supported by several other studies (385,696). Also, there is evidence that the serum antiprotease α2-macroglobulin might function in ovulation to restrict collagenolytic activity to the vicinity of the mature follicles that are destined to rupture (386,387,697). Further support for the hypothesis that collagenolytic enzymes are important in ovulation come from additional studies that demonstrate that other agents known to inhibit collagenase also inhibit ovulation (698–701). There are no data on whether these different inhibitory substances can effect the relaxin-induced collagenolytic activity that has been associated with ovulation (536,702,703).

The cytologic origin of ovarian collagenolytic activity has not been firmly established. Several studies suggest that such enzyme activity arises in the granulosa (385,692), whereas other work provides evidence that thecal fibroblasts may be the principal source (5,151, 153,154). It is possible that the enzymes that degrade the follicle wall arise from more than one cell type, but the fibroblast in particular must be considered as a probable source because it has been recognized for some time now that such connective tissue cells are not only the origin of collagen but also of the proteolytic enzymes that degrade this tenacious extracellular material (648,649,704–706). The cytologic structures that have been most frequently associated with ovarian collagenase activity are the multivesicular structures that protrude from the surface of follicular fibroblasts (5,151,153,154) and the limited number of lysosomes that are present within different cells in the follicle (29,64,142,707,708).

The relationship between collagenolytic activity and ovarian eicosanoid production is not clearly defined. A variety of experiments have demonstrated that indomethacin has an inhibitory effect on such proteolytic activity in gonadotropin-stimulated ovarian tissues, and this information suggests that eicosanoids may mediate the degradation of ovulatory tissue (18,152,385, 473,492,534,574). However, several other reports have concluded that prostaglandins have no effect on ovarian collagenolytic activity (535,536). This contradiction is not resolved by results obtained from other experimental models because, for example, one report claims that prostaglandin synthesis by bone cells may mediate collagenase activity (709), another concludes that prostaglandins of the E type enhance (but do not induce) macrophage collagenase production (710), and a more recent report shows that prostaglandin E_1 (but not E_2 or $E_{2\alpha}$) can selectively reduce collagenase mRNA levels in a dose-dependent fashion in rabbit synoviocytes and human fibroblasts (448).

With regard to the relationship between ovarian collagenolytic activity and steroid hormones, there is only limited information. Several studies have suggested that progesterone may have a negligible effect on such activity (18,536). Other reports have pointed to a positive correlation between the ovulatory increase in progesterone levels and the local production of TIMP by follicles (386,695). Besides this information, it is worth noting that progesterone is a potent inhibitor of collagenase expression by the uterus (711,712), the pubic symphysis ligament (713), and macrophages (714). In this same line, Espey (44) recently suggested that progesterone may have functions in the ovary that are comparable with the actions of this steroid in the uterus. Specifically, progesterone acts by inducing the formation of uteroglobin, which inhibits phospholipase A_2 activity and the metabolism of arachidonic acid in a manner that suppresses the proteolytic activity characteristic of inflammatory reactions (715,716). Thus, it is possible that, after exerting its acute pro-ovulatory effect during the first half of the ovulatory process, progesterone may impose a secondary effect that causes the decline in ovarian eicosanoid metabolism and proteolytic (including collagenolytic) activity within a few hours after a follicle ruptures. That is to say, the chronic effect of progesterone on reproductive tissues might be comparable with the anti-inflammatory actions of glucocorticoids that are mediated by lipocortins in other tissues (717–719).

Other Considerations

Follicular Inflammation

During the past 12 years, much of the work on ovulation has keyed on assessment of the hypothesis that ovulation is an inflammatory process. This idea that the ovulatory surge in gonadotropin induces an inflammatory reaction in mature follicles arose from a long pedigree of studies that reached maturity by the end of the 1970s. For more than a century, hyperemia and related vascular changes have been recognized as the cardinal signs of inflammation (45). In comparison, follicular hyperemia at the time of ovulation has been noted for at least one-half a century (8), and some of the more recent studies on this topic have been summarized in an earlier section of this chapter that keyed on the vascular system of the theca interna. Also, as early as 1951, Burr and Davies (180) noted the swelling and edema that occur in association with the ovulatory hyperemia in rabbit follicles. Likewise, Bjersing and Cajander (122) and Motta et al. (140) mentioned edema as a relevant factor in the final decomposition of ovulatory follicles. Historically, it is interesting to note that 32 years ago John Hammond, Jr., while comparing a follicle with the formation of a blister during discussions at a symposium on ovulation (720), stated, "You burn yourself, and a fluid is liberated from the blood vessels of the dermis, yet in like manner, the fluid accumulates in the epithelium of the epidermis." Thus, at least three decades ago, the ovulatory process was passingly compared with an inflammatory reaction.

Two of the more significant contributions to the "inflammation hypothesis" arose in the early 1970s when simultaneous experiments by innumerable investigators showed that prostaglandins increase markedly in ovulatory follicles and that indomethacin can block prostaglandin synthesis and ovulation. That work set the stage for some of the conclusions drawn from a series of studies by Parr (128,689,721). In his morphologic study, Parr (128) noticed that the walls of follicles about to rupture contained fibrin, which is commonly present in inflamed tissues. He coupled this observation with the previously overlooked fact that prostaglandins are an integral part of inflammatory reactions and that indomethacin is a potent anti-inflammatory agent. However, he did not consider the ovulatory process to be a complete inflammatory reaction. Instead, he concluded that ovarian prostaglandins might contribute to "the early vascular phase of an inflammatory response" but that the "inflammation never progresses to the cellular stage" (17). Consequently, he was unable to explain "the weakening of follicular tissue which precedes rupture" (17), especially because he concluded in several reports that "ovulation is not mediated by a proteolytic enzyme" (689) or by "a collagenase" (17). The latter deduction arose from his erroneous report that the thecal layers of the rat follicle do not contain any collagen for a collagenolytic enzyme to digest (128,150). Perhaps because of these erroneous deductions, Parr's highly relevant observations of inflammatorylike changes in ovulatory follicles received little attention, except in several review papers (18,19). Even Parr himself may not have realized the significance of his observations about inflammatorylike changes in ovulatory follicles, because in the concluding remarks of his review on ovulation, he did not mention this topic but instead stressed that future studies should key on "the possible role of ascorbic acid in follicle rupture" (17)—a point that had been made repeatedly throughout the 1970s (16,18,19,116). Several years later, Espey (45) reviewed the existing literature on ovulation and inflammation and concluded that both the vascular and the cellular (i.e., biochemical) changes in ovulatory follicles were comparable with an inflammatory reaction. A recent reassessment of this hypothesis summarizes a significant portion of the work that has been conducted on the mechanism of ovulation during the past 12 years and outlines the relationships among common mediators of inflammatory reactions (46) (Fig. 32).

Fibroblast Proliferation

As early as 1919, Corner (60) reported that the theca externa "is composed chiefly of collagenous fibrils and their associated fibroblasts." The existence of such connective tissue cells in the follicle wall has been confirmed by many other studies (32,64,95,128,144,152,222). However, the follicular fibroblasts have been given little attention in biochemical studies of the ovulatory process, probably because these cells are embedded in the collagen layers of the follicle and are relatively inaccessible to isolation compared with cells of the granulosa and theca interna. Nevertheless, the potentially prominent role of fibroblasts in the mechanism of ovulation should not be overlooked. It has been well established that fibroblasts produce collagenase and regulate collagen metabolism (704–706,709). Therefore, it is quite possible that the final stages of the ovulatory process involve activation and proliferation of the thecal fibroblasts. In this regard, it is interesting that, in his early observations of the morphologic changes during ovulation, Corner (60) also noted "just before rupture there are many mitotic figures in the cells of the theca externa, but only occasional signs of cell division in the theca interna and the granulosa."

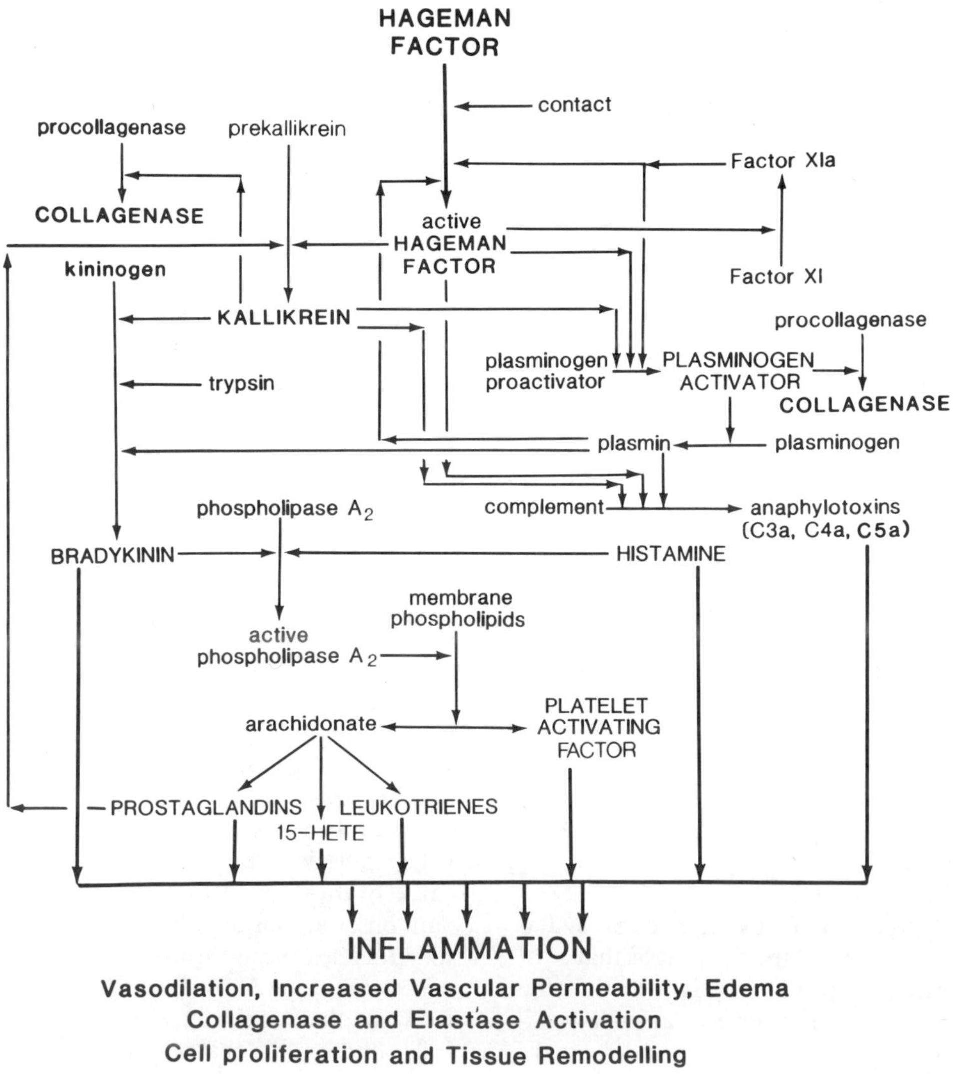

FIG. 32. Relationships among some of the common components of the inflammation "cascade." (From reference 46, with permission.)

Espey (32) also reported such mitotic activity and suggested that "the fibroblasts transform into actively proliferating cells and become quite long." O'Shea et al. (722) said that after ovulation the proliferating fibroblasts migrate "from their original sites into the deeper, granulosa-derived areas of the luteal tissue." Therefore, because the thecal fibroblasts are embedded in a framework of collagen, it seems almost inevitable that these cells must produce enzymes to weaken the extracellular matrix around them before they can migrate toward the luteinizing granulosa. The cytologic scenario may not be too unlike what happens in bone matrix, where, in response to low calcium levels and parathyroid hormone secretion, osteoblastic cells (which are closely related to fibroblasts) become motile and secrete collagenase to dissolve the connective tissue matrix in which bone salts are precipitated (157,723,724).

The important point is that within the mechanism of ovulation it appears quite likely that the thecal fibroblasts undergo transformation from a quiescent resting state to a motile proliferating state, yet there is virtually no information about the biochemical events that initiate this highly significant activity within the densest connective tissue in the follicle wall. In other experimental models, there are earlier reports that prostaglandins influence the proliferation of fibroblasts (725–728), with some evidence that prostaglandin $F_{2\alpha}$ in particular might initiate this activity (729). This information suggests that the fibroblasts in ovarian follicles might also be activated by the eicosanoids that increase so markedly during the ovulatory process. The prostaglandins could be generated by cells of the granulosa and/or theca interna, or they could arise from within the fibroblasts themselves (730). It is also possible that indomethacin and other nonsteroidal anti-inflammatory agents might inhibit ovulation by blocking such prostaglandin-induced activation of follicular fibroblasts. Espey (46) recently suggested that indomethacin may act by inhibiting "the transformation of the thecal fibroblasts from a dormant, resting state to a motile, proliferating stage" and that "without sufficient movement of the fibroblasts, ultimate dissociation of the thecal collagen may not occur." There is morphologic evidence to support this hypothesis (152).

Other ovarian factors that could influence proliferation of the thecal fibroblasts are steroid hormones (because fibroblasts contain sex steroid receptors [731–734]), cytokines such as interleukin 1 and lymphokines (735–737), proteolytic enzymes such as plasmin, trypsin, chymotrypsin, and elastase (649), and growth factors such as EGF and platelet-derived growth factor (PDGF), which are associated with the expression of protooncogenes to exert local mitogenic effects and promote collagenolytic activity (723,738–740). Also, blood serum contains factors that promote the proliferation of fibroblasts, and this relevant fact has been recognized for some time (741). More recent work has concentrated on identification of the genes that are expressed by serum-stimulated fibroblasts and some of these include the *fos, jun,* and *myc* proto-oncogenes (742–744). These actions of serum are particularly interesting because they raise the question of whether the gonadotropin-induced increase in vascular permeability and hyperemia (that were described earlier in this chapter) might permit serum factors to diffuse into the connective tissue layers of the follicle and transform the fibroblasts into proliferating cells.

Lastly, as mentioned earlier, fibroblasts transform into myofibroblasts under certain circumstances such as the development of granulation tissue in chronically inflamed areas (66,94,745). Ovarian luteal tissue has been compared with granulation tissue (45), but no experiments have been conducted to determine whether some of the fibroblasts in the follicle do indeed develop into myofibroblasts in the corpus luteum. The identification of actin and myosin contractile proteins alone will not confirm such a transition because contractile proteins such as actin and myosin are natural components of motile cells such as fibroblasts (68), and the genes for these proteins are expressed when quiescent fibroblasts are stimulated with serum (743). However, there is a recent report that the expression of a single gene may be all that is necessary to convert fibroblasts into myofibroblasts (746), and evidence of such expression in connective tissues in ovulatory or postovulatory follicles might help to clarify this issue.

Growth Factors and Ovulation

Growth factors are hormonelike peptides that have predominantly paracrine and autocrine functions in promoting mitogenic activity in local tissue proliferation and remodeling (323,747), such as that which occurs in the transformation of an ovarian follicle into a corpus luteum (44). In recent years, there has been considerable interest by Hsueh, Adashi, and others (393,657,748–751) in the action of growth factors on ovarian folliculogenesis. It has been suggested that ovarian thecal cells produce EGF and transforming growth factor-α (TGF-α), which exert a paracrine effect to promote the proliferation of granulosa cells in growing follicles (389,752). In comparison, it has been suggested that granulosa cells are the site of production, reception, and action of insulinlike growth factors (IGFs) (750), with activity being regulated by gonadotropins and local steroids (392). However, the follicular source of fibroblast growth factor (FGF) is uncertain, but it may not originate from granulosa cells (390,391,753). The potential role of growth factors in ovulation is especially intriguing because there is evidence these mitogenic agents may be involved in inflammatory processes (754–761), progesterone formation and other steroidogenic activity (338,393,749,750, 762–764), protease (including collagenase) synthesis

(384,723,738,739), angiogenesis (391,753,765,766), and possibly in prostanoid synthesis (767,768), all of which are events that are characteristic of ovulatory follicles.

Leukocytes and Ovulation

In inflamed tissues, the insulted cells produce chemotactic agents that attract a variety of leukocytes and migratory cells into the area as a line of defense against possible infection (45,46). There is also a local release of histamine, eicosanoids, PAF, and other vasoactive agents to increase the blood flow to the affected area. In some instances, the polymorphonuclear leukocytes that infiltrate the area may release stores of proteolytic enzymes including plasminogen activator, elastase, collagenase, and other neutral proteases that can soften the connective tissue elements and enhance proteolytic and phagocytic action against any invading microorganisms. Because these are physical and chemical changes that also occur during ovulation, some consideration has been given to the possible contributions of leukocytes and related cells in the ovulatory process. As early as 1958, Zachariae et al. (769) noted that basophils migrate into the ovary at the time of ovulation. Since that time, there has been additional direct and indirect evidence that different leukocytes, along with thrombocytes, might increase in ovulatory follicles (32,202,473,770–774). In support of these data, there are several recent reports that ovulatory follicles produce a chemotactic factor that attracts leukocytes into the area (473,775), and Murdoch and McCormick (772) may have isolated some such chemoattractant peptides. Also, Hellberg et al. (776) reported that the addition of leukocytes to the perfusion medium supplying rat ovaries slightly but significantly increased the number of LH-induced ovulations *in vitro.* However, Murdoch and Steadman (777) recently found that prednisolone-induced eosinopenia failed to impair ovulation in ewes, and they concluded that such leukocytes may not contribute to the mechanism of ovulation. Quantitative studies on the temporal and spacial distribution of these types of cells in mature follicles during ovulation would help elucidate the extent to which they might be involved in the degradation of the follicle wall. Although leukocytes might make some contribution to the process, it still appears more likely that the thecal fibroblasts are the principal source of proteolytic enzyme activity during ovulation.

OVERVIEW OF THE OVULATORY PROCESS

In a final analysis of the above information about ovulation, it is important, first, to key on luteinization as an ovarian process. When an ovulatory surge in gonadotropin(s) stimulates a mature ovarian follicle, the principal cellular response is luteinization of the theca interna and granulosa layers of the follicle wall. That is to say, the basic function of luteinizing hormone is, as the name implies, to initiate the luteinization process. The early events of membrane signal transduction generate cyclic AMP in the target cells, and this second messenger is an important mediator of the events that follow. Less is known about other second messengers and the protein kinases that may be generated during the early stages of luteinization, but it is becoming more and more evident that the signal transduction processes lead to a significant increase in cytochrome $P450_{scc}$ that promotes a substantial elevation in progesterone synthesis. Simultaneously, because of the rising progesterone levels or other unknown factors, there is a reciprocal decline in cytochromes $P450_{17\alpha}$ and $P450_{arom}$, and ovarian androgen and estrogen secretion drops quite sharply. Once $P450_{scc}$ mRNA has been expressed, cyclic AMP-independent mechanisms are established and progesterone synthesis and luteinization proceed as a single, self-perpetuating process. The luteinization process is virtually unaffected by antiovulatory agents such as indomethacin and is only transiently attenuated by antiovulatory agents such as epostane. Thus, it is difficult to interrupt the intrinsic, constitutive changes that are established during the earliest stages of luteinization. Furthermore, it is now rather clear that rupture of a follicle is not a prerequisite for luteal formation.

It is also now evident that a number of inflammatory-like changes occur in stimulated follicles during the early stages of the luteinization process. In particular, it is apparent that follicles become hyperemic within a few hours after the gonadotropin surge. This hyperemia is probably mediated by vasoactive agents such as histamine, kinins, prostaglandins, and possibly lipoxygenase products of arachidonate metabolism. The specific relationship between ovarian eicosanoid formation and progesterone synthesis has not been deciphered, but on the basis of the simultaneous onset of eicosanogenic and steroidogenic activities, it would appear that there is some interdependence in these two major metabolic events in the follicle. Also, there are several reports that serine proteases and metalloproteinases such as plasminogen activator, kallikrein, and collagenase activity increase in follicles as the luteinization process progresses. However, the interrelationships between these proteolytic enzymes and the eicosanoids and steroids mentioned above have not been worked out either. Nevertheless, more and more knowledge about the timing of these events is being gained in certain experimental models such as the gonadotropin-primed immature rat, and it should be only a matter of time before molecular techniques and other methods are successful in deciphering the relationships among ovarian progesterone, prostanoid, and protease metabolism.

In essence, the ovulatory process that has been referred to throughout this chapter is actually the first 10 to 40 h (depending on the species of mammal) of the luteinization process. Recognition of this duality, and separation of the two processes, may be important in further efforts to unravel the remaining questions about the mechanisms of ovulation. Realization of this duality raises the possibility that all the events of the luteinization process may not be essential to the ovulatory process, and vice versa. The existing data make it apparent that the early stages of progesterone synthesis (i.e., the principal aspect of the luteinization process) are necessary for ovulation but that progesterone synthesis can be inhibited during the second half of the ovulatory process without blocking ovulation. However, it is also now apparent that eicosanoid metabolism is required almost up to the time that a follicle ruptures, yet luteinization can occur in the absence of any elevation in ovarian eicosanoids.

In the past several decades, considerable knowledge has been gained about the timing of the biochemical events that occur during the ovulatory phase of the luteinization process. Although this "temporal" analysis of the ovulatory process has been very informative, it now may be appropriate to concentrate more on "spatial" analyses of the events of ovulation. That is to say, it may be important to key more on identifying the cellular locations of the different metabolic changes that arise during the ovulatory phase. It seems obvious enough that the principal events of luteinization are centered in the stratum granulosum and the theca interna (along with the vascular endothelial cells in the latter layer). However, it may be that the principal events that lead to degradation of the collagenous connective tissue and to ultimate rupture of a follicle may take place in the connective tissue cells themselves, namely, in the fibroblasts. If this is true, if the secret to understanding the mechanism of ovulation lies in decoding the events that convert quiescent fibroblasts into proliferating fibroblasts, it becomes equally imperative to distinguish the specific events that occur within luteinization of the granulosa and theca interna that lead to activation of the fibroblasts. Although it is obvious that progesterone is directly or indirectly involved, it is also feasible that activation of the fibroblasts could be induced either by serum factors within the exudate from hyperemic thecal capillaries or by action of eicosanoids of granulosa or thecal origin. This latter idea that eicosanoids might contribute to the activation of thecal fibroblast, if true, would help explain how anti-inflammatory agents such as indomethacin can block eicosanoid synthesis and ovulation without interfering in the luteinization process.

In summary, mammalian ovulation is considered to be an inflammatorylike process that occurs during the early stages of the luteinization process that is initiated by a surge in gonadotropic hormones from the pituitary gland. Although the luteinization process does not require ovulation, it appears that the ovulatory process is an integral part of the early stages of luteinization. Although both ovulation and luteinization are dependent on events in the theca interna and granulosa layers, ultimate rupture of a follicle may also depend on activation of the fibroblasts in the thecal connective tissue of a mature follicle. Therefore, any comprehensive analysis of the physiology of ovulation requires not only information about the timing of the principal events but also an assessment of the spatial distribution of these events within the different cellular components of a follicle.

ACKNOWLEDGMENTS

The more recent work reported by the authors has been supported in part by NIH grant HD21649 to Trinity University and by NIH grant HD10202 to the Center for Research in Reproductive Biology in the Department of Obstetrics and Gynecology at the University of Texas Health Science Center at San Antonio.

REFERENCES

1. Kelly GL. Direct observations of rupture of graafian follicles in the mammal. *J Fla Med Assoc* 1931;17:422–423.
2. Hill RT, Allen E, Kramer TC. Cinemicrographic studies of rabbit ovulation. *Anat Rec* 1935;63:239–245.
3. Blandau RJ. The mechanism of ovulation. In: Greenblatt RB, ed. *Ovulation: Stimulation Suppression Detection,* Philadelphia: JB Lippincott, 1966;3–15.
4. Walton A, Hammond J. Observations on ovulation in the rabbit. *Br J Exp Biol* 1928;6:190–204.
5. Espey LL. Evaluation of proteolytic activity in mammalian ovulation. In: Reich E, Rifkin DB, Shaw E, eds. *Proteases and Biological Control.* Cold Spring Harbor, NY: Cold Spring Harbor Laboratory, 1975;767–776.
6. Lipner H. Mechanism of mammalian ovulation. In: Knobil E, Neill JD, eds. *The Physiology of Reproduction,* Vol. 1. New York: Raven Press, 1988;447–488.
7. Hartman CG. Ovulation and the transport and viability of ova and sperm in the female genital tract. In: Allen E, ed. *Sex and Internal Secretions.* Baltimore: Williams & Wilkins, 1932;647–688.
8. Hisaw FL. Development of the graafian follicle and ovulation. *Physiol Rev* 1947;27:95–119.
9. Kraus SD. Observations on the mechanism of ovulation in the frog, hen and rabbit. *West J Surg Obstet Gynecol* 1947;55: 424–437.
10. Nalbandov AV. Mechanisms controlling ovulation of avian and mammalian follicles. In: Villee CA, ed. *Control of Ovulation.* New York: Pergamon, 1961;122–131.
11. Asdell SA. Mechanism of ovulation. In: Zuckerman S, ed. *The Ovary.* London: Academic Press, 1962;435–449.
12. Espey LL. *Mechanism of Mammalian Ovulation.* Doctoral dissertation. Tallahassee: Florida State University, 1964.
13. Espey LL, Lipner H. Enzyme-induced rupture of rabbit graafian follicle. *Am J Physiol* 1965;208:208–213.
14. Rondell P. Biophysical aspects of ovulation. *Biol Reprod* 1970;2(suppl):64–89.
15. Lipner H. Mechanism of mammalian ovulation. In: Greep RO, ed. *Handbook of Physiology—Endocrinology,* Vol II, part I. Washington, DC: American Physiological Society, 1973;409–437.
16. Espey LL. Ovarian proteolytic enzymes and ovulation. *Biol Reprod* 1974;10:216–235.

17. Parr EL. Rupture of ovarian follicles at ovulation. *J Reprod Fertil* 1975;22(suppl):1–22.
18. Espey LL, Coons PJ. Factors which influence ovulatory degradation of rabbit ovarian follicles. *Biol Reprod* 1976;14:233–245.
19. Espey LL. Ovulation. In: Jones RE, ed. *The Vertebrate Ovary.* New York: Plenum Press, 1978;503-532.
20. Tsafriri A, Braw RH, Reich R. Follicular development and the mechanism of ovulation. In: Insler V, Lunenfeld B, eds. *Infertility: Male and Female.* Edinburgh: Churchill Livingstone, 1986;73–100.
21. Yoshimura Y, Wallach EE. Studies of the mechanism(s) of mammalian ovulation. *Fertil Steril* 1987;47:22–34.
22. LeMaire WJ, Curry TE, Morioka N, et al. Regulation of ovulatory processes. In: Stouffer RL, ed. *The Primate Ovary.* New York: Plenum Press, 1987;91–111.
23. Thibault C, Levasseur MC. Ovulation. *Hum Reprod* 1988;3: 513–523.
24. Wallach EE, Atlas SJ, Dharmarajan AM, Oski JA, Santulli R. The periovulatory interval: physiologic and endocrinologic implications. *Prog Clin Biol Res* 1989;294:87–100.
25. LeMaire WJ. Mechanism of mammalian ovulation. *Steroids* 1989;54:455–469.
26. Morioka N, Zhu C, Brannstrom M, Woessner JF, LeMaire WJ. Mechanism of mammalian ovulation. *Prog Clin Biol Res* 1989;294:65–85.
27. Richards JS. Hormonal control of ovarian follicular development: a 1978 perspective. *Recent Prog Horm Res* 1979;35: 343–373.
28. Richards JS. Maturation of ovarian follicles: actions and interactions of pituitary and ovarian hormones on follicular cell differentiation. *Physiol Rev* 1980;60:51–89.
29. Bjersing L. Maturation, morphology, and endocrine function of the follicular wall in mammals. In: Jones RE, ed. *The Vertebrate Ovary.* New York: Plenum Press, 1978;181–214.
30. Balboni GC. Structural changes: ovulation and luteal phase. In: Serra BG, ed. *The Ovary.* New York: Raven Press, 1983;123–141.
31. Guraya SS. *Biology of Ovarian Follicles in Mammals.* Berlin: Springer-Verlag, 1985.
32. Espey LL. Ultrastructure of the ovulatory process. In: Familiari G, Makabe S, Motta PM, eds. *Ultrastructure of the Ovary,* Norwell, MA: Klewer, 1991;143–156.
33. LeMaire WJ, Clark MR, Marsh JM. Biochemical mechanism of ovulation. In: Hafez ESE, ed. *Human Ovulation.* Amsterdam: Elsevier/North Holland, 1979;159–175.
34. LeMaire WJ, Clark MR, Chainy GBN, Marsh JM. The role of prostaglandins in the mechanism of ovulation. In: Tozzini RI, Reaves G, Pineda RL, eds. *International Symposium on the Endocrine Physiopathology of the Ovary.* Amsterdam: Elsivier/ North Holland, 1980;207–217.
35. Tsafriri A, Abisogun AO, Reich R. Steroids and follicular rupture at ovulation. *J Steroid Biochem* 1987;27:359–363.
36. Espey LL. The role of steroids in mammalian ovulation. In: Tsafriri A, Dekal N, eds. *Follicular Development and the Ovulatory Process.* Rome: Ares-Serono Symposia, 1989;189–198.
37. Espey LL. Ovarian contractility and its relationship to ovulation: a review. *Biol Reprod* 1978;19:540–551.
38. Janson PO, Brannstrom M, Holmes PV, Sogn J. Studies on the mechanism of ovulation using the model of the isolated ovary. *Ann NY Acad Sci* 1988;541:22–29.
39. Adashi EY. The potential relevance of cytokines to ovarian physiology: the emerging role of resident ovarian cells of the white blood cell series. *Endocr Rev* 1990;11:454–464.
40. Mori T. Immuno-endocrinology of cyclic ovarian function. *Am J Reprod Immunol* 1990;24:80–89.
41. Richards JS, Jahnsen T, Hedin L, et al. Ovarian follicular development: from physiology to molecular biology. *Recent Prog Horm Res* 1987;43:231–276.
42. Richards JS, Hedin L. Molecular aspects of hormone action in ovarian follicular development, ovulation, and luteinization. *Annu Rev Physiol* 1988;50:441–463.
43. Richards JS. Gonadotropins—regulated gene expression in the ovary. In: Leung PK, Adashi E, eds. *The Ovary.* New York: Raven Press (in press).
44. Espey LL. A review of factors that could influence membrane potentials of ovarian follicular cells during mammalian ovulation. *Acta Endocrinol* 1992;2(suppl):1–31.
45. Espey LL. Ovulation as an inflammatory reaction: a hypothesis. *Biol Reprod* 1980;22:73–106.
46. Espey LL. Ovulation as an inflammatory process. In: Sjoberg N-O, Hamberger L, Janson PO, Owman Ch, Coelingh-Bennink HJT, eds. *Local Regulation of Ovarian Function.* Park Ridge, NJ: Parthenon Publishing Group, 1992;183–200.
47. Espey LL, Ben Halim IA. Characteristics and control of the normal menstrual cycle. *Obstet Gynecol Clin North Am* 1990;17: 275–298.
48. Irianni F, Hodgen GD. Mechanism of ovulation. *Endocrinol Metab Clin North Am* 1992;21:19–38.
49. Jocelyn HD, Setchell BP. Translation of Regnier de Graaf. *J Reprod Fertil* 1972;17(suppl):1–122.
50. Cruikshank WC. Experiments in which on the third day after impregnation the ova of rabbits were found in the fallopian tubes, on the fourth after, in the uterus with the first appearances of the fetus. *Philos Trans R Soc Lond (Biol)* 1797;87:197–214.
51. von Kolliker A. Beitrage zur kenntniss der glatten muskeln. *Abhandl Wiss Zool* 1849;1:48–87.
52. Rouget C. Recherches sur les organes erectiles de la femme et sur l'appareil musculataire tubo ovarien dans leurs rapports avec l'ovulation et la menstruation. *J Physiol (Paris)* 1858;1:320–343.
53. von Luschka H. Graafsche blaschen anatomie und physiologie. *Prager Vierteiljahrschrift Heilk* 1858;4:48–59.
54. Pfluger E. Ueber die bewegungen der ovarien. *Arch Anat* 1859;1:30–32.
55. Aeby C. Die glatten muskelfassen in den eierstocken der wirbelthiere. *Arch Anat Physiol Wissensch Med* 1961;1:635–645.
56. Grohe F. Uber den bau und das wachstum des menschlichen eierstocks. *Arch Pathol Anat Physiol* 1863;26:271–306.
57. Waldeyer W. *Eierstock und ei.* Leipzig: von Wilhelm Englemann, 1870.
58. von Winiwarter H, Sainmont G. Nouvelles recherches sur l'ovogenese et l'organogenese de l'ovaire des mammiferes chat. *Arch Biol Liege* 1909;24:627–651.
59. Thomson A. The ripe human graafian follicle, together with some suggestions as to its mode of rupture. *J Anat* 1919;54:1–40.
60. Corner GW. On the origin of the corpus luteum of the sow from both granulosa and theca interna. *Am J Anat* 1919;26:117–183.
61. Guttmacher MS, Guttmacher AF. Morphological and physiological studies of the musculature of the mature graafian follicle of the sow. *Johns Hopkins Hosp Bull* 1921;32:394–399.
62. Claesson L. Is there any smooth musculature in the wall of the graafian follicle? *Acta Anat* 1947;3:295–311.
63. Lipner H, Maxwell BA. Hypothesis concerning the role of follicular contractions in ovulation. *Science* 1960;131:1737–1738.
64. Espey LL. Ultrastructure of the apex of the rabbit graafian follicle during the ovulatory process. *Endocrinology* 1967;81:267–276.
65. Espey LL. Tenacity of porcine graafian follicle as it approaches ovulation. *Am J Physiol* 1967;212:1397–1401.
66. Gabbiani G, Badonnel M-C. Contractile events during inflammation. *Agents Actions* 1976;6:277–284.
67. Izzard CS, Izzard SL. Calcium regulation of the contractile state of isolated mammalian fibroblast cytoplasm. *J Cell Sci* 1975;18:241–256.
68. Small JV. Organisations of actin and fibroblast locomotion. In: Burger MM, Weber R, eds. *Embryonic Development: Part B, Cellular Aspects.* New York: Alan R. Liss, 1982;341–358.
69. Pendergrass PB, Talbot P. The distribution of contractile cells in the apex of the preovulatory hamster follicle. *Biol Reprod* 1979;20:205–213.
70. Martin GG, Talbot P. The role of follicular smooth muscle cells in hamster ovulation. *J Exp Zool* 1981;216:469–482.
71. Martin GG, Talbot P. Drugs that block smooth muscle contraction inhibit *in vivo* ovulation in hamsters. *J Exp Zool* 1981;216:483–491.
72. Talbot P, Chacon RS. *In vitro* ovulation of hamster oocytes depends on contraction of follicular smooth muscle cells. *J Exp Zool* 1982;224:409–415.
73. Talbot P. Videotape analysis of hamster ovulation *in vitro. J. Exp Zool* 1983;225:141–148.

74. Martin GG, van Steenwyk G, Miller-Walker C. The fate of thecal smooth muscle cells in postovulatory hamster follicles. *Anat Rec* 1983;207:267–277.
75. Self DA, Koch AR, Schroeder PC. Relaxation-induced contraction of smooth muscle surrounding hamster ovarian follicles. *J Reprod Fertil* 1989;85:593–603.
76. Amenta F, Allen DJ, Didio LJA, Motta P. A transmission electron microscopic study of smooth muscle cells in the ovary of rabbits, cats, rats and mice. *J Submicrosc Cytol* 1979;11:39–51.
77. Capps ML, Lawrence IE Jr, Burden HW. Cellular junctions in perifollicular contractile tissue of the rat ovary during the preovulatory period. *Cell Tissue Res* 1981;219:133–141.
78. Self DA, Schroeder PC, Gown AM. Hamster thecal cells express muscle characteristics. *Biol Reprod* 1988;39:119–130.
79. Rocereto T, Jacobowitz D, Wallach EE. Observations of spontaneous contractions of the cat ovary *in vitro*. *Endocrinology* 1969;84:1336–1341.
80. Morikawa H, Okamura H, Takenaka A, Morimoto K, Nishimura T. Histamine concentration and its effect on ovarian contractility in humans. *Int J Fertil* 1981;26:283–286.
81. Smith C, Perks AM. The effects of bradykinin on the contractile activity of the isolated rat ovary. *Acta Endocrinol* 1984;106:387–392.
82. Kannisto P, Batra S, Owman C, Walles B. Extracellular and intracellular calcium sources mediating contractile responses of smooth muscle in bovine ovarian follicle and ovarian artery. *Eur J Pharmacol* 1987;144:299–308.
83. Schroeder PC, Talbot P. Intrafollicular pressure decreases in hamster preovulatory follicles during smooth muscle cell contraction *in vitro*. *J Exp Zool* 1982;224:417–426.
84. Espey LL, Lipner H. Measurement of intrafollicular pressures in the rabbit ovary. *Am J Physiol* 1963;205:1067–1072.
85. Kobayashi Y, Kitai H, Santulli R, Wright KH, Wallach EE. Influence of calcium and magnesium deprivation on ovulation and ovum maturation in the perfused rabbit ovary. *Biol Reprod* 1984;31:287–295.
86. Lofman CO, Brannstrom M, Holmes PV, Janson PO. Ovulation in the isolated perfused rat ovary as documented by intravital microscopy. *Steroids* 1989;54:481–490.
87. Weiner S, Wright KH, Wallach EE. Lack of effect of ovarian denervation on ovulation and pregnancy in the rabbit. *Fertil Steril* 1975;26:1083–1087.
88. Markee JE. Rhythmic vascular uterine changes. *Am J Physiol* 1932;100:32–39.
89. Ford SP, Weber LJ, Kennick WH, Stormshak F. Response of bovine ovarian arterial smooth muscle to prostaglandin $F_{2\alpha}$ and neurotransmitter. *J Animal Sci* 1977;45:1091–1095.
90. Orgill D, Demling RH. Current concepts and approaches to wound healing. *Crit Care Med* 1988;16:899–908.
91. Sieggreen MY. Healing of physical wounds. *Nurs Clin North Am* 1987;22:439–447.
92. Laato M, Niinikoski J, Lundberg C, Arfors K-E. Effect of epidermal growth factor (EGF) on experimental granulation tissue. *J Surg Res* 1986;41:252–255.
93. Kingsnorth AN, Vowles R, Nash JRG. Epidermal growth factor increases tensile strength in intestinal wounds in pigs. *Br J Surg* 1990;77:409–412.
94. Garcia-Valdecasas JC, Garcia-Valdecasas F, Pera C. Pharmacological reactivity of granulation tissue. *J Pharm Pharmacol* 1981;33:650–654.
95. O'Shea JD. An ultrastructural study of smooth muscle-like cells in the theca externa of ovarian follicles in the rat. *Anat Rec* 1970;167:127–140.
96. Heape W. Ovulation and degeneration of the ova in the rabbit. *Proc R Soc Lond (Biol)* 1905;76:260–268.
97. Schochet SS. A suggestion as to the process of ovulation and ovarian cyst formation. *Anat Rec* 1916;10:447–457.
98. Wester J. *Eierstock und ei. Befruchtung und unfruchtbarkeit bei den haustieren.* Berlin: R Schoetz, 1921.
99. McKenzie FF, Terrill CE. Estrus, ovulation, and related phenomena in the ewe. *Res Bull Mo Agric Exp Sta* 1937;264:1–88.
100. Smith JT. Rupture of graafian follicles. *Am J Obstet Gynecol* 1937;33:820–827.
101. Smith JT, Ketteringham RC. Rupture of the graafian follicles. *Am J Obstet Gynecol* 1938;36:453–460.
102. Zachariae F. Studies on the mechanism of ovulation. Permeability of the blood-liquor barrier. *Acta Endocrinol* 1958;27:339–342.
103. Zachariae F, Jensen CE. Studies on the mechanism of ovulation. Histochemical and physico-chemical investigations on genuine follicular fluids. *Acta Endocrinol* 1958;27:343–355.
104. Blandau RJ, Rumery RE. Measurements of intrafollicular pressure in ovulatory and preovulatory follicles of the rat. *Fertil Steril* 1963;14:330–341.
105. Rondell P. Follicular pressure and distensibility in ovulation. *Am J Physiol* 1964;207:590–594.
106. Bronson RA, Bryant G, Balk MW, Emanuele N. Intrafollicular pressure within preovulatory follicles of the pig. *Fertil Steril* 1979;31:205–213.
107. Long JA, Evans HM. The maturation of the egg of the mouse. *Carnegie Inst Washington* 1911;142:1–72.
108. Rugh R. Ovulation in the frog. II. Follicular rupture to fertilization. *J Exp Zool* 1935;71:163–193.
109. Markee JE, Hinsey JC. Observations on ovulation in the rabbit. *Anat Rec* 1936;64:309–319.
110. Moricard R, Gothie S. Dissociation des cellules de la granulosa et probleme d'un mechanisme diastasique dans la rupture du follicule ovarien de lapine. *Compt Rend* 1946;140:249–272.
111. Jung G, Held H. Uber fermente in der follikelflussigkeit. *Arch Gynakol* 1959;192:146–150.
112. Jung G, Kides E. Proteolytische fermente im ovargewebe. *Arch Gynakol* 1959;192:151–154.
113. Unbehaun V, Jung G, Kides E. Enzymuntersuchungen im liquor folliculi. *Archiv Gynakol* 1965;202:225–228.
114. Reichert LE. Further studies on proteinases of the rat ovary. *Endocrinology* 1962;70:838–839.
115. Lee CY, Malvin R. Acid proteolytic activity in the sow ovarian follicle. *Fed Proc* 1970;29:643(abst).
116. Espey LL. Effect of various substances on tensile strength of sow ovarian follicles. *Am J Physiol* 1970;219:230–233.
117. Espey LL, Rondell P. Estimation of mammalian collagenolytic activity with a synthetic substrate. *J Appl Physiol* 1967;23:757–761.
118. Espey LL, Rondell P. Collagenolytic activity in the rabbit and sow graafian follicle during ovulation. *Am J Physiol* 1968;214:326–329.
119. Morales TI, Woessner JF, Howell DS, Marsh JM, LeMaire WJ. A microassay for the direct demonstration of collagenolytic activity in graafian follicles of the rat. *Biochim Biophys Acta* 1978;524:428–434.
120. Morales TI, Woessner JF Jr, Marsh JM, LeMaire WJ. Collagen, collagenase and collagenolytic activity in rat graafian follicles during follicular growth and ovulation. *Biochim Biophys Acta* 1983;756:119–122.
121. Harrison RJ. The structure of the ovary: C. Mammals. In: Zuckerman S, ed. *The Ovary.* New York: Academic Press, 1962;143–187.
122. Bjersing L, Cajander S. Ovulation and the mechanism of follicle rupture. I. Light microscopic changes in rabbit ovarian follicles prior to induced ovulation. *Cell Tissue Res* 1974;149:287–300.
123. Bjersing L, Cajander S. Ovulation and the mechanism of follicle rupture. II. Scanning electron microscopy of rabbit germinal epithelium prior to induced ovulation. *Cell Tissue Res* 1974;149:301–312.
124. Bjersing L, Cajander S. Ovulation and the mechanism of follicle rupture. III. Transmission electron microscopy of rabbit germinal epithelium prior to induced ovulation. *Cell Tissue Res* 1974;149:313–327.
125. Bjersing L, Cajander S. Ovulation and the mechanism of follicle rupture. IV. Ultrastructure of membrana granulosa of rabbit graafian follicles prior to induced ovulation. *Cell Tissue Res* 1974;153:1–14.
126. Bjersing L, Cajander S. Ovulation and the mechanism of follicle rupture. V. Ultrastructure of tunica albuginea and theca externa of rabbit graafian follicles prior to induced ovulation. *Cell Tissue Res* 1974;153:15–30.
127. Bjersing L, Cajander S. Ovulation and the mechanism of follicle

rupture. VI. Ultrastructure of theca interna and the inner vascular network surrounding rabbit graafian follicles prior to induced ovulation. *Cell Tissue Res* 1974;153:31–44.
128. Parr EL. Histological examination of the rat ovarian follicle wall prior to ovulation. *Biol Reprod* 1974;11:483–503.
129. Mossman HW, Duke KL. *Comparative Morphology of the Mammalian Ovary.* Madison: University of Wisconsin Press, 1973.
130. Lipner H, Cross NL. Morphology of the membrana granulosa of the ovarian follicle. *Endocrinology* 1968;82:638–641.
131. Mirecka J. Immunofluorescent localization of the female sex steroids in the porcine ovary. *Histochem J* 1975;7:249–257.
132. Schaar H. Functional morphology of the theca interna of the vesicular follicle in the human ovary. *Acta Anat* 1976;94: 283–298.
133. Espey LL, Stutts RH. Exchange of cytoplasm between cells of the membrana granulosa in rabbit ovarian follicles. *Biol Reprod* 1972;6:168–175.
134. McNatty KP. Follicular fluid. In: Jones RE, ed. *The Vertebrate Ovary.* New York: Plenum Press, 1978;215–259.
135. Cajander S, Janson PO, LeMaire WJ, et al. Studies on the morphology of the isolated perfused rabbit ovary. II. Ovulation *in vitro* after HCG-treatment *in vivo. Cell Tissue Res* 1984; 235:565–573.
136. Cherney DD, Liberato JA, Didio MD, Motta P. The development of rabbit ovarian follicles following copulation. *Fertil Steril* 1975;26:257–271.
137. Byskov AGS. Ultrastructural studies on the preovulatory follicle in the mouse ovary. *Z Zellforsch Mikrosk Anat* 1969;100: 285–299.
138. Cajander S. Structural alterations of rabbit ovarian follicles after mating with special reference to the overlying surface epithelium. *Cell Tissue Res* 1976;173:437–449.
139. Blandau RJ. Anatomy of ovulation. *Clin Obstet Gynecol* 1967;10:347–360.
140. Motta P, van Blerkom J. A scanning electron microscopic study of the luteo-follicular complex. II. Events leading to ovulation. *Am J Anat* 1975;143:241–263.
141. Rawson JMR, Espey LL. Concentration of electron dense granules in the rabbit ovarian surface epithelium during ovulation. *Biol Reprod* 1977;17:561–566.
142. Narimoto K, Okamura H, Mori T, Sakai M, Espey L, Ogawa K. Cytochemical localization of acid phosphatase in the rabbit ovarian follicle. *Acta Histochem Cytochem* 1985;18:525–537.
143. Cajander S. Structural alterations of rabbit ovarian follicles after mating with special reference to the overlying surface epithelium. *Cell Tissue Res* 1976;173:437–449.
144. Tsujimoto D, Katayama K, Tojo S, Mizoguti H. Scanning electron microscopic studies on stigmas in rat ovaries. *Acta Obstet Gynecol Scand* 1982;61:269–273.
145. Talbot P, Martin GG, Ashby H. Formation of the rupture site in preovulatory hamster and mouse follicles: loss of the surface epithelium. *Gamete Res* 1987;17:287–302.
146. Pendergrass PB, Reber M. Scanning electron microscopy of the graafian follicle during ovulation in the golden hamster. *J Reprod Fertil* 1980;59:21–24.
147. Danforth DN, Buckingham JC. Connective tissue mechanisms and their relation to pregnancy. *Obstet Gynecol Surv* 1964; 19:715–732.
148. Gross J. Evaluation of structural and chemical changes in connective tissue. *NY Acad Sci* 1953;56:674–683.
149. Rhodin JAG. *Histology: A Text and Atlas.* New York: Oxford University Press, 1974.
150. Espey LL. The distribution of collagenous connective tissue in rat ovarian follicles. *Biol Reprod* 1976;14:502–506.
151. Espey LL. Decomposition of connective tissue in rabbit ovarian follicles by multivesicular structures of thecal fibroblasts. *Endocrinology* 1971;88:437–444.
152. Espey LL, Coons PJ, Marsh JM, LeMaire WJ. Effect of indomethacin on preovulatory changes in the ultrastructure of rabbit graafian follicles. *Endocrinology* 1981;108:1040–1048.
153. Espey LL. Multivesicular structures in proliferating fibroblasts of rabbit ovarian follicles during ovulation. *J Cell Biol* 1971;48: 437–442.
154. Chihal HJ, Espey LL. Utilization of the relaxed symphysis pubis of the guinea pig for clues to the mechanism of ovulation. *Endocrinology* 1973;93:1441–1445.
155. Erickson GF, Magoffin DA, Dyer CA, Hofeditz C. The ovarian androgen producing cells: a review of structure/function relationships. *Endocr Rev* 1985;6:371–399.
156. Fawcett DW. *A Textbook of Histology.* Philadelphia: WB Saunders, 1986.
157. Hadley ME. *Endocrinology.* 3rd ed. Englewood Cliffs, NJ: Prentice Hall, 1992.
158. Yoshinaga K. Cyclic hormone secretion by the mammalian ovary. In: Jones RE, ed. *The Vertebrate Ovary.* New York: Plenum Press, 1978;691–729.
159. Guraya SS. Morphology, histochemistry, and biochemistry of human ovarian compartments and steroid hormone synthesis. *Physiol Rev* 1971;51:785–807.
160. Guraya SS. Morphology, histochemistry, and biochemistry of human oogenesis and ovulation. *Int Rev Cytol* 1974;37: 121–151.
161. Schwartz NB, Ely CA. Role of gonadotropins in ovulation. In: Moudgal NR, ed. *Gonadotropins and Gonadal Function.* New York: Academic Press, 1974;237–252.
162. Hay MF, Moor RM. Functional and structural relationships in the graafian follicle population of the sheep ovary. *J Reprod Fertil* 1975;45:583–593.
163. Moor RM, Hay MF, Seamark RF. The sheep ovary: regulation of steroidogenic, haemodynamic and structural changes in the largest follicle and adjacent tissue before ovulation. *J Reprod Fertil* 1975;45:595–604.
164. Falck B. Site of production of oestrogen in rat ovary as studied in microtransplants. *Acta Physiol Scand* 1959;47(suppl 163):1–101.
165. Bjersing L. On the morphology and endocrine function of granulosa cells in ovarian follicles and corpora lutea: biochemical, histochemical, and ultrastructural studies on the porcine ovary with special reference to steroid hormone synthesis. *Acta Endocrinol* 1967;125(suppl):1–23.
166. Hilliard J, Hayward JN, Sawyer CH. Postcoital patterns of secretion of pituitary gonadotropin and ovarian progestin in the rabbit. *Endocrinology* 1964;75:957–963.
167. Hilliard J, Eaton LW Jr. Estradiol-17β, progesterone and 20α-hydroxy-pregn-4-en-3-one in rabbit ovarian venous plasma. II. From mating through implantation. *Endocrinology* 1971;89: 522–527.
168. Younglai EV. Effect of mating on follicular fluid steroids in the rabbit. *J Reprod Fertil* 1972;30:157–159.
169. Kalra SP, Kalra PS. Temporal interrelationships among circulating levels of estradiol, progesterone, and LH during the rat estrous cycle: effects of exogenous progesterone. *Endocrinology* 1974;95:1711–1718.
170. Patwardhan VV, Lanthier A. Effect of an ovulatory dose of luteinizing hormone on the concentration of oestrone, oestradiol and progesterone in the rabbit ovarian follicle. *Acta Endocrinol* 1976;82:792–800.
171. Bahr JM. Simultaneous measurements of steroids in follicular fluid and ovarian venous blood in the rabbit. *Biol Reprod* 1978;18:193–197.
172. Goff AK, Henderson KM. Changes in follicular fluid and serum concentrations of steroids in PMS treated rats following LH administration. *Biol Reprod* 1979;20:1153–1157.
173. Saidapur SK, Greenwald GS. Regulation of 17β-estradiol synthesis in the proestrous hamster: role of progesterone and luteinizing hormone. *Endocrinology* 1979;105:1432–1439.
174. Hubbard CJ, Greenwald GS. Cyclic nucleotides, DNA, and steroid levels in ovarian follicles and corpora lutea of the cyclic hamster. *Biol Reprod* 1982;26:230–240.
175. Toorop AI, Gribling-Hegge L, Meijs-Roelofs HMA. Ovarian steroid concentrations in rats with spontaneous and with delayed or advanced ovulation. *J Endocrinol* 1982;95:287–292.
176. Espey LL, Norris C, Forman J, Siler-Khodr T. Effect of indomethacin, cycloheximide, and aminoglutethimide on ovarian steroid and prostanoid levels during ovulation in the gonadotropin-primed immature rat. *Prostaglandins* 1989;38: 531–539.

177. Mills TM, Savard K. Steroidogenesis in ovarian follicles isolated from rabbits before and after mating. *Endocrinology* 1973;92: 788–791.
178. Clark JG. The origin, development and degeneration of the blood vessels of the human ovary. *Johns Hopkins Hosp Rep* 1900;9:593–676.
179. Bassett DL. The changes in the vascular pattern of the ovary of the albino rat during the estrous cycle. *Am J Anat* 1943;73: 251–291.
180. Burr JH, Davies JI. The vascular system of the rabbit ovary and its relationship to ovulation. *Anat Rec* 1951;111:273–297.
181. Ellinwood WE, Nett TM, Niswender GD. Ovarian vasculature: structure and function. In: Jones RE, ed. *The Vertebrate Ovary.* New York: Plenum Press, 1978;583–614.
182. Kanzaki H, Okamura H, Okuda Y, Takenaka A, Morimoto K, Nishimura T. Scanning electron microscopic study of rabbit ovarian follicle microvasculature using resin injection-corrosion casts. *J Anat* 1982;134:697–704.
183. Kitai H, Yoshimura Y, Wright KH, Santulli R, Wallach EE. Microvasculature of preovulatory follicles: comparison of *in situ* and *in vitro* perfused rabbit ovaries following stimulation of ovulation. *Am J Obstet Gynecol* 1985;152:889–895.
184. Murakami T, Ikebuchi Y, Ohtsuka A, Kikuta A, Taguchi T, Ohtani O. The blood vascular wreath of rat ovarian follicle, with special reference to its changes in ovulation and luteinization: a scanning electron microscopic study of corrosion casts. *Arch Histol Cytol* 1988;51:299–313.
185. Macchiarelli G, Nottola SA, Vizza E, Kikuta A, Murakami T, Motta PM. Ovarian microvasculature in normal and hCG stimulated rabbits. A study of vascular corrosion casts with particular regard to the interstitium. *J Submicrosc Cytol Pathol* 1991;23:391–395.
186. Christiansen JA, Jensen CE, Zachariae F. Studies on the mechanism of ovulation. Some remarks on the effects of depolymerization of high-polymers on the pre-ovulatory growth of follicles. *Acta Endocrinol* 1958;29:115–117.
187. Okuda Y, Okamura H, Kanzaki H, Takenaka A. Capillary permeability of rabbit ovarian follicles prior to ovulation. *J Anat* 1983;137:263–269.
188. Murdoch WJ, Myers DA. Effect of treatment of estrous ewes with indomethacin on the distribution of ovarian blood to the periovulatory follicle. *Biol Reprod* 1983;29:1229–1232.
189. Murdoch WJ, Nix KJ, Dunn TG. Dynamics of ovarian blood supply to periovulatory follicles of the ewe. *Biol Reprod* 1983;28:1001–1006.
190. Brown BW, Cognie Y, Chemineau P, Poulin N, Salama OA. Ovarian capillary blood flow in seasonally anoestrous ewes induced to ovulate by treatment with GnRH. *J Reprod Fertil* 1988;84:653–658.
191. Blasco L, Wu C-H, Flickinger GL, Pearlmutter D, Mikhail G. Cardiac output and genital blood flow distribution during the preovulatory period in rabbits. *Biol Reprod* 1975;13:581–586.
192. Wu CH, Blasco L, Flickinger GL, Mikhail G. Ovarian function in the preovulatory rabbit. *Biol Reprod* 1977;17:304–308.
193. Lee W, Novy MJ. Effects of luteinizing hormone and indomethacin on blood flow and steroidogenesis in the rabbit ovary. *Biol Reprod* 1978;17:799–807.
194. Damber J-E, Cajander S, Gafvels M, Selstam G. Blood flow changes and vascular appearance in preovulatory follicles and corpora lutea in immature, pregnant mare's serum gonadotropin-treated rats. *Biol Reprod* 1987;37:651–658.
195. Wurtman RJ. An effect of luteinizing hormone on the fractional perfusion of the rat ovary. *Endocrinology* 1964;75:927–933.
196. Abisogun AO, Daphna-Iken D, Reich R, Kranzfelder D, Tsafriri A. Modulatory role of eicosanoids in vascular changes during the preovulatory period in the rat. *Biol Reprod* 1988;38:756–762.
197. Piacsek BE, Huth JF. Changes in ovarian venous blood flow following cannulation; effects of luteinizing hormone (LH) and antihistamine. *Proc Soc Exp Biol Med* 1971;138:1022–1024.
198. Makinoda S. Hemodynamical and histological studies on ovarian blood flow during ovulation. *Hokkaido J Med Sci* 1980;55:521–526.
199. Selstam G, Janson PO, Eden S. Effect of LH on the release of cyclic AMP by the rabbit ovary perfused *in vivo* and *in vitro. J Reprod Fertil* 1976;46:355–358.
200. Collins W, Jurkovic D, Bourne T, Kurjak A, Campbell S. Ovarian morphology, endocrine function and intra-follicular blood flow during the peri-ovulatory period. *Hum Reprod* 1991;6: 319–324.
201. Okamura H, Fukumoto M, Mori T. Prostaglandin-mediated changes of vasculature and collagen degradation/synthesis in the follicle wall during ovulation. In: Hayaishi O, Yamamoto S, eds. *Advances in Prostaglandin, Thromboxane, and Leukotriene Research,* Vol 15. New York: Raven Press, 1985;597–601.
202. Cavender JL, Murdoch WJ. Morphological studies of the microcirculatory system of periovulatory ovine follicles. *Biol Reprod* 1988;39:989–997.
203. Yoshimura Y, Dharmarajan AM, Gips S, et al. Effects of prostacyclin on ovulation and microvasculature of the *in vitro* perfused rabbit ovary. *Am J Obstet Gynecol* 1988;159:977–982.
204. Batta SK, Martini L. Influence of the estrous cycle and prostaglandins on utero-ovarian vein blood flow in the rat. *Prostaglandins* 1975;10:469–477.
205. Tanaka N, Espey LL, Okamura H. Increase in ovarian blood volume during ovulation in the gonadotropin-primed immature rat. *Biol Reprod* 1989;40:762–768.
206. Reed M, Burton FA, van Diest PA. Ovulation in the guinea-pig. I. The ruptured follicle. *J Anat* 1979;128:195–206.
207. Kranzfelder D, Korr H, Mestwerdt W, Maurer-Schultze B. Follicle growth in the ovary of the rabbit after ovulation-inducing application of human chorionic gonadotropin. *Cell Tissue Res* 1984;238:611–620.
208. Rose BI, Koos RD. The effect of human follicular fluid on endothelial cells: proliferation and DNA synthesis. *Biol Reprod* 1988;39:88–95.
209. Bjorkman N. A study of the ultrastructure of the granulosa cells of the rat ovary. *Acta Anat* 1962;51:125–147.
210. Guraya SS. Gonadotropins and functions of granulosal and thecal cells *in vivo* and *in vitro.* In: Moudgal NR, ed. *Gonadotropins and Gonadal Function.* New York: Academic Press, 1974;220–236.
211. Sobotta J. Uber die bildung des corpus luteum bei der maus. *Arch Mikrosk Anat* 1896;47:261–308.
212. Merk FB, McNutt NS. Nexus junctions between dividing and interphase granulosa cells of the rat ovary. *J Cell Biol* 1972;55:511–515.
213. Merk FB, Albright JT, Botticelli CR. The fine structure of granulosa cell nexuses in rat ovarian follicles. *Anat Rec* 1973;175: 107–126.
214. Coons LW, Espey LL. Quantitation of nexus junctions in the granulosa cell layer of rabbit ovarian follicles during ovulation. *J Cell Biol* 1977;74:321–325.
215. Albertini DF, Anderson E. The appearance and structure of intercellular connections during the ontogeny of the rabbit ovarian follicle with particular reference to gap junctions. *J Cell Biol* 1974;63:234–250.
216. Albertini DF, Anderson E. Structural modifications of lutein cell gap junctions during pregnancy in the rat and the mouse. *Anat Rec* 1975;181:171–194.
217. Amsterdam A, Josephs R, Lieberman ME, Lindner HR. Organization of intramembrane particles in freeze-cleaved gap junctions of rat graafian follicles: optical-diffraction analysis. *J Cell Sci* 1976;21:93–105.
218. Herr JC. Reflexive gap junctions: gap junctions between processes arising from the same ovarian decidual cell. *J Cell Biol* 1976;69:495–501.
219. Anderson E. Follicular morphology. In: Midgley AR Jr, Sadler WA, eds. *Ovarian Follicular Development.* New York: Raven Press, 1979;91–105.
220. Campbell KL, Albertini DF. Freeze-fracture analysis of gap junction disruption in rat ovarian granulosa cells. *Tissue Cell* 1981;13:651–668.
221. Larson WJ, Tung HN, Polking C. Response of granulosa cell gap junctions to human chorionic gonadotropin (hCG) at ovulation. *Biol Reprod* 1981;25:1119–1134.
222. Zuckerman S. The cellular components of the ovary. *Proc Soc Study Fertil* 1952;4:4–7.

223. Robinson A. The formation, rupture, and closure of ovarian follicles in ferrets and ferret-polecat hybrids and some associated phenomena. *Trans R Soc Edinb* 1918;52:303–362.
224. Bahr J, Kao L, Nalbandov AV. The role of catecholamines and nerves in ovulation. *Biol Reprod* 1974;10:273–294.
225. Burden HW. Ovarian innervation. In: Jones RE, ed. *The Vertebrate Ovary*. New York: Plenum Press, 1978;615–638.
226. Fink G, Schofield GC. Experimental studies on the innervation of the ovary in cats. *J Anat* 1971;109:115–126.
227. O'Shea JD. The ultrastructure, origin and fate of the theca externa of ovarian follicles in the sheep. *Res Vet Sci* 1973;14:273–278.
228. Walles B, Edvinsson L, Falck B, Owman C, Sjoberg NO, Svensson KG. Evidence for a neuromuscular mechanism involved in the contractility of the ovarian follicular wall: fluorescence and electron microscopy and effects of tyramine on follicle strips. *Biol Reprod* 1975;12:239–248.
229. Walles B, Edvinsson L, Owman C, Sjoberg NO, Sporrong B. Cholinergic nerves and receptors mediating contraction of the graafian follicle. *Biol Reprod* 1976;15:565–572.
230. Walles B, Owman C, Sjoberg NO. Contraction of the ovarian follicle induced by local stimulation of its sympathetic nerves. *Brain Res Bull* 1982;9:757–760.
231. McReynolds HD, Siraki CM, Bramson PH, Pollock RJ Jr. Smooth muscle-like cells in ovaries of the hamster and gerbil. *Z Zellforsch* 1973;140:1–8.
232. Burden HW. Ultrastructural observations on ovarian perifollicular smooth muscle in the cat, guinea pig, and rabbit. *Am J Anat* 1972;133:125-142.
233. Walles B, Edvinsson L, Falck B, et al. Modifications of ovarian and follicular contractility by amines. A mechanism involved in ovulation? *Europ J Obstet Gynecol* 1974;4:S103–S107.
234. Walles B, Falck B, Owman C, Sjoberg NO. Characterization of autonomic receptors in the smooth musculature of human graafian follicle. *Biol Reprod* 1977;17:423–431.
235. Kobayashi Y, Sjoberg NO, Walles B, et al. The effect of adrenergic agents on the ovulatory process in the *in vitro* perfused rabbit ovary. *Am J Obstet Gynecol* 1983;145:857–864.
236. Kannisto P, Owman C, Walles B. Involvement of local adrenergic receptors in the process of ovulation in gonadotrophin-primed immature rats. *J Reprod Fertil* 1985;75:357–362.
237. Schmidt G, Owman C, Sjoberg NO, Walles B. Influence of adrenoreceptor agonists and antagonists on ovulation in the rabbit ovary perfused *in vitro*. *J Auton Pharmacol* 1985;5:241–250.
238. Bahr JM, Ben-Jonathan N. Elevated catecholamines in porcine follicular fluid before ovulation. *Endocrinology* 1985;117:620–623.
239. Bodis J, Bognar Z, Hartmann G, Torok A, Csaba I, Halvax L. Analysis of noradrenaline, dopamine and serotonin levels in follicular fluid following superovulatory treatment. *Orv Hetil* 1991;132:2475–2477.
240. Jorgensen JC, Kannisto P, Liedberg F, Ottesen B, Owman C, Schmidt G. The influence of neuropeptide Y and norepinephrine on ovulation in the rat ovary. *Peptides* 1991;12:975–982.
241. Weiner S, Wright KH, Wallach EE. Selective ovarian sympathectomy in the rabbit. *Fertil Steril* 1975;26:353–362.
242. Weiner S, Wright KH, Wallach EE. Studies on the function of the denervated rabbit ovary: human chorionic gonadotropin-induced ovulation. *Fertil Steril* 1975;26:363–368.
243. Wylie SN, Roche PJ, Gibson WR. Ovulation after sympathetic denervation of the rat ovary produced by freezing its nerve supply. *J Reprod Fertil* 1985;75:369–373.
244. Higuchi Y, Espey LL. Pattern of ovarian steroid secretion during ovulation of *in vitro* perfused rat ovaries varies with method of sampling. *J Reprod Fertil* 1989;87:821–828.
245. Gruenberg ML, Steger RW, Peluso JJ. Follicular development, steroidogenesis and ovulation within ovaries exposed *in vitro* to hormone levels which mimic those of the rat estrous cycle. *Biol Reprod* 1983;29:1265–1275.
246. Scaramuzzi RJ, Blake CA, Papkoff H, Hilliard J, Sawyer CH. Radioimmunoassay of rabbit luteinizing hormone: serum levels during various reproductive states. *Endocrinology* 1972;90:1285–1291.
247. McFarland KC, Sprengel R, Phillips HS, et al. Lutropin-choriogonadotropin receptor: an unusual member of the G protein-coupled receptor family. *Science* 1989;245:494–499.
248. Schenken RS, Williams RF, Hodgen GD. Ovulation induction using "pure" follicle-stimulating hormone in monkeys. *Fertil Steril* 1984;41:629–634.
249. Armstrong DT, Opavsky MA. Superovulation of immature rats by continuous infusion of follicle-stimulating hormone. *Biol Reprod* 1988;39:511–518.
250. Nalbandov AV, Kao LWL, Jones EE. Effects of intrafollicular injection of hormones and drugs. *J Reprod Fertil* 1973;18 (suppl):15–22.
251. Greenwald GS, Papkoff H. Induction of ovulation in the hypophysectomized proestrous hamster by purified FSH or LH. *Proc Soc Exp Biol Med* 1980;165:391–393.
252. Galway AB, Lapolt PS, Tsafriri A, Dargan CM, Boime I, Hsueh AJW. Recombinant follicle-stimulating hormone induces ovulation and tissue plasminogen activator expression in hypophysectomized rats. *Endocrinology* 1990;127:3023–3028.
253. Eckholm C, Hillensjo I, Isaksson O. Gonadotropin releasing hormone agonists stimulate oocyte meiosis and ovulation in hypophysectomized rats. *Endocrinology* 1981;108:2022–2024.
254. Corbin A, Bex FJ. Luteinizing hormone releasing hormone agonists induce ovulation in hypophysectomized proestrous rats: direct ovarian effect. *Life Sci* 1981;29:185–192.
255. Dekel N, Sherizly A, Tsafriri A, Naor Z. A comparative study of the mechanism of action of luteinizing hormone and a gonadotropin releasing hormone analog on the ovary. *Biol Reprod* 1983;28:161–166.
256. Koos RD, LeMaire WJ. The effects of a gonadotropin-releasing hormone agonist on ovulation and steroidogenesis during perfusion of rabbit and rat ovaries *in vitro*. *Endocrinology* 1985;116:628–632.
257. Minegishi T, Leung PCK. Luteinizing hormone-releasing hormone stimulates arachidonic acid release in rat granulosa cells. *Endocrinology* 1985;117:2001–2007.
258. Davis JS, West LA, Farese RV. Gonadotropin-releasing hormone (GnRH) rapidly stimulates the formation of inositol phosphates and diacylglycerol in rat granulosa cells: further evidence for the involvement of Ca^{2+} and protein kinase C in the action of GnRH. *Endocrinology* 1986;118:2561–2571.
259. de la Lastra M, Leal J. Gonadotropin-releasing hormone (GnRH) inhibits ovulation induced with luteinizing hormone (LH) in proestrous hypophysectomized rats. *Life Sci* 1988;42:421–429.
260. Leung PCK, Steele GL. Intracellular signaling in the gonads. *Endocr Rev* 1992;13:476–498.
261. Rajaniemi HJ, Hirshfield AN, Midgley AR Jr. Gonadotropin receptors in rat ovarian tissue. I. Localization of LH binding sites by fractionation of subcellular organelles. *Endocrinology* 1974;95:579–588.
262. Han SS, Rajaniemi HJ, Cho MI, Hirshfield AN, Midgley AR Jr. Gonadotropin receptors in rat ovarian tissue. II. Subcellular localization of LH binding sites by electron microscopic radioautography. *Endocrinology* 1974;95:589–596.
263. DiZerega GS, Richardson CL, Davies TF, Hodgen GD, Catt KJ. Fluorescence localization of luteinizing hormone/human chorionic gonadotropin uptake in the primate ovary: characterization of the preovulatory ovary. *Fertil Steril* 1980;34:379–385.
264. Amsterdam A, Koch Y, Lieberman ME, Lindner HR. Distribution of binding sites for human chorionic gonadotropin in the preovulatory follicle of the rat. *J Cell Biol* 1975;67:894–900.
265. Uilenbroek JTJ, Richards JS. Ovarian follicular development during the rat estrous cycle: gonadotropin receptors and follicular responsiveness. *Biol Reprod* 1979;20:1159–1165.
266. Bogovich K, Richards JS, Reichert LE Jr. Obligatory role of luteinizing hormone (LH) in the initiation of preovulatory follicular growth in the pregnant rat: specific effects of human chorionic gonadotropin and follicle-stimulating hormone on LH receptors and steroidogenesis in theca, granulosa and luteal cells. *Endocrinology* 1981;109:860–867.
267. Oxberry BA, Greenwald GS. An autoradiographic study of the binding of ^{125}I-labeled follicle-stimulating hormone, human chorionic gonadotropin and prolactin to the hamster ovary throughout the estrous cycle. *Biol Reprod* 1982;27:505–516.

268. Richards JS, Bogovich K. Effects of human chorionic gonadotropin and progesterone on follicular development in the immature rat. *Endocrinology* 1982;111:1429–1438.
269. Webb R, England BG. Identification of the ovulatory follicle in the ewe: associated changes in follicular size, thecal and granulosa cell luteinizing hormone receptors, antral fluid steroids, and circulating hormones during the preovulatory period. *Endocrinology* 1982;110:873–881.
270. Dufau M, Ryan DW, Baukal AJ, Catt KJ. Gonadotropin receptors. Solubilization and purification by affinity chromatography. *J Biol Chem* 1975;250:4822–4824.
271. Mitsikko MK, Rajaniemi HJ. Immunoprecipitation of the lutropin receptor. *Biochem J* 1984;224:467–471.
272. Ascoli M, Segaloff DL. Effects of collagenase on the structure of the lutropin/chorionic gonadotropin receptor. *J Biol Chem* 1986;261:3807–3815.
273. Keinanen KP, Kellokumpu S, Metsikko MK, Rajaniemi HJ. Purification and partial characterization of rat ovarian lutropin receptor. *J Biol Chem* 1987;262:7920–7926.
274. Piquette GN, LaPolt PS, Oikawa M, Hsueh AJ. Regulation of luteinizing hormone receptor messenger ribonucleic acid levels by gonadotropins, growth factors, and gonadotropin-releasing hormone in cultured rat granulosa cells. *Endocrinology* 1991;128:2449–2456.
275. Lin KC, Kawamura N, Okamura H, Mori T. Inhibition of ovulation, steroidogenesis and collagenolytic activity in rabbits by sulpiride-induced hyperprolactinaemia. *J Reprod Fertil* 1988; 83:611–618.
276. Yoshimura Y, Maruyama K, Shiraki M, Kawakami S, Fukushima M, Nakamura Y. Prolactin inhibits plasminogen activator activity in the preovulatory follicles. *Endocrinology* 1990; 126:631–636.
277. Yoshimura Y, Nakamura Y, Yamada H, et al. Possible contribution of prolactin in the process of ovulation and oocyte maturation. *Horm Res* 1991;35(suppl 1):22–32.
278. Clausell DE, Soliman KFA. Ovarian serotonin content in relation to ovulation. *Experientia* 1978;34:410–411.
279. Schmidt G, Kannisto P, Owman C, Sjoberg N-O. Is serotonin involved in the ovulatory process of the rat ovary perfused *in vitro? Acta Physiol Scand* 1988;132:251–256.
280. Trzeciak WH, Ahmed CE, Simpson ER, Ojeda SR. Vasoactive intestinal peptide induces the synthesis of the cholesterol side-chain cleavage enzyme complex in cultured rat ovarian granulosa cells. *Proc Natl Acad Sci USA* 1986;83:7490–7494.
281. Schmidt G, Jorgensen J, Kannisto P, Liedberg F, Ottesen B, Owman C. Vasoactive intestinal polypeptide in the PMSG-primed immature rat ovary and its effect on ovulation in the isolated rat ovary perfused *in vitro. J Reprod Fertil* 1990;90:465–472.
282. Roca RA, Garofalo EG, Martino I, et al. Effects of oxytocin antiserum and of indomethacin on hCG-induced ovulation in the rabbit. *Biol Reprod* 1978;19:552–557.
283. Wathes DC, Guldenaar SE, Swann RW, Webb R, Porter DG, Pickering BT. A combined radioimmunoassay and immunocytochemical study of ovarian oxytocin production during the periovulatory period in the ewe. *J Reprod Fertil* 1986;78:167–183.
284. Marsh JM, Mills TM, LeMaire WJ. Cyclic AMP synthesis in rabbit graafian follicles and the effect of luteinizing hormone. *Biochim Biophys Acta* 1972;273:389–394.
285. Marsh JM, Mills TM, LeMaire WJ. Preovulatory changes in the synthesis of cyclic AMP by rabbit graafian follicles. *Biochim Biophys Acta* 1973;304:197–202.
286. Marsh JM, Yang NST, LeMaire WJ. Prostaglandin synthesis in rabbit graafian follicles *in vitro.* Effect of luteinizing hormone and cyclic AMP. *Prostaglandins* 1974;7:269–283.
287. Marsh JM. The role of cyclic AMP in gonadal function. In: Greengard P, Robison GA, eds. *Advances in Cyclic Nucleotide Research,* Vol 6. New York: Raven Press, 1975;137–199.
288. Ellsworth LR, Armstrong DT. Luteinization of transplanted ovarian follicles in the rat induced by dibutyryl cyclic AMP. *Endocrinology* 1973;92:840–843.
289. Mills TM. Effect of luteinizing hormone and cyclic adenosine 3′,5′-monophosphate on steroidogenesis in the ovarian follicle of the rabbit. *Endocrinology* 1975;96:440–444.
290. Mason NR, Marsh R. The effect of LH on cyclic AMP and progesterone in rat ovaries *in vivo. Endocr Res Commun* 1975;2:167–177.
291. Mason NR, Marsh R. Cyclic AMP in the rat ovary: effect of endogenous LH secretion. *Endocr Res Commun* 1975;2: 357–365.
292. Goff AK, Major PW. Concentrations of cyclic AMP in rabbit ovarian tissue during the preovulatory period and pseudopregnancy after induction of ovulation by administration of human chorionic gonadotrophin. *J Endocrinol* 1975;65:73–82.
293. Weiss TJ, Seamark RF, McIntosh JEA, Moor RM. Cyclic AMP in sheep ovarian follicles: site of production and response to gonadotrophins. *J Reprod Fertil* 1976;46:347–353.
294. Weiss TJ, Armstrong DT, McIntosh JEA, Seamark RF. Maturational changes in sheep ovarian follicles: gonadotrophic stimulation of cyclic AMP production by isolated theca and granulosa cells. *Acta Endocrinol* 1978;89:166–172.
295. Bergh C, Ahren K. Prolongation of the effects of gonadotrophins and prostaglandin E_2 on ovarian cyclic AMP formation by inhibitors of protein synthesis. *Acta Endocrinol* 1980;94:251–258.
296. Nordenstrom K, Hamberger L. Influence of gonadotrophins on cAMP formation in theca cells isolated from pre-ovulatory rat follicles. *Acta Endocrinol* 1981;96:534–540.
297. Holmes PV, Hedin L, Janso PO. The role of cyclic adenosine 3′,5′-monophosphate in the ovulatory process of the *in vitro* perfused rabbit ovary. *Endocrinology* 1986;118:2195–2202.
298. Hedin L, McKnight GS, Lifka J, Durica JM, Richards JS. Tissue distribution and hormonal regulation of mRNA for regulatory and catalytic subunits of cAMP-dependent protein kinases during ovarian follicular development and luteinization in the rat. *Endocrinology* 1987;120:1928–1935.
299. Hosoi Y, Yoshimura Y, Atlas SJ, Adachi T, Wallach EE. Effects of dibutyryl cyclic AMP on oocyte maturation and ovulation in the perfused rabbit ovary. *J Reprod Fertil* 1989;85:405–411.
300. Patwardhan VV, Lanthier A. Effect of luteinizing hormone on the concentration of cyclic GMP in rabbit ovaries. *J Endocrinol* 1978;79:251–252.
301. Richards JS, Hedin L, Caston L. Differentiation of rat ovarian thecal cells: evidence for functional luteinization. *Endocrinology* 1986;118:1660–1668.
302. Hedin L, Rodgers RJ, Simpson ER, Richards JS. Changes in content of cytochrome $P450_{17\alpha}$, cytochrome $P450_{scc}$ and 3-hydroxy-3-methylglutaryl CoA reductase in developing rat ovarian follicles and corpora lutea: correlation with theca cell steroidogenesis. *Biol Reprod* 1987;37:211–223.
303. Voutilainen R, Tapanainen J, Chung B-C, Matteson KJ, Miller WL. Hormonal regulation of $P450_{scc}$ (20,22-desmolase) and $P450_{c17}$ (17α-hydroxylase/17,20-lyase) in cultured human granulosa cells. *J Clin Endocrinol Metab* 1986;63:202–207.
304. Trzeciak WH, Waterman MR, Simpson ER. Synthesis of the cholesterol side-chain cleavage enzyme in cultured rat ovarian granulosa cells: induction by follicle-stimulating hormone and dibutyryl-adenosine 3′,5′-monophosphate. *Endocrinology* 1986; 119:323–330.
305. Goldring NB, Durica JM, Lifka J, et al. Cholesterol side-chain cleavage P450 ($P450_{scc}$) messenger ribonucleic acid: evidence for hormonal regulation in rat ovarian follicles and constitutive expression in corpora lutea. *Endocrinology* 1987;120:1942–1950.
306. Trzeciak WH, Duda T, Waterman MR, Simpson ER. Tetradecanoyl phorbol acetate suppresses follicle-stimulating hormone-induced synthesis of the cholesterol side-chain cleavage enzyme complex in rat ovarian granulosa cells. *J Biol Chem* 1987; 262:15246–15250.
307. Leung PCK, Minegishi T, Wang J. Inhibition of follicle-stimulating hormone- and adenosine-3′,5′-cyclic monophosphate-induced progesterone production by calcium and protein kinase C in the rat ovary. *Am J Obstet Gynecol* 1988;158: 350–356.
308. Miller WL. Molecular biology of steroid hormone synthesis. *Endocr Rev* 1988;9:295–318.
309. Hylka VW, Kaki MK, DiZerega GS. Steroidogenesis of porcine granulosa cells from small and medium-sized follicles: effects of follicle-stimulating hormone, forskolin, and adenosine 3′,5′-cyclic monophosphate versus phorbol ester. *Endocrinology* 1989; 124:1204–1209.

310. Oonk RB, Krasnow JS, Beattie WG, Richards JS. Cyclic AMP-dependent and -independent regulation of cholesterol side chain cleavage cytochrome P-450 (P-450_{scc}) in rat ovarian granulosa cells and corpora lutea. *J Biol Chem* 1989;264:21934–21942.
311. Oonk RB, Parker KL, Gibson JL, Richards JS. Rat cholesterol side-chain cleavage cytochrome P-450 (P-450_{scc}) gene: structure and regulation by cAMP *in vitro*. *J Biol Chem* 1990;265: 22392–22401.
312. Rhodes RC III, Fleming MW, Murdoch WJ, Inskeep EK. Formation of cyclic adenosine monophosphate (cAMP) in the preovulatory rabbit follicle: role of prostaglandins and steroids. *Prostaglandins* 1985;29:217–231.
313. Rhodes RC III, Inskeep EK. Ovarian 3′5′-cyclic adenosine monophosphate and prostaglandins: a sequential comparison of gonadotropin-stimulated events in small and large ovine follicles. *J Anim Sci* 1988;66:1453–1461.
314. Rigler GL, Peake GT, Ratner A. Effects of follicle-stimulating hormone and luteinizing hormone on ovarian cyclic AMP and prostaglandin E *in vivo* in rats treated with indomethacin. *J Endocrinol* 1976;70:285–291.
315. Tsang BX, Ainsworth L, Downey BR, Armstrong DT. Preovulatory changes in cyclic AMP and prostaglandin concentrations in follicular fluid of gilts. *Prostaglandins* 1979;17: 141–148.
316. Davis JS, Weakland LL, West LA, Farese RV. Luteinizing hormone stimulates the formation of inositol triphosphate and cyclic AMP in rat granulosa cells. Evidence for phospholipase C generated second messengers in the action of luteinizing hormone. *Biochem J* 1986;238:597–604.
317. Dimino MJ, Snitzer J, Brown KM. Inositol phosphates accumulation in ovarian granulosa after stimulation by luteinizing hormone. *Biol Reprod* 1987;37:1129–1134.
318. Veldhuis JD, Demers LM. Activation of protein kinase C is coupled to prostaglandin E_2 synthesis in swine granulosa cells. *Prostaglandins* 1987;33:819–829.
319. Veldhuis JD. Prostaglandin $F_{2\alpha}$ initiates polyphosphatidylinositol hydrolysis and membrane translocation of protein kinase C in swine ovarian cells. *Biochem Biophys Res Commun* 1987;149: 112–117.
320. Veldhuis JD, Klase PA. Calcium ions modulate hormonally stimulated progesterone production in isolated ovarian cells. *Biochem J* 1982;202:381–386.
321. Veldhuis JD, Klase PA. Mechanisms by which calcium ions regulate the steroidogenic actions of luteinizing hormone in isolated ovarian cells *in vitro*. *Endocrinology* 1982;111:1–6.
322. Veldhuis JD. Mechanisms subserving hormone action in the ovary: role of calcium ions as assessed by steady state calcium exchange in cultured swine granulosa cells. *Endocrinology* 1987;120:445–449.
323. Sibley DR, Benovic JL, Caron MG, Lefkowitz RJ. Phosphorylation of cell surface receptors: a mechanism for regulating signal transduction pathways. *Endocr Rev* 1988;9:38–56.
324. Hunzicker-Dunn M, Jungmann RA. Rabbit ovarian protein kinases. I. Effect of an ovulatory dose of human chorionic gonadotropin or luteinizing hormone on the subcellular distribution of follicular and luteal protein kinases. *Endocrinology* 1978;103: 420–430.
325. Hunzicker-Dunn M, Jungmann RA. Rabbit ovarian protein kinases. I. Effect of an ovulatory dose of human chorionic gonadotropin or luteinizing hormone on the multiplicity of follicular and luteal protein kinases. *Endocrinology* 1978;103:431–438.
326. Richards JS, Sehgal N, Tash JS. Changes in content and cAMP-dependent phosphorylation of specific proteins in granulosa cells of preantral and preovulatory ovarian follicles and in corpora lutea. *J Biol Chem* 1983;258:5227–5232.
327. Jahnsen T, Lohmann SM, Walter U, Hedin L, Richards JS. Purification and characterization of hormone-regulated isoforms of the regulatory subunit of type II cAMP-dependent protein kinase from rat ovaries. *J Biol Chem* 1985;260:15980–15987.
328. Jahnsen T, Hedin L, Lohmann SM, Walter U, Richards JS. The neural type II regulatory subunit of cAMP-dependent protein kinase is present and regulated by hormones in the rat ovary. *J Biol Chem* 1986;261:6637–6639.
329. Jahnsen T, Hedin L, Kidd VJ, et al. Molecular cloning, cDNA structure, and regulation of the regulatory subunit of type II cAMP-dependent protein kinase from rat ovarian granulosa cells. *J Biol Chem* 1986;261:12352–12361.
330. Ratoosh SL, Lifka J, Hedin L, Jahnsen T, Richards JS. Hormonal regulation of the synthesis and mRNA content of the regulatory subunit of cyclic AMP-dependent protein kinase type II in cultured rat ovarian granulosa cells. *J Biol Chem* 1987;262: 7306–7313.
331. Veldhuis JD, Demers LM. An inhibitory role for the protein kinase C pathway in ovarian steroidogenesis. *Biochem J* 1986; 239:505–511.
332. Ranta T, Huhtaniemi I, Jalkanen J, Koskimies A, Laatikainen T, Ylikorkala O. Activation of protein kinase-C stimulates human granulosa-luteal cell prostacyclin production. *J Clin Endocrinol Metab* 1986;63:513–515.
333. Veldhuis JD, Demers LM. Activation of protein kinase C is coupled to prostaglandin $F_{2\alpha}$ synthesis in the ovary: studies in cultured swine granulosa cells. *Mol Cell Endocrinol* 1987;49: 249–254.
334. Wang J, Leung PCK. Synergistic stimulation of prostaglandin E_2 production by calcium ionophore and protein kinase C activator in rat granulosa cells. *Biol Reprod* 1989;40:1000–1006.
335. Shinohara O, Knecht M, Feng P, Catt KJ. Activation of protein kinase C potentiates cyclic AMP production and stimulates steroidogenesis in differentiated ovarian granulosa cells. *J Steroid Biochem* 1986;24:161–168.
336. Roby KF, Terranova PF. Tumor necrosis factor-alpha alters follicular steroidogenesis *in vivo*. *Endocrinology* 1988;123:2952–2954.
337. Roby KF, Terranova PF. Effects of tumor necrosis factor-α *in vitro* on steroidogenesis of healthy and atretic follicles of the rat: theca as a target. *Endocrinology* 1990;126:2711–2718.
338. Sancho-Tello M, Terranova PF. Involvement of protein kinase C in regulating tumor necrosis factor α-stimulated progesterone production in rat preovulatory follicles *in vitro*. *Endocrinology* 1991;128:1223–1228.
339. Kaufman G, Dharmarajan AM, Takehara Y, Cropp CS, Wallach EE. The role of protein kinase-C in gonadotropin-induced ovulation in the *in vitro* perfused rabbit ovary. *Endocrinology* 1992;131:1804–1809.
340. Johnson GL, Dhanasekaran N. The G-protein family and their interaction with receptors. *Endocr Rev* 1989;10:317–331.
341. Simon MI, Strathmann MP, Gautam N. Diversity of G proteins in signal transduction. *Science* 1991;252:802–808.
342. Farese RV. Phosphoinositide metabolism and hormone action. *Endocr Rev* 1983;4:78–95.
343. Black AK, Barr RM, Wong E, et al. Lipoxygenase products of arachidonic acid in human inflamed skin. *Br J Clin Pharmacol* 1985;20:185–190.
344. Richmond R, Clarke SR, Watson D, et al. Generation of hydroxyeicosatetraenoic acids by human inflammatory cells: analysis by thermospray liquid chromatography-mass spectrometry. *Biochim Biophys Acta* 1986;881:159–166.
345. O'Flaherty JT. Phospholipid metabolism and stimulus-response coupling. *Biochem Pharmacol* 1987;36:407–412.
346. Samuelsson B, Dahlen S-E, Lindgren JA, Rouzer CA, Serhan CN. Leukotrienes and lipoxins: structures, biosynthesis, and biological effects. *Science* 1987;237:1171–1176.
347. Chilton FH, Ellis JM, Olson SC, Wykle RL. 1-*O*-Alkyl-2-arachidonoyl-*sn*-glycero-3-phosphocholine. A common source of platelet-activating factor and arachidonate in human polymorphonuclear leukocytes. *J Biol Chem* 1984;259:12014–12019.
348. Whatley RE, Nelson P, Zimmerman GA, et al. The regulation of platelet-activating factor production in endothelial cells. *J Biol Chem* 1989;264:6325–6333.
349. Pinckard RN, Farr RS, Hanahan DJ. Physiochemical and functional identity of platelet-activating factor (PAF) released *in vivo* during IgE anaphylaxis with PAF release *in vitro* from IgE sensitized rabbit basophils. *J Immunol* 1979;123:1847–1857.
350. Issekutz AC, Szpejda M. Evidence that platelet activating factor may mediate some acute inflammatory responses. Studies with the platelet-activating factor antagonist, CV3988. *Lab Invest* 1986;54:275–280.
351. McManus LM. Pathobiology of platelet-activating factors. *Pathol Immunopathol Res* 1986;5:104–117.

352. Showell HJ, Bray MA. Platelet activating factor (PAF), an inflammatory misnomer—where are we today? In: Lewis A, Capetola R, eds. *Advances in Inflammation Research,* Vol 11. New York: Raven Press, 1986;67–70.
353. Harper MJK. Platelet-activating factor: a paracrine factor in preimplantation stages of reproduction? *Biol Reprod* 1989;40: 907–913.
354. Mencia-Huerta JM, Lee CW, Lee TH, et al. Platelet-activating factor (PAF-acether): generation from a mast cell subclass by an IgE-dependent mechanism. In: Benveniste J, Arnoux B, eds. *Platelet-Activating Factor and Structurally Related Ether-Lipids.* Amsterdam: Elsevier, 1983;101–188.
355. Miwa M, Hill C, Kumar R, Sugatani J, Olson M, Hanahan DJ. Occurrence of an endogenous inhibitor of platelet-activating factor in rat liver. *J Biol Chem* 1987;262:527–530.
356. Henson PM. Extracellular and intracellular activities of platelet activating factor. In: Winslow CM, Lee ML, eds. *New Horizons in Platelet Activating Factor Research.* New York: John Wiley & Sons, 1987;3–10.
357. Michel L, Denizot Y, Thomas Y, et al. Biosynthesis of PAF-acether factor-acether by human skin fibroblasts *in vitro. J Immunol* 1988;141:948–953.
358. Humphrey DM, McManus LM, Hanahan DJ, Pinckard RN. Morphologic basis of increased vascular permeability induced by acetyl glyceryl ether phosphorylcholine. *Lab Invest* 1984;50: 16–25.
359. Archer CB, MacDonald DM, Morley J, Page CP, Paul W, Sanjar S. Effects of serum albumin, indomethacin and histamine H_1-antagonists on PAF-acether-induced inflammatory responses in the skin of experimental animals and man. *Br J Pharmacol* 1985;85:109–113.
360. Espey LL, Tanaka N, Woodard DS, Harper MJK, Okamura H. Decrease in ovarian platelet-activating factor during ovulation in the gonadotropin-primed immature rat. *Biol Reprod* 1989;40: 104–110.
361. Abisogun AO, Braquet P, Tsafriri A. The involvement of platelet activating factor in ovulation. *Science* 1989;243:381–383.
362. Kikukawa Y, Ishikawa M, Sengoku K, Kasamo M, Shimizu T. The effect of platelet activating factor on ovulation. *Prostaglandins* 1991;42:95–104.
363. Pool WR, Lipner H. Inhibition of ovulation in the rabbit by actinomycin D. *Nature* 1965;203:1385–1387.
364. Pool WR, Lipner H. Inhibition of ovulation by antibiotics. *Endocrinology* 1966;79:858–864.
365. Barros C, Austin CR. Inhibition of ovulation by systemically administered actinomycin D in the hamster. *Endocrinology* 1968;83:177–179.
366. Reel JR, Gorski J. Gonadotrophic regulation of precursor incorporation into ovarian RNA, protein, and acid-soluble fractions. I. Effects of pregnant mare serum gonadotrophin (PMSG), follicle-stimulating hormone (FSH), and luteinizing hormone (LH). *Endocrinology* 1968;83:1083–1091.
367. Reel JR, Gorski J. Gonadotrophic regulation of precursor incorporation into ovarian RNA, protein, and acid-soluble fractions. II. Changes in nucleotide labeling, nuclear RNA synthesis, and effects of RNA and protein synthesis inhibitors. *Endocrinology* 1968;83:1092–1100.
368. Clark MR, Marsh JM, LeMaire WJ. The role of protein synthesis in the stimulation by LH of prostaglandin accumulation in rat preovulatory follicles *in vitro. Prostaglandins* 1976;12:209–216.
369. Alleva JJ, Bonventre PF, Lamanna C. Inhibition of ovulation in hamsters by the protein synthesis inhibitors diphtheria toxin and cycloheximide. *Proc Soc Exp Biol Med* 1979;162:170–174.
370. Espey LL. Cycloheximide inhibition of ovulation, prostaglandin biosynthesis and steroidogenesis in rabbit ovarian follicles. *J Reprod Fertil* 1986;78:679–683.
371. Pool WR, Lipner H. Radioautography of newly synthesized RNA and protein in preovulatory follicles. *Endocrinology* 1969;84:711–716.
372. Mills TM. Protein and RNA synthesis in follicles isolated from rabbit ovaries. *Proc Soc Exp Biol Med* 1975;148:995–1000.
373. Hickey GJ, Chen S, Besman MJ, et al. Hormonal regulation, tissue distribution, and content of aromatase cytochrome P450 messenger ribonucleic acid and enzyme in rat ovarian follicles and corpora lutea: relationship to estradiol biosynthesis. *Endocrinology* 1988;122:1426–1436.
374. Fitzpatrick SL, Richards JS. Regulation of cytochrome P450 aromatase messenger ribonucleic acid and activity by steroids and gonadotropins in rat granulosa cells. *Endocrinology* 1991;129: 1452–1462.
375. Hedin, L, Gaddy-Kurten D, Kurten R, DeWitt DL, Smith WL, Richards JS. Prostaglandin endoperoxide synthase in rat ovarian follicles: content, cellular distribution, and evidence for hormonal induction preceding ovulation. *Endocrinology* 1987; 121:722–731.
376. Wong WYL, DeWitt DL, Smith WL, Richards JS. Rapid induction of prostaglandin endoperoxide synthase in rat preovulatory follicles by luteinizing hormone and cAMP is blocked by inhibitors of transcription and translation. *Mol Endocrinol* 1989; 3:1714–1723.
377. Wong WYL, Richards JS. Evidence for two antigenically distinct molecular weight variants of prostaglandin H synthase in the rat ovary. *Mol Endocrinol* 1991;5:1269–1279.
378. Sirois J, Richards JS. Purification and characterization of a novel, distinct isoform of prostaglandin endoperoxide synthase induced by human chorionic gonadotropin in granulosa cells of rat preovulatory follicles. *J Biol Chem* 1992;267:6382–6388.
379. Sirois J, Simmons DL, Richards JS. Hormonal regulation of messenger ribonucleic acid encoding a novel isoform of prostaglandin endoperoxide H synthase in rat preovulatory follicles. *J Biol Chem* 1992;267:11586–11592.
380. Kurten RC, Levy LO, Shey J, Durica JM, Richards JS. Identification and characterization of the GC-rich and cyclic adenosine 3′,5′-monophosphate (cAMP)-dependent inducible promoter of type IIβ cAMP-dependent protein kinase regulatory subunit gene. *Mol Endocrinol* 1992;6:536–550.
381. Clements JA, Mukhtar A, Erhlich A. Kallikrein gene expression in rat ovary. *The Endocrine Society 74th Annual Meeting, Program & Abstracts,* 1992.
382. O'Connell ML, Canipari R, Strickland S. Hormonal regulation of tissue plasminogen activator secretion and mRNA levels in rat granulosa cells. *J Biol Chem* 1987;262:2339–2344.
383. Hsueh AJ, Liu YX, Cajander S, et al. Gonadotropin-releasing hormone induces ovulation in hypophysectomized rats: studies on ovarian tissue-type plasminogen activator activity, messenger ribonucleic acid content, and cellular localization. *Endocrinology* 1988;122:1486–1495.
384. Galway AB, Oikawa M, Ny T, Hsueh AJW. Epidermal growth factor stimulates tissue plasminogen activator activity and messenger ribonucleic acid levels in cultured rat granulosa cells: mediation by pathways independent of protein kinases-A and -C. *Endocrinology* 1989;125:126–135.
385. Reich R, Iken D, Chun SY, et al. Preovulatory changes in ovarian expression of collagenases and tissue metalloproteinase inhibitor messenger ribonucleic acid: role of eicosanoids. *Endocrinology* 1991;129:1869–1875.
386. Curry TE Jr, Dean DD, Sanders SL, Pedigo NG, Jones PB. The role of ovarian proteases and their inhibitors in ovulation. *Steroids* 1989;54:501–521.
387. Curry TE Jr, Mann JS, Estes RS, Jones PB. Alpha$_2$-macroglobulin and tissue inhibitor of metalloproteinases: collagenase inhibitors in human preovulatory ovaries. *Endocrinology* 1990;127:63–68.
388. Mann JS, Kindy MS, Edwards DR, Curry TE Jr. Hormonal regulation of matrix metalloproteinase inhibitors in rat granulosa cells and ovaries. *Endocrinology* 1991;128:1825–1832.
389. Kudlow JE, Kobrin MS, Purchio AF, et al. Ovarian transforming growth factor-α gene expression: immunohistochemical localization to the theca-interstitial cells. *Endocrinology* 1987;121: 1577–1578.
390. Koos RD, Olson CE. Expression of basic fibroblast growth factor in the rat ovary: detection of mRNA using reverse transcription-polymerase chain reaction amplification. *Mol Endocrinol* 1989;3:2041–2048.
391. Koos RD, Seidel RH. Detection of acidic fibroblast growth factor mRNA in the rat ovary using reverse transcription-polymerase chain reaction amplification. *Biochem Biophys Res Commun* 1989;165:82–88.

392. Jesionowska H, Hemmings R, Guyda HJ, Posner BI. Determination of insulin and insulin-like growth factors in the ovarian circulation. *Fertil Steril* 1990;53:88–91.
393. Roy SK, Greenwald GS. *In vitro* effects of epidermal growth factor, insulin-like growth factor-I, fibroblast growth factor, and follicle-stimulating hormone on hamster follicular deoxyribonucleic acid synthesis and steroidogenesis. *Biol Reprod* 1991; 44:889–896.
394. Krishna A, Terranova PF. Alterations in mast cell degranulation and ovarian histamine in the proestrous hamster. *Biol Reprod* 1985;32:1211–1217.
395. Schmidt G, Owman C, Sjoberg NO. Cellular localization of ovarian histamine, its cyclic variations, and histaminergic effects on ovulation in the rat ovary perfused *in vitro. J Reprod Fertil* 1988;82:409–417.
396. Oriowo MA, Bevan JA. Characterization of histamine H_1 and H_2 receptors in the rabbit isolated ovarian artery and vein. *J Cardiovasc Pharmacol* 1987;10:76–81.
397. Szego CM, Gitin ES. Ovarian histamine depletion during acute hyperaemic response to luteinizing hormone. *Nature* 1964; 201:682–684.
398. Szego CM. Role of histamine in mediation of hormone action. *Fed Proc* 1965;24:1343–1352.
399. Wallach EE, Wright KH, Hamada Y. Investigation of mammalian ovulation with an *in vitro* perfused rabbit ovary preparation. *Am J Obstet Gynecol* 1978;132:728–738.
400. Knox E, Lowry S, Beck L. Prevention of ovulation in rabbits by antihistamine. In: Midgley AR Jr, Sadler WA, eds. *Ovarian Follicular Development and Function.* New York: Raven Press, 1979;159–163.
401. Schmidt G, Owman C, Sjoberg NO. Histamine induces ovulation in the isolated perfused rat ovary. *J Reprod Fertil* 1986;78: 159–166.
402. Krishna A, Terranova PF, Matteri RL, Papkoff H. Histamine and increased ovarian blood flow mediate LH-induced superovulation in the cyclic hamster. *J Reprod Fertil* 1986;76:23–29.
403. Kobayashi Y, Wright KH, Santulli R, Kitai HK, Wallach EE. Effect of histamine and histamine blockers on the ovulatory process in the *in vitro* perfused rabbit ovary. *Biol Reprod* 1983;28:385–392.
404. Schmidt G, Holmes PV, Owman C, Sjoberg NO, Walles B. The influence of prostaglandin E_2 and indomethacin on progesterone production and ovulation in the rabbit ovary perfused *in vitro. Biol Reprod* 1986;35:815–821.
405. Murdoch WJ. Localization and hormonal regulation of ovarian production of histamine in the sheep. *Life Sci* 1990;46: 1961–1965.
406. Lipner H. Ovulation from histamine depleted ovaries. *Proc Soc Exp Biol Med* 1971;136:111–114.
407. Espey LL, Stein VI, Dumitrescu J. Survey of antiinflammatory agents and related drugs as inhibitors of ovulation in the rabbit. *Fertil Steril* 1982;38:238–247.
408. Kitai H, Kobayashi Y, Santulli R, Wright KH, Wallach EE. The relationship between prostaglandins and histamine in the ovulatory process as determined with the *in vitro* perfused rabbit ovary. *Fertil Steril* 1985;43:646–651.
409. Halterman SD, Murdoch WJ. Ovarian function in ewes treated with antihistamines. *Endocrinology* 1986;119:2417–2421.
410. Koos RD, Clark MR. Production of 6-keto-prostaglandin $F_{1\alpha}$ by rat granulosa cells *in vitro. Endocrinology* 1982;111:1513–1518.
411. Regoli D, Barabe J. Pharmacology of bradykinin and related kinins. *Pharmacol Rev* 1980;32:1–46.
412. Straus DS, Pang KJ. Effects of bradykinin on DNA synthesis in resting NIL8 hamster cells and human fibroblasts. *Exp Cell Res* 1984;151:87–95.
413. Espey LL, Miller DH, Margolius HS. Ovarian increase in kinin-generating capacity in PMSG/hCG-primed immature rat. *Am J Physiol* 1986;251:E362–E365.
414. Carry F, Haworth D, Whalley ET. Pro-inflammatory effects of bradykinin, Σ-cyclo[lys^1,gly^6]bradykinin and Σ-cyclo-kallidine in the rat. *Eur J Pharmacol* 1988;156:161–164.
415. Chao J, Swain C, Chao S, Xiong W, Chao L. Tissue distribution and kininogen gene expression after acute-phase inflammation. *Biochim Biophys Acta* 1988;964:329–339.
416. Chao S, Chao L, Chao J. Sex dimorphism and inflammatory regulation of T-kininogen and T-kininogenase. *Biochim Biophys Acta* 1989;991:477–483.
417. Smith C, Perks AM. Plasma bradykininogen levels before and after ovulation: studies in women and guinea pigs, with observations on oral contraceptives and menopause. *Am J Obstet Gynecol* 1979;133:868–876.
418. Smith C, Perks AM. Changes in plasma kininogen levels in rats before ovulation, and after treatment with luteinizing hormone and oestradiol-17β. *Acta Endocrinol* 1983;104:123–128.
419. Smith C, Perks AM. The kinin system and ovulation: changes in plasma kininogens, and in kinin-forming enzymes in the ovaries and blood of rats with 4-day estrous cycles. *Can J Physiol Pharmacol* 1983;61:736–742.
420. Espey LL, Tanaka N, Winn V, Okamura H. Increase in ovarian kallikrein activity during ovulation in the gonadotropin-primed immature rat. *J Reprod Fertil* 1989;87:503–508.
421. Tanaka N, Espey LL, Stacy S, Okamura H. Epostane and indomethacin actions on ovarian kallikrein and plasminogen activator activities during ovulation in the gonadotropin-primed immature rat. *Biol Reprod* 1992;46:665–670.
422. Gao X, Greenbaum LM, Mahesh VB, Brann DW. Characterization of the kinin system in the ovary during ovulation in the rat. *Biol Reprod* 1992;47:945–951.
423. Yoshimura Y, Espey L, Hosoi Y, et al. The effects of bradykinin on ovulation and prostaglandin production by the perfused rabbit ovary. *Endocrinology* 1988;122:2540–2546.
424. Brannstrom M, Hellberg P. Bradykinin potentiates LH-induced follicular rupture in the rat ovary perfused *in vitro. Hum Reprod* 1989;4:475–481.
425. Hellberg P, Larson L, Olofsson J, Hedin L, Brannstrom M. Stimulatory effects of bradykinin on the ovulatory process in the *in vitro*-perfused rat ovary. *Biol Reprod* 1991;44:269–274.
426. Nasjletti A, Malik KU. Minireview: relationships between the kallikrein-kinin and prostaglandin systems. *Life Sci* 1979; 25:99–110.
427. Vio CP, Bednar MM, McGiff JC. Prostaglandins as mediators and modulators of the kallikrein-kinin system. *Adv Exp Med Biol* 1983;156:501–514.
428. Clements JA. The glandular kallikrein family of enzymes: tissue-specific expression and hormonal regulation. *Endocr Rev* 1989;10:393–419.
429. Inagami T, Murakami K. Prorenin. *Biomed Mater Res* 1980;1:456–475.
430. Itskovitz J, Sealey JE, Glorioso N, Rosenwaks Z. Plasma prorenin response to human chorionic gonadotropin in ovarian-hyperstimulated women: correlation with the number of ovarian follicles and steroid hormone concentrations. *Proc Natl Acad Sci* 1987;84:7285–7289.
431. Daud AI, Bumpus FM, Husain A. Characterization of angiotensin I-converting enzyme (ACE)-containing follicles in the rat ovary during the estrous cycle and effects of ACE inhibitor on ovulation. *Endocrinology* 1990;126:2927–2935.
432. Husain A, Bumpus FM, DeSilva P, Speth RC. Localization of angiotensin II receptors in ovarian follicles and the identification of angiotensin II in rat ovaries. *Proc Natl Acad Sci* 1987; 84:2489–2493.
433. Jentzsch KD, Hilse H, Siems WE, Heder G. Possible involvement of the renin-angiotensin system in reproduction. II. Occurrence and role in the female reproductive tract. *Zentralbl Gynakol* 1989;111:485–493.
434. Brunswig-Spickenheier B, Mukhopadhyay AK. Characterization of angiotensin-II receptor subtype on bovine thecal cells and its regulation by luteinizing hormone. *Endocrinology* 1992;131: 1445–1452.
435. Howard RB, Husain A. Rat ovarian angiotensin II receptors, renin, and angiotensin I-converting enzyme during pregnancy and the postpartum period. *Biol Reprod* 1992;47: 925–930.
436. Pellicer A, Palumbo A, DeCherney AH, Naftolin F. Blockage of ovulation by an angiotensin antagonist. *Science* 1988;240: 1660–1661.
437. Naftolin F, Andrade-Gordon P, Pellicer A, et al. Angiotensin II: does it have a direct obligate role in ovulation [Letter] *Science* 1989;245:871.
438. Andrade-Gordon P, Zreik T, Apa R, Naftolin F. Role of angioten-

sin II in the processes leading to ovulation. *Biochem Pharmacol* 1991;42:715–719.
439. Daud AI, Bumpus FM, Husain A. Angiotensin II: does it have a direct obligate role in ovulation [Letter] *Science* 1989;245: 870–871.
440. Espey LL, Tanaka N, Okamura H. Failure of the angiotensin antagonist saralasin and the angiotensin converting enzyme inhibitor captopril to inhibit ovulation in the gonadotropin-primed rat. *Proc Soc Exp Biol Med* 1990;193:249 (abst).
441. Dunn CJ, Willoughby DA, Giroud JP, Yamamoto S. An appraisal of the interrelationships between prostaglandins and cyclic nucleotides in inflammation. *Biomedicine* 1976;24:214–220.
442. Messina EJ, Weiner R, Kaley G. Prostaglandins and local circulatory control. *Fed Proc* 1976;35:2367–2375.
443. Bonta IL, Parnham MJ, Adolfs MJP. Reduced exudation and increased tissue proliferation during chronic inflammation in rats deprived of endogenous prostaglandin precursors. *Prostaglandins* 1977;14:295–307.
444. Bonta IL, Parnham MJ, Adolfs MJP, van Vliet L. Dual functions of E-type prostaglandins in models of chronic inflammation. In: Willoughby DA, ed. *Perspectives in Inflammation.* Baltimore: University Park Press, 1977;265–275.
445. Bonta IL, Parnham MJ. Prostaglandins and chronic inflammation. *Biochem Pharmacol* 1978;27:1611–1623.
446. Kunkel SL, Ogawa H, Conran PB, Ward PA, Zurier RB. Suppression of acute and chronic inflammation by orally administered prostaglandins. *Arthritis Rheum* 1981;24:1151–1158.
447. Schumert R, Towner J, Zipser RD. Role of eicosanoids in human experimental colitis. *Dig Dis Sci* 1988;33:58S–64S.
448. Salvatori R, Guidon PT Jr, Rapuano BE, Bockman RS. Prostaglandin E_1 inhibits collagenase gene expression in rabbit synoviocytes and human fibroblasts. *Endocrinology* 1992;131:21–28.
449. Labhsetwar AP. Luteolysis and ovulation induced by prostaglandin $F_{2\alpha}$ in the hamster. *Nature* 1971;230:528–529.
450. Labhsetwar AP. Luteolytic and ovulation-inducing properties of prostaglandin $F_{2\alpha}$ in pregnant mice. *J Reprod Fertil* 1972;28: 451–452.
451. Orczyk GP, Behrman HR. Ovulation blockade by aspirin or indomethacin—*in vivo* evidence for a role of prostaglandin in gonadotrophin secretion. *Prostaglandins* 1972;1:3–20.
452. Armstrong DT, Grinwich DL. Blockade of spontaneous and LH-induced ovulation in rats by indomethacin, an inhibitor of prostaglandin biosynthesis. *Prostaglandins* 1972;1:21–28.
453. O'Grady JP, Caldwell BV, Auletta FJ, Speroff L. The effects of an inhibitor of prostaglandin synthesis (indomethacin) on ovulation, pregnancy, and pseudopregnancy in the rabbit. *Prostaglandins* 1972;1:97–106.
454. Behrman HR, Orczyk GP, Greep RO. Effect of synthetic gonadotrophin-releasing hormone (Gn-RH) on ovulation blockade by aspirin and indomethacin. *Prostaglandins* 1972;1: 245–258.
455. Tsafriri A, Lindner HR, Zor U, Lamprecht SA. Physiological role of prostaglandins in the induction of ovulation. *Prostaglandins* 1972;2:1–10.
456. Diaz-Infante A Jr, Wright KH, Wallach EE. Effects of indomethacin and prostaglandin $F_{2\alpha}$ on ovulation and ovarian contractility in the rabbit. *Prostaglandins* 1974;5:567–579.
457. Armstrong DT, Grinwich DL, Moon YS, Zamecnik J. Inhibition of ovulation in rabbits by intrafollicular injection of indomethacin and prostaglandin F antiserum. *Life Sci* 1974;14:129–140.
458. Armstrong DT, Moon YS, Zamecnik J. Evidence for a role of ovarian prostaglandins in ovulation. In: Moudgal NR, ed. *Gonadotropins and Gonadal Function.* New York: Academic Press, 1974;345–356.
459. Armstrong DT, Zamecnik J. Pre-ovulatory elevation of rat ovarian prostaglandins F, and its blockade by indomethacin. *Mol Cell Endocrinol* 1975;2:125–131.
460. Armstrong DT, Dorrington JH, Robinson J. Effects of indomethacin and aminoglutethimide phosphate *in vivo* on luteinizing-hormone-induced alterations of cyclic adenosine monophosphate, prostaglandin F, and steroid levels in preovulatory rat ovaries. *Can J Biochem* 1976;54:796–802.
461. LeMaire WJ, Davies PJA, Marsh JM. The role of prostaglandins in the development of refractoriness to LH stimulation by graafian follicles. *Prostaglandins* 1976;12:271–279.
462. Hunzicker-Dunn M, Birnbaumer L. Adenylyl cyclase activities in ovarian tissues. II. Regulation of responsiveness to LH, FSH, and PGE_1 in the rabbit. *Endocrinology* 1976;99:185–189.
463. Ainsworth L, Tsang BK, Downey BR, Baker RD, Marcus GJ, Armstrong DT. Effects of indomethacin on ovulation and luteal function in gilts. *Biol Reprod* 1979;21:401–411.
464. Lau IF, Saksena SK. Inhibition of ovulation and fertilization by indomethacin and effect of prostaglandin-$F_{2\alpha}$ on early pregnancy in the rabbit. *Prostaglandin Med* 1979;2:425–432.
465. Downs SM, Longo FJ. Effects of indomethacin on preovulatory follicles in immature, superovulated mice. *Am J Anat* 1982;164:265–274.
466. Espey LL. Optimum time for administration of indomethacin to inhibit ovulation in the rabbit. *Prostaglandins* 1982;23: 329–335.
467. DeSilva M, Reeves JJ. Indomethacin inhibition of ovulation in the cow. *J Reprod Fertil* 1985;75:547–549.
468. Espey LL, Norris C, Saphire D. Effect of time and dose of indomethacin on follicular prostaglandins and ovulation in the rabbit. *Endocrinology* 1986;119:746–754.
469. Brannstrom M, Koos RD, LeMaire WJ, Janson PO. Cyclic adenosine 3′,5′-monophosphate-induced ovulation in the perfused rat ovary and its mediation by prostaglandins. *Biol Reprod* 1987; 37:1047–1053.
470. Espey LL, Kohda H, Mori T, Okamura H. Rat ovarian prostaglandin levels and ovulation as indicators of the strength of non-steroidal anti-inflammatory drugs. *Prostaglandins* 1988;36: 875–879.
471. Tamura K, Kogo H. The mode of action of indomethacin, aspirin and melatonin on the blockage of the first ovulation in immature rat pretreated with PMSG. *Jpn J Pharmacol* 1989; 50:491–494.
472. Tanaka N, Espey LL, Kawano T, Okamura H. Comparison of inhibitory actions of indomethacin and epostane on ovulation in rats. *Am J Physiol* 1991;260:E170–E174.
473. Murdoch WJ, McCormick RJ. Dose-dependent effects of indomethacin on ovulation in the sheep: relationship to follicular prostaglandin production, steroidogenesis, collagenolysis, and leukocyte chemotaxis. *Biol Reprod* 1991;45:907–911.
474. LeMaire WJ, Yang NST, Behrman HH, Marsh JM. Preovulatory changes in the concentration of prostaglandins in rabbit graafian follicles. *Prostaglandins* 1973;3:367–376.
475. Yang NST, Marsh JM, LeMaire WJ. Prostaglandin changes induced by ovulatory stimuli in rabbit graafian follicles. The effect of indomethacin. *Prostaglandins* 1973;4:395–404.
476. Yang NST, Marsh JM, LeMaire WJ. Post ovulatory changes in the concentration of prostaglandins in rabbit graafian follicles. *Prostaglandins* 1974;6:37–44.
477. LeMaire WJ, Leidner R, Marsh JM. Pre and post ovulatory changes in the concentration of prostaglandins in rat graafian follicles. *Prostaglandins* 1975;9:221–229.
478. Iesaka T, Sato T, Igarashi M. Role of prostaglandin $F_{2\alpha}$ in ovulation. *Endocrinol Jpn* 1975;22:279–285.
479. Ainsworth L, Baker RD, Armstrong DT. Pre-ovulatory changes in follicular fluid prostaglandin F levels in swine. *Prostaglandins* 1975;9:915–925.
480. Erickson GF, Challis JRG, Ryan KJ. Production of prostaglandin F by rabbit granulosa cells and thecal tissue. *J Reprod Fertil* 1977;49:133–134.
481. Aksel S, Schomberg DW, Hammond CB. Prostaglandin $F_{2\alpha}$ production by the human ovary. *Obstet Gynecol* 1977;50:347–350.
482. Clark MR, Marsh JM, LeMaire WJ. Mechanism of luteinizing hormone regulation of prostaglandin synthesis in rat granulosa cells. *J Biol Chem* 1978;253:7757–7761.
483. Murdoch WJ, Dailey RA, Inskeep EK. Preovulatory changes in prostaglandins E_2 and $F_{2\alpha}$ in ovine follicles. *J Anim Sci* 1981;53:192–205.
484. Darling M, Jogee M, Elder MG. Prostaglandin $F_{2\alpha}$ levels in the human ovarian follicle. *Prostaglandins* 1982;23:551–558.
485. Koos RD, Clark MR, Janson PO, Ahren KEB, LeMaire WJ. Prostaglandin levels in preovulatory follicles from rabbit ovaries perfused *in vitro*. *Prostaglandins* 1983;25:715–724.
486. Schlaff S, Kobayashi Y, Wright KH, Santulli R, Wallach EE. Prostaglandin $F_{2\alpha}$, an ovulatory intermediate in the *in vitro* perfused rabbit ovary model. *Prostaglandins* 1983;26:111–121.

487. Akinlosotu BA, Verma OP. Detection of ovulation in goats by blood prostaglandins concentrations. *Am J Vet Res* 1983;44: 1339–1343.
488. Brown CG, Poyser NL. Studies on ovarian prostaglandin production in relation to ovulation in the rat. *J Reprod Fertil* 1984;72:407–414.
489. LeMaire WJ, Koos RD, Clark MR, et al. Studies on the role of prostaglandins in ovulation using the isolated perfused ovary as a model. In: Hayaishi O, Yamamoto S, eds. *Advances in Prostaglandin, Thromboxane, and Leukotriene Research,* Vol 15. New York: Raven Press, 1985;589–591.
490. Lumsden MA, Kelly RW, Templeton AA, Van Look PFA, Swanston IA, Baird DT. Changes in the concentration of prostaglandins in preovulatory human follicles after administration of hCG. *J Reprod Fertil* 1986;77:119–124.
491. Carson R, Trounson A, Mitchell M. Regulation of prostaglandin biosynthesis by human ovarian follicular fluid: a mechanism for ovulation? *Prostaglandins* 1986;32:49–55.
492. Murdoch WJ, Peterson TA, Van Kirk EA, Vincent DL, Inskeep EK. Interactive roles of progesterone, prostaglandins, and collagenase in the ovulatory mechanism of the ewe. *Biol Reprod* 1986;35:1187–1194.
493. Kogo H, Tamura K, Satoh T, Taya K, Sasamoto S. Relationship between the production capacity of ovarian 13,14-dihydroprostaglandin $F_{2\alpha}$ and the process of ovulation in immature female rats pretreated with gonadotropin. *Prostaglandins Leukot Essent Fatty Acids* 1989;37:177–181.
494. Espey LL, Tanaka N, Adams RF, Okamura H. Ovarian hydroxyeicosatetraenoic acids compared with prostanoids and steroids during ovulation in rats. *Am J Physiol* 1991;260: E163–E169.
495. Algire JE, Srikandakumar A, Guilbault LA, Downey BR. Preovulatory changes in follicular prostaglandins and their role in ovulation in cattle. *Can J Vet Res* 1992;56:67–69.
496. LeMaire WJ, Marsh JM. Interrelationships between prostaglandins, cyclic AMP and steroids in ovulation. *J Reprod Fertil* 1975;22(suppl):53–74.
497. Armstrong DT. Prostaglandins and follicular functions. *J Reprod Fertil* 1981;62:283–291.
498. Batta SK, Stark RA, Brackett BG. Ovulation induction by gonadotropin and prostaglandin treatments of rhesus monkeys and observations of the ova. *Biol Reprod* 1978;18:264–278.
499. Thebault A, Lefevre B, Testart J. Role of the extra-follicular compartment in the ovulation of isolated rabbit ovarian follicles. *J Reprod Fertil* 1983;68:419–424.
500. Lamprecht SA, Zor U, Tsafriri A, Lindner HR. Action of prostaglandin E_2 and of luteinizing hormone on ovarian adenylate cyclase, protein kinase and ornithine decarboxylase activity during postnatal development and maturity in the rat. *J Endocrinol* 1973;57:217–233.
501. Kolena J, Channing CP. Stimulatory effects of LH, FSH and prostaglandins upon cyclic 3′,5′-AMP levels in porcine granulosa cells. *Endocrinology* 1972;90:1543–1550.
502. Bauminger S, Koch Y, Khan I, Hillensjo T, Nilsson L, Ahren K. Preovulatory changes in ovarian cyclic AMP and prostaglandins in immature rats injected with PMSG. *J Reprod Fertil* 1978;52:21–23.
503. Marsh JM, LeMaire WJ. The role of cyclic AMP and prostaglandins in the actions of luteinizing hormone. In: Moudgal NR, ed. *Gonadotropins and Gonadal Function.* New York: Academic Press, 1974;376–390.
504. Patwardhan VV, Lanthier A. Prostaglandis PGE and PGF in human ovarian follicles: endogenous contents and *in vitro* formation by theca and granulosa cells. *Acta Endocrinol* 1981;97: 543–550.
505. Evans G, Dobias M, King CJ, Armstrong DT. Production of prostaglandins by porcine preovulatory follicular tissue and their roles in intrafollicular function. *Biol Reprod* 1983;28:322–328.
506. Ainsworth L, Tsang BK, Marcus GJ, Downey BR. Prostaglandin production by dispersed granulosa and theca interna cells from porcine preovulatory follicles. *Biol Reprod* 1984;31:115–121.
507. Murdoch WJ, Slaughter RG, Ji TH. *In situ* hybridization analysis of ovarian prostaglandin endoperoxide synthase mRNA throughout the periovulatory period of the ewe. *Domest Anim Endocrinol* 1991;8:455–457.
508. Grinwich DL, Kennedy TG, Armstrong DT. Dissociation of ovulatory and steroidogenic actions of luteinizing hormone in rabbits with indomethacin, an inhibitor of prostaglandin biosynthesis. *Prostaglandins* 1972;1:89–96.
509. Bowring N, Earthy M, Mangan FR. Changes in prostaglandin content of the rabbit ovary associated with ovulation. *J Endocrinol* 1975;64:11(abst).
510. Phi LT, Moon YS, Armstrong DT. Effects of systemic and intrafollicular injections of LH, prostaglandins, and indomethacin on the luteinization of rabbit graafian follicles. *Prostaglandins* 1977;13:543–552.
511. Maia H, Barbosa I, Coutinho EM. Inhibition of ovulation in marmoset monkeys by indomethacin. *Fertil Steril* 1978;29:565–570.
512. Barbosa I, Maia H Jr, Lopes T, Elder MG, Coutinho EM. Effect of indomethacin on prostaglandin and steroid synthesis by the marmoset ovary *in vivo. Int J Fertil* 1979;24:142–144.
513. Kraeling RR, Rampacek GB, Kiser TE. Corpus luteum function after indomethacin treatment during the estrous cycle and following hysterectomy in the gilt. *Biol Reprod* 1981;25:511–518.
514. Murdoch WJ, Dunn TG. Luteal function after ovulation blockade by intrafollicular injection of indomethacin in the ewe. *J Reprod Fertil* 1983;69:671–675.
515. Holmes PV, Janson PO, Sogn J, et al. Effects of $PGF_{2\alpha}$ and indomethacin on ovulation and steroid production in the isolated perfused rabbit ovary. *Acta Endocrinol* 1983;104:233–239.
516. Satoh K, Kinoshita K, Tsutsumi O. Prostaglandins and ovulation. In: Hayaishi O, Yamamoto S, eds. *Advances in Prostaglandin, Thromboxane, and Leukotriene Research,* Vol. 15. New York: Raven Press, 1985;593–595.
517. Plas-Roser S, Kauffmann MT, Aron C. Prostaglandins involvement in the formation of luteinized unruptured follicles in the cyclic female rat. *Prostaglandins* 1985;29:243–253.
518. Schlegel W, Vancaillie T, Schneider HP. The influence of continuous intrauterine infusion of enzyme-inhibitors of the arachidonic acid cascade on ovulation and tubal ovum transport in the hyperstimulated rabbit. *Horm Metab Res* 1986;18:386–390.
519. Munalulu BM, Hillier K, Peddie MJ. Effect of human chorionic gonadotrophin and indomethacin on ovulation, steroidogenesis and prostaglandin synthesis in preovulatory follicles of PMSG-primed immature rats. *J Reprod Fertil* 1987;80:229–234.
520. YoungLai EV. Prostaglandins and steroidogenesis by isolated rabbit ovarian follicles. *Horm Res* 1978;9:31–40.
521. Plas-Roser S, Kauffmann MT, Aron C. Do luteinized unruptured follicles secrete progesterone in mature female rats? *Experientia* 1984;40:500–501.
522. Patwardhan VV, Lanthier A. Effect of prostaglandins on the *in vitro* biosynthesis of estrone, estradiol and progesterone by rabbit ovarian follicles. *J Steroid Biochem* 1977;8:777–780.
523. Mori T, Kohda H, Kinoshita Y, Ezaki Y, Morimoto N, Nishimura T. Inhibition by indomethacin of ovulation induced by human chorionic gonadotrophin in immature rats primed with pregnant mare serum gonadotrophin. *J Endocrinol* 1980;84: 333–341.
524. Kohda H, Mori T, Nishimura T, Kambegawa A. Cooperation of progesterone and prostaglandins in ovulation induced by human chorionic gonadotrophin in immature rats primed with pregnant mare serum gonadotrophin. *J Endocrinol* 1983;96:387–393.
525. Sogn JH, Curry TE Jr, Brannstrom M, et al. Inhibition of follicle-stimulating hormone-induced ovulation by indomethacin in the perfused rat ovary. *Biol Reprod* 1987;36:536–542.
526. Gould KG, Graham CE, Collins DC. Effects of prostaglandins on cultured granulosa cells from rhesus monkeys. *J Reprod Fertil* 1977;50:341–345.
527. Wehrenberg WB, Dierschke DJ, Wolf RC. The effect of prostaglandin $F_{2\alpha}$ on ovarian blood flow and progesterone concentrations in cyclic guinea pigs. *Biol Reprod* 1979;21:187–191.
528. Canipari R, Strickland S. Studies on the hormonal regulation of plasminogen activator production in the rat ovary. *Endocrinology* 1986;118:1652–1659.
529. Miyazaki T, Dharmarajan AM, Atlas SJ, Katz E, Wallach EE. Do prostaglandins lead to ovulation in the rabbit by stimulating proteolytic enzyme activity? *Fertil Steril* 1991;55:1183–1188.
530. Shimada H, Okamura H, Noda Y, Suzuki A, Tojo S, Takada A. Plasminogen activator in rat ovary during the ovulatory process:

independence of prostaglandin mediation. *J Endocrinol* 1983;97: 201–205.
531. Espey L, Shimada H, Okamura H, Mori T. Effect of various agents on ovarian plasminogen activator activity during ovulation in pregnant mare's serum gonadotropin-primed immature rats. *Biol Reprod* 1985;32:1087–1094.
532. Reich R, Miskin R, Tsafriri A. Follicular plasminogen activator: involvement in ovulation. *Endocrinology* 1985;116:516–521.
533. Tranquille N, Emeis JJ. Release of tissue-type plasminogen activator is induced in rats by leukotrienes C_4 and D_4, but not by prostaglandins E_1, E_2 and I_2. *Br J Pharmacol* 1988;93:156–164.
534. Reich R, Tsafriri A, Mechanic GL. The involvement of collagenolysis in ovulation in the rat. *Endocrinology* 1985;116:522–527.
535. Curry TE Jr, Clark MR, Dean DD, Woessner JF Jr, LeMaire WJ. The preovulatory increase in ovarian collagenase activity in the rat is independent of prostaglandin production. *Endocrinology* 1986;118:1823–1828.
536. Norstrom A, Tjugum J. Hormonal effects on collagenolytic activity in the isolated human ovarian follicular wall. *Gynecol Obstet Invest* 1986;22:12–16.
537. Dennefors B, Tjugum J, Norstrom A, et al. Collagen synthesis inhibition by PGE_2 within the human follicular wall—one possible mechanism underlying ovulation. *Prostaglandins* 1982;24: 295–302.
538. Himeno N, Kawamura N, Okamura H, Mori T, Fukumoto M, Midorikawa O. Collagen synthetic activity in rabbit ovary during ovulation and its blockage by indomethacin. *Acta Obstet Gynaecol Jpn* 1984;36:1930–1934.
539. Himeno N, Kawamura N, Okamura H, Mori T, Fukumoto M, Midorikawa O. The effect of prostaglandin F-2-alpha on collagen synthesis in rabbit ovary during the ovulatory process. *Acta Obstet Gynaecol Jpn* 1984;36:2494–2495.
540. Downs SM, Longo FJ. An ultrastructural study of preovulatory apical development in mouse ovarian follicles: effects of indomethacin. *Anat Rec* 1983;205:159–168.
541. Downs SM, Longo FJ. Prostaglandins and preovulatory follicular maturation in mice. *J Exp Zool* 1983;228:99–108.
542. Katz E, Dharmarajan AM, Sueoka K, Ghodgaonkar RB, Dubin NH, Wallach EE. Effects of systemic administration of indomethacin on ovulation, luteinization, and steroidogenesis in the rabbit ovary. *Am J Obstet Gynecol* 1989;161:1361–1366.
543. Espey LL, Tanaka N, Okamura H. Increase in ovarian leukotrienes during hormonally induced ovulation in the rat. *Am J Physiol* 1989;256:E753–E759.
544. Tanaka N, Espey LL, Okamura H. Increase in ovarian 15-hydroxyeicosatetraenoic acid during ovulation in the gonadotropin-primed immature rat. *Endocrinology* 1989;125: 1373–1377.
545. Espey LL, Tanaka N, Stacy S, Okamura H. Inhibition of ovulation in the gonadotropin-primed immature rat by exogenous prostaglandin E_2. *Prostaglandins* 1992;43:67–74.
546. Saksena SK, Lau IF, Shaikh AA. Cyclic changes in tissue content of F-prostaglandins and the role of prostaglandins in ovulation in mice. *Fertil Steril* 1974;25:636–641.
547. Murdoch WJ. Disruption of cellular associations within the granulosal compartment of periovulatory ovine follicles: relationship to maturation of the oocyte and regulation by prostaglandins. *Cell Tissue Res* 1988;252:459–462.
548. Downey BR, Ainsworth L. Reversal of indomethacin blockade of ovulation in gilts by prostaglandins. *Prostaglandins* 1980;19: 17–22.
549. Himeno N. Effect of prostaglandins on collagen synthesis in rabbit ovarian follicles during the ovulatory process. *Nippon Naibunpi Gakkai Zasshi* 1986;62:1181–1193.
550. Lerner LJ, Oldani C, Vitale A. Effects of prostaglandin E_2 and DL 204 IT, an inhibitor of prostaglandin degradation, on ovulation and ovum transport in the hamster. *Prostaglandins* 1978;15: 525–531.
551. Wallach EE, Bronson R, Hamada Y, Wright KH, Stevens V. Effectiveness of prostaglandin $F_{2\alpha}$ in restoration of hMG-hCG induced ovulation in indomethacin-treated rhesus monkeys. *Prostaglandins* 1975;10:129–138.
552. Hamada Y, Wright KH, Wallach EE. *In vitro* reversal of indomethacin-blocked ovulation by prostaglandin $F_{2\alpha}$. *Fertil Steril* 1978;30:702–706.
553. Chatterjee A, Chatterjee R. Inhibition of ovulation by indomethacin in rats. *Prostaglandins Leukot Med* 1982;9:235–240.
554. Chatterjee A. The possible mode of action of prostaglandins. IX. Prostaglandin $F_{2\alpha}$ involvement in the reversal of ovulation blockade by ergocornine in rats. *Prostaglandins* 1975;10:1067–1074.
555. Murdoch WJ. Effect of a steroidal (prednisolone) and nonsteroidal (indomethacin) antiinflammatory agent on ovulation and follicular accumulation of prostaglandin $F_{2\alpha}$ in sheep. *Prostaglandins* 1989;37:331–334.
556. Lau IF, Saksena SK, Chang MC. Prostaglandins F and ovulation in mice. *J Reprod Fertil* 1974;40:467–469.
557. Hellberg P, Brannstrom M. A prostacyclin analogue, iloprost, augments the ovulatory response of the LH-stimulated *in vitro* perfused rat ovary. *Prostaglandins* 1990;40:361–371.
558. Samuelsson B. Leukotrienes: mediators of immediate hypersensitivity reactions and inflammation. *Science* 1983;220:568–575.
559. Ford-Hutchinson AW. Leukotriene involvement in pathologic processes. *J Allergy Clin Immunol* 1984;74:437–440.
560. Ford-Hutchinson A, Letts G. Biological actions of leukotrienes: state of the art lecture. *Hypertension* 1986;8(suppl II):II44–II49.
561. Reich R, Kohen F, Naor Z, Tsafriri A. Possible involvement of lipoxygenase products of arachidonic acid pathway in ovulation. *Prostaglandins* 1983;26:1011–1020.
562. Reich R, Kohen F, Slager R, Tsafriri A. Ovarian lipoxygenase activity and its regulation by gonadotropin in the rat. *Prostaglandins* 1985;30:581–590.
563. Kranzfelder D, Reich R, Abisogun AO, Tsafriri A. Preovulatory changes in the perifollicular capillary network in the rat: role of eicosanoids. *Biol Reprod* 1992;46:379–385.
564. Yoshimura Y, Nakamura Y, Shiraki M, et al. Involvement of leukotriene B_4 in ovulation in the rabbit. *Endocrinology* 1991;129:193–199.
565. Hellberg P, Holmes PV, Brannstrom M, Olofsson J, Janson PO. Inhibitors of lipoxygenase increase the ovulation rate in the *in vitro* perfused luteinizing hormone-stimulated rabbit ovary. *Acta Physiol Scand* 1990;138:557–564.
566. Carvalho CB, Yeik BS, Murdoch WJ. Significance of follicular cyclooxygenase and lipoxygenase pathways of metabolism of arachidonate in sheep. *Prostaglandins* 1989;37:553–558.
567. Siegel MI, McConnell RT, Porter NA, et al. Aspirin-like drugs inhibit arachidonic acid metabolism via lipoxygenase and cyclo-oxygenase in rat neutrophils from carrageenan pleural exudates. *Biochem Biophys Res Commun* 1980;92:688–695.
568. Randall RW, Eakins KE, Higgs GA, Salmon JA, Tateson JE. Inhibition of arachidonic acid cyclo-oxygenase and lipoxygenase activities of leukocytes by indomethacin and compound BW755c. *Agents Actions* 1980;10:553–555.
569. Malmsten CL. Prostaglandins, thromboxanes, and leukotrienes in inflammation. *Am J Med* 1986;80(suppl 4B):11–17.
570. White RK, Montgomery S. Leukotrienes: inflammatory mediators—a review. *Oral Surg Oral Med Oral Pathol* 1986;61: 514–518.
571. Goetzl EJ, Burrall BA, Baud L, Scriven KH, Levine JD, Koo CH. Generation and recognition of leukotriene mediators of hypersensitivity and inflammation. *Dig Dis Sci* 1988;33(suppl):36S–40S.
572. Espey LL, Adams RF, Tanaka N, Okamura H. Effects of epostane on ovarian levels of progesterone, 17β-estradiol, prostaglandin E_2, and prostaglandin $F_{2\alpha}$ during ovulation in the gonadotropin-primed immature rat. *Endocrinology* 1990;127: 259–263.
573. Wang J, Yuen BH, Leung PCK. Stimulation of progesterone and prostaglandin E_2 production by lipoxygenase metabolites of arachidonic acid. *FEB Lett* 1989;244:154–158.
574. Reich R, Haberman S, Abisogun AO, et al. Follicular rupture at ovulation: collagenase activity and metabolism of arachidonic acid. In: Naftolin F, DeCherney AH, eds. *The Control of Follicle Development, Ovulation and Luteal Function: Lessons from In Vitro Fertilization.* New York: Raven Press, 1987;317–329.
575. Viggiano M, Franchi AM, Zicari JL, et al. The involvement of oxytocin in ovulation and in the outputs of cyclo-oxygenase and 5-lipoxygenase products from isolated rat ovaries. *Prostaglandins* 1989;37:367–378.
576. Pincus G, Merrill AP. The role of steroids in the control of mammalian ovulation. In: Villee CA, ed. *Control of Ovulation.* New York: Pergamon Press, 1961;37–55.

577. Hisaw FL. Endocrines and the evolution of viviparity among the vertebrates. In: *Physiology of Reproduction.* Proceedings of the Twenty-second Biology Colloquium. Corvallis: Oregon State University Press, 1961;119–138.
578. Lipner H, Greep RO. Inhibition of steroidogenesis at various sites in the biosynthetic pathway in relation to induced ovulation. *Endocrinology* 1971;88:602–607.
579. Ying S-Y, Greep RO. Prevention of aminoglutethimide phosphate (AGP) block of ovulation in PMS-treated immature rats. *Proc Soc Exp Biol Med* 1971;136:916–919.
580. Rondell P. Role of steroid synthesis in the process of ovulation. *Biol Reprod* 1974;10:199–215.
581. Shaykh M, LeMaire WJ, Papkoff H, Curry TE Jr, Sogn JH, Koos RD. Ovulations in rat ovaries perfused *in vitro* with follicle-stimulating hormone. *Biol Reprod* 1985;33:629–636.
582. Hilliard J, Scaramuzzi RJ, Pang CN, Penardi R, Sawyer CH. Testosterone secretion by rabbit ovary *in vivo. Endocrinology* 1974;94:267–271.
583. Waterston JW III, Mills TM. Peripheral blood steroid concentrations in the preovulatory rabbit. *J Steroid Biochem* 1976;7:15–17.
584. Janson PO, LeMaire WJ, Kallfelt B, et al. The study of ovulation in the isolated perfused rabbit ovary. I. Methodology and pattern of steroidogenesis. *Biol Reprod* 1982;26:456–465.
585. Koos RD, Jaccarino FJ, Magaril RA, LeMaire WJ. Perfusion of the rat ovary *in vitro:* methodology, induction of ovulation, and pattern of steroidogenesis. *Biol Reprod* 1984;30:1135–1141.
586. Holmes PV, Sogn J, Schillinger E, Janson PO. Effects of high and low preovulatory concentrations of progesterone on ovulation from the isolated perfused rabbit ovary. *J Reprod Fertil* 1985;75:393–399.
587. Brannstrom M, Johansson BM, Sogn J, Janson PO. Characterization of an *in vitro* perfused rat ovary model: ovulation rate, oocyte maturation, steroidogenesis and influence of PMSG priming. *Acta Physiol Scand* 1987;130:107–114.
588. Yoshimura Y, Hosoi Y, Bongiovanni AM, Santulli R, Atlas SJ, Wallach EE. Are ovarian steroids required for ovum maturation and fertilization? Effects of cyanoketone on the *in vitro* perfused rabbit ovary. *Endocrinology* 1987;120:2555–2561.
589. Stoklosowa S, Nalbandov AV. Luteinization and steroidogenic activity of rat ovarian follicles cultured *in vitro. Endocrinology* 1972;91:25–32.
590. Hillensjo T, Bauminger S, Ahren K. Effect of luteinizing hormone on the pattern of steroid production by preovulatory follicles of pregnant mare's serum gonadotropin-injected immature rats. *Endocrinology* 1976;99:996–1002.
591. Tsang BK, Ainsworth L, Downey BR, Marcus GJ. Differential production of steroids by dispersed granulosa and theca interna cells from developing preovulatory follicles of pigs. *J Reprod Fertil* 1985;74:459–471.
592. Moor RM. Sites of steroid production in ovine graafian follicles in culture. *J Endocrinol* 1977;73:143–150.
593. Ryan KJ. Granulosa-thecal cell interaction in ovarian steroidogenesis. *J Steroid Biochem* 1979;11:799–800.
594. Zoller LC. A comparison of rat and hamster preovulatory follicles: an examination of differences in morphology and enzyme activity using qualitative and quantitative analyses. *Anat Rec* 1984;210:279–291.
595. Bogovich K, Richards JS. Androgen biosynthesis in developing ovarian follicles: evidence that luteinizing hormone regulates thecal 17α-hydroxylase and $C_{17\text{-}20}$-lyase activities. *Endocrinology* 1982;111:1201–1208.
596. Bogovich K, Richards JS. Androgen synthesis during follicular development: evidence that rat granulosa cell 17-ketosteroid reductase is independent of hormonal regulation. *Biol Reprod* 1984;31:122–131.
597. Sirois J, Kimmich TL, Fortune JE. Steroidogenesis by equine preovulatory follicles: relative roles of theca interna and granulosa cells. *Endocrinology* 1991;128:1159–1166.
598. Rodgers RJ, Rodgers HF, Hall PF, Waterman MR, Simpson ER. Immunolocalization of cholesterol side-chain-cleavage cytochrome P-450 and 17α-hydroxylase cytochrome P-450 in bovine ovarian follicles. *J Reprod Fertil* 1986;78:627–638.
599. Johnson DC, Tsai-Morris C-H, Hoversland RC. Steroid 17α-hydroxylase activity of ovarian granulosa cells from hypophysectomized immature rats treated with pregnant mare's serum gonadotropin (PMS). *Steroids* 1981;38:581–592.
600. Amin H, Richart RM, Brinson AO. Preovulatory granulosa cells and steroidogenesis. An ultrastructural study in the rhesus monkey. *Obstet Gynecol* 1976;47:562–568.
601. Guraya SS. Histochemical study of granulosa and theca interna during follicular development, ovulation, and corpus luteum formation and regression in the human ovary. *Am J Obstet Gynecol* 1968;101:448–457.
602. Mori T, Takenaka A, Yoshida Y, Suzuki A, Fujita Y, Nishimura T. Preovulatory changes in morphology of rabbit ovarian follicles. *Endocrinol Jpn* 1979;26:379–388.
603. Erickson GF, Ryan KJ. The effect of LH/FSH, dibutyryl cyclic AMP, and prostaglandins on the production of estrogens by rabbit granulosa cells *in vitro. Endocrinology* 1975;97:108–113.
604. Terranova PF, Martin NC, Chien S. Theca is the source of progesterone in experimentally induced atretic follicles of the hamster. *Biol Reprod* 1982;26:721–727.
605. Makris A, Olsen D, Ryan KJ. Significance of the delta 5 and delta 4 steroidogenic pathways in the hamster preovulatory follicle. *Steroids* 1983;42:641–651.
606. Nakamura Y, Kato H, Terranova PF. Interleukin-1 alpha increases thecal progesterone production of preovulatory follicles in cyclic hamsters. *Biol Reprod* 1990;43:169–173.
607. Klinken SP, Stevenson PM. Changes in enzyme activities during the artificially stimulated transition from follicular to luteal cell types in rat ovary. *Eur J Biochem* 1977;81:327–332.
608. Hickey GJ, Krasnow JS, Beattie WG, Richards JS. Aromatase cytochrome P450 in rat ovarian granulosa cells before and after luteinization: adenosine 3′,5′-monophosphate-dependent and independent regulation. Cloning and sequencing of rat aromatase cDNA and 5′ genomic DNA. *Mol Endocrinol* 1990;4:3–12.
609. Koos RD, Feiertag MA, Brodie AMH, LeMaire WJ. Inhibition of estrogen synthesis does not inhibit luteinizing hormone-induced ovulation. *Am J Obstet Gynecol* 1984;148:939–945.
610. Morioka N, Brannstorm M, Koos RD, LeMaire WJ. Ovulation in the perfused ovary *in vitro:* further evidence that estrogen is not required. *Steroids* 1988;51:173–183.
611. Dierschke DJ, Braw RH, Tsafriri A. Estradiol-17β reduces number of ovulations in adult rats: direct action on the ovary? *Biol Reprod* 1983;29:1147–1154.
612. LeMaire WJ, Janson PO, Kallfelt BJ, et al. The preovulatory decline in follicular oestradiol is not required for ovulation in the rabbit. *Acta Endocrinol* 1982;101:452–457.
613. Swanson RJ, Lipner H. Mechanism of ovulation: effect of intrafollicular progesterone antiserum in rabbits. *Fed Proc* 1977;36:390(abst).
614. Saksena SK, Salmonsen R. Effects of cadmium chloride on ovulation and on induction of sterility in the female golden hamster. *Biol Reprod* 1983;29:249–256.
615. Snyder BW, Beecham GD, Schane HP. Inhibition of ovulation in rats with epostane, an inhibitor of 3β-hydroxysteroid dehydrogenase. *Proc Soc Exp Biol Med* 1984;176:238–242.
616. Brannstrom M, Janson PO. Progesterone is a mediator in the ovulatory process of the *in vitro*-perfused rat ovary. *Biol Reprod* 1989;40:1170–1178.
617. Iwamasa J, Shibata S, Tanaka N, Matsuura K, Okamura H. The relationship between ovarian progesterone and proteolytic enzyme activity during ovulation in the gonadotropin-treated immature rat. *Biol Reprod* 1992;46:309–313.
618. Bullock DW, Kappauf BH. Dissociation of gonadotropin-induced ovulation and steroidogenesis in immature rats. *Endocrinology* 1973;92:1625–1628.
619. Gosden RG, Everett JW, Tyrey L. Luteinizing hormone requirements for ovulation in the pentobarbital-treated proestrous rat. *Endocrinology* 1976;99:1046–1053.
620. Yoshimura Y, Hosoi Y, Atlas SJ, Bongiovanni AM, Santulli R, Wallach EE. The effect of ovarian steroidogenesis on ovulation and fertilizability in the *in vitro* perfused rabbit ovary. *Biol Reprod* 1986;35:943–948.
621. Webb R. Increasing ovulation rate and lambing rate in sheep by treatment with a steroid enzyme inhibitor. *J Reprod Fertil* 1987;79:231–240.

622. Roh SI, Batten BE, Friedman CI, Kim MH. The effects of progesterone antagonist RU486 on mouse oocyte maturation, ovulation, fertilization, and cleavage. *Am J Obstet Gynecol* 1988;159: 1584–1589.
623. Webb R, Baxter G, McBride D, McNeilly AS. 3β-Hydroxysteroid dehydrogenase inhibitor reduces ovarian steroid production but increases ovulation rate in the ewe: interactions with gonadotrophins and inhibin. *J Endocrinol* 1992;134:115–125.
624. Fu SL, Dial GD, Keister DM, Butler WR. Increased ovulation rate in gilts after oral administration of epostane. *J Reprod Fertil* 1990;90:297–304.
625. Hoefler WC, Holcombe DW, Blackwell JA, Hinrichs BD, Hallford DM. Reproductive responses, progesterone profiles and ovarian characteristics of cycling, fine-wool ewes treated with an inhibitor of progesterone synthesis (epostane). *J Anim Sci* 1986;63:1072–1077.
626. Potts GO, Creange JE, Harding HR, Schane HP. Trilostane, an orally active inhibitor of steroid biosynthesis. *Steroids* 1978;32: 257–267.
627. Bauminger S, Lieberman ME, Lindner HR. Steroid-independent effects of gonadotropins on prostaglandin synthesis in rat graafian follicles *in vitro*. *Prostaglandins* 1975;9:753–764.
628. Liu JH, Garzo G, Morris S, Stuenkel C, Ulmann A, Yen SS. Disruption of follicular maturation and delay of ovulation after administration of the antiprogesterone RU486. *J Clin Endocrinol Metab* 1987;65:1135–1140.
629. Luukkainen T, Heikinheimo O, Haukkamaa M, Lahteenmaki P. Inhibition of folliculogenesis and ovulation by the antiprogesterone RU486. *Fertil Steril* 1988;49:961–963.
630. Iwamasa J, Tajima C, Matsuura K, Okamura H. Role of progesterone in the ovulatory process of PMSG/hCG treated immature female rats. *Nippon Sanka Fujinka Gakkai Zasshi* 1989;41: 1551–1556.
631. Sanchez-Criado JE, Bellido C, Galiot F, Lopez FJ, Gaytan F. A possible dual mechanism of the anovulatory action of antiprogesterone RU486 in the rat. *Biol Reprod* 1990;42:877–886.
632. Loutradis D, Beltsa R, Aravantinos L, Kallianidis K, Michalas S. Preovulatory effects of the progesterone antagonist mifepristone (RU486) in mice. *Hum Reprod* 1991;6:1238–1240.
633. Zalanyi S Jr, Nemeth G. Ovulation inhibition with RU 486. *Orv Hetil* 1991;132:563–567.
634. Uilenbroek JT, Sanchez-Criado JE, Karels B. Decreased luteinizing hormone-stimulated progesterone secretion by preovulatory follicles isolated from cyclic rats treated with the progesterone antagonist RU486. *Biol Reprod* 1992;47:368–373.
635. Cheesman DW, Schlegel R. Effects of (1-(3-mercaptopropanoic acid))-vasopressin and -vasotocin on the pro-oestrous progesterone surge and ovulation in immature female rats. *J Endocrinol* 1983;97:389–394.
636. Ohno Y, Mori T. Correlation between progesterone and plasminogen activator in rat ovaries during the ovulatory process. *Nippon Sanka Fujinka Gakkai Zasshi* 1985;37:247–256.
637. Koshida M, Takenaka A, Okamura H, Mori T. Inhibition of ovulation in PMSG/hCG-treated rats by rotenone, a specific inhibitor of mitochondrial oxidation. *J Reprod Fertil* 1987;79: 391–395.
638. Check JH, Dietterich C, Nowroozi K, Wu CH. Comparison of various therapies for the luteinized unruptured follicle syndrome. *Int J Fertil* 1992;37:33–40.
639. Bomsel-Helmreich O, Vu-N-Huyen L, Durand-Gasselin I. Effects of varying doses of HCG on the evolution of preovulatory rabbit follicles and oocytes. *Hum Reprod* 1989;4:636–642.
640. Brann DW, Putnam CD, Mahesh VB. Corticosteroid regulation of gonadotropin secretion and induction of ovulation in the rat. *Proc Soc Exp Biol Med* 1990;193:176–180.
641. Hamada Y, Schlaff S, Kobayashi Y, Santulli R, Wright KH, Wallach EE. Inhibitory effect of prolactin on ovulation in the *in vitro* perfused rabbit ovary. *Nature* 1980;285:161–163.
642. Wang J, Leung PCK. Role of arachidonic acid in luteinizing hormone-releasing hormone action: stimulation of progesterone production in rat granulosa cells. *Endocrinology* 1988;122: 906–911.
643. Clarke CL, Sutherland RL. Progestin regulation of cellular proliferation. *Endocr Rev* 1990;11:266–301.
644. Latman NS, Kishore V, Bruot B. Progesterone secretion in the rat in response to an adjuvant arthritis challenge. *Arthritis Rheum* 1986;29:411–414.
645. Nakagawa H, Min KR, Nanjo K, Tsurufuji S. Anti-inflammatory action of progesterone on carrageenin-induced inflammation in rats. *Jpn J Pharmacol* 1979;29:509–514.
646. Nakagawa H, Min KR, Tsurufuji S. Anti-inflammatory action of progesterone and its possible mode of action in rats. *Biochem Pharmacol* 1981;30:639–644.
647. Campbell EJ, Senior RM, Welgus HG. Extracellular matrix injury during lung inflammation. *Chest* 1987;92:161–167.
648. Werb Z, Mainardi CL, Vater CA, Harris ED Jr. Endogenous activation of latent collagenase by rheumatoid synovial cells. *N Engl J Med* 1977;296:1017–1023.
649. Werb Z, Aggeler J. Proteases induce secretion of collagenase and plasminogen activator by fibroblasts. *Proc Natl Acad Sci* 1978;75:1839–1843.
650. Beers WH. Follicular plasminogen and plasminogen activator and the effect of plasmin on ovarian follicle wall. *Cell* 1975;6:379–386.
651. Beers WH, Strickland S, Reich E. Ovarian plasminogen activator: relationship to ovulation and hormonal regulation. *Cell* 1975;6:387–394.
652. Strickland S, Beers WH. Studies on the role of plasminogen activator in ovulation—*in vitro* response of granulosa cells to gonadotropins, cyclic nucleotides, and prostaglandins. *J Biol Chem* 1976;251:5694–5702.
653. Liu W-K, Burleigh BD, Ward DN. Steroid and plasminogen activator production by cultured rat granulosa cells in response to hormone treatment. *Mol Cell Endocrinol* 1981;21:63–73.
654. Too CKL, Weiss TJ, Bryant-Greenwood GD. Relaxin stimulates plasminogen activator secretion by rat granulosa cells *in vitro*. *Endocrinology* 1982;111:1424–1426.
655. Wang C, Leung A. Gonadotropins regulate plasminogen activator production by rat granulosa cells. *Endocrinology* 1983;112: 1201–1207.
656. Liu Y-X, Ny T, Sarkar D, Loskutoff D, Hsueh AJW. Identification and regulation of tissue plasminogen activator activity in rat cumulus-oocyte complexes. *Endocrinology* 1986;119:1578–1587.
657. Knecht M. Hormonal and immunological characterization of the cell-associated plasminogen activators produced by cultured rat granulosa cells. *Endocrinology* 1987;120:2174–2179.
658. Wang C, Leung A. Estrogens, progestogens, and androgens enhance the follicle-stimulating hormone-stimulated plasminogen activator production by cultured rat granulosa cells. *Endocrinology* 1987;120:2131–2136.
659. Liu Y-X, Hsueh AJW. Plasminogen activator activity in cumulus-oocyte complexes of gonadotropin-treated rats during the periovulatory period. *Biol Reprod* 1987;36:1055–1062.
660. Liu Y-X, Cajander SB, Ny T, Kristensen P, Hsueh AJ. Gonadotropin regulation of tissue-type and urokinase-type plasminogen activators in rat granulosa and theca-interstitial cells during the periovulatory period. *Mol Cell Endocrinol* 1987;54:221–229.
661. Cajander SB, Hugin MP, Kristensen P, Hsueh AJ. Immunohistochemical localization of tissue-type plasminogen activator in ovaries before and after induced and spontaneous ovulation in the rat. *Cell Tissue Res* 1989;257:1–8.
662. Maruyama K, Yoshimura Y, Kamiya T, et al. Involvement of plasminogen activator activity in the process of ovulation. *Nippon Sanka Fujinka Gakkai Zasshi* 1990;42:620–626.
663. Liu YX, Feng Q, Stefan C. A comparative study on involvement of tPA activity in ovulation induced by hCG and GnRH agonist in hypophysectomized rats. *Sci China* 1991;34:1215–1224.
664. Yoshimura Y, Nakamura Y, Oda T, et al. Effects of prolactin on ovarian plasmin generation in the process of ovulation. *Biol Reprod* 1992;46:322–327.
665. Mott DM, Fabisch PH, Sorof S. Cyclic AMP phosphodiesterase inhibitors depress production of plasminogen activator by Chinese hamster ovary cells. *Biochem Biophys Res Commun* 1976;70:1150–1154.
666. Reich R, Miskin R, Tsafriri A. Intrafollicular distribution of plasminogen activators and their hormonal regulation *in vitro*. *Endocrinology* 1986;119:1588–1601.
667. Smokovitis A, Kokolis N, Alexaki-Tzivanidou E. The plasmino-

gen activator activity is markedly increased mainly at the area of the rupture of the follicular wall at the time of ovulation. *Anim Reprod Sci* 1988;16:285–294.
668. Cajander SB. Periovulatory changes in the ovary. Morphology and expression of tissue-type plasminogen activator. *Prog Clin Biol Res* 1989;296:91–101.
669. Akazawa K, Mori N, Kosugi T, Matsuo O, Mihara H. Localization of fibrinolytic activity in ovulation of the rat follicle as determined by the fibrin slide method. *Jpn J Physiol* 1983;33:1011–1018.
670. Shimada H, Mori T, Takada A, et al. Use of chromogenic substrate S-2251 for determination of plasminogen activator in rat ovaries. *Thromb Haemost* 1981;46:507–510.
671. Akazawa K, Matsuo O, Kosugi T, Mihara H, Mori N. The role of plasminogen activator in ovulation. *Acta Physiol Lat Am* 1983;33:105–110.
672. Liu Y-X. Interaction and regulation of plasminogen activators and their inhibitor in rat follicles during periovulatory periods. *Sci Sin* 1988;31:47–57.
673. Liu Y-X, Peng XR, Ny-T. Tissue-specific and time-coordinated hormone regulation of plasminogen-activator-inhibitor type I and tissue-type plasminogen activator in the rat ovary during gonadotropin-induced ovulation. *Eur J Biochem* 1991;195:549–555.
674. Liu Y-X, Feng Q, Zou RJ. Changes of ovarian plasminogen activator and inhibitor during gonadotropin-induced ovulation in rhesus monkeys. *Sheng Li Hsueh Pao* 1991;43:472–479.
675. Yoshimura Y, Santulli R, Atlas SJ, Fujii S, Wallach EE. The effects of proteolytic enzymes on *in vitro* ovulation in the rabbit. *Am J Obstet Gynecol* 1987;157:468–475.
676. Woessner JF Jr, Morioka N, Zhu C, Mukaida T, Butler T, LeMaire WJ. Connective tissue breakdown in ovulation. *Steroids* 1989;54:491–499.
677. Tsafriri A, Bicsak TA, Cajander SB, Ny T, Hsueh AJW. Suppression of ovulation rate by antibodies to tissue-type plasminogen activator and α_2-antiplasmin. *Endocrinology* 1989;124:415–421.
678. Marceau F, Lussier A, Regoli D, Giroud JP. Pharmacology of kinins: their relevance to tissue injury and inflammation. *Gen Pharmacol* 1983;14:209–229.
679. Solomkin JS, Simmons RL. Cellular and subcellular mediators of acute inflammation. *Surg Clin North Am* 1983;63:225–243.
680. Sharma NJ, Zeitlen IJ, Deodhar SD, Buchana WW. Detection of kallikrein-like activity in inflamed synovial tissue. *Arch Int Pharmacodyn* 1983;262:279–286.
681. Fuller PJ, Funder JW. The cellular physiology of glandular kallikrein. *Kidney Int* 1986;29:953–964.
682. Eeckhout Y, Vaes G. Further studies on the activation of procollagenase, the latent precursor of bone collagenase—effects of lysosomal cathepsin B, plasmin and kallikrein, and spontaneous activation. *Biochem J* 1977;166:21–31.
683. Nagase H, Cawston TE, DeSilva M, Barrett AJ. Identification of plasma kallikrein as an activator of latent collagenase in rheumatoid synovial fluid. *Biochim Biophys Acta* 1982;702:133–142.
684. Espey LL, Rawson JMR. Regarding the role of plasminogen activator in ovulation. In: Midgley AR, Sadler WA, eds. *Ovarian Follicular Development and Function.* New York: Raven Press, 1979;155–158.
685. Yanker BA, Shooter EM. The biology and mechanism of action of nerve growth factor. *Annu Rev Biochem* 1982;51:845–868.
686. Bicsak TA, Michelson DS, Hsueh AJW. Rat granulosa cells produce a novel trypsin-like protease in response to gonadotropin treatment. *Biochem Biophys Res Commun* 1989;165:624–630.
687. Dhanju CKI, Dhanoa SK, Guraya SS. Effect of steroids on ovarian neutral proteinases during ovulation in cyclic albino rats. *Indian J Exp Biol* 1990;28:369–370.
688. Martin GG, Miller-Walker C. Visualization of the three-dimensional distribution of collagen fibrils over preovulatory follicles in the hamster. *J Exp Zool* 1983;225:311–319.
689. Parr EL. Absence of neutral proteinase activity in rat ovarian follicle walls at ovulation. *Biol Reprod* 1974;11:509–512.
690. Curry TE Jr, Dean DD, Woessner JF Jr, LeMaire WJ. The extraction of a tissue collagenase associated with ovulation in the rat. *Biol Reprod* 1985;33:981–991.
691. Puistola U, Salo T, Martikainen H, Ronnberg Lars. Type IV collagenolytic activity in human preovulatory follicular fluid. *Fertil Steril* 1986;45:578–585.
692. Fukumoto M, Yajima Y, Okamura H, Midorikawa O. Collagenolytic enzyme activity in human ovary: an ovulatory enzyme system. *Fertil Steril* 1981;36:746–750.
693. Himeno N, Kawamura N, Okamura H, Fukumoto M, Midorikawa O. Prolyl hydroxylase activity in rabbit ovary during ovulatory process. *Nippon Sanka Fujinka Gakkai Zasshi* 1983;35:1777–1782.
694. Curry TE Jr, Mann JS, Huang MH, Keeble SC. Gelatinase and proteoglycanase activity during the periovulatory period in the rat. *Biol Reprod* 1992;46:256–264.
695. Curry TE Jr, Sanders SL, Pedigo NG, Estes RS, Wilson EA, Vernon MW. Identification and characterization of metalloproteinase inhibitor activity in human ovarian follicular fluid. *Endocrinology* 1988;123:1611–1618.
696. Smith MF, Moor RM. Secretion of a putative metalloproteinase inhibitor by ovine granulosa cells and luteal tissue. *J Reprod Fertil* 1991;91:627–635.
697. Zhu C, Woessner JF Jr. A tissue inhibitor of metalloproteinases and α-macroglobulins in the ovulating rat ovary: possible regulators of collagen matrix breakdown. *Biol Reprod* 1991;45:334–342.
698. Ichikawa S, Ohta M, Morioka H, Murao S. Blockage of ovulation in the explanted hamster ovary by a collagenase inhibitor. *J Reprod Fertil* 1983;68:17–19.
699. Ichikawa S, Morioka H, Ohta M, Oda K, Murao S. Effect of various proteinase inhibitors on ovulation of explanted hamster ovaries. *J Reprod Fertil* 1983;68:407–412.
700. Brannstrom M, Woessner JF Jr, Koos RD, Sear CHJ, LeMaire WJ. Inhibitors of mammalian tissue collagenase and metalloproteinases suppress ovulation in the perfused rat ovary. *Endocrinology* 1988;122:1715–1721.
701. Butler TA, Zhu C, Mueller RA, Fuller GC, LeMaire WJ, Woessner JF Jr. Inhibition of ovulation in the perfused rat ovary by the synthetic collagenase inhibitor SC44463. *Biol Reprod* 1991;44:1183–1188.
702. Bryant-Greenwood GD, Jeffrey R, Ralph MM, Seamark RF. Relaxin production by the porcine ovarian graafian follicle *in vitro.* *Biol Reprod* 1980;23:792–800.
703. Evans G, Wathes C, King GJ, Armstrong DT, Porter DG. Changes in relaxin production by the theca during the preovulatory period of the pig. *J Reprod Fertil* 1983;69:677–683.
704. TenCate AR, Syrbu AS. A relationship between alkaline phosphatase activity and the phagocytosis and degradation of collagen by the fibroblast. *J Anat* 1974;117:351–359.
705. Bauer EA, Stricklin GP, Jeffrey JJ, Eisen AZ. Collagenase production by human skin fibroblasts. *Biochem Biophys Res Commun* 1975;64:232–240.
706. Birkedal-Hansen H, Cobb CM, Taylor RE, Fullmer HM. Synthesis and release of procollagenase by cultured fibroblasts. *J Biol Chem* 1976;251:3162–3168.
707. Dimino MJ, Reece RP. Effects of gonadotropic hormones on rat ovarian lysosomes. *Biol Reprod* 1973;8:523–530.
708. Okamura H, Takenaka A, Yajima Y, Nishimura T. Ovulatory changes in the wall at the apex of the human graafian follicle. *J Reprod Fertil* 1980;58:153–155.
709. Dowsett M, Eastman AR, Easty DM, Easty GC, Powles TJ, Neville AM. Prostaglandin mediation of collagenase-induced bone resorption. *Nature* 1976;263:72–74.
710. Wahl LM, Olsen CE, Sandberg AL, Mergenhagen SE. Prostaglandin regulation of macrophage collagenase production. *Proc Natl Acad Sci* 1977;74:4955–4958.
711. Jeffrey JJ, Coffey RJ, Eisen AZ. Studies on uterine collagenase in tissue culture II. Effect of steroid hormones on enzyme production. *Biochim Biophys Acta* 1971;252:143–149.
712. Koob TJ, Jeffrey JJ. Hormonal regulation of collagen degradation in the uterus: inhibition of collagenase expression by progesterone and cyclic AMP. *Biochim Biophys Acta* 1974;354:61–70.
713. Wahl LM, Blandau RJ, Page RC. Effect of hormones on collagen metabolism and collagenase activity in the pubic symphysis ligament of the guinea pig. *Endocrinology* 1977;100:571–579.
714. Wahl LM. Hormonal regulation of macrophage collagenase activity. *Biochem Biophys Res Commun* 1977;74:838–845.

715. Miele L, Cordella-Miele E, Mukherjee AB. Uteroglobin: structure, molecular biology, and new perspectives on its function as a phospholipase A_2 inhibitor. *Endocr Rev* 1987;8:474–490.
716. Kikukawa T, Cowan BD, Tejeda RI, Mukherjee AB. Partial characterization of a uteroglobin-like protein in the human uterus and its temporal relationship to prostaglandin levels in this organ. *J Clin Endocrinol Metab* 1988;67:315–321.
717. Fradin A, Rothhut B, Poincelot-Canton B, Errasfa M, Russo-Marie F. Inhibition of eicosanoid and PAF formation by dexamethasone in rat inflammatory polymorphonuclear neutrophils may implicate lipocortin(s). *Biochim Biophys Acta* 1988;963: 248–257.
718. Flower RJ. The mediators of steroid action. *Nature* 1986;320:20.
719. Wallner BP, Mattaliano RJ, Hession C, et al. Cloning and expression of human lipocortin, a phospholipase A_2 inhibitor with potential anti-inflammatory activity. *Nature* 1986;320:77–81.
720. Noyes RW, Clewe TH, Yamate AM. Follicular development, ovular maturation and ovulation in ovarian tissue transplanted to the eye. In: Villee CA, ed. *Control of Ovulation.* New York: Pergamon Press, 1961;24–36.
721. Parr E. β-Galactosidase in rat ovarian bursa fluid at ovulation. *Biol Reprod* 1974;11:504–508.
722. O Shea JD, Cran DG, Hay MF. Fate of the theca interna following ovulation in the ewe. *Cell Tissue Res* 1980;210:305–319.
723. Partridge NC, Jeffrey JJ, Ehlich LS, et al. Hormonal regulation of the production of collagenase and a collagenase inhibitor activity by rat osteogenic sarcoma cells. *Endocrinology* 1987;120: 1956–1962.
724. Civitelli R, Hruska KA, Jeffrey JJ, Kahn AJ, Avioli LV, Partridge NC. Second messenger signaling in the regulation of collagenase production by osteogenic sarcoma cells. *Endocrinology* 1989; 124:2928–2934.
725. Johnson GS, Pastan I. Change in growth and morphology of fibroblasts by prostaglandins. *J Natl Cancer Inst* 1971;47:1357–1364.
726. Perry CV, Johnson GS, Pastan I. Adenyl cyclase in normal and transformed fibroblasts in tissue culture. *J Biol Chem* 1971;246: 5785–5790.
727. Ko SD, Page RC, Narayanan AS. Fibroblast heterogeneity and prostaglandin regulation of subpopulations. *Proc Natl Acad Sci* 1977;74:3429–3432.
728. Hial V, DeMello MCF, Horakova Z, Beaven MA. Antiproliferative activity of anti-inflammatory drugs in two mammalian cell culture lines. *J Pharmacol Exp Ther* 1977;202:446–454.
729. DeAsua LJ, Clingan D, Rudland PS. Initiation of cell proliferation in cultured mouse fibroblasts by prostaglandin $F_{2\alpha}$. *Proc Natl Acad Sci* 1975;72:2724–2728.
730. Newcombe DS, Ishikawa Y. The effect of anti-inflammatory agents on human synovial fibroblast prostaglandin synthetase. *Prostaglandins* 1976;12:849–869.
731. Jung-Testas I, Bayard F, Baulieu EE. Two sex steroid receptors in mouse fibroblasts in culture. *Nature* 1976;259:136–138.
732. Corsina A, Granata A, Bernini F, Maggi FM, Fumagalli R, Catapano AL. Progesterone modulates the expression of HDL binding sites in human skin fibroblasts. *Atherosclerosis* 1988;74: 107–113.
733. Malet C, Gompel A, Yaneva H, et al. Estradiol and progesterone receptors in cultured normal human breast epithelial cells and fibroblasts: immunocytochemical studies. *J Clin Endocrinol Metab* 1991;73:8–17.
734. Gaben AM, Mester J. BALB/C mouse 3T3 fibroblasts expressing human estrogen receptor: effect of estradiol on cell growth. *Biochem Biophys Res Commun* 1991;176:1473–1481.
735. Kang AH. Fibroblast activation. *J Lab Clin Med* 1978;92:1–4.
736. Schmidt JA, Mizel SB, Cohen D, Green I. Interleukin 1, a potential regulator of fibroblast proliferation. *J Immunol* 1982;128: 2177–2182.
737. Mauviel A, Kahari VM, Evans CH, Uitto J. Transcriptional activation of fibroblast collagenase gene expression by a novel lymphokine, leukoregulin. *J Biol Chem* 1992;267:5644–5648.
738. Bauer EA, Cooper TW, Huang JS, Altman J, Deuel TF. Stimulation of *in vitro* human skin collagenase expression by platelet-derived growth factor. *Proc Natl Acad Sci* 1985;82:4132–4136.
739. Whitham SE, Murphy G, Angel P, et al. Comparison of human stromelysin and collagenase by cloning and sequence analysis. *Biochem J* 1986;240:913–916.
740. Ashcom G, Gurland G, Schwartz J. Growth hormone synergizes with serum growth factors in inducing c-fos transcription in 3T3-F442A cells. *Endocrinology* 1992;131:1915–1921.
741. Houck JC, Cheng RF, Sharma VK. Control of fibroblast proliferation. *Natl Cancer Inst Monogr* 1973;38:161–170.
742. Lau LF, Nathans D. Identification of a set of genes expressed during the G0/G1 transition of cultured mouse cells. *EMBO J* 1985;4:3145–3151.
743. Boeggeman E, Masibay AS, Qasba PK, Sreevalsan T. Identification and partial characterization of genes that are transactivated by different pathways in quiescent mouse cells stimulated with serum. *J Cell Physiol* 1990;145:286–294.
744. Mohn KL, Laz TM, Hsu J-C, Melby AE, Bravo R, Taub R. The immediate-early growth response in regenerating liver and insulin-stimulated H-35 cells: comparison with serum-stimulated 3T3 cells and identification of 41 novel immediate-early genes. *Mol Cell Biol* 1991;11:381–390.
745. Branwood AW. The fibroblast. In: Hall DA, ed. *International Review of Connective Tissue Research.* New York: Academic Press, 1963;1–28.
746. Davis RL, Weintraub H, Lassar AB. Expression of a single transfected cDNA converts fibroblasts to myoblasts. *Cell* 1987;51: 987–1000.
747. Deuel TF. Polypeptide growth factors: roles in normal and abnormal cell growth. *Annu Rev Cell Biol* 1987;3:443–492.
748. Hsueh AJW, Welsh TH, Jones PBC. Inhibition of ovarian and testicular steroidogenesis by epidermal growth factor. *Endocrinology* 1981;108:2002–2005.
749. Hsueh AJW, Adashi EY, Jones PBC, Welsh TH Jr. Hormonal regulation of the differentiation of cultured ovarian granulosa cells. *Endocr Rev* 1984;5:76–127.
750. Adashi EY, Resnick CE, D'Ercole AJ, Svoboda ME, Van Wyk JJ. Insulin-like growth factors as intraovarian regulators of granulosa cell growth and function. *Endocr Rev* 1985;6:400–420.
751. Hsu C-J, Holmes SD, Hammond JM. Ovarian epidermal growth factor-like activity. Concentrations in porcine follicular fluid during follicular enlargement. *Biochem Biophys Res Commun* 1987;147:242–247.
752. Skinner MK, Keski-Oja J, Osteen KG, Moses HL. Ovarian thecal cells produce transforming growth factor-β which can regulate granulosa cell growth. *Endocrinology* 1987;121:786–792.
753. Grothe C, Unsicker K. Immunocytochemical localization of basic fibroblast growth factor in bovine adrenal gland, ovary, and pituitary. *J Histochem Cytochem* 1989;37:1877–1883.
754. Ross R. Platelet-derived growth factor. *Lancet* 1989;May 27:1179–1182.
755. Desch CE, Dobrina A, Apparwal BB, Harlan JM. Tumor necrosis factor-α exhibits greater proinflammatory activity than lymphotoxin *in vitro. Blood* 1990;75:2030–2034.
756. Allen JB, Manthey CL, Hand AR, Ohura K, Ellingsworth L, Wahl SM. Rapid onset synovial inflammation and hyperplasia induced by transforming growth factor-β. *J Exp Med* 1990;171: 231–247.
757. Sano H, Forough R, Maier JAM, et al. Detection of high levels of heparin binding growth factor-1 (acidic fibroblast growth factor) in inflammatory arthritic joints. *J Cell Biol* 1990;110:1417–1426.
758. Bucala R, Ritchlin C, Winchester R, Cerami A. Constitutive production of inflammatory and mitogenic cytokines by rheumatoid synovial fibroblasts. *J Exp Med* 1991;173:569–574.
759. Raghow R. Role of transforming growth factor-β in repair and fibrosis. *Chest* 1991;99(suppl):61S–65S.
760. Mustoe TA, Pierce GF, Morishima C, Deuel TF. Growth factor-induced acceleration of tissue repair through direct and inductive activities in a rabbit dermal ulcer model. *J Clin Invest* 1991;87:694–703.
761. Gordon HM, Kucera G, Salvo R, Boss JM. Tumor necrosis factor induces genes involved in inflammation, Cellular and tissue repair, and metabolism in murine fibroblasts. *J Immunol* 1992;148:4021–4027.
762. Jones PBC, Welsh TH Jr, Hsueh AJW. Regulation of ovarian progestin production by epidermal growth factor in cultured rat granulosa cells. *J Biol Chem* 1982;257:11268–11273.

763. Cara JF, Fan J, Azzarello J, Rosenfield RL. Insulin-like growth factor-1 enhances luteinizing hormone binding to rat ovarian theca-intestitial cells. *J Clin Invest* 1990;86:560–565.
764. Pekonen F, Rutanen EM, Kurunmaki H, Hovatta O. Ovulation induction increases serum levels of insulin-like growth factor binding protein 1. *Int J Fertil* 1992;37:188–191.
765. Montesano R, Vassalli J-D, Baird A, Guillemin R, Orci L. Basic fibroblast growth factor induces angiogenesis *in vitro. Proc Natl Acad Sci* 1986;83:7297–7301.
766. Gonzalez A-M, Buscaglia M, Ong M, Baird A. Distribution of basic fibroblast growth factor in the 18-day rat fetus: localization in the basement membranes of diverse tissues. *J Cell Biol* 1990;110:753–765.
767. Nell A, Mailath G, Porteder H, Ulrich W, Sinzinger H, Matejka M. Enhancement of human dental cyst PGI_2 formation by platelet derived growth factor and its role in cyst growth and bone resorption. *Arch Oral Biol* 1989;34:187–190.
768. Wong WYL, Richards JS. Induction of prostaglandin H synthase in rat preovulatory follicles by gonadotropin-releasing hormone. *Endocrinology* 1992;130:3512–3521.
769. Zachariae F, Asboe-Hansen G, Boseila AWA: Studies on the mechanism of ovulation: migration of basophil leukocytes from blood to genital organs at ovulation in the rabbit. *Acta Endocrinol* 1958;28:547–552.
770. Mettler L, Shirwani D. The blood count during the ovarian cycle. *Am J Obstet Gynecol* 1974;119:1038–1043.
771. Murdoch WJ. Accumulation of thromboxane B_2 within periovulatory ovine follicles: relationship to adhesion of platelets to endothelium. *Prostaglandins* 1986;32:597–604.
772. Murdoch WJ, McCormick RJ. Sequence analysis of leukocyte chemoattractant peptides secreted by periovulatory ovine follicles. *Biochem Biophys Res Commun* 1992;184:848–852.
773. Gerdes U, Gafvels M, Bergh A, Cajander S. Localized increases in ovarian vascular permeability and leucocyte accumulation after induced ovulation in rabbits. *J Reprod Fertil* 1992;95:539–550.
774. Rajan P, Rao GS, Walter S. Blood basopenia as an indicator of ovulation. *Indian J Physiol Pharmacol* 1992;36:115–117.
775. Seow WK, Thong YH, Waters MJ, Walters M, Cummins JM. Isolation of a chemotactic protein for neutrophils from human ovarian follicular fluid. *Int Arch Allergy Appl Immunol* 1988;86:331–336.
776. Hellberg P, Thomsen P, Janson PO, Brannstrom M. Leukocyte supplementation increases the luteinizing hormone-induced ovulation rate in the *in vitro*-perfused rat ovary. *Biol Reprod* 1991;44:791–797.
777. Murdoch WJ, Steadman LE. Investigations concerning the relationship of ovarian eosinophilia to ovulation and luteal function in the sheep. *Am J Reprod Immunol* 1991;25:81–87.

The Physiology of Reproduction, Second Edition,
edited by E. Knobil and J.D. Neill,
Raven Press, Ltd., New York © 1994.

CHAPTER 14

Corpus Luteum and Its Control In Infraprimate Species[1]

Gordon D. Niswender and Terry M. Nett

The corpus luteum is a transient endocrine organ formed from cells of the follicle after ovulation (Fig. 1). That it is required for a successful pregnancy was first discovered early in the twentieth century by Frankel (1), who demonstrated that pregnancy in rabbits was terminated after removal of corpora lutea. Similar findings have since been reported in many different species of mammals. Even though the requirement for the corpus luteum during normal pregnancy was documented in 1903, the nature of the substance produced to maintain pregnancy remained unknown for more than two decades. In 1929, Allen and Corner (2) showed that a lipoidal extract of the corpus luteum could maintain pregnancy in rabbits ovariectomized a few days after mating. The component in the extract responsible for maintenance of pregnancy was subsequently called progesterone and was first crystallized in the laboratory of Allen and Wintersteiner in 1934 (3). Since that time, there has been a major interest in understanding the factors that regulate the life span and function of the corpus luteum. Development of methods to limit the function of this gland should have a major effect on limiting reproduction in humans, rodents, and pet animals. Also, 25% to 55% of all mammalian embryos are lost during early gestation, and much of this loss appears to be caused by inadequate luteal function. Development of procedures to prevent this loss would have a dramatic impact on increasing the production of food animals.

Department of Physiology, Colorado State University, Fort Collins, Colorado 80523

[1] See Chapter 49 for control of corpus luteum in primates.

BIOLOGIC FUNCTIONS OF PROGESTERONE

The primary function of the corpus luteum is to secrete progesterone. Progesterone has several biologic effects on target tissues in the reproductive system to prepare them for support of pregnancy or to provide nourishment to the conceptus. The following is a brief description of the general effects of progesterone on the reproductive organs of the female during the estrous cycle and in early pregnancy. It is not intended to provide a comparative description of the actions of progesterone in different species.

Reproductive Tract

A primary target for progesterone is the mucosal lining of the genital tract. For progesterone to affect the genital tract, the cells must first have been exposed to

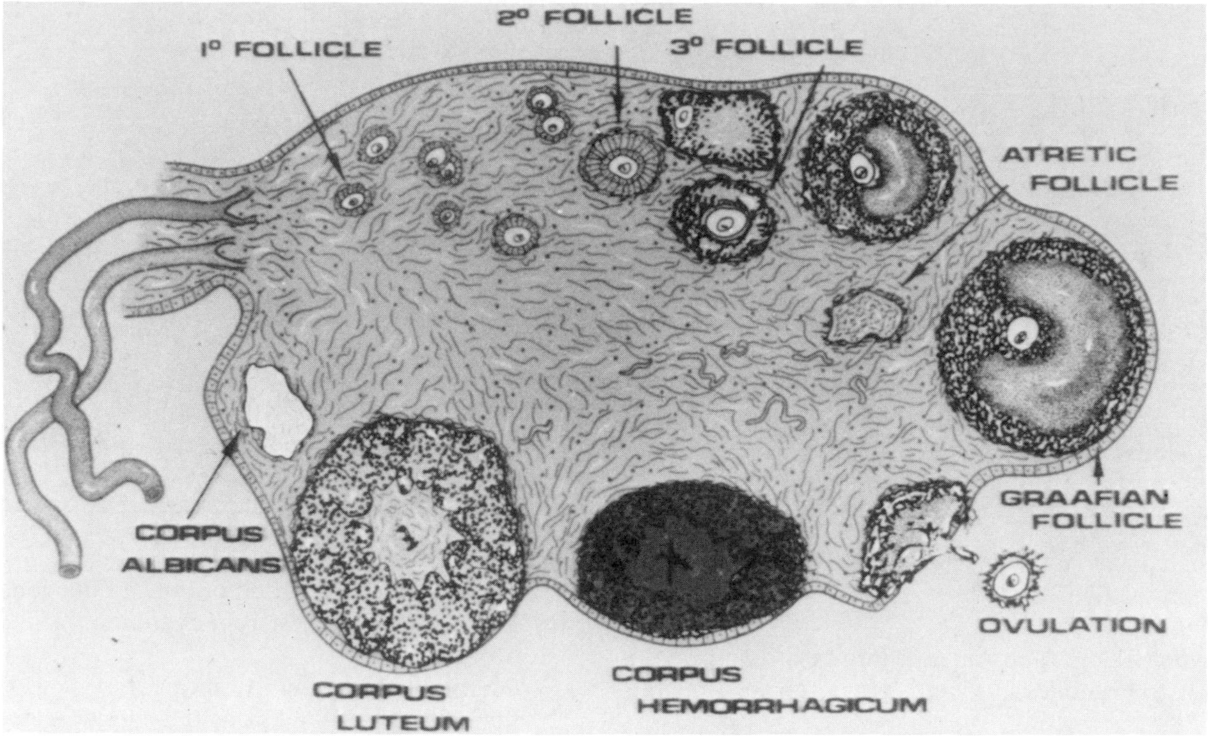

FIG. 1. Mammalian ovary. Progressive stages in follicular growth and development are depicted. Primary (1°) follicles have a single layer of granulosal cells surrounding the ovum. Secondary (2°) follicles have multiple layers of granulosal cells, and theca layers begin to differentiate. The tertiary (3°) follicle has fully developed granulosal, theca interna, and theca externa layers, and an antrum has formed and filled with follicular fluid. Graafian, or ovulatory, follicle continues to grow until ovulation occurs. Cavity of the ovulated follicle fills with blood (corpus hemorrhagicum), and the corpus luteum develops after several morphologic and biochemical changes that are described in text.

estradiol, which induces synthesis of receptors for progesterone (4). Estradiol acts on the oviductal epithelium to promote growth and proliferation of the cells and to induce ciliogenesis. After ovulation, ciliated cells in the fimbriated end of the oviduct appear to direct the ovum and associated cumulus cells into the infundibulum and then downward toward the ampulla. Together, estradiol and progesterone also regulate contractions of the oviduct that influence the rate of transport of the ovum to the uterus (5), resulting in delivery of the conceptus to the uterus at an appropriate time. Progesterone stimulates secretory activity of the oviductal epithelium to induce secretion of a fluid that supports early development of the conceptus. Finally, progesterone also plays a role in inducing regression of the oviductal epithelium (6).

One of the most significant actions of progesterone is to prepare the uterus for pregnancy. The uterine mucosa is composed of a surface layer of columnar epithelial cells overlying a stroma composed of spindle-shaped cells permeated by blood vessels. Many glands permeate the surface layer and dip into the stroma. These glands are lined by columnar epithelial cells, some of which are ciliated, whereas others are nonciliated and appear to be secretory. Under the influence of estradiol, the uterine mucosa thickens because of mitotic proliferation of the epithelium and stroma, and the tubular glands lengthen but remain straight. Progesterone, secreted by the developing corpus luteum, inhibits cell division, induces a marked coiling of the glands, and increases the vascularity of the stroma (7). There is also a dramatic increase in glycogen content of epithelial cells, the nuclei of epithelial cells become more basally oriented, and their cytoplasm becomes vacuolar. These changes prepare endometrial cells to provide nourishment and support to the conceptus until attachment (or implantation) and placentation occurs. In many species, progesterone also acts on cells of the myometrium to block organized contractions.

During nonfertile cycles, the progestational endometrium undergoes deterioration when serum levels of progesterone decrease as the corpus luteum ceases to function. Although the uteri of all species undergo regressive changes as serum levels of progesterone fall, it is most dramatic in primates in which the lining of the uterus actually is sloughed, resulting in menstruation. Under the influence of estradiol, the cervix secretes a mucus rich in glycoprotein that appears to align in filaments, facilitating passage of sperm through the cervical canal. Under the influence of progesterone, the consistency of the cervical mucus changes, and it becomes highly viscous. The glycoprotein filaments form networks that impede passage of materials either into or out of the uterus. Thus, when circulating levels of progesterone are high, the cervix provides an effective barrier between the uterus and the external environment (7).

Estradiol promotes proliferation and cornification of the vaginal epithelium. As the vaginal epithelium thickens, superficial layers that are not close to blood vessels keratinize and lose their nuclei. These cells are then sloughed off. This trend is reversed by progesterone. Under the influence of progesterone, the vaginal epithelium thins and is characterized by small nucleated cells. The thinness of the vaginal epithelium allows escape of leukocytes, which may appear in vaginal smears from animals under the influence of progesterone. These changes have been most completely characterized in rodents (8) and dogs (9) but occur to a lesser extent in other species as well.

Mammary Gland

Progesterone acts to promote lobuloalveolar development of the mammary glands after they have been exposed to estradiol. Anterior pituitary hormones must also be present (i.e., progesterone alone has little, if any, effect on mammary tissue) (10). During estrous (or menstrual) cycles, progesterone appears to have little effect on mammary gland growth. However, during the prolonged secretion of progesterone that occurs during pregnancy, there is considerable development of the lobuloalveolar system. Whether this can be credited to progesterone or placental lactogen and prolactin has not been resolved.

Hypothalamus and Anterior Pituitary Gland

Under the influence of estradiol during the follicular phase of the cycle, gonadotropin secretion is characterized by decreasing serum concentrations of follicle-stimulating hormone (FSH) and increasing concentrations of luteinizing hormone (LH) in most species. The increasing baseline concentrations of LH result from secretion of low-amplitude, high-frequency pulses of LH during the follicular phase of the cycle (11–14). During the luteal phase of the cycle, when serum levels of progesterone are elevated, the pattern of gonadotropin secretion changes dramatically. Pulses of LH are infrequent and are of higher amplitude than those observed during the follicular phase of the cycle. Secretion of FSH is not greatly affected by progesterone. As a result, in those species in which the corpus luteum does not secrete estradiol, the secretion of FSH is rather stable at a relatively high baseline during the luteal phase of the cycle. In primates, the corpus luteum does secrete estradiol, and basal concentrations of FSH remain suppressed during the luteal phase and do not increase until after regression of the corpus luteum (13,15).

Other Hormones Produced by the Corpus Luteum

Besides progesterone, the corpus luteum also secretes a variety of other hormones. In primates, the corpus luteum is a source of estradiol, but this does not appear to be the case in most other species. In several species, including human (16), pig (17), and rat (18), the corpus luteum produces relaxin. The function of ovarian relaxin is unclear. It may act synergistically with estradiol and progesterone to prepare the endometrium for implantation and may aid in development of the blood supply to the conceptus in primates. Near term, several changes in the birth canal that are required for parturition are induced by relaxin; however, in most species the fetoplacental unit appears to be the main source of relaxin in late gestation. Corpora lutea from a variety of species also contain oxytocin (19,20). Luteal oxytocin may play a role in luteolysis (21), and it may also function in a paracrine manner. There is also evidence that the corpus luteum from several species secretes prostaglandin (PG) $F_2\alpha$ (22,23). Finally, as will be discussed later, several peptidal hormones appear to be secreted from luteal cells and likely exert paracrine regulatory effects.

FORMATION OF THE CORPUS LUTEUM

Morphologic Changes Associated with Luteinization

Formation of the corpus luteum is initiated by a series of morphologic and biochemical changes in cells of the theca interna and membrana granulosa of the preovulatory follicle. These changes, termed *luteinization,* occur as a result of dramatic increases in serum levels of LH associated with the preovulatory surge of this hormone.

The most complete description of the morphologic changes associated with luteinization in the rat is that of Anderson and Little (24). After the ovulatory stimulus but before ovulation, there is hypertrophy of granulosal cells and nuclear activation. After ovulation, the basement membrane breaks down, and blood vessels from the theca interna invade the cavity of the ruptured follicle. The growth of these new vessels appears to be due to an angiogenic factor that must be secreted soon after rupture of the follicle. In rats, the number and size of gap junctions between granulosal cells increases as the follicle matures but then decreases just before ovulation. During luteinization, many gap junctions reappear between developing luteal cells in rats. The presence of gap junctions between luteal cells during the reproductive cycle is not a universal phenomenon. Gonadotropic hormones appear to amplify and modulate, rather than induce formation of gap junctions. The appearance of gap junctions may be dependent on intracellular levels of cyclic AMP (25). Cytoplasmic projections, which are characteristic of rat granulosal cells, are also found on luteal cells. These cytoplasmic projections contain receptors for LH (26,27) and have septatelike junctions between them (28). All cells of the follicle do not differentiate synchronously after ovulation. The amount of smooth endoplasmic reticulum and the number of mitochondria both increase during luteinization. Mitochondria in granulosal cells have lamellar cristae, whereas those in luteal cells have primarily tubular cristae. Luteal cells during early and midpregnancy in rats also contain lipid droplets and well-developed Golgi complexes.

In the ewe, the first signs of luteinization occur before ovulation. Dispersion of nuclear chromatin and formation of a nucleolus occurs with a concomitant increase in the number of polyribosomes. This suggests that RNA and protein synthesis are important at this stage. There are many gap junctions between adjacent granulosal cells in the preovulatory follicle, along with desmosome-like structures (29). Formation of smooth endoplasmic reticulum and alterations in mitochondria occur 30 to 40 hr after the ovulatory surge of LH. Smooth endoplasmic reticulum contains 3β-hydroxysteroid dehydrogenase, a critical steroidogenic enzyme produced by the granulosal cells within a few hours after ovulation (30). After ovulation, mitochondria become rounded and develop villiform cristae. Development of the smooth endoplasmic reticulum and mitochondria in granulosal-luteal cells is correlated with the initial rise in circulating concentrations of progesterone. Gap junctions are no longer apparent in the ovine corpus luteum 48 hr after ovulation. Based on detailed morphologic studies of the ovulatory follicle and developing corpus luteum, it has been concluded that granulosal cells differentiate into large steroidogenic luteal cells found in the mature corpus luteum in ewes (29,31) and cows (32).

Cells of theca interna in the preovulatory follicle of ewes possess abundant lipid droplets. Alkaline phosphatase and 3β-hydroxysteroid dehydrogenase are restricted to this cell type before ovulation (31). In contrast to granulosal cells, only occasional mitotic figures are seen in cells of the theca interna. Within 24 hr of ovulation, cells derived from theca interna begin migrating from their original sites into the deeper, granulosal-derived areas of luteal tissue (33). At later stages, cells derived from the theca interna are widely distributed throughout the corpus luteum.

Ontogeny of Luteal Receptors for Hormones

The induction and first appearance of receptors for LH during the course of follicular development has been intensely studied, particularly in granulosal cells. Granulosal cells obtained from immature rat or pig follicles possess few, if any, receptors for LH (34,35). However, as follicles mature and increase in size, the number of receptors for LH increases dramatically (36–40). On the basis of studies that have used estradiol-FSH-primed, hypophysectomized rats, it appears that the initial appearance and subsequent increase in the number of receptors for LH in granulosal cells is a result of the synergistic action of estradiol and FSH (39,41). According to Richards et al. (39): (a) estradiol-17β acts on granulosal cells to increase the concentration of its own receptor and induces receptors for FSH; (b) FSH then acts on estradiol-primed granulosal cells to increase receptors for both FSH and LH; and (c) finally LH acts on estradiol-FSH-primed cells to effect a decrease in receptors for estradiol, FSH, and LH and at the same time promote an increase in the number of receptors for prolactin. Data from intact, normally cycling rats also indicate that an increased number of receptors for LH is a result of the combined action of estradiol and FSH (42). Once granulosal cells acquire receptors for LH, they are capable of undergoing luteinization. As demonstrated by Richards et al. (43), LH induces luteinization by increasing the intracellular concentrations of cyclic AMP. In hypophysectomized rats, administration of LH or human chorionic gonadotropin (hCG) to cause ovulation and luteinization of follicular cells is followed by a decrease ("down-regulation") in the number of LH receptors on granulosal cells. These changes in the numbers of receptors for LH are paralleled by changes in levels of mRNA encoding the receptor (44).

The pattern of development of receptors for LH in follicular granulosal cells in pigs (37) and sheep (45) appears similar to that described for rats. There is little information regarding receptors for LH in follicular thecal cells. In sheep, it appears that receptors for LH appear first in thecal cells in small follicles and that as the follicle enlarges there is a slight decline in the capacity of thecal cells to bind LH concomitant with a dramatic increase in LH binding to granulosal cells (45).

In rats, prolactin is necessary to maintain normal numbers of receptors for LH in the developing corpus luteum (41). Prolactin treatment of pseudopregnant rats increases levels of mRNA encoding the LH receptor (44). This role is consistent with the known biologic effects of prolactin on luteal function in this species. However, the situation in other species is not so clear, because prolactin does not appear to influence luteal function in cattle (46–49) or sheep (48,49). Although receptors for prolactin have been reported in porcine luteal tissue (50), the exact role of this hormone in regulating luteal receptors for LH in species other than rodents will require additional experimentation. In porcine luteal cells, prolactin appears to influence the number of receptors for low-density lipoprotein (51), and therefore it may play a role in regulating substrate availability for steroidogenesis.

LUTEAL PHASE OF THE ESTROUS CYCLE

Morphology of Luteal Cells

In the late 1800s and early 1900s, there were two hypotheses concerning the follicular cell type responsible for formation of the corpus luteum. The first held that the corpus luteum was derived exclusively from granulosal cells of the follicle, and the cells from the theca interna degenerated shortly after ovulation. The second hypothesis held exactly the opposite view. In 1906, Loeb (52) performed a detailed morphologic analysis of the ovary in the guinea pig during the period of luteinization and concluded that cells from both the theca interna and granulosal layers of the ovarian follicle were involved in formation of the corpus luteum. Corner (53) came to the same conclusion concerning the corpus luteum of the sow, as have subsequent investigators examining corpora lutea in cows (32,54–56), ewes (31), rats (57), and women (58).

Because the cells of the corpus luteum appear to be derived from at least two different types of follicular steroid-secreting cells (thecal and granulosal cells), it is not surprising this gland consists of at least two distinct types of steroidogenic luteal cells in several species (53,59–61). The two types of steroidogenic cells are morphologically distinct. The so-called large luteal cells (32,33,56,62–66) also referred to as granulosa-lutein (60,67), Type II (68), and D cells (69) are the most readily distinguished cells in the corpus luteum (Fig. 2). They are the largest strictly endocrine cells in the body and range from approximately 20 μm in diameter in rodents to 40 μm or more in humans (70). Under the light microscope, large luteal cells appear polyhedral, with a lightly staining cytoplasm and a large, centrally located nucleus with a distinct nucleolus. In contrast, small luteal cells have a diameter of 22 μm or less and appear spindle-shaped with darkly staining cytoplasm, large lipid droplets, and an irregularly shaped nucleus that often contains what has been described as cytoplasmic inclusions. Alternative terms for small luteal cells include theca-lutein (60,67), Type I (68), and I cells (69). On a volume basis, large luteal cells comprise about 25% to 35% of the corpus luteum in sheep, whereas small luteal cells represent approximately 12% to 18% of the luteal volume (71,72). During the period of maximum secretion of progesterone, vascular elements account for approximately 11% of luteal volume (71). The remainder of the corpus luteum is composed of connective tissue (22–29%) and fibroblasts (7–11%) (71,72).

Ultrastructurally, large luteal cells contain all the elements of steroid-secreting cells (i.e., many mitochondria and an abundance of smooth endoplasmic reticulum) (73) (Fig. 3). Mitochondria in large luteal cells can take on a variety of shapes: spherical, cup-shaped, or elongated (70); in fact, it is not uncommon to find each of these shapes of mitochondria within a single cell. There is also considerable variation in the size of mitochondria in large luteal cells. In most species, mitochondria with tubular cristae predominate, but some with lamelliform cristae may also be observed. Clustering and regional exclusion of mitochondria are also common features noted in large luteal cells (70).

Large luteal cells have an abundance of smooth endoplasmic reticulum, primarily in the peripheral region of the cell. In fact, it is often the most abundant cytoplasmic component found at the cell's periphery. The smooth endoplasmic reticulum is in the form of branched tubules, tubular sheets, and fenestrated cisternae often centered around a mitochondrion or lipid droplet. The branched tubules may form an anastomotic network that traverses the entire cell.

The Golgi complex is quite extensive in large luteal cells and is usually located at one side of the nucleus and occupies a comparable volume. There is a paucity of tubular smooth endoplasmic reticulum and mitochondria in the area of the Golgi complex. Unlike other cell types, there is an indication that the smooth endoplas-

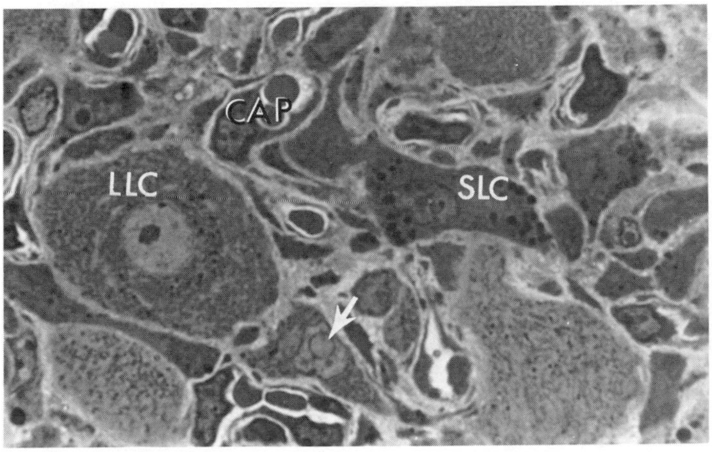

FIG. 2. Representative luteal tissue obtained during midluteal phase of estrous cycle from a ewe. Large luteal cells (*LLC*) can be easily distinguished from small luteal cells (*SLC*) in 1-μm-thick sections stained with toluidine blue. Small luteal cells are usually spindle-shaped, whereas LLC are typically spherical or polyhedral. Also, dark-staining cytoplasm of SLC contains large lipid droplets. Nuclei of SLC sometimes possess cytoplasmic inclusions (*arrow*). Both cell types are in close apposition to capillaries (*CAP*). ×800. (From ref. 61, with permission.)

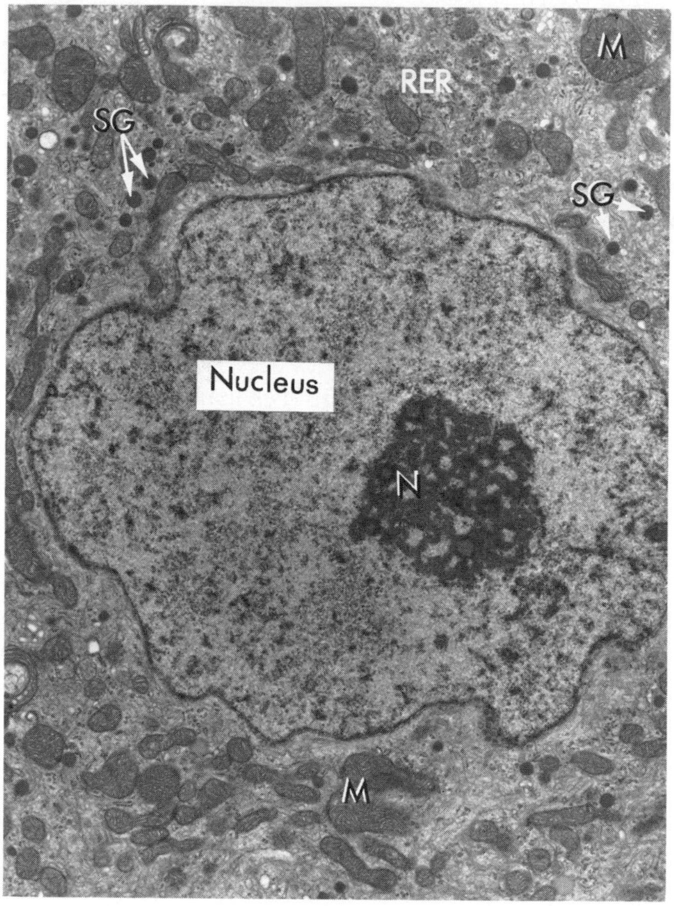

FIG. 3. Electron micrograph showing portion of large luteal cell (*LLC*) from a ewe. Presence of many electron-dense, membrane-bound secretory granules (*SG*) in the cytoplasm of LLC distinguishes these cells from small luteal cells (*SLC*) (see Fig. 5). Note absence of lipid droplets comparable with those found in SLC. *M,* Mitochondria; *N,* nucleolus; *RER,* rough endoplasmic reticulum. ×7,200. (From ref. 61, with permission.)

mic reticulum is in direct communication with the Golgi cisternae (74). There are abundant electron-dense, membrane-bound secretory granules in the cytoplasm of large luteal cells (Fig. 3). These granules are similar in size to lysosomes and peroxisomes, but they are a distinct form of granule (75) and their contents do not include acid phosphatase or catalase activity (75–77). Contents of the granules are released at the surface of the cell by exocytosis (78–80) (Fig. 4). At least one of the components in secretory granules in large luteal cells in cattle (81) and sheep (20,82) is oxytocin. Relaxin has also been identified in similar granules in rats (83,84), pigs (85–87), and cows (88). It is possible that the granules may contain more than one secretory product or that there are different types of granules within the same cell.

The ultrastructural appearance of small luteal cells is distinct from that of large luteal cells (Fig. 5). The nucleus is irregular in shape and, in approximately 10% of the cells, appears to contain areas of cytoplasm bounded by a completely inverted nuclear envelope (33) (Fig. 5). However, to date no one has serially sectioned the nucleus of the small luteal cell to establish whether these structures represent true cytoplasmic inclusions or, rather, whether they are simply cytoplasmic invaginations into the nucleus (Fig. 4). The characteristic small luteal cell contains a moderate number of mitochondria of variable size. Large amounts of endoplasmic reticulum are present in small luteal cells. The endoplasmic reticulum is predominantly of the smooth, tubular type, but scattered clusters of attached ribosomes are also present. The Golgi complex is less pronounced in the small luteal cell than in large luteal cells, is located perinuclearly, and is associated with many small coated or uncoated vesicles (33). A characteristic feature of the small luteal cell is the absence of secretory granules. Small lu-

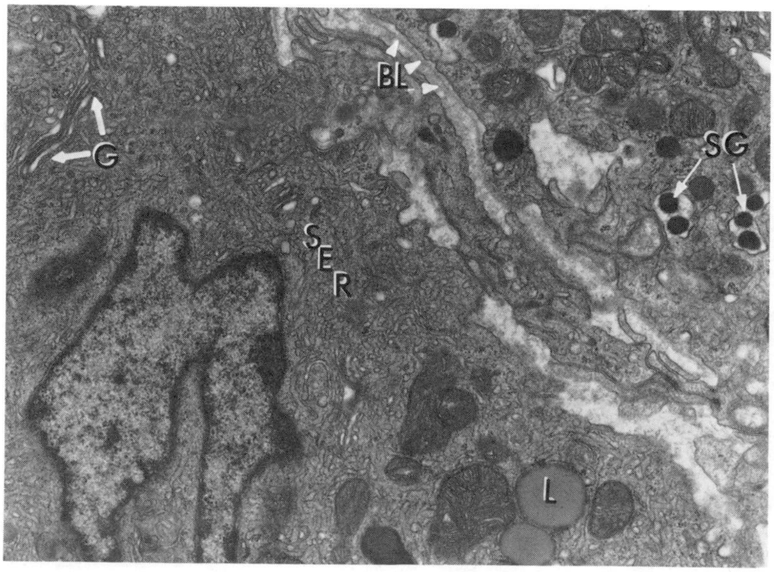

FIG. 4. Both small (*lower left*) and large (*upper right*) luteal cells possess fine structural characteristics consistent with a steroid-secreting function (i.e., extensive smooth endoplasmic reticulum [*SER*], lipid droplets [*L*], and Golgi apparatus [*G*]). However, LLC also have characteristics typical of protein-secreting cells, including secretory granules (*SG*), some of which have been exocytosed. Large luteal cells possess a more conspicuous basal lamina (*BL*) than do small luteal cells. ×14,800. (From ref. 61, with permission.)

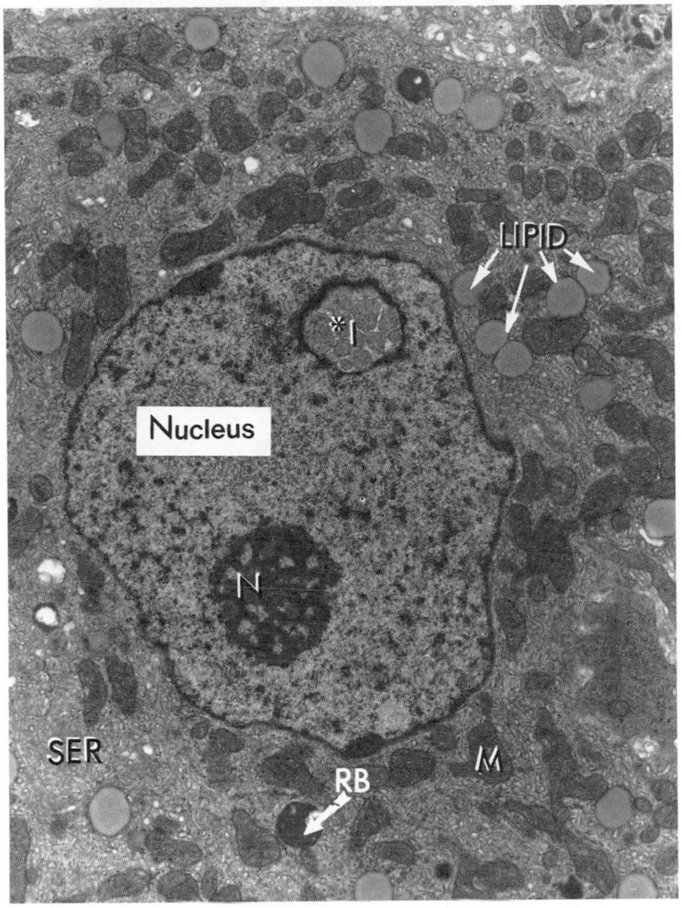

FIG. 5. Electron micrograph showing portion of small luteal cell from a ewe. Cytoplasm is characterized by an abundance of smooth endoplasmic reticulum (*SER*), many mitochondria (*M*), and lipid droplets. Residual bodies (*RB*) are often observed in these cells. Besides the nucleolus (*N*), the nucleus contains what appears to be cytoplasmic inclusion (*I*). ×7,200. (From ref. 61, with permission.)

teal cells also contain many lipid droplets, which are virtually absent in large luteal cells of ewes but are present in large cells of several other species.

Hypophyseal Regulation of Luteal Function

In most species, three organ systems regulate the function of the corpus luteum. The anterior pituitary gland secretes LH, which is the primary hormone responsible for stimulating the secretion of progesterone. In several rodent species, hypophyseal prolactin is also an important regulator of luteal function. In most nonprimate species, the uterus has a luteolytic effect during the late luteal phase of the estrous cycle. This luteolytic effect of the uterus is mediated via secretion of $PGF_2\alpha$ in most species (89). Finally, the conceptus has either direct luteotropic or antiluteotropic effects in most mammalian species.

Rats

Rothchild (90) reviewed the factors that regulate the function of the corpus luteum in most species, with particular attention to the rat. In rats, secretion of progesterone during the estrous cycle is short-lived and appears to be autonomous the first day of diestrus but requires prolactin during the second day (91). Postovulatory secretion of progesterone in rats has a pattern similar to the responsiveness of adenylate cyclase to LH (92). Although some minor differences may be present, it appears that the endocrine events controlling the life span and function of the corpus luteum during the estrous cycle in other rodents such as mice, hamsters, and gerbils are similar to those described here for the rat. One exception appears to be that prolactin, LH, and FSH are required for normal secretion of progesterone in hamsters (93).

Rabbits

Hormonal regulation of luteal function in the rabbit has been reviewed by Hilliard (94) and Keyes et al. (95). In rabbits, ovulation is induced by cervical stimulation, which causes the preovulatory surge of LH that results in ovulation. Maintenance of the structure and function of the corpus luteum requires estradiol (95). Despite a dependence on estradiol for maintenance of the corpus luteum, rabbit luteal tissue exhibits an acute steroidogenic response to LH (96), contains high-affinity receptors for LH (97), and possesses LH-sensitive adenylate cyclase (92). The corpus luteum of the rabbit contains two cell types: small luteal cells that are responsive to LH, and large cells that do not respond to LH with enhanced secretion of progesterone (98). There is no direct steroidogenic response to estradiol. Thus, the mechanisms whereby estradiol maintains the corpus luteum are not clear.

Domestic Ruminants

There has been considerable controversy regarding the requirement of the anterior pituitary gland for regulation of luteal function in ewes and cows. In 1963, Denamur and Mauleon (99) reported that formation and maintenance of an induced corpus luteum in prepubertal ewes was not influenced by hypophysectomy. However, Kaltenbach et al. (100) found that hypophysectomy on day 1 after a normal or induced ovulation resulted in failure of the corpus luteum to form, but hypophysectomy on day 5 resulted in regression of the partially formed corpus luteum. In subsequent studies, Denamur et al. (101) demonstrated that hypophysectomy of hysterectomized ewes also resulted in regression of the corpus luteum. Thus, there is agreement that hypophysectomy will prevent further luteal development and/or cause at least partial regression of existing luteal tissue. Infusion of LH, but not prolactin or estradiol, was followed by maintenance of the corpus luteum in hypophysectomized ewes with an intact uterus (102). Injections of LH to mimic the episodic patterns seen during the midluteal phase of the estrous cycle resulted in normal luteal function in hypophysectomized ewes (103). Based on these studies, it seems clear that LH is the primary luteotropic hormone in ewes.

The results of several additional studies are relevant regarding the roles of LH and prolactin in the regulation of luteal function. Constant infusions of LH prolonged the life span and function of corpora lutea in cyclic ewes (104), LH enhanced secretion of progesterone from the ovary *in situ* (105) or from luteal tissue *in vitro* (106,107), and daily injections of antiserum to LH caused luteal regression in cycling ewes (108). Similar data for cattle led Hansel et al. (46) to conclude that LH was the primary luteotropin in this species.

However, when serum concentrations of prolactin were reduced in ewes (49) or cows (47) for an entire estrous cycle, there was no effect on serum concentration of progesterone or length of the estrous cycle (49). Infusion of prolactin into intact ewes did not extend the life span of the corpus luteum (48), nor did infusion of prolactin into the ovarian artery result in enhanced secretion of progesterone (109). However, others (110) concluded that luteal receptors for prolactin are present and that their numbers change during pregnancy.

Pigs

Removal of the pituitary gland during the first 2 days of the estrous cycle did not affect corpora lutea in pigs (111). It was concluded that corpora lutea in cyclic pigs were capable of normal function without gonadotropic support after the initial stimulation of ovulation. Duncan et al. (112) were first to study progesterone synthesis by porcine luteal tissue *in vitro* and Cook et al. (113) demonstrated that LH stimulated synthesis of progesterone under these conditions.

Horses

Because of the unique structure of the equine ovary, ovulation occurs at only one site on the ovary, the ovulation fossa (60). As a result of this anatomic feature, essentially the entire structure of the corpus luteum is contained within the ovarian stroma (Fig. 6). Anatomically, the corpus luteum of the mare reaches its maximum diameter within approximately 3 days of ovulation (114), but maximum secretion of progesterone does not occur until about 9 days after ovulation (115).

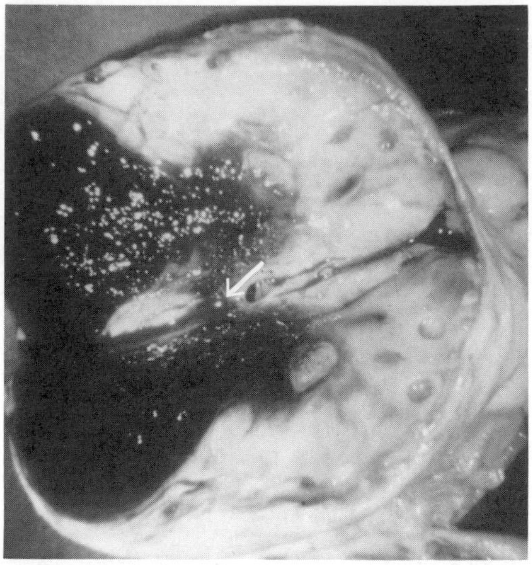

FIG. 6. Ovary from a mare cut midsagittally. Dark area is a developing corpus luteum. Note constricted portion of corpus luteum near center of ovary. This represents tract in which follicle grew from periphery of ovary to ovulation fossa (*arrow*).

Based on histologic studies (116,117), it appears that the secretory elements of the equine corpus luteum are derived primarily, if not exclusively, from granulosal cells. Thecal cells begin degenerating just before ovulation, and their degeneration is nearly complete by 24 hr after ovulation. In contrast, granulosal cells, which are approximately 10 μm in diameter at ovulation, have enlarged to 15 μm by 24 hr after ovulation and undergo cytologic changes characteristic of luteinization. Luteinization of the granulosal cells appears to be complete by 3 days postovulation, but they continue to hypertrophy until day 9 (average diameter, 37.5 μm), when maximal secretory activity is achieved. On day 9, besides the large, light-staining luteal cells, approximately 15% of the luteal cells are small cells. These small cells are eosinophilic and are thought to represent a resting stage that can be converted to the large, light-staining luteal cells. By 12 days postovulation, the large luteal cells begin to decrease in diameter, and by day 16, their diameter averages 20 μm. This reduction in size is correlated with a decrease in circulating concentrations of progesterone.

Endocrinologically, the corpus luteum of the mare appears to be primarily dependent on luteinizing hormone. Antisera raised against the gonadotropin fraction of equine pituitary extracts will induce luteal regression (118). Likewise, administration of hCG or equine pituitary extract can extend the life span of the corpus luteum in mares (114). Concentrations of receptors for LH in the corpus luteum of the mare parallel circulating concentrations of progesterone (119). Interestingly, the affinity of these receptors for LH also appears to increase when secretion of progesterone is maximal. This phenomenon appears to be unique to the equine corpus luteum.

Dogs

In the bitch, ovulation occurs 24 to 72 hr after the preovulatory LH surge. However, luteinization of ovarian follicles and secretion of progesterone begins before ovulation (120,121). There is a slight increase in secretion of progesterone concomitant with the onset of the LH surge. This increase is important for display of sexual receptivity by the bitch (120). Luteal growth continues for 10 to 20 days after ovulation, at which time secretion of progesterone is maximal. This is followed by decreasing luteal activity, with circulating concentrations of progesterone returning to basal levels by 55 to 90 days after ovulation in the pseudopregnant bitch. Concentrations of progesterone in the pregnant bitch appear to be similar to (122–124) or greater than those in the pseudopregnant bitch (125,126). Cessation of progesterone secretion is synchronous with the end of pregnancy, with a decrease to less than 1 ng/ml of blood occurring about 63 to 65 days after the LH surge.

Luteal function in the bitch requires the presence of pituitary hormones throughout pregnancy or pseudopregnancy because secretion of progesterone ceases after hypophysectomy (127). Two hypophyseal hormones, LH and prolactin, appear to be necessary for maintenance of the corpus luteum. Apparently, both hormones must be present continuously for normal luteal function. Administration of an antiserum to LH results in a dramatic decline in secretion of progesterone (128). Likewise, administration of ergocryptine to reduce circulating levels of prolactin results in a drastic reduction in circulating concentrations of progesterone.

Regulation of Progesterone Secretion

The mechanisms involved in the synthesis and secretion of progesterone are complex, although this hormone is the first biologically active compound produced in the steroid biosynthetic pathway (Fig. 7). Cholesterol bound to low-density lipoprotein (LDL) or, in some species, high-density lipoprotein (HDL) produced by the liver, is the primary substrate for progesterone synthesis. However, under some conditions, luteal cells also synthesize cholesterol from acetate for use in the steroidogenic pathway. The steroidogenic luteal cell contains LDL (or HDL) receptors that are involved in the transport of lipoprotein from outside to inside the cell. The occupied LDL receptor complex is internalized by endocytosis. Endocytotic vesicles combine with lysosomes, and cholesterol is liberated. Free cholesterol leaves the lysosome and is either esterified and stored as lipid droplets or is used for steroid biosynthesis or in membrane constituents of the cell. For biosynthesis of progesterone, cholesterol is transported to the mitochondria, where it is converted to pregnenolone by side-chain cleavage. The resultant pregnenolone is then converted to progesterone by 3β-hydroxysteroid dehydrogenase/Δ^5,Δ^4-isomerase (3β-HSD) in the smooth endoplasmic reticulum, and the progesterone is secreted. The luteal cell has a limited capacity to store progesterone. The most important endocrine factor, which acutely stimulates the synthesis and secretion of progesterone in the corpus luteum irrespective of species, appears to be LH. Luteiniz-

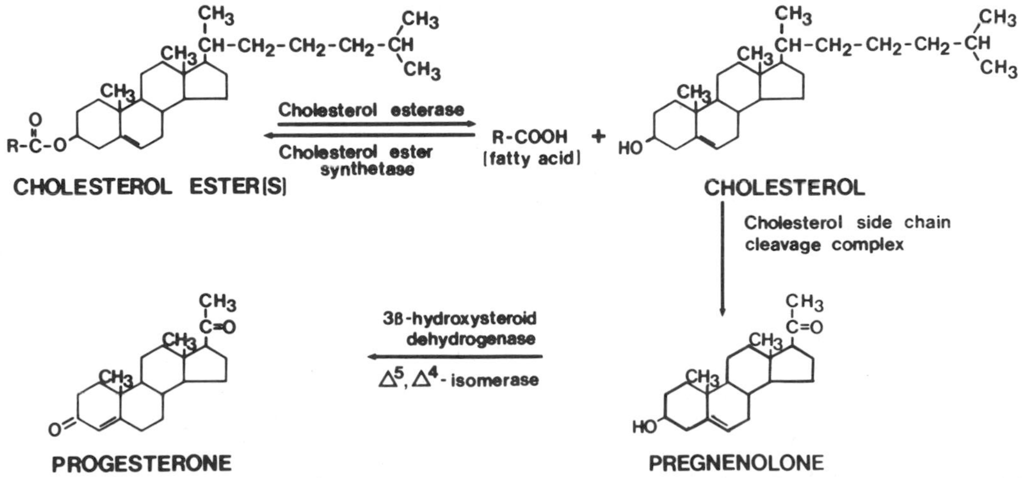

FIG. 7. Biosynthetic pathway for synthesis of progesterone from cholesterol ester. Conversion of cholesterol ester to cholesterol is a reversible reaction. Cholesterol side-chain cleavage complex within mitochondrion converts cholesterol to pregnenolone, which is converted to progesterone in smooth endoplasmic reticulum by 3β-hydroxysteroid dehydrogenase/Δ^5, Δ^4-isomerase.

ing hormone increases the synthesis and secretion of progesterone *in vivo* (129,130) or when incubated with luteal slices or cells *in vitro* (106,107,113,131,132). However, the hormone that appears to acutely inhibit progesterone synthesis and secretion is $PGF_{2}\alpha$ (133,134). Many growth factors also modulate both the positive and negative regulation of progesterone secretion from luteal cells.

Receptors for LH

The presence of specific receptors for LH in the ovary and testis was first demonstrated by the ability of these tissues to preferentially bind and concentrate radioactively labeled LH or hCG *in vivo* (34). Subsequent studies designed to determine the subcellular distribution of binding sites, the kinetics of hormone-receptor binding, and the physiochemical properties of the receptor molecule have used tissue slices (135), dispersed cells (136–138), homogenates or particulate fractions (139–142), and isolated membranes (143–145) prepared from target tissues. As a result of these early studies, the receptor for LH was purified and the molecular characteristics of this molecular elucidated.

The recent cloning of the gene encoding the receptor for LH from rats (146), pigs (147) and humans (148,149) has provided new insights into our understanding of how this critical luteal receptor is regulated (Fig. 8). The receptor contains a signal peptide of 26 or 27 amino acids, an N-terminal extracellular domain that contains the hormone binding site(s), seven putative transmembrane domains, and a C-terminal cytoplasmic tail responsible for G-protein activation. The rat receptor gene spans more than 70 kb, with a coding region of approximately 60 kb with 11 exons and ten introns (150). Exons 1 to 10 encode the extracellular domain (341 or 333 amino acids), whereas exon 11 encodes the transmembrane domains and the cytoplasmic tail (333 or 336 amino acids). It has been proposed that the LH receptor gene arose from the fusion of two genes. The transmembrane domain and cytoplasmic tail is thought to have evolved from an ancestral G-protein-coupled receptor. In contrast, the region encoding the extracellular portion of the receptor that contains ten exons and nine introns shares homology with the leucine-rich glycoprotein genes. The gene does not have a TATA box nor do there appear to be cyclic AMP response elements (151). This was surprising because hormones known to act through the cyclic AMP second-messenger system have been shown to influence the numbers of receptors for LH (152,153). The extracellular domain contains six potential N-linked glycosylation sites. The COOH-terminal intracellular tail contains potential phosphorylation sites for protein kinase C but does not contain the consensus site for phosphorylation by protein kinase A (147,154). The transmembrane domains and cytoplasmic tail exhibit sequence similarity with other receptors that activate G proteins.

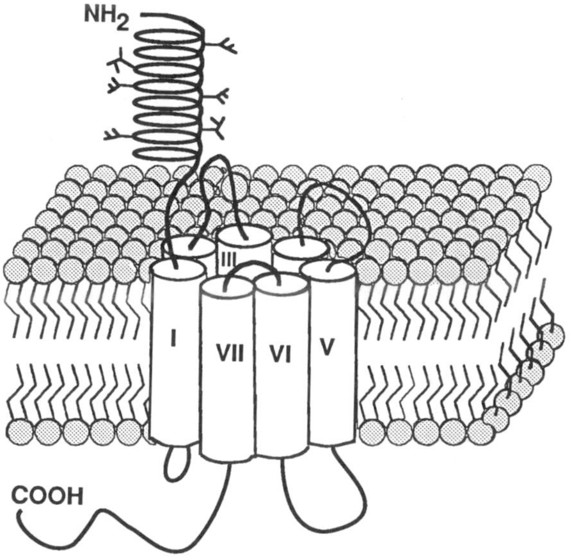

FIG. 8. Diagrammatic representation of receptor for luteinizing hormone. The receptor has a large extracellular (NH_2 terminus) domain that contains 333 to 341 amino acids and six potential glycosylation sites. There are seven proposed transmembrane segments terminating in a 70 amino acid cytoplasmic tail (COOH terminal).

To quantitate the number of receptors, these molecules have been labeled indirectly using LH or hCG coupled to different markers, such as ferritin (155), fluorescein (156), or radioiodine (157). It has been demonstrated repeatedly that hCG and LH compete for the same specific receptor, and hCG has been labeled most frequently. However, it has recently become clear that the steroidogenic response, the time required for internalization of the hormone-receptor complex, and the lateral mobility in the membrane of the occupied LH receptor are different for LH and hCG (61). Results from studies that have used LH covalently linked to ferritin (155) or agarose beads (158), as well as data from autoradiographic (27,159–161), immunocytochemical (161,162), and immunofluorescent studies (156,163), and cell fractionation (144,145,164) have clearly demonstrated that receptors for LH are localized in the plasma membrane of target cells. In rat luteal cells, most hCG binding sites are localized along regions of the cell surface facing capillaries, which are characterized by microvillus folds, whereas the basolateral surfaces of rat luteal cells are characterized by junctional complexes and contain very few binding sites (27). Thus, receptors for LH are localized in the plasma membrane and appear to be concentrated in specific regions and not distributed uniformly over the entire cell surface. Once the corpus luteum begins to develop, secretion of progesterone by this gland in women (165), rats (166), and cows (167) appears to be highly correlated with the number of receptors for LH. One of the most complete studies to date regarding the relationship between the total number of receptors, the number occupied by endogenous hormone, and secretion of progesterone by the corpus luteum is that of Diekman et al. (168). The total number of receptors for LH increased 40-fold between days 2 and 14 of the cycle in ewes (Fig. 9). There was a sixfold increase in both the number of receptors occupied by endogenous hormone and the weight of the corpus luteum and a tenfold increase in serum concentrations of progesterone during this same period. However, less than 0.5% of the total number of receptors was occupied by endogenous hormone. By day 16 (late luteal phase), both the total number of receptors and the number occupied by endogenous LH had decreased by 75%. During early pregnancy, the numbers of total and occupied receptors were very similar to those observed during the midluteal phase of the cycle (168). There was a high degree of correlation

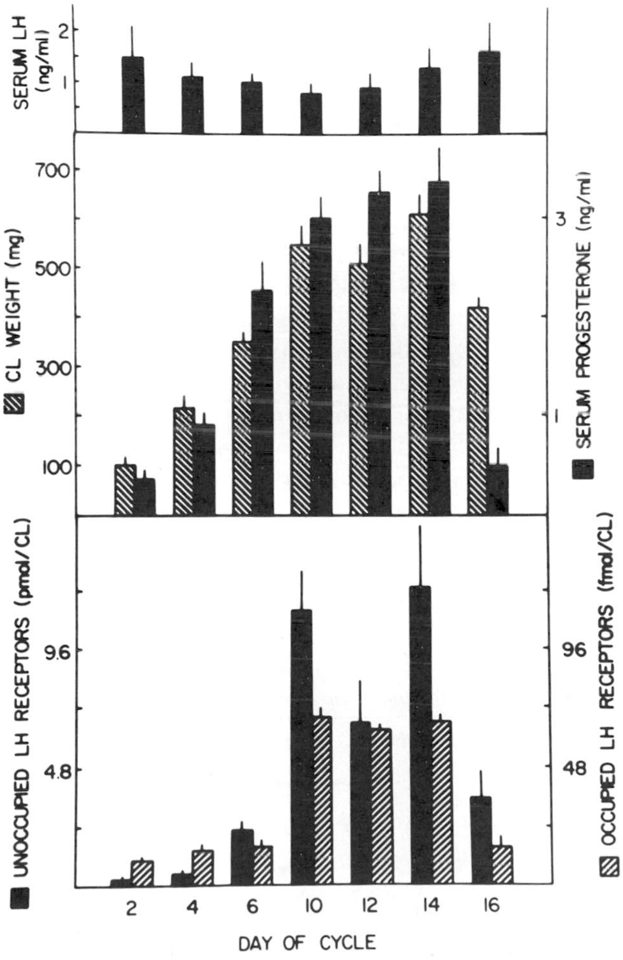

FIG. 9. Serum levels of LH (*top panel*) and progesterone (*middle panel*), weight of corpora lutea (*middle panel*), and number of occupied and unoccupied receptors for LH in ovine corpora lutea (*bottom panel*) collected throughout estrous cycle from ewes ($n = 6$). (From ref. 162, with permission.)

between the total number of LH receptors. the number occupied by endogenous LH, and serum concentrations of progesterone. However, the biologic significance of this finding has recently been questioned. There is little correlation between episodic peaks of LH in serum and systemic levels of progesterone during the midluteal phase of the estrous cycle in ewes (169). Also, when serum levels of LH were increased approximately 1,000-fold during the midluteal phase of the estrous cycle, the increase in serum levels of progesterone was less than twofold and lasted less than 6 hr (170). These findings can apparently be explained by the observation that in ewes more than 80% of progesterone secreted by the corpus luteum is derived from large steroidogenic luteal cells, which do not respond to LH with increased secretion of progesterone (61). However, it should not be inferred from these data that LH is not important for normal secretion of progesterone. Injections of hCG or LH increased the numbers of large luteal cells; concomitantly, the numbers of small luteal cells decreased (61). Thus, LH may regulate differentiation of small to large luteal cells, a suggestion originally presented by Donaldson and Hansel (32) for cattle. Therefore, although the secretion of progesterone by large luteal cells is not regulated directly by LH, the number of large luteal cells may depend, at least in part, on this hormone.

The observation that less than 1% of the receptors for LH in the ovary (168) are occupied under conditions of maximal steroid secretion has led to the concept of "spare" receptors for this tropic hormone. However, it seems unlikely that these receptors are really spare, because circulating levels of LH are so low (0.5–1.5 ng/ml) that the large number of receptors is required to ensure that sufficient numbers are occupied by endogenous hormone to stimulate steroidogenesis. Also, intracellular levels of cyclic AMP continue to increase with increased occupancy of LH receptors, even after steroidogenesis is maximal (171,172). This observation suggests that the receptors are coupled to adenylate cyclase and biologically functional. It may well be that cyclic AMP is important for aspects of luteal cell function not acutely related to secretion of progesterone. For example, cyclic AMP seems to be necessary for luteinization of granulosal cells (43) and maintenance of the characteristic morphology of luteal cells grown in culture (173). It is also possible that cyclic AMP may be the intracellular agent involved in differentiation of small luteal cells into large ones if such differentiation occurs (61).

A variety of factors may influence the concentration of LH receptors in the corpus luteum (35), but the primary factor appears to be LH itself. Exposure of luteal tissue to high concentrations of LH or hCG invariably results in a dramatic loss (up to 90% in some cases) of LH receptors, known as "down-regulation" (137,167,170, 174,175). The loss induced by homologous hormone is time- and dose-dependent, and it is accompanied by a concomitant loss in hCG-stimulated adenylate cyclase activity and/or steroid production (175,176). Although it is tempting to conclude that the loss of adenylate cyclase activity and tissue responsiveness is related to receptor loss, there may also be a secondary lesion involved, because the administration of dibutyryl cyclic AMP does not stimulate steroidogenesis in desensitized tissues (174).

Two mechanisms have been proposed to explain the loss of LH receptors after administration of a large dose of LH or hCG. Receptors for LH could be inactivated or sequestered within the plasma membrane and thus become inaccessible for binding (138,175) or the hormone receptor complex may be internalized (161). The latter possibility seems most likely because there is good evidence that the LH receptor complex enters the cell through small endocytotic vesicles (27,138,161,163), and the hormone is subsequently degraded by lysosomal enzymes (177–180). That internalization of the hormone is a degradatory process rather than a mechanism for action by the hormone is suggested by the fact that chloroquine, a lysosomal enzyme inhibitor, blocks degradation of the hormone by the target cell but does not reduce steroid secretion (178). Also, ovine luteal cells exposed to a 15-min pulse of LH secrete enhanced quantities of progesterone for 3 to 4 hr, whereas exposure to a 15-min pulse of hCG results in enhanced secretion of progesterone for more than 6 hr (181). Because the hCG-LH receptor complex is internalized approximately 50 times more slowly than the ovine LH-LH receptor complex, these data suggest that internalization of the hormone-receptor complex is the mechanism whereby the cell deactivates itself after stimulation (61).

Our current working hypothesis is that the functional life of the receptor for LH in ovine luteal cells is a single binding of hormone followed by internalization and degradation of the hormone. The receptor appears to be recycled to the plasma membrane (182), probably in a manner similar to that proposed for other peptide hormones (183). This suggests that regulation of the biologic effects of LH on luteal cells is a very precise phenomenon and may also explain how the hormone-stimulated cell returns to basal activity.

Data obtained *in vivo* by Suter et al. (170) provide additional insight into the mechanisms involved in the acute loss and renewal of receptors for LH in ewes administered a pharmacologic dose of LH during the midluteal phase of the estrous cycle. There was a dramatic increase in receptors occupied by LH within 10 min after the injection, after which the number of receptors occupied by LH decreased rapidly and returned to basal levels within 6 hr (Table 1). In contrast, the number of unoccupied receptors had decreased dramatically within 12 hr but had returned to preinjection levels within 48 hr. There were three interesting observations from this study. First, the total number of receptors (occupied plus unoccupied) for LH in the crude membrane fraction increased significantly within 10 min of the LH injection ("up-regulation"). Second, although the total number of receptors for LH was decreased within 12 to 24 hr after the injection of LH, at no time during the study did serum concentrations of progesterone fall below preinjection levels. Thus, the biologic significance of "down-regulation" of ovine luteal receptors is unclear. Finally, the number of receptors occupied at 10 min after injection of LH was almost perfectly correlated with the number of receptors lost by 24 hr. This finding certainly suggests that loss of receptors for LH in ovine luteal cells is a function of occupancy by hormone.

Recent evidence from rats has also indicated that down-regulation of the LH receptor involves decreased production of mRNA encoding the receptor (153). In this same system, prolactin increases mRNA encoding the receptor (44). Additional studies are required to determine the exact effects of the multiple endocrine signals known to influence the number of receptors for LH on transcription and translation of this gene. It seems clear that there will be differences between different species in this regard.

In rats, $PGF_{2}\alpha$ also appears to be involved in regulating the number of luteal receptors for LH (184). The number of receptors for LH in rats administered a luteo-

TABLE 1. *Number of receptors for LH in the corpus luteum (CL) after injection of 1 mg LH*[a]

Time after LH (hr)	Unoccupied receptors (mol/CL × 10^{12})	Occupied receptors (mol/CL × 10^{12})	Total receptors (mol/CL × 10^{12})
0	2.63 ± 0.48	0.41 ± 0.66	3.04 ± 0.88
0.17	2.48 ± 0.48	5.43 ± 0.73[a]	7.91 ± 0.99[b]
2	0.45 ± 0.48	1.51 ± 0.73	2.96 ± 0.99
6	1.54 ± 0.48	0.52 ± 0.66	2.06 ± 0.88
12	0.90 ± 0.48[a]	0.98 ± 0.66	1.88 ± 0.88
24	0.95 ± 0.48	0.21 ± 0.72	1.16 ± 0.98[b]
48	3.32 ± 0.54	0.41 ± 0.73	3.73 ± 0.99
72	3.92 ± 0.48	0.46 ± 0.73	3.75 ± 0.99

[a] Each value represents the least-squares mean ± SEM of seven determinations (170).
[b] Values significantly different from control (t = 0; P, .05).

lytic dose of $PGF_2\alpha$ decreases dramatically. However, $PGF_2\alpha$ does not appear to have the same effect in ewes (185).

Effects of LH on Steroidogenesis

Binding of LH to its receptor results in activation of adenylate cyclase in corpora lutea by a regulatory GTP-binding protein (186). The hormonal regulation of adenylate cyclase has been reviewed in detail by Birnbaumer et al. (187). Critical steps in activation of intracellular mechanisms through this process are outlined in Fig. 10. Most cell types have receptors for multiple regulatory hormones, some of which stimulate (Rs) adenylate cyclase and others are inhibitory (Ri). The stimulatory or inhibitory actions of the hormone receptor complexes are mediated by two transducing or coupling proteins. The protein complex involved in activating adenylate cyclase has been called the Gs (188) or Ns protein (187), whereas the protein that inhibits adenylate cyclase has been termed Gi (188) or Ni (187). These proteins will be referred to as Ns or Ni in this discussion. The activity of Ns is regulated by guanine nucleotide binding. The stimulatory, occupied hormone receptor interacts with Ns promoting GTP binding through a Mg-dependent process that results in activation of Ns. Dissociation of GDP from Ns is also a regulated component of the system. Activated Ns then stimulates the catalytic component of adenylate cyclase, resulting in conversion of Mg · ATP to cyclic AMP. Ns has inherent GTPase activity, which converts bound GTP to GDP, resulting in inactivation of Ns unless dissociation of GDP and further GTP binding occurs. Stimulatory hormones have been demonstrated to enhance the rate of exchange of GDP for GTP on Ns. Inhibitory hormones bind to their receptor, which activates Ni and results in an inhibition of the activity of adenylate cyclase. Oxytocin and vasopressin have been shown to activate Ni in rat Leydig cells and to prevent LH-stimulated increases in testosterone secretion. However, this phenomenon cannot be demonstrated in ovine luteal tissue.

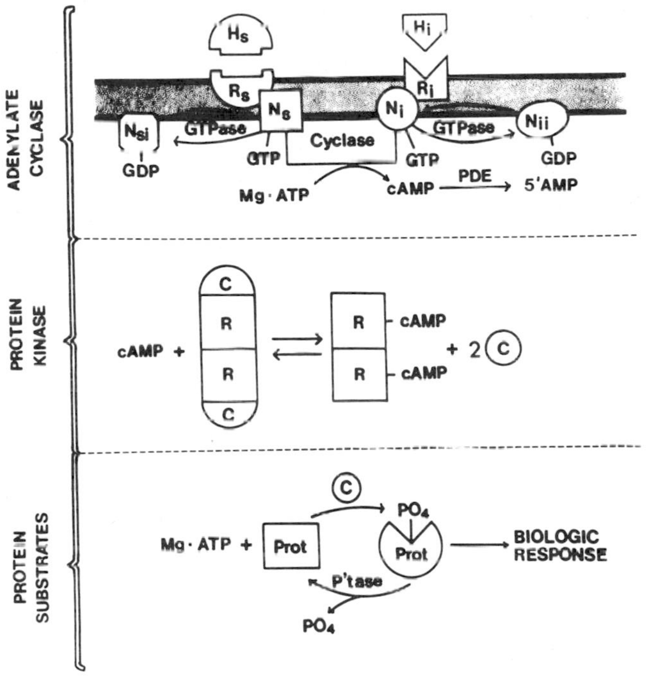

FIG. 10. Schematic representation of molecular events that occur as part of hormonal regulation of biologic responses of target cells. *Adenylate cyclase:* Hormone either stimulatory (*Hs*) or inhibitory (*Hi*) interacts with its cell membrane-bound receptor (*Rs* or *Ri*), which results in activation of appropriate regulatory component(s) of adenylate cyclase (*Ns* or *Ni*). Dissociation of GDP from inactive *Nsi* or *Nii* and binding of GTP activates Ns or Ni. This results in activation of catalytic subunit (cyclase), which converts ATP to cyclic AMP. *Protein kinase:* Cyclic AMP binds to receptor (*R*) subunit of cyclic AMP-dependent protein kinase, causing dissociation and activation of the catalytic subunit (*C*). *Protein substrate:* Catalytic subunit of protein kinase alters activity of different protein substrates (*Prot*) by phosphorylation, leading to activation of these proteins and modification of biologic response (see Fig. 11). Points for negative regulation of this system include activation of Ni, GTPase inactivation of Ns, phosphodiesterase (*PDE*) conversion of cyclic AMP to 5′AMP, dissociation of cyclic AMP from R, and dephosphorylation of phosphorylated protein substrate by phosphatase (*Ptase*).

In bovine and ovine corpus luteum, LH and epinephrine activate adenylate cyclase (172,186,189), but it is not clear whether they influence the same or different pools of the enzyme (172,189). Intracellular mediation of biologic responses by cyclic AMP involves several points of regulation (Fig. 10). Intracellular cyclic AMP that is produced binds to the regulatory subunit of the cyclic AMP-dependent protein kinase (190,191) or is degraded to 5′-AMP by a cyclic AMP-phosphodiesterase (186). The binding of cyclic AMP to the protein kinase promotes dissociation (activation) of the catalytic subunit of this enzyme. The activated catalytic subunit uses Mg · ATP to phosphorylate endogenous protein substrates, which results in altered activity (stimulated or inhibited) of these biologic regulators. Consequently, a biologic response ensues. These responses may be reversed by dephosphorylation of the protein substrate by a phosphoprotein phosphatase (192). It is generally accepted that all the intracellular effects of cyclic AMP are mediated by the cyclic AMP-dependent protein kinase (193).

The activity of protein kinase is enhanced in steroidogenic tissue at concentrations of LH that do not result in measurable increases in cyclic AMP (157,194). The increase in protein kinase activity and steroid secretion are highly correlated. Thus, it seems reasonable to assume that increased activity of protein kinase because of elevated intracellular levels of cyclic AMP in some compartments is involved in stimulation of steroidogenesis by LH. Increased protein kinase activity can influence the function of the luteal cell through several mechanisms (Fig. 11). (a) Protein kinases may influence nuclear events, gene expression, and protein synthesis (195), including steroidogenic enzymes and a cholesterol-binding protein (196), or they may enhance protein synthesis by phosphorylation of ribosomes (197). The exact sites in the steroidogenic pathway where protein synthesis is required have not been elucidated, but several have been suggested. (b) Phosphorylation of cholesterol esterase activates this steroidogenic enzyme (198,199). (c) It was suggested early that phosphorylation of a component (cytochrome P-450) of the cholesterol side-chain cleavage enzyme complex (200–202) is required for activation of this enzyme complex, but results of recent studies indicate that PK-A does not influence the activity of cholesterol side-chain cleavage complex (203). Rather the best evidence currently is that a specific protein(s) is involved in transport of cholesterol from the outer to the inner mitochondrial membrane. (d) Transport of cholesterol to the mitochondria has been suggested to involve microfilaments (204). (e) Microfilaments may also play a role in the transport of pregnenolone out of the mitochondria and/or (f) the internalization and transport of occupied lipoprotein receptors to lysosomes. Polymerization and activity of microfilaments is thought to be modified by protein kinase and phosphorylation. More recently, alterations in phospholipid turnover have been demonstrated after stimulation of steroidogenic tissues with 8-bromo-cyclic AMP or LH (205). Each of these sites of regulation of steroidogenesis will be discussed in more detail below.

The steroids and sterols involved in steroidogenesis are only slightly soluble in aqueous media; therefore, diffusion alone does not seem sufficient to shuttle substrates from one enzymatic site to another. This problem is partially alleviated by close association of several of the steroidogenic enzymes in linked complexes (e.g., cholesterol side-chain cleavage complex), and transport may be further assisted by close proximity of steroidogenically related organelles (206). Hepatocytes alleviate the problem of substrate transport by synthesizing sterol binding proteins, which render the otherwise insoluble sterols soluble in aqueous cytoplasm (207). Hepatic enzymes involved in synthesis of cholesterol appear to be

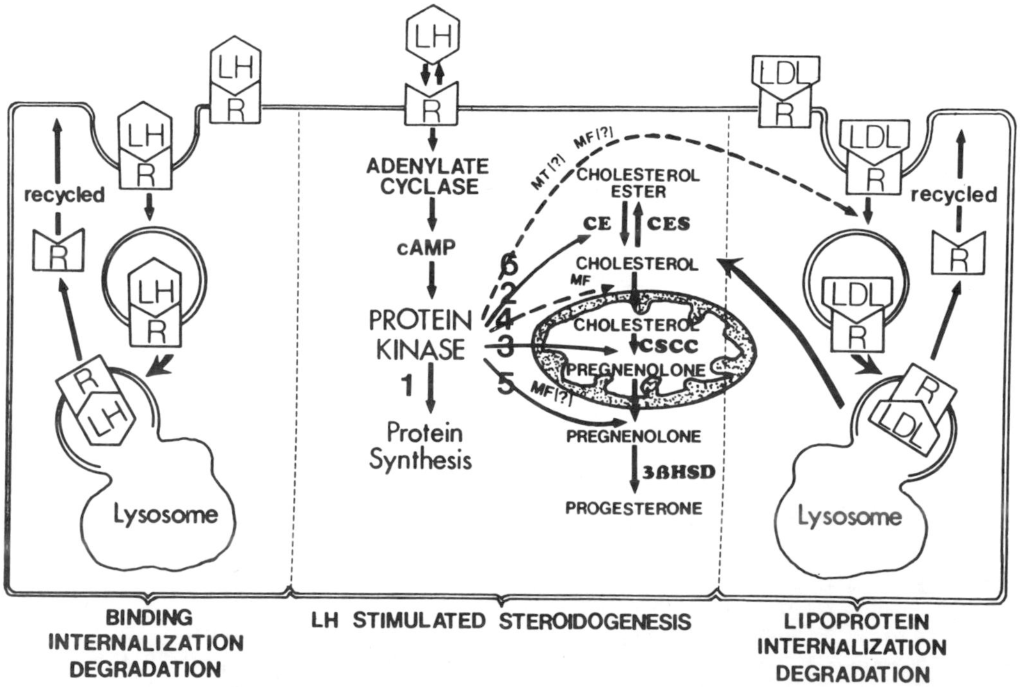

FIG. 11. Schematic representation of intracellular events involved in LH-stimulated steroidogenesis. LH binds to its receptor in cell membrane and activates adenylate cyclase, resulting in increased intracellular levels of cyclic AMP and activation of protein kinase (Fig. 9). Active protein kinase (1) stimulates protein synthesis; (2) activates cholesterol esterase (*CE*); (3) may stimulate cholesterol transport to mitochondria; (4) may stimulate transport of cholesterol from outer to inner mitochondrial membrane; (5) may stimulate transport of pregnenolone out of mitochondrion; and/or (6) may stimulate uptake of low-density lipoprotein (*LDL*), thus increasing cholesterol for substrate. In some species, high-density lipoprotein is preferred moiety for cholesterol uptake. See text for details of different actions of protein kinase. LDL is degraded in lysosome, providing cholesterol for steroidogenesis. LH and its receptor (*R*) is internalized, and LH is degraded in lysosomes. Receptors for LH and LDL are probably recycled to plasma membrane.

dependent on these proteins to facilitate substrate transport and transfer to successive enzymes in the pathway. A similar process appears to occur in luteal tissue because binding proteins for cholesterol (208,209) and pregnenolone (210) have been identified. Because ongoing protein synthesis is essential for the steroidogenic response (171,211–213) and the protein(s) synthesized has a very short half-life (213), it is possible that the protein(s) is a steroid carrier protein. In luteal cells, synthesis and/or activation of this carrier protein may be sensitive to stimulation by tropic hormones. It appears that ongoing protein synthesis is necessary for transport of cholesterol to the cytochrome P-450 component of the side-chain cleavage enzyme complex, and this may be one mechanism involved in stimulation of progesterone secretion in luteal tissue by LH (214).

All the enzymes involved in steroidogenesis in luteal tissue (cholesterol esterase, cholesterol side-chain cleavage complex, and 3β-HSD complex) are sensitive to end-product inhibition (215). This end-product inhibition is of such magnitude that it makes reliable measurement of 3β-HSD activity very difficult (216). In fact, the affinity of this enzyme complex for the end product, progesterone, is six times greater than for the precursor, pregnenolone (216). Reduced end-product inhibition of this enzyme would also be expected to decrease inhibitory effects exerted by other products synthesized previously in the steroidogenic pathway. Steroid binding proteins could provide a mechanism for reducing end-product inhibition of key steroidogenic enzymes.

Steroidogenesis in luteal tissue is less complex than in other steroidogenic tissues, because the main product, progesterone, is formed early in the steroidogenic pathway. Cholesterol is the initial substrate for luteal steroidogenesis. It may be extracted from the circulation, released from intracellular stores of cholesterol esters, or synthesized *de novo* from acetate. Although all three sources of cholesterol have been implicated in the steroidogenic response of luteal cells to LH (217–222), there are substantial quantities of cholesterol (both free and esterified) already present within luteal cells. Regulation of cholesterol uptake through the LDL- or HDL-receptor pathway is likely to involve microfilaments and may be regulated, at least to a degree, by LH. Release of cholesterol from pools of fatty acid esters is catalyzed by cholesterol esterase (222), which is activated by a cyclic AMP-dependent protein kinase (198,199). Therefore, this enzyme appears to be one important point for the regulation of steroidogenesis by LH.

Activation of cholesterol side-chain cleavage complex by a cyclic AMP-dependent protein kinase was suggested in 1975 (200), but more recent evidence indicates that activity of this enzyme is not regulated by PK-A (203,223). It now appears that cholesterol transport from the outer to the inner mitochondrial membrane is the rate-limiting step (224,225). The involvement of PK-A in this process is not clear. There is no evidence for acute hormonal regulation of the activity of 3β-HSD complex, and this enzyme appears to be present in considerable excess in luteal tissue (216). Enzyme synthesis does not appear to be involved in the acute response to stimulatory hormones in the case of cholesterol side-chain cleavage complex (mitochondria) or 3β-HSD complex (smooth endoplasmic reticulum), because both of these enzyme complexes are integral components of intracellular membranes (216,226). Turnover of these organelles is much too slow to account for the rapid, acute steroidogenic response that follows LH stimulation. However, synthesis of new enzyme might be expected as part of the chronic response to LH. Because cholesterol esterase is thought to be a cytoplasmic or soluble enzyme (216,222), its activity could be modified more easily as a result of increased synthesis or a decline in its degradation rate.

As a final consideration, cyclic AMP may be involved directly in the chronic response of luteal cells to LH. Gospodarowicz and Gospodarowicz (173) indicated that bovine luteal cells grown in culture tend to dedifferentiate with time but reform into luteal cells on addition of LH or cyclic AMP, apparently as a result of the effects of cyclic AMP on microtubules. Thus, it appears that cyclic AMP may be important for maintenance of normal morphology of luteal cells *in vivo* and for maintenance of intracellular components necessary for steroid synthesis and secretion. It has also been suggested that LH-stimulated cyclic AMP may be important for differentiation of small to large luteal cells in ewes (61) and cows (32).

Data presented above suggest that LH may stimulate synthesis of progesterone through several mechanisms, including protein kinase activation of cholesterol esterase, cholesterol transport to the inner mitochondrial membrane, and synthesis and/or activation of transport mechanisms responsible for enhancing substrate availability and/or relief of end-product inhibition. It is not necessary that the effects of LH be limited to one of these mechanisms. In fact, it seems likely that LH stimulates secretion of progesterone through several mechanisms.

The above discussion has dealt primarily with acute effects of LH on progesterone secretion from small luteal cells, which contain most of the LH receptors. However, in sheep—and probably in many other species—most of the progesterone is secreted by large luteal cells (61). Secretion of progesterone from large cells does not appear to be regulated by the cyclic AMP second-messenger system, although these cells contain adenylate cyclase (217). Treatment of large luteal cells with cholera toxin or forskolin to activate adenylate cyclase nonspecifically results in a dramatic increase in intracellular cyclic AMP, but there is no concomitant increase in progesterone production (227). This was true even though an enhanced occupancy of cyclic AMP-dependent protein kinase was demonstrated. In contrast, secretion of progesterone from large luteal cells is enhanced by PGE_2, although this response is not mediated by adenylate cyclase (227). Further studies are required to elucidate the mechanisms regulating synthesis of progesterone in large cells. It is possible that during differentiation these cells lose the ability to inhibit the cyclic AMP-dependent processes (i.e., they have reduced levels of phosphodiesterase or protein phosphatases). Because conversion of cyclic AMP to 5′-AMP and dephosphorylation of proteins by phosphatase are thought to be key mechanisms involved in limiting the stimulatory effect of increased intracellular levels of cyclic AMP, reduced levels or a total lack of these enzymes would be expected to permanently stimulate steroidogenesis. Further research is needed to unravel the mechanisms controlling secretion of progesterone by large cells.

To date there is little available information regarding the factors that regulate transcription and translation of the gene-encoding cholesterol esterase. However, recently there have been a large number of studies concerning regulation of cholesterol side-chain cleavage complex and 3β-HSD at the molecular level. The cholesterol side-chain cleavage complex consists of adrenodoxin reductase, adrenodoxin, and cytochrome P450 side-chain cleavage (cytochrome $P450_{scc}$), which are synthesized in the cytoplasm (229,230). The amino-terminal 15 to 20 amino acids of the peptides direct import of the protein into mitochondria (231). There is induction of all three proteins in response to cyclic AMP in rat granulosa cells (232). Rogers et al. (233) demonstrated that mRNAs encoding adrenodoxin and $P450_{scc}$ coordinately increased in bovine luteal tissue from ovulation until the late luteal phase and then decreased precipitously during luteolysis. In summary, there is evidence that the PK-A second-messenger system stimulates production of mRNAs encoding the components of the cholesterol side-chain cleavage complex in follicular steroidogenic tissues while activation of PK-C appears to be inhibitory to gene transcription (234,235). However, these long-term effects do not appear to be involved in the acute steroidogenic response of luteal cells to activation of second-messenger systems.

Activation of the PK-A second-messenger system also appears to increase mRNA encoding 3β-HSD in rat (236) and porcine (237) granulosa cells. In bovine (238) and ovine (239) luteal tissue, levels of mRNA for 3β-HSD were maximal during the midluteal phase and declined precipitously during luteolysis. Hawkins et al. (239) further demonstrated that a luteolytic regime of $PGF_2\alpha$ resulted in a rapid decline in levels of mRNA for 3β-HSD and speculated that the decrease was due to enhanced degradation.

The mechanisms responsible for transcriptional and translation control of steroidogenic enzyme activity should become more clear during the next few years. Essentially all the required molecular biological procedures are available, and progress in this area should be rapid.

LUTEOLYSIS

Uterine Involvement in Luteal Regression

The first evidence of uterine involvement in the luteolytic process was presented in 1923, when Loeb (240) reported that removal of the uterus (hysterectomy) lengthened the life span of the corpus luteum in guinea pigs. Extension of the life span of the corpus luteum after hysterectomy was later demonstrated in pseudopregnant rats (241,242), mice (243,244), hamsters (245–247), and rabbits (248–250). Maintenance of the corpus luteum also occurs after hysterectomy in cattle, sheep (251), swine (252), and horses (253,254).

In other species, presence of the uterus is not required for luteolysis. Most notably, in several species of primates including rhesus monkeys (255), cynomologus monkeys (256), and humans (257,258), removal of the uterus has no effect on normal cyclic activity. Also, hysterectomy has no effect on life span of the corpus luteum in the opossum (259), dog (124,260), or ferret (261). In contrast to pseudopregnant animals, the normal estrous cycle of the rat (262), mouse (263), and hamster (245,246) is not prolonged by hysterectomy.

Although there is variation among species in length of time that corpora lutea survive in hysterectomized animals, corpora lutea generally retain both structural and functional integrity for at least the duration of a normal pregnancy in guinea pigs (264–266), sheep (267–269), cattle (270,271), pigs (252,272–274), and rats (275). After hysterectomy of rabbits or horses, luteal function is maintained at levels lower than those established during the luteal phase (254,276–278).

In many species, effects of the uterus on luteal function are exerted locally. Unilateral hysterectomy (removal of one uterine horn) in sheep (279,280), cattle (281), swine (282), guinea pigs (283,284), pseudopregnant hamsters (285), and pseudopregnant rats (286) results in luteal regression in the ovary adjacent to the intact horn but prevents regression in the opposite ovary. The rabbit and horse are exceptions in that corpora lutea will undergo regression despite unilateral removal of the adjacent uterine horn (253,287). Thus, it is apparent that the luteolytic factor emanating from the uterus in most species exerts its effect only on the adjacent ovary. Therefore, it is unlikely that it is transported from uterus to ovary through the systemic circulation.

The mechanism of this transport is not clear. Corpora lutea are maintained when the connections (vascular and otherwise) between the ovary and uterus are severed in ewes (279), cows (288), guinea pigs (289–291), and pseudopregnant rats (283,286,292). Autotransplantation of either the uterus or ovary, while leaving the other organ *in situ*, results in extended luteal function in ewes (293,294) and guinea pigs (295–297). However, when the uterus and ovaries are transplanted to the neck as a unit, normal cyclic ovarian behavior continues in ewes (298). On the contrary, luteolysis is merely delayed after autotransplantation of the uterus or endometrial tissue in hamsters (245).

The uterine luteolytic factor appears to pass directly from the uterine vein to the ovarian artery in the ewe. This conclusion is based primarily on results of the elegant studies of Ginther and colleagues (for a review, see ref. 299). If the uterine vein draining the intact horn of unilaterally hysterectomized ewes is anastomosed to the uterine vein from the hysterectomized side, only corpora lutea on the hysterectomized side will regress (300,301). Reversal of the normal pattern of luteal regression in unilaterally hysterectomized ewes also occurs if the ovarian artery supplying the ovary on the uterine intact side is anastomosed to the artery on the hysterectomized side (300,301). A similar effect of uterine venous and ovarian arterial anastomoses has been described for cattle (302).

Although there do not appear to be vascular connections between the uterine vein and ovarian artery, there are regions of extensive contact between these two vessels throughout the broad ligament and up to their respective junctions with the vena cava and aorta (303,304). The ovarian artery is extremely tortuous, and collateral channels and venules separate from the uterine vein, wrapping around the artery and thus increasing the area of contact between the two vessels (305). The vessels share a common tunica adventitia and have thinner walls in regions where they make contact (306). Similar gross morphologic venoarterial relationships have been observed in guinea pigs, rats, hamsters (307), pigs (304), and cows (308). Interestingly, there is very little contact between the uterine vein and ovarian artery in the rabbit and horse, two species in which the uterine luteolytic effect is not exerted locally (304,307,309).

Identification of $PGF_2\alpha$ as the Uterine Luteolytic Factor

Although the luteolytic effect of the uterus was recognized more than 60 years ago, the biochemical signal(s) involved in this effect was difficult to elucidate. A major breakthrough occurred when the luteolytic actions of $PGF_2\alpha$ were demonstrated in pseudopregnant rats (310). This initial observation was rapidly extended to other species, and $PGF_2\alpha$ has been shown to exert a luteolytic effect in cattle (311–314), sheep (315–317), guinea pigs (318), goats (319), horses (320–322), pseudopregnant rodents (i.e., mice) (323), hamsters (324), and rabbits (325,326), and to a limited extent in swine (327–330). Interestingly, in rhesus monkeys (331,332), humans (333,334), and dogs (335), species in which the uterus has no clear luteolytic effect, there is a transitory suppression in the secretion of progesterone after short-term infusions (up to 12 hr) with $PGF_2\alpha$ during the luteal phase of the cycle. In fact, premature luteal regression can be induced in rhesus monkeys (336) and dogs (337) by more prolonged treatment regimens with high levels of $PGF_2\alpha$. Extremely high doses of $PGF_2\alpha$ are ineffective in causing luteal regression in the cat (338). If endogenous $PGF_2\alpha$ is involved in the normal luteolytic process in these species, it is probably not of uterine origin.

Although treatment of animals with $PGF_2\alpha$ caused premature luteolysis, this did not prove that it was the uterine factor involved in this process normally. However, considerable evidence has accumulated to suggest that $PGF_2\alpha$ is the factor of uterine origin responsible for luteolysis in both large domestic species and rodents. Treatment of intact animals with inhibitors of prostaglandin synthesis, such as indomethacin, will block spontaneous luteolysis in cattle, sheep, and guinea pigs. Length of pseudopregnancy can be prolonged in rabbits (339), rats, hamsters (340), and mice (341) by treatment with indomethacin. Thus, synthesis of prostaglandins (presumably $PGF_2\alpha$) appears to be required for normal luteolysis. Perhaps the best evidence that $PGF_2\alpha$ is the uterine luteolytic factor is the fact that spontaneous luteal regression can be prevented by active or passive immunization of sheep (342,343), cattle (344), and guinea pigs (266) to $PGF_2\alpha$.

Prostaglandin $F_2\alpha$ has been isolated from endometrial tissue of several species, and its concentration is maximal during the period of luteal regression in cattle (345), sheep (346), guinea pig (347), horses (348), swine (349), pseudopregnant rats (350), and pseudopregnant rabbits (351). Also, secretion of $PGF_2\alpha$ into the uterine vein is temporally associated with both spontaneous and hormonally induced luteal regression in several species. Concentrations of $PGF_2\alpha$ in uterine venous blood increase as spontaneous luteolysis commences in swine (352,353), horses (354), pseudopregnant rabbits (351), and rats (355).

Based on available data, it seems reasonable to conclude that $PGF_2\alpha$ is the factor, of uterine origin, responsible for luteolysis in large domestic species and pseudopregnant rodents.

Mechanism of Action of $PGF_2\alpha$

Several different mechanisms have been proposed to explain the luteolytic effects of $PGF_2\alpha$: (a) a rapid and dramatic decrease in luteal blood flow (71,130); (b) a reduction in the number of receptors for LH (356); (c) an uncoupling of the LH receptor from adenylate cyclase (357); (d) activation of protein kinase C (223); (e) influx of high levels of calcium (358,359); and (f) a cytotoxic effect (360). Although there is good evidence for all these actions, the effects of $PGF_2\alpha$ appear to differ among species, and the actions demonstrable *in vivo* often differ from those observed *in vitro.*

Injections of a luteolytic dose of $PGF_2\alpha$ into rats does not appear to decrease ovarian blood flow (184). However, it does dramatically decrease the binding of LH to luteal cells *in vivo* by an unexplained mechanism. There is a direct block of adenylate cyclase activation by LH in isolated rat luteal cells. Finally, there is an eventual loss of LH receptors after treatment with $PGF_2\alpha$ caused by inhibition of the actions of prolactin.

In ewes, the first effect of $PGF_2\alpha$ appears to be a rapid decrease in luteal blood flow (130). The decrease in blood flow is highly correlated with decreased levels of progesterone in serum. There is no decrease in the number of receptors for LH in ewes administered a luteolytic dose of $PGF_2\alpha$ until well after a dramatic decrease in serum levels of progesterone has occurred (185). Several effects of $PGF_2\alpha$ have also been demonstrated *in vitro.* There is a total block of LH-induced increases in the production of cyclic AMP and progesterone secretion (357). This observation is particularly interesting because most receptors for LH are on small steroidogenic cells, whereas receptors for $PGF_2\alpha$ are on large luteal cells (66). This suggests that there must be large cell–small cell communication in the corpus luteum. This concept is further substantiated by the observation that the number of large luteal cells and the levels of serum progesterone are reduced significantly within 12 hr of a luteolytic dose of $PGF_2\alpha$ but that the number of small cells does not decrease until 24 hr (361). Prostaglandin $F_2\alpha$ has been shown to be cytotoxic to large luteal cells *in vitro,* an effect that was reversed by coincubation in the presence of PGE_2 (360).

Recent data obtained in sheep demonstrated that $PGF_2\alpha$ acted through two distinct second-messenger systems (362). The hormonal and second-messenger pathways known to regulate secretion of progesterone and cellular degeneration in the two types of steoridogenic luteal cells are shown in Fig. 12. Prostaglandin $F_2\alpha$ activates PK-C in large luteal cells, which inhibits secretion of progesterone. However, activation of PK-C does not induce cytotoxic effects (362) or cause luteolysis (363). Treatment of large luteal cells with $PGF_2\alpha$ also results in a sustained increase in intracellular levels of free calcium (358), presumably through $PGF_2\alpha$-gated calcium channels. Increased intracellular Ca^{2+} appears to mediate the cytotoxic effects of $PGF_2\alpha$ probably by typical apoptotic changes (364). Interestingly, treatment of ewes with a luteolytic regime of $PGF_2\alpha$ also results in a rapid decrease in mRNA encoding 3β-HSD without an effect on levels of mRNA encoding cytochrome $P450_{scc}$ or tubulin (239). Thus, it appears that $PGF_2\alpha$ may have a specific

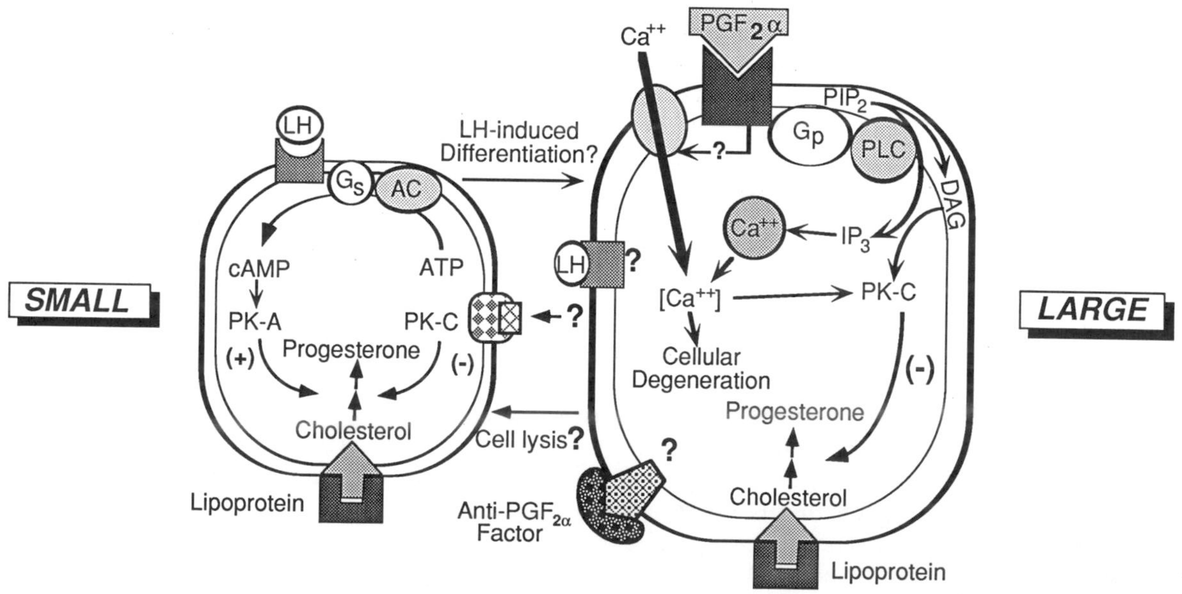

FIG. 12. Schematic diagram of some of hormonal and second-messenger systems that interact to regulate secretion of progesterone from small and large ovine luteal cells. LH binding to small luteal cells results in activation of protein kinase (*PK*)-A and stimulate (+) secretion of progesterone. Large luteal cells also contain receptors for LH, but binding of LH or increased intracellular levels of cyclic AMP does not stimulate progesterone secretion from large cells. $PGF_2\alpha$ activates PK-C system in large luteal cells, which inhibits (−) synthesis of progesterone. Activation of PK-C also inhibits LH-stimulated synthesis of progesterone from small luteal cells, but it is not clear what hormone activates this system. $PGF_2\alpha$ also stimulates Ca^{2+} influx, which appears to be responsible for degeneration of large luteal cells. Finally, conceptus may secrete a protein that prevents antisteroidogenic and cytotoxic effects of $PGF_2\alpha$ on large luteal cells.

effect on transcription of the gene for 3β-HSD or influence the rate of degradation of this mRNA. Although the cellular and molecular actions of $PGF_2\alpha$ in the sheep are becoming understood, this hormone may act differently in other species. For example, it has been suggested that activation of PK-C in bovine (365) and porcine (366) luteal tissue enhances secretion of progesterone. To determine whether these apparent differences are really fundamental differences in the actions of $PGF_2\alpha$ between species will require more research.

Morphologic Changes during Luteal Regression

During regression of the corpus luteum after pregnancy in rats, several distinct morphologic changes occur (24). The plasma membrane of cells from the regressing corpus luteum contain membrane specializations, including gap junctions, maculae adherents, coated invaginations, and microvilli similar to those of the corpus luteum of pregnancy. Many lipid droplets were found in the cytoplasm during early luteolysis, a time when luteal triglycerides have been shown to increase tenfold (24). There is a decrease in the quantity of smooth endoplasmic reticulum and an increase in the number of autophagic vacuoles and heterolysosomes. As regression progresses, many cells show an increased number of cytoplasmic vacuoles. Degenerating cells appear to be removed by macrophages (367).

Several morphologic changes appear to be common among several species during luteolysis. The increase in the number of lipid droplets and cytoplasmic vacuoles has also been observed in guinea pigs (367), rabbits (368), humans (369), and sheep (370). Other morphologic characteristics of degenerating cells also appear to be similar in several species. However, macrophages do not appear to be involved in removing the cell debris in regressing rabbit corpora lutea (368).

Degenerative changes in the ovine corpus luteum noted near the end of the estrous cycle and observed after treatment with $PGF_2\alpha$ have been studied extensively. The densely staining secretory granules observed during periods of maximal secretion of progesterone decrease in number throughout the period of luteal regression. Concurrent with the decrease in numbers of secretory granules is the appearance of autophagosomes (71). Autophagosomes appear to be sites of cytoplasmic involution, and their numbers increase as regression of the corpus luteum proceeds.

During regression of the corpus luteum, the percentage volume occupied by vascular elements decreases linearly during the last few days of the estrous cycle (130). Likewise, in sheep there is a rapid decrease in number of red blood cells and luminal volume of capillaries in the corpus luteum after treatment with $PGF_2\alpha$ (71). Swelling of endothelial cells appears to be responsible for the initial reduction in luminal volume. The decreased luminal volume most likely results in decreased perfusion of luteal tissue and probably causes blood to be shunted away from the corpus luteum (130,371,372).

As luteal regression continues, there is accumulation of lipid droplets in cells and steroidogenic cells decrease in size. Shrinkage of cells results in clumping of subcellular components, particularly mitochondria. Normally, there is little, if any, evidence of lipid accumulation in cells of the ovine corpus luteum; however, during regression there is a striking increase in intracellular lipid, with the lipid droplet becoming the most prominent organelle near the end of the estrous cycle.

Lysosomes are present in luteal cells throughout the estrous cycle; however, they appear to increase in number as regression of the corpus luteum progresses (77). During the midluteal phase of the cycle, acid phosphatase activity is restricted to lysosomes and inner cisternae of the Golgi apparatus. During regression, an increase in number of primary lysosomes appears to occur as a result of pinching off from the lateral margins of inner Golgi cisternae. As regression progresses, intracellular organelles become increasingly disorganized, and acid phosphatase activity is found with degenerating organelles. Cellular disorganization during luteal regression is not restricted to steroidogenic cells but involves essentially all cells comprising the corpus luteum.

LUTEAL FUNCTION DURING PREGNANCY

Maternal Recognition of Pregnancy

In most mammalian species, progesterone must be secreted throughout gestation to maintain a uterine environment conducive to pregnancy. In some species (e.g., carnivores and marsupials), gestation lasts no longer than a normal luteal phase. Therefore, there is no need for the conceptus to alter luteal function because the corpus luteum provides adequate progestational support. Most other mammalian species have developed a means of shortening the life span of the corpus luteum in event of a nonfertile cycle to increase reproductive efficiency. Along with development of a uterine luteolytic mechanism, some means of maintaining the uterus in a progestational state during pregnancy must also be developed if successful reproduction is to occur. The simplest solution would be for the conceptus itself to secrete progesterone and ensure its own survival. In many species, the placenta is a very active endocrine tissue, secreting several hormones, including progesterone. However, in most species, ability of the conceptus to secrete progesterone is not developed until after the corpus luteum of the estrous cycle would have normally regressed (e.g., sheep) (373). Thus, to maintain adequate progestational support for a developing pregnancy, it is necessary to prevent luteal regression. The process by which the conceptus acts to maintain luteal secretion of progesterone has been termed *maternal recognition of pregnancy.* The mechanism by which this process is accomplished differs from species to species, and a few representative examples will be considered in the following discussion.

Rat

The estrous cycle of the rat lasts only 4 to 5 days. The corpus luteum of the estrous cycle secretes progesterone for just 24 to 48 hr and never becomes fully functional (374,375). Sterile mating or cervical stimulation results in pseudopregnancy, and the corpus luteum continues to secrete progesterone for up to 12 days (269,275). Maintenance of the corpus luteum of gestation or pseudopregnancy appears to involve two separate endocrine effects. First, fertile mating (or cervical stimulation leading to pseudopregnancy) results in activation of a neural reflex arc, leading to a dramatic increase in serum concentrations of prolactin within 2 hr that persists as long as 48 hr (376). The increased serum levels of prolactin are dependent on stimulation of the pelvic nerve because bilateral resection of the pelvic nerve prevents the enhanced secretion of prolactin in mated rats. Freeman et al. (377) subsequently showed that cervical stimulation results in both diurnal and nocturnal surges of prolactin that last throughout pseudopregnancy. A similar phenomenon appears to exist during pregnancy because Butcher et al. (378) reported two surges of prolactin per day during early pregnancy. Thus, it seems clear that in rats, cervical stimulation on the morning of estrus leads to increased secretion of prolactin and enhanced concentrations of progesterone in serum. The increase in prolactin secretion appears to be responsible for prolongation of luteal function because daily injections of prolactin will maintain the corpus luteum in cycling rats (379) and because a single injection of ergocornine (an inhibitor of prolactin secretion) on days 6, 7, 8, or 9 terminates pseudopregnancy (380). The enhanced secretion of prolactin during pregnancy or pseudopregnancy is responsible for increasing the number of luteal receptors for LH and thus enhancing the steroidogenic responsiveness of this tissue to the hormone (41). These events appear sufficient to ensure that a proper endocrine environment is provided for implantation and normal development of the embryo during early pregnancy.

In the rat, gestation lasts about 22 days, and corpora lutea are required through day 17 to maintain pregnancy (381). The ovary is the primary source of progesterone throughout gestation, and replacement therapy with progesterone is all that is required to maintain pregnancy in ovariectomized rats (381). The process of maternal recognition of pregnancy in the rat involves prolonging the life span of the corpus luteum past normal pseudopregnancy.

The corpus luteum of early pregnancy is dependent on prolactin only through day 7 (382). Serum concentrations of progesterone during early pregnancy are very similar to those in pseudopregnancy; however, instead of decreasing on day 11, as in pseudopregnant rats, the concentration of progesterone in serum increases to about twice that seen in pseudopregnancy and is maintained at this higher level through day 20 (275). Corpora lutea of pseudopregnant rats are maintained after hysterectomy (241) or after induction of decidual tissue in the uterus (383,384); however, the concentration of progesterone in serum remains at the same lower level established early in pseudopregnancy in both of these situations (275).

A complete picture of uterine secretion of $PGF_2\alpha$ in pregnant and pseudopregnant rats is not available. Uterine content and uterine venous concentrations of $PGF_2\alpha$ are maximal on days 10 through 12 of pseudopregnancy (350,355), and this increase may initiate luteolysis. However, a similar increase in uterine venous concentrations of $PGF_2\alpha$ was observed on day 10 in pregnant rats (385). The ability of placental tissue from rats to synthesize $PGF_2\alpha$ is maximal on day 11 (386). Despite the increase in synthesis and secretion of $PGF_2\alpha$ from the uterus during pregnancy, the corpora lutea do not regress.

Maintenance of the corpus luteum during the second half of gestation in rats depends on the secretion of placental luteotropin (387,388). Luteotropic activity was first demonstrable by bioassay in serum on day 11 of pregnancy, reached peak levels on day 12, and had begun to decrease on day 13 (388). A substance with prolactinlike activity, rat placental lactogen (rPL) has been isolated and purified from placental tissue of rats (389,390). It is detectable in the serum of pregnant rats on days 8 through 15 (389,391). A similar lactogenic substance exists in decidual tissue of pseudopregnant rats (380). Placental tissue also secretes a substance with LH-like properties, a rat chorionic gonadotropin (rCG), whereas decidual tissue does not (392,393). These substances, secreted by the placenta and decidual endometrium, can account for all the endocrine changes associated with maternal recognition of pregnancy. The rPL, of placental or decidual origin, may provide adequate lactogenic support by day 8 such that prolactin is no longer necessary. Rat PL may also reduce the sensitivity of the corpus luteum to $PGF_2\alpha$. Behrman et al. (356) have shown that treatment of pseudopregnant rats with prolactin reduces the ability of exogenous $PGF_2\alpha$ to induce luteal regression. The rCG, secreted by the placenta, may be responsible for the increased secretion of progesterone observed during the second half of pregnancy. This substance is not present in hysterectomized or decidualized pseudopregnant rats, which maintain luteal function at a lower level than in pregnant rats.

Based on these observations, it appears that the conceptus alters luteal function in at least three ways: (a) It shortens the period over which the corpus luteum requires prolactin to maintain normal function; (b) it exerts a direct stimulatory effect on the corpus luteum not observed in hysterectomized pseudopregnant rats; and (c) it reduces the sensitivity of the corpus luteum to the luteolytic effect of $PGF_2\alpha$.

Rabbit

The rabbit is a reflex-ovulator; therefore, corpora lutea are found only after mating, cervical stimulation, or hormonal induction of ovulation. If the ovulatory stimulus is not a fertile mating, a pseudopregnancy results, and corpora lutea secrete progesterone for about 16 to 17 days (394). Follicular secretion of estrogens, stimulated by LH, is required to maintain normal luteal function throughout pseudopregnancy (395).

Chronic treatment of intact pseudopregnant rabbits with estradiol-17β stimulates luteal secretion of progesterone but has no effect on the life span of the corpus luteum (277,395). Hysterectomy has just the opposite effect. It lengthens the life span of the corpus luteum but only slows the reduction in luteal function, which begins about day 12. Luteal function is then maintained at a much lower level for several days (277,278,394). Maximal luteal function is maintained if hysterectomized, pseudopregnant rabbits are treated with estradiol-17β (277).

A significant increase in the concentration of $PGF_2\alpha$ in uterine tissue and uterine venous plasma occurs on day 17 of pseudopregnancy (278,351). Uterine production of $PGF_2\alpha$ may be stimulated by the decrease in concentrations of progesterone and/or increase in concentrations of estradiol-17β in serum that occurs during the last few days of pseudopregnancy (396). The increase in uterine secretion of $PGF_2\alpha$ is responsible for regression of the corpus luteum.

In the pregnant rabbit, corpora lutea continue to secrete progesterone for 31 days, the duration of gestation (396). Luteal progesterone is required throughout gestation to maintain pregnancy in the rabbit (397,398) because the placenta in this species does not produce progesterone (399).

Corpora lutea in the pregnant rabbit develop a dependence on some placental product around day 12. Removal of the conceptus before day 12 results in a temporal pattern in the concentration of progesterone very similar to that seen during pseudopregnancy (400,401). However, removal of the conceptus on day 12 or thereafter results in a very precipitous decline in the concentration of progesterone in serum. Removal of fetuses alone has very little effect (402,403). Unlike embryonic tissue from rats, the rabbit conceptus is devoid of LH-like activity throughout pregnancy (404,405).

The corpus luteum is dependent on follicular estrogens throughout pregnancy (406). Treatment of pregnant rabbits with very high doses of estradiol-17β after removal of the conceptus on day 18 results in maintenance of luteal function (403). However, physiologic doses of estradiol-17β are ineffective in maintaining the corpus luteum after hysterectomy on day 21 of pregnancy (406). These data imply that the presence of the embryo reduces the amount of estrogen required to maintain luteal function (i.e., it increases luteal sensitivity to estrogen).

There are dramatic changes in uterine secretion of PGs in pregnant rabbits (278,351). The increase in secretion of $PGF_2\alpha$ on day 17 of pseudopregnancy is absent in pregnancy, perhaps because secretion of progesterone is maintained at a very high level throughout pregnancy. Beginning on day 11 of pregnancy, there is an increase in uterine secretion of $PGF_2\alpha$, the amount secreted being proportional to the number of embryos in the uterus. The luteotropic properties of PGE_2 in rabbits have not been examined, but PGE_2 does stimulate luteal adenylate cyclase activity (407). The concentration of PGE_2 is extremely high in the fetal portion of the placenta (351), and rabbit blastocysts secrete PGE_2 during incubation *in vitro* (408). It is possible that PGE_2 is the placental factor that enhances luteal sensitivity to follicular estrogens.

Guinea Pig

As for all the remaining species to be discussed, the guinea pig is a spontaneous ovulator. It has recurrent estrous cycles about 16 days long. During the cycle, the concentration of progesterone in serum reaches a maximum on day 6 and is maintained at this level through day 11, after which levels fall as corpora lutea regress (409,410). As noted previously, uterine secretion of $PGF_2\alpha$ increases during the period of luteolysis (411,412).

Corpora lutea must continue to secrete progesterone through the first 30 days of gestation. Replacement therapy with progesterone will maintain pregnancy in ovariectomized guinea pigs (413,414). The placenta begins to synthesize some progesterone as early as day 15 and becomes the primary source from day 40 through the remainder of gestation (415).

Concentrations of progesterone in serum through the first 10 days of gestation are very similar to those observed during the estrous cycle; however, by day 20 the concentration of progesterone has increased nearly 100-fold (416), in part due to a reduction in the metabolic clearance rate for progesterone (417,418). The progesterone is primarily of luteal origin (415), and levels reached are much higher than in animals in which corpora lutea are maintained by hysterectomy or treatment with indomethacin (266). The corpora lutea also increase in size during this period (419,420). Thus, the conceptus appears to exert at least three effects: (a) It prevents luteal regression, (b) stimulates luteal growth and secretion of progesterone, and (c) reduces the metabolic clearance rate of progesterone.

The concentrations of $PGF_{2}\alpha$ in uterine venous plasma of pregnant guinea pigs on days 12 through 16 postestrus are lower than those in nonpregnant guinea pigs over the same period (421,422). Homogenates of uteri collected from pregnant guinea pigs on day 15 produced less $PGF_{2}\alpha$ *in vitro* than homogenates from nonpregnant guinea pigs (420). Thus, failure of the corpus luteum of early pregnancy to undergo luteal regression may be due to lack of synthesis and secretion of $PGF_{2}\alpha$ from the uterus.

An LH-like substance, a guinea pig CG, has been identified in placental tissue (423). The concentrations of the substance in placental tissue are maximal on day 18 postestrus, coinciding with the period of luteal growth and increased secretion of progesterone. Babra et al. (424) purified the substance and found it to be structurally similar and with comparable biological potency to hCG.

Domestic Ruminants

In the ewe, the corpus luteum must be present through the first 50 days of gestation to maintain pregnancy (425,426). Pregnancy can be maintained in ovariectomized ewes by treatment with progesterone (427,428). The placenta begins to secrete progesterone around day 50 of gestation (373) and provides adequate progestational support for the remainder of gestation. After removal of embryos on day 13 or thereafter, the life span of the corpus luteum is extended (429), indicating that the embryo has a luteotropic effect by this time. However, embryos can be successfully transferred to synchronized recipients as late as day 12 postestrus and the corpus luteum will be maintained (430). Thus, the critical period for maternal recognition of pregnancy in the ewe is days 12 to 13.

In ewes, homogenates of day 14 to 16 conceptuses maintain the corpus luteum when infused into the uterine lumen (431–433). The active component within the homogenate is heat labile and susceptible to proteolytic digestion. There is no LH- or prolactinlike bioactivity associated with these homogenates (432). Homogenates of 22-day-old embryos lack the ability to maintain the corpus luteum.

Concentrations of progesterone in serum of pregnant and nonpregnant ewes are similar through the first 14 days postestrus (434) and are maintained at this level through the first 50 days of gestation (435). Thus, it appears that the only effect of the conceptus is to prevent luteal regression. Investigations into the mechanism by which the conceptus maintains luteal function have centered around two possibilities. The first is that the conceptus suppresses uterine secretion of $PGF_{2}\alpha$. The second is that the conceptus reduces the sensitivity of the corpus luteum to the luteolytic effects of $PGF_{2}\alpha$. There is good evidence supporting both of these possibilities. With respect to the first possibility, concentrations of $PGF_{2}\alpha$ in uterine venous plasma of pregnant and nonpregnant ewes have been examined in many studies. It seems clear, from measurements of both $PGF_{2}\alpha$ and its major metabolite 13,14-dihydro-15-keto-$PGF_{2}\alpha$ (PGFM), that high-amplitude surges in secretion, which occur during and after luteolysis in nonpregnant ewes, are absent in pregnant ewes (436–439). However, basal levels of $PGF_{2}\alpha$ in uterine venous plasma collected at frequent intervals are higher in pregnant than in cycling ewes. Basal concentrations of PGFM in peripheral plasma are greater in pregnant animals, reaching a maximum value on day 14 or 15 (439,440). Before luteal regression, concentrations of $PGF_{2}\alpha$ in serum of pregnant ewes are similar to or greater than those in nonpregnant ewes (436,437,441–445).

Concentrations of $PGF_{2}\alpha$ in uterine tissue and uterine luminal flushings are greater in pregnant than in nonpregnant ewes (442,443,446,447). The ability of uterine tissue to secrete $PGF_{2}\alpha$ *in vitro* is also greater in pregnant ewes (443,448). Thus, the gravid uterus retains the ability to synthesize $PGF_{2}\alpha$; however, the pattern of secretion appears to be altered.

Although basal secretion of $PGF_{2}\alpha$ is higher on days 13 to 16 of pregnancy than during the estrous cycle, the main episodic peaks of $PGF_{2}\alpha$, which appear to be associated with luteolysis in cycling ewes, do not occur (449). Secretion of ovine trophoblast protein 1 from the day-13 to -17 sheep conceptus appears to be responsible for the lack of major peaks of $PGF_{2}\alpha$ in cycling ewes (450,451).

The ovine conceptus also secretes $PGF_{2}\alpha$ and PGE_{2} (452,453) but lacks the ability to form estrogens (454). Embryonic secretion of $PGF_{2}\alpha$ may account for the very high concentrations of $PGF_{2}\alpha$ in uterine flushings and for the increase in basal secretion of $PGF_{2}\alpha$ observed in early pregnancy.

Secretion of PGE_{2} by endometrial tissue *in vitro* is also greater in pregnant than in nonpregnant ewes (443,453,455,456). Therefore, both the uterus and conceptus may contribute to increased concentrations of PGE_{2} observed in pregnant ewes during the critical period for maternal recognition of pregnancy (443,445, 457). Infusion of PGE_{2} into the uterine lumen of nonpregnant ewes delays luteal regression (458,459) and suppresses the luteolytic action of exogenous estradiol-17β (460) and $PGF_{2}\alpha$ (461–463).

The luteotropic effect of the embryo is exerted locally (464). Anastomosis of the uterine vein draining the gravid horn to the opposite uterine vein results in luteal maintenance on the ovary, opposite the embryo (465). Similar cross-anastomosis of the ovarian arteries produces similar results, indicating that the embryonic sig-

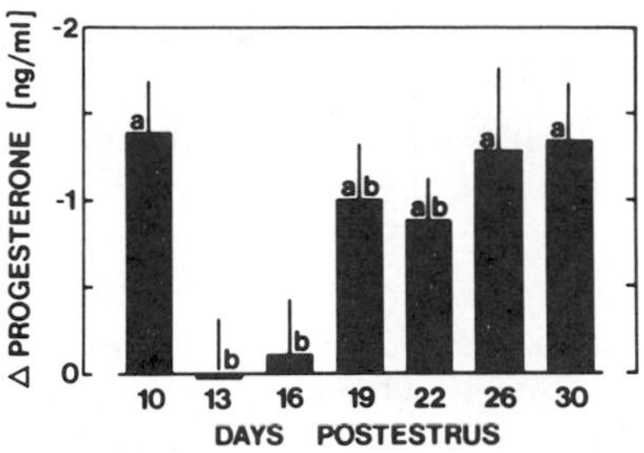

FIG. 13. Effect of treatment with $PGF_{2}\alpha$ (4 mg/58 kg body weight) on decrease in concentration of progesterone in serum (progesterone) of pregnant ewes treated on different days postbreeding. The corpus luteum was resistant to luteolytic effects of $PGF_{2}\alpha$ on days 13 and 16, as indicated by absence of decrease in serum levels of progesterone on these days. Groups with different superscripts are different ($P < .05$). (From ref. 468, with permission.)

nal is passed from the uterine vein to the ovarian artery (466). This does not seem to be compatible with transport of large molecular-weight proteins.

Sensitivity of the corpus luteum to luteolytic action of $PGF_{2}\alpha$ appears to be altered in early pregnancy. Intrafollicular or periarterial injections of $PGF_{2}\alpha$ were less effective in inducing luteal regression in pregnant than in nonpregnant ewes on day 12 or 13 (458,466,467). Also, the dose of $PGF_{2}\alpha$ required to induce continued luteolysis when given intramuscularly was less in cycling ewes than in pregnant ewes (468). Luteal resistance to $PGF_{2}\alpha$ was absent on day 10 after mating, was greatest from days 13 to 16, and was again absent by day 20 (Fig. 13). Thus, resistance to $PGF_{2}\alpha$ was transient and coincided with the time for maternal recognition of pregnancy. The factor responsible for this resistance to $PGF_{2}\alpha$ appeared to be of conceptal origin because corpora lutea from ewes with two embryos were more resistant to $PGF_{2}\alpha$ than corpora lutea from ewes with a single embryo. Wiltbank et al. (469) recently demonstrated that the day-15 sheep conceptus secretes a proteinaceous factor that is capable of preventing both the antisteroidogenic and the cytotoxic effects of $PGF_{2}\alpha$ (see Fig. 12). This factor does not bind $PGF_{2}\alpha$ or prevent it from binding to its luteal receptor. A similar factor is secreted from cow embryos. Because the molecular weight of this factor is approximately 30,000, it is hard to envision its being transported locally from the uterus to the ovary as the local embryonic luteotropic factor discussed above.

Based on these data, a model has been developed to describe how the conceptus might act to maintain the corpus luteum of early pregnancy (Fig. 14). In both pregnant and nonpregnant ewes, $PGF_{2}\alpha$ is secreted from the uterus beginning on days 12 to 13. In the nonpregnant ewe, luteolysis is initiated and secretion of progesterone declines. This allows increased follicular development

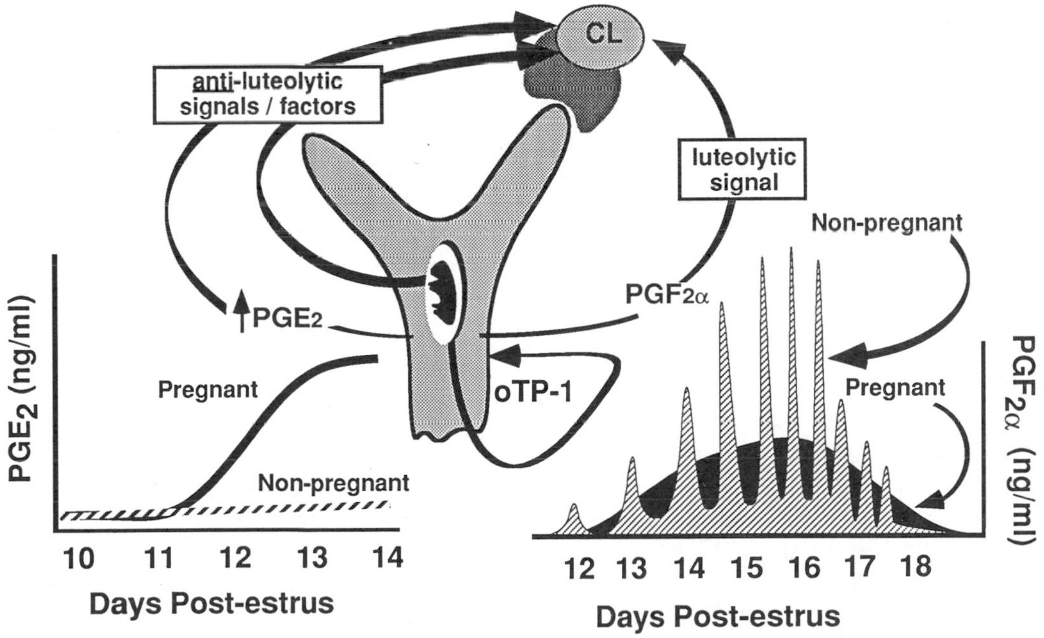

FIG. 14. Schematic representation of uterine and embryonic factors that interact to control life span and function of the ovine corpus luteum. Ovine trophoblastic protein-1 (oTP-1) secreted by the conceptus interacts with uterine endometrium to reduce secretion of luteolytic pulses of $PGF_{2}\alpha$ and change the pattern of $PGF_{2}\alpha$ secretion from that observed during the estrous cycle to that of early pregnancy as depicted in *lower right-hand corner.* Secretion of PGE_2 from pregnant uterus is increased during pregnancy (*lower left-hand corner*), which stimulates luteal progesterone secretion. The conceptus also secretes an anti-$PGF_{2}\alpha$ factor, which appears to block luteolytic actions of $PGF_{2}\alpha$ at large luteal cell level.

and, as a result, increased secretion of estradiol-17β. The combination of falling progesterone and increasing estradiol-17β results in the very high-amplitude surges of $PGF_2\alpha$ typically found during late luteolysis and the follicular phase. In the pregnant ewe, the conceptus secretes two proteins: ovine trophoblast protein-1, which reduces uterine secretion of $PGF_2\alpha$, and a proteinaceous factor, which prevents $PGF_2\alpha$ actions at the large luteal cell.

In the pregnant cow, the corpus luteum must be present for the first 200 days of gestation (470). Pregnancy can be maintained in ovariectomized cows by treatment with progesterone (471). The adrenal gland appears to secrete enough progesterone to maintain pregnancy after day 200 (472). The placental contribution to circulating concentrations of progesterone, even after day 200, appears to be negligible.

Embryos can be successfully transferred as late as day 16 postestrus (473), but the corpus luteum is maintained despite removal of embryos on day 17 or thereafter (474,475). Thus, the critical period for maternal recognition of pregnancy in the cow is days 16 to 17.

Some researchers have found that the concentrations of progesterone in serum are similar in pregnant and nonpregnant cows through days 17 to 18 postestrus (476,477). Others, using more frequent sampling protocols, have found significantly higher concentrations of progesterone in serum or milk of pregnant cows compared with both bred and nonbred nonpregnant animals as early as day 6 postestrus (478–481). Based on these reports, the existence of an embryonic luteotropin secreted by the bovine blastocyst has been proposed (482).

The concentration of $PGF_2\alpha$ in uterine venous plasma on day 18 postestrus is significantly lower in pregnant cows compared with nonpregnant cows (481). The high-amplitude surges of PGFM in peripheral plasma associated with luteolysis are absent in pregnant animals (483); however, basal concentrations increase during early pregnancy (484,485).

Homogenates of 17- or 18-day-old embryos have been infused into the uterine lumen, resulting in prolonged luteal function (474,475). Knickerbocker et al. (486) incubated 16- to 18-day-old conceptuses and infused the incubation medium (after dialysis) into the uterus to achieve similar results. Infusion of this mixture of large-molecular-weight, conceptus secretory products mimicked the suppressive effect of the embryo on secretion of $PGF_2\alpha$ from the uterus in response to treatment with estradiol-17β (487). The active factor(s) within this mixture appears to bovine trophoblast protein-1 analogous to oTP-1 in sheep.

Bovine conceptuses secrete $PGF_2\alpha$, PGE_2, progesterone, estradiol-17β, and 5-α-reduced steroids *in vitro* (454,488,489). Infusion of PGE_2 into the uterine lumen prolongs luteal life span for the duration of the infusion (475,490). Reynolds et al. (491) suggested that there may be some interaction between estradiol and PGE_2 in regulating luteal function in cows.

The conceptus prevents luteal regression through a local pathway similar to that used to transport the uterine luteolysin. If the uterine horns are surgically isolated from each other, only corpora lutea on the ovary adjacent to the gravid uterine horn are maintained (492). If the uterine vein draining the gravid uterine horn is anastomosed to the uterine vein draining the opposite horn, the corpus luteum on the ovary opposite the gravid horn is maintained (493). This type of preparation combines the uterine venous effluent from both the gravid and nongravid uterine horns. If the embryo acts primarily by reducing uterine secretion of $PGF_2\alpha$, maintenance of the corpus luteum must be due to a dilution of the $PGF_2\alpha$ coming from the nongravid horn. Alternatively, the gravid uterine horn may be actively secreting a substance that acts in a local fashion to reduce the luteolytic effectiveness of $PGF_2\alpha$. As with $PGF_2\alpha$, the physical properties and rapid metabolism of PGE_2 are compatible with the local nature of this effect. Thus, the ability of large-molecular-weight conceptus secretory products to prolong luteal function appears to be due to a direct inhibition of uterine secretion of $PGF_2\alpha$ but may also involve stimulation of uterine secretion of an antiluteolytic factor such as PGE_2. Prostaglandin E_2 stimulates secretion of progesterone by bovine luteal tissue *in vitro* (494,495). The biologic role, if any, of the embryonic protein that prevents the antisteroidogenic and cytotoxic effects of $PGF_2\alpha$ on large luteal cells remains to be elucidated.

Pigs

The corpus luteum of the sow must continue to secrete progesterone throughout gestation (115 days) to maintain pregnancy (496), and progesterone replacement therapy is sufficient to maintain pregnancy in ovariectomized sows (497). The increase in uterine secretion of $PGF_2\alpha$ associated with luteolysis in cycling pigs does not occur in pregnant pigs (353,498,499). Endometrial tissue from pregnant sows secretes less $PGF_2\alpha$ *in vitro* than similar tissue from nonpregnant sows (498,500). However, there is a very significant increase in the concentration of $PGF_2\alpha$ in flushings of the uterine lumen (501).

Treatment with estrogens, for as little as 5 days (days 11–15) will maintain normal luteal function in nonpregnant sows for up to 300 days (502–504). Uterine secretion of $PGF_2\alpha$, both *in vivo* and *in vitro,* is reduced by treatment of nonpregnant sows with estrogen *in vivo* (498,504,505). This treatment is also associated with an accumulation of $PGF_2\alpha$ in the uterine lumen (504,506). In these respects, treatment with estrogen mimics the effects of the conceptus.

The porcine conceptus synthesizes and secretes estrogens as early as day 12 (454,507,508). On the basis of these data, it has been proposed that the corpus luteum of early pregnancy in the pig is maintained by the secretion of estrogens from the conceptus. Besides the inhibitory effect that estrogens have on uterine synthesis of PGs, Bazer and Thatcher (509) proposed that estrogens alter the direction of secretion of $PGF_2\alpha$ so that $PGF_2\alpha$ moves into the uterine lumen rather than into the uterine vein. An essential role for embryonic synthesis of estrogens in the maintenance of corpora lutea of pregnancy remains to be demonstrated. No attempt has been made to prevent luteal maintenance by administering either inhibitors of estrogen synthesis or estrogen antagonists.

Besides estrogens, porcine embryos synthesize PGE_2 and $PGF_2\alpha$ (505,510), and concentrations of PGE_2 in the uterine lumen increase during early pregnancy (511). The role of PGE_2 in the process of maternal recognition of pregnancy in the sow has not been examined. Secretion of $PGF_2\alpha$ by the conceptus may contribute more to the accumulation of $PGF_2\alpha$ in the uterine lumen during early pregnancy than the proposed redirection of secretion of the limited amount of $PGF_2\alpha$ synthesized by the pregnant uterus.

Horse

The mechanism(s) responsible for maintenance of the primary corpus luteum during early pregnancy in the mare is not well understood. As in other species, $PGF_2\alpha$ appears to be responsible for regression of the corpus luteum at the end of the estrous cycle of the mare (329). On days 10 and 14 of pregnancy, the concentration of PGF in the uterine venous blood is lower than in nonpregnant mares (354).

There does not appear to be a redirecting of the secretion of $PGF_2\alpha$ into the uterine lumen. Further, there does not appear to be a reduction in the sensitivity of the corpus luteum to $PGF_2\alpha$ during early pregnancy. On the contrary, the ability of the corpus luteum to bind $PGF_2\alpha$ increases rather than decreases during early pregnancy (348).

The corpus luteum must continue to secrete progesterone through the first 50 to 70 days of gestation (512). During this period, pregnancy can be maintained in mares after ovariectomy by treatment with progesterone (512). The corpus luteum is maintained after removal of the embryo on day 16 or thereafter (513). The concentration of progesterone in serum of pregnant mares follows a temporal pattern similar to that of the nonpregnant mare through the first 12 days postestrus (276,514). From this point, the concentration of progesterone declines gradually, establishing a lower basal level between days 20 and 35 (515). About days 35 to 40, the concentration increases again, with maximal levels being achieved on day 100. This is in contrast to the pattern observed in hysterectomized mares (254,276). In that case, the gradual decline initiated on day 12 continues until luteal function is lost completely, sometime between days 100 and 200.

Certainly, the conceptus is involved in recognition of pregnancy and the subsequent maintenance of the primary corpus luteum. At least two different mechanisms seem to be involved. First, unfertilized ova are trapped in the oviduct of mares, where they degenerate over a period of months (516). In contrast, the fertilized ovum produces a substance that ensures its selective passage through the oviduct and into the uterus. Once in the uterus, the conceptus must come into contact with essentially the entire endometrial surface to prevent luteal regression. Because the equine conceptus does not elongate, but rather remains spherical until well into the second month of gestation, endometrial contact is achieved by migration of the conceptus throughout the uterus. In fact, the equine conceptus appears to traverse the entire uterus about every 2 hr during the critical period for recognition of pregnancy (517).

Interaction of conceptus with endometrium is speculated to prevent production and secretion of $PGF_2\alpha$ (517). The nature of the substance produced by the conceptus to inhibit production of $PGF_2\alpha$ has not been identified, but it is believed it may be estrogen. The equine conceptus is capable of synthesizing estradiol *in vitro* (518), and small quantities of estrogen induce a uterine tone characteristic of pseudopregnancy. Once the corpus luteum of pregnancy is established, secretion of progesterone gradually decreases until secretion of equine CG begins on about day 35 (515).

In the mare, increases in secretion of FSH occur at approximately 10-day intervals throughout early pregnancy (519), and this results in surges of follicular activity (520). Secretion of massive quantities of equine CG beginning around day 35 of gestation induces ovulation of these follicles and formation of secondary corpora lutea (521). Function of the primary corpus luteum is also stimulated by equine CG (522). Secondary corpora lutea appear similar to the primary corpus luteum in structure and function. They secrete progesterone until trophic support (equine CG) disappears from circulation at approximately day 150 of gestation, at which time they regress along with the primary corpus luteum. Progestational support for the remainder of pregnancy in the mare is provided by the feto-placental unit (523).

REFERENCES

1. Frankel L. Die function des corpus luteum. *Arch Gynaekol* 1903;68:438–443.
2. Allen WM, Corner GW. Physiology of the corpus luteum: production of special uterine reaction (progestational proliferation) by extracts of corpus luteum. *Am J Physiol* 1929;88:326–334.
3. Allen WM, Wintersteiner O. Crystalline progestin. *Science* 1934;80:190–191.

4. Muldoon TG. Regulation of steroid hormone receptor activity. *Endoc Rev* 1980;1:339–364.
5. Blandau RJ, Brackett B, Brenner RM, et al. The oviduct. In: Greep RO, Koblinsky MA, eds. *Frontiers in Reproduction and Fertility Control.* Cambridge, MA: MIT Press, 1977;132–145.
6. Brenner RM, Anderson RGW. Endocrine control of ciliogenesis in the primate oviduct. In: Greep, OR, Astwood EB, eds. *Handbook of Physiology.* Baltimore: Williams & Wilkins, 1973; 123–139.
7. Porter DG, Finn CA. The biology of the uterus. In: Greep RO, Koblinsky MA, eds. *Frontiers in Reproduction and Fertility Control.* Cambridge, MA: MIT Press, 1977;146–156.
8. Zarrow MX, Yochim JM, McCarthy JL. *Experimental Endocrinology.* New York: Academic Press, 1964.
9. Gier HT. Estrous cycle in the bitch; vaginal fluids. *Vet Scope* 1960;5:2–9.
10. Topper YJ, Freeman CS. Multiple hormone interactions in the developmental biology of the mammary gland. *Physiol Rev* 1980;60:1049–1106.
11. Baird DT, Scaramuzzi RJ. Changes in the secretion of ovarian steroids and pituitary luteinizing hormone in the periovulatory period in the ewe: the effect of progesterone. *J Endocrinol* 1976;70:237–245.
12. Karsch FJ, Foster DL, Legan SJ, Ryan KD, Peter GK. Control of the preovulatory endocrine events in the ewe: interrelationship of estradiol, progesterone and luteinizing hormone. *Endocrinology* 1979;105:421–426.
13. Knobil E. The neuroendocrine control of the menstrual cycle. *Recent Prog Horm Res* 1980;36:53–88.
14. Rahe CH, Owens RE, Fleeger JL, Newton HJ, Harms PG. Patterns of plasma luteinizing hormone in the cyclic cow: dependence upon period of the cycle. *Endocrinology* 1980;107: 498–503.
15. Midgley AR Jr, Jaffe RB. Regulation of human gonadotropins: IV. Correlation of serum follicle-stimulating hormone and luteinizing hormone during the menstrual cycle. *J Clin Endocrinol Metab* 1968;28:1699–1703.
16. Weiss G. Human relaxin: source and stimulus. In: Neill JD, Bryant-Greenwood GD, eds. *Relaxin.* New York: Elsevier North-Holland, 1981;167–168.
17. Sherwood OD, O'Byrne EM. Purification and characterization of porcine relaxin. *Arch Biochem Biophys* 1974;160:185–196.
18. Goldsmith LT, Grob HS, Scherer K, Surve A, Steinmetz GB, Weiss G. Placental control of ovarian immunoreactive relaxin secretion in the pregnant rat. *Endocrinology* 1981;109:548–552.
19. Wathes DC, Swann RW. Is oxytocin an ovarian hormone? *Nature* 1982;297:225–227.
20. Sawyer HR, Moeller CL, Kozlowski GP. Immunocytochemical localization of neurophysin and oxytocin in ovine corpora lutea. *Biol Reprod* 1986;34:543–548.
21. Flint APF, Sheldrick EL. Ovarian peptides and luteolysis. In: Edwards RG, Purdy JM, Steptoe PC, eds. *Implantation of the Human Embryo.* London: Academic Press, 1985;235–242.
22. Balmaceda J, Asch RM, Fernandez ED, Valenzuela G, Eddy CA, Pauerstein CJ. Prostaglandin production by rhesus monkey corpora lutea *in vitro. Fertil Steril* 1979;31:214–216.
23. Shutt DA, Shearman RP, Lyneham RC, Clark AH, McMahon AH, Goh P. Radioimmunoassay of progesterone, 17-hydroxy-progesterone, estradiol-17β and prostaglandin F in human corpus luteum. *Steroids* 1975;26:299–310.
24. Anderson E, Little B. The ontogeny of the rat granulosa cell. In: Toft DO, Ryan RJ, eds. *Proceedings of the Fifth Ovarian Workshop.* Champaign, IL: Ovarian Workshops, 1985;203–225.
25. Azamia R, Dahl G, Lowenstein WR. Cell junction and cyclic AMP: III. Promotion of junctional membrane permeability and junction membrane particles in a junction-deficient cell type. *J Membr Biol* 1981;63:133–146.
26. Amsterdam A, Tsafriri A. *In vitro* binding of ^{125}I-human chorionic gonadotropin (hCG) in the preovulatory follicle: absence of receptor sites on oocyte. *J Cell Biol* 1979;83:255.
27. Anderson W, Kang Y, Perotti ME, Bramley TA, Ryan RJ. Interactions of gonadotropins with corpus luteum membranes. III. Electron microscopic localization of [^{125}I]-hCG binding to sensitive and desensitized ovaries seven days after PMSG-hCG. *Biol Reprod* 1979;20:362–376.
28. Albertini D, Anderson E. Structural modifications of lutein cell gap junctions during pregnancy in the rat and the mouse. *Anat Rec* 1975;181:171–194.
29. McClellan MC, Diekman MA, Abel JH Jr, Niswender GD. Luteinizing hormone, progesterone and the morphological development of normal and superovulated corpora lutea in sheep. *Cell Tissue Res* 1975;164:291–307.
30. Hay MF, Moor RM. Distribution of Δ^5-3β-hydroxysteroid dehydrogenase activity in the Graafian follicle of the sheep. *J Reprod Fertil* 1975;43:313–322.
31. O'Shea JD, Cran DG, Hay MF. Fate of the theca interna following ovulation in the ewe. *Cell Tissue Res* 1980;210:305–319.
32. Donaldson L, Hansel W. Histological study of bovine corpora lutea. *J Dairy Sci* 1965;48:905–909.
33. O'Shea JD, Cran DG, Hay MF. The small luteal cell of the sheep. *J Anat* 1979;128:239–251.
34. Channing C, Kammerman S. Binding of gonadotropins to ovarian cells. *Biol Reprod* 1974;10:179–198.
35. Richards JS. Hormone regulation of hormone receptors in ovarian follicular development. In: Midgley AR, Sadler WA, eds. *Ovarian Follicular Development.* New York: Raven Press, 1979;225–242.
36. Zeleznik AJ, Midgley AR Jr, Reichert LE Jr. Granulosa cell maturation in the rat: increased binding of human chorionic gonadotropin following treatment with follicle-stimulating hormone *in vivo. Endocrinology* 1974;95:818–825.
37. Kammerman S, Ross J. Increase in numbers of gonadotropin receptors on granulosa cells during follicle maturation. *J Clin Endocrinol Metab* 1975;41:546–550.
38. Lee CY. The porcine ovarian follicle: III. Development of chorionic gonadotropin receptors associated with increase in adenyl cyclase activity during follicle maturation. *Endocrinology* 1976;99:42–48.
39. Richards JS, Ireland JJ, Rao MC, Bernath GA, Midgley AR Jr, Reichert LE Jr. Ovarian follicular development in the rat: hormone receptor regulation by estradiol. follicle stimulating hormone and luteinizing hormone. *Endocrinology* 1976;99: 1562–1570.
40. Chang SSC, Anderson W, Lewis JC, Ryan RJ, Kang YH. The porcine ovarian follicle. II. Electron microscopic study of surface features of granulosa cells at different stages of development. *Biol Reprod* 1977;16:349–357.
41. Richards JS, Williams JL. Luteal cell receptor content for prolactin (PRL) and luteinizing hormone (LH). Regulation by LH and PRL. *Endocrinology* 1976;99:1571–1581.
42. Nimrod A, Bedrak E, Lamprecht SA. Appearance of LH-receptors and LH-stimulable cyclic AMP accumulation in granulosa cells during follicular maturation in the rat ovary. *Biochem Biophys Res Commun* 1977;78:977–984.
43. Richards JS, Jonassen JA, Rolfes AI, Kersey K, Reichert LE Jr. Adenosine 3',5'-monophosphate, luteinizing hormone receptor, and progesterone during granulosa cell differentiation: effects of estradiol and follicle-stimulating hormone. *Endocrinology* 1979; 104:765–773.
44. Segaloff DL, Wang H, Richards JS. Hormonal regulation of luteinizing hormone/chorionic gonadotropin receptor mRNA in rat ovarian cells during follicular development and luteinization. *Mol Endocrinol* 1990;4:1856–1865.
45. Carson RS, Findlay JK, Burger HG. Receptors for gonadotrophins in the ovine follicle during growth and atresia. In: Channing CP, Marsh J, Sadler WA, eds. *Advances in Experimental Medicine and Biology,* Vol. 112: *Ovarian Follicular and Corpus Luteum Function.* New York: Plenum, 1979;89–94.
46. Hansel W, Concannon PW, Lukaszewska JH. Corpora lutea of the large domestic animals. *Biol Reprod* 1973;8:222–245.
47. Hoffman B, Schams D, Bopp R, Ender ML, Giminez T, Karg H. Luteotrophic factors in the cow: evidence for LH rather than prolactin. *J Reprod Fertil* 1974;40:77–85.
48. Karsch FJ, Cook B, Ellicott AR, Foster DL, Jackson GL, Nalbandov AV. Failure of infused prolactin to prolong the lifespan of the corpus luteum of the ewe. *Endocrinology* 1971;89:272–275.
49. Niswender GD. Influence of 2-Br-α-ergocryptine on the serum levels of prolactin and the estrous cycle in sheep. *Endocrinology* 1974;94:612–615.
50. Rolland R, Hammond JM, Schellekens LA, Lequin RM, deJong

FH. Prolactin and ovarian function. In: James VHT, Serio M, Giusti G, eds. *Endocrine Function of the Human Ovary.* New York: Academic Press, 1976;305–321.
51. Murphy BD, Rajkuman K. Prolactin as a luteotropin. *Can J Physiol Pharmacol* 1985;63:257–264.
52. Loeb L. The formation of the corpus luteum of the guinea pig. *J Vet Med Assoc* 1906;46:416–423.
53. Corner GW. On the origin of the corpus luteum of the sow from both granulosa and theca interna. *Am J Anat* 1919;26:117–183.
54. McNutt GW. The corpus luteum of the ox ovary in relation to the estrous cycle. *J Am Vet Med Assoc* 1924;65:556–597.
55. Lobel BL, Levy E. Enzymatic correlates of development, secretory function and regression of follicles and corpora lutea in the bovine ovary. *Acta Endocrinol Suppl* 1968;132:7–63.
56. Priedkalns J, Weber AF, Zemjanis R. Qualitative and quantitative morphological studies of the cells of the membrane granulosa, theca interna and corpus luteum of the bovine ovary. *Z Zellforsch* 1968;85:501–520.
57. Pederson ES. Histogenesis of lutein tissue of the albino rat. *Am J Anat* 1951;88:397–416.
58. Guraya S. Morphology, histochemistry and biochemistry of human ovarian compartments and steroid hormone synthesis. *Physiol Rev* 1971;51:785–897.
59. Warbritton V. The cytology of the corpora lutea of the ewe. *J Morphol* 1934;56:186–202.
60. Mossman HW, Duke KL. Some comparative aspects of the mammalian ovary. In: *Handbook of Physiology,* Sect. 7, Vol. 2, Pt. 1. Bethesda, MD: American Physiological Society, 1973; 389–402.
61. Niswender GD, Schwall RH, Fitz TA, Farin CE, Sawyer HR. Regulation of luteal function in domestic ruminants: new concepts. *Recent Prog Horm Res* 1985;41:101–142.
62. Deane HW, Hay MF, Moor RM, Rowson LEA, Short RV. The corpus luteum of the sheep: relationships between morphology and function during the oestrous cycle. *Acta Endocrinol* 1966;51:245–263.
63. Lemon M, Loir M. Steroid release *in vitro* by two luteal cell types in the corpus luteum of the pregnant sow. *J Endocrinol* 1977;72:351–359.
64. Ursely J, Leymarie P. Varying response to luteinizing hormone of two luteal cell types isolated from bovine corpus luteum. *Endocrinology* 1979;83:303–310.
65. Koos RD, Hansel W. The large and small cells of the bovine corpus luteum: ultrastructural and functional differences. In: Schwartz NB, Hunzicker-Dunn M, eds. *Dynamics of Ovarian Function.* New York: Raven Press, 1981;197–203.
66. Fitz TA, Mayan MH, Sawyer HR, Niswender GD. Characterization of two steroidogenic cell types in the ovine corpus luteum. *Biol Reprod* 1982;27:703–711.
67. Sinha AA, Seal JS, Doe RP. Ultrastructure of the corpus luteum of the white-tailed deer during pregnancy. *Am J Anat* 1971;132:189–206.
68. Foley RC, Greenstein JS. Cytological changes in the bovine corpus luteum during early pregnancy. In: Gassner FX, ed. *Reproduction and Infertility.* New York: Pergamon, 1958;88–96.
69. Wilkinson RF, Anderson E, Aalberg J. Cytological observations of dissociated rat corpus luteum. *J Ultrastruct Res* 1976;57: 168–184.
70. Enders AC. Cytology of the corpus luteum. *Biol Reprod* 1973;8:158–182.
71. Nett TM, McClellan MC, Niswender GD. Effects of prostaglandins on the ovine corpus luteum: blood flow, secretion of progesterone and morphology. *Biol Reprod* 1976;15:66–78.
72. Rodgers RJ, O'Shea JD, Bruce NW. Morphometric analysis of the cellular composition of the ovine corpus luteum. *J Anat* 1984;138:757–769.
73. Christensen AK, Gillim SW. The correlation of fine structure and function in steroid-secreting cells, with emphasis on those in the gonads. In: McKerns KW, ed. *The Gonads.* New York: Appleton-Century-Crofts, 1969;415–488.
74. Fawcett DT, Long JA, Jones AL. The ultrastructure of endocrine glands. *Recent Prog Horm Res* 1969;25:15–380.
75. Paavola LG, Christensen AK. Characterization of granule types in luteal cells of sheep at the time of maximum progesterone secretion. *Biol Reprod* 1981;25:203–215.
76. Gemmell RT, Stacy BD, Thorburn GD. Ultrastructural study of secretory granules in the corpus luteum of sheep during the estrous cycle. *Biol Reprod* 1974;16:499–512.
77. McClellan MC, Abel JH Jr, Niswender GD. Functions of lysosomes during luteal regression in normally cycling and $PGF_2\alpha$-treated ewes. *Biol Reprod* 1977;16:499–512.
78. Corteel M. Etude histologique de la transformation du follicle preovulatoire en corps jaune cyclique chez la brebis. *Annu Biol Anim Biochim Biophys Suppl* 1973;13:249–258.
79. Gemmell RT, Stacy BD. Granule secretion by the luteal cell of the sheep: the fate of the granule membrane. *Cell Tissue Res* 1979;197:413–419.
80. Sawyer HR, Abel JH Jr, McClellan MC, Schmitz M, Niswender GD. Secretory granules and progesterone secretion by ovine corpora lutea *in vitro. Endocrinology* 1979;104:476–486.
81. Wathes DC, Swann RW, Birkett SD, Porter DG, Pickering BT. Characterization of oxytocin, vasopressin and neurophysin from the bovine corpus luteum. *Endocrinology* 1983;113:693–698.
82. Rodgers RJ, O'Shea JD, Findlay JK, Flint APF, Sheldrick EL. Large luteal cells the source of oxytocin in sheep. *Endocrinology* 1983;113:2302–2304.
83. Anderson ML, Long JA. Localization of relaxin in the pregnant rat. Bioassay of tissue extracts and cell fractionation studies. *Biol Reprod* 1978;18:110–117.
84. Anderson MB, Sherwood OD. Ultrastructural localization of relaxin immunoreactivity in corpora lutea of pregnant rats. *Endocrinology* 1984;114:1124–1127.
85. Belt WD, Anderson LL, Cavazos LA, Mclampy RM. Cytoplasmic granules and relaxin levels in porcine corpora lutea. *Endocrinology* 1971;89:1–10.
86. Kendall JZ, Plopper CG, Bryant-Greenwood GD. Ultrastructural immunoperoxidase demonstration of relaxin in corpora lutea from a pregnant sow. *Biol Reprod* 1978;18:94–98.
87. Fields PA. Ultrastructural localization of relaxin in corpora lutea of pregnant, pseudopregnant and cycling gilts using porcine relaxin antiserum and goat anti-rabbit IgG-colloidal gold. *Biol Reprod* 1984;30(suppl 1):116A(abst).
88. Fields MJ, Fields PA, Castro-Hernandez A, Larkin LH. Evidence for relaxin in corpora lutea of late pregnant cows. *Endocrinology* 1980;107:869–876.
89. Knickerbocker JJ, Wiltbank MC, Niswender GD. Mechanisms of luteolysis in domestic livestock. *Dom Anim Endocrin* 1988;5:91–107.
90. Rothchild I. The regulation of the mammalian corpus luteum. *Recent Prog Horm Res* 1981;37:183–283.
91. Rothchild I. Interrelations between progesterone and the ovary, pituitary, and central nervous system in the control of ovulation and the regulation of progesterone secretion. *Vitam Horm* 1965;23:209–327.
92. Hunzicker-Dunn M, Birnbaumer L. Adenylyl cyclase activities in ovarian tissues. IV. Gonadotropin-induced desensitization of the luteal adenylyl cyclase throughout pregnancy and pseudopregnancy in the rabbit and the rat. *Endocrinology* 1976; 99:211–222.
93. Greenwald GS. Further observations on the luteotropic complex of the hamster. *Arch Anat* 1967;56:281–291.
94. Hilliard J. Corpus luteum function in guinea pigs, hamsters, rats, mice and rabbits. *Biol Reprod* 1973;8:203–211.
95. Keyes PL, Gadsby JE, Yuh K-C M, Bill CH II. The corpus luteum. In: Greep RO, ed. *International Review of Physiology. Reproductive Physiology,* Vol. 4. Baltimore, MD: University Park Press, 1983;57–97.
96. Damle S, LaBarbera AR, Hunzicker-Dunn M. Progesterone production by rabbit corpora lutea *in vitro:* regulation by LH and epinephrine. *Biol Reprod* 1984;30(suppl 1):115(abst).
97. Yuh K-CM, Bill C II, Keyes PL. Transient development and function of rabbit corpora lutea after hypophysectomy. *Am J Physiol* 1984;247:E808–814.
98. Hoyer PB, Keyes PL, Niswender GD. Size distribution and hormonal responsiveness of dispersed rabbit luteal cells during pseudopregnancy. *Biol Reprod* 1986;34:905–910.
99. Denamur R, Mauleon P. Effets de l'hypophysectomie sur la morphologie et l'histologie du corps jaune des ovins. *C R Acad Sci* 1963;257:264–267.
100. Kaltenbach CC, Graber JW, Niswender GD, Nalbandov AV. Ef-

fect of hypophysectomy on the formation and maintenance of corpora lutea in the ewe. *Endocrinology* 1968;82:753–759.
101. Denamur R, Martinet J, Short RV. Pituitary control of the ovine corpus luteum. *J Reprod Fertil* 1973;32:207–220.
102. Kaltenbach CC, Graber JW, Niswender GD, Nalbandov AV. Luteotrophic properties of some pituitary hormones in nonpregnant or pregnant hypophysectomized ewes. *Endocrinology* 1968;82: 818–824.
103. Farin CE, Nett TM, Niswender GD. Effects of luteinizing hormone on luteal cell populations in hypophysectomized ewes. *J Reprod Fertil* 1990;88:61–70.
104. Karsch FJ, Roche JF, Noveroske JW, Foster DL, Norton HW, Nalbandov AV. Prolonged maintenance of the corpus luteum of the ewe by continuous infusion of luteinizing hormone. *Biol Reprod* 1971;4:129–136.
105. Domanski E, Skrezczkowski L, Stupnicka E, Fitko R, Dobrowlski W. Effect of gonadotropins on the secretion of progesterone and oestrogens by the sheep ovary perfused *in situ. J Reprod Fertil* 1967;14:365–372.
106. Kaltenbach CC, Cook B, Niswender GD, Nalbandov AV. Effect of pituitary hormones on progesterone synthesis by ovine luteal tissue *in vitro. Endocrinology* 1967;81:1407–1409.
107. Simmons KR, Caffrey JL, Phillips JL, Abel JH Jr, Niswender GD. A simple method for preparing suspensions of luteal cells. *Proc Soc Exp Biol Med* 1976;152:366–371.
108. Fuller GB, Hansel W. Regression of sheep corpora lutea after treatment with antibovine luteinizing hormone. *J Anim Sci* 1970;31:99–103.
109. McCracken JA, Baird DT, Goding JR. Factors affecting the secretion of steroids from the transplanted ovary of the sheep. *Recent Prog Horm Res* 1971;27:537–582.
110. Jammes H, Schirar A, Djiane J. Differential patterns in luteal prolactin and LH receptors during pregnancy in sows and ewes. *J Reprod Fertil* 1985;73:27–35.
111. du Mesnil du Buisson F, Leglise PG. Effet de l'hypophysectomie sur les corps jaunes de la truie. Resultats preliminaires. *C R Acad Sci* 1963;257:261–263.
112. Duncan GW, Bowerman AM, Anderson LL, Hearn WR, Melampy RM. Factors influencing *in vitro* synthesis of progesterone. *Endocrinology* 1961;68:199–207.
113. Cook B, Kaltenbach CC, Norton HW, Nalbandov AV. Synthesis of progesterone *in vitro* by porcine corpora lutea. *Endocrinology* 1967;81:573–584.
114. Ginther OJ. *Reproductive Biology of the Mare. Basic and Applied Aspects.* Ann Arbor, MI: McNaughton and Gunn, 1979.
115. Nett TM, Pickett BW, Seidel GE Jr, Voss JL. Levels of luteinizing hormone and progesterone during the estrous cycle and early pregnancy in mares. *Biol Reprod* 1976;14:412–415.
116. Harrison RJ. The early development of the corpus luteum in the mare. *J Anat* 1946;80:160–166.
117. Van Niekerk CH, Morgenthal JC, Gerneke WH. Relationship between the morphology of and progesterone production by the corpus luteum of the mare. *J Reprod Fertil Suppl* 1975;23: 171–175.
118. Pineda MH, Ginther OJ, McShan WH. Regression of corpus luteum in mares treated with an antiserum against an equine pituitary fraction. *Am J Vet Res* 1972;33:1767–1773.
119. Roser JF, Evans JW. Luteal luteinizing hormone receptors during the postovulatory period in the mare. *Biol Reprod* 1983;29:499–510.
120. Concannon PW, Hansel W, McEntee K. Changes in LH, progesterone and sexual behavior associated with preovulatory luteinization in the bitch. *Biol Reprod* 1977;17:604–613.
121. Wildt DE, Panko WB, Chakraborty P, Seager SW. Relationship of serum estrone, estradiol-17β and progesterone to LH, sexual behavior and time of ovulation in the bitch. *Biol Reprod* 1979;20:648–658.
122. Nett TM, Akbar AM, Phemister RD, Holst PA, Reichert LE Jr, Niswender GD. Levels of luteinizing hormone estradiol and progesterone in serum during the estrous cycle and pregnancy in the beagle bitch. *Proc Soc Exp Biol Med* 1975;148:134–139.
123. Reimers TJ, Phemister RD, Niswender GD. Radioimmunological measurement of follicle-stimulating hormone and prolactin in the dog. *Biol Reprod* 1978;19:673–679.
124. Olson PN, Bowen RA, Behrendt MD, Olson JD, Nett TM. Concentrations of progesterone and luteinizing hormone in the serum of diestrous bitches before and after hysterectomy. *Am J Vet Res* 1984;45:149–153.
125. Smith MS, McDonald LE. Serum levels of luteinizing hormone and progesterone during the estrous cycle, pseudopregnancy and pregnancy in the dog. *Endocrinology* 1974;94:404–412.
126. Concannon PW, Hansel W, Visek WV. The ovarian cycle of the bitch: plasma estrogen, LH and progesterone. *Biol Reprod* 1975;13:112–121.
127. Concannon PW. Effects of hypophysectomy and of LH administration on luteal phase plasma progesterone levels in the beagle bitch. *J Reprod Fertil* 1980;58:407–410.
128. Concannon PW. Reproductive physiology and endocrine patterns of the bitch. In: Kirk RW, ed. *Current Veterinary Therapy VIII Small Animal Practice* Philadelphia: WB Saunders, 1983;886–901.
129. Schomberg DW, Coudert SP, Short RV. Effects of bovine luteinizing hormone and human chorionic gonadotrophin on the bovine corpus luteum *in vivo. J Reprod Fertil* 1967;14:277–285.
130. Niswender GD, Reimers TJ, Diekman MA, Nett TM. Blood flow: a mediator of ovarian function. *Biol Reprod* 1976;14: 64–81.
131. Armstrong DT, Black DL. Influence of luteinizing hormone on corpus luteum metabolism and progesterone biosynthesis throughout the bovine estrous cycle. *Endocrinology* 1966;78: 937–944.
132. Williams MT, Marsh JM. Estradiol inhibition of luteinizing hormone-stimulated progesterone synthesis in isolated bovine luteal cells. *Endocrinology* 1978;103:1611–1618.
133. Wiltbank MC, Diskin MG, Flores JA, Niswender GD. Regulation of the corpus luteum by protein kinase C. II. Inhibition of lipoprotein-stimulated steroidogenesis by prostaglandin $F_2\alpha$. *Biol Reprod* 1990;42:239–245.
134. Pate JL, Nephew KP. Effects of *in vivo* and *in vitro* administration of prostaglandin $F_2\alpha$ on lipoprotein utilization in cultured bovine luteal cells. *Biol Reprod* 1988;38:568–576.
135. Lee CY, Ryan RJ. The uptake of human luteinizing hormone (hLH) by slices of luteinized rat ovaries. *Endocrinology* 1971;89:1515–1523.
136. Papaionannou S, Gospodarowicz D. Comparison of the binding of human chorionic gonadotropin to isolated bovine luteal cells and bovine luteal plasma membranes. *Endocrinology* 1975;97: 114–124.
137. Conti M, Harwood JP, Dufau ML, Catt KJ. Effect of gonadotropin-induced receptor regulation on biological responses of isolated rat luteal cells. *J Biol Chem* 1976;252:8867–8874.
138. Conn PM, Conti M, Harwood JP, Dufau ML, Catt KJ. Internalisation of gonadotrophin-receptor complex in ovarian luteal slices. *Nature* 1978;274:598–600.
139. DeKrester DM, Catt KJ, Paulsen CA. Studies on the *in vitro* testicular binding of iodinated luteinizing hormone in rats. *Endocrinology* 1971;88:332–337.
140. Catt KJ, Dufau ML, Tsuruhara T. Studies of a radioligand-receptor assay system for luteinizing hormone and chorionic gonadotropin. *J Clin Endocrinol Metab* 1971;32:860–863.
141. Lee CY, Ryan RJ. Luteinizing hormone receptors. Specific binding of human luteinizing hormone to homogenates of luteinized rat ovaries. *Proc Natl Acad Sci USA* 1972;69:3520–3523.
142. Lee CY, Ryan RJ. Interaction of ovarian receptors with human luteinizing hormone and human chorionic gonadotropin. *Biochemistry* 1973;12:4609–4620.
143. Gospodarowicz D. Properties of the luteinizing hormone receptor of the isolated bovine corpus luteum plasma membrane. *J Biol Chem* 1973;248:5042–5049.
144. Bramley TA, Ryan RJ. Interactions of gonadotropins with corpus luteum membranes. I. Properties and distributions of some marker enzyme activities after subcellular fractionation of the superovulated rat ovary. *Endocrinology* 1978;103:778–795.
145. Bramley TA, Ryan RJ. Interactions of gonadotropins with corpus luteum membranes. II. The identification of two distinct surface membrane fractions from superovulated rat ovaries. *Endocrinology* 1978;103:796–804.
146. McFarland KC, Sprengel R, Phillips HS, et al. Lutropin-choriogonadotropin receptor: an unusual member of the G protein-coupled receptor family. *Science* 1989;245:494–499.
147. Loosfelt H, Misrahi M, Atger M, et al. Cloning and sequencing of

porcine LH-hCG receptor cDNA: variants lacking transmembrane domain. *Science* 1989;245:525–528.
148. Minigishi T, Nakamura K, Takakura Y, et al. Cloning and sequencing of human LH/hCG receptor cDNA. *Biochem Biophys Res Commun* 1990;172:1049–1054.
149. Jia X-C, Okawa M, Bo M, et al. Expression of human luteinizing hormone (LH) receptor: interaction with LH and chorionic gonadotropin from human but not equine, rat and bovine species. *Mol Endocrinol* 1991;5:759–768.
150. Ji I, Ji TH. Exons 1-10 of the rat LH receptor encode a high affinity hormone binding site and exon 11 encodes G-protein molecular and a potential second hormone binding site. *Endocrinology* 1991;128:2648–2650.
151. Ji TH, Koo YB, Ji I. The structure and regulation of the LH receptor gene and its transcripts. In: *Proc IX Ovarian Workshop, Ovarian Cell Interactions: Genes to Physiology.* Serono Symposium (in press).
152. Hu Z-Z, Tsai-Morris C-H, Buczko E, Dufau MI. Hormonal regulation of LH receptor mRNA and expression in the rat ovary. *FEBS Lett* 1990;274:181–184.
153. Hoffman YM, Peegel H, Sprock MJE, Zhang Q-Y, Menon KMJ. Evidence that human chorionic gonadotropin/luteinizing hormone receptor down-regulation involves decreased levels of receptor messenger ribonucleic acid. *Endocrinology* 1991;128: 388–393.
154. Koo YB, Ji H, Slaughter RG, Ji TH. Structure of the luteinizing hormone receptor gene and multiple exons of the coding sequence. *Endocrinology* 1991;128:2297–2308.
155. Luborsky JL, Slater WR, Behrman HR. Luteinizing hormone (LH) receptor aggregation: modification of ferritin-LH binding and aggregation by prostaglandin $F_2\alpha$, and ferritin-LH. *Endocrinology* 1984,115.2217–2226.
156. Hsueh AJ, Dufau ML, Katz SJ, Catt KJ. Immunofluorescence labeling of gonadotropin receptors in enzyme-dispersed interstitial cells. *Nature* 1976;261:710–711.
157. Dufau ML, Catt KJ. Gonadotropin receptors and regulation of steroidogenesis in the testis and ovary. *Vitam Horm* 1978;36: 462–592.
158. Dufau ML, Catt KJ, Tsuruhara T. Gonadotropin stimulation of testosterone production by the rat testis *in vitro. Biochim Biophys Acta* 1971;252:574–579.
159. Rajaniemi H, Vanha-Perttula T. Specific receptor for LH in the ovary: evidence by autoradiography and tissue fractionation. *Endocrinology* 1972;90:1–9.
160. Han SS, Rajaniemi H, Cho MI, Hirshfield AN, Midgley AR Jr. Gonadotropin receptors in rat ovarian tissue. II. Subcellular localization of LH binding sites by electron microscopic radioautography. *Endocrinology* 1974;95:589–598.
161. Chen TT, Abel JH, McClellan MC, Sawyer HR, Niswender GD. Localization of gonadotropic hormones in lysosomes of ovine luteal cells. *Cytobiologie* 1977;14:412–420.
162. Petrusz P, Sar M. Light microscopic localization of gonadotropin binding sites in ovarian target cells. In: Straub RW, Boles L, eds. *Cell Membrane Receptors for Drugs and Hormones.* New York: Raven Press, 1978;167–182.
163. Amsterdam S, Kohen F, Nimrod A, Lindner HR. Lateral mobility and internalization of hormone receptors to human chorionic gonadotropin in cultured rat granulosa cells. In: Channing CP, Marsh J, Sadler WA, eds. *Advances in Experimental Medicine and Biology,* Vol. 112: *Ovarian Follicular and Corpus Luteum Function.* New York: Plenum Press, 1979;69–75.
164. Rajaniemi HJ, Hirshfield AN, Midgley AR Jr. Gonadotropin receptors in rat ovarian tissue. I. Localization of LH binding sites by fractionation of subcellular organelles. *Endocrinology* 1974;95: 579–587.
165. Lee CY, Coulan CB, Jiang NS, Ryan RJ. Receptors for human luteinizing hormone in human corpora luteal tissue. *J Clin Endocrinol Metab* 1973;36:148–152.
166. Hacik T, Kolena J. Production of oestradiol, cAMP and ^{125}I-hCG binding by rat ovaries during the reproductive cycle. *Endokrinologie* 1975;66:15–23.
167. Rao CV, Estergreen VL, Carman FR, Moss GE, Frandle KA. Receptors for prostaglandin ($PGF_2\alpha$) and human choriogonadotropin (hCG) in cell membranes of bovine corpora lutea (CL) throughout estrous cycle. In: *Vth International Congress of Endocrinology.* Hamburg, Germany, 1976;322 (abst).
168. Diekman MA, O'Callaghan P, Nett TM, Niswender GD. Validation of methods and quantification of luteal receptors for LH throughout the estrous cycle and early pregnancy in ewes. *Biol Reprod* 1978;19:999–1009.
169. Baird DT, Swanston I, Scaramuzzi RJ. Pulsatile release of LH and secretion of ovarian steroids in sheep during the late luteal phase of the estrous cycle. *Endocrinology* 1976;98:1490–1496.
170. Suter DE, Fletcher PW, Sluss PM, Reichert LE Jr, Niswender GD. Alterations in the number of ovine luteal receptors for LH and progesterone secretion induced by homologous hormone. *Biol Reprod* 1980;22:205–210.
171. Mendelson C, Dufau M, Catt K. Gonadotropin binding and stimulation of cyclic adenosine 3′:5′-monophosphate and testosterone production in isolated Leydig cells. *J Biol Chem* 1975;250: 8818–8823.
172. Jordan AW III, Caffrey JL, Niswender GD. Catecholamine-induced stimulation of progesterone and adenosine 3′,5′-monophosphate production by dispersed ovine luteal cells. *Endocrinology* 1978;103:385–392.
173. Gospodarowicz D, Gospodarowicz F. The morphological transformation and inhibition of growth of bovine luteal cells in tissue culture induced by luteinizing hormone and dibutyryl cyclic AMP. *Endocrinology* 1975;96:458–467.
174. Conti M, Harwood JP, Dufau ML, Catt KJ. Regulation of luteinizing hormone receptors and adenylate cyclase activity by gonadotrophin in the rat ovary. *Mol Pharmacol* 1977;13:1024–1032.
175. Harwood JP, Conti M, Conn PM, Dufau ML, Catt KJ. Receptor regulation and target cell responses: studies in the ovarian luteal cells. *Mol Cell Endocrinol* 1978;11:121–135.
176. Catt KJ, Harwood JP, Richert NP, Conn PM, Conti M, Dufau ML. Luteal desensitization: hormone regulation of LH receptors, adenylate cyclase and responses in the luteal cell. In: Channing CP, Marsh J, Sadler WA, eds. *Ovarian Follicular and Corpus Luteum Function.* New York: Plenum Press, 1978;647–662.
177. Abel JH, Chen TT, Endres DB, et al. Sites of binding and metabolism of gonadotropic hormones in the mammalian ovary. In: Straub RW, Bolis L, eds. *Cell Membrane Receptors for Drugs and Hormones.* New York: Raven Press, 1978;183–202.
178. Ascoli M, Puett D. Inhibition of the degradation of receptor-bound human choriogonadotropin by lysosomotropic agents, protease inhibitors, and metabolic inhibitors. *J Biol Chem* 1978;253:7839–7843.
179. Chen TT, McClellan MC, Diekman MA, Abel JH, Niswender GD. Localization of human chorionic gonadotropin in the lysosomes of ovine luteal cells. In: McKerns KW, ed. *Structure and Function of the Gonadotropins.* New York: Plenum Press, 1981;591–612.
180. Ahmed CE, Sawyer HR, Niswender GD. Internalization and degradation of human chorionic gonadotropin in ovine luteal cells: kinetic studies. *Endocrinology* 1981;109:1380–1387.
181. Bourdage RJ, Fitz TA, Niswender GD. Differential steroidogenic response of ovine luteal cells to ovine luteinizing hormone and human chorionic gonadotropin. *Proc Soc Exp Biol Med* 1984;175:483–486.
182. Suter DE, Niswender GD. Internalization and degradation of human chorionic gonadotropin in ovine luteal cells: effects of inhibition of protein synthesis. *Endocrinology* 1983;112:838–845.
183. Willingham MC, Pastan I. Endocytosis and membrane traffic in cultured cells. *Recent Prog Horm Res* 1984;40:569–587.
184. Behrman HR, Luborsky-Moore JL, Pang CY, Wright K, Dorflinger LJ. Mechanisms of $PGF_2\alpha$ action in functional luteolysis. In: Channing CP, Marsh J, Sadler WA, eds. *Ovarian Follicular and Corpus Luteum Function, Advances in Experimental Medicine and Biology,* Vol. 112. New York: Plenum Press, 1979;557–571.
185. Diekman MA, O'Callaghan P, Nett TM, Niswender GD. Effect of prostaglandin $F_2\alpha$ on the number of LH receptors in ovine corpora lutea. *Biol Reprod* 1978;19:1010–1013.
186. Marsh J. The role of cAMP in gonadal function. *Adv Cyclic Nucleotide Res* 1975;6:137–199.
187. Birnbaumer L, Codina J, Mattera R, et al. Regulation of hormone receptors and adenylyl cyclases by guanine nucleotide binding N proteins. *Recent Prog Horm Res* 1985;41:41–94.
188. Gilman AG. G proteins and dual control of adenylate cyclase. *Cell* 1984;36:577–579.
189. Condon WA, Black DL. Catecholamine-induced stimulation of

progesterone by the bovine corpus luteum *in vitro*. *Biol Reprod* 1976;15:573–578.
190. Flockhart DA, Corbin JD. Regulatory mechanisms in the control of protein kinases. *CRC Crit Rev Biochem* 1982;12:133–186.
191. Nimmo HG, Cohen P. Hormonal control of protein phosphorylation. *Adv Cyclic Nucleotide Res* 1977;8:145–266.
192. Krebs EG, Beavo JA. Phosphorylation-dephosphorylation of enzymes. *Annu Rev Biochem* 1979;48:923–959.
193. Kuo JF, Greengard P. Cyclic nucleotide-dependent protein kinase. IV. Widespread occurrence of adenosine 3′,5′monophosphate-dependent protein kinase in various tissues and phyla of the animal kingdom. *Proc Natl Acad Sci USA* 1969;64:1349–1353.
194. Ling WY, Marsh JM. Reevaluation of the role of cyclic adenosine 3′,5′-monophosphate and protein kinase in the stimulation of steroidogenesis by luteinizing hormone in bovine corpus luteum slices. *Endocrinology* 1977;100:1571–1578.
195. Jungmann RA, Hunzicker-Dunn M. Mechanism of action of gonadotropins and the regulation of gene expression. In: McKerns KW, ed. *Structure and Function of the Gonadotropins*. New York: Plenum Press, 1978;1–29.
196. Simpson ER, McCarthy JL, Peterson FA. Evidence that the cycloheximide sensitive site of adrenocorticotropic hormone action is in the mitochondrion. Changes in pregnenolone formation, cholesterol content, and the electron paramagnetic resonance spectra of cytochrome P-450. *J Biol Chem* 1978;253:3135–3139.
197. Azhar S, Menon KMJ. Adenosine 3′,5′-monophosphate dependent phosphorylation of ribosomes and ribosomal subunits from bovine corpus luteum. *Biochim Biophys Acta* 1975;392:64–74.
198. Trzeciak WH, Boyd GS. Activation of cholesteryl esterase in bovine adrenal cortex. *Eur J Biochem* 1974;46:201–207.
199. Caffrey JL, Fletcher PW, Diekman MA, O'Callaghan PL, Niswender GD. The activity of ovine luteal cholesterol esterase during several experimental conditions. *Biol Reprod* 1979;21:601–608.
200. Caron MG, Goldstein S, Savard K, Marsh J. Protein kinase stimulation of a reconstituted cholesterol side chain cleavage enzyme system in the bovine corpus luteum. *J Biol Chem* 1975;250:5137–5143.
201. Downing JR, Dimino MJ. Studies on mitochondrial protein kinase activity of porcine corpora lutea. *Endocrinology* 1979;105:570–573.
202. Neymark MA, Biersyezad RR, Dimino MJ. Phosphorylation of mitochondrial proteins in isolated porcine ovarian follicles after treatment with luteinizing hormone. *Endocrinology* 1984;114:588–593.
203. Inaba T, Weist WG. Protein kinase stimulation of steroidogenesis in rat luteal cell mitochondria. *Endocrinology* 1985;117:315–322.
204. Hall PF. Trophic stimulation of steroidogenesis: in search of the elusive trigger. *Recent Prog Horm Res* 1985;41:1–31.
205. Lowitt S, Farese RV, Sabor MA, Root AW. Rat leydig cell phospholipid content is increased by luteinizing hormone and 8-bromo-cyclic AMP. *Endocrinology* 1982;111:1415–1417.
206. Ogle TF. Effects of ACTH on organelle interrelationships in the corpus luteum of the pregnant deermouse. *Cell Tissue Res* 1974;153:195–209.
207. Scallen TJ, Srikantaiah MV, Seetharam B, Hansbury E, Gavey KL. Sterol carrier protein hypothesis. *Fed Proc* 1974;33:1733–1746.
208. Erickson SK, Meyer DJ, Gould FT. Purification and characterization of a new cholesterol binding protein from rat liver cytosol. *J Biol Chem* 1978;253:1817–1826.
209. Strott CA, Lyons CD. Studies of cholesterol binding in the soluble fraction of the adrenal cortex of the guinea pig. *J Steroid Biochem* 1978;9:721–730.
210. Strott CA. A prenenolone-binding protein in soluble fraction of guinea pig adrenal cortex. *J Biol Chem* 1977;252:464–470.
211. Ferguson JJ Jr. Puromycin and adrenal responsiveness to adrenocorticotropic hormone. *Biochim Biophys Acta* 1962;57:616–617.
212. Garren LD. The mechanism of action of adrenocorticotropic hormone. *Vitam Horm* 1968;26:119–145.
213. Schulster D, Richardson MC, Palfreyman JW. The role of protein synthesis in adrenocorticotropin action: effects of cycloheximide and puromycin on the steroidogenic response of isolated adrenocortical cells. *Mol Cell Endocrinol* 1974;2:17–29.
214. Hermier C, Combarnous Y, Justisz M. Role of a regulating protein and molecular oxygen in the mechanism of action of luteinizing hormone. *Biochim Biophys Acta* 1971;244:625–633.
215. Hochberg RB, vader Hoeven TA, Welch S, Lieberman S. A simple and precise assay of the enzymatic conversion of cholesterol into pregnenolone. *Biochemistry* 1974;13:603–609.
216. Caffrey JL, Nett TM, Abel JH Jr, Niswender GD. Activity of 3β-hydroxy-Δ^5-steroid dehydrogenase/$\Delta^5\Delta^4$-isomerase in the ovine corpus luteum. *Biol Reprod* 1979;20:279–287.
217. Werbin H, Charkoff IL. Utilization of adrenal gland cholesterol for synthesis of cortisol by the intact normal and the ACTH-treated guinea pig. *Arch Biochem Biophys* 1961;93:474–482.
218. Armstrong DT, O'Brien J, Greep RO. Effects of luteinizing hormone on progestin biosynthesis in the luteinizing rat ovary. *Endocrinology* 1964;75:488–500.
219. Krum AA, Morris MD, Bennett LJ. Role of cholesterol in the *in vivo* biosynthesis of adrenal steroids by the dog. *Endocrinology* 1964;74:543–547.
220. Ichii S, Forchielli E, Dorfman RI. *In vitro* effect of gonadotropins on the soluble cholesterol side-cleaving enzyme of bovine corpus luteum. *Steroids* 1963;2:631–656.
221. Melby JC, Egdahl RH, Dale SL. Role of circulating free cholesterol of plasma in adrenal steroidogenesis. *Clin Res* 1967;15:263 (abst).
222. Behrman HR, Armstrong DT. Cholesterol esterase stimulation by luteinizing hormone in luteinized rat ovaries. *Endocrinology* 1969;85:474–480.
223. Wiltbank MC, Knickerbocker JJ, Niswender GD. Regulation of the corpus luteum by protein kinase C. I. Phosphorylation activity and steroidogenic action in large and small ovine luteal cells. *Biol Reprod* 1989;40:1194–1200.
224. Simpson ER, McCarthy JL, Peterson JA. Evidence that the cycloheximide-sensitive site of adrenocorticotropic hormone action is in the mitochondrion. *J Biol Chem* 1978;253:3135–3139.
225. Ghosh DK, Dunham WR, Sands RH, Menon KMJ. Regulation of cholesterol side-chain cleavage enzyme activity by gonadotropin in rat corpus luteum. *Endocrinology* 1987;121:21–27.
226. Koritz SB. On the regulation of pregnenolone synthesis. In: McKerns KM, ed. *Functions of the Adrenal Cortex*, Vol I. New York: Appleton-Century-Crofts, 1967;27–48.
227. Hoyer PB, Fitz TA, Niswender GD. Hormone independent activation of adenylate cyclase in large steroidogenic ovine luteal cells does not result in increased progesterone secretion. *Endocrinology* 1984;114:604–608.
228. Fitz TA, Hoyer PB, Niswender GD. Interactions of prostaglandins with subpopulations of ovine luteal cells. I. Stimulatory effects of prostaglandins E_1, E_2, and I_2. *Prostaglandins* 1984;28:119–126.
229. Kramer RE, Anderson CM, Peterson JA, Simpson ER, Waterman MR. Adrenodoxin biosynthesis by bovine adrenal cells in monolayer culture. *J Biol Chem* 1982;257:14921–14925.
230. Nabi N, Omura T. *In vitro* synthesis of adrenodoxin and adrenodoxin reductase: existence of a putative large precursor form of adrenodoxin. *Biochem Biophys Res Commun* 1980;97:680–686.
231. Omura T, Ito A. Biosynthesis and intracellular sorting of mitochondrial forms of cytochrome P450. *Methods Enzymol* 1991;206:75–77.
232. Trzeciak WH, Waterman MR, Simpson ER. Synthesis of the cholesterol side-chain cleavage enzymes in cultured rat ovarian granulosa cells: induction by follicle-stimulating hormone and dibutyryl adenosine 3′,5′-monophosphate. *Endocrinology* 1986;119:323–330.
233. Rogers RJ, Waterman MR, Simpson ER. Levels of messenger ribonucleic acid encoding cholesterol side-chain cleavage cytochrome P-450, 17α-hydroxylase cytochrome P-450, adrenodoxin, and low density lipoprotein receptor in bovine follicles and corpora lutea throughout the ovarian cycle. *Mol Endocrinol* 1987;1:274–279.
234. Trzeciak WH, Duda T, Waterman MR, Simpson ER. Tetradecanoyl phorbol acetate suppresses follicle-stimulating hormone-induced synthesis of the cholesterol side-chain cleavage enzyme complex in rat ovarian granulosa cells. *J Biol Chem* 1987;262:15246–15250.
235. Moore CC, Brentano ST, Miller WL. Human $P450_{scc}$ gene transcription is induced by cyclic AMP and repressed by 12-*O*-tetradecanoylphorbol-acetate and A23187 through independent *cis* elements. *Mol Cell Biol* 1990;10:6013–6023.

236. Martel C, Labrie C, Dupont E, et al. Regulation of 3β-hydroxysteroid dehydrogenase/Δ^5-Δ^4-isomerase expression and activity in the hypophysectomized rat ovary: interactions between the stimulatory effect of human chorionic gonadotropin and the luteolytic effect of prolactin. *Endocrinology* 1990; 127:2726–2737.
237. Chedrese PJ, Schott D, Zhang D, Murphy BD. The signal transduction system in luteotrophic stimulation of expression of the 3β-HSD gene in porcine granulosa cells in culture. In: Gibori G, ed. *Signaling Mechanisms and Gene Expression in the Ovary.* New York: Springer-Verlag, 1991;280–284.
238. Couet J, Martel C, Dupont E, et al. Changes in 3β-hydroxysteroid dehydrogenase/Δ^5-Δ^4 isomerase messenger ribonucleic acid, activity and protein levels during the estrous cycle in the bovine ovary. *Endocrinology* 1990;127:2141–2148.
239. Hawkins DE, Belfiore CJ, Niswender GD. Regulation of mRNA encoding 3β-hydroxysteroid dehydrogenase/Δ^5-Δ^4 isomerase (3β-HSD) in the ovine corpus luteum. *Biol Reprod,* 1993;48:1185–1190.
240. Loeb L. The effect of extirpation of the uterus on the life and function of the corpus luteum in the guinea pig. *Proc Soc Exp Biol Med* 1923;20:441–464.
241. Bradbury JT. Prolongation of the life of the corpus luteum by hysterectomy in the rat. *Anat Rec* 1937;70(suppl 1):51.
242. Bradbury JT, Brown WE, Gray LA. Maintenance of the corpus luteum and physiologic actions of progesterone. *Recent Prog Horm Res* 1950;5:151–194 (abst).
243. Bartke A. Influences of an IUD on the leucocytic content of the uterus and on the duration of pseudopregnancy in mice. *J Reprod Fertil* 1970;23:243–247.
244. Critser ES, Rutledge JJ, French RL. Role of the uterus and the conceptus in regulating luteal lifespan in the mouse. *Biol Reprod* 1980;23:558–563.
245. Caldwell BV, Mazer RS, Wright PA. Luteolysis as affected by uterine transplantation in the Syrian hamster. *Endocrinology* 1967;80:477–482.
246. Duby RT, McDaniel JW, Spilman CH, Black DL. Utero-ovarian relationships in the golden hamster. I. Ovarian periodicity following hysterectomy. *Acta Endocrinol* 1969;60:595–602.
247. Lukaszewska JH, Greenwald GS. Comparison of luteal function in pseudopregnant and pregnant hamsters. *J Reprod Fertil* 1969;20:185–187.
248. Asdell SA, Hammond J. The effect of prolonging the life of the corpus luteum in the rabbit by hysterectomy. *Am J Physiol* 1933;103:600–605.
249. Gillard JL. The effects of hysterectomy on mammary development in the rabbit. *Am J Physiol* 1937;120:300–303.
250. Chu JP, Lee CC, You SS. Functional relation between the uterus and the corpus luteum. *J Endocrinol* 1946;4:392–398.
251. Wiltbank JN, Casida LE. Alteration of ovarian activity by hysterectomy. *J Anim Sci* 1956;15:134–140.
252. Spies HG, Zimmerman DR, Self HL, Casida LE. Effect of exogenous progesterone on the corpora lutea of hysterectomized gilts. *J Anim Sci* 1960;19:101–108.
253. Ginther OJ, First NL. Maintenance of the corpus luteum in hysterectomized mares. *Am J Vet Res* 1971;32:1687–1691.
254. Stabenfeldt GH, Hughes JP, Wheat JD, Evans JW, Kennedy PC, Cupps PT. The role of the uterus in ovarian control in the mare. *J Reprod Fertil* 1974;37:343–351.
255. Neill JD, Johansson EDB, Knobil E. Failure of hysterectomy to influence the normal pattern of cyclic progesterone secretion in the rhesus monkey. *Endocrinology* 1969;84:464–465.
256. Castracane VD, Moore GT, Shaikh AA. Ovarian function in hysterectomized *Macaca fascicularis. Biol Reprod* 1979;20: 462–472.
257. Beling CG, Marcus SL, Markam SM. Functional activity of the corpus luteum following hysterectomy. *J Clin Endocrinol Metab* 1970;30:30–39.
258. Doyle LL, Barclay DL, Duncan GW, Kirton KT. Human luteal function following hysterectomy as assessed by plasma progestin. *Am J Obstet Gynecol* 1971;110:92–97.
259. Hartman CG. Hysterectomy and the oestrous cycle in the opossum. *Am J Anat* 1925;35:25–29.
260. Hadley JC. The effect of serial uterine biopsies and hysterectomy on peripheral blood levels of total unconjugated oestrogen and progesterone in the bitch. *J Reprod Fertil* 1975;45:389–393.
261. Deanesly R, Parkes AS. The effect of hysterectomy on the oestrous cycle of the ferret. *J Physiol (Lond)* 1933;78:80–84.
262. Durrant EP. Studies on vigor. XI. Relationship of hysterectomy to voluntary activity in the white rat. *Am J Physiol* 1927;82: 14–18.
263. Dewar AD. Effects of hysterectomy on corpus luteum activity in the cyclic, pseudopregnant and pregnant mouse. *J Reprod Fertil* 1973;33:77–89.
264. Rowlands IW, Short RV. The progesterone content of the guinea-pig corpus luteum during the reproductive cycle and after hysterectomy. *J Endocrinol* 1959;19:81–86.
265. Heap RB, Perry JS, Rowlands IW. Corpus luteum function in the guinea-pig; arterial and luteal progesterone levels, and the effects of hysterectomy and hypphysectomy. *J Reprod Fertil* 1967;13: 537–553.
266. Poser NL, Horton EN. Plasma progesterone levels in guinea-pigs actively immunized against prostaglandin $F_2\alpha$, hysterectomized or treated with intra-uterine indomethacin. *J Endocrinol* 1975;67:81–88.
267. Kiracofe GH, Spies HG. Length of maintenance of naturally formed and experimentally induced corpora lutea in hysterectomized ewes. *J Reprod Fertil* 1966;11:275–279.
268. Moor RM, Hay MF, Short RV, Rowson LEA. The corpus luteum of the sheep: effect of uterine removal during luteal regression. *J Reprod Fertil* 1970;21:319–326.
269. Sheldrick EL, Flint APF. Regression of the corpora lutea in sheep in response to cloprostenol is not affected by loss of luteal oxytocin after hysterectomy. *J Reprod Fertil* 1983;68:155–160.
270. Malven PV, Hansel W. Ovarian function in dairy heifers following hysterectomy. *J Dairy Sci* 1964;47:1388–1393.
271. Anderson LL, Bowerman AM, Melampy RM. Oxytocin on ovarian function in cycling and hysterectomized heifers. *J Anim Sci* 1965;24:864–868.
272. Anderson LL, Butcher RL, Melampy RM. Subtotal hysterectomy and ovarian function in gilts. *Endocrinology* 1961;68: 571–580.
273. Masuda H, Anderson LL, Henricks DM, Melampy RM. Progesterone in ovarian venous plasma and corpora lutea of the pig. *Endocrinology* 1967;80:240–246.
274. Moeljono MPE, Bazer FW, Thatcher WW. A study of prostaglandin $F_2\alpha$ as the luteolysin in swine. I. Effect of prostaglandin $F_2\alpha$ in hysterectomized gilts. *Prostaglandins* 1976;11:737–743.
275. Pepe GJ, Rothchild I. A comparative study of serum progesterone levels in pregnancy and in various types of pseudopregnancy in the rat. *Endocrinology* 1974;95:275–279.
276. Squires EL, Wentworth BC, Ginther OJ. Progesterone concentration in blood of mares during the estrous cycle, pregnancy and after hysterectomy. *J Anim Sci* 1975;39:759–767.
277. Miller JB, Keyes PL. A mechanism for regression of the rabbit corpus luteum: uterine induced loss of luteal responsiveness to 17β-estradiol. *Biol Reprod* 1976;15:511–518.
278. Lytton FDC, Poyser NL. Concentrations of $PGF_2\alpha$ and PGE_2 in the uterine venous blood of rabbits during pseudopregnancy and pregnancy. *J Reprod Fertil* 1982;64:421–429.
279. Inskeep EK, Butcher RI. Local component of utero-ovarian relationships in the ewe. *J Anim Sci* 1966;25:1164–1168.
280. Moor RM, Rowson LEA. Local uterine mechanisms affecting luteal function in sheep. *J Reprod Fertil* 1966;11:307–310.
281. Ginther OJ, Woody CO, Mahajan S, Janakiraman K, Casida LE. Effect of oxytocin administration on the oestrous cycle of unilaterally hysterectomized heifers. *J Reprod Fertil* 1967;14:225–229.
282. du Mesnil du Buisson F. Regression unilaterale des corpes jaunes apres hysterectomie partielle chez la truie. *Ann Biol Anim Biochim Biophys* 1961;1:105–112.
283. Fisher TV. Local uterine inhibition of the corpus luteum in the guinea pig. *Anat Rec* 1965;151:350 (abst).
284. Butcher RL, Barley DA, Inskeep EK. Local relationship between the ovary and uterus of rats and guinea pigs. *Endocrinology* 1969;84:476–481.
285. Duby RT, McDaniel JW, Spilman CH, Black DL. Utero-ovarian relationships in the golden hamster. II. Quantitative and local influences of the uterus on ovarian function. *Acta Endocrinol* 1969;60:603–610.
286. Barley DA, Butcher RL, Inskeep EK. Local nature of utero-ovarian relationships in the pseudopregnant rat. *Endocrinology* 1966;79:119–124.

287. Hunter GL, Casida LE. Absence of local effects of the rabbit uterus on weight of corpus luteum. *J Reprod Fertil* 1967;13: 179–181.
288. Hixon JE, Hansel W. Evidence for preferential transfer of prostaglandin $F_2\alpha$ to the ovarian artery following intrauterine administration in cattle. *Biol Reprod* 1974;11:543–552.
289. Bland KP, Donovan BT. Observations on the time of action and the pathway of the uterine luteolytic effect of the guinea pig. *J Endocrinol* 1969;43:259–264.
290. Ginther OJ. Utero-ovarian relationships in progesterone-treated guinea pig. *Am J Vet Res* 1969;30:261–267.
291. Fisher TV. Local pathway controlling luteal function in the guinea pig. *Biol Reprod* 1971;4:126–128.
292. O'Shea JD, Lee CS. Local uterine luteolysis in the rat. *J Reprod Fertil* 1972;28:155–156.
293. Goding JR, Harrison FA, Heap RB, Linzell JL. Ovarian activity in the ewe after autotransplantation of the ovary or uterus to the neck. *J Physiol (Lond)* 1967;191:129–130.
294. Baird DT, Goding JR, Ichikawa Y, McCracken JA. The secretion of steroids from the autotransplanted ovary in the ewe spontaneously and in response to systemic gonadotrophin. *J Endocrinol* 1968;42:283–299.
295. Butcher RL, Chow KY, Melampy RM. Effect of uterine autotransplants on the estrous cycle in the guinea pig. *Endocrinology* 1962;70:442–443.
296. Bland KP, Donovan BT. The effect of autotransplantation of the ovaries to the kidneys or the uterus on the oestrous cycle of the guinea pig. *J Endocrinol* 1968;41:95–103.
297. Bland KP, Donovan BT. Oestrogen and progesterone and the function of the corpora lutea in the guinea pig. *J Endocrinol* 1970;47:225–230.
298. Harrison FA, Heap RB, Linzell JL. Ovarian function in the sheep after autotransplantation of the ovary and the uterus to the neck. *J Endocrinol* 1968;40:viii.
299. Ginther OJ. Internal regulation of physiological processes through venoartenal pathways: a review. *J Anim Sci* 1974;39: 550–564.
300. Ginther OJ, Del Campo CH, Rawlings CA. Vascular anatomy of the uterus and ovaries and the unilateral luteolytic effect of the uterus: a local venoarterial pathway between uterus and ovaries in sheep. *Am J Vet Res* 1973;34:723–728.
301. Mapletoft R, Ginther OJ. Adequacy of main uterine vein and the ovarian artery in the local venoarterial pathway for uterine-induced luteolysis in ewes. *Am J Vet Res* 1975;36:957–963.
302. Mapletoft RJ, Del Campo MR, Ginther OJ. Local venoarterial pathway for uterine-induced luteolysis in cows. *Proc Soc Exp Biol Med* 1976;153:289–294.
303. Del Campo CH, Ginther OJ. Vascular anatomy of the uterus and ovaries and the unilateral luteolytic effect of the uterus: horses, sheep and swine. *Am J Vet Res* 1973;34:305–316.
304. Del Campo CH, Ginther OJ. Vascular anatomy of the uterus and ovaries and the unilateral luteolytic effect of the uterus: angioarchitecture in sheep. *Am J Vet Res* 1973;34:1377–1386.
305. Ginther OJ, Del Campo CH. Vascular anatomy of the uterus and ovaries and the unilateral luteolytic effect of the uterus: areas of close apposition between the ovarian artery and vessels which contain uterine venous blood in sheep. *Am J Vet Res* 1973;34:1387–1393.
306. Del Campo CH, Ginther OJ. Vascular anatomy of the uterus and ovaries and the unilateral luteolytic effect of the uterus: histologic structure of uteroovarian vein and ovarian artery in sheep. *Am J Vet Res* 1974;35:397–399.
307. Del Campo CH, Ginther OJ. Vascular anatomy of the uterus and ovaries and the unilateral luteolytic effect of the uterus: guinea pigs, rats, hamsters and rabbits. *Am J Vet Res* 1973;33: 2561–2578.
308. Ginther OJ, Del Campo CH. Vascular anatomy of the uterus and ovaries and the unilateral luteolytic effect of the uterus: cattle. *Am J Vet Res* 1974;35:193–203.
309. Ginther OJ, Garcia MC, Squires EL, Steffenhagen WP. Anatomy of uterus and ovaries in mares. *Am J Vet Res* 1972;33: 1687–1691.
310. Pharriss BB, Wyngarden L. The effect of prostaglandin $F_2\alpha$ on the progestogen content of ovaries from pseudopregnant rats. *Proc Soc Exp Biol Med* 1969;130:92–94.
311. Lauderdale JW. Effects of $PGF_2\alpha$ on pregnancy and estrous cycle of cattle. *J Anim Sci* 1972;35:246 (abst).
312. Liehr RA, Marion GB, Olson HH. Effects of prostaglandin on cattle estrous cycles. *J Anim Sci* 1972;35:247 (abst).
313. Louis TM, Hafs HD, Morrow DA. Estrus and ovulation after uterine prostaglandin $F_2\alpha$ in cows. *J Anim Sci* 1972;35:247.
314. Rowson LEA, Tervit HR, Brand A. The use of prostaglandins for synchronization of oestrus in cattle. *J Reprod Fertil* 1972;29:145.
315. McCracken JA, Glew ME, Scaramuzzi R. Corpus luteum regression induced by prostaglandin $F_2\alpha$. *J Clin Endocrinol Metab* 1970;30:544–546.
316. Barrett S, deB. Blockey MA, Brown JM, et al. Initiation of the oestrous cycle in the ewe by infusions of $PGF_2\alpha$ to the autotransplanted ovary. *J Reprod Fertil* 1971;24:136–137.
317. Thorburn GD, Nicol DH. Regression of the ovine corpus uteum after infusion of prostaglandin $F_2\alpha$ into the ovarian artery and uterine vein. *J Endocrinol* 1971;51:785–786.
318. Chaichareon DP, Mickley PE, Ginther OJ. Effect of prostaglandin $F_2\alpha$ on corpora lutea in guinea pigs and Mongolian gerbils. *Am J Vet Res* 1974;35:685–687.
319. Ott RS, Nelson DR, Hixon JE. Peripheral serum progesterone and luteinizing hormone concentrations of goats during synchronization of estrus and ovulation with prostaglandin $F_2\alpha$. *Am J Vet Res* 1980;41:1432–1434.
320. Douglas RH, Ginther OJ. Effect of prostaglandin $F_2\alpha$ on the length of diestrus in mares. *Prostaglandins* 1972;2:265–268.
321. Allen WR, Rowson LEA. Control of the mare's oestrous cycle by prostaglandins. *J Reprod Fertil* 1973;33:539–543.
322. Noden PA, Hafs HD, Oxender WD. Estrus, ovulation, progesterone and luteinizing hormone after prostaglandin $F_2\alpha$ in mares. *Proc Soc Exp Biol Med* 1974;145:145–150.
323. Bartke A, Merrill AP, Baker CF. Effects of prostaglandin $F_2\alpha$ on pseudopregnancy and pregnancy in mice. *Fertil Steril* 1972;23: 543–547.
324. Harris KH, Murphy BD. Luteolysis in the hamster: abrogation by gonadotropin and prolactin pretreatment. *Prostaglandins* 1981;21:177–187.
325. Scott RS, Rennie PIC. Factors controlling the lifespan of the corpora lutea in the pseudopregnant rabbit. *J Reprod Fertil* 1970;23: 415–422.
326. Gutknecht GD, Duncan GW, Wyngarden LJ. Inhibition of prostaglandin $F_2\alpha$ or LH induced luteolysis in the pseudopregnant rabbit by 17β-estradiol. *Proc Soc Exp Biol Med* 1972;139: 406–410.
327. Diehl JR, Day BN. Effect of prostaglandin $F_2\alpha$ on luteal function in swine. *J Anim Sci* 1973;37:307 (abst).
328. Gleeson AR. Luteal function of the cyclic sow after infusion of prostaglandin $F_2\alpha$ through a uterine vein. *J Reprod Fertil* 1974;36:518–522.
329. Douglas RH, Ginther OJ. Effect of prostaglandin $F_2\alpha$ on estrous cycles or corpus luteum in mares and gilts. *J Anim Sci* 1975;40:518–522.
330. Hallford DM, Wetteman RP, Turman EJ, Omtvedt IT. Luteal function in gilts after prostaglandin $F_2\alpha$. *J Anim Sci* 1975;41:1706–1710.
331. Kirton KT, Pharriss BB, Forbes AD. Luteolytic effect of prostaglandin $F_2\alpha$ in primates. *Proc Soc Exp Biol Med* 1970;133: 314–316.
332. Auletta FJ, Caldwell BV, Speroff L. Prostaglandin $F_2\alpha$ induced steroidogenesis and luteolysis in the primate corpus luteum. *J Clin Endocrinol Metab* 1973;36:405–407.
333. Lehmann F, Peters F, Breckholdt M, Bettendorf G. Plasma progesterone levels during infusion of prostaglandin $F_2\alpha$ in the human. *Prostaglandins* 1972;1:269–277.
334. Wentz AC, Jones GES. Transient luteolytic effect of prostaglandin $F_2\alpha$ in the human. *Obstet Gynecol* 1973;42:172–181.
335. Jochle W, Tomlinson RV, Andersen AC. Prostaglandin effects on plasma progesterone levels in the pregnant and cycling dog (beagle). *Prostaglandins* 1973;3:209–217.
336. Auletta FJ, Kamps DL, Pories S, Bisset J, Gibson M. An intracorpus luteum site for the luteolytic action of prostaglandin $F_2\alpha$ in the rhesus monkey. *Prostaglandins* 1984;27:285–298.
337. Concannon PW, Hansel W. Prostaglandin $F_2\alpha$ induced luteolysis hypothermia and abortions in beagle bitches. *Prostaglandins* 1977;13:533–542.

338. Wildt DE, Panko WB, Seager SWJ. Effect of prostaglandin $F_2\alpha$ on endocrine-ovarian function in the domestic cat. *Prostaglandins* 1979;18:883–892.
339. O'Grady JP, Caldwell BV, Auletta FJ, Speroff L. The effects of an inhibitor of prostaglandin synthesis (indomethacin) on ovulation, pregnancy and pseudopregnancy in the rabbit. *Prostaglandins* 1972;1:98–106.
340. Lau IF, Saksena SK, Chang MC. Effects of indomethacin, an inhibitor of prostaglandin biosynthesis on the length of pseudopregnancy in rats and hamsters. *Acta Endocrinol* 1975;78: 343–348.
341. Critser ES, Rutledge JJ, French LR. Effect of indomethacin on the interestrous interval of intact and hysterectomized pseudopregnant mice. *Biol Reprod* 1981;24:1000–1005.
342. Scaramuzzi RJ, Baird DT. The oestrous cycle of the ewe after active immunization against prostaglandin $F_2\alpha$. *J Reprod Fertil* 1976;46:39–47.
343. Fairclough RJ, Smith JF, Peterson AJ, McGowan L. Effect of oestradiol-17β progesterone and prostaglandin $F_2\alpha$ antiplasma on luteal function in the ewe. *J Reprod Fertil* 1976;46:523–524.
344. Fairclough RJ, Smith JF, McGowan LT. Prolongation of the oestrous cycle in cows and ewes after passive immunization with PGF antibodies. *J Reprod Fertil* 1981;62:213–219.
345. Shemesh M, Hansel W. Levels of prostaglandin F in bovine endometrium, uterine venous, ovarian arterial and jugular plasma during the estrous cycle. *Proc Soc Exp Biol Med* 1975;148: 123–126.
346. Wilson L Jr, Cenedella RJ, Butcher RL, Inskeep EK. Levels of prostaglandins in the uterine endometrium during the ovine estrous cycle. *J Anim Sci* 1972;34:93–99.
347. Poyser NL. Production of prostaglandins by the guinea-pig uterus. *J Endocrinol* 1972;54:147–159.
348. Vernon MW, Zavy MT, Aisquith RL, Sharp DC. Prostaglandin $F_2\alpha$ in the equine endometrium: steroid production and production capacities during the estrous cycle and early pregnancy. *Biol Reprod* 1981;25:581–589.
349. Guthrie HD, Rexroad CE Jr. Progesterone secretion and prostaglandin F release *in vitro* by endometrial and luteal tissue of cyclic pigs. *J Reprod Fertil* 1980;60:157–163.
350. Doebler JA, Wickersham EW, Anthony A. Uterine prostaglandin $F_2\alpha$ content and 20-α-hydroxy-steroid dehydrogenase activity in individual ovarian compartments during pseudopregnancy in the rat. *Biol Reprod* 1981;24:871–878.
351. Lytton FDC, Poyser NL. Prostaglandin production by the rabbit uterus and placenta *in vitro*. *J Reprod Fertil* 1982;66:591–599.
352. Gleeson AR, Thorburn GD, Cox RI. Prostaglandin F concentrations in the utero-ovarian vein plasma of the sow during the late luteal phase of the oestrous cycle. *Prostaglandins* 1974;5: 521–529.
353. Moeljono MPE, Thatcher WW, Bazer FW, Frank M, Owens LJ, Wilcox CJ. A study of prostaglandin $F_2\alpha$ as the luteolysin in swine: II. Characterization and comparison of prostaglandin F, estrogens and progestin concentrations in uteroovarian vein plasma of nonpregnant and pregnant gilts. *Prostaglandins* 1977;14:543–555.
354. Douglas RH, Ginther OJ. Concentrations of prostaglandin F in uterine venous plasma of anesthetized mares during the estrous cycle and early pregnancy. *Prostaglandins* 1976;11:251–260.
355. Castracane VD, Shaikh AA. Effect of decidual tissue on the uterine production of prostaglandins in pseudopregnant rats. *J Reprod Fertil* 1976;46:101–104.
356. Behrman H, Grinwich DH, Hichens M, MacDonald GJ. Effect of hypophysectomy, prolactin and prostaglandin $F_2\alpha$ on gonadotropin binding *in vivo* and *in vitro* in the corpus luteum. *Endocrinology* 1978;103:349–357.
357. Fletcher PW, Niswender GD. Effect of $PGF_2\alpha$ on progesterone secretion and adenylate cyclase activity in ovine luteal tissue. *Prostaglandins* 1982;20:803–818.
358. Wiltbank MC, Guthrie PB, Mattson MP, Kater SB, Niswender GD. Hormonal regulation of free intracellular calcium concentrations in small and large ovine luteal cells. *Biol Reprod* 1989;41:771–778.
359. Hoyer PB, Marion SL. Influence of agents that affect intracellular calcium regulation on progesterone secretion in small and large luteal cells of the sheep. *J Reprod Fertil* 1989;86:445–455.
360. Silvia WJ, Fitz TA, Mayan MH, Niswender GD. Cellular and molecular mechanisms involved in luteolysis and maternal recognition of pregnancy in the ewe. *Anim Reprod Sci* 1984;7:57–74.
361. Braden TD, Niswender GD. Differential loss of the two steroidogenic cell types in the ovine corpus luteum following prostaglandins (PG)$F_2\alpha$. *Biol Reprod* 1985;30(suppl 1):14 (abst).
362. Wiltbank MC, Diskin MG, Niswender GD. Differential actions of second messenger systems in the corpus luteum. *J Reprod Fertil* 1991; suppl 43:65–75.
363. McGuire WJ, Hawkins DE, Niswender GD. Activation of protein kinase (PK)-C inhibits progesterone production *in vivo*. *Biol Reprod* 1992;46(suppl 1):84 (abst).
364. Sawyer HR, Niswender KD, Braden TD, Niswender GD. Nuclear changes in ovine luteal cells in response to $PGF_2\alpha$. *Dom Anim Endocrinol* 1990;7:229–238.
365. Hansel W, Alila HW, Dowd JP, Yang X. Control of steroidogenesis in small and large bovine luteal cells. *Aust J Biol Sci* 1987;40:331–347.
366. Veldhuis JD. Prostaglandin $F_2\alpha$ initiates polyphosphatidylinositol hydrolysis and membrane translocation of protein kinase C in swine ovarian cells. *Biochem Biophys Res Commun* 1987;149: 112–117.
367. Paavola LG. The corpus luteum of the guinea pig. IV. Fine structure of macrophages during pregnancy and postpartum luteolysis and the phagocytosis of luteal cells. *Am J Anat* 1979;154: 337–364.
368. Koering MJ, Thor MJ. Structural changes in the regressing corpus luteum of the rabbit. *Biol Reprod* 1978;17:719–733.
369. VanLennys EW, Madden LM. Electron microscopic observations of the involution of the human corpus luteum of menstruation. *A Zellforsch Mikrosk Anat* 1965;66:365–380.
370. Corteel M. Luteolysis induced by prostaglandin $F_2\alpha$ compared with natural luteolysin in the ewe. *Ann Biol Anim Biochem Biophys* 1975;15:175–180.
371. Thorburn GD, Hales JRS. Selective reduction in blood flow to the ovine corpus luteum after infusion of prostaglandins $F_2\alpha$ into a uterine vein. *Proc Aust Physiol Pharmacol Soc* 1972;3:145 (abst).
372. Novy MJ, Cook MJ. Redistribution of blood flow by prostaglandin $F_2\alpha$ in the rabbit ovary. *Am J Obstet Gynecol* 1973;117: 381–385.
373. Ricketts AP, Flint APE. Onset of synthesis of progesterone by ovine placenta. *J Endocrinol* 1980;86:337–347.
374. Butcher RL, Collins WE, Fugo NW. Plasma concentration of LH, FSH, prolactin, progesterone and estradiol-17β throughout the 4-day estrous cycle of the rat. *Endocrinology* 1974;94: 1704–1708.
375. Smith MS, Freeman ME, Neill JD. The control of progesterone secretion during the estrous cycle and early pseudopregnancy in the rat: prolactin, gonadotropin and steroid levels associated with rescue of the corpus luteum of pseudopregnancy. *Endocrinology* 1975;96:219–226.
376. Spies HG, Niswender GD. Levels of prolactin, LH and FSH in the serum of intact and pelvic-neuroectomized rats. *Endocrinology* 1971;88:937–943.
377. Freeman ME, Smith MS, Nazian SJ, Neill JD. Ovarian and hypothalamic control of the daily surges of prolactin secretion during pseudopregnancy. *Endocrinology* 1974;94:875–882.
378. Butcher RL, Fugo NW, Collins WE. Semicircadian rhythm in plasma levels of prolactin during early gestation in the rat. *Endocrinology* 1972;90:1125–1127.
379. von Berswoldt-Wallabre I, Geller HF, Herlyn U. Temporal aspects of decidual cell reaction. I. Induction of decidual cell reaction in lactogenic hormone treated and in pseudopregnant rats. *Acta Endocrinol* 1964;45:349–352.
380. Gibori G, Rothchild I, Pepe GJ, Morishige WK, Lam P. Luteotropic action of decidual tissue in the rat. *Endocrinology* 1974;95:1113–1118.
381. Csapo AI, Wiest WG. An examination of the quantitative relationship between progesterone and the maintenance of pregnancy. *Endocrinology* 1969;85:735–746.
382. Morishige WK, Rothchild I. Temporal aspects of the regulation of corpus luteum function by luteinizing hormone, prolactin and placental luteotrophin during the first half of pregnancy in the rat. *Endocrinology* 1974;95:260–274.

383. Ershoff BH, Devel HI Jr. Prolongation of pseudopregnancy by induction of deciduomata. *Proc Soc Exp Biol Med* 1943;54: 167–168.
384. Peckham BM, Greene RR. Prolongation of pseudopregnancy by induction of deciduomata. *Proc Soc Exp Biol Med* 1948;69: 417–418.
385. Shaikh AA, Naqvi RH, Saksena SK. Prostaglandins E and F in uterine venous plasma in relation to peripheral plasma levels of progesterone and 20α-hydroxyprogesterone in the rat throughout pregnancy and parturition. *Prostaglandins* 1977;13:311–320.
386. Carminati P, Luzzani F, Soffientini A, Lemer L. Influence of day of pregnancy on rat placental, uterine and ovarian prostaglandin synthesis and metabolism. *Endocrinology* 1975;97:1071–1079.
387. Astwood EB, Greep RO. A corpus luteum-stimulating substance in the rat placenta. *Proc Soc Exp Biol Med* 1938;38:713–716.
388. Linkie DM, Niswender GD. Characterization of rat placental luteotropin: physiology and biochemical properties. *Biol Reprod* 1972;8:48–57.
389. Kelly PA, Shiu RPC, Robertson MC, Friesen HG. Characterization of rat chorionic mammotropin. *Endocrinology* 1975;96: 1187–1195.
390. Robertson MC, Friesen HG. The purification and characterization of rat placental lactogen. *Endocrinology* 1975;97:621–629.
391. Robertson MC, Gillespie B, Friesen HG. Characterization of the two forms of rat placental lactogen (rPL): rPL-I and rPL-II. *Endocrinology* 1982;111:1862–1866.
392. Haour F, Tell G, Sanchez P, Debre R. Mise en evidence et dosage d'une gonadotrophine chorionique chez le rat (rCG). *C R Acad Sci (D)* 1976;282:1183–1186.
393. Jayatilak PG, Glasser LA, Warshaw ML, Herz Z, Gruber JR, Gibori G. Relationship between luteinizing hormone and decidual luteotropin in the maintenance of luteal steroidogenesis. *Biol Reprod* 1984;31:556–564.
394. Hilliard J, Scaramuzzi RJ, Penardi R, Sawyer CH. Serum progesterone levels in hysterectomized pseudopregnant rabbits. *Proc Soc Exp Biol Med* 1974;145:151–153.
395. Bill CH II, Keyes PL. 17β-Estradiol maintains normal function of corpora lutea throughout pseudopregnancy in hypophysectomized rabbits. *Biol Reprod* 1983;28:608–617.
396. Browning JY, Keyes PL, Wolf RC. Comparison of serum progesterone, 20α-dihydroprogesterone and estradiol-17β in pregnant and pseudopregnant rabbits: evidence for postimplantation recognition of pregnancy. *Biol Reprod* 1980;23:1014–1019.
397. Wu DH, Allen WM. Maintenance of pregnancy in castrated rabbits by 17-α-hydroxy-progesterone caproate and by progesterone. *Fertil Steril* 1959;10:439–460.
398. Kwun JK, Emmens CW. Hormonal requirements for implantation and pregnancy in the ovariectomized rabbit. *Aust J Biol Sci* 1974;27:275–283.
399. Thau R, Lanman JT. Evaluation of progesterone synthesis in rabbit placentas. *Endocrinology* 1974;94:925–926.
400. Browning JY, Wolf RC. Maternal recognition of pregnancy in the rabbit: effect of conceptus removal. *Biol Reprod* 1981;24: 293–297.
401. Nowak RA, Bahr J. Maternal recognition of pregnancy in the rabbit. *J Reprod Fertil* 1983;69:623–627.
402. Klein M. Sur l'ablation des embryons chez la lapine gravid et sur les facteurs qui detemminent le maintien du corps jaune pendant la deuxieme partie de la grosesse. *C R Soc Biol* 1933;113: 441–443.
403. Lanman JT, Thau R. Effect of the fetal placenta and of a rabbit pituitary extract on plasma progesterone in fetectomized rabbits. *J Reprod Fertil* 1979;57:341–344.
404. Ellinwood WE, Seidel GE, Niswender GD. Secretion of gonadotropic factors by the preimplantation rabbit blastocyst. *Proc Soc Exp Biol Med* 1979;161:136–141.
405. Browning JY, Amis MA, Meller PA, Bridson WE, Wolf RC. Luteotropic and antiluteolytic activities of the rabbit conceptus. *Biol Reprod* 1982;27:665–672.
406. Gadsby JE, Keyes PL, Bill CH II. Control of corpus luteum function in the pregnant rabbit: role of estrogen and lack of a direct luteotropic role of the placenta. *Endocrinology* 1983;113: 2255–2262.
407. Abramowitz JA, Birnbaumer L. Prostacyclin activation of adenylyl cyclase in rabbit corpus luteum membranes: comparison with 6-keto-prostaglandin $F_2\alpha$ and prostaglandin E_1. *Biol Reprod* 1979;21:609–616.
408. Harper MJK, Norris CJ, Rajkumar K. Prostaglandin release by zygotes and endometria of pregnant rabbits. *Biol Reprod* 1983;28:350–362.
409. Croix D, Franchimont P. Changes in serum levels of gonadotropins, progesterone and estradiol during the estrous cycle of the guinea pig. *Neuroendocrinology* 1975;19:1–11.
410. Blatchley FR, Donovan BT, Ter Haar MB. Plasma progesterone and gonadotrophin levels during the estrous cycle of the guinea pig. *Biol Reprod* 1976;15:29–38.
411. Blatchley FR, Donovan BT, Horton EW, Poyser NL. The release of prostaglandins and progesterone into the utero-ovarian venous blood of guinea-pigs during the oestrous cycle and following oestrogen treatment. *J Physiol (Lond)* 1972;223:69–88.
412. Granstrom E, Kindahl H. Radioimmunoassay for urinary metabolites of prostaglandin $F_2\alpha$. *Prostaglandins* 1976;12:759–783.
413. Artunkal T, Colonge RA. Action de l'ovariectomie sur la gestation du cobaye. *C R Soc Biol* 1949;143:1590–1592.
414. Csapo AL, Puri CP, Tano S. Relationship between timing of ovariectomy and maintenance of pregnancy in the guinea-pig. *Prostaglandins* 1981;22:131–140.
415. Illingworth DV, Challis JRG. Concentrations of oestrogens and progesterone in the plasma of ovariectomized and ovariectomized norgestrel-treated pregnant guinea-pigs. *J Reprod Fertil* 1973;34:289–296.
416. Challis JRG, Heap RB, Willingworth DV. Concentrations of estrogen and progesterone in the plasma of nonpregnant, pregnant and lactating guinea-pigs. *J Endocrinol* 1971;51:333–345.
417. Heap RB, Deanesly R. The increase in plasma progesterone levels in the pregnant guinea-pig and its possible significance. *J Reprod Fertil* 1967;14:339–341.
418. Illingworth DV, Heap RB, Perry JS. Changes in the metabolic clearance rate of progesterone in the guinea pig. *J Endocrinol* 1970;48:409–417.
419. Moor RM. Effect of embryo on corpus luteum function. *J Anim Sci* 1968;27(suppl 1):97–118.
420. Maule-Walker FM, Poyser NL. Production of prostaglandins by the early pregnant guinea-pig uterus *in vitro*. *J Endocrinol* 1974;61:265–271.
421. Blatchley FR, Maule-Walker FM, Poyser NL. Progesterone, prostaglandin $F_2\alpha$ and oestradiol in the utero-ovarian venous plasma of nonpregnant and early, unilaterally pregnant guinea-pigs. *J Endocrinol* 1975;67:225–229.
422. Antonini R, Turner TT, Pauerstein CJ. The hormonal control of the guinea-pig corpus luteum during early pregnancy. *Fertil Steril* 1976;27:1322–1325.
423. Humphreys EM, Hobson BM, Wide L. Gonadotrophic activity of the guinea-pig placenta during pregnancy. *J Reprod Fertil* 1981;65:231–238.
424. Babra CS, Lynch SS, Foxcroft GR, Robinson G, Amoroso EC. Purification and characterization of guinea-pig chorionic gonadotrophin. *J Reprod Fertil* 1984;71:227–233.
425. Casida LE, Warwick EJ. The necessity of the corpus luteum for maintenance of pregnancy in the ewe. *J Anim Sci* 1945;4:34–36.
426. Denamur R, Martinet J. Effets de l'ovariectomie chez la brebis pendant la gestation. *C R Seanc Soc Biol* 1955;149:2105–2107.
427. Moore NW, Rowson LEA. Maintenance of pregnancy in ovariectomized ewes by means of progesterone. *Nature* 1959;184:1410.
428. Bindon BM. The role of progesterone in implantation in the sheep. *Aust J Biol Sci* 1971;24:149–158.
429. Moor RM, Rowson LEA. The corpus luteum of the sheep: effect of the removal of embryos on luteal function. *J Endocrinol* 1966;34:497–502.
430. Moor RM, Rowson LEA. The corpus luteum of the sheep: functional relationship between the embryo and corpus luteum. *J Endocrinol* 1966;34:233–239.
431. Rowson LEA, Moor RM. The influence of embryonic tissue homogenate infused into the uterus, on the lifespan of the corpus luteum in sheep. *J Reprod Fertil* 1967;13:511–516.
432. Ellinwood WE, Nett TM, Niswender GD. Maintenance of the corpus luteum of early pregnancy in the ewe. I. Luteotropic properties of embryonic homogenates. *Biol Reprod* 1979;21:281–288.
433. Martal J, LaCroix MC, Loudes C, Saunier M, Wintenberger-Torres S. Trophoblastin, an antiluteolytic protein present in early pregnancy in sheep. *J Reprod Fertil* 1979;56:63–73.

434. Bindon BM. Systematic study of preimplantation stages of pregnancy in the sheep. *Aust J Biol Sci* 1971;24:131–147.
435. Bassett IM, Oxborrow TJ, Smith ID, Thorburn GD. The concentration of progesterone in the peripheral plasma of the pregnant ewe. *J Endocrinol* 1969;45:449–457.
436. Thorburn GD, Cox RI, Currie WB, Restall BJ, Schneider W. Prostaglandin F concentration in the uteroovarian venous plasm of the ewe during the estrous cycle. *J Reprod Fertil* 1973;(suppl)18:151–158.
437. Barcikowski B, Carlson JC, Wilson L, McCracken JA. The effect of endogenous and exogenous estradiol-17β on the release of prostaglandin $F_2\alpha$ from the ovine uterus. *Endocrinology* 1974;95:1340–1349.
438. Peterson AJ, Tervit HR, Fairclough RJ, Havik PG, Smith JF. Jugular levels of 13,14-dihydro-15-keto-prostaglandin F and progesterone around luteolysis and early pregnancy in the ewe. *Prostaglandins* 1976;12:551–558.
439. Zarco L, Stabenfeldt GH, Kindahl H, Bradford GE, Basu S. A detailed study of prostaglandin $F_2\alpha$ release during luteolysis and establishment of pregnancy in the ewe. *Biol Reprod* 1984;(suppl 1)30:153 (abst).
440. Fincher KB, Hanson PJ, Thatcher WW, Roberts RM, Bazer FW. Ovine conceptus secretory proteins suppress induction of prostaglandins $F_2\alpha$ release by estradiol and oxytocin. *J Anim Sci* 1984;(suppl 1)59:369 (abst).
441. Nett TM, Staigmiller RB, Akbar AM, Diekman MA, Ellinwood WE, Niswender GD. Secretion of prostaglandin $F_2\alpha$ in cycling and pregnant ewes. *J Anim Sci* 1976;42:876–880.
442. Lewis GS, Wilson L Jr, Wilks JW, et al. Prostaglandin $F_2\alpha$ and its metabolites in uterine and jugular venous plasma and endometrium of ewes during early pregnancy. *J Anim Sci* 1977;45:320–327.
443. Ellinwood WE, Nett TM, Niswender GD. Maintenance of the corpus luteum of early pregnancy in the ewe. II. Prostaglandin secretion by the endometrium *in vitro* and *in vivo*. *Biol Reprod* 1979;21:845–856.
444. Ottobre JS, Vincent DL, Silvia WJ, Inskeep EK. Aspects of regulation of uterine secretion of prostaglandins during the oestrous cycle and early pregnancy. *Anim Reprod Sci* 1984;7:75–100.
445. Silvia WJ, Ottobre JS, Inskeep EK. Concentrations of prostaglandins E_2, $F_2\alpha$ and 6-keto-prostaglandin $F_1\alpha$ in the utero-ovarian venous plasma of nonpregnant and early pregnant ewes. *Biol Reprod* 1984;30:936–944.
446. Wilson L Jr, Butcher RL, Inskeep EK. Prostaglandin $F_2\alpha$ in the uterus of ewes during early pregnancy. *Prostaglandins* 1972;1:479–482.
447. Findlay JK, Colvin N, Swaney J, Doughton B. Prostaglandin F and 13-14-dihydro-15-keto prostaglandin F in the endometrium and uterine flushings of sheep before implantation. *J Reprod Fertil* 1983;68:343–349.
448. Findlay JK, Ackland N, Burton RD, et al. Protein, prostaglandin and steroid synthesis in caruncular endometrium of sheep before implantation. *J Reprod Fertil* 1981;62:361–377.
449. Silvia WJ. Maintenance of the corpus luteum of early pregnancy in the ewe. Doctoral dissertation, Colorado State University, Fort Collins, 1985.
450. Godkin JD, Bazer FW, Thatcher WW, Roberts RM. Proteins released by cultured day 15-16 conceptuses prolong luteal maintenance when introduced into the uterine lumen of cyclic ewes. *J Reprod Fertil* 1984;71:57–64.
451. Godkin JD, Bazer FW, Moffatt J, Sessions F, Roberts RM. Purification and properties of a major, low molecular weight protein released by the trophoblast of sheep blastocysts at day 13–21. *J Reprod Fertil* 1982;65:141–150.
452. Hyland JH, Manns JG, Humphrey WD. Prostaglandin production by ovine endometrium *in vitro*. *J Reprod Fertil* 1982;65:299–304.
453. LaCroix MC, Kann G. Comparative studies of prostaglandins $F_2\alpha$ and E_2 in late cyclic and early pregnant sheep: *in vitro* synthesis by endometrium and conceptus; effect of *in vivo* indomethacin treatment on establishment of pregnancy. *Prostaglandins* 1982;23:507–526.
454. Gadsby JE, Heap RB, Burton RD. Oestrogen production by blastocyst and early embryonic tissue of various species. *J Reprod Fertil* 1980;60:409–417.
455. Marcus GJ. Prostaglandin formation by the sheep embryo and endometrium as an indication of maternal recognition of pregnancy. *Biol Reprod* 1981;25:56–64.
456. LaCroix MC, Kann G. Discriminating analysis of "*in vitro*" prostaglandin release by myometrial and luminal sides of the ewe endometrium. *Prostaglandins* 1983;25:853–869.
457. Vincent DL, Inskeep EK. Effects of ovariectomy and progesterone replacement on uteroovarian venous prostaglandins (PG). *J Anim Sci* 1984;59(suppl 1):368 (abst).
458. Pratt BR, Butcher RL, Inskeep EK. Antiluteolyic effect of the conceptus and of PGE_2 in ewes. *J Anim Sci* 1977;45:784–791.
459. Magness RR, Huie JM, Weems CW. Effect of chronic ipsilateral or contralateral intrauterine infusion of prostaglandin E_2 (PGE_2) on luteal function of unilaterally ovariectomized ewes. *Prostagland Med* 1981;6:389–401.
460. Colcord ML, Hoyer GL, Weems CW. Effect of prostaglandin E_2 (PGE_2) as an anti-luteolysin in estrogen-induced luteolysis in ewes. *J Anim Sci* 1978;47(suppl 1):352 (abst).
461. Henderson KM, Scaramuzzi RJ, Baird DT. Simultaneous infusion of prostaglandin E_2 antagonizes the luteolytic action of prostaglandin $F_2\alpha$ *in vitro*. *J Endocrinol* 1977;72:379–383.
462. Mapletoft RJ, Miller KF, Ginther OJ. Effects of $PGF_2\alpha$ and PGE_2 on corpora lutea in ewes. *J Anim Sci* 1977;45(suppl 1):185.
463. Reynolds LP, Stigler J, Hoyer WL, et al. Effect of PGE_1 or PGE_2 of $PGF_2\alpha$-induced luteolysis in nonbred ewes. *Prostaglandins* 1981;21:957–972 (abst).
464. Moor RM, Rowson LEA. Local maintenance of the corpus luteum in sheep in embryos transferred to various isolated portions of the uterus. *J Reprod Fertil* 1966;12:539–550.
465. Mapletoft RJ, Del Campo MR, Ginther OJ. Unilateral luteotropic effect of uterine venous effluent of a gravid uterine horn in sheep. *Proc Soc Exp Biol Med* 1975;150:129–133.
466. Mapletoft RJ, Lapin DR, Ginther OJ. The ovarian artery as the final component of the local pathway between a gravid uterine horn and ovary in ewes. *Biol Reprod* 1976;15:414–421.
467. Inskeep EK, Smutny WJ, Butcher RL, Pexton JE. Effects of intrafollicular injections of prostaglandins in nonpregnant and pregnant ewes. *J Anim Sci* 1975;41:1098–1104.
468. Silvia WJ, Niswender GD. Maintenance of the corpus luteum of early pregnancy in the ewe. IV. Changes in luteal sensitivity to prostaglandin $F_2\alpha$ throughout early pregnancy. *J Anim Sci* 1986;63:1201–1207.
469. Wiltbank MC, Wiepz GJ, Knickerbocker JJ, Belfiore CJ, Niswender GD. Proteins secreted from the early ovine conceptus block the action of prostaglandin $F_2\alpha$ on large luteal cells. *Biol Reprod* 1992;46:275–282.
470. Estergreen VL, Frost OL, Gomes WR, Erb RE, Bullard JF. Effect of ovariectomy on pregnancy maintenance and parturition in dairy cows. *J Dairy Sci* 1967;50:1293–1295.
471. Tanabe TY, Hokanson JF, Griel LC. Minimal exogenous progesterone requirements for maintenance of pregnancy in dairy cows after corpus luteum removal via laparotomy. *Proceedings of the 2nd World Conference on Animal Productivity* 1968;370.
472. Wendorf GL, Lawyer MS, First NL. Role of the adrenals in maintenance of pregnancy in cows. *J Reprod Fertil* 1983;68:281–287.
473. Betteridge KG, Egglesome MD, Randall GCB, Mitchell D. Collection, description and transfer of embryos from cattle 10–16 days after oestrus. *J Reprod Fertil* 1980;59:205–216.
474. Northey DL, French LR. Effect of embryo removal and intrauteri infusion of embryonic homogenates on the lifespan of the bovine corpus luteum. *J Anim Sci* 1980;50:298–302.
475. Dalla Pona MA, Humblot P. Effect of embryo removal and embryonic extracts or PGE_2 infusions on luteal function in the bovine. *Theriogenology* 1983;19:122 (abst).
476. Shemesh M, Ayalon N, Lindner HR. Early effect of conceptus on plasma progesterone level in the cow. *J Reprod Fertil* 1968;15:161–164.
477. Pope GS, Gupta SK, Numro IB. Progesterone levels in systemic plasma of pregnant, cycling and ovariectomized cows. *J Reprod Fertil* 1969;20:369–381.
478. Henricks DM, Lamond DR, Hill JR, Dickey JF. Plasma progesterone concentrations before mating and in early pregnancy in the beef heifer. *J Anim Sci* 1971;33:450–454.
479. Erb RE, Garverick HA, Randel RD, Brown BL, Callahan CJ. Profiles of reproductive hormones associated with fertile and nonfertile inseminations of dairy cows. *Theriogenology* 1976;5:227–242.

480. Bulman DC, Lamming GE. Milk progesterone levels in relation to conception, repeat breeding and factors influencing acyclicity in dairy cows. *J Reprod Fertil* 1978;54:447–458.
481. Lukaszewska JH, Hansel W. Corpus luteum maintenance during early pregnancy in the cow. *J Reprod Fertil* 1980;59:485–493.
482. Hansel W. Plasma hormone concentrations associated with early embryo mortality in heifers. *J Reprod Fertil* 1981;30(suppl): 231–239.
483. Kindahl H, Edqvist LE, Bane A, Granstom E. Blood levels of progesterone and 15-keto-13,14-dihydro-prostaglandin $F_{2}\alpha$ during the normal estrous cycle and early pregnancy in heifers. *Acta Endocrinol* 1976;82:134–149.
484. Williams WF, Lewis GS, Thatcher WW, Underwood CS. Plasma 13,14-dihydro-15-keto-$PGF_{2}\alpha$ (PGFM) in pregnant and open heifers prior to and during laparotomy and following intrauterine injection of $PGF_{2}\alpha$. *Prostaglandins* 1983;25:891–899.
485. Thatcher WW, Wolfenson D, Curl JS, et al. Prostaglandin dynamics associated with development of the bovine conceptus. *Anim Reprod Sci* 1984;7:149–176.
486. Knickerbocker JJ, Thatcher WW, Bazer FW, et al. Proteins secreted by cultured day 17 bovine conceptuses extend luteal function in cattle. *Proceedings of The 10th International Congress on Animal Reproduction and Artificial Insemination,* 1984;88 (abst).
487. Knickerbocker JJ, Thatcher WW, Bazer FW, Barron DH, Roberts RM. Inhibition of estradiol-17β (E) induced uterine prostaglandin $F_{2}\alpha$ ($PGF_{2}\alpha$) production by bovine conceptus secretory proteins (CSP). *J Anim Sci* 1984;59(suppl 1):368 (abst).
488. Shemesh MF, Milaguir F, Ayalon N, Hansel W. Steroidogenesis and prostaglandin synthesis by cultured bovine blastocysts. *J Reprod Fertil* 1979;56:181–185.
489. Ely RM, Thatcher FW, Bazer FW, Fields MJ. Steroid metabolism by the bovine uterine endometrium and conceptus. *Biol Reprod* 1983;28:804–816.
490. Chenault JR. Response of bovine corpora lutea to intrauterine prostaglandin E_2 infusion. *J Anim Sci* 1983;57(suppl 1):323–324 (abst).
491. Reynolds LP, Robertson DA, Ford SP. Effects of intrauterine infusion of oestradiol-17β and prostaglandin E_2 on luteal function in nonpregnant heifers. *J Reprod Fertil* 1983;69:703–709.
492. Del Campo MR, Rowe RF, French LR, Ginther OJ. Unilateral relationship of embryos and the corpus luteum in cattle. *Biol Reprod* 1977;16:580–585.
493. Del Campo MR, Mapletoft RJ, Rowe RF, Critser JK, Ginther OJ. Unilateral utero-ovarian relationship in pregnant cattle and role of uterine vein. *Theriogenology* 1980;14:185–193.
494. Marsh JM. The stimulatory effect of PGE_2 on adenyl cyclase in the bovine corpus luteum. *FEBS Lett* 1970;7:283–286.
495. Speroff L, Ramwell PW. Prostaglandin stimulation of *in vitro* progesterone synthesis. *J Clin Endocrinol Metab* 1970;30: 345–350.
496. du Mesnil du Buisson F, Dauzier L. Influence de l'ovariectomie chez la truie pendant la gestation. *C R Soc Biol* 1957;151: 311–313.
497. Ellicott AR, Dzuik PJ. Minimum daily dose of progesterone and plasma concentration for maintenance of pregnancy in ovariectomized gilts. *Biol Reprod* 1973;9:300–304.
498. Guthrie HD, Rexroad CE Jr. Endometrial prostaglandin F release in vitro and plasma 13,14-dihydro-15-keto-prostaglandin F_2 in pigs with luteolysis blocked by pregnancy, estradiol benzoate or human chorionic gonadotropin. *J Anim Sci* 1981;52:330–339.
499. Schille WM, Karlbom I, Einarsson S, Larsson K, Kindahl H, Edqvist LE. Concentration of progesterone and 15-keto-13,14-dihydro-prostaglandin $F_{2}\alpha$ in peripheral plasma during the estrous cycle and early pregnancy in gilts. *Zentralbl Veterinaermed Reihe A* 1979;26:169–181.
500. Watson J, Pack CE. Steroid and prostaglandin secretion by the corpus luteum, endometrium and embryo of cyclic and pregnant gilts. *J Endocrinol* 1979;82:425–428.
501. Zavy MT, Bazer FW, Thatcher WW, Wilcox CJ. A study of prostaglandin $F_{2}\alpha$ as the luteolysis in swine. V. Comparison of prostaglandin F, progestins, estrone and estradiol in uterine flushings from pregnant and nonpregnant gilts. *Prostaglandins* 1980;20: 837–851.
502. Kidder HE, Casida LE, Grummer RH. Some effects of estrogen injections on the estrual cycle of gilts. *J Anim Sci* 1955;14: 470–474.
503. Gardner ML, First NL, Casida LE. Effect of exogenous estrogens on corpus luteum maintenance in gilts. *J Anim Sci* 1963;22: 132–134.
504. Frank M, Bazer FW, Thatcher WW, Wilcox CJ. A study of prostaglandin $F_{2}\alpha$ as the luteolysin in swine. III. Effects of estradiol valerate on prostaglandin F, progestin, estrone and estradiol concentration in the utero-ovarian veins of nonpregnant gilts. *Prostaglandins* 1977;14:1183–1196.
505. Guthrie HD, Lewis GS. Hormone production and [^{3}H]-$PGF_{2}\alpha$ metabolism by endometrium, lung and embryonal membranes of cyclic and pregnant gilts. *J Anim Sci* 1984;59(suppl 1):351 (abst).
506. Geisert RD, Thatcher WW, Roberts RM, Bazer FW. Establishment of pregnancy in the pig: III. Endometrial secretory response to estradiol valerate administered on day 11 of the estrous cycle. *Biol Reprod* 1982;27:957–965.
507. Perry JS, Heap RB, Amoroso EC. Steroid hormone production by pig blastocysts. *Nature* 1973;245:45–47.
508. Heap RB, Flint APF, Hartman PE, et al. Oestrogen production in early pregnancy. *J Endocrinol* 1981;89:77–94.
509. Bazer FW, Thatcher WW. Theory of maternal recognition of pregnancy in swine based on estrogen controlled endocrine versus exocrine secretion of prostaglandin $F_{2}\alpha$ by the uterine endometrium. *Prostaglandins* 1977;14:397–399.
510. Lewis GS, Waterman RA. Metabolism of arachidonic acid *in vitro* by porcine blastocysts and endometrium. *Prostaglandins* 1983;25:871–880.
511. Geisert RD, Renegar RH, Thatcher WW, Roberts RM, Bazer FW. Establishment of pregnancy in the pig: I. Interrelationships between preimplantation development of the pig blastocyst and uterine endometrial secretions. *Biol Reprod* 1982;27:925–939.
512. Holtan DW, Squires DL, Lapin DR, Ginther OJ. Effect of ovariectomy on pregnancy in mares. *J Reprod Fertil* 1979;27(suppl): 395–401.
513. Hershman L, Douglas RH. The critical period for the maternal recognition of pregnancy in pony mares. *J Reprod Fertil* 1979;27(suppl):395–401.
514. Holtan DW, Nett TM, Estergreen VL. Plasma progestins in pregnant, postpartum and cycling mares. *J Anim Sci* 1975;40: 251–260.
515. Nett TM, Pickett BW. Effect of diethylstilbestrol on the relationship between LH, PMSG and progesterone during pregnancy in the mare. *J Reprod Fertil* 1979;27(suppl):465–470.
516. van Niekerk CH, Gemeke WH. Persistence and parthogenetic cleavage of tubal ova in the mare. *Onderspoort J Vet Res* 1966;31:195–232.
517. Leith GS, Ginther OJ. Characterization of intrauterine mobility of the early equine conceptus. *Theriogeneology* 1984;22: 401–408.
518. Mayer RE, Vernon MW, Zavy MT, Bazer FW, Sharp DC. Estrogen production by the early equine conceptus. *Proceedings of the 69th Annual Meeting of The American Society of Animal Science,* 1977;186.
519. Evans MJ, Irvine CHG. Serum concentrations of FSH, LH and progesterone during the estrous cycle and early pregnancy in the mare. *J Reprod Fertil* 1975;23(suppl):193–200.
520. Allen WE. Ovarian changes during gestation in pony mares. *Equine Vet J* 1974;6:135–138.
521. Cole HH, Howell CE, Hart GH. Changes occurring in the ovary of the mare during pregnancy. *Anat Rec* 1931;49:199–210.
522. Squires EL, Stevens WB, Pickett BW, Nett TM. Role of pregnant mare serum gonadotropin in luteal function of pregnant mares. *Am J Vet Res* 1979;40:889–891.
523. Moss GE, Estergreen VL, Becker SR, Grant BD. The source of 5α-pregnanes that occur during gestation in the mare. *J Reprod Fertil* 1979;27:511–519.

The Physiology of Reproduction, Second Edition,
edited by E. Knobil and J.D. Neill,
Raven Press, Ltd., New York © 1994.

CHAPTER 15

Local Nonsteroidal Regulators of Ovarian Function

Alex Tsafriri[1] and Eli Y. Adashi[2]

> *"There should be no other motive for study except gaining knowledge, and there is no other purpose in truth than knowing it is the truth. Only man's ignorance makes him seek another aim for this ultimate aim."*
> RABBI MOSHE BEN MAIMON (MAIMONIDES, 1138–1204) INTRODUCTION TO COMMENTARY TO CHAPTER X OF SANHEDRIN

This thesis of Rabbi Moshe ben Maimon (Maimonides), a most prominent medieval referee of Jewish law, theologian, philosopher, and practicing physician, was originally formulated regarding theology but can be equally well adapted to any scientific endeavor. The quest for knowledge is, and should remain, the prime motivation of any scientific activity. It was argued that because complete understanding of any aspect of nature may be an unrealistic goal never to be attained, perhaps the best that we can hope for is to derive practical applications leading to the betterment of our society. Although the limitations of science and its asymptotic nature cannot be denied, overemphasis of the applied value of scientific inquiry may adversely affect both the advancement of our understanding and, in the long run, the use of this knowledge for human benefit.

In the first edition, it was stated: "The issue of local ovarian regulation, to be overviewed here, is in its forma-

[1] The Bernhard Zondek Hormone Research Laboratory, Department of Hormone Research, The Weizmann Institute of Science, Rehovot, 76100, Israel
[2] Division of Reproductive Endocrinology, Department of Obstetrics and Gynecology, University of Maryland School of Medicine, Baltimore, Maryland 21201

tive stage. This is evidenced by the rapid accumulation of new data and suggestions of additional local mechanisms. This makes it nearly impossible to avoid deletions and to overlook pertinent studies. Hence, this review should be considered merely as an interim account of intraovarian control mechanisms. As such, the emphasis is put on its comprehensiveness, rather than on selectiveness." During the time elapsed since then, the interest in local ovarian regulation increased even further and the attention focused on the possible role and actions of growth factors known from other organs and cell systems. Several reviews (1,2) and multiauthored books (3–8) have been recently published on paracrine regulation of gonadal function.

BACKGROUND

The concept of local gonadal regulators and regulation can be traced to the early days of ovarian research. Thus, differentiation of the gonads was hypothesized by Witchi (9) to result from the interaction of two morphogenetic substances termed *cortexine* and *medullarine.* Cortexine, which was later renamed cortecin (10), was postulated as the inducer of ovarian tissue and medullarine as the inducer of testicular tissue.

The rapid and impressive progress in the understanding of ovarian endocrine function, including production and secretion of steroids (early advances reviewed by refs. 11 and 12) and the regulation of ovarian activity by gonadotropins (reviewed by ref. 13) led to the widely accepted view that the ovary is the source of ova and of steroid hormones and that it is controlled by hypophyseal hormones. Relaxin remained for some time a disturbing and largely neglected exception in this outlook.

Development and application of more refined and sophisticated approaches to the study of reproductive processes and organs such as radioimmunoassays, the vast array of chromatographic techniques, and culture *in vitro* of ovarian follicles, corpora lutea, and isolated cells led to an increase in resolution and hence to a realization of a higher level of complexity in the control of ovarian activity. Studies revealed ovarian nonsteroidal substances exerting biologic effects on the ovary or ovarian cells and other organs. Also, it became increasingly difficult to explain all the fine details of ovarian function by the action of hypophyseal hormones alone. Thus, the initiation of meiosis in fetal ovaries, recruitment of primordial follicles, selection of ovulatory and atretic follicles, and follicular inhibition of precocious oocyte maturation cannot be attributed solely to changes in gonadotropin levels. Therefore, local factors were suggested to be superimposed and to modulate gonadotropin actions on these processes. Furthermore, analysis of ovarian activity revealed yet another type of local regulation, the coordinated production of steroids by granulosa and theca cells, known as the "two-cell hypothesis" (reviewed by ref. 14; Chapter 11 by Gore-Langton and Armstrong, this volume) on the one hand, and the regulatory functions of steroids within the ovary, probably exerted through variation in their local concentration on the other (reviewed in Chapter 11 by Gore-Langton and Armstrong, this volume).

ENDOCRINE, PARACRINE, AND AUTOCRINE REGULATION

The classical definition of endocrinology maintained that a group of cells located in endocrine glands releases chemical messengers, or hormones, which reach their target through the bloodstream and thereby affect other tissues, organs, or body functions (15). This system of communication was in contradistinction to the previously known nervous system. The line of demarcation between these two systems became obscured very early when neurotransmitters were first identified. Recent work revealed a wealth of intercellular communication systems that do not conform with the classical definitions set for either the endocrine or the nervous system (Fig. 1). Thus, for example, hormones were found in organs that were not considered endocrine glands or primary sources of the hormones. Conversely, many messenger molecules that cannot be considered as hormones according to the classical definition, because they reach their target cells without passing through the circulatory system, are indistinguishable from hormones in their structure, interaction with their target cells, and biologic actions. Furthermore, many *bona fide* hormones were also found to act locally without first being transported through the circulation. These and other considerations, including the finding of substances resembling vertebrate hormonal peptides in more primitive multicellular

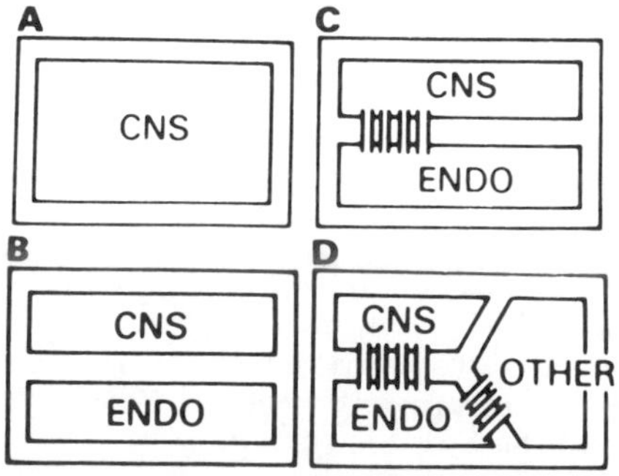

FIG. 1. Evolution of concepts about intercellular communication. **(A)** Central nervous system (*CNS*) was considered to be the unique coordinator among cells of multicellular animals; **(B)** integration and coordination were performed by two separate but equal systems, the CNS and the endocrine system (*ENDO*); **(C)** penetrations in the boundaries that separate the two systems became apparent, especially in recent years; **(D)** there are many examples of intercellular communication that we now recognize that do not fit either system, designated *OTHER.* (From ref. 16, with permission.)

or even unicellular organisms, led to the evolutionary approach unifying all modes of intercellular communication (16,17). According to this approach, intercellular communication by soluble messenger molecules was devised even before the appearance of multicellular organisms. The development of highly specialized cells devoted largely or exclusively to intercellular communication (i.e., nerves and endocrine glands) is the result of extreme cellular differentiation. Thus, the classical endocrine systems inherited their key molecular components (messenger and receptor mechanisms) from simpler unicellular ancestors.

These molecules, whether remaining conserved or undergoing substantial evolution, very often assumed new functions (18,19). Such a comprehensive view encompassing any intercellular chemical messenger molecules as hormones (Fig. 2) discerns three variations of endocrine regulation (Fig. 3). (a) The classical endocrine system—endocrine glands secreting their hormones into the circulation (including blood or lymph) through which they are transported to their target organs or cells. The specialized endocrine glands differ from other hormone secreting cells in their ability to produce large quantities of the hormone, store it, and release it into the circulation on the appropriate trigger. (b) Paracrine control mechanisms—which involve local diffusion of hormone to their target cells (20,21). In primitive organisms lacking a circulatory system or endocrine glands, this is the principal mode of humoral regulation. Paracrine regulation is probably important in vertebrates during early embryonic development before the establishment of circulation and endocrine glands. (c) Autocrine regulation, originally suggested by Sporn and Todaro (22) on the basis of studies with transformed cells "whereby a cell secretes a hormonelike substance for which the cell has functional external receptors." This definition warrants extension, to include not only peptides interacting with external membranal receptors, but to any regulatory molecule that interacts with cellular receptors. Thus, regulatory functions of steroid hormones in the gonads should be included in autocrine regulation, according to this view, provided that cellular production, interaction with receptors, and typical postreceptor responses can be discerned within the same cell type. The term *intracrine regulation* has been suggested, in the meantime, for eucaryotic cells whereby hormones are synthesized and act within a cell without exit and re-entry (23) (Fig. 4).

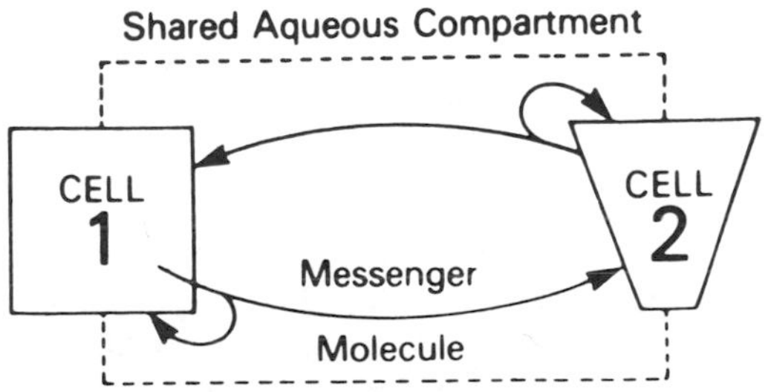

FIG. 2. Features of intercellular communication system. Secretory cell (*cell 1*) synthesizes and releases a soluble messenger (*signal*) into a shared aqueous compartment and acts on target cell (*cell 2*). In classical endocrine system, cell 1 is a glandular cell, signal molecule is a hormone, and shared aqueous compartment is blood, whereas in nervous system, cell 1 is a neuron, signal molecule a neurotransmitter, and shared aqueous compartment a synapse. Applying the term *hormone* to any intercellular messenger molecule extends endocrine interactions to include paracrine and endocrine regulation (see Fig. 3). (From ref. 16, with permission.)

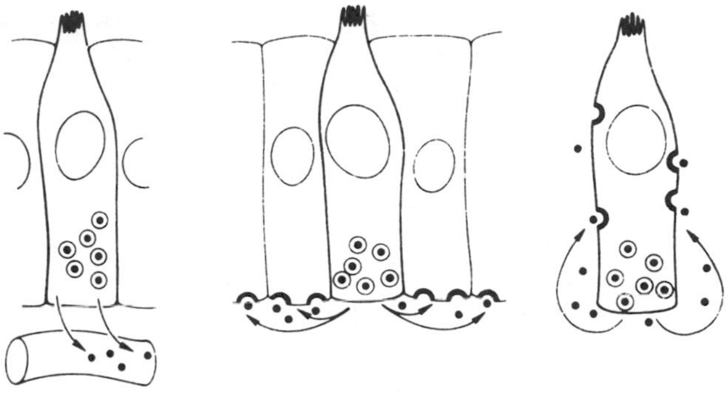

FIG. 3. Diagramatic representation of variants of communication used by hormonal system. Regulatory chemical messengers are shown in latent form within the cell. Thickened, semicircular regions of cell membrane represent receptor sites, but receptors to some hormones may be intracellular. (From ref. 22, with permission.)

Several terms were suggested for intercellular messenger molecules that do not conform to the classical definition of hormone regulatory or growth factors, regulins, chemitters (24), and cybernins (25). Except for the general term *factor,* none of the specific terms caught on. It will be most proper to extend our definition of hormone to all intercellular regulatory messenger molecules and adopt the radical suggestion of O'Malley (26) to concentrate on hormones and their functions, rather than glands and hormones. Hence, throughout this review, the term *hormone* will be applied to any regulatory messenger molecules.

OVARIAN, PARACRINE, AND AUTOCRINE REGULATION

Sharpe (2) suggested the following criteria for intragonadal hormones: (a) There is evidence that the hormone is produced within the gonad; (b) receptors for this hormone are present within the gonad; and (c) there are demonstrated biologic actions within the gonad. Ideally, only hormones that fulfill all three criteria should be considered as intragonadal hormones. Nevertheless, at present, most of the nonsteroidal hormones to be included in paracrine or autocrine regulation of ovarian function

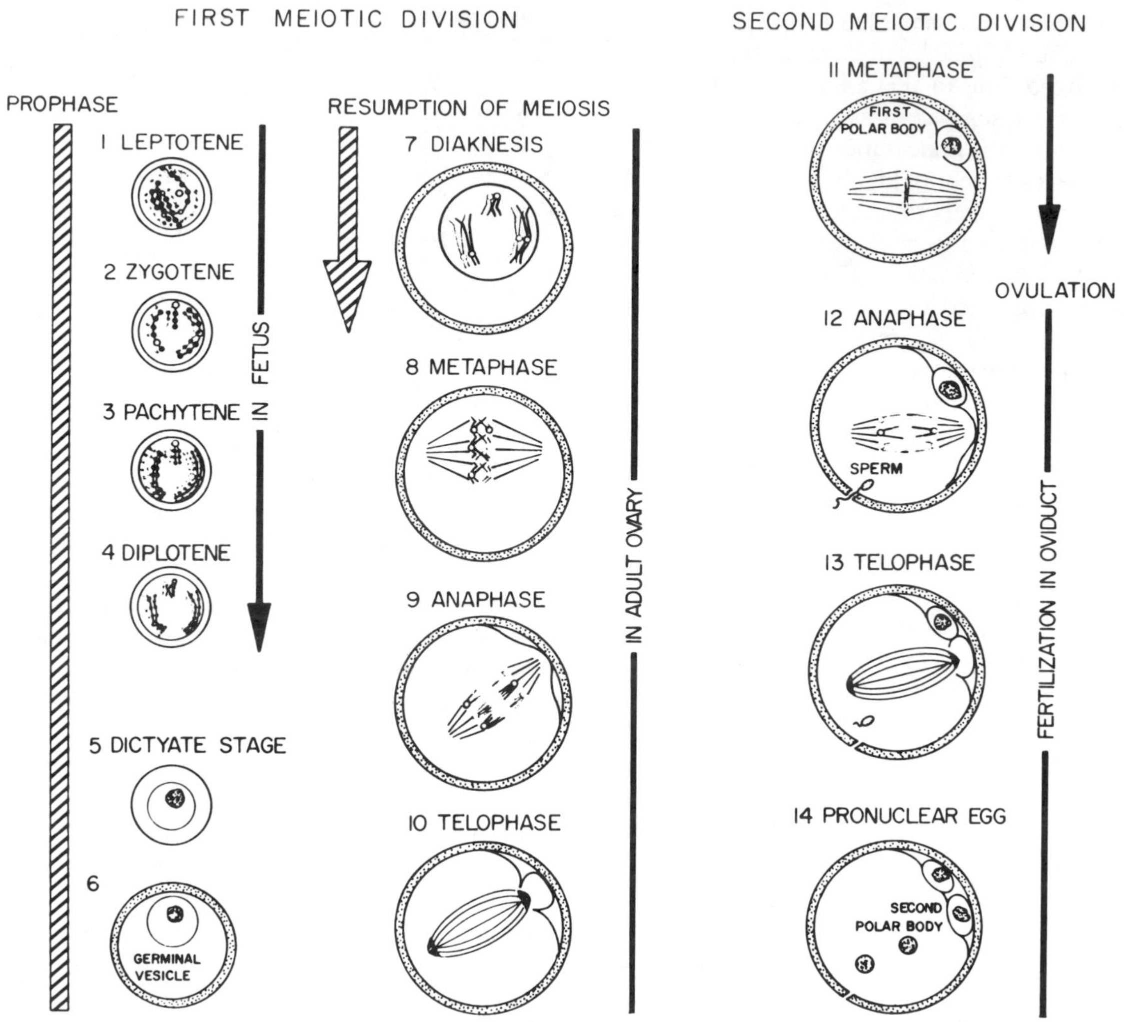

FIG. 4. Oocyte meiosis. For simplicity, only three pairs of chromosomes are depicted. (*1–4*) Prophase stages of first meiotic division that occur in most mammals during fetal life. At zygotene (*2*), homologous maternal and paternal chromosomes begin to pair. At pachytene (*3*), they are paired along their entire length, thus forming bivalents. During pachytene, each homolog cleaves longitudinally to form two sister chromatids, so that each bivalent forms a tetrad. During this stage, interchange of genetic material between maternal and paternal chromatids may occur by crossing over. At diplotene (*4*), chromosomes begin to separate, remaining united at chiasmata. Meiotic process is arrested at this stage (first meiotic arrest), and oocyte enters dictyate stage. When meiosis is resumed, first maturation division is completed (*7–11*). Ovulation usually occurs at metaphase II stage (*11*) (second meiotic arrest), and second meiotic division (*12–14*) is completed in oviduct after sperm penetration. (From ref. 37, with permission.)

cannot withstand rigorous examination by these three criteria. In most cases, the hormone has not been chemically characterized, and hence no receptor binding studies could be performed and unequivocal evidence for local production could be obtained. Furthermore, the intragonadal function is deduced in few cases from *in vivo* and in most cases from *in vitro* model systems that do not necessarily represent the physiologic situation. Therefore, we have included here as intraovarian hormones those fulfilling two more lenient criteria: (a) They are found in the ovary and there is no evidence of extraovarian origin; and (b) a biologic effect of the hormone can be demonstrated on the ovary *in situ* or *in vitro* or on ovarian cell preparations *in vitro*.

Adoption of these two criteria results in a chemically mixed group of substances, amines, peptides, steroids, and eicosanoids (Table 1). Some are chemically characterized and have, also, extraovarian source(s) and targets. In this group, we may name, for example, steroids, eicosanoids (prostaglandins and hydroperoxides), platelet-activating factor (PAF), oxytocin, vasopressin, and pro-opiomelanocortin-derived peptides. Another group, more difficult to deal with, is that of ovarian factors eliciting biologic responses in ovarian tissue and that are still in the process of chemical characterization and purification, such as follicular regulatory proteins (FRP); oocyte maturation inhibitor (OMI), luteinizing hormone (LH) and follicle-stimulating hormone (FSH)

TABLE 1. *Putative paracrine/autocrine regulators of ovarian function*

Hormone	Refer to[1]
Activin	(W.W. Vale) Characterization of OMI; TGFβ and Related Peptides
Adenosine	Adenosine and Other Purines
Angiogenic factor	Ovarian Angiogenesis, FGF and Other Growth Factors
Catecholamine	Neurotransmitters
Cytokine	Intraovarian Cytokines
Epidermal growth factor (EGF)	EGF and TGFα
Eicosanoid	Eicosanoids
Fibroblast growth factor (FGF)	Ovarian Angiogenesis, FGF and Other Growth Factors
Follicular regulatory protein(s) (FRP)	FOLLICULAR REGULATORY PROTEIN
Follistatin	(W.W. Vale) Characterization of OMI; TGFβ and Related Peptides
FSH binding inhibitor (FSH-BI); FSH receptor binding competitor (FRBC)	GONADOTROPIN BINDING INHIBITORS
γ-Aminobutyric acid (GABA)	Neurotransmitters
GnRH-like peptide	GnRH-LIKE PEPTIDES
Inhibin	(W.W. Vale) Characterization of OMI; TGTβ and Related Peptides
Insulinlike growth factor (IGF)	Intraovarian IGF System
Interleukin-1 (IL-1)	Intraovarian Cytokines
LH binding inhibitor (LH-BI)	GONADOTROPIN BINDING INHIBITORS
Luteinizing inhibitor (LI) or atretogenic factor	REGULATORS OF LUTEINIZATION
Luteinization stimulator (LS) or maturation stimulator	REGULATORS OF LUTEINIZATION
Müllerian inhibiting substance (MIS)/anti-Müllerian hormone (AMH)	(W.W. Vale) Characterization of OMI; TGTβ and Related Peptides
Oocyte maturation inhibitor (OMI)	OOCYTE MATURATION INHIBITOR
Ovarian growth stimulator(s)	Ovarian Growth Stimulating Actions
Oxytocin	Neurohypophyseal Hormones
Ovarian renin-angiotensin system (OVRAS)	The Ovarian Renin Angiotensin System
Pro-opiomelanocortin-derived hormones	Pro-Opiomelanocortin-Derived Hormones
Relaxin	(O.D. Sherwood)
Steroid	(R.E. Gore-Langton, DT) D.T. Armstrong & P. Leung; G.S. Greenwald & S. Roy)
Substance P	Neurotransmitters
Transforming growth factor α (TGFα)	EGF and TGFα
Transforming growth factor β	(W.W. Vale) Characterization of OMI; TGFβ and Related Peptides
Tumor necrosis factor (TNF)	Intraovarian Cytokines
Vasoactive intestinal peptide (VIP)	Neurotransmitters
Vasopressin	Neurohypophyseal Hormones
Vascular endothelial growth factor (VEGF)	Ovarian Angiogenesis, FGF and Other Growth Factors

[1] Refers to sections in this chapter; names in parens refer to other chapters in this volume.

binding inhibitors (LH-BI; FSH-BI) luteinization stimulator (LS) and inhibitor (LI). Because their chemical nature has not as yet been elucidated, some of them may turn out to be similar or identical to other hormones or some of their disparate activities may be assigned to the same molecule. The purification of these factors is proceeding very slowly partly because of the very nature of these factors and partly because of inadequacies in our assay and purification procedures. Acting locally, they are produced in minuscule quantities and act within discrete areas, some of them seemingly unstable and possibly subject to very rapid degradation. They appear to act in conjunction with other hormones, such as gonadotropins and steroids, and to assume a modulatory role. Therefore, their action may differ substantially according to the physiologic or endocrine status of the gonad. In comparison with the classical endocrine hormones, which can be considered as "macroregulators," the autocrine and paracrine hormones seem to be mainly involved in fine tuning. These biologic characteristics pose major practical difficulties for purification, particularly in two areas, the assay systems used to monitor purification and insufficient resolution of the purification procedures. Most of the *in vitro* assays are slow and cumbersome, and there is always the question of their relevance to physiologic regulation. Moreover, the lack of standard preparations and assay procedures makes it very difficult to compare results of different research groups. The sources of putative intraovarian regulators, follicular fluid (FF), ovarian extracts, and conditioned tissue culture media are extremely complex and variable according to subtle physiologic and endocrine conditions and impose high demands on the purification procedure. Finally, the factor isolated from FF or other biologic sources may not be the potent native hormone but a chemically modified product retaining some of the original activity or mimicking the action of an unrelated hormone. Because of these difficulties, relatively slow progress has been achieved in the research of these putative ovarian factors as compared with the evergrowing number of growth factors, well characterized in other cell systems, implicated in ovarian physiology. Nevertheless, such studies with growth factors, mostly based on *in vitro* actions on ovarian cells, should be extended to other model systems, and their physiologic relevance corroborated.

The present state of our knowledge does not permit a consistent classification of ovarian hormones according to either their precise chemical nature or ovarian function. Hence, they will be grouped as convenient, according to any of these criteria. Steroids are synthesized in the ovary, and their intraovarian receptors and actions have been convincingly demonstrated, in addition to their extragonadal effects. Steroids belong, therefore, to intraovarian hormones but will be dealt with elsewhere in this volume (Chapter 11 by Gore-Langton and Armstrong and Chapter 12 by Greenwald and Terranova). Likewise, eicosanoids (prostaglandins and hydroperoxides) are discussed in Chapter 13 by Espey and relaxin in Chapter 18 by Sherwood in this volume, and hence their intragonadal actions are described here only briefly.

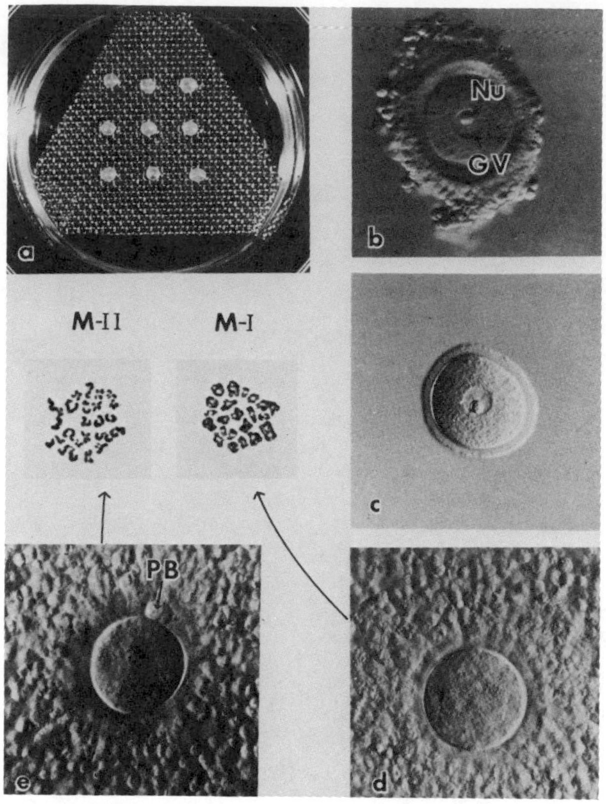

FIG. 5. Oocyte maturation in rat. (*a*) Explanted preovulatory follicles. (*b–e*) Oocytes viewed with Nomarski interference optics: isolated oocyte cultured with its intact cumulus mass (*b*). *GV*, germinal vesicle; *Nu*, nucleolus. (*c*) Denuded oocyte. (*d*) GVBD; *M-I* (**inset**), bivalents in metaphase I. (*e*) Secondary oocyte. *PB*, polar body; *M-II* (**inset**), chromosomes (dyads) seen at metaphase II. Chromosomes were prepared according to method of Tarkowski (1966) and photographed under phase contrast. (From ref. 37, with permission.)

OOCYTE MATURATION INHIBITOR

Life History of the Mammalian Ovum

Meiotic maturation in the mammalian female is a protracted process, subject to multiple stop–go controls. Meiotic maturation in mammalian oocytes is initiated during prenatal life or shortly after birth, but the process is arrested (*first meiotic arrest*) at the diplotene stage, usually referred to as the dictyate stage of the prophase of first meiotic division (Fig. 4). The meiotic arrest is maintained throughout oocyte and follicular development to the Graafian follicle stage. *In vivo* the meiotic process is resumed only in fully grown oocytes in follicles responding to the preovulatory surge of gonadotropins (27) or in follicles undergoing atresia (reviewed by ref. 28). At ovulation, in most mammalian species, a secondary oocyte arrested at the metaphase of the second meiotic division (*second meiotic arrest*) is released. The second meiotic division is completed only after fertilization or a parthenogenetic stimulus by abstriction of the second polar body.

The mechanism(s) involved in the regulation of meiosis in the fetus remains obscure. It has been proposed that meiosis in mammals is regulated by products of the somatic cells of the gonad: a meiosis-inducing substance (MIS) and a meiosis-promoting substance (MPS) (29). This suggestion is based on experiments in which MIS activity was demonstrated by the ability to promote meiosis in fetal mouse testis *in vitro,* whereas MPS retarded the initiation of meiosis in fetal mouse ovaries *in vitro* (29). That the somatic compartment of the ovary influences the meiotic behavior of germ cells is further supported by the observation that the first meiotic arrest coincides with folliculogenesis (i.e., enclosure of the germ cells with somatic cells) and that oocytes, which do not become enclosed with follicle cells, usually undergo further abortive meiotic changes and degenerate (30).

Here, the paracrine regulation of the progress of the dictyate oocyte to the metaphase of the second meiotic division is reviewed. We regard these changes as resumption of meiosis (or of maturation) or ovum maturation, even though it does encompass only a limited aspect of the meiotic process. The first change associated with preovulatory resumption of meiosis (i.e., the breakdown of the germinal vesicle [GVBD]) is most easily observed by microscopic observation of the ovum and hence frequently used as an experimental criterion for ovum maturation (Figs. 4 and 5). Being an early change, this seems to be a proper criterion when the study is aimed at the identification of mechanisms controlling the resumption of meiosis. However, GVBD should not be considered as an indicator of fertilizability of the ovum or of its competence to produce a viable embryo (31–33).

The resumption of meiosis in nonatretic follicles *in vivo* is critically dependent on the preovulatory surge of gonadotropins. Blocking the surge by pentobarbitone or similar drugs prevents ovum maturation as well as other ovulatory changes (27), and administration of exogenous LH to pentobarbitone-treated rats results in GVBD within 2.5 to 3.5 hr (34,35).

Three *in vitro* models have been used for investigating hormonal and follicular control of meiotic maturation in mammalian oocytes (Fig. 5). The simplest is that established by Pincus and Enzmann (36), who demonstrated that rabbit oocytes liberated from their follicles undergo spontaneous maturation in culture without any need for hormonal stimulation. Such spontaneous maturation of oocytes cultured either denuded of their cumulus cells or within their cumulus complex has been confirmed in all mammalian species examined (reviewed by ref. 37) and has been widely used for studying some physiologic aspects of oocyte maturation. However, oocytes isolated from preantral follicles do not resume meiosis spontaneously in culture. The ability to mature spontaneously *in vitro* ("meiotic competence") is acquired only when the oocyte enters its final stage of growth. Meiotic competence is gradually acquired at the age of 15 to 21 days in mice (38,39) and 20 to 26 days in rats (40). The development of meiotic competence appears to be regulated by FSH, an action that is at least partially mediated by follicular estrogen production (41). In the second model, consisting of explanted preovulatory follicles, resumption of meiosis is dependent on hormonal stimulation *in vivo* or *in vitro* (42). This model has been used extensively for studying the hormonal control of resumption of meiosis in a variety of mammalian species (37,42–48).

The finding that oocytes removed from their follicle mature spontaneously in culture whereas maturation in follicle-enclosed oocytes is dependent on hormonal stimulation led to the suggestion that within the follicle meiosis is prevented through follicular inhibitory action. To test this hypothesis, a third *in vitro* model was adopted: coculture of oocytes with different follicular components (49–58). Such studies corroborated the concept of follicular inhibitory action and led to partial characterization and purification of a factor, OMI (recently reviewed by refs. 1, 59, and 60). However, the coculture of oocytes with follicular components can hardly restore the precise follicular interactions between the ovum and its micromilieu. Furthermore, OMI, purified from the FF, may not necessarily be the native molecule regulating meiosis on direct transfer from follicle cells to the ovum through the gap junctions connecting these two follicular compartments. At the most, we can hope for an approximation and the gaining of some insight into the paracrine mechanisms participating in follicular control of meiosis *in situ*. Here, an overview of the present status of paracrine regulation of ovum maturation is presented.

Paracrine Regulation of Ovum Maturation

The spontaneous maturation of isolated oocytes in culture led Pincus and Enzmann (36) to suggest that follicle cells in mammals "supply to the ovum a substance or substances which directly inhibit nuclear maturation." This suggestion was supported by the inhibition of the resumption of meiosis of porcine oocytes cocultured with segments of follicle wall, but not with its theca layer (50,61) or ovarian bursa (53). Similarly, when porcine oocytes (up to 12) were transferred to host follicles and cultured in hormone-free medium, maturation was prevented (48,62) and maturation of rat oocytes injected into porcine follicles was markedly delayed (62). Further, coculture of porcine oocytes with porcine granulosa cells inhibited the spontaneous resumption of meiosis (51,63). The inhibitory effect of granulosa cells depended on their concentration in culture. Granulosa cells collected from small follicles inhibited meiosis more effectively than cells from medium or large follicles (51,64). Similarly, when rat oocytes were added to rat granulosa cells previously cultured for 24 or 48 hr, resumption of meiosis was suppressed and the degree of inhibition depended on the number of granulosa cells in the culture. This inhibitory effect of rat granulosa cells was reversed by the addition of LH to the cocultures (65,66).

Extracts of granulosa cells, as well as granulosa cell-conditioned medium (i.e., a medium in which granulosa cells were cultured previously), inhibited the resumption of meiosis (52,64,66–70). Collectively, these results suggest that within the follicle meiosis is kept in abeyance by an OMI produced by granulosa cells.

Follicular fluid from ovaries of rabbit, ovine, bovine, porcine, hamster, and human origin exerted an inhibitory effect on the spontaneous maturation of isolated oocytes (49,51,52,71,72). This inhibitory effect is not species-specific (52,65,72,73). The OMI activity in porcine FF appears to decline in the course of follicular growth. This was demonstrated by assaying FF freshly collected from small, medium, and large follicles (74) or fluid collected from pigs on specified days of their reproductive cycle (75). Similarly, in FF collected from women participating in *in vitro* fertilization-embryo transfer programs, the OMI activity was significantly lower in follicles yielding mature and fertilizable oocytes as compared with follicles yielding immature or atretic oocytes (73,76,77). The lower OMI activity in human FF from large follicles was recently associated with its epidermal growth factor (EGF) content (78), which has been shown to induce maturation of follicle-enclosed oocytes (79,80).

Characterization of OMI

Assays of OMI

Pig oocytes from either medium or large follicles were frequently used for bioassay of OMI (51,59,77,81). This assay requires a steady source of many porcine ovaries, a long incubation period (42–44 hr), and fixation and staining of the ova after the incubation. Rat (65,76) and mouse (82,83) oocytes were also used for assaying OMI. Murine oocytes are widely available, and the culture period is much shorter (up to 4–6 hr). Nevertheless, OMI assays involving mammalian ova are cumbersome and tedious, require experienced personnel, and can be applied only to a limited number of samples.

Recently, inhibitory effects of human FF on maturation of amphibian oocytes were demonstrated (84,85). It is postulated that the inhibition resulted from the presence of OMI in this fluid (73). Toad oocytes were used to monitor the purification of OMI from porcine FF (86).

At present, two biochemically different entities are proposed as putative follicular OMI, a yet unidentified peptide and hypoxanthine or other purine bases or metabolites. These studies are reviewed in the following sections.

Characterization and Purification of OMI

OMI as a Peptide

Tsafriri and colleagues (67) reported that OMI passed through an Amicon PM-10 filter that has a molecular weight cut-off of 10,000. Chromatography of the concentrated filtrate on Sephadex G-25 revealed that OMI had a molecular weight less than 2,000 and that two peaks of activity were present. OMI activity was lost on FF treatment with trypsin but was retained after freezing and thawing, treating with charcoal, and heating to 60°C for 20 min (67). Unpublished experiments (S. H. Pomerantz) showed that bacterial protease from *Streptomyces griseus* (Sigma) destroyed all of the OMI activity of a partially purified Biogel P2 fraction. Treatment of the same fraction with trypsin left no significant activity. These results are all consistent with OMI being a peptide of low molecular weight. Oocyte maturation inhibitor from bovine FF and granulosa cells appears to have similar properties (52,68,69).

The current procedure exploits the acidic nature of OMI. First, pig FF is filtered through an Amicon PM-10 filter and the filtrate passed through YC05 filter. The retentate is diluted to 50 mOsm/kg and passed onto a column of QAE-Sephadex. This strongly basic ion exchange resin binds OMI; the latter is eluted from the column with a steep gradient of NH_4HCO_3. Two peaks of OMI activity are detected by assays with pig oocytes. The combined active peaks are then treated by chromatography on reverse phase and gel filtration HPLC. Two active peaks were obtained. The purification from FF is about 20,000-fold, with a combined recovery of about 34% (86).

Recently several peptides, known from other systems, have been implicated in the regulation of meiosis. Thus, inhibition of spontaneous maturation of rat, but not mouse, oocytes by Müllerian inhibiting substance was reported (87). However, using a purified preparation, we could not detect any OMI-like activity (88). The inhibition of maturation by human recombinant Müllerian inhibiting substance was dependent on the presence of a detergent, Nonidet P-40 (89). Nevertheless, we have observed deleterious effects of the detergent on rat oocytes *in vitro* (90). Another member of the transforming growth factor (TGF) β family, inhibin, was shown to exert OMI-like activity with an ED_{50} of 4.0 nM (91). Using lower doses of inhibin (1.5 nM), we did not observe any inhibitory action on the spontaneous maturation of rat oocytes, but both TGFβ and inhibin attenuated the effect of LH on the maturation of follicle-enclosed rat oocytes (92). Buscaglia and colleagues (93) reported that the 35-kDa, but not 32-kDa follistatin, inhibited the maturation of rat oocytes. Furthermore, an antiserum toward the 27-amino-acid carboxy terminal of 35-kDa follistatin neutralized the OMI action of porcine FF. Although we could not confirm the inhibitory activity of 35-kDa follistatin, we confirmed the abolition of the inhibition of partially purified OMI by the antibody toward its carboxy-terminal peptide (Veljkovic, Ling, and Tsafriri, unpublished observations). In view of the recent demonstration that follistatin binds inhibin and activin (94,95), it is possible that members of the TGFβ family and follistatin are involved in the regulation of resumption of meiosis.

OMI as a Purine Base

By the use of mouse oocytes as an assay system, an inhibitory effect of porcine FF was demonstrated, and this inhibition was potentiated by cyclic AMP (82,83). By monitoring purification of OMI from porcine FF, Downs and colleagues (96) reached the conclusion that hypoxanthine is the predominant low-molecular-weight component of porcine FF that inhibits mouse oocyte maturation. This conclusion is based on the findings that the potent inhibitory fraction of porcine FF (a) had an absorption maximum (250 nm) identical to that of hypoxanthine; (b) had a retention time on HPLC of pure hypoxanthine; (c) inhibited oocyte maturation identical to that exhibited by a commercial preparation of hypoxanthine; and (d) hypoxanthine concentration of about 1.41

mM in porcine FF could account for most of the inhibitory activity of porcine FF on mouse oocytes. Likewise, Chari et al. (76), using human FF, did not find reduction in OMI activity by proteolytic treatment, thus supporting the notion that it is not a peptide. The concentrations of hypoxanthine (2–4 mM) and of adenosine (0.35–0.70 mM) in mouse FF could account for inhibition of oocyte maturation, because even lower concentration of these two purines combined inhibited the spontaneous maturation of mouse oocytes during a 24-hr incubation period *in vitro* (97). Nevertheless, the same authors were unable to detect a reduction in FF hypoxanthine and adenosine concentration 2 hr after human chorionic gonadotropin (hCG) administration (i.e., just before GVBD). It is possible that the concentration of these purines in FF does not necessarily reflect their levels within the oocyte, which are probably more relevant for maintenance of meiotic arrest. Hypoxanthine or adenosine were not detected in bovine FF, despite the presence of a low-molecular-weight component that was inhibitory for ovum maturation (Eppig, personal communication).

Purine bases were demonstrated to modulate levels of cyclic AMP, most probably by inhibiting cyclic AMP-phosphodiesterase activity (96). Furthermore, microinjection of oocytes with an inhibitor of cyclic AMP-dependent protein kinase (PKI) induced the resumption of meiosis in oocytes cultured in medium supplemented with hypoxanthine or guanosine (98). It seems, therefore, that purines affect resumption of meiosis by raising intraoocyte cyclic AMP to levels inhibitory for meiosis (see Role of cyclic AMP in Regulation of Meiosis). Such action of purine bases does not exclude the possibility of other follicular factors suppressing in parallel the resumption of meiosis. Indeed, Downs and colleagues (96) observed an additional inhibitory fraction that was not removed by charcoal extraction. The resistance of OMI activity to proteolytic activity cannot be taken as conclusive evidence that OMI is not a peptide. A small peptide may be a very poor substrate for proteases, and/or the appropriate sensitive peptide bonds may not be present. Hence, the final identification of OMI as a purine base or a peptide must await confirmation in several mammalian test systems. Furthermore, the recent identification of multiple mechanisms controlling ovarian cell activity supports the notion that resumption of meiosis may also be regulated by more than one factor. We discuss this issue further in the next section.

OMI as a Physiologic Regulator of Ovum Maturation

Reversibility of Inhibition by Follicular Factor(s)

To serve as a physiologic regulator of meiosis, a substance has to fulfill the following criteria: (a) It should be present in a compartment relevant to regulation of meiosis at the proper timing; (b) its action should be reversible with no adverse effects on further stages of ovum maturation, fertilization, and embryonic development; (c) the physiologic trigger of resumption of meiosis (gonadotropin) should be able to either bypass its inhibitory action or cause its degradation or removal from the relevant compartment. The inhibitory action of porcine FF and of its partially purified fractions could be reversed by either transferring the oocytes after an initial 24-hr incubation with the inhibitor to a medium without OMI (74,99) or by the addition of an antibody prepared against the low-molecular-weight fraction of porcine FF (66). Likewise, the inhibition of maturation of mouse oocytes by hypoxanthine and adenosine (96,100) was completely reversible by withdrawal of the purines; 47% of the ova were competent of fertilization and 30% of these developed to the expanded blastocyst stage (96,100). Thus, the inhibition of meiosis, by the apparently peptide OMI from porcine FF and by purine bases, appears not to be due to a toxic and irreversible action.

In vivo or in follicle-enclosed oocytes *in vitro*, resumption of meiosis is induced by LH. Hence, the ability of LH (or other gonadotropins) to overcome the inhibition of meiosis by FF or by coculture with granulosa cells lends support for the physiologic role of OMI in the regulation of meiosis. It was found that the addition of LH to cultures of porcine oocytes with porcine FF or its purified fractions overcame their inhibition of meiosis (51). Also, the inhibitory action of bovine or hamster FF (52), of porcine FF, and of rat granulosa cell "conditioned" medium as well as coculture with rat granulosa cells (65,66) were all alleviated by the addition of LH, closely resembling the regulation *in vivo* of oocyte maturation. Likewise, FSH induced the resumption of meiosis in the presence of hypoxanthine (101). Therefore, the peptide OMI and hypoxanthine fulfill the criteria of physiologic regulators of meiosis.

Role of cyclic AMP in Regulation of Meiosis

Many of the agents inducing the maturation of follicle-enclosed oocytes *in vitro* also stimulate production of cyclic AMP (42,102). Injection of the cyclic AMP derivative dibutyryl cyclic AMP (dbcAMP) into the follicular antrum (42) or short-term exposure of follicles to 8-bromo-cyclic AMP (103), dbcAMP, or isobutyl methyl xanthine (IBMX) (104) all triggered the resumption of meiosis. By contrast, the continuous presence of cyclic AMP derivatives or several inhibitors of phosphodiesterase prevented the induction of meiosis by LH (72,102,104). The spontaneous maturation of isolated oocytes from mice and rats was prevented in the presence of cyclic AMP derivatives or phosphodiesterase inhibitors (47,103,105,106).

It seems, therefore, that enhanced production of cyclic AMP in the somatic cell compartment of the follicle is involved in the mediation of the meiosis-inducing action of LH, whereas elevated cyclic AMP in the oocyte inhibits the resumption of meiosis. It has been suggested that cyclic AMP serves as a physiologic regulator of meiosis in mammalian oocytes (102,104,106,107). Indeed, a decrease in oocyte cyclic AMP precedes resumption of meiosis, and when this decrease is prevented, resumption of meiosis is blocked or substantially delayed (108–110). Likewise, incubation of rat oocytes with an invasive adenylate cyclase from bacteria of the genus *Bordetella* elevated oocyte cyclic AMP levels and inhibited resumption of meiosis; removal of the enzyme resulted in a drop of oocyte cyclic AMP levels and meiosis (111,112). These results support the notion that elevated levels of oocyte cyclic AMP maintain meiotic arrest and that an intraoocyte drop in cyclic AMP allows the resumption of meiosis.

Studies using forskolin, a potent and reversible activator of adenylate cyclase, provide further support for this hypothesis. Addition of forskolin to the medium induced resumption of meiosis in rat follicle-enclosed oocytes (113). By contrast, forskolin inhibited the spontaneous maturation of cumulus-enclosed oocytes and had no effect on the maturation of denuded oocytes (114,115). Similar results were obtained when cholera toxin was used (107). These results seem to indicate that (a) activation of adenylate cyclase in the whole follicle leads to the resumption of meiosis; (b) activation of adenylate cyclase in the cumulus–oocyte complex results in inhibition of meiosis; and (c) the oocyte is devoid of adenylate cyclase or the level of cyclic AMP produced by the oocyte is not sufficient to maintain meiotic arrest. Indeed, evidence for transfer of cyclic AMP from the cumulus cells to the ovum has been obtained in rat, mouse, hamster, and porcine oocytes (114–119). These studies leave little doubt regarding the important role of oocyte cyclic AMP in the resumption of meiosis in mammals. However, the question of whether the oocyte synthesizes a sufficient amount of cyclic AMP to inhibit meiosis and whether cyclic AMP is transferred from the cumulus to the oocyte was answered by contrasting experimental results. Thus, although forskolin did not affect the resumption of meiosis in denuded oocytes of the rat (114,115) and hamster (119), in other studies it was inhibitory in mouse (120), rat (121), and pig (116) denuded oocytes. The varying results may be related, at least in part, to species and strain differences, as well as to the experimental procedures used. Quantitative differences among species or even strains in oocyte adenylate cyclase, coupled with differences in cumulus cell–oocyte transport of cyclic AMP, can easily be envisioned. Examination of these parameters in several species supports this notion (see above). Nevertheless, the essential role of oocyte cyclic AMP and other cyclic nucleotides in the regulation of mammalian meiosis seems well established (see ref. 122). The observed synergism of cyclic AMP and OMI in inhibiting spontaneous maturation *in vitro* of isolated oocytes (59,123,124) is suggestive of interaction of cyclic-AMP and follicular OMI in the control of oocyte maturation. This concept further emphasizes the multifactorial control of resumption of meiosis.

Role of Cumulus Cells

The cumulus cells appear to have an important role in the regulation of meiosis. Whereas OMI from porcine FF inhibited the resumption of meiosis by oocytes cultured within their intact cumuli, it did not interfere with the maturation of denuded oocytes of the pig (125) or rat (126). By contrast, porcine FF attenuated maturation of mouse denuded oocytes. Nevertheless, in this study, too, the suppression of resumption of meiosis in mouse denuded oocytes was consistently less than in cumulus-enclosed oocytes (82). It appears, therefore, that the inhibitory action of OMI on meiosis is exerted, at least partially, through the mediation of cumulus cells.

The cumulus cells are, apparently, involved also in the mediation of the meiosis-inducing action of LH. Whereas it was not possible to demonstrate specific receptors of LH on the oocyte, specific LH/hCG receptors were demonstrated on cumulus cells (127,128). This finding was further supported by the response of the whole oocyte–cumulus complex to gonadotropins, involving enhanced steroidogenesis (128–130), lactate production (131), cumulus mucification (132,133), and activation of adenylate cyclase (134). Luteinizing hormone accelerated resumption of meiosis in mouse oocytes pretreated with dbcAMP and IBMX, and LH was effective only in oocytes cultured within their cumulus complex but not in denuded oocytes (106,107,135). It was suggested that acceleration of meiosis by LH is mediated by an increase in cumulus cell cyclic AMP levels, which promotes a decrease in maturation inhibitors.

That granulosa cells produce an inhibitor of resumption of meiosis has been suggested recently by the use of puromycin. Thus, although cycloheximide blocked the maturation of pig cumulus-enclosed oocytes even at low doses (1 μg/ml) (136,137), the inhibitory effect of puromycin was observed only at higher doses, whereas lower doses stimulated meiosis under certain conditions (138). In denuded or cumulus-enclosed oocytes, only 50 μg/ml and higher doses of puromycin inhibited the spontaneous resumption of meiosis. By contrast, cumulus-enclosed oocytes culture attached to their membrana granulosa—which remains immature unless stimulated by gonadotropin (139)—underwent GVBD in the presence of 17 to 25 μg/ml puromycin, and higher doses (50–75 μg/ml) were inhibitory (138). The stimulation of resumption of meiosis in the presence of granulosa cells by puromycin indicates that the inhibition of meiosis by granulosa cells entails protein synthesis.

Germinal vesicle breakdown in rat (66), mouse (140,141), and rabbit (142) isolated oocytes maturing spontaneously occurs 1 to 2 hr earlier than GVBD in follicle-enclosed oocytes stimulated by LH. This suggests that by isolating an oocyte from its follicle, some regulatory step(s) essential for triggering meiosis *in vivo* is bypassed. This may include merely the removal of the inhibitory signal (OMI) by decreased synthesis, increased degradation, or a combination of both or, alternatively, the generation of a positive signal that triggers the resumption of meiosis. Some of these alternative regulatory mechanisms of meiosis were reviewed and compared in mammalian, amphibian, and echinoderm oocytes (143).

Some investigators were unable to demonstrate OMI activity of follicular preparations. Granulosa cells did not inhibit maturation of cow, sow, or ewe oocytes, whereas FF showed such activity (71); porcine FF was inactive, whereas coculture with granulosa cells inhibited resumption of meiosis (63,68) and bovine and porcine FF as well as granulosa cells were inactive (54), but coculture with follicle hemisection prevented meiosis. This was overcome by addition of LH (53). Likewise, Racowsky and McGaughey (144) could not detect an inhibitory effect of porcine granulosa cells on the maturation of pig oocytes. These varying findings may be related, at least in part, to the low OMI activity of FF and of granulosa cell cultures, the finding that fluid and granulosa cells from large follicles are devoid of OMI activity, to the instability of OMI, and to differences in the methods of oocyte collection and culture. However, some of the researchers did later confirm OMI activity that could not be seen in earlier studies (55–58). The many studies from numerous laboratories demonstrating OMI activity attest to the paracrine regulation of the resumption of meiosis. Nevertheless, purification and chemical characterization of OMI are needed to further our understanding of the exact biochemical and cellular mechanisms controlling the preovulatory resumption of meiosis.

GONADOTROPIN BINDING INHIBITORS

A plausible mechanism for paracrine modulation of gonadotropin action could be interference with signal reception at the level of the receptor. Indeed, inhibitors of FSH and LH binding have been detected in ovarian tissues. It has already been indicated (145) that many factors may interfere with radioligand binding *in vitro;* hence, it is very difficult (especially when working on crude extracts) to distinguish between a regulatory gonadotropin binding inhibitor having a physiologic role and perturbation of the assay. The alternative assays, measuring biologic responses to gonadotropic challenge, may be misleading as far as binding is concerned, especially when tested *in vivo.* The recent cloning of the gonadotropin receptors and the elucidation of their structure–function relationship will allow detailed examination of the suggested role of binding inhibitors in ovarian function.

FSH Binding Inhibitor

Follicle stimulating hormone binding inhibitors were detected in ovarian extracts (146) and FF (145,147–155). Because many hormones and growth factors have been shown to modulate FSH actions at a point distal to the hormone-receptor binding, the FSH-BI are now referred to as FSH receptor binding competitors (FRBC) (156). Recent studies revealed that FSH-BI from porcine FF contains both stimulatory (agonistic) and inhibitory (antagonist) activities (157). Although the agonist FSH-BI activity of porcine and human FF was FSH immunoreactive, it was immunologically and biochemically distinguishable from pituitary FSH (158,159). Activity of FRBC from porcine and human FF was extracted by an α-inhibin immunoaffinity column. Conversely, α-inhibin precursor proteins inhibited FSH binding to its receptors, exerting antagonistic activity, and antisera to FRBC or α-inhibin identified a 57-kDa protein, suggesting that active FRBC is the α-inhibin precursor protein or a large molecular-weight fragment of it but not the mature α-inhibin (156).

The concentration of FSH-BI was higher in pools of bovine FF obtained from animals in the luteal phase of their cycle, as compared with that of pregnant animals (153). Furthermore, concentration of FSH-BI was correlated with the degree of follicular atresia (153). These findings suggest that FSH-BI may play a role in the induction or propagation of follicular atresia by attenuating the responsiveness of granulosa cells to FSH. Examination of FSH-BI in individual follicles at different stages of atresia as well as the ability of native or synthetic FSH-BI to induce atresia is required to confirm such a role of FSH-BI in follicular development.

LH Binding Inhibitor

Inhibitors of luteinizing hormone binding have been demonstrated in extracts of rat (160,161), pig (162,163), cat, dog, sheep, goat (164), and human (165) corpora lutea. This inhibition of LH binding could result from competition of tissue LH or of LH destruction by a protease present in the extract. Both of these possibilities seem unlikely, because boiling of rat corpora lutea extracts destroys only a small fraction (<20%) of LH-BI activity and exposure of LH to these extracts does not alter the physical and chemical properties of LH (166). Furthermore, several experimental approaches did not show appreciable binding of LH to LH-BI, thus supporting the notion that LH-BI activity is not due to solubilized LH receptors in the extracts (166).

Luteinizing hormone binding inhibitor activity is present in freshly collected corpora lutea of pregnant rat, dog, sheep, and goat (166,167) but not from fresh pseudopregnant rat and porcine corpora lutea (162,167). In all cases, storage at −20°C increased the LH-BI activity extractable from corpora lutea, but not in tissues other than luteinized ovary (166). This increase in LH-BI activity is thought to be related to the association of LH-BI with some cellular fraction. Storage appears to release (or to make readily extractable) LH-BI from these cellular sites. The finding that LH-BI could be extracted from fresh pseudopregnant rat ovaries with a nonionic detergent, Triton X-100, supports this notion (164).

Besides direct demonstration of inhibition of LH binding by LH-BI, studies were conducted to examine post-binding responses. Thus, LH-BI inhibited LH/hCG-stimulated, but not basal, progesterone synthesis by ovary slices of pseudopregnant rats (164,167). Likewise, Kumari and colleagues (168) demonstrated inhibition of progesterone synthesis by LH-BI preparations. *In vivo* effects of LH-BI preparations on ovulation were reported in rabbits (169), rats, and mice (170). However, because crude preparations were used, other than LH-BI activities cannot be excluded at present.

Aqueous extracts of rat luteinized ovaries contained LH-BI activity both in dialysate and in the nondialyzable fraction (160), whereas in the pig luteal extracts only nondialyzable activity was observed (166,171). The nondialyzable LH-BI from both rat and porcine extracts exhibited similar properties on gel filtration and ion-exchange chromatography. It seems that LH-BI exists in more than one molecular form, the main components with molecular mass of around 20 kDa (166).

FOLLICULAR REGULATORY PROTEIN

Using inhibition of aromatase activity in cultured granulosa cells led to the identification of FRP. This activity should not be confused with the FSH-releasing protein (172), now usually referred to as activin. Follicle regulatory protein was detected in human, ovine, bovine, porcine, and equine FF (173–178). Partially purified FRP from porcine FF was estimated as 15 kDa in its molecular mass, with an isoelectric point of 4.7 (179).

Follicle regulatory protein suppressed the ability of FSH to stimulate cyclic AMP and LH/hCG receptors in granulosa cells (180,181). It inhibited aromatase activity of porcine granulosa cells from small- and medium-sized but not large follicles (182). Progesterone secretion by rat and porcine granulosa cells was affected by FRP in a biphasic manner (183,184). It was stimulatory at low doses and inhibitory at high ones. Follicle regulatory protein inhibited hCG-stimulated 3β-hydroxysteroid dehydrogenase and aromatase in theca cells from medium- and large-sized pig follicles (185).

Studies with cultured porcine ovarian cells suggest that granulosa cells from small- and medium-sized follicles are the main source of FRP (186). Follicle regulatory protein content of FF from in vitro fertilization-embryo transfer (IVF-ET) patients was positively related with its prolactin, estradiol, and total protein levels. Because prolactin stimulated FRP accumulation in porcine granulosa cell cultures, it was suggested that some of the reported effects of prolactin on granulosa cells may be mediated by FRP (187).

The overall effects of FRP on granulosa cell function led to the suggestion that it may be involved, in concert with other hormones and growth factors, in follicle selection and atresia (177). Only following purification and full chemical characterization of FRP will it be possible to evaluate its putative role in follicular development and to distinguish it from other growth factors.

REGULATORS OF LUTEINIZATION

The findings that FF alters the *in vitro* responses of cultured granulosa cells to gonadotropins led to the suggestion that paracrine factors are involved in the differentiation of granulosa cells. Thus, responsiveness of granulosa cells to gonadotropins, according to this view, is not entirely dependent on gonadotropin receptors but modified also by locally produced hormonal regulators. One such activity was stimulation of the secretion of both progesterone and estrogens, enhancement of morphologic differentiation, and potentiation of FSH and LH action on granulosa cells from immature antral follicles. This activity is referred to as LS (and in later studies as maturation stimulator) (188,189). The other activity is consistently observed in fluid from small follicles and referred to as LI (and more recently as atretogenic factor) (188,189).

Most of the studies on LS and LI were performed using FF and conditioned media of granulosa cells obtained from pigs (163,188–191). But similar effects were reported using human (192,193), cow (194–196), and mare (197,198) FF.

The preponderance of LI activity in pools of fluid from small follicles and of LS in that from large follicles led Channing and colleagues (198) to suggest that the ratio between the stimulatory and inhibitory activity in the follicle plays an essential role in follicle selection. In agreement, it was found that fluid from midcycle bovine follicles decreased granulosa cell secretion of progesterone and prostaglandin *in vitro,* but fluid from preovulatory follicles was devoid of such inhibitory activity (196). Likewise, fluid from viable mare follicles enhanced FSH-stimulated steroidogenesis, but fluid from atretic follicles was inhibitory (198).

The most commonly applied approach to test for LS was to use fluid from large follicles and test its action on granulosa cells from small follicles, whereas LI activity was tested on the behavior of cells from large follicles.

Follicular fluid from large porcine follicles enhanced several aspects of granulosa cell behavior toward luteinization. Thus, it enhanced basal and gonadotropin-stimulated progesterone secretion (189,199–202), basal estrogen secretion (189), LH/hCG receptors (203–206), and morphologic changes indicative of luteinization (207). At least part of FF LS-like activity was ascribed to an ovarian gonadotropin-releasing hormone (GnRH)-related mechanism (208).

Granulosa cells explanted from porcine large follicles undergo *in vitro* a series of morphologic and endocrine changes commonly referred to as luteinization. Addition of FF from small- and medium-sized porcine follicles prevents these luteinizationlike changes (209) as well as FSH induction of LH/hCG receptors and progesterone synthesis from cells explanted from small follicles (1,203,204). Similar inhibitory activities were demonstrated in FF of other species (193,195,196).

Most of the studies on LI activity were performed with porcine FF. These revealed inhibitory action of FF from small follicles on morphologic luteinization (210) and basal and stimulated progesterone secretion (189, 209,211).

The question whether LS and LI activities of FF are due to specific molecules or the result of the action of the many hormones, growth factors, and metabolites accumulated in FF can be answered only on the purification and chemical characterization of the active principle(s). The overlapping activities exerted by some of the known growth factors and hormones pose serious obstacles for such an effort.

MITOGENIC AND GROWTH FACTORS

The ovarian follicle undergoes most impressive cell proliferation during its growth. Thus, it is estimated that a primordial follicle with approximately 50 granulosa cells (212) reaches more than 5×10^7 granulosa cells in preovulatory follicles in the human (213). These estimates may vary among species, different ovarian cell populations, and even researchers, but there is no question that cell replication is a major feature of ovarian activity.

The earliest stages of follicular growth seem to be independent of circulating gonadotropins (reviewed by refs. 214 and 215). Therefore, it is generally assumed that the initiation of follicular growth is regulated by ovarian autocrine and paracrine hormones. Furthermore, even after antrum formation, when follicular development is dependent on gonadotropins and estrogen, it is difficult to assign all aspects of follicular growth and selection solely to these hormones. The experiments demonstrating the ability of granulosa cells to reverse serum-attenuated cell differentiation *in vitro* and the dependence of this reversal on the density of the cultured granulosa cells (216) support this notion.

After antrum formation, there is a further 100- to 1,000-fold increase in follicular granulosa cell number (213). It has been demonstrated that FSH and estradiol enhance synergistically granulosa cell proliferation *in vivo* (217) and *in vitro* (218–220). In recent years, much work has been directed toward search of nongonadotropin and nonsteroidal growth-stimulating ovarian actions. This approach was complemented by testing the actions of known polypeptide growth factors on ovarian cells *in vivo* or *in vitro*. The studies involving ovarian tissues were reviewed recently (8,14,221). Much of the research on growth factors is centered on their growth-promoting actions. However, these factors may also modulate differentiation, and this action may be uncoupled from their effects on cellular proliferation. The following growth factors or growth factor families have been mostly considered regarding their putative involvement in ovarian physiology.

Insulin and insulinlike growth factors (IGFs): This is a family of serum-derived factors closely related to insulin. A gene duplication approximately 600 million years ago led to the diversion of a common precursor molecule into insulin and IGF as distinct hormones (222). The IGF family consists of several homologous, low-molecular-weight, single-chain polypeptide growth factors named after their remarkable similarity to insulin. These were originally isolated on the basis of their two different metabolic actions: (a) the ability to stimulate sulfate incorporation into cartilage (sulfation factor activity); and (b) nonsuppressible insulinlike activity (NSILA), demonstrating insulinomimetic actions originally tested in adipocytes (223,224). On the basis of net charge, the IGFs can be classed into two distinct groups: (a) basic IGFs (isoelectric points, 8.1–8.5), which include human IGF-I (hIGF-I), identified with somatomedin C (SmC) (225–227) and its suggested murine equivalent, basic rat somatomedin, labeled rat IGF-I (rIGF-I) (228); and (b) neutral IGFs, including IGF-II and its probable murine counterpart, multiplication stimulating activity (MSA), also referred to as IGF-II.

Epidermal growth factor: This was originally extracted from mouse submaxillary glands (229). It is mitogenic in ectodermal- and endodermal-derived cells *in vitro* (230–232). The closely related TGFα has been detected in culture media and extracts of rodent and human cells and subsequently shown to bind to EGF receptors and exert similar effects.

Fibroblast growth factor (FGF): This was originally purified from bovine pituitary (233). Fibroblast growth factor was purified to homogeneity and characterized (234,235). Fibroblast growth factor, among its multiple

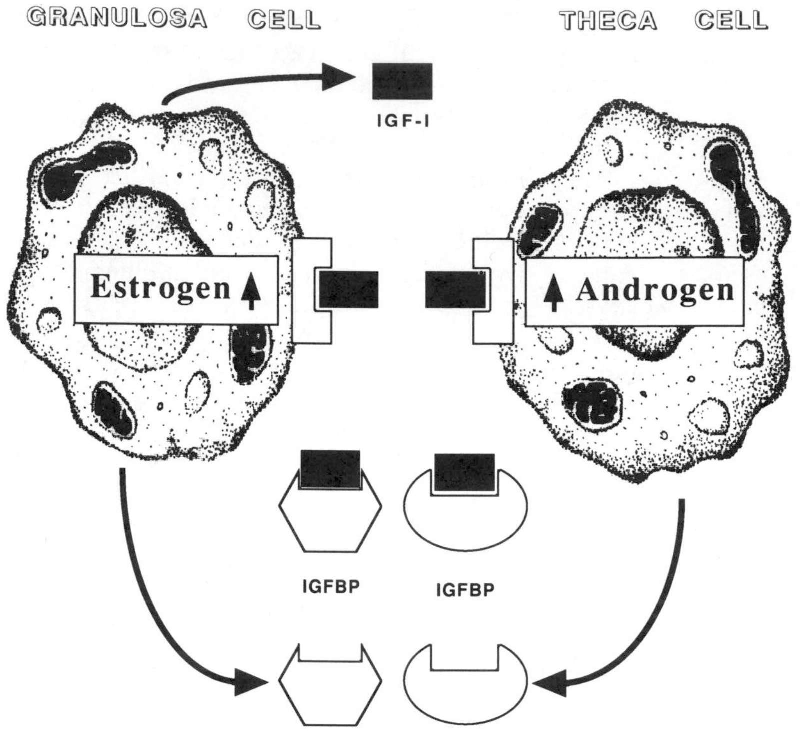

FIG. 6. Intraovarian IGF-I system. (From ref. 241a with permission.)

activities, is angiogenic (i.e., stimulates the growth of blood vessels).

Cytokines and lymphokines, originally described, characterized, and isolated on the basis of their autocrine and paracrine actions in the immune and blood systems, have been found to be produced and affect cells of other tissues. Here, the possible involvement of interleukin-1 (IL-1) and tumor necrosis factor (TNF) in ovarian physiology is reviewed.

Ovarian Growth Stimulating Actions

Under this subheading, a short review of unidentified ovarian growth activities is presented. This separation does not imply that they necessarily differ from the growth factors dealt with in the following sections.

Evidence suggesting that follicular theca components secrete substances that enhance granulosa cell proliferation *in vitro* was obtained by recombining *in vitro* thecal tissue and granulosa cells (236). Likewise, Makris and colleagues (237,238) have isolated a thecal factor stimulating porcine granulosa cell and BALB/3T3 cell proliferation. Using ornithine decarboxylase (ODC) activity as an indirect marker of mitogenic activity, Hammond and co-workers (239,240) found ODC stimulating activity in porcine FF.

Intraovarian IGF System

As the significance of putative intraovarian regulators became increasingly recognized, much of the attention has centered on IGFs. Indeed, a large body of evidence now suggests the existence of an intraovarian IGF system complete with ligands, receptors, and binding proteins (241) (Fig. 6). More importantly, IGFs have been shown to exert a variety of effects at the level of murine (242–250), porcine (251–261), and human (262–264) somatic ovarian cells, thereby raising the possibility of a meaningful *in vivo* role. Although, IGFs may be acting in their own right, their most important role appears contingent on their ability to synergize with pituitary gonadotropins and to amplify their impact (Fig. 7).

The above notwithstanding, there is at this time no compelling evidence to indicate that IGFs are indispensible to ovarian function. However, a large body of information of a somewhat indirect nature strongly suggests such a possibility. Nevertheless, much additional work would be required before unequivocal conclusions could be reached as to the *in vivo* relevance of IGFs to ovarian physiology. Indeed, limitations imposed by current experimental approaches may well require that definite proof await more sophisticated experimental paradigms. In particular, it is to be hoped that transgenic technology would develop to a level sufficient to allow selective ablation of IGFs at the level of the ovary. Such approach should yield critical information on the reproductive impact (if any) of intraovarian IGFs.

That the ovary is a site of (hormonally regulated) IGF-I gene expression has now been clearly established in several species including the murine (265–268), porcine (269–271), and possibly the human (272–277). Importantly, of all adult rat organs tested, the ovary displays the third highest level of IGF-I gene expression, second

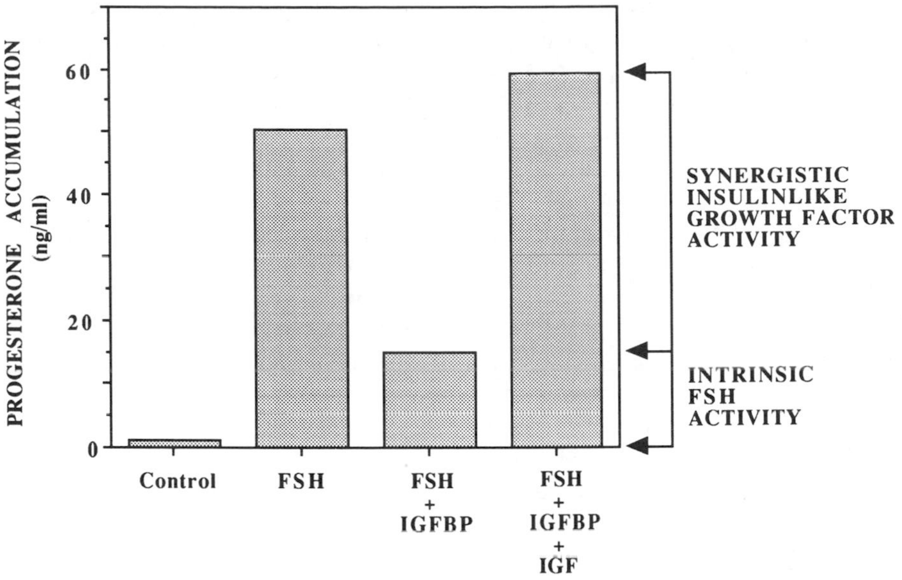

FIG. 7. Enhancing effect of IGF-I on FSH-stimulated progesterone accumulation. Optimal FSH action is dependent on availability of granulosa cell-derived IGF-I. Excess of exogenous IGFBPs revealed relatively modest intrinsic FSH activity. FSH activity was remarkably enhanced by adding IGF-I (320). (From ref. 241a with permission.)

only to the uterus and liver (265). In contrast, murine ovarian IGF-II gene expression, although clearly evident, appears much less pronounced (278). Cellular localization studies revealed the murine (266,268,279) and porcine (280–283) granulosa cells to be the main intraovarian cell concerned with IGF-I gene expression. In contrast, murine ovarian IGF-II gene expression proved virtually theca-interstitial cell exclusive (278). At the level of the human ovary, granulosa cells may be a site of IGF-II rather than IGF-I gene expression (284,285), thereby suggesting possible species specificity. Thus, at least in the murine and human models, IGF gene expression is highly compartmentalized, the two IGF species being expressed by two distinct somatic cell types.

Several reports now suggest that the ovary is not only a site of IGF production but that there exist specific and functional ovarian IGF receptors coupled to multiple critical end points. Murine (285–287), porcine (251,252), ovine (288), and human (289) granulosa cells have now been clearly shown to display high-affinity, low-capacity IGF-I binding sites. Studies limited to the murine granulosa cell have also established the existence of IGF-II receptors (290,291). Similarly, murine (292,293) and human (294,295) theca-interstitial cells appear to possess functional IGF-I receptors coupled to the promotion of ovarian androgen biosynthesis.

Besides ligands and receptors, the ovary is well endowed in IGF binding proteins, the exact role of which remains a matter of further study. Insulin growth factor binding proteins (IGFBPs) constitute a heterogeneous group of at least six distinct proteins capable of binding IGFs (but not insulin), with affinities in the 10^{-10} to 10^{-9} M range (296–299). The six known rat IGFBPs range in size from 21.5 to 29.6 kDa, as predicted from the nonglycosylated mature protein. It is assumed, although by no means proven, that the IGFBPs subserve different functions, thereby justifying the existence of multiple IGFBP species. Although the exact role of the IGFBPs remains a matter of study, general consensus supports a role in the transport of IGFs and in the regulation of their bioavailability (280,281,300–311).

Mapping studies carried out at the level of the rat ovary combined multiple approaches including molecular probing, immunoprecipitation, and deglycosylation. As a result of these efforts, it would appear that the rat granulosa cell is a site of IGFBP-4 and IGFBP-5 gene expression (311–314). In contrast, the theca-interstitial cell appears to be a site of IGFBP-2, IGFBP-3 (possibly IGFBP-4), and IGFBP-6 gene expression (313–316).

Preliminary regulatory studies at the level of the rat granulosa cell revealed a striking ability of FSH to substantially inhibit the release of otherwise constitutively elaborated IGFBPs (317,318). These observations are particularly noteworthy for the fact that FSH, by its very designation, is a FSH, rarely engaged in the inhibition of granulosa cell function. Re-evaluation, however, may suggest that this apparent inhibition may, in effect, constitute a net stimulatory gain provided one accepts the hypothesis that granulosa cell-derived IGFBPs are inhibitory to IGF hormonal action, the removal of which may well be conducive to granulosa cell differentiation. Specifically, diminishing the IGF binding capacity in granulosa cell environment may enhance the bioavailability of IGFs and hence their potency. Studies are currently underway to evaluate the above hypothesis.

Particularly noteworthy are observations made by several groups with respect to the antigonadotropic activity of IGFBPs. All told, these findings suggest highly specific antigonadotropic potential, which appears dependent on an intact IGF (but not FSH) binding site (319). As such, these observations suggest that IGFBPs may be acting as antigonadotropins by sequestering endogenously derived IGFs. These observations suggest that optimal FSH hormonal action is contingent on the bioavailability of granulosa cell-derived IGFs and the consequent amplification of the gonadotropic signal. According to this view, intrinsic FSH hormonal action is relatively limited. In contrast, augmented FSH hormonal action, as it is known *in vivo* or *in vitro,* consists of a modest intrinsic component complemented by a substantial portion contributed by synergistic interactions between FSH and IGFs. According to this view, FSH requires cooperation from tissue-based regulatory factors to realize its full potential (320). Preliminary findings suggest that similar statements can be made with respect to LH. Conceivably, this principle may prove generally applicable and perhaps of consequence to the action of other trophic principles, the optimal action of which may depend on interaction with tissue-based modulatory factors.

EGF and TGFα

Epidermal growth factor was initially discovered by the ability of a submandibular gland extract to stimulate precocious eyelid opening and incisor tooth eruption when injected into newborn mice (229). Mature EGF is a 53-amino-acid polypeptide single chain, with three internal disulfide bonds. Transforming growth factor α is an EGF-related single-chain 50-amino-acid polypeptide, first discovered from cultures of different tumor cells (321,322). Human TGFα has 40% sequence homology to human EGF. Epidermal growth factor and TGFα recognize the same cellular receptor and elicit similar, although not identical in all model systems, growth-promoting activities (323). Studies on EGF/TGFα in ovarian physiology were reviewed recently (324).

The initial studies of Gospodarowicz and colleagues (325–327) demonstrated the mitogenic activity of EGF on bovine, porcine, rabbit, guinea pig, and human granulosa cells *in vitro.* By contrast, granulosa cells of intact or hypophysectomized estrogen-treated rats or bovine luteal cells *in vitro* did not proliferate in response to EGF or FGF (327–329). Such seemingly disparate actions of EGF on granulosa cell proliferation may be related to differences in the stage of differentiation of the cells or to the need for additional growth factors, recently shown to be involved in granulosa cell proliferation. Thus, several growth factors enhanced the mitogenic action of EGF on granulosa cells, such as TGFβ (330), platelet-derived growth factor (PDGF), and α-fetoprotein (331–333).

The stimulatory action of EGF/TGFα on cellular proliferation is not limited to granulosa cells. Bovine theca cells respond to TGFα within 24 hr with increase in thymidine incorporation and increase in cell number during 4-day culture (334).

Besides the mitogenic action of EGF/TGFα on ovarian cells, they affect follicular cell differentiation. Thus, EGF attenuated FSH-induced LH receptors and aromatase activity in rat and porcine granulosa cells (262,329,335,336). Theca-interstitial cell steroidogenesis is also affected by EGF/TGFα. Luteinizing hormone-stimulated androgen secretion by rat theca-interstitial cells (337) and estrogen production by adult porcine preovulatory theca cells (338) was inhibited by EGF. In contrast to these inhibitory actions of EGF/TGFα, recently the induction of aromatase in prepubertal porcine granulosa and theca cells by TGFα was observed (339). These results underscore the complicated actions and interactions of growth factors in follicular cell function.

Epidermal growth factor (79) and TGFα (92) induce the resumption of meiosis in rat follicle-enclosed oocytes and mouse oocytes cultured in the presence of inhibitory purines (80). In the rabbit, EGF attenuated the hCG-

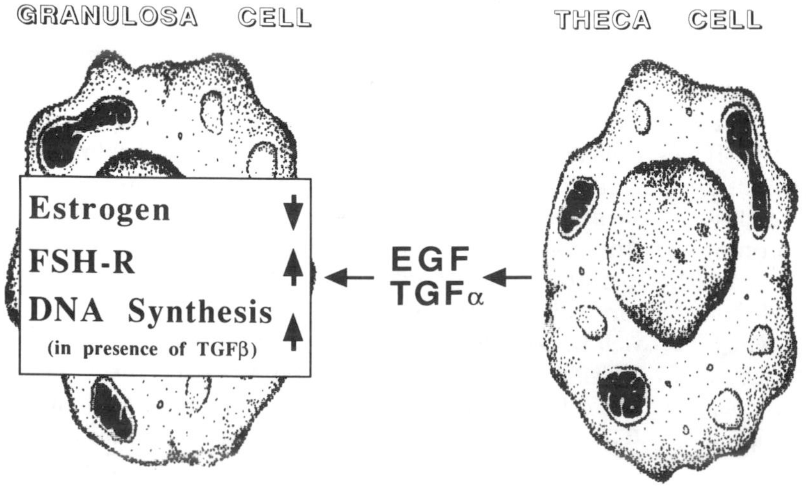

FIG. 8. Intraovarian EGF-TGFα system. (From ref. 241a with permission.)

stimulated steroid production and ovulation in perfused ovaries (340).

Receptors for EGF/TGFα have been demonstrated on bovine, ovine and murine granulosa cells (341,342) and bovine theca cells (343).

Transforming growth factor α has been localized by immunocytochemistry to the theca-interstitial cells in the rat (344). Likewise, TGFα was expressed only in bovine theca but not granulosa cells (343). Furthermore, in the bovine ovaries TGFα staining was most intense in theca cells of rapidly growing follicles (345). Accordingly, EGF-like activity was maximal in FF from small human antral follicles, and its levels were inversely related to follicular size (346). The exclusive localization of TGFα to the theca-interstitial compartment led to the suggestion that thecal TGFα acts as a paracrine regulator of adjacent granulosa cells (Fig. 8). The EGF/TGFα actions on thecal cells (337–339) allow also for autocrine regulation. Nevertheless, an EGF-like activity was localized immunocytochemically to both granulosa and theca cells of hamster growing follicles (347). Therefore, the source of follicular EGF/TGFα activity in different mammalian species and varying differentiation stages remains to be determined.

TGFβ and Related Peptides

Transforming growth factor β1, a homodimeric polypeptide composed of two identical 112-amino-acid chains is a polyfunctional regulator (348). Two mammalian related proteins, TGFβ2 and TGFβ3, have been cloned and sequenced. The identity between the mature form of these three protein sequences is 70% to 80%. The TGFβs are multifunctional, pleotropic molecules affecting cellular migration, proliferation, and elaboration of extracellular matrix. The three TGFβs seem to share similar, although not entirely identical in all cases, biologic activities. Additional mammalian proteins related to TGFβ are known. These include, among others, anti-Müllerian hormone (AMH) or Müllerian inhibiting substance (349,350), inhibin (351), and activin (172,352), which are involved in the regulation of reproduction. The role of inhibin and activin is reviewed in detail in this volume (Chapter 17 by Vale).

Transforming growth factor β has been shown to affect proliferation of follicular cells. Thus, it was reported to stimulate murine (353,354) and porcine (260) granulosa cells but suppressed the proliferative action of TGFα in bovine theca cells (334).

Differentiation of follicular cells in culture was markedly modified by TGFβ (355). Transforming growth factor β was shown to enhance FSH effects on granulosa cell differentiation (335,353,356–362). Likewise, TGFβ promoted the differentiation of rat theca-interstitial cells and inhibited androgen production (363,364).

Transforming growth factor β has been shown to be produced in the ovary by granulosa (365,366), theca-interstitial (353,354,367), as well as small luteal cells and the oocyte (368). Although rat theca cells expressed both TGFβ1 and TGFβ2, only TGFβ2 was regulated by the gonadotropin (369). In contrast, porcine granulosa cells seemed to secrete only low levels of TGFβ1 and possibly TGFβ but did not produce translatable TGFβ2 mRNA (370).

A most interesting concept was raised recently by Bendell and Dorrington (371). In view of the ability of estradiol-17β to stimulate granulosa cell DNA synthesis (and presumably proliferation), the similar action of TGFβ and FSH and, finally, the ability of TGFβ antiserum to block this effect of estradiol suggest that estrogen-induced growth of rat granulosa cells may be mediated by the production of TGFβ. Thus, both autocrine and paracrine actions of TGFβ may be involved in the regulation of ovarian action.

Transforming growth factor β was reported to accelerate the maturation of follicle-enclosed oocytes cultured within explanted ovarian fragments as well as in spontaneously maturing rat oocytes (372). However, spontaneous maturation of follicle-enclosed oocytes in these experiments reached 90% and higher within 8 hr of incubation. This is a very unique observation, contrasting the well-established need for hormonal stimulation of maturation in follicle-enclosed oocytes *in vivo* or *in vitro* (see Life History of the Mammalian Ovum above) (37,123,143). In contrast, TGFβ and inhibin partially suppressed the LH-induced maturation of rat follicle-enclosed oocytes and did not affect the spontaneous maturation of isolated oocytes (92). Likewise, TGFβ did not affect the spontaneous maturation of mouse oocytes blocked with hypoxanthine (373).

Müllerian inhibiting substance (89) and inhibin (91) were reported to act as OMI, whereas activin was found to stimulate resumption of meiosis (374). For further discussion of the possible role of inhibin-related peptides in the regulation of oocyte maturation, see OMI as a Peptide above.

Ovarian Angiogenesis, FGF, and Other Growth Factors

The cyclic changes associated with follicular growth and atresia, corpus luteum development and demise, include tissue remodeling, which is accompanied with generation of new blood vessels, angiogenesis (375). The role of angiogenesis in ovarian physiology has been reviewed recently (376,377).

Ovarian angiogenic activity was first demonstrated in bovine corpus luteum (378). This was followed by similar results using rabbit (379), pig (380), and rat (381–383) corpora lutea. These studies were extended also to nonluteinized ovarian tissue by testing angiogenic activity of ovarian extracts or fragments of pregnant male serum gonadotyopin (PMSG)-treated immature mice or rats (382,384). Both studies demonstrated PMSG-stimulated angiogenic activity and vascularization was most intense around follicles. Further studies demonstrated angiogenic activity in extracts of porcine nonluteal ovaries (385), rabbit (386), and primate (387) follicles and in FF of pigs (388) and of hormone-stimulated women (389). Ovarian origin of this angiogenic activity is suggested by the accumulation of such activity in media in which intact follicles (379), thecal tissue (385,387), granulosa cells (386), and luteal cells (390) were cultured previously. The studies reviewed demonstrate the presence of angiogenic activity in ovarian tissues of several mammalian species and in both early luteal and hormone-stimulated follicular tissues. The importance of follicular vasculature for supply of gonadotropins to monkey follicles has been suggested (391), and a decrease in follicular vasculature was associated with atresia (392–394). The bovine corpus luteum angiogenic factor has been purified to apparent homogeneity and found to be related to FGF (395).

Fibroblast growth factor exists in two closely related forms: basic (bFGF) and acidic (aFGF). They are products of two separate genes. The primary translation product of both genes is composed of 155 amino acids, which are further cleaved to produce the 146-amino-acid bFGF and 150-amino-acid aFGF (235,395,396). Both interact with common cell surface receptors and exert similar biologic effects on a wide range of cells of mesodermal and neuroectodermal origin. Fibroblast growth factor stimulates proliferation and differentiation of a wide variety of cells. Its activity appears to be closely regulated by TGFβ (397–399). One of the most notable of FGF actions is its angiogenic effect. Nevertheless, angiogenesis seems to be only one of the many actions of FGF on development and differentiation. Furthermore, angiogenesis seems to be regulated by additional factors, some of them still waiting for their identification and elucidation of their mode of action (396,400).

Fibroblast growth factor was shown to be mitogenic for cultured bovine, porcine, rabbit, guinea pig, and human granulosa cells (325,327) and to delay their differentiation (401). In porcine granulosa cells, bFGF suppressed the induction of LH/hCG receptors and progesterone secretion, and aFGF was much less effective (402). Although FGF does not increase the proliferation of rat granulosa cells in culture, it suppresses FSH induction of LH receptors and aromatase activity (403–406) but enhances progesterone synthesis. Furthermore, bFGF stimulates tissue-type plasminogen activator expression in cultured granulosa cells, and prostaglandin (PG) E synthesis and resumption of oocyte maturation in rat follicles *in vitro* (407). These latter are necessary components of the ovulatory response (408,409). Thus, although FGF seems to delay the earlier steps of granulosa cell differentiation stimulated by FSH, it seems to mimic some of the ovulatory actions of LH.

The two forms of FGF are synthesized in the ovary: Bovine granulosa cells in culture produced bFGF (410) and ovarian expression of aFGF mRNA was observed (411). The granulosa cells seemed to contribute only a small fraction of aFGF mRNA, as compared with the rest of ovarian tissue. Luteinizing hormone and angiotensin stimulated bovine luteal cell expression of bFGF mRNA (412).

As indicated above, most of the angiogenic activity of corpora lutea was ascribed to bFGF (395). Nevertheless, some doubts were raised whether FGF fulfills all the requirements of a diffusible angiogenic factor (413,414), and additional angiogenic factors, some of them also found in ovaries, were isolated (377,415). Of these, vascular endothelial growth factor (VEGF) (416,417) was expressed in rat corpora lutea (418) and in granulosa cells of late follicular phase and young corpora lutea in a primate (419). Therefore, ovarian angiogenic activity associated with follicular and luteal development may be related to several factors. Further understanding of angiogenesis in general and its regulation will allow understanding of the process in the ovaries.

Intraovarian Cytokines

Although most attention has been directed thus far at the somatic cellular components of the ovary, the potential role(s) and relative importance of the resident ovarian white blood cell and its cytokine product(s) have received relatively limited attention. Efforts are currently underway to reconcile traditional ovarian physiology with observations relevant to intraovarian components of the white blood cell series.

Interleukin-1 Example

Interleukin-1, a polypeptide cytokine (previously referred to as lymphocyte activating factor) predominantly produced and secreted by activated macrophages, has been shown to possess a wide range of biologic functions as well as to play a role as an immune mediator (420). Although the relevance of IL-1 to ovarian physiology remains uncertain, an increasing body of evidence supports such a possibility. First, measurable amounts of IL-1-like activity have been documented in both porcine (421) and human (422) FF. Second, *in vitro* studies at the level of the murine and porcine ovary revealed IL-1 to possess antigonadotropic (423–429) or steroidogenic (430) properties contingent on the experimental circumstances under study. Accordingly, it is tempting to speculate that locally derived IL-1, possibly originating from somatic ovarian cells or resident ovarian macrophages, may be the centerpiece of an intraovarian regulatory loop. Because IL-1 is an established mediator of inflammation (420) and because ovulation may constitute an inflammatorylike reaction, IL-1 may play an intermediary role in the preovulatory developmental cascade and the terminal ovulatory process (431). Such speculation is supported by the recognition that IL-1 has been shown in multiple (nonovarian) tissues to promote several ovulation-associated phenomena such as prostaglandin biosynthesis, plasminogen activator production, glycosaminoglycan generation, collagenase activation, and vascular permeability enhancement (420).

Tumor Necrosis Factor Example

The potential ovarian relevance of another macrophage product, TNF, has also been explored (432–439). Tumor necrosis factor, a 157-amino-acid polypeptide, was originally named for its oncolytic activity as displayed in the serum of Bacille Calmette-Guerin (BCG)-immunized, endotoxin-challenged mice (440–444). Indeed, TNF proved capable of inducing tumor necrosis *in vivo* and of exerting nonspecies-specific cytolytic or cytostatic effects on a broad range of transformed cell lines *in vitro*. Although TNF was initially thought to be tumor-selective, it has become clear that certain nontumor cells possess TNF receptors and that TNF may be a regulatory monkine with pleiotropic noncytotoxic activities in addition to its antitumor properties. Most importantly, TNF has been shown to engage in the differentiation of a variety of cell types.

At the level of the ovary, TNF was found capable of attenuating the differentiation of cultured granulosa cells from immature rats through virtual neutralization of FSH hormonal action at site(s) proximal but not distal to cyclic Amp generation (432). In other studies, TNF has been found to effect complex dose-dependent alterations in the elaboration of progesterone and androstenedione, but not estrogen, by explanted preovulatory follicles of murine origin (432,433,436). If TNF is to play a role in ovarian physiology, its *in vivo* origin(s) must be determined. In principle, two general possibilities are worthy of consideration. First, TNF may be locally derived from (activated) resident ovarian macrophages, as has been shown for regressing (but not young) corpora lutea (445,446). Although basal TNF activity was undetectable in corpora lutea of both pregnancy and pseudopregnancy, TNF activity was markedly stimulated in the presence of lipopolysacharide (LPS). However, the detection of TNF activity in some luteal tissue on day 5 and the scarcity of macrophages at this stage raise the possibility that cells other than macrophages may also produce TNF in the corpus luteum. Indeed, TNF may be of granulosa cell origin as suggested by immunohistochemical studies wherein antral or atretic granulosa cells have been implicated as a possible site of TNF gene expression. Given such strong association between TNF elaboration and follicular and luteal decline, it is tempting to speculate that TNF may play a role in the still enigmatic processes of atresia and/or luteolysis. In this capacity, TNF of intraovarian origin may exert its effect(s) at or adjacent to its site of synthesis, interacting with specific granulosa/luteal cell surface receptors to modulate gonadotropin hormonal action. Undoubtedly, future studies of the regulation of the TNF receptor and the elucidation of the *in vivo* source of its ligand will shed new light on the relevance of this system to the process of follicular development and/or demise.

GnRH-LIKE PEPTIDES

The direct effects of GnRH and of its synthetic analogs on the ovary are many and have been reviewed extensively (14,447–449). The suggestion that GnRH-like peptide is a gonadal hormone is based on the following findings, mostly obtained in the rat: (a) GnRH exerts both inhibitory and stimulatory actions on the ovary and ovarian cells; (b) receptors for GnRH were demonstrated within the ovary; and (c) several reports suggest the presence of a GnRH-like peptide in the ovary. The physiologic role of GnRH in regulating ovarian function was substantiated by the ability of GnRH antagonists to potentiate the action of FSH and enhance follicular development (450). It is unlikely that hypothalamic GnRH reaches the ovary in physiologically active concentrations because of its dilution in the circulation (451) and its rapid degradation in the pituitary, brain, kidney, liver, and serum (452,453). The rapid degradation of GnRH is the main reason for using GnRH agonistic analogs exhibiting higher resistance to degrading enzymes (454). Here, an overview of the direct actions of GnRH and of its analogs on the ovary, their binding, and suggested mechanism of action are presented. Also, the evidence for the suggested role of an ovarian GnRH-like peptide in regulating ovarian function is discussed.

Inhibitory Actions of GnRH on the Ovary

A direct ovarian effect of GnRH was demonstrated by Rippel and Johnson (455), who observed a decrease in hCG-augmented ovarian weight in immature hypophysectomized rats treated with GnRH. These findings were confirmed in hypophysectomized rats stimulated with PMSG (456) or FSH (457) and shown to be associated with inhibition of ovarian steroidogenesis (457).

In vitro studies demonstrated direct effects of GnRH on primary cultures of granulosa cells. These major effects are suppression of FSH-stimulated steroidogenesis and LH and (Prl) receptors (447). The action on granulosa cell steroidogenesis is exerted at multiple sites: inhibition of FSH-stimulated cyclic Amp production

(458,459); protein kinase activation (460); progesterone and estrogen production (457,461); inhibition of aromatase (462–464), 3β-hydroxysteroid dehydrogenase (465), and possibly the cholesterol side-chain cleavage enzyme (465); and stimulation of 20α-steroid dehydrogenase (466). The GnRH inhibition of FSH-enhanced steroidogenesis and LH- and Prl-receptor formation is blocked by concomitant treatment with GnRH antagonists (462,466–468). Likewise, PGE_2-, cholera toxin-, and cyclic Amp-derivative-stimulated estrogen production were all inhibited by GnRH (459,462,469–471).

The inhibitory action of GnRH on the ovary is exerted on other ovarian compartments in addition to the granulosa cells. Thus, GnRH inhibits basal- and LH-stimulated androgen synthesis by rat ovarian interstitial cells (472,473). Likewise, GnRH inhibits LH/hCG-stimulated progesterone secretion by rat luteal cells *in vitro* (461,469,474,475) or *in vivo* (469) and desensitizes the LH receptors of cultured luteal cells within 24 hr (476). It seems that as in granulosa cells, GnRH does not interfere with LH binding in luteal cells but prevents the activation of adenylate cyclase. In intact luteal cells, unlike the granulosa cells, the inhibition of progesterone secretion by GnRH is reversed by dibutyryl cyclic Amp (474,477).

Stimulatory Effects of GnRH on the Ovary

Gonadotropin-releasing hormone, given alone, stimulates some ovarian activities (13). Thus, GnRH stimulates granulosa cell production of estrogen, progesterone, 20α-hydroxyprogesterone, prostaglandin, and lactate (463–465,478–481). Nevertheless, the most consistent stimulatory action of GnRH on ovarian function is exerted on mature preovulatory follicles. Gonadotropin-releasing hormone induces ovulation in hypophysectomized rats (482,483). This action of GnRH, but not of LH, was blocked by GnRH antagonists (484,485). Hence, GnRH or ovarian GnRH-like peptide is capable of mimicking LH action on ovulation but does not seem to be involved in the mediation of LH action on ovulation. The action of GnRH on follicular rupture at ovulation seems to be related to its ability to stimulate *in vitro* granulosa cell and follicular prostaglandin (449,478, 479,484–487) and plasminogen activator (488–490) synthesis, both involved in follicular rupture at ovulation (see Chapter 13 by Espey, this volume). Thus, inhibitors of prostaglandins prevented the induction of ovulation by GnRH (484,485,491). Likewise, GnRH induced ovulation and stimulated progesterone secretion in perfused rat and rabbit ovaries, but it was much more effective in this respect in rat ovaries (492). Furthermore, rat oocytes matured in response to GnRH treatment were successfully fertilized *in vitro* and, on transfer to foster mothers, developed into live 20-day fetuses (493,494).

Explanation of preovulatory rat follicles *in vitro* allowed detailed analysis of GnRH effects. It induced resumption of ovum maturation, cumulus cell dispersion, and mucification and stimulated oocyte respiration (485,495–497). Unlike its effect on follicular rupture, the action of GnRH on the ovum is not prevented by indomethacin and hence does not seem to be mediated by follicular prostaglandin production (484). Recent studies seem to indicate that the action of GnRH on ovum maturation involves PKC. Thus, phospholipase (PL) C, phorbol ester, and diacylglycerol induced resumption of meiosis in follicle-enclosed oocytes and synergized with GnRH in this action (498). Likewise, GnRH-induced maturation of rabbit follicle-enclosed oocytes seemed to be mediated by PKC (499). Furthermore, inhibitors of the lipoxygenase pathway of arachidonic acid suppressed resumption of meiosis induced by GnRH, but not by LH, suggesting the involvement of this pathway in mediating GnRH action on ovum maturation (500). Gonadotropin-releasing hormone stimulated the accumulation in the medium of pregnenolone, progesterone, 20α-OH-progesterone, androstenedione, testosterone, and estradiol 17-β on short incubation (up to 6–8 hr) of rat preovulatory follicles (501,502). Although GnRH-induced accumulation of progestins continued beyond the initial 6 hr of incubation, androgen accumulation was reduced, in a similar pattern to that following stimulation with LH (502). Gonadotropin-releasing hormone mimicked several actions of LH on the rat preovulatory follicle, but not in all respects. Thus, the stimulatory effects of LH on steroidogenesis were expressed earlier and reached higher maximal response than with GnRH (502).

GnRH Binding and Mechanism of Action in the Ovary

Evidence for ovarian GnRH binding sites was obtained by ovarian uptake of ^{125}I-GnRH analog *in vivo* in intact and hypophysectomized rats (503). Detailed *in vitro* studies led to the conclusion that GnRH exerts its gonadal actions through membrane receptors showing similar specificity and affinity for GnRH and its analogs as GnRH receptors in the anterior pituitary (448,504). Conclusive evidence for specific high-affinity GnRH receptors has been obtained in granulosa and luteal cells of the rat (475,477,505–508). The number and affinity of GnRH receptors did not show conspicuous changes during the day stage of the estrous cycle or hypophysectomy, but the number of GnRH receptors in luteal membranes of cycling rats was half of that in granulosa cells (507). Ovarian GnRH binding sites are present already on day 10 of age to reach a maximum on day 20 (509) and decline during the early proestrous phase of puberty (510). Binding studies using fluorescent derivative of GnRH revealed initial uniform distribution on granulosa cell surface, followed by formation of patches and internalization (511). Photoaffinity labeling of ovarian GnRH receptors resulted in identification of two specific components with apparent molecular mass of 60 kDa and 54 kDa (511,512). Because only one component (60 kDa) was present in the pituitary (513), the extra component of the ovarian receptors may be related to different and specific functions of GnRH in the ovary.

Gonadotropin-releasing hormone binding sites decreased in PMSG- or FSH-treated rats after induction of ovulation by LH/hCG (505–507). By contrast, FSH maintains GnRH receptor content of granulosa cells *in vitro* (514) and GnRH *in vivo* may increase or decrease its own receptors, depending on the dose and time of treatment (505,507,514).

The earliest cellular response subsequent to GnRH binding to its ovarian receptor reported to date is an accumulation of labeled inositol triphosphate ($Insp_3$) and diphosphate ($Insp_2$) followed by an increase in phospholipid (phosphatidylinositol [PI] and phosphatidic acid [PA]) labeling in cultured granulosa and luteal cells (515–520). The antigonadotropic action of GnRH in rat ovarian cells appears to be dependent on and mediated by calcium (521–523). Indeed, GnRH stimulation is followed by a rapid and transient increase in free Ca^{2+} (499). Gonadotropin-releasing hormone stimulated arachidonic acid release from prelabeled granulosa cells in culture (524,525). Thus, GnRH action on the ovary (as in the pituitary) involves the mechanisms integrating PLC, calcium mobilization, protein phosphorylation, and arachidonic acid metabolism in signal transduction (449,526–529). Indeed, Dekel and colleagues (530) demonstrated that inhibitors of PKC blocked GnRH-induced maturation more effectively than that induced by LH. Also, GnRH was demonstrated to activate PLD (531) in rat granulosa cells (532). The actions of LH on the ovary are exerted primarily through the mediation of cyclic Amp (533), although there is cross talk with other signal transduction mechanisms (534). By contrast, no clear-cut stimulatory effects of GnRH on ovarian cyclic-AMP production could be detected (478,486,535). It seems, therefore, that despite the fact that GnRH mimics LH in triggering ovulation, its action is mediated through different mechanism(s) (Fig. 9). In explanted rat preovulatory follicles, inhibitors of cyclooxygenase and of lipoxygenase attenuated GnRH-induced progesterone

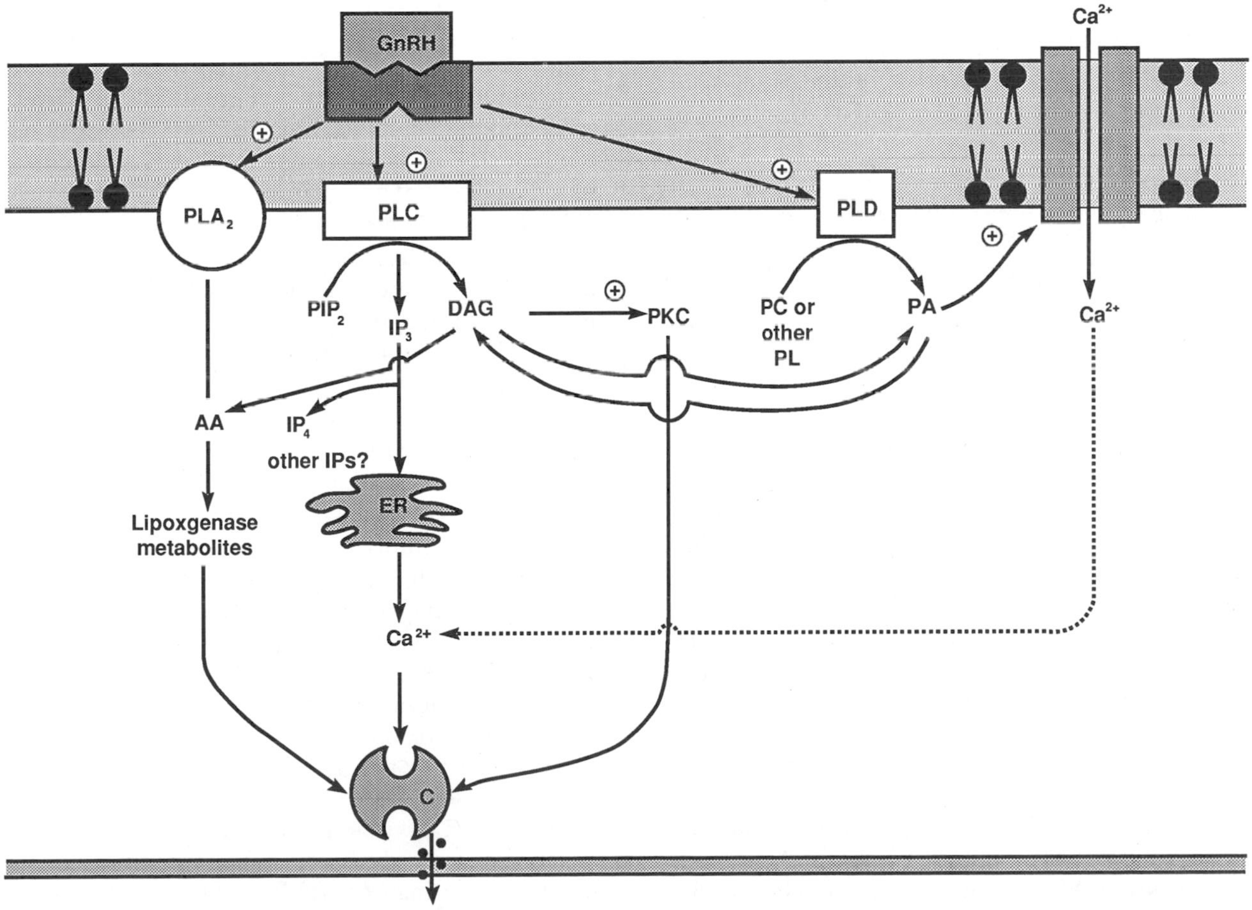

FIG. 9. Signaling mechanisms of GnRH in ovary. Three pathways appear to be involved: PLA_2, PLC, and PLD. (From ref. 529, with permission.)

synthesis and activity of plasminogen activator but had no effect on these parameters when LH was added to the medium (500). Likewise, lipoxygenase products were implicated in the mediation of GnRH effects on granulosa cell progesterone production (536,537). Thus, it is possible that at least part of the actions of GnRH on the follicle are exerted through changes in arachidonic acid metabolism and its active metabolites. Further studies are required to define the precise molecular mechanisms involved in the stimulatory as well as the inhibitory actions of GnRH in ovarian cells.

Possible Role of GnRH in Ovarian Physiology

Ovarian GnRH-like Peptides

The evidence reviewed in the previous sections of GnRH reception and action in the ovary needs complementary evidence for local production of the peptide to qualify as a paracrine/autocrine regulator of ovarian function. Recently, ovarian transcription of GnRH gene was observed by reverse transcription-polymerase chain reaction (RT-PCR) in the rat (538,539). Most of the ovarian GnRH gene transcripts retained intronic sequences (539).

Gonadotropin-releasing hormonelike molecules were detected by (RRA) from ovaries of rats, humans, cows, and ewes (540–543). This protein inhibited competitively and reversibly the binding of GnRH by rat ovarian membranes. This GnRH binding inhibitor was identified as histone H2A (544). Conversely, histone H2A exerted antigonadotropic effects on ovarian cells in culture (545), but this action did not seem to involve GnRH receptors (546). It remains, therefore, to examine the contribution, if any, of histone H2A in the observed actions of GnRH on ovarian cells.

GnRH Action and Reception in Different Species

Most of the studies on ovarian GnRH reception, production, and action were performed in the rat. Hence, if GnRH plays a regulatory role in ovarian physiology, it is important to see whether these findings can be extended to additional species. Attempts to demonstrate high-affinity ovarian GnRH receptors yielded, thus far, negative results in the sheep, cow and pig (547), monkey (548), and human (549), but low-affinity binding sites were demonstrated in human corpus luteum (550,551). Using radiographic approach, GnRH binding was limited to human granulosa cells of the dominant follicle (552). Other studies have demonstrated direct effects of GnRH on rabbit (492), pig (458), cow (553), monkey (554), and human (555) ovaries. In the two latter species, other authors under different experimental conditions did not observe any effects of GnRH agonists *in vitro* (548,556–558). Collectively, these studies seem to indicate that the rat is not the only species in which ovarian effects of GnRH could be demonstrated but, at the same time, suggest that rat ovaries are by far more responsive than other species to the agonists tested. The failure to demonstrate high-affinity binding sites in other species may be due to the poor ability of the labeled GnRH analogs used to interact with the gonadal GnRH-like peptide receptors in these species. Also, even in the rat ovaries, the number of GnRH receptors is low, and their demonstration poses many technical and methodologic difficulties.

Physiologic Attributes of GnRH Action on the Ovary

In general, the inhibitory effects of GnRH on nonluteal ovarian tissue make it likely that ovarian GnRH-like peptide may have a role in the regulation of follicular atresia. Furthermore, even some of GnRH stimulatory actions are compatible with such an atretogenic function. Thus, elevation of progestin secretion (prostesterone and 20α-hydroxyprogesterone) (see above) (559) and precocious maturation of the oocyte in preantral follicles (560) by GnRH may be indicative and associated with early atretic changes (28). In fact, the meiosis-inducing action of GnRH in immature, estrogen-primed hypophysectomized rats was limited to a subpopulation of atretic preantral follicles (561). The recent finding that antagonists of GnRH given concomitantly with FSH enhance its stimulatory action on follicular development and maturation of follicles to an ovulable stage (450) strongly supports the notion that an ovarian GnRH-like peptide may be involved in the regulation of follicular development and follicle selection as a physiologic atretic signal.

The inhibitory actions of GnRH on luteal cells are very similar to that of $PGF_{2\alpha}$, which serves as a natural luteolysin (558). Both GnRH and $PGF_{2\alpha}$ cause a rapid and marked increase in labeling of PA and PI of rat luteal cells in culture (518,520). Thus, it is possible that a GnRH-like peptide plays a physiologic role in regulating corpus luteum function.

In terms of physiologic function of an ovarian GnRH-like peptide, the ovulation inducing actions of GnRH seem difficult to interpret. One possible interpretation is that GnRH-like peptides mediate LH action on the preovulatory follicle. Inasmuch as LH action on the ovary could not be blocked by antagonistic analogs of GnRH, whereas the action of GnRH was blocked by such drugs (484,485) makes this interpretation unlikely. Alternatively, it is possible that the vital role of ovulation in reproduction resulted in the development of several parallel triggering or amplifying mechanisms. The findings that GnRH acts through cyclic Amp-independent pathways, whereas LH acts primarily through cyclic-

AMP, may be related to such a role. But, at the present time, there is no hard experimental evidence to support this notion. Nevertheless, it is possible that the action of GnRH on the preovulatory follicle is not physiologic and is related to the ability of GnRH to activate arachidonic acid metabolism and plasminogen activator production, which are also activated by LH and involved in ovulation (see GnRH Binding and Mechanism of Action in the Ovary and Chapter 13 by Espey, this volume). Further studies are required to distinguish between these alternative possibilities. In any case, GnRH has proved to be a powerful tool to probe into some of the normally obscured mechanisms of ovarian function, especially in the rat.

OTHER PUTATIVE LOCAL REGULATORS OF OVARIAN FUNCTION

In this section, the local regulatory actions in the ovary of hormones, neurotransmitters, and factors known from nonreproductive organs and tissues will be described. The list of such factors implicated in ovarian function by their action *in vivo* or *in vitro* is growing rapidly. Nevertheless, the scarcity of data supporting these claims by demonstrating their ovarian production and reception made it very difficult to decide which hormones or factors to include as ovarian regulators. Hence, it seems very likely that future research (and probably studies that we are not aware of at present) will extend the list of hormones included here, whereas some of these included will not withstand rigorous examination by the criteria set for local ovarian regulators. Also, enzymes or constitutive molecules were not included in this review, even if they may assume important functions in ovarian physiology. Thus, for example, plasminogen activator, which plays a central role in follicular rupture at ovulation (reviewed in Chapter 13 by Espey, this volume), or proteoglycans with their putative regulatory functions were not included. The role of relaxin as ovarian regulator is discussed elsewhere in this volume (Chapter 18 by Sherwood).

Neurotransmitters

Role of Catecholamines

The recent studies demonstrating biosynthesis of norepinephrine (NE) from its precursor tyrosine by ovarian slices (562) and its release from the rat ovaries (563–565), coupled with demonstration of its ovarian receptors (566–575) and actions (566,567,569,572,576–586) in the ovary, justify inclusion of catecholamines among ovarian regulators.

Most of the initial studies regarding the ovarian role of adrenergic agents were concerned with their involvement in ovulation and compensatory ovarian hypertrophy (reviewed in refs. 587 and 588). Such studies did not bring forward convincing evidence for the role of catecholamines in ovulation (589–592). However, these studies may be complicated by possible ingrowth of adrenergic nerves accompanying revascularization (593–595) and by local production of catecholamines. Furthermore, an increase in sensitivity of ovarian cells to adrenergic agents was associated with ovarian denervation (596). Likewise, culture of granulosa cells in the absence of catecholamines increased greatly their sensitivity to adrenergic stimuli, whereas addition of catecholamines down-regulated adrenergic receptors. It was suggested, therefore, that the adrenergic tone *in vivo* and *in vitro* may modulate ovarian cell responsiveness to adrenergic stimuli (596).

Local treatment of rat ovary with 6-hydroxydopamine (chemical sympathectomy) increased contralateral ovarian weight, and after unilateral ovariectomy, the treatment of the remaining ovary prevented compensatory changes in that ovary (597,598). As unilateral ovariectomy and the resulting compensatory ovarian hypertrophy were associated with increased uptake of ^{3}H-lysine and ^{3}H-uridine into the contralateral hypothalamic arcuate nucleus (599), the existence of a gonadal-hypothalamic neural axis or neural reflex mechanism necessary for the development of the hypotrophy was postulated (599). Nevertheless, in guinea pigs, a species with dense ovarian adrenergic innervation, chemical sympathectomy did not cause hypertrophy in the contralateral ovary, nor did 6-hydroxydopamine prevent hypertrophy of the remaining ovary (600). These species differences may be related to the varying density of ovarian adrenergic nerves. Sympathectomy somewhat impaired follicular development in mice (601) and guinea pigs (600,602). It is likely that ovarian catecholamines modulate follicular growth and response to gonadotropins, but the precise nature of its actions remains obscure.

The presence of α-adrenergic receptors in the ovary of immature rats, in both granulosa cells and residual tissue compartments, has been demonstrated (572). The concentration of these receptors increases between the late juvenile period and the morning of first proestrus and then decreases markedly at the first preovulatory surge of gonadotropins. Furthermore, adrenergic agonists elicit only a small increase in progesterone and marked increase in aromatizable androgens before ovulation. After ovulation, the action of the adrenergic agonist on progesterone release was enhanced and on androgens was reduced (572). Both ovarian content and biosynthesis of NE increased remarkably during the juvenile period (days 25–30) of rats (562). These data prompted Ojeda and Aguado (596) to suggest a modulatory action of catecholamines in prepubertal ovarian function. Nevertheless, bilateral section of the superior ovarian nerve

24 days of age did not alter the time of vaginal opening or of first ovulation (596). The superior ovarian nerve travels along the suspensory ligament and is one source of rat ovarian innervation, the other being the plexus nerve accompanying the ovarian artery.

By the use of double isotope radioenzymatic assay, a significant depletion of ovarian catecholamines following PMSG-treatment of immature rats was observed (603). The NE content of Graafian follicles is markedly reduced within 4 hr after the preovulatory surge of gonadotropins. Follicle-stimulating hormone, rather than LH or prolactin, seems to be responsible for follicular NE depletion (604,605). Catecholamines have been identified in porcine (606,607) and human (608) FF.

Activation of ovarian adenylate cyclase by catecholamines has been demonstrated. Studies in the pig (609), rabbit (583,610), and rat (585,611–614) agree that follicular tissues are relatively insensitive to catecholamines, whereas corpora lutea or its cells respond readily with enhanced adenylate cyclase activity. Norepinephrine was found to stimulate theca-interstitial cell androgen synthesis (575).

Catecholamine stimulation of corpus luteum progesterone secretion has been demonstrated in the rat (579,580,584,611,613), rabbit (571,583,608,615,616), ewe (578), and cow (576,577). The action of catecholamines to enhance progesterone accumulation is attributed, in part, to their reduction of 20α-hydroxysteroid-dehydrogenase (SDH) activity (582), and, in part, to enhanced pregnenolone production and stimulation of 3β-SDH activity (617).

The luteotropic action of catecholamines on the corpus luteum was found to be enhanced between day 2 and 4, and thereafter luteal response declines; this seems to be associated with changes in the content of adrenergic receptors (574). $PGF_{2\alpha}$, which exerts a luteolytic action in aging corpora lutea (618–621), inhibited the luteotrophic effect of epinephrine. This action, too, was dependent on the age of the corpus luteum; 1-day-old corpora lutea were not affected by $PGF_{2\alpha}$, whereas in 3-day-old ones, $PGF_{2\alpha}$ inhibited the stimulatory action of epinephrine on tissue levels of cyclic AMP and production of progesterone (622).

Besides the steroidogenic effects of adrenergic agents on luteinized granulosa cells and corpora lutea, stimulatory actions were also observed in interfollicular tissues of the rat. Thus, stimulation of the neural plexus in hypophysectomized rats caused interstitial cells to develop morphologic features of steroidogenically active cells (623). Likewise, adrenergic agents enhance hCG-induced rise in androgen secretion by ovarian theca-interstitial cells (586).

The studies reviewed seem to suggest a modulatory role of adrenergic agents in follicular development and corpus luteum function. However, the conflicting data obtained and several paradoxical observations make it very difficult at this time to draw a comprehensive mechanistic outline of the physiologic role of adrenergic agents in ovarian function. This will probably be achieved by additional studies in the future.

γ-Aminobutyric Acid

γ-Aminobutyric acid (GABA) is known as the main inhibitory neurotransmitter in the mammalian central nervous system (624). High GABA levels, comparable with those in the brain, have been demonstrated in the ovary (625–627). Both ovarian GABA concentration and content increased during days 3 to 14 of pregnancy and diminished on day 21 (628). Furthermore, the ovarian levels of glutamate decarboxylase, the primary enzyme responsible for GABA biosynthesis in the brain, correlated well with endogenous GABA concentrations (627,629–631). But in contrast to the high levels of GABA and its synthesizing enzyme in the whole ovary, both GABA and the enzyme are undetectable in granulosa cell preparations (627).

γ-Aminobutyric acid binding sites were described in ovarian tissue (629,630,632) and granulosa cells (627). Thus, granulosa cells have specific high-affinity binding sites but do not contain GABA or GABA biosynthesizing enzyme. The demonstrations of ovarian production and specific binding of GABA suggest a modulatory action of GABA in the ovary. Intrabursal administration of GABA to pseudopregnant rats increased ovarian blood flow, enhanced estradiol 17β release, and decreased progesterone secretion (633). Evidently, additional studies are needed for evaluating the physiologic role of GABA in ovarian function.

Vasoactive Intestinal Peptide

The possible role of vasoactive intestinal peptide (VIP) in ovarian physiology was reviewed recently (634). Vasoactive intestinal peptide and VIPergic nerve fibers were described in the ovarian stroma of laboratory animals and human ovaries (635–637), and even occasional association with antral follicles was noted in immature rat ovaries (638). Furthermore, a VIP encoding mRNA was located in ovarian tissue (639), which may suggest the presence of VIP-synthesizing cells within the ovary.

Vasoactive intestinal peptide enhanced both progestin and estrogen production *in vitro* by granulosa cells of hypophysectomized estrogen-treated rats. This effect was, at least partially, exerted through cyclic AMP-mediated mechanisms and entailed increased availability of pregnenolone, stimulation of 3β-hydroxysteroid-dehydrogenase (HSD), and decrease in 20α-hydroxysteroid-dehydrogenase (HSD) activities and stimulation of aromatase (640). On separation of granulosa cells on Metrizamide density gradient, VIP preferentially stimulated steroid production in cells with lower density as compared with FSH, which stimulated steroidogenesis in cells with the highest density (641). Similar results were obtained in granulosa cells of intact immature rats: VIP enhanced progesterone release from cells explanted from infantile (12-day-old), juvenile (30-day-old), and peripubertal rats, whereas estradiol release was stimulated by VIP during the two latter developmental stages and reached maximum during proestrous phases of puberty (638). Likewise, VIP mimicked the action of LH in stimulating cyclic AMP production, steroidogenesis, and oocyte maturation in explanted hamster and rat follicles (642,643). Finally, VIP induced ovulation in rat perfused ovaries, although less efficiently than LH (644).

These studies, indicating VIP production and action in ovarian tissues, should be extended to assess the possible modulatory role of VIP or VIPergic nerves in ovarian function.

Other Neurotransmitters

Studies using retrograde transport of horseradish peroxidase demonstrated vagal ovarian innervation (645; also see 645 for earlier literature). Abdominal vagotomy, which does not affect adrenergic innervation, decreased steroid secretion (646), delayed onset of puberty (647), and reduced the number of ovulated eggs (648). These studies suggest that additional neurotransmitters may be involved in modulating ovarian activity.

Fibers containing substance P have been observed by immunohistofluorescence in juvenile and prepubertal rat ovaries. These fibers were closely associated with the theca externa of antral follicles, interstitial tissue, and tunica adventitia of small blood vessels (649). Substance P was found in ovaries of mature hamsters (650) and in prepubertal rats (651). Nevertheless, addition of substance P to cultured granulosa cells had no effect on their steroidogenic activity, and hence involvement in the regulation of ovarian blood flow was suggested (649,651).

Neurohypophyseal Hormones

The role of oxytocin in luteal regression in ruminants through its action on the uterus has recently been reviewed (652) (see Chapter 14 by Niswender and Nett, this volume) and as such is not a local ovarian regulator. Nevertheless, paracrine and autocrine effects of oxytocin were suggested in follicles and corpora lutea of species with relatively low oxytocin production (653,654). Thus, oxytocin was detected in bovine (655–657), ovine (658,659), and human (660–663) follicles and corpora lutea. Bovine granulosa and luteal cells secreted oxytocin in culture (664–669).

In mice, oxytocin was found to affect follicular development (670). Infusion of oxytocin into ruminants shortened the luteal phase (671). Intraluteal perfusion of oxytocin into monkey corpora lutea resulted in early luteal regression (652). Likewise, the peptide inhibited progesterone (672) but stimulated estradiol (673) secretion by porcine luteal cells in culture. Using a microdialysis system to perfuse individual porcine corpora lutea, it was shown that oxytocin stimulated estradiol as well as progesterone secretion. The stimulatory effect of oxytocin on progesterone was prevented by tamoxifen, an estrogen receptor antagonist (674). This stimulating action of oxytocin was limited to young and middle-stage corpora lutea. At later stages of luteal development (luteal regression), oxytocin still slightly stimulated estradiol secretion, but the levels attained were insufficient to stimulate progesterone (674). Similarly, in fragments of human young corpora lutea microdialyzed *in vitro* responded to oxytocin with an increase in estradiol and progesterone release (675). It appears, therefore, that in both the sow and the human the inhibitory effect of oxytocin on young luteal cell progesterone is counteracted by the stimulation of estradiol production, which in turn increases progesterone secretion (674,675).

Arginine vasopressin was found in human ovaries and FF at concentrations significantly higher than in serum (655,658,662,676–678), suggesting local production. Arginine vasopressin was also present in rat and sheep ovaries (679), including demonstration of vasopressin-neurophysin II gene expression in the ovary (680). Although the data reviewed do implicate neourohypophyseal hormones in paracrine/autocrine modulation of ovarian activity, much more research is needed to define their precise role.

Pro-Opiomelanocortin-Derived Hormones

Pro-opiomelanocortin (POMC) is a precursor for a variety of peptide hormones including ACTH, melanocyte-stimulating hormones (MSHs), lipotropins, endorphins, enkephalins, and dynorphins (681,682). Immunoreactive β-endorphin, enkephalin, and dynorphin have been demonstrated in ovarian tissues of the rat (683–686), β-endorphin in the sheep (687) and the mouse (19,688), and enkephalin in the hamster and the cow (684). Human FF contains β-endorphin and enkaphalin (689). Local production in the ovary is suggested on the basis of mRNA identification in the tissue. Thus, mRNA transcripts for POMC (690–692), proenkephalin (684,691), and prodynorphin (685) were detected in rat and hamster ovaries. The ovarian content of immunoreactive β-endorphin (686) and POMC mRNA increased after PMSG administration to immature rats (691,693) or in pregnancy (690,691).

Thus, the ovaries, like other steroidogenic organs such as the adrenal and testis, contain POMC, and its ovarian production seems to be regulated by gonadotropins (694). At present, we do not have any clues regarding the physiologic role of POMC-derived peptides in ovarian physiology.

Adenosine and Other Purines

In the above sections on ovum maturation, the putative role of purine and pyrimidine bases in the regulation of meiosis has been discussed.

Adenosine and other purines have been shown to enhance gonadotropin-stimulated cyclic AMP accumulation in rat granulosa and luteal cells (695–698) and in periovulatory human granulosa cells (696). Adenosine exerted both stimulatory and inhibitory effects. Thus, acute stimulation with adenosine resulted in amplification of FSH-stimulated cyclic AMP production during the first 6 to 20 hr of culture. During the second 24 hr of culture, adenosine inhibited FSH-induced responses such as cyclic AMP and progesterone production and expression of FSH and LH receptors (699). In rat luteal cells, adenosine also enhances LH-stimulated progesterone synthesis. Adenosine amplification of cyclic AMP and of progesterone was a function of corpus luteum age, decreasing from days 4 to 11. Furthermore, adenosine antagonized the luteolytic actions of $PGF_{2\alpha}$ (700). These effects of adenosine led to the suggestion that adenosine may play a modulatory role in the ovary (701).

Granulosa cell ATP levels were rapidly and markedly increased by adenosine (697,701–704). This effect of adenosine occurred in the absence and presence of gonadotropins (703). By contrast, gonadotropins suppressed granulosa cell ATP levels both in cultures containing and devoid of adenosine (697,705). The finding that adenosine enhanced LH-dependent cyclic AMP to a greater extent than that stimulated by FSH implicated adenosine in promoting follicular atresia (705).

Adenosine may be involved in adenylate cyclase activity by dual mechanisms, direct regulation of enzyme activity through membranal adenosine receptors and as a substrate to the enzyme by conversion to ATP (706,707). Evidence for adenosine receptors in granulosa cells has been presented (708,709). The suggested role of adenosine as local ovarian regulator should be confirmed by direct demonstration of specific receptors on ovarian cells and by clarification of the physiologic role of adenosine in ovarian activity. The putative actions of adenosine include mediation of atresia, promotion and maintenance of corpora lutea, and regulation of oocyte maturation (705,709).

Eicosanoids

The role of arachidonic acid metabolites in ovarian physiology, and especially in follicular rupture at ovulation and in corpus luteum development and demise, is detailed in this volume (see Chapter 13 by Espey and Chapter 14 by Niswender and Nett).

Here, the role of eicosanoids, products of C_{20} fatty acids (710), as local ovarian regulators is outlined in brief. Ample evidence for ovarian production and action of cyclooxygenase-derived metabolites has been presented (see reviews by refs. 711–713). Recently, the activity of ovarian lipoxygenases has been demonstrated. Ovarian and follicular lipoxygenase activity was enhanced by LH/hCG stimulation *in vivo* or *in vitro* (714–716). Inhibitors of lipoxygenase prevented follicular rupture dose-dependently (717,718). Inhibitors of both pathways of arachidonic acid metabolism, namely, of cyclooxygenase and of lipoxygenase, did not affect follicular plasminogen activator but prevented LH-induced increase in ovarian collagenolytic activity and expression of interstitial collagenase mRNA (719,720). Furthermore, a specific inhibitor of 5-lipoxygenase, MK886, suppressed ovulation and attenuated follicular interstitial collagenase activity (721). Prostaglandins have been implicated in paracrine regulation of cumulus oophorus expansion (722,723). Thus, cumulus cells cocultured with granulosa cells or in a granulosa cell conditioned medium underwent cumulus expansion. Addition of cyclooxygenase inhibitors to the granulosa cell cultures prevented the action of conditioned media on cumulus expansion, whereas they did not prevent expansion of cumuli in response to hormonal stimuli (724). The evidence for arachidonic acid metabolite receptors in ovarian tissue is more limited. Nevertheless, the clear effects of these metabolites on ovarian function and their production in the ovary justify considering eicosanoids as local ovarian hormones. Further studies aimed at localization of ovarian receptors of eicosanoids and elucidation of cellular and molecular mechanisms underlying their involvement in follicular rupture and corpus luteum function are definitely required.

Ovarian Renin-Angiotensin System

The ovarian renin-angiotensin system (OVRAS) has been thoroughly reviewed recently (725,726). The original observations of high levels of prorenin, renin, and angiotensinlike immunoreactivity in human and bovine FF (727–729) lead to the suggestion of OVRAS. The levels of the constituents of OVRAS were markedly higher in gonadotropin-stimulated women and during the midcycle phase, and being higher in FF than in plasma, they seem to be produced locally. Follicular renin seems to be derived mainly from theca cells (729–733). Studies in both rat and human granulosa cells show dependence of angiotensin II (Ang II) and renin expression on the stage of follicular development. Thus, no Ang II immunoreactivity was found in granulosa cells of antral and preantral follicles of the rat (732), and in the human, only cells from preovulatory and atretic follicles stained for renin and Ang II (731). Renin activity in the rat ovary was highest between the afternoon of proestrus and estrus (734).

The OVRAS was implicated in ovulation by the use of an antagonist of Ang II receptor, saralasin, which blocked ovulation in approximately 50% of the hCG-treated rats (735). Later studies with saralasin *in vivo* resulted in variable results (736,737), but in perfused rat (738) and rabbit (739,740), ovary saralasin blocked ovulation and this was reversed by Ang II.

Angiotensin II has been implicated also in oocyte maturation. Thus, in the rat and the rabbit, saralasin attenuated hCG-induced resumption of meiosis (740,741).

Also, OVRAS has been implicated in ovarian steroidogenesis, angiogenesis during corpus luteum formation, and follicular atresia (725). Further studies are needed to elucidate the precise role of OVRAS in ovarian physiology.

CONCLUDING REMARKS

Throughout this review, we have considered a multitude of ovarian paracrine/autocrine hormones. Nevertheless, one cannot escape the feeling that the story of local ovarian regulation is probably, to a large measure, unknown as yet. This underlies the steadily increasing number of reports on new putative ovarian regulators and the additional data on previously described ones. This is one of the reasons why a comprehensive overview of local regulation of ovarian function was presented here, rather than a critical evaluation of each system. We believe that the data available at the present do not allow, in too many instances, a profound assessment. Another reason for the approach adopted is the implication of local regulators in a broad spectrum of ovarian activities, far beyond the area of our own research interests. Despite the intent to include any local regulators, some may have been overlooked due to our unawareness, the scarcity of information, and the difficulty of fitting them into proper perspective.

Most of the cell types considered regarding their ovarian regulatory function were those also having clear endocrine functions, granulosa, theca, and interstitial cells. The close proximity of additional cells in the ovary, such as nerve fibers, fibroblasts, macrophages, and mast cells, makes it likely that they also participate in paracrine regulation of ovarian activity. We have reviewed some of the putative paracrine actions of cytokines and neurotransmitters in ovarian function. In the future, we may learn more about the participation of the immune and nerve systems in the regulation of ovarian physiology.

In mammals, the evolution of cyclic ovulation of one (in monotocous species) or more (in polytocous species) ova has resulted in hierarchical development of follicles and oocytes. The coexistence of follicles and oocytes at different stages of development requires in mammals mechanisms allowing stage-specific responses to similar endocrine cues. Variability in sensitivity to hormones, because of stage-dependent changes in the repertoire of receptors and differential distribution of ovarian microcirculation, and hence exposure to varying hormone levels are among the mechanisms allowing differential responses. Paracrine and autocrine hormones play a most important role in localized responses of discrete ovarian structures, follicles, and corpora lutea, as well as in the integration of the activity within these physiologic units.

Finally, the very wide spectrum of agents modulating ovarian cell activity warrants special notice. Ovarian cells have both intracellular and plasma membrane receptors using all known modes of signal transduction. This wide spectrum of ovarian reception mechanisms, the integrated and well-concerted function of several cell types, and the multitude of endocrine, paracrine, and autocrine mechanisms involved in ovarian physiology warrant continued interest. This may lead to new insights into ovarian biology and also form the basis for novel approaches to fertility regulation in the human and in animal husbandry.

ACKNOWLEDGMENTS

The phrase of Judah HaNasi "I learned much from my teachers, more from my colleagues, and most from my students" (Talmud, Makot 10a) most properly reflects the pivotal role of our colleagues and students in our scientific undertakings. We are indebted to colleagues working in this field who have generously provided published and unpublished papers: their help is most appreciated. Dr. N. Dekel and Dr. Y. Koch have read part of the manuscript, and we thank them for their advice. Special thanks are due to our students, past and present, whose unquenched thirst for knowledge was a prime motivator. The meticulous secretarial help of Mrs. M. Kopelowitz is gratefully acknowledged. The studies at the WIS laboratory were supported by grants from the United States-Israel Binational Agricultural Research and Development Fund (BARD), the German-Israel Foundation for Scientific Research and Development (GIF), Jerusalem, Israel, and the Basic Science Research Foundation of the Israel Academy of Sciences and Humanities, Jerusalem, Israel.

REFERENCES

1. Channing CP, Anderson LD, Hoover DJ, et al. The role of nonsteroidal regulators in control of oocyte and follicular maturation. *Recent Prog Horm Res* 1982;38:331–408.
2. Sharpe RM. Bibliography on intragonadal hormones. *Bibliogr Reprod* 1984;44:C1–C16.

3. Channing CP, Segal S. Intraovarian control mechanisms. New York: Plenum Press. 1982;147:392.
4. Sairam MR, Atkinson LE. Gonadal proteins and peptides and their biological significance. Singapore: World Scientific Publishing Co., 1984;388.
5. Fujii T, Channing CP. Non-steroidal regulators in reproductive biology and medicine. Oxford: Pergamon Press., 1982;34.
6. Franchimont P. Clinics in endocrinology and metabolism. London: Saunders, 1986;15(1).
7. Hodgen GD, Rosenwaks Z, Spieler JM. Nonsteroidal gonadal factors. Physiological roles and possibilities in contraceptive development. *Conrad International Workshop.* 1988;374.
8. Hirshfield AN. Growth factors and the ovary. New York: Plenum, 1989;458.
9. Witschi E. Der Hermaphroditismus der Frösche und seine Bedentung fur das Geschlechts problem und Lehre von der inneren Sekretion der Keindrüsen. *Arch Entwicklungmesh Org* 1921;49: 316–358.
10. Witschi E. Biochemistry of sex differentiation in vertebrate embryos. In: Weber R, ed. *Biochemistry of Sex Differentiation in Vertebrate Embryos,* Vol 2. New York: Academic Press, 1968;193–225.
11. Marrian GF. Early work on the chemistry of pregnanediol and the oestrogenic hormones. *J Endocrinol* 1966;VI–XVI.
12. Parkes AS. The rise of reproductive endocrinology, 1926–1940. *J Endocrinol* 1966;34:XX–XXXII.
13. Greep RO. The sage and the science of the gonadotrophins. *J Endocrinol* 1967;39:ii–ix.
14. Hsueh AJW, Adashi EY, Jones PBC, Welsh TH. Hormonal regulation of the differentiation of cultured granulosa cells. *Endocr Rev* 1984;5:76–127.
15. Starling EH. The Croonian lectures. *Lancet* 1905;26:579–583.
16. Roth J, LeRoith D, Schiloach J, Rubinovitz C. Intercellular communication: an attempt at a unifying hypothesis. *Clin Res* 1983;31:354–363.
17. Roth J, LeRoith D, Schiloach J, Rabinowitz C. Hormones and other messenger molecules. In: McKerns KW, Naor Z, eds. *Hormonal Control of the Hypothalamo-Pituitary-Gonadal Axis.* New York: Plenum Press, 1984;71–87.
18. Medawar P. Some immunological and endocrinological problems raised by the evolution of viviparity in vertebrates. *Symp Soc Exp Biol Med* 1953;7:320–338.
19. Niall HD. The evolution of peptide hormones. *Annu Rev Physiol* 1982;44:616–624.
20. Feyrter F. Über die peripheren endokrinen (parakrinen). In: eds. *Drüsen des Menschen.* Leipsig: Ambrosius Barth, 1938.
21. Dockray GJ. Evolutionary relationships of the gut hormones. *Fed Proc* 1979;38:2295–2301.
22. Sporn MB, Todaro GJ. Autocrine secretion of malignant transformation of cells. *N Engl J Med* 1980;303:878–880.
23. O'Malley BW. Did eucaryotic steroid receptors evolve from intracrine gene regulators? *Endocrinology* 1989;125:1119–1120 (editorial).
24. Grossman MI. Chemical messengers: a view from the gut. *Fed Proc* 1979;38:2341–2343.
25. Guillemin R. Peptides of the brain: the new endocrinology of the neuron. *Science* 1978;202:390–402.
26. O'Malley IE. President's letter: endocrinology in the 1990's. *Endocr Soc Newslett* 1984;9:1–2.
27. Ayalon D, Tsafriri A, Lindner HR, Cordova T, Harrel A. Serum gonadotropin levels in proestrous rats in relation to the resumption of meiosis by the oocytes. *J Reprod Fertil* 1972;31:51–58.
28. Tsafriri A, Braw R. Experimental approaches to atresia in mammals. *Oxford Rev Reprod Biol* 1984;6:226–265.
29. Byskov AG. Regulation of meiosis in mammals. *Ann Biol Anim Biochem Biophys* 1979;19:1251–1261.
30. Ohno S, Smith JB. Role of fetal follicular cells in meiosis of mammalian oocytes. *Cytogenetics* 1964;3:324–333.
31. Moor RM, Polge C, Willadsen SM. Effect of follicular steroids on the maturation and fertilization of mammalian oocytes. *J Embryol Exp Morphol* 1980;56:319–335.
32. Crosby IM, Osborn JC, Moor RM. Follicle cell regulation of protein synthesis and developmental competence in sheep oocytes. *J Reprod Fertil* 1981;62:575–582.
33. Mattioli M, Bacci ML, Galeati G, Seren E. Developmental competence of pig oocytes matured and fertilized *in vitro. Theriogenology* 1989;31:1201–1207.
34. Vermeiden JPW, Zeilmaker GH. Relationship between maturation, division, ovulation and luteinization in the female rat. *Endocrinology* 1974;95:341–351.
35. Magnusson C, Hillensjö T, Tsafriri A, Hultborn R, Ahrén K. Oxygen consumption of maturing rat oocytes. *Biol Reprod* 1977;17:9–15.
36. Pincus G, Enzmann EV. The comparative behaviour of mammalian eggs *in vivo* and *in vitro. J Exp Med* 1935;62:655–675.
37. Tsafriri A. Oocyte maturation in mammals. In: Jones RE, ed. *The Vertebrate Ovary.* New York, London: Plenum Press, 1978;409–442.
38. Szybek K. *In vitro* maturation of oocytes from sexually immature mice. *J Endocrinol* 1972;54:527–528.
39. Sorensen RA, Wassarman PM. Relationship between growth and meiotic maturation of mouse oocyte. *Dev Biol* 1976;50:532–536.
40. Bar-Ami S, Tsafriri A. Acquisition of meiotic competence in the rat: role of gonadotropin and estrogen. *Gamete Res* 1981;4:463–472.
41. Bar-Ami S, Nimrod A, Brodie AMH, Tsafriri A. Role of FSH and oestradiol 17-β in the development of meiotic competence in rat oocytes. *J Steroid Biochem* 1983;19:965–971.
42. Tsafriri A, Lindner HR, Zor U, Lamprecht SA. *In vitro* induction of meiotic division in follicle-enclosed rat oocytes by LH, cyclic AMP and prostaglandin E_2. *J Reprod Fertil* 1972;31:39–50.
43. Moor RM, Trounson AO. Hormonal and follicular factors affecting maturation of sheep oocytes *in vitro* and their subsequent developmental capacity. *J Reprod Fertil* 1977;49:101–109.
44. Neal P, Baker TG. Response of mouse ovaries *in vivo* and in organ culture to pregnant mare's serum gonadotrophin and human chorionic gonadotrophin. I. Examination of critical time intervals. *J Reprod Fertil* 1973;33:399–410.
45. Thibault C, Gerard M. Cytoplasmic and nuclear maturation of rabbit oocytes *in vitro. Ann Biol Anim Biochem Biophys* 1973;13:145–155.
46. Thibault C. Are follicular maturation and oocyte maturation independent processes? *J Reprod Fertil* 1977;51:1–15.
47. Hillensjö T. Oocyte maturation and glycolysis in isolated preovulatory follicles of PMS-injected immature rats. *Acta Endocrinol (Copenh)* 1976;82:809–830.
48. Meinecke B, Meinecke-Tillman S. Induction and inhibition of meiotic maturation of follicle-enclosed porcine oocytes *in vivo. Theriogenology* 1981;216:205–209.
49. Chang MC. The maturation of rabbit oocytes in culture and their maturation, activation, fertilization and subsequent development in fallopian tube. *J Exp Zool* 1955;128:378–399.
50. Foote WD, Thibault C. Recherches experimentales sur la maturation *in vitro* des ovocytes de truie et de veau. *Ann Biol Anim Biochem Biophys* 1969;9:329–349.
51. Tsafriri A, Channing CP. Inhibitory influence of granulosa cells and follicular fluid upon porcine oocyte meiosis *in vitro. Endocrinology* 1975;96:922–927.
52. Gwatkin RBL, Andersen OF. Hamster oocyte maturation *in vitro*: inhibition by follicular components. *Life Sci* 1976;19: 527–536.
53. Leibfried L, First NL. Follicular control of meiosis in the porcine oocyte. *Biol Reprod* 1980;23:705–709.
54. Leibfried L, First NL. Effect of bovine and porcine follicular fluid and granulosa cells on maturation of oocyte *in vitro. Biol Reprod* 1980;23:699–704.
55. Sirard MA, First NL. *In vitro* inhibition of oocyte nuclear maturation in the bovine. *Biol Reprod* 1988;39:229–234.
56. Sirard MA, Bilodeau S. Effects of granulosa cell co-culture on *in-vitro* meiotic resumption of bovine oocytes. *J Reprod Fertil* 1990;89:459–465.
57. Sirard MA, Bilodeau S. Granulosa cells inhibit the resumption of meiosis in bovine oocytes *in vitro. Biol Reprod* 1990;43:777–783.
58. Racowsky C, Baldwin KV. *In vitro* and *in vivo* studies reveal that hamster oocyte meiotic arrest is maintained only transiently by follicular fluid, but persistently by membrana/cumulus granulosa cell contact. *Dev Biol* 1989;134:297–306.
59. Tsafriri A, Pomerantz SH. Oocyte maturation inhibitor. In:

Franchimont P, ed. *Clinics in Endocrinology and Metabolism,* Vol 15/1. London, Philadelphia, Toronto: WB Saunders, 1986;157–170.
60. Thibault C, Szollosi D, Gerard M. Mammalian oocyte maturation. *Reprod Nutr Dev* 1987;27:856–896.
61. Tsafriri A, Pomerantz SH, Channing CP. Follicular control of oocyte maturation. In: Crosignani PG, Michel DR, eds. *Ovulation in the Human.* New York: Academic Press, 1976;31–39.
62. Fleming AD, Kuehl TJ, Armstrong DT. Maturation of pig and rat oocytes transplanted into surrogate pig follicles *in vitro. Gamete Res* 1985;11:107–119.
63. Sato E, Ishibashi T. Meiotic arresting action of the substance obtained from cell surface to porcine ovarian granulosa cells. *Jpn J Zootech Sci* 1977;48:22–26.
64. Centola GM, Anderson LD, Channing CP. Oocyte maturation inhibitor (OMI) activity in porcine granulosa cells. *Gamete Res* 1981;4:451–461.
65. Tsafriri A, Channing CP, Pomerantz SH, Lindner HR. Inhibition of maturation of isolated rat oocytes by porcine follicular fluid. *J Endocrinol* 1977;75:285–291.
66. Tsafriri A. Mammalian oocyte maturation: model systems and their physiological relevance. In: Channing CP, Marsh JM, Sadler WJ, eds. *Ovarian Follicular and Corpus Luteum Function.* New York: Plenum Press, 1979:269–281.
67. Tsafriri A, Pomerantz SH, Channing CP. Inhibition of oocyte maturation by porcine follicular fluid: partial characterization of the inhibitor. *Biol Reprod* 1976;14:511–516.
68. Sato E, Ishibashi T, Iritani A. Meiotic arresting substance separated from porcine ovarian granulosa cells and hypothetical arresting mechanism of meiosis. In: Channing CP, Segal S, eds. *Intraovarian Control Mechanisms.* New York: Plenum Press, 1982;161–173.
69. Sato E, Koide SS. A factor from bovine granulosa cells preventing oocyte maturation. *Differentiation* 1984;26:59–62.
70. Anderson LD, Stone SL, Channing CP. Influence of hormones on the inhibitory activity of oocyte maturation present in conditioned media of porcine granulosa cells. *Gamete Res* 1985;12:119–130.
71. Jagiello G, Graffeo J, Ducayen M, Prosser R. Further studies of inhibitors of *in vitro* mammalian oocyte maturation. *Fertil Steril* 1977;28:476–481.
72. Hillensjö T, Batta SK, Schwartz-Kripner A, Wentz AC, Sulewski J, Channing CP. Inhibitory effect of human follicular fluid upon the maturation of porcine oocytes in culture. *J Clin Endocrinol Metab* 1978;47:1332–1335.
73. Channing CP, Liu CO, Jones GS, Jones H. Decline in follicular oocyte maturation inhibitor coincident with maturation and achievement of fertilizability of oocytes recovered at midcycle of gonadotropin-treated women. *Proc Natl Acad Sci USA* 1983;80:4184–4188.
74. Stone SL, Pomerantz SH, Schwartz-Kripner A, Channing CP. Inhibitor of oocyte maturation from porcine follicular fluid: further purification and evidence for reversible action. *Biol Reprod* 1978;19:585–592.
75. Van de Wiel DFM, Bar-Ami S, Tsafriri A, de Jong FH. Oocyte maturation inhibitor, inhibin and steroid concentrations in porcine follicular fluid at various stages of the oestrous cycle. *J Reprod Fertil* 1983;68:247–252.
76. Chari S, Hillensjo T, Magnusson C, Sturm G, Daume E. *In vitro* inhibition of rat oocyte meiosis by human follicular fluid fractions. *Arch Gynecol* 1983;233:155–164.
77. Hillensjö T, Brännström M, Chari S, et al. Oocyte maturation as regulated by follicular factors. *Ann NY Acad Sci* 1985;442:73–79.
78. Das K, Phipps WR, Hensleigh HC, Tagatz GE. Epidermal growth factor in human follicular fluid stimulates mouse oocyte maturation *in vitro. Fertil Steril* 1992;57:895–901.
79. Dekel N, Sherizly I. Epidermal growth factor induces maturation of rat follicle-enclosed oocytes. *Endocrinology* 1985;116: 406–409.
80. Downs SM, Daniel SAJ, Eppig JJ. Induction of maturation in cumulus cell-enclosed mouse oocytes by follicle-stimulating hormone and epidermal growth factor: evidence for a positive stimulus of somatic cell origin. *J Exp Zool* 1988;245:86–96.
81. Pomerantz S, Tsafriri A, Channing CP. Studies on purification and actions of an oocyte maturation inhibitor isolated from porcine follicular fluid. In: Gross E, Meienhofer J, eds. *Peptides, Structure and Biological Function.* Rockford, IL: Pierce Chemical Co., 1979;765–774.
82. Downs SM, Eppig JJ. Cyclic adenosine monophosphate and ovarian follicular fluid act synergistically to inhibit mouse oocyte maturation. *Endocrinology* 1984;114:418–427.
83. Downs SM, Eppig JJ. A follicular fluid component prevents gonadotropin reversal of cyclic adenosine monophosphate-dependent meiotic arrest in murine oocytes. *Gamete Res* 1985;11:83–97.
84. Schuetz AW, Rock J. Stimulatory and inhibitory effects of human follicular fluid on amphibian oocyte maturation and ovulation *in vitro. Differentiation* 1982;21:41–44.
85. Cameron IL, Lum JB, Nations C, Asch RH, Silverman AY. Assay for characterization of human follicular oocyte maturation inhibitor using *Xenopus* oocytes. *Biol Reprod* 1983;28:817–822.
86. Pomerantz SH, Bilello PA, Evans V. Recent developments in the purification of an inhibitor of oocyte maturation from pig follicular fluid. In: Tsafriri A, Dekel N, eds. *Follicular Development and the Ovulatory Response.* Rome: Ares-Serono Symposia, 1989;77–80.
87. Takahashi M, Koide SS, Donahue PK. Müllerian inhibiting substance as oocyte meiosis inhibitor. *Mol Cell Endocrinol* 1986;47:225–234.
88. Tsafriri A, Picard Y-Y, Josso N. Immunopurified anti-Müllerian hormone does not inhibit spontaneous maturation *in vitro* of rat oocytes. *Biol Reprod* 1988;38:481–485.
89. Ueno S, Manganaro TF, Donahoe PK. Human recombinant Müllerian inhibiting substance inhibition of rat oocyte meiosis is reversed by epidermal growth factor *in vitro. Endocrinology* 1988;123:1652–1659.
90. Tsafriri A, Veljkovic MV, Pomerantz SH, Ling N. The action of transforming growth factors and inhibin-related proteins on oocyte maturation. *Bull Assoc Anat* 1991;75:109–113.
91. O WS, Robertson DM, de Kretser DM. Inhibin as an oocyte meiotic inhibitor. *Mol Cell Endocrinol* 1989;62:307–311.
92. Tsafriri A, Vale W, Hsueh AJW. Effects of transforming growth factors and inhibin-related proteins on rat preovulatory Graafian follicles. *Endocrinology* 1989;125:1857–1862.
93. Buscaglia M, Fuller J, Mazzola T, et al. A new intra-ovarian function for follistatin: the inhibition of oocyte meiosis. *Proc Endocr Soc USA* 1989;71(Abst. 883).
94. Nakamura T, Takio K, Eto Y, Shibai H, Titani K, Sugino H. Activin-binding protein from rat ovary is follistatin. *Science* 1990;247:836–838.
95. Shimonaka M, Inouye S, Shimasaki S, Ling N. Follistatin binds to both activin and inhibin through the common beta-subunit. *Endocrinology* 1991;128:3313–3315.
96. Downs SM, Coleman DL, Ward-Bailey PF, Eppig JJ. Hypoxanthine is the principal inhibitor of murine oocyte maturation in a low molecular weight fraction of porcine follicular fluid. *Proc Natl Acad Sci USA* 1985;82:454–458.
97. Eppig JJ, Ward-Bailey PF, Coleman DL. Hypoxanthine and adenosine in murine ovarian follicular fluid: concentrations and activity in maintaining oocyte meiotic arrest. *Biol Reprod* 1985;33:1041–1049.
98. Eppig JJ. The participation of cyclic adenosine monophosphate (cAMP) in the regulation of meiotic maturation of oocytes in the laboratory mouse. *J Reprod Fertil Suppl* 1989;38:3–8.
99. Hillensjö T, Channing CP, Pomerantz SH, Schwartz-Kripner A. Intrafollicular control of oocyte maturation in the pig. *In Vitro* 1979;15:32–40.
100. Downs SM, Coleman DL, Eppig JJ. Maintenance of murine oocyte meiotic arrest: uptake and metabolism of hypoxanthine and adenosine by cumulus cell-enclosed and denuded oocytes. *Dev Biol* 1986;117:174–183.
101. Eppig JJ, Downs SM. The effect of hypoxanthine on mouse oocyte growth and development *in vitro:* maintenance of meiotic arrest and gonadotropin-induced oocyte maturation. *Dev Biol* 1987;119:313–321.
102. Lindner HR, Tsafriri A, Lieberman ME, et al. Gonadotropin action on cultured Graafian follicles: mechanism of induction of

maturation of the mammalian oocyte. *Recent Progr Horm Res* 1974;30:79–138.
103. Hillensjö T, Ekholm C, Ahrén K. Role of cyclic AMP in oocyte maturation and glycolysis in the pre-ovulatory rat follicle. *Acta Endocrinol (Copenh)* 1978;87:377–388.
104. Dekel N, Lawrence TS, Gilula NB, Beers WH. Modulation of cell-to-cell communication in the cumulus-oocyte complex and the regulation of oocyte maturation by LH. *Dev Biol* 1981;86:356–362.
105. Cho WK, Stern S, Biggers JD. Inhibitory effect of dibutyryl cAMP on mouse oocyte maturation *in vitro. J Exp Zool* 1974;187:383–386.
106. Dekel N, Beers WH. Rat oocyte maturation *in vitro:* relief of cyclic AMP inhibition by gonadotropins. *Proc Natl Acad Sci USA* 1978;75:3469–3473.
107. Dekel N, Beers WH. Development of rat oocyte *in vitro:* inhibition and induction of maturation in the presence or absence of the cumulus oophorus. *Dev Biol* 1980;75:247–252.
108. Schultz RM, Montgomery RR, Belanoff JR. Regulation of mouse oocyte meiotic maturation: implication of a decrease in oocyte cAMP and protein dephosphorylation in commitment to resume meiosis. *Dev Biol* 1983;97:264–273.
109. Schultz RM, Montgomery RR, Ward-Bailey PF, Eppig JJ. Regulation of oocyte maturation in the mouse: possible roles of intercellular communication, cAMP, and testosterone. *Dev Biol* 1983;95:294–304.
110. Vivarelli E, Conti M, DeFelici M, Siracusa G. Meiotic resumption and intracellular cAMP levels in mouse oocytes treated with compounds which act on cMP metabolism. *Cell Differ* 1983;12:271–276.
111. Dekel N, Aberdam E, Hanski E. Invasive bacterial adenylate cyclase maintains the meiotic arrest in isolated rat oocytes. In: Toft DO, Ryan RJ, eds. *Proceeding of the Fifth Ovarian Workshop.* Champaign, IL: Ovarian Workshops, 1985;65–69.
112. Aberdam E, Hanski E, Dekel N. Maintenance of meiotic arrest in isolated rat oocytes by the invasive adenylate cyclase of *Bordetella pertussis. Biol Reprod* 1987;36:530–535.
113. Dekel N, Sherizly I. Induction of maturation in rat follicle-enclosed oocyte by forskolin. *FEBS Lett* 1983;151:153–155.
114. Dekel N, Aberdam E, Sherizly I. Spontaneous maturation *in vitro* of cumulus-enclosed rat oocytes is inhibited by forskolin. *Biol Reprod* 1984;31:244–250.
115. Racowsky C. Effect of forskolin on the spontaneous maturation and cyclic AMP content of rat oocyte cumulus complexes. *J Reprod Fertil* 1984;72:107–116.
116. Racowsky C. Effect of forskolin on maintenance of meiotic arrest and stimulation of cumulus expansion, progesterone and cyclic AMP production by pig oocyte-cumulus complexes. *J Reprod Fertil* 1985;74:9–21.
117. Bornslaeger EA, Schultz RM. Regulation of mouse oocyte maturation: effect of elevating cumulus cell cAMP on oocyte cAMP levels. *Biol Reprod* 1985;33:698–704.
118. Sherizly I, Galiani D, Dekel N. Regulation of oocyte maturation: communication in the rat cumulus-oocyte complex. *Hum Reprod* 1988;3:761–766.
119. Racowsky C. Effect of forskolin on the spontaneous maturation and cyclic AMP content of hamster oocyte-cumulus complexes. *J Exp Zool* 1985;234:87–96.
120. Urner F, Herrman WL, Baullieu E-E, Schorderet-Saltkine S. Inhibition of denuded mouse oocyte meiotic maturation by forskolin, an activator of adenylate cyclase. *Endocrinology* 1983;113:1170–1172.
121. Olsiewski PJ, Beers WH. cAMP synthesis in the rat oocyte. *Dev Biol* 1983;100:287–293.
122. Törnell J, Billig H, Hillensjö T. Regulation of oocyte maturation by changes in ovarian levels of cyclic nucleotides. *Hum Reprod* 1991;6:411–422.
123. Eppig JJ, Downs SM. Chemical signals that regulate mammalian oocyte maturation. *Biol Reprod* 1984;20:1–12.
124. Törnell J, Brännström M, Chari S, Hillensjö T. Synergistic inhibitory effects by human follicular fluid and cAMP on spontaneous rat oocyte maturation. *Biol Reprod* 1984;(suppl 1)30:(abst. 228).
125. Hillensjö T, Kripner AS, Pomerantz SH, Channing CP. Action of porcine follicular fluid oocyte maturation *in vitro:* possible role of the cumulus cells. In: Channing CP, Marsh JM, Sadler WA, eds. *Ovarian Follicular and Corpus Luteum Function.* New York: Plenum Press, 1979;283–291.
126. Tsafriri A, Bar-Ami S. Oocyte maturation inhibitor: a 1981 perspective. In: Channing CP, Segal SJ, eds. *Intra-Ovarian Control Mechanisms, Advances in Experimental Medicine and Biology,* Vol 147. New York: Plenum Press, 1982;145–160.
127. Lawrence TS, Dekel N, Beers WH. Binding of human chorionic gonadotropin by rat cumuli oophori and granulosa cells: a comparative study. *Endocrinology* 1980;106:1114–1118.
128. Channing CP, Bae I-H, Stone SL, Anderson LD, Edelson S, Fowler SC. Porcine granulosa and cumulus cell properties: LH/hCG-receptors, ability to secrete progesterone and ability to respond to LH. *Mol Cell Endocrinol* 1981;22:359–370.
129. Hillensjö T, Pomerantz SH, Schwartz-Kripner A, Anderson LD, Channing CP. Inhibition of cumulus cell progesterone secretion by low molecular weight fractions of porcine follicular fluid which also inhibit oocyte maturation. *Endocrinology* 1980;106:584–591.
130. Nicosia SV, Mikhail G. Cumuli oophori in tissue culture: hormone production, ultrastructure and morphometry of early luteinization. *Fertil Steril* 1975;26:427–448.
131. Billig H, Hedin L, Magnusson C. Gonadotrophins stimulate lactate production by rat cumulus and granulosa cells. *Acta Endocrinol* 1983;103:562–566.
132. Dekel N, Kraicer PF. Induction *in vitro* of cumulus mucification by gonadotropins and cAMP. *Endocrinology* 1978;102:1797–1802.
133. Hillensjö T, Channing CP. Gonadotropin stimulation of steroidogenesis and cellular dispersion in cultured porcine cumuli oophori. *Gamete Res* 1980;3:233–240.
134. Eppig JJ, Freter RR, Ward-Bailey RF, Schultz RM. Inhibition of oocyte maturation in the mouse: participation of cAMP, steroid hormones, and a putative maturation-inhibitory factor. *Dev Biol* 1983;100:287–293.
135. Freter RR, Schultz RM. Regulation of murine oocyte meiosis: evidence for a gonadotropin-induced, cAMP-dependent reduction in maturation inhibitor. *J Cell Biol* 1984;98:1119–1128.
136. Fulka J Jr, Motlik J, Fulka J, Jilek F. Effect of cycloheximide on nuclear maturation of pig and mouse oocytes. *J Reprod Fertil* 1986;77:281–285.
137. Kubelka M, Motlik J, Fulka J Jr, Prochazka R, Rimkevicova Z, Fulka J. Time sequence of germinal vesicle breakdown in pig oocytes after cycloheximide and *p*-aminobenzamidine block. *Gamete Res* 1988;19:423–431.
138. Motlik J, Nagai T, Kikuchi K. Resumption of meiosis in pig oocytes cultured with cumulus and parietal granulosa cells: the effect of protein synthesis inhibition. *J Exp Zool* 1991;259:386–391.
139. Mattioli M, Galeati G, Seren E. Effects of follicle somatic cells during pig oocytes maturation on egg penetrability and male pronucleus formation. *Gamete Res* 1988;20:177–183.
140. Eppig JJ. The relationship between cumulus cell-oocyte coupling, oocyte meiotic maturation, and cumulus expansion. *Dev Biol* 1982;89:268–272.
141. Salustri A, Siracusa G. Metabolic coupling, cumulus expansion and meiotic resumption in mouse cumuli oophori cultured *in vitro* in the presence of FSH or dcAMP, or stimulated *in vivo* by hCG. *J Reprod Fertil* 1983;68:335–341.
142. Thibault C, Gerard M, Menezo Y. Nuclear and cytoplasmic aspects of mammalian oocyte maturation *in vitro* in relation to follicle size and fertilization. *Sperm Action Prog Reprod Biol* 1976;1:233–240.
143. Schuetz AW. Local control mechanisms during oogenesis and folliculogenesis. In: Browder LW, ed. *Developmental Biology. A Comprehensive Synthesis, Oogenesis,* Vol 1. New York: Plenum Press, 1985;3–83.
144. Racowsky C, McGaughey RW. Further studies of the effects of follicular fluid and membrana granulosa cells on the spontaneous maturation of pig oocytes. *J Reprod Fertil* 1982;66:505–512.
145. Reichert LE, Andersen TT, Branca AA, Fletcher PW, Sluss PM. FSH binding inhibitors of follicular fluid. In: Sairam MR, Atkinson LE, eds. *Gonadal Proteins and Peptides and their Biological Significance.* Singapore: World Scientific Publ. Co., 1984;153–160.

146. Krishnan KA, Vijayalakshmi S, Sheth AR. Presence of low molecular weight LH/hCG and FSH binding inhibitors in human and sheep ovaries. *Indian J Exp Biol* 1983;21:229.
147. Darga NC, Reichert LE Jr. Evidence for the presence of a low molecular weight follitropin binding inhibitor in bovine follicular fluid. *Adv Exp Med Biol* 1978;112:383–388.
148. Darga NC, Reichert LE Jr. Some properties of binding of follicle stimulating hormone to bovine granulosa cells and its inhibition of follicular fluid. *Biol Reprod* 1978;19:235–241.
149. Sato E, Miyamoto H, Ishibashi T, Iritani A. Identification, purification and immunohistochemical detection of the inhibitor from porcine ovarian follicular fluid to compensatory ovarian hypertrophy in mice. *J Reprod Fertil* 1978;54:263–267.
150. Fletcher PW, Dias JA, Sanzo MS, Reichert LE Jr. Inhibition of FSH action on granulosa cells by low molecular weight components of follicular fluid. *Mol Cell Endocrinol* 1982;25:303–315.
151. Sato E, Ishibashi T, Iritani A. Purification and action sites of a follicle stimulating hormone inhibitor from bovine follicular fluid. *J Anim Sci* 1982;55:873–877.
152. Sluss PM, Reichert LE Jr. Presence of bacteria in porcine follicular fluid and their ability to generate an inhibitor of follicle-stimulating hormone binding to receptor. *Biol Reprod* 1983;29:335–341.
153. Sluss PM, Fletcher PW, Reichert LE Jr. Inhibition of ^{125}I-human follicle-stimulating hormone binding to receptor by a low molecular weight fraction of bovine follicular fluid: inhibitor concentration is related to biochemical parameters of follicular development. *Biol Reprod* 1983;29:1105–1113.
154. Sluss PM, Reichert LE. Porcine follicular fluid contains several low molecular weight inhibitors of follicle-stimulating hormone binding to receptor. *Biol Reprod* 1984;30:1091–1104.
155. Sluss PM, Reichert LE. Secretion of an inhibitor of follicle-stimulating hormone binding to receptor by the bacteria *Serretia*, including a strain isolated from porcine follicular fluid. *Biol Reprod* 1984;31:520–530.
156. Schneyer AL, Sluss PM, Whitcomb RW, Martin KA, Sprengel R, Crowley WF Jr. Precursors of α-inhibin modulate follicle-stimulating hormone receptor binding and biological activity. *Endocrinology* 1991;129:1987–1998.
157. Sluss PM, Schneyer AL, Franke MA, Reichert LE Jr. Porcine follicular fluid contains both follicle-stimulating hormone agonist and antagonist activities. *Endocrinology* 1987;120:1477–1481.
158. Schneyer AL, Reichert LE Jr, Franke M, Ryan RJ, Sluss PM. Follicle-stimulating hormone (FSH) immunoactivity in porcine follicular fluid is not pituitary FSH. *Endocrinology* 1988;123: 487–491.
159. Lee DW, Butler WJ, Horvath PM, Shelden RM, Reichert LE Jr. Human follicular fluid contains a follicle-stimulating hormone (FSH) receptor binding inhibitor which has FSH agonist activity, is immunologically similar to FSH, but can be distinguished from FSH. *J Clin Endocrinol Metab* 1991;72:1102–1107.
160. Yang KP, Samaan NA, Ward DN. Characterization of an inhibitor of luteinizing hormone receptor site binding. *Endocrinology* 1976;98:233–241.
161. Yang KP, Samaan NA, Ward DN. Lutropin receptors from male and female tissues: different responses to a lutropin receptor inhibitor. *Proc Soc Exp Biol Med* 1976;152:606–609.
162. Sakai CN, Engel B, Channing CP. Ability of an extract of pig corpus luteum to inhibit binding of ^{125}I-labeled human chorionic gonadotropin to porcine granulosa cells. *Proc Soc Exp Biol Med* 1977;155:373–376.
163. Kumari GL, Channing CP. Intraovarian control of progesterone biosynthesis by granulosa cells and corpus luteum. *J Steroid Biochem* 1979;11:781–790.
164. Yang KP, Gray KN, Jardine JH, Yan HL, Samaan NA, Ward DN. LHRBI—an inhibitor of *in vitro* luteinizing hormone binding to ovarian receptors and LH-stimulated progesterone synthesis by ovary. In: Spilman CH, Wilks JW, eds. *Novel Aspects of Reproductive Physiology.* New York: SP Medical and Scientific Books, 1978;61–80.
165. Kumari GL, Kumar N, Duraiswami S, et al. Characterization of LH/hCG receptor binding inhibitor in corpora lutea of human and sheep ovaries. In: Channing CP, Segal SJ, eds. *Intraovarian Control Mechanisms,* Vol 147. New York: Plenum Press, 1982;283–301.
166. Yang KP, Neira ES, Yen HN, et al. Corpus luteum LH-receptor binding inhibitor (LH-RBI). In: Franchimont P, Channing CP, eds. *Intragonadal Regulation of Reproduction.* London: Academic Press, 1981;133–155.
167. Yang KP, Samaan VA, Ward DN. Effects of luteinizing hormone receptor-binding inhibitor on the *in vitro* steroidogenesis by rat ovary and testis. *Endocrinology* 1979;104:552–558.
168. Kumari GL, Tucker S, Channing CP. Changes in levels of a LH binding inhibitor in aqueous extracts of porcine corpora lutea as a function of aging of the corpus luteum. *Biol Reprod* 1979;21:1043–1050.
169. Channing CP, Batta SK, Bae IH. Inhibitory effect of charcoal treated aqueous porcine corpus luteum extract upon ovulation in the rabbit. *Proc Soc Exp Biol Med* 1981;166:479–483.
170. Kumari GL, Kumar N, Duraiswami S, Roy S. Ovarian lutropin receptor binding inhibitor. In: Sairam MR, Atkinson LE, eds. *Gonadal Proteins and Peptides and Their Biological Significance.* Singapore: World Scientific Publ. Co., 1984;161–175.
171. Ward DN. In pursuit of physiological inhibitors of and from the ovary. In: Jagiello G, Vogel HJ, eds. *Bioregulators of Reproduction.* New York: Academic Press, 1981;371–387.
172. Vale W, Rivier J, Vaughan J, et al. Purification and characterization of an FSH-releasing protein from porcine ovarian follicular fluid. *Nature* 1986;321:776–779.
173. diZerega GS, Campeau JD, Ujita EL, et al. The possible role for a follicular protein in the intraovarian regulation of folliculogenesis. *Semin Reprod Endocrinol* 1983;1:309–322.
174. diZerega GS, Marrs RP, Roche PC, Campeau JD, Kling OR. Identification of proteins in pooled human follicular fluid which suppress follicular response to gonadotropins. *J Clin Endocrinol Metab* 1983;56:35–41.
175. diZerega GS, Marrs RP, Campeau JD, Nakamura RM, Kling OR. Human granulosa cell secretion of protein(s) which suppress follicular response to gonadotropins. *J Clin Endocrinol Metab* 1983;56:147–155.
176. diZerega GS, Campeau JD, Lobo RA, Nakamura RM, Ujita EL, Marrs RP. Activity of a human follicular fluid protein(s) during normal and stimulated ovarian cycles. *J Clin Endocrinol Metab* 1983;57:838–846.
177. diZerega GS, Fujimori K, Tonetta SA, et al. Experience with follicle regulatory protein as an inhibitor of folliculogenesis and spermatogenesis *in vivo.* In: Hodgen GD, Rosenwaks Z, Spieler JM, eds. *Nonsteroidal Gonadal Factors: Physiological Roles and Possibilities in Contraceptive Development.* Norfolk, VA: The Jones Institute Press, 1988;235–248.
178. Westhof G, Fujimori K, Tonetta SA, et al. Follicle regulatory protein: an intraovarian regulatory of follicular response to gonadotropin stimulation. In: Stouffer R, ed. *The Primate Ovary.* New York: Plenum Press, 1987;49–60.
179. Ono T, Campeau JD, Holmberg EA, et al. Biochemical and physiological characterization of follicle regulatory protein: a paracrine regulator of folliculogenesis. *Am J Obstet Gynecol* 1986;154: 709–716.
180. diZerega GS, Goebelsmann U, Nakamura R. Identification of protein(s) secreted by the preovulatory ovary which suppress follicular response to gonadotropins. *J Clin Endocrinol Metab* 1982;54:1091–1096.
181. Montz FJ, Ujita EL, Campeau JD, deZerega GS. Inhibition of luteinizing hormone/human chorionic gonadotropin binding to porcine granulosa cells by a follicular fluid protein. *Am J Obstet Gynecol* 1984;148:436–441.
182. Kling OR, Roche PC, Campeau JD, Nishimura K, Nakamura RM, deZerega GS. Identification of a porcine follicular fluid fraction which suppresses follicular response to gonadotropins. *Biol Reprod* 1984;30:564–572.
183. Schreiber JR, diZerega GS. Porcine follicular fluid protein(s) inhibits rat ovary granulosa cell steroidogenesis. *Am J Obstet Gynecol* 1986;155:1281–1288.
184. Battin DA, deZerega GS. Effects of follicular fluid protein(s) on gonadotropin modulated secretion of progesterone in porcine granulosa cells. *Am J Obstet Gynecol* 1985;60:116–118.
185. Tonetta SA, DeVinna RS, DiZerega GS. Effects of follicle regulatory protein on thecal aromatase and 3β-hydroxysteroid dehydrogenase activity in medium- and large-sized pig follicles. *J Reprod Fertil* 1988;82:163–171.

186. Tonetta SA, Yanagihara DL, DeVinna RS, diZerega GS. Secretion of follicle-regulatory protein by porcine granulosa cells. *Biol Reprod* 1988;38:1001–1005.
187. Tonetta SA, Stone BA, Marrs RP, diZerega GS. Concentrations of follicle regulatory protein, steroids and gonadotrophins in antral fluids from women stimulated with metrodin and hCG. *J Reprod Fertil* 1990;88:389–397.
188. Ledwitz-Rigby F, Rigby BW. Ovarian inhibitors and stimulators of granulosa cell maturation and luteinization. In: Franchimont P, Channing CP, eds. *Intragonadal Regulation of Reproduction.* London: Academic Press, 1981;97–131.
189. Ledwitz-Rigby F, Rigby BW. The actions of follicular fluid factors on steroidogenesis by cultured ovarian granulosa cells. *J Steroid Biochem* 1983;19:127–131.
190. Vasilenko P, Mahajan DK. Stimulation and inhibition of granulosa cell progesterone secretion by porcine follicular fluids. In: Sairam MR, Atkinson LE, eds. *Gonadal Proteins and Peptides and Their Biological Significance.* Singapore: World Scientific Publ., 1984;229–237.
191. Kolena J, Channing CP. Stimulatory action of follicular fluid components on maturation of granulosa cells from small porcine follicles. *Horm Res* 1985;21:185–198.
192. Kraiem Z, Druker B, Lunenfeld B. Inhibitory action of human follicular fluid on the ovarian accumulation of cyclic AMP. *J Endocrinol* 1978;78:161–162.
193. Hillensjö T, Chari S, Nilsson L, Hamberger L, Daume E, Sturm G. Inhibition of progesterone secretion in cultured human granulosa cells by a low molecular weight fraction of human follicular fluid. *J Clin Endocrinol Metab* 1983;56:835–838.
194. Bernard J. Effect du liquide folliculaire sur la luteinisation *in vitro* des cellules granulosaires du rat. *C R Soc Biol (Paris)* 1973;6:882–885.
195. Bernard J, Psychoyos A. Inhibitory effect of follicular fluid on RNA synthesis of rat granulosa cells *in vitro. J Reprod Fertil* 1977;49:355–357.
196. Shemesh M. Inhibitory action of follicular fluid on progesterone and PG synthesis by bovine follicles. *J Endocrinol* 1979;82:27–31.
197. Younglai EV. The influence of follicular fluid and plasma on the steroidogenic activity of equine granulosa cells. *J Reprod Fertil* 1972;28:95–97.
198. Channing CP, Batta SK, Condon W, Ganjam VK, Kenney RM. Levels of inhibin activity and of atretogenic factor(s) in follicular fluid harvested from viable and atretic mare follicles. In: Schwartz NB, Hunzicker-Dunn M, eds. *Dynamics of Ovarian Function.* New York: Raven Press, 1981;73–78.
199. Ledwitz-Rigby F, Rigby BW. Follicular fluid stimulation of steroidogenesis in immature granulosa cells *in vitro. Mol Cell Endocrinol* 1979;14:73–80.
200. Stewart LE, Rigby BW, Ledwitz-Rigby F. Follicular fluid stimulation of progesterone secretion: time course, dose response and effect of inhibiting *de novo* cholesterol synthesis. *Biol Reprod* 1982;27:54–61.
201. Ledwitz-Rigby F, Petito SH, Tyner JK, Rigby BW. Follicular fluid effects on progesterone secretion are not due to follicle-stimulating hormone or steroids. *Biol Reprod* 1985;33:277–285.
202. Danisová A, Kolena J. Hormone-stimulated secretion of luteinization factor in porcine granulosa cells. *Reprod Nutr Dev* 1992;32:207–217.
203. Osteen KG, Loeken MR, Channing CP. Intraovarian control of granulosa cell luteinization. *Endocrinol Exp* 1982;16:301–309.
204. Osteen K, Anderson LD, Reichert LE, Channing CP. Follicular fluid modulation of functional LH receptor induction in porcine granulosa cells. *J Reprod Fertil* 1985;74:407–418.
205. Bar-Ami S, Haciski RC, Channing CP. Increasing ^{125}I-human chorionic gonadotrophin specific binding in human granulosa cells by follicle-stimulating hormone and follicular fluid. *Hum Reprod (Engl)* 1989;4:876–882.
206. Bar-Ami S, Channing CP. Inhibitory and stimulatory action of porcine follicular fluid on FSH-induced ^{125}I-hCG specific binding in rat granulosa cells. *Endocrinol Exp (Czech)* 1990;24:403–414.
207. McLean MP, Rigby WB, Hanzely L, Ledwitz-Rigby F. Morphological correlates of follicular fluid stimulation of steroidogenesis in immature granulosa cells. *Cytobios* 1986;47:115–128.
208. Ledwitz-Rigby F. A comparison of the actions of stimulatory follicular fluid and gonadotropin-releasing hormone analogs on progesterone secretion by porcine granulosa cells. *Biol Reprod* 1989;41:604–609.
209. Ledwitz-Rigby F, Rigby BW, Gay VL, Stetson M, Young J, Channing CP. Inhibitory action of porcine follicular fluid upon granulosa cell luteinization *in vitro:* assay and influence of follicular maturation. *J Endocrinol* 1977;74:175–184.
210. Alexander JS, Rigby BW, Ledwitz-Rigby F. Ultrastructural correlates of *in vitro* inhibition of luteinization of mature porcine ovarian granulosa cells by fluid from immature porcine follicles. *Biol Reprod* 1978;19:693–700.
211. Ledwitz-Rigby F. Reversal of follicular inhibition of granulosa cell progesterone secretion by manipulation of intracellular cyclic AMP. *Biol Reprod* 1980;23:324–333.
212. Lintern-Moore S, Peters H, Moore GPM, Faber M. Follicular development in the infant human ovary. *J Reprod Fertil* 1974;39:53–64.
213. McNatty KP, Moore-Smith D, Makris A, Osathanondh R, Ryan KJ. The microenvironment of the human antral follicle: interrelationships among the steroid levels in antral fluid, the population of granulosa cells, and the status of the oocyte *in vivo* and *in vitro. J Clin Endocrinol Metab* 1979;49:851–860.
214. Peters H, McNatty KP. *The Ovary.* London: Granada Publishing, 1980.
215. Richards JS. Maturation of ovarian follicles: actions and interactions of pituitary and ovarian hormones on follicular cell differentiation. *Physiol Rev* 1980;60:51–89.
216. May JV, Schomberg DW. The effect of plating density on granulosa cell growth and differentiation *in vitro. Mol Cell Endocrinol* 1984;34:201–213.
217. Rao MC, Midgley AR, Richards JS. Hormonal regulation of ovarian proliferation. *Cell* 1978;14:71–78.
218. McNatty KP, Sawers RS. Relationship between the endocrine environment within the Graafian follicle and the subsequent rate of progesterone secretion by human granulosa cells *in vitro. J Endocrinol* 1975;66:391–400.
219. Thanki KH, Channing CP. Influence of serum, estrogen, and gonadotropin upon growth and progesterone secretion by cultures of granulosa cells from small porcine follicles. *Endocr Res Commun* 1976;3:319–333.
220. Thanki KH, Channing CP. Effects of follicle-stimulating hormone and estradiol upon progesterone secretion by porcine granulosa cells in tissue culture. *Endocrinology* 1978;103:74–80.
221. Adashi EY, Resnick CE, D'Ercole AJ, Svoboda ME, VanWyk JJ. Insulin-like growth factors as intraovarian regulators of granulosa cell growth and function. *Endocr Rev* 1985;6:400–420.
222. Froesch ER, Schmid C, Schwander J, Zapf J. Actions of insulin-like growth factors. *Annu Rev Physiol* 1985;47:443–467.
223. Daughaday WH, Hall K, Raben MS, Salmon WD, Van Den Brande JL, Van Wyk JJ. Somatomedin: proposed designation for sulphation factor. *Nature* 1972;235:107.
224. Van Wyk JJ, Underwood LE, Hintz RL, Clemmons DR, Voina SJ, Weaver RP. The somatomedins: a family of insulin-like hormones under growth hormone control. *Recent Prog Horm Res* 1974;30:259–318.
225. Van Wyk JJ, Svoboda ME, Underwood LE. Evidence from radioligand assays that somatomedin-C and insulin-like growth factor-I are similar to each other and different from other somatomedins. *J Clin Endocrinol Metab* 1980;50:206–208.
226. Svoboda ME, Van Wyk JJ, Klapper DG, Fellows RE, Grissom FE, Schleuter RJ. Purification of somatomedin-C from human plasma: chemical and biological properties, partial sequence analysis and relationship to other somatomedins. *Biochemistry* 1980;19:790–797.
227. Klapper DG, Svoboda ME, Van Wyk JJ. Sequence analysis of somatomedin-C: confirmation of identify with insulin-like growth factor I. *Endocrinology* 1983;112:2215–2217.
228. Rubin JS, Mariz I, Jacobs JW, Daughaday WH, Bradshaw RA. Isolation and partial sequence analysis of rat basic somatomedin. *Endocrinology* 1982;110:734–740.
229. Cohen S. Isolation of a mouse submaxillary gland protein accelerating incisor eruption and eyelid opening in the newborn animal. *J Biol Chem* 1962;237:1555–1562.

230. Capenter G, Cohen S. Epidermal growth factor. *Annu Rev Biochem* 1979;48:193–216.
231. Gospodarowicz D, Moran JS. Growth factors in mammalian cell culture. *Annu Rev Biochem* 1976;45:531–558.
232. Gospodarowicz D, Greenburg G, Bialecki H, Zetter BR. Factors involved in the modulation of cell proliferation *in vivo* and *in vitro:* the role of fibroblast and epidermal growth factors in the proliferative response of mammalian cells. *In Vitro* 1978;14: 85–118.
233. Gospodarowicz D. Purification of a fibroblast growth factor from bovine pituitary. *J Biol Chem* 1975;250:2515–2520.
234. Böhlen P, Esch F, Baird A, Gospodarowicz D. Acidic fibroblast growth factor (FGF) from bovine brain: amino-terminal sequence and comparison with basic FGF. *EMBO J* 1985;4: 1951–1956.
235. Esch F, Baird A, Ling N, et al. Primary structure of bovine pituitary basic fibroblast growth factor (FGF) and comparison with the amino-terminal sequence of bovine brain acidic FGF. *Proc Natl Acad Sci USA* 1985;82:6507–6511.
236. McNatty KP, Makris A, De Grazia C, Osathanondh R, Ryan KJ. Steroidogenesis by recombined follicular cells from the human ovary *in vitro. J Clin Endocrinol Metab* 1980;51:1286–1292.
237. Makris A, Yasumizu T, Ryan KJ. A thecal protein growth factor which stimulates granulosa and BALBc 3T3 cell DNA synthesis. *Endocrinology* 1982;108(suppl):110.
238. Makris A, Klagsbrun MA, Yasumizu T, Ryan KJ. An endogenous ovarian growth factor which stimulates BALB/3T3 and granulosa cells. *Biol Reprod* 1983;29:1135–1141.
239. Veldhuis JB, Demers LM, Hammond JM. Regulation of ornithine decarboxylase in isolated granulosa cells *in vitro* by constituents of follicular fluid. *Endocrinology* 1979;105:1143–1151.
240. Hammond JM, Veldhuis JD, Seale TW, Rechler MM. Intraovarian regulation of granulosa cell replication. In: Channing CP, Segal SJ, eds. *Intraovarian Control Mechanisms, Adv. Exp. Biol. Med.,* Vol 147. New York: Plenum Press, 1982;341–356.
241. Adashi EY, Resnick CE, D'Ercole J, Svoboda ME, Van Wyk JJ. Insulin-like growth factors as intraovarian regulators of granulosa cell growth and function. *Endocr Rev* 1985;6:400–420.
242. Adashi EY, Resnick CE, Svoboda ME, Van Wyk JJ. Somatomedin-C synergizes with follicle stimulating hormone in the acquisition of progesterone biosynthetic capacity by cultured rat granulosa cells. *Endocrinology* 1985;116:2135–2142.
243. Adashi EY, Resnick CE, Brodie AMH, Svoboda ME, Van Wyk JJ. Somatomedin-C-mediated potentiation of follicle-stimulating hormone-induced aromatase activity of cultured rat granulosa cells. *Endocrinology* 1985;117:2313–2320.
244. Adashi EY, Resnick CE, Brodie AMH, Svoboda ME, Van Wyk JJ. Somatomedin-C enhances induction of luteinizing hormone receptors by follicle-stimulating hormone in cultured rat granulosa cells. *Endocrinology* 1985;116:2369–2375.
245. Davoren JB, Hsueh AJW, Li CH. Somatomedin C augments FSH-induced differentiation of cultured rat granulosa cells. *Am J Physiol* 1985;249:E26–E33.
246. Adashi EY, Resnick CE, Svoboda ME, Van Wyk JJ, Hascall VC, Yanagishita M. Independent and synergistic actions of somatomedin-C in the stimulation of proteoglycan biosynthesis by cultured rat granulosa cells. *Endocrinology* 1986;118: 456–458.
247. Bicsak TA, Tucker EM, Cappel S, et al. Hormonal regulation of granulosa cell inhibin biosynthesis. *Endocrinology* 1986;119: 2711–2719.
248. Zhiwen Z, Carson RS, Herington AC, Lee VWK, Burger HG. Follicle-stimulating hormone and somatomedin-C stimulate inhibin production by rat granulosa cells *in vitro. Endocrinology* 1987;120:1633–1638.
249. Cara JF, Rosenfeld R. Insulin-like growth factor I and insulin potentiate luteinizing hormone-induced androgen synthesis by rat ovarian thecal-interstitial cells. *Endocrinology* 1988;123: 733–739.
250. Magoffin DA, Kurtz KM, Erickson GF. Insulin-like growth factor-I selectively stimulates cholesterol side-chain cleavage expression in ovarian theca-interstitial cells. *Mol Endocrinol* 1990;4:489–496.
251. Baranao JLS, Hammond JM. Comparative effects of insulin and insulin-like growth factors on DNA synthesis and differentiation of porcine granulosa cells. *Biochem Biophys Res Commun* 1984;124:484–490.
252. Veldhuis JD, Furlanetto RW, Juchter D, J. G. Veldhuis P. Trophic actions of human somatomedin C/insulin-like growth factor I on ovarian cells: *in vitro* studies with swine granulosa cells. *Endocrinology* 1985;116:1235–1242.
253. Veldhuis JD, Demers LM. A role for somatomedin C as a differentiating hormone and amplifier of hormone action on ovarian cells: studies with synthetically pure human somatomedin C and swine granulosa cells. *Biochem Biophys Res Commun* 1985;130:234–240.
254. Veldhuis JD, Furlanetto RW, Juchte D, Garmey J, Veldhuis P. Trophic actions of human somatomedin-C/insulin like growth factor I on ovarian cells: *in vitro* studies with swine granulosa cells. *Endocrinology* 1985;116:1235–1242.
255. Veldhuis JD, Rodgers RJ, Furlanetto RW, Azimi P, Juchter D, Garmey J. Syntergistic actions of estradiol and the insulin-like growth factor somatomedin-C on swine ovarian (granulosa) cells. *Endocrinology* 1986;119:530–538.
256. Veldhuis JD, Rodgers RJ, Dee A, Simpson ER. The insulin-like growth factor, somatomedin C, induces the synthesis of cholesterol side-chain cleavage cytochrome P-450 and adrenodoxin in ovarian cells. *J Biol Chem* 1986;261:2499–2502.
257. Veldhuis JD, Nestler JE, Struass JF III, Azimi P, Garmey J, Juchter D. The insulin-like growth factor, somatomedin-C, modulates low density lipoprotein metabolism by swine granulosa cells. *Endocrinology* 1987;121:340–346.
258. Veldhuis JD, Rodgers RJ. Mechanisms subserving the steroidogenic synergism between follicle-stimulating hormone and insulin-like growth factor I (somatomedin C). *J Biol Chem* 1987;262:7658–7664.
259. Maruo T, Hayashi M, Matsuo H, Ueda Y, Morikawa H, Mochizuki M. Comparison of the facilitative roles of insulin and insulin-like growth factor I in the functional differentiation of granulosa cells: *in vitro* studies with the porcine model. *Acta Endocrinol* 1988;117:230–240.
260. May JV, Frost JP, Schomberg DW. Differential effects of epidermal growth factor, somatomedin-C/insulin-like growth factor I, and transforming growth factor-β on porcine granulosa cell deoxyribonucleic acid synthesis and cell proliferation. *Endocrinology* 1988;123:168–179.
261. Veldhuis JD, Gwynne JT. Insulin-like growth factor type I (somatomedin-C) stimulates high density lipoprotein (HDL) metabolism and HDL-supported progesterone biosynthesis by swine granulosa cells *in vitro. Endocrinology* 1989;124:3069–3076.
262. Steinkampf MP, Mendelson CR, Simpson ER. Effects of epidermal growth factor and insulin-like growth factor I on the levels of mRNA encoding aromatase cytochrome P-450 of human ovarian granulosa cells. *Mol Cell Endocrinol* 1988;59:93–99.
263. Erickson GF, Garzo VG, Magoffin DA. Insulin-like growth factor-I regulates aromatase activity in human granulosa and granulosa luteal cells. *J Clin Endocrinol Metab* 1989;69:716–724.
264. Erickson GF, Magoffin DA, Cragun JR, Chang RJ. The effects of insulin and insulin-like growth factors-I and -II on estradiol production by granulosa cells of polycystic ovaries. *J Clin Endocrinol Metab* 1990;70:894–902.
265. Murphy LJ, Bell GI, Friesen HG. Tissue distribution of insulin-like growth factor I and II messenger ribonucleic acid in the adult rat. *Endocrinology* 1987;120:1279–1282.
266. Hernandez ER, Roberts CH, LeRoith D, Adashi EY. Rat ovarian insulin-like growth factor I (IGF-I) gene expression is granulosa cell-selective: 5'UT mRNA variant representation and hormonal regulation. *Endocrinology* 1989;125:572–574.
267. Carlsson B, Carlsson L, Billig H. Estrus cycle-dependent co-variation of insulin-like growth factor-I (IGF-I) messenger ribonucleic acid and protein in the rat ovary. *J Mol Cell Endocrinol* 1989;64:271–275.
268. Hansson HA, Nilsson A, Isgaard J. Immunohistochemical localization of insulin-like growth factor I in the adult rat. *Histochemistry* 1988;89:403–410.
269. Hammond JM. Peptide regulators in the ovarian follicle. *Aust J Biol Sci* 1981;34:491–504.
270. Hammond JM, Hsu CJ, Klindt J, Tsang BK, Downey BR. Go-

nadotropins increase concentrations of immunoreactive insulin-like growth factor-I in porcine follicular fluid *in vivo*. *Biol Reprod* 1988;38:304–308.
271. Echternkamp SE, Spicer LJ, Gregory KE, Canning SF, Hammond JM. Concentrations of insulin-like growth factor-I in blood and ovarian follicular fluid of cattle selected for twins. *Biol Reprod* 1990;43:8–14.
272. Ramasharma K, Cabrera CM, Li CH. Identification of insulin-like growth factor-II in human seminal and follicular fluids. *Biochem Biophys Res Commun* 1986;140:536–542.
273. Eden JA, Jones J, Carter GD, Alaghband-Zadeh J. A comparison of follicular fluid levels of insulin-like growth factor-I in normal dominant and cohort follicles, polycystic and multicystic ovaries. *Clin Endocrinol* 1988;29:327–336.
274. Geisthoevel F, Moretti-Rojas IM, Rojas FJ. Immunoreactive insulin-like growth factor I in human follicular fluid. *Hum Reprod* 1989;4:35–38.
275. Jesionowska H, Hemmings R, Guyda H, Posner B. Determination of insulin and insulin-like growth factors in the ovarian circulation. *Fertil Steril* 1990;53:88–91.
276. Barreca A, Minuto F, Volpe A, et al. Insulin-like growth factor-I (IGF-I) and IGF-I binding protein in the follicular fluids of growth hormone treated patients. *Clin Endocrinol* 1990;32: 497–505.
277. Rabinovici J, Dandekar P, Angle MJ, Rosenthal S, Martin MC. Insulin-like growth factor I (IGF-I) levels in follicular fluid from human preovulatory follicles: correlation with serum IGF-I levels. *Fertil Steril* 1990;54:428–433.
278. Hernandez ER, Roberts CT, Hurwitz A, LeRoith D, Adashi EY. Rat ovarian insulin-like growth factor II gene expression is theca-interstitial cell-exclusive: hormonal regulation and receptor distribution. *Endocrinology* 1990;127:3249–3251.
279. Oliver JE, Aitman TJ, Powell JF, Wilson CA, Clayton RN. Insulin-like growth factor I gene expression in the rat ovary is confined to the granulosa cells of developing follicles. *Endocrinology* 1989;124:2671–2679.
280. Hammond JM, Lino J, Baranao S, et al. Production of insulin-like growth factors by ovarian granulosa cells. *Endocrinology* 1985;117:2553–2556.
281. Hsu CJ, Hammond JM. Gonadotropins and estradiol stimulate immunoreactive insulin-like growth factor-I production by porcine granulosa cells *in vitro*. *Endocrinology* 1987;120:198–207.
282. Mondschein JS, Canning SF, Hammond JM. Effects of transforming growth factor-β on the production of immunoreactive insulin-like growth factor I and progesterone and on [^{3}H]-thymidine incorporation in porcine granulosa cell cultures. *Endocrinology* 1988;123:1970–1976.
283. Mondschein JS, Hammond JM. Growth factors regulate immunoreactive insulin-like growth factor-I production by cultured porcine granulosa cells. *Endocrinology* 1988;123:463–468.
284. Geisthovel F, Moretti-Rojas I, Asch RH, Rojas FJ. Expression of insulin-like growth factor-II (IGF-II) messenger ribonucleic acid (mRNA), but not IGF-I mRNA, in human preovulatory granulosa cells. *Hum Reprod* 1989;4:899–902.
285. Adashi EY, Resnick CE, Hernandes ER, Svoboda ME, Van Wyk JJ. Characterization and regulation of a specific cell membrane receptor for somatomedin-C/insulin-like growth factor I in cultured rat granulosa cells. *Endocrinology* 1988;122:194–201.
286. Adashi EY, Resnick CE, Svoboda ME, Van Wyk JJ. Follicle-stimulating hormone enhances somatomedin-C binding to cultured rat granulosa cells: evidence for cAMP-dependence. *J Biol Chem* 1988;261:3923–3926.
287. Adashi EY, Resnick CE, Svoboda ME, Van Wyk JJ. *In-vivo* regulation of granulosa cells somadamedin-C/insulin-like growth factor-I receptors. *Endocrinology* 1988;122:1383–1389.
288. Monget P, Monniaux D, Durand P. Localization, characterization, and quantification of insulin-like growth factor-I-binding sites in the ewe ovary. *Endocrinology* 1989;125:2486–2493.
289. Gates GS, Bayer S, Seibel M, Poretsky L, Flier JS, Moses AC. Characterization of insulin-like growth factor binding to human granulosa cells obtained during *in-vitro* fertilization. *J Recept Res* 1987;7:885–902.
290. Davoren JB, Kasson BG, Li CH, Hsueh AJW. Specific insulin-like growth factor (IGF) I- and II-binding sites on rat granulosa cells: relation to IGF action. *Endocrinology* 1986;119: 2155–2162.
291. Adashi EY, Resnick CE, Rosenfeld RD. Insulin-like growth factor-I (IGF-I) and IGF-II hormonal action in cultured rat granulosa cells: mediation via I but not II IGF receptors. *Endocrinology* 1990;126:216–222.
292. Hernandez ER, Resnick CE, Svoboda ME, Van Wyk JJ, Payne DW, Adashi EY. Somatomedian-C/Insulin-like growth factor-I (Sm-C/IGF-I) as an enhancer of androgen biosynthesis by cultured rat ovarian cells. *Endocrinology* 1988;122:1603–1612.
293. Cara JF, Fan J, Azzarello J, Rosenfield RL. Insulin-like growth factor-I enhances luteinizing hormone binding to rat ovarian theca-interstitial cells. *J Clin Invest* 1990;86:560–565.
294. Poretsky L, Grigorescu F, Seibel M, Moses AC, Flier JS. Distribution and characterization of insulin and insulin-like growth factor I receptors in normal human ovary. *J Clin Endocrinol Metab* 1985;61:728–734.
295. Poretsky L, Bhargava G, Levitan E. Type I insulin-like growth factor receptors in human ovarian stroma. *Horm Res* 1990;33:22–26.
296. Rutanen E-M, Pekonen F. Insulin-like growth factors and their binding proteins. *Acta Endocrinol* 1990;123:7–13.
297. Ooi GT. At the cutting edge: insulin-like growth factor-binding protein (IGFBPs): more than just 1,2,3. *Mol Cell Endocrinol* 1990;71:C39–C43.
298. Sara VR, Hall K. Insulin-like growth factors and their binding proteins. *Physiol Rev* 1990;70:591–614.
299. Clemmons DR. Insulin-like growth factor binding proteins. *Trends Endocrinol Metab* 1990;1:412–417.
300. Seppala M, Wahlstrom T, Koskimies AI, et al. Human preovulatory follicular fluid, luteinized cells of hyperstimulated preovulatory follicles, and corpus luteum contain placental protein 12. *J Clin Endocrinol Metab* 1984;58:505–510.
301. Hartshorne GM, Bell SC, Waites GT. Binding proteins for insulin-like growth factors in the human ovary: identification, follicular fluid levels and immunohistological localization of the 29–32kd type 1 binding protein, IGF-bp1. *Hum Reprod* 1990;5:649–660.
302. Suikkari A-M, Jalkanen J, Koistinen R, et al. Human granulosa cells synthesize low molecular weight insulin-like growth factor-binding protein. *Endocrinology* 1981;124:1088–1090.
303. Jalkanen J, Suikkari A-M, Koistinen R, et al. Regulation of insulin-like growth factor-binding protein-1 production in human granulosa-luteal cells. *J Clin Endocrinol Metab* 1989;69: 1174–1179.
304. Koistinen R, Suikkari A-M, Tiitinen A, Kontula K, Seppala M. Human granulosa cells contain insulin-like growth factor binding protein (IGF-BP-1) mRNA. *Clin Endocrinol* 1990;32:635–640.
305. Hamori M, Blum WF, Torok A, et al. Immunoreactive insulin-like growth factor binding protein-3 in the culture of human luteinized granulosa cells. *Acta Endocrinol (Copenh)* 1991;24: 685–691.
306. Giudice IC, Milki AA, Milkowski DA, Danasouri IE. Human granulosa cells contain messenger ribonucleic acids encoding insulin-like growth factor-binding proteins (IGFBPs) and secrete IGFBPs in culture. *Fertil Steril* 1991;56:475–480.
307. Hsu C, Hammond JM. Concomitant effects of growth hormone on secretion of insulin-like growth factor I and progesterone by cultured porcine granulosa cells. *Endocrinology* 1987;121: 1343–1348.
308. Mondschein JS, Smith SA, Hammond JM. Production of insulin-like growth factor binding proteins (GFBPs) by porcine granulosa cells: identification of IGFBP-2 and -3 and regulation by hormones and growth factors. *Endocrinology* 1990;127: 2298–2306.
309. Grimes RW, Samaras SE, Barber JA, Shimasaki S, Ling N, Hammond JM. Gonadotropin and cAMP modulation of IGF binding protein production in ovarian granulosa cells. *Am J Physiol* 1992;262:E497–E503.
310. Samaras SE, Hagen DR, Shimasaki S, Ling N, Hammond JM. Expression of insulin-like growth factor-binding protein-2 and -3 messenger ribonucleic acid in the porcine ovary: localization and physiological changes. *Endocrinology* 1992;130:2739–2744.
311. Adashi EY, Resnick CE, Hernandez ER, Hurwitz A, Rosenfeld

RG. Ovarian granulosa cell-derived insulin-like growth factor (IGF) binding proteins: constitutive release of low molecular weight, high-affinity IGF-selective species. *Mol Cell Endocrinol* 1990;74:175–185.
312. Erickson GF, Nakatani A, Ling N, Shimasaki S. Localization of insulin-like growth factor-binding protein-5 messenger ribonucleic acid in rat ovaries during the estrous cycle. *Endocrinology* 1992;130:1867–1878.
313. Nakatani A, Shimasaki S, Erickson GF, Ling N. Tissue-specific expression of four insulin-like growth factor-binding proteins (1,2,3, and 4) in the rat ovary. *Endocrinology* 1991;129: 1521–1529.
314. Erickson GF, Nakatani A, Ling N, Shimasaki S. Cyclic changes in insulin-like growth factor-binding protein-4 messenger ribonucleic acid in the rat ovary. *Endocrinology* 1992;130:625–636.
315. Ricciarelli E, Hernandez ER, Hurwitz A, et al. The ovarian expression of the antigonadotropic insulin-like growth factor binding protein-2 is theca-interstitial cell-selective: evidence for hormonal regulation. *Endocrinology* 1991;129:2266–2268.
316. Ricciarelli E, Hernandez ER, Kokia E, et al. Rat ovarian insulin-like growth factor binding protein-3: a growth hormone-dependent theca-interstitial cell-derived antigonadotropin. *Endocrinology* 1992;130:3092–3094.
317. Adashi EY, Resnick CE, Hernandex ER, Hurwitz A, Rosenfeld RG. Follicle-stimulating hormone inhibits the constitutive release of insulin-like growth factor binding proteins by cultured rat ovarian granulosa cells. *Endocrinology* 1990;126:1305–1307.
318. Adashi EY, Resnick CE, Hurwitz A, Ricciarelli E, Hernandez ER, Rosenfeld RG. Ovarian granulosa cell-derived insulin-like growth factor-binding proteins: modulatory role of follicle-stimulating hormone. *Endocrinology* 1991;128:754–760.
319. Matsuo U, Motoyuki S, Shunichi S, Ling N. An insulin-like growth factor-binding protein in ovarian follicular fluid blocks follicle-stimulating hormone-stimulated steroid production by ovarian granulosa cells. *Endocrinology* 1989;125:912–916.
320. Adashi EY, Resnick CE, Ricciarelli E, et al. Local tissue modification of follicle stimulating hormone action. In: Genazzani GR, Petraglia F, eds. *Hormones in Gynecological Endocrinology.* Lancs, England: The Parthenon Publishing Group, 1992; 255–261.
321. Todaro GJ, Fryling C, DeLarco JE. Transforming growth factors produced by certain human tumor cells: polypeptides that interact with epidermal growth factor receptors. *Proc Natl Acad Sci USA* 1980;77:5258–5262.
322. DeLarco JE, Todaro GJ. Growth factors from murine sarcoma virus-transformed cells. *Proc Natl Acad Sci USA* 1978;75: 4001–4005.
323. Fisher DA, Lakshmanan J. Metabolism and effects of epidermal growth factor and related growth factors in mammals. *Endocr Rev* 1990;11:418–442.
324. May JV, Schomberg DW. The potential relevance of epidermal growth factor and transforming growth factor-alpha to ovarian physiology. *Semin Reprod Endocrinol* 1989;7:1–11.
325. Gospodarowicz D, Ill CR, Birdwell CR. Effect of fibroblast and epidermal growth factors on ovarian cell proliferation *in vitro.* I. Characterization of the response of granulosa cells for FGF and EGF. *Endocrinology* 1977;100:1108–1120.
326. Gospodarowicz D, Ill CR, Birdwell CR. Effect of fibroblast and epidermal growth factors on ovarian cell proliferation *in vitro.* II. Proliferative response of luteal cells to FGF but not EGF. *Endocrinology* 1977;100:1121–1128.
327. Gospodarowicz D, Bialecki II. Fibroblast and epidermal growth factors are mitogenic agents for cultured granulosa cells of rodent, porcine and human origin. *Endocrinology* 1979;104:757–764.
328. Vlodavsky I, Brown KD, Gospodarowicz D. A comparison of the binding of epidermal growth factor to cultured granulosa and luteal cells. *J Biol Chem* 1978;253:3744–3750.
329. Hsueh AJW, Welsh TH, Jones PBC. Inhibition of ovarian and testicular steroidogenesis by epidermal growth factor. *Endocrinology* 1981;108:2002–2004.
330. Bendell JJ, Dorrington JH. Epidermal growth factor influences growth and differentiation of rat granulosa cells. *Endocrinology* 1990;127:533–540.
331. May JV, Frost JP, Bridge AJ. Regulation of granulosa cell proliferation: facilitative roles of platelet-derived growth factor and low density lipoprotein. *Endocrinology* 1990;126:2896–2905.
332. Keel BA, Eddy KB, Cho S, May JV. Synergistic action of purified alpha-fetoprotein and growth factors on the proliferation of porcine granulosa cells in monolayer culture. *Endocrinology* 1991;129:217–225.
333. Keel BA, Eddy IB, Cho S, May JV. Human alpha-fetoprotein purified from amniotic fluid enhances growth factor-mediated cell proliferation *in vitro. Mol Reprod Dev* 1991;30:112–118.
334. Roberts AJ, Skinner MK. Transforming growth factor-alpha and -beta differentially regulate growth and steroidogenesis of bovine thecal cells during antral follicle development. *Endocrinology* 1991;129:2041–2048.
335. Adashi EY, Resnick CE. Antagonistic interactions of transforming growth factors in the regulation of granulosa cell differentiation. *Endocrinology* 1986;119:1879–1881.
336. Adashi EY, Resnick CE, Twardzik DR. Transforming growth factor-α attenuates the acquisition of aromatase activity by cultured rat granulosa cells. *J Cell Biochem* 1987;33:1–13.
337. Erickson GF, Case E. Epidermal growth factor antagonizes ovarian theca-interstitial cytodifferentiation. *Mol Cell Endocrinol* 1983;31:71–76.
338. Caubo B, DeVinna RS, Tonetta SA. Regulation of steroidogenesis in cultured porcine theca cells by growth factors. *Endocrinology* 1989;125:321–326.
339. Gangrade BK, Davis JS, May JV. A novel mechanism for the induction of aromatase in ovarian cells *in vitro:* role of transforming growth factor alpha-induced protein tyrosine kinase. *Endocrinology* 1991;129:2790–2792.
340. Endo K, Atlas SJ, Rone JD, et al. Epidermal growth factor inhibits follicular response to human chorionic gonadotropin: possible role of cell to cell communication in the response to gonadotropin. *Endocrinology* 1992;130:186–192.
341. Mock EJ, Niswender GD. Differences in the rates of internalization of ^{125}I-labeled human chorionic gonadotropin, luteinizing hormone, and epidermal growth factor by ovine luteal cells. *Endocrinology* 1983;113:259–264.
342. St. Arnaud R, Walter P, Kelly PA, Labrie F. Rat ovarian epidermal growth factor receptors: characterization and hormonal regulation. *Mol Cell Endocrinol* 1983;31:43–52.
343. Skinner MK, Coffey RJ Jr. Regulation of ovarian cell growth through the local production of transforming growth factor-α by theca cells. *Endocrinology* 1988;123:2632–2638.
344. Kudlow J, Kobrin MS, Purchio AF, et al. Ovarian transforming growth factor-α gene expression: immunohistochemical localization to the theca-interstitial cells. *Endocrinology* 1987;121: 1577–1579.
345. Lobb DK, Kobrin MS, Kudlow JE, Dorrington JH. Transforming growth factor-alpha in the adult bovine ovary: identification in growing ovarian follicles. *Biol Reprod* 1989;40:1087–1093.
346. Westergaard LG, Yding Andersen C, Byskov AG. Epidermal growth factor in small antral ovarian follicles of pregnant women. *J Endocrinol* 1990;127:363–367.
347. Roy SK, Greenwald GS. Immunohistochemical localization of epidermal growth factor-like activity in the hamster ovary with a polyclonal antibody. *Endocrinology* 1990;126:1309–1317.
348. Roberts AB, Sporn MB, Assoian DK, Smith JH, et al. TGFβ: rapid induction of fibrosis and angiogenesis *in vivo* and stimulation of collagen formation *in vivo. Proc Natl Acad Sci USA* 1986;83:4167–4171.
349. Cate RL, Mattaliano RJ, Hession C, et al. Isolation of the bovine and human genes for Müllerian inhibiting substance and expression of the gene in animal cells. *Cell* 1986;45:686–694.
350. Josso N. AntiMüllerian hormone: new perspectives for a sexist molecule. *Endocr Rev* 1986;7:421–433.
351. Mason AJ, Hayflick JS, Ling N, et al. Complementary DNA sequences of ovarian follicular fluid inhibin show precursor structure and homology with transforming growth factor-β. *Nature* 1985;318:659–663.
352. Ling N, Ying SY, Ueno N, et al. Pituitary FSH is released by a heterodimer of the β-subunits from the two forms of inhibin. *Nature* 1986;321:779–782.
353. Bendell JJ, Dorrington I. Rat theca/interstitial cells secrete a transforming growth factor β-like factor that promotes growth

and differentiation in rat granulosa cells. *Endocrinology* 1988;123:941–948.
354. Skinner MK, Keski-Oja J, Osteen KG, Moses HL. Ovarian theca cells produce transforming growth factor-β which can regulate granulosa cell growth. *Endocrinology* 1987;121:786–792.
355. Knecht M, Catt KJ. Transforming growth factor-beta: autocrine, paracrine, and endocrine effects in ovarian cells. *Semin Reprod Endocrinol* 1989;7:12–20.
356. Feng P, Catt KJ, Knecht M. Transforming growth factor-β regulates the inhibitory actions of epidermal growth factor during granulosa cell differentiation. *J Biol Chem* 1986;261:14167–14170.
357. Knecht M, Feng P, Catt KJ. Transforming growth factor-beta regulates the expression of luteinizing hormone receptors in ovarian granulosa cells. *Biochem Biophys Res Commun* 1986;139: 800–807.
358. Knecht M, Feng P, Catt KJ. Bifunctional role of transforming growth factor-β during granulosa cell development. *Endocrinology* 1987;120:1243–1249.
359. Ying SY, Becker A, Ling N, Ueno N, Guillemin R. Inhibin and beta type transforming growth factor (TGF-β) have opposite modulating effects on the follicle stimulating hormone (FSH)-induced aromatase activity of cultured rat granulosa cells. *Biochem Biophys Res Commun* 1986;136:969–975.
360. Dodson WC, Schomberg DW. The effect of transforming growth factor-beta on follicle-stimulating hormone-induced differentiation of cultured rat granulosa cells. *Endocrinology* 1987;120: 512–516.
361. Adashi EY, Resnick CE, Hernandez ER, May JV, Purchio AF, Twardzik DR. Ovarian transforming growth factor-β (TGFβ): cellular site(s), and mechanism(s) of action. *Mol Cell Endocrinol* 1989;61:247–256.
362. Zhiwen Z, Findlay JK, Carson RS, Herington AC, Burger HG. Transforming growth factor β enhances basal and FSH-stimulated inhibin production by rat granulosa cells *in vitro. Mol Cell Endocrinol* 1988;58:161–166.
363. Magoffin DA, Gancedo B, Erickson GF. Transforming growth factor-β promotes differentiation of ovarian thecal-interstitial cells but inhibits androgen production. *Endocrinology* 1989;125:1951–1958.
364. Hernandez ER, Hurwitz A, Payne DW, Dharmarajan AM, Purchio AF, Adashi EY. Transforming growth factor-β1 inhibits ovarian androgen production: gene expression, cellular localization, mechanism(s), and site(s) of action. *Endocrinology* 1990;127:2804–2811.
365. Kim IC, Schomberg DW. The production of transforming growth factor-β activity by rat granulosa cell cultures. *Endocrinology* 1989;124:1345–1351.
366. Mulheron GW, Schomberg DW. Rat granulosa cells express transforming growth factor-β type 2 messenger ribonucleic acid which is regulatable by follicle-stimulating hormone *in vitro. Endocrinology* 1990;126:1777–1779.
367. Gangrade B, May JV. The production of transforming growth factor-β in the porcine ovary and its secretion *in vitro. Endocrinology* 1990;127:2372–2380.
368. Chegini N, Flanders KC. Presence of transforming growth factor-β and their selective cellular localization in human ovarian tissue of various reproductive stages. *Endocrinology* 1992;130: 1707–1715.
369. Mulheron GW, Danielpour D, Schomberg DW. Rat theca/interstitial cells express transforming growth factor-β type 1 and 2, but only type 2 is regulated by gonadotropin *in vitro. Endocrinology* 1991;129:368–374.
370. Mulheron GW, Mulheron JG, Danielpour D, Schomberg DW. Porcine granulosa cells (pGC) do not express translatable TGF-β2 mRNA: molecular basis for their inability to produce TGF-β activity comparable to that of rat granulosa cells (rGC). *Biol Reprod* 1992;46(suppl 1):140(abst 357).
371. Bendell JJ, Dorrington I. Estradiol-17β stimulates DNA synthesis in rat granulosa cells: action mediated by transforming growth factor-β. *Endocrinology* 1991;128:2663–2665.
372. Feng P, Catt KJ, Knecht M. Transforming growth factor-β stimulates meiotic maturation of the rat oocyte. *Endocrinology* 1988;122:181–186.
373. Downs SM. Maturation of oocyte-cumulus cell complex in mice: specificity of epidermal growth factor activity. In: Hirshfield AN, ed. *Growth Factors and the Ovary.* New York: Plenum Press, 1989;221–225.
374. Itoh M, Igarashi M, Yamada K, et al. Activin-A stimulates meiotic maturation of the rat oocyte *in vitro. Biochem Biophys Res Commun* 1990;166:1479–1484.
375. Folkman J. How is blood vessel growth regulated in normal and neoplastic tissue? *Cancer Res* 1986;46:467–473.
376. Findlay JK. Angiogenesis in reproductive tissues. *J Endocrinol* 1986;111:357–366.
377. Koos RD. Potential relevance of angiogenic factors to ovarian physiology. *Semin Reprod Endocrinol* 1989;7:29–40.
378. Jakob W, Jentzsch KD, Mauersberger B, Oehme P. Demonstration of angiogenesis-activity in the corpus luteum of cattle. *Exp Pathol* 1977;13:231–236.
379. Gospodarowicz D, Thakral KK. Production of a corpus luteum angiogenic factor responsible for proliferation of capillaries and neovascularization of the corpus luteum. *Proc Natl Acad Sci USA* 1978;75:847–851.
380. Heder G, Jakob W, Halle W, et al. Influence of porcine corpus luteum extract on DNA synthesis and proliferation of cultured fibroblasts and endothelial cells. *Exp Pathol* 1979;17:493–497.
381. Koos RD, LeMaire WJ. Factors that may regulate the growth and regression of blood vessels in the ovary. *Semin Reprod Endocrinol* 1983;1:295–307.
382. Koos RD, LeMaire WJ. Evidence for an angiogenic factor from rat follicles. In: Greenwald GS, Terranova PF, eds. *Factors Regulating Ovarian Function.* New York: Raven Press, 1983;191–195.
383. Gaede SD, Sholley MM, Quattropani SL. Endothelial mitosis during initial stages of corpus luteum neovascularization in the cyclic adult rat. *Am J Anat* 1985;172:173–180.
384. Sato E, Ishibashi T, Koide SS. Inducement of blood vessel formation by ovarian extracts from mice injected with gonadotropins. *Experientia* 1982;38:1248–1249.
385. Makris A, Ryan KJ, Yasumizu T, Hill CL, Zetter BR. The nonluteal porcine ovary as a source of angiogenic activity. *Endocrinology* 1984;115:1672–1677.
386. Rone JD, Goodman AL. Detection of angiotropic activity from intact rabbit follicles cultured in serum-free media. *Biol Reprod* 1985;32(suppl 1):(abst 294).
387. Redmer DA, Rone JD, Goodman AL. Detection of angiotropic activity from primate dominant follicles. *Endocrinology* 1985;116(suppl 151A):(abst 604).
388. Frederick JL, Shimanuki T, diZerega GS. Initiation of angiogenesis by human follicular fluid. *Science* 1984;224:389–390.
389. Frederick JL, Campeau JD, Ono T, diZerega GS. Initiation of angiogenesis by a porcine follicular fluid factor. *Am J Obstet Gynecol* 1985;152:1073–1078.
390. Goodman AL, Rone JD. Detection of angiotropic (chemoattractant) activity released by rabbit luteal cells cultured in serum-free or serum-enriched media. *Biol Reprod* 1985;32(suppl 1):(abst 296).
391. Zeleznik AJ, Schuller HM, Reichert LE Jr. Gonadotropin-binding sites in the rhesus monkey ovary: role of the vasculature in the selective distribution of human chorionic gonadotropin to the preovulatory follicle. *Endocrinology* 1981;109:356–362.
392. Hay MF, Cran DG, Moor RM. Structural changes occurring during atresia in sheep ovarian follicles. *Cell Tissue Res* 1976;169:515–529.
393. O'Shea JD, Hay MF, Cran DG. Ultrastructural changes in the theca interna during follicular atresia in sheep. *J Reprod Fertil* 1978;54:183–187.
394. Kenney RM, Condon W, Ganjam VK, Channing CP. Morphological and biochemical correlates of equine ovarian follicles as a function of their state of viability or atresia. *J Reprod Fertil Suppl* 1979;27:163–171.
395. Gospodarowicz D, Cheng J, Lui GM, Bohlen P. Corpus luteum angiogenic factor is related to fibroblast growth factor. *Endocrinology* 1985;117:2283–2391.
396. Gospodarowicz D, Ferrara N, Schweigerer L, Neufeld G. Structural characterization and biological functions of fibroblast growth factor. *Endocr Rev* 1987;8:95–114.
397. Frater-Schröder M, Muller G, Burchmeier W, Bohlen P. Transforming growth factor β inhibits endothelial cell proliferation. *Biochem Biophys Res Commun* 1986;137:295–302.
398. Baird A, Durkin T. Inhibition of endothelial cell proliferation by

type β transforming growth factor: interactions with acidic and basic fibroblast factors. *Biochem Biophys Res Commun* 1986;138:476–482.
399. Globus RK, Patterson-Buckendahl P, Gospodarowicz D. Regulation of bovine bone cell proliferation by fibroblast growth factor and transforming growth factor β. *Endocrinology* 1988;123: 98–105.
400. Gospodarowicz D. Fibroblast growth factor and its involvement in developmental processes. In: Nilsen-Hamilton M, ed. *Growth Factors and Development,* Vol 24. San Diego, New York: Academic Press, 1990;57–93.
401. Gospodarowicz D, Bialecki H. The effects of the epidermal and fibroblast growth factors on the replicative lifespan of cultured bovine granulosa cells. *Endocrinology* 1978;103:854–865.
402. Biswas SB, Hammond RW, Anderson LD. Fibroblast growth factors from bovine pituitary and human placenta and their functions in the maturation of porcine granulosa cells *in vitro. Endocrinology* 1988;123:559–566.
403. Mondschein JS, Schomberg DW. Growth factors modulate gonadotropin receptor induction in granulosa cell cultures. *Science* 1981;211:1179–1180.
404. Baird A, Hsueh AJW. Fibroblast growth factor as an intraovarian hormone: differential regulation of steroidogenesis by an angiogenic factor. *Regul Pept* 1986;16:243–250.
405. Adashi EY, Resnick CE, Croft CS, May JV, Gospodarowicz D. Basic fibroblast growth factor as a regulator of ovarian granulosa cell differentiation: a novel non-mitogenic role. *Mol Cell Endocrinol* 1988;55:7–14.
406. Piquette GN, La Polt PS, Oikawa M, Hsueh AJ. Regulation of luteinizing hormone receptor messenger ribonucleic acid levels by gonadotropins, growth factors, and gonadotropin-releasing hormone in cultured rat granulosa cells. *Endocrinology* 1991;128:2449–2456.
407. LaPolt PS, Yamoto M, Veljkovic M, et al. Basic fibroblast growth factor induction of granulosa cell tissue-type plasminogen activator expression and oocyte maturation: potential role as a paracrine ovarian hormone. *Endocrinology* 1990;127:2357–2363.
408. Tsafriri A, Daphna-Iken D, Abisogun AO, Reich R. Follicular rupture during ovulation: activation of collagenolysis. In: Mashiach S, Ben-Rafael Z, Laufer N, Schenker JG, eds. *Advances in Assisted Reproductive Technologies.* New York: Plenum Press, 1991;103–112.
409. Tsafriri A, Reich R. Plasminogen activators in the preovulatory follicle: role in ovulation. In: Abbate R, Barni T, Tsafriri A, eds. *Plasminogen Activators: From Cloning to Therapy.* New York: Raven Press, 1991;81–93.
410. Neufeld G, Ferrara N, Mitchell R, Schweigerer L, Gospodarowicz D. Granulosa cells produce basic fibroblast growth factor. *Endocrinology* 1987;121:597–603.
411. Koos RD, Seidel RH. Detection of acidic fibroblast growth factor mRNA in the rat ovary using reverse transcription-polymerase chain reaction amplification. *Biochem Biophys Res Commun* 1989;165:82–88.
412. Stirling D, Magness RR, Stone R, Waterman MR, Simpson ER. Angiotensin II inhibits luteinizing hormone-stimulated cholesterol side-chain cleavage expression and stimulates basic fibroblast growth factor expression in bovine luteal cells in primary culture. *J Biol Chem* 1990;265:5–8.
413. Abraham JA, Whang JL, Tumolo A, et al. Human basic fibroblast growth factor: nucleotide sequence and genomic organization. *EMBO J* 1986;5:2523–2528.
414. Abraham JA, Mergia A, Whang JL, et al. Nucleotide sequence of a bovine clone encoding the angiogenic protein basic fibroblast growth factors. *Science* 1986;233:545–548.
415. Gospodarowicz D. Molecular characterization of fibroblast growth factor and possible role in early and late embryonic development. In: Hirshfield AN, ed. *Growth Factors and the Ovary.* New York: Plenum Press, 1989;75–92.
416. Ferrara N, Henzel WJ. Pituitary follicular cells secrete a novel heparin-binding growth factor specific for vascular endothelial cells. *Biochem Biophys Res Commun* 1989;161:851–858.
417. Leung DW, Cachianes G, Kuang WJ, Goeddel DV, Ferrara N. Vascular endothelial growth factor is a secreted angiogenic mitogen. *Science* 1989;246:1306–1309.
418. Phillips HS, Hains J, Leung DW, Ferrara N. Vascular endothelial growth factor is expressed in rat corpora *luteum. Endocrinology* 1990;127:965–967.
419. Ravindranath N, Little-Ihrig L, Phillips HS, Ferrary N, Zeleznik AJ. Vascular endothelial growth factor messenger ribonucleic acid expression in the primate ovary. *Endocrinology* 1992;131:254–260.
420. Dinarello CA. Biology of interleukin-1. *FASEB J* 1988;21: 108–115.
421. Takakura K, Taii S, Fukuoka M, et al. IL-2 Receptor/p55 (Tac)-inducing activity in porcine follicular fluid. *Endocrinology* 1989;125:618–623.
422. Khan SA, Schmid K, Hallin P, Paul RD, Geyter CD, Nieschlag E. Human testis cytosol and ovarian follicular fluid contains high amounts of interleukin-1-like factor(s). *Mol Cell Endocrinol* 1988;58:221–230.
423. Gottschall PE, Uehara A, Hoffman ST, Arimura A. Interleukin-1 inhibits FSH-induced differentiation in rat granulosa cells *in vitro. Biochem Biophys Res Commun* 1987;149:502–509.
424. Gottschall PE, Katsuura G, Arimura A. Interleukin-1 beta is more potent than interleukin-1 alpha in suppressing follicle-stimulating hormone-induced differentiation of ovarian granulosa cells. *Biochem Biophys Res Commun* 1989;163:764–770.
425. Kasson BG, Gorospe WC. Effects of interleukins 1, 2 and 3 on follicle stimulating hormone induced differentiation of rat granulosa cells. *Mol Cell Endocrinol* 1989;62:103–111.
426. Fukuoka M, Mori T, Taii S, Yasuda K. Interleukin-1 inhibits luteinization of porcine granulosa cells in culture. *Endocrinology* 1988;122:367–369.
427. Yasuda K, Fukuoka M, Taii S, Takakura K, Mori T. Inhibitory effects of interleukin 1 on follicle stimulating hormone induction of aromatase activity, progesterone secretion, and functional luteinizing hormone receptors in cultures of porcine granulosa cells. *Biol Reprod* 1990;43:905–912.
428. Fukuoka M, Taii S, Yasuda K, Takakura K, Mori T. Inhibitory effects of interleukin-1 on luteinizing hormone-stimulated adenosine 3′,5′-monophosphate accumulation by cultured porcine granulosa cells. *Endocrinology* 1989;125:136–143.
429. Gottschall PE, Katsuura G, Arimura A. Interleukin-1 suppresses follicle-stimulating hormone-induced estradiol secretion from cultured ovarian granulosa cells. *J Reprod Immunol* 1989;15:281–291.
430. Nakamura Y, Kato H, Terranova PF. Interleukin-α increases thecal progesterone production of preovulatory follicles in cyclic hamsters. *Biol Reprod* 1990;43:169–173.
431. Hurwitz A, Ricciarelli E, Botero L, Rohan RM, Hernandez ER, Adashi EY. Endocrine- and autocrine-mediated regulation of rat ovarian (theca-interstitial) interleukin-1β gene expression: gonadotropin-dependent preovulatory acquisition. *Endocrinology* 1991;129:3427–3429.
432. Emoto N, Baird A. The effect of tumor necrosis factor/cachectin on follicle-stimulating hormone-induced aromatase-activity in cultured rat granulosa cells. *Biochem Biophys Res Commun* 1988;153:792–798.
433. Roby KF, Terranova PF. Tumor necrosis factor alpha alters follicular steroidogenesis *in vitro. Endocrinology* 1988;123:2952–2954.
434. Adashi EY, Resnick CE, Croft CS, Payne DW. Tumor necrosis factor α inhibits gonadotropin hormonal action in non-transformed ovarian granulosa cells. *J Biol Chem* 1989; 264:11591–11597.
435. Adashi EY, Resnick CE, Packman JN, Hurwitz A, Payne DW. Cytokine-mediated regulation of ovarian function: tumor necrosis factor α inhibits gonadotropin-supported progesterone accumulation by differentiating and luteinized murine granulosa cells. *Am J Obstet Gynecol* 1990;162:889–899.
436. Sancho-Tello M, Terranova PF. Involvement of protein kinase C in regulating tumor necrosis factor-α-stimulated progesterone production in rat preovulatory follicles *in vitro. Endocrinology* 1991;128:1223–1228.
437. Veldhuis JD, Garmey JC, Urban RJ, Demers LM, Aggarwal BB. Ovarian actions of tumor necrosis factor-α (TNFα): pleiotropic effects of TNFα on differentiated functions of untransformed swine granulosa cells. *Endocrinology* 1991;129:641–648.
438. Zolti M, Meirom R, Shemesh M, et al. Granulosa cells as a source

and target organ for tumor necrosis factor-α. *FEBS Lett* 1990;261:253–255.
439. Darbon JM, Oury F, Laredo J, Bayard F. Tumor necrosis factor-α inhibits follicle-stimulating hormone-induced differentiation in cultured rat granulosa cells. *Biochem Biophys Res Commun* 1989;163:1038–1046.
440. Pennica D, Nedwin GE, Hayflick JS, et al. Human tumour necrosis factor: precursor structure, expression and homology to lymphotoxin. *Nature* 1984;312:724–729.
441. Old LJ. Tumor necrosis factor (TNF). *Science* 1985;230: 630–632.
442. Aggarwal B, Kohr W. Human tumor necrosis factors. *Methods Enzymol* 1985;116:448–456.
443. Beutler B, Cerami A. Cachectin and tumor necrosis factor as two sides of the same biological coin. *Nature* 1986;320:584–588.
444. Beutler B, Cerami A. Cachectin: more than a tumor necrosis factor. *N Engl J Med* 1987;316:379–385.
445. Bagavandoss P, Kunkel SL, Wiggins RC, Keyes PL. Tumor necrosis factor-α (TNF-α) production and localization of macrophages and T lymphocytes in the rabbit corpus luteum. *Endocrinology* 1987;122:1185–1187.
446. Bagavandoss P, Wiggins RC, Kunkel SL, Remick DJ, Keyes PL. Tumor necrosis factor production and accumulation of inflammatory cells in the corpus luteum of pseudopregnancy and pregnancy in rabbit. *Biol Reprod* 1990;42:367–376.
447. Hsueh AJW, Jones PBC. Extrapituitary actions of gonadotropin-releasing hormone. *Endocr Rev* 1981;2:437–461.
448. Clayton RN, Catt KJ. Gonadotropin-releasing hormone receptors: characterization, physiological regulation and relationship to reproductive function. *Endocr Rev* 1981;2:186–209.
449. Leung PCK, Wang J, Baimbridge KG. Mechanism of action of luteinizing hormone-releasing hormone in rat ovarian cells. *Can J Physiol Pharmacol* 1989;67:962–967.
450. Birnbaumer L, Shahabi N, Rivier Y, Vale W. Evidence for a physiological role of gonadotropin-releasing hormone (GnRH) or GnRH-like material in the ovary. *Endocrinology* 1985;116: 1367–1370.
451. Fink G. Control of the ovarian cycle in the rat. In: Crosignani PG, Mishell DR, eds. *Ovulation in the Human.* New York: Academic Press, 1976;95–114.
452. Bauer K, Horsthemke B. Degradation of LH-RH. In: McKerns KW, Naor Z, eds. *Hormonal Control of the Hypothalamo-Pituitary-Gonadal Axis.* New York: Plenum Press, 1984;101–114.
453. Koch Y, Elkabes S, Fridkin M. Degradation of luteinizing hormone-releasing hormone by rat pituitary plasma membrane associated enzymes. In: McKerns KW, Naor Z, eds. *Hormonal Control of the Hypothalamo-Pituitary-Gonadal Axis.* New York: Plenum Press, 1984;115–126.
454. Koch Y, Baram T, Hazum E, Fridkin M. Resistance to enzymic degradation of LHRH analogues possessing increased biological activity. *Biochem Biophys Res Commun* 1977;74:488–491.
455. Rippel RH, Johnson ES. Inhibition of hCG-induced ovarian and uterine weight augmentation in the immature rat by analogs of GnRH. *Proc Soc Exp Biol Med* 1976;152:432–436.
456. Ying SY, Guillemin R. (D-Trp^6-Pro^9-NEt)-luteinizing hormone-releasing factor inhibits follicular development in hypophysectomized rats. *Nature* 1979;280:593–595.
457. Hsueh AJW, Erickson GF. Extrapituitary action of gonadotropin--releasing hormone: direct inhibition of ovarian steroidogenesis. *Science* 1979;204:854–855.
458. Massicotte J, Veilleux R, Lavoie M, Labrie F. An LHRH agonist inhibits FSH-induced cyclic AMP accumulation and steroidogenesis in porcine granulosa cells in culture. *Biochem Biophys Res Commun* 1980;94:1362–1366.
459. Knecht M, Katz M, Catt KJ. GnRH inhibits cyclic nucleotide accumulation in cultured rat granulosa cells. *J Biol Chem* 1981;256:34–36.
460. Darbon JM, Knecht M, Ranta R, Dufau M, Catt KJC. Hormonal regulation of cyclic AMP-dependent protein kinase in cultured ovarian granulosa cells. *J Biol Chem* 1984;259:14778–14782.
461. Massicote J, Borgus JP, Lachance R, Labrie F. Inhibition of hCG-induced cyclic AMP accumulation and steroidogenesis in rat luteal cells by an LHRH agonist. *J Steroid Biochem* 1981;14:239–242.
462. Hsueh AJW, Wang C, Erickson GF. Direct inhibitory effect of gonadotropin-releasing hormone upon follicle-stimulating hormone induction of luteinizing hormone receptor and aromatase activity in rat granulosa cells. *Endocrinology* 1980;106: 1697–1705.
463. Dorrington J, McKeracher H, Munshi S, Gore-Langton R. LHRH independently stimulates steroidogenic enzymes in granulosa cell cultures. *Endocrinology* 1982;110(suppl):178.
464. Gore-Langton RE, Lacroix M, Dorrington JH. Differential effects of luteinizing hormone-releasing hormone on follicle-stimulating hormone-dependent responses in rat granulosa cells and Sertoli cells *in vitro. Endocrinology* 1981;108:812–818.
465. Jones PBC, Hsueh AJW. Pregnenolone biosynthesis by cultured rat granulosa cells: modulation by follicle-stimulating hormone and gonadotropin-releasing hormone. *Endocrinology* 1982;111: 713–721.
466. Jones PBC, Hsueh AJW. Direct stimulation of ovarian progesterone-metabolizing enzyme by gonadotropin-releasing hormone in cultured granulosa cells. *J Biol Chem* 1981;256:1248–1254.
467. Hsueh AJW, Ling NC. Effect of an antagonistic analog of gonadotropin releasing hormone upon ovarian granulosa cell function. *Life Sci* 1979;25:1223–1230.
468. Navickis RJ, Jones PBC, Hsueh AJW. Modulation of prolactin receptors in cultured rat granulosa cells by FSH, LH and GnRH. *Mol Cell Endocrinol* 1982;27:77–88.
469. Jones PBC, Hsueh AJW. Direct inhibitory effect of gonadotropin-releasing hormone upon luteal luteinizing hormone receptor and steroidogenesis in hypophysectomized rats. *Endocrinology* 1980;107:1930–1936.
470. Reddy PV, Azhar S, Menon KMJ. Multiple inhibitory actions of luteinizing hormone-releasing hormone agonist on luteinizing hormone/human chorionic gonadotropin receptor-mediated ovarian responses. *Endocrinology* 1980;107:930–936.
471. Hillier SG, Reichert LE Jr, van Hall EV. Modulation of FSH-controlled steroidogenesis in rat granulosa cells: direct *in vitro* effects of LHRH and ICI-118630. *Mol Cell Endocrinol* 1981;23:193–205.
472. Magoffin DA, Reynolds DS, Erickson GF. Direct inhibitory effect of GnRH on androgen secretion by ovarian interstitial cells. *Endocrinology* 1981;109:661–663.
473. Magoffin DA, Erickson GF. Mechanism by which GnRH inhibits androgen synthesis directly in ovarian interstitial cells. *Mol Cell Endocrinol* 1982;27:191–198.
474. Behrman HR, Preston SL, Hall AK. Cellular mechanism of the antigonadotropic action of LHRH in the corpus luteum. *Endocrinology* 1980;107:656–644.
475. Clayton RN, Harwood JP, Catt KJ. Gonadotropin-releasing hormone analogue binds to luteal cells and inhibits progesterone production. *Nature* 1979;282:90–92.
476. Hall AK, Behrman HR. Culture sensitization and inhibition of luteinizing hormone responsive production of cyclic AMP in luteal cells by luteinizing hormone, prostaglandin $F_{2\alpha}$ and [D-Trp^6]-luteinizing hormone-releasing hormone. *J Endocrinol* 1981;88: 27–38.
477. Harwood JP, Clayton RN, Catt KJ. Ovarian gonadotropin-releasing hormone receptors. I. Properties and inhibition of luteal cell function. *Endocrinology* 1980;107:407–413.
478. Clark MR, Thibier C, Marsh JM, LeMaire W. Stimulation of prostaglandin accumulation by luteinizing hormone-releasing hormone (LHRH) and LHRH analogs in rat granulosa cells *in vitro. Endocrinology* 1980;107:17–23.
479. Clark MR. Stimulation of progesterone and prostaglandin E_2 accumulation by luteinizing hormone-releasing hormone (LHRH) and LHRH analogs in rat granulosa cells. *Endocrinology* 1982;110:146–152.
480. Sheela Rani CS, Ekholm C, Billig H, Magnusson C, Hillensjö T. Biphasic effect of gonadotropin releasing hormone on progestin secretion by rat granulosa cells. *Biol Reprod* 1983;28:591–597.
481. Billig H, Sheela Rani CS, Ekholm C, Magnusson C, Hillensjö T. Effect of a GnRH analogue on rat granulosa cell lactate production *in vitro. Acta Endocrinol* 1984;105:112–118.
482. Corbin A, Bex FJ. Luteinizing hormone-releasing hormone agonists induce ovulation by hypophysectomized rats: direct ovarian effect. *Life Sci* 1981;29:185–192.

483. Ekholm C, Hillensjö T, Isaksson O. Gonadotropin releasing hormone agonists stimulate oocyte meiosis and ovulation in hypophysectomized rats. *Endocrinology* 1981;108:2022–2024.
484. Ekholm C, Clark MR, Magnusson C, Isaksson O, LeMaire WJ. Ovulation induction by a GnRH analog in hypophysectomized rats involves prostaglandins. *Endocrinology* 1982;110:288–290.
485. Dekel N, Sherizly I, Tsafriri A, Naor Z. A comparative study of the mechanism of action of luteinizing hormone and a gonadotropin releasing hormone analog on the ovary. *Biol Reprod* 1983;28:161–166.
486. Hillensjö T, LeMaire WJ, Clark MR, Ahrén K. Effect of GnRH and GnRH agonists upon accumulation of progesterone, cAMP and prostaglandin in isolated preovulatory rat follicles. *Acta Endocrinol (Copenh)* 1982;101:603–610.
487. Wong WYL, Richards JS. Induction of prostaglandin H synthase in rat preovulatory follicles by gonadotropin-releasing hormone. *Endocrinology* 1992;130:3512–3521.
488. Wang C. Luteinizing hormone releasing hormone stimulates plasminogen activator production by rat granulosa cells. *Endocrinology* 1983;112:1130–1132.
489. Ny T, Liu YX, Ohlsson M, Jones PBC, Hsueh AJW. Regulation of tissue-type plasminogen activator activity and messenger RNA levels by gonadotropin-releasing hormone in cultured rat granulosa cells and cumulus-oocyte complexes. *J Biol Chem* 1987;262:11790–11793.
490. Hsueh AJW, Liu YX, Cajander S, et al. Gonadotropin-releasing hormone induces ovulation in hypophysectomized rats: studies on ovarian tissue-type plasminogen activator activity, messenger ribonucleic acid content, and cellular localization. *Endocrinology* 1988;122:1486–1495.
491. Bex FJ, Corbin A. Cyclic response of hypophysectomized rats to ovulation induced by LHRH agonists. Mediation by prostaglandins. *Life Sci* 1984;35:969–979.
492. Koos RD, LeMaire WJ. The effects of gonadotropin-releasing hormone agonist on ovulation and steroidogenesis during perfusion of rabbit and rat ovaries *in vitro. Endocrinology* 1985;116:628–632.
493. Dekel N, Shalgi R. Fertilization *in vitro* of rat oocytes undergoing maturation in response to a GnRH analogue. *J Reprod Fertil* 1987;80:531–535.
494. Shalgi R, Dekel N. Embryonic development of fertilized rat oocytes induced to mature by an analogue of gonadotrophin-releasing hormone. *J Reprod Fertil* 1990;89:681–687.
495. Hillensjö T, LeMaire WJ. Gonadotropin-releasing hormone agonists stimulate meiotic maturation of follicle-enclosed rat oocytes *in vitro. Nature* 1980;287:145–146.
496. Magnusson C, LeMaire WJ. A gonadotrophin-releasing hormone agonist stimulated oxygen consumption and maturation of follicle-enclosed rat oocytes *in vitro. Acta Physiol Scand* 1981;111:377–379.
497. Dekel N, Sherizly I, Phillips DM, Nimrod A, Zilberstein M, Naor Z. Characterization of the maturational changes induced by a GnRH analogue in the rat ovarian follicle. *J Reprod Fertil* 1985;75:461–466.
498. Aberdam E, Dekel N. Activators of protein kinase C stimulate meiotic maturation of rat oocytes. *Biochem Biophys Res Commun* 1985;132:570–574.
499. Yoshimura Y, Nakamura Y, Ando M, et al. Protein kinase C mediates gonadotropin-releasing hormone agonist-induced meiotic maturation of follicle-enclosed rabbit oocytes. *Biol Reprod* 1992;47:118–125.
500. Tsafriri A, Reich R, Abisogun AO. Ovarian regulation of oocyte maturation. In: Genazzani AR, Volpe A, Facchinetti F, eds. *Gynecological Endocrinology.* Lancs: The Parthenon Publishing Group, 1986;109–115.
501. Popkin RM, Fraser HM, Jonassen J. Stimulation of androstenedione and progesterone release by LHRH agonist from isolated rat preovulatory follicles. *Mol Cell Endocrinol* 1983;29:169–180.
502. Hillensjö T, Ekholm C, Hedin L. Effect of gonadotrophin releasing hormone upon the pattern of steroidogenesis in isolated preovulatory rat follicles. *Acta Endocrinol* 1984;105:105–111.
503. Mayar MQ, Tarvansky GK, Reeves JJ. Ovarian growth and uptake of iodinated D-Leu^6,desGlyNH$_2^{10}$-LHRH ethylamide in hCG-treated rats. *Proc Soc Exp Biol Med* 1979;161:216–219.
504. Reeves JJ, Seguin C, Lefebvre FA, Kelly PA, Labrie F. Similar luteinizing hormone-releasing hormone binding sites in rat anterior pituitary and ovary. *Proc Natl Acad Sci USA* 1980;77:5567–5571.
505. Harwood JP, Clayton RN, Chen TT, Knox G, Catt KJ. Ovarian gonadotropin-releasing hormone receptors. II. Regulation and effects on ovarian development. *Endocrinology* 1980;107:414–421.
506. Jones PBC, Conn PM, Marian J, Hsueh AJW. Binding of gonadotropin-releasing hormone agonist to rat ovarian granulosa cells. *Life Sci* 1980;27:2125–2132.
507. Pieper DR, Richards JS, Marshall JC. Ovarian gonadotropin-releasing hormone (GnRH) receptors: characterization, distribution and induction by GnRH. *Endocrinology* 1981;108:1148–1155.
508. Smith-White S, Ojeda SR. Peripubertal decline in ovarian LHRH receptor content: characterization and distribution. *Neuroendocrinology* 1983;36:449–456.
509. Dalkin AC, Bourne GA, Pieper DR, Regiani S, Marshall JC. Pituitary and gonadal gonadotropin-releasing hormone receptors during sexual maturation in the rat. *Endocrinology* 1981;108:1658–1644.
510. White SS, Ojeda SR. Changes in ovarian LHRH receptor content during the onset of puberty in the female rat. *Endocrinology* 1981;108:347–349.
511. Hazum E, Nimrod A. Photoaffinity-labelling and fluorescence distribution studies on GnRH receptors in ovarian granulosa cells. *Proc Natl Acad Sci USA* 1982;79:1747–1750.
512. Hazum E. Nature of the GnRH receptor in the ovary. In: McKerns KW, Aakvag A, Hansson V, eds. *Regulation of Target Cell Responsiveness.* New York: Plenum Press, 1984;23–46.
513. Hazum E. Photoaffinity labeling of luteinizing hormone releasing hormone receptor of rat pituitary membrane preparations. *Endocrinology* 1981;109:1281–1283.
514. Ranta T, Knecht M, Kody M, Catt KJ. GnRH receptors in cultured rat granulosa cells: mediation of the inhibitory and stimulatory actions of GnRH. *Mol Cell Endocrinol* 1982;27:233–240.
515. Naor Z, Yavin E. Gonadotropin releasing hormone stimulates phospholipid labeling in cultured granulosa cells. *Endocrinology* 1982;111:1615–1619.
516. Davis JS, Farese RV, Clark MR. Gonadotropin-releasing hormone (GnRH) stimulates phosphatidylinositol metabolism in rat granulosa cells: mechanism of action of GnRH. *Proc Natl Acad Sci USA* 1982;80:2049–2053.
517. Leung PCK, Raymond V, Labrie F. Stimulation of phosphatidic acid and phosphatidylinositol labelling in luteal cells by LHRH. *Endocrinology* 1983;112:1138–1140.
518. Raymond V, Leung PCK, Labrie F. Stimulation by prostaglandin $F_{2\alpha}$ of phosphatidic acid-phsophatidylinositol turnover in rat luteal cells. *Biochem Biophys Res Commun* 1983;116:39–46.
519. Ma F, Leung PCK. Luteinizing hormone-releasing hormone enhances polyphosphoinositide breakdown in rat granulosa cells. *Biochem Biophys Res Commun* 1985;130:1201–1208.
520. Leung PCK. Mechanisms of gonadotropin-releasing hormone and prostaglandin action on luteal cells. *Can J Physiol Pharmacol* 1985;63:249–256.
521. Knecht M, Ranta T, Naor Z, Catt KJ. Direct effects of GnRH on the ovary. In: Greenwald GS, Terranova PF, eds. *Factors Regulating Ovarian Function.* New York: Raven Press, 1983;225–243.
522. Ranta T, Knecht M, Darbon JM, Baukal AJ, Catt KJ. Calcium dependence of the inhibitory effect of GnRH on LH-induced cyclic AMP production in rat granulosa cells. *Endocrinology* 1983;113:427–429.
523. Eckstein N, Eshel A, Eli Y, Ayalon D, Naor Z. Calcium-dependent actions of gonadotropin-releasing hormone agonist and luteinizing hormone upon cyclic AMP and progesterone production in ovarian granulosa cells. *Mol Cell Endocrinol* 1986;47:91–98.
524. Minegishi T, Leung PCK. Luteinizing hormone-releasing hormone stimulates arachidonic acid release in rat granulosa cells. *Endocrinology* 1985;117:2001–2007.
525. Wang J, Baimbridge KG, Leung PCK. Changes in cytosolic free calcium ion concentrations in individual rat granulosa cells: effect of luteinizing hormone-releasing hormone. *Endocrinology* 1989;124:1912–1917.
526. Naor Z, Molcho J, Zilberstein M, Zakut H. Phospholipid turn-

over in gonadotropin-releasing hormone target cells: comparative studies. In: McKerns KW, Naor Z, eds. *Hormonal Control of the Hypothalamo-Pituitary-Gonadal Axis.* New York, London: Plenum Press, 1984;493–508.
527. Naor Z, Molcho J, Hermon J, Zilberstein M, Zakut M, Dekel N. Phospholipid turnover and GnRH action in the pituitary and gonads. In: Labrie F, Belanger A, Dupont A, eds. *LHRH and Its Analogues: Basic and Clinical Aspects.* Amsterdam: International Congress Series 656, Excerpta Medica, 1984;245–260.
528. Leung PCK, Wang J. The role of inositol lipid metabolism in the ovary. *Biol Reprod* 1989;40:703–708.
529. Leung PCK, Steele GL. Intracellular signaling in the gonads. *Endocr Rev* 1992;13:476–498.
530. Dekel N, Galiani D, Aberdam E. Regulation of rat oocyte maturation: involvement of protein kinases. In: Bavister BD, Cummins J, Roldan ERS, eds. *Fertilization in Mammals.* Norwell, MA: Serono Symposia, 1990;17–24.
531. Liscovitch M. Signal-dependent activation of phosphatidylcholine hydrolysis: role of phospholipase D. *Biochem Soc Trans* 1991;19:402–407.
532. Liscovitch M, Amsterdam A. Gonadotropin-releasing hormone activates phospholipase D in ovarian granulosa cells. *J Biol Chem* 1989;264:11762–11768.
533. Marsh JM. The role of cyclic AMP in gonadal steroidogenesis. *Biol Reprod* 1976;14:30–53.
534. Gudermann T, Birnbaumer M, Birbaumer L. Evidence of dual coupling of the murine luteinizing hormone receptor of adenylyl cyclase and phosphoinositide breakdown and Ca^{2+} mobilization. *J Biol Chem* 1992;267:4479–4488.
535. Zilberstein M, Zakut H, Eli Y, Naor Z. Regulation of prostaglandin E, progesterone and cyclic AMP production in ovarian granulosa cells by LH and GnRH: comparative studies. *Endocrinology* 1984;114:2374–2381.
536. Wang J, Leung PCK. Role of arachidonic acid in luteinizing hormone-releasing hormone actions: stimulation of progesterone production in rat granulosa cells. *Endocrinology* 1988;122: 906–911.
537. Wang J, Ho-Yuen B, Leung PCK. Stimulation of progesterone and prostaglandin E_2 production by lipoxygenase metabolites of arachidonic acid. *FEBS Lett* 1989;244:154–158.
538. Oikawa M, Dargan C, Ny T, Hsueh AJW. Expression of gonadotropin-releasing hormone and prothymosin-a messenger ribonucleic acid in the ovary. *Endocrinology* 1990;127: 2350–2356.
539. Goubau S, Bond CT, Adelman JP, et al. Partial characterization of the gonadotropin-releasing hormone (GnRH) gene transcript in the rat ovary. *Endocrinology* 1992;130:3098–3100.
540. Aten RF, Williams AT, Behrman HR. Ovarian gonadotropin releasing hormone-like proteins: demonstration and characterization. *Endocrinology* 1986;118:961–967.
541. Aten RF, Ireland JJ, Weems CW, Behrman HR. Presence of gonadotropin releasing hormone-like proteins in bovine and ovine ovaries. *Endocrinology* 1987;120:1727–1733.
542. Aten RF, Polan ML, Bayless R, Behrman HR. A GnRH-like protein in human ovaries: similarity to the GnRH-like ovarian protein of the rat. *J Clin Endocrinol* 1987;64:1288–1293.
543. Ireland JJ, Aten RF, Behrman HR. GnRH-like proteins in cows: concentrations during corpora lutea development and selective localization in granulosal cells. *Biol Reprod* 1988;38:544–550.
544. Aten RF, Behrman HR. A GnRH binding inhibitor protein from bovine ovaries: purification and identification as histone H2A. *J Biol Chem* 1989;264:11065–11071.
545. Aten RF, Behrman HR. Antigonadotropic effects of the bovine ovarian GnRH binding inhibitor proteins/histone H2A in rat luteal and granulosal cells. *J Biol Chem* 1989;264:11072–11075.
546. Margolin Y, Aten RF, Behrman HR. Mechanisms for the antigonadotropic action of the ovarian gonadotropin-releasing hormone-binding inhibitor protein/histone H2A and ovarian cells. *Biol Reprod* 1992;46:1021–1026.
547. Brown JL, Reeves JJ. Absence of specific LHRH receptors in ovine, bovine and porcine ovaries. *Biol Reprod* 1983;29: 1179–1182.
548. Asch RH, Sickle MV, Rettori V, et al. Absence of LHRH binding sites in corpora lutea from rhesus monkeys (*Macaca mulatta*). *J Clin Endocrinol Metab* 1981;53:215–217.
549. Clayton RN, Huhtaniemi IT. Absence of gonadotropin-releasing hormone receptors in human gonadal tissue. *Nature* 1982;299: 56–59.
550. Popkin RM, Bramley TA, Currie AJ, Shaw RW, Baird DT, Fraser HM. Specific binding of luteinizing hormone-releasing hormone to human luteal tissue. *Biochem Biophys Res Commun* 1983;114:750–756.
551. Bramley TA, Menzies GC, Baird DT. Specificity of gonadotropin-releasing hormone binding sites of the human corpus luteum: comparison with receptors of rat pituitary gland. *J Endocrinol* 1986;108:323–328.
552. Latouche J, Crumeyrolle-Arias M, Jordan D, et al. GnRH receptors in human granulosa cells: anatomical localization by autoradiographic study. *Endocrinology* 1989;125:1739–1741.
553. Milvae RA, Murphy BD, Hansel W. Prolongation of the bovine estrous cycle with a gonadotropin-releasing hormone analog. *Biol Reprod* 1984;31:664–670.
554. Sharpe RM. Cellular aspects of the inhibitory actions of LHRH on the ovary and testis. *J Reprod Fertil* 1982;64:517–527.
555. Tureck RW, Mastroianni L Jr, Blasco L, Strauss JF. Inhibition of human granulosa cell progesterone secretion by a GnRH agonist. *J Clin Endocrinol Metab* 1982;54:1078–1083.
556. Casper RJ, Erickson GF, Rebar RW, Yen SSC. The effect of LHRH and its agonist on cultured human granulosa cells. *Fertil Steril* 1982;37:406–409.
557. Tan GJS, Biggs JSG. Absence of effect of LHRH on progesterone production by human luteal cells *in vitro*. *J Reprod Fertil* 1983;67:411–413.
558. Williams AT, Behrman HR. Paracrine regulation of the ovary by GnRH and other peptides. *Sem Reprod Biol* 1983;1:269–277.
559. Tsafriri A, Eckstein B. Changes in follicular steroidogenic enzymes following the preovulatory surge of gonadotropins and experimentally-induced atresia. *Biol Reprod* 1986;34:783–787.
560. Erickson GE, Hofeditz C, Hsueh AJW. GnRH stimulates meiotic maturation in pre-antral follicles of hypophysectomized rats. In: Greenwald GS, Terranova PF, eds. *Factors Regulating Ovarian Function.* New York: Raven Press, 1983;257–261.
561. Banka CL, Erickson GF. Gonadotropin-releasing hormone induces classical meiotic maturation in subpopulations of atretic preantral follicles. *Endocrinology* 1985;117:1500–1507.
562. Bahr JM, Ben-Jonathan N. Ovarian catecholamines during the pre-pubertal period and reproductive cycle of several species. In: Ben-Jonathan N, Bahr JM, Weiner RI, eds. *Catecholamines as Hormone Regulators.* New York: Raven Press, 1985;279–292.
563. Wolf R, Meier-Fleitmann A, Duker EM, Wuttke W. Intraovarian secretion of catecholamines, oxytocin, beta-endorphin, and gamma-amino butyric acid in freely moving rats: development of a push–pull tubing method. *Biol Reprod* 1986;35:599–607.
564. Ferruz J, Barria A, Galleguillos X, Lara HE. Release of norepinephrine from the rat ovary: local modulation of gonadotropins. *Biol Reprod* 1991;45:592–597.
565. Ferruz J, Ahmed CE, Ojeda SR, Lara HE. Norepinephrine release in the immature ovary is regulated by autoreceptors and neuropeptide-Y. *Endocrinology* 1992;130:1345–1351.
566. Coleman AJ, Paterson DS, Somerville AR. The β-adrenergic receptor of rat corpus luteum membranes. *Biochem Pharmacol* 1979;28:1003–1010.
567. Harwood JP, Richert ND, Dufau ML, Catt KJ. Gonadotropin-induced desensitization of epinephrine action in the luteinized rat ovary. *Endocrinology* 1980;107:280–288.
568. Jordan AW. Changes in ovarian β-adrenergic receptors during the oestrous cycle of the rat. *Biol Reprod* 1981;24:245–248.
569. Kliachko S, Zor U. Increase in catecholamine-stimulated cyclic AMP and progesterone synthesis in rat granulosa cells during culture. *Mol Cell Endocrinol* 1981;23:23–32.
570. Abramowitz J, Iyengar R, Birnbaumer L. Guanine nucleotides and magnesium ion regulation of the interaction of gonadotropic and β-adrenergic receptors with their hormones: a comparative study using a single membrane system. *Endocrinology* 1982;110:336–346.
571. Abramowitz J, Birnbaumer L. Temporal characteristics of gonadotropin interaction with rabbit luteal receptors and activation of adenylyl cyclase: comparison to the mode of action of catecholamine receptors. *Endocrinology* 1982;111:970–976.
572. Aguado LI, Petrovic SL, Ojeda SR. Ovarian β-adrenergic recep-

tors during the onset of puberty: characterization, distribution and coupling to steroidogenic responses. *Endocrinology* 1982;110:1124–1132.
573. Kirchick HJ, Iyengar R, Birnbaumer L. Human chorionic gonadotropin-induced heterologous desensitization of adenylyl cyclases from highly luteinized rat ovaries: attenuation of regulatory N component activity. *Endocrinology* 1983;113:1638–1646.
574. Norjavaara E, Rosberg S, Gafvels M, Selstam G. β-Adrenergic receptor concentration in corpora lutea of different ages obtained from PMSG-treated rat. *Endocrinology* 1984;114:2154–2159.
575. Hernandez ER, Jimenez JL, Payne DW, Adashi EY. Adrenergic regulation of ovarian androgen biosynthesis is mediated via β_2-adrenergic theca-interstitial cell recognition sites. *Endocrinology* 1988;122.1592–1602.
576. Condon WA, Black DL. Catecholamine induced stimulation of progesterone by the bovine corpus luteum *in vitro*. *Biol Reprod* 1976;15:573–578.
577. Godkin JD, Black DL, Duby RT. Stimulation of cyclic AMP and progesterone synthesis by LH, PGE_2 and isoproterenol in bovine corpus luteum *in vitro*. *Biol Reprod* 1977;17:514–518.
578. Jordan AW III, Caffrey JL, Niswender GD. Catecholamine-induced stimulation of progesterone and adenosine 3′,5′-monophosphate production by dispersed ovine luteal cells. *Endocrinology* 1978;103:385–392.
579. Ratner A, Sanborn CR, Weiss GK. β-Adrenergic stimulation of cAMP and progesterone in rat ovarian tissue. *Am J Physiol* 1980;239:E139–143.
580. Ratner A, Weiss GK, Sanborn CR. Stimulation by β_2-adrenergic receptors of the production of cyclic AMP and progesterone in rat ovarian tissue. *J Endocrinol* 1980;87:123–129.
581. Adashi EY, Hsueh AJW. Stimulation of β_2-adrenergic responsiveness by follicle-stimulating hormone in granulosa cells *in vitro* and *in vivo*. *Endocrinology* 1981;108:2170–2178.
582. Jones PBC, Hsueh AJW. Regulation of progesterone metabolizing enzyme by adrenergic agents, prolactin and prostaglandins in cultured rat ovarian granulosa cells. *Endocrinology* 1981;109: 1347–1354.
583. Hunzicker-Dunn M. Epinephrine-sensitive adenylyl cyclase activity in rabbit ovarian tissues. *Endocrinology* 1982;110:233–240.
584. Zsolnai B, Varga B, Horvath E. Increase of ovarian progesterone secretion by β_2-adrenergic stimulation in oestrous rats. *Acta Endocrinol (Copenh)* 1982;101:268–272.
585. Rani CS, Nordenström K, Norjavaara E, Ahrén K. Development of catecholamine responsiveness in granulosa cells from preovulatory rat follicles. Dependence on preovulatory luteinizing hormone surge. *Biol Reprod* 1983;28:1021–1031.
586. Dyer CA, Erickson GF. Norepinephrine amplifies human chorionic gonadotropin-stimulated androgen biosynthesis by ovarian theca-interstitial cells. *Endocrinology* 1985;116:1645–1652.
587. Burden HW. The adrenergic innervation of mammalian ovaries. In: Ben-Jonathan N, Bahr JM, Weiner RI, eds. *Catecholamines as Hormone Regulators*. New York: Raven Press, 1985;261–278.
588. Goetz FW, Berndtson AM, Ranjan M. Ovulation: mediators at the ovarian level. In: Pang PTK, Schreibman MP, Jones R, eds. *Vertebrate Endocrinology: Fundamentals and Biomedical Implications,* Vol 4. New York: Academic Press, 1991;127–203.
589. Burden HW, Lawrence IE. The effects of denervation on the localization of Δ^5-3β-hydroxysteroid dehydrogenase activity in the rat ovary during pregnancy. *Acta Anat* 1977;97:286–290.
590. Burden HW. Ovarian innervation. In: Jones RE, ed. *The Vertebrate Ovary*. New York: Plenum Press, 1978;616–638.
591. Owman CH, Sjöberg NO, Wallach EE, Walles B, Wright KH. Neuromuscular mechanisms of ovulation. In: Hafez ESE, ed. *Human Ovulation*. Elsevier, North-Holland: Biomedical Press, 1979;57–100.
592. Selstam G, Norjavaara E, Tegenfelt T, Lundberg S, Sandström C, Persson SA. Partial denervation of the ovaries by transection of the suspensory ligament does not inhibit ovulation in rats treated with pregnant mare serum gonadotropin. *Anat Rec* 1985;213: 392–395.
593. Deanesly R. Cyclic function in ovarian grafts. *J Endocrinol* 1956;13:211–220.
594. Jacobowitz D, Laties AM. Adrenergic reinnervation of the cat ovary transplanted to the anterior chamber of the eye. *Endocrinology* 1970;86:921–924.
595. Dominguez R, Riboni L. Failure of ovulation in autografted ovary of the hemispayed rat. *Neuroendocrinology* 1971;7: 164–170.
596. Ojeda SR, Aguado LI. Adrenergic control of the prepubertal ovary: involvement of local innervation and circulating catecholamines. In: Ben-Jonathan N, Bahr JM, Weiner RI, eds. *Catecholamines as Hormone Regulators*. New York: Raven Press, 1985;292–310.
597. Gerendai I, Marchetti B, Maugeri S, Amico-Roxas M, Scapagnini U. Prevention of compensatory ovarian hypertrophy by local treatment of the ovary with 6-OHDA. *Neuroendocrinology* 1978;27:272–278.
598. Gerendai I, Halasz B. Neural participation in ovarian control. *TINS* 1978,1.87–88.
599. Gerendai I, Halasz B. Hemigonadectomy-induced unilateral changes in the protein-synthesizing activity of the rat hypothalamic arcuate nucleus. *Neuroendocrinology* 1976;21:311–337.
600. Curry TE, Lawrence IE, Burden HW. Effect of ovarian sympathectomy on follicular development during compensatory ovarian hypertrophy in the guinea pig. *J Reprod Fertil* 1984;71:39–44.
601. Brink CE, Grob H. Response of the denervated mouse ovary to exogenous gonadotropins. *Biol Reprod* 1973;9:108(abstr 120).
602. Curry TE, Lawrence IE, Burden HW. Ovarian sympathectomy in the guinea pig. I. Effects on follicular development during the estrous cycle. *Cell Tissue Res* 1984;236:257–263.
603. Bahr JM, Ben-Jonathan N. Preovulatory depletion of ovarian catecholamines in the rat. *Endocrinology* 1981;108:1815–1821.
604. Ben-Jonathan N, Braw RH, Laufer N, Reich R, Bahr JM, Tsafriri A. Norepinephrine in Graafian follicles is depleted by FSH. *Endocrinology* 1982;110:457–461.
605. Morimoto K, Okamura H, Tanaka C. Developmental and preovulatory changes of ovarian norepinephrine in the rat. *Am J Obstet Gynecol* 1982;143:389–392.
606. Veldhuis JD, Harrison TS, Hammond JM. β_2-Adrenergic stimulation of ornithine decarboxylase activity in porcine granulosa cells *in vitro*. *Biochim Biophys Acta* 1980;627:123–130.
607. Bahr JM, Ben-Jonathan N. Elevated catecholamines in porcine follicular fluid before ovulation. *Endocrinology* 1985;117: 620–623.
608. Sosa A, Ortege-Corona B, Chargoy J, Rosado A. Presence and importance of biogenic amines in reproductive tract secretions. *Fertil Steril* 1980;33:235.
609. Birnbaumer L, Yang PC, Hunzicker-Dunn M, Bockaert J, Duran JM. Adenylyl cyclase activities in ovarian tissues. I. Homogenization and conditions of assay in Graafian follicles and corpora lutea of rabbits, rats and pigs: regulation by ATP, and some comparative properties. *Endocrinology* 1976;99:163–184.
610. Hunzicker-Dunn M, Day SL, Abramowitz J, Birnbaumer L. Ovarian responses of pregnant mare serum gonadotropin- and human chorionic gonadotropin-primed rats: desensitizing, luteolytic, and ovulatory effects of a single dose of human chorionic gonadotropin. *Endocrinology* 1979;105:442–451.
611. Norjavaara E, Selstam G, Ahrén K. Catecholamine stimulation of cyclic AMP and progesterone production in rat corpora lutea of different ages. *Acta Endocrinol* 1982;100:613–622.
612. Norjavaara E, Selstam G, Dambarg JE, Johansson BM. *In vivo* effect of noradrenaline on the cyclic AMP level in rat corpora lutea. *Acta Physiol Scand* 1983;119:113–116.
613. Zor U, Kliachko S. The β-adrenergic system in rat ovarian granulosa cells: hormonal and prostaglandin dependence *in vivo* and spontaneous development *in vitro*. In: Ben-Jonathan N, Bahr JM, Weiner RI, eds. *Catecholamines as Hormone Regulators*. New York: Raven Press, 1985;311–328.
614. Orly J, Farkash Y, Hershkovitz N, Mizrahi L, Weinberger O. Ovarian substance induces steroid production in cultured granulosa cells. *In Vitro* 1982;18:980–989.
615. Day SL, Birnbaumer L. The effect of estradiol on hormonally stimulable adenylyl cyclase activity and on progesterone production in normal and regressing corpora lutea from control and human gonadotropin-treated pseudopregnant rabbits. *Endocrinology* 1980;106:375–381.
616. Day SL, Birnbaumer L. Corpus luteum function and adenylyl cyclase stimulability in the rat after an estradiol benzoate-induced ovulatory surge of luteinizing hormone-induced ovula-

tory surge of luteinizing hormone: role of prolactin. *Endocrinology* 1980;106:382–389.
617. Jones PBC, Valk CA, Hsueh AJW. Regulation of progestin biosynthetic enzymes in cultured rat granulosa cells: effects of prolactin, β_2-adrenergic agonist, human chorionic gonadotropin and gonadotropin-releasing hormone. *Biol Reprod* 1983;29:572–585.
618. Lahav M, Freud A, Lindner HR. Abrogation by prostaglandin $E_{2\alpha}$ of LH-stimulated cyclic AMP accumulation in isolated rat corpora lutea of pregnancy. *Biochem Biophys Res Commun* 1976;68:1294–1300.
619. Khan I, Rosberg S. Acute suppression by $PGF_{2\alpha}$ on LH, epinephrine and fluoride stimulation of adenylate cyclase in rat luteal tissue. *J Cyclic Nucl Res* 1979;5:55–63.
620. Khan MI, Rosberg S, Lahav M, et al. Studies on the mechanism of action of the inhibitory effect of prostaglandin $F_{2\alpha}$ on cyclic AMP accumulation in rat corpora lutea of various ages. *Biol Reprod* 1979;21:1175–1183.
621. Thomas JP, Dorflinger LJ, Behrman HR. Mechanism of the rapid antigonadotropic action of prostaglandins in cultured luteal cells. *Proc Natl Acad Sci USA* 1978;75:1344–1348.
622. Ahrén K, Norjavaara E, Rosberg S, Selstam G. Prostaglandin $F_{2\alpha}$ inhibition of epinephrine stimulated cyclic AMP and progesterone production by rat corpora lutea of various ages. *Prostaglandins* 1983;25:839–850.
623. Capps ML, Lawrence IE, Burden HW. Ultrastructure of the cells of the interstitial gland in hypophysectomized rats. *Cell Tissue Res* 1978;193:433–442.
624. Krnjevitz K. Chemical nature of synaptic transmission in vertebrates. *Physiol Rev* 1974;54:418–540.
625. Martindelrio R, Caballero AL. Presence of gamma-aminobutyric acid in rat ovary. *J Neurochem* 1980;34:1584–1586.
626. Erdö SL, Rosdy B, Szporny L. Higher GABA concentrations in fallopian tube than in brain of the rat. *J Neurochem* 1982;38:1174–1176.
627. Schaeffer JM, Hsueh AJW. Identification of gamma-aminobutyric acid and its binding sites in the ovary. *Life Sci* 1982;30:1599–1604.
628. Erdö SL. Alteration of GABA levels in ovary and fallopian tube of the pregnant rat. *Life Sci* 1984;34:1879–1884.
629. Erdö SL, Lapis E. Bicuculline-sensitive GABA receptors in rat ovary. *Eur J Pharmacol* 1982;85:243–246.
630. Erdö SL, Lapis E. Presence of GABA receptors in rat oviduct. *Neurosci Lett* 1982;33:275–279.
631. Erdö SL, Joo F, Wolff JR. Immunohistochemical localization of glutamate decarboxylase in the rat oviduct and ovary: further evidence for non-neural GABA systems. *Cell Tissue Res* 1989;255:431–434.
632. Erdö SL. High affinity, sodium-dependent gamma-aminobutyric acid uptake by slices of rat ovary. *J Neurochem* 1983;40:582–584.
633. Erdö SL, Varga B, Horvath E. Effect of local GABA administration on rat ovarian blood flow, and on progesterone and estradiol secretion. *Eur J Pharmacol* 1985;111:397–400.
634. Ojeda SR, Lara H, Ahmed CE. Potential relevance of vasoactive intestinal peptide to ovarian physiology. *Semin Reprod Endocrinol* 1989;7:52–60.
635. Larsson LI, Fahrendrug J, Schaffalitzky de Muckadell OB. Vasoactive intestinal peptide occurs in nerves of the female genitourinary tract. *Science* 1977;197:1374–1375.
636. Alm P, Alumets J, Hakanson R, et al. Vasoactive intestinal polypeptide nerves in the human female genital tract. *Am J Obstet Gynecol* 1980;136:349–351.
637. Alm P, Alumets J, Hakanson R, et al. Origin and distribution of VIP (vasoactive intestinal peptide)-nerves in the genito-urinary tract. *Cell Tissue Res* 1980;205:337–347.
638. Ahmed CE, Dees WL, Ojeda SR. The immature rat ovary is innervated by vasoactive intestinal peptide (VIP)-containing fibers and responds to VIP with steroid secretion. *Endocrinology* 1986;118:1682–1689.
639. Gozes I, Tsafriri A. Detection of vasoactive intestinal peptide-encoding messenger ribonucleic acid in the rat ovaries. *Endocrinology* 1986;119:2606–2610.
640. Davoren JB, Hsueh AJW. Vasoactive intestinal peptide—a novel stimulator of steroidogenesis by cultured rat granulosa cells. *Biol Reprod* 1985;33:37–52.
641. Kasson BG, Meidan R, Davoren JB, Hsueh AJW. Identification of subpopulations of rat granulosa cells: sedimentation properties and hormonal responsiveness. *Endocrinology* 1985;117:1027–1034.
642. Törnell J, Carlsson B, Hillensjö T. Vasoactive intestinal polypeptide stimulates oocyte maturation, steroidogenesis, and cyclic adenosine 3′,5′-monophosphate production in *isolated* preovulatory rat follicles. *Biol Reprod* 1988;39:213–220.
643. Nakamura Y, Gangrade BK, Terranova IF. Vasoactive intestinal peptide (VIP) has a LH-like action on *in vitro* follicular steroidogenesis but not on ovulation in the cyclic hamster. In: Hirshfield AN, ed. *Growth Factors and The Ovary.* New York: Plenum Press, 1989;297–302.
644. Schmidt G, Jörgensen J, Kannisto P, Liedberg F, Ottensen B, Owman C. Vasoactive intestinal polypeptide in the PMSG-primed immature rat ovary and its effect on ovulation in the isolated rat ovary perfused *in vitro. J Reprod Fertil* 1990;90:465–472.
645. Burden HW, Leonard M, Smith CP, Lawrence IE. The sensory innervation of the ovary: a horseradish peroxidase study in the rat. *Anat Rec* 1983;207:623–627.
646. Lawrence IE, Burden HW, Lous TM. Effect of abdominal vagotomy of the pregnant rat on LH and progesterone concentrations and fetal resorption. *J Reprod Fertil* 1978;53:131–136.
647. Ojeda SR, White SS, Aguado LI, Advis JP, Andersen JM. Abdominal vagotomy delays the onset of puberty and inhibits ovarian function in the female rat. *Neuroendocrinology* 1983;36:261–267.
648. Nakamura Y, Kato H, Terranova PF. Abdominal vagotomy decreased the number of ova shed and serum progesterone levels on estrus in the cyclic hamster. *Endocrinol Jpn* 1992;39:141–145.
649. Dees WL, Kozlowski GP, Dey R, Ojeda SR. Evidence for the existence of substance P in the prepubertal rat ovary. II. Immunocytochemical localization. *Biol Reprod* 1985;33:471–476.
650. Makris A, Yazumizu T, Elkind-Hirsh K, Carraway R, Leeman SE, Ryan KJ. Substance P and neurotensin in the ovary and pituitary of the cycling golden hamster. *Biol Reprod* 1982;26:98A.
651. Ojeda SR, Costa ME, Katz KH, Hersh LB. Evidence for the existence of substance P in the prepubertal rat ovary. I. Biochemical and physiologic studies. *Biol Reprod* 1985;33:286–295.
652. Auletta FJ, Paradis DK, Wesley M, Duby RT. Oxytocin is luteolytic in the rhesus monkey (*Macaca mulatta*). *J Reprod Fertil* 1984;72:401–406.
653. Khan-Dawood FS, Dawood MY. Potential relevance of neurohypophysial hormones to ovarian physiology. *Semin Reprod Endocrinol* 1989;7:61–68.
654. Shukovski L. Is there a function for ovarian oxytocin in primates? *Reprod Fertil Dev* 1992;4:99–103.
655. Wathes DC, Swann RW, Birkett SD, Porter DG, Pickering BT. Characterization of oxytocin, vasopressin and neurophysin from the bovine corpus luteum. *Endocrinology* 1983;113:693–698.
656. Wathes DC, Swann RW, Pickering BT. Variations in oytocin, vasopressin and neurophysin concentrations in the bovine ovary during the oestrous cycle and pregnancy. *J Reprod Fertil* 1984;71:551–557.
657. Schams D, Kruip TAM, Koll R. Oxytocin determination in steroid producing tissues and *in vitro* production in ovarian follicles. *Acta Endocrinol (Copenh)* 1985;109:530–536.
658. Wathes DC, Swann RW. Is oxytocin an ovarian hormone? *Nature* 1982;297:225–227.
659. Wathes DC, Guldenaar SEE, Swann RW, et al. A combined radioimmunoassay and immunocytochemical study of ovarian oxytocin production during the periovulatory period in the ewe. *J Reprod Fertil* 1986;78:167–183.
660. Khan-Dawood FS, Dawood MY. Human ovaries contain immunoreactive oxytocin. *J Clin Endocrinol Metab* 1983;57:1129–1132.
661. Dawood MY, Khan-Dawood FS. Human ovarian oxytocin: its source and relationship to steroid hormones. *Am J Obstet Gynecol* 1986;154:756–763.
662. Schaeffer JM, Liu J, Hsueh AJW, Yen SSC. Presence of oxytocin and arginine vasopressin in human ovary, oviduct and follicular fluid. *J Clin Endocrinol Metab* 1984;59:970–973.

663. Peek JC, Choy VJ, Watkins WB, Graham FM. Levels of oxytocin-like activity and progesterone in follicular fluid from *in vitro* fertilization cycles. *J In Vitro Fert Embryo Transf* 1987;4:103–106.
664. Holtorf P, Furuya K, Ivell R, McArdle CA. Oxytocin production and oxytocin messenger ribonucleic acid levels in bovine granulosa cells are regulated by insulin and insulin-like growth factor-I: dependence on developmental status of the ovarian follicle. *Endocrinology* 1989;125:2612–2620.
665. McArdle CA, Holtrof AP. Oxytocin and progesterone release from bovine corpus luteal cells in culture: effects of insulin-like growth factor I, insulin, and prostaglandins. *Endocrinology* 1989;124:1278–1286.
666. Schams D, Koll R, Li CH. Insulin-like growth factor-I stimulated oxytocin and progesterone production by bovine granulosa cells in culture. *Endocrinology* 1988;116:97–100.
667. Shukovski, Fortune JE, Findlay JK. Oxytocin and progesterone secretion by bovine granulosa cells of individual preovulatory follicles cultured in serum-free medium. *Mol Cell Endocrinol* 1990;69:17–24.
668. Meidan R, Altstein M, Girsh E. Biosynthesis and release of oxytocin by granulosa cells derived from preovulatory bovine follicles: effects of forskolin and insulin-like growth factor-I. *Biol Reprod* 1992;46:715–720.
669. Furuya K, McArdle CA, Ivell R. The regulation of oxytocin gene expression in early bovine luteal cells. *Mol Cell Endocrinol* 1990;70:81–88.
670. Robinson G, Evans JJ, Forster ME. Oxytocin can affect follicular development in the adult mouse. *Acta Endocrinol* 1985;108:273–276.
671. Auletta FJ, Currie GN, Black DL. Effect of oxytocin and adrenergic drugs on bovine reproduction. I. Estrous cycle length and peripheral blood progesterone. *Acta Endocrinol (Copenh)* 1972;69:241–248.
672. Pitzel L, Probst I, Jarry H, Wuttke W. Inhibitory effect of oxytocin and vasopressin on steroid release of cultured porcine luteal cells. *Endocrinology* 1988;122:1780–1785.
673. Pitzel L, Jarry H, Wuttke W. Effects of oxytocin on *in vitro* steroid release of midstage small and large porcine luteal cells. *Endocrinology* 1990;126:2343–2349.
674. Jarry H, Einspanier A, Kanngießer L, et al. Release and effects of oxytocin on estradiol and progesterone secretion in porcine corpora lutea as measured by an *in vivo* microdialysis system. *Endocrinology* 1990;126:2350–2358.
675. Maas S, Jarry H, Teichmann A, Rath W, Kuhn W, Wuttke W. Paracrine actions of oxytocin, prostaglandin F2-alpha and estradiol within the human corpus luteum. *J Clin Endocrinol Metab* 1991;74:306–312.
676. Wathes DC, Pickering BT, Swann RW, Horter DG, Hull MGR, Drif GO. Neurohyperphasial hormones in the human ovary. *Lancet* 1982;2:410–412.
677. Wathes DC, Swann RW, Hull MGR, Drife JO, Porter DG, Pickering BT. Gonadal sources of the posterior pituitary hormones. *Prog Brain Res* 1983;60:513–520.
678. Verges B, Maurice C, Cornet D, et al. Arginine vasopressin in human follicular fluid. *J Clin Endocrinol Metab* 1986;63:928–930.
679. Lim ATW, Lolait SJ, Barlow JW, et al. Immunoreactive arginine-vasopressin in Brattleboro rat ovary. *Nature* 1984;310:61–64.
680. Fuller PJ, Clements JA, Tregear GW, Nikolaidis I, Whitfeld PL, Funder JW. Vasopressin-neurophysin II gene expression in the ovary: studies in Sprague-Dwaley, Long-Evans and Brattleboro rats. *J Endocrinol* 1985;105:317–321.
681. Akil H, Watson SJ, Young E, Lewis ME, Khachaturian H, Walker M. Endogenous opioids: biology and function. *Annu Rev Neurosci* 1984;7:223–255.
682. Smith AI, Funder JW. Proopiomelanocortin processing in the pituitary, central nervous system, and peripheral tissues. *Endocr Rev* 1988;9:159–179.
683. Lolait SJ, Autelitano DJ, Lim ATW, Smith AI, Toh BH, Funder JW. Ovarian immunoreactive β-endorphin and estrous cycle in the rat. *Endocrinology* 1985;117:161–168.
684. Kilpatrick DL, Howells RD, Noe M, Bailey LC, Udenfriend S. Expression of preproenkephalin-like mRNA and its peptide products in mammalian testis and ovary. *Proc Natl Acad Sci USA* 1985;82:7467–7469.
685. Douglass J, Cox B, Quinn B, Civelli O, Herbert E. Expression of the prodynorphin gene in male and female mammalian reproductive tissues. *Endocrinology* 1987;120:707–713.
686. Lovegren ES, Zimniski SJ, Puett D. Ovarian contents of immunoreactive β-endorphin and α-*N*-acetylated opioid peptides in rats. *J Reprod Fertil* 1991;91:91–100.
687. Lim AT, Lolait S, Barlow JW, et al. Immunoreactive β-endorphin in sheep ovary. *Nature* 1982;303:709–711.
688. Shaha C, Margioris A, Liotta AS, Krieger DT, Bardin CW. Demonstration of immunoreactive β-endorphin and γ-3-melanocyte-stimulating hormone-related peptides in the ovaries of neonatal, cyclic and pregnant mice. *Endocrinology* 1984;115:378–384.
689. Petraglia F, Segre A, Facchinetti F, Campanini D, Ruspa M, Genazzani AR. β-Endorphin and met-enkephalin in peritoneal and ovarian follicular fluids of fertile and postmenopausal women. *Fertil Steril* 1985;44:615–621.
690. Chen CLC, Chang CC, Krieger DT, Bardin CW. Expression and regulation of proopiomelanocortin-like gene in the ovary and placenta: comparison with the testis. *Endocrinology* 1986;118:2382–2389.
691. Jin DF, Muffy KE, Okulicz WC, Kilpatrick DL. Estrous cycle- and pregnancy-related differences in expression of the proenkephalin and proopiomelanocortin genes in the ovary and uterus. *Endocrinology* 1988;122:1466–1471.
692. Kew D, Jin DF, Kim F, Laddis T, Kilpatrick DL. Translation status of proenkephalin mRNA in the rat reproductive system. *Mol Endocrinol* 1989;3:1191–1196.
693. Melner MH, Young SL, Czerwiec FS, et al. The regulation of granulosa cell proopiomelanocortin messenger ribonucleic acid by androgens and gonadotropins. *Endocrinology* 1986;119:2082–2088.
694. Bardin CW, Chen CLC, Morris PL, et al. Proopiomelanocortin-derived peptides in testis, ovary, and tissues of reproduction. *Recent Prog Horm Res* 1987;43:1–28.
695. Hall AK, Preston SL, Behrman HR. Purine amplification of luteinizing hormone action in ovarian luteal cells. *J Biol Chem* 1981;256:10390–10398.
696. Polan ML, DeCherney AH, Haseltine FP, Mezer HC, Behrman HR. Adenosine amplifies follicle stimulating hormone action in granulosa cells and luteinizing hormone action in luteal cells of rat and human ovaries. *J Clin Endocrinol Metab* 1983;56:288–294.
697. Billig H, Rosberg S. Gonadotropin depression of ATP and interaction with adenosine in rat granulosa cells. *Endocrinology* 1986;118:645–652.
698. Soodak L, Musicki B, Behrman HR. Selective amplification of luteinizing hormone by adenosine in rat luteal cells. *Endocrinology* 1988;122:847–854.
699. Knecht M, Darbon JM, Ranta T, Baukal A, Catt KJ. Inhibitory actions of adenosine on follicle-stimulating hormone-induced differentiation of cultured rat granulosa cells. *Biol Reprod* 1984;30:1082–1090.
700. Behrman HR, Hall AK, Preston SL, Gore SD. Antagonistic interactions of adenosine and prostaglandin $F_{2\alpha}$ modulate acute response of luteal cells to luteinizing hormone. *Endocrinology* 1982;110:38–46.
701. Behrman HR, Polan ML, Ohkawa R, et al. Purine modulation of LH action in gonadal cells. *J Steroid Biochem* 1983;19:789–793.
702. Behrman HR, Ohkawa R, Preston SL, MacDonald GJ. Transport and selective utilization of adenosine as a prosubstrate for luteinizing hormone-sensitive adenylate cyclase in the luteal cell. *Endocrinology* 1983;113:1132–1140.
703. Brennan TJ, Ohkawa R, Gore SD, Behrman HR. Adenine-derived purines increase adenosine triphosphate (ATP) levels in the luteal cell: evidence that cell levels of ATP may limit the stimulation of adenosine 3′,5′-monophosphate accumulation by luteinizing hormone. *Endocrinology* 1983;112:499–508.
704. Soodak LK, Behrman HR. Mitochondria mediate amplification of luteinizing hormone action by adenosine in luteal cells. *Endocrinology* 1988;122:1308–1313.
705. Ohkawa R, Polan ML, Behrman HR. Adenosine differentially

amplifies luteinizing hormone over follicle-stimulating hormone-mediated effects in acute cultures of rat granulosa cells. *Endocrinology* 1985;117:248–254.
706. Fain JN, Malbon CC. Regulation of adenylate cyclase by adenosine. *Mol Cell Biochem* 1979;25:143–169.
707. Daly JW. Role of ATP and adenosine receptors in physiologic processes: summary and prospectus. In: Daly JW, Kuroda Y, Phillis JW, Shimiza H, Ui M, eds. *Physiology and Pharmacology of Adenosine Derivatives.* New York: Raven Press, 1983; 273–290.
708. Billig H, Thelander H, Rosberg S. Adenosine receptor-mediated effects by nonmetabolizable adenosine analogs in preovulatory rat granulosa cells: a putative local regulatory role of adenosine in the ovary. *Endocrinology* 1988;122:52–61.
709. Billig H, Rosberg S, Johanson C, Ahrén K. Adenosine as substrate and receptor agonist in the ovary. *Steroids* 1989;54: 523–542.
710. Corey EJ, Niwa H, Falck JR, Mioskowski C, Arai Y, Marfat A. Recent studies on the chemical synthesis of eicosanoids. *Adv Prostaglandin Thromboxane Res* 1980;6:19–26.
711. Behrman HR. Prostaglandins in hypothalamo-pituitary and ovarian function. *Annu Rev Physiol* 1979;41:685–700.
712. Lindner HR, Zor U, Kohen F, et al. Significance of prostaglandins in the regulation of cyclic events in the ovary and uterus. *Adv Prostaglandin Thromboxane Res* 1980;8:1371–1390.
713. Patrono C. Arachidonic acid metabolism in the ovary. In: Serra GB, ed. *The Ovary.* New York: Raven Press, 1983;45–56.
714. Reich R, Kohen F, Slager R, Tsafriri A. Ovarian lipoxygenase activity and its regulation by gonadotropin in the rat. *Prostaglandins* 1985;30:581–590.
715. Tanaka N, Espey LL, Okamura H. Increase in ovarian 15-hydroxyeicosatetraenoic acid during ovulation in the gonadotropin-primed immature rat. *Endocrinology* 1989;15:1373–1377.
716. Espey LL, Tanaka N, Adams RF, Okamura H. Ovarian hydroxyeicosatetraenoic acids compared with prostanoids and steroids during ovulation in rats. *Am J Physiol* 1991;260: E163–E169.
717. Reich R, Kohen F, Naor Z, Tsafriri A. Possible involvement of lipoxygenase products of arachidonic acid pathway in ovulation. *Prostaglandins* 1983;26:1011–1020.
718. Yoshimura Y, Nakamura Y, Shiraki M, et al. Involvement of leukotriene B_4 in ovulation in the rabbit. *Endocrinology* 1991;129:193–199.
719. Reich R, Tsafriri A, Mechanic GL. The involvement of collagenolysis in ovulation in the rat. *Endocrinology* 1985;116:521–527.
720. Reich R, Daphna-Iken D, Chun SY, et al. Preovulatory changes in ovarian expression of collagenases and tissue metalloproteinase inhibitor messenger ribonucleic acid—role of eicosanoids. *Endocrinology* 1991;129:1869–1875.
721. Tsafriri A, Chun SY, Reich R. Role of eicosanoids in the mediation of LH/hCG stimulation of ovarian collagenase and of ovulation. *The 8th International Conference on Prostaglandins and Related Compounds,* Montreal, Canada, 1992;130(abst 510).
722. Downs SM, Longo FJ. Effects of indomethacin on preovulatory follicles in immature, superovulated mice. *Am J Anat* 1982;164:265–274.
723. Downs SM, Longo FJ. Prostaglandins and preovulatory follicular maturation in mice. *J Exp Zool* 1983;228:99–108.
724. Salustri A, Petrungaro S, Siracusa G. Granulosa cells stimulate *in vitro* expansion of isolated mouse cumuli oophori: involvement of prostaglandin E_2. *Biol Reprod* 1985;33:229–234.
725. Pepperell JR, Nemeth G, Palumbo A, Naftolin F. Ovarian regulation and the renin-angiotensin system. In: Adashi EY, Leung PCK, eds. *The Ovary.* Raven Press (in press).
726. Sealey JE, Quimby FW, Itskovitz J, Rubattu S. The ovarian renin-angiotensin system. *Front Neuroendocrinol* 1990;11: 213–237.
727. Lightman A, Tarlatzis BC, Rzasa PJ, et al. The ovarian renin-angiotensin system: renin-like activity and angiotensin II/III immunoreactivity in gonadotrophin stimulated and unstimulated human follicular fluid. *Am J Obstet Gynecol* 1987;156:808–814.
728. Glorioso N, Atlas SA, Laragh JH, Jewelewicz R, Sealey JJE. Prorenin in high concentrations in human ovarian follicular fluid. *Science* 1986;233:1422–1424.
729. Schultze D, Brunswig B, Mukhopadhyay AK. Renin and prorenin-like activities in bovine ovarian follicles. *Endocrinology* 1989;124:1389–1398.
730. Do YS, Sherrod A, Lobo RA, et al. Human ovarian theca cells are a source of renin. *Proc Natl Acad Sci USA* 1988;85:1957–1961.
731. Palumbo A, Jones C, Lightman A, Carcangiu ML, DeCherney AH, Naftolin F. Immunohistochemical localization of renin and angiotensin II in human ovaries. *Am J Obstet Gynecol* 1989;160:8–14.
732. Lightman A, Jones C, McLusky NJ, Palumbo A, Naftolin F. Immunocytochemical localization of angiotensin II immunoreactivity and demonstration of angiotensin II binding in the rat ovary. *Am J Obstet Gynecol* 1988;159:526–530.
733. Itskovitz (Eldor) J, Bruneval P, Soubrier F, Thaler I, Corvol P, Sealey JE. Localization of renin gene expression to monkey ovarian theca cells by *in situ* hybridization. *J Clin Endocrinol Metab* 75:1374–1380.
734. Howard RB, Pucell AG, Bumpus FM, Husain A. Rat ovarian renin characterization and changes during the estrous cycle. *Endocrinology* 1988;123:2331–2340.
735. Pellicer A, Palumbo A, DeCherney AH, Naftolin F. Blockade of ovulation by an angiotensin antagonist. *Science* 1988;240: 1660–1661.
736. Daud AI, Bumpus FM, Husain A. Angiotensin II: does it have a direct obligate role in ovulation? *Science* 1989;245:870–871.
737. Naftolin F, Andrade-Gordon P, Pellicer A, et al. (Response to) Angiotensin II: does it have a direct obligate role in ovulation? *Science* 1989;245:870.
738. Petterson CM, Zhu C, Mukaido T, Butler TA, Woessner JF, Moire WJ. The angiotensin antagonist, saralasin inhibits ovulation in the perfused rat ovary. *Am J Obstet Gynecol* 1993;168:242–245.
739. Kuo TC, Endo K, Dharmarajan AM, Miyazaki T, Atlas SJ, Wallach EE. Direct effect of angiotensin II on *in vitro* perfused rabbit ovary. *J Reprod Fertil* 1991;92:469–474.
740. Yoshimura Y, Karube M, Koyama N, Shoikawa S, Nanno T, Nakamura Y. Angiotensin II directly induces follicle rupture and oocyte maturation in the rabbit. *FEBS Lett* 1992;307:305–308.
741. Palumbo A, Pellicer A, DeCherney AH, Naftolin F. Angiotensin action in oocyte maturation in the rat. *35th Annual Meeting of the Society for Gynecologic Investigation* 1988;(abst 107).

The Physiology of Reproduction, Second Edition,
edited by E. Knobil and J.D. Neill,
Raven Press, Ltd., New York © 1994.

CHAPTER 16

Relaxin

O. David Sherwood

F. L. Hisaw's interest in modifications of the pelvic girdle that many mammalian species undergo to facilitate giving birth to their young led to the discovery of relaxin. In 1926, Hisaw reported that the injection of serum from pregnant guinea pigs or rabbits into virgin guinea pigs shortly after estrus promoted a noticeable relaxation of the pubic ligament (460). The following year, he found the relaxative substance in sow corpora lutea and rabbit placentas (461). In 1930, Hisaw and co-workers obtained a crude aqueous extract of the relaxative hormone from sow corpora lutea, and the hormone was named relaxin (321).

During the 1930s and most of the 1940s, there was little interest in relaxin. Not much progress was made toward the isolation of relaxin; the few efforts to purify the hormone were hindered by limitations associated with the techniques available for its isolation and bioassay. Then, from the late 1940s through the 1950s, research on relaxin surged. Although researchers used impure porcine relaxin, they made pioneering discoveries concerning the biologic effects of relaxin on the female reproductive tract of nonpregnant animals. Relaxin was found to promote elongation of the interpubic ligament in estrogen-primed mice (422,423), inhibit spontaneous contractions of the uterine myometrium in estrogen-primed guinea pigs (575), and promote cervical softening in estrogen-primed cattle (408). These biologic effects, which have since been confirmed with highly purified relaxin preparations, provided valuable insight into probable physiologic roles of relaxin during pregnancy and at parturition in several species.

Interest in relaxin lagged again during the 1960s and until the mid-1970s when investigators began to describe straightforward techniques for isolating relaxin preparations of well-documented high purity. Since 1974, highly purified relaxin has been obtained from the pig, rat, shark, skate, whale, porpoise, rabbit, horse, and dog; and

Department of Physiology and Biophysics, College of Medicine, University of Illinois, Urbana, IL 61801 the availability of highly purified hormone preparations has triggered a sustained resurgence of research on relaxin. Highly purified relaxin was used to (a) determine the primary structure of pig (porcine), rat, shark, skate, whale, porpoise, horse (equine), and dog (canine) relaxin; (b) develop specific and sensitive homologous radioimmunoassays for porcine, rat, and equine relaxin and then determine the levels of relaxin in the blood of these species; (c) identify the source(s) and target tissues for relaxin in several species; (d) determine the biologic actions of relaxin in the female of many species; (e) develop monoclonal antibodies specific for equine, porcine, and rat relaxin that were used to expedite the isolation of equine relaxin, identify bioactive domains on porcine relaxin, and determine the biologic effects of endogenous rat relaxin, respectively; (f) investigate the mechanism of relaxin's action on myometrial cells and endometrial cells; (g) demonstrate that relaxin is essential for normal delivery in pigs and rats; (h) explore the possibility that relaxin may have clinical use at birth in women; and (i) demonstrate that relaxin may have a physiologic role(s) in the male. Additionally, information obtained with highly purified relaxin preparations was used with recombinant DNA techniques to determine the putative primary structures of human, rhesus monkey, and guinea pig relaxin as well as precursor forms of porcine, rat, human, rhesus monkey, and guinea pig relaxin.

No other polypeptide hormone has been demonstrated to be as rich as relaxin in the diversity of both its chemistry and physiology among species. This diversity, which includes relaxin's structure, source, regulation of synthesis and secretion, secretory profile during pregnancy, and physiologic effects during pregnancy, has influenced the organization and emphasis of this review. The review begins with a rather detailed description of both the isolation and chemistry of relaxin for the following three reasons. First, only the use of highly purified relaxin preparations provides a sound basis for the study of the physiology of relaxin; therefore, the reader should know the species for which relaxin isolation procedures have been reported and the yields obtained when reported. Second, the reader needs a good understanding of the unprecedented diversity of the structure of relaxin among species to recognize the importance of using relaxin from homologous species for physiologic studies of relaxin wherever possible. Third, although superficial features of relaxin are similar to those of insulin, it is important to appreciate that there are marked differences in the amino acid sequences of these two hormones.

In view of the marked differences that exist among species, relaxin's sources, secretion, and physiologic effects on the pubic symphysis, cervix, and mammary glands are described for individual species. Relaxin has long been considered a hormone produced only in the female, but this does not appear to be the case. This review will conclude with findings indicating that relaxin is also produced in the male and may have functions that enhance fertilization. Throughout the review initial discoveries and early studies that made major contributions to an understanding of the chemistry and biology of relaxin are described; furthermore, other early studies that contributed to this understanding are cited to provide a comprehensive reference to the relaxin literature. Emphasis, however, is on advances made after 1974 with highly purified or synthetic preparations of relaxin. For additional descriptions of the isolation, chemistry, measurement, and physiology of relaxin, the reader is referred to other reviews (20,138,139,329,512,542,638, 782–784,878,886,906,907,913,915,916,1106–1108) and conference proceedings (32,94,144,971).

ISOLATION OF RELAXIN

Efforts to Isolate Relaxin Before 1974

In 1930, Fevold et al. (321) reported the first effort to isolate and characterize porcine relaxin. Corpora lutea from unselected sows were ground and extracted with hydrochloric acid (HCl) in alcohol, and the relaxin was enriched by pH adjustment and fractionations with alcohol, acetone, and ether. Although the hormone preparation was impure, these workers discovered that relaxin was probably a peptide: It was soluble in aqueous media, amphoteric, and inactivated by digestion with trypsin (320,321).

For nearly 50 years, essentially all efforts to isolate relaxin used ovaries from pregnant pigs, because this source has a high content of relaxin bioactivity (15) and is relatively easy to acquire in large quantities. Until the late 1950s, efforts to isolate relaxin were hindered by the limited techniques available for isolating proteins. Relaxin was generally separated from other proteins on the basis of differential solubility after changes in pH, concentrations of salt, or concentrations of organic solvents (1,15,349,352). These techniques were laborious, and researchers generally obtained only modest enrichment of relaxin with each purification step. A second main obstacle was the lack of physicochemical techniques for determining the degree of purity of protein preparations. Instead, investigators relied heavily on the specific biologic activity of relaxin preparations to assess their degree of purity. The first quantitative bioassay for relaxin used ovariectomized, estrogen-primed guinea pigs and defined a "guinea pig unit" (GPU) as the dose of relaxin required to induce unmistakable mobility of the pubic symphysis of two-thirds of a group of 12 animals (1). This guinea pig pubic symphysis palpation bioassay had limited use for determining potency estimates because it was cumbersome and based on the subjective and imprecise assessment of the degree of relaxin-induced mobility of the pubic symphysis.

During the late 1950s, investigators developed improved quantitative bioassays for relaxin. In 1959, Kroc et al. (579) described a bioassay based on the ability of relaxin to inhibit spontaneous contractions of the mouse uterus *in vitro.* In 1960, Steinetz et al. (952) developed an objective bioassay in which the interpubic ligament formed in estrogen-primed female mice in response to relaxin is transilluminated and precisely measured with a dissecting microscope fitted with an ocular micrometer. Most efforts to isolate porcine relaxin after 1960 used one of these two mouse bioassays to locate relaxin-containing fractions and to determine the specific bioactivity of relaxin preparations.

Bioassay reference standards that made it possible to determine the relative potency (specific bioactivity) of relaxin preparations also became available during the 1950s. These standards included partially purified porcine relaxin preparations Warner-Lambert W1164-A lot 8 (150 GPU/mg), Warner-Lambert W1164, 48E-2103a (1,000 GPU/mg), and NIH-R-P1 (440 GPU/mg). These porcine relaxin reference standards enabled researchers to assess progress toward the isolation of porcine relaxin more reliably and to compare the biologic effects of impure relaxin preparations among laboratories.

During the 1960s, the laboratories of Frieden (346,357), Cohen (209), and Griss (413) used new protein isolation techniques such as countercurrent distribution, gel filtration, and ion-exchange chromatography to obtain preparations of porcine relaxin that contained high specific biologic activity. Although they did not precisely describe the physicochemical properties of their preparations, they determined correctly that porcine relaxin is a protein with a molecular weight between 4,000 and 10,000 (209,357,413), has a basic isoelectric point (209,413), and contains disulfide bonds essential for biologic activity (209,351).

Isolation of Relaxin Since 1974

Between 1974 and 1992, highly purified relaxin was isolated from the ovaries or corpora lutea of pregnant pigs, rats, sharks, skates, whales, porpoises, and humans; from the placentas of rabbits, horses, and dogs; and from the seminal plasma of humans.

Similarities exist in the procedures developed to isolate relaxin from these species. For extraction, nearly all the isolation procedures take advantage of relaxin's stability in acidic solvents, and most also use its solubility in 60% to 70% acetone. After extraction, relaxin is generally purified by a combination of gel filtration, ion-exchange chromatography, and in some cases, high-performance liquid chromatography (HPLC) and/or immunoaffinity chromatography. The mouse interpubic ligament bioassay (952) and *in vitro* mouse uterus bioassay (579) were used to locate relaxin bioactivity during the development of isolation procedures, but in some cases problems were encountered with the latter bioassay. The *in vitro* mouse uterus bioassay could not be used in the early stages of the isolation of relaxin from cow corpora lutea (323,324,330), rabbit placentas (335), or human placentas (330,331). This was because a small uterine "contraction factor" (thought to be oxytocin), which overrode relaxin's quiescent effect on uterine contractility, was present in the tissue extracts (330,331,335).

Yields of relaxin per kilogram equivalent of tissue source differ greatly among species. The concentrations of relaxin in pig and rat corpora lutea are much higher than they are in tissue sources in other species from which relaxin has been isolated. Therefore, with nearly all species, investigators developed isolation procedures applicable to kilogram quantities of the tissue source to obtain sufficient relaxin for chemical and/or physiologic studies. Physicochemical and biologic characterization studies of highly purified relaxin preparations not only revealed that superficial features of relaxin, such as its size and two-chain composition, are similar among species but also provided early indications that the primary structure of relaxin differed markedly among species. Distinct variation was found in the isoelectric points, amino acid contents, and specific bioactivities of relaxin preparations from different species.

This section describes nearly in the order of their publication the isolation and characterization of highly purified relaxin from the pig, rat, shark, rabbit, horse, skate, whale, dog, and human. A great majority of the recent research on the physiology of relaxin was conducted with highly purified pig, rat, and horse relaxin. Accordingly, the isolation and characterization of relaxin from these three species are described in sufficient detail to provide a good understanding of the nomenclatures and characteristics of these hormone preparations. A summary of yields, physicochemical characteristics, and biologic characteristics of highly purified relaxin preparations is given in Table 1. This section also contains a description of the partial purification of relaxin from the cow.

Isolation of Porcine Relaxin

In 1974, Sherwood and O'Byrne (924) described a procedure for isolating relaxin in high yields from the domestic pig (*Sus scrofa*). They extracted relaxin from 1 kg of frozen ovaries obtained from sows containing fetuses with a crown–rump length of 10 cm or greater with an acid–acetone method (0.15 N HCl, 70% acetone) patented in 1963 by Doczi (263). After gel filtration of the extract on Sephadex G-50 (Pharmacia, Piscataway, NJ), relaxin bioactivity was adsorbed to carboxymethyl cellu-

TABLE 1. *Summary of characteristics of highly purified relaxin preparations*

Species (source)	Preparation	Yield (mg/kg fresh tissue)	Molecular weight	Isoelectric point	Bioactivity (GPU/mg)	Reference
Pig (ovaries)	CMB	38	6,300	10.6	2,500–3,000[a]	924
	CMa	34	6,300	10.7		
	CMa′	36	6,300	10.8		
Rat (ovaries)	CM1	140	6,000	7.6	CM1 equivalent to CM2[a] and less than pig relaxin	905
	CM2	140	6,000	9.4		
Sand Tiger Shark (ovaries)		2–5	6,000	—	Not detected[a,b] and less than pig relaxin[c]	815
Spiny Dogfish Shark (ovaries)		3.5	6,000	—	Less than pig relaxin[a,c]	148
Skate (ovaries)	I	1	6,800	—	Less than pig relaxin[a,b]	157
	II	3.3	7,500			
Bryde's Whale (corpora lutea)					Equivalent to pig relaxin[a]	879
Minke Whale (corpora lutea)					Equivalent to pig relaxin[a]	879
Porpoise (corpora lutea)		—	6,050	—	—	1139
Rabbit (placenta)		12	7,200	6.8	23[b]	295
Horse (placenta)	R1	1.5	5,600	—	28[a]	982
	R2	0.2				
	R3	0.4				
	Four major isoforms AP-R-1,2,3,4	—	5,200–5,600	—	Less than pig relaxin[a]	981
Dog (placenta)	R2	—	6,800	—	—	979

[a] Mouse interpubic ligament bioassay (952).
[b] *In vitro* mouse uterus bioassay (317, 579, 591).
[c] Guinea pig pubic symphysis palpation bioassay and *in vitro* guinea pig uterus bioassay (951).

lose (CMC) and then eluted as three contiguous peaks designated CMB, CMa, and CMa′ by the addition of a linear salt gradient (Fig. 1A). The yields of each of the three relaxin preparations were about 35 mg/kg equivalent of ovarian tissue (924), and limited evidence indicated they may be increased by adding protease inhibitors to the extraction solvent (583). Characterization studies demonstrated that the three porcine relaxin preparations were essentially homogeneous and that their structures were nearly identical (i.e., they were microheterogeneous) (924). The specific bioactivities of CMB, CMa, and CMa′ were high and equipotent: They ranged from 2,500 to 3,000 GPU/mg when compared with Warner-Lambert Porcine Relaxin Reference Standard W1164, 48E-2103a (1,000 GPU/mg) in the mouse interpubic ligament bioassay. The amino acid compositions of CMB, CMa, and CMa′ were also in close agreement, and they contained no histidine, proline, or tyrosine. Sedimentation equilibrium analysis indicated that the molecular weights of the three relaxin preparations were about 6,000, and gel filtration of reduced and carboxymethylated CMB, CMa, and CMa′ showed they consisted of two chains of similar size (designated A and B) linked by disulfide bonds. The three porcine relaxin preparations had high isoelectric points, ranging from pH 10.6 to pH 10.8.

Additional procedures for isolating highly purified porcine relaxin have been described since 1974. Schwabe et al. (886) described a procedure for large-scale preparation of porcine relaxin that involved acid–acetone extraction of pig ovaries according to Doczi (263), followed by ion-exchange chromatography on CMC and gel filtration on Sephadex G-50. Frieden et al. (355,356) further purified a crude preparation of porcine relaxin (NIH-R-P1; 440 GPU/mg) by means of gel filtration on Bio-Gel P-10 (Bio-Rad Laboratories, Richmond, CA), followed by column electrophoresis on Sephadex G-25 (Pharmacia, Piscataway, NJ) to obtain three microheterogeneous preparations of porcine relaxin designated A, B, and C. Frieden et al. (354) later isolated porcine relaxin from pig ovaries according to a procedure nearly identical to that of Sherwood and O'Byrne (924) and discovered two additional relaxin preparations (designated C_1 and C_2) that eluted from the CMC ion exchange column before the three preparations CMB, CMa, and CMa′ shown in Fig. 1A.

A multiplicity of porcine relaxin components was observed by several workers when ovarian extracts were

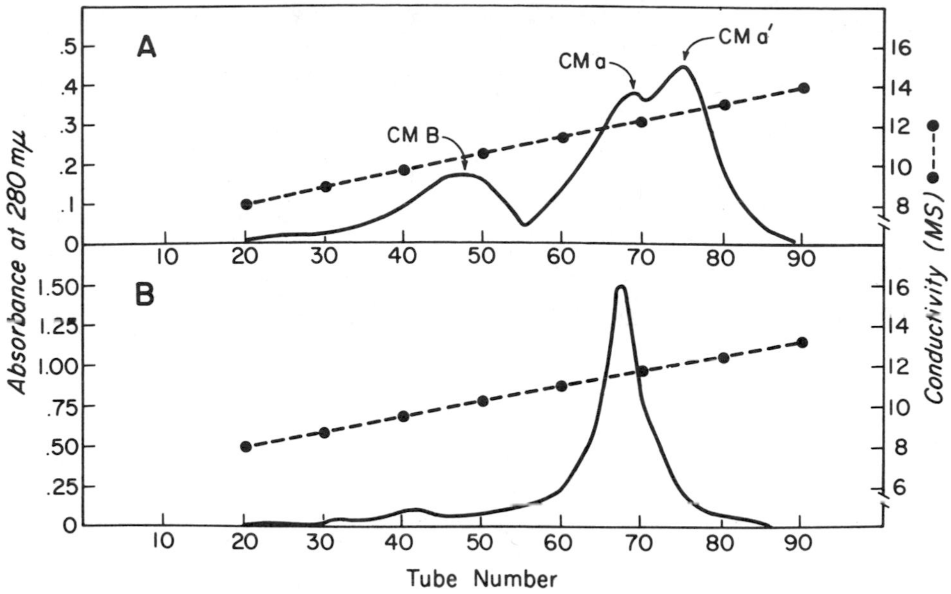

FIG. 1. Ion exchange chromatography of porcine relaxin on carboxymethyl cellulose. **A:** With the isolation procedure of Sherwood and O'Byrne (924), relaxin activity elutes in three contiguous preparations designated CMB, CMa, and CMa′ when a linear gradient of sodium chloride in equilibrating buffer is applied to the column. **B:** With the isolation procedure of Walsh and Niall (1093), nearly all relaxin activity elutes in one main component, which corresponds to CMa, when a linear gradient of ammonium acetate in equilibrating buffer is applied to the column. From ref. 1093, with permission.

subjected to countercurrent distribution (357), electrophoresis (209,346,356,590,737), or ion-exchange chromatography (149,150,354,886,924). This multiplicity was once thought attributable to the expression of more than one relaxin gene, but this is not the case. Complete amino acid sequence analysis of porcine relaxin preparations CMB, CMa, and CMa′ obtained by the isolation procedure of Sherwood and O'Byrne (924) demonstrated that the microheterogeneity among these three preparations was attributable to slight differences in the length of their B-chain C termini (701) (Fig. 2). Likewise, porcine relaxin components C_1 and C_2, identified by Frieden et al. (354) were found to be structurally identical to preparation CMB, except for the absence of two and three amino acid residues, respectively, on the C terminus of the B chain and arginine on the N terminus of the A chain. Walsh and Niall (1093) postulated that the differences in lengths of the B-chain C termini were attributable to limited proteolysis of a major stored form of porcine relaxin during its isolation. By modifying an extraction procedure applicable to small, acid-resistant peptides (84), Walsh and Niall nearly eliminated the multiplicity of forms of porcine relaxin (1093). Frozen ovaries were homogenized in a strongly acidic solvent (15% trifluoroacetic acid, 5% formic acid, 1% NaCl, 1 N HCl), and after adsorption to and elution from small octadecylsilica columns, the relaxin-containing fraction was further purified by gel filtration on Sephadex G-50 and ion-exchange chromatography on CMC. Nearly all the porcine relaxin eluted from the ion-exchange column as a single peak, that corresponded to peak CMa (Fig. 1B). It was postulated that the strongly acidic medium minimizes proteolysis both by the low pH *per se* and by precipitating high-molecular-weight proteases (84). Although Walsh and Niall's procedure (1093) has the apparent advantage of reducing the multiplicity of forms of porcine relaxin, it is not easily applied to the isolation of relaxin from kilogram batches of pig ovaries. There is reason to suspect that porcine relaxin is not normally processed to a major stored form within the corpora lutea. Büllesbach and Schwabe (150) used an isolation procedure that involved acid-acetone extraction, ion-exchange chromatography, gel filtration, and HPLC to obtain multiple fractions of porcine relaxin, and each fraction comprised a large portion of the porcine relaxin recovered. These fractions included not only CMa and CMa′ obtained by Sherwood and O'Byrne (924) but also forms with B chains (Leu^{B29}, Fig. 2) and/or A chains (Leu^{A-4}-Phe^{A-3}, Fig. 2) longer than the major form of porcine relaxin reported by Walsh and Niall (1093). Büllesbach and Schwabe (150) concluded that *in vivo* conversion of porcine prorelaxin to relaxin may be much less stringently controlled than the conversion of other prohormones to active hormones. Nearly all studies conducted with highly purified porcine relaxin used relaxin obtained by the procedures of Sherwood and O'Byrne (924) or Büllesbach and Schwabe (150) or modifications of those procedures.

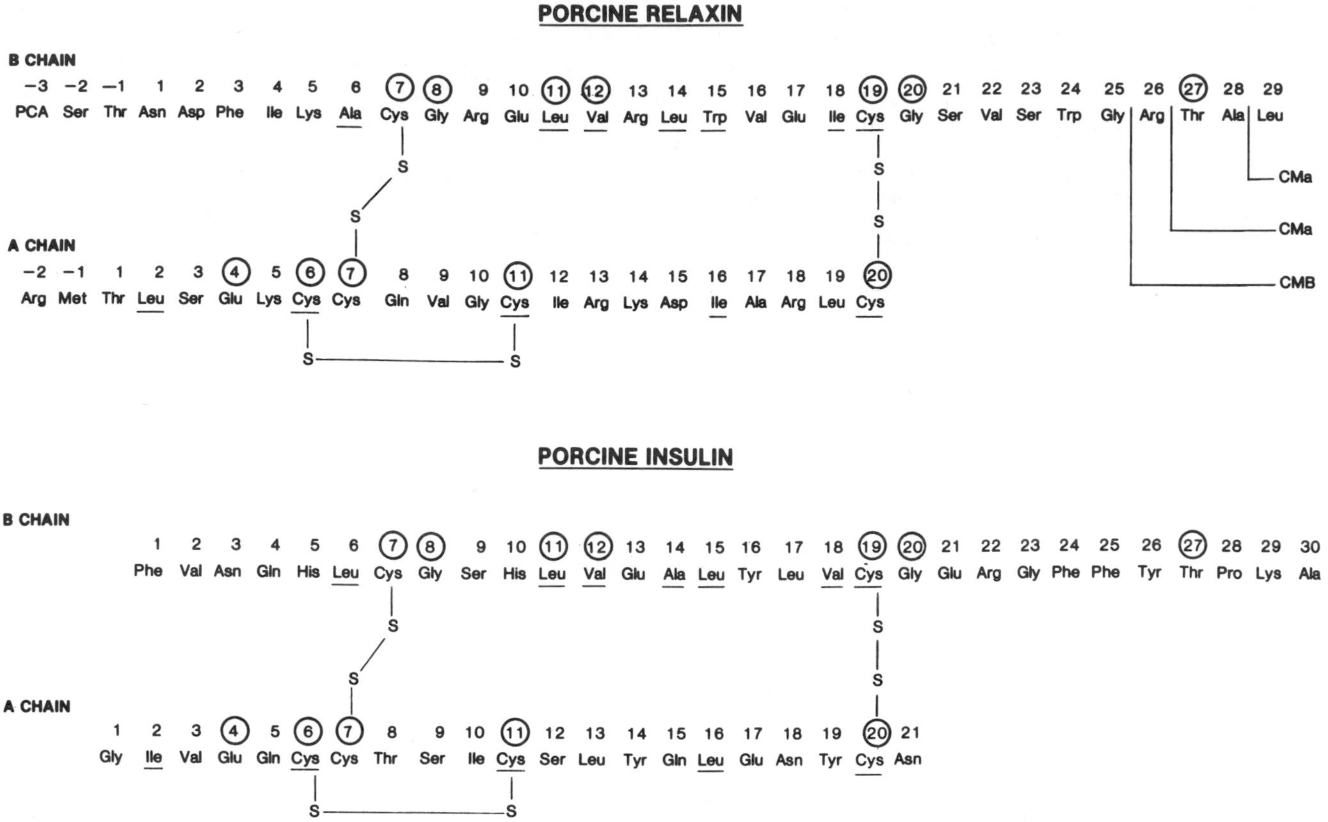

FIG. 2. Covalent structure of porcine relaxin (508,883–885) and porcine insulin (130). In this figure, residues are numbered with respect to the insulin sequence to facilitate comparison of the two hormones. CMB, CMa, and CMa′ forms of porcine relaxin shown in Fig. 1A (924) are attributable to small differences in the lengths of their B chains as shown with vertical lines (701). CMB, CMa, and CMa′ forms of porcine relaxin are sometimes designated B28, B31, and B29 porcine relaxin, respectively, to denote the numbers of amino acids in their B chains. The numbers of the residues that are identical in relaxin and insulin are circled. Residues that contribute to the hydrophobic core of insulin and those in comparable positions in relaxin are underlined (72,73).

Isolation of Rat Relaxin

In 1979, Sherwood described a method for the isolation of relaxin from the rat (*Rattus norvegicus*) (905). Approximately 3 g of frozen ovaries collected from 25 rats on day 20 of gestation, when ovarian relaxin levels are maximal (906), were extracted with phosphate-buffered saline. After gel filtration of the extract on Sephadex G-50, the relaxin bioactivity was adsorbed to CMC and then eluted as two preparations, designated CM1 and CM2, by the addition of a linear NaCl gradient. The yields of both CM1 and CM2 were about 140 mg/kg equivalent of ovarian tissue; therefore, the combined yield of rat relaxin was about 280 mg/kg equivalent of ovarian tissue. Characterization studies indicated that the two rat relaxin preparations were nearly homogeneous and microheterogeneous. No difference in biologic activity between CM1 and CM2 was found with the mouse interpubic ligament bioassay, and the amino acid compositions of the two preparations were similar. Superficial structural features of rat relaxin were similar to those of porcine relaxin. Sedimentation equilibrium analysis indicated the molecular weights of CM1 and CM2 to be about 6,000, and slab gel electrophoresis of reduced rat relaxin showed that it consisted of two chains of similar size linked by disulfide bonds. Other analyses, however, demonstrated differences between rat relaxin and porcine relaxin. Rat relaxin was much less bioactive, and its dose-response curve differed from that obtained with porcine relaxin in the mouse interpubic ligament bioassay (119,905). The amino acid composition of rat relaxin differed distinctly from that of porcine relaxin, and the isoelectric points of CM1 and CM2, pH 7.6 and 9.4, respectively, were lower than those of porcine relaxin preparations CMB, CMa, and CMa′.

The multiplicity of forms of rat relaxin appears to be attributable to limited proteolysis of a major stored form during the isolation procedure. Walsh and Niall (1093) found that when ovaries obtained from pregnant rats were quickly frozen, extracted in strongly acidic solvent, enriched by adsorption to octadecylsilica, and then further purified as described above for porcine relaxin, nearly all the rat relaxin eluted from the CMC as a single component. The yields of rat relaxin obtained with the isolation procedures of Sherwood (905) and Walsh and Niall (1093) are similar. In Sherwood's laboratory, the mean yields of relaxin obtained from ovaries collected on day 20 of gestation were 240 mg/kg equivalent of ovarian tissue ($N = 6$; O. D. Sherwood, *unpublished data*) with the isolation procedure of Walsh and Niall (1093) and 280 mg/kg equivalent of ovarian tissue with the procedure of Sherwood (905). In view of the minimal microheterogeneity associated with relaxin obtained by the procedure of Walsh and Niall (1093), it is the method of choice for the isolation of rat relaxin.

Isolation of Sand Tiger Shark Relaxin

Interest in the evolutionary origin of relaxin provided the motivation for its isolation from an ancient species —the shark. In 1981, Reinig et al. (815) isolated relaxin from the sand tiger shark (*Odontaspis taurus*). Ovaries obtained from pregnant sand tiger sharks were extracted with acid-70% acetone. The extract was further purified by gel filtration on Sephadex G-75, ion-exchange chromatography on CMC, and HPLC on octadecylsilica. The yield of highly purified sand tiger shark relaxin was low, 2 to 5 mg/kg equivalent of ovaries, but sufficient for chemical and biologic characterization. Gel filtration indicated the molecular weight of sand tiger shark relaxin to be about 6,000, and HPLC of the reduced shark relaxin showed that it consisted of two chains linked by disulfide bonds. The bioactivity of the sand tiger shark relaxin differed strikingly from that of porcine relaxin in both the guinea pig and the mouse. In guinea pigs, the sand tiger shark relaxin was only about 4% as bioactive as porcine relaxin in the pubic symphysis palpation bioassay, and it was also less effective than porcine relaxin in inhibiting the frequency of contractions of uterine segments. Sand tiger shark relaxin was even less active in the mouse, because high doses failed to either induce growth of the interpubic ligament or inhibit myometrial contractility. The amino acid composition of sand tiger shark relaxin differed distinctly from that of porcine and rat relaxin (815).

Isolation of Dogfish Shark Relaxin

In 1986, Büllesbach et al. (148) isolated relaxin from the dogfish shark (*Squalus acanthias*). Ovaries obtained from pregnant dogfish sharks were extracted with acid-70% acetone, and the extract was further purified by ion-exchange chromatography on CMC and gel filtration on Sephadex G-50. The yield of highly purified dogfish shark relaxin was 3.5 mg/kg equivalent of ovaries, and the molecular weight of dogfish shark relaxin was determined to be about 6,000 by gel filtration chromatography. Dogfish shark relaxin demonstrated activity in the guinea pig pubic symphysis palpation bioassay. Whereas dogfish shark relaxin promoted dose-dependent growth of the interpubic ligament in mice, it required approximately 1,000-fold more shark relaxin than porcine relaxin to induce this bioactivity.

Isolation of Rabbit Relaxin

In 1985, Eldridge and Fields (295) isolated relaxin from the domestic rabbit (*Oryctolagus cuniculus*). Placentas obtained from rabbits in unknown stages of pregnancy were extracted with a modified acid-acetone extraction medium (413) consisting of acetone:H_2O:HCl (5:2.83:0.17, v,v,v) plus protease inhibitors. The extract was further purified by gel filtration on Sephadex G-50, ion-exchange chromatography on CMC, and gel filtration on Sepharose CL-4B (Pharmacia, Piscataway, NJ). The yield of highly purified rabbit relaxin was about 12 mg/kg equivalent of placentas. Slab gel electrophoresis of unreduced and reduced relaxin indicated that the molecular weight of rabbit relaxin was about 7,200 and that it consisted of two chains of similar size linked by disulfide bonds. Rabbit relaxin was much less active than porcine relaxin in the *in vitro* mouse uterus bioassay—23 GPU/mg for rabbit relaxin compared with 2,500 to 3,000 GPU/mg for highly purified porcine relaxin. The isoelectric point of rabbit relaxin, pH 6.8, was lower than those of porcine and rat relaxin. The amino acid composition of rabbit relaxin was not reported.

Isolation of Equine Relaxin

In 1986, Stewart and Papkoff (982) isolated relaxin from the domestic horse (*Equus caballus*). Relaxin was extracted from placentas obtained at term with 0.5 N HCl-85% acetone, and the extract was further purified by stepwise elution from a CMC column, followed by gel filtration on Sephadex G-50. Relaxin in the fraction obtained from the Sephadex G-50 column was precipitated with 5% trichloroacetic acid, adsorbed to CMC, and then eluted in one major peak (designated R1) and two minor peaks (designated R2 and R3) with the addition of a linear NaCl gradient. The yield of the predominant equine relaxin preparation R1 was only about 1.5 mg/kg equivalent of placentas, but it was sufficient for characterization studies. Slab gel electrophoresis of unreduced and reduced R1 indicated that its molecular weight was about 6,000 and that it consisted of two chains of similar size linked by disulfide bonds. The specific bioactivity of R1 as determined in the mouse interpubic ligament bioassay was far lower than that of porcine relaxin—only 28 GPU/mg. The amino acid composition of equine relaxin differed from that of porcine, rat, and shark relaxin; it lacked phenylalanine and methionine.

Stewart et al. (981) generated a monoclonal antibody (5F-7A) against equine relaxin preparation R1. The monoclonal antibody was coupled to Sepharose 4B (Pharmacia, Piscataway, NJ) to form an affinity column that was used for rapid and efficient isolation of equine relaxin. In brief, acid-acetone extract of equine placentas was passed through the affinity column, and after unadsorbed proteins passed through the column, relaxin was eluted by a reduction in pH. Four major and two minor isoforms of equine relaxin were obtained by HPLC on octadecylsilica. Mass spectrometry indicated that the molecular weights of the isoforms ranged from 5,170 to 5,570, and the five most predominant isoforms displayed biologic activity in the mouse interpubic ligament bioassay. Sequence analysis demonstrated that the isoforms of equine relaxin are attributable to heterogeneity of the C termini of the B chains, and two of the isoforms (AP-R-1 and AP-R-4) were used to determine the amino acid sequence of horse relaxin.

Isolation of Skate Relaxin

In 1987, Büllesbach et al. (157) isolated relaxin from the skate (*Raja erinacea*). They extracted relaxin from 2 kg of frozen ovaries with the acid-acetone method of Doczi (263) and then further purified it by ion-exchange chromatography on CMC, followed by gel filtration on Sephadex G-50. Relaxin within the fraction obtained from Sephadex G-50 gave rise to two peaks designated relaxin I and relaxin II when subjected to HPLC on octadecylsilica. The yields of relaxin I and relaxin II were 1 mg and 3.3 mg/kg equivalent of ovaries, respectively. Amino acid composition of relaxin I and relaxin II indicated that their molecular weights were 6,800 and 7,500, respectively. The skate relaxin preparations demonstrated relaxin bioactivity in both the mouse interpubic ligament bioassay and *in vitro* mouse uterus bioassay. Büllesbach et al. (157) determined the amino acid sequence of the predominant skate relaxin II preparation.

Isolation of Whale Relaxin

In 1989, Schwabe et al. (879) isolated relaxin from the minke whale (*Balaenoptera acutorostrata*) and Bryde's whale (*Balaenoptera edeni*). Ground lyophilized powders of corpora lutea from the two species were extracted with 0.15 M HCl-85% acetone, and the extracts were further purified by ion-exchange chromatography on CMC, gel filtration on Sephadex G-50, and HPLC on octadecylsilica. The bioactivity of both whale relaxins reportedly did not differ from that of porcine relaxin in the mouse interpubic ligament bioassay. Schwabe et al. (879) found the amino acid contents of both whale relaxins to be almost identical to that of porcine relaxin, one exception being that whale relaxin lacked phenylalanine.

Isolation of Canine Relaxin

In 1992, Stewart et al. (979) isolated relaxin from the domestic dog (*Canis familiaris*). Term placentas and placentas obtained at spay were extracted with 15% trifluoroacetic acid, 5% formic acid, 1% NaCl, and 1 N HCl, as described by Walsh and Niall (1093). The extract was enriched by adsorption to octadecylsilica, eluted with 80% acetonitrile-0.1% trifluoroacetic acid, and dried. This enriched extract was further purified by stepwise elution from a CMC column, followed by gel filtration on Sephadex G-50. Relaxin obtained from the Sephadex G-50 column was adsorbed to CMC and then eluted in one minor peak (designated R1) and a major peak (designated R2) with the addition of a linear gradient of ammonium acetate. Slab gel electrophoresis of unreduced and reduced R2 indicated that its molecular weight was somewhat greater than porcine relaxin and that it consisted of two chains linked by disulfide bonds. Mass spectral analysis indicated that the molecular weight of canine relaxin R2 was 6,800.

Isolation of Human Relaxin

Four source tissues were used over several years in efforts to isolate relaxin from the human (*Homo sapiens*). Attempts were made during the early to mid-1980s to purify relaxin from human corpora lutea (725), placentas (294,305,306,308,334,1142), decidua (92, 96,97), and seminal plasma (1109). Although none of the human relaxin preparations were demonstrated to be highly purified, they displayed characteristics similar to those of porcine relaxin. Preparations from these tissues had molecular weights of about 6,000 (97,294,306,334, 725,1142); demonstrated activity in the guinea pig pubic symphysis palpation bioassay (721), mouse interpubic ligament bioassay (92,96,305,306,334), and/or rat uterine contractility bioassay (1109); and displayed immunologic cross-reactivity with antisera to highly purified porcine relaxin (97,306,334,721,725,1109,1142). Isolation and characterization of human relaxin did not occur until the late 1980s and early 1990s for three reasons. First, the quantities of relaxin in the corpus luteum of pregnancy, the richest source of relaxin in women, are low compared with those in the corpora lutea of pregnant pigs or rats during late pregnancy (721,725,1001,1067). Second, human corpora lutea of pregnancy are not readily available. Finally, the techniques generally available during most of the 1980s were not well suited for the isolation and characterization of extremely small quantities of protein.

In the late 1980s, Drolet et al. (278) and Winslow et al. (1132) isolated nanogram quantities of human relaxin from corpora lutea surgically removed from women with ectopic pregnancies. Relaxin was extracted from the corpora lutea with HCl-acetone containing protease inhibitors and the initial purification step was gel filtration on Bio Gel P-10. These workers (278,1132) then took advantage of the knowledge of the predicted amino acid sequence of human relaxin that was determined earlier by nucleotide sequence analysis (488,489): They conducted immunoaffinity chromatography of the Bio Gel P-10 preparation with a monoclonal antibody developed with chemically synthesized relaxin as immunogen. Reverse-phase HPLC on butyl silica was used as the last step in the isolation of relaxin from the human corpora lutea. In 1992, Winslow et al. (1131) isolated nanogram quantities of human relaxin from seminal plasma. Initially, 9 L of pooled seminal plasma were extracted with acid-acetone and hexane, subjected to two cycles of HPLC with octadecylsilica, and chromatographed on CM-Fractogel TSK (Merck, Rahway, NJ) by Weiss et al. (1109). This partially purified human relaxin preparation was then further purified (1131) by immunoaffinity chromatography using a monoclonal antibody to human relaxin followed by reverse-phase HPLC employing SynChropak C-4 (SynChrom Inc., Lafayette, IN). Yields of human luteal and seminal relaxin were sufficient for amino acid sequence analysis.

Isolation of Porpoise Relaxin

In 1991, Woods et al. (1139) reported that relaxin was extracted from the corpus luteum of the porpoise (*Phocaena phocaena*) with the acid-acetone method of Doczi (263) and isolated by reverse-phase HPLC. Details of the isolation procedure were not reported. The molecular weight of porpoise relaxin calculated from the amino acid composition was 6,060.

Purification of Bovine Relaxin

Relaxin has been purified from the domestic cow (*Bos taurus*). Fields et al. (323–326) extracted relaxin from cow ovaries obtained during late pregnancy with a modified acid-acetone extraction medium (413) consisting of a 3:5 volume ratio of 0.7 N HCl:acetone. When the extract was further purified by gel filtration on Sephadex G-50, three fractions that inhibited spontaneous contractions of the mouse uterus were eluted from the column. These fractions had molecular weights of 8,000, 6,000, and 1,400. The specific bioactivity of the 6,000-Da fraction determined with the mouse interpubic ligament bioassay was 71 GPU/mg, which is far lower than that of porcine relaxin. Electrofocusing of the 6,000-Da fraction demonstrated that it contained three basic forms that inhibited contractions of the mouse uterus and were immunologically cross-reactive with an antiserum to highly purified porcine relaxin (590). The chemical natures of the 8,000- and 1,400-Da fractions remain largely unexplained. The curiously small 1,400-Da fraction showed immunologic cross-reactivity with an antiserum to highly purified porcine relaxin and reportedly promoted growth of the mouse interpubic ligament (325). It was suggested that the 8,000- and 1,400-Da molecules may be partially degraded forms of prorelaxin or 6,000-Da relaxin, respectively; alternatively, they may be different gene products and members of a family of relaxinlike peptides (326,327). The yield of relaxin from cow ovaries was low, and the degree of purity of the bovine relaxin preparations was not described. Bovine relaxin remains largely uncharacterized.

CHEMISTRY OF RELAXIN

Covalent Structure of Relaxin

Investigators originally determined the amino acid sequences of the A and B chains of porcine, rat, shark, skate, whale, horse, dog, and porpoise relaxin by peptide sequence analysis of native hormone preparations (148,157,406,508,516,874,879,883–885,979,981,1139). Nucleotide sequence analysis not only confirmed the amino acid sequences of porcine and rat relaxin (417,418,487) but also predicted the amino acid sequences of two forms of human relaxin designated human relaxin 1 and human relaxin 2 (488,489) and single forms of both rhesus monkey (*Macaca mullata*) (218) and guinea pig (*Cavia porcellus*) relaxin (605) (Fig. 3). Human relaxin 2 is the main form, and perhaps the only form, of bioactive relaxin expressed in the human female and male. Conventional amino acid sequencing of the B chain of relaxin obtained from human corpora lutea (1001,1067,1132) and seminal plasma (1131) were in agreement with the predicted sequence of human relaxin 2. Fast-atom bombardment mass spectrometry indicated that the A chains of both relaxin preparations had the predicted 24 amino acids, whereas the B chain of luteal relaxin and seminal relaxin contained only 29 (B29) and 26 or 27 amino acids (B26-27), respectively (1131,1132). Throughout the remainder of this review where distinctions between the two forms of human relaxin 2 are made, the predicted form of human relaxin 2 shown in Fig. 3, which contains 33 amino acids in the B chain, will be designated human relaxin 2 (B33). The native form of human relaxin 2 isolated from the corpora lutea of pregnancy, which is devoid of Lys-Arg-Ser-Leu on the C terminus of its B chain (Fig. 3), will be designated human relaxin 2 (B29).

Locations of disulfide bonds (Fig. 2) were determined only for porcine relaxin (883) and human relaxin 2 (176,177). Nevertheless, it seems nearly certain that they are similar in other species, because in all species in which the amino acid sequences of relaxin are known, the half-cystine residues are found in positions comparable with those in porcine and human relaxin (Fig. 3).

Relaxin B Chains

	-7	-6	-5	-4	-3	-2	-1	1	2	3	4	(5)	6	7	8	(9)	10	11	12	(13)	14
Pig					PCA	Ser	Thr	Asn	Asp	Phe	Ile	Lys	Ala	Cys	Gly	Arg	Glu	Leu	Val	Arg	Leu
Rat	Arg	Val	Ser	Glu	Glu	Trp	Met	Asp	Gln	Val	Ile	Gln	Val	Cys	Gly	Arg	Gly	Tyr	Ala	Arg	Ala
Human 1					Lys	Trp	Lys	Asp	Asp	Val	Ile	Lys	Leu	Cys	Gly	Arg	Glu	Leu	Val	Arg	Ala
Human 2				Asp	Ser	Trp	Met	Glu	Glu	Val	Ile	Lys	Leu	Cys	Gly	Arg	Glu	Leu	Val	Arg	Ala
Monkey$_{R}$					Lys	Trp	Met	Asp	Asp	Val	Ile	Lys	Ala	Cys	Gly	Arg	Glu	Leu	Val	Arg	Ala
Shark$_{ST}$		PCA	Ser	Leu	Ser	Asn	Ala	Gly	Ser	Gly	Ile	Lys	Leu	Cys	Gly	Arg	Gly	Phe	Ile	Arg	Ala
Shark$_{D}$		PCA	Ser	Phe	Lys	Asn	Ala	Glu	Pro	Gly	Ile	Lys	Leu	Cys	Gly	Arg	Glu	Phe	Ile	Arg	Ala
Skate				Arg	Pro	Asn	Trp	Glu	Glu	Arg	Ser	Arg	Leu	Cys	Gly	Arg	Asp	Leu	Ile	Arg	Ala
Whale$_{B}$					PCA	Ser	Thr	Asn	Asp	Leu	Ile	Lys	Ala	Cys	Gly	Arg	Glu	Leu	Val	Arg	Leu
Whale$_{m}$					PCA	Ser	Thr	Asn	Asp	Leu	Ile	Lys	Ala	Cys	Gly	Arg	Glu	Leu	Val	Arg	Leu
Horse					Gln	Lys	Pro	Asp	Asp	Val	Ile	Lys	Ala	Cys	Gly	Arg	Glu	Leu	Ala	Arg	Leu
Dog						Thr	Asp	Asp	Lys	Lys	Leu	Lys	Ala	Cys	Gly	Arg	Asp	Tyr	Val	Arg	Leu
Guinea pig					Gly	Phe	Leu	Asp	Lys	Val	Ile	Lys	Val	Cys	Gly	Arg	Asp	Leu	Val	Arg	Ile
Porpoise					PCA	Arg	Thr	Asn	Asp	Phe	Ile	Lys	Ala	Cys	Gly	Arg	Glu	Leu	Val	Arg	Leu

	15	16	17	18	19	20	21	22	23	24	25	26	27	28	29	30	31	32	33	34	35	36
Pig	Trp	Val	Glu	Ile	Cys	Gly	Ser	Val	Ser	Trp	Gly	Arg	Thr	Ala	Leu							
Rat	Trp	Ile	Glu	Val	Cys	Gly	Ala	Ser	Val	Gly	Arg	Leu	Ala	Leu								
Human 1	Gln	Ile	Ala	Ile	Cys	Gly	Met	Ser	Thr	Trp	Ser	Lys	Arg	Ser	Leu							
Human 2	Gln	Ile	Ala	Ile	Cys	Gly	Met	Ser	Thr	Trp	Ser	Lys	Arg	Ser	Leu							
Monkey$_{R}$	Gln	Ile	Ala	Ile	Cys	Gly	Lys	Ser	Thr	Leu	Gly											
Shark$_{ST}$	Ile	Ile	Phe	Ala	Cys	Gly	Gly	Ser	Arg													
Shark$_{D}$	Val	Ile	Tyr	Thr	Cys	Gly	Gly	Ser	Arg	Trp												
Skate	Phe	Ile	Tyr	Leu	Cys	Gly	Gly	Thr	Arg	Trp	Thr	Arg	Leu	Pro	Asn	Phe	Gly	Asn	Tyr	Pro	Ile	Met
Whale$_{B}$	Trp	Val	Glu	Ile	Cys	Gly	Ser	Val	Ser	Trp	Gly	Arg	Thr	Ala	Leu							
Whale$_{m}$	Trp	Val	Glu	Ile	Cys	Gly	Ser	Val	Arg	Trp	Gly	Gln	Ser	Ala	Leu							
Horse	Arg	Ile	Glu	Ile	Cys	Gly	Ser	Leu	Ser	Trp	Lys											
Dog	Gln	Ile	Glu	Val	Cys	Gly	Ser	Ser	Trp	Trp	Gly	Arg	Lys	Ala	Gly	Gln	Leu	Arg	Glu			
Guinea pig	Lys	Ile	Asp	Ile	Cys	Gly	Lys	Ile	Leu	Leu	Gly	Asp	Met	Thr	Thr	Gly						
Porpoise	Trp	Val	Glu	Ile	Cys	Gly	Ser	Val	Ser	Trp	Gly	Arg	Thr	Ala								

Relaxin A Chains

	-4	-3	-2	-1	1	2	3	4	(5)	6	7	8	9	10	11	12	(13)	(14)	15	16	17	18	19	20
Pig			Arg	Met	Thr	Leu	Ser	Glu	Lys	Cys	Cys	Gln	Val	Gly	Cys	Ile	Arg	Lys	Asp	Ile	Ala	Arg	Leu	Cys
Rat	PCA	Ser	Gly	Ala	Leu	Leu	Ser	Glu	Gln	Cys	Cys	His	Ile	Gly	Cys	Thr	Arg	Arg	Ser	Ile	Ala	Lys	Leu	Cys
Human 1	Arg	Pro	Tyr	Val	Ala	Leu	Phe	Glu	Lys	Cys	Cys	Leu	Ile	Gly	Cys	Thr	Lys	Arg	Ser	Leu	Ala	Lys	Tyr	Cys
Human 2	PCA	Leu	Tyr	Ser	Ala	Leu	Ala	Asn	Lys	Cys	Cys	His	Val	Gly	Cys	Thr	Lys	Arg	Ser	Leu	Ala	Arg	Phe	Cys
Monkey$_{R}$	Gln	Leu	Tyr	Met	Thr	Leu	Ser	Asn	Lys	Cys	Cys	His	Ile	Gly	Cys	Thr	Lys	Lys	Ser	Leu	Ala	Lys	Phe	Cys
Shark$_{ST}$	Ala	Thr	Ser	Pro	Ala	Met	Ser	Ile	Lys	Cys	Cys	Ile	Tyr	Gly	Cys	Thr	Lys	Lys	Asp	Ile	Ser	Val	Leu	Cys
Shark$_{D}$	Glu	Gly	Ser	Pro	Gly	Met	Ser	Ser	Lys	Cys	Cys	Thr	Tyr	Gly	Cys	Thr	Arg	Lys	Asp	Ile	Ser	Ile	Leu	Cys
Skate	Glu	Glu	Lys	Met	Gly	Phe	Ala	Lys	Lys	Cys	Cys	Ala	Ile	Gly	Cys	Ser	Thr	Glu	Asp	Phe	Arg	Met	Val	Cys
Whale$_{B}$			Agr	Met	Thr	Leu	Ser	Glu	Lys	Cys	Cys	Gln	Val	Gly	Cys	Ile	Arg	Lys	Asp	Ile	Ala	Arg	Leu	Cys
Whale$_{m}$			Agr	Met	Thr	Leu	Ser	Glu	Lys	Cys	Cys	Gln	Val	Gly	Cys	Ile	Arg	Lys	Asp	Ile	Ala	Arg	Leu	Cys
Horse					Gln	Leu	Ser	His	Lys	Cys	Cys	Tyr	Trp	Gly	Cys	Thr	Arg	Lys	Glu	Leu	Ala	Arg	Gln	Cys
Dog	Asp	Asn	Tyr	Ile	Lys	Met	Ser	Asp	Lys	Cys	Cys	Asn	Val	Gly	Cys	Thr	Arg	Arg	Glu	Leu	Ala	Ser	Arg	Cys
Guinea pig	Gln	Leu	Asp	Met	Thr	Val	Ser	Glu	Lys	Cys	Cys	Gln	Val	Gly	Cys	Thr	Arg	Arg	Phe	Ile	Ala	Asn	Ser	Cys
Porpoise			Arg	Met	Thr	Leu	Ser	Glu	Lys	Cys	Cys	Gln	Val	Gly	Cys	Ile	Arg	Lys	Asp	Ile	Ala	Arg	Leu	Cys

FIG. 3. Amino acid sequences of relaxin B and A chains for those relaxin molecules whose complete sequences have been reported. Porcine (508,884,885), rat (516), sand tiger shark (148,406,874), dogfish shark (148), skate (157), Bryde's whale and minke whale (879), horse (981), dog (979), and porpoise (1139) sequences were determined by amino acid sequence analysis. Human (488,489), rhesus monkey (218), and guinea pig (605) sequences were predicted from nucleotide sequence analysis. Residues are numbered with respect to insulin as in Fig. 2. Residues common to the 14 sequences are shaded, and those in positions comparable with those that contribute to the hydrophobic core of insulin (72,73) are underlined. Numbers of basic amino acid residues postulated to be involved with the binding of porcine relaxin to its receptors are circled (72,102,154,160,265). Prorelaxins may not be processed *in vivo* to the single putative forms shown in this figure. Residues on the B-chain C termini of porcine relaxin (150,701) and human relaxin 2 (1001,1067) preparations that have been isolated from corpora lutea are boxed.

The structure of relaxin has apparently diverged considerably among species during evolution. Generally, only 30% to 60% amino acid sequence identity exists between species (Table 2), and the invariant positions in relaxin from all species are largely confined to the half-cystine residues and adjacent glycine residues (Fig. 3). The nearly identical structures of porcine, whale, and porpoise relaxin are a notable exception. The extensive differences in amino acid residues that generally exist on the surfaces of relaxin from different species form a structural basis for the observations that relaxin preparations display among-species differences in biologic activities in relaxin bioassays (905), immunologic cross-reactivity in radioimmunoassays (911), and self-association properties (929).

Relaxin as a Member of the Insulin Family

Structures of Relaxin, Insulin, and Insulinlike Growth Factors

Porcine relaxin and insulin have strikingly similar superficial structural features (Fig. 2): Their A and B chains are of similar length and their disulfide bridges have the same disposition. Discovery of the comparable cystine pairings in these two hormones stimulated the view that

TABLE 2. *Comparison of relaxin among species*

Species	Pig	Rat	Human 1	Human 2	$Monkey_R$	$Shark_{ST}$	$Shark_D$	Skate	$Whale_B$	$Whale_m$	Horse	Dog	Guinea pig	Porpoise
Pig	—	42	44	44	54	40	45	31	92	98	62	49	50	98
Rat	22/53	—	49	44	52	40	39	25	40	40	46	41	42	40
Human 1	24/54	26/53	—	77	73	42	43	32	43	45	54	44	44	43
Human 2	24/54	24/54	43/56	—	75	44	42	35	45	45	52	44	45	43
$Monkey_R$	27/50	27/52	38/52	39/52	—	42	43	33	55	51	56	49	58	54
$Shark_{ST}$	19/48	21/53	21/50	22/50	21/50	—	70	39	42	40	39	37	36	41
$Shark_D$	22/49	21/54	22/51	22/52	22/51	37/53	—	48	48	46	45	40	37	45
Skate	17/54	14/56	18/56	20/57	17/52	20/51	25/52	—	32	32	31	27	28	40
$Whale_B$	49/53	21/52	23/53	24/53	27/49	20/47	23/48	17/53	—	94	62	47	51	91
$Whale_m$	52/53	21/52	24/53	24/53	27/53	19/47	22/48	17/53	50/53	—	66	49	55	96
Horse	30/48	22/48	26/48	25/48	27/48	18/46	21/47	15/48	29/47	31/47	—	55	48	64
Dog	26/53	22/54	24/55	24/55	25/51	18/49	20/50	16/59	25/53	26/53	26/47	—	45	50
Guinea pig	27/54	23/55	24/55	25/56	30/52	18/50	19/51	16/57	27/53	27/49	23/48	25/56	—	51
Porpoise	52/53	21/53	23/53	23/53	27/50	20/49	22/49	21/53	48/53	51/53	30/47	26/52	27/53	—

Ratios are the number of identical amino acids to the total number of amino acid positions shared by each pair of relaxin molecules (lower left). These values are also given as percentages (upper right).

relaxin might have a tertiary structure similar to that of insulin. X-ray crystallographic analysis of porcine 2-zinc insulin (101) and 4-zinc insulin crystals (85) showed that each crystalline form exists as two independent molecules, designated protomers I and II. All four protomers are compact globular structures with a hydrophobic core. With the exception of protomer I of 4-zinc insulin, each protomer involves right-handed α-helical segments A2-8, A13-19, and B9-19; extended regions B1-7 and B24-30; and turns hinging on glycines at B8, B20, and B23, as shown schematically for 2-zinc insulin I in Fig. 4A (104). The B-chain C-terminal extended region con-

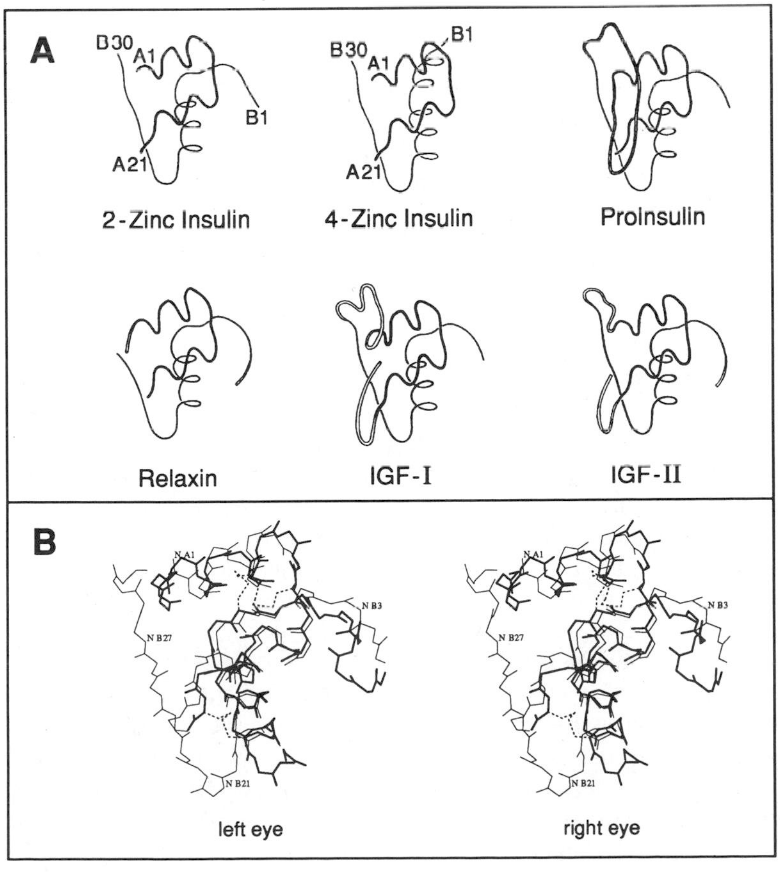

FIG. 4. A: Schematic representations of three-dimensional structures of protomer I forms of porcine insulin based on radiographic analysis of rhombohedral porcine 2-zinc insulin crystals (101) and 4-zinc insulin crystals (85). Proposed conformations of porcine proinsulin (937), porcine relaxin (73,498,499), and human IGF-I and IGF-II (100,103) were determined by model building. Modified from ref. 103. **B:** Stereo view of the radiographic crystal structure of human relaxin 2 (B29; protomer II) (*thick lines*) and 2-Zn porcine insulin (*thin lines*). Molecules in B are oriented approximately as those in A. Cystine residues are included for relaxin (*broken lines*). The relaxin sequence is four residues longer at the N terminus of both chains and five residues shorter at the B-chain C terminus. The C-terminal region of relaxin's B chain is coiled before becoming too disordered to be resolved in the electron density map, whereas insulin adopts a β-strand structure for the analogous sequence. From ref. 292, with permission.

tains a β turn (B20-23) and β strand (B24-28) (53,482). Protomer I of 4-zinc insulin is much like the other protomers except that the B-chain α-helix starts at residue 2 rather than at residue 9, as shown schematically for 4-zinc insulin (Fig. 4A), and it has a more open framework.

Although the extent of identity between porcine relaxin and porcine insulin is only 12 of 49 aligned amino acid residues, the common structural features shown in Fig. 2 permit porcine relaxin a theoretical three-dimensional conformation similar to either the 2-zinc or 4-zinc structure of insulin shown in Fig. 4A. Porcine relaxin has retained not only the six half-cystines but also the B8 and B20 glycines, which provide unique torsion angles for chain folding. Additionally, the residues corresponding to those packed into the hydrophobic core of insulin (indicated by underlining in Fig. 2) are nonpolar in porcine relaxin, with the exception of B15 tryptophan. Moreover, two pairs of these nonpolar residues, which would point toward the hydrophobic core from opposite sides in both insulin and relaxin (B6,B14 and A2,A16), have complementary changes in amino acid residues that enable maintenance of core volume (72,73, 104,499). Models of porcine relaxin obtained by model building (72,73,499) and interactive computer graphics (102,499,716) showed that all residues in the A chain and residues B6-20 in the B chain, including the burial of B15 tryptophan in the hydrophobic core, could be accommodated in a tertiary structure similar to that of 2-zinc insulin. Although the conformations of the N and C termini of porcine relaxin are presented schematically as being similar to those within 2-zinc insulin crystals as shown in Fig. 4A (99,100,103), they are not known.

The sequences of relaxin from species other than the pig (Fig. 3) provide supporting evidence for the similar folding of relaxin and insulin. The half-cystines involved in disulfide bridge formation and glycines at B8 and B20 needed for insulinlike chain folding are common to all relaxin molecules. Moreover, in most cases nonpolar residues are retained in positions comparable with those that contribute to the hydrophobic core of insulin.

There are indications that the hydrophobic core of relaxin in some species may be more open than that of 2-zinc insulin. First, predictions of protein structure on the basis of amino acid sequence indicate that the region of high probability of α-helix includes residues B9-16 in porcine, rat, and shark relaxin (102), and this region is shorter than the α-helical region in insulin, which extends from B9-19. Second, chymotrypsin produces cleavages in porcine relaxin at B15 tryptophan and B11 leucine, and this indicates that at least one of these core residues is sufficiently exposed to solvent to initiate a reaction with the proteolytic enzyme (109). Finally, the ring of B15 tryptophan in porcine relaxin, although in the hydrophobic core, is sufficiently exposed to form a charge transfer complex with the chemical probe *N*-methyl nicotinamide chloride (507). Dodson and co-workers (265) suggested that the relatively open hydrophobic core of porcine relaxin may indicate that it has a tertiary structure like the relatively open 4-zinc insulin protomer I, whereas Blundell and co-workers (102) suggested that the loosening of the core may derive from a degree of unwinding of the B-chain helix between B16-19 and between A17-20. Whereas computer-assisted model building indicated that shark relaxin residues can be accommodated in a tertiary structure similar to 2-zinc insulin (102,406), rat relaxin cannot because of close contacts produced by B6 valine, B11 tyrosine, and B15 tryptophan. Rat relaxin residues can be better accommodated in the more open framework of the 4-zinc insulin protomer I model (265) or the 2-zinc insulin model with limited unwinding of the B-chain helix between B16-19 and between A17-20 (102). Circular dichroic spectra of porcine, dogfish shark, sand tiger shark, and skate relaxin molecules in solution are similar to those of porcine insulin; thus, relaxin models based on insulin coordinates are realistic for these species (148,157,279,813,881).

The first direct analysis of the tertiary structure of relaxin was accomplished by Eigenbrot and co-workers in 1991 (292), and this work generally confirmed the predicted structural homology of relaxin to insulin. Crystals of synthetic human relaxin 2 (B29), which is the form isolated from human corpora lutea (1001,1067,1132), were grown in 150 mM NaCl, 10 mM citrate (pH 5.0), and 5 mg relaxin/ml by vapor diffusion. Radiographic structure analysis demonstrated that relaxin, like insulin, crystallizes in an asymmetric unit to form a dimer. Whereas the orientation of the two monomers in the relaxin dimer is completely different from the two monomers in the insulin dimer, the overall fold of relaxin is similar to that of insulin (Fig. 4B). Principal features of the molecule are a 24-residue A chain with two α-helices extending from A3-9 and from A13-20 and a 29-residue B chain containing one α-helix extending from B7-22. The relaxin model does not include the C terminus of the B chain, which appears to be disordered.

Insulinlike growth factor I (IGF-I) and IGF-II are single-chain polypeptides that have 70 and 67 amino acid residues, respectively, and structural features similar to those of insulin. The regions of structural similarity of IGF-I and IGF-II to insulin are confined to the B- and A-chain portions of the molecules where they are more homologous to insulin than relaxin is (Fig. 5). Models for IGF-I (100) and IGF-II (103) indicate that these two growth factors may have conformations similar to that of insulin (Fig. 4A). Considerable evidence indicates that the tertiary structure of relaxin differs from that of IGFs. Porcine relaxin failed to bind to IGF-I receptors on rat ovarian granulosa cells (9), IGF-I receptors on rat ovar-

B Chain

	-4	-3	-2	-1	1	2	3	4	5	6	7	8	9	10	11	12	13	14	15	16	17	18	19	20	21	22	23	24	25	26	27	28	29	30	31
Relaxin 1		Lys	Trp	Lys	Asp	Asp	Val	Ile	Lys	Leu	Cys	Gly	Arg	Glu	Leu	Val	Arg	Ala	Gln	Ile	Ala	Ile	Cys	Gly	Met	Ser	Thr	Trp	Ser	Lys	Arg	Ser	Leu		
Relaxin 2	Asp	Ser	Trp	Met	Glu	Glu	Val	Ile	Lys	Leu	Cys	Gly	Arg	Glu	Leu	Val	Arg	Ala	Gln	Ile	Ala	Ile	Cys	Gly	Met	Ser	Thr	Trp	Ser	Lys	Arg	Ser	Leu		
Insulin					Phe	Val	Asn	Gln	His	Leu	Cys	Gly	Ser	His	Leu	Val	Glu	Ala	Leu	Tyr	Leu	Val	Cys	Gly	Glu	Arg	Gly	Phe	Phe	Tyr	Thr	Pro	Lys	Thr	
IGF-I						Gly	Pro	Glu	Thr	Leu	Cys	Gly	Ala	Glu	Leu	Val	Asp	Ala	Leu	Gln	Phe	Val	Cys	Gly	Asp	Arg	Gly	Phe	Tyr	Phe	Asn	Lys	Pro	Thr...	
IGF-II			Ala	Tyr	Arg	Pro	Ser	Glu	Thr	Leu	Cys	Gly	Gly	Glu	Leu	Val	Asp	Thr	Leu	Gln	Phe	Val	Cys	Gly	Asp	Arg	Gly	Phe	Tyr	Phe	Ser	Arg	Pro	Ala...	

A Chain

	-4	-3	-2	-1	1	2	3	4	5	6	7	8	9	10	11	12	13	14	15	16	17	18	19	20	21	22	23	24	25	26	27	28	29
Relaxin 1	Arg	Pro	Tyr	Val	Ala	Leu	Phe	Glu	Lys	Cys	Cys	Leu	Ile	Gly	Cys	Thr	Lys	Arg	Ser	Leu	Ala	Lys	Tyr	Cys									
Relaxin 2	Gln	Leu	Tyr	Ser	Ala	Leu	Ala	Asn	Lys	Cys	Cys	His	Val	Gly	Cys	Thr	Lys	Arg	Ser	Leu	Ala	Arg	Phe	Cys									
Insulin					Gly	Ile	Val	Glu	Gln	Cys	Cys	Thr	Ser	Ile	Cys	Ser	Leu	Tyr	Gln	Leu	Glu	Asn	Tyr	Cys	Asn								
IGF-I	...	...	...	...	Gly	Ile	Val	Asp	Glu	Cys	Cys	Phe	Arg	Ser	Cys	Asp	Leu	Arg	Arg	Leu	Glu	Met	Tyr	Cys	Ala	Pro	Leu	Lys	Pro	Ala	Lys	Ser	Ala
IGF-II			...	...	Gly	Ile	Val	Gln	Glu	Cys	Cys	Phe	Arg	Ser	Cys	Asp	Leu	Ala	Leu	Leu	Glu	Thr	Tyr	Cys	Ala	Thr			Pro	Ala	Lys	Ser	Glu

FIG. 5. Amino acid sequences of the human hormones relaxin 1 (B32) (488), relaxin 2 (B33) (489), insulin (702), IGF-I (825), and IGF-II (824). The IGFs are single-chained peptides, and the positions of the 12 (IGF-I) and eight (IGF-II) amino acid residues that connect the B-chain-like and the A-chain-like regions of these molecules are indicated with *dots*. A gap has been placed at positions 23 and 24 of the A-chain-like region of IGF-II to illustrate better the homology of the C termini of IGF-I and IGF-II. Residues common to the five hormones are *shaded*.

ian thecal-interstitial cells (454), IGF-I receptors on pig endometrial membranes (470), IGF-I and IGF-II receptors on ewe mammary gland membranes (262), IGF-binding proteins secreted by rat skeletal muscle cells (685), or antisera to human IGF-I (441). IGF-I failed to displace human relaxin from relaxin-binding sites within the rat heart (742). Whereas IGF-I amplified synergistically the stimulatory actions of estrogen on progesterone biosynthesis in cultured swine granulosa cells, porcine relaxin did not (1078). IGF-I stimulated DNA synthesis in rat uterine cells, but porcine relaxin did not (70). Relaxin stimulated but IGF-I inhibited the release of insulinlike growth factor-binding protein I from human decidual cells (1042).

Evolutionary Origins of Relaxin

The similarity of their structures led to the postulation that relaxin, insulin, IGF-I, and IGF-II belong to a family of peptides (103,120). These hormones were proposed to be attributable to gene duplications of a primitive, insulinlike molecule followed by gene mutations encoding molecules with different functions (73,103, 508,883). Schwabe and co-workers (874,880) challenged the monophyletic hypothesis that relaxin and insulin are products of gene duplication on the basis of their observation that the amount of identity in the amino acid sequences of these two hormones remains relatively constant, about 25%, with no trend toward greater relatedness in the shark, which is thought to be an ancient species. Instead, they proposed a polyphyletic "genetic potential" hypothesis that places emphasis on deterministic chemical principles to account for the origin of the insulinlike family of proteins (874,887). According to the genetic potential hypothesis, prebiotic environmental conditions brought about abiotic synthesis of large but finite numbers of nucleotide polymers that, through self-replicating capabilities, mixed and spread throughout the primeval mud flats. When cells formed, they incorporated large numbers of informational polymers (genetic potential), and some of them coded for families of proteins such as insulin. If the genetic potential hypothesis is correct, genes present in higher forms of life should be present in some single cellular organisms. This may be the case. Schwabe et al. (882) reported the extraction of a molecule with the size and immunologic properties of porcine relaxin from the protozoan *Tetrahymena pyriformis.* Moreover, there is good evidence that relaxin is present in species more primitive than lower vertebrates. Georges and co-workers (385,386) identified both a 6,500-Da peptide with relaxin-like bioactivity and its messenger ribonucleic acid (mRNA) in the ovary of the tunicate *Herdmania momus,* and specific relaxin immunoreaction was localized in follicle cells surrounding mature oocytes in three species of tunicates.

Biologic and Immunologic Comparisons of Relaxin and Insulin

If relaxin and insulin originated from a common ancestral gene, considerable evolutionary divergence occurred between the two hormones. The limited amino acid sequence identity (about 25%) between relaxin and insulin is largely confined to the identical disposition of half-cystine residues involved in disulfide bridge formation and the glycine residues important for chain folding (Fig. 2).

Although stringent requirements to maintain similar tertiary structures appear to exist, four lines of evidence indicate that relaxin and insulin do not share common biologically active sites. First, amino acid residues within porcine insulin that are conserved among species (B12, B16, B24, B25, B26, A1, A4, A5, A19, A21) are in all but two cases (B12, A4) not shared by porcine relaxin. Dodson and co-workers (264) postulated that these surface invariant residues are important for insulin activity, and chemical modifications of several of them reduced insulin's activity. For example, high insulin biologic activity was reported to require conservation of residues B23-25, A19, and A21 on the surface of the molecule (798,1166). Amino acid A21 does not exist in relaxin. Second, the surface regions in insulin and relaxin that form dimer contacts differ. Amino acid residues B23-25 in porcine insulin form part of the β-sheet structure at its dimer interface (292). The C-terminal segment of the B chain in the human relaxin crystal is oriented in the opposite direction from that within the insulin crystal. Eigenbrot et al. (292) concluded that the marked differences in the dimer contacts of relaxin and insulin support the view that these two structurally related hormones evolved somewhat dissimilar mechanisms for receptor binding. Third, competitive binding studies indicated that relaxin and insulin do not share receptor-binding domains. Porcine relaxin did not displace porcine insulin from insulin receptors on rat brain cortex (372), human or rat adipocytes (509,736), and human mononuclear leukocytes (813). Likewise, porcine relaxin did not displace porcine insulin from chimeric receptors containing insulin receptor-related receptor (1162). Furthermore, porcine insulin did not displace porcine relaxin from relaxin receptors on human skin fibroblasts (689), rat uterine myometrium (663), or mouse uterine membranes (1143); and human insulin did not displace human relaxin from relaxin receptors on rat cervix (743), brain (744), or heart (742). Fourth, relaxin and insulin do not demonstrate common biologic activity in mammals. Unlike insulin, porcine relaxin failed to reduce blood glucose levels or increase diaphragm glucose levels in rats (1069), promote collagen synthesis in fetal rat bone (578), synergistically amplify gonadotropin or low-density lipoprotein-stimulation of progesterone secretion in pig granulosa cells (660,1076,1077), enhance luteinizing hormone stimulation of androstenedione production by porcine thecal cells (670), stimulate DNA synthesis in primary cultures of porcine granulosa cells (435), potentiate follicle-stimulating hormone (FSH) induction of aromatase activity in cultured rat granulosa cells (8), or stimulate androgen release from ovarian stromal tissue obtained from women with hyperandrogenism (66). Unlike porcine relaxin, insulin failed to increase uterine weight and uterine glycogen content in rats (1069), inhibit uterine contractions in rats (268), or increase aromatase activity in human endometrial cells (1053). Koob and co-workers (570) reported that relaxin and insulin demonstrate a common biologic activity in a lower vertebrate. They found that both porcine relaxin and bovine insulin promoted an increase in the cross-sectional area of the cervixlike constriction separating the uterus from the urogenital sinus of the spiny dogfish (*Squalus acanthias*); however, binding studies were not performed to determine whether the two hormones have the capacity to act through a common receptor in this species.

The surfaces of porcine relaxin and porcine insulin also appear to share no immunologic determinants. Studies that used polyclonal antibodies to porcine relaxin (412,925), polyclonal antibodies to synthetic human relaxin 2 (B33) (634), polyclonal antibodies to porcine insulin (813), monoclonal antibodies to rat relaxin (588), and monoclonal antibodies to porcine relaxin (158) showed no evidence of common antigenic domains between relaxin and insulin. Also supportive of the view that the surfaces of the two hormones differ extensively is the finding that relaxin interacts far less than insulin with insulin-degrading enzymes (261,771).

Structure–Activity Relationships

Structural features contributing to the biologic activity of relaxin were identified by determining the biologic activity of modified native porcine hormone and synthetic analogues of both porcine and human relaxin. Both chains, as well as the integrity of the putative hydrophobic core, appear to be essential for relaxin bioactivity. Shortly after the isolation of porcine relaxin, it was demonstrated that reduction and alkylation of the A and B chains (924) and oxidation of the tryptophan residue located at position B15 in Fig. 2 (877) abolished relaxin bioactivity. In the early 1980s, the basic amino acids that are invariant or that vary conservatively among species were postulated to be involved in bioactivity (72,102, 265,498). These amino acids (encircled in Fig. 3) include B5 Lys (Gln), B9 Arg, B13 Arg, A5 Lys (Gln), A13 Arg (Lys), and A14 Lys (Arg). In 1985, however, Büllesbach and Schwabe (151) found that biologic activity was reduced only about 70% in a derivative of porcine relaxin ($N^{\epsilon A5}$,$N^{\epsilon A14}$,$N^{\epsilon B5}$-tris[[(methyl-sulfonyl)ethyl]-

oxy]carbonyl]-B29 relaxin) where the ϵ amino groups of all three lysine residues (B5, A5, A14) were protected. In 1988, Büllesbach and Schwabe (154) demonstrated that modifying the six arginine residues in porcine relaxin with 1,2 cyclohexanedione essentially eliminated the hormone's bioactivity in both the mouse interpubic ligament bioassay and an *in vitro* mouse uterine contractility bioassay. These workers concluded at that time that it is one or both of the arginine residues B9 and B13 in the helix of the midregion of the B chain that are likely key receptor interaction sites for the following reasons. First, model building demonstrated that these two residues reside on the surface of the porcine relaxin molecule. Second, the B9 and B13 arginine residues are absolutely invariant among species. Third, removal of the arginine residues at the termini of the porcine relaxin molecule (A-2 and B26) does not reduce relaxin bioactivity. Finally, Thr-Glu in skate relaxin replaces the A13, A14 Arg (Lys) in porcine relaxin (Fig. 3), and skate relaxin has bioactivity in the mouse interpubic ligament bioassay (157). Büllesbach and co-workers (156,160) established in the early 1990s that both conserved arginine residues B9 and B13 in the midregion of the relaxin B chain are essential for relaxin bioactivity. They demonstrated that human relaxin derivatives in which either or both of the arginine residues in positions B9 and B13 were replaced with uncharged isosteric amino acid citrulline or positively charged lysine had little or no activity in the mouse interpubic ligament bioassay. These workers concluded that the two arginines B9 and B13 interact with the receptor like a prong and that binding is mediated by both a positive charge and by the hydrogen-binding network that can be induced by the guanidino groups.

The A chain forms a loop that contains an invariant A10 Gly. This A-chain loop is on the surface opposite that formed by the central portion of the B-chain helix that contains the two active arginine residues. Büllesbach et al. (159) obtained evidence that the invariant A10 Gly is also required for biologic activity. Synthetic human relaxin 2 (B29) derivatives in which L-alanine, D-alanine or L-isoleucine replaced A10 Gly were far less bioactive than human relaxin 2 (B29) in the mouse interpubic ligament bioassay. Büllesbach et al. (159) postulated that smallness is an important criteria for the A10 site. They further postulated that replacement of A10 Gly affects the conformation of the relaxin molecule in such a way that there is allosteric hindrance of the docking region of the molecule (B9 Arg and B13 Arg containing region of the B chain) or a steric hindrance on entrance of the relaxin into the binding pocket.

The complete C terminus of the B chain is not required for biologic activity. Porcine relaxin preparations CMB, CMa, and CMa′, which lack four, one, and three amino acids, respectively, at the C terminus of their B chains (Fig. 2), have full and equal activity in the mouse interpubic ligament bioassay (924), *in vitro* mouse uterine contractility bioassay (969), and *in vitro* rat uterine contractility bioassay (26). Also, oxidation of the tryptophan that is located six residues from the C terminus of the B chain (B24 in Fig. 2) did not reduce the activity of porcine relaxin in the mouse interpubic ligament bioassay (877). The numbers of residues on the C terminus of porcine relaxin that can be removed without influencing biologic activity remain to be established. Tregear and associates reported that a form of synthetic porcine relaxin that lacked seven amino acid residues on the C terminus of the B chain retained full biologic activity in the *in vitro* rat uterine contractility bioassay but that further reduction of the C terminus by one or two amino acids decreased bioactivity (1048,1049). Frieden et al. (354), however, reported that naturally occurring forms of porcine relaxin that lack six or seven amino acid residues on the C terminus of the B chain exhibit reduced bioactivity in the guinea pig pubic symphysis palpation bioassay and no bioactivity in the mouse interpubic ligament bioassay.

The N terminus of the A chain of porcine relaxin may be modified somewhat without complete loss of bioactivity. Full biologic activity was retained after the addition of polytyrosine residues to the N terminus (886,925), alkylation of the methionine residue adjacent to the N terminus (877), or removal of the first two amino acids on the N terminus (152). Some biologic activity was retained in synthetic porcine relaxin that lacked the three N-terminal amino acids of both the A and B chains (1048,1049). Porcine relaxin in which four or more amino acid residues were removed from the N terminus of the A chain were devoid of bioactivity in the mouse interpubic ligament bioassay (152). Büllesbach and Schwabe (153) found that replacement of the proposed N-terminal helix of the A chain (Arg-Met-Thr-Leu-Ser-Glu-Lys) by either the corresponding insulin segment or the strong helix promoter pentalanine restored about 30% of the bioactivity and concluded that it is the presence of a helix on the N terminus that is required for bioactivity.

The two methionine residues of human relaxin 2, which are located near the N and C termini of the B chain, are not required for bioactivity. Synthetic relaxin 2 (B33), that contained B-1 (Lys) and B21 (Ala) (Fig. 3) substitutions for methionine (523) or methionine residues oxidized by prolonged exposure to light (207) retained full bioactivity in the mouse interpubic ligament bioassay.

Whereas experiments involving deleting or altering amino acids provided insights about possible sites where relaxin interacts with its receptor, our knowledge of this interaction remains limited. Recent analyses of the structures of insulin and modified forms of insulin in both crystals and solution (256,482) provided strong evidence that the known crystal structure of insulin (Fig.

4A) reflects an inactive conformation and that a change in conformation is required for activity. Specifically, the C-terminal residues of the B chain (β strand B24-28 and perhaps the β turn B20-23) are proposed to separate from the amino terminal residues of the A chain exposing an alternate protein surface (256,482). We do not know the relevance of this finding, if any, to relaxin's interaction with its receptor. However, the observation that the C terminus of the B chain of porcine relaxin is not required for bioactivity is consistent with the possibility that relaxin and insulin may undergo similar conformational changes before or during interaction with their receptors.

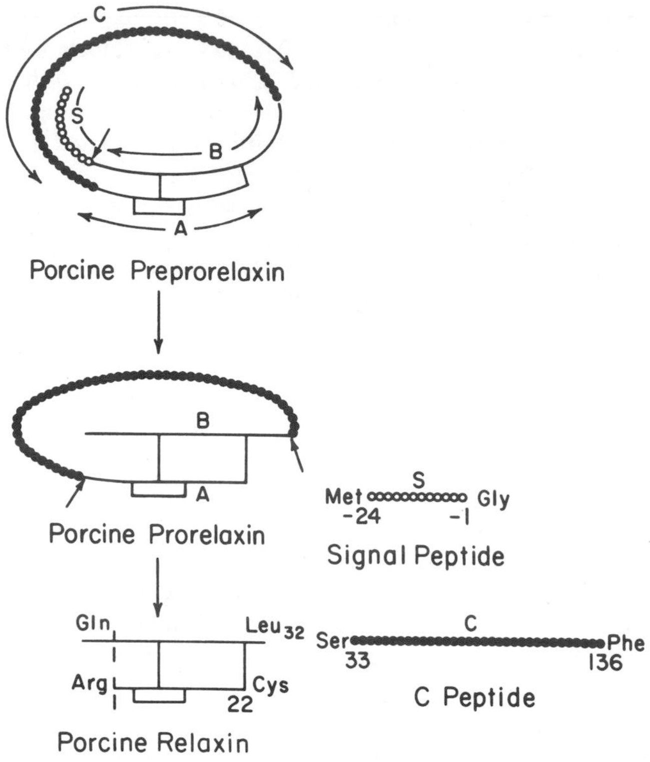

FIG. 6. Schematic summary of the processing of porcine preprorelaxin to relaxin by the successive removal of the signal peptide (*S*) and the connecting peptide (*C*) by proteolytic digestion. Modified from ref. 542.

Biosynthesis of Relaxin

Preprorelaxin Structure

Gel filtration of sow ovarian extracts provided the first indication that relaxin is synthesized originally in precursor forms and that the putative relaxin precursors are larger than preproinsulin and proinsulin, which are 11,000 and 9,000 Da, respectively (360,584). Frieden and Yeh (360) reported that about 5% to 10% of the relaxin bioactivity in an acid-acetone extract of porcine ovaries was associated with a biologically active fraction that had an apparent molecular weight of 42,000, as judged by its elution volume after gel filtration on Bio-Gel P-10. Similarly, Kwok et al. (584) reported that a small portion of the relaxin in an acid-acetone extract of porcine ovaries was associated with a biologically active fraction that had an apparent molecular weight of 19,000, as judged by its elution volume after gel filtration on Sephadex G-50. In both studies, treatment of the large, relaxinlike fraction with the proteolytic enzyme trypsin appeared to convert the putative precursor to 6,000-Da relaxin. The chromatographic (360,584) and electrophoretic characteristics (360) of the proteolytic digest were indicative of 6,000-Da relaxin formation, and relaxin bioactivity increased (360). Gast and co-workers (381–383) obtained more precise estimates of the size of the precursor(s) by synthesizing radiolabeled porcine relaxin precursors *in vitro* and then determining their size by sodium dodecylsulfate-polyacrylamide disk gel electrophoresis. Using a cell-free system, they demonstrated that pig luteal mRNA directed the synthesis of a 23,000-Da protein immunologically related to relaxin, whereas they obtained a 20,000-Da relaxin-related protein in the presence of ascites fluid (381–383). Gast (381,382) postulated that 23,000-Da preprorelaxin is the primary translation product and that the first step in relaxin biosynthesis is the membrane-dependent cleavage of a 3,000-Da signal peptide to form prorelaxin (Fig. 6).

Niall and co-workers (418,487) conducted detailed structural analyses of putative relaxin precursors in the early 1980s, and their findings are consistent with Gast's findings. These workers determined the complete amino acid sequences of porcine (418) and rat (487) preprorelaxin by cloning of relaxin cDNA. In general, this work involved (a) amino acid sequence analysis of porcine and rat relaxin, (b) synthesis of oligoribonucleotide primers complementary to the putative mRNA sequences predicted from the amino acid sequences of porcine and rat relaxin, (c) use of these synthetic DNA primers with mRNA isolated from pig and rat corpora lutea of pregnancy for the production of radiolabeled relaxin-specific cDNA probes, and (d) the identification of relaxin-specific clones in cDNA clone banks constructed from total pregnancy-derived corpus luteum mRNA (542). Relaxin, like insulin, is initially synthesized as a single-chained preprohormone with this overall structure: signal peptide/B chain/connecting peptide/A chain, as shown diagrammatically in Fig. 6. The signal peptides for porcine, rat, human, and monkey preprorelaxin contain 22 to 25 amino acid residues (Fig. 7).

The size difference between relaxin and insulin precursors is largely attributable to marked differences in the lengths of the connecting (C) peptides. The C peptides in porcine (418) and rat relaxin (487), for example, contain 104 or 105 residues, respectively; in porcine and

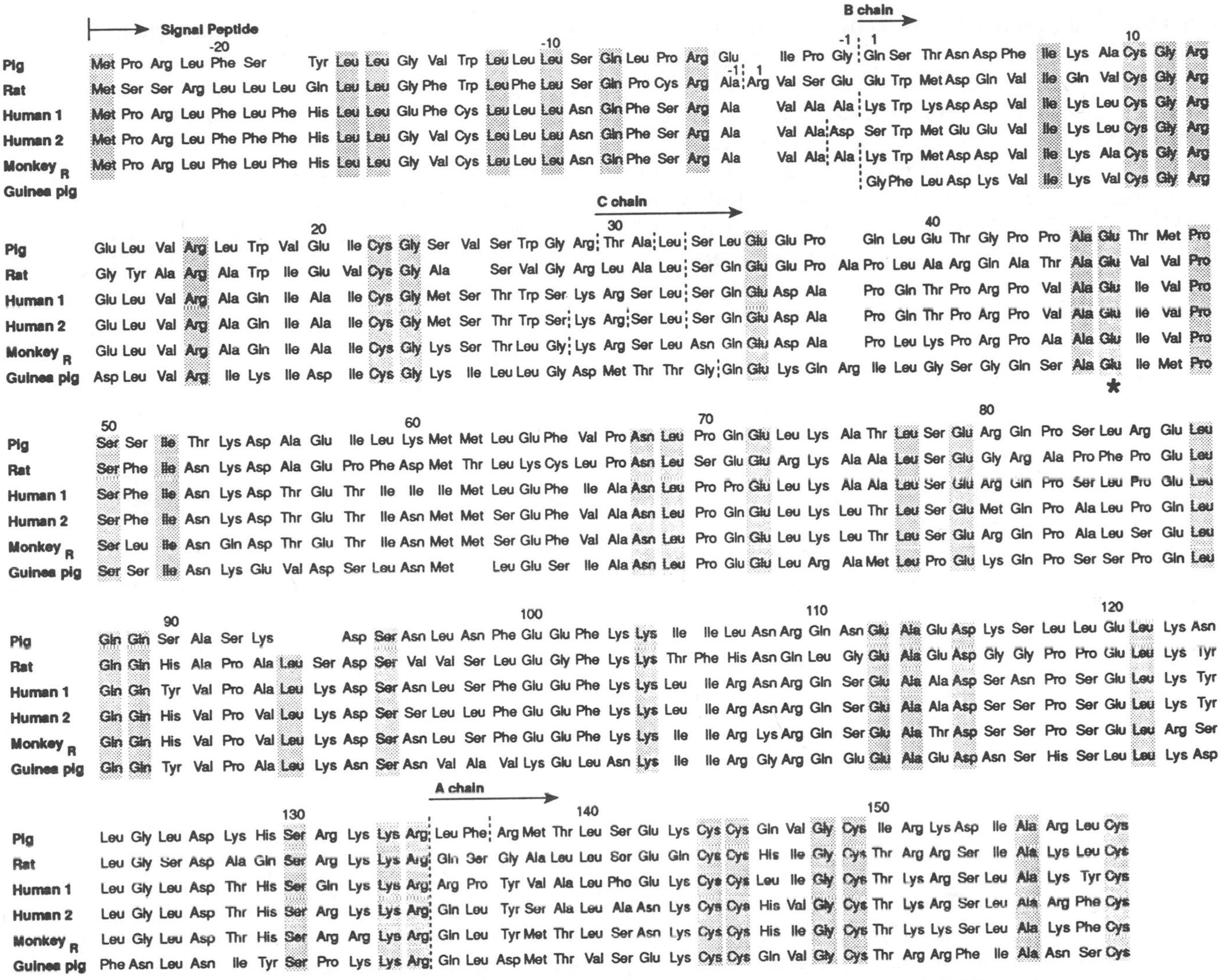

FIG. 7. Amino acid sequences of porcine (418), rat (487), human 1 (488), human 2 (489), and rhesus monkey (218) preprorelaxins, plus guinea pig prorelaxin (605). Sequences have been aligned to maximize homology, and amino acid identities are *shaded.* Amino acids are numbered from the N terminus of the porcine relaxin B chain. Putative cleavage sites (149,150,417,418,488,489,605) are indicated with *broken vertical lines.* The *asterisk* beneath Glu 46 in the C peptides denotes the site of the intron in human (489), monkey (218), and porcine (417) relaxin genes.

rat proinsulin, however, they contain only about 30 residues (1010). The function of the C peptide in relaxin is not known. One function presumably is to direct the folding of the precursors so the correct disulfide bonds are formed between the B and A chains. Furthermore, its large size, variety of amino acids, and reasonable level of conservation of primary structure among species led to the postulation that the C peptide may contain peptide sequences with hormonal activities (487,542). It remains to be demonstrated that the C peptide exhibits hormonal activity.

Knowledge of the structures of the C peptides of porcine and rat relaxin formed the basis of the strategy used by Hudson et al. in 1983 (488) to determine the structure of one form of human relaxin. Human relaxin had not been isolated, and its primary structure was not known; consequently, a radiolabeled cDNA probe complementary to its putative mRNA sequence could not be synthesized. Instead, Hudson et al. (488) constructed a specific probe consisting of a short fragment of porcine relaxin cDNA corresponding to amino acids 45 to 94 of the C peptide. This region had maximal homology (71% at the nucleotide level) between porcine and rat prorelaxin sequences and was postulated to be relatively homologous among species. By using this radiolabeled C peptide-specific probe to screen a human genomic library, a clone for one form of human relaxin (human relaxin 1) was obtained, and the complete coding sequence of human relaxin gene 1 was determined (488). In 1984, Hudson et al. (489) identified a clone for a second form of human relaxin (human relaxin 2) by screening a cDNA clone bank prepared from a human corpus luteum of pregnancy with radiolabeled relaxin-specific cDNA probes corresponding to exon I and exon II of the human preprorelaxin 1 gene. The amino acid sequences of human preprorelaxin 1 and preprorelaxin 2 are shown in Fig. 7. Although the four to six amino acid residues on the N termini of the B and A chains of putative human relaxin 1 and human relaxin 2 differ rather markedly, both chemically synthesized forms of the hormone had relaxinlike biologic activity, as judged by their ability to inhibit contractions of rat uterine strips *in vitro* (488,489).

In 1989, clones for rhesus monkey preprorelaxin were identified by screening a cDNA library prepared from corpora lutea of pregnancy with radiolabeled human relaxin-specific cDNA probes (218). The amino acid sequence of rhesus monkey relaxin (Fig. 7) displayed overall homologies of 77% and 83% with human relaxins 1 and 2, respectively. This is low in comparison with homologies between other primate peptides.

In 1992, Lee et al. (605) used a two-part strategy to determine the entire amino acid sequence of guinea pig prorelaxin (Fig. 7). Initially, they prepared a first strand cDNA pool from the endometrium of pregnant guinea pigs and determined the cDNA sequence of the B chain plus the 5′ end of the C peptide of relaxin by polymerase chain reaction using heterologous primers corresponding to partial sequences of mRNA from porcine preprorelaxin. Next, Lee et al. (605) determined the remaining sequence of guinea pig endometrial prorelaxin by rapid amplification of cDNA ends-polymerase chain reaction and subcloning using homologous primers. The complete amino acid sequence of the signal peptide on guinea pig relaxin remains to be determined.

Processing of Relaxin

In Fig. 6, a schematic summary of the processing of porcine preprorelaxin to porcine relaxin is shown. Figure 7 shows putative amino acids located at cleavage sites for the processing of porcine, rat, human, and monkey preprorelaxin. Cleavage of the signal peptides of preprorelaxin, like that of other peptide precursors (945), occurs at an amino acid with a small side chain. Subsequent cleavage of the C peptide in prorelaxin is less well defined and appears to be less stringently controlled than with proinsulin. Proinsulin is converted to insulin by trypsinlike enzymes that cleave at pairs of basic residues at both ends of the C peptide. This is not the case with porcine and rat relaxin. Cleavage at the C terminus of the B chain in porcine and rat relaxin appears to require an enzyme with chymotrypsinlike specificity that recognizes the neutral aliphatic side chains of leucine at position 32 (32 Leu) in prorelaxin (418). If this is the case with porcine relaxin, subsequent cleavage of 32 Leu and 30-31 Thr-Ala in prorelaxin (Fig. 7) must occur, because CMa porcine relaxin (Fig. 2), which has Ala at the C terminus of the B chain, and CMa′ porcine relaxin, which has Arg at the C terminus of the B chain, are major forms isolated from the ovaries under conditions designed to minimize autolysis (150,1093). Porcine relaxin CMa′ was also reported to be a major form of relaxin isolated from plasma obtained during the antepartum period (724). Hudson et al. (489) originally proposed that human relaxin 2 was also processed by a chymotrypsinlike enzyme at 32 Leu in Fig. 7, but human relaxin 2 (B29) isolated from corpus luteum of pregnancy is devoid of the four residues Lys-Arg-Ser-Leu thought to occur at the C terminus of the B chain of human relaxin 2 (B33) (1001,1067). Marriott et al. (654) recently obtained evidence that human relaxin 2 may be processed at both 30 Arg at the B/C-chain junction and at 134 Arg at the C/A-chain junction (Fig. 7). When they coexpressed the murine subtilisinlike serine protease called prohormone convertase 1 in human kidney 293 cells with human relaxin 2 preprorelaxin, a low-molecular-weight species with electrophoretic mobility similar to that of authentic mature human relaxin 2 (B29) was secreted. Marriott and co-workers (654) postulated that a similar enzyme might exist in human luteal cells and that the resultant basic amino acids Lys-Arg on the C terminus of the B chain may be cleaved subsequently by a carboxypeptidase enzyme within the luteal cells. There is limited evidence that metabolism of human relaxin within the blood may occur initially at the C terminus of the B chain. Within 60 min of intravenous administration of human relaxin 2 (B33) into rhesus monkeys, Ferraiolo et al. (319) identified up to 34% of the detectable relaxin as human relaxin 2 (B29). The physiologic significance of this observation is uncertain, because cleavage of human relaxin 2 (B33) to the human relaxin 2 (B29) form normally occurs within the corpora lutea before the hormone is released into the blood.

At the C-peptide/A-chain junction, the most likely cleavage point is C terminal to the three basic residues in positions 132–134, where a trypsinlike cleavage appears to occur. In porcine relaxin, subsequent cleavage of the 135-136 Leu-Phe of prorelaxin (Fig. 7) occurs, because most of the relaxin isolated from pig ovaries contains Arg on the N terminus of the A chain. Büllesbach and Schwabe (149,150) isolated small amounts of porcine relaxin with Leu-Phe or Phe extensions on the N terminus of A chains, and they postulated that these two forms of porcine relaxin were products of incomplete conversion of prorelaxin to relaxin.

Efforts to investigate the mechanisms that convert prorelaxin to relaxin are severely restricted by the limited amounts of prorelaxin present in source tissue as well as the difficulty of isolating the prohormone without modifying it. To overcome these problems, in 1983 Stewart et al. (973) prepared a gene coding for porcine prorelaxin that was cloned in the bacteria *Escherichia coli*, so that its expression was under the control of tryptophan promoter. After individual expression of the prohormone gene, more than 20% of the newly synthesized protein was associated with a molecule that appeared to be prorelaxin; its size was about 19,000 Da, and its antigenic determinants resembled those of relaxin. This group reported that sufficient amounts of the apparent porcine relaxin prohormone can be isolated from *E. coli* to study the process of cleavage of the C peptide and to isolate the enzymes involved. In 1992, Reddy et al. (814) produced and purified 19,000-Da recombinant porcine prorelaxin expressed in *E. coli*. Consistent with earlier findings with relaxin precursors in ovarian extracts (360,584), the purified recombinant prorelaxin could be converted to 6,000-Da relaxin by limited digestion with trypsin. The purified porcine prorelaxin was bioactive in an *in vitro* bioassay for relaxin (814).

Relaxin Genes

Partial or complete analysis of the genomic DNA from human, rhesus monkey, porcine, rat, and mouse relaxin genomic clones indicated that their general structures are consistent with that of the human relaxin gene shown in Fig. 8 (542). As indicated in Fig. 7, an intron interrupts the coding region at Glu in position 46 in the C peptide (218,417,489). The position of this intron corresponds closely to that of one of the two introns found in insulin genes (74). It is not known whether relaxin genes have a second intron corresponding to the position of the second insulin intron, which is located in the 5′ untranslated flanking region preceding the signal peptide. It was suggested that conservation of at least one

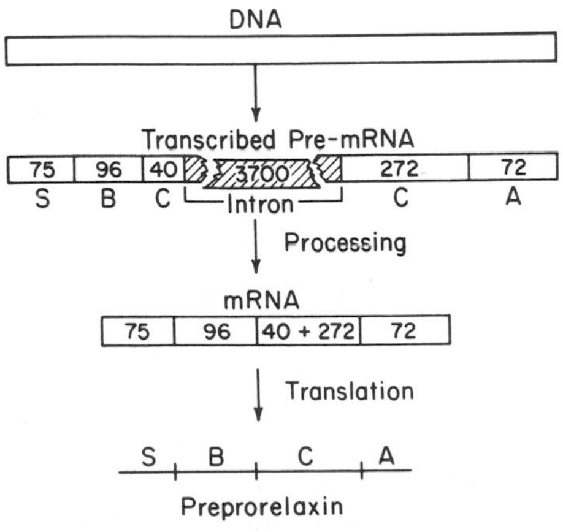

FIG. 8. Schematic illustration of the putative flow of information from human relaxin gene 1 to preprorelaxin. The relaxin gene is translated to give relaxin premessenger RNA, which contains a 3,700-base intron located at position 46 in the C peptide. After processing, the mRNA serves as a template for the translation of preprorelaxin. Modified from ref. 542.

intron site between relaxin and insulin genes supports the concept that these two hormones are related through a common ancestral gene (488,542).

In view of the apparent common ancestral origin of insulin and relaxin, the genes for these two hormones were presumed to be closely linked on the same chromosome after gene duplication. This does not appear to be the case. The human insulin gene is located on the short arm of chromosome 11 (748), whereas both relaxin genes are located on the short arm of chromosome 9 (219). Crawford et al. (219) suggested that after an original gene duplication, separation of the insulin-related and relaxin-related genes may have occurred by a chromosomal translocation, involving a breakpoint between the two genes, and that the two nonallelic human relaxin genes evolved by a second gene duplication event. Presumably, the second duplication occurred after the evolutionary divergence of pig, rat, mouse, and rhesus monkey genomes from the human genome, because only a single relaxin gene was found in these mammals (218,219,417).

The significance of two relaxin-related genes in the human is unknown. During pregnancy, the ovary synthesizes human relaxin 2 (278,489,1132), but ovarian expression of human relaxin gene 1 has not been detected (440,489). Winslow et al. (1131) determined that the relaxin found in human seminal plasma is also derived from the human relaxin gene 2. There is limited evidence that both human relaxin genes 1 and 2 are expressed in the decidua and placenta. Whereas one investigation failed to detect the biosynthesis of relaxin in either placental or decidual tissue (489), a more recent study detected both human relaxin 1 and human relaxin 2 mRNA in decidua and placental trophoblast (440). It remains to be demonstrated that bioactive forms of both human relaxin 1 and human relaxin 2 are produced in the decidua and/or placenta.

As in the human, the genes for relaxin and insulin in mice are located on different chromosomes. Mouse insulin 1 gene is on chromosome 6, and mouse insulin 2 gene is on chromosome 7 (636,837), whereas the mouse relaxin gene is on chromosome 19 (343).

Chemical and Recombinant Synthesis of Relaxin

Porcine relaxin was the first form of relaxin researchers chemically synthesized (1048,1049). Subsequent reports described methods for chemical synthesis of human relaxin 2 (B33) and human relaxin 2 (B29) (156,175,178,523,1047) and recombinant synthesis of human relaxin 2 (B29) (404,929,1001). Büllesbach and Schwabe (156) published the most detailed description of the chemical synthesis of human relaxin. These workers (156) used solid-phase synthesis of human relaxin 2 (B29), in combination with a novel thiol-protecting group strategy that synthesized the three disulfide bonds sequentially without error, to obtain a homogeneous and correct human relaxin 2 (B29) amino acid sequence. Several factors fuel great interest in the synthesis of human relaxin: the low nanogram yields of human relaxin 2 that can be obtained from corpora lutea of pregnancy, the potential clinical use of human relaxin in pregnant women and in humans with skin diseases, and the lack of information concerning the chemical and biologic characteristics of human relaxin. Chemically synthesized human relaxin 2 (B33) has been used to confirm the proposed amino acid sequence of human relaxin (156,523,1047), confirm that disulfide bonds are located as in insulin (175–177), demonstrate that exposure of human relaxin to intense light for several days oxidizes both methionine residues on the B chain without influencing bioactivity (207), show that both B9 Arg and B13 Arg in the midregion of the α-helix on the B chain (Fig. 3) are required for bioactivity (156,160), show that A10 Gly in the A chain (Fig. 3) is required for bioactivity and receptor binding (159), demonstrate that human relaxin is as active as porcine relaxin in the mouse interpubic ligament bioassay (156,159,160,234,523), and demonstrate that human relaxin increases both cyclic adenosine monophosphate (AMP) levels *in* and prolactin secretion *by* rat anterior pituitary cells in culture (234,235,943). Recombinant human relaxin 2 (B29) has been used to confirm that native human relaxin 2 contains four fewer amino acids on the C terminus of the B chain than originally proposed for human relaxin 2 (B33) (1001), demonstrate that a pyroglutamic acid residue is located on the N terminus of the A chain (1001), assign disulfide bond locations in human relaxin 2 (176,177,1001), determine the radiograph crystal structure of human relaxin 2 (292), demonstrate that human relaxin 2 self-associates to form a dimer in solution at high concentrations (929), and demonstrate that relaxin is active in the primary human uterine endometrial cell culture bioassay (176).

MEASUREMENT OF RELAXIN

Bioassays

The three types of relaxin bioassays used for more than 30 years are based on the original observations that relaxin causes the pubic bones in guinea pigs to separate when administered at estrus (460); promotes growth of the interpubic ligament in estrogen-primed mice (431); and inhibits myometrial contractility in estrogen-dominated guinea pigs, rats, and mice (575,863). Relaxin bioassays have indispensable applications. They identify and characterize relaxin preparations during the development of isolation procedures (148,157, 295,323,335,354,815,879,905,924,981,982), validate results obtained with radioimmunoassays (721,724,912, 926), determine structural requirements for biologic activity (151–153,156,159,160,207,354,523,877,924, 1048,1049), and determine whether putative forms of relaxin whose amino acid sequences have been deduced from gene nucleotide sequences are biologically active after chemical synthesis (156,488,489,523,1047,1048).

The extensive variation in relaxin's amino acid sequences among species has important implications for the investigator interested in bioassaying relaxin. First, it may be necessary to explore the bioactivity of relaxin from a given species in more than one bioassay to find a suitable response, because great differences in the bioactivity of highly purified relaxin preparations have been demonstrated in the commonly used bioassays (Table 1). Rat, shark, skate, and horse relaxin have less bioactivity than porcine relaxin in the mouse interpubic ligament bioassay (148,157,905,982). Rabbit and skate relaxin have less activity than porcine relaxin in the *in vitro* mouse uterine contractility bioassay (157,295). Shark relaxin promotes growth of the interpubic ligament and inhibits uterine contractions in guinea pigs, but not as effectively as porcine relaxin (815,969). Second, when researchers determine *levels of relaxin bioactivity,* they should use standard and unknowns from the same species, because in many cases, relaxin from different species will not provide the parallel dose-response curves needed for valid potency estimates. For example, rat relaxin has a lower dose-response curve than porcine relaxin in the mouse interpubic ligament bioassay (119,589,905). Porcine, whale, and human relaxins appear to be exceptions, as they were reported to have equivalent bioactivity in the mouse interpubic ligament bioassay (156,159,160,234,318,523,879). For additional information concerning the bioassay of relaxin, consult reviews by Steinetz et al. (951,965,967,969).

Interpubic Ligament Bioassays

Guinea Pig Pubic Symphysis Palpation Bioassay

The guinea pig pubic symphysis palpation bioassay, which was first described by Fevold et al. in 1930 (321), is based on the subjective assessment by palpation of the degree to which the pubic symphysis becomes movable after relaxin-induced separation of the pubic bones. In 1944, Abramowitz et al. (1) developed the first quantitative bioassay and defined a guinea pig unit as "that amount of hormone which induces, 6 h following injection, an unmistakable relaxation of the symphysis pubis in about two-thirds of a group of 12 castrated female guinea pigs weighing between 350 and 800 g and pretreated with 0.85 μg of estradiol daily for 4 days." This bioassay has limitations. GPUs based on response criteria are not valid because of variations in the judgment of investigators (969) and marked changes in the responsiveness of the pubic symphysis that occur when guinea pigs are used repeatedly for bioassay (345,347,349,709,1015,1016).

In the early 1950s, Talmage and Hurst (1016) described modifications of the bioassay that enabled more objective assessment of the influence of relaxin on the pubic symphysis. Using radiographic photography of the pubic symphysis, they found that the interpubic distance increased linearly as the dose of relaxin increased. Catchpole et al. (188), interpreting pubic symphysis relaxation as depolymerization or solubilization of the negatively charged matrix proteoglycans, used an electrometric method to determine the apparent density of immobile colloidal charge. Those workers found that as the dose of relaxin increased, there was a linear decrease in the density of negatively charged colloid in the pubic symphysis. Researchers have used neither of these objective guinea pig pubic symphysis bioassays (1,188), however. Instead, investigators have used a fast and relatively simple method described by Kroc et al. in 1959 (579). These workers described a revision of the guinea pig pubic symphysis palpation bioassay that largely overcomes limitations of the original quantitative bioassay (1). In this bioassay (579), two or more doses of unknowns and graded doses of reference standard are randomized, coded, and administered to estrogen-primed intact guinea pigs. Palpation is also performed under blind conditions by two or more independent operators who score the flexibility from 0 (no detectable flexibility) to 6 (extreme flexibility). Under these conditions, potency estimates with limits of error of less than 50% are obtained when 20 guinea pigs are used at each of two or more doses of standard and unknown (951). Although the guinea pig pubic symphysis palpation bioassay is cumbersome, imprecise, and expensive, it continues to be useful, because it is specific for relaxin and responsive to relaxin from a wide variety of species, including the pig, rat, shark, horse, rabbit, and human (148,467,721, 815,886,969).

Mouse Interpubic Ligament Bioassay

The mouse interpubic ligament bioassay is based on original observations of Hall and Newton in the mid-1940s. They found that the pubic symphysis of estrogen-primed mice responded to relaxin-containing extracts with a dose-dependent formation of a long interpubic ligament (422,431,433). The earliest bioassay procedures used radiographic examination of the pelvis to assess how much the interpubic ligament grew after relaxin treatment (266,423,433,558). In the late 1950s, Steinetz, Kroc, and co-workers devised a simpler direct measurement bioassay that enables researchers to determine objectively and rapidly the length of the interpubic ligament (579,951,952). Rapidly growing immature female mice weighing 18 to 21 g are first primed with a single injection of long-acting estrogen. Seven days later, three or more doses of the relaxin standard or unknown(s) are injected in the repository vehicle 1% benzopurpurine-4B. Between 18 and 24 h after the relaxin injection, the mice are killed, the pubic symphyses are cleaned of extraneous tissue, and the interpubic ligaments are measured using transillumination of the birth canal on a binocular dissecting microscope outfitted with an ocular micrometer (Fig. 9A). Considerable variation exists among animals, but when 20 mice are used per dose, potency estimates with limits of error of less than 50% can be obtained (924,951,952,969) (Fig. 9B). The repository vehicles, 5% beeswax in peanut oil (558) and 1% benzopurpurine-4B (an azo dye) in physiologic saline, potentiate the activity of porcine relaxin 100- to 300-fold and bring the mouse interpubic ligament bioassay for porcine relaxin to within the same range of sensitivity as the guinea pig pubic symphysis palpation bioassay (952). In 1989, the long-untested hypothesis that the repository vehicle benzopurpurine-4B potentiates relaxin bioactivity by mechanically retarding adsorption from the injection site (557) gained experimental support. When Ferraiolo and co-workers (318) injected chemically synthesized human relaxin 2 subcutaneously into estrogen-pretreated virgin female mice in a suspension of 1% benzopurpurine-4B, peak levels of relaxin were lower, but serum concentrations remained elevated far longer than when relaxin was administered without benzopurpurine-4B. We cannot presently rule out the possibility that benzopurpurine-4B may also bind strongly to relaxin and protect the relaxin from degradative metabolism (73). There is also limited evidence that the sensitivity of the mouse interpubic ligament bioassay may be increased further by using mice weighing 10 rather than 20 g (623).

The mouse interpubic ligament bioassay was used for the isolation and/or characterization of relaxin from the pig (149,150,152,153,193,354,724,924), rat (119,905), shark (148), skate (157), whale (879), rabbit (335), horse (982), cow (323,325), and human (96,156,159,160,207, 234,318,334,523). The low ability of both skate and shark relaxin to promote growth of the interpubic ligament in mice severely restricts the use of this bioassay with these species. Nevertheless, in view of its objectivity, specificity, and simplicity, the mouse interpubic ligament bioassay is the bioassay of choice when it can be used.

Uterine Contractility Bioassays

Uterine contractility bioassays are based on the original discovery by Krantz et al. (575) in 1950 that relaxin-containing extracts of swine corpora lutea diminished

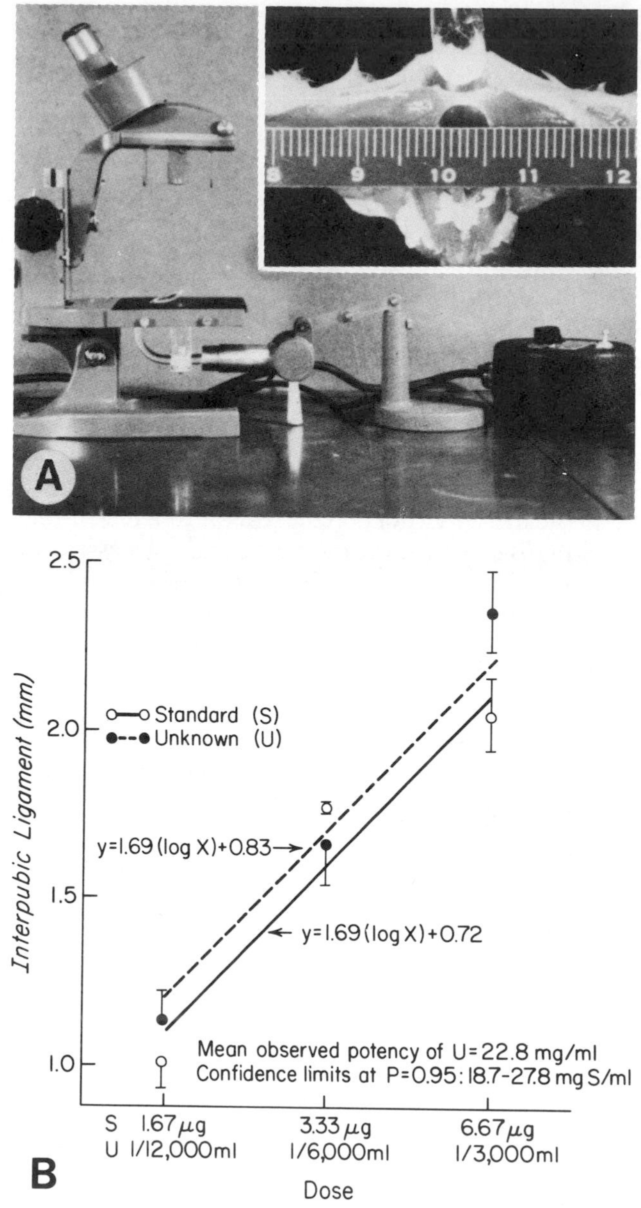

FIG. 9. A: Dissecting scope equipped with fixed transilluminating device and ocular micrometer for measurement of interpubic ligament length in mice. *Inset* shows the ventral view of a dissection of a mouse pelvis, showing the interpubic ligament positioned on the transilluminator. From ref. 579, with permission. **B:** Mouse interpubic ligament bioassay of an unknown porcine relaxin sample and a porcine relaxin reference standard designated Warner-Chilcott Relaxin Reference Standard W1164-A, lot 8. The unknown was made up to an estimated concentration of 20 mg reference standard/ml. From ref. 951, with permission.

spontaneous uterine contractility in guinea pigs. Since then, investigators have described both *in vivo* and *in vitro* methods for the bioassay of relaxin based on inhibition of uterine contractility in estrogen-dominated guinea pigs (317), rats (26,119,127,988,1137), and mice (579,591). The uterine contractility bioassays have desirable features. First, relaxin-induced inhibition of uterine contractility occurs rapidly—within minutes (Fig. 10). Second, relaxin from many species can be detected with the uterine contractility bioassays. For example, they were used for isolating or characterizing relaxin from the pig (26,193,354,413,969), rat (119), shark (815), skate (157), rabbit (295,335), cow (323), and human (96,294,334,523,721,1142). Finally, the uterine contractility bioassays may be somewhat more sensitive than the guinea pig and mouse pubic symphysis bioassays, because sensitivities lower than 100 ng were reported for porcine relaxin (26,127,193,859,860,969).

Uterine contractility bioassays also have limitations. They are not specific for relaxin. Oxytocin, which promotes uterine contractility, was present in extracts of cow corpora lutea (323,330,331), rabbit placentas (335), and human placentas (330,331) in levels sufficient to interfere with the quiescent effect of relaxin on uterine

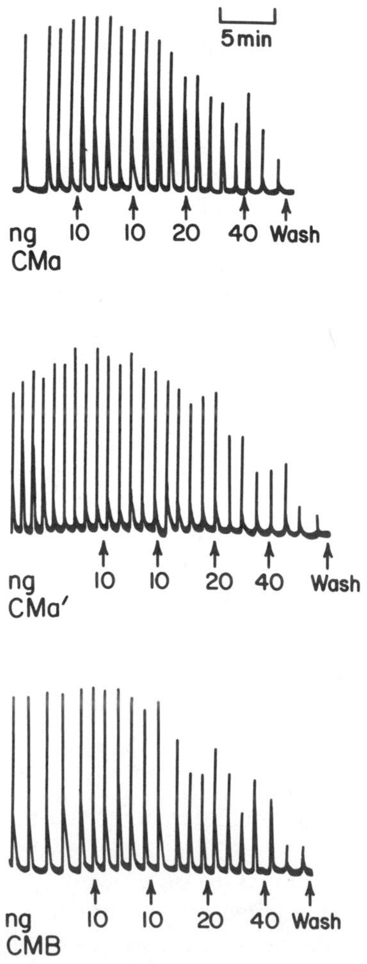

FIG. 10. Effects of increasing concentrations of highly purified porcine relaxin preparations CMa, CMa′, and CMB (924) on spontaneous contractility of estrous mouse uterine segment *in vitro.* Relaxin was added at 5-min intervals to baths containing uterine segments in Krebs-Ringer bicarbonate-buffered medium (pH 7.4) and aerated with 95% O_2/5% CO_2. Isotonic contractions; load 1 g. From ref. 969, with permission.

contractility. Also, several limitations restrict the use of these bioassays for quantitative determinations of relaxin bioactivity. First, there is considerable variation in sensitivity to relaxin among uteri; moreover, this sensitivity was reported to diminish after treatment with multiple doses of relaxin (863,1135). Second, relaxin influences both the frequency and amplitude of uterine contractions, and this makes quantitation of the response difficult (1137). Finally, spontaneous uterine contractions tend to be irregular, so they do not provide satisfactory baseline activity. Because of this irregularity, many of the early *in vitro* uterine contractility bioassays used a preliminary selection of tissue according to the frequency, regularity, and amplitude of spontaneous uterine contractions. Some investigators largely overcame the variability associated with spontaneous uterine contractions by using only total inhibition of uterine contractility as an end point (413).

In the early 1980s, researchers described several *in vitro* uterine contractility bioassays that used induced baseline uterine contractions rather than rely on irregular spontaneous uterine contractions. Nishikori et al. (706,707) induced contractions in isometrically suspended uteri from estrogen-primed rats by exposing them to a low dose of $PGF_{2\alpha}$ (0.28 μM) 10 min before the addition of relaxin. These workers determined the influence of relaxin on the amplitude of the $PGF_{2\alpha}$-induced uterine contractions. Bradshaw et al. (119) were the first to induce rat uterine segments to contract regularly by electrical stimulation. With this method, segments of uterine horn obtained from estrogen-dominated rats are suspended in an organ bath with one end attached to an isometric strain gauge. The uterine segments are then stimulated electrically (4–5 V, 50–60 Hz) for 4 or 5 sec at 45-sec (119) or 60-sec intervals (124,127,614,859,860), and the influence of relaxin on the amplitude of the electrically driven baseline uterine contractions is determined (Fig. 11A). St-Louis (988–990) described a procedure whereby a baseline tonic uterine contraction is obtained with a depolarizing solution of KCl. With this procedure, segments of uterine horn obtained from estrogen-primed rats are suspended in an organ bath with one end attached to an isotonic smooth-muscle transducer. A tonic contraction is then induced by partial (15% or 20%) replacement of the NaCl in physiologic saline with KCl. After the first tonic contraction and once a stable plateau is reached, relaxin is added to the organ bath. With this method, the degree to which relaxin induces a relaxation of the tonic contraction is determined by planimetry (988,990) (Fig. 11B).

In recent years, no single *in vivo* or *in vitro* method has emerged as the uterine contractility bioassay of choice. Both rats (253,268–270,272) and pigs (794) have been used to examine relaxin's effects on uterine contractility *in vivo*. Also, researchers have examined *in vitro* the influence of relaxin on both spontaneous contractility (388,394,622,641,687,740,769,799) and induced contractility (344,641,740,799) of uterine tissue obtained from rats, pigs, and humans.

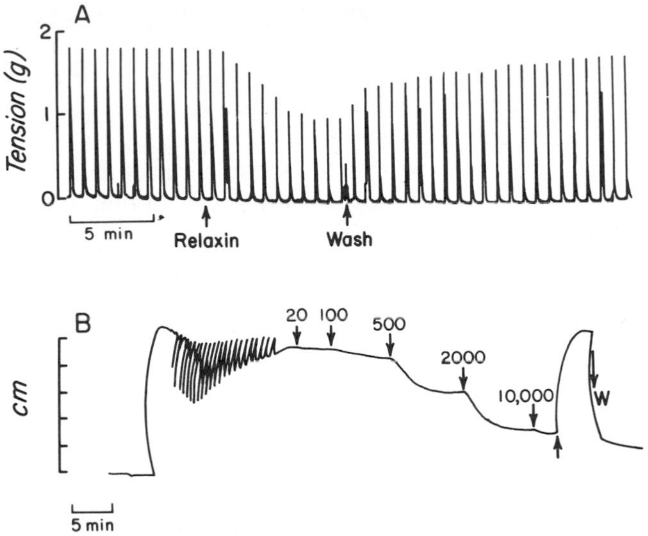

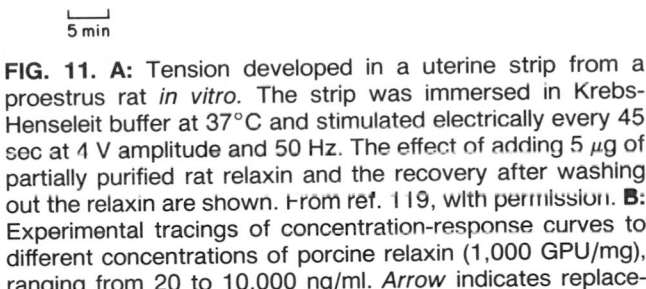

FIG. 11. A: Tension developed in a uterine strip from a proestrus rat *in vitro*. The strip was immersed in Krebs-Henseleit buffer at 37°C and stimulated electrically every 45 sec at 4 V amplitude and 50 Hz. The effect of adding 5 μg of partially purified rat relaxin and the recovery after washing out the relaxin are shown. From ref. 119, with permission. **B:** Experimental tracings of concentration-response curves to different concentrations of porcine relaxin (1,000 GPU/mg), ranging from 20 to 10,000 ng/ml. *Arrow* indicates replacement of bathing solutions by fresh KCl-substituted saline; *W* indicates replacement by normal saline. From ref. 988, with permission.

Cervical Extensibility Bioassay

It has been known since the 1950s that porcine relaxin increases cervical extensibility (408,409,1156). In 1980, Fields and Larkin (333) demonstrated that porcine relaxin promotes linear increases in cervical extensibility as well as growth of the interpubic ligament in estrogen-primed mice. Cervical extensibility, however, may not provide the basis for a useful relaxin bioassay, because they found slopes of dose-response curves to be shallow and the correlation between cervical extensibility and interpubic ligament length ($p < .08$) not highly significant.

Cell Culture Bioassays

We need improved methods for the bioassay of relaxin. Existing *in vivo* and *in vitro* methods lack precision. Also, they lack the sensitivity needed to measure readily relaxin bioactivity in peripheral blood or tissue extracts where the concentrations of relaxin are low. The limit of sensitivity for both the guinea pig pubic symphysis palpation bioassay and the mouse interpubic ligament bioassay is about 100 ng with highly purified porcine relaxin (151,924,969), and *in vitro* rat and mouse uterine contractility bioassays appear to be only moderately more sensitive (969). In 1990, two groups described relaxin bioassays based on the stimulation of increased cyclic AMP levels in established cultures of human endometrial cells (314) and newborn rhesus monkey uterine cells (574), respectively. They reported both cell culture bioassays to be specific for relaxin, more precise than previously used relaxin bioassays, and sufficiently sensitive to routinely measure less than 1 ng of human relaxin. These sensitive bioassays were used to determine the bioactivity of native human relaxin 2 isolated from corpora lutea of pregnancy (574), human relaxin 2 synthesized by chemical or recombinant methods (176,314,574), porcine relaxin (574), recombinant porcine prorelaxin (814), and rat relaxin (574). There are, however, important limitations to these cell culture bioassays for relaxin. The assays are neither practical nor economical for laboratories not equipped to conduct cell culture. Also, the cells are available in finite quantities and can only be distributed to a limited degree. Finally, the responsiveness to relaxin varied among different human endometrial cell lines (314) as well as among different passages (population doubling) of a given newborn rhesus monkey uterine cell line (574). A transformed cell line that is responsive to relaxin, stable, and widely available indefinitely would offer advantages over the two cell culture bioassays for relaxin that have been described (314,574).

Radioimmunoassays

The limits of sensitivity of bioassays restrict their applicability for the measurement of relaxin in the blood. Determination of relaxin bioactivity levels in ovarian venous blood during late pregnancy in the pig required concentration of the blood to attain the limits of assay sensitivity with the mouse interpubic ligament bioassay (81). Also pooled serum obtained from women during the third trimester was concentrated to attain the limits of assay sensitivity with the *in vitro* rat uterine contractility bioassay (124). Radioimmunoassays for relaxin have been developed to measure relaxin levels in small samples of blood. The first relaxin radioimmunoassay was developed in 1972 with the impure porcine relaxin preparation NIH-R-P1 (440 GPU/mg), which contains approximately 20% biologically active relaxin and 80% uncharacterized proteins (132,137). Using that radioimmunoassay, relaxin was reported to be present in sera of sheep and humans under many physiologic conditions (133–136,195).

When essentially pure preparations of relaxin became available, they were used for the development of homologous radioimmunoassays for porcine (12,316,416,546,604,630,723,817,907,925,983,984,1021), rat (514,785,911), and equine (974) relaxin. A synthetic analog of human relaxin 2 (B33) was used to develop a homologous radioimmunoassay for human relaxin (286,289). These homologous radioimmunoassays, which use relaxin from a single species for generation of antiserum, radioligand, and standard, are specific for relaxin and precise. Moreover, they are approximately 1,000-fold more sensitive than *in vivo* relaxin bioassays, because they generally detect 100 pg or less of relaxin (Fig. 12). During late pregnancy, relaxin levels in the peripheral blood of pigs, rats, and horses can be readily determined in serum volumes of 2 to 5 μl (910,912,974). Radioimmunoassays that use highly purified relaxin for radioligand and standard optimize the accuracy and specificity of relaxin immunoactivity determinations. All determinations of relaxin immunoactivity levels are now performed with radioimmunoassays that use highly purified relaxin preparations.

Because radioimmunoassays detect relaxin immunoactivity but not relaxin bioactivity, investigators must exercise caution with physiologic interpretations of relaxin immunoactivity levels. Nevertheless, where they were both measured, good correlations were demonstrated between levels of relaxin immunoactivity and relaxin bioactivity in the blood of pigs (81,724,910) and extracts of corpora lutea or ovaries from pigs (926), rats (912), and women (721).

The marked variation in the amino acid sequences of relaxin among species (Fig. 3) accounts for the limited immunologic cross-reactivity of purified relaxin preparations in homologous radioimmunoassays or enzyme-linked immunosorbant assays for relaxin of other species (286,416,634,815,907,911,974) (Fig. 12). It

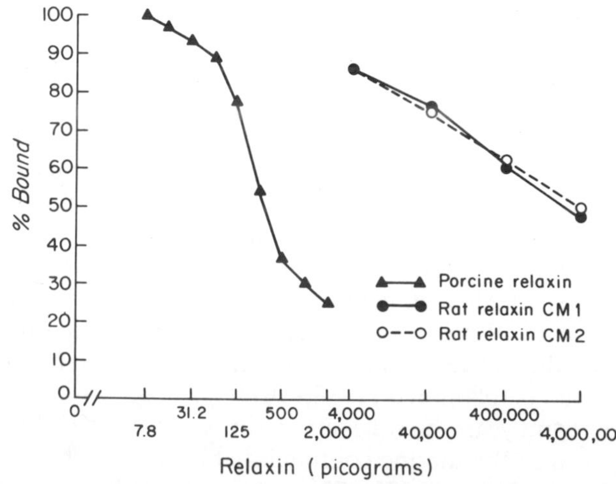

FIG. 12. Dose-response curves for highly purified porcine relaxin (924) and highly purified rat relaxin preparations CM1 and CM2 (905) in a homologous porcine relaxin radioimmunoassay (925). From ref. 911, with permission.

is advantageous to measure relaxin immunoactivity levels in a given species with a homologous radioimmunoassay for relaxin of that species, because there is an increased probability of high-affinity binding between relaxin and the relaxin antiserum. At present, however, homologous radioimmunoassays have been reported for only porcine, rat, equine, and human relaxin.

Antiporcine relaxin sera were shown to neutralize the biologic activity of relaxin from a wide variety of species (595,953). Several investigators took advantage of the species aspecificity of antiporcine relaxin sera and used homologous porcine relaxin radioimmunoassays to detect relaxin immunoactivity in tissues from species in which homologous radioimmunoassays were not available. Although these radioimmunoassays did not enable accurate measurement of relaxin levels, they provided an approximation of the profile of relaxin immunoactivity levels during pregnancy in the peripheral blood of the human (647,648,720,900), baboon (723), chimpanzee (970), monkey (708,747,1113), hamster (723,963), mouse (723), dog (955–957), rabbit (604), cat (10,984), horse (983), and cow (25,168).

Porcine Relaxin Radioimmunoassays

Table 3 summarizes the hormone preparations used, methods of radioiodination, and species applications for porcine relaxin radioimmunoassays developed with highly purified porcine relaxin. Because porcine relaxin lacks tyrosine and histidine, the commonly used chloramine T radioiodination procedure (492) cannot be used to radiolabel unmodified hormone. Instead, four methods have been described that involve conjugation of readily radioiodinated groups to porcine relaxin by amide bonds, followed by radioiodination of the modified relaxin by the chloramine T procedure. First, the reagent *N*-carboxy-L-tyrosine anhydride was used to incorporate one or more tyrosine residues primarily into the N terminus of the A chain (723,886,925). Second, the unlabeled Bolton and Hunter reagent (106) 3-(4-hydroxyphenyl) propionic acid *N*-hydroxysuccinimide ester was used to conjugate 3-(4-hydroxyphenol) propionic acid to porcine relaxin (12,690,983,1021). Third, the reagent *N*-formyltyrosine-*N*-hydroxysuccinimide ester was used to incorporate *N*-formyltyrosine largely into the N terminus of the A chain (875). Fourth, the reagent tertiary-butyl oxycarbonyl-tyrosine-*N*-succinimide ester was used to incorporate tyrosine into the N terminus of the A chain (420). An additional method in which unmodified porcine relaxin is radiolabeled directly with radioiodinated Bolton and Hunter reagent has also been described (416,546,604,630). All five procedures provide radioligand that is suitable for porcine relaxin radioimmunoassays. The sensitivity of the porcine relaxin radioimmunoassays summarized in Table 3 are comparable—100 pg of porcine relaxin or less.

Rat Relaxin Radioimmunoassays

Three homologous radioimmunoassays for rat relaxin have been described (514,785,911). Sherwood and Crnekovic (911) used equal amounts of the highly purified

TABLE 3. *Porcine relaxin radioimmunoassays developed with highly purified relaxin preparations*

Development reference	Relaxin used for generation of antiserum, radioligand, and standard	Method used for preparation of the radioligand	Species applied to
925	CMB + CMa + CMa′ [a] (2,500–3,000 GPU/mg)	Polytyrosyl relaxin: chloramine T	Pig
725, 946	CMB + CMa + CMa′ [b]	Polytyrosyl relaxin: chloramine T	Hamster, guinea pig, mouse, rat, cow, baboon, rhesus monkey, chimpanzee, human, dog, shark
630	CMa′	Radioiodinated Bolton and Hunter	Human
12	CMa′	Unlabeled Bolton and Hunter: chloramine T	Pig, guinea pig
983	CMB + CMa + CMa′	Unlabeled Bolton and Hunter: chloramine T	Horse, cat
1021	CMB + CMa + CMa′ [c]	Unlabeled Bolton and Hunter: chloramine T	Pig
546	CMB + CMa + CMa′	Radioiodinated Bolton and Hunter	Pig
875	CMB + CMa + CMa′	Monotyrosyl relaxin: chloramine T	Pig
416	CMa	Radioiodinated Bolton and Hunter	Pig, rat, human
604	Ref (327)	Radioiodinated Bolton and Hunter	Rabbit
370, 420	CMB + CMa + CMa′	Monotyrosyl relaxin: chloramine T	Pig

[a] The nomenclature of porcine relaxin preparations CMB, CMa, and CMa′ (924) is illustrated in Figs. 1 and 2.

[b] Subsequent to the original study (725) that used an antiserum to partially purified porcine relaxin (about 1,000 GPU/mg), antiserum R6 generated with CMB, CMa, and CMa′ has been used (946).

[c] Partially purified porcine relaxin (about 1,000 GPU/mg) was used to generate the antiserum.

microheterogeneous preparations of CM1 and CM2 obtained by the isolation procedure of Sherwood (905) for radioligand, standard, and generation of the antiserum. Porter (785) used highly purified rat relaxin obtained according to the isolation procedure of Walsh and Niall (1093) for the radioligand and standard and partially purified rat relaxin for generation of the antiserum. Jockenhövel et al. (514) used highly purified rat relaxin obtained by the isolation procedure of Walsh and Niall (1093) for the radioligand, standard, and generation of the antiserum. Three methods were used to radioiodinate rat relaxin. Rat relaxin was radiolabeled directly by either the chloramine T procedure (514) or the Bolton and Hunter procedure (911) or first conjugated with unlabeled Bolton and Hunter reagent and then radioiodinated by the chloramine T procedure (785). All three radioimmunoassays are sufficiently sensitive to measure 100 pg or less of rat relaxin.

Equine Relaxin Radioimmunoassay

Stewart developed a homologous equine relaxin radioimmunoassay (974). Highly purified hormone (982) was used for radioligand, standard, and generation of the antiserum. Equine relaxin was radiolabeled directly by the chloramine T procedure (492). The equine relaxin radioimmunoassay is sufficiently sensitive to detect approximately 25 pg of equine relaxin.

Human Relaxin Radioimmunoassay

Eddie et al. (286,289) described a homologous human relaxin radioimmunoassay in 1986. An analog of human relaxin 2 (B33) was prepared by chemical synthesis (523) and used for radioligand, standard, and generation of antiserum. The human relaxin 2 (B33) analog (designated DKA) contained two substitutions in the B chain to eliminate methionine residues: lysine at position −1 and alanine at position 21 in Fig. 3. The homologous human relaxin 2 radioimmunoassay, which is sufficiently sensitive to detect approximately 50 pg of human relaxin per milliliter, has been used to measure relaxin in the serum (75–78,288) and milk (289) of women.

Enzyme-Linked Immunosorbant Assays

Enzyme-linked immunosorbant assays for relaxin have potential advantages over radioimmunoassays. The enzyme-labeled antibody is more stable than radioiodinated hormone. Also, investigators can avoid problems associated with radioactive labeling of relaxin (875,925,1097), as well as handling and discarding radioactive waste.

Porcine Relaxin Enzyme-linked Immunosorbant Assays

In 1980, Bodsch and Struck (105) described the development of two types of enzyme-linked immunosorbant assays for porcine relaxin. A rabbit antiporcine relaxin antibody-horseradish peroxidase conjugate was used for a sandwich assay, and a mouse antirabbit Fab antibody-horseradish peroxidase conjugate was used for a combining-site blocking assay. The sensitivity of both enzyme-linked immunosorbant assays was approximately 200 pg porcine relaxin and comparable with porcine relaxin radioimmunoassays. Preliminary results indicated that relaxin was detectable with both assays in the blood of pregnant women (105).

Human Relaxin Enzyme-linked Immunosorbant Assay

In 1989, Lucas et al. (634) described the development of an enzyme-linked immunosorbant assay for human relaxin. The chemically synthesized human relaxin 2 analogue SKA (523), which is identical to human relaxin 2 analog DKA except for the deletion of aspartic acid from the N terminus of the B chain, was used for standard and generation of the antiserum. This enzyme-linked immunosorbant assay, which is specific for human relaxin and sufficiently sensitive to detect 2 pg of human relaxin, has been used to measure serum levels of relaxin in nonpregnant (976–978) as well as in pregnant women (519,522,976–978,1138).

Macaque Relaxin Enzyme-linked Immunosorbant Assay

Stewart et al. (987) developed a homologous macaque relaxin enzyme-linked immunosorbant assay. Synthetic rhesus monkey relaxin (218) was used for the standards and generation of rabbit antimacaque relaxin serum. This enzyme-linked immunoassay, which is specific for macaque relaxin and sufficiently sensitive to detect 10 pg relaxin, was used to measure relaxin levels in peripheral blood collected from cynomolgus and rhesus macaques during both nonconceptive menstrual cycles and the peri-implantation period (987).

SOURCES AND SECRETION OF RELAXIN IN THE FEMALE

Relaxin is produced in highest levels by female reproductive tract tissue(s) during pregnancy. Primary sources are the corpus luteum, placenta, and uterus. The tissue(s) that is the primary source of the relaxin circulating in the peripheral blood varies among species. Table 4 contains a summary of known sources of relaxin in several mammalian species. No clear pattern of pregnancy-related physiologic factors that might predict the source

TABLE 4. *Sources of relaxin in mammals*

Species	Ovary needed throughout pregnancy	Primary source of relaxin	Secondary source(s) of relaxin
Pig (*Sus scrofa*)	Yes	Corpus luteum (24, 332)	Uterus[a] (1164)
Horse (*Equus caballus*)	No	Placenta (982)	
Cow (*Bos taurus*)	Yes	Corpus luteum (323)	
Cat (*Felis catus*)	No	Placenta (10)	
Dog (*Canis familiaris*)	Yes	Placenta (956)	Ovaries[a] (956)
Rat (*Rattus norvegicus*)	Yes	Corpus luteum (328, 400)	Uterus[a] (336)
Mouse (*Mus musculus*)	Yes	Corpus luteum (31)	
Guinea pig (*Cavia porcellus*)	No	Uterus (750)	Mammary gland[a] (763)
Rabbit (*Oryctolagus cuniculus*)	Yes	Placenta (296, 297)	Uterus (296, 337)
Golden hamster (*Mesocricetus auratus*)	Yes	Placenta (816)	
Human (*Homo sapiens*)	No	Corpus luteum (992)	Decidua, placenta (145) Mammary gland[a] (661, 1020)

[a] Putative secondary sources of relaxin that are not well established.

of relaxin within species has emerged. With some species, such as the pig, rat, and mouse, where luteal progesterone production is required throughout pregnancy, the corpus luteum is the primary source of relaxin. However, in the dog, rabbit, and golden hamster where luteal progesterone is required throughout pregnancy, the placenta is the apparent primary source of relaxin. The horse, guinea pig, and human, species in which the corpora lutea are not the sole source of progesterone throughout pregnancy, produce most if not all their circulating relaxin in the placenta, uterus, and corpus luteum, respectively. There is also limited evidence that the corpora lutea produce relaxin in two marsupials, the opossum (*Didelphis virginiana*) (577,1056) and the tammar wallaby (*Macropus eugenii*) (1057,1098). The advent of sensitive techniques for localizing both relaxin and its mRNA has enabled the identification of secondary tissues that appear to produce small amounts of relaxin in some species. The relaxin produced in these so-called secondary sources may have local physiologic functions but appears to be produced in quantities unlikely to contribute appreciably to circulating relaxin levels. In this section, the tissue thought to be the source(s) of the relaxin secreted into the blood in each species is described before putative secondary tissue source(s) are described. Regulation of relaxin *synthesis* varies extensively among species. For example, rat ovarian relaxin levels remain low unless the animal is pregnant, whereas pig ovarian relaxin can increase to high levels in the absence of pregnancy. Regulation of relaxin *secretion* also varies among species; consequently, the profiles of relaxin levels in the peripheral blood throughout pregnancy differ strikingly among species. In this section, the sources and secretion of relaxin are described for individual domestic species, laboratory species, and primates. Emphasis is on the three species that were studied extensively in recent years—the pig, rat, and human.

Domestic Species

Pig

Estrous Cycle

Ovarian Source. Relaxin is produced within preovulatory follicles as well as in corpora lutea during the approximately 21-day estrous cycle in the pig (*Sus scrofa*) (Fig. 13). Day 0 of the estrous cycle is the first day of estrus. Investigators first detected relaxin immunoactivity in nonpregnant pigs in follicular fluid (143,659) and in media after culture of segments of follicle wall *in vitro* (143). Three lines of evidence support the view that theca interna cells produce relaxin in preovulatory follicles. First, theca tissue obtained from prepubertal pigs primed with pregnant mare serum gonadotropin/human chorionic gonadotropin (PMSG/hCG) secreted measurable levels of immunoactive relaxin *in vitro* (311). Second, immunohistochemical studies with both PMSG/hCG-primed prepubertal gilts (44,47) and sexually mature nonpregnant sows (255) demonstrated that relaxin immunoactivity was confined to the theca interna layer of the developing follicles before ovulation (Fig. 14A). Finally, a 1-kb relaxin transcript, which corresponds to the molecular size of the relaxin transcript in pregnant sow ovaries (417), was detected in ovarian extracts obtained from the ovaries of PMSG/hCG-primed prepubertal gilts; and *in situ* hybridization detected relaxin mRNA only in the theca interna layer of the developing follicle (50). The granulosa cells of preovulatory follicles produce little, if any, relaxin. Relaxin immunoactivity was not detected in the media bathing granulosa cells in culture (143,311). When granulosa cells obtained from preovulatory follicles were incubated for several days in the presence of luteinizing hormone (LH) (625) or LH plus FSH (293), small amounts of relaxin immunoactiv-

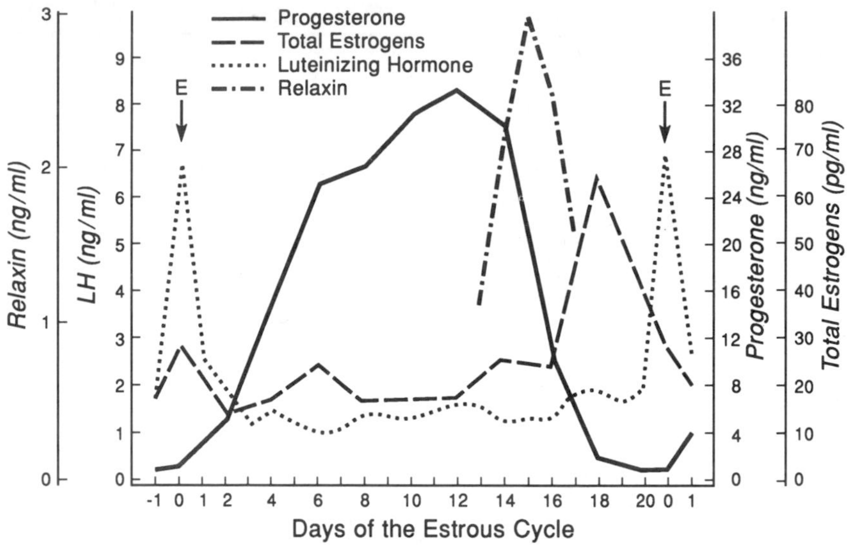

FIG. 13. Utero-ovarian vein plasma levels of relaxin (571) and peripheral plasma levels of LH, progesterone, and total estrogens during the porcine estrous cycle. *E*, estrus. Modified from ref. 438.

ity were secreted into the media (625), and small amounts of relaxin mRNA were detected in extracts from the granulosa cells (293). Bagnell and co-workers (44,47) postulated that the production of relaxin by granulosa cells in the presence of LH may be attributable to luteinization of the granulosa cells.

After ovulation and with differentiation of the theca cells and granulosa cells to form the corpus luteum, both cell types appear to produce relaxin. Bagnell et al. (44,51) reported that at 30 h after ovulation in PMSG/hCG-primed prepubertal gilts, relaxin immunostaining comparable with that in theca interna cells was evident in luteinizing granulosa cells (Fig. 14B) and that by 54 h postovulation, it became difficult to identify the cellular origin of the large luteal cells in which relaxin immunostaining became localized (Fig. 14C). A similar change in the immunohistochemical localization of relaxin during the development of the corpus luteum of adult nonpregnant sows was observed by Denning-Kendall et al. (255). Ultrastructural analysis indicated that at least a portion of the relaxin produced by the luteal cells during the estrous cycle appears to be packaged for storage. Using an antirelaxin serum and colloidal gold as marker, Fields and Fields (332) found that relaxin immunoactivity was associated with membrane-bound cytoplasmic granules in a small percentage of luteal cells obtained from pigs on day 14 of the cycle.

Several lines of evidence indicate that relaxin production is highest during the luteal phase of the estrous cycle (days 5 to 16) (Fig. 13) and declines to low levels after luteolysis. Extracts of corpora lutea contain relaxin bioactivity (24,950), and the levels of relaxin bioactivity in ovarian extracts are highest during the luteal phase of the estrous cycle (15,466,926). Relaxin immunostaining of corpora lutea (18) and levels of relaxin immunoactivity in luteal extracts (255) were reported to be maximal between days 11 to 15 of the estrous cycle. Relaxin mRNA transcript was demonstrated in the corpus luteum of the estrous cycle (49,293,624), and expression of relaxin mRNA was higher on day 13 than on days 3 or 19 of the cycle (49). Whereas relaxin is produced during the luteal phase of the estrous cycle, the content of relaxin within the corpora lutea during the cycle is much lower than it is during pregnancy (21). Fields and Fields (332) and Denning-Kendall et al. (255) reported that relaxin is produced by few luteal cells in cycling pigs (only 1–3%).

Blood levels. Levels of relaxin lower than those found during pregnancy were reported in blood obtained from the peripheral circulation (545) and utero-ovarian vein (571,666) during the luteal phase of the estrous cycle (Fig. 13). Levels of relaxin in utero-ovarian vein plasma were reported to increase by day 12, peak on days 15 to 16, and to be nearly undetectable by day 19 (666). The association of declining relaxin and progesterone levels between days 13 to 17 led Kotwica et al. (571) to postulate that relaxin secretion is associated with luteolysis in the cycling sow.

Pregnancy

Ovarian Source. The corpora lutea are the principal, and perhaps the sole, source of the relaxin secreted into the peripheral circulation during the approximately 114-day gestation period. Using immunohistochemical techniques, relaxin immunoactivity was found associated with the cytoplasm of cells from the corpora lutea but not other ovarian components (18,37,255,332,590) (Fig. 15A). Relaxin bioactivity levels within the corpora lutea were reported to increase steadily from about day 20 of pregnancy until about day 110 and then to decline rapidly within 16 h of birth (24,81) (Fig. 16). Consistent with these findings, ovarian relaxin mRNA levels were

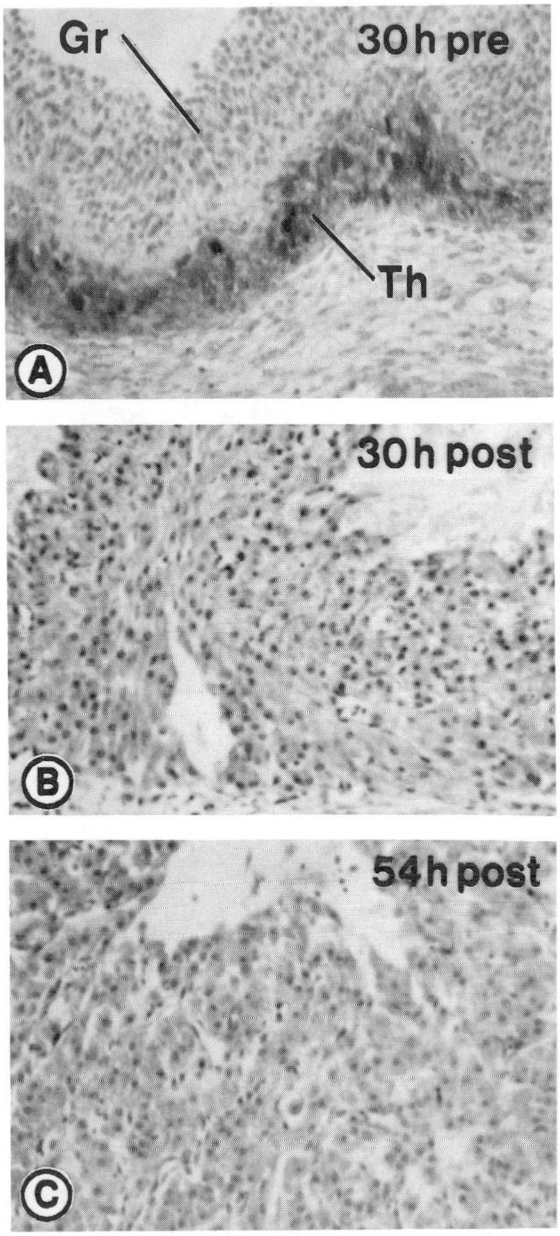

FIG. 14. Localization of relaxin immunoactivity in ovarian tissue of pregnant mare serum gonadotropin (PMSG)/human chorionic gonadotropin (hCG)-treated prepubertal pigs before and after ovulation. Light microscopy immunohistochemical localization of relaxin used rabbit antiporcine relaxin serum and the avidin-biotin immunoperoxidase method. **A:** Thirty hours before ovulation (84 h post-PMSG). Intense staining of theca interna (*Th*) layer of the follicle wall. (×200) **B:** Thirty hours after ovulation. Both theca interna and granulosa (*Gr*) cells demonstrate similar intensity of relaxin immunostaining. (×170) **C:** Fifty-four hours after ovulation. Relaxin immunostaining of luteal cells is homogeneous. Theca interna and granulosa cells are no longer distinguishable. (×170) Modified from ref. 44.

reported to be about 50-fold greater from day 40 to 90 of pregnancy than on day 13 of the estrous cycle and to decline about 1,000-fold by day 2 of lactation (49).

Although both theca interna and granulosa cells of the pig ovarian follicle contribute to the formation of the corpus luteum, the origin(s) of the cells that produce, store, and secrete relaxin in the fully developed corpus luteum of the pregnant pig are not known with certainty. It was postulated that the granulosa and theca layers give rise to the large and small luteal cells, respectively, which are found in the corpus luteum of the pregnant pig (189,213). Studies of immunohistochemical localization of relaxin in cycling gilts are consistent with this possibility. Bagnell et al. (44) found that the intensity of relaxin immunostaining in theca interna cells declined with luteinization (Fig. 14A and B), and large luteal cells, but not small luteal cells, show relaxin immunostaining (44,81,255,544,590). The large luteal cells have the organelles associated with both steroid and protein synthesis (19,81,82), and it seems likely that both progesterone and relaxin are produced by these cells.

Dense membrane-limited cytoplasmic granules (200–600 nm diameter) are observed within the luteal cells of pregnant pigs (Fig. 15B). Two lines of evidence indicate that relaxin is stored in these granules. First, the accumulation and disappearance of the cytoplasmic granules throughout pregnancy parallel that of relaxin bioactivity (24,81,484). Second, relaxin immunoactivity is associated with the cytoplasmic granules (214,332,544, 566,593) (Fig. 15C). The amount of relaxin stored within each granule may increase during pregnancy. Fields and Fields (332) reported that the apparent quantity of relaxin immunoactivity associated with each granule increased progressively from day 17 to day 106.

Ovarian sites other than the corpora lutea may produce small amounts of relaxin during pregnancy. Extremely low levels of relaxin bioactivity were found in follicular and interstitial tissue (24), and relaxin immunoactivity was found in follicular fluid in ovaries of pregnant animals (143,659). It was suggested that the relaxin in the follicles may result from transport of the hormone from adjacent corpora lutea or from *de novo* synthesis within the follicle (24,143). Consistent with the latter interpretation, intact follicles obtained from pregnant pigs secreted a relaxin-immunoactive substance(s) *in vitro* (143).

Regulation of Synthesis. The corpora lutea of the pregnant pig reach maximal size (≥450 mg) by day 8 (24) and produce not only relaxin but also the progesterone needed to maintain pregnancy throughout the approximately 114-day gestation period. Anderson and coworkers (23) demonstrated that maintenance of luteal function in the pig requires the secretion of pituitary gonadotropic hormones but not the presence of the conceptuses (21,24). In pigs with corpora lutea maintained beyond 100 days after either hysterectomy or the admin-

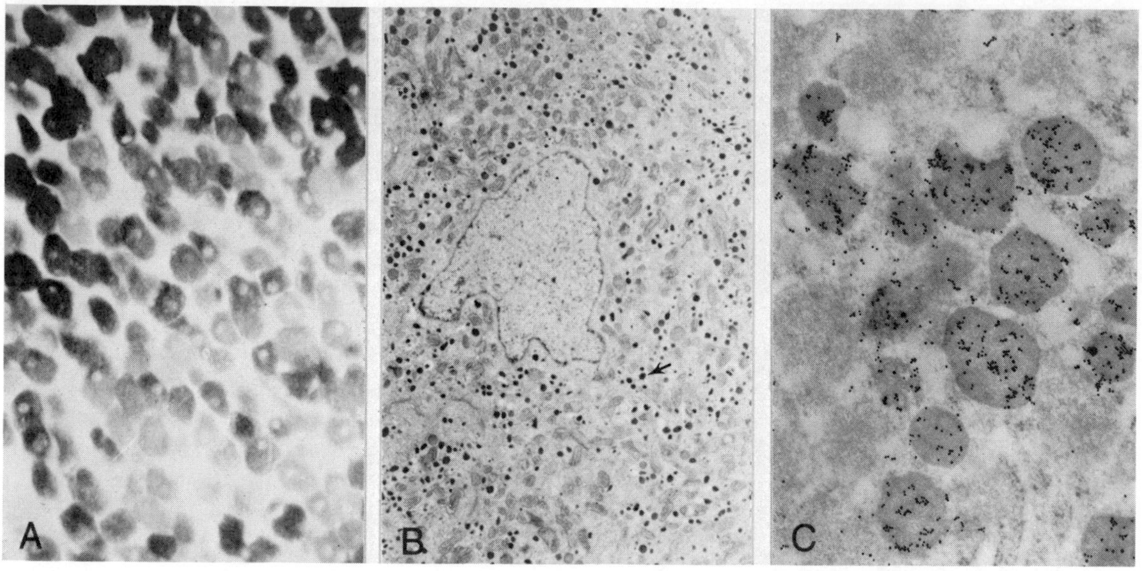

FIG. 15. A: Light microscopy immunohistochemical localization of relaxin in cytoplasm of pig luteal cells on day 106 of pregnancy using rabbit antiporcine relaxin serum and peroxidase–antiperoxidase as marker. Note that nuclei do not stain. From ref. 332, with permission. **B:** Electron microscopy of a portion of pig luteal cell on day 110 of pregnancy when granule content (*arrow*) is maximal. (×2,800) From ref. 81, with permission. **C:** Electron microscopy immunocytochemical localization of relaxin in pig luteal granules (200–600-nm diameter) on day 106 of pregnancy using rabbit antiporcine relaxin serum and goat antirabbit IgG-colloidal gold (10 nm) as marker. (×37,400) From ref. 332, with permission.

istration of estrogen during the luteal phase of the estrous cycle, the size (5), relaxin bioactivity levels (24), and relaxin immunoactivity levels of corpora lutea (21, 332,484), as well as serum progesterone levels (5), were similar to those of pregnant pigs. The observation that luteal relaxin levels are low during the estrous cycle (24,332,926,950) and increase steadily as the age of the corpora lutea increases in both hysterectomized and pregnant pigs (24,332), led to the postulation that the corpus luteum formed after ovulation is programmed for pregnancy and that luteal relaxin levels may be an indication

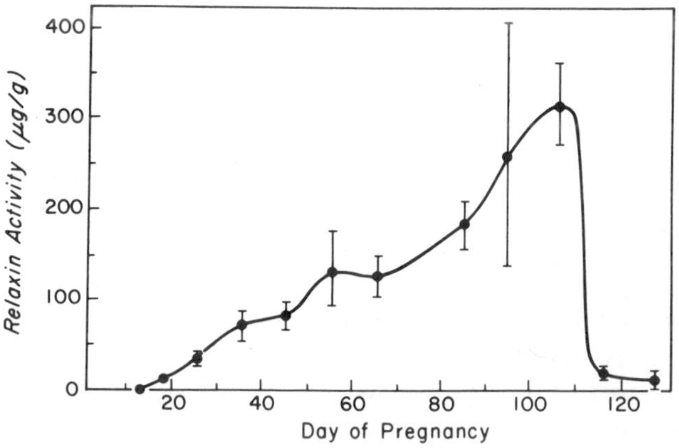

FIG. 16. Mean relaxin bioactivity levels (±SE) in corpora lutea throughout approximately 114-day pregnancy in the pig. From ref. 24, with permission.

of the luteal aging process (21,24,332). Consistent with this view, corpora lutea induced experimentally during late pregnancy had to be at least 15 days of age to release significant quantities of relaxin during the 2 days preceding birth (920).

There is recent evidence that luteal relaxin mRNA (624) and luteal relaxin immunoactivity levels (255) increase more than 100-fold between days 12 and 16 of pregnancy. The relationship, if any, between this dramatic amplification of relaxin gene expression and the presence of conceptuses remains to be demonstrated.

Blood Levels. The profile of relaxin levels in the peripheral blood throughout pregnancy is consistent with the view that relaxin accumulates within corpora lutea during most of pregnancy and is released during the rapid degranulation that occurs during the 2 days before birth (81). In 1971, Belt et al. (81) reported a sharp increase in relaxin bioactivity in plasma obtained from the ovarian vein between 44 and 26 h before birth. More recently, porcine relaxin radioimmunoassays were used to determine relaxin immunoactivity levels in peripheral blood during pregnancy (21,315,316,401,546,555,616, 809,910,923,993,1021,1040,1099,1102,1118). Plasma relaxin levels remain below 2 ng/ml until about day 100 and then increase gradually to approximately 10 ng/ml 3 days before delivery (21,910). During the 2 days before birth, relaxin levels increase markedly and attain maximal levels, which generally range from 50 to 250 ng/ml (315,316,401,546,555,616,809,908–910,922,923,927,

993,1021,1040,1099,1102,1118) (Fig. 17). In most cases, this antepartum surge in relaxin consists of two or three sustained peaks that last 10 to 20 h (555,809, 910,923,927,1099). The final peak, which has maximal relaxin levels, generally occurs 24 to 14 h before delivery (315,316,555,616,809,910,922,923,927,1021,1040, 1099,1102,1118). Relaxin levels then decline rapidly to about 10 ng/ml at birth (12,316,555,923,1102). It is not clear whether delivery influences the secretion of relaxin in the pig. Whereas one study found that peripheral blood relaxin immunoactivity levels fluctuated considerably during delivery (12), another study did not (923). More recently, Stone and co-workers (993) reported that levels of relaxin in utero-ovarian vein blood pulsed during delivery but did not coincide with expulsion of the piglets. Relaxin levels decline to less than 1 ng/ml by 24 to 48 h after delivery (316,791,910,922,923).

There has not been total agreement concerning the sizes of the relaxin-immunoactive components in the peripheral blood. One laboratory reported that 50% of the relaxin immunoactivity in serum obtained from pregnant sows was associated with components having greater than 40,000 molecular weight and that less than 30% was associated with a 6,300-Da component (143). In contrast, two other laboratories reported that essentially all the circulating relaxin had a molecular weight of approximately 6,300 (724,910). O'Byrne et al. (724) isolated circulating relaxin from 1 L of plasma obtained from sows on days 112 to 114 of pregnancy. The circulating relaxin had a molecular weight of 6,300, was equipotent with ovarian relaxin in the mouse interpubic ligament bioassay, and was microheterogeneous. The main form was CMa′ (Figs. 1 and 2), but other forms, including CMB, were also present. Thus, the forms of porcine relaxin in the peripheral blood appear to be those isolated from the ovary, and the levels of relaxin immunoactivity reflect levels of biologically active hormone.

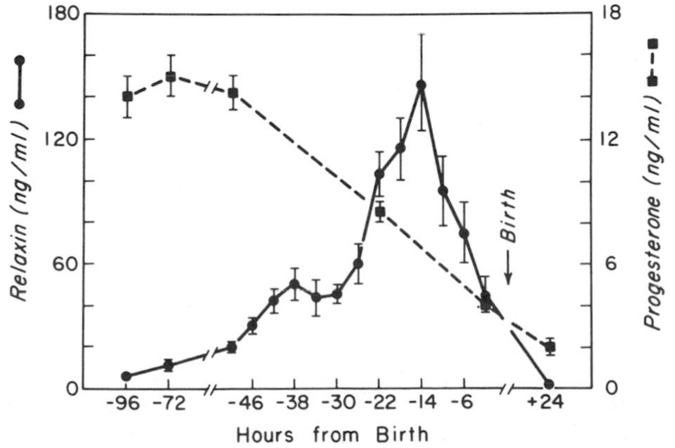

FIG. 17. Mean relaxin and progesterone immunoactivity levels (±SE) in peripheral blood plasma of pigs from 96 h before to 24 h after birth. From refs. 910 and 922, with permission.

In vivo *Studies of Regulation of Secretion.* Researchers have conducted little *in vivo* experimentation to understand the regulation of relaxin secretion throughout the first 110 days of pig pregnancy. We know more about the regulation of the antepartum surge in blood relaxin levels in the pig. The corpora lutea undergo functional regression during the 2 days that precede parturition as judged by a rapid fall in progesterone levels (38,669) (Fig. 17). Sherwood and co-workers (908,922,923) proposed that the simultaneous surge in blood relaxin levels is associated with luteal regression.

The factors that initiate functional luteolysis and the antepartum surge in relaxin levels are not known with certainty. There is evidence that the fetal pituitary-adrenal-placental system, which plays a role in the initiation of birth in the pig, may be involved. Destruction of the fetal pituitary (110) or fetal decapitation *in utero* (208,999) prolonged pregnancy and apparently did so by preventing the rapid and sustained luteolysis that normally occurs on approximately day 113 to day 115 (208). Fetal decapitation (908) and fetal hypophysectomy (543) also disrupted the normal close temporal association of the antepartum surge of relaxin levels and birth; the relaxin surge occurred at various intervals ranging up to 10 to 12 days before birth.

Anderson and co-workers (21,315,316,616,618,674) provided evidence that functional luteolysis and release of relaxin may occur, at least in part, independent of fetal control. When they prolonged the life-span of the corpora lutea by hysterectomizing pigs on day 6 of the estrous cycle, the timing of a decline in progesterone levels and surge in relaxin levels in the peripheral blood resembled the timing of these events in pregnant animals. There was a decline in progesterone levels from day 108 to day 114 (5,315,316,616,674) and an increase in relaxin to maximal levels on days 112 to 114 in the hysterectomized gilts (21,315,316,616) (Fig. 18). Anderson and co-workers (21,315,316,484) concluded that the initiation of the disappearance of cytoplasmic granules coincident with relaxin release in aging corpora lutea is, at least in part, a precisely timed, genetically controlled event related to the aging of the corpora lutea and independent of endocrine control by the conceptuses or uterus. Although genetic control may contribute to the timing of antepartum functional luteolysis and the antepartum release of relaxin, there are several indications that other factors are involved. First, both the duration of the antepartum relaxin surge and the apparent amounts of relaxin released into the plasma of pregnant pigs during the 4 days before birth were greater than those observed with hysterectomized gilts during the same period (315,316,616) (Fig. 18). Unlike pregnant pigs, in which peripheral blood progesterone and relaxin declined abruptly to basal levels by 1 day postpartum on about day 116, in hysterectomized gilts progesterone and relaxin levels declined less abruptly to reach basal levels

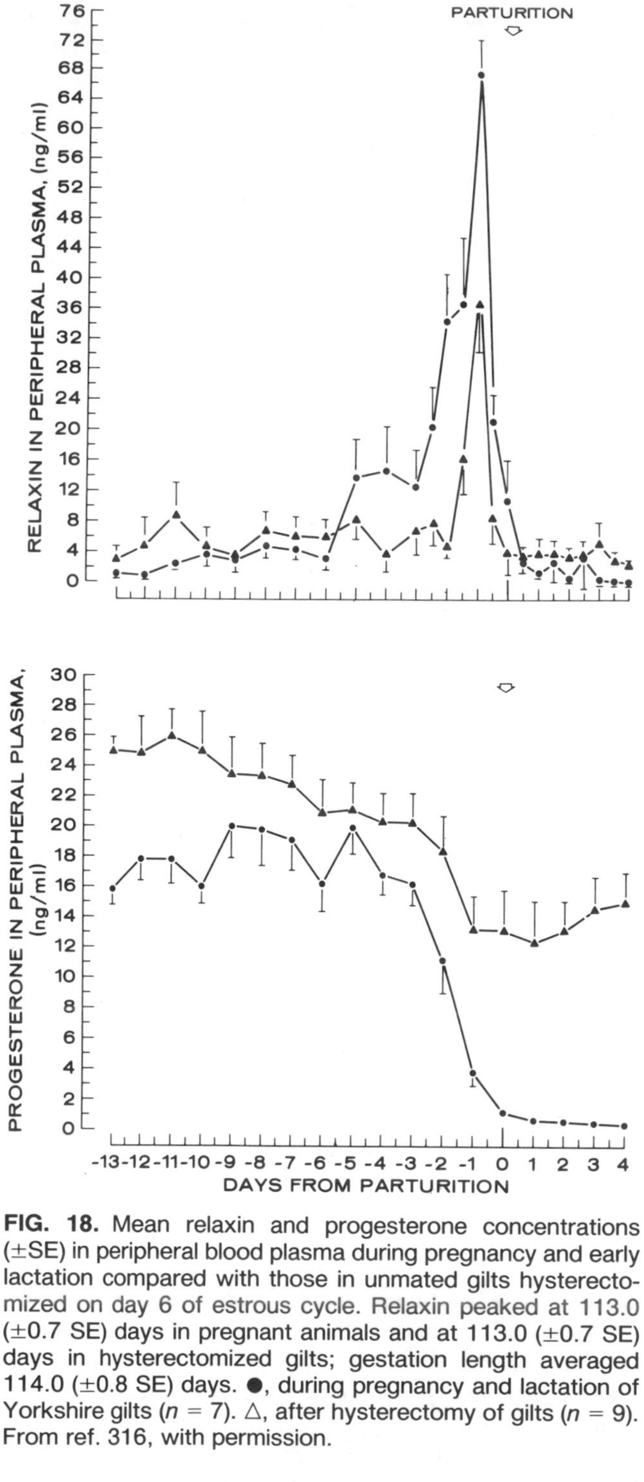

FIG. 18. Mean relaxin and progesterone concentrations (±SE) in peripheral blood plasma during pregnancy and early lactation compared with those in unmated gilts hysterectomized on day 6 of estrous cycle. Relaxin peaked at 113.0 (±0.7 SE) days in pregnant animals and at 113.0 (±0.7 SE) days in hysterectomized gilts; gestation length averaged 114.0 (±0.8 SE) days. ●, during pregnancy and lactation of Yorkshire gilts (*n* = 7). △, after hysterectomy of gilts (*n* = 9). From ref. 316, with permission.

after day 140 (5,21,315,316,484,616,674) (Fig. 18). Serum relaxin levels in hysterectomized gilts were higher than those in postpartum pigs until day 150 (21). Also, the corpora lutea in hysterectomized gilts (averaging greater than 450 mg) remained larger on days 124 and 136 than the corpora lutea in lactating gilts (averaging less than 75 mg) (5). Finally, the observation that there was an antepartum surge in plasma relaxin levels in pregnant pigs possessing only induced corpora lutea that were about 30 days of age supports the view that factors other than aging influence the release of relaxin from the corpora lutea during late pregnancy (920).

The putative factor(s) that promotes luteolysis, the antepartum surge in relaxin levels, and birth can be carried in the systemic circulation, because these events occurred at the appropriate time in pigs whose ovaries were transplanted to the external surface of the abdominal wall (656,921). Neither the nature nor the source of the blood-borne factor(s) that promotes the antepartum release of relaxin is known. Pituitary prolactin does not appear to be the factor. In fact, there is evidence that the antepartum surge in prolactin levels that coincides with the antepartum surge in relaxin levels (546,1021) has luteotropic rather than luteolytic effects on aging corpora lutea. Anderson and co-workers (618) demonstrated that corpora lutea undergo immediate luteolysis, as judged by both rapidly falling progesterone levels and a surge in relaxin levels, after hypophysectomy on day 110 in hysterectomized gilts, but that luteolysis does not occur in hypophyseal stalk transectioned gilts where plasma prolactin levels do not decline. Anderson and co-workers further demonstrated that administering porcine prolactin from days 110 to 120 to hysterectomized gilts (315) or hysterectomized plus hypophysectomized gilts increased plasma relaxin and plasma progesterone levels relative to controls throughout the 10-day treatment period (618). Also supportive of the view that prolactin does not promote luteolysis at term is the observation that the administration of bromocriptine prevented the antepartum prolactin surge but not the antepartum relaxin surge in pregnant pigs (1021). Whereas intravenous infusion of oxytocin for 6 h on day 110 elicited a rapid, sevenfold increase in relaxin levels in ovarian venous plasma (24), there is no evidence that endogenous oxytocin promotes the release of relaxin during late pregnancy in the pig. A most likely source of the luteolytic signal is the uterus and/or conceptuses, because luteal function terminates on about day 114 in pregnant gilts, whereas luteal function merely diminishes at this time in hysterectomized gilts (5,315).

Two lines of evidence indicate that prostaglandins (PGs) are factors that contribute to luteolysis and the antepartum surge in relaxin levels. First, prolonged infusion of $PGF_{2\alpha}$ on day 110 (922) or intramuscular injection of the synthetic PGs clinoprost tromethamine (Lutalyse, UpJohn, Kalamazoo, MI) or cloprostenol (Estrumate, Coopers Agrophorm, Willowdale, Ontario) on day 112 (555,1120) in quantities sufficient to induce delivery within 30 h triggered both a rapid drop in progesterone and a surge in relaxin levels in the peripheral plasma. Second, inhibition of prostaglandin synthesis by administration of the cyclooxygenase inhibitor indomethacin for 6 or 7 days during late pregnancy delayed luteolysis, the antepartum relaxin surge, and birth until 2 to 5 days after the termination of indomethacin administration (695,922,1021) (Fig. 19). Although administering the prostaglandin synthesis inhibitor meclofenamic acid daily from day 109 to day 113 failed to influence luteolysis and birth in pregnant pigs in one study, the authors concluded that a larger dose of the meclofenamic acid may have been required under the experimental conditions used (401).

There is reason to suspect that the main surge in PGs released by the uterus at term is not the luteolytic signal. Blood levels of the $PGF_{2\alpha}$ metabolite 13,14 dihydro-15-keto prostaglandin $F_{2\alpha}$ peak during the day of delivery and after the decline in progesterone levels and/or surge in relaxin levels that occur at luteolysis (401,695,809, 930,1102,1118). It was postulated that $PGF_{2\alpha}$ may reach the ovary through the mesosalpinx (572) or that repeated small pulses of $PGF_{2\alpha}$ that do not result in significantly increased PG metabolite levels in the peripheral blood may trigger luteolysis (809). Perhaps uterine PGs or other factors trigger PG synthesis in the ovary. Porcine corpora lutea can synthesize $PGF_{2\alpha}$ (415,758), and it has been postulated that intraluteal PGs may be responsible for regression of the corpora lutea (759,836) and release of relaxin (1102,1118). PGs do not appear to promote the release of relaxin through a reduction in progesterone production. Antepartum relaxin concentrations increase before progesterone declines in the maternal plasma (1021,1118). Moreover, elevation of blood progestin levels by administration of progesterone or medroxyprogesterone acetate from day 110 to 115 (927), day 111 to 116 (1021), or day 112 to 114 (1118) delayed delivery but not the time of occurrence of either the antepartum surge in relaxin levels (927,1021,1118) or, in the case of medroxyprogesterone acetate treatment, decline in progesterone levels (1118).

It is not known whether luteolysis and the antepartum release of relaxin are initiated by common or separate PG-mediated mechanisms. Brief infusions of low doses of $PGF_{2\alpha}$ by jugular vein (694) or ovarian artery (45) on day 108 of gestation caused an immediate surge in relaxin levels that lasted for 1 to 1.5 h but failed to reduce progesterone levels. This may indicate that luteolysis and the release of relaxin are mediated by separate mechanisms. Alternatively, both luteolysis and the release of relaxin may be mediated by common initial steps, perhaps at the level of the plasma membrane and beyond, with divergence at subsequent steps that influence cholesterol transport or pregnenolone synthesis (694). According to this hypothesis, brief infusion of a low dose of $PGF_{2\alpha}$ would be sufficient to trigger the release of relaxin from a portion of the cytoplasmic storage granules but would not be adequate to influence severely cellular mechanisms associated with steroid biosynthesis. Finally, it may be that luteal cells on day 108 of gestation release some relaxin in response to $PGF_{2\alpha}$ but have not undergone the maturational changes that make them as

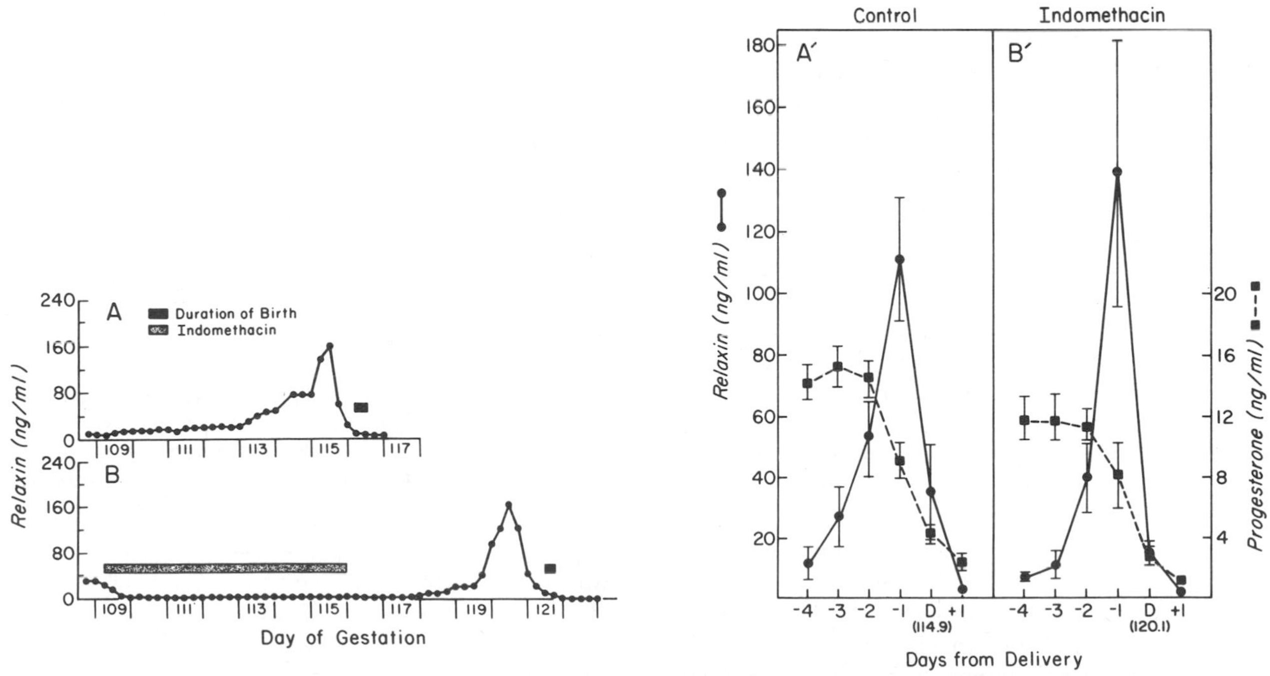

FIG. 19. Relaxin levels in peripheral blood plasma of (**A**) an untreated pig and (**B**) a pregnant pig injected intramuscularly twice each day from day 109 to day 116 with indomethacin at a dose of 4 mg/kg. Mean relaxin and progesterone concentrations (±SE; $n = 5$) in (**A′**) control pigs that delivered on day 114.9 ± 0.05 SE and (**B′**) indomethacin-treated pigs that delivered on day 120.1 ± 0.4 SE. From ref. 922, with permission.

susceptible to the luteolytic effects of $PGF_{2\alpha}$ as is the case on day 113 or 114 of gestation.

In vitro *Studies of Regulation of Secretion.* Beginning in 1987, Taylor and co-workers conducted a series of studies designed to not only identify the factors that influence the secretion of relaxin from porcine luteal cells but also to understand the intracellular pathways that transduce the secretion of relaxin (1023–1036). They used a reverse hemolytic plaque assay (RHPA) that detects the release of relaxin from individual luteal cells cultured in monolayer for these studies. With the RHPA (1035), monodispersed luteal cells, generally derived from pigs between day 26 and day 69 of gestation, are combined with protein A-labeled ovine erythrocytes, placed in a chamber on a microscope slide, and incubated overnight. The following day, the chamber is washed and filled with Dulbeco's modified Eagle's Medium—0.1% bovine serum albumin containing porcine relaxin antiserum and the secretagogue or other test substance of interest. After incubation periods ranging from 0.5 to 18 h, each chamber is filled with guinea pig serum as a source of complement and incubated for 50 min to allow hemolysis of ovine erythrocytes or so-called plaque formation around relaxin-releasing large luteal cells (Fig. 20A,B). Using the RHPA, small luteal cells do not release relaxin, but a maximum of approximately 50% of large luteal cells (20–70 μm) do (1033,1035,1036). The influence of compounds of interest on the amount of relaxin released over time is determined by measuring the rate of plaque formation (Fig. 20C), and in some cases, the total amount of relaxin released is determined by measuring total plaque area.

Using the RHPA, Taylor and co-workers found that hCG inhibited relaxin release from luteal cells, whereas oxytocin had no detectable effect (1023). In contrast, $PGF_{2\alpha}$, PGE_2, and prostacyclin (PGI_2) consistently stimulated the rate of plaque formation (1023–1025,1028, 1029,1031,1034,1035) (Fig. 20C). $PGF_{2\alpha}$, PGE_2, and/or PGI_2 could be produced locally to stimulate relaxin release, because luteal tissue possesses an active cyclooxygenase pathway, which is an obligatory enzyme in the conversion of arachidonic acid to PGs (439). Consistent with this possibility, either arachidonic acid or phospholipase A_2 and melittin, two agents that liberate endogenous arachidonic acid, stimulated relaxin release from luteal cells (1029,1033). Moreover, the stimulating effect of arachidonic acid on relaxin release was almost wholly blocked by the cyclo-oxygenase inhibitor ibuprofen (1029). It is not clear how to reconcile the findings described above with the observation that the cyclooxygenase inhibitors indomethacin, ibuprofen, and diclofenac sodium did not change the rate of basal relaxin release from luteal cells (1024). Basic fibroblast growth factor and transforming growth factor-β are produced in the corpora lutea (373,405), and both growth factors were reported to inhibit basal and PGE_2-stimulated relaxin release in the RHPA (1031,1032). Relaxin, but not

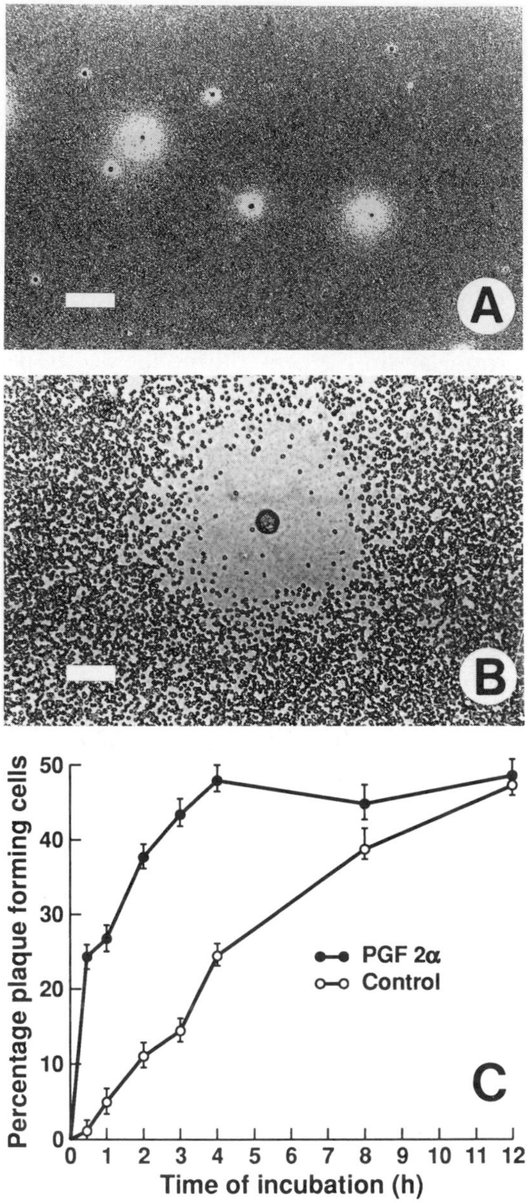

FIG. 20. A: Photomicrograph of monolayer containing sheep red blood cells and luteal cells derived from a day-26 pregnant pig, subjected to reverse hemolytic plaque assay for relaxin using 4-h incubation. Note presence of both plaque-forming and nonplaque-forming luteal cells. Magnification bar is 250 μm. **B:** Higher power view demonstrates typical plaque, a zone of hemolysis that contains ghosts of red blood cells around a relaxin-releasing large luteal cell. Magnification bar is 50 μm. **C:** Percentage of plaque-forming cells detected in monolayers incubated for 0.5 to 12 h in presence or absence of $PGF_{2\alpha}$ (1×10^{-6} M). Values are mean ± SE of triplicate slides from an individual experiment in which luteal cells were derived from a day-26 pregnant pig. Modified from ref. 1035.

progesterone, also inhibited basal relaxin release in the RHPA, and it was postulated that relaxin may have an autoregulatory influence on its own release (1026).

The second messengers that transduce the effect of secretogogues on relaxin secretion from luteal cells are poorly understood. There is limited evidence that activation of protein kinase C provides a mechanism that regulates relaxin secretion. The tumor-promoting agent phorbol 12-myristate 13-acetate and the synthetic 1,2-diacylglycerol 1-oleoyl-2-acetyl-rac-glycerol activate calcium-dependent protein kinase C, and both compounds stimulated relaxin release from luteal cells (1027,1033). There is also evidence that intracellular redistribution of calcium from endoplasmic reticulum may regulate relaxin release. The calcium mobilizing agent A23187 increased the rate of plaque formation, and this stimulatory effect on relaxin release was inhibited by the calcium channel blocker cobalt (1025). The source of calcium that influences relaxin secretion appears to be intracellular stores within the endoplasmic reticulum. Neither basal nor modulated relaxin secretion was found to be dependent on the presence of calcium in the medium (1025,1034). Also, incubation of luteal cells with hapsigargin, a compound thought to increase intracellular calcium by enhancing leakage of calcium from the endoplasmic reticulum, promoted a dose-dependent increase in relaxin secretion; whereas incubation with dantrolene, a compound thought to reduce calcium release from the endoplasmic reticulum, induced a dose-dependent inhibition of relaxin release (1034). In contrast to the above findings, treatment of luteal cells with dibutyryl cyclic AMP and dibutyryl cyclic guanosine monophosphate (GMP) resulted in a prompt inhibition in the rate of plaque formation (1028). Events triggered by second messengers to promote relaxin release are not known. Taylor and Clark (1030) postulated that microtubule-assisted transport may form an important intracellular mechanism that assists basal release of relaxin, because exposure of luteal cell monolayers to colchicine and vinblastine, two compounds that inhibit microtubule formation, reduced the rate of plaque formation in the RHPA.

Huang et al. (484) examined the effects of LH, prolactin, and dibutyryl cyclic AMP on relaxin secretion in cultured luteal cells obtained from gilts during late pregnancy. These workers (484) found that all three compounds promoted relaxin secretion from luteal cells obtained on day 110 of pregnancy, but not from luteal cells obtained on days 113 and 116. The findings that LH and prolactin promote relaxin secretion *in vitro* are consistent with this group's earlier *in vivo* findings (315,618), but the observation that LH and dibutyryl cyclic AMP promote relaxin secretion from luteal cells obtained on day 110 is not consistent with findings with the RHPA assay using corpora lutea obtained between days 26 and 69 of pregnancy (1023,1028). The reason for this apparent difference in findings is not known. Taylor et al. (1035) demonstrated that the rate of basal relaxin secretion from porcine luteal cells differs with the age of the cells. Perhaps the factors that regulate the secretion of relaxin from luteal cells differ with the stage of pregnancy.

Clearance of Relaxin from the Blood. The clearance half-life for porcine relaxin immunoactivity demonstrates characteristics of a multiexponential curve. From 60 to 180 min after the intravenous injection of highly purified porcine relaxin into an ovariectomized gilt, the terminal clearance half-life was about 70 min (907).

Extraovarian Production of Relaxin. There is limited evidence that small amounts of relaxin may also be produced by extraovarian sites during pregnancy. Anthony and co-workers (1164) reported the detection of pregnancy-dependent relaxin immunoactivity in uterine luminal and glandular epithelium and relaxin mRNA in endometrium obtained on day 16 in pregnant gilts (day 0 = first day of estrus; Fig. 13). Relaxin may also be produced in the pituitary. Relaxin immunoactivity was identified in the neurohypophysis of both male and female pigs (41) as well as in effluent from intact neural lobes immersed in normal Locke's solution (844,845).

Lactation

Levels of relaxin within the corpora lutea are extremely low during lactation (24). Bagnell et al. (49) detected low levels of a 1-kb relaxin transcript in ovaries obtained on day 2 of lactation by Northern analysis; and although the hybridization signal was markedly reduced compared with that before parturition, relaxin mRNA could still be detected. Consistent with the above observations, relaxin immunostaining was detected in a few cells within corpora lutea on day 2 or 4 of lactation (48,491). Thereafter, relaxin immunoactivity continued to decline steadily, and it was essentially nondetectable by day 14 of lactation on fixed ovarian sections (48,491) and in extracts of corpora lutea (491).

Small and diminishing amounts of relaxin appear to be secreted during the first few days of lactation in the pig. Two laboratories reported that plasma relaxin levels were less than 0.3 ng/ml by day 2 of lactation and not detectable by the fourth day of lactation (491,791,793). All laboratories are not in agreement concerning the influence of suckling on relaxin secretion. One group reported that acute and transient spikes in plasma relaxin occur with suckling or administration of oxytocin in lactating sows from day 6 to day 33 of lactation and that the source of the relaxin was the old corpora lutea of pregnancy (12,1119). Inconsistent with that finding, three laboratories reported that relaxin levels were extremely low to nondetectable in blood samples collected at intervals as short as 1 or 2 min during lactation and that relaxin levels were not influenced by suckling (545,793,923). Consistent with the latter finding, Hunter et al. (491) reported that oxytocin did not influence relaxin secretion from cultures of luteal cells obtained on days 4, 14, and 21 of lactation. It is hard to reconcile the reported acute and transient spikes in plasma relaxin levels between days 6 and 33 of lactation (12,1119) with the many reports of low relaxin levels in both the corpora lutea and blood during lactation (24,48,49,491,545,791, 793,923). Also, the apparent clearance half-life for relaxin immunoactivity in lactating pigs of less than 20 sec (1119) is exceedingly faster than the terminal clearance half-life of about 70 min reported for porcine relaxin (907,912).

Horse

The placenta is the main, and perhaps the sole, source of relaxin in the horse (*Equus caballus*) (982,986). Unlike corpora lutea of the pregnant pig, the placenta of the pregnant horse does not store much relaxin during pregnancy (see Table 1). Stewart and co-workers initially measured relaxin immunoactivity in the peripheral serum of horses throughout pregnancy and at parturition with a porcine relaxin radioimmunoassay (983, 985,986). Since 1986, however, they have used a homologous equine relaxin radioimmunoassay (649,974,975). Interestingly, the profiles of plasma relaxin immunoactivity throughout the approximately 350-day gestation period show marked among-breed differences in both amount and form (Fig. 21). Relaxin immunoactivity is detectable by about day 80 in standardbreds, thoroughbreds, and ponies, but concentrations rise from baseline earlier in standardbreds than in thoroughbreds or ponies. Peak concentrations on about day 175 are approximately 100 ng/ml in standardbreds, and they are higher than levels in thoroughbreds. Thoroughbred mares exhibit a nadir in relaxin concentrations around day 225 of gestation, but standardbred mares do not. In thoroughbred mares, relaxin immunoactivity levels increase throughout the last approximately 125 days of gestation, whereas relaxin levels decline gradually from about day 175 to foaling in standardbreds. Pony mares have much lower levels of relaxin immunoactivity than both standardbreds and thoroughbreds, and unlike these two breeds, relaxin immunoactivity levels in ponies increase gradually from day 115 to foaling. An antepartum elevation in relaxin levels may occur in horses. A surge in relaxin levels was reported to occur from a few hours before birth until the placenta is expelled with spontaneous or oxytocin-induced foaling in thoroughbred mares (974,980) and with oxytocin-induced foaling in domestic donkeys (*Equus asinus*) (975). No increase in plasma relaxin levels was observed when standardbred mares were induced to abort with oxytocin at midpregnancy (649). Plasma relaxin levels were low in each of three standardbred mares with abnormal termination of pregnancy, and it was postulated that relaxin may, as an indicator of placental function, be used to assess at-risk pregnancies in the mare (975).

Cow

Corpora lutea apparently produce relaxin in the pregnant cow (*Bos taurus*). Luteal cells from pregnant cows stained positively for relaxin with an immunohistochemical method that used an antiporcine relaxin serum (323). Unlike the pig, the corpora lutea in the cow store little relaxin. There is no evidence that luteal cells in the cow contain relaxin storage granules, and the levels of

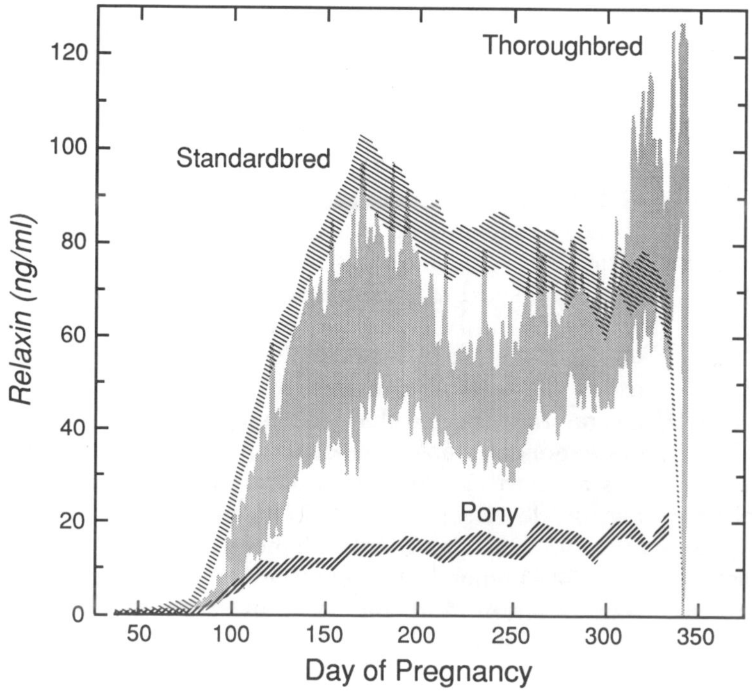

FIG. 21. Plasma relaxin concentrations throughout approximately 340-day pregnancy in thoroughbred mares (n = 4), standardbred mares (n = 21), and pony mares (n = 10). Modified from ref. 975.

relaxin bioactivity in extracts of corpora lutea obtained from pregnant cows were reported to be extremely low or nondetectable (19,323,324,327). The placenta in cows also produces little, if any, relaxin (19,323,324).

Limitations associated with the methods available for determining relaxin levels in the peripheral blood preclude a good understanding of the secretion of relaxin during pregnancy in the cow. In 1955, Wada and Yuhara (1083,1084) reported that relaxin bioactivity was present in the blood of pregnant cows. Using the guinea pig pubic symphysis palpation bioassay, relaxin levels were reported to increase steadily from the first month, plateau during the last trimester, and fall rapidly to nondetectable levels within a few days after parturition on about day 280 (1083,1084,1087). When porcine relaxin radioimmunoassays were used, however, relaxin immunoactivity levels were reported to be low (25,675,676,810) or nondetectable (168,925) during late pregnancy. Anderson and co-workers reported that relaxin levels generally peaked at concentrations ranging from 1 to 2 ng equivalents of porcine relaxin/ml between days 5 to 1 prepartum (25,676,810) and that there were breed differences in prepartum blood levels of relaxin (673,810).

Sheep

Porter and co-workers provided reason to think that the sheep (*Ovis aries*) produces relaxin when they demonstrated that the sheep uterus is responsive to the hormone. In 1981, Porter et al. (792) reported that the administration of porcine relaxin directly into the uterine artery of ovariectomized estrogen-primed ewes inhibited spontaneous uterine contractions. Nevertheless, a source of relaxin during the approximately 150-day gestation period in sheep remains to be established. Investigators are not in agreement concerning the possibility that low amounts of relaxin are produced by the ovary in pregnant ewes. It was reported that relaxin-specific immunofluorescence was observed in luteal cells of pregnant ewes (280) and that both crude ovarian extracts (792,1100) and partially purified ovarian extracts (817,1100) from pregnant ewes contained apparent low levels of a substance that cross-reacted in porcine relaxin radioimmunoassays. In contrast to these findings, relaxin immunoactivity was not detected in either sections of ovarian tissue with an antiserum to highly purified porcine relaxin using the avidin-biotin-immunoperoxidase localization technique or in sera collected in the ovarian vein draining the ovary containing the corpus luteum of pregnancy with a homologous porcine relaxin radioimmunoassay (817). Also, extracts of ovarian tissue obtained from ewes during late pregnancy demonstrated no relaxin bioactivity in mouse or rat uterine contractility bioassays (792,817).

Two groups also reported that low amounts of relaxin are produced in the placenta and endometrium in sheep. Fractions obtained after gel filtration of extracts of both placentomes and endometrium were reported to contain low levels of relaxin immunoactivity in porcine relaxin radioimmunoassays (817,1100), and most of the immunoactivity was associated with a 6,000-Da component (1100). Whereas early efforts to identify relaxin bioactivity in extracts of placentomes and endometrium were not successful (792,817), Wathes et al. (1100) reported that the 6,000-Da peak obtained after gel filtration of placentome extracts was bioactive in the *in vitro* mouse uterine contractility bioassay. Because the placentomes are larger by weight and contain higher apparent concentrations of relaxin immunoactivity (about 3 ng Eq porcine relaxin/g tissue) than endometrial or ovarian tissue (about 1 ng Eq porcine relaxin/g tissue), Wathes et al. (1100) postulated that the placentomes are the main source of relaxin in the pregnant ewe.

Recent findings appear to provide an explanation for the inability of many investigators to demonstrate convincingly the presence of relaxin in the sheep. Roche and co-workers (832) demonstrated the presence of a single copy gene that produces a relaxinlike mRNA. This mRNA, which is found in low abundance and only in the placenta, has many stop codons in the region corresponding to the C peptide (Fig. 8). Because there is no open reading frame that would allow translation through the C-peptide and A-chain regions, the mRNA transcript is not able to encode a functional relaxin molecule.

Reports concerning the secretion of relaxin in sheep are inconsistent. Using the guinea pig pubic symphysis palpation bioassay, blood relaxin levels were reported to increase steadily from the first month, plateau during the last month, and fall rapidly to nondetectable levels within a few days after parturition on about day 150 (1085). Inconsistent with this finding, relaxin bioactivity was not found in the blood of sheep during the last 2 months of pregnancy with the mouse interpubic ligament bioassay (430). Whereas one group that used a radioimmunoassay developed with crude porcine relaxin reported surges in relaxin immunoactivity during birth and suckling (141), a second group that used a radioimmunoassay developed with highly purified porcine relaxin found little or no relaxin immunoactivity in the serum during middle or late gestation (817).

This reviewer cannot with certainty account for the many inconsistencies in the literature concerning the presence or absence of relaxin in putative source tissues and blood in sheep. Collectively, however, the findings described above can be interpreted to indicate that the sheep placenta once produced bioactive relaxin but, during the course of evolution, ceased to do so.

Goat

Nearly nothing is known about relaxin in the domestic goat (*Capra hircus*). A source of relaxin in the goat has not been reported. In 1956, Wada and Yuhara (1085) reported that relaxin bioactivity was present in the blood of pregnant goats. Using the guinea pig pubic symphysis palpation bioassay, relaxin levels were reported to increase steadily from the first month, plateau during the last month, and fall rapidly to nondetectable levels within a few days after parturition on about day 150 (1085).

Chicken

An early report by Hisaw and Zarrow in 1950 (467) that extracts of chicken (*Gallus domesticus*) ovaries contain relaxinlike bioactivity in the guinea pig pubic symphysis palpation bioassay has received limited support. In 1985, Brackett et al. (114) reported that a peptide purified from active, deyolked hen ovaries had a molecular weight similar to that of porcine relaxin, exhibited relaxin immunoactivity in a homologous porcine relaxin radioimmunoassay, and had relaxin bioactivity in the mouse uterine contractility bioassay. Moreover, an immunocytochemical localization technique that used an antiserum to highly purified porcine relaxin demonstrated that relaxin immunoactivity was associated with granulosa cells (114).

Cat

In 1929, Hisaw (462) reported that the blood of pregnant cats (*Felix catus*) contained a substance that demonstrated relaxinlike bioactivity in the guinea pig pubic symphysis palpation bioassay. In 1985, Stewart and Stabenfeldt (984) determined the general profile of relaxin immunoactivity in the peripheral blood plasma of cats throughout the approximately 65-day gestation period with a homologous porcine relaxin radioimmunoassay

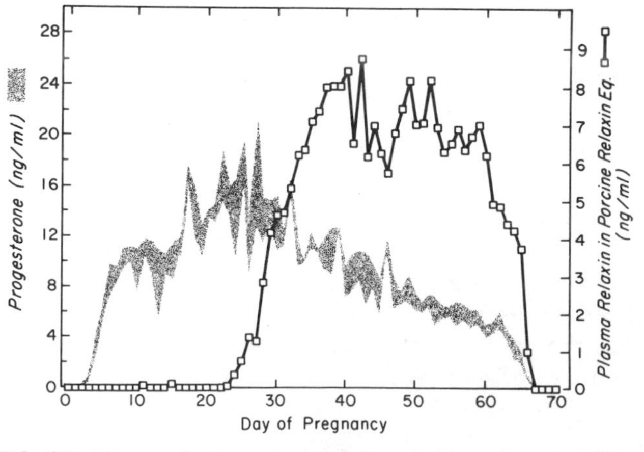

FIG. 22. Mean relaxin and progesterone immunoactivity levels (±SE; $n = 3$) in peripheral blood plasma during the approximately 65-day pregnancy in the cat. Relaxin immunoactivity was measured with a homologous porcine relaxin radioimmunoassay. From ref. 984, with permission.

(Fig. 22). Relaxin immunoactivity levels become detectable on about day 20, rise from about day 25 to maximal levels by about day 35, remain stable until just before parturition, and then decline sharply to undetectable levels by 24 h after delivery. The primary source of relaxin in the cat appears to be the placenta. Relaxin immunoactivity levels were higher in extracts of placentas obtained at days 28, 35, and near term than they were in uterine or luteal extracts (10). Moreover, ovariectomy on days 23 to 26 or days 40 to 44 did not influence relaxin levels in the peripheral blood (10). Placental relaxin levels may reflect the extent of placental sufficiency. In pregnant cats with dietary taurine deficiency, placental relaxin levels were reported to deviate from normal by day 25 in cats that aborted (259).

Dog

The placenta appears to be the main source of relaxin during the approximately 60- to 65-day pregnancy in dogs (*Canis familiaris*), but the ovary may also be a source. Relaxin bioactivity was detected in both homogenates of placentas obtained on day 60 of pregnancy and in homogenates of ovaries obtained on day 28 or 35 of pregnancy with the guinea pig pubic symphysis palpation bioassay (956). Relaxin immunoactivity was reported to be present in homogenates of placentas in greater amounts than in homogenates of corpora lutea when determined with homologous porcine relaxin radioimmunoassays (979,1055). Steinetz and co-workers (955–957) and Tsutsui and Stewart (1055) used porcine relaxin radioimmunoassays to demonstrate that relaxin immunoactivity becomes detectable in the peripheral serum during the fourth week of pregnancy and that relaxin levels remain elevated throughout the remainder of gestation (Fig. 23A). The secretion of relaxin in the dog is pregnancy-dependent; relaxin was not detected in the peripheral blood of cycling, hysterectomized, or pseudopregnant bitches (955,957,1055) (Fig. 23A). The observation that relaxin immunoactivity in the peripheral blood remains elevated after ovariectomy between days 28 to 50 of gestation was interpreted to indicate that the placenta secretes relaxin during pregnancy (955,1055) (Fig. 23B). Interestingly, serum levels of relaxin do not appear to decline as abruptly at term in dogs as they do in other species that have been investigated (957,1055). Serum relaxin levels were reported to decline gradually over several weeks of lactation in both Labrador retrievers and beagles (957). Steinetz and co-workers (955,956) postulated that both the placenta and the ovary secrete relaxin during pregnancy. Their observations that levels of serum relaxin in ovariectomized pregnant bitches were somewhat lower than in intact bitches and that circulating relaxin was detectable for several weeks during lactation were interpreted to indicate that the ovary secretes small quantities of relaxin during both

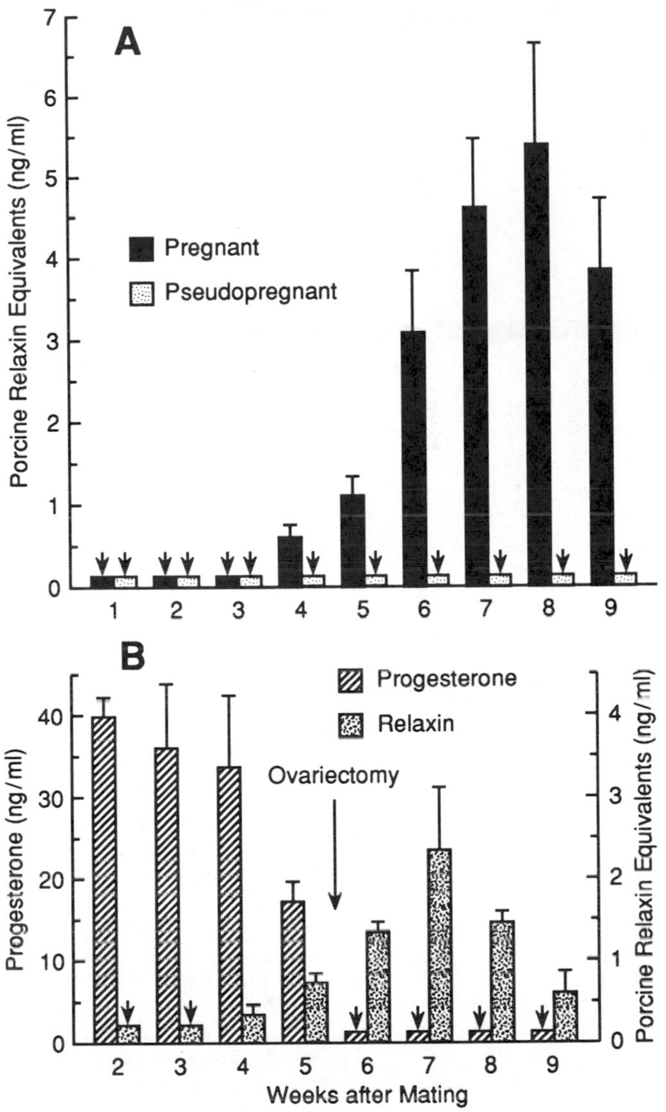

FIG. 23. A: Mean serum relaxin concentrations (±SE; n = 6–12) in pregnant and pseudopregnant bitches. ↓, less than minimal detectable concentration. **B:** Mean serum relaxin and progesterone concentrations (+SE; n = 3) in ovariectomized, pregnant bitches in which pregnancy was maintained by daily administration of 17α-ethyl-19-nortestosterone. ↓, less than minimal detectable concentrations. Modified from ref. 955.

pregnancy and lactation (957). The physiologic role of relaxin during lactation in the dog, if any, is unknown. Goldsmith et al. (395) provided limited evidence that relaxin is contained in the milk of lactating bitches and is absorbed into the circulation of suckling newborn pups.

Laboratory Species

Rat

Estrous Cycle

Both relaxin immunoactivity levels (926) and preprorelaxin mRNA levels (233) are extremely low, but detectable, in ovarian extracts obtained during the estrous cycle in rats (*Rattus norvegicus*). They are both maximal at estrus (233,926).

Pseudopregnancy

In deciduoma-bearing pseudopregnant rats, in which luteal function and elevated progesterone levels are maintained approximately 18 days, ovarian relaxin levels are approximately 20-fold greater than those in cycling rats (926), but they are extremely low compared with those in the ovaries of pregnant rats after day 10 (22,912,926).

Pregnancy

Ovarian Source. As in the pig, the corpora lutea in rats are the source of both the relaxin (28–30,328,336,400,487,565) and progesterone (457,1058) released into the peripheral blood during the approximately 23-day gestation period. Ovarian levels of relaxin bioactivity, relaxin immunoactivity, prorelaxin immunoactivity, and preprorelaxin mRNA increase from about day 10 to maximal levels 2 or 3 days before birth and then decline rapidly to low levels by 2 days postpartum (22,232,487,912,940) (Fig. 24A). Immunohistochemical localization of relaxin with an antiserum to rat relaxin (336,400,580) and hybridization-histochemical localization of rat relaxin mRNA with a rat relaxin-specific cDNA probe (487) identified the corpora lutea, but not other ovarian elements, as the ovarian source of relaxin during the second half of pregnancy. Unlike the pig, relaxin immunostaining was associated with both small (20–25-μm diameter) and large (>25-μm diameter) luteal cells (336,400). It is not clear whether rat luteal cells are derived from both granulosa and theca cells (764) or only from granulosa cells (671). As in the pig, both relaxin and progesterone are probably produced by the same cell, because the luteal cells have organelles associated with both protein and steroid synthesis (626).

Rat relaxin is stored in a manner similar to that of porcine relaxin. There is conclusive evidence that rat relaxin is stored in the cytoplasm of luteal cells in small, membrane-bound granules (100–270-nm diameter). These cytoplasmic granules, which are smaller than lysosomal granules, are first observed on day 14, occur in discrete clusters, become most abundant during the last third of gestation, and disappear within 3 days of parturition (336,626). This pattern of accumulation and disappearance of the small cytoplasmic granules during pregnancy parallels that of ovarian preprorelaxin mRNA (232), relaxin bioactivity (22,626,912), and relaxin immunoactivity (912,926,940), as well as that of serum relaxin immunoactivity (392,723,912) (Fig. 24A). Furthermore, luteal cell fractionation studies demonstrated that the greatest relaxin bioactivity was in the granule-rich

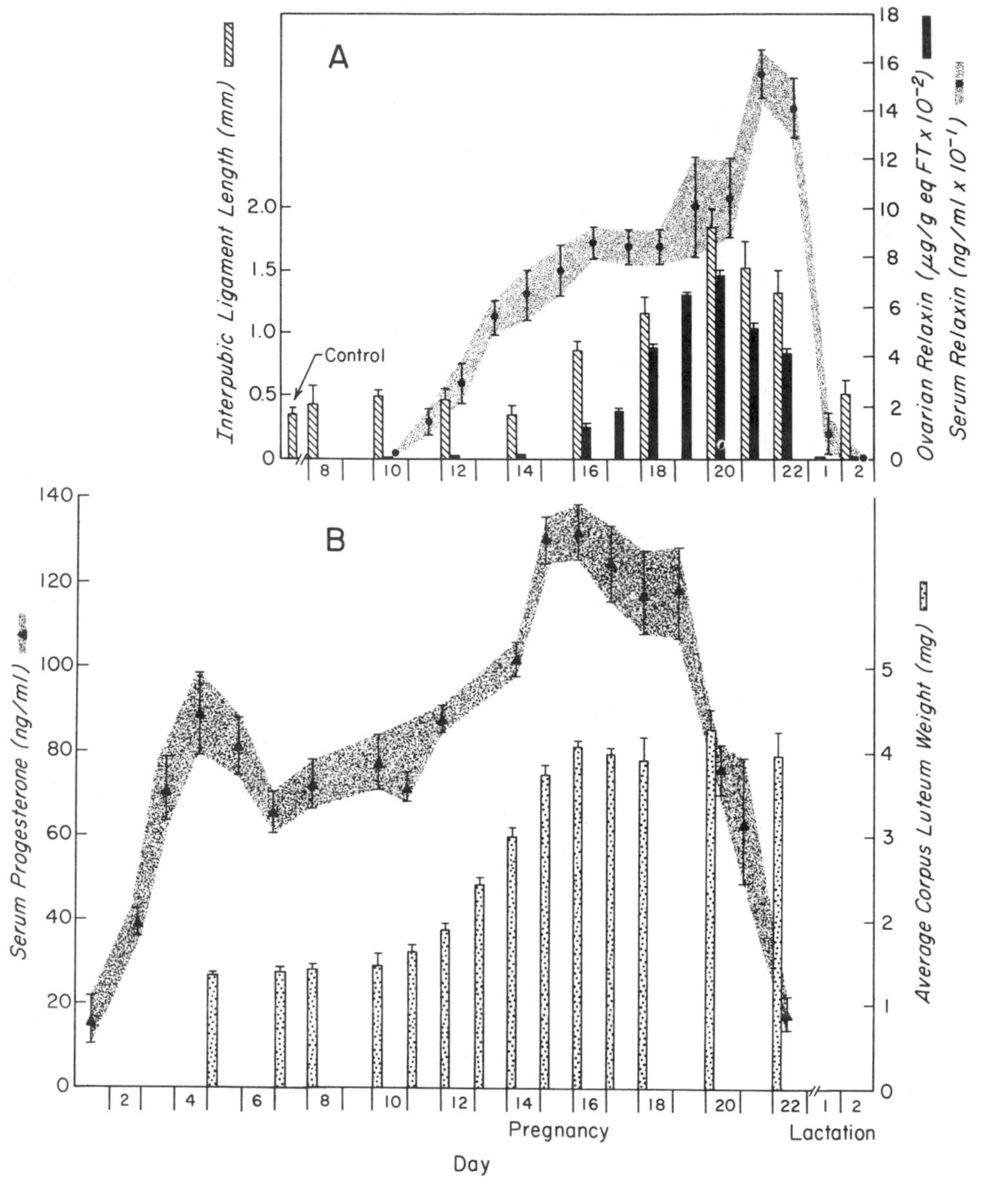

FIG. 24. A: Mean relaxin bioactivity and immunoactivity levels (+SE) in extracts of ovaries and mean relaxin immunoactivity levels (±SE) in peripheral blood sera obtained from rats on each of the days of pregnancy and lactation shown. From ref. 912, with permission. **B:** Mean progesterone levels in peripheral blood serum (±SE) and corpus luteum weights (+SE) during pregnancy in rats. Modified from refs. 765 and 1058.

fraction (28). Finally, immunocytochemical studies that used antisera to highly purified porcine relaxin (328) and rat relaxin (30,336,565) localized relaxin in the small cytoplasmic granules.

The processing of rat relaxin within luteal cells is poorly understood. There is evidence that relaxin may be stored primarily in precursor form. Soloff et al. (940) identified immunoactive bands of 18,000 Da and 16,500 Da in ovarian extracts with antisera against bacterially expressed rat prorelaxin. Changes in the combined concentrations of the 18,000-Da peptide (postulated to be intact prorelaxin) and the 16,500-Da peptide (postulated to be prorelaxin clipped at the C terminus) matched changes in the concentration of preprorelaxin mRNA (232), suggesting that relaxin synthesis is regulated at the transcriptional level and not by protein processing. On day 20, the combined concentrations of the two putative relaxin precursors were more than 30-fold that of relaxin (940).

Regulation of Synthesis. Unlike the pig, maintenance of corpora lutea throughout rat gestation requires the products of conception. After day 12 of pregnancy, maintenance of the corpora lutea is no longer dependent on the pituitary; instead, it is dependent on the placentas (39,836). Likewise, the synthesis of high levels of relaxin in the corpora lutea of the rat is pregnancy-dependent. Each conceptus appears to contribute to the promotion of relaxin synthesis, because a direct relationship was observed between the number of conceptuses and ovarian levels of relaxin immunoactivity and preprorelaxin mRNA from day 12 to day 20 (232,397,785) (Fig. 25).

There is evidence that the placentas stimulate relaxin synthesis (392,397), as well as progesterone synthesis and growth of the corpora lutea (39,539). After complete

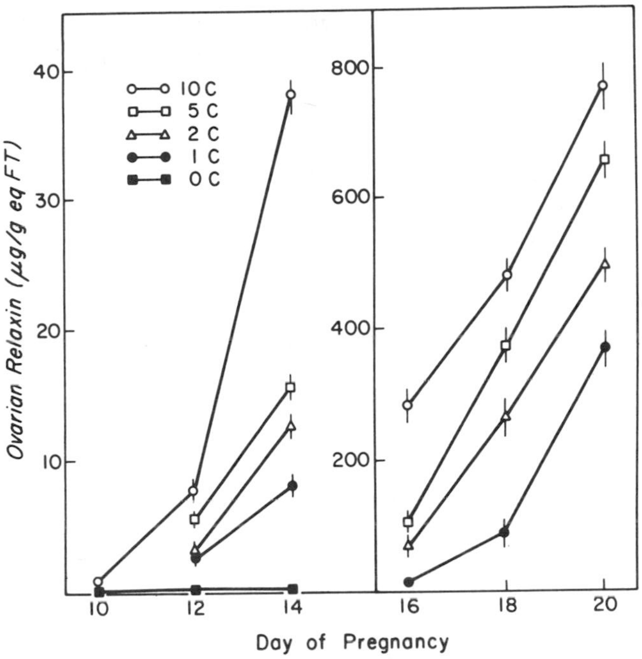

FIG. 25. Mean ovarian relaxin immunoactivity levels (±SE; $n = 5$–11) in pregnant rats with zero, one, two, five, or ten or more conceptuses (*C*) from day 10 through day 20. *FT*, fresh tissue. From ref. 397, with permission.

fetectomy on day 16 (392) or partial fetectomy on day 15 (397), with the placentas left undisturbed, ovarian relaxin levels and luteal weights did not differ from those in sham-operated controls. Also, the close temporal association of increasing ovarian relaxin levels, increasing luteal weights, and increasing serum progesterone levels between day 12 and day 15 is consistent with the view that relaxin synthesis, like the other two parameters of luteal function, is dependent on placental luteotropic support (Fig. 24). As is the case with progesterone synthesis (387,586,731,1011) and luteal weights (731,1011), placental support of relaxin synthesis appears to be mediated through estrogen (233,586).

Blood Levels from Day 10 to Day 20. Evaluation of the profile of both relaxin and progesterone immunoactivity levels in the peripheral serum throughout pregnancy led Sherwood and co-workers to postulate that the regulation of the release of relaxin from day 10 to day 20 differs from its regulation during the 3 days immediately before birth, which are designated the antepartum period (397,402,913). During the first period, relaxin immunoactivity becomes detectable in the serum by day 10, increases rapidly to 40 to 80 ng/ml by day 14, and remains relatively constant until day 20 (Fig. 24). Serum progesterone levels also remain high (>60 ng/ml) throughout this period (397,765).

Regulation of Secretion from Day 10 to Day 20. The placenta promotes the secretion as well as the synthesis of relaxin from day 10 to day 20 (392,397). Moreover, as with relaxin synthesis, progesterone synthesis, and luteal weights, there is evidence that placental support of relaxin secretion is mediated through estrogens. The decline in serum relaxin levels that followed hysterectomy on day 12 or day 15 was attenuated by administration of estradiol-17β or the estradiol-17β precursor testosterone (390,586). Furthermore, administration of the steroid biosynthesis inhibitor aminoglutethimide from day 10 to day 20 markedly reduced serum relaxin levels (966).

The placental factors that promote growth and activity of the corpora lutea during the second half of pregnancy in the rat have not been identified. Placental protein hormones may be involved. The rat placenta produces at least five hormones of the prolactin-growth hormone (PRL-GH) family. These hormones, which have molecular masses ranging from 25,000 to 30,000 Da, demonstrate 30% to 50% amino acid sequence homology with rat PRL (281–283,828,831). One of these hormones, designated rat placental lactogen-I (rPL-I) is produced in placental giant cells from about day 9 to day 14 of gestation (828). The other four known members of the PRL-GH family (rPL-I_v, rPL-II, rat PRL-like protein A, and rat PRL-like protein B) are produced in various placental sites after day 14 (281–283,831). The observations that these hormones have different amino acid sequences, have specific temporal appearances, and are expressed in different cell types led to the postulation that the PRL-GH family of hormones may have a variety of specific biologic functions during pregnancy (735). It is presently not known if one or more of the rat placental PRL-GH family of hormones is luteotropic during the second half of pregnancy. There is limited evidence that rPL-I may be luteotropic in the rat. First, its secretion from day 10 to day 14 (829,830) is coincidental with the period when relaxin secretion, progesterone secretion, and luteal weights increase markedly (Fig. 24). Also, administration of a partially purified fraction of day-12 serum that contained rPL-I, but not rPL-II, sustained progesterone synthesis and maintained pregnancy in rats after suppression of the pituitary luteotropic hormone prolactin on day 6 (389). Placental steroids may also promote luteal function. The placenta is a main source of androstenedione and testosterone in the peripheral blood during the second half of pregnancy (504,944), and the capacity of the ovary to convert these androgens to estrogen increases markedly between day 12 and day 16 (504).

The mechanisms whereby rat placental luteotropic factors promote relaxin synthesis, progesterone synthesis, luteal growth, and relaxin secretion are not well understood. The *in vivo* studies that demonstrated that the number of conceptuses is directly related to the rate or degree of increase of all four of these parameters of luteal function led to the postulation that placental support of these activities may be mediated, at least in part, through a common mechanism (397). Evidence obtained with *in vitro* studies, however, indicates that the secretion of relaxin and progesterone may not be mediated through a common mechanism. Although progesterone was secreted by rat luteal cell cultures treated with human chorionic gonadotropin (hCG), human placental lactogen, estradiol-17β, epinephrine, or dibutyryl cyclic AMP individually, relaxin was secreted only when hCG and progesterone (plus various combinations of human placental lactogen, prolactin, estradiol-17β, and epinephrine) were used in the presence of fetal calf serum (393).

The maternal pituitary first promotes and then suppresses luteal function during pregnancy in the rat. During the first half of pregnancy, the pituitary is luteotropic; it provides the prolactin and luteinizing hormone required to promote the secretion of progesterone (836). After day 12, however, the maternal pituitary suppresses luteal function. From day 14 through day 20, serum relaxin levels, serum progesterone levels, and luteal weights in rats bearing one conceptus were markedly lower than those in rats with a full complement of eight or more conceptuses (397,398) (Fig. 26). In contrast, when rats bearing one conceptus were hypophysectomized on day 13, all three parameters of luteal activity increased to values that were not significantly different from those of intact rats bearing a full complement of conceptuses (398,730) (Fig. 26). Neither the factor(s) nor the mechanism(s) whereby the pituitary suppresses relaxin secretion, progesterone secretion, and luteal weights is known. It appears that this effect is not mediated through nonluteal ovarian components. The suppressive effect of the maternal pituitary was demonstrable in ovariectomized pregnant rats whose pregnancy was maintained by ectopic corpora lutea located beneath the kidney capsule (399).

Blood Levels During the Antepartum Period. During the antepartum period, from day 20 until birth, there is an elevation of serum relaxin immunoactivity to maximal levels, which generally range from 120 to 220 ng/ml, and this surge in relaxin levels is followed by a rapid decline throughout the approximately 24 h before birth (402,819,912,914,917) (Fig. 27A).

Regulation of Secretion During the Antepartum Period. As in the pig, the antepartum surge in relaxin levels in the rat coincides temporally with functional luteolysis. Moreover, in the rat this surge is linked to photoperiod (914). The elevation in serum relaxin to maximal mean relaxin levels (M-MRL) occurs between 36 and 24 h before delivery, as does the marked antepartum decline in serum progesterone to basal mean progesterone levels (B-MPL) of less than 15 ng/ml (Fig. 27A). When the times of the light/dark phases of the conventional photoperiod were advanced 18 h on day 8, the times of occurrence of birth, M-MRL, and B-MPL were advanced; furthermore, they retained their close temporal association (cf. Fig. 27B to Fig. 27A).

The antepartum surge of relaxin levels consists of two phases that occur at 24-h intervals (see the vertical intermittent arrows in Fig. 27A). The first elevation (E1) begins approximately 60 h before birth, whereas the second elevation (E2), which produces maximal relaxin levels and coincides with functional luteolysis, begins 36 h be-

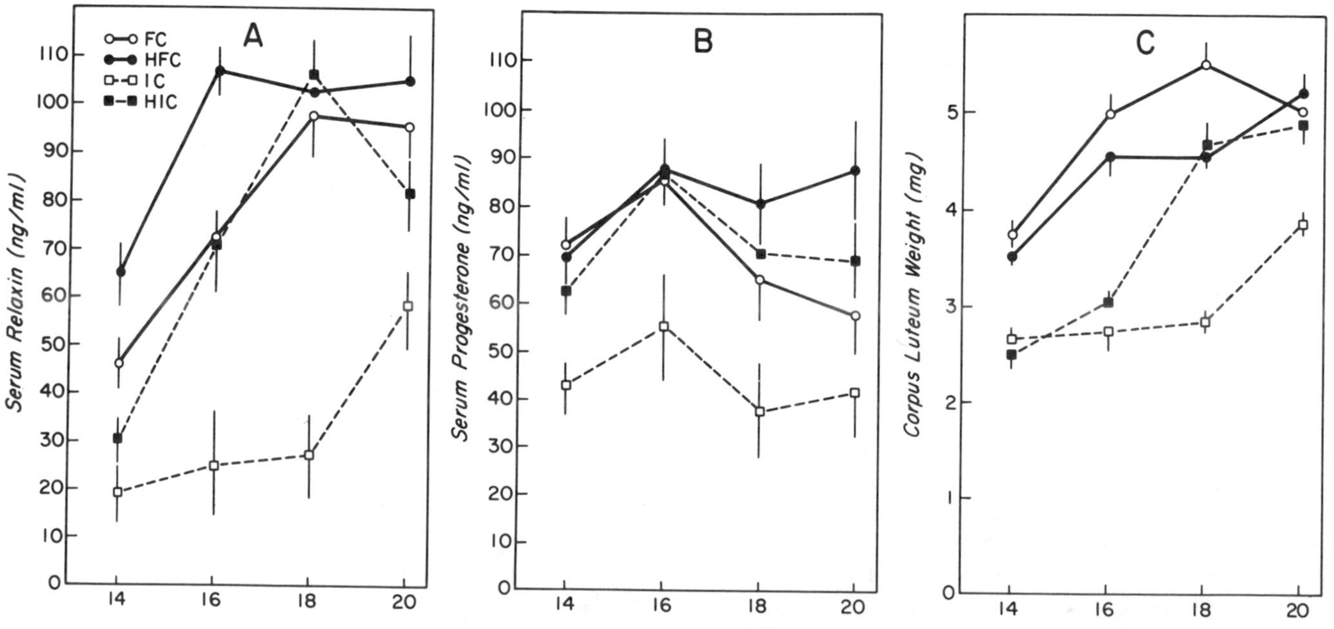

FIG. 26. Mean (±SE; $n = 5$–25) **(A)** levels of peripheral blood serum relaxin, **(B)** levels of peripheral blood serum progesterone, and **(C)** corpus luteum weights in full complement (*FC*), hypophysectomized full complement (*HFC*), one conceptus (*1C*), and hypophysectomized one conceptus (*H1C*) bearing rats. From ref. 398, with permission.

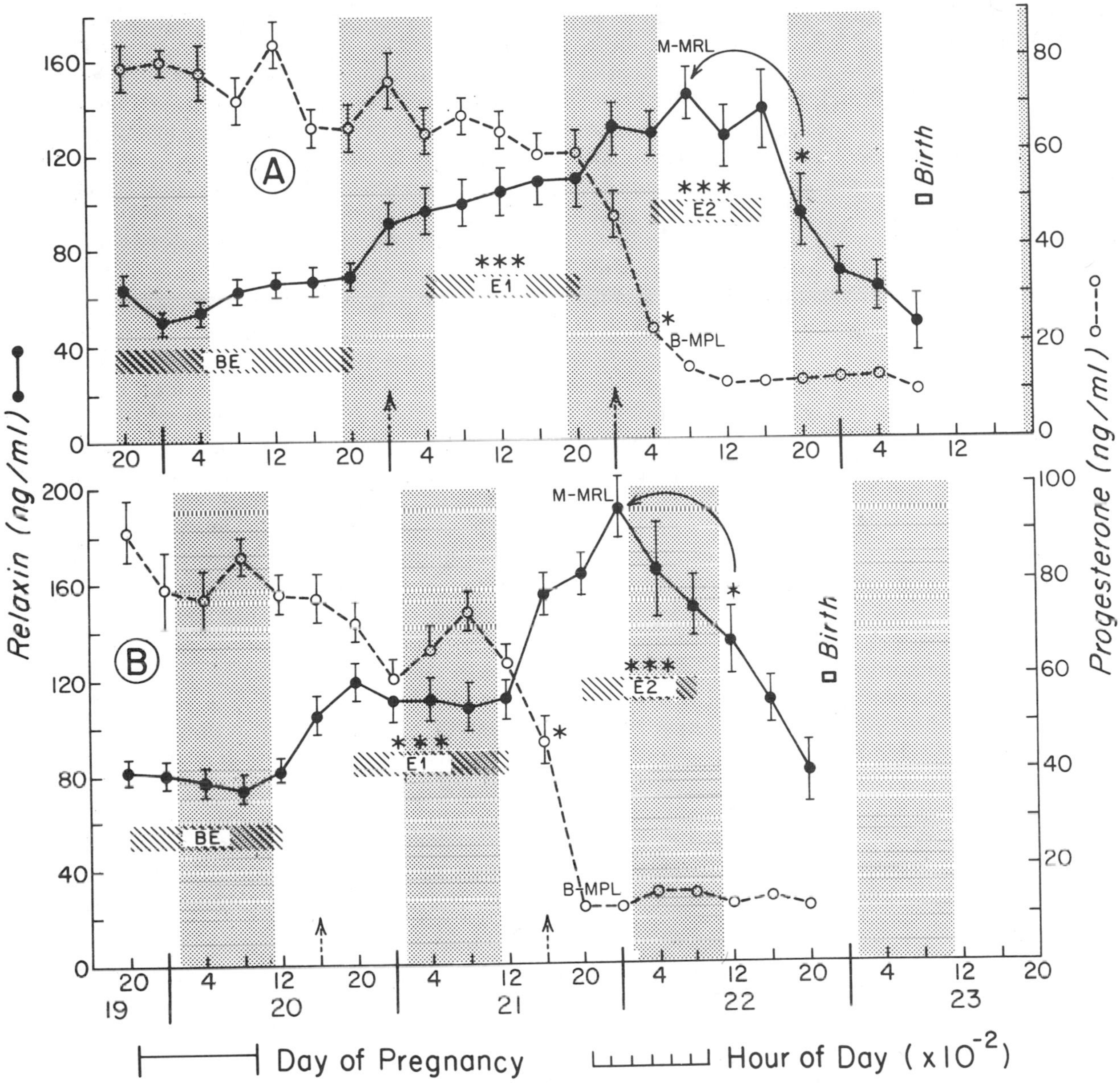

FIG. 27. Mean relaxin and progesterone immunoactivity levels (+SE) in peripheral blood serum of group A ($n = 10$) and group B ($n = 13$) pregnant rats throughout antepartum period. Times of light/dark phases of photoperiod were advanced by 18 h on day 8 in group B. Mean time of birth (±SE) for both groups is given (**box**). *Asterisks* denote levels that differ significantly (*$P < .05$; ***$P < .001$) from those that either immediately precede them or are indicated with an *arrow*. Times of occurrence of maximal mean relaxin levels (*M-MRL*) and basal mean progesterone levels (*B-MPL*) are beneath the corresponding abbreviation. *Left and right vertical dashed arrows* along the abscissas designate sampling times when first and second antepartum elevations of mean relaxin levels began, respectively. *Bars containing diagonal lines* indicate the before elevation (*BE*), elevation 1 (*E1*), and elevation 2 (*E2*) periods. From ref. 914, with permission.

fore birth. When the light/dark phases of the photoperiod were advanced, E1 and E2 were advanced; moreover, their advancement was comparable with that of birth, M-MRL, and B-MPL (cf. Fig. 27B to Fig. 27A). Sherwood et al. (914) hypothesized that these two phases in the antepartum surge of serum relaxin levels may indicate a progressively effective circadian luteolytic process, the time of occurrence of which is influenced by the photoperiod. That rats with small litters (three or fewer fetuses) show a strong tendency for a 24-h delay in the antepartum decline in serum relaxin levels and the antepartum decline in serum progesterone levels, and birth is consistent with this hypothesis (917).

The nature of the putative circadian luteolytic process is not well understood. The strong tendency for this process to be delayed 24 h in rats with small litters indicates that the conceptuses may be involved. Four lines of evidence indicate that maternal pituitary LH may also be associated with the luteolytic process in the rat (402). First, rats experience an antepartum surge in LH levels, and an experiment conducted with intact pregnant rats indicated that this surge in LH levels may promote the antepartum surge in serum relaxin levels. Highly purified ovine LH, when administered to intact rats early on day 20, caused an immediate and marked surge in serum relaxin levels, but ovine FSH and rat prolactin did not (Fig. 28A). Second, when rats were hypophysectomized on day 14, the antepartum elevation in relaxin levels was disrupted and delayed, the decline in progesterone to basal levels was protracted, and birth failed to occur. When LH was administered to similarly hypophysectomized rats on day 20, however, the antepartum elevation in relaxin levels, antepartum decline in progesterone levels, and birth occurred at the normal time. Third, administration of gonadotropin-releasing hormone to intact rats on day 20 resulted in prompt and marked elevations in serum relaxin levels. Finally, reduction of endogenous serum LH levels in intact rats by injection of an LH antiserum from day 19 through day 22 delayed both luteolysis and birth (402).

PGs may be associated with both functional luteolysis and the antepartum surge in relaxin in rats, as they appear to be in pigs. Administration of $PGF_{2\alpha}$ during late pregnancy caused an early decline in serum progesterone levels (147,997) and an early surge in relaxin levels (403) (Fig. 28B). Moreover, administration of indomethacin from day 19 to day 23 not only protracted luteolysis and delayed or prevented birth but also prevented the expected antepartum elevation of relaxin levels on days 21 and 22 (403).

The events within lutein cells that account for functional luteolysis and the surge in serum relaxin levels are not well understood. Levels of the enzyme 20α-hydroxysteroid dehydrogenase, which converts progesterone to a less active metabolite 20α-hydroxyprogesterone, increase during late pregnancy and appear to contribute to the reduction in progesterone levels (997). Although it seems likely that the surge in serum relaxin levels is attributable to accelerated release of relaxin from cytoplasmic storage granules, the mechanism that brings this phenomenon about is not understood.

Blood Levels During Delivery. Delivery in the rat normally lasts for about 90 min. During delivery, relaxin immunoactivity in the peripheral serum surges to high

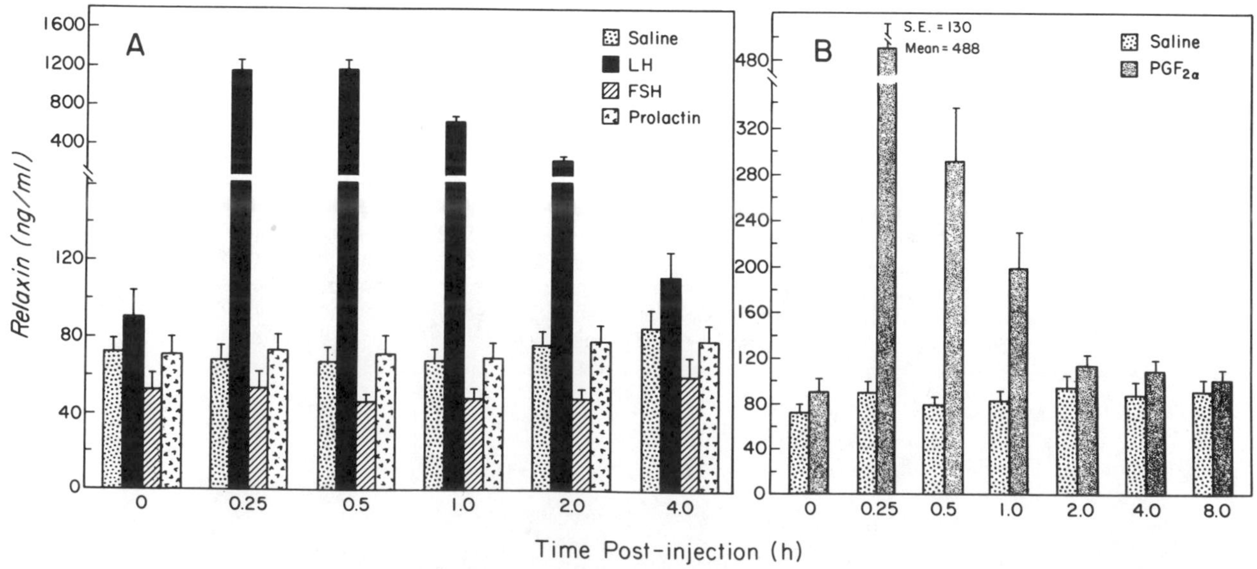

FIG. 28. Mean relaxin immunoactivity levels (±SE) in peripheral blood serum of pregnant rats given an intravenous injection of one of the following on day 20. **A:** Saline vehicle (n = 11), 10 μg LH (n = 5), 25 μg FSH (n = 4), or 25 μg prolactin (n = 5). From ref. 402, with permission. **B:** Saline vehicle (n = 8), or 50 μg $PGF_{2\alpha}$ (n = 10). From ref. 403, with permission.

levels (>100 ng/ml) for 1 hour or more (912). Neither the factor(s) that promotes this surge in relaxin levels nor the physiologic significance of the surge, if any, is known.

Multiple Forms of Relaxin in the Blood. Relaxin immunoactivity in the peripheral serum of pregnant rats is associated with three main components of different size, and the distribution of relaxin immunoactivity among these components changes in a progressive manner with the day of pregnancy (919). The three components, designated C1, C2, and C3, have molecular weights of about 60,000, 13,000, and 6,500, respectively. On day 15, essentially all relaxin immunoactivity is associated with C1 (Fig. 29). By day 17, approximately 20% of the total relaxin immunoactivity is in C2 plus C3, and by day 19 the proportion in each of these two components increases to about 25%. The nature of the three components is poorly understood. It was postulated (919) that C3 may be the 6,500-Da bioactive form of relaxin that has been isolated from the ovaries of rats (905,1093). Insights concerning the natures of C2 and C1 are more speculative. Because the molecular mass of C2, about 13,000, is less than the 20,000 Da reported for prorelaxin (487), it may be an intermediate in the conversion of the precursor to relaxin. The nature of C1 is particularly puzzling, because its apparent molecular weight of approximately 60,000 is considerably greater than that reported for rat prorelaxin (487) or prorelaxin immunoactive bands extracted from rat ovaries (940). Component C1 appears to possess the relaxinlike bioactivity of inhibiting uterine contractility. The frequency of intrauterine pressure cycles in nonpregnant rats declined during cross-circulation with day-15 rats, which have only the C1 component in their peripheral serum. Component C1 does not appear to be attributable to the binding of 6,000-Da relaxin to a binding protein: Relaxin immunoactivity remained associated with the large component(s) when serum obtained on day 15 was incubated and then filtered through Sephacryl S-200 in the presence of high concentrations of the conformation-destabilizing salt potassium thiocyanate (919).

There is evidence that the shift in the distribution of relaxin immunoactivity from C1 to the smaller components C2 and C3 during late pregnancy is promoted by the conceptuses but is not influenced by the maternal pituitary (918). In rats bearing a full complement of conceptuses, only about 50% of the total relaxin immunoactivity is associated with C1 on day 19, whereas in rats bearing a single conceptus, about 85% of the total relaxin immunoactivity is associated with C1 on day 19. The physiologic significance, if any, of this multiplicity of relaxin-immunoactive components is not known.

Clearance of Relaxin from the Blood. The clearance half-life for rat relaxin immunoactivity appears to be similar to that of porcine relaxin (912). After bilateral ovariectomy on day 21, the clearance half-life was approximately 20 min during the first half-hour and approximately 60 min thereafter (912). Interpretation of

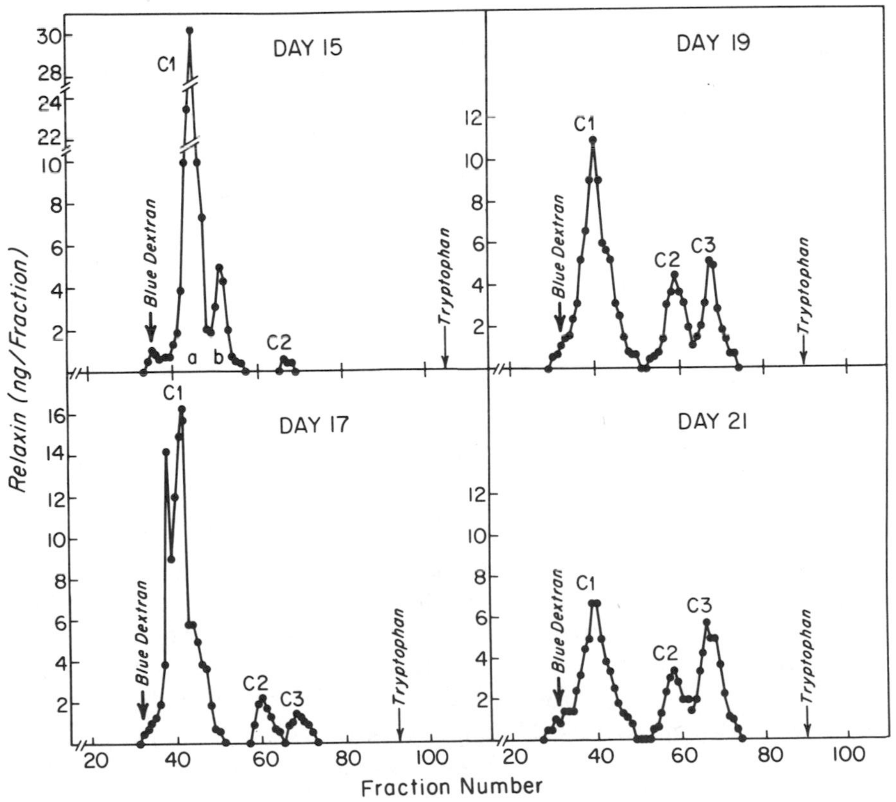

FIG. 29. Relaxin immunoactivity profiles obtained after gel filtration of peripheral blood serum from day-15, day-17, day-19, and day-21 pregnant rats on Sephacryl S-200 (Pharmacia, Piscataway, NJ). From ref. 919, with permission.

the apparent clearance for relaxin immunoactivity during late pregnancy is complicated, because it is influenced by the relative quantities and rates of clearance of the three relaxin immunoactive components C1, C2, and C3. There is limited evidence that the rate of clearance of C1 may be slower than that of C2 and C3 (919).

Extraovarian Production of Relaxin. Whereas studies that used bioassays consistently demonstrated that relaxin is found only in the ovary (22,98,589,912,950), investigations with more sensitive techniques provided indications that small amounts of relaxin may be produced in sites other than the corpora lutea during pregnancy. Early immunohistochemical localization studies using antisera to impure porcine relaxin indicated that relaxin may be found in uterine metrial glands (242) and placenta (1155). More recent research that used an antiserum to highly purified rat relaxin also identified low-intensity immunohistochemical staining in granulated metrial gland cells (580) but failed to find relaxin immunoactivity in placental tissue (336). In 1992, Fields et al. (336) detected relaxin immunostaining in endometrial epithelial cells during pregnancy with an antiserum to highly purified rat relaxin. Relaxin immunostaining, which was most pronounced in antimesometrial epithelial cells at implantation sites, was first evident on day 14 of pregnancy and continued through day 22 (Fig. 30A). The observation that relaxin immunoactivity was also present in the endometrial epithelial cells on day 22 in pregnant rats that had been ovariectomized on day 9 and given subsequent hormone replacement therapy with ovarian steroids (Fig. 30B) provided support for the view that the endometrium produces relaxin and does not simply sequester relaxin secreted by the corpora lutea. Finally, there is limited evidence that relaxinlike immunoactivity and relaxin mRNA are present in the brain of pregnant as well as nonpregnant female rats (54).

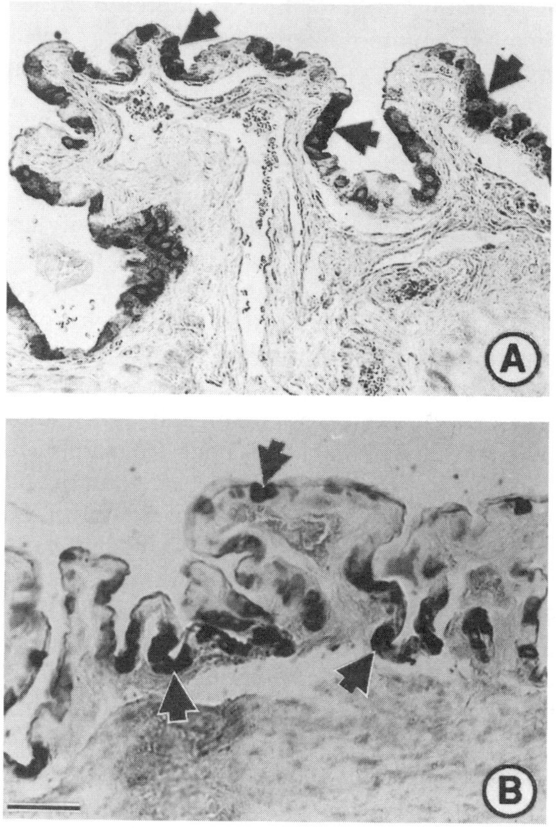

FIG. 30. Localization of relaxin immunostaining in endometrium obtained from pregnant rats. Light microscopy immunohistochemical localization of relaxin in rat uterine sections using rabbit antirat relaxin serum and avidin-biotin immunostaining technique. Note luminal epithelial cells (*closed arrows*). **A:** Intact day-22 pregnant rat. **B:** Day-22 pregnant rat in which ovariectomy was conducted on day 9. *Bar* = 80 μm for both A and B. Modified from ref. 336.

Lactation

Ovarian relaxin declines dramatically at term in the rat (24,912) but remains detectable in early lactation (48). Two types of corpora lutea are present in the rat ovary after parturition: the corpora lutea from the previous pregnancy and corpora lutea formed after postpartum ovulation, termed *corpora lutea of lactation.* Relaxin was detected only in a small and diminishing number of cells within the corpora lutea of the previous pregnancy during the first 9 days of lactation by immunohistochemistry, using an antiserum to highly purified rat relaxin (48). Relaxin immunoactivity was depleted from these corpora lutea within 12 h of intravenous injection of $PGF_{2\alpha}$ on day 3 of lactation and was not replaced 48 h after $PGF_{2\alpha}$ administration. It was concluded that the small amount of relaxin immunoactivity in the corpora lutea of the previous pregnancy is residual relaxin produced during that pregnancy (48). Relaxin immunostaining in endometrial epithelial cells was also reported to decline rapidly at delivery so that by day 2 of lactation immunostaining could be demonstrated in only a few epithelial cells (336). Relaxin immunoactivity has not been reported in the peripheral blood during lactation in the rat.

Mouse

In 1959, Steinetz et al. (950) detected relaxin bioactivity in the ovaries of pregnant mice (*Mus musculus*). More recent studies by Anderson and co-workers (31,1074) indicated that relaxin synthesis in the mouse is similar to that in the rat. Studies that used an antiserum to highly purified rat relaxin with either the unlabeled antibody peroxidase-antiperoxidase or the avidin-biotin immunoperoxidase cytochemical localization method demonstrated that immunostaining was confined to the corpora lutea of ovaries obtained during the second half of pregnancy, and no immunostaining was demonstrated in ovaries obtained throughout the estrous cycle (31,1074). Psalti et al. (797) used a rabbit antiporcine relaxin serum (968) with the avidin-biotin immunoperoxidase localization procedure to measure variations in luteal relaxin content throughout pregnancy by means of immunodensitometry. These workers found that relaxin immunostaining, which was localized in the perinuclear region of labeled cells, was first detected on day 11.5, increased progressively until day 18, dropped dramatically a few hours before delivery at day 18.5, and reached background levels shortly after delivery (797). The appearance and disappearance of membrane-bound cytoplasmic granules (200 nm in diameter) closely parallels that of relaxin immunostaining of luteal cells. Anderson and co-workers reported that granules appeared by day 12, were maximal between day 16 and day 18, and disappeared by 2 days postpartum (31). As with the rat, luteal relaxin production and secretion in the mouse may be regulated by a placental luteotropic factor(s). Hypophysectomized pregnant mice showed normal pubic relaxation if the placentas were retained, but not if they were removed (700).

O'Byrne and Steinetz (723) determined the general profile of relaxin immunoactivity in the peripheral blood serum of mice during the 20-day gestation period with a porcine relaxin radioimmunoassay. Relaxin immunoactivity levels rose from about day 12 to maximal levels a day or two before delivery and declined to low levels by 2 days postpartum (723).

Guinea Pig

Uterine Source

Unlike the pig, rat, and mouse, the primary source of relaxin in the guinea pig (*Cavia porcellus*) is the uterus. In 1928, Herrick (455) provided evidence that relaxin was produced in nonovarian tissue in the guinea pig when he reported that bilateral ovariectomy at midpregnancy did not prevent relaxation of the pubic symphysis during late pregnancy. Proof that the uterus was a main source of relaxin was first obtained in the 1940s when Hisaw et al. (465,468) and Zarrow (1151) demonstrated that the pelvic relaxation that occurred within 3 or 4 days after progesterone administration to castrated, estrogen-primed nonpregnant guinea pigs failed to occur if hysterectomy was performed at the same time as ovariectomy. It was not until the 1980s that the cellular source of relaxin in the guinea pig uterus was demonstrated to be the endometrial glands. These glands are simple tubular structures that open into the lumen of the uterus and extend deep into the endometrium where their most highly coiled parts lie adjacent to the innermost muscle layer of the uterus (Fig. 31A and B). Using antisera to highly purified porcine relaxin and either the peroxidase-antiperoxidase or avidin-biotin immunoperoxidase localization method, Larkin and co-workers (592,596, 750,751) and Bryant-Greenwood et al. (146) demonstrated that relaxin immunoactivity was confined to the endometrial gland cells during the second half of the approximately 65-day guinea pig pregnancy (Fig. 31A and B). Larkin and co-workers subsequently conducted ultrastructural immunocytochemical studies with an antiserum to highly purified porcine relaxin and either colloidal gold-antirabbit IgG or colloidal gold-protein A to localize the relaxin within the endometrial gland cells (592,594,596,752). These workers demonstrated that relaxin immunoactivity was located over large (0.5–1.5-μm diameter) granules located between the nucleus and luminal surface (apical region) of the endometrial gland cells (Fig. 31C and D) and that these granules were released, at least in part, into the lumen of the uterus (594).

Three lines of evidence make it seem likely that the relaxin immunostaining substance within the endometrial gland cells is relaxin. First, a close temporal association was found between the occurrence of relaxin immunostaining in uterine sections and the ability of uterine extracts to inhibit spontaneous contractions of the mouse uterus. Relaxin levels were detectable by day 30, but staining was heaviest on day 45 and during the last week of pregnancy (146,594,750), when bioactivity levels were maximal (750). After parturition on about day 65, uterine relaxin levels fell rapidly, and they were low by day 3 of lactation (750). Second, the biologically active substance in uterine extracts had a molecular weight of about 6,000—similar to that of relaxin from several species (751). Consistent with these studies, Nagao and Bryant-Greenwood (692) reported that relaxin immunoactivity levels were maximal in extracts of guinea pig uteri obtained during late pregnancy and that the relaxin-immunoactive substance had a molecular weight similar to that of porcine relaxin. Third, mRNA for guinea pig relaxin in extracts of endometrium obtained from guinea pigs during late pregnancy was detected by Northern analysis (146,1019), and a decline in the levels of relaxin immunoactivity was accompanied by an apparent reduction of the 1 kb relaxin transcript (146).

There is not total agreement concerning the reproductive states during which relaxin occurs in uterine endometrial gland cells. Whereas both Larkin and co-workers (594,750–752) and Bryant-Greenwood et al. (146) detected relaxin immunostaining in endometrial gland cells during the second half of pregnancy and lactation, only Bryant-Greenwood et al. (146) detected relaxin immunoactivity in these cells in cycling animals. Bryant-Greenwood and co-workers also reported low levels of relaxin immunoactivity in uterine extracts and peripheral blood plasma obtained during the estrous cycle with a porcine relaxin radioimmunoassay (112,692).

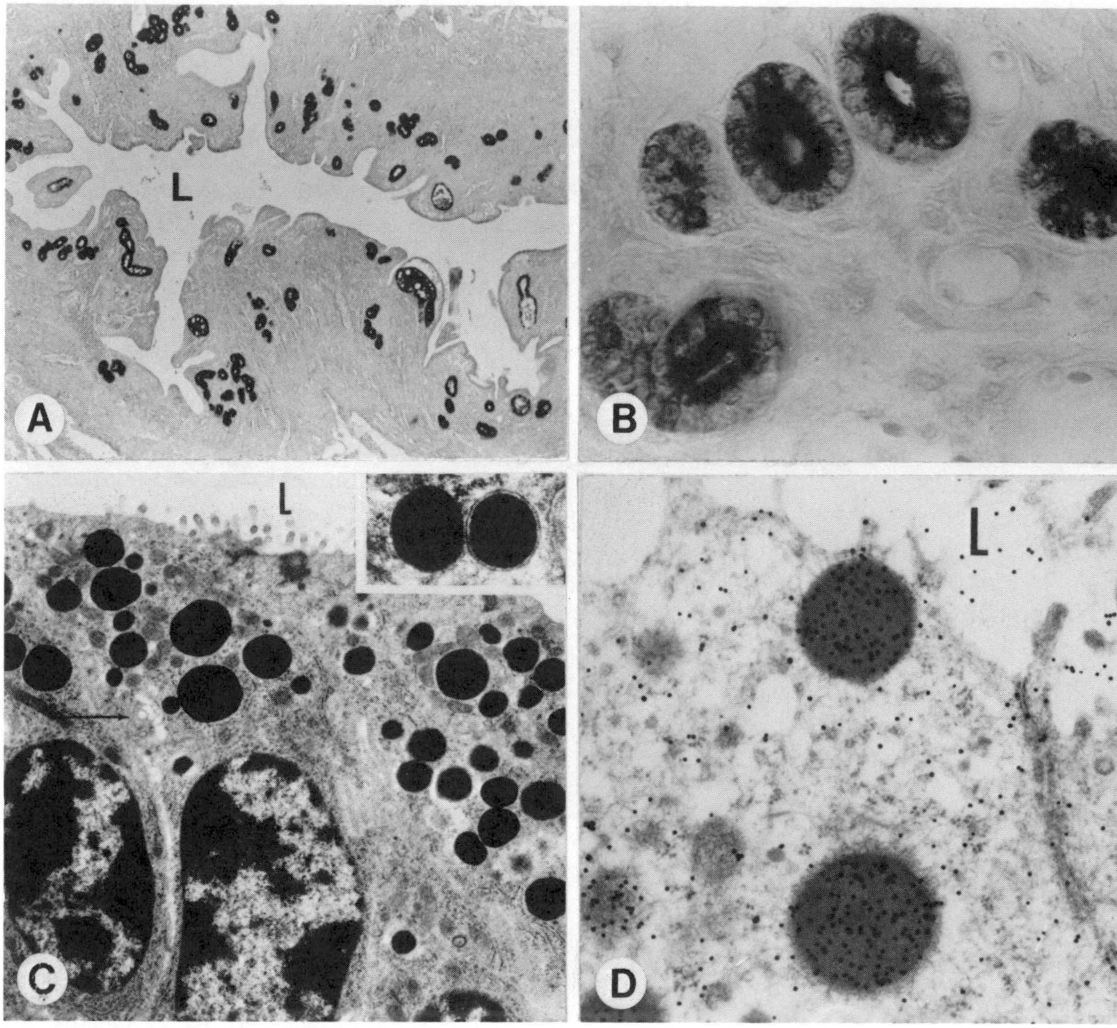

FIG. 31. **A:** Localization of relaxin immunoactivity in guinea pig uterus removed on day 60 of pregnancy. Light microscopy immunohistochemical localization of relaxin in a transverse section of a guinea pig uterus using rabbit antiporcine relaxin serum and peroxidase–antiperoxidase as marker. *L,* lumen. (×35) **B:** Higher magnification of a section of uterus (stained as in A), showing dense relaxin immunoactivity near luminal surfaces of endometrial gland cells. (×455) A and B from ref. 750, with permission. **C:** Electron micrograph showing many dense granules (500–1,000-nm diameter) in luminal portions of endometrial gland cells. Stacks of Golgi cisterne (*arrow*) are evident. (×900) **Inset:** Higher magnification of the dense granules. (×17,900) **D:** Electron microscopy immunocytochemical localization of relaxin in endometrial gland cell granules using rabbit antiporcine relaxin serum and goat antirabbit immunoglobulin G-colloidal gold as marker. Granules are labeled with many gold particles indicating presence of relaxin. (×30,000) C and D from ref. 752, with permission.

Regulation of Synthesis

It seems likely that it is the combination of elevated blood levels of both estrogen and progesterone that occurs during mid to late pregnancy (190) that most effectively stimulates relaxin synthesis in the endometrial gland cells. After the administration of both steroids to castrated nonpregnant guinea pigs, relaxation of the pelvic ligaments occurred (468,592,1151) and levels of relaxin immunoactivity in uterine extracts increased (692). Also, when ovariectomized guinea pigs were administered estrogen or progesterone individually for 14 days, most endometrial gland cells contained no relaxin immunoactivity, whereas when the two hormones were given in combination, all endometrial gland cells contained relaxin (592,750). Animals that received both estrogen and progesterone contained abundant large secretory granules that either contained relaxin alone or were composed of two portions: a central dense core that contained relaxin immunoactivity and a lighter-staining cortex that contained carbohydrate (592,596). A second and novel regulatory mechanism for relaxin synthesis in the guinea pig uterus has been postulated. In 1991, Bryant-Greenwood et al. (146) reported that relaxin synthesis within the endometrial gland cells may be regulated, at least in part, by the mammary glands. Endometrial gland cells from mastectomized cyclic and late pregnant guinea pigs showed a reduction in the amount of relaxin immunostaining compared with controls (146).

Blood Levels

The few reports describing blood levels of relaxin during pregnancy in the guinea pig are not in close agreement. In 1947, Zarrow (1150) determined relaxin bioactivity levels in the peripheral serum with the guinea pig pubic symphysis palpation assay. Relaxin bioactivity was reported to be detectable by day 21, maximal by day 28, and maintained at maximal levels until about day 63, when it began to drop gradually. Shortly after parturition, on about day 68, a precipitous decline occurred so that by 48 h after birth relaxin bioactivity was undetectable (1150). Two laboratories measured relaxin immunoactivity levels in peripheral blood with porcine relaxin radioimmunoassays. In one study, which determined relaxin levels in serum samples collected at 10 day intervals throughout pregnancy, relaxin immunoactivity was detectable on about day 20, rose steadily to maximal levels on about day 50 to day 60, and did not decline by the day after parturition (723). In the second investigation, which determined relaxin levels in plasma samples obtained at 24-h intervals from day 40 until birth, episodic surges in relaxin immunoactivity were detected, and there was no clear pattern among animals (112). Thus, a profile of relaxin levels in the peripheral blood throughout pregnancy in the guinea pig is not established.

Mammary Gland Production of Relaxin

In 1989, Peaker et al. (763) reported that the mammary gland produces relaxin in the guinea pig. When sections of mammary tissue were immunostained with the avidin-biotin immunoperoxidase technique using an antiserum to porcine relaxin, light immunostaining was observed in cuboidal epithelial cells forming the mammary duct system in both cyclic and pregnant animals. Intense immunostaining was observed throughout the epithelial cells of the alveoli on day 5 of lactation, and relaxin mRNA was detected in an extract from mammary tissue on day 6 of lactation (763).

Rabbit

Placental Source

Two lines of direct evidence indicate that the placenta is a main source of relaxin during the approximately 33-day gestation period in the rabbit (*Oryctolagus cuniculus*). First, extracts of rabbit placental tissue demonstrated relaxinlike bioactivity in the guinea pig pubic symphysis palpation bioassay (460–462,467,595,950, 1158), mouse uterine contractility bioassay (295, 335,595), and mouse interpubic ligament bioassay (335). Second, Fields and co-workers (295,296,337) localized relaxin in the multinucleated syncytiotrophoblast of placentas obtained on days 11, 16, 23, and 30 with an immunohistochemical method that used antisera to either highly purified rabbit relaxin or highly purified porcine relaxin and the avidin-biotin immunoperoxidase technique as marker (Fig. 32A). Furthermore, Eldridge and Fields (297) obtained evidence at the ultrastructural level that rabbit relaxin is stored in cytoplasmic membrane-bound granules (150–400-nm diameter) within the syncytiotrophoblast (Fig. 32B) where they migrate to the cell membrane and are released by exocytosis. Little is known concerning the regulation of the synthesis or secretion of relaxin from the rabbit placenta. There is limited evidence that progesterone and cyclic AMP increase relaxin production by trophoblast-derived cells in culture (602).

Uterine Source

There is evidence that the uterus is also a source of relaxin in the rabbit. Early reports indicated that extracts of uterine tissue obtained from pregnant (950) or castrated and steroid-treated rabbits (468) demonstrated relaxin bioactivity in the guinea pig pubic symphysis palpation bioassay. More recently, Fields and co-workers (296,337,603) found relaxin immunoactivity associated with the apical region of mononuclear endometrial gland cells and/or multinuclear luminal epithelial cells from day 4 of pregnancy until day 5 of lactation. They used the avidin-biotin immunoperoxidase method with an antiserum either to highly purified rabbit relaxin or highly purified porcine relaxin. The site(s) where relaxin immunoactivity was localized changed with the stage of pregnancy. During the preimplantation period on days 4 to 9, relaxin was found in the endometrial glands throughout the length of the uterus. After implantation and initiation of placental development (days 9–11), relaxin was localized in endometrial glandular and luminal epithelial cells on both the mesometrial and antimesometrial surfaces of the uterine horns adjacent to implantation sites but not between sites (337,603) (Fig. 32C). Fields and Lee (337) demonstrated that endometrial epithelial cells regressed and relaxin immunostaining was not found after day 7 in the sterile uterine horn of animals subjected to unilateral ligation of the oviduct. These workers postulated that a conceptus factor, acting in a paracrine manner, maintains endometrial epithelial cell integrity and enhances relaxin synthesis during pregnancy. Consistent with this possibility, relaxin immuno-

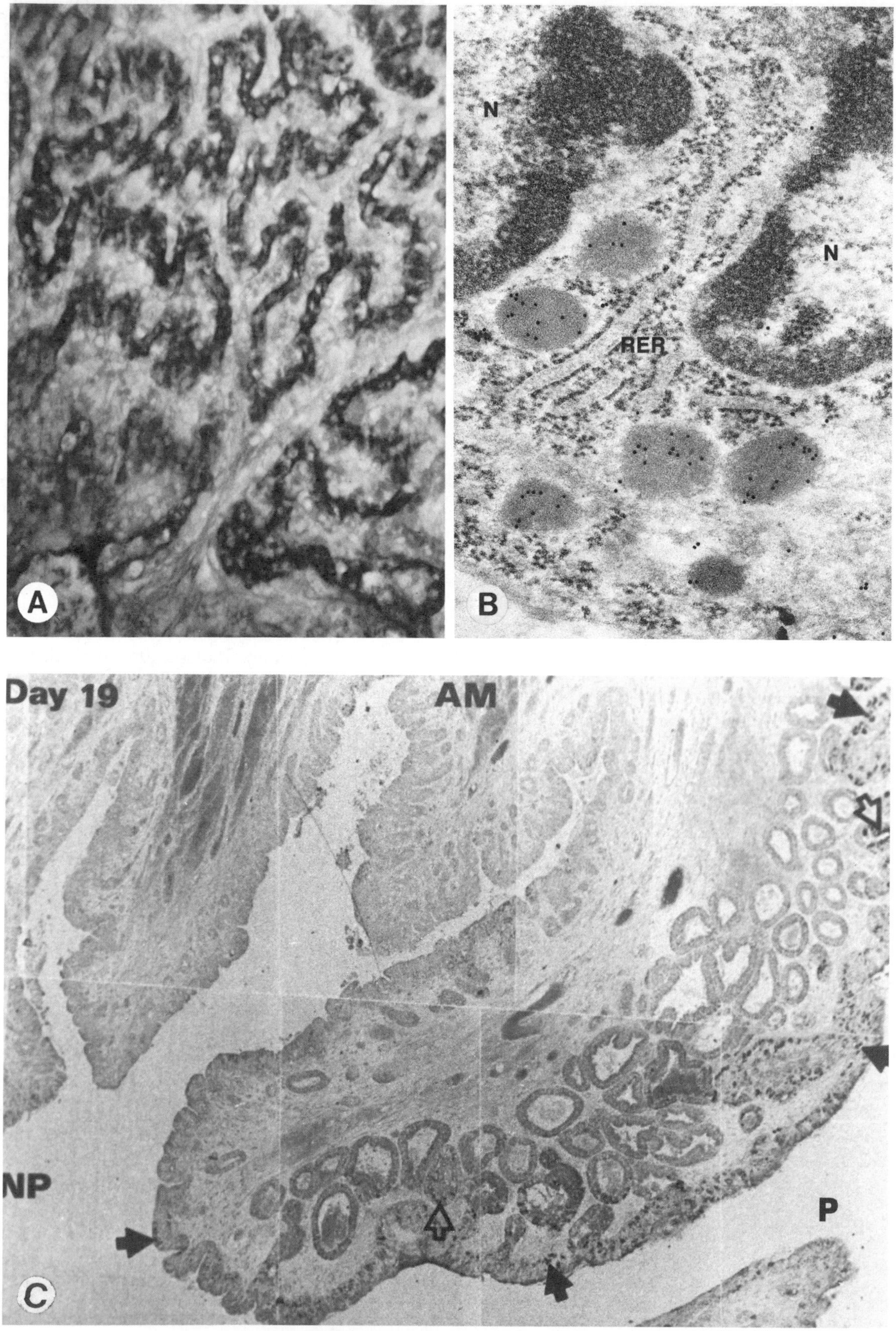
A
B
N
N
RER
Day 19
AM
NP
P
C

activity was detectable in antimesometrial glands in pseudopregnant rabbits only on day 7 (337). The nature of the putative conceptus factor(s) that enhances uterine relaxin synthesis in the rabbit is not known. There is limited evidence that estrogen and progesterone may promote relaxin synthesis in the rabbit uterus. Sera obtained from castrated adult female rabbits given pharmacologic doses of estradiol-17β and progesterone daily for several days promoted pelvic relaxation in guinea pigs, whereas sera obtained from castrated plus hysterectomized rabbits given the same steroid treatment did not (468).

Blood Levels

Relaxin bioactivity levels in the peripheral blood serum of rabbits throughout pregnancy were first determined in 1944 by Marder and Money (653), using a guinea pig pubic symphysis palpation bioassay. Relaxin levels were reported to remain low until day 12, increase about 50-fold by day 24, remain elevated and steady until delivery on day 32, and then decline precipitously. Similar results were reported in 1953 by Zarrow and Rosenberg (1158). In 1991, Lee and Fields (604) detected low relaxin immunoactivity levels in the peripheral blood of pregnant rabbits with a homologous porcine relaxin radioimmunoassay. During pregnancy, relaxin was detected during the preimplantation period (days 4–9), rose to maximal levels by day 15, remained elevated until delivery on day 32, declined abruptly on day 1 postpartum, and remained detectable during the first week postpartum (Fig. 33). Relaxin was not detected in pseudopregnant, cycling, or male rabbits. It seems likely that the placentas are the main source of the elevated relaxin in the peripheral blood during the second half of pregnancy in the rabbit. The marked increase in blood levels of relaxin on days 15 to 20 (604,653,1158) occurs during the period when major placental growth occurs and the precipitous decline in relaxin coincides with expulsion of the placenta at birth (604,653). It was postulated that the rabbit endometrium is the source of the low plasma relaxin concentrations during lactation (604). The observation that ovariectomy on day 13 of

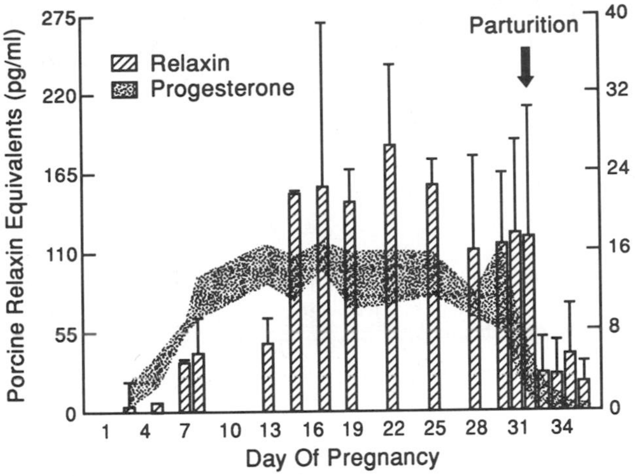

FIG. 33. Mean relaxin and progesterone immunoactivity levels (±SE; $n = 8$) in peripheral blood plasma in rabbits that delivered on day 32 of pregnancy. Relaxin was measured with a homologous porcine relaxin radioimmunoassay. From ref. 604, with permission.

pregnancy did not influence the profile or levels of relaxin immunoactivity is consistent with the view that the ovary is not a source of relaxin in the pregnant rabbit (604).

Ovarian Production of Relaxin

Reports are not entirely consistent, but it seems highly unlikely that the ovaries produce relaxin during pregnancy in the rabbit. Extracts of rabbit ovaries were reported to contain little relaxin bioactivity in the guinea pig pubic symphysis palpation bioassay (467,950,1158). When pregnant rabbits were ovariectomized on day 14 or day 15 and pregnancy was maintained by injecting progesterone daily, serum relaxin bioactivity levels remained similar to those in intact controls (1158). Using an immunohistochemical localization study that used an antiserum to impure porcine relaxin, Zarrow and O'Connor (1157) found immunofluorescence associated with the rabbit corpora lutea on days 23 to 28. More recent immunohistochemical localization studies by Fields and co-workers (295,297,603), however, which

FIG. 32. A: Light microscopy immunohistochemical localization of relaxin in syncytiotrophoblast cells of a rabbit placenta on day 23 of pregnancy using guinea pig antirabbit relaxin serum and avidin-biotin peroxidase as marker. (×218) **B:** Electron microscopy immunocytochemical localization of relaxin in rabbit placenta granules (150–400-nm diameter) on day 23 of pregnancy using guinea pig antirabbit relaxin and goat antiguinea pig immunoglobulin G-colloidal gold as marker. *N*, nucleus; *RER*, rough endoplasmic reticulum. (×56,600) From ref. 297, with permission. **C:** Montage showing light microscopy immunohistochemical localization of relaxin in uterus of a rabbit on day 19 of pregnancy using guinea pig antirabbit relaxin serum and avidin-biotin peroxidase as marker. Relaxin is seen in luminal epithelial cells (*large solid arrows*) and endometrial glands (*open arrows*) on the conceptus side (*P*) of valvelike structures that demarcate placental implantation sites. Relaxin immunostaining is absent on between-site side (*NP*). (×20) From ref. 603, with permission.

used an antiserum generated with highly purified rabbit relaxin at both the light and electron microscopy levels, failed to find relaxin immunoactivity associated with the corpora lutea of pregnant rabbits.

Hamster

The placenta synthesizes relaxin during the second half of the 16-day gestation period in the golden (Syrian) hamster (*Mesocricetus auratus*). Homogenates of placentas obtained on days 11, 14, and 15 were bioactive in the guinea pig pubic symphysis palpation bioassay (963). Also, Renegar and co-workers localized relaxin within the placenta from day 8 to day 15 by the avidin-biotin immunoperoxidase method using antiserum to porcine relaxin (517,816,818). Most of the relaxin immunoactivity was in fetal primary and secondary giant trophoblast cells found within the decidua capsularis and trophospongium, respectively (Fig. 34A, B, and C). These giant trophoblast cells possess the ability to migrate and were postulated to penetrate the uterine epithelium and participate in the enlargement of the decidual cavity, as well as in the destruction of maternal tissue (739). The giant

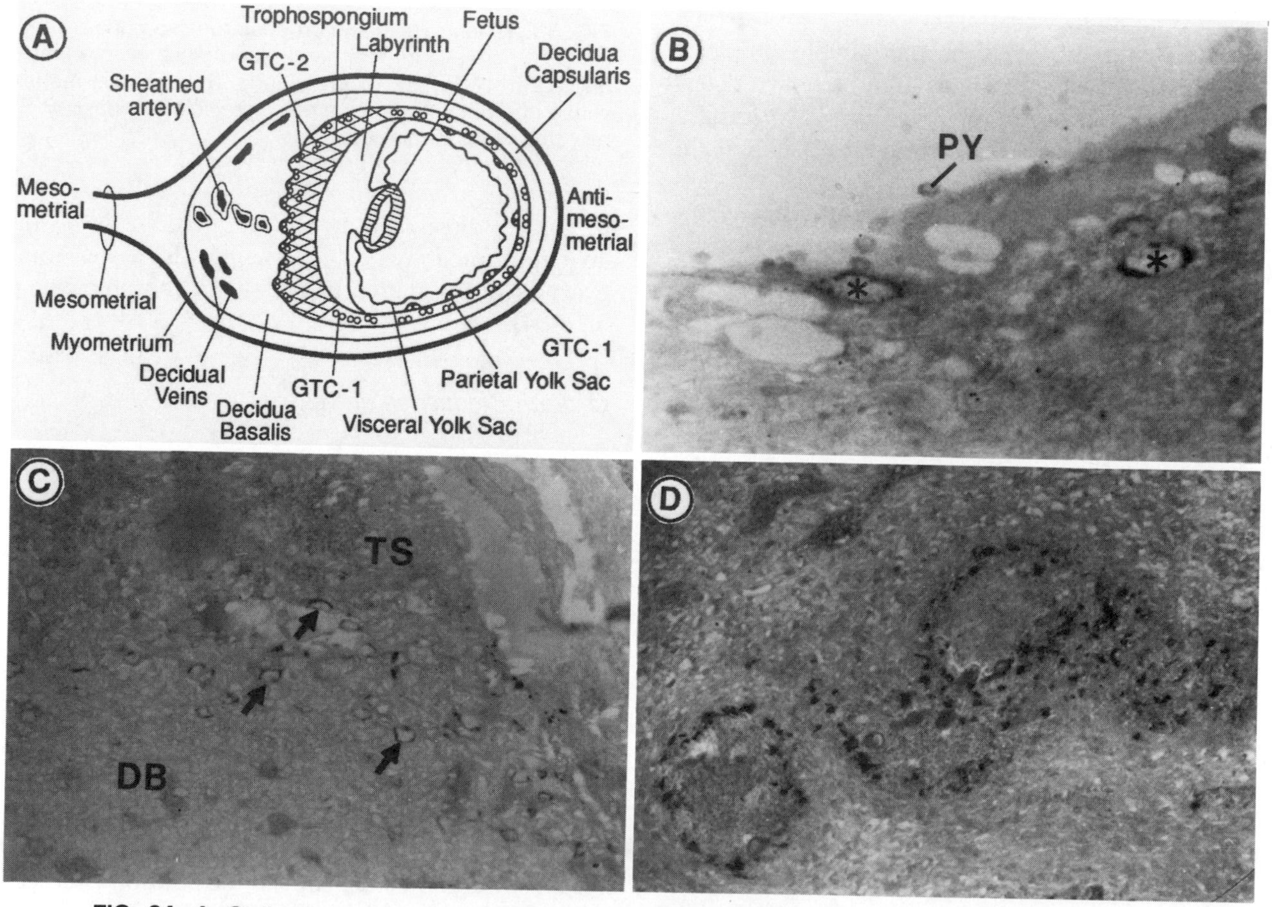

FIG. 34. A: Stylized drawing of cross-section of hamster implantation site on day 10 of gestation. *Allantoic placenta,* which consists of labyrinth and trophospongium, is forming on mesometrial side of uterus in part by proliferation of trophoblast cells. *Decidua capsularis* is reduced to a narrow zone surrounding the lateral and antimesometrial cavity. Primary giant trophoblast cells (*GTC-1*) lie between decidua capsularis and yolk sac and at reticular margins of developing allantoic placenta. Placental growth procedes by invasion by the *trophospongium,* with its leading edge of secondary giant trophoblast cells (*GTC-2*), into the decidua. The main maternal arterial blood supply to the placenta traverses the *decidua basalis* as the *sheathed artery.* **B, C, D:** Localization of relaxin immunostaining in hamster placenta using rabbit antiporcine relaxin serum and the avidin-biotin immunoperoxidase technique. **B:** Cross section of hamster implantation site on day 8 of gestation. Portion of antimesometrial decidual cavity showing parietal (*PY*) yolk sac. Note positive staining of relaxin immunoactivity in GTC-1 cells (*). (×280) **C:** Cross section of implantation site on day 10 of gestation. Portion of boundary between the decidua basalis (*DB*) and the trophospongium (*TS*). Note that relaxin immunoactivity is localized within GTC-2 cells (*arrows*) that precede invading trophoblast cells. (×103) **D:** Sheathed arteries located within the decidua basalis on day 10 of gestation. Note intense staining of cells within arterial sheath. (×103) Modified from ref. 816.

trophoblast cells appear to be the source of at least one other protein hormone during the second half of pregnancy: Hamster placental lactogen II was colocalized with relaxin in 75% of the primary and secondary giant trophoblast cells observed on day 14 (818). Relaxin immunoactivity was also localized in maternal endometrial granulocytes (816) (Fig. 34A and D). These cells, which are found in the wall of sheathed arteries in the decidua basalis, correspond to granulated metrial gland cells of the rat and may contribute to the dissolution of arterial wall before invasion by the trophoblast (816).

Relaxin is not stored in electron-dense cytoplasmic secretory granules in the hamster placenta as is the case in the pig corpus luteum (214,332,544,566,593), rat corpus luteum (30,328,336), human corpus luteum (992), guinea pig endometrium (594,596,752), and rabbit placental syncytiotrophoblast (297). Johns and Renegar (517) localized relaxin within the perinuclear Golgi complex of primary and secondary giant trophoblast cells by the avidin-biotin immunoperoxidase technique. Moreover, after differential centrifugation of hamster placental homogenates, most relaxin immunoactivity, detected by porcine relaxin radioimmunoassay, was in the postmicrosome fraction but not the mitochondria/granule fraction (517). It was postulated that relaxin may be secreted soon after synthesis in the hamster rather than being concentrated, packaged in membrane-bound storage granules, and released on stimulation by an appropriate secretogogue (517).

Apparently, the placenta is the sole source of relaxin in the hamster. Renegar et al. (816) did not detect relaxin in the corpora lutea or uterine glands with the avidin-biotin immunoperoxidase localization technique. Also, Steinetz et al. (963) demonstrated that peripheral serum levels of relaxin immunoactivity in hamsters ovariectomized on day 8 of gestation did not differ from those of intact controls on days 10 and 14.

O'Byrne and Steinetz (722) determined the general profile of relaxin immunoactivity in the blood of hamsters with a porcine relaxin radioimmunoassay. Consistent with its occurrence within the placenta (816), relaxin immunoactivity in peripheral serum appeared on day 8, rose to maximal levels by day 15, and dropped precipitously at parturition on day 16.

Primates

Human

With the isolation of porcine relaxin in 1974 (924), there came renewed interest in human relaxin. Since 1976, many studies concerning the source(s) of relaxin, blood levels of relaxin, and regulation of relaxin secretion in women have been conducted. From the late 1970s until the late 1980s, when a homologous human relaxin radioimmunoassay (286) and a homologous human relaxin enzyme-linked immunosorbant assay (634) were described, most studies used a rabbit antiporcine relaxin serum, designated R6, for both radioimmunoassay and immunohistochemical localization of human relaxin. Antiporcine relaxin serum R6 was generated by Steinetz and co-workers (968) with the three contiguous porcine relaxin peaks CMB, CMa, and CMa′ (924) shown in Fig. 1. Three lines of evidence indicate that antiserum R6 binds human relaxin. First, R6 bound to a molecule in human luteal extracts with a molecular weight that did not differ from that of porcine relaxin—about 6,300 (628). Second, R6 inhibited the ability of crude extracts of human corpora lutea of pregnancy to promote growth of the interpubic ligament in guinea pigs (968,969). Finally, when R6 was used with porcine relaxin radioimmunoassays, the concentration-dependent curves obtained with multiple volumes of both human corpora lutea extract and human pregnancy serum were reportedly parallel to those obtained with highly purified porcine relaxin (630,720). The homologous human relaxin radioimmunoassay (286,289) and homologous human relaxin enzyme-linked immunosorbant assay (87,634) developed in the late 1980s have advantages over porcine relaxin assays for measuring human relaxin: They are both more sensitive and more accurate. Nevertheless, many workers continue to use productively the generally available antiporcine relaxin sera for the study of relaxin in humans and other primates. Rabbit antiporcine relaxin serum R6, other antiporcine relaxin sera, antihuman relaxin sera, and monoclonal antibodies for human relaxin were used for the radioimmunoassays and immunohistochemical studies of human relaxin described in this section.

Menstrual Cycle

Ovarian Source. There are indications that small amounts of relaxin may be produced in extraluteal ovarian sites during the follicular phase of the menstrual cycle. Sufficient relaxin was reported to be present in follicular fluid obtained either during the late follicular phase of the normal cycle (710) or after ovarian stimulation with gonadotropins (1101) to inhibit contractions of the mouse and rat uterus, respectively. Moreover, most of the relaxin immunoactivity in follicular fluid obtained from artificially stimulated preovulatory follicles was associated with a 6,000-Da component (1101). Finally, detectable levels of relaxin immunoactivity were found in peripheral plasma before follicular rupture in women whose ovaries were hyperstimulated with exogenous gonadotropin treatment (1039). There is not total agreement on the cells that produce relaxin during the follicular phase of the menstrual cycle. Long-term cultures of granulosa cells were reported to release low amounts of relaxin in response to hCG stimulation (368,869,870). Moreover, an early study immunolocalized relaxin in granulosa cells from medium-sized cavitary follicles with an antiserum to porcine relaxin (56). A more recent investigation, however, identified mRNA for human relaxins 1 and 2 as well as immunoreactive relaxin in thecal cells (601).

Although extracts of the corpus luteum of the menstrual cycle contain insufficient relaxin to be readily detected with *in vivo* relaxin bioassays (720,1008), there is strong evidence that the corpus luteum of the cycle produces relaxin. Relaxin immunoactivity was found in luteal extracts (721), luteal cyst fluid (630), and culture medium bathing freshly dispersed luteal cells obtained during the menstrual cycle (867). The peritoneal fluid, which has been reported to be mainly an exudate of the active ovary in women (569), contains levels of relaxin that are detectable with porcine relaxin radioimmunoassays during the luteal phase of the cycle (629,1038). Whereas an investigation that used the peroxidase-antiperoxidase immunohistochemical method failed to locate relaxin immunoactivity in the corpora lutea during the early luteal phase (658), studies that used the more sensitive avidin-biotin immunoperoxidase method found specific staining associated with luteal cells (992,1145,1146,1149). Two laboratories reported that human relaxin gene 2, but not human relaxin gene 1, is expressed in the corpus luteum of the menstrual cycle in women (440,502). Both laboratories identified 1-kb and 2-kb relaxin mRNA transcripts by Northern analysis.

Blood Levels. There is now good evidence that the corpus luteum of the menstrual cycle releases relaxin into the circulation. The amount of relaxin released from the corpora lutea during the luteal phase of the menstrual cycle is not sufficient to be readily detected in the peripheral blood with porcine relaxin radioimmunoassays (367,553,720,804,806,894,1039), but it was detected in ovarian vein plasma draining the ovary that contained a corpus luteum (553). In the early 1990s, Stewart and co-workers (597,976) detected a small but consistent peak of relaxin immunoactivity in peripheral plasma about 9 to 10 days after ovulation in nonconceptive cycles by using a homologous human relaxin 2 enzyme-linked immunosorbant assay (634) (Fig. 35). Eddie et al. (288) also detected low levels of relaxin in the peripheral sera of nonpregnant women whose cycles were stimulated by clomiphene citrate and human menopausal gonadotropin by using a homologous human relaxin 2 radioimmunoassay.

Uterine Production of Relaxin. Human relaxin also appears to be synthesized by the endometrium during the menstrual cycle. Relaxin immunoactivity was initially detected within endometrial gland epithelial cells during the luteal phase of the menstrual cycle using anti-

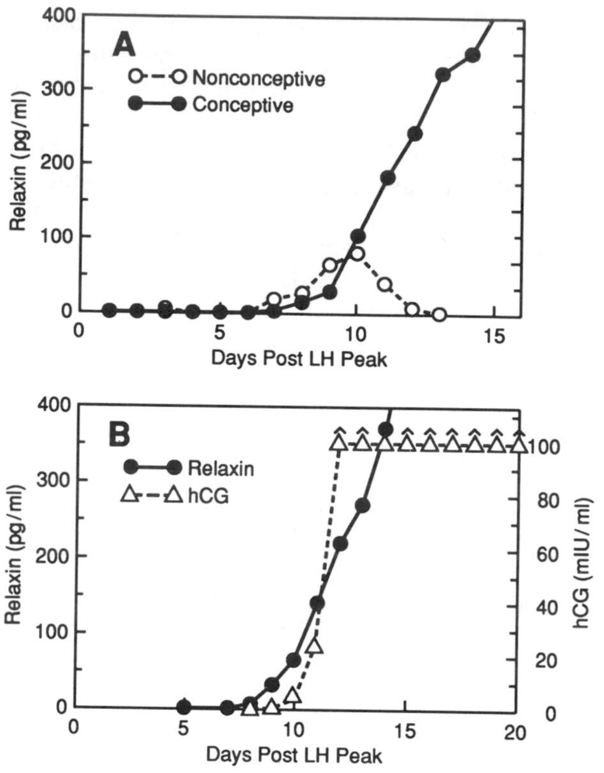

FIG. 35. A: Peripheral plasma relaxin concentrations in a nonconceptive cycle followed by a conceptive cycle in the same subject. **B:** Peripheral plasma relaxin and hCG concentrations from one pregnant subject. Values of hCG greater than 100 mIU/ml were off scale and are indicated by ^. From ref. 976, with permission.

porcine relaxin sera with the avidin-biotin immunoperoxidase method (1146,1148). More recently, relaxin immunostaining was detected in the endometrial glands during the luteal phase of the menstrual cycle by immunocytochemical localization with antibodies to human relaxin 2 and human relaxin C-peptide (113). The occurrence of relaxin in the human endometrium appears to be progesterone-dependent: It was found in postmenopausal women in an estrogen–progesterone replacement therapy program (1148) and in women in an *in vitro* fertilization program within 2 days of the administration of 17α-hydroxyprogesterone caproate at the time of follicle aspiration (1092). Perhaps endometrial relaxin accounts for the relaxin immunoactivity detected in cervical-vaginal secretions during the luteal phase of the menstrual cycle (366,367).

There were brief and isolated reports that relaxin immunoactivity is present in the myometrium (108), cervix (108,620), and cervicovaginal secretions (366,367).

Mammary Gland Production of Relaxin. Evidence that relaxin is produced within the human mammary gland regardless of the reproductive status of the woman is accumulating. Relaxin immunoactivity was detected in breast cyst fluid (697), milk (289), and mammary parenchyma in nonpregnant women (108). Bryant-

Greenwood and co-workers localized relaxin in normal lobular and ductal epithelial cells as well as myoepithelial cells in mammary tissue obtained from prepubertal, cyclic, gestational, lactational, and postmenopausal women, using antisera to both porcine relaxin (661) and human relaxin 2 (1020) with the avidin-biotin immunoperoxidase method. Strong relaxin immunostaining was also observed in ductal epithelial cells of both benign and atypical hyperplasia as well as epithelial and myoepithelial cells of fibroadenomas (661). Human relaxin 2 mRNA transcripts were also consistently present in extracts of benign and neoplastic breast tissue (1020).

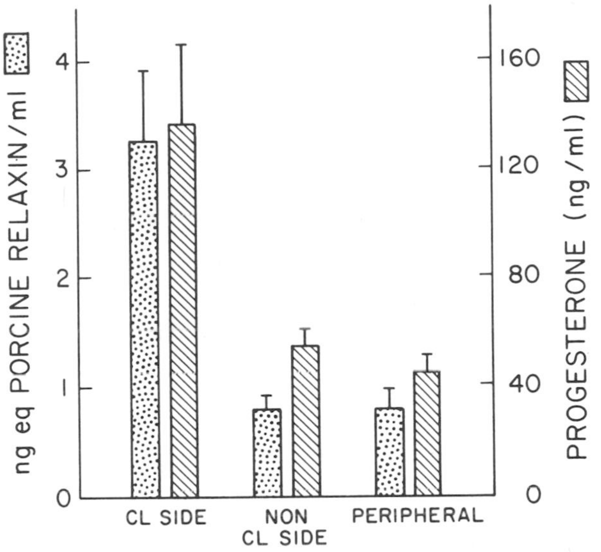

FIG. 36. Mean relaxin and progesterone immunoactivity levels (+SE; $n = 7$) in ovarian vein and peripheral blood plasma in women after term delivery by cesarean section. From ref. 1112, with permission.

Pregnancy

Ovarian Source. Many lines of evidence indicate that after conception the corpus luteum produces and secretes relaxin. First, extracts of corpora lutea of pregnancy were reported to contain relaxin immunoactivity (628,640,721,1111), to reduce the amplitude of spontaneous contractions of human myometrial strips (1008), and to be active in the guinea pig pubic symphysis palpation bioassay (721). Second, venous blood draining the ovary containing the corpus luteum had plasma relaxin levels three to four times higher during the sixth week of gestation than during the luteal phase of the cycle (553). Third, relaxin immunoactivity was present in the medium bathing collagenase-dispersed cells of human corpora lutea obtained at term (391,867). Fourth, large luteal cells displayed specific relaxin staining with studies that used the peroxidase-antiperoxidase and avidin-biotin immunoperoxidase localization methods (658, 992,1146). Moreover, immunocytochemical studies at the ultrastructural level indicated that, like the pig, most of the relaxin immunoactivity was associated with secretory granules (992). Further evidence of the luteal origin of relaxin is the presence of 1- and 2-kb mRNA molecules derived from human relaxin gene-2 in luteal tissue of pregnancy (502). Finally, Maclennan et al. (640) detected high levels of relaxin C peptide, which is present in prorelaxin, in purified extracts of human corpora lutea of pregnancy using a radioimmunoassay specific for human relaxin C-peptide.

The corpus luteum is the source of most, and perhaps all, circulating relaxin during pregnancy. Weiss et al. (1112) demonstrated that at term pregnancy relaxin immunoactivity was present in the ovarian vein draining the corpus luteum in far higher concentrations than in either the ovarian vein draining the contralateral ovary or the peripheral blood (Fig. 36). Moreover, these workers (1110) demonstrated that luteectomy produced a prompt disappearance of relaxin from the peripheral blood. Consistent with these findings, relaxin fell to undetectable levels after ovariectomy in molar pregnancies (893). Two laboratories reported that serum relaxin is not detectable in patients with premature ovarian failure who become pregnant with egg donation and do not have a corpus luteum (303,519).

Available evidence indicates that the levels of relaxin within the corpus luteum of pregnancy in women (721) are much lower than those in the corpora lutea of pigs (924) and rats (905). There is currently no evidence that the membrane-bound granules that store relaxin in the cytoplasm of human luteal cells accumulate during pregnancy (992) as they do in pigs (81,214,332,554), rats (30,328,626), and mice (31).

Blood Levels. Relaxin levels are elevated in the peripheral blood throughout nearly all gestation in the human (2,76,78,286,518,519,647,720,778,808,864,868,898, 1009,1154). The earliest indications that relaxin levels might be higher during early pregnancy than late pregnancy were obtained in the 1930s when Pommerenke (778) and Abramson et al. (2) reported that with advancing pregnancy, fewer and fewer human serum samples were capable of inducing pelvic relaxation in estrogen-primed guinea pigs. Consistent with these reports, subsequent radioimmunoassays, or enzyme-linked immunosorbant assays, which used antisera to either porcine relaxin (630,647,720,806,868,898,1009) or a synthetic analog of human relaxin 2 (76,78,286,518,519), demonstrated that relaxin immunoactivity levels are higher during the first trimester than during the second or third trimester (Fig. 37). Unlike the pig and rat, there is no antepartum surge in relaxin levels in women (720,805,808,897,1009). Perhaps this is a reflection of the apparent low level of relaxin that is stored in secretory granules in the corpus luteum of women during late pregnancy. There is limited evidence that relaxin con-

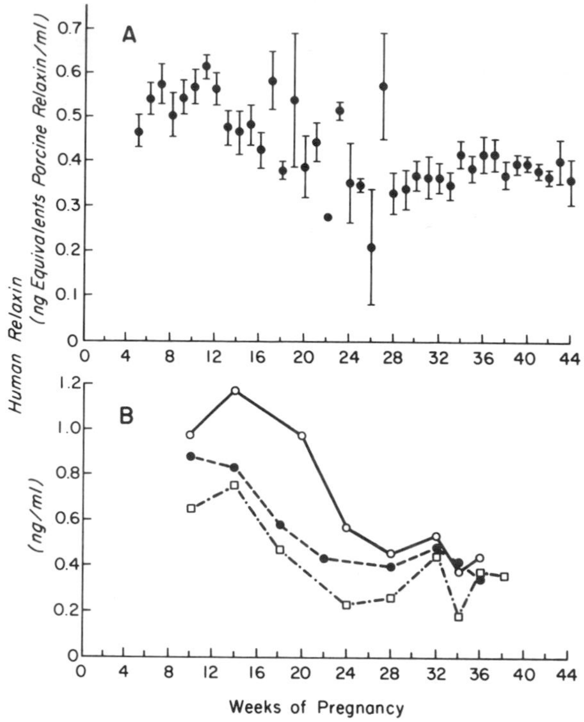

FIG. 37. Relaxin immunoactivity levels in peripheral blood of women throughout pregnancy. **A:** Relaxin levels (±SE) were determined with a homologous porcine relaxin radioimmunoassay that used rabbit antiporcine relaxin serum R6. From ref. 720, with permission. **B:** Relaxin levels were determined with a homologous human relaxin radioimmunoassay that used rabbit antihuman relaxin 2 serum. From ref. 286, with permission.

centrations change relatively rapidly and are somewhat elevated during labor (520,647).

Regulation of Secretion. Abundant evidence supports the hypothesis that hCG, which is secreted by the trophoblast and rescues the corpus luteum of the menstrual cycle, is a main stimulus for relaxin secretion during pregnancy. First, there is a good correlation between blood levels of endogenous hCG and blood levels of relaxin. The accelerated secretion of relaxin about 10 days postovulation coincides temporally with the appearance of hCG immunoactivity in the peripheral blood (288,668,806,976) (Fig. 35B). The subsequent blood level profiles of the two hormones are similar throughout pregnancy (76,78,286,522,647,720,808,898). Moreover, as in normal pregnancy (437,898,1138), blood levels of relaxin generally correlate with blood levels of endogenous hCG in women with ectopic pregnancy (374,891) as well as those with trophoblastic disease (893,895,899). Also, patients with twin pregnancies after *in vitro* fertilization and embryo transfer (75,76,78) or induction of ovulation with menotropins (437) had higher serum relaxin levels than patients with single pregnancies who had undergone similar preovulatory ovarian stimulation. It was postulated that higher hCG levels in the twin pregnancies may account for the elevated relaxin levels (75,76). Also, it was reported that spontaneously aborting women with low relaxin levels had low hCG levels, whereas those with normal hCG levels had normal relaxin levels (807,900).

Clinical or experimental procedures that alter the exposure of human luteal cells to hCG also provide evidence that hCG promotes relaxin secretion. Injection of hCG during the luteal phase of the menstrual cycle extended luteal function and induced relaxin secretion (693,804,1039). Also, women undergoing *in vitro* fertilization who were injected with hCG on the day of embryo transfer and 3 days thereafter had far higher plasma levels of relaxin on day 22 after embryo transfer than did women who did not receive the hCG (522). Consistent with these findings, removal of hydatidiform mole, where circulating hCG levels are higher than in normal pregnancy, brought about a decline in serum levels of both hCG and relaxin (893,899). Addition of hCG to long-term cultures of luteinized granulosa cells obtained from women undergoing controlled ovarian hyperstimulation for *in vitro* fertilization promoted the secretion of relaxin after a time lag of about 10 days (368). Finally, addition of hCG to monolayers of luteal cells collected at cesarean section increased relaxin immunoactivity levels in the media on day 2 of culture (391).

The secretion of relaxin also appears to be directly related to the number of corpora lutea in pregnant women. Relaxin immunoactivity levels were reported to be greater in spontaneous twin pregnancies than in singleton pregnancies (647) and also to be greater in two trizygotic triplet pregnancies than in either a monozygotic triplet pregnancy or singleton pregnancies during the third trimester (1009). Furthermore, both patients with singleton or multiple pregnancies after *in vitro* fertilization of their own ova (75,76,78) and patients with two or more fetuses after postmenopausal gonadotropin-induced ovulation (374,437) had significantly higher serum relaxin levels than normal antenatal patients who had a single corpus luteum of pregnancy. It was postulated that the multiple mature ovarian follicles induced in patients by a combination of clomiphene citrate and/or human menopausal gonadotropin form multiple corpora lutea (76,374,437). At the other extreme, serum relaxin was not detected in patients with premature ovarian failure who became pregnant with egg donation and did not have a corpus luteum (303,519). One study (519), which used the sensitive enzyme-linked immunosorbant assay for human relaxin, detected no relaxin in peripheral serum in 36 of 41 patients with premature ovarian failure throughout their ovum donation pregnancies. Moreover, serum relaxin was extremely low as compared with normal pregnancies in the remaining five women who also lacked a corpus luteum of pregnancy.

It is not known if hormones other than hCG influence relaxin secretion from the corpus luteum during pregnancy in women. The few reports concerning the influence of PGs on relaxin secretion are not in complete agreement. Vaginal administration of a synthetic derivative of PGE_1 during the first trimester reportedly increased serum relaxin concentrations (896). Efforts to induce the secretion of relaxin during late pregnancy with $PGF_{2\alpha}$ were not successful. The administration of sufficient $PGF_{2\alpha}$ or oxytocin (469) to induce delivery did not influence serum relaxin levels. Similarly, administration of sufficient PGE_2 to induce second trimester abortions did not alter serum relaxin levels (803).

Clinical Implications of Serum Relaxin Levels. Because serum levels of relaxin reflect both effective luteotropic stimulation and the amount of luteal tissue, investigators have examined the possibility that relaxin levels can be used for clinical diagnostic purposes. Luteal phase defect, which is characterized by a short luteal phase and inadequate action of progesterone on the endometrium, is a cause of infertility and pregnancy loss. Stewart et al. (978) used the human relaxin 2 enzyme-linked immunosorbant assay (634) to demonstrate that there is a marked reduction in both the duration of secretion and levels of relaxin during the luteal phase in women with luteal phase defect. After *in vitro* fertilization and embryo transfer, Eddie et al. (288) initially detected relaxin, but not hCG, in the peripheral serum of several nonpregnant women on days 6 to 8 postlaparoscopy. In contrast, both relaxin and hCG were first detected on days 10 to 12 postlaparoscopy in pregnant women. Because the maintenance of early pregnancy requires synchrony of factors from the embryo, endometrium, and corpus luteum, these workers (288) postulated that early secretion of relaxin in nonpregnant women could indicate asynchronous luteal function that results in loss of the embryo. Investigators have explored the possibility that atypically low peripheral serum relaxin levels can be used to predict abortions during the first trimester when maintenance of pregnancy is dependent on luteal support. Whereas all reports but one (900) indicated that serum relaxin levels were frequently low and/or declined before spontaneous abortion (76,78,374,977,1138), serum levels of relaxin offer no advantage over serum levels of hCG and/or progesterone in predicting early abortion.

It has also been postulated that atypically high serum relaxin levels during pregnancy may have clinical implications. There is limited but not entirely consistent evidence that elevated serum relaxin levels might be useful in predicting preterm labor. Petersen et al. (768) found that mean serum relaxin levels at 30 weeks of naturally occurring gestation were higher in patients that delivered preterm than in patients that delivered at term. In contrast, Bell et al. (77) reported that antepartum serum relaxin levels were within the normal range of values in women whose naturally occurring pregnancies ended preterm. Haning et al. (437) postulated that excessive secretion of relaxin may be a factor in the premature births with incompetent cervices associated with multiple gestation after postmenopausal gonadotropin administration. MacLennan et al. (648) reported that serum relaxin levels were higher in patients with pelvic pain and joint laxity than in controls. Steinetz et al. (972) reported that serum relaxin levels are significantly higher in all three trimesters in diabetic women than in nondiabetic controls. Neither the mechanism that accounts for the elevated relaxin levels in diabetic pregnancy nor the physiologic consequences is known. Steinetz et al. (972) postulated that relaxin may be a component in diabetic embryopathy.

Clearance of Relaxin from the Blood. The clearance of relaxin immunoactivity from humans has not been reported. The clearance of human relaxin from the serum of both pregnant and nonpregnant monkeys (319) and rats (215) was reported. There were no significant differences between nonpregnant and pregnant animals and, as with porcine relaxin and rat relaxin (912), the serum concentration–time data were described by multiple exponential terms. The terminal half-lives for clearance of human relaxin 2 in monkeys (319) and rats (215) were approximately 150 and 60 min, respectively. When human relaxin 2 was internally labeled with ^{35}S-cysteine and then injected into rats, the kidneys were the principal site of uptake and the liver was of secondary importance (215).

Decidual, Placental, and Mammary Production of Relaxin. Although reports are not entirely consistent, it seems likely that relaxin is produced in the decidua, cytotrophoblast of the chorionic laeve, and syncytiotrophoblast and may also be produced in the amnion (Fig. 38). In the early 1980s, several laboratories reported that extracts of term decidual tissue (92,94,96) or placental tissue (334,1142) contained sufficient relaxin to demonstrate bioactivity. These extracts were reported to inhibit spontaneous uterine contractions in guinea pigs (96), rats (96), and mice (334,1142); to produce growth of the interpubic ligament in mice (96,334) and guinea pigs (1154); and to promote morphologic changes in the mammary ducts in estrogen-pretreated mice (61–63). Schmidt et al. (871) failed to confirm the presence of sufficient relaxin in extracts of human placental or decidual tissue to promote growth of the interpubic ligament in mice or to inhibit contractions of rat uterine segments. They did, however, find that two partially purified fractions obtained from placental extract had limited bioactivity in the guinea pig pubic symphysis palpation bioassay and that extracts of both decidual and placental tissue contained relaxin immunoactivity. Two studies found little (1111) or no (630) relaxin immunoactivity in human placental extracts obtained at term.

Several workers used immunohistochemical techniques to localize relaxin in human decidual and placental tissues. The significance of an early investigation

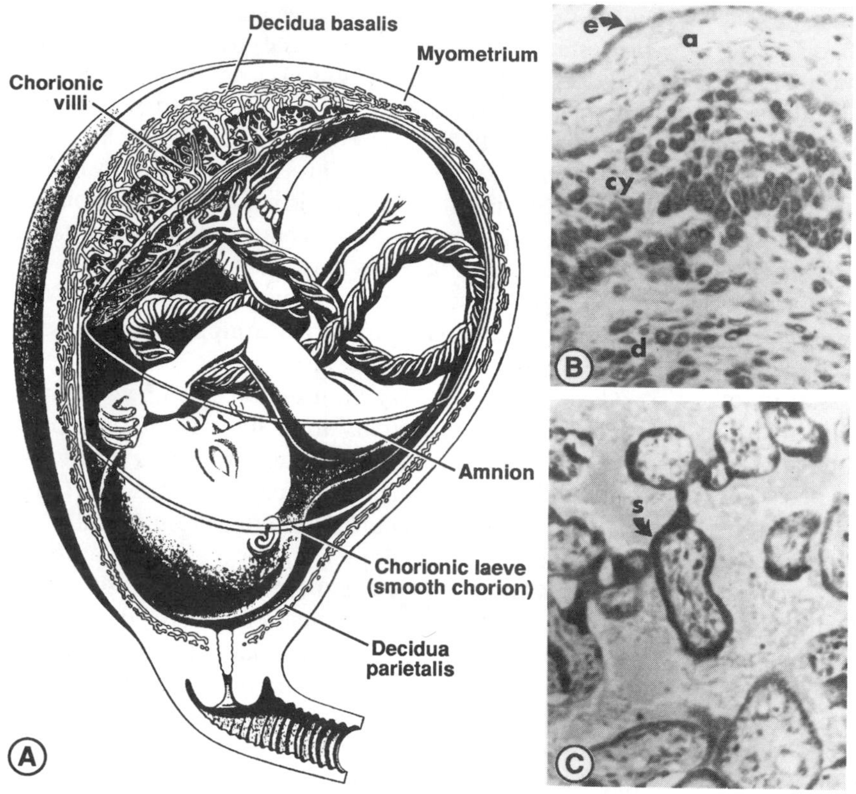

FIG. 38. **A:** Drawing of sagittal section of gravid uterus showing decidua parietalis, decidua basalis, chorionic laeve, placental trophoblast villi, and amnion. Modified from ref. 1127. **B, C:** Immunolocalization of human relaxin in decidual and placental tissue obtained after elective cesarean section at term by means of the avidin-biotin immunoperoxidase method using monoclonal antibodies against human relaxin 2. **B:** Amnion (*a*), amniotic epithelium (*e*), chorionic cytotrophoblast (*cy*), decidua parietalis (*d*). Note that relaxin immunostaining occurs in cytotrophoblast and decidua, with little, if any, in amnion. (×200) **C:** Syncytiotrophoblasts of placental villi. Note that dark syncytiotrophoblast relaxin immunostaining occurs in patches. (×200) B and C from ref. 847, with permission.

(241) that concluded that granulated cells in human decidua and basal trophoblast cells of the placenta contain relaxin was weakened by the impurity of the porcine relaxin used to generate the antiserum used for immunofluorescence localization of the hormone. Nevertheless, several more recent immunohistochemical studies that used a variety of antisera generated with highly purified porcine relaxin or monoclonal antibodies to synthetic human relaxin 2 also reported relaxin immunoactivity in decidual tissue (92,145,203,299,560,847,1146) and placental tissue (145,203,334,560,847,1144–1146).

Recently, Bryant-Greenwood and co-workers (139, 140,440,847,848) and MacLennan et al. (640) used immunohistochemical localization and/or Northern analysis to obtain evidence that the small amounts of relaxin identified within the decidua and placenta are produced locally and not attributable to bound circulating relaxin. Consistent with an earlier finding using antiporcine relaxin serum (1144), the decidua parietalis and cytotrophoblast of the chorionic laeve tissue obtained at term from a woman ovariectomized during the first half of pregnancy demonstrated relaxin immunostaining (847). Prorelaxin, as well as relaxin, was localized in both the decidua parietalis cells and cytotrophoblast of the chorionic laeve (smooth chorion) at term, using the avidin-biotin immunoperoxidase technique (Fig. 38A and B). Prorelaxin was localized with antisera to a synthetic 14-amino-acid protein of the C peptide (640,848), and relaxin was localized with monoclonal antibodies to human relaxin 2 (847). Finally, the detection of 1-kb mRNA for human relaxin in extracts of decidua parietalis and cytotrophoblast (139,440,847) by Northern analysis provides strong support for the view that relaxin is produced in these tissues. Interestingly, expression of human relaxin gene 1, as well as human relaxin gene 2, was detected in both decidua and placental trophoblast using reverse transcription polymerase reaction followed by selective amplification of the specific cDNA (440), and this provides the first indication that relaxin gene 1 may be expressed in the human female.

The syncytiotrophoblast of the placental villi may also produce relaxin. Efforts to immunolocalize relaxin or prorelaxin in this tissue site have provided positive (847,1144–1146), equivocal (203,560), or negative (640,848) findings. Immunolocalization of relaxin in the syncytiotrophoblast after a spontaneous delivery is shown in Fig. 38C. Also consistent with the possibility that the syncytiotrophoblast of placental villi produces relaxin is the observation that mRNA for human relaxin was extracted from the placental trophoblast (440,848).

Relaxin has been localized in the amnion by using the avidin-biotin immunoperoxidase technique with antiporcine relaxin serum (203,560), monoclonal antibody to human relaxin 2 (847), and human relaxin C peptide-specific serum (848). mRNA for human relaxin 2 was not found in extracts of the amnion, however, and it was postulated that the small amount of relaxin associated with the amnion may be receptor-bound (847,848).

Finally, Bryant-Greenwood and co-workers (661) recently reported the localization of relaxin immunoactivity in lobular and ductal epithelial cells as well as myoepithelial cells in mammary tissue obtained from a pregnant woman.

Relaxin in Compartments Other than the Maternal Blood During Pregnancy and Lactation. The amniotic fluid may contain low levels of relaxin immunoactivity (518,1111). Johnson et al. (518) found that the amniotic fluid contained detectable but far lower levels of relaxin than the maternal blood with an enzyme-linked immunosorbant assay for human relaxin 2. If the amniotic fluid contains relaxin, it is likely produced locally by decidual and/or placental tissue. Available evidence does not support the possibility that maternal relaxin produced by the corpus luteum of pregnancy passes freely through the placenta and enters the fetal blood.

Whereas there is not total agreement (304,518,521, 1111), it appears the fetal blood contains little, if any, relaxin. Little, if any, relaxin was detected in umbilical cord serum with a radioimmunoassay that used antiporcine relaxin serum R6 (1111), and no relaxin was detected with an enzyme-linked immunosorbant assay that used antihuman relaxin 2 serum (518). Moreover, when synthetic human relaxin 2 was infused into pregnant rhesus monkeys on gestational days ranging from 131 to 158, only small amounts passed into the fetal blood (216,634).

Relaxin immunoactivity was detected in the milk of lactating women from 3 days to 6 or more weeks of lactation with oral immunoassays that used either antiporcine relaxin serum R6 (621) or an antihuman relaxin 2 serum (289). The presence of relaxin in milk several weeks after both delivery and regression of the corpus luteum of pregnancy is consistent with the immunolocalization of relaxin in epithelial and myoepithelial cells of the mammary gland during lactation in women (661). There is also limited evidence that circulating levels of relaxin may increase in women during suckling (520).

Monkey, Baboon, and Chimpanzee

Menstrual Cycle

As is the case in the human, circulating relaxin levels rise in the late luteal phase of the menstrual cycle in rhesus monkeys (*Macaca mulatta*) (987) and chimpanzees (970).

Pregnancy

During pregnancy, the main source of relaxin, the profile of relaxin levels in the blood, and the control of relaxin secretion in monkeys (708,747,987,1113), baboons (*Papio ursinus*) (184,186), and chimpanzees (*Pan troglodytes*) (970) appear similar to those in the human. The corpus luteum of pregnancy has been demonstrated to be the main source of relaxin in monkeys and baboons. After bilateral ovariectomy of the monkey *Macaca mulatta* (rhesus monkey) during the first trimester (1113), luteectomy of the monkey *Macaca fascicularis* (cynomolgus monkey) during the first trimester (987) or on day 150 of pregnancy (708), and luteectomy of baboons on day 30 of pregnancy (184,186), serum relaxin immunoactivity levels fell abruptly. As in humans, it appears that chorionic gonadotropin is a major stimulus for the initiation of relaxin secretion during early pregnancy in monkeys and baboons. The rise of circulating relaxin levels paralleled the rise of monkey chorionic gonadotropin until 20 to 25 days postbreeding in cynomolgus macaque monkeys (987). When monkeys (746,747) and baboons (184) were administered hCG during the luteal phase of the nonfertile menstrual cycle, there was an increase in serum relaxin levels within a few days of the initiation of hCG treatment. Both the pattern and concentration of circulating relaxin in rhesus monkeys depend on the age of the corpus luteum at the onset of hCG treatment in rhesus monkeys (747), as is the case in women (804,1039). Circulating relaxin levels were detectable within 5 days when hCG treatment was initiated during the late luteal phase, whereas relaxin was not detected for 9 days when hCG treatment was initiated during the early luteal phase (747). Serum relaxin immunoactivity levels remain relatively constant in monkeys, baboons, and chimpanzees throughout most of pregnancy, with no evidence of a prelabor surge (186,708, 970,1113).

There is limited evidence that low levels of relaxin may be produced in nonluteal tissues in monkeys and baboons. Castration of monkeys during pregnancy did not interfere with the loosening of the pelvic ligaments near term (452). On about day 140 of the approximately 175-day gestation period, low levels of relaxin immunoactivity were found in the decidual, placental, and myometrial tissue of baboons in which the corpus luteum had been removed on day 30 (186). Because pregnancy proceeds normally after the first trimester in the absence of the corpus luteum in humans and baboons, Castracane and co-workers (186) suggested that relaxin produced in nonluteal tissue may have a physiologic role during late pregnancy and at parturition.

BIOLOGIC EFFECTS OF RELAXIN IN THE FEMALE VERTEBRATE

It was not possible to establish without doubt the biologic effects of relaxin until the late 1970s, when the hormone became available in highly purified form. Nevertheless, the multitude of earlier reports demonstrating that relaxin levels are elevated in the blood and ovaries (or other portions of the reproductive tract) in a variety of mammalian species during pregnancy, coupled with the observations that impure preparations of relaxin affect connective tissue in the pubic symphysis and cervix, as well as inhibit contractility of the uterus in estrogen-primed females, led to the view that relaxin was probably of considerable importance during pregnancy and at parturition (138,782,784,886,908,913,964). Recent studies with highly purified relaxin not only confirmed early findings concerning relaxin's effects on the pubic symphysis, cervix, and myometrium but also demonstrated that relaxin influences other reproductive tissues as well as nonreproductive tissues. This section emphasizes relaxin's effects on well-established target tissues: the pubic symphysis, cervix, uterus, and mammary glands. Also, it describes putative biologic effects of relaxin on other tissues that have received less attention and are not presently established target tissues—the vagina, ovary, amnion, chorion, pituitary, and brain. It should be recognized that some biologic effects of relaxin occur in certain species but not in others; for example, relaxin promotes growth of the interpubic ligament in guinea pigs (1), mice (422), Skomer bank voles (1160), and bats (732), but not in rats (226). Relaxin's effects on cervical extensibility and uterine contractility appear to be more widely distributed among mammals.

Most studies of the physiology of relaxin conducted after 1980 used highly purified porcine relaxin. Because these studies confirmed earlier results obtained with impure porcine relaxin, the degree of purity of porcine relaxin preparations will be described only where emphasis seems important. Whenever the effects of relaxin treatment are described, it may be assumed that porcine relaxin was used unless stated otherwise. Although the structure of porcine relaxin differs substantially from that of rat, human, and guinea pig relaxin, it is bioactive in all three species. Moreover, porcine relaxin is bioactive in the cow, in which the structure of relaxin has not been determined but probably differs from that of porcine relaxin. It seems likely that biologic effects induced by highly purified porcine relaxin in species other than the pig would normally be induced by endogenous relaxin in these species.

Optimally, at least three criteria should be met to establish that circulating relaxin has a direct biologic effect on a putative target tissue. First, the putative target tissue should either demonstrate the appropriate biologic response after treatment with highly purified relaxin or fail to respond after removal or neutralization of endogenous relaxin. Second, it should be demonstrated that the putative target tissue possesses finite numbers of high-affinity binding sites that are specific for relaxin. Third, a close temporal association should be demonstrated between the occurrence of the biologic effect and the presence of relaxin in the blood. All three criteria are seldom met for a putative target tissue in a given species.

Demonstrating that putative target tissues contain relaxin receptors (second criterion) has proved to be particularly difficult. Throughout the 1980s, binding of relaxin to putative target tissues, such as the pubic symphysis and uterus, was examined with ^{125}I-labeled porcine relaxin. Research conducted with this radiolabeled ligand did not demonstrate specific binding to target tissues consistently either *in vitro* (200,384,719) or *in vivo* (719); moreover, where binding was reported, the percentage of radioiodinated relaxin bound specifically to putative target tissues was low (200,663,665,690). The inconsistencies among investigations and the low percentage of specific binding may be attributable to (a) the employment of radioiodinated porcine relaxin with tissues from species other than the pig, (b) varying structural modifications of the porcine relaxin attributable to the different procedures used for radioiodination, (c) low numbers of relaxin receptors in target tissues, or (d) binding limitations associated with the method of preparation of the target tissue for *in vitro* studies. In recent years, techniques for preparing biologically active probes that enable progress toward the identification and characterization of relaxin receptors were described. Osheroff et al. (743) described the preparation and characterization of a radiolabeled probe with a single phosphorylated site on the B chain of human relaxin 2 (B33). The ^{32}P-human relaxin 2 (B33), which retained biologic activity in a primary human endometrial cell line (314), was used for *in situ* autoradiographic localization of relaxin binding sites in rat uterine, cervical, brain, and heart tissue sections (742–744). Büllesbach and Schwabe (155) described the preparation and characterization of monobiotinylated-porcine relaxin derivatives that retained full biologic activity in the mouse interpubic ligament bioassay and postulated that these derivatives could be used with the avidin-biotin system for relaxin receptor studies. In 1992, Yang et al. (1143) described the preparation of a monoiodinated ^{125}I-porcine relaxin tracer that retained biologic activity in the mouse interpubic ligament bioassay. These workers used that probe for *in situ* autoradiographic localization of relaxin binding sites in mouse pubic symphysis, uterus, and ovary.

It has also been difficult to demonstrate a close temporal association between the occurrence of biologic effects during pregnancy and the presence of relaxin in the blood (third criterion) in some cases. The available relaxin bioassays and radioimmunoassays may lack the specificity and/or sensitivity needed to determine relaxin levels in the peripheral blood of some species during pregnancy. Despite the present limitations associated with characterizing relaxin receptors and measuring blood levels of relaxin in most species, considerable progress has been made in recent years toward a better understanding of the biologic effects of relaxin.

Pubic Symphysis

In many species, modifications of the pelvic girdle occur to enable safe delivery of their young. Examples include mammals that use burrowing or flying for movement and that have streamlined bodies with narrow pelvic girdles or mammals whose fetal/maternal weight ratio is relatively large (782). Passage of young through the birth canal at delivery has been facilitated in many of these species by means of hormonally regulated adaptations of the pelvis. In nearly all mammals, these adaptations involve sexual dimorphism of the bony pelvis as well as increased flexibility of the sacroiliac and/or pelvic symphysis during late pregnancy. An additional adaptation that occurs in some species is transformation of pelvic joint cartilage to an elastic interpubic ligament, which enables considerable separation of the innominate bones.

A sexual dimorphism of the bony pelvis that causes the female to have a sufficiently large birth canal has been described in many mammals, including mice (224,375), rats (86,226), rabbits (632), free-tailed bats (231), and humans (225). It was demonstrated that pelvic dimorphism, which generally occurs between birth and puberty, is caused by exposure of the male pelvis to androgens during an early postnatal period. Both male and female mice and rats had female-type pelvises if they were castrated at birth, whereas treatment of both the male and female castrates with androgens led to development of male-type pelvises (86,224). Also, humans with testicular feminization syndrome, whose target tissues are insensitive to circulating androgens, have female-type bony pelvises (225). Although the ovary does not appear to influence prepubertal sexual dimorphism of the bony pelvis, it may have postpubertal influences on its structure. In mice, estrogens caused a partial resorption of the medial edges of the pubic bones (375).

Transformation of the pubic joint cartilage to a flexible and elastic interpubic ligament occurs during pregnancy in several species, including guinea pigs, mice, bats, and humans (732,962). It does not occur in species such as rats (226) and sheep (67). In the rat, there appears to be little adaptation of the pelvis at delivery. It was reported that the rat pelvis failed to relax during pregnancy (226,1013); moreover, injections of estrogen and relaxin promoted little, if any, increase in flexibility of the pubic symphysis (226).

Growth of the interpubic ligament can enable marked increases in the size of the birth canal. For example, in guinea pigs the length of the interpubic ligament increases so markedly during late pregnancy that a fetus with an average head diameter twice the average diameter of the pelvic canal is delivered (782). Extensive studies of the hormonal regulation of the transformation of the interpubic ligament have been conducted with only guinea pigs and mice, and these studies demonstrated that growth of the interpubic ligament is stimulated primarily by estrogen and relaxin. Although the emphasis of this section is on the roles estrogen and relaxin play in regulating the formation of the interpubic ligament during pregnancy, effects of other hormones are described briefly. For additional information concerning development of the bony pelvis and hormonal regulation of the connective tissues of the pubic symphysis, see other reviews (225,351,467,962).

Guinea Pig

Structure of the Pubic Symphysis During Pregnancy

The pubic symphysis of prepubertal male guinea pigs consists almost entirely of an uninterrupted plate of hyaline cartilage that is largely replaced by bone as adulthood is attained. Unlike the male, the cartilaginous pubic symphysis of the maturing female is gradually replaced by fibrous connective tissue that forms a ligament between the innominate bones (842). Development of the female-type pubic symphysis requires the presence of the ovary. Castration of females soon after birth results in retention of a male-type pubic symphysis that cannot be "relaxed" by estrogen plus relaxin treatment (462). Castration of adult females not only stops the removal of cartilage but also reverses the process and starts a gradual chondrification of the symphyseal tissue (1012).

The pubic symphysis of the estrogen-dominated adult female guinea pig consists largely of compact collagen fibers that are imbedded in an amorphous matrix that contains proteoglycans (206,962) (Fig. 39A). During approximately the last 4 weeks of the 9-week gestation period, transformation of the connective tissue of the pubic symphysis occurs, and this transformation becomes most dramatic during the week before birth. Grossly, there are marked increases in the vascularity (843,1013,1091), weight (1091), and length (1091) of the interpubic ligament during the last week of pregnancy (Fig. 40). Histologically, a rapid proliferation of connective tissue cells and resorption of the symphyseal faces of the pubic bones occur during the last 2 weeks of pregnancy (843).

Influence of Hormones on the Pubic Symphysis

Although the roles hormones play in transforming the pubic symphysis during pregnancy have not been established, available evidence indicates that estrogen and relaxin are the key hormones. Estrogen alone promotes growth of the interpubic ligament. Prolonged treatment of intact or ovariectomized guinea pigs with estradiol caused about a two- to threefold increase in interpubic distance after 10 to 24 days of treatment (257,1014,

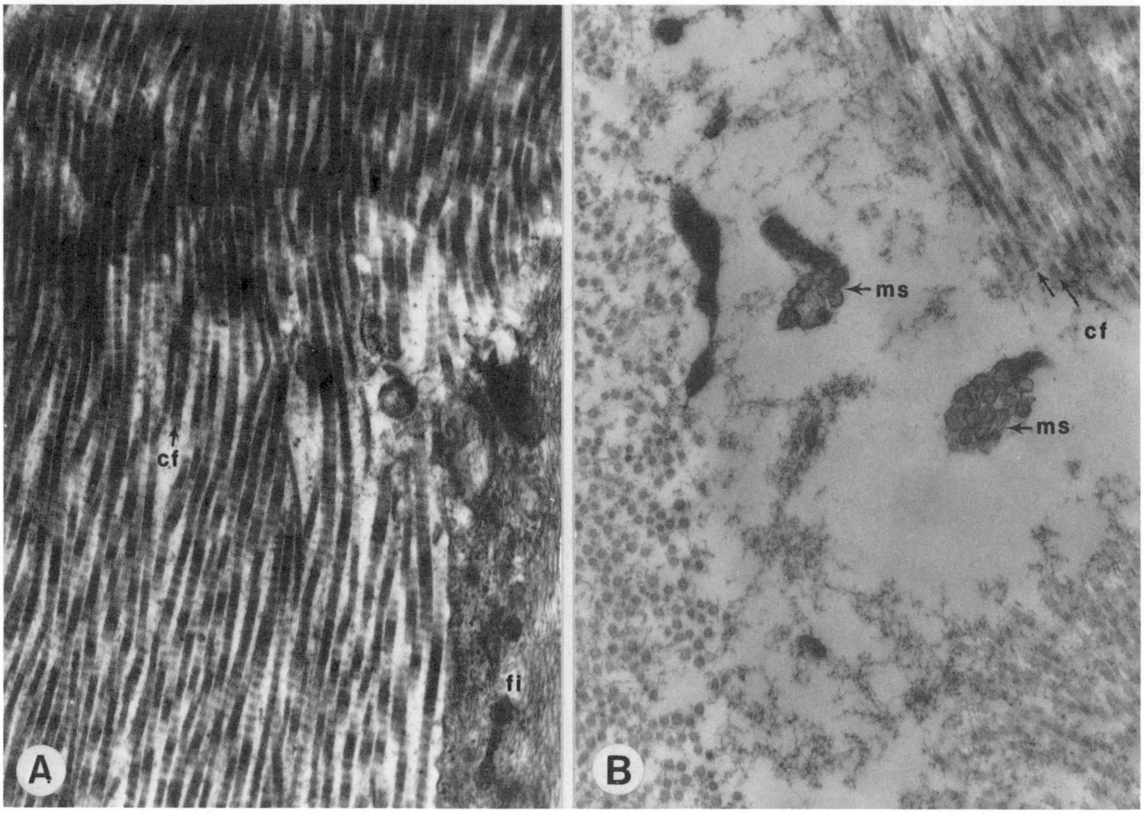

FIG. 39. **A:** Dense collagen (*cf*) in symphysis pubis of a guinea pig that has not received relaxin. A fibroblast (*fi*) appears in lower right portion of micrograph. (×25,500) **B:** Disrupted collagen fibers in the symphysis pubis of a guinea pig treated with porcine relaxin. Multivesicular structures (*ms*) are located near sites of collagen digestion. (×23,000) From ref. 206, with permission.

1015,1151). This estrogen-induced increase in interpubic ligament length was primarily attributable to proliferation of fibrous connective tissue, resorption of bone, and increased water content (467). Also important is the essential role estrogens play in conditioning the pubic symphysis for a response to relaxin. Whereas relaxin has little (353) or no (462,468) effect on symphyseal connective tissue in guinea pigs that have not been primed with estrogen, it has a marked and rapid effect in estrogen-pretreated animals. When relaxin was administered to castrated adult guinea pigs treated with estrogen for 4 or more days, the transformation of the symphyseal connective tissue was readily detected within 6 to 8 h (350, 468,1013,1151). The effects of relaxin on the connective tissue of the guinea pig pubic symphysis differ from those of estrogen. After relaxin treatment, extensive dissolution and disorientation of the collagen fibers occurred (206,1012,1013), and the pubic symphysis became a bloody, spongy, and highly flexible structure (350) (Fig. 39B). There is limited evidence that relaxin brings about its effects by acting directly on the guinea pig pubic symphysis. A time-dependent concentration of radioiodinated porcine relaxin occurred in the pubic symphyses of adult guinea pigs within 90 min of the administration of the hormone (384). Although ambiguity remains concerning the profile of relaxin levels in the peripheral blood of guinea pigs throughout pregnancy (112,723,1150), investigators agree that relaxin levels are elevated during late pregnancy, when growth of the interpubic ligament is most marked.

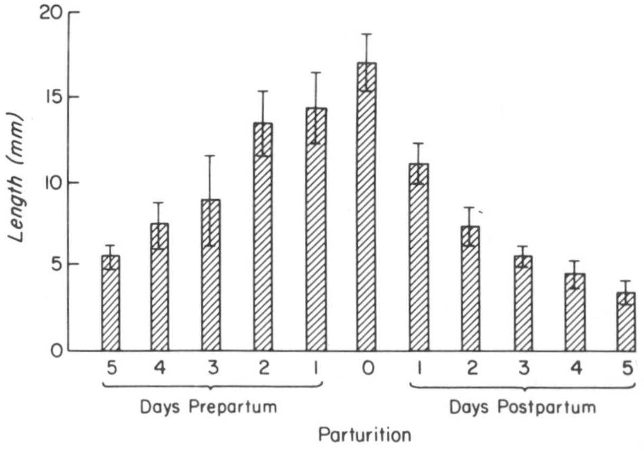

FIG. 40. Mean length (±SD; n = 8) of the guinea pig pubic symphysis ligament before and after parturition. From ref. 1091, with permission.

The mechanism(s) whereby relaxin promotes dissolution and disorientation of collagen in the guinea pig pubic symphysis is poorly understood. The cell type(s) that binds relaxin in the guinea pig pubic symphysis has not been determined, but it may be the fibroblasts. Chihal and Espey (206) suggested that the collagen breakdown may be caused by a substance released from multivesicular structures that are prominent at the end of cytoplasmic processes that protrude from the cell surface of fibroblasts located near sites of collagen digestion (Fig. 39B). If this is the case, the substance does not appear to be collagenase. Wahl et al. (1091) reported that collagenase levels remained low and that collagen synthesis increased about threefold during the last 5 days of pregnancy in the guinea pig. Another possibility is that relaxin exerts its effects, at least in part, by disaggregating complex proteoglycans within the matrix-ground substance. Perl and Catchpole (767) reported that highly polymerized proteoglycans in unrelaxed estrogen-dominated interpubic ligaments were insoluble in water and had little affinity for the dye Evans blue. After relaxin treatment, however, the proteoglycans became more water-soluble, and Evans blue dye was found in greatest concentrations in those areas of the symphyses that showed marked depolymerization (767). The localization of Evans blue was attributed to both increased availability of active groups on the depolymerized molecules and increased vascular permeability. Electrometric measurements that demonstrated that the charge density of matrix colloid was reduced in relaxin-treated guinea pigs (530) are also consistent with the view that relaxin exerts its effects through disaggregation of negatively charged proteoglycan aggregates. According to this hypothesis, the disaggregation of proteoglycans would somehow preclude the ordered arrangement of newly formed collagen into fibrils.

Progesterone also promotes relaxation of the interpubic ligament in guinea pigs. Unlike estrogen and relaxin, however, progesterone acts directly through the stimulation of relaxin secretion by the guinea pig uterus (467).

Mouse

Structure of the Pubic Symphysis During Pregnancy

In adult virgin female mice, the articular surfaces of the pubic bones are capped with hyaline cartilage and united by an interpubic disk of fibrocartilage (959) (Fig. 41A). During the last week of pregnancy, the pubic bones separate (Fig. 42). This separation of the pubic bones is attributable to resorption of the symphyseal surfaces of the pubic bones, swelling of the cartilaginous matrix, and transformation of the cartilage caps into a fibrous interpubic ligament that attains a maximum length of 3 to 6 mm at parturition (422,432,949,995). After parturition, the length of the interpubic ligament decreases rapidly and approaches nonpregnant dimensions by day 5 postpartum (225,432,949,995).

Influence of Hormones on the Pubic Symphysis

Although nearly all studies that have been conducted with mice used the species *Mus musculus,* the hormonal regulation of pelvic adaptations appears to be qualitatively similar among different strains and subspecies (1104,1153). As with guinea pigs, the combination of estrogen and relaxin promotes maximal relaxation of the pubic symphysis. After the administration of estrogen or relaxin alone to either intact or ovariectomized, nonpregnant mice, the increase in interpubic gap was smaller than that observed during pregnancy or after the

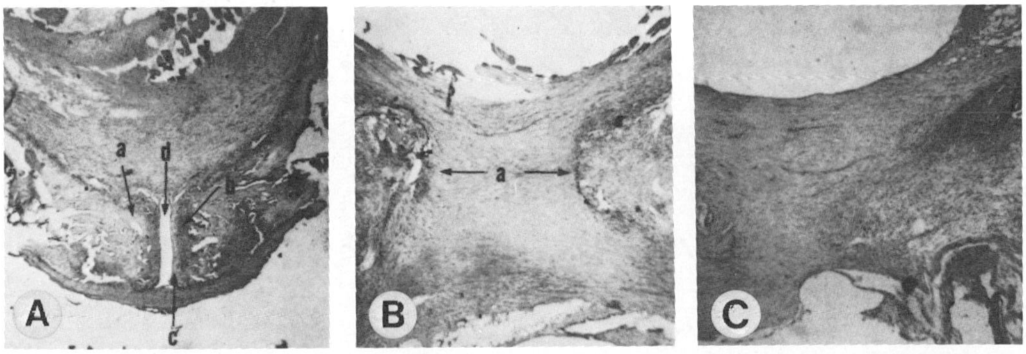

FIG. 41. A: Pubic symphysis of intact untreated control female mouse, demonstrating articular surfaces of pubic bones (*a*), capped with hyaline cartilage (*b*), and united by an interpubic disc of fibrocartilage (*c*). Note cleft (*d*). (×40) **B:** Pubic symphysis of intact mouse treated with estradiol cyclopentylpropionate. Bone and cartilage resorption occurred in area *a*, with replacement by connective tissue. (×40) **C:** Pubic symphysis of hypophysectomized mouse treated with estrogen, relaxin, and growth hormone. Extensive ligament formation is comparable with that found in intact mice treated with only estrogen and relaxin. (×40) From ref. 959, with permission.

administration of estrogen plus relaxin (222,228,375, 425,433,959).

Whereas many investigations have examined the individual and combined effects of estrogen and relaxin on the pubic symphysis in nonpregnant mice, it remains to be demonstrated directly that relaxin promotes the marked separation of the pubic bones that occurs during late pregnancy in mice. Nevertheless, the three criteria for establishing that relaxin promotes growth of the pubic symphysis in pregnant mice are largely met. First, it was demonstrated that relaxin administration to estrogen-primed mice promotes growth of the interpubic ligament similar to that which occurs during pregnancy (426,433,952,959). Second, it was reported that the mouse pubic symphysis contains binding sites for radioiodinated porcine relaxin (690,1143). Third, a close temporal association was demonstrated between increased pubic ligament length (422,949) and elevated levels of relaxin immunoactivity in the blood during pregnancy (723) (Fig. 42).

Estrogen's Effects on the Pubic Symphysis. In addition to conditioning the pubic symphysis to become responsive to relaxin (222), estrogen alone brings about initial stages of the transformation of the pubic symphysis (Fig. 41B). Specific actions that have been attributed to estrogen include (a) increased numbers of osteoclasts within the pubic bones (959), (b) resorption of the medial portions of the pubic bones (220,228,375,376,425, 426,959,995), (c) breakdown or "depolymerization" of the matrix proteoglycans polymers with a subsequent shift to a colloid-poor, water-rich phase (225,426,959, 962,995), (d) increased numbers of chondrocytes within the lacunae of both hyaline cartilage and fibrocartilage (223,959,960), and (e) swelling and transformation of hyaline cartilage caps to fibrocartilage (426,959,995). Steinetz et al. (959,962) postulated that estrogen may bring about its effects on the pubic symphysis, at least in part, by inducing cartilage and bone cells to produce catabolic enzymes that break down bone and matrix components. After estrogen treatment, the lysosomal enzyme acid phosphatase increased markedly in the pubic joints of ovariectomized mice (958), and histochemical studies demonstrated that acid phosphatase increased in osteoclasts, osteocytes, chondroclasts, and chondrocytes (652). Likewise, the lysosomal proteases cathepsin B and dipeptidyl peptidase I, which have the potential for degrading collagen and proteoglycans, were elevated in mouse pubic symphysis after estrogen treatment (686). Fluorescent histochemical staining indicated that both enzymes were primarily associated with chondrocytes and osteoclasts located along the periphery of the pelvic bones. Dipeptidylpeptidase I appeared to be associated with chondrocytes in the depolymerized cartilage caps and cathepsin B with osteoclastic cells inside the bone (686).

Relaxin's Effects on the Pubic Symphysis. When relaxin is administered to estrogen-primed nonpregnant mice, maximal swelling of the cartilage matrix occurs, there is increased release of fibroblasts and chondrocytes from their lacunae, and extensive growth of the interpubic ligament occurs within 6 to 12 h (426,959) (Fig. 41C). Relaxin may bring about its effects, in part, by augmenting estrogen-stimulated processes. Levels of the lysosomal enzymes acid phosphatase, cathepsin B, and dipeptidylpeptidase I, which increase in the pubic symphysis of nonpregnant mice after estrogen treatment, were further elevated moderately when porcine relaxin was administered to estrogen-treated mice (686,958).

There is evidence that relaxin also affects processes

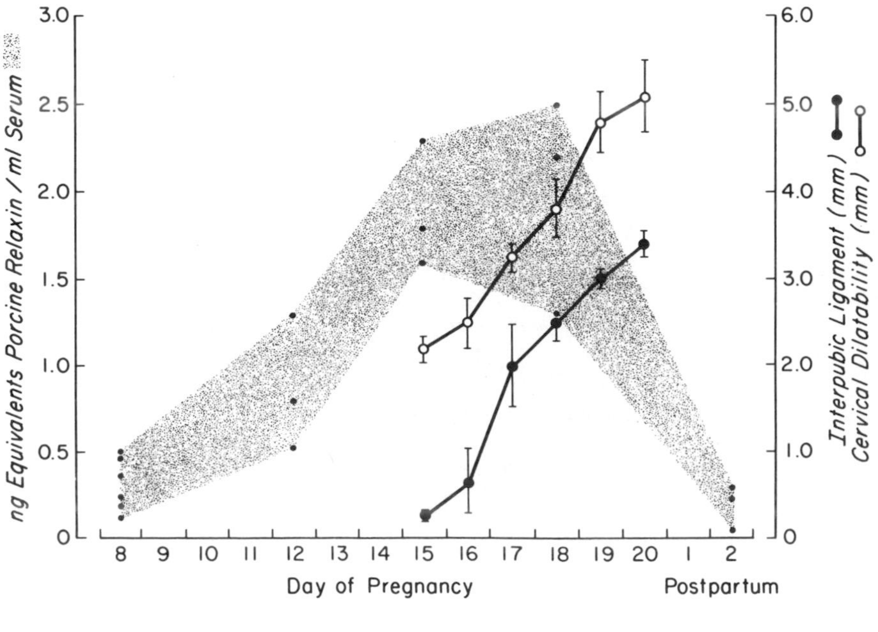

FIG. 42. Range of relaxin immunoactivity levels in sera of pregnant mice as determined with a homologous porcine relaxin radioimmunoassay and normal changes in interpubic ligament length and cervical dilatability in pregnant mice. Modified from refs. 723 and 949.

that are not obviously influenced by estrogen alone. Relaxin in combination with estrogen increased wet weight, dry weight, total collagen, soluble collagen, sialic acid, DNA, and glycosaminoglycans in pubic symphyseal tissue in immature mice (998,1079,1114). An apparent shift in the ratios of glycosaminoglycans with increasing hyaluronic acid and decreasing dermatan sulfate and chondroitin sulfate was reported (1079). Also, pubic symphyseal collagenase, serum collagen peptidase, and serum peptidase inhibitor levels were elevated after relaxin treatment in these estrogen-primed mice (1114). In view of these manifestations of relaxin-induced increases in enzyme activity, Steinetz et al. (962) postulated that relaxin may cause a rapid release of lysosomal enzymes that promote the breakdown of cartilage matrix proteoglycans and also attack collagen bonds in the pubic symphyses of estrogen-primed mice; thus, the lateral forces on the pelvic girdle could pull the pelvic bones apart and give the fibrogelatinous connective tissue joining them the aspects of a ligament.

There are many isolated findings concerning the mechanisms whereby relaxin may act on the mouse pubic symphysis, but the interrelationships and significance of these findings as they pertain to growth of the interpubic ligament remain unclear. It is not clear whether the effects of relaxin on the pubic symphysis are mediated by chondrocytes, fibroblasts, or both cell types (633,959). The effects of relaxin on chondrocytes obtained from the mouse pubic symphysis have not been examined *in vitro*. Porcine relaxin was reported to accelerate the natural tendency of cultured *rabbit* growth plate chondrocytes and articular chondrocytes to differentiate into cells producing higher amounts of type I and type III collagen (107). It was postulated that relaxin might remodel the connective tissue framework of the pubic symphysis by promoting the differentiation of cartilage to fibrous connective tissue (107). The relevance, if any, of these findings to the *mouse* pubic symphysis is uncertain. McMurtry et al. (689) reported that radioiodinated porcine relaxin bound to fibroblasts cultured from mouse pubic symphysis and that porcine relaxin stimulated growth of the fibroblasts *in vitro*. Yang et al. (1143) reported that ^{125}I-labeled porcine relaxin bound to the pubic ligament and not to the cartilage caps of the symphyseal bones in virgin female mice. Braddon (116,117) demonstrated that relaxin promotes an increase in the levels of cyclic AMP and ornithine decarboxylase in mouse pubic symphysis. The significance of Braddon's findings (116,117) is not clear, but it may be that stimulation of adenylyl cyclase and ornithine decarboxylase are early steps in the mechanism of relaxin's action on the mouse pubic symphysis. Ornithine decarboxylase promotes polyamine synthesis, and it is thought to function in the process of DNA, RNA, and protein synthesis in many hormonally stimulated tissues (116). Accordingly, ornithine decarboxylase may play a role in mediating the effects of relaxin on DNA synthesis (1079) in the mouse pubic symphysis. The mechanism whereby relaxin induces ornithine decarboxylase activity is unknown. Because ornithine decarboxylase activity is promoted by increasing cyclic AMP levels, ornithine decarboxylase elevation in the mouse pubic symphysis after relaxin treatment may be a reflection of relaxin-induced increases in intracellular cyclic AMP. Although estrogen priming is required for relaxin to induce a marked increase in the length of the interpubic ligament in nonpregnant mice (222), it may not be needed for initial steps in relaxin's action. Estrogen is not required for relaxin to bind to mouse pubic symphysis (690) or to increase levels of cyclic AMP (117) and ornithine decarboxylase (116) in the tissue.

Effects of Hormones Other than Estrogen and Relaxin on the Pubic Symphysis. Whereas progesterone indirectly promotes growth of the interpubic ligament in guinea pigs by inducing secretion of relaxin from the uterus, it has an inhibitory effect on the growth of the interpubic ligament in estrogen-treated (424,426,433, 1050) or estrogen plus relaxin-treated nonpregnant mice (958,959,1050), as well as in pregnant mice (229,959). Androgens also inhibit the symphyseal response to estrogen and relaxin in mice. Although significant pubic separation was obtained in castrate male mice given estrogen plus relaxin, the response was lower than in castrate females (221); moreover, the longer male mice retained their testes before puberty, the lower the response to hormonal treatment (227,230,442). When large doses of testosterone proprionate were administered to mice during the second half of pregnancy, growth of the interpubic ligament was inhibited (377). Thyroid hormone (477,478) and growth hormone (947,959) are required for pubic symphyseal relaxation, and there is evidence that growth hormone is needed for estrogen to bring about its "priming" effects (947,959).

Essentially nothing is known concerning hormonal control of regression of the interpubic ligament that occurs within 1 week after birth.

Human

Modest relaxation of the pelvic ligaments occurs during pregnancy in women. The pubic symphysis generally separates 3 to 10 mm before parturition (4,515,648, 1041) and frequently contains a gas-filled vertical fissure (173). Reports concerning the possible association of relaxin with modification of the pubic symphysis in women during pregnancy are limited and inconclusive. Pubic separation was reported to be detectable by the end of the first month, near maximal by the fifth to the seventh month, and relatively constant during the last 3 months of pregnancy (4,467,1041). Thus, pubic separation coincides temporally with the period when relaxin immunoactivity is elevated in the peripheral serum

(76,78,286,519,720,808,868,898) (Fig. 37). Reports concerning the effects of partially purified porcine relaxin on the pubic symphysis in women are not in total agreement. It was reported that partially purified porcine relaxin relieved the pain associated with symphyseolysis during pregnancy in five women (510). When separation of the pubic symphysis was determined with the aid of radiographs, one laboratory reported that impure porcine relaxin promoted separation of the pubic symphysis in 80% of the women (247), whereas two other laboratories reported that porcine relaxin had no effect on the separation of the pubic symphysis (932,1105). Finally, there is limited evidence that severe pelvic pain and excessive joint laxity that occur in some women during late pregnancy is attributable, at least in some cases, to relaxin levels significantly higher than those in controls (648).

Monkey

Relaxation of pelvic ligaments occurs during the $5\frac{1}{2}$ months of pregnancy in rhesus (*Macaca mulatta*) and bonnet (*Macaca radiata*) monkeys. There is spreading of the sacroiliac joints as well as the pubic symphysis, which increases from less than 2 mm to greater than 10 mm at parturition (452,996). Unlike guinea pigs and mice, in rhesus monkeys prepartum separation of the sacroiliac joints is more pronounced than that of the pubic symphysis. It remains to be established that relaxin plays an important role in the pelvic relaxation that occurs during pregnancy in rhesus monkeys (467,782,962). Little relaxation of the pelvic ligaments occurs until the last month of pregnancy (452), even though serum relaxin levels are elevated throughout nearly all of pregnancy (1113). Furthermore, removal of the source of relaxin in the rhesus monkey by means of bilateral ovariectomy was reported to have no influence on relaxation of the pelvis (452). Nevertheless, that prolonged treatment with estrogen, progesterone, and porcine relaxin (but not treatment with estrogen plus progesterone) increased flexibility of the pubic joint (463) supports the possibility that relaxin induces pelvic relaxation during late pregnancy in the rhesus monkey.

Cow

In cattle, the ratio of fetal birth weight to maternal weight is high (about 11%), and the pelvic canal expands rapidly during the last 4 days of pregnancy to facilitate birth of the relatively large calf (821). Although little is known concerning secretion of relaxin in the cow, there is reason to suspect that it may loosen the pelvic joints and particularly the sacroiliac articulations during late pregnancy. Elevation of the tail head (or "springing") is a recognized prepartum sign in cattle, and Anderson and co-workers (680,681,683,766) obtained evidence that relaxin may be implicated in that process. When 1 mg of highly purified porcine relaxin was placed in the cervical os of cattle 6 to 8 days before anticipated parturition, there was a rapid increase in pelvic height and width (680,681,766). These workers also reported that induction of parturition in beef heifers by injection of cloprostenol or dexamethasone intramuscularly on day 273 to 275 independently increased pelvic area and that this effect was potentiated by administering 1 mg of highly purified porcine relaxin (either intramuscularly or in the cervical os) in combination with either treatment (683).

Cervix

During the first half of pregnancy in mammals, the cervix is a relatively firm and inextensible structure, which not only protects the conceptuses from the external environment but also impedes premature delivery of the fetus. During the second half of pregnancy, however, the cervix increases in size and its consistency changes strikingly. The term *softens* is commonly used to refer to the changes in the tensile properties of the cervix that occur during late pregnancy. There is increased strain (increase in length divided by the original length) per unit of force, which is generally referred to as *distensibility*. During late pregnancy, cervical distensibility becomes a time-dependent process; that is, deformation of the tissue (strain) increases with time when a constant force (stress) is placed on the cervix (446,471). This slow deformation of the tissue under constant stress is referred to as cervical *creep* or *extensibility* (444,447). Histologic studies demonstrated that the cervices of mammals contain varying amounts of smooth muscle and extracellular matrix components within the predominant stroma. The extracellular matrix consists primarily of collagen and amorphous ground substance (471,1130). The tensile properties of the cervix are largely attributable to the connective tissue that predominates (444,474). In the firm cervix, collagen fibers are highly organized and arranged in dense parallel bands with little amorphous ground substance, which is rich in proteoglycans, glycosaminoglycans, and water, separating the collagen bundles. In the soft cervix, however, the collagen fibers are dispersed and randomly oriented within a considerably increased matrix (754).

A variety of methods have been used to measure cervical tensile properties (238,471). Cervical *dilatability* has generally been measured *in vivo* by inserting conical rods (probes or sounds) of different diameters into the cervix with a constant force until a diameter is recorded where a consistent resistance is encountered. An important limitation to this method is that it does not differentiate changes that occur in the internal diameter of the cervix from changes in the compliance of the cervical wall. Cervical *distensibility* has been determined *in vitro* by a variety of stress–strain measurements. Generally, the entire cervix (or a transverse section thereof) is suspended in a buffer bath and subjected to a progressively increasing load, and the increase in the inner circumference of the cervix (strain) against load (stress or tension) is plotted. Alternatively, the circumference of the cervix is increased (strain), and the tension (stress) produced within the tissue is measured with a strain gauge transducer. Cervical *creep* or *extensibility* is generally measured by subjecting the cervix to a constant load over time and measuring the rate of increase of the internal circumference of the cervix.

This section describes studies that provide convincing evidence that relaxin plays a major role in promoting the cervical modifications that occur during late pregnancy in several mammalian species. Although estrogen, prostaglandins, and, in some cases, progesterone also influence the tensile properties, morphology, and biochemical composition of the cervix (300,691,908,1129), evidence is accumulating that the mechanism(s) whereby relaxin interacts with these hormones to influence growth and softening of the cervix differs among species. Accordingly, the effects of these hormones on the cervix will receive modest attention. This section describes changes that occur in the physical properties, biochemical composition, and morphology of the cervix during pregnancy, as well as the influence of relaxin on these changes in individual species. The influence of relaxin on cervical softening appears to be a general phenomenon among mammalian species. Accordingly, the review of the literature concerning the mechanism of action of relaxin on the cervix combines information obtained from a variety of species to avoid redundancy and also to enable a comprehensive description of this topic in one section. The reader is referred to reviews concerning the influence of relaxin on the cervix for additional coverage of this topic (471,784,908,961,964).

Domestic Species

Pig

Structural Changes in the Pig Cervix that Occur During Pregnancy. The cervix in the pregnant pig is about 15 cm long, characterized by rounded prominences on its internal surface, and consists of a uterine portion (cephalic cervix) and vaginal portion (caudal cervix) (Fig. 43). Although there is no clear demarcation between the uterine and vaginal portions of the cervix, the prominences in the uterine portion are smaller and fit together more tightly than those in the vaginal portion of the cer-

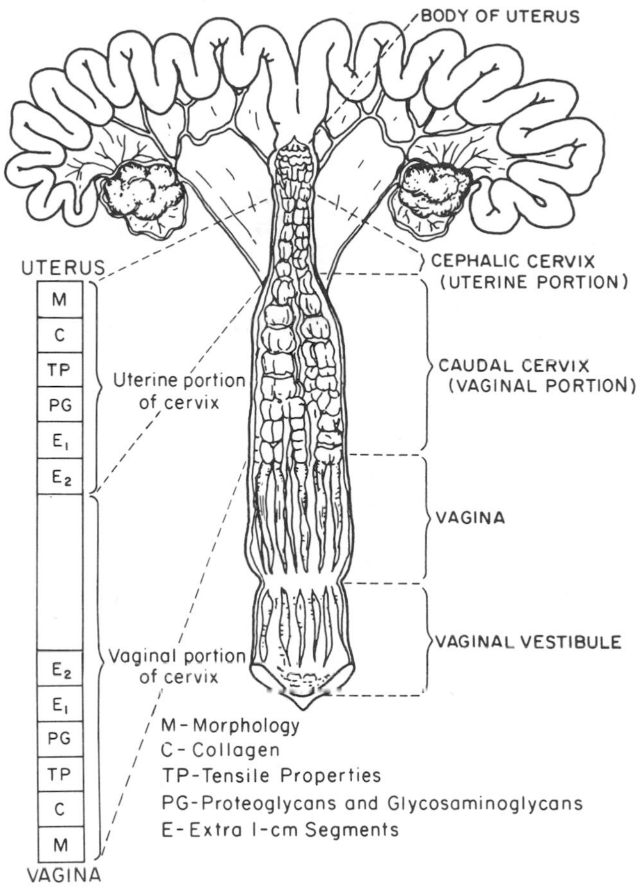

FIG. 43. Female pig reproductive tract. Adjacent 1-cm segments of both uterine and vaginal portions of the cervix were collected as indicated for analyses of physical characteristics, chemical characteristics, and morphology of cervix. From ref. 298, with permission.

vix. Eldridge-White et al. (298) determined the time-course of physical changes in both the uterine and vaginal portions of the cervix from day 40 until term by using 1-cm segments of cervical tissue collected as shown in Fig. 43. Throughout midpregnancy, wet weight, lumen diameter, and distensibility (softness) of the uterine portion of the cervix are less than those of the vaginal portion (Fig. 44A and B). After day 80, marked and sustained increases in these three physical parameters occur in the uterine portion of the cervix, whereas slight or moderate increases occur in the vaginal portion. By day 110 of the approximately 114-day gestation period, wet weight, lumen diameter, and distensibility of the uterine portion of the cervix are similar to those of the vaginal portion of the cervix. Because the uterine portion of the cervix has a relatively firm consistency and small lumen throughout most of pregnancy, it was concluded that it plays a more important role than the vaginal portion of the cervix in protecting the uterus and its contents during pregnancy (298).

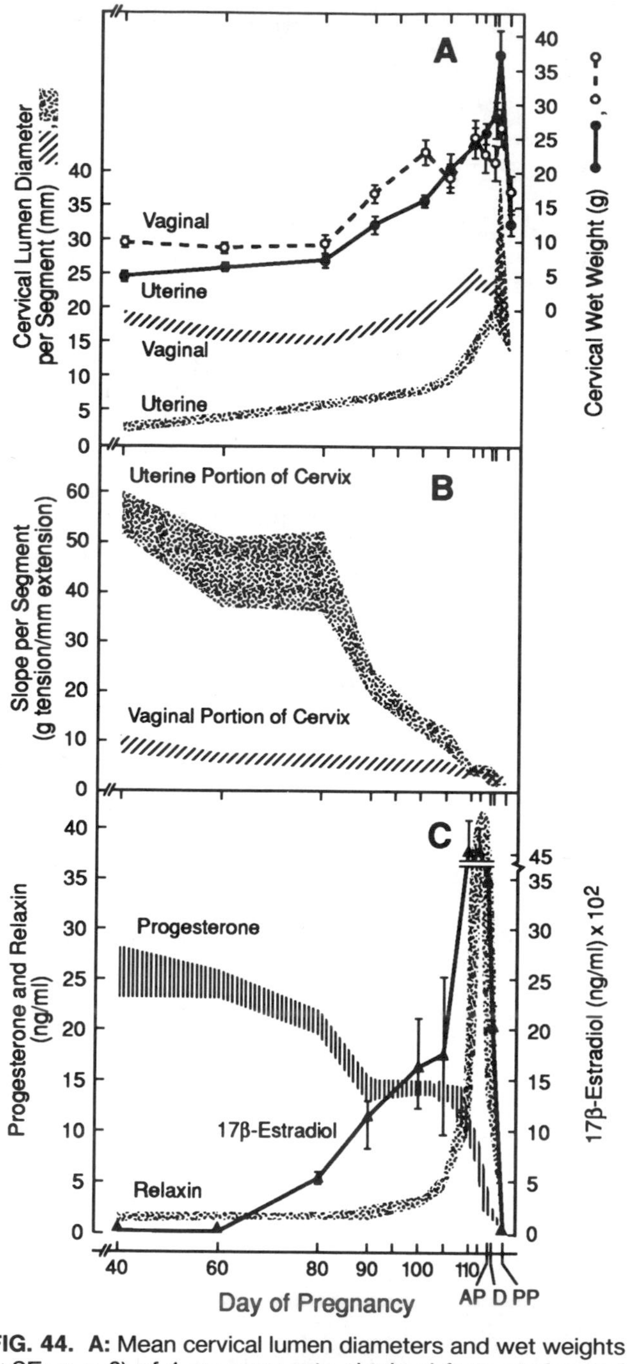

FIG. 44. **A:** Mean cervical lumen diameters and wet weights (±SE; n = 6) of 1-cm segments obtained from uterine and vaginal portions of pig cervix from day 40 until term. **B:** Mean slopes (±SE; n = 6) of linear regressions (grams of tension per millimeter extension) of 1-cm segments obtained from uterine and vaginal portions of cervix from day 40 until term. **C:** Mean peripheral serum levels (±SE) of relaxin, 17β-estradiol, and progesterone from day 40 until term. *AP*, antepartum; *D*, delivery or term; *PP*, postpartum. Modified from ref. 298.

Influence of Hormones on Growth of the Pig Cervix. The marked changes in the physical properties of the cervix that occur between day 80 and term are temporally correlated with rising levels of relaxin, rising levels of estrogen (which is produced by the placentas), and elevated levels of progesterone (298) (Fig. 44C). O'Day et al. (733) obtained direct evidence that relaxin plays a major role in promoting the growth of the cervix that occurs during late pregnancy. When gilts were ovariectomized on day 100 and given replacement therapy for 10 days with progesterone in doses selected to mimic physiologic levels between day 100 and 110 of pregnancy, cervical wet weight and lumen diameter did not increase (Fig. 45A and B). In contrast, when similarly ovariectomized gilts were given replacement therapy with progesterone plus highly purified porcine relaxin, cervical wet weight and lumen diameter did not differ from intact controls. To obtain a better understanding of the hormonal regulation of cervical growth in the pig, Winn et al. (1129) ovariectomized nonpregnant postpubertal gilts and administered highly purified porcine relaxin, estrogen, and progesterone alone or in various combina-

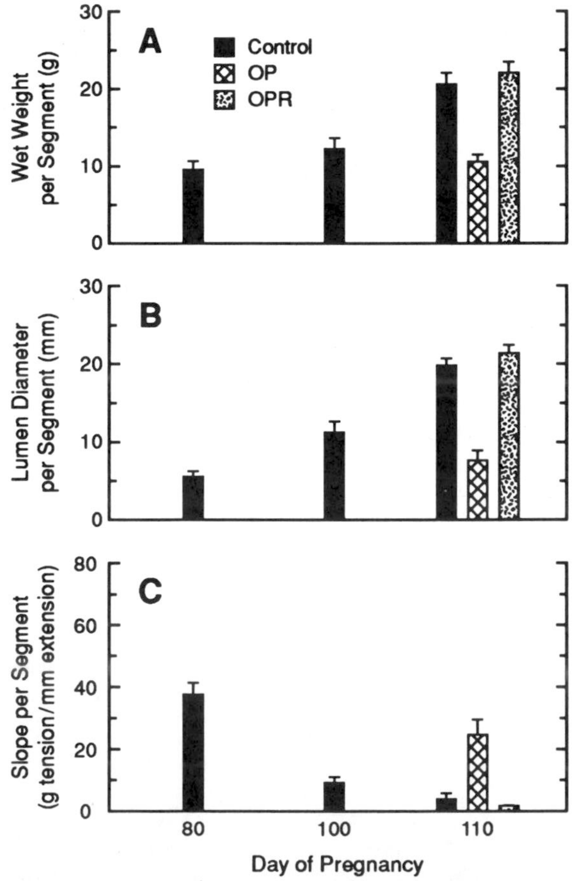

FIG. 45. Mean (+SE; n = 5 or 6) wet weights (*A*), lumen diameters (*B*), and slopes of linear regressions (g tension/mm extension) (*C*) of 1-cm segments from uterine portion of cervix of intact pregnant gilts (*control*) and ovariectomized (*O*) pregnant gilts treated with progesterone (*P*, 50 mg intramuscularly at 12-h intervals) or progesterone plus highly purified porcine relaxin (*R*, 1 mg intramuscularly at 6-h intervals) from day 100 to day 110 of pregnancy. Relaxin's effects on vaginal portion of cervix, which were similar but less dramatic, are not shown. Modified from ref. 733.

tions for 10 days at doses designed to resemble blood levels of these hormones from day 100 to day 110 of pregnancy. Whereas relaxin alone increased both the wet weight and lumen diameter of the uterine portion of the cervix, relaxin's effects were augmented markedly when it was given in combination with progesterone (Fig. 46A and B). Estrogen alone increased cervical wet weight but did not augment relaxin's effects on either wet weight or lumen diameter. Progesterone alone did not increase cervical wet weight or lumen diameter but did augment relaxin's effects on both of these physical properties.

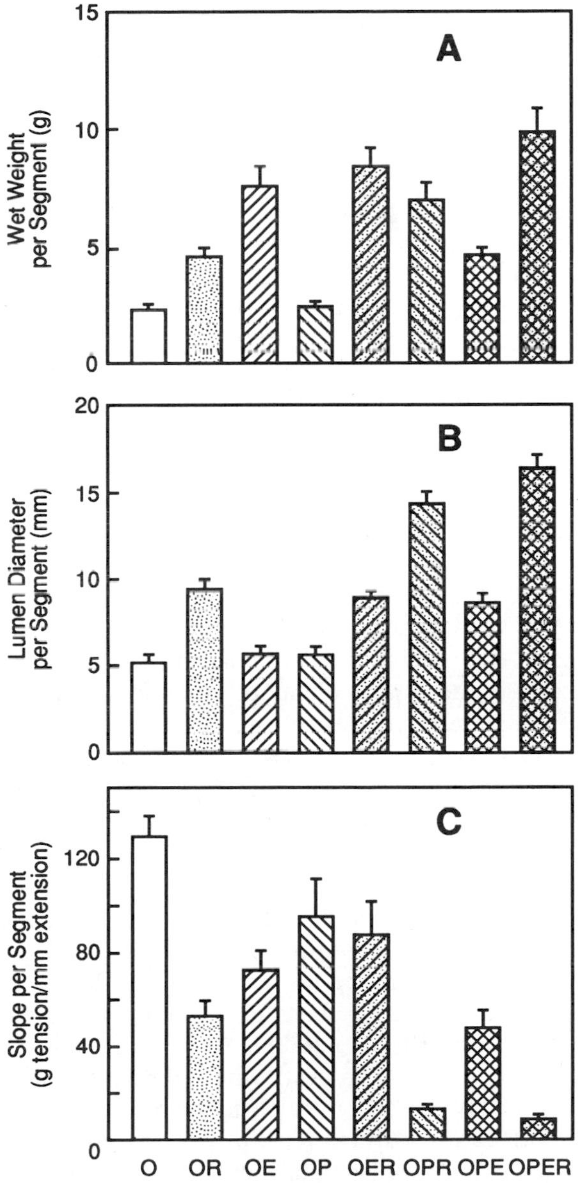

FIG. 46. Mean (±SE; n = 6–9) wet weights (*A*), lumen diameters (*B*), and slopes of linear regressions of tension versus extension (*C*) of 1-cm segments from uterine portion of cervix of ovariectomized nonpregnant control gilts (*O*) and ovariectomized gilts treated with progesterone (*P*, 50 mg intramuscularly at 12-h intervals), estrogen (*E*, 1 mg estradiol benzoate intramuscularly at 12-h intervals), and porcine relaxin (*R*, 0.5 mg intramuscularly at 6-h intervals), alone or in combination for 10 days. Modified from ref. 1129.

Influence of Hormones on Softening of the Pig Cervix. Zarrow and co-workers demonstrated in the 1950s that relaxin promotes cervical softening in pigs. With these early experiments, which examined the influence of partially purified porcine relaxin in both nonpregnant and pregnant gilts, cervical dilatability was determined by inserting rods into the cervix *in vivo.* Zarrow et al. (1156,1159) reported that three daily intramuscular injections of porcine relaxin (approximately 5 mg/day) for 4 days to ovariectomized, estrogen-primed sows increased dilatability of the cervix that was accompanied by an increase in water content and depolymerization of cervical glycoproteins. In 1979, Kertiles and Anderson (551) reported that daily intramuscular injections of partially purified porcine relaxin (approximately 250 μg relaxin) beginning on day 105 or day 107 increased cervical dilatability in pigs that were luteectomized on day 110. In 1989, O'Day et al. (733) demonstrated that relaxin plays a major role in promoting cervical softening in the pregnant gilt (Fig. 45C).

The roles that the steroids estrogen and progesterone play in influencing relaxin's effects on cervical softening in pigs have received little experimental attention, and the few investigations of their roles did not attain totally consistent findings. Hall et al. (419,421) reported that intramuscular administration of 500 μg porcine relaxin alone every 6 h for 54 h to intact (419) or ovariectomized prepubertal gilts (421) increased cervical distensibility and that its effects were greater when relaxin was given in combination with estrogen or estrogen plus progesterone (421). In agreement with these workers, Winn et al. (1129) found that administration of highly purified porcine relaxin alone for 10 days to ovariectomized postpubertal nonpregnant gilts promoted cervical distensibility (Fig. 46C). However, as with cervical wet weight and lumen diameter, progesterone, but not estrogen, augmented relaxin's effects on cervical softening. These data led Winn et al. (1129) to postulate that relaxin and estrogen have largely independent effects on the physical properties of the pig cervix, whereas relaxin's effects are augmented primarily by progesterone.

Influence of Relaxin on the Biochemical Changes that Occur in the Pig Cervix During Late Pregnancy. O'Day-Bowman et al. (734) found that relaxin plays a major role in promoting the changes in the biochemical composition of the cervix that occur after day 80 of gestation. In segments obtained from the uterine portion of the cervix from both intact control gilts and gilts that were ovariectomized on day 100 and given replacement therapy with relaxin plus progesterone for 10 days, the mean wet weight, percent hydration, dry weight, and glycosaminoglycans/collagen ratio increased, whereas mean collagen concentration decreased by day 110 of gestation

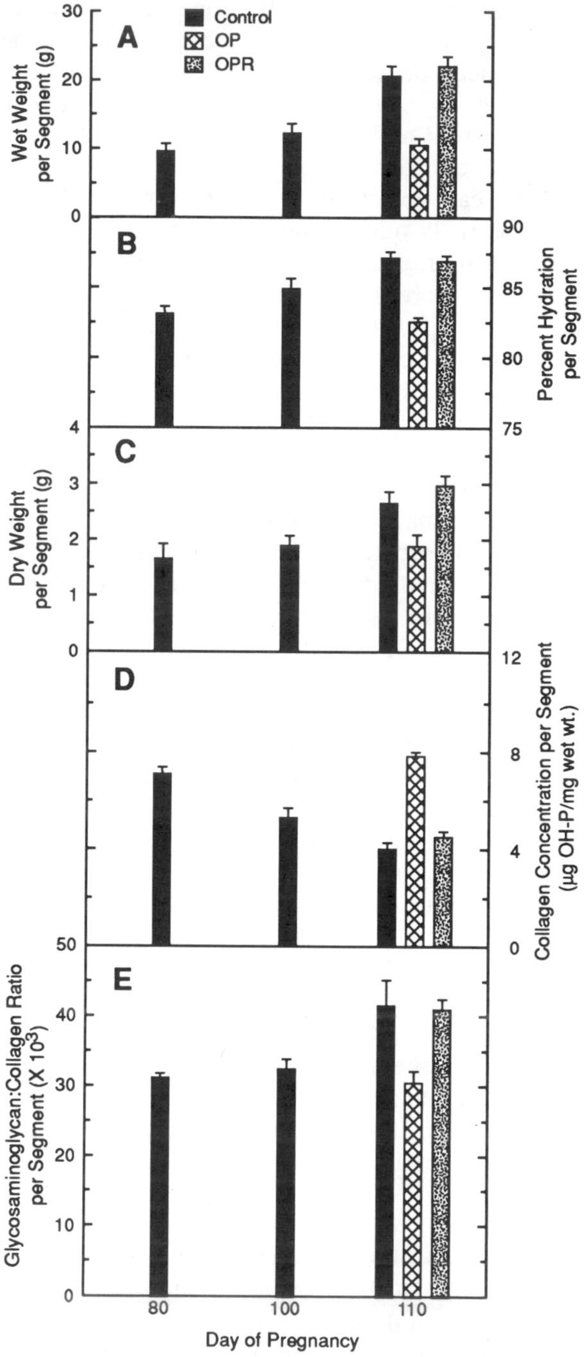

FIG. 47. Mean (+SE; $n = 5$ or 6) wet weight (*A*), percentage hydration (*B*), dry weight (*C*), collagen concentration (*D*), and glycosaminoglycans/collagen ratio (*E*) of 1-cm segments from uterine portion of cervix of intact pregnant gilts (*control*) and ovariectomized (*O*) pregnant gilts treated with progesterone (*P*, 50 mg intramuscularly at 12-h intervals) or progesterone plus highly purified porcine relaxin (*R*, 1 mg intramuscularly at 6-h intervals) from day 100 to day 110 of pregnancy. Relaxin's effects on vaginal portion of cervix, which were similar but less dramatic, are not shown. *OH-P*, hydroxy proline. Modified from ref. 734.

(Fig. 47). In contrast, these changes in biochemical composition of the uterine portion of the cervix did not occur when only progesterone was given to ovariectomized pregnant gilts (734). The main dermatan sulfate proteoglycan of the pig cervix, which increased during late pregnancy and in response to relaxin treatment, was found to be similar in size, immunoactivity, and amino acid sequence to that isolated from the cervices of rats (567).

Influence of Relaxin on the Histologic Changes that Occur in the Pig Cervix. The general organization of the cellular and extracellular components of the pig cervix is shown in Fig. 48. Near the lumen, it is characterized by a stroma that consists predominantly of collagen fiber bundles interspersed with fibroblasts, blood vessels, and varying amounts of amorphous ground substance. Farther from the lumen is a transition zone between the inner collagen-rich stromal layer and outer smooth-muscle layers. This transition layer is composed primarily of collagen fiber bundles of undefined orientation. Nearer the periphery, there is a dense layer of circular smooth muscle and an overlying layer of longitudinal smooth muscle. Unlike the sheep, rat, and human, where smooth muscle is found primarily at the uterine end of the cervix, smooth muscle is a predominant component (about 50%) throughout the length of the pig cervix. Throughout the first two-thirds of pregnancy, the collagen fiber bundles and smooth muscle fiber bundles in the uterine portion of the cervix are dense and highly organized (Fig. 49A). After day 80 of gestation, a remodeling of the cervix occurs. There is a reduction in the density and organization of collagen fiber bundles, reduction in the density of smooth-muscle fiber bundles, and an increase in the amorphous ground substance (Fig. 49B). Winn et al. (1130) found that relaxin plays an essential role in bringing about the changes in the histologic characteristics of the cervix that are associated with cervical softening during late pregnancy. When gilts were ovariectomized on day 100 and given replacement therapy with progesterone only for 10 days, the collagen fiber bundles and smooth-muscle fiber bundles in the uterine portion of the cervix were dense and highly organized on day 110. The histologic characteristics of the cervix in these gilts did not differ from intact controls on day 80 (Fig. 49C). In contrast, when gilts were ovariectomized on day 100 and given hormone replacement therapy with highly purified relaxin plus progesterone, the histologic characteristics of the cervix did not differ from intact controls on day 110 (Fig. 49D).

The three lines of evidence needed to support the view that relaxin acts directly on the pig cervix to promote the changes that occur after day 80 of gestation (Fig. 44) appear to be met. First, highly purified porcine relaxin was demonstrated to play a major role in promoting the changes in the physical properties (Fig. 45), biochemical composition (Fig. 47), and histologic characteristics (Fig.

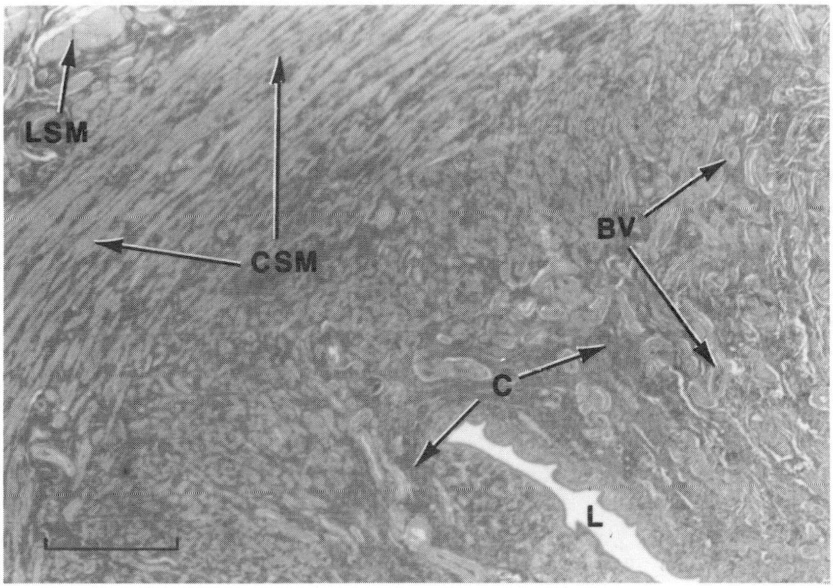

FIG. 48. General organization of pig cervix, as demonstrated by a section from vaginal portion of cervix obtained on day 80 of pregnancy. *L,* cervical lumen; *C,* collagen; *CSM,* circular smooth muscle; *LSM,* longitudinal smooth muscle; *BV,* blood vessel. Bar = 340 μm. Modified from ref. 1130.

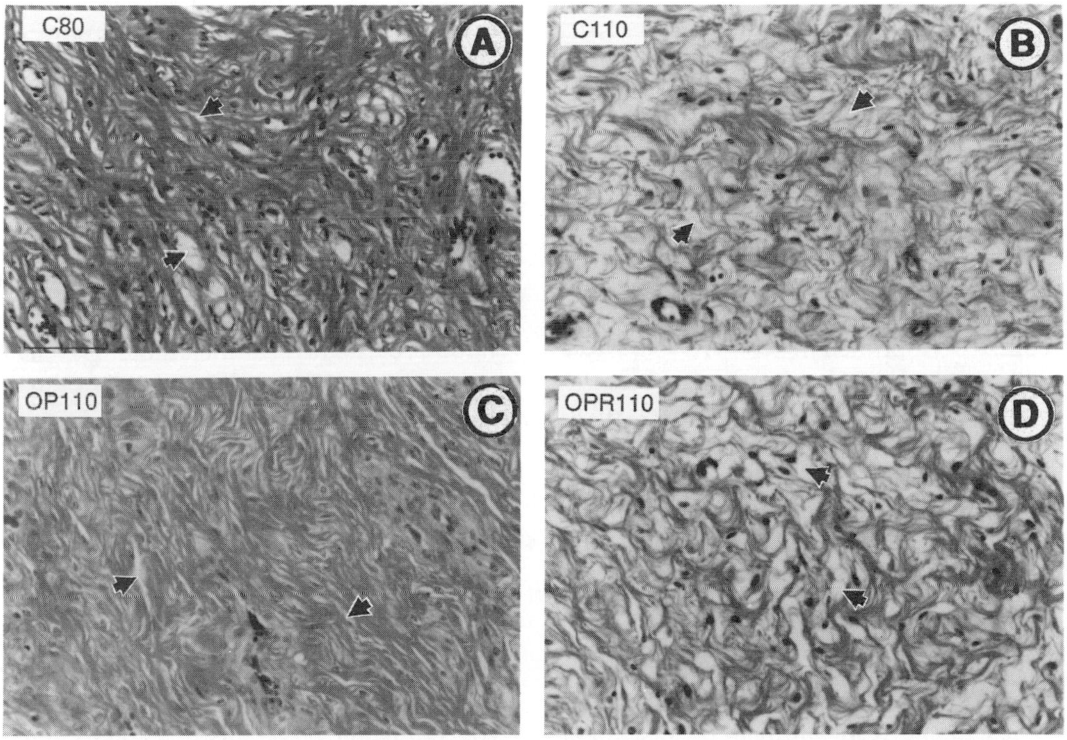

FIG. 49. Photomicrographs of organization of collagen in uterine portion of cervices obtained from intact control gilts on day 80 and day 110 of gestation (C80 and C110) and ovariectomized gilts on day 110 of gestation (OP110 and OPR110) treated as described in legend to Fig. 47. Tissues were stained with Gomori's trichrome to visualize collagen. In groups C80 (*A*) and OP110 (*C*), collagen fiber bundles near the cervical lumen are compact and highly organized. In groups C110 (*B*) and OPR110 (*D*), collagen fiber bundles located near cervical lumen are loosely organized, and there are many spaces containing amorphous ground substance (*filled arrows*) dispersed among collagen fiber bundles. Bar = 80 μm. The four photographs are the same magnification. Modified from ref. 1130.

49) of the cervix that occur after day 80 of pregnancy. Second, pig cervical tissue was reported to contain relaxin receptors. Cervical particulate membrane preparations obtained from gonadotropin-primed prepubertal or cycling pigs were reported to bind ^{125}I-labeled highly purified porcine relaxin with the characteristics of a hormone-receptor interaction (665). Third, there is a good temporal association between the progressive changes that occur in the cervix and elevated levels of progesterone coupled to rising levels of relaxin and estrogen in the serum between day 80 and term (298) (Fig. 44).

Cow

There are reasons to suspect that relaxin influences cervical softening in the cow. In cattle, dilatability of the cervix increases strikingly during late pregnancy—about 100-fold during the 3 days before birth (766). In the early 1950s, Graham and Dracy (408,409) discovered the influence of relaxin on cervical consistency in studies with nonpregnant cycling cattle. Aware of relaxin's effects on the pubic symphysis, these workers explored its use as a means of softening the cervix for ova recovery. Using a mechanical instrument for *in vivo* determination of cervical dilatability, they found that cervical dilatability increased within 12 h of the injection of porcine relaxin into diethylstilbestrol-primed cattle on day 5 postestrus, whereas the cervix remained firm in estrogen-primed controls (409). Within a year, the ability of porcine relaxin to promote cervical dilatability in cattle was confirmed by Zarrow and co-workers (1159), who used ovariectomized, estrogen-primed heifers. In 1966, Eggee and Dracy (290) obtained histologic evidence that progesterone as well as estrogen may interact with relaxin to promote cervical softening in cattle. These workers reported that, within 5 h of the administration of porcine relaxin, many changes occurred within cervical tissue obtained from nonpregnant cattle sensitized for 3 days with progesterone, estrogen, or combinations of the two steroids. The columnar epithelium showed light secretory activity, the stroma showed a tremendous increase in extracellular fluid, myometrial cells were separated and elongated, and muscle fibers appeared tangled and disrupted. Cervical tissue from animals primed for 3 days with estrogen and progesterone, then injected with relaxin, most closely resembled the natural condition of parturition (290). More recently, the effects of highly purified porcine relaxin on cervical dilatability in pregnant cattle were examined *in vivo* with a cervical probe (680,681,683,766). Anderson and co-workers (680,681, 766) reported that when porcine relaxin was placed in the cervical os on day 276 or day 278, about 5 to 7 days before anticipated birth, a premature increase in dilatability of the cervix occurred within 8 to 12 h of relaxin administration. Also, these workers (683) reported that induction of parturition in beef heifers on days 273 to 275 with either cloprostenol or dexamethasone increased cervical dilatability but that cervical dilatability was significantly potentiated by combining relaxin with each treatment. Although the above data support the possibility that relaxin plays a key role in promoting cervical softening during pregnancy in the cow, the lack of knowledge concerning the physiology of endogenous relaxin in the cow precludes this conclusion.

Sheep

In sheep, there is normally a striking increase in the compliance of the cervix at parturition (339,1002) that is accompanied by a disorganization of collagen fiber bundles and activation of fibroblasts (754). Failure of this process to occur in parturient ewes is called ringwomb or cervical dystocia, and the condition is of clinical interest. There is evidence that increased cervical compliance at parturition is hormone-dependent but independent of uterine contractility (599,1002). Several studies demonstrated that PGs (339,598,1003) and estrogens (339, 1002) promote cervical softening, but limited findings concerning the effects of relaxin on the sheep cervix are equivocal. An initial report indicated that relaxin did not influence the depth to which an inseminating pipet could be inserted into the cervical canal 12 h or 24 h after intramuscular injection of partially purified porcine relaxin into nonpregnant ewes at estrus (849). More recently, it was reported (14) that intramuscular administration of highly purified porcine relaxin permitted penetration of an inseminating pipet through the cervix within 20 to 30 h when 0.5 and 1.0 mg of relaxin were administered 24 h and 36 h, respectively, after PMSG-induced follicular development 30 days postpartum. When ewes received similar treatment between 90 and 120 days postpartum, relaxin did not enable penetration of the cervix (14). It was also reported that intramuscular administration of 0.5 mg of highly purified porcine relaxin increased within 12 h the efficacy of transcervical catheterization in ovariectomized ewes pretreated with estrogen (698). These studies provide little, if any, insight concerning the possibility that endogenous relaxin influences cervical consistency in sheep. Also, correlations between cervical softening and serum relaxin levels cannot be examined, because investigators (141,430,817, 1085) have not identified a consistent pattern of relaxin secretion during pregnancy in the sheep. Roche and co-workers' recent report (832) that the apparent single-copy relaxinlike gene in the sheep produces a relaxin-like mRNA that cannot encode a functional relaxin molecule can be interpreted to indicate that the sheep is devoid of relaxin. Thus the dramatic increase in cervical softening that occurs at parturition in sheep may be relaxin-independent.

Laboratory Species

Rat

Structural Changes in the Rat Cervix that Occur During Pregnancy. Cervical physical properties during pregnancy, as well as the influence of relaxin on these properties, have been studied most extensively in the rat. Moreover, the elegant studies of the Harknesses and their co-workers (238,443,444,446,447) in the 1950s and early 1960s not only contributed greatly to an understanding of cervical modifications in the pregnant rat but also provided reliable *in vitro* methods for measuring cervical tensile properties in any species. In the rat, both the size and tensile properties of the cervix change markedly during pregnancy. Cervical wet weight (444,475, 495,568,840,1045,1161) and the inner circumference of the cervix (447,568) increase from about day 13 until parturition (Fig. 50A). The inner circumference of the cervix increases approximately fivefold to be equivalent to the circumference of the fetal head at birth (475,568). This increase in inner circumference is attributable to both rapid cervical growth and a marked increase in cervical creep rate (447,568). Likewise, cervical softening increases progressively after day 13, as determined by increased cervical dilatability (579,950,1066,1161), distensibility (840), and extensibility (447,475,568) and decreased cervical tensile strength (277,1161). Cervical softening is a two-stage process in the rat. The first stage begins on about day 14 and increases progressively until the last day of pregnancy, when a second and more rapid stage occurs during the 3 h before birth (447,471,472) (Fig. 50A). During the 24 h after parturition, a rapid reduction in cervical creep rate (444,475,568) and an increase in cervical tensile strength (1161) occur (Fig. 50A). Hollingsworth and Gallimore (472) provided evidence that the first stage and perhaps the second stage of cervical softening are hormone-dependent and not dependent on uterine contractility. Cervical softening occurred normally during the second half of pregnancy in rats in which the cervix was separated surgically from the uterine horns on day 11 (472).

Influence of Hormones on Growth of the Rat Cervix. Maximal growth of the cervix in nonpregnant rats requires the combined effects of estrogen and relaxin. Administration of estrogen alone increased cervical wet weight in ovariectomized nonpregnant rats (238,579,846,1161), but cervical weight was greater after combined treatment with estrogen plus porcine relaxin (238,579,1161). Unlike the pig, the influence of relaxin

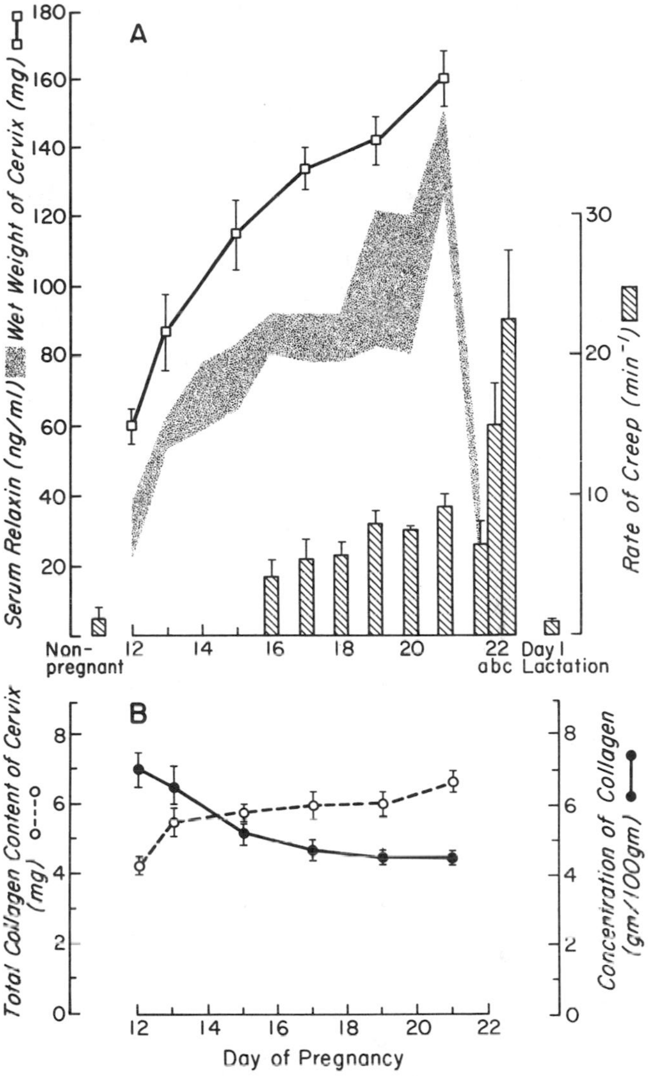

FIG. 50. Cervical changes and peripheral blood serum relaxin levels during second half of pregnancy in the rat. **A:** Mean wet weight (±SE) of cervix in pregnant rats and mean rate of creep (+SE) of cervix of nonpregnant, pregnant, and postpartum lactating rats. Day-22 rats were killed (*a*) at onset of nesting behavior, (*b*) 10 min after onset of continuous uterine contractility, and (*c*) 60 min after onset of continuous uterine contractility. Mean serum relaxin levels (±SE) in rats that gave birth on day 22. Modified from refs. 444, 471, and 912. **B:** Mean total collagen content and collagen concentration (±SE) of cervix during pregnancy in rats. From ref. 444, with permission.

on cervical growth is estrogen-dependent. There was little, if any, increase in cervical weight after treatment of ovariectomized nonpregnant rats with relaxin only (238,579,846). Relaxin's effects on wet weight of the cervix can be rapid. Vasilenko and Mead (1072) reported that the administration of as little as 1 μg of highly purified porcine relaxin in combination with the repository vehicle benzopurpurine-4B into ovariectomized estrogen-primed prepubertal rats induced a highly significant increase in wet weight within 6 h. Unlike the pig, progesterone has little apparent influence on cervical weight in rats (238,579).

There is also evidence that relaxin promotes cervical growth in pregnant rats (277,495,496,950). Pregnant rats were ovariectomized on day 9 and given replacement therapy throughout the remainder of pregnancy with progesterone plus estrogen in doses selected to mimic physiologic levels. In these animals, cervical wet weight was much lower than that of intact controls on days 18 and 22. In contrast, when similarly ovariectomized pregnant rats were given replacement therapy with progesterone, estrogen, and highly purified porcine relaxin, cervical wet weight did not differ from intact controls (277). Sherwood and co-workers also used a highly specific and noninvasive approach to examine the physiologic effects of endogenous relaxin on the cervix in intact pregnant rats. Lao Guico-Lamm et al. (587) produced a monoclonal antibody to rat relaxin, designated MCA1, that not only binds rat relaxin with high specificity and high affinity but also neutralizes rat relaxin's biological activity *in vivo.* When endogenous relaxin was neutralized by administering MCA1 daily either throughout the second half of pregnancy (days 12–22) or during the antepartum period (days 20–22), cervical wet weights on day 22 were markedly lower than in controls (495,496) (Fig. 51A).

Influence of Hormones on Softening of the Rat Cervix. Like cervical growth, cervical softening appears to be dependent on the combined effects of estrogen and relaxin. Whereas estrogen alone promoted *growth* of the cervix, administration of either estrogen or porcine relaxin alone to ovariectomized nonpregnant rats had little effect on cervical *softening* (238,579,1161). When porcine or rat relaxin was administered to ovariectomized nonpregnant rats pretreated with estrogen (or estrogen plus progesterone), there was marked cervical softening, as judged by increased cervical dilatability (579,1161), increased cervical extensibility (238), and decreased tensile strength (119,238,1161). Similarly, replacement therapy with progesterone, estrogen, and relaxin was much more effective than therapy with only progesterone and estrogen in promoting cervical softening in rats ovariectomized during the second half of pregnancy (276,475,579,950,1161). Downing and Sherwood (276) reported that when pregnant rats were ovariectomized on day 9 and given replacement therapy with progesterone and estrogen, cervical tension after extension was much greater than that of intact controls on days 18 and 22. When the ovariectomized rats were given replacement therapy with progesterone, estrogen, and highly purified porcine relaxin, however, cervical tension after extension was similar to that of intact control pregnant rats (276). Consistent with that study, when endogenous relaxin was neutralized with monoclonal antibody MCA1 for rat relaxin either throughout the second half of pregnancy (496) or during the antepartum period (495), the mean tension generated by extension of cervices obtained on day 22 from MCA1-treated rats was greater than controls (Fig. 51B).

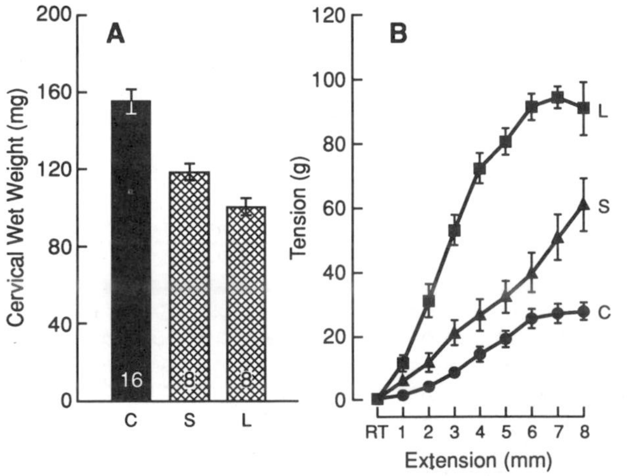

FIG. 51. Influence of neutralization of endogenous relaxin on weight and tensile properties of rat cervix on day 22 of pregnancy. **A:** Mean wet weight (±SE) of cervices obtained from phosphate-buffered saline-treated controls (*C; n* = 16) and rats treated with monoclonal antibody MCA1 for rat relaxin either throughout second half of pregnancy (long treatment, *L; n* = 8) or during 3-day antepartum period (short treatment; *S; n* = 8). **B:** Mean tension (±SE) at extension of cervices of three groups for eight successive 1-mm extensions at 30-min intervals. *RT,* resting tension. Modified from refs. 495 and 496.

The role, if any, that progesterone plays in promoting cervical softening in rats is not presently clear. The cervices of ovariectomized nonpregnant rats remained inextensible after the administration of progesterone or progesterone plus porcine relaxin (238,579). In contrast, Downing and Sherwood (276) found that cervices in ovariectomized pregnant rats that received replacement therapy with progesterone plus relaxin from day 9 were nearly as distensible on days 18 and 22 as those from ovariectomized pregnant rats that received replacement therapy with progesterone, estrogen, and relaxin. This observation may indicate that progesterone influences cervical softening in the pregnant rat, as appears to be the case in the pig (Fig. 46). Alternatively, it may be that peripheral aromatization of the high levels of androgens secreted by the placentas during the second half of rat pregnancy (504,944) provide systemic estrogen levels sufficient to act in combination with relaxin to promote cervical softening.

PGs may be associated with cervical softening in the pregnant rat. Cervical softening increased dramatically within 24 h after the administration of PGE_2, $PGF_{2\alpha}$, or the $PGF_{2\alpha}$ analog fluprostenol to intact rats on day 18 (473,1126). When pregnant rats were ovariectomized on day 16 (pregnancy was maintained by replacement therapy with progesterone and estrogen), administration of

PGE_2 on day 18 promoted increased cervical extensibility by day 19, but administration of $PGF_{2\alpha}$ or fluprostenol did not (473,1126). Hollingsworth and co-workers (473,1126) concluded that PGE_2 may act directly on the cervix, whereas $PGF_{2\alpha}$ and fluprostenol may promote cervical softening indirectly through the ovaries by promoting luteolysis. In addition to a rapid and sustained drop in progesterone levels (147), a rapid, but transient (less than 2 h) surge in serum relaxin immunoactivity levels occurs after the administration of $PGF_{2\alpha}$ during late pregnancy (403). Hollingsworth et al. (473) hypothesized that $PGF_{2\alpha}$-induced cervical softening might be attributable to the release of relaxin. The failure of Williams et al. (1126) to observe elevated serum relaxin immunoactivity levels after fluprostenol administration on day 18 may be attributable to the long interval (14 h or more) between administration of the $PGF_{2\alpha}$ analog and collection of the serum. The observation that indomethacin, a PG synthesis inhibitor, blocked the ability of relaxin to dilate the cervix of estrogen-primed nonpregnant rats (548,549) is consistent with the view that PGs may be associated with relaxin-induced cervical softening in the rat.

Biochemical Changes that Occur in the Rat Cervix During Pregnancy. Changes in the biochemical composition of the rat cervix are similar to the changes that occur in the pig cervix during pregnancy. Cervical water content (495,579,950,1125,1161), collagen content (166,277,396,444,568,1125,1161), and collagen solubility (277,459,568) increase during the second half of pregnancy, whereas cervical collagen concentration decreases (166,277,396,444,459,568,840,1125,1161) (see Figs. 50B and 52). Increased synthesis of matrix proteoglycans also occurs in the rat cervix during the second half of pregnancy (Fig. 52). The combined concentration of the three primary glycosaminoglycans—dermatan sulfate, hyaluronic acid, and heparan sulfate—does not appear to change, but changes in the concentrations of individual glycosaminoglycans were reported. During late pregnancy, the cervical concentration of hyaluronic acid increases (166,277,396), whereas that of the principal dermatan sulfate proteoglycan was reported to decrease somewhat (166), to show little change (277,396), or to increase slightly (568).

Influence of Relaxin on the Biochemical Changes that Occur in the Rat Cervix. Although estrogen alone has been shown to increase the water and collagen content of the cervix (238,1161), studies with both ovariectomized nonpregnant rats and ovariectomized pregnant rats indicate that relaxin normally plays a main role in promoting several of the changes in the biochemical composition of the cervix that occur during the second half of pregnancy. Early work with ovariectomized estrogen-treated nonpregnant rats showed that cervical water (579,1161) and collagen (238) content increased, whereas cervical collagen concentration decreased (238,1161) after administration of partially purified porcine relaxin. Similar results were obtained with pregnant rats. When pregnant rats were ovariectomized on day 9 and given replacement therapy throughout the remainder of pregnancy with progesterone and estrogen, cervical collagen and glycosaminoglycans parameters had not changed by day 22; that is, they resembled those of day-9 intact control rats (Fig. 52). When similarly ovariectomized pregnant rats were administered progesterone, estrogen, and highly purified porcine relaxin,

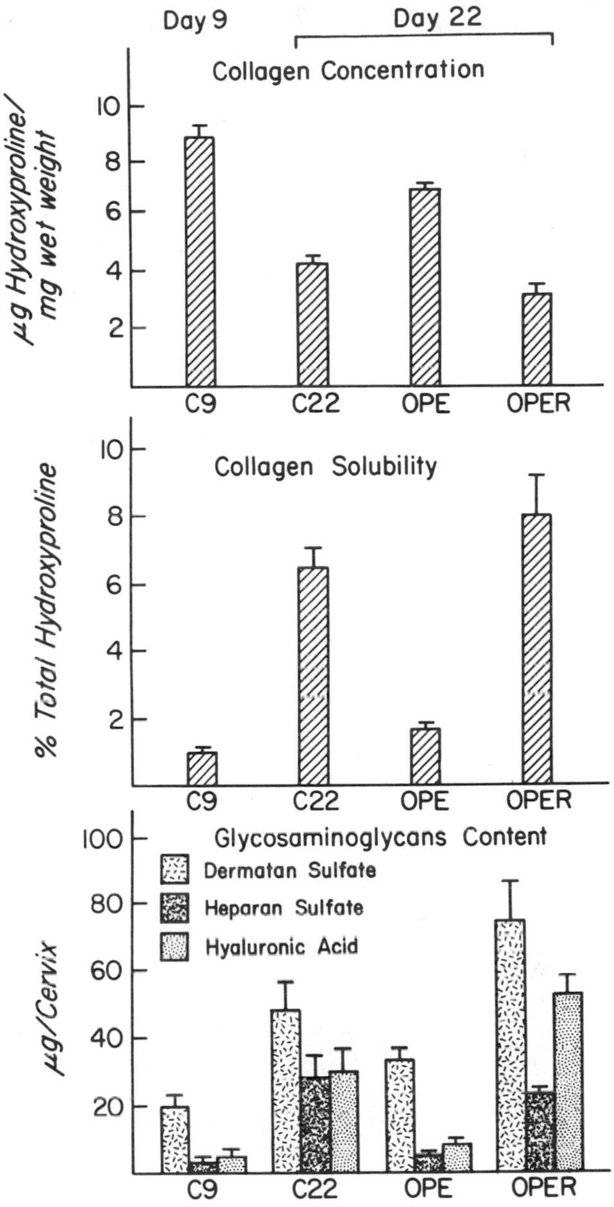

FIG. 52. Mean (+SE) collagen concentration, collagen solubility, and glycosaminoglycans content on day 9 of pregnancy in intact control rats (*C9*), on day 22 in intact control rats (*C22*), on day 22 in ovariectomized rats treated with progesterone and estrogen (*OPE*), and on day 22 in ovariectomized rats treated with progesterone, estrogen, and highly purified porcine relaxin (*OPER*). From ref. 277, with permission.

however, cervical collagen concentrations were reduced, and cervical collagen solubility was increased by day 22 to levels comparable with those of day-22 intact controls. Similarly, relaxin treatment increased glycosaminoglycan contents to levels as high as those of day-22 controls (277) (Fig. 52).

Influence of Relaxin on the Histologic Changes that Occur in the Rat Cervix. The dense and highly organized collagen fiber bundles found throughout the cervical stroma in early pregnancy become dispersed and disorganized by late pregnancy (Fig. 53A and C). Also, the vascularity increases and luminal epithelium undergoes stratification and folding (245). Until recently, hormonal regulation of the histologic changes associated with cervical softening in the rat received little experimental attention. In an isolated report, Saito et al. (846) reported that a single injection of either estradiol-17β or partially purified porcine relaxin to ovariectomized nonpregnant rats promoted both dissociation of collagen fiber bundles and dilatation of capillaries. In 1992, Lee et al. (600) demonstrated that relaxin plays a main role in bringing about the histologic changes in the cervix that occur during late pregnancy by specifically neutralizing endogenous relaxin with monoclonal antibody MCA1 for rat relaxin from day 12 to day 22 of pregnancy. Whereas the collagen fiber bundles within cervices obtained on day 22 from control rats were dispersed and disorganized, those of MCA1-treated rats were densely

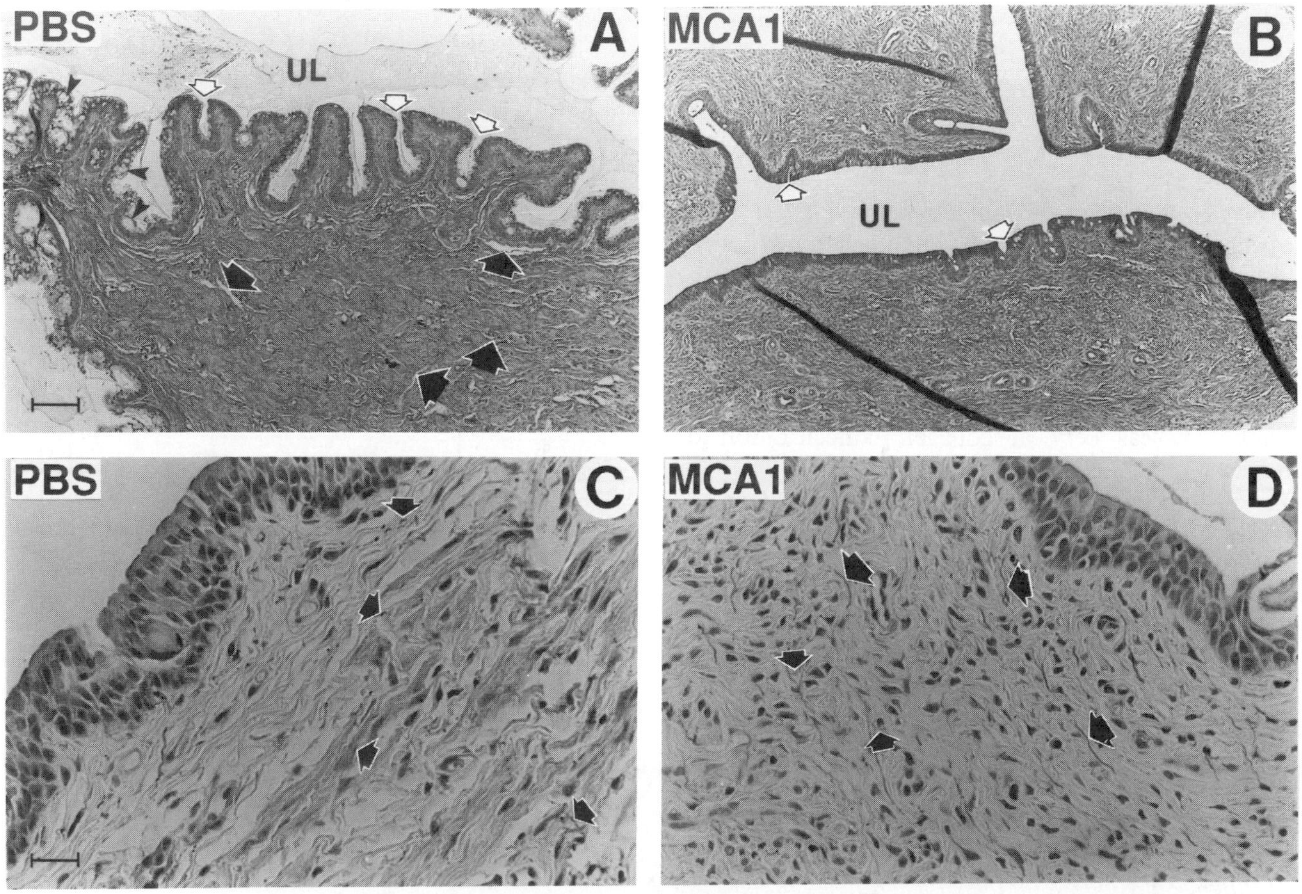

FIG. 53. Influence of neutralization of endogenous relaxin with monoclonal antibody MCA1 for rat relaxin throughout second half of pregnancy on histologic characteristics of rat cervix on day 22 of pregnancy. *UL,* cervical lumen. **A:** Phosphate-buffered saline-treated control. Disruption of connective tissue matrix is indicated by many spaces between collagen fiber bundles (*large closed arrows*). Note large luminal epithelial cell involutions (*open arrows*) and large vacuolated epithelial cells that appear to be secreting a mucouslike material (*closed arrow heads*). **B:** MCA1-treated. Connective tissue matrix is more compact, luminal epithelial cell involutions are smaller, and epithelial cells are less vacuolated than seen in A. Bar in A = 400 μm. A and B are the same magnification. **C:** PBS control. Note many small pieces of elastin fibers (*closed arrows*) and scant amount of long elastin fibers. Interdigitation of elastin fibers is not apparent. Disruption of connective tissue matrix is more apparent than in D. **D:** MCA1-treated. Long strands of elastin fibers (*large closed arrows*) and interdigitation of elastin fibers (*small closed arrows*) are more numerous than in C. Bar in C = 40 μm. C and D are the same magnification. From ref. 600, with permission.

packed and displayed similar orientation (compare Fig. 53A with Fig. 53B). The elastin fibers of controls were sparser, shorter, and exhibited less interdigitation than did those in MCA1-treated rats (compare Fig. 53C with Fig. 53D). The cross-sectional area of arteries in the cervices of control rats was greater than that in MCA1-treated rats. Although the number of luminal involutions did not differ, the area of luminal involutions was greater in controls than in MCA1-treated animals. (compare Fig. 53A with Fig. 53B).

The three lines of evidence required to support the view that relaxin promotes cervical growth and softening in the pregnant rat appear to be met. First, the administration of porcine relaxin to ovariectomized pregnant rats promotes changes in the tensile properties and biochemical components of the cervix that are similar to those that occur in intact rats during late pregnancy (276,277). Also, neutralization of endogenous relaxin throughout the second half of pregnancy with a monoclonal antibody for rat relaxin prevents changes in the growth, tensile properties, and histologic characteristics of the cervix that occur in control rats (Figs. 51 and 53). Second, apparent receptors for relaxin have been reported in the rat cervix (743,1115). Finally, cervical growth and softening occurs between day 14 and parturition in pregnant rats (447,471,950,1066), when relaxin levels are elevated (912) (Fig. 50).

Mouse

Available data indicate that cervical softening and its hormonal control in the mouse are similar to those in the rat. The wet weight and dilatability of the mouse cervix increase throughout most of the second half of pregnancy, with the most pronounced increases occurring during the last 4 or 5 days before birth (608,822,949), when serum relaxin levels are maximal (723) (Fig. 42). When partially purified porcine relaxin was administered to ovariectomized estrogen-primed mice, it synergized with the estrogen to promote maximal cervical growth and cervical dilatability (579,608). Consistent with these findings, a single injection of highly purified porcine relaxin increased cervical wet weight (1018) and extensibility (333) in intact estrogen-primed mice. Moreover, the response was rapid—It occurred within 24 h (333,1018). Biochemical analyses of the mouse cervix demonstrated that the total collagen content increases during the second half of pregnancy, but the collagen concentration decreases (822). The influence of relaxin on the biochemical composition of the mouse cervix has not been described. Leppi and Kinnison (609) reported that the ultrastructural changes that occurred in the connective tissue of the mouse cervix after treatment with estrogen and relaxin were similar to those that occur during pregnancy. The cervix in control mice consisted of a compact array of interlacing collagenous fiber bundles interspersed with fibroblasts that contained little cytoplasm and appeared inactive. After treatment with estrogen or estrogen plus porcine relaxin, there was a change in the appearance of the extracellular matrix. More abundant amorphous ground substance aggregates were observed among the collagen fiber bundles, which became smaller and more widely scattered. The fibroblasts, which are thought to secrete extracellular collagen and proteoglycans, became more active in appearance and had an abundance of rough endoplasmic reticulum.

Hamster

O'Byrne et al. (722) reported a close temporal association between elevated serum relaxin levels and increased cervical dilatability during the second half of pregnancy in hamsters. As with pigs and rats, collagen fibers were reported to disperse during the second half of pregnancy and to be randomly oriented at parturition (52). The effects of relaxin on the hamster cervix have not been described.

Rabbit

MacLennan et al. (645) compared the effects of relaxin and $PGF_{2\alpha}$ on the cervix in pregnant rabbits in an effort to gain insight concerning their mechanism(s) of action. Either highly purified porcine relaxin or $PGF_{2\alpha}$ was mixed in a cellulose gel and administered intravaginally on day 27. Within 15 h, each hormone induced cervical growth and softening. Moreover, the histologic changes in the cervix produced by porcine relaxin and $PGF_{2\alpha}$ were comparable with those seen in the cervix of control rabbits in labor on day 30: There was a dissolution of collagen fiber bundles and increase in amorphous ground substance (645). These workers concluded that relaxin and $PGF_{2\alpha}$ may bring about identical effects in cervical connective tissue rather than act in parallel to produce separate or complementary structural changes (645).

Primate

Human

Changes that Occur in the Human Cervix During Pregnancy. Knowledge concerning the role of relaxin in cervical softening in primates is limited. The only primate in which cervical softening has been studied is the human. Data concerning cervical softening in the human are necessarily fragmentary, because cervical tensile properties are generally determined *in vivo,* and analysis of cervical biochemistry is restricted to the use of small tissue samplings. Nevertheless, it appears that changes occurring in the tensile properties and biochemical composition of the human cervix during pregnancy are similar to those described in pigs, rats, and mice. It was reported that cervical consistency decreases progressively from early pregnancy until delivery (55), whereas cervical dilatation progresses slowly from about 1 month before birth until the last few hours of pregnancy when, along with cervical effacement, it occurs rapidly (361).

More than 85% of the human cervix consists of fibrous connective tissue (244) with the remainder consisting primarily of smooth-muscle cells and epithelial cells. The main components of the connective tissue are collagen types I and III. Also, proteoglycans and elastin are present (607,1060). As with pigs and rats, the main proteoglycan is a small dermatan sulfate (1060). During pregnancy, changes in the biochemical composition of the cervix occur. Cervical water content is higher (244,1060), collagen concentration is lower (244,1060), and collagen solubility in acetic acid is higher (501,1060) in tissue obtained at delivery than in cervices obtained during early pregnancy or prepregnancy. Data concerning the proteoglycan composition of the human cervix during pregnancy are limited. It was reported that both the rate of proteoglycan synthesis (711) and the total proteoglycan content increase during late pregnancy (244,650) but that there is a modest decline in the concentration of proteoglycan (650,1060). Thus, as in pigs (734) and rats (277), the ratio of proteoglycan to collagen increases during late pregnancy.

Influence of Hormones on the Changes that Occur in the Human Cervix. Regulation of cervical softening in the human is complex, because several factors, including estrogens, PGs, relaxin, oxytocin, catecholamines, progesterone, and uterine contractions, may be involved directly (167,340,458,556,610,637,643) (Fig. 54). At present, it is not established that relaxin plays a major role in this process in the human. It is known that relaxin levels

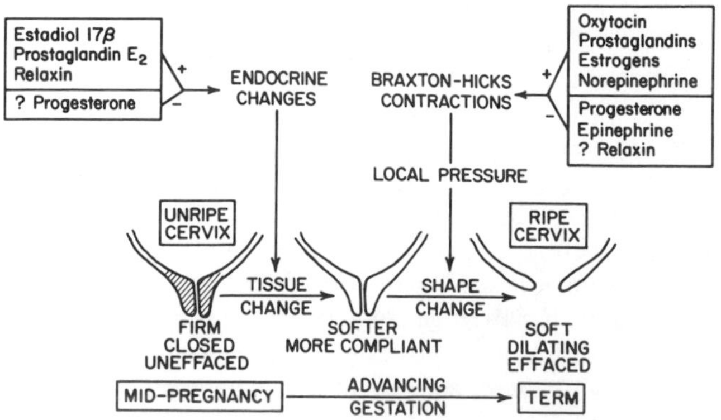

FIG. 54. Schematic representation of factors that may control cervical ripening in the human. *Plus signs* indicate stimulation; *minus signs,* inhibition. Modified from ref. 167.

are elevated when cervical softening occurs, because the corpus luteum of pregnancy secretes relaxin throughout pregnancy (76,78,286,519,647,720,898). Nevertheless, there is reason to suspect that the secretion of luteal relaxin is not essential for cervical softening in women. In women with premature ovarian failure, pregnancy can be achieved by *in vitro* fertilization with a donated ovum, and the pregnancy progresses normally to term in the absence of a corpus luteum and elevated serum relaxin levels (287,303,519). Eddie et al. (287) reported that cervical dilatation occurred in an ovum donation pregnancy in which serum relaxin levels were not detectable. Perhaps relaxin produced by the decidua and/or placenta contributes to cervical softening in the human. Entenmann et al. (307) reported that relaxin immunoactivity was detectable in partially purified extracts of placentas obtained from women with normal deliveries but not detectable in a partially purified extract of a placenta obtained from a woman with severe cervical dystocia.

Regardless of whether endogenous human relaxin is required for cervical softening during pregnancy in the human, there is evidence that the hormone may be administered at term to enhance cervical softening. The results of early efforts to determine the effects of impure porcine relaxin on cervical softening in the human were inconsistent. In one investigation, where a large dose of porcine relaxin (18,000 GPU) was administered intravenously to 16 nonpregnant women during a stage in the menstrual cycle when estrogen levels were elevated, no increase in the diameter of the internal cervical os was observed with cervical rods within 24 h (933). Two other investigations were clinical efforts to prepare the cervix for labor in patients who required delivery but had an inextensible (unripe) cervix (291,994), and in both cases cervical softening was reported to occur within 24 h of parenteral administration of impure porcine relaxin. However, like the study in nonpregnant women (933), these two studies (291,994) were compromised not only by the impurity of the porcine relaxin preparations but also by the subjective methods used for determining cervical softening.

More recent research, which applied highly purified porcine relaxin either to the vagina or to the cervix to prepare the cervix for labor induction, strengthened the view that relaxin may induce cervical softening in women. MacLennan et al. (642) conducted one double-blind experiment in which 2 mg of highly purified porcine relaxin were mixed in a cellulose gel and placed in the posterior vaginal fornix the evening before the surgical induction of labor. Compared with controls, the relaxin-treated group had a greater number of patients with improved cervical score; furthermore, fewer relaxin-treated women required augmentation in labor with oxytocin. Similar results were obtained in a subsequent experiment in which 2 mg of porcine relaxin were again placed in the vagina (643). In a double-blind study,

Evans et al. (313) incorporated 2 or 4 mg of highly purified porcine relaxin into polyethylene glycol pellets that were inserted as a suppository into the cervical canal at the time of the initiation of oxytocin-induced labor. Compared with controls, the two relaxin-treated groups had faster rates of both cervical effacement and dilatation as well as shorter intervals from the initiation of labor induction to delivery. In an outpatient study in which 2 or 4 mg of highly purified porcine relaxin were similarly placed in the cervical canal, 2 mg of relaxin induced greater cervical changes than the placebo control, but for unknown reasons 4 mg of relaxin did not (313). MacLennan et al. (644) also examined the efficacy of placing relaxin directly into the cervix. A double-blind investigation was conducted in which 1 or 2 mg of highly purified porcine relaxin were mixed in a cellulose gel and placed in the cervix by means of a plastic cannula the evening before the surgical induction of birth. Compared with controls, only the group treated with 2 mg of relaxin had a significant improvement of cervical score 15 h after treatment. MacLennan et al. (644) also reported that porcine relaxin was absorbed into the peripheral circulation after its intracervical application. Five of six patients given 2 mg of porcine relaxin showed a rise in serum relaxin levels within 1 hour of treatment. Although these studies (313,642–644) provide some encouragement for the prospect that relaxin may have clinical use, the known differences in the structure of human and porcine relaxin make it seem advisable to use synthetic human relaxin rather than porcine relaxin for either experimental or clinical purposes in women. The use of human relaxin may not only increase the efficacy of treatment but also reduce the risk of inducing the formation of relaxin antibodies.

Monkey

Nearly nothing is known concerning the influence of relaxin on cervical ripening in primates other than humans. A brief report (655) indicated that repeated intravenous infusion of synthetic human relaxin increased cervical ripening in rhesus monkeys during the last third of gestation.

Mechanism of Action of Relaxin on the Cervix

It now appears established that relaxin plays a main role in promoting the growth and softening of the cervix that occur in both pregnant pigs (298,733,734,1130) and rats (276,495,496,600). Moreover, it seems likely that relaxin has a comparable role in many other mammalian species. To obtain a good understanding of the mechanism whereby relaxin promotes growth and softening of the cervix, an understanding of the mechanisms whereby the steroids estrogen and/or progesterone influence the response of the cervix to relaxin will be required. Not only is knowledge on this subject generally lacking, available evidence indicates these steroids may not influence relaxin's effects on growth and/or softening of the cervix in a constant way in all species. For example, relaxin's effects on *growth* of the cervix are dependent on estrogen in rats (238,579,846) and mice (1018) but not in pigs (1129) (Fig. 46). Paradoxically, in rats, estrogen alone may bring about effects on *softening* of the cervix that are opposite to those it brings about in concert with relaxin. There is limited evidence that exogenously administered estrogen increases the density and promotes the organization of cervical collagen fiber bundles in pregnant rats when relaxin is removed by ovariectomy (198,199,202,276). Consistent with that finding, cervical fiber bundles remained dense and cervices remained inextensible during late pregnancy in relaxin deficient rats (496,600) that had normal elevated endogenous estrogen levels. How might estrogen enable relaxin to bring about its effects on growth and softening of the cervix in species such as rats? The target cells for relaxin that influence cervical connective tissue metabolism have not been identified, but they may include fibroblasts. There is limited evidence that the estrogen dependence of relaxin's effects on cervical softening may be mediated, at least in part, through fibroblasts. Leppi and Kinnison (609) demonstrated at the ultrastructural level that estrogen activates mouse cervical fibroblasts. Estrogen may prepare the fibroblasts for relaxin by inducing the synthesis of relaxin receptors or other molecules required for relaxin's effects. There is reason to suspect that progesterone may also augment relaxin's effects on the weight and/or tensile properties of the cervix in pigs (1129) (Fig. 46) and rats (276). No experimental attention has been given to the mechanisms whereby progesterone interacts with relaxin on the cervix.

The mechanism whereby relaxin brings about its effects on the cervix has received limited attention, and the early events whereby relaxin promotes cervical softening remain poorly understood. Three lines of evidence indicate that relaxin acts directly on cervical tissue. First, finite numbers of high-affinity binding sites for radioiodinated porcine relaxin were reported in cervical tissue of the pig (664), guinea pig (384,690), rat (1115), and rabbit (338). Second, levels of cyclic AMP increased in rat, pig, and human cervical tissue after *in vitro* incubation with porcine relaxin (200,536,715,854). Third, highly purified porcine relaxin inhibited ^{3}H-proline incorporation into human cervical tissue and, in combination with estrogen, promoted collagen secretion by collagenase-dispersed porcine uterine-cervical fibroblasts (485,1134) under *in vitro* incubation conditions. The first two lines of evidence must be interpreted with caution, because they may reflect the interaction of relaxin with smooth-muscle cells, which generally comprise at least 10% of cervical tissue, rather than with other cervical cells that influence connective tissue composition. It is known that relaxin promotes increased cyclic AMP levels in rat and pig uterine strips (200,536,854) and rat myometrial cells (479). Moreover, highly purified porcine relaxin was reported to inhibit smooth-muscle cell activity in human cervical tissue *in vitro* (713).

Our understanding of the means whereby relaxin-dependent changes in the histologic characteristics and biochemical composition of the cervix contribute to the alterations in the tensile properties of the cervix is extremely limited. Whereas the general features of the histologic and ultrastructural changes of the cervix that occur during pregnancy appear to be similar among species where they have been examined (244,600,609,645,754, 1130), it is not clear that common hormone-induced mechanisms operate among mammalian species to bring these changes about. The reader should keep in mind that this brief description of mechanisms at the cellular and molecular level whereby relaxin contributes to modifications of the cervix during pregnancy is largely based on observations obtained with pregnant pigs, rats, and humans; and it is speculative. The increased solubility of collagen, which occurs during pregnancy (277,459,501,568,1060) or after relaxin treatment (277), may reflect either increased collagen synthesis or collagen degradation. Alternatively, it may indicate that collagen is organized in smaller fiber bundles (277). The greater separation, reduction in size, and more random orientation of the collagen fiber bundles may allow the fibers to be pulled past one another so that the tissue becomes sufficiently pliable to permit rapid dilatation during labor. The mechanisms that account for the changes in collagen may differ among species. Collagenase increases in the cervix of pregnant women at term (812) but not in rats (568,1045). It is presently not known whether elastin fibers assist in maintaining a rigid connective tissue matrix. If that is the case, the relaxin-dependent reduction in length and interdigitation of elastin fibers observed in the rat cervix (600) would reasonably be expected to contribute to increased cervical softening.

The increase in the ratio of glycosaminoglycans to collagen may contribute to the remodeling of cervical collagen that occurs during late pregnancy. It was postulated that the highly hydrated hyaluronic acid may accumulate in the interstices among collagen fibrils and disperse or prevent aggregation of the fibrils (396). It has also been suggested that the predominant cervical proteoglycan in rats, pigs, and humans, which is the small dermatan sulfate proteoglycan designated decorin (568,711, 734), may, through interaction with collagen, influence cervical softening. Decorin, which has a molecular weight of 95,000, consists of a core protein of molecular weight 45,000 and a single glycosaminoglycan chain (567). It has been demonstrated that dermatan sulfate proteoglycan binds at specific binding sites (so-called d bands) at regular intervals along the surface of insoluble collagen fibrils in tendon and skin (718,888,890). During late pregnancy, there is an increase in the ratio of dermatan sulfate proteoglycan (decorin) to collagen in the rat and pig cervix, and it was postulated that this may lead to increased coating of newly synthesized collagen fibrils (277,568,734). The high charge density of the sulfated glycosaminoglycans tends to cause mutual repulsion of the molecules (453), which in turn could contribute to increasing separation and random orientation of collagen fibrils during late pregnancy. Limited evidence obtained from *in vitro* experimentation suggests that this may not be the case. Uldbjerg and Danielson (1059) demonstrated that a highly purified small dermatan sulfate proteoglycan isolated from the human cervix failed to influence the rate of collagen fibrillogenesis; moreover, it *enhanced* the alignment and density of collagen fibrils *in vitro*. There is more recent evidence that proteoglycans are associated with regular subfibrillar structures within collagen fibrils, and Scott (889) postulated that disaggregation and reaggregation of the so-called protofibrils may remodel collagen fibrils in tissues. Finally, it may not be solely the changing ratio of dermatan sulfate to collagen that accounts for remodeling of collagen fibrils. A new class of large dermatan sulfate was reported to appear both in the sheep and human cervix during pregnancy (342,711).

Also unknown is the physiologic importance of the relaxin-dependent changes that occur in the vasculature, lumen involutions, and epithelial cells that line the cervical lumen in the rat during late pregnancy (Fig. 53). Enlargement of the cervical arteries, which would more easily be accomplished in a disrupted connective tissue matrix with low spacial constraints, might contribute to the increase in cervical water concentration that occurs during the second half of pregnancy (600). Also, enlargement of the blood vessels may enhance migration of nonresident cells that are involved in modification of the extracellular matrix into the cervix. Osmers et al. (745) provided evidence that the increase in cervical collagenase that occurs during parturition in humans originates in polymorphonuclear leukocytes that migrate into the cervix from blood vessels and does not originate in resident fibroblasts. It may be that enlarged luminal involutions provide sufficient luminal surface area to enable the expansion of the surface to a diameter required for safe delivery of the pups at parturition (600). During late pregnancy, many of the luminal epithelial cells contain enlarged vacuoles and apparently release a polysaccharide-rich secretion into the cervical lumen. Thus, in addition to its effects on cervical growth and softening, relaxin may expedite delivery by promoting the secretion of a lubricant into the cervical lumen (600).

Uterus

Relaxin's Effects on Uterine Metabolism

General Effects

It has been known for more than 30 years that relaxin causes several rapid changes in the biochemical composition of rat and mouse uteri. In 1957, Steinetz et al. (948) reported that uterine water content, wet weight, dry weight, glycogen content, and nitrogen content increased to maximal levels within 6 to 12 h after the administration of crude porcine relaxin to ovariectomized estrogen-primed immature rats (Fig. 55). The general metabolic effects of relaxin were confirmed in rats and mice with studies that used not only partially purified porcine relaxin (123,129,428,429,503,579,872,1082, 1152,1160) and crude human relaxin extract (770) but also highly purified porcine relaxin (7,165,348,1068–1073,1088). The physiologic effects of relaxin on uterine metabolism in rats appear to be less dependent on prior sensitization with estrogen than are its effects on the cervix. Relaxin treatment induced increased uterine growth, glycogen content, and protein synthesis in ovariectomized rats that were not pretreated with estrogen (6,7,348,1070). Although estrogen pretreatment is not essential for relaxin to exert these effects on the rat uterus, a synergistic effect was obtained between the two hormones (6,7,348,1070). The influence of progesterone on relaxin's metabolic effects has received little experimental attention. In one study, progesterone was reported to inhibit the uterotropic effect of porcine relaxin in both estrogen-primed and unprimed ovariectomized immature rats (7).

In the early 1990s, it was demonstrated that relaxin also has uterotropic effects in pigs (370,371,419,420, 483), and as is the case with rats, these effects are not dependent on prior sensitization with estrogen. Anthony and co-workers reported that the administration of 0.5 mg of highly purified porcine relaxin to prepubertal gilts (419) or ovariectomized prepubertal gilts (420) at 6-h intervals for 54 h induced increased uterine wet weight, dry weight, water content, protein content, and DNA content. Whereas estrogen does not appear to be essential for relaxin's uterotropic effects on the pig uterus, a synergistic effect was reported when both hormones were administered to intact (483) or ovariectomized (420) gilts. Uterotropic effects were also reported when 0.5 mg of highly purified porcine relaxin was administered to gilts at 6-h intervals on days 6 to 11 of pregnancy: The wet weight, water content, volume, and circumference of the uterus increased, but its length did not (370). Increased water content accounts for most of the increase in uterine wet weight that occurs after relaxin treatment in rats, mice, and pigs, but there is evidence that hyperplasia also occurs in pigs. Uterine DNA content increased after administration of highly purified porcine relaxin in estrogen-pretreated prepubertal intact and ovariectomized gilts (419,420).

Specific Effects

Vasculature. Relaxin appears to increase the blood flow to the uterus. Vasilenko et al. (1073) reported that within 6 h of the injection of relaxin to ovariectomized estrogen-primed rats, there was a significant increase in vascularization of the vascular connective tissue layer located between the circular and longitudinal smooth-muscle layers of the uterus.

Glycogen. Limited studies indicate that relaxin may regulate glycogen metabolism during late pregnancy in rats and mice. Glycogen is stored primarily in the myometrium of rats during pregnancy (1068) and after re-

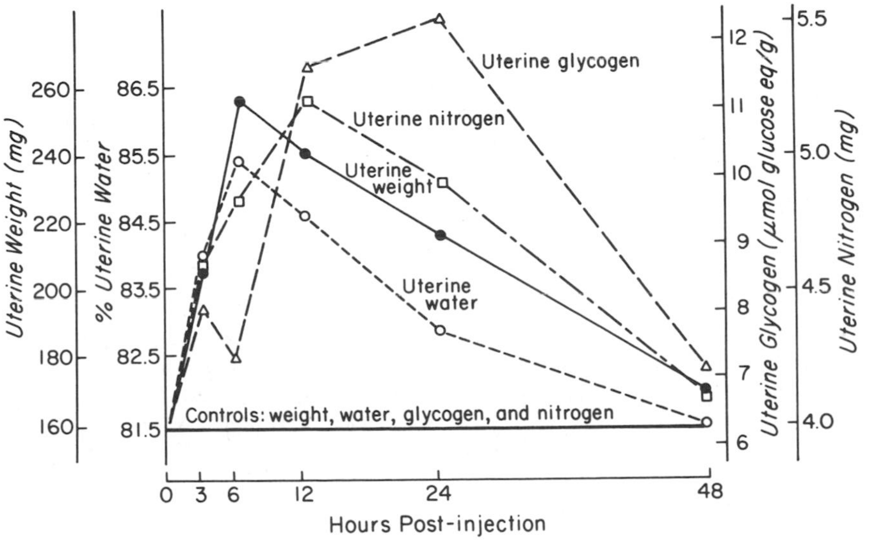

FIG. 55. Changes in uterine composition after a single injection of 100 μg of impure porcine relaxin (equivalent to approximately 5–10 μg highly purified porcine relaxin) to ovariectomized rats primed 8 days previously with 5 μg estradiol cyclopentylpropionate. Control rats received vehicle only (0.1 ml 1% benzopurpurine-4B in physiologic saline). From ref. 948, with permission.

laxin administration (428,429). Moreover, glycogen accumulates during late pregnancy in rats with a profile resembling that of relaxin levels in the peripheral serum (205,912,1068) (Fig. 56). Because the glycogen levels, which increase in the myometrium of rats during the second half of pregnancy, fall after birth, it was postulated that this glycogen may provide a source of energy for the strong, highly coordinated uterine contractions that occur at delivery (205,1068). The mechanism(s) whereby relaxin promotes glycogen accumulation is not known. It may involve induction of enzymes associated with glycogen metabolism. Early reports indicated that crude porcine relaxin either increased uterine concentrations or decreased the rate of loss of glycogen phosphorylase activity in estrogen-primed mice (429) and rats (823,872). A more recent report indicated that highly purified porcine relaxin, as well as partially purified relaxin obtained from human decidua, increased uterine concentrations of hexokinase, phosphoglucomutase, and glycogen phosphorylase activities in estrogen-primed mice (131). Moreover, the stimulatory effect of partially purified human relaxin on hexokinase and phosphoglucomutase activities in estrogen-primed mice was confirmed (770). This reviewer does not know how to reconcile the glycogenic effect of relaxin with its putative capacity to increase glycogen phosphorylase activity in the uteri of estrogen primed mice and rats, because this enzyme catalyzes the breakdown of glycogen. Perhaps relaxin's glycogenic effect is not mediated through the induction of enzymes. It has been postulated that relaxin may promote glycogen accumulation indirectly; that is, by inhibiting uterine contraction, relaxin may have a glycogen-sparing effect (851,1068).

Connective Tissue Remodeling. Relaxin may also influence connective tissue remodeling of the uterine horns during pregnancy through actions that are analogous to those on the cervix. In the rat, the profile of uterine growth and involution coincides closely with the rise and fall in serum relaxin levels (912); that is, both the weight and collagen content of the uterine horns increase markedly during the second half of pregnancy and then decline rapidly after parturition (443,1068) (Fig. 56). In 1964, Cullen and Harkness (239) reported that the collagenous framework of the uterine horns of ovariectomized rats increased maximally when partially purified porcine relaxin was administered in combination with estrogen and progesterone. More recent morphometric and histologic analyses of uteri obtained from immature and mature ovariectomized estrogen-primed rats are consistent with these findings. Vasilenko et al. (1073) reported that within 6 h after relaxin treatment, the connective tissue framework of the endometrium and circular layer of the myometrium changed from dense, wavy bundles of collagen fibers to a more loosely arranged and widely separated collagen network that contained thinner collagen fibers and more intrafibrillar space. Cullen and Harkness (239) postulated that, independent of the distending forces exerted by the fetuses, hormone-induced cellular activity within the uterine wall may promote an increase in the collagenous framework of the uterus in the pregnant rat. Thus, relaxin might form a part of the mechanism(s) whereby pregnancy is maintained by facilitating the accommodation of the growing conceptuses. Although relaxin may influence the connective tissue framework of the uterus, it is not clear that relaxin promotes an increase in the distensibility of the uterine horns as it does in the cervix. Supportive of the possibility, Wiqvist (1136) reported that uterine resistance to distension with fluid was lower in ovariectomized rats treated with estrogen, progesterone, and relaxin than in animals treated with only the steroids. However, Harkness and Harkness (445) found that in contrast to the cervix, the extensibility of the uterine horns was consistently low throughout pregnancy in rats. These workers (445) concluded that the differences in extensibility of the two portions of the reproductive tract fit their func-

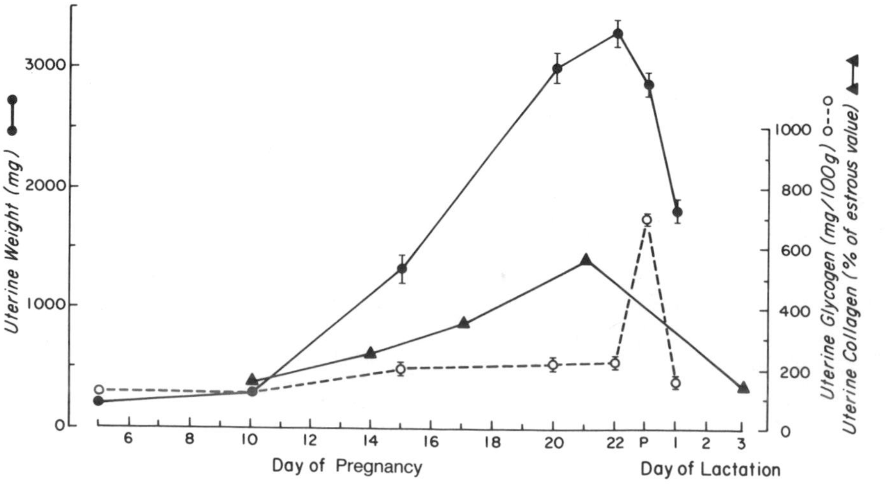

FIG. 56. Mean (±SE; $n = 6$) total uterine weight and uterine glycogen composition (myometrium plus endometrium) of gravid horns of unilaterally pregnant rats. Mean total collagen content (±SE; $n = 6$ or 7) as percentage of estrous value. *P*, parturition. Modified from refs. 443 and 1068.

tions, because the strong contractions of the uterine horn at delivery must extend the cervix rather than its own tissue.

Mechanism(s) of Relaxin's Metabolic Effects on the Uterus. The mechanism whereby relaxin influences connective tissue remodeling of the uterine horns during pregnancy is not known. There are only a few isolated reports concerning the influence of relaxin on uterine collagen metabolism, and they are not in agreement. Frieden, Adams, and co-workers reported that highly purified porcine relaxin not only stimulated the synthesis of uterine collagen to a greater extent than uterine noncollagen protein in unprimed (7) or estrogen-primed ovariectomized rats (348) but also inhibited uterine involution and collagenolysis in the postpartum rat (6). These workers concluded that relaxin may act as an anabolic and anticatabolic modulator of uterine collagen metabolism (348). Consistent with this finding, Bylander et al. (165) reported that 6 h after the administration of highly purified porcine relaxin to ovariectomized and estrogen-primed mice, collagen synthesis increased. Relaxin may promote collagen synthesis in the uterus through direct effects on fibroblasts. Porcine relaxin, as well as estrogen, increased tritiated thymidine incorporation into fibroblasts from the uteri of guinea pigs during *in vitro* culture (902).

There are reports that are inconsistent with the hypothesis that relaxin promotes uterine collagen synthesis. Six hours after administration of highly purified porcine relaxin to ovariectomized and estrogen-primed immature rats, there was no change in uterine collagen content, but both the content and concentration of glycosaminoglycan increased (1072). Likewise, highly purified porcine relaxin did not influence significantly either collagen or glycosaminoglycan content in uterine tissue obtained from estrogen- and/or progesterone-primed ovariectomized gilts (420) or glycosaminoglycan synthesis in uterine tissue obtained from women at term (1133). Also, highly purified porcine relaxin was reported to decrease incorporation of tritiated proline into uterine tissue cultures obtained from women at cesarean section (1134) and to increase collagenase activity in medium bathing cultures of whole uteri obtained from estrogen-primed rats (1043).

Braddon (116) found that uterine levels of ornithine decarboxylase activity increased within 2 h of the administration of highly purified porcine relaxin to mice. The physiologic significance of this observation is not known. Ornithine decarboxylase may play a role in mediating the effects of relaxin on uterine growth, glycogen synthesis, and connective tissue metabolism. The mechanism whereby relaxin induces uterine ornithine decarboxylase activity is unknown. It may be a reflection of relaxin-induced increases in intracellular cyclic AMP, because relaxin treatment was shown to increase cyclic AMP levels in rat and pig uterine tissue (200,536,854). The influence of relaxin on uterine ornithine decarboxylase activity does not require estrogen priming, and this may mean that estrogen either plays no role in the mechanism of action of relaxin or does so at a stage beyond the induction of relaxin receptors (116). Unlike pigs (419,420), there is presently no evidence that the acute metabolic effects of relaxin are accompanied by hyperplasia in rats. Whereas insulin and insulinlike growth factor stimulated DNA synthesis in primary cultures of rat "uterine cells," porcine relaxin did not (70).

Physiologic Significance of Relaxin's Metabolic Effects on the Uterus. It remains to be established that endogenous relaxin has general metabolic effects on the uterus in any species. To the contrary, there is reason to suspect that the endogenous rat relaxin found in high levels in the peripheral blood during the second half of pregnancy does not have tropic effects on the uterus during pregnancy. Neutralization of endogenous relaxin throughout the second half of pregnancy with sufficient monoclonal antibody MCA1 for rat relaxin to inhibit markedly the growth and softening of the cervix did not influence uterine wet weight on day 22 (496). Nevertheless, the possibility that relaxin promotes uterine growth during pregnancy cannot be ruled out. It is possible that endogenous relaxin produced in the uterine endometrium during the second half of rat pregnancy (336) acts locally through paracrine mechanisms to bring about changes in the biochemical composition of the uterus. The observation that uterine growth in the gravid horn of a unilaterally pregnant rat was far greater than in the nongravid horn during the second half of rat pregnancy (1068) is consistent with this possibility.

Relaxin's Effects on Myometrial Contractile Activity

The myometrium is relatively inactive throughout most of pregnancy; thus, the developing fetus is maintained within a tranquil uterine cavity. Normally at term, the uterine myometrium contracts rhythmically and forcefully, and this highly coordinated pattern of contractions aids in dilating the cervix and expelling the fetus and placenta. The changes in the contractile properties of the uterus during pregnancy are regulated, at least in part, by changing levels of (a) hormones that stimulate or inhibit uterine contractility, (b) hormone receptors on myometrial cells, and (c) gap junctions between adjacent myometrial cells. This section largely consists of a description of the influence of relaxin on uterine contractility in the rat, because this is the species with which most of the research has been conducted. Emphasis is placed on recent studies conducted with highly purified relaxin, which not only encourage the view that relaxin plays a role in the regulation of uterine contractility during pregnancy but also provide considerable insight concerning the mechanism(s) of action of relaxin on the myometrial cells in the rat.

The effect of relaxin on uterine contractility was discovered in 1950, when Krantz et al. (575) found that intravenous administration of a crude extract of porcine relaxin to estrogen-primed guinea pigs diminished spontaneous uterine activity *in situ*. Shortly thereafter, Sawyer et al. (863) reported that crude porcine relaxin inhibited spontaneous and electrically stimulated uterine contractions in excised uteri obtained from estrogen-primed rats. Most subsequent investigations of the influence of relaxin on uterine contractility examined the effects of porcine relaxin on uterine contractility in the rat. The few investigations that examined its influence in species other than the rat encourage the view that relaxin's quiescent effect on uterine contractility is a widely distributed phenomenon.

Pharmacologic Effects of Relaxin on Uterine Contractility

Studies of the influence of impure relaxin preparations on uterine contractility in nonpregnant mammals contributed a great deal toward our present understanding of relaxin's role in this process. Partially purified porcine relaxin was reported to reduce the frequency and/or amplitude of uterine contractions in the rat (127,192, 267,413,614,667,783,789,790,859,860,863,988–990, 1086,1135–1137), mouse (579,863,1135,1136), guinea pig (317,575,779,780,1086), hamster (552), sheep (792), and human (540,795). Partially purified rat relaxin reduced the amplitude of electrically driven contractions of rat uterine strips *in vitro* (119). It was also reported that crude extracts obtained from the human corpus luteum of pregnancy reduced the amplitude of spontaneous contractions of human uterine strips *in vitro* (71,1008) and that a relaxin preparation obtained from human term placenta inhibited spontaneous contractions of mouse myometrial strips *in vitro* (334).

Many studies with highly purified porcine relaxin that examined uterine contractility either *in vivo* or *in vitro* confirmed that relaxin renders the uterus quiescent in nonpregnant rats (95,193,194,201,268–270,272,344, 388,394,410,497,622,641,687,706,707,740,769,854–856). Moreover, highly purified porcine relaxin inhibited contractions of the mouse (591), pig (641,794,799), and turtle (170,941) uterus. Highly purified preparations of relaxin from species other than the pig also influence uterine contractility in mammals and lower vertebrates. Rat relaxin (253) and skate relaxin (157) inhibited contractions of the rat uterus (253); rabbit relaxin inhibited contractions of the mouse uterus (295); shark relaxin inhibited contractions of both the shark uterus (171,942) and guinea pig uterus (815); and synthetic human relaxin 2 (B29) inhibited contractions of the rat (769) and pig uterus (639). There is reason to suspect that relaxin is not a potent inhibitor of uterine contractions in women. Both highly purified porcine relaxin (641) and synthetic human relaxin 2 (B29) (639,769) had either no effect or only a slight effect on spontaneous contractility of human myometrial strips obtained from pregnant women at cesarean section or from nonpregnant women at hysterectomy. It was reported that human cervical smooth muscle responds to relaxin, but that its response depends on the reproductive status of the woman. Whereas cervical strips obtained from nonpregnant women generally failed to respond to porcine relaxin, spontaneous contractility in approximately half of the strips obtained during the first trimester of pregnancy and in all the strips obtained at term pregnancy was inhibited by porcine relaxin (712,713). The putative differences in response of human uterine and cervical smooth muscle to relaxin are presently not understood.

Experimentation with nonpregnant animals also demonstrated that relaxin can inhibit spontaneous uterine contractility over a sustained period of time. Impure porcine relaxin reduced the frequency of spontaneous uterine contractions in nonpregnant guinea pigs throughout a 20-h infusion (780); furthermore, highly purified porcine relaxin inhibited both the frequency and amplitude of spontaneous uterine contractions in conscious and unrestrained ovariectomized rats (both estrogen-treated and steroid-untreated) throughout a 2-day infusion of the hormone (201) (Fig. 57A).

Studies of an unphysiologic nature involving the administration of porcine relaxin during early pregnancy in rats before endogenous relaxin levels are elevated, provided indirect evidence that the uterus of the pregnant rat is responsive to relaxin. Porcine relaxin was infused intravenously for 16 h (802) or 41 h (833) during the peri-implantation period (beginning at 5 PM on day 4) to determine if the even distribution of implanted blastocysts is dependent on spontaneous myometrial activity. Apparently it is. A preponderance of preimplantation blastocysts (802) and implantation sites (833) were found in the cranial half of the uterine horns in relaxin-treated rats. Also, it was observed that the implanted blastocysts were no longer invariably positioned antimesometrially within the uterine lumen and that embryonic disc orientation was frequently abnormal after prolonged infusion of relaxin from day 4 to day 6 (833). Abnormal positioning of the implantation sites may account for the high rate of fetal resorption that occurred during the second half of pregnancy, when highly purified porcine relaxin was administered to rats during the peri-implantation period (954).

Reports of relaxin's quiescent effect on uterine contractility in nonpregnant mammals provided the stimulus for several clinical efforts during the late 1950s to use relaxin to prevent threatened premature labor or to inhibit the early stages of labor at term. These experiments, which generally used (a) crude and poorly characterized porcine relaxin preparations; (b) variations in doses,

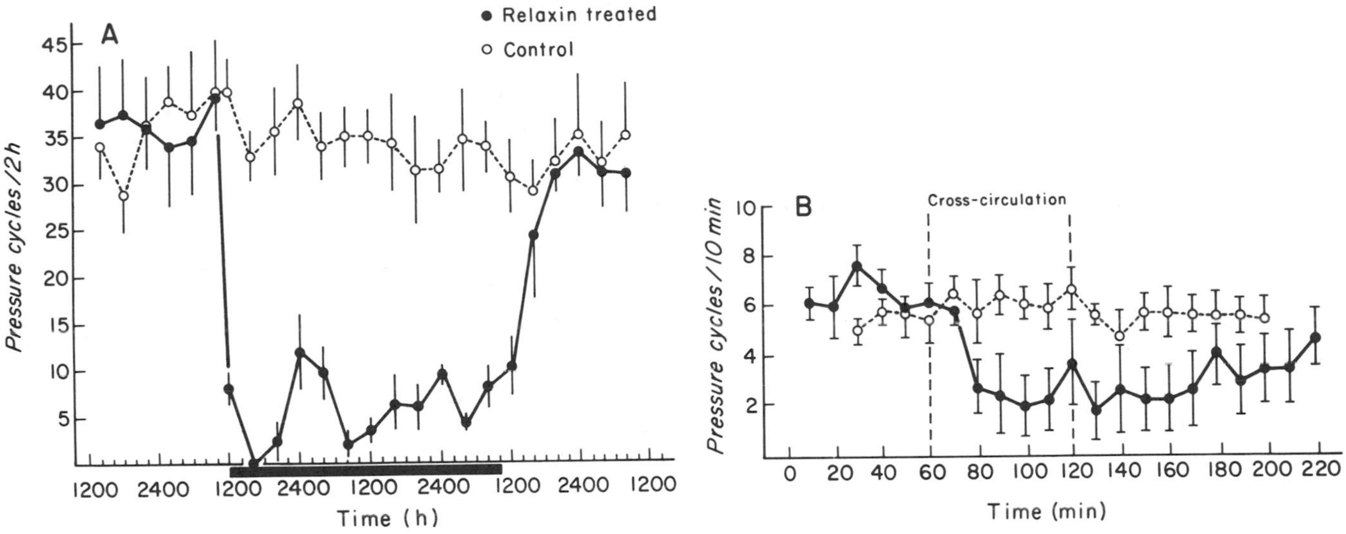

FIG. 57. A: Frequency of intrauterine pressure cycles of estrogen-dominated ovariectomized rats infused with saline (n = 3) or porcine relaxin (20 μg/h; n = 4) for 46 h. From ref. 201, with permission. **B:** Frequency of intrauterine pressure cycles of postpartum untreated rats linked by cross-circulation to day-21 pregnant rats (—●—) (n = 8) or postpartum rats (---○---) (n = 6). From ref. 788, with permission.

routes of administration, and duration of relaxin treatment; (c) inadequate controls; and (d) inadequately described and subjective means of determining the status of labor, were confusing and in some cases conflicting. Although several investigators reported that porcine relaxin inhibited uterine contractions and/or delayed birth when given to women in premature labor (3,128,291, 341,476,651,684), the most rigorous, double-blind study, which used many women and appropriate controls, reported relaxin had little, if any, effect on premature labor (248). There was general agreement that relaxin had little effect on the course of term labor (248,260,302,540), and two of these investigations used internal tocometric devices for objective determination of uterine contractility (302,540). The recent finding that both highly purified porcine relaxin (641) and synthetic human relaxin 2 (B29) (639,769) have little or no influence on the contractility of human myometrial tissue *in vitro* provides support for the view that relaxin's putative quiescent effect on the myometrium is of little physiologic or clinical importance in the human.

Relaxin's Effects on Uterine Contractility During Pregnancy

Three lines of evidence support the view that relaxin restrains uterine contractile activity during pregnancy in rats, pigs, and other mammalian species. First, studies in which the blood of a pregnant donor was cross-circulated with that of a nonpregnant recipient demonstrated the presence of a myometrial inhibitor(s) with a more rapid onset of activity than estrogen or progesterone (which require about 12 h) in the blood of the pregnant rat, guinea pig, and rabbit (780,781,788,919) (Fig. 57B). Second, there is evidence in rats and pigs that the uterine myometrium is relatively quiescent during the stage of pregnancy when relaxin levels are elevated. In pregnant rats, the frequency of uterine contractions diminishes throughout the second half of pregnancy (275), when relaxin levels in the blood are elevated (723,912) (Fig. 58A). In pregnant pigs, the electrical activity and myometrial contractile activity of the myometrium remain low as late as the period between 24 and 10 h before expulsion of the first piglet despite a decline in serum progesterone levels (809,1022,1102), and this is the time when pigs experience the antepartum surge in serum relaxin levels (315,316,401,546,555,616,809,909,910, 922,923,993,1021,1099,1102,1118). Finally, in ovariectomized pregnant rats, replacement of endogenous relaxin with exogenous relaxin reduces the frequency of uterine contractility. When rats were ovariectomized on day 9 and given replacement therapy with progesterone and estrogen throughout the remainder of pregnancy, the frequency of intrauterine pressure cycles was considerably greater than that of intact controls, whereas when replacement therapy consisted of progesterone, estrogen, and highly purified porcine relaxin, the frequency of intrauterine pressure cycles declined to levels that did not differ from those of intact controls (275) (Fig. 58B).

Characterization of Relaxin's Effects on Uterine Contractility

Desensitization. Desensitization of the rat uterus may occur with prolonged exposure to relaxin. Several investigators reported that the effectiveness with which por-

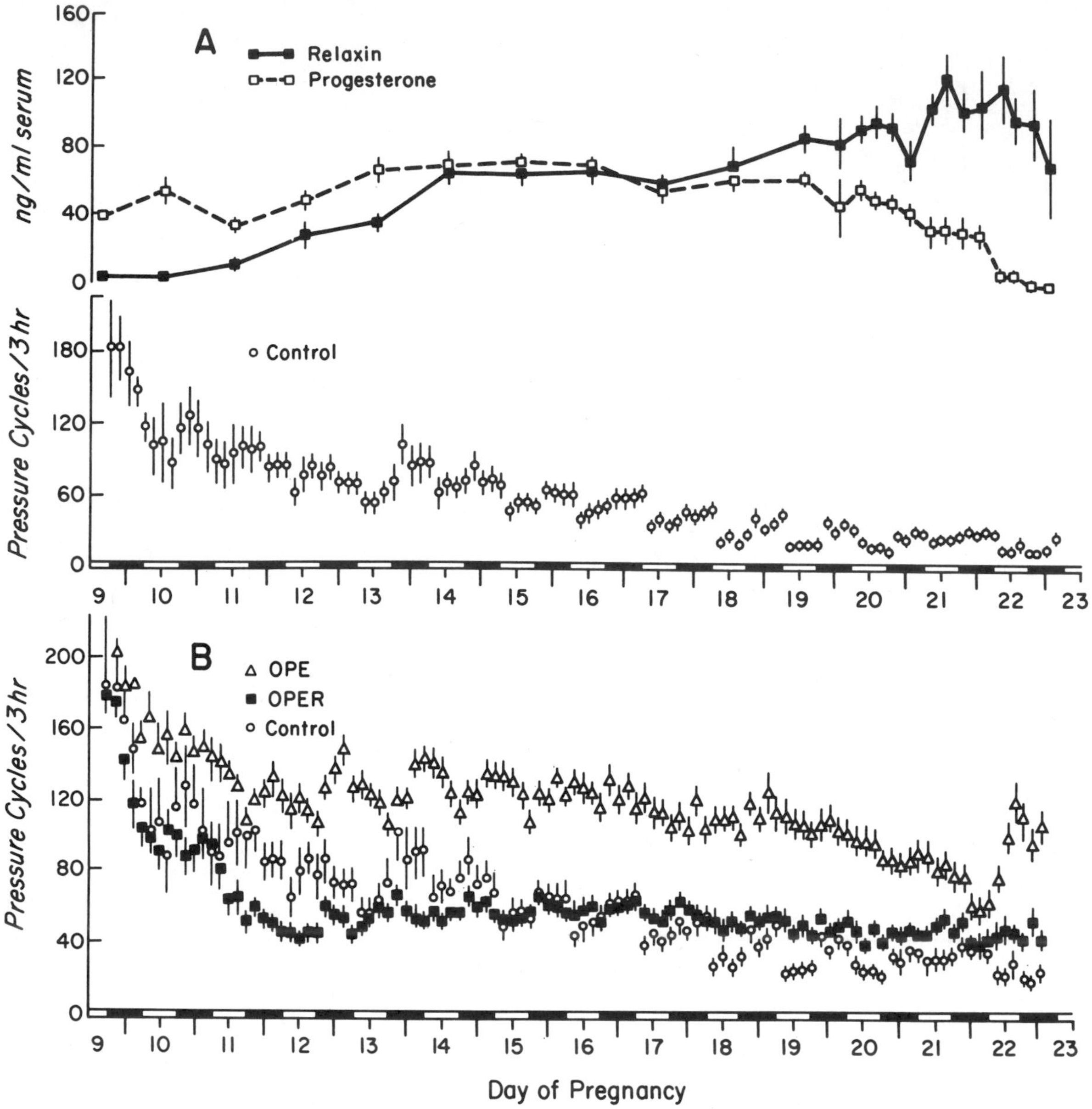

FIG. 58. A: Mean frequency (±SE) of intrauterine pressure cycles from day 9 until day 23 in intact pregnant rats. Mean peripheral blood serum relaxin and progesterone levels are from the same animals. **B:** Mean frequency (±SE) of intrauterine pressure cycles from day 9 until day 23 in intact pregnant rats (*control*), ovariectomized pregnant rats treated with progesterone and estrogen (*OPE*), and ovariectomized pregnant rats treated with progesterone, estrogen, and highly purified porcine relaxin (*OPER*). Means are from 25 or more rats. From ref. 275, with permission.

cine relaxin inhibited uterine contractility in uteri of estrogen-primed nonpregnant rats diminished after prolonged exposure to elevated relaxin levels *in vivo* (201,269,1135) or *in vitro* (194,667,1135) (Fig. 59A). One study, however, failed to observe this tachyphylaxis. After KCl-induced *in vitro* contraction of uterine segments obtained from estrogen-primed nonpregnant rats, the tonus of the uterine contractures declined continuously with prolonged exposure to porcine relaxin (989). It is not clear whether the uteri of pregnant rats become refractory to endogenous relaxin. Whereas four laboratories reported that uteri obtained from rats become refractile to relaxin during late pregnancy when treated with porcine relaxin (194,641,785,1135), one laboratory reported that uteri obtained from rats during late pregnancy were far more responsive to highly purified porcine relaxin than uteri obtained from either rats during early pregnancy or rats that were not pregnant (928). The demonstration that hormone replacement therapy in ovariectomized pregnant rats with physiologic levels of porcine relaxin from day 10 to day 23 reduced the frequency of intrauterine pressure cycles to levels found in

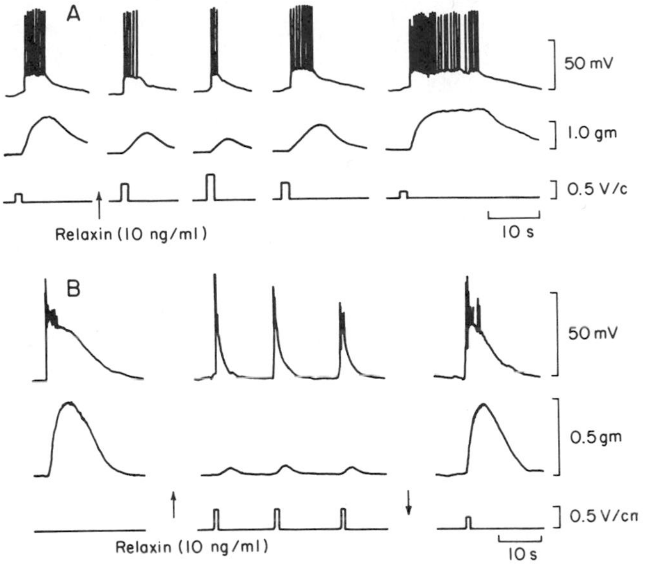

FIG. 59. Effect of addition of highly purified porcine relaxin (↑) on the electrical activity (*upper trace*) and mechanical activity (*middle trace*) evoked by depolarizing current pulses (*lower trace*) in longitudinal myometrium (**A**) and circular myometrium (**B**) of the estrogen-treated rat. In longitudinal muscle (A), duration of electrical burst and hence amplitude and duration of contraction were initially decreased in presence of relaxin; however, activity recovered within 8 to 15 min despite continual presence of relaxin. In circular muscle (B), relaxin selectively blocked the plateau component of electrical activity, and the effect was reversed 20 to 30 min after removal of peptide (↓). From ref. 194, with permission.

intact controls throughout the 13-day treatment period (Fig. 58B) does not encourage the view that desensitization, if it exists, is a physiologically important phenomenon in the rat. Limited data indicate that the pig uterus does not become refractory to relaxin during pregnancy (641,799).

Physical Characteristics of Contractions. In vivo analyses of the influence of relaxin on uterine contractility—which may have more physiologic relevance than experimentation conducted *in vitro*—demonstrated that the primary influence of relaxin is to reduce the frequency rather than the amplitude of uterine contractility. Whereas the frequency of spontaneous uterine contractions in nonpregnant guinea pigs (779,780), rabbits (781), pigs (794), sheep (792), sharks (171,942), and rats (201,268,667,788,789) was reduced dramatically during cross-circulation with pregnant animals or after administration of highly purified relaxin, the reduction in the amplitude of uterine contractions in these species was less marked. In addition, there is evidence that the coordination of rat uterine contractile activity may be improved during recovery from relaxin-induced quiescence. The rate of rise of intrauterine pressure cycles recorded from conscious (267) or anesthetized (119,267) ovariectomized rats was significantly elevated during recovery from the total myometrial quiescence imposed by treatment with porcine (267) or rat (119) relaxin.

A variety of *in vitro* methods have been used to examine the characteristics of relaxin's action on uterine contractility. Despite the important limitation that they are relatively unphysiologic, these methods have advantages over *in vivo* methods for some research objectives. For example, they require less relaxin, enable more than one treatment with uterine tissue from a single animal, permit more accurate measurement of parameters of uterine contractility, and enable direct correlations between the contractile state and biochemical composition of the uterus. *in vitro* methods were used to examine the site(s) and physical characteristics of relaxin's action on the rat myometrium. A radioautographic localization study with ^{125}I-labeled porcine relaxin led Weiss and Bryant-Greenwood (1115) to conclude that relaxin binding sites are present on both the longitudinal and circular smooth-muscle layers of the myometrium, with the preponderance of binding sites on the circular layer. In subsequent *in vitro* investigations, porcine relaxin was reported to inhibit the contractility of segments of both longitudinal and circular smooth muscle (194,497,740, 786). Chamley and Parkington (194) and Osa et al. (740) obtained evidence that relaxin may act, at least in part, through inhibition of action potentials in both smooth-muscle layers. When strips of rat uterine longitudinal smooth muscle were mounted in organ baths and stimulated electrically to induce electronic depolarization of the membrane, bursts of spike-type action potentials occurred that outlasted the stimulus (Fig. 59A). Addition of highly purified porcine relaxin to the electrically stimulated longitudinal muscle tissue decreased the number of action potentials per burst with a consequent decrease in the amplitude and duration of the accompanying contractions (194,740). When strips of uterine circular smooth muscle were stimulated electrically, there was an initial spike-type or short burst of spike-type action potentials followed by a long plateau of depolarization (Fig. 59B). Application of porcine relaxin to the circular-muscle tissue bath eliminated the plateau component of the action potential (194). Consistent with these findings, the burst frequency of uterine action potentials in sheep was reduced *in vivo* after intravenous administration of highly purified porcine relaxin (796).

Interaction of Relaxin with Other Hormones. The response of the uterus to relaxin is influenced by other hormones that act on the uterine myometrium during pregnancy, such as progesterone, estrogen, oxytocin, PGs, and endothelin. The way in which relaxin interacts with these hormones to influence uterine contractility is not well understood for any species, but it has been examined to some extent in the rat and pig. Whereas progesterone alone markedly reduces the frequency or amplitude of intrauterine pressure cycles in species such as the sheep, rabbit, and pig (786,794), it does not in the rat

(271,273,787). Instead, progesterone desynchronizes the electrical activity of the rat uterus, thus rendering the uterus unresponsive to oxytocin-induced contractions and preventing strong, highly coordinated uterine contractions such as those that occur at delivery. Progesterone in combination with estrogen was reported to influence the characteristics of spontaneous contractions of the rat uterus *in vitro.* When immature rats were treated with both progesterone and estrogen *in vivo,* uteri demonstrated a decrease in the contraction cycle length, an increase in the frequency of contractions, and an increase in the duration of peak force of contraction *in vitro* relative to uteri obtained from rats treated with estrogen only (394). There is evidence that progesterone may also increase the sensitivity of the rat uterus to relaxin. Exposure of the uteri of estrogen-primed nonpregnant rats to progesterone *in vivo* (127) or *in vitro* (859,860) was reported to reduce by about half the dose of porcine relaxin needed to decrease the amplitude of electrically stimulated contractions of uterine segments *in vitro.* Also, exposure of myometrial strips obtained from both nonpregnant and pregnant rats and pigs to progesterone for 45 min *in vitro* reduced markedly the amounts of relaxin required to inhibit spontaneous uterine contractions and KCl-induced tetanic contractions (641). Progesterone may enhance the response of myometrial cells to relaxin at the level of the plasma membrane. There is limited evidence that uteri from immature rats pretreated with both progesterone and estrogen produce more cyclic AMP in response to relaxin treatment *in vitro* than do uteri from rats primed with only estrogen (410).

Estrogen has been demonstrated to inhibit the frequency of intrauterine pressure cycles in ovariectomized postpartum rats (271). It may be, however, that estrogen has little effect on uterine contractility during most of pregnancy, because peripheral blood levels of estrogen are low until late pregnancy. Moreover, blood levels of progesterone are elevated throughout nearly all of pregnancy, and they probably override or moderate whatever effects the low estrogen levels might have on uterine contractility in the absence of progesterone. However, the low levels of estrogen may be sufficient to influence relaxin's effects on uterine contractility during the second half of pregnancy. Although relaxin has the capacity to inhibit spontaneous myometrial activity in the absence of estrogen treatment in ovariectomized nonpregnant rats (201,789,790), several workers reported that the sensitivity of the uterus to relaxin increases markedly with prior estrogen treatment (269,667,839,1135). The mechanism whereby estrogen enhances the sensitivity of the uterus to relaxin is not known. It may do so by inducing the formation of relaxin receptors. Estrogen administration was reported to induce uterine relaxin receptors in ovariectomized rats (664,742) and pigs (665). It seems likely that estrogen has its most profound effects on uterine contractility during the antepartum period, when estrogen levels increase. As the uterus comes under progressively greater estrogen domination during late pregnancy, its capacity for highly coordinated contractions increases (363). In the presence of elevated estrogen levels, there is an increase in uterine gap junctions (931), uterine electrical conductivity (662), PG production (179), oxytocin production (606), oxytocin receptors (16,17), and relaxin receptors (664,665).

It is not presently clear whether relaxin blocks or attenuates uterine contractions induced by endogenous stimuli such as oxytocin, PGs, and endothelin. Available evidence indicates that under normal physiologic conditions, oxytocin and PGs override relaxin's effects on uterine contractility. Oxytocin (119,192,201,639, 667,779,780,788,789,792,794,799,990,1136), $PGF_{2\alpha}$ (119,192,792,799,990), and PGE_2 (799) stimulated myometrial contractions in rat, pig, guinea pig, and sheep uteri that were under the quiescent influence of relaxin. Nevertheless, evidence obtained both *in vivo* and *in vitro* indicated that pharmacologic doses of relaxin inhibited oxytocin- and PG-driven uterine contractions in the rat (194,201,269,394,480,706,707,789,790,990) and pig (799). Thus, the response of the uterus to relaxin or the contractile stimulants oxytocin and $PGF_{2\alpha}$ appears to depend, at least in part, on their relative concentrations in the extracellular fluid. There is limited evidence that the ability of relaxin to inhibit oxytocin- and PG-driven contractions may require prior estrogen treatment (269,740,789,790). Endothelin, which is a 21-amino-acid peptide produced by vascular endothelial cells, is found in higher concentrations in human amniotic fluid than in peripheral plasma (1094) and in higher concentrations in women in labor compared with third trimester controls not in labor (1065). Endothelin stimulates rhythmic contractions of the rat uterus (573) and may play a role in the control of uterine contractility at the initiation of labor. Similar to findings with oxytocin- and PG-stimulated uterine contractions, McGovern et al. (687) demonstrated that endothelin and relaxin interacted in a reversible and antagonistic way to control the contractility of isolated rat uterine horn segments *in vitro.*

Postulated Role of Relaxin on Uterine Contractility During the Antepartum Period

The role of relaxin on the normal progression of antepartum and parturient uterine contractile activity has not been determined with certainty for any species. Porter (783) postulated that relaxin may provide a mechanism that protects the fetuses and placentas during the antepartum period of progesterone withdrawal in species such as rats and pigs in which high blood levels of progesterone prevent highly coordinated uterine contractility until just before birth. In these species, relaxin may restrain uterine contractile activity during the antepartum period of progesterone withdrawal until overridden by stimulating agents, such as oxytocin and PGs, or other mechanisms that bring about the onset of strong, highly coordinated uterine contractions and the delivery of the fetuses. Downing and Sherwood (275) obtained evidence that is consistent with this hypothesis. In the pregnant rat, the myometrium is almost completely quiescent from day 20 until about 3 h before the onset of labor, when there is an abrupt increase in uterine contractility that lasts until labor is completed (275) (Fig. 60A). When pregnant rats were ovariectomized on day 9 and administered hormone replacement therapy with progesterone and estrogen, the frequency of intrauterine pressure cycles was far greater than in controls throughout the 24-h prelabor and postlabor periods. However, when similarly ovariectomized pregnant rats were given replacement therapy with progesterone, estrogen, and highly purified porcine relaxin, the frequency of intrauterine pressure cycles was close to that in intact controls throughout this period (275) (Fig. 60B).

Although much has been learned concerning relaxin's direct effects on myometrial cells, little is known concerning the process whereby relaxin interacts with other hormones to influence the coordinated contractile activity of the entire uterus. Summerlee and co-workers obtained limited and indirect evidence that relaxin may

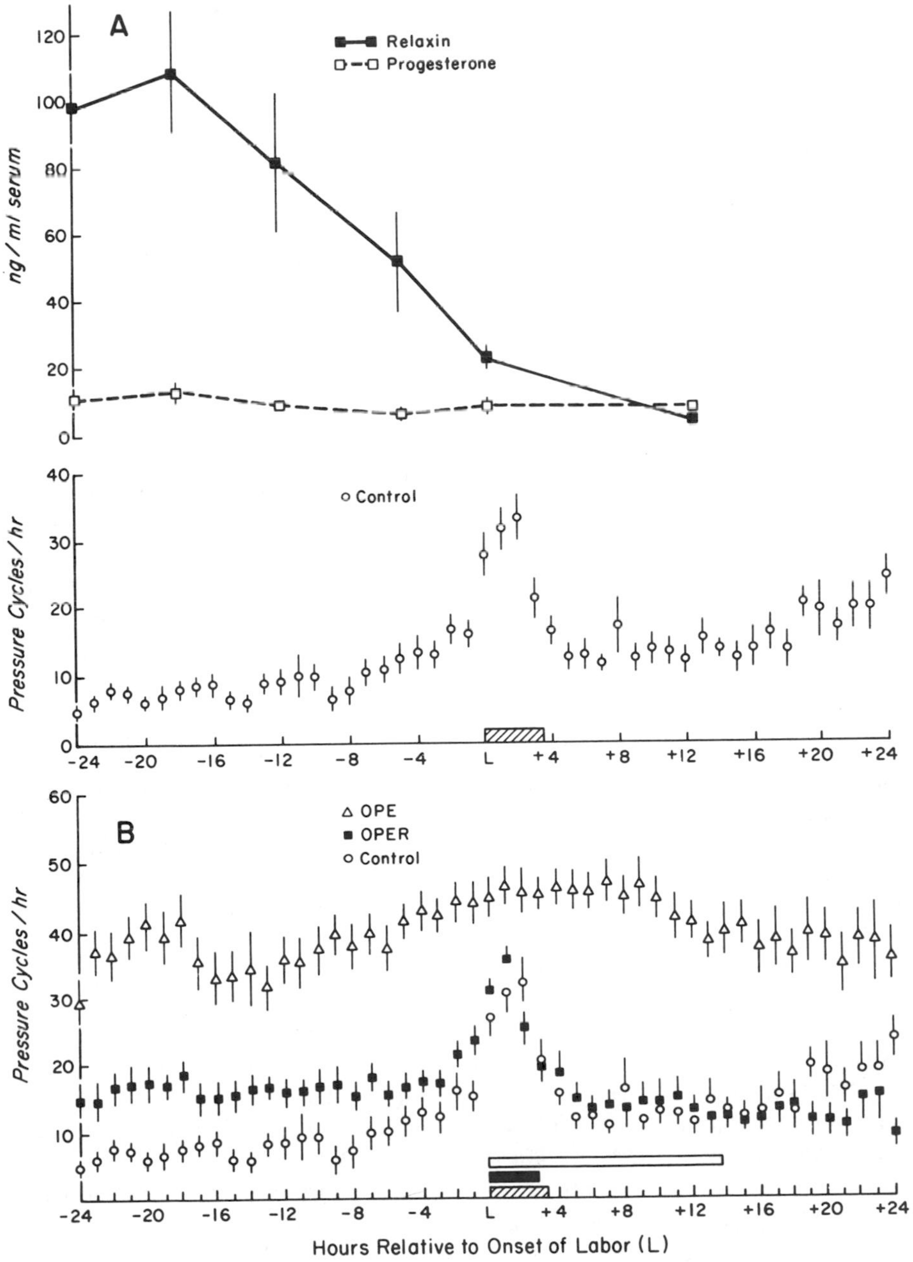

FIG. 60. A: Mean frequency (±SE; n = 18) of intrauterine pressure cycles from 24 h before onset of labor until 24 h after onset of labor in rats. Mean (±SE) serum relaxin and progesterone levels are from same animals. **B:** Mean frequency (±SE; n = 18–25) of intrauterine pressure cycles from 24 h before onset of labor until 24 h after onset of labor in intact pregnant rats (*control*), ovariectomized pregnant rats treated with progesterone and estrogen (*OPE*), and ovariectomized pregnant rats treated with progesterone, estrogen, and highly purified porcine relaxin (*OPER*). Mean durations of labor are indicated: ▨, intact controls; □, group OPE; ■, group OPER. From ref. 275, with permission.

reduce antepartum myometrial activity in pregnant rats not only through effects on the uterine myometrium but also through a central action to prevent oxytocin release from the posterior pituitary (524,526,527,529,726–729,1004,1006,1007). It was postulated that under normal physiologic conditions, endogenous relaxin may influence the time of onset of delivery and/or progress of labor by inhibiting oxytocin secretion prepartum (524,526,527,1007). Evidence obtained in pregnant rats is not supportive of that hypothesis. Passive immunization of endogenous relaxin with a monoclonal antibody for rat relaxin, either throughout the second half of pregnancy (587) or during the antepartum period (495), did not influence the time of onset of labor. Moreover, the putative inhibitory effect of relaxin on oxytocin secretion from the posterior pituitary is hard to understand in the light of the fact that serum relaxin surges to high levels during delivery (912) when serum oxytocin levels are also elevated (527). Finally, there is strong evidence that oxytocin is produced in the rat uterus in high levels near term, and it was postulated that it is local oxytocin rather than circulating oxytocin that participates in the induction of labor (606). Whereas these findings in intact pregnant rats do not rule out the possibility that endogenous relaxin reduces antepartum myometrial activity by reducing the availability of oxytocin to the rat uterus, they make it seem unlikely.

Mechanism of Action of Relaxin on Myometrial Cells

Since 1980, considerable progress has been made at the molecular level toward an understanding of the mechanism(s) whereby relaxin inhibits contractility of the uterine myometrium, and this progress, made primarily with studies in the rat, has been reviewed (542,851,853).

Relaxin Receptors on Myometrial Cells. It is clear that relaxin acts directly on the myometrium. Studies at both the whole-animal level and tissue level demonstrated that relaxin receptors are present in the uterus. Finite numbers of high-affinity binding sites for radioiodinated porcine relaxin were reported in rat (663,664, 690,1115), guinea pig (384), pig (665), and mouse (1143) uterine horns. Also, ^{32}P-labeled human relaxin 2 was found associated with rat myometrium when used for *in situ* localization of relaxin binding sites (743). Examination of ^{125}I-labeled porcine relaxin binding by radioautography demonstrated that the uterine binding sites in the rat are located in both the longitudinal and circular muscle layers (1115). As with other protein hormone receptors, relaxin receptors appear to be associated with the plasma membrane. Mercado-Simmen et al. (663–665) reported that high-affinity binding sites with $K_a = 10^9$ to 10^{10} M^{-1} were located in plasma membrane-enriched particulate fractions of rat and pig uterine tissue. These relaxin binding sites were reported to be elevated during the estrogen-dominated stages of the estrous cycle in rats (664) and after estrogen administration to ovariectomized rats and pigs (663–665). Mercado-Simmen et al. (664) postulated that modulation of relaxin receptors in the uterus may be part of the mechanism whereby estrogen increases the sensitivity of the uterus to relaxin. These workers (663,664) also reported that relaxin binding sites are elevated during the second half of pregnancy in the rat uterus and that endogenous relaxin and exogenously administered porcine relaxin may reduce their number.

Efforts to examine the mechanism of action of relaxin on the rat uterus at the cellular level are consistent with the view that relaxin acts directly on the myometrium. Sanborn and co-workers (35,36,479–481,811,852) demonstrated that porcine relaxin acts directly on rat myometrial cells in culture to alter their oxytocin-induced shape and also to influence levels of intracellular molecules thought to mediate relaxin's effects on uterine contractility. The influence of estrogen, relaxin, or other factors on relaxin receptors has not been measured directly, because relaxin receptors have not been isolated or characterized.

Molecular Basis for Smooth Muscle Contraction. A brief summary of the molecular basis for the regulation of smooth-muscle contraction (11,542,851,852) seems appropriate to facilitate understanding the intracellular mechanism(s) whereby relaxin may inhibit uterine contractility. The reader is encouraged to refer to Fig. 61 throughout this description of the mechanism of action on myometrial cells. Contraction of smooth muscle occurs as a result of actomyosin interaction in a process that involves the hydrolysis of ATP. The actin-activated myosin ATPase activity requires phosphorylation of the 20,000-Da light chains that are associated with the globular head of myosin. Activation of the enzyme myosin light-chain kinase (MLCK), which catalyzes myosin light-chain phosphorylation, is a sequential process requiring an elevation of the intracellular calcium levels. Calcium first binds to the calcium-regulatory protein calmodulin, which is found in high concentrations and is not limiting in the uterus, to form a $Ca^{2+}\cdot$calmodulin complex. The $Ca^{2+}\cdot$calmodulin complex then binds to the inactive MLCK to form the active holoenzyme complex $Ca^{2+}\cdot$calmodulin$\cdot$MLCK. Phosphorylation of MLCK, which is catalyzed by cyclic AMP-dependent protein kinase (protein kinase A), reduces the capacity of the MLCK to combine with $Ca^{2+}\cdot$calmodulin. Thus, phosphorylation of MLCK inhibits formation of the active $Ca^{2+}\cdot$calmodulin$\cdot$MLCK complex.

Possible Mediation Through Activation of Protein Kinase A. The mechanism(s) whereby relaxin brings about the inhibition of uterine contractions is not known. It seems likely that it does so, at least in part, through protein kinase A–mediated phosphorylation of proteins

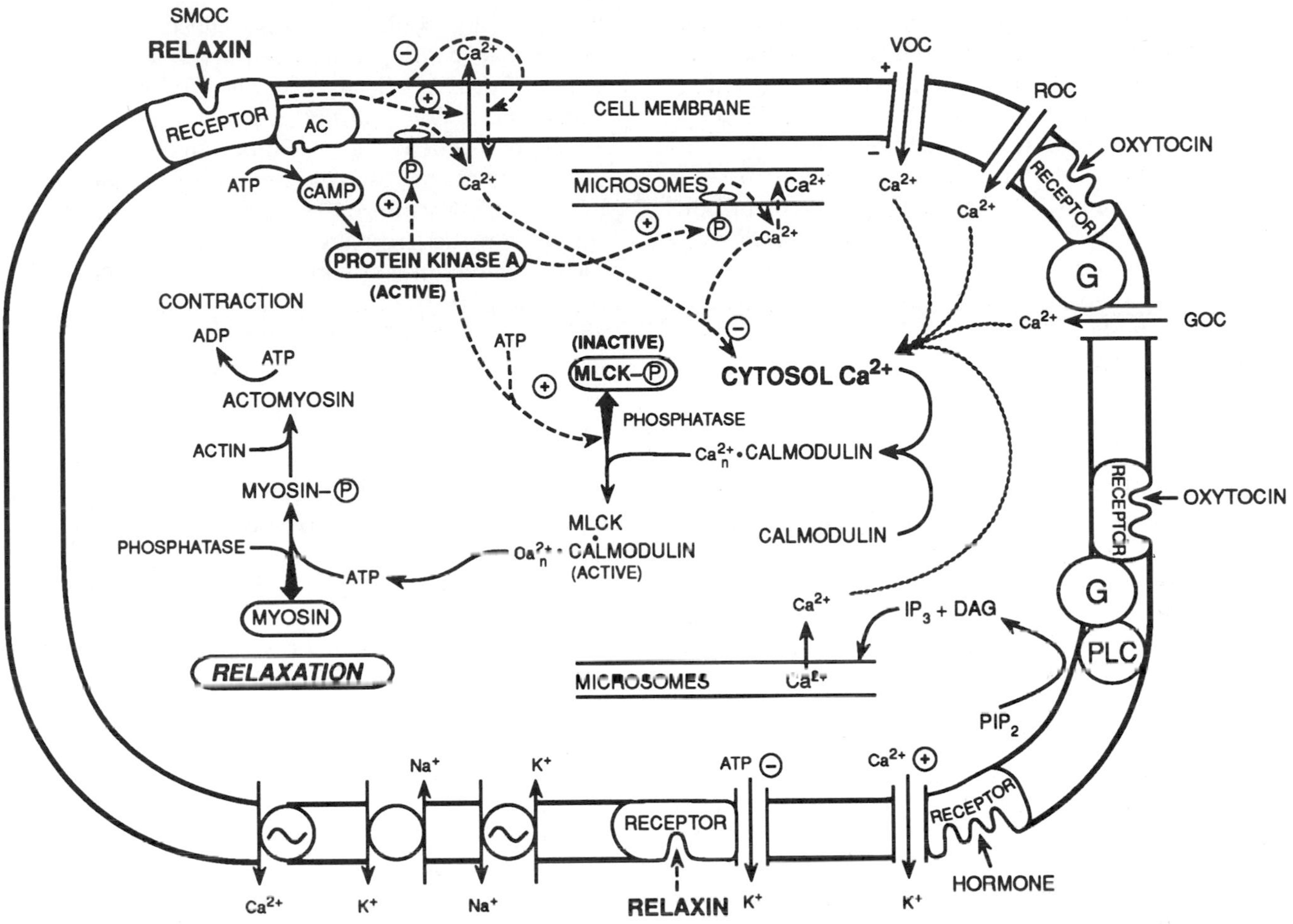

FIG. 61. Intracellular mechanisms whereby relaxin may inhibit contractions of uterine myometrial cells. Putative effects of relaxin that are supported by experimental data in rat myometrial tissue are enclosed by *solid lines* and preceded by *solid arrows.* Possible effects of relaxin that have not been demonstrated are shown with *dashed lines. AC,* adenylyl cyclase; *protein kinase A,* cyclic AMP-dependent protein kinase; *MLCK,* myosin light-chain kinase; *G,* guanosine triphosphate-binding protein; *PLC,* phospholipase C; *PIP_2*, phosphoinositol 4,5-biphosphate; *DAG,* diacylglycerol; *IP_3*, inositol triphosphate. Ion channels that control influx of calcium at the level of plasma membrane are second-messenger-operated (*SMOC*), receptor-operated (*ROC*), gated (*GOC*), and voltage-operated (*VOC*). Protein kinase A dissociates in presence of cyclic AMP into a regulatory subunit–cyclic AMP complex and an active protein kinase A subunit that promotes phosphorylation of intracellular proteins. After relaxin treatment, cyclic AMP increases, protein kinase A activity increases, affinity of MLCK for the Ca^{2+} · calmodulin complex decreases, MLCK activity decreases, myosin light-chain phosphorylation decreases, actomyosin ATPase activity decreases, and there is a relaxation of uterine contractility. It is not clear whether relaxin brings about its effects through phosphorylation of MLCK. Relaxin also acts, at least in part, by reducing intracellular Ca^{2+} levels, thus decreasing MLCK activity and myosin light-chain phosphorylation. There is evidence that relaxin not only promotes increased Ca^{2+} efflux from myometrial cells but also inhibits mobilization of Ca^{2+} from intracellular stores. Finally, there is evidence that relaxin may mediate its effects by opening ATP-dependent K^+ channels. References that describe these relaxin are cited in the text. Modified from refs. 851 and 853.

within myometrial cells. After treatment with highly purified porcine relaxin in the presence of phosphodiesterase inhibitors, there was a time- and dose-dependent increase in cyclic AMP levels in rat and pig uterine tissue (200,410,536,854) and rat myometrial cells (479). Consistent with these findings, synthetic human relaxin 2 provoked time- and dose-dependent increases in both intracellular and extracellular levels of cyclic AMP when a newborn rhesus monkey uterine cell line with characteristics of smooth muscle was incubated in the presence of a phosphodiesterase inhibitor (574). Two reports have described a positive correlation between relaxin's capacity to inhibit rat uterine contractions and the elevation of intrauterine cyclic AMP. In one investigation, the effectiveness with which porcine relaxin inhibited rat uterine contractions *in vitro* was found to increase when the phosphodiesterase inhibitor theophylline was present in the organ bath (990). A second study demonstrated that the addition of magnesium to rat uterine longitudinal muscle strips in culture increased relaxin's capacity to both elevate intracellular cyclic AMP levels and inhibit uterine contractions (740). A preliminary experiment showed that relaxin may elevate cyclic AMP levels in rat uterine myometrium by increasing adenylyl cyclase activity (855).

There is evidence that the relaxin-induced elevation in cyclic AMP may activate protein kinase A, which then triggers subsequent events that inhibit uterine contractions. Binding of cyclic AMP to a protein presumed to be the regulatory subunit of protein kinase A occurred after treatment of rat uterine tissue with porcine relaxin in the presence of a phosphodiesterase inhibitor (856). It was reported that relaxin activated rat uterine protein kinase A within 30 sec in the absence of phosphodiesterase inhibitors, and the effects of relaxin on the activation of protein kinase A paralleled those on muscle contraction in terms of time-course and dose response (541). Anwer et al. (36) reported that preincubation of rat uterine myometrial cells with the protein kinase A inhibitor *N*-[2-(methylamino)ethyl]-5-isoquinolinesulfonamide dihydrochloride (H8) prevented relaxin's capacity to inhibit both oxytocin-induced uptake of Ca^{2+} and oxytocin-induced stimulation of [^{3}H] inositol phosphate formation.

Nishikori et al. (706,707) reported that relaxin inhibited MLCK activity and myosin light-chain phosphorylation in isometrically suspended strips of uteri obtained from estrogen-primed rats; furthermore, the time-course and concentration response of these biochemical effects of relaxin paralleled hormone-induced inhibition of uterine contractility. The reduction of MLCK activity was attributed to a decrease in the affinity of MLCK for its modulator Ca^{2+} · calmodulin as well as a reduction in the affinity of the active Ca^{2+} · calmodulin · MLCK complex for its substrate myosin (707). Hsu and Sanborn (481) obtained results with myometrial cells in culture that partially confirmed these effects of relaxin on MLCK. Reduction in myometrial cell MLCK activity was attributed to a decrease in the affinity of MLCK for its modulator Ca^{2+} · calmodulin (481). A decrease in the affinity of the active Ca^{2+} · calmodulin · MLCK complex for its substrate myosin was not observed with the myometrial cells in culture (481). The mechanism that accounts for the reduction in affinity of MLCK for Ca^{2+} · calmodulin is not known with certainty. There is reason to postulate that it may be attributable to phosphorylation of MLCK by protein kinase A. In the absence of calmodulin, two sites on MLCK can be phosphorylated, and phosphorylation of one of these sites reduces the affinity of MLCK for calmodulin (705). Furthermore, it was demonstrated that Forskolin-induced elevation of cyclic AMP levels in tracheal smooth-muscle cells resulted in increased MLCK phosphorylation and a relaxation of the contracted muscle (252). There are criteria that must be met before it can be concluded that relaxin inhibits uterine contractility through the phosphorylation of MLCK. These include demonstrating that relaxin promotes phosphorylation of MLCK and that there is a stoichiometric relationship between the degree of MLCK phosphorylation and changes in the affinity of MLCK for Ca^{2+} · calmodulin (542).

Perhaps relaxin-induced elevation in cyclic AMP influences uterine contractility through mechanisms in addition to its putative effect on MLCK activity. Relaxin-induced cyclic AMP may influence gap junctions, which are intercellular channels that link cells to their neighbors by allowing the passage of inorganic ions and small molecules. There is a dramatic increase in both the numbers and sizes of gap junctions between uterine smooth-muscle cells before labor in rats and other mammalian species (379). The increase in junctional area is thought to improve electrical interactions between smooth-muscle fibers and permit a more extensive cell-to-cell spread of action potentials from pacemaker regions, thus permitting normal and effective development of intrauterine pressure and delivery of the young. Cole and Garfield (210) demonstrated relaxin and other agents that elevate cyclic AMP reduce the rate of cell-to-cell diffusion of the intracellular marker 2[^{3}H] deoxy-D-glucose in strips of longitudinal myometrium obtained from rats in labor. Whereas no difference in the area of gap junctions was observed after relaxin treatment, large electron-opaque deposits were found associated with the surface of many gap junctions in the myometrial tissue (Fig. 62). The deposits, which were not observed in controls, were occasionally observed to be precisely paired in position and size on opposite sides of the region of cell-to-cell contact as shown in Fig. 62. The relationship between the formation of electron-dense deposits at the gap junctions in the myometrium and the uncoupling of intercellular communication produced by relaxin remains

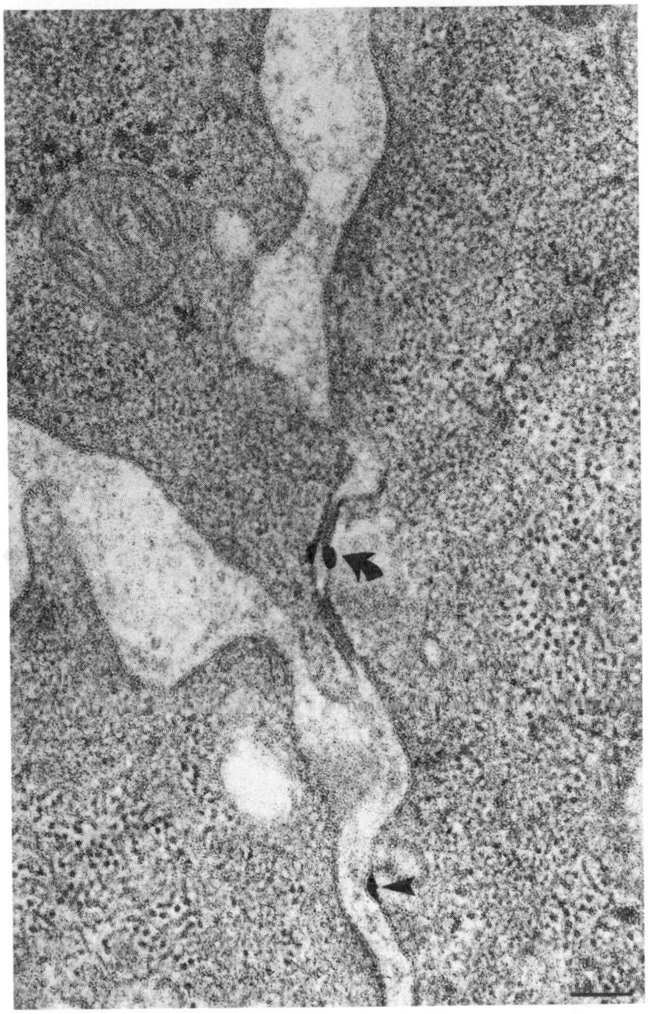

FIG. 62. Electron micrograph of a gap junction in parturient rat myometrial tissue. Two small electron opaque deposits occur on membrane beside a gap junction (*arrow*) and a single deposit is observed at some distance from any junction (*arrowhead*) in a tissue exposed to porcine relaxin (0.1 μg/ml). ($\times$76,000) From ref. 210, with permission.

to be determined. It was postulated that relaxin may reduce gap junction permeability and thereby render the myometrium incapable of generating sufficient intrauterine pressure for effective expulsion of fetuses.

A few observations raise questions concerning the role of cyclic AMP in relaxin's actions on rat uterine contractility. Relaxin elevates uterine and myometrial cell cyclic AMP levels *in vitro* with a slower time-course than that seen for either the physical effects or the activation of protein kinase A after relaxin treatment (479,856). Downing and co-workers (272,688) examined the relationship between relaxin-induced elevation of cyclic AMP levels and uterine contractility *in vivo*. When ovariectomized rats were administered a low bolus dose of the β-adrenergic agonist salbutamol, which is thought to inhibit uterine contractions by activation of adenylyl cyclase, there was a 19-fold increase in uterine cyclic AMP levels within 1 minute of treatment. The salbutamol produced an initial inhibition of uterine contractions of about 80%, which declined to about 30% inhibition over 60 min. In contrast, when rats were administered a low bolus dose of porcine relaxin, there was a similar reduction in uterine contractility but no detectable increase in tissue cyclic AMP levels (272,688).

Possible Mediation Through Reduction of Intracellular Ca^{2+} Levels. Relaxin may reduce MLCK activity, at least in part, through reduction of intracellular Ca^{2+} levels. Formation of the Ca^{2+} · calmodulin complex needed for MLCK activation is inhibited through reduction of intracellular Ca^{2+} levels. Potential means whereby relaxin can reduce intracellular Ca^{2+} levels are to increase Ca^{2+} sequestration in microsomes, increase efflux of Ca^{2+} from myometrial cells, decrease influx of Ca^{2+} into the cell, or promote combinations of these processes. The extracellular environment is a main source of Ca^{2+} for myometrial smooth-muscle cells. At the level of the plasma membrane receptor-operated (ROC), voltage-operated (VOC), second-messenger-operated (SMOC), GTP-binding protein (G-protein), and gated (GOC) ion channels control the influx of calcium (835). Activation of Ca^{2+}-activated K^+ channels and ATP-dependent K^+ channels resulting in membrane repolarization influences VOC and is thought to be involved in termination of the Ca^{2+} signal in smooth muscle (853).

There is evidence that relaxin enhances the efflux of Ca^{2+} from rat myometrial cells (811) and rat myometrial tissue (388). The mechanism whereby relaxin stimulates the efflux of Ca^{2+} is not known, but it does not appear to be attributable to increased Na^+/Ca^{2+} exchange coupled to indirect stimulation of Na^+/K^+-ATPase activity (851).

Relaxin has little detectable effect on resting intracellular Ca^{2+} concentrations (35). In contrast, the uterine contractant oxytocin not only increases the influx of Ca^{2+} but also stimulates the release of Ca^{2+} from intracellular stores within microsomes (68,180). Acting through its receptors, oxytocin enhances activity of the enzyme phospholipase C, which hydrolyzes phosphatidylinositol 4,5-biphosphate (PIP_2), to generate two second messengers—inositol triphosphate (IP_3) and diacylglycerol (DAG). The IP_3 interacts with receptors in microsomes to release Ca^{2+}. Anwer et al. (35) examined the influence of relaxin in combination with oxytocin on rat myometrial cells in culture to obtain evidence that relaxin influences intracellular levels of Ca^{2+} by mechanisms in addition to enhanced Ca^{2+} efflux. In the absence of extracellular Ca^{2+}, when Ca^{2+} is presumably mobilized only from internal stores, the ability of oxytocin to increase intracellular free Ca^{2+} from those stores was almost totally inhibited by relaxin. Also, when the mobilization of Ca^{2+} from internal stores was inhibited by preventing IP_3 formation with pertussis toxin, the ability of oxytocin to increase intracellular Ca^{2+} levels by enhancing Ca^{2+} influx was inhibited by relaxin. Thus, relaxin appears to attenuate the effects of oxytocin on rat myometrial cells by inhibiting both Ca^{2+} mobilization from internal stores and Ca^{2+} influx. It appears the action of relaxin versus oxytocin is mediated through protein kinase A. Preincubation of rat myometrial cells with the protein kinase A inhibitor H8 reversed relaxin's inhibitory effects on oxytocin-stimulated increase in intracellular Ca^{2+} and IP_3 formation (36). Moreover, activation of endogenous protein kinase A was demonstrated to inhibit phospholipase C activity in rat myometrial plasma membranes (1117).

Possible Mediation Through Opening of K^+ Channels. There is evidence that relaxin may mediate its effects, at least in part, by opening K^+ channels. Downing and Hollingsworth (268) examined the influence of glibenclamide, a relatively selective blocker of ATP-dependent K^+ channels, and apamin, a selective blocker of low conductance calcium-activated K^+ channels, on porcine relaxin's capacity to inhibit spontaneous uterine contractions in ovariectomized rats. Glibenclamide treatment *in vivo* reduced markedly uterine sensitivity to relaxin, but apamin had no effect. Whereas the results obtained with this *in vivo* study indicate that glibenclamide-sensitive ATP-dependent K^+ channels may play a role in relaxin's mechanism of action, a subsequent study that examined the influence of glibenclamide on relaxin's capacity to inhibit rat uterine contractions *in vitro* did not demonstrate an effect (490).

Possible Mediation Through Activation of Protein Kinase C. There is evidence that relaxin does not regulate uterine contractility through activation of protein kinase C. The potent protein kinase C inhibitor H7 only partially attenuated the inhibition by relaxin of oxytocin-induced increase in Ca^{2+} levels and IP_3 formation in rat myometrial cells. Moreover, preincubation of myometrial cells with the protein kinase C stimulator phorbol myristate acetate did not alter the ability of oxytocin to increase Ca^{2+} or the capacity of relaxin to inhibit the effect of oxytocin on Ca^{2+} (36).

Possible Indirect Mediation Through the Release of Catecholamines. Relaxin may influence uterine contractions, at least in part, through a completely different and indirect mechanism. In the early 1960s, Rudzik and Miller (838,839) examined the mechanism whereby crude porcine relaxin inhibits uterine contractility in estrogen-primed rats. They concluded that relaxin may act indirectly through the release of the catecholamine epinephrine, because (a) the sensitivity of the myometrium to relaxin was parallel to the epinephrine content, (b) relaxin treatment reduced the epinephrine content, and (c) the influence of relaxin on uterine contractility was inhibited by adrenergic neuron blocking agents. Subsequent investigations have in some cases been consistent with those of Rudzik and Miller (838,839). For example, the observations that β-adrenergic receptor agonists stimulate cyclic AMP levels (479,536,854) and inhibit uterine contractility (839,854,858,989,990) are consistent with the possibility that the effects of relaxin on uterine contractility are mediated indirectly through β-adrenergic agonist activation of adenylyl cyclase. For the most part, however, experimentation supports the view that relaxin acts independently or only partially through stimulation of β-adrenergic receptors. Several studies demonstrated that levels of β-adrenergic receptor antagonists that block the effects of β agonists do not block relaxin's inhibitory effect on uterine contractility (344,622,760,789,989,990,1135) or relaxin's stimulatory effect on cyclic AMP levels in estrogen-dominated rats (536,857). Also, in contrast to the early work of Rudzik and Miller (838), Sanborn et al. (857,858) reported that highly purified porcine relaxin did not reduce uterine catecholamine levels in estrogen-primed rats; moreover, depletion of nearly all the epinephrine from the uteri of reserpine-treated rats did not prevent relaxin from relaxing potassium-depolarized uterine strips in the absence or presence of the β-adrenergic receptor antagonist propranolol. Finally, St-Louis (989) reported that the β-adrenergic receptor antagonist propranolol abolished the relaxing effects of the β-adrenergic receptor agonist isoproterenol but that it only inhibited about 45% of the action of relaxin on potassium-contracted rat uterine strips.

Possible Mediation Through Prostaglandins. The prostaglandins $PGF_{2\alpha}$ and PGE_2 are potent stimulants of uterine contractility in many mammalian species. The effects of the PGI_2 on uterine contractility appear to vary among species. PGI_2 was reported to stimulate uterine contractility and to potentiate the effects of oxytocin on strips of rat pregnant uterus *in vitro* (1124). In contrast, PGI_2 was reported to inhibit spontaneous and $PGF_{2\alpha}$-induced contractile activity in strips of human myometrium *in vitro* (738) and to reduce uterine electromyographical and contractile activity *in vivo* in nonpregnant ovariectomized sheep (635). Circumstantial evidence indicates that increased PGI_2 synthesis may be associated with the mechanisms that control uterine contractility at parturition in the rat. In pregnant rats, myometrial levels of the predominant prostaglandin PGI_2 increase sharply at birth, and synthesis of PGI_2 is promoted by oxytocin (1121,1122). Williams and El Tahir (1123) reported that relaxin inhibited both spontaneous and oxytocin-induced synthesis of PGI_2 and appeared to do so by inhibiting the enzyme phospholipase A_2, which is obligatory for the synthesis of PGI_2 as well as other PGs. These workers (1123) concluded that relaxin might act through inhibitory effects on PG synthesis. In contrast, there are studies that indicate that relaxin's effects are not dependent on its capacity to reduce PG synthesis. Indomethacin in concentrations sufficient to block PG synthesis did not inhibit the stimulatory effects of relaxin on uterine cyclic AMP levels (854). Moreover, the ability of relaxin to relax KCl-contracted uterine segments was reported to be potentiated by the presence of indomethacin in the organ bath (990).

Relaxin's Effects on the Endometrium

Rat

Isolated reports indicate that relaxin may have effects on the uterine endometrium in rats, but those effects remain poorly understood. In 1952 and 1960, Frieden and Velardo (358,359) reported that partially purified porcine relaxin inhibited deciduoma formation in ovariectomized pseudopregnant rats treated with progesterone; however, an effect on deciduoma formation was not confirmed when more highly purified porcine relaxin was used (1071,1075,1160). Nevertheless, studies conducted after 1980 indicate that relaxin may act directly on the rat endometrium and have profound effects on its growth and metabolism. There is limited evidence that the endometrium in rats contains relaxin receptors. Weiss and Bryant-Greenwood (1115) reported finite numbers of binding sites for radioiodinated porcine relaxin in the endometrium as well as the myometrium of gonadotropin-primed rats. Morphometric and histologic analyses of uterine tissue obtained from ovariectomized estrogen-primed rats demonstrated that highly purified porcine relaxin had a rapid effect on the endometrium. Vasilenko et al. (1073) reported that within 6 h of the administration of 100 μg porcine relaxin, there was a dramatic increase in the volume of both the endometrium and the myometrium; moreover, the collagen network became more loosely arranged and widely scattered, resulting in more intrafibrillar space in both uterine compartments. The physiologic significance of relaxin's putative effects on the growth and metabolism of the endometrium in pregnant rats during pregnancy is unknown. They may be important for uterine accommodation of the rapidly growing fetuses. Steinetz et al. (954) hypothesized that the fetal resorption that accompanies the administration of large doses of purified porcine relaxin during the peri-implantation period may be attributable, at least in part, to relaxin-induced disruption of endometrial function.

Rhesus Monkey

Early investigations with impure porcine relaxin indicated that relaxin may influence growth of the endometrium and differentiation of its vasculature in the rhesus monkey. In the 1960s, Hisaw and co-workers (243,463,464) conducted histologic studies of the influence of prolonged administration of estrogen, progesterone, and partially purified porcine relaxin on the endometrium of juvenile or ovariectomized rhesus monkeys. Growth of the endometrial stroma was reported to be maximal when the monkeys were treated with a combination of estrogen, progesterone, and relaxin (243,463). Relaxin appeared to intensify the differentiation of stromal cells into granulocytes that accumulated around the spiral arteries in the basal endometrium (243,464). Relaxin was also reported to stimulate proliferation of the endothelial cells located in the distal portions of the spiral arteries in a manner similar to the formation of sinus-like channels below an implanted embryo during early pregnancy in the rhesus monkey (243,464). This latter biologic effect of relaxin, called endothelioid cytomorphosis (464), led Dallenbach-Hellweg et al. (243) to hypothesize that one of the functions of relaxin during early pregnancy in primates is to assist in the preparation of the endometrial blood vessels for implantation and embryonic nourishment.

Human

Endometrial Stromal Cells. Extensive studies conducted since 1986 provide evidence that relaxin acts directly on the human endometrium. Tseng and coworkers demonstrated that highly purified porcine relaxin exerts a synergistic effect in the presence of the progestin medroxyprogesterone acetate on human endometrial stromal cells in primary culture. Prolactin production (83,486,834,1054,1165), prolactin mRNA production (1052), and both aromatase activity and production (485,1053) were increased in stromal cell cultures maintained from 5 to 40 days in the presence of both porcine relaxin and progestin. Production of prolactin was greater in primary cell cultures obtained during the secretory phase of the cycle than during the proliferative phase (1165) and production of prolactin (486) and aromatase activity (1053) were enhanced when estrogen was also placed in the medium. Also, porcine relaxin and progestin induced estrone sulfate sulfatase production (83) and morphologic changes (1165) in human endometrial cells maintained in culture. It was postulated that these hormone-induced events represent differentiation of the stromal cells into decidual cells and that the finding that relaxin synergizes with progestin to bring about this differentiation may have relevance to early pregnancy when both relaxin and progesterone are elevated (79,834).

Insulinlike growth factor-binding protein 1 (IGFBP-1) is the main soluble protein synthesized and secreted *in vitro* by decidualized explants of the gestational endometrium (80). Tseng and co-workers reported that progestin promotes the synthesis and secretion of IGFBP-1 by endometrial stromal cells obtained from cycling women after about 10 to 16 days in culture and that inclusion of porcine relaxin tended to increase and sustain IGFBP-1 (79) and IGFBP-1 mRNA (1052) synthesis. In endometrial stromal cells treated with progestin plus porcine relaxin, the concentration of phosphorylated IGFBP-1 was also reported to be elevated above controls (362). It was suggested that the influence of relaxin in combination with progestin on IGFBP-1 synthesis supports the view that relaxin may be a regulator of decidualization during early pregnancy (79). There is evidence that relaxin also stimulates fully differentiated decidual cells to produce and secrete IGFBP-1. Highly purified porcine relaxin stimulated in a time- and dose-dependent manner a 16-fold increase in the secretion of IGFBP-1 from human decidual cells after 120 h in culture. It appears relaxin stimulates IGFBP-1 production as well as secretion because relaxin's effects on IGFBP-1 secretion were blocked by the protein synthesis inhibitor cycloheximide (1042). Porcine relaxin has also been reported to increase the synthesis and secretion of prorenin from human decidual cells in culture (777) and superfused decidual tissue (776).

There is limited evidence that highly purified porcine relaxin promotes the synthesis and secretion of human relaxin from decidual cells obtained at term cesarean section, and it was suggested that human decidual relaxin may regulate its own secretion through an autocrine effect (456).

There may be differences among species in the regulation of endometrial cells in culture. Whereas progestin stimulated aromatase activity in rabbit endometrial stromal cells in culture, as it does in the human, porcine relaxin did not (1051). A second interpretation of this finding is that porcine relaxin is not active in the rabbit.

Endometrial Epithelial Cells. Human endometrial epithelial cells may also be target cells for relaxin. Porcine relaxin promoted a marked accumulation of cyclic AMP in human endometrial epithelial cells obtained during either the proliferative or secretory phase of the cycle when the cells were incubated for 30 min in the presence of a phosphodiesterase inhibitor (204).

Mechanism of Action of Relaxin on Endometrial Cells. Little is known concerning the mechanism whereby relaxin brings about effects on human endometrial cells in culture. Moreover, the few reports do not always differentiate between stromal and epithelial cells. Relaxin may increase intracellular levels of cyclic AMP. Whereas Tseng and co-workers (1053) initially reported that porcine relaxin had little or only a moderate effect on cyclic AMP levels in human endometrial stromal cells in culture, they later indicated that the addition of porcine relaxin to stromal cells results in a large increase in cyclic AMP (362). Consistent with the latter observation, Fei et al. (314) reported that human relaxin 2 caused a time- and dose-dependent stimulation of cyclic AMP in endometrial cells obtained from a premenopausal woman. Relaxin may also bring about its effects on human endometrial cells, at least in part, through activation of protein kinase C. Kalbag et al. (538) reported that treatment of secretory phase endometrial cells, but not proliferative phase endometrial cells, with synthetic human relaxin 2 caused a translocation of protein kinase C from cytosol to membranes.

Vagina

There are isolated reports that relaxin has effects on the vagina. Relaxin-containing extracts obtained from the serum of pregnant rabbits or ovaries of pregnant sows were reported to potentiate the action of estrogen in inducing vaginal cornification in mice and rats (258,428,866,1160). Also, crude preparations of porcine relaxin were reported to induce opening of the vaginal membrane in ovariectomized or hysterectomized guinea pigs (505,506). More recently, highly purified porcine relaxin was reported to stimulate within 6 h dose-dependent increases in wet weight, dry weight, percentage water content, total soluble protein, and total glycogen and glycogen concentration within vaginas removed from ovariectomized and estrogen-pretreated rats (1072).

Mammary Glands

Effects of Relaxin on Growth and Development of the Mammary Glands

The second biologic effect of relaxin to be reported was its putative growth-promoting effect on mammary glands. In 1945, Hamolsky and Sparrow (436) reported that, when administered together with estrogen and progesterone, a crude preparation of porcine relaxin promoted growth and lobulation of the mammary glands of ovariectomized immature rats beyond that obtained with steroids alone. Relaxin's effects on mammary gland growth and development were examined only sporadically from 1945 until the early 1980s. Most of this research, which used either examination of whole mounts of mammary glands or total DNA content as an index of mammary gland development in rats (448,935), guinea pigs (380), rabbits (380), and mice (1080,1081), supported the original findings of Hamolsky and Sparrow (436). Impure porcine relaxin was reported to be relatively ineffective by itself (448,1080,1081); in fact, its effects on growth of the mammary tissue were reported to be dependent on not only ovarian mammotropic steroids but also pituitary mammotropic hormones (436,935,1080) such as prolactin and growth hormone (449,450). Not all investigators, however, found that relaxin promoted growth of the mammary glands. In one study, multiple injections of crude porcine relaxin over a period of several days failed to promote alveolar growth in ovariectomized steroid-treated mice (1050), and in a second investigation, similar treatment reportedly inhibited mammary gland growth in ovariectomized goats (217).

The influence of partially purified porcine relaxin on mammary tumor induction in rats was examined before the mid-1980s. These early studies also produced seemingly contradictory results, which, although difficult to interpret, appear to support the view that relaxin influences mammary tissue. Cutts (240) reported that when rats bearing estrone-induced mammary tumors were administered crude porcine relaxin for a sustained period, both the growth and numbers of tumors increased markedly. Similarly, Plunkett and Gammal (773) found that crude porcine relaxin increased the induction of mammary tumors in rats when administered 6 weeks after carcinogen treatment. Paradoxically, these workers (773) reported that relaxin inhibited tumor induction when administration of the hormone was begun 1 week before carcinogen treatment. Segaloff (892) reported that prolonged administration of partially purified porcine relaxin initially accelerated and then diminished the rate of mammary tumor growth in intact or ovariectomized estrogen-primed rats. The influence of highly purified relaxin on mammary tumor growth has not been reported. Other findings from pathologic studies are consistent with the possibility that relaxin influences mammary gland growth and differentiation. A relaxin-like immunoactive substance was reportedly found in the mammary gland cyst fluid of women with fibrocystic disease using a homologous porcine relaxin radioimmunoassay (697).

Whereas collectively these early studies provided reason to suspect that relaxin influences growth and development of the mammary glands, findings were neither consistent nor definitive. Definitive conclusions were not possible because of the lack of purity of relaxin preparations, the use of porcine relaxin in a wide variety of species, and extensive variations in both the physiologic state of the animals and experimental protocols used. Since the mid-1980s, investigators have used highly purified porcine and rat relaxin preparations to provide strong evidence that relaxin has effects on mammary gland growth and development in at least three mammalian species—the mouse, pig, and rat.

Mouse

Bani, Bigazzi, and co-workers (64) examined the influence of highly purified porcine relaxin on the morphology of the mammary glands in intact (61) and ovariectomized (58,60,62,63,65,88) virgin female mice at both the light and electron microscope levels. Animal treatment followed closely that described for the mouse interpubic ligament bioassay (951,952) except that a control group was not pretreated with estrogen. Abdominal and inguinal mammary glands were removed 18 to 20 h after a single subcutaneous injection of 1 μg (3 GPU) porcine relaxin in the repository vehicle 1% benzopurpurine-4B. Relaxin had little or no effect in the absence of estrogen. When relaxin was administered to estrogen-pretreated mice, changes occurred in both the parenchyma and stroma. The changes in the parenchyma included elongation and branching of lactiferous ducts (61–63,65,88) and proliferation of both the epithelial cells that line the lumen of the ducts and the myoepithelial cells that lie between the inner epithelial cells and basement membrane (61–63). Relaxin-induced changes in the stroma included growth of both the blood capillary bed and fat-pad (61,65,88). Morphometric analysis of the mammary gland microvasculature indicated that relaxin induced striking dilatation of the lumen of arterioles, capillaries, and venules. Ultrastructural analysis revealed an increase in the pinocytotic vesicles in blood capillary endothelial cells that was interpreted to indicate that relaxin enhances transendothelial transport of substances. Relaxin-induced growth of the fat pad appeared to be due to both hypertrophy and hyperplasia of adipose cells (65,88). Bani and co-workers (60) also reported that porcine relaxin promotes lipid deposition in parametrial fat and postulated that relaxin may contribute to the deposition of lipid stores during pregnancy that are depleted during lactation.

Pig

Like cervical modifications, mammary lobuloalveolar tissue proliferation begins to occur rapidly about day 80 in primiparous pigs (550). Between days 80 and 110 of pregnancy, mammary parenchyma invades and largely replaces the fat pad (Fig. 63). Hurley et al. (493) demonstrated that relaxin plays a major role in promoting growth of mammary parenchymal tissue between day 80 and 110 of pregnancy. When gilts were bilaterally ovariectomized on day 100 and given progesterone only, development of the mammary parenchyma was markedly impaired. In contrast, the mammary parenchyma appeared as well developed as that in intact controls on day 110 of pregnancy when replacement therapy consisted of both progesterone and highly purified porcine relaxin (Fig 63). The striking effects of porcine relaxin on growth of mammary parenchymal tissue in pregnant pigs are consistent with the effects of porcine relaxin in nonpregnant estrogen-pretreated mice (61–63,65,88). The hormonal requirements for growth of the mammary gland parenchyma in gilts are not well understood. It seems likely relaxin acts in concert with estrogen, progesterone, glucocorticoids, pituitary mammotropins, insulin, and perhaps other hormones to bring about its effects. Buttle and Lin (164) reported that insulin, but not relaxin, promoted the incorporation of ^{3}H-thymidine into the DNA of mammary gland explants *in vitro*. It is possible that all

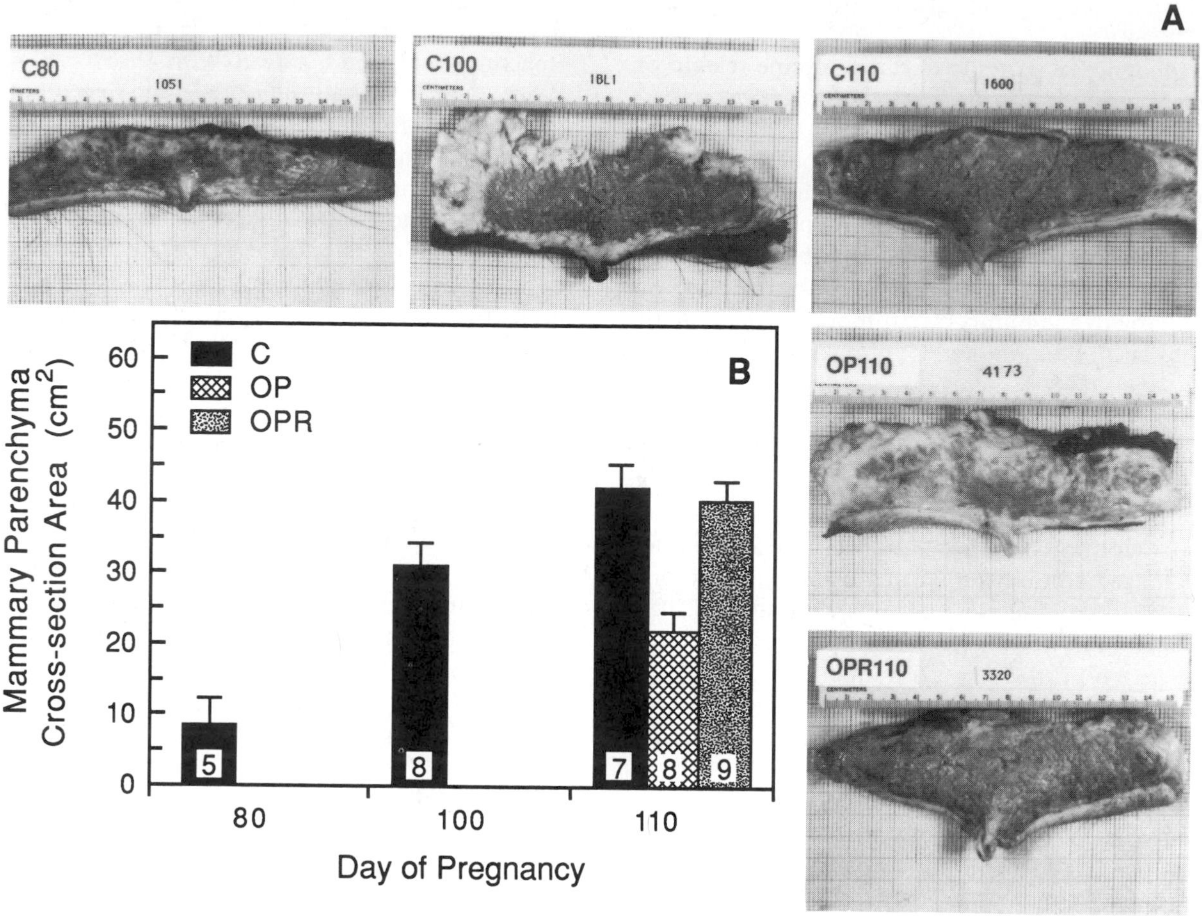

FIG. 63. **A:** Photographs of transverse cross sections of mammary glands from gilts during late gestation. Representative mammary glands are from intact control gilts on days 80 (*C80*), 100 (*C100*), and 110 (*C110*); ovariectomized progesterone-treated gilts on day 110 (*OP110*); and ovariectomized progesterone plus relaxin-treated gilts on day 110 (*OPR110*). Sham surgery or ovariectomy was performed on day 100 of gestation, and ovariectomized gilts were treated with either progesterone (50 mg/intramuscularly at 12-h intervals) or progesterone plus highly purified porcine relaxin (1 mg intramuscularly at 6-h intervals) from day 100 to day 110 of pregnancy. **B:** Mean cross-section areas (±SE) of mammary parenchymal tissue from the five groups of gilts in A. Number of animals is given at base of each bar. Modified from ref. 493.

components that synergize with relaxin to promote development of mammary parenchyma were not present in that *in vitro* experimental model.

Rat

Anderson and co-workers (1090,1140) conducted experiments with highly purified porcine relaxin in nonpregnant rats to obtain evidence that supports the view that relaxin promotes growth of mammary tissue. When porcine relaxin was administered to hypophysectomized immature rats in combination with ovarian and/or pituitary hormones known to contribute to mammary growth, it promoted growth of the mammary ducts, end buds, and lobule-alveoli (1140). Also, 10 days of administration of highly purified porcine relaxin promoted increased wet weight, dry fat-free tissue, total DNA, total RNA, total protein, and total collagen in ovariectomized rats (1090).

In 1991, Hwang et al. (494) demonstrated that endogenous relaxin is required for normal mammary development during the second half of pregnancy in rats. When rat relaxin was neutralized by daily administration of monoclonal antibody MCA1 for rat relaxin throughout the second half of pregnancy, the mammary glands of MCA1-treated rats on day 22 of pregnancy weighed the same as those in controls. Surprisingly, however, the mammary nipples in MCA1-treated rats were strikingly smaller than in controls (Figs. 64 and 65A and B). Whereas neutralization of endogenous relaxin with MCA1 throughout the second half of pregnancy does not influence the wet weight of the mammary glands, it does influence the histologic characteristics of both the

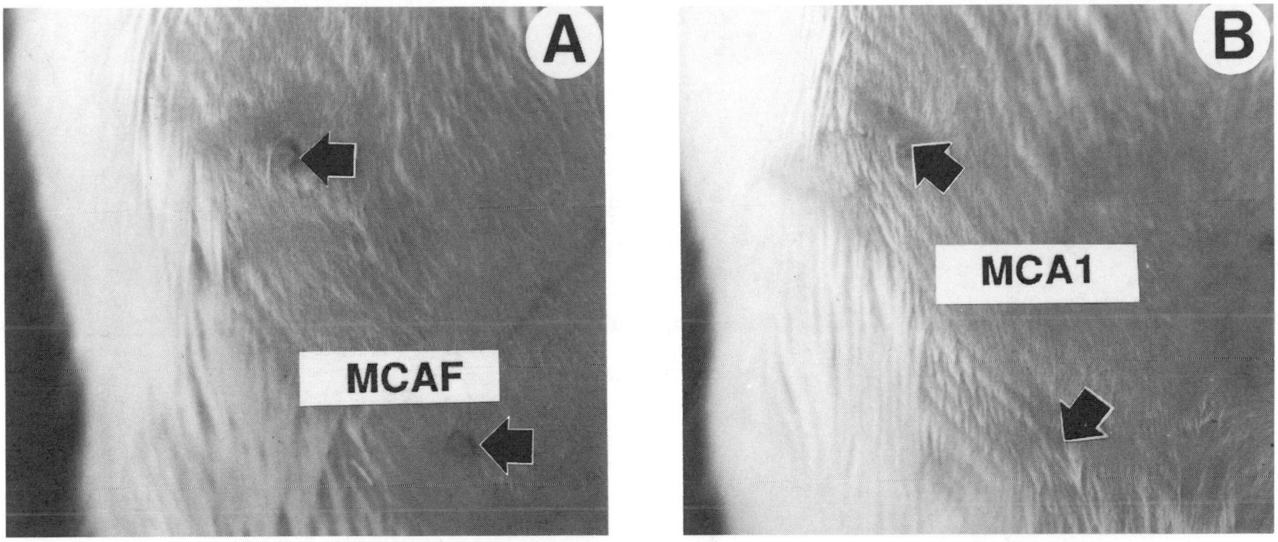

FIG. 64. Influence of neutralization of endogenous relaxin throughout second half of pregnancy on mammary nipple development in rats. Photographs of representative abdominal and first inguinal mammary nipples on day 22 of pregnancy in rats treated with control monoclonal antibody MCAF for fluorescein (**A**) and monoclonal antibody MCA1 for rat relaxin (**B**). From ref. 581, with permission.

mammary glands and nipples (494,581). Moreover, the effects of endogenous relaxin on the histologic characteristics of both components of the mammary apparatus are similar to relaxin's effects on the histologic characteristics of the cervix described previously (Fig. 53). In both the mammary glands and nipples of MCA1-treated rats, collagen fiber bundles were more compact and elastin fibers were longer than in controls (Fig. 65C and D). Also, in mammary nipples the cross-sectional areas of the blood vessels in MCA1-treated rats were smaller than in controls (581).

Mechanism of Action of Relaxin on the Mammary Glands

The mechanism(s) whereby relaxin promotes growth and differentiation of the mammary glands and/or mammary nipples is not known. It may do so through direct effects on connective tissue remodeling. Fibroblasts obtained from rat mammary glands during late pregnancy were reported to contain sites that bound radioiodinated porcine relaxin (690). Also, it was reported that when fibroblasts obtained from postpubertal guinea pig mammary glands were grown in culture for 2 days with estrogen and/or highly purified porcine relaxin, both hormones (individually and in combination) promoted synthesis of DNA and RNA beyond that achieved in controls (903). The nature of the proteins synthesized by the guinea pig mammary gland fibroblasts in response to relaxin treatment is unknown. It was reported that estrogen promoted the synthesis of both collagen and noncollagen protein, whereas relaxin had no apparent effect on collagen synthesis and decreased noncollagenous protein synthesis (904). The observation that highly purified porcine relaxin had a direct effect on proliferation of the human breast adenocarcinoma cell line MCF-7 (91) is also consistent with the view that mammary tissue contains relaxin receptors.

Effects of Relaxin on the Function of the Mammary Glands

Relaxin-dependent development of the mammary apparatus is required for normal postpartum lactational performance in rats. The mean pup weight and number of live pups declined markedly during days 1 to 5 of fosterage when pups born of untreated donor rats were fostered to rats that were relaxin-deficient throughout the second half of pregnancy (494). Nipples were extremely small when endogenous relaxin was neutralized with monoclonal antibody MCA1 for rat relaxin throughout the second half of pregnancy (494,581) (Fig. 64). Lactational failure in these animals was found to be attributable to the inability of the pups to attach to the nipple, stimulate prolactin release, and obtain milk from the dams (494,581). It remains to be demonstrated that endogenous relaxin's mammotropic effects during the second half of pregnancy are required for normal lactational performance in pigs or other species.

Unlike prolactin, relaxin does not appear to be a lactogenic hormone (64). Sporadic early reports that used crude relaxin preparations suggested that extended treatment over several days with relaxin diminishes lactational capacity. Prolonged treatment with porcine re-

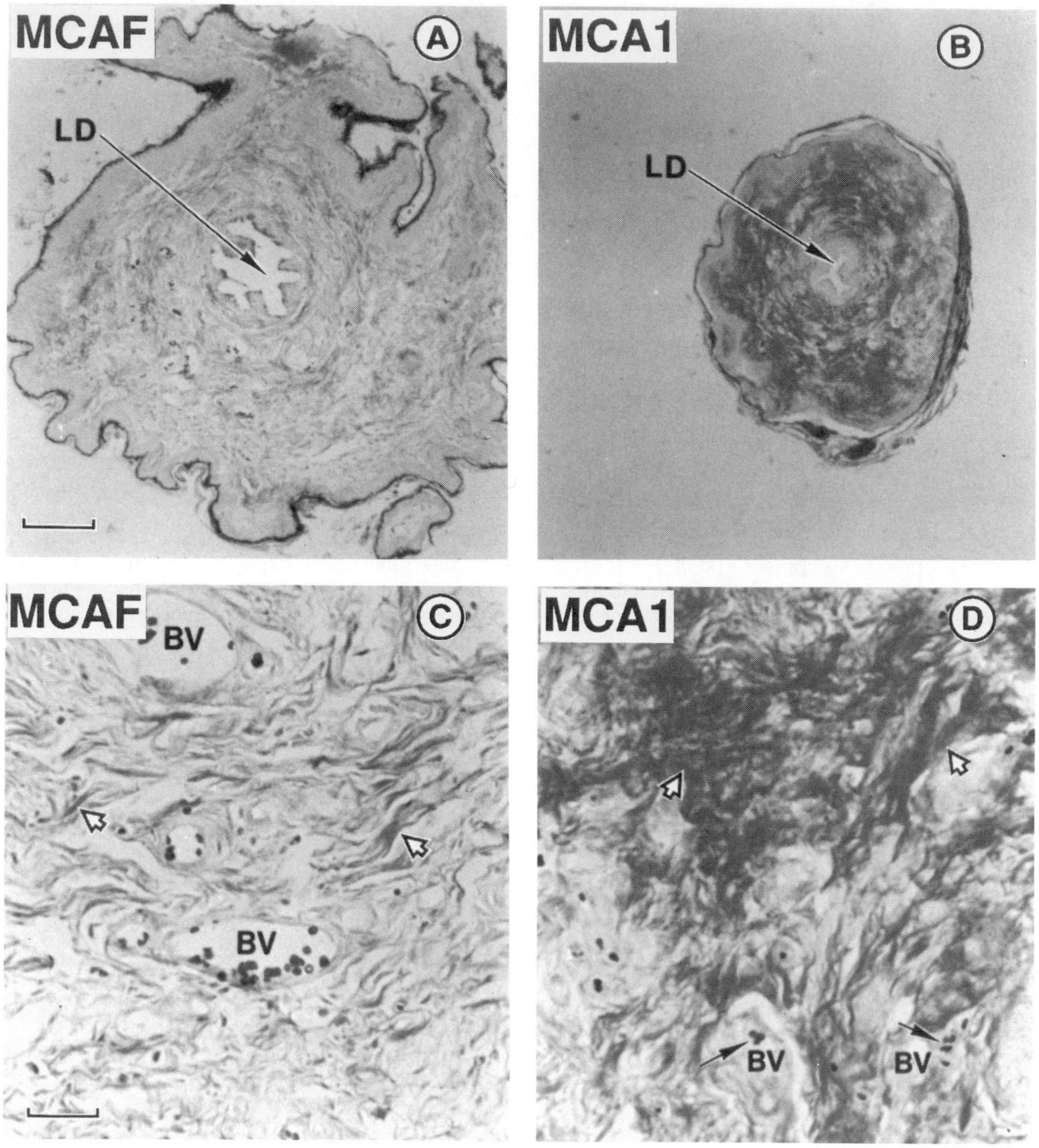

FIG. 65. Photomicrographs of representative cross sections of abdominal nipples obtained on day 22 of pregnancy from monoclonal antibody for fluorescein (*MCAF;* **A, C**) and monoclonal antibody for rat relaxin (*MCA1;* **B, D**) treated rats. Tissue sections were stained with Gomori's trichrome stain to visualize collagen and amorphous ground substance. *LD,* lactiferous duct; *BV,* blood vessel; *white arrows,* collagen fiber bundles. Bar in A = 270 μm. A and B are the same magnification. Bar in C = 54 μm. C and D are the same magnification. From ref. 581, with permission.

laxin, administered in combination with ovarian steroids, reduced milk yield in ovariectomized goats (217) and depressed both milk yield and litter weights in ovariectomized rats (559). Also, porcine relaxin was reported to reduce nursing capabilities and litter survival to weaning when administered for an extended period during late pregnancy in both intact and luteectomized pigs (551). Cowie et al. (217) attributed the reduced milk secretion to a deficiency in growth of alveolar tissue in relaxin-treated goats.

Relaxin may influence milk ejection, but the limited experimentation, diversity of experimental conditions, and inconsistency of results preclude firm conclusions. In 1954, Shaffhausen et al. (901) reported that intravenous injection of a crude porcine relaxin preparation *increased* milk ejection in lactating ewes. Grosvenor and Turner (414) shortly thereafter reported that intravenous injection of impure porcine relaxin was *without effect* on milk ejection in lactating rats. Knox and Griffith (559) suggested that the reduced milk secretion they observed in rats may be attributable to *interference* with milk ejection, because the mammary glands contained a copious amount of milk after the nursing period, and exogenous oxytocin had no influence on milk removal. Consistent with the latter mechanism, Summerlee et al. (1007) reported that highly purified porcine relaxin inhibited reflex milk ejection in lactating rats. Moreover, Summerlee and co-workers (529,726,727,729,1007) reported that relaxin appeared to inhibit reflex milk ejection through a dual mechanism—that is, by acting centrally to reduce the release of oxytocin through a direct effect on the brain and by acting peripherally to inhibit the influence of oxytocin on the myoepithelial cells of the mammary gland. Relaxin does not appear to influence milk ejection in the pig. Porter and co-workers (793,844) found that highly purified porcine relaxin did not affect the output of oxytocin from the porcine neural lobe *in vitro* or in lactating sows *in vivo.* Furthermore, these workers reported that neither poor lactational performance nor hypogalactia were associated with inappropriate plasma relaxin levels during early lactation (791).

Crop Sac

The crop sac of the columbine birds—pigeons and doves—is functionally analogous to the mammary gland and hormone responsive. Prolactin, which stimulates mammalian milk secretion, acts directly on the pigeon crop sac to produce crop milk. After local intradermal injection of prolactin, the lateral lobes of the crop sac undergo enlargement, thickening of the mucosa, and increased vascularization, accompanied by desquamation of lipid-laden superficial cells of the lining epithelium. The production of crop "milk" occurs in both parents, and the young are fed through a process of regurgitation (69,585). The local injection of prolactin into the crop sac is a sensitive and repeatable bioassay for prolactin (703).

Beginning in 1987, Bani, Bigazzi, and co-workers (57,59,64,89,90) examined the influence of a single intradermal injection of 1 μg highly purified porcine relaxin into the pigeon (*Columba livia*) crop sac. Six hours after injection, 3-cm disks of crop sac mucosa were resected around the site of injection. Highly purified porcine relaxin caused a significant dose-related increase in wet and dry weight of the crop sac, ^{3}H-thymidine and ^{3}H-uridine uptake of the mucosa, and DNA content of the mucosal epithelium.

Thickening of the crop sac mucosa with formation of convoluted ridges visible on macroscopic examination occurred after relaxin treatment. Histologically, the squamous epithelium of the crop sac mucosa became deeply folded, and pegs and down growths from the basal layer invaded the underlying connective tissue (Fig. 66A and B). Many mitoses occurred in the basal cells and empty spaces appeared between the outer layers of the epithelium (57,59,90). Relaxin produced an enlargement of the blood capillaries in the crop sac mucosa (89) (Fig. 66C and D). Relaxin was found to have a greater effect than prolactin on the growth of the crop sac in short exposure times, whereas prolactin had a greater effect in long exposure times (57). The ability of relaxin to influence crop sac cells directly was further shown by demonstrating a dose-dependent mitogenic effect of porcine relaxin on crop cells in culture (121). The finding that relaxin has marked local effects on the crop sac in the pigeon provides the first evidence of a direct mammotropic effect of relaxin. Furthermore, these findings, by providing evidence that the crop sac in columbine birds contains functional relaxin receptors, raise the possibility of a physiologic role of relaxin in birds.

There is disagreement concerning the effects of relaxin alone on the pigeon crop sac. Anderson et al. (33,34) reported that the local administration of highly purified porcine relaxin alone to the crop sac of pigeons over a 2-day treatment period had no effect on growth of mucosal epithelial cells but that porcine relaxin caused a striking augmentation of the prolactin response.

Local Effects on the Female Reproductive System

The identification of relaxin production in developing ovarian follicles in cycling pigs and rats, endometrium in pregnant pigs, rats, and humans, and mammary glands in guinea pigs and humans led to postulations that relaxin may contribute to the regulation of reproductive processes through local control (42,43,139,140, 142,631).

Intraovarian Effects of Relaxin

It will be recalled that relaxin is produced in preovulatory follicles of the pig (143,659) and rat (233,926) and that the theca interna is the site of relaxin production in the preovulatory follicle of the pig (47,49,50,311). In view of relaxin's well-established effects on collagen remodeling in the interpubic ligament and uterine cervix, it was postulated that follicular connective tissue may be a target tissue for the biologic actions of relaxin (138). Consistent with this possibility, Bryant-Greenwood and co-workers (138,1044,1046) obtained evidence that relaxin influences the activity of three enzymes that may contribute to ovarian connective tissue remodeling during follicular development and/or ovulation—plasminogen activator (PA), collagenase, and proteoglycanase. Plasminogen activator is a protease that catalyzes conversion of plasminogen to plasmin, and the plasmin in turn activates latent collagenase and thereby promotes

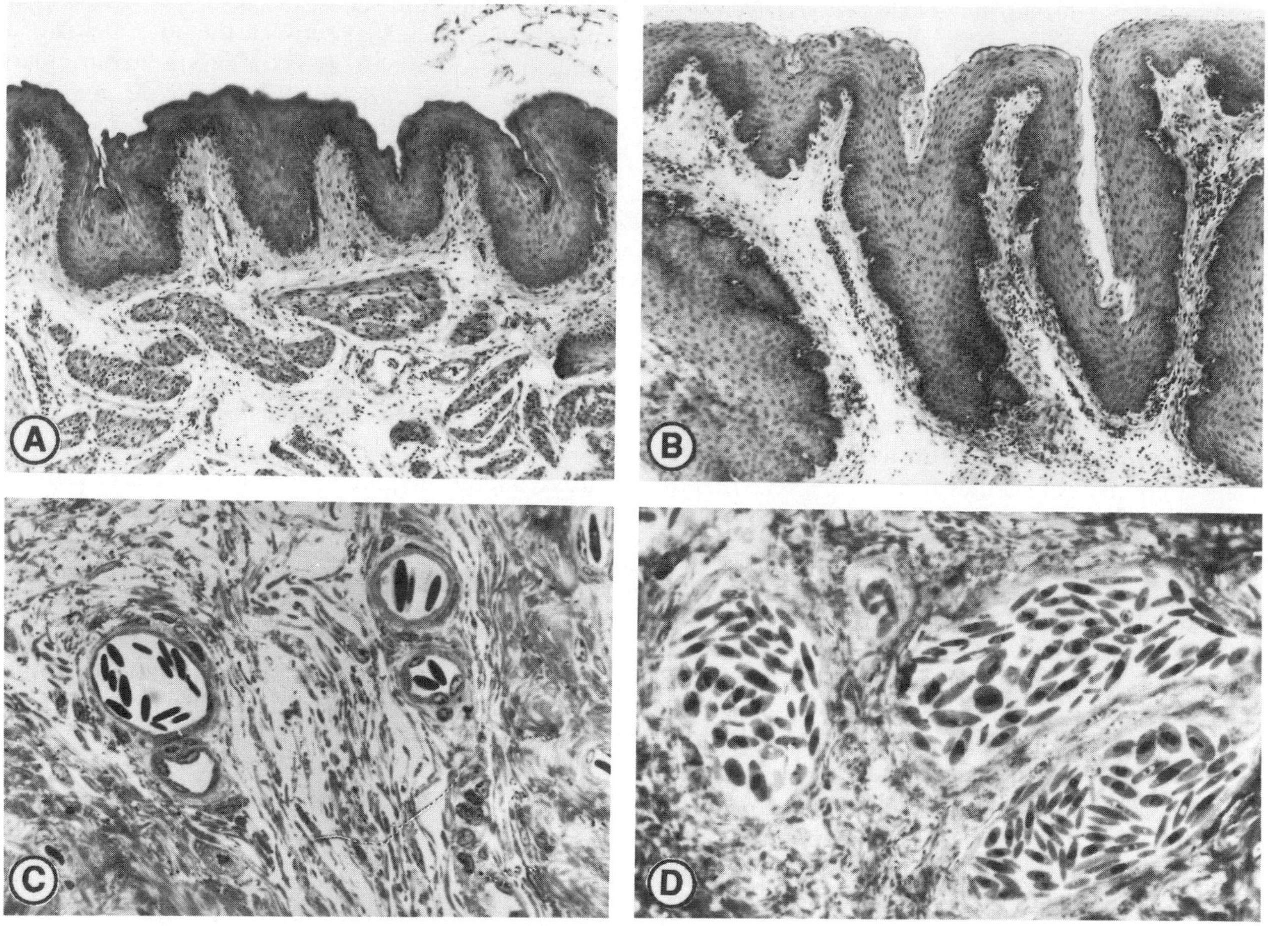

FIG. 66. Photomicrographs of hemicrops from pigeons. **A:** Untreated hemicrop. Epithelium forms short folds and its junction with lamina propria is linear. (×130) **B:** Relaxin-treated hemicrop. Note increased length of epithelial folds and presence of down growths into lamina propria. (×130) A and B were stained with hematoxylin and eosin. **C:** Untreated hemicrop. Blood capillaries in lamina propria. (×800) **D:** Relaxin-treated hemicrop. Striking enlargement of blood capillaries, which are now filled with erythrocytes. (×800) C and D were stained with toluidine blue-Na tetraborate. Modified from ref. 59.

collagen breakdown. Both plasmin and proteoglycanase degrade proteoglycans. It is known that ovarian PA activity is, at least in part, regulated by the gonadotropins that are required for follicular development and ovulation. In the rat ovary, as in other mammalian tissues, there are two types of PA, designated u-PA and t-PA, and it was reported that ovarian u-PA and t-PA activities are stimulated *in vitro* by LH and FSH, respectively (174,717). Relaxin may also promote one or both of these forms of PA in cycling rats. Highly purified porçine relaxin promoted PA, as well as collagenase, and proteoglycanase activities *in vitro* when added to granulosa cells obtained from gonadotropin-primed rats (Fig. 67). Relaxin-stimulated PA activity was maximal when granulosa cells obtained from preantral and antral follicles rather than preovulatory follicles were used (46,1044,1046); therefore, it was postulated that relaxin's main paracrine function may be associated with connective tissue remodeling of the follicular wall and surrounding stroma as the antrum forms and the follicle enlarges rather than with follicular rupture (46,138,1044). There is limited evidence that porcine relaxin also influences enzymes associated with remodeling in rabbit, pig, and human ovarian tissue. Porcine relaxin increased t-PA immunostaining in primary cultures of rabbit ovarian granulosa cells and ovarian surface epithelium (772). Whereas porcine relaxin alone had no effect on plasminogen activator activity in porcine granulosa cells in culture, it enhanced FSH-stimulated plasminogen activity (42). Collagenase activity was reported to be elevated in tissue pieces from the wall (tunica albuginea with adjacent theca externa) of human follicles after 4-h incubation in the presence of porcine relaxin (714). There is also limited evidence that porcine relaxin may contribute to granulosa cell and theca cell growth during porcine follicular development (1163). Evidence for relaxin receptors in ovarian tissue is largely inferred from responses of granulosa and/or theca cells to relaxin *in vitro*. An iso-

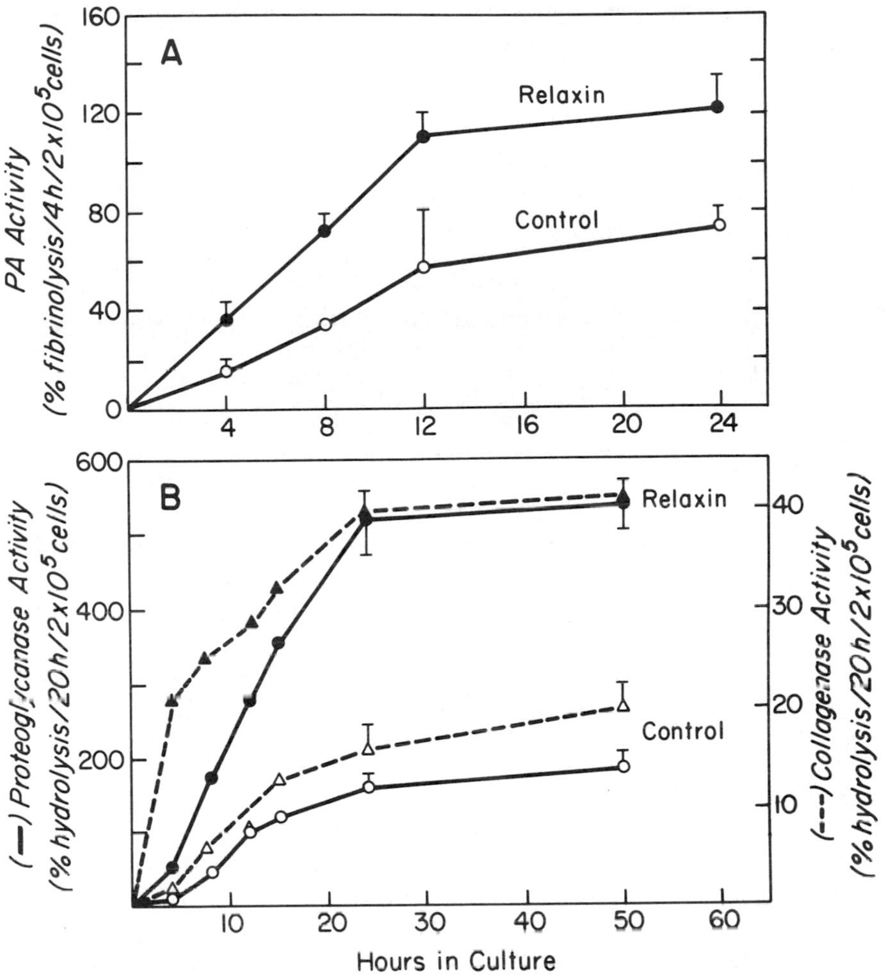

FIG. 67. Influence of relaxin on the secretion of plasminogen activator (*PA*) activity, proteoglycanase activity, and collagenase activity from rat granulosa cells *in vitro.* Immature rats were primed with 5 IU of pregnant mare serum gonadotropin, and granulosa cells were harvested 48 h later and treated with highly purified porcine relaxin (5 μg/ml) or left untreated. **A:** PA activity in the medium is shown as the mean of cumulative activities (+SD; $n = 3$). **B:** Proteoglycanase and collagenase activities in the medium are shown as the mean of cumulative activities (+SD; $n = 4$). From ref. 1044, with permission.

lated report localized specific binding sites for radioiodinated porcine relaxin in the ovary of prepubertal mice where the putative relaxin receptors appeared to be confined to the theca layer (1143).

It is also possible that relaxin has autocrine effects on luteal function in species that produce relaxin within the corpus luteum. The limited research that examined the influence of relaxin on luteal function generally determined its effects on progesterone secretion. *In vivo* studies in cattle indicated that during late pregnancy, highly purified porcine relaxin has a biphasic effect on progesterone secretion. Intravenous infusion of relaxin in low dosages (i.e., <500 μg/h) was associated with greater peripheral blood concentrations of progesterone, whereas high dosages (i.e., >600 μg/h) or intramuscular injections of 1 or 2 mg of relaxin resulted in an acute decrease in progesterone secretion (676,681,934). The influence of porcine relaxin on bovine luteal cells obtained from cattle during late pregnancy was also studied *in vitro.* It was reported that porcine relaxin induced a dose- and time-dependent increase in progesterone levels (678) after 24 or 48 h of cell culture. An effect of relaxin on progesterone secretion was not found after culture of human luteinizing granulosa cells with human relaxin 2 (411). Oxytocin is also produced by bovine luteal cells (322), and Musah et al. (679) obtained evidence that relaxin may regulate the release of oxytocin from luteal cells. Porcine relaxin suppressed both basal- and PG-induced release of oxytocin when bovine luteal cells obtained at different stages of pregnancy were incubated 2 to 4 days in culture.

Intrauterine Effects of Relaxin at Parturition in the Human

The localization of relaxin within human decidual and placental tissue during late pregnancy (92,96,145, 203,334,560,847,1142,1144,1146) stimulated interest in its possible function. Bryant-Greenwood and co-workers (561,563) obtained evidence that relaxin may act directly to influence connective tissue remodeling in human fetal membranes. They reported that the secretion of plasminogen activator and collagenase into the medium increased when highly purified porcine relaxin was added to cultures of human amnion and chorion cells that were dispersed from placentas obtained at elective cesarean section (561,563) (Fig. 68). Also, porcine relaxin influenced PGE production by human amnion *in vitro* (627). Also, particulate fractions from the amnion and chorion contained high-affinity sites that bound radiolabeled porcine relaxin with considerable specificity (561). Bryant-Greenwood and co-workers (139,140,142, 560–562) postulated that the human decidual and placental relaxin may have autocrine and/or paracrine roles that contribute to connective tissue remodeling in fetal membranes during the last weeks of pregnancy and at birth.

Central Effects

In 1984, Summerlee et al. (1007) reported that relaxin may act within the central nervous system to control oxytocin secretion in female rats. That finding motivated Summerlee and others to conduct subsequent studies that collectively support the possibility that relaxin has several effects on the central nervous system. There is limited evidence that peripherally circulating relaxin enters the cerebrospinal fluid in rats (756), and therefore production of relaxin within the brain may not be required for the hormone to have central effects. Also, specific binding of ^{125}I-labeled porcine relaxin was observed in crude membrane preparations of mouse brain (1143), and relaxin binding sites were identified by autoradiographic localization of bioactive ^{32}P-labeled human relaxin in several anatomic regions within the rat brain (744). Although it remains to be established that endogenous relaxin has physiologic effects on the central nervous system, there is evidence that relaxin may regulate the secretion of hormones from the posterior pituitary, the secretion of hormones from the anterior pituitary, and water intake.

Effects of Relaxin on Secretion of Hormones from the Posterior Pituitary

Oxytocin

Oxytocin Secretion in Rats. Summerlee and co-workers reported that either systemic or central administration of porcine relaxin suppresses reflex-stimulated or electrically stimulated milk ejection (301,525,529,726, 727,1006,1007,1128) and prolongs gestation and labor by acting centrally to suppress oxytocin secretion (526, 527). These workers' conclusion that relaxin acts centrally to inhibit oxytocin secretion was based on three primary observations. First, it was thought likely that the relaxin-induced block in reflex intramammary pressure cycles was attributable, at least in part, to inhibition of the release of oxytocin rather than to inhibition of oxytocin's effects on mammary myoepithelial cells because exogenously administered oxytocin produced intramammary pressure cycles in relaxin-treated rats (726, 727,1006,1007). Second, intravenous administration of porcine relaxin inhibited oxytocin release evoked by electrical stimulation of the neurohypophysis *in vivo* (729). Third, plasma oxytocin levels were reported to be lower than controls during delivery in rats infused with porcine relaxin (527) and to rise significantly within 30 min of stopping a 3-day infusion of porcine relaxin during lactation (529). Furthermore, Jones and Summerlee claimed, as an unpublished observation, that electrical activity of oxytocin neurons was suppressed after intravenous administration of porcine relaxin (527,1006).

The site(s) within the brain that mediates relaxin's putative suppressive effects on oxytocin secretion is not

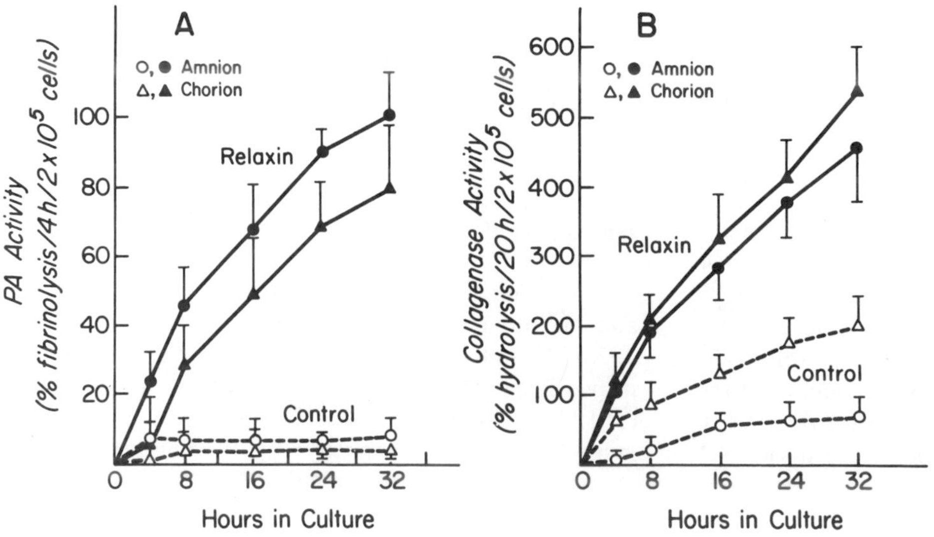

FIG. 68. A: Pattern of accumulation of plasminogen activator (*PA*) activity in serum-free culture medium bathing amnion cells or chorion cells treated with highly purified porcine relaxin (10 μg/ml) or untreated over a 32-h period. Values are the mean of cumulative activities (±SD; *n* = 3). **B:** Pattern of accumulation of total collagenase (latent plus active) in serum-free culture medium bathing amnion cells or chorion cells treated with highly purified porcine relaxin (10 μg/ml) or untreated over a 32-h period. Values are the mean of cumulative activities (±SD; *n* = 3). From ref. 563, with permission.

known with certainty. The subfornical organ, one of the so-called circumventricular organs, is located in the roof of the third ventricle at the interface between the blood, brain, and cerebrospinal fluid. This organ has many fenestrated capillaries that allow movement of circulating molecules between the blood and brain, and it is thought to be an important site for haemo–neural interaction (115). Three lines of evidence indicate that relaxin may mediate its effects on oxytocin secretion, at least in part, through the subfornical organ. First, injection of porcine relaxin into the third ventricle inhibited the pattern of reflex milk ejection to suckling young more profoundly than injection into other sites in the cerebroventricular system (727). Second, lesions of the subfornical organ completely negated the suppressive effects of centrally or peripherally administered porcine relaxin on reflex milk ejection in rats (1006). Third, Osheroff and Phillips (744) localized relaxin binding sites in the subfornical organ and other circumventricular organs.

In vivo experiments conducted to determine the influence of porcine relaxin on oxytocin secretion in the rat are not in total agreement. In agreement with Summerlee and co-workers (726,727,1006,1007), Way and Leng (1103) found that porcine relaxin inhibited reflex milk ejection in lactating rats, but the latter workers (1103) reported that porcine relaxin *increased* both plasma oxytocin concentrations and the firing rate of oxytocin neurons in the supraoptic nucleus of the hypothalamus in ovariectomized and lactating rats.

In vitro studies to determine if relaxin acts directly on the posterior pituitary to influence oxytocin release are also not in agreement. Dayanithi et al. (246) reported that porcine relaxin *inhibited* the release of oxytocin from both isolated neural lobes and isolated neurosecretory nerve endings of the neurohypophysis of male rats. In contrast, these workers (246) found that porcine relaxin *potentiated* potassium-stimulated release of oxytocin from both the isolated nerve endings and neural lobes. O'Byrne et al. (726) reported that porcine relaxin *failed to inhibit* the release of oxytocin from electrically stimulated rat posterior pituitary lobes *in vitro.*

The mechanism whereby relaxin influences oxytocin secretion is not known. Summerlee and co-workers obtained evidence that endogenous opioids may mediate relaxin's putative effects on oxytocin secretion in rats. Pretreatment with the opioid antagonist naloxone negated relaxin's inhibitory effects on both reflex-stimulated and electrically stimulated milk ejection (529,726–728) and delivery (527). The origin(s) of the opioids is not known with certainty, but there is evidence that they are not produced locally within the posterior pituitary (246,726) and that they may originate in the adrenals (301,726). In contrast to these findings, Way and Leng (1103) reported that the effect of intravenously administered porcine relaxin on the firing rate of supraoptic neurons was not influenced by the opioid antagonist naloxone in lactating rats. Dayanithi et al. (246) reported that the direct effects of relaxin on rat posterior pituitary neurosecretosomes *in vitro* are attributable to interference with Ca^{2+} entry preceding the release of oxytocin. The type of Ca^{2+} channel(s) inhibited by relaxin is not known, but studies with isolated rat neurosecretory nerve terminals from the rat posterior pituitary indicate relaxin's actions do not include direct effects on Ca^{2+} influx mediated by voltage-sensitive L-type Ca^{2+} channels or mobilization of Ca^{2+} from intraterminal stores (1000).

Putative Physiologic Significance of Relaxin's Effects on Oxytocin Secretion in Rats. It has been postulated that under normal physiologic conditions, endogenous relaxin may influence the time of onset of delivery and/or progress of labor by inhibiting oxytocin secretion from the posterior pituitary prepartum (526,527,1004, 1007). There is evidence that does not support this hypothesis. Passive neutralization of endogenous relaxin with monoclonal antibody MCA1 for rat relaxin either throughout the second half of pregnancy (587) or during the antepartum period (495) did not influence the time of onset of labor.

Oxytocin Secretion in Species Other than Rats. The possible central effects of relaxin on oxytocin secretion in species other than rats have received little experimental attention. Porcine relaxin did not affect oxytocin release from either porcine neurosecretosomes or porcine neural lobes *in vitro* (793). Moreover, administration of porcine relaxin 6–10 days postpartum immediately before a suckling episode did not affect the plasma oxytocin profile in lactating sows (793). Anderson and co-workers reported that the administration of large doses of porcine relaxin to beef heifers during late pregnancy provoked acute release of oxytocin (677), but it was not determined if the source of the oxytocin was the corpus luteum or posterior pituitary. It seems unlikely relaxin induced oxytocin secretion from the corpus luteum since these workers (679) reported that relaxin suppressed oxytocin secretion from bovine luteal cells *in vitro.*

Vasopressin

Influence of Relaxin on Vasopressin Secretion and Blood Pressure in Nonpregnant Rats. It was reported that acute administration of porcine relaxin, either intravenously (528,755,757,1103) or within the third or a lateral cerebral ventricle (672,757) increased plasma vasopressin levels (528,672,1103) and caused a prolonged increase in systemic arterial blood pressure (528,672, 755,757) in urethane-anesthetized nonpregnant rats. Two lines of evidence indicate that the pressor effects of intravenously administered porcine relaxin are mediated predominantly by the release of vasopressin. Parry and co-workers reported that pretreatment with a specific vasopressin (V1) receptor antagonist before porcine relaxin treatment nearly completely blocked the pressor effects of relaxin (755,757). Also, acute administration of porcine relaxin was reported to increase the firing rate of vasopressin neurons (524,1103).

Two central locations have been implicated as sites for relaxin's pressor effects. Relaxin may promote the secretion of vasopressin, at least in part, through a direct effect on the neurohypophysis. Dayanithi et al. (246) reported that porcine relaxin enhanced the release of vasopressin from electrically stimulated neural lobes and potassium-depolarized neural lobe neurosecretosomes obtained from male rats *in vitro.* O'Byrne et al. (726), however, failed to detect relaxin-induced release of vasopressin from electrically stimulated neural lobes obtained from lactating rats *in vitro.* Relaxin also binds directly to two circumventricular organs (subfornical organ and organum vasculosum of the lamina terminalis) that are known to be involved with the control of blood pressure (744). Relaxin may bind directly to these circumventricular organs to promote the release of vasopressin. Lesion of the subfornical organ negated the pressor effect of relaxin injected into the dorsal region of the third ventricle (672). The pressor effect of relaxin appears to be mediated, at least in part, by the brain angiotensin system. Continuous infusion of an angiotensin II receptor antagonist into the left lateral cerebral ventricle almost completely blocked the pressor response to intracerebroventricular injection of porcine relaxin and partially blocked the pressor response to intravenous injection of relaxin (757).

There is not total agreement concerning the influence of relaxin on blood pressure in nonpregnant rats. Porter et al. (789) reported that acute administration of impure porcine relaxin into sodium pentobarbitone-anesthetized ovariectomized rats did not influence carotid arterial pressure. Consistent with this finding, Ward et al. (1096) reported that subcutaneous infusion of synthetic human relaxin 2 over a 14-day period in quantities sufficient to produce circulating blood levels ranging from 4 to 8 ng/ml did not influence mean arterial pressure in either normotensive or spontaneously hypertensive nonpregnant adult female rats. St-Louis, Massicotte, and co-workers reported that infusion of highly purified rat relaxin into virgin spontaneously hypertensive rats for 2 days (657) or 6 days (991) caused a decline in arterial blood pressure, whereas the same treatment in normotensive nonpregnant rats was without effect (991). A subsequent investigation of the mechanism whereby relaxin reduces blood pressure in spontaneously hypertensive nonpregnant rats provided evidence that relaxin blunts the vascular response of the mesenteric vasculature to vasoconstrictor agents (657).

Influence of Relaxin on Blood Pressure and Vasopressin Secretion in Pregnant Rats. Total peripheral vascular resistance and blood pressure decrease during pregnancy in rats. During the 2 or 3 days that precede delivery, there is a rapid decline in arterial blood pressure in both spontaneously hypertensive and normotensive rats (13,991). Because a surge in relaxin occurs during this antepartum period (912), it was postulated that relaxin might contribute to the decline in arterial blood pressure that occurs near term (13). This does not appear to be the case. Ahokas et al. (13) reported that both a decrease in vascular reactivity to angiotensin II and a fall in blood pressure occurred near term in rats in which the ovaries were removed on day 13 of pregnancy, and therefore concluded that endogenous relaxin does not cause vasodilation or decreased sensitivity to angiotensin II during rat pregnancy. Consistent with this finding, Ward et al. (1095) found that intravenous administration of synthetic human relaxin 2 to unanesthetized rats on day 19 of pregnancy had no effect on arterial blood pressure or plasma vasopressin concentrations. Thus, the limited data available indicate relaxin probably does not play a major role in the pregnancy-induced decline in blood pressure.

Effects of Relaxin on Secretion of Hormones from the Anterior Pituitary

Relaxin may have direct effects on the anterior pituitary. A brief report indicated that administration of porcine relaxin for 20 days increased pituitary weights in intact (but not ovariectomized) female rats (1089). Cronin and co-workers (234,235) reported that human relaxin 2 stimulates increased cyclic AMP in cultured rat anterior pituitary cells in a dose-dependent manner. This response was specific for relaxin, more pronounced in anterior pituitary cells obtained from female than male rats, and inhibited by dopamine and somatostatin, the predominant hypothalamic inhibitors of prolactin and growth hormone secretion, respectively (234). These findings stimulated subsequent efforts to determine if relaxin influences the secretion of prolactin, growth hormone, and LH.

Prolactin

Sortino et al. (943) reported that human relaxin 2 stimulated the release of prolactin *in vitro* from enzymatically dispersed anterior pituitary cells obtained from cycling rats and that dopamine suppressed the stimulatory action of relaxin on prolactin release. Consistent with this finding, intravenous infusion of human relaxin 2 into rhesus monkeys provoked the release of prolactin during both the midluteal phase of the cycle and the period from day 120 to day 140 of pregnancy (87). Also, intracerebroventricular administration of porcine relaxin on days 111 and 113 of gestation in pigs was reported to cause an increase in prolactin secretion (617). Inconsistent with these findings, a brief report indicated that porcine relaxin and human relaxin 2 failed to stimulate prolactin secretion in both rat anterior pituitary cell cultures and intact adult female rats (850).

Growth Hormone

Two reports are consistent with the possibility that relaxin promotes growth hormone secretion. It was reported that growth hormone levels in the peripheral blood increased markedly when human relaxin 2 was infused into rhesus monkeys during the midluteal phase of the menstrual cycle (87). Also, growth hormone levels were reported to be lower than in controls in pregnant women who lacked a corpus luteum of pregnancy and had undetectable peripheral plasma relaxin levels (303). Inconsistent with these findings, a brief report indicated that human relaxin did not induce growth hormone secretion in cycling rats (850).

Luteinizing Hormone

Summerlee et al. (1005) reported that acute intravenous administration of porcine relaxin reduced mean plasma LH levels and the frequency of LH pulses in ovariectomized rats; whereas the same treatment promoted the secretion of LH in ovariectomized rats pretreated with both estrogen and progesterone. The effects of relaxin were blocked when the central angiotensin system was compromised with an angiotensin II receptor antagonist, thus indicating that relaxin's influence on LH secretion may be mediated through the central angiotensin II system (1005). In contrast to this finding, human relaxin 2 failed to influence LH secretion in cycling rats (850), in midluteal phase monkeys (87), or from female rat pituitary cells in culture (943).

Effects of Relaxin on Drinking

Robertson and Summerlee (827) reported that central administration of as little as 10 ng porcine relaxin into the left lateral cerebral ventricle in conscious unrestrained female rats induced a significant increase in water intake. Moreover, the effect of porcine relaxin on drinking behavior was dose-dependent. Because this finding is similar to the well-known angiotensin II drinking response, it complements earlier findings concerning the possible mechanism whereby relaxin regulates vasopressin and LH secretion through angiotensin II (757,1005). Ward et al. (1096) reported that subcutaneous infusion of synthetic human relaxin 2 over a 14-day period did not consistently or significantly alter drinking in nonpregnant female rats and postulated that the putative effects of relaxin on drinking could be attributable to an autocrine or paracrine effect of relaxin produced within the blood–brain barrier.

Miscellaneous Effects on Nonreproductive Tissues

Effects of Relaxin on the Integumentary System

Extensive clinical studies were conducted in the late 1950s and early 1960s to examine relaxin's putative effects on the integumentary system in humans (876). In 1956, it was reported that rats receiving prolonged administration of impure porcine relaxin showed a marked increase in the elasticity of the skin *in vivo* (111). This observation led Casten and co-workers (182,183) to explore the use of porcine relaxin in patients with two chronic debilitating connective tissue diseases characterized by severe reductions in cutaneous elasticity and blood flow to the peripheral vascular beds—scleroderma and obliterative peripheral arterial disease. These workers (182,183) reported that when impure porcine relaxin was injected intramuscularly at 1- or 3-day intervals for periods ranging from 6 to 30 months in combination with estrogen, dramatic curative effects were observed. Ulcers on the fingers and toes healed, the blood flow and temperature of the toes increased, and in patients with Raynaud's phenomenon the tolerance to cold increased.

Although similar curative effects were reported by several others after the administration of partially purified porcine relaxin to patients with scleroderma (118,191, 312,407,500,820,826), some investigators reported that porcine relaxin had little or no curative value (511, 1116). Relaxin's putative therapeutic effects on the peripheral vascular beds appeared to require continual treatment. Several workers reported that after relaxin withdrawal there was a return of the Raynaud's phenomenon and skin tightness (182,183,407,826). Repeated injections of crude porcine relaxin preparations into humans proved to be extremely dangerous. An anaphylactic shock was fatal to a patient after the intravenous administration of impure porcine relaxin (312).

Treatment of patients with integumentary connective tissue disease or restrictive peripheral vascular disease has not been reported since the 1960s. Efforts to examine further the influence relaxin might have on the human integumentary connective tissue have been hindered for more than 25 years by (a) skepticism concerning the putative curative effects of relaxin, (b) uncertainties that accompany the use of impure and poorly characterized hormone preparations, (c) expense and physical discomfort associated with prolonged intramuscular administration of relaxin, (d) fear of adverse reactions to prolonged administration of porcine relaxin, and (e) unavailability of human relaxin. At the present time, there are no reports of the influence of human relaxin on human integumentary connective tissue *in vivo.*

Recent efforts to examine the influence of human relaxin on human dermal fibroblasts *in vitro* encourage the view that relaxin may have the ability to modulate connective tissue remodeling in the human integumentary system. Unemori and Amento (1061) reported that physiologic levels of human relaxin 2 down-regulated the collagen secretory phenotype of normal human dermal fibroblasts, especially when the cells were stimulated to overproduce collagen by the cytokines transforming growth factor β or IL-1 β. This occurred in conjunction with a dose-dependent elevation in procollagenase secretion and a small decrease in tissue inhibitor of metalloproteinase expression and a marked decrease in the expression of interstitial collagens, indicating relaxin may favor net collagen breakdown in situations of overexpression. Consistent with this hypothesis, Unemori and co-workers found that human relaxin 2 decreased collagen accumulation in two rodent models of fibrosis *in vivo* (1063,1064) and also decreased collagen synthesis by human scleroderma fibroblasts *in vitro* (1062). In scleroderma, fibroblasts from four of seven patients, combination of relaxin with interferon-γ resulted in a cooperative effect in decreasing collagen expression, and it was postulated that human relaxin might be administered systemically alone or in combination with interferon-γ for the treatment of scleroderma (1062). Inconsistent with Unemori and co-workers, a brief report indicated that human dermal fibroblasts failed to proliferate or produce collagen, proteoglycan, fibronectin, or collagenase in response to a wide range of doses of recombinant human relaxin 2 in culture (284). There is evidence that highly purified relaxin can modify the dermal collagenous framework *in vivo.* Porcine relaxin was reported to alter *ex vivo* the mechanical properties of mouse skin (285). Pigs were chosen in two studies because of the similarities of pig skin to that of humans (554). A brief report indicated that highly purified porcine relaxin increased the rate of tissue expansion in pigs when administered into the skin over tissue expanders for 7 days (741). Likewise, intravenous infusion of sufficient recombinant human relaxin to maintain serum relaxin levels of about 1 ng/ml into piglets facilitated tissue expansion without affecting dermal thickness (554).

Effects of Relaxin on the Heart

The reader will recall that Summerlee and co-workers (528,672,755,757) obtained evidence that the acute administration of porcine relaxin increases blood pressure in urethane-anesthetized nonpregnant rats and that it may do so, at least in part, through effects on the central nervous system. These workers also claimed that either acute intravenous or intracerebroventricular administration of porcine relaxin increased heart rate in urethane-anesthetized rats. Subsequent work by other investigators provided evidence that relaxin has the ability to act directly on the heart. Osheroff et al. (742) demonstrated that the heart atrium of both female and male rats contains sites that bind ^{32}P-labeled human relaxin 2 with both specificity and high affinity. The dissociation constant for relaxin in the atrium was similar to that in the uterus, but unlike the uterus, relaxin binding in the heart was not affected by castration or estrogen administration (742). Kakouris et al. (537) and Ward et al. (1096) examined the effects of human relaxin 2 on contractility of isolated right and left atrium of male rat hearts *in vitro* to obtain evidence that relaxin has direct, potent, and concentration-dependent effects on the heart. Both laboratories (537,1096) reported that human relaxin 2 produced dose-dependent and marked increases in both the rate of spontaneous contractions of the right atrium and the force of electrically stimulated contractions of the left atrium. The physiologic significance, if any, of relaxin's putative effects on the rate and force of contractions of the rat heart remain to be demonstrated. Ward and co-workers reported that intravenous injection of human relaxin 2 on day 19 of rat pregnancy did not influence heart rate (1095), whereas subcutaneous infusion of human relaxin 2 for 1 to 2 weeks increased heart rate in nonpregnant female rats regardless of whether they were normotensive or spontaneously hypertensive (1096).

Effects of Relaxin on Adipocytes

Olefsky et al. (736) reported that highly purified porcine relaxin enhanced the ability of adipocytes obtained from adult female rats (but not those obtained from adult male or immature female rats) to bind to porcine insulin and that the enhanced binding of insulin was attributable to an increase in the affinity of its receptor. It was postulated that the relaxin-induced increase in insulin binding may have biologic significance, because physiologic levels of relaxin potentiated the ability of submaximal concentrations of insulin to promote glucose transport and glucose oxidation in the adipocytes (736). An enhancing effect of relaxin on both the binding and biologic activity of insulin was also observed in a similar study that used human adipocytes obtained at cesarean section (509). The mechanism(s) whereby relaxin modifies the interaction of insulin with its receptor is not known. Jarrett et al. (509) postulated that this heterologous hormone–receptor interaction may make insulin-responsive cells more sensitive to insulin during pregnancy, when women develop relative insulin resistance.

The reader will recall that there is evidence that relaxin promotes the differentiation of preadipocytes during mammary development in mice (65,88). There is evidence that relaxin inhibits the differentiation of mouse 3T3-L1 preadipocyte cells to adipocytes *in vitro.* Before confluency, 3T3-L1 cells exhibit the characteristics of fibroblasts. Once confluent, insulin-treated cells undergo two rounds of cell division during the first 2 days of induction followed by accumulation of lipid and expression of insulin-stimulated glucose transport (761). Pawlina et al. (761,762) reported that both porcine relaxin and human relaxin 2 blocked the normal course of cell division during the induction phase but did not interfere with expression of the adipocyte phenotype as indicated by lipid accumulation and insulin-sensitive glucose transport.

Other Effects of Relaxin

There are isolated reports that relaxin has additional effects on nonreproductive tissues. Claims that crude porcine relaxin increased thyroid weights, radioactive iodine uptake, and protein-bound iodine in rats (774,775) were not confirmed (122). The influence of highly purified relaxin on thyroid growth or function has not been reported. A brief report indicated that low doses of impure porcine relaxin activated human and rat gastric mucosal adenylyl cyclase (841); however, more extensive studies that use highly purified relaxin are needed before the gastric mucosa can be considered a target tissue for relaxin. There is limited evidence that relaxin's quiesent effects on smooth-muscle contractility are not confined to the uterus. Highly purified rat relaxin, but not insulin, was reported to inhibit spontaneous contractions of the rat ileum both *in vivo* and *in vitro* (253). Relaxin may also have direct effects on the microcirculation in the gastrointestinal tract. Topical administration of porcine relaxin and human decidual extract produced a rapid dilatation of the veins of the rat mesocecum (93,254).

INFLUENCE OF RELAXIN ON PARTURITION

Physiologic Role at Parturition

The early reports that relaxin levels are elevated in the blood of several mammals during pregnancy and that impure preparations of relaxin affect collagenous and muscular tissues in the estrogen-dominated reproductive tract of the nonpregnant female led to the view that relaxin may have an important physiologic role(s) during pregnancy and/or at parturition. Efforts to demonstrate such a role have used ablation of the source of relaxin and subsequent hormone replacement therapy in pregnant mice, rats, and pigs. These three species were used because the source of circulating relaxin, the ovaries, is readily removed. Moreover, in all three cases, porcine relaxin, which is available in relatively large quantities, is bioactive. Data obtained with these three species indicate that progesterone, but not relaxin, is essential for maintenance of pregnancy, whereas relaxin in combination with estrogen is essential for normal parturition.

Mouse

When pregnant mice were ovariectomized and treated with progesterone only, pregnancy was maintained, but parturition was delayed, prolonged, and difficult; furthermore, there was a low incidence of live births (427,579,936,950). When similarly ovariectomized mice were treated with progesterone plus partially purified relaxin, delivery generally occurred at or near the appropriate time, but the incidence of live births remained low (579,936,950). Finally, when ovariectomized mice were treated with partially purified relaxin in combination with both progesterone and estrogen, delivery was punctual, and unlike ovariectomized animals treated with steroids only, the uterine evacuation was generally complete (427,579). Mice homozygous for a mutant allele *an* have lifelong macrocytic anemia (Hertwig's anemia) and demonstrate reproductive deficiencies including the inability to deliver their young. The recent findings (1018) that the interpubic ligaments in Hertwig's anemia not only demonstrated a response deficit to estrogen and estrogen plus relaxin but also failed to become as long as those of controls during pregnancy are consistent with the view that relaxin in combination with estrogen is essential for normal parturition in mice.

Rat

Influence of Relaxin Before Term on Rat Parturition

In 1959, Kroc et al. (579) provided the first direct evidence that relaxin is not required for maintenance of pregnancy but that it is likely essential for normal delivery in rats. These workers demonstrated that rats ovariectomized on day 15 of pregnancy and given partially purified porcine relaxin in combination with both progesterone and estrogen did not experience the prolonged pregnancy or incomplete uterine evacuation experienced by ovariectomized steroid-treated animals. Advances made since the mid-1970s gave recent experimental efforts to understand relaxin's role during pregnancy advantages over the earlier work; the availability of highly purified relaxin, knowledge of blood levels of relaxin during pregnancy, and development of methods for producing large quantities of monoclonal antibodies for rat relaxin made it possible to determine the effects of relaxin under physiologic conditions that closely mimic those of normal pregnancy.

Sherwood and co-workers used two experimental approaches to demonstrate that relaxin is required for normal delivery in rats. In 1985, Downing et al. (274) examined the influence of relaxin on birth in rats that were bilaterally ovariectomized on day 9 before plasma levels of relaxin are elevated (Fig. 24). Throughout the remainder of pregnancy, the ovariectomized rats were given progesterone plus estrogen and/or highly purified porcine relaxin in doses selected to provide serum levels similar to those observed in intact pregnant rats. Ovariectomized rats given hormone replacement therapy with progesterone plus estrogen exhibited prolonged gestation, prolonged delivery, and reduced fetal survival (Fig. 69A). In contrast, ovariectomized rats given relaxin in combination with progesterone and estrogen exhibited birth parameters that did not differ from intact controls. In 1988, Lao Guico-Lamm and Sherwood (587) used a highly specific and noninvasive approach to determine the influence of endogenous relaxin on birth in intact pregnant rats. Unanesthetized pregnant rats were injected once daily with highly purified monoclonal antibody MCA1 for relaxin, monoclonal antibody for fluorescein control, or phosphate buffered saline vehicle

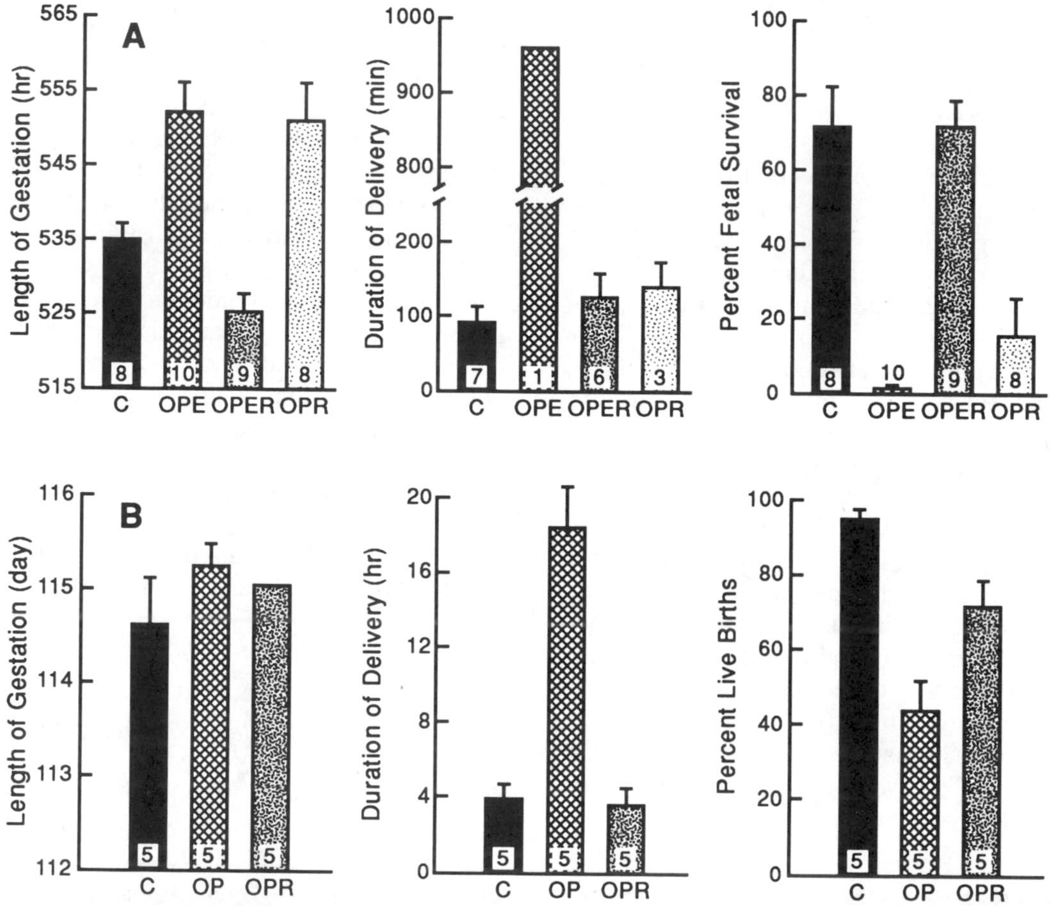

FIG. 69. A: Influence of estrogen and relaxin on birth in rats. Pregnant rats were bilaterally ovariectomized (*O*) on day 9 and given progesterone (*P*) implants (two silastic implants each containing 60 mg P) and, in addition, one of the following injection regimens: estrogen (*E;* group *OPE*); E and highly purified porcine relaxin (*R;* group *OPER*); or porcine relaxin (group *OPR*). Estrogen was administered once daily from day 9 until birth in 0.1 ml sesame oil subcutaneously, and R was administered twice daily from day 9 until birth in 0.2 ml 5% beeswax in corn oil subcutaneously. E and R were administered in various doses designed to mimic peripheral blood serum levels of hormones during pregnancy. P implants were removed on the evening of day 21 to mimic decline in serum progesterone levels that normally occurs at luteolysis. Control group (*C*) was sham-ovariectomized on day 9 and treated with vehicle controls from day 9 until birth. Means (+SE) are for numbers of animals shown at base of each histogram. From ref. 274, with permission. **B:** Influence of relaxin on birth in pigs. Pregnant pigs were bilaterally ovariectomized (*O*) on day 105 and given 100 mg progesterone (*P*) intramuscularly in 4 ml of corn oil at 12-h intervals from day 105 through day 112 and, in addition, one of the following injection regimens: highly purified porcine relaxin (*R;* group *OPR*) or R vehicle (group *OP*). Group OPR received 1 mg of highly purified porcine R intramuscularly in 1 ml of 0.9% saline at 6-h intervals from day 105 until birth. The control group (*C*) was sham-ovariectomized on day 105 and received the P and R vehicles thereafter. Means (±SE) are for the five animals used for each group. From ref. 696, with permission.

control from day 12 through day 22. Whereas the administration of neither monoclonal antibody for fluorescein nor phosphate buffered saline had effects on birth, neutralization of endogenous relaxin with MCA1 did (Fig. 70). The onset of delivery in MCA1-treated rats was delayed relative to controls, and this appeared to be caused by the prolonged duration of straining. The duration of litter delivery in MCA1-treated rats was approximately 12-fold longer than in controls, and the incidence of live pups at birth was approximately 50% of that in controls. About 20% of the fetuses and placentas were retained *in utero* on day 24 in MCA1-treated rats. Passive immunization of rats against relaxin had no apparent effect on ovarian function; the time of occurrence of functional luteolysis as determined by rapidly declining serum progesterone levels in MCA1-treated rats did not differ from that in control rats (587).

Removal of endogenous relaxin during just the last day or two of pregnancy, by either bilateral ovariectomy (202) or neutralization with monoclonal antibody MCA1 for rat relaxin (495), also markedly prolonged delivery in rats. Nevertheless, there is evidence that relaxin's important effects are not confined to the antepartum period. The deleterious effects on birth observed after neutralization of endogenous relaxin during just the antepartum period were not as severe as those that followed neutralization of endogenous relaxin throughout the second half of pregnancy. The observations that neutralization of rat relaxin throughout the second half of pregnancy not only disrupts birth but also inhibits growth and softening of the cervix more profoundly than does deprivation of relaxin during just the antepartum period led Sherwood and co-workers (915,916) to postulate that endogenous relaxin plays a role throughout the second half of pregnancy in preparing the mother rat for a rapid and safe delivery and that it does so largely through its effects on the cervix.

Relaxin's effects on parturition are estrogen-dependent. Ovariectomized rats given hormone replacement with progesterone plus relaxin exhibited prolonged gestation and markedly reduced fetal survival (275) (Fig. 69A). At least five mechanisms have been postulated whereby estrogen may influence myometrial contractility and thus promote normal parturition in rats. First, estrogen induces oxytocin receptors on the rat myometrium (16,17,364) and thereby increases the responsiveness of the myometrium to oxytocin at parturition (364,873). Second, it was reported that estrogen induced relaxin receptors in the rat myometrium (664). Third, estrogen increases the capacity of the rat myometrium and endometrium to synthesize PGs (185). There is evidence that PGs may be required for luteolysis (403) as well as for mediating oxytocin-stimulated myometrial contractility at delivery in rats (197). Fourth, estrogen induces the formation of gap junctions, and these specialized contacts between adjacent myometrial cells are thought to permit coordinated and synchronized contractions during labor (378,801). Finally, estrogen pro-

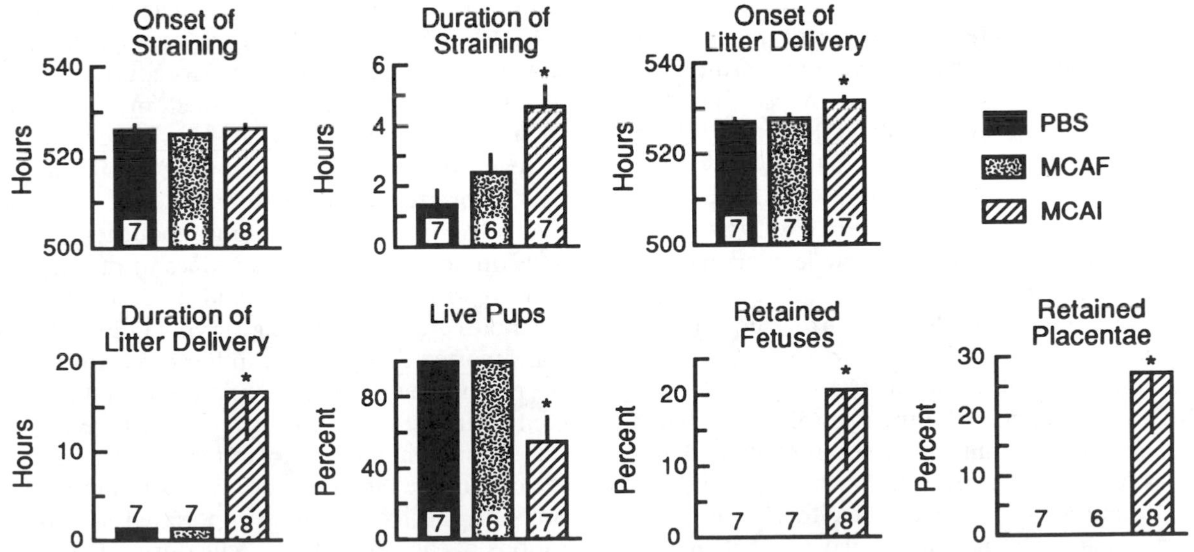

FIG. 70. Influence of neutralization of endogenous relaxin throughout second half of pregnancy on delivery in rats. Unanesthetized pregnant rats were injected once daily (days 12–22) through tail vein with 5 mg of monoclonal antibody MCA1 for rat relaxin, 5 mg of monoclonal antibody for fluorescein (*MCAF;* monoclonal antibody control) or phosphate-buffered saline (*PBS;* vehicle control). Each *bar* represents the mean (+ or − SE), and the number of animals is shown at base of (or above) each bar. *Asterisks* denote mean values in MCA1-treated rats that differ ($P \leq .05$) from those in PBS- and MCAF-treated control rats. Modified from ref. 587.

motes the formation of the contractile proteins actin and myosin, which are associated with uterine myometrial activity (236).

Estrogen also acts on the cervix in pregnant rats, and its effects on cervical tensile properties appear to be particularly interesting. On the one hand, estrogen enhances relaxin's effects on cervical softening. Maximal cervical extensibility was obtained in ovariectomized pregnant rats that received hormone replacement therapy with estrogen, progesterone, and porcine relaxin (274). In the absence of relaxin, however, the rat cervix becomes increasingly inextensible (198) and the duration of straining and delivery are increasingly prolonged with increasing doses of estrogen (202). The mechanism(s) whereby estrogen enhances relaxin's effects on cervical softening in the rat is not known. It may promote relaxin receptors (665,742) or promote the synthesis of PGs (185), which have been reported to reduce collagen concentrations near term in the rat cervix (459).

The mechanism whereby relaxin acts in combination with estrogen to promote normal parturition (see Fig. 69A) in rats is not known with certainty. Relaxin may promote normal parturition by increasing the extensibility of the cervix, preventing excessive myometrial activity until time for delivery, and enhancing the responsiveness of the uterus to oxytocics (274).

Influence of Relaxin at Term on Rat Parturition

Whereas it is now well established that elevated levels of relaxin in the peripheral blood of rats during the second half of pregnancy are required for normal parturition, it is not clear whether the decline in relaxin levels that occurs during the 24 h before birth (see Fig. 24) is also of importance. Elevated blood levels of relaxin throughout the anticipated time of delivery may interfere with normal delivery. When highly purified porcine relaxin was infused intravenously from day 19 to day 23 at a rate that maintained plasma relaxin levels more than 20-fold higher than maximal endogenous levels during pregnancy, gestation was prolonged; furthermore, in rats that gave birth during relaxin infusion, there was an increase in the interval between successive deliveries (524,526,527). Jones and Summerlee (527) postulated that the exogenously administered relaxin inhibited parturition, at least in part, by acting centrally to inhibit oxytocin secretion, because plasma oxytocin levels were lower during delivery in relaxin-treated rats than in controls. Moreover, the opioid antagonist naloxone, which has been reported to negate relaxin's inhibitory effects on oxytocin secretion (529,726–728) reversed the inhibitory effect of relaxin on delivery when treatment was given immediately after delivery of the first fetus. There is also reason to suspect that the antepartum decline of relaxin is not essential for delivery in the rat. The reader will recall that during normal delivery, relaxin in the peripheral blood surges to high levels for more than 1 hour without an apparent effect on the progress of delivery (912).

Pig

The reader will recall that the corpus luteum is the source of both relaxin and progesterone throughout pregnancy in the pig and that the placenta is the primary source of estrogen in the peripheral blood during late pregnancy in this species. Nara et al. (696) demonstrated that relaxin is required for normal delivery in pigs. The elevated levels of relaxin and progesterone normally experienced during late pregnancy were abolished by bilaterally ovariectomizing pigs on day 105. The pregnancy was maintained by progesterone administration. When parturition was induced by progesterone withdrawal on day 112, the duration of delivery was prolonged, and the incidence of live births was only 50% of that in intact controls (Fig. 69B). Replacement therapy with progesterone plus highly purified porcine relaxin restored the duration of delivery and the incidence of live births to values similar to those of controls. The hormonal milieu bathing target tissues in pigs treated with progesterone and relaxin (group OPR) was most nearly like that of rats treated with progesterone, estrogen, and relaxin (group OPER)—thus, the identical stippling of the histograms for these two groups in Fig. 69.

The importance of estrogen and progesterone at parturition in pigs has not been clearly demonstrated (187,237,274) (Fig. 69B). Progesterone cannot be withdrawn from the pregnant pig. Moreover, because estrogen is not withdrawn after ovariectomy of pregnant pigs (696), as it is in pregnant rats (274), the importance of estrogen at delivery in pigs cannot be examined with the ovariectomized pregnant animal model. Nevertheless, it seems likely that relaxin brings about its beneficial effects on delivery in pigs, as it does in rats, by acting in concert with both estrogen and progesterone. Estrogen promotes growth of the pig cervix (1129). Moreover, it was reported that estrogen induced relaxin receptors in the pig myometrium (665), and it may influence uterine contractility through effects on PG synthesis, gap junction formation, and oxytocin receptor production, as is the case in the rat. A recent investigation indicated that progesterone likely plays an important role in the modifications of the cervix that occur during late pregnancy. Winn et al. (1129) obtained evidence in nonpregnant pigs that progesterone may play a more important role than estrogen in augmenting relaxin's effects on cervical growth and softening in the pregnant pig (Fig. 46).

Kertiles and Anderson (551) also obtained evidence that relaxin facilitates birth in pigs. They reported that daily intramuscular injections of partially purified porcine relaxin from day 105 or day 107 until luteectomy on day 110 reduced both the interval from surgery to the delivery of the first neonate and the duration of delivery compared with luteectomized controls (551). Also, intramuscular administration of highly purified porcine relaxin for 1 or 2 days before the induction of parturition with $PGF_{2\alpha}$ on day 112 reportedly improved the synchrony of onset of farrowing in pigs (163).

The influence, if any, of endogenous relaxin levels on the rate of delivery is not known for any species. Wathes et al. (1099) reported that high relaxin concentrations during the last 14 h before the onset of parturition were associated with increased farrowing time in pigs, and these workers postulated that the elevated relaxin levels may have retarded the progress of delivery.

Human

Whereas there is now strong evidence that circulating levels of relaxin, progesterone, and estrogen play predominating roles in controlling parturition in rats and pigs, circulating hormones appear to modulate, but not control, human parturition. In humans, the entire conceptus including the placenta, fetal membranes, amniotic fluid, and fetus itself play the major role in controlling parturition by interacting with contiguous uterine tissue by means of a local (paracrine) system (619). It will be recalled that circulating relaxin in the human is produced in the corpus luteum (Fig. 36) (303,519,553, 1110,1146) but that relaxin is also produced in the decidua and chorionic cytotrophoblast (Fig. 38) (96,145, 203,334,440,560,847,848). There is good evidence that circulating relaxin of luteal origin is not required during pregnancy. Women with premature ovarian failure who become pregnant with oocyte donation have normal pregnancies (862) despite the fact that they have no corpus luteum and serum relaxin levels are undetectable (303,519). Bryant-Greenwood and co-workers (139,140, 142,560,561) postulated that relaxin produced by the decidua and chorionic cytotrophoblast acts locally to influence the cervix, myometrium, and fetal membranes. On the basis of *in vitro* studies that showed that porcine relaxin induced chorion and amnion cells to secrete plasminogen activator and collagenolytic enzymes (Fig. 68), these workers postulated that relaxin is one of the hormones that remodels human fetal membranes (561). They also provided evidence that relaxin might influence PGE synthesis in the amnion (627) and thereby contribute to the onset of parturition. Presently techniques are not available to establish whether relaxin produced by the decidua and/or chorionic cytotrophoblast has physiologic functions. Accordingly, it remains to be demonstrated that endogenous relaxin contributes to normal parturition in the human. Nevertheless, consideration of the essential and dramatic effects relaxin has on the cervix in pregnant rats and pigs, as well as knowledge of the early reports that porcine relaxin contributes to ripening of the cervix in women, makes attractive the possibility of using human relaxin as a clinical tool to promote cervical softening in women.

Pharmacologic Induction of Parturition

Cow

Anderson and co-workers reported that intramuscular (40,675) or intracervical (680,681,766) administration of 1 mg (3,000 units) of highly purified porcine relaxin into cattle 4 to 5 days (40,680,681,766) or about 10 days (675) before anticipated parturition induced early calving (40,675,681,766) that was accompanied by premature dilatation of the cervix (40,681,766), increased pelvic area (40,680,681,766) and decreased incidence of dystocia (40). Likewise, these workers reported that when 1 mg porcine relaxin was administered intracervically 4 to 5 days before birth in combination with the PG agonist cloprostenol or the glucocorticoid agonist dexamethasone, the interval between treatment and calving was shortened, both cervical dilatability and pelvic area were increased, and there was a reduction in both dystocia and retention of placentas relative to cloprostenol- and dexamethasone-treated controls (682,683). Anderson and co-workers postulated that exogenously administered porcine relaxin probably induces premature delivery through a luteolytic action (40,676). These workers reported that after the administration of porcine relaxin into pregnant cattle, there is a decline in progesterone (40,675,676,681,682), increase in estrogen (676,681), and increase in $PGF_{2\alpha}$ (675) levels in the peripheral plasma. Moreover, Anderson and co-workers reported that the profile of these hormones after relaxin treatment (40,675,676,681,682) is similar to that observed during normal luteal regression near term (676).

That porcine relaxin influences the course of pregnancy in cattle has not been observed with all studies. The administration of 1 mg of highly purified porcine relaxin intramuscularly either 4 to 7 days (168,766) or 10 days (169) before delivery did not induce luteolysis or advance delivery in beef heifers. The reason for the discrepancy among studies is not apparent.

A discrepancy also remains concerning the effectiveness with which porcine relaxin enters the peripheral circulation after being placed intracervically in cellulose gel (KY, Johnson and Johnson Co., New Brunswick, NJ). Musah et al. (676) reported that after placement of 1 mg of highly purified porcine relaxin into the cervix of beef heifers during late pregnancy, peripheral plasma levels of relaxin rose acutely to maximal levels of approximately 30 ng/ml within 1 h of relaxin administration. Moreover, the plasma profile and blood levels of relaxin in cattle administered relaxin intracervically did not differ markedly from cattle that received 1 mg porcine relaxin intramuscularly. Whereas Paccamonti et al. (749) obtained results similar to those of Musah et al. (676) when 1 mg porcine relaxin was administered intramuscularly to cycling cattle at estrus, they reported that systemic relaxin was marginally detectable when relaxin was administered intracervically in KY gel during either estrus or late pregnancy.

Human

The reader will recall that it has been reported that intravaginal or intracervical administration of highly purified porcine relaxin at term increased the rate of cervical dilatation and facilitated birth in women (313,637,642–644). There is also evidence that local administration of relaxin at term accelerates the onset of delivery. When MacLennan et al. (642) mixed 2 mg of highly purified porcine relaxin in a cellulose gel and placed the mixture into the posterior vaginal fornix the evening before the surgical induction of labor, ten of the 30 relaxin-treated patients, but none of the 30 control patients, entered labor spontaneously between treatment and the proposed time of induction of labor. Similar results were obtained when 2 mg porcine relaxin were placed in the cervix by means of a plastic cannula the evening before the surgical induction of birth (644). In agreement with the study of Musah et al. (676) in cattle, MacLennan et al. (644) found that peripheral serum relaxin levels increased within 1 hour of placing 2 mg porcine relaxin into the cervix of women during late pregnancy. Peripheral serum levels of porcine relaxin peaked at between 1 and 3 ng/ml 2 to 3 h after relaxin administration.

Spiny Dogfish

After administration of partially purified porcine relaxin to estrogen-treated spiny dogfish when their pregnancy was more than 75% completed, there was a premature loss of developing fetuses that was accompanied by an expansion of the cross-sectional area of the cervix-like constriction between the uterus and urogenital sinus (570). It was concluded that a relaxinlike molecule may be involved during normal parturition in the spiny dogfish (570). The spiny dogfish is the most ancient vertebrate in which relaxin has been demonstrated to influence the female reproductive tract.

RELAXIN IN THE MALE VERTEBRATE

Sources of Relaxin in the Male

In 1959, Steinetz et al. (950) reported that a bioactive equivalent of relaxin was present in rooster testicular extracts and subsequently reported that its growth-promoting effect on the mouse pubic symphysis was neutralized with an antiserum to impure porcine relaxin (953). With the advent of sensitive and specific techniques for identifying relaxin in the late 1970s, workers examined the male reproductive tract of several species for the presence of relaxin. There is now good evidence that small amounts of relaxin are produced within the reproductive tract in male mammals, birds, and elasmobranchs. The male does not appear to produce relaxin in all species. Moreover, the source of relaxin varies among species in males as it does in females.

Mammals

Human

Relaxin immunoactivity was reported in human seminal plasma by many workers (126,212,249,250,310,451, 576,628,865,1109). There were considerable differences among laboratories, but relaxin immunoactivity levels in seminal plasma were generally reported to be at least one order of magnitude greater than peripheral plasma levels in females during pregnancy. Because porcine relaxin radioimmunoassays were used in all investigations and it was demonstrated in one case that the human semen samples did not provide a curve parallel to the porcine relaxin standard (451), reported relaxin levels in human seminal plasma should not be regarded as uniformly accurate. Initial efforts to characterize the relaxinlike immunoactive substance in human seminal plasma indicated that it was associated with a 6,000-Da fraction (161,628). Moreover, seminal plasma extracts or partially purified fractions of these extracts reportedly displayed relaxin bioactivity in the guinea pig pubic symphysis palpation bioassay (251,310), in the rat uterine *in vitro* bioassay (251,1109), and on the mouse cervix (161). In only one case, however, was the claim that human seminal plasma contained relaxin bioactivity supported by data (1109). That the human male produces relaxin was established when Winslow et al. (1131) isolated human relaxin from human seminal plasma and found that its structure is the same as human relaxin 2 (B29) produced by the human corpus luteum.

The preponderance of available evidence indicates that the prostate is the source of relaxinlike activity in human seminal plasma. Elevated levels of relaxin immunoactivity were found in the seminal fluid when the ejaculated fluid was essentially of pure prostatic origin—that is, after vasectomy and in cases of bilateral congenital vas deferens agenesis (249,250). Also, low but detectable levels of relaxin immunoactivity and bioactivity were reported in human prostate extracts (547). Relaxin immunoactivity was localized in the glandular epithelium of the prostate with the avidin-biotin immunoperoxidase method using antisera for both porcine relaxin (1147) and the human relaxin analogue SKA (939) (Fig. 71). Finally, the prostate has been reported to contain low amounts of mRNA for human relaxin (440,502). Hansell et al (440) reported that both the human relaxin 1 and 2 genes are expressed in the prostate. It remains to be proved that the prostatic relaxin consists of both human relaxin 1 and human relaxin 2 proteins. There is limited evidence that the seminal vesicle and ampullary part of the vas deferens may be additional sources of relaxin in the human. When reproductive tract tissues from adult human males were stained for relaxin using rabbit antiporcine relaxin sera with the avidin-biotin immunoperoxidase technique, relaxin immunoactivity was localized in the glandular epithelium of the seminal vesicles and ampullary part of the vas deferens as well as in the prostate (1147).

In the human male, it appears likely that relaxin is released primarily, and perhaps solely, into the prostatic fluid. Whereas relaxin was detected in the blood plasma with an early porcine relaxin radioimmunoassay developed with crude porcine relaxin (132), radioimmunoassays that used pure relaxin for development of antisera provide no evidence that relaxin is found in the peripheral plasma in the human male (634,720).

Pig, Armadillo, and Dog

There is limited evidence that relaxin is produced in boars. The source of relaxin in the boar is not known with certainty, but it appears to be the seminal vesicles. Relaxin immunoactivity was first reported to be associated with both the interstitial and sertoli cells of the testis (37,280), but when an antiserum against highly purified porcine relaxin was used, specific fluorescence was not observed in the testis (37). Moreover, the extremely low levels of relaxin immunoactivity found in tissue extracts indicate that the boar testis is probably not a source of relaxin (1141). A study that used antiporcine relaxin serum with the peroxidase–antiperoxidase immunocytochemical localization technique at the light microscope level provided evidence that the secretory epithelial cells of the seminal vesicles of intact boars produce relaxin (564). Moreover, electron microscope immunocytochemistry using the protein A-gold technique and rabbit antiporcine serum demonstrated that relaxin immunoactivity was associated with 200- to 600-nm cytoplasmic granules in these cells (565). Production and storage of relaxin in the seminal vesicles may be androgen-dependent. A brief report indicated the cytoplasm of the seminal vesicle epithelial cells did not dem-

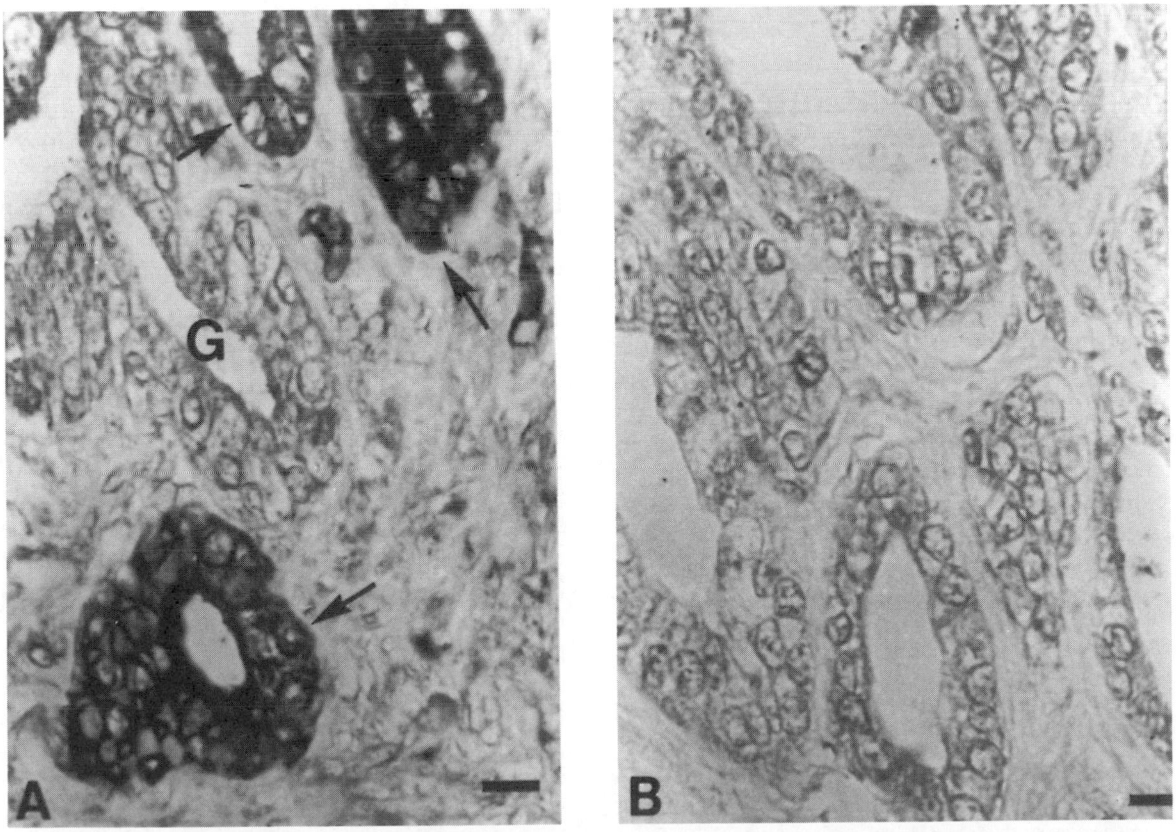

FIG. 71. Human prostate immunostained with rabbit antihuman relaxin 2 analog SKA. **A:** At 1:3200 dilution of the antiserum, three glands (*arrows*) are positive, whereas one (*G*) is negative. **B:** Similar area in same specimen treated with same dilution of antibody preincubated with excess relaxin analog. Note that all immunostaining was blocked. Bars = 10 μm. From ref. 939, with permission.

onstrate relaxin immunoactivity in castrate boars (564). Relaxin immunostaining was not found in the boar testis, epididymis, ductus deferens, or prostate (565), and relaxin mRNA was not found in the boar prostate (624). Brief reports (532,533,535) that low levels of relaxin are found within the peripheral plasma of boars and that they decline after mating (533) require confirmation. In armadillos (*Dasypus novemcinctus*), relaxin may only be produced by postpubertal animals and appears to be confined to the prostate. Relaxin immunostaining was localized only within cells of the prostatic secretory epithelium of adult animals (172). The prostate in dogs may also produce relaxin. Cysts associated with cystic prostatic hypertrophy were reported to contain immunopositive components with molecular weights characteristic of prorelaxin and preprorelaxin (704).

Rat and Mouse

There is no evidence that male rats and mice produce relaxin. Relaxin immunostaining was absent from the testes, prostate, seminal vesicles, and epididymides of both the rat and mouse when rabbit antirat relaxin sera and rabbit antiporcine relaxin sera were used with the avidin-biotin immunoperoxidase technique for immunolocalization (27).

Birds

Almost nothing is known concerning relaxin in males in nonmammalian species. As previously mentioned, the detection of relaxin bioactivity within extracts of rooster testes by Steinetz and co-workers (950) was the first report of relaxin production in a male of any species.

Biologic Effects of Relaxin in the Male

The presence of relaxin in seminal plasma led many workers to examine the influence of relaxin on the motility of spermatozoa as well as the capacity of spermatozoa to fertilize oocytes *in vitro* (615,1107). Experimentation was conducted under a wide variety of experimental conditions with spermatozoa from several species, and findings were not consistent.

Influence of Relaxin on Sperm Motility

There is evidence that *endogenous* relaxin within the seminal plasma of humans and pigs contributes to normal motility of the spermatozoa, which will hereafter be referred to as sperm. When added to samples *in vitro,* rabbit antiporcine relaxin sera caused a rapid and marked decline in the percentage of motile washed human sperm (861) and of both fresh and washed porcine sperm (531,534). Also, a monoclonal antibody for human relaxin 2 analog SKA decreased the percentage of motile washed human sperm (938); whereas anti-insulin antiserum had no effect on human sperm motility (613). A brief report indicated that active immunization of rabbits with porcine relaxin inhibited the overall forward grade motility of sperm, overall percentage motility of sperm, and percentage live sperm (369), whereas a second report indicated that active immunization of rabbits with porcine relaxin did not influence objectively determined sperm motility characteristics (513). The reason for the discrepancy between these two studies is not known. Juang et al. (532) reported sperm motility was correlated with levels of relaxin immunoactivity in boars, but similar correlations were not obtained with human semen samples (126,865).

A second experimental approach has been to examine the effects of *exogenous* relaxin on sperm motility characteristics such as percentage of motile sperm, rate of loss of motility, and grade of forward progression. Generally, the addition of relaxin did not influence sperm motility when added to *whole fresh* semen. In one case, the addition of porcine relaxin to diluted fresh boar semen was reported to retard the rate of loss of sperm motility (534), whereas porcine relaxin did not influence the percentage of motile sperm within whole normal human semen samples (212,611) or human semen diluted in *in vitro* fertilization medium (699). Likewise, equine relaxin did not influence the motility of fresh whole equine sperm diluted with an extender and cooled to 4°C (181). In contrast, several workers reported that the addition of porcine relaxin to *washed* human sperm delayed the loss of forward motion and the decline in the grade of forward progression (212,309,611,753). One report (196) indicated that porcine relaxin did not influence the motility of washed human sperm.

A decrease in fertility occurs with semen that are frozen (cryopreserved) and then thawed, and this has been largely attributed to the 25% to 75% reduction in sperm motility that occurs during freezing and thawing of human semen (434). Several workers have explored the possibility that relaxin enhances the motility of thawed sperm. Porcine relaxin was reported to increase the motility and grade of forward progression of thawed human (612), porcine (534), and equine (162) sperm. Equine relaxin was also reported to increase the motility of cryopreserved equine sperm (181). Two laboratories failed to observe an improvement in sperm motility when porcine relaxin was added to cryopreserved human (434) and bovine (365) semen. Finally, two reports indicated that highly purified porcine relaxin (125) and synthetic human relaxin 2 (211) increased the ability of washed human sperm to penetrate human cervical mucus and bovine cervical mucus, respectively, whereas a third investigation found that only high doses of porcine relaxin influenced the ability of washed human sperm to penetrate human cervical mucus and that relaxin inhibited penetration (451).

Because circulating relaxin levels in males are low or nondetectable (532,533,634,720), it seems doubtful that endogenous relaxin influences testicular function. Whereas it was reported that adding supraphysiologic levels of porcine relaxin to the microsomal fraction obtained from adult macaque (*Macaca fascicularis*) testes inhibited testosterone production (582), porcine relaxin did not influence testosterone production when added to minced macaque testicular tissue that contained intact cells (1017).

Influence of Relaxin on Fertility

Physiologic levels of highly purified porcine relaxin were reported to have little or no effect on *in vitro* fertilization of hamster oocytes with human sperm obtained from fertile donors (196,753). Porcine relaxin treatment, however, was reported to increase the percentage of hamster oocytes fertilized *in vitro* with sperm from men with low sperm count and poor sperm motility (753). Also, physiologic levels of porcine relaxin increased the proportion of mouse oocytes fertilized *in vitro* by suboptimal concentrations of sperm (800). These latter studies led to the postulation that relaxin might be useful as a tool for the treatment of male infertility (753). Two studies have examined the influence of relaxin on fertility *in vivo*, and both obtained negative results. The addition of porcine relaxin to fresh-extended and frozen-thawed semen did not affect pregnancy rate or litter size in sows (1037). Also, porcine relaxin given in a vaginal gel on the day of embryo transfer did not influence pregnancy rate in humans (646).

In view of the many inconsistencies among existing findings and the lack of experimentation under rigorously physiologic conditions, it remains to be established that relaxin has a physiologic role in the male in any species.

SUMMARY AND CONCLUSIONS

The isolation of porcine relaxin in high yields in the mid-1970s triggered a sustained resurgence of research on relaxin. Considerable progress has been made toward a better understanding of the chemistry and physiology of relaxin during the past two decades, but much research on this hormone remains to be accomplished. Accordingly, this section not only summarizes principal recent advances but also includes this reviewer's perception of important unsolved problems that will likely constitute a main portion of the research effort on relaxin in the foreseeable future.

Structural studies of relaxin from 11 species (pig, rat, human, monkey, shark, skate, whale, horse, dog, guinea pig, porpoise) demonstrated that relaxin has superficial structural features similar to those of insulin. The two hormones have molecular weights of about 6,000, contain A and B chains of similar length, and contain disulfide bridges that have the same disposition. Early studies that used model building and computer-assisted graphics indicated that relaxin can be accommodated into a three-dimensional structure similar to that of insulin, and more recent radiographic analysis of human relaxin 2 demonstrated that the overall fold of relaxin is similar to that of insulin. The similarities in their superficial structural features led to the postulation that relaxin and insulin (as well as IGF-I and IGF-II) evolved from a common ancestral gene. The process whereby relaxin is biosynthesized is consistent with this hypothesis. Relaxin, like insulin, is originally synthesized as a preprohormone containing the following sequence: signal peptide/B chain/connecting peptide/A chain. After cleavage of the signal peptide, the connecting peptide is cleaved to form the active 6,000-Da hormone. Also supportive of the view that relaxin and insulin evolved from a common gene is the observation that an intron interrupts the coding region of the connecting peptide in human, porcine, and monkey relaxin genes at a position that corresponds closely to one of two introns in the human insulin gene.

If relaxin and insulin evolved from a common ancestral gene, considerable evolutionary divergence occurred. The molecular weight of prorelaxin is approximately 19,000, whereas that of proinsulin is only 9,000; the connecting peptide of prorelaxin contains about 100 amino acids, whereas the connecting peptide of proinsulin contains about 30 amino acids. The processing of prorelaxin is less stringently controlled than proinsulin. With proinsulin, paired basic residues flanking the mature hormone are cleavage sites; whereas with the exceptions of human and monkey prorelaxin, there are no paired basic amino acid residues flanking mature relaxin. Also, the primary structures of relaxin and insulin differ extensively. There is only about 25% homology in their amino acid sequences, and this homology is largely attributable to those amino acids involved in cross-linking of the A and B chains or chain folding. The surfaces of relaxin and insulin differ markedly, and these hormones share neither immunologic determinants nor biologic effects. If the receptors for relaxin and insulin evolved from a common ancestral gene, they too diverged extensively during evolution (as did their function): neither relaxin nor insulin has biologically active sites that are capable of interacting with receptors for both hormones.

The variation in the primary structure of relaxin among species is striking. Generally, only 30% to 60% amino acid sequence homology exists among species. The nearly identical structures of porcine, whale, and porpoise relaxin are a notable exception. The apparent low degree of evolutionary constraint that permitted the divergence of relaxin's structure among species is extraordinary, and we do not understand it from either an evolutionary or physiologic perspective. The extreme variation of the primary structure of relaxin among species has at least four important implications to the researcher studying relaxin. First, to have anything beyond a superficial understanding of the structure of relaxin for a given species, its amino acid sequence must be determined. Second, the demonstrated or implicit variation in the structure of relaxin among species as well as the possibility that relaxin receptors have undergone evolutionary divergence may make it necessary to explore the bioactivity of relaxin from a given species in more than one bioassay to find a suitable response. Regardless of the bioassay used, when specific bioactivities are determined, standard and unknown relaxin preparations from the same species should be used to optimize the chances that parallel dose-response curves are obtained. Third, it is advisable to determine relaxin immunoactivity levels in a given species with a homologous radioimmunoassay or enzyme-linked immunosorbant assay for relaxin in that species wherever feasible. With a totally homologous immunoassay, the antiserum will bind relaxin with high affinity, so the sensitivity of the immunoassay will be high. Moreover, accurate measurements of relaxin immunoactivity are dependent on the standard and unknown dose-response curves being parallel. One obvious implication is that, when rigorous studies of the secretion of relaxin in a given species are to be conducted, it may be necessary to isolate relaxin from that species so that a homologous immunoassay for relaxin can be developed. Finally, the diversity of relaxin's structure among species provided valuable insight concerning the structural features of the hormone required for bioactivity. The premise that amino acids that contribute to relaxin's bioactivity are conserved among species led to experimentation demonstrating that disulfide bonds, the two invariant arginine residues in the β chain and the invariant glycine residue in the A chain are required for bioactivity.

Progress has been made in recent years toward the development of improved methods for both the bioassay and immunoassay of relaxin. For more than 30 years, the commonly used guinea pig pubic symphysis palpation bioassay, mouse interpubic ligament bioassay, and mouse and rat uterine contractility bioassays provided indispensable information concerning the biologic activity of relaxin preparations or tissue samples, but these bioassays have important limitations. They are neither precise nor sensitive, and they are expensive. Two recently described *in vitro* relaxin bioassays that are based on the stimulation of cyclic AMP in established primary cultures of either human endometrial cells or newborn rhesus monkey uterine cells are specific, precise, and at least 100-fold more sensitive than previously used relaxin bioassays. Nevertheless, even these *in vitro* relaxin bioassays have important limitations. The responsiveness to relaxin varied among different cell lines as well as among different passages (population doubling) and the cells are available in finite quantities. A transformed cell line that is responsive to relaxin, stable, and widely available indefinitely would be an important contribution to the relaxin field. Recently developed enzyme-linked immunosorbant assays for human and macaque relaxin are sufficiently sensitive ($\leq$10 pg/ml) to measure low circulating levels of relaxin in humans and monkeys during the luteal phase of nonconceptive menstrual cycles. Moreover, enzyme-linked antibody is more stable than radioiodinated relaxin, and problems associated with handling and disposing of radioactivity are avoided with enzyme-linked immunosorbant assays. In view of the demonstrated advantages of enzyme-linked immunosorbant assays for primate relaxin over radioimmunoassays, it seems advantageous to develop enzyme-linked immunosorbant assays for relaxin from other species.

When considering the source of *circulating* relaxin in mammalian species, it can be stated that most if not all the hormone is produced in a single tissue in the female reproductive tract and that the highest levels are produced during pregnancy. The specific tissue that is the source of circulating relaxin, however, varies among species. It may be the corpus luteum, placenta, or uterus. No clear pattern of pregnancy-related physiologic factors that predicts the source of relaxin within a given species has emerged.

Although little is known concerning the factors that influence the synthesis of relaxin in any species, limited evidence indicates that striking differences exist among species. The synthesis of high levels of relaxin in the corpora lutea is dependent on placental luteotropic support in rats and women, whereas the corpora lutea appear to have an inherent capacity to produce high levels of relaxin for a period at least as long as pregnancy in pigs. Steroids have been demonstrated to promote relaxin synthesis in two species. Estrogen promotes luteal relaxin synthesis in rats hysterectomized during the second half of pregnancy, and estrogen in combination with progesterone promotes uterine relaxin synthesis in ovariectomized nonpregnant guinea pigs. After its synthesis, at least a portion of the relaxin is stored in dense, membrane-limited cytoplasmic granules within the source tissue in several species. These relaxin-containing granules have been identified in pig, rat, and human luteal cells, rabbit placental syncytiotrophoblast cells, guinea pig uterine endometrial gland cells, and pig seminal vesicle secretory epithelial cells. Relaxin may not be stored within cytoplasmic granules in all species. For example, there is no evidence that relaxin is stored in granules within the hamster placenta. The levels of relaxin that are stored in tissue sources vary tremendously among species. For example, the yields of highly purified relaxin per gram equivalent of fresh tissue from pig and rat ovaries are approximately 100-fold greater than those from shark ovaries, skate ovaries, and horse placentas. Neither the mechanisms responsible for the great differences in tissue levels of relaxin among species nor the physiologic significance of these differences is understood.

Studies with the pig, rat, horse, human, and monkey have provided limited insight concerning the factors that influence relaxin secretion in these species. As with relaxin synthesis, the regulation of relaxin secretion varies greatly among species. Pigs secrete relatively little relaxin throughout the first 100 days of the 114-day gestation period, but there is a massive release of relaxin from the corpora lutea during the 2 to 3 days before birth. There is evidence that this surge in relaxin levels, which appears to reflect both the age of the corpora lutea and the luteolytic process that precedes parturition, depends on endogenous PG biosynthesis. There is no evidence of placental involvement in the regulation of relaxin secretion in pigs.

Rats secrete little relaxin from the corpora lutea until midpregnancy. Relaxin levels in the peripheral blood rise rapidly from about day 12 until day 15 and remain elevated until day 20, when, as in the pig, there is a surge in relaxin levels during the antepartum period. Available evidence indicates that relaxin secretion during the period from day 15 to day 20 is promoted by a placental luteotropic factor (which acts in combination with estrogen) and inhibited by a pituitary suppressive factor(s). The chemical natures and mechanisms of action of the placental and pituitary factors remain completely unknown. The antepartum surge in relaxin levels in the rat is associated with an apparent luteolytic process that occurs at 24-h intervals and is linked to both the photoperiod and the numbers of fetuses. The factors that promote the antepartum surge in relaxin levels in the rat are not known; however, there is limited evidence that PGs and LH may be involved.

In horses, relaxin levels are elevated from about day 80 until term on about day 350. Interestingly, there are marked among-breed differences in both the amount and form of circulating relaxin in horses. For example, relaxin levels in standardbreds rise rapidly to maximal levels of about 100 ng/ml on day 175 and then decline gradually to foaling. In contrast, relaxin levels in ponies rise gradually to maximal levels of about 20 ng/ml at foaling. The factors that influence the secretion of relaxin from the horse placenta have not been determined.

Relaxin is secreted from the corpora lutea of humans and monkeys throughout nearly all of pregnancy. Relaxin levels are higher during the first trimester than during the second or third, and unlike in the pig and rat, there is no evidence of an antepartum surge in relaxin levels in the human and monkey. It appears that chorionic gonadotropic hormones play a major role in promoting relaxin secretion in both the human and monkey.

Until recently, nearly all efforts to identify the factors that influence relaxin synthesis and secretion have involved surgical or pharmacologic manipulations of pregnant animals. The use of *in vivo* methods has three important advantages. First, *in vivo* methods can identify various organs (the placenta and pituitary, e.g., in the rat) that are involved with the regulation of relaxin synthesis and secretion. Second, with *in vivo* methods, studies can be conducted with confidence that tissue sources for relaxin are being maintained in a viable and potentially responsive state. Finally, by using *in vivo* methods, the chance that clear findings have physiologic significance is optimized.

There is an important advantage to *in vitro* methods for examining relaxin secretion. *In vitro* methods permit the examination of factors thought to act directly on source tissues to influence relaxin secretion under more rigidly controlled conditions than *in vivo* methods. Since 1987, a reverse hemolytic plaque assay that examines the secretion of relaxin from individual pig luteal cells has not only implicated PGs and growth factors as possible factors that influence the secretion of relaxin from pig luteal cells, it has also provided indications that mobilization of intracellular calcium and activation of protein kinase C may promote relaxin secretion from luteal cells obtained during the first half of pregnancy in pigs.

Relaxin immunoactivity in the peripheral blood of rats has been demonstrated to be associated with multiple components. The relaxin immunoactivity is associated with three main components of different size during late pregnancy, and the distribution of relaxin immunoactivity among these components changes progressively with the day of pregnancy. The chemical nature and physiologic significance of these multiple relaxin-immunoactive components in the rat remain to be determined. Rigorous studies of the chemical nature of relaxin immunoactivity within the blood at various stages of pregnancy have not been conducted with species other than rats.

Studies with highly purified relaxin have confirmed earlier findings that relaxin induces growth of the interpubic ligament, promotes softening of the cervix, promotes growth of the uterus, and inhibits contractility of the uterus. Whereas relaxin's effects on the cervix and uterus appear to be generally distributed among mammalian species, its effects on the interpubic ligament are not. Relaxin promotes growth of the interpubic ligament in guinea pigs and mice but not in rats, rabbits, or sheep. It cannot be concluded, however, that relaxin does not have generally distributed effects on pelvic ligament softening, of which growth of the interpubic ligament may be only one manifestation. Important fundamental questions remain unanswered concerning relaxin's effects on the interpubic ligament, cervix, and uterus. It appears clear that relaxin's effects on the growth of the interpubic ligament in rodents is dependent on estrogen, but the influence of estrogen on relaxin's more generally distributed effects on the cervix and uterus are not so well understood. For example, in rats and pigs in which the individual and combined effects of the two hormones have been examined most extensively, there are apparent between-species differences. Relaxin's effects on both growth and softening of the *cervix* are dependent on and augmented by estrogen in rats but not in pigs. In both species, relaxin's effects on *uterine* growth are not dependent on, but are augmented by, estrogen. Nothing is known concerning the interactive roles of estrogen and relaxin on uterine contractility in pigs. In rats relaxin's inhibitory effect is not dependent on estrogen exposure, but the sensitivity of the uterus is increased by exposure to this steroid.

Limited studies indicate that progesterone may influence relaxin's effects on the interpubic ligament, cervix, and uterus in ways that differ among tissues. Progesterone was reported to inhibit relaxin's effects on growth of the interpubic ligament in mice as well as growth and softening of the cervix in rats but to increase the sensitivity of the uterus to the quiescent effect of relaxin on uterine contractility in both rats and pigs. The physiologic role of progesterone on a given tissue may also differ among species. Whereas there is no evidence that progesterone synergizes with relaxin to promote growth and softening of the cervix in rats, it appears to do so in pigs. Clearly, the effects of the sex steroids estrogen and progesterone on the cervix and uterus are complex and poorly understood. Because blood levels of both estrogen and progesterone are elevated when relaxin levels are elevated during pregnancy, and one or both of these steroids very likely influence relaxin's effects on the cervix and uterus, much work is needed to understand the roles of estrogen and progesterone as well as relaxin to gain a good understanding of the malfunctions of the female reproductive tract that occur during pregnancy.

During recent years, studies of the influence of relaxin on the histologic characteristics and biochemical composition of the cervix have contributed to a better understanding at the cellular and molecular levels of the mechanism(s) whereby relaxin contributes to growth and softening of the cervix of both pregnant pigs and pregnant rats. In both species, relaxin plays a major role in promoting the reduction in the density and organization of collagen fiber bundles, the accumulation of amorphous ground substance among collagen fiber bundles, and the increase in blood vessel diameter that occur during late pregnancy. Moreover, there is evidence that relaxin reduces the length and degree of interdigitation of elastin fibers in the rat cervix. In both pregnant rats and pregnant pigs, relaxin promotes increased water concentration, dry weight, and glycosaminoglycans/collagen ratio. Much additional experimentation is needed. Rigorous studies that provide definitive answers to the following questions are needed. What are the target cells for relaxin in the cervix? Can these target cells be examined in culture in an appropriately differentiated state? Does relaxin influence the cellular composition of the cervix—either by stimulating hyperplasia or promoting migration of leukocytes into the cervical stroma? What is the biochemical nature of the changes relaxin induces in the collagen, proteoglycans, and/or elastin, and how do these changes contribute to softening of the cervix? What molecules are secreted by relaxin-responsive cells to trigger the remodeling of the cervical stroma and smooth muscle? Studies of the mechanism of relaxin's actions on the cervix are in their infancy. Available data provide no clear hypothesis concerning the chain of molecular events between interaction of relaxin with target cells and cervical softening. It seems certain that the molecular events associated with cervical softening are complex and that a good understanding of this phenomenon and its hormonal control will require many years of research effort.

Considerable progress has been made in recent years with intact uteri or uterine segments toward an understanding of relaxin's effects on uterine contractility in the rat. Available data indicate that relaxin not only inhibits the frequency and, to a lesser degree, the amplitude of spontaneous uterine contractions but also attenuates oxytocin- and PG-induced contractions when the concentrations of these contractile agents are low. The sensitivity of the uterus to the quiescent effects of relaxin is enhanced by prior estrogen treatment (and perhaps progesterone treatment), but the mechanism whereby estrogen brings about this effect is largely unexplored. Considerable advances have been made at the molecular level toward an understanding of the mechanism(s) whereby relaxin inhibits contractility of the rat uterine myometrium. There is good evidence that relaxin decreases the activity of the enzyme MLCK, which promotes smooth-muscle contraction by catalyzing the phosphorylation of myosin light chains. The mechanism(s) whereby relaxin decreased MLCK activity is not known with certainty. There is evidence that can be interpreted to infer that relaxin's effects are mediated, at least in part, through protein kinase A–mediated phosphorylation of MLCK (which reduces MLCK activity) and/or other proteins that reduce intracellular Ca^{2+} to levels inadequate to form the active Ca^{2+}·calmodulin·MLCK complex. Further studies are needed to provide a more detailed understanding of the mechanism whereby relaxin reduces MLCK activity. Although it appears clear that relaxin inhibits the contractility of myometrial cells through a direct relaxin-induced reduction in MLCK activity, relaxin may bring about its effects, at least in part, through additional mechanisms. For example, there is evidence that relaxin-induced elevation of cyclic AMP may inhibit uterine contractile activity by reducing the permeability of gap junctions between adjacent myometrial cells. There are also isolated and conflicting reports that relaxin may inhibit uterine contractility indirectly by activating β-adrenergic receptors (presumably through relaxin-induced release of endogenous catecholamines from myometrial cells). Finally, there are recent but not entirely consistent reports that relaxin may mediate its effects by opening ATP-dependent K^+ channels. Studies that clarify the putative involvement of catecholamines and/or K^+ channels with the mechanism of action of relaxin on myometrial cells would contribute substantially to this area.

Besides inhibiting myometrial contractility, relaxin has general metabolic effects on rat, mouse, and pig uteri (increased uterine water content, wet weight, dry weight, glycogen content, and protein content) that are similar to the metabolic changes that occur in the uterine composition during the second half of pregnancy, when relaxin levels are elevated in the peripheral blood. It was postulated that myometrial glycogen stores may provide a source of energy for the strong, highly coordinated uterine contractions that occur at birth and that the increases in the size and collagenous framework of the uterus during the second half of pregnancy may accommodate the rapidly growing fetuses. Whereas it is well established that administration of porcine relaxin to rats, pigs, and mice promotes uterine growth, it remains to be established that endogenous relaxin promotes growth of the uterus in any species. The observation that neutralization of endogenous rat relaxin within the peripheral blood did not influence uterine growth is not supportive of an important role of circulating relaxin on uterine growth in rats. It is possible that relaxin produced within the rat endometrial epithelial cells during pregnancy exerts general metabolic effects on the rat uterus through paracrine mechanisms.

Evidence is accumulating that relaxin may have effects on the uterine endometrium as well as the uterine myometrium. Highly purified porcine relaxin was reported to promote not only growth of the rat uterine endometrium *in vivo,* but also, when given in combination with progesterone, the production of prolactin, IGFBP-1, aromatase, and estrone sulfate sulfatase by human endometrial stromal cells *in vitro.* Whereas it was postulated that relaxin may be a regulator of decidualization in the human, it remains to be established that endogenous relaxin influences endometrial function during pregnancy in any species.

Studies since 1990 have established that relaxin plays a major role in promoting growth and development of mammary tissue during pregnancy in both rats and pigs. Interestingly, the main effects of relaxin are targeted on the nipples in rats, whereas they are targeted on the glandular parenchyma in pigs. Relaxin-dependent growth of the nipples in rats is required for normal lactational performance. The observations that highly purified relaxin promoted growth of mammary parenchymal and stromal elements in estrogen-pretreated mice and growth of the pigeon crop sac (a structure analogous to the mammary gland in mammals) encourages the view that relaxin's mammotropic effects may be widely distributed among species. Many fundamental questions concerning the influence of relaxin on mammary tissue remain unanswered. Does endogenous relaxin have effects on mammary tissue in a given species? If so, what are those effects and are they important? Does relaxin act directly on mammary tissue to bring about its effects? If so, what are the target cells for relaxin? What are the mechanisms whereby relaxin brings about its effects on mammary tissue? In this regard, there are early indications that relaxin may have actions in mammary tissue that are similar to those in the cervix. In rats, relaxin promotes a reduction in the density and organization of collagen fiber bundles, a reduction in the length and degree of interdigitation of elastin fibers, and an increase in the diameter of blood vessels in the cervix, mammary glands, and nipples.

The possibility that relaxin may act locally to influence connective tissue remodeling in female reproductive tissues where small quantities of relaxin have been detected has received increasing attention in recent years. The following conditions would provide strong indications that a paracrine regulatory mechanism exists: (a) local production of relaxin, (b) biologic action of relaxin on cells adjacent to the site of relaxin production, (c) relaxin receptors on relaxin-responsive cells, and (d) developmental alterations in the above elements of the paracrine system that correlate with the changing physiologic state (43). The first condition has been met in several cases. There is evidence that low amounts of relaxin are produced in developing ovarian follicles in cycling pigs and rats; endometrium in pregnant pigs, rats, and humans; and mammary duct epithelial cells in guinea pigs and humans. There is also evidence that relaxin stimulates the activity of enzymes associated with collagen and proteoglycan metabolism in ovarian granulosa and/or thecal cells obtained from rats, pigs, and humans, as well as in amnion and chorion cells obtained from women. Finally, a recent report identified binding sites for relaxin within the ovarian thecal cells of prepubertal mice. To date, a close temporal correlation of developmental alterations in the production of relaxin and/or relaxin receptors with a putative paracrine activity of relaxin has not been demonstrated. Finally, to *establish* that a paracrine mechanism is operative, it should be demonstrated that the putative paracrine process fails to occur in the absence of relaxin. Unfortunately, experimental techniques that block production or local availability of relaxin are not presently available. Therefore, it remains to be established that relaxin exerts paracrine control in any tissue.

Among the most fascinating concepts to emerge since

the mid-1980s is the possibility that relaxin acts centrally to bring about physiologic effects. The two most prominent hypotheses that relaxin influences the time of delivery in rats through effects on oxytocin secretion and that relaxin influences blood pressure in rats through effects on vasopressin secretion emerged from studies that largely involved the acute administration of porcine relaxin to surgically and/or pharmacologically manipulated nonpregnant rats. These hypotheses received experimental support when apparent relaxin-binding sites were identified in several locations within the rat brain including the circumventricular organs thought to mediate relaxin's effects on oxytocin and vasopressin secretion. Nevertheless, it is not established that relaxin has centrally mediated physiologic effects. There are conflicting reports in the literature regarding the influence of porcine relaxin on oxytocin secretion and blood pressure in rats, and there is no evidence that endogenous relaxin has central effects in any species. There are many fundamental questions to be answered concerning the putative central effects of relaxin. Does endogenous relaxin have central effects? If so, is it circulating relaxin or relaxin produced within the brain that acts on the brain? What are the physiologic effects of relaxin on the brain, and are they of vital importance to the animal? Are central effects of relaxin found in males? How widely distributed are central effects of relaxin among species?

The putative effects of relaxin on diverse nonreproductive tissues are not established. Claims that relaxin has effects on integumentary connective tissue and peripheral vascular tissue largely arose from studies that used crude porcine relaxin in humans in the late 1950s and early 1960s for the treatment of chronic debilitating connective tissue diseases. Whereas studies that used either highly purified porcine relaxin or synthetic human relaxin provided limited evidence that relaxin reduces collagen production by human dermal fibroblasts *in vitro* and increases the elasticity of mouse and pig skin *in vivo,* not all recent studies are supportive of an effect of human relaxin on human dermal fibroblasts. Moreover, it remains to be demonstrated that endogenous relaxin influences the integumentary system in any species. Regardless of whether endogenous human relaxin has a normal physiologic role on the integumentary system, a resurgence of interest in the possibility of using relaxin for the treatment of chronic diseases such as scleroderma and obliterative peripheral arterial disease would occur if treatment with human relaxin is demonstrated to be therapeutic and synthetic human relaxin can be made available in quantities sufficient for chronic treatment at a reasonable cost. Accordingly, additional experimentation on the possible effects of relaxin on integumentary connective tissue and peripheral vasculature seems important. The heart has recently emerged as a possible target organ for relaxin. The observation that both female and male rat atria contain relaxin binding sites and that human relaxin 2 increases heart rate in both sexes provides strong evidence that the heart has the capacity to respond to relaxin in this species. Even so, it remains to be demonstrated that endogenous relaxin influences heart rate in rats or other species. If it does, are its effects confined to the female during pregnancy? If not, what is the source of relaxin that influences heart rate in the rat? There are isolated reports of putative effects of relaxin on other nonreproductive tissues such as rat thyroid; rat, human, and mouse adipocytes; human and rat gastric mucosa; rat ileum; and rat mesocecum. Additional work is needed to establish that relaxin acts on these tissues, and it if does, it should be proved that endogenous relaxin has important effects on their function.

For 50 years after its discovery in 1926, there was a general lack of interest in relaxin among both reproductive biologists and clinicians. A key reason for this apathy was a lack of information concerning relaxin's physiologic importance during pregnancy in any species. Although there were those who believed relaxin to be of importance, studies that substantiated that view were few in number and they used crude porcine relaxin. Research conducted since the early 1980s has established that the hormone relaxin is essential during pregnancy in at least two species—rats and pigs. Two vital roles during pregnancy have been identified. Relaxin promotes growth and softening of the cervix and thereby enables rapid and safe delivery in both rats and pigs. Relaxin also promotes growth and development of the mammary apparatus in both species, and it has been established that relaxin-dependent growth of the nipples is required for normal lactational performance in rats. It remains to be established that relaxin's profound effects on mammary parenchymal tissue in the pregnant pig are required for normal lactational performance. The fact that relaxin has effects on cervical and mammary gland development in both rats and pigs encourages the view that relaxin may have similar effects during pregnancy in other species. Nevertheless, one must keep in mind that there is great diversity in the physiology of relaxin among species. This diversity includes not only relaxin's source, regulation of synthesis and secretion, and secretory profiles during pregnancy, but also its physiologic effects. It is possible that endogenous relaxin may have little or no physiologic significance during pregnancy in some species. Accordingly, there is need to investigate the physiologic importance of relaxin in additional laboratory rodents, domestic species, and primates including the human. Regardless of whether endogenous relaxin plays a major role in promoting cervical growth and softening in the human, the clinical studies that demonstrated intravaginal or intracervical administration of highly purified porcine relaxin before induced delivery of women at term increased the rate of cervical effacement and dilatation encourage the view that synthetic human relaxin may have clinical use. It remains to be demonstrated that synthetic human relaxin is an effective cervical softening agent in the human. If it is and human relaxin can be made available at reasonable cost, relaxin will likely be of considerable clinical interest.

Sufficient evidence has accumulated since the late 1970s to discard the long-held view that relaxin in mammals is produced only by the female. Moreover, as in the female, the apparent source of relaxin in the male varies among species. Relaxinlike immunoactivity has been localized in the human, armadillo, and dog prostate; pig seminal vesicles; and chicken testes. That the human male produces relaxin was established when human relaxin 2 was isolated from human seminal plasma, and it was demonstrated that the seminal plasma contained relaxin bioactivity. Whereas several studies provided indications that relaxin may enhance sperm motility and thereby enhance the capacity of sperm to fertilize oocytes, many studies do not provide support for this hypothesis. Accordingly, it remains to be established that relaxin has a physiologically important function in the male in any species.

In conclusion, many advances have been made toward a better understanding of the chemistry and physiology of relaxin since the mid-1970s. These studies have demonstrated that relaxin has diverse and vital physiologic roles during pregnancy and at parturition in the pig and rat. Consequently, the status of relaxin has been rapidly elevated from a poorly understood and frequently ignored hormone to one that requires substantive attention when the hormonal regulation of pregnancy and parturition in mammalian and other species is being considered.

The chemistry and physiology of relaxin are richly diverse among species. The primary structure, source, regulation of synthesis and secretion, quantities stored in source tissue(s), and target tissue vary extensively among species. This diversity has important implications. Sweeping statements concerning the chemistry and physiology of relaxin among species cannot be made. Understanding the chemistry and physiology of relaxin for a given species is dependent on detailed study of relaxin in that species. Although considerable progress has been made toward an understanding of the physiology of relaxin in a few species, accumulation of knowledge concerning this hormone is in its infancy. It is this reviewer's expectation that the many unexplored opportunities for further discoveries with relaxin will sustain the present high level of interest in this fascinating hormone for many years to come.

ACKNOWLEDGMENTS

I am grateful to the following persons for reviewing this manuscript and providing helpful advice for its improvement: Ms. L. L. Burger, Mr. M. J. Kuenzi, Dr. K. J. Lilley, Mr. G.-S. Min, Dr. D. G. Porter, Mr. J. E. Whaley, Mr. R. J. Winn, Dr. H. M. Zaleski, and Ms. S. Zhao. A special thanks to my wife Julie and sister Dr. Rhoda I. Sherwood for editorial assistance with this review. I also wish to thank Mrs. A. M. Roberts for the patience and high standards she maintained in typing this manuscript. I am indebted to Mrs. A. A. Prickett for her expert help in preparing illustrations.

REFERENCES

1. Abramowitz AA, Money WL, Zarrow MX, Talmage RVN, Kleinholz LH, Hisaw FL. Preparation, biological assay and properties of relaxin. *Endocrinology* 1944;34:103–114.
2. Abramson D, Hurwitt E, Lesnick G. Relaxin in human serum as a test of pregnancy. *Surg Gynecol Obstet* 1937;65:335–339.
3. Abramson D, Reid DE. Use of relaxin in treatment of threatened premature labor. *J Clin Endocrinol Metab* 1955;15: 206–209.
4. Abramson D, Roberts SM, Wilson PD. Relaxation of the pelvic joints in pregnancy. *Surg Gynecol Obstet* 1934;63:595–613.
5. Adair V, Stromer MH, Anderson LL. Progesterone secretion and mitochondrial size of aging porcine corpora lutea. *Anat Rec* 1989;223:252–256.
6. Adams WC, Frieden EH. Inhibition of post-partum uterine involution in the rat by relaxin. *Biol Reprod* 1985;33:1168–1173.
7. Adams WC, Hanousek CA, Frieden EH. Progesterone inhibits the uterotrophic effect of relaxin in immature rats. *Proc Soc Exp Biol Med* 1989;191:159–162.
8. Adashi EY, Resnick CE, Brodie AMH, Svoboda ME, Van Wyk JJ. Somatomedin-C-mediated potentiation of follicle-stimulating hormone-induced aromatase activity of cultured rat granulosa cells. *Endocrinology* 1985;117:2313–2320.
9. Adashi EY, Resnick CE, Hernandez ER, Svoboda ME, Van Wyk JJ. *In vivo* regulation of granulosa cell somatomedin-C/insulin-like growth factor I receptors. *Endocrinology* 1988; 122:1383–1389.
10. Addiego LA, Tsutsui T, Stewart DR, Stabenfeldt GH. Determination of the source of immunoreactive relaxin in the cat. *Biol Reprod* 1987;37:1165–1169.
11. Adelstein RS, Pato MD, Conti MA. The role of phosphorylation in regulating contractile proteins. *Adv Cyclic Nucleotide Res* 1981;14:361–373.
12. Afele S, Bryant-Greenwood GD, Chamley WA, Dax EM. Plasma relaxin immunoactivity in the pig at parturition and during nuzzling and suckling. *J Reprod Fertil* 1979;56:451–457.
13. Ahokas RA, Sibai BM, Anderson GD. Lack of evidence of a vasodepressor role for relaxin in spontaneously hypertensive and normotensive pregnant rats. *Am J Obstet Gynecol* 1989;161:618–622.
14. Akinbami MA, Meredith S, Warren JE Jr, Anthony RV, Day BN. Cervical dilation, conception rate, and concentrations of progesterone and estradiol-17β in postpartum ewes treated with porcine relaxin. *Theriogenology* 1990;34:927–940.
15. Albert A, Money WL, Zarrow MX. An improved method of extraction and purification of relaxin from fresh whole ovaries of the sow. *Endocrinology* 1947;40:370–374.
16. Alexandrova M, Soloff MS. Oxytocin receptors and parturition. I. Control of oxytocin receptor concentration in the rat myometrium at term. *Endocrinology* 1980;106:730–735.
17. Alexandrova M, Soloff MS. Oxytocin receptors and parturition. II. Concentrations of receptors for oxytocin and estrogen in the gravid and nongravid uterus at term. *Endocrinology* 1980;106:736–738.
18. Ali SM, McMurtry JP, Bagnell CA, Bryant-Greenwood GD. Immunocytochemical localization of relaxin in corpora lutea of sows throughout the estrous cycle. *Biol Reprod* 1986;34: 139–143.
19. Anderson LL. Relaxin localization in porcine and bovine ovaries by assay and morphological techniques. *Adv Exp Med Biol* 1982;143:1–67.

20. Anderson LL. Regulation of relaxin secretion and its role in pregnancy. *Adv Exp Med Biol* 1987;219:421–463.
21. Anderson LL, Adair V, Stromer MH, McDonald WG. Relaxin production and release after hysterectomy in the pig. *Endocrinology* 1983;113:677–686.
22. Anderson LL, Bast JD, Melampy RM. Relaxin in ovarian tissue during different reproductive stages in the rat. *J Endocrinol* 1973;59:371–372.
23. Anderson LL, Dyck GW, Mori H, Henricks DM, Melampy RM. Ovarian function in pigs following hypophyseal stalk transection or hypophysectomy. *Am J Physiol* 1967;212: 1188–1194.
24. Anderson LL, Ford JJ, Melampy RM, Cox DF. Relaxin in porcine corpora lutea during pregnancy and after hysterectomy. *Am J Physiol* 1973;225:1215–1219.
25. Anderson LL, Perezgrovas R, O'Byrne EM, Steinetz BG. Biological actions of relaxin in pigs and beef cattle. *Ann NY Acad Sci* 1982;380:131–150.
26. Anderson MB. Bioassay of porcine relaxin components by *in vitro* inhibition of rat uterine contractions. *Endocrinology* 1984;114:364–368.
27. Anderson MB, Collado-Torres M, Vaupel MR. Absence of relaxin immunostaining in the male reproductive tracts of the rat and mouse. *J Histochem Cytochem* 1986;34:945–948.
28. Anderson MB, Long JA. Localization of relaxin in the pregnant rat. Bioassay of tissue extracts and cell fractionation studies. *Biol Reprod* 1978;18:110–117.
29. Anderson MB, Long JA, Hayashida T. Immunofluorescence studies on the localization of relaxin in the corpus luteum of the pregnant rat. *Biol Reprod* 1975;13:499–504.
30. Anderson MB, Sherwood OD. Ultrastructural localization of relaxin immunoreactivity in corpora lutea of pregnant rats. *Endocrinology* 1984;114:1124–1127.
31. Anderson MB, Vaupel MR, Sherwood OD. Pregnant mouse corpora lutea: Immunocytochemical localization of relaxin and ultrastructure. *Biol Reprod* 1984;31:391–397.
32. Anderson RR, ed. Relaxin. *Adv Exp Med Biol* 1982;143.
33. Anderson TR, Mayer GL, Hebert N, Nicoll CS. Interactions among prolactin, epidermal growth factor and proinsulin on the growth and morphology of the pigeon crop-sac mucosal epithelium *in vivo*. *Endocrinology* 1987;120:1258–1264.
34. Anderson TR, Rodriguez J, Nicoll CS, Spencer EM. The synlactin hypothesis: Prolactin's mitogenic action may involve synergism with a somatomedin-like molecule. In: Spencer EM, ed. *Insulin-Like Growth Factors/Somatomedins.* Berlin: Walter de Gruyter, 1983;71–78.
35. Anwer K, Hovington JA, Sanborn BM. Antagonism of contractants and relaxants at the level of intracellular calcium and phosphoinositide turnover in the rat uterus. *Endocrinology* 1989;124:2995–3002.
36. Anwer K, Hovington JA, Sanborn BM. Involvement of protein kinase A in the regulation of intracellular free calcium and phosphoinositide turnover in rat myometrium. *Biol Reprod* 1990;43:851–859.
37. Arakaki RF, Kleinfeld RG, Bryant-Greenwood FC. Immunofluorescence studies using antisera to crude and to purified porcine relaxin. *Biol Reprod* 1980;23:153–159.
38. Ash RW, Heap RB. Oestrogen, progesterone and corticosteroid concentrations in peripheral plasma of sows during pregnancy, parturition, lactation, and after weaning. *J Endocrinol* 1975;64:141–154.
39. Astwood EB, Greep RO. A corpus luteum-stimulating substance in the rat placenta. *Proc Soc Exp Biol Med* 1938;38:713–716.
40. Bagna B, Schwabe C, Anderson LL. Effect of relaxin on facilitation of parturition in dairy heifers. *J Reprod Fertil* 1991;91:605–615.
41. Bagnell CA. Identification of immunoreactive relaxin in the neurohypophysis of the pig. *Biol Reprod* 1990;42(suppl 1):102 (abst).
42. Bagnell CA. Production and biologic action of relaxin within the ovarian follicle: An overview. *Steroids* 1991;56:242–246.
43. Bagnell CA, Ainsworth L, Bryant-Greenwood GD, Greenwood FC. Follicular relaxin. A role in the paracrine control of ovarian function. In: Naftolin F, De Cherney AH, eds. *The Control of Follicle Development, Ovulation and Luteal Function: Lessons from In Vitro Fertilization.* New York: Raven Press, 1987;35–44.
44. Bagnell CA, Ayau E, Downey BR, Tsang BK, Ainsworth L. Localization of relaxin during formation of the porcine corpus luteum. *Biol Reprod* 1989;40:835–841.
45. Bagnell CA, Baker NK, McMurtry JP, Brocht DM, Lewis GS. Control of luteal relaxin release by prostaglandin F2α: Differences in the sow cycle and pregnancy. *Proc Soc Exp Biol Med* 1990;194:125–130.
46. Bagnell CA, Domondon MC, Bryant-Greenwood GD. Plasminogen activator (PA) activity in rat and pig follicles during follicular development. In: Ryan RJ, Tofts DO, eds. *Proceedings of the 5th Ovarian Workshops.* Champaign, IL: Ovarian Workshops. 1984;233–238.
47. Bagnell CA, Frando LB, Downey BR, Tsang BK, Ainsworth L. Localization of relaxin in the pig follicle during preovulatory development. *Biol Reprod* 1987;37:235–240.
48. Bagnell CA, McMurtry JP, Baker NK, Timtim JK, Bryant-Greenwood GD. Detection of relaxin by immunohistochemistry in the corpus luteum during lactation. *Biol Reprod* 1987;37:1317–1325.
49. Bagnell CA, Tashima L, Tsark W, Ali SM, McMurtry JP. Relaxin gene expression in the sow corpus luteum during the cycle, pregnancy, and lactation. *Endocrinology* 1990;126:2514–2520.
50. Bagnell CA, Tsark W, Tashima L, Downey BR, Tsang BK, Ainsworth L. Relaxin gene expression in the porcine follicle during preovulatory development induced by gonadotrophins. *J Mol Endocrinol* 1990;5:211–219.
51. Bagnell CA, Zhang Q, Ohleth K, Downey BR, Ainsworth L. Developmental expression of the relaxin gene in the porcine corpus luteum. *Biol Reprod* 1991;44(suppl 1):100 (abst).
52. Bailey SB, Vaupel MR, Steinetz BG, Anderson MB. Morphological changes in the cervix of the pregnant hamster and correlation with serum relaxin levels. *Anat Rec* 1987;218:13 (abst).
53. Baker EN, Blundell TL, Cutfield JF, et al. The structure of 2 Zn pig insulin crystals at 1.5 Å resolution. *Philos Trans R Soc Lond [Biol]* 1988;319:369–456.
54. Bakhit C, Kado-Fong H, Lewis D, Tregear G, Malfroy B. Presence of relaxin-like peptides in rat brain. *17th Annual Meeting of the Society for Neuroscience,* New Orleans, LA, 1987;1660 (abst).
55. Bakke T, Gytre T. Ultrasonic and mechanical measurement of human cervical consistency. In: Naftolin F, Stubblefield PG, eds. *Dilatation of the Uterine Cervix.* New York: Raven Press, 1980;219–232.
56. Balboni GC, Denkova R, Vannelli GB, Zecchi S. Immunofluorescent localization of relaxin-like molecules in the granulosa cells of cavitary follicles of human and porcine ovary. In: Bigazzi M, Greenwood FC, Gasparri F, eds. *Biology of Relaxin and Its Role in the Human.* Amsterdam: Excerpta Medica, 1983;216–218.
57. Bani G, Bani Sacchi T, Bigazzi M. Response of the pigeon crop sac to mammotropic hormones: Comparison between relaxin and prolactin. *Gen Comp Endocrinol* 1990;80:16–23.
58. Bani G, Bani Sacchi T, Bigazzi M, Bianchi S. Effects of relaxin on the microvasculature of mouse mammary gland. *Histol Histopathol* 1988;3:337–343.
59. Bani G, Bani Sacchi T, Cecchi R, Bigazzi M. The effects of relaxin on the pigeon crop-sac mucosa. Light and electron microscopic study. *Z Mikrosk-Anat Forsch (Leipz)* 1987;101: 577–596.
60. Bani G, Bianchi S, Formigli L, Bigazzi M. Responsiveness of mouse parametrial fat to relaxin. *Acta Anat* 1989;134:128–132.
61. Bani G, Bigazzi M. Morphological changes induced in mouse mammary gland by porcine and human relaxin. *Acta Anat* 1984;119:149–154.
62. Bani G, Bigazzi M, Bani D. Effects of relaxin on the mouse mammary gland. I. The myoepithelial cells. *J Endocrinol Invest* 1985;8:207–215.
63. Bani G, Bigazzi M, Bani D. The effects of relaxin on the mouse mammary gland. II. The epithelium. *J Endocrinol Invest* 1986;9:145–152.

64. Bani G, Bigazzi M, Bani Sacchi T. Relaxin as a mammotrophic hormone. *Exp Clin Endocrinol* 1991;10:143–150.
65. Bani Sacchi T, Bianchi S, Bani G, Bigazzi M. Ultrastructural studies on white adipocyte differentiation in the mouse mammary gland following estrogen and relaxin. *Acta Anat* 1987;129:1–9.
66. Barbieri RL, Makris A, Randall RW, Daniels G, Kistner RW, Ryan KJ. Insulin stimulates androgen accumulation in incubations of ovarian stroma obtained from women with hyperandrogenism. *J Clin Endocrinol Metab* 1986;62:904–910.
67. Bassett EG, Phillipps DSM. Changes in the pelvic region of the ewe during pregnancy and parturition. *N Z Vet J* 1955;3:20–25.
68. Batra S. Effect of oxytocin on calcium influx and efflux in the rat myometrium. *Eur J Pharmacol* 1986;120:57–62.
69. Beams HW, Meyer RK. The formation of pigeon "milk." *Physiol Zool* 1931;4:486–500.
70. Beck CA, Garner CW. Stimulation of DNA synthesis in rat uterine cells by growth factors and uterine extracts. *Mol Cell Endocrinol* 1992;84:109–118.
71. Beck P, Adler P, Szlachter N, Goldsmith LT, Steinetz BG, Weiss G. Synergistic effect of human relaxin and progesterone on human myometrial contractions. *Int J Gynaecol Obstet* 1982;20:141–144.
72. Bedarker S, Blundell T, Gowan LK, McDonald JK, Schwabe C. On the three-dimensional structure of relaxin. *Ann NY Acad Sci* 1982;380:22–33.
73. Bedarker S, Turnell WG, Blundell TL, Schwabe C. Relaxin has conformational homology with insulin. *Nature* 1977;270: 449–451.
74. Bell GI, Pictet RL, Rutter WJ, Cordell B, Tischer E, Goodman HM. Sequence of human insulin gene. *Nature* 1980;284:26–32.
75. Bell RJ, Eddie LW, Lester AR, Wood EC, Johnston PD, Niall HD. Levels of relaxin in *in vitro* fertilization pregnancies in the first trimester measured with an homologous radioimmunoassay for human relaxin. *J In Vitro Fert Embryo Transfer* 1986;3:184.
76. Bell RJ, Eddie LW, Lester AR, Wood EC, Johnston PD, Niall HD. Relaxin in human pregnancy serum measured with an homologous radioimmunoassay. *Obstet Gynecol* 1987;69: 585–589.
77. Bell RJ, Eddie LW, Lester AR, Wood EC, Johnston PD, Niall HD. Antenatal serum levels of relaxin in patients having preterm labor. *Br J Obstet Gynaecol* 1988;95:1264–1267.
78. Bell RJ, Sutton B, Eddie LW, Healy DL, Johnston PD, Tregear GW. Relaxin levels in antenatal patients following *in vitro* fertilization. *Fertil Steril* 1989;52:85–87.
79. Bell SC, Jackson JA, Ashmore J, Zhu HH, Tseng L. Regulation of insulin-like growth factor-binding protein-1 synthesis and secretion by progestin and relaxin in long term cultures of human endometrial stromal cells. *J Clin Endocrinol Metab* 1991;72:1014–1024.
80. Bell SC, Patel SR, Jackson JA, Waites GT. Major secretory protein of human decidualized endometrium in pregnancy is an insulin-like growth factor-binding protein. *J Endocrinol* 1988;118:317–328.
81. Belt WD, Anderson LL, Cavazos LF, Melampy RM. Cytoplasmic granules and relaxin levels in porcine corpora lutea. *Endocrinology* 1971;89:1–10.
82. Belt WD, Cavazos LF, Anderson LL, Kraeling RR. Fine structure and progesterone levels in the corpus luteum of the pig during pregnancy and after hysterectomy. *Biol Reprod* 1970;2:98–113.
83. Benedetto MT, Tabanelli S, Gurpide E. Estrone sulfate sulfatase activity is increased during *in vitro* decidualization of stromal cells from human endometrium. *J Clin Endocrinol Metab* 1990;70:342–345.
84. Bennett HPJ, Hudson AM, Kelly L, McMartin C, Purdon GE. A rapid method, using octadecasilyl-silica for the extraction of certain peptides from tissues. *Biochem J* 1978;175:1139–1141.
85. Bentley G, Dodson E, Dodson G, Hodgkin D, Mercola D. Structure of insulin in 4-zinc insulin. *Nature* 1976;261: 166–168.
86. Bernstein P, Crelin ES. Bony pelvic sexual dimorphism in the rat. *Anat Rec* 1967;157:517–526.
87. Bethea CL, Cronin MJ, Haluska GJ, Novy MJ. The effect of relaxin infusion on prolactin and growth hormone secretion in monkeys. *J Clin Endocrinol Metab* 1989;69:956–962.
88. Bianchi S, Bani G, Bigazzi M. Effects of relaxin on the mouse mammary gland. III. The fat pad. *J Endocrinol Invest* 1986;9:153–160.
89. Bianchi S, Petrucci F, Bani G. The effects of relaxin on the blood capillaries of the pigeon crop sac. *Z Mikrosk-Anat Forsch (Leipz)* 1988;102:221–227.
90. Bigazzi M, Bani G, Bani Sacchi T, Petrucci F, Bianchi S. Relaxin: A mammotropic hormone promoting growth and differentiation of the pigeon crop sac mucosa. *Acta Endocrinol* 1988;117:181–188.
91. Bigazzi M, Brandi ML, Bani G, Bani Sacchi T. Relaxin influences the growth of MCF-7 breast cancer cells. Mitogenic and antimitogenic action depends on peptide concentration. *Cancer* 1992;70:639–643.
92. Bigazzi M, Bruni P, Nardi E, et al. Human decidual relaxin. *Ann NY Acad Sci* 1982;380:87–99.
93. Bigazzi M, Del Mese A, Petrucci F, Casali R, Novelli GP. The local administration of relaxin induces changes in the microcirculation of the rat mesocaecum. *Acta Endocrinol* 1986;112: 296–299.
94. Bigazzi M, Greenwood FC, Gasparri F, eds. *Biology of Relaxin and Its Role in the Human.* Amsterdam: Excerpta Medica, 1983.
95. Bigazzi M, Nardi E. Prolactin and relaxin: Antagonism on the spontaneous motility of the uterus. *J Clin Endocrinol Metab* 1981;53:665–667.
96. Bigazzi M, Nardi E, Bruni P, Petrucci F. Relaxin in human decidua. *J Clin Endocrinol Metab* 1980;51:939–941.
97. Bigazzi M, Petrucci F, Nardi E, Scarselli G. Decidua and other extraluteal sources of human relaxin. In: Bigazzi M, Greenwood FC, Gasparri F, eds. *Biology of Relaxin and Its Role in the Human.* Amsterdam: Excerpta Medica, 1983;377–388.
98. Bloom G, Paul K-G, Wiqvist N. A uterine-relaxing factor in the pregnant rat. *Acta Endocrinol (Copenh)* 1958;28:112–118.
99. Blundell T. Conformation and molecular biology of polypeptide hormones. I. Insulin, insulin-like growth factor, and relaxin. *Trends Biochem Sci Rev* 1979;4:51–54.
100. Blundell TL, Bedarker S, Rinderknecht E, Humbel RE. Insulin-like growth factor: A model for tertiary structure accounting for immunoreactivity and receptor binding. *Proc Natl Acad Sci USA* 1978;75:180–184.
101. Blundell TL, Dodson GG, Hodgkin DC, Mercola DA. Insulin: The structure in the crystal and its reflection in chemistry and biology. *Adv Protein Chem* 1972;26:279–402.
102. Blundell T, Gowan LK, Schwabe C. Relaxin—a member of the insulin family? In: Bigazzi M, Greenwood FC, Gasparri F, eds. *Biology of Relaxin and Its Role in the Human.* Amsterdam: Excerpta Medica, 1983;14–21.
103. Blundell TL, Humbel RE. Hormone families: Pancreatic hormones and homologous growth factors. *Nature* 1980;287: 781–787.
104. Blundell T, Wood S. The conformation, flexibility, and dynamics of polypeptide hormones. *Annu Rev Biochem* 1982;51:123–154.
105. Bodsch W, Struck H. Enzyme-immunoassay for the peptide hormone relaxin. *Fresenius Z Anal Chem* 1980;301:133–134.
106. Bolton AE, Hunter WM. The labelling of proteins to high specific radioactivities by conjugation to a ^{125}I-containing acylating agent. *Biochem J* 1973;133:529–539.
107. Bonaventure J, De La Tour B, Tsagris L, Eddie LW, Tregear G, Corvol MT. Effect of relaxin on the phenotype of collagens synthesized by cultured rabbit chondrocytes. *Biochim Biophys Acta* 1988;972:209–220.
108. Bongers-Binder S, Burgardt A, Seeger H, Voelter W, Lippert TH. Distribution of immunoreactive relaxin in the genital tract and in the mammary gland of nonpregnant women. *Clin Exp Obstet Gynecol* 1991;18:161–164.
109. Borjesson BW, John MJ, Niall HD. The topographical mapping of porcine relaxin: Accessibility of hydrophobic residues and amino groups. In: Bryant-Greenwood GD, Niall HD, Green-

wood FC, eds. *Relaxin.* New York: Elsevier/North-Holland, 1981;93–95.

110. Bosc MJ, du Mesnil du Buisson F, Locatelli A. Mise en évidence d'un controle foetal de la parturition chez la truie. Interactions avec la fonction lutéale. *C R Acad Sci Paris* 1974;278: 1507–1510.
111. Boucek RJ. Biochemical and histological aspects of *in vivo* cultivated connective tissue. In: *Lectures on Orthopedics and Rheumatic Diseases.* Dedication volume, Hospital for Special Surgery. New Haven, CT: Quinnipiak Press, 1956;155–158.
112. Boyd S, Kendall JZ, Mento N, Bryant-Greenwood GD. Relaxin immunoactivity in plasma during the reproductive cycle of the female guinea pig. *Biol Reprod* 1981;24:405–41.
113. Boyers SP, Stewart DR, Douglas GC, et al. Immunocytochemical localization of relaxin and prorelaxin in endometrial biopsies from normal and out-of-phase cycles. *Program of the 39th Annual Meeting of the Society for Gynecological Investigation,* San Antonio, TX, 1992;300 (abst).
114. Brackett KH, Dubois W, Mather FB, Roberts RF, Fields PA, Fields MJ. Relaxin: An ovarian peptidyl hormone in an avian species (*Gallus domesticus*). *Biol Reprod* 1985;32(suppl 1):43 (abst).
115. Bradbury MWB. The blood-brain barrier, transport across the cerebral endothelium. *Circ Res* 1985;57:213–222.
116. Braddon SA. Stimulation of ornithine decarboxylase by relaxin. *Biochem Biophys Res Commun* 1978;80:75–80.
117. Braddon SA. Relaxin-dependent adenosine 3′,5′-monophosphate concentration changes in the mouse pubic symphysis. *Endocrinology* 1978;102:1292–1299.
118. Bradham GB, Stallworth JM, Brailsford LE, Threatt BA. Clinical evaluation of relaxin in ulcerative ischemic vascular or collagen diseases. *Angiology* 1962;13:418–420.
119. Bradshaw JMC, Downing SJ, Moffatt A, Hinton JC, Porter DG. Demonstration of some of the physiological properties of rat relaxin. *J Reprod Fertil* 1981;63:145–153.
120. Bradshaw RA, Niall HD. Insulin-related growth factors. *Trends Biochem Sci Rev* 1978;3:274–278.
121. Brandi ML, Bigazzi M, Bani G, Bani Sacchi T. Mitogenic effect of relaxin on pigeon crop mucosa and human breast cancer cells in culture. *J Endocrinol Invest* 1990;13(suppl 2):301 (abst).
122. Braverman LE, Ingbar SH. Effects of preparations containing relaxin on thyroid function in the female rat. *Endocrinology* 1963;72:337–341.
123. Brennan DM, Zarrow MX. Water and electrolyte content of the uterus of the intact and adrenalectomized rat treated with relaxin and various steroid hormones. *Endocrinology* 1959;64: 907–913.
124. Brenner SH, Lessing JB, D'Eletto RD, Weiss G. Relaxin-like bioactivity in pooled human pregnancy serum. *Obstet Gynecol* 1985;66:46–49.
125. Brenner SH, Lessing JB, Schoenfeld C, Amelar RD, Dubin L, Weiss G. Stimulation of human sperm cervical mucus penetration *in vitro* by relaxin. *Fertil Steril* 1984;42:92–96.
126. Brenner SH, Lessing JB, Schoenfeld C, et al. Human semen relaxin and its correlation with the parameters of semen analysis. *Fertil Steril* 1987;47:714–716.
127. Brenner SH, Lessing JB, Weiss G. The effect of *in vivo* progesterone administration on relaxin-inhibited rat uterine contractions. *Am J Obstet Gynecol* 1984;148:946–950.
128. Bret AJ, Coiffard P, Motamedi. Releasine: Son emploi et ses résultats au cours de la gravidité dans les manaces d'avortement et d'accouchement prématuré. *Rev Fr Gynecol Obstet* 1963;58:649–668.
129. Brody S, Wiqvist N. Ovarian hormones and uterine growth: Effects of estradiol, progesterone, and relaxin on cell growth and cell division in the rat uterus. *Endocrinology* 1961;68:971–977.
130. Brown H, Sanger F, Kitai R. The structure of pig and sheep insulins. *Biochem J* 1955;60:556–565.
131. Bruni P, Bigazzi M, Farnararo M. The interaction of porcine and human relaxin with the mouse uterus: Effect on some carbohydrate-metabolizing enzymes. *Mol Physiol* 1982;2: 357–362.
132. Bryant GD. The detection of relaxin in porcine, ovine, and human plasma by radioimmunoassay. *Endocrinology* 1972;91: 1113–1117.
133. Bryant GD, Chamley WA. Changes in relaxin and prolactin immunoactivities in ovine plasma following suckling. *J Reprod Fertil* 1976;46:457–459.
134. Bryant GD, Chamley WA. Plasma relaxin and prolactin immunoactivities in pregnancy and at parturition in the ewe. *J Reprod Fertil* 1976;48:201–204.
135. Bryant GD, Panter MEA, Stelmasiak T. Immunoreactive relaxin in human serum during the menstrual cycle. *J Clin Endocrinol Metab* 1975;41:1065–1069.
136. Bryant GD, Sassin JF, Weitzman ED, Kapen S, Frantz A. Relaxin immunoactivity in human plasma during a 24-hr period. *J Reprod Fertil* 1976;48:389–392.
137. Bryant-Greenwood GD. Radioimmunoassay of relaxin. In: Abraham GE, ed. *Handbook of Radioimmunoassay.* New York: Marcel Dekker, 1977;243–273.
138. Bryant-Greenwood GD. Relaxin as a new hormone. *Endocr Rev* 1982;3:62–90.
139. Bryant-Greenwood GD. The human relaxins: Consensus and dissent. *Mol Cell Endocrinol* 1991;79:C125–C132.
140. Bryant-Greenwood GD. Human decidual and placental relaxins. *Reprod Fertil Dev* 1991;3:385–389.
141. Bryant-Greenwood GD, Greenwood FC. Specificity of radioimmunoassays for relaxin. *J Endocrinol* 1979;81:239–247.
142. Bryant-Greenwood GD, Greenwood FC. Postulated roles for luteal or decidual relaxins at parturition in the pregnant sow and woman. In: Mitchell BF, ed. *The Physiology and Biochemistry of Human Fetal Membranes.* Ithaca, NY: Perinatology Press, 1988;141–156.
143. Bryant-Greenwood GD, Jeffrey R, Ralph MM, Seamark RF. Relaxin production by the porcine ovarian Graafian follicle *in vitro. Biol Reprod* 1980;23:792–800.
144. Bryant-Greenwood GD, Niall HD, Greenwood FC, eds. *Relaxin.* New York: Elsevier/North-Holland, 1981.
145. Bryant-Greenwood GD, Rees MCP, Turnbull AC. Immunohistochemical localization of relaxin, prolactin and prostaglandin synthase in human amnion, chorion and decidua. *J Endocrinol* 1987;114:491–496.
146. Bryant-Greenwood GD, Tashima L, Greenwood FC, Taylor E, Peaker M. Endometrial relaxin: Effects of mastectomy in the cyclic and pregnant guinea pig. *Endocrinology* 1991;129: 2119–2125.
147. Buckle JW, Nathanielsz PW. The effect of low doses of prostaglandin $F_{2\alpha}$ infused into the aorta of unrestrained pregnant rats: Observations on induction of parturition and effect on plasma progesterone concentration. *Prostaglandins* 1973;4:443–457.
148. Büllesbach EE, Gowan LK, Schwabe C, Steinetz BG, O'Byrne E, Callard IP. Isolation, purification and the sequence of relaxin from spiny dogfish *Squalus acanthias. Eur J Biochem* 1986;161:335–341.
149. Büllesbach EE, Schwabe C. [Å-phenylalanyl] relaxin (porcine): An active intermediate. *Biochem Biophys Res Commun* 1985;126:130–135.
150. Büllesbach EE, Schwabe C. Naturally occurring porcine relaxins and large-scale preparation of the B29 hormone. *Biochemistry* 1985;24:7717–7722.
151. Büllesbach EE, Schwabe C. Preparation and properties of α- and ϵ-amino-protected porcine relaxin derivatives. *Biochemistry* 1985;24:7722–7728.
152. Büllesbach EE, Schwabe C. Preparation and properties of porcine relaxin derivatives shortened at the amino terminus of the A chain. *Biochemistry* 1986;25:5998–6004.
153. Büllesbach EE, Schwabe C. Relaxin structure. Quasi allosteric effect of the NH_2-terminal A-chain helix. *J Biol Chem* 1987;262:12496–12501.
154. Büllesbach EE, Schwabe C. On the receptor binding site of relaxins. *Int J Pept Protein Res* 1988;32:361–367.
155. Büllesbach EE, Schwabe C. Monobiotinylated relaxins: Preparation and chemical properties of the mono(biotinyl-ϵ-aminohexanoyl) porcine relaxin. *Int J Pept Protein Res* 1990; 35:416–423.
156. Büllesbach EE, Schwabe C. Total synthesis of human relaxin

and human relaxin derivatives by solid-phase peptide synthesis and site-directed chain combination. *J Biol Chem* 1991; 266:10754–10761.

157. Büllesbach EE, Schwabe C, Callard IP. Relaxin from an oviparous species, the skate (*Raja erinacea*). *Biochem Biophys Res Commun* 1987;143:273–280.
158. Büllesbach E, Warr G, Schwabe C. Antigenically important regions of the relaxin molecule: Studies with monoclonal antibodies. *Life Sci* 1987;41:989–994.
159. Büllesbach EE, Yang S, Schwabe C. On the native conformation of human relaxin-II. Sensitive dependence upon glycine A14 in the A chain loop. (*In press*).
160. Büllesbach EE, Yang S, Schwabe C. The receptor-binding site of human relaxin II: A dual prong-binding mechanism. *J Biol Chem* 1992;267:22957–22960.
161. Burgardt A, Bauer H, Lippert TH, Voelter W. Purification and biological activity of relaxin from human seminal fluid. In: Bigazzi M, Greenwood FC, Gasparri F, eds. *Biology of Relaxin and Its Role in the Human.* Amsterdam: Excerpta Medica, 1983;399–401.
162. Burns PJ, Fleming SA. Computerized analysis of sperm motion: Effects of relaxin on cryopreserved equine spermatozoa. *Program of the 14th Annual Meeting of the American Society of Andrology,* New Orleans, LA, 1989;31 (abst).
163. Butler WR, Boyd RD. Relaxin enhances synchronization of parturition induced with prostaglandin $F_{2\alpha}$ in swine. *Biol Reprod* 1983;28:1061–1065.
164. Buttle HL, Lin CL. The effect of insulin and relaxin upon mitosis (*in vitro*) in mammary tissue from pregnant and lactating pigs. *Domest Anim Endocrinol* 1991;8:565–571.
165. Bylander JE, Frieden EH, Adams WC. Effects of porcine relaxins upon uterine hypertrophy and protein metabolism in mice. *Proc Soc Exp Biol Med* 1987;185:76–80.
166. Cabrol D, Huszar G, Romero R, Naftolin F. Gestational changes in the rat uterine cervix: Protein, collagen, and glycosaminoglycan content. In: Ellwood DA, Anderson ABM, eds. *The Cervix in Pregnancy and Labour.* New York: Churchill Livingstone, 1981;34–39.
167. Calder AA. The human cervix in pregnancy: A clinical perspective. In: Ellwood DA, Anderson ABM, eds. *The Cervix in Pregnancy and Labour.* New York: Churchill Livingstone, 1981;103–122.
168. Caldwell RW, Bellows RA, Hall JA, Anthony RV. Administration of pig relaxin to beef heifers 4 to 7 days prepartum. *J Reprod Fertil* 1990;90:165–174.
169. Caldwell RW, Whittier JC, Smith MF, Morrow RE, Anthony RV. Parturition in beef cows following administration of porcine relaxin at ten days prepartum. *Theriogenology* 1990;33:613–625.
170. Callard IP, Abrams-Motz V. Hormonal regulation of myometrial activity in the turtle *Chrysemys picta. Am Zool* 1985;25:117 (abst).
171. Callard IP, Klosterman LL, Sorbera LA, Fileti LA, Reese JC. Endocrine regulation of reproduction in elasmobranchs: Archetype for terrestrial vertebrates. *J Exp Zool* 1989;2(suppl):12–22.
172. Cameron DF, Corton GL, Larkin LH. Relaxin-like antigenicity in the armadillo prostate gland. *Ann NY Acad Sci* 1982;380:231–240.
173. Camiel MR. Relaxin and the radiolucent fissure in the symphysis pubis during pregnancy: The gas phenomenon. *Am J Obstet Gynecol* 1986;154:1104–1105.
174. Canipari R, Strickland S. Plasminogen activator in the rat ovary. *J Biol Chem* 1985;260:5121–5125.
175. Canova-Davis E, Baldonado IP, Teshima GM. Characterization of chemically synthesized human relaxin by high-performance liquid chromatography. *J Chromatogr* 1990;508:81–96.
176. Canova-Davis E, Kessler TJ, Lee P-J, et al. Use of recombinant DNA derived human relaxin to probe the structure of the native protein. *Biochemistry* 1991;30:6006–6013.
177. Canova-Davis E, Kessler TJ, Ling VT. Transpeptidation during the analytical proteolysis of proteins. *Anal Biochem* 1991;196:39–45.
178. Canova-Davis E, Teshima GM, Kessler TJ, Lee P-J, Guzzetta AW, Hancock WS. Strategies for an analytical examination of biological pharmaceuticals. In: Horvath C, Nikelly JG, eds. *Analytical Biotechnology: Capillary Electrophoresis and Chromatography.* Washington, DC: American Chemical Society, 1990;90–112.
179. Carminati P, Luzzani F, Soffientini A, Lerner LJ. Influence of day of pregnancy on rat placental, uterine, and ovarian prostaglandin synthesis and metabolism. *Endocrinology* 1975;97: 1071–1079.
180. Carsten ME, Miller JD. Effects of prostaglandins and oxytocin on calcium release from a uterine microsomal fraction. *J Biol Chem* 1977;252:1576–1581.
181. Casey PJ, Liu IKM, Stewart DR, Scott MA. The effects of equine relaxin on sperm longevity and motility in chilled and cryopreserved equine semen. *J Reprod Fertil* 1992; 44(suppl):645–646.
182. Casten GG, Boucek RJ. Use of relaxin in the treatment of scleroderma. *JAMA* 1958;166:319–324.
183. Casten GG, Gilmore HR, Houghton FE, Samuels SS. A new approach to the management of obliterative peripheral arterial disease. *Angiology* 1960;11:408–414.
184. Castracane VD, D'Eletto R, Weiss G. Relaxin secretion in the baboon (*Papio cynocephalus*). In: Greenwald GS, Terranova PF, eds. *Factors Regulating Ovarian Function.* New York: Raven Press, 1983;415–419.
185. Castracane VD, Jordon VC. The effect of estrogen and progesterone on uterine prostaglandin biosynthesis in the ovariectomized rat. *Biol Reprod* 1975;13:587–596.
186. Castracane VD, Lessing J, Brenner S, Weiss G. Relaxin in the pregnant baboon: Evidence for local production in reproductive tissues. *J Clin Endocrinol Metab* 1985;60:133–136.
187. Catala S, Deis RP. Effect of estrogen upon parturition, maternal behavior and lactation in ovariectomized pregnant rats. *J Endocrinol* 1973;56:219–225.
188. Catchpole HR, Joseph NR, Engel MB. The action of relaxin on the pubic symphysis of the guinea-pig, studied electrometrically. *J Endocrinol* 1952;8:377–385.
189. Cavazos LF, Anderson LL, Belt WD, Henricks DM, Kraeling RR, Melampy RM. Fine structure and progesterone levels in the corpus luteum of the pig during the estrous cycle. *Biol Reprod* 1969;1:83–106.
190. Challis JRG, Heap RB, Illingworth DV. Concentrations of oestrogen and progesterone in the plasma of nonpregnant, pregnant and lactating guinea pigs. *J Endocrinol* 1971;51:333–345.
191. Chalmers TM, Hearnshaw JR. A case of scleroderma treated with relaxin. *Ann Rheum Dis* 1961;20:202.
192. Chamley WA, Bagoyo MM, Bryant-Greenwood GD. *In vitro* response of relaxin-treated rat uterus to prostaglandins and oxytocin. *Prostaglandins* 1977;14:763–769.
193. Chamley WA, Bagoyo MM, Bryant-Greenwood GD. Potencies of porcine relaxins using two bioassays. *J Endocrinol* 1981;88:89–96.
194. Chamley WA, Parkington HC. Relaxin inhibits the plateau component of the action potential in the circular myometrium of the rat. *J Physiol* 1984;353:51–65.
195. Chamley WA, Stelmasiack T, Bryant GD. Plasma relaxin immunoactivity during the oestrus cycle of the ewe. *J Reprod Fertil* 1975;45:455–461.
196. Chan SYW, Tang LCH. Lack of effect of exogenous relaxin on the fertilizing capacity of human spermatozoa. *IRCS Med Sci* 1984;12:879–880.
197. Chan WY. Uterine and placental prostaglandins and their modulation of oxytocin sensitivity and contractility in the parturient uterus. *Biol Reprod* 1983;29:680–688.
198. Cheah SH, Lingam VTJ, Ragavan M. Effects of 17 β-estradiol (E) and relaxin (R) on cervical extensibility in the rat. *Program of the 17th International Union of Physiological Sciences,* Helsinki, Finland, 1989;183 (abst).
199. Cheah SH, Ng KH, Johgalingam VT, Ragavan M. Effects of estradiol (E) and relaxin (R) on collagen organization in the rat cervix: Light and electron microscope studies. *Biol Reprod* 1992;46(suppl 1):172 (abst).
200. Cheah SH, Sherwood OD. Target tissues for relaxin in the rat:

Tissue distribution of injected ^{125}I-labeled relaxin and tissue changes in adenosine 3′,5′-monophosphate levels after *in vitro* relaxin incubation. *Endocrinology* 1980;106:1203–1209.
201. Cheah SH, Sherwood OD. Effects of relaxin on *in vivo* uterine contractions in conscious and unrestrained estrogen-treated and steroid-untreated ovariectomized rats. *Endocrinology* 1981;109: 2076–2083.
202. Cheah SH, Sherwood OD. Effect of preparturient 17 β-estradiol and relaxin on parturition and pup survival in the rat. *Endocrinology* 1988;122:1958–1963.
203. Chen G, Elias JM, Steinetz BG, Tseng L. Immunocytochemical localization of relaxin in human decidua and fetal membrane by colloidal gold labeled antibody. *J Histotechnol* 1987;10:99–100.
204. Chen G, Huang JR, Tseng L. The effect of relaxin on cyclic adenosine 3′5′-monophosphate concentrations in human endometrial glandular epithelial cells. *Biol Reprod* 1988;39:519–525.
205. Chew CS, Rinard GA. Glycogen levels in the rat myometrium at the end of pregnancy and immediately postpartum. *Biol Reprod* 1979;20:1111–1114.
206. Chihal HJ, Espey LL. Utilization of the relaxed symphysis pubis of guinea pigs for clues to the mechanism of ovulation. *Endocrinology* 1973;93:1441–1445.
207. Cipolla DC, Shire SJ. Analysis of oxidized human relaxin by reverse phase HPLC, mass spectrometry and bioassays. In: Villafranca JJ, ed. *Techniques in Protein Chemistry II*. New York: Academic Press, 1991;543–555.
208. Coggins EG, First NL. Effect of dexamethasone, methallibure, and fetal decapitation on porcine gestation. *J Anim Sci* 1977;44:1041–1049.
209. Cohen H. Relaxin: Studies dealing with isolation, purification, and characterization. *Trans NY Acad Sci* 1963;25:313–330.
210. Cole WC, Garfield RE. Evidence for physiological regulation of myometrial gap junction permeability. *Am J Physiol* 1986;20:C411–C420.
211. Colon JM, Gagliardi C, Schoenfeld C, Amelar RD, Dubin L, Weiss G. Human relaxin stimulates human sperm penetration of bovine cervical mucus. *Fertil Steril* 1989;52:340–342.
212. Colon JM, Ginsburg F, Lessing JB, et al. The effect of relaxin and prostaglandin E_2 on the motility of human spermatozoa. *Fertil Steril* 1986;46:1133–1139.
213. Corner GW. On the origin of the corpus luteum of the sow from both granulosa and theca interna. *Am J Anat* 1919;26:117–183.
214. Corteel M, Lemon M, Dubois M. Evolution de la réaction immunocytologique du corps jaune de truie au cours de la gestation. *J Physiol (Paris)* 1977;73:63A–64A.
215. Cossum PA, Dwyer KA, Roth M, et al. The disposition of a human relaxin (hRlx-2) in pregnant and nonpregnant rats. *Pharm Res* 1992;9:419–424.
216. Cossum PA, Hill DE, Bailey JR, Anderson JH, Slikker W Jr. Transplacental passage of a human relaxin administered to rhesus monkeys. *J Endocrinol* 1991;130:339–345.
217. Cowie AT, Cox CP, Folley SJ, Hosking ZD, Tindal JS. Relative efficiency of crystalline suspensions of hexoestrol and of oestradiol monobenzoate in inducing mammary development and lactation in the goat; and effects of relaxin on mammogenesis and lactation. *J Endocrinol* 1965;31:165–172.
218. Crawford RJ, Hammond VE, Roche PJ, Johnston PD, Tregear GW. Structure of rhesus monkey relaxin predicted by analysis of the single-copy rhesus monkey relaxin gene. *J Mol Endocrinol* 1989;3:169–174.
219. Crawford RJ, Hudson P, Shine J, Niall HD, Eddy RL, Shows TB. Two human relaxin genes are on chromosome 9. *EMBO J* 1984;3:2341–2345.
220. Crelin ES. The effect of estrogen and relaxin on intact and transplanted pubic symphyses in mice. *Anat Rec* 1954;118:380–381.
221. Crelin ES. The effects of androgen, estrogen, and relaxin on intact and transplanted pelves in mice. *Am J Anat* 1954;95:47–73.
222. Crelin ES. Response of the pubic symphysis in castrated mice to relaxin alone. *Anat Rec* 1956;124:397 (abst).
223. Crelin ES. Mitosis in adult cartilage. *Science* 1957;125:650.
224. Crelin ES. The development of bony pelvic sexual dimorphism in mice. *Ann NY Acad Sci* 1960;84:481–511.
225. Crelin ES. The development of the bony pelvis and its changes during pregnancy and parturition. *Trans NY Acad Sci* 1969;31:1049–1058.
226. Crelin ES, Brightman MW. The pelvis of the rat: Its response to estrogen and relaxin. *Anat Rec* 1957;128:467–484.
227. Crelin ES, Grillo MA. The conditioning effect of puberty on the response of the pubic symphysis in mice to estrogen and relaxin. *Anat Rec* 1957;127:407 (abst).
228. Crelin ES, Haines AL. The effects of locally applied estrogen on the pubic symphysis and knee joint in castrated mice. *Endocrinology* 1955;56:461–470.
229. Crelin ES, Honeyman MS. The inhibition of interpubic ligament formation by progesterone in pregnant mice. *Anat Rec* 1957;127:407 (abst).
230. Crelin ES, Levin J. The prepuberal pubic symphysis and uterus in the mouse: Their response to estrogen and relaxin. *Endocrinology* 1955;57:730–747.
231. Crelin ES, Newton EV. The pelvis of the free-tailed bat: Sexual dimorphism and pregnancy changes. *Anat Rec* 1969;164: 349–358.
232. Crish JF, Soloff MS, Shaw AR. Changes in relaxin precursor mRNA levels in the rat ovary during pregnancy. *J Biol Chem* 1986;261:1909–1913.
233. Crish JF, Soloff MS, Shaw AR. Changes in relaxin precursor messenger ribonucleic acid levels in ovaries of rats after hysterectomy, removal of conceptuses, and during the estrous cycle. *Endocrinology* 1986;119:1222–1228.
234. Cronin MJ, Malaska T. Characterization of relaxin-stimulated cyclic AMP in cultured rat anterior pituitary cells: Influence of dopamine, somatostatin and gender. *J Mol Endocrinol* 1989;3:175–182.
235. Cronin MJ, Malaska T, Bakhit C. Human relaxin increases cyclic AMP levels in cultured anterior pituitary cells. *Biochem Biophys Res Commun* 1987;148:1246–1251.
236. Csapo AI. Actomyosin formation by estrogen action. *Am J Physiol* 1950;162:406–410.
237. Csapo AI, Currie WB, Erdos T, Resch BA. Effect of passive immunization against estradiol on the regulatory profile and character of labor in the rat. *Am J Obstet Gynecol* 1978;132:464–470.
238. Cullen BM, Harkness RD. The effect of hormones on the physical properties and collagen content of the rat's uterine cervix. *J Physiol* 1960;152:419–436.
239. Cullen BM, Harkness RD. Effects of ovariectomy and of hormones on collageneous framework of the uterus. *Am J Physiol* 1964;206:621–627.
240. Cutts JH. Estrogen-induced breast cancer in the rat. *Can Cancer Conf* 1966;65:50–68.
241. Dallenbach FD, Dallenbach-Hellweg G. Immunohistologische untersuchungen zur lokalisation des relaxins in menschlicher placenta und decidua. *Virchows Arch Pathol Anat* 1964; 337:301–316.
242. Dallenbach-Hellweg G, Battista JV, Dallenbach FD. Immunohistological and histochemical localization of relaxin in the metrial gland of the pregnant rat. *Am J Anat* 1965;117:433–444.
243. Dallenbach-Hellweg G, Dawson AB, Hisaw FL. The effect of relaxin on the endometrium of monkeys. Histological and histochemical studies. *Am J Anat* 1966;119:61–71.
244. Danforth DN. Early studies of the anatomy and physiology of the human cervix—and implications for the future. In: Naftolin F, Stubblefield PG, eds. *Dilatation of the Uterine Cervix*. New York: Raven Press, 1980;3–15.
245. Datta IC, Karkun JN, Kar AB. Studies on physiology and biochemistry of the cervix: Changes in cervix of rats during pregnancy and post-partum periods. *Acta Biol Med Ger* 1968;20:163–172.
246. Dayanithi G, Cazalis M, Nordmann JJ. Relaxin affects the release of oxytocin and vasopressin from the neurohypophysis. *Nature* 1987;325:813–816.
247. De Camillis L, Pozzi V. Radiological study of the pubic symphysis after administration of relaxin. *Minerva Ginecol* 1961;13:19–21.
248. Decker WH, Thwaite W, Bordat S, Kayser R, Harami T, Camp-

bell J. Some effects of relaxin in obstetrics. *Obstet Gynecol* 1958;12:37–46.
249. De Cooman S, Gilliaux P, Thomas K. Immunoreactive relaxin-like substance in human split ejaculates. *Fertil Steril* 1983;39:111–113.
250. De Cooman S, Loumaye E, Thomas K. IR-relaxin in human seminal plasma. In: Bigazzi M, Greenwood FC, Gasparri F, eds. *Biology of Relaxin and Its Role in the Human.* Amsterdam: Excerpta Medica, 1983;350–360.
251. D'Eletto RD, Schoenfeld C, Weiss G. Partial purification of relaxin from human semen plasma using only reversed-phase liquid chromatography. In: Bigazzi M, Greenwood FC, Gasparri F, eds. *Biology of Relaxin and Its Role in the Human.* Amsterdam: Excerpta Medica, 1983;397–398.
252. De Lanerolle P, Nishikawa M, Yost DA, Adelstein RS. Increased phosphorylation of myosin light chain kinase after an increase in cyclic AMP in intact smooth muscle. *Science* 1984;223:1415–1417.
253. Del-Angel-Meza AR, Beas-Zárte C, Alfaro FL, Morales-Villagran A. A simple biological assay for relaxin measurement. *Comp Biochem Physiol* 1991;99:35–39.
254. Del Mese A, Casali R, Novelli GP. Relaxin induced dilatation of the venous wall and reduction of the venous blood flow. In: Bigazzi M, Greenwood FC, Gasparri F, eds. *Biology of Relaxin and Its Role in the Human.* Amsterdam: Excerpta Medica, 1983;291–293.
255. Denning-Kendall PA, Guldenaar SEF, Wathes DC. Evidence for a switch in the site of relaxin production from small theca-derived cells to large luteal cells during early pregnancy in the pig. *J Reprod Fertil* 1989;85:261–271.
256. Derewenda U, Derewenda Z, Dodson EJ, Dodson GG, Bing X, Markussen J. X-ray analysis of the single chain B29-A1 peptide-linked insulin molecule. A completely inactive analogue. *J Mol Biol* 1991;220:425–433.
257. Dessau F. Effect of crystalline female sex hormones on the pelvic ligaments of the guinea pig. *Act Brev Neerl* 1935;5:138–139.
258. Dewar AD, Hall K, Newton WH. Potentiation of the vaginal response to oestrone by the "relaxin" fraction of pregnant rabbit serum. *J Physiol* 1946;105:37 (abst).
259. Dieter JA, Stewart DR, Haggarty MA, Stabenfeldt GH. Pregnancy failure in cats associated with dietary taurine deficiences. *Biol Reprod* 1988;38(suppl 1):139 (abst).
260. Dill LV, Chanatry JC. Effect of relaxin on normal labor. *JAMA* 1958;167:1910–1912.
261. Ding L, Becker AB, Suzuki A, Roth RA. Comparison of the enzymatic and biochemical properties of human insulin-degrading enzyme and *Escherichia coli* protease III. *J Biol Chem* 1992;267:2414–2420.
262. Disenhaus C, Belair L, Djiane J. Characterization and physiological variations of IGFs receptors in the ewe mammary gland. *Reprod Nutr Dev* 1988;28(2A):241–252.
263. Doczi J. 1963. Process for the extraction and purification of relaxin. U.S. Patent 3,096,246.
264. Dodson EJ, Dodson GG, Hubbard RE, Reynolds CD. Insulin's structural behavior and its relation to activity. *Biopolymers* 1983;22:281–291.
265. Dodson GG, Eliopoulos EE, Isaacs NW, McCall MJ, Niall HD, North ACT. Rat relaxin: Insulin-like fold predicts a likely receptor binding region. *Int J Biol Macromol* 1982;4:399–405.
266. Dorfman RI, Marsters RW, Dinerstein J. Bioassay of relaxin. *Endocrinology* 1953;52:204–214.
267. Downing SJ, Bradshaw JMC, Porter DG. Relaxin improves the coordination of rat myometrial activity *in vivo. Biol Reprod* 1980;23:899–903.
268. Downing SJ, Hollingsworth M. Antagonism of relaxin by glibenclamide in the uterus of the rat *in vivo. Br J Pharmacol* 1991;104:71–76.
269. Downing SJ, Hollingsworth M. Influence of ovarian steroids on myometrial sensitivity and tolerance to relaxin in the rat *in vivo:* Lack of cross-tolerance between relaxin, salbutamol and cromakalim. *J Endocrinol* 1992;135:17–28.
270. Downing SJ, Hollingsworth M. Interaction between myometrial relaxants and oxytocin: A comparison between relaxin, cromakalim and salbutamol. *J Endocrinol* 1992;135:29–36.
271. Downing SJ, Lye SJ, Bradshaw JMC, Porter DG. Rat myometrial activity *in vivo:* Effects of oestradiol-17β and progesterone in relation to the concentration of cytoplasmic progesterone receptors. *J Endocrinol* 1978;75:103–117.
272. Downing SJ, McIlwrath A, Hollingsworth M. Cyclic adenosine 3′5′-monophosphate and the relaxant action of relaxin in the rat uterus *in vivo. J Reprod Fertil* 1992;96:857–863.
273. Downing SJ, Porter DG, Redstone CD. Myometrial activity in rats during the oestrus cycle and pseudopregnancy: Interaction of oestradiol and progesterone. *J Physiol* 1981;317:425–433.
274. Downing SJ, Sherwood OD. The physiological role of relaxin in the pregnant rat. I. The influence of relaxin on parturition. *Endocrinology* 1985;116:1200–1205.
275. Downing SJ, Sherwood OD. The physiological role of relaxin in the pregnant rat. II. The influence of relaxin on uterine contractile activity. *Endocrinology* 1985;116:1206–1214.
276. Downing SJ, Sherwood OD. The physiological role of relaxin in the pregnant rat. III. The influence of relaxin on cervical extensibility. *Endocrinology* 1985;116:1215–1220.
277. Downing SJ, Sherwood OD. The physiological role of relaxin in the pregnant rat. IV. The influence of relaxin on cervical collagen and glycosaminoglycans. *Endocrinology* 1986;118: 471–479.
278. Drolet DW, Henzel WJ, Johnston PD. Purification, amino-terminal sequencing and demonstration of biological activity of human relaxin from corpora lutea. *Program of the 69th Annual Meeting of the Endocrine Society,* Indianapolis, IN, 1987;196 (abst).
279. Du Y-C, Minasian E, Tregear GW, Leach SJ. Circular dichroism studies of relaxin and insulin peptide chains. *Int J Pept Protein Res* 1982;20:47–55.
280. Dubois MP, Dacheux JL. Relaxin, a male hormone? *Cell Tissue Res* 1978;187:201–214.
281. Duckworth ML, Kirk KL, Friesen HG. Isolation and identification of a cDNA clone of rat placental lactogen II. *J Biol Chem* 1986;261:10871–10878.
282. Duckworth ML, Peden LM, Friesen HG. Isolation of a novel prolactin-like cDNA clone from developing rat placenta. *J Biol Chem* 1986;261:10879–10884.
283. Duckworth ML, Peden LM, Friesen HG. A third prolactin-like protein expressed by the developing rat placenta: Complementary deoxyribonucleic acid sequence and partial structure of the gene. *Mol Endocrinol* 1988;2:912–920.
284. Duncan MR, Berman B. Recombinant human relaxin does not modulate the proliferation or biosynthetic functions of cultured human adult dermal fibroblasts. *Cin Res* 1989;37:349 (abst).
285. Dylewski JR, Larkin LH, Beatty CL. Effects of relaxin on the mechanical properties of collagen-rich tissues. *Mater Res Soc Symp Proc* 1986;55:341–348.
286. Eddie LW, Bell RJ, Lester A, et al. Radioimmunoassay of relaxin in pregnancy with an analogue of human relaxin. *Lancet* 1986;1(No. 8494):1344–1346.
287. Eddie LW, Cameron IT, Leeton JF, Healy DL, Renou P. Ovarian relaxin is not essential for dilatation of the cervix. *Lancet* 1990;336:243.
288. Eddie LW, Martinez F, Healy DL, Sutton B, Bell RJ, Tregear GW. Relaxin in sera during the luteal phase of *in vitro* fertilization cycles. *Br J Obstet Gynaecol* 1990;97:215–220.
289. Eddie LW, Sutton B, Fitzgerald S, Bell RJ, Johnston PD, Tregear GW. Relaxin in paired samples of serum and milk from women after term and preterm delivery. *Am J Obstet Gynecol* 1989;161:970–973.
290. Eggee CJ, Dracy AE. Histological study of effects of relaxin on the bovine cervix. *J Dairy Sci* 1966;49:1053–1057.
291. Eichner E, Waltner C, Goodman M, Post S. Relaxin, the third ovarian hormone: Its experimental use in women. *Am J Obstet Gynecol* 1956;71:1035–1047.
292. Eigenbrot C, Randal M, Quan C, et al. X-ray structure of human relaxin at 1.5 Å: Comparison to insulin and implications for receptor binding determinants. *J Mol Biol* 1991;221:15–21.
293. Einspanier R, Pitzel L, Wuttke W, et al. Demonstration of

mRNAs for oxytocin and prolactin in porcine granulosa and luteal cells. *FEBS Lett* 1986;204:37–40.
294. Eldridge RK, Fields PA. Isolation of human placental relaxin with octadecylsilica. In: Bigazzi M, Greenwood FC, Gasparri F, eds. *Biology of Relaxin and Its Role in the Human.* Amsterdam: Excerpta Medica, 1983;389–391.
295. Eldridge RK, Fields PA. Rabbit placental relaxin: Purification and immunohistochemical localization. *Endocrinology* 1985; 117:2512–2519.
296. Eldridge RK, Fields PA. Immunohistochemical localization of relaxin in the placenta and endometrial glands of pregnant rabbits. *Biol Reprod* 1985;32(suppl 1):152 (abst).
297. Eldridge RK, Fields PA. Rabbit placental relaxin: Ultrastructural localization in secretory granules of the syncytiotrophoblast using rabbit placental relaxin antiserum. *Endocrinology* 1986;119:606–615.
298. Eldridge-White R, Easter RA, Heaton DM, et al. Hormonal control of the cervix in pregnant gilts. I. Changes in the physical properties of the cervix correlate temporally with elevated serum levels of estrogen and relaxin. *Endocrinology* 1989; 125:2996–3003.
299. Elias J, Chen GA, Tseng L, Steinetz BG. Immunocytochemical localization of relaxin in human fetal membrane by colloidal gold-labeled antibody. *Acta Histochem Cytochem* 1986;19:381 (abst).
300. Ellwood DA, Anderson ABM, eds. *The Cervix in Pregnancy and Labour.* London: Churchill Livingstone, 1981.
301. Eltringham L, O'Byrne KT, Summerlee AJS. Opioids from the adrenal glands may mediate relaxin inhibition of oxytocin release in lactating rats. *J Physiol (Lond)* 1986;371:183P (abst).
302. Embrey MP, Garrett WJ. The effect of relaxin on the contractility of the human pregnant uterus. *J Obstet Gynaecol Br Emp* 1959;66:594–597.
303. Emmi AM, Skurnick J, Goldsmith LT, et al. Ovarian control of pituitary hormone secretion in early human pregnancy. *J Clin Endocrinol Metab* 1991;72:1359–1363.
304. Entenmann AH, Lippert TH, Seeger HM, Kieback DG, Voelter W. Identification of immunologically active relaxin in fetal blood. *IRCS Med Sci* 1984;12:881.
305. Entenmann AH, Lippert TH, Voelter W. Isolation of relaxin from human placenta and its biological activity. In: Bigazzi M, Greenwood FC, Gasparri F, eds. *Biology of Relaxin and Its Role in the Human.* Amsterdam: Excerpta Medica, 1983;392–394.
306. Entenmann AH, Lippert TH, Voelter W. Menschliches relaxin aus placenta: Isolierung und biologische aktivität im vergleich zu schweinerelaxin. *Chemiker-Zeitung* 1987;111:263–268.
307. Entenmann AH, Seeger H, Voelter W, Lippert TH. Relaxin deficiency in the placenta as possible cause of cervical dystocia. *Clin Exp Obstet Gynecol* 1988;15:13–17.
308. Entenmann AE, Voelter W, Lippert TH. Isolation and biological standardization of relaxin from human placenta. *Acta Endocrinol [Suppl] (Copenh)* 1984;105:70–71.
309. Essig M, Schoenfeld C, Amelar RD, Dubin L, Weiss G. Stimulation of human sperm motility by relaxin. *Fertil Steril* 1982;38:339–343.
310. Essig M, Schoenfeld C, D'Eletto R, et al. Relaxin in human seminal plasma. *Ann NY Acad Sci* 1982;380:224–230.
311. Evans G, Wathes DC, King GJ, Armstrong DT, Porter DG. Changes in relaxin production by the theca during the preovulatory period of the pig. *J Reprod Fertil* 1983;69:677–683.
312. Evans JA. Relaxin (releasin) therapy in diffuse progressive scleroderma: A preliminary report. *AMA Arch Dermatol* 1959;79:150–158.
313. Evans MD, Dougan M-B, Moawad AH, Evans WJ, Bryant-Greenwood GD, Greenwood FC. Ripening of the human cervix with porcine ovarian relaxin. *Am J Obstet Gynecol* 1983;147:410–414.
314. Fei DTW, Gross MC, Lofgren JL, Mora-Worms M, Chen AB. Cyclic AMP response to recombinant human relaxin by cultured human endometrial cells—A specific and high throughput *in vitro* bioassay. *Biochem Biophys Res Commun* 1990; 170:214–222.
315. Felder KJ, Klindt J, Bolt DJ, Anderson LL. Relaxin and progesterone secretion as affected by luteinizing hormone and prolactin after hysterectomy in the pig. *Endocrinology* 1988; 122:1751–1760.
316. Felder KJ, Molina JR, Benoit AM, Anderson LL. Precise timing for peak relaxin and decreased progesterone secretion after hysterectomy in the pig. *Endocrinology* 1986;119:1502–1509.
317. Felton LC, Frieden EH, Bryant HH. The effects of ovarian extracts upon activity of the guinea pig uterus *in situ. J Pharmacol Exp Ther* 1953;107:160–164.
318. Ferraiolo BL, Cronin M, Bakhit C, Roth M, Chestnut M, Lyon R. The pharmacokinetics and pharmacodynamics of a human relaxin in the mouse pubic symphysis bioassay. *Endocrinology* 1989;125:2922–2926.
319. Ferraiolo BL, Winslow J, Laramee G, Celniker A, Johnston P. The pharmacokinetics and metabolism of human relaxins in rhesus monkeys. *Pharm Res* 1991;8:1032–1038.
320. Fevold HL, Hisaw FL, Leonard SL. The hormones of the corpus luteum. The separation and purification of three active substances. *J Am Chem Soc* 1932;54:254–263.
321. Fevold HL, Hisaw FL, Meyer RK. The relaxative hormone of the corpus luteum. Its purification and concentration. *J Am Chem Soc* 1930;52:3340–3348.
322. Fields MJ, Fields PA. Luteal neurophysin in the nonpregnant cow and ewe: Immunocytochemical localization in membrane-bounded secretory granules of the large luteal cell. *Endocrinology* 1986;118:1723–1725.
323. Fields MJ, Fields PA, Castro-Hernandez A, Larkin LH. Evidence for relaxin in corpora lutea of late pregnant cows. *Endocrinology* 1980;107:869–876.
324. Fields MJ, Fields PA, Larkin LH. Chemistry of bovine relaxin. *Adv Exp Med Biol* 1982;143:191–207.
325. Fields MJ, Roberts R, Castro-Hernandez A. Two cow relaxins: A comparison. In: Bryant-Greenwood GD, Niall HD, Greenwood FC, eds. *Relaxin.* New York: Elsevier/North-Holland, 1981;119–125.
326. Fields MJ, Roberts RF, Dubois W, Ganz NI, Weber DM. Bovine relaxin: Isolation of luteal peptides with biological and immunological activity. In: Bigazzi M, Greenwood FC, Gasparri F, eds. *Biology of Relaxin and Its Role in the Human.* Amsterdam: Excerpta Medica, 1983;56–58.
327. Fields MJ, Roberts R, Fields PA. Octadecylsilica and carboxymethyl cellulose isolation of bovine and porcine relaxin. *Ann NY Acad Sci* 1982;380:36–46.
328. Fields PA. Intracellular localization of relaxin in membrane-bound granules in the pregnant rat luteal cell. *Biol Reprod* 1984;30:753–762.
329. Fields PA. Relaxin and other luteal secretory peptides: Cell localization and function in the ovary. In: Familiari G, Makabe S, Motta PM, eds. *Ultrastructure of the Ovary.* Norwell, MA: Kluwer Academic Publishers, 1991;177–198.
330. Fields PA, Eldridge RK, Fuchs A-R, Fields MJ. Oxytocin contamination of bovine corpora lutea and human placental relaxin extracts: Problems encountered with the *in vitro* mouse uterus relaxin bioassay. In: Bigazzi M, Greenwood FC, Gasparri F, eds. *Biology of Relaxin and Its Role in the Human.* Amsterdam: Excerpta Medica, 1983;185–187.
331. Fields PA, Eldridge RK, Fuchs A-R, Roberts RF, Fields MJ. Human placental and bovine corpora lutea oxytocin. *Endocrinology* 1983;112:1544–1546.
332. Fields PA, Fields MJ. Ultrastructural localization of relaxin in the corpus luteum of the nonpregnant, pseudopregnant, and pregnant pig. *Biol Reprod* 1985;32:1169–1179.
333. Fields PA, Larkin LH. Enhancement of uterine cervix extensibility in oestrogen-primed mice following administration of relaxin. *J Endocrinol* 1980;87:147–152.
334. Fields PA, Larkin LH. Purification and immunohistochemical localization of relaxin in the human term placenta. *J Clin Endocrinol Metab* 1981;52:79–85.
335. Fields PA, Larkin LH, Pardo RJ. Purification of relaxin from the placenta of the rabbit. *Ann NY Acad Sci* 1982;380:75–86.
336. Fields PA, Lee AB, Haab LM, Hwang J-J, Sherwood OD. Evidence for a dual source of relaxin in the pregnant rat: Immunolocalization in the corpora lutea and endometrium. *Endocrinology* 1992;130:2985–2990.
337. Fields PA, Lee VH. Conceptus-mediated integrity of endome-

trial epithelial cells and maintenance of relaxin synthesis in pregnant rabbits: Effects of unilateral oviduct ligation. *Biol Reprod* 1991;44:364–374.

338. Fields PA, Lee VH, Ellerman AB. Rabbit relaxin: *In vivo* uptake of ^{125}I-relaxin in the pregnant rabbit. *Biol Reprod* 1987;36(suppl 1):97 (abst).
339. Fitzpatrick RJ, Dobson H. Softening of the ovine cervix at parturition. In: Ellwood DA, Anderson ABM, eds. *The Cervix in Pregnancy and Labour.* New York: Churchill Livingstone, 1981;40–56.
340. Fitzpatrick RJ, Liggins GC. Effects of prostaglandins on the cervix of pregnant women and sheep. In: Naftolin F, Stubblefield PG, eds. *Dilatation of the Uterine Cervix.* New York: Raven Press, 1980;287–300.
341. Folsome CE, Harami T, Lavietes SR, Massell GM. Clinical evaluation of relaxin. *Obstet Gynecol* 1956;8:536–544.
342. Fosang AJ, Handley CJ, Santer V, Lowther DA, Thorburn GD. Pregnancy-related changes in the connective tissue of the ovine cervix. *Biol Reprod* 1984;30:1223–1235.
343. Fowler KJ, Clouston WM, Fournier REK, Evans BA. The relaxin gene is located on chromosome 19 in the mouse. *FEBS Lett* 1991;292:183–186.
344. Fox D, Handberg GM, Hartley ML, Monagle J, Pennefather JN. Actions of some autocoids and peptides, including relaxin, on costo-uterine muscle from rats. *Clin Exp Pharmacol Physiol* 1989;16:561–569.
345. Frieden EH. Non-steroid ovarian hormones: Observations on the mechanism of the acquisition of relaxin resistance in guinea pigs. *Endocrinology* 1958;62:41–46.
346. Frieden EH. Purification and electrophoretic properties of relaxin preparations. *Trans NY Acad Sci* 1963;25:331–336.
347. Frieden EH, Adams WC. The response to endogenous relaxin of guinea pigs refractory to porcine relaxin. *Proc Soc Exp Biol Med* 1977;155:558–561.
348. Frieden EH, Adams WC. Stimulation of rat uterine collagen synthesis by relaxin. *Proc Soc Exp Biol Med* 1985;180:39–43.
349. Frieden EH, Hisaw FL. The purification of relaxin. *Arch Biochem Biophys* 1950;29:166–178.
350. Frieden EH, Hisaw FL. The mechanism of symphyseal relaxation. The distribution of reducing groups, hexoseamine, and proteins in symphyses of normal and relaxed guinea pigs. *Endocrinology* 1951;48:88–97.
351. Frieden EH, Hisaw FL. The biochemistry of relaxin. *Rec Prog Horm Res* 1953;8:333–378.
352. Frieden EH, Layman NW. Non-steroid ovarian hormones: An improved method for the preparation of relaxin. *J Biol Chem* 1957;229:569–573.
353. Frieden EH, Martin AS. Uptake of glycine-1-C^{14} by connective tissue. I. Effects of estrogen and relaxin. *J Biol Chem* 1954;207:133–142.
354. Frieden EH, Pollock HG, Steinetz BG, Rawitch AB. Structure of a porcine relaxin inactive on the mouse pubic ligament. *Arch Biochem Biophys* 1988;266:334–342.
355. Frieden EH, Rawitch AB. Isolation and chemical properties of relaxin subspecies. In: Bryant-Greenwood GD, Niall HD, Greenwood FC, eds. *Relaxin.* New York: Elsevier/North-Holland, 1981;21–26.
356. Frieden EH, Rawitch AB, Wu L-HC, Chen S-WC. The isolation of two proline-containing relaxin species from a porcine relaxin concentrate. *Proc Soc Exp Biol Med* 1980;163:521–527.
357. Frieden EH, Stone NR, Layman NW. Nonsteroid ovarian hormones. III. The properties of relaxin preparations purified by counter-current distribution. *J Biol Chem* 1960;235:2267–2271.
358. Frieden EH, Velardo JT. Effect of relaxin upon decidual reactions in the rat. *Proc Soc Exp Biol Med* 1952;81:98–103.
359. Frieden EH, Velardo JT. Reversal of the decidual-inhibiting effect of relaxin by an inactive derivitive. *Acta Endocrinol (Copenh)* 1960;34:312–316.
360. Frieden EH, Yeh L-A. Evidence for a "pro-relaxin" in porcine relaxin concentrates. *Proc Soc Exp Biol Med* 1977;154:407–411.
361. Friedman EA. Cervical function in human pregnancy and labor. In: Naftolin F, Stubblefield PG, eds. *Dilatation of the Uterine Cervix.* New York: Raven Press, 1980;17–26.
362. Frost RA, Tseng L. Insulin-like growth factor-binding protein-1 is phosphorylated by cultured human endometrial stromal cells and multiple protein kinases *in vitro. J Biol Chem* 1991;266:18082–18088.
363. Fuchs A-R. Hormonal control of myometrial function during pregnancy and parturition. *Acta Endocrinol* [*Suppl*] *(Copenh)* 1978;221:1–70.
364. Fuchs A-R, Periyasamy S, Alexandrova M, Soloff MS. Correlation between oxytocin receptor concentration and responsiveness to oxytocin in pregnant rat myometrium: Effect of ovarian steroids. *Endocrinology* 1983;113:742–749.
365. Fuchs U. The effect of relaxin on sperm motility. *In vitro* experiments with bull sperm. *Andrologia* 1988;21:297–300.
366. Fuchs U, Seeger H, Völter W, Lippert TH. Immunoreactive relaxin in human cervicovaginal secretion. *Arch Gynecol Obstet* 1988;243:37–39.
367. Fuchs U, Seeger H, Völter W, Lippert TH. Investigation into the hormone profile of serum and cervical-vaginal secretion throughout a menstrual cycle. *Geburtshilfe Frauenheilkd* 1989;49:125–126.
368. Gagliardi CL, Goldsmith LT, Saketos M, Weiss G, Schmidt CL. Human chorionic gonadotropin stimulation of relaxin secretion by luteinized human granulosa cells. *Fertil Steril* 1992;58:314–320.
369. Galhotra MM, Nieschlag E. Active immunization against relaxin inhibits sperm motility. *J Reprod Fertil Abstr Series* 1989;3:43 (abst).
370. Galvin JM, Anthony RV, Day BN. Effects of purified porcine relaxin on the uterus of gilts during early pregnancy. *Anim Reprod Sci* 1991;26:293–301.
371. Galvin JM, Cantley TC, Hall JA, Anthony RV, Day BN. Uterine response to increasing doses of relaxin in ovariectomized gilts. *J Anim Sci* 1991;69(suppl 1):415 (abst).
372. Gammeltoft S, Staun-Olsen P, Ottesen B, Fahrenkrug F. Insulin receptors in rat brain cortex. Kinetic evidence for a receptor subtype in the central nervous system. *Peptides* 1984;5:937–944.
373. Gangrade BK, May JV. The production of transforming growth factor β in the porcine ovary and its secretion *in vitro. Endocrinology* 1990;127:2372–2380.
374. Garcia A, Skurnick JH, Goldsmith LT, Emmi A, Weiss G. Human chorionic gonadotropin and relaxin concentrations in early ectopic and normal pregnancies. *Obstet Gynecol* 1990;75:779–783.
375. Gardner WU. Sexual dimorphism of the pelvis of the mouse, the effect of estrogenic hormones upon the pelvis and upon the development of scrotal hernias. *Am J Anat* 1936;59:459–483.
376. Gardner WU, Pfeiffer CA. Skeletal changes in mice receiving estrogens. *Proc Soc Exp Biol Med* 1938;37:678–679.
377. Gardner WU, Van Heuverswyn J. Inhibition of pelvic changes occurring during pregnancy in mice by testosterone propionate. *Endocrinology* 1940;26:833–836.
378. Garfield RE, Kannan MS, Daniel EE. Gap junction formation in myometrium: Control by estrogens, progesterone and prostaglandins. *Am J Physiol* 1980;238:C81–C89.
379. Garfield RE, Tabb T, Thilander G. Intercellular coupling and modulation of uterine contractility. In: Garfield RE, ed. *Uterine Contractility.* Norwell, MA: Serono Symposia, 1990;21–40.
380. Garrett FA, Talmage RV. The influence of relaxin on mammary gland development in guinea-pigs and rabbits. *J Endocrinol* 1952;8:336–341.
381. Gast MJ. Studies of luteal generation and processing of the high molecular weight relaxin precursor. *Ann NY Acad Sci* 1982;380:111–125.
382. Gast MJ. Characterization of preprorelaxin by tryptic digestion and inhibition of its conversion to prorelaxin by amino acid analogs. *J Biol Chem* 1983;258:9001–9004.
383. Gast MJ, Mercado-Simmen R, Niall H, Boime I. Cell-free synthesis of a high molecular weight relaxin-related protein. *Ann NY Acad Sci* 1980;343:148–154.
384. Gates GS, Flynn JJ, Ryan RJ, Sherwood OD. *In vivo* uptake of ^{125}I-relaxin in the guinea pig. *Biol Reprod* 1981;25:549–554.

385. Georges D, Tashima L, Yamamoto S, Bryant-Greenwood GD. Relaxin-like peptide in ascidians I. Identification of the peptide and its mRNA in ovary of *Herdmania momus*. *Gen Comp Endocrinol* 1990;79:423–428.
386. Georges D, Viguier-Martinez MC, Poirier JC. Relaxin-like peptide in ascidians II. Bioassay and immunolocalization with anti-porcine relaxin in three species. *Gen Comp Endocrinol* 1990;79:429–438.
387. Gibori G, Antczak E, Rothchild I. The role of estrogen in the regulation of luteal progesterone secretion in the rat after day 12 of pregnancy. *Endocrinology* 1977;100:1483–1495.
388. Ginsburg FW, Rosenberg CR, Schwartz M, Colon JM, Goldsmith LT. The effect of relaxin on calcium fluxes in the rat uterus. *Am J Obstet Gynecol* 1988;159:1395–1401.
389. Glaser LA, Kelly PA, Gibori G. Differential action and secretion of rat placental lactogens. *Endocrinology* 1984;115:969–976.
390. Goldsmith LT, De la Cruz JL, Weiss G, Castracane VD. Steroid effects on relaxin secretion in the rat. *Biol Reprod* 1982;27:886–890.
391. Goldsmith LT, Essig M, Sarosi P, Beck P, Weiss G. Hormone secretion by monolayer cultures of human luteal cells. *J Clin Endocrinol Metab* 1981;53:890–892.
392. Goldsmith LT, Grob HS, Scherer KJ, Surve A, Steinetz BG, Weiss G. Placental control of ovarian immunoreactive relaxin secretion in the pregnant rat. *Endocrinology* 1981;109:548–552.
393. Goldsmith LT, Grob HS, Weiss G. *In vitro* induction of relaxin secretion in corpora lutea from nonpregnant rats. *Ann NY Acad Sci* 1982;380:60–71.
394. Goldsmith LT, Skurnick JH, Wojtczuk AS, Linden M, Kuhar MJ, Weiss G. The antagonistic effect of oxytocin and relaxin on rat uterine segment contractility. *Am J Obstet Gynecol* 1989;161:1644–1649.
395. Goldsmith LT, Steinetz BG, Lust G. Relaxin in the milk of lactating bitches is transferred into the circulation of newborn pups. *Program of the 72nd Annual Meeting of the Endocrine Society,* Atlanta, GA, 1990;205 (abst).
396. Golichowski AM, King SR, Mascaro K. Pregnancy-related changes in rat cervical glycosaminoglycans. *Biochem J* 1980;192:1–8.
397. Golos TG, Sherwood OD. Control of corpus luteum function during the second half of pregnancy in the rat: A direct relationship between conceptus number and both serum and ovarian relaxin levels. *Endocrinology* 1982;111:872–878.
398. Golos TG, Sherwood OD. Evidence that the maternal pituitary suppresses the secretion of relaxin in the pregnant rat. *Endocrinology* 1984;115:1004–1010.
399. Golos TG, Sherwood OD. The suppressive effect of the maternal pituitary on relaxin secretion during the second half of pregnancy in rats does not require the presence of the nonluteal ovarian tissue. *Biol Reprod* 1986;34:595–601.
400. Golos TG, Weyhenmyer JA, Sherwood OD. Immunocytochemical localization of relaxin in the ovaries of pregnant rats. *Biol Reprod* 1984;30:257–261.
401. Gooneratne AD, Bryant-Greenwood GD, Walker FM, Nottage HM, Hartmann PE. Pre-partum changes in the plasma concentrations of progesterone, relaxin, prostaglandin $F_{2\alpha}$ and 13,14-dihydro-15-keto prostaglandin $F_{2\alpha}$ in meclofenamic acid-treated sows. *J Reprod Fertil* 1983;68:33–40.
402. Gordon WL, Sherwood OD. Evidence that luteinizing hormone from the maternal pituitary gland may promote antepartum release of relaxin, luteolysis, and birth in rats. *Endocrinology* 1982;111:1299–1310.
403. Gordon WL, Sherwood OD. Evidence for a role of prostaglandins in the antepartum release of relaxin in the pregnant rat. *Biol Reprod* 1983;28:154–160.
404. Gorman CM, Ross MJ, Niall HD. 1988. Human prorelaxin, its preparation and use. European Patent Application 0 260 149.
405. Gospodarowicz D, Ferrara N. Fibroblast growth factor and the control of pituitary and gonad development and function. *J Steroid Biochem* 1989;32:183–192.
406. Gowan LK, Reinig JW, Schwabe C, Bedarker S, Blundell TL. On the primary and tertiary structure of relaxin from the sand tiger shark. *FEBS Lett* 1981;129:80–82.
407. Graciansky P de, Boulle S. Essais de traitement de la sclérodermie par la relaxine. *Bull Soc Fr Derm Syph* 1961;68:83–86.
408. Graham EF, Dracy AE. The effects of relaxin on the cow's cervix. *J Dairy Sci* 1952;35:499 (abstract).
409. Graham EF, Dracy AE. The effect of relaxin and mechanical dilatation of the bovine cervix. *J Dairy Sci* 1953;36:772–777.
410. Grazi RV, Goldsmith LT, Schmidt CL, Von Hagen S, Weiss G. Synergistic effect of relaxin and progesterone on cyclic adenosine 3′5′-monophosphate levels in the rat uterus. *Am J Obstet Gynecol* 1988;159:1402–1406.
411. Greenberg LH, Stouffer RL, Brenner RM, Molskness TA, Hild-Petito SA, Yu Q. Are human luteinizing granulosa cells a site of action for progesterone and relaxin? *Fertil Steril* 1990;53:446–453.
412. Greenwood FC, Mercado-Simmen RC, Greenwood GD. Insulin-related peptides examined by radioimmunoassay and radioreceptor assay: A note. In: Bryant-Greenwood GD, Niall HD, Greenwood FC, eds. *Relaxin.* New York: Elsevier/North-Holland, 1981;97–98.
413. Griss G, Keck J, Engelhorn R, Tuppy H. The isolation and purification of an ovarian polypeptide with uterine-relaxing activity. *Biochim Biophys Acta* 1967;140:45–54.
414. Grosvenor CE, Turner CW. Milk let-down activity of synthetic oxytocin (syntocinon) and relaxin in lactating rats. *Proc Soc Exp Biol Med* 1958;97:189–190.
415. Guthrie HD, Rexroad CR, Bolt DJ. *In vitro* synthesis of progesterone and prostaglandin F by luteal tissue and prostaglandin by endometrial tissue from the pig. *Prostaglandins* 1978;16:433–440.
416. Gutkowska J, St-Louis J, Genest J. Solid-phase radioimmunoassay for relaxin. *Clin Invest Med* 1985;8:133–138.
417. Haley J, Crawford R, Hudson P, et al. Porcine relaxin: Gene structure and expression. *J Biol Chem* 1987;262:11940–11946.
418. Haley J, Hudson P, Scanlon D, et al. Porcine relaxin: Molecular cloning and cDNA structure. *DNA* 1982;1:155–162.
419. Hall JA, Cantley TC, Day BN, Anthony RV. Uterotropic actions of relaxin in prepubertal gilts. *Biol Reprod* 1990;42:769–774.
420. Hall JA, Cantley TC, Galvin JM, Day BN, Anthony RV. Influence of ovarian steroids on relaxin-induced uterine growth in ovariectomized gilts. *Endocrinology* 1992;130:3159–3166.
421. Hall JA, Day BN, Anthony RV. Influence of steroids on relaxin-induced changes in distensibility and composition of the cervix in gilts. *Biol Reprod* 1991;44(suppl 1):164 (abst).
422. Hall K. The effects of pregnancy and relaxin on the histology of the pubic symphysis of the mouse. *J Endocrinol* 1947;5:174–185.
423. Hall K. Further notes on the action of oestrone and relaxin on the pelvis of the spayed mouse, including a single-dose test of potency of relaxin. *J Endocrinol* 1948;5:314–321.
424. Hall K. The role of progesterone in the mechanism of pelvic relaxation in the mouse. *Q J Exp Physiol* 1949;35:65–75.
425. Hall K. The effect of various combinations of progesterone and oestrogen on the symphysis pubis of ovariectomized mice. *J Endocrinol* 1955;12:247–251.
426. Hall K. An evaluation of the roles of oestrogen, progesterone and relaxin in producing relaxation of the symphysis pubis of the ovariectomized mouse, using the technique of metachromatic staining with toluidine blue. *J Endocrinol* 1956;13:384–393.
427. Hall K. The effect of relaxin extracts, progesterone and oestradiol on maintenance of pregnancy, parturition, and rearing of young after ovariectomy in mice. *J Endocrinol* 1957;15:108–117.
428. Hall K. Modification by relaxin of the response of the reproductive tract of mice to oestradiol and progesterone. *J Endocrinol* 1960;20:355–364.
429. Hall K. Histochemical investigation of the effects of oestrogen, progesterone and relaxin on glycogen, amylophosphorylase, transglycosylase, and uridine diphosphate glucose-glycogen transferase in uteri of mice. *J Endocrinol* 1965;32:245–257.
430. Hall K, Hoare M, Turner CB. Relaxin in the blood of prepartu-rient ewes. *J Endocrinol* 1962;28:271–278.

431. Hall K, Newton WH. The action of relaxin in the mouse. *Lancet* 1946;1:54–55.
432. Hall K, Newton WH. The normal course of separation of the pubes in pregnant mice. *J Physiol* 1946;104:346–352.
433. Hall K, Newton WH. The effect of oestrone and relaxin on the X-ray appearance of the pelvis of the mouse. *J Physiol* 1947;106:18–27.
434. Hammitt DG, Bedia E, Rogers PR, Syrop CH, Donovan JF, Williamson RA. Comparison of motility. Stimulants of cryopreserved human semen. *Fertil Steril* 1989;52:495–502.
435. Hammond JM, English HF. Regulation of deoxyribonucleic acid synthesis in cultured porcine granulosa cells by growth factors and hormones. *Endocrinology* 1987;120:1039–1046.
436. Hamolsky M, Sparrow RC. Influence of relaxin on mammary development in sexually immature female rats. *Proc Soc Exp Biol Med* 1945;60:8–9.
437. Haning RV Jr, Steinetz BG, Weiss G. Elevated serum relaxin levels in multiple pregnancy after menotropin treatment. *Obstet Gynecol* 1985;66:42–45.
438. Hansel W, Concannon PW, Lukaszewska JH. Corpora lutea of the large domestic animals. *Biol Reprod* 1973;8:222–245.
439. Hansel W, Dowd JP. New concepts of the control of corpus luteum function. *J Reprod Fertil* 1986;78:755–768.
440. Hansell DJ, Bryant-Greenwood GD, Greenwood FC. Expression of the human relaxin H1 gene in the decidua, trophoblast and prostate. *J Clin Endocrinol Metab* 1991;72:899–904.
441. Hansson HA, Nilsson A, Isgaard J, et al. Immunohistochemical localization of insulin-like growth factor I in the adult rat. *Histochemistry* 1988;89:403–410.
442. Harkey ME, Crelin ES. Hormonal response of the pubic symphysis in adult mice gonadectomized at different times before puberty. *Anat Rec* 1963;145:323.
443. Harkness MLR, Harkness RD. The collagen content of the reproductive tract of the rat during pregnancy and lactation. *J Physiol* 1954;123:492–500.
444. Harkness MLR, Harkness RD. Changes in the physical properties of the uterine cervix of the rat during pregnancy. *J Physiol* 1959;148:524–547.
445. Harkness MLR, Harkness RD. The mechanical properties of the uterus compared to those of the birth canal of the rat in pregnancy. *Acta Physiol Acad Sci Hung* 1965;27:101–109.
446. Harkness RD. The physiology of the connective tissues of the reproductive tract. *Int Rev Connect Tissue Res* 1964;2:155–211.
447. Harkness RD, Nightingale MA. The extensibility of the cervix uteri of the rat at different times of pregnancy. *J Physiol* 1962;160:214–220.
448. Harness JR, Anderson RR. Effect of relaxin on mammary gland growth and lactation in the rat. *Proc Soc Exp Biol Med* 1975;148:933–936.
449. Harness JR, Anderson RR. Effects of relaxin in combination with prolactin and ovarian steroids on mammary growth in hypophysectomized rats. *Proc Soc Exp Biol Med* 1977;156:354–358.
450. Harness JR, Anderson RR. Effect of relaxin and somatotropin in combination with ovarian steroids on mammary glands in rats. *Biol Reprod* 1977;17:599–603.
451. Harris MA, Rees JM, McLaughlin EA, Ford WCL, Wardle PG, Hull MGR, Wathes DC. An evaluation of the role of relaxin in the penetration of cervical mucus by spermatozoa. *Hum Reprod* 1988;3:856–860.
452. Hartman CG, Straus WL. Relaxation of the pelvic ligaments in pregnant monkeys. *Am J Obstet Gynecol* 1939;37:498–500.
453. Hascall VC, Hascall GK. Proteoglycans. In: Hay ED, ed. *Cell Biology of the Extracellular Matrix.* New York: Plenum, 1981;39–63.
454. Hernandez ER, Resnick CE, Svoboda ME, Van Wyk JJ, Payne DW, Adashi EY. Somatomedin-C/Insulin-like growth factor I as an enhancer of androgen biosynthesis by cultured rat ovarian cells. *Endocrinology* 1988;122:1603–1612.
455. Herrick EH. The duration of pregnancy in guinea-pigs after removal and also after transplantation of the ovaries. *Anat Rec* 1928;39:193–200.
456. Hijazi M, Bryant-Greenwood GD. An autocrine action of relaxin on human decidual cell relaxin secretion. *Biol Reprod* 1991;44(suppl 1):166 (abst).
457. Hilliard J. Corpus luteum function in guinea pigs, hamsters, rats, mice and rabbits. *Biol Reprod* 1973;8:203–221.
458. Hillier K, Wallis RM. Prostaglandins, steroids and the human cervix. In: Ellwood DA, Anderson ABM, eds. *The Cervix in Pregnancy and Labour.* New York: Churchill Livingstone, 1981;144–162.
459. Hillier K, Wallis RM. Collagen solubility and tensile properties of the rat uterine cervix in late pregnancy: Effects of arachidonic acid and prostaglandin $F_{2\alpha}$. *J Endocrinol* 1982;95:341–347.
460. Hisaw FL. Experimental relaxation of the pubic ligament of the guinea pig. *Proc Soc Exp Biol Med* 1926;23:661–663.
461. Hisaw FL. Experimental relaxation of the symphysis pubis of the guinea-pig. *Anat Rec* 1927;37:126.
462. Hisaw FL. The corpus luteum hormone. I. Experimental relaxation of the pelvic ligaments of the guinea pig. *Physiol Zool* 1929;2:59–79.
463. Hisaw FL, Hisaw FL. Effect of relaxin on the uterus of monkeys (*Macaca mulatta*) with observations on the cervix and symphysis pubis. *Am J Obstet Gynecol* 1964;89:141–155.
464. Hisaw FL, Hisaw FL, Dawson AB. Effects of relaxin on the endothelium of endometrial blood vessels in monkeys (*Macaca mulatta*). *Endocrinology* 1967;81:375–385.
465. Hisaw FL, Talmage RVN, Money WL, Abramowitz AA. Relation of progesterone to the formation of relaxin. *Anat Rec* 1942;84:457.
466. Hisaw FL, Zarrow MX. Relaxin in the ovary of the domestic sow. *Proc Soc Exp Biol Med* 1948;69:395–398.
467. Hisaw FL, Zarrow MX. The physiology of relaxin. *Vitam Horm* 1950;8:151–178.
468. Hisaw FL, Zarrow MX, Money WL, Talmage RVN, Abramowitz AA. Importance of the female reproductive tract in the formation of relaxin. *Endocrinology* 1944;34:122–134.
469. Hochman J, Weiss G, Steinetz BG, O'Byrne EM. Serum relaxin concentrations in prostaglandin- and oxytocin-induced labor in women. *Am J Obstet Gynecol* 1978;130:473–474.
470. Hofig A, Michel FJ, Simmen FA, Simmen RCM. Constitutive expression of uterine receptors for insulin-like growth factor-I during the peri-implantation period in the pig. *Biol Reprod* 1991;45:533–539.
471. Hollingsworth M. Softening of the rat cervix during pregnancy. In: Ellwood DA, Anderson ABM, eds. *The Cervix in Pregnancy and Labour.* New York: Churchill Livingstone, 1981;13–33.
472. Hollingsworth M, Gallimore S. Evidence that cervical softening in the pregnant rat is independent of increasing uterine contractility. *J Reprod Fertil* 1981;63:449–454.
473. Hollingsworth M, Gallimore S, Isherwood CNM. Effects of prostaglandins $F_{2\alpha}$ and E-2 on cervical extensibility in the late pregnant rat. *J Reprod Fertil* 1980;58:95–99.
474. Hollingsworth M, Gallimore S, Williams LM. Creep testing of isolated cervix from pregnant rats. In: Vincent JFV, Currey JD, eds. *Mechanical Properties of Biological Materials.* Symposia of the Society for Experimental Biology, Vol. 34. Cambridge: Cambridge University Press, 1980;477–478.
475. Hollingsworth M, Isherwood CNM, Foster RW. The effects of oestradiol benzoate, progesterone, relaxin, and ovariectomy on cervical extensibility in the late pregnant rat. *J Reprod Fertil* 1979;56:471–477.
476. Holmstrom EG. The prevention of prematurity. *W Va Med J* 1958;54:343–344.
477. Horn EH. Effects of feeding thiouracil and/or thyroid powder upon pubic symphyseal separation in female mice. *Endocrinology* 1958;63:481–486.
478. Horn EH. Interpubic ligament regression in relaxin-treated virgin and primiparous, post-partum mice. *Endocrinology* 1960;67:668–673.
479. Hsu CJ, McCormack SM, Sanborn BM. The effect of relaxin on cyclic adenosine 3′5′-monophosphate concentrations in rat myometrial cells in culture. *Endocrinology* 1985;116:2029–2035.
480. Hsu CJ, Sanborn BM. Relaxin affects the shape of rat myometrial cells in culture. *Endocrinology* 1986;118:495–498.
481. Hsu CJ, Sanborn BM. Relaxin treatment alters the kinetic prop-

erties of myosin light chain kinase activity in rat myometrial cells in culture. *Endocrinology* 1986;118:499–505.
482. Hua QX, Shoelson SE, Kochoyan M, Weiss MA. Receptor binding redefined by a structural switch in a mutant human insulin. *Nature* 1991;354:238–241.
483. Huang CJ, Li Y, Anderson LL. Growth-promoting effects of relaxin on the uterus of prepubertal pigs are estrogen dependent. *J Anim Sci* 1991;69(suppl 1):414 (abst).
484. Huang CJ, Stromer MH, Anderson LL. Abrupt shifts in relaxin and progesterone secretion by aging luteal cells: Luteotropic response in hysterectomized and pregnant pigs. *Endocrinology* 1991;128:165–173.
485. Huang JR, Bellino FL, Osawa Y, Tseng L. Immunologic identification of the aromatase enzyme system in human endometrium. *J Steroid Biochem* 1989;33:1043–1047.
486. Huang JR, Tseng L, Bischof P, Jänne OA. Regulation of prolactin production by progestin, estrogen, and relaxin in human endometrial stromal cells. *Endocrinology* 1987;121:2011–2017.
487. Hudson P, Haley J, Cronk M, Shine J, Niall H. Molecular cloning and characterization of cDNA sequences coding for rat relaxin. *Nature* 1981;291:127–131.
488. Hudson P, Haley J, John M, et al. Structure of a genomic clone encoding biologically active human relaxin. *Nature* 1983; 301:628–631.
489. Hudson P, John M, Crawford R, et al. Relaxin gene expression in human ovaries and the predicted structure of a human preprorelaxin by analysis of cDNA clones. *EMBO J* 1984; 3:2333–2339.
490. Hughes SJ, Downing SJ, Hollingsworth M. Relaxin, a potassium channel opener in the isolated rat uterus? *Br J Pharmacol* 1992;106:80P (abst).
491. Hunter MG, Denning-Kendall P, Boulton MI, DeRensis F, Wild ML, Foxcroft GR. Lack of stimulation of relaxin secretion in lactating sows by suckling *in vivo* or by oxytocin *in vitro*. *J Reprod Fertil* 1992;94:121–128.
492. Hunter WM, Greenwood FC. Preparation of iodine-131 labelled human growth hormone of high specific activity. *Nature* 1962;194:495–496.
493. Hurley WL, Doane RM, O'Day-Bowman MB, Winn RJ, Mojonnier LE, Sherwood OD. Effect of relaxin on mammary development in ovariectomized pregnant gilts. *Endocrinology* 1991;128:1285–1290.
494. Hwang J-J, Lee AB, Fields PA, Haab LM, Mojonnier LE, Sherwood OD. Monoclonal antibodies specific for rat relaxin. V. Passive immunization with monoclonal antibodies throughout the second half of pregnancy disrupts development of the mammary apparatus and, hence, lactational performance in rats. *Endocrinology* 1991;129:3034–3042.
495. Hwang J-J, Shanks RD, Sherwood OD. Monoclonal antibodies specific for rat relaxin. IV. Passive immunization with monoclonal antibodies during the antepartum period reduces cervical growth and extensibility, disrupts birth, and reduces pup survival in intact rats. *Endocrinology* 1989;125:260–266.
496. Hwang J-J, Sherwood OD. Monoclonal antibodies specific for rat relaxin. III. Passive immunization with monoclonal antibodies throughout the second half of pregnancy reduces cervical growth and extensibility in intact rats. *Endocrinology* 1988;123:2486–2490.
497. Inoue H, Osa T, Okabe K. Effects of porcine relaxin on contraction, membrane response, and cyclic AMP content in rat myometrium. *Jpn J Pharmacol* 1992;58:353.
498. Isaacs N, Dodson G. Models of relaxin. In: Bryant-Greenwood GD, Niall HD, Greenwood FC, eds. *Relaxin.* New York: Elsevier/North-Holland, 1981;101–106.
499. Isaacs N, James R, Niall H, et al. Relaxin and its structural relationship to insulin. *Nature* 1978;271:278–281.
500. Ismay G. Relaxin: Its effects in a case of acrosclerosis. *Br J Dermatol* 1958;70:171–175.
501. Ito A, Kitamura K, Mori Y, Hirakawa S. The change in solubility of type I collagen in human uterine cervix in pregnancy at term. *Biochem Med* 1979;21:267–270.
502. Ivell R, Hunt N, Khan-Dawood F, Dawood MY. Expression of the human relaxin gene in the corpus luteum of the menstrual cycle and in the prostate. *Mol Cell Endocrinol* 1989; 66:251–255.
503. Jablonski WJA, Velardo JT. Effects of relaxin on uterine weight of immature rats. *Endocrinology* 1957;61:474–475.
504. Jackson JA, Albrecht ED. The development of placental androstenedione and testosterone production and their utilization by the ovary for aromatization to estrogen during rat pregnancy. *Biol Reprod* 1985;33:451–457.
505. Jagiello G. Effects of selected hormones on the closed vaginal membrane of the ovariectomized guinea pig. *Proc Soc Exp Biol Med* 1965;118:412–414.
506. Jagiello G. The effect of several relaxin preparations on the hysterectomized guinea-pig. *J Reprod Fertil* 1967;13:175–177.
507. James R, Niall HD, Bradshaw RA. The topographical mapping of porcine relaxin: Location of the tryptophan residues. In: Bryant-Greenwood GD, Niall HD, Greenwood FC, eds. *Relaxin.* New York: Elsevier/North-Holland, 1981;85–90.
508. James R, Niall H, Kwok S, Bryant-Greenwood G. Primary structure of porcine relaxin: Homology with insulin and related growth factors. *Nature* 1977;267:544–546.
509. Jarrett JC, Ballejo G, Saleem TH, Tsibris JCM, Spellacy WN. The effect of prolactin and relaxin on insulin binding by adipocytes from pregnant women. *Am J Obstet Gynecol* 1984;149:250–255.
510. Järvinen PA, Luukkainen T. Treatment of symphyseolysis with relaxin. *Ann Chir Gynaecol* 1963;52:251–254.
511. Jefferis JE, Dixon AStJ. Failure of relaxin in the treatment of scleroderma. *Ann Rheum Dis* 1962;21:295–297.
512. Jockenhövel F. Relaxin, ein wiederendecktes hormon für Geburtshilfe und reproduktionsmedizin. *Geburtshilfe Frauenheilkd* 1989;49:127–139.
513. Jockenhövel F, Altensell A, Nieschlag E. Active immunization with relaxin does not influence objectively determined sperm motility characteristics in rabbits. *Andrologia* 1990;22:171–178.
514. Jockenhövel F, Peterson MA, Johnston PD, Swerdloff RS. Directly iodinated rat relaxin as a tracer for use in radioimmunoassays. *Eur J Clin Chem Clin Biochem* 1991;29:71–75.
515. Johanson C-E, Järvinen PA. Factors affecting relaxation of the pelvis during normal pregnancy, delivery, and the puerperium. *Acta Obstet Gynecol Scand* 1957;36:179–193.
516. John MJ, Borjesson BW, Walsh JR, Niall HD. Limited sequence homology between porcine and rat relaxins: Implications for physiological studies. *Endocrinology* 1981;108: 726–729.
517. Johns TC, Renegar RH. Ultrastructural morphology and relaxin immunolocalization in giant trophoblast cells of the golden hamster placenta. *Am J Anat* 1990;189:167–178.
518. Johnson MR, Abbas A, Nicolaides KH, Lightman SL. Distribution of relaxin between human maternal and fetal circulations and amniotic fluid. *J Endocrinol* 1992;134:313–317.
519. Johnson MR, Abdalla H, Allman ACJ, Wren ME, Kirkland A, Lightman SL. Relaxin levels in ovum donation pregnancies. *Fertil Steril* 1991;56:59–61.
520. Johnson MR, Allman ACJ, Pickering SJ, Ulthayakumar S, Steer PS, Lightman SL. Plasma relaxin concentrations during pregnancy, labour and breast feeding. *J Endocrinol* 1991;(suppl 1):129 (abst).
521. Johnson MR, Nicolaides KH, Thorpe-Beeston G, Siderist I, Lightman SL. Feto-maternal levels of relaxin. *J Endocrinol (Suppl)* 1990;127:34 (abst).
522. Johnson MR, Okokon E, Collins WP, Sharma V, Lightman SL. The effect of human chorionic gonadotropin and pregnancy on the circulating level of relaxin. *J Clin Endocrinol Metab* 1991;72:1042–1047.
523. Johnston PD, Burnier J, Chen S, et al. Structure/function studies of human relaxin. In: Deber CM, Hruby VJ, Kopple KD, eds. *Peptides, Structure and Function.* Rockford, IL: Pierce Chemical Co., 1985;683–686.
524. Jones SA. 1986. Birth in the rat: A central role for relaxin. Ph.D. Thesis. University of Bristol, England.
525. Jones SA, Kelly SA, Summerlee AJS. Evidence that chronic treatment with intravenous (i.v.) relaxin induces relaxin tolerance and opioid dependence in the oxytocin system of the lactating rat. *J Physiol* 1987;382:40P (abst).

526. Jones SA, Summerlee AJS. Effects of porcine relaxin on the length of gestation and duration of parturition in the rat. *J Endocrinol* 1986;109:85–88.
527. Jones SA, Summerlee AJS. Relaxin acts centrally to inhibit oxytocin release during parturition: An effect that is reversed by naloxone. *J Endocrinol* 1986;111:99–102.
528. Jones SA, Summerlee AJS. Relaxin increases blood pressure and vasopressin levels in anaesthetized rats. *J Physiol (Lond)* 1986;381:37P (abst).
529. Jones SA, Summerlee AJS. Effects of chronic infusion of porcine relaxin on oxytocin release in lactating rats. *J Endocrinol* 1987;114:241–246.
530. Joseph NR, Engel MB, Catchpole HR. Interaction of ions and connective tissue. *Biochim Biophys Acta* 1952;8:575–587.
531. Juang HH, Musah AI, Anderson LL. Ethylenediaminetetraacetic acid (EDTA) and caffeine are antagonistic to antirelaxin serum inhibition of porcine sperm motility. *Anim Reprod Sci* 1990;22:253–260.
532. Juang HH, Musah AI, Schwabe C, Anderson LL. Relaxin in peripheral plasma and seminal plasma of mature and prepubertal boars and its correlation with sperm motility. *Biol Reprod* 1988;38(suppl 1):89 (abst).
533. Juang HH, Musah AI, Schwabe C, Anderson LL. Relaxin in peripheral plasma of boar during development after castration and HCG administration. *J Anim Sci* 1988;66(suppl 1):396 (abst).
534. Juang HH, Musah AI, Schwabe C, Anderson LL. Effect of relaxin and antirelaxin serum on porcine sperm motility. *Anim Reprod Sci* 1989;20:21–29.
535. Juang HH, Musah AI, Schwabe C, Anderson LL. Immunoactive relaxin in boar seminal plasma and its correlation with sperm motility. *Anim Reprod Sci* 1990;22:47–53.
536. Judson DG, Pay S, Bhoola KD. Modulation of cyclic AMP in isolated rat uterine slices by porcine relaxin. *J Endocrinol* 1980;87:153–159.
537. Kakouris H, Eddie LW, Summers RJ. Cardiac effects of relaxin in rats. *Lancet* 1992;339:1076–1078.
538. Kalbag SS, Roginsky MS, Jelveh Z, Sulimovici S. Phorbol ester, prolactin, and relaxin cause translocation of protein kinase C from cytosol to membranes in human endometrial cells. *Biochim Biophys Acta* 1991;1094:85–91.
539. Kato H, Morishige WK, Rothchild I. A quantitative relation between the experimentally determined number of conceptuses and corpus luteum activity in the pregnant rat. *Endocrinology* 1979;105:846–850.
540. Kelly JV, Posse N. The hormone relaxin in labor. *Obstet Gynecol* 1956;8:531–535.
541. Kemp BE. Activation of rat uterine cAMP-dependent protein kinase by relaxin. *Program of the 63rd Annual Meeting of the Endocrine Society,* Cincinnati, OH, 1981;200 (abst).
542. Kemp BE, Niall HD. Relaxin. *Vitam Horm* 1984;41:79–115.
543. Kendall JZ, Dziuk PJ, Nelson DR, Sherwood OD, Thurmon JC, Frankowski RF. The effect of fetal hypophysectomy and fetal death in gilts with small litters on concentrations of relaxin, progesterone and estradiol-17β. *Anim Reprod Sci* 1988;16: 107–123.
544. Kendall JZ, Plopper CG, Bryant-Greenwood GD. Ultrastructural immunoperoxidase demonstration of relaxin in corpora lutea from a pregnant sow. *Biol Reprod* 1978;18:94–98.
545. Kendall JZ, Richards GE, Shih L-N. Effect of haloperidol, suckling, oxytocin, and hand milking on plasma relaxin and prolactin concentrations in cyclic and lactating pigs. *J Reprod Fertil* 1983;69:271–277.
546. Kendall JZ, Richards GE, Shih L-N, Farris TS. Plasma relaxin concentrations in the pig during the periparturient period: Association with prolactin, estrogen, and progesterone concentrations. *Theriogenology* 1982;17:677–687.
547. Kendall JZ, Smith RG, Shih L-N, Webb PD, Tate WH. Characterization of prostatic relaxin. In: Bigazzi M, Greenwood FC, Gasparri F, eds. *Biology of Relaxin and Its Role in the Human.* Amsterdam: Excerpta Medica, 1983;363–366.
548. Kennedy TG. Effect of relaxin on oestrogen-induced uterine luminal fluid accumulation in the ovariectomized rat. *J Endocrinol* 1974;61:347–353.
549. Kennedy TG. Does prostaglandin $F_{2\alpha}$ ($PGF_{2\alpha}$) mediate the effect of relaxin on cervical tone in the rat? *Proc Can Fed Biol Soc* 1976;19:69 (abst).
550. Kensinger RS, Collier RJ, Bazer FW, Ducsay CA, Becker HN. Nuclei acid, metabolic and histological changes in gilt mammary tissue during pregnancy and lactogenesis. *J Anim Sci* 1982;54:1297–1308.
551. Kertiles LP, Anderson LL. Effect of relaxin on cervical dilatation, parturition and lactation in the pig. *Biol Reprod* 1979;21:57–68.
552. Khaligh HS. Inhibition by relaxin of spontaneous contractions of the uterus of the hamster *in vitro. J Endocrinol* 1968;40:125–126.
553. Khan-Dawood FS, Goldsmith LT, Weiss G, Dawood MY. Human corpus luteum secretion of relaxin, oxytocin, and progesterone. *J Clin Endocrinol Metab* 1989;68:627–631.
554. Kibblewhite D, Larrabee WF, Sutton D. The effect of relaxin on tissue expansion. *Arch Otolaryngol Head Neck Surg* 1992;118:153–156.
555. King GJ, Wathes DC. Relaxin, progesterone and estrogen profiles in sow plasma during natural and induced parturitions. *Anim Reprod Sci* 1989;20:213–220.
556. Kirton KT. Use of prostaglandins for dilatation of the cervix. In: Naftolin F, Stubblefield PG, eds. *Dilatation of the Uterine Cervix.* New York: Raven Press, 1980;355–361.
557. Kliman B, Greep RO. The enhancement of relaxin-induced growth of the pubic ligament in mice. *Endocrinology* 1958;63:586–595.
558. Kliman B, Salhanick HA, Zarrow MX. The response of the pubic symphysis of the mouse to extracts of pregnant rabbit serum and pregnant sow ovaries and its application as an assay method. *Endocrinology* 1953;53:391–409.
559. Knox FS, Griffith DR. Effect of ovarian hormones upon milk yield in the rat. *Proc Soc Exp Biol Med* 1970;133:135–137.
560. Koay ESC, Bagnell CA, Bryant-Greenwood GD, Lord SB, Cruz AC, Larkin LH. Immunocytochemical localization of relaxin in human decidua and placenta. *J Clin Endocrinol Metab* 1985;60:859–863.
561. Koay ESC, Bryant-Greenwood GD, Yamamoto SY, Greenwood FC. The human fetal membranes: A target tissue for relaxin. *J Clin Endocrinol Metab* 1986;62:513–521.
562. Koay ESC, Greenwood FC, Bryant-Greenwood GD. Relaxin: A local hormone in human parturition. In: Jaffe RB, Dell'Acqua S, eds. *The Endocrine Physiology of Pregnancy and the Peripartal Period.* New York: Raven Press, 1985;247–253.
563. Koay ESC, Too CKL, Greenwood FC, Bryant-Greenwood GD. Relaxin stimulates collagenase and plasminogen activator secretion by dispersed human amnion and chorion cells *in vitro. J Clin Endocrinol Metab* 1983;56:1332–1334.
564. Kohsaka T, Kawarasaki T, Sone M, Muraki T, Bamba K. Electron microscopical and immunocytochemical approach on the production of relaxin-like peptide in boar seminal vesicle. *J Histochem Cytochem* 1988;36:932 (abst).
565. Kohsaka T, Sasada H, Masaki J. Subcellular localization of the antigenic sites of relaxin in the luteal cells of the pregnant rat using an improved immunocytochemical technique. *Anim Reprod Sci* 1992;29:123–132.
566. Kohsaka T, Takahara H, Sasada H, et al. Evidence for immunoreactive relaxin in boar seminal vesicles using combined light and electron microscope immunocytochemistry. *J Reprod Fertil* 1992;95:397–408.
567. Kokenyesi R, Woessner JF Jr. Purification and characterization of a small dermatan sulphate proteoglycan implicated in the dilatation of the rat uterine cervix. *Biochem J* 1989; 260:413–419.
568. Kokenyesi R, Woessner JF Jr. Relationship between dilatation of the rat uterine cervix and a small dermatan sulphate proteoglycan. *Biol Reprod* 1990;42:87–97.
569. Koninckx PR, Renaer M, Brosens IA. Origin of peritoneal fluid in women: An ovarian exudation product. *Br J Obstet Gynaecol* 1980;87:177–183.
570. Koob TJ, Laffan JJ, Callard IP. Effects of relaxin and insulin on reproductive tract size and early fetal loss in squalus acanthias. *Biol Reprod* 1984;31:231–238.

571. Kotwica G, Dusza L, Ciereszko R, Okrasa S, Schams D. Evidence for relaxin and progesterone synchronous secretion on days 13 to 17 of the oestrous cycle in sows. *Exp Clin Endocrinol* 1991;98:3–8.
572. Kotwica J, Krzymowski T, Stefanczyk S, Koziorowski M, Czarnocki J, Ruszczyk T. A new route of prostaglandin F-2α transfer from the uterus into the ovary in swine. *Anim Reprod Sci* 1983;5:303–309.
573. Kozuka M, Ito T, Hirose S, Takahashi K, Hagiwara H. Endothelin induces two types of contractions of rat uterus: Phasic contractions by way of voltage-dependent calcium channels and developing contractions through a second type of calcium channels. *Biochem Biophys Res Commun* 1989;159:317–323.
574. Kramer SM, Gibson UEM, Fendly BM, Mohler MA, Drolet DW, Johnston PD. Increase in cyclic AMP levels by relaxin in newborn rhesus monkey uterus cell culture. *In Vitro Cell Dev Biol* 1990;26:647–656.
575. Krantz JC, Bryant HH, Carr CJ. The action of aqueous corpus luteum extract upon uterine activity. *Surg Gynecol Obstet* 1950;90:372–375.
576. Krassnigg F, Töpfer-Petersen E, Frick J, Schill W-B. Functional role of relaxin in the human seminal fluid. In: Thompson W, Harrison RF, Bonnar J, eds. *The Male Factor in Human Infertility. Diagnosis and Treatment.* Boston, MA: MTP Press, 1984;69–72.
577. Krause WJ, Sherman DM. Immunohistochemical localization of relaxin in the reproductive system of the female opossum (*Didelphis virginiana*). *Ann Anat Anatom Anzeiger* 1992; 174:341–344.
578. Kream BE, Smith MD, Canalis E, Raisz LG. Characterization of the effect of insulin on collagen synthesis in fetal rat bone. *Endocrinology* 1985;116:296–302.
579. Kroc RL, Steinetz BG, Beach VL. The effects of estrogens, progestagens, and relaxin in pregnant and nonpregnant laboratory rodents. *Ann NY Acad Sci* 1959;75:942–980.
580. Kubota M, Mizuhira V. Fine structure and functions of the rat metrial gland: I. Effect of prostaglandin $F_{2\alpha}$ on the granulated metrial gland cells. *Acta Chem Cytochem* 1988;21:1–13.
581. Kuenzi MJ, Sherwood OD. Monoclonal antibodies specific for rat relaxin. VII. Passive immunization with monoclonal antibodies throughout the second half of pregnancy prevents development of normal mammary nipple morphology and function in rats. *Endocrinology* 1992;131:1841–1847.
582. Kwan TK, Cheah SH, Tan GJS, Gower DB. Effect of relaxin on macaque testicular microsomal steroidogenesis. *Med Sci Res* 1989;17:353–354.
583. Kwok SCM, Bryant-Greenwood GD, Niall HD. Evidence for proteolysis during purification of relaxin from pregnant sow ovaries. *Endocr Res Commun* 1980;7:1–12.
584. Kwok SCM, Chamley WA, Bryant-Greenwood GD. High molecular weight forms of relaxin in pregnant sow ovaries. *Biochem Biophys Res Commun* 1978;82:997–1005.
585. Lahr EL, Riddle O. Proliferation of crop-sac epithelium in incubating and in prolactin-ingested pigeons studied with the colchicine method. *Am J Physiol* 1938;123:614–619.
586. Lao Guico MS, Sherwood OD. Effect of oestradiol-17β on ovarian and serum concentrations of relaxin during the second half of pregnancy in the rat. *J Reprod Fertil* 1985;74:65–70.
587. Lao Guico-Lamm ML, Sherwood OD. Monoclonal antibodies specific for rat relaxin II. Passive immunization with monoclonal antibodies throughout the second half of pregnancy disrupts birth in intact rats. *Endocrinology* 1988;123:2479–2485.
588. Lao Guico-Lamm ML, Voss EW Jr, Sherwood OD. Monoclonal antibodies specific for rat relaxin I. Production and characterization of monoclonal antibodies that neutralize rat relaxin's bioactivity *in vivo. Endocrinology* 1988;123:2472–2478.
589. Larkin LH. Bioassay of rat metrial gland extracts for relaxin using the mouse interpubic ligament technique. *Endocrinology* 1974;94:567–570.
590. Larkin LH, Fields PA, Oliver RM. Production of antisera against electrophorectically separated relaxin and immunofluorescent localization of relaxin in the porcine corpus luteum. *Endocrinology* 1977;101:679–685.
591. Larkin LH, Fields PA, Pardo R. Mouse uterus bioassay for relaxin. In: Bryant-Greenwood GD, Niall HD, Greenwood FC, eds. *Relaxin.* New York: Elsevier/North-Holland, 1981; 321–328.
592. Larkin LH, Ogilvie S, Wubbel L, Welch DE. Effects of estradiol and progesterone on accumulation of relaxin- and carbohydrate-containing granules in endometrial gland cells of the guinea pig. *Am J Anat* 1987;179:333–341.
593. Larkin LH, Pardo RJ, Renegar RH. Sources of relaxin and morphology of relaxin-containing cells. In: Bigazzi M, Greenwood FC, Gasparri F, eds. *Biology of Relaxin and Its Role in the Human.* Amsterdam: Excerpta Medica, 1983;191–205.
594. Larkin LH, Renegar RH. Immunochemical and cytochemical studies of relaxin-containing cells in the guinea pig uterus. *Am J Anat* 1986;176:353–365.
595. Larkin LH, Suarez-Quian CA, Fields PA. *In vitro* analysis of antisera to relaxin. *Acta Endocrinol (Copenh)* 1979;92:568–576.
596. Larkin LH, Welch DE, Ogilvie S, Wubbel L. Cytochemical detection of carbohydrate and immunocytochemical detection of relaxin in the same secretory granule. *J Histochem Cytochem* 1987;35:693–697.
597. Lasley BL, Overstreet JW, Stewart DR, Boyers SP, Cragun JR, Taylor CA. Biomarkers for assessing environmental hazards to female reproduction. In: Carpenter RA, Cirillo RR, eds. *From Cradle to Grave. Trends in Hazardous Waste Management.* Honolulu, Hawaii: Pacific Basin Consortium for Hazardous Waste Research, 1992;411–417.
598. Ledger WL, Webster MA, Anderson ABM, Turnbull AC. Effect of inhibition of prostaglandin synthesis on cervical softening and uterine activity during ovine parturition resulting from progesterone withdrawal induced by epostane. *J Endocrinol* 1985;105:227–233.
599. Ledger WL, Webster MA, Harrison LP, Anderson ABM, Turnbull AC. Increase in cervical extensibility during labor induced after isolation of the cervix from the uterus in pregnant ewes. *Am J Obstet Gynecol* 1985;151:397–402.
600. Lee AB, Hwang J-J, Haab LM, Fields PA, Sherwood OD. Monoclonal antibodies specific for rat relaxin. VI. Passive immunization with monoclonal antibodies throughout the second half of pregnancy disrupts histological changes associated with cervical softening at parturition in rats. *Endocrinology* 1992; 130:2386–2391.
601. Lee HL, Tashima L, Bryant-Greenwood GD. Immunolocalization and relaxin gene expression in the human preovulatory follicle. *Program of the 38th Annual Meeting of the Society for Gynecological Investigation,* San Antonio, TX, 1991;293 (abst).
602. Lee VH, Fields PA. Rabbit placental relaxin: Progesterone and cyclic AMP effects on *in vitro* production. *Biol Reprod* 1989;40(suppl 1):87 (abst).
603. Lee VH, Fields PA. Rabbit endometrial relaxin: Immunohistochemical localization during preimplantation, pregnancy and lactation. *Biol Reprod* 1990;42:737–745.
604. Lee VH, Fields PA. Rabbit relaxin: The influence of pregnancy and ovariectomy during pregnancy on the plasma profile. *Biol Reprod* 1991;45:209–214.
605. Lee YA, Bryant-Greenwood GD, Mandel M, Greenwood FC. The complementary deoxyribonucleic acid sequence of guinea pig endometrial prorelaxin. *Endocrinology* 1992;130:1165–1172.
606. Lefebvre DL, Giaid A, Bennett H, Larivière R, Zingg HH. Oxytocin gene expression in rat uterus. *Science* 1992;256: 1553–1555.
607. Leppert PC, Yu SY, Keller S, Cerreta J, Mandl I. Decreased elastic fibers and desmosine content in incompetent cervix. *Am J Obstet Gynecol* 1987;157:1134–1139.
608. Leppi TJ. A study of the uterine cervix of the mouse. *Anat Rec* 1964;150:51–66.
609. Leppi TJ, Kinnison PA. The connective tissue ground substance in the mouse uterine cervix: An electron microscopic histochemical study. *Anat Rec* 1971;170:97–118.
610. Lerner U. The uterine cervix and the initiation of labour: Action of estradiol 17-β. In: Naftolin F, Stubblefield PG, eds. *Dilatation of the Uterine Cervix.* New York: Raven Press, 1980;301–316.
611. Lessing JB, Brenner SH, Colon JM, et al. Effect of relaxin on human spermatozoa. *J Reprod Med* 1986;31:304–309.

612. Lessing JB, Brenner SH, Schoenfeld C, et al. The effect of relaxin on the motility of sperm in freshly thawed human semen. *Fertil Steril* 1985;44:406–409.
613. Lessing JB, Brenner SH, Schoenfeld C, et al. The effect of an anti-insulin antiserum on human sperm motility. *Fertil Steril* 1984;42:309–311.
614. Lessing JB, Brenner SH, Weiss G. Effect of prolactin and relaxin on *in vitro* rat uterine contractions and prolactin interaction with relaxin. *Obstet Gynecol* 1984;64:97–100.
615. Lessing JB, Paz GF, Peyser MR, Homonnai ZT, Brenner SH, Weiss G. Laboratory efforts to improve motility of human sperm. *Semin Reprod Endocrinol* 1987;5:91–98.
616. Li Y, Huang C, Klindt J, Anderson LL. Divergent effects of antiprogesterone, RU 486, on progesterone, relaxin, and prolactin secretion in pregnant and hysterectomized pigs with aging corpora lutea. *Endocrinology* 1991;129:2907–2914.
617. Li Y, Huang C, Klindt J, Anderson LL. Stimulation of prolactin secretion in the pig: Central effects of antiprogesterone, RU 486, and relaxin. *Program of the 74th Annual Meeting of the Endocrine Society,* San Antonio, TX, 1992;245 (abst).
618. Li Y, Molina JR, Klindt J, Bolt DJ, Anderson LL. Prolactin maintains relaxin and progesterone secretion by aging corpora lutea after hypophysial stalk transection or hypophysectomy in the pig. *Endocrinology* 1989;124:1294–1304.
619. Liggins GC. The paracrine system controlling human parturition. In: Jaff RB, Dell'Acqua S, eds. *The Endocrine Physiology of Pregnancy and the Peripartal Period.* New York: Raven Press, 1985;205–221.
620. Lippert TH, Burghardt A, Seeger H, Reus W, Völter W. Presence of immune reactive relaxin in uterus and ovaries of non-pregnant humans. *Program of the 11th World Congress of Gynecology and Obstetrics,* Berlin, West Germany, 1985 (abst 383).
621. Lippert TH, God B, Vöelter W. Immunoreactive relaxin-like substance in milk. *IRCS J Med Sci* 1981;9:295.
622. Lippert TH, Schneider-Zeh S, Vöelter W. The action of relaxin, fenoterol and etilefrine on uterine motility of the rat. *Int J Clin Pharmacol Ther Toxicol* 1987;25:565–566.
623. Lippert TH, Steinberg A, Seeger H, Völter W, Ruoff HJ. Dose response relationship of relaxin on the pubic ligament of the mouse. *Clin Exp Obstet Gynecol* 1987;14:80–83.
624. Lobb DK, Porter DG. Rapid increase in relaxin gene expression in early pregnancy in the pig. *Mol Cell Endocrinol* 1992;89:R5–R8.
625. Loeken MR, Channing CP, D'Eletto R, Weiss G. Stimulatory effect of luteinizing hormone upon relaxin secretion by cultured porcine preovulatory granulosa cells. *Endocrinology* 1983; 112:769–771.
626. Long JA. Corpus luteum of pregnancy in the rat—Ultrastructural and cytochemical observations. *Biol Reprod* 1973; 8:87–99.
627. López Bernal A, Bryant-Greenwood GD, Hansell DJ, Hicks BR, Greenwood FC, Turnbull AC. Effect of relaxin on prostaglandin E production by human amnion: changes in relation to the onset of labor. *Br J Obstet Gynaecol* 1987;94:1045–1051.
628. Loumaye E, De Cooman S, Thomas K. Immunoreactive relaxin-like substance in human seminal plasma. *J Clin Endocrinol Metab* 1980;50:1142–1143.
629. Loumaye E, Depreester S, Donnez J, Thomas K. Immunoreactive relaxin surge in the peritoneal fluid of women during the midluteal phase. *Fertil Steril* 1984;42:856–860.
630. Loumaye E, Teuwissen B, Thomas K. Characterization of relaxin radioimmunoassay using Bolton-Hunter reagent. *Gynecol Obstet Invest* 1978;9:262–267.
631. Loumaye E, Thomas K. Relaxin, a para-hormone of the ovary. *Contracept Fertil Sex (Paris)* 1987;15:585–587.
632. Lovell AP. Bony pelvic dimorphism in rabbits. *Anat Rec* 1965;151:462 (abst).
633. Lowther DA. Molecular aspects of connective tissue remodelling. In: Bryant-Greenwood GD, Niall HD, Greenwood FC, eds. *Relaxin.* New York: Elsevier/North-Holland, 1981;277–292.
634. Lucas C, Bald LN, Martin MC, et al. An enzyme-linked immunosorbant assay to study human relaxin in human pregnancy and in pregnant rhesus monkeys. *J Endocrinol* 1989;120:449–457.
635. Lye SJ, Challis JRG. Inhibition by PGI-2 of myometrial activity *in vivo* in non-pregnant ovariectomized sheep. *J Reprod Fertil* 1982;66:311–315.
636. Lyons MF, Searle AG. *Genetic Variants and Strains of the Laboratory Mouse,* Ed 2. Oxford: Oxford University Press, 1989;187–188.
637. MacLennan AH. Cervical ripening and the induction of labour by vaginal prostaglandin $F_{2\alpha}$ and relaxin. In: Ellwood DA, Anderson ABM, eds. *The Cervix in Pregnancy and Labour.* London: Churchill Livingstone, 1981;187–195.
638. MacLennan AH. The role of the hormone relaxin in human reproduction and pelvic girdle relaxation. *Scand J Rheumatol Suppl* 1991;88:7–15.
639. MacLennan AH, Grant P. Human relaxin: *In vitro* response of human and pig myometrium. *J Reprod Med* 1991;36:630–634.
640. MacLennan AH, Grant P, Borthwick AC. Relaxin and relaxin c-peptide levels in human reproductive tissues. *Reprod Fertil Dev* 1991;3:577–583.
641. MacLennan AH, Grant P, Ness D, Down A. Effect of porcine relaxin and progesterone on rat, pig and human myometrial activity *in vitro. J Reprod Med* 1986;31:43–49.
642. MacLennan AH, Green RC, Bryant-Greenwood GD, Greenwood FC, Seamark RF. Ripening of the human cervix and induction of labour with purified porcine relaxin. *Lancet* 1980;1:220–223.
643. MacLennan AH, Green RC, Bryant-Greenwood GD, Greenwood FC, Seamark RF. Cervical ripening with combinations of vaginal prostaglandin $F_{2\alpha}$, estradiol, and relaxin. *Obstet Gynecol* 1981;58:601–604.
644. MacLennan AH, Green RC, Grant P, Nicolson R. Ripening of the human cervix and induction of labor with intracervical purified porcine relaxin. *Obstet Gynecol* 1986;68:598–601.
645. MacLennan AH, Katz M, Creasy R. The morphologic characteristics of cervical ripening induced by the hormones relaxin and prostaglandin $F_{2\alpha}$ in a rabbit model. *Am J Obstet Gynecol* 1985;152:691–696.
646. MacLennan AH, Kerin JFP, Kirby C, et al. The effect of porcine relaxin vaginally applied at human embryo transfer in an *in vitro* fertilization programme. *Aust N Z J Obstet Gynaecol* 1985;25:68–71.
647. MacLennan AH, Nicolson R, Green RC. Serum relaxin in pregnancy. *Lancet* 1986;2:241–244.
648. MacLennan AH, Nicolson R, Green RC, Bath M. Serum relaxin and pelvic pain of pregnancy. *Lancet* 1986;2:243–245.
649. Madej A, Kindahl H, Nydahl C, Edqvist L-E, Stewart DR. Hormonal changes associated with induced late abortions in the mare. *J Reprod Fertil (Suppl)* 1987;35:479–484.
650. Maillot K von. Changes in the glycosaminoglycans distribution pattern in the human uterine cervix during pregnancy and labor. *Am J Obstet Gynecol* 1979;135:503–506.
651. Majewski JT, Jennings T. A uterine relaxing factor for premature labor. *Obstet Gynecol* 1955;5:649–652.
652. Manning JP, Steinetz BG, Butler MC, Priester S. The effect of steroids and relaxin on acid phosphatase in the pubic symphysis of the ovariectomized mouse. *J Endocrinol* 1965;33:501–506.
653. Marder SN, Money WL. Concentration of relaxin in the blood serum of pregnant and postpartum rabbits. *Endocrinology* 1944;34:115–121.
654. Marriott D, Gillece-Castro B, Gorman CM. Prohormone convertase-1 will process prorelaxin, a member of the insulin family of hormones. *Mol Endocrinol* 1992;6:1441–1450.
655. Martin MC, Johnston PD, Rudman C. Human relaxin causes cervical ripening in primate pregnancy without change in uterine activity. *Program of the 33rd Annual Meeting of the Society for Gynecological Investigation,* Toronto, 1986;19 (abst).
656. Martin PA, BeVier GW, Dziuk PJ. The effect of disconnecting the uterus and ovary on the length of gestation in the pig. *Biol Reprod* 1978;18:428–433.
657. Massicotte G, Parent A, St-Louis J. Blunted responses to vasoconstrictors in mesenteric vasculature but not in portal vein of spontaneously hypertensive rats treated with relaxin. *Proc Soc Exp Biol Med* 1989;190:254–259.
658. Mathieu P, Rahier J, Thomas K. Localization of relaxin in hu-

man gestational corpus luteum. *Cell Tissue Res* 1981;219: 213–216.
659. Matsumoto D, Chamley WA. Identification of relaxins in porcine follicular fluid and in the ovary of the immature sow. *J Reprod Fertil* 1980;58:369–375.
660. May JV, Schomberg DW. Granulosa cell differentiation *in vitro:* Effect of insulin on growth and functional integrity. *Biol Reprod* 1981;25:421–431.
661. Mazoujian G, Bryant-Greenwood GD. Relaxin in breast tissue. *Lancet* 1990;335:298–299.
662. Melton CE, Saldivar JT. Impulse velocity and conduction pathways in rat myometrium. *Am J Physiol* 1964;207:279–285.
663. Mercado-Simmen RC, Bryant-Greenwood GD, Greenwood FC. Characterization of the binding of ^{125}I-relaxin to rat uterus. *J Biol Chem* 1980;255:3617–3623.
664. Mercado-Simmen RC, Bryant-Greenwood GD, Greenwood FC. Relaxin receptor in the rat myometrium: Regulation by estrogen and relaxin. *Endocrinoloy* 1982;110:220–226.
665. Mercado-Simmen RC, Goodwin B, Ueno MS, Yamamoto SY, Bryant-Greenwood GD. Relaxin receptors in the myometrium and cervix of the pig. *Biol Reprod* 1982;26:120–128.
666. Messine O, Barros C, Chang SM, Thatcher WW, Fields MJ. Relaxin secretion during the cycle and early pregnancy in the pig. *Biol Reprod* 1989;40(suppl 1):58 (abst).
667. Miller JW, Kisley A, Murray WJ. The effects of relaxin-containing ovarian extracts on various types of smooth muscle. *J Pharmacol Exp Ther* 1957;120:426–437.
668. Mishell DR, Nakamura RM, Barberia JM, Thorneycroft IH. Initial detection of human chorionic gonadotropin in serum in normal human gestation. *Am J Obstet Gynecol* 1974;118: 990–991.
669. Molokwu ECI, Wagner WC. Endocrine physiology of the puerperal sow. *J Anim Sci* 1973;36:1158–1163.
670. Morley P, Calaresu FR, Barbe GJ, Armstrong DT. Insulin enhances luteinizing hormone-stimulated steroidogenesis by porcine theca cells. *Biol Reprod* 1989;40:735–743.
671. Mossman HW, Duke KL. *Comparative Morphology of the Mammalian Ovary.* Madison: University of Wisconsin Press, 1973;209–220.
672. Mumford AD, Parry LJ, Summerlee AJS. Lesion of the subfornical organ affects the haemotensive response to centrally administered relaxin in anaesthetized rats. *J Endocrinol* 1989;122:747–755.
673. Musah AI, Bellows RA, Schwabe C, Anderson LL. Relaxin and progesterone secretion are breed dependent in Bos-Taurus and Bos-Indicus cattle. *Program of the Combined Meeting of the American Dairy Science Association and the American Society of Animal Science,* Lexington, KY, 1989;391 (abst).
674. Musah AI, Ford JJ, Anderson LL. Progesterone secretion as affected by 17β-estradiol after hysterectomy in the pig. *Endocrinology* 1984;115:1876–1882.
675. Musah AI, Huang CJ, Bagna B, Schwabe C, Anderson LL. Peripheral plasma progesterone, prostaglandin $F_{2\alpha}$ ($PGF_{2\alpha}$), prostaglandin E2 (PGE2), 6-keto prostaglandin (6-keto PG) and calving after relaxin administration in heifers. *Biol Reprod* 1989;40(suppl 1):70 (abst).
676. Musah AI, Schwabe C, Anderson LL. Acute decrease in progesterone and increase in estrogen secretion caused by relaxin during late pregnancy in beef heifers. *Endocrinology* 1987; 120:317–324.
677. Musah AI, Schwabe C, Anderson LL. Relaxin regulates oxytocin secretion in late-pregnant beef heifers. *Proc Soc Exp Biol Med* 1989;191:124–129.
678. Musah AI, Schwabe C, Anderson LL. Relaxin, oxytocin, and prostaglandin effects on progesterone secretion from bovine luteal cells during different stages of gestation. *Proc Soc Exp Biol Med* 1990;195:255–260.
679. Musah AI, Schwabe C, Anderson LL. Relaxin and prostaglandin on oxytocin secretion from bovine luteal cells during different stages of gestation. *Acta Endocrinol* 1990;122:396–402.
680. Musah AI, Schwabe C, Willham RL, Anderson LL. Pelvic development as affected by relaxin in three genetically selected frame sizes of beef heifers. *Biol Reprod* 1986;34:363–369.
681. Musah AI, Schwabe C, Willham RL, Anderson LL. Relaxin on induction of parturition in beef heifers. *Endocrinology* 1986;118:1476–1482.
682. Musah AI, Schwabe C, Willham RL, Anderson LL. Induction of parturition, progesterone secretion, and delivery of placenta in beef heifers given relaxin with cloprostenol or dexamethasone. *Biol Reprod* 1987;37:797–803.
683. Musah AI, Schwabe C, Willham RL, Anderson LL. Dystocia, pelvic and cervical dilatation in beef heifers after induction of parturition with relaxin combined with cloprostenol or dexamethasone. *Anim Reprod Sci* 1988;16:237–248.
684. McCarthy JJ, Erving HW, Laufe LE. Preliminary report on the use of relaxin in the management of threatened premature labor. *Am J Obstet Gynecol* 1957;74:134–138.
685. McCusker RH, Camacho-Hübner C, Clemmons DR. Identification of the types of insulin-like growth factor-binding proteins that are secreted by muscle cells *in vitro. J Biol Chem* 1989;264:7795–7800.
686. McDonald JK, Schwabe C. Relaxin-induced elevations of cathepsin B and dipeptidyl peptidase I in the mouse pubic symphysis, with localization by fluorescence enzyme histochemistry. *Ann NY Acad Sci* 1982;380:178–186.
687. McGovern PG, Goldsmith LT, Schmidt CL, von Hagen S, Linden M, Weiss G. Effects of endothelin and relaxin on rat uterine segment contractility. *Biol Reprod* 1992;46:680–685.
688. McIlwrath A, Downing SJ, Hollingsworth M. Relaxin and cAMP in rat uterus *in vivo. Biochem Soc Trans* 1991;19:356S (abst).
689. McMurtry JP, Floersheim GL, Bryant-Greenwood GD. Characterization of the binding of ^{125}I-labeled succinylated porcine relaxin to human and mouse fibroblasts. *J Reprod Fertil* 1980;58:43–49.
690. McMurtry JP, Kwok SCM, Bryant-Greenwood GD. Target tissues for relaxin identified *in vitro* with ^{125}I-labeled porcine relaxin. *J Reprod Fertil* 1978;53:209–216.
691. Naftolin F, Stubblefield PG, eds. *Dilatation of the Uterine Cervix.* New York: Raven Press, 1980.
692. Nagao R, Bryant-Greenwood GD. Evidence for a uterine relaxin in the guinea pig. In: Bryant-Greenwood GD, Niall HD, Greenwood FC, eds. *Relaxin.* New York: Elsevier/North-Holland, 1981;61–69.
693. Nakajima ST, Stewart DR, Brumsted JR, Lasley BL, Gibson M. The luteal and endometrial response to human pseudopregnancy. *Program of the 74th Annual Meeting of the Endocrine Society,* San Antonio, TX, 1992;278 (abst).
694. Nara BS, Ball GD, Rutherford JE, Sherwood OD, First NL. Release of relaxin by a nonluteolytic dose of prostaglandin $F_{2\alpha}$ in pregnant swine. *Biol Reprod* 1982;27:1190–1195.
695. Nara BS, First NL. Effect of indomethacin and prostaglandin $F_{2\alpha}$ on parturition in swine. *J Anim Sci* 1981;52:1360–1370.
696. Nara BS, Welk FA, Rutherford JE, Sherwood OD, First NL. Effect of relaxin on parturition and frequency of live births in pigs. *J Reprod Fertil* 1982;66:359–365.
697. Nardi E, Bigazzi M, Agrimonti F, et al. Relaxin and fibrocystic disease of the mammary gland. In: Bigazzi M, Greenwood FC, Gasparri F, eds. *Biology of Relaxin and Its Role in the Human.* Amsterdam: Excerpta Medica, 1983;417–419.
698. Nemec LA, Loskutoff NM, Lasley BL, Fields MJ, Bowen MJ, Kraemer DC. The influence of relaxin, with steroid pretreatment, on cervical dilatation in ovariectomized ewes. *Theriogenology* 1988;29:282 (abst).
699. Neuwinger J, Jockenhövel F, Nieschlag E. The influence of relaxin on motility of human sperm *in vitro. Andrologia* 1990;22:335–339.
700. Newton WH, Beck N. Placental activity in the mouse in the absence of the pituitary gland. *J Endocrinol* 1939;1:65–75.
701. Niall HD, James R, John M, et al. Chemical studies on relaxin. *Adv Exp Med Biol* 1982;143:163–169.
702. Nicol DSHW, Smith LF. The amino acid sequence of human insulin. *Nature* 1960;187:483–485.
703. Nicoll CS. Bio-assay of prolactin. Analysis of the pigeon crop-sac response to local prolactin injection by an objective and quantitative method. *Endocrinology* 1967;80:641–655.
704. Niebauer GW, Ritter C, Wolf B. The potential role of relaxin in canine perineal hernia. *FASEB* 1991;5:A1639 (abst).

705. Nishikori K, Burroughs M, Sanborn BM. cAMP-dependent phosphorylation on rat uterine myosin light chain kinase activity partially mimics the effects of relaxin treatment. *Program of the 65th Annual Meeting of the Endocrine Society,* San Antonio, TX, 1983;291 (abst).
706. Nishikori K, Weisbrodt NW, Sherwood OD, Sanborn BM. Relaxin alters rat uterine myosin light chain phosphorylation and related enzymatic activities. *Endocrinology* 1982;111 1743–1745.
707. Nishikori K, Weisbrodt NW, Sherwood OD, Sanborn BM. Effects of relaxin on rat uterine myosin light chain kinase activity and myosin light chain phosphorylation. *J Biol Chem* 1983;258:2468–2474.
708. Nixon WE, Reid R, Abou-Hozaifa BM, Williams RF, Steinetz BG, Hodgen GD. Origin and regulation of relaxin secretion in monkeys: Effects of chorionic gonadotropin, luteectomy, fetectomy, and placentectomy. In: Greenwald GS, Terranova PF, eds. *Factors Regulating Ovarian Function.* New York: Raven Press, 1983;427–431.
709. Noall MW, Frieden EH. Variations in sensitivity of ovariectomized guinea pigs to relaxin. *Endocrinology* 1956;58:659–664.
710. Noci I, Nardi E, Scarselli G, et al. Immuno- and bio-active relaxin in human ovarian follicles. In: Bigazzi M, Greenwood FC, Gasparri F, eds. *Biology of Relaxin and Its Role in the Human.* Amsterdam: Excerpta Medica, 1983;270–272.
711. Norman M, Ekman G, Ulmsten U, Barchan K, Malmström A. Proteoglycan metabolism in the connective tissue of pregnant and non-pregnant human cervix. *Biochem J* 1991;275:515–520.
712. Norström A, Bryman I. Adenosine 3′,5′-monophosphate in relation to inhibition of cervical smooth muscle activity in early pregnant women. *Acta Endocrinol* 1991;125:122–125.
713. Norström A, Bryman I, Wiqvist N, Sahni S, Lindblom B. Inhibitory action of relaxin on human cervical smooth muscle. *J Clin Endocrinol Metab* 1984;59:379–382.
714. Norström A, Tjugum J. Hormonal effects on collagenolytic activity in the isolated human ovarian follicular wall. *Gynecol Obstet Invest* 1986;22:12–16.
715. Norström A, Wiqvist I. Relaxin-induced changes in adenosine 3′5′-monophosphate levels in the human cervix. *Acta Endocrinol* 1985;109:122–125.
716. North ACT, Denson AK, Evans AC, Ford LO, Willoughby TV. The use of an interactive computer graphics system in the study of protein conformations. *Biomol Struct Conform Funct Evol Proc Int Symp* 1981;1:59–72.
717. Ny T, Bjersing L, Hseuh AJW, Loskutoff DJ. Cultured granulosa cells produce two plasminogen activators and an antiactivator, each regulated differently by gonadotropins. *Endocrinology* 1985;116:1666–1668.
718. Obrink B. A study of the interactions between monomeric tropocollagen and glycosaminoglycans. *Eur J Biochem* 1973;33 387–400.
719. O'Byrne EM, Brindle S, Quintavalla J, Strawinski C, Tabachnick M, Steinetz BG. Tissue distribution of injected ^{125}I-labeled porcine relaxin: Organ uptake, whole-body autoradiography, and renal concentration of radiometabolites. *Ann NY Acad Sci* 1982;380:187–197.
720. O'Byrne EM, Carriere BT, Sorensen L, Segaloff A, Schwabe C, Steinetz BG. Plasma immunoreactive relaxin levels in pregnant and nonpregnant women. *J Clin Endocrinol Metab* 1978;47: 1106–1110.
721. O'Byrne EM, Flitcraft JF, Sawyer WK, Hochman J, Weiss G, Steinetz BG. Relaxin bioactivity and immunoactivity in human corpora lutea. *Endocrinology* 1978;102:1641–1644.
722. O'Byrne EM, Sawyer WK, Butler MC, Steinetz BG. Serum immunoreactive relaxin and softening of the uterine cervix in pregnant hamsters. *Endocrinology* 1976;99:1333–1335.
723. O'Byrne EM, Steinetz BG. Radioimmunoassay of relaxin in sera of various species using an antiserum to porcine relaxin. *Proc Soc Exp Biol Med* 1976;152:272–276.
724. O'Byrne EM, Tabachnick M, Anderson LL, Steinetz BG. Characterization of the circulating form of porcine relaxin: Biological activity and terminal amino acids. *Endocrinology* 1989;124: 2920–2927.
725. O'Byrne EM, Weiss G, Steinetz BG. The isolation of human relaxin from the corpus luteum. In: Bigazzi M, Greenwood FC, Gasparri F, eds. *Biology of Relaxin and Its Role in the Human.* Amsterdam: Excerpta Medica, 1983;370–376.
726. O'Byrne KT, Eltringham L, Clarke G, Summerlee AJS. Effects of porcine relaxin on oxytocin release from the neurohypophysis in the anesthetized lactating rat. *J Endocrinol* 1986;109: 393–397.
727. O'Byrne KT, Eltringham L, Summerlee AJS. Central inhibitory effects of relaxin on the milk ejection reflex of the rat depends upon the site of injection into the cerebroventricular system. *Brain Res* 1987;405:80–83.
728. O'Byrne KT, Summerlee AJS. Naloxone reverses relaxin inhibition of oxytocin release in the rat. *Neurosci Lett* 1985;22:S573 (abst).
729. O'Byrne KT, Summerlee AJS. Relaxin suppression of oxytocin release occurs at the neurohypophysis in the rat. *J Physiol (Lond)* 1985;365:49P (abst).
730. Ochiai K, Kato H, Kelly PA, Rothchild I. The importance of a luteolytic effect of the pituitary in understanding the placental control of the rat's corpus luteum. *Endocrinology* 1983;112: 1687–1695.
731. Ochiai K, Rothchild I. The relation between conceptus number and the luteotropic effect of estrogen in rats after hypophysectomy and hysterectomy on day 12 of pregnancy. *Endocrinology* 1981;109:1111–1116.
732. O'Connor WB, Cain GD, Zarrow MX. Elongation of the interpubic ligament in the little brown bat (*Myotis lucifugus*). *Proc Soc Exp Biol Med* 1966;123:935–937.
733. O'Day MB, Winn RJ, Foster RA, Dziuk PJ, Sherwood OD. Hormonal control of the cervix in pregnant gilts. II. Relaxin promotes changes in the physical properties of the cervix in ovariectomized hormone-treated pregnant gilts. *Endocrinology* 1989;125:3004–3010.
734. O'Day-Bowman MB, Winn RJ, Dziuk PJ, Lindley ER, Sherwood OD. Hormonal control of the cervix in pregnant gilts. III. Relaxin's influence on cervical biochemical properties in ovariectomized hormone-treated pregnant gilts. *Endocrinology* 1991;129:1967–1976.
735. Ogilvie S, Duckworth ML, Larkin LH, Buhi WC, Shiverick KT. *De novo* synthesis and secretion of prolactin-like protein-B by rat placental explants. *Endocrinology* 1990;126:2561–2566.
736. Olefsky JM, Sackow M, Kroc RL. Potentiation of insulin binding and insulin action by purified porcine relaxin. *Ann NY Acad Sci* 1982;380:200–215.
737. Oliver RM, Fields PA, Larkin LH. Separation of relaxin activities in extracts of ovaries of pregnant sows by polyacrylamide gel electrophoresis. *J Endocrinol* 1978;76:517–525.
738. Omini G, Pasargiklian R, Folco GC, Fano M, Berti F. Pharmacological activity of PGI2 and its metabolite 6-oxo-PGF$_{1\alpha}$ on human uterus and fallopian tubes. *Prostaglandins* 1978;15: 1045–1054.
739. Orsini MW. The trophoblastic giant cells and endovascular cells associated with pregnancy in the hamster, *Cricetus auratus. Am J Anat* 1954;94:273–331.
740. Osa T, Inoue H, Okabe K. Effects of porcine relaxin on contraction, membrane response and cyclic AMP content in rat myometrium in comparison with the effects of isoprenaline and forskolin. *Br J Pharmacol* 1991;104:950–960.
741. Osetinsky GV, Marion MS, McCaffrey TV. Modification of collagen in tissue expansion. *Surg Forum* 1988;39:559–561.
742. Osheroff PL, Cronin MJ, Lofgren JA. Relaxin binding in the rat heart atrium. *Proc Natl Acad Sci* 1992;89:2384–2388.
743. Osheroff PL, Ling VT, Vandlen RL, Cronin MJ, Lofgren JA. Preparation of biologically active ^{32}P-labeled human relaxin. Displaceable binding to rat uterus, cervix and brain. *J Biol Chem* 1990;265:9396–9401.
744. Osheroff PL, Phillips HS. Autoradiographic localization of relaxin binding sites in rat brain. *Proc Natl Acad Sci USA* 1991;88:6413–6417.
745. Osmers R, Rath W, Adelmann-Grill BC, et al. Origin of cervical collagenase during parturition. *Am J Obstet Gynecol* 1992;166: 1455–1460.
746. Ottobre AC, Ramsey KR, Ottobre JS. Acute versus chronic ef-

fects of human chorionic gonadotrophin on relaxin secretion in rhesus monkeys. *J Reprod Fertil* 1991;91:313–320.
747. Ottobre JS, Nixon WE, Stouffer RL. Induction of relaxin secretion in rhesus monkeys by human chorionic gonadotropin: Dependence on the age of the corpus luteum of the menstrual cycle. *Biol Reprod* 1984;31:1000–1006.
748. Owerbach D, Bell GI, Rutter WJ, Shows TB. The insulin gene is located on chromosome 11 in humans. *Nature* 1980;286:82–84.
749. Paccamonti DL, Chang ST, Dubois W, et al. Circulating concentrations of porcine relaxin in cows: Evaluation of vehicles and routes of administration. *Theriogenology* 1991;35:1131–1146.
750. Pardo RJ, Larkin LH. Localization of relaxin in endometrial gland cells of pregnant, lactating, and ovariectomized hormone-treated guinea pigs. *Am J Anat* 1982;164:79–90.
751. Pardo R, Larkin LH, Fields PA. Immunocytochemical localization of relaxin in endometrial glands of the pregnant guinea pig. *Endocrinology* 1980;107:2110–2112.
752. Pardo RJ, Larkin LH, Renegar RH. Immunoelectron microscopic localization of relaxin in endometrial gland cells of the pregnant guinea pig. *Anat Rec* 1984;209:373–379.
753. Park JM, Ewing K, Miller F, Friedman CI, Kim MH. Effects of relaxin on the fertilization capacity of human spermatozoa. *Am J Obstet Gynecol* 1988;158:974–979.
754. Parry DM, Ellwood DA. Ultrastructural aspects of cervical softening in the sheep. In: Ellwood DA, Anderson ABM, eds. *The Cervix in Pregnancy and Labour.* New York: Churchill Livingstone, 1981;74–84.
755. Parry LJ, Poterski RS, Summerlee AJS, Jones SA. Mechanism of the haemotensive action of porcine relaxin in anaesthetized rats. *J Neuroendocrinol* 1990;2:53–58.
756. Parry LJ, Poterski RS, Wasnidge C, Summerlee AJS. Relaxin in the cerebrospinal fluid of female rats. *Program of the 21st Annual Meeting of the Society of Neuroscience,* New Orleans, LA, 1991;1196 (abst).
757. Parry LJ, Summerlee AJS. Central angiotensin partially mediates the pressor action of relaxin in anesthetized rats. *Endocrinology* 1991;129:47–52.
758. Patek CE, Watson J. Prostaglandin F and progesterone secretion by porcine endometrium and corpora lutea *in vitro. Prostaglandins* 1976;12:97–111.
759. Patek CE, Watson J. Factors affecting steroid and prostaglandin secretion by reproductive tissues of cycling and pregnant sows *in vitro. Biochim Biophys Acta* 1983;755:17–24.
760. Paterson G. The nature of the inhibition of the rat uterus by relaxin. *J Pharm Pharmacol* 1965;17:262–264.
761. Pawlina W, Larkin LH, Frost SC. Effect of relaxin on differentiation of 3T3-L1 preadipocytes. *Endocrinology* 1989;125:2049–2055.
762. Pawlina W, Larkin LH, Ogilvie S, Frost SC. Human relaxin inhibits division but not differentiation of 3T3-L1 cells. *Mol Cell Endocrinol* 1990;72:55–61.
763. Peaker M, Taylor E, Tashima L, Redman TL, Greenwood FC, Bryant-Greenwood GD. Relaxin detected by immunocytochemistry and northern analysis in the mammary gland of the guinea pig. *Endocrinology* 1989;125:693–698.
764. Pederson ES. Histogenesis of lutein tissue of the albino rat. *Am J Anat* 1951;88:397–427.
765. Pepe GJ, Rothchild I. A comparative study of serum progesterone levels in pregnancy and in various types of pseudopregnancy in the rat. *Endocrinology* 1974;95:275–279.
766. Perezgrovas R, Anderson LL. Effect of porcine relaxin on cervical dilatation, pelvic area and parturition in beef heifers. *Biol Reprod* 1982;26:765–776.
767. Perl E, Catchpole HR. Changes induced in the connective tissue of the pubic symphysis of the guinea pig with estrogen and relaxin. *Arch Pathol Lab Med* 1950;50:233–239.
768. Petersen LK, Skajaa K, Uldbjerg N. Serum relaxin as a potential marker for preterm labour. *Br J Obstet Gynaecol* 1992;99:292–295.
769. Petersen LK, Svane D, Uldbjerg N, Forman A. Effects of human relaxin on isolated rat and human myometrium and uteroplacental arteries. *Obstet Gynecol* 1991;78:757–762.
770. Petrucci F, Goed B, La Malfa A, et al. Metabolism of the uterus after administration of relaxin from human decidua. In: Bigazzi M, Greenwood FC, Gasparri F, eds. *Biology of Relaxin and Its Role in the Human.* Amsterdam: Excerpta Medica, 1983;137–139.
771. Pilistine SJ, Varandani PT. Degradation of porcine relaxin by glutathione-insulin transhydrogenase and a neutral peptidase. *Mol Cell Endocrinol* 1986;46:43–52.
772. Piquette GN, Timms BG. Immunohistochemical localization of tissue-type plasminogen activator (t-PA) in primary cultures of rabbit ovarian surface epithelium, granulosa cells and peritoneal mesothelium. *Biol Reprod* 1988;38(suppl 1):183 (abst).
773. Plunkett ER, Gammal EB. The effect of relaxin upon DMBA-induced mammary cancer in female rats. *Br J Cancer* 1967;21:592–600.
774. Plunkett ER, Squires BP, Heagy FC. Effect of relaxin on thyroid function in the rat. *J Endocrinol* 1963;26:331–338.
775. Plunkett ER, Squires BP, Richardson SJ. The effect of relaxin on thyroid weights in laboratory animals. *J Endocrinol* 1960;21:241–246.
776. Poisner AM, Poisner R, Downing G, Relaxin, calcium and oxygenation influence prorenin release from superfused human placenta and decidua. *Program of the 74th Annual Meeting of the Endocrine Society,* San Antonio, TX, 1992;408 (abst).
777. Poisner AM, Thrailkill K, Poisner R, Handwerger S. Relaxin stimulates the synthesis and release of prorenin from human decidual cells: Evidence for autocrine/paracrine regulation. *J Clin Endocrinol Metab* 1990;70:1765–1767.
778. Pommerenke WT. Experimental ligamentous relaxation in the guinea pig pelvis. *Am J Obstet Gynecol* 1934;27:708–713.
779. Porter DG. The action of relaxin on myometrial activity in the guinea-pig *in vivo. J Reprod Fertil* 1971;26:251–253.
780. Porter DG. Myometrium of the pregnant guinea pig: The probable importance of relaxin. *Biol Reprod* 1972;7:458–464.
781. Porter DG. Inhibition of myometrial activity in the pregnant rabbit: Evidence for a "new" factor. *Biol Reprod* 1974;10:54–61.
782. Porter DG. Relaxin: Old hormone, new prospect. In: Finn CA, ed. *Oxford Reviews of Reproductive Biology.* Oxford: Clarendon Press, 1979;1–57.
783. Porter DG. The myometrium and the relaxin enigma. *Anim Reprod Sci* 1979;2:77–96.
784. Porter DG. Relaxin and cervical softening: A review. In: Ellwood DA, Anderson ABM, eds. *The Cervix in Pregnancy and Labour.* New York: Churchill Livingstone, 1981;85–99.
785. Porter DG. Unsolved problems of relaxin's physiological role. *Ann NY Acad Sci* 1982;380:151–162.
786. Porter DG. The possible involvement of relaxin in the regulation of uterine contraction. In: Bigazzi M, Greenwood FC, Gasparri F, eds. *Biology of Relaxin and Its Role in the Human.* Amsterdam: Excerpta Medica, 1983;114–124.
787. Porter DG, Challis JRG. Failure of high uterine concentrations of progesterone to inhibit myometrial activity *in vivo* in the postpartum rat. *J Reprod Fertil* 1974;39:157–162.
788. Porter DG, Downing SJ. Evidence that a humoral factor possessing relaxin-like activity is responsible for uterine quiescence in the late pregnant rat. *J Reprod Fertil* 1978;52:95–102.
789. Porter DG, Downing SJ, Bradshaw JMC. Relaxin inhibits spontaneous and prostaglandin-driven myometrial activity in anaesthetized rats. *J Endocrinol* 1979;83:183–192.
790. Porter DG, Downing SJ, Bradshaw JMC. Inhibition of oxytocin- or prostaglandin $F_{2}\alpha$-driven myometrial activity by relaxin in the rat is oestrogen-dependent. *J Endocrinol* 1981;89:399–404.
791. Porter DG, Friendship RM, Ryan PL, Wasnidge C. Relaxin is not associated with poor milk yield in the postpartum sow. *Can J Vet Res* 1992;56:204–207.
792. Porter DG, Lye SJ, Bradshaw JMC, Kendall JZ. Relaxin inhibits myometrial activity in the ovariectomized non-pregnant ewe. *J Reprod Fertil* 1981;61:409–414.
793. Porter DG, Ryan PL, Norman L. Lack of effect of relaxin on oxytocin output from the porcine neural lobe *in vitro* or in lactating sows *in vivo. J Reprod Fertil* 1992;96:251–260.
794. Porter DG, Watts AD. Relaxin and progesterone are myometrial inhibitors in the ovariectomized non-pregnant mini-pig. *J Reprod Fertil* 1986;76:205–213.
795. Posse N, Kelly JV. A study of the effect of relaxin on contractil-

ity of the non-pregnant uterus by internal tocometry. *Surg Gynecol Obstet* 1956;103:687–694.

796. Prud'Homme M-J, Martinat N, Picaper G. The effect of relaxin on *in vivo* uterine electromyographic activity in the conscious ovariectomized ewe is oestrogen-dependent. *Reprod Nutr Dev* 1983;23:493–499.
797. Psalti I, Rahier J, Loumaye E, Haumont S, Thomas K. Changes of relaxin concentrations determined by immunodensitometry in ovaries of NMRI mice during pregnancy. *Gynecol Obstet Invest* 1990;30:133–138.
798. Pullen RA, Lindsay DG, Wood SP, et al. Receptor-binding region of insulin. *Nature* 1976;259:369–373.
799. Pupula M, MacLennan AH. Effect of porcine relaxin on spontaneous, oxytocin-driven and prostaglandin-driven pig myometrial activity *in vitro*. *J Reprod Med* 1989;34:819–823.
800. Pupula M, Quinn P, MacLennan A. The effect of porcine relaxin on the fertilization of mouse oocytes *in vitro*. *Clin Reprod Fertil* 1986;4:383–387.
801. Puri CP, Garfield RE. Changes in hormone levels and gap junctions in the rat uterus during pregnancy and parturition. *Biol Reprod* 1982;27:967–975.
802. Pusey J, Kelly WA, Bradshaw JMC, Porter DG. Myometrial activity and the distribution of blastocysts in the uterus of the rat: Interference by relaxin. *Biol Reprod* 1980;23:394–397.
803. Quagliarello J, Cederqvist L, Steinetz B, Weiss G. Serum relaxin levels in prostaglandin E_2 induced abortions. *Prostaglandins* 1978;16:1003–1006.
804. Quagliarello J, Goldsmith L, Steinetz BG, Lustig DS, Weiss G. Induction of relaxin secretion in nonpregnant women by human chorionic gonadotropin. *J Clin Endocrinol Metab* 1980;51:74–77.
805. Quagliarello J, Lustig DS, Steinetz BG, Weiss G. Absence of a prelabor relaxin surge in women. *Biol Reprod* 1980;22:202–204.
806. Quagliarello J, Steinetz BG, Weiss G. Relaxin secretion in early pregnancy. *Obstet Gynecol* 1979;53:62–63.
807. Quagliarello J, Szlachter N, Nisselbaum JS, Schwartz MK, Steinetz BG, Weiss G. Serum relaxin and human chorionic gonadotropin concentrations in spontaneous abortions. *Fertil Steril* 1981;36:399–401.
808. Quagliarello J, Szlachter N, Steinetz BG, Goldsmith LT, Weiss G. Serial relaxin concentrations in human pregnancy. *Am J Obstet Gynecol* 1979;135:43–44.
809. Randall GCB, Taverne MAM, Challis JRG, Kendall JZ, Tsang BK. Interrelationships between endocrine changes in peripheral and uterine-venous blood and uterine activity at parturition in the pig. *Anim Reprod Sci* 1986;11:283–294.
810. Randel RD, Stanko RL, Musah AI, Anderson LL. Temporal relationship between peripheral plasma relaxin, estradiol-17β and progesterone in Brahman cows near parturition. *J Anim Sci* 1988;66(suppl 1):64 (abst).
811. Rao MR, Sanborn BM. Relaxin increases calcium efflux from rat myometrial cells in culture. *Endocrinology* 1986;119:435–437.
812. Rath W, Adelmann-Grill BC, Pieper U, Kuhn W, Osmers R. Collagenase activity in cervical tissue of the non-pregnant and pregnant human cervix. *Acta Physiol Hung* 1988;71:491–496.
813. Rawitch AB, Moore WV, Frieden EH. Relaxin-insulin homology: Predictions of secondary structure and lack of competitive binding. *Int J Biochem* 1980;11:357–362.
814. Reddy GK, Gunwar S, Green CB, Fei OTW, Chen AB, Kwok SCM. Purification and characterization of recombinant porcine prorelaxin expressed in *Escherichia coli*. *Arch Biochem Biophys* 1992;294:579–585.
815. Reinig JW, Daniel LN, Schwabe C, Gowan LK, Steinetz BG, O'Byrne EM. Isolation and characterization of relaxin from the sand tiger shark (*Odontaspis taurus*). *Endocrinology* 1981;109:537–543.
816. Renegar RH, Cobb AD, Leavitt WW. Immunocytochemical localization of relaxin in the golden hamster (*Mesocricetus auratus*) during the last half of gestation. *Biol Reprod* 1987;37:925–934.
817. Renegar RH, Larkin LH. Relaxin concentrations in endometrial, placental, and ovarian tissues, and in sera from ewes during middle and late pregnancy. *Biol Reprod* 1985;32:840–847.
818. Renegar RH, Southard JN, Talamantes F. Immunohistochemical co-localization of placental lactogen II and relaxin in the golden hamster (*Mesocricetus auratus*). *J Histochem Cytochem* 1990;38:935–940.
819. Renegar RH, Steel M, Burden HW, Hodson CA. Endocrine parameters associated with disruption of parturition after bilateral pelvic neurectomy. *Proc Soc Exp Biol Med* 1992;201:28–33.
820. Reynolds H, Livingood CS. Use of relaxin in management of ulceration and gangrene due to collagen disease. *AMA Arch Dermatol* 1959;80:407–409.
821. Rice LE, Wiltbank JN. Factors affecting dystocia in beef heifers. *JAMA* 1972;161:1348–1358.
822. Rimmer DM. The effect of pregnancy on the collagen of the uterine cervix of the mouse. *J Endocrinol* 1973;57:413–418.
823. Rinard GA. Phosphorylase a activity in rat uterine homogenates: Loss of activity related to *in vivo* treatment with estrogen, progesterone, relaxin, and CaEDTA. *Biochim Biophys Acta* 1970;222:455–464.
824. Rinderknecht E, Humbel RE. Primary structure of human insulin-like growth factor II. *FEBS Lett* 1978;89:283–286.
825. Rinderknecht E, Humbel RE. The amino acid sequence of human insulin-like growth factor I and its structural homology with proinsulin. *J Biol Chem* 1978;253:2769–2776.
826. Rivelis AL, Traeger C, Rogoff B. The use of relaxin in progressive systemic sclerosis and other connective tissue diseases. A clinical study. *Arch Interam Rheumatol* 1965;8:19–31.
827. Robertson GF, Summerlee AJS. Porcine relaxin induces drinking responses in conscious rats. *Program of the 73rd Annual Meeting of the Endocrine Society,* Washington, DC, 1991;154 (abst).
828. Robertson MC, Croze F, Schroedter IC, Friesen HG. Molecular cloning and expression of rat placental lactogen-I complementary deoxyribonucleic acid. *Endocrinology* 1990;127:702–710.
829. Robertson MC, Friesen HG. Two forms of rat placental lactogen revealed by radioimmunoassay. *Endocrinology* 1981;108:2388–2390.
830. Robertson MC, Gillespie B, Friesen HG. Characterization of the two forms of rat placental lactogen (rPL): rPL-I and rPL-II. *Endocrinology* 1982;111:1862–1866.
831. Robertson MC, Schroedter IC, Friesen HG. Molecular cloning and expression of rat placental lactogen-I_V, a variant of rPL-I present in late pregnant rat placenta. *Endocrinology* 1991;129:2746–2756.
832. Roche PJ, Crawford RJ, Tregear GW. A single-copy relaxin-like gene sequence is present in the sheep. *Mol Cell Endocrinol* 1993;91:21–28.
833. Rogers PAW, Murphy CR, Squires KR, MacLennan AH. Effects of relaxin on the intrauterine distribution and antimesometrial positioning and orientation of rat blastocysts before implantation. *J Reprod Fertil* 1983;68:431–435.
834. Rosenberg M, Mazella J, Tseng L. Relative potency of relaxin, insulin-like growth factors, and insulin on the prolactin production in progestin-primed human endometrial stromal cells in long-term culture. *Ann NY Acad Sci* 1991;622:138–144.
835. Rosenthal W, Hescheler J, Trautwein W, Schultz G. Receptor- and G-protein-mediated modulations of voltage-dependent calcium channels. *Cold Spring Harbor Symp Quant Biol* 1988;53:247–254.
836. Rothchild I. The regulation of the mammalian corpus luteum. *Rec Prog Horm Res* 1981;37:183–283.
837. Rotwein P, Hall LJ. Evolution of insulin-like growth factor II: Characterization of the mouse IGF-II gene and identification of two pseudo-exons. *DNA Cell Biol* 1990;9:725–735.
838. Rudzik AD, Miller JW. The mechanism of uterine inhibitory action of relaxin-containing ovarian extracts. *J Pharmacol Exp Ther* 1962;138:82–87.
839. Rudzik AD, Miller JW. The effect of altering the catecholamine content of the uterus on the rate of contractions and the sensitivity of the myometrium to relaxin. *J Pharmacol Exp Ther* 1962;138:88–95.
840. Rundgren A. Physical properties of connective tissue as in-

fluenced by single and repeated pregnancies in the rat. *Acta Physiol Scand* 1974;92(suppl 417):1–138.
841. Ruoff HJ, Lippert TH, Seeger H, Voelter W. Immunoreactive relaxin-like substance and relaxin sensitive adenylate cyclase in the gastric mucosa. *IRCS Med Sci* 1984;12:224–225.
842. Ruth EB. Metamorphosis of the pubic symphysis. II. The guinea pig. *Anat Rec* 1936;67:69–79.
843. Ruth EB. Metamorphosis of the pubic symphysis. III. Histological changes in the symphysis of the pregnant guinea pig. *Anat Rec* 1937;67:409–421.
844. Ryan PL, Norman L, Porter DG. Relaxin does not affect oxytocin release from the porcine neural lobe in vitro or in lactating sows *in vivo*. *Biol Reprod* 1991;44(suppl 1):105 (abst).
845. Ryan PL, Summerlee AJS, Porter DG. Does the pig neurointermediate lobe secrete relaxin? *J Reprod Fertil Abstract Series* 1992;9:37 (abst).
846. Saito Y, Takahashi S, Maki M. Effects of some drugs on ripening of uterine cervix in nonpregnant castrated and pregnant rats. *Tohoku J Exp Med* 1981;133:205–220.
847. Sakbun V, Ali SM, Greenwood FC, Bryant-Greenwood GD. Human relaxin in the amnion, chorion, decidua parietalis, basal plate, and placental trophoblast by immunocytochemistry and Northern analysis. *J Clin Endocrinol Metab* 1990;70:508–514.
848. Sakbun V, Koay ESC, Bryant-Greenwood GD. Immunocytochemical localization of prolactin and relaxin C-peptide in human decidua and placenta. *J Clin Endocrinol Metab* 1987;65: 339–343.
849. Salamon S, Lightfoot RJ. Fertility of ram spermatozoa frozen by the pellet method. III. The effects of insemination technique, oxytocin and relaxin on lambing. *J Reprod Fertil* 1970;22: 409–423.
850. Samson WK, Anthony RV. Is relaxin a prolactin releasing factor in the rat? *Program of the 72nd Annual Meeting of the Endocrine Society,* Atlanta, GA, 1990;318 (abst).
851. Sanborn BM. The role of relaxin in uterine function. In: Huszar G, ed. *Physiology and Biochemistry of the Uterus in Pregnancy and Labor.* Boca Raton, FL: CRC Press, 1986;225–238.
852. Sanborn BM. Rat myometrial Na/K ATPase is increased by serum but not by isoproternol and relaxin. *Comp Biochem Physiol C* 1989;93:341–344.
853. Sanborn BM, Anwer K. Hormonal regulation of myometrial intracellular calcium. In: Garfield RE, ed. *Uterine Contractility.* Norwell, MA: Serono Symposia, 1990;69–82.
854. Sanborn BM, Kuo HS, Weisbrodt NW, Sherwood OD. The interaction of relaxin with the rat uterus. I. Effect on cyclic nucleotide levels and spontaneous contractile activity. *Endocrinology* 1980;106:1210–1215.
855. Sanborn BM, Kuo HS, Weisbrodt NW, Sherwood OD. Effect of relaxin on cyclic nucleotide levels and spontaneous contractions of the rat uterus. *Adv Exp Med Biol* 1982;143:273–282.
856. Sanborn BM, Sherwood OD. Effect of relaxin on bound cAMP in rat uterus. *Endocrin Res Commun* 1981;8:179–192.
857. Sanborn BM, Sherwood OD, Kuo HS, Evidence against the primary role for catecholamine release or prostaglandin synthesis in the effect of relaxin on uterine cyclic AMP levels. *Program of the 62nd Annual Meeting of the Endocrine Society,* Anaheim, CA, 1980;85 (abst).
858. Sanborn BM, Weisbrodt NW, Sherwood OD. Evidence against an obligatory role for catecholamine release in the effects of relaxin on the rat uterus. *Biol Reprod* 1981;24:987–992.
859. Sarosi P, Schmidt CL, Essig M, Steinetz BG, Weiss G. The effect of relaxin and progesterone on rat uterine contractions. *Am J Obstet Gynecol* 1983;145:402–405.
860. Sarosi P, Schmidt CL, Steinetz BG, Weiss G. Progesterone relaxin synergism and $PGF_{2\alpha}$-relaxin antagonism in electrostimulated isolated rat uterine horn segments. In: Bigazzi M, Greenwood FC, Gasparri F, eds. *Biology of Relaxin and Its Role in the Human.* Amsterdam: Excerpta Medica, 1983;180.
861. Sarosi P, Schoenfeld C, Berman J, et al. Effect of anti-relaxin antiserum on sperm motility *in vitro. Endocrinology* 1983;112: 1860–1861.
862. Sauer MV, Paulson RJ, Lobo RA. A preliminary report on oocyte donation extending reproductive potential to women over 40. *N Engl J Med* 1990;323:1157–1160.
863. Sawyer WH, Frieden EH, Martin AC. *In vitro* inhibition of spontaneous contractions of the rat uterus by relaxin-containing extracts of sow ovaries. *Am J Physiol* 1953;172:547–552.
864. Scarselli G, Bigazzi M, Acanfora L, Cozzi C, Branconi F, Nardi M. RIA assay of relaxin in human pregnancy. In: Bigazzi M, Greenwood FC, Gasparri F, eds. *Biology of Relaxin and Its Role in the Human.* Amsterdam: Excerpta Medica, 1983;318–320.
865. Schieferstein G, Vöelter W, Seeger H, Lippert TH. Immunoreactive relaxin in seminal plasma of men. *Int J Fertil* 1989;34: 215–218.
866. Schink W, Struck H. Relaxin in Allen-Doisy test. *Zentralbl Gynakol* 1968;90:675–678.
867. Schmidt CL, Black VH, Sarosi P, Weiss G. Progesterone and relaxin secretion in relation to the ultrastructure of human luteal cells in culture: Effects of human chorionic gonadotropin. *Am J Obstet Gynecol* 1986;155:1209–1219.
868. Schmidt CL, Goldsmith LT, Carr BR, Weiss G, Parker CR Jr, Illingworth DR. Peripheral relaxin levels during pregnancy in a woman with homozygous familial hypobetalipoproteinemia. *Fertil Steril* 1988;50:815–817.
869. Schmidt CL, Goldsmith LT, Weiss G. Relaxin production in long-term monolayer cultures of luteinized human granulosa cells is determined by the follicle stimulation regimen. *Program of the 33rd Annual Meeting of the Society for Gynecological Investigation,* Toronto, 1986;150 (abst).
870. Schmidt CL, Kendall JZ, Dandekar PV, Quigley MM, Schmidt KL. Characterization of long-term monolayer cultures of human granulosa cells from follicles of different size and exposed *in vivo* to clomiphene citrate and hCG. *J Reprod Fertil* 1984;71:279–287.
871. Schmidt CL, Sarosi P, Steinetz BG, et al. Relaxin in human decidua and term placenta. *Eur J Obstet Gynaecol Reprod Biol* 1984;17:171–182.
872. Schmidt JE, Leonard SL. The effect of relaxin on uterine phosphorylase in the rat. *Endocrinology* 1960;67:663–667.
873. Schreifer JA, Lewis PR, Miller JW. Role of fetal oxytocin in parturition in the rat. *Biol Reprod* 1982;27:362–368.
874. Schwabe C. Relaxin sequences. In: Bigazzi M, Greenwood FC, Gasparri F, eds. *Biology of Relaxin and Its Role in the Human.* Amsterdam: Excerpta Medica, 1983;22–31.
875. Schwabe C. *N*-α-formyl-tyrosyl-relaxin. A reliable tracer for relaxin radioimmunoassays. *Endocrinology* 1983;113:814–815.
876. Schwabe C. Relaxin in connective tissue diseases. In: Bigazzi M, Greenwood FC, Gasparri F, eds. *Biology of Relaxin and Its Role in the Human.* Amsterdam: Excerpta Medica, 1983;402–409.
877. Schwabe C, Braddon SA. Evidence for one essential tryptophan residue at the active site of relaxin. *Biochem Biophys Res Commun* 1976;68:1126–1132.
878. Schwabe C, Büllesbach EE. Relaxin. *Comp Biochem Physiol B* 1990;96:15–21.
879. Schwabe C, Büllesbach EE, Heyn H, Yoshioka M. Cetacean relaxin. Isolation and sequence of relaxins from *Balaenoptera acutorostrata* and *Balaenoptera edeni. J Biol Chem* 1989;264: 940–943.
880. Schwabe C, Gowan LK, Reinig JW. Evolution, relaxin, and insulin: A new perspective. *Ann NY Acad Sci* 1982;380:6–12.
881. Schwabe C, Harmon SJ. A comparative circular dichroism study of relaxin and insulin. *Biochem Biophys Res Commun* 1978;84:374–380.
882. Schwabe C, LeRoith D, Thompson RP, Shiloach J, Roth J. Relaxin extracted from protozoa (*Tetrahymena pyriformis*). *J Biol Chem* 1983;258:2778–2781.
883. Schwabe C, McDonald JK. Relaxin: A disulfide homolog of insulin. *Science* 1977;197:914–915.
884. Schwabe C, McDonald JK, Steinetz BG. Primary structure of the A chain of porcine relaxin. *Biochem Biophys Res Commun* 1976;70:397–405.
885. Schwabe C, McDonald JK, Steinetz BG. Primary structure of the B chain of porcine relaxin. *Biochem Biophys Res Commun* 1977;75:503–510.
886. Schwabe C, Steinetz BG, Weiss G, et al. Relaxin. *Recent Prog Horm Res* 1978;34:123–199.
887. Schwabe C, Warr GW. A polyphyletic view of evolution: The

genetic potential hypothesis. *Perspect Biol Med* 1984;27: 465–485.
888. Scott JE. Proteoglycan-fibrillar collagen interactions. *Biochem J* 1988;252:313–324.
889. Scott JE. Proteoglycan: Collagen interactions and subfibrillar structure in collagen fibrils. Implications in the development and ageing of connective tissues. *J Anat* 1990;169:23–35.
890. Scott JE, Orford CR. Dermatan sulphate-rich proteoglycan associates with rat tail-tendon collagen at the d band in the gap region. *Biochem J* 1981;197:213–216.
891. Seeger H, Zwirner M, Völter W, Lippert TH. Relaxin and human chorionic gonadotropin concentrations in blood serum during the first trimester of normal and pathological pregnancy. *Gynecol Obstet Invest* 1988;25:209–212.
892. Segaloff A. The role of the ovary in the synergism between radiation and estrogen in the production of mammary cancer in the rat. In: Bigazzi M, Greenwood FC, Gasparri F, eds. *Biology of Relaxin and Its Role in the Human.* Amsterdam: Excerpta Medica, 1983;410–416.
893. Seki K, Kato K. Evidence for the luteal source of circulating relaxin in molar pregnancy. *Acta Obstet Gynecol Scand* 1987;66:319–320.
894. Seki K, Kato K, Tabei T. Serum immunoreactive relaxin in women during a 24-h period. *J Reprod Fertil* 1987;79:363–365.
895. Seki K, Uesato T, Kato K. Serum relaxin in patients with invasive mole choriocarcinoma and persistent trophoblastic disease. *Endocrinol Jpn* 1986;33:727–733.
896. Seki K, Uesato T, Kato K. Serum relaxin concentrations in women following the administration of 16,16-dimethyl-trans-Δ-2-PGE_1 methyl ester during early pregnancy. *Prostaglandins* 1987;33:739–742.
897. Seki K, Uesato T, Kato K, Tabei T. Decline in serum relaxin levels before labor in women. *Acta Obstet Gynaecol Jpn* 1987;39:2073–2074.
898. Seki K, Uesato T, Tabei T, Kato K. The secretory patterns of relaxin and human chorionic gonadotropin in human pregnancy. *Endocrinol Jpn* 1985;32:741–744.
899. Seki K, Uesato T, Tabei T, Kato K. Serum relaxin in patients with hydatidiform mole. *Obstet Gynecol* 1986;67:381–383.
900. Seki K, Uesato T, Tabei T, Kato K. Serum relaxin and steroid hormones in spontaneous abortions. *Acta Obstet Gynecol Scand* 1988;67:483–486.
901. Shaffhausen DD, Jordan RM, Dracy AE. The effect of relaxin upon milk ejection. I. The let-down effect upon sheep. *J Dairy Sci* 1954;37:1173–1175.
902. Sheffield LG, Anderson RR. Effect of porcine relaxin and estradiol-17β on the incorporation of tritiated thymidine by fibroblasts isolated from guinea pig uteri. *Life Sci* 1983;33: 543–546.
903. Sheffield LG, Anderson RR. Effect of estradiol and relaxin on growth of fibroblastic cells isolated from guinea pig mammary glands. *Biol Reprod* 1984;30:338–343.
904. Sheffield LG, Anderson RR. Effect of estradiol and relaxin on collagen and non-collagen protein synthesis by mammary fibroblasts. *Life Sci* 1984;35:2199–2203.
905. Sherwood OD. Purification and characterization of rat relaxin. *Endocrinology* 1979;104:886–892.
906. Sherwood OD. Isolation and characterization of porcine and rat relaxin. *Adv Exp Med Biol* 1982;143:115–147.
907. Sherwood OD. Radioimmunoassay of relaxin. *Adv Exp Med Biol* 1982;143:221–248.
908. Sherwood OD. Relaxin at parturition in the pig. In: Cole DJA, Foxcroft GR, eds. *Control of Pig Reproduction.* London: Butterworth Scientific, 1982;343–375.
909. Sherwood OD, Chang CC, BeVier GW, Dial JR, Dziuk PJ. Relaxin concentrations in pig plasma following the administration of prostaglandin $F_2\alpha$ during late pregnancy. *Endocrinology* 1976;98:875–879.
910. Sherwood OD, Chang CC, BeVier GW, Dziuk PJ. Radioimmunoassay of plasma relaxin levels throughout pregnancy and at parturition in the pig. *Endocrinology* 1975;97:834–837.
911. Sherwood OD, Crnekovic VE. Development of a homologous radioimmunoassay for rat relaxin. *Endocrinology* 1979;104: 893–897.
912. Sherwood OD, Crnekovic VE, Gordon WL, Rutherford JE. Radioimmunoassay of relaxin throughout pregnancy and during parturition in the rat. *Endocrinology* 1980;107:691–698.
913. Sherwood OD, Downing SJ. The chemistry and physiology of relaxin. In: Greenwald GS, Terranova PF, eds. *Factors Regulating Ovarian Function.* New York: Raven Press, 1983;381–410.
914. Sherwood OD, Downing SJ, Golos TG, Gordon WL, Tarbell MK. Influence of light-dark cycle on antepartum serum relaxin and progesterone immunoactivity levels and on birth in the rat. *Endocrinology* 1983;113:997–1003.
915. Sherwood OD, Downing SJ, Lao Guico-Lamm M, Hwang JJ. Relaxin promotes diverse physiological processes in the pregnant rat. In: Garfield RE, ed. *Uterine Contractility.* Norwell, MA: Serono Symposia, 1990;237–252.
916. Sherwood OD, Downing SJ, Lao Guico-Lamm M, Hwang JJ, O'Day-Bowman MB, Fields PA. The physiological effects of relaxin during pregnancy: Studies in rats and pigs. In: Milligan S, ed. *Oxford Review of Reproductive Biology,* vol 15. Oxford: Oxford Press, 1993;143–189.
917. Sherwood OD, Downing SJ, Rieber AJ, et al. Influence of litter size on antepartum serum relaxin and progesterone immunoactivity levels and on birth in the rat. *Endocrinology* 1985;116: 2554–2562.
918. Sherwood OD, Golos TG, Key RH. Influence of the conceptuses and the maternal pituitary on the distribution of multiple components of serum relaxin immunoactivity during pregnancy in the rat. *Endocrinology* 1986;119:2143–2147.
919. Sherwood OD, Key RH, Tarbell MK, Downing SJ. Dynamic changes of multiple forms of serum immunoactive relaxin during pregnancy in the rat. *Endocrinology* 1984;114:806–813.
920. Sherwood OD, Martin PA, Chang CC, Dziuk PJ. Plasma relaxin levels in pigs with corpora lutea induced during late pregnancy. *Biol Reprod* 1977;17:97–100.
921. Sherwood OD, Martin PA, Chang CC, Dziuk PJ. Plasma relaxin levels during late pregnancy and at parturition in pigs with altered utero-ovarian connections. *Biol Reprod* 1977;17:101–103.
922. Sherwood OD, Nara BS, Crnekovic VE, First NL. Relaxin concentrations in pig plasma after the administration of indomethacin and prostaglandin $F_{2}\alpha$ during late pregnancy. *Endocrinology* 1979;104:1716–1721.
923. Sherwood OD, Nara BS, Welk FA, First NL, Rutherford JE. Relaxin levels in the maternal plasma of pigs before, during, and after parturition and before, during, and after suckling. *Biol Reprod* 1981;25:65–71.
924. Sherwood OD, O'Byrne EM. Purification and characterization of porcine relaxin. *Arch Biochem Biophys* 1974;160:185–196.
925. Sherwood OD, Rosentreter KR, Birkhimer ML. Development of a radioimmunoassay for porcine relaxin using ^{125}I-labeled polytyrosyl-relaxin. *Endocrinology* 1975;96:1106–1113.
926. Sherwood OD, Rutherford JE. Relaxin immunoactivity levels in ovarian extracts obtained from rats during various reproductive states and from adult cycling pigs. *Endocrinology* 1981;108:1171–1177.
927. Sherwood OD, Wilson ME, Edgerton LA, Chang CC. Serum relaxin concentrations in pigs with parturition delayed by progesterone administration. *Endocrinology* 1978;102:471–475.
928. Shimizu Y, Ochiai K, Terashima H, Mineya S, Maruyama R. Effect of relaxin on the contractile mechanism of uterine muscles. *Jpn J Smooth Muscle Res* 1986;22:312–314.
929. Shire SJ, Holladay LA, Rinderknecht E. Self-association of human and porcine relaxin as assessed by analytical ultracentrifugation and circular dichroism. *Biochemistry* 1991;30:7703–7711.
930. Silver M, Barnes RJ, Comline RS, Fowden AL, Clover L, Mitchell MD. Prostaglandins in the foetal pig and prepartum endocrine changes in mother and foetus. *Anim Reprod Sci* 1979;2:305–322.
931. Sims SM, Daniel EE, Garfield RE. Improved electrical coupling in uterine smooth muscle is associated with increased numbers of gap junctions at parturition. *J Gen Physiol* 1982;80:353–375.
932. Slate WG. Pelvic girdle relaxation. *Obstet Gynecol* 1960;16: 625–627.
933. Slate WG. Effect of relaxin on the cervix of nonpregnant women. *Obstet Gynecol* 1961;17:294–296.
934. Smith KH, Musah AI, Schwabe C, Anderson LL. Continuous

infusion of porcine relaxin affects peripheral plasma levels of progesterone in late pregnant beef heifers. *J Anim Sci* 1988;66(suppl 1):417 (abst).
935. Smith TC. The action of relaxin on mammary gland growth in the rat. *Endocrinology* 1954;54:59–70.
936. Smithberg M, Runner M. The induction and maintenance of pregnancy in prepuberal mice. *J Exp Zool* 1956;133:441–457.
937. Snell CR, Smyth DG. Proinsulin: A proposed three-dimensional structure. *J Biol Chem* 1975;250:6291–6295.
938. Sokol RZ, Okuda H, Johnston PD, Swerdloff RS. Videomicrographic analysis of the effects of antihuman relaxin antibody on human sperm motility. *Fertil Steril* 1988;49:729–731.
939. Sokol RZ, Wang XS, Lechago J, Johnston PD, Swerdloff RS. Immunohistochemical localization of relaxin in human prostate. *J Histochem Cytochem* 1989;37:1253–1255.
940. Soloff MS, Shaw AR, Gentry LE, Marquardt H, Vasilenko P. Demonstration of relaxin precursors in pregnant rat ovaries with antisera against bacterially expressed rat prorelaxin. *Endocrinology* 1992;130:1844–1851.
941. Sorbera L, Giannoukos G, Callard I. Progesterone and relaxin inhibit turtle myometrium. *Am Zool* 1988;28:145 (abst).
942. Sorbera LA, Schwabe C, Callard IP. The effect of homologous relaxin and neurointermediate lobe extracts on *in vivo* and *in vitro* myometrial activity in the viviparous dogfish, *Squalus acanthias. Mount Desert Island Biol Lab Bull* 1986;26: 133–135.
943. Sortino MA, Cronin MJ, Wise PM. Relaxin stimulates prolactin secretion from anterior pituitary cells. *Endocrinology* 1989;124: 2013–2015.
944. Sridaran R, Basuray R, Gibori G. Source and regulation of testosterone secretion in pregnant and pseudopregnant rats. *Endocrinology* 1981;108:855–861.
945. Steiner DF, Quinn PS, Chan SJ, Marsh J, Tager HS. Processing mechanisms in the biosynthesis of proteins. *Ann NY Acad Sci* 1980;343:1–16.
946. Steinetz BG. Specificity and reliability of radioimmunoassays, radioreceptor assays, and bioassays: Round table discussion summary. *Ann NY Acad Sci* 1982;380:51–59.
947. Steinetz BG, Beach VL. Hormonal requirements for interpubic ligament formation in hypophysectomized mice. *Endocrinology* 1963;72:771–776.
948. Steinetz BG, Beach VL, Blye RP, Kroc RL. Changes in the composition of the rat uterus following a single injection of relaxin. *Endocrinology* 1957;61:287–292.
949. Steinetz BG, Beach VL, Kroc RL. The influence of progesterone, relaxin and estrogen on some structural and functional changes in the pre-parturient mouse. *Endocrinology* 1957;61: 271–280.
950. Steinetz BG, Beach VL, Kroc RL. The physiology of relaxin in laboratory animals. In: Lloyd CW, ed. *Recent Progress in the Endocrinology of Reproduction.* New York: Academic Press, 1959;389–423.
951. Steinetz BG, Beach VL, Kroc RI. Bioassay of relaxin. In: Dorfman RI, ed. *Methods in Hormone Research.* New York: Academic Press, 1969;481–513.
952. Steinetz BG, Beach VL, Kroc RL, et al. Bioassay of relaxin using a reference standard: A simple and reliable method utilizing direct measurement of interpubic ligament formation in mice. *Endocrinology* 1960;67:102–115.
953. Steinetz BG, Beach VL, Tripp LV, DeFalco RJ. Reactions of antisera to porcine relaxin with relaxin-containing tissues of other species *in vivo* and *in vitro. Acta Endocrinol* 1964;47: 371–384.
954. Steinetz BG, Butler MC, Sawyer WK, O'Byrne EM. Effects of relaxin on early pregnancy in rats. *Proc Soc Exp Biol Med* 1976;152:419–422.
955. Steinetz BG, Goldsmith LT, Harvey HJ, Lust G. Serum relaxin and progesterone concentrations in pregnant, pseudopregnant and ovariectomized, progestin-treated pregnant bitches: Detection of relaxin as a marker of pregnancy. *Am J Vet Res* 1989;50:68–71.
956. Steinetz BG, Goldsmith LT, Hasan SH, Lust G. Diurnal variation of serum progesterone, but not relaxin, prolactin or estradiol-17β in the pregnant bitch. *Endocrinology* 1990;127: 1057–1063.
957. Steinetz BG, Goldsmith LT, Lust G. Plasma relaxin levels in pregnant and lactating dogs. *Biol Reprod* 1987;37:719–725.
958. Steinetz BG, Manning JP. Influence of growth hormone, steroids and relaxin on acid phosphatase activity of connective tissue. *Proc Soc Exp Biol Med* 1967;124:180–184.
959. Steinetz BG, Manning JP, Butler M, Beach V. Relationships of growth hormone, steroids and relaxin in the transformation of pubic joint cartilage to ligament in hypophysectomized mice. *Endocrinology* 1965;76:876–882.
960. Steinetz BG, Matthews JR, Butler MT, Thompson SW. Inhibition by thyrocalcitonin of estrogen-induced bone resorption in the mouse pubic symphysis. *Am J Pathol* 1973;73:735–741.
961. Steinetz BG, O'Byrne EM. Speculations on the probable role of relaxin in cervical dilation and parturition in rats. *Semin Reprod Endocrinol* 1983;1:335–342.
962. Steinetz BG, O'Byrne EM, Butler MC, Hickman LB. Hormonal regulation of the connective tissue of the symphysis pubis. In: Bigazzi M, Greenwood FC, Gasparri F, eds. *Biology of Relaxin and Its Role in the Human.* Amsterdam: Excerpta Medica, 1983;71–92.
963. Steinetz BG, O'Byrne EM, Goldsmith LT, Anderson MB. The source of relaxin in pregnant Syrian hamsters. *Endocrinology* 1988;122:795–798.
964. Steinetz BG, O'Byrne EM, Kroc RL. The role of relaxin in cervical softening during pregnancy in mammals. In: Naftolin F, Stubblefield PG, eds. *Dilation of the Uterine Cervix.* New York: Raven Press, 1980;157–177.
965. Steinetz BG, O'Byrne EM, Sarosi P, Weiss G. Bioassay of relaxin: Present status and future prospects. In: Bigazzi M, Greenwood FC, Gasparri F, eds. *Biology of Relaxin and Its Role in the Human.* Amsterdam: Excerpta Medica, 1983;140–147.
966. Steinetz BG, O'Byrne EM, Sawyer WK, Butler MC, Munigle J, Steele RE. Effects of aminoglutethimide on cervical dilatability and serum immunoreactive relaxin in pregnant rats. *Proc Soc Exp Biol Med* 1985;178:101–104.
967. Steinetz BG, O'Byrne EM, Schwabe C. Specificity and applications of biological assays for porcine relaxin. In: Bryant-Greenwood GD, Niall HD, Greenwood FC, eds. *Relaxin.* New York: Elsevier/North-Holland, 1981;331–335.
968. Steinetz BG, O'Byrne EM, Weiss G. Measurement of "relaxin" in human plasma and serum samples using a homologous porcine radioimmunoassay. In: Bryant-Greenwood GD, Niall HD, Greenwood FC, eds. *Relaxin.* New York: Elsevier/North-Holland, 1981;373–375.
969. Steinetz BG, O'Byrne EM, Weiss G, Schwabe C. Bioassay methods for relaxin: Uses and pitfalls. *Adv Exp Med Biol* 1982;143:79–104.
970. Steinetz BG, Randolph C, Mahoney CJ. Serum concentrations of relaxin, chorionic gonadotropin, estradiol-17β, and progesterone during the reproductive cycle of the chimpanzee (*Pan troglodytes*). *Endocrinology* 1992;130:3601–3607.
971. Steinetz BG, Schwabe C, Weiss G, eds. Relaxin: Structure, function, and evolution. *Ann NY Acad Sci* 1982;380.
972. Steinetz BG, Whittaker PG, Edwards JRG. Maternal relaxin concentrations in diabetic pregnancy. *Lancet* 1992;340: 752–755.
973. Stewart AG, Richards H, Roberts S, et al. Cloning and expression of porcine prorelaxin gene in *E. coli. Nucleic Acids Res* 1983;11:6597–6609.
974. Stewart DR. Development of a homologous equine relaxin radioimmunoassay. *Endocrinology* 1986;119:1100–1104.
975. Stewart DR, Addiego LA, Pascoe DR, Haluska GJ, Pashen R. Breed differences in circulating equine relaxin. *Biol Reprod* 1992;46:648–652.
976. Stewart DR, Celniker AC, Taylor CA Jr, Cragun JR, Overstreet JW, Lasley BL. Relaxin in the peri-implantation period. *J Clin Endocrinol Metab* 1990;70:1771–1773.
977. Stewart DR, Celniker AC, Taylor CA Sr, Cragun JR, Overstreet JW, Lasley BL. Relaxin in transient early human pregnancies. *Program of the 72nd Annual Meeting of the Endocrine Society,* Atlanta, GA, 1990;204 (abst).

978. Stewart DR, Cragun JR, Boyers SP, Oi R, Overstreet JW, Lasley BL. Serum relaxin concentrations in patients with out-of-phase endometrial biopsies. *Fertil Steril* 1992;57:453–455.
979. Stewart DR, Henzel WJ, Vandlen R. Purification and sequence determination of canine relaxin. *J Protein Chem* 1992;11:247–253.
980. Stewart DR, Kindahl H, Stabenfeldt GH, Hughes JP. Concentrations of 15-keto-13,14-dihydroprostaglandin $F_{2\alpha}$ in the mare during spontaneous and oxytocin-induced foaling. *Equine Vet J* 1984;16:270–274.
981. Stewart DR, Nevins B, Hadas E, Vandlen R. Affinity purification and sequence determination of equine relaxin. *Endocrinology* 1991;129:375–383.
982. Stewart DR, Papkoff H. Purification and characterization of equine relaxin. *Endocrinology* 1986;119:1093–1099.
983. Stewart DR, Stabenfeldt GH. Relaxin activity in the pregnant mare. *Biol Reprod* 1981;25:281–289.
984. Stewart DR, Stabenfeldt GH. Relaxin activity in the pregnant cat. *Biol Reprod* 1985;32:848–854.
985. Stewart DR, Stabenfeldt GH, Hughes JP. Relaxin activity in foaling mares. *J Reprod Fertil* 1982;32(suppl):603–609.
986. Stewart DR, Stabenfeldt GH, Hughes JP, Meagher DM. Determination of the source of equine relaxin. *Biol Reprod* 1982;27:17–24.
987. Stewart DR, Stouffer R, Overstreet JW, Hendrickx A, Lasley BL. Measurement of periimplantational relaxin concentrations in the macaque using a homologous assay. *Endocrinology* 1992;132:6–12.
988. St-Louis J. Relaxin inhibition of KCl-induced uterine contractions *in vitro:* An alternative bioassay. *Can J Physiol Pharmacol* 1981;59:507–512.
989. St-Louis J. Pharmacological studies on the action of relaxin upon KCl-contracted rat uterus. *Pharmacology* 1982;25:327–337.
990. St-Louis J. Pharmacological studies of the effect of porcine relaxin on rat uterus *in vitro.* In: Bigazzi M, Greenwood FC, Gasparri F, eds. *Biology of Relaxin and Its Role in the Human.* Amsterdam: Excerpta Medica, 1983;128–133.
991. St-Louis J, Massicotte G. Chronic decrease of blood pressure by rat relaxin in spontaneously hypertensive rats. *Life Sci* 1985;37:1351–1357.
992. Stoelk E, Chegini N, Lei ZM, Rao CHV, Bryant-Greenwood G, Sanfilippo J. Immunocytochemical localization of relaxin in human corpora lutea: Cellular and subcellular distribution and dependence on reproductive state. *Biol Reprod* 1991;44:1140–1147.
993. Stone BA, Petrucco OM, Seamark RF, MacLennan AH. Concentrations of steroid hormones, and of relaxin, in utero-ovarian venous plasma of periparturient sows. *Anim Reprod Sci* 1987;15:227–239.
994. Stone ML. Effects of relaxin in the human. In: Lloyd CW, ed. *Recent Progress in the Endocrinology of Reproduction.* New York: Academic Press, 1959;429–439.
995. Storey E. Relaxation in the pubic symphysis of the mouse during pregnancy and after relaxin administration, with special reference to the behavior of collagen. *J Pathol Bacteriol* 1957;74:147–162.
996. Straus WT. Pelvic relaxation in the pregnant rhesus macaque. *Anat Rec* 1932;52:38.
997. Strauss JF, Stambaugh RL. Induction of 20α-hydroxysteroid dehydrogenase in rat corpora lutea of pregnancy by prostaglandin $F2_{\alpha}$. *Prostaglandins* 1974;5:73–85.
998. Struck H, Viell B. Metabolic responses to relaxin in the mouse symphysis pubis. *Horm Metabol Res* 1987;19:669.
999. Stryker JL, Dziuk PJ. Effects of fetal decapitation on fetal development, parturition, and lactation in pigs. *J Anim Sci* 1975;40:282–287.
1000. Stuenkel EL. Effects of membrane depolarization on intracellular calcium in single nerve terminals. *Brain Res* 1990;529:96–101.
1001. Stults JT, Bourell JH, Canova-Davis E, et al. Structural characterization by mass spectrometry of native and recombinant human relaxin. *Biomed Environ Mass Spectrom* 1990;19:655–664.
1002. Stys SJ, Clark KE, Clewell WH, Meschia G. Hormonal effects on cervical compliance in sheep. In: Naftolin F, Stubblefield PG, eds. *Dilatation of the Uterine Cervix.* New York: Raven Press, 1980;147–156.
1003. Stys SJ, Dresser BL, Otte TE, Clark VE. Effect of prostaglandin E_2 on cervical compliance in pregnant ewes. *Am J Obstet Gynecol* 1981;140:415–419.
1004. Summerlee AJS. Relaxin, opioids, and the timing of birth in rats. In: Dyer RG, Bicknell RJ, eds. *Brain Opioid Systems in Reproduction.* Oxford: Oxford University Press, 1989;257–270.
1005. Summerlee AJS, Mumford AD, Smith MS. Porcine relaxin affects the release of luteinizing hormone in rats. *J Neuroendocrinol* 1991;3:133–138.
1006. Summerlee AJS, O'Byrne KT, Jones SA, Eltringham L. The subfornical organ and relaxin-induced inhibition of reflex milk ejection in lactating rats. *J Endocrinol* 1987;115:347–353.
1007. Summerlee AJS, O'Byrne KT, Paisley AC, Breeze MF, Porter DG. Relaxin affects the central control of oxytocin release. *Nature* 1984;309:372–374.
1008. Szlachter BN, O'Byrne E, Goldsmith L, Steinetz BG, Weiss G. Myometrial inhibiting activity of relaxin-containing extracts of human corpora lutea of pregnancy. *Am J Obstet Gynecol* 1980;136:584–586.
1009. Szlachter BN, Quagliarello J, Jewelewicz R, Osathanondh R, Spellacy WN, Weiss G. Relaxin in normal and pathogenic pregnancies. *Obstet Gynecol* 1982;59:167–170.
1010. Tager HS, Steiner DF. Primary structures of the proinsulin connecting peptides of the rat and the horse. *J Biol Chem* 1972;247:7936–7940.
1011. Takayama M, Greenwald GS. Direct luteotropic action of estrogen in the hypophysectomized-hysterectomized rat. *Endocrinology* 1973;92:1405–1413.
1012. Talmage RV. Changes produced in the symphysis pubis of the guinea pig by the sex steroids and relaxin. *Anat Rec* 1947;99:91–113.
1013. Talmage RV. A histological study of the effects of relaxin on the symphysis pubis of the guinea pig. *J Exp Zool* 1947;106:281–297.
1014. Talmage RV. The role of estrogen in the estrogen-relaxin relationship in symphyseal relaxation. *Endocrinology* 1950;47:75–82.
1015. Talmage RV, Garrett FA. Effects of repeated injections of the steroids and relaxin on the symphysis pubis of the guinea pig as studied by X-ray. *Endocrinology* 1951;48:162–168.
1016. Talmage RV, Hurst WR. Variability in the response of the symphysis pubis of the guinea-pig to relaxin. *J Endocrinol* 1950;7:24–30.
1017. Tan GJS, Kwan TK, Cheah SH. Testosterone production by the macaque testis: Lack of effect of oxytocin and relaxin. *Med Sci Res* 1988;16:531.
1018. Taney FH, Vasilenko P, Steinetz BG, Weiss G, Cole D, Goldsmith LT. The role of estrogen and relaxin in the reproductive abnormalities of mice with Hertwig's anemia. *Biol Reprod* 1991;45:719–726.
1019. Tashima L, Greenwood FC, Bryant-Greenwood GD, Peaker M. Identification of mRNA for relaxin in the endometrium of the pregnant guinea pig. *J Endocrinol* 1988;118:R9–R11.
1020. Tashima LS, Mazoujian G, Bryant-Greenwood GD. The expression of relaxin gene(s) in human benign and neoplastic breast tissue. *Program of the 73rd Annual Meeting of the Endocrine Society,* Washington, DC, 1991;177 (abst).
1021. Taverne M, Bevers M, Bradshaw JMC, Dieleman SJ, Willemse AH, Porter DG. Plasma concentrations of prolactin, progesterone, relaxin, and oestradiol-17β in sows treated with progesterone, bromocriptine or indomethacin during late pregnancy. *J Reprod Fertil* 1982;65:85–96.
1022. Taverne MAM, Naaktgeboren C, Elsaesser F, et al. Myometrial electrical activity and plasma concentrations of progesterone, estrogens and oxytocin during late pregnancy and parturition in the miniature pig. *Biol Reprod* 1979;21:1125–1134.
1023. Taylor MJ, Clark CL. Detection of relaxin release by porcine

luteal cells using a reverse hemolytic plaque assay: Effect of prostaglandins E_2 and $F_{2\alpha}$, human chorionic gonadotropin, and oxytocin. *Biol Reprod* 1987;37:377–384.
1024. Taylor MJ, Clark CL. Prostacyclin stimulates relaxin release from cultured porcine luteal cells. *Biol Reprod* 1987;37: 1241–1247.
1025. Taylor MJ, Clark CL. Regulation of relaxin release from monodispersed porcine luteal cells: Effect of calcium ionophore A23187 and calcium channel blockers. *Endocrinology* 1988; 123:1893–1901.
1026. Taylor MJ, Clark CL. Analysis of release of porcine relaxin by reverse haemolytic plaque assay: Evidence for autoregulation. *J Endocrinol* 1988;116:287–291.
1027. Taylor MJ, Clark CL. Stimulatory effect of phorbol diester on relaxin release by porcine luteal cells in culture. *Biol Reprod* 1988;39:743–750.
1028. Taylor MJ, Clark CL. Inhibitory effect of analogues of cyclic nucleotides and cholera toxin on relaxin release from cultured porcine luteal cells. *Biol Reprod* 1988;38:315–323.
1029. Taylor MJ, Clark CL. Analysis of relaxin release by cultured porcine luteal cells using a reverse hemolytic plaque assay: Effects of arachidonic acid, cyclo- and lipoxygenase blockers, phospholipase A_2 and melittin. *Endocrinology* 1989;125: 1389–1397.
1030. Taylor MJ, Clark CL. Effect of antimicrotubule agents on secretion of relaxin by large luteal cells derived from pregnant swine. *Endocrinology* 1990;126:1790–1795.
1031. Taylor MJ, Clark CL. Basic fibroblast growth factor inhibits basal and stimulated relaxin secretion by cultured porcine luteal cells: Analysis by reverse hemolytic plaque assay. *Endocrinology* 1992;130:1951–1956.
1032. Taylor MJ, Clark CL. Transforming growth factor-β is a potent inhibitor of basal and stimulated relaxin secretion by porcine luteal cells maintained in monolayer culture. *J Endocrinol* 1992;135:543–550.
1033. Taylor MJ, Clark CL. Discordant secretion of relaxin by individual porcine large luteal cells: Quantitative analysis by a reverse haemolytic plaque assay. *J Endocrinol* 1992;134:77–83.
1034. Taylor MJ, Clark CL. Evidence that basal secretion of relaxin by individual cultured large luteal cells is influenced by mobilization of intracellular calcium: Analysis by a reverse hemolytic plaque assay. *Cell Calcium* 1992;13:571–580.
1035. Taylor MJ, Clark CL, Frawley LS. Analysis of relaxin release from cultured porcine luteal cells by reverse hemolytic plaque assay: Influence of gestational age and prostaglandin $F_{2\alpha}$. *Endocrinology* 1987;120:2085–2091.
1036. Taylor MJ, Clark CL, Frawley LS. Evidence for the existence of a luteal cell type that is steroidogenic and releases relaxin. *Proc Soc Exp Biol Med* 1987;185:469–473.
1037. Thacker PA, Gooneratne AD, Kirkwood RN. The influence of purified porcine relaxin on the reproductive performance of sows following artificial insemination with fresh or frozen semen. *Can J Anim Sci* 1991;71:237–239.
1038. Thomas K, Loumaye E, Donnez J. Immunoreactive relaxin in the peritoneal fluid during spontaneous menstrual cycle in women. *Ann NY Acad Sci* 1982;380:126–130.
1039. Thomas K, Loumaye E, Ferin J. Relaxin in nonpregnant women during ovarian stimulation. *Gynecol Obstet Invest* 1980;11:75–80.
1040. Thomford PJ, Sander HKL, Kendall JZ, Sherwood OD, Dziuk PJ. Maintenance of pregnancy and levels of progesterone and relaxin in the serum of gilts following a stepwise reduction in the number of corpora lutea. *Biol Reprod* 1984;31:494–498.
1041. Thoms H. Relaxation of the symphysis pubis in pregnancy. *JAMA* 1936;106:1364–1366.
1042. Thrailkill KM, Clemmons DR, Busby WH Jr, Handwerger S. Differential regulation of insulin-like growth factor-binding protein secretion from human decidual cells by IGF-1, insulin, and relaxin. *J Clin Invest* 1990;86:878–883.
1043. Too CKL, Bryant-Greenwood GD, Greenwood FC. The effect of relaxin on the release of collagenase from rat uterine and granulosa cells *in vitro. Program of the 64th Annual Meeting of the Endocrine Society,* San Francisco, CA, 1982;162 (abst).
1044. Too CKL, Bryant-Greenwood GD, Greenwood FC. Relaxin increases the release of plasminogen activator, collagenase, and proteoglycanase from rat granulosa cells *in vitro. Endocrinology* 1984;115:1043–1050.
1045. Too CKL, Kong JK, Greenwood FC, Bryant-Greenwood GD. The effect of oestrogen and relaxin on uterine and cervical enzymes: collagenase, proteoglycanase and β-glucuronidase. *Acta Endocrinol* 1986;111:394–403.
1046. Too CKL, Weiss TJ, Bryant-Greenwood GD. Relaxin stimulates plasminogen activator secretion by rat granulosa cells *in vitro. Endocrinology* 1982;111:1424–1426.
1047. Tregear G, Du Y-C, Wang K, et al. The synthesis of human relaxin. *Peptide Chem* 1985;22:13–18.
1048. Tregear GW, Du Y-C, Wang K-Z, et al. The chemical synthesis of relaxin. In: Bigazzi M, Greenwood FC, Gasparri F, eds. *Biology of Relaxin and Its Role in the Human.* Amsterdam: Excerpta Medica, 1983;42–55.
1049. Tregear GW, Fagan C, Reynolds H, et al. Porcine relaxin: Synthesis and structure activity relationships. In: *Peptides, Synthesis, Structure, Function: Proceedings of the Seventh American Peptide Symposium.* Rockford, IL: Pierce Chemical Co., 1982;249–252.
1050. Trentin JJ. Relaxin and mammary growth in the mouse. *Proc Soc Exp Biol Med* 1951;78:9–11.
1051. Tseng JK, Sun B, Tseng L. The effect of progestin on rabbit endometrial aromatase activity. *J Steroid Biochem* 1988;29: 9–13.
1052. Tseng L, Gao J-G, Chen R, Zhu H-H, Mazella J, Powell DR. Effect of progestin, antiprogestin, and relaxin on the accumulation of prolactin and insulin-like growth factor-binding protein-1 messenger ribonucleic acid in human endometrial stromal cells. *Biol Reprod* 1992;47:441–450.
1053. Tseng L, Mazella J, Cheng G. Effect of relaxin on aromatase activity in human endometrial stromal cells. *Endocrinology* 1987;120:2220–2226.
1054. Tseng L, Zhu HH, Mazella J, Bell SC. Differential regulation of IGFBP-1 and prolactin by insulin, IGF-1 and relaxin in progestin-primed human endometrial stromal cells. *Program of the 73rd Annual Meeting of the Endocrine Society,* Washington, DC, 1991;296 (abst).
1055. Tsutsui T, Stewart DR. Determination of the source of relaxin immunoreactivity during pregnancy in the dog. *J Vet Med Sci* 1991;53:1025–1029.
1056. Tyndale-Biscoe CH. Relaxin activity during the oestrous cycle of the marsupial, *Trichosurus vulpecula* (Kerr). *J Reprod Fertil* 1969;19:191–193.
1057. Tyndale-Biscoe CH. Evidence for relaxin in marsupials. In: Bryant-Greenwood GD, Niall HD, Greenwood FC, eds. *Relaxin.* New York: Elsevier/North Holland, 1981;225–231.
1058. Uchida K, Kadowaki M, Nomura Y, Miyata K, Miyake T. Relationship between ovarian progestin secretion and corpora lutea function in pregnant rats. *Endocrinol Jpn* 1970;17:499–507.
1059. Uldbjerg N, Danielsen CC. A study of the interaction *in vitro* between type I collagen and a small dermatan sulphate proteoglycan. *Biochem J* 1988;251:643–648.
1060. Uldbjerg N, Ulmsten U, Ekman G. The ripening of the human uterine cervix in terms of connective tissue biochemistry. *Clin Obstet Gynecol* 1983;26:14–26.
1061. Unemori EN, Amento EP. Relaxin modulates synthesis and secretion of procollagenase and collagen by human dermal fibroblasts. *J Biol Chem* 1990;265:10681–10685.
1062. Unemori EN, Bauer EA, Amento EP. Relaxin alone and in conjunction with interferon-γ decreases collagen synthesis by cultured human scleroderma fibroblasts. *J Invest Dermatol* 1992;99:337–342.
1063. Unemori EN, Beck S, Siegel M, Keller G, Liggit D, Amento EP. Relaxin decreases collagen accumulation *in vivo* in two rodent models of fibrosis. *Arthritis Rheum* 1990;33(suppl 9):S66 (abst).
1064. Unemori EN, Siegel M, Keller G, Liggitt D, Amento EP. Relaxin decreases collagen accumulation *in vivo* in a murine model of fibrosis. *Clin Res* 1990;38:233 (abst).
1065. Usuki S, Saitoh T, Sawamura T, et al. Increased maternal plasma concentration of endothelin-1 during labor pain or on

delivery and the existence of a large amount of endothelin-1 in amniotic fluid. *Gynecol Endocrinol* 1990;4:85–97.
1066. Uyldert IE, De Vaal OM. Relaxation of the rat's uterine ostium during pregnancy. *Acta Brev Neerl Physiol* 1947;15:49–53.
1067. Vandlen RL, Winslow JW, Kohr WJ, Bourell JH, Stults JT, Canova-Davis E. Instrumentation needs for the biotechnology laboratory. In: Burlingame AL, McCloskey JA, eds. *Biological Mass Spectrometry.* Amsterdam: Elsevier Science Publishers, 1990;579–598.
1068. Vasilenko P, Adams WC, Frieden EH. Uterine size and glycogen content in cycling and pregnant rats: Influence of relaxin. *Biol Reprod* 1981;25:162–169.
1069. Vasilenko P, Adams WC, Frieden EH. Comparison of systemic and uterine effects of relaxin and insulin in alloxan-treated, hyperglycemic rats. *Proc Soc Exp Biol Med* 1982;169:376–379.
1070. Vasilenko P, Frieden EH, Adams WC. Effect of purified relaxin on uterine glycogen and protein in the rat. *Proc Soc Exp Biol Med* 1980;163:245–248.
1071. Vasilenko P, Mahajan DK. Anabolic effects of relaxin in the uterus and cervix of the rat: Comparison with insulin, estrogen, and progesterone. In: Bigazzi M, Greenwood FC, Gasparri F, eds. *Biology of Relaxin and Its Role in the Human.* Amsterdam: Excerpta Medica, 1983;134–136.
1072. Vasilenko P, Mead JP. Growth-promoting effects of relaxin and related compositional changes in the uterus, cervix, and vagina of the rat. *Endocrinology* 1987;120:1370–1376.
1073. Vasilenko P, Mead JP, Weidmann JE. Uterine growth promoting effects of relaxin: A morphometric and histological analysis. *Biol Reprod* 1986;35:987–995.
1074. Vaupel MR, Sherwood OD, Anderson MB. Immunocytochemical studies of relaxin in ovaries of pregnant and cycling mice. *J Histochem Cytochem* 1985;33:303–308.
1075. Velardo JT. Inability of purified relaxin to inhibit progesterone in decidual tissue formation. *Anat Rec* 1958;130:445–446.
1076. Veldhuis JD, Kolp LA, Toaff ME, Strauss JF, Demers LM. Mechanisms subserving the trophic actions of insulin on ovarian cells. *J Clin Invest* 1983;72:1046–1057.
1077. Veldhuis JD, Nestler JE, Strauss JF, III, Gwynne JT. Insulin regulates low density lipoprotein metabolism by swine granulosa cells. *Endocrinology* 1986;118:2242–2253.
1078. Veldhuis JD, Rodgers RJ, Furlanetto RW. Synergistic actions of estradiol and the insulin-like growth factor somatomedin-C on swine ovarian (granulosa) cells. *Endocrinology* 1986;119: 530–538.
1079. Viell B, Struck H. Effects of the hormone relaxin on the metabolism of the glycosaminoglycans in the mouse symphysis pubis. *Horm Metab Res* 1987;19:415–418.
1080. Wada H, Turner CW. Role of relaxin in stimulating mammary gland growth in mice. *Proc Soc Exp Biol Med* 1958;99:194–197.
1081. Wada H, Turner CW. Effect of relaxin on mammary gland growth in female mice. *Proc Soc Exp Biol Med* 1959;101: 707–709.
1082. Wada H, Turner CW. Interaction of relaxin and ovarian steroid hormones on uterus of rat. *Endocrinology* 1961;68:1059–1063.
1083. Wada H, Yuhara M. Studies on relaxin in ruminants. (1) Relaxin content of the blood serum of pregnant and postpartum dairy cows. *Jpn J Zootech Sci* 1955;26:215–220.
1084. Wada H, Yuhara M. Studies on relaxin in ruminants. (2) Relaxin content of the blood serum of pregnant and postpartum cows of the Japanese black breed of cattle. *Sci Rep Fac Agric Okayama Univ* 1955;7:13–21.
1085. Wada H, Yuhara M. Studies on relaxin in ruminants. (4) Concentration of relaxin in the blood serum of pregnant and postpartum goats and ewes. *Sci Rep Fac Agric Okayama Univ* 1956;8:31–37.
1086. Wada H, Yuhara M. Inhibitory effect of relaxin preparation upon spontaneous uterine contractions of the rat and guinea pig *in vitro. Sci Rep Fac Agric Okayama Univ* 1956;9:11–20.
1087. Wada H, Yuhara M. Concentration of relaxin in the blood serum of pregnant cow and cow with ovarian cyst. *Proc Silver Jubilee Lab Anim Husbandry Kyoto Univ* 1961;61–66.
1088. Wahab IM, Anderson RR. Relaxin alone and in conjunction with ovarian steroid hormones on growth of the uterus in ovariectomized and intact female rats. *J Dairy Sci* 1988;71(suppl 1):191 (abst).
1089. Wahab IM, Anderson RR. Exogenous porcine relaxin on adrenal and pituitary weights in male and female rats. *J Dairy Sci* 1988;71(suppl 1):191 (abst).
1090. Wahab IM, Anderson RR. Physiological role of relaxin on mammary gland growth in rats. *Proc Soc Exp Biol Med* 1989;192:285–289.
1091. Wahl LM, Blandau RJ, Page RC. Effect of hormones on collagen metabolism and collagenase activity in the pubic symphysis ligament of the guinea pig. *Endocrinology* 1977;100:571–579.
1092. Wahlström T, Koskimies AI, Tenhunen A, et al. Pregnancy proteins in the endometrium after follicle aspiration for *in vivo* fertilization. In: Seppälä M, Edwards RG, eds. *In Vitro Fertilization and Embryo Transfer. NY Acad Sci* 1985;442:402–407.
1093. Walsh JR, Niall HD. Use of an octadecylsilica purification method minimizes proteolysis during isolation of porcine and rat relaxins. *Endocrinology* 1980;107:1258–1260.
1094. Wang YN, Chou JC, Chang D, Chang JK, Avila C, Romero R. Endothelin-1 in human plasma and amniotic fluid. In: Rubanyi GM, Vanhoutte PM, eds. *Endothelium-Derived Constricting Factors.* Basel: Karger, 1990;143–148.
1095. Ward DG, Cronin MJ, Baertschi AJ. Lack of cardiovascular and vasopressin responses to human relaxin in conscious late-pregnant rats. *Am J Physiol* 1991;261:H206–H211.
1096. Ward DG, Thomas GR, Cronin MJ. Relaxin increases rat heart rate by a direct action on the cardiac atrium. *Biochem Biophys Res Commun* 1992;186:999–1005.
1097. Wasnidge C, Porter DG. Is there a season for iodinating relaxin? *J Immunoassay* 1992;13:315–320.
1098. Wathes DC, Denning-Kendall PA, Renfree MB, Porter DG. Identification of neurohypophysial-like and relaxin-like peptides in the corpus luteum of the Tammar wallaby (*Macropus eugenii*). *Program of the 6th Joint Meeting of the British Endocrine Societies,* Warwick, England, 1987;175 (abst).
1099. Wathes DC, King GJ, Porter DG, Wathes CM. Relationship between pre-partum relaxin concentrations and farrowing intervals in the pig. *J Reprod Fertil* 1989;87:383–390.
1100. Wathes DC, Rees JM, Porter DG. Identification of relaxin in the placenta of the ewe. *J Reprod Fertil* 1988;84:247–257.
1101. Wathes DC, Wardle PG, Rees JM, et al. Identification of relaxin immunoreactivity in human follicular fluid. *Hum Reprod* 1986;1:515–517.
1102. Watts AD, Flint APF, Foxcroft GR, Porter DG. Plasma steroid, relaxin and dihydro-keto-prostaglandin F-2α changes in the minipig in relation to myometrial electrical and mechanical activity in the pre-partum period. *J Reprod Fertil* 1988;83: 553–564.
1103. Way SA, Leng G. Relaxin increases the firing rate of supraoptic neurones and increases oxytocin secretion in the rat. *J Endocrinol* 1992;132:149–158.
1104. Wedemeyer PP. Response of four inbred types of mice to relaxin. *Yale J Biol Med* 1964;37:153–157.
1105. Weinberg A. An X-ray pelvimetric study of relaxin extract in pelvic expansion. *Surg Gynecol Obstet* 1956;103:303–306.
1106. Weiss G. Relaxin in human pregnancy. In: Jaffe RB, Dell'Acqua S, eds. *The Endocrine Physiology of Pregnancy and the Peripartal Period.* New York: Raven Press, 1985;241–246.
1107. Weiss G. Relaxin in the male. *Biol Reprod* 1989;40:197–200.
1108. Weiss G. The physiology of human relaxin. *Contrib Gynecol Obstet* 1991;18:130–146.
1109. Weiss G, Goldsmith LT, Schoenfeld C, D'Eletto R. Partial purification of relaxin from human seminal plasma. *Am J Obstet Gynecol* 1986;154:749–755.
1110. Weiss G, O'Byrne EM, Hochman JA, Goldsmith LT, Rifkin I, Steinetz BG. Secretion of progesterone and relaxin by the human corpus luteum at midpregnancy and at term. *Obstet Gynecol* 1977;50:679–681.
1111. Weiss G, O'Byrne EM, Hochman J, Steinetz BG, Goldsmith L, Flitcraft JG. Distribution of relaxin in women during pregnancy. *Obstet Gynecol* 1978;52:569–570.
1112. Weiss G, O'Byrne EM, Steinetz BG. Relaxin: A product of the

human corpus luteum of pregnancy. *Science* 1976;194: 948–949.
1113. Weiss G, Steinetz BG, Dierschke DJ, Fritz G. Relaxin secretion in the rhesus monkey. *Biol Reprod* 1981;24:565–567.
1114. Weiss M, Nagelschmidt M, Struck H. Relaxin and collagen metabolism. *Horm Metab Res* 1979;11:408–410.
1115. Weiss TJ, Bryant-Greenwood GD. Localization of relaxin binding sites in the rat uterus and cervix by autoradiography. *Biol Reprod* 1982;27:673–679.
1116. Wells RS. Relaxin in the treatment of localized scleroderma. *Trans St John Hosp Derm Soc* 1963;49:149–151.
1117. Wen Y, Khursheed A, Singh SP, Sanborn BM. Protein kinase-A inhibits phospholipase-C activity and alters protein phosphorylation in rat myometrial plasma membranes. *Endocrinology* 1992;131:1377–1382.
1118. Whitely JL, Hartmann PE, Willcox DL, Bryant-Greenwood GD, Greenwood FC. Initiation of parturition and lactation in the sow: effects of delaying parturition with medroxyprogesterone acetate. *J Endocrinol* 1990;124:475–484.
1119. Whitely JL, Willcox DL, Hartmann PE, Yamamoto SY, Bryant-Greenwood GD. Plasma relaxin levels during suckling and oxytocin stimulation in the lactating sow. *Biol Reprod* 1985;33:705–714.
1120. Widowski TM, Curtis SE, Dziuk PJ, Wagner WC, Sherwood OD. Behavioral and endocrine responses of sows to prostaglandin F2α and cloprostenol. *Biol Reprod* 1990;43:290–297.
1121. Williams KI, El Tahir KEH. Spatial and temporal variations in prostacyclin production by the pregnant rat uterus. *Adv Prostaglandin Thromboxane Res* 1980;8:1413–1417.
1122. Williams KI, El Tahir KEH. Effect of uterine stimulant drugs on prostacyclin production by the pregnant rat myometrium. I. Oxytocin, bradykinin and $PGF_{2\alpha}$. *Prostaglandins* 1980;19: 31–38.
1123. Williams KI, El Tahir KEH. Relaxin inhibits prostacyclin release by the rat pregnant myometrium. *Prostaglandins* 1982;24: 129–136.
1124. Williams KI, El Tahir KEH, Marcinkiewicz E. Dual actions of prostacyclin (PGI2) on the rat pregnant uterus. *Prostaglandins* 1979;17:667–672.
1125. Williams LM, Hollingsworth M, Dixon JS. Changes in the tensile properties and fine structure of the rat cervix in late pregnancy and during parturition. *J Reprod Fertil* 1982;66:203–211.
1126. Williams LM, Hollingsworth M, Dukes M, Morris ID. Fluprostenol-induced softening of the cervix of the pregnant rat. *J Endocrinol* 1983;97:283–290.
1127. Williams PL, Warwick R. *Gray's Anatomy,* Ed. 36. Philadelphia: WB Saunders, 1980.
1128. Wilson BC, Mingram W, Parry LJ, et al. Could relaxin act via vasopressin to suppress reflex milk-ejection in anaesthetized rats. *J Endocrinol* 1991;129(suppl):314.
1129. Winn RJ, Baker MD, Sherwood OD. Progesterone augments relaxin's effects on cervical softening in ovariectomized gilts. *Biol Reprod* 1992;46(suppl 1):153 (abst).
1130. Winn RJ, O'Day-Bowman MB, Sherwood OD. Hormonal control of the cervix in pregnant gilts: IV. Relaxin promotes changes in the histological characteristics of the cervix that are associated with cervical softening during late pregnancy in gilts. *Endocrinology* 1993;133:121–128.
1131. Winslow JW, Shih A, Bourell JH, et al. Human seminal relaxin is a product of the same gene as human luteal relaxin. *Endocrinology* 1992;130:2660–2668.
1132. Winslow J, Shih A, Laramee G, Bourell J, Stults J, Johnston P. Purification and structure of human pregnancy relaxin from corpora lutea, serum and plasma. *Program of the 71st Annual Meeting of the Endocrine Society,* Seattle, WA, 1989;245 (abst).
1133. Wiqvist I, Linde A. Hormonal influence of glycosaminoglycan synthesis in uterine connective tissue of term pregnant women. *Hum Reprod (Oxford)* 1987;2:177–182.
1134. Wiqvist I, Norström A, O'Byrne E, Wiqvist N. Regulatory influence of relaxin on human cervical and uterine connective tissue. *Acta Endocrinol (Copenh)* 1984;106:127–132.
1135. Wiqvist N. Desensitizing effect of exo- and endogenous relaxin on the immediate uterine response to relaxin. *Acta Endocrinol [Suppl] (Copenh)* 1959;46:3–14.
1136. Wiqvist N. The effect of prolonged administration of relaxin on some functional properties of the non-pregnant mouse and rat uterus. *Acta Endocrinol [Suppl] (Copenh)* 1959;46:15–32.
1137. Wiqvist N, Paul K-G. Inhibition of the spontaneous uterine motility *in vitro* as a bioassay of relaxin. *Acta Endocrinol (Copenh)* 1958;29:135–146.
1138. Witt BR, Wolf GC, Wainwright CJ, Johnston PD, Thorneycroft IH. Relaxin, CA-125, progesterone, estradiol, Schwangerschaft protein, and human chorionic gonadotropin as predictors of outcome in threatened and nonthreatened pregnancies. *Fertil Steril* 1990;53:1029–1036.
1139. Woods AS, Cotter RJ, Yoshioka M, Büllesbach E, Schwabe C. Enzymatic digestion on the sample foil as a method for sequence determination by plasma desorption mass spectrometry: The primary structure of porpoise relaxin. *Int J Mass Spectrom Ion Processes* 1991;111:77–88.
1140. Wright LC, Anderson RR. Effect of relaxin on mammary growth in the hypophysectomized rat. *Adv Exp Med Biol* 1982;143:341–353.
1141. Yamamoto S, Bryant-Greenwood GD. The isolation of relaxin from boar testis. In: Bryant-Greenwood GD, Niall HD, Greenwood FC, eds. *Relaxin.* New York: Elsevier/North-Holland, 1981;71–74.
1142. Yamamoto S, Kwok SCM, Greenwood FC, Bryant-Greenwood GD. Relaxin purification from human placental basal plates. *J Clin Endocrinol Metab* 1981;52:601–604.
1143. Yang S, Rembiesa B, Büllesbach EE, Schwabe C. Relaxin receptors in mice: Demonstration of ligand binding in symphyseal tissues and uterine membrane fragments. *Endocrinology* 1992;130:179–185.
1144. Yki-Järvinen H, Wahlström T. Immunohistochemical demonstration of relaxin in the placenta after removal of the corpus luteum. *Acta Endocrinol (Copenh)* 1984;106:544–547.
1145. Yki-Järvinen H, Wahlström T, Seppälä M. Immunohistochemical demonstration of relaxin in gynecological tumors. *Cancer* 1983;52:2077–2080.
1146. Yki-Järvinen H, Wahlström T, Seppälä M. Immunohistochemical demonstration of relaxin in the genital tract of pregnant and nonpregnant women. *J Clin Endocrinol Metab* 1983;57: 451–454.
1147. Yki-Järvinen H, Wahlström T, Seppälä M. Immunohistochemical demonstration of relaxin in the genital tract of men. *J Reprod Fertil* 1983;69:693–695.
1148. Yki-Järvinen H, Wahlström T, Seppälä M. Human endometrium contains relaxin that is progesterone-dependent. *Acta Obstet Gynecol Scand* 1985;64:663–665.
1149. Yki-Järvinen H, Wahlström T, Tenhunen A, Koskimies AI, Seppälä M. The occurrence of relaxin in hyperstimulated human preovulatory follicles collected in an *in vitro* fertilization program. *J In Vitro Fertil Embryo Transf* 1984;1:180–182.
1150. Zarrow MX. Relaxin content of blood, urine and other tissues of pregnant and postpartum guinea pigs. *Proc Soc Exp Biol Med* 1947;66:488–491.
1151. Zarrow MX. The role of steroid hormones in the relaxation of the symphysis pubis of the guinea pig. *Endocrinology* 1948;42: 129–140.
1152. Zarrow MX, Brennan DM. Increased concentration of water in uterus of the rat following treatment with relaxin. *Proc Soc Exp Biol Med* 1957;95:745–747.
1153. Zarrow MX, Eleftheriou BE, Whitecotten GL, King JA. Separation of the pubic symphysis during pregnancy and after treatment with relaxin in two subspecies of *Peromyscus maniculatus. Gen Comp Endocrinol* 1961;1:386–391.
1154. Zarrow MX, Holmstrom EG, Salhanick HA. The concentration of relaxin in the blood serum and other tissues of women during pregnancy. *J Clin Endocrinol Metab* 1955;15:22–27.
1155. Zarrow MX, McClintock JA. Localization of ^{131}I-labelled antibody to relaxin. *J Endocrinol* 1966;36:377–387.
1156. Zarrow MX, Neher GM, Sikes D, Brennan DM, Bullard JF. Dilatation of the uterine cervix of the sow following treatment with relaxin. *Am J Obstet Gynecol* 1956;72:260–264.
1157. Zarrow MX, O'Connor WB. Localization of relaxin in the corpus luteum of the rabbit. *Proc Soc Exp Biol Med* 1966;121: 612–614.

1158. Zarrow MX, Rosenberg B. Sources of relaxin in the rabbit. *Endocrinology* 1953;53:593–598.
1159. Zarrow MX, Sikes D, Neher GM. Effect of relaxin on the uterine cervix and vulva of young, castrated sows, and heifers. *Am J Physiol* 1954;179:687.
1160. Zarrow MX, Wilson ED. Hormonal control of the pubic symphysis of the Skomer bank vole (*Clethrionomys skomerensis*). *J Endocrinol* 1963;28:103–106.
1161. Zarrow MX, Yochim J. Dilation of the uterine cervix of the rat and accompanying changes during the estrous cycle, pregnancy and following treatment with estradiol, progesterone, and relaxin. *Endocrinology* 1961;69:292–304.
1162. Zhang B, Roth RA. Binding properties of chimeric insulin receptors containing the cysteine-rich domain of either the insulin-like growth factor 1 receptor or the insulin receptor related receptor. *Biochemistry* 1991;30:5113–5117.
1163. Zhang Q, Ohleth K, Bagnell CA. Biological action of relaxin in the developing pig follicle: Effects on cell proliferation and deoxyribonucleic acid (DNA) synthesis *in vitro. Biol Reprod* 1992;46(suppl 1):105 (abst).
1164. Zhang Z, Day BN, Samson WK, Anthony RV. Relaxin is expressed by pregnant uterine epithelium during early pregnancy in swine. *Program of the 74th Annual Meeting of the Endocrine Society,* San Antonio, TX, 1992;417 (abst).
1165. Zhu HH, Huang JR, Mazella J, Rosenberg M, Tseng L. Differential effects of progestin and relaxin on the synthesis and secretion of immunoreactive prolactin in long term culture of human endometrial stromal cells. *J Clin Endocrinol Metab* 1990;71: 889–899.
1166. Zimmerman AE, Moule ML, Yip CC. Guinea pig insulin. II. Biological activity. *J Biol Chem* 1974;249:4026–4029.

The Physiology of Reproduction, Second Edition,
edited by E. Knobil and J.D. Neill,
Raven Press, Ltd., New York © 1994.

CHAPTER 17

Actions of Ovarian Steroid Hormones

James H. Clark and Shailaja K. Mani

INTRODUCTION

Ovarian steroid hormones (estrogen and progesterone) control or influence every aspect of reproductive function. The purpose of this chapter is to discuss the mechanism by which these two hormones accomplish these tasks. To provide some perspective and to set the stage for a contemporary discussion of this problem, it is important to examine the historical background for our current understanding of ovarian hormone action.

Discovery and Identification

It has been known from ancient times that removal of the ovaries from animals resulted in the loss of sexual activity and infertility. However, several centuries passed before the concept evolved that these processes were controlled by the hormones produced by the ovary. Knauer (1) demonstrated this convincingly by removing the ovaries from guinea pigs and grafting ovarian pieces back to the same animals at new sites. He noted that this prevented the occurrence of castrate atrophy and concluded that the ovary was secreting substances responsible for uterine growth. Marshall and Jolly (2) showed that estrus could be induced in ovariectomized dogs by injecting extracts of the ovary removed from another dog during estrus. These investigators recognized that the ovary produced two different hormones and that the secretion causing estrus was different from that of the corpora lutea. The work of Allen and Doisy (3,4), who discovered that follicular fluid from the pig ovary caused vaginal cornification in the rat, led the way to the isolation and identification of estrone (5,6). This was followed by the demonstration by Corner and Allen (7) that extracts from the corpora lutea of pigs would cause progestational proliferation of the rabbit uterus. This observation led to the isolation and identification of progesterone (8–12).

Department of Cell Biology, Baylor College of Medicine, Houston, Texas 77030

Early Studies on Permeability Changes and Enzymatic Activity

During the years that followed these extremely important findings, many investigators engaged in descriptive studies that defined the multiple functions of the ovarian hormones. Much of the work on the actions of estrogen and progesterone centered on the uterus, and it became clear that these two hormones regulated the growth of this organ by stimulating hypertrophy and hyperplasia of uterine cells (13–16). It was also established that progesterone was effective only when the uterus had been activated by previous exposure to estrogen (14,17,18). The ability of ovarian steroids to regulate the growth and development of all female sex accessory organs and tissues was carefully documented by many investigators during the 2 decades following their discovery (for reviews, see refs. 14,16, and 18). Early work on the mechanism of action of ovarian steroids suggested that the hyperemia and vasodilation that occurred after estrogen treatment might be involved with the stimulation of uterine growth (19,20). Although many investigators considered such mechanisms, Szego and Roberts (21) were the first to suggest that alterations in uterine vascularity and permeability might play a role in the primary events that result in uterotropic responses. Such changes in permeability were thought to be caused by the local mobilization and release of histamine (22–24). There is no question that such changes in uterine permeability occur and undoubtedly are important for the full expression of estrogen-induced uterine growth. However, these changes do not appear to be the primary cause of uterine growth, but instead provide the optimal environment for growth by maximizing substrate availability and ionic constituents. The relationships between these early supportive events and the biosynthetic events that result in true uterine growth will be discussed in detail below under Control of Gene Expression and Growth.

The increased metabolic activity stimulated by estrogen was considered by some investigators to result from direct effects of estrogen on enzymes. Villee (25) proposed that estrogen interacted with transhydrogenase in the placenta to stimulate the formation of high-energy phosphates and thioesters, which were used in the biosynthesis of proteins, lipids, and nucleic acids. Talalay (26,27) proposed that the oxidation-reduction of estradiol and estrone by estradiol dehydrogenase was involved in the production of triphosphopyridine nucleotides, which were responsible for the physiological effects of estrogen. Although the concepts of Villee and Talalay created considerable interest and investigation, their hypothesis that such enzymatic interactions were the primary cause of estrogenic stimulation have not received support. The studies on transhydrogenase were done in the placenta, and it was subsequently demonstrated that this enzyme was not found in other estrogen target organs (28). Also, low levels of diethylstilbestrol (DES), a very potent estrogen, had no effect on this enzyme (29); therefore, direct interaction of estrogen with transhydrogenase seemed not to be a primary event in estrogen action.

It is clear that estrogens do undergo oxidation-reduction reactions during their metabolism; however, these reactions do not appear to be directly involved in the mechanism of action of estrogens. One of the first experiments with [^{3}H]estradiol demonstrated that no conversion to estrone took place in the rat uterus, and that [^{3}H]estradiol could be recovered from uterine tissue (30). Since uterotropic stimulation was observed under these conditions, it was concluded that metabolism is not involved in any primary or direct way.

Early Studies on the Stimulation of Biosynthetic Activity

Although the idea that estrogen acts through direct enzyme interaction appeared to be unlikely as a primary event in the mechanism of action of estrogen, it was clear that estrogen administration elevated enzyme activity in target tissues. Mueller and his colleagues (31–34) demonstrated that estrogen enhanced the synthesis of phospholipids, nucleic acids, and proteins in the rat uterus. They proposed that estrogen controlled the production of templates composed of nucleic acids and that estrogen may act as an inducer or antiinducer of this biosynthetic activity (34,35). These important studies were followed by experiments demonstrating that puromycin, an inhibitor of protein synthesis, blocked the stimulatory effects of estrogen (36–38). Thus the idea evolved that estrogen increased enzymatic activity in the uterus by stimulating the synthesis of enzymes. Further experiments demonstrated that the incorporation of [^{3}H]RNA precursors into all classes of RNA was elevated during the first few hours after estrogen treatment and that actinomycin-D, an RNA synthesis inhibitor, would block this effect (36–42). Estrogen and progesterone were also shown to regulate RNA and protein synthesis in the chick oviduct (43). These experiments, along with others that will be discussed later in this chapter, led to the conclusion that estrogens had a direct effect at the level of RNA transcription that resulted in increased synthesis of specific proteins (43,44).

Current Model of Ovarian Hormone Action

Steroid hormones enter most cells by diffusion, although in some cases active uptake may be involved (Fig. 1). In target cells (i.e., cells sensitive to hormone) the steroid binds to macromolecules called receptors. These molecules are relatively large proteins that have specific binding sites for the hormone found in both the cytoplasm and nuclear fractions of the cell. Binding of the steroid to its receptor molecule results in ill-defined

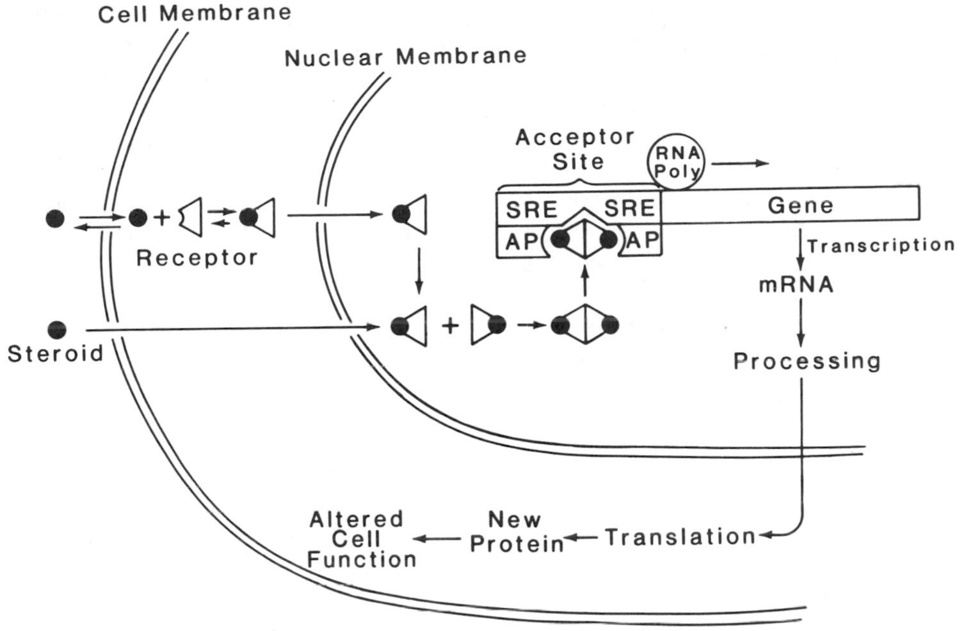

FIG. 1. General model for the mechanism of steroid hormone action.

conformational (allosteric) changes in structure that convert the receptor from an inactive to an active conformation. These changes result in the formation of an "activated or transformed" receptor steroid complex that has a high affinity for various nuclear binding sites. Figure 1 shows the receptor-steroid complexes binding as a dimer to regulatory DNA sequences called steroid response elements (SRE) in the 5′-end of a responsive gene. Receptor steroid complexes are thought to form dimers when they interact and bind to SREs. Receptor-hormone complexes also bind to other nuclear sites (which have been called acceptor proteins [AP]) such as the nuclear matrix, nonhistone proteins, and nuclear membranes. The combination of the SRE and the AP probably form a specific recognization unit to which the receptor hormone complex binds. In the past it was thought that the activation or transformation step occurred in the cytoplasm (this possibility is shown in Fig. 1); however, recent evidence indicates that this process may also occur in the nuclear compartment (also shown in Fig. 1). The binding of the receptor hormone complex to regulatory elements usually results in gene activation, i.e., transcription of the gene by RNA polymerase to produce messenger RNA. The mRNA is translated on cytoplasmic ribosomes to produce the appropriate protein, which alters cell function, growth, or differentiation. In some cases receptor-gene interaction causes gene activity to be decreased rather than increased.

Once the receptor-hormone complex has interacted with a gene, the protein undergoes reactions that are not well understood; they result in the reestablishment of unoccupied receptor (recycling) and elimination of the steroid from the cell. These steps may involve dissociation of the steroid from the receptor and conversion of the receptor to a form that can subsequently rebind hormone again and recycle. The steroid may be metabolized to forms that do not bind tightly to the receptor and hence diffuse out of the cell.

RECEPTORS AND HORMONE ACTION

The Receptor Hypothesis

The concept of receptors for drugs and hormones is an old one; it was first proposed by Langley (45) and extended by Ehrlich (46), who stated that "drugs do not act unless they bind." However, no experimental evidence existed for this concept until the demonstration by Glasscock and Hoekstra (47) and Jensen and Jacobsen (30) that [^{3}H]estrogens were preferentially accumulated and retained by target organs. Jensen's laboratory succeeded in synthesizing [^{3}H]estradiol labeled to a high specific activity and showed that the uterus, vagina, and pituitary retained significant quantities of the hormone against a marked concentration gradient. Since nontarget tissues such as diaphragm, muscle, and kidney did not retain [^{3}H]estradiol, the assumption was made that specific molecules that bind estradiol must be present in target tissues. The concept of steroid receptors was extended by King et al. (48), who proposed that [^{3}H]estradiol was localized in nuclei of target cells and in association with chromatin (49–52). The existence of specific steroid receptors was verified by Talwar et al. (53) and Toft and Gorski (54), who showed that cytosol fractions of the rat uterus contained a macromolecule with the characteristics expected of an estradiol receptor. Experiments with [^{3}H]progesterone established that receptors with similar characteristics also exist for this hormone (55–59).

The important demonstration of specific receptors present in target organs for ovarian hormones and the growing knowledge concerning the ability of estrogen to stimulate RNA and protein synthesis led to the concept that these hormones were acting at the genomic level through a receptor-mediated mechanism. This concept was an important step in our understanding of the mechanism of ovarian hormone action. The binding of a steroid hormone to a receptor and the subsequent interactions of this receptor hormone complex with cellular components are considered to be primary events in the mechanism of action of ovarian steroids. Thus a knowledge of ovarian steroid hormone receptors forms the foundation for understanding the action of these hormones.

Definition and Characteristics of Steroid Receptors

Based on theoretical considerations, steroid hormone receptors are expected to display certain characteristics. These were first formalized by Clark and Peck (60), who outlined the basic mathematical formulation that describes receptor-binding characteristics. These considerations, along with others that will be discussed later, constitute the basic criteria for ovarian hormone receptors.

Finite Binding Capacity

The biological response to steroid hormones is a saturable phenomenon. Assuming that the formation of receptor-hormone complexes is obligatory for the production of biological responses, then the number of receptors per unit mass of tissue should be limited; hence there should exist a finite number of receptor sites. This criterion is met by the demonstration that the steroid-binding system under study can be saturated. This is usually accomplished by exposing the receptor to various concentrations of radioactive steroid and subsequently measuring the amount of bound and/or free steroid after equilibrium is achieved.

High Affinity

Steroid receptors should possess a high affinity for their respective hormones. This is expected because the circulating levels of steroid are usually 10^{-10} to 10^{-8} M. Thus the existence of receptor-mediated responses of physiologic importance demands that the receptors have an affinity for the hormone that is in the range of the blood hormone levels; otherwise the response would not occur. These considerations have proved true for a variety of target tissue receptors; however, they do not preclude receptor interactions of weaker affinity if blood or tissue levels of steroids or receptors are elevated.

The affinity of a receptor for a hormone is in general an indication of the relative potency of the hormone; however, a number of factors determine the ultimate expression of hormonal activity, and these considerations will be discussed later in this chapter.

Hormone Specificity

Generally speaking, receptors are expected to display high affinities for a specific hormone or class of hormones. This "specificity" enables a given target cell to respond to a hormonal signal without interference from other signals. Thus, hormones of the same class, as well as their agonists and antagonists, should compete effectively for a given class of receptor, while not affecting other receptor systems.

It should be noted that steroid receptor sites do not display absolute stereospecificity, that is, the binding or recognition site on the receptor has a limited capacity for the recognition and differentiation of various steroid structures. Estrogen receptors have some affinity for all steroids, as has been shown for androgens (61–64). These *in vitro* and *in vivo* studies have demonstrated that extremely high concentrations of androgen (3 to 10 mg *in vivo;* 1 to 10 M *in vitro*) will promote nuclear accumulation of the estrogen receptor as well as stimulate both general protein synthesis and the synthesis of the so-called induced proteins (IP). Under these conditions testosterone also binds to androgen receptors that are present in the uterus. These receptors are distinct from the estrogen receptor and do not appear to be involved in the observed estrogenic stimulation (65).

The binding of progesterone to its receptor appears to be less specific than that of estrogen. High concentrations of progesterone bind to both androgen and glucocorticoid receptors (66,67); likewise, glucocorticoids at high concentrations are known to bind to progesterone receptors (68). Therefore, the progesterone receptor must be measured with particular attention to competitive binding analysis.

Tissue Specificity

Only certain tissues and organs appear to be stimulated by the sex steroids. Classically these have been termed target organs, e.g., uterus, vagina, mammary gland, etc. It is generally accepted that if responses of these target organs result from receptor steroid interactions, then the number of receptors in these tissues should be higher than that of nontarget tissues. Although there is no established minimum for the number of receptors required to define a target cell, tissue specificity should be part of any receptor validation scheme. For example, the number of soluble estrogen receptors is very high in uterus, vagina, and pituitary and low but not totally absent in other tissues (60). Some target tissues such as hypothalamus possess low densities of receptor because of the heterogeneity of cell types within their anatomic boundary. Thus, not all cells in the hypothalamus are estrogen targets, but those that are estrogen responsive probably possess receptors in numbers equivalent to other target cells. When receptors are fewer than one per cell, one must presume that the tissue is either not a target or that the target is more circumscribed than the tissue.

Correlation with Biological Response

Implicit in all studies of macromolecules that bind steroids and meet the above criteria is the assumption that this binding results in a biological response. Thus, binding of hormone to putative receptors must precede or accompany tissue responses, and the extent of response should relate to some function of receptor occupancy. The relationship between receptor occupancy and response will be discussed further in a subsequent portion of this chapter.

The preceding discussion of receptor characteristics and criteria provide only the basic principles for defining receptors. A complete consideration of these concepts, as well as the complex interactions of hormones with other binding sites and the methods which can be used to resolve these interactions, is presented elsewhere (60).

Hormone Uptake and Cellular Localization of Receptors

The uptake of ovarian steroids is a necessary step before hormone receptor binding can occur. Considerations of how this occurs in relation to cellular localization of receptors has been and still is a much discussed area of research.

Cellular Uptake

The experiments of Jensen and Jacobsen (30) demonstrated that [^{3}H]estradiol was taken up very rapidly after injection by both target and nontarget organs in the rat. Retention of the [^{3}H]hormone for several hours was noted only in the target organs, while the hormone was lost rather rapidly from nontarget organs. This initial and very important observation not only provided evidence for the presence of receptors in target organs but also demonstrated that all tissues could take up the hormone readily. Thus, there appears to be no impediment to cellular uptake by any cell, and the retention of the hormone in target cells is due to the presence of receptors. Also, since the uptake is rapid (within minutes) by all organs, it seems unlikely that any active uptake process is involved. However, the mechanism of cellular uptake and its possible involvement with receptors has concerned several investigators.

Some of the confusion in early studies concerning cellular uptake arose from a failure to differentiate between uptake and retention. Uptake is defined as the initial rate of movement of steroid into cells, whereas retention is defined as the amount of steroid found in the cells under equilibrium conditions. Two experimental approaches have been employed to counter the difficulty of entry versus retention. In an elegant series of experiments employing steady-state perfusion of two isotopes, Gurpide and co-workers (69,70) showed that various steroids can enter target and nontarget cells with equal facility at rates linearly related to their steady-state concentration over a rather wide range of concentrations (0.2 to 5,000 ng/ml). Although it is not possible to rule out a carrier-mediated process completely, these results are most easily interpreted in terms of the diffusion of steroid across cell membranes.

The more direct approach to this problem is to examine the initial rate of uptake of the steroid. Peck et al. (71) demonstrated that the uptake of [^{3}H]estradiol under initial velocity conditions was linear over a wide range of steroid concentration at physiologic temperatures. In addition, this rate was the same for both target and nontarget tissues in the presence or absence of N-ethylmaleimide or excess DES. Either of these compounds would interfere with carrier-mediated transport and/or processes employing cytoplasmic receptor as a carrier. The entry of steroid is not dependent on metabolic energy, as demonstrated by preincubation with 2,4-dinitrophenol for 30 minutes at 37°C prior to the study of uptake. Thus, estradiol enters uterine cells by passive diffusion. The same conclusion was reached by Muller and Wotiz (72), who performed similar experiments with rat uterine cell suspensions. These investigators also found no evidence for the presence of estrogen receptors in purified uterine plasma membranes (73), as had been proposed by Pietras and Szego (74). Recent work by King and Greene (75) using monoclonal antibodies to the estrogen receptor demonstrates that estrogen receptors are absent in plasma membranes. Therefore it appears that estradiol is not taken up by a plasma membrane-mediated process in uterine cells. However, membrane-mediated effects of estrogens cannot be excluded in the central nervous system. Electrophysiological responses induced by direct application of steroid hormones have latencies that are too short to be the result of nuclear mediated events (76), and steroids are known to have anesthetic properties that probably result from steroid membrane interactions (77). Whether these effects on the nervous system are membrane receptor-mediated or the consequence of non-receptor-membrane interactions remains to be resolved.

The studies of initial rate of uptake discussed above were done at 37°C and appear to reflect the rapid uptake *in vivo* by target and nontarget tissues as first shown by Jensen and Jacobsen (30). Several investigators have suggested a pump or carrier-mediated uptake because steroid uptake is a temperature-dependent process (78–80). At low temperatures estradiol enters cells very slowly; however, uptake is rapid at elevated temperature. This finding is consistent with a carrier-mediated transport process; however, it is not sufficient to establish such a process. In fact, activated diffusion (as opposed to facilitated diffusion) may result from the chemical properties of solutes and their affinities for the lipid matrix of the cellular membrane (81). In activated diffusion, transport rate is linearly related to solute concentration and shows a temperature dependence indicative of activated states (kinetic properties similar to carrier-mediated diffusion or transport). The diffusion of steroids is expected to be "activated" since they are lipophilic and likely to encounter a diffusional barrier before entering the aqueous environment of the cytoplasm from the hydrophobic environment of the membrane matrix. In addition, the state of lipid bilayers is temperature dependent, undergoing transition from a liquid to more solid state with decreasing temperature (82,83). Finally, the mobility within bilayers of optical probes is restricted by these phase transitions (84,85). Thus, transitions of membrane state may impose a temperature dependence on estrogen entry. However, such observations appear to have little application to the *in vivo* situation, since (as discussed above) uptake is by passive diffusion at 37°C. Therefore, it is generally believed that ovarian steroid hormones enter cells by passive diffusion and bind to receptors present inside the cell.

Cellular Localization of Receptors and the Nuclear Translocation Model

The exact subcellular localization of receptors for steroid hormones may never be known with certainty because the exposure of tissues to experimental manipulations is likely to alter the distribution of the receptor. However, early experiments indicated that the estrogen receptor existed as a macromolecule with a sedimentation coefficient of 8S in the high-speed cytosol prepared from non-estrogen-treated rat uteri (54). Following exposure to estrogen, the receptor was found predominantly in the uterine nuclear fraction that could be partially extracted with 0.4 M KCl to yield a macromolecule with a sedimentation coefficient of 5S (86–88). Jensen et al. (86) proposed that the 8S form of the receptor was made up of 4S subunits and that the binding of estradiol to the 4S form of the receptor resulted in a transformed 5S receptor hormone complex that migrated (translocated) to the nucleus. Similar, but not identical, generalizations concerning the progesterone receptor were also made by O'Malley et al. (56) and Schrader and O'Malley (57). In contrast to these findings, Siiteri et al. (89) and Linkie and Siiteri (90) suggested that the 4S to 5S transformation was an intranuclear event and that estrogen first binds to a 4S form of the receptor, which undergoes translocation to the nucleus before the transformation step takes place.

The nuclear translocation or two-step model of Jensen et al. (86) and Gorski et al. (91) was widely accepted and appeared to be applicable to all steroid hormone receptors (92–95). Notable and important studies that support this hypothesis were done in the laboratories of Munck and Katzenellenbogen. In these experiments the kinetics of the formation of the cytosol receptor steroid complex were compared with the kinetics of nuclear accumulation of the complex (96–98). These authors concluded that the cytosol receptor hormone complex forms before nuclear accumulation occurs. Even though these experiments were done under conditions that seemed to preclude an artifactual relocation of the receptor, such an artifact cannot be excluded, and will be discussed in the following section.

Williams and Gorski (80) made the important observation that the amount of occupied nuclear-bound receptor relative to the amount of occupied cytosol receptor maintained a constant ratio of approximately 95% to 5%, respectively, over a wide range of [^{3}H]estradiol concentrations. They suggested that these results probably reflected an equilibrium state of the receptor in which most of the unoccupied receptor was nuclear and very little was cytoplasmic. Such a proposal was a prelude to the work discussed below suggesting that unoccupied receptors are found exclusively in the nuclear compartment.

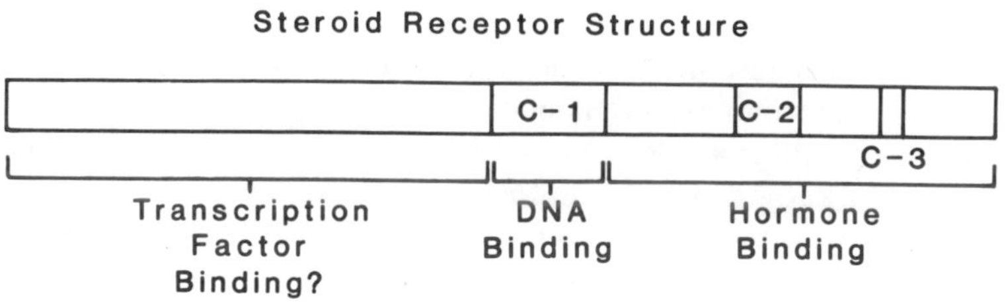

FIG. 2. Steroid receptor structure.

Nuclear Localization Model

Most of the experiments cited above suggest that receptor steroid complexes undergo translocation to the nucleus of target cells; however, they do not prove that such translocation occurs. Indeed, it has been suggested that steroid receptors reside predominantly in the nucleus *in vivo* and that cytoplasmic receptor may represent an artifact found only after cellular disruption during homogenization of tissues (99). According to this hypothesis, receptor is observed in the cytosol fraction after homogenization because it is readily solubilized from the nucleus, where it resides as an unoccupied nuclear receptor *in vivo*. Steroid treatment would result in an apparent translocation because nuclear receptor estrogen complexes are tightly bound or stabilized in the nucleus and are not readily dislodged upon homogenization. In this manner, exposure to steroid would appear to decrease the quantity of cytosol receptor while increasing the quantity of nuclear receptor.

The presence of unoccupied nuclear estrogen receptors has been reported by several investigators (99–109) Nuclear localization of estrogen receptors has been reported by Martin and Sheridan (110), who used autoradiography to detect receptors in uteri incubated *in vitro* at 4°C. Under these conditions the temperature-dependent transformation step (4S to 5S transition) would not take place. Also, unoccupied nuclear receptors have been reported for thyroxine, ecdysteroids, and vitamin D (111–114).

Two important experimental approaches have been taken recently in an attempt to resolve the cellular localization problem. Welshons et al. (115) have shown that cytocholasin enucleation of GH_3 cells results in the formation of cytoplasts (cytoplasm plus intact plasma membrane), which contain few unoccupied estrogen receptors, whereas the majority of the receptors were found in the nucleoplasts (nuclei plus small amounts of cytoplasm surrounded by intact membrane). In contrast, unoccupied receptors were found predominantly in the cytosol fraction following homogenization and fractionation of GH_3 cells. These authors conclude that unoccupied estrogen receptors are found *in situ* predominantly in the nucleus and that the homogenization artifact accounts for the previous observations of unoccupied receptors in the cytosol.

In another approach to this problem, King and Greene (75) used immunocytochemistry with monoclonal antibodies to the estrogen receptor and reached the same conclusion. They showed that unoccupied receptor could be found only in the nuclei and not in the cytoplasm of human and rabbit endometrium, human breast tumor, and MCF-7 cells. Also, their studies indicate that the estrogen receptor is distributed throughout the nucleus and is not localized on the nuclear membrane or any specific nuclear compartment. Similar observations have been made in the reproductive tract of the macaque (116).

The progesterone receptor also appears to be localized in the nucleus of target cells. Perrot-Applanat et al. (117) demonstrated nuclear localization in several target tissues of the rabbit and guinea pig by immunocytochemical methods using monoclonal antibodies to the progesterone receptor.

These experiments lead one to the tentative conclusion that unoccupied estrogen receptors are loosely bound to nuclear sites in situ prior to hormone exposure and become tightly bound following the hormone binding and transformation interaction. Such a new model of receptor localization has perplexed many investigators because of the widely held belief that cytoplasmic receptors were necessary for the transport of hormones to the nucleus. However, as pointed out earlier, there appears to be no barrier to estradiol uptake by target or nontarget cells or tissues. Likewise, no impediment exists to nuclear accumulation in nontarget organs. Peck et al. (71) showed that nonspecific accumulation of [^{3}H]estradiol by diaphragm and uterine nuclei are identical. Also, nonspecific nuclear localization of [^{3}H]estradiol has been demonstrated by autoradiography (118). Therefore, estradiol appears to be able to diffuse readily into the nuclear compartment of all cells, but is accumulated and retained in this compartment only when receptors are present. The finding that most of the receptor is found in nucleoplast after cytocholasin exposure could reflect some unknown effect of this drug on redistribution of the receptor. Such results would argue against a drug-induced artifact; however, one can still argue about the possible effects of centrifugation on receptor redistribution.

The nuclear localization of receptor with antibodies would appear to be free of the above-mentioned experimentally induced artifacts. However, the results of King and Greene (75) are in conflict with several reports, including one from their own laboratory that showed cytoplasmic or perinuclear localization (119). Cytoplasmic localization of receptor has been reported by Lee (120), Pertschuk et al. (121), and Rao et al. (122), who used histochemical methods, and by Pertschuk et al. (123) and Nenci et al. (124), who used immunohistochemical methods. These studies have all been criticized on the basis that the estrogen derivatives used were binding to lower affinity or type II estrogen binding sites and thus do not reflect an accurate measurement of estrogen receptors (125).

Recent work from Blaustein's laboratory indicates that the estrogen receptor is located in the cytoplasmic processes of neurons in the guinea pig brain (126,127). It is possible that different antibodies used in these studies recognize different activated states of the receptor, i.e., antibodies such as H-222 used by King and Greene (75) may recognize only activated receptors localized only in the nucleus, whereas other antibodies may recognize activated and unactivated receptors and localize them in the cytoplasmic and nuclear compartments. In contrast to these findings, Brink et al. (128) concluded that steroid receptors are not localized in the cytoplasm in either the unactivated or activated state.

Nuclear localization of proteins has been shown to occur by two mechanisms: by diffusion of proteins through the nuclear membrane or by interaction of proteins with the nuclear pore, a process mediated by a translocation signal in the protein (129). In the former case, the exclusion limit for spherical proteins is a molecular weight of 67 kDa (130), although the elliptic shape of steroid receptors (131) might facilitate their diffusion despite their larger size. Furthermore, amino acid sequences located on the C-terminal side of the DNA-binding (C1) region found in several steroid receptors bear strong homology to the nuclear translocation signal of (SV40) simian virus 40 T antigen (132,133), suggesting that the localization could be mediated via the latter process. Nearly identical sequences are found in the glucocorticoid, progesterone, androgen, and mineralocorticoid receptors from various species. In contrast, sequences in this region of the estrogen, vitamin D, thyroid, and retinoic acid receptors do not exhibit strong homology to the T-antigen nuclear localization signal. Vitamin D and thyroid receptors are tightly associated with the nucleus even in the absence of hormone and therefore may differ from the larger receptors in their subcellular localization mechanisms (134–136).

Receptor sequences have been shown to function as nuclear translocation signals in the rabbit progesterone (137) and rat glucocorticoid receptors by analyses of deletion mutants (138,139). For the rabbit progesterone receptor, this sequence was the primary signal, but a second minor signal was observed that required activation of the DNA binding domain to function. Unlike the progesterone receptor, the primary signal for nuclear localization of rat glucocorticoid receptor deletion mutants was located in the steroid-binding domain of the molecule and was unrelated to sequences found in T antigen (140,141). The progesterone receptor is clearly capable of shuttling from the nuclear to the cytoplasmic compartment in heterokaryons (142). Thus, not only can the progesterone receptor be imported into the nucleus, but it can also be exported to the cytoplasm.

It is difficult to imagine the thermodynamic properties that would permit exclusive nuclear localization of loosely associated receptor molecules. Therefore, it is likely that an equilibrium exists between unoccupied receptors that maintain most but not all receptors in the nucleus. Such an equilibrium state was first suggested by Williams and Gorski (80,143) and extended by Sheridan et al. (118). Such a circumstance may reflect the reason that a small number of receptors (5% to 10%) was observed in cytoplast in the enucleation studies of Welshons et al. (115). Therefore, it seems likely that unoccupied receptors are present predominantly in the nucleus loosely bound to nuclear sites (a more detailed discussion of this topic can be found in Biochemistry and Molecular Biology of Steroid Receptors, below). The nuclear sites are in a state of equilibrium with the cytoplasmic compartment, which results in a small percentage of receptors being located in the cytoplasm. The controversy concerning cellular localization of estrogen receptors remains a hot topic for debate, and the reader is referred to refs. 144 to 148 for interesting discussions of this problem.

It has been suggested that unoccupied nuclear receptors are active and that binding of hormone simply increases their activity. It is well known that antiestrogens suppress the activity of MCF-7 cells in the absence of estrogen, and thus the unoccupied estrogen receptor may be active in maintaining basal cell regulation (149,150). The concept of active unoccupied receptors may at first glance seem surprising; however, it is generally held that hormones are substances that do not initiate new events, but instead, act as modulators or regulators of physiological processes already in operation. Therefore, unoccupied nuclear receptors may be involved in the control of basal cellular activity and are able to stimulate enhanced activity when they are occupied by hormone.

Receptor States: Occupied and Unoccupied Binding Sites

The measurement of cytosol and nuclear receptors has been used extensively to assess the responsive state of target cells. These observations must be considered in the light of the discussions above concerning the true cellular localization of a receptor; however, regardless of the precise localization, it is clear that receptors exist in at least two binding states in the cell: occupied and unoccupied sites. Unoccupied sites are measured by exposing the receptor to [^{3}H]steroid and assessing the amount of bound and free [^{3}H]steroid (151,152). Occupied receptors are measured by [^{3}H]steroid exchange assays that employ methods resulting in the dissociation of the bound ligand from occupied receptor sites and the reassociation of [^{3}H]steroid (67,78,153–156); for a review of these various methods, see Clark and Peck (60).

The actual binding state in situ and relationship between occupied and unoccupied estrogen receptor sites was first demonstrated by Williams and Gorski (80) in their study of the cytoplasmic estrogen receptor. This investigation, since confirmed by our own laboratory [Clark and Peck (60)], demonstrated that a constant and very low percentage of total occupied estrogen receptors remain in the cytoplasmic compartment of uterine cells despite the level of estrogen present. Furthermore, the number of occupied cytoplasmic sites could be artifactually high unless precautions are taken to prevent the association of estrogen with unoccupied cytosol receptors following tissue disruption.

Target tissue contains several pools of estrogen: free hormone in the intercellular and intracellular spaces, loosely associated hormone bound to nonspecific sites (lipids, hydrophobic proteins), hormone bound to higher affinity type II sites, and hormone bound to the receptor. Occupied receptors are present primarily in the nuclear compartment, and unoccupied sites are found primarily in the cytosol fraction (60,80). If tissues are homogenized, estrogen previously in the intercellular space and unavailable for interaction with the cytosol receptor is free to occupy previously unoccupied sites. In addition, estrogen previously bound to nonspecific, low-affinity sites is likely to dissociate and be available for interaction with unoccupied receptor sites. Thus, the act of homogenization, with its attendant disruption of cellular compartments and dilution of pools, results in an artifactually high estimate of occupied cytosol sites. The correction introduced by Williams and Gorski (80) to avoid this artifact consisted of tissue homogenization in the presence of excess unlabeled estrogen. This manipulation allows the estimation of receptor sites occupied with [^{3}H]estradiol under various *in vitro* conditions. The procedure has been modified for *in vivo* studies (68).

These experimental manipulations are absolutely required for valid assessment of the binding state of steroid receptors, and since they are rarely performed, most studies concerning this point must be viewed with caution. This stipulation, plus the problems involved with the determination of the in situ localization of receptor, makes it difficult to draw concrete conclusions about receptor localization and receptor binding state in most studies.

Biochemistry and Molecular Biology of Steroid Receptors

Estrogen and progesterone receptors are members of a family of ligand-activated transcription factors, including, for instance, the thyroid hormone and vitamin D receptors. Many of the known steroid receptors have been cloned, and, as a result, we now know a great deal about steroid receptor structure (progesterone receptor [157–159]; estrogen receptor [160,161]; androgen receptor [162–164]; glucocorticoid receptor [164–166]; mineralocorticoid receptor [167,168]; thyroid receptor [140,169,170]; retinoic acid receptor [171–174]; vitamin D_3 receptor [175–177]; and see refs. 140, 178, and 179 for review). Steroid receptors are thought to mediate all known activities of steroid hormones. Modulation of the effective concentration of these proteins constitutes the first likely step in control of cellular responses.

Structural Organization of Receptor Proteins

Estrogen and progesterone receptors, like other steroid receptors, are present in small amounts, ranging in abundance from about 0.001% (aldosterone receptor) to 0.1% (progesterone receptors) of total cellular soluble protein. Receptor proteins for all the common steroid hormones have now been purified to apparent homogeneity. Sequence comparisons of the cloned receptors reveal three regions of consensus homology, referred to as C1, C2, and C3, and shown in Fig. 2. The first region of homology, C1, is the most highly conserved, and is a cysteine-rich DNA binding domain. C2 and C3 are less highly conserved, and yet have significant homology. The C-terminal region has been associated with ligand binding, transcriptional activation, and potential protein-protein interactions with other steroid receptors as well as potential inhibitory factors. These structural observations suggest that the steroid receptor supergene family represents an old family of transcription factors that can be regulated. One can speculate that the early forms of these receptors were regulated by intracellular metabolic ligands, in an intracrine fashion (179). Some of the receptors may have lost the ligand-binding domain, and hence became constitutive transcription factors, such as v-erb-A (180). Other receptors may have acquired the ligand specificity for steroids, thyroid hormones, retinoic acid, and perhaps even other unidentified ligands. Low-stringency Southern blot hybridization analysis with the DNA-binding domain of the glucocorticoid receptor has suggested an abundance of related receptor proteins (181). Some of these receptor proteins have been cloned, but the ligands are yet to be identified (181–183). These "orphan receptors" or receptor variants may represent the earliest forms of the steroid receptor gene family.

Steroid Receptor Gene Family

A number of structural features are similar among all of the steroid receptors, suggesting that they are considered correctly as members of a class of regulatory proteins. These features include (a) a structurally separate hormone-binding site comprising a fraction of the total receptor polypeptide chain; (b) the presence of a high-affinity, DNA-binding site distinct from the hormone site; (c) a tendency to aggregate in low ionic strength to form either dimers or tetramers of the subunits; and (d) enhanced affinity for the cell nucleus in the presence of bound hormone. These four characteristics can be observed in both crude extracts and purified preparations, and hence are probably characteristics of the proteins in situ.

Even before the steroid receptors were cloned, it was clear that they were organized into functional domains.

Proteolytic cleavage analysis first revealed receptor fragments that separated DNA-binding activity from steroid binding (184). Once the receptors were cloned, these domains were better defined (185–190). Functionally, the steroid receptors are known to interact with certain inhibitory proteins like heat shock protein 90 (hsp90), to bind to ligand, to dimerize, to bind to specific sequences of DNA with high affinity, and to activate transcription. These various functions ascribed to receptor proteins will be discussed by structure and putative locations.

General Features

Steroid receptor proteins have molecular weights of about 80 to 100,000. Each monomeric unit binds a single steroid molecule, but the receptors are thought to dimerize when bound to the genes they regulate. They are acidic, asymmetric, and present in low abundance in cells. With the exception of phosphorylation, no other covalent posttranslational modifications are known. There is no evidence for either lipid, carbohydrate, or nucleic acid in their structures, and no confirmed evidence that any receptor possesses an intrinsic enzymatic activity. Rather, the proteins are thought to function primarily by virtue of their DNA-binding activity (see below).

Molecular Parameters of Steroid Receptor Subunits

Certain features of steroid receptors are common to all of the known cases studied in detail. The subunits are asymmetric, rather than globular, proteins with axial ratios (long axis: short axis) of about 10:1. This asymmetry is not as evident in the receptor 8S aggregate, suggesting an arrangement of subunits lying with their long axes parallel to each other.

The hormone-binding properties of the proteins are sometimes perturbed by dissociation to individual subunits, as in the case of estrogen receptor, in which the binding constant changes about twofold in high ionic strength. However, the chick progesterone receptor's hormone site is unaffected by subunit dissociation.

Steroid Receptor Organization of Functional Elements

Organization of the Hormone-Binding Domain

The structure of the hormone-binding site itself on a receptor protein has not been determined yet by x-ray crystallography or other precise means. Rather, relative binding activity measurements of both agonists and antagonists have been used. When a large number of substituted steroids of a particular class are tested, a pattern of preferred structures and side groups can be discerned.

A hormone-binding site consists of a hydrophobic pocket, generally contacting the steroid A-ring with great precision, and with greater structural flexibility at the D-ring end of the molecule. Substituents at the latter end are also recognized. However, progesterone and testosterone, for example, differ only at the D-ring, but each hormone's receptor is selective for the proper hormone. No cofactors are known to participate in the hormone site. Unlike the DNA-binding domain, the steroid-binding domain is less well localized, and has only limited homology among the various receptors. Early proteolytic studies with affinity-labeled receptors suggested that steroid-binding activity resided in so-called meroreceptor polypeptides with Mr 27,000 to 34,000 (191–194). Progesterone, glucocorticoid, estrogen, and vitamin D receptor mutants that lacked C-terminal residues were also unable to bind steroid, suggesting that this steroid-binding domain was C-terminal (158,164,186,195–198). More direct evidence was obtained by insertional mutagenesis studies (199,200). These experiments revealed that mutations in roughly the last 200 to 250 amino acids of the glucocorticoid and progesterone receptors abolished steroid-binding activity. Moreover, chimeric proteins involving these C-terminal residues fused to E1A (201) or c-myc (202) conferred hormone-dependent regulation of transcription and transformation, respectively.

Receptor DNA-Binding Domain

Sequence comparisons of the earliest cloned steroid receptors suggested that the conserved 66 to 68 amino acid C1 region coded for the DNA-binding domain (195,203,204). However, direct evidence was not obtained until receptor chimeras were constructed containing the 66-amino acid DNA-binding domain of the human glucocorticoid receptor (hGR) cloned in place of the homologous sequence of the human estrogen receptor (172,205,206). This estrogen receptor-GR chimera was stimulated by estrogen to activate a glucocorticoid-responsive reporter gene, but was unable to stimulate an estrogen-inducible gene. These experiments verified that the C1 domain contained all the information necessary for the sequence-specific recognition of target DNA. In the C1 domain there are nine invariant cysteine residues that have the potential to coordinate Zn^{2+} in a structure analogous to the transcription factor TFIIIA (207). Extensive structural analyses of this region suggest the occurrence of two fingers that might interact with DNA (208,209) and act as the region of the receptor that binds to the regulatory regions of the target gene.

Transcription Activation Regions

The ultimate function of receptors is to modulate specific effects at the transcriptional level. This function has been analyzed extensively in cultured cells using receptor-deficient cell lines into which expression vectors are introduced. These vectors contain cDNAs encoding receptors together with a reporter vector containing specific response elements linked to a gene whose product is readily assayable, such as chloramphenicol acetyltransferase (CAT) or luciferase. These analyses demonstrate that receptors contain two or more activation domains. The chicken and human progesterone receptors provide a unique system to analyze the function of the N terminus of the protein since the A protein lacks more than 100 amino acids, including a highly acidic region found in the N terminus of the B protein. Differential activation of transcription was reported for the chicken progesterone receptors. The receptor A protein, but not the B protein, was able to activate transcription from the ovalbumin promoter, whereas both proteins activated transcription from a reporter plasmid containing a GRE/PRE fused to the thymidine kinase promoter and the CAT gene (210,211). The lack of activation of ovalbumin by PR_B was further investigated using a chimera of the human estrogen receptor and the N-terminal 128 amino acids of the progesterone receptor B protein. This fusion protein did not induce ovalbumin gene transcription, whereas the estrogen receptor alone did (211). These results suggest an inhibitory role for the N-terminal domain that is independent of DNA binding specificity. In addition, this region may help to determine gene specificity.

Regulatory elements do not exist as isolated pieces of DNA but rather are arranged in complex chromatin structures. In order to achieve appropriate gene activation, it is probable that receptors must interact with other transcription factors or with structural components of chromatin. However, very little is known about these interactions.

Nuclear Binding of Receptor Hormone Complexes

The binding of occupied receptor hormone complexes to nuclear sites is thought to be an important step in the mechanism of action of steroid hormones. This concept was derived from studies of nuclear binding done before and after the molecular biological revolution. The purpose of this section is to describe the older studies and to relate these to the modern observations.

Receptor Transformation and Nuclear Binding

As discussed in previous sections, unoccupied receptors have a relatively low affinity for nuclear sites and are more easily solubilized, whereas occupied receptors have a high affinity for nuclear sites. This change from low affinity to high affinity has been called activation or transformation.

Estrogen Receptor

Jensen et al. (86) suggested that the 4S form of the estrogen receptor was converted to a 5S form that had a high affinity for nuclear binding sites. This reaction was thought to occur in the cytosol; however, as pointed out earlier, it probably occurs in the nucleus (89). Regardless of the cellular localization of this reaction, it is clear that receptor estrogen complexes undergo a change in affinity for nuclear sites. This receptor activation or transformation reaction has been examined in detail by several investigators. Notides and Nielsen (212) have suggested that the formation of the 5S complex (mol. wt. 130,000 to 140,000) involves the dimerization of two 4S subunits (*f* 75,000 mol. wt.). When transformation occurs, the dissociation of estradiol from the receptor changes from a rapid to a slow rate (213). Thus, the transformed receptor is a dimer of 4S subunits that binds estradiol with high affinity (slow dissociation rate) and has a high affinity for nuclear binding sites. Bailly et al. (214) suggested that the 4S to 5S conversion step was not synonymous with transformation but instead represented a second order dimerization that takes place after the transformation step. The exact molecular interactions involved in these conversions are a matter of debate, and their relationship to binding and response studies done in transfected cells containing known response elements is not known.

Müller et al. (73,215) presented a model in which the 4S monomers undergo a pretransformation step that results in a shift from a low-affinity 4S form to a high-affinity 4S form. The high-affinity 4S monomers then combine to form a 5S dimer. Evidence for this model is based on the observation that 4S monomers immobilized on hydroxylapitite undergo a temperature-induced transition from a rapidly dissociating to a slowly dissociating state that remains as a 4S form when it is eluted from the hydroxylapitite and analyzed by sucrose density centrifugation (73). Similar findings have been reported by Sakai and Gorski (216).

Notides et al. (217) have shown that estradiol-modulated equilibrium between low- (4S) and high-affinity states (5S) of the cytosol receptor results in a positively cooperative equilibrium binding of estradiol. This finding is in contrast to the findings of others, who showed that estradiol binding is noncooperative in intact tissues and cells (71,80,143,218). In addition, 4S receptor immobilized on hydroxylapitite does not display this cooperative binding behavior. The immobilized 4S forms of the receptor are not free to form dimers; therefore, dimerization is not required for transformation of the receptor from a low-affinity to a high-affinity form. Gorski et al. (219a) suggest that these divergent results can be explained if the unoccupied receptor is immobilized in the nuclear compartment and as such would not display cooperative behavior. However, when receptors are solubilized, as they were in the studies of Notides et

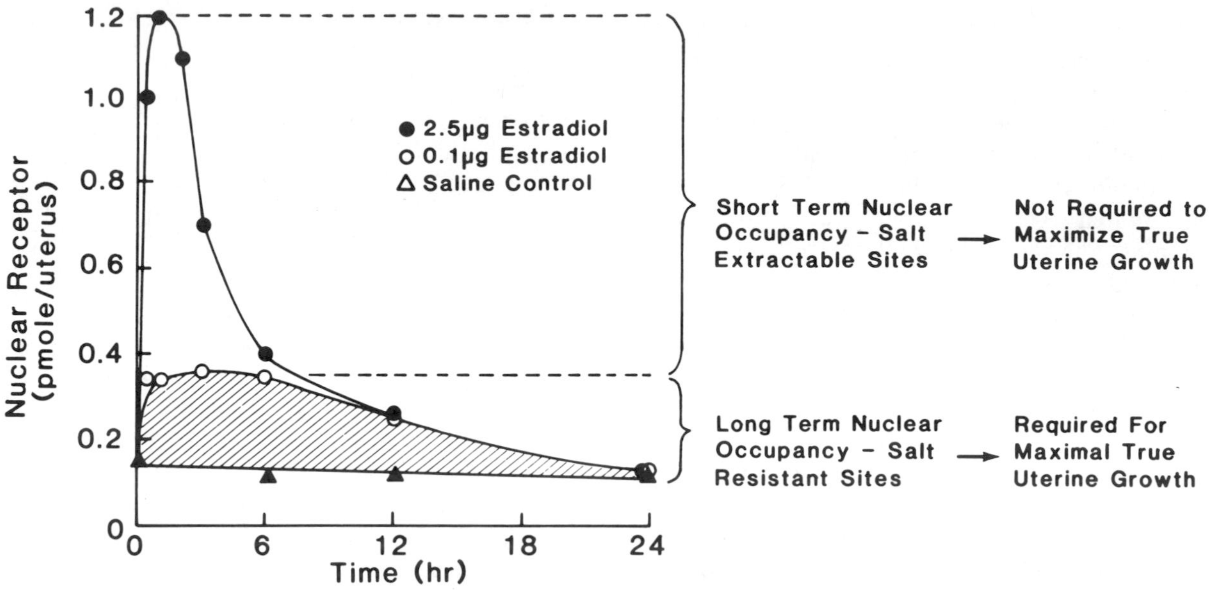

FIG. 3. The relationship between nuclear occupancy of the estrogen receptor and uterine growth.

al., they are free to form dimers and to undergo a shift from a lower to higher affinity state; this is observed as cooperative binding.

Notides et al. (217) observed apparent cooperativeness only when the concentration of receptor was relatively high. Under such conditions the concentration of receptor is equal to or greater than the K_d of the binding reaction, and will result in a linear saturation curve at the lowest concentrations of ligand, which becomes curvilinear at higher concentrations. Such saturation data, when transformed by Scatchard analysis, will give a straight line that is parallel to the x-axis at low concentrations of bound ligand and that gradually curves downward at higher concentration of bound ligand. Such a curve can mistakenly be considered to represent a cooperative binding interaction. Whether cooperativeness exists is still open to question; however, some recent experiments suggest that the formation of homodimers is a requirement for steroid hormone action. These are discussed in the following section.

Receptor Dimerization

Although the dimerization of the estrogen receptor has been suggested and argued for more than a decade (193,194), the relevance of this phenomenon has only been recently determined for the other steroid receptors, namely, dimerization facilitates the binding of steroid receptor complexes to target DNA enhancer sequences (218).

Interactions with Nonreceptor Proteins

Certain steroid receptors bind to hsp90 (90 kDa). This molecule has been identified as a prominent component of the *in vitro* heteromeric untransformed 8S receptor complex for the progesterone, glucocorticoid, estrogen, and androgen receptors (see refs. 219–222 and references therein). Because of the relatively high abundance of hsp90 in the cell (1% to 2% of cytosolic proteins [223,224]), many investigators have been concerned that the hsp90-receptor complex represents a nonspecific *in vitro* artifact. Although the preponderance of the early studies conducted were performed *in vitro*, more recent data have shown that these complexes can form in cultured cells. Pulse-chase experiments performed in cells revealed a time lag between the synthesis of hsp90 and the association with the glucocorticoid receptor (225). Moreover, chemical crosslinking of the receptors in intact cells resulted in the covalent association of hsp90 (226). Thus, it appears that certain steroid receptors can interact with hsp90 under physiological conditions.

When a steroid receptor is complexed to hsp90, the 8S complex is unable to bind to calf thymus DNA. Binding of the steroid ligand, high salt, and high temperature, as well as a variety of other treatments, has been shown to facilitate the dissociation of this 8S complex to the 4S to 5S receptor forms. Thus, one physiological implication is that hsp90 may be involved in the hormone-induced activation of certain steroid receptors. However, this point still remains to be proved.

Deletion mutagenesis mapping studies have been performed on the glucocorticoid and progesterone receptors to try to determine the hsp90 interaction site (227,228). Both studies have localized a fairly large C-terminal region that includes a large portion of the steroid-binding domain. Interestingly, small deletions created throughout this entire region do not disrupt the formation of an 8S complex (228). Thus, it appears that the receptor may have multiple hsp90 contact sites. Monospecific polyclonal antibodies generated against peptide fragments within the DNA-binding domain (229,230) and the linker region (231) are sterically prohibited from binding when the receptor is in the 8S form.

In addition to hsp90, a number of other proteins have been described in association with the untransformed 8S receptor complex. A 59-kDa protein has also been found associated with the progesterone, estrogen, androgen, and glucocorticoid receptors (232). Although less is known about p59, it does appear to be predominantly an intranuclear phosphoprotein (233).

Another nonreceptor component of the untransformed 8S complex is hsp70 (234), a highly conserved protein present in all cells from bacteria to higher eukaryotes. Normally hsp70 is found in the cytoplasm. However, under stress it is concentrated into the nucleus of the cell, where it specifically activates certain target genes involved in the heat shock response (235). Unlike hsp90, hsp70 binds ATP and may be a member of the energy-dependent "chaperonin" class of proteins, which are thought to be involved in protein folding (236). Although salt and heat treatment alone are not sufficient to cause hsp70 to dissociate from the progesterone receptor, high concentrations of ATP do cause dissociation (234).

Estradiol induces hsp70 mRNA and hsp90 protein in the uterus and in the ventral medial hypothalamus (237–240). Since estradiol also induces the synthesis of the progesterone receptor, one can imagine that the function of the estrogen-induced hsp70 and -90 may be to prevent nonspecific interactions of the progesterone receptor with DNA. However, as noted previously, since these two proteins are found in great abundance, their role (if any) in mediating steroid receptor function is still unknown.

Receptor Activity Modifications by Phosphorylation

All steroid receptors studied to date are phosphoproteins. This type of posttranslational covalent modification is another potential pathway for hormone action, particularly if a phosphorylation is hormone dependent. However, the functional significance of steroid receptor phosphorylation has yet to be determined.

Phosphorylation has been implicated in the hormone-binding capacity of the androgen (241), estrogen (242), and glucocorticoid receptors (243). Phosphatase studies of the androgen receptor suggest that hormone binding is enhanced by the presence of phosphotyrosine (244). In the case of the estrogen receptor, studies show that hormone-binding activity requires the presence of phosphotyrosine (245). Moreover, treatment of estrogen receptor synthesized *in vitro* with a purified tyrosine kinase increases the hormone binding capacity from 1% to 4% to near maximal levels (246). Other work has shown no evidence for this pathway. In contrast, the progesterone receptor appears to be phosphorylated exclusively on serine residues (247), while the glucocorticoid receptor contains 89% phosphoserine, and 11% phosphotyrosine (248). Thus, it is not clear that the phosphorylation-dependent hormone-binding requirements of the estrogen and androgen receptors can be extended to all steroid receptors.

Hormone-dependent phosphorylation of the steroid receptors results in a characteristic decrease of mobility by sodium dodecyl sulfate-polyacrylamide gel electrophoresis (SDS-PAGE) (249). This characteristic upshift has been used successfully as a means of correlating receptor modification with function. The human progesterone B receptor in breast tumor cells in culture has a nascent molecular mass of 114 kDa. About 6 to 10 hours after hormone treatment of the cells, the receptor undergoes a phosphorylation maturation step that results in an increased apparent molecular mass of 117 kDa and 120 kDa by SDS-PAGE (250). Studies using [^{35}S]methionine pulse-chase labeling and immunoaffinity purification demonstrated that the phosphorylation maturation was not necessary for hormone-binding activity (251). Similarly, progesterone receptor purified from hormone-treated cells could be used for DNA binding filter assays. In that analysis, the hormone-induced phosphorylation of the progesterone receptor had no effect on the absolute affinity for DNA (252). In contrast, other studies of hormone-dependent receptor processing have indicated that crude preparations of the progesterone receptor isolated from cells treated with hormone have an enhanced affinity for DNA (253,254). Because similar hormone treatments have been shown to increase the phosphorylation of the progesterone (255–257) and glucocorticoid receptors (258), it is widely held that phosphorylation may regulate the DNA-binding and/or transcriptional activation functions of steroid receptors (259).

Progesterone Receptor

The early experiments on the progesterone receptor indicated that transformation of the receptor from chick oviduct involved a dissociation of subunits rather than an association or dimerization, as is currently thought (see discussion on dimerization above). The native progesterone receptor was thought to exist as a 6S to 8S dimer made up of two nonidentical subunits. The complex can be dissociated to 4S A and B monomers by any of the treatments known to cause transformation of other receptors, i.e., heat, salt, dialysis, etc. (260,261). The A monomer exhibits high-affinity binding to DNA, and its binding site is apparently occluded when it is complexed with the B monomer (262,263). Thus, transformation appears to involve the dissociation of A-B dimer as an obligatory step before the binding of the A monomer to DNA can take place. Under some conditions the B form of the receptor from oviduct can bind to DNA (264), and both A and B forms of the receptor from rabbit uterus and MCF-7 cells bind to DNA (265,266). Also, the A form of the receptor, but not the B form, is able to activate transcription from an ovalbumin promoter, whereas both proteins activated transcription from a reporter plasmid containing a progesterone response element. How these more recent observations relate to the older observations must await further consideration.

These considerations of transformation of the progesterone receptor are based on DNA binding as an end point, and it should be pointed out that, unlike the estrogen receptor, the 6S dimer of the progesterone receptor will bind to nuclei without transformation (267), that is, the 6S dimer binds to nuclei at 4°C under low salt conditions. Therefore it appears that the 6S dimer is already in a transformed state with respect to its ability to bind to nuclei. It is possible that the 6S dimer does not represent the native nontransformed receptor but instead a dissociated product of larger aggregates that are not transformed (268). The topic of nuclear binding will be discussed in detail below.

Nuclear Binding In Vivo

Studies of nuclear binding of steroid receptor complexes *in vivo* have revealed complexities that require consideration and that will eventually have to be integrated into our understanding of *in vitro* analyses of nuclear-receptor interactions.

Estrogen Receptor

An injection of estradiol results in the rapid accumulation of the estrogen receptor complex in rat uterine nuclei (Fig. 3; 30,48,51,153,269–271). This is accompanied by a stoichiometric depletion of cytosol receptors and probably reflects increased nuclear affinity of occupied receptor for nuclear binding sites. Nuclear accumulation and cytosol depletion of the receptor probably reflects the relative affinity of the receptor hormone complex for nuclear binding sites and not a real accumulation and depletion. Cellular localization and homogenization artifacts were discussed previously. Following nuclear accumulation, 10% to 20% of the estrogen receptor is occupied for several hours in the nuclear compartment. Thus, *in vivo* nuclear binding has a temporal as well as a quantitative aspect that requires consideration.

The most straightforward relationship that could exist between nuclear binding of receptor steroid complexes and biological response would be that these parameters were proportional and that occupancy of all receptors would be correlated with maximal response. Such rela-

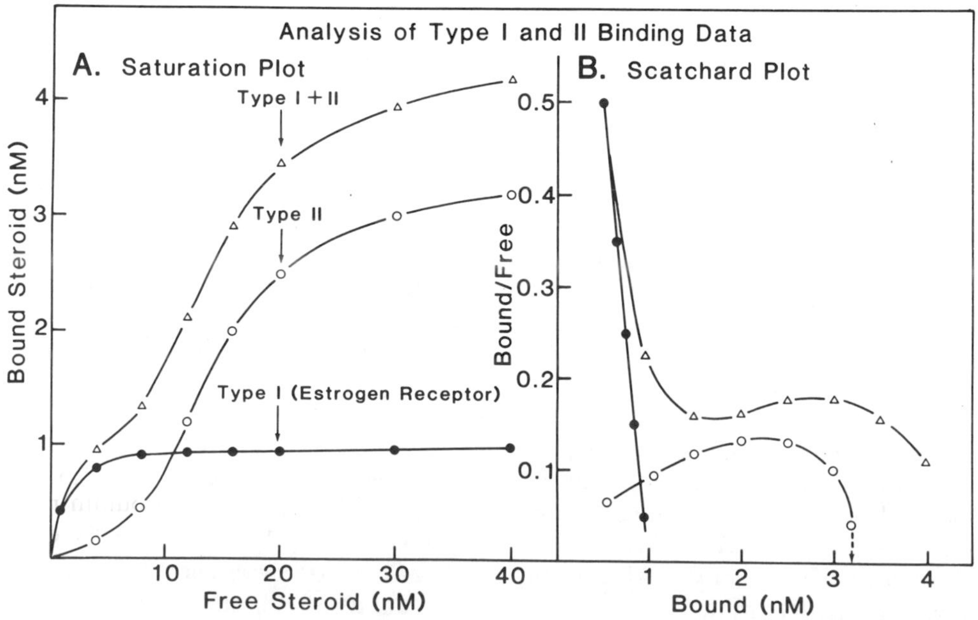

FIG. 4. Saturation (**A**) and Scatchard (**B**) analysis of types I and II binding sites. W, total specific binding; { binding due to type I site (estrogen receptor); O, specific binding due to type II sites; arrow in B, number of type II sites.

tionships have been shown for several responses but not for others. For example, early uterotropic responses, such as water inhibition, stimulation of uterine IP, and early activation of RNA polymerase are proportional to receptor occupancy (269,270,272–274). In contrast, glucose oxidation is maximal in the rat uterus when only 5% to 10% of the receptors are occupied (272). Late uterotropic responses, such as sustained RNA polymerase activity, cellular hypertrophy, and hyperplasia, are correlated with the nuclear occupancy of 10% to 20% of the total number of receptors present (for review see Clark and Peck [60]). These receptor hormone complexes that are occupied for long periods of time (6 hours and longer) are resistant to extraction by high salt and probably represent a population of complexes that are tightly bound to nuclear acceptor sites (Fig. 3; 68,275). The complexes that are extractable with salt may represent more loosely attached complexes that are either bound to nonspecific nuclear sites or are only associated with the stimulation of early uterotropic responses.

Long-term nuclear occupancy of other steroid hormone receptors has been correlated with biological response in other systems. Pajunen et al. (276) demonstrated that androgen receptor occupancy was correlated with the magnitude and timing of enzyme stimulation in the mouse kidney.

Barrack et al. (277) have suggested that salt-insoluble receptor sites are bound to the nuclear matrix and that

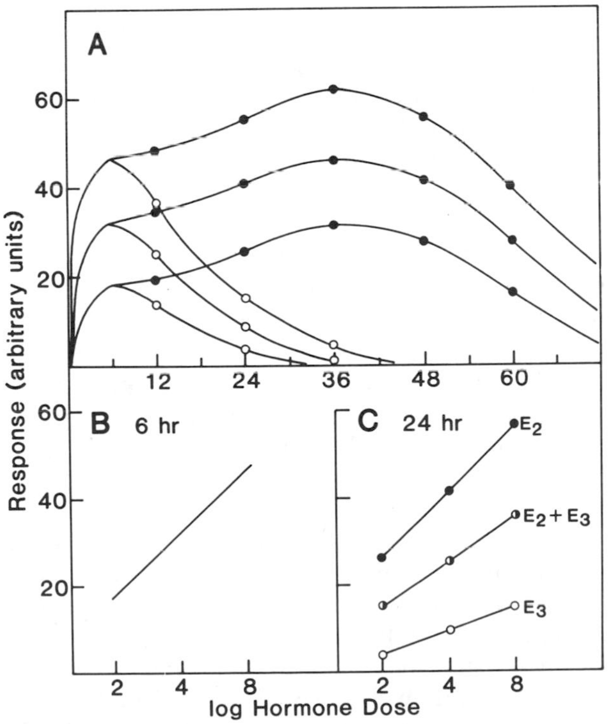

FIG. 5. Relationship between the uterotropic response and dose-response curves obtained with estradiol (E_2, ●, and estriol E_3, ○). See text for discussion.

they may be involved in the control of DNA and RNA synthesis (278). The binding of receptor hormone complexes to the nuclear matrix will be discussed in more detail under DNA Binding and Acceptor Sites, below.

Long-term nuclear occupancy of estrogen receptors has also been described for the mouse uterus; however, an additional second nuclear elevation occurs between 7 and 8 hours after an injection of estradiol (279). Although the reason for this second nuclear peak of receptor occupancy is not clear, it is also correlated with true uterine growth in the mouse (280). Roselli and Fasasi (281) have shown that estradiol increases the duration of nuclear androgen receptor occupation in the preoptic area of the male rat treated with dihydrotestosterone.

Subsequent to the initial accumulation of receptor hormone complexes in nuclei, there is a gradual loss of the receptor from the nucleus, which may involve an active processing step rather than a simple dissociation of the complex and the hormone from nuclear sites (282). This processing step may involve the inactivation of the receptor by a specific nuclear phosphatase (283). Whether receptor loss occurs under all experimental circumstances is debatable. Jakesz et al. (284) have suggested that no receptor loss occurs following continuous estrogen exposure in the rat uterus and that a portion of cytosol receptors and salt-resistant receptor estrogen complexes do not dissociate overtime. Although we have never observed nondissociable receptor forms, we have shown that continuous estrogen exposure leads to receptor loss after 24 h exposure, but not before (285). During the period of receptor loss, uterine growth becomes maximal, and this response is maintained for up to 16 days. Whether this receptor loss is due to the formation of nonexchangeable receptor forms is unknown. As explained above, all studies of receptor processing or loss are compounded by the failure of most investigators to assess the loss of nuclear bound receptors during the preparation of nuclei. In addition, artifactual loss of receptors can be observed in crude nuclear fractions due to endogenous nuclease activity, which results in the release of receptors from nuclear sites (286).

In the chick oviduct system an injection of estradiol is followed by nuclear accumulation of the estrogen receptor (287). If occupancy is maintained by long-acting estrogens such as estradiol benzoate, the rate of conalbumin mRNA production is directly proportional to the concentration of nuclear receptors, with a half-maximal induction occurring at 50% occupancy. In contrast, half-maximal induction of ovalbumin mRNA occurs when nuclear receptor levels are 80% of maximum (288). These authors suggest that these differential responses may be related either to different numbers of specific binding sites regulating the production of each mRNA, or to different affinities of regulatory sites for estrogen receptors.

Progesterone Receptor

An injection of [^{3}H]progesterone in estrogen-primed chicks will result in the nuclear binding of receptor progesterone complexes in the oviduct (56,289). In contrast to the long-term nuclear occupancy of the receptor estrogen, progesterone receptor complexes accumulate rapidly (peak at 8 minutes) and decline significantly by 45 minutes after the injection. In addition, a large proportion of the total receptor remains in the cytosol during the entire time following injection. Apparently receptor progesterone complexes are readily solubilized from their nuclear sites during the preparation of nuclei. Although this possibility has not been examined in the chick oviduct, it is likely in view of the results that have been obtained from studies in the rat uterus. In contrast to these observations, progesterone receptor occupancy in oviduct nuclei can be observed for several hours after large doses of progesterone in oil (290). However, even under these circumstances, only 15% to 20% of the cytosol receptors are recovered in the nuclear fraction. Within 30 minutes after the injection the number of nuclear receptors increases fivefold (1,500 molecules/cell); however, the induction of ovalbumin and conalbumin mRNA is delayed for 2 hours. Half-maximal induction of conalbumin mRNA occurs when nuclear occupancy is 50% of maximum, while half-maximal induction of ovalbumin mRNA occurs at 80% occupancy. Mulvihill and Palmiter (290) suggest that the lag period in mRNA induction is due to intermediate events between receptor localization in the nucleus and an activation of transcription and that different numbers of regulatory sites account for the differences in receptor numbers required to give half-maximal responses.

Rat uterine nuclei also show a rapid accumulation of the progesterone receptor; however, the number of nuclear receptors accumulated is considerably lower than the number of depleted cytosol receptors (155,291). This lack of stoichiometry is due to the loss of loosely bound receptor complexes during nuclear preparation and washing (156,292). These results indicate that progesterone receptor complexes are less tightly associated with nuclear binding sites and do not undergo long-term nuclear occupancy, as do estrogen receptor complexes. Therefore, it is likely that nuclear binding of progesterone and estrogen receptor complexes may differ in significant ways.

In T47D human breast cancer cells, exposure to micromolar levels of progesterone does cause a stoichiometric nuclear accumulation and cytosol depletion of the progesterone receptor (293). This is also a very rapid process (5 minutes) and is followed by a loss of receptors in both cellular compartments. This loss has been attributed to nuclear processing of the receptor; however, it is also possible that the loosely bound nuclear receptor is being lost during the nuclear washing procedures.

Specificity of Nuclear Binding In Vitro

A great deal of effort has gone into the analysis of receptor binding to cellular components *in vitro.* These experiments have been done in order to define the specific acceptors for receptor hormone complexes. Most investigators have concentrated on the examination of acceptor sites in nuclei, chromatin, DNA and the nuclear matrix. Each of these will be discussed below; however, before detailing these findings, a general discussion of the specificity of acceptor site-binding will be presented.

The demonstration of acceptor sites in the nucleus has been the subject of considerable controversy (294–296). Several investigators have shown that nuclear binding of receptor steroid complexes is a saturable phenomenon, thus suggesting that specific acceptor sites exist (50,100, 287,294,297–302), while others claim that limited numbers of specific nuclear sites do not exist and that nuclear saturation is an artifact (143,295,296). Much of this conflict probably stems from the difficulties inherent in the detection of a low number of specific binding sites in the presence of a large number of nonspecific sites (303). This is especially true in view of the very "sticky" nature of the receptor estrogen complex after it has been exposed to elevated temperatures (20 to 30°C) at physiologic salt concentrations (304). This process has been observed by many investigators and is generally called transformation, a topic discussed previously. Thus, studies of the binding of the receptor estrogen complex to nuclei, chromatin, and/or DNA in cell-free systems are susceptible to the error introduced by the masking effect on nonspecific binding to many surfaces. The problem of nonspecific binding is not easily overcome; however, certain basic criteria and principles outlined in the following discussion should be followed.

The principles involved in the study of specific binding of receptor steroid complexes (RS) to acceptor sites are identical to those encountered in the examination of the binding of a steroid to its receptor. These principles have been carefully worked out, and criteria for specific binding have been established. Although these principles and concepts have been discussed above for receptor hormone interactions, they will be reiterated here as they apply to receptor steroid complex binding to acceptor sites.

The binding of RS to acceptor sites should be a saturable function from which a dissociation constant (K_d) can be determined. Such analysis must be done under conditions that maintain the concentration of DNA sequences at approximately the K_d of the binding interaction. If the DNA concentration greatly exceeds the K_d of the interaction, which is likely to be the case, then DNA binding sites will act as a "sink" for RS binding, and a normal saturation curve will not be obtained. Therefore, no determination of K_d can be determined.

The binding of RS to acceptor sites should be a specific interaction, that is, labeled complexes (RS*) should be competitively inhibited by nonlabeled complexes (RS). This can be accomplished by adding increasing concentrations of nonlabeled RS complexes to a fixed quantity of RS* plus acceptor sites or by saturation analysis with different concentrations of nonlabeled RS complexes. These two methods provide data that can be analyzed via competitive inhibition curves or by double reciprocal analysis, respectively. Usually the only assessment of specificity that is performed consists of adding nonlabeled steroid to the RS* plus acceptor sites mixture, with subsequent analysis of the amount of RS* bound to acceptor sites. This procedure only tests the specificity of RS* interaction, *not* the specificity of the RS* binding to acceptor sites.

Chromatin Binding and Chromatin Proteins

The specific binding of receptor steroid complexes to acceptor sites probably involves binding interactions between chromosomal proteins, DNA, and the receptor steroid complex. Such interactions were first suggested by Schrader et al. (267), who showed that the A-subunit of the progesterone receptor binds to DNA, and the B-subunit binds to chromatin. These authors have suggested that the A-B dimeric form of the receptor first binds to chromatin protein acceptors, probably specified by the B-component, and results in the dissociation of the A-subunit, which subsequently binds to DNA (268).

Putative chromatin acceptor proteins have been studied extensively by Spelsberg and his collaborators (302,305–307). Referred to as nucleoacidic proteins (NAP), they are acidic and bound to DNA. NAP bind the progesterone receptor in a saturable fashion, with a dissociation constant of nM (308). Similar acceptor sites have been described for the estrogen receptor complex from the avian oviduct (309,310).

Whether these NAP are true nuclear acceptors for the progesterone receptor is open to question; indeed, Littlefield and Spelsberg (311) have recently discussed several of the problems and artifacts that can arise from such binding analyses. For example, a highly purified receptor loses its capacity to bind to NAP under some conditions; assay conditions employing pH of 6.0 to 6.5 greatly increase the binding to NAP, and unmasking of chromatin by high salt exposure increases the number of apparent NAPs. Thus, one can obtain false estimates of acceptor site-binding depending on assay conditions and receptor preparation. A major consideration in all acceptor site studies, which is usually not addressed, is the evaluation of the specificity of acceptor sites interactions, as explained under Nuclear Binding In Vivo, above. In any evaluation of putative acceptor sites the specificity of binding must be examined by competitive inhibition analysis with nonlabeled receptor steroid complexes. If this were done many of the artifacts might disappear.

DNA Binding and Acceptor Sites

Most steroid-regulated genes share one important structural feature, the presence of steroid receptor binding sites referred to above as SREs. These elements have all the characteristics of a classical enhancer element (312). They are position and orientation independent, and their presence has a profound effect on transcriptional activity when stimulated by hormones (313,314).

Binding to the SRE DNA sequence involves receptor dimerization on the DNA. Coordinate regulation of gene networks is achieved through the appropriate combination of SREs, silencers, tissue-specific promoter elements, and basal promoter elements, for each individual gene (315–317). Thus, different genes can be regulated to varying extents in the same cell by a single concentration of activated steroid receptors. Transcriptional response to steroids in different tissues and cells is additionally controlled by limiting the tissue-specific expression and concentration of the various different steroid receptors (318).

For each of the known ligand-activated nuclear receptors, SREs have been described. In general, they are characterized by an imperfect hexanucleotide palindrome separated by a spacer, suggesting that receptors bind these sequences as functional dimers (319). Negatively regulated steroid response elements (nSREs) have also been described. In most cases, however, nSREs appear to be essentially SREs that have been positioned so that binding of a steroid receptor sterically prevents the formation of an active transcription complex (320–322).

The SREs for progesterone and glucocorticoids are identical and will also act as response elements for mineralocorticoids and androgens (323–326). These findings are problematic because if such circumstances existed *in vivo,* steroid hormone specificity would be lost, that is, glucocorticoids could regulate those genes in the uterus that are under the physiological control of progesterone, and vice versa. Since this is not the case, it is likely that tissue and hormonal specificity is maintained by the presence of tissue-specific transcription factors that interact with steroid receptor complexes to activate transcription. Also, the conformation of the N-terminal portion of the receptor may dictate whether a specific gene will be transcribed.

The estrogen response element (ERE) (327–329) is similar to, but structurally distinct from, the canonical GRE (330). The consensus ERE is more closely related to the thyroid response element (TRE) (331). The sequences are identical, but the ERE contains a trinucleotide spacer in the exact center of the recognition sequence.

Although these are interesting and important findings, they were drawn from *in vitro* observations or from transfected cells in culture and therefore may not reflect the situation in the animal. As discussed above, studies *in vivo* indicate that receptor steroid complexes bind to chromatin and probably result from binding interactions of the receptor with DNA and chromosomal proteins. How these chromosomal proteins influence the binding to steroid response elements is not known.

Nuclear Matrix

The nuclear matrix is a fibrillar network of proteins that contains the residual nucleus and lies within the nuclear membrane (278). Several actively transcribed genes and repeated DNA sequences are anchored to the nuclear matrix, and it is the site of synthesis and processing of heterogeneous nuclear RNA and DNA replication (332–337). Barrack et al. (277) demonstrated that the estrogen receptor is tightly bound to the nuclear matrix of rat uterine nuclei after an injection of estradiol. These matrix-bound receptor estrogen complexes are probably identical to the fraction of receptor complexes that are not extractable with high salt and have correlated with true growth of the uterus (68).

The binding of estrogen and androgen receptor complexes to the nuclear matrix from several hormone-responsive tissues has been demonstrated *in vivo* (338–340) and *in vitro* (341,342). Nuclear type II estrogen binding sites are also tightly associated with the nuclear matrix of uterine, prostatic, and liver nuclei (343–345). Since both the nuclear binding of the estrogen receptor and the elevation of type II binding sites are thought to be involved in the regulatory mechanisms that control biosynthetic activity of target tissues, it is tempting to conclude that nuclear matrix-receptor binding is involved in this mechanism. This point will be discussed further under Molecular Mechanism of Steroid Receptor Action, below.

Synthesis and Replenishment of Receptors

The intracellular concentration of steroid receptors is an important factor in determining the responsive state of the target cells. The control of the cellular concentration of steroid receptors is influenced by several interacting factors, which will be discussed in this section. As in previous sections of this chapter, the term cytosol receptor is used to define the soluble unoccupied form of the receptor regardless of its actual site of cellular localization.

Although many aspects of receptor replenishment and control are not known, a general picture of the possible pathways will be discussed and in subsequent sections specific receptor control mechanism will be examined. Following transformation and nuclear binding there are at least three ways that receptor regulation may occur. The receptor steroid complex may stimulate the transcription of its own mRNA, which will result in the synthesis of new receptor molecules. These may be either hormone-binding forms or non-hormone-binding forms that have to be converted to hormone-binding forms. The receptor may be reutilized by either being converted to a non-binding form, which is subsequently activated to a binding form, or be recycled directly as an activated binding form. In addition to these replenishment mechanisms, the receptor may undergo degradation to an inactive form. Associated with each of these receptor pathways is the loss or elimination of the steroid from the cell.

Control of Estrogen Receptor Concentration

Estrogen-responsive cells in the uterus of a castrate rat maintain levels of receptor that enable it to respond to administered estrogen. This basal level of receptor is probably controlled by genetic mechanisms programmed for the constitutive synthesis of the cytosol receptor. Thus estrogen target tissues can usually detect and respond to estrogens. This is also true of estrogen target tissues in the male animal, which will respond readily to exogenous estrogen and which have estrogen receptor levels equal to those of the female (346–350).

Although estrogen target cells appear capable of maintaining a constitutive level of cytosol receptor, this does not imply that sex hormones have no influence on the level of cytosol receptor. On the contrary, it is well known that steroid receptor levels are influenced by endogenous and exogenous steroids. As pointed out earlier, an injection of estradiol causes a rapid depletion of cytosol receptors, which bind tightly in the nucleus as receptor estrogen complexes. This is followed by a period during which the cytosol receptor is replenished. This replenishment involves at least two processes, the reactivation or reutilization of nuclear bound receptor and the de novo synthesis of receptor molecules. In tissues that do not grow in response to hormone, replenishment may involve only reactivation or recycling. This notion was first suggested by Munck et al. (351) for glucocorticoid receptors in thymus cells. In fact, replenishment of cytosol receptors for glucocorticoids does not depend on protein and RNA synthesis (66,352,353).

In tissues that grow in response to hormone stimulation, such as uterus, vagina, and mammary gland, it is easy to envision the involvement of both reactivation and synthesis in the replenishment process. It follows that synthesis of more cytosol receptor molecules is required in cells that will undergo cell division after hormone stimulation. In this manner a constant amount of receptor per cell is maintained. Cells that grow in size and do not divide may also require receptor synthesis to counteract the dilution effect brought about by cellular hypertrophy. The involvement of protein synthesis in the replenishment process has been suggested by several investigators (289,347,354,355). In these experiments protein synthesis inhibitors, such as cycloheximide, were shown to block replenishment of the estrogen receptor partially. All of these results are subject to question, since long periods of cycloheximide exposure are required to observe inhibitory effects, and nonspecific toxic side effects of this drug cannot be ruled out. Kassis and Gorski (356) demonstrated that the short-acting estrogen 16α-estradiol will cause complete replenishment of cytosol receptor within 4 hours after an injection that is not blocked by cycloheximide. Thus, reutilization or recycling of the estrogen receptor can occur when short-acting estrogens are used to cause nuclear accumulation. Such short-acting estrogens do not cause true uterine growth and therefore may not stimulate the necessary biosynthetic events associated with cell hypertrophy and hyperplasia. This point will be discussed in more detail under Antagonism of Hormone Action, below.

The replenishment of cytosol receptors following hormone-induced depletion is an important factor in determining the ability of the uterus to respond to subsequent hormone stimulation. Within the first 6 hours after an injection of estradiol, a time during which very little replenishment has taken place, a second injection of estradiol does not stimulate uterotropic responses above those obtained with the first injection (357), whereas a second injection at 12 hours, when cytosol receptors have been replenished, will cause nuclear accumulation of the newly replenished receptor and elevated uterotropic responses.

It is well known that estrogen pretreatment increases the level of estrogen receptors in various target tissues, and this is correlated with an increased sensitivity to subsequent estrogen treatment (60). This priming effect has also been observed for sexual behavior (358; we have also observed this phenomenon in our laboratory). However, recent reports on estrogen-induced expression of estrogen receptor have indicated that estrogen receptor gene expression is downregulated rather than upregulated in the hypothalamus and uterus (359,360). Such a result would indicate that the level of estrogen receptor was decreased by estrogen treatment and that responsiveness to subsequent estrogen treatment would be reduced, which is clearly not the case. The resolution of this paradox awaits further experimentation.

Control of the Progesterone Receptor by Estrogen

The uterus is relatively insensitive to progesterone unless first exposed to estrogen. Thus progesterone treatment in the nonestrogenized uterus will not produce a secretory uterine epithelium (16); however, with estrogen priming, progesterone treatment has dramatic effects on the production of secretory responses. These observations may be explained a priori by assuming that estrogen priming stimulates the synthesis of the progesterone receptor, thereby enhancing the ability of the uterus to respond to progesterone. Several investigators have shown that estrogen treatment does increase the quantity of progesterone receptors (78,122,361–370). These effects of estrogen occur in both the endometrium and myometrium of the guinea pig uterus and hence there does not appear to be any differential cell effect of estrogen (367,371). The ability of estradiol to increase the level of the cytosol progesterone receptor also occurs in the neurons of the hypothalamus (372–374).

Other investigators have observed that not only does estrogen treatment increase the quantity of cytosol progesterone receptor but it also causes a shift in the sedimentation coefficient. Castrate animals contain primarily the 4S form of the receptor, and estrogen treatment causes a shift to the 7-8S form. This observation has been made in endometrium and myometrium of the monkey (375,376), in the human uterus (377), in the guinea pig uterus (363), and in the chick oviduct (369). Estrogen also stimulates the transcription of the progesterone receptor gene in the reproductive tract and in regions of the hypothalamus, resulting in an increase in progesterone receptor mRNA (378–380). From these observations it can be concluded that estrogen stimulates the uterus to produce qualitative, as well as quantitative, changes in the progesterone receptor. Thus, estrogen sets the stage for the binding of progesterone that is prerequisite for progesterone action.

Effects of Progesterone on Progesterone Receptors

Milgrom et al. (78) and Freifeld et al. (363) demonstrated that progesterone causes a rapid decline in the quantity of cytosol progesterone receptors in the guinea pig uterus. Progesterone also causes a downregulation of progesterone receptor mRNA (378,379). Thus, progesterone exposure leads to a condition that would appear to make target organs insensitive to subsequent effects of progesterone. During pregnancy such a situation would lead to termination since pregnancy is dependent on the action of progesterone. The resolution of this dilemma must await further experimentation. Regardless of the ultimate interpretation of these paradoxical results, it is clear that the presence of estrogen is required to maintain progesterone receptor levels (112). If rats are maintained on estrogen, no decline of progesterone receptors occurs after progesterone administration, whereas in estrogen-withdrawn animals a rapid decline appears to take place. Therefore, it is possible that the observed downregulation of the progesterone receptor by progesterone is related to estrogen withdrawal.

Estrogen withdrawal implies a lack of estrogen action

that could result from either declining serum levels of estrogen or declining levels of estrogen receptor. Since progesterone suppresses the synthesis of the estrogen receptor (see below), and since the synthesis of the progesterone receptor is dependent on the action of estrogens via the estrogen receptor, it is possible for progesterone to suppress the synthesis of its own receptor by desensitizing the uterus to estrogen.

The level of cytosol progesterone receptor is correlated with the ability of the uterus to respond to progesterone. When cytosol progesterone receptors are low, an injection of progesterone has no antagonistic effect on estrogen-induced early uterotropic events. Thus, the ability of the uterus to respond to progesterone depends on the presence of its receptor.

Control of the Estrogen Receptor by Progesterone

Progesterone acts on the estrogen-primed uterus to alter cell function and reproductive competence. Often this ability of progesterone is considered to be antagonistic to estrogen; however, it probably should be referred to as a modifier of estrogen action. Nevertheless, progesterone will reduce the ability of estrogens to cause uterine growth and vaginal cornification (for reviews, see refs. 199 and 283). This ability of progesterone to modify or antagonize estrogen action is generally considered to involve receptor mechanisms.

Progesterone does not interfere with the initial binding of estradiol to the cytosol estrogen receptor or to the subsequent nuclear binding of the complex (54,153, 380). Thus, the source of its antagonism does not lie at these levels. Instead, progesterone has the ability to decrease the level of cytosol estrogen receptor concentration (289,364,381,382). This decline in receptor level is correlated with a decreased ability of estradiol to stimulate uterine growth (364). In addition to this decrease in cytosol estrogen receptors, progesterone also reduces the level of nuclear bound receptor estrogen complexes in the hamster uterus (383–385). This reduction may be due to the induction of an estrogen receptor regulatory factor by progesterone (90,383,384,386). Such a factor may be involved in the dephosphorylation-inactivation mechanisms reported by Aurricchio et al. (283). Under conditions of continuous exposure of the animal to estrogen, progesterone causes a temporary reduction of nuclear estrogen receptor complexes that is followed by a return to elevated levels (387). The involvement of the control of estrogen receptor levels by progesterone, as well as other proposed antagonistic functions of progesterone, will be discussed below in more detail under Antagonism of Hormone Action.

Non-Receptor-Binding Proteins

In addition to steroid hormone receptors, there are several nonreceptor proteins that bind estrogen and progesterone. These are found in both cytosol and nuclear fractions.

Cytosol Non-Receptor-Binding Sites

The cytosol from immature rat uteri contains a proteinaceous macromolecule, which is observed when saturation analysis by [^{3}H]estradiol exchange is performed on uterine cytosol obtained from immature rats. These type II estrogen binding sites have a 4S sedimentation coefficient on postlabeled sucrose density gradients and, unlike the estrogen receptor, they do not appear to undergo translocation to the nucleus (388,389), that is, an injection of estradiol that causes cytoplasmic depletion and concomitant nuclear accumulation of the estrogen receptor does not deplete type II sites from the cytosol. Type II sites have a somewhat lower affinity (K_d 20 nM) than the receptor (K_d 1 nM), but the number of sites may greatly exceed type I sites. Type II sites display stereospecificity for estrogenic compounds and are present in other estrogen targets such as the vagina (38), mouse (390) and human mammary tumors (391), MCF-7 cells (125), rabbit endometrial cells (392), and Müllerian ducts of the chick embryo (393). Similar secondary binding sites have been observed in the prostate (344,345), seminal vesicle (394), and rabbit corpus luteum (395). Thus, the presence of secondary binding sites for estrogenic hormones appears to be a general phenomenon.

The presence of type II sites complicates the interpretation of receptor assays. The quantity of these sites varies with many factors and may range from two to ten times the quantity of estrogen receptor. The influence of these kinds of variation on the determination of the type I receptor can be significant. As the quantity of type II sites increases, the error introduced in the estimation of the K_d and the number of type I sites progressively increases. This only becomes apparent when saturation analysis is run over a wide range of hormone concentrations. Consequently, assays that are limited to a single concentration of hormone (1 to 10 nM) will measure both sites and may lead to overestimates of the affinity and numbers of type I sites. These points have been discussed in detail in Clark and Peck (60).

A steroid-binding protein that is somewhat similar to cytosol type II sites has been reported from the chick oviduct (396). This protein, called the Z protein, does not display stereospecificity for estrogens, but instead, binds estrogens, progestins, and androgens with similar affinities. Therefore, the Z protein is different from cytosol type II sites; however, it is similar in that it does not undergo translocation to the nucleus and has approximately the same affinity for estradiol (K_d, 20 nM). Also the Z protein is in excess (15-fold) of the estrogen receptor in the oviduct cytosol (397).

The relationship of the Z protein to the steroid receptor is unknown; however, the Z protein does have certain characteristics in common. These include a sedimentation coefficient of 8S, tissue specificity, stabilization by molybdate, and similar chromatographic behavior on diethyl aminoethyl (DEAE) cellulose (396,397). Thus, it is possible that this protein may be a precursor of other sex steroid receptors in the oviduct (396). It is also possible that the Z protein could act as a general mechanism for concentrating steroids in oviduct tissue. This function has also been suggested for type II sites (60). However, currently it is thought that type II sites are more likely involved in binding an endogenous ligand that is involved in the control of cell proliferation.

Nuclear Type II Estradiol-Binding Sites

In addition to nuclear bound estrogen receptor (type I sites), a second estrogen binding site is found in nuclei of various tissues. These are called nuclear type II estradiol binding sites and are located on the nuclear matrix (343,398,399). The relationship between cytosol and nuclear type II sites is not known; however, as explained above, cytosol type II sites do not appear to undergo nuclear translocation and therefore the cytosol and nuclear forms may be separate forms of related macromolecules. Nuclear type II sites are specific for estrogenic molecules and are elevated by estrogen treatment (93,400).

Nuclear type II sites appear to bind estrogen in a cooperative manner and display a sigmoid saturation curve. Figure 4 shows an example of this type of curve and its relationship to the type of curve obtained with the estrogen receptor (type I). Type I sites display the usual saturation curve, which has the shape of a rectangular hyperbola and can be analyzed by a Scatchard plot to yield a linear component. Nuclear type II sites, however, have a more complex binding function that is sigmoidal and curvilinear by saturation and Scatchard analysis, respectively (Fig. 4A and B). Complex curves such as these are difficult to resolve into their individual components; however, we have observed that dithiothreitol (DTT) exposure causes the disappearance of type II sites and permits the independent measurement of the estrogen receptor (401).

CONTROL OF GENE EXPRESSION AND GROWTH

Estrogen and progesterone stimulate many biosynthetic events in their respective target organs. As discussed in the introduction to this chapter, early work by several investigators suggested that ovarian steroids stimulated RNA and protein synthesis in the uterus and chick oviduct. This stimulation of biosynthetic events, which leads to changes in cell function and proliferation, are thought to involve the interactions of receptor hormone complexes with the genome. The purpose of this section is to discuss these interactions and to present the more recent work on the control of gene expression and growth by ovarian steroids.

Hormone Effects on Protein and RNA Synthesis

Early experiments suggested that general protein synthesis could be stimulated by steroid hormones, and subsequent studies with antibodies to specific proteins confirmed this concept. Since it was first determined that RNA plays a central role in the control of protein synthesis in microorganisms, a large body of experimental evidence accumulated suggesting that animal hormones also regulate the amount of cell enzymes and secretory proteins via RNA mediators. Although there were doubts concerning the primacy of these studies, the advent of nucleic acid hybridization methods permitted studies showing that estrogen or progesterone stimulated the production of new RNA species. These findings suggested strongly that steroid hormones could exert a qualitative influence on DNA transcription (402).

Regulation of Messenger RNA Levels

The initial indication that steroid hormones lead to elevated cellular mRNA levels was the result of studies in the uterus and chicken oviduct using RNA translated *in vitro* with ribosomes from rabbit reticulocytes. The synthesis of radiolabeled ovalbumin was shown to be dependent on prior administration of estrogen (403–407). Following purification of the ovalbumin mRNA to near homogeneity, a radioactive complementary DNA (cDNA) probe was synthesized using reverse transcriptase and employed in hybridization studies to quantify the number of ovalbumin mRNA molecules per cell. In the absence of hormone, oviduct cells contained less than five copies of ovalbumin mRNA. Within 4 hours following stimulation with sex steroid hormone (DES), the mRNA reached levels greater than 2,000 molecules/cell, and by 24 hours the level approached 20,000 molecules/cell. These results are consistent with an effect of steroid hormones on ovalbumin gene transcription.

Increase in Rate of mRNA Synthesis

Although these and other results were consistent with the primary effect of steroid hormones being at the level of gene transcription, it could be argued that the rate of transcription remains relatively constant during induction and that the accumulation of mRNA is due simply to the prevention of RNA degradation by steroid hormone. In fact, evidence exists that in certain cases sex steroid hormones can indeed decrease the turnover of mRNA. Definitive answers to these questions required synthetic analyses of pulse-labeled RNA obtained in "nuclear runoff assays."

In studies in the chick oviduct, nuclei were obtained prior to and following hormonal stimulation of target cells. The nuclei were incubated with radioactive precursors to RNA, and the labeled RNA so obtained was hybridized to cloned ovalbumin cDNA or natural gene fragments. In the absence of hormone, no detectable synthesis of radiolabeled mRNA was detected, but within 1 hour following the exposure of cells to steroid hormones, an induction of synthesis was observed. Under these conditions, an accurate assessment of the rate of mRNA synthesis could be obtained (405,408). This rapid response was consistent with a more direct effect of the hormone-receptor complex on DNA transcription rather than with a complex set of intermediate reactions or with a requirement for a newly synthesized intermediate protein. These results were subsequently confirmed for the actions of additional steroid hormones on the synthesis of a variety of mRNAs in other systems (409,410).

It should be noted, however, that all steroid responses at the level of DNA may not be inductive. For example, evidence exists that glucocorticoid actions on proopiomelanocortin mRNA and prolactin mRNA and on thymus cell function may depress activity, that is, transcription of specific mRNAs is decreased in the presence of hormone. Nevertheless, most studies have provided definitive evidence that the primary effect of steroid hormones is to induce the accumulation of specific mRNAs in target cells, and for the most part, the effect is at the level of gene transcription.

Regulation of Messenger RNA Stability

The majority of inducible proteins are synthesized from inducible mRNAs. In the case of steroid hormones, for instance, it is rare that increased protein does not result from increased mRNA via stimulation of gene transcription. If such mRNAs and proteins were totally stable they would soon reach an infinite concentration. Therefore, differential stability is a fundamental property of mRNAs and proteins that make biological regulation possible (411). Average half-lives of eucaryotic mRNAs range from 8 to 20 hours; the average half-life for protein is about 48 to 72 hours. Labile mRNAs contain structural features that make them unstable in cells via nuclease degradation.

In addition to their well-known effects on gene transcription, hormones can coordinately lead to stabilization of mRNA and protein products emanating from their target genes. This is a powerful combination in that a 5-fold increase in transcription coupled with a 5-fold increase in both mRNA and protein half-lives can result in a 125-fold increase in the protein product of that gene (412). The half-life of total poly (A) mRNA in these cells is unaffected by hormone.

Organization of Eucaryotic Chromosomes

Active Domains in Chromosomes

Numerous studies in recent years have established firmly that expressible genes are packaged into chromatin differently, compared with regions of the DNA that are genetically repressed (413–415). In particular, genes that are transcriptionally active, or that have the potential for rapid expression in response to appropriate inducers, have been shown to exhibit a preferential susceptibility to cleavage by nucleases. Such genes include globin, ovalbumin, vitellogenin, insulin, immunoglobulin, histone, and a variety of integrated genes for viral proteins. It is thought that nuclease sensitivity is the result of accessibility to this enzyme because the DNA exists in a more unraveled or "open" superstructure.

The chromosomal domains appear to be related to molecular differentiation since they are not only tissue-specific but irreversible. The DNA that is not contained in these domains appears to be passively packaged into a more complex and inaccessible chromatin structure by histones. The DNA in such higher order structures, the majority of DNA in each cell type, would be unavailable for subsequent interactions with regulatory molecules. In contrast, DNA included in an "expressible" domain, would contain genes accessible to regulatory factors such as hormone receptor complexes.

Nuclear Matrix

Finally, it is appropriate to conclude a discussion of higher order structure by consideration of an even more complex structural interaction of cellular genes and genomic domains with the nuclear skeleton (matrix) itself. The nuclear matrix is a dense fibrillar network of proteins that contains a residual nucleus and lies within the nuclear membrane (416). This newly emerging and potentially important structure acts as a framework or skeleton for many nuclear processes and may form continuous communication with certain cytoskeleton proteins. The structure of the matrix is not yet understood, although we do know that it is rather complex since it is composed of a large number of different proteins. The chromatin itself is intermittently attached to the nuclear matrix, and it is likely that the primary RNA transcripts of genes become attached soon after or even during their transcription.

The ovalbumin gene was found to be attached to matrix during hormonal stimulation. In contrast, when hormone is withdrawn from the tissue and ovalbumin gene transcription ceases, the gene is no longer found attached to the matrix. Constitutively expressed genes are always attached to the matrix, and the attachment is independent of the absolute rate of transcription. This close relationship between the transcription of genes and their association with the nuclear matrix indicates that the nuclear matrix is a likely site for cellular DNA transcription.

It is interesting to note that steroid hormone receptors have also been found in association with the nuclear matrix. Upon hormonal withdrawal, the cellular receptors are no longer associated with the nuclear matrix. Although receptors may play some role in the attachment of inducible genes to the nuclear matrix, it appears unlikely that the hormone receptor is the sole protein responsible for binding an active gene to the matrix structure.

Structural Requirements for Gene Expression

In conclusion, it is fair to speculate that the cellular forces involved in steroid hormone induction of transcription are complex indeed. Our best guess on the major structural determinants for induction of gene expression is as follows:

1. The steroid receptor is activated by hormone, dimerizes, and binds DNA. It is the obligatory and active intermediate required for steroid hormone action. It acts as a transducer to transfer the informational signal inherent in a steroid hormone molecule to the regulatable gene. It is clear now that steroid hormone receptors are only members of a larger, and as yet undefined, class of nuclear transcription factors.
2. The primary sequence of the gene itself is of obvious importance since it not only contains the inherited structural code for the protein, but it appears to contain distinct "promoter" and "enhancer" elements, both of which bind transcription factors and receptors and determine the maximal rate of hormone-induced gene expression. An enhancer element is the cognate DNA binding site for the receptor dimer.
3. Inducible genes are contained within large structurally distinct (DNAse I-sensitive) domains that are an index of molecular differentiation and that are likely to maintain the capacity of genes to respond to inductive influences.
4. The chromatin itself undergoes a specific attachment to the nuclear matrix so that the actively expressed regions of these domains appear to be more firmly bound, and perhaps more easily transcribed by the nuclear transcription apparatus.

Molecular Mechanism of Steroid Receptor Action

The pathway of steroid receptor action has been known for the past decade. It has been generally accepted that the primary regulatory interactions occur at the level of nuclear DNA. Over the past 5 years, a large number of mutational analyses using cloned receptor cDNAs have been carried out to determine the structure-function relationships of steroid hormone receptors. A more precise description of the mechanism(s) of receptor action, however, has required *in vitro* studies of receptor function in a cell-free (reconstituted) transcription system. Until recently, such a system has not been available.

Hormone-dependent transcription of the vitellogenin gene in crude extracts of *Xenopus* nuclei has been observed (417), and it has been demonstrated that bacterially expressed truncated glucocorticoid receptor fragment (418) and native progesterone receptor (419,420) are capable of enhancing RNA synthesis in an *in vitro* transcription assay. These findings suggest that enhancer binding proteins may interact with one or a subset of general transcription factors to recruit and stabilize the formation of preinitiation complexes at distal proximal promoters and thus enhance the initiation of transcription. Preliminary investigations using other steroid receptors (e.g., glucocorticoid and estrogen) indicate that this may be a general mechanism by which all receptors act to regulate the expression of their respective target genes.

Steroid hormone response elements are often found in multiple copies in the 5′-flanking regions of hormone-responsive genes (329,420–423). Transient transfection studies demonstrate that deletion or mutation of one of two SREs lead to a dramatic decrease in the inducibility of a target gene, suggesting that the SREs cooperate with one another to confer synergistic induction. Cooperative binding of receptors to progesterone receptor elements (PREs) appears to contribute to the hormone-induced synergism in gene expression observed *in vivo*. Taken together, these results demonstrate that complex regulation of eucaryotic gene expression can be achieved by assembling unique subsets of cis elements. Through either cooperative binding or cooperative interactions of specific activation domains with other transcription factors at target genes, expression of a given gene can be regulated over a wide range.

Role of Ligand in Steroid Receptor Function

It is well documented that steroid receptor-mediated induction of target gene expression *in vivo* depends on the presence and concentration of steroid hormone (149,321,424,433). Consistent with this model, specific hypersensitive sites, which correlate well with the state of expression of hormone-responsive genes, are detected in and around the SREs in the presence of the cognate hormone (174). A nuclear genomic footprint, demonstrating receptor binding to the PRE/GRE element of the tyrosine aminotransferase gene, is only observed in the presence of hormone (175). Furthermore, estrogen or progesterone (425) receptors in crude nuclear extracts bind to their respective SRE DNAs only when the extracts are prepared from hormone-treated cells. Recent results of *in vitro* transcription experiments have revealed that highly purified progesterone receptors bind and function to enhance the expression of PRE-containing target genes in a hormone-independent manner. In contrast, less pure nuclear extracts isolated from T47D cells contain ligand-free progesterone receptors that do not bind to PRE sites; these receptors also fail to enhance transcription of PRE-containing test genes. Upon treatment with progesterone ligand, either *in vitro* or *in vivo,* the receptors in such extracts now bind specifically to their respective PREs and enhance transcription of PRE-containing test genes. This transcriptional stimulation is specific for progestins and is inhibited by 70% when the antiprogestin RU 486 is added to the reaction.

Such evidence indicates that hormone is needed to effect an additional structural alteration(s) in the receptor molecule, an event not induced completely by antihormones or steroid antagonists. In situ, this event could be represented by dissociation of additional inhibitory proteins, by inducing a specific conformation change in the receptor, via covalent modifications such as phosphorylation, or likely by a combination of these parameters. Following such an alteration, the receptor gains the capacity to bind and activate hormone-responsive genes. Steroid antagonists are inefficient in affecting this process. In highly purified forms of receptor, this "active" conformation may be achieved via the purification process itself.

In summary, steroid-activated receptor dimers bind to SRE elements and further stabilize crucial transcription factors bound at the distal and proximal promoter elements. Receptor tetramers, bound to two SREs, are most efficient in this process. When these transcription factors are bound stably, they are able to recruit RNA polymerase repeatedly to that gene, and a high rate of transcription is achieved.

Relationship of Receptor-Response Element Binding and Biological Response

The simplest relationship between the binding of receptor-steroid complexes to their response elements is one in which a linear relationship exists between receptor-response element binding and biological response. This has proved difficult to demonstrate, and divergent results have been published. Relatively low occupancy of EREs by the estrogen receptor is associated with maximal vitellogenin expression (434). In contrast, the ERE of chicken apolipoprotein very low-density lipoprotein (VLDL) II gene is nearly completely occupied under similar circumstances (435). In cell lines stably expressing high concentrations of the estrogen receptor, the ability of estrogen to induce reporter gene expression is directly related to the cellular concentration of the estrogen receptor (436). These authors estimate that half-maximal response occurs in these cells at a concentration of occupied receptor approximately equal to 100 nM. This figure is considerably higher that an estimate made *in vivo* of 0.5 nM (437).

The reasons for this disparity are not clear, but it seems likely that they reflect differences in receptor binding to DNA when it is complexed with chromatin proteins compared with naked DNA. Using the assumption that the K_d for estrogen receptor-ERE binding is 100 nM, Webb et al. (436) estimate that only 10% of EREs are occupied *in vivo* in cells that contain normal quantities of estrogen receptor (10,000 to 50,000 site/cell). Considering the fact that receptors exhibit only a 10% to 20% occupancy *in vivo* (see Nuclear Binding of Receptor Hormone Complexes), this would mean that only 1% or 2% of EREs would be occupied in a target tissue. Although these estimates may be correct, it seems more likely that other chromosomal proteins in association with EREs increase the affinity with which receptor hormone complexes bind to these chromosomal acceptor sites.

The question that is usually not examined in these experiments with transfected cells is: Do transfected receptors regulate endogenous genes? In human osteosarcoma cell stably transfected with estrogen receptor, Watts et al. (438) failed to observe regulation of alkaline phosphatase by estrogen. However, Migliaccio et al. (439) were able to detect stimulation of this enzyme activity in an osteoblast cell-like stably transfected with estrogen receptor. In both studies a cotransfected reporter gene was responsive to estrogen. The reasons for this discrepancy are not clear; however, it is evident that more studies are needed concerning the hormonal control on endogenous genes.

Hormone-Induced Response Patterns and Cellular Growth

In the preceding section, the mechanism of action of ovarian steroids has been discussed from the molecular biological or reductionist approach. It is clear from the work of many investigators that these hormones have a multiplicity of effects, not all of which may be mediated by genomic interactions. In addition, the biological responses of a target organ to an ovarian hormone involves interactions at many levels of biological organization. The purpose of this section is to present a more integrated synthesis of the existing data on these complex interactions.

Early and Late Responses

Many hormones induce responses that occur within minutes after hormone exposure (60). The relationship between these early responses and later events that culminate in cellular hypertrophy and hyperplasia (true growth) have received considerable study. Uterotropic responses to estrogen will be used as an example of such relationships. Other growth-promoting hormones also stimulate similar pleiotropic response patterns, and these have been reviewed by Tata (440).

Uterotropic responses to estrogen can be classified according to their time of appearance and functional relationship. Early responses include both biosynthetic and metabolic activities. The relationship between these events can be visualized in the following way. Hyperemia, calcium influx, histamine release, eosinophil infiltration, increased RNA and protein precursor uptake, and enhanced glucose oxidation are due to the ability of estrogen to mobilize many physiological functions in order to optimize biosynthetic activity. Early responses also include increased RNA and protein synthesis, which are components of the biosynthetic machinery that eventually causes the uterus to grow. However, as discussed below, the stimulation of these biosynthetic events is not necessarily obligatory in the stimulation of uterine growth. Late responses, some of which are simply extensions of those begun during the early period, include increased and sustained RNA and protein synthesis. This biosynthetic activity results in cellular hypertrophy and eventual DNA synthesis and hyperplasia. These late responses are considered to be true growth responses of the uterus. Obviously true growth would occur most readily in an environment in which substrate availability has been optimized.

Very rapid elevations in cyclic adenosine monophosphate (cAMP) levels have been reported following estrogen treatment in the uterus, and it has been suggested that cAMP is a mediator of estradiol effects (441,442). Other investigators have not confirmed this effect, and it remains to be shown that activation of adenylate cyclase is involved in estrogen action (443,444). Several investigators have demonstrated that estrogen treatment *in vivo* and *in vitro* stimulates cyclic guanosine monophosphate (cGMP) accumulation in the rat uterus (445–447). This response appears to depend on RNA and protein synthesis since it can be blocked by cycloheximide and actinomycin D administration (448,449). Szego (450) has suggested that estrogen causes nuclear accumulation of lysosomes and that enzymes released into the nucleus control gene activity. Because of the uncertain role of lysosomes in the mechanism of hormone action, they have been included in both categories of early responses. Tchernitchin and Tchernitchin (451) have suggested that estrogen causes eosinophils to be attracted to uterine capillaries, where they migrate into the extracellular spaces of the uterus. The eosinophils then release hydrolytic enzymes that depolymerize the uterine ground substance (452). Eosinophils may also cause mast cells to release histamine, and this, coupled with the hydrolysis of mucopolysaccharides, increases vascular permeability and creates an osmotic environment that favors waters inhibition and precursor uptake.

It has been suggested that some of these early events are involved in the primary mechanism of action of estrogen. Spaziani and Szego (22,23) and Szego and Lawson (453) have suggested that uterine growth is mediated by estrogen-induced histamine release, which causes increased capillary permeability and hyperemia. Although these events undoubtedly maximize the ability of the uterus to grow, most investigators do not consider them as primary events. Eosinophil infiltration and its attendant responses can be blocked with glucocorticords without having any significant effect on DNA, RNA, and protein synthesis in the uterus (452,454). Early uterotropic responses can be induced by estradiol in rats pretreated with nafoxidine, an antiestrogen that blocks late responses; however, no stimulation of late responses is observed (455,456). Zor et al. (444) showed that estrogen-induced uterine growth was independent of cAMP, prostaglandins, and β-adrenergic mediation. Even the estrogen-induced elevation in the activity of ornithine decarboxylase, an enzyme assumed to be involved in cell proliferation, can be blocked, and estrogen-induced uterine growth still takes place (457).

Early uterotrophic responses also include the estrogen-induced expression of creatine kinase (458), epidermal growth factor (EGF) and its receptor (459), insulinlike growth factor I (460), tissue factor (a factor involved in the coagulation of blood) (461), and alterations in the structure of collagen (462). In addition, protooncogenes have been added to this list of early responses induced by estrogen (463–465). c-Fos, c-jun, and jun-B expression occurs very rapidly and reaches a peak by 2 to 3 hours, while c-myc is somewhat slower and exhibits a broad peak between 4 and 6 hours (463,466). It has also been suggested that oncogenes interact with steroid receptors to regulate expression of the ovalbumin gene (467). Since protooncogenes are thought to be involved in the regulation of cell division, these findings are of considerable interest; however, their relationship to the later events that culminate in true uterine growth awaits determination.

The relationship of estrogen action to EGF is especially interesting. Not only does estrogen induce EGF and its receptor, but EGF administration also mimics the effects of estrogen on the proliferation and differentiation of the mouse reproductive tract (468). The effects of EGF appear to occur as a result of its ability to activate the estrogen receptor via its membrane receptor, which signals a phosphorylation cascade and estrogen receptor activation (469). The effects of hormones that act at the membrane level on steroid receptor activation are just beginning to be realized. Power et al. (470,471) have reported that dopamine transcriptionally activates estrogen receptor, progesterone receptor, and the chicken ovalbumin up-stream promoter (COUP) in transfected cells. Thus, it is possible that hormones that bind to cell membranes are involved in the transcriptional activation of steroid hormone receptors.

Generally it has been difficult to show that early events are sufficient to cause true uterine growth (68,270, 271,472). For example, estriol causes transient nuclear binding of the estrogen receptor and stimulates all the early uterotropic responses, including expression of several protooncogenes (473); however, it fails to stimulate uterine hyperplasia and growth. Estriol apparently fails in this regard because it does not maintain the estrogen receptor in an occupied state for a sufficient length of time, and, as a consequence, it does not maintain the necessary biosynthetic events (late responses) that culminate in cell proliferation and growth.

From the above results it is concluded that early uterotropic responses are supportive, but not obligatory for the stimulation of uterine hypertrophy and hyperplasia. Also, it is likely that separate regulatory mechanisms are involved in the control of some early and late events in the rat uterus (452,456,474,475).

The sustained stimulation of RNA and protein synthesis that ultimately culminates in cell proliferation appears to depend on the nuclear occupancy of 10% to 20% of estrogen receptors for longer than 4 to 6 hours (68,269–271). This long-term nuclear occupancy of receptor is correlated with elevations in total cellular RNA, sustained RNA polymerase I and II activity, sustained chromatin template activity, DNA synthesis, and cellular growth. Sustained levels of estrogen are required for mRNA stability and continued synthesis of several proteins (476–484). Long-term nuclear occupancy estrogen receptors is also associated with an elevation of nuclear type II estrogen binding sites that is correlated with the late uterotropic growth responses (41,93,399,400).

These results suggest that a sustained occupancy of estrogen receptors is required for the complete sequence of events that ultimately produce uterine hypertrophy and hyperplasia. Therefore, the examination of initial binding interactions of hormone receptor complexes with acceptor sites may give only a limited amount of information concerning the full sequence of events necessary to elicit growth responses. Also, the number of receptor-acceptor sites appears to be small and involves only 10% to 20% of the total number of receptors available. This observation will also eventually have to be integrated into the overall scheme of binding and response studies done at the molecular level.

Direct and Indirect Actions of Ovarian Steroids

In addition to the direct hormone receptors pathway, which leads to changes in cellular function and proliferation, indirect pathways have been suggested to account for some of the actions of ovarian steroids.

In Vivo Studies

Kirland et al. (485) and Sonnenschein and Soto (486) proposed that a factor from the pituitary was necessary to obtain a full growth response of the oviduct and uterus. In their experiments, a single injection of estradiol failed to stimulate the complete growth response in the absence of the pituitary. However, Huggins and Jensen (487) showed that a full uterotropic response could be obtained in hypophysectomized rats if estradiol were given for several days. Therefore, it seems that the pituitary plays a permissive role, probably because growth hormone and perhaps other pituitary hormones are required to maintain the integrity of the metabolic machinery necessary to maximize response to a single estrogen injection. Other experiments making it unlikely that pituitary or other extrauterine factors are involved include the stimulation of epithelial proliferation following direct local application of estrogen to the vagina (488). These and other experiments involving direct applicants to target organs will be discussed below.

It has also been proposed that the liver responds to estrogen and acts as an intermediary in the stimulation of the quail oviduct (489). In these experiments estradiol was infused into the hepatoportal circulation and was completely metabolized by the liver. Under these circumstances no estrogen receptor accumulation by oviduct nuclei was observed, yet the DNA content of the oviduct was elevated to the same extent as in animals receiving systemic treatment with estradiol. Although these are interesting findings, the same investigators did not observe a similar liver-mediated effect on the rat uterus (490). Therefore, the general applicability of this effect is questionable.

Sirbasku and Benson (491) have proposed that estrogens stimulate the synthesis of specific polypeptide growth factors that act as mitogens on estrogen-responsive cells. These growth factors are produced by the rat uterus and kidney and have been proposed to act in one of three ways: (a) As endocrine factors secreted into the circulation, (b) as paracrine factors produced by cells in close proximity to the target cell, and (c) as autocrine factors produced by the same cell in which they act. Certainly there is evidence for a paracrine function of uterine stromal tissue on the epithelium of this organ (492). Whether these stromal epithelial interactions involve specific factors remains to be determined.

ANTAGONISM OF HORMONE ACTION

The subject of ovarian steroid hormone antagonism is very broad and complex; therefore, no attempt will be made in this section to present a comprehensive treatment of this subject (for reviews, see refs. 493–496). Instead, the salient features of hormone antagonism and their relationship to reproductive function will be presented.

Short-Acting Estrogen Antagonists

Short-acting estrogens are estrogenic compounds that display mixed agonist-antagonistic properties when they are injected in saline. Such a mixed estrogenic function results from the rapid clearance of these compounds from target tissues. In contrast, when short-acting estrogens are administered by pellet implant, which results in sustained blood and tissue levels, they act as full agonists.

Uterotropic Responses

Short-acting estrogens have the ability to stimulate early uterotropic responses while having little effect on true uterine growth when they are administered in saline by injection. This pattern of activity was first observed by Hisaw (497) for estriol and has been shown to occur for other estrogens such as dimethystilbestrol (DMS), and estradiol-17α (269,271,380,498). Early uterotropic responses are usually made by simply measuring the 4- to 6-hour gain in wet weight of the uteri, following an injection (Fig. 5). This parameter is easy to measure and seems to reflect a multitude of complex events.

The activities of RNA polymerase I and II increase during early periods following an injection of either estradiol or estriol. However, estriol fails to sustain the stimulation of RNA polymerase I and to cause a secondary stimulation in RNA polymerase II, whereas estradiol maintains both of these parameters over long periods of time. A similar pattern of differences was also observed for RNA polymerase initiation sites (499). We concluded from these experiments that estriol is able to initiate the early biosynthetic events but is not able to maintain them; consequently, early uterotropic events are stimulated, but late events are not.

Such a pattern of early stimulation followed by minimal to no long-term stimulation produces dose-response curves in the classical uterine growth assay that are attenuated and not similar to those obtained with estradiol (500). Uterine growth assays are usually done after 3 to 4 days of daily injections of the hormone and thus involve primarily the late uterotropic events. Under such conditions short-acting estrogens will not produce similar dose-response curves. However, during the first few hours after injection the dose-response curves for long- and short-acting estrogens will be identical. This point is examined further below. Such differences in response pattern and intensity have often been ignored and have lead to considerable confusion concerning relative potencies and biological activity. It should be noted that the differentiation of early and late responses depends on the administration of the hormone in saline or some vehicle which permits rapid absorption and dissemination. If oil is used as an injection vehicle, the hormone will be absorbed and cleared more slowly and hence will act as an intermediate to long-acting hormone. This probably explains the observation of Fagg and Martin (501) that estriol injected in oil will cause late uterotropic events such as DNA synthesis and cell division with half the effectiveness of estradiol (see below for further discussion).

Receptor Interactions and Uterotropic Responses

Short-acting estrogens such as estriol and DMS bind to the cytosol form of the estrogen receptor with an affinity similar to or slightly less than that of estradiol (K_d 1 to 10 nM; 57,151). Therefore, it is possible that if they formed a receptor complex that did not undergo nuclear binding they would act as estradiol antagonists. This does not appear to be the case, since it has been shown by many investigators that short-acting estrogens are highly effective in this regard (269,271,498). The mechanism of action of short acting estrogens as agonist and antagonist appears to involve steps subsequent to nuclear binding, and these interactions are the subject of the following discussion.

Pollard and Martin (502), Martin (503), Miller and Emmens (504), and Terenius and Ljungkvist (505) were the first to suggest that the pattern of estrogenic response observed with short-acting estrogens was due to a failure of these compounds to occupy receptors for sufficient periods of time to elicit full responses. This concept has been confirmed and extended by several investigators. The uterotropic response patterns observed with estriol are correlated with short-term occupancy of estrogen receptors in uterine nuclei (269,270). Estriol and estradiol are equally capable of causing early nuclear accumulation of receptor hormone complexes; however, the quantity of receptor estriol complexes declined rapidly following the initial accumulation. In contrast, the quantity of receptor estradiol complexes was maintained for considerably longer periods of time. Similar findings have been observed in the mouse uterus by Korach et al. (280); however, in these studies a second small elevation in nuclear bound receptor estradiol sites was noted between 7 and 9 hours after hormone treatment. These observations led to the conclusion that long-term retention of the receptor in the nucleus is required for the late uterotropic responses that involve true uterine growth (60). These observations have been confirmed by several investigators in the rat (271,472,506) and in the guinea pig. The concept predicts that short-acting estrogens would be full agonists if they were administered in a continuous fashion (see Antagonistic Effects of Short-Acting Estrogens, below, for further discussion of this point).

The reasons why short-acting estrogens occupy nuclear bound receptors for short periods of time following an injection are manifold and not completely clear. It is known that the dissociation rate of estriol from the receptor is more rapid than estradiol (507), and Bouton and Raynard (508) have suggested that this differential in dissociation rate accounts for short-term nuclear retention. Estriol is also cleared from the body more rapidly than estradiol (509). Therefore, the equilibrium between tissue and blood levels would result in more rapid dissociation of nuclear bound receptor estriol complexes. It is also possible that receptor estriol complexes dissociate from their nuclear binding sites more rapidly than receptor estradiol complexes. This could result in a more rapid turnover or processing of receptor and loss of hormone from the tissues.

Antagonistic Action of Short-Acting Estrogens

As explained in the previous sections, short-acting estrogens have the ability to stimulate early uterotropic responses while having little effect on true uterine growth when they are administered by injection in saline. This explains why they have no antagonistic action when examined by short-term uterotropic assays but display partial antagonism when long-term uterine growth assays are used. This dichotomy is easily explained by examining the idealized data shown in Fig. 5. The response patterns for estradiol and estriol at three dose levels are plotted as a function of time after a single injection. If uterotropic responses are measured at 6 hours after an injection of either estradiol or estriol, they are identical (Fig. 5B) and therefore no antagonism will be noted. However, measurements made at 24 hours do show antagonism (Fig. 5C). This inhibition is shown in the form of dose-response curves and results from the reduced capacity of estriol to stimulate true uterine growth. When the effects of estradiol and estriol are summed at 24 hours, the overall uterotropic effect is reduced.

The antagonistic effects of short-acting estrogens do not appear to be due to a failure of these hormones to induce the replenishment of cytosol receptors (356,380, 498,510,511). Instead, the antagonistic effects are due to competitive interaction of the estriol and estradiol receptor complexes at the nuclear level. Both estrogens cause a rapid accumulation of receptor by the nucleus. Estradiol treatment results in long-term nuclear reaction of the receptor, whereas a rapid decline in nuclear bound receptor is observed following estriol. When estradiol and estriol are given simultaneously, the number of receptor rats exhibiting long-term nuclear retention is reduced (380). These results indicate that the partial antagonistic effects of estriol probably result from competition between estradiol and estriol receptor complexes for nuclear acceptor sites, and from the rapid clearance of estriol from uterine tissue (509). Thus, estradiol and estriol promote the nuclear binding of receptors, and receptor estriol complexes compete with receptor estradiol complexes for those nuclear sites that are involved in long-term occupancy and promotion of uterotropic response (269,270,272). Since estriol is cleared rapidly and because estriol receptor complexes are in equilibrium with receptor and estriol, the competition between estradiol and estriol receptor complexes reduces the number of receptor-estrogen complexes retained in the nuclear compartment. Because long-term retention of estrogen receptor complexes is related to the stimulation of true uterine growth, this reduction in the number of effective receptor estrogen complexes could account for the observed antagonism. These pharmacokinetic properties of estriol explain why some investigators have considered this hormone to be impeded or inadequate (487,512–514). The rapid loss of estriol receptor complexes from the nuclear compartment may be due in part to the rapid rate of dissociation of estriol receptor complexes when compared with estradiol receptor complexes. Bouton and Raynaud (508) have suggested that the degree of antagonism observed with any estrogen antagonist is related to the dissociation rate of the hormone from the receptor. This is probably true for short-acting estrogens of the estriol type; however, it does not seem to be the case with triphenylethylenes such as tamoxifen and clomiphene (64,493).

Agonistic Effects of Short-Acting Estrogens

The results discussed above suggest that short-acting estrogens would not be antagonists if they were present in a continuous fashion, which would result in constant or long-term occupancy of the estrogen receptor. Pollard and Martin (502) showed that frequent administration of DMS stimulated full estrogenic responses in the mouse vagina. They suggested that this effect was the result of continuous occupancy of receptors. This suggestion was confirmed in the rat by injecting estriol every 3 hours for 15 hours or by implanting estriol (270,380). These treatments stimulated full uterine growth and continuous occupancy of nuclear estrogen receptors. No antagonism was observed in animals implanted with estriol plus estradiol. Martucci and Fishman (506) have confirmed these observations with estriol and demonstrated that estrone is also capable of causing true uterine growth under these conditions. Gulino et al. (515) have made similar observations with repeated estriol administration in the fetal guinea pig uterus. A similar effect has been observed by Lan and Katzenellenbogen (271) with 17α ethinyl estriol and estriol cyclopentylether. These steroid derivatives extend the biological half-life of the estrogen and result in long-term nuclear occupancy and true uterine growth. Thus, they are analogous to the hormone implant system. Likewise, DMS acts as a full uterotropic agent when its biological half-life is extended by derivitizing it with the dimethyl ether (510). When injected in oil, which acts to extend its half-life, DMS is also an agonist (389). Continuous administration of estriol has also been shown to cause implantation in the rat (516), whereas a single injection will block this process (517). Implantation in the rat is dependent on elevated levels of estradiol on days 3 to 4 of pregnancy, and a bolus administration of estriol apparently interferes with estradiol action by reducing the effective level of receptor estradiol complexes. However, if estriol is given continuously, it acts as an estrogen and causes implantation.

In addition to these animal studies, Lippman et al. (66) have shown that estriol is fully capable of stimulating metabolic activity of human breast cancer cells (MCF-7) in culture. Likewise, estradiol-17α has also been shown to elicit full estrogenic responses in MCF-7 cells (518). In these experiments the hormone was maintained at a constant level in the culture medium, which results in continuous occupancy of the estrogen receptor and thereby simulates pellet implant conditions in the animal.

These results demonstrate that short-acting estrogens are neither ineffectual nor antagonistic when present in a continuous or chronic fashion. However, estriol does manifest these properties when injected. This paradox relates to the concept, previously suggested by Emmens and Miller (519), Martin (503), and Miller and Emmens (504), that "weak" estrogenicity correlates with short-term nuclear receptor occupancy. What is clear from the present results is that "weak" estrogenicity in the case of estriol arises from competition between estradiol and estriol receptor complexes for nuclear retention sites and from the rapid clearance of estriol from uterine tissue (509). Thus, estradiol and estriol promote the accumulation of receptors in the nuclear compartment, where estriol receptor complexes compete with estradiol receptor complexes for those nuclear sites involved in long-term occupancy and promotion of uterotropic responses (269,270,272). The competition between estradiol and estriol receptor complexes reduces the number of receptor-estrogen complexes retained in the nuclear compartment. Because long-term retention appears to be necessary for the stimulation of true uterine growth, this reduction in the number of effective receptor-estradiol complexes could account for the observed antagonism. However, when estriol is present in a continuous fashion, as in the pellet implant experiments presented here, estriol, by continually binding to receptor sites, promotes long-term nuclear retention and true uterine growth equivalent to that of estradiol. Since long-term retention of the receptor-estrogen complex by the nucleus appears to cause true growth regardless of the estrogen occupying the receptor, estriol acts as an estrogen agonist under these conditions.

Nonsteroidal Antiestrogens

Nonsteroidal antiestrogens are triphenylethylene derivatives, such as tamoxifen and clomiphene. These drugs have been used extensively in women for the induction of ovulation (clomiphene) or in the treatment of breast cancer (tamoxifen) (493,495,496). They are generally considered to be antiestrogens; however, their agonistic or antagonistic properties depend on the species, organ, tissue, and experimental condition used to test those activities.

Agonistic and Antagonistic Properties

Mixed agonism-antagonism is very common among the antisteroid hormones; therefore, an explanation of this term will be offered here as a general example. An agonist is a compound that stimulates a response (Fig. 6A), while an antagonist will completely inhibit the action of an agonist. A mixed agonist-antagonist will partially inhibit the action of an agonist, but because it has inherent agonistic properties it will partially mimic the response of the agonist. The degree of agonist or antagonist activity observed depends on the species, organ, tissue, or cell type being examined and upon the end-point assay chosen (493). For example, clomiphene and tamoxifen stimulate the rat uterus to grow when administered alone, but they inhibit the growth-promoting effects of estradiol when both substances are given simultaneously (68,520,521). These stimulatory and inhibitory functions are the result of the ability of these drugs to stimulate cellular hypertrophy of the epithelial cells of the endometrium while having little effect on hypertrophy of the stromal or myometrial cells. Curiously, RU 486—the well-known antiprogestational drug—also preferentially stimulated the uterine epithelium in a fashion similar to estradiol (522). Estradiol, on the other hand, stimulates cellular hypertrophy and hyperplasia in all three tissue layers and hence produces a uterus that is considerably larger than that seen with clomiphene alone. The elevation in uterine weight caused by clomiphene or tamoxifen alone is due primarily to the hypertrophy of epithelial cells and some slight, but insignificant, stimulation of the stroma and myometrium. The inhibition of estradiol action on uterine growth results from the antagonism of cellular hypertrophy in the stromal and myometrial compartments. Therefore, triphenylethylene drugs act like partial estrogen agonists in the epithelial cells and primarily as estrogen antagonists in other uterine cells *in vivo*.

The estrogenic properties of clomiphene have also

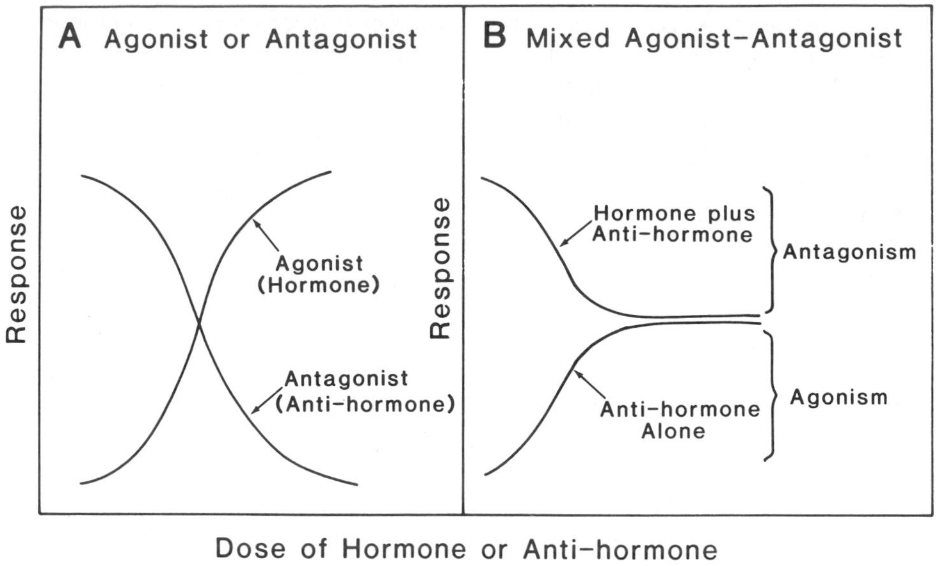

FIG. 6. Comparison of dose-response curves for agonists, antagonists, and mixed agonist-antagonists.

been observed in vaginal epithelium. Both the cis and trans isomers of clomiphene stimulate vaginal epithelial cell proliferation and keratin synthesis comparable to that seen with estradiol during the first 24 hours after treatment (523). No further stimulation is observed with longer exposure to clomiphene, whereas longer estradiol exposure stimulates full vaginal cornification and keratin synthesis.

The ability of triphenylethylene drugs to manifest any estrogen antagonism is difficult to understand in light of their estrogenlike actions during the first 12 to 24 h after administration in the rat. During this time, these drugs cause nuclear binding of the estrogen receptor and stimulate RNA and protein synthesis, specific uterine IP, RNA polymerase I and II activity, and DNA synthesis (93,273,499,524–529). Thus the uterus and vagina of the rat display a response profile as though they had been exposed to an estrogen. It is only after 24 hours that antiestrogens begin to exert their antagonistic effects, even though they maintain a significant level of estrogenic stimulation. Thus, by 3 to 4 days after the beginning of such treatment, both antagonistic and agonistic effects can be observed. Obviously, triphenylethylene drugs must have some indirect action that accounts for their antagonistic effects, and these are associated with events that require at least 24 hours. At the present time the mechanisms involved are not known, but some suggestions will be presented in Antiestrogen Binding Sites, below.

In contrast to the mixed agonistic-antagonistic function of nonsteroidal antiestrogens in the rat, in the adult mouse these compounds are estrogenic, with little if any antiestrogenic activity (500,502,530), whereas in the chick oviduct and liver these compounds are estrogen antagonists, with virtually no detectable agonist activity under most circumstances (531–534). However, it has been shown by Binart et al. (531) that tamoxifen when administered with progesterone will induce cytodifferentiation of oviduct tubular gland cells and stimulate the synthesis of conalbumin and ovalbumin, while tamoxifen alone has no effect. The interactions of these two compounds that bring about these effects are not known. In primates, clomiphene and tamoxifen are primarily antiestrogenic; however, estrogenicity has been noted depending on the species and endpoint used (493, 535). The effects of clomiphene at the hypothalamic-hypophyseal level in primates will be discussed below under Ovulation and Hypothalamic Hypophyseal Interactions. Other species manifest a broad spectrum of agonistic-antagonistic responses to nonsteroidal antiesrogens, discussion of which goes beyond the scope of this chapter (for review, see refs. 493 and 495).

These species differences in response to nonsteroidal antiestrogens are not as evident when these compounds are tested in some types of cells in culture. Tamoxifen and 4-hydroxytamoxifen block the estrogen-stimulated increases in several specific proteins in MCF-7 cells and have no agonistic activity (536,537). Tamoxifen and nafoxidine inhibit [^{3}H]thymidine incorporation and DNA polymerase activity and reduce cell number in MCF-7 cell cultures (150,538,539). In contrast, tamoxifen has been reported to stimulate cell proliferation in pituitary cells in culture (540), while other investigators have found no effect on proliferation (541,542). Estrogen-stimulated prolactin synthesis is inhibited by tamoxifen, and no agonistic effect is seen with the drug alone (543,544), yet others report a stimulation of prolactin expression by tamoxifen in pituitary cell cultures

(541,542,545). Although it is difficult to reconcile these differences, it is clear that tamoxifen can act as an agonist or an antagonist depending on the cell type and culture conditions.

Another estrogen antagonist that was originally reported to be without agonistic activity, ICI 164,384, has prompted some interesting work. Recent studies with ICI 164,384 in yeast cells expressing the estrogen receptor indicate that the drug binds to the receptor and does not antagonize the effect of estrogen on the stimulation of the β-galactosidase gene, yet it has agonistic activity when used alone (546).

Molecular characterization of the events associated with nonsteroidal antiestrogens has suggested that antiestrogens do not inhibit the association of the receptor with DNA but rather appear to hinder the interactions of the receptor with the transcriptional machinery (547–550). How these observations translate into an understanding of antiestrogen action in the animal is not clear.

Ovulation and Hypothalamic-Hypophyseal Interactions

Clomiphene and its closely related analog ethamoxytriphetol (MER-25) were initially described as inhibitors of gonadotropin secretion in the rat (282) and were considered to be likely candidates for agents that would block fertility. However, when they were tried in women, the opposite situation was observed (551). This difference between the effects of clomiphene in the rodent and human may be due to species differences; however, it is more likely to be due to differences in treatment protocols (reviewed by Clark and Markaverich [493]).

As originally observed by Holtkamp et al. (552), clomiphene inhibits reproduction in the cycling rat. This inhibition was attributed to decreased secretion of gonadotropins; however, these studies were done with high doses of clomiphene and over long periods of time relative to the short cycle length of the rat. Schally et al. (553) suggested that high doses of clomiphene inhibit follicle-stimulating hormone (FSH) and luteinizing hormone (LH) release and lower doses either stimulate release or facilitate LH reducing hormone (LHRH) action. Recently Hseuh et al. (554) have shown that enclomiphene sensitizes the pituitary to LHRH. Several studies have shown that low doses of clomiphene increase gonadotropin secretion and cause ovulation in the intact rat (555–557). As pointed out by Docke (558), the cycling rat is not comparable to an ovulatory woman, and he demonstrated that clomiphene did induce ovulation in either androgen-sterilized rats or in rats in persistent estrus due to constant light.

In humans, clomiphene induces ovulation in anovulatory women (551). The drug is usually administered for 5 days beginning on the fifth day of cycle following either spontaneous or progesterone-induced menstrual bleeding. The blood levels of gonadotropins increase during the time of clomiphene treatment, which correlates with follicular growth and a gradual elevation in estrogen secretion (559–561). Ovulation occurs approximately 7 days after the end of treatment.

The mechanisms and sites of action of clomiphene are not completely understood. Igarashi et al. (562) showed that implantation of clomiphene directly into the anterior hypothalamus or median eminence caused increased gonadotropin levels in the blood of rats, which suggested that the hypothalamus was the site of action. Indirect evidence for central nervous system effects was shown by Coppola et al. (563), who demonstrated that phenobarbital would block gonadotropin secretion in clomiphene-treated Pregnant Mare Serum (PMS) primed immature rats. Likewise, clomiphene was shown to cause ovulation when implanted in the hypothalamus, implying a direct stimulatory effect in the brain (564).

In addition to the effects of clomiphene at the hypothalamic level, the pituitary also appears to be a primary target of this compound. The work of Docke (564) with bilaterial implants of clomiphene in the brain indicates that the drug blocks ovulation induction by estrogen at the pituitary level. The pituitary is much more sensitive to clomiphene than the hypothalamus (565–567). In addition, Hseuh et al. (554) have shown that enclomiphene sensitizes the pituitary to LHRH in a fashion similar to estradiol (568). Enclomiphene also stimulates the secretion of prolactin and suppresses growth hormone secretion in pituitary cell cultures (GH-cells), while zuclomiphene is without effect (569). Suppression of blood levels of growth hormone has also been reported in normal men (570).

From the above discussion it can be concluded that both the hypothalamus and pituitary are involved in the action of clomiphene. The mechanisms by which clomiphene exerts its effects are not fully understood and are undoubtedly more complex than the normal mechanisms by which endogenous hormones function. The usual explanation given, however, is based on the antiestrogenic properties of the drug and is focused on the ability of clomiphene to bind to estrogen receptors, thus blocking the negative feedback effects of estrogen. This inhibition of negative feedback presumably results in gonadotropin secretion and ovulation. This explanation seems to hold for some circumstances; however, it is incomplete and ignores some of the basic pharmacology of clomiphene.

It should be remembered that clomiphene is both estrogenic and antiestrogenic to varying degrees in all mammals including humans; therefore, this mixed function must be considered in any model. As mentioned above, some investigators have attempted to explain these mixed agonistic/antagonistic properties by proposing that clomiphene is antagonistic at low concentrations and agonistic at high concentrations (553,556, 557,571,572). In this scheme, clomiphene binds to estrogen receptors at low doses and blocks the negative feedback of endogenous estrogens. This results in the release of gonadotropins and subsequent ovulation. At high doses the drug also binds estrogen receptors but acts as an estrogen and blocks gonadotropin secretion because of its inherent estrogenicity at these high levels. However, clomiphene is estrogenic and antiestrogenic over the same dose range in uterotropic assays (573). Therefore, unless one is willing to envoke a special case for the brain, the above explanation of positive and negative effects on gonadotropic secretion do not hold. It is possible, however, to propose a scheme whereby stimulatory and inhibitory effects could be observed. Perhaps clomiphene at low doses interacts only with estrogen receptors in the pituitary, and this effect is positive, i.e., gonadotropin secretion is stimulated. At higher doses the drug binds to hypothalamic estrogen receptor sites, which has a negative effect on gonadotropin-releasing hormone secretion. These differential effects seem quite likely in view of the previously noted steroid-binding affinity of pituitary and hypothalamic estrogen receptors for clomiphene (565,566,567).

A positive feedback role for clomiphene on gonadotropin release in humans is not usually considered; however, it seems as likely an explanation as the inhibition of the negative feedback effects of estrogens. Indeed, it has been demonstrated that estradiol administration for 3 days of the menstrual cycle results in an increase in blood levels of LH and FSH (561,574). These changes in gonadotropin secretion are highly similar, although not identical, to those seen following clomiphene administration. These changes in gonadotropin levels have been attributed to the positive feedback effects of estrogens and are similar to those described for the rat (for review, see ref. 575).

It is thus possible to envision clomiphene acting, at least in some anovulatory syndromes, as an extra estrogenic-positive stimulus to gonadotropin secretion. This action may explain the ability of zuclomiphene to cause ovulation in patients with Chiari-Frommel syndrome who have very low to nondetectable levels of estrogen (535). It is difficult to fit this finding with the concept of a blockade of the negative feedback of endogenous estrogen, since zuclomiphene is considered to be primarily estrogenic. A positive action of clomiphene is also possible in women with polycystic ovarian disease. The ovarian follicles of these women synthesize large quantities of androstenedione but fail to convert this precursor to estradiol. Since clomiphene can be estrogenic under some circumstances, perhaps the drug is acting directly at the ovarian level as an estrogen. This estrogenicity of clomiphene may be a necessary requirement for ovulation in these patients.

Ethynyl estradiol is known to have negative feedback effects on gonadotropin secretion in humans, and clomiphene will block this effect under some circumstances (576). These results are usually cited as evidence that clomiphene acts by blocking the negative feedback effects of estrogen. However, it is also known that clomiphene will suppress gonadotropin secretion in ovariectomized or postmenopausal women (577–579). Therefore, under some circumstances, clomiphene can mimic the negative feedback effects of estrogens. In addition to these estrogenic effects of clomiphene, it has been shown that high doses of ethynyl estradiol do not interfere with the ovulation-inducing effects of clomiphene (580). If clomiphene were acting only to block the negative feedback effects of estrogens, then high doses of ethynyl estradiol should overcome this effect and block gonadotropin secretion.

These observations appear contradictory and difficult to reconcile; however, it must be remembered that the various effects of estrogen or clomiphene on ovulation are being observed under two different physiological circumstances. Negative feedback effects are seen after castration or menopause when gonadotropin blood levels are very high. Conversely, the positive effects are observed when gonadotropin secretion is operating at a much reduced level and is under the control of endogenous steroids. These two hypothalamic-hypophyseal states are probably not comparable with respect to control mechanisms. For example, in the ovariectomized animal the gonadotropin control centers in the brain have been operating in the absence of estrogen for several days to weeks before experiments are performed. Thus, it is possible that a positive feedback center might not operate optimally under these conditions and only the negative functions would be intact. A decline in the function of a positive center could reflect a dependency on continuous exposure to some level of estrogen. Therefore, when either estradiol or clomiphene is given to a castrate animal or postmenopausal woman, a suppression of gonadotropin secretion is observed. However, under normal physiological circumstances, the presence of estrogen maintains the positive feedback control centers at an operative level, and when a sufficient estrogenic stimulus is detected, ovulatory levels of gonadotropins are secreted. Czygan and Schulz (577) demonstrated that clomiphene had a positive effect on gonadotropin secretion in the presence of estrogen, while, as mentioned earlier, it suppressed gonadotropin in the absence of estrogen. These results support the concept that estrogen is required for maintenance of the positive control centers.

Receptor Binding

Nonsteroidal antiestrogens bind to the cytosol form of the estrogen receptor and will cause nuclear accumulation of the receptor antiestrogen complex (64,373, 510,581–583). This is expected because, as discussed previously, these compounds stimulate biosynthetic activity in target tissues during the first 24 hours in a fashion similar to estradiol. Obviously there is a paradox, since one would expect that antiestrogens would block the action of estrogens, yet during these initial hours of interaction they appear to be estrogenic. Therefore, differences must exist at some level or at some time that account for the mixed agonistic and antagonistic properties of these drugs.

One difference is that triphenylethylene antiestrogens, such as nafoxidine, clomiphene and tamoxifen cause long term occupancy of the nuclear bound receptor and a sustained depletion of cytosol receptors (582). Such an effect could be caused by the long half-life of these compounds with the resultant continuous nuclear occupancy of receptors or a defect in nuclear receptor processing (60). Defective nuclear processing of the receptor nafoxidine complex has been observed in MCF-7 cells (282,584,585). In these experiments the long term occupancy of the nuclear receptor induced by nafoxidine continued in the absence of nafoxidine in the culture media, thus eliminating the possibility that sustained occupancy results from the continuous presence of nafoxidine as might be the case *in vivo*. Continuous occupancy of nuclear estrogen receptor by estradiol does not produce inhibitory effects on uterine growth responses (380,511). Therefore, it is likely that defective nuclear processing is somehow involved in the failure of these non-steroidal antiestrogens to elicit the entire spectrum of true uterine growth.

Some investigators have reported specific but subtle differences in the physicochemical characteristics of receptor antiestrogen and receptor estradiol complexes (586–588). However, it is not clear how such differences relate to hormone antagonism. No difference between receptor antiestrogen and receptor estradiol complexes has been found with respect to their recognization by monoclonal antibodies to the receptor, or binding to their DNA or polynucleotides (589–591). Evans et al. (586) did show that estradiol receptor complexes bind more tightly to calf thymus DNA than antiestrogen receptor complexes. Perhaps this observation relates to the finding that nuclear bound receptor antiestrogen complexes can be readily extracted by high salt, whereas a portion of estrogen receptor complexes cannot (275). These salt-extracted forms of the receptor do not differ significantly from those of the estradiol receptor complex (588,592,593). Differential extraction of estrogen and tamoxifen receptors has also been observed with the nonionic detergent Nonidet P-40 (594). All of the nuclear tamoxifen receptor complex from MCF-7 cells is extracted with this detergent and sediments as 7S and 5S peaks on sucrose density gradients. In contrast, nuclear estradiol complexes resist extraction. These results suggest that the interactions of these two receptor complex forms with chromatin differ in some way.

Although there are some differences between the receptor binding interactions of estrogens and antiestrogens, it is difficult to fit these into a unifying scheme to explain the antagonistic activity of these compounds. Considering the ability of these compounds to cause nuclear accumulation of the estrogen receptor and to stimulate uterine DNA, RNA, and protein synthesis during the first 24 hours after exposure, it seems likely that mechanisms other than those mediated by the estrogen receptor may be involved. Some of these mechanisms will be discussed in the following sections.

Antiestrogen Binding Sites

In addition to the estrogen receptor, many tissues contain triphenylethylene antiestrogen binding sites (TABS), which bind antiestrogens such as tamoxifen and clomiphene with high affinity (K_d, 1 nM) and are present in estrogen target and nontarget tissues (595,596). In addition, somewhat similar sites with lower affinity (K_d, 10 nM) are associated with low-density lipoprotein in rat serum (597). The binding specificity of TABS spans a rather broad range; however, it is generally agreed that triphenylethylene derivatives that contain the alkylaminoethoxy side chain are bound with the highest affinity, and steroids are not bound by these sites (598–600). Other compounds such as chlorpromazine, ketocholesterol, and cholesterol have a reduced affinity; however, as discussed below, these may be significant (601).

The subcellular localization of TABS appears to vary with species and/or cell type. Several laboratories have reported the presence of TABS in high-speed cytosols of the chick oviduct, guinea pig and rat uterus, human mammary carcinoma, and nontarget human tissues (595,596,602–606); Sudo et al. (599) found TABS predominantly in the microsomal fraction of tissues from the rat. Cytosol and nuclear localization in the guinea pig uterus has been reported by Gulino and Pasqualini (598), and it has been suggested that the level of these sites is modulated by estradiol and progesterone (597,607). Nuclear localization has also been reported in human breast cancer tissue and in chicken and rat liver (601,604,608).

The physiological function of TABS has not been defined, and although it is tempting to suggest that these sites are antiestrogen receptors, in general the data do not support this hypothesis. The estrogenic and antiestrogenic properties of nonsteroidal antiestrogens correlate with their relative binding affinities for the estrogen receptor and not for TABS (582,590). The *cis* and *trans* isomers of clomiphene bind to TABS with similar affinities, yet they have dissimilar agonist-antagonist profiles (597,599). Tamoxifen resistance has been described in a cell line of MCF-7 breast cancer cells that contained very low levels of TABS and normal levels of estrogen receptor (609). However, Miller and Katzenellenbogen (610) were unable to relate the levels of TABS to tamoxifen sensitivity but instead showed that sensitivity was correlated with estrogen receptor levels. Some indication that TABS are involved in antiestrogen action comes from the work of Brandes (611), who showed that a diphenylmethane derivative that binds to TABS, but not to the estrogen receptor, inhibits the growth of MCF-7 cells.

The possible involvement of TABS in the mechanism of action of antiestrogen is suggested by the observation that estrogen administration and the physiological state of the ovary have effects on the level of TABS in both liver and uterus (600). At the time of puberty, the liver TABS concentration increased significantly in the female when compared with both mature males or immature females. TABS levels in rat uterine cytosol increase significantly in mature females when compared with either castrated or younger animals. In addition, both uterine and liver TABS levels fluctuated throughout the estrous cycle and reached a peak approximately on the day of estrus. Treatment of ovariectomized rats with physiological amounts of estradiol caused a twofold increase in TABS levels in the uterus, thus mimicking the midcycle peak of TABS. Gulino and Pasqualini (568) have shown that the level of TABS is modulated in the guinea pig uterus by estradiol and progesterone.

The presence of TABS associated with the serum low-density lipoprotein (LDL) fraction from the rat is of interest since LDL cholesterol is involved in the control of cellular cholesterol synthesis (597,612). Triphenylethylene antiestrogens are inhibitors of cholesterol synthesis, and Tabacik et al. (613) showed that tamoxifen inhibited cholesterol synthesis in MCF-7 cells. Murphy et al. (601) demonstrated that 7-ketocholesterol acts as an endogenous ligand that binds to tissue TABS. 7-Ketocholesterol is a potent inhibitor of cholesterol synthesis and cell growth in human fibroblasts (612), and its half-maximal concentration (1 nM) for inhibition is in the range of its binding affinity for TABS (601). These results suggest that TABS may be involved in some aspect of cholesterol synthesis or metabolism. Since cellular growth is dependent on cholesterol synthesis, it is possible that these sites are somehow involved. However, triparanol (MER-25) is a potent inhibitor of cholesterol synthesis, yet it has little to no antiestrogenic properties (unpublished observations).

The binding of 7-ketocholesterol to TABS may be fortuitous since many other compounds inhibit the binding of [^{3}H]tamoxifen with the same relative affinities. Cholesterol, chlorpromazine, various ligands and W-13, a calmodulin inhibitor, act as competitive inhibitors of the binding of [^{3}H]tamoxifen to TABS (unpublished observations). The inhibition by W-13 is of special interest since it has been demonstrated that tamoxifen is an inhibitor of calmodulin-mediated phosphodiesterase activity (614). Calmodulin is thought to be involved in the control of cell proliferation, and inhibitors of calmodulin will block the cell cycle at the G1 phase (615–617). Since nonsteroidal antiestrogens block cellular proliferation, it is possible that calmodulin inhibition is involved in this effect. However, such an inhibition of cell proliferation appears to occur primarily in estrogen-responsive cells, and therefore must somehow be linked to estrogen sensitivity.

In estrogen-sensitive tissues (such as the liver) that contain high concentrations of TABS, antiestrogens do not inhibit the action of estrogens (618). A similar condition develops in some breast cancers, and the tissue is resistant to the action of antiestrogens while retaining the ability to respond to estrogen (619). Thus these sites may be important modulators of antiestrogen action under some circumstances.

Physiological Estrogen Antagonists

The blood levels of estrogen fluctuate according to the stage of the reproductive cycle, and this is accompanied by changing levels of estrogen receptor binding (348,385). Thus the effects of estrogen wax and wane as a result of these changes in ovarian secretion of estrogens. In addition to the influence of estrogen alone, other hormones act to alter the actions of estrogen at the cellular level and modify estrogen-directed functions.

Progesterone

Progesterone acts on the estrogen-primed uterus to alter cell function and reproductive competence. Often this ability of progesterone is considered to be antagonistic to estrogen; however, it probably should be referred to as a modifier of estrogen action rather than an antagonist. Nevertheless, progesterone will reduce the ability of estrogens to cause uterine growth and vaginal cornification (487,620). This ability of progesterone to modify or antagonize estrogen action is generally considered to involve receptor mechanisms that have been discussed previously (under Synthesis and Replenishment of Receptors). These effects of progesterone involve decreasing the number of cytosol and nuclear bound estrogen receptor complexes. Such reductions in receptor number have been correlated with a reduced sensitivity of the uterus to estradiol (365,380).

Most of the studies concerned with progesterone effects on estrogen receptor levels have been done under nonphysiological circumstances. However, in the elegant studies of Brenner et al. (381), physiological conditions were maintained by creating artificial menstrual cycles in ovariectomized rhesus monkeys. Under these conditions estradiol blood levels were maintained at a constant level throughout the cycle, and progesterone was elevated during the second half of the cycle. Cytosol estrogen receptor levels were elevated during the first half of the cycle and dramatically decreased during the second half. These data suggest that progesterone does lower cytosol estrogen receptor even when estradiol is present. Although nuclear estrogen receptors were not examined in this study, progesterone does decrease their level in the hamster uterus under physiological circumstances (385).

Modulated estrogen receptor levels are correlated with striking changes in the morphology of the uterine luminal epithelium (385). When nuclear receptor levels are elevated the epithelium is hypertrophied and mitotic, whereas when receptor levels are suppressed, the epithelium is atrophied and shows degenerative changes. Such changes in morphology and functional state of uterine cells probably reflect the normal cyclic interaction of estrogen and progesterone on the reproductive tract.

In addition to these effects on the estrogen receptor, progesterone also inhibits the stimulation of nuclear type II estrogen binding sites (93). This inhibition is correlated with reduced uterotropic response to estrogen, and does not appear to be related to any effects of progesterone on estrogen receptor levels. The inhibitory effects of progesterone do appear to be mediated by the progesterone receptor, since estrogen priming is necessary in order to observe the inhibitory effects of progesterone.

Androgens

Androgenic steroids are known to inhibit the actions of estrogen on the growth of estrogen target tissues (63). Indeed, androgen therapy is used in the treatment of estrogen-dependent breast cancer (621). This treatment is based on the rationale that androgens should block or antagonize the estrogen-stimulated growth of breast cancer cells. The mechanisms by which androgens antagonize estrogenic functions are not known; however, it is known that androgen receptors are present in estrogen target tissues. Physiological concentrations of androgens do not cause growth or stimulate other known functions of MCF-7 breast cancer cells, even though nuclear binding of the receptor androgen complex is readily observed (63). Likewise, in the rat uterus there appears to be no biological response to nuclear binding of the receptor androgen complex. However, chronic exposure to physiological levels of androgens in the rat does depress uterine weight, an indication that androgens are antiestrogenic by some mechanism (63).

In contrast, high doses of androgens stimulate growth of the rat uterus, mammary tumors, and MCF-7 cells (61,109,150,514,622). Thus androgens appear to have the capacity to both inhibit and stimulate estrogen target tissues depending on the dose used. The low-dose inhibition may be mediated directly by the androgen receptor or it may operate indirectly via interactions at the hypothalmic-pituitary level or some other pathway. The high-dose stimulation effect is mediated by the estrogen receptor, since it is known that high concentrations of androgens will bind to the estrogen receptor, cause nuclear accumulation, and produce an estrogenlike response (64,65).

Type II Estrogen Binding Sites and Estrogen Antagonism

One of the pleiotropic events stimulated by exposure to estrogen is an elevation of type II estrogen binding sites (399). These sites are present in the cytosol and nuclei and are different from the estrogen receptor (type I; see ref. 388 for review). Nuclear type II sites are occupied by an endogenous ligand that appears to be an inhibitor of cell proliferation and, as such, may constitute a new class of antiestrogens (623). Since estrogen-induced uterine cell proliferation is observed only when nuclear type II sites are elevated, this may mean that the inhibitory ligand has dissociated from these sites. Such dissociation would open up sites that are measured by the binding of labeled estradiol. Nuclear type II sites are tightly associated with the nuclear matrix and may be coupled to the regulatory components involved with DNA synthesis. Therefore, the dissociation of an inhibitory ligand from these sites may act as a positive regulation signal that initiates DNA synthesis and cell proliferation.

Inhibitors of Progesterone Action

Although there are several exogenous and endogenous antiestrogens, antiprogestational compounds are rare. Many progesterone derivatives have been synthesized; however, only one compound appears to have antagonistic properties (624–626). 17β-Hydroxy-11β-[-4-dimethlaminophenyl]-17α-[1-propynyl] estra-4, 9-dien-3-one (RU 38486), which was synthesized by Roussel Uclaf, has been shown to interrupt the luteal phase of the menstrual cycle and terminate pregnancy in women (625). RU 38486 induces early onset of vaginal bleeding when administered during the luteal phase of cycling monkeys (624,627). Such actions are considered to be due to a direct antagonistic effect of RU 38486 at the receptor level in the uterine endometrium (628). This compound binds to progesterone receptors in the rabbit uterus and glucocorticoid receptors in the thymus, where it acts as an antiglucocorticoid (625,627). It also has a very slight estrogenic activity, which manifests as cellular hypertrophy of uterine epithelium (522). In T47D cells, RU 38486 binds to the progesterone receptor and inhibits cellular proliferation, as does R5020, a synthetic progesterone (629). Thus, RU 38486 is an agonist by this criterion; however, it does antagonize the stimulation of insulin receptors by R5020. Therefore, in T47D cells RU 38486 manifests mixed agonist-antagonist properties.

RU 486 binds well to all mammalian progesterone receptors except those of the hamster (630). In this species the drug also has no antiprogestational effects. Progesterone receptors from the chick oviduct also do not bind this compound. Such loss of affinity in the hamster and chicken indicates that some important structural differences exist in the receptors in these animals.

The mechanism by which RU 486 exerts its antagonistic activity does not involve any differences in activation and transformation of the drug-receptor complex (631,632). Both progesterone and RU 486 form complexes that bind to hormone response elements in a qualitative and quantitatively similar manner. This binding even involves the same G nucleotides. The only difference appeared to be in the sedimentation properties and the gel retardation characteristics of the two receptor-hormone-response element complexes. The antagonistic effect of RU 486 does appear to result from the inability of the hormone binding domain to act as a transcription activator (633). Thus it seems likely that the binding of the receptor-RU 486 complex to hormone response elements results in a conformation that is different from that of the receptor-progesterone complex. This different conformation does not permit the protein-protein interactions necessary for induction of gene transcription.

In hamster and chicken, RU 486 does not bind to the progesterone receptor and is not an antagonist (634). Substitution of cysteine at position 575 by glycine in the hormone-binding domain of the chicken progesterone receptor produces a receptor that binds RU 486; under these circumstances, RU 486 acts as an antagonist (635). All receptors that bind RU 486 have a glycine at the corresponding position; therefore, this amino acid appears to be necessary for the hormone-binding domain to bind the antagonist and to interfere with normal agonist function.

As pointed out earlier for antiestrogens, the actions of antisteroid hormone drugs *in vitro* in cells in culture are not necessarily identical to their actions *in vivo.* Obviously more work *in vivo* is needed on this important class of antiprogestins before definitive statements can be made regarding their mechanism of action and their true pharmacologic and physiological actions.

An inhibitor of progesterone receptor binding has been described in the cytosol from rat placenta (636). This inhibitor is a macromolecule that decreases the affinity of the receptor for progesterone but has no effect on the number of receptor sites. The function of this inhibitor is not known; however, inhibitory activity in trophoblast cytosol is greatest on days 9 and 12 of pregnancy and declines thereafter (636). By day 18 inhibitory activity is no longer detectable, which coincides with a sharp decrease in the progesterone receptor. The presence of such inhibitors in other systems has not been described; however, their potential physiological significance in the regulation of progesterone action is considerable.

ACKNOWLEDGMENTS

This work was supported by NIH grant HD 08436. We thank Dr. Barry Markaverich for his unconventional wisdom, deep insight, and philosophical discussions, David Scarff for his help with the figures, and Carolyn Armijo for her secretarial assistance.

REFERENCES

1. Knauer E. Die ovarientransplantation. *Arch Gynakol* 1900; 60:322–376.
2. Marshall FHA, Jolly WA. Contributions to the physiology of mammalian reproduction. *Philos Trans R Soc* [*Biol*] 1095; 198:99–142.
3. Allen E, Doisy EA. An ovarian hormone. *JAMA* 1923; 81:819–821.
4. Allen E, Doisy EA. The induction of a sexually mature condition in immature females by injection of the ovarian follicular hormone. *Am J Physiol* 1924;69:577–588.
5. Doisy EA, Veler CD, Thayer S. Folliculin from urine of pregnant women. *Am J Physiol* 1929;90:329–330.
6. Butenandt A. Untersuchungen über das weibliche sexual hormon. *Dtsch Med Wochenschr* 1929;55:2171–2173.
7. Corner GW, Allen WM. Physiology of the corpus luteum. *Am J Physiol* 1929;88:326–339.
8. Allen WM, Wintersteiner OS. Crystalline progestin. Science 1934;80:190–191.
9. Butenandt A, Dannenbaum H. Uber androsteron: isolierung eines neuen, physiologisch unwirksamen sterioderivatives ans mannernarn, seine verknutsung mit dehydroandrosterone und androsterone bin beitrag vurk constitution des androsterone. *Z Physiol Chem* 1934;229:192–208.
10. Hartmann M, Wettstein A. Zur Kenntnis der corpus-luteum hormone. *Helv Chim Acta* 1934;17:1365–1372.
11. Hartmann M, Wettstein A. Ein krystallisiertes hormon aus corpus luteum. *Helv Chim Acta* 1934b;17:878–882.
12. Slotta KH, Ruschig H, Fels E. Die reindarstellung der hormone aus dem corpus luteum. *Bev Dtsch Chem Ges* 1934;67: 1207–1208.
13. Allen E, Smith GM, Gardner WV. Accentuation of the growth effect of theelin on genital tissues of the ovariectomized mouse by arrest of mitosis with colchicine. *Am J Anat* 1937;61:321–341.
14. Burrows H. *Biological actions of sex hormones.* 2nd ed. Cambridge: Cambridge University Press, 1949.
15. Crandall WR. Effect of progesterone on cell division in circular muscle of rabbit's uterus. *Anat Rec* 1938;72:195–210.
16. Reynolds SRM. Determinants of uterine growth and activity. *Physiol Rev* 1951;1:244–273.
17. Hisaw FL, Greep RO, Ferold HL. Effects of progesterone on female genital tract after castration atrophy. *Proc Soc Exp Biol Med* 1937;36:840–842.
18. Reynolds SRM. *Physiology of the uterus.* 2nd ed. New York: Hoeber, 1949.
19. Markee JE. Rhythmic vascular uterine changes. *Am J Physiol* 1932;100:32–39.
20. Markee JE. Analysis of rythmic vascular changes in uterus of rabbit. *Am J Physiol* 1932;100:374–382.
21. Szego CM, Roberts S. Steroid action and interaction in uterine metabolism. *Recent Prog Horm Res* 1953;8:419–469.
22. Spaziani E, Szego CM. The influence of estradiol and cortisol on uterine histamine of the ovariectomized rat. *Endocrinology* 1958;63:669–678.
23. Spaziani E, Szego CM. Early effects of estradiol and cortisol on

water and electrolyte shifts in the uterus of the immature rat. *Am J Physiol* 1958;197:355–359.
24. Spaziani E. Relationship between early vascular responses and growth in the rat uterus: stimulation of cell division by estradiol and vasodilating amines. *Endocrinology* 1963;72:180–191.
25. Villee CA. The role of steroid hormones in the control of metabolic activity. In: Allen JM, ed. *The molecular control of cellular activity.* New York: Allen McGraw-Hill, 1962;297–213.
26. Talalay P. Enzymatic interactions between steroid hormones and pyridine nucleotides. In: Harris RJC, ed. *Biological approaches to cancer chemotherapy.* New York: Academic Press, 1961;59–75.
27. Talalay P. Studies on the placental 17β-hydroxy steroid dehydrogenase. In: *On Cancer and Hormones: Essays in Experimental Biology.* Chicago: University of Chicago Press, 1962. 271–289.
28. Mueller GC. Discussion of a paper: Hagerman DD, Villee CA: A mechanism of action for estrogenic steroid hormones, pp. 169–181. In: Villee CA, Engel LL, eds. *Mechanism of action of steroid hormones.* New York: Pergamon Press, 1961;181–187.
29. Glass R, Loring J, Spencer J, Villee CA. The estrogenic properties in vitro of diethylstilbestrol and substances related to estradiol. *Endocrinology* 1961;68:327–333.
30. Jensen EV, Jacobsen HI. Basic guides to the mechanism of estrogen action. *Recent Prog Horm Res* 1962;18:387–414.
31. Aizawa Y, Mueller GC. The effect in vivo of estrogens on lipid synthesis in the rat uterus. *J Biol Chem* 1961;236:281–286.
32. McCorquodale DJ, Mueller GC. Effect of estradiol on the level of amino acid-activating enzymes in the rat uterus. *J Biol Chem* 1958;232:31–42.
33. Mueller GC. A discussion of the mechanism of action of steroid hormones. *Cancer Res* 1957;17:490–506.
34. Mueller GC, Herranen AM, Jervell K. Studies on the mechanisms of action of estrogens. *Recent Prog Horm Res* 1958; 14:95–139.
35. Mueller GC. Biochemical parameters of estrogen action. In: Pincus G, Vollmer EP, eds. *Biological activities of steroids in relation to cancer.* New York: Academic Press, 1960;129–145.
36. Hamilton H. Inhibition of protein synthesis and some quantifications of early estrogen action and response. *Science* 1962; 138:989.
37. Hamilton TH. Isotopic studies on estrogen-induced accelerations of ribonucleic acid and protein synthesis. *Proc Natl Acad Sci USA* 1963;49:373–379.
38. Mueller GC, Gorski J, Aizawa Y. The role of protein synthesis in early estrogen action. *Proc Natl Acad Sci USA* 1961;47:164–169.
39. Gorski J, Mueller GC. Early effects of estrogen and acid soluble nucleotides of the rat uterus. *Arch Biochem Biophys* 1963; 102:21–25.
40. Hamilton TH. Sequences of RNA and protein synthesis during early estrogen action. *Proc Natl Acad Sci USA* 1964;51:83–89.
41. Noteboom WD, Gorski J. An early effect of estrogen on protein synthesis. *Proc Natl Acad Sci USA* 1963;50:250–255.
42. Wilson JD. The nature of the RNA response to estradiol administration by the uterus of the rat. *Proc Natl Acad Sci USA* 1963;50:93–100.
43. O'Malley BW, McGuire WL, Kohler PO, Korenman SG. Studies on the mechanism of steroid hormone regulation of synthesis of specific proteins. *Recent Prog Horm Res* 1969;25:105–160.
44. Hamilton TH. Control by estrogen of genetic transcription and translation. *Science* 1968;161:649–660.
45. Langley JN. On the reaction of cells and of nerve-endings to certain poisons chiefly as regards the reaction of striated muscle to nicotine and to curare. *J Physiol* 1905;33:374–413.
46. Ehrlich P. Chemotherapeutics: scientific principles, methods, and results. Lancet 1913;II:445–451.
47. Glasscock RF, Hoekstra WG. Selective accumulation of tritium-labeled hexosterol by the reproductive organs of immature female goats and sheep. *Biochem J* 1959;72:673–682.
48. King RJB, Gordon J, Inman DR. The intracellular localization of oestrogen in rat tissues. *J Endocrinol* 1965;32:9–15.
49. King RJB, Cowan DM, Inman DR. The uptake of ^{3}H-oestradiol by dimethyl-benzanthracene in induced rat mammary tumors. *J Endocrinol* 1965;32:83–90.
50. King RJB, Gordon J. The localization of ^{3}H-oestradiol-17β in rat uterus. *J Endocrinol* 1966;34:431–437.
51. King RJB, Gordon J, Cowan DM, Inman DR. The intranuclear localization of ^{3}H-oestradiol in dimethylbenzanthracene induced rat mammary adenocarcinoma and other tissues. *J Endocrinol* 1966;36:139–150.
52. King RJB, Gordon J, Martin L. The association of (6,7-$^{3}H_2$) oestradiol with nuclear chromatin. *Biochem J* 1965;97:28P.
53. Talwar GP, Segal SJ, Evans A, Davidson OW. The binding of estradiol in the uterus: a mechanism for derepression of RNA synthesis. *Proc Natl Acad Sci USA* 1964;52:1059–1066.
54. Toft D, Gorski J. A receptor molecule for estrogens: isolation from the rat uterus and preliminary characterization. *Proc Natl Acad Sci USA* 1966;55:1574–1581.
55. Laumas KR, Farooq A. The uptake in vivo of [1,2-^{3}H]-progesterone by the brain and genital tract of the rat. *J Endocrinol* 1966;36:95–96.
56. O'Malley BW, Toft DO, Sherman MR. Progesterone binding components of chick oviduct. II. Nuclear components. *J Biol Chem* 1971;246:1117–1122.
57. Schrader TW, O'Malley BW. Progesterone-binding components of chick oviduct. IV. Characterization of purified subunits. *J Biol Chem* 1972;247:51–59.
58. Sherman MR, Corval PL, O'Malley BW. Progesterone-binding components of chick oviduct. I. Preliminary characterization of cytoplasmic components. *J Biol Chem* 1970;245:6085–6096.
59. Wiest WG, Rao BR. Progesterone binding proteins in rabbit uterus and human endometrium. In: Raspe G, ed. *Advances in the biosciences, no. 7.* New York: Pergamon Press, 1971; 251–266.
60. Clark JH, Peck EJ, Jr. *Female sex steroids: Receptors and function.* Berlin: Springer-Verlag, 1979.
61. Garcia M, Rochefort H. Androgen effects mediated by estrogen receptor in 7,12 dimethylbenz(a)anthracene-induced rat mammary tumors. *Cancer Res* 1978;38:3922–3929.
62. Garcia M, Rochefort H. Evidence and characterization of the binding of two ^{3}H androgens to the estrogen receptor. *Endocrinology* 1979;104:1797–1804.
63. Rochefort H, Garcia G. The estrogenic and antiestrogenic activities of androgens in female target tissues. *Pharmacol Ther* 1984;23:193–216.
64. Ruh TS, Wassilak SG, Ruh MF. Androgen-induced nuclear accumulation of the estrogen receptor. *Steroids* 1975;25:257–273.
65. Rochefort H, Lignon F, Capony F. Formation of estrogen nuclear receptor in uterus: effects of androgen, estrone and nafoxidine. *Biochem Biophys Res Commun* 1972;47:662–670.
66. Lippman M, Monaco ME, Bolan G. Effects of estrone, estradiol and estriol on hormone-responsive human breast cancer in long-term tissue culture. *Cancer Res* 1977;37:1901–1907.
67. Rousseau GG, Baxter JD, Higgins SJ, Tomkins GM. Steroid-induced nuclear binding of glucocorticoid receptors intact hepatoma cells. *J Mol Biol* 1973;79:539–544.
68. Walters MR, Clark JH. Cytosol progesterone receptors of the rat uterus: assay and receptor characteristics. *J Steroid Biochem* 1977;8:1137–1144.
69. Gurpide E, Stolee A, Tseng L. Quantitative studies of tissue uptake and disposition of hormones. In: *Karolinska symposia on research methods in reproductive endocrinology.* 3rd Symposium. In: *In vitro methods in reproductive cell biology.* 1971;247–278.
70. Gurpide E, Welch M. Dynamics of uptake of estrogens and androgens by human endometrium. *J Biol Chem* 1969;224: 5159–5167.
71. Peck EJ Jr, Burgner J, Clark JH. Estrophilic binding sites of the uterus. Relation to uptake and retention of estradiol in vitro. *Biochemistry* 1973;12:4596–4603.
72. Müller RE, Wotiz HH. Kinetics of estradiol entry into uterine cells. *Endocrinology* 1979;105:1107–1114.
73. Müller RE, Traish AM, Hirota T, Bercel E, Wotiz HH. Conversion of estrogen receptor from a state with low affinity for estradiol into a state of higher affinity does not require 4S to 5S dimerization. *Endocrinology* 1985;116:337–345.
74. Pietras RJ, Szego CM. Specific binding sites for oestrogen at the outer surfaces of isolated endometrial cells. *Nature* 1977; 265:68–71.
75. King WJ, Greene GL. Monoclonal antibodies localize oestrogen receptor in the nuclei of target cells. *Nature* 1984;307:745–747.

76. Kelly MJ, Moss RL, Dudley CA, Fawcett CP. The specificity of the response of preoptic-septal area neurons to estrogen: 17β-estradiol versus 17α-estradiol and the response of extra hypothalamic neurons. *Exp Brain Res* 1977;30:43–52.
77. Holzbauer M. Physiological aspects of steroids with anesthetic properties. *Med Biol* 1976;54:227–242.
78. Milgrom E, Thi L, Atger M, Baulieu EE. Mechanisms regulating the concentration and the conformation of progesterone receptor(s) in the uterus. *J Biol Chem* 1973;248:6366–6374.
79. Terenius L. Oestrogen binding in the mouse uterus. *Acta Endocrinol* 1968;57:669–682.
80. Williams D, Gorski J. A new assessment of subcellular distribution of bound estrogen in the uterus. *Biochem Biophys Res Commun* 1971;45:258–264.
81. Giese AC. *Cell physiology.* 4th ed. Philadelphia: WB Saunders, 1973;289–292.
82. Overath P, Trauble H. Phase transitions in cells, membranes, and lipids of *Escherichia coli.* Detection by fluorescent probes, light scattering, and dilatometry. *Biochemistry* 1973;12:2625–2634.
83. Singer SJ. The molecular organization of membranes. *Annu Rev Biochem* 1974;43:805–833.
84. Tsong TW. Effect of phase transition on the kinetics of dye transport in phospholipid bilayer structures. *Biochemistry* 1975; 14:5409–5414.
85. Tsong TW. Transport of 8-anilino-1-papthalenesulfunate as a probe of the effect of cholesterol on the phospholipid bilayer structure. *Biochemistry* 1975;14:5415–5417.
86. Jensen EV, Suzuki T, Kawashima T, Stumpf WE, Jungblut P, DeSombre ER. A two-step mechanism for the interaction of estradiol with rat uterus. *Proc Natl Acad Sci USA* 1968; 59:623–638.
87. Shyamala G, Gorski J. Estrogen receptors in the rat uterus. Studies on the interaction of cytosol and nuclear binding sites. *J Biol Chem* 1979;244:1097–1103.
88. Toft D, Shyamala G, Gorski J. A receptor molecule for estrogens: studies using a cell-free system. *Proc Natl Acad Sci USA* 1967;57:1740–1743.
89. Sitteri PK, Schwartz BE, Moriyama I, Ashby R, Linkie D, MacDonald PC. Estrogen binding in the rat and human. In: O'Malley BW, Means AR, eds. *Receptors for reproductive hormones.* New York: Plenum Press, 1973;97–112.
90. Linkie DM, Sitteri PK. A re-examination of the interaction of estradiol with target receptors. *J Steroid Biochem* 1978;9: 1071–1078.
91. Gorski J, Toft D, Shyamala G, Smith D, Notides A. Hormone receptors: studies on the interaction of estrogen with the uterus. *Recent Prog Horm Res* 1968;24:45–80.
92. Pavlik EJ, Rutledge S, Eckert RL, Katzenellenbogen BS. Localization of estrogen receptors in uterine cells: an appraisal of translocation. *Exp Cell Res* 1979;123:177–189.
93. Markaverich BM, Upchurch S, McCormack SA, Glasser SR, Clark JH. Differential stimulation of uterine cells by nafoxidine and clomiphene: relationship between nuclear estrogen receptors and type II estrogen binding sites and cellular growth. *Biol Reprod* 1981;24:171–181.
94. Tomkins GM, Martin DW, Stillwagen RH, Baxter JD, Mamont P, Levinson BB. Regulation of specific protein synthesis in eucaryotic cells. *Cold Spring Harbor Symp Quant Biol* 1970;35: 635–640.
95. Wilson JD, Glozna RE. The intranuclear metabolism of testosterone in the accessory organs of reproduction. *Recent Prog Horm Res* 1970;26:309–336.
96. Liao S, Fang S. Receptor-proteins for androgens and the mode of action of androgens on gene transcription in ventral prostate. *Vitam Horm* 1970;27:17–90.
97. Munck A, Foley R. Kinetics of glucocorticoid-receptor complexes in rat thymus cells. *J Steroid Biochem* 1976;7:1117–1122.
98. Wira CR, Munck A. Glucocorticoid receptor complexes in rat thymus cells. *J Biol Chem* 1974;249:5328–5336.
99. Sheridan PJ. Is there an alternative to the cytoplasmic receptor model for the mechanism of action of steroids. *Life Sci* 1975;17:497–502.
100. Alberga A, Massol N, Raynaud J-P, Baulieu E-E. Estradiol binding of exceptionally high affinity by a nonhistone chromatin fraction. *Biochemistry* 1971;10:3835–3843.
101. Jackson V, Chalkley R. The binding of estradiol-17β to the bovine endometrial nuclear membrane. *J Biol Chem* 1974;249: 1615–1626.
102. McCormack SA, Glasser SR. Differential response of individual uterine cell types from immature rats treated with estradiol. *Endocrinology* 1980;106:1634–1649.
103. Mester J, Baulieu EE. Nuclear estrogen receptor of chick liver. *Biochim Biophys Acta* 1972;261:236–244.
104. Mester J, Brunelle R, Tung I, Sonnenschein C. Estrogen-sensitive cells. *Exp Cell Res* 1973;81:447–452.
105. Panko WB, Macleod RM. Uncharged nuclear receptors for estrogen in breast cancers. *Cancer Res* 1978;38:1948–1951.
106. Pietras RJ, Szego CM. Partial purification and characterization of oestrogen receptors in subfractions of hepatocyte plasma membranes. *Biochem J* 1980;191:743–760.
107. Satyswaroop PG, Fleming H, Bressler RS, Gurpide E. Human endometrial cancer cell cultures for hormonal studies. *Cancer Res* 1978;38:4367–4375.
108. Snow LD, Eriksson H, Hardin JW, et al. Nuclear estrogen receptor in the avian liver: correlation with biologic response. *J Steroid Biochem* 1978;9:1017–1026.
109. Zava DT, McGuire WL. Androgen action through estrogen receptor in a human breast cancer cell line. *Endocrinology* 1978;103:624–631.
110. Martin PM, Sheridan PJ. Towards a new model for the mechanism of action of steroids. *J Steroid Biochem* 1982;16:215–229.
111. Oppenheimer JH, Schwartz HL, Surks MI, Koeruer D, Dillman WH. Nuclear receptors and the initiation of thyroid hormone action. *Recent Prog Horm Res* 1976;32:529–565.
112. Walters MR, Hunziker W, Clark JH. Hydroxylapatite prevents nuclear receptor loss during the exchange assay of progesterone receptors. *J Steroid Biochem* 1980;13:1129–1132.
113. Walters MR, Hunziker W, Norman AW. Unoccupied 1,25-dihydroxy vitamin D_3 receptors. *J Biol Chem* 1980;255: 6799–6805.
114. Yand MA, King DS, Fristrom P. Ecdysteroid receptors in imaginal discs of *Drosophilia melanogaster. Proc Natl Acad Sci USA* 1978;75:6039–6043.
115. Welshons WV, Lieberman ME, Gorski J. Nuclear localization of unoccupied estrogen receptors: cytochalasin enucleation of GH_3 cells. *Nature* 1984;307:747–749.
116. McClellan MC, West NB, Tacha DE, Greene GL, Brenner RM. Immunochemical localization of estrogen receptors in the macaque reproductive tract with monoclonal antiestrophilins. *Endocrinology* 1984;114:2002–2014.
117. Perrot-Applanat M, Logeat F, Groyer-Picard MT, Milgrom E. Immunocytochemical study of mammalian progesterone receptor using monoclonal antibodies. *Endocrinology* 1985;116: 1473–1484.
118. Sheridan PJ, Buchanan JM, Anselmo VC, Martin PM. Equilibrium: the intracellular distribution of steroid receptors. *Nature* 1979;282:579–582.
119. Jensen EV, Greene GL, Closs LE, DeSombre ER, Nadji M. Receptors reconsidered: a 20-year perspective. *Recent Prog Horm Res* 1982;38:1–40.
120. Lee SH. Cytochemical study of estrogen receptor in human mammary cancer. *Am J Clin Pathol* 1978;70:197–203.
121. Pertschuk LP, Gatejens EG, Carter AC, Brigati DJ, Kim DS, Fealey TE. An improved histochemical method for detection of estrogen receptors in mammary cancer. *Am J Clin Pathol* 1979;71:504–508.
122. Rao BR, Fry GC, Hunt S, Kuhnel R, Dandliker WB. A fluorescent probe for rapid detection of estrogen receptors. *Cancer* 1980;46:2902–2906.
123. Pertschuk LP, Tobin EH, Brigati DJ, et al. Immunofluorescent detection of estrogen receptors in breast cancer. *Cancer* 1978;41:907–911.
124. Nenci I, Beccatti MD, Piffanelli A, Lanza G. Detection and dynamic localization of estradiol-receptor complexes in intact target cells by immunofluorescent technique. *J Steroid Biochem* 1976;7:505–510.
125. Mercer WD, Edwards DP, Chamness GC, McGuire WL. Failure of estradiol immunofluorescence in MCF-7 breast cancer cells to detect estrogen receptors. *Cancer Res* 1981;41(11 Pt 1): 4644–4652.

126. Blaustein JD, Turcotte JC. Estrogen receptor-immunostaining of neuronal cytoplasmic processes as well as cell nuclei in guinea pig brain. *Brain Res* 1989;495:75–82.
127. Blaustein JD, Lehman MN, Turcotte JC, Greene G. Estrogen receptors in dendrites and axon terminals in the guinea pig hypothalamus. *Endocrinology* 1992;131:281–290.
128. Brink M, Humbel BM, De Kloet ER. The unliganded glucocorticoid receptor is localized in the nucleus, not in the cytoplasm. *Endocrinology* 1992;130:3575–3581.
129. Dingwall C, Laskey RA. Protein import into the nucleus. *Annu Rev Cell Biol* 1986;2:367–390.
130. Paine PL, Moore LC, Horowitz SB. Nuclear envelope permeability. *Nature* 1975;254:109–114.
131. Sherman MR, Corvol PL, O'Malley BW. Progesterone-binding components of chick oviduct. *J Biol Chem* 1970;245:6085–6096.
132. Kalderon D, Roberts BL, Richardson WD, Smith AE. A short amino acid sequence able to specify nuclear location. *Cell* 1984;39:499–509.
133. Lanford RE, Kanda P, Kennedy RC. Induction of nuclear transport with a synthetic peptide homologous to the SV40 antigen transport signal. *Cell* 1986;46:575–582.
134. Clemens TL, Garrett KP, Zhou XY, Pike JW, Haussler MR, Dempster DW. Immunocytochemical localization of the 1,25-dihydroxyvitamin D_3 receptor in target cells. *Endocrinology* 1988;122:1224–1230.
135. Oppenheimer JH. Thyroid hormone action at the cellular level. *Science* 1979;203:971–979.
136. Walters MR, Hunziker W, Norman AW. 1,25 dihydroxyvitamin D_3 receptors: intermediates between triiodothyronine and steroid hormone receptors. *Trends Biochem Sci* 1981;6:268–271.
137. Picard D, Salser SJ, Yamamoto KR. A movable and regulatable inactivation function within the steroid binding domain of the glucocorticoid receptor. *Cell* 1988;54:1073–1080.
138. Picard D, Yamamoto KR. Two signals mediate hormone-dependent nuclear localization of the glucocorticoid receptor. *EMBO J* 1987;6:3333–3340.
139. Gorski J, Noteboom WD, Nicollette JA. Estrogen control of the synthesis of RNA and protein in the uterus. *J Cell Comp Physiol* 1965;66[Suppl 1]:91.
140. Evans RE. The steroid and thyroid hormone receptor superfamily. *Science* 1988;240:889–895.
141. Maxwell BL, McDonnell DP, Conneely OM, Schulz TZ, Greene GL, O'Malley BW. Structural organization and regulation of the chicken estrogen receptor. *Mol Endocrinol* 1987;1:25–35.
142. Chandran UR, DeFranco DB. Internuclear migration of chicken progesterone receptor, but not simian virus-40 large tumor antigen, in transient heterokaryons. *Mol Endocrinol* 1992;6:837–844.
143. Williams D, Gorski J. Equilibrium binding of estradiol by uterine cell suspensions and whole uteri in vitro. *Biochemistry* 1974;13:5537–5542.
144. Gorski J. Gorski replies. *Nature* 1985;318:89.
145. Greene GL, King WJ. Greene and King reply. *Nature* 1985;317:88–89.
146. Jensen EV. Editorial: intracellular localization of estrogen receptors, implications for interaction mechanism. *Lab Invest* 1984;51:11.
147. Schrader WT. New model for steroid hormone receptors? *Nature* 1984;308:17.
148. Szego CM, Pietras RJ. Subcellular distribution of oestrogen receptors. *Nature* 1985;317:88.
149. Katzenellenbogen JA, Johnson HJ, Carlson KE. Studies on the uterine, cytoplasmic estrogen binding protein. Thermal stability and ligand dissociation rate. An assay of empty and filled sites by exchange. *Biochemistry* 1973;12:4092–4099.
150. Lippman M, Bolan G, Huff K. The effects of androgens and anti-androgens on hormone-responsive human breast cancer in long term tissue culture. *Cancer Res* 1976;36:4595–4601.
151. Korenman SG, Perrin LE, McCallum TP. A radio-ligand binding assay system for estradiol measurement in human plasma. *J Clin Endocrinol* 1969;29:879–883.
152. Erdos T, Best-Belpomme M, Bessada R. A rapid assay for binding estradiol to uterine receptor(s). *Anal Biochem* 1970;37:244–252.
153. Anderson JN, Clark JH, Peck EJ, Jr. Oestrogen and nuclear binding sites: determination of specific sites by ^{3}H-oestradiol exchange. *Biochem J* 1972;126:561–567.
154. Katzenellenbogen BS, Norman MJ, Eckert RL, Peltz SW, Mangel WF. Bioactivities, estrogen receptor interactions, and plasminogen activator-inducing activities of tamoxifen and hydroxytamoxifen isomers in MCF-7 human breast cancer cells. *Cancer Res* 1984;44:112–119.
155. Walters MR, Clark JH. Cytosol and nuclear compartmentalization of progesterone receptors of the rat uterus. *Endocrinology* 1978;103:601–609.
156. Walters MR, Clark JH. Stoichiometric translocation of the rat uterine progesterone receptor. *Endocrinology* 1978;103:1952–1955.
157. Conneely OM, Sullivan WP, Toft DO, et al. Molecular cloning of the chicken progesterone receptor. *Science* 1986;233:767–770.
158. Gronemeyer H, Turcotte B, Quirin-Stricker C, et al. The chicken progesterone receptor: sequence, expression and functional analysis. *EMBO J* 1987;6:3985–3994.
159. Misrahi M, Atger M, d'Auriol L, et al. Complete amino acid sequence of the progesterone receptor deduced from cloned cDNA. *Biochem Biophys Res Commun* 1987;143:740–748.
160. Koike S, Masaharu S, Maramatsu M. Molecular cloning and characterization of rat estrogen receptor cDNA. *Nucl Acids Res* 1987;15:2499–2513.
161. Walter PW, Green S, Greene G, et al. Cloning of the human estrogen receptor cDNA. *Proc Natl Acad Sci USA* 1985;82:7889–7893.
162. Chang C, Kokontis J, Liao S. Molecular cloning of human and rat complementary DNA encoding androgen receptors. *Science* 1988;240:324–327.
163. Lubahn DB, Joseph DR, Sullivan PM, Willard HF, French FS, Wilson EM. Cloning of human androgen receptor complementary DNA and localization to the X chromosome. *Science* 1988;240:327–330.
164. Hollenberg SM, Weinberger C, Ong ES, et al. Primary structure and expression of a functional human glucocorticoid receptor cDNA. *Nature* 1985;318:635–641.
165. Miesfeld R, Rusconi S, Godowski PJ, et al. Genetic complementation of a glucocorticoid receptor deficiency by expression of cloned receptor cDNA. *Cell* 1986;46:389–399.
166. Murray JC, Smith RF, Ardinger HA, Weinberger C. RFLP for the glucocorticoid receptor (GRL) located at 5q11-5q13. *Nucl Acids Res* 1987;15:6765.
167. Arriza JL, Weinberger C, Cerelli G, et al. Cloning of human mineralocorticoid receptor complementary DNA: structural and functional kinship with the glucocorticoid receptor. *Science* 1987;237:268–274.
168. Patel PD, Sherman TG, Goldman DJ, Watson SJ. Molecular cloning of a mineralocorticoid (type I) receptor complementary DNA from rat hippocampus. *Mol Endocrinol* 1989;3:1877–1885.
169. Thompson CC, Weinberger C, Lebo R, Evans RM. Identification of a novel thyroid hormone receptor expressed in the mammalian central nervous system. *Science* 1987;237:1610–1614.
170. Benbrook D, Pfahl M. A novel thyroid hormone receptor encoded by a cDNA clone from a human testis library. *Science* 1987;238:788–791.
171. Giguere V, Ong ES, Segui P, Evans RM. Identification of a receptor for the morphogen retinoic acid. *Nature* 1987;330:624–629.
172. Petkovich M, Brand NJ, Krust A, Chambon P. A human retinoic acid receptor which belongs to the family of nuclear receptors. *Nature* 1987;330:444–450.
173. Zelent A, Krust A, Petkovich M, Kastner P, Chambon P. Cloning of murine alpha and beta retinoic acid receptors and a novel receptor gamma predominantly expressed in skin. *Nature* 1989;339:714–717.
174. Krust A, Kastner P, Petkovich M, Zelent A, Chambon P. A third human retinoic acid receptor, hRAR-gamma. *Proc Natl Acad Sci USA* 1989;86:5310–5314.
175. Hughes MR, Malloy PJ, Kieback DG, et al. Point mutations in the human vitamin D receptor gene associated with hypocalcemic rickets. *Science* 1988;242:1702–1705.
176. McDonnell DP, Mangelsdorf DJ, Pike JW, Haussler MR, O'Malley BW. Molecular cloning of cDNA encoding the avian receptor for vitamin D. *Science* 1987;235:1214–1217.

177. Baker AR, McDonnell DP, Hughes M, et al. Cloning and expression of full-length cDNA encoding human vitamin D receptor. *Proc Natl Acad Sci USA* 1988;85:3294–3298.
178. Green S, Chambon P. A superfamily of potentially oncogenic hormone receptors. *Nature* 1986;324:615–617.
179. O'Malley BW. Did eucaryotic steroid receptors evolve from intracrine gene regulators? *Endocrinology* 1989;25:1119–1120.
180. Debuire B, Henry C, Banaissa M, et al. Sequencing the erbA gene of avian erythroblastosis virus reveals a new type of oncogene. *Science* 1984;224:1456–1459.
181. Giguere V, Yang N, Segui P, Evans RM. Identification of a new class of steroid hormone receptors. *Nature* 1988;331:91–94.
182. Wang LH, Tsai SY, Cook RG, Beattie WG, Tsai M-J, O'Malley BW. COUP transcription factor is a member of the steroid receptor superfamily. *Nature* 1989;340:163–166.
183. Watson MA, Milbrandt J. The NGFI-B gene, a transcriptionally inducible member of the steroid receptor gene superfamily: genomic structure and expression in rat brain after seizure induction. *Mol Cell Biol* 1989;9:4213–4219.
184. Vedeckis WV, Schrader WT, O'Malley BW. Progesterone-binding components of chick oviduct: analysis of receptor structure by limited proteolysis. *Biochemistry* 1980;2:343–349.
185. de Boer W, Bolt J, Kuiper GG, Brinkman AO, Mulder E. Analysis of steroid- and DNA-binding domains of the calf uterine androgen receptor by limited proteolysis. *J Steroid Biochem* 1987;28:9–19.
186. Rusconi S, Yamamoto KR. Functional dissection of the hormone and DNA binding activities of the glucocorticoid receptor. *EMBO J* 1987;6:1309–1315.
187. Green S, Kumar V, Krust P, Walter P, Chambon P. Structural and functional domains of the estrogen receptor, *Cold Spring Harbor Symp Quant Biol* 1986;51:751–758.
188. Carlstedt-Duke J, Stromstedt P-E, Wrange O, Bergman T, Gustafsson J-A, Jornvall H. Domain structure of the glucocorticoid receptor protein. *Proc Natl Acad Sci USA* 1987;84:4437–4440.
189. White R, Lees JA, Needham M, Ham J, Parker M. Structural organization and expression of the mouse estrogen receptor. *Mol Endocrinol* 1987;1:735–744.
190. Haussler MR, Mangelsdorf DJ, Komm BS, et al. Molecular biology of the vitamin D hormone. *Recent Prog Horm Res* 1988;44:263–305.
191. Reichman ME, Foster CM, Eisen LP, Eisen HJ, Torain BF, Simons SS, Jr. Limited proteolysis of covalently labeled glucocorticoid receptors as a probe of receptor structure. *Biochemistry* 1984;23:5376–5384.
192. Wrange O, Okret S, Radojcic M, Carlsted-Duke J, Gustaffson J-A. *J Biol Chem* 1984;259:4534–4541.
193. Weichman BM, Notides AC. Estradiol-binding kinetics of the activated and nonactivated estrogen receptor. *J Biol Chem* 1977;252:8856–8862.
194. Gorden MS, Notides AC. Computer modeling of estradiol interactions with the estrogen receptor. *J Steroid Biochem* 1986;25:177–181.
195. Kumar V, Green S, Staub A, Chambon P. Localization of the oestradiol-binding and putative DNA-binding domains of the human oestrogen receptor. *EMBO J* 1986;5:2231–2236.
196. Dobson ADW, Conneely OM, Beattie W, et al. Mutational analysis of the chicken progesterone receptor. *J Biol Chem* 1989;264:4207–4211.
197. Carson MA, Tsai M-J, Conneely OM, et al. Structure-function properties of the chicken progesterone receptor. A synthesized from complementary deoxyribonucleic acid. *Mol Endocrinol* 1987;1:791.
198. McDonnell DP, Scott RA, Kerner SA, O'Malley BW, Pike JW. Functional domains of the human vitamin D_3 receptor regulate osteocalcin gene expression. *Mol Endocrinol* 1989;3:635–644.
199. Giguere V, Hollenberg SM, Rosenfeld MG, Evans RM. Functional domains of the human glucocorticoid receptor. *Cell* 1986;46:645–652.
200. Conneely OM, Dobson AD, Carson MA, et al. Structure-function relationships of the chicken progesterone receptor. *Biochem Soc Trans* 1988;16:683–687.
201. Picard D, Salser SJ, Yamamoto KR. A movable and regulable inactivation function within the steroid binding domain of the glucocorticoid receptor. *Cell* 1988;54:1073–1080.
202. Eilers M, Picard D, Yamamoto KR, Bishop JM. Chimeras of Myc oncoprotein and steroid receptors cause hormone-dependent transformation of cells. *Nature* 1989;340:66–68.
203. Conneely OM, Dobson ADW, Carson MA, et al. Structure-function relationships of the chicken progesterone receptor. *Biochem Soc Trans* 1988;16:683–687.
204. Weinberger C, Hollenberg SM, Rosenfeld MG, Evans RM. Domain structure of human glucocorticoid receptor and its relationship to the v-erb-A oncogene product. *Nature* 1985;318:668–672.
205. Green S, Chambon P. Oestradiol induction of a glucocorticoid-responsive gene by a chimaeric receptor. *Nature* 1987;325:75–78.
206. Kumar V, Green S, Stack G, Berry M, Jin J-R, Chambon P. Functional domains of the human estrogen receptor. *Cell* 1987;51:941–951.
207. Miller J, McLachlan AD, Klug A. Repetitive zinc-binding domains in the protein transcription factor IIIA from *Xenopus* oocytes. *EMBO J* 1985;4:1609–1614.
208. Green S, Chambon P. Chimeric receptors used to probe the DNA-binding domain of the estrogen and glucocorticoid receptors. *Cancer Res* 1989;49[Suppl]:2282s–2285s.
209. Severne Y, Wieland S, Schaffner W, Rusconi S. Metal binding 'finger' structures in the glucocorticoid receptor defined by site-directed mutagenesis. *EMBO J* 1988;7:2503–2508.
210. Tora L, Gronemeyer H, Turcotte B, Gaub MP, Chambon P. The N-terminal region of the chicken progesterone receptor specifies target gene activation. *Nature* 1988;333:185–188.
211. Conneely OM, Kettelberger D, Tsai M-J, O'Malley BW. Promoter specific activating domains of the chicken progesterone receptor. In: Roy AK, Clark JH, eds. *Gene regulation by steroid hormones IV.* New York: Springer-Verlag, 1989;221.
212. Notides AC, Nielsen S. The molecular mechanism of the in vitro 4S to 5S transformation of the uterine estrogen receptor. *J Biol Chem* 1974;249:1866–1873.
213. Weichman BM, Notides AC. Estradiol-binding kinetics of the activated and nonactivated estrogen receptor. *J Biol Chem* 1977;252:8856–8862.
214. Bailly A, Le Fevre B, Savouret JF, Milgrom E. Activation and changes in sedimentation properties of steroid receptors. *J Biol Chem* 1980;10:255:2729–2734.
215. Müller RE, Beebe DM, Bercel E, Traish AM, Wotiz HH. Estriol and estradiol interactions with the estrogen receptor in vivo and in vitro. *J Steroid Biochem* 1984;20:1039–1046.
216. Sakai D, Gorski J. Estrogen receptor transformation to a high-affinity state without subunit-subunit interactions. *Biochemistry* 1984;23:3541–3547.
217. Notides AC, Lerner N, Hamilton DE. Positive cooperativity of the estrogen receptor. *Proc Natl Acad Sci USA* 1981;78:4926–4930.
218. McKnight GS, Kingsbury R. Transcriptional control signals of a eucaryotic protein-coding gene. *Science* 1982;217:316–324.
219. Joab I, Radanyi C, Renoir M, et al. Common non-hormone binding component in nontransformed chick oviduct receptors of four steroid hormones. *Nature* 1984;308:850–853.
219a. Gorski J, Welshons W, Sakai D. Remodeling the estrogen receptor model. *Med Cell Endocrinol* 1984;36:11–15.
220. Schuh S, Yonemoto W, Brugge J, et al. A 90,000-dalton binding protein common to both steroid receptors and the Rous sarcoma virus transforming protein, pp60v-src. *J Biol Chem* 1985;260:14292–14296.
221. Aranyi P, Radanyi C, Renoir M, Devin J, Baulieu E-E. Covalent stabilization of the nontransformed chick oviduct cytosol progesterone receptor by chemical cross-linking. *Biochemistry* 1988;27:1330–1336.
222. Baulieu E-E. Steroid hormone antagonists at the receptor level: a role for the heat-shock protein MW 90,000 (hsp90). *J Cell Biochem* 1987;35:161–174.
223. Craig EA. The heat shock response. *CRC Crit Rev Biochem* 1985;18:239–280.
224. Riehl RM, Sullivan WP, Vroman BT, Bauer VJ, Pearson GR, Toft DO. Immunological evidence that the nonhormone binding component of avian steroid receptors exists in a wide range of tissues and species. *Biochemistry* 1985;24:6586–6591.
225. Howard KJ, Distelhorst CW. Evidence for intracellular associa-

tion of the glucocorticoid receptor with the 90-kDa heat shock protein. *J Biol Chem* 1988;263:3474–3481.
226. Rexin M, Busch W, Gehring U. Chemical cross-linking of heteromeric glucocorticoid receptors. *Biochemistry* 1988;27: 5593–5601.
227. Pratt WB, Jolly DJ, Pratt DV, et al. A region in the steroid binding domain determines formation of the non-DNA-binding, 9S glucocorticoid receptor complex. *J Biol Chem* 1988;263: 267–273.
228. Carson-Jurica MA, Lee AT, Dobson AW, Conneely OM, Schrader WT, O'Malley BW. Interaction of the chicken progesterone receptor with heat shock protein (HSP)-90. *J Steroid Biochem* 1989;34:1–8.
229. Smith DF, McCormick DJ, Toft DO. Studies with antibodies against the conserved cysteine region of progesterone receptor. *J Steroid Biochem* 1988;30:1–7.
230. Smith DF, Lubahnm DB, McCormick DJ, Wilson EM, Toft DO. The production of antibodies against the conserved cysteine region of steroid receptors and their use in characterizing the avian progesterone receptor. *Endocrinology* 1988;122:2816–2825.
231. Weigel NL, Schrader WT, O'Malley BW. Antibodies to chicken progesterone receptor peptide 523–536 recognize a site exposed in receptor-deoxyribonucleic acid complexes but not in receptor-heat shock protein-90 complexes. *Endocrinology* 1989;125: 2494–2501.
232. Tai PK, Maeda Y, Nakao K, Wakim NG, Duhring JL, Faber LE. A 59-kilodalton protein associated with progestin, estrogen, androgen, and glucocorticoid receptor. *Biochemistry* 1986;25: 5269–5275.
233. Gasc JM, Renoir JM, Faber LE, Delahaye F, Baulieu EE. Nuclear localization of 2 steroid receptor-associated proteins, hsp90 and p59. *Exp Cell Res* 1990;186:362–367.
234. Kost SL, Smith DF, Sullivan WP, Welch WJ, Toft DO. Binding of heat shock proteins to the avian progesterone receptor. *Mol Cell Biol* 1989;9:3829–3838.
235. Velazquez JM, Lindquist S. hsp70: nuclear concentration during environmental stress and cytoplasmic storage during recovery. *Cell* 1984;36:655–662.
236. Cheng MY, Hart F-U, Martin J, et al. Mitochondrial heatshock protein hsp60 is essential for assembly of proteins imported into yeast mitochondria. *Nature* 1989;337:620–625.
237. Mobbs CV, O'Malley KL, Lauber A, Romano GJ, Pfaff DW. Heat-shock-70 mRNA induced by estrogen in uterine secretory cells: analysis by northern and slot blots and in situ hybridization. In: *Program of the 71st annual meeting of the Endocrine Society* 1989;725(abst).
238. Mobbs CV, O'Malley KL, Lauber A, Pfaff DW. Constitutive heat-shock-70 mRNA in brain is primarily neuronal and is increased by estrogen in hypothalamus. In: *Program of the 19th annual meeting of the Society of Neuroscience* 1989;1128(abst).
239. Olazabal UE, Pfaff DW, Mobbs CV. Estrogenic regulation of heat shock protein 90 kd in the rat ventromedial hypothalamus and uterus. *Mol Cell Endocrinol* 1992;84:175–183.
240. Ramachandran C, Catelli MG, Schneider W, Shyamala G. Estrogenic regulation of uterine 90-kilodalton heat shock protein. *Endocrinology* 1988;123:956–961.
241. Liao S, Rossini GP, Hiipakka RA, Chen C. Factors that can control the interaction of the androgen-receptor complex with the genomic structure in the rat prostate. In: Bresciani F, ed. *Perspectives in steroid receptor research.* New York: Raven Press, 1980;99–112.
242. Auricchio R, Migliaccio A, Castoria G, Rotondi A, Lastoria S. Direct evidence of in vivo phosphorylation-dephosphorylation of the estradiol-17β receptor. Role of Ca^{2+}-calmodulin in the activation of hormone binding sites. *J Steroid Biochem* 1984;20:31–35.
243. Grandics P, Miller A, Schmidt TJ, Litwack G. Phosphorylation in vivo of rat hepatic glucocorticoid receptors. *Biochem Biophys Res Commun* 1984;120:59–65.
244. Goldsteyn EJ, Graham JS, Goren HJ, Lefebvre YA. Phosphorylation status of nuclear and cytosolic androgen receptors in the rat ventral prostate. *Prostate* 1989;4:91–101.
245. Auricchio F, Migliaccio A, Castoria G, et al. Phosphorylation of estradiol receptor on tyrosine and interaction of estradiol and glucocorticoid receptors with antiphosphotyrosine antibodies. *Adv Exp Med Biol* 1988;231:519–539.
246. Migliaccio A, Di Domenicio M, Green S, et al. Phosphorylation on tyrosine of in vitro synthesized human estrogen receptor activates its hormone binding. *Mol Endocrinol* 1989;3:1061–1069.
247. Sheridan PL, Evans RM, Horwitz KB. Phosphotryptic peptide analysis of human progesterone receptors. New phosphorylated sites formed in nuclei after hormone treatment. *J Biol Chem* 1989;264:6520–6528.
248. Rao KV, Fox CF. Epidermal growth factor stimulates tyrosine phosphorylation of human glucocorticoid receptor in cultured cells. *Biochem Biophys Res Commun* 1987;144:512–519.
249. Logeat F, Le Cunff M, Pamphile R, Milgrom E. The nuclear-bound form of the progesterone receptor is generated through a hormone-dependent phosphorylation. *Biochem Biophys Res Commun* 1985;131:421–427.
250. Horwitz KB, Alexander PS. *Endocrinology* 1983;113:2195–2201.
251. Sheridan PL, Francis MD, Horwitz KB. Synthesis of human progesterone receptors in T47D cells. Nascent A- and B-receptors are active without a phosphorylation-dependent post-translational maturation step. *J Biol Chem* 1989;264:7054–7058.
252. Bailly A, Le Page C, Rauch M, Milgrom E. Sequence-specific DNA binding of the progesterone receptor to the uteroglobin gene: effects of hormone, antihormone, and receptor phosphorylation. *EMBO J* 1986;5:3235–3241.
253. Edwards DP, Kuhnel B, Estes PA, Nordeen SK. Human progesterone receptor binding to mouse mammary tumor virus deoxyribonucleic acid: dependence on hormone and nonreceptor nuclear factor(s). *Mol Endocrinol* 1989;3:381–391.
254. Denner LA, Weigel NL, Schrader WT, O'Malley BW. Hormone dependent regulation of chicken progesterone receptor deoxyribonucleic acid binding and phosphorylation. *Endocrinology* 1989;125:3051–3058.
255. Sullivan WP, Madden BJ, McCormick DJ, Toft DO. Hormone-dependent phosphorylation of the avian progesterone receptor. *J Biol Chem* 1989;263:14717–14723.
256. Sullivan WP, Smith DF, Beato TG, Krco CJ, Toft DO. Hormone-dependent processing of the avian progesterone receptor. *J Cell Biochem* 1988;36:103–119.
257. Denner LA, Bingman WE, Greene GL, Weigel NL. Phosphorylation of the chicken progesterone receptor. *J Steroid Biochem* 1987;27:235–243.
258. Hoeck W, Rusconi S, Groner B. Down-regulation and phosphorylation of glucocorticoid receptor in cultured cells. Investigations with a monospecific antiserum against a bacterially expressed receptor fragment. *J Biol Chem* 1989;264:14296–14402.
259. Sheridan PL, Krett NL, Gorden JA, Horwitz KB. Human progesterone receptor transformation and nuclear down-regulation are independent of phosphorylation. *Mol Endocrinol* 1988;2: 1329–1342.
260. Schrader WT, Coty WA, Smith RG, O'Malley BW. Purification and properties of progesterone receptors from chick oviduct. *Ann NY Acad Sci* 1977;286:64–80.
261. Schrader WT, Heuer SS, O'Malley BW. Progesterone receptors of chick oviduct: identification of 6S receptor dimers. *Biol Reprod* 1975;12:134–142.
262. O'Malley BW, Schrader WT. Progesterone receptor components: identification of subunits binding to the target-cell genome. *J Steroid Biochem* 1972;3:617–629.
263. O'Malley BW, Schrader WT, Spelsberg TC. Hormone receptor interactions with the genome of eukaryotic target cells. *Adv Exp Med Biol* 1973;36:174–196.
264. Gronemeyer H, Govindan MV, Chambon P. Immunological similarity between the chick oviduct progesterone receptor forms A and B. *J Biol Chem* 1985;260:6916–6925.
265. Horwitz KB, Alexander PS. In situ photolinked nuclear progesterone receptors of human breast cancer cells: subunit molecular weights after transformation and translocation. *Endocrinology* 1983;113:2195–2201.
266. Lamb DL, Bullock SW. Heterogeneous deoxyribonucleic acid-binding forms of rabbit uterine progesterone receptor. *Endocrinology* 1984;114:1833–1840.
267. Schrader WT, Toft DO, O'Malley BW. Progesterone-binding protein of chick oviduct: VI. Interaction of purified progesterone-receptor components with nuclear constituents. *J Biol Chem* 1972;247:2401–2407.

268. Grody WW, Schrader WT, O'Malley BW. Activation, transformation and subunit structure of steroid hormone receptors. *Endocrine Rev* 1982;3:141–163.
269. Anderson JN, Clark JH, Peck EJ, Jr. The relationship between nuclear receptor estrogen binding and uterotrophic responses. *Biochem Biophys Res Commun* 1972;48:1460–1468.
270. Anderson JN, Peck EJ, Jr, Clark JH. Estrogen-induced uterine responses and growth: relationship to receptor estrogen binding by uterine nuclei. *Endocrinology* 1975;96:160–167.
271. Lan NC, Katzenellenbogen BS. Temporal relationships between hormone receptor binding and biological responses in the uterus: studies with short- and long-acting derivatives of estriol. *Endocrinology* 1976;98:220–227.
272. Anderson JN, Peck EJ, Jr, Clark JH. Nuclear receptor estrogen complex: relationship between concentration and early uterotrophic responses. *Endocrinology* 1973;92:1488–1495.
273. Hardin JW, Clark JH, Glasser SR, Peck EJ, Jr. Estrogen receptor binding by uterine nuclei: relationship to endogenous nuclear RNA polymerase activity. *Biochemistry* 1976;15:1370–1374.
274. Katzenellenbogen BS, Katzenellenbogen JA, Ferguson ER, Krauthammer N. Antiestrogen interaction with uterine estrogen receptors: studies with a radiolabeled anti-estrogen (CI 628). *J Biol Chem* 1978;253:697–707.
275. Ruh TS, Baudendistel LJ. Different nuclear binding sites for antiestrogen and estrogen receptor complexes. *Endocrinology* 1977;100:420–426.
276. Pajunen *et al.*
277. Barrack ER, Hawkins EF, Allen SL, Hicks LL, Coffey DS. Concepts related to salt resistant estradiol receptors in rat uterine nuclei: nuclear matrix. *Biochem Biophys Res Commun* 1977;79:829–836.
278. Barrack ER, Coffey DS. Biological properties of the nuclear matrix: steroid hormone binding. *Recent Prog Horm Res* 1982; 38:133–195.
279. Korach KS, Ford EB. Estrogen action in the mouse uterus: an additional nuclear event. *Biochem Biophys Res Commun* 1978;83:327–333.
280. Korach KS, Fox-Davies C, Baker V. Differential response to estriol and estradiol in the mouse uterus: correlation to an additional nuclear event. *Endocrinology* 2980;106:1900–1906.
281. Roselli CE, Fasasi TA. Estradiol increases the duration of nuclear receptor occupation in the preoptic area of the male rat treated with testosterone. *J Steroid Biochem Mol Biol* 1992;42:161–168.
282. Horwitz KB, McGuire WL. Actinomycin D prevents nuclear processing of estrogen receptor. *J Biol Chem* 1978;253:6319–6322.
283. Aurricchio F, Migliaccio A, Castoria G, Rotondi A, Lastoria S. Direct evidence of in vitro phosphorylation-dephosphorylation of the estradiol-17β receptor, role of Ca^{2+}-calmodulin in the activation of hormone binding sites. *J Steroid Biochem* 1984; 20:31–35.
284. Jakesz R, Kasid A, Lippman ME. Continuous estrogen exposure in the rat does not induce loss of uterine estrogen receptor. *J Biol Chem* 1983;258:11798–11806.
285. Markaverich BM, Roberts RR, Alejandro M, Clark JH. The effect of low dose continuous exposure to estradiol on the estrogen receptor (type I) and nuclear type II sites. *Endocrinology* 1984;114:814–820.
286. Schoenberg DR, Clark JH. Effect of intercalating drugs on the release of uterine nuclear estrogen receptors. *J Biol Chem* 1979;254:8270–8275.
287. Kalimi M, Beato M, Feigelson P. Interaction of glucocorticoids with rat liver nuclei. I. Role of the cytosol proteins. *Biochemistry* 1973;2:3365–3371.
288. Mulvihill ER, Palmiter RD. Relationship of nuclear estrogen receptor levels to induction of ovalbumin and conalbumin mRNA and chick oviduct. *J Biol Chem* 1977;252:2060–2068.
289. Mester J, Baulieu EE. Dynamics of oestrogen-receptor distribution between the cytosol and nuclear fractions of immature rat uterus after oestradiol administration. *Biochem J* 1975;146: 617–623.
290. Mulvihill ER, Palmiter RD. Relationship of nuclear progesterone receptors to induction of ovalbumin and conalbumin mRNA in chick oviduct. *J Biol Chem* 1980;255:2085–2091.
291. Milgrom E, Vu Hai MT, Logeat F. Use of ^{3}H-R5020 for the assay of cytosol and nuclear progesterone receptor in the rat uterus. In: McGuire WL, Raynaud M-P, Baulieu E-E, eds. *Progesterone receptors in normal and neoplastic tissues.* New York: Raven Press, 1977;261–270.
292. Walters MR, Clark JH. Relationship between the quantity of progesterone receptor and the antagonism of estrogen induced uterotropic response. *Endocrinology* 1979;105:382–386.
293. Mockus MB, Howitz KB. Progesterone receptors in human breast cancer. Stoichiometric translocation and nuclear receptor processing. *J Biol Chem* 1983;258:4778–4783.
294. Buller RE, Schrader WT, O'Malley BW. Progesterone-binding components of chick oviduct. IX. The kinetics of nuclear binding. *J Biol Chem* 1975;250:809–818.
295. Chamness GC, Jennings AW, McGuire WL. Oestrogen receptor binding is not restricted to target nuclei. *Nature* 1973;241: 458–460.
296. Chamness GC, Jennings AW, McGuire W. Estrogen receptor binding to isolated nuclei. A nonsaturable process. *Biochemistry* 1974;13:327–331.
297. Fang S, Liao S. Steroid and tissue specific retention of a 17β-hydroxy-5α-androstan-3-one-protein complex by the cell nuclei of ventral prostate. *J Biol Chem* 1979;246:16–24.
298. Higgins SJ, Rousseau GG, Bacter JD, Tomkins GM. Nature of nuclear acceptor sites for glucocorticoid- and estrogen-receptor complexes. *J Biol Chem* 1973;248:5873–5879.
299. Leclercq G, Hulin N, Heuson JC. Interaction of activated estradiol-receptor complex and chromatin in isolated uterine nuclei. *Eur J Cancer* 1973;9:681–685.
300. Mainwaring WIP, Peterken BM. A reconstituted cell-free system for the specific transfer of steroid-receptor complexes into nuclear chromatin isolated from rat ventral prostate gland. *Biochem J* 1971;125:285–295.
301. O'Malley BW, Sherman MR, Toft DO. Progesterone "receptors" in the cytoplasm and nucleus of chick oviduct target tissue. *Proc Natl Acad Sci USA* 1970;67:501–511.
302. Spelsberg TC. Nuclear binding of progesterone in chick oviduct: multiple binding sites in vivo and transcriptional response. *Biochem J* 1976;156:391–398.
303. Yamamoto K, Alberts B. The interaction of estradiol-receptor protein with the genome: an argument for the existence of undetected specific sites. *Cell* 1975;4:301–310.
304. Clark JH, Gorski J. Estrogen receptors: an evaluation of cytoplasmic-nuclear interactions in a cell-free system and a method for assay. *Biochim Biophys Acta* 1969;192:5-8–515.
305. Spelsberg TC, Steggles AW, O'Malley BW. Progesterone-binding components of chick oviduct. *J Biol Chem* 1971;246:4188–4197.
306. Spelsberg TC, Steggles AW, Chytil F, O'Malley BW. Progesterone binding components of chick oviduct. V. Exchange of progesterone binding capacity from target to nontarget tissue chromatin. *J Biol Chem* 1972;247:1368–1374.
307. Spelsberg TC, Webster R, Pickler G, Thrall C, Wells D. Role of nuclear proteins as high affinity sites ("acceptors") for progesterone in the avian oviduct. *J Steroid Biochem* 1976;7:1091–1101.
308. Spelsberg TC, Littlefield BA, Seelke R, et al. Role of specific chromosomal proteins and DNA sequences in the nuclear binding sites for steroid receptors. *Recent Prog Horm Res* 1983; 39:463–517.
309. Kon OL, Spelsberg TC. Nuclear binding of estrogen-receptor complex: receptor-specific nuclear acceptor sites. *Endocrinology* 1982;111:1925–1935.
310. Ruh TS, Spelsberg TC. Acceptor sites for the oestrogen receptor in hen oviduct chromatin. *Biochem J* 1983;210:905–912.
311. Littlefield BA, Spelsburg TC. Problems and artifacts in the identification of nuclear acceptor sites for avian oviduct progesterone receptor. *Endocrinology* 1985;17:412–414.
312. Maniatis T, Goodbourn S, Fischer JA. Regulation of inducible and tissue-specific gene expression. *Science* 1987;236:1237–1244.
313. Chandler VL, Maler BA, Yamamoto KR. DNA sequences bound specifically by glucocorticoid receptor in vitro render a heterologous promoter hormone responsive in vivo. *Cell* 1983;33: 489–499.
314. Ponta H, Kennedy N, Skroch P, Hynes NE, Groner B. Hormonal response region of the mouse mammary tumor virus long termi-

nal repeat can be dissociated from the proviral promoter and has enhancer properties. *Proc Natl Acad Sci USA* 1985;84: 1020–1024.
315. Bradshaw MS, Tsai M-J, O'Malley BW. A steroid response element can function in the absence of a distal promoter. *Mol Endocrinol* 1988;2:1286–1293.
316. Dynan WS. Modularity in promoters and enhancers. *Cell* 1989;58:1–4.
317. Tremea F, de Medeiros SRB, Heggeler-Bordier BT, et al. Identification of two steroid-responsive promoters of different strength controlled by the same estrogen-responsive element in the 5'end region of the *Xenopus laevis* vitellogenin gene A1. *Mol Endocrinol* 1989;3:1596–1609.
318. Vanderbilt JN, Miesfeld R, Maler BA, Yamamoto KR. Intracellular receptor concentration limits glucocorticoid-dependent enhancer activity. *Mol Endocrinol* 1987;1:68–74.
319. Chalepakis G, Postma JPM, Beato MA. Model for hormone receptor binding to the mouse mammary tumour virus regulatory element based on hydroxyl radical footprinting. *Nucl Acids Res* 1988;16:10237–10247.
320. Drouin J, Chamberland M, Charron J, et al. Pro-opiomelanocortin gene: a model for negative regulation of transcription by glucocorticoids. *J Cell Biochem* 1987;35:293–304
321. Akerblom IE, Slater EP, Beato M, Baxter JD, Mellon PL. Negative regulation by glucocorticoids through interference with a cAMP responsive enhancer. *Science* 1988;241:350–353.
322. Sakai DD, Helms S, Carlstedt-Duke J, Gustafsson J-A, Rottman FM, Yamamoto KR. Hormone-mediated repression: a negative glucocorticoid response element from the bovine prolactin gene. *Genes Dev* 1988;2:1144–1154.
323. Cato ACB, Miksicek R, Schutz G, Arnemann J, Beato M. The hormone regulatory element of mouse mammary tumour virus mediates progesterone induction. *EMBO J* 1986;5:2237–2240.
324. von der Ahe D, Janich S, Scheidereit C, Renkawitz R, Schutz G, Beato M. Glucocorticoid and progesterone receptors bind to the same sites in two hormonally regulated promoters. *Nature* 1985;313:706–709.
325. Parker MG, Webb P, Needham M, White R, Ham J. Identification of androgen response elements in mouse mammary tumour virus and the rat prostate C3 gene. *J Cell Biochem* 1987; 35:285–292.
326. Ham J, Thomson A, Needham M, Webb P, Parker M. Characterization of response elements for androgens, glucocorticoids, and progestins in mouse mammary tumour virus. *Nucl Acids Res* 1988;16:5263–5276.
327. Otten AD, Sanders MM, McKnight GS. The MMTV LTR promoter is induced by progesterone and dihydrotestosterone but not by estrogen. *Mol Endocrinol* 1988;2:143–147.
328. Peale FV, Ludwig LB, Zain S, Hilf R, Bambara RA. Properties of a high-affinity DNA binding site for estrogen receptor. *Proc Natl Acad Sci USA* 1988;85:1038–1042.
329. Klein-Hitpass L, Tsai SY, Greene GL, Clark JH, Tsai M-J, O'Malley BW. Specific binding of estrogen receptor to the estrogen response element. *Mol Cell Biol* 1989;9:43–49.
330. Klock G, Struhle U, Schutz G. Oestrogen and glucocorticoid responsive elements are closely related but distinct. *Nature* 1987;329:734–736.
331. Brent GA, Harney JW, Chen Y, Warne RL, Moore DD, Larsen PR. Mutations of the rat growth hormone promoter which increase and decrease response to thyroid hormone define a consensus thyroid hormone response element. *Mol Endocrinol* 1989;3:1996–2004.
332. Ciejek EM, Nordstrom JL, Tsai M-J, O'Malley BW. Ribonucleic acid precursors are associated with the chick oviduct nuclear matrix. *Biochemistry* 1982;21:4945–4953.
333. Jackson DA, McCready SJ, Cook PR. RNA is synthesized at the nuclear cage. *Nature* 1981;292:552–555.
334. Pardoll DM, Vogelstein B, Coffey DS. A fixed site of DNA replication in eukaryotic cells. *Cell* 1980;19:527–536.
335. Robson JM, Adler J. Site of action of oestrogens. *Nature* 1940;146–160.
336. Small D, Nelkin B, Vogelstein B. Nonrandom distribution of repeated DNA sequences with respect to supercoiled loops and the nuclear matrix. *Proc Natl Acad Sci USA* 1982;79:5911–5915.
337. Vogelstein B, Pardoll DM, Coffey DS. Supercoiled loops and eukaryotic DNA replication. *Cell* 1980;22:79–85.
338. Barrack ER, Bujnovszky P, Walsh PC. Subcellular distribution of androgen receptors in human normal, benign hyperplastic, and malignant prostatic tissues: characterization of nuclear salt-resistant receptors. *Cancer Res* 1983;43:1107–1116.
339. Barrack ER, Coffey DS. The specific binding of estrogens and androgens to the nuclear matrix of sex hormone responsive tissues. *J Biol Chem* 1980;255:7265–7275.
340. Simmen RCM, Means AR, Clark JH. Estrogen modulation of nuclear matrix associated steroid hormone binding. *Endocrinology* 1984;115:1197–1202.
341. Barrack ER. The nuclear matrix of the prostate contains acceptor sites for androgen receptors. *Endocrinology* 1983;113:430–432.
342. Buttyan R, Olsson CA, Sheard B, Kallos J. Steroid receptor-nuclear matrix interactions: the role of DNA. *J Biol Chem* 1983;258:14366–14370.
343. Clark JH, Markaverich BM. Heterogeneity of estrogen binding sites and the nuclear matrix. In: Manul B, ed. *The nuclear envelope and the nuclear matrix.* New York: Alan R Liss, 1982;259.
344. Ekman P, Barrack ER, Greene GL, Jensen EV, Walsh PC. Estrogen receptors in human prostate: evidence for multiple binding sites. *J Clin Endocrinol Metab* 1983;57:166–176.
345. Swaneck GE, Alvarez JM, Sufrin G. Multiple species of estrogen binding sites in the nuclear fraction of the rat prostate. *Biochem Biophys Res Commun* 1982;106:1441–1447.
346. Anderson JN, Peck EJ, Clark JH. Nuclear receptor estrogen complex: accumulation, retention and localization in the hypothalamus and pituitary. *Endocrinology* 1973b;93:711–717.
347. Cidlowski JA, Muldoon TG. Sex-related differences in the regulation of cytoplasmic estrogen receptor levels in responsive tissues of the rat. *Endocrinology* 1976;94:833–841.
348. Clark JH, Campbell PS, Peck EJ, Jr. Receptor estrogen complex in the nuclear fraction of the pituitary and hypothalamus of male and female immature rats. *Neuroendocrinology* 1972;77: 218–228.
349. Muldoon TG. Regulation of steroid hormone receptor activity. *Endocrine Rev* 1981;1:339–364.
350. Muldoon TG. Role of receptors in the mechanism of steroid hormone action in the brain. In: Motta M, ed. *The endocrine functions of the brain.* New York: Raven Press, 1981;51–93.
351. Munck A, Wira C, Young DA, Mosher KM, Hallahan C, Bell PA. Glucocorticoid-receptor complexes and the earliest steps in the action of glucocorticoids on thymus cells. *J Steroid Biochem* 1972;3:567–578.
352. Ishii DN, Aronow L. In vitro degradation and stabilization of the glucocorticoid binding component from mouse fibroblasts. *J Steroid Biochem* 1973;4:593–603.
353. Middlebrook JL, Wong MD, Ishii DN, Aronow L. Subcellular distribution of glucocorticoid receptors in mouse fibroblasts. *Biochemistry* 1975;14:180–186.
354. Jensen EV, Suzuki T, Numata M, Smith S, DeSombre ER. Estrogen binding substances of target tissues. *Steroids* 1969;13: 417–427.
355. Sarff M, Gorski J. Control of estrogen-binding protein concentration under basal conditions and after estrogen administration. *Biochemistry* 1971;10:2557–2563.
356. Kassis JA, Gorski J. Estrogen receptor replenishment: evidence for receptor recycling. *J Biol Chem* 1984;256:7378–7382.
357. Anderson JN, Peck EJ, Jr, Clark JH. Nuclear receptor estradiol complex: a requirement for uterotropic responses. *Endocrinology* 1974;95:174–178.
358. Whalen RE, Nakayama K. Induction of oestrus behavior: facilitation by repeated hormone treatments. *J Endocrinol* 1965; 33:525–526.
359. Simerly RB, Young BJ. Regulation of estrogen receptor messenger ribonucleic acid in rat hypothalamus by sex steroid hormones. *Mol Endocrinol* 1991;5:424–432.
360. Shupnik MA, Gordon MS, Chin WW. Tissue-specific regulation of rat estrogen receptor mRNAs. *Mol Endocrinol* 1989;3: 660–665.
361. Faber LE, Sandmann ML, Stavely HE. Progesterone-binding

proteins of the rat and rabbit uterus. *J Biol Chem* 1972;247: 5648–5649.
362. Feil PD, Glasser SR, Toft DO, O'Malley BW. Progesterone binding in the mouse and rat uterus. *Endocrinology* 1972;1:738–746.
363. Freifeld ML, Feil PD, Bardin CW. The in vivo regulation of the progesterone "receptor" in guinea pig uterus: dependence on estrogen and progesterone. *Steroid* 1974;23:93–103.
364. Hsueh AJ, Peck EJ, Jr, Clark JH. Progesterone antagonism of the oestrogen receptor and oestrogen-induced uterine growth. *Nature* 1975;254:337–339.
365. Hsueh AJ, Peck EJ, Jr, Clark JH. Control of uterine estrogen receptor levels by progesterone. *Endocrinology* 1976;98:438–444.
366. Leavitt WW, Toft DO, Strott CA, O'Malley BW. A specific progesterone receptor in the hamster uterus: physiologic properties and regulation during the estrous cycle. *Endocrinology* 1974; 94:1041–1053.
367. Luu Thi MT, Baulieu EE, Milgrom E. Comparison of the characteristics and of the hormonal control of endometrial and myometrial progesterone receptors. *J Endocrinol* 1975;66:349–356.
368. Reel JR, Shih Y. Oestrogen-inducible uterine progesterone receptors. Characteristics in the ovariectomized immature and adult hamster. *Acta Endocrinol (Copenh)* 1975;80:344–354.
369. Toft D, O'Malley BW. Target tissue receptors for progesterone: the influence of estrogen treatment. *Endocrinology* 1972;9: 1041–1045.
370. Vanderbilt JN, Bloom KS, Anderson JN. Endogenous nuclease: properties and effects on transcribed genes in chromatin. *J Biol Chem* 1982;257:13009–13017.
371. Warembourg M, Milgrom E. Radioautography of the uterus and after [^{3}H] progesterone injection into guinea pigs at various periods of the estrous cycle. *Endocrinology* 1977;100:175–181.
372. Kato J, Onouchi T. Specific progesterone receptors in the hypothalamus and anterior hypophysis of the rat. *Endocrinology* 1977;101:920–928.
373. Jordan VC, Prestwich G. Binding of [^{3}H]tamoxifen in rat uterine cytosols: a comparison of swinging bucket and vertical tube rotor sucrose density gradient analysis. *Mol Cell Endocrinol* 1977;8: 179–188.
374. Sar M, Stumpf WE. Neurons of the hypothalamus concentrate (^{3}H) progesterone or its metabolites. *Science* 1973;182: 1266–1268.
375. Elsner CW, Illingworth DV, De Groot K, Flickinger GL, Mikhail G. Cytosol and nuclear estrogen receptor in the genital tract of the rhesus monkey. *J Steroid Biochem* 1977;8:151–155.
376. Illingworth DV, Elsner C, De Groot K, Flickinger GL, Mikhail G. A specific progesterone receptor of myometrial cytosol from the rhesus monkey. *J Steroid Biochem* 1977;8:157–160.
377. Jänne O, Kontula K, Vihko R. Progestin receptors in human tissues: concentrations and binding kinetics. *J Steroid Biochem* 1976;7:1061–1068.
378. Weil L, Krett NL, Francis MD, et al. Multiple human progesterone receptor messenger ribonucleic acids and their autoregulation by progestin agonists and antagonists in breast cancer cells. *Mol Endocrinol* 1988;2:62–72.
379. Read LD, Snider CE, Miller JS, Greene GL, Katzenellenbogen BS. Ligand-modulated regulation of progesterone receptor messenger ribonucleic acid and protein in human breast cancer cell lines. *Mol Endocrinol* 1988;2:263–271.
380. Romano GJ, Krust A, Pfaff DW. Expression and estrogen regulation of progesterone receptor mRNA in neurons of the mediobasal hypothalamus: an in situ hybridization study. *Mol Endocrinol* 1989;3:1295–1300.
381. Brenner RM, Resko JA, West NB. Cyclic changes in oviductal morphology and residual cytoplasmic estradiol binding capacity induced by sequential estradiol-progesterone treatment of spayed rhesus monkeys. *Endocrinology* 1974;95:1094–1104.
382. Pavlik EJ, Coulson PB. Modulation of estrogen receptors in four different target tissues: differential effects of estrogen vs. progesterone. *J Steroid Biochem* 1976;7:369–376.
383. Okulicz WC, Evans RW, Leavitt WW. Progesterone regulation of the occupied form of nuclear estrogen receptor. *Science* 1981;213:1503–1505.
384. Olge FF. Kinetic and physiochemical characteristics of an endogenous inhibitor to progesterone-receptor binding in rat placental cytosol. *Biochem J* 1981;199:371–381.
385. West NB, Norman RL, Sandow BA, Brenner RM. Hormonal control of nuclear estradiol receptor content and the luminal epithelium in the uterus of the golden hamster. *Endocrinology* 1978;103:1732–1741.
386. MacDonald RG, Okulicz WC, Leavitt WW. Progesterone-induced inactivation of nuclear estrogen receptor in the hamster uterus is mediated by acid phosphatase. *Biochem Biophys Res Commun* 1982;104:570–576.
387. Okulicz WC, Evans RW, Leavitt WW. Progesterone regulation of estrogen receptor in the rat uterus: a primary inhibitory influence on the nuclear fraction. *Steroids* 1981;37:463–470.
388. Clark JH, Hardin JW, Upchurch S, Eriksson H. Heterogeneity of estrogen binding sites in the cytosol of the rat uterus. *J Biol Chem* 1978;253:7630–7634.
389. Etgen AM, Whalen RE. Dimethystilbestrol is not antiestrogenic for rat sexual behavior or gonadotropin secretion. *Biol Reprod* 1978;19:454–458.
390. Watson CS, Clark JH. Heterogeneity of estrogen binding sites in mouse mammary cancer. *J Recept Res* 1980;1:91–111.
391. Panko WB, Watson CS, Clark JH. The presence of a second, specific estrogen binding site in human breast cancer. *J Steroid Biochem* 1981;14:1311–1316.
392. Murai JT, Lieberman RC, Yang JJ, Gerschenson LE. Decrease of estrogen receptors induced by 17β-estradiol and progesterone in cultured rabbit endometrial cells. *Endocrinol Res Commun* 1979;6:235–247.
393. MacLaughlin DT, Hudson JM, Donoahue PK. Specific estradiol binding in embryonic mullerian ducts: a potential modulator of regression in the male and female chick. *Endocrinology* 1983;113:144–145.
394. Weinberger MJ. Heterogeneity and distribution of estrogen binding sites in guinea pig seminal vesicle. *J Steroid Biochem* 1984;20:1327–1332.
395. Yuh K-C, Keyes PL. Properties of nuclear and cytoplasmic estrogen receptor in the rabbit corpus luteum: evidence for translocation. *Endocrinology* 1979;105:690–696.
396. Taylor RN, Smith RG. Identification of a novel sex steroid binding protein. *Proc Natl Acad Sci USA* 1982;79:1742–1746.
397. Pasqualini JR, Gulino A, Nguyen BL, Partois MC. Receptor and biological response to estriol in the fetal uterus of guinea pig. *J Recept Res* 1980;1–261.
398. Eriksson H, Upchurch S, Hardin JW, Peck EJ, Jr, Clark JH. Heterogeneity of estrogen receptors in the cytosol and nuclear fractions of the rat uterus. *Biochem Biophys Res Commun* 1978;81:1–7.
399. Markaverich BM, Clark JH. Two binding sites for estradiol in rat uterine nuclei: relationship to uterotropic response. *Endocrinology* 1979;105:1458–1462.
400. Markaverich BM, Williams M, Upchurch S, Clark JH. Heterogeneity of nuclear estrogen-binding sites in the rat uterus: a simple method for the quantitation of the type I and type II sites by [^{3}H]estradiol exchange. *Endocrinology* 1981;109:62–69.
401. Markaverich BM, Upchurch S, Clark JH. Progesterone and dexamethasone antagonism of nucleus growth: a role for a second nuclear binding site for estradiol in estrogen action. *J Steroid Biochem* 1981;4:125–132.
402. O'Malley BW, McGuire WL, Middleton PA. Altered gene expression during differentiation: population changes in hybridizable RNA after stimulation of the chick oviduct with oestrogen. *Nature* 1968;218:1249.
403. Means AR, Comstock JP, Rosenfeld GC, et al. Ovalbumin messenger RNA of chick oviduct: partial characterization, estrogen dependence and translation in vitro. *Proc Natl Acad Sci USA* 1972;69:1146.
404. Chan L, O'Malley BW. Mechanism of action of the sex steroid hormones. *N Engl J Med* 1976;294:1322–1328.
405. LeMeur M, Glanville N, Mandell JL, et al. The ovalbumin gene family: hormonal control of X and Y gene transcription and mRNA accumulation. *Cell* 1981;23:561–571.
406. McKnight GS, Palmiter RD. Transcriptional regulation of the ovalbumin and conalbumin genes by steroid hormones in chick oviduct. *J Biol Chem* 1979;254:9050–9058.
407. Rhoads RE, McKnight GS, Schmike RT. Synthesis of ovalbumin in a rabbit reticulocyte cell-free system programmed with hen oviduct ribonucleic acid. *J Biol Chem* 1971;246:7407–7410.

408. Swaneck GE, Nordstrom JL, Kreutzaler F, et al. Effect of estrogen on gene expression in chicken oviduct: evidence for transcriptional control of ovalbumin gene. *Proc Natl Acad Sci USA* 1979;76:1049–1053.
409. Tomkins GM, Gelehrter TD, Granner D, et al. Control of specific gene expression in higher organisms. *Science* 1969; 166:1474.
410. Zubay G. *Biochemistry* Reading, MA: Addison-Wesley, 1983.
411. Hargrove JL, Schmidt FH. The role of mRNA and protein stability in gene expression. *FASEB J* 1989;3:2360–2370.
412. Brock ML, Shapiro DJ. Estrogen stabilizes vitellogenin mRNA against degradation. *Cell* 1983;34:207–214.
413. Weintraub H, Groudine M. Chromosomal subunits in active genes have an altered conformation. *Science* 1976;193:848–856.
414. Lamb MM, Daneholt B. Characterization of active transcription units in Balbiani rings of *Chironomus tentans*. *Cell* 1979;17: 835–848.
415. Lawson GM, Knoll BJ, March CJ, et al. Definition of 5′ and 3′ structure boundaries of the chromatin domain containing the ovalbumin multigene family. *J Biol Chem* 1981;257:1501–1507.
416. Barrack ER, Coffey DS. Biological properties of the nuclear matrix: steroid hormone binding. *Recent Prog Horm Res* 1982;28:133–195.
417. Corthesy B, Hispking R, Theulaz I, Wahli W. Estrogen-dependent in vitro transcription from the vitellogenin promoter in liver nuclear extracts. *Science* 1988;239:1137–1139.
418. Freedman L, Yoshinaga S, Vanderbilt J, Yamamoto K. In vitro transcription enhancement by purified derivatives of the glucocorticoid receptor. *Science* 1989;245:298–300.
419. Klein-Hitpass L, Tsai SY, Weigel NL, et al. The progesterone receptor stimulates cell-free transcription by enhancing the formation of a stable preinitiation complex. *Cell* 1990;60:247–257.
420. Bagchi MK, Tsai SY, Weigel NL, Tsai MJ, O'Malley BW. Regulation of in vitro transcription by progesterone receptor-characterization and kinetic studies. *J Biol Chem* 1990;265: 5129–5134.
421. Chalepakis G, Arnemann J, Slater E, Bruller H-J, Gross B, Beato M. Differential gene activation by glucocorticoids and progestins through the hormone regulatory element of mouse mammary tumor virus. *Cell* 1988;53:371–382.
422. Glass CK, Holloway JM, Devary OV, Rosenfeld MG. The thyroid hormone receptor binds with opposite transcriptional effects to a common sequence motif in thyroid hormone and estrogen response elements. *Cell* 1988;54:313–323.
423. Jantzen K, Fritton HP, Igo-Kemenes T, et al. Partial overlapping of binding sequences for steroid hormone receptors and DNase I hypersensitive sites in the rabbit uteroglobin gene region. *Nucl Acid Res* 1987;15:4535–4552.
424. Hwung YP, Crowe DT, Wang L-H, Tsai SY, Tsai M-J. The COUP transcription factor binds to an upstream promoter element of the rat insulin II gene. *Mol Cell Biol* 1988;8:2070–2077.
425. Scatchard G. The attractions of proteins for small molecules and ions. *Ann NY Acad Sci* 1949;51:660–672.
426. O'Malley BW, Roop DR, Lai EC, et al. The ovalbumin gene: organization, structure, transcription and regulation. *Recent Prog Horm Res* 1979;35:1–46.
427. Yamamoto, KR. Steroid receptor-regulated transcription of specific genes and gene networks. *Annu Rev Genet* 1985;19:209–252.
428. Beato M. Gene regulation by steroid hormones. *Cell* 1989; 56:335–344.
429. Fritton HP, Igo-Kemenes TI, Nowock J, Strech-Jurk U, Theisen M, Sippel AE. Alternative sets of DNase I-hypersensitive sites characterize the various functional states of the chicken lysozyme gene. *Nature* 1984;311:163–165.
430. Becker PB, Gloss B, Schmid W, Strahle V, Schutz G. In vivo protein DNA interactions in a glucocorticoid response element require the presence of the hormone. *Nature* 1986;324:686–688.
431. Kumar V, Chambon P. The estrogen receptor binds tightly to its responsive element as a ligand induced homodimer. *Cell* 1988;55:145–156.
432. Bagchi MK, Elliston JF, Tsai SY, Edwards DP, Tsai M-J, O'Malley BW. Steroid hormone-dependent interaction of human progesterone with its target enhancer element. *Mol Endocrinol* 1988;2:1221–1229.
433. O'Malley BW. The steroid receptor superfamily: more excitement predicted for the future. *Mol Endocrinol* 1990;4:363–369.
434. Philipsen JNJ, Hennis BC, Ab G. In vivo footprinting of the estrogen inducible vitellogennin II gene from chicken. *Nucleic Acids Res* 1988;15:2255–2274.
435. Wijnholds J, Philipsen JNJ, Ab G. Tissue-specific and steroid dependent interaction of transcription factors with the estrogen inducible apoVLDL II promoter in vivo. *EMBO J* 1988;7: 2757–2663.
436. Webb P, Lopez GN, Greene GL, Baxter JD, Kushner PJ. The limits of the cellular capacity to mediate an estrogen response. *Mol Endocrinol* 1992;6:157–167.
437. Peale FV, Ludwig LB, Zain S, Hilf R, Bambera RA. Properties of a high affinity DNA binding site for the estrogen receptor. *Proc Natl Acad Sci USA* 1988;85:1038–1042.
438. Watts CK, Parker MG, King RJB. Stable transfection of the estrogen receptor gene into a human osteosarcoma cell line. *J Steroid Biochem* 1990;34:483–490.
439. Migliaccio S, Davis VL, Gibson MK, Gray TK, Korach KS. Estrogen modulates the responsiveness of osteoblast-like cells (ROS 17/2.8) stably transfected with estrogen receptor. *Endocrinology* 1992;130:2617–2624.
440. Tata JR. The action of growth and developmental hormones: evolutionary aspects. In: Goldberger RF, Yamamoto KR, eds. *Biological regulation and development*. New York: Plenum Press, 1984;1–58.
441. Szego CM, Davis JS. Adenosine 3′5′-monophosphate in rat uterus (1967): acute elevation by estrogen. *Proc Natl Acad Sci USA* 1967;58:1711–1718.
442. Szego CM, Davis JS. Inhibition of estrogen-induced elevation of cyclic 3′,5′-adenosine monophosphate in rat uterus. I. By β-adrenergic receptor blocking drugs. *Mol Pharmacol* 1969; 5:470–480.
443. Korenman SG, Sanborn BM, Bhalla RC. Adenyl cyclase and the cyclic AMP responsive systems in the uterus. In: O'Malley BW, Means AR, eds. *Receptors for reproductive hormones*. New York: Plenum Press, 1973;241–262.
444. Zor U, Koch Y, Lamprecht SA, Ausher J, Lindner HR. Mechanism of oestradiol action on the rat uterus: independence of cyclic AMP, prostaglandin E_2 and β-adrenergic mediation. *J Endocrinol* 1973;58:525–533.
445. Flandroy L, Fastrez-Boute A, Galand P. Oestrogen induced changes in uterine cGMP: relationship with other parameters of hormonal stimulation. *Arch Int Physiol Biochim* 1976;84: 1072–1078.
446. Flandroy L, Galand P. Oestrogen related changes in uterine and vaginal cAMP and cGMP. *Arch Int Physiol Biochim* 1975;83: 965–971.
447. Kuehl FA, Ham EA, Zanetti ME, Sanford C, Nicol SE, Goldberg ND. Estrogen-related increases in uterine guanosine 3′:5′-cyclic monophosphate levels. *Proc Natl Acad Sci USA* 1974;71: 1866–1870.
448. Flandroy L, Galand P. Changes in cGMP and cAMP content in the estrogen stimulated rat uterus: temporal relationship with other parameters of hormonal stimulation. *J Cycle Nucleotide Res* 1978;4:145–151.
449. Nicol SE, Goldberg ND. Inhibition of estrogen induced changes in uterine cGMP: relationship with other parameters of hormonal stimulation. *Arch Int Physiol Biochim* 1976;84: 1072–1078.
450. Szego CM. The lysosomal membrane complex as a proximate target for steroid hormone action. In: McKerns KW, ed. *The sex steroids*. New York: Appleton-Century-Crofts, 1971;1–51.
451. Tchernitchin A, Tchernitchin X. Characterization of the estrogen receptors in the uterine and blood eosinophil leukocytes. *Experientia* 1976;32:1240–1242.
452. Tchernitchin A, Tchernitchin X, Galand P. New concepts on the actions of oestrogens in the uterus and the role of the eosinophil receptor system. *Differentiation* 1976;5:145–150.
453. Szego CM, Lawson DA. Influence of histamine on uterine metabolism: stimulation of incorporation of radioactivity from amino acids into protein, lipid and purines. *Endocrinology* 1964;74: 372–381.
454. Tchernitchin A, Roorijck J, Tchernitchin X, Van den Hende J,

Galand P. Effects of cortisol on uterine eosinophilia and other oestrogenic responses. *Mol Cell Endocrinol* 1975;2:331–337.
455. Galand P, Mairesse N, Roorijck J, Fandroy L. Differential blockade of estrogen induced uterine responses by the antiestrogen nafoxidine. *J Steroid Biochem* 1983;19:1259–1263.
456. Gardner RM, Kirkland JL, Stancel GM. Selective blockade of estrogen-induced uterine responses by the antiestrogen nafoxidine. *Endocrinology* 1978;103:1583–1589.
457. Rorke EA, Katzenellenbogen BS. Dissociated regulation of growth and ornithine decarboxylase activity by estrogen in the rat uterus. *Biochem Biophys Res Commun* 1984;122:1186–1193.
458. Pentecost BT, Mattheiss L, Dickerman HW, Kumar SA. Estrogen regulation of creatine kinase-B in the rat uterus. *Mol Endocrinol* 1990;4:1000–1010.
459. Lingham RB, Stancel GM, Loose-Mitchell DS. Estrogen regulation of EGF receptor mRNA. *Mol Endocrinol* 1988;2:230–235.
460. Murphy LJ, Murphy LC, Friesen HG. Estrogen induces insulin-like growth factor-I expression in the rat uterus. *Mol Endocrinol* 1987;1:445–450.
461. Henrikson KP, Greenwood JA, Penticost BT, Jazin EE, Dickerman HW. Estrogen control of uterine tissue factor messenger ribonucleic acid levels. *Endocrinology* 1992;130:2669–2674.
462. Pastore GN, Dicola LP, Doooahon NR, Gardner RM. Effect of estriol on the structure and organization of collagen in the lamina propria of the immature rat uterus. *Biol Reprod* 1992;47:83–91.
463. Weisz A, Bresciani F. Estrogen induces expression of c-fos and c-myc protoocogenes in rat uterus. *Mol Endocrinol* 1988;2:816–824.
464. Loose-Mitchell DS, Chiappetta C, Stancel GM. Estrogen regulation of c-fos messenger ribonucleic acid. *Mol Endocrinol* 1988;2:946–951.
465. Papa M, Mezzogiorno V, Bresciani F, Weisz A. Estrogen induces c-fos expression specifically in the luminal and glandular epithelia of adult rat uterus. *Biochem Biophys Res Commun* 1991;175:480–485.
466. Chiappetta C, Kirkland JL, Loose-Mitchell DS, Murthy L, Stancel GM. Estrogen regulates expression of the jun family of protooncogenes in the uterus. *J Steroid Biochem Mol Biol* 1992;41:113–123.
467. Gaub MP, Bellard M, Scheuer I, Chambon P, Sassone-Corsi P. Activation of the ovalbumin gene by the estrogen receptor involves the fos-jun complex. *Cell* 1990;63:1267–1276.
468. Nelson KG, Takahashi T, Bossert NL, Walmer DK, McLachlan JA. *Proc Natl Acad Sci USA* 1991;88:21–25.
469. Ignar-Trowbridge DM, Belson KG, Bidwell MC, et al. Coupling of dual signaling pathways: epidermal growth factor action involves the estrogen receptor. *Proc Natl Acad Sci USA* 1992;89:4658–4662.
470. Power RF, Lydon JP, Conneely OM, O'Malley BW. *Science* 1991;252:1546–1547.
471. Power RF, Mani SK, Codina J, Conneely OM, O'Malley BW. *Science* 1991;254:1636–1639.
472. Harris J, Gorski J. Evidence for a discontinuous requirement for estrogen in stimulation of deoxyribonucleic acid synthesis in the immature rat uterus. *Endocrinology* 1978;103:240–245.
473. Persico E, Scalona M, Cicatiello L, Sica V, Bresciani F, Weisz A. Activation of immediate early genes by estrogen is not sufficient to achieve stimulation of DNA synthesis in rat uterus. *Biochem Biophys Res Commun* 1990;171:287–292.
474. Galand PN, Tchernitchin X, Tchernitchin AN. Time course of the effects of nafoxidine and oestradiol on separate groups of responses in the uterus of the immature rat. *J Steroid Biochem* 1984;21:43–47.
475. Tchernitchin A, Tchernitchin X, Galand P. Dissociation of separate mechanisms of estrogen action by actinomycin D. *Experientia* 1982;38:511–512.
476. Baker HJ, Shapiro DJ. Kinetics of estrogen induction of *Xenopus laevis* vitellogenin messenger RNA as measured by hybridization to complementary DNA. *J Biol Chem* 1977;252:8428–8434.
477. Farmer SR, Henshaw EC, Berridge MV, Tata JR. Translation of *Xenopus* vitellogenin mRNA during primary and secondary induction. *Nature* 1978;273:401–403.
478. Guyette WA, Matusik RJ, Rosen JM. Prolactin-mediated transcriptional and post-transcriptional control of casein gene expression. *Cell* 1979;17:1013–1023.
479. Hobbs AA, Richards DA, Kessler DJ, Rosen JM. Complex hormonal regulation of rat casein gene expression. *J Biol Chem* 1982;257:3598–3605.
480. Palmiter RD. Quantitation of parameters that determine the rate of ovalbumin synthesis. *Cell* 1975;4:189–197.
481. Palmiter RD, Mulvihill ER, McKnight GS, Senear AW. Regulation of gene expression in the chick oviduct by steroid hormones, *Cold Spring Harbor Symp Quant Biol* 1978;42:639–647.
482. Schutz G, Nguyen-Huu MC, Giesecke K, et al. Hormonal control of egg white protein messenger RNA synthesis in the chicken oviduct. *Cold Spring Harbor Symp Quant Biol* 1977;42:617–624.
483. Searle PF, Tata JR. Vitelloginin gene expression in male *Xenopus* hepatocytes during primary and secondary stimulation with estrogen in cell cultures. *Cell* 1981;23:741–746.
484. Swanson LV, Barker K. Antagonistic effects of progesterone on estradiol-induced synthesis and degradation of uterine glucose-6-phosphate dehydrogenase. *Endocrinology* 1983;112:459–465.
485. Kirland JL, Gardner RM, Ireland JS, Stancel GM. The effect of hypophysectomy on the uterine response to estradiol. *Endocrinology* 1977;101:403–410.
486. Sonnenschein C, Soto AM. Pituitary uterotrophic effect in the estrogen-dependent growth of the rat uterus. *J Steroid Biochem* 1978;9:533–537.
487. Huggins C, Jensen EV. The depression of estrone-induced uterine growth by phenolic estrogens with oxygenated functions at positions 6 or 16; the impeded estrogens. *J Exp Med* 1955;102:335–346.
488. Robinson SI, Nelkin BD, Vogelstein B. The ovalbumin gene is associated with the nuclear matrix of chicken oviduct cells. *Cell* 1982;28:99–106.
489. Langier C, Pageaux JF, Soto AM, Sonnenschein C. Mechanisms of estrogen action: indirect effect of estradiol on proliferation of quail oviduct cells. *Proc Natl Acad Sci USA* 1983;80:1621–1625.
490. Schatz R, Soto AM, Sonnenschein C. Estrogen induced cell multiplication: direct or indirect effect on rat uterine cells. *Endocrinology* 1984;115:501–506.
491. Sirbasku DA, Benson RH. Estrogen-inducible growth factors that may act as mediators (estromedins) of estrogen promoted tumor cell growth. *Cold Spring Harbor Conf Cell Prolif* 1979;6:477–497.
492. Cunha GR, Chung LWK, Shannon JM, Taguchi O, Fujii H. Hormone induced morphogenesis and growth: role of mesenchymal-epithelial interactions. *Recent Prog Horm Res* 1983;39:559–598.
493. Clark JH, Markaverich BM. Agonist and antagonist properties of clomiphene: a review. *Pharmacol Ther* 1982;15:467–519.
494. Clark JH, Markaverich BM. The agonistic and antagonistic effects of short acting estrogens: a review. *Pharmacol Ther* 1983;21:429–453.
495. Furr BJA, Jordon VC. The pharmacology and clinical uses of tamoxifen. *Pharmacol Ther* 1984;25:127–205.
496. Jordan VC. Biochemical pharmacology of antiestrogen action. *Pharmacol Rev* 1984;36:245–276.
497. Hisaw FL, Jr. Comparative effectiveness of estrogens on fluid inhibition and growth of the rat's uterus. *Endocrinology* 1959;64:276–289.
498. Capony F, Rochefort H. In vitro and in vivo interaction of ^{3}H-dimethylstilbestrol with the estrogen receptor. *Mol Cell Endocrinol* 1977;8:47–64.
499. Markaverich BM, Clark JH, Hardin JW. RNA transcription and uterine growth: differential effects of estradiol, estriol and nafoxidine on chromatin RNA initiation sites. *Biochemistry* 1978;17:3146–3152.
500. Terenius L. Structure-activity relationships of anti-oestrogens with regard to interaction with 17 beta-oestradiol in the mouse uterus and vagina. *Acta Endocrinol* 1971;66:431–447.
501. Fagg B, Martin L. Oestrogen content of the uterine tissues of mice and their relationship to epithelial cell proliferation after subcutaneous and intraluminal administration of hormones. *J Endocrinol* 1979;83:295–304.
502. Pollard I, Martin L. The oestrogenic and anti-oestrogenic activity of some synthetic steroids and non-steroids. *Steroids* 1968;11:897–907.
503. Martin L. Dimethylstilbestrol and 16-oxo-estradiol: antiestrogens or estrogens. *Steroids* 1969;13:1–10.
504. Miller BG, Emmens CW. The oestrogenic potency in the mouse

of several substances closely related to diethylstilboestrol and mesohexoestrol. *J Endocrinol* 1969;45:9–15.
505. Terenius L, Ljungkvist I. Aspects on the mode of action of antiestrogens and anti-progestogens. *Gynecol Invest* 1972;3:96–107.
506. Martucci C, Fishman J. Direction of estradiol metabolism as a control of its hormonal action—uterotrophic activity of estradiol metabolites. *Endocrinology* 1977;101:1709–1715.
507. Brecher PI, Wotiz HH. *Proc Soc Exp Biol Med* 1968;128: 470–472.
508. Bouton M, Raynaud JP. The relevance of interaction kinetics in determining biological responses to estrogens. *Endocrinology* 1979;105:509–515.
509. Jensen EV, Jacobson HI, Flesher JW, et al. Estrogen receptors in target tissues. In: Pincus G, Nakao T, Tait JF, eds. *Steroid dynamics.* New York: Academic Press, 1966;133–157.
510. Katzenellenbogen JA, Carlson KE, Heiman DF, Robertson DW, Wai LL, Katzenellenbogen BS. Efficient and highly selective covalent labeling of the estrogen receptor with [^{3}H]tamoxifen aziridine. *J Biol Chem* 1983;258:3487–3495.
511. Clark JH, Williams M, Upchurch S, Eriksson H, Helton E, Markaverich BM. Effects of estradiol 17α on nuclear occupancy of the estrogen receptor stimulation of nuclear type II sites and uterine growth. *J Steroid Biochem* 1982;16:323–328.
512. Cole P, MacMahon B. Oestrogen fractions during early reproductive life in the etiology of breast cancer. *Lancet* 1969;i:604–606.
513. Lemon H. Pathophysiologic considerations in the treatment of menopausal patients with oestrogens; the role of oestriol in the prevention of mammary carcinoma. *Acta Endocrinol (Suppl)* 1980;23:17–27.
514. Lerner LJ, Hilt R, Turkheimer AR, Michel I, Engle SL. Effects of hormone antagonists on morphological and biochemical changes induced by hormonal steroids in the immature rat uterus. *Endocrinology* 1966;78:111–124.
515. Gulino A, Sumida C, Gelley C, Giambiagi N, Pasqualini JR. Comparative dynamic studies of the biological responses to estriol and estradiol in the fetal uterus of guinea pig: relationship to circulating estrogen concentration. *Endocrinology* 1981;109: 748–756.
516. Kapetanakis M, Dnowski WP, Scommegna A. Induction of delayed implantation in rats with continuous but not with bolus administration of estriol. *Biol Reprod* 1980;23:88–91.
517. Wotiz HH, Scublinsky A. The contraceptive action of impeding oestrogens. *J Reprod Fertil* 1971;26:143–148.
518. Edwards DP, McGuire WL. 17α-Estradiol is a biologically active estrogen in human breast cancer cells in tissue culture. *Endocrinology* 1980;107:884–891.
519. Emmens CW, Miller BG. Estrogens, progestogens and antiestrogens. *Steroids* 1969;13:723–750.
520. Jordan VC, Dix CJ, Prestwich G. Inhibition of cell division and stimulation of progesterone receptor synthesis in rat oestrogen target tissues by non-steroidal anti-oestrogens. In: Leavitt WW, Clark JH, eds. *Steroid hormone receptor systems.* New York: Plenum Press, 1979;133–156.
521. Kang Y-H, Anderson WA, DeSombre ER. Modulation of uterine morphology and growth by estradiol-17β and an estrogen antagonist. *J Cell Biol* 1975;64:682–691.
522. Secchi J, Lecaque D, Tournemie C, Philibert D. Histopathology of RU 486. In: Baulieu EE, Segal SJ, eds. *The antiprogestin steroid, RU 486, and human fertility control.* New York: Plenum Press, 1985;49–68.
523. Kornberg RD. Structure of chromatin. *Annu Rev Biochem* 1977;46:931.
524. Baudendistel LJ, Ruh MF, Nadel EM, Ruh TS. Cytoplasmic oestrogen receptor replenishment: oestrogens versus antioestrogens. *Acta Endocrinol (Copenh)* 1978;89:599–611.
525. Clark JH, Anderson JN, Peck EJ, Jr. Oestrogen receptors and antagonism of steroid hormone action. *Nature* 1974;251: 446–448.
526. Gasde K, Kramer G, Schulz KO. Effects of oestradiol-17β on uterine ribosomes: altered sedimentation profile and enhanced protein-synthesizing activity. *Hoppe-Seylers Z Physiol Chem* 1971;352:318–320.
527. Kurl RN, Borthwick NM. Clomiphene and tamoxifen action in the rat uterus. *J Endocrinol* 1980;85:519–524.
528. Mairesse N, Galand P. Comparison between the action of estradiol and that of the antiestrogen U11-100A on the induction in the rat uterus of a specific protein (the induced protein). *Endocrinology* 1979;105:1248–1253.
529. Martin L. Estrogens, anti-estrogens and the regulation of cell proliferation in the female reproductive tract in vivo. In: McLachlan J, ed. *Estrogens in the environment.* North Holland: Elsevier, 1980;103–130.
530. Emmens CW. Oestrogenic, anti-oestrogenic and anti-fertility activity. *Acta Med Philip* 1965;1:220–224.
531. Binart N, Catelli MH, Geynet C, et al. Monohydroxytamoxifen: an antiestrogen with high affinity for the chick oviduct oestrogen receptor. *Biochem Biophys Res Commun* 1979;91:812–818.
532. Capony F, Williams DL. Antiestrogen action in avian liver: the interaction of estrogens and antiestrogens in the regulation of apolipoproteins b synthesis. *Endocrinology* 1981;108: 1862–1868.
533. Lazier CB, Capony F, Williams DL. Antioestrogen action in chick liver: effects on oestrogen receptors and oestrogen-induced proteins. In: Sutherland RL, Jordan VC, eds. *Non-steroidal antioestrogens.* Sydney: Academic Press, 1981;215–230.
534. Sutherland RL. Estrogen antagonists in chick oviduct: antagonist activity of eight synthetic triphenylethylene derivatives and their interactions with cytoplasmic and nuclear estrogen receptors. *Endocrinology* 1981;109:2061–2068.
535. Natrajan PK, Greenblatt RB. Clomiphene citrate: induction of ovulation. In: Greenblatt RB, ed. Philadelphia: Lea & Febiger, 1979;35–76.
536. Westley BR, Rochefort H. Estradiol-induced proteins in the MCF-7 human breast cancer cell line. *Biochem Biophys Res Commun* 1979;90:410–416.
537. Westley B, Rochefort H. A secreted glycoprotein induced by estrogen in human breast cancer cell lines. *Cell* 1980;20:353–362.
538. Coezy E, Borgna JL, Rochefort H. Tamoxifen and metabolites in MCF-7 cells. *Corr* 1982;42:317–323.
539. Edwards DP, Murphy SR, McGuire WL. Effects of estrogen and antiestrogen on DNA polymerase in human breast cancer. *Cancer Res* 1980;40:1722–1726.
540. Amara JF, Dannies PS. Characterization of antiestrogen stimulation of cell number and prolactin production. *Mol Cell Endocrinol* 1986;47:183–189.
541. Prysor-Jones RA, Silverlight JJ, Jenkins JS. Effect of tamoxifen on growth and prolactin secretion of rat pituitary tumours. *J Endocrinol* 1983;97:261–266.
542. Shull JD, Beams FE, Baldwin TM, Gilchrist CA, Hrbek MJ. The estrogenic and antiestrogenic properties of tamoxifen in GH4C1 pituitary tumor cells are gene specific. *Mol Endocrinol* 1992;6:529–535.
543. Lieberman ME, Gorski J, Jordan VC. An estrogen receptor model to describe the regulation of prolactin synthesis by antiestrogens in vitro. *J Biol Chem* 1983a;258:4741–4745.
544. Lieberman ME, Jordan VC, Fritsch M, Santos MA, Gorski J. Direct and reversible inhibition of estradiol-stimulated prolactin synthesis by antiestrogen in vitro. *J Biol Chem* 1983;258: 4734–4740.
545. Martinez-Campos A, Amara JF, Dannies PS. Anti-estrogens are partial estrogen agonists for prolactin production in primary pituitary cultures. *Mol Cell Endocrinol* 1986;48:127–133.
546. Lyttle RC, Damian-Matsumura P, Juul H, Butt TR. Human estrogen receptor regulation in a yeast model system and studies on receptor agonists and antagonists. *J Steroid Biochem Mol Biol* 1992;42:677–685.
547. Green S. Modulation of estrogen receptor activity by estrogens and antiestrogens. *J Steroid Biochem Mol Biol* 1990;37:747–751.
548. Pham TA, Elliston JF, Nawaz Z, McDonnell DP, Tsai MJ, O'Malley BW. Antiestrogen can establish nonproductive receptor complexes and alter chromatin structure at target enhancers. *Proc Natl Acad Sci USA* 1991;88:3125–3129.
549. Pham TA, Hwung YP, Santiso-Mere D, McDonnell DP, O'Malley BW. Ligand dependent and independent function of the transactivation regions of the human estrogen receptor in yeast. *Mol Endocrinol* 1992;6:1043–1050.
550. Berry M, Metzger D, Chambon P. Role of the two activating domains of the estrogen receptor in the cell type and promoter context dependent agonist activity of the antiestrogen 4-hydroxytamoxifen. *EMBO J* 1990;9:2811–2818.

551. Greenblatt RB, Barfield WE, Jungck EC, Ray AW. Induction of ovulation with MRL/41. Preliminary report. *JAMA* 1961;178: 101–104.
552. Holtkamp DE, Greslin JG, Root CA, Lerner LJ. Gonadotrophin inhibiting and anti-fecundity effect of chloramiphene. *Proc Soc Exp Biol Med* 1960;105:197–201.
553. Schally AV, Carter WH, Parlow AF, et al. Alteration of LH and FSH release in rat treated with clomiphene and its isomers. *Am J Obstet Gynecol* 1970;107:1156–1167.
554. Hsueh AJW, Erickson GF, Yen SSC. Sensitization of pituitary cells to luteinizing hormone releasing hormone by clomiphene citrate in vitro. *Nature* 1978;273:57–59.
555. Coppola JA, Perrine JW. Influence of two nonsteroidal antiestrogens on vaginal opening and PMS-induced ovulation in rats. *J Reprod Fertil* 1965;13:373–374.
556. Koch Y, Dikstein S, Superstine E, Sulman FG. The effect of promethazine and clomiphene on gonadotrophin secretion in the rat. *J Endocrinol* 1971;49:13–17.
557. Nagel S, Baier H, Taubert H-D. Contrasting actions of cis and trans-clomiphene on the release of FSH and FSH-RF in the female rat. *Horm Metab Res* 1970;2:344–348.
558. Docke F. Ovulation-inducing action of clomiphene citrate in the rat. *J Reprod Fertil* 1969;18:135–139.
559. Rebar R, Judd HL, Yen SSC, Rakoff J, Vandenberg G, Naftolin F. Characterization of the inappropriate gonadotropin secretion in polycystic ovary syndrome. *J Clin Invest* 1976;57:1320–1329.
560. Ross GT, Cargille CM, Lipsett MB, et al. Pituitary and gonadal hormones in women during spontaneous and induced ovulatory cycles. *Recent Prog Horm Res* 1970;26:1–62.
561. Adashi EV, Hsueh AJW, Yen SSC. Alterations induced by clomiphene in the concentrations of oestrogen receptors in the uterus, pituitary gland and hypothalamus of female rats. *J Endocrinol* 1980;87:383–392.
562. Igarashi M, Ibuki Y, Kubo H, et al. Mode and site of action of clomiphene. *Am J Obstet Gynecol* 1967;97:120–123.
563. Coppola JA, Leonardi RG, Ringler I. Reversal of the effects of anti-oestrogens and norethynodrel on gonadotropin-induced ovulation in rats. *J Reprod Fertil* 1966;11:65–71.
564. Docke F. Studies on the anti-ovulatory action of clomiphene citrate in the rat. *J Reprod Fertil* 1971;24:45–54.
565. Yen SSC, Vela P, Ryan KJ. Effect of clomiphene citrate in polycystic ovary syndrome: relationship between serum gonadotropin and corpus luteum function. *J Clin Endocrinol* 1970;31: 7–13.
566. Kato J, Kobayashi T, Villee CA. Effect of clomiphene on the uptake of estradiol by the anterior hypothalamus and hypophysis. *Endocrinology* 1968;82:1049–1052.
567. Kurl RN, Morris ID. Differential depletion of cytoplasmic high affinity oestrogen receptors after the in vitro administration of the antioestrogen clomiphene, MER-25 and tamoxifen. *Br J Pharmacol* 1978;62:487–493.
568. Labrie F, Drouin J, Ferland L, et al. Mechanism of action of hypothalamic hormones in the anterior pituitary gland and specific modulation of their activity by sex steroids and thyroid hormones. *Recent Prog Horm Res* 1978;34:25–93.
569. Dannies PS, Yen PN, Tashjian AH, Jr. Anti-estrogenic compounds increase prolactin and growth hormone synthesis in clonal strains of rat pituitary cells. *Endocrinology* 1977;101: 1151–1156.
570. Perlow M, Sassin J, Boyar R, Hellman L, Weitzman ED. Reduction of growth hormone secretion following clomiphene administration. *Metabolism* 1973;22:1269–1275.
571. Boyar RM. Effects of clomiphene citrate on pituitary FSH, FSH-RF, and release of LH in immature and mature rats. *Endocrinology* 1970;86:629–633.
572. Schulz KD, August S, Gasde K, Kramer G. Studies on the anti-oestrogenic and oestrogen-like action of clomiphene citrate. Animal experiments. *Gynecol Invest* 1972;3:135–141.
573. Clark JH, Guthrie SC. The agonistic and antagonistic effects of clomiphene citrate and its isomers. *Biol Reprod* 1981;25: 667–672.
574. Thompson IE, Karam KS, Taymor ML. Positive feedback effects of estrogen in amenorrheic women. *Am J Obstet Gynecol* 1974;118:788–792.
575. Knobil E. The neuroendocrine control of the menstrual cycle. *Recent Prog Horm Res* 1980;36:53–88.
576. Vaitukaitis JL, Bermudez JA, Cargille CM, Lipdryy MB, Ross GT. New evidence for an anti-estrogenic action of clomiphene citrate in women. *J Clin Endocrinol* 1971;32:503–508.
577. Czygan P-J, Schulz KD. Studies on the anti-oestrogenic and oestrogen-like action of clomiphene citrate in women. *Gynecol Invest* 1972;3:126–134.
578. Hashimoto T, Miyai K, Izumi K, Kumahara Y. Effect of clomiphene citrate on basal and LRH-induced gonadotropin secretion in postmenopausal women. *J Clin Endocrinol Metab* 1976;42: 593–594.
579. Ravid R, Jedwab G, Persitz E, et al. Gonadotrophin release in ovariectomized patients. I. Suppression by clomiphene or low doses of ethinyl oestradiol. *Clin Endocrinol* 1977;6:333–338.
580. Taubert H-D, Dericks-Tan JSE. High doses of estrogens do not interfere with the ovulation-inducing effect of clomiphene citrate. *Fertil Steril* 1976;27:375–382.
581. Capony F, Rochefort H. High affinity binding of the antiestrogen [^{3}H]tamoxifen to the 8S estradiol receptor. *Mol Cell Endocrinol* 1978;11:181–198.
582. Clark JH, Anderson JN, Peck EJ, Jr. Estrogen receptor-antiestrogen complex: atypical binding by uterine nuclei and effects on uterine growth. *Steroids* 1973;22:707–718.
583. Jordan VC, Naylor KE. The binding of ^{3}H-oestradiol in the immature rat uterus during the sequential administration of anti-oestrogens. *Br J Pharmacol* 1979;65:167–173.
584. Horwitz KB, Koseki Y, McGuire WL. Estrogen control of progesterone receptor in human breast cancer: role of estradiol and antiestrogen. *Endocrinology* 1978;103:1742–1751.
585. Horwitz KB, McGuire WL. Nuclear mechanisms of estrogen action. Effects of estradiol and anti-estrogens on estrogen receptors and nuclear receptor processing. *J Biol Chem* 1978;253: 8185–8191.
586. Evans E, Baskevitch PP, Rochefort H. Estrogen receptor DNA ineractions: difference between activation by estrogen and antiestrogen. *Eur J Biochem* 1982;128:185–191.
587. Rochefort H, Borgna JL. Differences between oestrogen receptor activation by oestrogen and antioestrogen. *Nature* 1981;292: 257–259.
588. Tate AC, Greene GL, DeSombre ER, Jensen EV, Jordan VC. Differences between estrogen- and antiestrogen-estrogen receptor complexes from human breast tumors identified with an antibody raised against the estrogen receptor. *Cancer Res* 1984; 44:1012–1018.
589. Borgna JL, Rochefort H. High affinity binding to the estrogen receptor of [^{3}H]4-hydroxytamoxifen, an active antiestrogen metabolite. *Mol Cell Endocrinol* 1980;20:71–85.
590. Murphy LC, Sutherland RL. Antitumor activity of clomiphene analogs in vitro: relationship to affinity for the estrogen receptor and another high affinity antiestrogen-binding site. *J Clin Endocrinol Metab* 1983;57:373–379.
591. Tate AC, DeSombre ER, Greene GL, Jensen EV, Jordan VC. Interaction of [^{3}H]monohydroxytamoxifen-estrogen receptor complexes with a monoclonal antibody. *Breast Cancer Res Treat* 1983;3:267–277.
592. Ruh TS, Ruh MF. The agonistic and antagonistic properties of the high affinity antiestrogen H1285. *Pharmacol Ther* 1983; 21:247–264.
593. Tate AC, Lieberman ME, Jordan VC. The inhibition of prolactin synthesis in GH_3 rat pituitary tumor cells by monohydroxytamoxifen is associated with changes in the properties of the estrogen receptor. *J Steroid Biochem* 1984;20:391–395.
594. Ikeda M, Omukai Y, Hosokawa K, Senoo T. Differences in extractability of estradiol and tamoxifen receptor complex in the nuclei from MCF-7 cells with Nonidet P-40. *Steroids* 1984; 43:481–489.
595. Sutherland RL, Foo MS. Differential binding of antiestrogens by rat uterine and chick oviduct cytosol. *Biochem Biophys Res Commun* 1979;91:183–191.
596. Sutherland RL, Murphy LC, Foo MS, Green MD, Whybourne AM, Krozowski AS. High affinity anti-oestrogen binding site distinct from the oestrogen receptor. *Nature* 1980;288:273–275.
597. Winneker RC, Guthrie SC, Clark JH. Characterization of a

triphenyethylene-antiestrogen-binding site on rat serum low density lipoprotein. *Endocrinology* 1983;112:1823–1827.
598. Gulino A, Pasqualini JR. Heterogeneity of binding sites for tamoxifen and tamoxifen derivatives in estrogen target and nontarget fetal organs of guinea pig. *Cancer Res* 1982;42:1913–1921.
599. Sudo K, Monsma FJ, Jr, Katzenellenbogen BS. Antiestrogen-binding sites distinct from the estrogen receptor: subcellular localization, ligand specificity, and distribution in tissues of the rat. *Endocrinology* 1983;112:425–434.
600. Winneker RC, Clark JH. Estrogen stimulation of the antiestrogen specific binding site in rat uterus and liver. *Endocrinology* 1983;112:1910–1915.
601. Murphy PR, Breckenridge WC, Lazier CB. Binding of oxygenated cholesterol metabolites to antiestrogen binding sites from chicken liver. *Biochem Biophys Res Commun* 1985;127:786–792.
602. Faye JC, Lasserre B, Bayard F. Antiestrogen specific, high affinity saturable binding sites in rat uterine cytosol. *Biochem Biophys Res Commun* 1980;93:1225–1231.
603. Gulino A, Pasqualini JR. Specific binding and biological response of antiestrogens in the fetal uterus of the guinea pig. *Cancer Res* 1980;40:3821–3826.
604. Kon OL. An antiestrogen-binding protein in human tissues. *J Biol Chem* 1983;258:3173–3177.
605. Murphy LC, Sutherland RL. A high-affinity binding site for the antioestrogen, tamoxifen and CI628, in immature rat uterine cytosol which is distinct from the oestrogen receptor. *J Endocrinol* 1981;91:155–161.
606. Sutherland RL, Murphy LC. The binding of tamoxifen to human mammary carcinoma cytosol. *Eur J Cancer* 1980;16:1141–1148.
607. Gulino A, Pasqualini JR. Modulation of tamoxifen specific binding sites and estrogen receptors by estradiol and progesterone in the neonatal uterus of guinea pig. *Endocrinology* 1983;112:1871–1873.
608. Clark JH, Guthrie SC. Subcellular localization of triphenylethylene and antiestrogen binding sites (TABS) in rat liver. *J Steroid Biochem* 1986;(*In press*).
609. Faye JC, Jozan S, Redewith G, Baulieu EE, Bayard F. Physicochemical and genetic evidence for specific antiestrogen binding sites. *Proc Natl Acad Sci USA* 1983;80:3158–3162.
610. Miller MA, Katzenellenbogen BS. Characterization and quantitation of antiestrogen binding sites in estrogen receptor-positive and -negative human breast cancer cell lines. *Cancer Res* 1983;43:3094–3100.
611. Brandes LJ. A diphenylmethane derivative selective for the antiestrogen binding site may help define its biological role. *Biochem Biophys Res Commun* 1984;124:244–249.
612. Goldstein JL, Brown MS. The LDL receptor locus and the genetics of familial hypercholesterolemia. *Annu Rev Genet* 1979;13:259–291.
613. Tabacik C, Cypriani B, Alian S, Crastes de Paulet A. Cholesterol biosynthesis in MCF-7 cell line in relation to cell division: stimulation by estradiol and inhibition by tamoxifen. In: Bresciani F, King RJB, Lippman ME, Namer M, Raynaud J-P, eds. *Progress in cancer research and therapy 31.* New York: Raven Press, 1984;213–222.
614. Lam PH-Y. Tamoxifen is a calmodulin antagonist in the activation of cAMP phosphodiesterase. *Biochem Biophys Res Commun* 1984;118:27–32.
615. Chafouleas JG, Lagace L, Boulton WE, Boyd AE, Means AR. Changes in calmodulin and its mRNA accompany re-entry of quiescent (G_0) cells in the cell cycle. *Cell* 1984;36:73–81.
616. Ito H, Hidaka H. Antitumor effect of a calmodulin antagonist on the growth of solid sarcoma-180. *Cancer Lett* 1983;19:215–220.
617. Willingham MC, Wehland J, Klee CB, Richert NO, Rutherford AV, Pastan IH. Ultrastructural immunocytochemical localization of calmodulin in cultured cells. *J Histochem Cytochem* 1984;31:445–461.
618. Kneifel MA, Katzenellenbogen BS. Comparative effects of estrogen and antiestrogen on plasma renin substrate levels and hepatic estrogen receptors in the rat. *Endocrinology* 1981;108:545–552.
619. Pavlik EJ, Nelson K, Srinivasan S, et al. Resistance to tamoxifen with persisting sensitivity to estrogen: possible mediation by excessive antiestrogen binding site activity. *Cancer Res* 1992;52:4106–4112.
620. Lerner LJ. Hormone antagonists: inhibitors of specific activities of estrogen and androgen. *Recent Prog Horm Res* 1964;20:435–490.
621. McGuire WL, Carbone PP, Sears ME, Escher GC. Estrogen receptors in human breast cancer: an overview. In: McGuire WL, Carbone PP, Vollmer EP, eds. *Estrogen receptors in human breast cancer.* New York: Raven Press, 1975;1–7.
622. Heise E, Gorlich M. Growth and therapy of mammary tumors induced by 7,12-dimethylbenzanthracene in rats. *Br J Cancer* 1966;20:539–545.
623. Markaverich BM, Roberts RR, Finney RW, Clark JH. Preliminary characterization of an endogenous inhibitor of [^{3}H]estradiol binding in rat uterine nuclei. *J Biol Chem* 1983;258:11663–11671.
624. Asch RH, Rojas FJ. The effects of RW 486 on the luteal phase of the rhesus monkey. *J Steroid Biochem* 1985;22:227–230.
625. Herrmann W, Wyss R, Riondel A, et al. The effects of an antiprogesterone steroid in women: interruption of the menstrual cycle and of early pregnancy. *CR Sci Acad Sci (III)* 1982;294:933–938.
626. Raynaud J-P, Ojasco T. The relevance of structure affinity relationships in the study of steroid hormone action. In: Eriksson H, Gustafsson JA, eds. *Steroid hormone receptors: structure and function.* Amsterdam: Elsevier Science, 1983.
627. Healy DL, Baulieu EE, Hodgen GD. Induction menstruation by an antiprogesterone steroid (RU 486) in primates: site of action, dose-response relationships, and hormonal effects. *Fertil Steril* 1983;40:253–257.
628. Philibert D, Moguilewske M, Mary I, et al. Pharmacological profile of RU 486 in animals. In: Baulieu EE, Segal SJ, eds. *The antiprogestin steroid RU 486 and human fertility control.* New York: Plenum Press, 1985;49–68.
629. Horwitz KB. The antiprogestin RW 38486: receptor-mediated progestin versus antiprogestin actions screened in estrogen-insensitive T47D human breast cancer cells. *Endocrinology* 1985;116:2236–2245.
630. Gray OG, Leavitt WW. RU 486 is not an antiprogestin in the hamster. *J Steroid Biochem* 1987;28:493–497.
631. El-Ashry D, Onate SA, Nordeen SK, Edwards DP. Human progesterone receptor complexed with the antagonist RU 486 binds to hormone response elements in a structurally altered form. *Mol Endocrinol* 1989;3:1545–1558.
632. Bagchi MK, Tsai SY, Tsai MJ, et al. Progesterone-dependent cell free transcription: identification of a functional intermediate in receptor activation. *Nature* 1990;345:547–550.
633. Meyer ME, Pornon A, Ji JW, Bocquel MT, Chambon P, Gronemeyer H. Agonistic and antagonistic activities of RU 486 on the functions of the human progesterone receptor. *EMBO J* 1990;12:3923–3932.
634. Okulicz WC. Effect of the antiprogestin RU-486 on progesterone inhibition of occupied nuclear estrogen receptor in the uterus. *J Steroid Biochem* 1987;28:117–122.
635. Benhamou B, Garcia T, Lerouge T, et al. A single amino acid that determines the sensitivity of progesterone receptors to RU 486. *Science* 1992;255:206–209.
636. Okulicz WC. Temporal limitation of progesterone inhibition of occupied nuclear estrogen receptor retention in the rat uterus. *Prog Endocr Soci* 1985;81, abst 322.

The Reproductive System

The Male

The Physiology of Reproduction, Second Edition,
edited by E. Knobil and J.D. Neill,
Raven Press, Ltd., New York © 1994.

CHAPTER 18

Anatomy, Vasculature, Innervation, and Fluids of the Male Reproductive Tract

Brian P. Setchell, S. Maddocks, and the late D. E. Brooks

ANATOMY

The male reproductive tract consists of two testes, two epididymides, each with its ductus deferens, and the accessory glands, as shown in Figs. 1 and 2. The reproductive organs of the male rat, which is a species in which all the main accessory glands are present, are shown in Fig. 3. The testes are formed from the primordial germ cells, which migrate from the yolk sac to the genital ridge of the mesonephros, where they form the primary epithelial or medullary cords in association with somatic cells from the genital ridge. This gonad then appropriates the duct system of the degenerating mesonephros or wolffian duct to form the epididymis, ductus deferens, ampulla, and seminal vesicles (vesicular glands). The prostate and bulbourethral (Cowper's) glands are derived from the urogenital sinus or urethra. The main portion of the wolffian duct develops into the epididymis, a single tubule of considerable length that is coiled on itself and comes to lie around one margin of the testis. It leads sperm from the efferent ducts of the testis to the ductus deferens. The lower end of the ductus deferens may possess a glandular wall to form the ampullary gland. In primates, the duct of the seminal vesicle joins the ductus deferens to form a common duct, the ejaculatory duct, which opens into the urethra. However, in most mammals the seminal vesicles have separate openings into the

Department of Animal Sciences, Waite Agricultural Research Institute, University of Adelaide, South Australia

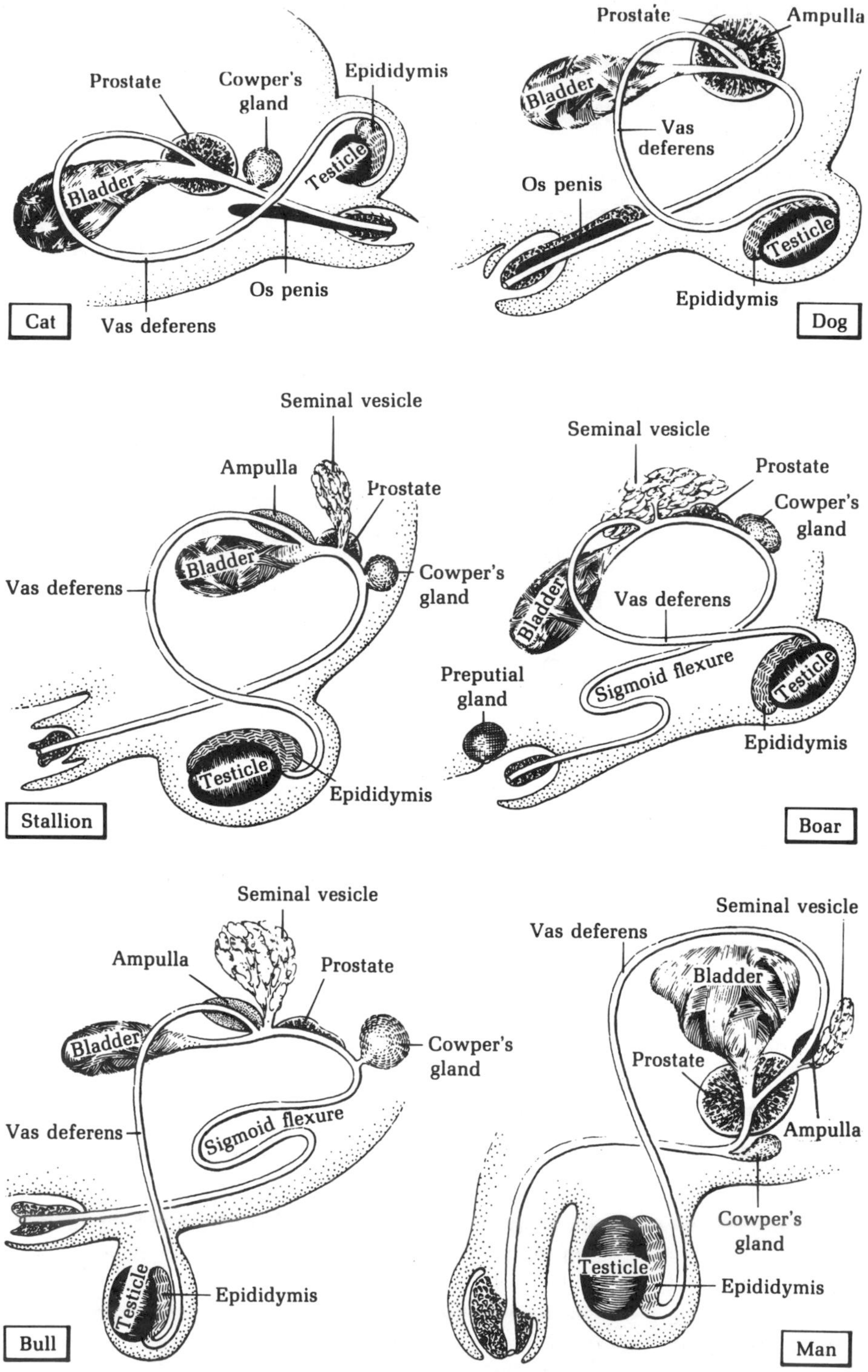

FIG. 1. Schematic representation of the genital tracts of man, dog, stallion, boar, bull, and tom cat. Where a common duct drains the contents of the ductus deferens and the seminal vesicles into the urethra, as occurs in man, it is known as the ejaculatory duct. (From ref. 833.)

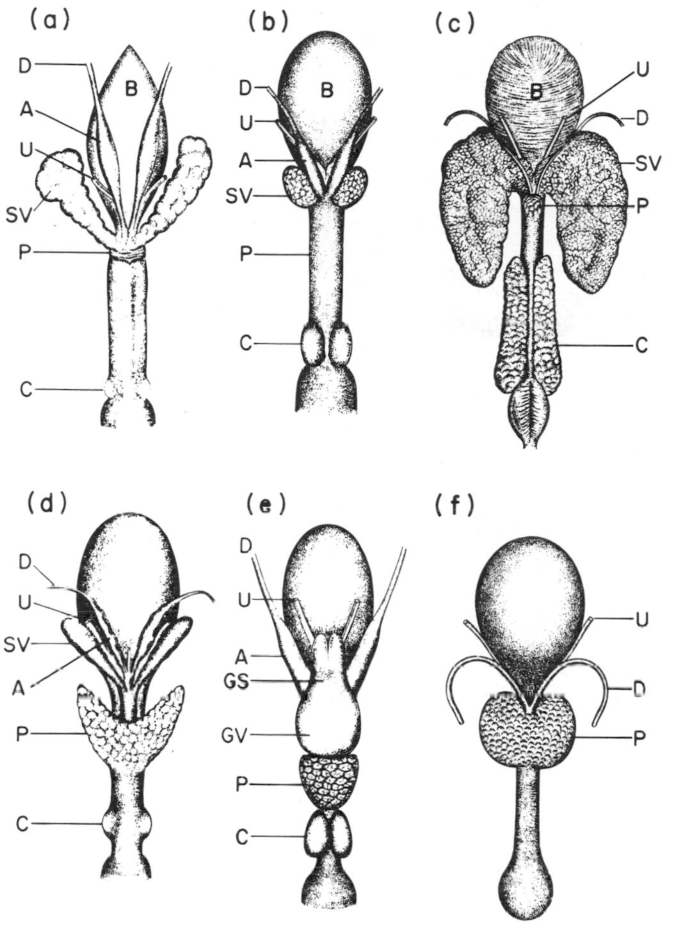

FIG. 2. Diagrammatic view of the dorsal aspect of the male accessory glands in various species. **(a):** bull; **(b):** ram; **(c):** boar; **(d):** stallion; **(e):** rabbit; **(f):** dog. SV, seminal vesicle; P, prostate (disseminate in ram); C, Cowper's glands; A, ampulla; D, ductus deferens; U, ureter; B, bladder; GS, glandula seminalis; GV, glandula vesiculàris. (From ref. 1040.)

urethra, close to the openings of the deferent ducts. The prostate glands are associated with the proximal urethra and generally drain into it through multiple ducts at the level of the colliculus seminalis. The bulbourethral glands drain into the distal urethra in the region of the urethral bulb. Besides these principal male accessory glands, there are small mucus-secreting glands (glands of Littré) that open into the urethra along its length, as well as preputial glands that are modified sebaceous glands, of ectodermal origin, emptying into the prepuce.

There is considerable variation between and within orders of mammals with respect to the range of accessory glands that are represented (Table 1). Apart from the excurrent duct system of the testis (i.e., the epididymis and ductus deferens), which is present in all species, the only other accessory gland present in virtually all mammals is the prostate gland. In some mammals, such as cetaceans and carnivores, the prostate is the only male accessory gland. Practically all other mammals have at least one pair of bulbourethral glands, which are especially well developed in certain insectivores (e.g., moles) and squirrels.

However, it should be remembered that nomenclature of glands in early descriptive studies was based on anatomic relationships and gross morphologic appearance and does not necessarily reflect the functional relationships of the glands. This is exemplified by somewhat confusing differences in chemical composition of secretions from similarly named glands in various species (746).

Testis

The testes in all mammals are paired encapsulated ovoid organs consisting of seminiferous tubules separated by interstitial tissue. Their size varies, depending on the species; in rodents and ungulates, they can be as much as 1% or more of body weight (see ref. 1032), whereas in the human and some apes, they are considerably smaller (444). The largest testes, as a proportion of body weight are to be found in a tiny Australian marsupial, *Tarsipes spenceri,* whose testes can reach 5% of body weight (619). There are two similar, closely related genera of Australian rodents (*Pseudomys* and *Notomys*) between which testis size differs by a factor of 20! (113). Testis weight increases manyfold at puberty and in some species at the beginning of each breeding season (see refs. 706,1032). In humans, it decreases slightly with age (578,1123).

Descent of the Testis

In most mammals, the testes migrate from their original site, and in many, they pass through the abdominal wall into an evagination of the peritoneum to form a scrotum. In some species (e.g., sheep and cattle), the testis has reached the scrotum by the time of birth (in cattle, descent is complete by 18 to 20 weeks of pregnancy) (1403), but in others such as rats and dogs, the testis reaches its final position only after birth. This process of testicular descent has been divided into three stages: nephric displacement, transabdominal movement, and inguinal passage (398,546,1277; but cf ref. 1213). The last phase involves a structure known as the gubernaculum, which develops in the caudal end of the nephrogenic cord. It was formerly believed that the gubernaculum played no active role in testicular descent, merely providing a space into which the testis descended (52,53), but later evidence suggested that outgrowth of the gubernaculum through the inguinal canal and its enlargement in what is effectively a nondistensible tube forces it outward, with the testis following; regression of the gubernaculum completes the process of testicular descent (1277) (Fig. 4). It is probably incorrect to speak of contraction of the gubernaculum, as it contains no con-

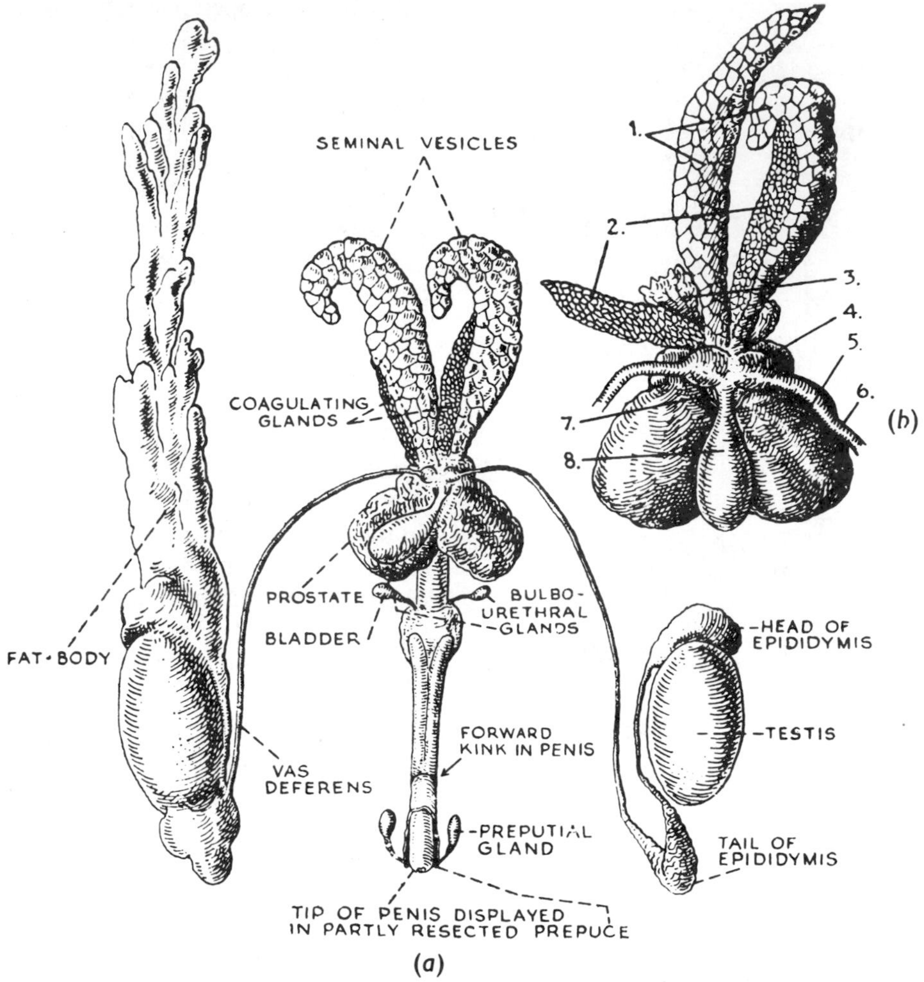

FIG. 3. Reproductive organs of the male rat. **(a):** Anterior view with the epididymal fat body removed on the left side; **(b):** magnified view of the prostatic lobes and seminal vesicles with the right lobe of the coagulating gland drawn away from the seminal vesicle to display the dorsolateral lobe of the prostate. 1, Seminal vesicles; 2, coagulating glands; 3, lobe of dorsolateral prostate; 4, ampullary gland; 5, lobe of ventral prostate; 6, ductus deferens; 7, ureter; 8, bladder (displaced downwards). (From ref. 306.)

tractile elements, and in any case, its distal insertion into the subcutaneous tissue is hardly a secure base from which to apply traction. Some authors believe that an intact hypothalamic-pituitary-testis axis is necessary for descent (945), but in pigs decapitated *in utero* before testicular descent has begun, the gubernaculum develops normally and initially the testis descends normally (214). Androgens appear to be responsible for the regression of the cranial gonadal suspensory ligament; in rats treated with flutamide, the ligament persists and the testis moves back up the abdominal cavity with the kidney as the ovary does normally between days 19 and 22 of gestation (1212,1214). Outgrowth of the gubernaculum in the dog certainly requires the presence of a testis (65), but it does not appear to involve androgens in this species (66) or in the rat (1214), although it may in the rabbit (318). There is no doubt that regression of the gubernaculum and hence the final stage of testicular descent do involve androgens (66). If the gubernaculum is cut near its cutaneous end in newborn rats, the testis on that side never descends; whereas if the cut is made nearer the testis, the vaginal process of the peritoneum forms normally, but it often remains empty as there is nothing to hold the testis and epididymis in the scrotum (71,90,375,1275). If one gubernaculum is removed or the distal attachment severed unilaterally, the testis on that side often descends into the contralateral scrotal sac, even when the contralateral testis has also descended there normally (375).

It has been suggested (548) that this is because the genital branch of the genitofemoral nerve passes downward behind the spermatic cord and testis and enters the gubernaculum from its distal end (1162). Certainly, division of this nerve leads to cryptorchidism (70,699), and this nerve supplies the scrotal area before testicular descent occurs; the nuclei in the spinal cord from which it arises appear to be sexually dimorphic. The nerves in the gubernaculum contain calcitonin gene-related peptide (CGRP) (670), and injection of an antagonist to

TABLE 1. *Occurrence of male accessory reproductive glands in various mammalian orders*[a]

Mammalian order	Ampulla	Seminal vesicle	Prostate	Bulbo-urethral
Monotremata	−	−	−[b]	+
Marsupiala	−	−	+	+
Insectivora	±	±	+	+
Chiroptera	±	±	+	+
Primates	±	±	+	+
Carnivora	±	−	+	±
Perissodactyla	+	+	+	+
Artiodactyla	±	+	+	+
Hyraciodea	−	+	+	+
Proboscidea	+	+	+	+
Sirenia	−	+	+	−
Cetacea	−	−	+	−
Edentata	−	+	+	±
Pholidota	−	+	+	−
Rodentia	±	+	+	+
Lagomorpha	+	±	+	+

[a] + = The presence of a well-developed functioning gand; − = either a small vestigial gland or the absence of any rudiment.

[b] More recent opinion considers that glands lining the urethra of monotremes corresponds to the disseminate prostate found in marsupials and many eutherian mammals (163).

From ref. 936.

CGRP into the scrota of neonatal mice delays testicular descent (991).

It has been suggested that mullerian inhibiting substance (MIS), also known as antimullerian hormone (AMH), is responsible for the transabdominal migration of the testis (544,546,548). There is no doubt that in persistent mullerian duct syndrome, which is due to either a deficiency in or a failure to respond to AMH (425), the testes do not descend normally (545), but some believe that this is because the persistent mullerian duct mechanically hinders testicular descent (598). Further doubt has arisen from the observations that a female rabbit immunized against AMH gave birth to three litters, in which the males had persistent mullerian ducts but normally situated testes (918), and that some male transgenic mice chronically expressing high levels of AMH had undescended testes (75). Also, normal AMH levels are found in blood of cryptorchid boys (599). However, estrogen-treated fetal mice have cryptorchid testes and persistent mullerian ducts (547), and in patients with primary testicular agenesis, gonadal descent is proportional to the degree of mullerian duct regression (548,1014).

Cryptorchism occurs spontaneously in many mammals and is relatively common in pigs, horses, and men. When the testis does not descend properly, spermatogenesis does not proceed, and although some androgens are produced, the secretion rate is lower than normal (see ref. 1032), particularly if the condition is unilateral (263), because then there is no compensatory stimulation by the increased levels of luteinizing hormone (LH) (958). Spermatogenesis can be initiated in an abdominal testis by cooling it artificially, so it appears that temperature is the key (362).

The reason for the testis making this remarkable journey is not clear. Although a scrotal testis is damaged by warming to body temperature, movement to a cooler environment cannot be the prime motive because testicular migration within the abdominal cavity occurs in many mammals without any change in temperature (164). It has been suggested that the epididymis initiates the process and the testis just follows (72), but experiments in which the epididymis was returned to the abdominal cavity leaving the testis in the scrotum gave somewhat equivocal results (73), and in any case, these results are open to alternative explanation because of the disruption of lymphatic communications between the testis and epididymis during this procedure (1036).

Capsule

The capsule of the testis is often referred to as the tunica albuginea. It is a tough fibrous covering, which is really composed of three layers: an outer layer of visceral peritoneum, the tunica vaginalis, then the tunica albuginea proper, and on the inside, the tunica vasculosa (Fig. 5.), which is really a subtunical extension of the interstitial tissue, consisting of blood vessels and some Leydig cells in a loose connective tissue (see ref. 1032). In humans, the tunica albuginea and the rete together comprise about 20% of the testis of young men, and this value increases with age (1123). The tunica albuginea itself consists of fibroblasts and bundles of collagen, but in some species, there are appreciable numbers of smooth-muscle cells. These cells are particularly well developed in the rabbit (286,521) and horse (173) (Fig. 6) but can also be found in the dog and cat (684), man (521,667), and pig (173). In the rat (409,683) and sheep (173), these cells are mainly "myofibroblasts" rather than typical smooth-muscle cells. In the boar, the large- and medium-sized vessels are sandwiched between two layers, the outer consisting of dense collagenous tissue and the inner layer of collagen fibres, fibroblasts, Leydig cells, and small blood and lymph vessels; in this layer near the epididymal margin of the testis, myoid cells can be found also (864). The tunic is well innervated (78,668,996), although there appear to be few nerve terminals among the actual muscle cells (684) and the contractile activity is probably myogenic (445). The capsule also contains a few peptidergic nerves (19,663,1135) and also contains significant amounts of serotonin (5-HT) (158). The muscle cells are capable of rhythmic contractions (284,285), which seem to be more important in the rabbit than in the rat, mouse, hamster, or squirrel. These contractions may be important for the transport of sper-

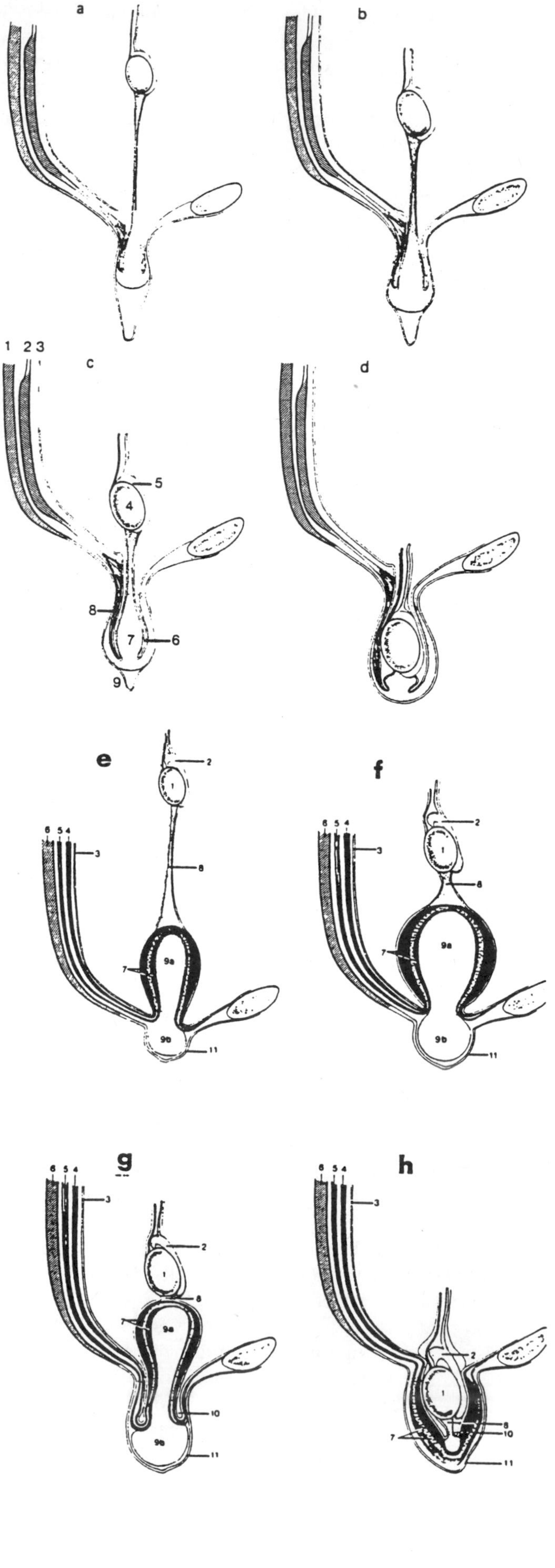

FIG. 4. a–d: Schematic drawings of 4 phases in the process of testicular descent in the pig fetus: a) 60 days post coitum: b) 70 days p.c.: c) 80 days p.c.: d) term, 114 days. 1) external oblique muscle. 2) internal oblique muscle. 3) parietal peritoneum. 4) testis. 5) epididymis. 6) cavity of the vaginal process. 7) gubernaculum. 8) cremaster muscle. 9) external spermatic fascia. **e–h:** Schematic drawings summarising testicular descent in the rat: e) 20 days post coitum. f) 20 days p.c. g) day of birth. h) 10 to 15 days after birth. 1) testis. 2) epididymis. 3) parietal peritoneum. 4) transverse abdominal muscle. 5) internal oblique muscle. 6) external oblique muscle. 7) cremaster muscle, divided into two layers. 8) gubernacular cord. 9a) mesenchyme of intra-abdominal segment of gubernaculum, forming with 7 the gubernacular cone. 9b) extra-abdominal segment of caudal part of gubernaculum. 10) vaginal process. (From ref. 1277).

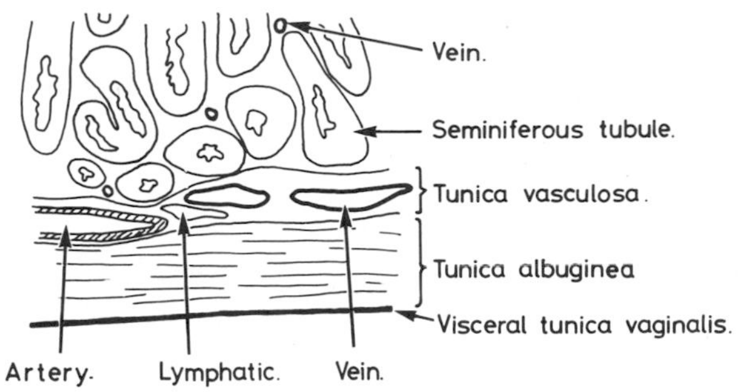

FIG. 5. Diagram (based on an actual section) of the tunics of the testis of a ram. The parenchyma of the testis is at the top of the drawing. (From ref. 1032.)

matozoa out of the testis into the epididymis (322), although in the rat, the flow of fluid from the rete testis is unaffected by removal of the capsule (370). Capsular contractions in the rabbit are maximal at a temperature of 32°C and are inhibited at higher or lower temperatures (281). The capsule contracts in response to acetylcholine, noradrenaline, adrenaline, and prostaglandin (PG) F_1, as well as to sympathetic nerve stimulation, and it relaxes when exposed to isopropylnoradrenaline and PGE_1 (282,283,285,446-448,575,955,956,1177). Histamine also stimulates contraction of the capsule, probably due, at least in part, to the secondary release of PGs (835). In man, the capsule contracts spontaneously at a frequency of about once every 14 min and in response to acetylcholine, noradrenaline, tetramethylammonium, and barium salts (284,346). In the pig, there were regular spontaneous contractions (five to 30 per 10 min) and noradrenaline, acetylcholine, and oxytocin all produced an increase in contractility (Fig. 7.), mainly in the form of a rise in tone (864). The myoid cells in the capsule are not apparent at birth but appear in the rat shortly before and in the rabbit at about the time of puberty (680,683).

As well as its influence on sperm transport, the capsule probably plays an important role in maintaining the interstitial pressure inside the testis. This pressure has been measured in dogs (957) and rats (365,524), and it increases after the administration of cadmium salts (638), but otherwise, little attention has been directed to this particular aspect. It was also suggested many years ago that the capsule may control the flow of blood through the testis because the testicular artery passes through the capsule at a very oblique angle (1013), but this interesting suggestion does not appear to have been followed up. In the capsule of the testis, particularly in the vicinity of the testicular artery, there are appreciable numbers of mast cells (848,1125), which may release vasoactive materials that influence the blood vessels of the testis.

Interstitial Tissue

The interstitial tissue (Fig. 8.) fills up the spaces between the seminiferous tubules and contains all the blood and lymph vessels and nerves of the testicular parenchyma (200,339–341). Also found there are the hormone-secreting Leydig cells, as well as appreciable numbers of mast cells (193,488,848) and macrophages (191,192,760,792,843) (Fig. 9). The close association of these macrophages with Leydig cells suggests some functional association, and the macrophages can be seen to endocytose portions of Leydig cell cytoplasm (791). In unilaterally cryptorchid rats, a reduction in macrophage cell size is correlated with a reduction in Leydig cell size (84). In bilaterally cryptorchid mice, the number of Leydig cells increases, but the size of each cell is reduced, so that the total volume of Leydig cells does not change as an absolute value, although as a percentage of the whole testis or of interstitial tissue, there is an increase; the absolute total and relative volumes of the macrophages show no consistent changes (781). The macrophages may respond to endocrine stimuli as they are reported to have receptors for follicle-stimulating hormone (FSH) (878) and to increase their production of lactate and other biochemical activities when stimulated with this hormone (1323–1325). However, their role(s) in the testis is yet to be established. They possess a number of the attributes required for immunologic activity (Fc receptors, expression of MHC II) but appear to be deficient in the secretion of immunologically important cytokines such as interleukin-1 (IL-1) (620). They may play a role in Leydig cell steroidogenesis, and their depletion from the testis leads to a reduction in testosterone secretion (732). Macrophages such as those found in the testis of the rat are not found in the testis of the ram, suggesting species differences in the occurrence and significance of this interstitial cell type (929). Some of the Leydig cells appear to be associated with blood vessels (339,341); others are found nearer to the walls of the seminiferous tubules, and these latter cells show variations in size and structure depending on the spermatogenic stage of the adjacent tubules (82,83). The connective tissue of the interstitial tissue, as well as the peritubular tissue, is rich in fibrinonectin (1128).

The amount of interstitial tissue varies between species (335) (Fig. 8), from about 10% of the tissue in guinea pigs and dogs, about 15% in sheep and most rodents and marsupials, 25% to 30% in man to about 30% in stallions and almost 40% in pigs (64,113,577,688,806,808,902, 1124,1215) and didelphid and peramelid marsupials (see ref. 1031). In the pig, Leydig cells appear to fill almost the entire space between the tubules (341), and by morphometric measurements, they occupy about 50% of the interstitial tissue (1215); there are about 90×10^6 Leydig cells per gram of testis, each cell about 2,000 μm^3 in volume (18,719). In mature stallions, there are about 25×10^6 Leydig cells per gram of testis, occupying about 60% of the interstitial tissue, each cell being about 7,000 μm^3 in volume (577), whereas in rats, there are about 14×10^6 Leydig cells in each gram of testis, occupying only 17% of the interstitial tissue, each cell being about

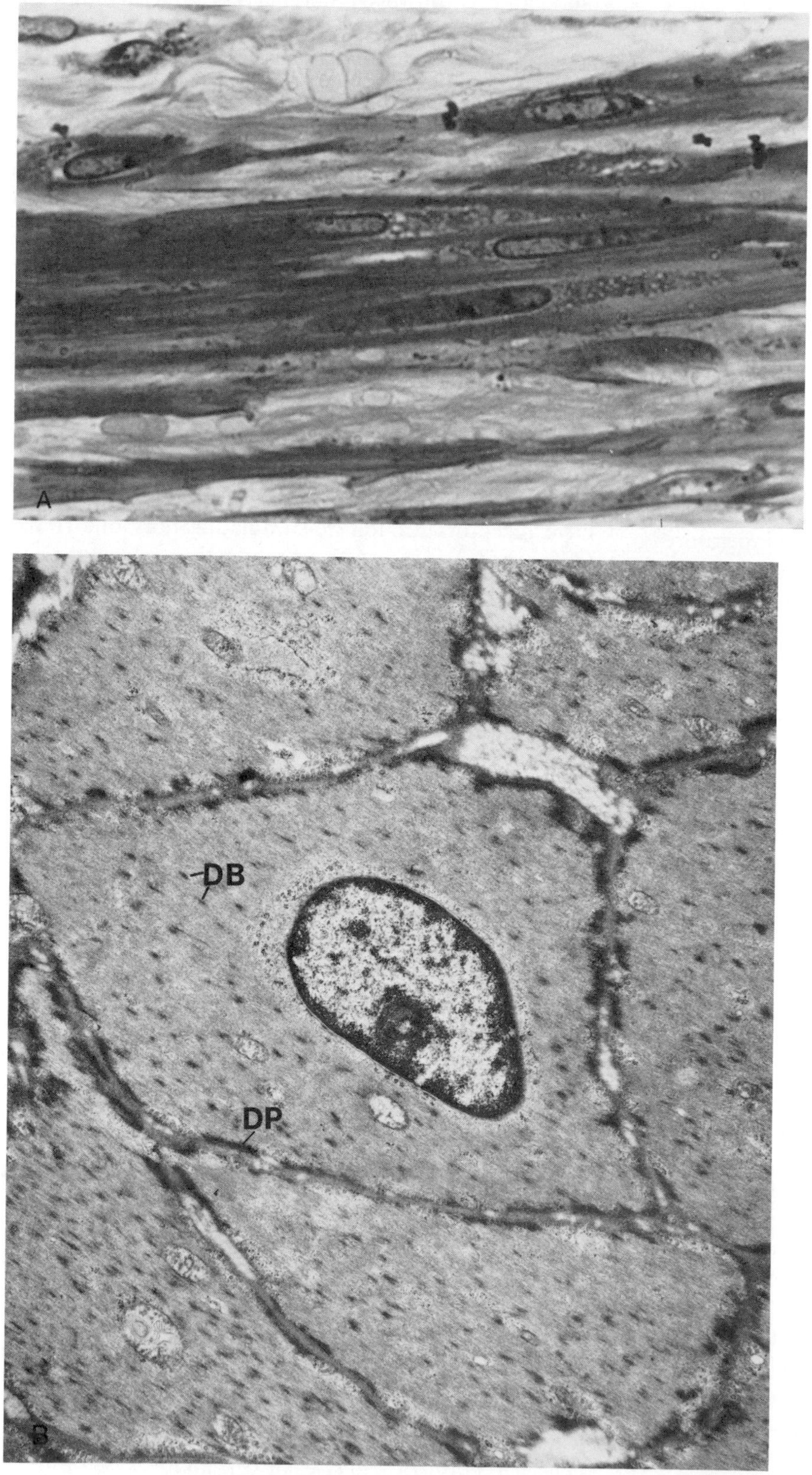

FIG. 6. The structure of the testicular capsule of the horse. **(A):** Section at right angles to the surface of the capsule showing a group of smooth muscle cells lying somewhat obliquely to the longitudinal axis. The cytoplasm beyond the poles of the nuclei is characteristically more granular. (Toluidine blue stain, ×1,120.) **(B):** Section parallel to the surface, showing the typical distribution of organelles including dense bodies (DB) and dense plaques (DP). There are numerous intercellular junctions involving opposing dense plaques with an intervening condensation of extracellular matrix; no gap junctions could be found. (×992.) (From ref. 173.)

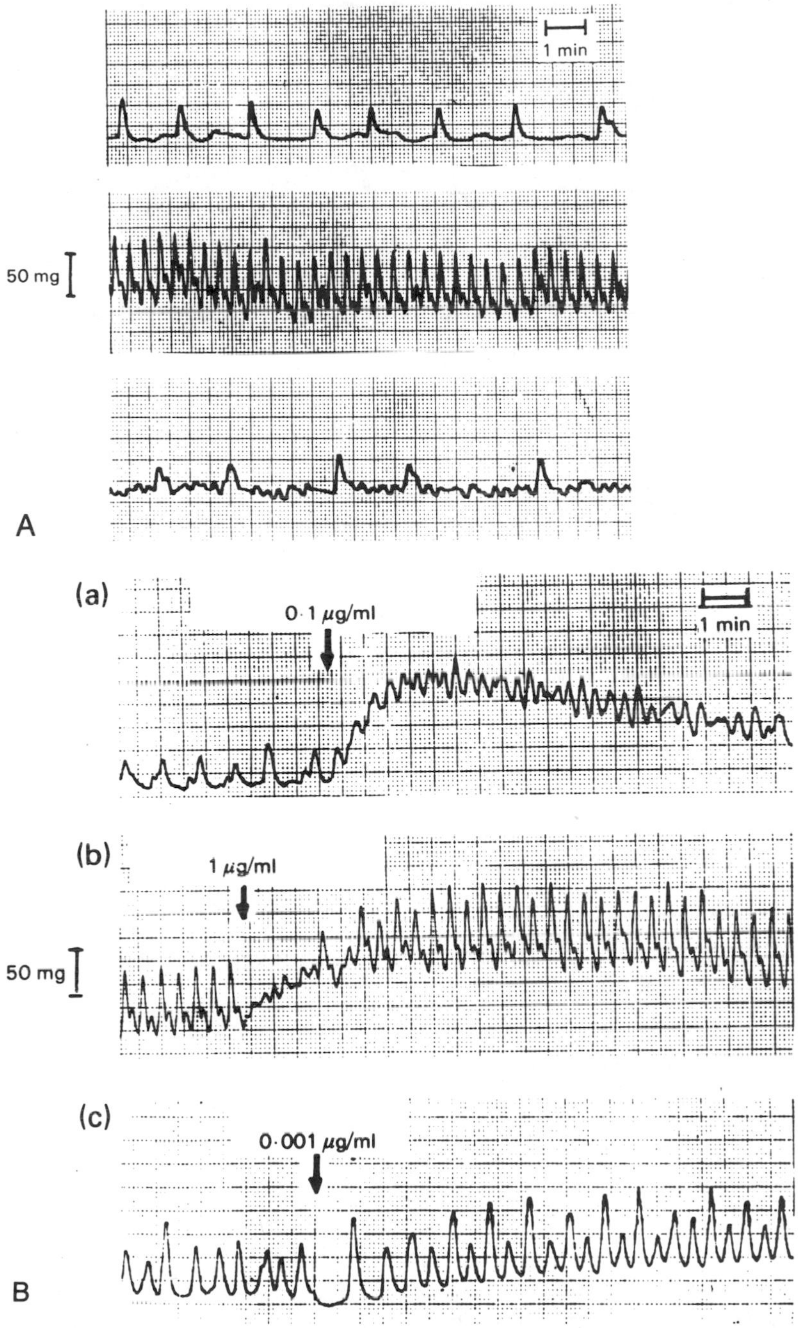

FIG. 7. Contractions of the testicular capsule of the boar. **A:** Different patterns of spontaneous contractions of part of the capsule from the mid-posterior border. **B:** The effect of (a) norepinephrine, (b) acetylcholine, and (c) oxytocin on the contractions. (From ref. 864.)

1,200 μm³ in volume (806); in mice, there are 25 × 10⁶ Leydig cells per gram of testis, occupying 35% of the interstitial tissue, each cell being about 1,500 μm³ in volume (808). The corresponding values in another study are 13.2 × 10⁶/g, 60%, and 4,000 μm³ (781). In hamsters, there are 15 × 10⁶ Leydig cells per gram of testis, each cell about 1,100 μm³ in volume (1108), and in guinea pigs, there are 6 × 10⁶ Leydig cells per gram, about 10% of interstitial tissue, and each cell about 1,400 μm³ (807); in an Australian rodent (*Notomys alexis*) with very small testes, the Leydig cells occupy about 50% of the interstitial tissue (902). In rams, there are about 30 × 10⁶ Leydig cells per gram of testis, but they make up only about 8% of the interstitial tissue, as each cell has a volume of only about 350 μm³ (510,1070). In stallions, the numbers of Leydig cells increase from 1.4 to 4.7 × 10⁹ with age between 2 and 20 years (577). No explanation has been advanced for this difference in Leydig cell numbers or volume, but it is interesting that in two species with abundant large Leydig cells, the pig and the horse, the testis secretes large amounts of oestrogens (1042,1073).

Seminiferous Tubules

Most of the testis is made up by the seminiferous tubules (Fig. 10.), where the spermatozoa are formed. In

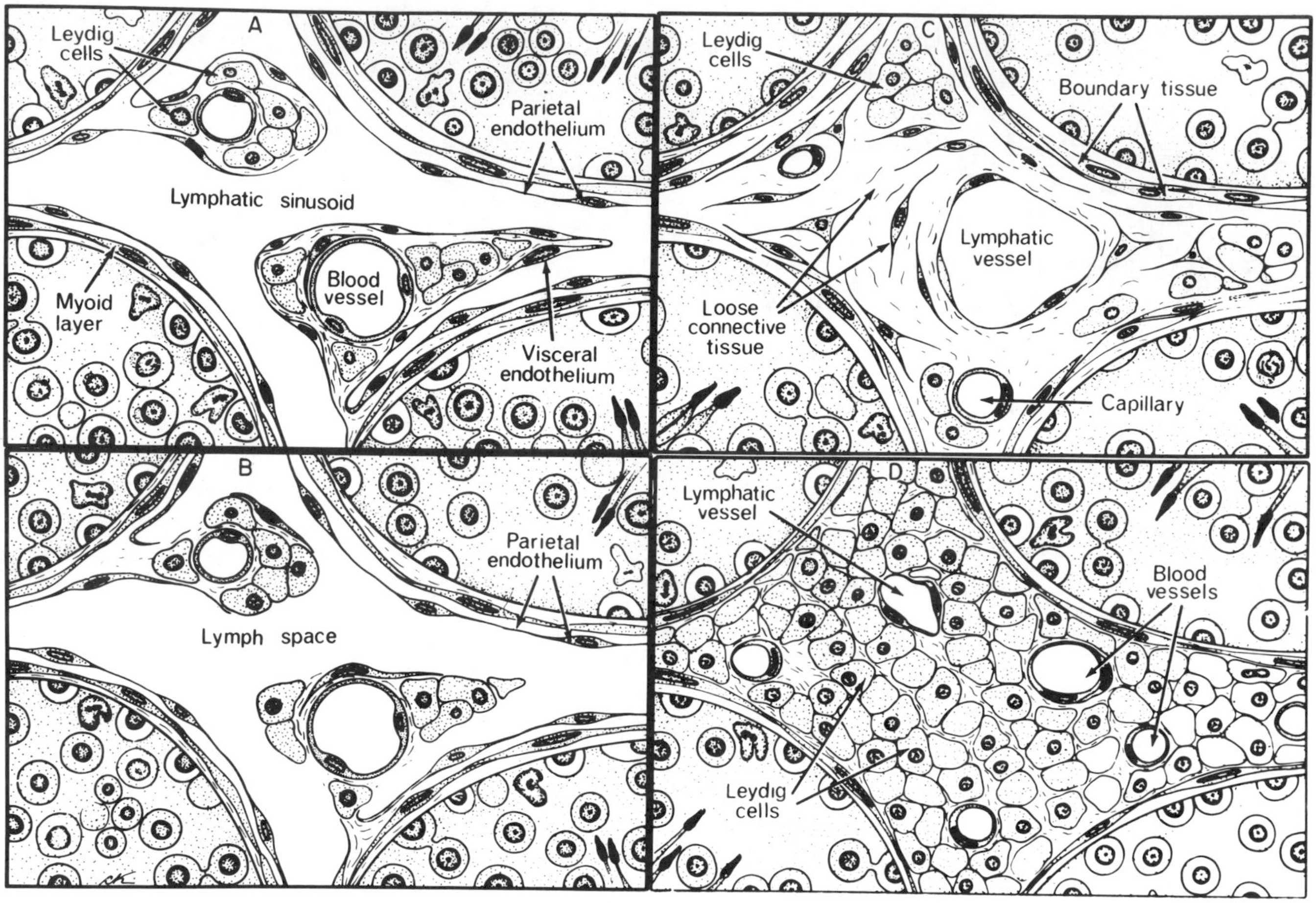

FIG. 8. Diagram of the interstitial tissue of various species. **A:** Guinea pig, showing the Leydig cells clustered around the blood vessels, with the groups of cells completely surrounded by endothelial cells and "floating" in a fluid-filled lymphatic sinusoid. **B:** Rat, similar to the guinea pig, but with an incomplete investment of endothelial cells around the groups of Leydig cells. **C:** Sheep and man, with the Leydig cells either in groups near a blood vessel or in a loose connective tissue. **D:** Pig, with the interstitial tissue packed with numerous Leydig cells, with very inconspicuous blood and lymph vessels. (From ref. 335.)

most species, these tubules are between 200 and 350 μm in diameter. However, in some Australian marsupials, in particular the dasyurids and peramelids, the tubules are almost twice this diameter (1122,1394), but the significance of this difference is obscure. In the rat, there are about 12 m of tubules per gram of testis, with a surface area of about 120 cm/g (1382).

In rams, the tubules are about 3,000 m in total length, about 11 m/g, with a basal area of about 85 cm^2/g (600). In stallions, there are about 15 m of tubules per gram of testis parenchyma (667). In man, the tubules are slightly smaller in diameter, and there are between 15 and 25 m/g of testis (64,668,779); the length of the seminiferous tubules decreases with age, as testis weight falls (668). Hemicastration of piglets at 10 days after birth produced a doubling of seminiferous tubule length between 20 and 122 days of age (730). In most mammalian species, the tubules are two-ended, convoluted loops, with both ends opening into the rete testis (Fig. 11.). In rats, it has been shown that there are normally about 30 tubules (302), but there are many more in humans and in farm animals. There may be as few as five in some of the dasyurid marsupials (1303) and even fewer in *Sminthopsis crassicaudata* (W. G. Breed and E. J. Pierce, *personal communication*). In humans, the tubules are arranged in about 300 lobules, each containing between one and four tubules (676), and lobulation is much more obvious than in some other animals (e.g., bulls) (474). It has been suggested that in humans, hypercurvature of the seminiferous tubules may be a cause of infertility (48,49). In mature rats, each tubule has a lumen with a diameter of between 50 and 100 μm along most of its length (1027,1291), although this value does increase to about double in the area where the spermatozoa are just about to be released (621,985,1089). The lumen in rats first appears at about 15 days of age in some tubules and is present in all tubules by 25 days but continues to enlarge until the rat is at least 60 days old (985,1075). Its formation seems to depend on the formation and integrity of Sertoli cell–Sertoli cell tight junctions, rather than the

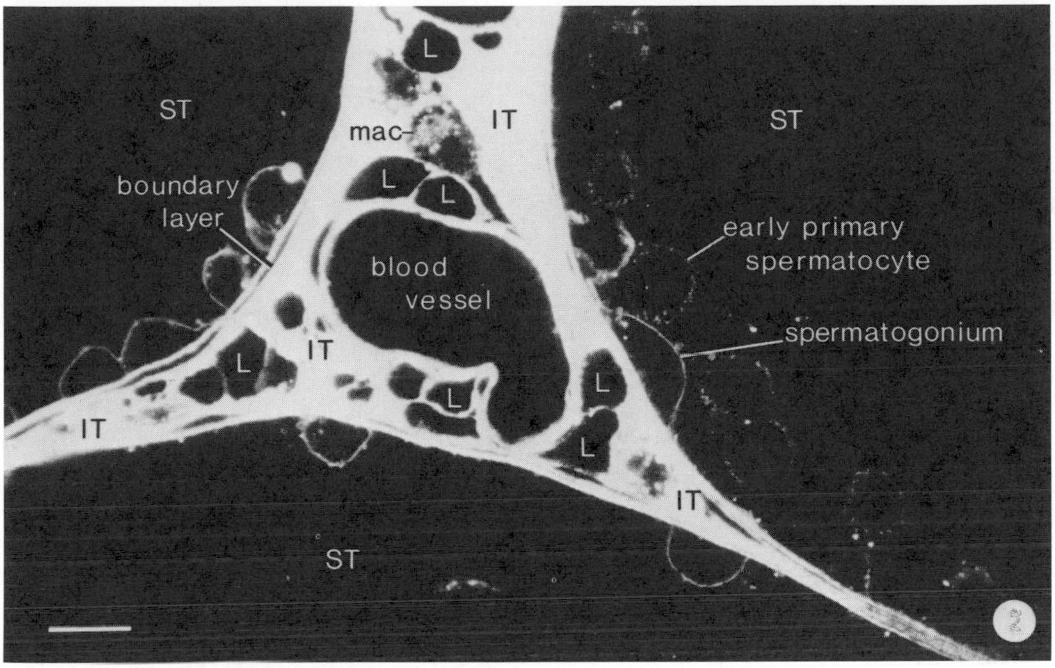

FIG. 9. A fluorescent light micrograph of the interstitial tissue of a frozen section of a rat testis which had been treated with a fluorescein-coupled antibody to rat serum albumin. Albumin fills the interstitial tissue (IT) except for the Leydig cells (L); a macrophage (mac) has taken up some of the albumin. The seminiferous tubules (ST) contain no detectable albumin, except around the spermatogonia and early primary spermatocytes. (From ref. 193.)

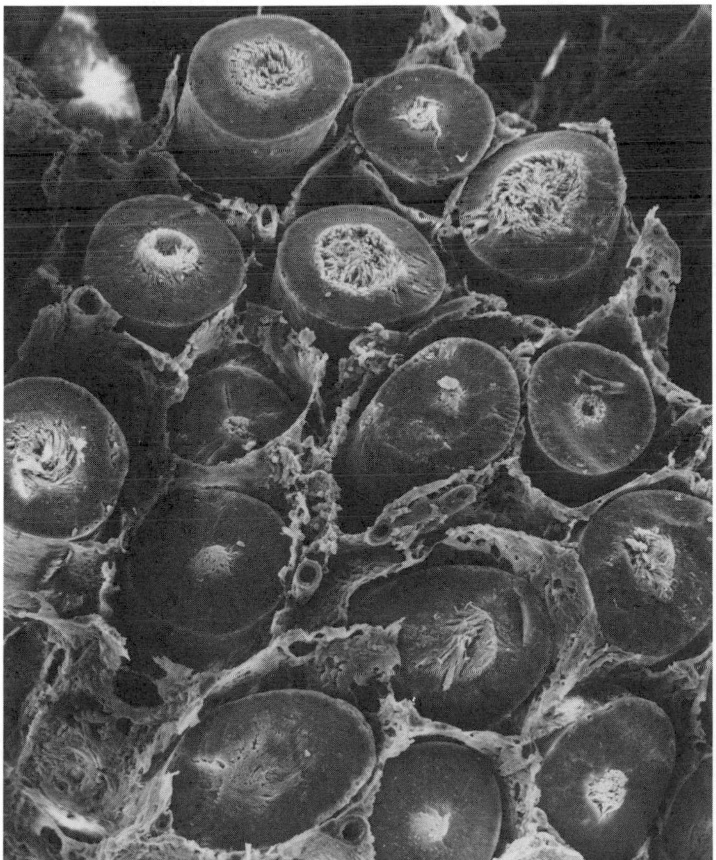

FIG. 10. A scanning electron micrograph of a cut surface of a rat testis. Note the individual seminiferous tubules embedded in the interstitial tissue. (Electron micrograph supplied by Dr. A. K. Christensen, Department of Anatomy and Cell Biology, The University of Michigan Medical School, Ann Arbor, MI.)

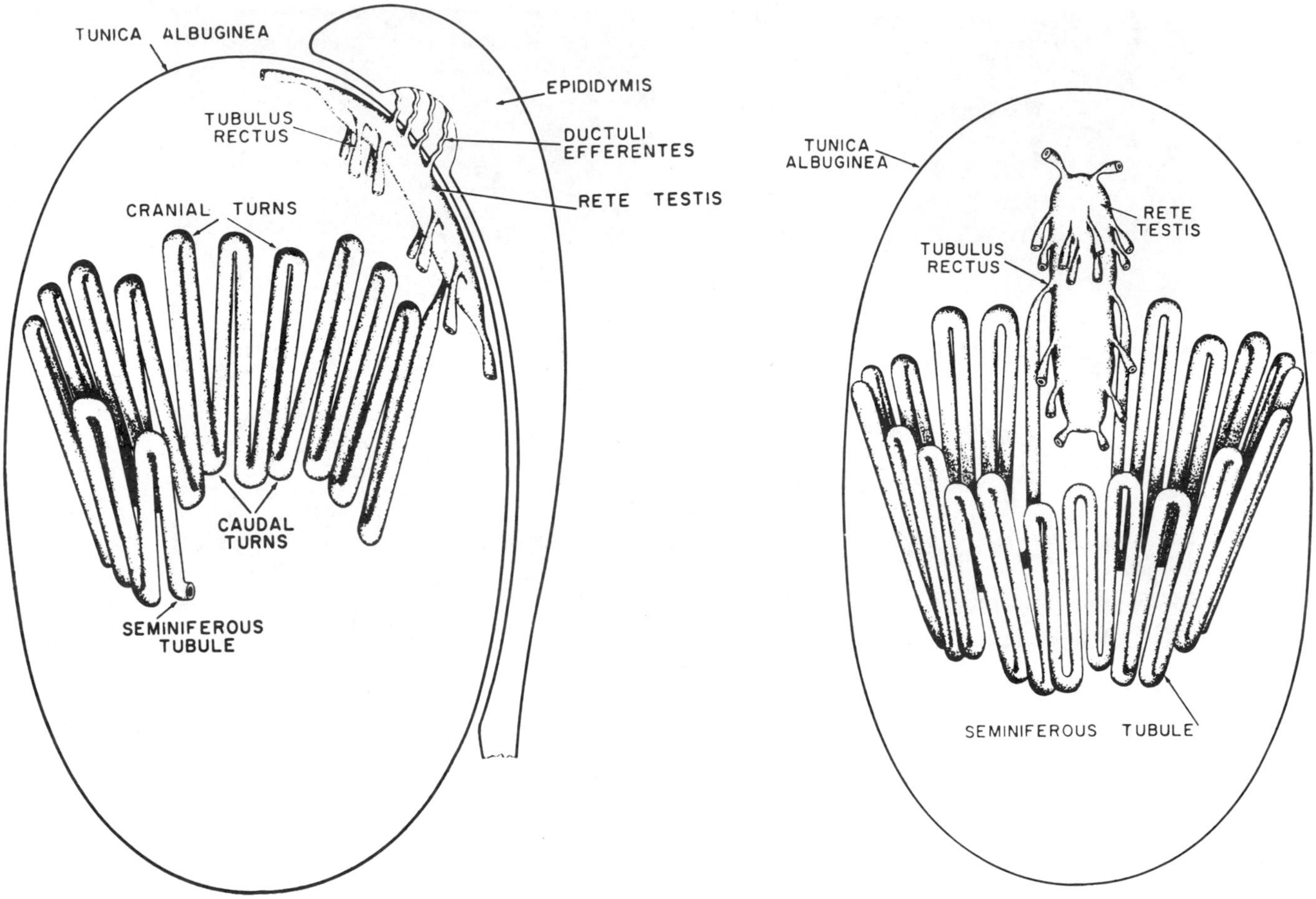

FIG. 11. A diagram of the anatomy of an individual seminiferous tubule and the rete testis of a rat. **Left:** Only part of one tubule is shown, and only some of the junctions of seminiferous tubules with the rete testis are depicted. (From ref. 212.)

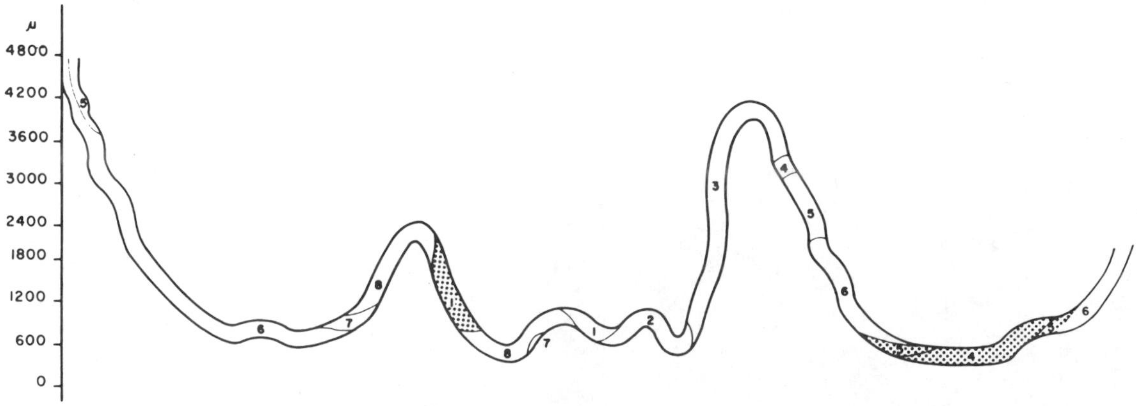

FIG. 12. A diagram of seminiferous tubule of a rat, showing a complete spermatogenic wave. The stages are arranged from left to right, and the wave includes two modulations (*dotted shading*). (From ref. 509.)

presence of germ cells (731,905,906,1169). During seasonal regression of the testis in hamsters, the lumen shows a greater proportional decrease in size than the tubule as a whole (1108). The lumen of the seminiferous tubules in humans is larger near the poles of the testis than in the equatorial region (1124). For some unexplained reason, successive stages of the spermatogenic cycle are arranged in descending order along the tubule, beginning at the rete (Fig. 12.). Consequently, these two "waves" meet at a point along the length of the tubule, the "site of reversal," and there are modulations of the wave, where for short stretches, the order of the stages is reversed (509,909). In man, the wave is arranged helically (1011,1012).

The walls of the tubules of rodents are composed of four layers: an innermost layer of noncellular material, surrounded by a layer of smooth muscle-like or myoid cells, which are probably responsible for the peristaltic movements of the tubules (211,975); then there is a layer of collagen fibers; and finally on the outside, a layer of endothelial cells, which line the lymphatic sinusoids in the interstitial tissue (211; see ref. 1032 for earlier references). The myoid cells are extremely flat and are arranged in a single virtually continuous layer (821). A similar arrangement is found in rabbits (242,680), but in humans and monkeys (Fig. 13), there are multiple layers of myoid cells (147,490,647,982). There are five to seven cellular layers separated by laminae of connective tissue components; the innermost three or four layers are myofibroblasts, the outermost two or three ordinary fibroblasts, probably of interstitial origin (276), which possess receptors for nerve growth factor (1019). There are several layers of myoid cells in the ram (146) and cat (141), and in the ram and boar, the inner noncellular layer consists of several concentric layers (146,297). In the ram lamb, the myoid cells are apparent as early as 1 week after birth (146), but in the mouse (980), rat (635,681) and rabbit (680), they do not appear until about the time of puberty. Under scanning electron microscopy, the basal surface of the basement membrane of the seminiferous tubule appears like a tiled floor, with a meshwork of collagen fibres evident (1320). The development of the myoid cells in the mouse depends on the presence of pituitary hormones (114), but it is not clear whether these hormones act directly. Testosterone receptors seem to be present in these cells (998), and the contractility in organ culture of tubules from immature rats was enhanced by the addition of testosterone and inhibited by the antiandrogen, cyproterone acetate (528). In adult animals, testosterone, dihydrotestosterone, and estradiol added *in vitro* inhibited tubular contractions at low concentrations, whereas higher concentrations were without effect; pretreatment of the rats had a similar effect except that estradiol was inhibitory at all doses used (1202). Cyproterone acetate also impaired differentiation and the appearance of alkaline phosphatase in the myoid cells, whereas treatment with human chorionic gonadotrophin stimulated their division; this latter effect was not produced by testosterone (997). Myoid cells persist in hypophysectomized adult rodents (114,981), suggesting that the hormonal control of their differentiation may be different from that of their maintenance. Actin, myosin, tubulin, desmin, vimentin, and fibronectinlike proteins have been demonstrated in peritubular cells (276,422, 986,1128,1176,1184,1238).

Isolated tubules from rats older than 15 days contract

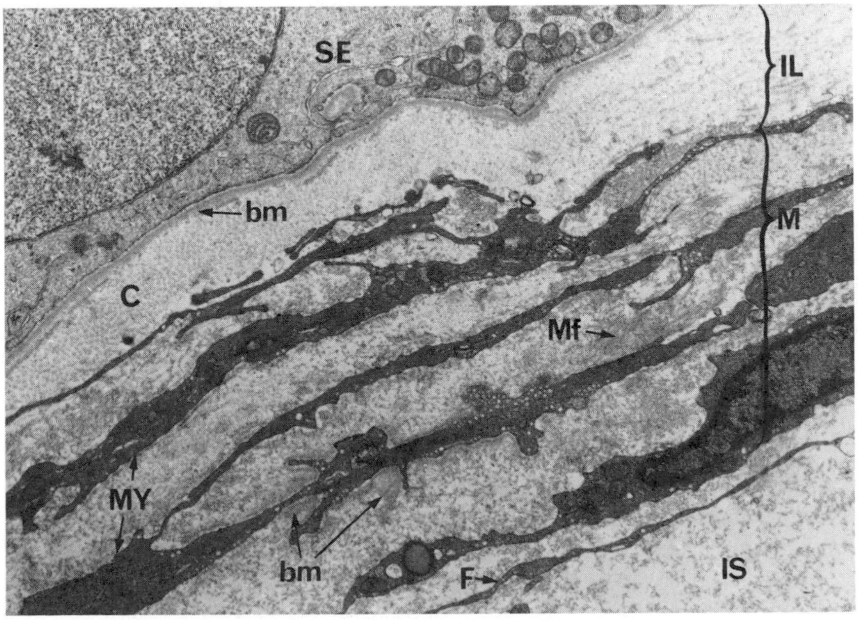

FIG. 13. A low-power electron micrograph of the peritubular tissue in a human testis. The seminiferous epithelium (SE) is towards the *top* and the interstitial tissue (IS) towards the *bottom*. The peritubular tissue shows three distinct zones; a thick inner lamella (IL) containing a large amount of collagen (C), poorly stained in this preparation; a myoid layer (M) composed of several layers of myoid cells (MY) interspersed with connective tissue lamellae, and an adventitial layer of fibrocytes (F). The myoid cells contain many more filaments than the fibrocytes, which show only a few caveolae associated with the plasma membrane. The connective tissue lamellae contain abundant microfibrils (Mf) as well as collagen. There is a continuous basement membrane (bm) underlying the seminiferous epithelium, and similar material (bm) is also seen over small areas of the surfaces of the myoid cells. (From ref. 490.)

spontaneously *in vitro* (636) and respond to oxytocin (841); in very young rats at about the age when oxytocin levels in the testis are at a peak, there are no spontaneous contractions but the response to oxytocin is increased (1304). Melatonin, cyclic adenosine monophosphate (AMP), and theophylline decreased the frequency and depth of the contractions. PGE_1 had a stimulatory effect at low concentrations but was inhibitory at higher levels (321). The frequency and depth of contraction do not appear to be associated with any particular stages of the seminiferous cycle (1142) but increase if the temperature of incubation is increased (1141).

Contractility persists for about 3 weeks in cultured fragments of seminiferous tubules from adult rats, as does the enzyme alkaline phosphatase, which appears at about the age at which the tubules begin to contract (527,636). However, addition of cyproterone acetate to the culture medium eliminates contractions within 1 week, without affecting the enzyme levels (109). Contractions disappear from the fifth day after the testis has been made cryptorchid (1141), and the peritubular tissue becomes noticeably thickened as spermatogenesis becomes affected (622,685,987,1141), as seen during aging (578) after hypophysectomy and aspermatogenesis, but not after irradiation (647,659,1174). Myoid cells have been kept in culture and, under these conditions, secrete several proteoglycans and extracellular matrix, especially when cocultured with Sertoli cells (1110,1111,1184); the myoid cells also exercise important influences on Sertoli cells in cocultures (1202,1273).

Transitional Zone and Tubuli Recti

At each end of the seminiferous tubules, where they open into the rete testis (Fig. 14), there is a short transitional zone lined only with cells resembling Sertoli cells (301,332,487,712,819,881,884–886,1235,1310). These cells appear to form a valve or plug (see refs. 635,1028 for early references), which may prevent the passage of fluid from the rete into the tubules (976), although the effectiveness of this valve would depend on the state of the cells in the living animal. In later studies, it was found that in most of the tubules there was a narrow open channel (301,861), and the passage of injected dyes from the rete into the tubules (208) and the opening up of the channels after efferent duct ligation (862,883) would suggest that if they do act as valves, they are reasonably ineffective. The transitional zone is joined to the rete testis by a tubulus rectus, which is really a narrow extension of the rete proper and is lined with similar cells (883). In the human, up to six seminiferous tubules can join a single tubulus rectus (978). In the horse, junctions between seminiferous epithelium and transitional tubules can be found throughout the parenchyma (26). In bulls, the terminal segment of each seminiferous tubule is surrounded by a vascular plexus and consists of three parts, a transitional region, an intermediate portion, and a terminal plug; this terminal segment develops at between 25 and 40 weeks of age, just after the seminiferous tubules develop a lumen (1311).

Some dyes and horseradish peroxidase infused into an individual seminiferous tubule appear to be taken up by the cells of the tubulus rectus (501,1069), and the cells there appear to have phagocytic activity (487,819). The cells of the tubuli recti and the proximal part of the rete testis in the guinea pig are rich in glycogen (337).

Rete Testis

The rete testis is a complicated network of intercommunicating channels, in the bull about 30 in number (472); the channels are lined with cells that range from squamous to columnar, with comparatively few organelles; the cells are joined near their luminal boundaries by specialized junctions (80,148,302,586,635,661,682, 882,978,1309). The rete in the buffalo has a stratified epithelium (296), but in most other species, the cells are a mixture of columnar, cuboidal, and squamous, with a few intraepithelial lymphocytes and macrophages (413, 415,473,1234,1315). The cells lining the bull rete show an unusually high leucine aminopeptidase activity (473, 1308). The cells lining the rete in the rat are involved in both adsorptive and fluid-phase endocytosis (805). The rete can undergo cystic transformation after renal failure (850; see also 442).

Through this network, the spermatozoa and the fluid in which they are suspended are carried to the epididymis. In humans and monkeys, the rete lies along the epididymal edge of the testis (302,715,978). In the rat, it is a fairly simple sac just under the tunica albuginea near where the efferent ducts run to the epididymis (976). In some marsupials, it extends down both surfaces of the testis under the superficial arteries and veins (1031), whereas in ungulates, carnivores, rabbits, and guinea pigs, the rete is located near the center of the testis (Fig. 15), extending along about two-thirds of its long axis (see refs. 80,472,473,675,1028,1234). In the horse, there is a recognizable rete adjacent to the central vein, but other tubuli recti led individually to the dorsocranial pole of the testis, where they join the efferent ducts (26).

In all species, the rete testis appears to be located close to the testicular artery in part of its course on the surface of the testis or where the main branches of the testicular artery turn back into the parenchyma and begin to branch, and in the rat, it is covered by the veins of the intra-albugineal plexus (364). This significance of this arrangement is not yet fully understood, although it has been suggested that pulsatile blood flow through the arte-

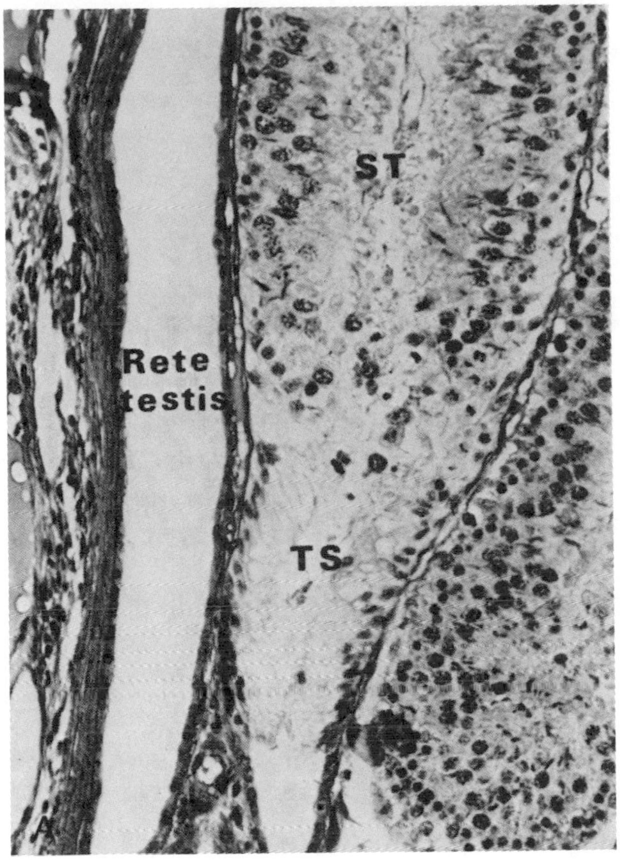

FIG. 14. The structure of the terminal segment of the seminiferous tubule. **A:** Photomicrograph (×300) of a longitudinal section through the terminal segment (TS) of a seminiferous tubule (ST) in a rat testis. The lumen appears to be completely occluded by vacuolated cytoplasmic processes of modified Sertoli cells. (From ref. 884.) **B:** Semi-schematic drawing of the transitional zone of a seminiferous tubule in a human, based on numerous semi-thin sections, with a similar valvelike structure formed by modified Sertoli cells, and a May'scher Pfropf consisting of a basal lamina and myoid cells protruding into the lumen of the tubulus rectus. (From ref. 713.)

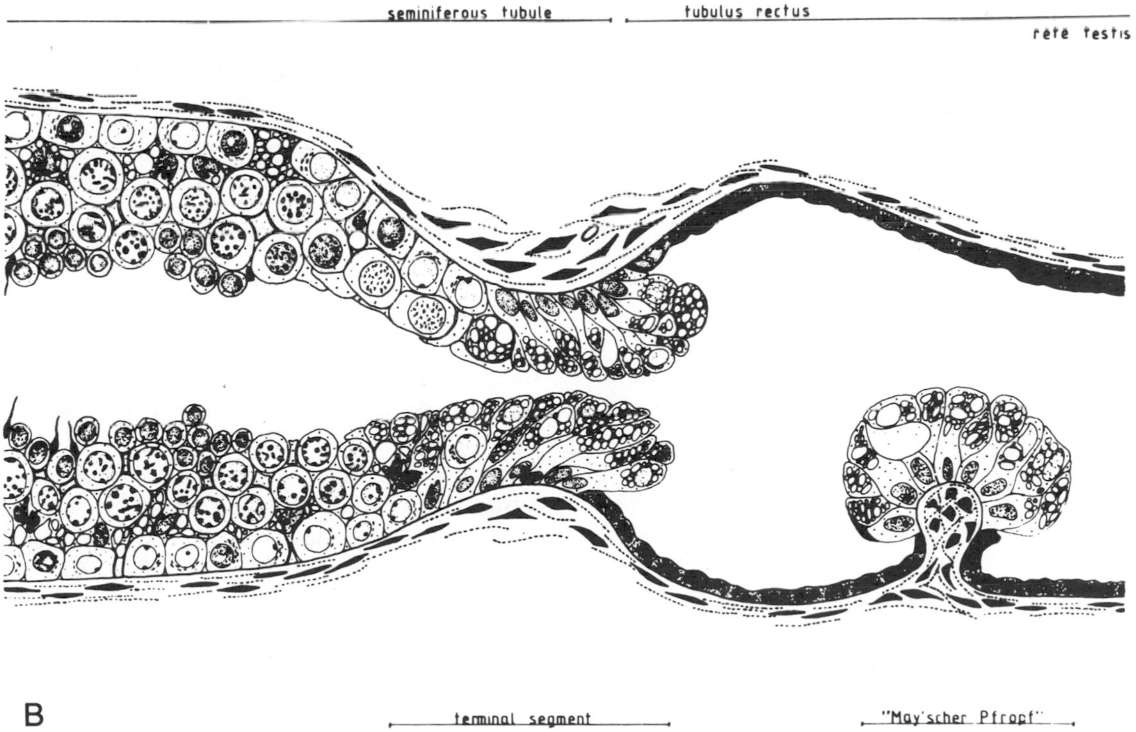

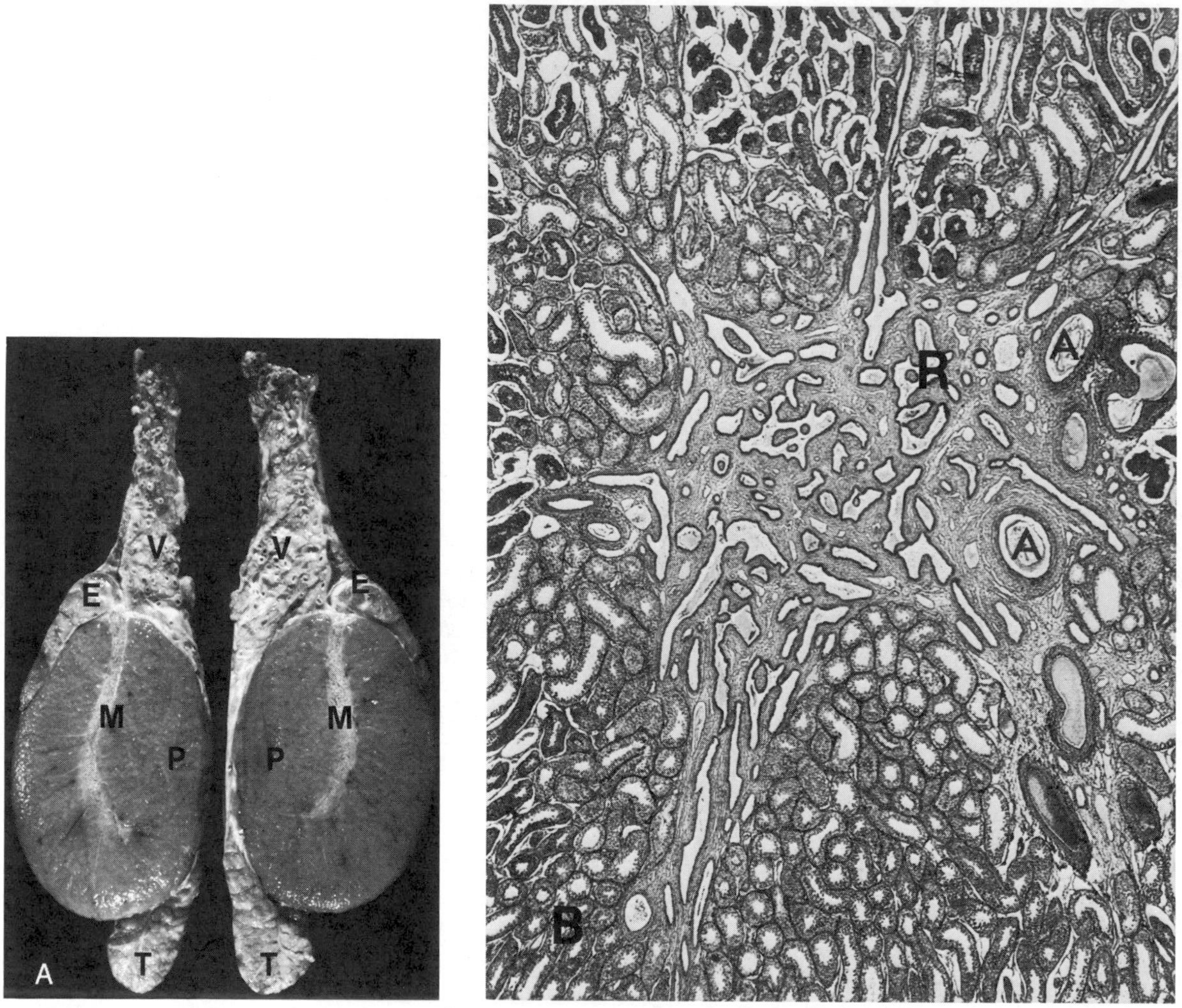

FIG. 15. The anatomy of the rete testis in the ram. **A:** A ram testis has been cut longitudinally to show the rete testis, which is situated in a fibrous mediastinum (M) along the long axis of the testis, surrounded by parenchyma (P); E: head of epididymis; T: tail of epididymis; V: vascular cone. **B:** A transverse section through a ram testis, showing the multiple channels of the rete (R) in a fibrous mediastinum, with arterial branches (A) cut in cross-section where they run near the rete. (From ref. 1032.)

rial coils near the rete may assist in transport of fluid and sperm into the epididymis (472,473). This idea is hard to reconcile with the fact that much of the pulse is removed from the arterial blood during its passage down the spermatic cord.

Efferent Ducts

The rete testis is linked to the epididymis by the efferent ducts. The position and dimensions of these depend on the relationship between the testis and epididymis; in rats and marsupials, the ducts are comparatively long because the epididymis is only loosely attached to the testis, whereas in man and the domestic animals, the epididymis is much more closely applied to the testis and the efferent ducts are correspondingly shorter. In humans, there are five or six efferent ducts (595,988), whereas in monkeys, there are between eight and 16 (715,948). In the rat, there are between two and nine ducts (80,220,302,432,592,701,1153), whereas in the domestic animals, there are between 13 and 20 efferent ducts (472,473,483,876), which show evidence of fluid resorption and acid phosphatase, esterase, β-glucuronidase, and carbonic anhydrase activity (414,1307). Some of these ductules may coalesce before they join the epididymal duct proper (cf ref. 595) (Fig. 16). Blind-ending ducts and other ducts that make no connection with the rete testis (abberrant ductuli) are not uncommon (432,483). At the testicular end, the ducts are only slightly convoluted but then become more convoluted to form the bulbous coni vasculosi, which then extend by a narrow isthmus to connect with the epididymal duct (Fig. 16). In pigs, the efferent ducts can be divided into a proximal or intratesticular and distal or epididymal segments, the former being thicker and the latter, long and flexuous (876).

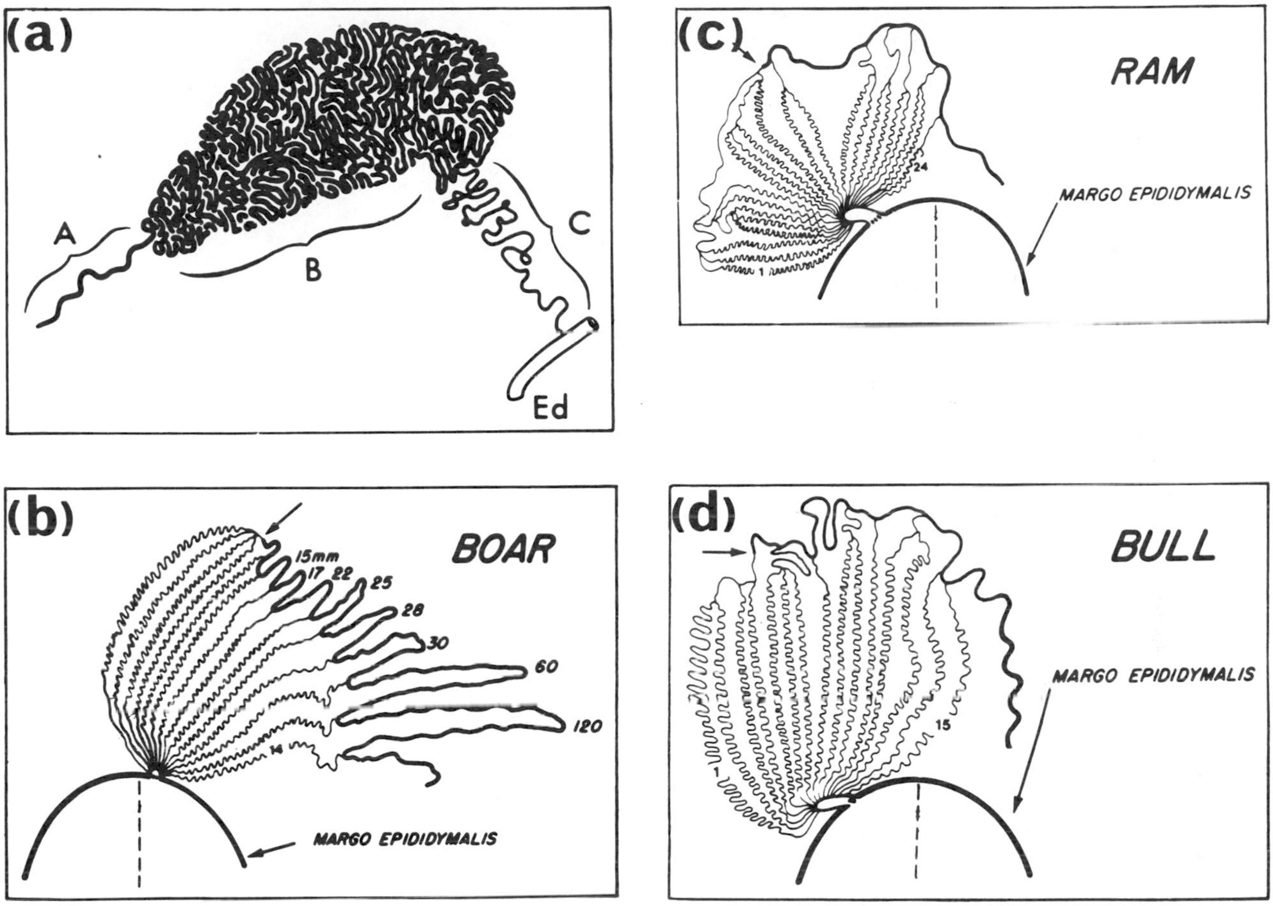

FIG. 16. Arrangement of ductuli efferentes in various species. **(a):** A single efferent ductule of a bull showing the slightly undulating testicular segment (A); the highly coiled cone segment (B); the moderately coiled epididymal segment (C); the epididymal duct (Ed). **(b), (c),** and **(d)** show the ductuli efferentes of the boar, ram, and bull, respectively. The ductuli are drawn to scale to show the relative coiled lengths of the ductuli. The first and last ductuli have numerals and the *arrow* marks the beginning of the epididymal duct. (From ref. 170.)

The epithelium of the efferent ducts is composed of two main cells types in most species, namely, principal and ciliated cells, along with intraepithelial lymphocytes; the principal cells are columnar, with prominent intercellular junctions near their luminal borders and a thick basal lamina. The ultrastructural features of the cells suggest only a low capacity for protein synthesis and secretion, but the nonciliated cells appear to be actively involved in fluid resorption (414,436,515,520,586,592, 660,661,715,809,876,948,988,1121,1316) and in fluid-phase and adsorptive endocytosis (489,804). In the horse, there is a sharp transition between the simple cuboidal cells of the rete and the columnar epithelium of the ducts; the efferent ducts are also surrounded by many more peritubular capillaries (26).

Epididymis

The epididymal duct is a single highly convoluted duct, closely applied to the surface of the testis extending from the anterior to the posterior pole of that organ and held more or less firmly, depending on the species, to the tunica albuginea by connective tissue. The duct is coiled into segments demarcated by connective tissue septula and the organ is contained within a fibrous tissue capsule. The segment into which the ductuli efferentes empty is usually referred to as the initial segment, and the remainder of the epididymis is loosely divided into three parts termed the caput, corpus, and cauda epididymidis (Fig. 17). An alternative subdivision, based on histologic and functional criteria, has been proposed (407). In this system, the epididymis is subdivided into three regions: the initial, middle, and terminal segments (Fig. 18). The initial and middle segments are primarily concerned with sperm maturation, whereas the terminal segment coincides with the region where mature sperm are stored before ejaculation or voidance into the urine.

These subdivisions of Glover and Nicander (407) do not necessarily coincide with the more traditional subdivision of initial segment, caput, corpus, and cauda. This is particularly apparent in the case of the guinea pig in which the corpus region should be classified as part of the

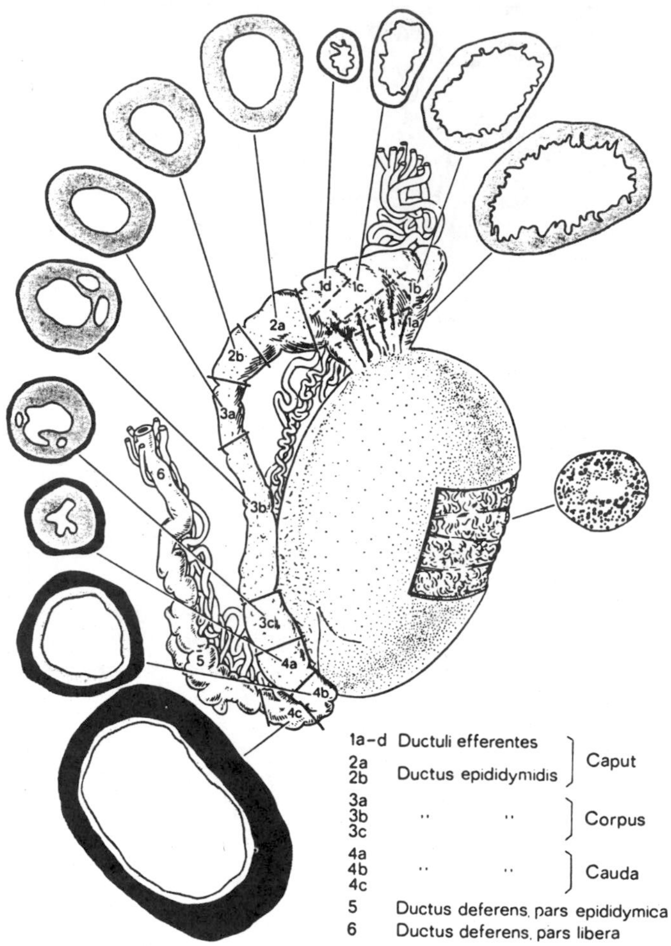

FIG. 17. Semi-schematic diagram of a human testis and epididymis. The shaded area represents the epithelial lining of the duct, the black area represents the muscle layer. (From ref. 69).

initial segment (Fig. 18). In certain rodents, such as the rat, large accumulations of fat surround the proximal regions of the epididymis and constitute the "epididymal fatpad" (Fig. 3). The location of the epididymis together with the testis in the scrotum results in the maintenance of epididymal, as well as testicular temperature, several degrees below that of core body temperature (117,354, 686,1134).

Perhaps the most comprehensive histologic descriptions of the epididymis have been carried out in the rat (950), the rabbit (536), and the stallion, ram, and bull (837), although some studies have also been undertaken in humans (522,1329) and some American and Australian marsupials (133,185,248,593,875,901,966,1150). These descriptions subdivided the epididymis into between six and 12 histologic zones. The epididymal epithelium is complex in that it contains a variety of cell types (436,950,1316), each cell type varying as a proportion of the total population at different points along the duct. In contrast to the ductuli efferentes, ciliated cells are absent from the epithelium of the epididymal duct. The predominant cell type is the principal cell, which bears apical stereocilia. Other cell types described include apical cells, basal cell, clear cells, and halo cells (intraepithelial lymphocytes). Many detailed descriptions of the ultrastructure of these cells have been published (e.g., rat [436], mouse [2], hamster [349], rabbit [586], monkey [947], bull [412]). In general terms, the first part of the epididymis or initial segment is characterized by a high epithelium with long straight stereocilia that almost obliterate a lumen that is sparsely populated with spermatozoa. The middle segment has a wider lumen, and the stereocilia are usually bent and sometimes branched, whereas supranuclear vacuoles are prominent in the epithelium. The terminal segment has a lower epithelium; stereocilia are shorter and less dense and the lumen of the tubule is wider and densely packed with sperm. The epididymis of testicond mammals, such as the elephant, follows the same basic structure as that of the scrotal mammals (590).

The epididymal duct is surrounded by connective tissue that contains fibroblasts, collagen, elastic fibers, blood vessels, lymphatic vessels, nerve fibers, macrophages, wandering leucocytes, and concentric layers of smooth-muscle fibers. The amount of intertubular connective tissue varies considerably between species.

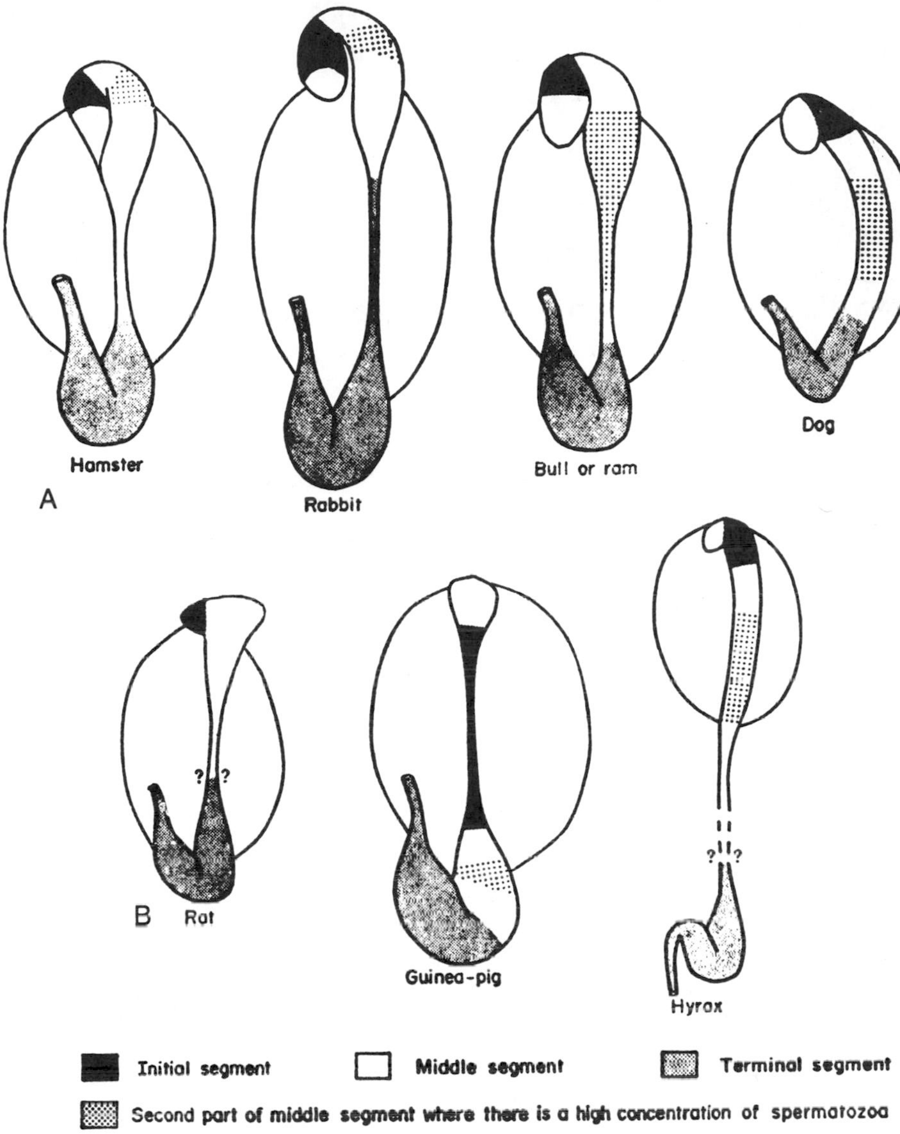

FIG. 18. Diagrammatic representation of a scheme for the subdivision of the epididymis into three segments in a variety of species. The subdivision into initial, middle, and terminal segments is based on histological and cytological features which do not necessarily occupy the same gross morphological position in different species. (From ref. 407.)

Within a species, the thickness of the smooth-muscle layer surrounding the tubules increases from the initial segment to the terminal segment.

Ductus Deferens

The ductus (or vas) deferens is a continuation of the epididymal duct beginning at the point where the duct of the epididymis straightens and reverses direction toward the inguinal canal. The ductus deferens is approximately 25 cm long in the human man and 6 cm in the rat and is suspended in a mesentery that is continuous with that over the epididymis. The ductus deferens should not be considered as a simple conduit leading sperm from the epididymis to the urethra, because it has a complex epithelium that has both absorptive and secretory functions.

In the rat, the ductus deferens can be subdivided into three sections (439). The proximal vas deferens, located primarily in the scrotum, is flattened due to an asymmetric distribution of longitudinal muscle layers but contains a tubule that is circular in cross section. The distal vas deferens, in the inguinal region, is circular in cross section because of the presence of thick longitudinal layers, but the epithelium of the duct becomes crenelated with two to six infoldings, and the structural features of the epithelial cells differ from those in the proximal vas. The terminal region of the vas deferens lies in the abdominal pelvis and terminates in humans where it is joined by the duct of the seminal vesicles to form the short ejaculatory duct. It is characterized by replacement of columnar principal cells, in some areas, by pockets of smaller cells that can be seen actively to phagocytose spermatozoa. The epithelium of the human vas deferens is crenelated in more distal regions as in the rat, and this

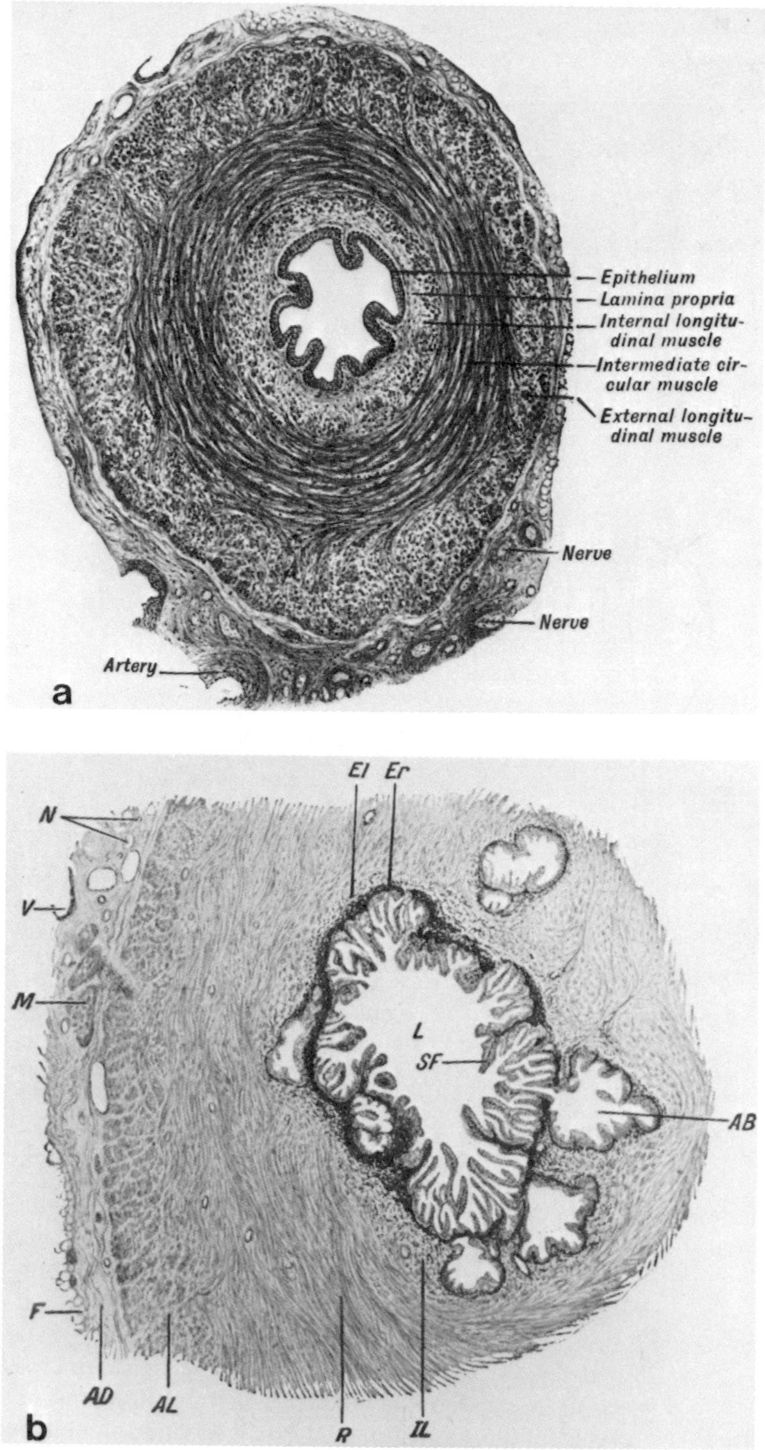

FIG. 19. Cross-section of **(a)** the ductus deferens, and **(b)** a portion of the ampulla of man. F, fat tissue; M, smooth muscle bundles in adventitia; N, nerves; V, veins; AD, adventitia; AL, external longitudinal muscle; R, intermediate circular muscle; IL, internal longitudinal muscle; El, longitudinal elastic fibers; Er, ring-shaped elastic fibers; L, main lumen; AB, gland-like outpouching of the main lumen; SF, folds of mucosa. (From ref. 103.)

produces a stellate shape in cross section (Fig. 19A). Four different cell types are recognized in the epithelium, namely principal cells, pencil cells, mitochondrion-rich cells, and basal cells (892). The muscle coat is composed of three layers, an inner longitudinal layer, a middle oblique or circular layer, and an outer longitudinal layer (Fig. 19A). In contrast to the rat, there is a progressive decrease in the development of the epithelium and muscle layers in moving from the proximal to terminal regions. Elastic fibers are prominent in the lamina propria, where they form two layers, and they are also present among the smooth-muscle cells of the inner muscle layer (893).

Ampulla

The ampulla, when present, exists as a spindle-shaped thickening of the terminal portion of the ductus deferens. It is particularly well developed in the stallion, where it may measure 25 cm long and 2 cm in diameter. Dimensions in other species have been reported as follows: bull (10 × 1.5 cm), ram (7 × 0.6 cm), red deer (6 × 0.6 cm), elephant (8 × 6 cm), and camel (13 × 0.5 cm) (43,306,323,1104). Details of the structure of the ampulla are scant. In the human, the epithelium lining the ampulla is thrown into many irregular branching folds (Fig. 19B). Between the folds, there are many branched outpocketings that reach deep into the surrounding muscular layer, which is less regularly arranged than in the rest of the ductus deferens. A single layer of columnar cells with secretory function line the surface of the ampullary glands. A similar arrangement appears to exist in the bull (602), red deer (43), and rabbit (97,526). In the last-mentioned species, the glands consist of large fluid-filled vesicles connecting with the lumen where the mucosa is thrown into irregular folds. The ampulla in the elephant consists of many, simple tubular glands containing large eosinophilic bodies of homogenous but concretionary appearance, as well as spermatozoa (1104). In the camel, two types of ampullary glands are present (15). Central submucosal glands are relatively small with narrow lumina lined by a low columnar epithelium; larger peripheral glands with wide lumina are lined by tall slender columnar cells with a brush border. The luminal fluid contains globular bodies, oval concretions, and spermatozoa. Ampullary glands have been described in the rat, mouse, and hamster, where they are located on the dorsal wall of the urethra. They consist of acini lined with cuboidal to columnar epithelial cells with the epithelium being thrown into deep longitudinal folds (537,569). Tubules leading from the acini to the wide vestibule of the ampulla are surrounded by a thin layer of smooth-muscle cells and are held together by a thin connective tissue membrane.

Seminal Vesicles

Seminal vesicles are so-named because of an early misconception that they were receptacles or reservoirs for sperm (1035). The glands are absent from monotremes, marsupials, carnivores, cetaceans, and from some primates, insectivores, chiropterans, and lagomorphs (306) (Table 1). Some confusion originally surrounded the homology of the vesicular glands in the rabbit, but it is now considered that the glandula seminalis and glandula vesicularis, both being derived from the wolffian duct, correspond to the seminal vesicles (277). The seminal vesicles are paired, bag-shaped glands in man, stallion, rat, and guinea pig, although the internal surface may be thrown into an intricate system of folds to form irregular diverticula (Fig. 20). In other mammals, such as the bull, ram, and boar (750), the seminal vesicles consist of compact glandular tissue arranged in multiple lobes and containing a system of ramified secretory ducts. The epithelium is generally pseudostratified, consisting of a row of round basal cells and a row of larger low columnar cells. The remainder of the gland is completed by loose connective tissue, a layer of smooth muscle, and an external sheet of connective tissue. The guinea pig seminal vesicle has been used as a model system for studies of the differential action of hormones on the epithelium versus the stroma, because of the ease of stripping the epithelium from the underlying tissue (691,756).

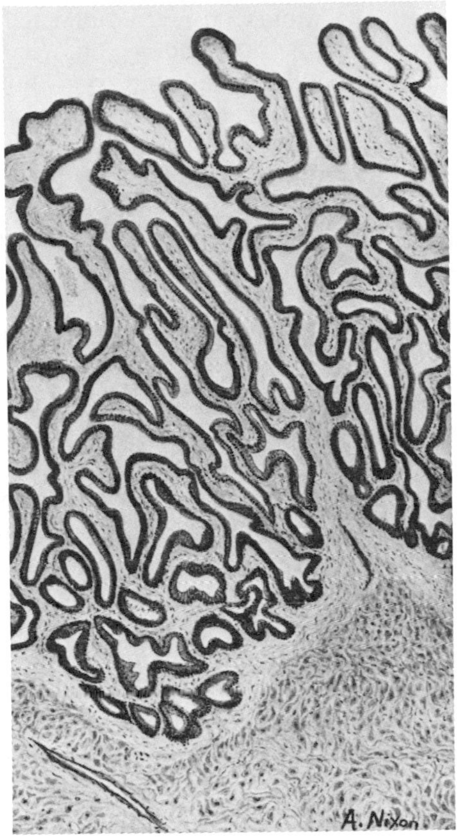

FIG. 20. Section through the wall of the human seminal vesicle. The mucosa is thrown into an intricate system of folds with the epithelium overlying the lamina propria. The smooth muscle layer occupies the lower part of the tissue section. (From ref. 103.)

Prostate

The prostate, apparently so-named because of its location anterior to the bladder and seminal vesicles, is present apparently in all mammalian species (Table 1) but has a widely varying morphology. It is not our intention to make an exhaustive review of the prostate in various species, and the reader is referred to the more extensive systematic coverage by Eckstein and Zuckerman (306). The prostate is a compound tubuloalveolar gland. It is classified as disseminate or diffuse if the glandular acini remain within the lamina propria around the urethra without penetrating the surrounding voluntary muscle. However, if the gland forms a definite body outside the urethral muscle, it is classified as discrete. In some species, such as the bull and boar, both types of prostatic tissue may be present. The prostate may frequently be referred to as "lobed," although some confusion surrounds the use of this term. It may refer to separate and distinct anatomic structures, to histologically discrete areas within a given structure, to zones that respond differentially to hormones, or to zones with differential propensity to metastasis. The human prostate is a compact gland about the size of a chestnut, weighing approximately 20 g. It is unusual in that it surrounds the urethra at the base of the bladder with the two ejaculatory ducts penetrating the gland through its posterior surface close to its upper border. The organ contains between 30 and 50 tubuloalveolar glands, which empty into the prostatic urethra through 15 to 30 ducts. Calcified concretions, which may exceed 1 mm in diameter, exist in the secretion within the lumen of the acini (Fig. 21). The gland was considered by early anatomists to be reasonably homogeneous, but more recent studies have shown this not to be correct. There is, nevertheless, still some dispute as to the precise subdivision of the gland (e.g., ref. 1170). Detailed anatomic studies (44,377,775, 776,1233) recognized three glandular regions, the peripheral zone, central zone, and preprostatic region, surrounded by a thick anterior fibromuscular stroma. Benign prostatic hyperplasia is specifically restricted to the preprostatic region. The ferret prostate consists of tubuloalveolar glands surrounded by fibromuscular connective tissue (552). The dog prostate has been a popular experimental system for studies of prostatic function for several reasons. It is the only accessory gland in this species, and when stimulated with pilocarpine hydrochloride, large quantities of pure prostatic secretion can be obtained (534,535). Moreover, the canine prostate has a tendency to hypertrophy and thus provides a suitable model system in which to study this aspect of human pathology.

The rat prostate is also a popular experimental system, particularly for studies of androgenic control of male accessory glands, and its size and the appearance of its cells are determined by the level of androgenic stimulation (625,737,924), although from studies involving grafts of anterior pituitaries into the prostate, prolactin may also have a direct effect (1044). Prostate size and activity are also greater in sexually active rats (45), although it is not clear how much of this is due to changes in androgen levels. The rat prostate is a complex structure with several distinct anatomic lobes (Fig. 3). Some confusion surrounded the classification of these lobes in early descriptions. The currently accepted classification encompasses the ventral prostate, which is a bilobed structure situated ventral to the urethra, and the dorsolateral prostate, which comprises a clearly separate medial portion and two lateral lobes located over the dorsolateral aspect of the urethra. The coagulating gland is an additional lobe of the prostate and was previously known as the anterior prostate. It lies adjacent to the seminal vesicles, with which it shares a common peritoneal sheath. In a detailed morphologic and histologic study of the rat prostatic complex (569), it was shown that the ventral, lat-

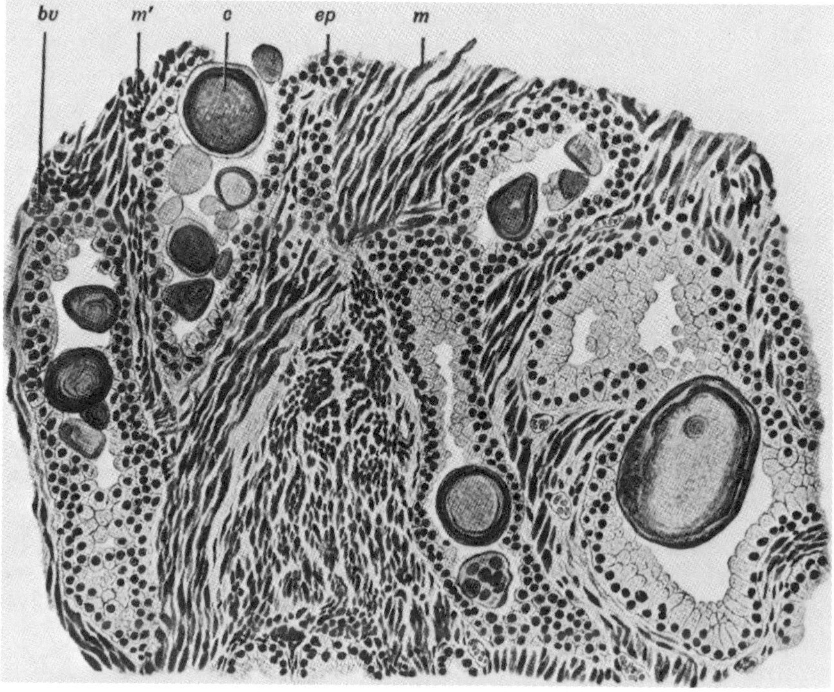

FIG. 21. Section through portion of the human prostate. bv, Blood vessels; c, concretions; ep, epithelium lining the glandular acini; m, smooth muscle in longitudinal section; m′, smooth muscle in cross-section. (From ref. 103.)

eral, and dorsal lobes of the prostate are each drained into the urethra by multiple ducts, whereas each coagulating gland is drained by a single duct. The guinea pig has a prostatic complex and coagulating gland complex, each consisting of six to seven lobes bound closely together by loose areolar tissue and discharging by individual ducts into a common ejaculatory chamber. Each major lobe is subdivided peripherally into fingerlike lobules (278). These authors consider that subdivision of the prostatic lobes into discrete dorsal, ventral, and lateral entities cannot be justified. Histologically, the prostatic lobes can be seen to be simple tubular glands, whereas the coagulating glands are tubuloalveolar in type. The epithelium is described as stratified, consisting of a superficial columnar secretory layer overlying a basal layer. In all probability, fine structural studies may reveal that the superficial columnar cells extend to the basement membrane, in which case the epithelium would be more correctly described as pseudostratified. In hamsters, the lumen of each acinus is lined by columnar cells (1173). The prostate of the musk shrew (*Suncus murinus*) has many unusual features, including spontaneous release of secretory granules and the presence of secretory and clear cells in the glandular epithelium (493). The disseminate prostate of marsupials is generally carrot-shaped, except in bandicoots and the koala in which it is described as heart-shaped and surrounded by a thick striated muscle coat (851,967,1031). The prostate may attain considerable size during the breeding season when it may be the largest organ in the body cavity after the liver (106). Histologically, the prostate of marsupials can be divided into two to three segments arranged along the urethra or ventral and dorsal to it (967). The segments contain many simple branched tubular glands lined by a single layer of columnar cells and empty through collecting ducts into the urethra.

Bulbourethral Glands

Bulbourethral glands or Cowper's glands are multilobular compound, tubular, or tubuloalveolar glands (98) present in most mammals but absent in aquatic mammals, mustelids, bears, and dogs (306) (Table 1). The glands are especially large in the boar (774). A single pair of glands is usually present, but there may be as many as three pairs in some marsupials (133,967,1031). The glands are compact and smooth-surfaced, being located near the bulb of the penis and connected to the urethra by a duct (1106). The glands are divided by connective tissue septa containing a net of elastic fibers together with both smooth and striated muscle fibers, and the whole gland is surrounded by a fibroelastic capsule and a thick striated compressor muscle. Striated muscle fibers are apparently absent from the septa in ruminants (cattle, goats, and sheep), which also have an exceptionally thick collagenous capsule (98). The alveoli of the glands are lined with mucous-like cells (Fig. 22) and the ducts by a single layer of cuboidal or squamous cells (11,839,964).

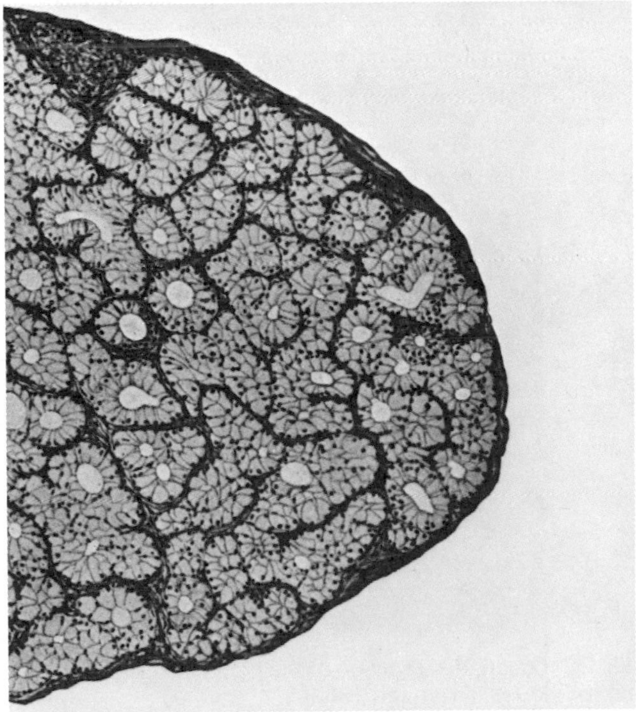

FIG. 22. Section through portion of the human bulbourethral (Cowper's) gland. The gland in man is about the size of a pea and is divided into lobules, a portion of which is shown in the figure. The section shows individual acini surrounded by a thin layer of smooth muscle. (From ref. 103.)

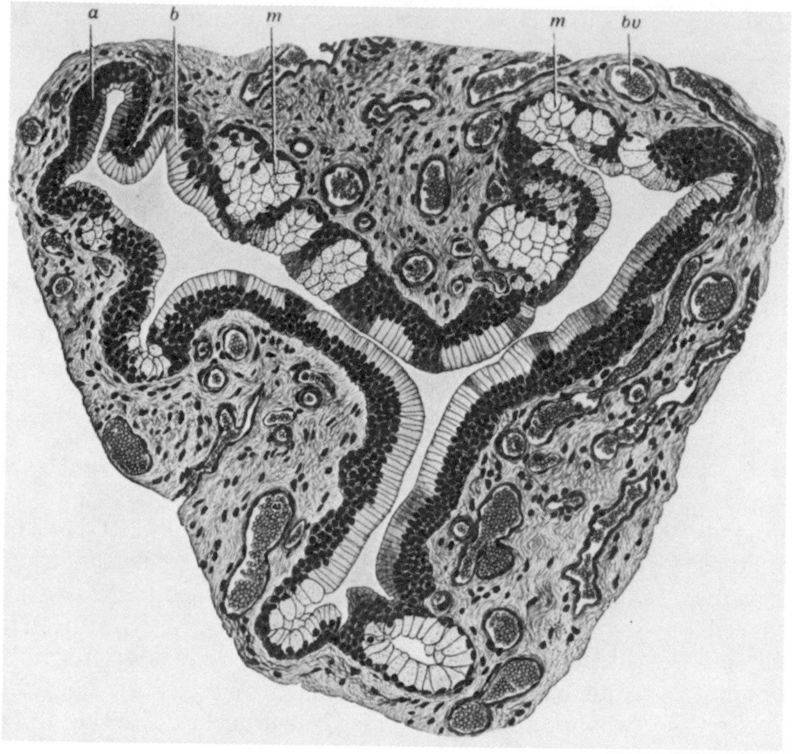

FIG. 23. Section through human urethral glands (glands of Littré) from the cavernous part of the urethra. The glands run obliquely in the lamina propria and may penetrate deep into the spongy body of the penis. The lumen is lined with the same epithelium as the mucus membrane of the urethra, but containing intraepithelial nests of clear mucous cells. a, Darkly staining stratified columnar epithelium; b, epithelium with clear cells; bv, blood vessels; m, outpocketings with clear mucous cells. (From ref. 103.)

Urethral Glands

The urethral glands or glands of Littre are multiple mucosal glands opening into the cavernous portion of the urethra in man (Fig. 23). Some of the glands are simple outpocketings of the urethral mucosa, whereas others are more globular and connected to the urethra by a short duct. Earlier reports of the presence of urethral glands in the bull have since been refuted (602), but they are clearly present in the boar (774).

Preputial Glands

Preputial glands are found in rodents, where they lie beneath the preputial skin, and open, each by a main secretory duct, into the preputial sac near its free margin (Fig. 3). A homologous gland occurs in female rodents. The gross morphology of the gland has been described as "flasklike" in the rat and "leaflike" in the mouse. The gland is usually regarded as a hypertrophied and modified sebaceous gland, but on a histologic basis, this may be an oversimplification. Histologic studies (803,894, 1005) show the gland to contain dense epithelioid acini supported by thin connective tissue trabeculae, which are continuous with the capsule of the organ. The rat gland has a dense parenchyma and a ramifying system of ductules (Fig. 24A). In comparison, the parenchyma of the mouse gland is much less dense with fewer acini and large cavernous ductular spaces (Fig. 24B). There is evidence that the preputial gland of the rat, but not the mouse, produces a nonlipid secretion in addition to the normal lipid secretion characteristic of sebaceous glands. Smaller glands, but of similar structure, can be found surrounding the prepuce of the rabbit (526).

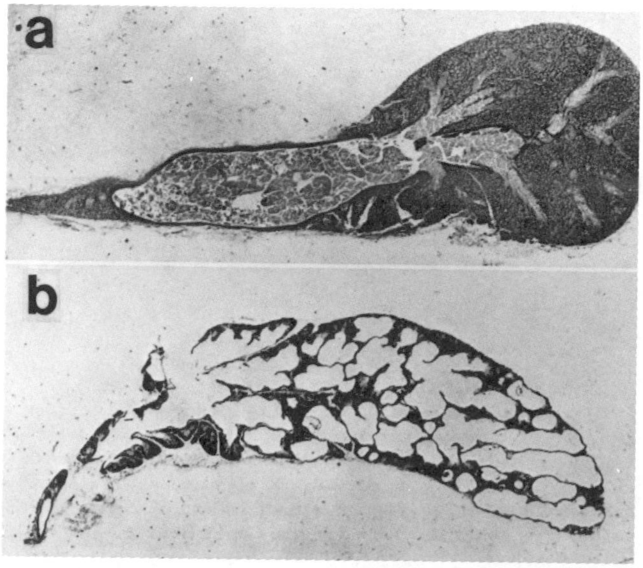

FIG. 24. Longitudinal section of the preputial gland of **(a)** rat and **(b)** mouse. (From ref. 136.)

BLOOD VASCULAR SYSTEM

Spermatic Cord and Pampiniform Plexus

In those mammals whose testes descend into a scrotum, the testicular arteries retain their origin from the abdominal aorta and become elongated as thc testes migrates. The elongation is greater than is necessary to allow for the movement of the testis, with the result that in the eutherian mammals, the artery also becomes extensively coiled, particularly in the section outside the inguinal canal (Figs. 25 and 26A). The artery has been divided into a straight part (inside the abdomen), a convoluted part (in the cord), and a marginal part on the

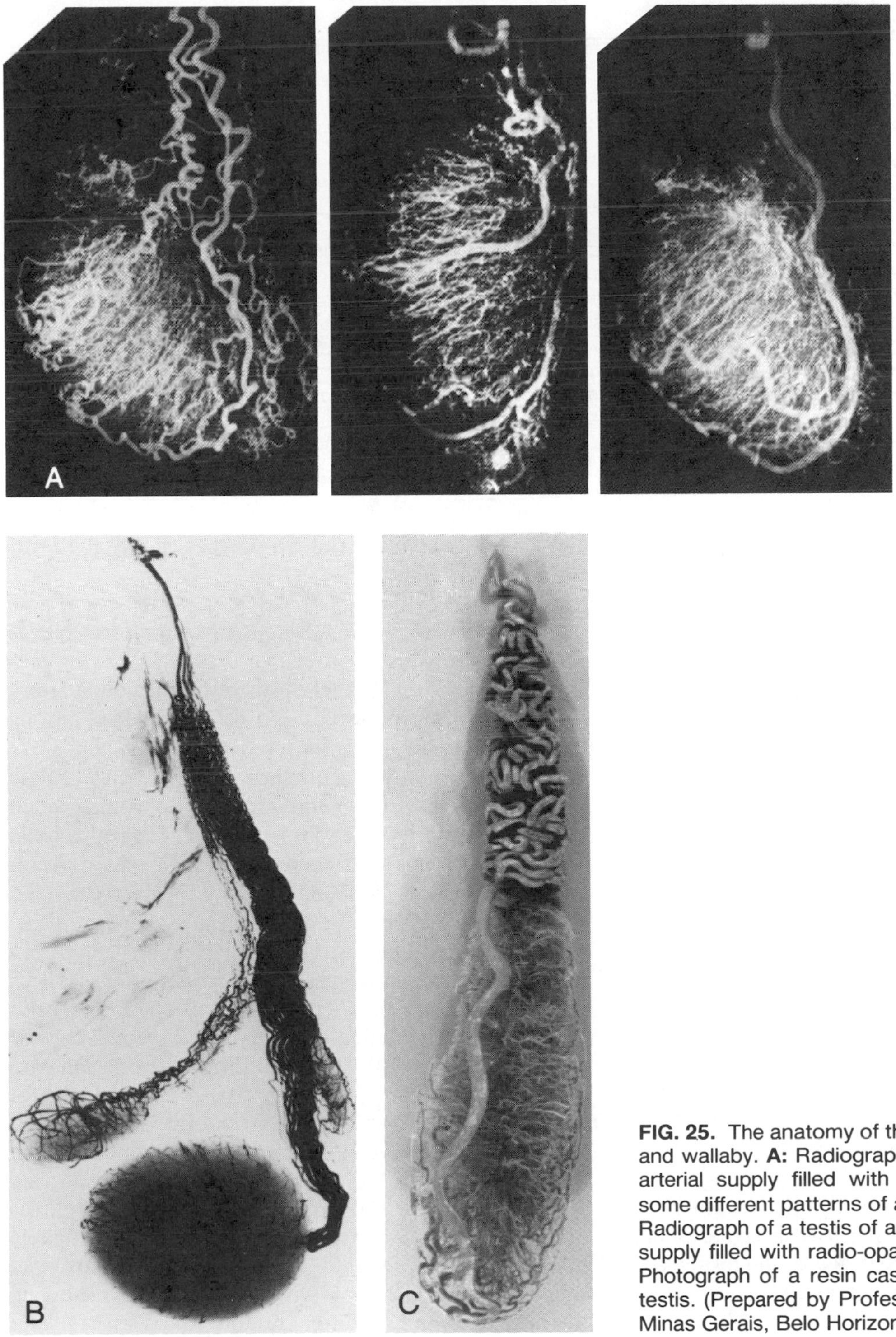

FIG. 25. The anatomy of the testicular artery of human, bull, and wallaby. **A:** Radiograph of three human testes with the arterial supply filled with radio-opaque medium, showing some different patterns of arterial supply. (From ref. 999.) **B:** Radiograph of a testis of a tammar wallaby, with the arterial supply filled with radio-opaque medium. (From ref. 457.) **C:** Photograph of a resin cast of the arterial supply to a bull testis. (Prepared by Professor H. P. Godinho, University of Minas Gerais, Belo Horizonte, Brazil.)

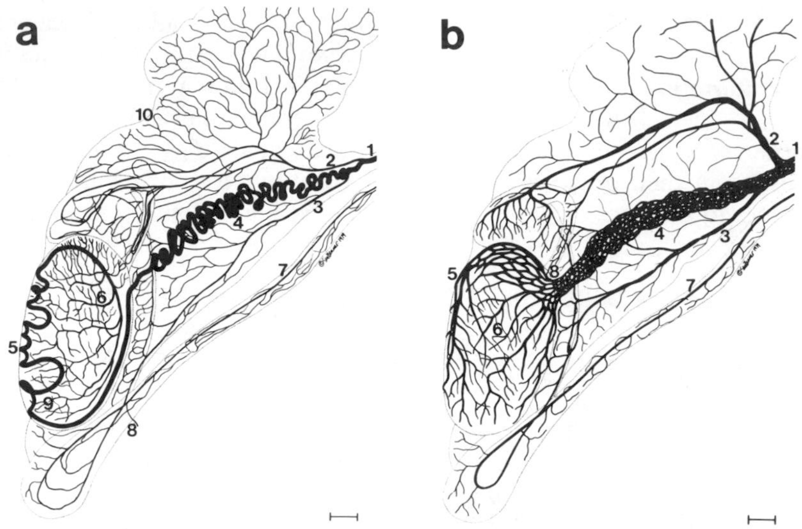

FIG. 26. Arrangement of arteries and veins supplying the rat testis and epididymis. The margins of the organs are shown in *stippled outline.* Blood vessels are drawn to accurately reflect relative dimensions and to provide a three-dimensional view. *Solid black lines* designate blood vessels closest to the medial surface whereas vessels coursing near the lateral surface appear as *discontinuous lines.* **a:** Arterial system: 1, spermatic artery; 2, superior epididymal artery; 3, inferior epididymal artery; 4, testicular artery; 5, capsular artery; 6, intratesticular artery; 7, vas deferential artery; 8, cremasteric artery; 9, intratesticular artery-artery anastomosis; 10, epididymal fat pad artery-artery anastomosis. **b:** Venous system: 1, spermatic vein; 2, superior epididymal vein; 3, inferior epididymal vein; 4, pampiniform plexus; 5, testicular surface vein; 6, intratesticular vein; 7, vas deferential vein; 8, anastomosis between testicular surface and efferent ductule veins. Scale bar = 2.7 mm. (From ref. 194.)

testis surface (1313). In the large domestic ruminants and in the pig, as much as 5 m of the convoluted part of the artery can be tightly coiled up into about 10 cm of spermatic cord (see refs. 30,108,455,518,1028,1032), and in most species the artery does not normally divide until it reaches the testis. However, in humans, the artery often has branched by the level of the inguinal ring (561). The thickness of the wall and the number of layers of smooth-muscle cells decreases along the length of the artery (471). The arterial convolutions are much less obvious in rats (326,455,866,1032,1272) and hamsters (951,952), but in the latter species, there is a capillary network from the epididymal artery between the testicular artery and the veins of the pampiniform plexus, and lymphatic vessels and mast cells are distributed within the connective tissue of the vascular wall (952). In the pampiniform plexus of the guinea pig, there are many endothelial bridges, strands, and trabeculae projecting into the lumen and attached to the opposite or adjacent wall, as well as a frequently discontinuous smooth-muscle layer. Around the testicular artery, there are abundant nerve fibers containing neuropeptide Y and dopamine β-hydroxylase, and a few containing substance P; there are also many lymphatic capillaries coursing through the interstitium between the arterial and venous walls (420). In marsupials, as the testicular artery passes through the inguinal canal, it divides into an arterial rete of up to 200 parallel branches, which run in the spermatic cord to the testis, where they reunite to form two or three arterial trunks that supply the testis (454,1031).

The veins leaving the testis divide near the dorsal pole to form a venous plexus, called the pampiniform plexus (Fig. 26B) from its resemblance to a mass of vine tendrils. These venous branches surround the coiled artery in the eutherian mammals and lie interspersed among the branches of the arterial rete in the marsupials until about the level of the inguinal canal, where they reunite progressively to form several large venous trunks, which eventually empty either into the vena cava, the renal vein, or the hypogastric or common iliac vein, depending on species (389,700,866,921,922,949,1028,1032, 1294,1295). Within the plexus in bulls, there are three classes of veins: The first type is large (about 200 μm in diameter), with four to six layers of smooth muscles cells in the walls, running parallel to one another, and surrounding the testicular artery. The second class is smaller (40 to 70 μm), lack smooth-muscle cells, and are arranged in a less-organized pattern. The third class of veins occupy a periarterial or intramural location, often at the junction between the media and adventitia of the artery (Fig. 27). Veins of the three classes communicate with one another, and none of the veins in the plexus have valves (471), in contrast to those immediately above it (1053). A slightly simpler, but similar arrangement is found in the rat, with the larger veins showing sac-like pouching and constriction bands in the wall; there are two types of venules, long smooth-surfaced and

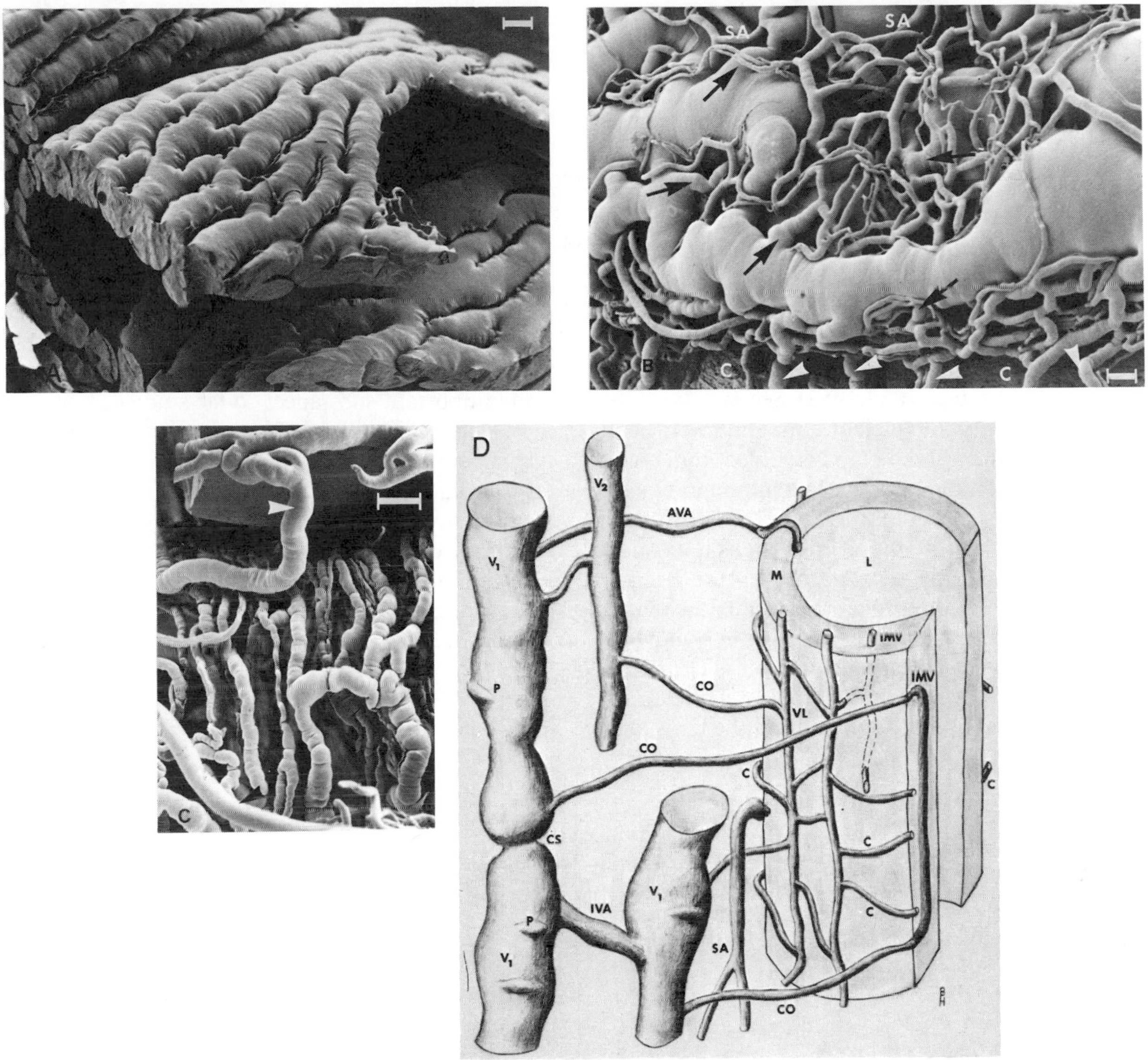

FIG. 27. The anatomy of the veins of the pampiniform plexus in the bull. **A:** Cast of the large veins of the first network, which run parallel and anastomose frequently, forming a venous covering to the testicular artery, which lies in the central empty space. Where the artery reaches the surface of the spermatic cord, the covering of veins is absent. Bar = 200 μm. **B:** Venous cast showing the first and intermediate networks of the pampiniform plexus. The large veins show varicose pouches. The *arrows* indicate connections between the two networks and the *arrowheads* point to connecting veins joining the periarterial venous network (C), seen faintly in the background. SA, small branches of the testicular artery. Bar = 100 μm. **C:** Cast of the third periarterial venous network, consisting of venules and venous capillaries. The venules show characteristic constrictions along their course. The *arrowhead* shows a connecting vein running from the periarterial network to the first venous network at the top. Bar = 100 μm. **D:** A diagram illustrating the arrangement of the three venous networks (V1, V2, and VL, respectively). A small arterial branch (SA) of the testicular artery and an arteriovenous anastomosis (AVA) are also shown. L, lumen of testicular artery; M, media of wall of testicular artery; C, venous capillaries of the third venous network; CO, connecting veins linking the periarterial and the other venous networks; IVA, anastomosis between veins of the first and second network; IMV, intramural venule of the periarterial network; P, pouches; and CS, constrictions in the veins. (From ref. 471.)

short saccular ones (866,1272). Around the outside of this vascular complex, there are several sizeable lymphatic vessels that originate from the testis and epididymis. The whole cord is encased in a peritoneal covering, with the cremaster muscle on one side in ungulates but surrounding it in rodents (1277). The ductus deferens and its associated deferential artery and veins run in a separate fold of peritoneum into the abdominal cavity (389). Both the arterial coils and the venous plexus are formed during fetal life in cattle (1313,1314). This curious arrangement has several consequences (Fig. 28). First, the pulse is almost eliminated from the arterial blood as it flows through the cord, with only minor changes in mean pressure (1054,1252). Second, the spermatic cord acts as a very efficient countercurrent heat exchanger, so that the arterial blood is cooled from body temperature to scrotal temperature by the venous blood, which leaves the testis at a temperature similar to that under the scrotal skin; at the same time, the venous blood is warmed to body temperature by the arterial blood (256,1054,1253). A similar arrangement is found in the extremities of several animals living in cold environments, but in these cases, the function is clearly to prevent heat loss to the surroundings (see ref. 1028). In the testis, it is probably more to maintain the testis and epididymis at a temperature lower than that of the abdominal cavity, although why this should be an advantage is not clear. The system does ensure that an even temperature is maintained throughout the testis, and there is no doubt that the function of the testis is deranged if its temperature is raised to body temperature for more than a short period (see ref. 1032). There is also evidence that substances can cross from the arterial blood to the venous blood by diffusion or transport through the vessel walls. Although this undoubtably occurs for several marker substances such as inert gases (311,313,402) and tritiated water (551), it appears to be of trivial quantitative significance for all the physiologically important substances so far studied. Unless active transport against a concentration gradient is invoked, the system would only operate for a substance produced or utilized by the testis, producing a locally increased or decreased concentration in the tissue respectively. An obvious candidate is testosterone, but the increase in the concentration in the arterial blood as it passes through the cord (363) is insignificant when compared with the difference between venous and arterial blood (see section *Composition of Testicular Venous Blood*). However, the transfer of testosterone to the epididymis or the fatpad may be of much greater importance.

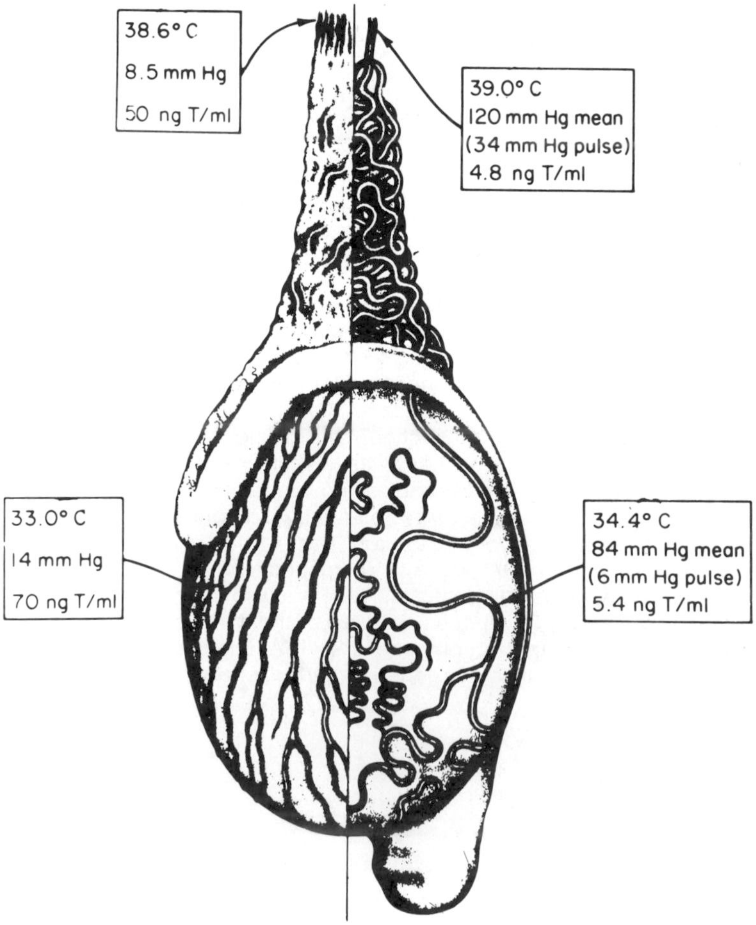

FIG. 28. The effects of the spermatic cord on blood temperature, pressure, and concentrations of testosterone. A composite diagram with the arterial system shown on the *right* and the venous drainage on the *left*. The figures in the boxes give the values for blood at the point in the vascular system indicated by the *arrow tip.* (From ref. 722.)

One of the most interesting findings of recent years has been the demonstration of arteriovenous anastomoses in the spermatic cord of sheep and pigs. Experimental evidence for these was first sought by de Graaf more than 300 years ago, but he could find none. Several later authors suggested that these anastomoses did exist (see ref. 1028 for early references), but it was only recently that conclusive anatomic (471,1278) and functional evidence for their existence in bulls, rams, and boars has been obtained. It now seems that as much as 40% of the blood flowing through the testicular artery into the cord in rams and boars may return to the venous system without passing through the testis, even when all the vessels to the epididymis are ligated (348,857,858). The significance and control of these anastomoses require further study, and they cannot be seen in rats (1272) or hamsters (951,952) but are apparent in tree shrews (*Tupaia*) (953). Furthermore, when radioactive microspheres 15 ± 5 μm in diameter were injected into the arterial system of rats, only about 1% of those lodging in the right testis, epididymis, and epididymal fat were found in venous blood collected from a catheter in the right spermatic vein about 5 mm from its entry into the vena cava (259).

However, studies of hormone secretion from the testis provide physiologic evidence for the existence of such anastomoses in rats, rams, boars, guinea pigs, monkeys, and humans (728,733). These studies show a consistent reduction in testosterone concentrations of some 40% to 60% when levels in venous blood sampled from below the pampiniform plexus are compared with the levels in blood sampled from higher up the spermatic cord (Fig. 34). This reduction is unaffected by the removal of the epididymis, and the magnitude of this reduction cannot be accounted for by passive venous-arterial diffusion of testosterone (728). The only explanation at present is for arterial-venous anastomoses providing a transfer of arterial blood to the venous drainage in the pampiniform plexus, thereby "diluting" the venous concentrations measured above the pampiniform plexus.

In mammals whose testes do not descend into a scrotum, there is no spermatic cord, but the artery does show some elongation and coiling in those species in which the testis migrates within the abdominal cavity. In animals such as the elephant and hyrax, in which the testis does not migrate at all, the artery is simple and runs straight into the parenchyma of the testis (see ref. 1028). In seals, which do not form a scrotum but in which the testis does migrate down through the abdominal wall, venous blood from the hind flippers forms a secondary plexus overlying the testis (101), resulting in testicular temperatures of about 30°C (140). In dolphins, in which the testis migrates to the caudal end of the abdominal cavity but does not pass through the body wall, there is a lumbocaudal venous plexus, which drains blood from the dorsal fin and caudal flukes. This plexus lies on either side of the dorsal aorta, between the kidney and the origin of the caudal artery. Each venous plexus is juxtaposed to a spermatic arterial plexus made up by about 40 arteries, each of which arises from the aorta and runs to form a single testicular artery near the caudal pole of the testis (Fig. 29). The testicular veins also run through the same region (1065). Although no measurements of temperature have been reported, it seems likely that this arrangement also acts as countercurrent heat exchanger and that the testis in cetacea is also kept at a lower temperature than the rest of the abdominal organs. In birds, the arterial supply and venous drainage is simple and direct (646,845).

Varicocele

In humans, there is a common condition known as varicocele, which is a varicosity of the veins of the paminiform plexus. It is usually found on the left side but may be bilateral and is probably caused by incompetence of the valves in the main vein near where it opens into the renal vein. This can lead to retrograde flow of blood down the plexus, returning to the general circulation through anastomoses with the cremasteric or scrotal vessels. Many authors believe that this condition is associated with lowered fertility (see refs. 215,216,1002, 1185,1229,1230), but a detailed statistical study of the fertility of normal men and men with varicocoele found no evidence that men with varicocoele were less fertile or that their fertility was improved by ligation of the varicocoele (56). Why varicocoele should cause infertility is not certain, although several possible mechanisms have been suggested. One suggestion is that dilated veins in the mediastinum cause obstruction to the excurrent ducts (847). There is some evidence that the left or both testes are smaller in men with varicocele (171,433), and there may be changes in the ultrastructure of the cells in the adluminal compartment (157). There also appear to be changes in the blood vessels and stagnation of blood inside the testis (177,492), and testicular venous blood pressure is increased (1001,1081,1322,1333). Reflux of blood down the spermatic veins could be demonstrated with Doppler recording (295). An experimental model for varicocele has been developed in rats, dogs, and monkeys, by ligating the left renal vein medial to the entrance of the internal spermatic vein. In rats, this produces varicosity of the left spermatic vein (946,1197), which sometimes extends to the right vein (829). There is no effect on testis weight, an irregular disruption of spermatogenesis, and a slight decrease in epididymal sperm numbers and motility, but there is a consistent bilateral increase in testis blood flow and temperature (418,419,542,543,829, 946,1003,1187,1188,1197), with a loss of vasomotion (829) and decreased concentrations of testosterone in the testis (946) and probably also in testis venous blood (1200). The contralateral changes in blood flow still hap-

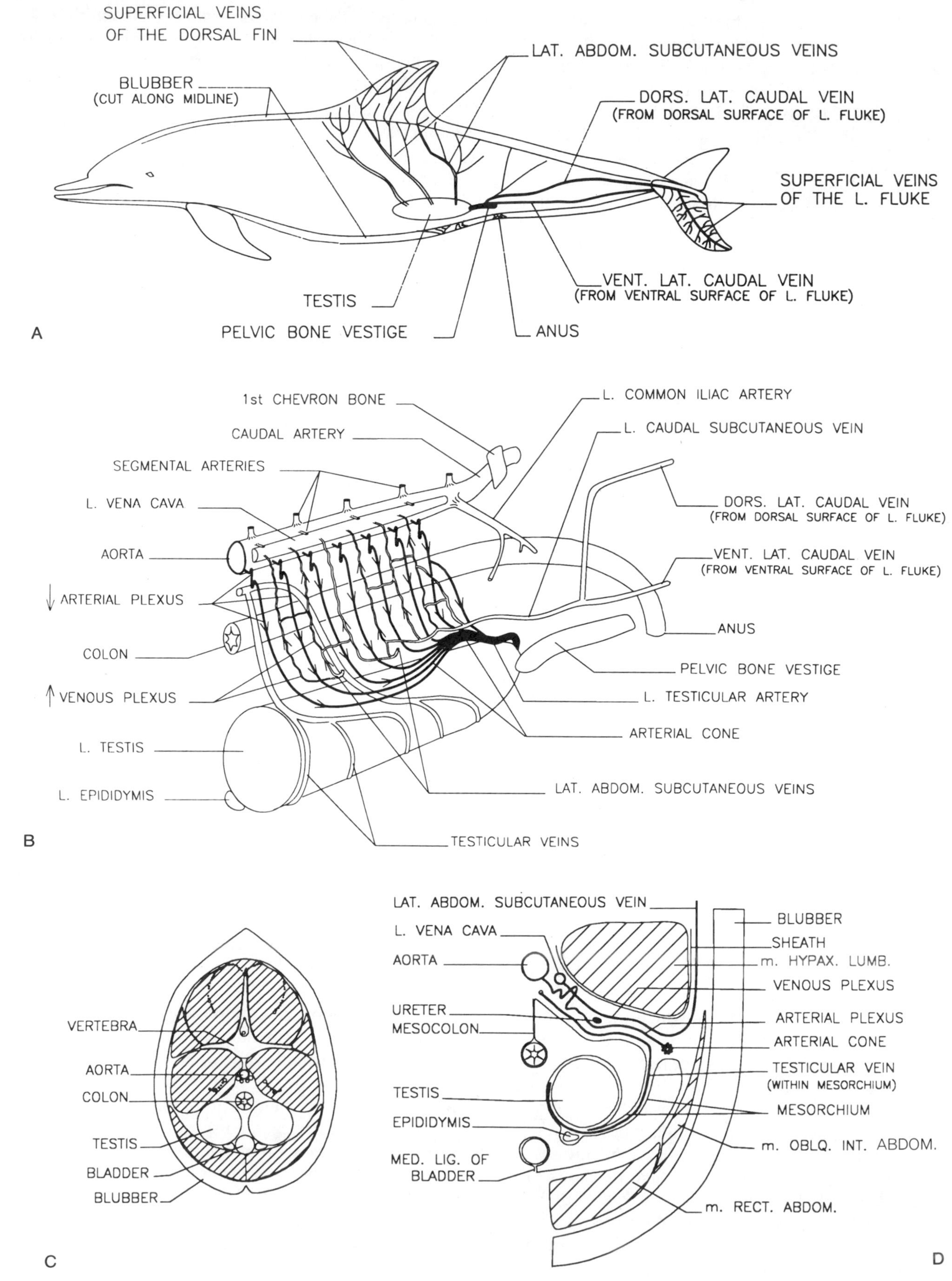

SUPERFICIAL VEINS OF THE DORSAL FIN
LAT. ABDOM. SUBCUTANEOUS VEINS
BLUBBER (CUT ALONG MIDLINE)
DORS. LAT. CAUDAL VEIN (FROM DORSAL SURFACE OF L. FLUKE)
SUPERFICIAL VEINS OF THE L. FLUKE
VENT. LAT. CAUDAL VEIN (FROM VENTRAL SURFACE OF L. FLUKE)
TESTIS
PELVIC BONE VESTIGE
ANUS
A
1st CHEVRON BONE
CAUDAL ARTERY
SEGMENTAL ARTERIES
L. VENA CAVA
AORTA
↓ ARTERIAL PLEXUS
COLON
↑ VENOUS PLEXUS
L. TESTIS
L. EPIDIDYMIS
L. COMMON ILIAC ARTERY
L. CAUDAL SUBCUTANEOUS VEIN
DORS. LAT. CAUDAL VEIN (FROM DORSAL SURFACE OF L. FLUKE)
VENT. LAT. CAUDAL VEIN (FROM VENTRAL SURFACE OF L. FLUKE)
ANUS
PELVIC BONE VESTIGE
L. TESTICULAR ARTERY
ARTERIAL CONE
LAT. ABDOM. SUBCUTANEOUS VEINS
TESTICULAR VEINS
B
VERTEBRA
AORTA
COLON
TESTIS
BLADDER
BLUBBER
C
LAT. ABDOM. SUBCUTANEOUS VEIN
L. VENA CAVA
AORTA
URETER
MESOCOLON
TESTIS
EPIDIDYMIS
MED. LIG. OF BLADDER
BLUBBER
SHEATH
m. HYPAX. LUMB.
VENOUS PLEXUS
ARTERIAL PLEXUS
ARTERIAL CONE
TESTICULAR VEIN (WITHIN MESORCHIUM)
MESORCHIUM
m. OBLQ. INT. ABDOM.
m. RECT. ABDOM.
D

pen if the left testis (418,543) or adrenal (1187) is removed at the time of vein ligation, although it has been suggested that excessive production of progestagens by the adrenal may be involved in the production of the changes in the testis (769). In dogs, there is a bilateral decrease in testis weight and an increase in testis blood flow (1003), and sperm numbers and motility decreased, without any change in semen volume in an uncontrolled study (12). In monkeys, in other uncontrolled experiments, semen quality and sperm numbers decreased after the induction of a left varicocele (461,607) and ultrastructural changes have been reported (382). However, in this species, testis blood flow appears to be decreased, even after removal of the left adrenal (461), consistent with increased testosterone concentrations in spermatic vein blood, although testis temperature is still increased (607). None of these studies report the results of any fertility trials, although the models have been studied for more than 10 years, and therefore their relevance to the human condition must be open to question.

Testis

Testicular Artery

By the time the artery reaches the surface of the scrotal testis, it is comparatively thin-walled, so that in its course along the surface of the testis, it has a flattened profile. Instead of penetrating directly into the parenchyma, in many species the artery runs for a considerable distance in the tunic, often running along the epididymal margin to the caudal pole before branching. In humans, this results in a risk of arterial occlusion if sutures are placed through the tunic for traction during orchidopexy (559,560). In the rabbit, the artery encircles the testis completely before branching, and the two initial branches then make a further half-circuit before branching again. In the rat, the artery runs straight down the epididymal margin of the testis, around the caudal pole, and then winds along the free surface (Fig. 26A) to enter the parenchyma near the rete before beginning to branch (see refs. 194,820,1028,1032). In many larger animals, the artery begins to branch near the caudal pole, and the convoluted branches run along the surface for some distance before turning sharply to run without further branching to near the rete; there they often form a tight coil before turning back on themselves to begin branching (108,472,474,1028,1032). In marsupials, several arteries are formed at the end of the arterial rete in the cord, and these run down one face of the testis, on the opposite side to the veins (see refs. 1028,1031,1032). In the rat, there are frequent arterioarterial anastomotic arcades and occasional arteriovenous anastomoses within the testis (820,1272). In birds, the testicular arteries pass through the capsule and then penetrate to the center of the testis and terminate as branching centrifugal radiate arteries (646).

It has been suggested that a myogenic response of the subcapsular artery to increases in blood pressure may have an important role in the autoregulation of testicular blood supply (280). The sensitivity of the arterial wall to the vasoconstrictor activity of noradrenaline decreases along the length of the testicular artery in the ram, with the artery on the surface of the testis being almost unresponsive even to very large doses (1260). The characteristics of the artery can be modified by implantation of a Walker carcinoma into the testis (899). The endothelial cells of the artery in the spermatic cord and on the surface of the postpubertal rat testis, as well as those lining the arterioles inside the testis, contain a high concentration of the enzyme γ-glutamyl transpeptidase (842); in other tissues, this enzyme is associated with amino acid transport, and the endothelial cells of the arterioles within the testis have been shown to transport leucine in a selective and saturable manner (145).

When the testicular artery was transected above the spermatic cord in young pigs, anastomoses between the testicular and vasal arteries opened up, both in the cord and on the surface of the testis. When the animals were examined 4 months later, the testes had developed normally, testicular blood flow was only slightly reduced, and testosterone concentrations in peripheral blood were normal (855). Similar results have been reported for immature rats (898). This suggests that during orchidopexy for treatment of cryptorchidism in boys, transection of the artery might be an acceptable alternative to imposing excessive tension on the testis and the artery.

FIG. 29 A. Pattern of subcutaneous venous return from the surface of the dorsal fin and flukes of a common dolphin (*Delphinus delphis*). Subcutaneous veins feed into the lumbo-caudal venous plexus. **B.** Schematic representation of the left countercurrent heat exchanger of a sexually mature male dolphin. Venous blood from subcutaneous veins flows from the lateral and ventro-lateral margin of the lumbo-caudal plexus towards the vena cava (arrows show the direction of flow). Arterial blood flows from the aorta, through the vessels of the spermatic arterial plexus, towards the ventro-lateral margin of the plexus. Here the vessels turn to run caudally and form a cone-shaped structure from which a single testicular artery passes through the tunic of the testis. Venous blood from the testis flows through veins underneath the arterial plexus to the vena cava. **C.** Cross-section through a male dolphin at the level of the middle of the testis, showing relationship of testis, colon and muscle (hatched). **D.** Expanded view of the cross-section in C, showing the course of the vessels. (From ref. 974).

Testicular Capillaries

The capillaries of the rat testis are of two types (Fig. 30): the Zwickelcapillaren, which run parallel to the seminiferous tubules, and the Quercapillaren, which run around the tubular walls at approximately right angles to their long axes (Fig. 31A,B) (631,818,820,1143,1153, 1272). This arrangement appears in rats only at puberty (632) but is much less obvious in bulls (31,474) and is absent from human testes (1143; but cf. ref. 1151), although it is present in some birds (646) and fish (662). Both peritubular and intertubular capillaries in the rat testis are permeable to lanthanum, but in humans the capillaries appear to be less permeable (1151). The capillaries in the rat testis also develop a high level of alkaline phosphatase activity at puberty (632) and have receptors for insulin-like growth factor (465).

Important changes also occur in the ultrastructure of the testicular capillaries as the animal passes through puberty (763) and during seasonal regression and recrudescence (765). The walls of the testicular capillaries, in contrast to those of all other endocrine tissues, are unfenestrated, being of the A-1-α type (540,1296), similar to those found in muscle (339), although capillaries in the testis restrict the movement of horseradish peroxidase much more than muscle capillaries do (1273). Fenestrations can be induced in testicular capillaries in dogs by treatment with a gonadotrophin-releasing hormone (GnRH) agonist (764). The capillaries and postcapillary venules in rats comprise 6.2% of the interstitial tissue and 0.6% of the whole rat testis and have a total volume of 5.8 μl/g and an endothelial surface area of 27 cm^2/g (267), while the total blood volume in the rat testis is about 10 μl/g (1052). In rams, the blood plus lymphatic

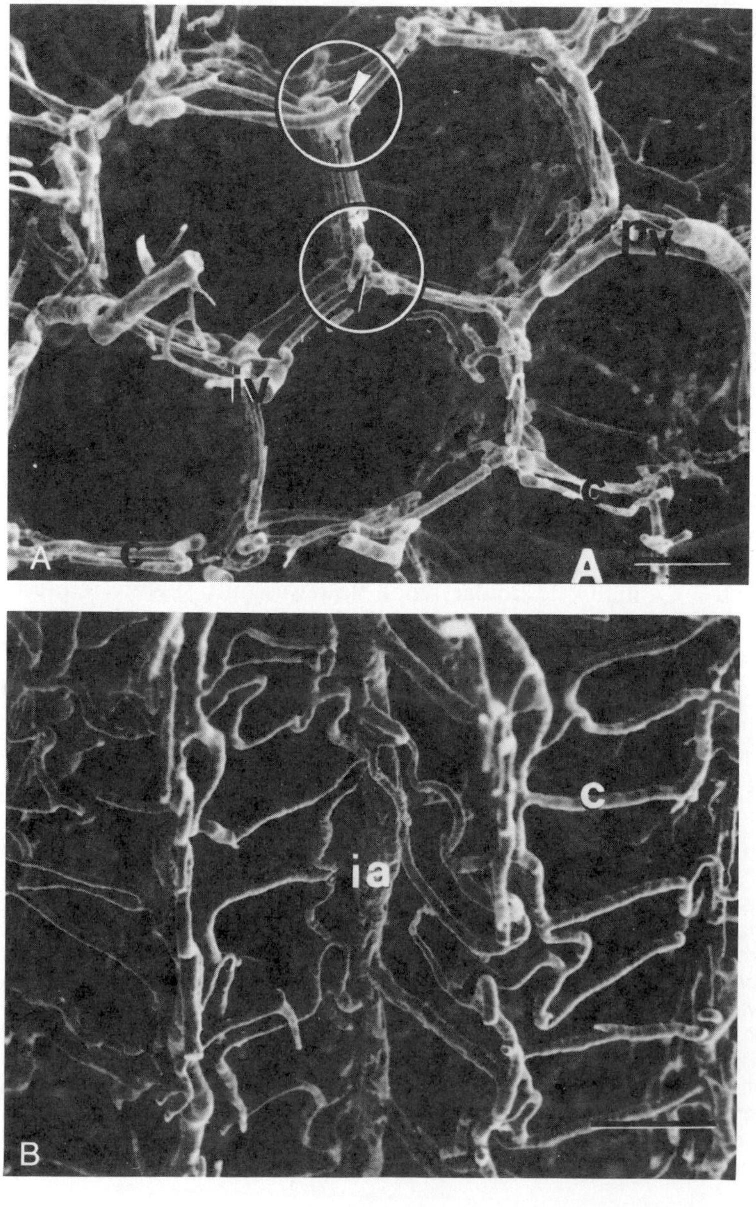

FIG. 30. The anatomy of the blood vessels in the rat testis. **A:** Cast of the blood vessels inside the testis sectioned at right angles to the seminiferous tubules, showing the three-dimensional arrangement of the intertubular and peritubular vessels. Note the clear hexagonal pattern of the vessels, with only one intertubular vessel (*arrowhead*) at each interstitial space (*circled*). iv, intertubular venule; pv, peritubular venule; c, peritubular capillaries; A, artery. Bar = 100 μm. **B:** Cast of the blood vessels cut parallel to the seminiferous tubules. Note the wavy intertubular vessels connected by short peritubular capillaries (c) to give the appearance of a rope-ladder. ia, Intertubular arteriole. Bar = 100 μm. (From ref. 1272.)

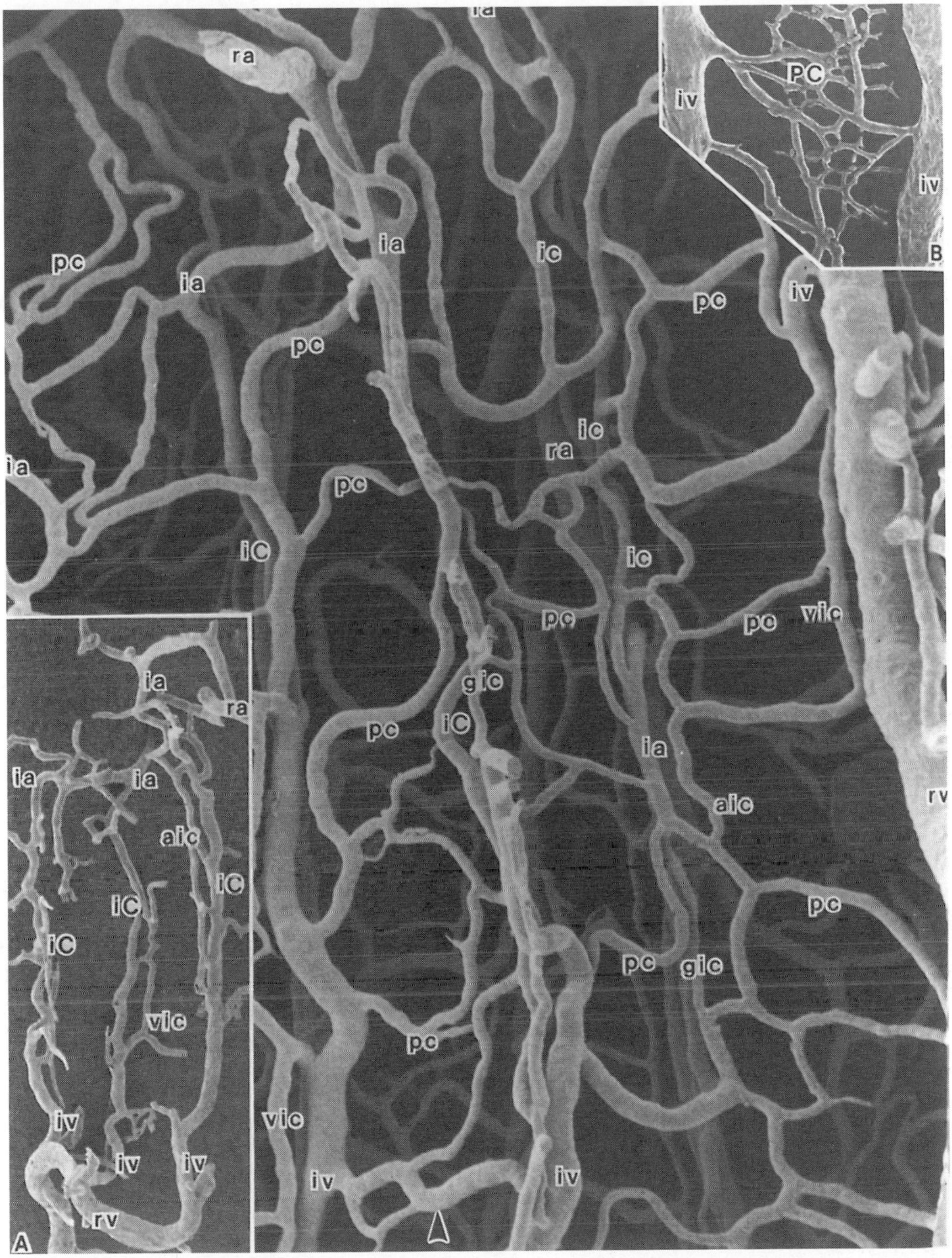

FIG. 31 A. Longitudinally freeze-cut aspect of the capillary networks surrounding the seminiferous tubules of an adult rat. Intertubular arterioles (ia), originating from terminal branches of a radiate artery (ra), give off intertubular (ic) and peritubular (pc) capillaries, which converge into intertubular veins (iv), which empty into a branch of a radiate vein (rv). Some of the peritubular capillaries continue into perivenular intertubular capillaries (vic), which run along the intertubular venules or larger veins before emptying into them. Some intertubular arterioles are accompanied by a periarteriolar intertubular capillary (aic). There are also intertubular arteriolar-venular thick capillary channels (iC). Some genuine intertubular capillaries (gic) drain into intertubular venules. The arrowhead indicates a venulo-venular anastomosis between intertubular venules. Inset A shows a dissected network from which the peritubular capillaries have been removed. Insert B shows a dense capillary meshwork (PC) between thick segments of intertubular venules.

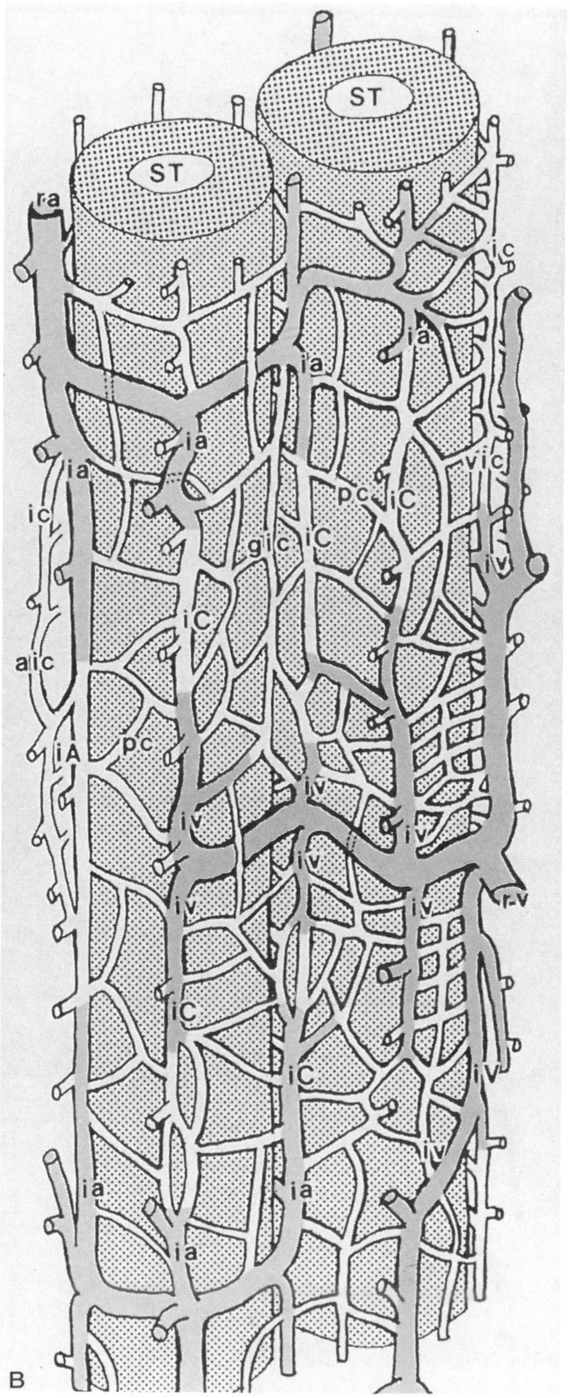

FIG. 31 B. Diagram showing the arrangement of the blood vascular bed of the testis of an adult rat. ST: seminiferous tubules, iA: arteriolo-arteriolar capillary channel, iC: intertubular arteriolo-venular capillary channel, iV: venulo-venular capillary channel, ia: intertubular arteriole, ic: intertubular capillary, iv: intertubular venule, pc: peritubular capillary, ra: branch of radiate artery, rv: branch of radiate vein, aic: periarterioar intertubular capillary, gic: genuine intertubular capillary, pic: perivenular intertubular capillary. (From ref. 820).

vessels comprise 5.6% of the whole testis and about 14% of the interstitial tissue (1078). In hamsters, the blood vessels comprise about 1.5% of the testis in the active phase and about 24% of the interstitial tissue (1108), and the volume density of the blood vessels does not change during seasonal regression and recrudescence (765). The pressure inside capillaries in the capsule of the hamster testis is about 10 mm Hg, which is appreciably lower than in other tissues (1146).

The permeability of the capillaries in the perfused rat testis to sodium, mannitol, and Cr-EDTA (144) can be estimated by injecting a bolus into the arterial inflow and estimating the fraction that is extracted by the testis during a single passage. The permeability-surface area product (PS) can then be calculated from the formula:

$$\mathrm{PS} = -Q \cdot \mathrm{Ln}\,(1 - E),$$

where Q is the blood or perfusate flow and E is the fraction extracted by the tissue. In the rat testis, PS for sodium, mannitol, or Cr-EDTA does not appear to be very different from that of capillaries in other tissues (144,1074).

By contrast, the entry and exit of larger hydrophilic molecules are largely determined by two factors, namely, vascular permeability and net fluid flux. Permeability in the strict sense is bidirectional and is determined by the properties of the walls of the blood vessels. Net fluid flux, however, is unidirectional and is influenced by the properties of the interstitial tissue as well as those of the vessel wall. In many other tissues, the interstitial barrier, and not the vascular wall, is the rate-limiting step in plasma-to-lymph albumin transport (81). PS area product for albumin can be calculated over a period of time (minutes or hours) from the rate at which radioactive albumin accumulates in the testis (Fig. 32)

$$\mathrm{PS} = k \cdot V_{\mathrm{final}},$$

where V_{final} is the volume of distribution of albumin at equilibrium, usually at between 5 and 10 h and k is the slope of the line $Ln\,(1 - V_t/V_{\mathrm{final}})$, where V_t is the volume of distribution of albumin at time t. This value is really a measure of permeability of the vessel wall plus the interstitial tissue and is influenced by both net fluid flux and vessel wall permeability and will be referred to as "apparent permeability." It is approximately equivalent to and has the same units (μl/g/min) as the albumin "clearance," as determined by Haraldsson et al. (443) from the change in albumin space with time between 3 and 120 min after injection of the marker into the bloodstream. Immediate or "true" permeability of the vessel wall to albumin can be determined by the same formula as for small molecules [$\mathrm{PS} = -Q \cdot \mathrm{Ln}\,(1 - E)$] from the single pass extraction (E) of radioactive albumin and flow rate (Q). Values for "true" permeability are much higher than those for "apparent" permeability determined under comparable conditions, emphasizing the impor-

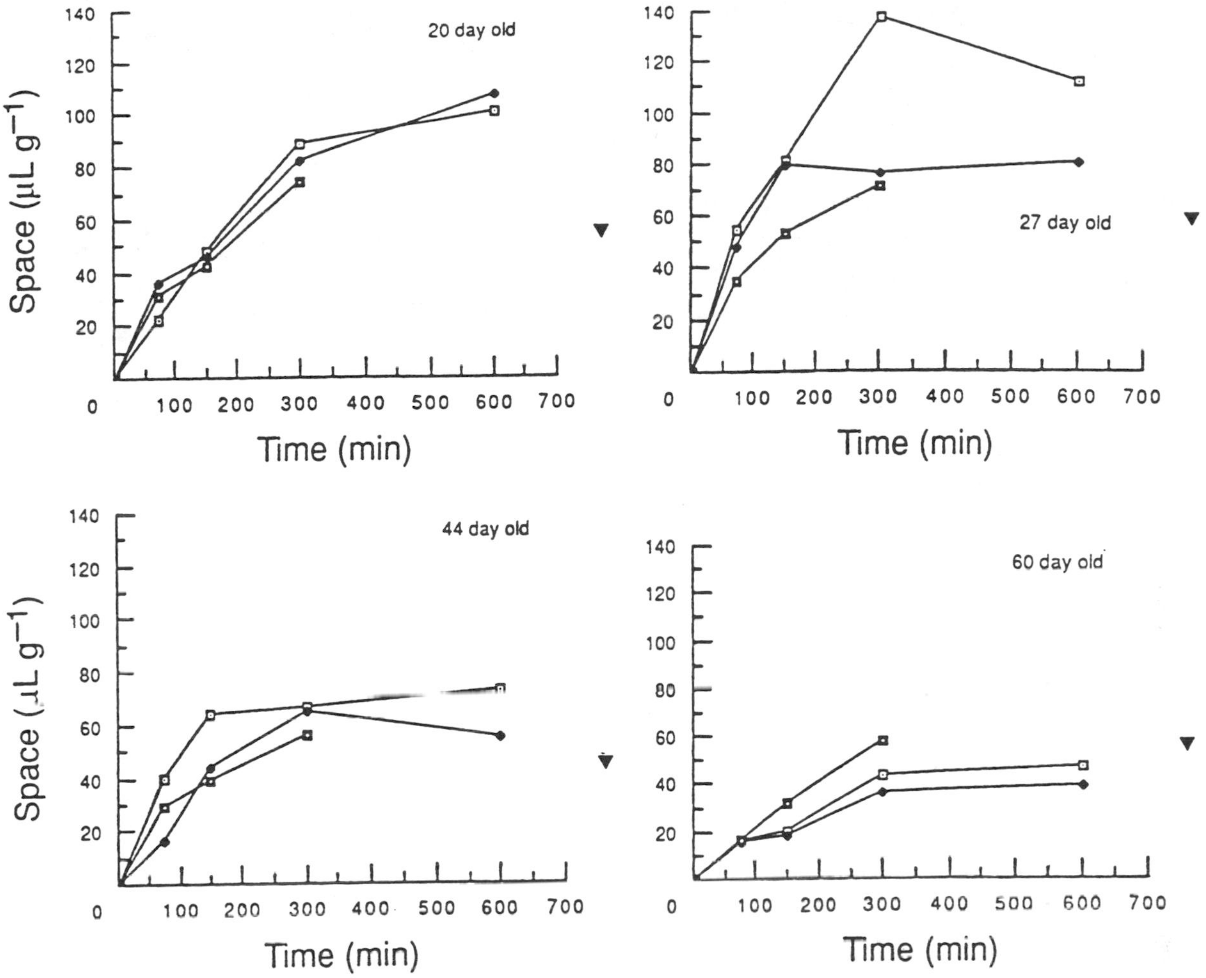

FIG. 32. Increments of the albumin space (open squares: data from ref. 1075, diamonds, unpublished observations) or of gamma globulin spaces (solid squares, data from ref. 930) at the times shown after intravenous injection of the marker, over the 3-min. albumin space, which is assumed to represent vascular volume, in rats of different ages. The triangles off the horizontal scale show the gamma globulin space increments at 1200 min. Mean apparent PS for albumin, calculated as described in the text, was 0.510, 1.706, 0.554 and 0.379 μl/g/min for the 20, 27, 44 and 60 day-old rats respectively, while the equivalent figures for gamma-globulin apparent PS were 0.418, 0.657, 0.440 and 0.313 μl/g/min. (From ref. 1039).

tance of net fluid flux and the interstitial tissue in determining the access of peptides to the cells in the testis. Furthermore, the calculated PS for γ-globulin, albumin, and human chorionic gonadotropin (hCG) are comparable (724,930), despite the differences in molecular size, supporting the idea that this measurement is more related to net fluid flux than to true permeability of the vessel wall.

Apparent permeability to albumin increases dramatically in the testes of rats after a single injection of hCG, beginning at about 8 h after injection (1052) and reaching a maximum after about 30 h. This effect seems to be mediated to some extent by 5-hydroxytryptamine (1125) and can be inhibited by treatment with the β-adrenergic agonist terbutaline (86). It does not appear to involve androgens, estrogens, PGs, histamine, or bradykinin (1125,1224) but depends on the presence of the Leydig cells (1051,1225), presumably because these are the cells that express the LH/hCG receptor, and appears to involve the accumulation of polymorph neutrophils (85,91,92,1284). Depletion of the macrophage population within the testis enhances the inflammatory response to hCG (94). However, it is striking that after hCG, there is only a small temporary increase in true permeability to albumin (339), and therefore, the rise in apparent permeability after hCG must involve primarily changes in net fluid flux.

Similarly, there is a large increase in apparent permeability to albumin and γ-globulin in rats at the age of about 30 days (930,1075) but no increase in true permeability at about this time (L. Tao, J. L. Zupp, and B. P. Setchell, *unpublished observations*). In contrast, after a single injection of a nontoxic dose of cadmium salts, both apparent and true permeability rise sharply (206,429,1055,1079), leading in a few hours to a virtual stoppage of blood flow (1255). Ultrastructural changes in the endothelial cells can be seen within hours of the administration of cadmium (34,190), and again it is only the capillaries of the postpubertal testis that show this peculiarity (209,844). Furthermore, the perfusion pressure needed to maintain normal flow rate also rises (1160). It is also interesting that neither histamine nor serotonin (5-hydroxytryptamine), which increases permeability in many other tissues, has any effect on apparent permeability in the testis (89,623,1076), although IL-1β does cause accumulation of leukocytes and an increase in vascular permeability, as studied by the accumulation of colloidal carbon in the tissue after injection into the bloodstream (89). In cryptorchid testes, apparent permeability is lower than normal, but there is a greater increase in interstitial fluid volume after injection of hCG (267,1086). There is clearly an important role for permeability and/or net fluid flux in regulating the access of peptide hormones to cells in the testis. The claim that a close "temporal coordination between pulses of luteinizing hormone and testosterone in the systemic circulation imply that peptides such as LH (mol wt = 28,000) are transferred across testicular capillaries remarkably fast" (383) cannot be sustained with the present evidence. It may be normal for a Leydig cell to "see" only 1% of an LH pulse, but obviously the extent to which the Leydig cells "see" any pulse will depend heavily on the permeability of the vessels.

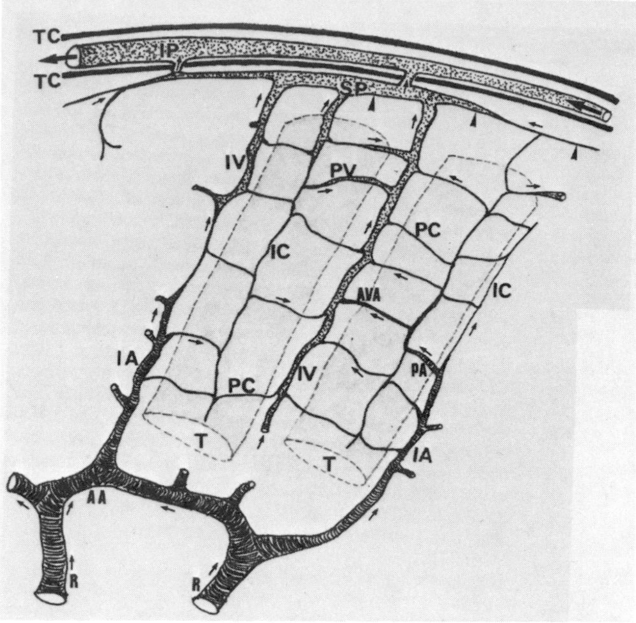

FIG. 33. A diagram of the blood vessels in the testis of a rat, in a plane parallel to the seminiferous tubules. The direction of blood flow is indicated by the *arrows*. T, seminiferous tubules; R, radiate arteries; AA, arterioarterial anastomotic arcade; IA, intertubular arteriole; IC, intertubular capillary; PA, peritubular arteriole; PC, peritubular capillary; PV, peritubular venule; AVA, arteriovenous anastomosis; IP, intra-albugineal plexus within the testicular capsule (TC); SP, subalbugineal plexus, with *arrowheads* indicating its component vein, venule, and capillary, respectively, from left to right. Venovenous anastomoses in this area are not shown. (From ref. 1272.)

Testicular Veins

The veins of the testis are also unusual in that they do not run with a corresponding artery. The small veins in the parenchyma open either into small veins on the surface of the testis (Fig. 33) or into a group of veins near the mediastinum. The balance between these two routes depends on species (e.g., the capsular veins take most of the blood in the ram and bull, whereas in the stallion, the mediastinal veins are more important; in human, the two routes are of approximately equal importance). In the rat, there are two large veins on the free face of the testis that unite just where the artery enters the parenchyma; they then divide again to form over the rete a small plexus that is really an extension of the pampiniform plexus (Fig. 34A and B). This intra-albugineal venous plexus has a "pore" (Fig. 35) where the veins part to run around a protusion of the rete testis and the efferent ducts (820). This smaller rete-associated plexus in the rat has recently been implicated in the resorption of fluids and substances from the seminiferous tubular fluid as it passes through the rete testis and appears to be an important site for the transport of substances from the seminiferous tubules into blood (see *Testis Blood Flow and Composition*). The existence of a rete testis–vascular association is harder to demonstrate physiologically in other mammals in which the rete testis is positioned mediastinally, because comparable blood samples cannot be obtained. However, there are anatomic descriptions of the vascular–rete associations in other species (454, 472,474,1311). Veins from the epididymal face join the pampiniform plexus near the point where the testicular artery reaches the testis (194,389,474,820,949,1028, 1032,1272). Valves are a rare feature of the testicular veins (474,1295). In marsupials, the veins drain to several main veins on the opposite side of the testis to the arteries (1028,1031,1032). In birds, the venous drainage is principally through surface veins, which unite to form two veins from each testis, and these enter the vena cava directly (646). No values have been reported for the pressure in the testicular veins of humans, but in the internal spermatic veins, the pressure reported ranges from 10 to 60 mm Hg (1001,1081,1322,1333). The mean pressure in the veins on the surface of the testes of rams and boars was between 10 and 40 mm Hg, depending on position of the animal, approximately twice that in the testicular vein above the spermatic cord (856,1252). In rats, testis vein pressure was about 12 mm Hg in conscious ani-

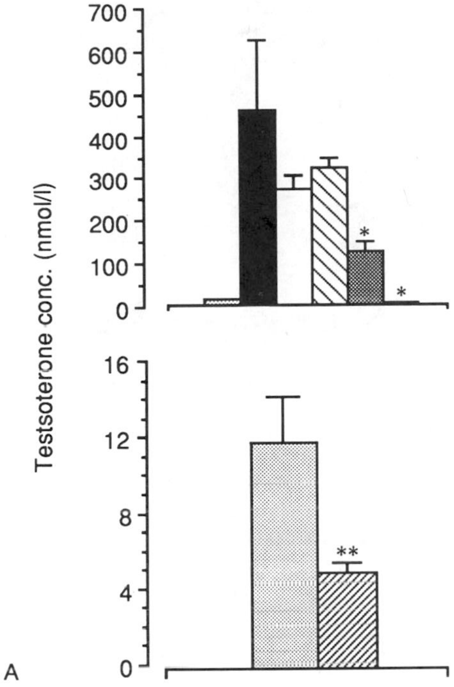

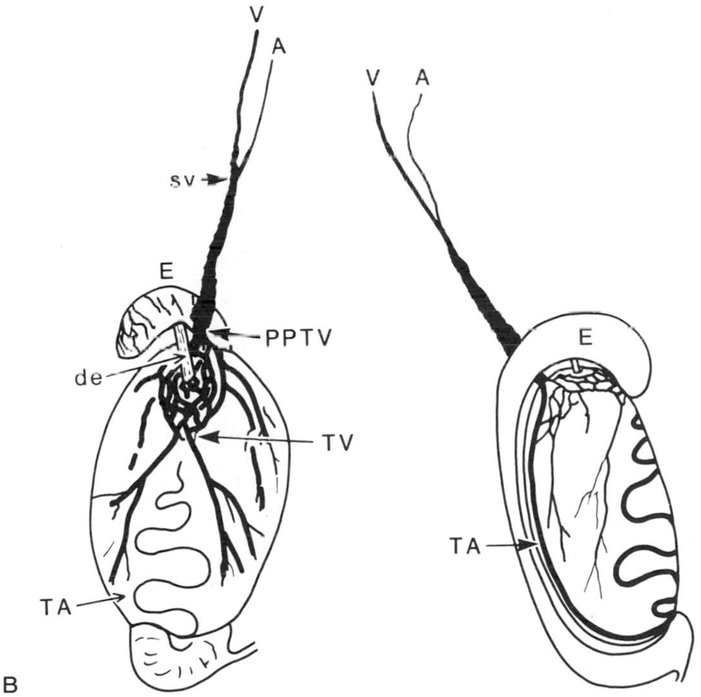

FIG. 34. A: The concentrations of testosterone in blood plasma from various sites around the testis of adult rats ($n = 5$), as illustrated in **B,** and in interstitial fluid (IF) collected by the drip technique. A: internal spermatic artery. TA: testicular artery on surface of testis. TV: testicular vein on surface of testis. PPTV: testicular veins at distal end of pampiniform plexus. SV and V: internal spermatic vein above the pampiniform plexus. PV: posterior vena cava. E: epididymis. de: efferent ducts. *: $P < 0.05$ compared with values in preceding column; **: $P < 0.01$ compared with TA values, by paired t-test. (From ref. 728).

mals, with little effect of anesthesia (365). The values given in a recent study in hamsters (1146), with pressures of 12.7 mm Hg in arterioles, 10.1 mm Hg in capillaries, and 9.9 mm Hg in small venules in the capsule, may be underestimates because of the position of the animal, on its back with its legs and scrotum above the heart. However, the small difference between arteriolar and venular pressure and the high pre- to postcapillary resistance ratio are most unusual and may have important consequences in fluid movement in the testis (see section *Interstitial Fluid of the Testis; Volume, Turnover Rate, and Composition*). It also makes capillary pressure particularly sensitive to increases in venous pressure (1146), and venous pressure has been reported to be elevated in vari-

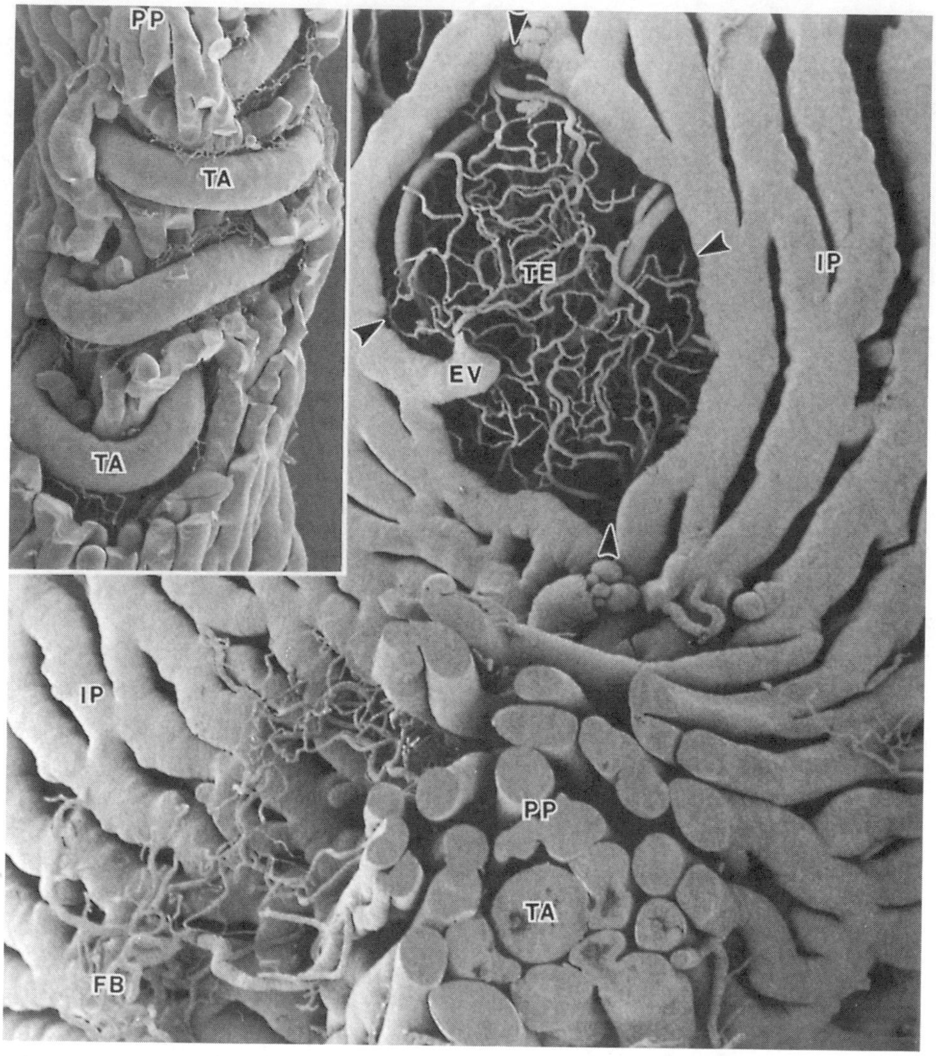

FIG. 35. Scanning electron microscope picture of a methacrylate corrosion cast of the intra-albugineal venous plexus (IP) of a testis of an adult rat. The pampiniform plexus (PP) has been cut off at its base, along with the testicular artery (TA). As the venous plexus converges towards the pampiniform plexus, there is an intra-albugineal venous "pore". (arrowheads) through which the rete testis is joined to the efferent ducts. TE: the testicular capillay bed, seen through the intra-albugineal pore. EV: a venous branch from the epididymis joining the intra-albugineal plexus. FB: remnants of blood vessels in the fatty tissue surrounding the spermatic cord. The inset show the testicular artery (TA) and the pampiniform plexus (PP) in the thickest part of the spermatic cord. (From ref. 820).

cocele (see above), possibly contributing to the pathogenesis of this condition. Testicular venous pressure would almost certainly be reduced during caudal elevation and in simulated and real space flights, which may help explain the lesions in the testes of rats subjected to these procedures (28,76,289).

Epididymis

The epididymis receives its blood from two main arterial routes (Fig. 28A). The caput, corpus, and proximal cauda epididymidis are supplied by arteries that branch from the spermatic artery just before, or soon after, it reaches thc pampiniform plexus (e.g., mouse [3,194, 1143], rat [194,456,633,866], rabbit [194,202], dog [456], ram [558], boar [1132,1133], camel [887], and man [456,721]), whereas the cauda epididymidis is supplied from the deferential artery, a branch from the internal iliac (hypogastric) artery. The lemur does not conform to this general pattern in that vessels supplying the caput and corpus epididymidis branch from the testicular artery after it has gained the surface of the testis rather than branching in the spermatic cord (455). There are usually two branches of the epididymal artery (Fig. 28A). The superior epididymal artery supplies the ductuli efferentes, caput, and proximal corpus, whereas the inferior epididymal artery serves the corpus and proximal cauda epididymidis. Anastomoses exist between the epididymal arteries and deferential artery on the surface of the epididymis (3,194,202,344,456,458,633,721,865, 887,1143). Functional anastomoses between the superior epididymal artery and the testicular artery and between the deferential artery and the testicular artery have also been reported (108,344,456,596,631,721,840,1133). The epididymal arteries ramify on the surface of the epididymis and enter the organ centripetally within the connective tissue septula, which divide the epididymis into zones. Each septal artery provides branches to both adjacent zones to form capillary networks around the tubule. The epididymal veins follow the same route as their respective arteries (Fig. 28B). As with the arterial system, extensive anastomoses occur among the epididymal veins. In the rat, the inferior epididymal vein forms a plexus, which completely surrounds the proximal portion of the inferior epididymal artery (866). A similar arrangement has been described in the rabbit for the superior and inferior epididymal veins and the deferential vein (194). These plexus systems may function as a countercurrent heat exchange system to cool the epididymal blood supply in an analogous fashion to the pampiniform plexus. Veins have also been shown to form vascular connections between the testis and ductuli efferentes in the mouse, rat, and rabbit (194); in the rat, rabbit, and human, there is also a venous connection between the posterior pole of the testis and the cauda epididymidis (194,389,631). The microvascular structure of the epididymis has been the subject of several studies using a variety of techniques. In the now classical study of Kormano (633), the microangiographic technique revealed significant differences in the capillary arrangement in different regions of the epididymis. In the initial segment of the epididymis, capillaries form a dense and tortuous network around the tubules. In the middle segment of the epididymis, the density and tortuosity of the capillaries is reduced, and the capillaries follow the wall of the epididymal duct more closely. As the muscle wall thickens in the terminal segment of the epididymis, the capillaries tend to form two separate networks around the epididymal duct. One network is located in the interductular connective tissue, and this sends branches to a second network surrounding the lamina propria. A similar study of the human epididymis (637) reveals some differences when compared with the rat. The principal differences concern a thick, densely vascularized connective tissue sheath surrounding the human epididymis and an extensive degree of coiling of the arteries, which penetrate into the organ among the connective tissue septula. Few branches are given off before the septal arteries disperse into the fine microvascular bed. The human ductuli efferentes are supplied by a relatively dense subepithelial capillary bed. The capillary bed of the epididymis is less extensive, and in contrast to the rat, the organization of the capillary network does not show much variation along the length of the epididymis.

A more recent technique of casting coupled with scanning electron microscopy has been applied to examine the microvasculature of the mouse epididymis (1143), which largely confirms the features described in the rat (633). The ductuli efferentes are supplied with vessels that run longitudinally and give off peritubular capillaries analogous to the arrangement seen within the testis (Fig. 30, 31). A similar arrangement is present in the middle segment of the epididymis (Figs. 36A and 37A). By contrast, in the initial segment, peritubular capillaries penetrate the thin muscular layer and form a dense cylindrical subepithelial network with frequent intercon-

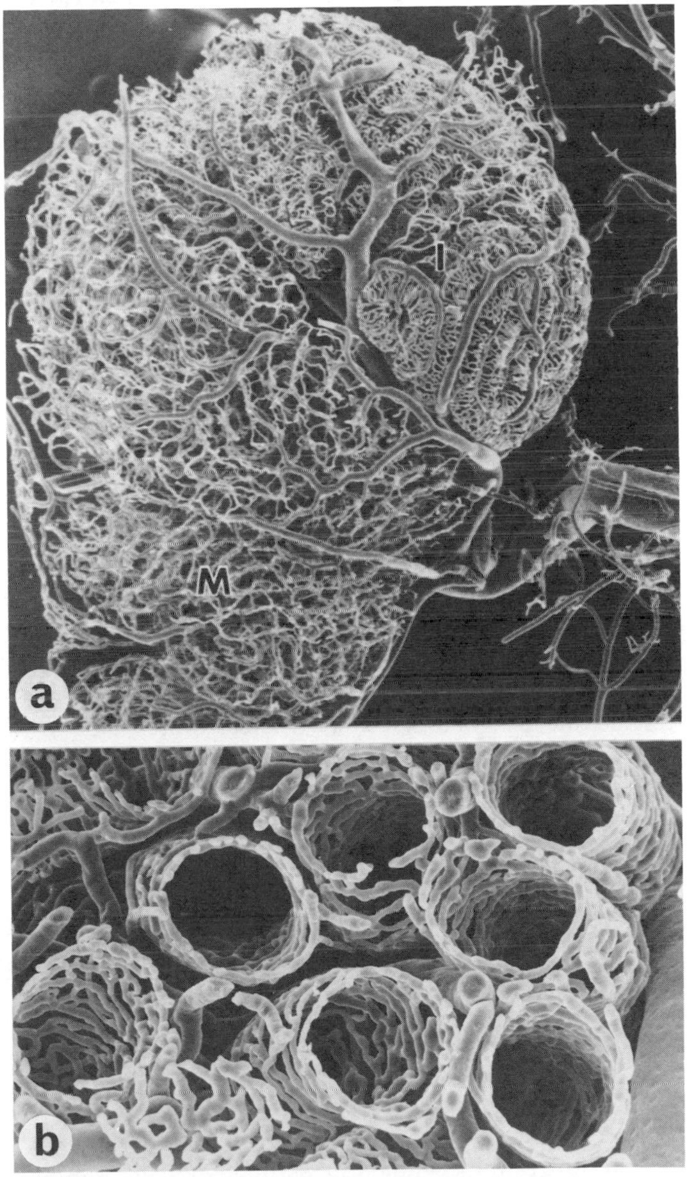

FIG. 36. Microvasculature of the initial and middle segments of the mouse epididymis. **a:** In the initial segment (I) peritubular capillaries form a dense cylindrical subepithelial network with frequent interconnections, while in the middle segment (M) peritubular capillaries branch from longitudinal vessels and do not interconnect. **b:** View of the cut surface of the initial segment to reveal the dense network of interconnected peritubular capillaries. Larger vessels can be seen running in the interstitial spaces. (From ref. 1143.)

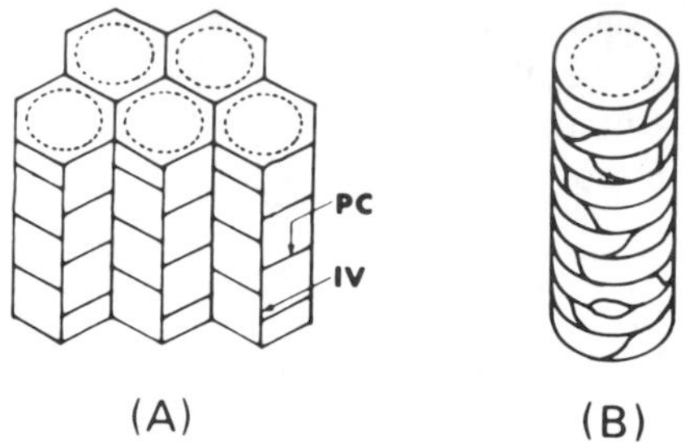

FIG. 37. Diagrammatic representation of the two fundamental types of peritubular capillaries seen in the mouse testis and excurrent duct system. The arrangement in the testis and middle segment of the epididymis is depicted in **(A),** whereas **(B)** represents the arrangement in the initial segment and ductus deferens. The tubule is depicted by the *dotted line* and the intertubular vessels (IV) are simplified as a single straight line joined by peritubular capillars (PC). (From ref. 1143.)

nections (Figs. 36A,B and 37B). In rats, there is a decrease in capillary size and in the percentage of capillaries within the interstitial region from the initial segment to the cauda (758). The dense peritubular capillary network of the initial segment is absent in XXSxr "pseudomale" mice (678). In the boar epididymis, there are two superimposed vascular networks; the outer consists of feeding and draining vessels, and the inner comprises periductal capillaries. The arrangement of these varies along the epididymis, with polygonal meshes around the efferent ducts and circularly distributed capillaries around the duct in the caput. The arrangement changes back to a polygonal network as one passes from the caput to the cauda (1132). In the fowl, the rete testis has a sparse microvasculature, but the efferent ducts and the rest of the epididymis have a dense peritubular network located just beneath the epithelium. The capillaries in the rete are nonfenestrated, whereas those in the rest of the excurrent duct system are fenestrated (831). By contrast, in mammals, the capillaries of the initial segment are fenestrated, whereas those in the remainder of the epididymis are not (3,1143). The presence of fenestrated capillaries in the initial segment may be an adaptation to the specific role of this region of the epididymis in the reabsorption of the bulk of the rete testis fluid that enters the epididymis. Indeed, the development and continued presence of fenestrated capillaries is dependent on the efferent ducts being patent, because the fenestrations are markedly reduced after section or ligation of the ducts (3). This specific role of the initial segment in fluid reabsorption is also reflected by the fact that the blood flow to this region is substantially greater than in any other part of the epididymis (1059). Moreover, the enhanced blood flow in the initial segment is abolished after efferent duct ligation or castration (138).

Ductus Deferens

Blood travels to the ductus deferens by way of the internal iliac, hypogastric, and finally the deferential artery. The returning venous blood travels in the deferential vein, which returns along the ductus deferens and empties into the hypogastric vein. It is clear from microangiographic studies that the microvascular bed surrounding the ductus deferens forms two separate networks (633,637). The outer network is located within the connective tissue surrounding the muscle layers, and from this, small arteries penetrate through the muscle to the lamina propria, where they form a dense subepithelial capillary network. More sophisticated corrosion casting and scanning electron microscopy have confirmed this arrangement and revealed additional features (439,865,1143). In the distal two-thirds of the rat ductus deferens and also in the mouse ductus deferens, a sinusoidal layer is found beneath the muscle layer (Fig. 38). Arterial branches penetrate from the adventitial layer centripetally through the muscle layer supplying capillaries to the muscular tissue *en route.* When they reach the lamina propria, these arteries break up into arterioles, some of which end in a sinusoidal layer while others penetrate through this network to form a subepithelial capillary network (Fig. 38A) reminiscent of that seen in the initial segment of the epididymis (Fig. 36). The subepithelial capillary network drains into the sinusoidal network, which is in turn drained by venules that pass through the muscle layers, collecting capillaries from the muscle layers on the way, and joining veins in the adventitia. Conspicuous constrictions are present in the venules at the point at which they leave the sinusoidal network (Fig. 38B). The exact function of the sinusoidal layer in the ductus deferens is unknown at present. It is possible that engorgement of the sinusoidal network could be achieved by further contraction of the sphincter-like constrictions present in the venules that drain the system. Thus, the sinusoidal layer may function as a device to increase pressure within the lumen of the ductus deferens during ejaculation.

Prostate and Seminal Vesicles

The blood supply to the accessory glands of the rat has been described by Jesik et al. (569). The arterial supply can be traced from the aorta to the common iliac arteries, which divide to form the internal and external iliac arteries. The internal iliac artery, otherwise known as the hypogastric artery, supplies the prostate, bladder, coagulating glands, seminal vesicles, and vasa deferentia (Fig. 39). The superior vesical artery leaves from the ventral surface of the internal iliac and supplies branches to the seminal vesicles and coagulating glands and continues to supply branches to the dorsal, lateral, and ventral prostatic lobes and to the vasa deferentia (deferential arteries) and ureters (ureteral arteries). The inferior vesical artery leaves the superior vesical artery at the point where it meets the urinary bladder. It supplies blood to the dorsal surface of the prostate and the bladder, anastomosing with the superior vesical artery. The venous drainage of

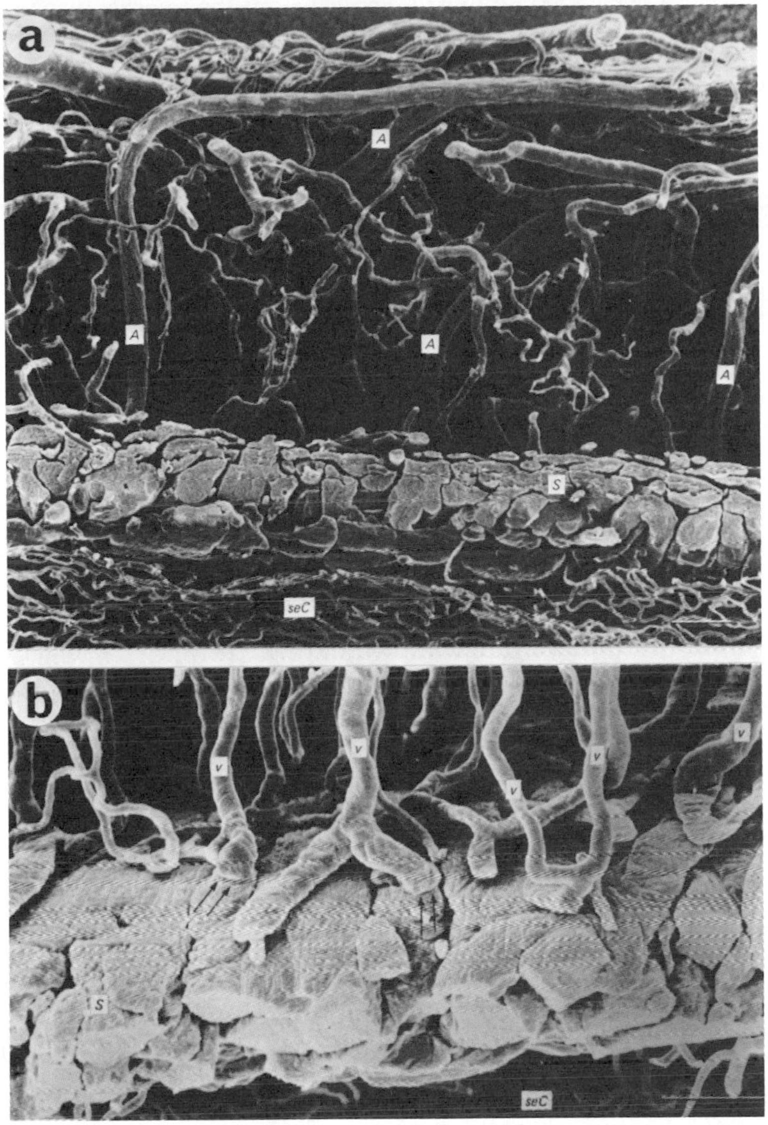

FIG. 38. Corrosion cast of the vascular supply to the rat ductus deferens. **a:** The major blood vessels run in the adventitia and send arterial branches (A) through the muscle layer where they supply a sinusoidal layer (S) and a subepithelial network (seC). **b:** Detailed view of the sinusoidal layer (S) being drained by venules (V) with prominent constrictions (*arrows*) located at the point of departure of these vessels from the sinusoidal layer. (From ref. 865.)

the rat accessory glands has been studied in detail by Lewis and Moffat (700), and the organization described by them has been largely confirmed by Ohtani and Gannon (865). The general arrangement is depicted in Fig. 40. The deferential vein draining the cauda epididymidis and ductus deferens empties into the hypogastric vein, as does the left spermatic vein from the testis and veins from the seminal vesicle and coagulating gland. The hypogastric vein drains at one end into the external iliac vein, but as its other end it joins a single large circular anastomosis formed by dorsal and ventral veins surrounding the base of the bladder. The ventral prostatic lobes drain by straight veins directly into this venous circle around the bladder and the term *prostatic veins* has been suggested for them. Lewis and Moffat (700) considered that veins from the dorsolateral prostate also drain into the venous circle, but Ohtani and Gannon (865) claimed that the drainage of this gland and of the distal vas deferens is into the vein leaving the seminal vesicle. The particular anatomy of the venous system may allow intermittent reversed flow from the hypogastric vein, thus carrying the drainage from the cauda epididymidis and ductus deferens into the prostatic complex. A similar vascular arrangement would allow retrograde flow from the deferential vein into the canine prostate (294). Such an event may explain the observed local control of the accessory sex glands by the epididymis and ductus deferens (920). It is assumed that the local factors responsible are androgens traveling in the deferential vein. In fact, the concentration of steroid hormones measured in the deferential vein of the dog are an order of magnitude greater than in peripheral plasma (109). The arterial supply to the seminal vesicles and prostate of man has been the subject of several studies (204,205,350,825). There is considerable variation between specimens in the arrangement of the blood vessels, and some confusion has arisen because of differences in the nomenclature used to describe the vessels. It seems

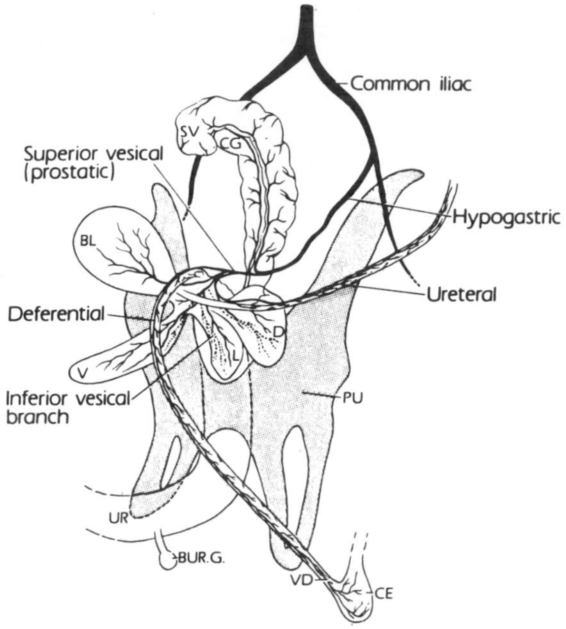

FIG. 39. Arterial supply to the male accessory glands of the rat. SV, seminal vesicle; CG, coagulating gland; V, ventral prostate; L, lateral prostate; D, dorsal prostate; BL, bladder; UR, urethra; PU, pubic bones; BUR.G., bulbourethral gland; VD, vas deferens; CE, cauda epididymidis. (From ref. 569.)

that the main arterial supply is derived from the anterior division of the internal iliac (hypogastric) artery. From this vessel arise the umbilical, vesiculodeferential, and prostatovesical arteries. The superior vesical branches from the umbilical artery near its junction with the internal iliac artery, whereas the origin of the vesiculodeferential and prostatovesical arteries is variable. The seminal vesicles and ductus deferens are supplied by branches from the vesiculodeferential artery, whereas the prostatovesical artery divides to form the inferior vesical and prostatic arteries. The prostatic artery further subdivides into a urethral and capsular group of blood vessels. The urethral group supplies the periurethral regions of the prostate and the urethra, whereas the capsular group supplies the ventral and dorsal regions of the prostatic capsule and approximately two-thirds of the parenchyma. A particular feature of the prostatic arteries is a tortuosity or "corkscrew" pattern on the surface of the organ and also in the stroma (204). Greater detail of the arrangement of vessels within the gland can be found in the article by Clegg (205). Venous blood leaves the prostate through a plexus (plexus of Santorini) situated at the base of the gland, particularly on the anterior and lateral surface. The seminal vesicle also drains into the prostatic plexus and the inferior vesical plexus. Blood from these plexuses then enters the internal iliac veins. The arterial supply to the prostate of the dog differs from that in man in that the glandular tissue of the prostate is supplied solely from the capsular group of arteries (513). The capsular arteries are derived from branches of the umbilical artery, urogenital artery, and internal pudendal arteries, which are ultimately derived from the internal iliac artery. The venous drainage takes the form of a densely branching network within the radial septa of the gland, which converge to form larger vessels within the septa and pass toward the periphery to form a venous plexus beneath the capsule. Prostatic veins leave this plexus accompanying prostatic arteries and unite to form the prostatica-vesical vein, which may unite with the prostatica-urethral vein to become the urogenital vein, which drains into the external iliac vein (294,513,1145).

Bulbourethral Glands

The main arterial supply to the human bulbourethral glands is derived from the artery to the bulb of the penis with subsidiary supplies from the internal pudendal artery, the urethral artery, the perineal artery, or an anastomosis between the cystic inferior artery and the internal pudendal artery (673). Arteries within the capsule of the gland send arterioles into the septa between the lobules of the gland.

LYMPHATIC DRAINAGE

The general arrangement of the lymphatic drainage from the testis and accessory glands is shown in Fig. 41. Lymphatic vessels that originated from the testis and epididymis run in the spermatic cord to the lumbar or para-aortic lymph nodes (709,773,800,811). In pigs, there may sometimes be a small lymph node in the spermatic cord itself. It has been claimed that in rats, testicular lymph reached the thoracic duct without passing through a lymph node (325,612,613), but other studies using the movement of carbon particles (467,1168), fluorescein-labeled lymph node cells (467), radio-opaque media (771), or colloidal radiopharmaceuticals (1326) injected into the testis showed that the lymphatic vessels in the cord run to iliac and renal lymph nodes, with some drainage to para-aortic, lumbar, and posterior gastric nodes. These findings were supported by observations on regional hypertrophy of draining lymph nodes after a graft-versus-host reaction induced by the injection of foreign lymph node cells into the testis (467).

Testis

The lymphatic drainage of the testis was described and illustrated by the early anatomists (see refs. 541,1028), but there was a lively controversy about the nature of the system inside the testis. One group believed that there were no true lymphatic vessels there but only lymphatic spaces surrounding the tubules. Another series of authors believed that in the interstitial spaces they could see discrete lymphatic vessels, which joined larger vessels in

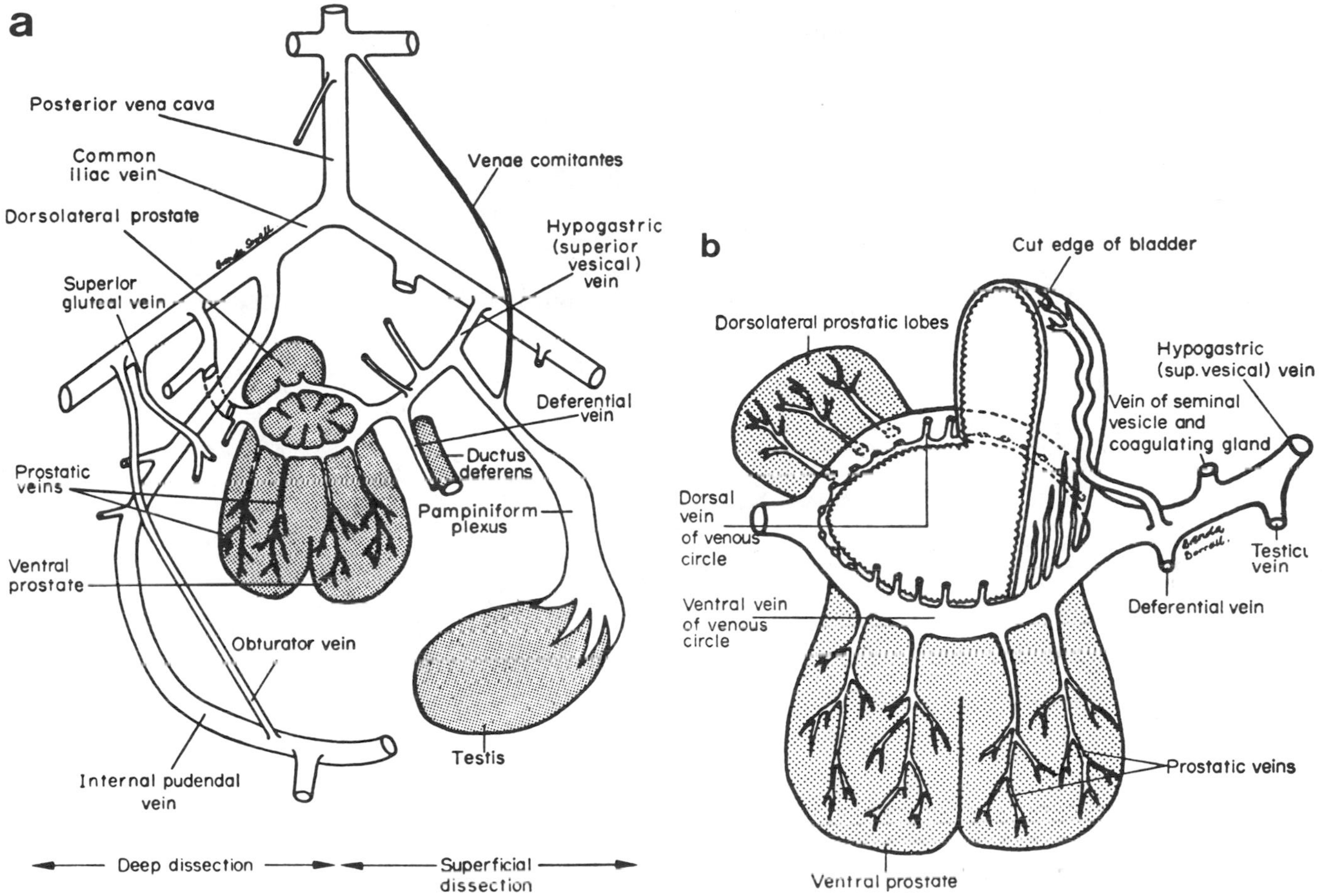

FIG. 40. Venous drainage of the male accessory glands of the rat. **(a):** General representation of the pelvic venous system showing vessels seen by superficial dissection on the right and deep dissection on the left. **(b):** Details of the venous drainage from the bladder and prostatic lobes. (From ref. 700.)

the septa and a network of vessels in the capsule, giving rise to the lymphatic trunks in the spermatic cord. Later studies with the electron microscope showed that in rodents, there were indeed large lymphatic sinusoids surrounding the tubules, so that these were virtually floating in a sea of lymph; however, in man and in many of the larger mammals, there were definite lymphatic vessels that lay in a fibrous interstitial tissue (339,341) (Figs. 8 and 9). In birds, there are prelymphatic spaces between the seminiferous tubules, communicating with discrete vessels that carry the lymph to a narrow-mesh network on the surface of the testis; collecting vessels converge on the hilus and carry the lymph to the thoracoabdominal trunk (645). The lymphatic vessels of the rabbit testis run in the tunica albuginea toward the epididymal margin and over the epididymis to join the epididymal lymphatics and form large lymphatic vessels in the cord (203). The lymphatic drainage of the rat testis has been examined in some detail (913,914). There are three groups of lymphatic vessels leaving the surface of the testis, from the cranial pole, the epididymal margin, and the caudal pole (Fig. 42), but all three join the epididymal lymphatics in the spermatic cord (Figs. 43 and 44). Other studies have confirmed that the lymphatic vessels leaving the rat testis pass over the surface of the epididymis and showed that, in the ram, much of the lymphatic drainage from the caudal pole of the testis runs in a vessel that passes under the tail of the epididymis and then between the ductus deferens and the body of the epididymis to the spermatic cord (1036). This arrangement may have important physiologic implications in the transfer of substances from the testis to the epididymis (see *Significance of Testicular Lymph*). In bulls, there is an intimate association between the cranial part of the rete and adjacent large, thin-walled lymphatics, and it has been suggested that this arrangement may facilitate transfer of androgen into rete testis fluid (472). Ligation of the testicular lymphatic vessels in the rabbit led to degenerative changes in the testis and substantial falls in the testosterone levels in blood from the internal spermatic vein (644). In the rat, less obvious, but nonetheless appreciable changes in the testis and epididymis have been reported after interruption of the lymphatic drainage (912).

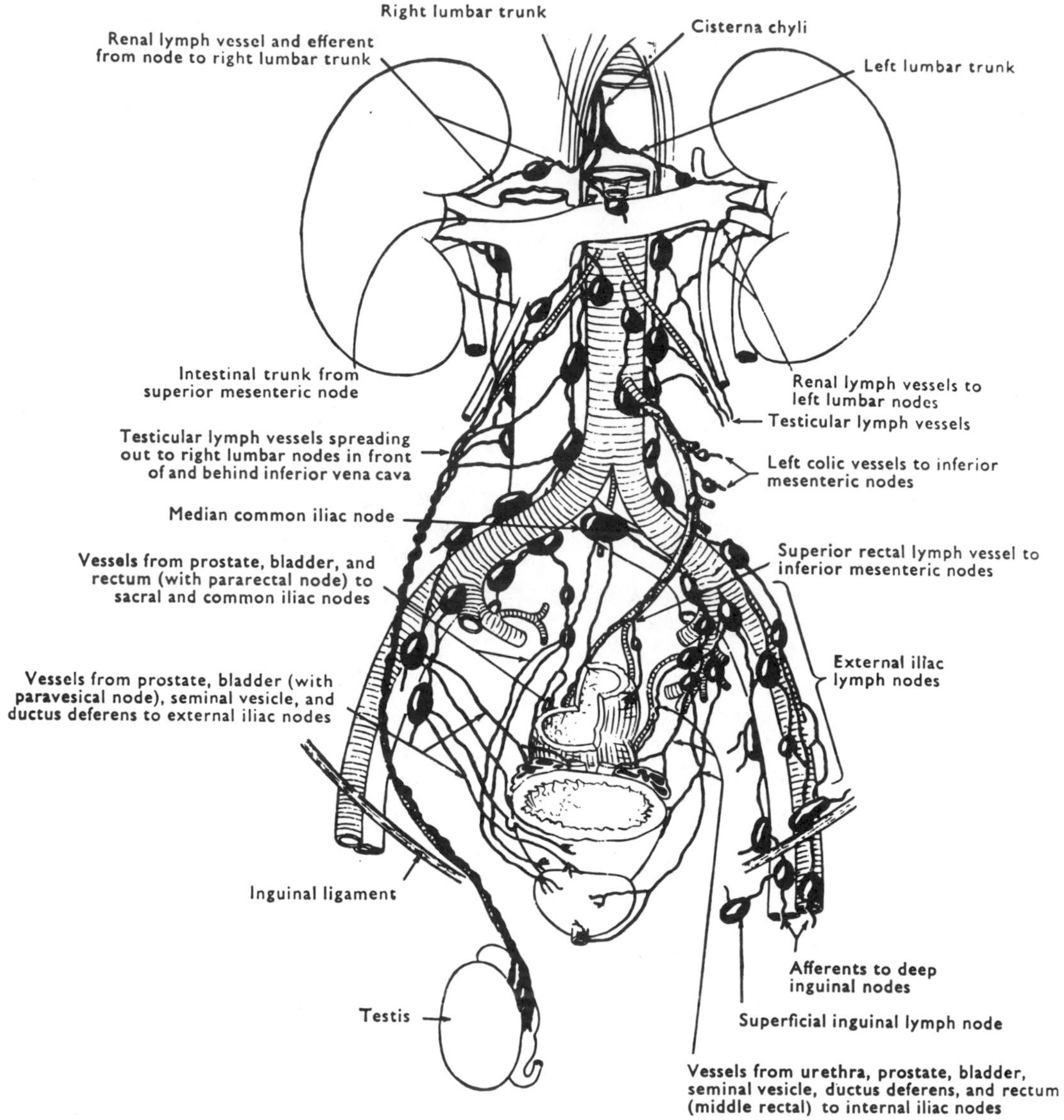

FIG. 41. Distribution of lymph vessels and lymph nodes in the human pelvis and abdomen. (From ref. 1264.)

Epididymis

Lymphatic sinusoids can be seen in the intertubular spaces in tissue sections prepared for electron microscopy (e.g., refs. 436,611). Details of the arrangement of lymphatic vessels within the organ as a whole have not, however, been elucidated. The only species in which there has been any detailed investigation of the lymphatic drainage system leaving the epididymis has been the rat (772,914). Lymphatic vessels leave the epididymis at various points along its length. The caput epididymidis has the greatest number of vessels leaving it, one or two vessels leave the corpus, and a single vessel emanates from the cauda. There is little anastomosis between the vessels, with the exception of a channel running along the medial face of the caput and proximal corpus, but the vessels gradually coalesce and join the main testicular lymphatic trunk, which accompanies the spermatic artery to reach the para-aortic group of lymph nodes. The lymphatic vessels leaving the epididymis form a so-called lymphatic triangle (Fig. 43), occupying a plane posterolateral to the testicular vascular bundle, which intervenes between the lymphatic drainage system of the testis and the epididymis. Nevertheless, there are several connections between the lymphatic drainage of the testis and epididymis, apart from the final convergence of the main testicular and lymphatic trunks (Fig. 44).

Prostate

The only male accessory organ that has received any attention with regard to lymphatic drainage is the prostate. The lymphatic drainage system is conceived as a

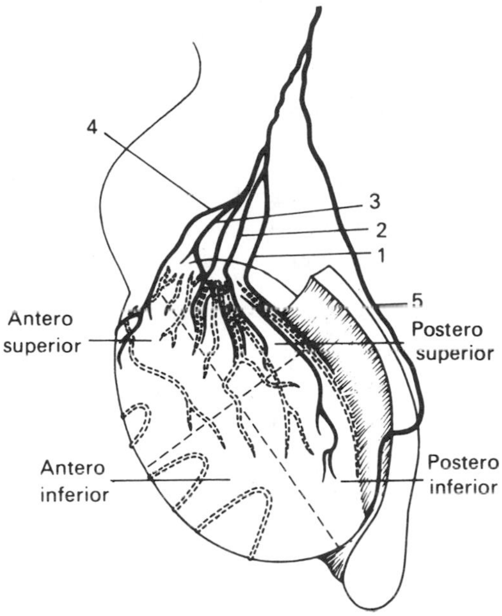

FIG. 42. The lymphatic drainage of the testis of a rat. This drawing was made from a rat that had received an intratesticular injection of India ink. The testicular artery and veins are shown by *dotted lines,* and the testis has been divided into four quadrants. The superficial lymphatic vessels are shown draining the anterosuperior, posterosuperior, and posteroinferior quadrants. The numbers on the diagram show the order in which the vessels were filled with the ink when injection was made into the lower pole of the testis. (From ref. 913.)

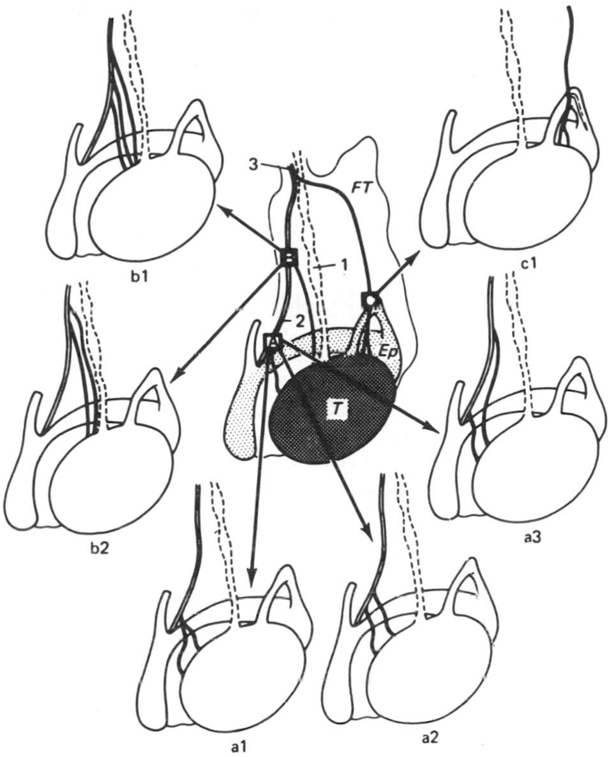

FIG. 44. Diagrammatic representation of various patterns of communication between the lymphatic drainage of the testis and the lymphatic drainage of the epididymis in the rat. T, testis; Ep, epididymis; FT, epididymal fat pad. In the central drawing, note (1) the pampiniform plexus in *dotted outline,* (2) the inferior epididymal trunk, (3) the main testicular lymphatic trunk and other testicular lymphatics in *black.* Sites at which testicular lymphatics join epididymal lymphatics are indicated by A, B, and C; variations in the communication of testicular lymphatics with epididymal lymphatics at the three sites are depicted in the peripheral drawings (a_1, a_2, a_3, b_1, b_2, c_1). (From ref. 914.)

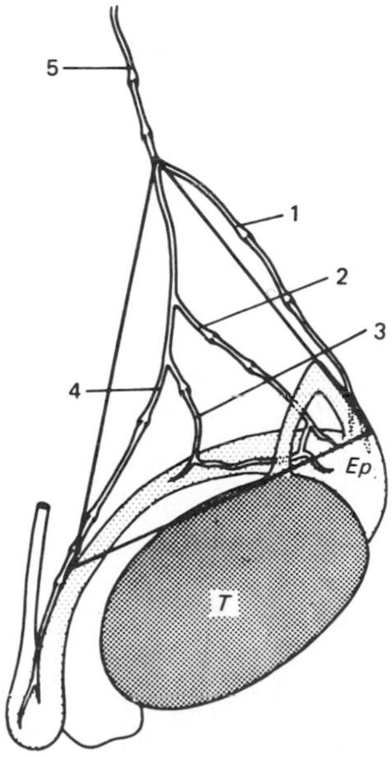

FIG. 43. Diagrammatic representation of the basic pattern of lymphatic drainage of the rat epididymis. 1, Ductular lymphatic trunk; 2, superior epididymal trunk; 3, corporeal epididymal trunk; 4, inferior epididymal trunk; 5, main testicular lymphatic trunk; T, testis; Ep, epididymis. Note the epididymal "lymphatic triangle" subtended on the epididymis and bounded by the lymphatic trunk (1) and the inferior epididymal trunk (4). (From ref. 914.)

possible route for the spread of tumor cells derived from carcinoma of the prostate, whereas the possible absence of intraprostatic lymphatics could render the prostate an immunologically privileged site favoring growth of malignantly transformed cells. The existence of a pericapsular lymphatic system, which drains toward the external iliac, internal iliac, and common iliac lymph nodes, is well established (see ref. 1105), but the existence of intraprostatic lymphatics has been open to more controversy (771). The debate has perhaps arisen because the methods chosen to demonstrate intraprostatic lymphatics have not always been appropriate, such as the use of vital stains that leach out during processing of tissue for light microscopy (1119). There has also been some confusion as to whether spaces that are observed to surround some prostatic neurons in tissue sections are perineural spaces or lymphatic channels (971), but the absence of an endothelium indicates that such spaces are not lymphatic vessels. However, the weight of evidence from studies using precipitable dyes and direct ultrastructural studies

(218,381,782,834,1201) would support the existence of intraprostatic lymphatics located in the connective tissue of the gland parenchyma and radiating to the capsule of the organ through the fibrous trabeculae.

INNERVATION

For an historical account of the study of the innervation of the internal male genital organs, the reader is referred to the article by Sjostrand (1109). The testis, epididymis, and male accessory glands are devoid of somatic innervation but receive dual innervation from branches of the autonomic nervous system and possess, in addition, a sensory afferent system. The visceral efferent (motor) supply to these organs is derived from prevertebral nerve plexuses surrounding the arteries. There are five main interconnecting prevertebral plexuses: the celiac (solar), intermesenteric (aortic), caudal (inferior, posterior) mesenteric, hypogastric, and pelvic plexuses. The celiac plexus obtains its sympathetic supply from the thoracic and lumbar splanchnic nerves, whereas the other plexuses receive only lumbar splanchnics. The celiac plexus also receives a parasympathetic supply from the vagus nerve. The intermesenteric plexus, which lies on the ventral and ventrolateral aspects of the aorta, connects the celiac plexus with the more caudal plexuses (caudal mesenteric, hypogastric, and pelvic plexuses). In most species, most of the nerves pass from the intermesenteric plexus to the caudal mesenteric plexus, but in man some of the outermost nerves pass directly to the hypogastric plexus. The caudal mesenteric plexus surrounds the caudal mesenteric artery and contains one or more ganglia. A net of nerves located distal to the bifurcation of the aorta constitutes the hypogastric plexus in man, but in other species the hypogastric nerve is a single discrete nerve arising from the posterior border of the caudal mesenteric ganglion. The hypogastric nerves, which are fused for a short distance in the rabbit, supply the right and left pelvic plexuses. In addition to the sympathetic supply from the hypogastric nerve, the pelvic plexus receives parasympathetic fibers from the pelvic nerve, which arises from the sacral nerves. Various peripheral ganglia have been recognized in different species (316). There is often a small ganglion, the spermatic ganglion, near the origin of the testicular artery from the aorta; this ganglion is supplied by branches from several other ganglia, the intermesenteric and celiac plexuses, and in many mammals, but not man, the caudal mesenteric plexus. The spermatic ganglion also receives fibers directly from the lumbar sympathetic nerves. In some species, the spermatic ganglion is fused with the caudal mesenteric plexus (514). The "hypogastric ganglion" occurs only in man and monkey and is located at the junction of the hypogastric and pelvic nerve trunks. In the rat, the "major pelvic ganglion" lies on the posterosuperior surface of the lateral prostatic lobe. Its equivalent in the guinea pig is the "anterior pelvic ganglion" located on the posterolateral aspect of the coagulating gland and a smaller "posterior pelvic ganglion" behind the caudal portion of the gland. The "pelvic plexus ganglia" are present in all species associated with branch nerves of the pelvic plexus but can only be seen under magnification. The ganglia vary in number, being most numerous in the cat, and are freely interconnected. Visceral afferent (sensory) fibers are present among all the nerve tracts described above. These fibers either travel in the pelvic nerve to enter the spinal cord through the sacral nerves or pass by way of the hypogastric nerve and more proximal prevertebral plexuses, and thence through the splanchnic nerves and sympathetic chain ganglia, to enter the spinal cord through the dorsal roots of the spinal nerves.

Testis

The nerves to the testis run from the spermatic ganglion alongside the testicular artery, in some species as a sheath of nerves (spermatic plexus) surrounding the artery and in others as a discrete nerve, the superior spermatic nerve (514). In the testis, adrenergic nerves can be found in the interstitial tissue in association with blood vessels, particularly in and near the capsule (see p. 1067); the cat and man have a much greater density of nerves than the other species studied (rats, rabbits, and guinea pigs) (67,68,78,859,1137). There is no doubt that vascular tone in the testis is under nervous control, as stimulation of the nerves in the spermatic cord of isolated perfused ram testes led to sudden increases in pressure during isovolumetric perfusions (713), but unilateral lumbar sympathectomy produced a bilateral increase in testicular blood flow (419). Treatment with guanethidine, a sympathetic-blocking agent, has no effect on testicular blood flow in rats (257) and α-adrenergic blockade had no effect in rams (1061). It was originally believed that the testis had no cholinergic fibers (960), but later studies revealed that there were acetylcholinesterase-containing fibers in the testicular capsule of several species of mammal, including monkey, rat, rabbit, and ram (78,668). In the cat, there are also vasoactive intestinal polypeptide (VIP)-containing terminals in the capsule and around the blood vessels of the cat and guinea pig but not in the rat (23,672,996). There may be associations between the nerve fibers and the cells of the peritubular tissue (67,1102,1319), and some authors have suggested that the Leydig cells may also be in contact with nerve terminals (67,523,867,1137,1210). Testosterone secretion by the perfused guinea pig and rabbit testis was stimulated by adrenocorticotropic hormone (ACTH) but not by other pro-opiomelanocortin-derived peptides (601). It is probably relevant that Leydig cells appear to have β-adrenergic binding sites (32) and that cultured Leydig cells and fragments of testis tissue increase their production of testosterone when stimulated with catecholamines (219,766,768,798,799). Blockade of sympathetic activity with guanethidine reduced testosterone levels and the response to hCG (257). Furthermore, nicotinic cholinergic agonists inhibit androgen biosynthesis by cultured testicular cells from hypophysectomized rats (606). There appear to be α- and β-adrenergic receptors as well as muscarinic receptors on myoid cells, and the contractions of these cells may be influenced by adrenergic nerves (794). Catecholamines also stimulate cyclic AMP production and aromatization in Sertoli cells (1228), and these cells also contain β-adrenergic receptors (475). The interstitial cells and interstitial fluid, as well as the capsule but not the seminiferous tubules, contain appreciable amounts of 5-HT (serotonin), and the levels are reduced by denervation, suggesting that serotinergic innervation may be important in the control of testicular functions. The mature testis contains many fewer neuropeptide-Y-containing nerves than the ovary, and these are confined largely to the capsule and subcapsular blood vessels (19). No nerves penetrate the seminferous tubules, but axons bearing synaptic vesicles are found on the basal lamina in humans (846), and nerve growth factor and its messenger ribonucleic acid (mRNA) are found in the tubules of rats (50). Sensory receptors with fibers in the spermatic nerve are probably responsible for the sensation of the pain commonly experienced after trauma to the testis. Studies with local anesthetics applied to the outside of the testis suggest that these receptors are present in the parenchyma as well as in the capsule (915), but there is a higher density of receptors near the surface (1321). Several possible nociceptor-related thin axons have been identified in the capsule (1107). In the cat and dog, the receptors appear to be of three types: mechanoreceptors, chemical receptors, and thermal receptors. As judged by electrical recording from fibers in the superior spermatic nerve, the mechanical receptors respond to a degree of compression of the testis that does not invoke a pseudoaffective response in lightly anesthetized subjects, but a different response, possibly from different receptors, is obtained if the intensity of the stimulus is increased. The chemical receptors respond to hypertonic sodium chloride, potassium chloride, bradykinin, sodium citrate, substance P, acetylcholine, and histamine (Fig. 45), and their sensitivity is increased when the temperature is raised; the response to bradykinin is blocked by indomethacin, so PGs are probably involved. The discharge from the thermal receptors increased roughly in parallel to the temperature rise, with an average threshold of approximately 42°C. However, more than 90% of the receptors respond to all three stimuli and therefore probably should be classified as polymodal receptors (648–655,915). The receptors were not suppressed by opoids but were instead excited by these drugs (656). The fibers in the spermatic nerve are largely unmyelinated, but the myelinated fibers have diameters ranging from 1.4 to 6 μm, with conduction velocities of electrically evoked potentials typical of A-fibers, ranging from 3 to 52 m/sec (Fig. 46). A large compound potential representing C-fibers could also be evoked, with conduction velocities ranging from 0.5 to 2.3 m/sec (649–651,653,915). Single units responding to compression of the testis have been identified in the spinal cord (604), and respiratory changes can be evoked by activation of testicular afferents (795). There were some suggestions in the early literature that removal of part of the lumbar sympathetic chain and/or the thoracic splanchnic nerves, or the celiac plexus, or the caudal mesenteric ganglion and spermatic plexus caused vasodilatation and degeneration in the testis (see refs. 514,1032). However, the effects were slow to appear, and the degeneration may have been secondary to the vascular effects or to interference with transport of sperm and fluid through the epididymis. Transection of the main vascular and nervous supply to the testes of young pigs had no effect on their subsequent development (852), although re-innervation could not be excluded. Similarly, section of the testicular nerves to the testes of adult rams caused no deterioration in seminal characteristics during the next 6 weeks (759). Testicular denervation in young rats caused severe degeneration and reduced testis weight, and a similar effect was produced by local injection of 6-hydroxydopamine, which induces local destruction of sympathetic nerve terminals (827). In adult rats, 6-hydroxydopamine injected directly into one testis caused derangement of spermatogenesis, a small decrease in testis weight, and a slight increase in testis testosterone concentrations (767). Injection of a high dose of 6-hydroxydopamine in immature (5-day-old) rats caused decreases in testis weight, reduced compensatory hypertrophy after unilateral castration, and decreased testosterone production *in vitro,* but a low dose increased compensatory hypertrophy (394,395). Testicular atrophy is common in men with spinal lesions in the T12 region (181), and lesions in the mesencephalic reticular formation in rats caused testicular atrophy (16); however, as no values for LH or FSH were reported, an indirect effect could not be excluded. Testicular innervation appears to be necessary for the response of plasma testosterone concentrations to acute stress in rats (360), and although denervation has no effect of the endocrine response to hemicastration (359,797), this is suppressed by vasectomy on the side of the remaining testis, suggesting that the inferior spermatic nerves may be involved (361). It has recently been suggested that the short-term effects of vasoligation or unilateral castration on plasma FSH, LH, and prolactin provide evidence for a direct neural connection between the testes and the central nervous system (796,935). The effect of section of the genitofemoral nerve on testicular descent has already been discussed (see p. 1065).

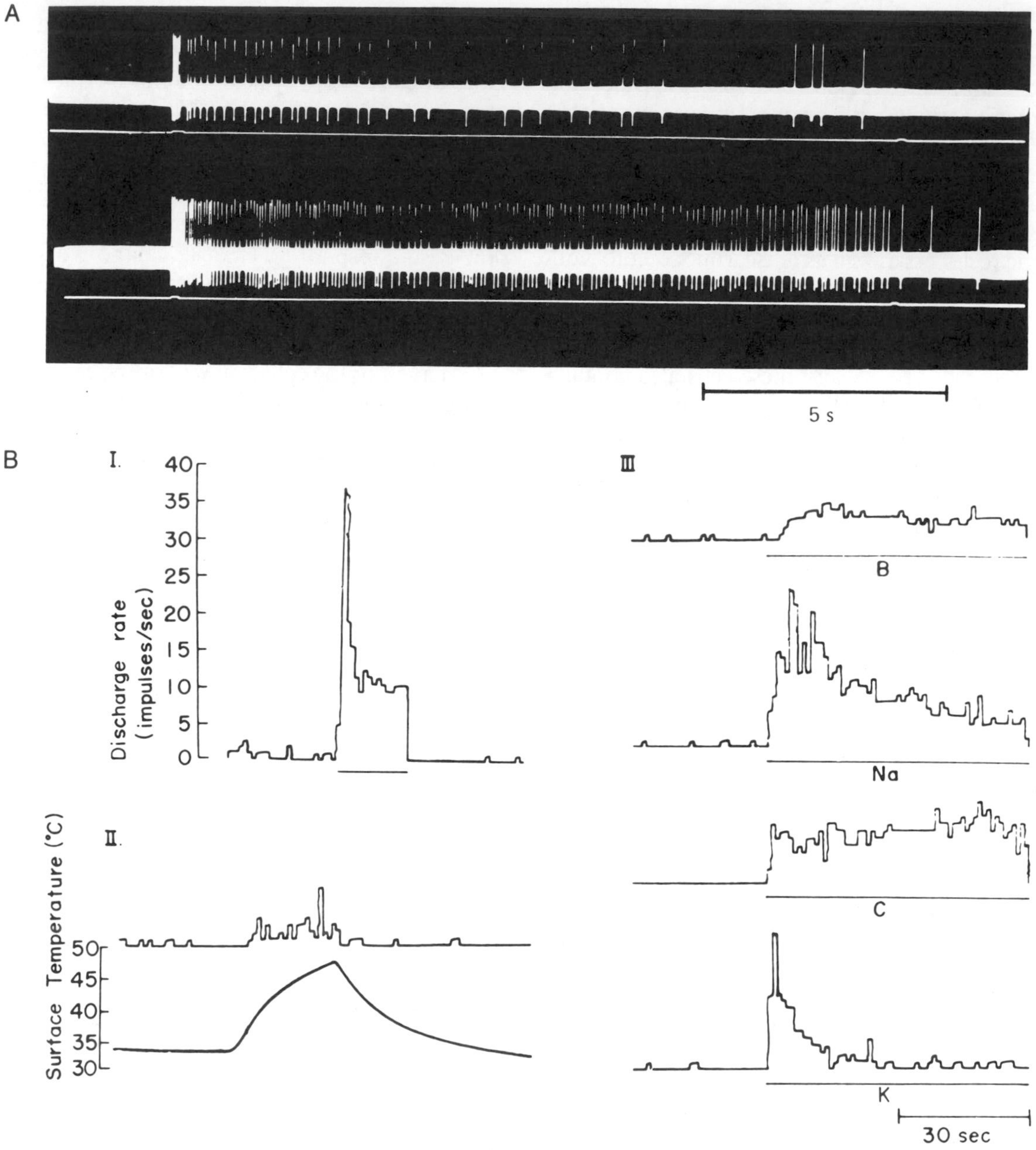

FIG. 45. Response of nerve bundles or filaments in the superior spermatic nerve in the abdominal cavity of dogs to mechanical, chemical, and thermal stimuli. **A:** Discharge pattern in response to mechanical stimulation of a polymodal unit with a conduction velocity of 10.5 m/sec. During the period between the two upward deflections of the lower line, a weight was applied to the testis using a falling type mechanostimulator, 500 g in the *upper panel* and 1,000 g in the *lower;* the upper line shows the action potential. **B:** Response of an Ad fiber unit with a conduction velocity of 5.6 m/sec to various stimuli. I: the receptive point was pressed with a von Frey hair (2 g, 420-μm diameter), for the period shown by the lower line. II: the surface of the testis around the receptive area was heated by radiant heat, while the surface temperature (*lower trace*) was recorded with a thermistor. III: Chemical stimulation was applied to the receptive area by applying a cotton ball (1.5-mm diameter) soaked in bradykinin (10 μg/ml, B), sodium chloride (4.5%, Na), sodium citrate (18%, C) or potassium chloride (60 mM, K) for the period shown by the lower line. (From refs. 651 and 648, respectively.)

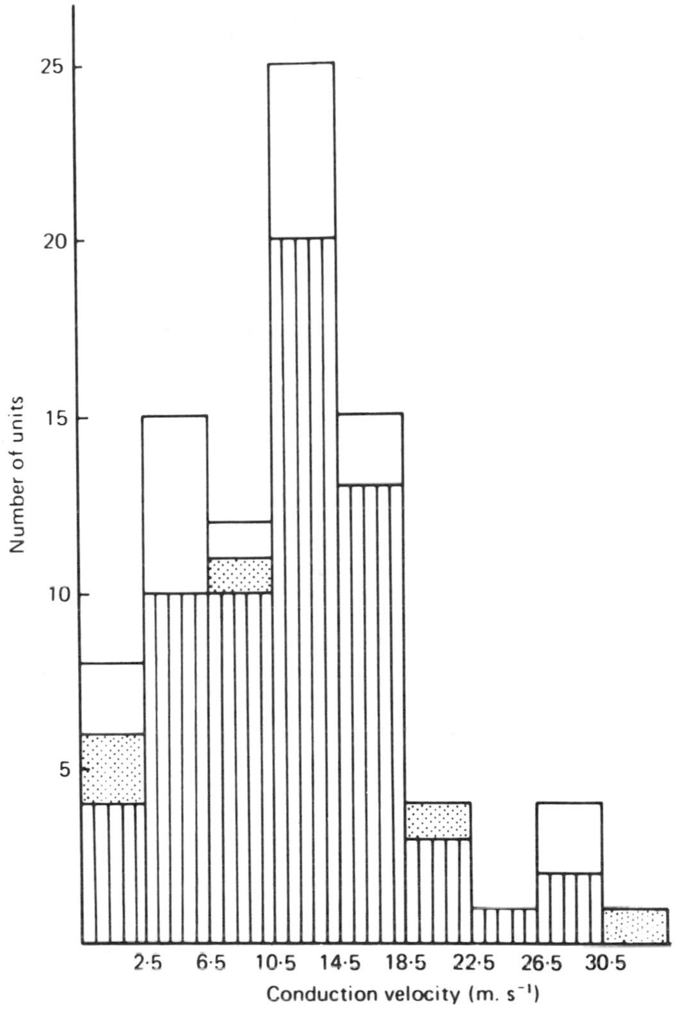

FIG. 46. The conduction velocities of all units responding to mechanical stimulation studied in the superior spermatic nerves of dogs. The histograms show the total number of units with conduction velocities in the ranges shown. The *hatched columns* represent units which were also sensitive to heat, the *stippled columns* the units which were not also sensitive to heat, and the *open columns* units whose response to heat was not tested. (From ref. 650.)

Epididymis and Ductus Deferens

The epididymis is supplied by the middle spermatic and inferior spermatic nerves (514). The route of the middle spermatic nerves depends on species. In man and cat (859), the nerves originate from the hypogastric plexus and accompany the spermatic artery to the epididymis, whereas in other species a group of nerves leaves the termination of the hypogastric nerve and passes to a group of ganglia located near the termination of the ductus deferens from where they travel to the epididymis along the ductus deferens. The inferior spermatic nerves arise from the pelvic plexus and contain both sympathetic and parasympathetic fibers. These nerves form a plexus around the ductus deferens after synapsing with a group of ganglia near the prostate (657). The nerves supply the muscle of the ductus deferens and continue to the cauda epididymidis. Throughout the epididymis, there are rich adrenergic and cholinergic perivascular plexuses (317). The distribution of interstitial and peritubular adrenergic and cholinergic nerves, however, varies considerably in different anatomic regions of the epididymis and in different species. Thus, the ductuli efferentes and the caput and corpus epididymidis are sparsely innervated in the rat, rabbit, guinea pig, and man (68,69,317, 859; but cf refs. 1007,1008,1136,1137), but a richer innervation exists in these regions in the cat and dog (317). The innervation of the cauda epididymidis becomes progressively more prominent as the layer of smooth muscle increases toward the ductus deferens. Ganglia have been seen only in the caput epididymidis of the cat, whereas cholinergic and adrenergic fibers have been reported in the lamina propria and epithelium by light microscopy in the caput and cauda, but not the corpus of all species studied except the rat (317,859,860,1007,1008,1136). However, intraepithelial localization of neurons has never been observed in ultrastructural studies (421).

The ductus deferens has been a favorite system for neuropharmacologic studies, for which a voluminous literature exists. The extensive adrenergic innervation of the smooth-muscle layers, which becomes prominent in the cauda epididymidis, continues in the three layers of the ductus deferens (1109). The particular exception appears to be the dog, and possibly the fox, in which the outer and middle muscle layers of the proximal portion of the duct lack a rich adrenergic innervation (77,1109); the smooth muscle of the terminal portion of the duct has a more normal adrenergic innervation (77,1226). The adrenergic innervation to the human vas deferens is also relatively sparse in comparison with most other species (20). The presence of cholinergic neurons in the ductus deferens has been adequately demonstrated by histochemical and ultrastructural techniques in several species (13,77,380,410,553,960), although the cholinergic innervation is largely confined to the subepithelial mucosa. Specific purinergic terminals that may use adenosine triphosphate (ATP) or other purines as a cotransmitter with norepinephrine have also been described (20,343,770,1226), and short circuit current in epididymal cells in culture is affected by ATP (1388) and adrenaline (1297). Nerve fibers showing immunoreactivity to CGRP were particularly numerous in the cauda, where the nerves were found in the capsular and interstitial connective tissue, and in the smooth muscle layer and the subepithelial tissue surrounding the duct (1317).

Scrotum

The nervous supply of the scrotal skin is quite separate from that of the testis and epididymis, but in view of the importance of the scrotum in keeping the testis and epididymis cool, some consideration of its nerve supply seems appropriate. The scrotum is supplied by fibers in the pudendal, inguinal, and ilio-inguinal nerves, and these contain sensory, sympathetic (vasomotor, sudomotor, and piloerector), and somatic efferent fibers (see refs. 504,1032). Scrotal skin also contains many thermal receptors that transmit information about the temperature of the scrotal skin through the spinal cord to the thalamus, the hypothalamus, and cortex through the raphe magnus. Some neurons increase their firing rate dramatically as scrotal skin temperature rises by about 2°C, whereas other neurons increase their firing rate as the temperature falls by a similar amount, although different neurons have different transition temperatures, above and below which the rate of firing is reasonably constant (477–482,549,832,919,1009,1163).

These thermal receptors provide the input through the pudendal nerve, which enables the brain to control the important systemic responses (1248), the increase in scrotal sweating (1257), and the relaxation of the tunica dartos (356), which follow an increase in scrotal skin temperature. The response of the dartos muscle was not dependent on the normal functioning of these scrotal nerves, because contraction of the dartos muscle could still be induced by exposure to low temperatures in rams with denervated scrotal skin (759). The pudendal nerve also carries the efferent fibers to the tunica dartos (356) and the sweat glands, although the latter also respond to catecholamines in the blood (1257). Branches of the genitofemoral nerve pass through the scrotal area to reach the gubernaculum, where they contain CGRP (670) (see also p. 1065).

Accessory Glands

Nerves supplying the accessory glands arise on each side from the pelvic plexus. The nerves supply the ipsilateral organs, but there is also crossing of the midline ventrally and dorsally to provide innervation to the contralateral organ. Peripheral ganglia are located along the neural pathway to the accessory organs distal to the pelvic plexus and at a short distance from, adjacent to, or within the organs they innervate (Fig. 47). The existence of short postganglionic fibers with their cell bodies located in ganglia close to the innervated organ is a feature of the male accessory organs that differs from that associated with the sympathetic adrenergic innervation of most other organs. Collectively, these nerves have been termed the *short adrenergic neuron system* (1109) or the *urogenital short neuron system* (316). The existence of the short adrenergic neuron system is revealed by the persistence of unchanged neurons after total extrinsic denervation (e.g., refs. 888,1109). The short adrenergic neuron system seems largely to be responsible for innervation of the smooth muscle. The vasculature would appear to be supplied by long postganglionic nerves that travel with the blood vessels and bypass the short adrenergic neuron system, because lumbosacral sympathectomy results in marked depletion of adrenergic vascular neuroplexuses within the accessory glands (1109). Many "intrinsic preterminal ganglia" are present in most species. These individual or clustered ganglion cells are associated with intrinsic nerves supplying the terminal ramifications of the nerve fibers within the accessory glands. They are particularly abundant in the organ capsule or adventitia; some are present in the muscle layer; and a few are located in the subepithelial connective tissue. These ganglia may also be classified as "epineural" or "intraneural" (beside or within major nerve bundles), "paravascular" (next to major intrinsic blood vessels), or "neuroterminal" (within neuroplexuses such as those supplying the smooth muscle of the organ). Catecholamine-containing neurons are distinguishable by fluorescence microscopy of formaldehyde-fixed tissue, whereas cholinergic neurons are detected by histochemical staining for acetylcholinesterase. The adrenergic neurons are postganglionic sympathetic fibers characterized by many intracytoplasmic granules of moderate fluorescence. The nonadrenergic neurons are nonfluorescent, but most are acetylcholinesterase-positive and represent postganglionic parasympathetic fibers. Persistence of the staining reactions after extrinsic denervation has frequently been used to confirm the identity of neurons as postganglionic elements of the short neuron system (e.g.,

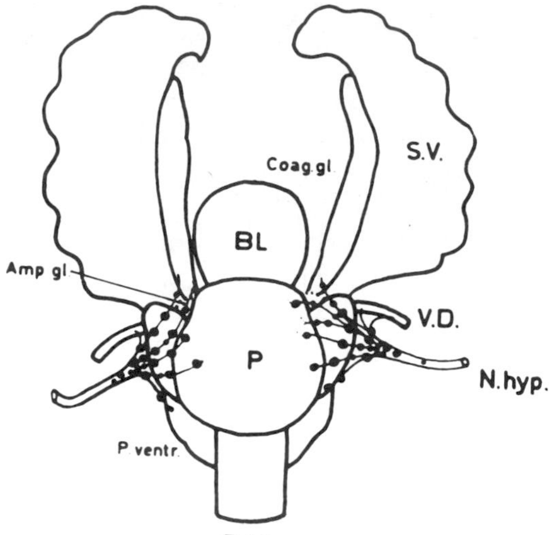

FIG. 47. Diagrammatic representation of the localization of sympathetic ganglia innervating the male accessory glands of the rat. Dorsal view with adrenergic ganglia indicated by *black dots.* BL, bladder; S.V., seminal vesicle; Coag. gl., coagulating gland; Amp. gl., ampullary gland; V.D., vas deferens; P, dorsal prostate with lateral lobes at each side; P. ventr., ventral prostate; N. hyp., hypogastric nerve. (From ref. 1109.)

ref. 1109). A third type of neuronal element, termed the *small intensely fluorescent cell* (*SIF*) or *chromaffin cell,* is also present in the male accessory glands. These cells are characterized by an intense homogeneous cytoplasmic fluorescence caused by their content of both epinephrine and norepinephrine. The SIF cells are believed to be interneurons that establish efferent synapses with juxtaposed sympathetic or parasympathetic neurons. The different types of neurons can also be distinguished by their ultrastructure (954). The general structure and arrangement of the intrinsic innervation of the male accessory glands is similar to that of the excurrent duct system (316,317). Nerve bundles, containing both adrenergic and cholinergic fibers, travel in the adventitia or capsule of the organ or gland in association with blood vessels and their perivascular neuroplexuses (944). These adventitial nerves branch and penetrate the gland, where they ramify in the fibromuscular stroma to form adrenergic and cholinergic perivascular plexuses around arteries and veins. Some stromal nerves do not associate with blood vessels but innervate smooth muscle of the glandular and ductal components of the gland (1222,1223). Also, prominent neuroplexuses may also form below the epithelium lining the ducts and acini. These neuroplexuses are predominantly cholinergic, whereas the innervation to the musculature is mainly adrenergic. The density of the adrenergic innervation is very variable in different glands and in different species but correlates to a large degree with the extent of the development of the smooth musculature (151,1109). The extent of the sparse cholinergic innervation of the smooth muscle is also variable but is unrelated to the amount of smooth muscle (316,1222,1223). Adrenergic innervation of the smooth muscle in the seminal vesicles has been clearly demonstrated in several species (859,1109), the innervation being particularly rich in the case of the rabbit. Ultrastructural identification of fibers with the characteristics of adrenergic and cholinergic neurons has been made in the guinea pig (13,210). The smooth muscle of the proximal 1.5 cm of the gland is in two layers, an outer longitudinal and inner circular layer. Adrenergic neurons are abundant throughout both muscle layers, whereas cholinergic neurons are largely restricted to the inner circular layer. Both types of neurons arise from mixed ganglia located in the adventitia located on the lateral sides of the proximal part of the seminal vesicle. Below the muscle layers, acetylcholinesterase-positive neurons form a rich submucosal complex and the presence of a few intraepithelial fibers has been reported (13). Catecholamine-containing neurons are rare in the submucosa, and those that are present are associated with blood vessels, occasionally forming perivascular plexuses. The pattern of adrenergic innervation of the prostate is similar to that observed in the other accessory glands (1109). The extent of innervation is proportional to the amount of smooth muscle present in the organ. This is evident both in cases in which there are separate and distinct morphologic lobes (e.g., rat) as well as histologically demonstrable lobes (e.g., dog, monkey). Dual innervation of the rat and human prostate has been confirmed (151,1203–1205). β-Adrenergic receptors can be demonstrated in the rat ventral prostate (299) and α-adrenergic and muscarinic receptors in the human prostate (470,910,911). Cholinergic neurons are more sparsely distributed than the adrenergic neurons in the rat prostate and do not make such intimate contact with the smooth-muscle cells. Cholinergic neurons are more numerous in the human compared with the rat prostate, and they outnumber adrenergic neurons in the fibrous capsule and fibromuscular stroma. Some cholinergic neurons are present near the base of the epithelium. However, no evidence has been found for direct contact of neurons with epithelial cells in either the rat or human prostate, but the sympathetic nerves may be important in the control of prostatic muscle tone (183,1122), including benign prostatic hypertrophy (155). The adrenergic innervation of the bulbourethral glands, which has been examined in the rabbit and guinea pig, is relatively sparse commensurate with the thin layer of smooth muscle (888,1109). Innervation of the vasculature is unexceptional. The preputial gland of the rat has been shown to contain both adrenergic and cholinergic fibers located in the connective tissue capsule and in the trabeculae that separate the acini; some association of neurons with blood vessels has also been demonstrated (29). Little is known about the afferent (sensory) innervation of the male accessory glands because there is currently no way to identify unequivocally afferent neurons by their morphology in autonomically innervated visceral organs. One can merely make predictions that free terminals located in a subepithelial position and separate from blood vessels (910,911) could serve a sensory function. Fibers of this type have been shown to degenerate in the rabbit seminal vesicle after extrinsic denervation (292), although this was not the case for other fibers presumably belonging to the short adrenergic neuron system. The variety of sensory functions that might be represented include pressure, pain, and temperature.

Peptidergic Neurons

Peptide neurotransmitter substances have been extracted from different parts of the male reproductive tract (e.g., refs. 671,904,928,1000), and immunohistochemical techniques have been used to localize putative peptidergic neurons within these structures. It is possible that the peptide transmitters are costored in adrenergic or cholinergic neurons (421,1131). Alternatively, the peptidergic neurons may correspond to the nonadrenergic noncholinergic neurons, which are characterized by a predominance of large granular vesicles when viewed in the electron microscope (1205), but such an assignation remains entirely speculative at present. Within the human genital tract, neuropeptide Y is found in highest concentration in the seminal vesicles (7,1131), and many neuropeptide Y, VIP, and tyrosine hydroxylase reactive nerve fibers were observed in the rat seminal vesicle (1332). Immunohistochemical staining showed this substance to be associated primarily with the connective tissue in the seminal vesicles and prostate (184,665) and with the smooth-muscle layer and vascular smooth muscle of the ductus deferens. Enkephalin immunoreactive nerves have been demonstrated in the distal ductus deferens and in the prostate of man in close relation to smooth-muscle cells, but these fibers are absent or very rare in the ampulla and seminal vesicles (47,184,290,600,1206). They are also present in the dog prostate (47) but have not been detected in guinea pig ductuli efferentes or epididymis (421). Nerves positive for methionine-enkephalin are more numerous than those that stain for leucine-enkephalin in the human prostate (1206). However, Gu et al. (423) were unable to demonstrate enkephalin-positive fibers in any of the human accessory glands. A few nerves staining for somatostatin have been found in the interstitium and smooth muscle of the human prostate and in the muscle of the vas deferens (184,423) and in sheep prostate (1237). Scattered fibers staining for gastrin-releasing peptide have been found in the vas deferens and seminal vesicles of mice, guinea pigs, and rabbits (1130). Nerves containing substance P have been found in parts of the male reproductive tract of the mouse, guinea pig, rabbit, and cat but are totally absent from the rat (22,421,1130). In man, the ductus deferens is devoid of fibers (20), but occasional nerves have been found in the connective tissue of the seminal vesicle (423) and prostate (184; but cf ref. 665). In the ductuli efferentes and epididymis of the guinea pig, fibers are present in the interstitial connective tissue mostly adjacent to blood vessels and also in muscle layers of more distal regions of the epididymis (421). The ductus deferens of the guinea pig and cat has fibers beneath the epithelium, in the muscle layer, and in the adventitia (23). Positive fibers have been located in the seminal vesicle of the mouse, guinea pig, and rabbit, particularly in the smooth muscle, but not in the seminal vesicle of rat or cat nor in the prostate of any of these species (23,1130). VIP nerves have been demonstrated in the testis, epididymis, ductus deferens, seminal vesicles, prostate, and bulbourethral glands of several species (21,23,184,421,423,665,672,1206). However, the distribution of VIP-positive fibers within any particular organ or gland is somewhat variable between species, and in some instances, conflicting results have been reported by different authors. In the testis, VIP fibers are associated almost exclusively with the organ capsule in the guinea pig and cat but are totally absent in the rat (23,672). In the cat epididymis, fibers are much more numerous than in the testis and are located immediately below the basement membrane and in the connective tissue between the tubules (672). A similar localization below the basement membrane exists in the human epididymis (423); in the guinea pig, positive fibers are found only in the terminal segment, where they are present in large numbers in the subepithelial and muscular layers (421). The distribution of VIP fibers in the ductus deferens of rat, guinea pig, cat, and man is predominantly in the submucosa with a few scattered fibers in the smooth muscle and around blood vessels in the adventitia (20,23,423). However, Larsson et al. (672) reported that in the cat they are mainly associated with the smooth muscle with only a few fibers in the submucosa and around adventitial blood vessels, although Alm et al. (21) found an approximately equal density of fibers in the submucosa and muscle. The seminal vesicles of man and guinea pig contain a dense plexus of VIP fibers just below the epithelium with other fibers in the muscle layer (7,23,423). In the cat prostate, fibers are present in the smooth muscle, connective tissue, and around adventitial arteries (21,672). In man, the distribution is rather variable in different regions of the prostate, but fibers with a thin-beaded appearance can be found around the acini, in the interstitial tissue, and in the perivascular plexuses of arteries (1206). In the cat, VIP nerves form a dense plexus in the prostatic capsule and give off branches to the stroma (23). VIP fibers are less numerous in the guinea pig prostate, whereas they are absent from the rat prostate (23). CGRP has also been demonstrated in nerves in human prostate in one study (184) but not in another (665).

Functional Significance of Innervation to the Male Accessory Organs

Motor innervation to the male accessory glands can be considered as subserving the following principal functions, namely, motor control of smooth muscle contraction, vascular activity, and epithelial secretory activity (Fig. 48). Most visceral organs are considered to be in a state of tonic activity, which can be excited or inhibited by activity of the autonomic nervous system. Thus, smooth-muscle systems exhibit spontaneous activity, have extensive electrotonic coupling and abundant muscle to muscle nexus-type close contact, and demonstrate slow, graded responses to neural stimulation. By contrast, the smooth muscle of the male accessory glands, as typified by the vas deferens, does not establish nexuslike close contacts and shows limited electrotonic coupling. Direct innervation of individual muscle cells is usually associated with only limited or no spontaneous activity but allows a fast, powerful, and coordinated response to neural stimulation. A gradation between the two forms of smooth-muscle activity can be observed along the

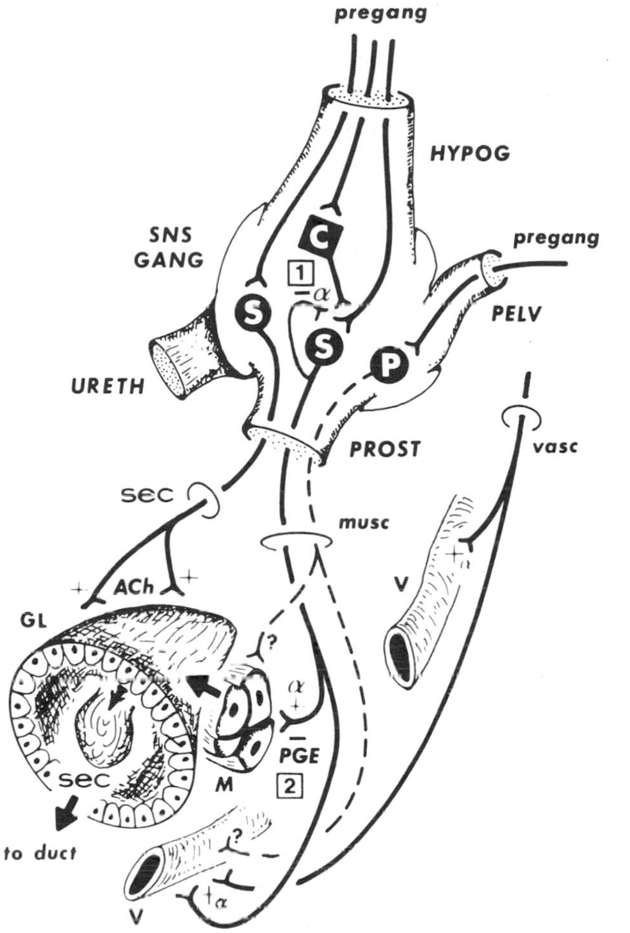

FIG. 48. Model of proposed pathways involved in the neural control of glands (GL), muscle (M), and vasculature (V) of the prostate. Prostatic nerves (PROST) originate together with urethral nerves (URETH) from ganglia of the short neuron system (SNS GANG). Sympathetic and parasympathetic preganglionic nerve fiber (*pregang*) input to the ganglion is provided by pelvic plexus branches of the hypogastric (HY-POG) and pelvic (PELV) nerves, respectively. Prostatic nerves are composed of sympathetic secretory nerves (*sec*) which supply the glands (GL), and muscular nerves (musc) which innervate both musculature (M) and vessels (V). These nerves are derived from cell bodies of postganglionic sympathetic (S) and parasympathetic (P) neurons located within the short neuron system ganglion. Sympathetic secretory nerves are cholinergic, stimulating secretion by release of acetylcholine (ACh). The secretion is expelled into the draining duct by contraction of related musculature (*arrows*) under the α-adrenergic excitatory effect of sympathetic adrenergic muscular nerves, which also have an α-adrenergic excitatory effect on blood vessels. The functional significance of parasympathetic cholinergic muscular nerves (*dashed line*) is still not fully resolved (?). Prostatic vessels are also supplied by vascular nerves (*vasc*), which are derived directly from the sympathetic chain and reach the organ along its vessels, independently of the pelvic plexus and short neuron system ganglia. Two inhibitory mechanisms probably modulate sympathetic muscular action: 1, α-adrenergic influence of SIF cell (C) terminals and/or collateral postganglionic adrenergic fibres on the sympathetic ganglion cell (S); and 2; prostaglandin E (PGE) released indigenously in the vicinity of the sympathetic neuromuscular junction. (From ref. 316.)

male excurrent duct system (69,779,1154). Thus, the ductuli efferentes and proximal regions of the epididymis, which are sparsely innervated, display spontaneous contraction (959,1153,1211), which can be increased by adrenergic agents acting on α-receptors (627,823,824, 916), whereas the distal cauda epididymidis and vas deferens are normally quiescent until neural stimulation is received during the ejaculatory process (491,627). Contraction of the smooth muscle of the cauda epididymidis, vas deferens, and accessory sex glands occurs in response to stimulation of the hypogastric nerve (245). The response is adrenergic because seminal emission can be induced by intravenous injection of epinephrine (245, 1082) or norepinephrine (1268) and inhibited by selective chemical sympathectomy (486,1207) or appropriate antagonists (1082). The bulbourethral glands may be an exception to this generalization because atropine, which acts as a blocker of muscarinic receptors, selectively and substantially reduces the liberation of bulbourethral gland secretion during ejaculation in the boar (305). There is evidence that release of norepinephrine at the neuromuscular junction in the vas deferens is subject to inhibitory or braking influences at the postganglionic synapse and the neuromuscular junction (316). The role of parasympathetic innervation to the musculature of the excurrent ducts and accessory glands is not entirely clear. It is suggested that it is preferentially involved in basal muscular activity in the parasympathetic-dependent erection phase before ejaculation and during the process of urination (316). Stimulation of intramural nerves or application of noradrenaline or acetyl choline caused contraction of smooth muscle in the capsule and outermost layers of the rabbit prostate (1022).

Regulation of vascular tonus of the male accessory glands is probably mediated both by direct neural stimulation and by indirect humoral control from the adrenal gland. This dual control is indicated by the demonstration that either direct nervous stimulation or intravenous injection of epinephrine can decrease testicular and epididymal oxygen tension presumably caused by reduction in capillary blood flow (246). Further evidence for neural control of the vascular system in the excurrent duct system is seen by removal of the lumbar sympathetic chain together with the posterior mesenteric ganglion and the hypogastric nerves from rabbits, which results in considerable vasodilation and vascular stagnation in certain regions of the epididymis and ductus deferens (512). The effect of autonomic innervation on secretory activity of the male accessory glands has been studied extensively in the dog prostate (1114). Copious secretion can be induced above the low basal rate, which is independent of the autonomic nervous system, by electrical stimulation of the hypogastric nerve. The secretory rate depends on the frequency of stimulation, with a maximal effects at 20/sec, and the response can be blocked with atropine (1115,1269). Pilocarpine, which is a powerful cholinomimetic drug, can also induce the formation of copious amounts of secretion when administered systemically. Other cholinomimetics also induce secretion, although sympathomimetics and cholinesterase inhibitors have only a weak effect. The use of a variety of blocking drugs and the absence of any involvement of the pelvic nerve indicate that the nerves responsible for stimulating secretion are postganglionic cholinergic sympathetic neurons and not parasympathetic neurons (316,1114). The role of nerves in regulating the secretory activity of glandular epithelia in the accessory glands of other species is far from clear. Denervation of the rat prostate leads to lower weight, decreased cell height, and reduced secretory activity (1268). Removal of the posterior mesenteric ganglion plus hypogastric nerves or removal of the lumbar sympathetic chain has no effect on the secretory activity of the prostate and seminal vesicles in the rabbit (511). However, when all these components are removed, secretory activity is markedly disrupted (512). Although this result may implicate direct neuronal involvement in secretion, the observation may also be explained as an indirect consequence of reduced testosterone synthesis by the concomitantly damaged testes (512). The adrenergic, cholinergic, and peptidergic innervation and activity of the prostate and seminal vesicles in rats are reduced in streptozotocin-induced diabetes (247,814).

The urethral glands, or glands of Littre, do not store secretion but produce it during coitus. Control of secretion by these glands has been studied in the boar (305), which has a protracted ejaculatory period of 15 to 30 min. Secretory activity appears to be under cholinergic control because administration of atropine, a muscarinic receptor antagonist, causes marked inhibition of secretion from these glands.

FLUIDS OF THE MALE REPRODUCTIVE TRACT

Testis

Blood Flow

In any organ, the amount of arterial blood entering must equal the sum of the amount of venous blood and lymph leaving; otherwise, the size of the organ would change. Under most circumstances, the flow of lymph is small compared with blood flow, and therefore it is usual to equate arterial and venous blood flow. It is also important to make a distinction between total blood flow and nutrient blood flow (i.e., the fraction of the total that exchanges with the tissue through the capillaries). Each of these components can be measured, and the testis has the added complication of the spermatic cord, which can introduce errors in some of the measurements.

Arterial inflow can be measured by an electromagnetic flowmeter, either applied to the outside of the vessel or introduced into the circuit by cannulation of the vessel. It is difficult with either procedure to ensure that measurements are made under physiologic conditions, but it is a useful technique for following rapid changes in flow and can be useful for calibrating other methods (722,854,857). A friction flowmeter introduced into the course of the vessel has also been used (365). The flow-velocity of arterial blood can be measured using a Doppler flowmeter (27) (not to be confused with a laser-Doppler probe; see p. 1116), but this method is also most useful for recording rapid changes in flow and showing testicular arterial anatomy by imaging intra-arterial blood flow (788). Arterial inflow can also be measured by dilution of a suitable marker infused into the arterial system, knowing the amount infused and its concentration in venous blood when equilibrium has been attained. Suitable markers used have been iodinated albumin, Cr-EDTA, sodium, and glucose. Usually radioactively labeled material is used (408,722,1044), but with Cr-EDTA, the chromium can be measured by atomic absorption spectroscopy; β-Aminohippurate (PAH), which is a suitable marker for venous infusion, does not appear to be suitable for intra-arterial infusion, presumably because it is metabolized to some extent in the tissue. Unless an arterial catheter is being introduced for some other reason, probably the most physiologic way of measuring total testicular blood flow is to infuse a suitable marker into a testicular vein on the surface of the testis and to measure its concentration in blood from the testicular or internal spermatic vein above the spermatic cord. This uses the pampiniform plexus as a mixing unit and can give successive measurements of venous flow every minute, or even more frequently depending on how little blood is necessary for the estimation of the marker. In this instance, PAH is probably the best marker to use, as it does not build up in the arterial blood because it is cleared from the circulation by the kidneys (179,180,675,789). The marker must not cross from the vein to the artery in the spermatic cord, otherwise errors could result. Overestimation from this source is a problem in the use of tritiated water and the Fick principle, which states that the amount of a marker taken up or produced by a tissue is a product of blood flow and the integrated arteriovenous difference over the period of study. The amount of tritiated water taken up is derived from the equilibrium concentration at the end of a 20-min infusion of the marker into the jugular or any other suitable peripheral vein, and the arteriovenous difference is calculated from the concentrations in a series of testicular venous and peripheral arterial blood samples (1053,1060,1254). As well as being difficult to carry out and being possible only once or at most twice in any one animal because of accumulation of the marker, this method gives a slight overestimate because tritiated water does cross from artery to vein and vice versa in the spermatic cord. A marker that did not do so would probably not come into equilibrium quickly enough with the tissue. In measurements of total blood flow, there is still a place for the simplest method of all, the collection of the total venous outflow over a given time. This is obviously unphysiologic because of the surgery involved and disturbances to venous pressure, but it does have value for calibration of more physiologic methods.

Total blood flow is what should be measured if production or uptake is being estimated, but if one is interested in the fluid dynamics in the tissue, then a measurement of nutrient or capillary blood flow is probably more appropriate. One technique for measuring this depends on measurement of the rate of clearance or accumulation of a suitable marker in the tissue. The markers used have been radioactive inert gases (259,262,312,376,572,573, 594,826,925,926,1061,1270) and radioactive sodium (408), but the former suffer from difficulty in knowing their lipid solubility and therefore their partition coefficient and also probably give a slight underestimate because they cross readily from vein to artery and therefore recirculate back to the testis; with sodium, the difficulty is to determine its volume of distribution accurately. Alternatively, one can measure the amount of microspheres or an appropriate soluble marker, which lodges in the tissue after introduction into the circulation. Microspheres have become very popular (260,854,925,942, 1052,1265), but their use does require cannulation either of the left side of the heart or the aorta above the testicular arteries for their injection, and if absolute values are to be obtained instead of a fraction of the cardiac output, then this must be measured separately or arterial blood must be sampled at a known and constant rate from an artery near the tissue under investigation. Furthermore, although several estimates can be made in an individual animal by using microspheres labeled with different isotopes, the method is expensive and does not lend itself to repeated measurements. Although the technique using soluble markers (99,138,357,816,1059,1216,1255) is easier to use, requiring only intravenous injection of marker, the animal must be killed or the tissue removed soon after injection, and there is some doubt about the precision of the quantitative values obtained because of the loss of marker from the tissue back into the circulation. As with microspheres, it is necessary to measure cardiac output at the same time if the values are to be in absolute terms. Nevertheless, this technique has been useful in demonstrating differences within a tissue or between organs. The most recent introduction has been the laser-Doppler probe (258,265,266,268,271), which gives a semiquantitative index of capillary flow, either recorded with a probe placed against the surface of the testis or a needle probe inserted into the parenchyma. As well as its use in experimental animals, it has been used to monitor testis blood flow during orchidopexy of cryptorchid testes (453) or during repair of inguinal hernia (658). In rats, testis blood flow recorded with the laser-Doppler system shows periodic fluctuations, referred to as vasomotion, during which the blood flow changes by about 30% rhythmically at about ten cycles per second (258,271). Fluctuations in total blood flow measured with a friction flowmeter with a frequency of about six per minute had been previously reported by Free and Jaffe (365). The significance of these fluctuations is not known, but they are unaffected by unilateral orchidectomy (88) or treatment with estradiol (1285), are not seen before puberty, and disappear after treatment of the rats with hCG (271,1282) or a luteinizing hormone-releasing hormone (LHRH) agonist (269,1283), when the temperature of the testis is raised to about body temperature (Setchell, Damber, Bergh, *unpublished observations*; see also 1079) and when the Leydig cells are removed by treatment with ethane dimethane sulphonate (EDS); in the last case, vasomotion can be restored by treatment of the animals with testosterone (272). Vasomotion is seen in the testes of rams (Setchell, Damber, and Bergh, *unpublished observations*) but is not apparent in mice (87).

Representative values for testicular blood flow obtained by the various techniques in a variety of species are given in Table 2. Blood flow through the testis is relatively low, compared with other tissues, but this may be due at least in part to a physical limitation imposed by the dimensions of the testicular artery in the spermatic

TABLE 2. *Blood flow through the testes of various mammals estimated by different techniques*[a]

Techniques	Rat	Rabbit	Dog	Monkey	Ram	Boar
Direct collection	6	15	7–20		10	
Friction flowmeter	22					
Electromagnetic flowmeter					12	12
Dilution of intra-arterial marker					11	
Dilution of intravenous marker					11–26	4–18
Fick principle with TOH or iodoantipyrine					10	
Microspheres	14–38	28				9
Indicator fractionation	23	24			9	
Inert gas clearance	18–24		22	16	8	

[a] Blood flow in ml/100 g/min.

cord (363,1028). Testicular blood flow (TBF) does not show any change during a spontaneous peak of LH (Fig. 49; 675) nor any immediate increase when the testis is stimulated by trophic hormones (27) or shows only a small rise (261) or an initial fall and then a small rise (1286), in contrast to other endocrine tissues such as ovary, adrenal cortex, and thyroid. However, when the stimulation is prolonged, as by the use of hCG instead of LH, TBF initially falls (1217) but subsequently does increase (Fig. 50; 254,264,267,384,942,1052,1217,1265). Repeated doses of hCG appear to have a similar effect on TBF (391). A hyperaemia, presumably caused by dilatation of the testicular veins, eventually becomes apparent (462). As already discussed (see p. 1095), these changes in flow are preceded by a dramatic increase in "apparent" vascular permeability, and both the initial fall and the subsequent rise in blood flow are absent if the Leydig cells have been removed with EDS, although EDS-treated rats had normal levels of blood flow (270,1217). TBF is lower than normal in hypophysectomised rats and mice (99,254,1065,1217), but it is also reduced in hypophysectomized rams treated with high doses of pituitary extract (1078). In adult rams there was no response in TBF to hCG during the first 2 h after injection; in rams, immunized against testosterone, in which gonadotrophin levels and testosterone production were increased, TBF was reduced (Fig. 51; 42). The changes in TBF found at the time of puberty were unexpected; although there was no change in capillary flow (240), there was a decrease in total flow per gram of testis, although total flow per testis increased (41). This would suggest a difference in the fraction of total flow passing through arteriovenous anastomoses as the animal matures.

Vasodilatory drugs such as acetylcholine and isopropylnoradrenaline are without marked effects (854,1061), although there is a marked vasodilation after adenosine (348). Increases in TBF have been reported after systemic treatment with kallikrein (989) or an LHRH agonist given intratesticularly (1283), although a similar compound given systemically caused vasodilation and congestion of erythrocytes in the vessels (434). The response to vasoconstrictors seems to depend on the mode of administration. When adrenaline or noradrenaline was given into the testicular artery, a marked reduction in TBF followed in rams and rats (365,1061); if the drug was administered peripherally, a reduction was reported in some studies but not in others (260,365,854). Blockage of α-adrenergic receptors (1061) or sympathetic blockade (257) has no effect on TBF, suggesting that there is little resting sympathetic tone, although unilateral lumbar sympathectomy caused a bilateral increase in TBF in rats (419). VIP, which produces rises in blood flow through several tissues, has no effect in the testis (523). PGs (366), 5-hydroxytryptamine (368), and arginine vasopressin (1287) produce reductions in TBF. The testis shows a reactive hyperaemia after a short period of ischaemia (102,722) and after release of torsion (778).

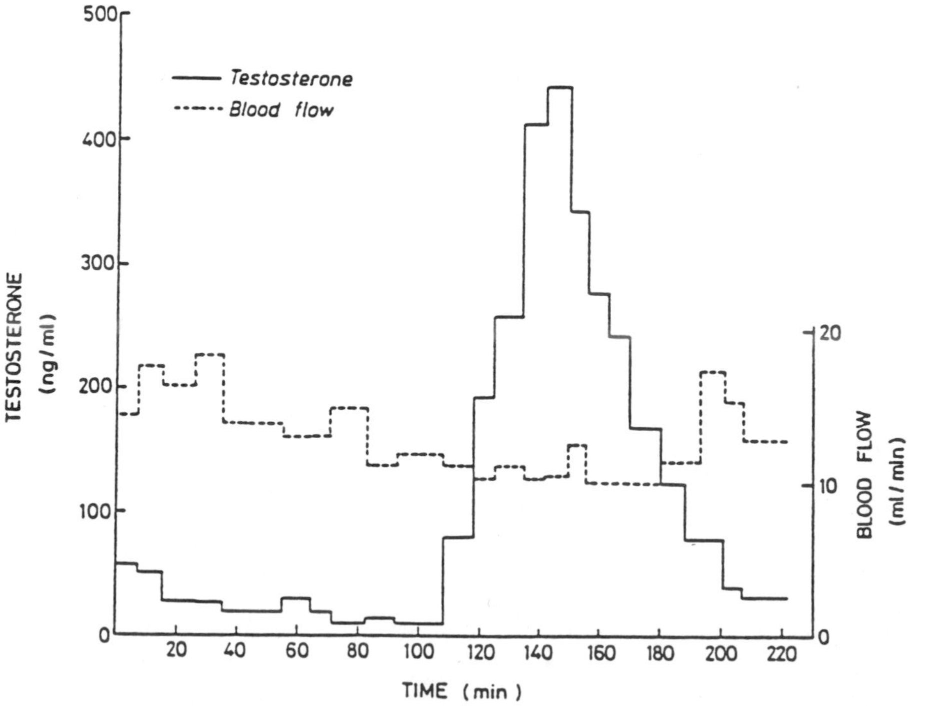

FIG. 49. Testosterone concentrations (solid line) in blood plasma from the internal spermatic vein of a conscious ram and blood flow (dashed line) determined in the same samples by the infusion of PAH at a constant rate into a vein on the surface of the testis. Note that there is very little change in blood flow during the spontaneous peak of testosterone, caused presumably by a peak of LH secretion from the pituitary. (Data from ref. 675, see ref. 1037).

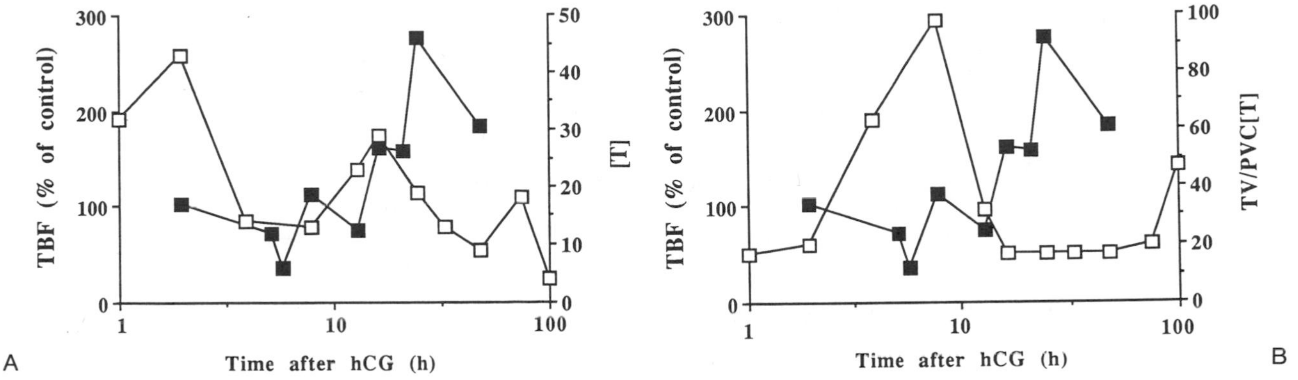

FIG. 50 A. The effect of a single injection in rats of hCG on plasma testosterone concentrations in peripheral blood plasma (open squares) and on various measurements of blood flow through the testis (solid squares, for original refs. see ref. 1039). **B.** The effect of a single injection of hCG on blood flow (solid squares, as above) and on the ratio (open squares) of the concentration of testosterone in plasma from the internal spermatic vein (TV) to that from a peripheral vein (PVC, Data from ref. 1125, see ref. 1039). The rise in ratio, assuming no change in clearance of the secreted steroid, would indicate a fall in blood flow through the testis.

The testis does not vary its capillary blood flow with temperature unless the heating is frankly unphysiologic (263,267,357,404–406,822,1061,1259), and in early studies on total blood flow, there also appeared to be no increase if the testis was heated inside the scrotum (408, 1254). However, more extensive measurements of total TBF made with the scrotal skin removed indicated that flow rose as temperature increased from 33° to 36°C but showed no further change as the temperature rose to 39°C (Fig. 52; 789). Cadmium salts in subtoxic doses cause a catastrophic fall in blood flow (1055,1255), which is probably secondary to an increase in vascular permeability (see p. 1095). If spermatogenesis is disrupted by heat (384,1078), cryptorchidism (267), or irradiation (1265) or after efferent duct ligation (1266), TBF falls proportionately with testis weight (see Fig 53A and B); it therefore appears that the seminiferous tubules, because of their greater mass, are a more important determinant of TBF than are the Leydig cells (1037, 1039,1043). However, androgen does appear to be important in maintaining normal TBF, possibly through actions on the seminiferous tubules (272). Conversely, unilateral orchidectomy led to an increase in the volume density of Leydig cells and blood vessels, without a change in testis weight or blood flow (88,262). Treatment with estrogens had no direct effect on TBF but reduced the response to hCG (254,264).

Ischemia

Considerable interest has been shown in the effects of ischemia on the testis because of concerns about the subsequent effects on the testis of torsion of the spermatic cord (237,238,476,571,1112), damage to the blood vessels during orchidopexy of cryptorchid testes (358,897,

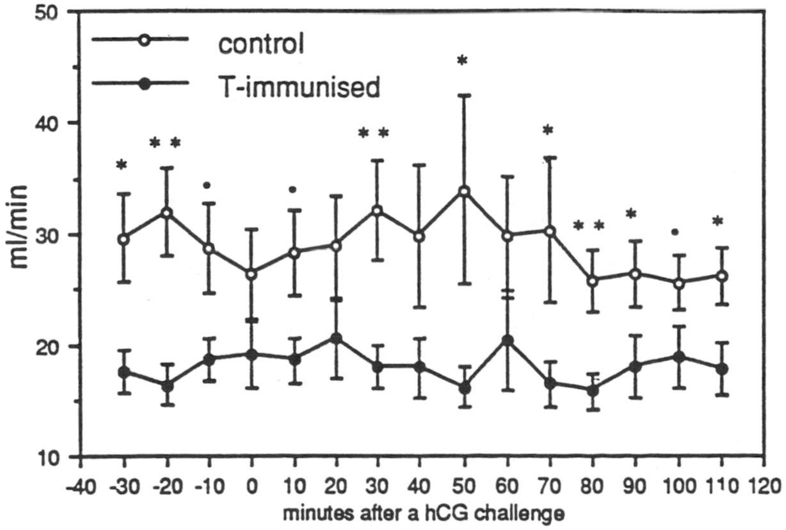

FIG. 51. Blood plasma flow (determined by the infusion of PAH) in one internal spermatic vein of adult rams, five of which had been immunized against a conjugate of testosterone with bovine serum albumin (BSA) and 5 controls immunized against BSA. All rams were given an intravenous injection of hCG (20 units/kg body weight) at time 0, which caused an increase of about 70% in the concentration of testosterone in peripheral blood of both groups of rams, and in blood from the internal spermatic vein of control rams, but a somewhat larger (about 250%) increase in blood from the internal spermatic vein of immunised rams. (Data from ref. 42).

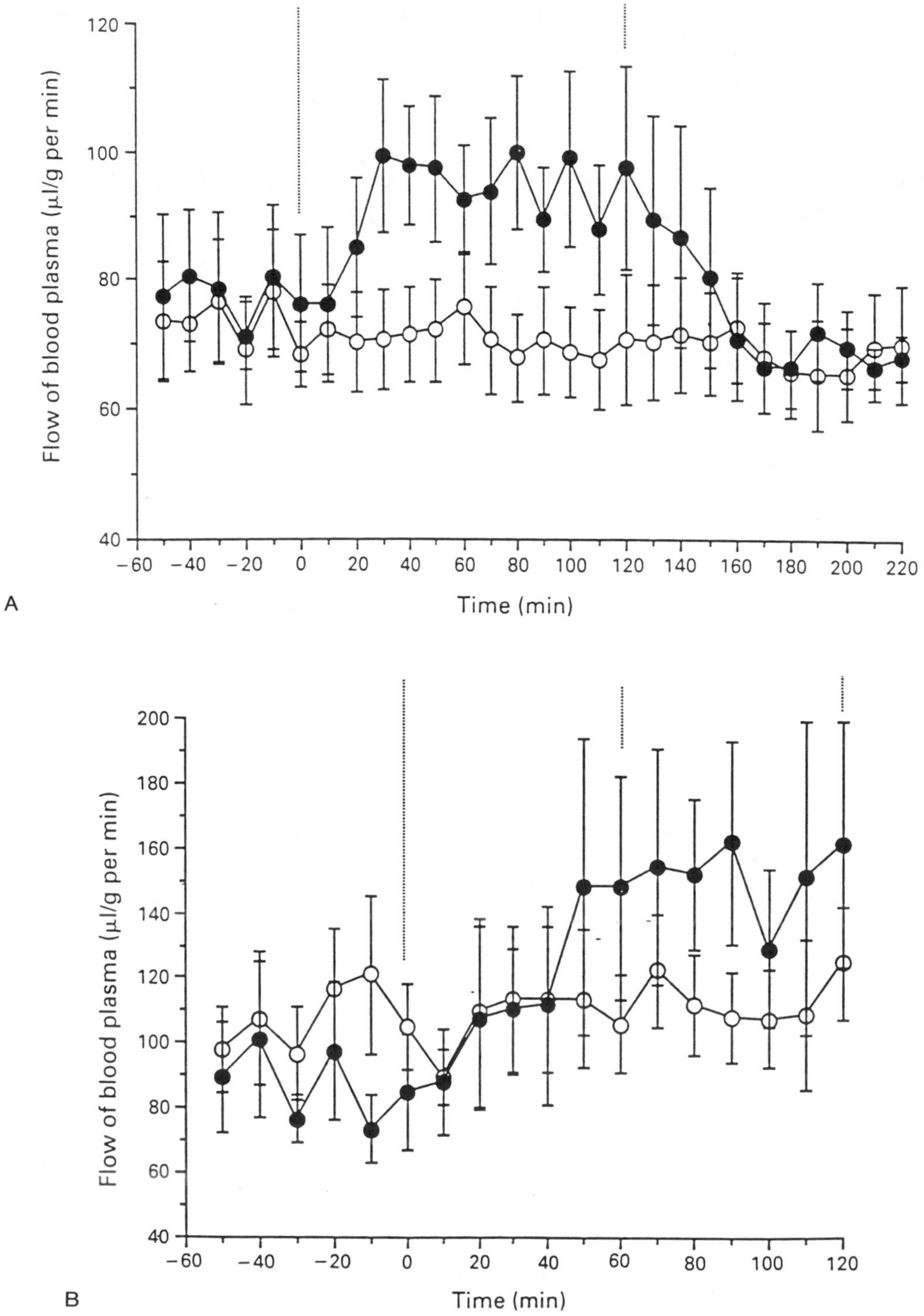

FIG. 52. Blood plasma flow (determined by infusion of PAH) in the internal spermatic vein of anaesthetised rams, one testis of each being maintained at 33°C throughout as a control, while the temperature of the other testis was raised to 36°C for 120 min, and then returned to 33°C for 100 min **(A),** or to 36°C for 60 min and 39°C for 60 min **(B).** (From ref. 789).

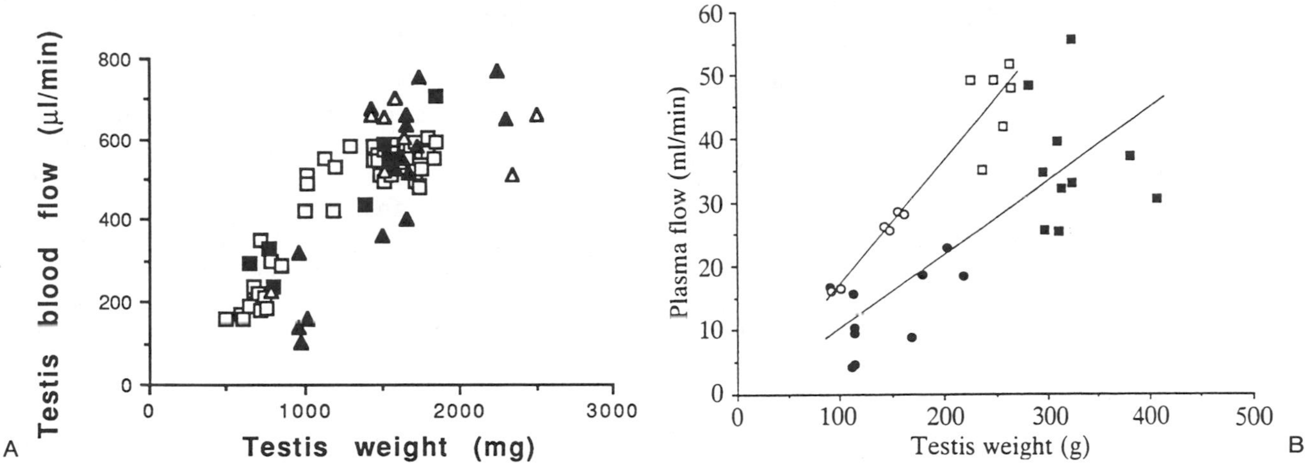

FIG. 53. **A.** Blood flow (determined by radioactive microspheres) in the testes of rats, some of which had been subjected to local heating (open squares) or gamma-irradiation (solid squares) of the testes or to efferent duct ligation (EDL, triangles) at various times previously. Note that except for those animals in which the testis was enlarged to more than 2g, in the first 36 h after EDL, there was a close relationship between testis weight and blood flow. Each point is the mean for a group of a group of 4 to 10 rats; r = 0.896, n = 47 for heating, r = 0.955, n = 7 for irradiation, and r = 0.826, n = 23 for EDL where testis weight was normal or reduced. Data from refs. 384 (open squares), 1265 (solid squares), 1266 (open triangles) and our unpublished data (solid triangles). **B.** Blood plasma flow in the internal spermatic vein of intact rams (open symbols) and surgically hypophysectomized rams treated with pituitary extract (Solid symbols); the testes of half of the rams (circles) had been heated at the time of hypophysectomy or at an equivalent time by immersion in a temperature controlled water bath so that subcutaneous scrotal temperature rose to about 42°C for 45 min. There was a close relationship between testis weight and blood flow, r = 0.956 for the intact rams and 0.803 for the hypophysectomised, hormone-treated rams. (From ref. 1078).

990), or during repair of inguinal hernia (386,494,849), or deliberate temporary obstruction of the blood supply to the testes during drug therapy (717). The blood vessels of the testis may also be affected by hypersensitivity angitis (54).

Conflicting results have been given by several experimental studies of the effects of ischemia on the testes of experimental animals. Some of the differences are due to differences in technique (e.g., ligation of the artery on the surface of the testis, clamping of the spermatic cord, or ligation of the individual vessels near their origin); others are more difficult to explain, although uncertainty about completeness of obstruction and re-establishment of flow seems widespread. Ligation of the artery on the surface of the rat testis is likely to minimize the possibility that an alternative arterial supply can take over, as the artery at this point is an end artery. Significant damage to the seminiferous epithelium has been reported after 10 to 20 min ligation by one group (459,609,610,863), but only after more than 60 min by another (93,1127,1171). When the spermatic cord was clamped, some damage to the testis was seen in one study if the ischemia lasted for 1 h, but greater effects were seen after 3 h or longer; the fertility of the rats, judged from their ability to get a female pregnant over a 21-day period, was decreased only if the ischemia lasted for 9 h or longer (239); in another study, effects on spermatogenesis were obvious after 15-min ischemia (399). If the spermatic cord and the gubernaculum were clamped, testis weight and sperm count fell only if the ischemia lasted for 45 min or longer (716,718), although complete recovery had occurred by 72 weeks (1129). In another study in which the testicular artery and vein were clamped separately, no effects on testis weight, seminiferous tubule diameter, or biopsy score were apparent after 30 min ischemia, but reductions were produced by 60- or 120-min ischemia, and clamping either vessel was as effective as clamping both (531) (Figs. 2 and 6 in this paper appear to have been transposed). Ligation and transection of the testicular artery and vein within 1 cm of the great vessels led to an 80% reduction in TBF immediately afterward, but flow had recovered to normal 30 days later; ventral prostate and seminal vesicle weights at that time were normal, although testis weight was slightly reduced and more variable (897). In another study, ligation and transection of the testicular vessels in the abdomen produced a fall in testis weight, seminiferous tubule diameter, and biopsy score and in blood testosterone levels 3 weeks later (990). Other studies showed that ligation of the spermatic vessels in the abdomen had a smaller effect than if the deferential and gubernacular vessels were ligated as well (880) or if the vasal veins and arteries were ligated as well as the spermatic vein in the abdomen or if the ligature was placed distally near the testis (973). In dogs, application of a torniquet to the spermatic cord for 2 h was without effects, whereas ischemia for 4 h or longer caused disruption of spermatogenesis (1117). Intra-abdominal transection of the testicular vessels invariably had a deleterious effect on the testes of adult rats (863) and pigs (853), whereas the same operation in young animals had no effect (852,898). In adult rams, ligation of one arterial branch on the surface of the testis produced a focal area of necrosis in the testis (Jequier, Zupp, and Setchell, *unpublished observations*); semen characteristics were affected by occlusion of the spermatic vessels for 30 or 60 min (994), but reversible occlusion of the artery above the cord for up to 60 min was without long-term effect on spermatogenesis in this species (1216). Surgical restriction of the growth of the testicular artery in young bulls reduced final testis size and affected spermatogenesis (608).

There is also disagreement about the influence of hypothermia on the effects of ischemia on the testis. Several groups claim that subjecting the testes to temperature reduction during ischemia reduces the effects on spermatogenesis (615,790), and "cold ischemia" has been suggested as a way of producing Sertoli cell-only testes (1331). Another study (716,718) reported that the effects of ischemia on testis weight and sperm count were greater if the testis was cooled in crushed ice while the spermatic cord and gubernaculum were occluded.

A deleterious effect of unilateral ischemia on the contralateral testis was demonstrated in humans (175, 176,178,460,828), guinea pigs (174,175,571), and rabbits (172), but in rats, the response seemed to be variable (238,531,990) and depended on the age of the animals used, affecting rats between 35 and 50 days old but not those younger or older (476). Torsion of one testis can affect the contralateral testis, causing a decrease in blood flow in rabbits (1158) and stagnation of blood in humans (176).

Lesions resembling those seen in men with higher epididymal obstruction can be produced in rams by ligation of the superior epididymal artery just above the testis (757).

Composition of Testicular Venous Blood

Changes in composition of the blood passing through the testis are caused both by the production and uptake of substances by the testis. The most important substances produced by the testis and secreted into blood are hormones, both steroid and peptide, although other substances may also be removed this way. From the interstitial tissue, peptides larger than a few amino acids will probably leave the testis largely in lymph. However, other routes of secretion are used within the seminiferous tubules. The Sertoli cells in the seminiferous epithelium are known to secrete many products bidirectionally, both through the base of the seminiferous tubules into the interstitium and apically into the tubule lumen. Factors secreted basally can pass into lymph or venous blood within the interstitial tissue, depending largely on their physicochemical properties. However, factors secreted into the seminiferous tubule lumen (apical secretion by Sertoli cells) also appear able to contribute to the venous blood leaving the testis. Inhibin is a high-molecular-weight peptide secreted bidirectionally by the Sertoli cell, and recent studies in the rat demonstrated that inhibin secreted into the seminiferous tubule lumen fluid and passing through the rete testis is resorbed into testicular venous blood as the blood passes through the small vascular plexus overlying the rete testis (see page 35) (726). This route of secretion becomes increasingly important from puberty to adulthood, as the Sertoli cell increases the apical secretion of this peptide postpubertally, and most of the inhibin leaving the adult testis is secreted into blood by this route (729) (Fig. 54). This has enormous significance for our ability to define and to develop sensitive assays for suitable markers of normal or abnormal spermatogenesis (1090).

However, the most significant changes in blood composition occurring within the testis and the changes most investigated to date involve the secretion of steroid hormones by the testis into the venous blood. The one usually associated with the testis is testosterone, first isolated from the testis in 1935 and shown to be secreted into the blood in the mid-1950s (see ref. 1035), but several other steroids, including some such as pregnenolone, which do not appear to be androgens, are secreted by the testis, the exact pattern depending on the species (Table 3). Testosterone is the steroid secreted in largest amount by most mammalian testes into the testicular venous blood (25,162,329,351,441,614,687,707,708, 801,1010,1155,1164), with the exception of the pig testis, which secretes as much of the "boar-taint" steroid, 5a-androstenone as testosterone (201,411). Stallion testes secrete 19-nortestosterone (79), as well as testosterone (1042). The testes of men (687,1274,1293), dogs (785), pigs (1073), bulls (485), and ram lambs (932) secrete significant amounts of unconjugated estrogens, and the pig testis secretes almost as much dehydroepiandrosterone sulfate and estrone sulfate as testosterone (201,1073) into the venous blood (Fig. 47). Sulfated steroids are also secreted by the human testis into venous blood (687,983), but in the pig, the lymph appears to be a more important route than the venous blood for the secretion of conjugated steroids (1073) (see p. 1121). The concentration of testosterone in the testicular venous blood varies by a factor of ten between species; the human with a small testis in relation to body size has the highest reported concentration of testosterone in testicular venous blood. Testosterone is also the main steroid secreted by the maximally stimulated perfused testis of several species, although the rabbit testis secretes appreciable amounts of 5α-reduced androgens and the rat testis produces almost as much pregnenolone as testosterone under these conditions (Table 4; 195–197,329–331, 1334).

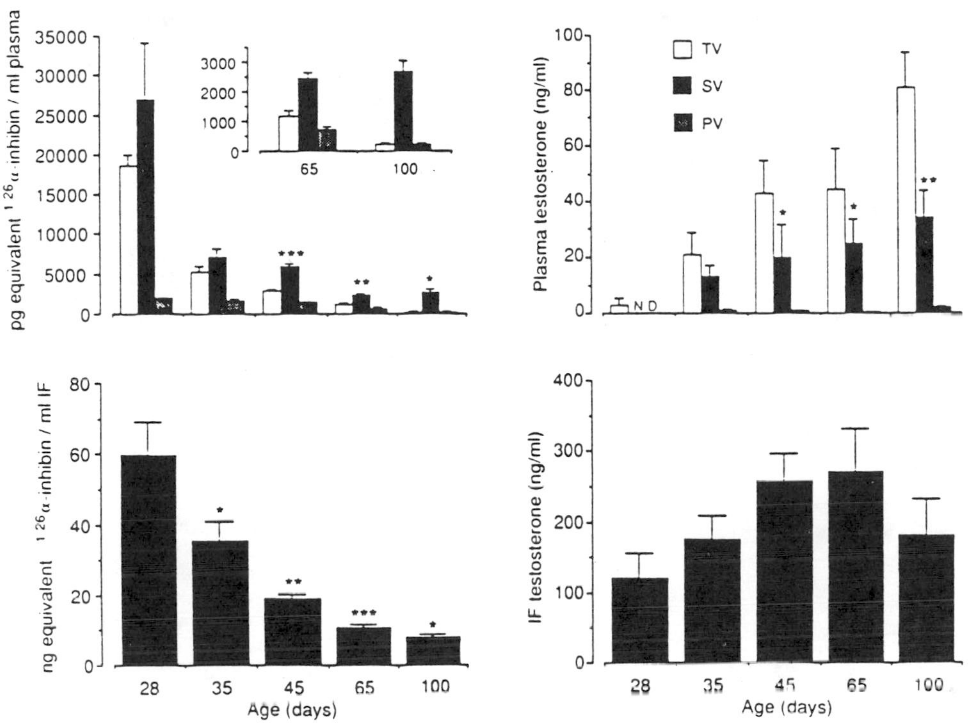

FIG. 54. The concentrations of inhibin and testosterone in testicular (TV) and spermatic (SV) venous blood plasma (see Fig. 34 for sites of sampling) and in peripheral blood plasma (PV) and testicular interstitial fluid collected by the drip technique. Note that the concentration of testosterone is always higher in the TV than in the SV, presumably because of dilution of the venous blood in the spermatic cord by flow through arteriovenous anastomoses, whereas the concentration of inhibin is higher in SV than TV, presumably because of absorption of inhibin from the excurrent ducts into the venous blood as it passes nearby. (From ref. 729).

In some species, the pattern of steroid secretion changes with age. The greatest rises in secretion during puberty in boys are found in testosterone and androstenediol, but a substantial part of these rises takes place in the early stages of puberty, so that dehydroepiandrosterone and androstendione show the greatest difference between midpuberty and adulthood (353). In young bulls, there is more androstenedione secreted than testosterone, but as the animal matures, the arteriovenous difference for androstenedione falls and that for testosterone rises, so that in mature bulls, more than 90% of the androgen secreted by the testis is testosterone (25,707,711). In the rat, the ratio between 3α-androstanediol and testosterone falls as the animal matures (351), whereas in the rabbit, whose testes also secrete appreciable amounts of 5α-reduced androgens, the proportion does not change with age (198,199). In the pig, testosterone secretion approximately doubles at puberty, compared with increases of about fivefold in the sulfated steroids (1073).

Inhibin is present in higher concentrations in testicular or spermatic venous blood than in arterial blood in men (550,733,1292), monkeys (733), rats (726,729), guinea pigs (733), and rams (1167), although still higher concentrations are present in testicular interstitial fluid in the rats and testicular lymph in the rams. There is also a higher concentration of an LH-inhibiting activity in testicular venous than arterial blood from rams (895). Plasma renin activity is higher in blood from the internal spermatic vein than from the cubital vein in men but only after treatment with hCG, and angiotensin levels were also higher in internal spermatic vein blood (630,869–871). Other studies (1017) suggested that it is prorenin rather than active renin that is released. The markers for testicular cancer, α-fetoprotein and hCG, are also released into spermatic venous blood (704). Perifused rat testes release β-endorphin and dynorphin (755), but this cannot be taken as evidence of secretion into the blood, as rat testes with pancreatic islet implants release insulin into a perifusate but not into a vascular perfusate (730).

Testicular venous blood contains about half as much oxygen as arterial blood (495,1050), so that if metabolism increases without a corresponding increase in blood flow, the testis can become hypoxic; this may happen if the temperature of the testis is increased (1254). The testis releases significant amounts of carbon dioxide and lactate into the venous blood and removes about 20% of the glucose and ketone bodies and about one-third of the acetate from the arterial blood (1028,1044).

The concentration of testosterone in the effluent from isolated perfused rat testes does not change significantly if perfusate flow is changed from the normal value of 500

TABLE 3. *Differences between the concentrations (ng/ml) of steroids in the spermatic venous blood and arterial blood in various species*

Steroid	Rat	Rabbit	Man	Sheep	Bull	Pig	Horse
Pregnenolone			10				
Progesterone			5–23		3–7		
17α-Hydroxyprogesterone			60–340				
Dehydroepiandrosterone			38			0.3–0.8	1.5
Androstenedione			10–40		1.8–8		
Androstenediol			47		5–23		
Testosterone	50–200	140	200–680	30–80	75–340	40–60	4–26
Dihydrotestosterone	6	40	3.5–22				
3α-Androstanediol	25	5	0.9–1.7		2–11		
3β-Androstanediol	4	25	7.5		4–16		
Estradiol-17β			0.6–3.4		0.003–0.015	0.25	
Estrone			49			62	
5α-Androstenone						62	
Pregnenolone sulphate			140				
Dehydroepiandrosterone sulphate			96–155			34–120	2.7
Dehydroepiandrosterone glucuronide						2	
5-Androstene-3β,17β-diol sulphate			34–102				
Testosterone sulphate			28–53				
Testosterone glucosiduronate							
Estrone sulphate						0.53	200

References are given in the text.

μl/min (about 300 μl/g/min) to values between 125 to 900 μl/g/min (Fig 55; 1079), and testosterone secretion is closely related to blood flow in the autoperfused dog testis (308) and in the rat testis *in vivo* (261,369). It would therefore appear that flow is an important factor in determining the amount of testosterone being secreted by the testes.

Lymph Flow and Composition

Flow of testicular lymph has been estimated in three ways: by cannulation of one or more of the lymphatic vessels in the spermatic cord and ligation of the rest, by measuring the degree of hemoconcentration as the blood passes through the testis, or by measuring the half-time of clearance of radioactive albumin injected directly into the testis, when this marker will be removed almost entirely in the lymph. There is considerable variation between species in the flow of lymph, with animals such as the rat with the largest lymphatic sinusoids in the testis having the slowest flow (about 0.5 μl/g/h), the ram and ferret being intermediate (about 1 μl/g/h), whereas the boar, which has very inconspicuous lymphatic vessels in the testis, has the highest lymph flow of up to 10 μl/g/h. (241,385,709,734,810,811,1034,1052,1073). Lymph flow can be increased by increasing venous pressure (1034), by warming the testis, and during exercise; flow is decreased by cooling the scrotum (241).

TABLE 4. *Difference between the concentrations (ng/ml) of steroids in perfusion fluid leaving and entering the maximally stimulated testis in various species*

Steroid	Rat	Rabbit	Mouse	Hamster	Guinea Pig	Dog
Pregnenolone	135	100	20			
Progesterone	20	4	10			
17α-Hydroxypregnenolone	130	60	50			
17α-Hydroxyprogesterone	40	45	6			
Dehydroepiandrosterone	10	65	53			
Androstenedione	5	20	100			
Androstenediol	undetectable	65	10			
Testosterone	165–180	370–660	600	40	450	370–400
Dihydrotestosterone	0.5	210	5			6
3α-Androstanediol	0.5	17	10			4.5
3β-Androstanediol	0.5	40	5			55

References are given in the text.

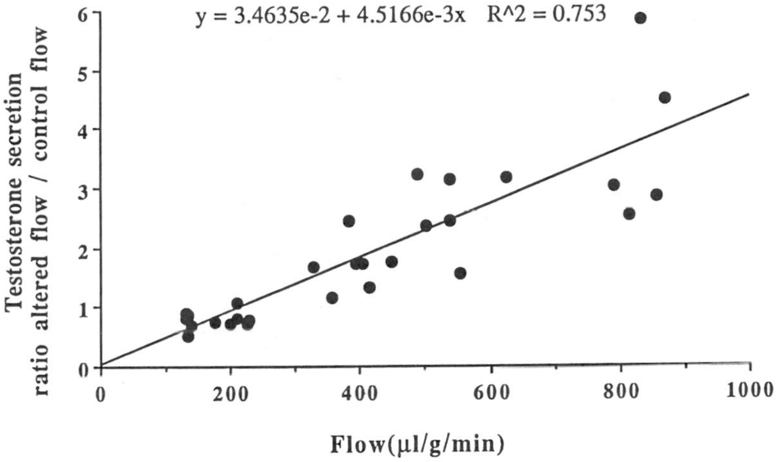

FIG. 55. The relationship between perfusate flow and testosterone secretion (flow × venous-arterial concentration) in isolated perfused testes of adult rats. Each point is the ratio of the secretion by one testis in which the perfusate flow rate was changed for 15 min after a control period of 30 min, to the contralateral testis in which flow was maintained at 300 μl/g/min for the whole 45 min period. (From ref. 1079).

Testicular lymph collected from a catheter in a lymphatic vessel in the spermatic cord of rams (241,1262) and boars (1034) is in general very similar to testicular venous blood plasma; the ionic composition is virtually identical whereas the glucose concentration is somewhat lower, presumably because of use by the testis. The protein concentration is between two-thirds and three-quarters as high as blood plasma and surprisingly does not vary with lymph flow (1034); the difference in the protein concentration between lymph and blood plasma is much less for testicular lymph than for lymph from other sites in the body with the exception of liver lymph. The proteins in blood plasma and testicular lymph are similar, although the albumin/globulin ratio in lymph is higher (74,810), and there is a lower concentration of α_2-macroglobulin there (709). The amino acid composition of testicular lymph is very similar to that of blood plasma (1062). There are no red cells in testicular lymph, but there are between 100 and 400 white cells/μl, of which about 80% are lymphocytes; the concentration of cells is at the lower end of the range for afferent lymph, and the proportion of different cell types is typical (1118,1262). After vasectomy, significant numbers of spermatozoa can be found in lymph collected from a vessel in the spermatic cord of sheep and pigs (57).

The concentration of testosterone and androstenedione in testicular lymph from rams was about two-thirds of that in testicular venous blood, even when the animals were injected with hCG (273,709–711). In men, the fluid within the tunica vaginalis contained about 20 times as much testosterone as peripheral blood (605); this ratio is much lower than the testicular vein to peripheral ratio of 260:1 (733), and the fluid is probably derived from several sources besides testicular lymph. In pigs and horses, there is appreciably more testosterone, dehydroepiandrosterone, and total unconjugated estrogens in lymph than in venous blood, and very much more estrone sulfate and dehydroepiandrosterone sulfate (1042,1073). Because lymph flow is also high in pigs, this means that in this species, most of these conjugated steroids are secreted through the lymph (Fig. 56). Inhibin is also present in testicular lymph from rams in concentrations about six times higher than in spermatic venous blood and more than ten times those in peripheral blood (1167). Consequently, testicular lymph, like rete testis fluid, has been used as a standard for inhibin bioassays (532).

Significance of Testicular Lymph

With its comparatively high concentration of steroids, testicular lymph probably exerts an important influence on the lymph nodes to which it drains. This may be at least a partial explanation for the persistence of grafts in the rodent testis (730). However, neither the testes of sheep (723) nor monkeys (Setchell, Granholm, Ploen, and Ritzen, *unpublished observations*) show any evidence of being immunologically privileged sites, so this cannot be the entire explanation. Spermatozoa in the lymph (57) and in abdominal lymph nodes (58) after vasectomy will obviously be an important source of antigen in the immunologic reactions seen under these conditions (14). There is some evidence for another target for testicular lymph. Radioactive albumin injected into one testis or into a lymphatic vessel on the surface of a testis is preferentially transferred to the ipsilateral epididymis (and to the ipsilateral fatpad in rats) (1036). This provides an alternative route by which hormones could reach the epididymis and may provide another explanation for the seminal abnormalities seen in rabbits whose epididymides were separated from the testes and reflected into the inguinal canal (73), because effects on semen quality were also seen in some but not all rams in which the testis and epididymis were separated but left in the scrotum (Quintana Casares, Zupp, and Setchell, *unpublished observations*). Transfer through the fluid in the tunica vaginalis may also be important, especially in

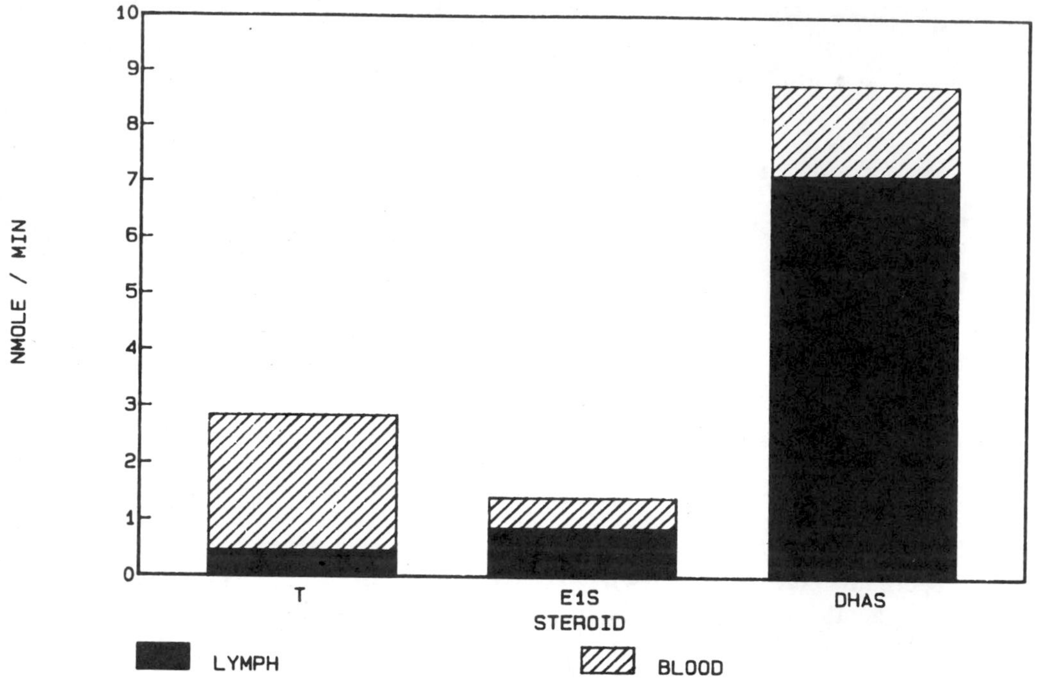

FIG. 56. The secretion of free and conjugated steroids into venous blood and lymph by the pig testis. The steroids shown are testosterone (T), estrone sulphate (E1S), and dehydroepiandrosterone sulphate (DHAS); the secretion rates were calculated from measurements of blood and lymph flow and the concentrations of these steroids in testicular lymph and venous blood and in arterial blood. (From ref. 1073.)

humans (605) where this cavity becomes separate from the peritoneal cavity.

There have also been several studies on the effects on the testis of lymphatic obstruction. Ligature of the lymphatics accompanying the spermatic artery and vein at the level of the common iliac artery in rabbits was followed by a fall in the testosterone levels in testicular venous blood and serious degenerative changes in the seminiferous epithelium (644). In rats, ligature of the lymphatic vessels either near or at a distance from one testis produced degeneration of the tubules and interstitial edema, with some abnormalities on the control side; the latter were attributed to immunologic damage (912). The lymphatics are an important route for the spread of metastases from testicular tumors (815,937).

Interstitial Fluid of the Testis; Volume, Turnover Rate, and Composition

The seminiferous tubules and the cells of the interstitial tissue are surrounded by an interstitial extracellular fluid. It appears from electron micrographs (339) that the fluid has a high protein concentration, and it gives a strong reaction to a fluorescent-labeled antiserum to albumin (193). The volume of this fluid can be estimated from the volume of distribution or "space" in the testis of a marker for extracellular fluid, which is excluded from the tubules (e.g., chromium-EDTA infused intravenously), provided that an infusion schedule is chosen so that the concentration rises rapidly and then remains constant until the tissue is sampled; this concentration profile is often referred to as a "square wave." As a less satisfactory alternative, the mean concentration between the beginning of the infusion and the time of sampling can be used. A single intravenous injection into rats whose ureters had been ligated or severed has also been used, as this prevents excretion of the marker in the urine. Values of about 60 μl/g are obtained for the parenchyma of rat testes, with higher values for some reason in animals with severed ureters (1039,1159). Values for the whole testis are higher than for the parenchyma, as the capsule appears to have a much higher Cr-EDTA space (930). Radioactive albumin introduced into the blood stream of rams reaches equilibrium with lymph from a lymphatic vessel in the spermatic cord within 2 to 3 h (241), and its volume of distribution of albumin within the rat testis (again calculated from mean concentrations between injection and sampling) reaches values similar to those for the usual markers for interstitial fluid within 3 to 6 h (1039,1052), (Fig. 32). Consequently, albumin space also gives a reasonable estimate of the volume of interstitial fluid and is much simpler to use, not requiring a continuous intravenous infusion or severing of the ureters as Cr-EDTA does. The volume of interstitial fluid can also be approximated from the volume of fluid collected from the testes of rats kept in a refrigerator overnight with a cut in the tunica (see, e.g., ref. 1085). This technique may be useful for indicating changes in volume (see, e.g., refs. 557,563), but it is not certain that all the extracellular interstitial fluid and nothing other than this fluid is collected. The values obtained do come close to the 24-h albumin space (1085,1091,1093), but the latter are likely to be overestimates, as plasma levels at the time of sampling were used in the calculations, with no correction for the fall between the time of injection and sampling. The volume of interstitial fluid is decreased after hypophysectomy or treatment with estradiol (1285) or ethanol, and ethanol treatment reduces the response to hCG (6). Fluid volume is also decreased in prepubertal rats (1093) or adult rats in which the Leydig cells are removed by treatment with EDS (270); in the last instance, the reduction can be reversed by treatment of the animals with testosterone (727). The volume of interstitial fluid is increased after treatment with hCG (1052,1085) or LHRH agonist (1098,1208) and in several conditions in which spermatogenesis is deranged (e.g., after heating of the testes [383,563], cryptorchidism [267,557,1086], efferent duct ligation [557,1159], irradiation [1265], or treatment with methoxyacetic acid [1099]). Although this may be due to a direct effect of the tubular cells on the testicular microvasculature, it would seem more likely to be due to a change in the pressure within the testis, as a result of shrinkage of the damaged tubules, and in all instances where it has been studied, the volume of fluid in the testes with arrested spermatogenesis still increases after treatment with hCG (1072).

Knowing the volume of the interstitial fluid, its turnover rate can be estimated from the half-time of clearance of albumin injected directly into the testis, as albumin injected in this way is almost exclusively removed in the lymph (385). The results obtained with this technique are discussed in the section on lymph flow.

Interstitial fluid can be collected from isolated testes for analysis by making an incision in the capsule and allowing the fluid to drip out into a container in the cold room (889–891,1084) or collecting it by gentle centrifugation (435,1195,1196). A more physiologic approach is to use a micropipette (496,1181) or a push–pull cannula in anesthetized animals, the degree of dilution of the infused fluid with interstitial fluid being determined by loading the animal previously with an appropriate marker (722). When the "drip" technique was used, interstitial fluid appeared to contain higher concentrations of potassium and certain intracellular enzymes than blood plasma and much higher levels of testosterone than in testicular venous blood plasma (Fig. 34). This would imply that testosterone was not crossing the endothelial lining of the capillaries as readily as one would expect (see ref. 1037), but analysis of fluid collected with the push–pull cannula indicates that the testosterone concentration is certainly no higher than that in venous blood plasma and may be somewhat lower; the protein and potassium concentrations are, as expected, similar to plasma (722,724). The similarity of the potassium concentrations in interstitial fluid and blood plasma have been confirmed by direct measurements in the testes of anesthetized rats with ion-sensitive microelectrodes (1335).

Interstitial fluid collected by a micropipette from anesthetised rats after removing a portion of the tunic contained amino acids, the concentrations of some of which differed slightly but significantly from arterial or testicular venous blood plasma (496). Interstitial fluid collected by the drip technique contains an LHRH-like substance (1095–1097), which may influence testosterone secretion by the Leydig cells (1087,1088,1091,1094,1098), as well other steroidogenesis-stimulating activities (468, 469,557,780). There is also a report that testicular interstitial fluid from rats contains more than ten times as much ABP as testicular venous blood (1195) and about 100 times as much arginine vasopressin as blood plasma, the level falling if the testes are made cryptorchid or the efferent ducts are ligated to disrupt spermatogenesis (931). Again, these values may be somewhat suspect because of the unphysiologic technique used for the fluid collection. The Leydig cells of several species have also been shown to contain β-endorphin or other proopiomelanocortin-derived peptides (60,396,754,1083, 1178,1179), and as judged by the localization of the mRNA, the highest concentrations are found in the Leydig cells adjacent to tubules in which a generation of spermatozoa had just been shed (401). It has been suggested that this peptide may exert a paracrine effect on the function of Sertoli cells or an autocrine effect on the Leydig cells themselves, presumably by secretion into the interstitial fluid, and β-endorphin and dynorphin can be detected in rat testis perifusion effluent (755), which would include some interstitial fluid. Appreciable concentrations of β-endorphin and ACTH have been found in interstitial fluid collected postmortem from rat testes, severalfold higher than in blood plasma; hypophysectomy has no effect on the concentrations in interstitial fluid, while reducing those in plasma, hCG causes an increase, and LHRH agonist a decrease (1208). The levels of β-endorphin in testicular interstitial fluid are increased after intraperitoneal injections of ethanol, whereas testosterone levels fall (6). There are also appreciable concentrations of IL-like material in interstitial fluid, collected either by the drip technique or by push–pull (431), similar to the peptide found in extracts of whole testis (1120,1147); surprisingly, no such activity could be detected in thoracic duct lymph (Setchell, Froysa, Soder, and Ritzen, *unpublished results*), although the extent of dilution should not have been sufficient to reduce the levels below the limit of detection of the assay. Interstitial fluid also contains a mediator of vasopermeability, probably originating from polymorphonuclear leucocytes (1161).

The amount of interstitial fluid is determined by the balance between formation and removal. Fluid is removed both by resorption (i.e., re-entry into the venous ends of the capillaries or the venules) or through the lymph, the flow of which will be influenced by the volume of fluid but also contractions of the walls of the lymphatic vessels (1330). The fluid is presumably formed, as in other tissues, by filtration of blood plasma at the arterial ends of the capillaries. The amount of fluid produced or resorbed in unit time (J_v) is determined by the formula:

$$J_v = L_p S[P_c - P_i - \sigma(\pi_p - \pi_i)]$$

where L_p is the hydraulic conductivity of the vessel wall, S is its surface area, P_c and P_i are the hydrostatic pressure in the capillary and the interstitial tissue, respectively, π_p and π_i are the colloid osmotic pressures of the plasma and intersitial fluid, respectively, and σ is the reflection coefficient of the vessel wall for protein. S is not likely to change in the short term, unless a substantial proportion of the testicular vessels are normally closed. The low extraction of albumin during a single passage suggests that σ is near 1. However, in contrast to other tissues, π_i must be close to π_p, because the protein concentration in interstitial extracellular fluid in the testis is almost the same as that in plasma. Therefore, the principal factors determining whether fluid is filtered (positive J_v) or reabsorbed (negative J_v) will be the hydrostatic pressures in the capillaries and the interstitial tissue. As already mentioned, capillary pressure appears to be lower in the blood vessels in the capsule of the hamster testis than in other tissues (1146) and indeed is not much higher than one value of 10 mm Hg for tissue pressure in the rat reported by Free and Jaffe (365), although there are other lower values in the literature (524,638). Tissue pressure may rise as high as 40 mm Hg in the cryptorchid testes rats treated with hCG (508). It is also relevant that testicular venous pressure, and therefore presumably capillary pressure is elevated in varicocele (see p. 1092), which may be a significant factor in pathogenesis of this condition.

Seminiferous Tubule Fluid: Flow and Composition

The lumina of the seminiferous tubules are filled with a fluid that carries the spermatozoa away when they have been released. Some studies have been made of the electrophysiology of isolated tubules in relation to fluid secretion (249,403), and a technique has been described for measuring fluid secretion *in vitro;* the rates found were approximately three times higher than those for the whole testis and could be reduced by cooling, removal of glucose or potassium from the bathing medium, or the addition of the inhibitors 2,4-dinitrophenol, ouabain, or acetazolamide; removal of calcium from the bathing fluid caused an increase in secretory rate (188). The amount of fluid being secreted *in vivo* by all the tubules plus the rete testis can be estimated by measuring the weight gain of a testis after ligation of the efferent ducts; the weight of the testis increases linearly for approximately 36 h in rats and hamsters and for approximately 72 h in sheep and goats, and histologic examination of the ligated testes shows that the increase is due to distention of the seminiferous tubules and rete testis (503,1027,1067). There is evidence from some but not all studies that some fluid secretion can be demonstrated as early as 20 or 25 days of age, at about the time that the first spermatids appear in the testis. However, it is clear that fluid secretion increases dramatically after 30 days of age and continues to increase when expressed per testis, and therefore per Sertoli cell, up to about 70 days of age (Fig. 57). The flow rate per gram of testis, however, reaches a maximum at about 40 days of age, when the first spermatozoa are shed into the tubular lumen. In adult golden hamsters, fluid secretion measured by weight gain after EDL decreases from about 550 mg/24 h per testis to about 50 mg/24 h per testis when the testes regress under short daylengths (62).

The question of the effects of hormones or drugs on fluid secretion must be separated into two components: direct effects, and effects secondary to changes in cell populations in the testis. The latter becomes important if the studies involve administration of the treatment for periods greater than the time needed to measure fluid secretion.

Surgical hypophysectomy has no immediate effect on fluid secretion (38,1027), but there were small falls between 2 and 3 days posthypophysectomy before the weight of the testis begins to decrease in one experiment (564) but not in another (38). Subsequently, as the testis decreases in size because of disruption of spermatogenesis, fluid secretion falls in absolute terms (μl/h) but not in relation to testis weight, whether measured by weight gain after EDL (38,564,1027) or cannulation of the efferent ducts (370).

LH from sheep pituitaries had no immediate effect on fluid secretion by testes of intact rats or hamsters (1067) but did produce an increase in fluid production when given for 3 days (564). hCG, which has mainly LH-like effects, had no significant effect on fluid production when administered to rats for 3 or 9 weeks (1067); treatment for 2 days was without effect in mice (59) and a single intramuscular injection of hCG and pregnant mare serum gonadotrophin (PMS-G) was without effect on flow of rete testis fluid in conscious rams (1047). In young (20- to 25-day-old) rats, a single injection (563) or treatment for 3 days (1067) with ovine follicle-stimulating hormone (FSH) produced increases in fluid secretion, whereas growth hormone, prolactin, or LH were without effect. Treatment of hypophysectomized adult rats with ovine FSH had no significant effect, but

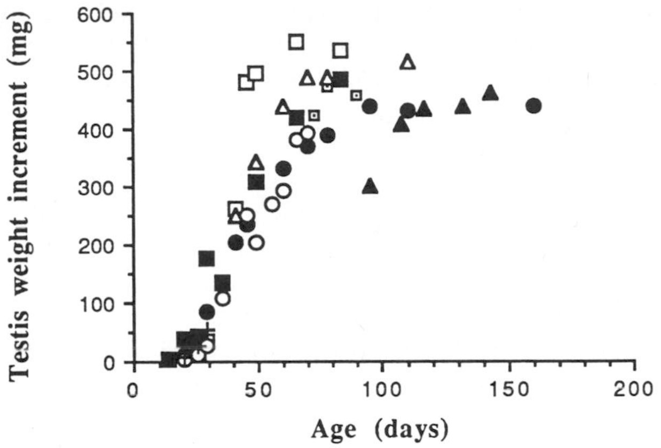

FIG. 57. The secretion of fluid (measured by the gain in weight during 16h after efferent duct ligation) in rats of various ages. (From ref. 503, data from refs. 1027 (open squares), 1056 (solid squares), 563 and 564 (solid circles), 39 (open circles), 985 (crosses), 669 (solid triangles), 530 (open triangles) and our unpublished observations (open squares with central dot).

injection with LH or testosterone propionate for 3 days beginning 4 days after operation (564) or with high-dose testosterone implants before and for 50 days after operation (40) returned fluid production to the levels seen in intact animals when measured by weight gain after EDL. Treatment with testosterone propionate increased fluid flow from the testes of hypophysectomized rats but did not restore it to normal vales (370). Treatment with low-dose implants of testosterone, which cause decreases in testis size by suppressing gonadotrophin secretion, reduced fluid secretion by the testes of intact rats and did not maintain fluid secretion by the testes of hypophysectomized rats (39).

Making the testis cryptorchid has no immediate effect on fluid production (1027), and no effect was apparent in testes made cryptorchid 8 h before efferent duct ligation (shown as 1-day cryptorchidism in ref. 565; G. Risbridger, *personal communication*). Falls were apparent by 2 and 3 days after the testis had been placed at the higher temperature inside the abdominal cavity. This fall preceded any change in testis weight (37,565), but an additional fall in fluid secretion occurred with the fall in testis weight (37,565,1027). In rats made cryptorchid when they were 14 days old, fluid secretion was depressed when they had reached 35 and 130 days of age, but if the testes were returned to the scrotum at 35 days, fluid secretion was normal at 130 days (567). However, fluid secretion by testes of adult rats made cryptorchid for 10 days did not recover during the subsequent 3-month period (566).

However, when the testes of rats were heated either to 41°C for 1 or 1.5 h (1056) or to 43°C for 15 min (567), there were falls in fluid secretion, in the former study in parallel with testis weight, and in the latter, only at 26 days after heating, although testis weight was reduced at 7 and 14 days as well; as testis weight recovered, so did fluid secretion (Fig. 58).

However, when spermatogenesis was disrupted by treatment of adult rats with busulphan, fluid secretion increased as testis weight fell (669). In rats fed a vitamin A-deficient diet from 20 days of age, fluid secretion remained normal while testis weight was similar to controls, but fell by 80 and 110 days of age, when testis weight had fallen below control (530). Single doses of the phthalate esters, di-*n*-pentyl phthalate (DPP) or mono-2-pentyl phthalate (MEHP) caused decreases in fluid production by the testes of 4- to 5-week-old rats, but three daily doses of DPP were needed to produce a fall in adult 10-week-old rats, and MEHP was without effect (417). By contrast, treatment of rats with ethylene glycol monomethyl ether for up to 10 days caused significant decreases in testis weight without having any consistent effect on fluid secretion (182) and reserpine treatment of rats increased viscosity of the fluid in the epididymal lumen without having any effect on fluid secretion by the testis (1276). Colchicine given intraperitoneally in doses that should have blocked cell division had no effect

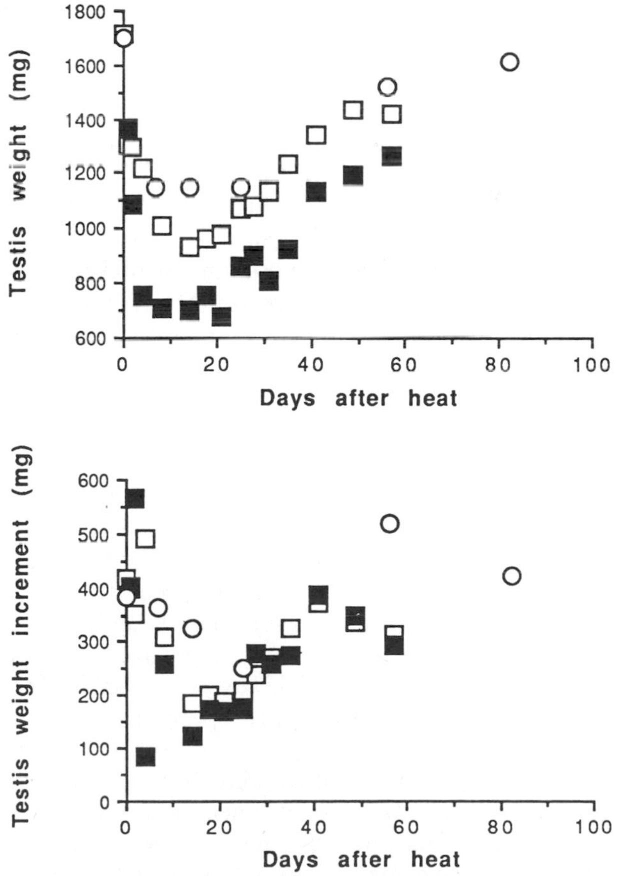

FIG. 58. The secretion of fluid, measured by the gain in weight during 16h after efferent duct ligation, by the testes of rats following a single period of local heating, to 41°C for 60 min (open squares), 41°C for 90 min (solid squares, ref. 1056) or 43°C for 15 min (open circles, ref. 566). (From ref. 503).

on fluid secretion in testes of mice (59), but injections given directly into the testis at doses sufficient to cause disruption of the cytoskeleton of the Sertoli cells reduced fluid secretion immediately afterward to practically zero (17). Addition of 2,5-hexanedione to the drinking water of rats for 5 weeks initially has no effect on fluid secretion, although it caused changes in Sertoli cells and elongated spermatids after 3 weeks 3 days exposure; there was no change in fluid secretion up to 3 weeks 4 days of dosage, but by 3 weeks 6 days, there were also changes in the round spermatids and fluid secretion had fallen to about half, remaining at about the same low level up to 3 weeks after the end of treatment (576).

Acetazolamide, an inhibitor of carbonic anhydrase, has also been shown to decrease fluid secretion from catheters in the rete testis of rams (1047), and after EDL in rats, when administered intravenously. Ethoxyzolamide, another inhibitor of the enzyme, was effective when given intraperitoneally, but neither inhibitor was effective if given orally. Metabolic alkalosis induced by the infusion of sodium acetate or sodium bicarbonate also reduced fluid secretion in rats (1041).

Fluid secretion can also be demonstrated in the testes of rats treated prenatally with busulphan or irradiation to destroy the germ cells (ref. 1025; B. P. Setchell and B. T. Hinton, *unpublished results*) and in the testes of rats treated with ethanedimethane sulfonate to eliminate the Leydig cells (812).

The dynamics of fluid flow in individual tubules is more difficult to study, but from the infusion of concentrated dye solutions into individual superficial tubules or the introduction of small droplets of colored oil, it appears that the flow is irregular both in rate and direction. Each tubule did appear to have a preferred direction of flow, but whether this was toward or away from the rete testis could not be determined. By sampling as much fluid as possible from a single tubule over approximately 1 h and by estimating the degree of dilution of infused dye, it did appear that the flow along each tubule is probably between 0.5 and 1 μl/h (1069), and as there are approximately 30 tubules in the rat, this would correspond reasonably well with the estimates of total flow.

Small samples of fluid can be removed by micropuncture from individual tubules for analysis, although the samples are so small that the range of possible analyses is limited (Tables 5 and 6). Originally, it was believed that there was a higher concentration of spermatozoa in seminiferous tubule fluid (STF) than in rete testis fluid (1181), but when the numbers were obtained by counting the cells (1069) rather than centrifuging the samples, it became clear that the "spermatocrit" values for STF were too high (spermatocrit is analogous to hematocrit and measures the proportion of the luminal fluid occupied by spermatozoa after centrifugation in a small capillary tube). STF is appreciably hypertonic in the hamster (574) but not in the rat (1181). There is almost ten times as much potassium in STF as in blood plasma (568,692,1181). However, in rats made aspermatogenic by treatment *in utero* with busulphan or irradiation, the potassium concentration in STF was serumlike (693,1069,1180; but cf. ref. 817). Chloride concentration in STF is similar to plasma (568,1181) and so is calcium and sulfur, whereas magnesium and total phosphorus are higher in STF (568). The protein concentration is less in STF than in blood plasma or interstitial fluid (501,1069), but there are several proteins in tubular fluid that cannot be seen in blood plasma (639,641–643) and high concentrations of androgen-binding protein (1192,1195). There are also low concentrations of transferrin in STF, approximately 25 times less than in blood plasma or testicular interstitial fluid (1148). The amino acid composition of STF is quite different from blood plasma or interstitial fluid; it contains much higher concentrations of aspartic acid, glutamic acid, glycine, and alanine (496). Glucose cannot be detected in STF, but there is more than 100 times as much inositol as in blood plasma (505). The concentration of testosterone in STF (Table 7) is slightly lower than that in interstitial fluid, and both increase similarly if the animal is stimulated for 4 days with hCG (217). Larger samples of less pure fluid can be collected by decapsulating the testis, disrupting the seminiferous tubules by forcing the parenchyma through a hypodermic needle, and centrifuging the cell dispersion. Contamination with interstitial fluid can be minimized by rinsing the tubules before disrupting them (1195) or by applying a correction obtained by ligating the efferent ducts of one testis 16 h previously to increase the proportion of tubular fluid in that testis and assuming that both have the same amount of interstitial fluid (1048,1068,1070). With the latter variant, the potassium and inositol content of the fluid are identical to those of fluid obtained by micropuncture, and with both variants, the testosterone concentrations are similar. However, with the former variant, the protein content is clearly higher, suggesting that there is appreciable contamination with cell contents or interstitial fluid; androgen-binding protein concentrations, however, are appreciably lower than in micropuncture fluid. When the testosterone concentration in the blood was raised by parenteral injection of the steroid in oil or hCG, the concentration of testosterone in tubular fluid did increase but not to the same extent; this was taken as evidence that testosterone was entering the tubules by a process involving facilitated diffusion (1033,1070).

Rete Testis Fluid: Flow and Composition

Rete testis fluid (RTF) has been collected from catheters chronically implanted into the rete testis of rams (1241,1242), bulls (1243), and boars (251,328) and acutely from rats (367,1181), rhesus monkeys (1250),

TABLE 5. *Concentration (mM) of ionic constitutents in secretions of the male reproductive tract*[a]

Male reproductive tract secretions	Sodium	Potassium	Calcium	Magnesium	Chloride	Phosphate	Bicarbonate
Seminiferous tubule fluid							
Rat	108	50	0.44	1.2	120	<0.1	20
	(±7)	(±5)	(±0.02)	(±0.18)	(±5)		
Rete testis fluid							
Wallaby	118	14			137		
Rat	143	14	0.81	0.39	140	<0.1	21
	(±4)	(±1)	(±0.09)	(±0.09)	(±2)		
Rabbit	147	7.8	0.8	0.5			
Ram	121	11.2	1.0	0.4	128	0.025	8
Bull	133	9.1	0.4	0.4	122	0.017	7
Boar	116	8.8	1.2		134	0.22	
Monkey	136	7.4					
Cauda epididymidis or ductus deferens							
Rat	26	47	0.18	1.1	24	13	6.7
	(15–37)	(43–55)	(0.11–0.25)	(0.9–1.3)	(20–27)	(9.5–16)	
Hamster	16	31	0.1	1.3	11	29	
	(6.1–25)	(24–38)					
Guinea pig	17	18	0.1	2.2	10	5.4	
Rabbit	17	22	0.47	7.2	14	3.9	
	(15–20)	(18–25)			(8–23)		
Dog	22	38	0.85	1.1	16	7.2	
Goat	50	30	1.3				
Ram	40	29	0.61	0.7	22	8.3	
	(22–57)	(24–39)	(0.48–0.95)	(0.3–1.3)	(9.4–34)	(7.6–9)	
Bull	34	26	1.35	1.2	30	17.5	0
	(30–38)	(22–28)	(0.35–1.1)		(12–65)	(14–21)	
Boar	30	35	1.8	0.8	13	5.3	4
	(24–38)	(35–48)	(0.9–2.8)	(0–1.2)	(3.4–23)	(2.2–12)	
Stallion	41	32	0.55	1.2	12	4.3	
Elephant	103	37					
Monkey	18	49		2	10.5	1.7	
Man	30	111			103	24	
Ampulla							
Goat	50	31	1.9				
Bull	84	28	8.8	3.1			
	(60–108)		(8–9.6)	(2.7–3.5)			
Stallion					36		
Seminal vesicles							
Rat						4.8	
Guinea pig						1.6	
Goat	87	61	3				
Ram	93	37	3.4	3.2			
Bull	109	64	15	5.6		2.3	
		(27–100)	(12.6–17.5)	(3.9–7.2)			
Boar	26	126	3	28	12	1	
	(22–30)	(24–300)			(3–20)	(0.7–1.3)	
Stallion					59		
Man		19			28	8.9	
		(18–20)				(3.2–14.5)	
Prostate							
Dog	157	6.3	0.5	0.6	160	1	4.2
	(154–159)	(5.1–8.7)	(0.3–1.1)				
Man	155	53	26	19	45	1	8
	(153–157)	(45–67)	(15–32)	(17–20)	(38–61)		
Cowper's gland							
Boar	90	28			105	2.3	

[a] Where several values were available, the mean was calculated and the SEM or the range is shown in parentheses.

From refs. 128 and 1028.

TABLE 6. *Concentration (mM) of low-molecular-weight organic compounds and of total protein (mg/ml) in secretions of the male reproductive tract[a]*

Male reproductive tract secretions	Glucose	Fructose	Inositol	Citric acid	Carnitine	Glycerophosphocholine	Phosphocholine	Ergothioneine	Ascorbic acid	Protein
Semininferous tubule fluid										
Rat	<1		1.8		<1	<0.1	<0.1			6
Hamster			3.2		<1					
Rabbit			2.1							
Rhesus monkey			9.5							
Rete testis fluid										
Rat	<0.1		2.5		<1	<0.1	<0.1			
Hamster			3.1		<1					
Ram	0.1		5.7		0.028					1
Boar			5.7		0.012					1.1
Cauda epididymidis or ductus deferens										
Rat			31		54 (16–82)	32 (21–41)	20			32 (27–41)
Hamster			90		30 (11–48)	41				37 (24–49)
Guinea pig					67	39 (27–51)				34 (25–42)
Rabbit		0	0		43 (19–69)	41 (19–59)				42 (35–62)
Dog					20	34				30
Ram			2.1 (1–3.2)		17 (15–19)	65 (21–97)				19 (13–27)
Bull			2.5	0	2	36 (17–54)				31 (29–33)
Boar		0.2	2.8 (1–5.3)	0.3 (0–0.6)	11 (6–16)	72 (48–111)		0.06 (0–0.13)		35 (19–100)
Jackass				0						
Stallion					11	45 (43–46)				32
Elephant										36
Monkey			17		80	87				74
Man			5.9		5.8 (5.5–6)	<5	<5			29
Ampulla										
Rat				0						
Bull				29		3.4				
Jackass				0				3.8 (2.2–5)		
Zebra			0	0						
Stallion		0.15	1.1	0.04 (0.02–0.05)				3.6 (1.9–6.1)		
Elephant		4.3		0						
Seminal vesicles										
Hedgehog		28		0				2		
Rat	0.4	0.2		6		22 (16–25)		0	0.23	250 (200–300)
Mouse	1.1	31								
Vole	0.3	0								
Hamster	trace	0								
Guinea pig	9 (6.5–11)	5.8 (3.5–6.9)	1.1 (6–18)	12		10		0	0.5	
Coypu		3		5						
Rabbit				43						
Ram		99								55
Bull		46	1.6	35		trace		0	0.8	
Buffalo		54		15						
Boar		4.3 (3.1–6.2)	117 (100–134)	30 (29–32)		6.9		2.9 (1.8–3.8)	0.23	99 (80–112)

TABLE 6. *Continued.*

Male reproductive tract secretions	Glucose	Fructose	Inositol	Citric acid	Carnitine	Glycero-phospho-choline	Phospho-choline	Ergo-thioneine	Ascorbic acid	Protein
Jackass				3.3 (2.7–3.8)				0.09		
Stallion		trace		13 (6.6–19)		trace		0.49 (0.26–0.71)		
Zebra				27						
Elephant		4		0.01						
Monkey			8.1			0				
Man		22		3.8 (1–6.5)				0	0.28	
Coagulating glands										
Rat	9	28 (23–34)		0						240
Guinea pig		0		0						
Coypu		0.2		19						
Prostate										
Rat		0				0				95
Guiena pig		0								
Dog				0.14					0.04	8
Boar								0		44
Jackass				0				0		
Stallion				trace				trace		
Elephant		2.1		0.15						
Man	0.9	0	8.2	91 (45–176)					0.03	24 (22–26)
Cowper's glands										
Coypu		0.1		0.2						
Hedgehog		0		4.5				0		
Rabbit		0								
Boar		0	0	0				0		5
Elephant		0.06		0.26						

[a] Where several values were available, the mean was calculated and the range is shown in parentheses.
From refs. 128 and 1028.

rabbits (225,230,425,664), and wallabies (1026). In some studies, the efferent ducts were ligated for some hours beforehand to allow some fluid to accumulate, but this does not appear to make much difference to the flow of the fluid once the accumulated fluid has gone (367). Flow rate of fluid from a catheter was usually in the range of 4 to 20 μl/g/h, with the smaller animals tending to have faster flows (see refs. 793,1028,1032,1249,1251, 1256). The flow of fluid in rams is steady and shows no apparent diurnal rhythm. Administration of gonadotropins does not have any obvious effect, nor did atropine or pilocarpine. Oxytocin had no effect in one study (1047), although there was a small short-lived increase in another (1239). PG injections into the intertubular tissue of rat testes also caused short-term increases in flow of rete testis fluid, but this effect was blocked by incising the capsule (370), so it was probably also due to contractions of capsular cells induced by the drug.

Fluid flow from a catheter in the rete testis of isolated perfused ram testes fell if glucose concentration in the perfusate fell to low levels or if the temperature was raised to 39°C or above (713). Fluid secretion from the testes of conscious rams was unaffected by halothane, pentobarbitone, or spinal anesthesis or the administration of atropine or pilocarpine (1047). Reducing the concentration of spermatozoa by locally heating the testis had no effect on the flow of fluid (1066), and fluid flow increased first, followed by sperm concentration, at the beginning of the breeding season of rams in France (252).

RTF is a dilute suspension of immature, immotile spermatozoa, the concentration ranging from approximately 30 million/ml in rats and rabbits to between 100 and 300 million/ml in rams, boars, and monkeys (see refs. 1028,1032,1064,1249,1251,1256). In rams, there is a seasonal variation in concentration (252), and locally heating the testis causes a drop in sperm concentration approximately 20 days later, without any apparent effect on flow or composition of the fluid (1066). In rats, a similar but slightly earlier fall in sperm concentration can be detected (1056). As well as being immotile, the testicular spermatozoa differ from sperm from the tail of the epididymis in composition, metabolism, and surface properties (see Chapter 23 by Robaire and Hermo in the first edition of this volume). The ionic composition of RTF is different from blood plasma, lymph, and testicu-

TABLE 7. *Concentration (ng/ml) of steroids in the testicular excurrent duct system*[a]

Steroid	Peripheral blood plasma	Seminiferous tubule fluid	Rete testis fluid	Caput epididymal fluid	Cauda epididymal fluid
Pregnenolone					
Rabbit	2.8		3.3–22.4		
Ram			0.85		9.9
Progesterone					
Rabbit			1.2		
Bull	0.3–0.6		3.7		7.4
Dehydroepiandrosterone					
Rabbit	0.4		0.5–4.2	4.2	
Ram			6.4	33.8	25.8
Bull	0.65–0.71		21	8	
5-Androstene-3,17-dione					
Rabbit	0.1		1.1–5.2		
Dog				2	
Ram			1.5		1.3
Bull	0.38–0.57		7.6–17		1.7
Testosterone					
Rat	0.8–7.7	40–115	22–46.5	5	2–4
Rabbit	0.5–10		47.8–69		
Dog	0.8–1.9				2.5
Ram	0.7–26		3–88	24.8	10.8
Bull	2–24		20.4–33		6.2–11.5
Boar	2.9–7		13.3		
Monkey	3.2–10.3		2.5–10.5		
Dihydrotestosterone					
Rat	0.24	1.0–1.5	1.9–32.7	40	5–7
Rabbit	0.5		11.2–28.5		
Dog				3	
Ram	0.14		1		4.4–17
Bull	<0.03–0.10		1.3		13.6–20.3
5α-Androstan-3α,17β-diol					
Rat			26		9.2
Dog					2.1
Bull	<0.03		1.6		4.0
5α-Androstan-3β,17β-diol					
Rat			8		7.8
Dog					1.8
Bull	<0.03		2.4		6.5
5-Androstene-3β,17β-diol					
Bull	0.12–0.16		4.0		4.2
Estradiol or total estrogens					
Rat			0.248		
Rabbit			<0.02–0.027		
Bull	0.009–0.010		0.012		0.026
Boar	0.050		0.10		
Monkey			0.066		

[a] From ref. 128. Values for peripheral blood plasma are from refs. 387, 430, 675, 938, 1006 and 1043.

lar interstitial fluid on the one hand and from STF on the other; its potassium and sodium concentrations are intermediate, and it contains more chloride and less bicarbonate than any of the other fluids (Table 5). The concentrations of calcium and magnesium in ram RTF are about half of the total in blood plasma but similar to the concentrations of the free ions (see refs. 1028,1032,1064, 1249,1251,1256), although measurements in rats using electron probe microanalysis gave serumlike values for magnesium and higher than serum for calcium, with calcium higher and magnesium less than in STF (568). Inorganic phosphate was undetectable in rat RTF (502), and much lower than blood plasma in the rat (1064); total phosphorus was slightly lower in RTF than in serum but much lower than in STF. Total sulfur concentrations were comparable in all three fluids (568). There is practically no glucose in RTF, but inositol is to be found there in concentrations up to 100 times those in blood plasma (505,1063) (Table 6). The inositol appears to be formed by synthesis within the tubules from glucose, not accumulated as such from the blood (787), and if rats are given galactose in their diet, RTF contains galactitol as well as inositol (786). Ram RTF contains about as much glycerol as does testicular venous blood, and this substrate, in contrast to inositol, can be used by testicular spermatozoa (250). Lactate and pyruvate are present in RTF in similar concentrations to those in blood plasma, and there are slightly lower concentrations of acetate (1028). Most of the free amino acids are found in RTF in lower concentrations than in blood, but glutamate, aspartate, glycine, and alanine are present in much higher concentrations (496,713,1064). RTF contains very little protein (Table 6), approximately 1 mg/ml, even less than STF, although the reason for this latter difference is not clear (501,1069). Many of the proteins of blood plasma appear to be present in RTF, but this fluid is proportionately richer in α_2-macroglobulin, which is less abundant in lymph (see *Lymph Flow and Composition,* p. 1121), although immunoglobulins are proportionately even lower than total protein (583, 1029). Using step-gel electrophoresis, it was shown that several blood plasma proteins were not present in RTF, and conversely, there were proteins in RTF that could not be found in blood plasma; however, the concentrations of these specific proteins appeared to be less in RTF than in STF (639). Using polyvalent antisera, it was found that RTF contained nine specific proteins and 12 proteins identical to those in serum; however, even the latter were probably also synthesized by the Sertoli cells and not derived from the blood (1306). Rat RTF contains an ABP (371,372), which can only be detected in blood at very much lower concentrations, and is probably derived from the testis (426,427); the concentration in RTF is very similar to that found in micropuncture samples of STF (1195). ABP is also present in ram RTF, but in this species a very similar protein is found in blood plasma, even in castrated animals (562). Boar RTF contains no detectable ABP (B. Jegou and J.-L. Dacheux, quoted in ref. 562). Transferrin is found in rat RTF in concentrations approximately one-third of those in STF and approximately 75 times less than those in blood plasma and lymph (1148). Several enzymes are found in higher concentrations in ram RTF than in blood plasma, and one isozyme of malate dehydrogenase and one of aspartate aminotransferase are found in RTF but not in blood plasma; the isozymes of lactate dehydrogenase found in RTF are those found in many tissues, but isozyme X, which is specific to the testis, is not present in RTF (1139). Rat RTF also contains different forms of esterase, acid phosphatase (641), and uridine 5′-diphosphate (UDP)galactose: *N*-acetylglucosamine galactosyltransferase (437) from those found in blood serum; this last enzyme is believed to transfer galactose from UDP-galactose to glycoproteins in epididymal fluid or spermatozoa, and it was reported that its receptor specificity is changed from *N*-acetylglucosamine to glucose or inositol by an α-lactalbumin-like material in epididymal fluid (438); however, later studies suggest that this may not be so (519,1156). RTF from rams and boars contains high concentrations of a peptide inhibitor of trypsin and acrosin, which may be important in neutralizing the effect of any of the latter enzyme released prematurely from the spermatozoa (1139,1140). A nonglycosylated peptide mitogenic growth factor, which stimulates the division of mouse 3-T-3 cells in culture has been found in ram RTF; this factor appears to be different from other better known growth factors (137) and from the growth factor derived from Sertoli cells (345). Another peptide has been described in RTF that inhibits spermatogonial mitoses (107). There is also a highly acidic glycoprotein there that has been named *clusterin* and that elicits clustering of Sertoli and other cells in culture; this substance comprises approximately 18% of the total protein in ram RTF and may be involved in influencing cell interactions in the testis or epididymis at some stage of germ cell development or maturation (100,378,1183). Ram RTF is a potent source of inhibin-like activity (279,1046), although the endocrino logic significance of this hormone to the male animal is still obscure; and mullerian duct-inhibiting factor, usually considered to be a secretory product of fetal Sertoli cells, can be found in boar RTF (597). RTF in the ram carries into the epididymis approximately 22 ng/day oxytocin, most of which is reabsorbed by the epithelium of the caput epididymidis (626,1219).

Testosterone was shown to be present in some of the first samples of RTF collected from conscious rams (1241), and since then several analyses of fluids from a variety of species have been reported (Table 7). In general, most of the free steroids present in interstitial fluid or testicular venous blood are present in RTF, although usually in slightly lower concentrations if the concentrations outside the tubules are normal or elevated (217, 226,230,352,387,424,449,450,674,963,1066,1071, 1073). Conjugated steroids are present in much lower concentrations in RTF than in venous blood or lymph (1073). However, in hypophysectomized rats, especially if they were treated with pregnenolone, 17-hydroxypregnenolone, progesterone, or 17-hydroxyprogesterone, the concentrations of androgens in the RTF are higher than those in testicular venous blood (450,1196). The concentration of testosterone in RTF is lower than that in STF, whereas the concentration of dihydrotestosterone (DHT) is higher in RTF (217,1195). The concentration of testosterone is similar in fluid collected after ligation of the efferent ducts and in fluid collected without ligation, whereas estradiol concentrations are much higher in samples collected from unligated testes (367). The earlier observations on ionic composition and on spermatocrit (484,1181) were interpreted as evidence for two types of secretion, one in the tubules and one in the rete. However, later evidence on the similar numbers of spermatozoa and the similar concentrations of inositol in the two fluids, led to a revision of this two-fluid theory, and it was suggested that the composition of tubular fluid was altered when it reached the rete (1069). This conclusion has been supported by the observation that the concentration of ABP was similar in the two fluids (1195) but is difficult to reconcile with the differences in total protein and steroids, although it is possible that these compounds and others may be resorbed in the rete. There is some evidence that the rete and the tubules may have different permeabilities to sodium and potassium ions (1069), and it has been suggested that substances can exchange directly between the superficial testicular veins and the fluid in the rete (364). Whereas the STF is of interest primarily as a reflection of the complex cell interaction involved in spermatogenesis, RTF has the added interest of being a possible route of communication between the testis and epididymis, although many of the functions of the epididymis are unaffected by interrupting the flow of RTF by ligating the efferent ducts (see ref. 917). However, the cells in the first part of the epididymis do appear to alter after efferent duct ligation (1,3,275,291,338,416,802,838), and specific changes in intermediary metabolism (121) and in protein synthesis (129,587,588) are evident. Thus, further investigation on the significance of RTF in the control of epididymal function would appear to be warranted.

Epididymis

Blood Flow

Blood flow through the epididymis has been measured using indicator dilution with soluble markers or microspheres, with comparable results. Mean values for the whole organ of about 15 ml/100 g/min have been reported in rats (264,1059,1259), 24 ml/100 g/min in rabbits (138) and 11 ml/100 g/min in rams (1059). However, blood flow is not uniform throughout the tissue, and areas of higher flow, corresponding to areas of fluid resorption or secretory activity, can be demonstrated in rat, ram (1059), and rabbit (138). These peaks of flow are eliminated by unilateral orchidectomy or efferent duct ligation, with a slight overall reduction in average flow (138). Hypophysectomy led to a halving of average flow, which could be restored by treatment with hCG (254), although this hormone had no effect in intact animals (264). Raising the temperature of the scrotum and its contents had no effect on epididymal blood flow, unless the temperature rose above 40°C (1259). Injection of cadmium salts, which cause a catastrophic fall in TBF, had only minor effects in the epididymis (1255).

Luminal Fluid

The RTF, which passes to the epididymis by way of the ductuli efferentes, is the initial source of luminal fluid for the epididymis. A cilioperistaltic model for the flow of the fluid and spermatozoa through the efferent ducts has been proposed (1290). It is now well established that the epididymis has both a secretory and absorptive function, and thus, the composition of the RTF is extensively modified as it makes its progress through the epididymal duct. Originally, the extent of these modifications was assessed by cannulating the rete testis and distal cauda epididymidis or vas deferens and comparing the composition of the fluids thus obtained. Greater insight into which regions of the epididymis are responsible for making specific changes to the composition of the intraluminal fluid has been gained by the use of the micropuncture technique. The most extensive studies of this type have been carried out in the laboratory rat and are presented in Fig. 59. The absorptive capacity of the epididymal epithelium, which results in the bulk removal of fluid, is reflected by the increase in spermatocrit (Fig. 59) and slowing of the movement along the duct (1199). The proximal caput and the efferent ducts are the principal regions involved in fluid resorption (592), but because of the technical difficulties of cannulating this region of the epididymal duct, the cauda epididymidis has been used more extensively to study the mechanism of fluid resorption. Here, it has been shown that resorption is an energy-dependent process that can be modified by hormones and sympathetic agents (36,1299–1302). It has been suggested that sodium ions are passively transported from the luminal fluid at the luminal surface of the epithelial cells and actively transported at the serosal surface to establish a standing osmotic gradient that draws water and chloride ions from the luminal fluid. Transcytosis may also be important, particularly in reabsorbing proteins (236,1328). In contrast, potassium and phosphate ions are retained or secreted into the luminal fluid with the result that their concentration increases as the fluid travels down the epididymal duct (see ref. 591) (Fig. 59). Osmotic pressure of the luminal fluid is consistently slightly higher than that of plasma in rats (692), appreciably higher in hamsters (574), and two to four times higher than blood plasma in hibernating bats (244).

However, the bulk of the replacement of sodium chloride is with various low-molecular-weight organic molecules, which, together with the remaining ions, sustain a constant fluid osmolarity. The principal organic molecules involved in this replacement are glycerophosphocholine, phosphocholine, carnitine, and inositol (Fig. 59). The other feature brought out in Fig. 59 is the marked acidification of the epididymal fluid (152–154,161,972) that occurs in the proximal portion of the epididymis. This is achieved by the removal of bicarbonate and is possibly aided by the addition or retention of substantial quantities of glutamic acid (128,496). It is now recognized that the low pH of epididymal fluid and the presence of permeant organic acids are important contributing factors to the maintenance of sperm in a

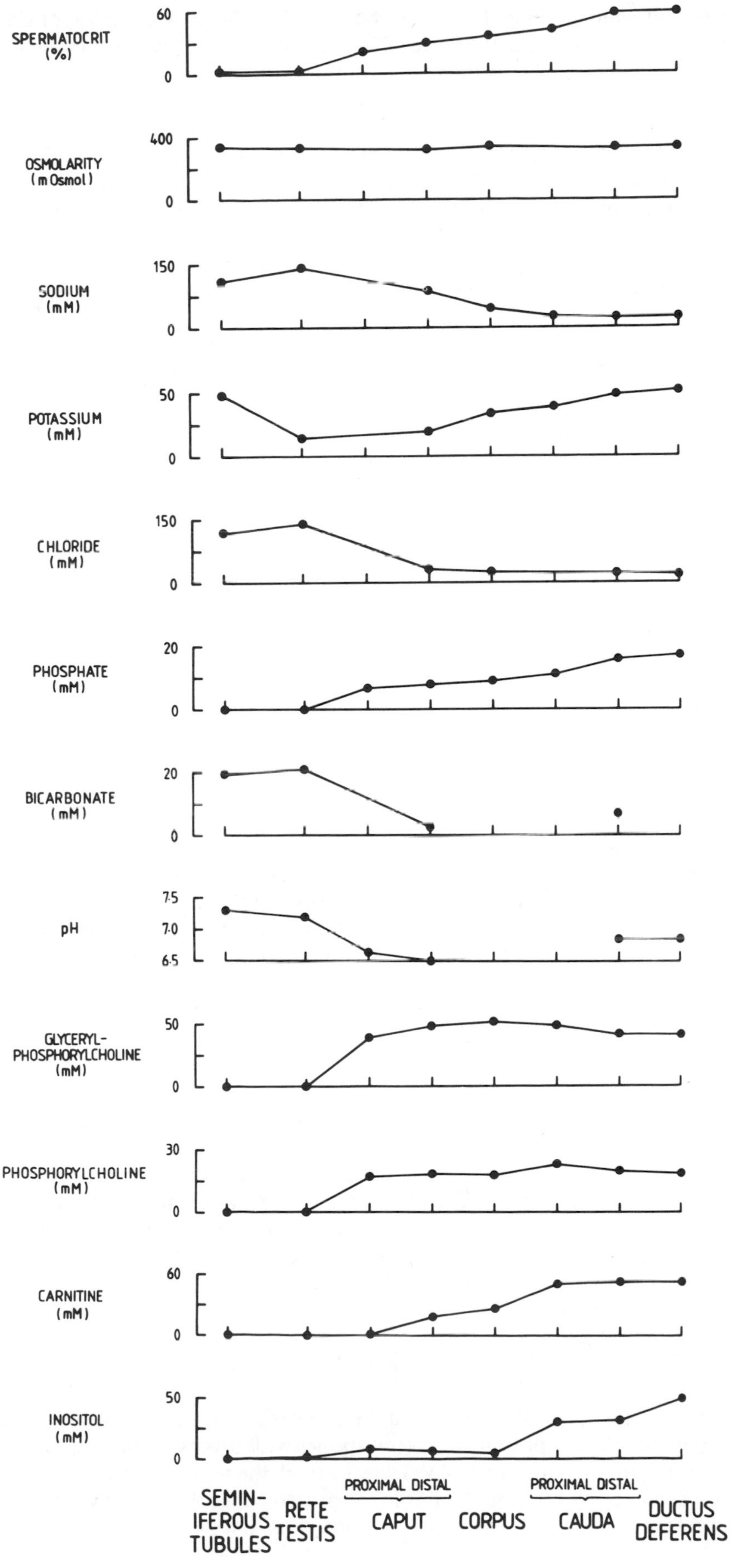

FIG. 59. Characteristics of the fluid sampled at various points within the testis and excurrent duct system of the rat. (From ref. 126.)

quiescent condition within the epididymal environment (5,160). There is a general lack of reducing sugar in epididymal fluid. However, a facilitated transport system for glucose does exist in epididymal cells (119), and glucose can be shown to appear in the epididymal lumen when the normal luminal contents are removed (222,229). Transport of the nonmetabolizable glucose analog 3-*O*-methylglucose from the bloodstream to the epididymal lumen *in vivo* has also been demonstrated (1193). It has been suggested that metabolic disposal of glucose by sperm within the epididymal lumen normally accounts for the failure of reducing sugar to accumulate in the epididymal fluid (118). Lactate concentrations *in vivo* (161,213,1244) were comparable with those found in blood plasma, although the levels rose almost tenfold in samples collected postmortem. The high concentration of inositol in cauda epididymal fluid is a specific feature of the rat, hamster, and monkey (505) (Table 6); in other species, such as bull and rabbit, inositol concentrations are greater in proximal than in distal regions of the duct (1240). The testis actively synthesizes inositol from glucose (314,315) and the secreted inositol passes into the epididymis with the RTF (505,1063,1181, 1240). It has been calculated that additional inositol must be added to the epididymal fluid (1045). This could occur by synthetic activity of the epididymal tissue (464, 965) and by transport from the bloodstream (222,235, 500,696–698,1138). High concentrations of glycerophosphocholine are encountered in the epididymal plasma of all species studied except man (Table 6). Epididymal tissue itself is responsible for the synthesis of this compound (1016,1263). Current evidence favors epididymal lecithin as the immediate precursor (281,1015, 1016), which may, in turn, be derived from lecithin associated with blood lipoproteins (440). Another major constituent of epididymal fluid, except in the bull, is carnitine (Table 6). This compound is transported into the epididymal lumen against a concentration gradient of more than 2,000:1 (122,132,497,504,1327) by a saturable uptake process (126,232,233,498,555). The epididymis itself appears unable to synthesize carnitine (166). Epididymal fluid contains a broad range of amino acids (139,496,579,584,1062,1080) with particularly high levels of glutamic acid (10–30 mM) in the ram, bull, and boar; asparagine plus glutamine (21 mM) in the ram; and taurine plus hypotaurine (50 mM) in the boar and rabbit. In rats, there is about 50 mM glutamate in the caput fluid, about 20 mM in the corpus, but only less than 1 mM in the caudal fluid (496). The high concentration of glutamate in the caput is reduced by about 70% after efferent duct ligation (1101), suggesting that most of it or a precursor originates in the testis. The presence in the caput of high concentrations of the enzyme-γ-glutamyl transpeptidase, which forms glutamic acid from glutathione, may be relevant (9,10,507). There is also evidence for selective absorption of neutral amino acids from luminal fluid into blood (498). The concentration of urea is in the range of 7 to 19 mM (579,584), which is comparable with the concentration in blood serum (1–10 mM) (24). High concentrations of sialic acid are present in epididymal luminal fluid in rats and hamsters, with little difference between caput, corpus, and cauda (1227).

Epididymal fluid contains substantial quantities of steroid hormones and their metabolites (Table 7). The RTF entering the epididymis is undoubtably a main source of these steroids, at least for fluid from proximal regions of the epididymal duct (Table 7). Testosterone is the predominant androgen in RTF but is converted to the reduced form of dihydrotestosterone on entering the epididymal duct, due presumably to the activity of 5α-reductase in the epididymal epithelium. The bloodstream is the other main route for the supply of androgens to the epididymis; uptake of systemic androgens into the epididymal lumen has been amply demonstrated (51,221,228,1194).

It is not our intention to discuss in any depth the protein components of epididymal fluid; for this the reader is referred to Chapter 23 by Robaire and Hermo in the first edition of this volume and the reviews by Brooks (128), Jones (585), and Cooper (223,224). There has been a particular interest in recent years in analyzing various androgen-dependent secretory proteins (123) that are synthesized and secreted by the epididymal epithelium and that are implicated in effecting the functional maturation of sperm during their passage through the epididymis. This functional maturation is thought to be brought about by an incorporation of the proteins into the sperm plasma membrane or through enzymatic activity of the proteins producing changes to existing membrane components. The most intensively studied species has been the rat, in which several of these epididymal proteins have been purified (124,125,127,342,388, 587,677), and for two of the proteins, the complete amino acid sequence has been derived by cloning their cDNA (134,135). The use of antibody and cDNA probes has in general established that the secretory proteins are tissue-specific and species-specific (134,135,629). The precise physiologic role of any particular protein, however, remains to be established. Other proteins, such as ABP (1221), transferrin (298), and clusterin (761,762), are reduced in concentration as the fluid passes along the epididymis (see also refs. 253,589,872), probably by endocytosis (392,393,1220).

Blood Flow through the Accessory Glands

Blood flow has been measured in seminal vesicles and prostate of several species with several techniques. In intact rats, blood flow through the seminal vesicles is about 17 ml/100 g/min, measured with soluble indicators, and decreases slightly during the first 24 h after an injection of cadmium salts at a dose sufficient to cause virtual stoppage of TBF (1255). Flow in the seminal vesicles of hypophysectomized rats measured with microspheres is about the same as the above figure and is increased if the animals are treated with hCG; the increase is virtually abolished if they are also given estrogens (254). Blood flow through the seminal vesicles of rabbits is somewhat higher than in rats (about 30 ml/100 g/min) (138).

Blood flow through the rat ventral prostate is about 50 ml/100 g/min, whether measured with a soluble indicator (112,1255) or microspheres (1023), somewhat higher than through the seminal vesicles. Intermediate flows (26 ml/100 g/min) have been reported for the dorsolateral prostate (255,1255). Flow through the ventral prostate increases after treatment with hCG and decreases after estrogen treatment, even in castrated animals; castration itself causes a slight nonsignificant reduction (1023). In another study, testosterone supplementation decreased vascular resistance in both ventral and dorsolateral prostate, and treatment also with estrogens caused an increase (255). Hypophysectomy reduces flow to levels that are impossible to measure accurately with microspheres, but hCG still produces a rise, partially blockable with estrogens (254).

Blood flow through the dog prostate has been measured by radioactive Xenon clearance (33), and in humans, blood flow has been determined in prostates with adenocarcinoma, using the hydrogen gas clearance technique. Flow before treatment was about 30 ml/100 g/min and surprisingly increased after treatment with estrogens, despite a decrease in testis size (1172).

Fluids of the Accessory Glands

The male accessory glands contain a rather bewildering array of chemical constituents, and we still remain rather ignorant of the specific physiologic function of many of the components. Accessory glands were originally classified on the basis of their gross morphology and anatomic relationship to other parts of the male reproductive tract. Unfortunately, this classification does not always coincide with functional relationships from the point of view of the nature of the chemical constituents present in the secretion (746). For instance, fructose, which is the principal glycolyzable substrate for sperm in seminal plasma, may, depending on species, have its origin in either the seminal vesicles, coagulating glands, or ampullary glands. Moreover, particular chemical constituents are present almost universally in mammalian semen but are notably absent from the semen of certain species without any obvious physiologic explanation. This is the case with fructose, for example, which is completely lacking in the semen of the dog, stallion, and jackass. For these reasons, a global description of the composition of the chemical constituents of the secretions of the male accessory glands is difficult. However, a comprehensive catalog of the concentration of identified constituents in the accessory gland secretions of various animals is presented in Tables 5 and 6, and a description of the more salient features is attempted. For more detailed and comprehensive historical accounts, and in particular for a review of the protein components of these fluids, the reader is referred to Mann (744), Mann and Lutwak-Mann (747), and Brooks (128).

Ampulla

There have been only scattered reports on the composition of the secretion of the ampulla perhaps because of the problem of obtaining pure ampullary secretion without contamination from fluid arriving at the ampulla from the ductus deferens. In the goat, there is little difference in fluid composition between the epididymis and ampulla (Table 5), but in the bull, the concentration of sodium, calcium, and magnesium ions are two to ten times greater in fluid from the ampulla than from the epididymis (243,943). Fluid from the bovine ampulla contains a high concentration of citric acid (539), whereas the stallion and jackass are noted for the substantial quantities of ergothionine present in this secretion (690,753).

Seminal Vesicles

The secretions of the seminal vesicles are usually collected postmortem, but a technique for their continuous collection from rats *in vivo* has been described (1166). Sodium and potassium are the predominant cations in seminal vesicle secretion (Table 5). Unusually high concentrations of calcium and magnesium are found in the vesicular secretion of bull and boar, respectively (243,309,943). Chloride and phosphate concentrations are relatively low (Table 5), indicating that some other moiety must be the main anion. The usual alkaline pH of vesicular secretion may indicate that bicarbonate is an important anion, and undoubtably citrate also fulfills a role as a major anion (Table 6). The seminal vesicle is the principal accessory gland responsible for synthesis of fructose from blood glucose in most species. Glucose itself is also present in the vesicular secretion of some species, attaining a concentration equivalent to that of blood plasma in the guinea pig (355,934). Fructose is lacking in stallion and jackass semen, which implies that these sugars are not secreted by the seminal vesicles (or any other gland) in these species. The synthesis of fructose, like many other secretory products of the male accessory glands, is strictly regulated by androgenic hormones, and the concentration of seminal fructose can serve as a simple test of the androgenic status of an animal. Inositol, a cyclic polyol, is present in the vesicular secretion of several species (Table 6), attaining extraordinarily high concentrations in the case of the boar (309,743). High concentrations are also found in extracts of rat seminal vesicles (315,777). Most of the inositol is present as myoinositol, but approximately 6% of the total occurs as scylloinositol (1018). Other compounds that are present in high concentrations in a few species include glycerophosphocholine (rat, guinea pig, and boar [287,288,1288]), ergothioneine (boar, stallion, and hedgehog [690,742,743,752]), and hypotaurine and taurine (guinea pig [628]). The PG content of seminal plasma, which is particularly high in the case of man and the ram, is probably derived principally from the seminal vesicle secretion (319,397).

The secretions of rat seminal vesicles contain a number of specific proteins (SVS I to VIII, also known as RVS or SV), some of which, particularly SVS II, serve as a substrate for enzymes secreted by the coagulating glands to form the copulatory plug (1020,1247). A protein resembling SVS II appears to be present also on the head and principal piece of epididymal sperm (1021). Another of these proteins (SVS IV), the gene which is largely unmethylated in the seminal vesicles, prostate, and coagulating gland, in contrast to other tissues (603), has strong immunosuppressive and anti-inflammatory properties (783), possibly in association with SVS V (741); it also inhibits phagocytosis and chemotaxis of human polymorph neutrophils (784). SVS IV is present on ejaculated but not on epididymal spermatozoa (740). Mouse seminal vesicle secretion also contains a nondialysable substance that inhibits the blastogenic response of splenocytes to concanavalin A or phytohemagglutanin (324). Seminal vesicle fluid alters sperm motility in mice (903).

Boar seminal vesicle fluid contains a specific proteinase inhibitor (1231). The principal basic proteins in bull seminal vesicle secretion are a proteinase inhibitor, a ribonuclease, an antimicrobial protein, and a fourth protein (PG) of unknown function (1100). A neutral protein, molecular mass about 15 kD, makes up about 40% of the secretion of bull seminal vesicles; its secretion is androgen-dependent, it binds to the sperm neck and midpiece (46,618), and its DNA sequence is known (617). Several enzymes are also found in bull seminal vesicle secretion (9,1218).

Coagulating Glands

In the rat, the coagulating glands, rather than the seminal vesicles, are responsible for fructose secretion (355,538,539,720), and the secretion of the coagulating gland also contains high concentrations of basic fibroblast growth factor (FGF) (1113). In the mouse, this activity is shared by the coagulating glands and the seminal vesicles, whereas the coagulating gland secretion is devoid of fructose in the guinea pig and coypu (749,879). Glucose and citric acid are found in the secretions of the rat and coypu, respectively (355,539,694,720). The mechanism of secretion of proteins and glucoproteins appears to be merocrine (992,993).

Prostate

The composition of prostatic secretion has largely been gleaned from the dog, because in this species, neither seminal vesicles nor bulbourethral glands are present. A surgical procedure has been developed to divert the urinary outflow, which allows pure prostatic secretion to be collected directly from the urethra (535,536). Moreover, the rate of production of secretion can be enhanced from 0.1 to 2 ml/h to 60 ml/h by administration of pilocarpine hydrochloride (534,535) or hypogastric nerve stimulation (1115). Secretion appears to involve a Na^+/K^+-coupled active Cl transporting system (1116). However, there are significant differences in the composition of canine prostatic secretion when "resting fluid" is compared with "active secretion" produced under the influence of pilocarpine or hypogastric nerve stimulation or during ejaculation (1114). A technique involving perfusion of the prostatic urethra has been developed to collect prostatic secretion in rats; the collected material contained EGF, the secretion of which was stimulated by α-adrenergic and cholinergic agonists (554).

The predominant ionic constituents of canine prostatic active secretion are sodium and chloride (Table 5). In contrast, human prostatic secretion contains considerably more calcium and potassium, and the principal anion is citrate rather than chloride. Prostatic secretion is usually slightly acid, with a pH of about 6.5 (534). Citric acid also occurs in the prostate of human, rat, mole, and hedgehog (538,539,743,747), whereas inositol is an important component of the rat prostate (777) and possibly the human prostate (695). The prostate in man and rat is also a rich source of polyamines, particularly spermine and spermidine (451,452,900,979). The concentration of spermine and spermidine in rat prostatic secretion has been measured as 6 mM and 7 mM, respectively (694), whereas in blood serum these compounds are essentially undetectable. Human prostatic secretion contains high concentrations of acid phosphatase, which is often used as a marker for prostatic contribution to semen (747). Two other specific proteins in human prostatic fluid have attracted attention recently, prostatic specific antigen and prostatic binding protein (679). There is also a glucoprotein that is identical to serum Zn-α_2-glycoprotein (373) and a β-microseminoprotein or β-inhibin (705). The latter appears in normal serum from both sexes at about the same concentration but is often greatly elevated in men with prostatic cancer (4). A 22-kDa secretory protein has also been demonstrated in rat ventral prostate (159).

Bulbourethral Glands

The ionic composition of the secretion of the bulbourethral glands has been reported only for the boar (Table 5). The secretion generally lacks any of the unusual low-molecular-weight organic compounds encountered in the other accessory glands (Table 6). The principal component of the secretion is a sialomucin, which is responsible for the gelation reaction in boar semen (110,111). The composition of the mucin has been analyzed (111,463) and found to contain on a dry weight basis 27% sialic acid, 13% galactose (probably as *N*-acetylgalactosamine), and 4% neutral sugars. The extraordinarily high content of sialic acid accounts for the very low isoelectric point ($pI = 1.1$) of the mucin. The approximate molecular weight of the mucin has been estimated as 6.5×10^6 D.

Preputial Glands

Preputial glands differ from other accessory glands in that they do not produce a copious watery secretion. Rather, these glands are modified sebaceous glands, and as such they produce a fatty secretion that seems to be primarily associated with pheromonal functions (e.g., refs. 115,189,877). The precise structure of these pheromones has not been determined, but in the rat they are possibly volatile seven- and eight-carbon alcohols (390). Nine main water-soluble proteins have been identified in rat preputial glands (666).

Seminal Plasma

Seminal plasma is the fluid portion of the ejaculate and results from the admixture of secretions from the various male accessory glands during seminal emission. Several points should be borne in mind when analyzing the composition of seminal plasma. For instance, there is a temporal sequence among the glands with respect to voidance of their respective secretions; complete mixing of the secretions may not take place for semen deposited normally within the female reproductive tract. In the case of semen collected artificially by electroejaculation, the contribution of any particular accessory gland is critically dependent on the positioning of the stimulating electrodes. There is also considerable variation in seminal plasma composition between individual males as well as for the same individual between successive ejaculates, which may reflect seasonal differences and the time intervening since the previous ejaculation. Apart from this form of variability, there are also changes brought about in seminal plasma composition after ejaculation through the agency of enzymes in the seminal plasma and metabolic activity of the sperm suspended in the seminal plasma. Particular examples of enzymatic activity in seminal plasma include proteolytic activity, which results in liberation of peptides and amino acids, and in human seminal plasma, the hydrolysis of phosphocholine to release free phosphate, which interacts with spermine to form insoluble crystals of spermine phosphate. The most obvious change induced by spermatozoa is the metabolic conversion of fructose to lactic acid.

A detailed account of the composition of seminal plasma can be found in the monographs by Mann (744) and Mann and Lutwak-Mann (747). A summary of the most salient features is presented in Table 8. Our coverage is restricted to inorganic ions and low-molecular-weight organic molecules, as a detailed examination of the proteins in seminal plasma had recently appeared (1103). Sodium is the principal cation in seminal plasma, but its concentration is considerably below that encountered in blood plasma and interstitial fluid. The deficit is, to some extent, accounted for by potassium. Calcium and magnesium concentrations in seminal plasma are generally similar to those of blood plasma, although there are exceptions, such as the high concentration of calcium in the case of bull, stallion, and man and of magnesium in rabbit and boar (Table 8). However, the proportion of these ions that are free in solution as against that proportion that is complexed with low-molecular-weight organic molecules (e.g., citrate) and proteins has not generally been ascertained. Chloride is the principal anion, and bicarbonate concentrations are relatively low, although postejaculatory changes in bicarbonate concentration have generally not been taken into account.

Fructose rather than glucose is the principal reducing sugar in seminal plasma, although small amounts of glucose are also encountered. It thus serves as the main glycolyzable substrate for spermatozoa in semen. Fructose concentrations are particularly high in bull and ram seminal plasma but are considerably lower in other species, whereas fructose is essentially absent from dog and stallion semen (Table 8). In certain Australian marsupials, the chief seminal carbohydrate is not fructose but *N*-acetylglucosamine (968,969). The concentration of *N*-acetylglucosamine in kangaroo seminal plasma is in the range of 15 to 23 mM; glucose is also present at a concentration of 1.6 to 6.2 mM (969). The origin of the *N*-acetylglucosamine in marsupial semen is the prostate (970). *N*-acetylglucosamine may not, however, be the characteristic sugar of the semen of all marsupials (133). Sorbitol also occurs in seminal plasma. The sperm of some species such as rams, but not boars, possess a sorbi-

TABLE 8. *Concentration of various substances in the seminal plasma of several species*[a]

Seminal plasma	Rabbit	Dog	Ram	Goat	Boar	Bull	Stallion	Man
Volume (ml)	0.4–6	2–15	0.7–2	0.2–2.5	150–500	2–10	30–300	2–6
Sperm concentration ($\times 10^{-6}$/ml)	50–350	60–300	2,000–5,000	1,000–5,000	25–300	300–2,000	30–800	50–150
Sodium	61–82	72–180	77		125–252	65–161	112	43–112
Potassium	20–29	8	23		17–46	13–97	26	14–28
Calcium	1.5–2	0.2–1.2	1.6–2.3		1.5–4.6	6–15	6.5	5–7
Magnesium	11	0.15–1.5	2.4		2.5–24	3.3	3.7	1.2–5
Chloride	99	152	51		85–105	42–110	23–113	28–56
Phosphate		0.3	2.5		0.4	2.8	0.6	
Bicarbonate		2.9	7			7	11	8
Fructose	2.2–18	<0.03	8–37		0.5	17–56	<0.06	2–33
Glucose	1.6				0.06–0.3		0.7	0.4
Sorbitol	4.4	<0.05	1.4–6.6		0.4	0.6–7.5	1.1–3.3	0.6
Inositol			0.6–0.8		28	1.3–2.6	1.1–2.6	3–3.5
Lactic acid		1.2–3.3	3.9		2.2	2.2–5.6	1–2.8	2.2–5.6
Pyruvic acid			1.1			0.6	0.3	3.4
Citric acid	5.2–26		16–42		2.6–10.4	18–52	0.5–2.6	5.2–73
Glutamic acid			4.5–5.2		2	1–8		6.5
Ascorbic acid			0.3			0.3	0.3	0.6
Carnitine			4.5					0.2–1.3
Acetylcarnitine			2.8					0.06–0.28
Glycerophosphocholine	7.6–14	6.6	58–73	51–58	4	4–18	1.4–4	2.0–3.3
Phosphocholine	0		0	0	0	0	0	14–21
Glycerophosphoinositol			1.5		0.26	1.4	0.25	
Spermine						0.1		3
Spermidine								0.1
Putrescine								0.2
Creatine	0.15	0	0.15–1.2			0.9	0.4	1.5
Arginine	0	0.11	0.53–1.2		0.01	0.2		5.2
Creatine					0.03	1.1	0.3	
Ergothionine			trace	absent	0.7	trace	0.2–0.7	trace
Uric acid			0.24–1.4					0.1–0.4
Protein (mg/ml)	22	24			30	55		35–50

[a] Concentration is given in mM unless stated otherwise.
From refs. 61, 63, 116, 122, 139, 310, 320, 347, 525, 579, 745, 746, 748, 749, 873, 943, 1062 and 1279.

tol dehydrogenase that enables sorbitol to be converted to fructose and used as a metabolic substrate (130,624). Inositol is another polyol that is present in seminal plasma, particularly in the boar, in which it is derived from the seminal vesicle secretion. However, unlike sorbitol, inositol cannot be used as a metabolic substrate for spermatozoa. Both lactic and pyruvic acids, which are the end products of glycolysis, are found in seminal plasma. These acids presumably accumulate in accessory gland secretions because of glycolytic activity within the glandular tissue. Additional lactic acid accumulates in seminal plasma because of the fructolytic activity of the spermatozoa after ejaculation. Spermatozoa are also capable of carrying out a dismutation reaction with pyruvate under aerobic and anaerobic conditions. The products of this reaction under anaerobic conditions include lactate, acetate, succinate, acetoacetate, and CO_2 (131). The other organic acids that occur in seminal plasma cannot, in general, serve as metabolic substrates for spermatozoa. Citric acid is the principal organic acid and is usually derived from the seminal vesicle secretion, except in man, in whom it is produced in the prostate (Table 6); its function still remains obscure. There is a broad range of amino acids in seminal plasma, and their concentration increases after ejaculation because of the extensive proteolytic activity that takes place in semen. Glutamic acid is particularly notable for its relatively high concentration in RTF, epididymal plasma, and seminal plasma. The carnitine and acetylcarnitine found in seminal plasma is derived entirely from the epididymal secretion (120), except possibly in man, in whom other accessory glands may contribute up to half of the carnitine in seminal plasma (333,374). The acetylcarnitine in seminal plasma, unlike that within the sperm, cannot be used as a metabolic substrate (120) owing to its inability to permeate the sperm plasma membrane (104,105, 156). There is some suggestion that exogenous acetylcarnitine can influence sperm motility through a pharmacologic effect (506,570,1157). Glycerophosphocholine is a common constituent of seminal plasma, attaining substantial concentrations, particularly in ram seminal plasma (Table 8). Like carnitine, glycerophosphocholine is derived principally from the epididymal fluid, but other accessory glands, especially the seminal vesicles, also make a contribution in some species (e.g., rat, man). A related compound, glycerophosphoinositol, has been found at somewhat lower concentrations in the seminal plasma of domestic livestock (116). Whereas choline exists in bound form in seminal plasma principally as glycerophosphocholine, in human seminal plasma the predominant form is phosphocholine (288). In contrast to glycerophosphocholine, which is relatively stable in seminal plasma, phosphocholine is rapidly degraded after ejaculation to free choline and inorganic phosphate, owing to its exposure to phosphatase enzymes. The liberated phosphate can complex with spermine to form insoluble crystals of spermine phosphate (Boettcher's crystals). The concentration of spermine is normally approximately 1 to 3 mM in human seminal plasma, whereas the concentration of the other polyamines (spermidine, putrescine) are at least ten times lower (334, 556). Seminal plasma polyamines in men and rats are derived from the prostatic secretion (452,694). Polyamines are involved in the clotting reaction of rat and guinea pig seminal plasma (1289). A variety of other functions has been ascribed to the polyamines with regard to their influence on spermatozoa (see ref. 128). Whereas spermine can considerably enhance the glycolytic rate of epididymal rat sperm (940), oxidized spermine is extremely toxic to spermatozoa (939,941,1149). Oxidation of the polyamines is brought about by a polyamine oxidase that is particularly active in human seminal plasma (556). A variety of reducing substances such as ascorbic acid, ergothioneine, hypotaurine, and uric acid is found in seminal plasma. Ascorbic acid is present in ram, bull, stallion, and human seminal plasma (Table 8). Ergothioneine occurs predominantly in the seminal plasma of boar, stallion, jackass, and zebra (744,751). Hypotaurine has been identified in boar, bull, and dog seminal plasma (579,1209) but undoubtedly occurs in the seminal plasma of other species, as it has been found in epididymal plasma (e.g., ram and rabbit) (584) and in seminal vesicles and prostate (guinea pig) (628). Uric acid exists in ram, bull, boar, and human seminal plasma (744); in the bull, it is derived from the seminal vesicle secretion (689). The seminal plasma of some primates contains the highest concentration of PGs of any biologic fluid, principally 19-hydroxylated derivatives of the E series: 19-OH PGE_1 + 19-OH PGE_2 amounts to 53 to 1,094 μg/ml in man (1065) and 474, 504, and 930 μg/ml in the semen of chimpanzee, rhesus monkey, and stump-tailed monkey, respectively (616). However, these high levels of 19-OH PGEs are not found in gorilla or orangutan semen or in the semen of various nonprimates (stallion, bull, ram, boar, rabbit) (616). Quantitatively, the next most important PGs in man are PGE_1 + PGE_2, 19-OH PGFs, and $PGF_{1\alpha}$ + $PGF_{2\alpha}$. The concentration of PGs in ram seminal plasma is somewhat less than for the primates (150), whereas the concentration in other species is very much lower (<1 μg/ml) (933). It seems unlikely that PGs have any direct effect on spermatozoa (170), and suggestions that they aid in sperm transport within the female reproductive tract by stimulating smooth-muscle activity likewise have no firm foundation (747).

THE BLOOD–TESTIS AND BLOOD–EPIDIDYMAL BARRIERS

The remarkable differences in composition between STF and RTF on the one hand and blood plasma and testicular lymph and interstitial fluid on the other imply that substances do not diffuse readily into or out of the semiferous tubules and rete; otherwise, these concentration differences would be dissipated. This suggestion has been abundantly substantiated by measurements of the rates at which a range of marker substances infused into the circulation appears in the fluids. Studies of this nature have been done for RTF in rams (787,1024,1029, 1058,1065), boars (1030), and rats (227,307,736,868, 1048,1049,1069,1070,1258) and for STF in rats using micropuncture (529) and the difference technique (1048,1049,1068–1070). Various markers enter the fluids at widely differing rates, ranging from almost instantaneous entry to virtual exclusion. The main factor that determines the entry rate is lipid solubility; molecular size is much less important (Fig. 60). Lipid-soluble substances probably pass through the cells, whereas water-soluble compounds would enter through the spaces between them (see refs. 1028,1033,1037,1057, 1251). Two substances enter STF and RTF more rapidly than one would predict from their lipid solubility, glucose (or rather its nonmetabolized analog 3-*O*-methylglucose), and testosterone. Glucose enters many cells by facilitated diffusion, and therefore it is perhaps not surprising that it should enter the luminal fluids of the testis in a similar way (786). However, it is usually assumed that steroids enter cells readily, and it was rather surprising to find that testosterone entered the luminal fluids more rapidly than dihydrotestosterone, which is marginally more lipid-soluble (227,1048,1194); progesterone, which is much more lipid-soluble than either of the other two steroids, entered only slightly more quickly than testosterone (1194). Furthermore, the entry rate of radioactive testosterone into STF or RTF was depressed by injecting the animal with hCG to stimulate testosterone production or with nonradioactive testosterone, but not dihydrotestosterone (735,1070). In hamsters, when radioactive testosterone was infused intravenously (1194) or by microperifusion (1186), the radioactivity in the tubular fluid collected by micropuncture or centrifugation rose to about 15% of the level in interstitial fluid during the first hour and then remained there; when the concentration of testosterone in the interstitial fluid was raised, the concentration in the

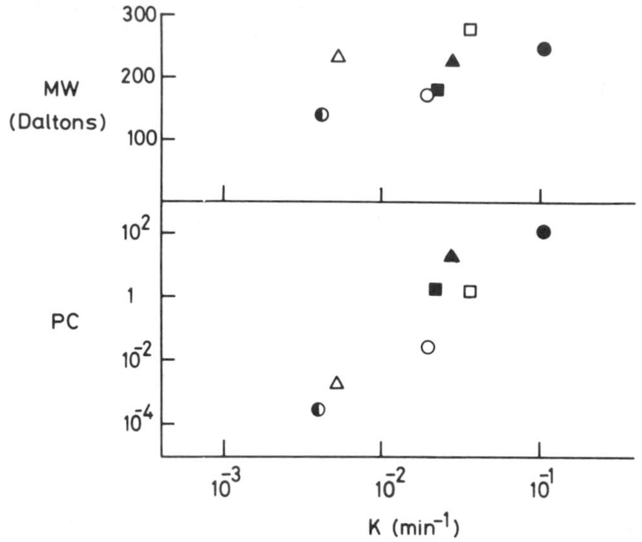

FIG. 60. The relationships between lipid solubility or molecular size and the rate of entry of some barbiturates and sulphonamides into rete testis fluid of rats. The entry rate has been calculated as a transfer constant ($K = -(l/t) \log e[Cp - (C_{rtf}/C_p)$ where C_p and C_{rtf} are the concentrations in plasma and rete testis fluid, respectively, at time t. The lipid solubility is given as a partition coefficient between chloroform and phosphate buffer and the molecular weight (MW) is given in Daltons. The compounds shown are thiopental (*solid circle*), pentobarbital (*solid triangle*), barbital (*solid square*), sulphanamide (*open circle*), sulphaguanidine (*open triangle*), sulphamethoxypyridazine (*open square*), and salicylic acid (*half-filled circle*). (From ref. 868 as plotted by Setchell [1033]).

tubular fluid rose but maintained the same ratio of about 15% of interstitial fluid (1190). The data presented are too scattered to sustain the authors' statement that there is "no evidence of a plateau," and a sustained discrepancy between the concentration in the STF and the interstitial fluid is not compatible with their conclusion that their results "confirm movement by diffusion," unless androgen is being bound **outside** the tubule (i.e., the reverse of what one would expect from the presence of ABP **inside** the tubule). In contrast to glucose, the entry of radioactive testosterone into rat tubules incubated *in vitro* cannot be depressed by the addition of the nonradioactive form (Setchell and Laurie, *unpublished observations*), so details of the transport mechanism have not yet been elucidated. The situation with urea is rather puzzling. In rams, this substance passes reasonably freely from blood to RTF, reaching equilibrium in about 2 h (1065). In hamsters, the level of ^{14}C-urea in STF never exceeds 25% of blood levels even during experiments lasting up to 4 h (529). In nephrectomized rats, however, radioactivity in STF reached values comparable with those in blood by 90 min but then continued to increase, reaching 150% of blood levels after 19 h; this apparent concentration of urea inside the tubules was inhibited by dinitrophenol and ouabain, suggesting that urea was being actively transported into the tubules (1191), but the identity of the radioactivity was not established.

Some studies have also been conducted in which the marker substances were infused into the lumen of one seminiferous tubule by micropuncture and the appearance of radioactivity measured in the circulating blood. Using this technique, it was confirmed that albumin did not cross the tubular wall, but the rate of appearance of inositol and testosterone in the blood was much reduced if the efferent ducts were ligated, suggesting that these markers were leaving the tubules rapidly and being resorbed in the efferent ducts or the epididymis. The exit rates for testosterone, with the ducts ligated or not, were reduced by the inclusion of nonradioactive compound in the infusate, supporting the idea of a saturable transport system (142,143).

The location of the barrier was established in a series of studies, first with dyes (632,634; see ref. 1057 for early references), then with labeled proteins (192,429,582, 738,739) and finally and most precisely with electron-opaque markers (300,304,340). There is some slight restriction of movement at the capillary wall and some at the peritubular myoid cells, but the most complete barrier to these molecules is at the junctions between pairs of adjacent Sertoli cells (Fig. 61). These junctions have a very elaborate structure (149,336,908, see refs. 503,927 for early references) and form only at puberty when the barrier is established (95,400,466,1232,1236). When new junctions form below the developing germ cells, it has been suggested that the zygotene spermatocytes are in an "intermediate compartment," with Sertoli cell junctions on both their basal and luminal sides (203,984). However, when lanthanum or peroxidase was injected into the seminiferous tubule lumen, markers appeared around these cells, casting doubt on the functional existence of an intermediate compartment (168). All the molecules that can be visualized either under the light or the electron microscope are fairly large hydrolophilic molecules that must enter the tubules by a paracellular route. Smaller, lipophilic molecules enter through the cells, and their entry is regulated by the cells themselves, not by the junctions between them.

As already stated, the junctions form at about the time of puberty, in the rat at about 18 days of age (400,1236), and it is at about this age that the barrier to dyes develops (632). However, the establishment of a functional barrier to smaller molecules is less sudden, and the barrier to chromium-EDTA is still not complete even at 25 days of age in rats (1071,1075). This gradual development of a barrier is consistent with the pattern of fluid secretion, which in rats rises suddenly at about 30 days but continues to increase until the animal is about 70 days of age (see section *Seminiferous Tubule Fluid: Flow and Composition*). A lumen first appears in the tubules at about 20 days but continues to enlarge beyond 40 days of age (985,1075,1169). Androgen binding protein concentra-

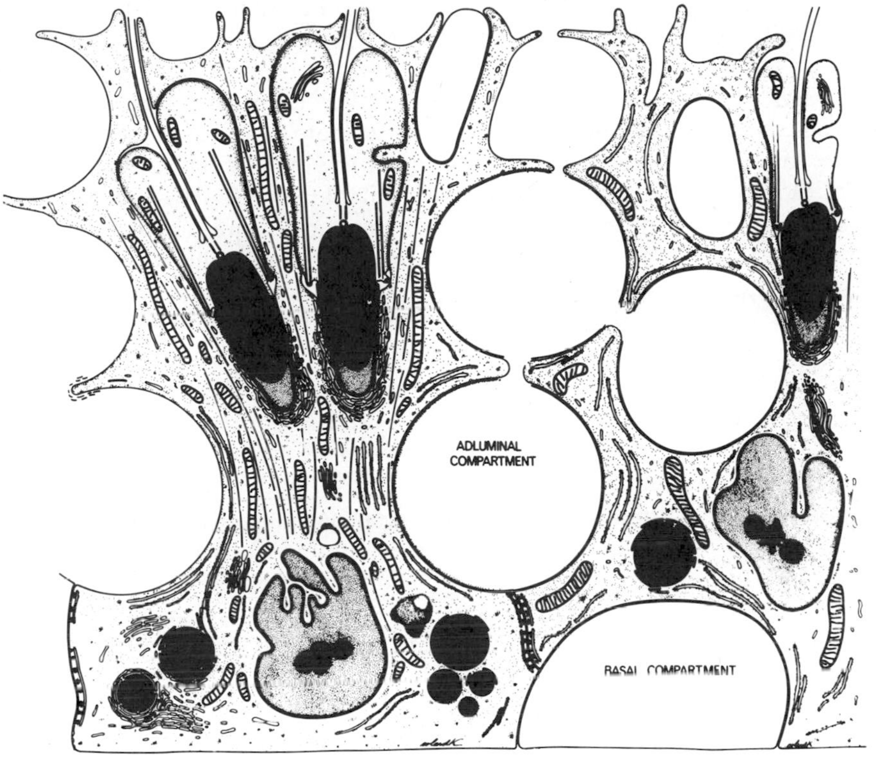

FIG. 61. A diagram of the junctional complexes between Sertoli cells and their role in forming the blood-testis barrier. A section of the wall of a seminiferous tubule is represented, with the lumen at the top and the peritubular tissue at the bottom. Late spermatids embedded in the luminal surfaces of the Sertoli cells are the only germ cells shown. The basal compartment between the Sertoli cells and the peritubular tissue is filled with spermatogonia and preleptotene primary spermatocytes, and the adluminal compartment between adjacent pairs of Sertoli cells is filled with later primary and secondary spermatocytes and round spermatids. The junctional complexes between the Sertoli cells prevent electron-opaque markers from penetrating any further into the tubule. (From ref. 336.)

tions in the testes of rats peaks at 20 days of age and then falls away to reach adult levels at about 40 days of age, whereas epididymal levels rise steadily until about 50 days of age (274,1169). Plasma ABP concentrations also peak at 20 days of age and then fall away again, but the concentrations at 40 days of age are still considerably higher than adult levels (274,426,427), suggesting that the barrier is still not fully functional even at that age. In seasonal breeding animals, such as mink (905–907), the barrier is not functional outside the breeding season and its establishment or re-establishment is better correlated with the formation of a lumen than the presence of any particular type of germ cell.

Once established, the blood–testis barrier apparently cannot be easily disrupted. Heat (736,1065) or irradiation (1265) is without effect, and the only treatments that do appear to cause a breakdown are treatment with cadmium salts (580,1055) and distention of the tubules after efferent duct ligation; in the latter case, evidence includes an increase in the space of distribution of Cr-EDTA to values greater than the volume of the interstitial tissue (1037,1159) and in increased levels of ABP in blood (426). Both treatments are certainly followed by degeneration of the seminiferous epithelium, but cadmium salts also produce virtual cessation of blood flow within 8 h. Interpretation of the effects of ligation of the efferent ducts is complicated by the very similar tubular lesions seen if the lumen of a single tubule is blocked with a plug of nontoxic latex (923); it is likely that efferent duct ligation and the consequent turgidity of the testis would also interfere with fluid movement along the tubules. Intratesticular injection of cytochalasin, which disrupts ectoplasmic specialization microfilaments, allows markers to penetrate past the Sertoli cell junctions, shrinkage of cells in the adluminal compartment when the tubules are exposed to hypertonic fixative, and an increase in the entry of radioactive inulin into the luminal fluid (1271). The barrier is deficient in the testes of mice with testicular feminization and sex reversal, but not in several other genetically defective mice (379). More ABP appears in the blood and less in the epididymis of rats homozygous for the grc complex (428), as in animals irradiated prenatally or treated with EDS (813), methoxyacetic acid (MAA) (1092), or medroxyprogesterone acetate (714), but it is not clear whether this is due to changes in directional secretion by the Sertoli cells, as the authors suggest (187), or effects on the barrier or fluid secretion.

The significance of the barrier is difficult to define, but it seems likely that it is involved in creating the right conditions for meiosis in the tubules. The barrier develops at about the time the first cells are entering the meiotic prophase and the exclusion of lanthanum is clearest in those parts of the seminiferous tubules of 15-day-old rats where the germ cells have reached pachytene (95,169), although it may be different in seasonal breeders (908). Meiosis fails in cultured fragments of seminiferous tubules (1126), in which the barrier is not maintained (I. B. Fritz, *personal communication*). However, it is difficult to say just what the right conditions are, as complete spermatogenesis has never been achieved *in vitro* with mammalian cells in contrast to the success achieved in amphibia (961). Some progress has recently been reported (896,1175), but there are still several steps that apparently cannot progress outside the animal. However, a blood–testis barrier has been described in a range of vertebrate and invertebrate animals (see refs. 96,908,1050), and a close association of somatic and germ cells is found in a wide range of animals (977).

Other consequences of the blood–testis barrier, although not its primary function, may nevertheless be of considerable significance (see refs. 1033,1057). The barrier ensures that the body does not recognize the haploid germ cells, or the spermatocytes from midpachytene onward as self (see ref. 1077). A male animal can therefore become immune to his own spermatozoa, and this does often happen in vasectomised men (14). This could be due to the spermatozoa found in spermatic cord lymph after vasectomy (57) or to spermatozoal proteins absorbed from the ligated portion of the ductus deferens, where many of the sperm break down. The barrier would normally also restrict the access of circulating antibodies to the cells on the luminal side, although in "sympathetic orchiopathia," in which the contralateral testis is affected after damage to one testis, IgM and IgG antibodies breach the barrier at different times after the initial damage (702). The environment created by the barrier may also be important in allowing pathogenic (165,1281) or leukemic cells (962) to persist in the testis, although the immune privilege offered by the testis is not confined to the tubular compartment (see refs. 725,1038).

The barrier also regulates the movement of peptide hormones such as inhibin and the gonadotrophins, maintaining a high concentration of the former in the luminal fluids and excluding the latter (1068), although the main site of action of FSH is the Sertoli cell; it was therefore of considerable interest that the receptors for FSH appear to be on the basal surfaces of these cells (878). Other peptides formed inside the tubules would be largely retained there, as indeed are smaller molecules such as inositol. The blood–testis barrier should also be considered in any toxicologic investigations involving the testis. The entry of a substance into the tubule is an essential first step for it to have a direct effect on the later germ cells (see ref. 1049). For example, it has recently been shown that although colchicine and vinblastine have similar effects in arresting mitosis in many tissues, colchicine is much more effective in the testis (703). It would be interesting to know whether both compounds enter the tubules.

From immunologic studies, it has been claimed that the barrier in the rete is less complete than in the tubules (581,1261), and the permeability of the rete to potassium but not sodium is higher than that of the tubules (1069). The even greater concentration difference between epididymal luminal fluid and blood plasma suggests that a permeability barrier exists there as well as in the seminiferous tubules, and again this suggestion has been confirmed in studies with suitable tracers. Two preparations have been used. With micropuncture techniques, it is possible to remove samples of luminal fluid during intravenous infusion of suitable markers in rats and hamsters; tritiated water enters the epididymal luminal fluid (ELF) readily, urea enters only slightly slower, and inulin, polyethylene glycol, and iodinated bovine serum albumin are virtually excluded (499,529 but see 234). The entry of 3-*O*-methylglucose into ELF from the caput is much faster than that of L-glucose and can be reduced by making the animal hyperglacaemic either with streptozotocin or urethane; saturable carriers can also be demonstrated for the nonmetabolized amino acid α-aminobutyric acid and inositol (500), although the difference in level of inositol between RTF and ELF from the caput could be explained by concentration of the fluid by absorption (1045) and the epididymis also contains the enzymes for synthesizing this compound from glucose (965). With both markers, fluid-to-plasma ratios greater than 1 are found in the caput (for inositol, values greater than 10 are found after 24 h), whereas much lower fluid-to-plasma ratios for inositol (0.3 after 3 h) are found in the cauda (500), although this is an area where the rise in inositol concentration cannot be explained by fluid resorption (1045). Radioactivity appears in ELF from the cauda when labeled testosterone, 5α-dihydrotestosterone, or progesterone was infused into the bloodstream, but the total radioactivity in ELF was only about 20% of that in plasma; furthermore, as less than half of the radioactivity in the blood was associated with DHT and progesterone, respectively, when these steroids were infused and only 4% of the radioactivity in the caudal ELF chromatographed with authentic testosterone (1194), these results are difficult to interpret. However, when ^{3}H-labeled testosterone was presented to the epididymal tubules by microperifusion in the interstitial fluid, radioactivity, which mostly comigrated with testosterone and DHT, was present in both caput and cauda luminal fluid at greater concentrations than in the interstitial fluid (1186,1318). This process was susceptible to competitive inhibition with nonradioactive steroid, was reduced by metabolic inhibitors (1190,1198), and was enhanced by the presence of ABP in the lumen (1189,1190).

An alternative technique to study the entry of substances into the epididymal lumen involves the perfusion of sections of the epididymal duct during infusion of marker into the blood or its incorporation in the perfusate (229). Unfortunately, this technique can be applied only to the cauda, which is probably less active in transport than the caput or corpus, but it has been shown that tritiated water in the perfusate reaches values almost equal to blood within 30 min, no radioactivity was detected when inulin or carboxydextran were infused into the bloodstream, and no cholesterol, protein, or sialic acid appeared in the perfusate, although appreciable amounts were present in the blood. Small amounts of radioactivity appeared in the perfusate when radioactive glucose or 3-*O*-methylglucose was infused into the blood (229). Radioactive inositol entered the perfusate, reaching 26% of blood levels after 3 h of perfusion without reaching a plateau, and this value was not affected by the inclusion of nonradioactive inositol in the perfusate; radioactive inositol perfused through the lumen was not absorbed by the tissue. Inositol could be detected in perfusate at concentrations about five times those in blood, suggesting either that there is a large intracellular pool of inositol accumulated from the blood or that local synthesis from glucose is an important source (222). Using this technique, it was also shown that the entry of testosterone into the cauda depended very much on the protein content of the perfusate; the inclusion of albumin (38 mg/ml) increased entry rate by about ten times, and the addition of protein from ovine RTF increased it even farther (221,229). Radioactive DL-carnitine also appears in perfusate, reaching a plateau after 2 to 4 h of about 0.5% of blood values per centimeters of duct perfused in the distal cauda, 1%/cm for proximal cauda, and 2%/cm for corpus. The addition of DL- or L-carnitine, phosphocholine, or inositol was without effect on these values, but the addition of glycerophosphocholine, choline, or betaine to the perfusion fluid increased carnitine entry, whereas the addition of albumin decreased it; glycine and γ-butyrobetaine were without effect. L-Carnitine entered the perfusate 14 times faster than D-carnitine (1327). However, it is only in the caput where it is necessary to invoke carnitine transport to explain the differences in concentration in the luminal fluid (1045), and therefore these studies using the cauda should be extended with experiments on the caput. Radioactive inositol enters a section of epididymal duct from the cauda or corpus in which the lumen was perfused *in vitro;* the rate of entry could be reduced by the inclusion of nonradioactive inositol in the bath fluid but was unaffected by increasing the luminal concentration to physiologic levels. The amount of radioactivity in the perfusate reached about 25% of bath values after 3 h of perfusion (231).

The site of the barrier in the epididymis to intravascularly perfused lanthanum nitrate was located at the zonula occludens at the apicolateral surface of the epididymal epithelial cells; the movement of the marker was not impeded by the vascular endothelium, the peritubular myoid layer, or other lateral cell surface specializations (517). The barrier to lanthanum develops in rats between the ages of 14 and 18 days (8). Similar tight junctions are found between the epithelial cells in the excurrent ducts of fowls (830).

REFERENCES

1. Abe K, Takano H. Cytological response of the principal cells in the initial segment of the epididymal duct to efferent duct cutting in mice. *Arch Histol Cytol* 1989;52:321–326.
2. Abe K, Takano H, Ito T. Ultrastructure of the mouse epididymal duct with special reference to the regional differences of the principal cells. *Arch Histol Jpn* 1983;46:51–68.
3. Abe K, Takano H, Ito T. Microvasculature of the mouse epididymis, with special reference to fenestrated capillaries localized in the initial segment. *Anat Rec* 1984;209:209–218.
4. Abrahamsson PA, Andersson C, Bjork T, et al. Radioimmunoassay of β-microseminoprotein, a prostatic-secreted protein present in era of both men and women. *Clin Chem* 1989;35:1497–1503.
5. Acott TS, Carr DW. Inhibition of bovine spermatozoa by caudal epididymal fluid: 11. Interaction of pH and a quiescence factor. *Biol Reprod* 1984;30:926–935.
6. Adams ML, Little PJ, Bell B, Cicero TJ. Alcohol affects rat testicular interstitial fluid volume and testicular secretion of testosterone and β-endorphin. *J Pharmacol Exp Ther* 1991;258: 1008–1014.
7. Adrian TE, Gu J, Allen IM, Tatemoto K, Polak JM, Bloom SR. Neuropeptide Y in the human male genital tract. *Life Sci.* 1984;35:2643–2648.
8. Agarwal A, Hoffer AP. Ultrastructural studies on the development of the blood–epididymis barrier in immature rats. *J Androl* 1989;10:425–431.
9. Agrawal Y, Vanha-Perttula T. Effect of secretory particles in bovine seminal vesicle secretion on sperm motility and acrosome reaction. *J Reprod Fertil* 1987;79:409–419.
10. Agrawal YP, Peura T, Vanha-Perttula T. Distribution of gamma-glutamyl transpeptidase in the mouse epididymis and its response to acivicin. *J Reprod Fertil* 1989;86:185–193.
11. Aitken RNC. A histochemical study of the accessory genital glands of the boar. *J Anat* 1960;94:130–142.
12. Al Juburi A, Pranikoff K, Dougherty KA, Urry RL, Cockett ATK. Alteration of semen quality in dogs after creation of varicocele. *Urology* 1979;13:535–539.
13. Al-Zuhair A, Gosling JA, Dixon JS. Observations on the structure and autonomic innervation of the guinea-pig seminal vesicle and ductus deferens. *J Anat* 1975;120:81–93.
14. Alexander NJ. Immunological aspects of vasectomy. In: Boettcher B ed. *Immunological Influences on Human Fertility* Sydney: Academic Press, 1977;25–46.
15. Ali HA, Tingari MD, Moniem KA. On the morphology of the accessory male glands and histochemistry of the ampulla ductus deferentis of the camel (*Camelus dromedarius*). *J Anat* 1978;125:277–292.
16. Ali MA. Effects of mesencephalic lesion on the histomorphology of testis and spermatogenesis. *Indian J Physiol Pharmacol* 1986;30:11–21.
17. Allard EK, Johnson KJ, Boekelheide K. Colchicine disrupts the cytoskeleton of rat testis seminiferous epithelium in a stage-dependent manner. *Biol Reprod* 1993;48:143–153.
18. Alldrich RD, Christenson RK, Ford JJ, Zimmerman DR. Pubertal development of the boar: age-related changes in testicular morphology and *in vitro* production of testosterone and estradiol-17β. *Biol Reprod* 1983;28:902–909.
19. Allen LG, Wilson FJ, Macdonald GJ. Neuropeptide Y-containing nerves in rat gonads: sex difference and development. *Biol. Reprod* 1989;40:371–378.
20. Alm P. On the autonomic innervation of the human vas deferens. *Brain Res Bull* 1982;9:673–677.

21. Alm P, Alumets J, Hakanson R, Sundler F. Peptidergic (vasoactive intestinal peptide) nerves in the genito-urinary tract. *Neuroscience* 1977;2:751–754.
22. Alm P, Alumets J, Brodin E, et al. Peptidergic substance P nerves in the genitourinary tract. *Neuroscience* 1978;3:419–425.
23. Alm P, Alumets J, Hakanson R, et al. Origin and distribution of VIP (vasoactive intestinal polypeptide)-nerves in the genito-urinary tract. *Cell Tiss Res* 1980;205:337–347.
24. Altman PL, Dittmer DS, ed. *Biology Data Book,* Ed 2, Vol III. Bethesda, MD: Federation of American Societies for Experimental Biology, 1974;1433–2123.
25. Amann RP, Ganjam VK. Steroid production by the bovine testis and steroid transfer across the pampiniform plexus. *Biol Reprod* 1976;15:695–703.
26. Amann RP, Johnson L, Pickett BW. Connection between the seminiferous tubules and the efferent ducts in the stallion. *Am J Vet Res* 1977;38:1571–1579.
27. Amann RP, Nett TM, Niswender GD. Effects of LH, FSH, prolactin and PGF2α on testicular blood flow and testosterone secretion in the ram. *J Anim Sci* 1978;47:1307–1313.
28. Amann RP, Deaver DR, Zirkin BR, et al. Effects of microgravity or simulated launch on testicular function in rats. *J Appl Physiol* 1992;73(Suppl):174S–185S.
29. Ambadkar PM, Vyas DM. Innervation of the rat preputial gland. *Acta Anat* 1981;110:98–102.
30. Amselgruber W, Sinowatz F. Zur Bezeihung zwischen der Arteria testicularis und den Venen des Plexus pampiniformis beim Bullen. *Anat Histol Embryol* 1987;16:363–370.
31. Amselgruber W, Sinowatz F, Spanel-Borowski K. Rasterelektronenmikroskopische Untersuchungen zur Mikrovascularisation der Tubuli seminiferi contorti des Bullenhodens. *Berl Munch Tierarztl Wochensch* 1986;99:166–170.
32. Anakwe OO, Murphy PR, Moger WH. Characterization of β-adrenergic binding sites on rodent Leydig cells. *Biol Reprod* 1985;33:815–826.
33. Andersson L, Dahn I, Nelson CE, Norgren A. Method for measuring prostatic blood flow with Xenon-133 in the dog. *Invest Urol* 1967;5:140–148.
34. Aoki A, Hoffer AP. Reexamination of the lesions in rat testis caused by cadmium. *Biol Reprod* 1978;18:579–591.
35. Archer FL, Beck IS, Melvin JMO. Localization of smooth muscle protein in myoepithelium by immunofluorescence. *Am J Pathol* 1971;63:109–118.
36. Au CL, Ngai HK, Yeung CH, Wong PYD. Effect of adrenalectomy and hormone replacement on sodium and water transport in the perfused rat cauda epididymidis. *J Endocrinol* 1978;77:265–266.
37. Au CL, Robertson DM, de Kretser DM. An *in-vivo* method for estimating inhibin production by adult rat testes. *J Reprod Fertil* 1984;71:259–265.
38. Au CL, Robertson DM, de Kretser DM. Effects of hypophysectomy and subsequent FSH and testosterone treatment on inhibin production by adult rat testes. *J Endocrinol* 1985;105:1–6.
39. Au CL, Robertson DM, de Kretser DM. Measurement of inhibin and an index of inhibin production by rat testes during postnatal development. *Biol Reprod* 1986;35:37–43.
40. Au CL, Irby DC, Robertson DM, de Kretser DM. Effects of testosterone on inhibin and fluid production in intact and hypophysectomized adult rats. *J Reprod Fertil* 1986;76:257–266.
41. Auclair D, Sowerbutts SF, Setchell BP. Testicular blood flow during pubertal development in merino lambs. *Abstracts, 11th North American Testis Workshop* 1991; p. 110.
42. Auclair D, Sowerbutts SF, Setchell BP. Active immunization against testosterone in adult merino rams: a one year-duration study. *Proc Aust Soc Reprod Biol* 1992;24:83.
43. Aughey E. Histology and histochemistry of the male accessory glands of the red deer, *Cervus elaphus* L. *J Reprod Fertil* 1969;18:399–407.
44. Aumuller G. Morphologic and regulatory aspects of prostatic function. *Anat Embryol (Berl.)* 1989;179:519–531.
45. Aumuller G, Braun BE, Seitz J, Muller T, Heyns W, Krieg M. Effects of sexual rest or sexual activity on the structure and function of the ventral prostate of the rat. *Anat Rec* 1985;212:345–352.
46. Aumuller G, Vesper M, Seitz J, Kemme M, Scheit KH. Binding of a major secretory protein from bull seminal vesicles to bovine spermatozoa. *Cell Tissue Res* 1988;252:377–384.
47. Aumuller G, Jungblut T, Malek B, Konrad S, Weihe E. Regional distribution of opioidergic nerves in human and canine prostates. *Prostate* 1989;14:279–288.
48. Averback P. Histopathological diagnosis of hypercurved seminiferous tubules. *Histopathology* 1980;4:75–82.
49. Averback P, Wight DGD. Seminiferous tubule hypercurvature: a newly recognized common syndrome of human male infertility. *Lancet* 1979;I:81–183.
50. Ayer-LeLievre C, Olson L, Ebendal T, Hallbook F, Persson H. Nerve growth factor mRNA and protein in the testis and epididymis of mouse and rat. *Proc Natl Acad Sci USA* 1988;85:2628–2632.
51. Back DJ. The presence of metabolites of ^{3}H-testosterone in the lumen of the cauda epididymidis of the rat. *Steroids* 1975;25:413–420.
52. Backhouse KM. The gubernaculum testis Hunteri, testicular descent and maldescent. *Ann R Coll Surg Engl* 1964;35:15–32.
53. Backhouse KM, Butler H. The gubernaculum testis of the pig (*Sus scrofa*). *J Anat* 1960;94:107–120.
54. Baer HM, Gerber WL, Kendall AR, Locke JL, Putong PB. Segmental infarct of the testis due to hypersensitivity angiitis. *J Urol* 1989;142:125–127.
55. Baker HW, Sonstein FM, Eichner GJ, Santen RJ, Jefferson LS, Bardin CW. Perfusion of rat testes and accessory sex organs: a new method. *Endocrinology* 1977;100P:699–708.
56. Baker HWG, Burger HG, de Kretser DM, Hudson B, Rennie GC, Straffon WGE. Testicular vein ligation and fertility in men with varicoceles. *Br Med J* 1985;291:1678–1680.
57. Ball RY, Setchell BP. The passage of spermatozoa to regional lymph nodes in testicular lymph following vasectomy in rams and boars. *J Reprod Fertil* 1983;68:145–153.
58. Ball RY, Naylor CPE, Mitchinson MJ. Spermatozoa in an abdominal lymph node after vasectomy in a man. *J Reprod Fertil* 1982;66:715–716.
59. Barack BM. Transport of spermatozoa from seminiferous tubules to epididymis in the mouse: a histological and quantitative study. *J Reprod Fertil* 1968;16:35–48.
60. Bardin CW, Shaha C, Mather J, et al. Identification and possible function of pro-opiomelanocortin-derived peptides in the testis. *Ann NY Acad Sci* 1984;438:346–364.
61. Baronos S. Seminal carbohydrate in boar and stallion. *J Reprod Fertil* 1971;24:303–305.
62. Bartke A, Amador AG, Chandrashekar V, Klemcke HG. Seasonal difference in testicular receptors and steroidogenesis. *J Steroid Biochem* 1987;27:81–587.
63. Bartlett DT. Studies on dog semen. II. Biochemical characteristics. *J Reprod Fertil* 1962;3:190–205.
64. Bascom KF, Osterud HL. Quantitative studies of the testicle. II. Pattern and total tubule length in the testicles of certain common mammals. *Anat Rec* 1925;31:159–169.
65. Baumans V, Dijkstra G, Wensing CJG. The effect of orchidectomy on gubernacular outgrowth and regression in the dog. *Int J Androl* 1982;5:387–400.
66. Baumans V, Dijkstra G, Wensing CJG. The role of a nonandrogenic testicular factor in the process of testicular descent in the dog. *Int J Androl* 1983;6:541–552.
67. Baumgarten HG, Holstein AF. Catecholaminhaltige Nervenfasern im Hoden des Menschen. *Z Zellforsch* 1967;79:389–395.
68. Baumgarten HG, Falck B, Holstein A-F, Owman C, Owman T. Adrenergic innervation of the human testis, epididymis, ductus deferens and prostate: a fluorescence microscopic and fluorimetric study. *Z Zellforsch* 1968;90:81–95.
69. Baumgarten HG, Holstein AF, Rosengren E. Arrangement, ultrastructure, and adrenergic innervation of smooth musculature of the ductuli efferentes, ductus epididymidis and ductus deferens of man. *Z Zellforsch* 1971;120:37–79.
70. Beasely SW, Hutson JM. Effect of division of the genitofemoral nerve on testicular descent in the rat. *Aust NZJ Surg* 1987;57:49–51.
71. Beasely SW, Hutson JM. The role of the gubernaculum in testicular descent. *J Urol* 1988;140:1191–1193.

72. Bedford JM. Anatomical evidence for the epididymis as the prime mover in the evolution of the scrotum. *Am J Anat* 1978;152:483–508.
73. Bedford JM. Influence of abdominal temperature on epididymal function in the rat and rabbit. *Am J Anat* 1978; 152:509–522.
74. Beh KJ, Watson DL, Lascelles AK. Concentrations of immunoglobulins and albumin in lymph collected from various regions of the body of the sheep. *Aust J Exp Biol Med Sci* 1974;52:81–86.
75. Behringer RR, Cate RL, Froelick GJ, Palmiter RD, Brinster RL. Abnormal sexual development in transgenic mice chronically expressing mullerian inhibiting substance. *Nature* 1990;345: 167–170.
76. Belkin VSh, Kaiumov AK. Vascularization of the testes of the white rat in the high altitude conditions of the Pamir and Antartica (in Russian). *Arkh Anat Gistol Embriol* 1986;91:67–70.
77. Bell C, McLean JR. The distribution of cholinergic and adrenergic nerve fibres in the retractor penis and vas deferens of the dog. *Z Zellforsch* 1970;106:516–522.
78. Bell C, McLean JR. The autonomic innervation of the rat testicular capsule. *J Reprod Fertil* 1973;32:253–258.
79. Benoit E, Garnier F, Courtot D, Delatour P. Radioimmunoassay of 19 nortestosterone. Evidence of its secretion by the testis of the stallion. *Ann Rech Vet* 1985;16:379–383.
80. Benoit J. Recherches anatomiques, cytologiques et histophysiologiques sur les voies excretrices du testicule chez les mammiferes. *Arch Anat Histol Embryol* 1926;5:173–414.
81. Bent-Hansen L. Whole body capillary exchange of albumin. *Acta Physiol Scand* 1991;143(Suppl 603):5–11.
82. Bergh A. Local differences in Leydig cell morphology in the adult rat testis: evidence for a local control of Leydig cells by adjacent seminiferous tubules. *Int J Androl* 1982;5:325–330.
83. Bergh A. Paracrine regulation of Leydig cells by the seminiferous tubules. *Int J Androl* 1983;6:57–65.
84. Bergh A. Effect of cryptorchidism on the morphology of testicular macrophages: evidence for a Leydig cell macrophage interaction in the rat testis. *Int J Androl* 1985;8:86–96.
85. Bergh A. Treatment with human chorionic gonadotrophin induces inflammation-like changes in the testicular microcirculation in adult unilaterally cryptorchid rats. *Horm Res* 1988;30:207–209.
86. Bergh A, Damber JE. Terbutaline treatment inhibits the hCG-induced increase in venular permeability in the rat testis. *J Reprod Fertil* 1987;80:623–627.
87. Bergh A, Damber JE. Treatment with an LHRH agonist or hCG increases interstitial fluid volume and permeability to Evans blue in the mouse testis. *Int J Androl* 1988;11:449–456.
88. Bergh A, Damber JE. Does unilateral orchidectomy influence blood flow, microcirculation and vascular morphology in the remaining testis? *Int J Androl* 1991;14:453–460.
89. Bergh A, Soder O. Interleukin-1 beta but not interleukin-1 alpha, induces acute inflammation-like changes in the testicular microcirculation of adult rats. *J Reprod Immunol* 1990;17: 155–165.
90. Bergh A, Helander HF, Wahlqvist L. Studies on factors governing testicular descent in the rat—particularly the role of gubernaculum testis. *Int J Androl* 1982;1:42–356.
91. Bergh A, Widmark A, Damber JE, Cajander S. Are leukocytes involved in the human chorionic gonadotrophin-induced increase in testicular vascular permeability? *Endocrinology* 1986;119:586–590.
92. Bergh A, Rooth P, Widmark A, Damber JE. Treatment of rats with hCG induces inflammation-like changes in the testicular microcirculation. *J Reprod Fertil* 1987;79:135–143.
93. Bergh A, Damber JE, Marklund SL. Morphologic changes induced by short-term ischemia in the rat testis are not affected by superoxide dismutase and catalase. *J Androl* 1988;9:15–20.
94. Bergh A, Damber JE, van Rooijen N. The hCG-induced inflammatory response is enhanced in macrophage-depleted testes. *Miniposters of the VIIth European Workshop on Molecular and Cellular Endocrinology of the Testis* 1992; p. 103.
95. Bergmann M, Dierichs R. Postnatal formation of the blood–testis barrier in the rat with special reference to the initiation of meiosis. *Anat Embryol* 1983;168:269–275.
96. Bergmann M, Schindelmeiser J, Greven H. The blood–testis barrier in vertebrates having different testicular organization. *Cell Tissue Res* 1984;228:145–150.
97. Bern HA, Krichesky B. Anatomic and histological studies of the sex accessories of the male rabbit. *Univ Calif Publ Zool* 1943;47:175–196.
98. Bharadwaj MB, Calhoun ML. Histology of the bulbo-urethral gland of the domestic animals. *Anat Rec* 1962;142:216.
99. Bindon BM, Waites GMH. Discrepancy in weight and blood flow of the testis and epididymis of the mouse before and after hypophysectomy. *J Endocrinol* 1968;40:385–386.
100. Blaschuk O, Burdzy K, Fritz IB. Purification and characterization of a cell-aggregating factor (clusterin), the major glycoprotein in ram rete testis fluid. *J Biol Chem* 1983;258:7714–7720.
101. Blix AS, Fay FH, Ronald K. On testicular cooling in phocid seals. *Polar Res* 1983;1:231–233.
102. Blombery PA, Waites GMH. Non-uniform blood flow in the testis of sheep and dog and preliminary observations on reactive hyperaemia. *Aust J Exp Biol Med Sci* 1968;46:25.
103. Bloom W, Fawcett DW. *A Textbook of Histology* Ed 8. Philadelphia: WB Saunders, 1962.
104. Bøhmer T, Johansen L. Inhibition of sperm maturation through intervention of the carnitine system. *Int J Androl* 1978;2 (*Suppl*):565–573.
105. Bøhmer T, Johansen L, Kjekshus E. Carnitine-acetyl-transferase transferase in human spermatozoa and seminal plasma determined by a sensitive radioisotope method. *Int J Androl* 1978;1:262–269.
106. Bolliger A. Presidential address. *Proc R Soc NSW* 1946;80:1–13.
107. Bolonge R, Demoulin A, Hustin J, Verstraelen-Proyard J, Gysen P, Franchimont P. Etude de l'incorporation de la thymidine tritieé dans l'acide desoxyribonucleique testiculaire du rat. Influence de l'inhibine. *CR Soc Biol* 1979;173:654–659.
108. Bottcher M, Lange W. Untersuchungen am arteriellen Gefasssystem des Eberhodens. *Arch Exp Veterinarmed* 1987;41: 58–64.
109. Boulanger P, Desaulniers M, Bleau G, Roberts KD, Chapdelaine A. Sex steroid concentrations in plasma collected from the canine deferential vein. *J Endocrinol* 1983;96:223–228.
110. Boursnell JC, Butler EJ. Studies on properties of the seminal gel of the boar using natural gel and gel formed *in vitro*. *J Reprod Fertil* 1973;34:457–465.
111. Boursnell JC, Hartree EF, Briggs PA. Studies of the bulbo-urethral (Cowper's)-gland mucin and seminal gel of the boar. *Biochem J* 1970;117:981–988.
112. Braunschweiger PG, Glode LM, Maring EM, Mahus K, Reynolds K. Biological implications of androgen dependent changes in proton-NMR relaxation times in rat ventral prostate. *Prostate* 1986;9:283–294.
113. Breed WG. Morphological variation in the testes and accessory sex organs of Australian rodents in the genera *Pseudomys* and *Notomys*. *J Reprod Fertil* 1982;66:607–613.
114. Bressler RS, Ross MH. Differentiation of peritubular myoid cells of the testis: effects of intratesticular implantation of newborn mouse testes into normal and hypophysectomised adults. *Biol Reprod* 1972;6:148–159.
115. Bronson FH, Caroom D. Preputial gland of the male mouse: attractant function. *J Reprod Fertil* 1971;25:279–282.
116. Brooks DE. Acid-soluble phosphorus compounds in mammalian semen. *Biochem J* 1970;118:851–857.
117. Brooks DE. Epididymal and testicular temperature in the unrestrained conscious rat. *J Reprod Fertil* 1973;35:157–160.
118. Brooks DE. Biochemical environment of sperm maturation. In: Fawcett DW, Bedford JM, eds. *The Spermatozoon,* Baltimore: Urban & Schwarzenberg, 1979;23–34.
119. Brooks DE. Carbohydrate metabolism in the rat epididymis: evidence that glucose is taken up by tissue slices and isolated cells by a process of facilitated transport. *Biol Reprod* 1979;21:19–26.
120. Brooks DE. Carnitine, acetylcarnitine and the activity of carnitine acyltransferases in seminal plasma and spermatozoa of men, rams and rats. *J Reprod Fertil* 1979;56:667–673.

121. Brooks DE. Influence of testicular secretions on tissue weight and on metabolic and enzyme activities in the epididymis of the rat. *J Endocrinol* 1979;82:305–313.
122. Brooks DE. Carnitine in the male reproductive tract and its relation to the metabolism of the epididymis and spermatozoa. In: Frenkel RA, McGarry JD, eds. *Carnitine Biosynthesis, Metabolism, and Functions.* New York: Academic Press, 1980;219–235.
123. Brooks DE. Metabolic activity in the epididymis and its regulation by androgens. *Physiol Rev* 1981;61:515–555.
124. Brooks DE. Secretion of proteins and glycoproteins by the rat epididymis: regional differences, androgen-dependence, and effects of protease inhibitors, procaine, and tunicamycin. *Biol Reprod* 1981;25:1099–1117.
125. Brooks DE. Purification of rat epididymal proteins 'D' and 'E', demonstration of shared immunological determinants, and identification of regional synthesis and secretion. *Int J Androl* 1982;5:513–524.
126. Brooks DE. Epididymal functions and their hormonal regulation. *Aust J Biol Sci* 1983;36:205–221.
127. Brooks DE. Characterization of a 22kDa protein with widespread tissue distribution but which is uniquely present in secretions of the testis and epididymis and on the surface of spermatozoa. *Biochim Biophys Acta* 1985;841:59–70.
128. Brooks DE. Biochemistry of the male accessory glands. In: Lamming GE, ed. *Marshall's Physiology of Reproduction, Vol 2.* Edinburgh: Churchill Livingstone, 1990;569–690.
129. Brooks DE, Higgins SJ. Characterization and androgen-dependence of proteins associated with luminal fluid and spermatozoa in the rat epididymis. *J Reprod Fertil* 1980;59: 363–375.
130. Brooks DE, Mann T. Relation between the oxidation state of nicotinamide-adenine dinucleotide and the metabolism of spermatozoa. *Biochem J* 1972;129:1023–1034.
131. Brooks DE, Mann T. Pyruvate metabolism in boar spermatozoa. *J Reprod Fertil* 1973;34:105–119.
132. Brooks DE, Hamilton DW, Mallek AH. The uptake of L-[methyl-^{3}H]carnitine by the rat epididymis. *Biochem Biophys Res Commun* 1973;52:1354–1360.
133. Brooks DE, Gaughwin M, Mann T. Structural and biochemical characteristics of the male accessory organs of reproduction in the hairy-nosed wombat (*Lasiorhinus latifrons*). *Proc R Soc London (B.)* 1978;201:191–207.
134. Brooks DE, Means AR, Wright EJ, Singh SP, Tiver KK. Molecular cloning of the cDNA for androgen dependent sperm-coating glycoproteins secreted by the rat epididymis. *Eur J Biochem* 1986;161:13–18.
135. Brooks DE, Means AR, Wright EJ, Singh SP, Tiver KK. Molecular cloning of the cDNA for two major androgen-dependent secretory proteins of 18.5 kilodaltons synthesized by the rat epididymis. *J Biol Chem* 1986;261:4956–4962.
136. Brown JC, Williams JD. A histochemical study of the preputial glands of male laboratory rat and mouse. *Acta Anat* 1972;81:270–285.
137. Brown KD, Blakely DM, Henville A, Setchell BP. Rete testis fluid contains a growth factor for cultured fibroblasts. *Biochem Biophys Res Commun* 1982;105:371–379.
138. Brown PDC, Waites GMH. Regional blood flow in the epididymis of the rat and rabbit: effect of efferent duct ligation and orchidectomy. *J Reprod Fertil* 1972;28:221–233.
139. Brown-Woodman PDC, White IG. Amino acid composition of semen and the secretions of the male reproductive tract. *Aust J Biol Sci* 1974;27:415–422.
140. Bryden MM. Testicular temperature in the southern elephant seal. *J Reprod Fertil* 1967;13:583–584.
141. Burgos MH, Vitale-Calpe R, Aoki A. Fine structure of the testis and its functional significance. In: Johnson AD, Gomes WR, Vandemark NL, eds. *The Testis, Vol I.* New York: Academic Press, 1970;551–649.
142. Burrow P, Setchell BP. The fate of radioactive substances infused into a single seminiferous tubule in anaesthetised rats. *Proceedings of the Winter Meeting of the Society for the Study of Fertility,* London. (abst 32). 1980.
143. Burrow PV, Pholpramool C, Setchell BP. The movement of substances out of the seminiferous tubules and epididymal duct during microinfusion. *J Physiol* 1981;319:15P–16P.
144. Bustamante JC, Setchell BP. Measurement of capillary permeability-surface area products in the isolated perfused rat testis. *J Physiol* 1981;319:16P–17P.
145. Bustamante JC, Jarvis LG, Setchell BP. Role of the endothelium in the uptake of amino acids by the isolated perfused testis. *J Physiol* 1982;330:62P–63P.
146. Bustos-Obregon E, Courot M. Ultrastructure of the lamina propria in the ovine seminiferous tubule. *Cell Tiss Res* 1974;150:481–492.
147. Bustos-Obregon E, Holstein AF. Ultrastructure and function of the lamina propria of human seminiferous tubules. *Z Zellforsch* 1973;141:413–425.
148. Bustos-Obregon E, Holstein AF. The rete testis in man: ultrastructural aspects. *Cell Tiss Res* 1976;175:1–15.
149. Byers S, Pelletier RM. Sertoli–Sertoli cell tight junctions and the blood–testis barrier. In: Cereijido M, ed. *Tight Junctions.* Boca Raton, FL: CRC Press, 1991;279–304.
150. Bygdeman M, Holmberg O. Isolation and identification of prostaglandins from ram seminal plasma. *Acta Chem Scand* 1966;20:2308–2310.
151. Cabo-Tomargo JA, Lopez-Muniz A, Bengoechea ME, Vega-Alvarez JA, Perez-Casas A. Contribicion al conocimiento de la inervacion microscopica de la prostata (I): La formacion vegativa distal, *Arch Esp Urol* 1989;38:231–241.
152. Caflisch CR, DuBose TD Jr. Effect of alpha-chlorhydrin on in situ pH in rat testis and epididymis. *Contraception* 1990;41: 207–212.
153. Caflisch CR, Dubose TD. Direct evaluation of acidification by rat testis and epididymis: role of carbonic anhydrase. *Am J Physiol* 1990;258:E143–E150.
154. Caflisch CR, DuBose TD Jr. Cadmium-induced changes in luminal fluid pH in testis and epididymis of the rat in vivo. *J Toxicol Environ Health* 1991;32:49–57.
155. Caine M. Alpha-adrenergic mechanisms in dynamics of benign prostatic hypertrophy. *Urology* 1988;32, Suppl 6:16–20.
156. Calvin J, Tubbs PK. A carnitine: acetylcarnitine exchange system in spermatozoa. *J Reprod Fertil* 1976;48:417–420.
157. Cameron DF, Snydle FE, Ross MH, Drylie DM. Ultrastructural alterations in the adluminal testicular compartment in men with varicocele. *Fert Steril* 1989;33:526–533.
158. Campos MB, Vitale ML, Calandra RS, Chiocchio SR. Serotonergic innervation of the rat testis. *J Reprod Fertil* 1990;88:475–479.
159. Carmo-Fonesca M, Vaz Y. Immunocytochemical localization and lectin-binding properties of the 22kDa secretory protein from rat ventral prostate. *Biol Reprod* 1989;40:153–164.
160. Carr DW, Acott TS. Inhibition of bovine spermatozoa by caudal epididymal fluid: I. Studies of a sperm motility quiescence factor. *Biol Reprod* 1984;30:913–925.
161. Carr DW, Usselman MC, Acott TS. Effects of pH, lactate and viscoelastic drag on sperm motility: a species comparison. *Biol Reprod* 1985;33:588–595.
162. Carrick FN, Cox RI. Testicular endocrinology of marsupials and monotremes. In: *Reproduction and Evolution,* edited by JH Calaby and CH Tyndale-Biscoe, Australian Academy of Sciences, Canberra. 1977; pp. 137–141.
163. Carrick FN, Hughes RL. Reproduction in male monotremes. *Aust Zool* 1978;20:211–231.
164. Carrick FN, Setchell BP. The evolution of the scrotum. In: *Reproduction and Evolution,* edited by JH Calaby and CH Tyndal-Biscoe, Australian Academy of Sciences, Canberra. 1977; pp. 165–170.
165. Carvalho TL, Ribiero RD, Lopes RA. The male reproductive organs in experimental Chagas' disease. I. Morphometric study of the vas deferencs in the acute phase of the disease. *Exp Pathol* 1991;41:203–214.
166. Casillas ER, Erickson BJ. Studies on carnitine synthesis in the rat epididymis. *J Reprod Fertil* 1975;44:287–291.
167. Cavicchia JC, Burgos MH. Tridimensional reconstruction and histology of the intratesticular seminal pathway in the hamster. *Anat Rec* 1977;187:1–10.
168. Cavicchia JC, Sacerdote FL. Topography of the rat blood-testis

barrier after intratubular administration of intercellular tracers. *Tissue Cell* 1988;20:577–586.
169. Cavicchia JC, Sacerdote FL. Correlation between blood-testis barrier development and onset of the first spermatogenic wave in normal and Busulphan-treated rats: a lanthanum and freeze-fracture study. *Anat Rec* 1991;230:361–368.
170. Cenedella RJ. Prostaglandins and male reproductive physiology. In: *Molecular Mechanisms of Conadal Hormone Action,* edited by JA Thomas and RL Singhall, University Park Press, Baltimore. 1975; pp. 325–328.
171. Centola GM, Lee K, Cockett AT. Relationship between testicular volume and presence of varicoceles. *Urology* 1987;30: 479–481.
172. Cerasaro TS, Nachtsheim DA, Otero F, Parsons CL. The effect of testicular torsion on contralateral testis and the production of antisperm antibodies in rabbits. *J Urol* 1984;132:577–579.
173. Chacon-Arellano JT, Woolley DM. Smooth muscle in the testicular capsule of the horse, pig and sheep. *J Anat* 1980;131: 263–273.
174. Chakraborty J, Jhunjhunwala J. Experimental unilateral torsion of the spermatic cord in guinea pigs: effects on the contralateral testis. *J Androl* 1982;3:117–123.
175. Chakraborty J, Jhunjhunwala J, Nelson L, Young M. Effects of unilateral torsion of the spermatic cord on the contralateral testis in human and guinea pig. *Arch Androl* 1980;4:95–108.
176. Chakraborty J, Sinha-Hikim AP, Jhunjhunwala JS. Stagnation of blood in the microvasscculature of the affected and contralateral testes of men with short-term torsion of the spermatic cord. *J Androl* 1985;6:291–299.
177. Chakraborty J, Sinha Hikim AP, Jhunjhunwala JS. Stagnation of blood in the microcirculatory vessels in the testes of men with varicocele. *J Androl* 1985a;6:117–126.
178. Chakraborty J, Sinha Hikim AP, Jhunjhunwala JS. Quantitative evaluation of testicular biopsies from men with unilateral torsion. *Urology* 1985;25:145–150.
179. Chandrasekhar Y, D'Ochhio MJ, Holland MK, Setchell BP. Activity of the hypothalamo-pituitary axis and testicular development in prepubertal ram lambs with induced hypothyroidism or hyperthyroidism. *Endocrinology* 1985;117:1645–1651.
180. Chandrasekhar Y, Holland MK, D'Ochhio MJ, Setchell BP. Spermatogenesis, seminal characteristics and reproductive hormone levels in mature rams with induced hypothyroidism and hyperthyroidism. *J Endocrinol* 1985;105:39–46.
181. Chapelle PA, Roby-Brami A, Yakovleff A, Bussel B. Neurological correlations of ejaculation and testicular size in men with a complete spinal cord section. *J Neurol Neurosurg Psychiatry* 1988;51:197–202.
182. Chapin RE, Dutton SL, Ross MD, Sumrell BM, Lamb JC. The effects of ethylene glycol monomethyl ether on testicular histology in F344 rats. *J Androl* 1984;5:369–380.
183. Chapple CR, Aubry ML, James S, Greengrass PM, Burnstock G, Turner-Warwick RT, Milroy EJ, Davey MJ. Characterisation of human prostatic adrenoreceptors using pharmacology receptor binding and localisation. *Br J Urol* 1989;63:487–496.
184. Chapple CR, Crowe R, Gosling J, Burnstock G. The innervation of the human prostate gland—the changes associated with benign enlargement. *J Urol* 1991;146:1637–1644.
185. Chaturapanich G, Jones RC. Morphometry of the epididymis of the tammar wallaby, *Macropus eugenii,* and estimation of some physiological parameters. *Reprod Fertil Dev* 1991;3:651–658.
186. Chaturapanich G, Jones RC, Clulow J. Role of androgens in survival of spermatozoa in epididymis of tammar wallaby (Macropus eugenii). *J Reprod Fertil* 1992;95:421–429.
187. Cheng CY, Gunsalus GL, Morris ID, Turner TT, Bardin CW. The heterogeneity of rat androgen binding protein (rABP) in the vascular compartment differs from that in the testicular tubular lumen. Further evidence for bidirectional secretion of rABP. *J Androl* 1986;7:175–179.
188. Cheung YM, Hwang JC, Wong PYD. *In vitro* measurement of rate of fluid secretion in rat isolated seminiferous tubules: effects of metabolic inhibitors and ions. *J Physiol* 1977;269:115.
189. Chipman RK, Albrecht ED. The relationship of the male preputial gland to the acceleration of oestrus in the laboratory mouse. *J Reprod Fertil* 1974;38:91–96.
190. Chiquoine AD. Observations on the early events of cadmium necrosis of the testis. *Anat Rec* 1964;149:23–35.
191. Christensen AK. Leydig cells. In: *Handbook of Physiology,* Vol. V, edited by Hamilton DW, Greep RO, eds. Washington, DC., American Physiological Society, 1975; pp. 57–94.
192. Christensen AK, Gillim SW. The correlation of fine structure and function in steroid-secreting cells, with emphasis on those of the gonads. In: *The Gonads,* edited by KW McKems, Appleton-Century Crofts, New York, 1969; pp. 415–488.
193. Christensen AK, Komorowski TE, Wilson B, Ma SF, Stevens RW. The distribution of serum albumin in the rat testis, studied by electron microscope immunocytochemistry on ultrathin sections. *Endocrinology* 1985;116:1983–1996.
194. Chubb C, Desjardins C. Vasculature of the mouse, rat and rabbit testis-epididymis. *Am J Anat* 1982;165:357–372.
195. Chubb C, Desjardins C. Steroid secretion by mouse testes perfused *in vitro. Am J Physiol* 1983;244:E575–E580.
196. Chubb C, Ewing LL. Steroid secretion by *in vitro* perfused testes: secretions of rabbit and rat testes. *Am J Physiol* 1979;237: E231–E238.
197. Chubb C, Ewing LL. Steroid secretion by *in vitro* perfused testes: testosterone biosynthetic pathways. *Am J Physiol* 1979;237: E247–E254.
198. Chubb C, Ewing LL. Steroid secretion by sexually immature rat and rabbit testes perfused *in vitro. Endocrinology* 1981;109: 1999–2003.
199. Chubb C, Ewing L, Irby D, Desjardins C. Testicular maturation in the rabbit: secretion of testosterone, dihydrotestosterone, 5α-androstan-$3\alpha,17\beta$-diol and 5α-androstan-$3\beta,17\beta$-diol by perfused rabbit testes-epididymides and spermatogenesis. *Biol Reprod* 1978;18:212–218.
200. Clark RV. Three-dimensional organization of testicular interstitial tissue and lymphatic space in the rat. *Anat Rec* 1976;184:203–226.
201. Claus R, Hoffmann B. Oestrogens, compared to other steroids of testicular origin, in blood plasma of boars. *Acta Endocrinol* 1980;94:404–411.
202. Clavert A, Cranz C, Brun B. Etude de la vascularisation de l'epididyme. *Bull Assoc Anat* 1980;64:539–546.
203. Clavert A, Cranz C, Brun B. Epididymal vascularization and microvascularization. *Prog Reprod Biol* 1981;8:48–57.
204. Clegg EJ. The arterial supply of the human prostate and seminal vesicles. *J Anat* 1955;89:209–216.
205. Clegg EJ. The vascular arrangements within the human prostate gland. *Br J Urol* 1956;28:428–435.
206. Clegg EJ, Carr I. Increased vascular permeability in the reproductive organs of cadmium chloride-treated male rats. *J Anat* 1966;100:696–697.
207. Clegg EJ, Carr I. Changes in the blood vessels of the rat testis and epididymis produced by cadmium salts. *J Pathol Bacteriol* 1967;94:317–322.
208. Clegg EJ, MacMillan EW. The uptake of vital dyes and particulate matter by the Sertoli cells of the rat testis. *J Anat* 1965;99:219–229.
209. Clegg EJ, Niemi M, Carr I. The age at which the blood vessels of the rat testis become sensitive to cadium salts. *J Endocrinol* 1969;43:445–449.
210. Clementi F, Naimzada KM, Mantegazza P. Study of the nerve endings in the vas deferens and seminal vesicle of the guinea pig. *Int J Neuropharmacol* 1969;8:399–403.
211. Clermont Y. Contractile elements in the limiting membrane of the seminiferous tubules of the rat. *Exp Cell Res* 1958; 15:438–440.
212. Clermont Y, Huckins C. Microscopic anatomy of the sex cords and seminiferous tubules in growing and adult male albino rats. *Am J Anat* 1961;108:79–97.
213. Clulow J, Jones RC, Murdoch RN. Maturation and regulation of the motility of spermatozoa in the epididymis of the tammar wallaby (*Macropus eugenii*). *J Reprod Fertil* 1992;94:295–303.
214. Colenbrander B, van Rossum-Kok CMJE, van Straaten HWM, Wensing CJG. The effect of fetal decapitation on the testis and other endocnne organs in the pig. *Biol Reprod* 1979;20: 198–204.

215. Comhaire FH. Varicocele and its role in male infertility. *Oxf Rev Reprod Biol* 1986;8:165–213.
216. Comhaire FH. Varicocele infertility: an enigma. *Int J Androl* 1983;6:401–404.
217. Comhaire FH, Vermeulen A. Testosterone concentration in the fluids of seminiferous tubules, the interstitium and the rete testis of the rat. *J Endocrinol* 1976;70:229–235.
218. Connolly JG, Thomson A, Jewett MAS, Hartman N, Webber M. Intraprostatic lymphatics. *Invest Urol* 1968;5:371–378.
219. Cooke BA, Golding M, Dix CJ, Hunter MG. Catecholamine stimulation of testosterone production via cyclic AMP in mouse Leydig cells in monolayer culture. *Mol Cell Endocrinol* 1982;27:221–231.
220. Cooper ERA, Jackson H. The vasa efferentia in the rat and mouse. *J Reprod Fertil* 1972;28:317–319.
221. Cooper TG. The general importance of proteins and other factors in the transfer of steroids into the rat epididymis. *Int J Androl* 1980;3:333–348.
222. Cooper TG. Secretion of inositol and glucose by the perfused rat cauda epididymidis. *J Reprod Fertil* 1982;64:373–379.
223. Cooper TG. The Epididymis, Sperm Maturation and Fertilisation. Springer-Verlag, Heidelberg, 1986;1–281.
224. Cooper TG. Secretory proteins from the epididymis and their clinical relevance. *Andrologia* 22 Suppl 1990;1:155–165.
225. Cooper TG, Orgebin-Crist MC. The effect of epididymal and testicular fluids on the fertilising capacity of testicular and epididymal spermatozoa. *Andrologia* 1975;7:85–93.
226. Cooper TG, Waites GMH. Testosterone in rete testis fluid and blood of rams and rats. *J Endocrinol* 1974;62:619–629.
227. Cooper TG, Waites GMH. Steroid entry into rete testis fluid and the blood-testis barrier. *J Endocrinol* 1975;65:195–205.
228. Cooper TG, Waites GMH. Factors affecting the entry of testosterone into the lumen of the cauda epididymis of the anaesthetized rat. *J Reprod Fertil* 1979;56:165–174.
229. Cooper TG, Waites GMH. Investigation by luminal perfusion of the transfer of compounds into the epididymis of the anaesthetized rat. *J Reprod Fertil* 1979;56:159–164.
230. Cooper TG, Danzo BJ, Dipietro DL, McKenna TJ, Orgebin-Crist MC. Some characteristics of rete testis fluid from rabbits. *Andrologia* 1976;8:87–94.
231. Cooper TG, Yeung CH, Lui W, Yang CZ. Luminal secretion of myo-inositol by the rat epididymis perfused in vitro. *J Reprod Fertil* 1985;74:135–144.
232. Cooper TG, Gudermann TW, Yeung CH. Characteristics of the transport of carnitine into the cauda epididymis of the rat as ascertained by luminal perfusion in vitro. *Int J Androl* 1986;9:348–358.
233. Cooper TG, Yeung CH, Weinbauer GF. Transport of carnitine by the epididymis of the cynamologous macaque (Macaca fascicularis). *J Reprod Fert* 1986;77:297–301.
234. Cooper TG, Yeung CH, Bergmann M. Protein transport to the epididymal lumen. *Cell Tissue Res* 1987;248:527–530.
235. Cooper TG, Gudermann TW, Yeung CH. Transport of inositol into the distal cauda epididymis of the rat. *J Androl* 1988;9:403–407.
236. Cooper TG, Yeung CH, Bergmann M. Transcytosis in the epididymis studied by local arterial perfusion. *Cell Tissue Res* 1988;253:631–637.
237. Cosentino MJ, Rabinowitz R, Valvo JR, Cockett ATK. The effect of prepubertal spermatic cord torsion on subsequent fertility in rats. *J Androl* 1984;5:93–98.
238. Cosentino MJ, Nishida M, Rabinowitz R, Cockett ATK. Histological changes occurring in the contralateral testes of prepubertal rats subjected to various durations of unilateral spermatic cord torsion. *J Urol* 1985;133:906–911.
239. Cosentino MJ, Nishida M, Rabinowitz R, Cockett ATK. Histopathology of prepubertal rat testes subjected to various durations of spermatic cord torsion. *J Androl* 1986;7:23–31.
240. Courot M, Joffre M. Testicular capillary blood flow in the impubertal and the ram during the breeding and non-breeding seasons. *Andrologia* 1977;9:332–336.
241. Cowie AT, Lascelles AK, Wallace JC. Flow and protein content of testicular lymph in conscious rams. *J Physiol* 1964;171:176–187.
242. Crabo B. Fine structure of the interstitial cells of the rabbit testis. *Z Zellforsch Mikroskop Anat* 1963;61:587–604.
243. Cragle RG, Salisbury GW, Muntz JH. Distribution of bulk and trace minerals in bull reproductive tract fluids and semen. *J Dairy Sci* 1972;41:1273–1277.
244. Crichton EG, Hinton BT, Hammerstedt RH. Cauda epididymal storage of sperm in hibernating bats requires a hyperosmolar environment. *Biol Reprod* 1992;46 Suppl. 1:149.
245. Cross BA, Glover TD. The hypothalamus and seminal emission. *J Endocrinol* 1958;16:385–395.
246. Cross BA, Silver IA. Neurovascular control of oxygen tension in the testis and epididymis. *J Reprod Fertil* 1962;3:377–395.
247. Crowe R, Milner R, Lincoln J, Burnstock G. Histochemical and biochemical investigation of adrenergic, cholinergic and peptidergic innervation of the rat ventral prostate 8 weeks after streptozotocin diabetes. *J Auton Nerv Syst* 1987;20:103–112.
248. Cummins JM, Temple-Smith PD, Renfree MB. Reproduction in the male honey possum (Tarsipes rostratus; Marsupialia): the epididymis. *Am J Anat* 1986;177:385–401.
249. Cuthbert AW, Wong PYD. Intracellular potentials in cells of seminiferous tubules of rats. *J Physiol* 1975;248:173–191.
250. Dacheux JL. Interactions de l'environment sur l'activite metabolique, la motilite et le pouvoir fecondant des sperrnatozoides en fonction de leur etat de maturation. *D. Sc. Thesis,* Universite Francois-Rabelais, Tours, France. 1980.
251. Dacheux JL, O'Shea T, Paquinon M. Effects of osmolality, bicarbonate and buffer on the metabolism and motility of testicular, epididymal and ejaculated spermatozoa of boars. *J Reprod Fertil* 1979;55:287–296.
252. Dacheux JL, Pisselet C, Blanc MR, Hochereau-de Reviers MT, Courot M. Seasonal variations in rete testis fluid secretion and sperm production in different breeds of ram. *J Reprod Fertil* 1981;61:363–371.
253. Dacheux JL, Dacheux F, Paquignon M. Changes in sperm surface membrane and luminal protein fluid content during epididymal transit in the boar. *Biol Reprod* 1989;40:635–651.
254. Daehlin L, Damber JE, Selstam G, Bergman B. Effects of human chorionic gonadotrophin, oestradiol and estromustine on testicular blood flow in hypophysectomized rats. *Int J Androl* 1985;8:58–68.
255. Daehlin L, Damber JE, Selstam G, Bergman B. Testosterone-induced decrement of prostatic vascular resistance in rats is reversed by estrogens. *Prostate* 1985;6:351–359.
256. Dahl EV, Herrick JF. A vascular mechanism for maintaining testicular temperature by counter-current exchange. *Surg Gynecol Obstet* 1959;108:697–705.
257. Damber JE. The effect of guanethidine treatment on testicular blood flow and testosterone production in rats. *Experientia* 1990;46:486–487.
258. Damber JE, Bergh A. Testicular microcirculation—a forgotten essential in andrology? *Int J Androl* 1992;15:285–292.
259. Damber JE, Janson PO. Methodological aspects of testicular blood flow measurements in rats. *Acta Physiol Scand* 1977;101:278–285.
260. Damber JE, Janson PO. Testicular blood flow and testosterone concentrations in spermatic venous blood of anaesthetized rats. *J Reprod Fertil* 1978;52:265–269.
261. Damber JE, Janson PO. The effects of LH, adrenaline and noradrenaline on testicular blood flow and plasma testosterone concentrations in anaesthetized rats. *Acta Endocrinol* 1978;88:391–396.
262. Damber JE, Lindgren S, Nasman B. Testicular blood flow and oxygen tension in unilaterally orchidectomized rats. *Experientia* 1977;33:635–636.
263. Damber JE, Bergh A, Janson PO. Testicular blood flow and testosterone concentration in the spermatic venous blood in rats with experimental unilateral cryptorchidism. *Acta Endocrinol* 1978;88:611–618.
264. Damber JE, Selstam G, Wang J. Inhibitory effect of estradiol-17β on human chorionic gonadotropin-induced increment of testicular blood flow and plasma testosterone concentrations in rats. *Biol Reprod* 1981;25:555–559.
265. Damber JE, Lindahl O, Selstam G, Tenland T. Testicular blood flow measured with a laser Doppler flowmeter: acute effects of catecholamines. *Acta Physiol Scand* 1982;115:209–215.

266. Damber JE, Lindahl O, Selstam G, Tenland T. Rhythmical oscillations in rat testicular microcirculation as recorded by laser Doppler flowmetry. *Acta Physiol Scand* 1983;118:117–123.
267. Damber JE, Bergh A, Daehlin L. Testicular blood flow, vascular permeability and testosterone production after stimulation of unilaterally cryptorchid adult rats with human chorionic gonadotropin. *Endocrinology* 1985;117:1906–1913.
268. Damber JE, Bergh A, Fagrell B, Lindahl O, Rooth P. Testicular microcirculation in the rat studied by videophotometric capillaroscopy, fluorescence microscopy and laser Doppler flowmetry. *Acta Physiol Scand* 1986;126:371–376.
269. Damber JE, Bergh A, Widmark A. Effect of an LHRH-agonist on testicular microcirculation in hypophysectomized rats. *Int J Androl* 1987;10:785–791.
270. Damber JE, Bergh A, Widmark A. Testicular blood flow and microcirculation in rats after treatment with ethane dimethyl sulfonate. *Biol Reprod* 1987;37:1291–1296.
271. Damber JE, Bergh A, Widmark A. Age-related differences in testicular microcirculation. *Int J Androl* 1990;13:197–206.
272. Damber JE, Maddocks S, Widmark A, Bergh A. Testicular blood flow and vasomotion can be maintained by testosterone in Leydig cell-depleted rats. *Int J Androl* 1992;15:385–393.
273. Daniel PM, Gale MM, Pratt OE. Hormones and related substances in the lymph leaving four endocrine glands - the testis, ovary, adrenal and thyroid. *Lancet* 1963;1:1232–1234.
274. Danzo BJ, Eller BC. The ontogeny of biologically active androgen-binding protein in rat plasma, testis and epididymis. *Endocrinology* 1985;117:1380–1388.
275. Danzo BJ, Cooper TG, Orgebin-Cnst MC. Androgen binding protein (ABP) in fluids collected from the rete testis and cauda epididymis of sexually mature and immature rabbits and observations on morphological changes in the epididymis following ligation of the ductuli efferentes. *Biol Reprod* 1977;17:64–77.
276. Davidoff MS, Breucker H, Holstein AF, Seidl K. Cellular architecture of the lamina propria of human seminiferous tubules. *Cell Tiss Res* 1990;262:253–261.
277. Davies DV, Mann T. Functional development of accessory glands and spermatogenesis. *Nature* 1947;160:295.
278. Davies J, Danzo BJ. Hormonally responsive areas of the reproductive system of the male guinea pig. 1. Morphology. *Biol Reprod* 1981;25:1135–1147.
279. Davies RV, Main SJ, Setchell BP. Inhibin in ram rete testis fluid. *J Reprod Fertil Suppl* 1979;26:87–95.
280. Davis JR. Myogenic tone of the rat testicular subcapsular artery has a role in autoregulation of testicular blood supply. *Biol Reprod* 1990;42:727–735.
281. Davis JR, Horowitz AM. Effect of various exposure times to hyperthermia and hypothermia on spontaneous contractions of the adult rabbit isolated testicular capsule. *Biol Reprod* 1979;21:413–417.
282. Davis JR, Langford GA. Response of the testicular capsule to acetylcholine and noradrenaline. *Nature* 1969;222:386–387.
283. Davis JR, Langford GA. Response of the isolated testicular capsule of the rat to autonomic drugs. *J Reprod Fertil* 1969;19:595–598.
284. Davis JR, Langford GA. Pharmacological studies on the testicular capsule in relation to sperm transport. Adv. *Exp Med Biol* 1970;10:495–514.
285. Davis JR, Langford GA. Comparative responses of the isolated testicular capsule and parenchyma to autonomic drugs. *J Reprod Fertil* 1971;26:241–246.
286. Davis JR, Langford GA, Kirby PJ. The testicular capsule. In: Johnson AD, Gomes WR, Vandemark NL eds, *The Testis, Vol. 1,* New York: Academic Press, 1970; pp.281–337.
287. Dawson RMC, Rowlands IW. Glycerylphosphorylcholine in the male reproductive organs of rats and guinea pigs. *Q J Exp Physiol* 1959;44:26–34.
288. Dawson RMC, Mann T, White IG. Glycerylphosphorylcholine and phosphorycholine in semen, and their relation to choline. *Biochem J* 1957;65:627–634.
289. Deaver DR, Amann RP, Hammerstedt RH, Ball R, Veeramachneni DNR, Musacchia XJ. Effects of caudal elevation on testicular function in rats. Separation of effects on spermatogenesis and steroidogenesis. *J Androl* 1992;13:224–231.
290. Del Fiacco M. Enkephalin-like immunoreactivity in the human male genital tract. *J Anat* 1982;135:649–656.
291. Delongeas JL, Gelly JL, Leheup B, Grignon G. Influence of testicular secretions on differentiation in the rat epididymis: ultrastructural studies after castration, efferent duct ligation and cryptorchidism. *Exp Cell Biol* 1987;55:74–82.
292. Dent J, Hodson N, Selhi H. Ultrastructural differentiation of fibre types in rabbit seminal vesicles. *J Physiol* 1971;217:7P–9P.
293. Desjardins C. The microcirculation of the testis. *Ann NY Acad Sci* 1989;64:243–249.
294. Dhabuwala CB, Pierrepoint CG. Venous drainage and functional control of the canine prostate gland. *J Endocrinol* 1977;75:105–108.
295. Dhabuwala CB, Kumar AB, Kerkar PD, Bhutwala A, Pierce J. Patterns of Doppler recordings and its relationship to varicocele in infertile men. *Int J Androl* 1989;12:430–438.
296. Dhingra LD. Mediastinum testis. In: Johnson D, Gomes WR, eds. *The Testis, Vol. IV,* New York: Academic Press, 1977; pp. 451–460.
297. Dierachs R, Wrobel KH. Licht-und elektronenenmikroskopische Untersuchungen an der peritubularen Zellen des Schweinhodens wahrend der postnatalen Entwicklung. *Z Anat Entwickl* 1973;143:49–64.
298. Djakiew D, Griswold MD, Lewis DM, Dym M. Micropuncture studies of receptor-mediated endocytosis of transferrin in the rat epididymis. *Biol Reprod* 1986;34:691–699.
299. Dube D, Poyet P, Pelletier G, Labrie F. Radioautographic localization of beta adrenergic receptors in the rat ventral prostate. *J Androl* 1986;7:169–174.
300. Dym M. The fine structure of the monkey (*Macaca*) Sertoli cell and its role in maintaining the blood-testis barrier. *Anat Rec* 1973;175:639–656.
301. Dym M. The fine structure of monkey Senoli cells in the transitional zone at the junction of the seminiferous tubules with the tubuli recti. *Am J Anat* 1974;140:1–26.
302. Dym M. The mammalian rete testis a morphological examination. *Anat Rec* 1976;186:493–524.
303. Dym M, Cavicchia JC. Further observations on the blood-testis barrier in monkeys. *Biol Reprod* 1977;17:390–403.
304. Dym M, Fawcett DW. The blood-testis barrier in the rat and the physiological compartmentation of the seminiferous epithelium. *Biol Reprod* 1970;3:308–326.
305. Dziuk PJ, Mann T. Effect of atropine on the composition of semen and secretory function of male accessory organs in the boar. *J Reprod Fertil* 1963;5:101–108.
306. Eckstein P, Zuckerman S. Morphology of the reproductive tract. In: Parkes AS, ed. *Marshall's Physiology of Reproduction, 3rd ed Vol 1,* London: Longmans, 1956; pp. 43–155.
307. Edwards EM, Jones AR, Waites GMH. The entry of α-chlorhydrin into body fluids of male rats and its effect upon incorporation of glycerol into lipids. *J Reprod Fertil* 1975;43:225–232.
308. Eik-Nes KB. On the relationship between testicular blood flow and secretion of testosterone in anesthetized dogs stimulated with human chorionic gonadotrophin. *Can J Physiol Pharmacol* 1964;42:671–677.
309. Einarsson S. Studies on the composition of epididymal content and semen in the boar. *Acta Vet Scand (Suppl)* 1971;36:1–80.
310. Einarsson S, Crabo B, Ekman L. A comparative study on the chemical composition of plasma from the cauda epididymidis, semen fractions, and whole semen in boars. *Acta Vet Scand* 1970;11:156–180.
311. Einer-Jensen N. Local recirculation of ^{133}-xenon and ^{85}-krypton to the testes and caput epididymidis in rats. *J Reprod Fertil* 1974;37:55–60.
312. Einer-Jensen N, Soofi G. Decreased blood flow through rat testis after intratesticular injection of PGF-2α. *Prostaglandins* 1974;7:377–382.
313. Einer-Jensen N, Waites GMH. Testicular blood flow and a study of the testicular venous to arterial transfer of radioactive krypton and testosterone in the rhesus monkey. *J Physiol* 1977;267:1–15.
314. Eisenberg F, Bolden AH. Biosynthesis of inositol in rat testis homogenate. *Biochem Biophys Res Commun* 1963;12:7277.
315. Eisenberg F, Bolden AH. Reproductive tract as site of synthesis

and secretion of inositol in the male rat. *Nature* 1964;202: 559–560.

316. El-Badawi A, Goodman DC. Autonomic innervation of accessory male genital glands. In: Spring-Mills E, Hafez ESE, eds. *Male Accessory Sex Glands,* Amsterdam: Elsevier/North-Holland, 1980;101–128.
317. El-Badawi A, Schenk EA. The distribution of cholinergic and adrenergic nerves in the mammalian epididymis. A comparative histochemical study. *Am J Anat* 1967;121:1–14.
318. Elder JS, Isaacs JT, Walsh PC. Androgenic sensitivity of the gubernaculum testis: evidence for hormonal/mechanical interactions in testicular descent. *J Urol* 1982;127:170–176.
319. Eliasson R. Studies on prostaglandin. Occurrence, formation and biological actions. *Acta Physiol Scand (Suppl)* 1959;46: 158–173.
320. Eliasson R. Accurate determination of glucose in human semen. *J Reprod Fertil* 1965;9:325–330.
321. Ellis LC, Buhrley LE. Inhibitory effects of melatonin, prostaglandin E-1, cyclic AMP, dibutyryl cyclic AMP and theophyline on rat seminiferous tubular contractility in vitro. *Biol Reprod* 1978;19:217–222.
322. Ellis LC, Buhrley LE, Hargrove JL. Species differences in contractility of seminiferous tubules and tunica albuginea as related to sperm transport through the testis. *Arch Androl* 1978;1:139–146.
323. Elwishy AB, Mobarak AM, Fouad SM. The accessory genital organs of the one-humped male camel (*Camelus dromedarius*). *Anat Anz* 1972;131:1–12.
324. Emoto M, Kita E, Nishikawa F, Katsui N, Yagyu Y, Kashiba S. Biological functions of mouse seminal vesicle fluid I. Suppression of blastogenic responses of lymphocytes. *Arch Androl* 1990;24:35–40.
325. Engeset A. The route of peripheral lymph to the blood stream. An X-ray study of the barrier theory. *J Anat* 1959;93:96–100.
326. Esperanca-Pina JA, Pais D, Goyri-O'Neill JE. Arter spermatique du rat albimos segment spirale. *Bull Assoc Anat (Nancy)* 1985;69:377–388.
327. Esponda P, Bedford JM. The influence of body temperature and castration on the protein composition of fluid in the rat cauda epididymis. *J Reprod Fert* 1986;78:505–514.
328. Evans RW, Setchell BP. Lipid changes in boar spermatozoa during epididymal maturation, with some observations on the flow and composition of boar rete testis fluid. *J Reprod Fertil* 1979;57:189–196.
329. Ewing L, Brown B, Irby DC, Jardine J. Testosterone and 5α-reduced androgen secretion by rabbit testes-epididymides perfused *in vitro. Endocrinology* 1975;96:610–617.
330. Ewing LL, Zirkin BR, Cochran RC, Kromann N, Peters C, Ruiz-Bravo N. Testosterone secretion by rat, rabbit, guinea pig, dog, and hamster testes perfused *in vitro:* correlation with Leydig cell mass. *Endocrinology* 1979;15:1135–1142.
331. Ewing LL, Thompson DL, Cochran RC, Lasley BL, Thompson MA, Zirkin BR. Testicular androgen and estrogen secretion and benign prostatic hyperplasia in the beagle. *Endocrinology* 1984;14:1308–1314.
332. Ezeasor DN. Ultrastructural observations on the terminal segment epithelium of the seminiferous tubule of West African dwarf goats. *J Anat* 1986;144:167–179.
333. Fahimi F, Bieber L, Lewin LM. The sources of carnitine in human semen. *J Androl* 1981;2:339–342.
334. Fair WR, Clark RB, Wehner N. A correlation of seminal polyamine levels and semen analysis in the human. *Fertil Steril* 1972;23:38–42.
335. Fawcett DW. Observations on the organization of the interstitial tissue of the testis and on the occluding cell junctions in the seminiferous epithelium. *Adv Biosci* 1973;10:83–99.
336. Fawcett DW. Ultrastructure and function of the Sertoli cell. In: Hamilton DW, Greep RO, eds. *Handbook of Physiology, Section 7-Endocrinology Vol V.,* Washington, D.C.: American Physiological Society, 1975;21–55.
337. Fawcett DW, Dym M. A glycogen-rich segment of the tubuli recti and proximal portion of the rete testis in the guinea pig. *J Reprod Fertil* 1974;38:401–409.
338. Fawcett DW, Hoffer AP. Failure of exogenous androgen to prevent regression of the initial segments of the rat epididymis after efferent duct ligation or orchidectomy. *Biol Reprod* 1979;20: 162–181.
339. Fawcett DW, Heidger PJ, Leak LV. The lymph-vascular system of the interstitial tissue of the testis as revealed by electron microscopy. *J Reprod Fertil* 1969;19:109–119.
340. Fawcett DW, Leak LV, Heidger PM. Electron microscopic observations on the structural components of the blood-testis barrier. *J Reprod Fertil* 1970; Suppl. 10:105–119.
341. Fawcett DW, Neaves WB, Flores MN. Comparative observations on intertubular lymphatics and the organization of the interstitial tissue of the mammalian testis. *Biol Reprod* 1973;9:500–512.
342. Faye JC, Duguet L, Mazzuca M, Bayard F. Purification, radioimmunoassay, and immunohistochemical localization of a glycoprotein produced by the rat epididymis. *Biol Reprod* 1980;23:423–432.
343. Fedan JS, Hogaboom GK, O'Donnell JP, Colby J, Westfall DP. Contribution by purines to the neurogenic response of the vas deferens of the guinea pig. *Eur J Pharmacol* 1981;69:41–53.
344. Fehlings K, Pohlmeyer K. Die Arteria testicularis und ihre Aufzweigung im Hoden und Nebenhoden des Esels (*Equus africanus f. asinus*). Korrosionsanatomische und rontgenologische Untersuchungen. *Anat Histol Embryol* 1978;7:74–78.
345. Feig LA, Bellve AR, Erickson NH, Klagsbum M. Sertoli cells contain a mitogenic polypeptide. *Proc Natl Acad Sci USA* 1980;77:4774–4778.
346. Firlit CF, King LR, Davis IR. Comparative responses of the isolated human testicular capsule to autonomic drugs. *J Urol* 1975;113:500–504.
347. Fjellstrom D, Kihlstrom JE. On the concentrations of some inorganic ions and protein nitrogen in rabbit seminal fluid. *J Reprod Fertil* 1975;44:559–560.
348. Fleet IR, Laurie MS, Noordhuizen-Stassen EN, Setchell BP, Wensing CJG. The flow of blood from artery to vein in the spermatic cord of the ram, with some observations on reactive hyperaemia in the testis and the effects of adenosine and noradrenaline. *J Physiol* 1982;332:44P–45P.
349. Flickinger CJ, Howards SS, English HF. Ultrastructural differences in efferent ducts and several regions of the epididymis of the hamster. *Am J Anat* 1978;152:557–586.
350. Flocks RH. The arterial distribution within the prostate gland: its role in transurethral prostatic resection. *J Urol* 1937;37: 524–548.
351. Foldesy RG, Leathem JH. Simultaneous measurements of testosterone and three 5a-reduced androgens in the venous effluent of immature rat testes *in situ. Steroids* 1980;35:621–631.
352. Foldesy RG, Leathem JH. Pubertal changes in androgen composition of rat rete testis and cauda epididymal fluids. *J Ster Biochem* 1981;14:109–110.
353. Forti G, Toscano V, Casilli D, Maroder M, Balducci R, Adamo MV, Santoro S, Grisolia GA, Pampaloni A, Serio M. Spermatic and peripheral venous plasma concentrations of testosterone, 17-hydroxyprogesterone, androstenedione, dehydroepiandrosterone, Δ5-androstene-3β,17β-diol, dihydrotestosterone, 5α-androstane-3α,17β-diol, 5α-androstane-3β,17β-diol, and estradiol in boys with idiopathic varicocele in different stages of puberty. *J Clin Endocrinol Metabol* 1985;61:322–327.
354. Foster ME, Jones AS, Eccles R. Epididymal and testicular temperature in the anaesthetized rat. *IRCS Med Sci* 1983;11: 234–235.
355. Fouquet JP. Secretion of free glucose and related carbohydrates in the male accessory organs of rodents. *Comp. Biochem Physiol* 1971;40A:305–317.
356. Fowler DG. The relationship between air temperature and scrotal surface area and testis temperature in rams. *Aust J Exp Agric Anim Husb* 1969;9:258–261.
357. Fowler DG, Setchell BP. Selecting Merino rams for ability to withstand infertility caused by heat. 2. Effect of heat on scrotal and testicular blood flow. *Aust J Exp Agric Anim Husb* 1971;11:143–147.
358. Fowler R, Stephens FD. The role of testicular vascular anatomy in the salvage of high undescended testes. *Aust N Z J Surg* 1959;29:92–106.

359. Frankel AI, Mock EJ. A study of the first eight hours in the stabilization of plasma testosterone concentration in the hemicastrated rat. *J Endocrinol* 1982;92:225–229.
360. Frankel AI, Ryan EL. Testicular innervation is necessary for the response of plasma testosterone levels to acute stress. *Biol Reprod* 1981;24:491–495.
361. Frankel AI, Mock EJ, Chapman JC. Hypophysectomy and hemivasectomy can inhibit the testicular hemicastration response of the mature rat. *Biol Reprod* 1984;30:804–808.
362. Frankenhuis MT, Wensing CJG. Induction of spermatogenesis in the naturally cryptorchid pig. *Fertil Steril* 1979;31:428–433.
363. Free MJ. Blood supply to the testis and its role in local exchange and transport of hormones. In: Johnson AD, Gomes WR eds. *The Testis, Vol IV,* New York: Academic Press. 1977; 39–90.
364. Free MJ. "Leaky" membranes in the male reproductive tract: a discussion of unusual molecular exchanges between different fluid compartments. In: Steinberger A, Steinberger E. eds. *Testicular Development, Structure and Function* New York: Raven Press. 1980;281.
365. Free MJ, Jaffe RA. Dynamics of circulation in the testis of the conscious rat. *Am J Physiol* 1972;223:241–248.
366. Free MJ, Jaffe RA. Effect of prostaglandins on blood flow and pressure in the testis of the conscious rat. *Prostaglandins* 1972;I:483–498.
367. Free MJ, Jaffe RA. Collection of rete testis fluid from rats without previous efferent duct ligation. *Biol Reprod* 1979;20: 269–278.
368. Free MJ, Nguyen Duc Kien. Venous arterial interactions involving serotonin in the pampiniform plexus of the rat. *Proc Soc Exp Biol Med* 1973;143:284–288.
369. Free MJ, Tilson SA. Secretion rate of testicular steroids in the conscious and halothane anesthetized rat. *Endocrinology* 1973;93:874–878.
370. Free MJ, Jaffe RA, Morford DE. Sperm transport through the rete testis of anesthetized rats: role of the testicular capsule and effect of gonadotropins and prostaglandins. *Biol Reprod* 1980;22:1073–1078.
371. French FS, Ritzen EM. A high affinity androgen binding protein (ABP) in rat testis. Evidence for secretion into efferent duct fluid and absorption by the epididymis. *Endocrinology* 1973;93: 88–95.
372. French FS, Ritzen EM. Androgen-binding protein in efferent duct fluid of rat testis. *J Reprod Fertil* 1973;32:479–483.
373. Frenette G, Dube JY, Lazure C, Paradis G, Chretien M, Tremblay RR. The major 40-kDa glycoprotein in human prostatic fluid is identical to Zn-α2-glycoprotein. *Prostate* 1987;11: 257–270.
374. Frenkel G, Peterson RN, Davis JE, Freund M. Glycerylphosphorylcholine and carnitine in normal human semen and in postvasectomy semen: differences in concentrations. *Fertil Steril* 1974;25:84–87.
375. Frey HL, Rajfer J. Role of the gubernaculum and intraabdominal pressure in the process of testicular descent. *J Urol* 1984;131:574–579.
376. Fritjofsson A, Persson JE, Pettersson S. Testicular blood flow in man measured with xenon-133. *Scand J Urol Nephrol* 1969;3:276–280.
377. Fritjofsson A, Kvist U, Ronquist G. Anatomy of the prostate. Aspects of the secretory function in relation to lobar structure. *Scand J Urol Nephrol* 1988;Suppl. 107:5–13.
378. Fritz IB, Burdzy K, Setchell BP, Blaschuk O. Ram rete testis fluid contains a protein (clusterin) which influences cell-cell interactions *in vitro. Biol Reprod* 1983;28:1173–1188.
379. Fritz IB, Lyon MF, Setchell BP. Evidence for a defective seminiferous tubular barrier in the testes of Tfm and Sxr mice. *J Reprod Fertil* 1983;67:359–363.
380. Furness JB, Iwayama T. The arrangement and identification of axons innervating the vas deferens of the guinea-pig. *J Anat* 1972;113:179–196.
381. Furusato M, Mostofi FK. Intraprostatic lymphatics in man: light and ultrastructural observations. *Prostate* 1980;1:15–23.
382. Fussell EN, Lewis RW, Roberts JA, Harrison RM. Early ultrastructural findings in experimentally produced vaicocele in the monkey testis. *J Androl* 1981;2:111–119.
383. Galil KAA. Effects of high environmental temperature on the testis. *PhD Thesis,* University of Cambridge, Cambridge. 1982.
384. Galil KAA, Setchell BP. Effects of local heating of the testis on testicular blood flow and testosterone secretion in the rat. *Int J Androl* 1988;11:73–85.
385. Galil KAA, Laurie MS, Main SJ, Setchell BP. The measurement of the flow of lymph from the testis. *J Physiol* 1981;319:17P.
386. Gamble WG, Keller GA. Testicular infarction associated with incarcerated inguinal hernia. *Minn Med* 1987;70:529–532.
387. Ganjam VK, Amann RP. Steroids in fluids and sperm entering and leaving the bovine epididymis, epididymal tissue and accessory sex gland secretions. *Endocrinology* 1976;99:1618–1630.
388. Garberi JC, Kohane AC, Cameo MS, Blaquier JA. Isolation and characterization of specific rat epididymal proteins. *Mol Cell Endocrinol* 1979;13:72–82.
389. Gaudin J, Lefevre C, Person H, Nguyen-Huu, Senecail B. The venous hilum of the testis and epididymis: anatomic aspect. *Surg Radiol Anat* 1988;10:233–242.
390. Gawienowski AM, Orsulak PJ, Stacewicz-Sapuntzakis M, Joseph BM. Presence of sex pheromone in preputial glands of male rats. *J Endocrinol* 1975;67:283–288.
391. Geesaman B, Villanueva-Meyer J, Bluestein D, Miller L, Mena I, Rajfer J. Effects of multiple injections of HCG on testicular blood flow. *Urology* 1992;40:81–83.
392. Gerard A, Khanfri J, Gueant JL, Fremont S, Nicolas JP, Grignon G, Gerard H. Electron microscopc radioautorgraphic evidence of in vivo androgen-binding protein internalization in the rat epididymis principal cells. *Endocrinology* 1988;122: 1297–1307.
393. Gerard H, Gueant JL, Gerard A, Fremont S, el Harate A, Nicolas JP, Grignon G. Endocytosis of the androgen-binding protein (ABP) by the principal cells of rat epididymis. *Reprod Nutr Dev* 1988;28:1257–1266.
394. Gerendai I, Nemeskeri A, Csernus V. Depending on the dose 6-OHDA stimulates of inhibits thee testis of immature rats. *Exp Clin Endocr* 1984;84:27–36.
395. Gerendai I, Nemeeskeri A, Csernus V, Halasz B. Effect of simultaneous local injection of 6-hydroxydopamine and naloxone on the testis of neonatal rats. *Andrologia* 1989;21:449–455.
396. Gerendai I, Shaha C, Thau R, Bardin CW. Do testicular opiates regulate Leydig cell function? *Endocrinology* 1984;115: 1645–1647.
397. Gerozissis K, Jouannet P, Soufir JC, Dray F. Origin of prostaglandins in human semen. *J Reprod Fertil* 1982;65:401–404.
398. Gier HT, Marion GB. Development of the mammalian testis. In: *The Testis Vol. I,* edited by A. D. Johnson, W. R. Gomes, and N. L. Vandemark, pp. 1–45. Academic Press, New York.
399. Gilbert P, Wetterauer U, Wokalek H. Histological changes in rat testicles after short-term ischaemia. *Urol Int* 1986;41:145–148.
400. Gilula NB, Fawcett DW, Aoki A. The Sertoli cell occluding junctions and gap junctions in mature and developing mammalian testes. *Dev Biol* 1976;50:142–168.
401. Gizang-Ginsberg E, Wolgemuth DJ. Localization of mRNAs in mouse testes by *in situ* hybridization: distribution of (αtubulin and developmental stage specificity of pro-opiomelanocortin transcripts. *Dev Biol* 1985;111:293–305.
402. Glad-Sorensen H, Lambrechtsen J, Einer-Jensen N. Efficiency of the countercurrent transfer of heat and ^{133}Xenon between the pampiniform plexus and testicular artery of the bull under invitrop conditions. *Int J Androl* 1991;14:232–240.
403. Gladwell RT. The effect of temperature on the potential difference and input resistance of rat seminiferous tubules. *J Physiol* 1977;268:111–121.
404. Glode LM, Robinson J, Horwitz LD. Scrotal hypothermia and testicular blood flow in the dog. *J Androl* 1984;5:227–229.
405. Glover TD. Changes in blood flow in the testis and epididymis of the rat following artificial cryptorchidism. *Acta Endocrinol (Suppl)* 100:38.
406. Glover TD. The influence of temperature on flow of blood in the testis and scrotum of rats. *Proc R Soc Med* 1966;59:765–766.
407. Glover TD, Nicander L. Some aspects of structure and function

in the mammalian epididymis. *J Reprod Fertil (Suppl)*, 1971;13:39–50.
408. Godinho HP, Setchell BP. Total and capillary blood flow through the testes of anaesthetized rams. *J Physiol* 1975; 251:19P.
409. Gorgas K, Bock P. Myofibroblasts in the rat testicular capsule. *Cell Tiss Res* 1974;154:533–541.
410. Gosling JA, Dixon JS. Differences in the manner of autonomic innervation of the muscle layers of the guinea-pig ductus deferens. *J Anat* 1972;112:81–91.
411. Gower DB, Hamson FA, Heap RB. The identification of C19-16-unsaturated steroids and estimation of 17-oxosteroids in boar spermatic vein plasma and urine. *J Endocrinol* 1970;47:357–368.
412. Goyal HO. Morphology of the ovine epididymis. *Am J Anat* 1985;172:155–172.
413. Goyal HO, Williams CS. The rete tesits of the goat, a morphological study. *Acta Anat (Basel).* 1987;130:151–157.
414. Goyal HO, Hrudka F. Ductuli efferentes of the bull—a morphological, experimental and developmental study. *Andrologia* 1981;13:292–306.
415. Goyal HO, Hutto V, Robinson DD. Reexamination of the morphology of the extratesticular rete and ductuli efferentes in the goat. *Anat Rec* 1992;233:53–60.
416. Gray BW, Brown BG, Ganjam VK, Whitesides JF. Effect of deprival of rete testis fluid on the morphology of efferent ductules. *Biol Reprod* 1983;29:525–534.
417. Gray TJB, Gangalli SD. Aspects of the testicular toxicity of phthalate esters. *Environ Health Persp* 1986;65:229–235.
418. Green KF, Turner TT, Howards SS. Varicocele: reversal of the testicular blood flow and temperature effects by varicocele repair. *J Urol* 1984;131:1208–1211.
419. Green KF, Turner TT, Howards SS. Effects of varicocele after unilateral orchidectomy and sympathectomy. *J Urol* 1985;134: 378–383.
420. Greenberg J, Forssmann WG, Gorgas K. Morphology and innervation of a testicular 'rete mirabile' in the guinea pig. *Anat Embryol (Berlin)* 1985;173:225–235.
421. Greenberg J, Schubert W, Metz J, Yanaihara N, Forssmann W-G. Studies of the guinea-pig epididymis. III. Innervation of epididymal segments. *Cell Tiss Res* 1985;239:395–404.
422. Groschel-Stewan U, Unsicker K. Direct visualization of contractile proteins in peritubular cells of the guinea-pig testis using antibodies against highly purified actin and myosin. *Histochemistry* 1977;51:315–319.
423. Gu J, Polak JM, Probert L, Islam KN, Marangos PJ, Mina S, Adrian TE, McGregor GP, O'Shaughnessy DJ, Bloom SR. Peptidergic innervation of the human male genital tract. *J Urol* 1983;130:386–391.
424. Guerrero R, Ritzen EM, Purvis K, Hansson V, French FS. Concentration of steroid hormones and androgen binding protein (ABP) in rabbit efferent duct fluid. *Curr Top Mol Endocrinol* 1975;2:213–221.
425. Guerrier D, Tran D, Vanderwinden JM, Hideux S, van Outryve L, Legeai L, Bouchard M, van Vliet G, de Laet MH, Picard JY, Kahn A, Josso N. The persistent Mullerian duct syndrome: A molecular approach. *J Clin Endocr Metab* 1989;68:46–52.
426. Gunsalus GL, Musto NA, Bardin CW. Factors affecting blood levels of androgen binding protein in the rat. *Int J Androl* 1978;Suppl. 2:482–493.
427. Gunsalus GL, Musto NA, Bardin CW. Bidirectional release of a Sertoli cell product, androgen binding protein, into the blood and seminiferous tubule. In: Steinberger A and Steinberger E, eds. *Testicular Development, Structure and Function.* New York: Raven Press, 291–297.
428. Gunsalus GL, Musto NA, Bardin CW, Kunz HW, Gill TJ. Rats homozygous for the grc complex have defective transport of androgen-binding protein to the epididymis, but normal secretion into the blood. *Biol Reprod* 1985;33:1057–1063.
429. Gupta RK, Barnes GW, and Skelton FR. Light microscopic and immunopathologic observations of cadmium chloride-induced injury in mature rat testis. *Am J Pathol* 1967;51:191–205.
430. Gustafson AW, Shemesh M. Changes in plasma testosterone levels during the annual reproductive cycle of the hibernating bat, *Myotis lucifugus lucifugus* with a survey of plasma testosterone levels in adult male vertebrates. *Biol Reprod* 1976;15:9–24.
431. Gustafsson K, Soder O, Pollanen P, Ritzen M. Isolation and partial characterization of an interleukin-1-like factor from rat interstitial fluid. *J Reprod Immunol* 1988;14:139–150.
432. Gutroff RF, Cooke PS, Hess RA. Blind ending tubules and branching patterns of the rat ductuli efferentes. *Anat Rec* 1992;232:423–431.
433. Haans LCF, Laven JSE, Mali WPTM, te Velde ER, Wensing CJG. Testis volume, semen quality, and hormonal patterns in adolescent with and without a varicocele. *Fertil Steril* 1991;56:731–736.
434. Habenicht UF, Neumann F, El Etreby MF. Short-term effects of an LHRH-agonist alone or in combination with testosterone propionate or indomethacin on rat testes. Evidences of testosterone independent effects. I. *Andrologia* 1987;19:602–613.
435. Hagenas L, Ritzen EM, Suginami H. Hormonal milieu of the seminiferous tubules in the normal and cryptorchid rat. *Int J Androl* 1978;1:477–484.
436. Hamilton DW. Structure and function of the epithelium lining the ductuli efferentes, ductus epididymidis and ductus deferens in the rat. In: Hamilton DW and Greep RO, eds. *Handbook of Physiology, Vol. V.* Washington, D.C: American Physiological Society, 1975;259–301.
437. Hamilton DW. UDP-galactose: N-acetylglucosamine galactosyltransferase in fluids from rat rete testis and epididymis. *Biol Reprod* 1980;23:377–385.
438. Hamilton DW. Evidence for α-lactalbumin-like activity in rat male reproductive fluids. *Biol Reprod* 1981;25:385–392.
439. Hamilton DW, Cooper TG. Gross and histological variations along the length of the rat vas deferens. *Anat Rec* 1978;190:795–810.
440. Hammerstedt RH, Rowan WA. Phosphatidylcholine of blood lipoprotein is the precursor of glycerophosphorylcholine found in seminal plasma. *Biochim Biophys Acta* 1982;710:370–376.
441. Hammond GL, Ruokonen A, Kontturi M, Koskela E, Vikho R. The simultaneous radioimmunoassay of seven steroids in human spermatic and penpheral venous blood. *J Clin Endocrinol* 1977;45:16–24.
442. Handelsman DJ, Spaliviero JA, Turtle JR. Testicular function in experimental uremia. *Endocrinology* 1985;117:1974–1983.
443. Haraldsson B, Reger L, Weiss L, Jansson I, Hultborn R. Blood-to-tissue transport of albumin in rat fibrosarcomas at two different implantation sites. *Acta Physiol Scand* 1987;131:93–101.
444. Harcourt AH, Harvey PH, Larson SG, Short RV. Testis weight, body weight and breeding systems in primates. *Nature* 1981;293:55–57.
445. Hargrove JL, Ellis LC. Autonomic nerves versus prostaglandins in the control of rat and rabbit testicular capsular contractions *in vivo* and *in vitro*. *Biol Reprod* 1976;14:651–657.
446. Hargrove JL, Johnson JM, Ellis LC. Prostaglandin E-1 induced inhibition of rabbit testicular contractions *in vitro*. *Proc Soc Exp Biol Med* 1971;136:958–961.
447. Hargrove JL, Seeley RR, Johnson JM, Ellis LC. Prostaglandin-like substances: initiation and maintenance of rabbit testicular contraction *in vitro*. *Proc Soc Exp Biol Med* 1973;142:205–209.
448. Hargrove JL, Seeley RR, Ellis LC. Rabbit testicular contractions: bimodal interaction of prostaglandin E-1 with other agonists. *Am J Physiol* 1975;228:810–814.
449. Harris ME, Bartke A. Concentration of testosterone in testis fluid of the rat. *Endocrinology* 1974;95:701–706.
450. Harris ME, Bartke A. Maintenance of rete testis fluid testosterone and dihydrotestosterone level by pregnenolone and other C21 steroids in hypophysectomized rats. *Endocrinology* 1975;96:1396–1402.
451. Harrison GA. Spermine in human tissues. *Biochem J* 1931;25:1885–1892.
452. Harrison GA. The approximate determinations of spermine in single human organs. *Biochem J* 1933;27:1152–1156.
453. Harrison JD, Tweedie J, Wilson C, Rance C, Kapila L. Measurement of testicular blood flow at orchipexy with a solid state laser. *Surgery* 1991;109:160–162.
454. Harrison RG. Vascular patterns in the testis, with particular reference to *Macropus*. *Nature* 1948;161:399–400.

455. Harrison RG. The comparative anatomy of the blood supply of the mammalian testis. *Proc Zool Soc Lond* 1949;19:325–343.
456. Harrison RG. The distribution of the vasal and cremasteric arteries to the testis and their functional importance. *J Anat* 1949;83:267–282.
457. Harrison RG. Applications of microradiography: The testis. In: *Microarteriography,* edited by AE Barclay, Blackwell, Oxford. 1951:89–90.
458. Harrison RG, Barclay AE. The distribution of the testicular artery (internal spermatic artery) to the human testis. *Br J Urol* 1948;20:5–66.
459. Harrison RG, Oettle AG. Pathologic changes in the rat testis following ischaemia. *Proc Soc Study Fertil* 1950;2:6–11.
460. Harrison RG, Lewis-Jones DI, Moreno deMarval MJ, Connolly RC. Mechanism of damage to the contralateral testis in rats with an ischaemic testis. *Lancet II* 1981:723–725.
461. Harrison RM, Lewis RW, Roberts JA. Pathophysiology of varicocele in nonhuman primates: long-term seminal and testicular changes. *Fertil Steril* 1986;46:500–510.
462. Hartmann CG, Millman N, Stavorski J. Vasodilatation of the rat testis in response to human chorionic gonadotropin. *Fertil Steril* 1950;1:443–453.
463. Hartree EF. Sialic acid in the bulbo-urethral glands of the boar. *Nature* 1962;196:483–484.
464. Hasegawa R, Eisenberg F. Selective hormonal control of myoinositol biosynthesis in reproductive organs and liver of the male rat. *Proc Natl Acad Sci* 1981;78:4863–4866.
465. Haskell JF, Myers RB. Insulin-like growth factor receptors in testicular vascular tissue from normal and diabetic rats. *Adv Exp Med Biol* 1991;293:297–309.
466. Hatier R, Grignon G. Ultrastructural study of Sertoli cells in rat seminiferous tubules during intrauterine life and the postnatal period. *Anat Embryol* 1980;160:11–27.
467. Head JR, Neaves WB, Billingham RE. Reconsideration of the lymphatic drainage of the rat testis. *Transplantation* 1983;35:91–95.
468. Hedger M, Robertson DM, de Kretser DM, Risbridger GP. The quantification of steroidogenesis-stimulating activity in testicular interstitial fluid by an in vitro bioassay employing adult rat Leydig cells. *Endocrinology.* 1990;127:1967–1977.
469. Hedger M, Leung A, Robertson DM, de Kretser DM, Risbridger GP. Steroidogenesis-stimulating activity in the gonalds: comparison of rat testicular interstitial fluid with bovine and human ovarian follicular fluids. *Biol Reprod* 1991;44:937–944.
470. Hedlund H, Andersson KE, Larsson B. Alpha-adrenoreceptors and muscarinic receptors in the isolated human prostate. *J Urol* 1985;134:1291–1298.
471. Hees H, Leiser R, Kohler T, Wrobel KH. Vascular morphology of the bovine spermatic cord and testis 1. Light and scanning electron-microscopic studies on the testicular anery and pampiniform plexus. *Cell Tiss Res* 1984;237:31–38.
472. Hees H, Wrobel KH, Kohler T, Leiser R, Rothbacher I. Spatial topography of the excurrent duct system in the bovine testis. *Cell Tissue Res* 1987;248:143–151.
473. Hees H, Wrobel KH, Kohler T, Abou Elmagd A, Hees I. The mediastinum of the bovine testis. *Cell Tissue Res* 1989; 255:29–39.
474. Hees H, Kohler T, Leiser R, Hees I, Lips T. Gefass-Morphologie des Rinderhodens. Licht- und rasterelektonenmikroskopische Studien. *Anat Anz* 1990;170:119–132.
475. Heindel JJ, Steinberger A, Strada JJ. Identification and characterization of a β_1-adrenergic receptor in the rat Sertoli cell. *Mol Cell Endocrinol* 1981;22:349–358.
476. Heindel RM, Pakyz RE, Cosentino MJ. Spermatic cord torsion. Contralateral testicular degeneration at various ages in the rat. *J Androl* 1990;11:506–513.
477. Hellon RF, Misra NK. Neurones in the dorsal horn of the rat responding to scrotal skin temperature changes. *J Physiol* 1973;232:375–388.
478. Hellon RF, Misra NK. Neurones in the ventrobasal complex of the rat responding to scrotal skin temperature changes. *J Physiol,* 1973;232:389–399.
479. Hellon RF, Mitchell D. Convergence in a thermal afferent pathway in the rat. *J Physiol* 1975;248:359–376.
480. Hellon RF, Taylor DCM. An analysis of a thermal afferent pathway in the rat. *J Physiol* 1973;326:319–328.
481. Hellon RF, Misra NK, Provins KA. Neurones in the somatosensory cortex of the rat responding to scrotal skin temperature changes. *J Physiol* 1973;232:401–411.
482. Hellon RF, Hensel H, Schafer K. Thermal receptors in the scrotum of the rat. *J Physiol* 1975;248:349–357.
483. Hemeida NA, Sack WO, McEntee K. Ductuli efferentes in the epididymis of boar, goat, ram, bull and stallion. *Am J Vet Res* 1978;39:1892–1900.
484. Henning RD, Young JA. Electrolyte transport in the seminiferous tubules of the rat studied by the stopped-flow microperfusion technique. *Experientia,* 1971;27:1037–1039.
485. Henricks DM, Hoover JL, Gimenez T, Grimes LW. A study of the source of estradiol-17 beta in the bull. *Horm Metab Res* 1988;20:494–497.
486. Hepp R, Kreye VAW. Effect of long-term treatment with high doses of guanethidine on sperm transport and fertility of rats. *Br J Pharmacol* 1973;48:30–35.
487. Hermo L, Dworkin J. Transitional cells at the junction of seminiferous tubules with the rete testis of the rat: their fine structure, endocytic activity and basement membrane. *Am J Anat* 1988;181:111–131.
488. Hermo L, Lalli M. Monocytes and mast cells in the limiting membrane of human seminiferous tubules. *Biol Reprod* 1978;19:92–100.
489. Hermo L, Morales C. Endocytosis in non-ciliated cells of the ductuli efferentes in the rat. *Am J Anat* 1984;171:59–64.
490. Hermo L, Lalli M, Clermont Y. Arrangement of connective tissue components in the walls of seminiferous tubules of man and monkey. *Am J Anat* 1977;148:433–446.
491. Hib J, Ponzio R, Vilar O. Contractility of the rat cauda epididymidis and vas deferens during seminal emission. *J Reprod Fertil* 1982;66:47–50.
492. Hienz HA, Voggenthaler J, Weissbach L. Histological findings in testes with varicocele during childhood and their therapeutic consequences. *Eur J Pediatr* 1980;133:139–146.
493. Hijikata T, Saito H, Yohro T. Anatomy and histology of the musk shrew (Suncus murinus) prostate. *Prostate* 1986;8: 277–291.
494. Hill MR, Polock WF, Sprong DH. Testicular infarction and incarcerated inguinal hernias. *Arch Surg* 1962;85:351–354.
495. Himwich HE, Nahum LH. The respiratory quotient of the testicle. *Am J Physiol* 1929;88:680–685.
496. Hinton BT. The testicular and epididymal luminal amino-acid microenvironment in the rat. *J Androl* 1990;11:498–505.
497. Hinton BT, Hernandez H. Selective luminal absorption of L-carnitine from the proximal regions of the rat epididymis. Possible relationships to development of sperm motility. *J Androl* 1985;6:300–305.
498. Hinton BT, Hernandez H. Neutral amino acid absorption by the rat epididymis. *Biol Reprod* 1987;37:288–292.
499. Hinton BT, Howards SS. Permeability characteristics of the epithelium in the rat caput epididymidis. *J Reprod Fertil* 1981;63:95–99.
500. Hinton BT, Howards SS. Rat testis and epididymis can transport [^{3}H]3-O-methyl-D-glucose, [^{3}H]inositol and [^{3}H]-amino-isobutyric acid across its epithelia *in vivo. Biol Reprod* 1982;27:1181–1189.
501. Hinton BT, Keefer DA. Evidence for protein absorption from the lumen of the seminiferous tubule and rete of the rat testis. *Cell Tiss Res* 1983;230:367–375.
502. Hinton BT, Setchell BP. Concentration of glycerophosphocholine, phosphocholine and free inorganic phosphate in the luminal fluid of the rat testis and epididymis. *J Reprod Fenil* 1980;58:401–406.
503. Hinton BT, Setchell BP. Fluid secretion and movement. In: *The Sertoli Cell,* edited by LD Russell and MD Griswold, Cache River Press, Clerwater Fl., (in press).
504. Hinton BT, Snoswell AM, Setchell BP. The concentration of carnitine in the luminal fluid of the testis and epididymis of the rat and some other mammals. *J Reprod Fertil* 1979;56: 105–111.
505. Hinton BT, White RW, Setchell BP. Concentrations of myoino-

sitol in the luminal fluid of mammalian testes and epididymides. *J Reprod Fertil* 1980;58:395–399.
506. Hinton BT, Brooks DE, Dott HM, Setchell BP. Effects of carnitine and some related compounds on the motility of rat spermatozoa from the caput epididymidis. *J Reprod Fertil* 1981;61:59–64.
507. Hinton BT, Palldino MA, Mattmueller DR, Bard D, Good K. Expression and activity of gamma-glutamyl transpeptidase in the rat epididymis. *Mol Reprod Dev* 1991;28:40–46.
508. Hjertkvist M, Bergh A, Damber JE. HCG treatment increases intratesticular pressure in the abdominal testis of unilaterally cryptorchid rats. *J Androl* 1988;9:116–120.
509. Hochereau MT. Etude comparee de la vague spermatogenetique chez le taureau et chez le rat. *Ann Biol Anim Biochim Biophys* 1963;3:5–20.
510. Hochereau de Reviers MT, Perreau C, Piesselet C, Fontaine I, Monet-Kuntz C. Comparisons of endocrinological and testis parameters in 18-month-old Ille de France and Romanov rams. *Domest Anim Endocrinol* 1990;7:63–73.
511. Hodson N. Role of the hypogastric nerves in seminal emission in the rabbit. *J Reprod Fertil* 1964;7:113–122.
512. Hodson N. Sympathetic nerves and reproductive organs in the male rabbit. *J Reprod Fertil* 1965;10:209–220.
513. Hodson N. On the intrinsic blood supply to the prostate and pelvic urethra in the dog. *Res Vet Sci* 1968;9:274–280.
514. Hodson N. The nerves of the testis, epididymis, and scrotum. In: *The Testis, Vol. 1,* edited by AD Johnson, WR Gomes and NL Vandemark, 1970:47–99. Academic Press, New York.
515. Hoffer AP. The fine structure of the ductuli efferentes in mouse and rat. *Anat Rec* 1972;172:331–332.
516. Hoffer AP, Greenberg J. The structure of the epididymis, efferent ductules and ductus deferens of the guinea pig: a light microscope study. *Anat Rec* 1978;190:659–678.
517. Hoffer AP, Hinton BT. Morphological evidence for a blood-epididymis barrier and the effects of gossypol on its integrity. *Biol Reprod* 1984;30:991–1004.
518. Hofmann R. Die Gefassarchitektur des Bullenhodens, zugleich ein Versuch ihrer funktionellen Deutung. *Zentrabl Veterinaermed* 1960;7:59–63.
519. Holpert M, Cooper TG. Re-examination of the presence of α-lactalbumin in the epididymis of the rat. *J Reprod Fertil* 1990;90:503–514.
520. Holstein AF. Elektronenemikroskopische Untersuchungen an den Ductuli-Efferentes des normalen und kastrieten Kaninchens. *Z Zellforsch* 1964;64:767–777.
521. Holstein AF. Die glatte Muskulatur in der Tunica albuginea des Hodens und ihr Einfluss auf den Spermatozoentransport in den Nebenhoden. *Anat Anz Ergeb* 1967;121:103–108.
522. Holstein AF. Die Morphologie des Nebenhodens beim Menschen. In: Physiologie und Pathophysiologie des Nebenhodens und der Samenblase, edited by T Senge, F Neumann, UW Tunn, Georg Thieme, Stuttgart, 1980:1–14.
523. Holstein AF. Die mannlichen Geschlechtsorgane. In: *Benninghoff Anatomie. Makroskopische und microskopische Anatomie des Menschen, Band 2. Kreislauf ind Eingeweide,* edited by K. Fleischhauer, Urban & Schwarzenberg, Munich. 1985:460–514.
524. Holstein AF, Weiss C. Uber die Wirkung der glatten Muskulatur in der Tunica Albuginea im Hoden des Kaninchens; Messungen des interstitiellen Druckes. *Z Ges Exp Med* 1967; 142:334–337.
525. Holtz W, Foote RH. Composition of rabbit semen and the origin of several constituents. *Biol Reprod* 1978;18:286–292.
526. Holtz W, Foote RH. The anatomy of the reproductive system in male dutch rabbits (*Oryctolagus cuniculus*) with special emphasis on the accessory sex glands. *J Morphol* 1978;158:1–20.
527. Hovatta O. Contractility and structure of adult rat seminiferous tubules in organ culture. *Z Zellforsch* 1972;130:171–179.
528. Hovatta O. Effect of androgens and antiandrogens on the development of the myoid cells of the rat seminiferous tubules (organ culture): *Z Zellforsch* 1972;131:299–308.
529. Howards SS, Jesse SJ, Johnson AL. Micropuncture studies of the blood-seminiferous tubule barrier. *Biol Reprod* 1976; 14:264–269.
530. Huang HFS, Gould S, Boccabella AV. Modification of Sertoli cell function in vitamin A-deficient rats. *J Reprod Fertil* 1989;85:273–281.
531. Huang EJ, Kelly RE, Masuda H, Bjerke HS, Fonkalsrud EW. Deleterious effects of testicular venous occlusion in young rats. *Surg Gynecol Obstet* 1990;171:382–387.
532. Hudson B, Baker HWG, Eddie LW, Higginson RE, Burger HG, de Kretser DM, Dobos M, Lee VWK. Bioassays for inhibin: a critical review. *J Reprod Fertil Suppl* 1979;26:17–29.
533. Huffman LJ, Connors JM, Hedger GA. VIP and its homologues increase vascular conductance in certain endocrine glands. *Am J Physiol* 1988;254:E435–442.
534. Huggins C. The physiology of the prostate gland. *Physiol Rev* 1945;25:281–295.
535. Huggins C. The prostatic secretion. *Harvey Lect* 1947;42: 148–193.
536. Huggins C, Masina MH, Eichelberger L, Wharton JD. Quantitative studies of prostatic secretion. 1. Characteristics of the normal secretion; the influence of thyroid, suprarenal, and testis extirpation and androgen substitution on the prostatic output. *J Exp Med* 1939;70:543–556.
537. Hummel KP, Richardson FL, Fekete E. Anatomy. In: *Biology of the Laboratory Mouse, 2nd ed.,* edited by EL Green, McGraw-Hill, New York, 1966:247–307.
538. Humphrey GF, Mann T. Citric acid in semen. *Nature* 1948;161:352–353.
539. Humphrey GF, Mann T. Studies on the metabolism of semen. 5. Citric acid in semen. *Biochem J* 1949;44:97–105.
540. Hundeiker M. Die Capillaren im Hodenparenchym. *Arch Klin Exp Dermatol* 1971;239:426–435.
541. Hundeiker M, Keller L. Die Gefassarchitektur des menschlichen Hodens. *Morphol Jb* 1963;105:26–73.
542. Hurt GS, Howards SS, Turner TT. Repair of experimental varicocele in the rat. Long-term effects on testicular blood flow and temperature and cauda epididymal sperm concentration and motility. *J Androl* 1986;7:271–276.
543. Hurt GS, Howards SS, Turner TT. The effects of unilateral experimental varicocele are not mediated through the ipsilateral testis. *J Androl* 1987;8:402–406.
544. Hutson JM, Donahoe PK. The hormonal control of testicular descent. *Endocr Rev* 1986;7:270–283.
545. Hutson JM, Chow CW, Ng WD. Persistent Mullerian duct syndrome with transverse testicular ectopia. An experiment of nature with clues for understanding testicular descent. *Pediat Surg Int* 1987;2:191–194.
546. Hutson JM, Williams MPL, Fallat ME, Attah A. Testicular descent: new insights into its hormonal control. *Oxf Rev Reprod Biol* 1990;12:1–56.
547. Hutson JM, Watts LM, Montalto J, Greco S. Both gonadotropin and testosterone fail to reverse estrogen-induced cryptorchidism in fetal mice: further evidence for non-androgenic control of testicular descent in the fetus. *Pediat Surg Int* 1990;5:13–18.
548. Hutson JM, Baker ML, Griffiths AL, Momose Y, Goh DW, Middlesworth W, Yun ZB, Cartwright E. Endocrine and morphological perspectives in testicular descent. *Reprod Med Rev* 1992;1:165–177.
549. Iggo A. Cutaneous thermoreceptors in primates and subprimates. *J Physiol* 1969;200:403–430.
550. Ishida H, Tashiro H, Watanabe M, Fujii N, Yoshida H, Imamura K, Minowada S, Shinohara M, Fukutani K, Aso Y, de Kretser DM. Measurement of inhibin concentrations in men: study of changes after castration and comparison with androgen levels in testicular tissue, spermatic venous blood, and peripheral venous blood. *J Clin Endocrinol Metab* 1990;70: 1019–1022.
551. Jacks F, Setchell BP. A technique for studying the transfer of substances from venous to anerial blood in the spermatic cord of wallabies and rams. *J Physiol* 1973;233:17P–18P.
552. Jacob S, Poddar S. Morphology and histochemistry of the ferret prostate. *Acta Anat (Basel)* 1986;125:268–273.
553. Jacobowitz D, Koelle GB. Histochemical correlations of acetylcholinesterase and catecholamines in postganglionic autonomic nerves of the cat, rabbit, and guinea pig. *J Pharmacol Exp Ther* 1965;148:225–237.

554. Jacobs SC, Story MT. Exocrine secretion of epidermal growth factor by the rat prostate: effect of adrenergic agents, cholinergic agents and vasoactive intestinal peptide. *Prostate* 1988;13: 79–87.
555. James MJ, Brooks DE, Snoswell AM. Kinetics of carnitine uptake by rat epididymal cells. Androgen-dependence and lack of stereospecificity. *FEBS Lett.* 1981;126:53–56.
556. Janne J, Holtta E, Haaranen P, Elfving K. Polyamines and polyamine-metabolizing enzyme activities in human semen. *Clin Chim Acta* 1973;48:393–401.
557. Jansz GF, Pomerantz DK. The effect of spermatogenic disruption on the ability of testicular fluid to stimulate androgen production by normal Leydig cells. *Biol Reprod* 1987;36:807–815.
558. Jantosovicova J. Topographisch-anatomische Angaben uber die A. testicularis, A. ductus deferentis und A. cremasterica beim Widder. *Gegenbaurs Morphol Jahrb* 1977;123:914–923.
559. Jarow JP. Intratesticular arterial anatomy. *J Androl* 1990;11:255–259.
560. Jarow JP. Clinical significance of intratesticular arterial anatomy. *J Urol* 1991;145:777–779.
561. Jarow JP, Ogle A, Kaspar J, Hopkins M. Testicular artery ramification within the inguinal canal. *J Urol* 1992;147:1290–1292.
562. Jegou B, Dacheux JL, Garnier DH, Terqui M, Colas G, Courot M. Biochemical and physiological studies of androgen-binding protein in the reproductive tract of the ram. *J Reprod Fertil* 1979;57:311–318.
563. Jegou B, Le Gac F, de Kretser DM. Seminiferous tubule fluid and interstitial fluid production. 1. Effects of age and hormonal regulation in immature rats. *Biol Reprod* 1982;27:590–595.
564. Jegou B, Le Gac F, Irby DC, de Kretser DM. Studies on seminiferous tubule fluid production in the adult rat: effect of hypophysectomy and treatment with FSH, LH and testosterone. *Int J Androl* 1983;6:249–260.
565. Jegou B, Risbridger GP, de Kretser DM. Effects of experimental cryptorchidism on testicular function in adult rats. *J Androl* 1983;4:88–94.
566. Jegou B, Laws AO, de Kretser DM. Changes in testicular function induced by short-term exposure of the rat testis to heat: further evidence for interation of germ cells, Sertoli cells and Leydig cells. *Int J Androl* 1984;7:244–257.
567. Jegou B, Peake RA, Irby DC, de Kretser DM. Effects of induction of experimental cryptorchidism and subsequent orchidopexy on testicular function in immature rats. *Biol Reprod* 1984;30:179–187.
568. Jenkins AD, Lechene CP, Howards SS. Concentration of seven elements in the intraluminal fluids of the rat seminiferous tubules, rete testis and epididymis. *Biol Reprod* 1980;23:981–987.
569. Jesik CJ, Holland JM, Lee C. An anatomic and histologic study of the rat prostate. *Prostate* 1982;3:81–97.
570. Jeulin C, Soufir JC, Jouannet P. The effects of L-carnitine and D,L-acetylcarnitine on human sperm motility as measured by laser doppler velocimetry. *IRCS Med Sci* 1981;9:722–723.
571. Jhunjhunwala JS, Sinha-Hikim AP, Budd CA, Chakraborty J. Germ cell degeneration in the contralateral testis of the guinea pig with unilateral torsion of the spermatic cord. Quantitative and ultrastructural studies. *J Androl* 1986;7:16–22.
572. Joffre J, Joffre M. Seasonal changes in the testicular blood flow of seasonally breeding mammals: dormouse (*Glis glis*), ferret (*Mustela furo*) and fox (*Vulpes vulpes*). *J Reprod Fertil* 1973;34:227–233.
573. Joffre M. Relationship between testicular blood flow, testosterone secretion and spermatogenic activity in young and adult wild red foxes (*Vulpes vulpes*). *J Reprod Fertil* 1977;51:35–40.
574. Johnson AL, Howards SS. Hyperosmolarity in intraluminal fluids from hamster testis and epididymis: a micropuncture study. *Science* 1977;195:492–493.
575. Johnson JM, Hargrove JL, Ellis LC. Prostaglandin F-1α induced stimulation of rabbit testicular contractions *in vitro*. *Proc Soc Exp Biol Med* 1971;138:378–381.
576. Johnson KJ, Hall ES, Boekelheide K. 2,5-Hexadione exposure alters the rat Sertoli cell cytoskeleton. I. Microtubules and seminiferous tubule fluid secretion. *Toxicol Appl Pharmacol* 1991;111:432–442.
577. Johnson L, Neaves WB. Age-related changes in the Leydig cell population, seminiferous tubules, and sperm production in stallions. *Biol Reprod* 1981;24:703–712.
578. Johnson L, Petty CS, Neaves WB. Age-related variation in seminiferous tubules in men. A stereologic evaluation. *J Androl* 1986;7:316–322.
579. Johnson LA, Pursel VG, Gerrits RJ, Thomas CH. Free amino acid composition of porcine seminal, epididymal and seminal vesicle fluids. *J Anim Sci* 1972;34:430–434.
580. Johnson MH. The effect of cadmium chloride on the blood-testis barrier of the guinea-pig. *J Reprod Fertil* 1969;19: 551–553.
581. Johnson MH. Changes in the blood-testis barrier of the guinea-pig in relation to histological damage following isoimmunization. *J Reprod Fertil* 1970;22:119–127.
582. Johnson MH. The distribution of immunoglobulin and spermatozoal autoantigen in the genital tract of the male guinea pig. *Fertil Steril* 1972;23:383–392.
583. Johnson MH, Setchell BP. Protein and immunoglobulin content of rete testis fluid of rams. *J Reprod Fertil* 1968;17: 403–406.
584. Jones R. Comparative biochemistry of mammalian epididymal plasma. *Comp Biochem Physiol* 1978;61B:365–370.
585. Jones R. Membrane remodelling during sperm maturation in the epididymis. *Oxf Rev Reprod Biol* 1989;11:285–337.
586. Jones R, Hamilton DW, Fawcett DW. Morphology of the epithelium of the extratesticular rete testis, ductuli efferentes and ductus epididymidis of the adult male rabbit. *Am J Anat* 1979;156:373–400.
587. Jones R, Brown CR, von Glós KI, Parker MG. Hormonal regulation of protein synthesis in the rat epididymis. Characterization of androgen-dependent and testicular fluid-dependent proteins. *Biochem J* 1980;188:667–676.
588. Jones R, von Glós KI, Brown CR. The synthesis of a sperm-coating protein in the initial segment of the rat epididymis is stimulated by factors in testicular fluid. *IRCS Med Sci* 1980;8:56.
589. Jones RC. Changes in protein composition of the luminal fluids along the epididymis of the tammar, Macropus eugenii. *J Reprod Fertil* 1987;80:193–199.
590. Jones RC, Brosnan MF. Studies of the deferent ducts from the testis of the African elephant, *Loxodonta africana*. 1. Structural differentiation. *J Anat* 1981;132:371–386.
591. Jones RC, Clulow J. Regulation of the elemental composition of the epididymal fluids in the tammar, Macropus eugenii. *J Reprod Fertil* 1987;81:583–590.
592. Jones RC, Jurd KM. Structural differentiation and fluid reabsorption in the ductuli efferentes testis of the rat. *Aust J Biol Sci* 1987;40:79–90.
593. Jones RC, Hinds LA, Tyndale-Biscoe CH. Ultrastructure of the epididymis of the tammar, *Macrous eugenii*, and its relationship to sperm maturation. *Cell Tiss Res* 1984;237:525–535.
594. Jones T. Blood flow and volume measurements in the radiation depopulated testis of the rat. *Br J Radiol* 1971;44:841–849.
595. Jonte G, Holstein AF. On the morphology of the transitional zones from the rete testis into the ductuli efferentes and from the ductuli efferentes into the ductus epididymidis. *Andrologia* 1987;19:398–412.
596. Joranson Y, Emmel VE, Pilka HJ. Factors controlling the arterial supply of the testis under experimental conditions. *Anat Rec* 1929;41:157–176.
597. Josso N, Picard JY, Dacheux JL, Courot M. Detection of anti-Müllerian activity in boar rete testis fluid. *J Reprod Fertil* 1979;57:397–400.
598. Josso N, Fekete C, Cachin O, Nezelof C, Rappaport R. Persistence of Mullerian ducts in male pseudohermaphroditism, and its relationship to cryptorchidism. *Clin Endocr* 1983;19: 247–258.
599. Josso N, Jegeai L, Forest MG, Chaussain JL, Brauner R. An enzyme linked immunoassay for anti-Mullerian hormone: a new tool for the evaluation of testicular function in infants and children. *J Clin Endocr Metab* 1990;70:23–27.
600. Jungblut T, Aumuller G, Malek B, Melchior H. Age-dependency and regional distribution of enkephalinergic nerves in human prostate. *Urol Int* 1989;44:352–356.

601. Juniewicz PE, Keeney DS, Ewing LL. Effect of adrenocorticotropin and other proopiomelanocortin-derived peptides on testosterone secretion by the in vitro perfused testis. *Endocrinology* 1988;122:891–898.
602. Kainer RA, Faulkner LC, Abdel-Raouf M. Glands associated with the urethra of the bull. *Am J Vet Res* 1969;30:963–974.
603. Kandal JC, Kistler WS, Kistler MK. Methylation of the rat seminal vesicle secretory protein IV gene. Extensive demethylation occurs in several mae sex accessory glands. *J Biol Chem* 1985;260:15959–15964.
604. Kanui TI. Responses of spinal cord neurone to noxious and nonnoxious stimulation of the slin and testicle of the rat. *Neurosci Lett* 1985;58:315–319.
605. Karpe B, Fredricsson B, Svensson J, Ritzen EM. Testosterone concentration within the tunica vaginalis of boys and adult men. *Int J Androl* 1982;5:549–556.
606. Kasson BG, Hsueh AJW. Nicotinic cholinergic agonists inhibit androgen biosynthesis by cultured rat testicular cells. *Endocrinology,* 1985;117:1874–1880.
607. Kay R, Alexander NJ, Baugham WL. Induced varicocele in rhesus monkeys. *Fertil Steril* 1979;31:195–199.
608. Kay GW, Grobbelaar JAN, Hattingh J. Effect of surgical restriction of growth of the testicular artery on testis size and histology in bulls. *J Reprod Fertil* 1992;96:549–553.
609. Kaya M. Sertoli cells and various types of multinucleates in the rat seminiferous tubules following temporary ligation of the testicular artery. *J Anat* 1986;144:15–29.
610. Kaya M, Harrison RG. An analysis of the effect of ischaemia on testicular ultrastructure. *J Path* 1975;117:105–117.
611. Kazeem AA. The assessment of epididymal lymphatics within the concept of immunologically privileged sites. *Lymphology* 1983;16:168–171.
612. Kazeem A. Reexamination of testicular lymphatic drainage in the rat. *Lymphology* 1986;19:172–174.
613. Kazeem AA. Species variation in the extrinsic lymphatic drainage of the rodent testis: its role within the context of an immunologically privileged site. *Lymphology* 1991;24:140–144.
614. Kelch RP, Jenner MR, Weinstein R, Kaplan SL, Grumbach MM. Estradiol and testosterone secretion by human, simian and canine testes, in males with hypogonadism and in male pseudohermaphrodites with the feminizing testes syndrome. *J Clin Invest* 1972;51:824–830.
615. Kelly MJ, Wheatley R, Smith JH, Thomas WE. Cooling prevents ischaemic damage after spermatic cord clamping in rats. *Int J Androl* 1987;10:721–726.
616. Kelly RW, Taylor PL, Hearn JP, Short RV, Martin DE, Marston JH. 19-Hydroxyprostaglandin E, as a major component of the semen of primates. *Nature* 1976;260:544–545.
617. Kemme M, Scheit KH. Cloning and sequence analysis of a cDNA from seminal vesicle tissue encoding the precursor of the major protein of bull semen. *DNA* 1988;7:595–599.
618. Kemme M, Madiraju MV, Krauhs E, Zimmer M, Scheit KH. The major protein of bull seminal plasma is a secretory product of seminal vesicle. *Biochim Biophys Acta* 1986;884:282–290.
619. Kenagy GJ, Trombulak SC. Size and function of mammalian testes in relation to body size. *J Mammalogy* 1986;67:1–22.
620. Kern S, Robertson SA, Maddocks S. Cytokine secretion by macrophages isolated from the rat testis. *Proc Aust Soc Reprod Biol* 1992;24:87.
621. Kerr JB. A light microscopic and morphometric analysis of the Sertoli cells during the spermatogenic cycle of the rat. *Anat Embryol* 1988;177:341–348.
622. Kerr JB, Rich KA, de Kretser DM. Effects of experimental cryptorchidism on the ultrastructure and function of the Sertoli cell and peritubular tissue of the rat testis. *Biol Reprod* 1979;21:823–838.
623. Kilzer P, Chang C, Marvel J, Kilo C, Williamson JR. Tissue differences in vascular permeability changes induced by histamine. *Microvasc Res* 1985;30:270–285.
624. King TE, Mann T. Sorbitol metabolism in spermatozoa. *Proc R Soc Lond (B)* 1959;151:226–243.
625. Kiplesund KM, Halgunset J, Fjosne HE, Sunde A. Light microscopic morphometric analysis of castration effects in the different lobes of the rat prostate. *Prostate* 1988;13:221–232.
626. Knickerbocker JJ, Sawyer HR, Amann RP, Tekpetey FR, Niswender GD. Evidence for the presence of oxytocin in the ovine epididymis. *Biol Reprod* 1988;39:391–397.
627. Knight TW. A qualitative study of factors affecting the contractions of the epididymis and ductus deferens of the ram. *J Reprod Fertil* 1974;40:19–29.
628. Kochakian CD. Hypotaurine: regulation of production in seminal vesicles and prostate of guinea-pig by testosterone. *Nature* 1973;241:202–203.
629. Kohane AC, Garberi JC, Cameo MS, Blaquier JA. Quantitative determination of specific proteins in rat epididymis. *J Steroid Biochem* 1979;11:671–674.
630. Kondoh N, Koh E, Takeyama M, Fujioka H, Nonomura N, Nakamura M, Namiki M, Okuyama A. Induction of plasma renin activity in human internal spermatic vein after treatment of HCG (in Japanese). *Hinyokika Kiyo* 1989;35:997–1000.
631. Kormano M. An angiographic study of the testicular vasculature in the postnatal rat. *Z Anat Entwickl* 1967;126:138–153.
632. Kormano M. Dye permeability and alkaline phosphatase activity of testicular capillaries in the postnatal rat. *Histochemie* 1967;9:327–338.
633. Kormano M. Microvascular structure of the rat epididymis. *Ann Med Exp Fenn* 1968;46:113–118.
634. Kormano M. Penetration of intravenous trypan blue into the rat testis and epididymis. *Acta Histochem* 1968;30:133–136.
635. Kormano M. The rete testis. In: *The Testis, Vol. IV,* edited by AD Johnson and WR Gomes, Academic Press, New York. 1977:461–479.
636. Kormano M, Hovatta O. Contractility and histochemistry of the myoid cell layer of the rat seminiferous tubules during postnatal development. *Z Anat Entwickl* 1972;137:239–248.
637. Kormano M, Reijonen K. Microvascular structure of the human epididymis. *Am J Anat* 1976;145:23–32.
638. Kormano M, Suvanto O. Cadmium-induced changes in the intratesticular pressure in the rat. *Acta Pathol Microbiol Scand* 1968;72:444–445.
639. Kormano M, Koskimies AL, Hunter RL. The presence of specific proteins in the absence of many serum proteins in the rat seminiferous tubule fluid. *Experentia* 1971;27:1461–1463.
640. Kosco MS, Loseth KJ, Crabo BG. Development of the seminiferous tubules after neobnatal hemicastration in the boar. *J Reprod Fertil* 1989;87:1–11.
641. Koskimies AJ, Kormano M. Proteins in fluids from the seminiferous tubules and rete testis in the rat. *J Reprod Fertil* 1973;34:433–444.
642. Koskimies AJ, Kormano M, Lahti A. A difference in the immunoglobulin content of seminiferous tubule fluid and rete testis fluid of the rat. *J Reprod Fenil* 1971;27:463–465.
643. Koskimies AJ, Kormano M, Alfthan O. Proteins of the seminiferous tubule fluid in man—evidence for a blood-testis barrier. *J Reprod Fertil* 1973;32:79–86.
644. Kotani M, Seiki K, Hattori M. Retardation of spermatogenesis and testosterone secretion after ligature of lymphatics draining the testes of rabbits. *Endocrinol Jpn* 1974;21:1–8.
645. Kremer A, Budras KD. Lymphsystem und lymphdrainage im Hoden des Pekingerpels (*Anas platyrhynchos,* L.). *Anat Histol Embryol* 1988;17:246–257.
646. Kremer A, Budras KD. Zur Blutgefassversorgung des Hodens beim Pekingerpel (*Anas platyhynchos* L.). Makroskopische, lichtmikroskopische und rasterelektonenmikroskopische Untersuchingen. *Anat Anz* 1990;171:73–87.
647 de Kretser DM, Kerr JB, Paulsen CA. The peritubular tissue in the normal and pathological human testis. An ultrastructural study. *Biol Reprod* 1975;12:317–324.
648. Kruger L, Kumazawa T, Mizumura K, Sato J, Yeh Y. Observations on electrophysiologically characterized receptive fields of thin testicular afferent axons: a preliminary note on the analysis of fine structural specializations of polynodal receptors. *Somatosens Res* 1988;5:373–380.
649. Kumazawa T, Mizumura K. The polymodal receptors in the testis of dog. *Brain Res* 1977;136:553–558.
650. Kumazawa T, Mizumura K. Effects of synthetic substance P on unit-discharges of testicular nociceptors of dogs. *Brain Res* 1979;170:553–557.

651. Kumazawa T, Mizumura K. Chemical responses of polymodal receptors of the scrotal contents in dogs. *J Physiol* 1980;299:219–231.
652. Kumazawa T, Mizumura K. Mechanical and thermal responses of polymodal receptors recorded from the superior spermatic nerve of dogs. *J Physiol* 1980;299:233–245.
653. Kumazawa T, Mizumura K. Temperature dependency of the chemical responses of the polymodal receptor units in vitro. *Brain Res* 1983;278:305–307.
654. Kumazawa T, Mizumura K, Sato J. Response properties of polymodal receptors studied using in vitro superior spermatic nerve preparations of dogs. *J Neurophysiol* 1987;57:702–711.
655. Kumazawa T, Mizumura K, Sato J. Thermally potentiated responses to algesis substances of visceral nociceptors. *Pain* 1987;28:255–264.
656. Kumazawa T, Mizumura K, Sato J, Minagawa M. Facilitatory effects on the discharges of visceral nociceptors. *Brain Res* 1989;497:231–238.
657. Kuntz A, Morris RE. Components and distribution of the spermatic nerves and the nerves of the vas deferens. *J Comp Neurol* 1946;85:33–44.
658. Kupczyk-Joeris D, Kalb A, Hofer M, Toens C, Schumpelick V. Doppler sonography of testicular circulation following reconstruction of inguinal hernia (in German). *Chirurg.*, 1989; 60:536–540.
659. Lacy D, Rotblat J. Study of normal and irradiated boundary tissue of the seminiferous tubules of the rat. *Exp Cell Res* 1960;21:49–70.
660. Ladman AJ. The fine structure of the ductuli efferentes of the opossum. *Anat Rec* 1967;157:559–576.
661. Ladman AJ, Young WC. An electron microscopic study of the ductuli efferentes and rete testis of the guinea pig. *J Biophys Biochem Cytol* 1958;4:219–226.
662. Lahnsteiner F, Lametschwandtner A, Patzner RA, Adam H. Vascularization of male gonads in Blennius pavo (Teleostei, Blenniidae) as revealed by scanning electron microscopy of vascular corrosion casts. *Scanning Microsc* 1988;2:2077–2086.
663. Lamano-Carvalho TL, Hodson NP, Blank MA, Watson PF, Mulderry PK, Bishop AE, Gu J, Bloom SR, Polak JM. Occurrence, distribution and origin of peptide containing nerves of guinea pig and rat male genitalia and the effects of denervation on sperm characteristics. *J Anat* 1986;149:121–141.
664. Lambiase JT, Amann RP. Infertility of rabbit testicular spermatozoa collected in their native fluid environment. *Fertil Steril* 1973;24:65–67.
665. Lange W, Unger J. Peptidergic innervation within the prostate gland and seminal vesicle. *Urol Res* 1990;18:337–340.
666. Langeland A. Characterization of the secretory proteins of rat preputial gland in relation to urinary proteins. *J Exp Zool* 1986;238:401–408.
667. Langford GA, Heller CG. Fine structure of muscle cells of the human testicular capsule: basis of testicular contractions. *Science* 1973;179:573–575.
668. Langford GA, Silver A. Histochemical localization of acetylcholinesterase-containing nerve fibres in the testis. *J Physiol* 1974;242:9P–10P.
669. Laporte P, Gillet J. Influence de la spermatogenese sur la secretion du fluide testiculaire chez le rat adulte. *C R Acad Sci (Paris)* 1975;281:1397–1400.
670. Larkins SL, Hutson JM. Fluorescent antegrade labelling of the genitofemoral nerve shows that it supplies the scrotal region before migration of the gubernaculum. *Pediatr Surg Int* 1991;6:167–171.
671. Larsen J-J, Ottesen B, Fahrenkrug J, Fahrenkrug L. Vasoactive intestinal polypeptide (VIP) in the male genitourinary tract. Concentration and motor effect. *Invest Urol* 1981;19:211–213.
672. Larsson LI, Fahrenkrug J, Schaffalitsky de Muckadell OB. Occurrence of nerves containing vasoactive intestinal polypeptide immunoreactivity in the male genital tract. *Life Sci* 1977;21:503–508.
673. Lasinski W, Sikorski A. La vascularisation arterielle des glandes bulbo-uretrales humaines. *Bull Assoc Anat* 1975;59:911–918.
674. Lau IF, Saksena SK. Steroids in the rete testis fluid of fertile male rabbits. *Arch Androl* 1979;2:49–52.
675. Laurie MS, Setchell BP. The continuous measurement of testicular blood flow in the ram, in relation to the pulsatile secretion of testosterone. *J Physiol* 1979;287:10P.
676. Lauth EA. Memoire sur le testicule humaine. *Mem Soc Hist Nat (Strasbourg)* 1830;1:1–42.
677. Lea OA, Petrusz P, French FS. Purification and localization of acidic epididymal glycoprotein (AEG): a sperm coating protein secreted by the rat epididymis. *Int J Androl Suppl* 1978;2:592–607.
678. LeBarr DK, Blecher SR. Decreased arterial vasculature of the epididymal head in XXSxr pseudomale ('sex-reversed') mice. *Acta Anat (Basel)* 1987;129:123–126.
679. Lee C, Tsai Y, Sensibar J, Oliver L, Grayhack JT. Two-dimensional characterization of prostatic acid phosphatase, prostatic specific antigen and prostate binding protein in expressed prostatic fluid. *Prostate* 1986;9:135–146.
680. Leeson CR, Forman DE. Postnatal development and differentiation of contractile cells within the rabbit testis. *J Anat* 1981;132:491–511.
681. Leeson CR, Leeson TS. The postnatal development and differentiation of the boundary tissue of the seminiferous tubule of the rat. *Anat Rec* 1963;147:243–259.
682. Leeson TS. Electron microscopy of the rete testis of the rat. *Anat Rec* 1962;144:57–67.
683. Leeson TS. Smooth muscle cells in the rat testicular capsule: a developmental study. *J Morphol* 1975;147:171–186.
684. Leeson TS, Cookson FB. The mammalian testicular capsule and its muscle elements. *J Morphol* 1974;14:237–254.
685. Leeson TS, Leeson CR. Experimental cryptorchidism in the rat. A light and electron microscope study. *Invest Urol* 1970;8: 127–144.
686. Leidl W, Schefels W. Thermographische Registrierung der Temperaturveteilung am Skrotum. *Fortpfl Haust* 1970;6: 207–212.
687. Leinonen P, Ruokonen A, Kontturi M, Vikho R. Effects of estrogen treatment on human testicular unconjugated steroid and steroid sulfate production *in vivo*. *J Clin Endocrinol Metabol* 1981;53:569–573.
688. Lennox B, Ahmad KN, Mack WS. A method for determining the relative total length of the tubules in the testis. *J Pathol* 1970;102:229–238.
689. Leone E. Acido urico e xantinossidasi in vescichette seminali. *Boll Soc Ital Biol Sper* 1953;29:513–516.
690. Leone E. Ergothioneine in the equine ampullar secretion. *Nature* 1954;174:404–405.
691. Levey HA, Szego CM. Metabolic characteristics of the guinea-pig seminal vesicle. *Am J Physiol* 1955;182:507–512.
692. Levine N, Marsh DJ. Micropuncture studies of the electrochemical aspects of fluid and electrolyte transport in individual seminiferous tubules, the epididymis and vas deferens in rats. *J Physiol* 1971;213:557–570.
693. Levine N, Marsh DJ. Micropuncture study of the fluid composition of 'Sertoli cell-only' seminiferous tubules in rats. *J Reprod Fertil* 1975;43:547–549.
694. Levy BJ, Fair WR. The location of antibacterial activity in the rat prostatic secretions. *Invest Urol* 1973;11:173–177.
695. Lewin LM, Beer R. Prostatic secretion as the source of myoinositol in human seminal fluid. *Fertil Sterl* 1973;24:666–670.
696. Lewin LM, Sulimovici S. The distribution of radioactive myoinositol in the reproductive tract of the male rat. *J Reprod Fertil* 1975;43:355–358.
697. Lewin LM, Yannai Y, Kraicer P. The effect of cyproterone acetate on myo-inositol uptake and secretion in the reproductive tract of the male rat. *Int J Androl* 1979;2:171–181.
698. Lewin LM, Yannai Y, Sulimovici S, Kraicer PF. Studies on the metabolic role of myo-inositol. Distribution of radioactive myoinositol in the male rat. *Biochem J* 1976;156:375–380.
699. Lewis LG. Cryptorchidism. *J Urol* 1948;60:345–356.
700. Lewis MH, Moffat DB. The venous drainage of the accessory reproductive organs of the rat with special reference to prostatic metabolism. *J Reprod Fertil* 1975;42:497–502.
701. Lewis-Jones DI, Harrison RG, MacMillan EW. A reexamination of rat ductuli efferentes. *Anat Rec* 1982;203:461–462.
702. Lewis-Jones DI, Richards RC, Lynch RV, Jouglin EC. Immuno-

cytochemical localization of the antibody which breaches the blood-testis barrier in sympathetic orchiopathia. *Br J Urol* 1987;59:452–457.
703. Liang IC, Hsu TC, Gay M. Response of murine spermatocytes to the metaphase-arresting effect of several mitotic arrestants. *Experientia* 1985;41:1586–1588.
704. Light PA, Tyrrell CJ. Testicular tumour markers in spermatic vein blood. *Br J Urol* 1987;59:74–75.
705. Lilja H, Abrahamsson PA. Three predominant proteins secreted by the human prostate gland. *Prostate* 1988;12:29–38.
706. Lincoln GA. Seasonal aspects of testicular function. In: *The Testis, Second Edition,* edited by H Burger and D de Kretser, Raven Press, New York, 1989:329–385.
707. Lindner HR. Androgens and related compounds in the spermatic vein blood of domestic animals 1. Neutral steroids secreted by the bull testis. *J Endocrinol* 1961;23:139–159.
708. Lindner HR. Androgens and related compounds in the spermatic vein blood of domestic animals IV. Testicular androgens in the ram, boar and stallion. *J Endocrinol* 1961;23:171–178.
709. Lindner HR. Partition of androgen between the lymph and venous blood of the testis in the ram. *J Endocrinol* 1963; 25:483–494.
710. Lindner HR. Participation of lymph in the transport of gonadal hormones. *Excerpta Med Found Int Congr Ser* 1967;132: 821–827.
711. Lindner HR. The androgenic secretion of the testis in domestic ungulates. In: *The Gonads,* edited by KW McKerns, Appleton-Century-Crofts, New York. 1969:615–648.
712. Lindner SG. On the morphology of the transitional zone of the seminiferous tubule and the rete testis in man. *Andrologia* 1982;14:352–362.
713. Linzell JL, Setchell BP. Metabolism, sperm and fluid production of the isolated perfused testis of the sheep and goat. *J Physiol* 1969;201:129–143.
714. Lobl TJ, Musto NA, Gunsalus GL, Bardin CW. Medroxyprogesterone has opposite effects on the androgen-binding protein concentrations in serum and epididymis. *Biol Reprod* 1983;29:697–712.
715. Lohiya NK, Sharma RS, Ansari AS, Anand Kumar TC. Structure of rete testis, vas efferens, epididymis and vas deferens of langur monkey (Presbytis entellus entellus Dufresne). *Acta Eur Fertil* 1988;19:167–173.
716. Lui RC, LaRegina MC, Herbold DR, Johnson FE. Tolerance of the rat testis to graded periods of total ischemia. *Curr Surg* 1986;43:403–406.
717. Lui RC, LaRegina MC, Herbold DR, Stern LA, Johnson FE. Regional doxorubicin delivery reduces testicular toxicity. *J Surg Res* 1987;43:286–295.
718. Lui RC, LaRegina MC, Herbold DR, Johnson FE. Tolerance of rat testis to graded periods of total circulatory isolation. *J Surg Oncol* 1988;39:264–268.
719. Lunstra DD, Ford JJ, Christenson RK, Allrich RD. Changes in Leydig cell ultrastructure and function during pubertal development in the boar. *Biol Reprod* 1986;34:145–158.
720. Lutwak-Mann C, Mann T, Price D. Metabolic activity in tissue transplants. Hormone-induced formation of fructose and citric acid in transplants from accessory glands of reproduction. *Proc Roy Soc Lond (Biol)* 1949;136:461–471.
721. MacMillan EW. The blood supply of the epididymis in man. *Br J Urol* 1954;26:60–71.
722. Maddocks S, Setchell BP. The composition of extracellular interstitial fluid collected with a push-pull cannula from the testes of adult rats. *J Physiol* 1988;407:363–372.
723. Maddocks S, Setchell BP. The failure of thyroid allografts in the ovine testis. *Immunol Cell Biol* 1988;66:1–8.
724. Maddocks S, Setchell BP. The physiology of the endocrine testis. *Ox Rev Reprod Biol* 1988;10:53–123.
725. Maddocks S, Setchell BP. Recent evidence for immune privilege in the testis. *J Reprod Immunol* 1990;18:9–18.
726. Maddocks S, Sharpe RM. The route of secretion of inhibin from the rat testis. *J Endocrinol* 1989;120:R5–R8.
727. Maddocks S, Sharpe RM. Interstitial fluid volume in the rat testis: androgen-dependent regulation by the seminiferous tubules? *J Endocrinol* 1989;120:215–222.
728. Maddocks S, Sharpe RM. Dynamics of testosterone secretion by the rat testis: implications for measurement of the intratesticular levels of testosterone. *J Endocrinol* 1989;122:323–329.
729. Maddocks S, Sharpe RM. The effects of sexual maturation and altered steroid synthesis on the production and route of secretion of inhibin from the rat testis. *Endocrinology* 1990; 126:1541–1550.
730. Maddocks S, Oliver JR, Setchell BP. The survival and function of isolated pancreatic islets of Langerhans transplanted into the testis of adult rats and their effect on the testis. *Coll INSERM* 1984;123:497–502.
731. Maddocks S, Kerr JB, Allenby G, Sharpe RM. Evaluation of the role of germ cells in regulating the route of secretion of immunoactive inhibin from the rat testis. *J Endocrinol* 1992;132: 439–448.
732. Maddocks S, Sowerbutts S, van Rooijen N, Kerr JB. Macrophage depletion in the rat testis and its effect on the hCG response. *Miniposters of the VIIth European Workshop on Molecular and Cellular Endocrinology of the Testis,* 104.
733. Maddocks S, Hargreave TB, Reddie K, Fraser HM, Kerr JB, Sharpe RM. Intratesticular hormone levels and the route of secretion of hormones from the testis of the rat, guinea pig, monkey and human testis. *Int J Androl,* in press. 1993.
734. Main SJ. The blood-testis barrier and temperature. *Ph.D. Thesis,* University of Reading, Reading, England.
735. Main SJ, Setchell BP. The facilitated diffusion of testosterone into the rete testis of the ram. *J Physiol* 1978;284:17P–18P.
736. Main SJ, Waites GMH. The blood-testis barrier and temperature damage to the testis of the rat. *J Reprod Fertil* 1977;51:439–450.
737. Mainwaring WIP, Haining SA, Harper B. The functions of testosterone and its metabolites. In: Hormones and their Actions, Part I, edited by BA Cooke, RJB King, HJ van der Molen, Elsevier, Amsterdam, 1988:169–196.
738. Mancini RE, Vilar O, Alvarez B, Seiguer AC. Extravascular and intratubular diffusion of labelled serum proteins in the rat testis. *J Histochem Cytochem* 1965;13:376–385.
739. Mancini RE, Castro A, Seiguer AC. Histological localization of follicle-stimulating and luteinizing hormones in the rat testis. *J Histochem Cytochem* 1967;15:516–525.
740. Manco G, Abrescia P. A major secretory protein from rat seminal vesicle binds ejaculated spermatozoa. *Gamete Res* 1988;21:71–84.
741. Manco G, Sansone G, Abrescia P. Interaction of proteins RSV IV and RSV V in rat seminal vesicle secretion. *J Exp Zool* 1989;249:193–202.
742. Mann T. On the presence and role of inositol and certain other substances in the seminal vesicle secretion of the boar. *Proc R Soc Lond (B),* 1954;142:21–32.
743. Mann T. Male sex hormone and its role in reproduction. *Rec Prog Horm Res* 1956;12:353–376.
744. Mann T. *The Biochemistry of Semen and of the Male Reproductive Tract,* Methuen, London. 1964:493.
745. Mann T. Physiology of semen and of the male reproductive tract. In: *Reproduction in Domestic Animals, 2nd ed.,* edited by HH Cole and PT Cupps, Academic Press, New York. 1969:277–312.
746. Mann T, Lutwak-Mann C. Evaluation of the functional state of male accessory glands by the analysis of seminal plasma. *Andrologia* 1976;8:237–242.
747. Mann T, Lutwak-Mann C. *Male Reproductive Function and Semen,* Springer-Verlag, Berlin. 1981:495.
748. Mann T, Parsons U. Studies on the metabolism of semen. 6. Role of hormones, effect of castration, hypophysectomy and diabetes. Relation between blood glucose and seminal fructose. *Biochem J* 1950;46:440–450.
749. Mann T, Wilson ED. Biochemical observations on the male accessory organs of nutria, *Myocastor coypus* (Molina). *J Endocrinol* 1962;25:407–408.
750. Mann T, Davies DV, Humphrey GF. Fructose and citric acid assay in the secretions of the accessory glands of reproduction as indicator tests of male sex hormone activity. *J Endocrinol* 1949;6:75–85.

751. Mann T, Leone E, Polge C. The composition of the stallion's semen. *J Endocrinol* 1956;13:279–290.
752. Mann T, Short RV, Walton A, Archer RK, Miller WC. The 'tail-end sample' of stallion semen. *J Agric Sci (Camb),* 1957;49:301–312.
753. Mann T, Minotakis CS, Polge C. Semen composition and metabolism in the stallion and jackass. *J Reprod Fertil* 1963;5:109–122.
754. Margioris AN, Liotta AS, Vaudry H, Bardin CW, Krieger DT. Characterization of immunoreactive propiomelanocortin-related peptides in rat testes. *Endocrinology* 1983;113:663–671.
755. Margioris AN, Koukoulis G, Grino M, Chrousos GP. In vitro-perifused rat testes secrete beta-endorphin and dynorphin: their effect on testosterone secretion. *Biol Reprod* 1989;40:776–784.
756. Mariotti A, Mawhinney M. The hormonal maintenance and restoration of guinea pig seminal vesicle fibromuscular stroma. *J Urol* 1982;128:852–857.
757. Markey CM, Jequier AM. Effects of ischaemia on the caput epididymidis and its relationship to higher epididymal obstruction: A qualitative ultrastructural study in the ram. *J Androl* (in press) 1993.
758. Markey CM, Meyer GT. A quantitative description of the epididymis and its microvasculature i: an age-related study in the rat. *J Anat* 1992;180:255–262.
759. Martin ICA, Lapwood KR, Kitchell RL. The effects of specific neurectomies and cremaster muscle sectioning on semen characteristics and scrotal thermoregulatory responses of rams. In: *Reproduction in Sheep,* edited by DR Lindsay and DT Pearce, Australian Academy of Science, Canberra. 1984:73–75.
760. Maseki Y, Miyake K, Mitsuya H, Kitamura H, Yamada K. Mastocytosis occurring in the testes from patients with idiopathic male infertility. *Fertil Steril* 1981;36:814–817.
761. Mattmueller DR, Hinton BT. In vivo secetion and association of clusterin (SGP-2) in luminal fluid with spermatozoa in the rat testis and epididymis. *Mol Reprod Devel* 1991;30:62–69.
762. Mattmueller DR, Hinton BT. Clusterin (SGP-2) in epididymal luminal fluid and its association with epididymal spermatozoa in androgen-deprived rats. *Mol Reprod Dev* 1992;32:73–80.
763. Mayerhofer A, Bartke A. Developing testicular microvasculature in the golden hamster, Mesocricetus auratus: a model for angiogenesis under physiological conditions. *Acta Anat (Basel)* 1990;139:78–85.
764. Mayerhofer A, Dube D. Chronic administration of a gonadotropin-releasing hormone (GnRH) agonist affects testicular microvasculature. *Acta Endocrin (Copenh)* 1989;120:75–80.
765. Mayerhofer A, Sinha Hikim AP, Bartke A, Russell LD. Changes in the testicular microvasculature during photperiod-related seasonal transition from reproductive quiescence to reproductive activity in the adult golden hamster. *Anat Rec* 1989;224:495–507.
766. Mayerhofer A, Bartke A, Steger RW. Catecholamine effects on testicular testosterone production in the gonadally active and the gonadally regresses adult golden hamster. *Biol Reprod* 1989;40:752–761.
767. Mayerhofer A, Amador AG, Steger RW, Bartke A. Testicular function after local injection of 6-hydroxydopamine or norepinephrine in the golden hamster (*Mesocricetus auratus*). *J Androl* 1990;11:301–311.
768. Mayerhofer A, Steger RW, Gow G, Bartke A. Catechoamines stimulate testicular testosterone release of the immature golden hamster via inter action with alpha- and beta-adrenergic receptors. *Acta Endocr* 1992;127:526–530.
769. Mazo EB, Koriakin MV, Evseev LP, Akopian AS. The role of the functional interrelation of the adrenals and testes in the pathogenesis of sterility in patients with left-sided varicocele. (in Russian) *Urol Nefrol (Mosk)* 1990;(2):50–58.
770. McConnell J, Benson GS, Wood JG. Autonomic innervation of the urogenital system: adrenergic and cholinergic elements. *Brain Res Bull* 1982;9:679–694.
771. McCullough DL. Experimental lymphangiography. Experience with direct medium injection into the parenchyma of the rat testis and prostate. *Invest Urol* 1975;13:211–219.
772. McDonald SW, Scothorne RJ. The lymphatic drainage of the epididymis and of the ductus deferens of the rat, with reference to the immune response to vasectomy. *J Anat* 1988;158:57–64.
773. McIntosh GH. Lymphatics of the urogenital system of the sheep. *Ph.D. Thesis,* Australian National University, Canberra, 1969.
774. McKenzie FF, Miller JC, Bauguess LC. The reproductive organs and semen of the boar. *Bull Univ Miss Agric Exp Sta.,* No. 279. 1938.
775. McNeal JE. The zonal anatomy of the prostate. *Prostate* 1981;2:35–49.
776. McNeal JE. Normal histology of the prostate. *Am J Surg Pathol* 1988;12:619–633.
777. Melampy RM, Mason RB. Androgen and the myoinositol content of male accessory organs of the rat. *Proc Soc Elp Biol Med* 1957;96:405–408.
778. Melikoglu M, Guntekin E, Erkilic M, Karaveli S. Contralateral testicular blood flow in unilateral testicular torsion measured by the ^{133}Xe clearance technique. 1992.
779. Melin P. *In vivo* recording of contractile activity of male accessory genital organs in rabbits. *Acta Physiol Scand* 1970;79: 109–113.
780. Melsert R, Hoogerbrugge JW, Rommerts FFG. The albumin fraction of rat testicular fluid stimulates steroid production by isolated Leydig cells. *Molec Cell Endocr* 1988;59:221–231.
781. Mendis-Handagama SMLC, Kerr JB, de Kretser DM. Experimental cryptorchidism in the adult mouse: I. Qualitative and quantitative light microscopic morphology. *J Androl* 1990;11: 539–547.
782. Menon M, Menon S, Strauss HW, Catalona WJ. Demonstration of the existence of canine prostatic lymphatics by radioisotope techniques. *J Urol* 1977;118:274–277.
783. Metafora S, Peluso G, Persico P, Ravagnan G, Esposito C, Porta R. Immunosuppressive and anti-inflammatory properties of a major protein secreted from the epithelium of the rat seminal vesicles. *Biochem Pharmacol* 1989;38:121–131.
784. Metafora S, Porta R, Ravagnan G, Peluso G, Tufano MA, de Martino L, Ianello R, Galdiero F. Inhibitory effect of SV-IV, a major protein secreted from the rat seminal vesicle epithelium, on phagocytosis and chemotaxis of human polymophonuclear leukocytes. *J Leukoc Biol* 1989;46:409–416.
785. Metheeuws D, Comhaire FH. Concentrations of oestradiol and testosterone in peripheral and spermatic venous blood of dogs with unilateral cryptorchidism. *Domest Anim Endocrinol* 1989;6:203–209.
786. Middleton A. Glucose metabolism in rat seminiferous tubules. *Ph.D. Thesis,* University of Cambridge, Cambridge. 1973:90.
787. Middleton A, Setchell BP. The origin of inositol in rete testis fluid. *J Reprod Fertil* 1972;30:473–475.
788. Middleton WD, Thorne DA, Melson GL. Color doppler ultrasound of the normal testis. *Am J Roentgenol* 1989;152:293–297.
789. Mieusset R, Sowerbutts SF, Zupp JL, Setchell BP. Increased testicular blood plasma flow during local heating of the testes of rams. *J Reprod Fertil* 1992;94:345–352.
790. Miller DC, Peron SE, Keck RW, Kropp KA. Effects of hypothermia on testicular ischemia. *J Urol* 1990;143:1046–1048.
791. Miller SC, Bowman BM, Rowland HG. Structure, cytochemistry, endocytotic activity and immunoglobulin (Fc): receptors of rat testicular interstitial-tissue macrophages. *Am J Anat* 1983;168:1–13.
792. Miller SC, Bowman BM, Roberts LK. Identification and characterization of mononuclear phagocytes isolated from rat testicular interstitial tissues. *J Leucocyt Biol* 1984;36:679.
793. Mirando MA, Hoagland TA, Woody CO Jr, Riesen JW. The influence of unilateral castration on testicular morphology and function in adult rams. *Biol Reprod* 1989;41:798–806.
794. Miyake K, Yamamoto M, Mitsuya H. Pharmacological and histological evidence for adrenergic innervation of the myoid cells in the rat seminiferous tubule. *Tohoku J Exp Med* 1986;149:79–87.
795. Mizamura K, Tadaki E, Kumazawa T. Respiratory changes induced by activation of testicular afferents in dogs. *Pflugers Arch* 1988;411:27–33.
796. Mizunuma H, Palatis L, McCann SM. Effect of unilateral orchidectomy on plasma FSH concentration: evidence for a direct

neural connection between testes and CNS. *Neuroendocrinology* 1983;37:291–296.
797. Mock EJ, Frankel AI. Response of testosterone to hemicastration in the testicular vein of the mature rat. *J Endocrinol* 1982;92:231–236.
798. Moger WH, Murphy PR. β-Adrenergic agonist induced androgen production during primary culture of mouse Leydig cells. *Arch Androl* 1983;10:135–142.
799. Moger WH, Murphy PR, Casper RF. Catecholamine stimulation of androgen production by mouse interstitial cells in primary culture. *J Androl* 1982;3:227–231.
800. Moller R. Arrangement and fine structure of lymphatic vessels in the human spermatic cord. *Andrologia* 1980;12:564–576.
801. Moneti G, Pazzagli M, Fiorelli G, Serio M. Measurement of 5α-androstane-3α,17β-diol in human spermatic venous plasma by mass-fragmentography. *J Steroid Biochem* 1980;13:623–627.
802. Moniem KA, Glover TD, Lubicz-Nawrocki CW. Effect of duct ligation and orchidectomy on histochemical reactions in the hamster epididymis. *J Reprod Fertil* 1978;54:173–176.
803. Montagna W, Noback CR. The histology of the preputial gland of the rat. *Anat Rec* 1946;96:111–128.
804. Morales C, Hermo L. Intracellular pathways of endocytosed transferrin and non-specific tracers in epithelial cells lining the rete testis of the rat. *Cell Tissue Res* 1986;245:323–330.
805. Morales C, Hermo L, Clermont Y. Endocytosis in epithelial cells lining the rete testis of the rat. *Anat Rec* 1984;209:185–195.
806. Mori H, Christensen AK. Morphometric analysis of Leydig cells in the normal rat testis. *J Cell Biol* 1980;84:340–354.
807. Mori H, Shimizu D, Takeda A, Takioka Y, Fukunishi R. Stereological analysis of Leydig cells in normal guinea pig testis. *J Electron Microsc* 1980;29:8–21.
808. Mori H, Shimizu D, Fukunishi R, Christensen AK. Morphometric analysis of testicular Leydig cells in normal adult mice. *Anat Rec* 1982;204:333–339.
809. Morita I. Some observations on the fine structure of the human ductuli efferentes testis. *Arch Histol Jpn* 1966;6:341–365.
810. Morris B, McIntosh GH. The lymphatic drainage of the testis and scrotal serous cavity in the ram. In: *Progress in Lymphology 11,* edited by M Viamonte PR Kochler M Witte, C Witte, Stuttgart: Georg Thieme Verlag, 1970:173–176.
811. Morris B, McIntosh GH. Techniques for the collection of lymph with special reference to the testis and ovary. *Acta Endocrinol., Suppl* 1971;158:145–168.
812. Morris ID. Effect on gonadotrophin secretion of blockage of ductuli efferentes in the normal and androgen-deprived rat. *J Reprod Fertil* 1979;57:469–475.
813. Morris ID, Bardin CW, Musto NA, Thau RB, Gunsalus GL. Evidence suggesting that germ cells influence the bidirectional secretion of androgen binding protein by the seminiferous epithelium demonstrated by selective impairment of spermatogenesis with busulphan. *Int J Androl* 1987;10:691–700.
814. Moss HE, Crowe R, Burnstock G. The seminal vesicle in eight and 16 week streptozotocin-induced diabetic rats: adrenergic, cholinergic and peptidergic innervation. *J Urol* 1987;138: 1273–1278.
815. Mostofi FK. Testicular tumors. *Cancer* 1973;32:1186–1201.
816. Motola JA, Hoory S, Smith AD, Mellinger BC. RP-30A: new tracer for detection of changes in testicular blood flow in rat torision model. *Urology* 1992;39:194–198.
817. Muffly KE, Turner TT, Brown M, Hall PF. Content of K^+ and Na^+ in seminiferous tubule and rete testis fluids from Sertoli cell-enriched testes. *Biol Reprod* 1985;33:1245–1251.
818. Muller I. Kanalchen- und Capillararchitektonik des Rattenhodens. *Z Zellforsch* 1957;45:522–537.
819. Murakami M, Yokoyama R, Nishida T, Shiromoto M, Sato H. Scanning and transmission electron microscope observations of the terminal segment of the cat seminiferous tubule: epithelial phagocytosis of spermatozoa and latex beads. *Arch Histol Cytol* 1988;51:185–192.
820. Murakami T, Uno Y, Ohtsula A, Taguchi T. The blood vascular architecture of the rat testis: a scanning electron microscopic study of corrosion casts followed by light microscopy of tissue sections. *Arch Histol Cytol* 1989;52:151–172.
821. Muramaki M, Hamasaki M, Okitas S, Abe I. SEM surface morphology of the contractile cells in the rat seminiferous tubules. *Experientia,* 1979;35:1099–1101.
822. Murashev AN, Medvedev OS, Meertsuk FE, Milakova GS. Hemodynamics in waking rats undergoing testicular exposure to elevated temperature. (in Russian) *Fiziol Zh SSSR.,* 1988;74: 1433–1437.
823. Muratori G. Osservazioni preliminari sull'azione dell'adrenalina e dell'acetilcolina sui movimenti del canale dell'epididimo del ratto. *Boll Soc Ital Biol Sper* 1956;32:248–249.
824. Muratori G. Bewegungen des Ductus epididymidis der Ratte (film). *Acta Anat* 1961;47:393.
825. Myers RP. Anatomical variation of the superficial preprostatic veins with respect to radical retropubic prostatectomy. *J Urol* 1991;145:992–993.
826. Myren CJ, Einer-Jensen N, Bennett P. The physiology of the testes in the Gottingen mini pig. *Z Versuchstierkd* 1989;32: 183–187.
827. Nagai K, Murano S, Minokoshi Y, Okuda H, Kinutani M. Effects of denervation and local 6-hydroxydopamine injection on testicular growth in rats. *Experientia* 1982;38:592–594.
828. Nagler HM, White R deV. The effect of testicular torsion on the contralateral testis. *J Urol* 1982;128:1343–1348.
829. Nagler HM, Lizza EF, House SD, Tomashefsky P, Lipowsky HH. Testicular hemodynamic changes after a surgically induced varicocele in the rat. Intravital microscopic observations. *J Androl* 1987;8:292–298.
830. Nakai M, Nasu T. Ultrastructural study on junctional complexes of the excurrent duct epithelia in the epididymal region in the fowl. *J Vet Med Sci* 1991;53:677–681.
831. Nakai M, Hashimoto Y, Kitagawa H, Kon Y, Kudo N. Microvasculature of the epididymis and ductus deferens of domestic fowls. *Nippon Juigaku Zasshi* 1988;50:371–381.
832. Nakayama T, Ishikawa Y, Tsurutani T. Projection of scrotal thermal afferents to the preoptic and hypothalamic neurons in rats. *Pfluegers Arch* 1979;380:59–64.
833. Nalbandov AV. *Reproductive Physiology of Mammals and Birds,* 3rd ed., W. H. Freeman and Company, San Francisco. 1976:334.
834. Neaves WB, Billingham RE. The lymphatic drainage of the rat prostate and its status as an immunologically privileged site. *Transplantation,* 1979;27:127–132.
835. Nemetallah BR, Howell RE, Ellis LC. Histamine H1 receptors and prostaglandin-histamine interactions modulating contractility of rabbit and rat testicular capsules *in vitro. Biol Reprod* 1983;28:632–635.
836. Nicander L. On the regional histology and cytochemistry of the ductus epididymidis in rabbits. *Acta Morphol Neerl Scand* 1957;1:99–118.
837. Nicander L. Studies on the regional histology and cytochemistry of the ductus epididymidis in stallions, rams and bulls. *Acta Morphol Neerl Scand* 1957;1:337–362.
838. Nicander L, Osman DL, Ploen L, Bugge HP, Kvisgaard KN. Early effects of efferent ductule ligation on the proximal segment of the rat epididymis. *Int J Androl* 1983;6:91–102.
839. Nielsen EH. The bulbourethral gland of the rat. Fine structure and histochemistry. *Anat Anz* 1976;139:254–263.
840. Niemi M, Kormano M. An angiographic study of cadmium-induced vascular lesions in the testis and epididymis of the rat. *Acta Pathol Microbiol Scand* 1965;63:513–521.
841. Niemi M, Kormano M. Contractility of the seminiferous tubule of the postnatal rat testis and its response to oxytocin. *Ann Med Exp Fenn* 1965;43:40–42.
842. Niemi M, Setchell BP. Gamma-glutamyl transpeptidase in the vasculature of the rat testis. *Biol Reprod* 1987;35:385–391.
843. Niemi M, Sharpe RM, Brown WRA. Macrophages in the interstitial tissue of the rat testis. *Cell Tiss Res* 1986;243:337–344.
844. Niewenhuis RJ, Meineke HA. Sensitivity of locally regenerated testicular vessels to cadmium. *Arch Androl* 1986;16:13–18.
845. Nishida T. Comparative and topographical anatomy of the fowl. XLII. Blood vascular system of the male reproductive organs (in Japanese). *Nippon Jugaku Zasshi* 1964;26:211–221.
846. Nistal M, Paniagua R, Abaurrea MA. Varicose axons bearing "synaptic" vesicles on the basal lamina of the human seminiferous tubules. *Cell Tiss Res* 1982;226:75–82.

847. Nistal M, Paniagua R, Regadera J, Santamaria L. Obstruction of the tubuli recti and ductuli efferentes by dilated veins in the testes in men with variococele and its possible role in causing atrophy of the seminiferous tubules. *Int J Androl* 1984;7: 309–323.
848. Nistal M, Santamaria L, Paniagua R. Mast cells in the human testis and epididymis from birth to adulthood. *Acta Anat* 1984;119:155–160.
849. Nistal M, Palacios J, Refadera J, Paniagua R. Postsurgical focal testicular infarction. *Urol Int* 1986;41:149–151.
850. Nistal M, Santamaria L, Paniagua R. Acquired cyctic transformation of the rete testis secondary to renal failure. *Hum Pathol* 1989;20:1065–1070.
851. Noguiera JC, Ribiero MG, Campos PA. Histology and carbohydrate histochemistry of the prostate gland of the Brazilian four-eyed opossum (Philander opossum Linnaeus, 1758). *Anat Anz* 1985;159:241–252.
852. Noordhuizen-Stassen EN, Wensing CJG. The effect of transection of the main vascular and nervous supply of the testis on the development of spermatogenic epithelium in the pig. *J Pediatr Surg* 1983;18:601–606.
853. Noordhuizen-Stassen EN, Wensing CJG. Age-related effects of transection of the testicular blood vessels on subsequent testicular development in the pig. *Int J Androl* 1986;9:141–151.
854. Noordhuizen-Stassen EN, Beijer HIM, Charbon GA, Wensing CJG. The effect of norepinephrine, isoprenaline and acetylcholine on the testicular and epididymal circulation in the pig. *Int J Androl* 1983;6:44–56.
855. Noordhuizen-Stassen EN, Dijkstra G, Schanhardt HC, Wensing CJG. Compensatory development of a patent vascular supply to the testis after intra-abdominal transection of its main blood vessels. *Int J Androl* 1983;6:509–519.
856. Noordhuizen-Stassen EN, Buwalda G, Wensing CJG. Testicular, arterial, and venous blood pressure patterns in ram and boar. *In: Functional and Morphological Aspects of Testicular Blood Supply* [Doctoral thesis]. EN Noordhuizen-Stassen. Utrecht, Netherlands: Rijksuniversiteit, Amsterdam: Offsetdrukkerij Kanters BV, 1984;73–80.
857. Noordhuizen-Stassen EN, Charbon GA, de Jong FH, Wensing CJG. Functional arterio-venous anastomoses between the testicular artery and the pampiniform plexus in the spermatic cord of rams. *J Reprod Fertil* 1985;75:193–201.
858. Noordhuizen-Stassen EN, de Jong FH, MacDonald AA, Schamhardt HC, Wensing CJG. Investigations of arteriovenous anastomoses in the spermatic cords and blood supply, oxygen consumption and testosterone production of scrotal and abdominal testes in the pig. *Int J Androl* 1988;11:493–505.
859. Norberg KA, Risley PL, Ungerstedt U. Adrenergic innervation of the male reproductive ducts in some mammals. 1. The distribution of adrenergic nerves. *Z Zellforsch* 1967;76:278–286.
860. Nouhaouayi Y, Negulesco I. Histochemical and ultrastructural data on the adrenergic and cholinergic innervation of the epididymis in the mouse. *Acta Anat (Basel)* 1987;128:23–26.
861. Nykanen M. Fine structure of the transitional zone of the rat seminiferous tubule. *Cell Tiss Res* 1979;198:441–454.
862. Nykanen M, Kormano M. Early effects of efferent duct ligation on the rat rete testis. *Int J Androl* 1978;1:225–234.
863. Oettle AG, Harrison RG. The histological changes produced in the rat testis by temporary and permanent occlusion of the testicular artery. *J Path Bact* 1952;64:273–29.
864. Ohanian C, Rodriguez H, Piriz H, Martino I, Rieppi G, Garafalo EG, Roca RA. Studies on the contractile activity and ultrastructure of the boar testicular capsule. *J Reprod Fertil* 1979;57:79–85.
865. Ohtani O, Gannon BJ. The microvasculature of the rat vas deferens: a scanning electron and light microscopic study. *J Anat* 1982;135:521–529.
866. Ohtsuka A. Microvascular architecture of the pampiniform plexus-testicular artery system in the rat: a scanning microscope study of corrosion casts. *Am J Anat* 1984;169:285–293.
867. Okkels H, Sand K. Morphological relationship between testicular nerves and Leydig cells in man. *J Endocrinol* 1940;2:38–46.
868. Okumura K, Lee IP, Dixon RL. Permeability of selected drugs and chemicals across the blood testis barrier of the rat. *J Pharmacol Exptl Ther* 1975;194:89–95.
869. Okuyama A, Nakamura M, Namiki M, Takeyama M, Fujioka H, Matsuda M, Matsumoto K, Sonoda T. Demonstration of gonadotropin-induced plasma renin activity in human internal spermatic vein. *Acta Endocrinol (Copenh)* 1988;117:268–272.
870. Okuyama A, Nonomura N, Koh E, Kondoh N, Takeyama M, Nakamura M, Namiki M, Fujioka H, Matsumoto K, Matsuda M. Induction of renin-angiotensin system in human testis in vivo. *Arch Androl* 1988;21:29–35.
871. Okuyama A, Kondoh N, Koh E, Takeyama M, Fujioka H, Matsuda M, Matsumoto K. Correlative changes of plasma renin activity and serum testosterone in human internal spermatic vein after surgical administration of human chorionic gonadotrophin. *Int Urol Nephrol* 1989;21:659–665.
872. Olson GE, Hinton B. Regional difference in luminal fluid polypeptides of the rat testis and epididymis revealed by two-dimensional gel electrophoresis. *J Androl* 1985;6:20–34.
873. Oltjen RR, Bond J, Gerrits RJ, Johnson LA. Growth and reproductive performance of bulls and heifers fed purified and natural diets. V. Free amino acids in the semen and blood plasma of bulls (puberty to 148 weeks of age). *J Anim Sci* 1971;33:814–818.
874. Ong DE, Chytil F. Presence of novel retinoic acid-binding proteins in the lumen of rat epididymis. *Arch Biochem Biophys* 1988;267:474–478.
875. Orsi AM, Ferreira AL, de Mello VR, Oliviera MC. Regional histology of the epididymis in the South American opossum. Light microscope study. *Anat Anz* 1981;150:521–528.
876. Orsi AM, Dias SM, Seullner G, Guazzelli-Filho J, Vicentini CA. Structure des canaux efferents du porc domestique (*Sus scrofa domestica*). *Anat Anz* 1987;163:249–254.
877. Orsulak PJ, Gawienowski AM. Olfactory preferences for the rat preputial gland. *Biol Reprod* 1972;6:219–223.
878. Orth J, Christensen AK. Localization of 125-I-labelled FSH in the testes of hypophysectomized rats by autoradiography at the light and electronmicroscope levels. *Endocrinology* 1977;101: 262–278.
879. Ortiz E, Price D, Williams-Ashman HG, Banks J. The influence of androgen on the male accessory reproductive glands of the guinea pig: studies of growth, histological structure and fructose and citric acid secretion. *Endocrinology* 1956;59:479–492.
880. Ortolano V, Nasrallah PF. Spermatic vein ligation (Fowler-Stephens maneuver): experimental results with regard to fertility. *J Urol* 1986;136:211–213.
881. Osman DI. On the ultrastructure of modified Sertoli cells in the terminal segment of seminiferous tubules in the boar. *J Anat* 1978;127:603–613.
882. Osman DI. The ultrastructure of the rete testis and its permeability barrier before and after efferent duct ligation. *Int J Androl* 1978;1:357–370.
883. Osman DI, Ploen L. The mammalian tubuli recti: ultrastructural study. *Anat Rec* 1978;192:1–18.
884. Osman DI, Ploen L. The terminal segment of the seminiferous tubules and the blood-testis barrier before and after efferent ductule ligation in the rat. *Int J Androl* 1978;1:234–249.
885. Osman DI, Ploen L. Fine structure of the modified Sertoli cells in the terminal segment of the seminiferous tubules of the bull, ram and goat. *Anim Reprod Sci* 1979;2:343–351.
886. Osman DI, Ploen L, Hagenas L. On the postnatal development of the terminal segment of the seminiferous tubules in normal and germ cell depleted rat testes. *Int J Androl* 1979;2:419–431.
887. Osman DI, Tingari MD, Moniem KA. Vascular supply of the testis of the camel (*Camelus dromedarius*). *Acta Anat* 1979;104:16–22.
888. Owman C, Sjostrand NO. Short adrenergic neurons and catecholamine-containing cells in vas deferens and accessory male genital glands of different mammals. *Z Zellforsch* 1965;66: 300–320.
889. Pande JK, Chowdhury SR, Dasgupta PR, Chowdhury AR, Kar AB. Biochemical composition of the rat testis fluid. *Proc Soc Exp Biol Med* 1966;121:899–902.
890. Pande JK, Dasgupta PR, Kar AB. Biochemical composition of human testicular fluid collected post mortem. *J Clin Endocrinol Metabol* 1967;27:892–894.

891. Pande JK, Dasgupta PR, Kar AB. Chemical composition of fluid collected from testis of the rhesus monkey and goat. *Ind J Exp Biol* 1967;5:65–67.
892. Paniagua R, Regadera J, Nistal M, Abaurrea MA. Histological, histochemical and ultrastructural variations along the length of the human vas deferens before and after puberty. *Acta Anat* 1981;111:190–203.
893. Paniagua R, Regadera J, Nistal M, Santamaria L. Elastic fibres of the human ductus deferens. *J Anat* 1983;137:467–476.
894. Pannese E. Osservazioni morfologiche e istochemiche sulle ghiandole preputiale del ratto. *Arch Ital Anat Embriol* 1954;59:57–82.
895. Papadopoulos V, Kamtchouing P, Boujrad N, Pisselet C, Perreau C, Locatelli A, Drosdowsky MA, Hochereau-de Reviers MT, Carreau S. Evidence for LH-inhibiting activity in ovine peripheral and testicular blood. *Acta Endocr* 1990;123:345–352.
896. Parvinen M, Wright WW, Phillips DM, Mather JP, Musto NA, Bardin CW. Spermatogenesis *in vitro:* completion of meiosis and early spermiogenesis. *Endocrinology* 1983;112:1150–1152.
897. Pascual JA, Villanueva-Meyer J, Salido E, Ehrlich RM, Mena L, Rajfer J. Recovery of testicular blood flow following ligation of testicular vessels. *J Urol* 1989;142:549–552.
898. Pascual JA, Villanueva-Meyer J, Rutgers JL, Lemmi CA, Sikka SC, Ehrlich RM, Mena L, Rajfer J. Long-term effects of prepubertal testicular vessel ligation on testicular function in the rat. *J Urol* 1990;144:466–468.
899. Paskins-Hurlburt AJ, McCracken S, Hollenberg NK. Autonomy extends to the arterial supply of rapidly growing tumors. Studies on the feeder vessels to carcinoma in rat testis. *Invest Radiol* 1986;21:455–458.
900. Pegg AE, Lockwood DH, Williams-Ashman HG. Concentrations of putrescine and polyamines and their enzymic synthesis during androgen-induced prostatic growth. *Biochem J* 1970; 117:1731.
901. Peirce EJ, Breed WG. Light microscopical structure of the excurrent ducts and distribution of spermatozoa in the Australian rodents Pseudomys australis and Notomys alexis. *J Anat* 1989;162:195–213.
902. Peirce EJ, Breed WG. Organization of testicular interstitial tissue of an Australian rodent the spinifex hopping mouse, *Notomys alexis. Cell Tiss Res* 1990;260:469–477.
903. Peitz B. Effects of seminal vesicle fluid components onsperm motility in the house mouse. *J Reprod Fertil* 1988;83:169–176.
904. Pekary AE, Yamada T, Sharp B, Bhasin S, Swerdloff RS, Hershman IM. Somatostatin-14 and -28 in the male rat reproductive system. *Life Sci* 1984;34:939–945.
905. Pelletier RM. Cyclic formation and decay of the blood-testis barrier in the mink (Mustela vison), a seasonal breeder. *Am J Anat* 1986;175:91–117.
906. Pelletier RM. Cyclic modulation of Sertoli cell junctional complexes in a seasonal breeder: The mink (*Mustela vison*). *Am J Anat* 1988;183:68–102.
907. Pelletier RM. A novel perspective: The occluding zonule encircles the apex of the Sertoli cell as observed in birds. *Am J Anat* 1990;188:87–108.
908. Pelletier RM, Byers SW. The blood-testis barrier and Sertoli cell junctions: Structural considerations. *Microsc Res Tech* 1992;20:3–22.
909. Perey B, Clermont Y, Leblond CP. The wave of the seminiferous epithelium in the rat. *Am J Anat* 1961;108:47–77.
910. Perez-Casas A, Cabo-Tomargo JA, Bengoechea-Gonzalez E, Lopez-Muniz A, Vega-Alvarez JA. Contribicion al conocimiento de la inervacion microscopica de la prostata (II): Los microganglios intramurales. *Arch Esp Urol* 1985;38:365–373.
911. Perez-Casas A, Cabo-Tamargo JA, Begoechea-Gonzalez E, Lopez-Muniz A, Vega-Alvarez JA. Contribucion al conocimiento de la prostata III. Los corpusculos sensitivos terminales. *Arch Esp Urol* 1985;38:433–438.
912. Perez-Clavier R, Harrison RG. The effect of interruption of lymphatic drainage from the rat testis. *J Pathol* 1978;124:219–225.
913. Perez-Clavier R, Harrison RG. The pattern of lymphatic drainage of the rat testis. *J Anat* 1978;127:93–100.
914. Perez-Clavier R, Harrison RG, MacMillan EW. The pattern of the lymphatic drainage of the rat epididymis. *J Anat* 1982;134:667–675.
915. Peterson DF, Brown AM. Functional afferent innervation of testis. *J Neurophysiol* 1973;36:425–433.
916. Pholpramool C, Triphrom N. Effects of cholinergic and adrenergic drugs on intraluminal pressures and contractility of the rat testis and epididymis *in vivo. J Reprod Fertil* 1984;71:181–188.
917. Pholpramool C, White RW, Setchell BP. Influence of androgens on inositol secretion and sperm transport in the epididymis of rats. *J Reprod Fertil* 1982;66:547–553.
918. Picard JV, Tran D, Vigier B, Josso N. Maintien des canaux de Muller chez le lapin male par immunisation passive contre l'hormone antimullerienne pendant la vie foetale. *C R Acad Sc Paris* 1983;297:567–570.
919. Pierau FK, Torrey P, Carpenter DO. Afferent nerve fiber activity responding to temperature changes of scrotal skin of the rat. *J Neurophysiol* 1975;38:601–612.
920. Pierrepoint CG, Davies P, Lewis MH, Moffat DB. Examination of the hypothesis that a direct control system exists for the prostate and seminal vesicles. *J Reprod Fertil* 1975;44:395–409.
921. Piffer CR, Piffer MI. Anatomical observations of the testicular veins. *Anat Anz* 1988;166:249–255.
922. Piffer CR, Piffer MI, Zorzetto NL. Structural features of the human testicular veins walls. *Anat Anz* 1988;166:257–266.
923. Pilsworth LMC, Hinton BT, Setchell BP. Effects of obstruction of the flow of seminiferous tubule fluid on the germinal epithelium of the rat. *J Reprod Fertil* 1981;63:347–353.
924. Pinelli P, Trivulzio S, Colombo R, Cocchi D, Faravelli R, Ciavezel F, Galmozzi G, Cavallaro R. Antiprostatic effect of cimetidine in rats. *Agents Actions* 1987;22:197–201.
925. Pirke KM, Bofilas I, Sintermann R, Langhammer H, Wolf I, Pabst HW. Relative capillary blood flow and Leydig cell function in old rats. *Endocrinology* 1979;105:842–845.
926. Pirke KM, Bofilas I, Spyra B, Langhammer H, Pabst HW. Capillary blood flow in the testes and testosterone secretion in the starved rat. *Experientia* 1982;38:516–517.
927. Ploen L, Setchell BP. Blood-testis barriers revisited. A homage to Lennart Nicander. *Int J Androl* 1992;15:1–4.
928. Polak JM, Gu I, Mina S, Bloom SR. VIPergic nerves in the penis. *Lancet* 1981;2:217–219.
929. Pollanen P, Maddocks S. Macrophages, lymphocytes and MHC II antigen in the ram and rat testis. *J Reprod Fert* 1988;82:437–445.
930. Pollanen P, Setchell BP. Microvascular permeability to IgG in the rat testis at puberty. *Int J Androl* 1989;12:206–218.
931. Pomerantz DK, Jansz GF, Wilson N. Disruption of spermatogenesis is associated with decrease concentration of immunoreactive arginine vasopressin in testicular fluid. *Biol Reprod* 1988;39:610–616.
932. Pope GS, Cunningham JM, Jenkins N, Waites GMH, Watts GE. Oestradiol-17β in testis and jugular venous plasma of intact and hemicastrated prepubertal lambs and in jugular venous plasma of castrated prepubertal lambs. *Anim Reprod Sci* 1990;22:9–19.
933. Poyser NL. Some aspects of prostaglandins in reproduction. *Biochem Soc Trans* 1974;2:1196–1200.
934. Prendergast FG, Veneziale CM. Control of fructose and citrate synthesis in guinea pig seminal vesicle epithelium. *J Biol Chem* 1975;250:1282–1289.
935. Preslock JP, McCann SM. Short-term effects of vasoligation upon plasma follicle-stimulating hormone, luteinizing hormone and prolactin in the adult rat: further evidence for a direct neural connection between the testes and the central nervous system. *Biol Reprod* 1985;33:1120–1125.
936. Price D, Williams-Ashman HG. (1961): The accessory reproductive glands of mammals. In: *Sex and Internal Secretions, 3rd ed., Vol. 1,* edited by WC Young, pp. 366–448. Williams & Wilkins, Baltimore.
937. Pugh RCB. (1976): *Pathology of the Testis.* Blackwells, Oxford, 487 pp.
938. Pujol A, Bayard F, Louvet J-P, Boulard C. Testosterone and dihydrotestosterone concentrations in plasma, epididymal tissues, and seminal fluid of adult rats. *Endocrinology* 1976;98:111–113.
939. Pulkkinen P. Specific inhibition of spermatozoal energy metabolism by oxidized spermine. *Contraception* 1978;17:423–433.

940. Pulkkinen P, Sinervirta R, Janne J. Modification of the metabolism of the rat epididymal spermatozoa by spermine. *Biochem Biophys Res Commun* 1975;67:714–722.
941. Pulkkinen P, Sinervirta R, Janne J. Mechanism of action of oxidized polyamines on the metabolism of human spermatozoa. *J Reprod Fertil* 1977;51:399–404.
942. Punjabi U, Van Hoecke L, Verdonck L, Vermeulen A. Testicular blood flow in young and old rats and influence of hCG. *J Androl* 1984;5:223–226.
943. Quinn PJ, White IG, Wirrick BR. Studies of the distribution of the major cations in semen and male accessory secretions. *J Reprod Fertil* 1965;10:379–388.
944. Ragimov Z. Adrenergic and cholinergic innervation of the prostate in laboratory animals (in Russian). *Arkh Anat Gistol Embriol* 1988;94:47–53.
945. Rajfer J, Walsh PC. Hormonal regulation of testicular descent: experimental and clinical observations. *J Urol* 1977;118: 985–990.
946. Rajfer J, Turner TT, Rivera F, Howards SS, Sikka SC. Inhibition of testicular testosterone biosynthesis following experimental varicocele in rats. *Biol Reprod* 1987;36:933–937.
947. Ramos AS, Dym M. Fine structure of the monkey epididymis. *Am J Anat* 1977;149:501–532.
948. Ramos AS, Dym M. Ultrastructure of the ductuli efferentes in monkeys. *Biol Reprod* 1977;17:339–349.
949. Redondo E, Regadera J, Nistal M, Rey A, Espana G, Regadera-Sejas FJ, Codesal J. Anatomia y desarrollo del sistema venoso testicular. *Arch esp Urol* 1988;41:171–178.
950. Reid BL, Cleland KW. The structure and function of the epididymis. I. The histology of the rat epididymis. *Aust J Zool* 1957;5:223–246.
951. Rerkamnuaychoke W, Kuromaru M, Nishida T. Microvascular architecture of the pampiniform plexus and testicular artery in the golden hamster. *Nippon Juigaku Zasshi* 1988;50:273–275.
952. Rerkamnuoychoke W, Nishida T, Kuromaru M, Hayashi Y. Vascular morphology of the golden hamster spermatic cord. *Arch Histol Cytol* 1989;52:183–190.
953. Rerkamnuaychoke W, Nishida T, Kurohmaru, Hayashi Y. Evidence for a direct arteriovenous connection (A-V shunt) between the testicular artery and pampiniform plexus in the spermatic cord of the tree shrew. *J Anat* 1991;178:1–9.
954. Richardson KC. Electron microscopic identification of autonomic nerve endings. *Nature* 1966;210:756.
955. Rikimaru A, Shirai M. Responses of the human testicular capsule to electrical stimulation and to autonomic drugs. *Tohoku J exp Med* 1972;108:303–304.
956. Rikamaru A, Suzuki T. Mechanical responses of the isolated rabbit testis to electrical stimulation and autonomic drugs. *Tohoku J exp Med* 1972;103:283–289.
957. Rikimaru A, Maruyama T, Shirai M, Dendo I. Pressure recording of contraction of the dog testis. *Tohoku J Exp Med* 1972;108:305–306.
958. Risbridger GP, Kerr JB, de Kretser DM. Evaluation of Leydig cell function and gonadotropin binding in unilateral and bilateral cryptorchidism: evidence for local control of Leydig cell function by the seminiferous tubule. *Biol Reprod* 1981;24: 534–540.
959. Risley PL. The contractile behavior *in vivo* of the ductus epididymidis and vasa efferentia of the rat. *Anat Rec* 1958;130:471.
960. Risley PL, Skrepetos CN. Histochemical distribution of cholinesterases in the testis, epididymis and vas deferens of the rat. *Anat Rec* 1964;148:231–249.
961. Risley MS, Miller A, Bumcrot DA. *In vitro* maintenance of spermatogenesis in *Xenopus laevis* explants culture in serum-free media. *Biol Reprod* 1987;36:985–997.
962. Ritzen EM. Testicular relapse of acute lymphoblastic leukemia. *J Reprod Immunol* 1990;18:117–121.
963. Ritzen EM, Hagenas L, Purvis K, Guerrero T, Johnsonbaugh RE, Dym M, French FS, Hansson V. Androgens and androgen binding protein (ABP) in testicular fluids. In: Bierich JR, Raher K, Ranke MB. *Maldescensus Testis.* Heidelberg: Urban and Schwarzenberg, 1976;79–97.
964. Riva A, Usai E, Cossu M, Scarpa R, Testa-Riva F. The human bulbo-urethral glands. A transmission electron microscopy and scanning electron microscopy study. *J Androl* 1988;9:133–141.
965. Robinson R, Fritz IB. Myoinositol biosynthesis by Sertoli cells, and levels of myoinositol biosynthetic enzymes in testis and epididymis. *Can J Biochem* 1979;57:962–967.
966. Rodger JC. The testis and its excurrent ducts in American caenolestid and didelphid marsupials. *Am J Anat* 1982;163: 269–282.
967. Rodger JC, Hughes RL. Studies of the accessory glands of male marsupials. *Aust J Zool* 1973;21:303–320.
968. Rodger JC, White IG. Free N-acetylglucosamine in marsupial semen. *J Reprod Fertil* 1974;39:383–386.
969. Rodger JC, White IG. Electroejaculation of Australian marsupials and analyses of the sugars in the seminal plasma from three macropod species. *J Reprod Fertil* 1975;43:233–239.
970. Rodger JC, White IG. Source of seminal N-acetylglucosamine in Australian marsupials and further studies of free sugars of the marsupial prostate gland. *J Reprod Fertil* 1976;46:467–469.
971. Rodin AE, Larson DL, Roberts DK. Nature of the perineural space invaded by prostatic carcinoma. *Cancer* 1967;20: 1772–1779.
972. Rodriguez-Martinez H, Ekstedt E, Einarsson S. Acidification of the epididymal fluid in the boar. *Int J Androl* 1990;13:238–243.
973. Romero-Maroto J, Verdu-Tartajo F, Garcia-Gonzalez P, Cacicedo L. The functional value of collateral vascularisation. An experimental study. *Br J Urol* 1986;58:553–556.
974. Rommel SA, Pabst DA, McLellan WA, Mead JG, Potter CW. Anatomical evidence for a countercurrent heat exchanger associated with dolphin testes. *Anat Rec* 1992;232:150–156.
975. Roosen-Runge EC. Motions of the seminiferous tubules of rat and dog. *Anat Rec* 1951;109:413.
976. Roosen-Runge EC. The rete testis in the albino rat: its structure, development and morphological significance. *Acta Anat* 1961;45:1–30.
977. Roosen-Runge EC. *The Process of Spermatogenesis in Animals,* Cambridge: Cambridge University Press; 1977:214.
978. Roosen-Runge EC, Holstein AF. The human rete testis. *Cell Tiss Res* 1978;189:409–433.
979. Rosenthal SM, Tabor CW. The pharmacology of spermine and spermidine. Distribution and excretion. *J Pharmacol Exp Ther* 1956;116:131–138.
980. Ross MH. The fine structure and development of the peritubular contractile cell component in the seminiferous tubules of the mouse. *Am J Anat* 1967;121:523–558.
981. Ross MH, Grant L. On the structural integrity of the basement membrane. *Exp Cell Res* 1968;50:277–285.
982. Ross MH, Long IR. Contractile cells in human seminiferous tubules. *Science* 1966;153:1271–1273.
983. Ruokonen A, Lukkarinen O, Vihko R. Secretion of steroid sulphates from human testis and their response to a single intramuscular injection of 5000 IU hCG. *J Ster Biochem* 1981;14: 1357–1360.
984. Russell LD. Movement of spermatocytes from the basal to the adluminal compartment of the rat testis. *Am J Anat* 1977;148:313–328.
985. Russell LD, Bartke A, Goh JC. Postnatal development of the Sertoli cells barrier, tubular lumen and cytoskeleton of Sertoli and myoid cells in the rat, and their relationship to tubular fluid secretion and flow. *Am J Anat* 1989;184:179–189.
986. Russell LD, Saxena NK, Turner TT. Cytoskeletal involvement in spermiation and sperm transport. *Tissue Cell* 1989;21: 361–379.
987. Saba P, Gon Z, Carnicelli A, Todeschini G, Marescotti V. An electron microscopic study of the rat testis in experimental cryptorchidism. *Endokrinologie* 1972;60:103–116.
988. Saithoh K, Terada T, Hatakeyama S. A morphological study of the efferent ducts of the human epididymis. *Int J Androl* 1990;13:369–376.
989. Saito S, Kumamoto Y. Effect of kallikrein on testicular blood circulation. *Arch Androl* 1988;20:51–65.
990. Salman FT, Fonkalsrud EW. Effects of spermatic vascular division for correction of the high undescended testis on testicular function. *Am J Surg* 1990;160:506–510.
991. Samarakkody UKS, Hutson JM. Intrascrotal CGRP 8-37 causes a delay in testicular descent in mice. *J Pediatr Surg* (in press) 1992.
992. Samuel LH, Flickinger CJ. Incorporation of ^{3}H-fucose and the

secretion of glycoproteins in the coagulating gland of the mouse. *Anat Rec* 1986;214:53–60.
993. Samuel LH, Flickinger CJ. Intracellular pathway and kinetics of protein secretion in the coagulating gland of the mouse. *Biol Reprod* 1986;34:107–117.
994. Sand RS, Dutt RH. Semen characteristics in rams following occlusion of testis blood flow. *J Anim Sci* 1973;36:215.
995. Sand RS, Dutt RH, Preston DF. Effects of local heating on ram testis blood flow. *J Anim Sci* 1971;32:391.
996. Santamaria L, Reoyo A, Regadera J, Paniagua R. Histochemistry and ultrastructure of nerve fibres and contractile cells in the tunica albuginea of the rat testis. *Acta Anat (Basel)* 1990;139:126–133.
997. Santiemma V, Francavilla S, Santucci R, Onori D, Bellocci M, Fabbrini M. Development and hormone dependence of peritubular smooth muscle cells of the rat testis. In: Fabbrini A, Steinberger E. *Recent Progress in Andrology.* London: Academic Press, 1978:185–199.
998. Sar M, Stumpf WE, McLean WS, Smith AA, Hansson V, Nayfeh SN, French FS. Localization of androgen target cells in the rat testis: autoradiographic studies. *Curr Top Mol Endocrinol* 1975;2:311–319.
999. Sasano N, Ichijo S. Vascular patterns of the human testis with special reference to its senile changes. *Tohoku J Exp Med* 1969;99:269–280.
1000. Sastry BVR, Lanson VE, Owens LK, Tayeb OS. Enkephalin- and substance P-like immunoreactivities of mammalian sperm and accessory sex glands. *Biochem Pharmacol* 1982;31: 3519–3522.
1001. Sayfan J, Adams YG. Varicocele subfertility and venous pressure in the left internal spermatic vein. *Fertil Steril* 1978;29:366–367.
1002. Saypol DC. Varicocele. *J Androl* 1981;2:61–71.
1003. Saypol DC, Howards SS, Turner TT, Miller ED. Influence of surgically induced varicocele on testicular blood flow, temperature and histology in adult rats and dogs. *J Clin Invest* 1981;68:39–45.
1004. Schacht MJ, Niederberger CS, Garnett JE, Sensibar JA, Lee C, Grayhack JT. A local direct effect of pituitary graft on growth of the lateral prostate in rats. *Prostate* 1992;20:51–58.
1005. Schaffer J. Die Vorhautdrusen von Maus und Ratte. *Z Mikrosk Anat Forsch* 1933;34:1–22.
1006. Schanbacher BD. Rapid chromatography for quantitation of radioimmunoassayable 5α-androstane-17β-ol-3-one and testosterone in ram, bull and boar serum. *Endocr Res Commun* 1976;3:71–82.
1007. Schindelmeiser J, Kindermann EM, Hoffmann K. Photoperiodic influence on the innervation of the ductus epididymidis and ductus deferens of Phodopus sungorus-light microscopic studies. *Anat Anz* 1989;168:347–353.
1008. Schindelmeiser J, Kutzner M, Rolf LH, Hoffmann K. Photoperiodic influence on the innervation of the ductus epididymidis and ductus deferens of the Djungarian hamster, Phodopus sungorus: electron-microscopic and biochemical results. *Cell Tissue Res* 1989;256:175–181.
1009. Schingnitz G, Werner J. Responses of thalamic neurons to thermal stimulation of the limbs, scrotum and tongue in the rat. *J Therm Biol* 1980;5:53–61.
1010. Scholler R, Nahoul K, Grenier J, Charles JF, Netter A. Concentrations de sept steroides dans la veine spermatique de l'homme. Comparaison aux taux peripheriques. *Ann Endocrinol* 1975;36:353–354.
1011. Schulze W. Evidence of a wave of spermatogenesis in human testis. *Andrologia* 1982;14:200–207.
1012. Schulze W, Salzbrunn A. Spatial and quantitative aspects of spermatogenetic tissue in primates. In: Nieschlag E, Habenicht UF, eds. *Spermatogenesis, Fertilization, Conception.* Berlin: Springer-Verlag, 1992;267–283.
1013. Schweitzer R. Uber die Bedeutung der Vascularisation, der Binnendruckes und der Zwischenzellen fur die Biologie des Hodens. *Z Anat Entwickl* 1929;89:775–796.
1014. Scott JES. The Hutson hypothesis. *Br J Urol* 1987;60:74–76.
1015. Scott TW, Dawson RMC, Rowlands IW. Phospholipid interrelationships in rat epididymal tissue and spermatozoa. *Biochem J* 1963;87:507–512.
1016. Scott TW, Wales RG, Wallace JC, White IG. Composition of ram epididymal and testicular fluid and the biosynthesis of glycerylphosphorylcholine by the rabbit epididymis. *J Reprod Fertil* 1963;6:49–59.
1017. Sealy JE, Goldstein M, Pitarresi T, Kudlak TT, Glorioso N, Fiamengo SA, Laragh JH. Prorenin secretion from human testis: no evidence for secretion of active renin or angiotensinogen. *J Clin Endocrinol Metab* 1988;66:974–978.
1018. Seamark RF, Tate ME, Smeaton TC. The occurrence of scylloinositol and D-glycerol l-(L-myoinositol l-hydrogen phosphate) in the male reproductive tract. *J Biol Chem* 1968;243:2424–2428.
1019. Seidl K, Holstein AF. Evidence for the presence of nerve growth factor (NGF) and NGF receptor in human testis. *Cell Tiss Res* 1990;261:549–554.
1020. Seitz J, Aumuller G. Biochemical properties of secretory proteins from rat seminal vesicles. *Andrologia* 1990;22 Suppl. 1. 25–32.
1021. Seitz J, Enderle-Schmitt U, Scheit KH, Aumuller G. Immunological relationships between specific sperm proteins and secretory polypeptides from seminal vesicles. *Acta Histochem* 1989;37 Suppl.:231–233.
1022. Seki N, Suzuki H. Electrical and mechanical activity of rabbit prostate smooth muscles in response to nerve stimulation. *J Physiol (Lond)* 1989;419:651–663.
1023. Selstam G, Damber JE. Measurement of blood flow to the ventral prostate in the rat with radioactive microspheres: Effects of estradiol-17β and human chorionic gonadotrophin. *Acta Physiol Scand* 1983;119:209–212.
1024. Setchell BP. The blood-testicular fluid barrier in sheep. *J Physiol* 1967;189:63P.
1025. Setchell BP. Do Sertoli cells secrete fluid into the seminiferous tubules? *J Reprod Fertil* 1969;19:391–392.
1026. Setchell BP. Fluid secretion by the testes of an Australian marsupial *Macropus eugenii. Comp Physiol Biochem* 1970;36:411–414.
1027. Setchell BP. The secretion of fluid by the testes of rats, rams, and goats with some observations on the effect of age, cryptorchidism and hypophysectomy. *J Reprod Fertil* 1970;23:79–85.
1028. Setchell BP. Testicular blood supply, lymphatic drainage and secretion of fluid. In: Johnson AD, Gomes WR, Vandemark NL, eds. *The Testis, vol. 1.* New York: Academic Press, 1970;101–239.
1029. Setchell BP. Secretions of the testis and epididymis. *J Reprod Fertil* 1974;37:165–177.
1030. Setchell BP. The entry of substances into the seminiferous tubules. In: Mancini RE, Martini L, eds. *Male Fertility and Sterility,* New York: Academic Press; 1974:37–57.
1031. Setchell BP. Reproduction in male marsupials. In: Stonehouse B, Gilmore D, eds. *The Biology of Marsupials,* London: Macmillan; 1975:411–457.
1032. Setchell BP. *The Mammalian Testis,* London, Elek Books; and Ithaca: Cornell University Press; 1978.
1033. Setchell BP. The functional significance of the blood-testis barrier. *J Androl* 1980;1:3–10.
1034. Setchell BP. The flow and composition of lymph from the testes of pigs with some observations on the effect of raised venous pressure. *Comp Biochem Physiol* 1982;73A:201–205.
1035. Setchell BP. Male Reproduction. *Benchmark Papers in Human Physiology,* New York: Van Nostrand Reinhold; 1984;17.
1036. Setchell BP. Physiological communications between the testis and epididymis. *Proceedings of the International Union of Physiological Sciences,* 1986;16:494.
1037. Setchell BP. The movement of fluids and substances in the testis. *Aust J Biol Sci* 1987;39:193–207.
1038. Setchell BP. The testis and tissue transplantation; historical aspects. *J Reprod Immunol* 1990;18:1–8.
1039. Setchell BP. Local control of testicular fluids. *Reprod Fertil Dev* 1990;2:291–309.
1040. Setchell BP. Male reproductive organs and semen. In: Cupps PT, ed. *Reproduction in Domestic Animals, 4th ed.* New York: Academic Press; 1991:221–249.

1041. Setchell BP, Brown BW. The effect of metabolic alkalosis, hypotension and inhibitors of carbonic anhydrase on fluid secretion by the rat testis. *J Reprod Fertil* 1972;28:235–240.
1042. Setchell BP, Cox JE. Secretion of free and conjugated steroids by the horse testis into lymph and venous blood. *J Reprod Fertil* 1982;Suppl. 32:123–127.
1043. Setchell BP, Galil KAA. Limitations imposed by testicular blood flow on the function of Leydig cells in rats *in vivo. Aust J Biol Sci* 1983;36:285–293.
1044. Setchell BP, Hinks NT. The importance of glucose in the oxidative metabolism of the testis of the conscious ram and the role of the pentose cycle. *Biochem J* 1967;102:623–631.
1045. Setchell BP, Hinton BT. The effects of spermatozoa of changes in the composition of luminal fluid as it passes along the epididymis. *Prog Reprod Biol* 1981;8:58–66.
1046. Setchell BP, Jacks F. Inhibin-like activity in rete testis fluid. *J Endocrinol* 1974;62:675–676.
1047. Setchell BP, Linzell JL. Effects of some drugs, hormones and physiological factors on the flow of rete testis fluid in the ram. *J Reprod Fertil* 1968;16:320–321.
1048. Setchell BP, Main SJ. The blood-testis barrier and steroids. *Curr Top Mol Endocrinol* 1975;2:223–233.
1049. Setchell BP, Main SJ. Drugs and the blood-testis barrier. *Environ Health Perspect* 1978;24:61–64.
1050. Setchell BP, Pilsworth LM. Functions of the testes of vertebrate and invertebrate animals. In: Burger H, de Kretser D, eds. *The Testis, 2nd Edition,* New York: Raven Press; 1989:1–66.
1051. Setchell BP, Rommerts FFG. The importance of the Leydig cells in the vascular response to hCG in the rat testis. *Int J Androl* 1986;8:436–440.
1052. Setchell BP, Sharpe RM. Effect of injected human chorionic gonadotrophin on capillary permeability, extracellular fluid volume and the flow of lymph in the testes of rats. *J Endocrinol* 1981;91:245–254.
1053. Setchell BP, Waites GMH. Blood flow and the uptake of glucose and oxygen in the testis and epididymis of the ram. *J Physiol* 1964;171:411–425.
1054. Setchell BP, Waites GMH. Pulse attenuation and countercurrent heat exchange in the internal spermatic artery of some Australian marsupials. *J Reprod Fertil* 1969;20:165–169.
1055. Setchell BP, Waites GMH. Changes in the permeability of the testicular capillaries and of the "blood-testis barrier" after injection of cadmium chloride in the rat. *J Endocrinol* 1970;47:81–86.
1056. Setchell BP, Waites GMH. The effects of local heating of the testis on the flow and composition of rete testis fluid in the rat, with some observations on the effects of age and unilateral castration. *J Reprod Fertil* 1972;30:225–233.
1057. Setchell BP, Waites GMH. The blood-testis barrier. In: Hamilton DW, Greep RO, eds. *Handbook of Physiology, Section 7, Vol. V.* Washington, D.C.: American Physiological Society; 1975:143–172.
1058. Setchell BP, Wallace AL. The penetration of iodine-labelled FSH and albumin into the seminiferous tubules of sheep and rats. *J Endocrinol* 1972;54:67–77.
1059. Setchell BP, Waites GMH, Till AR. Variations in flow of blood within the epididymis and testis of the sheep and rat. *Nature* 1964;203:317–318.
1060. Setchell BP, Waites GMH, Lindner HR. Effect of undernutrition on testicular blood flow and metabolism and the output of testosterone in the ram. *J Reprod Fertil* 1965;9:149–162.
1061. Setchell BP, Waites GMH, Thorburn GD. Blood flow in the testis of the conscious ram measured with krypton-85; effects of heat catecholamines and acetylcholine. *Circ Res* 1966;18:755–765.
1062. Setchell BP, Hinks NT, Voglmayr JK, Scott TW. Amino acids in ram testicular fluid and semen and their metabolism by spermatozoa. *Biochem J* 1967;105:1061–1065.
1063. Setchell BP, Dawson RMC, White RW. The high concentration of free myo-inositol in rete testis fluid from rams. *J Reprod Fertil* 1968;17:219–221.
1064. Setchell BP, Scott TW, Voglmayr JK, Waites GMH. Characteristics of testicular spermatozoa and the fluid which transports them into the epididymis. *Biol Reprod Suppl* 1969;1:40–66.
1065. Setchell BP, Voglmayr JK, Waites GMH. A blood-testis barrier restricting passage from blood into rete testis fluid but not into lymph. *J Physiol* 1969;200:73–85.
1066. Setchell BP, Voglmayr JK, Hinks NT. The effect of local heating on the flow and composition of rete testis fluid in the conscious ram. *J Reprod Fertil* 1971;25:81–89.
1067. Setchell BP, Duggan MC, Evans RW. The effects of gonadotrophins on fluid secretion and production of spermatozoa by the rat and hamster testis. *J Endocrinol* 1973;56:27–36.
1068. Setchell BP, Hinton BT, Jacks F, Davies RV. Restricted penetration of iodinated follicle-stimulating and luteinizing hormone into the seminiferous tubules of the rat testis. *Mol Cell Endocrinol* 1976;6:59–69.
1069. Setchell BP, Davies RV, Gladwell RT, Hinton BT, Main SJ, Pilsworth L, Waites GMH. The movement of fluid in the seminiferous tubules and rete testis. *Ann Biol Anim Biochim Biophys* 1978;18:623–632.
1070. Setchell BP, Laurie MS, Main SJ, Goats GC. The mechanism of transport of testosterone through the walls of the seminiferous tubules of the rat testis. *Int J Androl (Suppl)* 1978;2:506–512.
1071. Setchell BP, Laurie MS, Jarvis LG. The blood-testis barrier at puberty. *Excerpta Med Int Cong Ser* 1981;559:186–190.
1072. Setchell BP, Bustamante JC, Galil KAA, Laurie MS, Sharpe RM. Changes in capillary permeability in the testis after injection of hCG in normal and apermatogenic rats. *Ann NY Acad Sci* 1982;383:499.
1073. Setchell BP, Laurie MS, Flint APF, Heap RB. Transport of free and conjugated steroids from the boar testis in lymph, venous blood and rete testis fluid. *J Endocrinol* 1983;96:127–136.
1074. Setchell BP, Bustamante JC, Niemi M. The microcirculation of the testis. In: Courtice FC, Garlick DG, Perry MA, eds. *Progress in Microcirculation Research, 11.* Committee in Postgraduate Medical Education, Sydney: University of New South Wales; 1984:291–296.
1075. Setchell BP, Pollanen P, Zupp JL. The development of the blood-testis barrier and changes in vascular permeability at puberty in rats. *Int J Androl* 1988;11:225–233.
1076. Setchell BP, Sowerbutts SF, Zupp JL. The failure of 5'-hydroxytryptamine (serotonin) or histamine to increase vascular permeability in the rat testis. *Biol Reprod* 1988;38 Suppl. 1:86.
1077. Setchell BP, Uksila J, Maddocks S, Pollanen P. Testis physiology relevant to immunoregulation. *J Reprod Immunol* 1990;18:19–32.
1078. Setchell BP, Locatelli A, Perreau C, Pisselet C, Fontaine I, Kuntz C, Saumande J, Fontaine J, Hochereau-de Reviers MT. Form and function of the Leydig cells in hypophysectomized rams treated with pituitary extract when spermatogenesis is disrupted by heating the testis. *J Endocrinol* 1991;131:101–112.
1079. Setchell BP, Maddocks S, Tao L, Zupp JL. Vascular functions in the testis and infertility. In: Whitcomb RW, Zirkin B, eds. *Understanding Male Infertility: Basic and Clinical Approaches.* New York: Raven Press; (in press) 1993.
1080. Sexton TJ, Amann RP, Flipse RJ. Free amino acids and protein in rete testis fluid, vas deferens plasma, accessory sex gland fluid, and seminal plasma of the conscious bull. *J Dairy Sci* 1971;54:412–416.
1081. Shafik A, Bedeir GAM. Venous tension patterns in cord veins I. In normal and varicocele individuals. *J Urol* 1980;123:383–385.
1082. Shapiro E, Tsitlik JE, Lepor H. Alpha-2 adrenergic receptors in canineprostate: biochemical and functional correlations. *J Urol* 1987;137:565–570.
1083. Sharp B, Pekary AE, Meyer NV, Hershman JM. β-Endorphin in male rat reproductive organs. *Biochem Biophys Res Commun* 1980;95:618–623.
1084. Sharpe RM. Gonadotrophin-induced accumulation of 'interstitial fluid' in the rat testis. *J Reprod Fertil* 1979;55:365–371.
1085. Sharpe RM. The importance of testicular interstitial fluid in the transport of injected hCG to the Leydig cells. *Int J Androl* 1981;4:64–74.
1086. Sharpe RM. Impaired gonadotrophin uptake *in vivo* by the cryptorchid rat testis. *J Reprod Fertil* 1983;67:379–387.
1087. Sharpe RM. Local control of testicular function. *Q J Exp Physiol* 1983;68:265–287.

1088. Sharpe RM. Intratesticular factors controlling testicular function. *Biol Reprod* 1984;30:29–49.
1089. Sharpe RM. Possible role of elongated spermatids in control of stage-dependent changes in the diameter of the lumen of the rat seminiferous tubule. *J Androl* 1989;10:304–310.
1090. Sharpe RM. Monitoring of spermatogenesis in man—measurement of Sertoli cell- or germ cell-secreted proteins in semen or blood. *Int J Androl* 1992;15:201–210.
1091. Sharpe RM, Bartlett JMS. Intratesticular distribution of testosterone in rats and the relationship to the concentrations of a peptide that stimulates testosterone secretion. *J Reprod Fertil* 1985;73:223–236.
1092. Sharpe RM, Bartlett JM. Changes in the secretion of ABP into testicular interstitial fluid with age and in situations of impaired spermatogenesis. *Int J Androl* 1987;10:701–710.
1093. Sharpe RM, Cooper I. Testicular interstitial fluid as a monitor for changes in the intratesticular environment in the rat. *J Reprod Fertil* 1983;69:125–135.
1094. Sharpe RM, Cooper I. Intratesticular secretion of a factor(s) with major stimulatory effects on Leydig cell testosterone secretion *in vitro. Mol Cell Endocrinol* 1984;37:159–168.
1095. Sharpe RM, Fraser HM. HCG stimulation of testicular LHRH-like activity. *Nature* 1980;290:642–643.
1096. Sharpe RM, Fraser HM, Cooper I, Rommerts FFG. Sertoli-Leydig cell communications via an LHRH-like factor. *Nature* 1981;290:785–787.
1097. Sharpe RM, Fraser HM, Cooper I, Rommerts FFG. The secretion, measurement and function of a testicular LHRH-like factor. *Ann NY Acad Sci* 1982;383:272–294.
1098. Sharpe RM, Doogan DG, Cooper I. Direct effects of a luteinizing hormone-releasing hormone agonist on intratesticular levels of testosterone and interstitial fluid formation in intact male rats. *Endocrinology* 1983;113:1306–1313.
1099. Sharpe RM, Maddocks S, Kerr JB. Cell-cell interactions in the control of spermatogenesis as studied using Leydig cell destruction and testosterone replacement. *Am J Anat* 1990;188:3–20.
1100. Scheit KH. The major basic proteins of bull seminal vesicle secretion. *Biol Chem Hoppe Seyler* 1986;367:229–233.
1101. Shimazaki J, Yamanaka H, Taguchi I, Shida K. Free amino acids in the caput and the cauda epididymis of adult rats. *Endocrin Jpn* 1976;23:149–156.
1102. Shioda T, Nishida S. Innervation of the bull testis. *Jpn J Vet Sci* 1966;28:251–257.
1103. Shivaji S, Scheit KH, Bhargava PM. Proteins of Seminal Plasma. New York: John Wiley & Sons; 1990.
1104. Short RV, Mann T, Hay MF. Male reproductive organs of the African elephant, *Loxodonta africana. J Reprod Fertil* 1967;13:517–536.
1105. Shvarko MG, Borziak EI. Anatomy and topography of extraorganic lymphatic vessels and regional lymph nodes of human prostate (in Russian). *Arkh Anat Gistol Embriol* 1990;99:72–77.
1106. Sikorski A. Comparative anatomy of the bulbourethral glands. *Folia Morphol (Warsz)* 1978;37:151–156.
1107. Silvermann JD, Kruger L. Lectin and neuropeptide labeling of separate populations of dorsal root ganglion neurons and associated "nociceptor" thin axons in rat testis and cornea whole-mount preparations. *Somatosens Res* 1988;5:259–267.
1108. Sinha Hikim AP, Bartke A, Russell LD. Morphometric studies on hamster testes in gonadally active and inactive states: light microscope findings. *Biol Reprod* 1988;39:1225–1237.
1109. Sjostrand NO. The adrenergic innervation of the vas deferens and the accessory male genital glands. *Acta Physiol Scand* 1965;65, Suppl. 257:1–82.
1110. Skinner MK, Fritz IB. Structural characterization of proteoglycans produced by testicular peritubular cells and Sertoli cells. *J Biol Chem* 1985;260:11874–11883.
1111. Skinner MK, Tung PS, Fritz IB. Cooperativity between Sertoli cells and testicular peritubular cells in the production and deposition of extracellular matrix components. *J Cell Biol* 1985;100:1941–1947.
1112. Skoglund RW, McRoberts JW, Ragde H. Torsio of the spermatic cord: a review of the literature and analysis of 70 new cases. *J Urol* 1970;104:604–607.
1113. Smith EP, Russell WE, French FS, Wilson EM. A form of basic fibroblast growth factor is secreted into the adluminal fluid of the rat coagulating gland. *Prostate* 1989;14:353–365.
1114. Smith ER. The canine prostate and its secretion. In: Thomas JA, Singhal RL, eds. *Molecular Mechanisms of Gonadal Hormone Action, Vol. 1,* Baltimore: University Park Press; 1975:167–204.
1115. Smith ER, Lebeaux MI. The mediation of the canine prostatic secretion provoked by hypogastric nerve stimulation. *Invest Urol* 1970;7:313–318.
1116. Smith ER, Miller TB, Palermo NJ, Donovan DW. Effects on canine prostatic secretion of some drugs that modify ion transport. *J Pharmacol exp Ther* 1986;238:26–31.
1117. Smith GI. Cellular changes from graded testicular ischemia. *J Urol* 1955;73:355–362.
1118. Smith JB, McIntosh GH, Morris B. The traffic of cells through tissues: a study of peripheral lymph in sheep. *J Anat* 1970;107:87–100.
1119. Smith MJV. The lymphatics of the prostate. *Invest Urol* 1966;3:439–444.
1120. Soder O, Syed V, Callard GV, Toppari J, Pollanen P, Parvinen M, Froysa B, Ritzen M. Production and secretion of an interleukin-1-like factor is stage dependent and correlates with spermatogonial DNA synthesis in the rat seminiferou epithelium. *Int J Androl* 1990;14:223–231.
1121. Soler C, Blasquez C, Pertusa J, Nunez M, Nunez J, Nunez A. A comparison of the effects of bilateral efferent duct ligation and of partial epididymectomy on the testes of rats. *Reprod Fert Dev* 1990;2:321–326.
1122. Somers WJ, Felsen D, Chou TC, Marion DN, Chernesky CE, Vaughan ED. An in vivo evaluation of alpha adrenergic receptors in canine prostate. *J Urol* 1989;141:1230–1233.
1123. Sosnik H. Studies on the participation of tunica albuginea and rete testis (TA and RT) in the quantitative structure of human testis. *Gegenbaurs Morphol Jahrb* 1985;131:347–356.
1124. Sosnik H. Quantitative investigations on the topography of twelve structural elements of the male gonad. *Gegenbaurs Morphol Jahrb* 1986;132:154–169.
1125. Sowerbutts SF, Jarvis LG, Setchell BP. The increase in testicular vascular permeability induced by human chorionic gonadotrophin involves 5-hydroxytryptamine and possibly oestrogens, but not testosterone, prostaglandins, histamine or bradykinin. *Ausl J Exp Biol Med Sci* 1986;64:137–147.
1126. Steinberger A. *In vitro* techniques for the study of spermatogenesis. *Meth Enzymol* 1975;39:283–296.
1127. Steinberger E, Tjioe DY. Spermatogenesis in rat testes after experimental ischemia. *Fertil Steril* 1969;20:639–649.
1128. Stenman S, Vaheri A. Distribution of a major connective tissue protein, fibronectin, in normal human tissues. *J Exp Med* 1978;147:1054–1064.
1129. Stern JA, Lui RC, LaRegina MC, Herbold DR, Tolman KC, Johnson FE. Long-term outcome following testicular ischemia in the rat. *J Androl* 1990;11:390–395.
1130. Stjernquist M, Hakanson R, Leander S, Owman C, Sundler F, Uddman R. Immunohistochemical localization of substance P, vasoactive intestinal polypeptide and gastrin-releasing peptide in vas deferens and seminal vesicle, and the effect of these and eight other neuropeptides on resting tension and neurally evoked contractile activity. *Reg Pep* 1983;7:67–86.
1131. Stjernquist M, Owman C, Sjoberg NO, Sundler F. Coexistence and cooperation between neuropeptide Y and norepinephrine in nerve fibers of guinea pig vas deferens and seminal vesicle. *Biol Reprod* 1987;36:149–155.
1132. Stoffel M, Friess AE, Kohler T. Die Vaskularisation des Eberne-benhodens unter besonderer Berucksichtigung der Perfusionfixation. *Schweiz Arch Tierheilkd* 1990;132:571–579.
1133. Stoffel M, Kohler T, Friess AE, Zimmermann W. Microvasculature of the epididymis in the boar. *Cell Tissue Res* 1990;259:495–501.
1134. Stone BA. Thermal characteristics of the testis and epididymis of the boar. *J Reprod Fertil* 1981;63:551–557.
1135. Suarez-Garnacho S, Vega JA. Inervacion microscopica de las vias espermaticas y testicolo. IV. Testis. *Arch Esp Urol* 1990;43:443–447.

1136. Suarez-Garnacho S, Vega JA, Alvarez-Arenal A, Bengoechea ME, del Valle ME, Zubizarreta JJF. Inervacion microscopica de las vias espermaticas y testicolo II Ductus epididymidis. *Arch Esp Urol* 1989;42:499–504.
1137. Suarez-Garnacho S, Vega JA, Alvarez-Arenal A, Perez-Casas A. Inervacion microscopia de las vias espermaticas y testicolo. III. Tubuli semimiferi recti, rete testis y ductuli efferentes testis. *Arch Esp Urol* 1989;42:727–732.
1138. Sujarit S, Chaturapanich G, Pholpramool C. Evidence for blood myo-inositol as a source of the epididymal secretion in the perfused cauda epididymis of the rat. *Andrologia* 1985;17:321–326.
1139. Suominen J, Setchell BP. Enzymes and trypsin inhibitor in the rete testis fluid of rams and boars. *J Reprod Fertil* 1972;30:235–245.
1140. Suominen JJO, Setchell BP. Proteinase inhibitors in testicular and epididymal fluid. In: Peeters H, ed. *Protides of the Biological Fluids,* Oxford: Pergamon Press; 1976:171–175.
1141. Suvanto O, Kormano M. Effect of experimental cryptorchidism and cadmium injury on the spontaneous contractions of the seminiferous tubules of the rat testis. *Virchows Arch Abt B Zellpath* 1970;4:217–224.
1142. Suvanto O, Kormano M. The relation between *in vitro* contractions of the rat seminiferous tubules and the cyclic stage of the seminiferous epithelium. *J Reprod Fertil* 1970;21:227–232.
1143. Suzuki F. Microvasculature of the mouse testis and excurrent duct system. *Am J Anat* 1982;163:309–325.
1144. Suzuki F, Nagano T. Microvasculature of the human testis and excurrent duct system. Resin-casting and scanning electron-microscopic studies. *Cell Tissue Res* 1986;243:79–89.
1145. Suzuki T, Kurokawa K, Okabe K, Ito K, Hatori T, Imai K, Yamanaka H. Correlation between the prostatic vessels and vertebral venous system of the dog (in Japanese). *Nippon Hinyokika Gakkai Zasshi* 1991;82:1742–1747.
1146. Sweeney TE, Rozum JS, Desjardins C, Gore RW. Microvascular pressure distribution in the hamster testis. *Am J Physiol* 1991;260:H1581–H1589.
1147. Syed V, Soder O, Arver S, Lindh M, Khan S, Ritzen M. Ontogeny and cellular origin of an interleukin-1-like factor in the reproductive tract of the male rat. *Int J Androl* 1988;11:437–447.
1148. Sylvester SR, Griswold MD. Localization of transferrin and transferrin receptors in rat testes. *Biol Reprod* 1984;31:195–203.
1149. Tabor CW, Rosenthal SM. Pharmacology of spermine and spermidine. Some effects on animals and bacteria. *J Pharmacol Elp Ther* 1956;116:139–155.
1150. Taggart DA, Temple-Smith PD. Structural features of the epididymis in a dasyurid marsupial (Antechinus stuartii). *Cell Tissue Res* 1989;258:203–210.
1151. Takayama H. Ultrastructure of testicular capillaries as a permeability barrier (in Japanese). *Nippon Hinyokika Gakkai Zasshi* 1986;77:1840–1850.
1152. Takayama H, Tomoyoshi T. Microvascular architecture of rat and human testes. *Invest Urol* 1981;18:341–344.
1153. Talo A. *In vitro* spontaneous electrical activity of rat efferent ductules. *J Reprod Fertil* 1981;63:17–20.
1154. Talo A, Jaakkola U-M, Markkula-Vittanen M. Spontaneous electrical activity of the rat epididymis *in vitro. J Reprod Fertil* 1979;57:423–429.
1155. Tamm J, Volkwein U, Becker H, Klosterhalfen H. Comparison of steroid concentrations in venous and arterial blood across the human testis. Unconjugated 5-androstane-3,17-diol: an important androgen metabolite of the human testicular-epididymal unit. *J Steroid Biochem* 1982;16:567–571.
1156. Tang Y. No α-lactalbumin-like activity can be detected in a small molecular mass protein fraction of rat epididymal extract. *Reprod Fert Dev* (in press).
1157. Tanphaichitr N. *In vitro* stimulation of human sperm motility by acetylcarnitine. *Int J Fertil* 1977;22:85–91.
1158. Tanyel FC, Buyukpamukcu N, Hicsonmez A. Contralateral testicular blood flow during unilateral testicular torsion. *Br J Urol* 1989;63:522–524.
1159. Tao L, Setchell BP. The blood-testis barrier after efferent duct ligation. *Miniposters, 7th European Workshop on the Testis,* 1992:45.
1160. Tao L, Zupp JL, Setchell BP. Changes in vascular permeability to albumin in the rat testis after treatment with hCG or cadmium. *Proc Aust Soc Reprod Biol* 1992;24:89.
1161. Tapainenen JM, Paloneva T, Veijola M, Rajaniemi H. Rat testicular interstitial fluid contains mediators of vasopermeability. *J Reprod Fertil* 1990;89:723–728.
1162. Tayakkononta K. The gubernaculum testis and its nerve supply. *Aust N Z J Surg* 1963;33:61–67.
1163. Taylor DCM. The effects of nucleus raphe magnus lesions on an ascending thermal pathway in the rat. *J Physiol* 1982;326: 309–318.
1164. Tcholakian RK, Eik-Nes KB. Δ^5-Pregnenolone and testosterone in spermatic venous blood of anaesthetized dogs. *Am J Physiol* 1971;221:1824–1826.
1165. Templeton AA, Cooper I, Kelly RW. Prostaglandin concentrations in the semen of fertile men. *J Reprod Fertil* 1978;52:147–150.
1166. Terasaki T, Kojima M, Kitamori T, Yuri K, Azuma Y, Kaneko H, Watanabe H. A continuous sampling model of the seminal vesicle fluid in rat. *Tohoku J exp Med* 1987;153:395–396.
1167. Tilbrook AJ, de Kretser DM, Clarke IJ. Studies on the testicular source of inhibin and its route of secretion in rams: failure of the Leydig cell to secrete inhibin in response to a human chorionic gonadotropin/LH stimulus. *J Endocrinol* 1991;130:107–114.
1168. Tilney NL. Patterns of lymphatic drainage in the adult laboratory rat. *J Anat* 1971;109:369–383.
1169. Tindall DJ, Vitale R, Means AR. Androgen binding protein as a biochemical marker of formation of the blood-testis barrier. *Endocrinology* 1975;97:636–648.
1170. Tisell LE, Salander H. Anatomy of the human prostate and its three paired lobes. *Prog Clin Biol Res* 1984;145:55–65.
1171. Tjioe DY, Steinberger E. A quantitative study of the effect of ischaemia on the germinal epithelium of rat testes. *J Reprod Fertil* 1970;21:489–494.
1172. Toma H, Nakamura R, Onitsuka S, Goya N, Nakazawa H. Effect of endocrine treatment on prostatic blood flow inpatients with prostatic adenocarcinoma. *J Urol* 1988;140:91–95.
1173. Toma JG, Buzzell GR. Fine structure of the ventral and dorsal lobes of the prostate in the young adult Syrian hamster, Mesocricetus auratus. *Am J Anat* 1988;181:132–140.
1174. Tonutti E. Uber die Strukturelemente des Hodens und ihr Verhalten unter experimentellen Bedingungen. In: 1. *Symposium Deutsche Gesellschaft Endokrinologie,* Hamburg, Berlin: Springer; 1955:146–158.
1175. Toppari J, Parvinen M. *In vitro* differentiation of rat seminiferous tubular segments from defined stages of the epithelial cycle: morphological and immunolocalization analysis. *J Androl* 1985;6:334–343.
1176. Toyama Y. Actin-like filaments in the myoid cell of the testis. *Cell Tiss Res* 1977;177:221–226.
1177. Tso ECF, Lacy D. Effects of prostaglandin F-2α on the reproductive system of the male rat. *J Reprod Fertil* 1975;44: 545–550.
1178. Tsong SD, Phillips DM, Halmi N, Krieger D, Bardin CW. t3-Endorphin is present in the male reproductive tract of five species. *Biol Reprod* 1982;27:755–764.
1179. Tsong SD, Phillips D, Halmi N, Liotta AS, Margioris A, Bardin CW, Krieger D. ACTH and β-endorphin-related peptides are present in multiple sites in the reproductive tract of the male rat. *Endocrinology* 1982;110:2204–2206.
1180. Tuck RR. An investigation of the fluid secreted by the seminiferous tubules and the rete testis of the rat. *B Sc Thesis,* Sydney: University of Sydney; 1969.
1181. Tuck RR, Setchell BP, Waites GMH, Young JA. The composition of fluid collected by micropuncture and catheterization from the seminiferous tubules and rete testis of rats. *Pfluegers Arch* 1970;318:225–243.
1182. Tung PS, Fritz IB. Interactions of Sertoli cells with myoid cells *in vitro. Biol Reprod* 1980;23:207–217.
1183. Tung PS, Fritz IB. Immunolocalization of clusterin in the ram testis, rete testis and excurrent ducts. *Biol Reprod* 1985;33: 177–186.
1184. Tung PS, Skinner MK, Fritz IB. Fibronectin synthesis is a

marker for peritubular cell contaminants in Sertoli cell-enriched cultures. *Biol Reprod* 1984;30:199–211.
1185. Turner TT. Varicocele: still an enigma. *J Urol* 1983;129: 695–699.
1186. Turner TT. Transepithelial movement of ^{3}H-androgen in seminiferous and epididymal tubules: a study using micropuncture and in vivo microperfusion. *Biol Reprod* 1988;39:399–408.
1187. Turner TT, Lopez TJ. Effects of experimental varicocele require neither adrenal contribution nor venous reflux. *J Urol* 1989;142:1372–1375.
1188. Turner TT, Lopez TJ. Testicular blood flow in peripubertal and older rats with unilateral experimental varicocele and investigation into the mechanism of the bilateral response to the unilateral lesion. *J Urol* 1990;144:1018–1021.
1189. Turner TT, Roddy MS. Intraluminal androgen binding protein alters ^{3}H-androgen uptake by rat epididymal tubules in vitro. *Biol Reprod* 1990;43:414–419.
1190. Turner TT, Yamamoto M. Different mechanisms are responsible for ^{3}H-androgen movement across the rat seminiferous and epididymal epithelia in vivo. *Biol Reprod* 1991;45:358–364.
1191. Turner TT, Hartmann PK, Howards SS. Urea in the seminiferous tubule: evidence for active transport. *Biol Reprod* 1979;20:511–515.
1192. Turner TT, Plesums JL, Cabot CL. Luminal fluid proteins of the male reproductive tract. *Biol Reprod* 1979;21:883–890.
1193. Turner TT, D'Addario DA, Howards SS. [^{3}H]3-*O*-methyl-D-glucose transport from blood into the lumina of the seminiferous and epididymal tubules in intact and vasectomized hamsters. *J Reprod Fertil* 1980;60:285–289.
1194. Turner TT, Cochran RC, Howards SS. Transfer of steroids across the hamster blood testis and blood epididymal barrier. *Biol Reprod* 1981;25:342–348.
1195. Turner TT, Jones CE, Howards SS, Ewing LL, Zegeye B, Gunsalus GL. On the androgen microenvironment of maturing spermatozoa. *Endocrinology* 1984;115:1925–1932.
1196. Turner TT, Ewing LL, Jones CE, Howards SS, Zegeye B. Androgens in male reproductive tract fluids: hypophysectomy and steroid replacement. *Am J Physiol* 1985;248:E274–E280.
1197. Turner TT, Jones CE, Roddy MS. Experimental varicocele does not affect the blood-testis barrier, epididymal electrolyte concentrations or testicular blood gas concentrations. *Biol Reprod* 1987;36:926–932.
1198. Turner TT, Jones CE, Roddy MS. On the proluminal movement of ^{3}H-androgens across the rat epidiymal epithelium. *Biol Reprod* 1989;41:143–152.
1199. Turner TT, Gleavy JL, Harris JM. Fluid movement in the lumen of the rat epididymis: effect of vasectomy and subsequent vasovasostomy. *J Androl* 1990;11:422–428.
1200. Turner TT, Evans WS, Lopez TJ. Gonadotroph and Leydig cell responsiveness in the male rat. Effects of experimental left varicocele. *J Androl* 1990;11:555–562.
1201. Uemura Y. The fine distribution of the lymph vessels in the prostate of the dog. *Acta Anat Nippon* 1976;51:17–31.
1202. Urry RL, Asay RW, Cockett ATK. Hormonal control of seminiferous tubule contractions; a hypothesis of sperm transport from the testicle. *Invest Urol* 1976;14:194–197.
1203. Vaalasti A, Hervonen A. Autonomic innervation of the human prostate. *Invest Urol* 1979;17:293–297.
1204. Vaalasti A, Hervonen A. Innervation of the ventral prostate of the rat. *Am J Anat* 1979;154:231–244.
1205. Vaalasti A, Hervonen A. Nerve endings in the human prostate. *Am J Anat* 1980;157:41–47.
1206. Vaalasti A, Linnoila I, Hervonen A. Immunohistochemical demonstration of VIP, [Met5]- and [Leu5]-enkephalin immunoreactive nerve fibres in the human prostate and seminal vesicles. *Histochemistry* 1980;66:89–98.
1207. Vaalasti A, Alho AM, Tainio H, Hervonen A. The effect of sympathetic denervation with 6-hydroxydopamine othe ventral prostate of the rat. *Acta Histochem* 1986;79:49–54.
1208. Valenca MM, Negro-Vilar A. Proopiomelanocorin-derived peptides in testicular interstitial fluid: Characterization and cganges in secretion after human chorionic gonadotrophin or luteinizing hormone-releasing hormone analog treatment. *Endocrinology* 1986;118:32–37.
1209. Van der Horst CJG, Grooten HJG. The occurrence of hypotaurine and other sulfur-containing amino acids in seminal plasma and spermatozoa of boar, bull and dog. *Biochim Biophys Acta* 1966;117:495–497.
1210. van Campenhout E. Les relations nerveuses de la glande interstitielle des glandes genitales chez les mammiferes. *Rev Can Biol* 1949;8:374–429.
1211. van de Velde RL, Risley PL. The origin and development of smooth muscle and contractility in the ductus epididymidis of the rat. *J Embryol Exp Morphol* 1963;11:369–382.
1212. van der Schoot P. Disturbed tesicular descent in the rat after prenatal exposure to the antiandrogen flutamide. *J Reprod Fertil* 1992;96:483–496.
1213. van der Schoot P. Doubts about the "first phase of testis descent" in the rat as a valid concept. *Anat Embryol* 1993;187:203–208.
1214. van der Schoot P, Elger W. Androgen-induced prevention of the outgrowth of cranial suspensory ligaments in fetal rats. *J Androl* 1992;13:534–542.
1215. van Straaten HWM, Wensing CJG. Histomorphometric aspects of testicular morphogenesis in the pig. *Biol Reprod* 1977;17:467–472.
1216. van Vliet J, de Ruiter-Bootsma AL, Oei YH, Hoekstra A, de Rooij DG, Wensing CJG. Reversible harmless interruption of testicular blood supply in the ram. *J Androl* 1987;8:108–115.
1217. van Vliet J, Rommerts FF, de Rooij DG, Buwalda G, Wensing CJ. Reduction of testicular blood flow and focal degeneration of tissue in the rat after administration of human chorionic gonadotrophin. *J Endocrinol* 1988;117:51–57.
1218. Vanha-Perttula T, Ronkko S, Lahtinen R. Hydrolases from bovine seminal vesicle, prostate and Cowper's gland. *Andrologia* 1990;22 Suppl 1.:10–24.
1219. Veeramachaneni DN, Amann RP. Oxytocin in the ovine ductuli efferentes and caput epididymis: immunolocalization and endocytosis from the luminal fluid. *Endocrinology* 1990;126: 1156–1164.
1220. Veeramachaneni DN, Amann RP. Endocytosis of androgen-binding protein, clusterin and transferin in the efferent ducts and epididymis of the ram. *J Androl* 1991;12:288–294.
1221. Veeramachaneni DN, Amann RP, Palmer JS, Hinton BT. Proteins in luminal fluid of the ram excurrent ducts: changes in composition and evidence for differential endocytosis. *J Androl* 1990;11:140–154.
1222. Vega-Alvarez JA, Marinez-Telleria A, Coalla C, Bengoechea ME, Perez-Casas A. Inervacion colinergica de la prostata en la rat blanca (*Rattus norvegicus*). *Arch Esp Urol* 1989;42:297–304.
1223. Vega-Alvarez JA, Marinez-Telleria A, del Valle ME, Coalla C, Bengoechea ME, Perez-Casas A. Inervacion de la prostat ventral de la rata: estudio ultrestructural. *Arch Esp Urol* 1989;42:397–400.
1224. Veijola M, Rajaniemi H. The hCG-induced increase in hormone uptake and interstitial fluid volume in the rat testis is not mediated by steroids, prostaglandins or protein synthesis. *Int J Androl* 1985;8:69–79.
1225. Veijola M, Rajaniemi H. Luteinising hormones activate a factor(s) in testicular interstitial fluid which increases testicular vascular permeability. *Mol Cell Endocrinol* 1986;45:113–118.
1226. Ventura S, Pennefather JN. Sympathetic co-transmission to the cauda epidiymidis of the rat: characterization of postjunctional adrenpreceptors and purinoreceptors. *Br J Pharmacol* 1991; 102:540–544.
1227. Verawatnapakul V, Pholpramool C. Free and bound sialic acid in rat and hamster epididymal fluid. *Andrologia* 1988;20: 389–395.
1228. Verhoeven G, Dierickx P, de Moor P. Stimulation effect of neurotransmitters on the aromatization of testosterone by Sertoli cell-enriched cultures. *Mol Cell Endocrinol* 1979;13:241–253.
1229. Verstoppen GR, Steeno OP. Varicocele and the pathogenesis of the associated subfertility: a review of the various theories. I. Varicocelogenesis. *Andrologia* 1977;9:133–140.
1230. Verstoppen GR, Steeno OP. Varicocele and the pathogenesis of the associated subfertility: a review of the various theories. II. Results of surgery. *Andrologia* 1977;9:293–305.
1231. Veselsky L, Jonakova V, Cechova D. A kunitz type of protein-

ase inhibitor isolated from boar seminal vesicle fluid. *Andrologia* 1985;17:352–358.

1232. Vignon X, Terquem A, Dadoune JP. The postnatal development of the junctional complexes of hamster Sertoli cells as revealed by HRP and freeze-fracture. *J Submicrosc Cytol* 1987;19:303–309.
1233. Villers A, Steg A, Boccon-Gibod L. Anatomy of the prostate: review of the different models. *Eur Urol* 1991;20:261–268.
1234. Viotto MJ, Orsi AM, Mello Dias S, Newmann HK. Structure of the rete testis of the cat (Felis domestica, L). *Anat Anz* 1991;172:341–349.
1235. Vitale-Calpe R, Aoki A. Fine structure of the intratesticular excretory pathway in the guinea pig. *Z Anat Entwicklung* 1969;129:135–153.
1236. Vitale-Calpe R, Fawcett DW, Dym M. The normal development of the blood-testis barrier and the effects of clomiphene and estrogen treatment. *Anat Rec* 1973;176:333–344.
1237. Vittoria A, LaMura E, Cocca T, Cecia A. Serotonin-, somatostain- and chromogranin A-containing cells of the urethroprostatic complex in the sheep. An immunocytochemical and immunofluorescent study. *J Anat* 1990;171:169–178.
1238. Vogl AW, Soucy LJ, Lew GJ. Distribution of actin in isolated seminiferous epithelia and denuded tubule walls of the rat. *Anat Rec* 1985;213:63–71.
1239. Voglmayr JK. Output of spermatozoa and fluid by the testis of the ram and its response to oxytocin. *J Reprod Fertil* 1975;43:119–122.
1240. Voglmayr JK, Amann RP. The distribution of free myo-inositol in fluids, spermatozoa, and tissues of the bull genital tract and observations on its uptake by the rabbit epididymis. *Biol Reprod* 1973;8:504–513.
1241. Voglmayr JK, Waites GMH, Setchell BP. Studies on spermatozoa and fluid collected directly from the testis of the conscious ram. *Nature* 1966;210:861–863.
1242. Voglmayr JK, Scott TW, Setchell BP, Waites GMH. Metabolism of testicular spermatozoa and characteristics of testicular fluid collected from conscious rams. *J Reprod Fertil* 1967;14:87–99.
1243. Voglmayr JK, Larsen LH, White IG. Metabolism of spermatozoa and composition of fluid collected from the rete testis of living bulls. *J Reprod Fertil* 1970;21:449–460.
1244. Voglmayr JK, Musto NA, Saksena SK, Brown-Woodman PDC, Marley PB, White IG. Characteristics of semen collected from the cauda epididymis of conscious rams. *J Reprod Fertil* 1977;49:245–251.
1245. Voglmayr JK, Roberson C, Musto NA. Comparison of androgen levels in ram rete testis fluid, testicular lymph and spermatic venous blood plasma: evidence for a regulatory mechanism in the seminiferous tubules. *Biol Reprod* 1980;23:29–39.
1246. Vreeburg JTM. Distribution of testosterone and 5α-dihydrotestosterone in rat epididymis and their concentrations in efferent duct fluid. *J Endocrinol* 1975;67:203–210.
1247. Wagner CL, Kistler WS. Analysis of the major large polypeptides of rat seminal vesicle secretions: SVS I, II and III. *Biol Reprod* 1987;36:501–510.
1248. Waites GMH. The effect of heating the scrotum of the ram on respiration and body temperature. *Q J Exp Physiol* 1962;47:314–323.
1249. Waites GMH. Fluid secretion. In: Johnson AD, Gomes WR, eds. *The Testis, Vol. IV.* New York: Academic Press, 1977;91–123.
1250. Waites GMH, Einer-Jensen N. Collection and analysis of rete testis fluid from Macaque monkeys. *J Reprod Fertil* 1974;41:505–508.
1251. Waites GMH, Gladwell RT. Physiological significance of fluid secretion in the testis and blood-testis barrier. *Physiol Rev* 1982;62:624–671.
1252. Waites GMH, Moule GR. Blood pressure in the internal spermatic artery of the ram. *J Reprod Fertil* 1960;1:223–229.
1253. Waites GMH, Moule GR. Relation of vascular heat exchange to temperature regulation in the testis of the ram. *J Reprod Fertil* 1961;2:213–224.
1254. Waites GMH, Setchell BP. Effect of local heating on blood flow and metabolism of the testes of the conscious ram. *J Reprod Fertil* 1964;8:339–344.
1255. Waites GMH, Setchell BP. Changes in blood flow and vascular permeability of the testis, epididymis and accessory reproductive organs of the rat after the administration of cadmium chloride. *J Endocrinol* 1966;34:329–342.
1256. Waites GMH, Setchell BP. Physiology of the mammalian testis. In: Lamming GE, ed. *Marshall's Physiology of Reproduction, Vol. B,* London: Churchill Livingstone; 1990:1–105.
1257. Waites GMH, Voglmayr JK. The functional activity and control of the apocrine sweat glands of the scrotum of the ram. *Aust J Agric Res* 1963;14:839–851.
1258. Waites GMH, Jones AR, Main SJ, Cooper TG. The entry of antifertility and other drugs into the testis. *Adv Biosci* 1973;10:101–116.
1259. Waites GMH, Setchell BP, Quinlan D. The effect of local heating of the scrotum, testes and epididymides on cardiac output and regional blood flow. *J Reprod Fertil* 1973;34:41–49.
1260. Waites GMH, Archer V, Langford GA. Regional sensitivity of the testicular artery to noradrenaline in the ram, rabbit, rat and boar. *J Reprod Fertil* 1975;45:159–163.
1261. Waksman BH. A histologic study of the auto-allergic testis lesion in the guinea-pig. *J Exp Med* 1959;109:311–324.
1262. Wallace JC, Lascelles AK. Composition of testicular and epididymal lymph in the ram. *J Reprod Fertil* 1964;8:235–242.
1263. Wallace JC, Wales RG, White IG. The respiration of the rabbit epididymis and its synthesis of glycerylphosphorylcholine. *Aus J Biol Sci* 1966;19:849–856.
1264. Walls EW. The blood vascular and lymphatic systems. In: Romanes GJ, ed.*Cunningham's Textbook of Anatomy, 12th ed.* Oxford: Oxford University Press; 1981:871–1037.
1265. Wang J, Galil KAA, Setchell BP. Changes in testicular blood flow and testosterone production during aspermatogenesis after irradiation. *J Endocrinol* 1983;98:35–46.
1266. Wang JM, Gu CH, Tao L, Wu XL, Qiu JP. Electrolyte composition of rete testis fluid and cauda epididymal plasma and spermatozoa from rats following gossypol treatment. *Andrologia* 1986;18:43–49.
1267. Wang JM, McKenna KE, Lee C. Determination of prostatic secretion in rats: effect of neurotransmitters and testosterone. *Prostate* 1991;18:289–301.
1268. Wang JM, McKenna KE, McVary KT, Lee C. Requirement of innervation for maintenance of structural and functional integrity in the rat prostate. *Biol Reprod* 1991;44:1171–1176.
1269. Watanabe H, Shima M, Kojima M, Ohe H. Dynamic study of nervous control on prostatic contraction and fluid excretion in the dog. *J Urol* 1988;140:1567–1570.
1270. Wax SH, Peterson N. Measurement of testicular blood flow by intratesticular injection of xenon-133. *Surg Forum* 1967;18:544–546.
1271. Weber JE, Turner TT, Tung KS, Russell LD. Effects of cytochalasin D on the integrity of the Sertoli cell (blood-testis) barrier. *Am J Anat* 1988;182:130–147.
1272. Weerasooriya TR, Yamamoto T. Three-dimensional organization of the vasculature of the rat spermatic cord and testis. A scanning electron-microscopic study of vascular corrosion casts. *Cell Tiss Res* 1985;241:317–323.
1273. Weihe E, Nimmrich H, Metz J, Forssmann WG. Horseradish peroxidase as a tracer for capillary permeability studies. *J Histochem Cytochem* 1986;27:1357–1359.
1274. Weinstein RL, Kelch RP, Jenner MR, Kaplan SL, Grumbach MM. Secretion of unconjugated androgens and estrogens by the normal and abnormal testis before and after human chorionic gonadotropin. *J Clin Invest* 1977;53:1–6.
1275. Wells LJ. Descensus testiculorum: descent after severance of gubernaculum. *Anat Rec* 1944;88:465.
1276. Wen RQ, Wong PYD. Reserpine treatment increases viscosity of fluid in the epididymis of rats. *Biol Reprod* 1988;38:969–974.
1277. Wensing CJG, Colenbrander B. Normal and abnormal testicular descent. *Oxf Rev Reprod Biol* 1986;8:125–130.
1278. Wensing CJG, Dijkstra G, Frankenhuis MT. The intricate morphological relations between testicular artery and pampiniform plexus. *Int J Androl* 1981;Suppl. 3:77–78.

1279. White IG, Griffiths DE. Guanidines and phosphagens of semen. *Aust J Exp Biol Med Sci* 1958;36:97–102.
1280. White IG, Hudson B. The testosterone and dehydroepiandrosterone concentration in fluids of the mammalian male reproductive tract. *J Endocrinol* 1968;41:291–292.
1281. Wicher V, Wicher K. Immunocompetence of inflammatory cells in rabbit testes infected with *Treponema pallidum*. *J Reprod Immunol* 1990;18:105–116.
1282. Widmark A, Damber JE, Bergh A. Relationship between human chorionic gonadotrophin-induced changes in testicular microcirculation and the formation of testicular interstitial fluid. *J Endocrinol* 1986;109:419–425.
1283. Widmark A, Damber JE, Bergh A. Testicular vascular resistance in the rat after intratesticular injection of an LRH-agonist. *Int J Androl* 1986;9:416–423.
1284. Widmark A, Bergh A, Damber JE, Smedegard G. Leucocytes mediate the hCG-induced increase in testicular venular permeability. *Mol Cell Endocrinol* 1987;53:25–31.
1285. Widmark A, Damber JE, Bergh A. Effects of oestradiol-17 beta on testicular microcirculation in rats. *J Endocrinol* 1987;115: 489–495.
1286. Widmark A, Damber JE, Bergh A. High and low doses of luteinizing hormone induce different changes in testicular microcirculation. *Acta Endocrinol (Copenh)* 1989;121:621–627.
1287. Widmark A, Damber JE, Bergh A. Arginine-vasopressin induced changes in testicular blood flow. *Int J Androl* 1991;14:58–65.
1288. Williams-Ashman HG, Banks J. Participation of cytidine coenzymes in the metabolism of choline by seminal vesicle. *J Biol Chem* 1956;223:509–521.
1289. Williams-Ashman HG, Canellakis ZN. Polyamines in mammalian biology and medicine. *Perspect Biol Med* 1979;22:421–453.
1290. Winet H. On the mechanism of flow in the efferent ducts. *J Androl* 1980;1:304–311.
1291. Wing TY, Christensen AK. Morphometric studies on rat seminiferous tubules. *Am J Anat* 1982;165:13–25.
1292. Winters SJ. Inhibin is released together with testosterone by the human testis. *J Clin Endocrinol Metab* 1990;70:548–550.
1293. Winters SJ, Troen P. Testosterone and estradiol are co-secreted episodically by the human testis. *J Clin Invest* 1986;78:870–873.
1294. Wishashi MM. Detailed anatomy of the internal spermatic vein and the ovarian vein. Human cadaver study and operative spermatic venography: clinical aspects. *J Urol* 1991;145:780–784.
1295. Wishashi MM. Anatomy of the venous drainage of the human testis: testicular vein cast, microdissection and radiographic demonstration. A new anatomical concept. *Eur Urol* 1991;20:154–160.
1296. Wolff J, Merker HJ. Ultrastruktur und Bildung von Poren im Endothel von porosen und geschlossen Kapillaren. *Z Zellforsch* 1966;73:174–191.
1297. Wong PY. Control of anion and fluid secretion by apical Ps-purinoreceptors in the rat epididymis. *Br J Pharmacol* 1988;95:1315–1321.
1298. Wong PY. Mechanism of adrenergic stimulation of anion secretion in cultured rat epididymal epithelium. *Am J Physiol* 1988;243:F121–F133.
1299. Wong PYD, Yeung CH. Inhibition by amiloride of sodium-dependent fluid reabsorption in the rat isolated caudal epididymis. *Br J Pharmacol* 1976;58:529–531.
1300. Wong PYD, Yeung CH. Fluid reabsorption in the isolated duct of the rat cauda epididymis. *J Reprod Fertil* 1977;49:77–81.
1301. Wong PYD, Yeung CH. Absorptive and secretory functions of the perfused rat cauda epididymidis. *J Physiol* 1978;275:1326.
1302. Wong PYD, Yeung CH. Effects of catecholamines and adrenergic blockage on fluid reabsorption in isolated rat cauda epididymidis. *Jpn J Pharmacol* 1978;28:115–123.
1303. Woolley P. The seminiferous tubules in Dasyurid marsupials. *J Reprod Fertil* 1975;45:255–261.
1304. Worley RTS, Nicholson HD, Pickering BT. Testicular oxytocin: an initiator of seminiferous tubule movement? *Coll INSERM* 1984;123:205–212.
1305. Wright WW, Luzarrage ML. Isolation of cyclic protein-2 from rat seminferous tubule fluid and Sertoli cell culture medium. *Biol Reprod* 1986;35:762–772.
1306. Wright WW, Musto NA, Mather JP, Bardin CW. Sertoli cells secrete both testis-specific and serum proteins. *Proc Natl Acad Sci USA* 1981;78:7565–7569.
1307. Wrobel KH. Zur Morphologie der Ductuli efferentes des Bullen. *Z Zellforsch* 1972;135:129–148.
1308. Wrobel KH, El Etreby MF. Enzymhistochemie an der mannlichen Keimdruse des Rindes wahrend ihres fetalen und postnatalen Entwicklung. *Histochemie* 1971;26:160–179.
1309. Wrobel KH, Sinowatz F, Kugler P. Zur funktionellen Morphologie des Rete testis, der Tubuli recti und der Terminalsegmente der Tubuli seminiferi des geschlechtsreifen Rindes. *Anat Histol Embryol* 1978;7:320–335.
1310. Wrobel KH, Sinowatz F, Mademann R. The fine structure of the terminal segment of the bovine seminiferous tubule. *Cell Tiss Res* 1982;225:29–44.
1311. Wrobel KH, Schilling E, Zwack M. Postnatal development of the connexion between tubulus seminiferous and tubulus rectus in the bovine testis. *Cell Tissue Res* 1986;246:387–400.
1312. Wyrost P, Radek J, Radek T. Some aspects of development and homology of the genital glands arteries in cattle. *Pol Arch Weter* 1989;29(1–2):95–106.
1313. Wyrost P, Radek J, Radek T. Morphology and development of the bovine testicular artery during fetal and neonatal periods (in Polish). *Pol Arch Weter* 1990;30(1–2):39–56.
1314. Wyrost P, Radek J, Radek T. Morfologia i rowoj zyly jadrowej (V. testicularis) bydla w okresie plodowym i neonatalnym. *Pol Arch Weter* 1990;30(3–4):17–38.
1315. Wystub T, Branscheid W, Paufler S. Scanning electron and light microscopic studies of the surface epithelium of the rete testis and epididymis of the boar. I. Rete testis and efferent ducts. *DTW Dtsch Tierarztl Wochenschr* 1989;96:384–389.
1316. Wystub T, Branscheid W, Paufler S. Scanning electron and light microscopic studies of the surface epithelium of the rete testis and epididymis in the boar. II. Ductus epididymis. *DTW Dtsch Tierarztl Wochenschr* 1989;96:452–459.
1317. Yamamoto M, Kondo H. Occurrence of a dense plexus of sensory nerve fibers immunoreactive to calcitonin-gene-related peptide in the cauda epididymidis of rats. *Acta Anat (Basel)* 1988;132:169–176.
1318. Yamamoto M, Turner TT. Transepithelial movement of nonpolar and polar compounds in male rat trproductive tubule examined by in vivo microperfusion and in vivo micropuncture. *J Urol* 1990;143:853–856.
1319. Yamamoto M, Takaba H, Hashimoto J, Miyake K. Evidence for innervation of the myoid cells in the human seminiferous tubule. *Urol Int* 1987;42:137–139.
1320. Yamamoto M, Miyake K, Takaba H, Hashimoto J, Sahashi M. Overall morphology of basement membrane of rat seminiferous tubule as revealed by scanning electron microscopy. *Urol Int* 1987;42:140–142.
1321. Yamashita K. Histological studies on the innervation of human testis and epididymis (in Japanese). *J Orient Med* 1939;30: 367–394.
1322. Yasumoto R, Asakawa M, Kakinoki K, Kawashima H, Moriya K, Maekawa T, Kobayakawa H. Clinical studies of varicocele 2: Radiographic examination and measurement of spermatic venous pressure in varicocele patients. (in Japanese) *Hinyokika Kiyo* 1988;34:312–315.
1323. Yee JB, Hutson JC. Testicular macrophages: isolation, characterization and hormonal responsiveness. *Biol Reprod* 1983;29: 1319–1326.
1324. Yee JB, Hutson JC. Biochemical consequences of follicle-stimulating hormone binding to testicular macrophages in culture. *Biol Reprod* 1985;32:872–879.
1325. Yee JB, Hutson JC. *In vivo* effects of follicle-stimulating hormone on testicular macrophages. *Biol Reprod* 1985;32: 880–883.
1326. Yeh SD, Morse MJ, Grando R, Kleinert EL, Whitmore WF. Lymphoscintigraphic studies of lymphatic drainage from the testes. *Clin Nucl Med* 1986;11:823–827.
1327. Yeung CH, Cooper TG, Waites GMH. Carnitine transport into the perfused epididymis of the rat: regional differences, stereospecificity, stimulation by choline, and the effect of other luminal factors. *Biol Reprod* 1980;23:294–304.

1328. Yeung CH, Coper TG, Weinbauer GF, Bergmann M, Kleinhns G, Schulze H, Nieschlag E. Fluid-phase transcytosis in the primate epididymis in vitro and in vivo. *Int J Androl* 1989;12:384–394.

1329. Yeung CH, Cooper TG, Bergmann M, Schulze H. Organization of tubules in the human caput epididymidis and the ultrastructure of their epithelia. *Am J Anat* 1991;191:261–279.

1330. Yoffey JM, Courtice FC. *Lymphatics, Lymph and the Lymphomyeloid Complex,* London: Academic Press.

1331. Young GP, Goldstein M, Phillips DM, Sundaram K, Gunsalus GL, Bardin CW. Sertoli cell-only syndrome produced by cold testicular ischemia. *Endocrinology* 1988;122:1974–1082.

1332. Yuri K. Immunohistochemical and enzyme histochemical localization of peptidergic, aminergic and cholinergic nerve fibers in the rat seminal vesicle. *J Urol* 1990;143:194–198.

1333. Zerhouni EA, Siegelman SS, Wapsh PC, White RI. Elevated pressure in the left renal vein in patients with varicocele: preliminary observations. *J Urol* 1980;123:512–513.

1334. Zirkin BR, Ewing LL, Kromann N, Cochran RC. Testosterone secretion by rat, rabbit, guinea pig, dog, and hamster testes perfused in vitro: correlation with Leydig cell ultrastructure. *Endocrinology* 1980;107:1867–1874.

1335. Zupp JL, Maddocks S, Setchell BP. K and Na in interstitial extracellular fluid (IEF) in rat testes. *J Reprod Fertil Abstract Ser* 1988;1:37.

The Physiology of Reproduction, Second Edition,
edited by E. Knobil and J.D. Neill,
Raven Press, Ltd., New York © 1994.

CHAPTER 19

The Cytology of the Testis

D. M. de Kretser and J. B. Kerr

HISTORICAL ASPECTS

Although the effects of castration were recognized in antiquity, probably dating back to the Neolithic age (ca. 7000 B.C.) (1), the association of the testis with fertility did not emerge until the 17th century. Reasonably accurate diagrammatic representations of the testicular anatomy can be attributed to Aristotle in 400 B.C. (2), but the necessity of the testes for fertility did not emerge at that time. De Graaf's (3) treatise recorded accurately the general structure and functions of the testis, and his observations were soon followed by the observation of spermatozoa in seminal fluid by van Leeuwenhoek in 1667 (4). The link between the seminiferous tubules and the production of spermatozoa did not fully emerge until the studies of von Köelliker (5), who concluded that spermatozoa were formed by a process of cellular development within the tubules. The cellular changes resulting in the production of spermatozoa thus constituted spermatogenesis. Accurate descriptions of the hormonal effects of castration were also available in Aristotle's time, but experimental proof emerged from the studies of Berthold (6), who showed that the loss of comb size and crowing that occurred in roosters after castration could be reversed by transplantation of the testes. The site of production of the masculinizing factor was subsequently attributed to the Leydig cells by Bouin and Ancel (7), but the isolation of testosterone did not occur until 1935 by David et al. (8). The improvements in microscopy in the late 19th century expanded our knowledge of the light microscopic features of spermatogenesis and the identification of chromosomes and the processes of mitosis and meiosis greatly improved our understanding of gamete production in the male. The results of those studies provide the foundation of our knowledge.

Institute of Reproduction and Development and Department of Anatomy, Monash University, Victoria 3168, Australia

GENERAL STRUCTURE OF THE TESTIS

The testis is surrounded by a dense connective tissue capsule, the tunica albuginea, which is covered on its anterior and lateral aspects with the remnants of the process vaginalis, forming the visceral and parietal layers of the tunica vaginalis (9). From the internal surface of the tunica albuginea connective tissue septa extend posteriorly toward a region of the testis termed the mediastinum. This area consists of connective tissue within which an anastomotic network of ducts can be identified—the rete testis.

The tunica albuginea is formed by dense connective tissue within which smooth muscle fibers can be found (10), the latter being responsible for the capacity of the capsule to contract in response to pharmacological stimuli (11). The inner surface of the tunica albuginea is apposed to loose, highly vascular connective tissue sometimes termed the tunica vasculosa. The degree of lobulation of the testis varies between species, and within these lobules lie the seminiferous tubules within which spermatogenesis occurs. The tubules extend as loops from the mediastinum testis, both ends of each loop communicating via single straight tubules, the tubuli recti (12). In the majority of mammals this simple arrangement is obscured in the adult testis (Fig. 1), since the tubule forming each loop becomes extensively folded, thereby extending its surface area (13–15). The extensive lengthening of the tubule loops that occurs during development is the result principally of the mitotic activity of immature Sertoli cells.

The organization of the intertubular tissue varies dramatically between species (16), but it contains the blood vessels, lymphatics, and nerve fibers (see later discussion). The Leydig cells are scattered in groups in the intertubular tissue in relation to the vasculature and the lamina propria of the seminiferous tubules, the outer layers of which consist of modified smooth muscle cells termed myoid cells (Fig. 1).

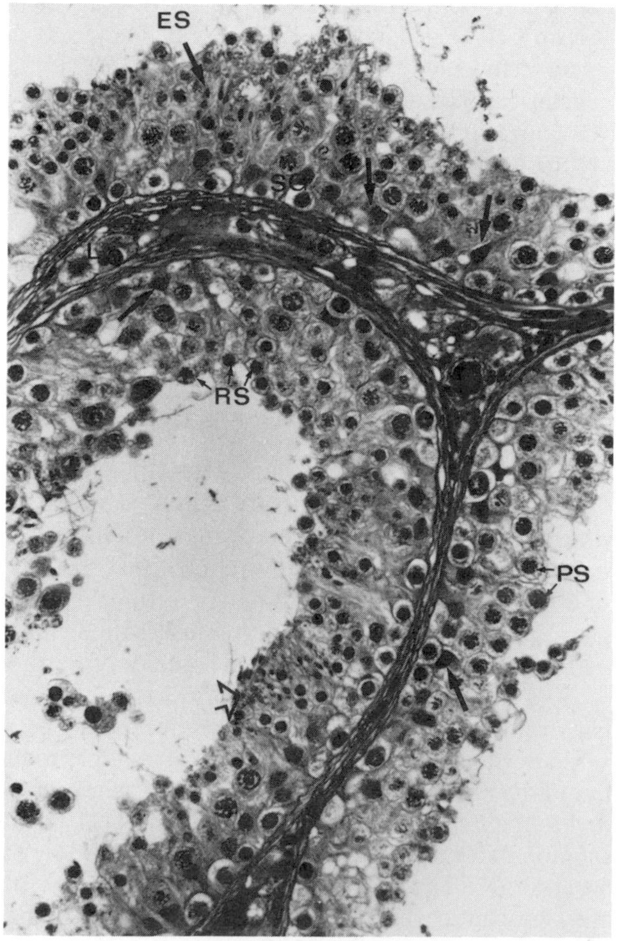

FIG. 1. This light micrograph of the normal human testis illustrates spermatogonia (SG), primary spermatocytes (PS), round spermatids (RS), and elongating spermatids (ES). Note residual bodies (*open arrows*), Sertoli cells (*arrows*), and Leydig cells (L).

INTRATESTICULAR DUCTS

Transitional Distal Segment of Seminiferous Tubule

The segment of the seminiferous tubule that establishes continuity with the rete testis is lined by an epithelium devoid of germ cells. The segment, termed the transitional distal seminiferous segment (Fig. 2), narrows, forming an "epithelial plug" that projects slightly into the tubuli recti, which has a wider lumen. The epithelium consists of Sertoli cells, which contain more extensive rough endoplasmic reticulum and lipid inclusions but less smooth endoplasmic reticulum. Prominent bundles of filaments are present in the cells and may confer some structural rigidity to this region, which may function as a plug to regulate the movement of cells and fluid into the rete testis (14). Dym (17) suggested that the slope of the apices of the cells toward the rete testis made it unlikely that reflux could occur into the seminiferous tubules.

Rete Testis

This represents an anastomotic series of ducts into which the transitional distal segment of the seminiferous tubules opens and that drain at their cranial pole via the ductuli efferentes to form the duct of the epididymis. It lies in the mediastinum of the testis parallel to the axis of the epididymis and has been divided into several zones (Fig. 2) by Roosen-Runge and Holstein (18): (a) septal rete, (b) mediastinal rete, and (c) extratesticular rete. The septal rete consists of the zone of the straight ducts, the tubule recti, which drain the seminiferous tubules. The mediastinal rete can be subdivided further into a deep zone consisting of an anastomotic maze of tubules drain-

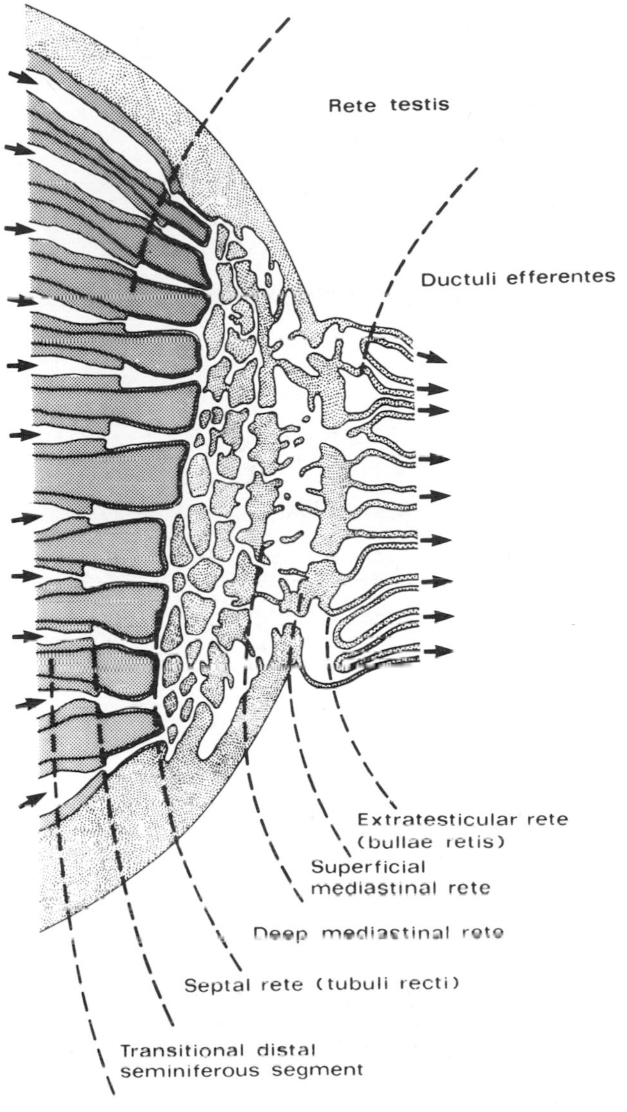

FIG. 2. The method by which the seminiferous tubules terminate in the rete testis is shown. The zones of the rete testis are denoted. (From de Kretser et al., ref. 890, with permission.)

ing the septal rete and opening into a superficial zone, a series of relatively wide longitudinal channels emptying into the extratesticular rete or bullae retis. The latter is characterized by macroscopically visible dilated spaces drained by the ductuli efferentes.

The region of the mediastinal rete is characterized by an irregular network of cylindrical strands, the chordae retis, which range in diameter from 5 to 40 μm (18). The thinner cords are avascular, but each contains a fibroelastic matrix containing myofibroblastic cellular elements, the myoid cells showing similar features to those surrounding the seminiferous tubules. It is postulated that their strutlike features may prevent overdistension of the thin-walled rete channels and, together with the contractile properties of the myoid elements, may provide a mechanism for raising intrarete pressure, thereby forcing fluid into the extratesticular ducts. Two distinct cell types are present, the squamous cells lining most of the rete and the prismatic cells, which occur in clusters at bends and corners in the channels (19). The squamous cells are studded with short microvilli and contain a long single cilium, cytoplasm-containing lipid inclusions, glycogen, and a few areas of smooth endoplasmic reticulum. The prismatic cells stain lightly, contain an irregular nucleus with fine granular chromatin, and also contain a single cilium. Their cytoplasmic organelles are polarized, with prominent basal collections of lipid and glycogen and a supranuclear Golgi complex, the surface showing a few thick microvilli that are shorter than the squamous cells. External to the epithelium is a connective tissue layer containing fibroblasts and smooth muscle cells and bundles of collagen and elastin fibers. The extratesticular rete is characterized by vesicular dilatations that are visible macroscopically and act as the vestibules for the excurrent duct system, which extends as the ductuli efferentes.

SPERMATOGENESIS

The sequence of cytological events that result in the formation of mature spermatozoa from precursor cells is known as spermatogenesis (Figs. 3 and 4). In many mammals this process takes place within the seminiferous tubule throughout the reproductive life span of the male. In some species it is interrupted or subdivided into a series of distinct phases based on environmental cues that are transduced into hormonal signals stimulating or inhibiting spermatogenesis, e.g., seasonal breeders (20). In others, unique processes occur such that a single wave of spermatogenic development is seen within the testis, subsequent to which the animal is sterile; such a process occurs in the marsupial mouse, *Antechinus strudii* and *swainsonii,* wherein the stem cells, after a burst of mitotic activity, differentiate and proceed through the spermatogenic process, resulting in a single wave of reproductive activity (21). Thus, it is possible to see within a seminiferous tubule spermatids of varying maturity without any other basally placed germ cells (Figs. 5–10).

Spermatozoa can be viewed as the "secretory product" of the spermatogenic process. To enable a continuous production of "cells" as a product, the process of spermatogenesis must involve a continuous replication of stem cells to produce cohorts of cells that can proceed through the subsequent changes. Furthermore since the nucleus of the sperm fuses with that of the oocyte to form the zygote, a reduction of the number of chromosomes to the haploid state must occur in gametogenesis such that the diploid state is restored on syngamy. There are three major elements that together constitute spermatogenesis: (a) stem cell renewal by the process of mitosis,

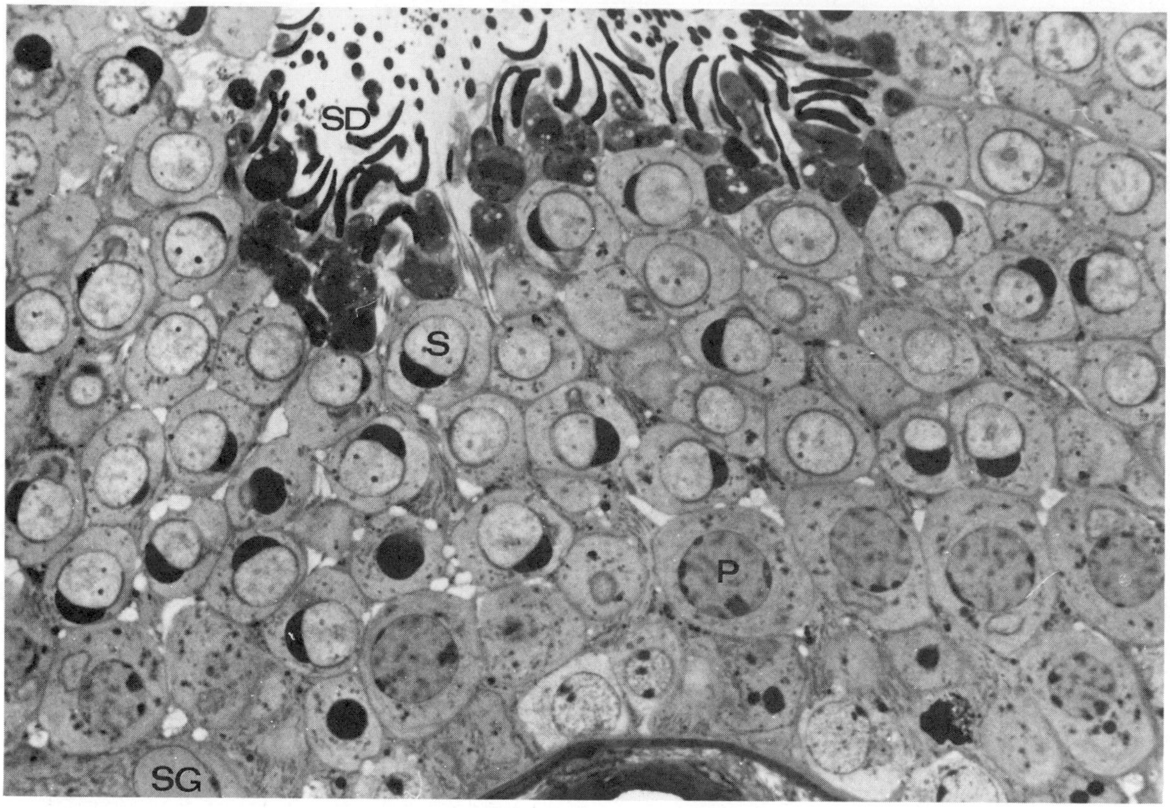

FIG. 3. Guinea pig seminiferous epithelium showing spermatogonia (SG), primary spermatocytes (P), round spermatids (S), and mature spermatids (SD).

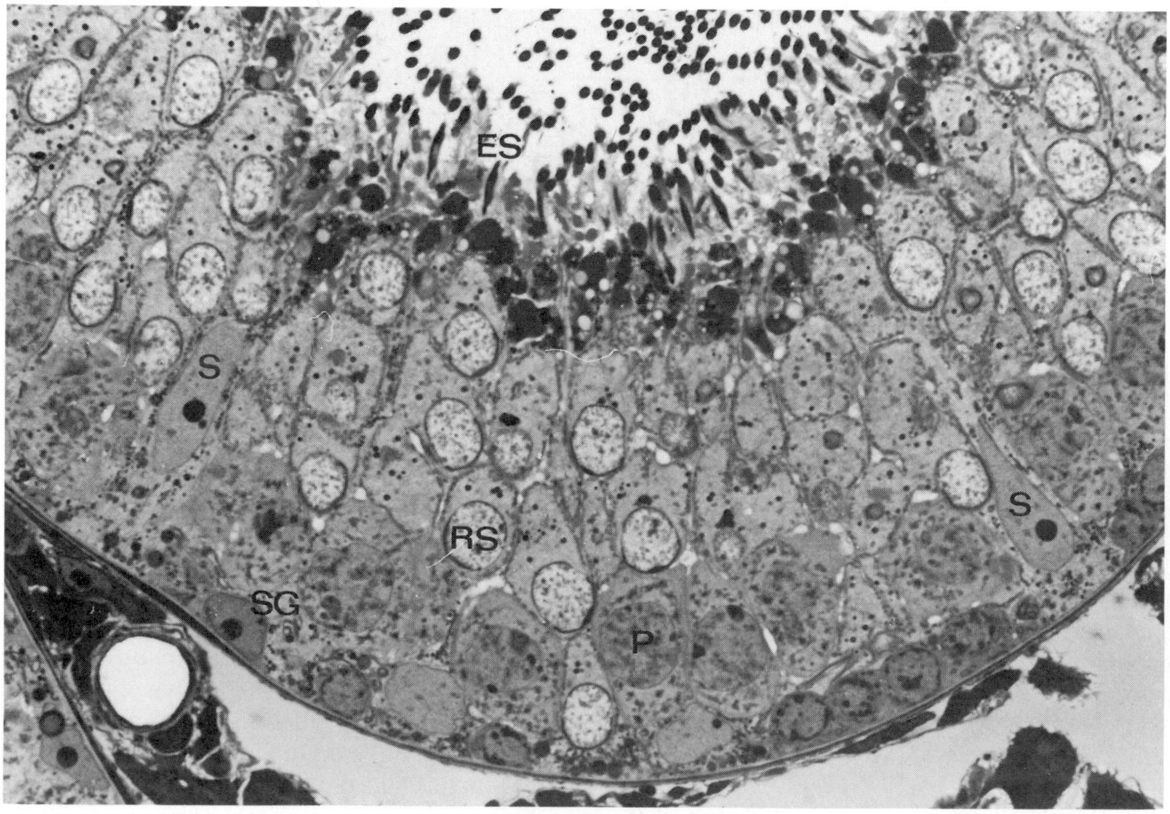

FIG. 4. Rat seminiferous epithelium showing Sertoli cells (S), spermatogonia (SG), primary spermatocytes (P), and round (RS) and elongated spermatids (ES).

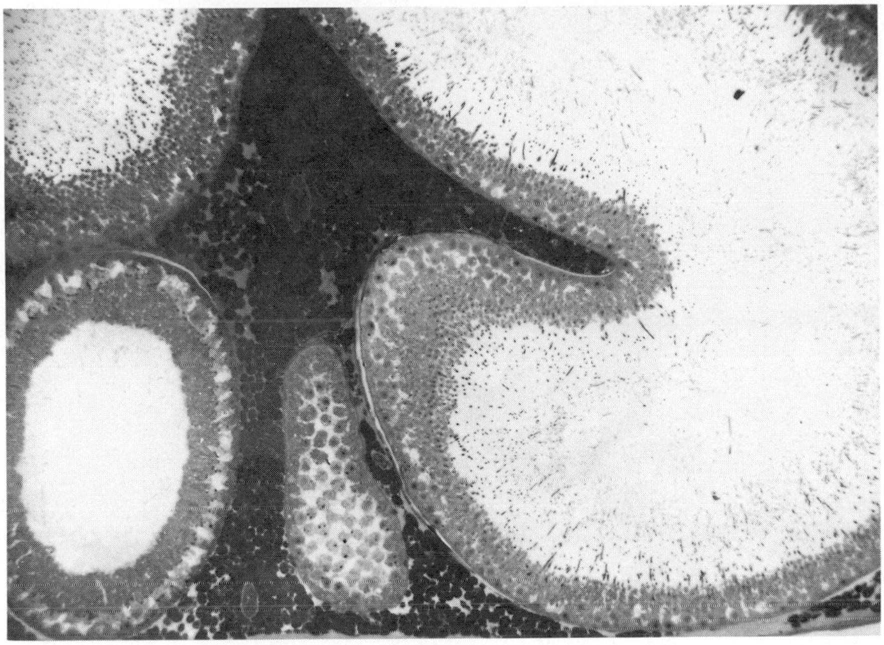

FIG. 5. *Antechinus* testis, illustrating the shallow depth of the seminiferous epithelium in relation to the dimensions of the seminiferous tubules.

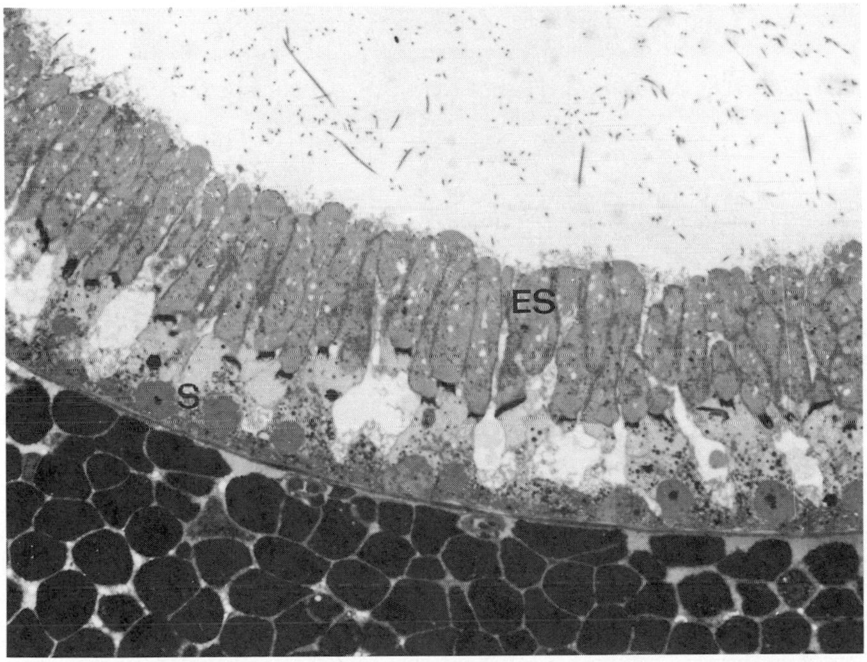

FIG. 6. *Antechinus* testis in June, showing a shallow epithelium containing Sertoli cells (S) and elongated spermatids (ES). Other germ cell types are rarely seen.

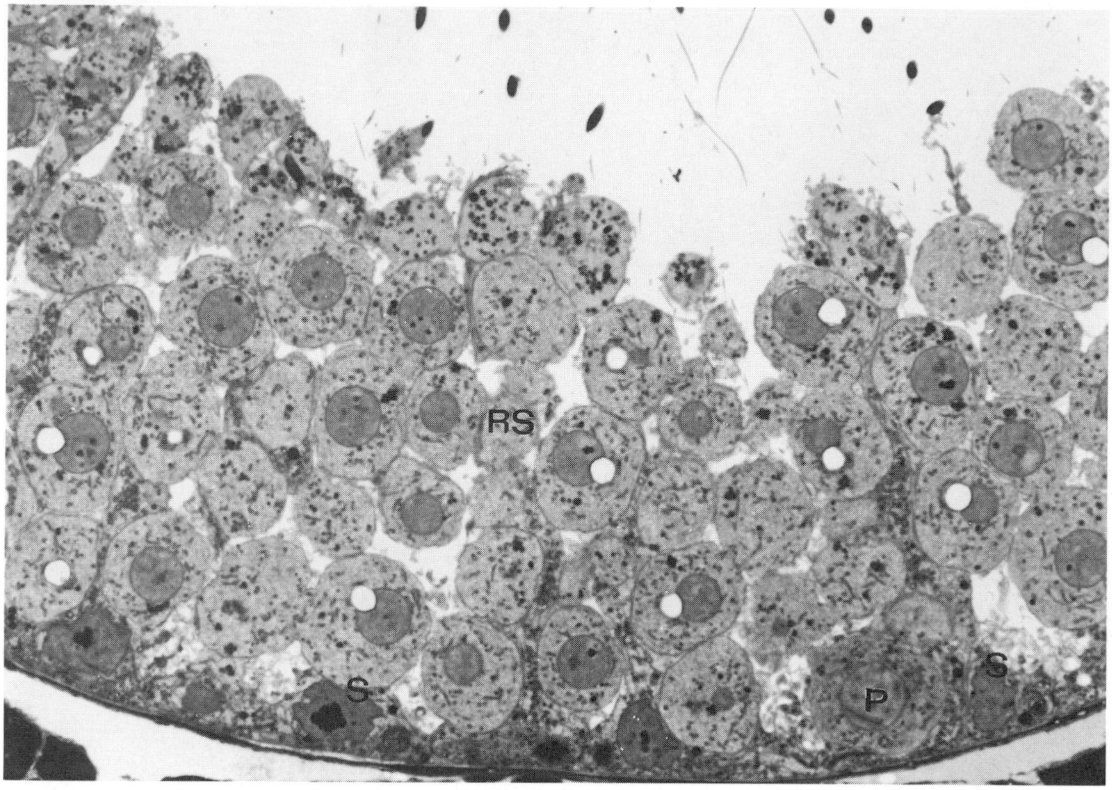

FIG. 7. *Antechinus* seminiferous epithelium in late June showing Sertoli cells (S) and round spermatids (RS). Only one primary spermatocyte (P) is visible.

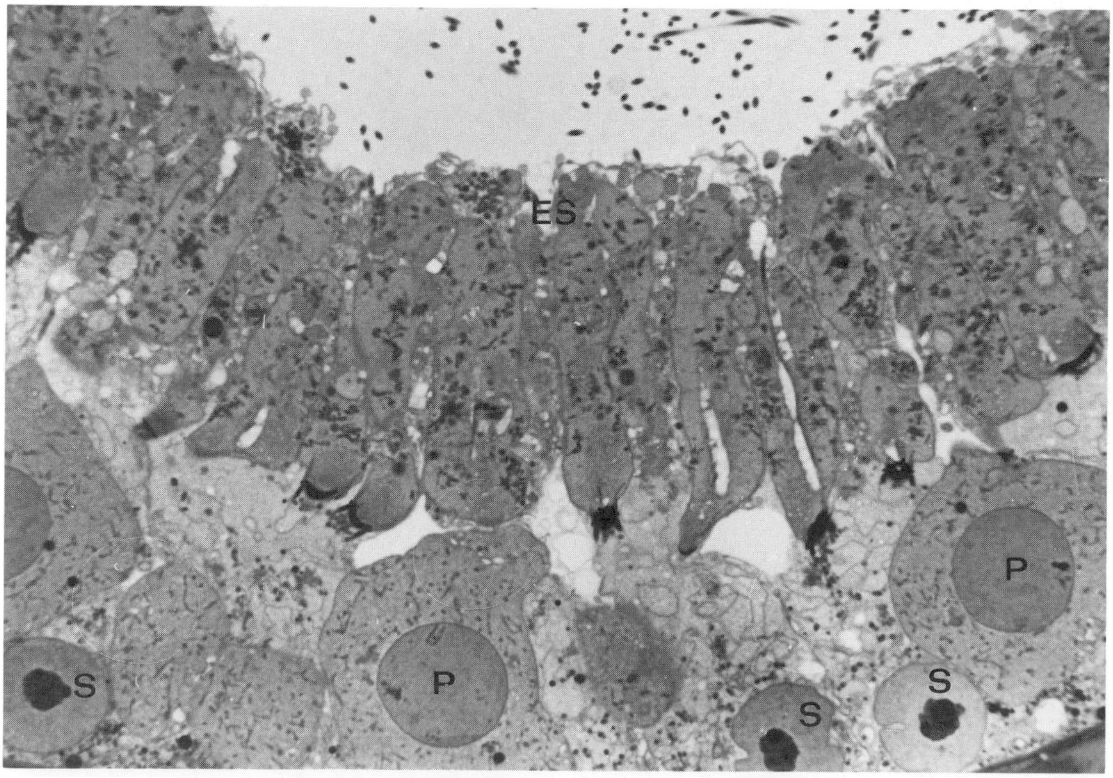

FIG. 8. *Antechinus* seminiferous epithelium in late June showing Sertoli cells (S), pachytene primary spermatocytes (P), and elongated spermatids (ES). Spermatogonia and early spermatocytes not visible.

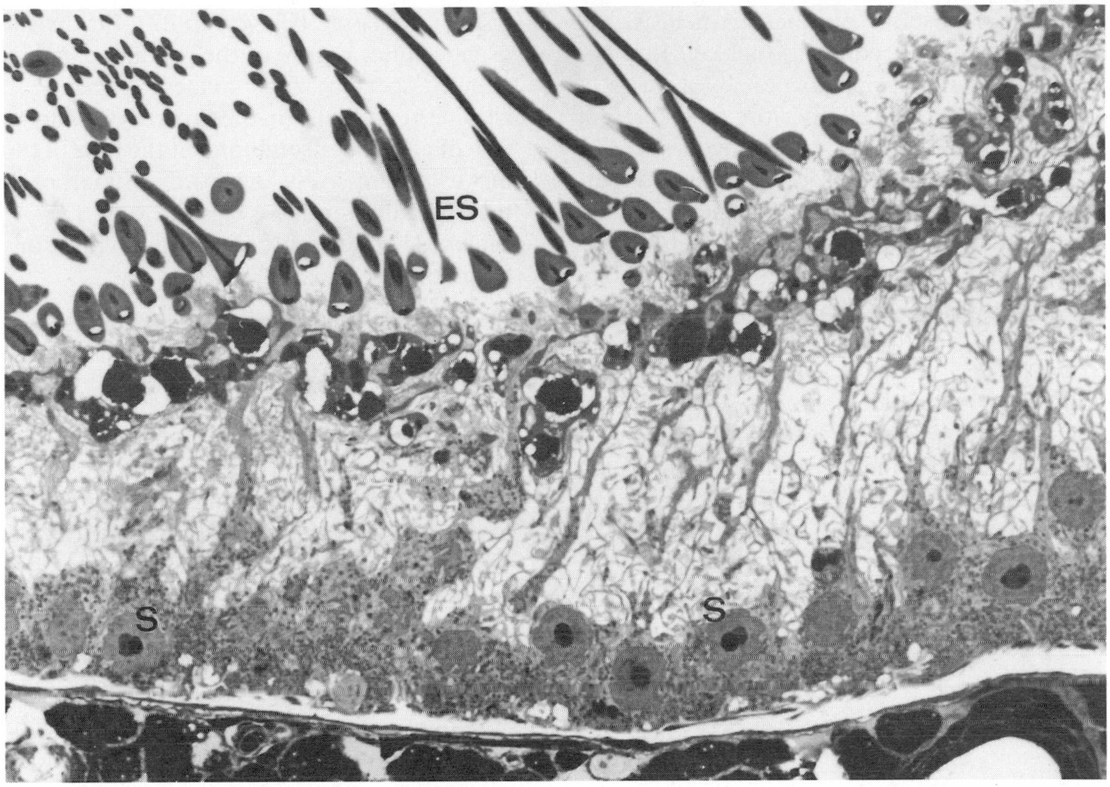

FIG. 9. *Antechinus* seminiferous epithelium in July. Sertoli cells (S) and elongated spermatids (ES) are noted, but other germ cell types are not present.

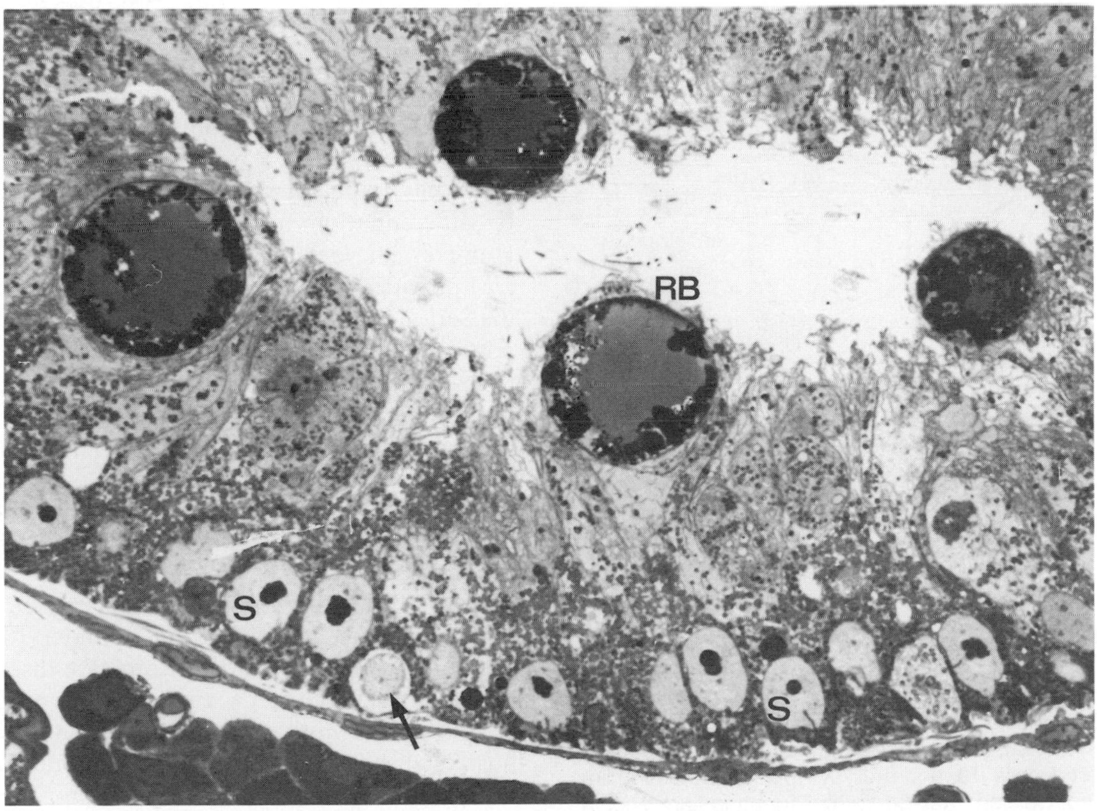

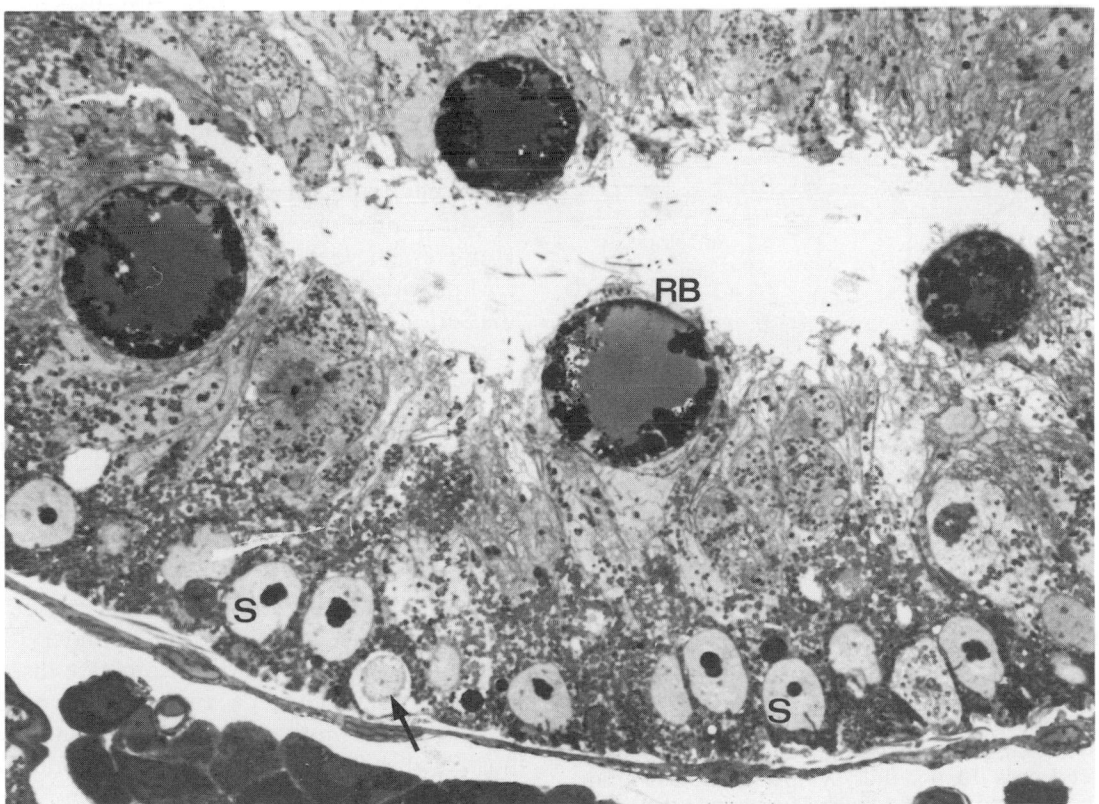

FIG. 10. *Antechinus* seminiferous epithelium in August at the time of breeding. Sertoli cells (S) and spermatid residual bodies (RB) are noted, together with a single basally located spermatogonium (*arrow*).

(b) reduction of chromosomal number by meiosis, and (c) the transformation of a conventional cell into the complex structure of the spermatozoon by a series of changes involving no further cell division; this represent a metamorphic process termed spermiogenesis. The stem cells for the spermatogenic process are termed spermatogonia and undergo mitotic division (Figs. 1 and 3). Groups of spermatogonia then proceed to enter meiosis and are termed primary spermatocytes and secondary spermatocytes. The latter divide to form spermatids, which are transformed during spermatogenesis into spermatozoa.

The conditions under which spermatogenesis is successfully completed are relatively specialized and necessitate the creation of a unique environment within the seminiferous tubule. This is achieved by the organization of the non-germ-cell elements within the tubules, namely, the Sertoli cells (Fig. 11), which form the blood–testis barrier (see below; ref. 22). Furthermore, the unusual cellular nature of the product of spermatogenesis, namely spermatozoa, creates a specific requirement within the epithelium, the support of a migratory population of cells that proliferates at the base of the tubule and moves progressively toward the lumen of the tubule as the cells differentiate (Figs. 12 and 13). Again, this is achieved by the nature of the nondividing or stable population of Sertoli cells.

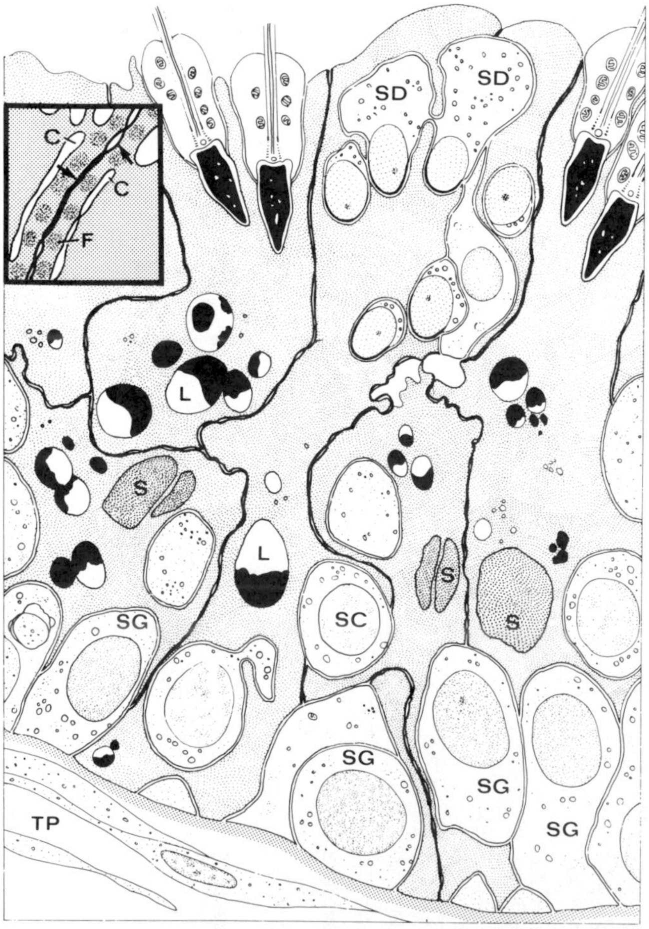

FIG. 11. The relationships between germ cells and Sertoli cells are shown for the human seminiferous epithelium. Note spermatogonia (SG), primary spermatocytes (SC), spermatids (SD), Sertoli cells (S), and their cytoplasm containing lipids (L). The specialized inter-Sertoli-cell junctions are shown by a *heavy line* and diagrammatically illustrated at higher magnification in the **inset.** C, cisternae; F, fibrils.

Developmental Considerations

Although a detailed development of the testis is the subject of Chapter 8 (this volume), a brief consideration is of value in understanding the relationships of the two populations of cells, the germ cells and the Sertoli cells. The development of the testis is associated with the formation of a series of sex cords, arranged as a series of C-shaped arches running at right angles to the long axis of the testis, each end of the arch connecting with developing rete testis (12,13). With further development, the orientation of the plane of the cords perpendicular to the longitudinal axis of the testis changes, and elongation is achieved by infolding of the cords to form a series of convolutions, mostly in a craniocaudal orientation (12). The mechanisms by which these cords arise from their mesenchymal precursors is complex and still the subject of debate (see review ref. 23). Nevertheless, there is general agreement that the cords are composed of two types of cells, the supporting cells and the primordial germ cells (Fig. 14). Though it is now accepted that these two cell types remain distinct in terms of origin and subsequent development, earlier studies suggested that the germ cells degenerated in fetal life and were reestablished by differentiation from the supporting cells (24–27). However, the detailed studies of Clermont and Perey (28) provided strong evidence to support the view that the Sertoli cells are formed by differentiation of the supporting cells and that the primordial germ cells give rise to spermatogonia. The number of supporting cells in the fetal testis greatly outnumbers the primordial germ cells. Though this balance changes as a result of mitotic multiplication of the primordial germ cells, even at birth in the majority of mammalian species, the number of supporting cells is considerably greater than the number of germ cells (28).

Before birth, the primitive Sertoli cells are predominantly arranged adjacent to the boundary tissue of the seminiferous cords, although some are displaced more centrally by the close packing of cells within the cords (23,29–37). Primitive Sertoli cells exhibit a conical or polygonal shape, with their cytoplasm often oriented radially within the seminiferous cord (Fig. 14). Their nuclei are variable in shape and seldom show deep indentations. A nucleolus is often present, together with

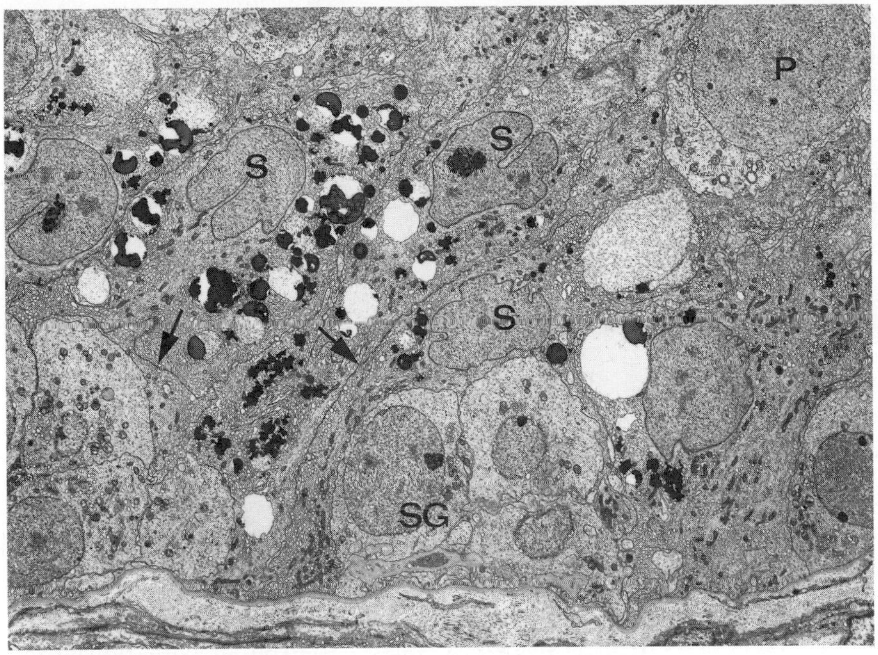

FIG. 12. Ultrastructure of human seminiferous epithelium showing Sertoli cell nuclei (S), spermatogonia (SG), pachytene primary spermatocyte (P), and inter-Sertoli-cell junctional complexes (*arrows*).

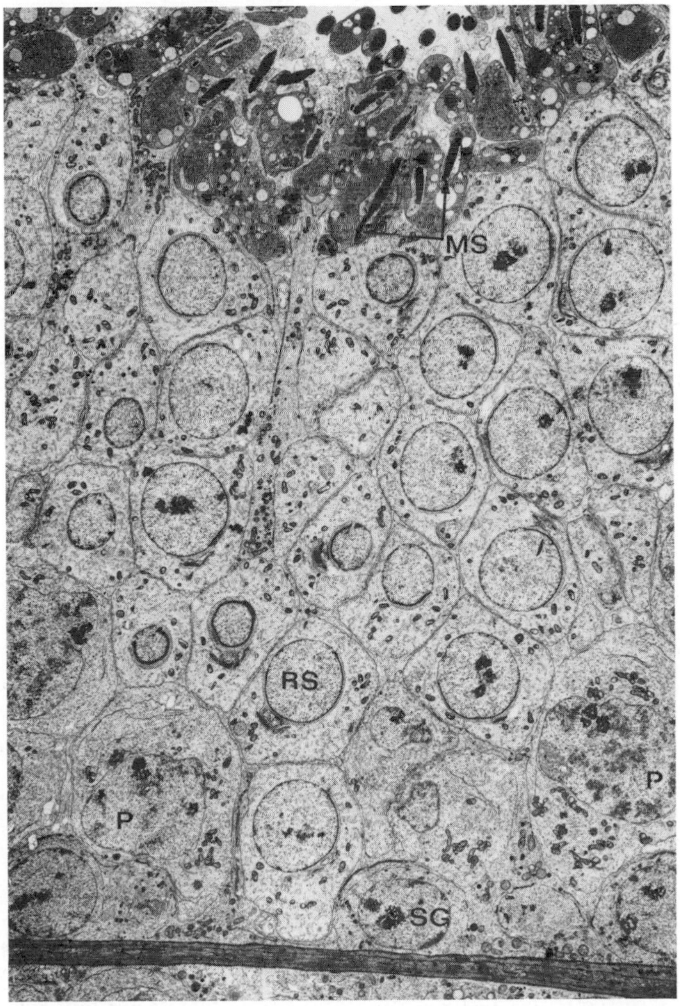

FIG. 13. Mouse seminiferous epithelium showing spermatogonia (SG), pachytene primary spermatocytes (P), and round (RS) and mature (MS) spermatids.

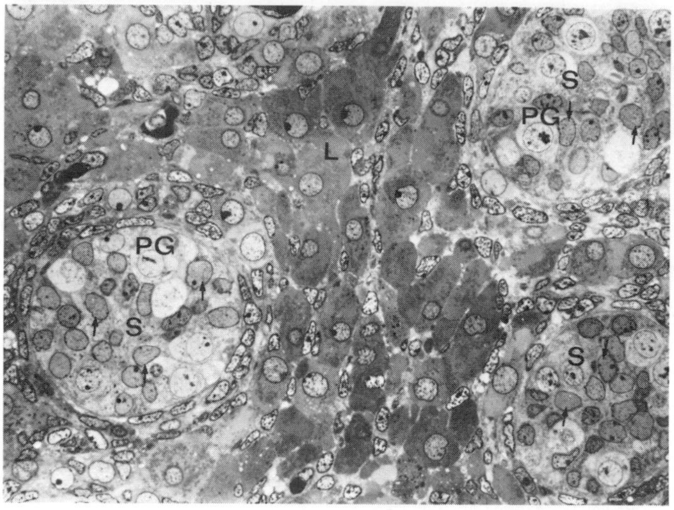

FIG. 14. Leydig cells (L) seminiferous cords (S) from a 16-week human fetus. Note primordial germ cells (PG) and immature Sertoli cells (*arrows*).

peripheral clumps of heterochromatin associated with the nuclear membrane. The cytoplasm of primitive Sertoli cells in the fetus is unremarkable, but tubular membranes of endoplasmic reticulum are well represented, often bearing variable amounts of ribosomes (29,38), and for this reason, these organelles are referred to as a transitional form between conventional smooth and rough endoplasmic reticulum.

A gradual expansion in the diameter of seminiferous cords during fetal life is a reflection of the changing internal organization caused by proliferation of primitive Sertoli cells and the gonocytes (38). For instance, the number of Sertoli cells increases from 1.5 ± 0.4 million/testis at birth to 30 ± 2.5 million/testis at 20 days (39). As the gonocytes proliferate and differentiate into spermatogonia, they often form groups of cells that are accommodated in recesses provided by the Sertoli cells, indicating that the fetal Sertoli cells are deformable. This presumably allows the immature germ cells to gain attachment to the boundary tissues of the seminiferous cords, a location that, in postnatal life, becomes their exclusive domain. Information on the proliferative behavior of Sertoli cells in the fetus has been gained from morphometric assessment of their numbers in the pig and from autoradiographic studies in rodents examining the incorporation of tritiated thymidine into the DNA of primitive Sertoli cell nuclei (30,31,38). It was found that the numbers of fetal Sertoli cells increase steadily until shortly before birth, and thereafter their proliferative capacity declines to produce a stable population of nondividing Sertoli cells. Cessation of Sertoli cell proliferation has been much studied in laboratory rodents and occurs on day 10 to 12 after birth in the mouse (28,40–45) and on day 14 to 16 in the immature rat. In the human, Sertoli cell numbers increase from 250 million to 1500 million/testis between 3 months and 10 years and further increase to 3700 million during puberty (46).

The peak of proliferative activity of Sertoli cells just prior to parturition has implicated the production of mitogenic factors capable of controlling expansion of the fetal Sertoli cell population. Not unexpectedly, the involvement of gonadotrophic hormones has been favored as the mechanism governing the mitotic activity of fetal Sertoli cells. This idea has gained support not only by inference from the known trophic actions of FSH on the seminiferous epithelium in postnatal life (47) but also from evidence gained from studies of the male fetus suggesting a functional relationship between the fetal pituitary and testis. The pituitary–testicular axis appears to be activated by day 17 of fetal life in the rat, since at or before this time the hypothalamus contains GnRH (48), and FSH and LH are detectable in the pituitary (48–50). The role of FSH in development of fetal Sertoli cells has been highlighted further by the demonstration of maximum FSH binding to fetal testes at precisely the time of maximum proliferation of Sertoli cells (51). Furthermore, addition of FSH to cultures of Sertoli cells derived from postnatal testes results in increased mitotic activity (52,53).

A significant step forward in elucidation of the factors that control proliferation of fetal Sertoli cells was provided by Orth (31), who showed that removal of the fetal pituitary or treatment with an antiserum to FSH produced a dramatic reduction in Sertoli cell mitosis. Orth further showed that this effect, at least in utero, was mediated via cAMP. Another collection of data indicates that local interactions within the fetal testis may be involved with cell proliferation prior to birth. Coincident with maximum mitoses of fetal Sertoli cells shortly before parturition, the fetal Leydig cells attain their maximum numbers at or slightly prior to this time (54,55). Levels of circulating testosterone (56), the activity of Leydig cell steroidogenic enzymes (57), the production of testicular testosterone, and total steroid content per

Leydig cell are greatest during this period (55,58,59). These data raise the possibility that a paracrine relationship exists between fetal Sertoli and Leydig cells and emphasize that, in addition to the demonstrated role of FSH, other factors may be of importance in influencing the expansion of the Sertoli cell population.

The attainment of adequate numbers of Sertoli cells achieved during their proliferative phase in the fetal and neonatal growth periods has important implications for the subsequent spermatogenic potential of the mature testis. Administration of the antimitotic agent cytosine arabinoside to neonatal rats partly arrests Sertoli cell proliferation, and the reduced number of Sertoli cells is accompanied by a significant decline in the production of spermatids by the developing testis (60). Conversely, experimental induction of transient hypothyroidism in neonatal rats results in an extended period of Sertoli cell proliferation (up to 30 days postnatally) in which the maturation of the testis and growth of the seminiferous tubules is suppressed up to 60 days of age (61). However in these rats, the testes contain approximately twice the normal number of Sertoli cells (62), and at 160 days of age testis weight is increased by 80% and daily sperm production by 140% (61,63,64). Paradoxically, circulating gonadotropin and testosterone levels were similar or lowered compared to age-matched control animals, yet TSH levels were markedly elevated coincident with the expansion of Sertoli cell numbers. Thus, nongonadotropic factors may play a crucial role in the developmental capacity of the Sertoli cell population, which ultimately affects the spermatogenic potential of the fully mature testis. This concept has been extended by recent studies using recombinant inbred mouse strains that suggest that at least two autosomal genes regulate the number of Sertoli cells and associated testis size (65).

During postnatal growth of the testis, the immature Sertoli cells continue to proliferate, albeit at a steadily declining rate, until the adult population is established. The appearance of pachytene primary spermatocytes in the rat testis is associated with this restriction of Sertoli cell division, which, according to numerous studies, provides for a stable Sertoli cell population during adult life (66–68). With the initiation of spermatogenesis soon after birth in rodents and at various later times in domestic, ruminant, and primate species, the immature Sertoli cells undergo morphological maturation to attain the adult-type structural features seen in the mature testis (68–72). These changes include a large increase in cell size, the movement of the nucleus to a basal position within the cell, the development of a complex nuclear shape and a tripartite nucleolus, and the proliferation of organelles, particularly the smooth endoplasmic reticulum. A much studied aspect of Sertoli cell maturation in the developing testis has focused on the morphological differentiation of the blood–testis barrier. Light microscopic analysis had earlier indicated that the barrier detected by the admittance or exclusion of acridine dyes appears at the onset of spermatogenesis (73). Electron microscopic studies (69,72–77) confirm that electron-opaque tracers freely penetrate into the seminiferous cords of newborn animals but are subsequently restricted from entry concurrent with the appearance of inter-Sertoli-cell junctional complexes. In the immature rat the barrier forms during the 16th to 19th postnatal day, which is after the cessation of Sertoli cell mitoses and the commencement of the meiotic maturation of germ cells. Because pachytene primary spermatocytes are formed prior to the effective establishment of the blood–testis barrier (72), it seems that the meiotic maturation process during the initiation of spermatogenesis is not dependent on the formation of an adluminal epithelial compartment.

The factors controlling the formation of the blood–testis barrier are not known, although the possible involvement of gonadotropins remains under discussion. Certainly the appearance of inter-Sertoli-cell junctions is not dependent on spermatogenesis, since the elimination of germ cells from the testis (47,78–80) cannot prevent development of the junctions. A similar conclusion can be drawn from studies of the permeability of the Sertoli cell junctional complexes in seasonally breeding species such as the mink (81), in which the barrier undergoes structural decay and reformation in association with respective phases of testicular regression and recrudescence. The fact that germ cells survive and are capable of development in the absence of a functional permeability barrier suggests that the tightness or leakiness of the junctional complexes is related more to the fluid secretory properties of the Sertoli cell than to the extent of germ cell development. However, the appearance of the blood–testis barrier in immature rats was delayed when rats were treated daily from birth with clomiphene citrate or estradiol benzoate, agents that are thought to suppress gonadotropin secretion (74). This finding has remained difficult to evaluate, since measurements of gonadotropin levels were not available, and the possible direct effects of clomiphene or estradiol on the testis were not considered. It was concluded that the formation of inter-Sertoli-cell junctions was not directly dependent on gonadotropins.

Similar views were expressed when it was found that long-term hypophysectomy failed to disrupt the blood–testis barrier in rats (82–85). In the human testis, however, it has been shown (86) that the formation of inter-Sertoli-cell junctions in men with hypogonadotropic hypogonadism is related to the administration of exogenous gonadotropins. The morphological changes that appear in the Sertoli cells during sexual maturation require further study with particular emphasis on the role of the gonadotropic and steroid hormones. The primordial germ cells migrate from endoderm and dorsal yolk sac epithelium via the dorsal mesentery into the gonadal ridge (87,88). Recent studies suggest that the migration is under the control of the tyrosine kinase receptor, *c-kit,* and its ligand, variably called stem cell factor or mast cell growth factor (89,90). Whether they arise from endoderm or the underlying mesoderm is still in question; Clark and Eddy (91) noted that their fine-structural features resembled underlying mesodermal cells rather than the surrounding endoderm. The histochemical presence of alkaline phosphatase in these primordial germ cells enabled their identification during this migratory phase (92). These germ cells become associated with the precursors of the Sertoli cells to form primitive testicular cords, an association that is thought to be important in establishing the different behavior of male primordial germ cells from those in the female. Evidence exists that if the structure of the cords is disrupted, or if male germ cells lodge in aberrant sites such as the adrenal gland (93), they will commence meiosis during fetal life—a characteristic of germ cells in the developing ovary (94).

Subsequently, the primordial germ cells undergo a defined period of mitotic cell division, during which daughter cells remain connected by intercellular bridges (95,96). In the rat, the period of cell division occurs for 48 hours from days 14 to 16 of fetal life, and, since the daughter cells differ slightly in structure from the primordial germ cells, they have been called M-prospermatogonia (97). Hilscher and colleagues identified yet another period of fetal mitotic activity that gave rise to T-prospermatogonia, in turn giving rise to the adult A-spermatogonial stage. In other species the sequence of changes is less well defined, and the terminology confusing. However, there is general agreement that a period of mitotic activity occurs within the prenatal testis that increases germ cell numbers, but they still remain the minority cell population within the seminiferous cords, usually lying in a central position. The numbers of gonocytes and spermatogonia decrease in fetal life as a result of a degenerative process that has been estimated to reduce numbers between 30% and 40% (98). The degenerating cells are phagocytosed by the immature Sertoli cells.

Gondos (99) has suggested a simpler terminology, dividing the germ cells in the fetal testis into (a) primitive germ cells, which are part of the undifferentiated gonad, (b) gonocytes, when the germ cells are located within the seminiferous cords in a central position, and (c) spermatogonia, when they move to the periphery of the tubule. The primordial germ cells are relatively large rounded cells with an irregular horseshoe-shaped nucleus and filamentous centrally placed nucleolus (91). The mitochondria are large, rounded, and contain few cristae. There is sparse endoplasmic reticulum, plentiful free ribosomes, and characteristic membrane-bounded granules with a central dense core separated from the membrane by a flocculent zone (91). In the human, the gonocytes have similar features with globular mitochondria whose cristae are dilated (100). Apart from perinuclear smooth-membraned vesicles, there is paucity of other organelles. Gondos and colleagues (95,100) noted that processes extend from the gonocytes as they migrate toward the basement membrane of the cords to become spermatogonia. The processes contain microtubules, presumably aiding the migratory process. The spermatogonia have similar cytological features during fetal life but differ in being peripherally placed and being interconnected by cytoplasmic bridges as a result of incomplete cytokinesis during mitosis.

In the testes of newborn rats, gonocyte proliferation occurs prior to their movement toward the basement membrane of the seminiferous cord. Since both events can occur *in vitro* in the absence of serum- and hormone-supplemented media, it seems likely that local intratesticular factors regulate the initial maturation of these cells (101).

The pattern of development in the sex cords after birth varies considerably in mammals depending on the time span between birth and the acquisition of sexual maturity. In species such as the rat, spermatogenesis effectively commences at birth since the duration of spermatogenesis in this species is 49 days (102) and spermatozoa are present in the testis at about 50 days (103). Hence, the seminiferous tubules undergo rapid development after birth, sequentially demonstrating the stages of germ cell development constituting spermatogenesis. In other species such as man, there is an extensive prepubertal period during which the testes show little change from their appearance at birth. Recent detailed morphometric studies of testes from children dying suddenly have shown that little change occurs until 7 to 9 years, following which mitotic activity of the gonocytes occurs, populating the base of the seminiferous tubules with spermatogonia in numbers equal to those of the Sertoli cells (104). The spermatogonia subsequently undergo the spermatogenic process, with spermatozoa being released into the lumen between 11 and 13 years.

Spermatogonia

The cells that divide by mitosis and constitute the pool of cells from which meiosis and spermatogenesis proceed are termed spermatogonia. They were first identified as separate entities from the Sertoli cells by von Ebner in 1871 (105), but the term spermatogonia was first applied to this class of cells by La Valette St. George in 1876 (106). The first detailed study of these cells was performed by Regaud (27), who defined two types of spermatogonia in the rat, the "dusty" cells and "crusty" cells, on the basis of differences in the chromatin patterns of their nuclei. The "dusty" cells showed a nucleus with fine palely stained chromatin granulation, whereas the "crusty" cells had nuclei with coarse granules of heavily stained chromatin close to the nuclear membrane. Regaud (27) subdivided the "dusty" spermatogonia into two classes based on nuclear morphology and staining with safranin and also clearly distinguished early primary spermatocytes from the "crusty" spermatogonia.

Allen (25) used a different terminology, which persists today, calling the equivalent of "dusty" spermatogonia type A, and the "crusty" cells type B spermatogonia. In the rat, spermatogonia with nuclear characteristics intermediate between type A and type B could be identified principally on the presence of fine plaques of chromatin close to the nuclear membrane; these were termed intermediate spermatogonia (41). Similar subtypes can also be identified in other species such as the mouse (107), ram (42), bull (108), and guinea pig (109). More recent studies in the rat identified further spermatogonial types on the basis of their nuclear morphology, separating four classes of type A spermatogonia as well as the intermediate and type B (110). Similar types of observations are now available for other species, the number of generations of spermatogonia varying significantly (see review, ref. 102).

The ability to differentiate different classes of spermatogonia is critically dependent on the fixation employed, since identification is based on the morphological characteristics of the nuclei. The type of fixation precipitates chromatin to varying degrees: Zenker-formol provides optimal chromatin patterns for identification, since the chromatin remains widely dispersed (102); on the other hand, Bouin's fixative creates larger chromatin clumps close to the nuclear membrane, rendering spermatogonial classification more difficult. Additionally, the characteristic features of the nuclei that are used to identify each type are only present at certain phases of the cell cycle, usually acquiring the typical nuclear morphology at the S and G_2 phases (41,111). In man and in some primate species, somewhat different nuclear characteristics were noted. Branca (112) reported great variability in the morphology of human spermatogonia, describing palely staining areas in some nuclei, termed nuclear vacuoles. Subsequently types A and B spermatogonia were identified in man, with the type A being subdivided into the dark and pale types (113–115). The A dark spermatogonia are characterized by a densely staining chromatin usually containing a central pale-stained area termed the nuclear vacuole. Close to the nuclear membrane one or more nucleoli are found. In contrast, the A pale spermatogonia contain an ovoid nucleus with palely staining granular chromatin and exhibit one or two nucleoli lying close to the nuclear membrane. The type B spermatogonia exhibit the characteristics described for other species, although the human cells are somewhat smaller. Similar spermatogonial types have also been identified in monkeys (*Macacus rhesus; Ceropithecus aethiops*) but do not show the nuclear vacuole (116,117).

It is self-evident that to enable spermatogenesis to proceed as a continuous process, the spermatogonia must not only provide the precursors for the meiotic process but must also renew themselves. The mechanisms by which this is achieved are discussed later in this review, together with the cycle of spermatogenesis. The cytoplasmic features of spermatogonia by light microscopy are relatively unremarkable. They have a poorly staining cytoplasm, and studies of whole mounts of seminiferous tubules demonstrate that they remain connected by intercellular bridges such that large numbers are effectively linked together (118–120). By the periodic-acid–Schiff reaction, glycogen is found in the A dark spermatogonia.

Fine Structure

There have been relatively few detailed ultrastructural studies of spermatogonia, and in these investigators have often had difficulty in identifying the ultrastructural counterparts of the subclasses of spermatogonia identified by light microscopy. The basal position of spermatogonia within the epithelium (Figs. 12, 13, and 15) and their extensive contact with the basement membrane of the tubule are clearly evident by electron microscopy (121,122). The extent of this contact decreases in type B spermatogonia, which will eventually lose all contact with the basement membrane to become preleptotene primary spermatocytes (123). All types of spermatogonia are characterized by a relatively electron-lucent cytoplasm and a paucity of cytoplasmic organelles (122–125). Furthermore, because of incomplete cytokinesis during mitosis, spermatogonia remain connected by intercellular bridges originally identified by Watson (126). These bridges are 2 to 3 μm in width and do not usually contain organelles or microtubules; they are limited by the cell membrane, which is more electron-dense in this region, and separated from the adjacent Sertoli cell membrane by an intercellular space of approximately 200 Å (120,127). Occasionally microtubules can be observed crossing these intercellular bridges, and Fawcett (128) has observed membranous partitions that can appear transiently across the bridge separating the cells without breaking down the connections.

Attempts have been made to classify spermatogonia at the electron microscopic level, particularly in the human (123,129,130). Most investigators agree that it is possible in man to identify the type A dark, A pale, and B spermatogonia, though intermediate forms were noted to occur (131). The classification (123) is based on (a) the nuclear and nucleolar features, (b) the presence of aggregations of mitochondria, (c) the presence or absence of glycogen granules, and (d) the presence of crystalloids known as the Lubarsch crystal found in human spermatogonia (132).

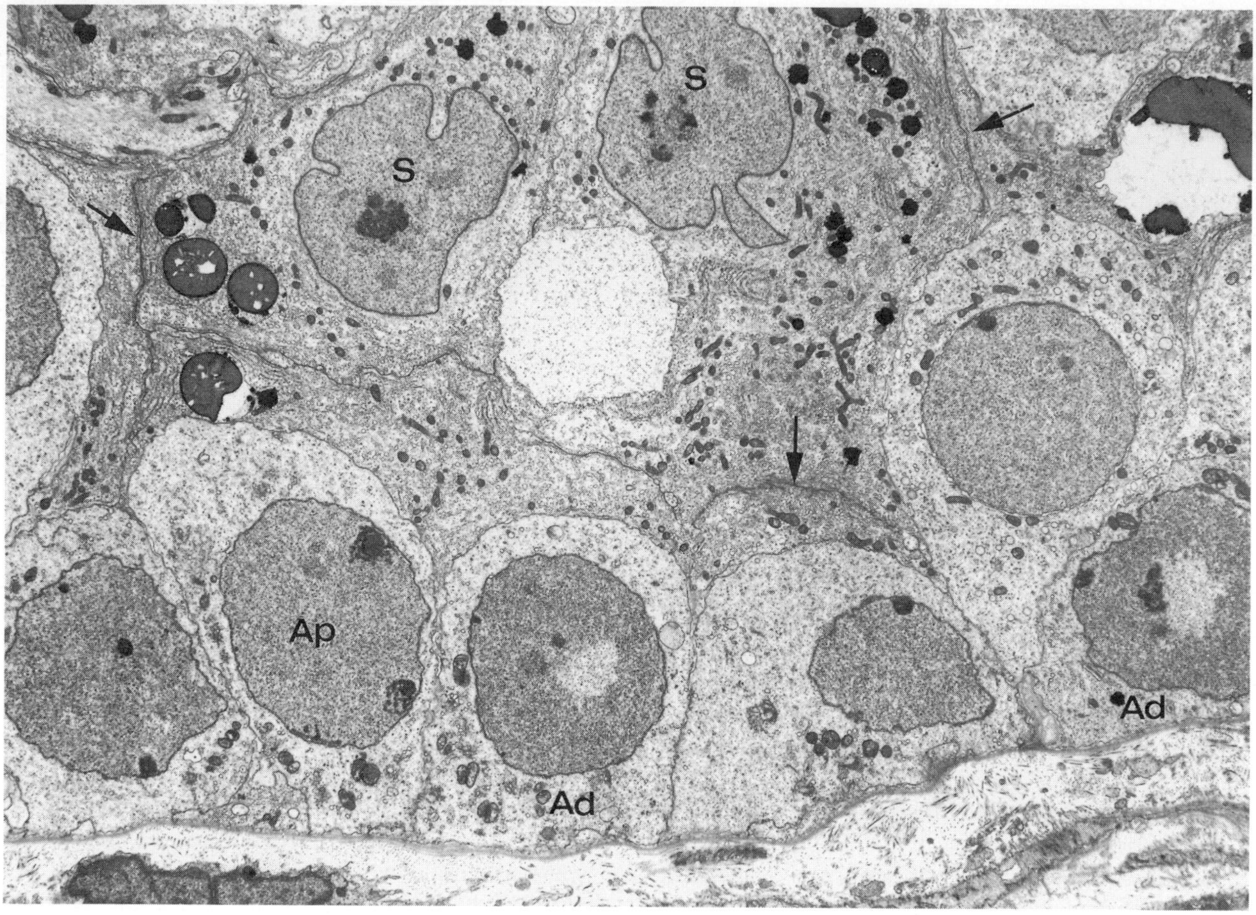

FIG. 15. Human seminiferous epithelium showing type A dark (Ad) and type A pale (Ap) spermatogonia. Note Sertoli cell nuclei (S) and inter-Sertoli-cell junctional complexes (*arrows*).

The A dark spermatogonia have an oval-shaped nucleus and demonstrate a relatively electron-translucent region consistent with the appearance of the nuclear vacuole by light microscopy. The nucleoli are small and peripherally placed adjacent to the nuclear membrane and consist of a nucleolonema; occasionally they are surrounded by the nuclear vacuole. The decreased electron density of these regions results from the absence of chromatin fibrils from the area. The mitochondria lie close to the nucleus, and between the mitochondria finely granular moderately electron-dense material is found. The cristae extend transversely across the matrix, although some areas of the mitochondria are devoid of cristae; in some mitochondria the intracristal space is dilated. Profiles of rough endoplasmic reticulum are largely seen, although some smooth-membraned vesicles are present. The Golgi complex is poorly developed. Glycogen granules are present, often forming aggregations (123). The crystalloids of Lubarsch are present, represented by collections of fibrils and tubules aligned along the long axis of the structure, which may be up to 3 μm in length. Linear arrays of small electron-dense granules separate the fibrillar elements, and small collections of similar granular material are sometimes present in the adjacent cytoplasm (125,133,134). Their function is unknown, though they show some similarities to the structure of the crystals of Charcot Bottcher found in Sertoli cells.

The A pale spermatogonia have a less extensive contact with the basement membrane of the tubule, and their nuclei do not show nuclear vacuoles (Fig. 16). Their nucleoli are peripherally placed and consist of a nucleolonema and pars amorpha. The mitochondria rarely form perinuclear collections, often lying together as pairs separated by the granular intermitochondrial material found in A dark spermatogonia. Glycogen granules are infrequently found although Lubarsch crystals can be present.

Type B spermatogonia have the least contact with the basement membrane and contain peripherally placed nuclear chromatin aggregations that, because of the thin sections, are not as prominent as visualized by light microscopy. The nucleolus is centrally placed and consists of nucleolonema and pars amorpha. The mitochondria are scattered singly in the cytoplasm with an apparent disappearance of the intermitochondrial material seen in

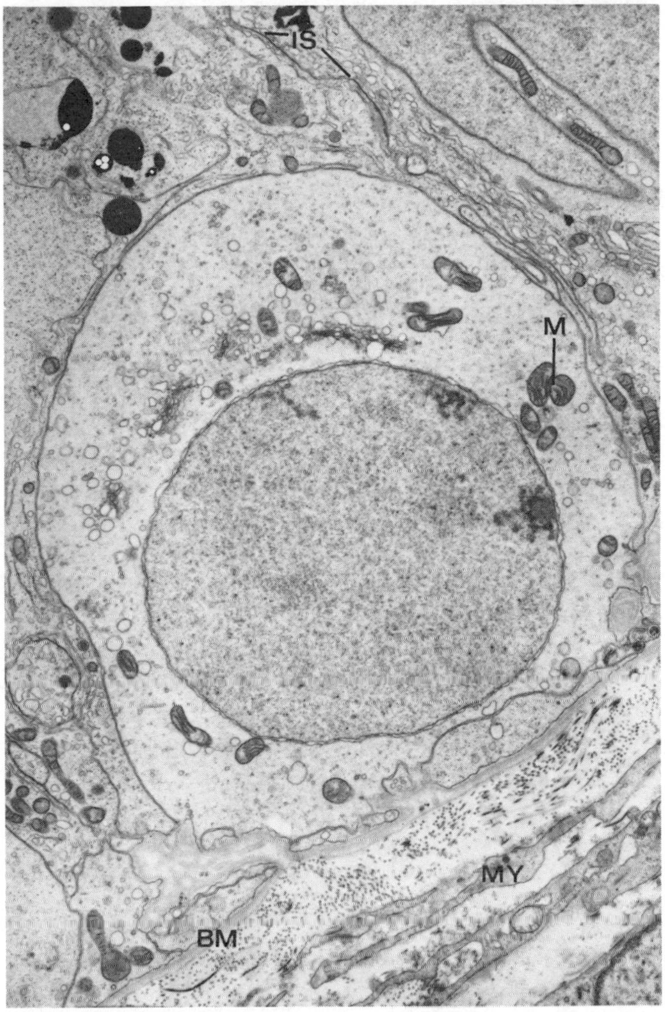

FIG. 16. This electron micrograph illustrates a type A pale spermatogonium situated on the basement membrane (BM) of a seminiferous tubule from the human testis. Note the paucity of organelles and the mitochondria (M) sometimes clustered around an intermitochondrial electron-dense matrix. The adjacent Sertoli cells show specialised inter-Sertoli-cell junctions (IS). Note myoid cell processes (MY).

type A cells. This is of interest because it reappears in primary spermatocytes and has been linked to the perinuclear dense bodies or nuage of invertebrate and amphibian oogenesis (see review, ref. 135). Scanty profiles of smooth and rough endoplasmic reticulum are present, and the Golgi complex, although not dramatic, is better developed than in the type A spermatogonia.

Rowley et al. (123) identified yet another type characterized by its shape—long, very flat, with contact to the basal lamina extending up to 30 μm in length. The nucleus was irregular in shape with a peripherally placed nucleolus. The mitochondria occurred in large collections (up to ten) in the perinuclear region and were joined together by the granular intermitochondrial material. Glycogen and Lubarsch crystalloids were noted. They comment that this type may correspond to the A_0 spermatogonial type of other species (111).

Spermatocytes

The cells in the spermatogenic process that are involved in meiosis are the primary and secondary spermatocytes. The term spermatocyte was first used by von La Valette St. George (109) to designate the cells previously termed growing cells by other investigators. Although the drawings of Brown (136) are remarkably accurate in depicting the nuclear patterns in these cells, true appreciation of their significance did not become apparent until the studies of Winiwater (137) and Montgomery (138).

The process of meiosis actually involves two cell divisions (Fig. 17). In the first, which involves the primary spermatocytes, the chromosomes appear as pairs of chromatids, subsequent to which heterologous chromosomes pair by synapsis to form bivalents. Each member of the bivalent pair subsequently moves to the daughter cells termed secondary spermatocytes, which contain half the number of chromosomes (haploid number), but since each chromosome is composed of a pair of daughter chromatids, the actual total DNA content is equivalent to that of somatic cells. The second division occurs after a relatively short duration, and during this the chromatids of each chromosome separate to daughter cells by

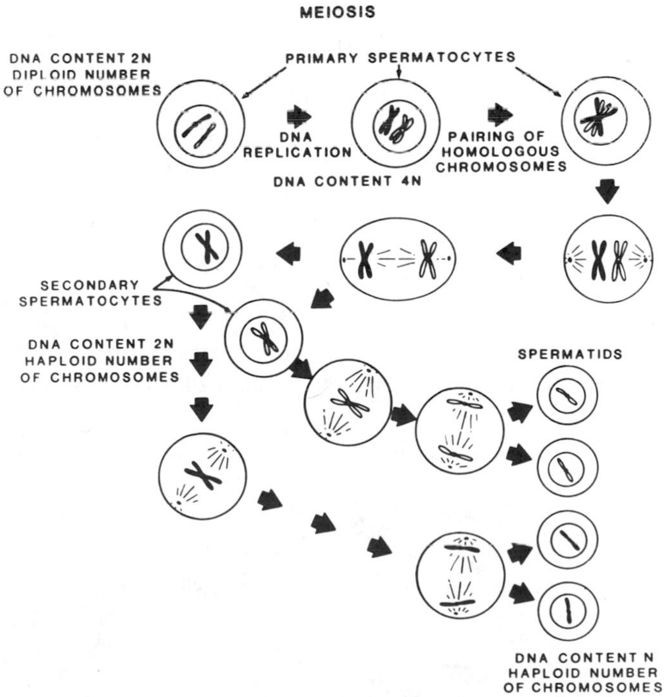

FIG. 17. This diagram illustrates the changes occurring during the meiotic divisions involving primary and secondary spermatocytes.

mechanisms similar to those of mitotic division. The daughter cells, termed spermatids, contain the haploid number of chromosomes and half the DNA content of somatic cells.

Primary Spermatocytes

These cells demonstrate the features of the first meiotic division in terms of nuclear morphology. Early studies by Montgomery (138) showed that distinct pairs of chromosomes were visible in primary spermatocytes and suggested that each pair was composed of a chromosome of maternal or paternal origin. Their pairing was originally suggested to be end to end (138,139) but was subsequently shown to be side to side (137). The primary spermatocytes arise from type B spermatogonia that lose contact with the basement membrane of the seminiferous tubule. They are characterized by a spherical nucleus with features similar to the type B spermatogonia lacking any details of chromosomal structure. During this phase they are termed preleptotene spermatocytes and are actively engaged in DNA synthesis (140). This DNA synthesis is the mechanism by which each chromosome, when it condenses, is composed of a pair of chromatids, the total DNA content representing twice the diploid content (Fig. 17). The period of DNA synthesis represents the last in the process of spermatogenesis, and these cells represent the most mature cells capable of being labeled with markers such as [^{3}H]thymidine, which is incorporated into the DNA.

The primary spermatocytes are the cells that undergo the first meiotic division, and their nuclear morphology reflects the events associated with this process. The prophase of the first division is characteristically of long duration, and cells in the phases of this process demonstrate nuclear features based on the appearance and morphology of the chromosomes. Condensation of chromosomes results in their appearance in the leptotene stage (Fig. 18) as single filamentous strands that have been shown by electron microscopic studies to be attached at each end to the nuclear membrane by attachment plaques (141). These attachments probably represent the reasons for the bouquet arrangement of chromosomes seen in leptotene. Though at this stage the chromosomes are already composed of two chromatids, these do not become evident until later in prophase. The zygotene stage is characterised by thickening of the chromosomal elements, which commences the process of pairing known as synapsis (Fig. 18). The mechanisms whereby homologous chromosomes recognize each other to pair as bivalents are still unknown.

The long pachytene stage commences with the completion of synapsis and is associated with further thickening and shortening of the chromosomes, which by careful study can be shown to be paired (142). During this phase, exchange of chromosomal material between maternal and paternal homologous chromosomes occurs by crossing over, the chromosomes being linked at such sites by chiasmata. The pachytene phase is characterized by nuclear and cytoplasmic growth resulting in these cells becoming the largest of the germ cell line. As desynapsis occurs during the next phase known as diplotene, the paired chromosomes partially separate but remain joined at their chiasmata. Subsequently in the diakinetic phase, further shortening of chromosomes occurs, and they detach from the nuclear membrane. It is at this stage that each chromosome can be seen to be composed of two chromatids.

Diakinesis is rapidly followed by the dissolution of the nuclear membrane, appearance of the spindle, and the attachment of the bivalents to equator of the spindle during metaphase. Anaphase subsequently results in the movement of the members of each bivalent to opposite poles of the spindle, resulting in daughter cells termed secondary spermatocytes that contain the haploid number of chromosomes, each composed of two chromatids. As with other cell divisions within the seminiferous epithelium, cytokinesis is incomplete, and the secondary spermatocytes remain joined by intercellular bridges.

Fine Structure

Electron microscopy has added greatly to our knowledge of events in these cells. Moses (143) and Fawcett (144) independently described the existence of elements termed synaptinemal complexes in the nuclei of primary

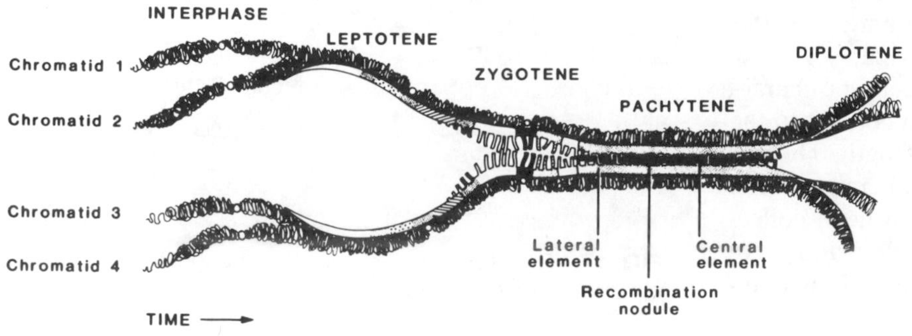

FIG. 18. The manner in which pairs of homologous chromosomes undergo synapsis during meiosis is shown. Note how the lateral elements of the synaptinemal complex come together at pachytene, separating at the diplotene stage.

spermatocytes from a number of species. This complex consisted of two lateral elements that appeared as electron-dense fibrils equidistant from a central element consisting of a delicate linear region of increased electron density (Figs. 18 and 19). Woolam and Ford (145) suggested that the lateral elements represented cores of the paired chromosomes and that the central element was composed of microfibrillar processes that extend inwards from each lateral element. These views were supported by the observations, from serial electron microscopic reconstructions of the spermatocyte nucleus, that the number of synaptinemal complexes was equal to the number of bivalents (141). Each lateral element first appears in the leptotene stage, representing elements of the single unpaired chromosomes that attach to the nuclear membrane at each end (146,147). Pairing of the elements commences in zygotene, and fully formed synaptinemal complexes over the entire length of the chromosomes are seen in pachytene. Study of these events has been greatly facilitated by the observation that the protein that forms the lateral elements of the complex stains with silver (148). The DNA of each chromosome forms a series of loops extending away from the lateral element, and the process of synapsis is associated with the assembly of the central component, probably by a recognition process involving proteins of the microfibrillar elements projecting centrally from the lateral elements (149,150).

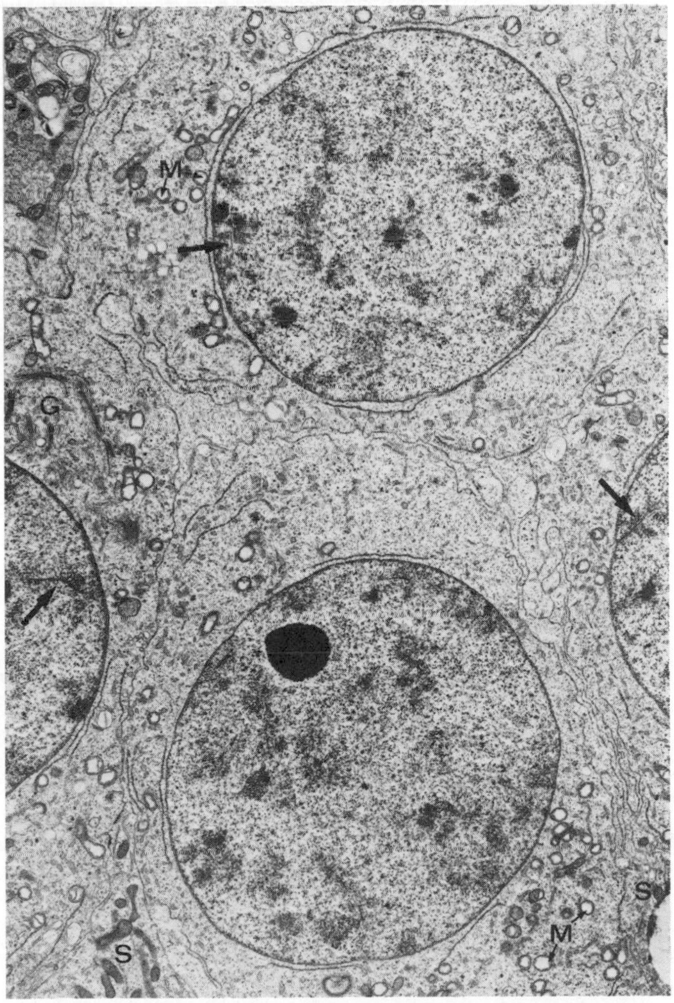

FIG. 19. Two human primary spermatocytes are shown. Note mitochondria (M), Golgi complex (G), leptotene synaptinemal threads (*arrows*), and Sertoli cell cytoplasm (S).

In recent studies Heyting and colleagues (151,152) have undertaken biochemical characterization of the synaptinemal complexes following their initial isolation (150) and the development of several monoclonal antibodies. These studies demonstrated that the complexes are not assesembled from preexisting components but are synthesized during zygotene. Using one of these monoclonal antibodies these investigators have isolated a cDNA encoding a protein involved in the lateral elements of the synaptinemal complex (153). This protein, SCP1, shares several features with nuclear laminins and some nuclear matrix proteins. It contains long stretches capable of forming amphipathic α helices, and these regions show amino acid sequence similarities to the coiled coil region of myosin heavy chain. Although the synaptinemal complex provides the framework necessary for synapsis, it is thought that the recombination nodules are the vital component in crossing over of genetic material. These represent ellipsoidal to spherical protein globules approximately 90 nm in diameter that sit along the central portion of the synaptinemal complexes at a number of sites consistent with the number of chiasmata (Fig. 18). Events in diplotene result in disruption of the synaptinemal complexes and separation of the bivalents, which still remain connected at chiasmata.

During meiosis, the sex chromosomes were noted by Painter (142) to be associated with a "chromatin nucleolus," a structure subsequently termed the sex vesicle since it was shown not to represent a true nucleolus (154). It is formed at the end of leptotene and disappears after diakinesis. It is ovoid in shape with a diameter of 2 to 3 μm. It consists of an area of increased electron density composed of chromatin fibrils through which linear elements similar in appearance to the lateral elements of synaptinemal complexes are scattered (155–158). These take the form of linear arrays or circular profiles, and only occasional short full-formed synaptinemal complexes are seen. This is consistent with the behavior of the sex chromosomes, which only pair over relatively short portions of their length (159).

Nucleoli are frequently seen in primary spermatocytes and consist of peripherally placed collections of extremely electron-dense granules. These are sometimes associated with chromatin collections close to synaptinemal complexes. A structure termed the "round body" has been found in spermatocyte nuclei (156,160), occurring as a spherical electron-dense structure adjacent to the nuclear membrane. It is composed of nonhistone protein, appears in leptotene, and increases in size to 1.6

μm in diameter in diplotene. It persists in secondary spermatocytes and spermatids, decreasing in size progressively and disappearing at step 8 spermatids (160). Schultz and colleagues noted that nucleoli actively incorporated [^{3}H]thymidine while they were associated with a round body that was increasing in size but not during its decline, thereby suggesting that the round body may be a controller of nucleolar activity in meiotic cells.

The cytoplasm of primary spermatocytes is more electron dense than that of spermatogonia and contains evenly scattered polysomes and ribosomes (161). Profiles of rough or smooth endoplasmic reticulum are sparse, although as prophase progresses, the Golgi complex progressively enlarges. It is perinuclear in position and consists of concentric arrays of membranous lamellae and vesicles, some of which contain a prominent electron-dense core. A detailed analysis of the Golgi complex of rat pachytene spermatocytes has been performed recently and demonstrated a marked increase in size of this organelle late in pachytene (162). This increase was shown to result predominantly from the accumulation of *trans* Golgi. It is unclear whether this increase is associated with secretory activity of late pachytene spermatocytes or whether it represents an unusual mechanism to ensure that partitioning of this organelle with secondary spermatocytes and subsequently spermatids occurs without a disassembly. The mitochondria are ovoid (Fig. 19) and in the leptotene and zygotene stages are frequently aggregated into groups of two or three with electron-dense mitochondrial material similar to that seen in spermatogonia (163,164). The intracristal spaces are dilated, and later in meiosis the cristae are often displaced toward the periphery as concentric membranous layers, leaving a central electron-lucid area. Other types of collections of finely granular electron-dense material have also been seen in spermatocytes and termed nuage; Russell and Frank (164) identified six types. Their exact role remains unclear, though one type is similar in appearance to the chromatoid body (165); Russell and Frank suggest that this structure disappears in late diplotene, reforming by coalescence in secondary spermatocytes.

Unusual aggregations of parallel membranous lamellae or cisternae are seen, the adjacent lamellae sometimes joined to each other at regular intervals by annuli. These resemble the structures termed annulate lamellae that are found in oocytes of many species (166). Similar aggregations have been observed, adjacent to or often attached to the nuclear membrane, supporting views that they originate from that site (167,168).

Primary spermatocytes are joined to each other by intercellular bridges similar to those found between spermatogonia. They are separated from adjacent Sertoli cells by a distinct intercellular space that is modified in some regions by desmosomelike structures (169,170). As preleptotene spermatocytes lose their contact with the basement membrane, the processes of Sertoli cell cytoplasm that intervene develop specialized inter-Sertoli-cell junctions, discussed later in this review (171).

Secondary Spermatocytes

These are the cells that undertake the second meiotic division, and the first description of their characteristics is credited to Von Ebner (172). The relatively infrequent appearance of these cells in sections of the testis (173) indicates that they have a short life span before they complete meiosis to form spermatids. Montgomery (174) correctly noted that the secondary spermatocytes have the haploid number of chromosomes, although their DNA content is still diploid (Fig. 17), and when they complete meiosis the resultant spermatids have both the haploid DNA and chromosomal content. The cells are spherical, intermediate in size between primary spermatocytes and spermatids, with a diameter of 10 to 12 μm. They are situated close to the lumen of the seminiferous tubules, and their spherical nuclei contain a homogeneous chromatin network throughout which large globular chromatin masses are dispersed. Centrally placed nucleoli are often seen. Light and electron microscopic studies have shown that these cells are joined by intercellular bridges identical to those found between other germ cells (120,175,176).

Fine Structure

There have been few detailed studies of the ultrastructure of secondary spermatocytes, partly because of the difficulty of identifying sections of tubules within which they are present (163,176,177). Their cytoplasm contains scattered cisternal profiles of endoplasmic reticulum arranged concentrically around the nucleus. The Golgi complex is prominent and often contains vesicles demonstrating electron-dense granules. Collections of membranes with the features of annulate lamellae are found sometimes embedded in electron-dense granular material (167,176). The mitochondria are dispersed within the cytoplasm and show dilated intracristal spaces, which result in the cristal membranes being pushed to the periphery of the organelle.

Spermiogenesis

The transformation of spermatids to spermatozoa involves a fascinating but complex sequence of events that constitute the process of spermiogenesis. No cell division is involved, but the process is in essence a metamorphosis in which a conventional cell is converted into a highly organized motile structure. The major features of spermiogenesis are common to all species, but the details differ in each species since there are distinguishing morphological features between spermatozoa determined by genetic factors. Many aspects are visible by light microscopy, but the finer details require the magnification of the electron microscope. Hence, in this section of the review, the light and electron microscopic features are described together (Figs. 20 and 21). For convenience, it is possible to divide the cytological changes during spermiogenesis into a series of developmental steps involving different cellular organelles, but it is important to recognize that some steps occur contemporaneously. The changes can be grouped into (a) formation of the acrosome, (b) nuclear changes, (c) development of the flagellum, (d) reorganization of the cytoplasm and cell organelles, and (e) spermiation relationships of the Sertoli cell and spermatids.

Spermatids, like other germ cells, were named by von La Valette (178), and some investigators use the term spermateliosis as an alternative to spermiogenesis. A number of early studies described the general changes characterizing spermiogenesis (112,138,179–181), and these were expanded and utilized by Clermont (182–184) in developing a classification for the stages of spermiogenesis. This classification was aided by the demonstration that the acrosome stained clearly with the periodic acid–Schiff (PAS) reaction. Recently formed spermatids are spherical cells that are smaller in size than secondary spermatocytes and are found at the luminal aspect of the seminiferous epithelium. They have a centrally placed spherical nucleus, a well-developed Golgi complex, and adjacent centrioles. The mitochondria are dispersed and lie peripherally close to the plasma membrane. Additionally, a chromophilic electron-dense mass, the chromatoid body, can be observed adjacent to the Golgi complex in a perinuclear location (182,185).

Formation of the Acrosome

This structure arises from the Golgi complex, a fact established early this century by Bowen (186–188) from studies in mammals and other classes. Gatenby and Beams (181) identified proacrosomic granules in the Golgi regions of primary spermatocytes, though it is still

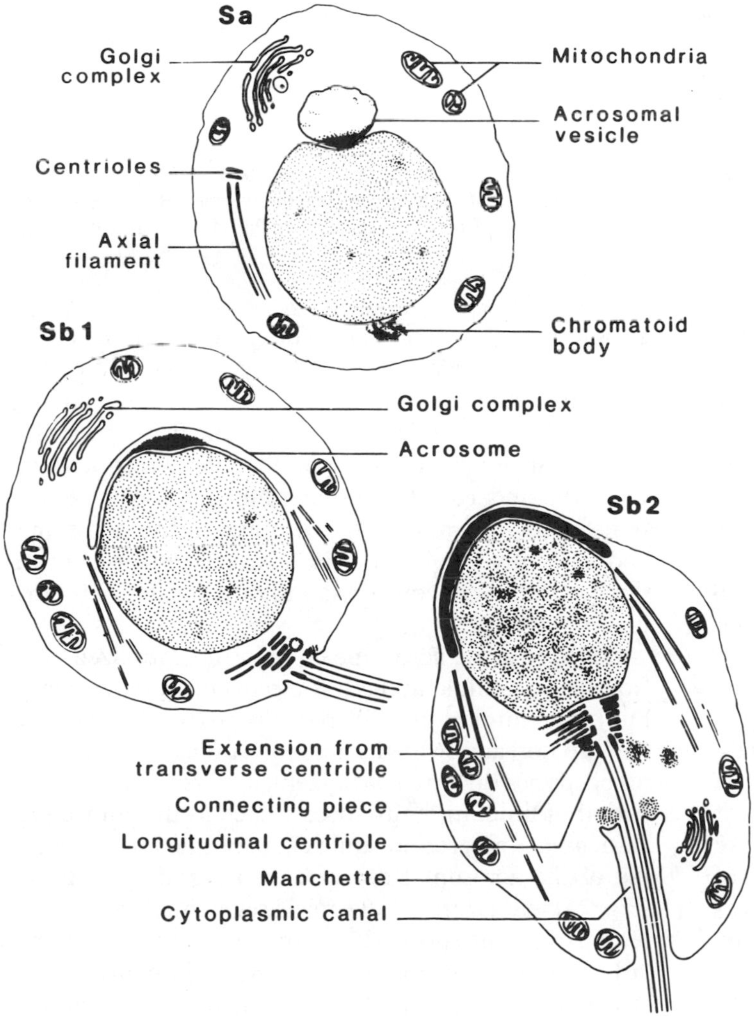

FIG. 20. The electron microscopic features of the stages of human spermatogenesis (Sa to Sb_2) are shown. (From de Kretser, ref. 891, with permission.)

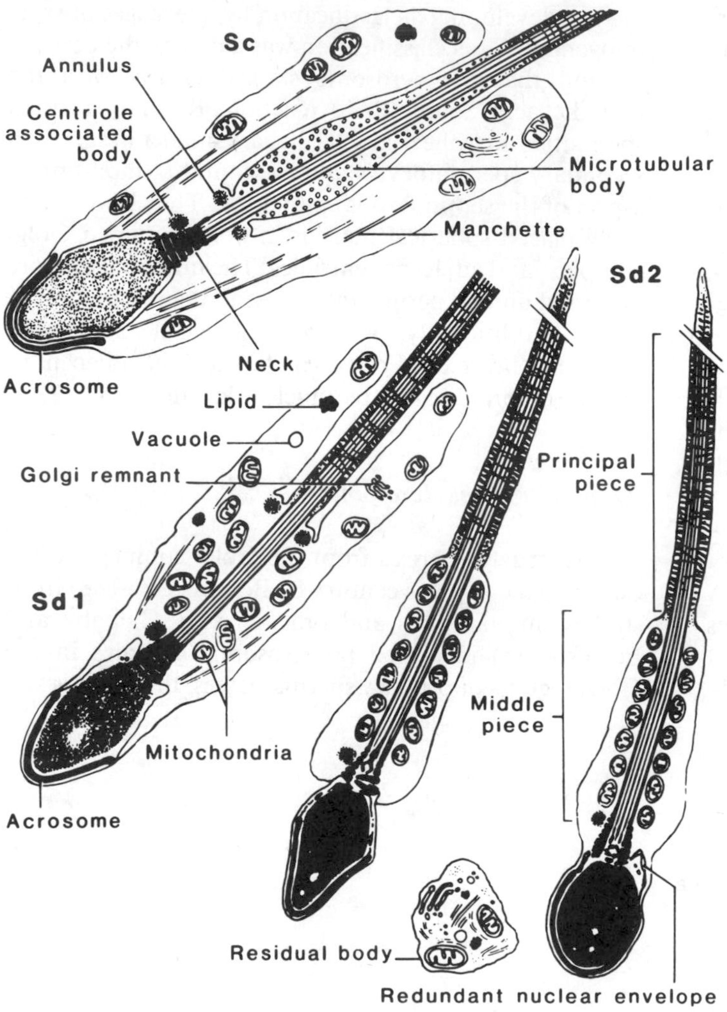

FIG. 21. The electron microscopic features of the stages of human spermatogenesis (Sc to Sd_2) are shown. (From de Kretser, ref. 891, with permission.)

unclear today whether the granules in these cells are transmitted to daughter cells; more likely they represent some form of secretory protein that is packaged in the Golgi complex (Figs. 22 and 23). These investigators noted that similar granules were elaborated in the Golgi apparatus of newly formed spermatids, and the vacuole and granule were deposited at one pole of the nucleus, where they spread out to form the acrosome cap. Gatenby and Beams (181) noted that once the acrosomal cap had been formed, the remainder of the Golgi complex passed to the opposite pole of the spermatid.

This view concerning the formation of the acrosome was confirmed by early electron microscopic studies (188–190). Several proacrosomic granules are often elaborated in the Golgi complex, coalescing to form a single large granule that comes into contact with the nuclear membrane (Fig. 22). It is closely applied as a caplike structure spreading over approximately 25% to 60% of the nuclear surface. During this phase, additional material appears to be transferred from Golgi to the acrosome by vesicles, a process recently analyzed in considerable detail (191–193). They have divided the Golgi into cortical and medullary zones, the cortex being limited externally by cisternae of rough endoplasmic reticulum. The transition from cortex to medulla is marked by a change from cisternal profiles to vesicles, and it is from this aspect that vesicles are transported to the acrosomal cap. Clermont and Tang (193) showed that glycoproteins are transferred from the Golgi complex to the acrosome, and, in contrast to other cells, this accumulation occurs slowly (1 hour) in comparison to other cells (2–10 minutes) (194,195).

For a time the acrosome contains a centralized electron-dense granule and a less electron-dense periphery, but in the human this difference is progressively lost as the cap spreads over the nuclear surface (Fig. 24). In other species this zonal arrangement persists for a longer period of time. In many species, such as the guinea pig, chinchilla, and ground squirrel, a conspicuous thickening of the acrosomal cap extends beyond the nucleus (Fig. 25) and is termed the apical segment (196), but the reasons for this specialization remain unknown. Similarly, the caudal region of the acrosome in many species is partly attenuated and is termed the equatorial seg-

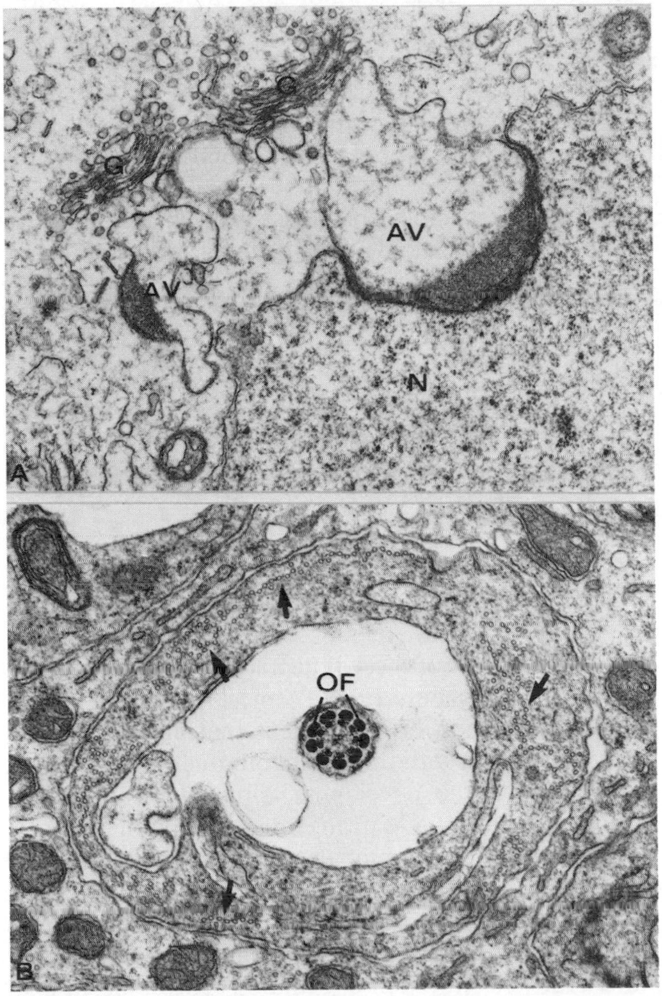

FIG. 22. A: The developing acrosomal cap of a human spermatid is illustrated. Note nucleus (N), Golgi complex (G), and acrosomal vesicle (AV). **B:** The axial filament of a spermatid is shown. Note outer dense fibers (OF) surrounding the 9 + 2 microtubular structure. The surrounding spermatid cytoplasm contains the microtubules of the manchette (*arrows*).

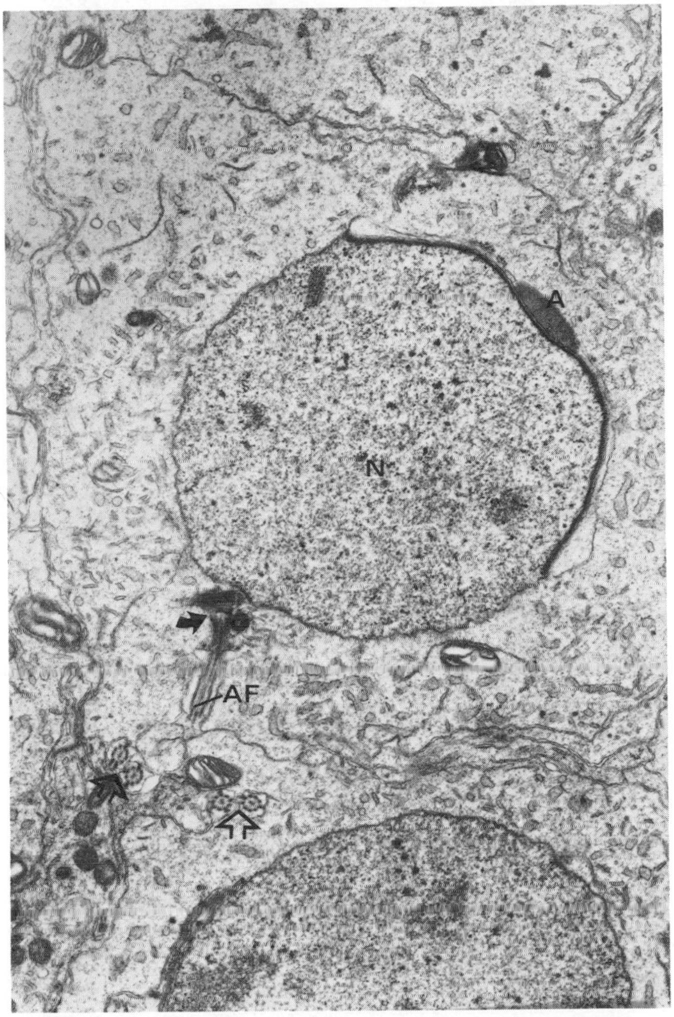

FIG. 23. A human spermatid (stage Sb_1) shows acrosome (A), nucleus (N), developing connecting piece (*arrow*), and axial filament (AF, *open arrow*).

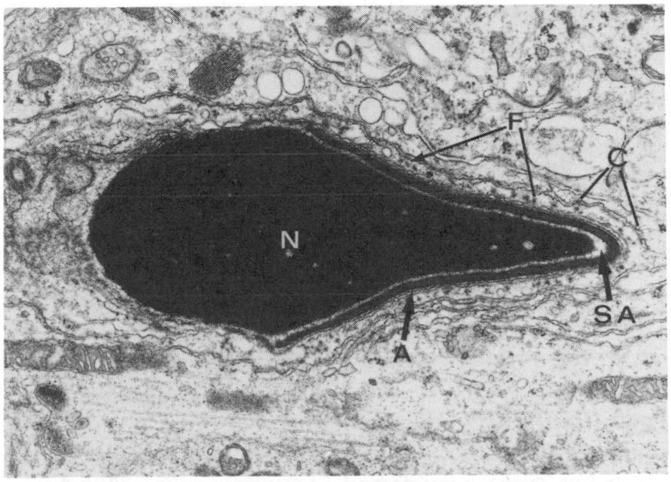

FIG. 24. This view illustrates the human spermatid head composed of the nucleus (N), acrosome (A), and subacrosomal space (SA). Note the cisternae (C) delineating a zone of Sertoli cell cytoplasm containing fibrils (F).

ment, and in the human some lamination has been noted in this area (197,198). Although the reason for this specialization is unknown, this region of the acrosome persists after the remainder of the acrosomal contents are lost following the acrosomal reaction (199). Furthermore, it represents the region in which binding occurs to the cell membrane of the oocyte during fertilization (200). The size of the acrosome varies significantly between species, being closely applied to the nucleus in man but being very large and elaborate in species such as the guinea pig (201,202). Furthermore, modifications to this structure may occur after spermatozoa leave the epithelium and pass through the epididymis (201). The glycoprotein nature of the acrosome is consistent with the observation that it contains a variety of lysosomal enzymes important for penetration of the zona pellucida of

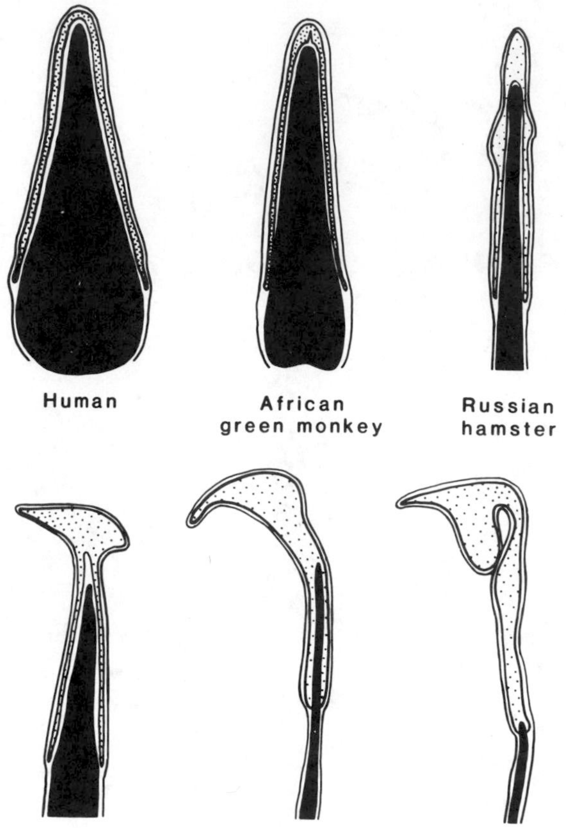

FIG. 25. The variation in the shape of the components of the head of spermatozoa from a number of species is illustrated. Some views are drawn from micrographs in refs. 205 and 230.

the ovum and other specific proteins such as acrosin (203,204).

With subsequent changes in nuclear position, the acrosome is closely applied to the cell membrane of the spermatid. Between the inner acrosomal membrane and nuclear membrane, the human spermatid contains a thin layer of moderately electron-dense material (Fig. 24), which Bedford (205) has suggested represents the perforatorium. The subacrosomal space contains a variable amount of electron-dense material whose organization differs markedly between species. In rodents, this space is extensive, particularly at the cranial aspect, and the material is organized to form a rodlike perforatorium that appears to be prolonged backwards over the nucleus as three prongs, possibly thickenings of the nuclear membrane (206,207) (Figs. 26 and 27). In the toad, the perforatorium consists of strands of electron-dense material in the subacrosomal space (208), and a similar structure has since been found in many species (209,210). The protein composition of the perforatorium in the rat has been partially characterized by Oko and Clermont (211), who identified a number of components. Using antibodies to these components, they have demonstrated regional difficulties in the protein composition of the perforatorium (212). Furthermore, although they could not identify actin in the perforatorium, they noted actin and seven perforatorium proteins in the subacrosomal space prior to the condensation of the perforatorium.

Some investigators postulated a mechanical role for the perforatorium, and others have suggested that it carries a lysin distinct from that found in the acrosome (213). Actin has been identified as a component of the subacrosomal space in a number of species (214–216). The number of actin filaments increases during steps 9 to 13 in the rat and decreases in the later stages of spermiogenesis (215). It is important to note that in men in whom the acrosome is absent, the head of the sperm takes on a globular appearance (217).

Nuclear Changes

In the majority of species the nucleus changes position during spermiogenesis from a central to an eccentric position. The region of the nucleus that first comes into close apposition with the cell membrane is that segment covered with the developing acrosomal cap. Subsequently, during the rearrangement of spermatid cytoplasm, larger segments of the nucleus come into close association with the plasma membrane.

Associated with the change in nuclear position there is a progressive condensation of chromatin to form larger and more electron-dense granules. These increase in number and condense eventually to form an osmiophilic electron-dense homogeneous mass. The degree of condensation can vary with species and is particularly variable in human spermiogenesis (191,218,219). In different species the temporal linkage between the changes in nuclear shape and chromatin condensation vary. In the rat and the mouse the phase of nuclear elongation precedes the principal condensation events (220). In the rat there is a progressive pattern of development that is not complete until late in spermiogenesis (Figs. 26 and 27). Together with the acrosomal modifications, the final structure of the head of the rat spermatid takes some time to evolve (207). Additionally, in man, electron-lucid spaces occur with the nucleus that, though not limited by a membrane, are termed nuclear vacuoles (208). The coalescence of chromatin granules is associated with ill-defined chemical changes in the DNA, which is stabilized and is resistant to digestion by the enzyme DNase (185,221). This stabilization occurs at a time when lysine-rich histones are being replaced by arginine-rich, testis-specific histones in the spermatid nuclei, the lysine-rich protein accumulating subsequently in the sphere chromatophile, a component of the residual body of spermatids (222).

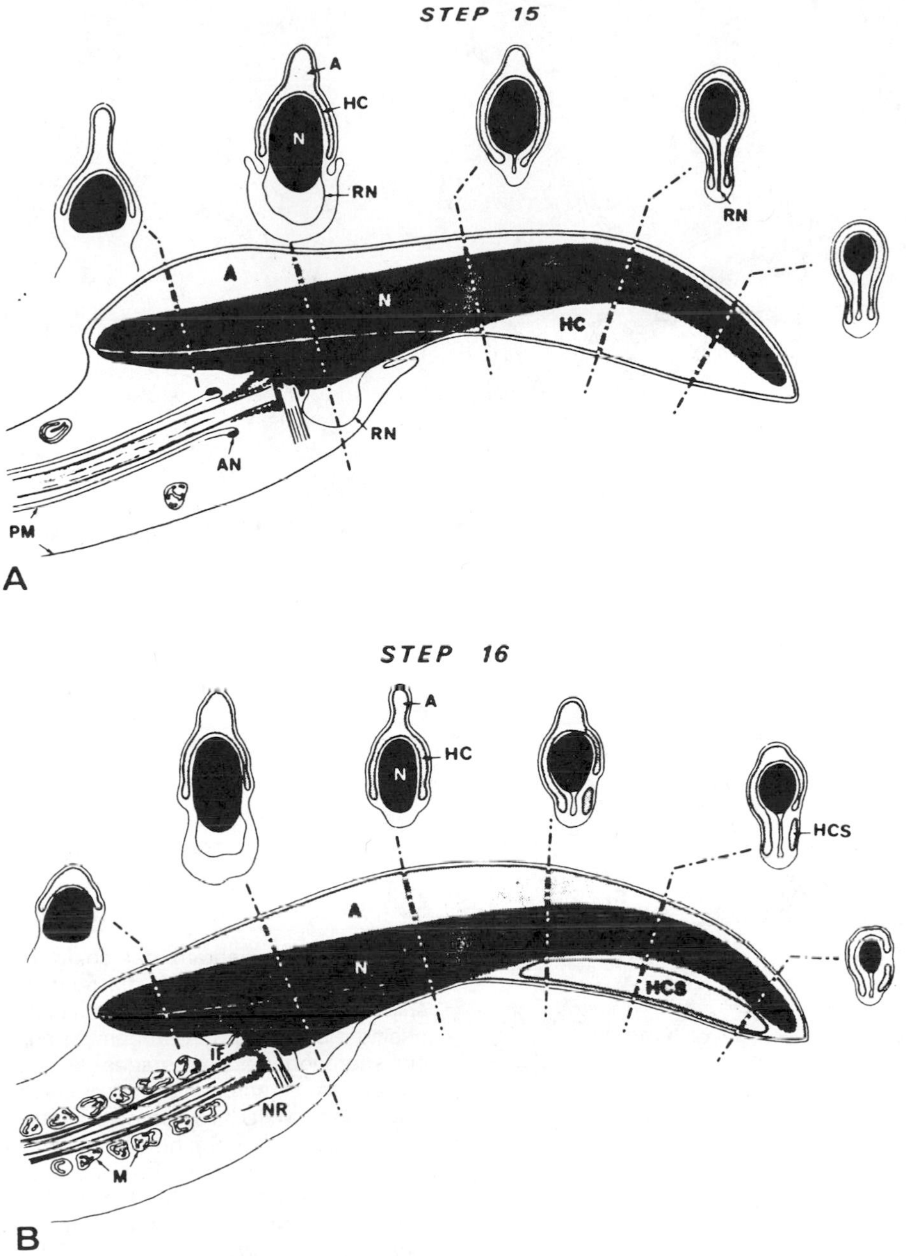

FIG. 26. This diagram demonstrates the changes occurring in the relationships and shape of the structures composing the head of the rat spermatid during spermatogenesis at stages 15 and 16. Labels: A, acrosome; AN, annulus; AX, axoneme; HC, headcap; HCS, separated head cap segment; IF, implantation fossa; M, mitochondria; N, nucleus; NR, neck region; P, perforatorium; PM, plasma membrane; RN, redundant nuclear envelope; VS, ventral spur. (From Lalli and Clermont, ref. 207, with permission.)

Several studies of nuclear proteins have shown dramatic changes during spermiogenesis with the appearance of species-specific protamine rich in arginine and cysteine, the presence of several nonprotamine proteins, and the transient appearance of several basic nuclear proteins (transition proteins) (223–225). In all eutherian mammals, sperm protamines are encoded by two genes termed P_1 and P_2, with the majority of species containing P_1, whereas the hamster, mouse, stallion, and human have principally P_2 (226). The transition proteins, found in elongated spermatids, consist of two major types, TP_1 and TP_2 (227,228), and appear to occupy the nucleus between the removal of the histones and their replacement by the protamines. It is possible that the posttranslational modification of the histones such as the acetylation of H_4 in the rat may, through decompaction of nucleosomes and chromatin, facilitate displacement of histones (220,229). These changes and the loss of virtually all nonhistone nuclear proteins late in spermiogenesis occur at a time of complete repression of gene transcription and shaping of the sperm nucleus (230,231).

During the chromatin condensation, there is a progressive reduction in nuclear volume and, in some species, dramatic changes in shape to result in sperm heads with shapes characteristic for each species (230,232). These striking differences in head shape have prompted investigators to seek the mechanisms responsible. The appearance of a microtubular sheath termed the manchette (see below) close to the nucleus at a time when significant

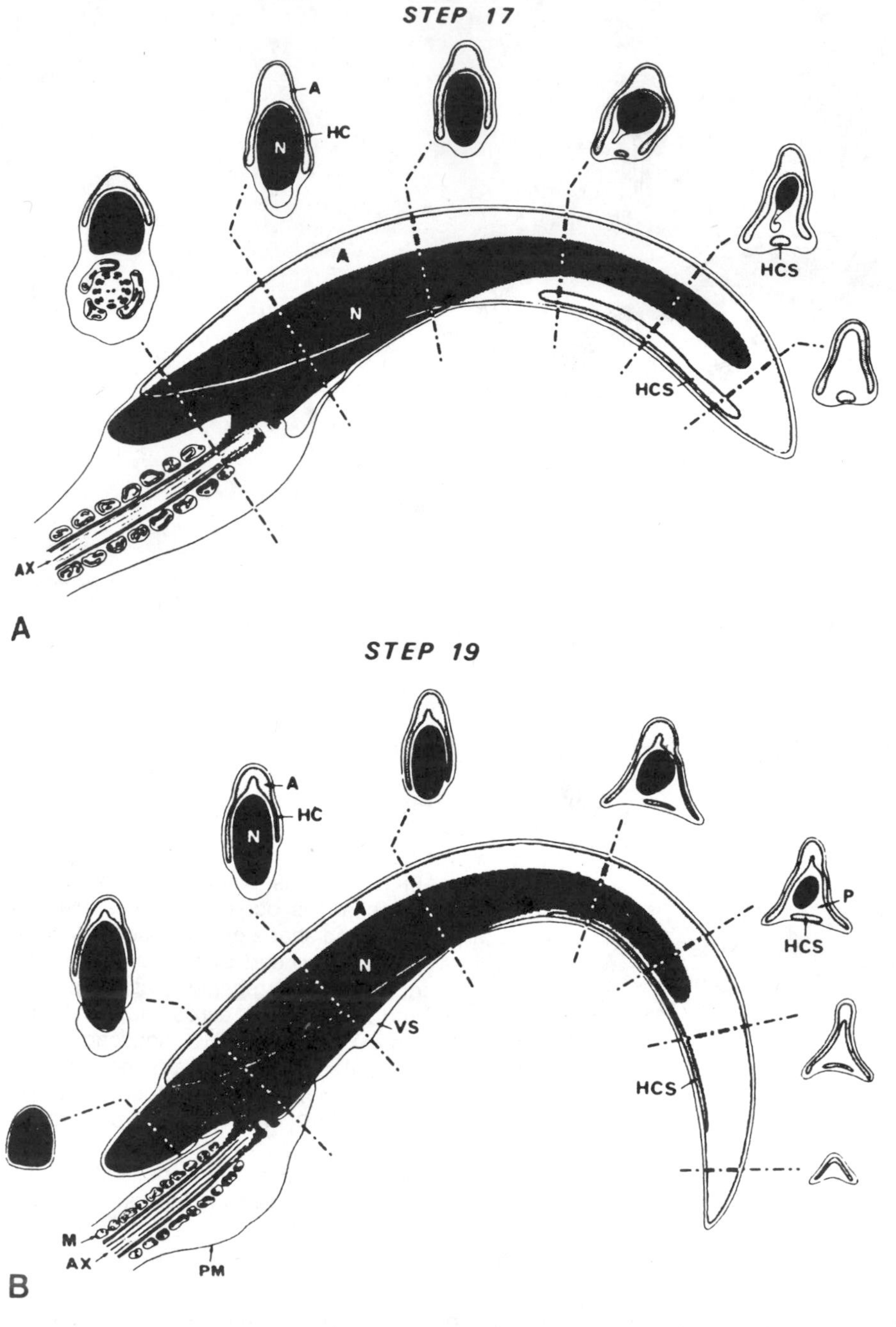

FIG. 27. This diagram demonstrates the changes occurring in the relationships and shape of the structures comprising the head of the rat gamete during spermiogenesis at stages 17 and 19. Labels: A, acrosome; AN, annulus; AX, axoneme; HC, head cap; HCS separated head cap segment; IF, implantation fossa; M, mitochondria; N, nucleus; NR, neck region; P, perforatorium; PM, plasma membrane; RN, redundant nuclear envelope; VS, ventral spur. (From Lalli and Clermont, ref. 207, with permission.)

elongation and shaping occur (Fig. 28) led a number of investigators to suggest a causal relationship (233,234). However, from their detailed studies, Fawcett and colleagues (230) could not support this view. They noted that significant variations in the form of the manchette did not occur, a fact that would be necessary to explain the nuclear changes if they were causally related. They noted the observations of Beatty (235) that head shape could vary between strains of the same species and could be varied experimentally by selective breeding. In view of this and their own observations, they proposed that the remarkable diversity of head shape is the result of genetically determined patterns of the molecular aggregation that takes place during chromatin condensation.

In contrast, Meistrich and colleagues (236), from their studies of abnormal spermiogenesis in *azh* mutant mice, concluded that the abnormal head shape may in part relate to the abnormal shape and size of the manchette. Russell and colleagues (237) carried out extensive investigations of the structures involved in nuclear elongation in mice and rats. They used observations on normal and abnormal animals, the latter representing experimental treatments designed to alter head shape such as cytoxan, 5-fluorouracil, and taxol treatments. They noted the pres-

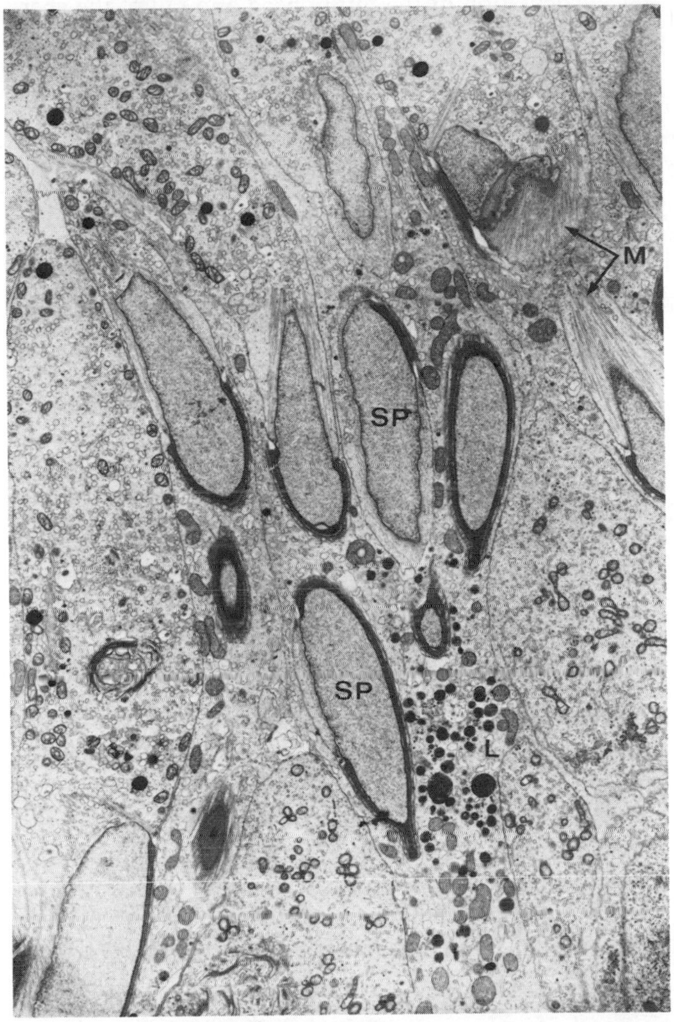

FIG. 28. Rat seminiferous epithelium, illustrating elongated spermatids (SP) and the manchette (M). The Sertoli cell cytoplasm contains numerous lysosomes (L).

ence of rodlike elements extending between the innermost microtubules of the manchette and the outer nuclear envelope and raised the possibility that these structures may represent a mechanism by which the microtubules of the manchette could exert a deforming force on the nucleus. They also suggested that the chromatin condensation reinforces the changes in shape already brought about by the manchette.

The reduction in nuclear volume is associated with the probable loss of materials from the nucleus via nuclear pores (218) and also results in the formation of redundant folds of nuclear membrane (219,238). This is most evident at the abacrosomal pole of the nucleus, where these folds are separated from the condensed chromatin by an electron-lucid zone containing flocculent material. In this region the nuclear membrane is studded with nuclear pores and frequently exhibits the formation of lamellae and vesicles, the latter containing flocculent material (Fig. 24).

Formation of the Tail

The concept that the sperm tail arose from the centrioles of spermatids was recognized by Meves (179,180), who noted that the two centrioles moved to the periphery of the cell, where the axial filament arose from the more peripherally placed centriole. These observations were substantiated by other investigators early this century (117,174,181). However, Gatenby and Beams (181) implicated both centrioles in the formation of the axial filament and noted that the flagellum moved inward toward the nucleus, where the complex lodged at its caudal pole opposite the developing acrosome. Some confusion, however, arose from these early studies, since the structures involved in development of the tail were difficult to observe because they are at the limit of resolution of the light microscope.

The early electron microscopic studies confirmed that the central core of the sperm tail, the axial filament, arose from the pair of centrioles lodged at the periphery of the spermatid cytoplasm and subsequently moved centrally to be lodged at the caudal pole of the nucleus (200). Both Anberg (239) and Fawcett (240) noted the presence of a centriole within the connecting piece of the neck of human spermatozoa and termed it the proximal or transverse centriole. However, they failed to find evidence of the distal or longitudinal centriole. Fawcett (240) also showed that the structure termed the ring centriole by light microscopists appears in ultrastructural studies as the annulus that marks the caudal limit of the middle piece of the tail.

More recent studies have confirmed that the axial filament arises from the distal or longitudinal centriole and that this basic structure is modified by specialization in the different regions of the sperm tail. The subsequent description of cytological events is most easily subdivided into (a) development of the axial filament, (b) formation of the neck or connecting piece, (c) formation of the dense fiber system, (d) development of the principal piece, and (e) formation of the middle piece.

Development of the Axial Filament

Several studies have shown that the axial filament develops from the centriole that is aligned to the axis of the flagellum and is termed the longitudinal or distal centriole (219,241,242). The other centriole is oriented perpendicular to the axial filament and is termed the proximal or transverse centriole. The basic structure of the axial filament is common to flagella and cilia and consists of nine peripheral doublet microtubules arranged equidistant from each other around a circle at whose center two single microtubules are found (Figs. 22 and 29).

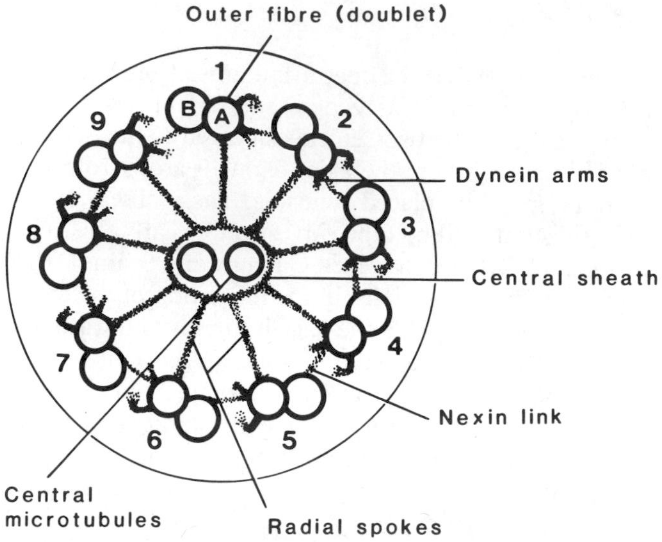

FIG. 29. This diagram illustrates the components of the axial filament when cut in perfect cross section.

The doublets consist of two subfibers, one of which (subfiber A) is a complete microtubule and is circular in cross section whereas the other (subfiber B) is C-shaped with its concavity attached to subfiber A (232). The walls of both subfibers are composed of protofilaments of tubulin (243–245). The axoneme demonstrates a highly organized substructure, which is considered in more detail elsewhere (see E. M. Eddy, Chapter 2, Volume 1). Briefly, subfiber A extends a pair of hooklike arms that project toward subfiber B of the adjacent doublet; these extensions, termed dynein arms, are composed of a protein, dynein, with ATPase activity (246).

Additional links between the doublets are provided by nexin links (247), and the doublets are connected to the helical sheath surrounding the two central microtubules by radial spokes (248). The nature of the substructure of the flagellum has taken on additional significance because of genetically determined abnormalities in its structure that result in immotility of sperm and consequent infertility (249,250). Fawcett (232) proposed a numbering system for the doublets, designating the doublet bisected by a plane passing between the central two microtubules as 1 and the others sequentially in a clockwise direction.

Development of the axial filament commences early in spermiogenesis and projects from the surface of round spermatids, the microtubular core being separated from a fingerlike protrusion of the cell membrane by a thin layer of cytoplasm. An invagination of the cell membrane forms a cleft, the cytoplasmic canal, which surrounds the proximal portion of the axial filament and whose proximal limit is formed by the attachment of the annulus (241). Later the centriolar complex and axial filament become lodged at the abacrosomal pole of the nucleus to form the neck or connecting piece, the complex articulation of the future head and tail of the spermatozoon (Fig. 23). Recently, flagellum formation has been successfully initiated by *in vitro* culture of spermatids (251).

Formation of the Neck or Connecting Piece

The final form of the connecting piece varies significantly between species, but in all mammalian forms a basic structural organization can be discerned. The connecting piece can be regarded as a truncated cone, modified to contain the proximal and distal centrioles (Fig. 30). The truncated apex points distally, and from it emerges the tail of the sperm. The base forms an arched sheet, termed the capitulum, composed of electron-dense material, which is lodged in a shallow depression called the implantation fossa in the caudal pole of the nucleus. The truncated apex of the cone surrounds the distal or longitudinal centriole, from which the axial filament of the tail is derived. Superior or rostral to the distal centriole, the conical structure surrounds the proximal centriole, which lies at an angle of 75° to 90° to the longitudinal axis of the sperm tail, except in one region opposite distal end of the proximal centriole from which an extension, termed the centriolar adjunct, emerges (Figs. 30 and 31). The actual structure of the wall of the truncated cone is dependent on the level at which it is examined. The truncated apex at the level of the distal centriole is composed of nine longitudinal cross-striated columns that cranially fuse to varying degrees. Those

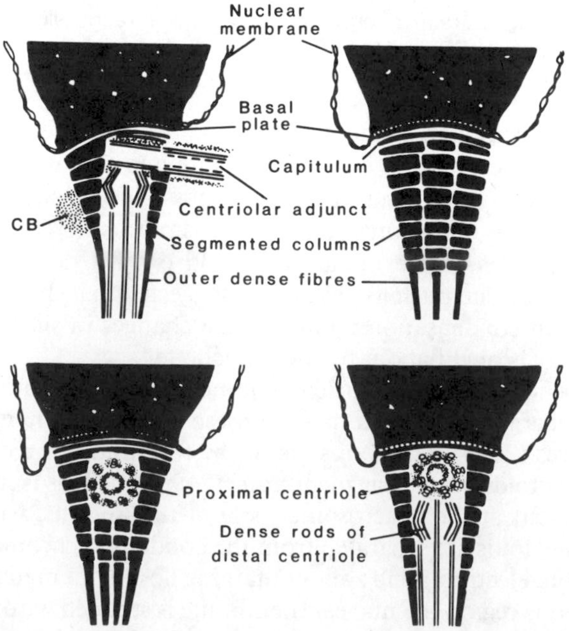

FIG. 30. This diagram illustrates the relationships of the components of the neck of the human spermatid during spermiogenesis. The different appearances represent views seen from different planes of section.

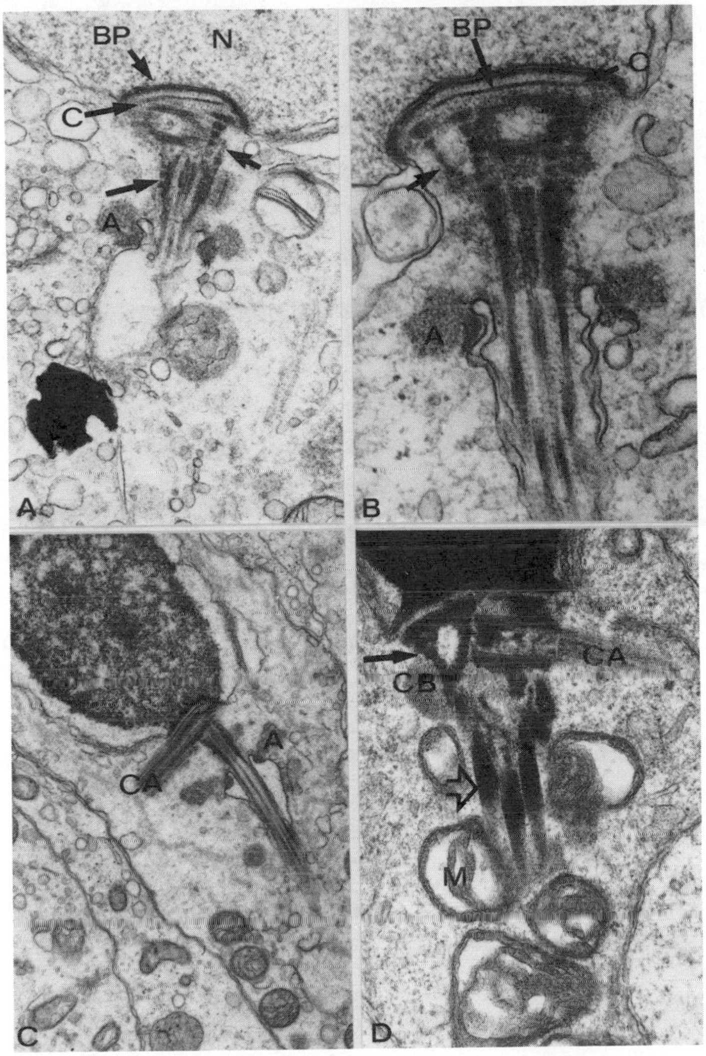

FIG. 31. The developing connecting piece of the human spermatid is shown at the Sb_2 (**A, B**), Sc (**C**), and Sd_2 stages (**D**). Note progressive condensation of the nucleus (N); also, basal plate (BP), capitulum (C), segmented columns of connecting piece (*arrows*), annulus (A), centriolar adjunct (CA), centriole-associated body (CB), mitochondrial sheath (M), and outer dense fibers of midpiece (*open arrow*).

columns opposite the centriolar extension coalesce and lose their individuality and, together with the others except those interrupted by the centriolar adjunct or extension, extend cranially to fuse with the capitulum.

The development of the connecting piece commences in round or Golgi-phase spermatids prior to the association of the developing axial filament with the nucleus. Although the ultimate structure of the connecting piece differs considerably between species, there is general agreement as to the roles played by the proximal and distal centrioles during its formation. This has arisen from the detailed studies of this region during spermatogenesis in a number of different species (176,219,242). During formation of the connecting piece, the nine cross-striated columns arise from electron-dense material that accumulates adjacent to the triplets of the distal centriole (Fig. 32). This material is augmented by material of similar appearance that develops adjacent to the triplets of the proximal centriole and also extends to contribute to the capitulum. The cross banding of these fibers is relatively imprecise early in spermatogenesis but becomes very evident later in the process (242). The dimensions of the cross-striated columns are usually smaller in the region of the distal centriole, expanding to varying degrees depending on the species as they pass rostrally to insert into the basal plate of the implantation fossa. The latter occurs except for those columns that are interrupted by the extension from the proximal centriole, termed the centriolar adjunct, which takes the form of a "miniflagellum" extending into the cytoplasm adjacent to the neck of the spermatid (Fig. 33). The cross-striated columns adjacent to the proximal centriole opposite the centriolar adjunct tend to lose their individuality, fusing together to variable degrees.

The centriolar adjunct is preferred as the term to denote the structure that emerges from the distal end of the proximal centriole, since it is not a direct extension of the triplet structure of the centriole (242). The centriolar adjunct extends into the cytoplasm adjacent to the neck of the spermatid (219). This extension retains the basic organization of the centriole with the nine triplets forming a major part of the adjunct (Figs. 32 and 33). How-

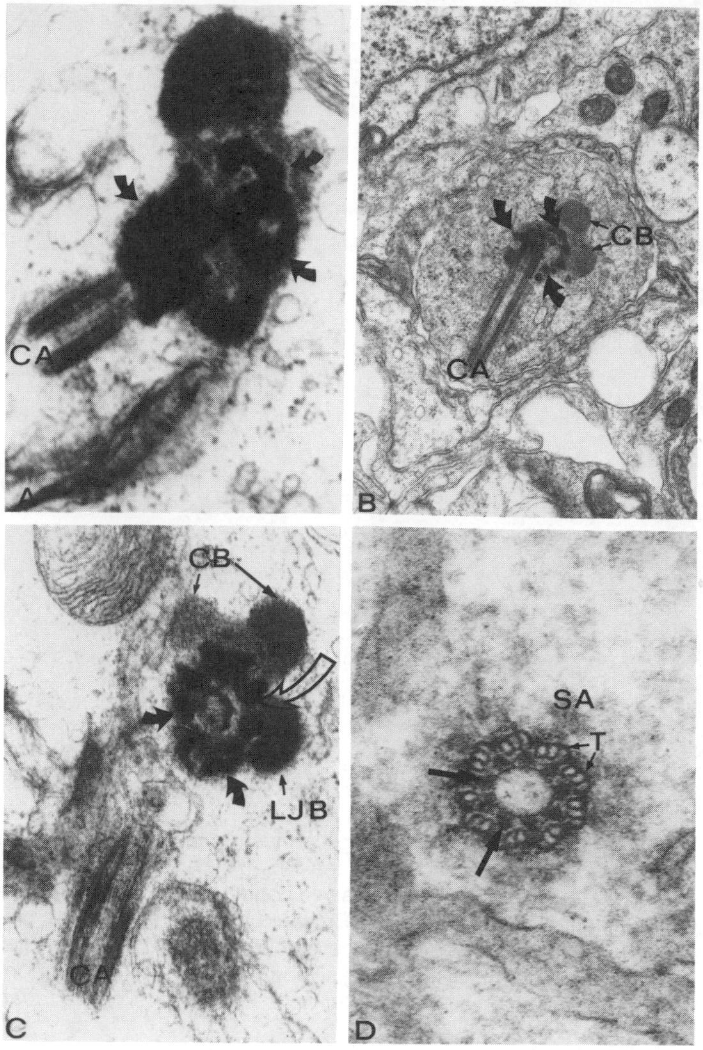

FIG. 32. These micrographs (**A–C**) illustrate sections taken at approximately right angles to the axial filament at progressively descending levels of the connecting piece of the spermatid. Note the columns of the connecting piece (*large arrows*), centriolar adjunct (CA), triplets of longitudinal centrile (*open arrow,* **C**), centriole-associated body (CB), and lateral junctional body (LJB). **D** represents a section at right angles through the centriolar adjunct (CA), triplets of longitudinal centrile (*open arrow,* **C**), centriole-associated body (CB), and lateral junctional body (LJB). **D** represents a section at right angles through the centriolar adjunct showing triplets (T) of proximal centriole satellite arms (S) and the inner ring (*arrows*).

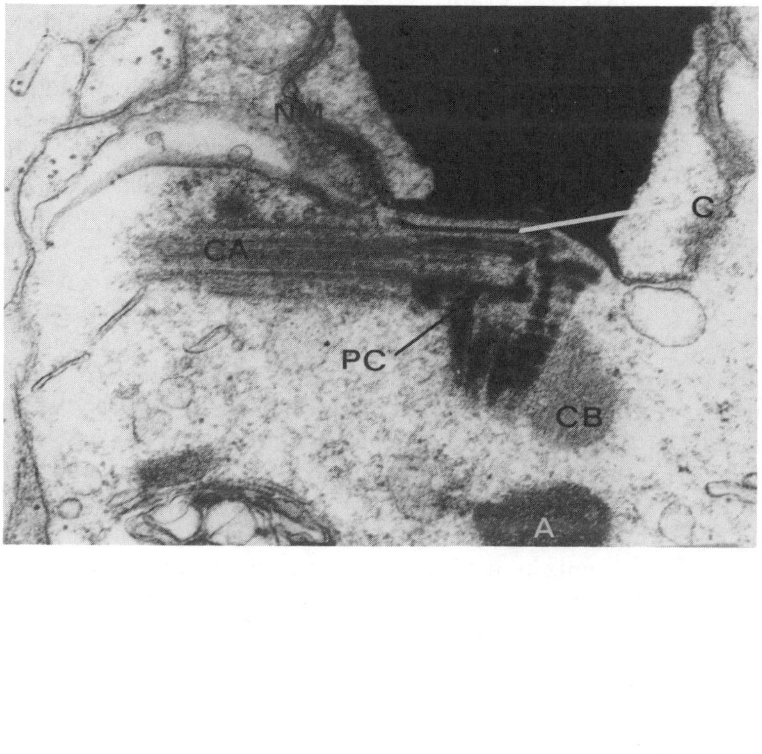

FIG. 33. The neck of the developing human spermatid at the Sd_1 stage shows the proximal centriole (PC), centriolar adjunct (CA), capitulum (C), centriole-associated body (CB), annulus (A), and nuclear membrane (NM).

ever, the outer pair of subunits, termed B and C, of the triplets are incomplete, presenting a J-shaped profile (242). Within this ring of nine modified triplets, a second ring of nine collections of minute tubular units is found (176,219). These collections are not continuous, as longitudinal views of the centriolar adjunct demonstrate distinct breaks, suggesting a series of 10 to 14 rings in human spermatids (176). Internal to these collections a circular rim of tubular profiles surrounds an empty cylindrical space.

External to the modified triplets, a moderately electron-dense material is organized to form satellite arms (176). Despite its structural similarity to a centriole, the centriolar adjunct appears to lack the capacity to organize cross-striated material (242). The purpose of forming a centriolar adjunct remains obscure, but it may represent a response of the proximal centriole to influences that cause the distal centriole to form the axial filament. Later in spermatogenesis, the adjunct disappears, since it is only occasionally observed in ejaculated spermatozoa.

The structure of the distal centriole is significantly modified during spermatogenesis, and in some species no evidence of its structure is discernible in mature spermatozoa (219,252). Early in spermatogenesis, periodic densities can be observed in the walls of the distal centriole and adjacent cytoplasm that are the precursors of the distal ends of the longitudinal cross-striated columns of the connecting piece (Fig. 23). The electron-dense material accumulates around the triplets of the centriole and appears to expand the diameter of the centriole (242). The dense material extends outward between the triplets, forming the longitudinal columns of the connecting piece (Fig. 32). Additionally, a pair of rodlike masses develop between the centriole wall and the central pair of microtubules of the axial filament and traverse this region to make contact with the proximal centriole (242). In man, these dense rods appear to consist of two electron-dense laminae separated by an electron-lucent region and to bow symmetrically (176).

There is general agreement that the distal centriole does not give rise to the nine outer dense fibers that characterize the middle piece of spermatozoa (242,253). They arise in continuity with the doublet microtubules of the axial filament and diverge cranially to appear as separate entities (242,254). They develop out of synchrony with the longitudinal striated columns of the connecting piece, but the two systems are closely apposed at an oblique junction at the level of the distal centriole.

Although the method of formation of the connecting piece has been elucidated, the actual mechanisms remain unknown. Fawcett and Phillips (242) proposed that the centrioles act as sites of assembly of precursor molecules formed by normal mechanisms of ribosomal protein synthesis and that the nine striated columns originally present in the developing connecting piece are an expression of the nine-part symmetry of the centriole established by the nine triplets. Fawcett and Phillips (242) have suggested that the cross-striated appearance of the columns arises from the alignment of successive segments of cross-striated fibers composed of a fibrous protein with a repeating period of 665 Å measured from the middle of one light band to the corresponding next light band. The dark segments demonstrate less obvious banding, each exhibiting ten minor bands similar to the cross-striated elements of goshopod spermatozoa (255). The source of precursor material remains conjectural, but several electron-dense aggregations of fibrillar granular material are seen in the vicinity of the developing connecting piece. In human spermatozoa one of these consists of electron-dense granular material that is found associated with one side of the distal centriole and often exhibits a less dense central zone (219). It is also present in bandicoot spermatids (*Perameles nasuta*) and was termed the lateral junctional body by Sapsford and coworkers (241).

The lateral junctional body appears early in spermatogenesis, prior to the articulation of the developing tail with the nucleus (Figs. 30–32). A second roughly spherical body, slightly less electron dense than the lateral junctional body, is seen at the same level, closely associated with the distal centriole; this has been termed the centriole-associated body (219). In some views, the finely granular material demonstrates periodicity, giving the appearance of linear arrays (176). Both the centriole-associated body and lateral junctional body disappear very late in spermatogenesis.

A third structure of moderate electron density is the annulus, which also appears early in spermatogenesis at the stage in which the intracytoplasmic portion of the axial filament is largely exteriorized. This occurs by the formation of a cleft termed the cytoplasmic canal, which results in an invagination of the cell membrane around the flagellum. The annulus forms a ring-shaped structure that limits the proximal boundary of the cytoplasmic canal. Early in spermatogenesis it is relatively small, but it is augmented later by yet another structure, the chromatoid body, which has migrated from the vicinity of the Golgi complex to the region of the annulus (165). Here it forms a relatively large ring-shaped electron-dense granular structure that is in contact with the annulus and in some views appears to contribute material to that structure. The combined annulus and ring-shaped chromatoid body correspond to what was termed by early investigators the ring centriole. Fawcett et al. (165) note a progressive decrease in size of the chromatoid body with its eventual disappearance, whereas others suggested it was lost in the residual body (257). The actual nature of the chromatoid body is under debate. Early work suggested that it contained basic proteins and may be a source of RNA (185,258,259); however, Eddy (259) was not able to confirm this conclusion. More recently, Walt and Armbuster (260) again proposed that RNA is found in the chromatoid body and also demonstrated that it contained actin, perhaps reflecting its remarkable motility in spermatids.

The form of the annulus varies between species (253). In some such as man, guinea pig, chinchilla, mouse, and ram, the ring-shaped electron density has a convex outer border in contact with the cell membrane in a fold at the proximal limit of the cytoplasmic canal (Fig. 34). Its free edge is in contact rostrally with the lower edge of the mitochondrial helix of the midpiece. In other species (dormouse, Chinese hamster, suni antelope), the annulus is wedge-shaped, is located at the proximal limit of the cytoplasmic canal, and its apex extends toward the axial filament.

The articulation of the connecting-piece with the nucleus occurs at the implantation fossa. In this region the nuclear membranes are closely apposed and separated by a space of 60 to 80 Å that in favorable views is crossed by uniformly spaced densities possibly indicating structures that bind the membranes together (254). The outer nuclear membrane appears thickened by the deposition of electron-dense material to form the basal plate (Figs. 30 and 31). The anlage of the connecting piece lodges in the implantation fossa in such a manner that the capitulum is aligned parallel to the basal plate but separated from it by an electron-lucent space approximately 40 Å wide. Fawcett and Phillips (242) observed many fine filaments traversing this zone, oriented perpendicular to the capitulum and basal plate, and suggested that they were responsible for attaching the flagellum to the head.

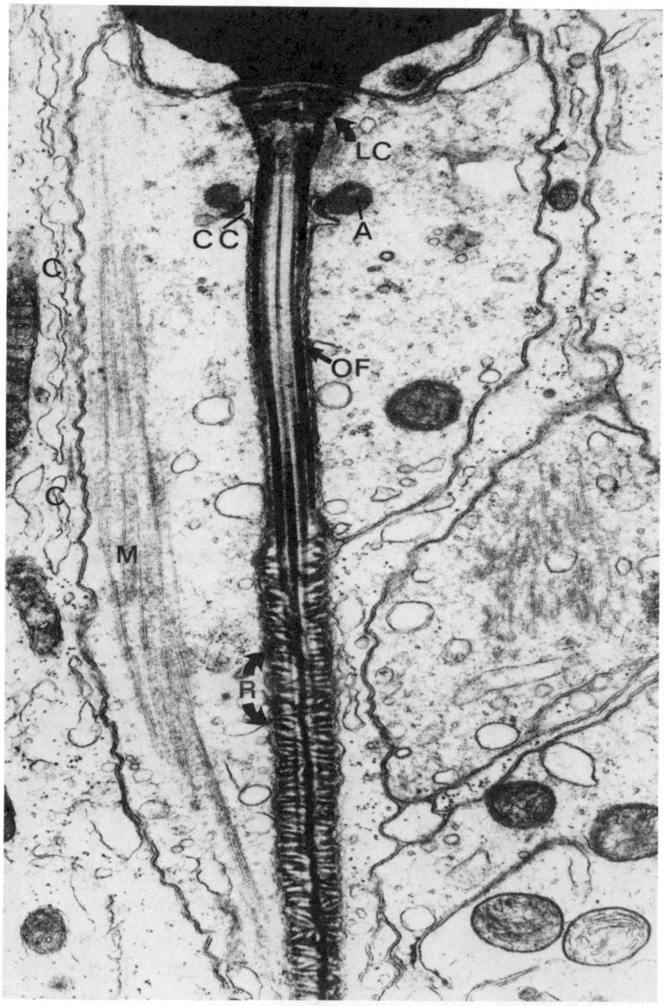

FIG. 34. The structure of the developing human spermatid at the Sd_1 stage is shown, illustrating the longitudinal segmented columns (LC), annulus (A), cytoplasmic canal (CC), outer dense fibers (OF), ribs (R) of principal piece, and manchette (M). Note the cisternae (C) delineating a mantle of Sertoli cell cytoplasm containing fibrils.

Formation of the Dense Fiber System

Over a large portion, the axial filament is modified by the development of a set of nine electron-dense fibers termed the outer dense fiber system (Figs. 22 and 34). They appear to develop as very thin fibers that are attached to the outer wall of the doublet microtubules of the axial filament (242) and seem to separate proximally to develop further as independent fibers by further accretion of material. This relationship to the doublets of the axoneme persists, the outer dense fibers being separated by a greater distance from the doublets cranially while distally they retain their close association with the doublets and taper to eventually disappear. Irons and Clermont (261) have shown that [^{3}H]proline and [^{3}H]cystine are incorporated into the outer dense fiber system over an extensive period of spermatid development from step 8 to 19, indicating the presence of a peak of protein synthetic activity in midspermiogenesis. This view is supported by the studies of O'Brien and Bellve (262), who approached the problem in the mouse by different techniques. Recently, Oko (263) undertook a comparative analysis of the proteins forming the outer dense fibers and produced polyclonal antibodies to some of the major fractions. Using these antibodies raised against components of 32, 26, and 14.4 kD, they noted that granular cytoplasmic localization was present over spermatids from steps 9 to 19 with peak activity at step 16 (264). At the electron microscopic level, the antibodies reacted positively to components of the granulated bodies that appear in relationship to the cisternal of endodoplasmic reticulum from stages 10 to 14, increasing to a peak at stages 15 to 17 and decreasing thereafter. These results support the view that the granulated bodies represent transitory stores of proteins en route to the outer dense fibers (265).

There are significant differences in the size and length of the outer dense fiber system between species (232,239). In human sperm the outer fibers end in the proximal part of the principal piece, fibers 3 and 8 being the first to terminate. In some they are prominent and extend throughout the midpiece and principal piece, whereas in others they terminate more proximally. Unlike the doublets of the axial filament, which are similar in size and appearance, the outer dense fiber system, numbered according to the adjacent doublet, show significant differences in size (232). Fibers 1, 5, and 6 are usually larger in many species.

Telkka et al. (265) showed that the outer dense fibers possess cortical and central zones that differ in electron density. The portion of the cortical zone immediately adjacent to axial filament consists of electron-dense punctate granules in guinea pig spermatozoa, leading Fawcett (232) to call them satellite fibrils. The outer dense fiber system must be considered an independent set of structures to the striated fibers of the connecting piece, since they develop independently and asynchronously (242). However, they do join each other at the lower level of the connecting piece at an oblique junction.

Development of the Principal Piece

The region of the tail between the annulus and the termination of the fibrous sheath or tail helix is termed the principal piece (240). The presence of a fibrous sheath is peculiar to mammalian spermatozoa, and early ultrastructural studies demonstrated that the sheath was not helical but consisted of riblike structures joined to two longitudinal columns (240,267,268) (Fig. 35). The closely spaced ribs sometimes branch, attaching to adjacent ribs. Proximally the longitudinal columns consist of the outer dense fibers 3 and 8, but these terminate distally, and the ribs are attached to a thin electron-dense ridge that projects from doublets 3 and 8. The longitudinal columns vary in prominence with species, being well developed in rodents but insignificant in man (239,240,267).

In the human, the analage of the fibrous sheath appears to be a system of transversely oriented microtubules (219). The hollow cores of these tubules are progressively obliterated by an electron-dense material, a process that gives rise to the transversely oriented ribs (Fig. 36). Progressive addition of electron-dense material thickens the ribs. More extensive studies of the development of the principal piece in human spermatids have confirmed the microtubular origin of the ribs (268). They showed that a large accumulation of microtubules occurs in the region of the developing principal piece (Fig. 37) to form a microtubular body at the equivalent of Sc spermatids (184). Subsequently, with elongation of the axial filament and distal migration of the annulus, this collection of microtubules is diminished and eventually disappears (176). A microtubular body similar to that in human spermatids was described by Nicander

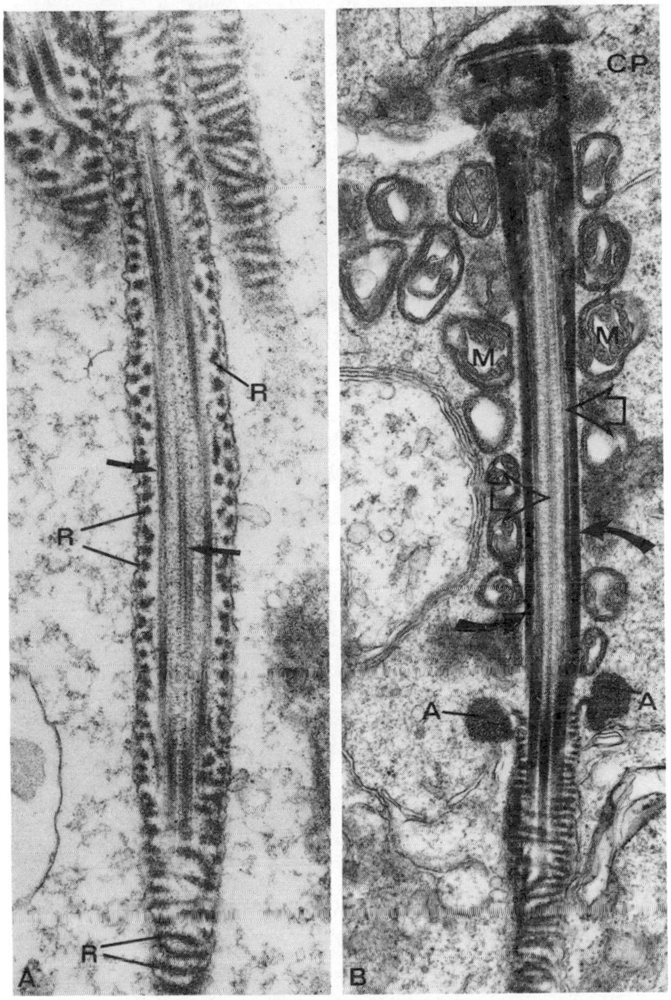

FIG. 35. Two longitudinal sections through developing spermatid tails in the region of the midpiece (**B**) and principal piece (**A**). Note the ribs (R), microtubules of axial filament (*arrows* in **A**, *open arrows* in **B**), annulus (A), connecting piece (CP), mitochondria (M), and outer dense fibers (*arrows* in **B**).

(269) in cat and rabbit spermatids; it occurred at the anterior extremity of the principal piece and eventually disappeared.

An alternative method of formation of the ribs of the principal piece was proposed by Sapsford and colleagues (270) from their studies of the bandicoot (*Perameles nasuta*). They could find no evidence of microtubules forming the analage of the ribs; instead they observed that a series of fine filaments joined the longitudinal columns that had appeared as electron-dense thickenings adjacent to doublets 5 and 8. These filaments aggregate and converge to form the definitive ribs. Similar fine filaments were also noted in the lizard (271) and in the mouse (272). The two methods of rib formation are strikingly dissimilar, and further studies in other species are required to determine which process is more common. Recently, Irons and Clermont (273) demonstrated by the use of [^{3}H]proline incorporation into proteins that

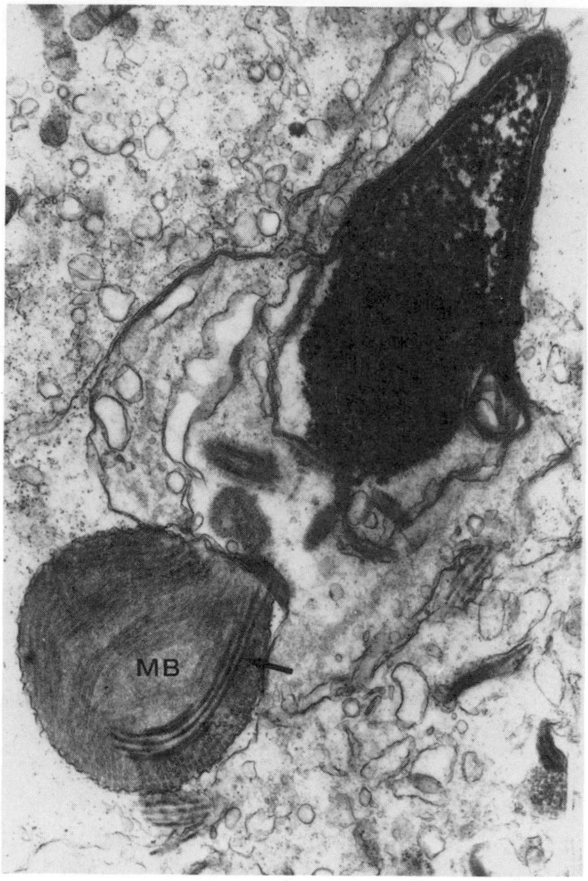

FIG. 36. A human spermatid at the Sc stage shows the axial filament (*arrow*) surrounded by the microtubular body (MB).

the longitudinal columns of the principal piece take 15 days to be formed. They also showed that in the rat, the ribs develop independently and asychronously from the longitudinal columns over a period of 4 to 5 days from proteinacious filaments. Recent studies using immunocytochemical techniques localized fibrous sheath proteins to the cytoplasm of spermatids at steps 9 to 19 (264,265). This diffuse cytoplasmic material did not appear in granulated bodies and did not localize at the electron microscopic level over dense material that accumulates in the regions where the ribs of the fibrous sheath form (265). However, positive immunocytochemical localization was noted over the ribs of the fibrous sheath, suggesting a direct transfer of the cytoplasmic protein to the ribs.

The Mitochondrial Sheath

Jensen (274) and Benda (275) described the aggregation of mitochondria in spermatids around the axial filament in the region now called the middle piece. Similar findings were noted for the human testis. Early ultrastructural studies demonstrated that the mitochondria actually form a spiral sheath that in mammalian spermatozoa was of variable length (240,276). The number of spirals forming the sheath varies from 5 to 14 for man (277,278) and up to 40 in the guinea pig (232). The mouse (up to 90), bat (up to 15), and rat (up to 350) represent the largest number of spirals encountered (196). Andre (163) has drawn attention to the fact that the helical configuration provides the least resistance to bending.

The actual formation of the middle piece occurs late in spermiogenesis (241). Earlier, the mitochondria are distributed evenly in the cytoplasm in some species, and in others, such as man, they are peripherally placed close to the cell membrane (188,218). Formation of the mitochondrial sheath is preceded by caudal migration of the annulus, and the mitochondria associate with the axial filament between the connecting piece and the annulus (Figs. 34 and 35). The mechanisms involved in the migration and aggregation of mitochondria remain unknown. However, the organization of the manchette, a cylindrical collection of microtubules extending from the nuclear region to the caudal region of the spermatid, excludes the mitochondria from the region of the flagellum. When this collection of microtubules disperses late in spermatogenesis, the mitochondria are free to aggregate to form helical arrays (230). The end-to-end arrangement of mitochondria is usually random, but Fawcett (196) has drawn attention to the observation that in some species there is a remarkable regularity in spacing (230).

In many species the organization of the cristae of mitochrondria in germ cells takes on certain unique features. As described earlier, the intracristal space of mitochondria in primary and secondary spermatocytes is dilated, often giving a vacuolated appearance to these organelles (163). This process persists in spermatids and results in peripheral margination of the cristae such that in some species a central clear zone appears in the mitochondria (277). In other species the entire mitochondrion appears to be filled by membranes that are concentrically orientated (254,278,279).

Reorganization of Cytoplasm and Organelles and Spermiation

The process of spermatogenesis is characterized by dramatic changes in the relationship of the nucleus and cytoplasm and the remarkable movements of organelles within spermatids. Many of these changes were described by the classical cytologists and were used by Le Blond and Clermont (182) to stage the process of spermatogenesis. The changes in nuclear shape and position were described earlier, but the movement of cytoplasm towards the caudal end of the spermatid requires some discussion.

It was noted that when the caudal movement of cytoplasm occurred, a system of cytoplasmic filaments ap-

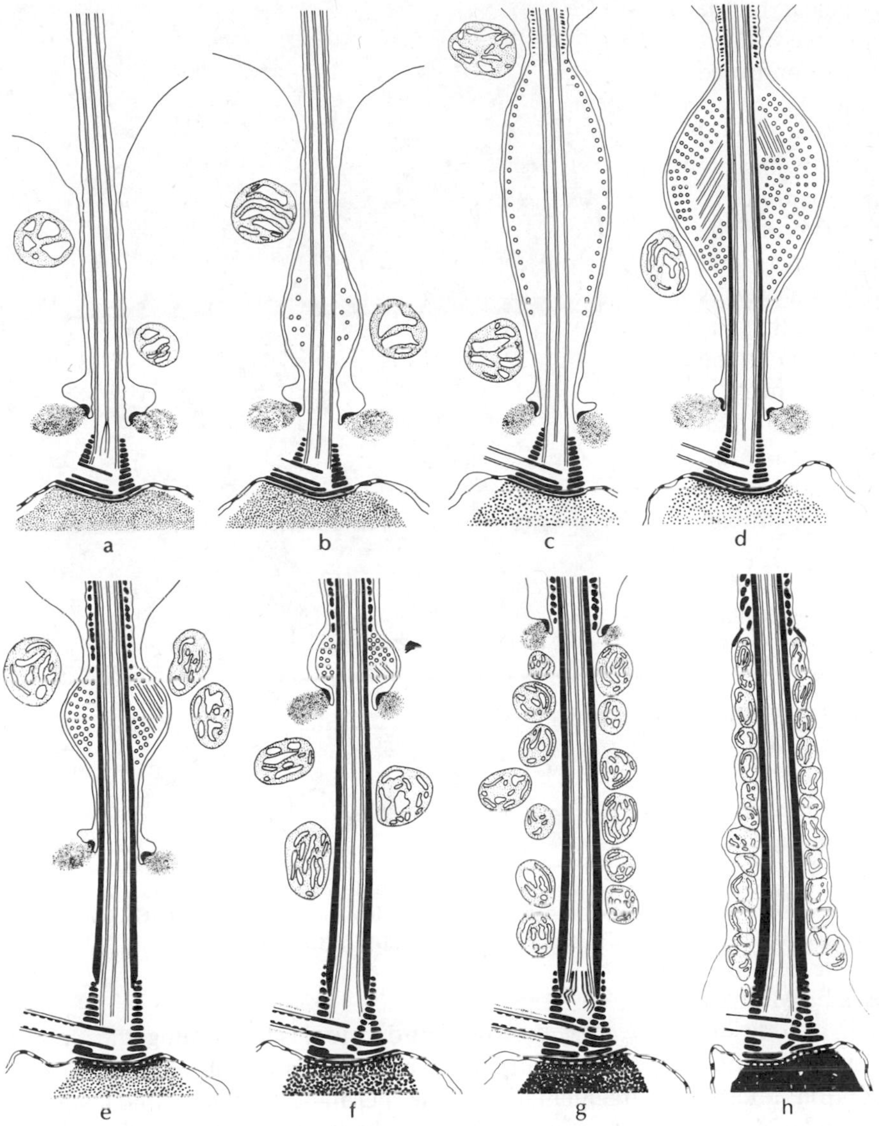

FIG. 37. This diagram illustrates the contribution of the "microtubular body" to the formation of the principal piece in human spermiogenesis. (From Holstein and Roosen-Runge, ref. 176, with permission.)

peared, extending from the nuclear membrane and terminating freely in the caudal cytoplasm (182). This system was given the name manchette by Lenhossek (280). Subsequently Zlotnik (281) described the origin of the manchette as the nuclear membrane caudal to the acrosome, a view confirmed by later electron microscopic studies. These early studies also observed that the manchette disappeared later in spermatogenesis.

McIntosh and Porter (233) demonstrated that the manchette actually was composed of a cylindrical array of microtubules that was noted to arise from a ring-like structure surrounding the postacrosomal region of spermatids in the cat (188). This nuclear ring, originally described by Gresson and Zlotnik (282), consists of electron-dense material that appears to thicken the cell membrane adjacent to the postacrosomal region of the nuclear membrane (230). The proximal ends of the microtubules of the manchette are embedded in this dense fibrillar material. However, this electron-dense deposit has not been observed in all species, being absent in man and the bandicoot (219,241). The microtubular nature of the manchette (Figs. 24 and 28) has led numerous investigators to suggest that it is responsible for shaping of the nucleus and reorganization of the cytoplasm (233). However, from a detailed study of spermatogenesis in a number of species, Fawcett and co-workers (230) produced evidence to indicate that nuclear shape was dependent on genetic factors rather than the manchette. They also suggested that rather than being involved in the physical movement of cytoplasm, the microtubules of the manchette may act as a framework or conveyor for the transport of cytoplasmic vesicles. These vesicles were closely associated with the manchette and sometimes were physically linked by slender linear densities (230). These linear densities are similar in appearance to those linking adjacent microtubules composing the manchette

(Fig. 24). The fate of the manchette was unclear, but de Kretser (219) suggested that the microtubules were incorporated in the residual body, a view recently confirmed by studies of equine spermatogenesis (283).

Associated with the caudal movement of the cytoplasm, the Golgi complex and chromatoid body migrate to the abacrosomal pole. The former can be identified as a component of the residual body, that portion of the spermatid cytoplasm that is shed when the spermatid leaves the seminiferous epithelium (Fig. 3) in a process called spermation. Early studies demonstrated that the greater part of the spermatid cytoplasm is shed as the residual body, which, in the majority of instances, is phagocytosed by the adjacent Sertoli cells (284,285). The term residual body (corps residuel) was originally applied to these structures by Regaud (27), who noted their formation. Some cytoplasm remains to form a droplet that surrounds the middle piece and contains a few vesicular profiles. Lacy (285) noted that the residual body contained remnants of the Golgi complex and endoplasmic reticulum, and a number of studies have confirmed their phagocytosis by the Sertoli cell (286–289).

The method by which the spermatid sheds the residual body and leaves the epithelium has emerged from the results of a number of ultrastructural studies (219, 290,291). de Kretser (219) noted that late in spermatogenesis, the caudal spermatid cytoplasm is invaginated by processes of Sertoli cell cytoplasm and postulated that these processes actually were responsible for pulling off the residual body (Figs. 38 and 39). Similar processes of Sertoli cell cytoplasm within spermatids have been observed in the studies of rat spermatogenesis by Morales and Clermont (291). The residual cytoplasm, in addition to containing remnants of the Golgi complex, also contains ribosomes, lipid inclusions, mitochondria, microtubular remnants of the manchette, and electron-dense remnants of the chromatoid body. The residual bodies from human spermatids were also noted to contain flowerlike structures noted in the cytoplasm of spermatids earlier in spermatogenesis (292). These consist of a core of densely packed osmiophilic granules surrounded by a translucent vesicle and originally appear near the nucleus in association with the chromatoid body. Their function within the spermatid remains unclear. Associated with the invagination of spermatid cytoplasm by Sertoli cell processes, there is progressive movement of the spermatid toward the lumen; the cytoplasm attached to the Sertoli cell is linked to the spermatid by progressively attenuating connections (290). All connections are lost eventually, the majority of the residual bodies being retained with the Sertoli cell. Breucker et al. (293), however, suggest that in the human many residual bodies are shed into the tubule lumen. Recent studies by Sakai and colleagues (294,295) showed that late in spermatogenesis intertwining tubules of Sertoli cells could be found invading the spermatid cytoplasm, forming the "mixed body." Later the lumina of these tubules enlarge, causing fragmentation of the spermatid cytoplasm and leading to engulfment of the residual cytoplasm by the Sertoli cell.

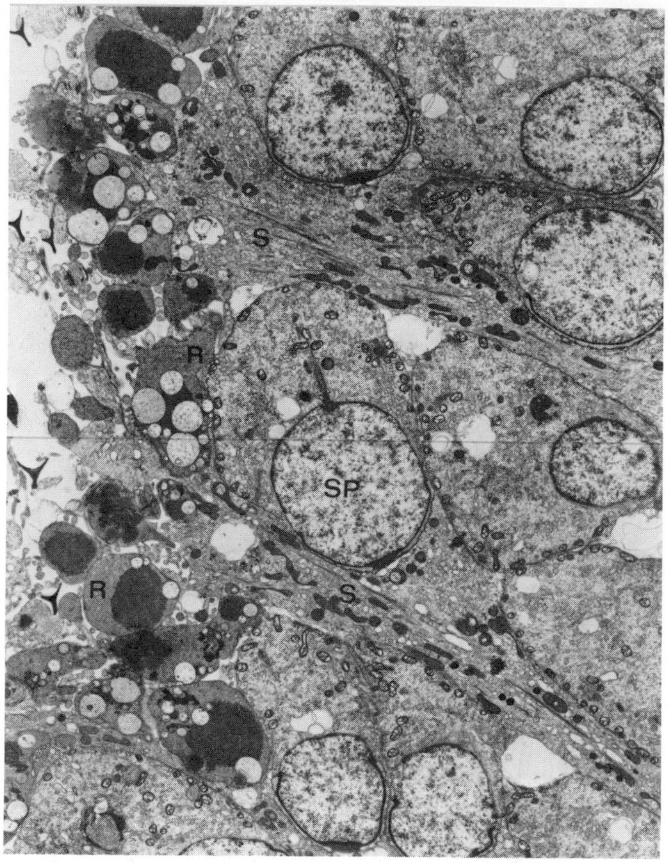

FIG. 38. Adluminal aspect of the seminiferous epithelium of the rat testis, illustrating Sertoli cell cytoplasm (S), spermatids (SP), and lobes of residual cytoplasm (R).

The mechanisms involved in spermiation remain unclear. In mammals, the late spermatids appear to progressively lose their contact with the Sertoli cell, being anchored by a special device in the region of the head described originally in the rat by Russell and Clermont (296). The structure of this device is described later, but it represents the final attachment device by which the spermatid retains contact with the Sertoli cell; although originally described in the rat, it has also been found in man (176). Loss of this final contact represents the completion of spermatogenesis, and by definition, the cell is now termed a spermatozoon (290,297). In amphibians, Burgos and Vitale-Calpe (298,299) suggested that spermiation resulted in a swelling of the terminal cytoplasmic processes of the Sertoli cells, resulting in the evagination of the lacunae that housed the spermatids, thereby shedding them into the lumen of the tubule. This was suggested to be a response to hCG or LH, but similar actions have not been confirmed in mammals.

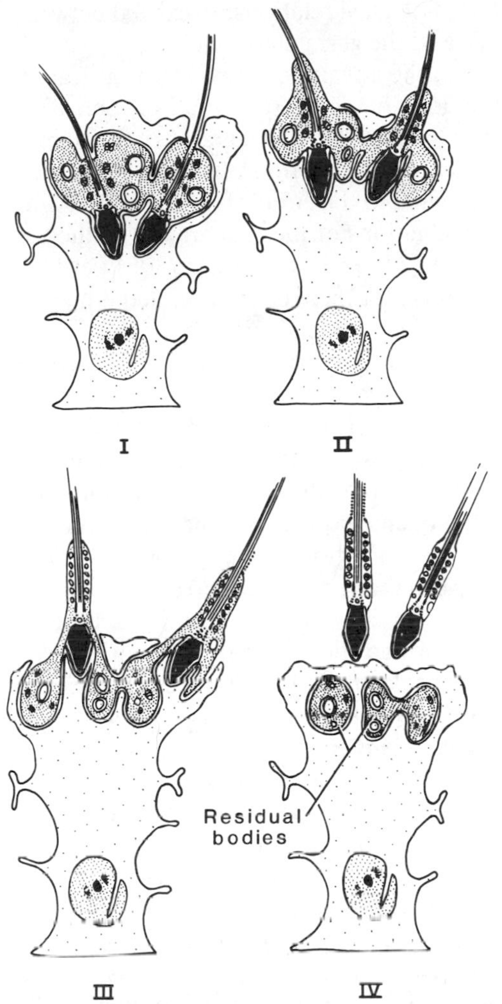

FIG. 39. The final stages of human spermiogenesis are illustrated diagrammatically. Note the manner in which processes of Sertoli cell cytoplasm essentially "pull off" the residual cytoplasm (residual body) and retain it within their cytoplasm.

Relationships Between the Sertoli Cell and Spermatids

During the early stages of spermatogenesis, the spermatids lie centrally immediately adjacent to the lumen of the seminiferous tubules, surrounded by processes of Sertoli cell cytoplasm. At this time small punctate desmosomelike cell junctions occur with the adjacent Sertoli cell (169). The spermatids do not demonstrate any specific orientation to the Sertoli cell, but in later stages they are deeply embedded within the epithelium, oriented such that their heads, covered by the acrosomal cap, point toward the basement membrane of the tubule. Subsequently, as described above, they are progressively moved toward the lumen of the tubule, eventually to lose all contact after spermiation. Studies in procarbazine-treated rats have shown that acrosome formation is disrupted but that this process did not alter the movement of the nucleus into its eccentric position (300). However, the altered acrosome formation disrupted alignment of the heads of the spermatid within the epithelium, possibly by altering the distribution of the Sertoli-cell–spermatid junctional specializations described below.

The formation of certain specialized junctions with the adjacent Sertoli is probably related to the specific orientation taken by the spermatids in midspermatogenesis. Early studies noted that the cytoplasm of the Sertoli cell adjacent to the heads of spermatids late in spermatogenesis (Fig. 24) was separated into a mantle layer by the presence of an array of vesicles (218,301). Nagano (302) confirmed these findings and noted the presence of thick filaments in this mantle layer of Sertoli cell cytoplasm. A number of studies in different species have demonstrated the existence of these specialized cell attachments in which there is no reduction in the intercellular space but the demarcation of a thin zone of Sertoli cell cytoplasm by the presence of a series of cisternae, the cytoplasmic layer so defined demonstrating the presence of numerous fibrils (175,303,304). The cell junctions have some similarity to the inter-Sertoli-cell junctions, but there is no modification of the intercellular space. In

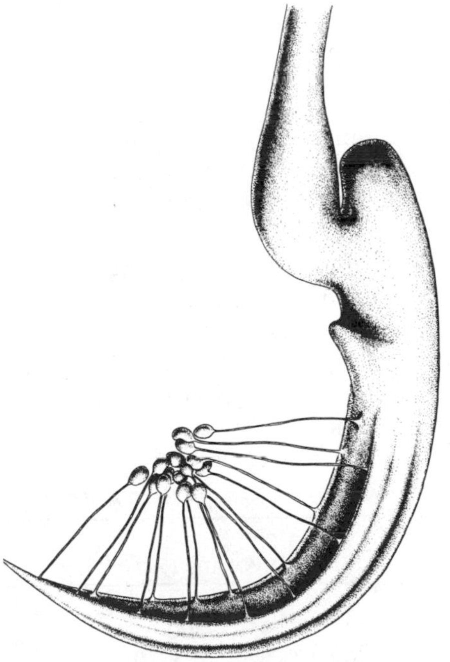

FIG. 40. A diagrammatic representation of the three-dimensional features of a step 19 spermatid of the rat. The concave aspect of the sperm head extends elaborate tubulobulbar complexes into the surrounding Sertoli cell cytoplasm, the latter not shown here. The complexes are congregated together and form bulbous terminal dilations. They are said to act as an anchoring device to temporarily retain the spermatid head within apical extensions of Sertoli cell cytoplasm. (From Russell and Clermont, ref. 296, with permission.)

many species these specialized Sertoli cell–spermatid cell junctions are located only in the region of the head, but in the human they can be demonstrated over larger areas of the spermatid cell surface (Fig. 34). The cell junctions first appear when the spermatid nucleus takes up an eccentric position with the cell coming into close association with the cell membrane.

A further junctional specialization occurs between late spermatids and the Sertoli cells wherein the cell membrane in the region of the head of the spermatid projects into the surrounding Sertoli cell cytoplasm (304). These tubulobulbar processes provide a mechanism of anchoring spermatids immediately prior to spermiation (Fig. 40). In the rat, they appear to be limited to the cell membrane in relation to the concave portion of the nucleus (304,305), but in man they are more irregularly distributed (176).

Reference was made earlier to the processes of Sertoli cell cytoplasm that appears to invaginate the caudal spermatid cytoplasm immediately preceding spermiation. Morales and Clermont (291) have described two types of Sertoli cell processes in the rat, one that is essentially devoid of organelles and the other, which contains vesicles. From these observations they propose that the latter may represent a mechanism of transferring materials between these two cell types.

SERTOLI CELL

The nongerminal component of the seminiferous epithelium was originally described in 1865 by the Italian physiologist Enrico Sertoli (306). He identified the cells that now bear his name as being individual elements extending from the basement membrane to the lumen of the seminiferous tubule and, in doing so, envelop the many clusters of associated germ cells. Within the mammalian testis the Sertoli cell is a tall columnar cell extending perpendicularly through the seminiferous epithelium (Fig. 11), and von Ebner (105,172) first proposed that a physiological relationship existed between the Sertoli cells and the germ cells.

Without the advantage of modern optical equipment and methods of tissue preservation, Sertoli (307) and Brown (136) constructed diagrams of the shape of Sertoli cells indicating the pronounced length of the centripetal axis compared to the circumferential axis. Although further investigations of the topography of the Sertoli cells by Regaud (27) and von Ebner (308) verified Sertoli's observations that these cells presented a highly irregular nucleus and elaborate ramifying cytoplasmic processes, the limited resolution of their light microscopes raised a point of controversy regarding the existence of the Sertoli cell as a syncitium or as an individual cell. It had been Sertoli's earlier contention that the Sertoli cells were independent cellular units and did not form a syncitial relationship with each other, but von Ebner (105) put forward the notion that a symbiotic relationship existed between the Sertoli cells and the more mature generations of germ cells, thereby forming a functional unit, which he termed the spermatoblast. In the same study, he also considered the Sertoli cells to form a complex syncitium, a concept he later discarded (172) in favor of their independent existence.

The precise morphological organization of the Sertoli cell remained poorly understood for many years thereafter (126,309–313). With the greatly improved resolution of the electron microscope, Watson (126,314) and Challice (315) provided the first descriptions of the fine structure of the seminiferous epithelium, but it was not until 1956 that Fawcett and Burgos demonstrated that each Sertoli cell had distinct cellular boundaries. The recent ultrastructural investigations contributed by Fawcett (see reviews, refs. 316–320) have greatly increased our appreciation of the central role played by this cell in the regulation of spermatogenesis. Detailed studies of the topography of the Sertoli cell, its relationship to germ cells, and the changes in Sertoli cell morphology in health and disease (321–328) have each added substantially to a deeper understanding of Sertoli cell histology (Table 1).

TABLE 1. *Quantitative morphology of Sertoli cells*

Species	Volume (μm^3)	Surface area (μm^2)	Numerical density ($10^6/cm^3$ testis)	References
Opossum	7000			864
Mouse	3300		36	864
Rat	5–8000	9–20,000	26–28	324–326
Guinea pig	3300		55	864
Hamster	4200–4700	13,000	35–44	864,540,518
Woodchuck	3000		47	864
Degu	2000		80	864
Rabbit	4500		25	864
Dog	5000		43	864
Water buffalo	7–9000	11–14,000		361
Stallion	3300		24–60	528,864
Monkey	2600–4100	2,400	102	483,864
Human	4800		33–49	351,864

Sertoli Cell Shape

The early histologists recognized that the unusual columnar shape of the Sertoli cell reflected a three-dimensional configuration of great complexity (136, 307). In their studies defining the seminiferous cycle, Le Blond and Clermont (183) noted that the Sertoli cells alter their shape in relation to the 14 stages of the spermatogenic cycle. With a silver staining method applied to paraffin sections, Elftman (329) concluded that in the rat testis, the Sertoli cells were tall, columnar in shape, and their distribution within the seminiferous epithelium resembled the pattern of trees planted in an orchard. On the basis of this and earlier studies on the mouse testis (313) the basal aspect of the Sertoli cells, most readily visible by light microscopy, was likened to a trunk of a tree (Fig. 41), the many cytoplasmic ramifications between the surrounding germ cells being analogous to the branches of a tree. This simple description has largely stood the test of time, and many subsequent ultrastructural studies of thin sections have confirmed that although this appealing topographical description may not be entirely applicable to all species so far studied, a better portrayal has not emerged.

The strategic position of the Sertoli cell within the seminiferous epithelium and its intrinsic relationships to neighboring Sertoli cells and germ cells (Figs. 41–45) has reputedly been emphasized in fine structural analysis of a great variety of vertebrate and invertebrate species (318,330–335). Recent ultrastructural studies in the rat have shown that Sertoli cell shape is more complex than was appreciated previously and stress that the cytoplasmic extensions of the Sertoli cell characterize the topography of the cell as possibly the most complex yet described in any epithelium. The Sertoli cells must continually alter their shape to accommodate the structural transformations and mobilization of germ cells from the base to the free surface of the seminiferous epithelium. Wong and Russell (324) serially sectioned a single Sertoli cell from a stage V rat seminiferous tubule and showed that the cell was best characterized as a short body resting on the basal lamina with many upward-projecting sheetlike cytoplasmic extensions forming cone, cup, and cylindrical configurations in relation to germ cells and adjacent Sertoli cells. When the seminiferous epithelium was viewed perpendicular to the basal lamina, the Sertoli cells were reported to form a hexagonal array; i.e., they presented six membrane surfaces near their base (307,312,336). More recent studies suggest that the basal regions of the Sertoli cells are more likely packed in the seminiferous tubule in a pentagonal arrangement (325,337).

Ultrastructural studies of rat Sertoli cells at stages II, VII, VIII, IX–XI, and XIII–XIV of the spermatogenic cycle depicted variations in shape (Fig. 42) that seem at first to indicate highly irregular and disordered configurations (338). However, the margins of the Sertoli cell are obliged to undergo transformations to remain in association with (a) the expanding spherical volumes exemplified by spermatogonia, spermatocytes, and spermatids,

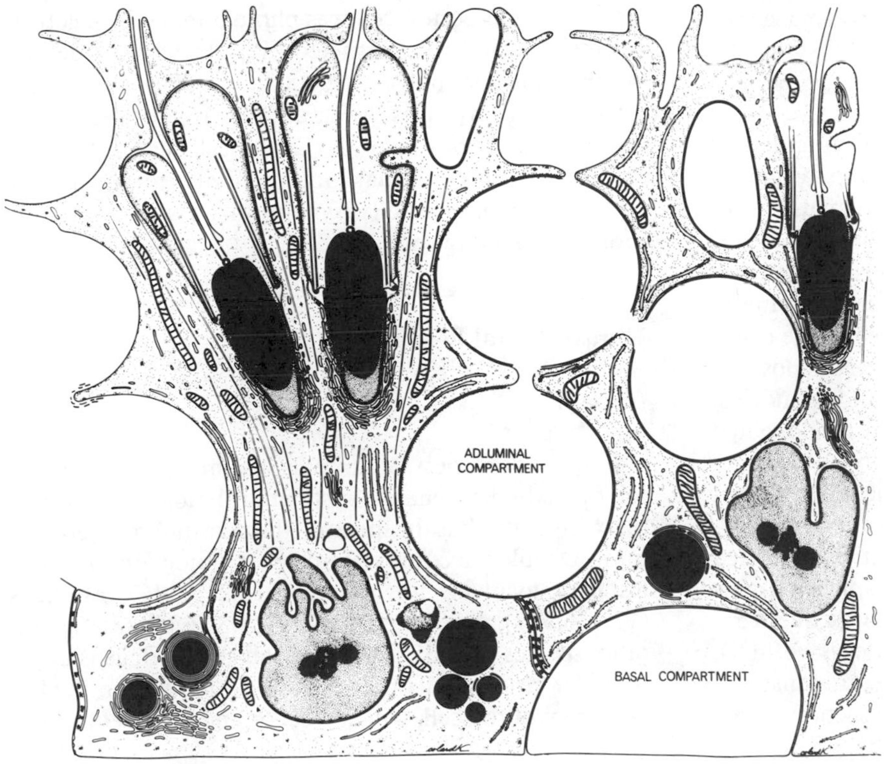

FIG. 41. A diagram illustrating how the occluding inter-Sertoli-cell junctions divide the seminiferous epithelium into a basal compartment (containing spermatogonia and early primary spermatocytes) and an adluminal compartment (containing more advanced germ cells). (From Fawcett, ref. 318, with permission.)

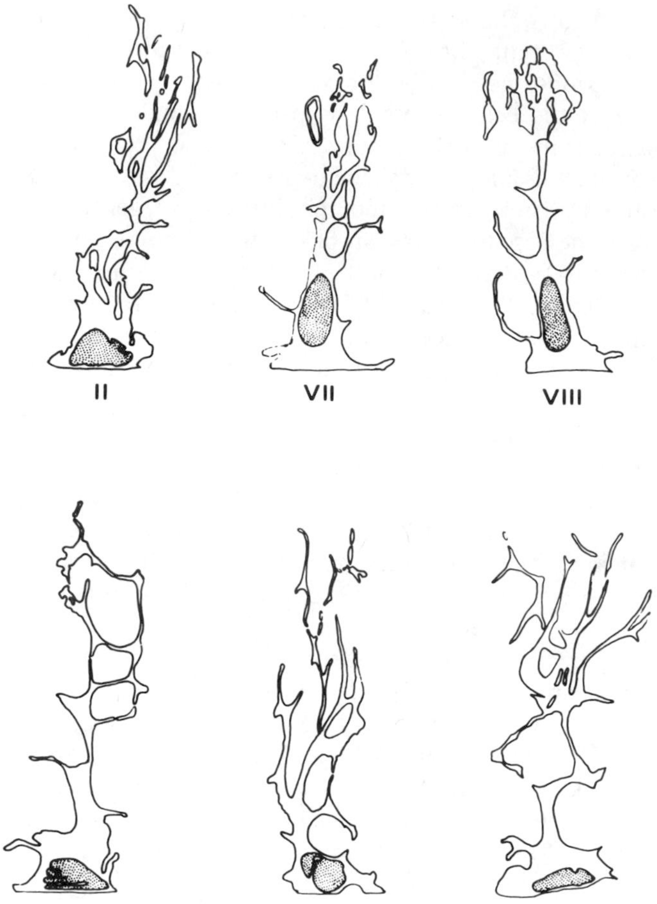

FIG. 42. India ink tracings of the plasma membrane of individual Sertoli cells at various stages of the rat spermatogenic cycle. The surface of each Sertoli cell was identified from assembled electron micrograph montages and emphasizes the complex and varying shape of the Sertoli cell.

(b) mature spermatids, (c) spermatogonial mitoses and the meiotic maturation divisions, and (d) the formation and subsequent resolution of the excess spermatid residual cytoplasm. Reconstruction of entire profiles of Sertoli cells from many smaller micrographs of each cell reveal that for the major proportion of the rat spermatogenic cycle (Figs. 43–45), the overall shape of the cell is best described as tall, irregularly columnar, and possessing numerous very thin lateral processes and cylindrical recesses to accommodate the penetration of elongated spermatids. Similar findings were noted by Wong and Russell (324), who emphasized that for the remainder of the spermatogenic cycle, these extremely attenuated cytoplasmic processes are absent because the elongated spermatids adopt positions at the extreme apical margins of the Sertoli cells and because of their subsequent release from the seminiferous epithelium (stages VII–IX).

Cyclic variations in Sertoli cell shape commensurate with the changing composition and cross-sectional area of the seminiferous epithelium (339) logically lead to a consideration of changes in Sertoli cell volume that may also reveal morphological alterations in the internal composition of the Sertoli cell, a subject dealt with in detail later in this section. Although morphometric techniques have been used to estimate the numerical density and total number of Sertoli cells in the perfused, fixed rat testis (339), efforts to obtain additional quantitative information on Sertoli cell shape and volume during the spermatogenic cycle have met with considerable difficulty because of the intricate topography of the Sertoli cells. Earlier quantitative studies on rat seminiferous tubules reported a 10% to 13% occupancy of the seminiferous epithelium by the Sertoli cells (340). In the human and rat testis, Sertoli cells were reported to occupy 36% and 11%, respectively, of the seminiferous epithelium (341). However, these data are difficult to evaluate since they were based on light microscopic analysis of Sertoli cells in semithin sections of seminiferous tubules, where the limits of optical resolution possibly fail to detect the thin ramifying processes of the Sertoli cell. Ultrastructural examination of monkey Sertoli cells revealed that the relative volume of the Sertoli cell within the seminiferous epithelium ranged from 24% at stage I to 32% at stage VII of the monkey spermatogenic cycle (342,343). Morphometric analysis of the rat seminiferous epithelium in our laboratory (344,345) has shown that the proportion occupied by Sertoli cells during the spermatogenic cycle ranges from 20% to 29%, representing a cyclical volume change, lowest during stages VI to VIII (5300–5500 μm^3) and increasing to maximum volume during stages XII to XIV (7000–7700 μm^3. When a single stage V rat Sertoli cell was photographed by electron microscopy and reconstructed as a plexiglas model, its volume was estimated at 6000 μm^3 (324). Taken together, these advances in our appreciation of the changing shape and volume of the Sertoli cell suggest that the cell engages in continual motor activity and exhibits a high degree of plasticity synchronized with the ever-mobile population of germ cells.

Ultrastructural Features

Nucleus

For a wide variety of animals, the nucleus of the Sertoli cell exhibits a characteristic morphology readily visible within the basal aspect of the seminiferous epithelium. Detailed accounts of nuclear cytology in the adult testis are available for rodents (318,319,346), monkeys (17,346,347), the human (125,321,322,348–352), and other species (318,327). The Sertoli cell nucleus is large, irregular, and usually occupies a position within the basal aspect of the cell, which rests on the basement mem-

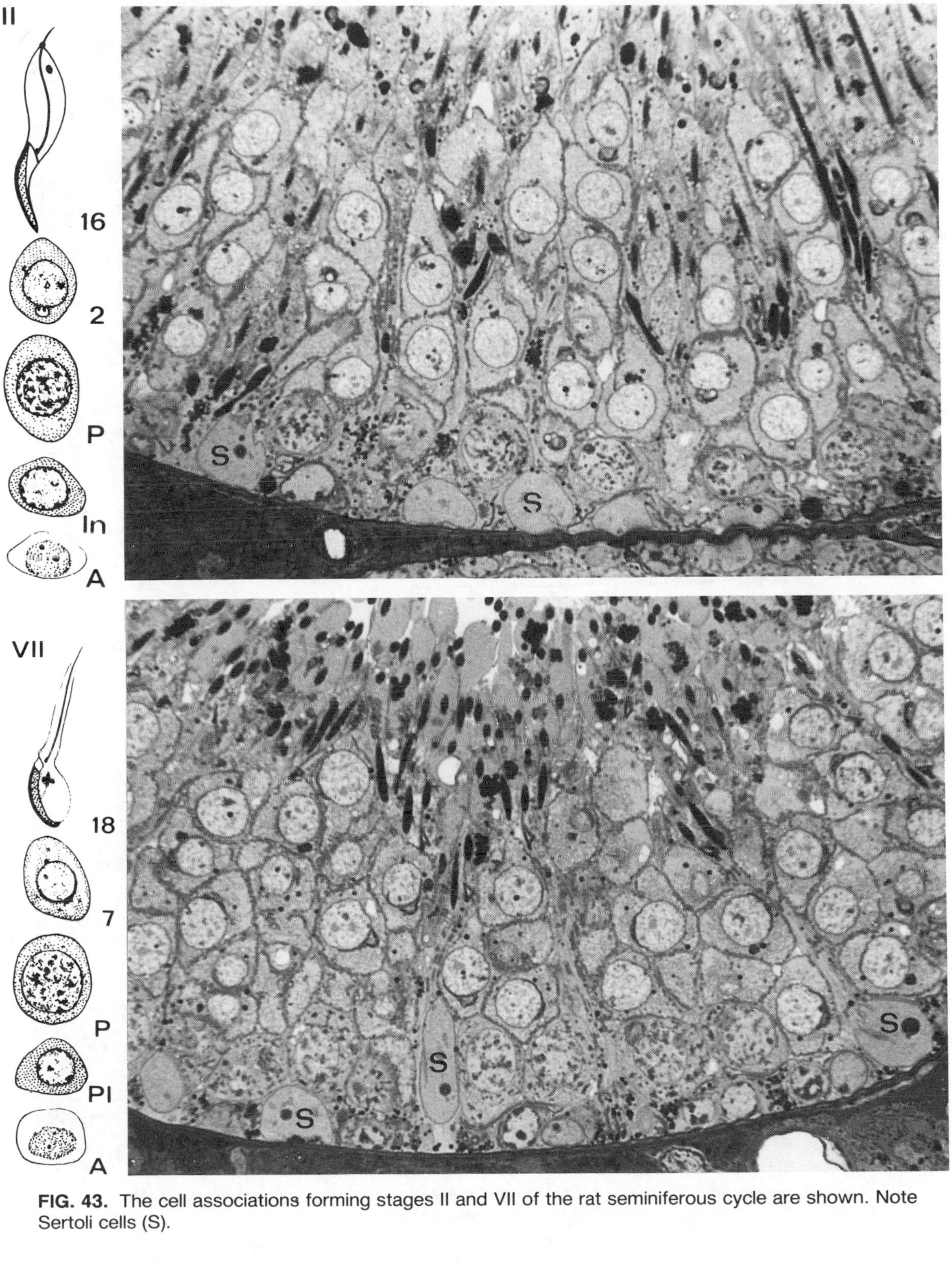

FIG. 43. The cell associations forming stages II and VII of the rat seminiferous cycle are shown. Note Sertoli cells (S).

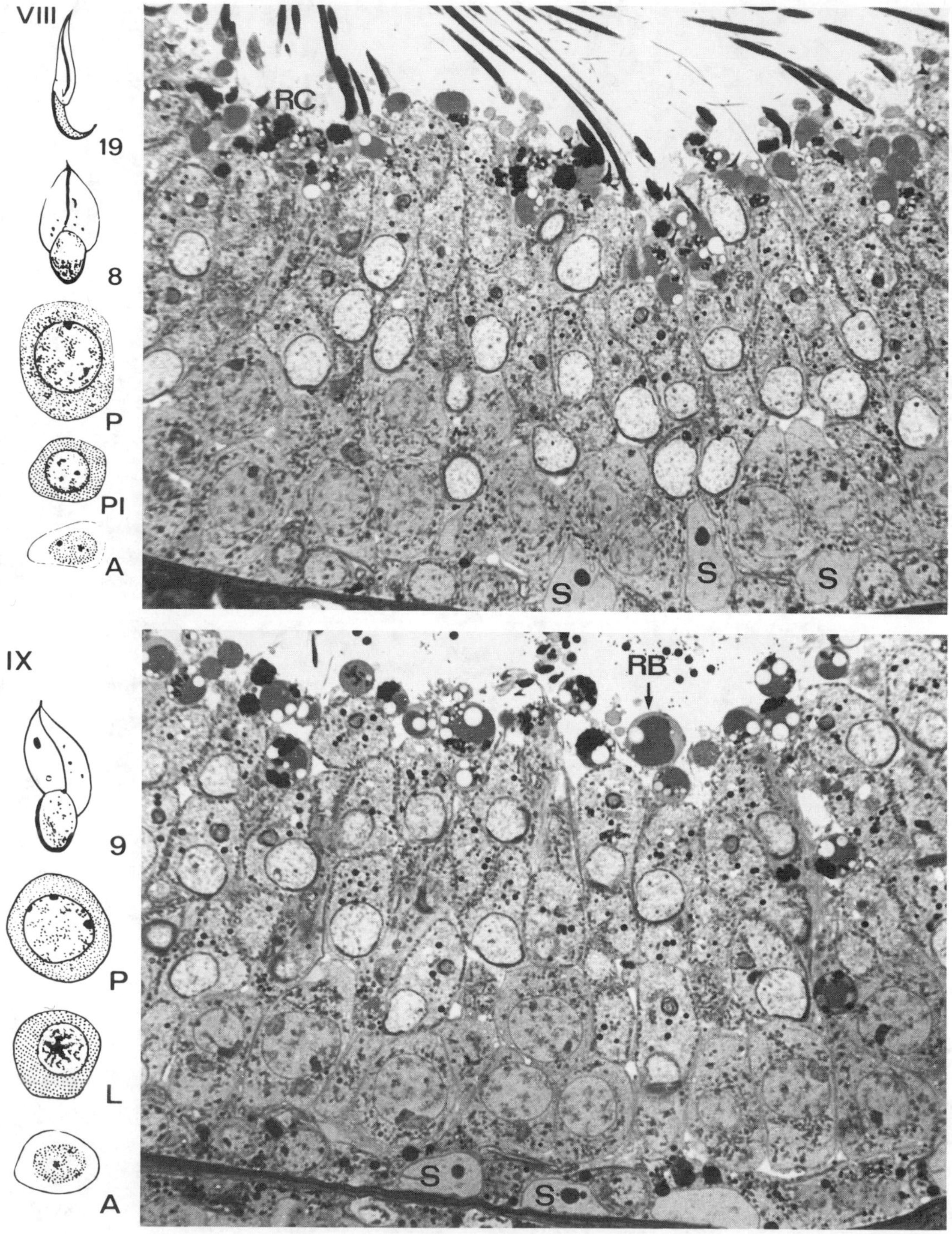

FIG. 44. Cell associations forming stages VIII and early IX of the rat seminiferous cycle. Note residual cytoplasm (RC) and residual bodies (RB). For symbols see Fig. 43.

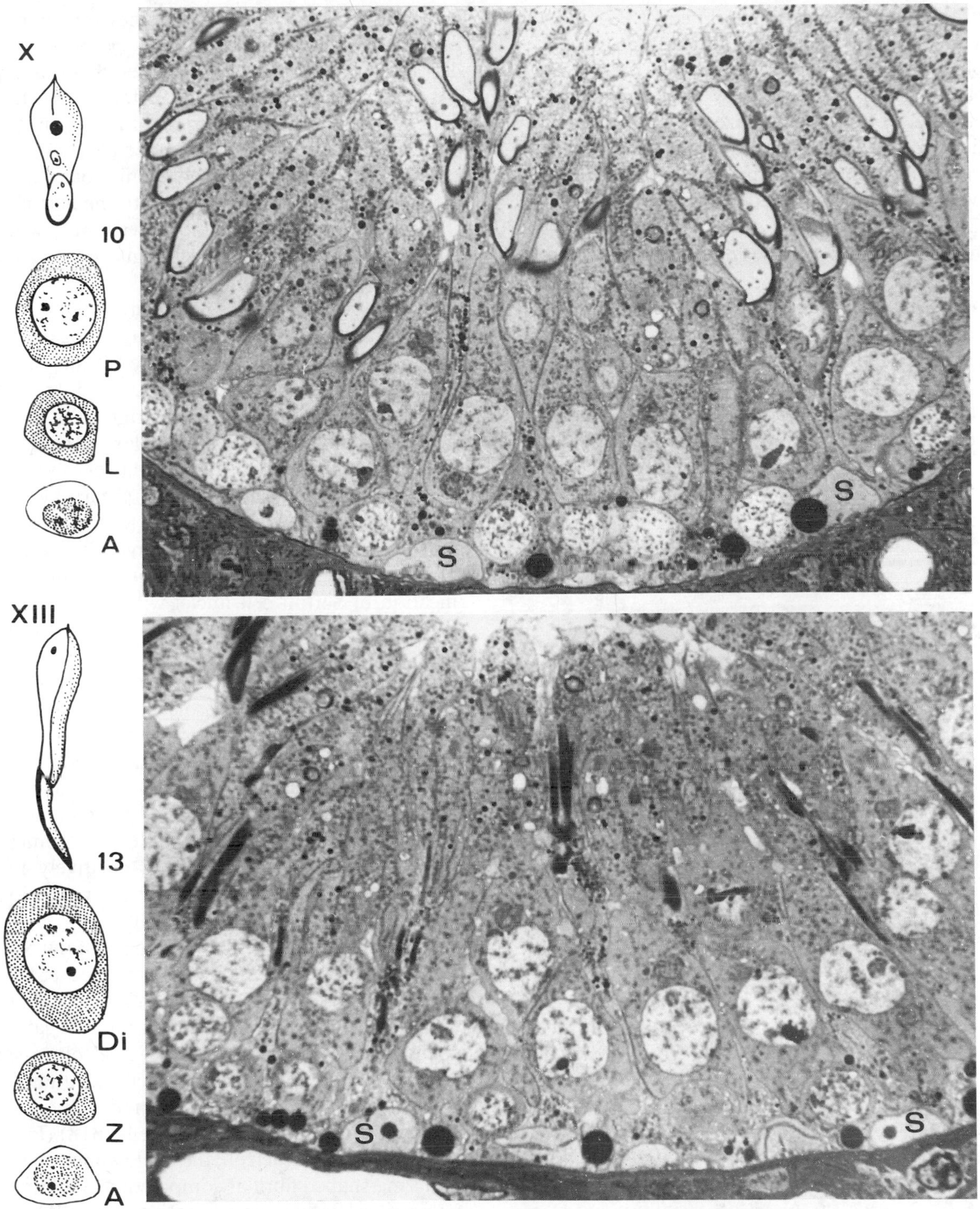

FIG. 45. Cell associations forming stages X and XIII of the rat seminiferous cycle. For symbols see Fig. 43.

brane of the seminiferous tubule (Figs. 12, 13, and 46). Usually they form a single row, although at times they are displaced toward the luminal regions of the seminiferous tubule (Figs. 43–45). Often the nuclear membrane is highly infolded, a feature recognized by light microscopy of plastic-embedded sections, and numerous electron microscope studies of many divergent species have revealed extensive nuclear membrane infoldings (318,327,347, 350,352).

Neither the position nor the many lobulations of the monkey Sertoli cell nucleus exhibited any variations throughout the spermatogenic cycle (347). Similar results were reported for the human Sertoli cell (321,348, 349). However, in rodents, the shape and position of the Sertoli cell nucleus vary according to the stage of the spermatogenic cycle. The nucleus may often be triangular or polygonal in appearance following release of mature spermatids, or alternatively they may appear elongated as the developing elongated spermatids penetrate deeply into the basal aspects of the epithelium (288; Figs. 34–45). Generally, most of the Sertoli cell nuclei remain flattened along the basal lamina of the seminiferous tubule throughout the spermatogenic cycle (167). Within the terminal portions of the seminiferous tubules near their junctions with the tubuli recti, the Sertoli cells exclusively occupy these terminal segments, where their nuclei become closely packed, elongated, and highly irregular in profile (17,353).

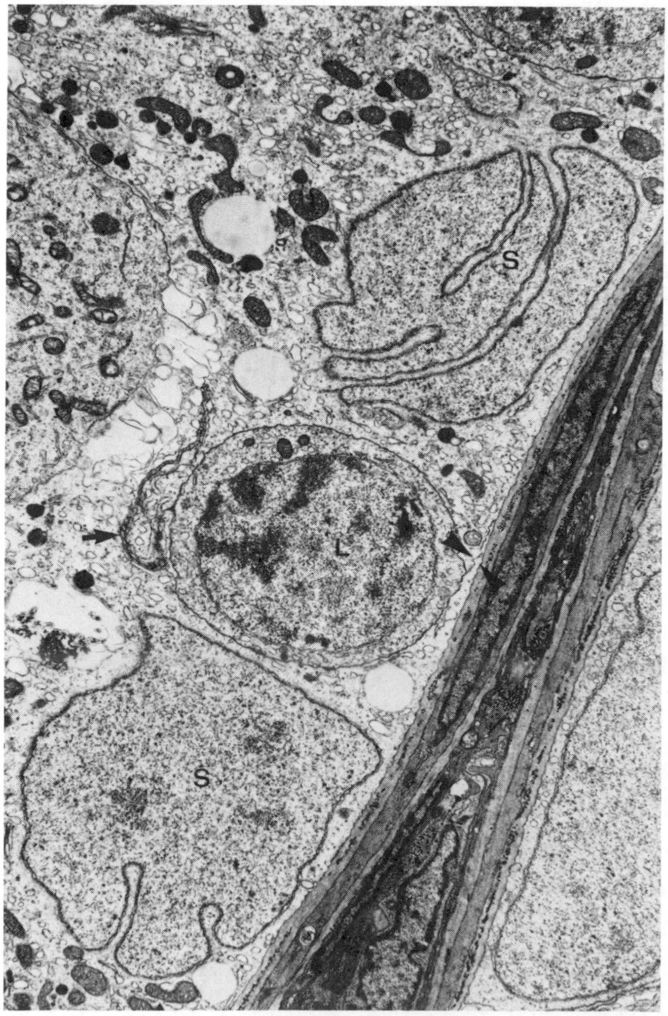

FIG. 46. Basal aspects of two Sertoli cells (S) showing an inter-Sertoli-cell tight junction (*arrow*) above a leptotene primary spermatocyte (L). Note that below the germ cell the opposing surfaces of the Sertoli cells are not associated with specialized junctional complexes (*arrowheads*).

The fine structure of the adult Sertoli cell nucleoplasm in all species so far studied reveals a homogeneous distribution of euchromatin with a fine fibrillogranular texture. Clumps of more densely stained and compact masses of heterochromatin are principally confined to the region of the nucleolar complex, although on rare occasions small heterochromatic masses may occur elsewhere within the nucleoplasm or associated with the nuclear membrane (69,324,338,347). Sertoli cells of the human testis contain a relatively large nucleolus, and its intense staining with basophilic dyes facilitates the identification of Sertoli cell nuclei within the seminiferous epithelium (Fig. 12). Its usual configuration (322,354, 355) resembles a tripartite structure with a central dense compact nucleolar mass, the nucleolonemma proper. From this body, variable projections often extend outward to gain association with two patches of heterochromatin material that flank the central nucleolonemma in a symmetrical relationship. These two laterally associated bodies are at times referred to as the pars amorpha, perinucleolar spheres, satellite karyosomes, or heteropyknotic bodies, which stain positively for DNA with the Feulgen reaction, whereas the nucleolonemma material remains negative (68,318).

Although the tripartite arrangement of the Sertoli cell nucleolus is maintained in rodents and other laboratory species, no close association or contact is established between the central nucleolonemma and the satellite heterochromatin. Nevertheless, the nucleolus is readily identified in rat Sertoli cell nuclei and attains special prominence in size and electron density in mouse, guinea pig, and hamster Sertoli cells (318) (Fig. 41). In mouse Sertoli cell nucleoli, the nucleolonemma contains serial ring-shaped fibrillar components (356) that rapidly incorporate [^{3}H]uridine, indicating sites of RNA synthesis. With the passage of time, the incorporation of labeled uridine occurred within clusters of interchromatin granules at sites distant from the nucleolus, and at later intervals evidence of labeling disappears from the nucleus. More recent studies of mouse nucleoli (357) showed that hybridization with [^{3}H]rRNA has localized to the central nucleolar mass, within which were many fibrillar centers (26% to 41% cell). The latter, together with an interconnecting nucleolar fibrillar network, constitute the site of nucleolus-organizing regions. Autoradiographic studies after [^{3}H]uridine incorporation indicated that rDNA transcription occurred only in the fibrillar nucleolar network, implying that the above-mentioned fibrillar centers are not the site of rRNA gene transcription. Bustos-Obregon and Esponda (349) described unusual granular nuclear bodies, termed sphaeridia, in human Sertoli cells, 0.4 to 1.9 μm in diameter and surrounded by a clear halo 0.08 to 0.1 μm in width (355). Their functional significance remains unknown.

A highly unusual nucleolar morphology has been described for the Sertoli cells of the bull (358–361), which display an aggregation of many membrane-limited vesicles averaging 0.2 to 0.35 μm in diameter and bearing 150-Å granules on their outer surface. Similar structures have been noted in the Sertoli cells of the ram, African buffalo, and gerenuk (a rare antelope of East Africa), and it has been suggested (318) that other ruminant species may display these multivesicular nucleolar bodies. Although these membranous forms of the nucleolus in Sertoli cells resemble those observed in the human endometrium (362) and dark type A spermatogonia (123), their functional duties remain unclarified. Sertoli cell nuclei of the seasonally breeding mallard duck contain bundles of intermediate-size filaments, which have also been observed in mouse and pig Sertoli cells when spermatogenesis is quiescent (363). Many nuclear pores traverse the nuclear membrane (364), which itself is invested with a thin zone of 70-Å cytoplasmic filaments, forming a sheath 150 to 250 nm in thickness, thought to confer structural rigidity to the nucleus and prevent close incursion of cytoplasmic organelles.

Cytoplasm

In general the cytoplasmic components of the Sertoli cell show a polarized distribution: The basal and lower trunk regions of the cytoplasm contain an abundance of organelles and inclusions, whereas the apical extensions usually exhibit a paucity of such structures. Exceptions to this role can be illustrated by preferential distribution of mitochondria, smooth endoplasmic reticulum, and glycogen to the uppermost apical extensions of Sertoli cell cytoplasm in the mouse, squirrel, and human (321,365,366), although it must be emphasized that these arrangements are not often encountered. Sertoli cell mitochondria in the past have been considered to adopt slender or spherical shapes in ultrathin sections (318,319,321), although cup-shaped forms have been noted (321). Analysis of Sertoli cells throughout the rat spermatogenic cycle reveals a greater diversity of mitochondrial form than was previously described (Fig. 46). The mitochondria of this species exhibit S shapes and irregular dumbbell or doughnut-type profiles in addition to the usual elongated and round forms. In all of the species so far examined, the mitochondria have transversely oriented foliate cristae, but the tubular form is often encountered, particularly in the spherical varieties.

Detailed ultrastructural studies of the three-dimensional morphology of the Golgi apparatus have been achieved by high-voltage electron microscopic analysis of semithin and thick (1–7 μm) sections stained with a variety of heavy metal salts (367,368). In rat and mouse testes, the Sertoli cell Golgi apparatus consists of a primary network, visible only by electron microscopy, of perforated membrane sheets interconnected by narrow bridges. When considered in its entirely, the secondary network, detectable by light microscopy, forms a large three-dimensional structure adopting the overall shape of a cylinder that extends in the main body of Sertoli cell cytoplasm from the juxtanuclear region toward the lumen of the seminiferous epithelium. These findings were chiefly confined to stages V–VIII of the spermatogenic cycle, so it is possible that the general architecture of the Golgi apparatus is modified in other stages.

Despite these elegant descriptions of the Golgi membranes of the Sertoli cell, they appear to be devoid of any appreciable numbers of vesicles or condensing vacuoles usually associated with cells actively engaged in the synthesis of proteins destined for transport or secretion (318,319). Similarly, the Sertoli cells contain only limited amounts of rough or granular endoplasmic reticulum, which occurs as several short lengths of parallel cisternae or alternatively takes the form of small individual tubules principally in the base or trunk of the Sertoli cell cytoplasm (321,322,347,354). This is surprising in view of the increasing evidence that the Sertoli cells produce numerous proteins (195,369–371), some of which, such as androgen binding protein, are secreted into the lumen of the tubules. Others, such as the glycoprotein hormone inhibin, must be secreted by the Sertoli cells to circulate in plasma and influence FSH secretion (372–375).

The occurrence of smooth or agranular endoplasmic reticulum has been exhaustively described in studies of the fine structure of the Sertoli cell in vertebrate and invertebrate animals (see reviews, refs. 321,322,327,330, 334,347,350). There is no general morphological pattern that can be applied to a description of the Sertoli cell smooth endoplasmic reticulum, since it has been referred to as vesicular, tubular, cisternal, fenestrated, or lamellar (Figs. 46–48). Species differences may account for such variations in fine structure, but equally, the differential effects of tissue fixation probably contribute substantially to the observed changes in vesicular structure. The true morphology of smooth endoplasmic reticulum is often difficult to preserve faithfully (376–379), making it likely that the descriptions of this organelle derived from some studies merely reflect random ultrastructural alterations.

The most striking arrangements of Sertoli cell smooth endoplasmic reticulum occur in several artiodactyl species (even-toed quadrupeds such as the bull, boar, ram,

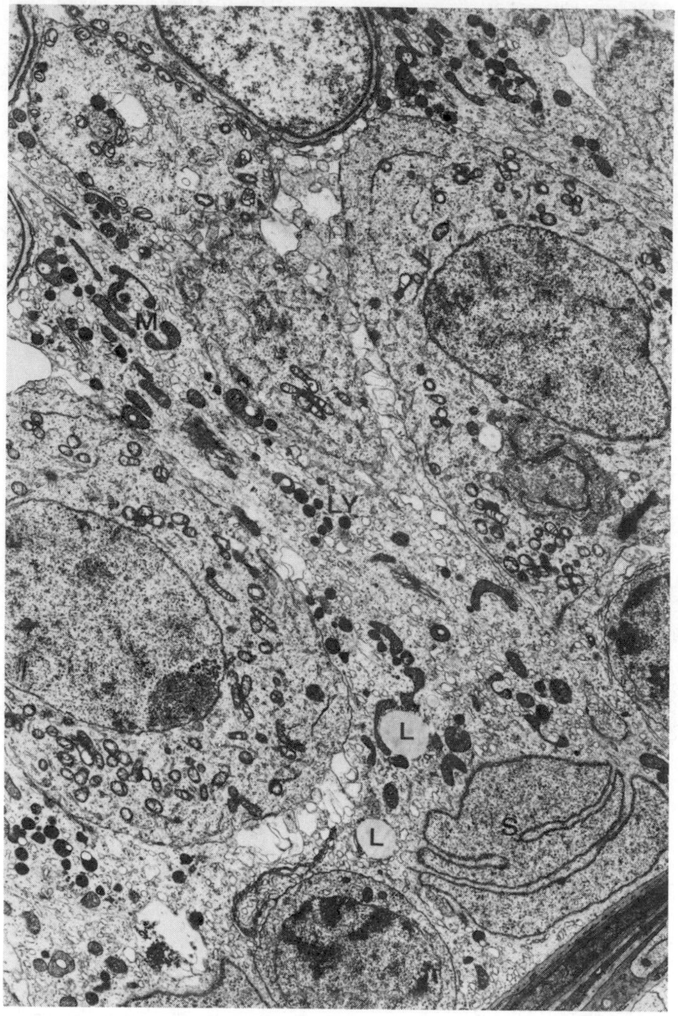

FIG. 47. Stage IX of the rat spermatogenic cycle illustrating the Sertoli cell nucleus (S) and the columnar trunk of the Sertoli cell containing lysosomes (LY), mitochondria (M), and lipid inclusions (L).

antelope, and gazelle), where large compacted masses of smooth membranes invest and surround the developing heads of elongating spermatids (321,322,361,380). A remarkable development of the smooth endoplasmic reticulum in relation to the maturation of spermatids is illustrated by the squirrel, where just prior to sperm release, the spermatid head is retained by the Sertoli cell via its association with very large bulbous projections of Sertoli cell cytoplasm filled with smooth endoplasmic reticulum. After spermiation these membranous masses are transported toward the base of each Sertoli cell (366,381). Multiple concentric layers of smooth endoplasmic reticulum have also been described in the basal aspects of ruminant Sertoli cells, where they surround lipid inclusions (321) or form whorls adjacent to the basement membrane (361,380). In rat Sertoli cells, smooth endoplasmic reticulum undergoes cyclic change in morphology, from tubular to vesicular, in association with the spermatogenic cycle (382,383). To date, however, nothing is known about the functional significance of the often rich supplies of smooth endoplasmic reticulum within the Sertoli cells. However, the ubiquitous occurrence of many or large lipid inclusions within the Sertoli cell cytoplasm has reinforced a long-standing view that in some way the metabolism or synthesis of certain steroid compounds known to occur in isolated Sertoli cells (384,385) is mediated via their distinctive cytoplasmic components, characteristically found in accredited steroidogenic cells.

In parallel to the general uncertainty regarding the role of smooth endoplasmic reticulum in the Sertoli cell, some confusion exists as to the formation, distribution, and fate of Sertoli cell lipid inclusions. A readily recognizable and striking variation in Sertoli cell morphology between different species and between Sertoli cells in different stages of the spermatogenic cycle in a given species is seen in the size and content of their cytoplasmic lipid inclusions (Figs. 43–45). Von Ebner (172) was the first to suggest that the seminiferous epithelium exhibited a cyclic variation in lipid content, and interest in Sertoli cell lipids has received increasing attention in more recent investigations (285,289,318,321,386–389). Recently, these observations have been confirmed by morphometric analysis of Sertoli cells during the spermatogenic cycle in the rat, where a cyclic accumulation and decline in Sertoli cell lipid inclusions has been described (338). Dramatic increases in Sertoli cell lipid content are evident in situations of spermatogenic arrest (e.g., seasonal breeders) or conditions that cause germ cell damage (20,330,390–392), but with the reinitiation of spermatogenesis, the lipids gradually disappear, and the inclusions return to their normal size and number.

Degenerating germ cells and the end products of degenerate lobes of spermatid residual cytoplasm have been considered to provide the source of lipid inclusions (Fig. 49) that accumulate within the Sertoli cell (285,390,393). However, no definite link between the phagocytosis of residual cytoplasm and the content of Sertoli cell lipid inclusions has been demonstrated. In the mouse (286), rat (394), bandicoot (287), human (321), and other species (318), the lipid components of degenerating residual bodies do not appear to be released into the Sertoli cell but are probably degraded entirely. Following the destruction of residual bodies, Sertoli cells in the rat testis actually begin to accumulate lipid inclusions (338).

In support of the notion that cyclic variations in Sertoli cell lipid inclusions represent a balance between lipolysis and synthesis, Bergh (79) found that an increase in Sertoli cell lipid inclusions in the cryptorchid rat testis preceded the phase of germ cell degeneration. Accumulation of Sertoli cell lipid also occurred following induction of cryptorchidism in testes lacking germ cells as a result of prior fetal irradiation (79). It therefore seems

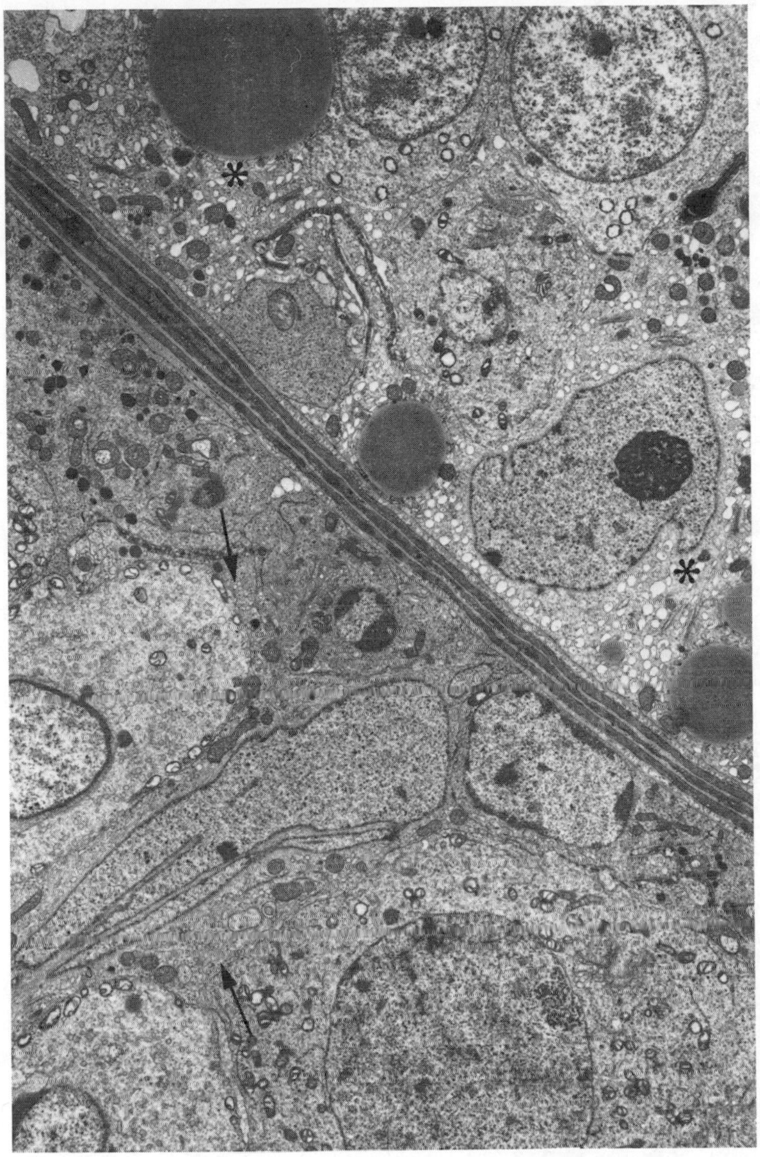

FIG. 48. Rat seminiferous epithelium showing stage 1 (**upper**) with dilated Sertoli cell smooth endoplasmic reticulum (*asterisks*) and stage VII (**lower**) exhibiting tubulovesicular profiles (*arrows*) of Sertoli cell smooth endoplasmic reticulum.

that Sertoli cells are capable of synthesizing lipid in the absence of a contribution of substrates from degenerating germ cells. In this connection, the smooth endoplasmic reticulum enzymes are perhaps responsible for lipid synthesis from glycerol and fatty acids, which, on esterification within the Sertoli cell, become visible as lipid inclusions. This hypothesis is supported by the finding that in mammals and a variety of vertebrate species, Sertoli cell lipid inclusions contain a higher ratio of esterified to unesterified cholesterol than germ cells (305,395, 396). However, none of the above studies have determined a role for lipid within the Sertoli cell, and there is a need for further work to clarify their function.

An unusual type of inclusion body found within the human Sertoli cell is the Charcot–Bottcher crystal. Such filamentous inclusions are of two main types, originally classified according to their length and thickness. Stieve (397) reported that Lubarsch (132) discovered large crystals up to 25 μm in length within the Sertoli cell cytoplasm, which he termed crystals of Charcot–Bottcher. Later Spangaro (398) observed much smaller crystals within the Sertoli cell, and all of these inclusions are now collectively referred to as Charcot–Bottcher crystals (399,400). Readily visible by light microscopy, their ultrastructural features can be summarized as follows: (a) perinuclear, often obliquely oriented in relation to the basal lamina; (b) elongated, fusiform shape, up to 5 μm in width and 10 to 25 μm long; (c) often form simple bifurcations, between which are found glycogen or 10-nm filaments; (d) consist of dense parallel filaments, approximately 150 Å in diameter, that in cross section exhibit zig-zag or meandering profiles; (e) their terminal spikelike ends may be continuous with 9- to 12-nm cytoplasmic filaments (293,294,297). Crystalloids are also

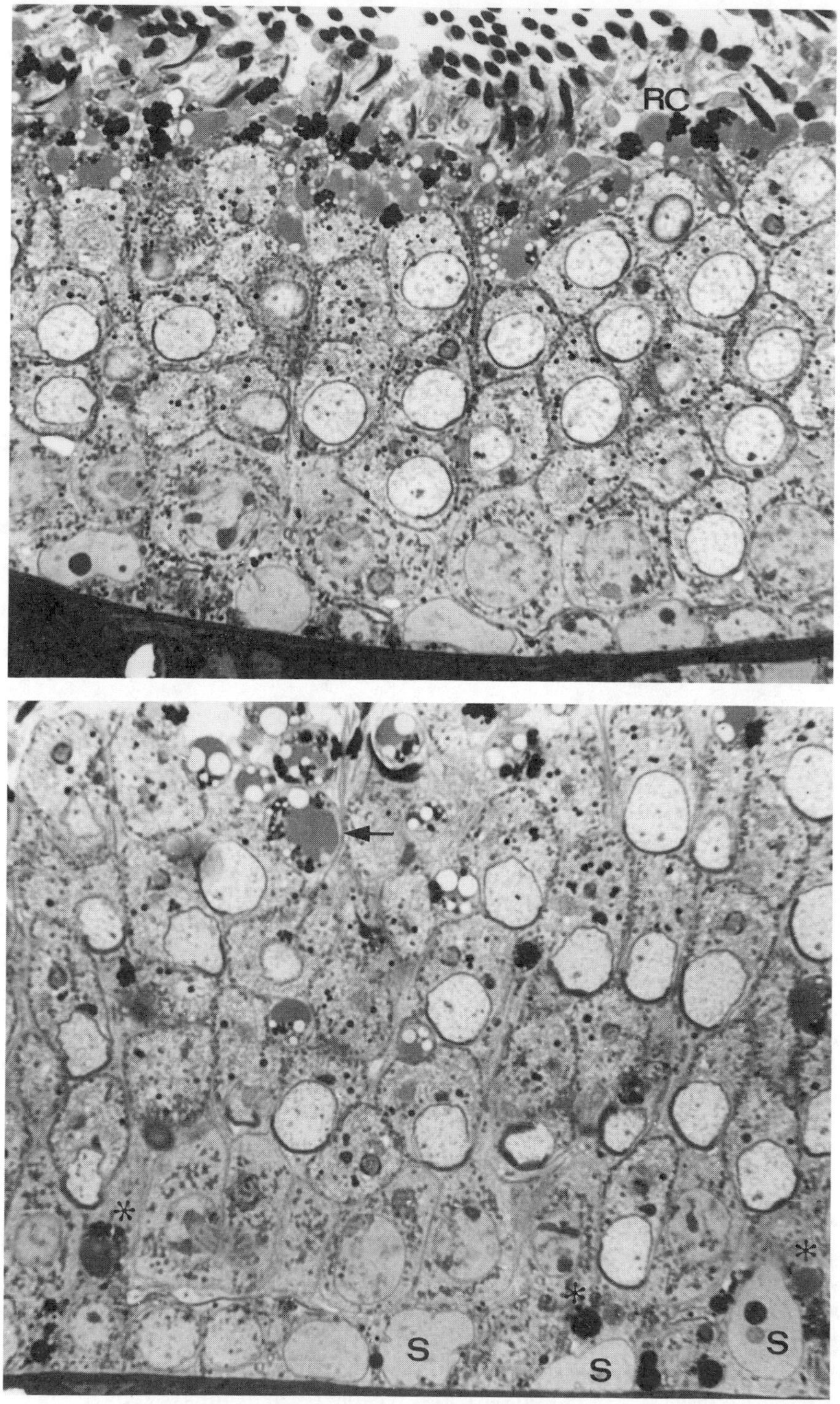

FIG. 49. A: Late stage VII of the rat spermatogenic cycle showing extensive lobes of excess residual cytoplasm (RC) retained by the epithelium as the elongated spermatids are preparing for release into the tubule lumen. **B:** Early stage IX of the rat spermatogenic cycle showing intact (*arrows*) and disintegrating residual bodies (*asterisks*) at various levels within the epithelium. Note Sertoli cell nuclei (S).

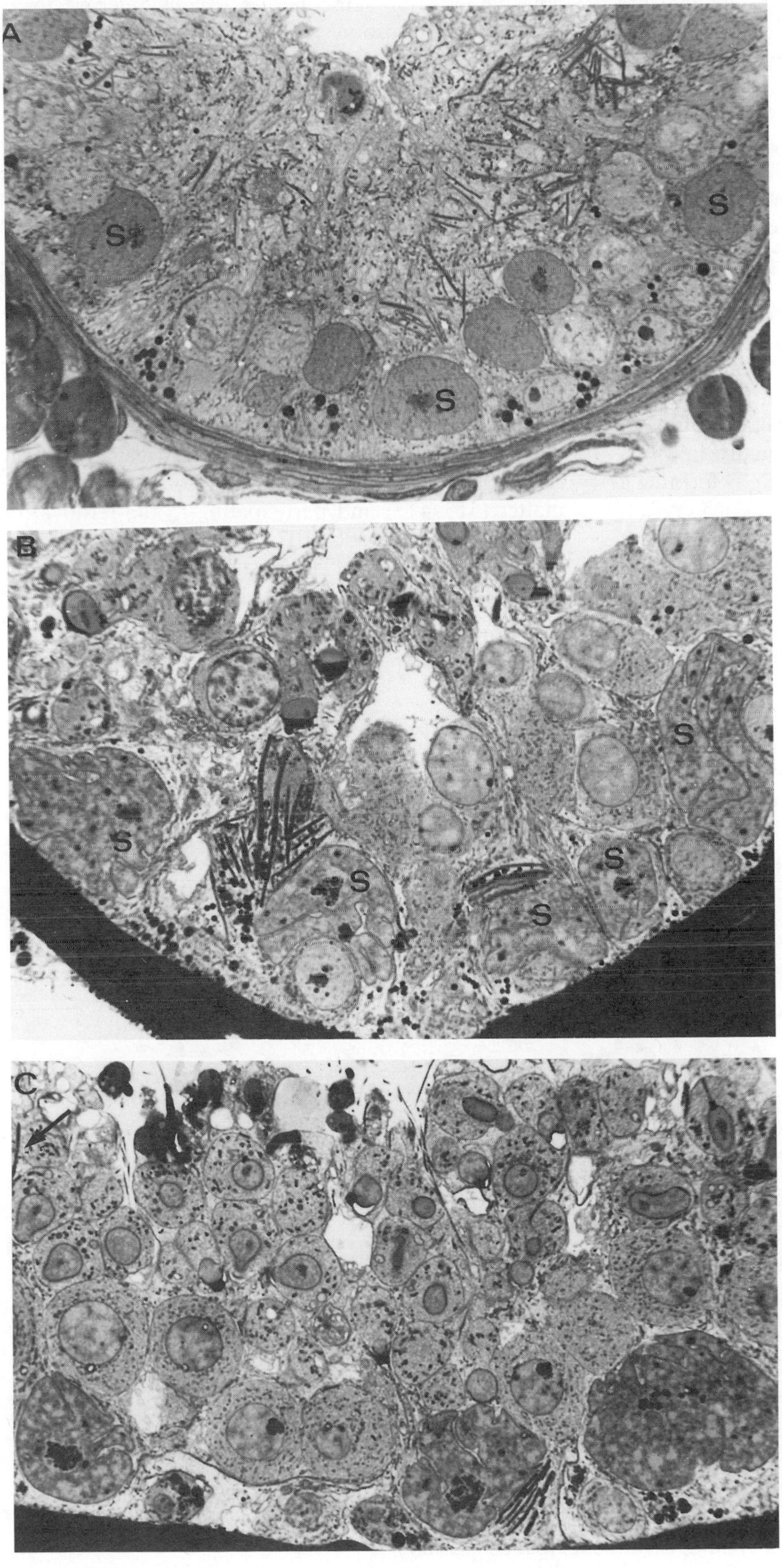

FIG. 50. A: Juvenile koala testis, showing oval-shaped Sertoli cell nuclei (S) and needle-type inclusions in the adluminal cytoplasm. **B:** Late pubertal koala testis showing large Sertoli cell nuclei (S) with clusters of crystalloids in the juxtanuclear cytoplasm. **C:** Adult koala testis showing crystalloid inclusions in the basal Sertoli cell cytoplasm and near the lumen (*arrow*) in association with spermatids. (From Kerr et al., ref. 892, with permission.)

found in Sertoli cells of the pig (401), although they are smaller than those seen in the human and consist of parallel filaments, 50 Å in diameter. These filaments contain actin (402) and thus may be derivatives of the cytoskeleton of the Sertoli cell.

Rodlike crystalloid inclusions have also been described in Sertoli cells of some marsupials, notably the koala (403–405) and the American opossum (406). Recently ultrastructural analysis of koala Sertoli cells (407) confirmed these earlier observations and showed that koala Sertoli cells exhibit extraordinary cytoplasmic crystals, often aligned perpendicular to the basal lamina and in the vicinity of the Sertoli cell nucleus. They are easily visible by light microscopy and occur in prepubertal and adult specimens (Fig. 50). Ultrastructurally they resemble human Charcot–Bottcher crystals, although they exhibit a more highly ordered substructure in which the filaments are arranged in tubules, thereby forming a regular latticework (Figs. 51 and 52). Although crystalloids of koala Sertoli cells are at times associated with cytoplasmic filaments in various configurations, suggesting assembly of or dissociation from the major crystalloid body, their functional duties in this species, the pig, and the human are not clear. Sertoli cells contain variable amounts of dense bodies usually referred to as collections of lysosomes, multivesicular bodies, and heterophagic vacuoles (318,321,347,350). Often these components of the lysosomal system are sequestered in the deepest regions of the Sertoli cell, where they flank the nucleus, but, alternatively, they are seen in large numbers within the upward columnar trunk of the Sertoli cell, where they lie close to developing spermatids (Figs. 46 and 47).

Historically, Maximow (408) originally suggested that the Sertoli cell is active in the phagocytosis of germ cells, and more recent histochemical analysis has revealed the presence of strong hydrolytic enzyme activity in the Sertoli cell (394,409–414), which is principally localized within membrane-limited dense bodies (lysosomes) (394). Sertoli cells are thus equipped with a well-developed cytoplasmic digestive system capable of ingesting injected dyes and certain foreign particulate matter (415–417) and participating in the removal of degenerating germ cells (107,270).

The disposal of the excess spermatid cytoplasm left behind by the mature sperm as they are released from the luminal surface of the Sertoli cells (Fig. 49) has received much attention ever since it was recognized by Regaud

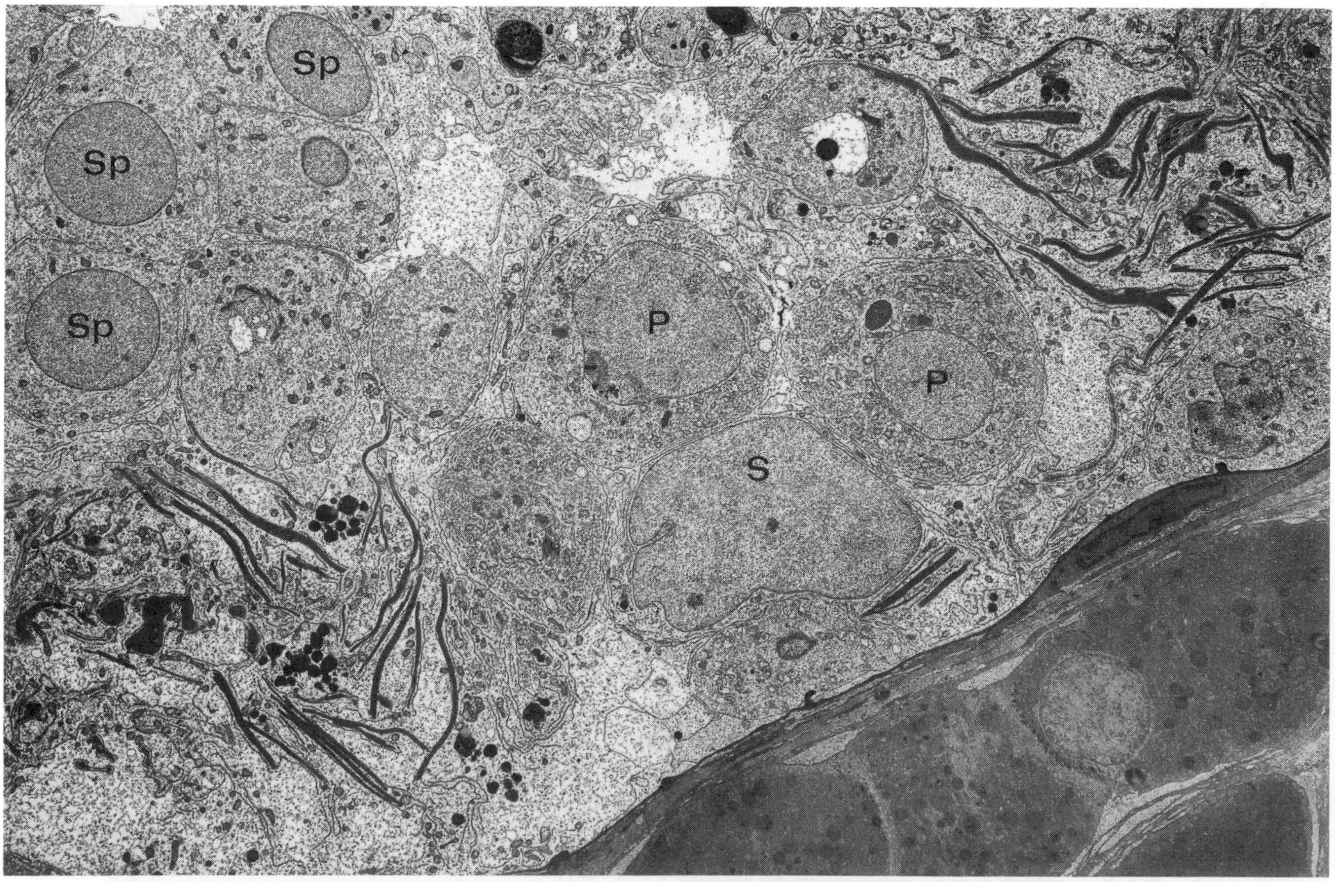

FIG. 51. Ultrastructure of koala seminiferous epithelium showing numerous crystalloid inclusions within the basal Sertoli cell cytoplasm. Sertoli cell nucleus (S), pachytene primary spermatocytes (P), and round spermatids (Sp) are shown. (From Kerr et al., ref. 892, with permission.)

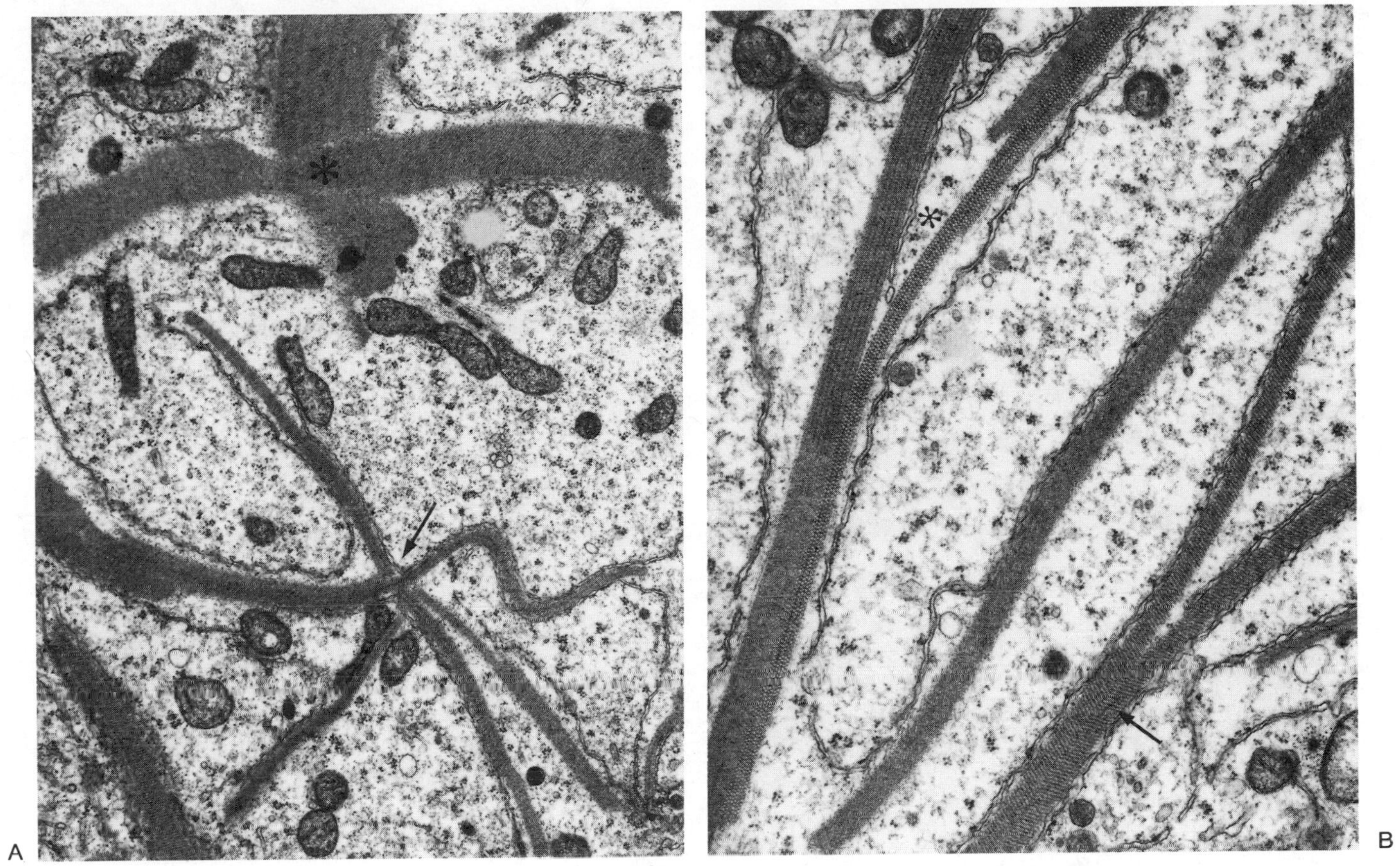

FIG. 52. **A:** Koala Sertoli cell crystalloids exhibiting cross (*asterisk*) and star-like configurations (*arrow*). **B:** Bifurcation of crystalloids showing that their individual arms may present differing substructures (*asterisk*). A bipennate crystalloid is shown (*arrow*). (From Kerr et al., ref. 892, with permission.)

in 1901 (27) that the Sertoli cells were probably responsible for the phagocytosis and destruction of the excess residual cytoplasm. Regaud described their disposal in four steps: (a) release into the lumen; (b) resorption within the Sertoli cells; (c) peripheral migration deep into the epithelium; (d) transformation into "Sertoli hyaline" spheres that blacken in the presence of osmic acid. Since then the formation (Figs. 53–57) and fate of residual bodies has been studied by light and electron microscopy (285,286,318,338,347,382,418), but the mechanisms by which the residual bodies are eliminated by the Sertoli cells was not resolved by these studies.

Recent examination of the lysosomal apparatus of the Sertoli cells has now shed light on this process. When electron-dense tracers were introduced into the lumen of seminiferous tubules, they were actively incorporated into the apical regions of the Sertoli cells by means of small vesicles formed at the cell surface (419,420), suggesting a process of fluid-phase endocytosis (pinocytosis). The tracers internalized by this process are eliminated by the lysosomes in the columnar and basal regions of Sertoli cell cytoplasm (424). These studies have been extended (422) to an investigation of the endocytic and phagocytic properties of the Sertoli cell using native ferritin and protein–gold complexes to demonstrate fluid-phase endocytosis and cationic ferritin and concanavalin A ferritin to identify absorptive endocytosis. The latter process occurs when molecules initially bind to the cell surface prior to internalization by small vesicles. The results indicate that fluid-phase endocytosis by rat Sertoli cells occurs in all stages of the spermatogenic cycle. At stages VIII and IX the lysosomes formed as a consequence of this process fuse with the newly formed residual bodies and transform them into phagolysosomes, whereupon they disintegrate at the base of the Sertoli cell (Fig. 58). The formation of lysosomes and their participation in the dissolution of residual bodies thus provide a link between the endocytic and phagocytic activities of the Sertoli cell. Adsorptive endocytosis occurred principally during stage VII, when various phagocytic vacuoles form close to the heads of late spermatids, where they probably play a role in resorption of the specialized tubulobulbar complexes that anchor the spermatid head to the apical cytoplasmic processes of the Sertoli cells.

Scant attention has been accorded to the presence of concentric layers of smooth membranes usually confined to the basal aspects of the human Sertoli cell

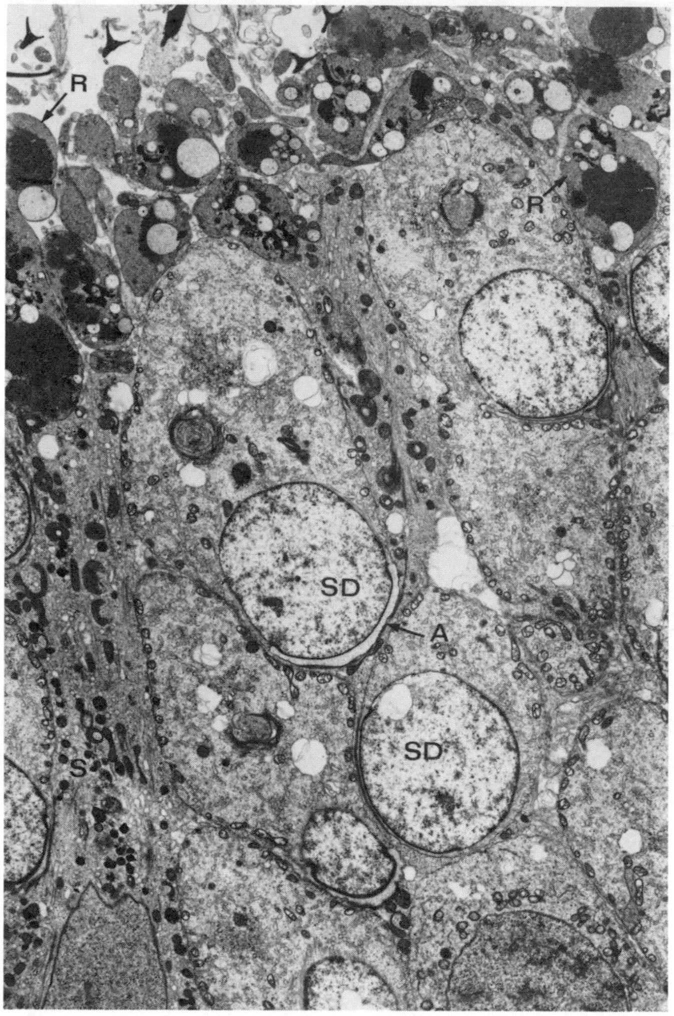

FIG. 53. Stage VIII of the rat spermatogenic cycle illustrating a tall columnar Sertoli cell (S), spermatids (SD) with acrosomal cap (A), and many lobes of residual cytoplasm (R).

(218,296,297,351,400). Because of the presence of pore-like complexes that form a bridgework between parallel profiles of these membranes (321,350), they have been likened to annulate lamellae that have been described in other tissues (423–426). Although their function in the Sertoli cell remains unknown, the annulate lamellae have been implicated in RNA transport from the nucleus (427), protein synthesis (425,426,428), and the site of tubulin synthesis or polymerization of microtubules (429).

As would be expected for a cell that is obliged to alter its shape radically in conforming to the ever-changing events within the seminiferous epithelium, all Sertoli cells so far studied are endowed with an elaborate cytoskeleton together with contractile elements occupying most parts of the cytoplasmic matrix (285,286). The former component, responsible for maintenance of cell shape and the redistribution of the cytostolic gel matrix, is attributed to an often extensive and intricate system of micro- (60–70 Å) and intermediate filaments (100 Å). Together these dense filamentous networks are thought to play a major role in structural support of the Sertoli cell when rigidity is necessary, and at other times it is thought that they engineer changes in cell matrix viscosity, allowing variable degrees of plasticity that are essential to accommodate the constant mobility of the germ cells. These filaments are rich in actin (430–432) and vimentin (431–434). Concentrations of filaments occur at the very base of the Sertoli cell adjacent to the basal lamina, around the Sertoli cell nucleus in the columnar cytoplasm, where they course parallel to the cell axis, and also in association with numerous ectoplasmic specializations. The latter attain a close proximity to developing spermatids and form junctional complexes between neighboring Sertoli cells in the basal aspects of the epithelium.

Especially rich supplies of filaments are seen to fill the cytoplasm of many monkey Sertoli cells in the terminal segments of the seminiferous tubules (17), although the reason for their abundance is not clear. Study of the structure–function relationships of the Sertoli cell cytoskeleton in the ground squirrel has added much to an understanding of the mechanisms underlying shape change (337). The Sertoli cells of the squirrel were chosen for investigation because the seminiferous epithelium contains relatively small numbers of germ cells compared to other species (320), and the Sertoli cells undergo dramatic shape changes. It now seems likely, based on the results obtained from squirrel Sertoli cells (337,381), that actin-rich filaments in ectoplasmic specializations are devoid of myosin and, rather than fulfilling a contractile role, probably stabilize the cortical cytoplasm of Sertoli cells at the sites where they occur. Perhaps the filaments maintain the shape of Sertoli cell crypts embracing the penetrating clones of spermatids (298,435) and may add reinforcement to the zone of Sertoli cell ectoplasm at the level of the basal junctional complexes between adjacent Sertoli cells.

If filaments associated with ectoplasmic specializations are not contractile, then what generates the forces necessary for alterations in Sertoli cell shape? New light has been shed on this problem following the recent demonstration that exposure of Sertoli cells to colchicine causes severe disruption of germ cell movements and blocks intracellular transport of membranous organelles (366). Administration of colchicine *in vivo* destroyed virtually all Sertoli cell microtubules, indicating that they play a significant part in molding and sculpturing the Sertoli cell cytoplasm to facilitate upward and downward movements of germ cells. Additionally, these studies offered a new interpretation of the mechanism by which Sertoli cells participate in sperm release. Earlier studies (436–438) favored the view that microtubules were involved with shedding of spermatids from the apex of the Sertoli cell. Others (439) proposed that the

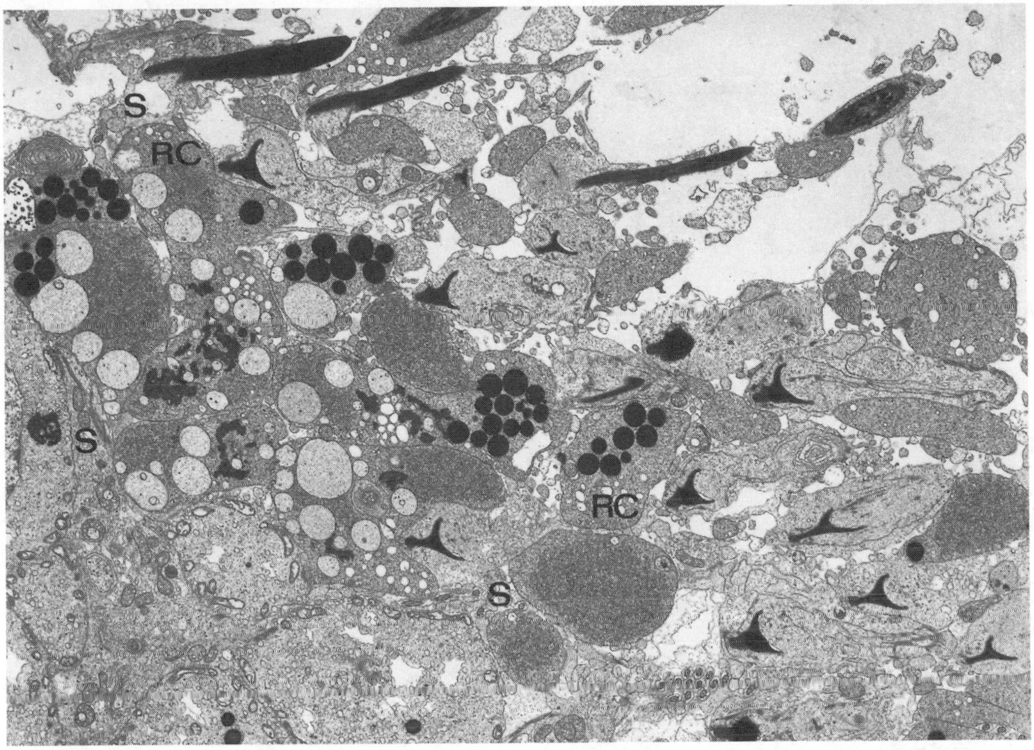

FIG. 54. Stage VII of the rat spermatogenic cycle, showing formation of many lobes of excess spermatid residual cytoplasm (RC) lodged between extensions of Sertoli cell cytoplasm (S).

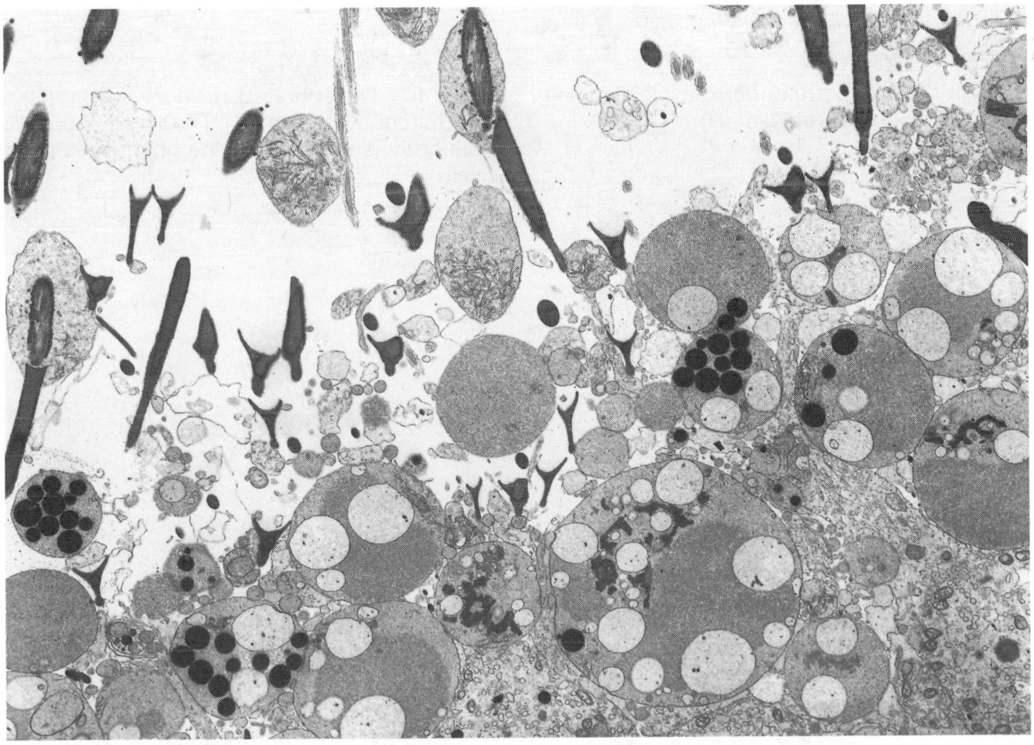

FIG. 55. At stage VIII of the rat spermatogenic cycle, lobes of residual cytoplasm adopt spherical shapes, which characterize the formation of residual bodies.

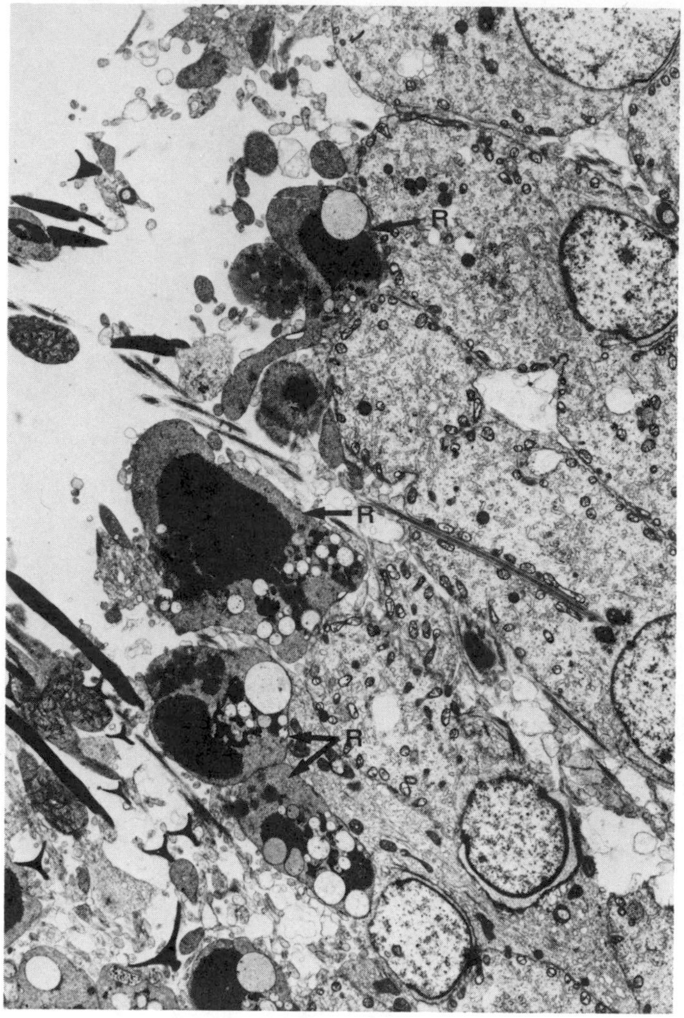

FIG. 56. Stage VIII of the rat spermatogenic cycle showing large irregular lobes of residual cytoplasm (R).

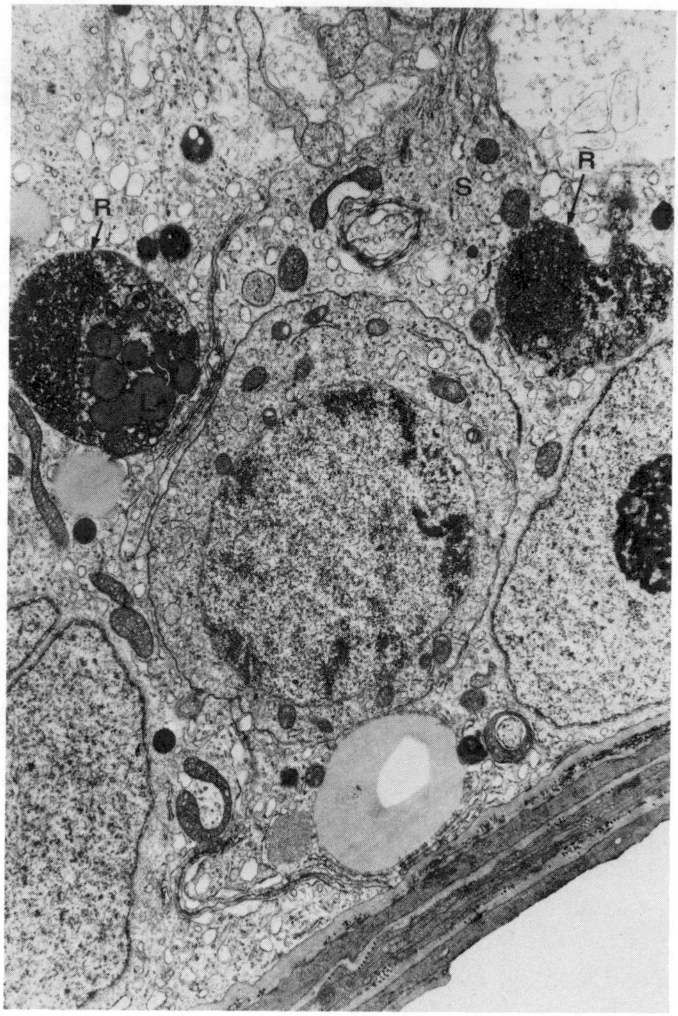

FIG. 57. Degenerated residual bodies (R) deep within the Sertoli cell cytoplasm (S). The lipid component (L) of the residual body is resistant to the phagocytic action of the Sertoli cell.

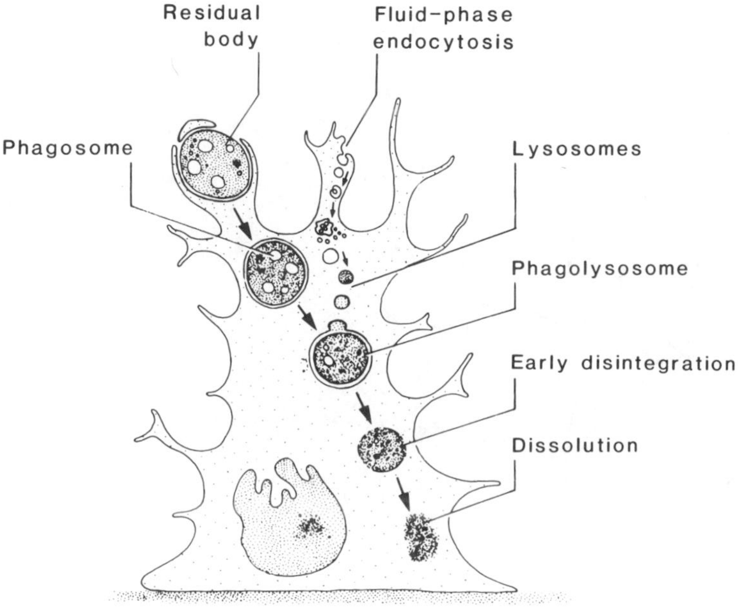

FIG. 58. Representation of phagocytosis of residual bodies and fluid-phase endocytosis by the Sertoli cell. These processes may be integrated to allow disintegration of the residual bodies as they proceed through the body of the Sertoli cell. (Modified from Morales et al., ref. 422.)

sloughing of many spermatids into the lumen of the seminiferous tubule after colchicine treatment was caused by Sertoli cell disruption rather than a selective interference with Sertoli cell microtubules. When the effects of colchicine were reinvestigated (366), late spermatids were not shed from the Sertoli cells, and the special ectoplasmic regions adjacent to spermatid heads remained intact, as did those subjacent to basal tight junctions between Sertoli cells.

As yet no adequate explanation has been offered to account for the role of those filaments that are found in random orientations throughout the Sertoli cell cytoplasm. The role of microtubules in generating shape changes within the Sertoli cells has been more clearly defined following the demonstration of regional variations in their intracellular distribution. In the rat Sertoli cell, microtubules are abundant in the deep crypts that accommodate elongating spermatids but are absent in regions associated with early germ cells (440). Running parallel to the long axis of the Sertoli cell trunk, microtubules also conform to the contours of the developing spermatid heads (440,441), and electrophoretic studies of isolated preparations of microtubule-associated proteins have shown the presence of dyneinlike proteins similar to those with axons (442). It seems likely, therefore, that Sertoli cell microtubules are potential candidates for intracellular transport of organelles and provide the motor pathways for translocation of germ cells within the seminiferous epithelium.

Surface Specializations

A well-recognized property of the testis is the maintenance, within the seminiferous tubules, of a highly specialized microenvironment created by the Sertoli cells that partitions young and more mature germ cells into two compartments within the seminiferous epithelium. At this point it is pertinent to acknowledge the contribution of earlier studies to this topic. Together these numerous observations led to the discovery of a blood–testis barrier that exists in the testes of phylogenetically distant species and thus reinforces the fundamental importance of the Sertoli cell in the regulation of spermatogenesis.

Early this century physiological studies by Ribbert (443), Bouffard (404), and Pari (445) indicated that the testis was one of the few organs into which intravenously injected dyes did not gain entry. No significance was assigned to these initial observations or to more recent work reporting similar results (446,447). The vascular network of the testicular interstitial tissue is highly permeable to large molecules, as demonstrated by Everett and Simmons (448) when they noted that intravenously injected serum albumin had a rapid rate of extravascular transfer and readily permeated into the interstitium. Many other substrates were found to diffuse readily from the testicular blood vessels into the interstitial lymphatics but did not appear in the fluid collected from the rete testis. Thus, a blood–testis permeability barrier seemed to be anatomically located either surrounding or actually within the wall of the seminiferous tubules (71,449–453).

In common laboratory rodents, the penetration of electron-dense markers from the blood vasculature into the seminiferous tubules is partly retarded by peritubular myoid cells. This incomplete barrier is not found in the ram, bull, boar, or primate (318,319), and in all species, the effective component of the blood–testis barrier resides within the seminiferous epithelium. In the light of this evidence, closer examination of the ultrastructural features of the seminiferous epithelium revealed the presence of various types of tight junctions or desmosome-like structures associated with the plasma membrane of the Sertoli cell (177,218,358,400). Brokelmann (189) originally provided a clear illustration of these inter-Sertoli-cell junctions in a variety of animals. We noted that whenever the boundaries of the Sertoli cell were apposed, they formed complex cytoplasmic membranes immediately adjacent to and parallel with the limiting plasma membrane. These profiles were apparently cisternae of endoplasmic reticulum, and in a study of the postnatal development of the mouse testis, Flickinger (70) again observed a similar type of junction and noted that these specializations between Sertoli cells increased in numbers with the onset of meiosis and the formation of a tubule lumen.

Junctional specializations were not seen in the testes of fetal or neonatal cattle or dogs, and Nicander (175) proposed that in adult testes the junctions might restrict the intercellular passage of substances to germ cells. These morphological studies were complemented by physiological work indicating that the barrier was absent at birth, but with sexual maturation, the previously unrestricted transport of acriflavine dyes was prevented concomitant with meiotic maturation of the primary spermatocytes (71). Since then, the ultrastructural features of inter-Sertoli-cell junctions have been documented in many excellent descriptions (74,303,317–319,347,454–457) and are summarized in Figs. 59–61 and as follows: (a) Junctional specializations between Sertoli cells are particularly prominent in the basal regions, the seminiferous epithelium, and usually occur when adjacent Sertoli cell cytoplasmic processes meet. (b) Sometimes, at the very base of the Sertoli cell adjacent to the basal lamina, the meeting of two apposed Sertoli cell cytoplasmic processes may be devoid of junctional specialization. (c) The basal location of junctional specializations circumscribing the lateral margins of Sertoli cells is anatomically reversed compared to tight junctional specializations present in many other epithelia. (d) Normally a space of 150 to 200 Å separates the outer leaflets of adjacent Sertoli cell membranes. (e) Occasionally this space

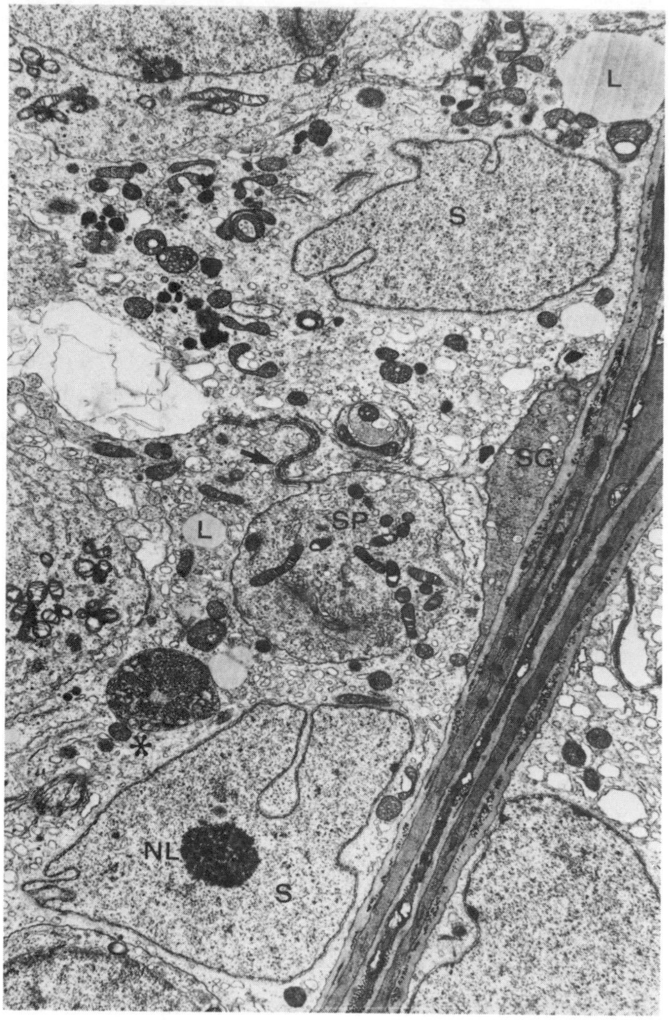

FIG. 59. Basal aspects of the rat seminiferous epithelium illustrating two Sertoli cells (S), one containing a large nucleolus (NL). Note inter-Sertoli-cell junction (*arrow*) and cytoplasm of an early primary spermatocyte (SP) and a basally situated spermatogonium (SG). A degenerated residual body (*asterisk*) and lipid inclusions (L) are shown.

is narrowed to 20 Å similar to the traditional gap junction or nexus of other cells. (f) In thin sections studied by transmission electron microscopy, multiple sites of fusion of the outer membrane leaflets are seen at regular intervals along the cell-to-cell interfaces. (g) Sertoli cell junctions are often flanked by parallel cisternae of endoplasmic reticulum, irregularly fenestrated and exhibiting ribosomes toward the cell body, but are agranular on the ectoplasmic face. (h) Sandwiched between the cisternae and cell surface, bundles of fine filaments are oriented parallel to the cell surface and, in transverse views, are packed in hexagonal arrays.

With the advent of freeze-cleaving methods, the multiple focal sites of fusion between Sertoli cell membranes were shown to extend entirely around the circumference of the cell and consisted of long parallel rows of intramembranous particles intercalated with matching grooves (74,317–319,364,458,459). This collar of junctional specialization occupies approximately 4% of the surface area of the plasma membrane in the rat Sertoli cell (325). Up to 50 parallel lines of membrane fusion between adjacent surfaces of Sertoli cells together constitute a highly effective barrier against the intraepithelial penetration of the spaces between cells residing in the base of the seminiferous epithelium (347,454,456). The capacity of inter-Sertoli-cell junctions to maintain cell adhesion was convincingly demonstrated after ligation of the efferent ductules, a procedure causing marked distention of the seminiferous tubules. Junctions between Sertoli cells fail to separate regardless of the degree of tubular distension (455). Recent studies of the permeability properties of inter-Sertoli-cell tight junctions have shown a progressive loss of impermeability from the base

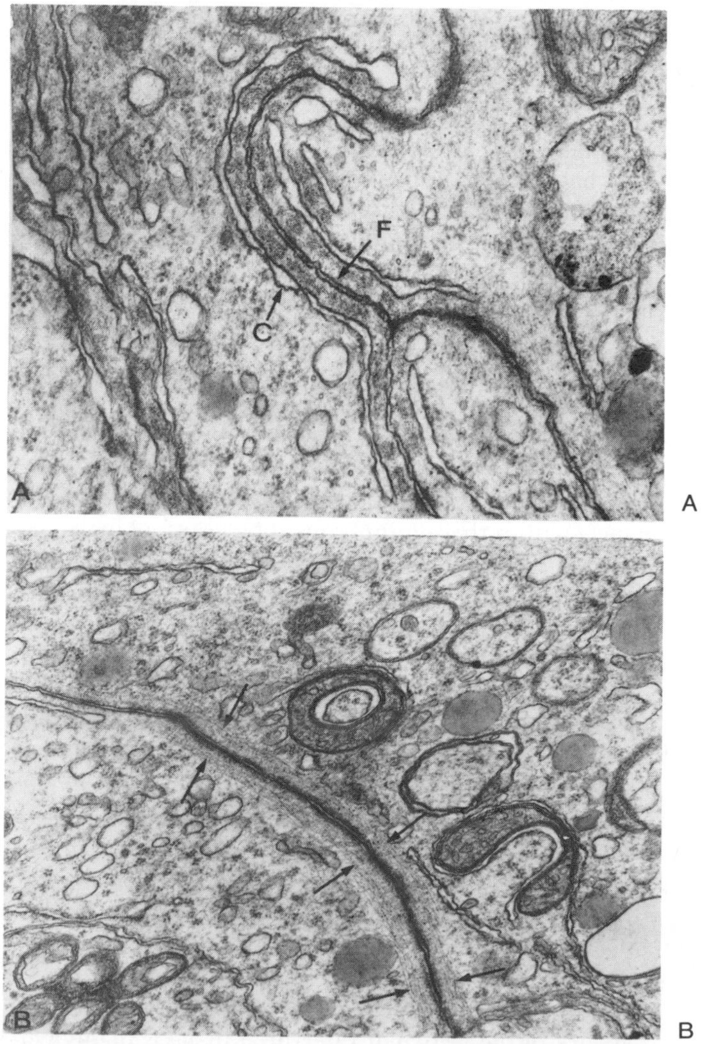

FIG. 60. A: Inter-Sertoli-cell junction illustrating bundles of filaments (F) adjacent to the Sertoli cell plasma membrane. Smooth-surfaced cisternae (C) run parallel to the opposed surfaces of the Sertoli cells. **B:** Longitudinal profile of an inter-Sertoli-cell junction showing parallel arrays of filaments (*arrows*).

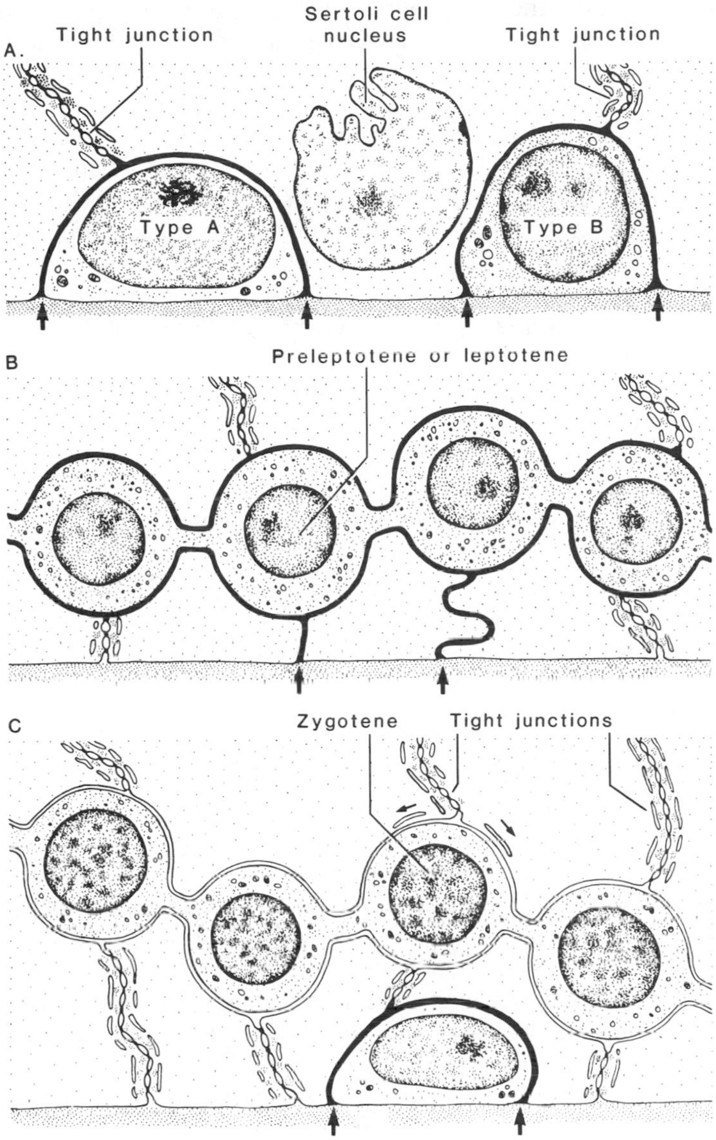

FIG. 61. Diagram illustrating the upward migration of germ cells from the basal aspect of the seminiferous epithelium toward the lumen. In each diagram, tracer entry into the intercellular spaces is shown by *large arrows*. (Modified from Dym and Cavicchia, ref. 460.) **A:** The entry of tracers into the seminiferous epithelium is prevented by the occluding inter-Sertoli-cell tight junctions. **B:** Preleptotene and lepototene primary spermatocytes are displaced above the basal lamina. Tight junctions are seen below, above, or both below and above these cells, and consequently tracers are able to surround the interconnected cells via cytoplasmic bridges. Tight junctions above the germ cells prevent further passage of tracers into the seminiferous epithelium. **C:** When leptotene primary spermatocytes enter the zygotene phase of meiotic prophase, tracers do not surround zygotene spermatocytes, since tight junctions are formed beneath these cells. Dissociation of inter-Sertoli-cell junctions into hemijunctions has been suggested and is indicated by *small arrows*.

to the lumen of the seminiferous tubule, which is correlated with increasing incidence of disintegration of the junctional complex (75).

The strategic and unusual location of Sertoli cell tight junctions in relation to the germ cells has given rise to the concept of an anatomic and functional subdivision of the seminiferous epithelium into (a) a basal compartment containing spermatogonia, preleptotene, and leptotene primary spermatocytes and (b) an adluminal component beyond the level of the tight junctions that sequesters the more differentiated germ cells into a unique physiological environment (317,347,456). Some species differ in the precise manner in which germ cells ascend from the basal to the adluminal compartment, thereby breaching the barrier maintained by the Sertoli cell tight junctions. In the macaque testis, leptotene primary spermatocytes reside in the basal subdivision and, with their upward mobilization, mature into zygotene primary spermatocytes on reaching the adluminal compartment (460). In the rat, the transition from basal to adluminal regions has been suggested to occur through the agency of a short-lived intermediate compartment embodying some leptotene primary spermatocytes (461). This transit chamber is flanked above and below by tight junctional complexes, i.e., neither truly basal (permeable to blood-borne substances) nor adluminal (impermeable to blood-borne substances). Further research will be necessary to establish if the so-called intermediate compartment provides a special physiological milieu different from either the basal or the adluminal compartment.

Whatever the histological organization of the testis, some form of intraepithelial junctional specialization is always localized in the somatic cells surrounding the germ cells, suggesting that the blood–testis barrier is an ancient evolutionary trait of central importance for the successful development of viable gametes. In broad terms the ultrastructural organization of the inter-Sertoli-cell junctions can be classified into three main types based principally on the type of membrane specialization. The testes of mammals show a complex organization of the blood–testis barrier, and in species described to date, the arrangement described above is virtually unchanged. Examples can be found in studies of rodents (mouse, rat, guinea pig, squirrels), ruminants (bull, ram, goat), domesticated carnivores (dog and cat), and primates (macaque and human). A group exhibiting somewhat simpler organization of the junctional complexes in that they often lack the bundles of actin-rich filaments and subsurface membranous cisternae is illustrated by birds and reptiles (322,334,462). A simple arrangement serving the function of a blood–testis barrier is peculiar to amphibians and fish, where only desmosomelike and short tight junctions are observed between Sertoli cells (298,331,463–468). In other groups, however, the form of barrier is less well defined, and in nematodes and insects, the occurrence of small septate, desmosomelike, and tight junctions is seen as the structural basis of the blood–testis barrier (465, 469–471).

Despite all the abovementioned studies, very little is known about the actual physiological role of the blood–testis barrier (82). The formation of inter-Sertoli-cell junctions coincides with the cessation of Sertoli cell proliferation in the immature testis (44), and junctions make their appearance as germ cells proceed through the zygotene to pachytene steps of meiotic maturation (72,74,76,460). However, the junctions also appear in the absence of germ cells (47,78,79) or in response to gonadotropic stimulation of the Sertoli cells (86), but their formation is dependent on the transformation of Sertoli cells from an immature to an adult-type morphology. Since early primary spermatocytes (leptotene or zygotene) reside in the basal compartment of the mammalian seminiferous epithelium, and similar observations are reported in lower orders of animals (331), then evidently the initiation of meiotic maturation does not require the specialized intratubular milieu provided within the confines of the adluminal epithelial compartment. In the rat testis as the primary spermatocytes enter prophase, cell surface antigens specific to germ cells appear on pachytene primary spermatocytes and all subsequent stages of germ cell differentiation (472–475). Specific antigens also appear on the surface of Sertoli cells (476), and it has been suggested that the processes of meiotic maturation and differentiation of spermatids occurs in an immunologically privileged adluminal microenvironment via the inter-Sertoli-cell tight junctions (82,477). Isolation of these germ cells by the blood–testis barrier either restricts leakage of antigen or prevents entry of antibodies or immune cells from the vascular system.

That the germ cells are not absolutely dependent on an intact blood–testis barrier has recently been demonstrated in the seasonally breeding mink, where the blood–testis barrier appears to undergo cyclic formation and decay related to tubular lumen formation in association with respective periods of activity and inactivity of the seminiferous epithelium (478). The relationship between the formation of Sertoli cell junctional complexes and the establishment of spermatogenesis during postnatal growth of the testis has been studied using recent physiological and histological techniques. Permeability of the blood–testis barrier appears to be related to the progressive development of a lumen within the growing seminiferous tubules in which the capacity of the junctional complexes to restrict entry of exogenous hypertonic fluids or water-soluble markers is attained gradually rather than abruptly (480,481). The tightness of the barrier is maximally efficient coincident with the complete canalization of the seminiferous tubules with a recognizable lumen, which in the rat testis occurs at about day 30 of postnatal development.

The upward movement of early spermatocytes into the adluminal compartment requires that some mechanism be available to allow the migrating germ cells to traverse the specialized inter-Sertoli-cell junctions. These junctions have been observed both above and below young spermatocytes (175,460), and an orderly breakdown and formation of tight junctions has been proposed to permit cell transfer from the basal to the adluminal compartment (175,456). Further studies have indicated that new tight junctions between Sertoli cells form below young spermatocytes, whereas those previously above these cells are thought to dissociate, thus ensuring the patency of the permeability barrier (435,460,461). Thus, the barrier is flexible and deformable and compatible with the movements of migrating germ cells. Early stages of formation of tight junctions beneath migrating germ cells are characterized by increasing numbers of intramembranous junctional strands, which increase in length and begin to assume parallel orientations, thus collectively contributing to an increasing degree of continuity, culminating in a typical junctional complex (75).

The complex yet highly ordered arrangement of multiple clones of germ cells, each embraced by the highly branched Sertoli cell, demands not only that the Sertoli cell should be capable of conforming to the remarkable shape changes of the germ cells but also that it play a role in conferring stability throughout the seminiferous epithelium. In reviewing this topic a wealth of morphological information is now available from comparative studies of Sertoli-cell–germ-cell relationships that together indicates the central role played by the Sertoli cell in maintaining an attachment to germ cells in addition to providing potential avenues of intercellular communication. The literature concerned with this aspect of the biology of Sertoli cells is voluminous, but the reader is directed to a number of excellent papers that provide the basis for our present understanding (318,325,337,365, 366,381,457,479,482,483).

Prevention of premature disengagement and sloughing of germ cells into the lumen of the seminiferous tubule is thought to rely, at least in part, on regions of ectoplasmic specializations of the Sertoli cell that face the surface of certain germ cells. These structures consist of a dense band of actin-rich filaments sandwiched between the Sertoli cell plasma membrane and a cistern of endoplasmic reticulum and thus resemble one half of the paired ectoplasmic specializations that constitute the inter-Sertoli-cell tight junctions at the base of the Sertoli cells. Originally described between adjacent Sertoli cells and spermatids in the lumen testis (189,301), their widespread occurrence in other species has subsequently been confirmed (318,335,365,431,435,484,485).

Visualization of the sites of apposition of germ cells to ectoplasmic specializations at the lateral and apical surfaces of the Sertoli cell is dependent on the orientation and plane of section when the seminiferous epithelium is examined with the electron microscope. This limitation not only restricts an objective appraisal of what type and how many germ cells are associated with ectoplasmic specialization, but it also seems likely that this relationship is variable between species. In the hamster, monkey, and human testis, regions of ectoplasmic specialization have been reported facing zygotene primary spermatocytes (95,322,347,485), but other studies of a number of species have suggested that this association occurs very rarely (484). Where most reports seem to be in agreement is in the occurrence of ectoplasmic specializations facing midpachytene primary spermatocytes (Fig. 62) and round spermatids, but as the spermatids begin to elongate (Figs. 24 and 62) and undergo their final phase of maturation, a mantle of ectoplasmic specialization is always positioned around the spermatid head (29,435, 484). Whenever elongated spermatids are seen to penetrate the Sertoli cell deeply, the resultant recess that contains the spermatid head is lined by ectoplasmic specialization that is preferentially associated with the acrosome.

The function of Sertoli cell ectoplasmic specializations adjacent to germ cells is, however, unknown. Differences in the adhesive properties between Sertoli cells and various germ cells have provided circumstantial evidence that ectoplasmic specializations may actually bind to adjacent germ cells. Round germ cells (spermatocytes and early round spermatids) are easily separated from Sertoli cells (431,435,486), but elongated germ cells (maturing spermatids) are more resistant to dislodgement, and enzymatic digestion with trypsin is required to separate them from the Sertoli cell (68,486). Since desmosomes are not observed between elongated spermatids and Sertoli cells, the adhesive property that exists between them has implicated the ectoplasmic specialization in partly fulfilling this role. Additional theories of the activities of the ectoplasmic specializations include (a) structural support for the Sertoli cell during germ cell mobilization (323,435), (b) participation in sperm release and acrosome shaping (320,365,479,486), (c) a contractile role (430,487), and (d) sites of intercellular attachment (365,431,486,488). Actin is especially abundant within ectoplasmic specializations associated with junctional complexes and flanks the spermatids that form recesses within the plasma membrane of the Sertoli cell (489–491). Vinculin is codistributed with bundles of actin (492,493), adding support to the concept that ectoplasmic specializations serve as sites for intercellular adhesion between adjacent Sertoli cells and between Sertoli cells and spermatids.

A general concept of the origin of ectoplasmic specializations and their role in sperm release was put forward by Ross and Dobler (335) and Ross (365). Based on their observations on the mouse Sertoli cell, they suggested that as primary spermatocytes begin to ascend through the area of the blood–testis barrier, the inter-Sertoli-cell tight junctions disengage, and each intact, free ectoplasmic specialization so formed would gain attachment to the spermatocyte on entering the adluminal compartment of the seminiferous epithelium. This hypothesis has been questioned (323) on the grounds that (a) in the rat testis, no ectoplasmic specializations were observed in association with the ascending young spermatocytes, and (b) such round germ cells are not actually attached to ectoplasmic specializations as discussed above. Further studies will be necessary to clarify the origin and early location of ectoplasmic specializations.

There is no doubt that ectoplasmic specializations are seen facing midpachytene primary spermatocytes and round spermatids (322,323,365,460), where they occupy approximately 1% of the surface area of the Sertoli cell in the rat testis at stage V of the spermatogenic cycle (325). All elongated and maturing spermatids are associated with ectoplasmic specializations, which comprise approximately 3% of Sertoli cell membrane surface area. The participation in sperm release and ultimate fate of ectoplasmic specializations are the subject of some discussion. Following elongation of mature spermatids and their ascent toward the lumen of the seminiferous tubule, the spermatid head disengages from the ectoplasmic specializations and allows the release of sperm from the apical surface of the Sertoli cells. Profiles of ectoplasmic specialization are retained by the Sertoli cell, and in studies of the mouse Sertoli cell (365) they were seen facing the engulfed lobes of excess spermatid residual cytoplasm; they were also found free at the surface of the Sertoli cell or as isolated nonsurface elements within the

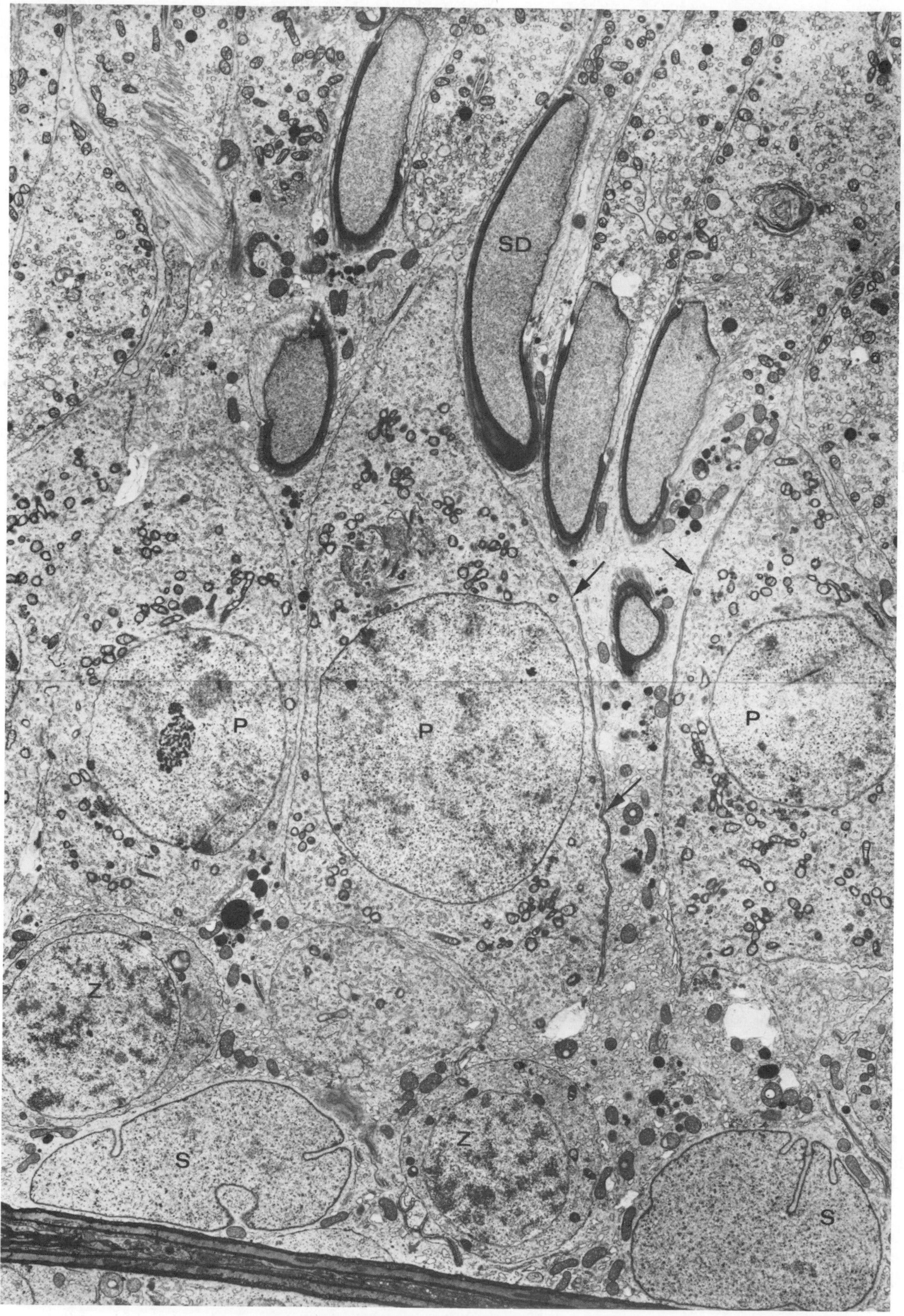

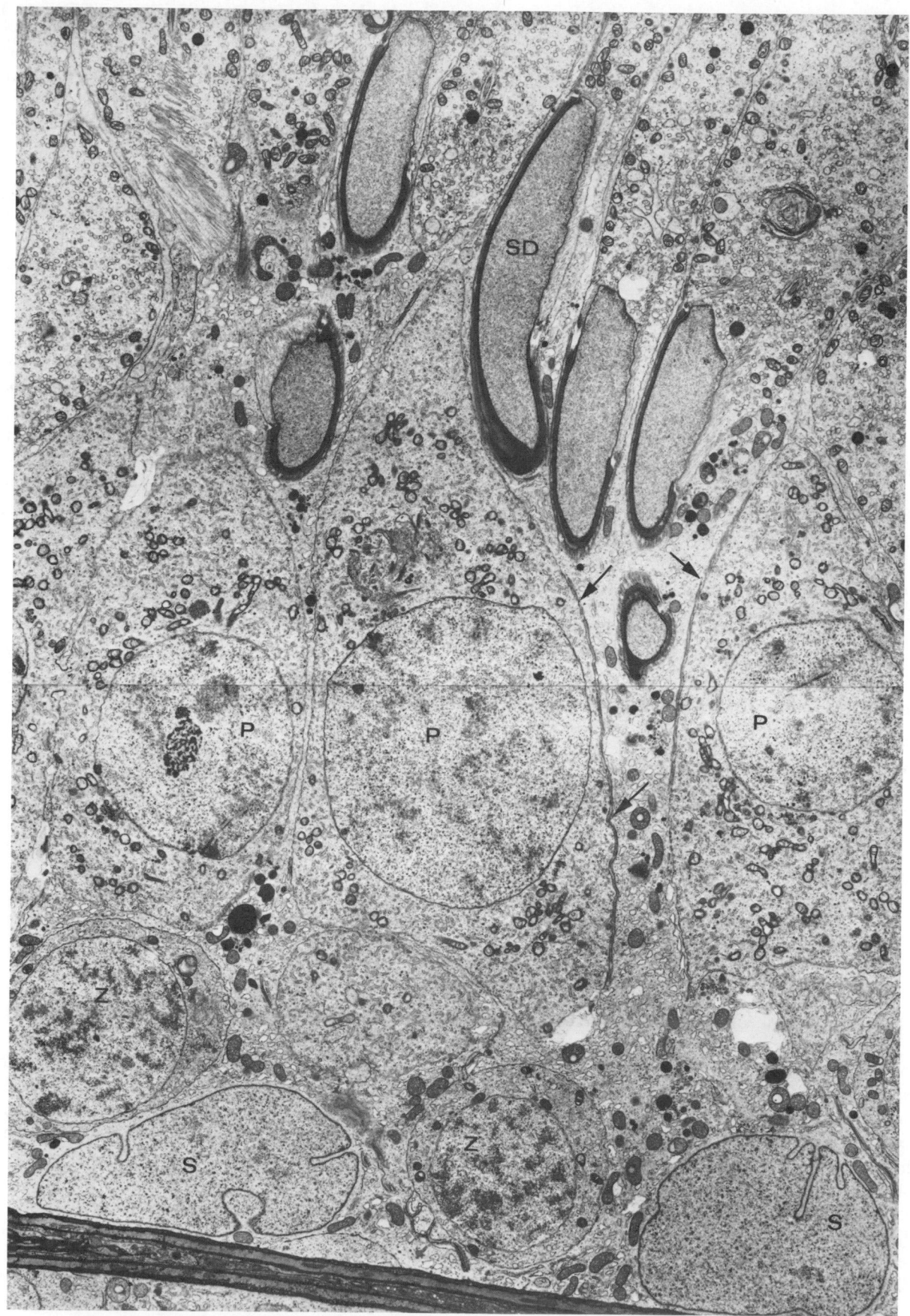

FIG. 62. Stage XI of the rat spermatogenic cycle illustrating Sertoli cells (S), zygotene primary spermatocytes (Z), pachytene primary spermatocytes (P), and elongated spermatids (SD). Note hemijunctions (*arrows*) associated with the plasma membrane of the pachytene primary spermatocytes.

cytoplasm. It was inferred from these observations that the occurrence of ectoplasmic specializations free within the cytoplasm signaled an early stage in their disintegration and subsequent disappearance. These findings have formed the basis for additional study of the ectoplasmic specializations (435,461,479,484,494), and three theories have been advanced to account for the origin, behavior, and fate of ectoplasmic specializations. These events are depicted in Fig. 63: (a) they may degenerate and, following internalization by the Sertoli cell, then disappear (365,484,487,495,496); (b) they become adherent to the cytoplasmic lobe of the sperm and thus selectively retain the lobes of residual cytoplasm (485); (c) they are removed intact from the Sertoli cell surface and, when free in the cytoplasm, became available for reutilization by the next generation of germ cells. Recycling of ectoplasmic specializations could occur by their distribution from a common pool or by intercellular transfer, e.g., from round spermatids to pachytene spermatocytes (435,484,497).

As yet, the factors regulating the formation and degradation of ectoplasmic specializations and their suggested role in germ cell movement, sperm release, and structural support of the Sertoli cell remain to be determined. As the mature spermatids are released from their attachments to Sertoli cell ectoplasmic specializations, they are retained at the surface of the seminiferous epithelium via very slender upward projections of the apical Sertoli cell cytoplasm. In this position they await their release into the lumen of the seminiferous tubule (Figs. 40 and 64). In favorable semithin sections examined by light microscopy, spermatid heads lie at the very tip of the seminiferous epithelium, and their flagellum projects into the lumen. The recent study by Palombi and colleagues (498) provides immunocytochemical evidence that β_1 integrins maybe involved in the formation of these ectoplas-

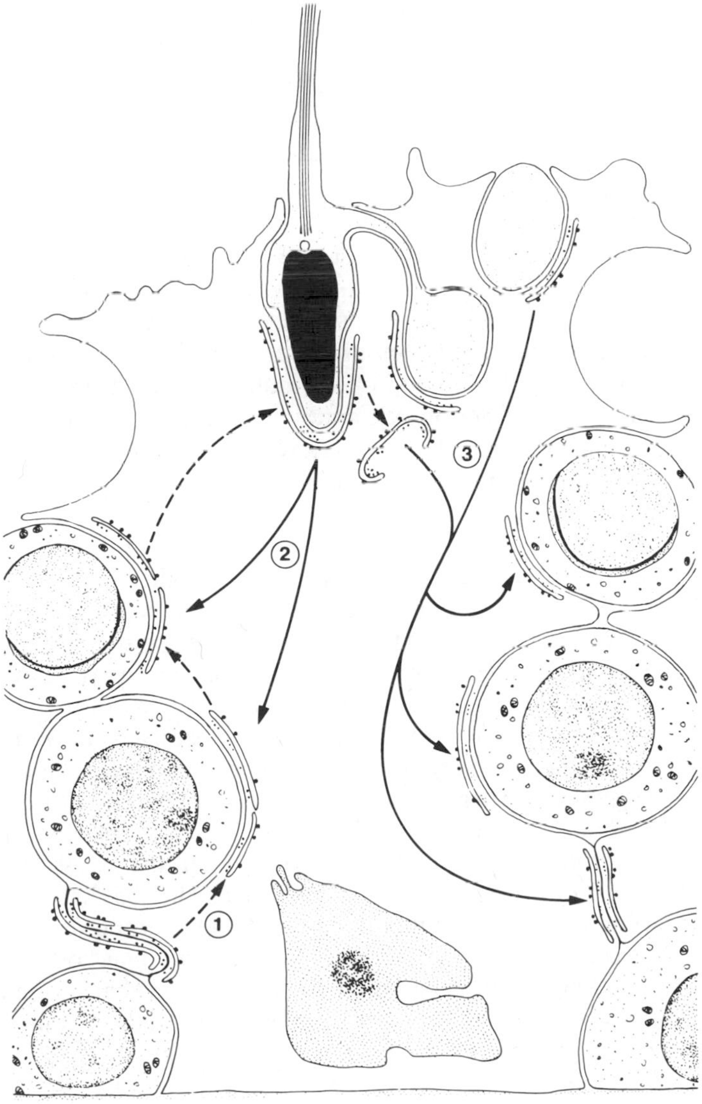

FIG. 63. Diagram demonstrating possible pathways for redistribution of inter-Sertoli-cell junctions. In route 1, basally situated junctions may separate to form hemijunctions associated with the surface of primary spermatocytes and early and late spermatids. Route 2 indicates proposed recycling of crypt-shaped hemijunctions from the late spermatids back to earlier generations of germ cells. Route 3 illustrates possible formation of pools of free hemijunctions, which recycle to earlier germ cells and may be involved in the formation of basal inter-Sertoli-cell junctions. (Based on Ross, ref. 365, and Russell, ref. 484.)

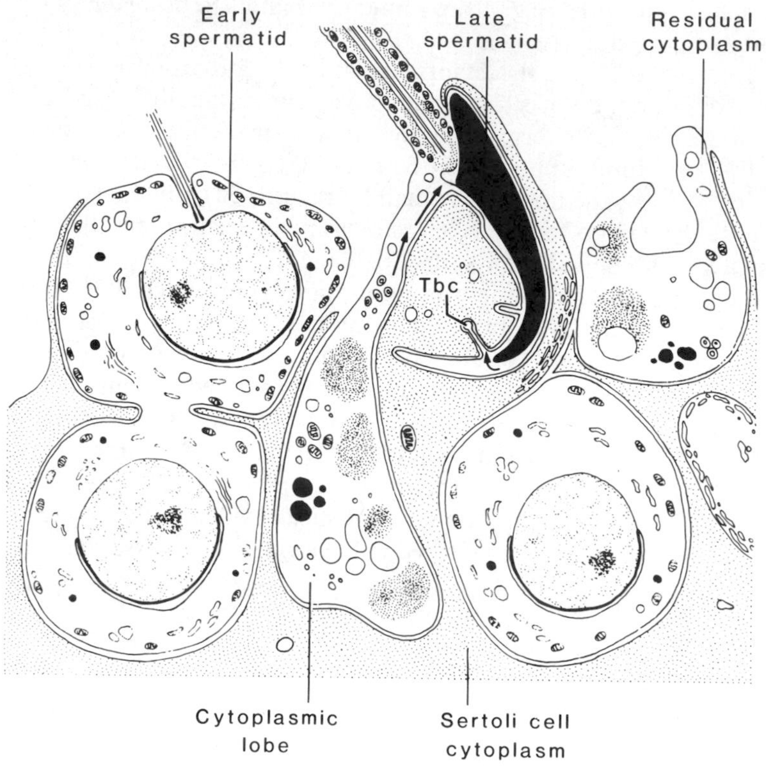

FIG. 64. Relationship between the mature generation of spermatids and the apical surface of the Sertoli cell. Tubulobulbar complexes (Tbc) extend from the concave surface of the spermatid head into the Sertoli cell cytoplasm. Cytoplasm within the cytoplasmic lobe of the spermatid is thought to flow into tubulobulbar complexes as indicated by *arrows*. (Modified from Russell and Clermont, ref. 296.)

mic specializations. They noted that the stage-specific identification of β_1 integrins and their cellular localization fit with the above description. The sperm appear to retain contact with the seminiferous epithelium via two structures. First, and well illustrated in the rat, the apical stalk of Sertoli cell cytoplasm balloons out within the concave aspect of the spermatid head, and second, the cytoplasm of the elongated spermatid becomes progressively attenuated along the long axis of the sperm and thus forms a slender cytoplasmic lobe (future residual cytoplasm) extending from the neck of the spermatid and coursing toward the apical regions of the Sertoli cell.

Returning to the delicate Sertoli cell cytoplasmic stalk associated only with the head and neck of the spermatid, faint striations are observed within the concave recess of Sertoli cell cytoplasm. In a series of excellent studies of this relationship between the two cells (296,304,305,323, 479,482), these radially oriented spokes (Figs. 40 and 65) form a so-called tubulobulbar complex. This region of specialization consists of a series of long, narrow cytoplasmic stalks that protrude, in the case of rat spermatids, from the spermatid head and invaginate the recess of Sertoli cell cytoplasm that fills out the concave environs of the spermatid head (Fig. 65). As the spermatid tubular evaginations penetrate into the Sertoli cell, the Sertoli cell plasma membrane closely conforms to that of the spermatid except at the tips of the projections, where small bulbous knobs are formed. Tubulobulbar complexes are described in numerous mammals (482); their number ranges from 4 to 24 per spermatid head, and they attain lengths of 1 to 8 μm. The complexes are not formed from round spermatids, nor are they seen emanating from elongated spermatids located deep within recesses of Sertoli cell cytoplasm. However, when spermatids rise to the very tips of the Sertoli cell, they lose their relationship to ectoplasmic specializations, whereupon tubulobulbar complexes make their initial appearance. As the Sertoli cell gradually withdraws from the spermatid head, these complexes are maintained until only the extreme tip of the late spermatid head is related to the slender processes of the Sertoli cell. This finding has led to the suggestion that the complexes anchor the spermatid head and participate in its stabilization.

Because several generations of tubulobulbar complexes are formed and then degraded in succession by the Sertoli cells (305), it seems plausible that a proportion of spermatid cytoplasm is resorbed through the degradation of numerous tubulobulbar complexes. The flow of spermatid cytoplasm into these complexes has also been suggested to trigger the sperm release mechanism (497). Although the mechanism by which the Sertoli cell is able to selectively retain, sculpture, and engulf the excess residual cytoplasm remains unclear, Russell (305) has advanced the concept that the tubulobulbar complexes indirectly engineer the formation of the residual bodies. This suggestion is based on his observation that in the period immediately preceding sperm release, the volume of the spermatid cytoplasm is reduced as much as 70%, and this disposal of cytoplasm coincides with the successive formation and degradation of tubulobulbar com-

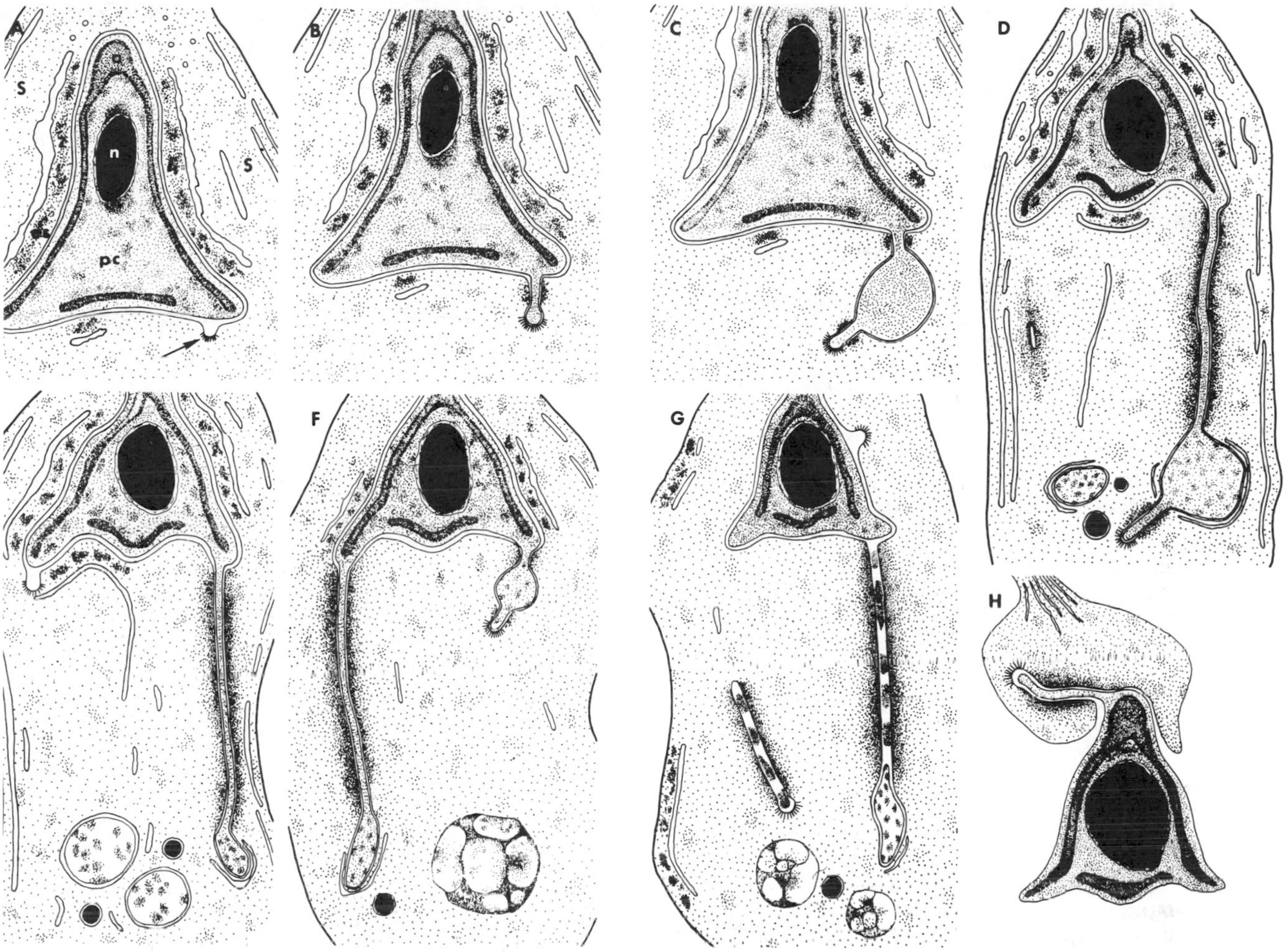

FIG. 65. Illustrations demonstrating the temporal sequence in the formation and disappearance of tubulobulbar complexes in the rat testis. Sertoli cell cytoplasm is *stippled;* spermatid head drawn in transverse section. **A:** A coated pit (*arrow*) of the Sertoli cell occurs in areas devoid of junctional specialization. Perinuclear cytoplasm (pc) is indicated. **B:** A tube forms by evagination of spermatid into the Sertoli cell. **C:** Midportion of the tube develops a bulbous dilatation. **D:** Proximal elongation of the tube, with the distal portion associated with lysosomes. **E:** Separation of bulbs from the tube with an associated increase in their watery consistency. **F:** Individual bulbs sequestered into Sertoli cell phagocytic vacuoles. New tubulobular complexes form. **G:** Dissolution of tubular portions. **H:** Prior to sperm release, the Sertoli cell cytoplasm withdraws from the spermatid head, and new tubulobulbar complexes develop at the convex margin of the spermatid head. These are subsequently resorbed, and the sperm is released (323).

plexes. The cytoplasm eliminated with the resorption of the tubulobulbar complexes by the Sertoli cell is usually watery and lacks organelles, suggesting that the remaining spermatid cytoplasm could become progressively more condensed and filled with spermatid organelles and inclusion bodies. In all species so far studied, the excess cytoplasmic lobes always exhibit these features, and after the sperm are shed, they form deeply staining residual bodies (Figs. 58 and 64). It is not yet known how the Sertoli cell releases the sperm but selectively retains the excess residual cytoplasm, although a recent report (366) has shown that the Sertoli cell cytoplasmic projections that surround and invaginate the residual cytoplasm are richly supplied with filaments and microtubules, which probably pull the residual cytoplasm from the lumen to the apical trunk of the Sertoli cell.

Tubulobulbar complexes also occur between adjacent Sertoli cells at the level of the blood–testis barrier and occasionally give rise to tight and gap junctions in the region of interdigitation (296,494). The tubulobulbar complex is a protrusion of cytoplasm of one Sertoli cell into a neighboring Sertoli cell and resembles a narrow tube, 2 to 4 μm in length terminating in a bulbous dilation. The complexes undergo a cyclic variation in number during the spermatogenic cycle in the rat, and their degradation and disappearance at stages VI to VII may represent a mechanism for the development or turnover of junctional contacts between the Sertoli cell.

Other types of specialized junctional regions found within the seminiferous epithelium include desmosomes, hemidesmosomes, and gap junctions. Desmosomes (or macula adherens) are traditionally recognized as small apposed plaques on adjacent cells flanked by a thin dense layer just beneath the plaque and represent strong adhesion sites between cells. They have been described between Sertoli cells and all round germ cells but are absent at the interface with elongated spermatids (75,169,170,175,189,322,499). In the rat they are oriented toward the body of the Sertoli cell and are often seen toward the base of the seminiferous tubule, suggesting that they could resist any force tending to dislodge germ cells into the lumen (326). Their general function is believed to be to assist the surface of the Sertoli cell in the orderly upward movement of germ cells during their maturation. A recent quantitative analysis of desmosome gap junctions between Sertoli cells and germ cells of the rat testis has shown that germ cells early in the meiotic maturation process exhibit larger numbers of these junctions than those in more advanced phases of development (500). The finding suggests that whatever their functional significance, desmosome gap junctions are possibly more important for the initiation of meiosis than for its continuence.

Hemidesmosomes occupy the site where the base of the Sertoli cell rests on the basal lamina of the seminiferous tubule (461,501) and probably confer firm anchoring of the Sertoli cell necessary for them to maintain their pentagonal or hexagonal relationships to each other. Gap junctions (or nexus) are represented as extremely close sites of apposition (20 Å) between adjacent cell membranes and are thought to offer the capability of ionic flux and exchange of small molecules. They also confer sites of firm adhesion between cells. Gap junctions occur between Sertoli cells in laboratory species (74,318,456,502) but are not present on human Sertoli cells (322,364). Their presence has also been noted between Sertoli cells and round germ cells (231,503), although they are often seen in association with desmosomes and are occasionally referred to as desmosome gap junctional complexes (326). Gap junctions are not observed between Sertoli cells and elongating spermatids. At present their function is unknown, although potentially they play a role in intercellular communication.

Changes Associated with Seasonal Breeding and Age

The great majority of mammals are subjected to wide variations in the environmental conditions in which they live, and thus seasonal variations in photoperiod, ambient temperatures, and the availability of food and water together contribute to seasonal cycles of reproductive activity of many wild and domestic animals. Seasonally breeding animals, unlike their laboratory-bred counterparts, provide an opportunity to investigate the structure and function of the Sertoli cell during the cyclic waxing and waning of spermatogenesis. A great deal of information has accumulated over many years that attests to the annual regression and recovery of spermatogenic activity within the testes of a wide range of vertebrates (20,330,390,504–507).

Histological investigations of the changes in testicular activity among seasonally breeding fish, amphibians, reptiles, birds, and mammals have demonstrated that regression of the seminiferous epithelium is often accompanied by an accumulation of lipid inclusions within the Sertoli cells (330). With reactivation of spermatogenesis, the Sertoli cell lipid inclusions disappear, although the precise role of lipid in the presumed alterations of Sertoli cell function remain unknown. Examples of the changing structure of the Sertoli cell in a seasonally breeding wild rat have been documented at the light and electron microscopic level (391,506,507). In seasonally breeding mammals the arrest of spermatogenesis is accompanied by a marked reduction in Sertoli cell volume and its content of organelles (508–510). Simultaneous accumulation of lipid inclusions is also a common feature, possibly relating to deposition and storage of lipid-rich substances contributed in part from the degeneration of many germ cells (511–513). These structural changes in Sertoli cells during the nonbreeding season are thought to occur in response to a decline in the levels of FSH, LH, and testosterone (514–516) and resemble the morphological changes in Sertoli cells seen after hypophysectomy (517,518).

Little is known concerning the integrity of the blood–testis barrier in seasonally breeding mammals, and although the inter-Sertoli-cell junctions remain during the regression of the seminiferous epithelium (487,506,519), their effectiveness as a permeability barrier requires additional study. However, in lower orders of vertebrates such as reptiles and amphibians (331,334), tight junctions between Sertoli cells disappear during the nonbreeding season. In testes exhibiting regional differences in spermatogenic activity, germ cell maturation is accompanied by Sertoli cell junctions, whereas in regressive zones of the testis not associated with germ cell activity, tight junctions disappear. Thus, at least in some species, the formation of the barrier is correlated with spermatogenic activity.

The basic tenet that Sertoli cell numbers remain stable in the adult testis (28,44) has been brought into question in recent years. Because sperm production in many animals may vary with season, and because daily sperm production is subject to an age-related decline, the effect of variation in Sertoli cell numbers offers a theoretical mechanism to allow these changes to occur. Variation in the Sertoli cell population has been documented, although this phenomenon has in the past attracted little attention, possibly for lack of statistical significance or because of large changes in the dimensions of the seminiferous tubules. Nevertheless, when mouse testes were X-irradiated to partially destroy the germ cell population, the restoration of testicular function was associated with an increased number of Sertoli cells per seminiferous tubule cross section (520).

When rat testes were made artificially cryptorchid (521,522), the Sertoli cells were reported to transiently increase in number, and with prolonged periods of cryptorchidism, Sertoli cells disappear from the seminiferous tubules (523). Sertoli cells of the immature rat testis apparently continue their division processes for longer than is otherwise indicated by their mitotic index (524), and in the absence of germ cells Sertoli cells in prepubertal rats continue to proliferate beyond day 20, when their numbers normally stabilize (79). Increases in the Sertoli cell population have been reported to occur during FSH treatment of rats following hypophysectomy (525). The lack of rigid quantitative assessment of Sertoli cell numbers in some of these and other studies has been voiced as a criticism of their conclusions. However, other studies of seasonally breeding red deer (526) and stallions (522,528) have presented clear evidence that the Sertoli cell population is capable of increasing in the adult by fluctuating with season. Seasonal differences in Sertoli cell numbers of 60 adult stallions were characterized by a 36% increase in the breeding versus the nonbreeding season. Since the horse Sertoli cells only have a limited capacity to alter the ratio of germ cells to single Sertoli cells, a seasonal variation in total numbers of Sertoli cells provides an additional mechanism for increased daily sperm production per testis, which is known to occur in the breeding season.

The source of additional Sertoli cells found in the breeding season and the factors promoting their appearance and disappearance remain unclear. Mitotic figures at the base of the seminiferous epithelium in the stallion were seen at stages II–III of the spermatogenic cycle, whereas spermatogonia are thought to divide only between stages V and VIII. Concentrations of FSH, LH, and testosterone measured in the same study (528) were altered not only by season but also with age, and no clear relationship has emerged to link hormone changes with Sertoli cell numbers. The numbers of type A spermatogonia also exhibit changes with season in adult stallions (529), and it seems possible that the Sertoli cells may influence these cells through hormonal action (530) or perhaps directly via mitogenic peptides secreted by the Sertoli cells (531). Although the adult stallion appears to be an exception to the rule that Sertoli cell numbers remain stable after puberty, additional research may well indicate that Sertoli cells are a dynamic rather than sessile population.

A very different account of the biology of Sertoli cells has been revealed when their numbers are related to increasing age. With morphometric techniques to evaluate cell numbers (532) it was shown that the number of Sertoli cells in the human testis exhibits an age-related decline. In a study of men aged 20 to 85 years who were in apparent good health prior to sudden death, young adult men (20 to 48 years, n = 37) had approximately 500 million Sertoli cells per testis, and this number declined significantly to a mean of 300 million per testis for older men (50 to 85 years, n = 34). When the relationship between age and numbers of Sertoli cells per testis was examined, there was a significant age-related decline in the Sertoli cell population (351). In addition, the same study reported a significant correlation between Sertoli cell numbers and daily sperm production, although the numbers of germ cells accommodated by the Sertoli cells at any age remain unchanged. Taken together the analysis of changes in spermatogenesis and Sertoli cell numbers in the special examples of old age and in seasonal breeders indicate that variation in daily sperm production can be attributable to alterations in the total numbers of Sertoli cells and/or to changes in the numbers of germ cells that are associated with an individual Sertoli cell.

Response to Injury

In the past, the persistence of Sertoli cells following damage or elimination of the germ cells was taken to indicate that the Sertoli cells were resistant to a wide variety of treatments that otherwise caused spermatogenic disruption. This belief was based on light microscopic observations of Sertoli cells following testicular damage in which their morphology appeared little changed from normal. However, as pointed out by Fawcett (318,319), the availability of semithin sections of testicular tissues embedded in plastic has revealed far more morphological details of the Sertoli cell than previously appreciated from studies on paraffin sections. The sensitivity of the Sertoli cell to damage has been emphasized by the early ultrastructural and functional changes of this cell in response to a great range of unrelated treatments that exert adverse effects on the testis (392).

The literature relating to morphological alterations of Sertoli cells is voluminous and encompasses a wide range of treatments too numerous to describe in this chapter. We have chosen, therefore, to discuss and illustrate changes in Sertoli cell structure in a general manner, since it seems likely that the reaction of this cell to injury is often reflected by very similar morphological alterations. An early indication of altered Sertoli cell cytology is the appearance of many clear, watery vacuoles or vesicles within the basal aspects of the cell. These are readily visible by light microscopy (Fig. 66), and, when examined by electron microscopy, they consist of membrane-limited vacuoles arising from three locations. First, the basal cytoplasm exhibits intracellular vac-

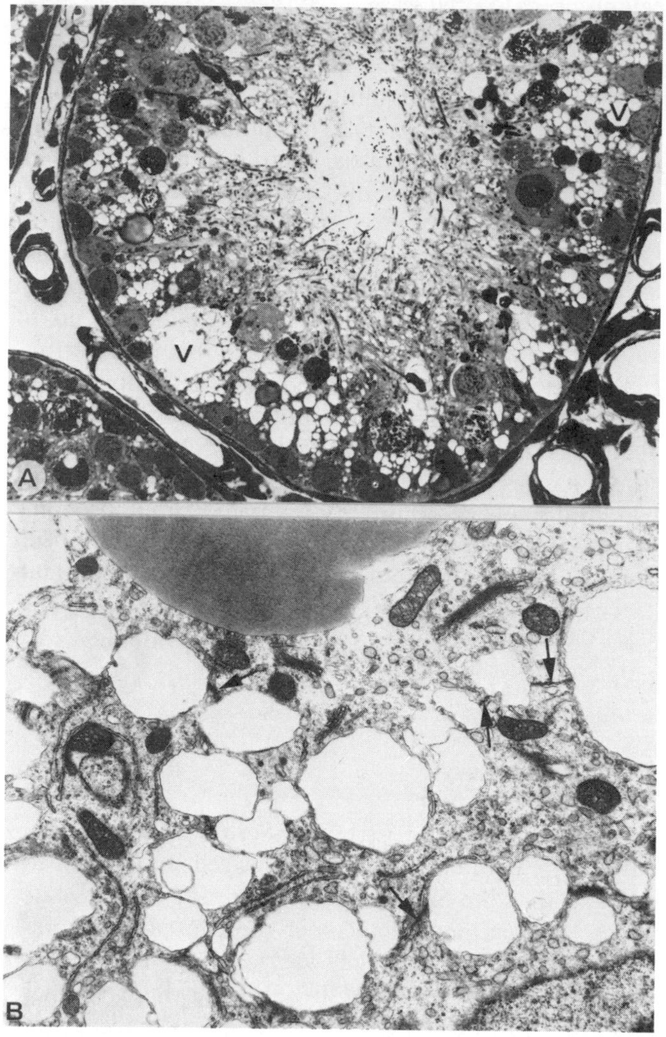

FIG. 66. **A:** Five-day experimentally cryptorchid rat testis showing many vacuoles (V) within the seminiferous epithelium. **B:** Many of these vacuoles in the 5-day cryptorchid testis are interconnected (*arrows*) by junctional specializations between adjacent Sertoli cells.

uoles of variable configuration (Fig. 66), but whether these form by dilation of endoplasmic reticulum or endocytosis of fluids has not been clarified. Second, vacuoles occasionally appear in the intercellular spaces between Sertoli cells and neighboring germ cells, and third, vacuoles clearly visible by light microscopy are associated with the regions of junctional specialization between adjacent Sertoli cells (Fig. 67). These vacuoles are of particular interest since they involve radical disorganization of the inter-Sertoli-cell junctions in which progressive expansion of the intercellular spaces at the site of junctional complexes gives rise to multiple extracellular vacuoles along the pathway of each junctional complex. The formation of these vacuoles in relation to seminiferous tubule damage has been closely studied after the induction of experimental cryptorchidism (533), in which it was suggested that they contribute to complex membranous bodies within the Sertoli cells. The sequence of morphological changes to the inter-Sertoli-cell junctions during cryptorchidism is illustrated by light and electron micrographs (Fig. 68) and summarized diagrammatically in Fig. 69. Vacuolization is probably a nonspecific response to the Sertoli cells to injury, since it occurs in unrelated conditions of experimental damage to the seminiferous epithelium (79,83,439,534–542).

An additional sign of morphological disturbance to the Sertoli cell is the rapid accumulation of cytoplasmic lipid droplets, which very often accompany impairment of spermatogenesis. Although lipid inclusions are a common feature of Sertoli cells in the normal testis, they appear to increase in size and number coincident with morphological evidence of germ cell degeneration, suggesting that the degradation products of effete germ cells contribute to ever-increasing numbers of Sertoli cell lipid inclusions. However, the autolysis and phagocytosis of germ cells by Sertoli cells may not be the exclusive source of these lipid droplets, since they are known to accumulate within the Sertoli cell in the absence of germ cells (79). In conditions of prolonged atrophy of the seminiferous tubules, some Sertoli cells retain their content of lipid, whereas others exhibit few if any lipid inclusions. The latter situation of complete degeneration and disappearance of germ cells from the seminiferous epithelium results in further structural modifications to the Sertoli cells, which involve retraction and convolution of their apical cytoplasm. Such seminiferous tubules exhibit a thin rim of flattened Sertoli cells. Alternatively, removal of the germ cells allows for shrinkage of the seminiferous tubule, whereupon the Sertoli cell cyto-

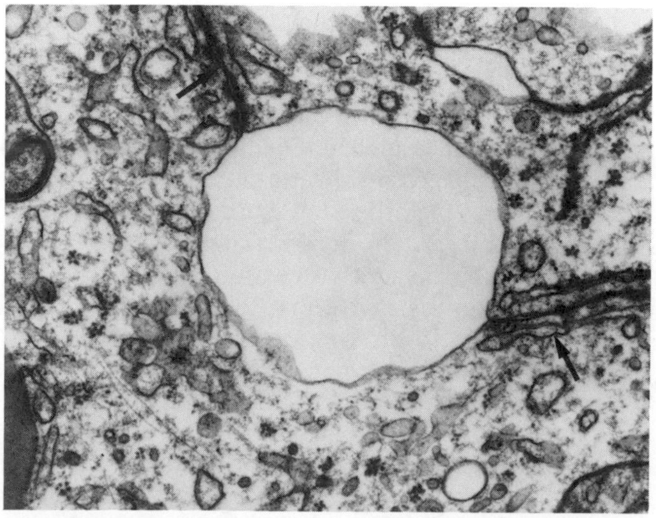

FIG. 67. Five-day experimentally cryptorchid testis showing a dilation of the intercellular space between two Sertoli cells. At opposite sides of the extracellular space, the pathway of inter-Sertoli-cell junctional complexes can be noted (*arrows*).

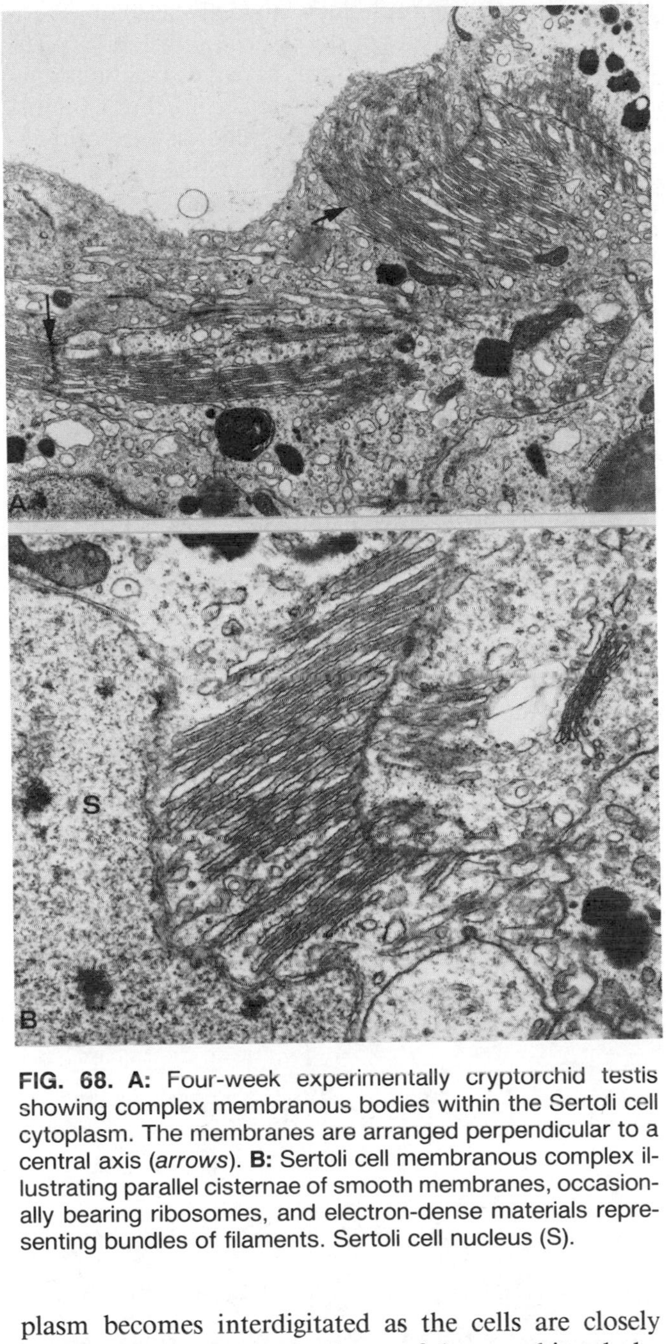

FIG. 68. A: Four-week experimentally cryptorchid testis showing complex membranous bodies within the Sertoli cell cytoplasm. The membranes are arranged perpendicular to a central axis (*arrows*). **B:** Sertoli cell membranous complex illustrating parallel cisternae of smooth membranes, occasionally bearing ribosomes, and electron-dense materials representing bundles of filaments. Sertoli cell nucleus (S).

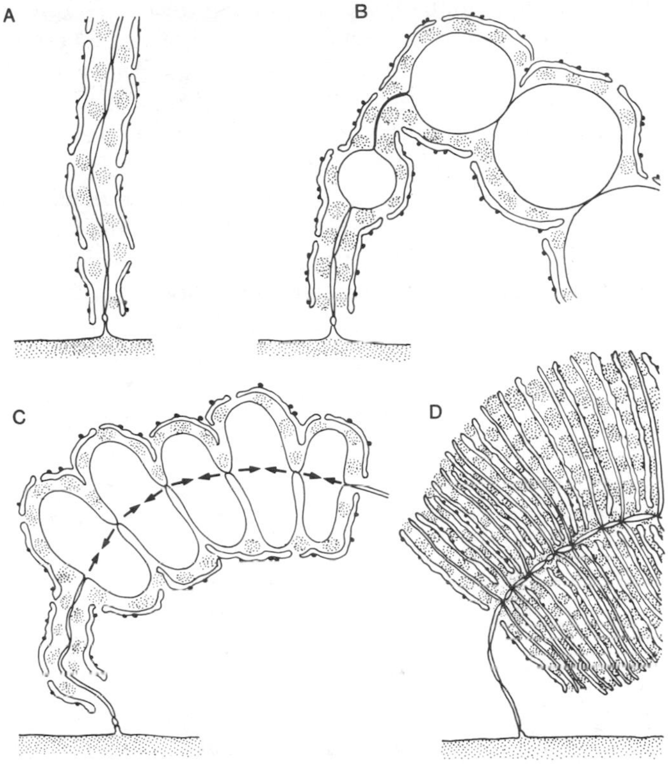

FIG. 69. Suggested sequence of formation of extracellular vacuoles and complex membranous cisternae in the seminiferous epithelium of the experimentally cryptorchid rat testis. **A:** Inter-Sertoli-cell junction in normal testis. **B:** In short-term cryptorchidism, vacuoles develop in the intercellular regions between sites of membrane occlusion. **C:** At later time intervals, the degeneration of germ cells allows shrinkage of the seminiferous tubule and progressive collapse of the vacuoles, as indicated by *arrows*. **D:** With continued compression of the Sertoli cells, it is suggested that the rows of collapsing vacuoles undergo a "connective-type" compression, forming elaborate parallel stacks of flattened vacuoles interposed between the cisternae associated with the tight junctions.

plasm becomes interdigitated as the cells are closely packed into the reduced volume of the atrophic tubule.

Destruction of Sertoli cells has not often been reported, although this was clearly demonstrated some years ago (543) when it was shown that cadmium salts were acutely toxic to the seminiferous epithelium, causing the destruction of germ cells and Sertoli cells. Other agents that bring about Sertoli cell necrosis include LH, LH plus LHRH agonists, and hCG (544,545), although the mechanism by which these hormones destroy the Sertoli cells has not been studied. All of the above-mentioned alterations to the Sertoli cell have been described in disorders of the human testis (322,352,354, 546–548) and in testes of men of advanced age (532,549).

THE PERITUBULAR TISSUE

The seminiferous tubules are supported by a circumferential layer of attenuated cells (fibroblasts and myoid cells) and extracellular materials (collagen and glycoproteins), collectively termed the lamina propria, whose ultrastructure features have been extensively documented (Fig. 46) (454,456,533,550–555). To date our knowledge of the functional duties of the lamina propria can be summarized as follows: (a) provision of mechanical support and contractile function for the seminiferous tubule, (b) passive paracrine influence on spermatogenesis via secretory products stimulated by testosterone, (c) partial and species-specific restriction of macromolecules entering the seminiferous tubules via the intertubular tissues, (d) a source of precursor cells capable of differentiating into Leydig cells (556–561). Recent work has focused on the contractile properties of peritubular tissues, which for the rat are capable of induced or spontaneous contractions between days 4 and 7 of postnatal life (562). These myoid-type cells contain actin, desmin, and vimentin filaments (481,489,490,557,558,563), and it has been suggested that the outermost peritubular cells in the human testis are probably derived from the intertubular fibroblastic tissue, since they contain vimentin but lack desmin (559). More information on the receptor, synthetic, and secretory properties of the peritubular tissue is required to gain a better understanding of its role in the physiology of the testis.

CYCLE OF THE SEMINIFEROUS EPITHELIUM

The organization of the cell types that comprise the process of spermatogenesis within the seminiferous epithelium is not random but in fact highly organized. This fact was elucidated toward the end of the 19th century by a number of investigators (27,105,136,172,564). They noted that the germ cells at different developmental phases formed easily identifiable collections termed cell associations. Subsequent studies (565,566) were extended by the detailed investigations of Le Blond and Clermont (182,183), who defined the cycle of the seminiferous epithelium as the series of changes in a given area of the seminiferous epithelium between two appearance of the same developmental stage. These studies utilized the periodic acid–Schiff (PAS) reaction to stain the acrosome of spermatids and, on the basis of this structure and nuclear morphology, divided spermatogenesis in the rat into 14 stages or cell associations (Fig. 70). The complete sequence of 14 stages or cell associations constitutes one cycle of the seminiferous epithelium. Should we have the ability to observe a segment of the seminiferous epithelium by time-lapse photography over a period of days, the organization of spermatogenesis in this cyclic manner would result in the epithelium passing through the 14 stages with the eventual appearance of stage 1. They also established that the transformation of a type A spermatogonium into a mature spermatid, which is released at stage 7 of the cycle, occupied four such cycles. In the rat, the entire tubule cross section is in the same stage of the seminiferous cycle, which, in fact, extends over several millimeters of adjacent seminiferous tubule.

Investigation in other mammals subsequently established a seminiferous cycle in the mouse (107,567), the ram (568), and the monkey (104). Since spermatogenesis is a continuous sequence of changes, the subdivision into stages is artificial, and the number of stages will depend on the criteria used. The more extensive the criteria used, the more specific and detailed become the stages that can be identified. For light microscopic studies, the conventional staging of Clermont (116) is usually applied to kinetic studies of the seminiferous epithelium. The cycle has been studied and defined in a number of mammalian species, each of which has a characteristic pattern and number of stages (Table 2).

In the human, considerable difficulty was experienced

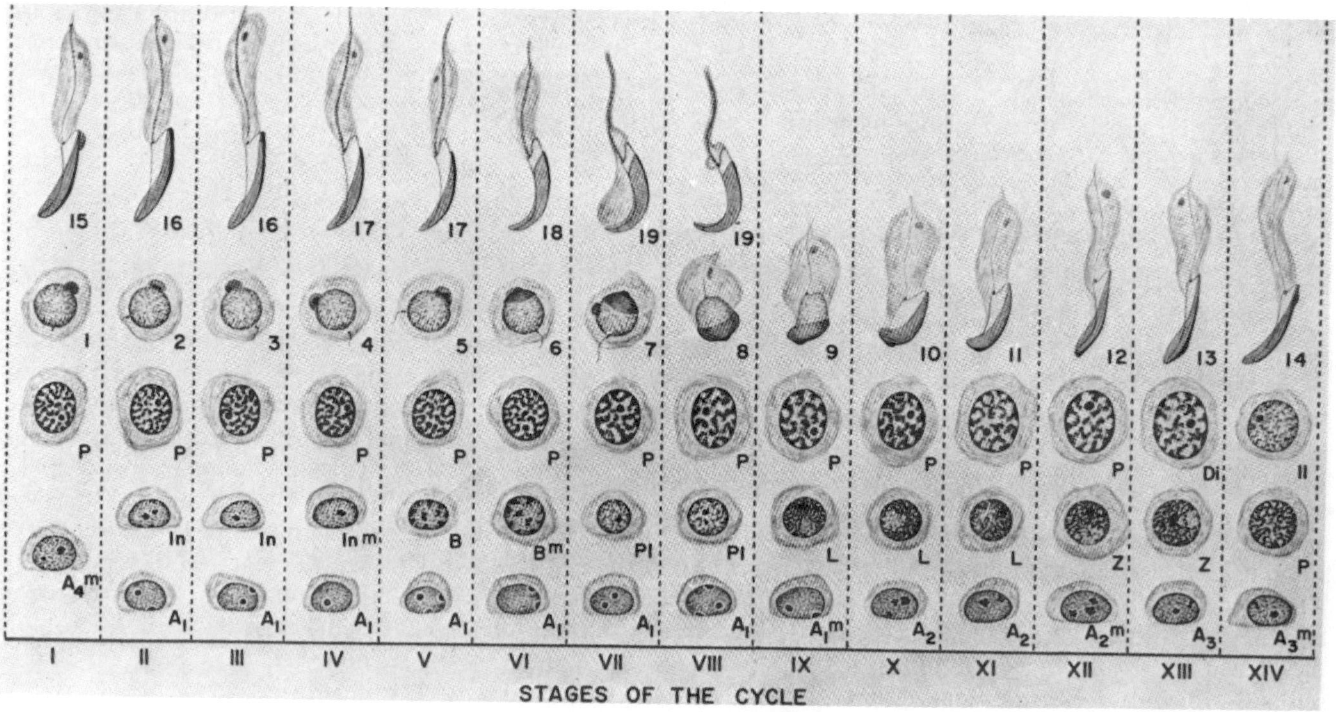

FIG. 70. This diagram illustrates the stages of the rat seminiferous cycle and the cell associations comprising them. (From Dym and Clermont, ref. 579, with permission.)

TABLE 2. *Duration of seminiferous cycle*

Species	Days	References
Mouse	34–35	880
Hamster (*Cricetus auratus*)	35–36	880,881
Boar	34–35	882
Rat	48–53	883,884
Ram	49	572,885
Bull	54	595
Rabbit	48–51	886,887
Monkey		
Macaca speciosa	45	888
Macaca mulatta	70	889
Human	64	173

in identifying the cell associations or stages because multiple stages could be seen in a single cross section of a tubule and because of inadequate care in the fixation and handling of tissue. However, by detailed studies, Clermont (184) identified six cell associations as stages that formed the cycle of the human seminiferous epithelium (Fig. 71). Of the species examined to date, the only one demonstrating multiple stages in a seminiferous tubule cross section is the baboon, *Papio anubis* (569). Recently, Schulze and Reheder (570) analyzed the human seminiferous epithelium in a different manner and proposed that germ cells at the same stage of development are distributed in a helical pattern. As they progress through spermatogenesis, the diameter of the helix decreases such that they are overlapped on the external surface by a gyration from another helical sequence (Fig. 72). They propose that this concept of an Archimedian spiral provides the best explanation of the human data. They also suggest that the greater spermatogonal mitotic rate in species other than man provides a larger spermatocyte population and hence the conventional appearance of stages of a seminiferous cycle. Further studies are clearly necessary to demonstrate whether this concept extends to all species or whether it may be limited to

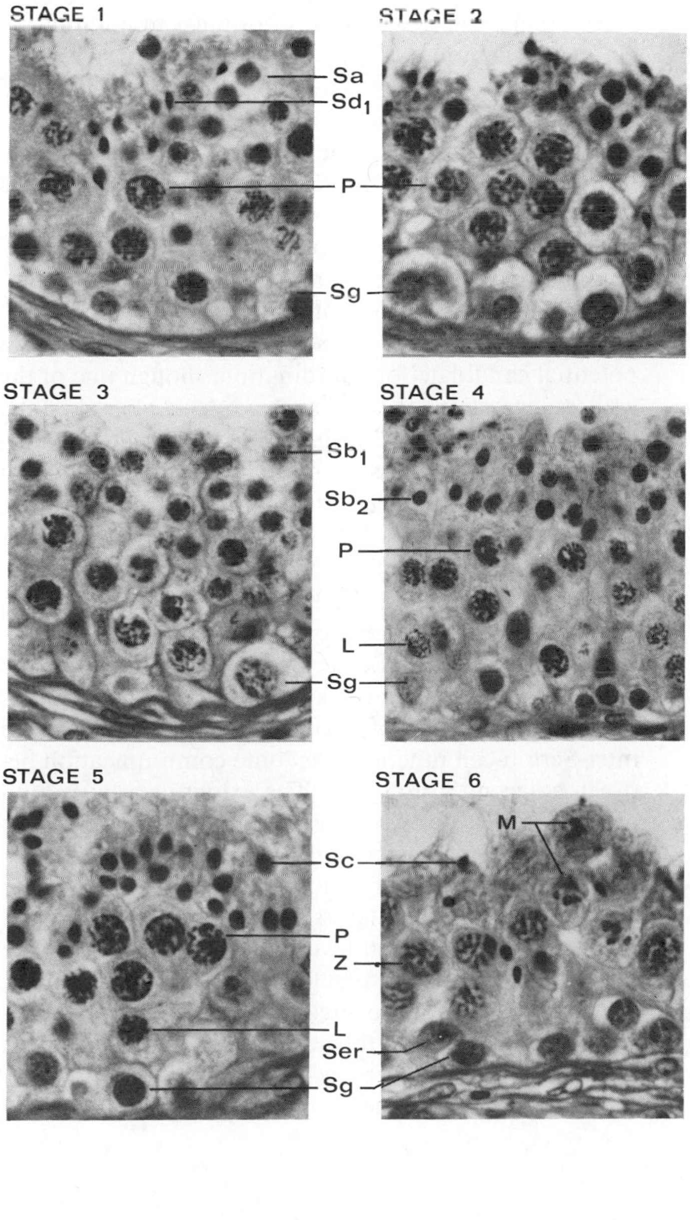

FIG. 71. This series of light micrographs illustrates the stages of the human seminiferous cycle as defined by Clermont (124). (From de Kretser et al., ref. 890, with permission.)

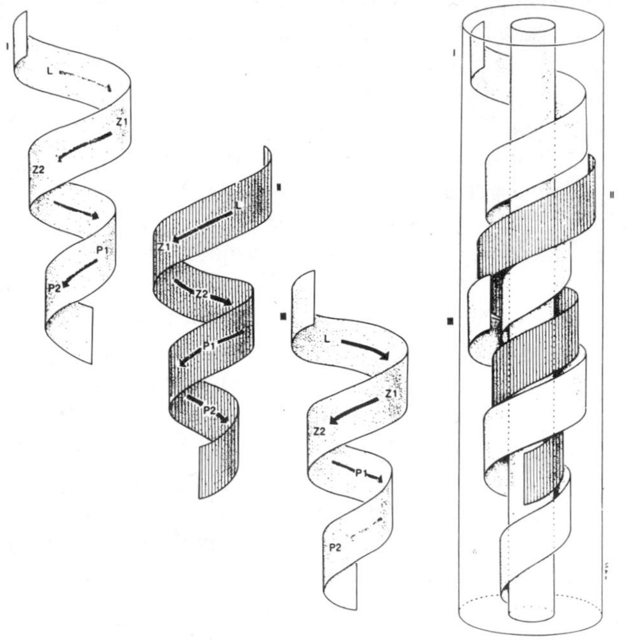

FIG. 72. This illustrates the proposed three-dimensional model for the arrangement of primary spermatocytes in the human seminiferous tubule. Populations of successive degrees of development occupy helically running strip-shaped areas of the epithelium. As development proceeds the strip approaches the lumen. L, leptotene; Z, early zygotene; Z_2, late zygotine; P, early/mid-pachytene; P_2, late pachytene. (From Schulze and Rehder, ref. 570, with permission.)

species such as the baboon, which has a similar seminiferous epithelium to man (569).

Duration of Spermatogenesis

Studies to determine the duration of spermatogenesis centered initially on attempts to destroy sensitive germ cell stages and analyze the rate of depletion of the seminiferous epithelium. Such approaches defined the duration of the cycle in the mouse as 8.6 days, with the entire process taking 34.6 days (567). Alternative approaches emerged with the availability of radioactive tracers such as ^{32}P and ^{3}H-labeled thymidine. Using ^{32}P, Ortavant (571,572) demonstrated that the cycle in the ram lasted 10.4 days, the entire process occupying 49 days. Subsequently, the incorporation of tritiated thymidine into the DNA of dividing cells has been used in studies of spermatogenesis in a number of species and demonstrated a specific duration for each species (Table 2). The duration of spermatogenesis appears to be specific for each species, and attempts to influence this biological constant by numerous factors have been unsuccessful. Ortavant (568) showed that although photoperiod could affect the yield of spermatozoa, it could not affect the rate of spermatogenesis. Removal of the pituitary to assess the influence of the hypophyseal hormones was shown to be without effect (573), and similar conclusions were reached in studies in the ram (574). It appears that the germ cells progress through the spermatogenic process at predetermined rates or subsequently degenerate. This view has recently been challenged by Russell et al. (575), who noted that spermatids in procarbazine-treated rats were found out of phase with the normal cycle of the seminiferous epithelium. The existence of a fixed rate of development of the germ cells results in an important corollary, namely, the volume occupancy (or absolute volume if referring to the testis) of a germ cell in sections of the epithelium is a reflection of the length that that cell occupies in the spermatogenic process. Thus, secondary spermatocytes have a short life span, and they and the stage of the cycle at which they are seen (stage 14 in the rat; stage 6 in human) are represented infrequently in sections of the seminiferous epithelium.

Coordination Within the Seminiferous Epithelium

The remarkable organization of the seminiferous cycle and the demonstration that the duration of spermatogenesis in many species is a biological constant have led to speculation as to the method by which this coordination is achieved. Two basic concepts of the method of synchronization were proposed by Roosen-Runge and Giesel (566): (a) that the regulated development depended on the precise rate of each stage of cell development because of inherent timing devices or (b) that synchronization was dependent on external factors.

Of external factors, the Sertoli cell has emerged as a potential candidate for coordination, though one of the earliest suggestions (576) of such a role was based on the concept that the Sertoli cells formed a syncytium, now known to be a false assumption. The demonstration of the existence of specialized inter-Sertoli-cell junctions (303) forming the blood–testis barrier (456) emphasizes the close relationship of this cell to the germ cells, particularly those located on the luminal side of the barrier. Though favorably placed to exert a coordinating influence based in a radial direction in the epithelium, the Sertoli cell is less able to extend its coordinating influence along the length of the tubule unless the specialized inter-Sertoli-cell junctions facilitate communication between adjacent Sertoli cells. The extensive arborization of the Sertoli cell extends a potential influence over a number of germ cells in various phases of development, raising the potential of it influencing these cells by the secretion of local regulators, a hypothesis put forward many years ago but still lacking evidence (285). The phagocytosis of the residual bodies of spermatids led numerous investigators to suggest that this action constituted a signal to the Sertoli cell that may be important in controlling spermatogenesis (285,577). Clermont (102), however, discounted the Sertoli cell as a factor based on

(a) the fact that cyclic activity is established within the epithelium prior to the Sertoli cells attaining their mature cytological characteristics (578), and (b) the observation that in hypophysectomized rats, the Sertoli cells are regressed, yet the germ cell stages that are present in the epithelium maintain their characteristic cell associations (574). Furthermore, he noted that coordination within the epithelium also existed in the absence of residual bodies either prior to their formation (578) or subsequent to irradiation (579). He concluded that the cycle of the epithelium is the direct consequence of the entrance, at fixed intervals, of spermatogonial stem cells in spermatogenesis and of the fixed duration of the various steps of spermatogenesis.

The nature of such inherent timing devices has not been resolved, but more recent studies have emphasized the extensive links between synchronously developing germ cells through the formation of cytoplasmic bridges associated with incomplete cytokinesis (120). These bridges, which link adjacent cells at all stages of germ cell development, effectively create a syncytium, and, based on calculations, up to 512 spermatids may be linked in such a manner (120). The existence of large numbers of cells joined in this manner was amply demonstrated by Moens and Hugenholtz (580), who observed 80 spermatocytes joined by cytoplasmic bridges. By incomplete cytokinesis of spermatogonial stem cells, cohorts of cells remain linked in a syncytium enabling coordinated subsequent cell division.

In an extensive reexamination of this hypothesis, Ren and Russell (581) examined the number of germ cells linked by intercellular bridges by treating rat testis *in vitro* with cytochalasin D, leading to the formation of symplasts (582). They concluded that since the clone size so determined was greater than the smallest known unit of synchrony within the epithelium, the intercellular bridges were the likely mechanism to allow coordination. This coordination is likely to result from the relative ease of cytoplasmic transport of coordinating molecules, and in fact, "cytoplasmic flow" was found to occur in some of the changes noted after cytochalasin treatment (582). In other studies they demonstrated that the intercellular bridges are not static structures but vary considerably in form during spermatogenesis (583).

Spermatogonial or Stem Cell Renewal

Because it is likely that one of the major factors responsible for the coordination seen in spermatogenesis is the regular division of spermatogonia, it seems pertinent to consider their pattern of division in more detail. Spermatogonial renewal is also of importance for the continuation of spermatogenesis throughout adult life, as there must be a mechanism by which they are renewed and yet provide a pool of cells to enter the later stages of the process. Early studies proposed that this was achieved by the products of spermatogonial division being different, i.e., bivalent, with one daughter cell remaining a spermatogonium and the other a primary spermatocyte (584). This concept ignored the fact that there were different types of spermatogonia as described by Regaud (27). Further studies by Roosen-Runge and Giesel (566) recognized that multiple spermatogonial divisions occur throughout the seminiferous cycle. Subsequently Clermont and Le Blond (41) proposed a scheme to account for the five peaks of mitoses observed in the epithelium during the seminiferous cycle. In their view, some type A spermatogonia divided in "bivalent" fashion to form stem cells, which remained dormant throughout the cycle, and type A spermatogonia, which entered the cycle.

Subsequent development of concepts in this field was the direct result of improved methods of identifying spermatogonial cell types and the study of spermatogonia in whole mounts of seminiferous tubules (110,111,119). In the rat five different types of spermatogonia were identified, A_0 and A_1 through A_4, the A_0 being viewed as a reserve stem cell that did not divide unless the epithelium was damaged by agents such as irradiation (110,111). The renewing stem cells were proposed to arise by one of the A_4 spermatogonia dividing to form two A_1 spermatogonia. This proposal seemed unlikely in view of the observation that groups of dividing spermatogonia remained linked by cytoplasmic bridges, making it difficult to accept that one member of such a cohort could act independently of the rest (120).

A new theory emerged from the studies of Huckins (119,585–587) using whole mounts of rat seminiferous tubules in combination with autoradiography with [^{3}H]thymidine. She recognized three spermatogonial compartments (Fig. 73), the stem cells (As), the proliferating cells (Apr and Aal), and the differentiating cells (A_{1-4}, In, B). The stem cells divide sporadically to replicate themselves as isolated entitles and to provide pairs of spermatogonia (Apr). The latter engage in a series of synchronous divisions leading to the formation of chains

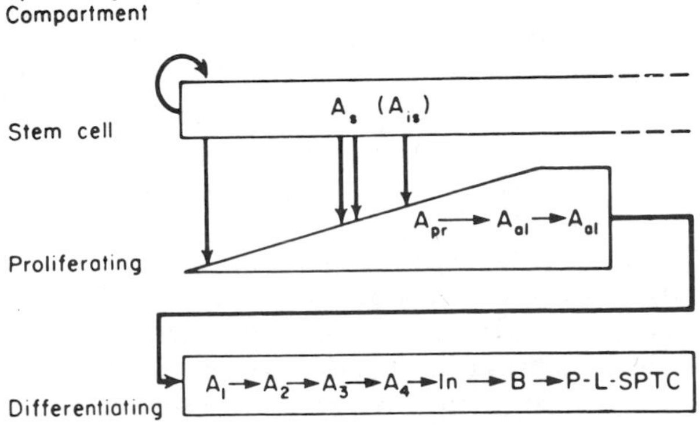

FIG. 73. This figure diagrammatically illustrates the proposed model for renewal and differentiation of spermatogonia. (From Huckins, ref. 119, with permission.)

of spermatogonia joined by intercellular bridges, the aligned spermatogonia (Aal). The proliferating compartment, on approaching its final size, ceases mitotic division, and the Aal cells differentiate synchronously into A_1 spermatogonia, which resume, again synchronously, their maturation into the more differentiated spermatogonial types (A_2, A_3, A_4, In, B). The type B subsequently differentiate to form preleptotene spermatocytes. This view has been supported by studies in the mouse (588,589), the Chinese hamster (590,591), and the ram (592). The concept proposed by Huckins (119) fits well with the observed data of increased numbers of proliferating cells joined by intercellular bridges (120).

Numerous studies were performed in the era 1960 to 1970 in different species, quantifying the number of spermatogonial divisions and proposing schemes of spermatogonial multiplication (Table 2). These have been extensively reviewed by Clermont (102), and readers are referred to that paper for details. Although they may be inaccurate in terms of the method of stem cell renewal, they do provide a data base for each species.

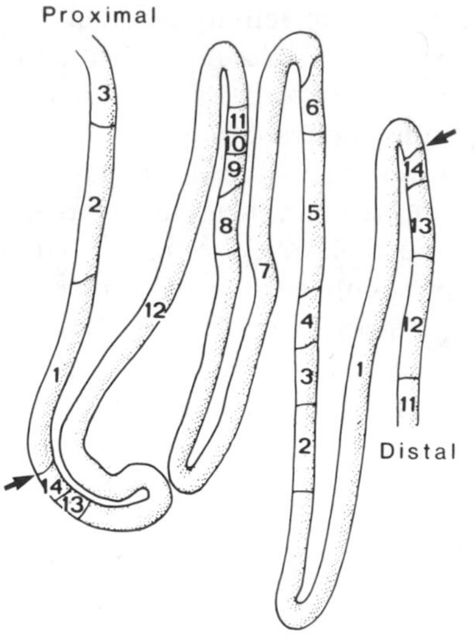

FIG. 74. The distribution of the stages of the rat seminiferous cycle that constitute the seminiferous wave along the tubule. (Redrawn from Perey et al., ref. 578.)

Spermatogonial Wave

Von Ebner (105) recognized that the stages of the seminiferous cycle were distributed along the length of the seminiferous tubule in an orderly sequence, thus introducing the concept of the spermatogenic wave. Regaud (27) correctly interpreted the significance of this wave by the statement that the wave is in space what the cycle is in time. Detailed histological studies have analyzed the distribution of stages along the length of the seminiferous tubule (Fig. 74) and found that the subdivisions between stages are irregular but distinct (578). Each rat seminiferous tubule contains approximately 12 complete spermatogenic waves, each approximately 2 to 6 cm in length (578). Studies using autoradiography of whole mounts of seminiferous tubules demonstrated orderly mitotic activity of spermatogonia according to the stage of the cycle, providing further evidence to support the concept that the cycle of the seminiferous epithelium is coordinated by the mitotic activity of the spermatogonia (593). The wave has been identified in a number of mammalian species such as the mouse, bull, mink, guinea pig, rabbit, boar, dog, cat, and marsupials (564,578,594–596).

The orderly distribution of stages of the seminiferous cycle along the tubule is the basis for the innovative studies of Parvinen (597), which involved dissection of the tubule into lengths according to the stage of the cycle present. This was achieved by transillumination of the tubule, the stages providing particular appearances based principally on the light scattering achieved by the condensing spermatid nucleus. The studies of Parvinen (598) have demonstrated that the nature of the germ cells surrounding the Sertoli cell can significantly influence certain metabolic activities of the Sertoli cells. Additional evidence has been provided by the studies of Jegou et al. (599), which showed that modification of Sertoli cell function following exposure of the rat testis to a single episode of heat did not occur until a loss of spermatids occurred. During recovery, Sertoli cell function remained abnormal until the return of spermatids. Furthermore, the studies of Kerr and colleagues (289,338) have shown significant changes in the morphology of the Sertoli cell according to the stage of the cycle of the rat. These studies emphasize the fact that the seminiferous tubule compartment cannot be viewed as homogeneous tissue in terms of either structure or function.

Germ Cell Degeneration

Several quantitative studies in a number of species have shown that a significant degree of germ cell degeneration occurs during spermatogenesis (600–602). The cell types involved in the degeneration have been shown to include spermatogonia, spermatocytes, and spermatids. The degree of degeneration can be translated into the efficiency of spermatogenesis, which can be measured as daily sperm production per gram testis (603) and in humans has been shown to be 25–35% of other species (604). In a recent study Johnson et al. (605) suggest that this degeneration is evidenced by the paucity of cells within each generation and may contribute to the relatively disorganized appearance of the human seminiferous epithelium.

LEYDIG CELLS

In reviewing the cytology of the Leydig cells and the intertubular tissues in which they reside, we recognized that for the purposes of this chapter it was not possible to acknowledge the work supplied by every contributor to this field of study. Readers will appreciate the difficulties faced when one considers that a review of the same topic in 1921 by Stieve (606) was based on approximately 1000 earlier studies. Thus, the literature on Leydig cell morphology and its functional significance is vast. Our objectives are subsequently directed toward two major topics. The first is to provide a review of Leydig cells based on authoritative accounts that together form an accurate survey of the light and electron microscopic features of the Leydig cells and the interstitial tissue. Particularly useful dissertations are available in the literature (16,378,397,454,606–616). Second, we discuss and provide new illustrations on the morphology of Leydig cells, which we hope will add to an increased understanding of the biology of these cells.

Historical Background

The earliest description of the histology of the intertubular tissue of the testis was provided by Leydig in 1850 (617), who reported that the spaces between the seminiferous tubules were occupied by conspicuous masses of cells containing fatty vacuoles and pigment inclusions. Kolliker, another student of testicular histology, who some years earlier had concluded that spermatozoa originate from the seminiferous tubules, also provided a similar description of the cellular composition of the intertubular tissue (5). Both investigators considered the cells to be a specialized form of connective tissue.

Although Berthold (6) demonstrated that the testis secreted substances into the bloodstream to influence the growth of anatomically distant tissues, the question of which tissue in the testis contributed to this secretion remained unanswered for many years. The prevailing view of Leydig cells as connective tissue was extended by von Ebner (105) and Hofmeister (618). But thereafter a new concept gained favor in which Leydig cells were thought to produce fats, nutrients, or other substances for consumption by the seminiferous tubules (27,619, 620). Because of the well-recognized occurrence of lipid inclusions within the Leydig cells of many species, several investigators put forward the view that Leydig cell lipid droplets provided the substrate from which testicular hormones were synthesized. This idea received support from the studies of Bouin and Ancel (7,624) and Ancel and Bouin (625), who coined the term "la glande interstitielle" and offered convincing evidence that the Leydig cells of both normal and cryptorchid testes provided the hormonal stimulus for the production of sperm and for maintenance of secondary sexual characteristics.

Leydig cell lipid inclusions later were shown to contain cholesterol esters (626–628) and led to the demonstration by McGee (629) that lipid extracts from bovine testes could stimulate masculine development when administered to other animals. Testosterone was finally identified in these extracts (8,630) and soon was synthesized using cholesterol as the starting material (631,632). Pathways for steroidogenesis and their control by various hormones are reviewed elsewhere in this volume, although it is important to emphasize that many years passed by until it became clear that the Leydig cells represented the predominant site for steroidogenic enzymes (633–635) and the chief source of testicular androgens (636,637).

Organization of Intertubular Tissue

In routine histological sections of the testes of common laboratory rodents (rat, mouse, guinea pig, hamster), a clear space of variable extent is commonly observed separating individual seminiferous tubules. Within this space are found numerous blood vessels of variable caliber, often forming a central core around which are deployed numerous Leydig cells and other cellular constituents of the intertubular tissue. Thus, a cursory examination of the intertubular tissue confirms that its histological organization is consistent with an endocrine function, namely, a rich vascular supply and a close association between Leydig cells and blood vessels, the latter facilitating the passage of steroids into the circulation. Empty spaces surrounding the seminiferous tubules have often been interpreted as preparation artifacts brought about by shrinkage during tissue fixation and dehydration prior to paraffin embedding. Although this is no doubt correct, we now recognize that these clear spaces, at least in the above-mentioned species, are not entirely exaggerated in their extent but in fact represent species variation in the size and architecture of intertubular lymphatic vessels. For many years the intertubular tissue was regarded simply as loose connective tissue harboring Leydig cells, fibroblasts, and extracellular elements. The concept of a system of lymphatic channels penetrating beyond the regions of the septula, rete, and tunica albuginea and into the interior of the testis had long been supported (638–644) but was doubted (645–648). Improvements in tissue preservation for subsequent ultrastructural examination have shown that the intertubular tissue is in fact supplied by a lymph vascular system, and its relative volume, architecture and relationship to Leydig cells are unique for a given species (320,454,614,649,650).

The claim that in the mammalian testis, Leydig cells are usually clustered around blood vessels is somewhat misleading in the light of an excellent comparative study by Fawcett, Neaves, and Flores (16) of the organization of the testicular intertubular tissue in 14 species of mammals. Four more-or-less distinct patterns of organization were distinguished (Figs. 75–79). In rodents such as the guinea pig and chinchilla, only a small fraction of the testicular volume is taken up by the Leydig cells, which are commonly clustered together around blood vessels. The remaining and greater part of the intertubular area is occupied by extensive peritubular lymphatic sinusoids, whose limiting walls consist of a delicate layer of endothelium. To accommodate the intervening blood vessels and Leydig cells, the lymphatic endothelium invests the perivascular Leydig cells in what has been termed visceral (16) or interstitial (649) endothelium. Closely applied and coursing parallel to the boundary tissues of the seminiferous tubules, the lymphatic endothelial wall here is termed parietal (16) or peritubular (649) endothelium. In general the endothelial walls of the lymphatic sinusoids are continuous, although on some occasions small gaps or discontinuities have been noted in the visceral wall flanking the Leydig cells. Structural support between the seminiferous tubules and the Leydig cell vascular entities is provided by bundles of collagen fibers and occasional fibroblastlike cells forming a bridge linking the clusters of Leydig cells with the peritubular tissues.

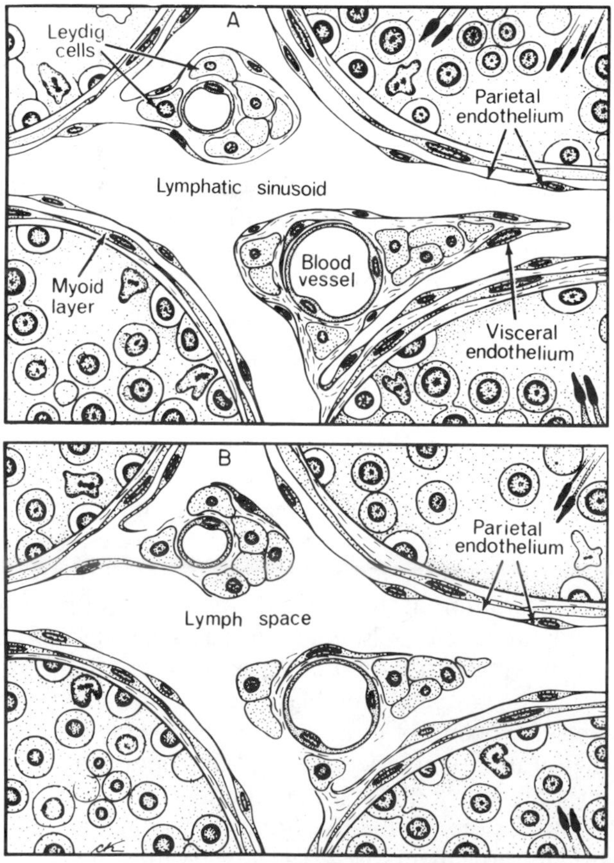

FIG. 75. Architecture of the intertubular tissue from a variety of species. **A:** Chincilla and guinea pig. Leydig cells associated with blood vessels and enclosed by lymphatic endothelium. **B:** Rat and mouse, showing discontinuities of the lymphatic endothelium partly surrounding perivacular Leydig cells (317).

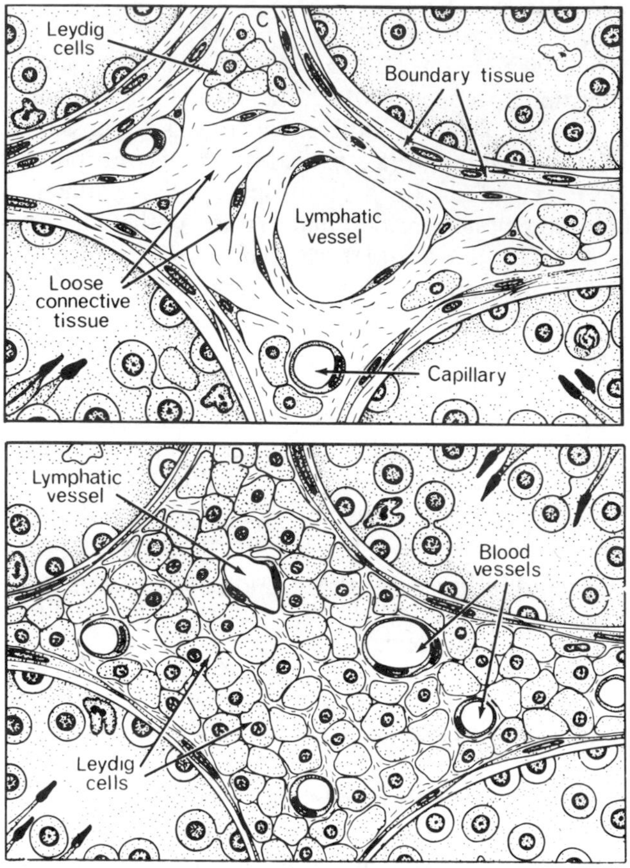

FIG. 76. Architecture of the intertubular tissue from a variety of species. **C:** Larger animals including ram, bull, monkey, and man. Randomly scattered clusters of Leydig cells appear within loose connective tissue rich in interstitial fluid. Lymphatic vessels are also demonstrated. **D:** Boar, wart hog, zebra, naked mole, rat, and numerous marsupial species. Many large Leydig cells occupy the intertubular space. Connective tissue and lymphatic vessels are not prominent. (From Fawcett, ref. 317, with permission.)

A similar organization of the intertubular tissue is seen in the rat and mouse, although a significant difference occurs in the extent to which Leydig cells are exposed to the fluids within the lymphatic sinusoids. Thus, the visceral layer of lymphatic endothelium is usually absent from the surface of Leydig cell clusters, permitting a direct communication between loose connective tissues containing collagen and the lymph space (Figs. 80 and

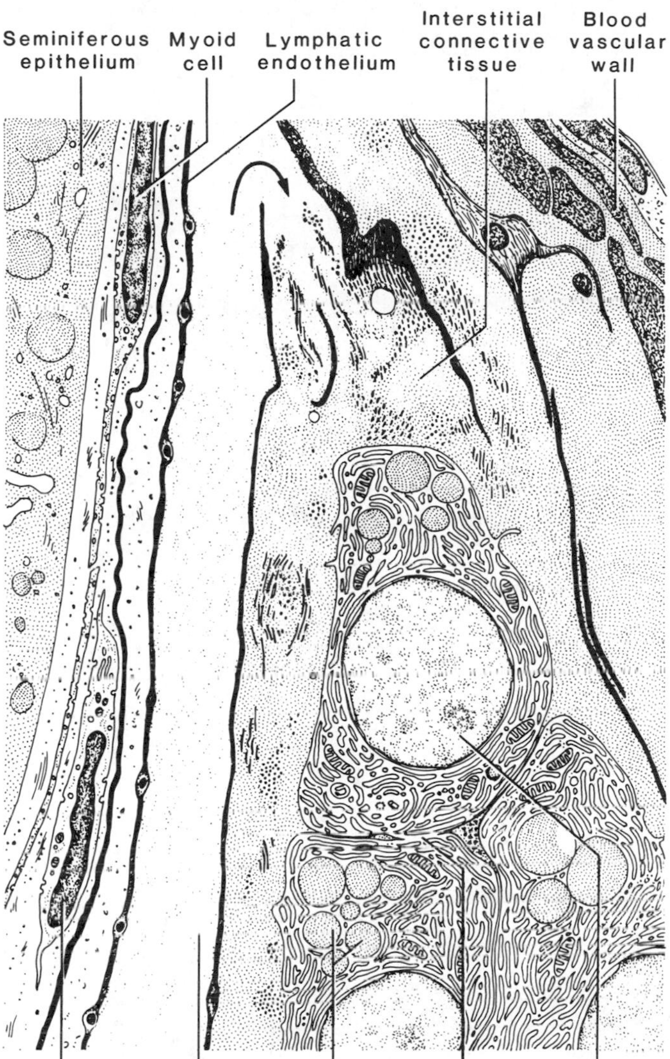

FIG. 77. Schematic representation of the intertubular tissue of the testis. Note the discontinuity in the endothelial wall of a lymphatic vessel, allowing its contents of interstitial fluid to gain access to the loose connective tissues containing the Leydig cells. (Based on micrographs from Fawcett et al., refs. 454 and 614.)

81). In these species the architecture of the intertubular lymphatic channels has been aptly classified as lymphatic sinusoids (Fig. 81), implying a continuous admixture of lymph fluids and the ground substance of perivascular connective tissues. It should be mentioned here that in addition to the schema described (16), Leydig cells of the rat and mouse are not constantly confined to perivascular locations but are often seen in peritubular positions or, alternatively, in more central regions of the intertubular tissue, where they appear to lack any association with connective tissue and are in fact almost entirely bathed by lymph (Fig. 80). This observation emphasizes the role played by the lymphatic sinusoids in providing the medium by which Leydig cells receive and secrete substances carried by the bloodstream. However, these special features of the histology of intertubular tissues in rat and mouse are quite different from those of many other mammals and raise a note of caution in extrapolating their associated physiological properties to cover other species in general.

In the second category described by Fawcett and colleagues (16), the intertubular tissue is characterized by large areas of very loose connective tissues containing small aggregations of Leydig cells often associated with blood vessels or, less often, occupying positions rather distant from the vascular supply. Lymphatic drainage is achieved through prominent lymphatic vessels placed

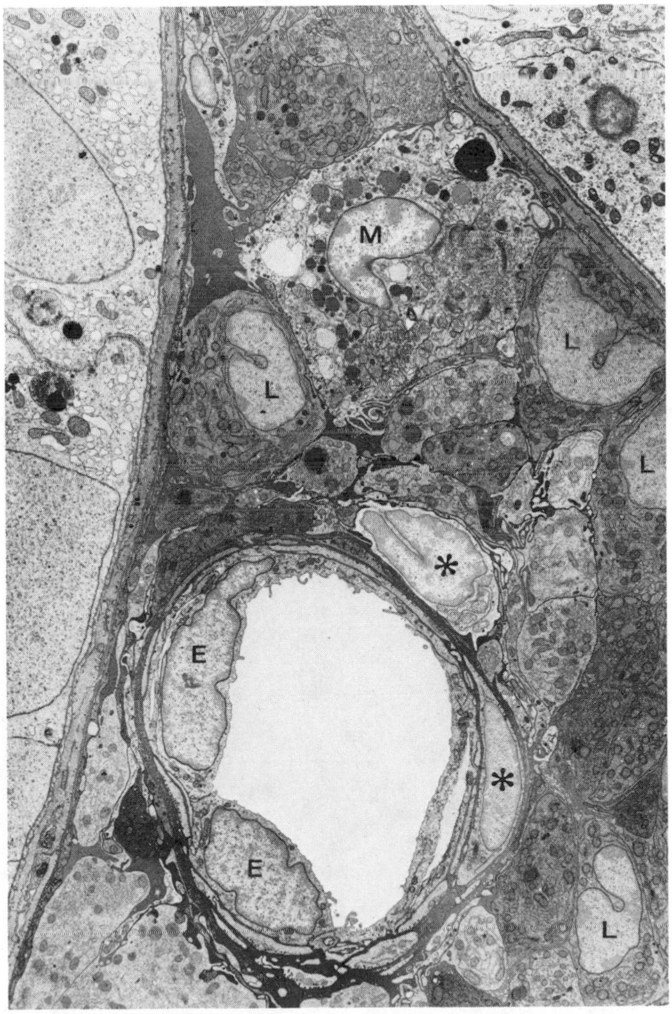

FIG. 78. Ultrastructure of the intertubular tissue of the adult rat testis, showing Leydig cell nuclei (L), a macrophage (M), vascular endothelial cell nuclei (E), and perivascular interstitial cells (*asterisks*) traditionally classified as pericytes or adventitial cells. Tissue fixed with collidine-buffered glutaraldehyde.

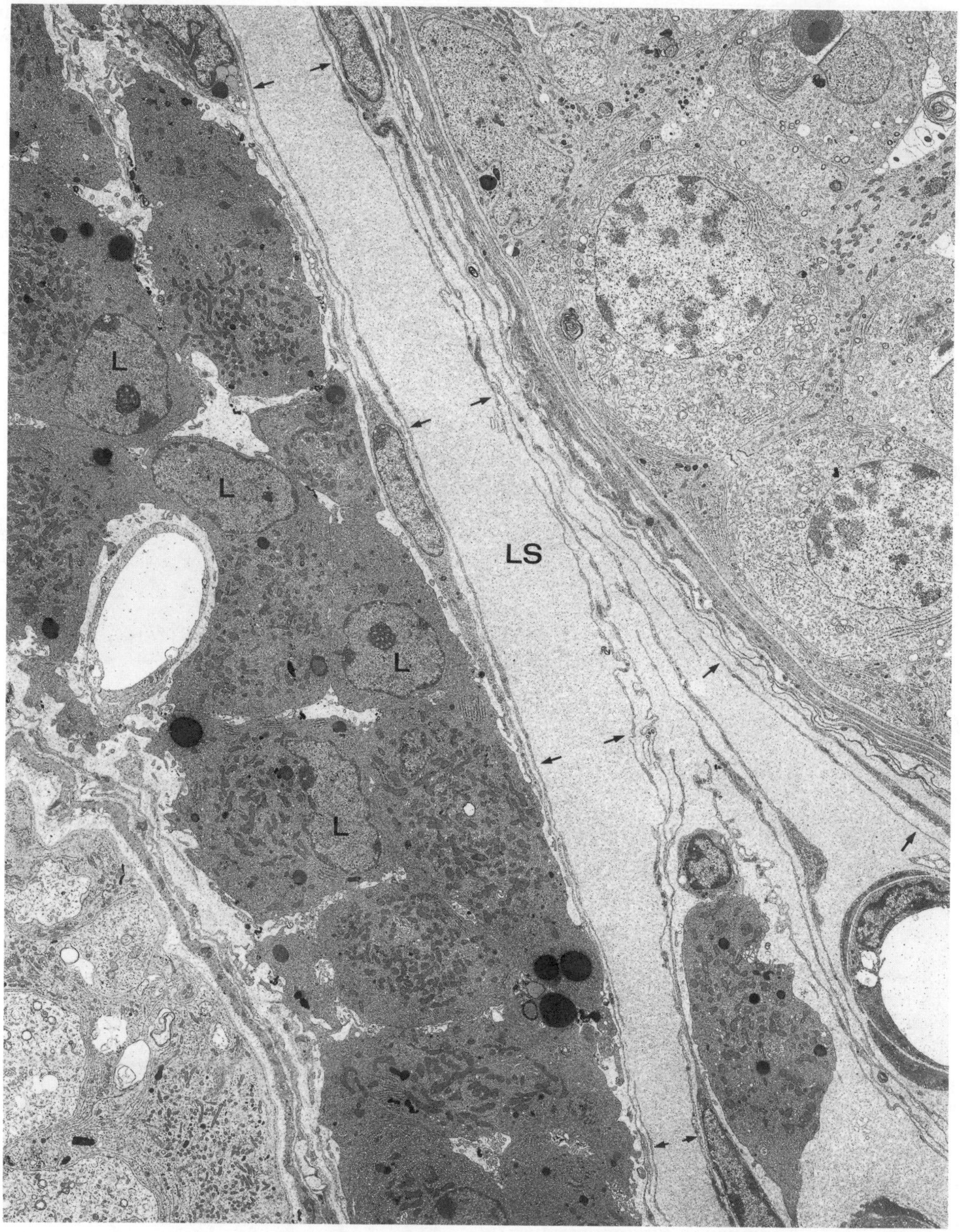

FIG. 79. Ultrastructure of guinea pig intertubular tissue, showing a lymphatic sinusoid (LS) bordered by visceral and parietal endothelium (*arrows*). Leydig cell nuclei (L) are indicated.

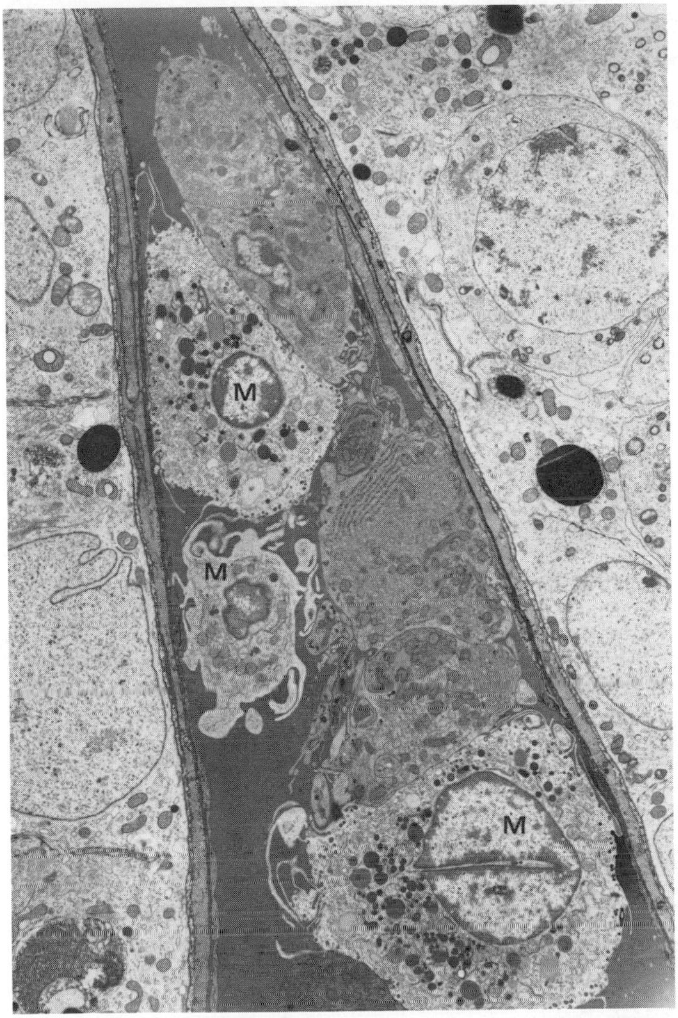

FIG. 80. Ultrastructure of macrophages in the intertubular tissue of the rat testis. The macrophages (M) show many cytoplasmic organelles and inclusions and possess numerous filopodial surface extensions. Tissue fixed with collidine-buffered glutaraldehyde.

centrally or eccentrically within each intertubular area. These lymphatic vessels are bounded by continuous, unbroken endothelial cells and, together with the Leydig cells, are supported by variable quantities of collagen and fibroblasts. To this broad but distinct category belong species such as the ram, bull, hydrax, elephant, monkey, and man (Fig. 76). The relative paucity of Leydig cells in this group together with their often wide separation from blood vessels suggest that steroids secreted from the Leydig cells must gain access to the seminiferous tubules and venous system via diffusion through the edematous loose connective tissues. When the intertubular architecture of the rat and mouse (with extensive lymphatic sinusoids) is compared to that found in these larger mammals (exhibiting much connective tissue), it can be appreciated why Christensen and Mason (636) found that manual separation of seminiferous tubules in rats and mice could be achieved with ease but were unsuccessful in their attempts to tease out fresh specimens obtained from the cat and the human. The lack of extensive peritubular sinusoids in the latter examples thus prevents a clean separation of the two testicular compartments.

A third variation in the composition of the intertubular tissue is exemplified by those animals displaying an extraordinary abundance of Leydig cells but very little intertubular connective tissue. Examples falling into this category include the zebra, domestic boar, wart hog, dog, opossum, and naked mole rat, where Leydig cells occupy 20% to 60% of the testis volume (Fig. 76). To this group we can now add some Australian marsupials, the brush and ring-tailed possum and two marsupial mice, *Antechinus stuartii* and *A. swainsonii,* belonging to the dasyurid group, and the koala (Fig. 82). Small lymphatic vessels are encountered infrequently, and it is remarkable that many Leydig cells, by virtue of their large numbers and close packing, are often positioned at considerable distances from the nearest blood vessel. Why these animals develop large masses of Leydig cells is not understood, although some interesting speculations have been put forward by Fawcett (16,317). These authors reject as unlikely that such a large volume of endocrine tissue is necessary to offset a relative insensitivity of the seminiferous epithelium or to compensate for relatively inefficient mechanisms for delivery of androgens to the tubules. In their view the appreciable numbers of Leydig cells may be related to a systemic requirement for products of the interstitial tissue other than testosterone, such as the secretion of hormone-binding globulins or pheromones. A further possibility of an androgen-dependent enhancement of aggression and courtship behavior exhibited by male marsupial mice has also been considered (21).

Turning now to other cytological features of the intertubular tissue, the presence of macrophages, fibroblasts, lymphocytes, plasma cells, and more rarely mast cells have been recognized for many years, but very little is known of their function. Because of their capacity for phagocytosis, macrophages have been readily identified in the interstitial tissue following application of various dyes such as pyrrol blue, chlorazol fast pink, and acid fuchsin and thionin (651,652). Subcutaneous injection of trypan blue had been a favored method with which to identify macrophages (616,653–656). Additional methods have recently become available to demonstrate macrophages using nonspecific esterase histochemistry (657) and the uptake of latex beads (658). Numerous ultrastructural descriptions of testicular macrophages (Fig. 80; for review see ref. 659) have stimulated renewed interest in their function, and it is known that testicular macrophages are endocytotically active, avidly incorporating

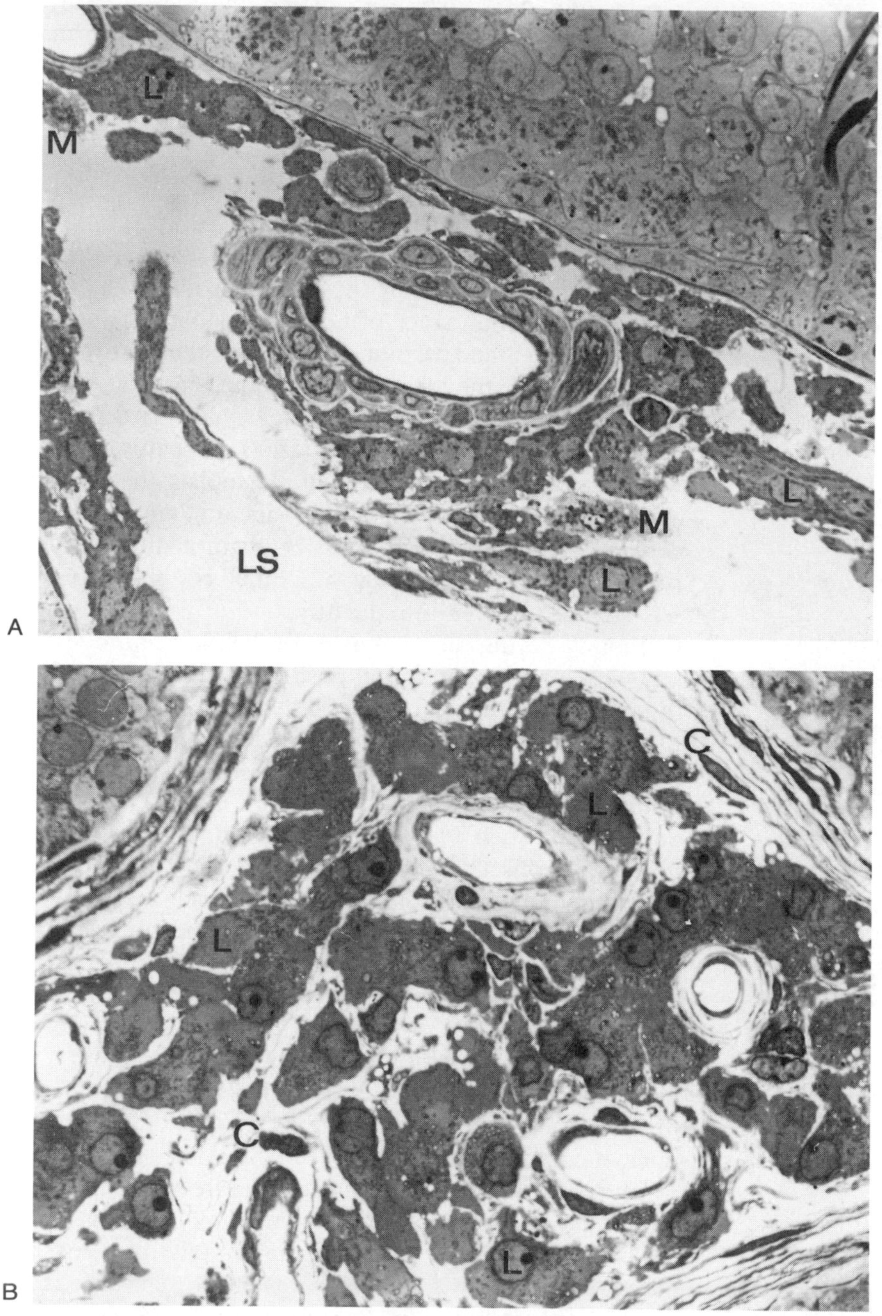

FIG. 81. **A:** Rat intertubular tissue showing Leydig cells (L), macrophages (M), and extensive lymphatic sinusoid (LS). **B:** Human intertubular tissue containing Leydig cells (L) and various connective tissue cells (C).

a variety of exogenous dyes, radiolabeled plutonium, and FSH (659–662).

Recently macrophages in rat intertubular tissue were shown to take up albumin (663). The presence of coated residues beneath the surface membrane of macrophages (Fig. 83) has been linked to a receptor-mediated transport of specific proteins, since plutonium is known to bind to transferrin. Alternatively, fluid-phase endocytosis (pinocytosis) is thought to be the mechanism by which macrophages incorporate albumin from the interstitial lymphatics (663). Specialized contacts have been noted between Leydig cells and macrophages (659,664), and Bergh (663) has shown that an approximate ratio of four to one between these cells occurs in the normal rat testis and following destruction of the seminiferous epithelium induced by artificial cryptorchidism. These findings suggest a functional coupling of these cell types. Rat testicular macrophages express class II MHC androgens (666) and are increased in numbers in response to hCG stimulation (541,542,667); in the developing rat testis they are abundant in fetal life and again at 3 weeks postpartum (668). Macrophages have been difficult to detect

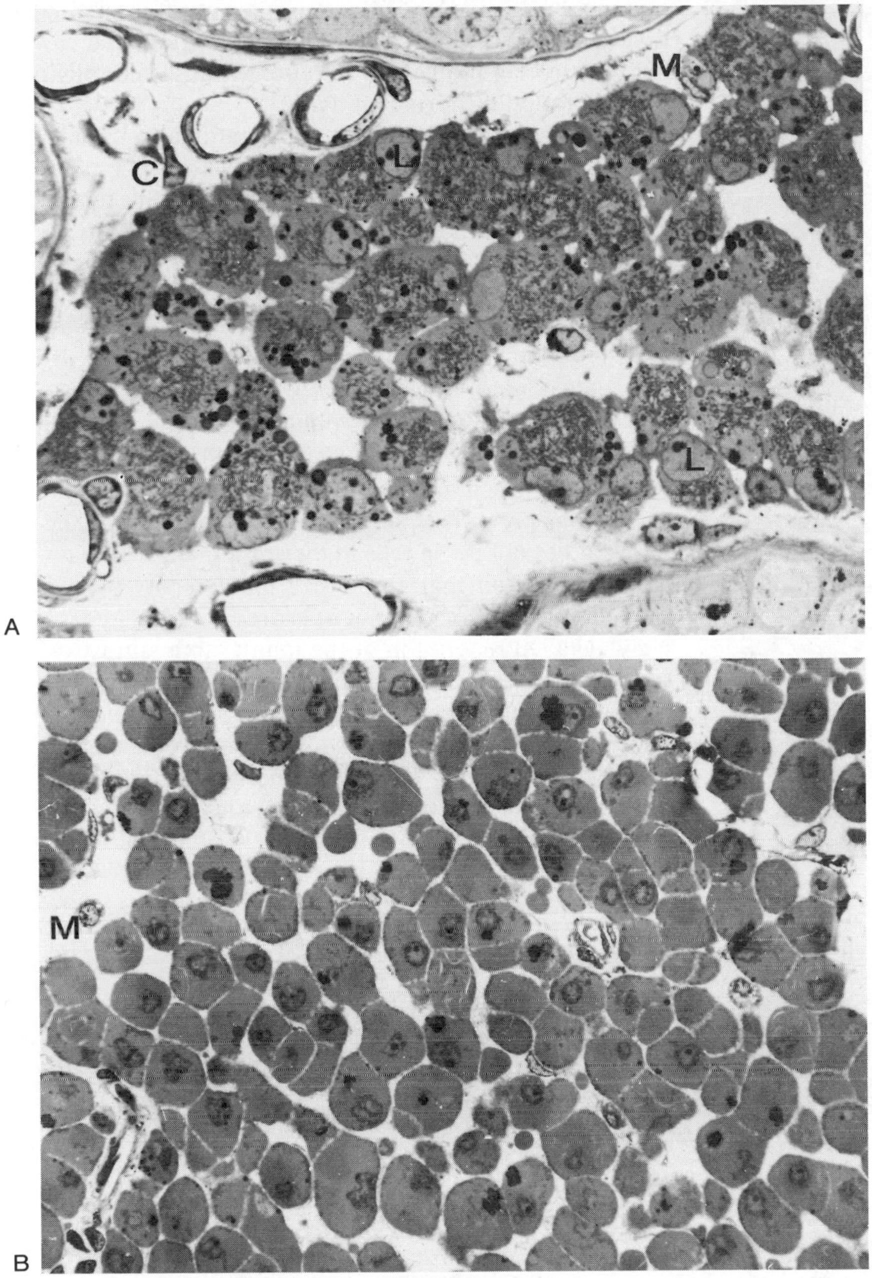

FIG. 82. A: Guinea pig intertubular tissue showing Leydig cells (L) with many mitochondria, macrophages (M), and connective tissue cells (C). **B:** Marsupial mouse Leydig cells whose homogeneous cytoplasm represents smooth endoplasmic reticulum. Macrophages (M) also shown.

in ram testes (669) because of their paucity and small slender morphology, which has likened them to histiocytes or dendritic-type cells.

Additional data on the function of interstitial macrophages have indicated that under special circumstances, they engulf and phagocytose the Leydig cells (561,670). The participation of macrophages in the destruction of the Leydig cells has been verified by ultrastructural studies (671) showing that once this activity has commenced, all Leydig cells disappear from the testis, leaving the interstitial volume practically empty save for the presence of the macrophages and connective tissue cells. These findings are discussed more fully in the section dealing with response of the Leydig cells to testicular damage.

The supporting connective tissues of the interstitial space have received little attention in the past, principally because of their unremarkable morphology and relative scarcity compared to the often much larger size and numbers of Leydig cells (616). However, their importance is highlighted when consideration is given to the mechanisms by which Leydig cells develop within the testis and the question of dedifferentiation of Leydig

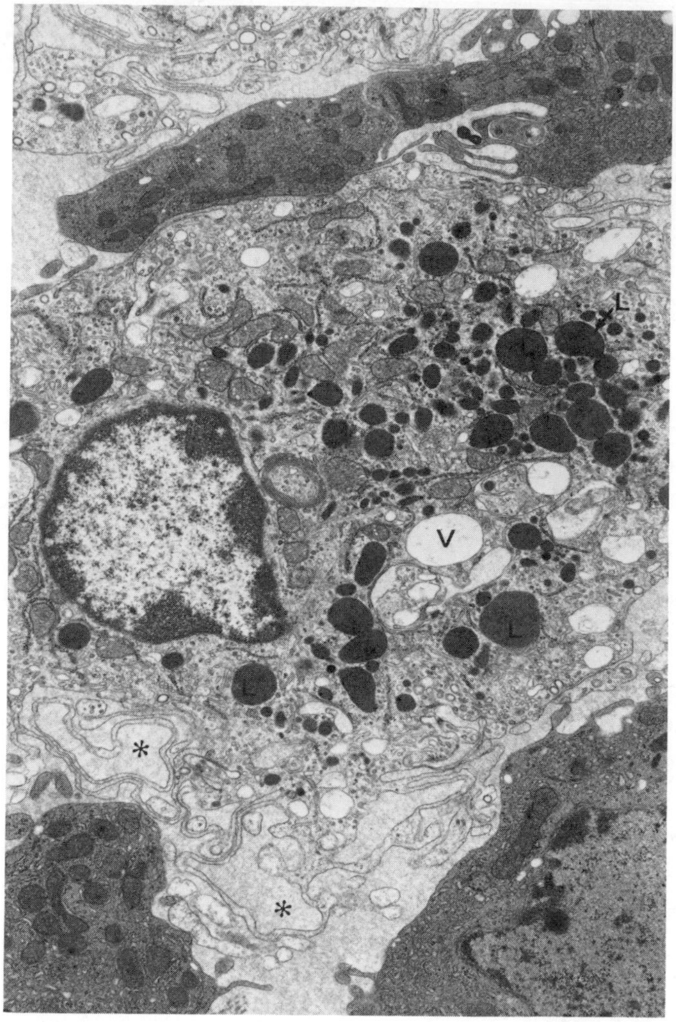

FIG. 83. Intertubular macrophage from the rat testis, showing cytoplasmic lysosomes and dense bodies (L), vacuoles (V), and long surface filopodia and lamellipodia (*asterisks*).

cells into fibroblastlike cells (322,646). A fuller account of the morphology of fibroblastic tissue and its proposed relationship to Leydig cell differentiation is given below in the section concerned with the life history of Leydig cells.

Mononucleated wandering cells such as monocytes together with infrequently encountered lymphocytes and plasma cells have been accorded scant attention in studies of the morphology of the intertubular tissue. At present we can add little to this topic beyond mentioning that severe insults to the testis are unmistakably accompanied by increased numbers of these cells (670,672). Mast cells are occasionally observed in human intertubular tissues (673,674) but rarely encountered in species such as the rat except in the peripheral margins of the intertubular tissue, where it joins within the subtunical arerolar tissues. Most cells may be functionally linked to Leydig cells, since steroidogenesis by hamster Leydig cells is enhanced in the presence of mast cells (675). In the normal testis their functional significance remains obscure, but their plentiful occurrence in rat interstitial tissue following recovery of testicular function after earlier impairment indicates a hitherto unsuspected role in the restoration of normal activity.

Although this resume of the organizational patterns of intertubular tissues has been confined to mammalian species, a substantial body of information on this topic is available for nonmammalian vertebrates and many invertebrates (505,676–682).

Ultrastructure

Detailed descriptions of Leydig cell structure in relation to function have been published in the excellent reviews by Christensen and Gillim (378) and Christensen (616) in which information on some 46 mammalian species was presented. Since then additional ultrastructural studies of Leydig cells in the adult mammalian testis have emerged that emphasize the diversity of their internal composition (for examples, see Table 3). Accordingly, detailed reiteration of the many subtle ultrastructural features of Leydig cells unique to a given species would be largely redundant and add little to advance our understanding or identify gaps in our knowledge of the biology of these cells. Therefore emphasis is directed toward a review of the subcellular structure of Leydig cells in relation to known or suggested physiological activities. A summary of selected species indicating quantitative morphological features of their Leydig cells is presented in Table 4.

Nucleus

Leydig cell nuclei are often eccentrically placed within the cell and usually display a round or irregularly oval

TABLE 3. *Selected examples of Leydig cell ultrastructure in adult mammalian testis since 1975*

Species	References
Mouse	693,702,712
Rat	688,899,711,729
Bush rat	507,718
Guinea pig	690,871,872
Hamster	690,815,873,874
Squirrel	512
Hare	675
Hyrax	812
Mole	816
Armadillo	695
Iranian vole	876
Bat	723
Seal	877
Boar	878
Ox	712
Dog	615,694
Monkey	786
Human	322,350,692,879

TABLE 4. *Quantitative morphology of Leydig cells*

Species	Volume (μl/cm³ testis)	Numerical density (10⁶/cm³ testis)	Volume/ cell (μm³)	Volume smooth ER (% cytoplasm)	Volume smooth ER (μm³/cell)	Surface area of plasma membrane (μm²/cell)	Surface area smooth ER (μm²/cell)	Surface area smooth ER (% cell membrane)	References
Mouse	38–52	25	1500–4000	6	1240	1150	10–12,000	60	693,866,869
Rat	22–34	14–22	1200–2400	13–44	160–750	1500	30–70,000	54–64	702,735,786
Guinea pig	19–30	22	1600	62	900		135,000	68	702,705
Hamster	10–23	15	970–1100	18–20	160–180	960	22,000	19–65	508,510,518, 705
Rock hyrax			3000–5000						811
Woodchuck	480	89	5300						818
Rabbit	22			42					702
Dog	32			37					702
Stallion	120–170	21–25	5800–7000						527
Monkey	8	6	1300	14	165				776
Human	32	8	3000–4500	15	550	2400	32,000	71	690,692,830, 866,870

shape. Alternatively, the nucleus may present as irregularly polygonal in thin sections with numerous indentations of the nuclear envelope. When seen in proximity to the walls of blood vessels or the tunica propria of the seminiferous tubules, the nucleus usually conforms to the elongated configuration of the cell by displaying an elliptical profile. In the human testis, Leydig cells with two or more nuclei have been noted (322). An inner mantle of peripheral heterochromatin associated with the nuclear envelope is a universal feature of Leydig cells, at times forming small dense clumps of electron-dense material at irregularly spaced intervals along the inner aspect of the nuclear membrane (Fig. 84). The nucleolus is usually conspicuous and exhibits a conventional fine structure comprising the nucleolonemma and dense granular and amorphous areas. Leydig cells of the human testis frequently show duplicate nucleoli, and in the nuclei of adult mouse Leydig cells, an annular nucleolus is commonly noted (683). This unusual configuration in mouse Leydig cells has been correlated with Leydig cell development, since they do not appear in immature animals. Extrapolating from their occurrence in other cell types (684), it has been suggested that the central core of annular nucleoli is associated with partial cessation of RNA synthesis. The suppression of RNA synthesis in the annular nucleolus may be reflected by a maturational shift in the conversion of rough to smooth endoplasmic reticulum in the cytoplasm, since the cistrons of rRNA exist in the nucleolus.

Cytoplasm

The dominant organelle within the cytoplasm of mammalian Leydig cells is the smooth endoplasmic reticulum, which provides binding sites on its surface for numerous enzymes necessary for a variety of steroidogenic conversions. Great diversity in the architecture of the smooth endoplasmic reticulum has been indicated in reviews of its ultrastructure (378,616). The qualitative and quantitative differences in the morphology of membranes of smooth endoplasmic reticulum have been described in common laboratory species such as the guinea pig and mouse, in which it is most abundant (616,685), and the rat and human, where it may vary considerably in amount and concentration (378,686,687). Examples of these between-species ultrastructural differences are illustrated in Figs. 84–86.

Our own studies of the internal organization of the Leydig cell were the first to examine quantitatively the proportion of cytoplasm that was occupied by smooth endoplasmic reticulum (688), and for the rat, approximately 39% of Leydig cell volume was taken up by the internal cavities of this organelle. Since then the volume occupancy and surface area of this and all other cytoplasmic components in Leydig cells of the rat, mouse, hamster, dog, rabbit, guinea pig, and human have been documented (689–693). All of these studies indicate that the surface area of smooth endoplasmic reticulum is vast. For example, if a single rat Leydig cell were represented as a golf ball, then an unraveling of its membranes of smooth endoplasmic reticulum would generate a square approximately three feet on a side. In situ, therefore, the membranes of smooth endoplasmic reticulum appear as a vast concentration of tubules interconnected in various patterns to form a meshwork extending throughout the entire cytoplasm of the Leydig cell. The membranes thus enclose a cavity constituting an intracellular compartment separated from the ground cytoplasm.

A scheme suggesting possible interconversions of the different ultrastructural configurations of smooth endoplasmic reticulum was based on electron microscopic analysis of guinea pig Leydig cells (376). The common form of smooth endoplasmic reticulum consists of a random network of interconnected tubules (Fig. 85), which may transform into loosely packed sheets of tubules or form more regular arrays of fenestrated cisternae. Leydig cells of the mouse exhibit all these various forms and in

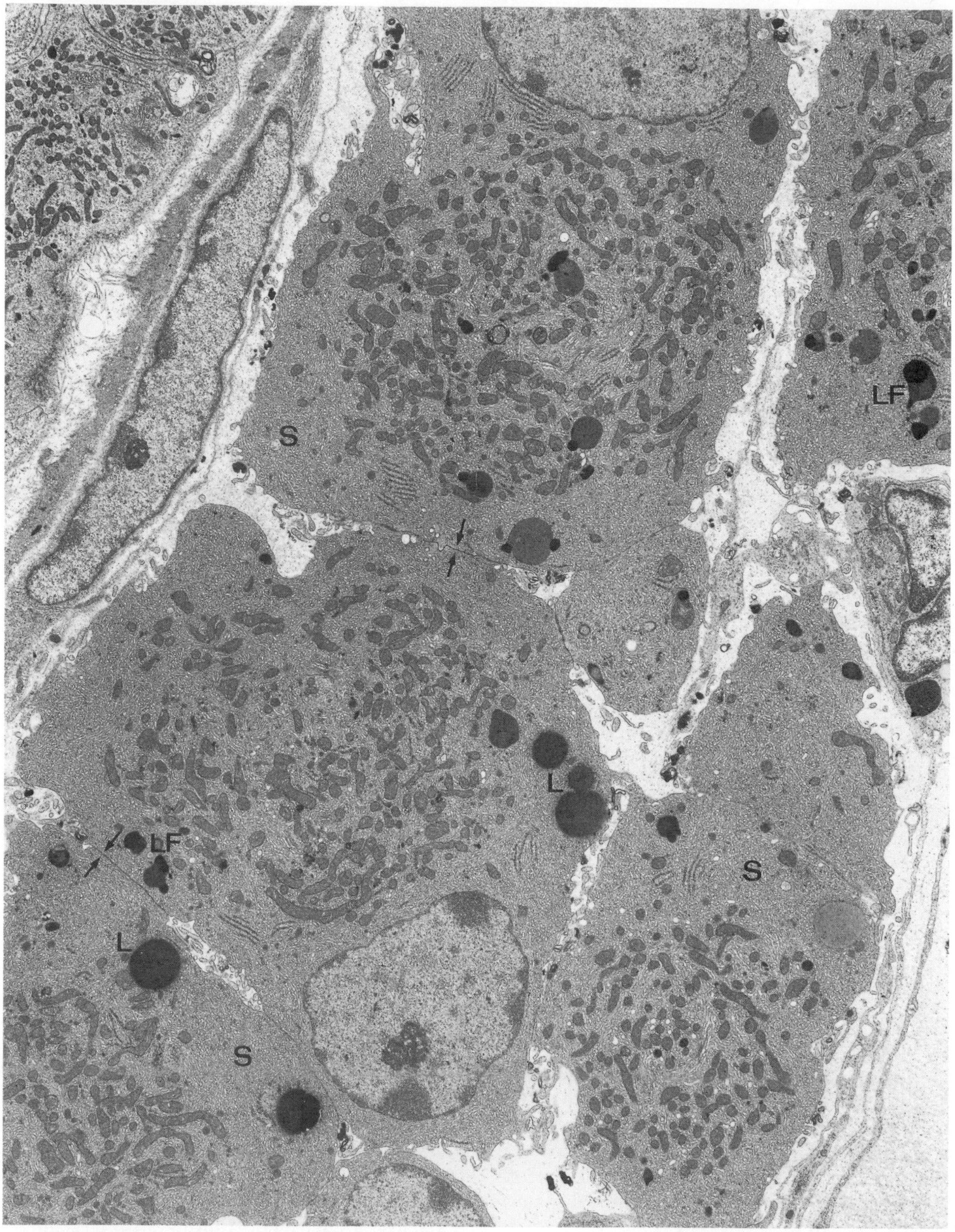

FIG. 84. Guinea pig Leydig cells illustrating central aggregations of mitochondria and peripheral concentrations of smooth endoplasmic reticulum (S). Lipid inclusions (L) and lipofuscin bodies (LF) are shown. Note close apposition of adjacent Leydig cells (*arrows*).

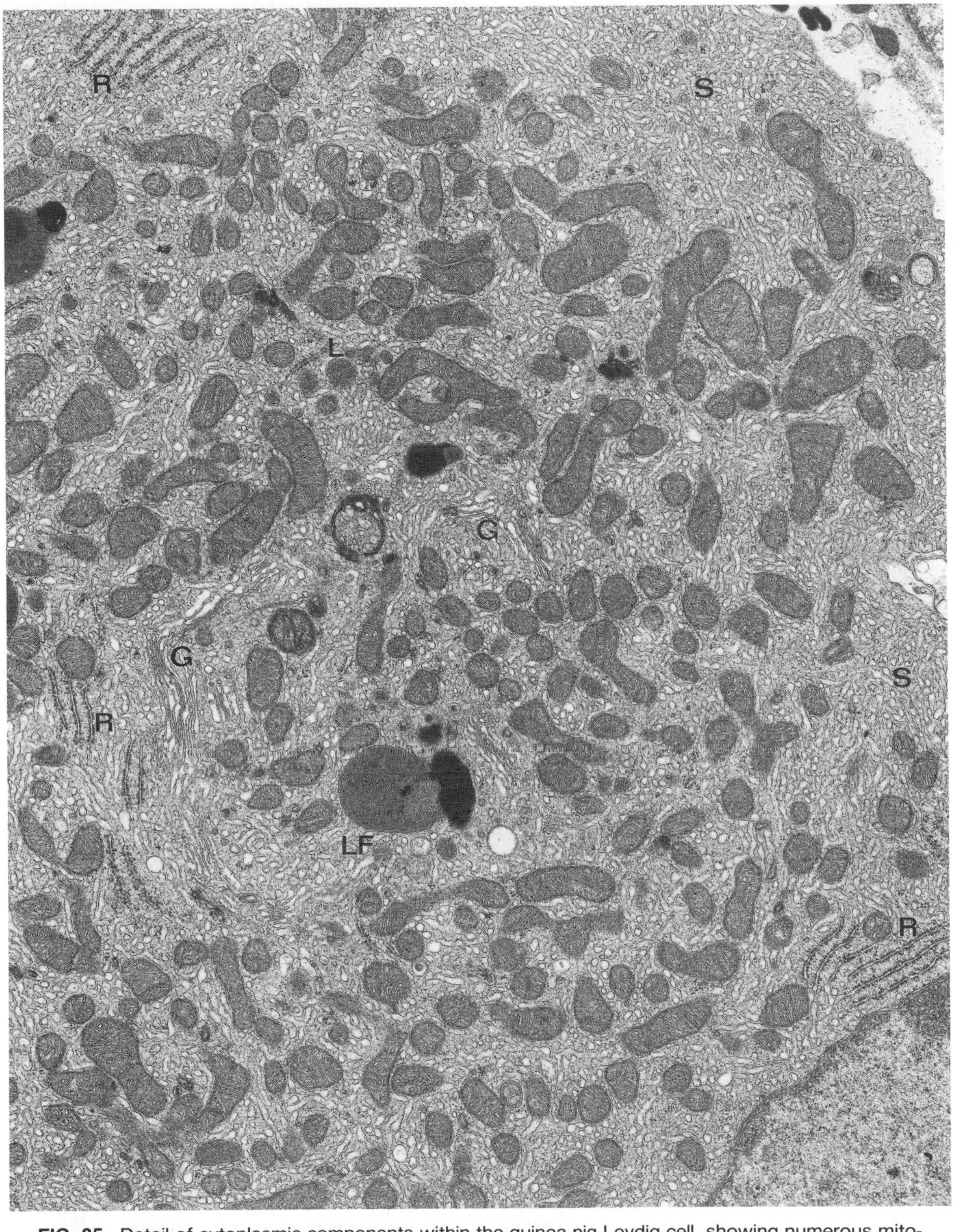

FIG. 85. Detail of cytoplasmic components within the guinea pig Leydig cell, showing numerous mitochondria, tubules of smooth endoplasmic reticulum (S), Golgi membranes (G), rough endoplasmic reticulum (R), lysosomal bodies (L), and lipofuscin inclusions (LF).

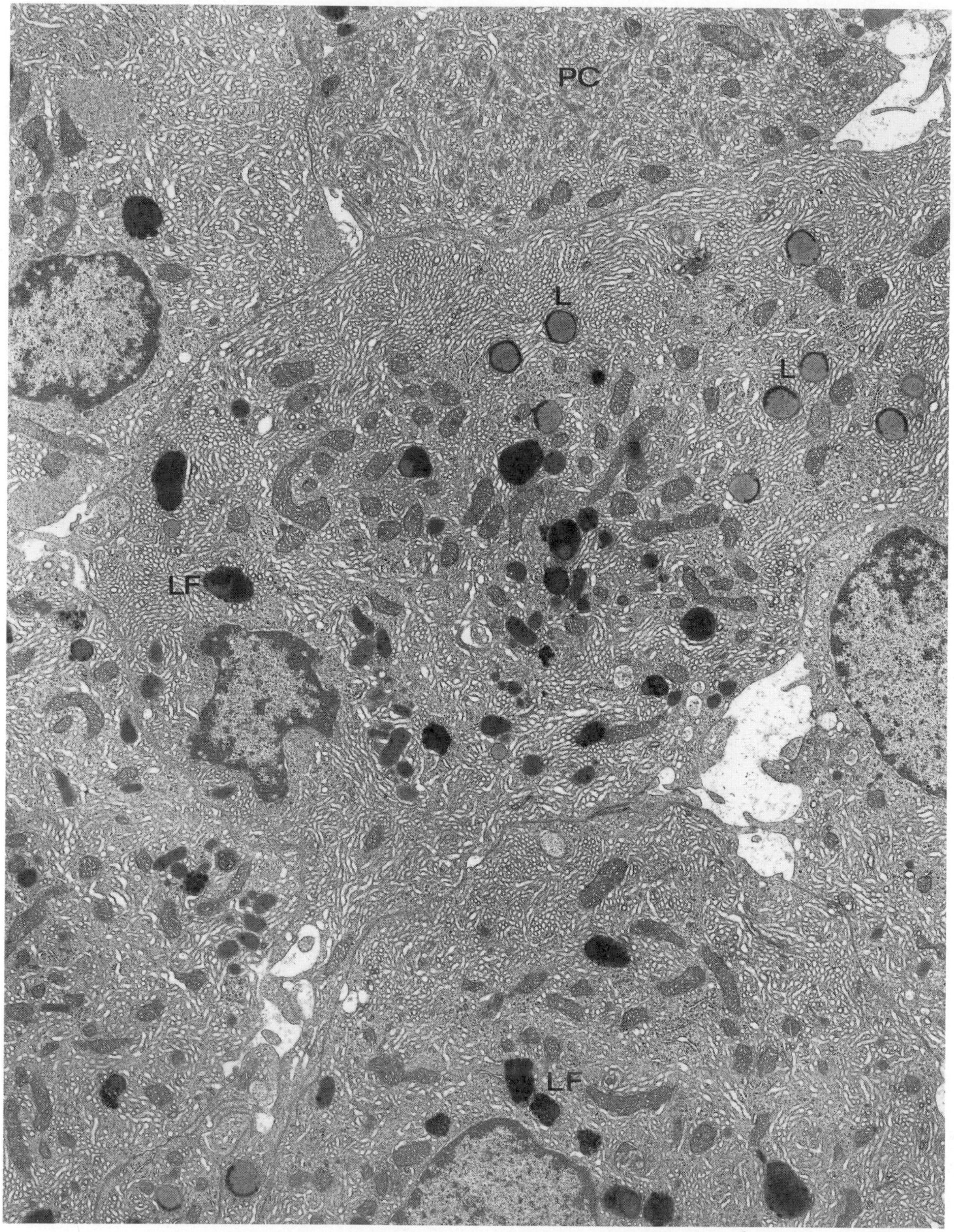

FIG. 86. In human Leydig cells fixed via perfusion, the smooth endoplasmic reticulum is the dominant organelle and presents as tightly packed anastomotic tubules. Lipofuscin pigments (LF) are common, and small lipid inclusions (L) are noted. Paracrystalline inclusions (PC) are shown.

addition show a marked segregation of their cytoplasmic membranes, a spectacular example being seen in the appearance of extensive concentric whorls of smooth membranes. These may surround lipid inclusions, mitochondria, or dense membrane-bound bodies, and similar whorls are observed in the guinea pig, rat, dog, armadillo, and monkey (378,533,694–696). The absence of these whorled membranes in many other species raises the possibility that they provide a specific function to meet the biochemical requirements of these particular cells.

A similar concept could be used to explain the infrequent occurrence of other unusual membranous bodies such as single- or double-walled tubules, which occur in the mouse, opossum, and rat (683,685,697,698), and structures resembling annulate lamellae, seen in adult mouse and rabbit Leydig cells (697–701). The functional significance of these organelles remains unknown. However, the morphological diversity of Leydig cell smooth membranes emphasizes the role of quantitative methods designed to estimate what proportion of the cytoplasm is occupied by a particular organelle. A major objective of stereological analysis of the Leydig cell has been to correlate the relative abundance of cellular components with the amount of steroid compounds synthesized and secreted by the same cells (689).

One approach adopted by Ewing and co-workers has attempted to link Leydig cell ultrastructure and various pathways of steroidogenesis. They have examined changes in Leydig cell morphology and the capacity to synthesize various steroids by manipulating the degree to which LH is available to act on the Leydig cell (690,702–705). A summary of their findings is presented. When different species were examined, the production of testosterone after LH stimulation was significantly different between species but was not related to the total mass of Leydig cells within the testis. Instead they found a strong correlation between testosterone secretion and the amount of smooth endoplasmic reticulum and Golgi membranes within the Leydig cell cytoplasm, indicating the central role played by these organelles in determining how much testosterone is provided by a single Leydig cell. Furthermore, they have shown that there is a subdivision of enzyme function in the steroidogenic pathway that exists within the membranes of smooth endoplasmic reticulum, raising the interesting possibility that certain conversions such as pregnenolone to progesterone may be sequestered to specialized regions of the Leydig cell. These findings implicate the concentric whorls and other varieties of smooth cytoplasmic membranes in subserving this function. The levels of testosterone in plasma during the development of the monkey testis are also correlated with the volume of smooth endoplasmic reticulum within the Leydig cell or whole testis rather than the total volume or numbers of these cells (706). A similar study of the Leydig cells of the human testis has shown that the volume of smooth endoplasmic reticulum within the Leydig cells is positively correlated with daily sperm production (707).

Mitochondria vary in size and form both in a given Leydig cell and between different species, and their ultrastructure has been well described in earlier studies (378,616,708). Cholesterol is known to undergo side-chain cleavage within the mitochondrion, possibly on the surface of the cristae, which exhibit various profiles ranging from foliate, tubular, or intermediate forms, and details of the reactions and enzyme systems with Leydig cell mitochondria appear elsewhere in this volume. Electron-dense mitochondrial granules often occur within the matrix of the mitochondrion, but that function is obscure (378,616,708).

Depending on the species, Leydig cells may exhibit an abundance of lipid inclusions or may not. Some confusion may exist about the occurrence of lipid inclusions in Leydig cells, since even within a single section of a testis, Leydig cells may show differing amounts of lipid (Fig. 87) (687), suggesting variable degrees of functional activity. When an estimation of the lipid content of mouse Leydig cells was averaged over many cells (692), each Leydig cell contained about 147 lipid inclusions, diameter approximately 1 μm, and collectively occupying about 6% of cytoplasmic volume. However, when mouse Leydig cells are centrifuged in Percoll density gradients (709), they separate according to buoyant density, and cells of low and high specific gravity show, respectively, a great many or very few cytoplasmic lipid inclusions (Fig. 87). Similar observations may be made for rat Leydig cells, of which the greatest majority are devoid of lipid inclusions, although occasionally some Leydig cells contain an abundance of these inclusions. The latter are possibly the few surviving fetal-type Leydig cells, which are known to persist within the adult rat testis (710).

Obvious differences in the extent of lipid inclusions occur between species. The Leydig cells of the dog, cat, mole, rat, mouse, elephant, and rhesus monkey often contain a high proportion of lipid (16,590,694); guinea pig, rabbit, and boar exhibit somewhat less (16,376,690), and Leydig cells of the human, rat, hamster, opossum, ox, African green monkey, squirrel monkey, and several marsupial species found in Australia contain very few lipid inclusions (689,690,692,698,711–713). A discussion of the likely functional role of Leydig cell lipid inclusions (378,616) has reviewed the evidence that they represent sites of cholesterol storage and/or synthesis. The belief that lipid inclusions are intimately involved in fatty metabolism and, by inference, certain steroidogenic reactions has been supported by morphological data. In rat fetuses, for example, one of the principal structural features enabling identification of the fetal Leydig cells is their rich supply of lipid inclusions, but in postnatal life, adult Leydig cells rarely contain lipid. That these changes in lipid content reflect alterations in

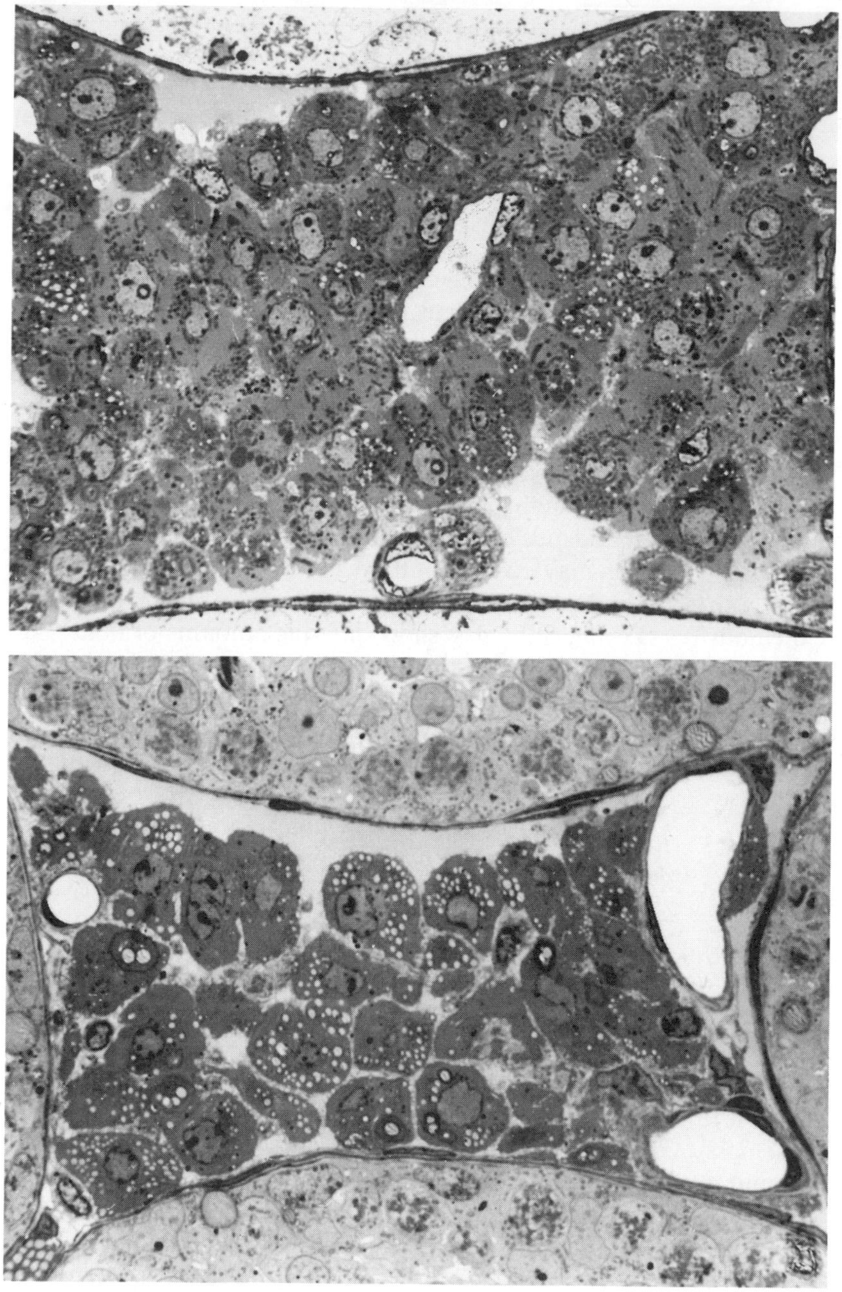

A

B

FIG. 87. A: Adult mouse testis showing a large cluster of Leydig cells containing numerous dense inclusions representing mitochondria together with homogeneously stained cytoplasmic regions filled with smooth endoplasmic reticulum. **B:** Adult mouse testis showing Leydig cells with prominent aggregations of pale-staining cytoplasmic lipid inclusions.

Leydig cell function is further emphasized, since trophic stimulation (with LH/hCG) of Leydig cells rapidly depletes their stores of morphologically recognizable lipid droplets (714–718) and heralds an increase in testosterone secretion. Animals fed a cholesterol-rich diet showed a significant depletion of lipid inclusions in the Leydig cells, indicating that if available, cholesterol is taken up by the Leydig cell, which obviates the need for lipid storage in the cytoplasm (691). Opposite changes occur when Leydig cells were examined after withdrawal of gonadotropins, where lipid inclusions became plentiful (711,719), but replacement therapy with exogenous LH resulted in a marked depletion of the accumulated lipid.

The Golgi apparatus of Leydig cells is moderately well developed (Fig. 85), and although its peripheral vesicles are usually devoid of any internal material, under conditions of Leydig cell hyperactivity, the saccules of the Golgi complex often appear swollen and contain distinct electron-dense flocculent material (Fig. 84). Nothing is at present known about the role played by the Golgi apparatus, except its participation in the intracellular passage of radiolabeled fucose, traced by electron microscope autoradiography (720,721). It was tentatively concluded from a brief summary of this study that Leydig cells secrete glycoproteins, with the Golgi complex featuring prominently in their early synthesis.

The uncertainty that surrounds the precise functional duties of Leydig cell organelles is no more apparent than in relation to the question, often posed, of the mechanism by which testosterone or any other secretory product is transported through the cytoplasm and released into the extracellular space. This intriguing topic has been discussed many times (see ref. 616) but at present remains only speculative. However, in other steroid-secreting tissues such as the luteal cells of the ovary, evidence has been put forward to suggest that progesterone is secreted in granule form (721). Secretion of corticosteroids from the adrenal tissue is thought to occur in a similar fashion (722). For most species, Leydig cells do not exhibit typical secretory granules or vacuoles in their cytoplasm. However, in a species of seasonally breeding bat, maximum testosterone secretion in the breeding season is accompanied by a marked increase in the abundance of small, dense, membrane-bound granules, whereas in periods of Leydig cell quiescence, the granules largely disappear from the cytoplasm (723). Since the majority of these granules do not share the enzymatic or morphological properties attributable to lysosomes or peroxisomes, they were thought to be involved in the transport of testosterone through the cytoplasm prior to its secretion. More recent studies (724) on cytoplasmic granules in luteal cells of guinea pigs failed to detect granule exocytosis and could show no relationship between the abundance of small granules and maximum progesterone secretion. The functional significance of Leydig cell granules in particular species thus requires further clarification. Furthermore, there is increasing evidence that the ovary secretes relaxin and oxytocin, which, being peptides, are more likely to be stored as secretory granules (725,726).

Lysosomes are commonly observed in Leydig cells. These organelles are about 0.5 μm in diameter, bounded by a single membrane, and show circular or irregular profiles by electron microscopy. They are also referred to as dense bodies because of their notable staining properties. The lysosomes present in Leydig cells conform to their usual pleomorphic occurrence in other cells, exhibiting various states of fusion with cytoplasmic vacuoles, thus categorizing them as secondary lysosomes as distinct from the individual primary lysosome (616). Multivesicular bodies are regarded as structural variations within the lysosomal system and probably represent packaging of recently internalized vesicles destined for lysosomal disposal. The involvement of elements of the lysosomal family of organelles within the Leydig cell has been investigated by studying the response of Leydig cells to exogenous tracers known to be incorporated into lysosomes of other cell types (727). In this study, Leydig cells were active endocytic cells using both fluid-phase and adsorptive endocytic mechanisms to take up extracellular macromolecules. The destruction of the internalized tracers followed different routes of transport within the Leydig cell cytoplasm, depending on the ionic charge of the individual tracer. As seen diagrammatically in Fig. 88, fluid-phase endocytosis involved the lysosomal tracers following this same route or, alternatively, were carried to the Golgi region, whereupon they ultimately disappeared. The existence of these separate pathways for internalized macromolecules suggests that the disposal of unwanted material can be dealt with in a variety

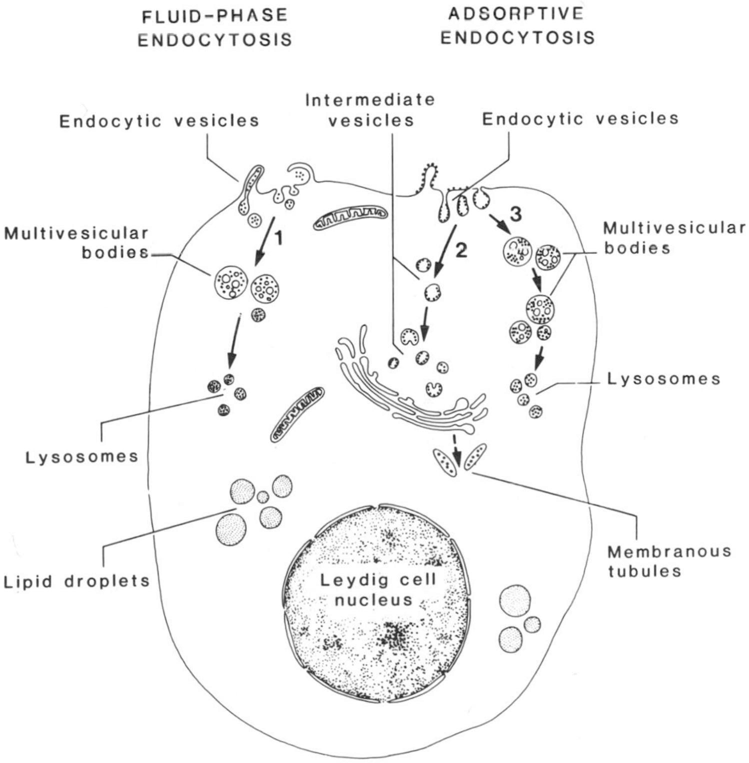

FIG. 88. Diagram illustrating intracellular pathways of endocytosed tracers in the Leydig cell. Pathway 1 shows tracers destined for lysosomal incorporation. Pathway 2 illustrates absorptive endocytosis of molecules initially bound to the cell surface and ultimately transported to the Golgi region via intermediate vesicles. In pathway 3, these molecules follow an intracellular route involving only the lysosomes. Some tracer molecules also appear in membranous tubules associated with the Golgi membranes, although their subsequent fate is not known. (Data from Hermo et al., ref. 727.)

of ways. Leydig cells contain autophagolysosomes (728), which arise independently within the cytoplasm and acquire lysosomal enzymes from secondary lysosomes by fusion with them. They are eliminated from the cell by exocytosis.

Poorly digested substances often remain within the Leydig cell lysosomal system and are recognized as dense membrane-bound granules referred to as lipofuscin pigment granules. They are commonly seen in human Leydig cells as heterogeneous conglomerates of myelin figures and particulate matter (616,686,729–731). Stimulation of Leydig cells with hCG tended to increase their abundance (687,719). Although the biochemistry of lipofuscin granules is unclear, they contain acid phosphatases (687,719), suggesting a derivation from lysosomes. Their appearance in other species is reviewed by Ohata (701). The studies of Reddy and Svoboda (732) and Hruban et al. (743) identified the peroxisome within Leydig cells as a homogeneous pale-staining granule, approximately 0.2 μm in diameter. These organelles contain catalase and oxidases, and although they increase in number following hCG stimulation (625), their functional role has remained unclear until recent morphometric and immunolabeling studies suggested their involvement in steroidogenesis. The relationship between testosterone secretory capacity and cellular organelles has identified a positive correlation between steroid secretion and the volume and surface area of peroxisomes (705). Stimulation of Leydig cells with LH is followed rapidly by a three- to fivefold increase in total volume of peroxisomes, whereas other organelles are unchanged (734,735). Peroxisomes contain a sterol carrier protein thought to be involved with the transport of cholesterol to the inner mitochondrial membrane for subsequent side-chain cleavage reactions in the steroid pathway.

Centrioles at times associated with the Golgi complex have been identified, and cilia may be noted developing from the paired centrioles (694,701,736). Since the fibril pattern of the cilium has a 9 + 0 pattern, it could reflect a sensory or chemoreceptor property (737). Microtubules and filaments are present within the Leydig cell cytoplasm; the latter occur throughout the cytoplasm and at times form a network subjacent to the plasma membrane (322). When microtubular systems of steroid-secreting cells are disrupted with inhibitors such as colchicine or vinblastine (738,739), an increase in steroidogenesis is observed. In isolated rat Leydig tumor cell lines, the resting cells exhibit tubulin in discrete granular units distributed throughout the cytoplasm, but when steroidogenesis was induced by treatment with cAMP, vast microtubular networks appear, forming radial patterns around the central cell nucleus (740). The small cytoplasmic granules in unstimulated cells were rich in tubulin and cholesterol, indicating that one role of microtubular organization is to make intracellular cholesterol freely available for conversion into pregnenolone. An additional role of microtubular–microfilamentous systems in Leydig cells is in the process of LH/hCG receptor down-regulation, which does not occur following treatment with microtubule inhibitors (741). When vinblastine was administered, the Leydig cells showed remarkable increases in Golgi-associated vesicles and cytoplasmic filamentous material, suggesting alterations of the transport mechanisms within the cytoplasm. Filaments with diameters of 5 to 7 nm or 10 to 12 nm are always seen in Leydig cells, and their ultrastructure has been reviewed earlier (616,694).

A remarkable specialization of human Leydig cells is the crystal of Reinke, originally described by Reinke (742). Readily visible by light microscopy, they frequently present as rod-shaped structures up to 20 μm in length, although they may exhibit triangular, rhombic, or polygonal shapes (Fig. 89). Not every Leydig cell contains these crystals. Their ultrastructure and crystalline nature have been repeatedly documented (686,687,729, 730,743–746). Although they are known to contain protein (745) and to increase in size and number in aging testes (746), their functional role is unclear. A variety of other crystalline structures, termed paracrystalline inclusions, have also been noted in human Leydig cells (322). Since the subunits of Reinke crystals are similar to the paracrystalline inclusions, the latter have been considered precursors of the much larger Reinke crystals (686). Occasionally, either type of crystalline material may occur in the Leydig cell nucleus (685,744,747).

Reinke crystals were commonly believed to be unique to human Leydig cells until similar cytoplasmic crystalloids were described in Leydig cells of the sexually regressed wild bush rat, *Rattus fuscipes* (391). These rats are seasonal breeders, and in the nonbreeding season, serum gonadotropins and testosterone are decreased. Using modified laboratory conditions mimicking the natural environment of the nonbreeding season, Irby et al. (507) induced Leydig cell atrophy in the same species, whereupon many large crystalloid inclusions made their appearance in the Leydig cell cytoplasm (Figs. 90 and 91). Again serum hormone levels declined significantly compared to breeding rats that do not display these crystalloid inclusions. When gonadotropin secretion was experimentally suppressed by hypophysectomy or testosterone implants (748), the Leydig cells atrophied, and many crystalloids appeared in the cytoplasm (Fig. 92). Formation of nuclear vesicles, their subsequent transfer to the Leydig cell cytoplasm, and the concurrent development of paracrystalline material within the vesicles have been suggested as a mechanism to explain the growth of crystalloids by assembly and fusion of smaller subunits (Fig. 91). Because these crystals occur only in regressive forms of Leydig cells that produce very little testosterone, they may represent a storage facility of steroid precursors and enzymes, although further work will be necessary to elucidate their precise function.

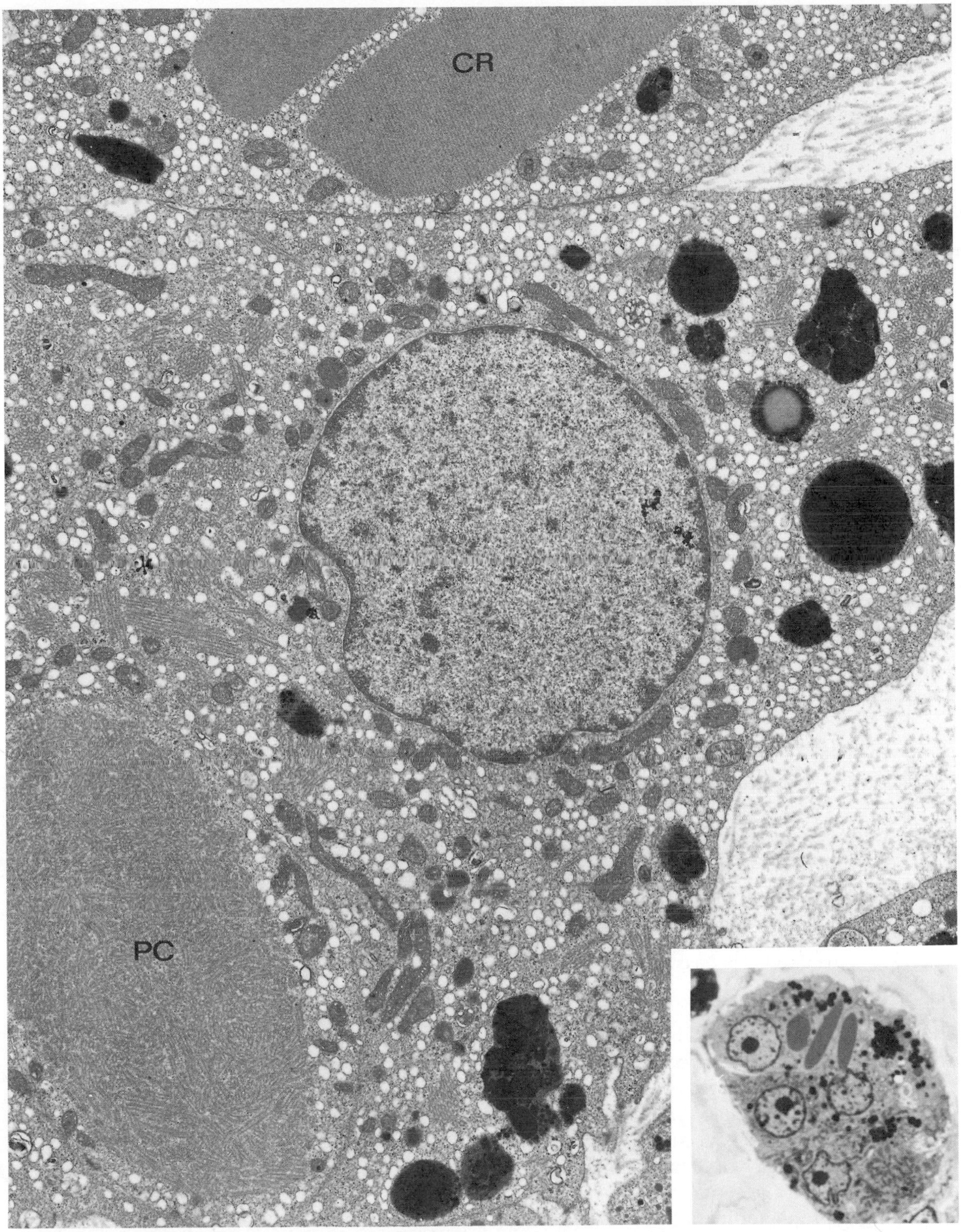

FIG. 89. Leydig cells of the human testis prepared by immersion fixation of biopsy material. The smooth endoplasmic reticulum shows individual vesicles. Crystals of Reinke (CR) are seen, together with paracrystalline inclusions (PC), forming large aggregations or scattered within the cytoplasm (*asterisk*). **Inset:** Crystals of Reinke observed by light microscopy.

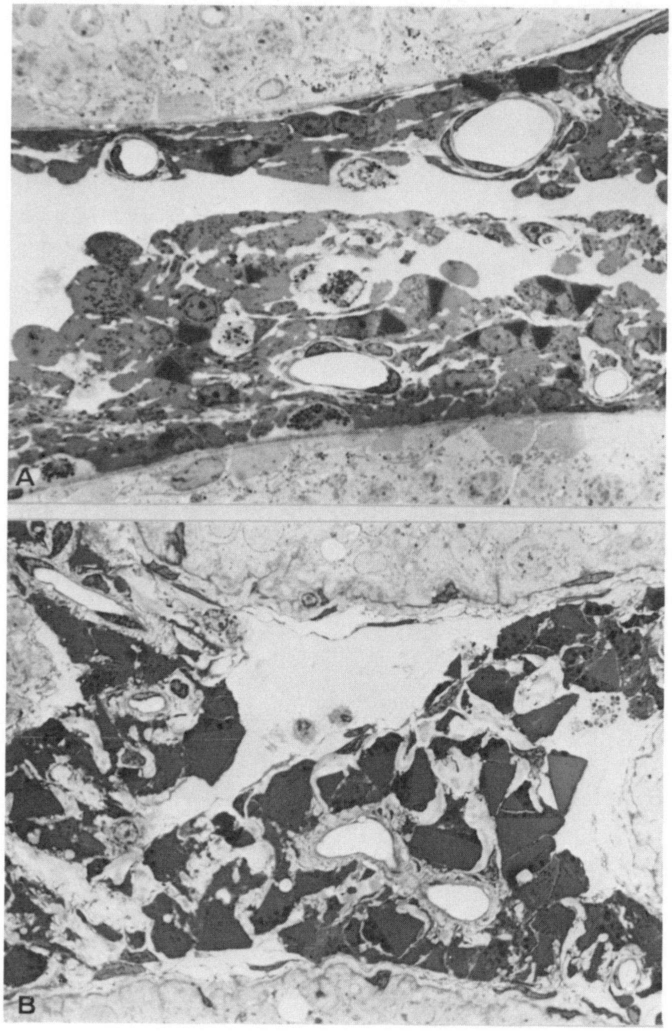

FIG. 90. A: Leydig cells in the testis of the bush rat, *R. fuscipes,* showing triangular and polygonal crystalloid inclusions that appear as the process of spermatogenesis begins to undergo regression. **B:** In the fully regressed testis of *R. fuscipes,* the Leydig cells develop large crystalloid inclusions.

The surface area of Leydig cell plasma membrane is very large because of extensive surface projections of filopodia and microvilli (615,616,701,711). In a morphometric analysis of rat Leydig cells (689), their volume was estimated to be about 1200 μm^3, and if considered to be spherical their surface area would have been approximately 500 μm^2. However, the actual figure is 1500 μm^2, reflecting the complex topography of its surface. Leydig cells found in clusters form junctions with neighboring Leydig cells and occasionally form junctions with themselves (615). Gap junctions are frequently observed where the intercellular space is narrowed to 20 Å (616,694). These junctions are normally 0.2 to 2 μm in greater diameter (364) and in thin sections appear as ring-shaped, circular, or double-circle structures (Fig. 93). Septatelike junctions have occasionally been described (616), and these are partially permeable to electron-dense tracers such as lanthanum. Tight junctions or desmosomes are generally not considered to form between Leydig cells, although rudimentary desmosomes have been observed in canine Leydig cells (694). Special sites of contact between Leydig cells and macrophages occur frequently (659,664) and consist of short projections of Leydig cell cytoplasm that invaginate nearby macrophages. The plasma membrane of the macrophage develops an inner bristle coat, suggesting the possibility that small amounts of Leydig cell cytoplasm may be endocytosed by the macrophage. A thin, discontinuous layer of basal-lamina-type material may partly surround the surface of the Leydig cell (616,694,701,730) and may provide structural support to the cell in conjunction with scattered bundles of collagen fibers. Autonomic nerves have been observed in close association with Leydig cells of the immature hu-

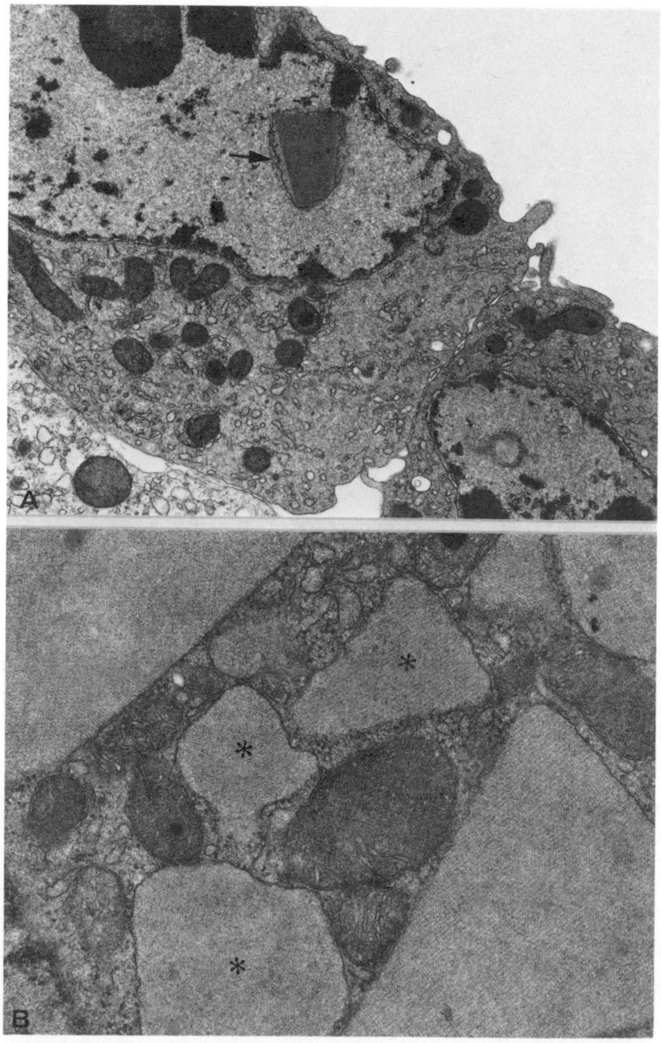

FIG. 91. A: *R. fuscipes* Leydig cells illustrating intranuclear formation of a crystalloid (*arrow*). **B:** *R. fuscipes* Leydig cell showing angular and pleomorphic (*asterisks*) cytoplasmic crystalloid inclusions.

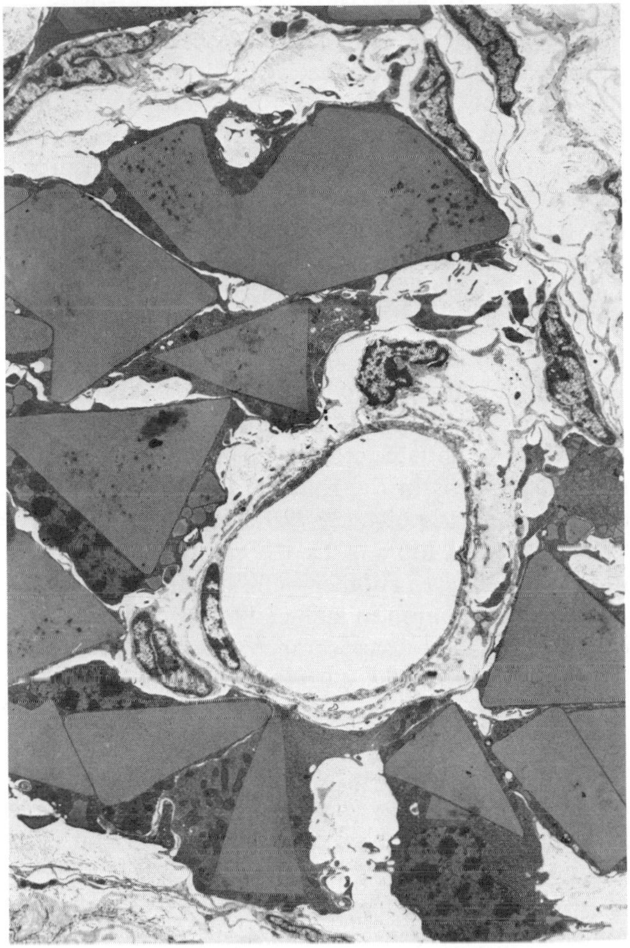

FIG. 92. Leydig cells in the testis of the hypophysectomized bush rat, *R. fuscipes,* showing the striking formation of crystalloid inclusions.

man testis (749), but their functional significance is not clear.

Life History

The origin, differentiation, proliferation, and attrition of Leydig cells has been the subject of hundreds of investigations, and yet many unsolved problems remain. A comprehensive review of this morphology and function of Leydig cells from the initiation of testicular differentiation proceeding through puberty and adult life and terminating with the seniscent testis is quite beyond the range of this review, and therefore we intend to emphasize some of the fundamental aspects of Leydig cell biology available from selected earlier studies and some very recent investigations. The history of Leydig cell life in the normal mammalian testis can be temporally subdivided into six categories: (a) the development of fetal Leydig cells, (b) changes in Leydig cells at birth, (c) pubertal development, (d) the adult population, (e) sessional alterations in Leydig cell biology, and (f) the status of Leydig cells in old age.

In those species so far studied, the fetal testis develops a spectacularly high proportion of active Leydig cells whose morphology and secretory function are unique to this phase of their growth. The debate concerning the precise embryological derivation of fetal Leydig cells has been amply discussed in the past (23,750–755), with two concepts being put forward to explain their origin. First, the most generally accepted theory favors a mesenchymal origin, although alternative evidence is available (756) favoring their derivation from mesonephric cells. A good deal of uncertainty surrounds the validity of both of these theories because the process of gonadal differentiation is extremely complex, and repeated attempts to identify the origin and cell type giving rise to histologically recognizable Leydig cells have fallen short of pro-

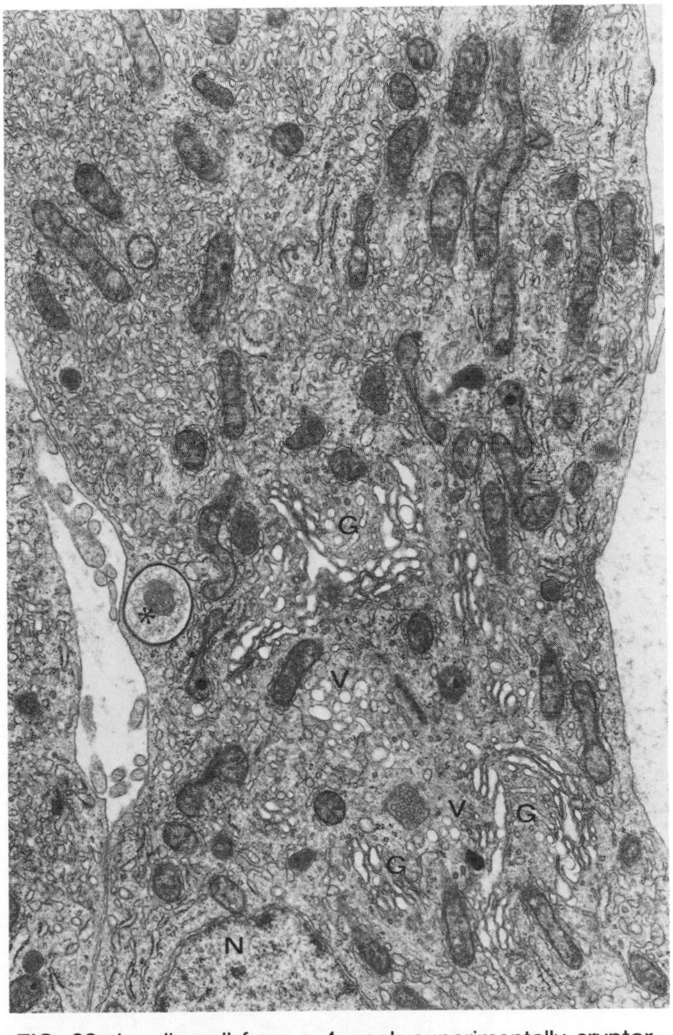

FIG. 93. Leydig cell from a 4-week experimentally cryptorchid rat testis illustrating numerous stacks of Golgi membranes (G) and associated vesicles (V). Note circular junctional specialization (*asterisk*) formed by a penetrating piece of cytoplasm. Leydig cell nucleus (N) is shown.

viding clear answers. A useful review of this problem has recently been provided (23).

The notion of a mesenchymal origin of Leydig cells has gained acceptance on a number of grounds. Ultrastructural analysis of the early fetal testis reveals numerous mesenchymallike interstitial cells between the seminiferous cords that are believed to differentiate into fetal Leydig (Figs. 14 and 94) cells (29,35,757,758). Similar observations have been presented many times for the postnatal development of Leydig cells, where they are thought to arise chiefly by differentiation from simple bipolar interstitial cells within the interstitial tissue and to a lesser extent by mitotic proliferation of fully formed Leydig cells (378,610,611,616,752,759–762). Some confusion still exists as to the precise histological classification of these Leydig stem cells (see refs. 762,763). They have been designated as pure mesenchymal cells (especially in the fetus) or fibroblasts, myofibroblasts (having affinity with peritubular smooth muscle contractile cells), fibroblastic mesenchymal cells, and many other classifications. A further complication pertaining to Leydig cell differentiation concerns the dual site of their origin, some arising in peritubular positions and others developing in association with capillaries and in more central regions of the interstitial tissue, a feature well illustrated in the pig testis (764–767).

Which cell type(s) represent the Leydig cell precursor? The answer to this question is not yet available, but here we return to the alternative theory of Leydig cell differentiation, namely, their development from mesonephrogenic tissues. During early gonadal differentiation, mesenchymelike cells of mesonephric origin invade the entire testis and occupy the presumptive interstitial tissue (23). These cells, together with others migrating in from the gonadal blastema, could thus form the stem cells for later development of Leydig cells. Because mesonephric cells exhibit the capacity to "transdifferentiate" into completely different cells during fetal life, then in theory this behavior may be retained by the intertubular tissue beyond intrauterine life. Examples of transdifferentiation of testicular interstitial cells are available. At birth, the seminiferous cords are surrounded by a homogeneous population of fibroblasts, but as the tubules expand during testicular enlargement, these cells transform into an inner peritubular myoid cell, acquiring epitheloid characteristics, and an outer fibroblastic layer of similar ultrastructure to the newborn situation (768). Alternatively, cells lining the seminiferous tubules are known to differentiate into Leydig cells (769,770), and intermediate steps in the route of differentiation have been suggested (124,694,729,770–772).

This intriguing topic of Leydig cell differentiation is intimately related to another well-known feature of the Leydig cell population in late fetal life and shortly after birth, namely, their disappearance from the testis. A biphasic pattern of Leydig cell growth has been recognized for many years. Among the first to describe peaks of Leydig cell development in the fetus and in postnatal life was Whitehead (783,784), who studied the pig testis. In fact, the pig testis its a special case, since it exhibits three consecutive stages of Leydig cell development: fetal, perinatal, and postpubertal, whereas the common laboratory rodents and other species show a spurt of Leydig cell proliferation in late fetal life and postnatally coincident with initiation of spermatogenesis (54,762,763,775,776). The stimulus for rapid proliferation of fetal Leydig cells is chorionic gonadotropin and, possibly to a lesser extent, pituitary LH, which result in large elevations of

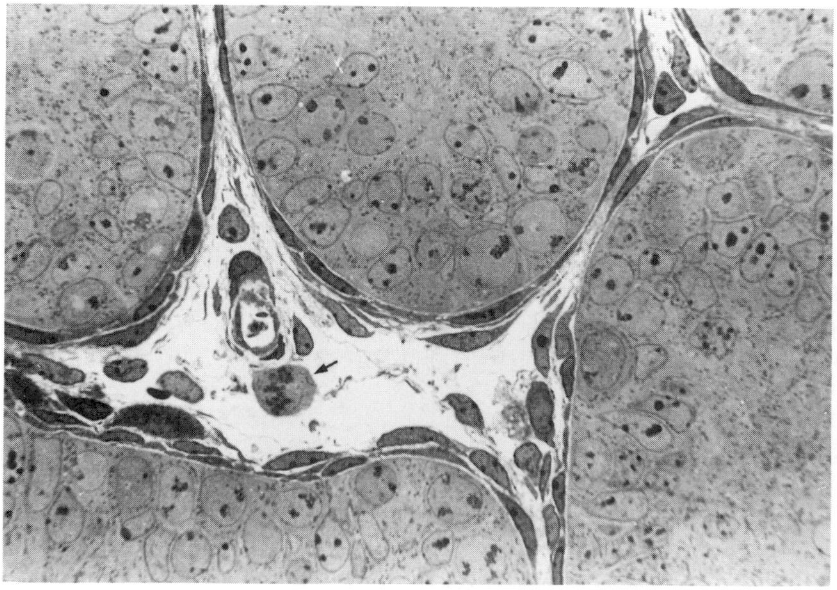

FIG. 94. Seven-day-old mouse testis showing numerous mesenchymal cells in peritubular locations. Note mitotic figure probably representing a dividing immature Leydig cell (*arrow*).

intratesticular testosterone and other steroids, reflected a short time later by raised serum levels of testosterone (55,777,778). A sharp decline in the amount of steroids secreted by each fetal Leydig cell occurs just before birth in the rat, and thereafter a further fall is a reflection of a considerable loss of Leydig cells from the testis (55).

Two suggestions have been offered to account for the dramatic perinatal decline in Leydig cell numbers: (a) a process of cell death (35,762,770,771,779) or (b) dedifferentiation back to fibroblastic-type cells (780,781). Because the morphology of the fetal Leydig cells is well recognized, it has been possible to trace their fate within the developing testis using morphometric analysis (710). Contrary to the notion of cell differentiation or degeneration, fetal Leydig cells persist in the postnatal testis and survive in small numbers within the adult testis, suggesting that they are a distinct line of cell development not related to the development of immature and adult-type Leydig cells. At this time it is also not clear if changes in the pituitary–testicular hormonal axis and/or alterations in the cellular composition of the fetal testis may influence this pattern of Leydig cell survival, at least in the rat testis.

A great many studies have concentrated on the morphological features of the intertubular tissue during the period between birth and puberty. The point of interest here has been to characterize, in morphological terms, the process of Leydig cell differentiation and proliferation that parallels the establishment of spermatogenesis and to ascertain the identity and mechanisms of action of hormones that support renewed growth of Leydig cells at puberty (see reviews, refs. 782–784). When the developing testis is studied by light and electron microscopy, there is general agreement that the resident population of interstitial fibroblasts or mesenchymal cells is stimulated by LH to differentiate into the adult-type generation of Leydig cells (616,686,759,760,762,767). Differentiation of adult-type Leydig cells in postnatal life is thought to occur as the numbers of mesenchymal cells decline (752,759,760), with the latter signaling their transformation into Leydig cells by synthesizing increasing amounts of smooth endoplasmic reticulum (751,762,763,765). New information on the dynamics of Leydig cell development is now available (786–788). Leydig cells become increasingly apparent within the intertubular tissue soon after birth, and studies using tritiated thymidine methods to trace the pattern of cell proliferation among intertubular cells of the rat show that mesenchymal cells provide the source of new Leydig cells up to 4 weeks of postnatal development. Thereafter the greatly increased numbers of Leydig cells seen in more mature testes arise via one or two rounds of mitoses of existing Leydig cells. The previously high proportion of mesenchymal cells in fetal and neonatal testes (greater than 50%) is subject to a significant decline to around 3% within the mature testis. Approximately one-third of the normal adult Leydig cell population arise by development from mesenchymal cells. Morphological maturation of mesenchymal cells into accredited Leydig cells is accompanied by their acquisition of receptors for LH and androgen (789).

The complex hormonal control of sexual maturation has been the subject of intensive clinical and experimental investigations, which have been continually updated as new information has become available (790–794). However, some data relating to the physiology of testicular maturation have been difficult to interpret. First, mature or partly differentiated Leydig cells in humans were thought to be absent from the testis from about 1 year after birth until puberty (23,35,770,771,795–798). However, the concentration of testosterone in spermatic venous blood of boys is five times higher than in peripheral blood (798). Second, acute hCG treatment of prepubertal boys induces a rapid increase in serum testosterone levels (799), which can probably be explained by the recent observation that differentiated Leydig cells do exist in the neonatal human testis (800). Third, elevation of serum FSH levels during sexual maturation is known to increase testis weight via stimulation of spermatogenesis. Some data favoring a stimulatory effect of FSH on the interstitial tissue have demonstrated FSH-induced enhancement of LH receptors (801–803) and increased testosterone secretion in response to LH *in vivo* and *in vitro* (801,804–806). Furthermore, these findings have been difficult to evaluate because Leydig cells and the primitive mesenchymal cells lack receptors for FSH.

The results of recent investigations have provided additional information on the structure–function relationships of Leydig cells in the immature testis. Ultrastructural analysis of testicular biopsies collected from 30 boys aged 3 to 8 years has revealed the presence of immature Leydig cells comprising about 9% of the total interstitial cell population (762). Furthermore, acute hCG stimulation of the testes of cryptorchid boys caused a precocious secretion of testosterone within the testis and induced rapid differentiation of immature Leydig cells from primitive fibroblastic cells (763).

The role of FSH in induction of Leydig cell function during testicular maturation has been studied in immature rats, where FSH treatment induces rapid hypertrophy and hyperplasia of interstitial cells that transform into mature Leydig cells (807,808). These effects could not be duplicated with LH given in an amount thought to contaminate the FSH preparation. Similar findings in the immature rat have been repeated using highly purified GSH (809). With FSH treatment, numerous Leydig cells appeared to arise from the peritubular tissues, again implicating a reserve stock of mesenchymal or fibroblastic cells capable of differentiation into Leydig cells. Since the target tissue for FSH is the seminiferous epithelium, the effects on Leydig cells of FSH treatment suggest that secretion of factors by the seminiferous tubules may mediate the maturation of Leydig cells.

Very recently, studies with a single dose of the substance ethane dimethane sulfonate have demonstrated that the Leydig cells in the adult rat testis can be totally destroyed, but they subsequently regenerate 2 to 3 weeks later (561,670,810). This regeneration appears to occur from a multifocal differentiation of connective tissue cells consisting of pericytes, fibroblasts and lymphatic endothelial cells. These data indicate that with appropriate stimulation the connective tissue of the intertubular region and the testis can be induced to develop into Leydig cells (670). During adult life, very little is known about the dynamics of the total Leydig cell population, since in the common laboratory species (mouse, rat, guinea pig) the histology of the interstitial tissue appears unchanged during the reproductive lifetime of the animal. However, most mammalian species do not remain reproductively active throughout the year and show varying degrees of seasonal regression of spermatogenesis and Leydig cell function (20,507). Studies of the morphological and functional changes in Leydig cells of pronounced seasonal breeders have not been prolific, and additional work is warranted. Examples of a combined ultrastructural–functional investigation of changes in the Leydig cells of seasonal breeders include amphibians (682), the rock hyrax (811–813), wild rats (391,507,748), bats (723,814), hamsters (815), squirrels (512), moles (816), and monkeys (713).

It is known that Leydig cells usually undergo some degree of atrophy during periods of diminished sperm production; in the hamster, Leydig cell volume may vary two- to threefold (509,510,815). Morphometric studies also show significant changes in Leydig cell numbers in the hamster (509,817) and woodchuck (819), although this does not seem to occur in the ram testis (819). The source of new Leydig cells accompanying the restoration of spermatogenic activity is the mesenchymal cell (817). Involution of the Leydig cells is often marked by accumulation of cytoplasmic lipid inclusions, suggestive of Leydig cell inactivity (713,812), whereas in seasonally breeding white-tailed deer and European moles, Leydig cell lipid content is maximal in the sexually active phase (820,821). Clearly the morphological features of Leydig cells in seasonal breeding species represent a spectrum of changes that emphasize caution in extrapolating observations from a given species to another. The effects of season on numerous Leydig cell parameters was recently reported in adult stallions (527), 48 of which were selected at the onset and during the midphase of the breeding season. The latter stallions exhibited a 30% increase in testis weight and 50% increase in daily sperm production per testis, compared to the values obtained in the nonbreeding period. When the interstitial compartment was analyzed by quantitative light microscopy and electron microscopy, the total volume of Leydig cells per testis also showed a corresponding 50% increase, yet the numbers of Leydig cells remain unchanged, indicating, at least for this species, that hypertrophy rather than hyperplasia characterizes the Leydig cell response to seasonal changes in testis function. However, in a further reexamination of the stallion testis, evidence is available that in the nonbreeding season, Leydig cell numbers per testis decline by 36% compared to the fully active testis (822).

The fate of Leydig cells with increasing age has been discussed for many years (322,608). A considerable degree of controversy over the morphological and functional status of the Leydig cell population, particularly in the human, has been evident from conflicting reports claiming an age-related increase (823,824) or decline in Leydig cell numbers or mass (532,825,826). Other claims have been put forward favoring no change in Leydig cell abundance with increasing age (770,827) or a progressive atrophy in elderly men (828) commonly characterized by increasing degrees of vacuolization, lipid accumulation, and pigmentation (see ref. 322 for a review). In a reinvestigation of this subject in 25 men ranging from 18 to 87 years of age in whom spermatogenesis was normal, it was shown that a significant negative correlation existed between age and total Leydig cell number (829). Young adult men, 20 years of age on average, contained over 700 million Leydig cells in paired testes and by 60 this figure had declined to about 200 million per paired testes, representing a loss of 8 million Leydig cells per annum beyond the age of 20. These findings were confirmed and extended (830) in a subsequent study of 30 men aged between 20 and 76 years in which the average 60-year-old man had fewer than half as many Leydig cells as an average 20-year-old individual. However, the question remained as to the mechanism of attrition, either through Leydig cell death or via dedifferentiation back to a primitive interstitial cell. If the latter process occurred, then the abundance of primitive (or fibroblastic-type) cells might be expected to increase as the Leydig cells declined. When this idea was tested by morphometric examination of cell types in the interstitial tissue of testes from the above-mentioned group (831), the population of interstitial cells (neither Leydig cells nor macrophages) decreased significantly with increasing age. This finding thus makes it unlikely that the loss of Leydig cells from aging results from Leydig cell regression into other interstitial cells. Still unresolved, however, is the process by which Leydig cells undergo a slow yet continual loss from the testis.

Although Leydig cells in the aging human testis may develop abundant lipid inclusions, lysosomes, and lipofuscin bodies (322), there is no evidence to suggest that these morphological features reflect an exhausted functional state, nor have there been any data to show that the disappearance of Leydig cells might occur by autolysis, culminating in self-destruction. It seems more likely that dysfunctional Leydig cells would be disposed of by cells equipped to fulfill this role, namely, the interstitial macrophages. At present, nothing is known about the functional duties of testicular macrophages, but from evidence reviewed in the next section, it is clear that their phagocytic capacity can be directed toward the Leydig cells. These observations may help to explain the age-related disappearance of the Leydig cell.

No such attrition of the Leydig cell population has been recorded in aging rats (832), but in distinct contrast to this species and the human, the aging stallion testes show a striking increase in Leydig cell numbers (527). A two- to threefold increase in Leydig cell number per testis occurred in stallions between 2 to 3 years and 20 years of age, yet in the examination of 48 testes in this study, no mitotic figures were observed. A similar failure to observe mitotic figures in the interstitial tissue of rats was reported in a study in which Leydig cell number per testis was tripled during 5 weeks of chronic hCG stimulation (656). However, as mentioned in the study of Leydig cells in stallions (527), if mitosis were responsible for Leydig cell proliferation at the measured rate, no more than one Leydig cell of every 20,000 observed should exhibit a mitotic figure. Hence, failure to detect mitosis of Leydig cells was not considered as supporting the notion that cell division does not occur. An alternative mechanism of Leydig cell proliferation from other interstitial cells has been reviewed earlier in this section and remains a viable possibility to account for these age- and treatment-related changes in Leydig cell populations.

Response to Testicular Damage

Impairment of testicular function can be manifested by changes in either seminiferous tubules or the interstitial tissue, and for many years it was thought that treatments compromising one particular compartment of the testis were virtually without harmful effect on the adjacent compartment. This conclusion seemed valid at the time because microscopists had to rely heavily on the relatively imprecise technique of histological evaluation of the testis in paraffin section, and on the other hand, biochemists and physiologists interested in pathological changes to the testis had very few methods available with which to monitor alterations in testicular function. Significant advances in the morphological sciences together with an ever-increasing number of sensitive and specific assays of cell and tissue function in the testis have together greatly improved our understanding of testicular pathology (392,833–836). In this section we present an overview of the morphological changes of Leydig cells in three broad areas where testicular damage is sustained. First, we discuss nonspecific and unrelated treatments that precipitate impairment of spermatogenesis in varying degrees of severity; second, the deleterious effects on spermatogenesis of endogenous hormones or their synthetic analogs are contrasted with alterations of the Leydig cell population; and third, the extreme sensitivity of Leydig cells to selected toxic compounds is reviewed.

A considerable body of evidence is now available that clearly indicates that disruption of spermatogenesis induced by unrelated agents is accompanied by morphological and function changes of the Leydig cells indicative of a state of stimulation (Figs. 95 and 96). Those treatments that result in this peculiar response of the Leydig cells share a common feature, namely, the induction of varying degrees of seminiferous tubule damage. Some examples of these experimental models of spermatogenic damage include surgical cryptorchidism, ligation of the efferent ducts, temporary heat treatment, a vitamin-A-deficient diet, treatment with the cytostatic agent hydroxyurea, and irradiation in utero; the details of these

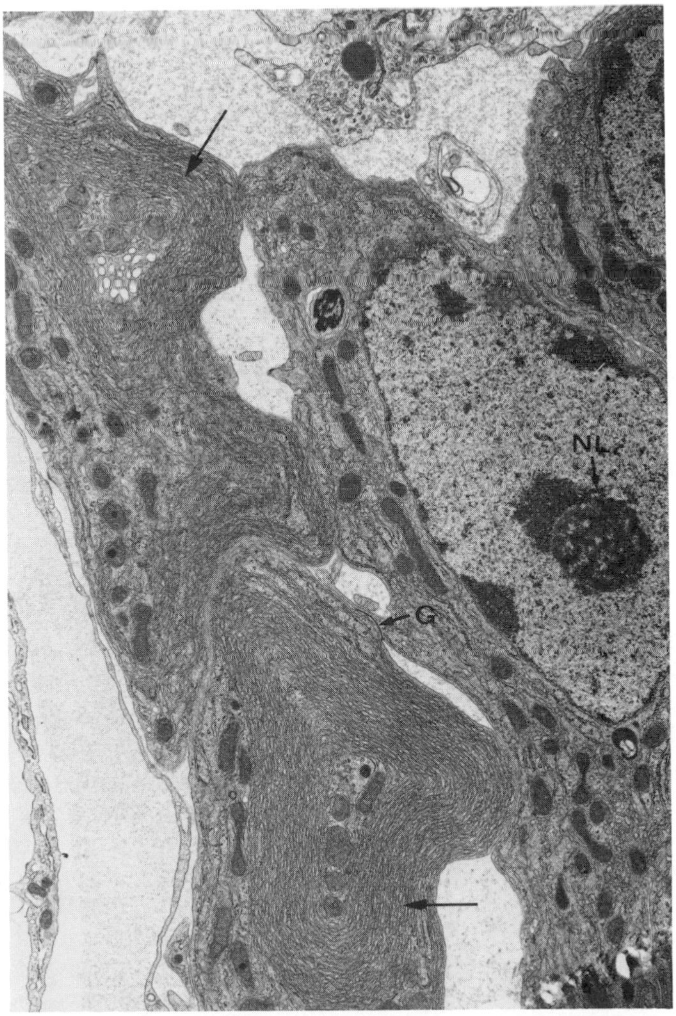

FIG. 95. Leydig cells from a 7-day experimentally cryptorchid rat testis showing large concentric whorls of smooth endoplasmic reticulum. The Leydig cell nucleus contains a prominent nucleolus (NL), and a gap junction (G) is shown.

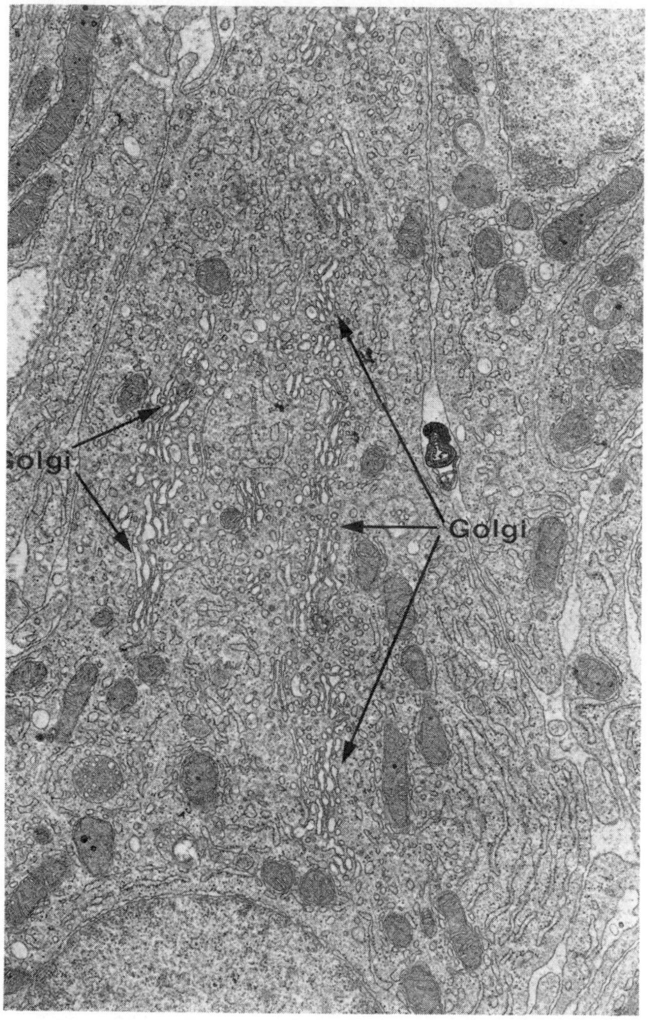

FIG. 96. Rat Leydig cell of the 4-week experimentally cryptorchid testis, illustrating proliferation of the Golgi apparatus and associated vesicles.

experiments have been reviewed elsewhere (392,597, 598,783,784,837). The stimulated condition of Leydig cells is reversible (598), can occur independently of any involvement by their known endogenous trophic hormone (838–840), and in addition, this same response is confined only to the immediate vicinity of damaged seminiferous tubules (841). Thus, the concept has emerged of a paracrine relationship between the seminiferous tubules and the Leydig cells, a subject that is attracting increasing attention (784,842,843). Judging from the morphological response of the Leydig cells to spermatogenic damage, it seems likely that their enlargement and proliferation of organelles are a reflection of the actions of some potent intratesticular factor(s) that, for reasons not yet understood, constitute a pathway of a short-loop feedback mechanism within the testis.

It is a little known fact that the naturally occurring gonadotropic hormones LH and hCG can exert a deleterious effect on the testis (541,542,844) in direct contrast to their usual mode of action, namely, the stimulation of intertubular tissue with subsequent support or enhancement of spermatogenesis. Data in support of these findings are new, and examples of the toxic effects of hCG on spermatogenesis in immature rats and guinea pigs are available (718,845). However, the impairment of spermatogenesis in these experimental situations is again accompanied by hypertrophy and/or hyperplasia of the Leydig cells, an effect similar to that described above for nonspecific induction of spermatogenic damage. This phenomenon is not confined to hCG treatment, since hCG and PMSG given to adult rats for 1 to 2 weeks caused degeneration of the seminiferous epithelium (845,846), and in investigations of the antispermatogenic effects of LH and LHRH agonists in adult hypophysectomized rats (544) it was shown that LH alone or in combination with LHRH agonist can focally inhibit spermatogenesis and, in certain areas of the testis, destroy all the cells of the seminiferous epithelium. When the intertubular tissue was examined using morphometric techniques, the adjacent Leydig cells exhibited significant hyperplasia compared to saline-treated controls not experiencing seminiferous tubular damage. The observations emphasize that agents that disrupt the spermatogenic process also interfere with the Leydig cells.

The number of substances known to be specifically toxic to the intertubular tissue is large, and relevant reviews are available (672,836,847–849). Of particular interest is the influence of cadmium salts and the group of alkylating agents, diesters of methane sulfonic acid. For many years cadmium administration, even in minute doses, has been recognized to cause acute testicular necrosis by rapid disturbance of the testicular circulation (543,847). Within several hours after cadmium exposure, morphological signs of intertubular disruption are noted, including edema, hemorrhage, and infiltration of mononucleated cells. Finally, complete testicular necrosis occurs in which the seminiferous tubules degenerate totally and the intertubular tissue resembles loose connective tissue mainly containing extracellular materials. A surprising long-term consequence of cadmium-induced testicular degeneration is the slow but unmistakable regeneration of Leydig cells within the intertubular tissue. The new generation of Leydig cells are functionally active, as indicated by restoration of previously reduced weights of seminal vesicles and prostate (543,672). It is of interest that regeneration of Leydig cells occurs initially just beneath the tunica albuginea and is accompanied by regeneration of blood vessels and intertubular macrophages. Continued proliferation of Leydig cells gives rise to interstitial cell tumors, but the seminiferous tubules remain permanently sclerosed. This observation raises the possibility that Leydig cell differentiation and hyperplasia may be dependent on vascular proliferation. The blood vessels that regenerate within those testes are evidently quite different from those in the nontreated stis, since they do not react to a second cadmium treatment (850–852), thus conferring resistance on the regenrated Leydig cells to further cadmium insult.

In many aspects, the toxic effects of ethane dimethane sulfonate (EDS) on the intertubular tissue of the rat testis bear some resemblance to those described above for cadmium: EDS specifically destroys Leydig cells within 3 days after a single treatment (Figs. 97 and 98) (561,670,671,853–856). Macrophages phagocytose the degenerating Leydig cells and bring about the complete elimination of Leydig cells from the testis (Figs. 99 and 100). However, beginning several weeks after initial treatment with EDS, new Leydig cells regenerate within the intertubular tissue and bear a striking morphological resemblance to Leydig cells seen in the fetal rat testis (Fig. 101). The fetal-type Leydig cells arise from perivascular and peritubular positions within the intertubular tissue (Fig. 98) and, over 8 to 10 weeks post-EDS treatment, transform into adult-type Leydig cells occupying these above-mentioned positions and more centrally placed locations.

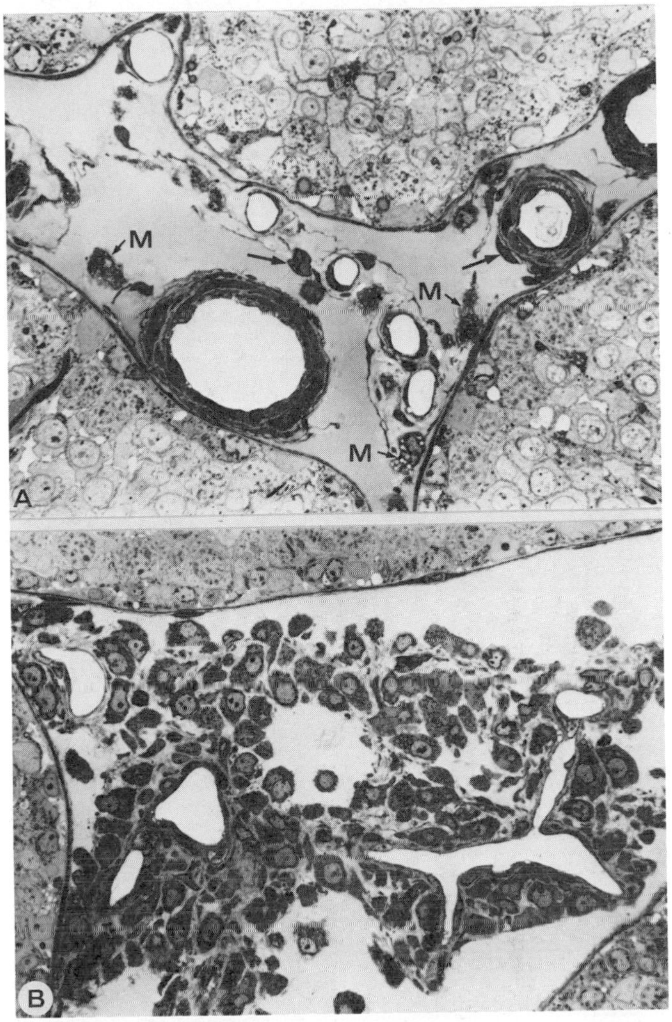

FIG. 98. A: Seven days after ethane dimethanesulfonate treatment, illustrating macrophages (M) and irregularly shaped interstitial cells (*arrows*). **B:** Four weeks after ethane dimethanesulfonate treatment, showing the regenerated population of Leydig cells.

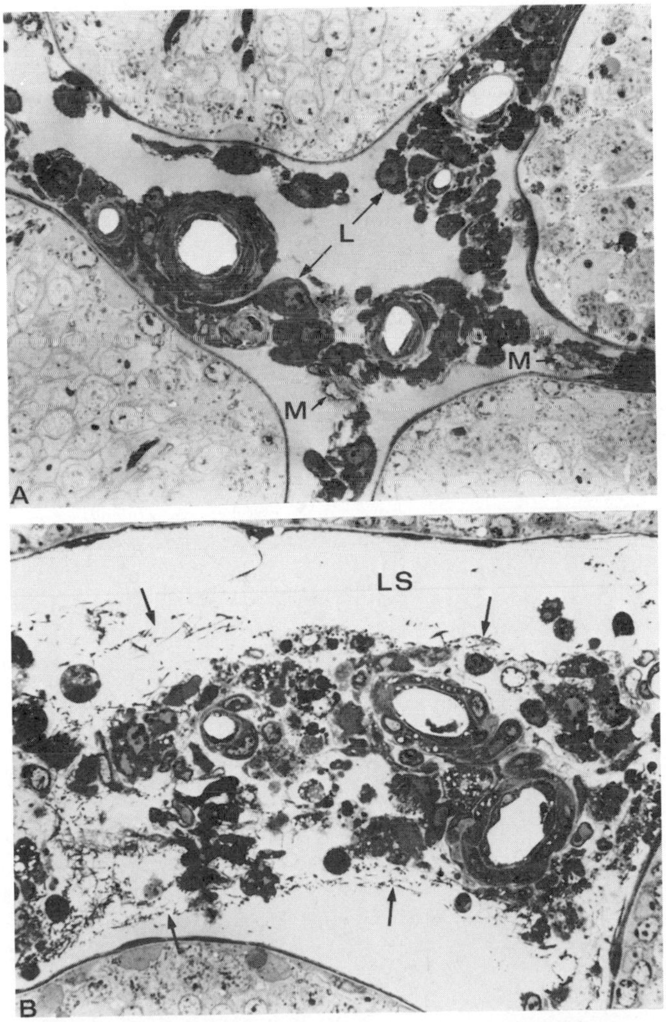

FIG. 97. A: Intertubular tissue of the normal rat testis, illustrating Leydig cells (L) and macrophages (M). **B:** Marked degeneration of Leydig cells of the rat testis 1 day after treatment with ethane dimethanesulfonate. Widening of the lymphatic space (LS) and formation of fibrillar material (*arrows*) are noted.

In a series of experiments aimed at identifying the hormonal control and cellular dynamics of Leydig cell regeneration in the rat testis it has been shown that hCG causes rapid proliferation and differentiation of precursor mesenchymal cells into Leydig cells. New Leydig cells arise from perivascular regions in response to hCG treatment, whereas in EDS-treated testes not stimulated with hCG, the preferred origin of Leydig cells seems to be a peritubular location (857,858). The same laboratory has also shown that proliferation of putative Leydig cell precursor cells can occur in association with suppressed endogenous LH (858), suggesting that local intratesticular or paracrine factors are involved in the early phases of Leydig cell development. Following the establishment of

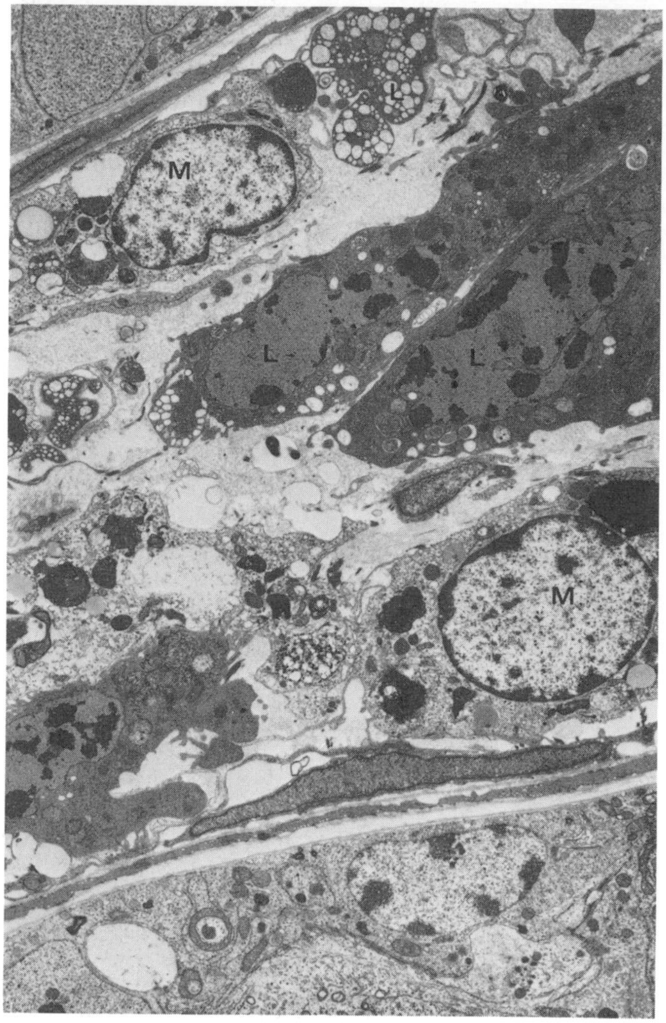

FIG. 99. Degenerative changes in Leydig cells (L) and accumulation of Leydig cell debris within the interstitial macrophages (M) 1 day after treatment with ethane dimethanesulfonate.

a pool of precursors destined to provide an initial wave of Leydig cell development, further expansion of the Leydig cell population occurs via Leydig cell mitosis, which is dependent on LH stimulation (859). Clearly there must be some mechanism to regulate this proliferative activity in order to attain, but not exceed, the normal number of 28 to 30 million Leydig cells per testis. Recent studies have shown that administration of 17β-estradiol plus hCG blocks Leydig cell regeneration in the EDS-treated rat if given between 5 and 16 days post-EDS (860), implicating the Leydig precursor cell as the estrogen target.

Since Leydig cells produce estrogen themselves, perhaps estrogen acts locally within the testes as a paracrine regulator of precursor cell differentiation. However, it has also been shown (856) that the fetal-type Leydig cells are resistant to additional EDS exposure when it is given at weekly intervals up to 6 weeks from initial treatment. The inability of EDS to destroy these Leydig cells ha also been shown for the Leydig cells of the immature ra testis (853), suggesting that only the adult-type Leydi cell is sensitive to the toxic effects of EDS. Data available from the response of Leydig cells to indirect or direct assaults on them therefore indicate that although Leydig cells are actually sensitive to many agents causing testicular damage, the intertubular tissue retains the capacity to ensure their persistence in the testis (560).

Interesting results supporting the presence of a paracrine regulation of Leydig cells are also available from studies using EDS. If given to cryptorchid rats, EDS causes a destruction of Leydig cells as seen in normal animals, but the recovery of the Leydig cells is more rapid in the cryptorchid testes (861–863). These results support the view that factors are present in testes with damaged seminiferous tubules that not only cause Leydig cell hypertrophy (688,839,840) but also stimulate a more rapid regeneration of Leydig cells following their destruction.

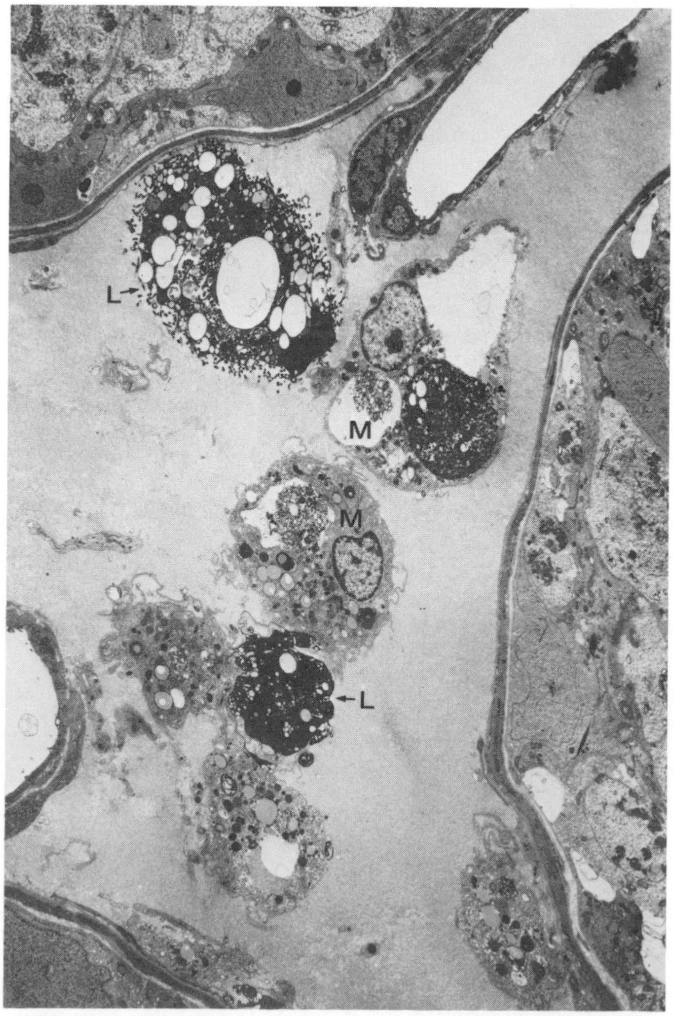

FIG. 100. Degeneration of Leydig cells (L) and their phagocytosis by macrophages (M) 2 days after treatment with ethane dimethanesulfonate.

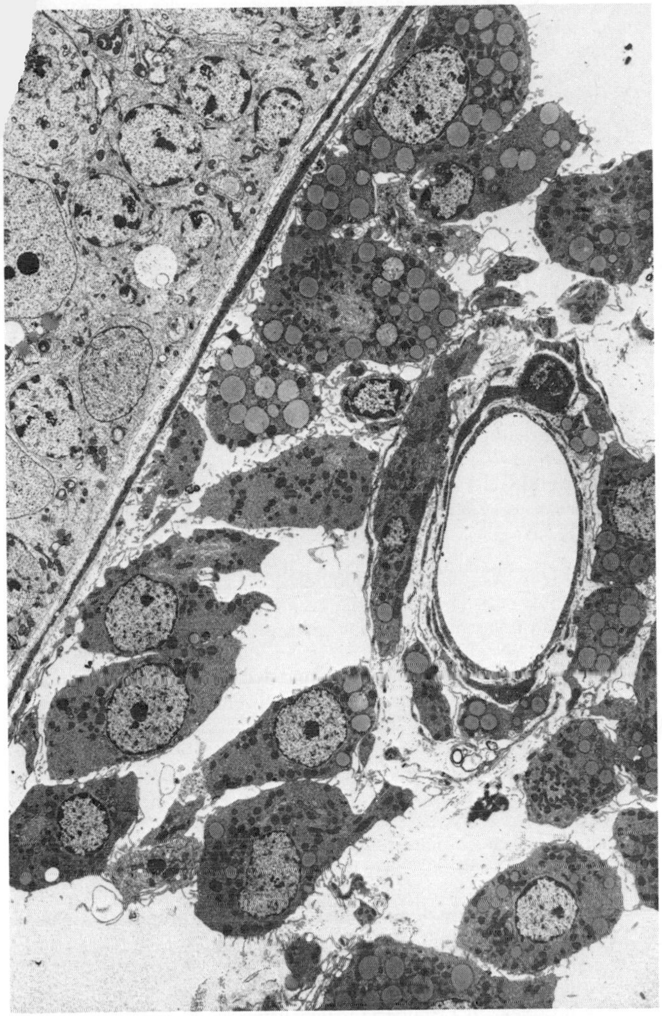

FIG. 101. Regeneration of fetal-type Leydig cells in the rat testis 4 weeks after treatment with ethane dimethanesulfonate. Note the abundance of cytoplasmic lipid inclusions.

REFERENCES

1. Steinach E. *Sex and Life: Forty Years of Biological and Medical Experiments.* New York: Viking Press; 1940.
2. Aristotle. Historia animalium. In: *The Works of Aristotle,* Vol. IV. Oxford: Clarendon Press; 1910. Thompson DW, translator.
3. de Graaf, R. On the human reproductive organs. *J Reprod Fertil Suppl* 1972;17. Jocelyn ND, Setchell BP, translators.
4. van Leeuwenhoek A. Observations de natis e semine genitali animaliulis. *Phil. Trans.* 1667;12:1040. Cited in: *Marshall's Physiology of Reproduction.* London: Longmans & Green; 1960:1–129.
5. von Köellicker RZ. *Bertrage zur Kenntniss der Geschlechtverhaltsmisse und der Samen-flussigkeit wirbelloser Thiere und die Bedeutung de sogenannten Samenthiere,* Berlin: 1841.
6. Berthold AA. Transplantation der Hoden. *Arch Anat Physiol Wiss Med* 1849;16:42–46.
7. Bouin P, Ancel P. Recherches sur les cellules interstitielles de testicule des mammifères. *Arch Zool (Stockh)* 1903;1:437–523.
8. David K, Dingemanse E, Freud J, Laquer F. Ueber krystallinisches mannliches Hormon aus Hoden (Testosterone), wirksamer als aus Harn oder aus Cholesterin hereites Androsteron. *Z Physiol Chem* 1935;233:281–282.
9. Leeson CR, Adamson L. The mammalian tunica vaginalis testis and its fine structure and function. *Acta Anat* 1962;51:226–240.
10. Holstein AF, Weiss C. Über die Wirkung der glatten Muskulatur in der Tunica Albuginea in Hoden des Kaninchens Messungen des interstitiellen Druckes. *Z Ges Exp Med* 1967;142:334–337.
11. Davis JR, Langford GA. Pharmacological studies on the testicular capsule in relation to sperm transport. In: Rosenberg E, Paulsen CA, eds. The *Human Testis.* New York: Plenum Press; 1970:495–514.
12. Clermont Y, Huckins C. Microscopic anatomy of the sex cords and seminiferous tubules in growing and adult male albino rats. *Am J Anat* 1961;108:79–97.
13. Bremer JTJ. Morphology of the tubules of the human testis and epididymis. *Am J Anat* 1911;11:393–417.
14. Roosen-Runge EC. The rete testis in the albino rat: its structure, development and morphological significance. *Acta Anat* 1961; 45:1–30.
15. Scott UG, Scott PP. Postnatal development of the testis and epididymis in the cat. *J Physiol (Lond)* 1957;136:40–45.
16. Fawcett DW, Neaves WR, Flores MN. Comparative observations on intertubular lymphatics and the organisation of the interstitial tissue of the mammalian testis. *Biol Reprod* 1973;9:500–532.
17. Dym M. The fine structure of monkey Sertoli cells in the transitional zone at the junction of the seminiferous tubules with the tubuli recti. *Am J Anat* 1974;140:1–6.
18. Roosen-Runge EC, Holstein AF. The human rete testis. *Cell Tissue Res* 1978;189:409–433.
19. Bustos Obregon E, Holstein AF. The rete testis in man: Ultrastructural aspects. *Cell Tissue Res* 1976;175:1–15.
20. Lincoln GA. Seasonal aspects of testicular function. In: Burger HG, de Kretser DM, eds. *The Testis,* 2nd ed. New York: Raven Press; 1989:329–385.
21. Kerr JB, Hedger MP. Spontaneous spermatogenic failure in the marsupial mouse *Antechinus stuartii.* Macleay (*dasyuride: Marsupialia*). *Aust J Zool* 1983;31:445–466.
22. Setchell BP, Waites GMH. The blood–testis barrier. In: Hamilton DW, Greep RO, eds. *Handbook of Physiology* Section 7. 143–172. Baltimore: Williams & Wilkins; 1975:143–172.
23. Wartenberg H. Differentiation and development of the testis. In: Burger HG, de Kretser DM, eds. *The Testis.* 2nd ed. New York: Raven Press; 1989:67–118.
24. Kirkham WB. The germ cell cycle in the mouse. *Anat Rec* 1915;10:217–219.
25. Allen E. Studies on cell division in the albino rat. *J Morphol* 1918;31:133–185.
26. Hargitt GT. The formation of the sex gland and germ cells of mammals. 1. The origin of the germ cells in the albino rat. *J Morphol Physiol* 1926;40:517–558.
27. Regaud C. Etudes sur la structure des tubes seminiferes et sur la spermatogenese chez les mammiferes. *Arch Anat Microsc* 1901;4:101–156.
28. Clermont Y, Perey B. Quantitative study of the cell population of the seminiferous tubules in immature rats. *Am J Anat* 1957; 100:241–267.
29. Black V, Christensen AK. Differentiation of interstitial cells and Sertoli cells in fetal guinea pig testes. *Am J Anat* 1969; 124:211–238.
30. Orth J. Proliferation of Sertoli cells in fetal and postnatal rats: a quantitative autoradiographic study. *Anat Rec* 1982;203: 485–492.
31. Orth JM. The role of follicle stimulating hormone in controlling Sertoli cell proliferation in testes of fetal rats. *Endocrinology* 1984;115:1248–1255.
32. Magre S, Jost A. The initial phases of testicular organogenesis in the rat. *Arch Anat Microsc Morphol Exp* 1980;69:297–317.
33. Pelliniemi LJ. Ultrastructure of the indifferent gonad in male and female pig embryos. *Tissue Cell* 1975;8:162–174.
34. Pelliniemi LJ. Ultrastructure of the gonadal ridge in male and female pig embryos. *Anat Embryol* 1975;147:19–43.
35. Pelliniemi LJ, Niemi M. Fine structure of the human foetal testis. *Z Zellforsch* 1969;99:507–522.
36. Jost A, Vigier B, Prepin J, Perchelet JP. Studies on sex differentiation in mammals. *Recent Prog Horm Res* 1973;29:1–35.
37. Almond GD, Singh RP. Development of the Sertoli cell in the fetal mouse. *Acta Anat* 1980;106:276–280.
38. van Vorstenbosch CJAHV, Spek E, Colenbrander R, Wensing

CJG. Sertoli cell development of pig testis in the fetal and neonatal period. *Biol Reprod* 1984;31:565–577.
39. Zhengwei Y, Wreford NG, de Kretser DM. A quantitative study of spermatogenesis in the developing rat testis. *Biol Reprod* 1990;43:629–625.
40. Kluin PM, Kramer MF, de Rooij DG. Proliferation of spermatogonia and Sertoli cells in maturing mice. *Anat Embryol* 1984;169:73–78.
41. Clermont Y, Le Blond CP. Renewal of spermatogonia in the rat. *Am J Anat* 1953;93:475–502.
42. Ortavant R. Spermatogenesis and morphology of the spermatozoon. In: Cole HH, Cupps PT, eds. *Reproduction in Domestic Animals,* Vol 2. New York: Academic Press; 1959.
43. Hilscher W, Makoski HB. Histollogisch und Autoradiographische Untersuchungen zur "Praspermatogenese" und "Spermatogenese" der Ratte. *Z Zellforsch* 1968;86:327–350.
44. Steinherger A, Steinberger E. Replication pattern of Sertoli cells in maturing rat testis *in vivo* and in organ culture. *Biol Reprod* 1971;4:84–87.
45. Steinberger A, Steinberger E. The Sertoli cell. In: AD Johnson, WR Gomes, eds. *The Testis,* Vol 4. New York: Academic Press; 1977:371–399.
46. Cortes D, Muller J, Skakkebaek NE. Proliferation of Sertoli cells during development of the human testis assessed by stereological methods. *Int J Androl* 1987;10:589–596.
47. Means AR, Fakunding JL, Huckins C, Tindall DJ, Vitale R. Follicle-stimulating hormone, the Sertoli cell, and spermatogenesis. *Recent Prog Horm Res* 1976;32:477–522.
48. Chiappa S, Fink G. Releasing factor and hormonal changes in the hypothalamic–pituitary–gonadotrophin and adrencorticotrophin systems before and after birth and puberty in male, female and androgenized female rats. *J Endocrinol* 1977;72:211–224.
49. Chowdhury J, Steinberger E. Pituitary and plasma levels of gonadotropin in fetal and newborn male and female rats. *J Endocrinol* 1976;69:381–384.
50. Begeot M, Dupouy JP, Dubois MP, Dubois PM. Immunocytological determination of gonadotrophic and thyrotrophic cells in fetal rat anterior pituitary during normal development and under experimental conditions. *Neuroendocrinology* 1981;32:285–294.
51. Warren D, Huhtaniemi I, Tapanainen J, Dufau M, Catt K. Ontogeny of gonadotrophin receptors in the fetal and neonatal rat testis. *Endocrinology* 1984;114:470–476.
52. Griswold M, Solari A, Tung P, Fritz I. Stimulation by FSH of DNA synthesis and of mitosis in cultured Sertoli cells prepared from testes of immature rats. *Mol Cell Endocrinol* 1977; 7:151–165.
53. Solari AJ, Fritz IB. The ultrastructure of immature Sertoli cells. Maturation-like changes during culture and the maintenance of mitotic potentiality. *Biol Reprod* 1978;18:329–345.
54. Lording DW, de Kretser DM. Comparative ultrastructural and histochemical studies of the interstitial cells of the rat testis during fetal and postnatal development. *J Reprod Fertil* 1972;29: 261–269.
55. Tapanainen J, Kuopio T, Pelliniemi LJ, Huhtaniemi I. Rat testicular endogenous steroids and number of Leydig cells between the fetal period and sexual maturity. *Biol Reprod* 1984;31: 1027–1035.
56. Weisz J, Ward I. Plasma testosterone and progesterone titres of pregnant rats, their male and female fetuses and neonatal offspring. *Endocrinology* 1980;106:306–316.
57. Orth J, Weisz J. Development of Δ_5-3β hydroxysteroid dehydrogenase and glucose-6-phosphate dehydrogenase activity in Leydig cells of the fetal rat testis: A quantitative cytochemical study. *Biol Reprod* 1980;22:1201–1209.
58. Nomura T, Weisz J, Lloyd CW. *In vitro* conversion of 7-^{3}H progesterone to androgens by the rat testis during the second half of fetal life. *Endocrinology* 1966;78:245–253.
59. Warren C, Haltmeyer GC, EikNes KR. Testosterone in the fetal testis. *Biol Reprod* 1973;8:560–565.
60. Orth JM, Gunsalus GL, Lamperti AA. Evidence from Sertoli cell-depleted rats indicates that spermatid number in adults depends on numbers of Sertoli cells produced during perinatal development. *Endocrinology* 1988;122:787–794.
61. Kirby JD, Jetton AE, Cooke PS, et al. Developmental hormonal profiles accompanying the neonatal hypothyroidism-induced increase in adult-testicular size and sperm production in the , *Endocrinology* 1992;131:559–565.
62. van Haaster LH, de Jong FH, Docter R, de Rooij DG. The effe of hypothyroidism on Sertoli cell proliferation and differentiatio and hormone levels during testicular development in the rat. *Endocrinology* 1992;131:1574–1576.
63. Cooke PS, Meisami E. Early hypothyroidism in rats causes increased adult testis and reproductive organ size but does not change testosterone levels. *Endocrinology* 1991;129:237–243.
64. Cooke PS, Hess RA, Porcelli J, Meisami E. Increased sperm production in adult rats after transient neonatal hypothyroidism. *Endocrinology* 1991;129:244–248.
65. Chubb C. Genes regulating testis size. *Biol Reprod* 1992; 47:29–36.
66. Bishop MWH, Walton A. Spermatogenesis and the structure of mammalian spermatozoa. In: *Marshall's Physiology of Reproduction,* Vol 1. London: Longmans Green; 1960:1–29.
67. Attal J, Courot M. Development testiculaire et establissement de la spermatogenese chez le taureau. *Ann Biol Anim Biochem Biophys* 1963;3:219–241.
68. Sapsford CS. The development of the Sertoli cell of the rat and mouse: its existence as a mononucleate unit. *J Anat* 1963;97: 225–238.
69. Ramos AS, Dym M. Ultrastructural differentiation of rat Sertoli cells. *Biol Reprod* 1979;21:909–922.
70. Flickinger CJ. The postnatal development of the junctional complexes of the mouse Sertoli cells of the mouse. *Z Zellforsch* 1967;78:92–113.
71. Nagano T, Suzuki F. The postnatal development of the junctional complexes of the mouse Sertoli cells as revealed by freeze-fracture. *Anat Rec* 1976;185:403–418.
72. Vitale R, Fawcett DW, Dym M. The normal development of the blood–testis barrier and the effects of clomiphene and estrogen treatment. *Anat Rec* 1973;176:333–344.
73. Kormano M. Dye permeability and alkaline phosphatase activity of testicular capillaries in the postnatal rat. *Histochemie* 1967;9:327–338.
74. Gilula WB, Fawcett DW, Aoki A. The Sertoli cell occluding junctions and gap junctions in mature and developing mammalian testis. *Dev Biol* 1976;50:142–168.
75. Pelletier RM, Friend DS. The Sertoli cell junctional complex: structure and permeability to filipin in the neonatal and adult guinea pig. *Am J Anat* 1983;168:213–228.
76. Connell CJ. Blood–testis barrier formation and the initiation of meiosis in the dog. In: Steinberger A, Steinberger E, eds. *Testicular Development, Structure and Function.* New York: Raven Press; 1980:71–78.
77. Hägenas L, Ploen L, Ritzén EM, Ekwall H. Blood–testis barrier: maintained function of inter-Sertoli cell junctions in experimental cryptorchidism in the rat, as judged by a simple lanthanum-immersion technique. *Andrologia* 1977;9:250–254.
78. Vitale R. The development of the blood–testis barrier in Sertoli cell only rats. *Anat Rec* 1975;181:501–508.
79. Bergh A. Morphological signs of a direct effect of experimental cryptorchidism on the Sertoli cells in rats irradiated as fetuses. *Biol Reprod* 1981;24:145–152.
80. Rich KA, Kerr JB, de Kretser DM. Evidence for Leydig cell dysfunction in rats with seminiferous tubule damage. *Mol Cell Endocrinol* 1979;13:123–135.
81. Pelletier RM. Cyclic formation and decay of the blood–testis barrier in the mink (*Mustela ison*): a seasonal breeder. *Am J Anat* 1986;175:91–117.
82. Waites GMH, Gladwell RT. Physiological significance of fluid secretion in the testis and blood–testis barrier. *Physiol Rev* 1982;62:624–671.
83. Setchell BP, Voglmayr JK, Waites GMH. A blood–testis barrier restricting passage from blood into rete testis fluid but not into lymph. *J Physiol (Lond)* 1969;200:73–85.
84. Hagenas L, Ploen L, Ekwall H. Blood–testis barrier: Evidence for intact inter-Sertoli cell junctions after hypophysectomy in the adult rat. *J Endocrinol* 1978;76:87–91.
85. Johnson MH. The role of the pituitary in the development of the blood–testis barrier in mice. *J Reprod Fertil* 1973;32:509–511.
86. de Kretser DM, Burger HG. Ultrastructural studies of human Sertoli cells in normal men and males with hypogonadotrophic

hypogonadism before and after gonadotrophic treatment. In: Saxena BB, Beling CG, Gandy HM, eds. *Gonadotropins.* New York: Wiley Interscience; 1972:640–656.

87. Fuss A. Über die Geschlechtzellen des Menschen und der Saugetiere. *Arch Mikrosc Anat* 1912;81:1–23.
88. Witschi E. Migration of the germ cells of human embryos from the yolk sac to the primitive gonadal fold. *Carnegie Inst Wash Contrib Embryol* 1948;209:67–80.
89. Yoshinaga K, Nishikawa S, Ogawa M, et al. Role of *c-kit* in mouse spermatogenesis: Identification of spermatogonia as a specific site of *c-kit* expression and function. *Development* 1991;113:689–699.
90. Brannan CI, Bedell MA, Resnick JL, et al. Developmental abnormalities in Steel^{17H} mice result from a splicing defect in the steel factor cytoplasmic tail. *Genes Dev* 1992;6:1832–1842.
91. Clark JM, Eddy EM. Fine structural observations on the origin and associations of primordial germ cells of the mouse. *Dev Biol* 1975;47:136–155.
92. McKay DG, Hertig AT, Adams EC, Danziger S. Histochemical observations on the germ cells of human embryos. *Anat Rec* 1953;117:201–291.
93. Zamboni L, Upadhyay S. Germ cell differentiation in mouse adrenal glands. *J Exp Zool* 1983;228:173–193.
94. McLaren A. Studies on mouse germ cells inside and outside the gonad. *J Exp Zool* 1983;228:167–171.
95. Gondos B, Conner LA. Ultrastructure of developing germ cells in the fetal rabbit testis. *Am J Anat* 1973;136:23–42.
96. Wartenburg H. Comparative cytomorphologic aspects of the male germ cells especially of the "gonia." *Andrologia* 1976; 8:117–130.
97. Hilscher B, Hilscher W, Bulthoff-Obnolz B, et al. Kinetics of gametogenesis. I. Comparative histological and autoradiographic studies of oocytes and transitional prospermatogonia during oogenesis and prespermatogenesis. *Cell Tissue Res* 1974;154: 443–470.
98. Roosen-Runge EC, Leik J. Gonocyte degeneration in the postnatal male rat. *Am J Anat* 1975;122:275–300.
99. Gondos B. Testicular development. In: Johnson AD, Gomes WR, eds. *The Testis,* Vol IV. New York: Academic Press; 1977:1–25.
100. Gondos B, Hobel CJ. Ultrastructure of germ cell development in the human fetal testis. *Z Zellforsch* 1971;119:1–20.
101. McGuiness MP, Orth JM. Reinitiation of gonocyte mitosis and movement of gonocytes to the basement membrane in testes of newborn rats *in vivo* and *in vitro. Anat Rec* 1992;233:527–537.
102. Clermont Y. Kinetics of spermatogenesis in mammals: seminiferous epithelium cycle and spermatogonial renewal. *Physiol Rev* 1972;52:198–236.
103. Lee VWK, de Kretser DM, Hudson BH, Wang C. Variations in serum FSH, LH and testosterone levels in male rats from birth to sexual maturity. *J Reprod Fertil* 1975;42:121–126.
104. Muller J, Skakkebaek NE. Quantification of germ cells and seminiferous tubules by stereological examination of testicles from 50 boys who suffered from sudden death. *Int J Androl* 1983;6:143–156.
105. von Ebner V. Untersuchungen über den Bau der Samenkanalchen und die Entwicklung der Spermtozoiden bei den Sangentieren und beim Menschen. *Rollet Untersuch Inst Physiol Histol,* 1871;2:200–236.
106. von La Valette, St George AJH. Ueber die Genese der Samenkorper. *Arch Mikrosk Anat* 1876;12:797–825.
107. Oakberg EF. A description of spermiogenesis in the mouse and its use in analysis of the cycle of the seminiferous epithelium and germ cell renewal. *Am J Anat* 1956;99:391–413.
108. Hochereau MT. Étude des divisions spermatogiales et du renouvellement de la spermatogonie souche chez le taureau. *Int Cong Anim Reprod* 1968;1:149–152.
109. Clermont Y. Cycle of the seminiferous epithelium of the guinea pig. A method for identification of stages. *Fertil Steril* 1960;11:563–573.
110. Clermont Y. Quantitative analysis of spermatogenesis of the rat: a revised model for the renewal of spermatogonia. *Am J Anat* 1962;111:111–129.
111. Clermont Y, Bustos Obregon E. Re-examination of spermatogonial renewal in the rat by means of seminiferous tubules mounted "in toto." *Am J Anat* 1968;122:237–247.
112. Branca A. Les canilicules testiculaires et spermatogénèse de l'homme. *Arch Zool Exp Genet* 1924;62:53–252.
113. Roosen-Runge EC, Barlow FD. Quantitative studies on human spermatogenesis. I. Spermatogonia. *Am J Anat* 1953;93:143–169.
114. Clermont Y. Renewal of spermatogonia in man. *Am J Anat* 1966;118:509–524.
115. Clermont Y. Spermatogenesis in man. A study of the spermatogonial population. *Fertil Steril* 1966;17:705–721.
116. Clermont Y, Le Blond CP. Differentiation and renewal of spermatogonia in the monkey *Macacus rhesus. Am J Anat* 1959;104:237–272.
117. Clermont Y. Two classes of spermatogonial stem cells in the monkey (*Ceropithecus aethiops*). *Am J Anat* 1969;126:57–72.
118. Fawcett DW, Ito S, Slautterback DB. The occurrence of intercellular bridges in groups of cells exhibiting synchronous differentiation. *J Biophys Biochem Cytol* 1959;5:453–458.
119. Huckins C. The spermatogonial stem cell population in adult rats. I. Their morphology, proliferation and maturation. *Anat Rec* 1971;169:533–558.
120. Dym M, Fawcett DW. Further observations on the numbers of spermatogonia, spermatocytes and spermatids connected by intercellular bridges in the mammalian testis. *Biol Reprod* 1971;4:195–215.
121. Vilar O, Perez del Cerro, Mancini RE. The Sertoli cell as a "Bridge cell" between the basal membrane and the germinal cells. *Exp Cell Res* 1962;27:158–161.
122. Nicander L, Abdel-Raouf M, Crabo B. On the ultrastructure of the seminiferous tubules in bull calves. *Acta Morphol Neerl Scand* 1961;4:127–135.
123. Rowley MJ, Berlin JD, Heller CG. The ultrastructure of four types of human spermatogonia. *Z Zellforsch* 1971;112:139–157.
124. Leeson CR. An electron microscopic study of cryptorchid and scrotal human testes, with special reference to pubertal maturation. *Invest Urol* 1966;3:498–511.
125. de Kretser DM. The fine structure of the immature human testis in hypogonadotrophic hypogonadism. *Virchows Arch Zellpathol* 1968;1:283–296.
126. Watson ML. Spermatogenesis in the albino rat as revealed by electron microscopy. *Biochim Biophys Acta* 1952;8:369–374.
127. Moens PB, Go VLW. Intercellular bridges and division patterns of rat spermatogonia. *Z Zellforsch* 1972;127:201–208.
128. Fawcett DW. The cell biology of gametogenesis in the male. *Perspect Biol Med* 1979;2:S56–S73.
129. Tres LL, Solari AJ. The ultrastructure of the nuclei and the behaviour of the sex chromosomes of human spermatogonia. *Z Zellforsch* 1968;91:75–89.
130. Schulze W. Licht und elektronen-mikroskopische Studien an den A-Spermatogonien von Mannern mit intakter Spermatogenese und bei Patienten nach Behandlung mit Antiandrogenen. *Andrologia* 1978;10:307–320.
131. Schulze W. Zum Problem der morphologischen Characterisierung von Spermatogonien typen beim Erwachsenen. *Verh Anat Ges* 1978;72:539–540.
132. Lubarsch O. Ueber da Vorkommen krystallinischer und krystalloider Bildungen in den Zellen des menschilchen Hodens. *Virchows Arch Pathol Anat* 1896;145:316–338.
133. Sohval AR, Suzuki Y, Gabrilove JL, Churg J. Ultrastructure of crystalloids in spermatogonia and Sertoli cells of normal human testis. *J Ultrastruct Res* 1971;34:83–102.
134. Nagano T. The crystalloid of Lubarsch in the human spermatogonium. *Z Zellforsch* 1969;97:491–501.
135. Fawcett DW. Observations on cell differentiation and organelle continuity in spermatogenesis. In: Beatty RA, Gluecksohn-Waelsch S, eds. *Proceedings International Symposium on the Genetics of Spermatozoon.* Copenhagen: Bogtrykkeriet Forum; 1972:37–67.
136. Brown HH. On spermatogenesis in the rat. *Q J Microsc Sci* 1885;25:343–370.
137. Winiwater H. Réchèrche sur l'ovogenese et l'organogenese de l'ovaire des mamiferes. *Arch Biol* 1901;17:33–199.
138. Montgomery TH. A study of the chromosomes of the germ cells of the metazoa. *Trans Am Phil Soc* 1901;20:154–236.

139. Sutton WS. The chromosomes in heredity. *Biol Bull* 1903; 4:231–251.
140. Swift HH. The desoxyribose nucleic acid content of animal nuclei. *Physiol Zool* 1950;23:169–200.
141. Wettstein R, Sotelo JR. Electron microscope serial reconstruction of the spermatocyte 1 nuclei at pachytene. *J Microsc* 1967;6:557–576.
142. Painter TS. Studies in mammalian spermatogenesis. II. The spermatogenesis of man. *J Exp Zool* 1923;37:291–338.
143. Moses MJ. Chromosomal structures in crayfish spermatocytes. *J Biophys Biochem Cytol* 1956;12:215–218.
144. Fawcett DW. The fine structure of chromosomes in the meiotic prophase of vertebrate spermatocytes. *J Biophys Biochem Cytol* 1956;2:403–406.
145. Woollam DHM, Ford EHR. The fine structure of the mammalian chromosome in meiotic prophase with special reference to the synaptinemal complex. *J Anat (Lond)* 1956;98:163–173.
146. Moses MJ. Synaptinemal complex. *Annu Rev Genet* 1968; 2:363–412.
147. Comings DE, Okada TA. Fine structure of the synaptonemal complex. *Exp Cell Res* 1971;65:104–116.
148. Dresser ME, Moses MJ. Silver staining of synaptonemal complexes in surface spreads for light and electron microscopy. *Exp Cell Res* 1979;121:416–419.
149. Moses MJ, Solari AJ. Positive contrast staining and protected drying of surface spreads: electron microscopy of the synaptinemal complex by a new method. *J Ultrastruct Res* 1976; 54:109–114.
150. Heyting C, Dietrich AJ, Redeker EJ, Vink AC. Structure and composition of synaptonemal complexes isolated from rat spermatocytes. *Eur J Cell Biol* 1985;36:307–314.
151. Heyting C, Dettmers RJ, Dietrich AJJ, Redeker EJW, Vink ACG. Two major components of synaptonemal complexes are specific for meiotic prophase nuclei. *Chromosoma* 1988; 96:325–332.
152. Offenberg HH, Dietrich AJJ, Heyting C. Tissue distribution of two major components of synaptonemal complexes of the rat. *Chromosoma* 1991;101:83–91.
153. Meuwissen RLJ, Offenberg HH, Dietrich AJJ, Riesewijk A, van Lersel M, Heyting C. A coiled-coil related protein specific for synapsed regions of meiotic prophase chromosomes. *Embo* 1992;11:5091–5100.
154. Sachs L. Sex linkage and sex chromosomes in man. *Ann Eugen (Lond)* 1954;18:255–261.
155. Solari AJ. The morphology and ultrastructure of the sex vesicle in the mouse. *Exp Cell Res* 1964;36:160–168.
156. Solari AJ, Tres L. The ultrastructure of the human sex vesicle. *Chromosoma* 1967;22:16–31.
157. Solari AJ. The behaviour of the XY pair in mammals. *Int Rev Cytol* 1974;38:273–317.
158. Moses MJ, Counce SJ, Paulson DF. Synaptonemal complex complement of man in spreads of spermatocytes with details of the sex chromosome pair. *Science* 1975;187:363–365.
159. Chandley AC, Gaetz P, Hargreave TB, Joseph AM, Speed RM. On the nature and extent of XY pairing at meiotic prophase in man. *Cytogenet Cell Genet* 1984;38:241–247.
160. Schultz MC, Hermo L, Le Blond CP. Structure, development and cytochemical properties of the nucleolus-associated "round body" in rat spermatocytes and early spermatids. *Am J Anat* 1984;171:41–57.
161. Nicander L, Ploen L. Fine structure of spermatogonia and primary spermatocytes in rabbits. *Z Zellforsch* 1969;99:221–234.
162. Suarez-Quian CA, Qu A, Jelesoff N, Dym M. The Golgi apparatus of rat pachytene spermatocytes during spermatogenesis. *Anat Rec* 1991;229:16–26.
163. André J. Contribution a la connaissance du chondriome. Étude de ses modifications la spermatogénèse. *J Ultrastruct Res* 1962;Suppl 3:1–185.
164. Russell LD, Frank B. Ultrastructural characterization of nuage in spermatocytes in the rat testis. *Anat Rec* 1978;190:79–98.
165. Fawcett DW, Eddy E, Phillips DM. Observations on the fine structure and relationships of the chromatoid body in mammalian spermatogenesis. *Biol Reprod* 1970;2:129–153.
166. Rehbun LI. Some electron microscope observations on membranous basophilic elements of invertebrate eggs. *J Ultrastruct Res* 1961;5:208–225.
167. Smith PE, Berlin JD. Cytoplasmic annulate lamellae in human spermatogenesis. *Cell Tissue Res* 1977;176:235–242.
168. Chemes HE, Fawcett DW, Dym M. Unusual features of the nuclear envelope in human spermatogenic cells. *Anat Rec* 1978;192:495–512.
169. Russell LD. Desmosome-like junctions between Sertoli and germ cells in the rat testis. *Am J Anat* 1977;148:301–312.
170. Kaya M, Harrison RG. The ultrastructural relationships between Sertoli cells and spermatogenic cells in the rat. *J Anat* 1976;121:279–290.
171. Russell LD. The blood–testis barrier and its formation relative to spermatocyte maturation in the adult rat: A lanthanum study. *Anat Rec* 1978;190:99–112.
172. von Ebner V. Zur Spermatogenese bei den Saugethieren. *Arch Mikr Anat* 1888;31:236–292.
173. Heller CG, Clermont Y. Kinetics of the germinal epithelium in man. *Recent Prog Horm Res* 1964;20:545–575.
174. Montgomery TH. Human spermatogenesis, spermatocytes and spermiogenesis. A study in inheritance. *J Acad Natl Sci Phil* 1912;15:1–22.
175. Nicander L. An electron microscopical study of cell contacts in the seminiferous tubules of some mammals. *Z Zellforsch* 1967;83:375–397.
176. Holstein AF, Roosen-Runge EC. *Atlas of Human Spermatogenesis.* Berlin: Grosse Verlag; 1981:1–224.
177. Gardner PH, Holyoke EA. Fine structure of the seminiferous tubule of Swiss mouse, I. The limiting membrane, Sertoli cell, spermatogonia and spermatocytes. *Anat Rec* 1964;150:391–404.
178. von La Valette, St George AJH. Spermatologische Beitrage. *Arch Mikr Anat* 1885;25:581–593.
179. Meves F. Uber das Verhalten der Zentralkorper bei der histogenese der Samenfaden von Mensch und Ratte. *Arch Mikr Anat* 1898;54:329–402.
180. Meves F. Zur Entstehung der Achsenfaden menschlicher Spermatozoen. *Anat Anz* 1898;14:168–170.
181. Gatenby JB, Beams HW. The cytoplasmic inclusions in the spermatogenesis of man. *Q J Microsc Sci* 1936;78:1–33.
182. Le Blond CP, Clermont Y. Spermiogenesis of rat, mouse, hamster and guinea pig as revealed by the "periodic acid-fuschin sulphurous acid" technique. *Am J Anat* 1952;90:167–206.
183. Le Blond CP, Clermont Y. Definition of the stages of the cycle of the seminiferous epithelium in the rat. *Am NY Acad Sci* 1952;55:548–573.
184. Clermont Y. The cycle of the seminiferous epithelium in man. *Am J Anat* 1963;112:35–51.
185. Daoust R, Clermont Y. Distribution of nucleic acids in germ cells during the cycle of the seminiferous epithelium in the rat. *Am J Anat* 1955;96:255–283.
186. Bowen RH. On the idiosome, Golgi apparatus and acrosome in the male germ cells. *Anat Rec* 1922;24:158–180.
187. Bowen RH. On the acrosome of the animal sperm. *Anat Rec* 1924;28:1–13.
188. Burgos MH, Fawcett DW. Studies of the fine structure of the mammalian testis. I. Differentiation of the spermatids in the cat (*Felis domestica*). *J Biophys Biochem Cytol* 1955;2:223–240.
189. Brökelmann J. Fine structure of germ cells and Sertoli cells during the cycle of the seminiferous epithelium in the rat. *Z Zellforsch* 1963;59:820–850.
190. Gardner P. Fine structure of the seminiferous epithelium of the Swiss mouse. The spermatid. *Anat Rec* 1966;155:235–250.
191. Holstein AF. Ultrastructural observations on the differentiation of spermatids in man. *Andrologia* 1976;8:157–165.
192. Hermo L, Rambourg A, Clermont Y. Three-dimensional architecture of the cortical region of the Golgi apparatus in the rat spermatids. *Am J Anat* 1980;157:357–373.
193. Clermont Y, Tang XM. Glycoprotein synthesis in the Golgi apparatus of spermatids during spermiogenesis of the rat. *Anat Rec* 1985;213:33–43.
194. Sandoz D. Étude autoradiographique de l'incorporation *in vitro* de galactose-^{3}H dans les spermatides de souris. *J Microsc* 1972;15:403–408.
195. Lalli MF, Tang XM, Clermont Y. Glycoprotein synthesis in Ser-

toli cells during the cycle of the seminiferous epithelium of adult rats. A radioautographic study. *Biol Reprod* 1984;30:493–505.
196. Fawcett DW. The mammalian spermatozoon. *Dev Biol* 1975;44:394–436.
197. Pederson H. The postacrosomal region of man and *Macaca artoides. J Ultrastruct Res* 1972;40:366–377.
198. Pederson H. Further observations of the fine structure of the human spermatozoon. *Z Zellforsch* 1972;123:305–315.
199. Bedford JM. Ultrastructural changes in the sperm head during fertilization in the rabbit. *Am J Anat* 1968;123:329–358.
200. Stefanini M, Oura C, Zamboni L. Ultrastructure of fertilization in the mouse. 2. Penetration of sperm into the ovum. *J Submicrosc Cytol* 1969;1:1–23.
201. Fawcett DW, Hollenberg RD. Changes in the acrosome of guinea pig spermatozoa during passage through the epididymis. *Z Zellforsch* 1963;60:276–292.
202. Harding HR, Carrick FN, Shorey CD. Ultrastructural changes in spermatozoa of the brush-tailed possum *Trichosurus vulpecula* (Marsupialia) during epididymal transit. Part II. The acrosome. *Cell Tissue Res* 1976;171:61–73.
203. Allison AC, Hartree EF. Lysosomal enzymes in the acrosome and their possible role in fertilization. *J Reprod Fertil* 1970; 21:501–515.
204. Chang MC, Hunter RHF. Capacitation of mammalian sperm: biological and experimental aspects. In: Hamilton DW, Greep RO, eds. *Handbook of Physiology,* Section 7, vol 5. Baltimore: Williams & Wilkins; 1975:339–352.
205. Bedford JM. Observations on the fine structure of spermatozoa of the bush baby (*Galago senegalensis*), the African green monkey (*Cercopithecus aethiops*) and man. *Am J Anat* 1967; 121:443–460.
206. Clermont Y, Einberg E, Le Blond CP, Wagner S. The perforatorium—an extension of the nuclear membrane of the rat spermatozoon. *Anat Rec* 1955;121:1–12.
207. Lalli MF, Clermont Y. Structural changes of the head components of the rat spermatid during spermatogenesis. *Am J Anat* 1981;160:419–434.
208. Burgos MH, Fawcett DW. An electron microscope study of spermatid differentiation in the toad, *Bufo arenarium hensel. J Biophys Biochem Cytol* 1956;2:223–240.
209. Bedford JM. Fine structure of the sperm head in ejaculate and uterine spermatozoa of the rabbit. *J Reprod Fertil* 1964; 7:221–228.
210. Bane A, Nicander L. The structure and formation of the perforatorium in mammalian spermatozoa. *Int J Fertil* 1963;8:865–869.
211. Oko R, Clermont Y. Isolation, structure and protein composition of the perforatorium of rat. *Biol Reprod* 1988;39:673–687.
212. Oko R, Moussakova L, Clermont Y. Regional differences in composition of the perforatorium and outer periacrosomal layer of the rat spermatozoon as revealed by immunocytochemistry. *Am J Anat* 1990;188:64–73.
213. Austin CR, Bishop MWH. Role of the rodent acrosome and perforatorium in fertilization. *Proc R Soc Lond* [*Biol*] 1958;149: 234–240.
214. Welch JE, O'Rand MG. Identification and distribution of actin in spermatogenic cells and spermatozoa of the rabbit. *Dev Biol* 1985;109:411–417.
215. Russell LD, Weber JE, Vogl AW. Characterisation of filaments within the subacrosomal space of rat spermatids during spermiogenesis. *Tissue Cell* 1986;18:887–898.
216. Fouquet JP, Kahn ML. Species specific isolation of actin in mammalian spermatozoa: Fact or artifact. *Micro Res Tech* 1992;20:251–258.
217. Holstein AF, Roosen-Runge EC, Schirren C. *Illustrated Pathology of Human Spermatogenesis.* Grosse Verlag: Berlin; 1988: 1–278.
218. Horstmann E. Electronemikroskopische Untersuchungen zur Spermiohistogenese beim menschen. *Z Zellforsch* 1961;54: 68–89.
219. de Kretser DM. Ultrastructural features of human spermiogenesis. *Z Zellforsch* 1969;98:477–505.
220. Meistrich M. Nuclear morphogenesis during spermiogenesis. In: de Kretser DM, ed. *Molecular Biology of Male Reproduction,* New York: Academic Press [*in press*].
221. Gledhill BL, Gledhill MP, Rigler R, Ringertz NR. Changes in deoxyribonucleoprotein during spermatogenesis in the bull. *Exp Cell Res* 1966;41:652–665.
222. Vaughn JC. The relationship of the sphere chromatophile to the fate of displaced histones following histone transition in rat spermiogenesis. *J Cell Biol* 1966;31:257–278.
223. Bellve AR, Anderson E, Hanley-Bowdoin I. Synthesis and amino acid composition of basic proteins in mammalian sperm nuclei. *Dev Biol* 1975;47:349–365.
224. Kistler WS, Nayes C, Hsu R, Heinrikson RL. The amino acid sequence of a testis-specific basic protein that is associated with spermatogenesis. *J Biol Chem* 1975;250:1847–1853.
225. Loir M, Lanneau M. Partial characterization of ram spermatidal basic nuclear proteins. *Biochem Biophys Res Commun* 1978;80:975–982.
226. Balhorn R. Mammalian protamines. In: Adolph KW, ed. *Molecular Biology of Chromosome Function.* New York: Springer Verlag; 1989:366–395.
227. Meistrich M. Histone and basic nuclear protein transections in mammalian spermatogenesis: In: Hnilica LS, Stein GS, Stein JL, eds. *Histones and Other Basic Nuclear Proteins.* Boca Raton, FL: CRC Press; 1989:165–182.
228. Alfonso PJ, Kistler WS. Immuno-histochemical localization of spermatid nuclear transition protein 2 (TP2) in the testes of rats and mice. *Biol Reprod* [*in press*].
229. Meistrich ML, Trostle-Weige PK, Lin R, Bhatnager YM, Allis CD. Highly acetylated H_4 is associated with histone displacement in rat spermatids. *Mol Reprod Dev* 1992;31:170–181.
230. Fawcett DW, Anderson WA, Phillips DM. Morphogenetic factors influencing the shape of the sperm head. *Dev Biol* 1971;26:220–251.
231. Bellve AR. The molecular biology of mammalian spermatogenesis. In: Finn CA, ed. *Oxford Reviews in Reproductive Biology,* Vol 1. Oxford: Clarendon Press; 1979:159–261.
232. Fawcett DW. The anatomy of the mammalian spermatozoon with particular reference to the guinea pig. *Z Zellforsch* 1965;67:279–296.
233. McIntosh JR, Porter KR. Microtubules in the spermatids of the domestic fowl. *J Cell Biol* 1967;35:153–173.
234. Clark AW. Some aspects of spermiogenesis in a lizard. *Am J Anat* 1967;121:369–400.
235. Beatty RA. The genetics of the mammalian gamete. *Biol Rev* 1970;45:73–119.
236. Meistrich ML, Trostle-Weige PK, Russell LD. Abnormal manchette development in spermatids of *azh/azh* mutant mice. *Am J Anat* 1990;188:74–86.
237. Russell LD, Russell JA, MacGregor GR, Meistrich ML. Linkage of manchette microtubules to the nuclear envelope and observations of the role of the manchette in nuclear shaping during spermiogenesis in rodents. *Am J Anat* 1991;192:97–120.
238. Franklin LE. Formation of the redundant nuclear envelope in monkey spermatids. *Anat Rec* 1968;161:149–162.
239. Anberg A. The ultrastructure of the human spermatozoon. *Acta Obstet Gynaecol* 1957:XXXVI,Suppl 2:1–133.
240. Fawcett DW. The structure of the mammalian spermatozoon. *Int Rev Cytol* 1958;7:195–234.
241. Sapsford CS, Rae CA, Cleland KW. Ultrastructural studies on spermatids and Sertoli cells during early spermiogenesis in the Bandicoot *Perameles nasuta geoffroy* (Marsupialia). *Aust J Zool* 1967;15:881–909.
242. Fawcett DW, Phillips DM. The fine structure and development of the neck region of the mammalian spermatozoon. *Anat Rec* 1969;165:153–184.
243. Grimstone AV, Klug A. Observations on the substructure of flagella fibres. *J Cell Sci* 1966;1:351–362.
244. Warner FD. New observations on flagella fine structure: The relationship between matrix structure and the microtubule component of the axoneme. *J Cell Biol* 1970;47:159–182.
245. Tilney L, Bryan J, Bush DJ, et al. Microtubules: Evidence for 13 protofilaments. *J Cell Biol* 1973;59:267–275.
246. Gibbons IR. Studies on the ATP-base activity of 14S and 30S dynein from cilia of tetrahymena. *J Biol Chem* 1966;241: 5590–5596.
247. Stephens RE. Isolation of nexin—the linkage protein responsible

for the maintenance of the 9-fold configuration of flagellar axonemes. *Biol Bull* 1970;139:438–442.
248. Hopkins JM. Subsidary components of the flagellar of *Chlamydomonas reinhardtii. J Cell Sci* 1970;7:823–839.
249. Afzelius BA. A human syndrome caused by immotile cilia. *Science* 1976;193:317–319.
250. Sturgess JM, Chao J, Wong J, Aspin N, Turner JAP. Cilia with defective radial spokes—a cause of human respiratory disease. *N Engl J Med* 1979;300:53–56.
251. Gerton GL, Millette CG. Generation of flagella by cultured mouse spermatids. *J Cell Biol* 1984;98:619–628.
252. Woolley DM, Fawcett DW. The degeneration and disappearance of the centrioles during the development of the rat spermatozoon. *Anat Rec* 1973;177:289–301.
253. Fawcett DW. A comparative view of sperm ultrastructure. *Biol Reprod* 1970;2:90–127.
254. Fawcett DW, Ito S. The fine structure of bat spermatozoa. *Am J Anat* 1965;116:567–610.
255. Anderson WA, Personne P. The fine structure of the neck region of spermatozoa of *Helix aspersa. J Microsc* 1967;6:1033–1042.
256. Austin CR, Sapsford CS. The development of the rat spermatid. *J R Microsc Soc* 1951;71:397–406.
257. Sud BN. Morphological and histochemical studies of the chromatoid body and related elements in spermatogenesis of the rat. *Q J Microsc Sci* 1961;102:495–505.
258. Maillet PL, Gouranton J. Sur l'expulsion de l'acide ribonucleique nucleaire par les spermatides de *Philaenus spumarius* L (*Hamoptera cucopidae*). *Comp Rendue* 1965;261:1417–1419.
259. Eddy EM. Cytochemical observations on the chromatoid body of the male germ cell. *Biol Reprod* 1970;2:114–119.
260. Walt H, Armbruster BL. Actin and RNA are components of the chromatoid body in spermatids of the rat. *Cell Tissue Res* 1984;236:487–490.
261. Irons MJ, Clermont Y. Formation of the outer dense fibres during spermiogenesis in the rat. *Anat Rec* 1982;202:463–471.
262. O'Brien DA, Bellve AR. Protein constituents of the mouse spermatozoon. II. Temporal synthesis during spermatogenesis. *Dev Biol* 1980;75:405–418.
263. Oko R. Comparative analysis of proteins from the fibrous sheath and outer dense fibres of rat spermatozoa. *Biol Reprod* 1988;39:169–182.
264. Oko R, Clermont Y. Light microscopic immunocytochemical study of fibrous sheath and other dense fibre formation in the rat spermatid. *Anat Rec* 1989;225:46–55.
265. Clermont Y, Oko R, Hermo L. Immunocytochemical localization of proteins utilized in the formation of outer dense fibres and fibrous sheath in rat spermatids: An electron microscopic study. *Anat Rec* 1990;227:447–457.
266. Telkka A, Fawcett DW, Christensen AK. Further observations on the structure of the mammalian sperm tail. *Anat Rec* 1961;141:231–246.
267. Bradfield JRG. Fibre patterns in animal flagella and cilia. *Symp Soc Exp Biol* 1955;9:306–322.
268. Wartenberg H, Holstein AF. Morphology of the "spindle-shaped body" in the developing tail of human spermatids. *Cell Tissue Res* 1975;159:435–443.
269. Nicander L. Development of the fibrous sheath of the mammalian sperm tail. In: *Proceedings 5th International Conference for Electron Microscopy,* New York: Academic Press, 1962:M4.
270. Sapsford CS, Rae CA, Cleland KW. Ultrastructural studies on the development and form of the principal piece sheath of the bandicoot spermatozoon. *Aust J Zool* 1970;18:21–48.
271. Sotelo JR, Trujillo-Cenoz O. Electron microscope study of the kinetic apparatus in animal sperm cells. *Z Zellforsch* 1958; 565–601.
272. Illison L. *Studies on the Genetics and Development of Spermatozoon Head Shape in the Mouse.* PhD thesis, University of Sydney, Australia.
273. Irons MJ, Clermont Y. Kinetics of fibrous sheath formation in the rat spermatid. *Am J Anat* 1982;165:121–130.
274. Jensen OS. Untersuchungen über die Samenkorper du Saugethiere, Vogel und Amphibien. I. Saugethiere, *Arch Mikrosk Anat* 1887;30:379–425.
275. Benda C. Uber die Spermatogenese der Vertebraten und hoherer Evertebraten. II Die Histogenese der Spermien. *Arch Physiol* 1898;30:385–393.
276. Yasuzumi G. Spermatogenesis in animals as revealed by electron microscopy. I. Formation and submicroscopic structure of the middle-piece of the albino rat. *J Biophys Biochem Cytol* 1956;2:445–449.
277. Reed RI, Reed BP. Comparative study of human and bovine sperm by electron microscopy. *Anat Rec* 1948;100:1–7.
278. Schultz-Larsen J. The morphology of the human sperm. *Acta Pathol Microbiol Scand* 1958;Suppl 128:1–121.
279. Phillips DM. Development of spermatozoa in the wooly opossum with special reference to the shaping of the sperm head. *J Ultrastruct Res* 1970;33:369–380.
280. Lenhossek M von. Untersuchungen uber Spermatogenese. *Arch Mikrosk Anat* 1898;51:215–318.
281. Zlotnik I. Nuclear ring in developing male germ cells of dog and cat. *Nature* 1943;151:670.
282. Gresson RAR, Zlotnik I. A comparative study of the cytoplasmic components of the male germ cells of certain mammals. *Proc R Soc Edinburgh* [*Biol*] 1945;62:137–170.
283. Goodrowe KL, Heath E. Disposition of the manchette in the normal equine spermatid. *Anat Rec* 1984;290:177–183.
284. Kingsley-Smith BV, Lacy D. Residual bodies of seminiferous tubules of the rat. *Nature* 1959;184:249–251.
285. Lacy D. Light and electron microscopy and its use in the study of factors influencing spermatogenesis in the rat. *J Microsc Soc* 1960;79:290–225.
286. Diertert SE. Fine structure of the formation and fate of the residual bodies and degenerating germ cells and the lipid cycle in Sertoli cells in the bandicoot *Perameles nasuta Geoffrey* (Marsupialia). *Aust J Zool* 1966;120:317–346.
287. Sapsford CS, Rae CA, Cleland KW. The fate of residual bodies and degenerating germ cells and the lipid cycle in Sertoli cells in the bandicoot *Perameles nasuta Geoffrey* (Marsupialia). *Aust J Zool* 1969;17:729–753.
288. Fouquet JP. La spermiation et la formation des corpus residuels chez la hamster: role des cellules de Sertoli. *J Microsc* 1974;19:161–168.
289. Kerr JB, de Kretser DM. Cyclic variations in Sertoli cell lipid content throughout the spermatogenic cycle in the rat. *J Reprod Fertil* 1975;43:1–8.
290. Fawcett DW, Phillips DM. Observations on the release of spermatozoa and on changes in the head during passage through the epididymis. *J Reprod Fertil* 1969;Suppl 6:405–418.
291. Morales C, Clermont Y. Evolution of Sertoli cell processes invading the cytoplasm of rat spermatids. *Anat Rec* 1982;203:233–244.
292. Holstein AF, Schafer E. A further type of transient cytoplasmic organelle in human spermatids. *Cell Tissue Res* 1978; 192:359–361.
293. Breucker H, Schafer E, Holstein AF. Morphogenesis and fate of the residual body in human spermiogenesis. *Cell Tissue Res* 1985;240:303–309.
294. Sakai Y, Nakamoto T, Yamashina SC. Dynamic changes in Sertoli cell processes invading spermatids cytoplasm during mouse spermiogenesis. *Anat Rec* 1988;220:51–57.
295. Sakai Y, Yamashina S. Mechanism for the removal of residual cytoplasm from spermatids during mouse spermiogenesis. *Anat Rec* 1989;223:43–48.
296. Russell LD, Clermont Y. Anchoring device between Sertoli cells and late spermatids in rat seminiferous tubules. *Anat Rec* 1976;185:259–278.
297. Vitale-Calpe R. Ultrastructural studies of spontaneous spermiation in the guinea pig. *Z Zellforsch* 1970;105:222–223.
298. Burgos MH, Vitale-Calpe R. The fine structure of the Sertoli cell–spermatozoon relationship in the toad. *J Ultrastruct Res* 1967;19:221–237.
299. Burgos MH, Vitale-Calpe R. The mechanism of spermiation in the toad. *Am J Anat* 1967;120:227–252.
300. Russell LD, Lee IP, Ettlin R, Peterson RN. Development of the acrosome and alignment, elongation and entrenchment of spermatids in procarbazine-treated rats. *Tissue Cell* 1983;15: 615–626.
301. Brökelmann J. Surface modifications of Sertoli cells at various stages of spermatogenesis in the rat. *Anat Rec* 1961;139:211.

302. Nagano T. Fine structure relation between the Sertoli cell and the differentiating spermatid in the human testis. *Z Zellforsch* 1968;89:39–43.
303. Flickinger CJ, Fawcett DW. The junctional specialization of Sertoli cells in the seminiferous epithelium. *Anat Rec* 1967; 158:207–222.
304. Russell LD. Spermatid–Sertoli tubulobulbar complexes as devices for elimination of cytoplasm from the head region of late spermatids of the rat. *Anat Rec* 1979;194:233–246.
305. Russell LD. Further observations on tubulobular complexes formed by later spermatids and Sertoli cells in the rat testis. *Anat Rec* 1979;194:213–232.
306. Sertoli E. Dell'esistenza di particulari cellule ramificate nei canalicoli seminiferi dell'testicolo umano. *Morgagni* 1865;7:31–39.
307. Sertoli E. Sulla struttura dei canalicoli seminiferi dei testiculo. *Arch Sci Med* 1878;2:267–295.
308. von Ebner V. Mannliche geschlechtsorgne. In: Kolliker A, ed. *Handbuch de Gewebelchre des Menschen,* Leipzig: Englemann; 1902:402.
309. von La Valette, St. George AJH. Über die Genese der Samenkorper. *Arch Mikrosk Anat Entwickl* 1878;15:261–314.
310. Hoven H. Histogenese du testicule des mammiferes. *Anat Anz* 1914;47:90–109.
311. Stieve H. Die Entwicklung der Keimzellen und der Zwischenzellen in der Hodenaniage des Menschen. Ein Beitrag zur Keimbahufrage. *Z Mikrosk Anat Forsch* 1927;10:225–285.
312. Rolshoven E. Die funktionelle polymorphie des Sertolisyncytioms und ihr Zumsammenhang mit der Spermatogenese. *Z Zellforsch* 1940;31:156–164.
313. Elftman H. The Sertoli cell cycle in the mouse. *Anat Rec* 1950;106:381–393.
314. Watson ML. Spermatogenesis in the albino rat as revealed by tissue sections in the electron microscope. *University of Rochester Atomic Energy Project, Atomic Energy Report,* UR 185, unclassified, 1955.
315. Challice CE. Electron microscope studies of spermiogenesis in some rodents. *J R Microsc Soc* 1953;73:115–127.
316. Fawcett DW. Interrelationships of cell types within the seminiferous epithelium and their implications for control of spermatogenesis. In: Segal SJ, Crozier R, Corfman PA, Condliffe PG, eds. *The Regulation of Mammalian Reproduction.* Springfield, IL: Charles C Thomas; 1973:116–138.
317. Fawcett DW. Observations on the organization of the interstitial tissue of the testis and on the occluding cell junctions in the seminiferous epithelium. *Adv Biosci* 1973;10:83–99.
318. Fawcett DW. Ultrastructure and function of the Sertoli cell. In: Hamilton DW, Greep RO, eds. *Handbook of Physiology,* Sect 7, vol 5. Washington: American Physiological Society; 1975:21–55.
319. Fawcett DW. The ultrastructure and functions of the Sertoli cell. In: Green RO, Koblinsky MA, eds. *Frontiers in Reproduction and Fertility.* Cambridge, MA: MIT Press; 1977:302–320.
320. Fawcett DW. Comparative aspects of the organization of the testis and spermatogenesis. In: Alexander NJ, ed. *Animal Models for Research on Contraception and Fertility.* Gaithersburg, MD: Harper & Row; 1979:84–104.
321. Schulze C. On the morphology of the human Sertoli cell. *Cell Tissue Res.* 1974;153:339–355.
322. Schulze C. Sertoli cells and Leydig cells in man. *Adv Anat Embryol Cell Biol* 1984;88:1–104.
323. Russell LD. Sertoli-germ cell interrelations: a review. *Gamete Res* 1980;3:179–202.
324. Wong V, Russell LD. Three-dimensional reconstruction of a rat stage V Sertoli cell: I. Methods, basic configuration and dimensions. *Am J Anat* 1983;167:143–161.
325. Weber JE, Russell LD, Wong V, Peterson RN. Three-dimensional reconstruction of a rat stage V Sertoli cell: II. Morphometry of Sertoli–Sertoli and Sertoli–germ cell relationships. *Am J Anat* 1983;167:163–179.
326. Russell LD, Tallon-Doran M, Weber JE, Wong V, Peterson RN. Three-dimensional reconstruction of a rat stage V Sertoli cell: III. A study of specific cellular relationships. *Am J Anat* 1983; 167:181–192.
327. Ploen L, Ritzén EM. Fine structural features of Sertoli cells. In: Van Berkom J, Motta PM, eds. *Ultrastructure of Reproduction.* Boston: Martinus Nijhoff; 1984:67–74.
328. Tindall DJ, Rowley DR, Murthy L, Lipshultz LI, Chang CH. Structure and biochemistry of the Sertoli cell. *Int Rev Cytol* 1985;94:127–149.
329. Elftman H. Sertoli cells and testis structure. *Am J Anat* 1963; 113:25–33.
330. Lofts B. The Sertoli cell. *Gen Comp Endocrinol* 1972;Suppl 3:636–648.
331. Bergmann M, Greven R, Schindelmeiser J. Observations on the blood–testis barrier in a frog and a salamander. *Cell Tissue Res* 1983;232:189–200.
332. Cooksey EJ, Rothwell B. The ultrastructure of the Sertoli cell and its differentiation in the domestic fowl (*Gallus domesticus*). *J Anat* 1973;114:329–345.
333. Dufaure JP. L'ultrastructure du testicule de lezard vivipare (Reptile, Lacertilien). II. Les cellules de Sertoli. Étude du glycogene. *Z Zellforsch* 1971;115:565–578.
334. Baccetti B, Bigliardi E, Vegni Talluri M, Burrini AG. The Sertoli cells in lizards. *J Ultrastruct Res* 1983;85:11–23.
335. Ross MR, Dobler J. The Sertoli cell junctional specializations and their relationship to the germinal epithelium as observed after efferent ductule ligation. *Anat Rec* 1975;183:267–292.
336. Rolshoven E. Spermatogenese und Sertoli Syncitium. *Z Zellforsch* 1975;33:439–460.
337. Vogl AW, Soucy LJ. Arrangement and possible function of actin filament bundles in ectoplasmic specializations of gonad squirrel Sertoli cells. *J Cell Biol* 1985;100:814–825.
338. Kerr JB, Mayberry RA, Irby DC. Morphometric studies on lipid inclusions in Sertoli cells during the spermatogenic cycle in the rat. *Cell Tissue Res* 1984;236:699–709.
339. Wing TY, Christensen AK. Morphometric studies on rat seminiferous tubules. *Am J Anat* 1982;165:13–25.
340. Roosen-Runge EC. Quantitative studies on spermatogenesis in the albino rat. III. Volume changes in the cells of the seminiferous tubules. *Anat Rec* 1955;123:385–398.
341. Johnson L, Petty CS, Neaves WB. A comparative study of daily sperm production and testicular composition in humans and rats. *Biol Reprod* 1980;22:1233–1243.
342. Cavicchia JC, Dym M. Relative volume of Sertoli cells in monkey seminiferous epithelium. *Am J Anat* 1977;150:501–503.
343. Dym M, Cavicchia JC. Functional morphology of the testis. *Biol Reprod* 1978;18:1–15.
344. Kerr JB. A light microscopic and morphometric analysis of the Sertoli cell during the spermatogenic cycle of the rat. *Anat Embryol* 1988;177:341–348.
345. Kerr JB. An ultrastructural and morphometric analysis of the Sertoli cell during the spermatogenic cycle of the rat. *Anat Embryol* 1988;179:191–203.
346. Chung KW. Fine structure of Sertoli cells and myoid cells in mice with testicular feminization. *Fertil Steril* 1974;25:325–335.
347. Dym M. The fine structure of the monkey (*Macaca*) Sertoli cell and its role in maintaining the blood–testis barrier. *Anat Rec* 1973;175:639–656.
348. Nagano T. Some observations on the fine structure of the Sertoli cell in the human testis. *Z Zellforsch* 1966;73:89–106.
349. Bustos-Obregon E, Esponda P. Ultrastructure of the nucleus of human Sertoli cells in normal and pathological testes. *Cell Tissue Res* 1974;152:467–475.
350. Kerr JB, de Kretser DM. The cytology of the human testis. In: Burger HG, de Kretser DM, eds. *The Testis.* New York: Raven Press; 1981:141–170.
351. Johnson L, Zane RS, Petty GS, Neaves WB. Quantification of human Sertoli cell population: Its distribution, relation to germ cell numbers, and age-related decline. *Biol Reprod* 1984; 31:785–795.
352. de Kretser DM, Kerr JB, Paulsen CA. Evaluation of the ultrastructural changes in the human Sertoli cells in testicular disorders and the relationship of the changes to the levels of serum FSH. *Int J Androl* 1981;4:124–144.
353. Dym M, Romrell LJ. Intraepithelial lymphocytes in the male reproductive tract of rats and rhesus monkeys. *J Reprod Fertil* 1975;42:1–7.
354. Chemes HE, Dym M, Fawcett DW, Javadpour N, Sherins RJ.

Patho-physiological observations of Sertoli cells in patients with germinal aplasia or severe germ cell depletion. Ultrastructural findings and hormone levels. *Biol Reprod* 1977;17:108–123.
355. Kerr JB. Ultrastructure of the seminiferous epithelium and intertubular tissue of the human testis. *J Electron Microsc Tech* 1991;19:215–240.
356. Kierszenbaum AL. RNA synthetic activities of Sertoli cells in the mouse testis. *Biol Reprod* 1974;11:365–376.
357. Mirre C, Knibiehler B. A re-evaluation of the relationships between the fibrillar centrs and the nucleolus-organising regions in reticulated nucleoli: Ultrastructural organisation, number and distribution of the fibrillar centres in the nucleolus of the mouse Sertoli cells. *J Cell Sci* 1982;55:247–259.
358. Nicander L. Some ultrastructural features of mammalian Sertoli cells. *J Ultrastruct Res* 1963;8:190–191.
359. Zibrin M. Some ultrastructural aspects of nuclear morphology in developing spermatids and mature spermatozoa of the bull. *Mikroskopie* 1971;27:10–16.
360. Zibrin M. Multivesicular nuclear body with nucleolar activity in Sertoli cells of bulls. An ultrastructural study. *Z Zellforsch* 1972;135:155–164.
361. Pawar HS, Wrobel KH. The Sertoli cell of the water buffalo (*Bubalus bubalis*) during the spermatogenic cycle. *Cell Tissue Res* 1991;265:45–30.
362. Tersakis JA. The nucleolar channel system in the human endometrium. *J Cell Biol* 1965;166:37–48.
363. Pelletier RM. A novel perspective: The occluding zonule encircules the apex of the Sertoli cell as observed in birds. *Am J Anat* 1993;235:191–205.
364. Nagano T, Suzuki F. Freeze-fracture observations on the intercellular junctions of Sertoli cells and of Leydig cells in the human testis. *Cell Tissue Res* 1976;166:37–48.
365. Ross MH. The Sertoli cell junctional specialization during spermiogenesis and at spermiation. *Anat Rec* 1976;186:79–104.
366. Vogl AW, Linck RW, Dym M. Colchicine-induced changes in the cytoskeleton of the golden mantled ground squirrel (*Spermophilus lateralis*) Sertoli cells. *Am J Anat* 1983;168:99–108.
367. Rambourg A, Clermont Y, Marrand A. Three-dimensional structure of the osmium-impregnated Golgi apparatus as seen in the high voltage electron microscope. *Am J Anat* 1974;140:27–46.
368. Rambourg A, Clermont Y, Hermo L. Three-dimensional architecture of the Golgi apparatus in Sertoli cells of the rat. *Am J Anat* 1979;154:455–476.
369. Gunsalus GL, Musto NA, Bardin CW. Bidirectional release of a Sertoli cell product, androgen binding protein, into the blood and seminiferous tubule. In: Steinberger A, Steinberger E, eds. *Testicular Development, Structure and Function,* New York: Raven Press; 1980:291–298.
370. Wright WW, Parvinen M, Musto NA, et al. Identification of stage-specific proteins synthesized by rat seminiferous tubules. *Biol Reprod* 1983;29:257–270.
371. Ritzen EM, Boitani C, Parvinen M. Cyclic secretion of proteins by the rat seminiferous tubule, depending on the stage of spermatogenesis. *Int J Androl* 1981;Suppl 3:57–58.
372. Robertson DM, Foulds LM, Leversha L, et al. Isolation of inhibin from bovine follicular fluid. *Biochem Biophys Res Commun* 1985;126:220–226.
373. Forage RG, Ring JM, Brown RW, et al. Cloning and sequence analysis of cDNA species coding for the two subunits of inhibin from bovine follicular fluid. *Proc Natl Acad Sci USA* 1986;83:3091–3095.
374. Mason AJ, Hayflick JS, Ling N, et al. Complementary DNA sequences of ovarian follicular fluid inhibin show precursor structure and homology with transforming growth factor B. *Nature* 1985;318:659–663.
375. McLachlan RI, Robertson DM, Burger HG, de Kretser DM. The radioimmunoassay of bovine follicular fluid inhibin. *Mol Cell Endocrinol* 1986;46:175–185.
376. Christensen AK. The fine structure of testicular interstitial cells in guinea pigs. *J Cell Biol* 1965;26:911–935.
377. Blanchette EJ. Ovarian steroid cells: II. The lutein cell. *J Cell Biol* 1966;31:517–542.
378. Christensen AK, Gillim SW. The correlation of fine structure and function in steroid-secreting cells, with emphasis on those of the gonads. In: McKerns WW, ed. *The Gonads.* New York: Appleton-Century-Crofts; 1972:415–488.
379. Abrunhosa R. Microperfusion fixation of embryos for ultrastructural studies. *J Ultrastruct Res* 1972;41:176–184.
380. Wrobel KH, Schimmel M. Morphology of the bovine Sertoli cell during the spermatogenic cycle. *Cell Tissue Res* 1989; 257:93–103.
381. Vogl AW, Lin YC, Dym M, Fawcett DW. Sertoli cells of the golden-mantled ground squirrel (*Spermophilus lateralis*): a model system for the study of shape change. *J Reprod Fertil* 1983;168:83–98.
382. Kerr JB, de Kretser DM. The role of the Sertoli cell in phagocytosis of the residual bodies of spermatids. *J Reprod Fertil* 1974;36:439–440.
383. Olvik NM, Dahl E. Stage-dependent variation in volume density and size of Sertoli cell vesicles in the rat testis. *Cell Tissue Res* 1981;221:311–320.
384. Welsh MJ, Wiebe JP. Sertoli cell capacity to metabolize C19 steroids. Variation with age and the effect of FSH. *Endocrinology* 1978;103:838–844.
385. Tcholakian RK, Steinberger A. Progesterone metabolism by cultured Sertoli cells. *Endocrinology* 1978;103:1335–1343.
386. Lacy D. Certain aspects of testis structure and function. *Br Med Bull* 1962;18:205–208.
387. Lacy D. The seminiferous tubules in mammals. *Endeavour* 1967;26:101–108.
388. Lacy D, Pettitt AJ. Transmission electron microscopy and the production of steroids by the Leydig and Sertoli cells of the human testis. *Micron* 1969;1:15–53.
389. Lacy D, Pettitt AJ. Sites of hormone production in the mammalian testis and their significance in the control of male fertility. *Br Med Bull* 1970;26:87–91.
390. Johnson AD. Testicular lipids. In Johnson AD, Gomes WR, van Demark NL, eds. *The Testis,* Vol II. New York: Academic Press; 1970:193–258.
391. Kerr JB, Keogh EJ, Hudson B, Whipp GT, de Kretser DM. Alterations in spermatogenic activity and hormonal status in a seasonally breeding rat, *Rattus fuscipes. Gen Comp Endocrinol* 1980;40:78–88.
392. de Kretser DM, Kerr JB. The effect of testicular damage on Sertoli and Leydig cell function. In: de Kretser DM, Burger HG, Hudson B, eds. *The Pituitary and Testis. Clinical and Experimental Studies.* Berlin: Springer Verlag; 1983:133–154.
393. Collins PM, Lacy D. Studies on the structure and function of the mammalian testis. II. Cytological and histochemical observations on the testis of the rat after a single exposure of heat applied for different lengths of time. *Proc R Soc Lond [Biol]* 1969; 172:17–38.
394. Posalaki Z, Szabo D, Bacsi E, Okros I. Hydrolytic enzymes during spermatogenesis in rat. An electron microscopic and histochemical study. *J Histochem Cytochem* 1968;16:249–262.
395. Beckman JK, Conigliio JG. A comparative study of the lipid composition of isolated rat Sertoli and germinal cells. *Lipids* 1979;14:262–267.
396. Fleeger JL, Bishop JP, Gomes WR, van Demark NL. Testicular lipids. I. Effect of unilateral cryptorchidism on lipid classes. *J Reprod Fertil* 1968;15:1–7.
397. Stieve H. Mannliche Genitalorgane. In: Mollendorf W, ed. *Handbuch der Mikroskopischen Anatomie des Menschen,* Vol 7, Part 2. Berlin: Springer; 1930:1–399.
398. Spangaro S. Über die histologischen Veranderungen des Hodens, Nebehodens, und Samenleiters von Geburt an biz zum Griersalter, mit besonderer Berucksichtigung der Hodenatrophie, des elastischen Gewebes und des Vorkommens von Krystallen in Hoden. *Anat Rec* 1902;18:593–771.
399. Fawcett DW, Burgos MH. The fine structure of Sertoli cells in the human testis. *Anat Rec* 1956;124:401.
400. Bawa SR. The fine structure of the Sertoli cell of the human testes. *J Ultrastruct Res* 1963;9:459–474.
401. Toyama Y. Ultrastructure study of crystalloids in Sertoli cells of the normal, intersex and experimental cryptorchid swine. *Cell Tissue Res* 1975;158:205–213.
402. Toyama Y, Obinata T, Holtzen H. Crystalloids of actin-like filaments in the Sertoli cell of the swine testis. *Anat Rec* 1979;195:47–62.

403. von Bardeleben K. Die Zwischenzellen des Saugetierhodens. *Anat Anz* 1897;13:529–536.
404. Benda C. Die spermiogenese der marsupialier. *Denkschr Mednatur Ges Jena* 1906;6:441–458.
405. Greenwood AW. Marsupial spermatogenesis. *Q J Microsc Sci* 1923;64:203–218.
406. Duesberg J. On the interstitial cells of the testicle in *Didelphys. Biol Bull* 1918;35:175–198.
407. Harding HR, Carrick FN, Shorey CD. Crystalloid inclusions in the Sertoli cell of the koala. *Phascolarctos cinereus* (Marsupialia). *Cell Tissue Res* 1982;221:633–642.
408. Maximow A. Die histologische Vorgange bei der Heilung von Hodenvertetzungen und die Regenerationsfahigkeit des Hodengwebes. *Beitr Pathol Anat* 1899;26:230–319.
409. Niemi M, Harkonen H, Kokko A. Localisation and identification of testicular esterases in the rat. *J Histochem Cytochem* 1962;10:186–193.
410. Posalaki Z. Histochemische untersuchungen der spermiogenese. *Symp Biol Hung* 1964;4:83–87.
411. Posalaki Z. Activity of different dehydrogenases and diaphorases in the spermatogenesis of the rat and its relation to motility. *Acta Histochem* 1965;20:86–90.
412. Niemi M, Kormano M. Cyclical changes in and significance of lipids and acid phosphatase activity in the seminiferous tubules of the rat testis. *Anat Rec* 1965;157:159–170.
413. Parvinen M, Vanha-Pertulla T. Identification and enzyme quantification of the stages of the seminiferous epithelial wave in the rat. *Anat Rec* 1972;174:435–450.
414. Barham SS, Berlin JD. Fine structure and cytochemistry of testicular cells in men treated with testosterone propionate. *Cell Tissue Res* 1974;148:159–182.
415. Clegg EJ, MacMillan EW. Uptake of vital dyes and particulate matter by the Sertoli cells of the rat testis. *J Anat* 1965;99:219–229.
416. Carr I, Clegg EJ, Meek GA. Sertoli cells as phagocytes: an electron microscopic study. *J Anat* 1968;102:501–509.
417. Soares Pessoa JF, David-Ferreira JF. Bidirectional transport of horseradish peroxidase by rat Sertoli cells. An *in vitro* study. *Biol Cell* 1980;39:301–304.
418. Reddy JK, Svoboda DJ. Lysosomal activity in Sertoli cells of normal and degenerating seminiferous epithelium of rat testis. *Am J Pathol* 1967;51:1–17.
419. Morales C, Hermo L. Demonstration of fluid phase endocytosis in epithelial cells of the male reproductive system by means of horseradish peroxidase colloidal gold complex. *Cell Tissue Res* 1983;230:503–510.
420. Hinton BT, Keefer DA. Evidence for protein absorption from the lumen of the seminiferous tubuli and rete testis of the rat testis. *Cell Tissue Res* 1983;230:367–375.
421. Hermo L, Morales CR, Clermont Y. Endocytic activity of Sertoli cells in the rat. *J Cell Biol* 1982;95:434a.
422. Morales C, Clermont Y, Hermo L. Nature and function of endocytosis in Sertoli cells of the rat. *Am J Anat* 1985;173:203–217.
423. Golyas BJ. The rabbit zygote: formation of annulate lamellae. *J Ultrastruct Res* 1971;35:112–126.
424. Maul GG. On the relationship between the Golgi apparatus and annulate lamellae. *J Ultrastruct Res* 1970;30:368–384.
425. Wischmitzer S. The annulate lamellae. *Int Rev Cytol* 1970; 27:65–100.
426. Sun CN, White HJ. Annulate lamellae in human tumour cells. *Tissue Cell* 1979;11:139–146.
427. Kessel RG. Annulate lamellae. *J Ultrastruct Res* 1968;Suppl 10:1–82.
428. Merkow L, Leighton J. Increased numbers of annulate lamellae in myocardium of chick embryo incubated at abnormal temperatures. *J Cell Biol* 1966;28:127–137.
429. de Brabander M, Borgers M. The formation of annulated lamellae induced by the disintegration of microtubules. *J Cell Sci* 1975;19:331–340.
430. Toyama Y. Actin-like filaments in the Sertoli cell junctional specializations in the swine and mouse testis. *Anat Rec* 1976;186:477–492.
431. Franke WW, Grund C, Fink A, et al. Location of actin in the microfilament bundles associated with the junctional specializations between Sertoli cells and spermatids. *Biol Cell* 1978; 31:7–14.
432. Oko R, Hermo L, Hecht NB. Distribution of actin isoforms within cells of the seminiferous epithelium of the rat testis: evidence for a muscle form of actin in spermatids. *Anat Rec* 1991;231:63–81.
433. Franke WW, Grund C, Schmid E. Intermediate-sized filaments present in Sertoli cells are of the vimentin type. *Eur J Cell Biol* 1979;19:269–275.
434. Paranko J, Kallajoki M, Pelliniemi LJ, Lehto VP, Virtanen I. Transient co-expression of cytokeratin and vimentin in differentiating rat Sertoli cells. *Dev Biol* 1986;117:35–44.
435. Russell LD. Observations on rat Sertoli ectoplasmic ('junctional') specializations in their association with germ cells of the rat testis. *Tissue Cell* 1977;9:475–498.
436. Aoki A. Induction of sperm release by microtubule inhibitors in rat testis. *Eur J Cell Biol* 1980;22:467.
437. Roosen-Runge EC. Quantitative studies on spermatogenesis in the albino rat. II. The duration of spermatogenesis and some effects of colchicine. *Am J Anat* 1951;88:163–176.
438. Parvinen LM, Soderstrom KO, Parvinen M. Early effects of vinblastine and vincristine on the rat spermatogenesis: analysis by a new transillumination-phase contrast microscopic method. *Exp Pathol* 1978;15:85–96.
439. Russell LD, Malone JP, MacCurdy DS. Effect of the microtubule disrupting agents, colchicine and vinblastine, on seminiferous tubule structure in the rat. *Tissue Cell* 1981;13:349–367.
440. Vogl AW. Changes in the distribution of microtubules in rat Sertoli cells during spermatogenesis. 1988;222:34–41.
441. Amlani S, Vogl AW. Changes in the distribution of microtubules and intermediate filaments in mammalian Sertoli cells during spermatogenesis. *Anat Rec* 1988;220:143–160.
442. Neely MD, Boekelheide K. Sertoli cell processes have axoplasmic features: An ordered microtubule distribution and an abundant high molecular weight microtubule-associated protein (cytoplasmic dynein). *J Cell Biol* 1988;107:1767–1776.
443. Ribbert H. Die abscheidung intravenos injizierten gelosten Karmins in den Geweben. *Z Allg Physiol* 1904;4:201–214.
444. Bouffard G. Injection des couters de benzidine aux animaux normaux. *Ann Inst Pasteur* 1906;20:539–546.
445. Pari G. Uber die Verwendbarkeit vitaler Karmineinspritzungen fur die pathologische Anatomie. *Frank Z Pathol* 1910;4:1–29.
446. Goldacre RJ, Sylven B. A rapid method for studying tumour blood supply using systemic dyes. *Nature* 1959;184:63–64.
447. Goldacre RJ, Sylven B. On the access of blood-borne dyes to various tumor regions. *Br J Cancer* 1962;16:306–322.
448. Everett NB, Simmons B. Measurement and radioautographic localization of albumin in rat tissues after intravenous injection. *Circ Res* 1958;6:307–313.
449. Kormano M. Penetration of intravenous trypan blue into the rat testis and epididymis. *Acta Histochem* 1968;30:133–136.
450. Setchell BP. The blood–testicular fluid barrier in sheep. *J Physiol (Lond)* 1967;189:63P–65P.
451. Cowie AT, Lascelles AK, Wallace JC. Flows and protein content of testicular lymph in conscious rams. *J Physiol (Lond)* 1964;171:176–187.
452. Waites GMH, Setchell BP. Changes in blood flow and vascular permeability of the testis, epididymis and accessory reproductive organs of the rat after administration of cadmium chloride. *J Endocrinol* 1966;34:329–342.
453. Waites GMH, Setchell BP. Some physiological aspects of the function of the testis. In: McKerns WW, ed. *The Gonads.* New York: Appleton-Century-Crofts; 1965:649–714.
454. Fawcett DW, Leak LV, Heidger PM. Electron microscopic observations on the structural components of the blood–testis barrier. *J Reprod Fertil* (Suppl) 1970;10:105–122.
455. Ross MH. The Sertoli cell and the blood–testicular barrier: an electronmicroscopic study. In: Hostein AF, Horstmann E, eds. *Morphological Aspects of Andrology.* Berlin: Grosse Verlag; 1970:83–86.
456. Dym M, Fawcett DW. The blood–testis barrier in the rat and the physiological compartmentation of the seminiferous epithelium. *Biol Reprod* 1970;3:308–326.
457. Russell LD, Peterson RN. Sertoli cell junctions: morphological and functional considerations. *Int Rev Cytol* 1985;94:177–211.

458. Nagano T. Freeze-fracture observations on the rat Sertoli cell junctions by metal contact freezing. *J Electron Microsc* 1980;29:250–255.
459. Connell CJ. A freeze-fracture and lanthanum tracer study of the complex junction between the Sertoli cells of the canine testis. *J Cell Biol* 1978;76:57–75.
460. Dym M, Caviccia JC. Further observations on the blood–testis barrier in monkeys. *Biol Reprod* 1977;17:390–403.
461. Russell LD. Movement of spermatocytes from the basal to the adluminal compartment of the rat testis. *Am J Anat* 1977;148:313–328.
462. Osman D, Ekwall H, Ploen L. Specialized cell contacts and the blood–testis barrier in the seminiferous tubules of the domestic fowl (*Gallus domesticus*). *Int J Androl* 1980;3:553–562.
463. Franchi E, Camatini M, de Curtis I. Morphological evidence of a permeability barrier in urodele testis. *J Ultrastruct Res* 1982;80:253–263.
464. Abraham M, Rahamim E, Tibika H, Golenser E, Kieselstein M. The blood–testis barrier in *Aphanius dispar* (Teleostei). *Cell Tissue Res* 1980;211:207–214.
465. Marcaillou C, Szollosi A. The blood–testis barrier in a nematode and a fish: a generalizable concept. *J Ultrastruct Res* 1980;70:128–136.
466. Mattei X, Mattei C, Marcand B, Leung TKD. Ultrastructure des cellules de Sertoli d'un teleosteen: *Abudefduf marginatus. J Ultrastruct Res* 1982;81:333–340.
467. Billard R. La spermatogenese de *Poecilia reticulata*. III. Ultrastructure des cellules de Sertoli. *Ann Biol Anim Biochem Biophys* 1980;10:37–50.
468. Parmentier HK, van den Boogaart JGM, Timmermans LPM. Physiological compartmentation in gonadal tissue of the common carp (*Cyprinus carpio L*). A study with horseradish peroxidase and monoclonal antibodies. *Cell Tissue Res* 1985; 242:75–81.
469. Szollosi A, Reimann J, Marcaillou C. Localization of the blood–testis barrier in the testis of the moth, *Anagasta kuehnilla. J Ultrastruct Res* 1980;72:189–199.
470. Toshimori K, Iwashata T, Oura C. Cell junctions in the cyst envelope in the silkworm testis, *Bombyx mori Linne. Cell Tissue Res* 1979;202:63–73.
471. Lane NJ, Skaer HL. Intercellular junctions in insect tissues. *Adv Insect Physiol* 1980;15:35–213.
472. O'Rand MG, Romrell LH. Appearance of cell surface auto- and isoantigens during spermatogenesis in the rabbit. *Dev Biol* 1977;55:347–358.
473. Millette CF, Bellve AR. Temporal expression of membrane antigens during mouse spermatogenesis. *J Cell Biol* 1977;74:86–97.
474. Romrell LH, O'Rand MG. Capping and ultrastructural localization of sperm surface isoantigens during spermatogenesis. *Dev Biol* 1978;63:76–93.
475. Tung PS, Fritz IB. Specific surface antigens on rat pachytene spermatocytes and successive classes of germ cells. *Dev Biol* 1978;64:297–315.
476. Tung PS, Fritz IB. A maturation surface antigen of rat Sertoli cells. *J Cell Biol* 1977;75:165a.
477. Fritz IB. Sites of action of androgens and follicle-stimulating hormone on cells of the seminiferous tubule. In: Litwak G, ed. *Biochemical Actions of Hormones,* Vol V. New York: Academic Press; 1978:249–281.
478. Pelletier RM. Cyclic formation and decay of the blood–testis barrier in the mink (*Mustela vison*), a seasonal breeder. *Am J Anat* 1986;175:91–117.
479. Russell LD. Spermiation—the sperm release process: ultrastructure observations and unresolved problems. In: van Berkom J, Motta PM, eds. *Ultrastructure of Reproduction.* Boston: Martinus Nijhoff; 1984:46–66.
480. Setchell BP, Pollanen P, Zupp JL. Development of the blood–testis barrier and changes in vascular permeability at puberty in rats. *Int J Androl* 1988;11:225–233.
481. Russell LD, Bartke A, Goh JC. Postnatal development of the Sertoli cell barrier, tubular lumen, and cytoskeleton of Sertoli and myoid cells in the rat, and their relationship to tubular fluid secretion and flow. *Am J Anat* 1989;184:179–189.
482. Russell LD, Malone JP. A study of Sertoli–spermatid tubulobular complexes in selected mammals. *Tissue Cell* 1980;12:263–285.
483. Russell LD, Gardner RJ, Weber JE. Reconstruction of a type-B configuration monkey Sertoli cell: size, shapes and configurational and specialized cell-to-cell relationships. *Am J Anat* 1986;175:73–90.
484. Russell LD, Myers P, Ostenburg J, Malone J. Sertoli ectoplasmic specializations during spermatogenesis. In: Steinberger A, Steinberger E, eds. *Testicular Development, Structure and Function,* New York: Raven Press; 1980:53–63.
485. Gravis CJ. Interrelationships between Sertoli cells and germ cells in the Syrian hamster. *Z Mikrosk Anat Forsch (Leipzig)* 1979;93:321–342.
486. Romrell LH, Ross MH. Characterization of Sertoli cell–germ cell junctional specialization in dissociated testicular cells. *Anat Rec* 1979;193:23–42.
487. Gravis CJ. Inhibition of spermiation in the Syrian hamster using dibutyryl cyclic AMP. *Cell Tissue Res* 1978;192:241–248.
488. Ross MH. Sertoli–Sertoli junctions and Sertoli–spermatid junctions after efferent ductule ligation and lanthanum treatment. *Am J Anat* 1977;148:49–56.
489. Oko R, Hermo L, Hecht NB. Distribution of actin isoforms within cells of the seminiferous epithelium of the rat testis: Evidence for a muscle form of actin in spermatids. *Anat Rec* 1991;231:63–81.
490. Russell LD, Saxena NK, Turner TT. Cytoskeletal involvement in spermiation and sperm transport. *Tissue Cell* 1989;21:361–379.
491. Weber JE, Turner TT, Tung K, Russell LD. Effect of cytochalasin D on the integrity of the Sertoli cell barrier. *Am J Anat* 1988;182:130–147.
492. Pfeiffer DC, Vogl AW. Evidence that vinculin is co-distributed with actin bundles in ectoplasmic (junctional) specializations of mammalian Sertoli cells. *Anat Rec* 1991;231:89–100.
493. Grove BD, Pfeiffer DC, Allen S, Vogl AW. Immunofluorescence localization of vinculin in ectoplasmic (junctional) specializations of rat Sertoli cells. *Am J Anat* 1990;188:44–56.
494. Russell LD. Observations on the interrelationships of Sertoli cells at the level of the blood–testis barrier: Evidence for formation and resorption of Sertoli–Sertoli tubulobulbar complexes during the spermatogenic cycle of the rat. *Am J Anat* 1979;155:259–280.
495. Clermont Y, McCoshen J, Hermo L. Evolution of the endoplasmic reticulum in the Sertoli cell cytoplasm encapsulating the heads of late spermatids in the rat. *Anat Rec* 1980;196:83–99.
496. Cooper CW, Bedford JM. Asymmetry of spermiation and sperm surface charge patterns over the giant acrosome in the musk shrew *Suncus murinus. J Cell Biol* 1976;69:415–428.
497. Gravis CJ. Ultrastructural observations on spermatozoa retained within the seminiferous epithelium after treatment with dibutyryl cyclic AMP. *Tissue Cell* 1980;12:309–322.
498. Palombi F, Salanova M, Tarone G, Farini D, Stefanini M. Distribution of β_1 integrin subunit in rat seminiferous epithelium. *Biol Reprod* 1992;47:1173–1182.
499. Altorfer J, Fukuda T, Hedinger C. Desmosomes in human seminiferous epithelium. *Virchows Arch (Cell Pathol)* 1974;16: 181–194.
500. Ren HP, Russell LD. Quantitation of Sertoli cell–germ cell desmosome–gap junctions in relation to meiotic divisions in the male rat. *Tissue Cell* 1992;24:565–573.
501. Connell CJ. The Sertoli cell of the sexually mature dog. *Anat Rec* 1974;178:333.
502. McGinley D, Pozalaky Z, Porvanznik M. Intercellular junctional complexes of the rat seminiferous tubules: a freeze-fracture study. *Anat Rec* 1977;189:211–232.
503. McGinley DM, Pozalaky Z, Porvaznik M, Russell LD. Gap junctions between Sertoli and germ cells of rat seminiferous tubules. *Tissue Res* 1979;11:741–754.
504. Lodge JR, Salisbury GW. Seasonal variation and male reproductive efficiency. In: Johnson AD, Gomes AD, van Denmark NL, eds. *The Testis,* Vol III. New York: Academic Press; 1970: 139–167.
505. Lofts B, Bern HA. The functional morphology of steroidogenic tissues. In: Idler DR, ed. *Steroids in Non-Mammalian Vertebrates,* New York: Academic Press; 1972:37–125.
506. Hodgson YM, Irby DC, Kerr JB, de Kretser DM. Studies of the structure and function of the Sertoli cell in a seasonally breeding rodent. *Biol Reprod* 1979;21:1091–1098.
507. Irby DC, Kerr JB, Risbridger GP, de Kretser DM. Seasonally and

experimentally induced changes in testicular function of the Australian bush rat, *Rattus fuscipes*. *J Reprod Fertil* 1984;70: 657–666.
508. Sinha Hikim AP, Bartke A, Russell LD. The seasonal breeding hamster as a model to study structure–function relationships in the testis. *Tissue Cell* 1988;20:63–78.
509. Sinha Hikim AP, Bartke A, Russell LD. Morphometric studies on hamster testes in gonadally active and inactive states: light microscopic findings. *Biol Reprod* 1988;39:1225–1237.
510. Sinha Hikim AP, Amador AG, Klemcke HG, Bartke A, Russell LD. Correlative morphology and endocrinology of Sertoli cells in hamster testes in active and inactive states of spermatogenesis. *Endocrinology* 1989;125:1829–1843.
511. Zamboni L, Conaway CH, van Pelt L. Seasonal changes in production of semen in free-ranging rhesus monkeys. *Biol Reprod* 1974;11:251–267.
512. Pudney J, Lacy D. Correlation between ultrastructure and biochemical changes in the testes of the American grey squirrel, *Sciurus carolinesis,* during the reproductive cycle. *J Reprod Fertil* 1977;49:5–16.
513. Vendreley E, Guerillot C, Da Lage C. Variations saisonnieres des cellules de Sertoli et de Leydig dans le testicule du hamster dore. Etude caryometrique. *CR Acad Sci (Paris)* 1972;275:1143–1146.
514. Berndston WE, Desjardins C. Circulating LH and FSH in hamsters during light deprivation and subsequent photoperiodic stimulation. *Endocrinology* 1974;95:195–205.
515. Lincoln GA. Seasonal variation in the episodic secretion of luteinizing hormone and testosterone in the ram. *J Endocrinol* 1976;69:213–226.
516. Michael RP, Bonsall RW. A 3-year study of an annual rhythm in plasma androgen levels in male rhesus monkey (*Macaca mulatta*) in a constant laboratory environment. *J Reprod Fertil* 1977;49:129–131.
517. Vilar O. Ultrastructural changes observed after hypophysectomy in rat testis. In: Rosemberg E, ed. *Gonadotrophins.* Los Angeles: Geron-X; 1968:205–211.
518. Ghosn S, Bartke A, Grasso P, Reichert LE, Russell LD. The structural response of the hamster Sertoli cell to hypophysectomy: A correlative morphometric and endocrine study. *Anat Rec* 1992;234:513–529.
519. Gravis CJ, Weaker FJ. Testicular involution following optic enucleation. *Cell Tissue Res* 1977;184:67–77.
520. Nebel BR, Murphy CJ. Damage and recovery of mouse testis after 1000r acute localized X-irradiation, with reference to restitution cells, Sertoli cell increase, and type A spermatogonial recovery. *Radiat Res* 1960;12:626–641.
521. Clegg EJ. Studies on artificial cryptorchidism: degenerative and regenerative changes in germinal epithelium of rat testis. *J Endocrinol* 1963;27:241–251.
522. Clegg EJ. Studies on artificial cryptorchidism: degenerative and regenerative changes in germinal epithelium of rat testis. *J Endocrinol* 1963;26:567–574.
523. Felizet G, Branca A. Histologie du testicule ectopique. *J Anat Physiol* 1898;34:589–641.
524. Nagy F. Cell division kinetics and DNA synthesis in the immature Sertoli cells of the rat testis. *J Reprod Fertil* 1972;28: 389–395.
525. Murphy HD. Sertoli cell stimulation following intratesticular injections of FSH in the hypophysectomized rat. *Proc Soc Exp Biol Med* 1965;118:1202–1205.
526. Hochereau-de Reviers MT, Lincoln GA. Seasonal variation in the histology of the testis of the red deer, *Cervus elaphus*. *J Reprod Fertil* 1978;54:209–213.
527. Johnson L, Neaves WB. Age-related changes in the Leydig cell population, seminiferous tubules and sperm production in stallions. *Biol Reprod* 1981;24:703–712.
528. Johnson L, Thompson DL. Age-related and seasonal variation in the Sertoli cell population, daily sperm production and serum concentrations of follicle-stimulating hormone, luteinizing hormone and testosterone in stallions. *Biol Reprod* 1983; 29:777–789.
529. Johnson L. Increased daily sperm production in the breeding season of stallions is explained by an elevated population of spermatogonia. *Biol Reprod* 1985;32:1181–1190.
530. Hochereau-de Reviers MT. Control of spermatogonial multiplication. In: McKerns KW, ed. *Reproductive Processes and Contraception,* New York: Plenum Press; 1981:307–331.
531. Feig LA, Bellve AR, Erickson NH, Klagsbrun M. Sertoli cells contain a mitogenic polypeptide. *Proc Natl Acad Sci USA* 1980;77:4774–4778.
532. Harbitz TB. Morphometric studies of the Sertoli cells in elderly men with special reference to the histology of the prostate. *Acta Pathol Microbiol Scand* 1973;81A:703.
533. Kerr JB, Rich KA, de Kretser DM. Effects of experimental cryptorchidism on the ultrastructure and function of the Sertoli cell and peritubular tissue of the rat testis. *Biol Reprod* 1979; 21:823–838.
534. Hoffer AP. Effects of gossypol on the seminiferous epithelium in the rat: a light and electron microscopy study. *Biol Reprod* 1983;28:1007–1020.
535. Flickinger CJ. Effects of clomiphene on the structure of the testis, epididymis and sex accessory glands of the rat. *Am J Anat* 1981;149:533–562.
536. Kreuger PM, Hodgen GD, Sherins RJ. New evidence for the role of the Sertoli cell and spermatogonia in feedback control of FSH secretion in male rats. *Endocrinology* 1974;95:955–962.
537. Chapin RE, Dutton SL, Ross MD, Sumrell BM, Lamb JC. The effects of ethylene glycol monomethyl ether on testicular histology in rats. *J Androl* 1984;5:369–380.
538. Hildebrandt-Stark HE, Fawcett DW. Effects of deficiency of essential fatty acids and treatment with prostaglandin E_2 on the ultrastructure of the rat testis. *Biol Reprod* 1978;19:736–746.
539. Kierszenbaum AL. Effect of trenimon on the ultrastructure of Sertoli cells in the mouse. *Vichows Arch (Cell Pathol)* 1970; 5:1–12.
540. Zhuang LZ, Phillips DM, Gunsalus GL, Bardin CW, Mather JP. Effects of gossypol on rat Sertoli and Leydig cells in primary culture and established cell lines. *J Androl* 1983;4:336–344.
541. Kerr JB, Sharpe RM. Macrophage activation enhances the human chorionic gonadotrophin-induced disruption of spermatogenesis in the rat. *J Endocrinol* 1989;121:285–292.
542. Kerr JB, Sharpe RM. Focal disruption of spermatogenesis in the testis of adult rats after a single administration of human chorionic gonadotrophin. *Cell Tissue Res* 1989;257:163–169.
543. Parizek J. Sterilization of the male by cadmium salts. *J Reprod Fertil* 1960;1:294–309.
544. Kerr JB, Sharpe RM. Effects and interactions of LH and LHRH agonist on testicular morphology and function in hypophysectomized rats. *J Reprod Fertil* 1986;76:175–192.
545. Vickery B, McRae GI, Bergstrom K, Briones W, Worden A, Seidenberg R. Inability of long-term administration of D-Nal(2)^6-LHRH to abolish fertility in male rats. *J Androl* 1983;4:283–291.
546. Schulze W, Schulze C. Multinucleate Sertoli cells in aged human testis. *Cell Tissue Res* 1981;217:259–266.
547. Schulze C, Holstein AF, Schirren C, Korner F. On the morphology of the human Sertoli cells under normal conditions and in patients with impaired fertility. *Andrologia* 1976;8:167–178.
548. Nistal M, Paniagua R, Abaurrea MA, Santamaria L. Hyperplasia and the immature appearance of Sertoli cells in primary testicular disorders. *Hum Pathol* 1982;13:1.
549. Paniagua R, Amat R, Nistal M, Martin A. Ultrastructural changes in Sertoli cells in ageing humans. *Int J Androl* 1985;8:295–312.
550. Bustos-Obregon E. Ultrastructure and function of the lamina propria of mammalian seminiferous tubules. *Andrologia* 1976;8:179–185.
551. Bustos-Obregon E. Ultrastructure and function of the lamina propria of human seminiferous tubules. *Z Zellforsch* 1976; 141:413–425.
552. de Kretser DM, Kerr JB, Paulsen CA. The peritubular tissue in the normal and pathological human testis. An ultrastructural study. *Biol Reprod* 1975;12:317–324.
553. Christl HW. The lamina propria of vertebrate seminiferous tubules: A comparative light and electron microscopic investigation. *Andrologia* 1990;22:85–94.
554. Hermo L, Lalli M, Clermont Y. Arrangement of connective tissue components in the walls of seminiferous tubules of man and monkey. *Am J Anat* 1977;148:433–436.
555. Chan FL, Inoue S, Le Blond CP. Cryofixation of basement mem-

branes followed by freeze substitution or freeze drying demonstrates that they are composed of a tridimensional network of irregular cords. *Anat Rec* 1993;235:199–205.
556. de Kretser DM, Risbridger GP, Kerr JB. In: de Groot LJ, ed. *The Basic Endocrinology of the Testis.* Philadelphia: WB Saunders; 1993 (In press).
557. Virtanen I, Kallajoki M, Narvanen O, et al. Peritubular myoid cells of human and rat testis are smooth muscle cells that contain desmin-type intermediate filaments. *Anat Rec* 1986;215:10–20.
558. Palombi F, Farini D, Salanova M, De Grossi S, Stefanini M. Development and cytodifferentiation of peritubular myoid cells in the rat testis. *Anat Rec* 1992;233:32–40.
559. Davidoff MS, Breucker H, Holstein AF, Seidl K. Cellular architecture of the lamina propria of human seminiferous tubules. *Cell Tissue Res* 1990;262:253–261.
560. Kerr JB, Knell CM. The regenerative capacity of testicular interstitial tissue. *Wilhelm Roux Arch Dev Biol* 1987;196:467–471.
561. Jackson AE, O'Leary P, Ayers MM, de Kretser DM. The effects of ethylene dimethane sulphonate (EDS) on rat Leydig cells: Evidence to support a connective tissue origin of Leydig cells. *Biol Reprod* 1986;35:425–437.
562. Worley RTS, Nicholson HD, Pickering BT. Testicular oxytocin: an initiator of seminiferous tubule movement? In: Saez JM, Forest MG, Dazoid A, Bertrand J, eds. *Recent Progress in Cellular Endocrinology of the Testis.* Paris: INSERM; 1984:205–212.
563. Paranko J, Kallajoki M, Pelliniemi LJ, Lehto VP, Virtanen I. Transient co-expression of cytokeratin and vimentin in differentiating rat Sertoli cells. *Dev Biol* 1986;117:35–44.
564. Benda C. Untersuchunger über den Bau des funktionierenden Samenkanalchens einiger Saugetiere und Folgerungen fur die Spermatogenese dieser Wirbeltierklasse. *Arch Mikrosk Anat* 1887;30:49–110.
565. Curtis GM. The morphology of the mammalian seminiferous tubule. *Am J Anat* 1918;24:339–394.
566. Roosen-Runge EC, Giesel LO. Quantitative studies on spermatogenesis in the albino rat. *Am J Anat* 1950;87:1–30.
567. Oakberg EF. Duration of spermatogenesis in the mouse and timing of stages of the cycle of the seminiferous epithelium. *Am J Anat* 1956;99:507–516.
568. Ortavant R. *La cycle spermatogénètique chez le Belier.* Thesis, Paris; 1958.
569. Chowdhury AK, Marshall G. Irregular pattern of spermatogenesis in the baboon (*Papio anubis*) and its possible mechanism. In: Steinberger A, Steinberger E, eds. *Testicular Development, Structure and Function,* New York: Raven Press; 1980:129–137.
570. Schulze W, Rehder U. Organization and morphogenesis of the human seminiferous epithelium. *Cell Tissue Res* 1984;237: 395–407.
571. Ortavant R. Étude des generations spermatogoniales chez le Belier. *C R Soc Biol* 1954;148:1958–1961.
572. Ortavant R. Autoradiographie des cellules germinales du testicule de Belier. Duree des phenomenes spermatogénètiques. *Arch Anat Microsc Morphol Exp* 1956;45:1–10.
573. Clermont Y, Harvey SG. Duration of the cycle of the seminiferous epithelium of normal hypophysectomized and hypophysectomized-hormone treated albino rats. *Endocrinology* 1965; 76:80–89.
574. Desclin J, Ortavant R. Influences des hormones gonadotropes sur la duree des processus spermatogénètiques chez le rat. *Ann Biol Anim Biochem Biophys* 1963;3:329–342.
575. Russell LD, Lee IP, Ettlin R, Malone JP. Morphological pattern of response after administration of procarbazine: Alteration of specific cell associations during the cycle of the seminiferous epithelium of the rat. *Tissue Cell* 1983;15:391–404.
576. Cleland KW. The spermatogenic cycle of the guinea pig. *Aust J Biol Sci* 1951;4:344–369.
577. Johnsen SG. Studies on the testicular–hypophyseal feedback mechanism in man. *Acta Endocrinol (Kbh)* 1964;Suppl 90: 99–124.
578. Perey B, Clermont Y, Le Blond GP. The wave of the seminiferous epithelium in the rat. *Am J Anat* 1961;108:47–77.
579. Dym M, Clermont Y. Role of spermatogonia in the repair of the seminiferous epithelium following X-irradiation of the rat testis. *Am J Anat* 1970;128:265–282.
580. Moens PB, Hugenholtz AD. The arrangement of germ cells in the rat seminiferous tubule: An electron microscopic study. *J Cell Sci* 1975;19:487–507.
581. Ren HP, Russell LD. Clonal development of interconnected germ cells in the rat and its relationship to the segmental and subsegmental organization of spermatogenesis. *Am J Anat* 1991;192:121–128.
582. Russell LD, Vogl AW, Weber JE. Actin localization in male germ cells intercellular bridges in the rat and ground squirrel and disruption of bridges by cytochalasin D. *Am J Anat* 1987;180:25–40.
583. Weber JE, Russell LD. A study of intercellular bridges during spermatogenesis in the rat. *Am J Anat* 1987;180:1–24.
584. Rolshoven E. Zur Frage des "Alterns" der generativen Elemente in den Hodenkanalchen. *Anat Anz* 1941;91:1–8.
585. Huckins C. Cell cycle properties of differentiating spermatogonia in adult Sprague Dawley rats. *Cell Tissue Kinet* 1971;4:139–154.
586. Huckins C. The spermatogonial stem cell population in adult rats. III. Evidence for a long-cycling population. *Cell Tissue Kinet* 1971;4:335–349.
587. Huckins C. The spermatogonial stem cell population in adult rats. II. A radioautographic analysis of their cell cycle properties. *Cell Tissue Kin* 1971;4:313–334.
588. Oakberg EF. Spermatogonial stem-cell renewal in the mouse. *Anat Rec* 1971;169:515–531.
589. Huckins C, Oakberg EF. Morphological and quantitative analysis of spermatogonia in mouse testes using whole mounted seminiferous tubules. I. The normal testes. *Anat Rec* 1978;192:519–528.
590. Oud JL, de Rooij DG. Spermatogenesis in the Chinese hamster. *Anat Rec* 1977;187:113–124.
591. de Rooij DG, Lok D, Weenk D. Feedback regulation of the proliferation of the undifferentiated spermatogonia in the Chinese hamster by the differentiating spermatogonia. *Cell Tissue Kinet* 1985;18:71–81.
592. Lok D, Weenk D, de Rooij DG. Morphology, proliferation and differentiation of undifferentiated spermatogonia in the Chinese hamster and the ram. *Anat Rec* 1982;203:83–99.
593. Chowdhury AK, Steinberger E. A radioautography technique for human and rat seminiferous tubules mounted *in toto. Exp Cell Res* 1971;64:450–456.
594. Fuerst C. Über die Entwicklung der Samenkoerperchen bei den Beteltieren. *Arch Mikrosk Anat* 1887;81:1–23.
595. Hochereau MT. Constance des frequences relatives des etudes du cycle de l'epithelium seminifere chez lez taureau et chez le rat. *Ann Biol Anim Biochem Biophys* 1963;3:93–102.
596. Tiba T, Ishikawa T, Murakami A. Histologische Untersuchung der Kinetik des Spermatogenese beim Mink. II. Samenepithelwelle in der Paarungszeit. *Jpn J Vet Res* 1968;16:159–187.
597. Parvinen M. Regulation of the seminiferous epithelium. *Endocr Rev* 1982;3:404–417.
598. Parvinen M, Vihko KK, Toppari J. Cell interactions during the seminiferous epithelial cycle. *Int Rev Cytol* 1987;104:115–151.
599. Jegou B, Laws AO, de Kretser DM. Changes in testicular function in the rat testis to heat: further evidence for interaction of germ cells, Sertoli cells and Leydig cells. *Int J Androl* 1984;7:244–257.
600. Roosen-Runge EC. Untersuchungen uber die degeneration samenbilender zellen in der normalen spermatogenese der ratte. *Z Zellforsch* 1955;41:221–225.
601. Amann RP. Reproductive capacity of dairy bulls. IV Spermatogenesis and testicular germ cell degeneration. *Am J Anat* 1962;110:69–78.
602. Barr AB, Moore DJ, Paulsen CA. Germinal cell loss during human spermatogenesis. *J Reprod Fertil* 1971;25:75–80.
603. Amann RP. Sperm production rates. In: Johnson AD, Gomes WR, van Denmark NL, eds. *The Testis,* Vol 1. New York: Academic Press; 1970:433–482.
604. Johnson L. Spermatogenesis and aging in the human. *J Androl* 1986;7:331–354.
605. Johnson L, Chaturvedi PK, Williams JD. Missing generations of spermatocytes and spermatids in seminiferous epithelium contribute to low efficiency of spermatogenesis in humans. *Biol Reprod* 1992;47:1091–1098.
606. Stieve H. *Entwickelung Bau und Bedeutung der Keimdrusenzwischenzellen.* Munich: JF Bergmann; 1921.
607. Hanes FM. The relations of the interstitial cells of Leydig to the

production of an internal secretion by the mammalian testis. *J Exp Med* 1911;13:338–354.
608. Rasmussen AT. Interstitial cells of the testis. In: Cowdrey EV, ed. *Special Cytology,* Vol 3, Sect XLII. New York: Hafner; 1932:1675–1725.
609. Hooker CW. The postnatal history and function of the interstitial cells of the testis of the bull. *Am J Anat* 1944;74:1–37.
610. Hooker CW. The biology of the interstitial cells of the testis. *Recent Prog Horm Res* 1948;3:173–195.
611. Hooker CW. The intertubular tissue of the testis. In: Johnson AD, Gomes WR, van Demark NL, *The Testis,* Vol 1. New York: Academic Press; 1970:483–550.
612. Albert A. The mammalian testis. In: Young WC, ed. *Sex and Internal Secretions,* Vol 1. Baltimore: Williams & Wilkins; 1961:305–365.
613. Burgos MH, Vitale-Calpe R, Aoki A. Fine structure of the testis and its functional significance. In: Johnson AD, Gomes WR, van Demark NL, eds. *The Testis,* Vol 1. New York: Academic Press; 1970:551–649.
614. Fawcett DW, Heidger DM, Leak LV. Lymph vascular system of the interstitial tissue of the testis as revealed by electron microscopy. *J Reprod Fertil* 1969;19:109–119.
615. Connell CG, Connell GM. The interstitial tissue of the testis. In: Johnson AD, Gomes WR, eds. *The Testis,* Vol 4. New York: Academic Press; 1977:333–370.
616. Christensen AK. Leydig cells. In: Hamilton DW, Greep RO, eds. *Handbook of Physiology,* Sect 7, Vol 5. Washington: American Physiological Society; 1975:57–94.
617. Leydig F. Zur anatomie der mannlichen Geschlechtsorgane und Analdrusen der Saugetiere. *Z Wiss Zool* 1850;2:1–57.
618. Hofmeister H. Untersuchungen uber die Zwischensubstanz im Hoden der Saugethiere. *Sitzungsber Acad Wiss Mathnatur Classe Wien* 1872;5:77.
619. Plato J. Die interstitiellen Zellen des Hodens und ihre physiologische Bedeutung. *Arch Mikrosk Anat* 1896;48:280.
620. Lenhossek M. Beitrage zur Kenntniss der Zwischenzellen des Hodens. *Arch Anat Physiol Anat Abt* 1897;51:65.
621. Loisel G. Etudes sur le spermatogénèse chez le moineau domestique. *Anat Physiol* 1902;33:112.
622. Bovin P, Ancel P. Recherches sur les cellules interstitielles du testicule des mammiferes. *Arch Zool* 1903;1:437–523.
623. Ganfini C. Struttura e sviluppo delle cellule interstiziali del testicolo. *Arch Ital Anat Embriol* 1902;1:233.
624. Bouin P, Ancel P. La glande interstitielle a seule dans le testicule une action generale sur l'organisme. *Demonstr Exp CR Acad Sci (Paris)* 1904;138:110.
625. Ancel P, Bouin P. L'apparition des caracteres sexuels secondaires est sous la dependance de la gland interstitielle. *CR Acad Sci (Paris)* 1903;138:168.
626. Ciaccio C. Contributo alla distribuzione ed alla fisiopathologia cellulare dei lipoidi. *Arch Zellforsch* 1910;5:235.
627. Whitehead RH. On the chemical nature of certain granules in the interstitial cells of the testis. *Am J Anat* 1912;14:63.
628. Lotz A, Jaffe R. Die Hoden bei Allgemeinerkrankungen. *Z Konstit* 1924;10:99.
629. McGee LC. Effect of injections of lipid fraction of bull testicle in capons. *Proc Inst Med Chicago* 1972;6:242.
630. Gallagher TF, Koch FC. The testicular hormone. *J Biol Chem* 1929;84:495–500.
631. Butenandt A, Hanisch G. Uber Testosteron. Umwandlung des Dehydroandrosterons in Androstenediol und Testosteron: ein Weg zur Darstellung des Testosterons ans Cholesterin. *Z Physiol Chem* 1935;237:89–97.
632. Ruzicka L, Wettstein A. Kunstliche Herstellung des mannlichen sexual Hormones. Transdehydro-androsten-3,17-dions. *Helv Chim Acta* 1935;18:986–994.
633. Wattenberg LW. Microscopic histochemical demonstration of steroid-3β-ol dehydrogenase in tissue sections. *J Histochem Cytochem* 1958;6:225–232.
634. Levy H, Dean HW, Rubin BL. Visualization of steroid-3β-ol-dehydrogenase activity in tissues of intact and hypophysectomized rats. *Endocrinology* 1959;65:932–943.
635. Baillie AH. Further observations on the growth and histochemistry of the Leydig tissue in the postnatal prepubertal mouse testis. *J Anat* 1964;98:403–419.
636. Christensen AK, Mason NR. Comparative ability of seminiferous tubules and interstitial tissue of rat testes to synthesize androgens from progesterone-4-^{14}C *in vitro. Endocrinology* 1965;76: 646–656.
637. Hall PF, Irby DC, de Kretser DM. Conversion of cholesterol to androgens by rat testes: comparison of interstitial cells and seminiferous tubules. *Endocrinology* 1969;84:488–496.
638. Ludwig C, Tomsa W. Die Lymphwerge des Hodens und ihr Verhaltnis zu den Blut- und Samengefassen. *S Ber Akad Wiss Wein Math Klin* 1862;46:221.
639. Freg H. Zur kenntnis der Lymphbahnen in Hoden. *Virchows Arch* 1963;28:563–569.
640. Regaud C. Les vaisseaux lymphatiques de testicule. *CR S Soc Biol* 1897;14:695.
641. Testut L. *Traite d'Anatomie Humanie* Paris: Octave Doin; 1902.
642. Mihalkovics V. Beitrage zur Anatomie und Histologie des Hodens. *Ber Verbandl K Sachs Gesellsch Wiss Math (Leipzig)* 1873;25:217.
643. Gerster R. Über die lymphgefasse des hodens. *Z Anat Entwickl Gesch* 1876;2:36.
644. Hasumi S. Anatomische untersuchungen über die lymphgefasse des mannlichen urogenital-system. *Jpn J Med Sci Anat* 1930;11:159–186.
645. Renyi Vamos F. Das lymphsystem des hodens und nebenhodens. *Z Urol* 1955;48:355–372.
646. Renyi Vamos F. Beitrage und richlinien zur anatomie des lymphgefassystems. *Virchows Arch Pathol Anat Physiol* 1956;328:503.
647. Brzezinski VDK. Nene befunde mit einer verbesserten darstellung experimentell anfgefullter lymphkapillaren an niere, hoden bebenhoden, darm- und dickdaom. *Anat Anz* 1963;113:289–306.
648. Staudt J, Wenzel J. Untersuchungen über das lymphgefassystem des kaninchenhodens. *Z Mikrosk Anat Forsch* 1965;73:203–226.
649. Clark RV. Three-dimensional organization of testicular interstitial tissue and lymphatic space in the rat. *Anat Rec* 1976;184:203–226.
650. Holstein AF, Orlandini GE, Moller R. Distribution and fine structure of the lymphatic system in the human testis. *Cell Tissue Res* 1979;200:15–27.
651. Wagner K. Sind die Zwischenzellen des Saugetierhodens Drusenzellen? Ein Beitrag zur Zytologie und Zygotogenese. *Biol Gen* 1925;1:22.
652. Hooker CW, Pfieffer CA, de Vita J. The significance of the diameter of the interstitial cells of the testis in the aged dog. *Anat Rec* 1946;94:471–472.
653. Stein AA. Experimentelle Untersuchungen uber die Zellformen des interstitiellen Hodengewebes. *Z Zellforsch* 1931;12:483.
654. Esaki S. Uber kulturen des Hodengewebes der Saugthiere und über die Nater der interstitiellen Hodengewebes und des Zwischenzellen. *Z Mikrosck Anat Forsch* 1928;15:368–404.
655. Evans HM, Schulemann W. The action of vital stains belonging to the benzidine group. *Science* 1914;39:443.
656. Christensen AK, Peacock KC. Increase in Leydig cell number in testis of adult rats treated chronically with an excess of human chorionic gonadotrophin. *Biol Reprod* 1980;22:383–392.
657. Ennist DL, Jones KH. Rapid method for identification of macrophages in suspension by acid alpha-naphthyl acetate esterase activity. *J Histochem Cytochem* 1983;31:960–963.
658. Molenaar R, Rommerts FFG, van der Molen HJ. Non-specific esterase: a specific and useful marker enzyme for Leydig cells from mature rats. *J Endocrinol* 1986;108:229–334.
659. Miller SC, Bowman BM, Rosland HG. Structure, cytochemistry, endocytic activity and immunoglobulin (Fc) receptors of rat testicular interstitial-tissue macrophages. *Am J Anat* 1983;168: 1–13.
660. Miller SC. Localization of plutonium-241 in the testis. An interspecies comparison using light and electron microscope autoradiography. *Int J Radiat Biol* 1982;41:633–643.
661. Miller SC, Bowman BM. Tissue, cellular and subcellular distribution of ^{241}Pu in the rat testis. *Radiat Res* 1983;94:416–426.
662. Orth J, Christensen AK. Localization of ^{125}I-labelled FSH in the testes of hypophysectomized rats by autoradiography at the light and electron microscope levels. *Endocrinology* 1977;101: 262–278.
663. Christensen AK, Komorowski TE, Wilson B, Ma SF, Stevens RW. The distribution of serum albumin in the rat testis, studied

by electron microscope immunocytochemistry on ultrathin frozen sections. *Endocrinology* 1985;116:1983–1996.
664. Hutson JC. Development of cytoplasmic digitations between Leydig cells and testicular macrophages of the rat. *Cell Tissue Res* 1992;267:385–389.
665. Berg A. Effect of cryptorchidism on the morphology of testicular macrophages: evidence for a Leydig cell–macrophage interaction in the rat testis. *Int J Androl* 1985;8:86–96.
666. Niemi M, Sharpe RM, Brown WRA. Macrophages in the interstitial tissue of the rat testis. *Cell Tissue Res* 1986;243:337–344.
667. Raburn DJ, Coquelin A, Hutson JC. Human chorionic gonadotrophin increases the concentration of macrophages in neonatal rat testis. *Biol Reprod* 1991;44:172–177.
668. Hutson JC. Changes in the concentration and size of testicular macrophages during development. *Biol Reprod* 1990;43: 885–890.
669. Pollanen P, Maddocks S. Macrophages, lymphocytes and MHC II antigen in the ram and rat testis. *J Reprod Fertil* 1988;82:437–445.
670. Kerr JB, Donachie KI, Rommerts FFG. Selective destruction and regeneration of rat Leydig cells *in vivo.* A new method for the study of seminiferous tubular–interstitial tissue interaction. *Cell Tissue Res* 1985;242:145–156.
671. Kerr JB, Bartlett JMS, Donachie K. Acute response of testicular interstitial tissue in rats to the cytotoxic drug ethane dimethane sulfonate. *Cell Tissue Res* 1986;243:405–414.
672. Gunn SA, Gould TC. Vasculature of the testes and adnexa. In: Hamilton DW, Greep RO, eds. *Handbook of Physiology,* Sect 7, Part 5. Washington: American Physiological Society; 1975: 117–142.
673. Maseki Y, Miyake K, Mitsuya H, Kitamura H, Yamada K. Mastocytosis occurring in the testes from patients with idiopathic male infertility. *Fertil Steril* 1981;36:814–817.
674. Nistal M, Santamaria L, Paniagua R. Mast cells in the human testis and epididymis from birth to adulthood. *Acta Anat* 1984;119:155–160.
675. Mayerhofer A, Bartke A, Amador AG, Began T. Histamine affects testicular steroid production in the golden hamster. *Endocrinology* 1989;125:560–562.
676. Pilsworth LM, Setchell BP. Spermatogenic and endocrine function of the testes of invertebrate and vertebrate animals. In: Burger HG, de Kretser DM, eds. *The Testis.* New York: Raven Press; 1981:9–38.
677. Roosen-Runge EC. *The Process of Spermatogenesis in Animals.* Cambridge: Cambridge University Press; 1977.
678. Lofts B. Patterns of testicular activity. In: Barrington EJW, Jorgensen CB, eds. *Perspectives in Endocrinology. Hormones in the Lives of Lower Vertebrate.* London: Academic Press; 1968: 239–304.
679. Lofts B. Reproduction. In: Lofts B, ed. *Physiology of the Amphibia,* Vol II. New York: Academic Press; 1974:107–218.
680. Pudney J, Canick JA, Mak P, Callard GV. The differentiation of Leydig cells, steroidogenesis and the spermatogenic wave in the testis of *Necturus maculosus. Gen Comp Endocrinol* 1983; 50:43–66.
681. Ucci AA. A fine structural study of interstitial cell changes in the testis of *Necturus maculosus* during a portion of the annual cycle, and possible evidence for local feedback control by seminiferous epithelium. *Am J Anat* 1982;165:22–38.
682. Schulze C. Saisonbedingte Veranderungen in der Morphologie der Leydigzellen von Rana esculenta. *Z Zellforsch* 1973; 142:367–386.
683. Terao K. Annular nucleolus in Leydig cells of mouse. *Z Zellforsch* 1973;137:167–175.
684. Terao L, Sakaibara Y, Yamazaki M, Miyaki K. Annular nucleolus in chicken embryonal hepatocyte induced by aflatoxin B. *Exp Cell Res* 1971;66:81–89.
685. Christensen AK, Fawcett DW. The fine structure of testicular interstitial cells in mice. *Am J Anat* 1966;118:551–572.
686. de Kretser DM. The fine structure of the testicular interstitial cells in men of normal androgenic status. *Z Zellforsch* 1967;80:594–609.
687. de Kretser DM. Changes in the fine structure of human testicular interstitial cells after treatment with human gonadotrophins. *Z Zellforsch* 1967;83:344–358.
688. Kerr JB, Rich KA, de Kretser DM. Alteration of the fine structure and androgen secretion of the interstitial cells in the experimentally cryptorchid rat testis. *Biol Reprod* 1979;20:409–422.
689. Mori H, Christensen AK. Morphometric analysis of Leydig cells in the normal rat testis. *J Cell Biol* 1980;84:340–354.
690. Zirkin BR, Ewing LL, Kromann N, Cochran RC. Testosterone secretion by rat, rabbit, guinea pig, dog and hamster testes perfused *in vitro:* Correlation with Leydig cell ultrastructure. *Endocrinology* 1980;107:1867–1874.
691. Mori H, Kadota A, Fukunishi R, Kukita H, Takeuchi N, Matsumoto K. Effects of a cholesterol-rich diet and a hypolipidemic drug (Clofibrate, CP1B) on Leydig cells in rats. Stereological and biochemical analysis. *Andrologia* 1980;12:271–291.
692. Mori H, Hiromoto N, Nakahara M, Shiraishi T. Stereological analysis of Leydig cell ultrastructure in aged humans. *J Clin Endocrinol Metab* 1982;55:634–641.
693. Mori H, Shimizu D, Fukunishi Y, Christensen AK. Morphometric analysis of testicular Leydig cells in normal adult mice. *Anat Rec* 1982;204:333–339.
694. Connell CJ, Christensen AK. The ultrastructure of the canine testicular interstitial tissue. *Biol Reprod* 1975;12:368–382.
695. Weaker FJ. The fine structure of the interstitial tissue of the testis of the nine-banded armadillo. *Anat Rec* 1977;187:11–28.
696. Camatini M, Franchi E, de Curtis I. Ultrastructure of Leydig cells in the African green monkey. *J Ultrastruct Res* 1981;76:224–234.
697. Murakami M, Kitahara Y. Cylindrical bodies derived from endoplasmic reticulum in Leydig cells of the rat testis. *J Electronmicrosc* 1971;20:318–323.
698. Christensen AK, Fawcett DW. The normal fine structure of opossum testicular interstitial cells. *J Biophys Biochem Cytol* 1961;9:653–670.
699. Nakai Y. Adult interstitial cell. In: Kurosumi K, Fujita H, eds. *An Atlas of Electron Micrographs. Functional Morphology of Endocrine Glands.* Tokyo: Igaku Shoin; 1974:178–179.
700. Emura S. Electron microscopic studies on annulate lamellae in Leydig cells of rabbit. *Cell* 1978;10:752–756.
701. Ohata M. Electron microscopic study on the testicular interstitial cells in the mouse. *Arch Histol Jpn* 1979;42:51–79.
702. Ewing LL, Zirkin BR, Cochran RC, Kromann N, Peters C, Ruiz-Bravo N. Testosterone secretion by rat, rabbit, guinea pig, dog, and hamster testes perfused *in vitro:* correlation with Leydig cell mass. *Endocrinology* 1979;105:1135–1142.
703. Wing TY, Ewing LL, Zirkin BR. Effects of luteinizing hormone withdrawal on Leydig cell smooth endoplasmic reticulum and steroidogenic reactions which convert pregnenolone to testosterone. *Endocrinology* 1984;115:2290–2296.
704. Wing TY, Ewing LL, Zegeye B, Zirkin BR. Restoration effects of exogenous luteinizing hormone on the testicular steroidogenesis and Leydig cell ultrastructure. *Endocrinology* 1985;117: 1779–1787.
705. Mendis-Handagama SMLC, Zirkin BR, Ewing LL. Comparison of components of the testis interstitium with testosterone secretion in hamster, rat, and guinea pig testes perfused *in vitro. Am J Anat* 1988;181:12–22.
706. Fouquet JP, Meusy-Dessolle N, Dang DC. Relationships between Leydig cell morphometry and plasma testosterone during postnatal development of the monkey, *Macaca fascicularis. Reprod Nutr Dev* 1984;24:281–296.
707. Johnson L, Grumbles JS, Chastain S, Goss HF, Petty CS. Leydig cell cytoplasmic content is related to daily sperm production in men. *J Androl* 1990;11:155–160.
708. Russell LD, Burguet S. Ultrastructure of Leydig cells as revealed by secondary tissue treatment with a ferrocyanide–osmium mixture. *Tissue Cell* 1977;9:751–766.
709. Kerr JB, Robertson DM, de Kretser DM. Morphological and functional characterization of interstitial cells from mouse testes fractionated on Percoll density gradients. *Endocrinology* 1985;116:1030–1043.
710. Kerr JB, Knell CM. The fate of fetal Leydig cells during the development of the fetal and postnatal rat testis. *Development* 1988;103:535–544.
711. Aoki A, Massa EM. Early responses of testicular interstitial cells to stimulation by interstitial cell stimulating hormone. *Am J Anat* 1972;134:239–262.

712. Wrobel KH, Sinowatz F, Mademann R. Intertubular topography in the bovine testis. *Cell Tissue Res* 1981;217:289–310.
713. Belt WD, Cavazos LF. Fine structure of the interstitial cells of Leydig in the squirrel monkey during seasonal regression. *Anat Rec* 1971;169:115–128.
714. Russo J, Sacerdote FC. Ultrastructural changes induced by hCG in the Leydig cell of the adult mouse testis. *Z Zellforsch* 1971;112:363–370.
715. Nussdorfer GG, Robba C, Mazzocchi G, Rebuffat P. Effects of chorionic gonadotrophins on the interstitial cells of the rat testis: a morphometric and radioimmunological study. *Int J Androl* 1980;3:319–332.
716. Neaves WB. The pattern of gonadotropin-induced changes in plasma testosterone, testicular esterified cholesterol and Leydig cell lipid droplets in immature mice. *Biol Reprod* 1978;19:864–871.
717. Aoki A. Hormonal control of Leydig cell differentiation. *Protoplasma* 1970;71:209–225.
718. Merkow L, Acevedo H, Slifkia M, Caito M. Studies on the interstitial cells of the testis: I. The ultrastructure of the immature guinea pig and the effect of stimulation with human chorionic gonadotropin. *Am J Pathol* 1968;33:47–62.
719. Aoki A, Massa EM. Subcellular compartmentation of free and esterified cholesterol in the interstitial cells in the mouse testis. *Cell Tissue Res* 1975;165:49–62.
720. Lalli MF, Clermont Y. Leydig cells and their role in the synthesis and secretion of glycoproteins. *Anat Rec* 1975;181:403–404.
721. Gemmell RT, Stacy BD. Ultrastructural study of granules in the corpora lutea of several mammalian species. *Am J Anat* 1979;155:1–14.
722. Gemmell RT, Laychock SG, Rubin RP. Ultrastructural and biochemical evidence for a steroid-containing secretory organelle in the perfused cat adrenal gland. *J Cell Biol* 1977;72:209–215.
723. Loh HS, Gemmell RT. Changes in the fine structure of the Leydig cells of the seasonally breeding bat, *Myotis adversus. Cell Tissue Res* 1980;210:339–347.
724. Paavola LG, Boyd CO. Cytoplasmic granules in luteal cells of pregnant and nonpregnant guinea pigs. A cytochemical study. *Anat Rec* 1981;201:127–140.
725. Porter DG. Relaxin: old hormone, new prospect. *Oxf Rev Reprod Endocrinol* 1979;1:1–45.
726. Fields PA, Eldrige RK, Fuchs AR, Roberts RF, Fields MJ. Human placental and bovine corpora luteal oxytocin. *Endocrinology* 1983;112:1544–1546.
727. Hermo L, Clermont Y, Lalli M. Intracellular pathways of endocytosed tracers in Leydig cells of the rat. *J Androl* 1985;6:213–224.
728. Tang XM, Clermont Y, Hermo L. Origin and fate of autophagosomes in Leydig cells of normal adult rats. *J Androl* 1988;9:284–293.
729. Fawcett DW, Burgos MH. Studies on the fine structure of the mammalian testis. II. The human interstitial tissue. *Am J Anat* 1960;107:245–269.
730. Yamada E. Some observations on the fine structure of the interstitial cells and Sertoli cells of the human testis. *Gunma Symp Endocrinol* 1965;2:1–17.
731. Nagano T. Some observations on the structure of interstitial cells and Sertoli cells of the human testis. *Gunma Symp Endocrinol* 1965;2:19–28.
732. Reddy J, Svoboda D. Microbodies (peroxisomes) in the interstitial cells of rodent testes. *Lab Invest* 1972;26:657–665.
733. Hruban Z, Vigil EL, Steasers A, Hopkins E. Microbodies, constituent organelles of animals. *Lab Invest* 1972;27:184–191.
734. Mendis-Handagama SMLC, Zirkin BR, Scallen TJ, Ewing LL. Studies on peroxisomes of the adult rat Leydig cells. *J Androl* 1990;11:270–278.
735. Mendis-Handagama SMLC, Watkins PA, Gelber SJ, Scallen TJ, Zirkin BR, Ewing LL. Luteinizing hormone causes rapid and transient changes in rat Leydig cell peroxisome volume and intraperoxisomal sterol carrier protein-2 content. *Endocrinology* 1990;127:2947–2954.
736. Usui N. Fine structure of interstitial cells and macrophages in immature rat testes. *J Tokyo Womens Med Coll* 1976;46:809–825.
737. Tanuma Y, Ohata M. Transmission electron microscopic observation of epithelial cells with single cilia in intrahepatic biliary ductules of bats. *Arch Histol Jpn* 1978;41:367–376.
738. Temple R, Wolff J. Stimulation of steroid secretion by antimicrotubular agents. *J Biol Chem* 1973;248:2691.
739. Ray P, Strott CA. Stimulation of steroid synthesis by normal rat adrenocortical cells in response to antimicrotubular agents. *Endocrinology* 1978;103:1281–1288.
740. Clark MA, Shay JW. The role of tubulin in the steroidogenic response of murine adrenal and rat Leydig cell. *Endocrinology* 1981;109:2261–2263.
741. Laws AO, Kerr JB, de Kretser DM. The role of the microtubular system in LH/hCG receptor downregulation in rat Leydig cells. *Mol Cell Endocrinol* 1984;38:39–51.
742. Reinke F. Beitrage zur Histologie des Menschen. *Arch Mikrosk Anat* 1896;47:34–44.
743. Nagano T, Ohtsuki I. Reinvestigation of the fine structure of Reinke's crystals in the human testicular interstitial cell. *J Cell Biol* 1971;51:148–161.
744. Yasuzumi G, Nakai Y, Tsubo I, Yasuda M, Sugioka T. The fine structure of nuclei as revealed by electronmicroscopy: IV. The intranuclear inclusion formation of Leydig cells of ageing human testes. *Exp Cell Res* 1967;45:261–276.
745. Janko AB, Sandberg EC. Histochemical evidence for the protein nature of the Reinke crystalloid. *Obstet Gynaecol* 1970;35:493–503.
746. Mori H, Fukunishi R, Fujii M, Hataji K, Shiraishi T, Matsumoto K. Stereological analysis of Reinke crystals in human Leydig cells. *Virchows Arch (Pathol Anat)* 1978;380:1–10.
747. Sohval AR, Gabrilove JL, Chung L. Ultrastructure of Leydig cell paracrystalline inclusions, possibly related to Reinke crystals, in the normal human testis. *Z Zellforsch* 1973;142:13–26.
748. Kerr JB, Abbenhuys DC, Irby DC. Crystalloid formation in rat Leydig cells. An ultrastructural and hormonal study. *Cell Tissue Res* 1986;245:91–100.
749. Prince FP. Ultrastructural evidence of indirect and direct autonomic innervation of human Leydig cells: comparison of neonatal, childhood and pubertal ages. *Cell Tissue Res* 1992;269:383–390.
750. Satoh M. The histogenesis of the gonads in the rat embryos. *J Anat* 1985;143:17–37.
751. Pelliniemi LJ, Dym M. The fetal gonad and sexual differentiation. In: Tulchinsky D, Ryan KJ, eds. *Maternal–Fetal Endocrinology.* Philadelphia: WR Saunders; 1980:252–280.
752. Mancini RE, Vilar O, Lavieri JC, Andrada JA, Heinrich JJ. Development of Leydig cells in the normal human testis. *Am J Anat* 1963;112:203–214.
753. Pelliniemi L, Dym M, Crigler J, Retik A, Fawcett DW. Development of Leydig cells in human fetuses and in patients with androgen insensitivity. In: Steinberger A, Steinberger E, eds. *Testicular Development, Structure and Function.* New York: Raven Press; 1980:49–54.
754. Gondos B. Development and differentiation of the testis and male reproductive tract. In: Steinberger A, Steinberger E, eds. *Testicular Development, Structure and Function.* New York: Raven Press; 1980:3–20.
755. Gondos B. Cellular interrelationships in the human foetal ovary and testis. *Proc Clin Biol Res* 1981;59B:373–381.
756. Witschi E. Embryogenesis of the adrenal and the reproductive gland. *Recent Prog Horm Res* 1951;6:1–27.
757. Holstein AF, Wartenburg H, Vossmeyer J. Zur Cytologie de pranatalen Gonadenentwicklung beim Menschen. III. Die Entwicklung der Leydig-zellen im Hoden von embrynon und Feten. *Z Anat Entwickl Gesch* 1971;135:43–66.
758. Gondos B, Paup D, Ross J, Gorski R. Ultrastructural differentiation of Leydig cells in the fetal and postnatal hamster testis. *Anat Rec* 1974;178:551–566.
759. Gondos B, Renston R, Goldstein D. Postnatal differentiation of Leydig cells in the rabbit testis. *Am J Anat* 1976;145:167–182.
760. Gondos B, Morrison K, Renston R. Leydig cell differentiation in the prepubertal rabbit testis. *Biol Reprod* 1977;17:745–748.
761. Niemi M, Kormano M. Cell renewal in the interstitial tissue of postnatal prepubertal rat testis. *Endocrinology* 1964;74:996–998.
762. Prince FP. Ultrastructure of immature Leydig cells in the human prepubertal testis. *Anat Rec* 1984;209:165–176.

763. Chemes HE, Gottlieb SE, Pasqualini T, Domenichini E, Rivarola MA, Bergada C. Response to acute hCG stimulation and steroidogeneic potential of Leydig cell fibroblastic precursors in humans. *J Androl* 1985;6:102–112.
764. Dierichs R, Wrobel KH, Schilling E. Licht und elektronenmikroskopische Untersuchungen an den Leydigzellen des Schweines wahrend der postnatalen Entwicklung. *Z Zellforsch* 1973;143:203–277.
765. Dierichs R, Wrobel KH. Licht und electronenmikroskopische Untersuchnugen an den peritubularen Zellen des Schweinhoden wahrend der postnatalen Entwicklung. *Z Anat Entwickl Gesch* 1973;143:49–64.
766. van Straaten HWM, Wensing CJG. Histomorphometric aspect of testicular morphogenesis in the pig. *Biol Reprod* 1977; 17:467–472.
767. van Straaten HWM, Wensing CJG. Leydig cell development in the testis of the pig. *Biol Reprod* 1978;18:86–93.
768. Bressler RS, Ross MH. Differentiation of peritubular myoid cells of the testis: effects of intratesticular implantation of newborn mouse testes into normal and hypophysectomized adult. *Biol Reprod* 1972;6:148–159.
769. Mori H, Shiraishi T, Matsumoto K. Leydig cells within the lamina propria of seminiferous tubules in four patients with azoospermia. *Andrologia* 1978;10:444–452.
770. Sniffen RC. The testis. I. The normal testis. *Arch Pathol* 1950;50:259–284.
771. Vilar O. Histology of the human testis from neonatal period to adolescence. In: Rosenburg E, Paulsen CA, eds. *The Human Testis,* New York: Plenum Press; 1970;95–108.
772. Hadziselimovic F. Cryptorchidism: Ultrastructure of normal and cryptorchid testis development. *Adv Anat Embryol Cell Biol* 1977;53:1–17.
773. Whitehead RH. The embryonic development of the interstitial cells of Leydig. *Am J Anat* 1904;3:167.
774. Whitehead RH. Studies on the interstitial cells of Leydig. No. 2. Their post-embryonic development in the pig. *Am J Anat* 1905;4:193.
775. Roosen-Runge EC, Anderson D. The development of the interstitial cells in the testis of the albino rat. *Acta Anat* 1959;37:125–137.
776. Fouquet JP, Meusy-Dessolle N, Dang DC. Relationships between Leydig cell morphometry and plasma testosterone during postnatal development of the monkey, *Macaca fascicularis. Reprod Nutr Dev* 1984;24:281–286.
777. Winter JSD, Faiman C, Reyes FI. Sex steroid production by the human fetus: its role in morphogenesis and control by gonadotrophins. *Birth Defects* 1977;13:41–52.
778. Faiman C, Winter JSD, Reyes FI. Endocrinology of the fetal testis. In: Burger HG, de Kretser DM, eds. *The Testis,* 2nd ed. New York: Raven Press; 1989:119–142.
779. Niemi M, Ikonen M, Hervonen A. Histochemistry and fine structure of the interstitial tissue in the human foetal testis. In: Wolstenholme GEW, O'Connor M, eds. *Endocrinology of the Testis.* London: Churchill; 1967;31–55.
780. Gruenwald P. Structure of the testis in infancy and in childhood. *Arch Pathol* 1946;42:35–48.
781. Ottowicz J. The stadial development of Leydig cells. *Acta Med Pol* 1963;4:1–13.
782. Sharpe RM. The hormonal regulation of the Leydig cell. In: Finn CA, ed. *Oxford Reviews of Reproductive Biology.* Oxford: Oxford University Press; 1982:241–317.
783. Sharpe RM. Local control of testicular function. *Q J Exp Physiol* 1983;68:265–287.
784. Sharpe RM. Intratesticular factors controlling testicular function. *Biol Reprod* 1984;30:24–49.
785. Ichihara I. The fine structure of testicular interstitial cells in mice during postnatal development. *Z Zellforsch* 1970;108:475–486.
786. Zirkin BR, Ewing LL. Leydig cell differentiation during maturation of the rat testis: a stereological study of cell number and ultrastructure. *Anat Rec* 1987;219:157–163.
787. Hardy MP, Zirkin BR, Ewing LL. Kinetic studies on the development of the adult population of Leydig cells of the pubertal rat. *Endocrinology* 1989;124:762–770.
788. Vergouwen R, Jacobs S, Huiskamp R, Davids J, de Rooij D. Proliferative activity of gonocytes, Sertoli cells and interstitial cells during testicular development in mice. *J Reprod Fertil* 1991;93:233–243.
789. Shan LX, Hardy MP. Developmental changes in levels of luteinizing hormone receptor and androgen receptor in rat Leydig cells. *Endocrinology* 1992;131:1107–1114.
790. Faiman C, Winter JSD. Gonadotropins and sex hormone patterns in puberty: clinical data. In: Grumbach MM, Grave GD, Mayer FE, eds. *The Control of the Onset of Puberty.* New York: Wiley; 1974:32.
791. Swerdloff RS, Heber D. Endocrine control of testicular function from birth to puberty. In: Burger HG, de Kretser DM, eds. *The Testis.* New York: Raven Press; 1981:107–126.
792. Odell WD, Swerdloff RS. The role of the gonads in sexual maturation. In: Grumbach MM, Grave GD, Mayer FE, eds. *The Control of the Onset of Puberty.* New York: Wiley; 1974:313.
793. Odell WD, Swerdloff RS. Etiologies of sexual maturation: A model system based on the sexually maturing rat. *Recent Prog Horm Res* 1976;32:245.
794. Lee VWK, Burger HG. Pituitary testicular axis during pubertal development. In: de Kretser DM, Burger HG, Hudson B, eds. *The Pituitary and Testis. Clinical and Experimental Studies.* Berlin: Springer-Verlag; 1983:44–83.
795. Charny C, Conston A, Meranze D. Development of the testis. *Fertil Steril* 1952;3:461–479.
796. de la Balze F, Mancini R, Arrillaga F, Andrada J, Vilar O. Pubertal maturation of the human testis. A histologic study. *J Clin Endocrinol Metab* 1960;20:266–285.
797. Hayashi H, Harrison R. The development of the interstitial tissue of the human testis. *Fertil Steril* 1971;22:351–355.
798. Forti G, Santoro S, Grisolla GA, et al. Spermatic and peripheral plasma concentrations of testosterone and androstenedione in prepubertal boys. *J Clin Endocrinol Metab* 1981;53:883–886.
799. Rivarola MA, Bergada C, Cullen M. hCG stimulation test in prepubertal boys with cryptorchidism, in bilateral anorchia and in male pseudohermaphroditism. *J Clin Endocrinol Metab* 1970; 31:526–530.
800. Prince FP. Ultrastructural evidence of mature Leydig cells and Leydig cell regression in the neonatal human testis. *Anat Rec* 1990;228:405–417.
801. Chen YDI, Shaw MJ, Payne AP. Steroid and FSH action on LH receptors and LH-sensitive testicular responsiveness during sexual maturation of the rat. *Mol Cell Endocrinol* 1977;8:291–299.
802. Odell WD, Swerdloff RS, Jacobs HS, Hescox MA. FSH induction of sensitivity to LH: one cause of sexual maturation in the male rat. *Endocrinology* 1973;92:160–165.
803. van Beurden WMO, Roodnat B, de Jong FH, Mulder E, van der Molen HJ. Hormonal regulation of LH stimulation of testosterone production in isolated Leydig cells of immature rats: the effects of hypophysectomy, FSH and estradiol-17β. *Steroids* 1976;28:847–866.
804. Chen YDI, Payne AP, Kelch RP. FSH stimulation of Leydig cell function in the hypophysectomized immature rat. *Proc Soc Exp Biol Med* 1976;153:473–475.
805. Odell WD, Swerdloff RS. The role of testicular sensitivity to gonadotrophins in sexual maturation of the male rat. *J Steroid Biochem* 1975;6:853–857.
806. Selin LK, Moger WH. The effect of FSH on LH induced testosterone secretion in the immature hypophysectomized male rat. *Endocrinol Res Commun* 1977;4:171–182.
807. Kerr JB, Sharpe RM. Follicle-stimulating hormone induction of Leydig cell maturation. *Endocrinology* 1985;116:2592–2604.
808. Kerr JB, Sharpe RM. Stimulatory effect of follicle-stimulating hormone on rat Leydig cells. A morphometric and ultrastructural study. *Cell Tissue Res* 1985;239:405–415.
809. Teerds KJ, Closset J, Rommerts FFG, et al. Effects of pure FSH and LH preparations on the number and function of Leydig cells in immature hypophysectomized rats. *J Endocrinol* 1989; 120:97–106.
810. Kerr JB, Bartlett JMS, Donachie K, Sharpe RM. Origin of regenerating Leydig cells in the testis of the adult rat. An ultrastructural, morphometric and hormonal assay study. *Cell Tissue Res* 1987;249:367–377.
811. Neaves WB. Changes in testicular Leydig cells and in plasma testosterone levels among seasonally breeding rock hyrax. *Biol Reprod* 1973;8:451–466.

812. Neaves WB. The annual testicular cycle in an equatorial colony of lesser rock hyrax, *Heterohyrax brucei*. *Proc R Soc Lond [Biol]* 1979;206:183–189.
813. Neaves WB. Asynchronous testicular cycles among equatorial colonies of rock hyrax (*Procavia habessinica*). In: Steinberger E, Steinberger A, eds. *Testicular Development, Structure and Function,* New York: Raven Press; 1980:411–418.
814. Gustafson AW. Observations on the hydroxysteroid dehydrogenase and lipid histochemistry and ultrastructure of the Leydig cells in adult *Myotis lucifugus* during the annual reproductive cycle. *Anat Rec* 1975;181:366–367.
815. Wing TY, Lin HS. The fine structure of testicular interstitial cells in the adult golden hamster with special reference to seasonal changes. *Cell Tissue Res* 1977;183:385–393.
816. Suzuki F, Racey PA. The organization of testicular interstitial tissue and changes in the fine structure of the Leydig cells of European moles (*Tulpa europaea*) throughout the year. *J Reprod Fertil* 1978;52:189–194.
817. Hardy MP, Mendis-Handagama SMLC, Zirkin BR, Ewing LL. Photoperiodic variation of Leydig cell numbers in the testis of the golden hamster: A possible mechanism for their renewal during recrudescence. *J Exp Zool* 1987;244:269–276.
818. Sinha Hikim AP, Sinha Hikim I, Amador AG, Bartke A, Woolf A, Russell LD. Reinitiation of spermatogenesis by exogenous gonadotrophins in a seasonal breeder, the woodchuck (*Marmota monax*), during gonadal activity. *Am J Anat* 1991;192:194–213.
819. Hochereau-de Reviers MT, Perreau C, Lincoln GA. Photoperiodic variations of somatic and germ cell populations in the Soay ram testis. *J Reprod Fertil* 1985;74:329–334.
820. Wislocki GB. Seasonal changes in the testes, epididymides and seminal vesicles of deer investigated by histochemical methods. *Endocrinology* 1949;44:167–189.
821. Lofts B. Cyclical changes in the distribution of the testis lipids of a seasonal mammal (*Talpa europaea*). *J Microsc Sci* 1960; 101:199–205.
822. Johnson L, Thompson DL. Seasonal variation in the total volume of Leydig cells in stallions is explained by variation in cell number rather than cell size. *Biol Reprod* 1986;35:971–979.
823. Kothari LK, Gupta AS. Effect of ageing on the volume, structure and total Leydig cell content of the human testis. *Int J Fertil* 1974;19:140–146.
824. Honore LH. Ageing changes in the human testis: a light microscopic study. *Gerentology* 1978;24:58–65.
825. Teem MVB. The relation of the interstitial cells of the testis to prostatic hypertrophy. *J Urol* 1935;34:692–713.
826. Sargent JW, McDonald JR. A method for the quantitative estimate of Leydig cells in the human testis. *Proc Staff Meet Mayo Clin* 1948;23:249–254.
827. Sokal Z. Morphology of the human testis in various periods of life. *Folia Morphol* 1964;23:102–111.
828. Vermeulen A. Leydig cell function in old age. In: Burgess JA, ed. *Hypothalamus, Pituitary and Aging,* Springfield, IL: Charles C Thomas; 1976:458–463.
829. Kaler LW, Neaves WB. Attrition of the human Leydig cell population with advancing age. *Anat Rec* 1978;192:513–518.
830. Neaves WB, Johnson L, Porter JC, Parker CR, Petty CS. Leydig cell numbers, daily sperm production and serum gonadotrophin levels in ageing men. *J Clin Endocrinol Metab* 1984;59:756–763.
831. Neaves WB, Johnson L, Petty CS. Age-related change in numbers of other interstitial cells in testes of adult men: Evidence bearing on the fate of Leydig cells lost with increasing age. *Biol Reprod* 1985;33:259–269.
832. Kaler LW, Neaves WB. The androgen status of ageing male rats. *Endocrinology* 1981;108:712–719.
833. Kerr JB, de Kretser DM. Techniques for detecting and evaluating abnormalities in testicular function. In: Vouk VB, Sheehan PJ, Scientific Committee on Problems of the Environment, eds. *Methods for Assessing the Effects of Chemicals on Reproductive Functions.* New York: Wiley; 1983:247–262.
834. Russell LD. Normal testicular structure and methods of evaluation under experimental and disruptive conditions. In: Clarkson TW, Nordberg GF, Sager PR, eds. *Reproductive and Developmental Toxicity of Metals.* New York: Plenum Press; 1983:227–252.
835. Mann T, Lutwak-Mann C. *Male Reproductive Function and Semen. Themes and Trends in Physiology, Biochemistry and Investigative Andrology,* Suppl 5. Berlin: Springer-Verlag; 1981.
836. Vermeulen A. Effects of drugs on Leydig cell function. *Int J Androl* 1982;Suppl 5:163–182.
837. de Kretser DM. Sertoli cell–Leydig cell interaction in the regulation of testicular function. *Int J Androl* 1982;Suppl 5:11–17.
838. Wilton LJ, de Kretser DM. The influence of luteinizing hormone on the Leydig cells of cryptorchid rat testes. *Acta Endocrinol (Kbh)* 1984;107:110–116.
839. Risbridger GP, Kerr JB, de Kretser DM. Evaluation of Leydig cell function and gonadotrophin binding in unilateral and bilateral cryptorchidism: evidence for local control of Leydig cell function by the seminiferous tubule. *Biol Reprod* 1981;24:534–540.
840. Risbridger GP, Kerr JB, Peake RA, de Kretser DM. An assessment of Leydig cell function after bilateral or unilateral efferent duct ligation: further evidence for local control of Leydig cell function. *Endocrinology* 1981;109:1234–1241.
841. Aoki A, Fawcett DW. Is there a local feedback from the seminiferous tubules affecting activity of the Leydig cell? *Biol Reprod* 1978;19:144–158.
842. Sharpe RM. Intragonadal hormones. *Bibl Reprod* 1985; 133:C1–C5.
843. Sharpe RM. Paracrine control of the testis. *Clin Endocrinol Metab* 1986;15:185–207.
844. van Vlliet J, Rommerts FFG, de Rooij DG, Buwalda G, Wensing CJG. Reduction of testicular blood flow and focal degeneration of tissue in the rat following administration of human chorionic gonadotrophin. *J Endocrinol* 1988;117:51–57.
845. Chemes HE, Rivarola MA, Bergada C. Effect of gonadotrophins and testosterone on the seminiferous tubules of the immature rat. *J Reprod Fertil* 1976;46:283–288.
846. Rivier C, Rivier J, Vale W. Chronic effects of [D-Trp^6, Pro^9-NET]-luteinizing hormone-releasing factor on reproductive processes in the male rat. *Endocrinology* 1979;105:1191–1201.
847. Johnson AD. The influence of cadmium on the testis. In: Johnson AD, Gomes WR, eds. *The Testis,* Vol IV. New York: Academic Press; 1977:1191–1201.
848. Patanelli DJ. Suppression of fertility in the male. In: Hamilton DW, Greep RO, eds. *Handbook of Physiology,* Sect 7. Washington: American Physiological Society; 1975:245–258.
849. Jackson H, Ericsson RJ. Effect of chemical agents and hormones on spermatogenesis and the epididymis. *Bibl Reprod* 1970; 14:453–600.
850. Gunn SA, Gould TC, Anderson WAD. Loss of selective injurious vascular response to cadmium in regenerated blood vessels of testis. *Am J Pathol* 1966;48:959–969.
851. Gunn SA, Gould TC. Specificity of the vascular system of the male reproductive tract. *J Reprod Fertil Suppl* 1970;10:75–95.
852. Gunn SA, Gould TC. Cadmium and other mineral elements. In: Johnson AD, Gomes WR, van Demark NL, eds. *The Testis,* Vol III. New York: Academic Press; 1970:377–481.
853. Rommerts FFG, Grootenhuis AJ, Hoogerbrugge JW, van der Molen HJ. Ethane dimethane sulphonate specifically inhibits LH stimulated steroidogenesis in Leydig cells isolated from mature rats but not in cells from immature rats. *Mol Cell Endocrinol* 1985;42:105–111.
854. Molenaar R, de Rooji DG, Rommerts FFG, Reuvers PJ, van der Molen HJ. Specific destruction of Leydig cells in mature rats after *in vivo* administration of ethane dimethane sulphonate. *Biol Reprod* 1985;33:1213–1222.
855. Bartlett JMS, Kerr JB, Sharpe RM. The effect of selective destruction and regeneration of rat Leydig cells on seminiferous tubule morphology and the intratesticular distribution of testosterone. *J Androl* 1986;7:240–253.
856. Morris ID. Leydig cell resistance to the cytotoxic effect of ethylene dimethanesulphonate in the adult rat testis. *J Endocrinol* 1985;105:311–316.
857. Teerds KJ, de Rooij DG, Rommerts FFG, Wensing CJG. The regulation of the proliferation and differentiation of rat Leydig cell precursor cells after EDS administration or daily hCG treatment. *J Androl* 1988;9:343–351.
858. Teerds KJ, de Rooij DG, Rommerts FFG, van den Hurk R, Wensing CJG. Proliferation and differentiation of possible Leydig cell precursors after destruction of the existing Leydig cells

with ethane dimethylsulphonate: the role of LH/human chorionic gonadotrophin. *J Endocrinol* 1989;122:689–696.
859. Teerds KJ, de Rooij DG, Rommerts FFG, Wensing CJG. Development of a new Leydig cell population after the destruction of existing Leydig cells by ethane dimethane sulphonate in rats: an autoradiographic study. *J Endocrinol* 1990;126:229–236.
860. Abney TO, Myers RB. 17β-Estradiol inhibition of Leydig cell regeneration in the ethane dimethylsulphonate-treated mature rat. *J Androl* 1991;12:295–304.
861. O'Leary PO, Jackson AE, Averill S, de Kretser DM. The effects of ethane dimethanesulphonate (EDS) on bilaterally cryptorchid rat testes. *Mol Cell Endocrinol* 1986;45:183–190.
862. Kerr JB, Donachie K. Regeneration of Leydig cells in unilaterally cryptorchid rats: evidence for stimulation by local testicular factors. *Cell Tissue Res* 1986;243:405–414.
863. Sharpe RM, Maddocks S, Kerr JB. Cell–cell interactions in the control of spermatogenesis as studied using Leydig cell destruction and testosterone replacement. *Am J Anat* 1990;188:3–20.
864. Russell LD, Ren HP, Sinha Hikim I, Schulze W, Sinha Hikim AP. A comparative study in twelve mammalian species of volume densities, volumes, and numerical densities of selected testis components, emphasizing those related to the Sertoli cell. *Am J Anat* 1990;188:21–30.
865. Johnson L, Nguyen HB. Annual cycle of the Sertoli cell population in adult stallions. *J Reprod Fertil* 1986;76:311–316.
866. Mori H. Ultrastructure and stereological analysis of Leydig cells. In: Motta P, ed. *Ultrastructure of Endocrine Cells and Tissues,* The Hague: Martinus Nijhoff; 1984:225–237.
867. Mendis-Handagama SMLC, Kerr JB, de Kretser DM. Experimental cryptorchidism in the adult mouse. I. Quantitative and qualitative light microscopic morphology. *J Androl* 1990;11: 539–547.
868. Mendis-Handagama SMLC, Kerr JB, de Kretser DM. Experimental cryptorchidism in the adult mouse. II. A hormonal study. *J Androl* 1990;11:548–554.
869. Mendis-Handagama SMLC, Kerr JB, de Kretser DM. Experimental cryptorchidism in the adult mouse. III. Quantitative and qualitative electron microscopic morphology of Leydig cells. *J Androl* 1991;12:335–343.
870. Sinha Hikim AP, Chakraborty J, Jhunjhunwala JS. Unilateral torsion of spermatic cord in men: effect on Leydig cell. *Urology* 1987;29:40–44.
871. Mori H, Shimizu D, Takeda A, Takioka Y, Fukuhishi R. Stereological analysis of Leydig cells in normal guinea pig testes. *J Electron Microsc* 1980;29:8–21.
872. Ewing LL, Zirkin BR. Leydig cell structure and steroidogenic function. *Recent Prog Horm Res* 1983;39:599.
873. Lin HS, Wing TY. A dense-cored filamentous body in Leydig cells of the golden hamster. *Cell Tissue Res* 1979;201:369–376.
874. Payer AF, Parkening TA. Membrane-bound intranuclear inclusions in the Leydig cell of the Chinese hamster (*Cricetulus griseus*). *J Ultrastruct Res* 1983;84:317–325.
875. Mugisha-Girasi H, Radke B, Schwarz R. Observations on the Leydig cells in the male East African spring hare (*Pedetes surdaster larvalis*). *Z Mirkrosk Anat Forsch* 1979;93:65–73.
876. Stefan Y, Steimer T. The Leydig cell of a hypogonadic rodent (*Ellobius lutescens Th*): correlation between ultrastructure and biosynthetic activity. *Biol Reprod* 1978;19:913–921.
877. Sinha AA, Erickson AW, Seal US. Fine structure of Leydig cells in crabeater, leopard and Ross seals. *J Reprod Fertil* 1977; 49:51–54.
878. Osman DJ, Ploen L. The ultrastructure of Sertoli cells in the boar. *Int J Androl* 1978;1:162–179.
879. Gotoh M, Miyake K, Mitsuya H, Hoshino T, Yamada K. Cytoplasmic inclusion bodies in Leydig cells from the testes of postpubertal cryptorchid patients. *Int J Androl* 1983;6:221–228.
880. Clermont Y, Troh M. Duration of the cycle of the seminiferous epithelium in the mouse and hamster determined by means of ^{3}H-thymidine and radioautography. *Fertil Steril* 1969;20: 805–817.
881. de Rooij DG. Stem cell renewal and duration of spermatogonial cycle in the golden hamster. *Z Zellforsch* 1968;89:133–136.
882. Swierstra EE. Cytology and duration of the seminiferous epithelium of the boar. Duration of spermatozoon transit through the epididymis. *Anat Rec* 1968;161:171–186.
883. Clermont Y, Le Blond CP, Messier B. Durée du cycle de l'epithelium seminal du rat. *Arch Anat Microsc Morphol Exp* 1959; 48:37–56.
884. Hilscher W. Beitrage zur Orthologie und Pathologie des "Spermatogoniogenese" der Ratte. *Beitr Pathol Anat* 1964;130: 69–132.
885. Hochereau MT, Courot M, Ortavant R. Marquage des cellules germinales du belier et du taureau par injection de thymidine tritee dans l'artere spermatique. *Am Biol Anim Biochem Biophys* 1964;2:157–161.
886. Orgebin-Crist MC. Passage of spermatozoa labelled with ^{3}H-thymidine through the ductus epididymis of the rabbit. *J Reprod Fertil* 1965;10:241–251.
887. Swierstra EE, Foote RH. Cytology and kinetics of spermatogenesis in the rabbit. *J Reprod Fertil* 1963;5:309–322.
888. Antar M. Duration of the cycle of the seminiferous epithelium and of spermatogenesis in the monkey (*Macaca speciosa*). *Anat Rec* 1971;169:268–269.
889. Arsenieva NA, Dubinin NP, Orlova NN, Bakulina ED. A radiation analysis of the duration of meiotic phases in the monkey (*Macaca mulatta*). *Dokl Akad Nauk SSSR* 1961;141:1486–1489.
890. de Kretser DM, Temple-Smith PD, Kerr JB. Anatomical and functional aspects of the male reproductive organs. In: Bandhauer K, Frick J, eds. *Disturbances in Male Fertility.* Berlin: Springer Verlag; 1982:1–131.
891. de Kretser DM. The light and electron microscope anatomy of the normal human testis. In: Santen RJ, Swerdloff R, eds. *Male Sexual Dysfunction: Diagnosis and Management of Hypogonadism, Infertility and Impotence.* New York: Marcel Dekker; 1986:3–28.
892. Kerr JB, Knell CM, Irby DC. Ultrastructure and possible function of giant crystalloids in the Sertoli cell of the juvenile and adult koala (*Phascolarctos cinereus*). *Anat Embryol* 1987;176: 213–244.

The Physiology of Reproduction, Second Edition,
edited by E. Knobil and J.D. Neill,
Raven Press, Ltd., New York © 1994.

CHAPTER 20

The Sertoli Cell[1]

C. Wayne Bardin, C. Yan Cheng, Neal A. Mustow, and Glen L. Gunsalus

THE SERTOLI CELL

The testis can be divided functionally into interstitium and seminiferous tubules, which are responsible for the production of testosterone and spermatozoa, respectively. In the 1960s, assays for luteinizing hormone (LH) and testosterone as well as for other androgens were developed which permitted investigators to define the physiology and pathophysiology of Leydig cells, a major component of the interstitium. By contrast, an understanding of the function of cells in the seminiferous tubules did not advance as rapidly. This was due primarily to the complexity of spermatogenesis, a process involving interactions of multiple cells with several hormones over a relatively long period of time, which could be studied only *in vivo*. In addition, spermatozoa, the major product of the germinal epithelium, could be quantified only in testicular biopsies of the seminiferous tubular epithelium or after their appearance in the ejaculate following passage through the epididymis. In view of the difficulties in studying the seminiferous tubules, many investigators sought other products that could be measured more easily than spermatozoa. It was appreciated that Sertoli cells were the major secretory element of the germinal epithelium and that their proteins might be useful for studying this portion of the testis. Accordingly, a large number of Sertoli cell products were identified and used to monitor the function of Sertoli cells and intact seminiferous tubules, both *in vivo* and *in vitro* (Table 1). Identification of new Sertoli cell products also led to a better understanding of how testicular cells interact with each other.

A second major advance in the study of Sertoli cells was the development of procedures for *in vitro* studies, which involved the identification of factors required for their growth and differentiation (28–31). Although cells grown in this way do not mimic the morphological features of Sertoli cells *in vivo,* defined culture techniques provide a method for examining many aspects of Sertoli cell function not previously amenable to study. Techniques were also developed for culturing small segments of seminiferous tubules that corresponded to defined stages of the seminiferous tubular cycle (32). This per-

Center for Biomedical Research, The Population Council, New York, New York 10021

[1] Reprinted from *The Physiology of Reproduction,* edited by Ernst Knobil and Jimmy D. Neill, et al. Raven Press, Ltd., New York © 1988, pp. 933–974.

TABLE 1. *Sertoli cell proteins*

Protein	Investigators (reference)
ABP	Hansson et al., 1975 (1)
	Bardin et al., 1981 (2)
	Ritzén et al., 1981 (3)
Inhibin	de Jong and Robertson, 1985 (4)
Growth factors	Feig et al., 1980 (5)
	Feig et al., 1983 (6)
	Brown et al., 1982 (7);
	Holmes et al., 1986 (8)
Somatomedin	Hall et al., 1983 (9)
Transferrin	Skinner and Griswold, 1980 (10)
	Skinner et al., 1984 (11)
Ceruloplasmin	Skinner and Griswold, 1983 (12)
Retinol-binding protein	Huggenvik and Griswold, 1981 (13)
	Carson et al., 1984 (14)
H-Y antigen	Brunner et al., 1984 (15)
Plasminogen activator	Lacroix et al., 1977 (16)
	Vihko et al., 1984 (17)
Clusterin	Fritz et al., 1983 (18)
	Blaschuk et al., 1984 (19)
	Tung and Fritz, 1985 (20)
Cyclic proteins	Wright et al., 1983 (21)
Dimeric acid glycoprotein	Sylvester et al., 1984 (22)
Scm proteins	DePhilip and Kierszenbaum, 1982 (23)
CMB proteins	Cheng et al., 1986 (24)
Testibumin	Cheng and Bardin, 1986 (25)
FSH- and testosterone-responsive protein (CMB-21)	Cheng, 1986 (26)
Testosterone-responsive proteins	Cheng et al., 1985 (27)

mitted experiments on Sertoli cells with germ cells still attached. More recently, the growth of Sertoli cells on filters and matrices allowed media to be presented from the top and bottom (33,34). Cells grown in this way become confluent, establish junctional complexes, and assume an epitheliallike appearance reminiscent of Sertoli cells *in vivo.* These coupled cells appear to function as a polarized epithelium, which permits more complex studies of Sertoli cell biology.

Recent studies of the Sertoli cell focused on: (a) identification of Sertoli cell secretory products and investigation of their possible functions, both in the seminiferous tubule and in other parts of the testis; (b) definition of the humoral factors regulating Sertoli cell function *in vitro* and examination of their mechanisms of action; (c) determination of how other cells in the testis interact with and regulate Sertoli cells; and (d) definition of Sertoli cells as functional components of the seminiferous tubular epithelium *in vivo.* Although this review will focus on these recent studies, we will attempt to refer to earlier experiments covered in other reviews.

THE STRUCTURAL FEATURES OF SERTOLI CELLS

In his now classic review of Sertoli cell ultrastructure, Fawcett (35) point out that nuclei of these cells contain very little heterochromatin in comparison to other somatic cells. The nucleoplasm contains primarily euchromatin, consistent with the postulate that Sertoli cells express a large portion of their genome in accordance with their highly versatile functions. The structure of the multiple Golgi elements in this cell type is also consistent with a highly active mechanism for processing newly synthesized proteins; however, there appeared to be insufficient rough endoplasmic reticulum to account for appreciable protein synthesis. These observations, coupled with (a) the lack of large vacuoles or membrane-bound secretory granules in association with Golgi, (b) the paucity of morphologic evidence for exocytosis, and (c) the small number of vesicles opening into the lateral surfaces of Sertoli cells, suggested that this cell type did not release a significant amount of protein into the seminiferous tubular lumen. Although these morphological observations at first seemed contradictory to many investigators, they now appear to be consistent with the growing body of knowledge regarding Sertoli cell secretory products. That is, Sertoli cells may secrete up to 100 proteins, a finding consistent with the structures of nuclear chromatin and Golgi complex. It now appears that these proteins are not stored, but rather are secreted immediately after synthesis. This would account for the lack of obvious secretory granules. Even though Sertoli cells, like hepatocytes, synthesize multiple proteins, the total production per Sertoli cell per day may be much less than that produced by liver cells, especially when one considers the relative protein concentrations in seminiferous tubular fluid as compared to plasma (36).

In addition to the morphologic evidence for protein secretion, there are other structural features of Sertoli cells which relate to their function in the seminiferous tubular epithelium. These include: (a) numerous primary lysosomes, autophagic vacuoles, and heterophagic vacuoles, which are believed to participate in the phagocytosis and digestion of germ cells that degenerate during development; (b) large amounts of smooth endoplasmic reticulum in some species, suggestive of steroid synthesis; (c) specific alterations in Sertoli cell morphology along the length of the seminiferous tubule, suggesting that these cells participate, along with germinal elements, in forming the spermatogenic cycle; (d) unique junctional specializations between Sertoli cells which maintain the structural integrity of the tubular epithelium, provide low-resistance pathways for electrical coupling of adjacent cells, and constitute the epithelial component of the blood-testis barrier. These junctional complexes divide the epithelium of the seminiferous tubule into two separate physical compartments: (i) an exterior or basal compartment containing spermatogonia and preleptotene spermatocytes and (ii) an interior compartment containing the remaining spermatocytes and spermatids. The basal compartment is contiguous with the basal lamina, myoid cells, and the blood as well as with lymphatic vessels in the interstitial space. For the purposes of anatomical description, the interior compartment is further subdivided into two contiguous compartments: the adluminal and luminal compartments (see, e.g., ref. 35). The luminal space is continuous with the rete testis, efferent ducts, and epididymis. In general, substances present in the basal compartment can only enter the adluminal and luminal compartments by traversing Sertoli cell cytoplasm and vice versa. In the following discussion, we will emphasize the physical separation between the exterior and interior compartments of the seminiferous epithelium, which is provided by the Sertoli-Sertoli tight junctional complexes. These unique morphological features provide the background for present and future studies of Sertoli cell biology.

THE FUNCTIONS OF SERTOLI CELLS

Maintenance of the Blood-Testis Barrier and Secretion of Tubular Fluid

The seminiferous tubules compose the proximal portion of a continuous ductal system that comprises the male reproductive tract. Although there is considerable variation among different mammalian species, the general plan is similar for all. The seminiferous tubules of each testis empty by way of tubuli recti into the rete testis, which, in turn, empties by several efferent ducts into the proximal portion of the epididymis. The seminiferous tubule is a complex epithelium composed of Sertoli and germ cells which rests on the basal lamina. The junctional contacts between adjacent Sertoli cells form the structural basis of the most important portion of the blood-testis barrier (for a review see ref. 36) (37–40).

Part of the evidence indicating the existence of a blood-testis barrier is that the fluid composition inside the seminiferous tubule and rete testis is dramatically different from that found in testicular lymph and blood. The fluid secreted into the tubular epithelium by Sertoli cells contains five to seven times more potassium than does the fluid in the rete testis, which, in turn, contains two to three times more potassium than does the serum (41). Both testicular fluids contain proportionally less sodium and chloride (36). Seminiferous tubular fluid contains more protein than that of rete testis, but both have much less than serum (36,42,43). Fluid is produced in the testis of most species at a rate of 10 to 20 μl per gram of testis per hour (44–48) and is continuous without diurnal variation. This fluid drive provides a mechanism by which sperm are moved from the testis to the epididymis, where they become fully mature.

Fluid production begins when the first spermatozoa are released from the Sertoli cells (49). In immature animals, it is increased by follicle-stimulating hormone (FSH) but not by other pituitary hormones (50). Following hypophysectomy of adult animals, fluid secretion does not decrease until regression of the seminiferous tubule begins. Fluid secretion continues after the loss of germ cells, but at a reduced rate; the potassium concentration of such fluid is similar to that of plasma (51–53). Normal fluid production is dependent on the lower temperature found in the scrotum and a continuous supply of glucose (54,55). In his review on testicular fluid secretion, Setchell concluded that fluid production is dependent on hormones because of their ability to maintain the structural integrity of the seminiferous tubular epithelium (36).

In view of the unusual ion composition of tubular fluid, it is easy to understand that small molecules in lymph and serum do not readily enter into the seminiferous tubules and vice versa. This was first realized when it was noted that dyes injected into the blood did not enter into the lumen of the seminiferous tubules (56,57). The differential transport of various factors from the serum into tubular and rete testis fluids has been extensively reviewed (36). It would appear from a variety of studies that the rete testis is slightly more permeable to a variety of small molecules than are the seminiferous tubules. Furthermore, since protein concentrations in tubular and rete testis fluids are much lower than in blood, free movement of proteins into the testis does not occur. Thus, one functional consequence of the blood-testis barrier is to maintain a gradient of ions, small molecules, and proteins between blood and tubular fluid.

Although many studies suggest the potassium gradient is maintained by ion pumps, it is not clear how the complex protein composition of tubular fluid is maintained. It is possible that some proteins are moved into tubular fluid by selective transport mechanisms, analogous to those used to transport γ-globulins across epithelia in the gut (58). However, such transport mechanisms have not been demonstrated in Sertoli cells. As shall be discussed in the next section, it appears more likely that most of the proteins in tubular fluid are secreted by Sertoli cells (59). Thus, Sertoli cells secrete products that provide developing germ cells with a unique environment which is maintained by the blood-testis barrier (59). The ability to exclude small molecules allows the blood-testis barrier to protect developing germ cells from mutagenic agents. Since sperm are immunogenic, the blood-testis barrier also serves to sequester this population of cells from the immune system.

Secretion of Proteins, Peptides, and Other Products

Androgen-binding protein (ABP) was one of the first Sertoli cell-specific proteins to be identified and extensively studied (60–62). This product is important since it provides a prototype for other Sertoli cell secretory proteins. Studies in the rat indicate that approximately 80%

of rABP is secreted into the lumen of the seminiferous tubule and then is transported to the epididymis, where it is taken into cells and degraded (1,63–65). The remaining 20% is released into the blood, probably from the base of Sertoli cells (66). These early observations gave rise to the concept that seminiferous tubular physiology can be monitored by measuring Sertoli cell secretory products in the peripheral blood and reproductive tract (66).

Another important concept regarding Sertoli cell secretory products derives from a series of observations in rats demonstrating that these cells secrete not only testis-specific proteins such as rABP, but also proteins that are normally found in the serum. Skinner and Griswold (10) first demonstrated that Sertoli cells secrete transferrin. Subsequently Wright et al. (67) showed that in addition to secreting transferrin, cultured Sertoli cells synthesize and secrete multiple serum proteins, including ceruloplasmin and acidic glycoprotein (Table 1).

It had long been known that serumlike proteins are present in tubular and rete testis fluids, and it had been proposed that these proteins are transported by some unknown mechanism across the seminiferous tubular epithelium. The demonstration that Sertoli cells can synthesize serum proteins provides an alternative explanation for the presence of such products in the adluminal compartment. These observations also set forth the concept that Sertoli cells can secrete the essential proteins necessary for maintenance and maturation of germ cells in the adluminal compartment. Thus, many proteins that are delivered to somatic cells by serum are provided to late spermatocytes and spermatids by tubular fluid.

Androgen-Binding Protein

This protein was first identified in the epididymis (60,61) and was later shown to be of testicular origin (68). The speculation that rABP is of Sertoli cell origin derives from observations that: (a) tubules depleted of germ cells by prenatal x-ray treatment secrete rABP; and (b) peritubular interstitial fluid contains little rABP compared to rete testis fluid, where the concentration is high (69). In addition, Sertoli cell-enriched cultures secrete large quantities of this binding protein into the media (70,71), confirming that rABP is derived from Sertoli cells. The development of methods for quantifying rABP by steady state polyacrylamide gel electrophoresis (SS-PAGE) (72), dextran-coated charcoal (73), and radioimmunoassay (74) allowed many investigators to study its hormonal regulation, tissue distribution, and physiologic function. The development of a photoaffinity ligand, [^{3}H]-Δ^6-testosterone, also facilitated studies of the physical properties of this protein in biological fluids without extensive purification (75–77). Studies with antibodies to ABP show that this protein is immunologically related to the testosterone-estradiol-binding globulin (TeBG) from the same species (78–81).

Rat ABP (rABP). The ability to obtain highly purified rABP in good yield depends on the development of a stable androgen-affinity chromatographic matrix, as well as a procedure for eluting the protein in high yield (82). The rat is an ideal species in which ABP can be identified unambiguously since there is no possibility of contaminating the purified protein with the serum protein, TeBG, because the latter protein is not present in serum of adult rats (83). Native rABP is a heterogeneous dimeric glycoprotein with a native molecular weight of 85,000. It is composed of two kinds of monomers with apparent molecular weights of 45,000 and 41,000. These monomers are designated heavy (H) and light (L), respectively ($rABP_H$; $rABP_L$), according to their electrophoretic mobilities in SDS-polyacrylamide gels. Since $rABP_H$ and $rABP_L$ are present in the native molecule in a ratio of 3:1, the dimer could not be composed of stoichiometric amounts of H and L. It was, therefore, concluded that H and L might be different forms, or protomers, of the same molecule. This conclusion is supported by observations that the H and L monomers have similar amino acid compositions, peptide maps, immunodeterminants, and binding sites (84–86). The structural basis for this size heterogeneity of promoters and how they are assembled to form the native molecule is not clearly understood, but there are several possibilities (59). Either variations in the lengths of the polypeptide chains or differences in glycosylation, or both, could be responsible for the size differences in $rABP_H$ and $rABP_L$. It is reasonable to suggest that $rABP_L$ is a proteolytic product of $rABP_H$, since this protein is usually isolated from the epididymis, a site of rABP degradation. If this were the case, then one would expect a preponderance of $rABP_H$ in rABP isolated from testes. This is not the case, however, since rABP purified from testes and rABP newly synthesized *in vitro* have H:L ratios of 3:1. These observations suggest that $rABP_L$ is not likely to be a degradation product of the H protomer (85). Thus, if one protomer is derived from the other, it is probably formed in Sertoli cells prior to secretion. This hypothesis is supported by recent studies showing that cDNA encoding for rABP hybridizes to a single-size mRNA species in testis and Sertoli cell poly(A) RNA (Fig. 1) (87). In addition to heterogeneity based on protomer size, the ABPs of rat and other species exhibit heterogeneity secondary to carbohydrate structure based on differential binding to Con A (88,89).

Further understanding of rABP structure will provide insight not only into this unique secretory product from rat testis, but also into ABP and TeBG of other species. The physical properties of all the androgen-binding proteins isolated to date are similar to rABP in that they all are dimeric glycoproteins which exhibit protomeric heterogeneity. In addition, within a given species, ABP and

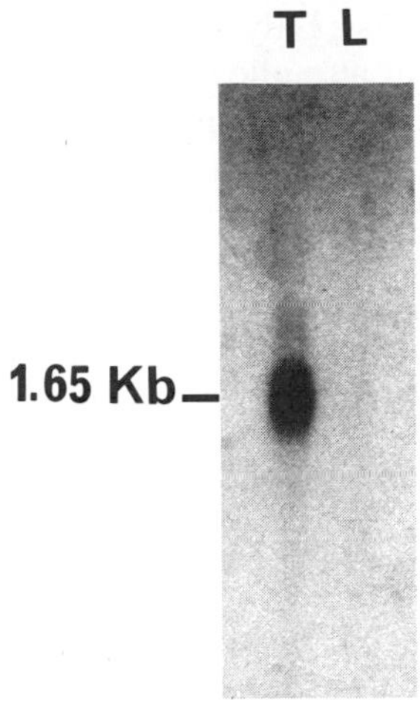

FIG. 1. Northern blot analysis of mRNA, isolated from testis and liver of a 20-day-old rat, probed with rABP cDNA. A single 1.65-kilodalton rABP mRNA is present in testis, but not in liver.

TeBG proteins bear strong resemblance to each other with regard to physicochemical and immunological properties. Furthermore, the amino acid sequence of rABP, recently predicted from a cDNA sequence, is greater than 65% homologous with the protein sequence of human TeBG (hTeBG) (P. H. Petra, *personal communication*). Because of the striking resemblance of ABPs to TeBGs, it is relevant to review the current knowledge of these latter proteins.

Rat TeBG (rTeBG). As noted previously, this protein is not detected in the serum of adult rats (83). However, a relatively large amount of rABP is secreted by Sertoli cells into the blood of male rats at the time of puberty, and this protein has been confused with TeBG (90). The basis for the distinction between these proteins rests upon the observation that rABP is present only in males and is clearly of testicular origin (74). By contrast, in those species that make TeBG, this protein is present in the serum of both males and females. Unexpectedly, an immunoreactive rABP-like material was detected in the serum and amniotic fluid of male and female fetuses (91–93). The concentrations of this material in these fluids decline during the last few days of fetal life and disappear from the blood of female rats by the fifth postnatal day. The fetal ABP-like material is in highest concentration in brain and liver. Studies using immunoprecipitation of radiolabeled proteins suggest that this material is synthesized in the liver but not the brain. Furthermore, the immunoprecipitated product produced by fetal hepatocytes contains two immunoreactive proteins in the ratio of 3:1; these proteins are slightly larger than the H and L protomers of rABP of testicular origin. When these observations are interpreted in light of extensive comparative studies performed on rabbit and human ABPs and TeBGs, they suggest that the protein of hepatic origin in fetal rats should be designated rTeBG. We conclude, therefore, that the rat does produce rTeBG and that this molecule, like rat alphafetoprotein, is synthesized during fetal life. Studies to date cannot distinguish whether rABP and rTeBG are the same or similar proteins.

Rabbit ABP and TeBG. In the rabbit, ABP (rbABP) is in the lumen of the male reproductive tract. In this species, studies of rbABP are complicated by the presence of another extracellular binding protein, rbTeBG, which is presumably of hepatic origin. Early studies using partially purified rbABP suggested that it shared immunodeterminants with rbTeBG (78). This observation, coupled with the desire to measure rbABP in the presence of rbTeBG, led to an extensive characterization of these proteins (79,94,95). Even though these two purified proteins have many similar physicochemical properties, including native molecular weights, isoelectric points, and binding constants, rbABP differs from rbTeBG with regard to the molecular weight and distribution of the two protomers, carbohydrate composition, and peptide composition. Similar results on the composition of these two proteins were obtained using unfractionated samples studied by photoaffinity labeling techniques (76,96). In addition, comparison of displacement curves using multiple dilutions of each protein in homologous and heterologous radioimmunoassays demonstrated that rbABP and rbTeBG have both common and unique immunodeterminants (81,97).

The above observations indicate that monospecific polyclonal antisera against rbABP and rbTeBG will recognize, but not distinguish between, the reciprocal protein. Monoclonal antibodies against highly purified rbABP do not interact with highly purified rbTeBG. It is of note, however, that this antibody does not distinguish between these proteins in freshly prepared tissue extracts. This suggests that highly purified rbABP has antigenic sites that are not exposed in biological fluids (N. A. Musto, *unpublished observations*). These latter observations suggest it may not be possible to produce antibodies that measure ABP in the presence of TeBG using highly purified proteins as antigens.

Studies using monospecific antiserum against rbTeBG localize the antigenic sites of this protein at the junction of the head and midpiece of ejaculated rabbit spermatozoa. By contrast, epididymal spermatozoa do not stain (98). The intracellular location of this protein is suggested, since the intensity of the staining is maximal following permeabilization of the plasma membrane with cold acetone. Such findings are used to support the postulate that rbABP and rbTeBG function as steroid carriers across the plasma membrane of the ejaculated spermatozoa (98).

Human ABP and TeBG. The presence of proteins in human serum that bind testosterone and estradiol was identified by Mercier et al. (99) and Rosenbaum et al. (100), respectively. Subsequent studies indicated that the same protein binds androgens as well as estrogens, and thus was designated testosterone-estradiol-binding globulin (hTeBG), sex steroid-binding globulin (SBG), or sex hormone-binding globulin (SHBG) by different groups of investigators (2,101). The highly purified protein is a dimer (102–106). Studies on purified photolabeled hTeBG indicate that it is composed of two types of monomers (Fig. 2), as is the case with the ABPs and TeBGs of other species (107). These monomers, designated $hTeBG_H$ and $hTeBG_L$ after the nomenclature established for rABP and rbABP, occur at a ratio of 10:1 (H:L) in multiple preparations using two different purification schemes (107–109). By contrast, protomers have many of the same epitopes because both polyclonal and monoclonal antibodies developed against hTeBG reacted with both protomers on immunoblots (110). Moreover, the size differences of the hTeBG protomers may not be entirely due to differential carbohydrate content, since removal of this moiety from the molecule, both by enzymatic and chemical treatment, did not abolish or alter the distribution of the protomeric forms of hTeBG (108).

The development of sensitive radioimmunoassays for hTeBG (111,112) not only enhanced the ability to study its physiology, but also allowed investigation of its relationship to similar proteins present in human testicular extracts. Soon after the identification of rABP, many investigators attempted to demonstrate the presence of a similar protein in primate testes. Studies using conventional fractionation procedures and binding assays were unable to conclusively distinguish the androgen-binding protein in human and monkey testes from primate TeBGs (113–115). However, these studies suggested that the androgen-binding activity in testicular cytosol was greater than might be expected from serum contamination (116). Subsequently, it was shown that hABP in testicular extracts could be distinguished from hTeBG in serum using Con A chromatography (117). The binding activity in testicular extracts resolves into two fractions: Form 1 hABP, which does not bind to Con A, and Form II hABP, which does (117,118). By contrast, hTeBG is bound quantitatively by this lectin (Fig. 3). In addition, both forms of hABP cross-react in a hTeBG radioimmunoassay (Fig. 4) using antiserum raised against hTeBG (80). Based on these studies, it was not possible to distinguish Form II hABP from hTeBG.

To further study the subtle differences between hABP

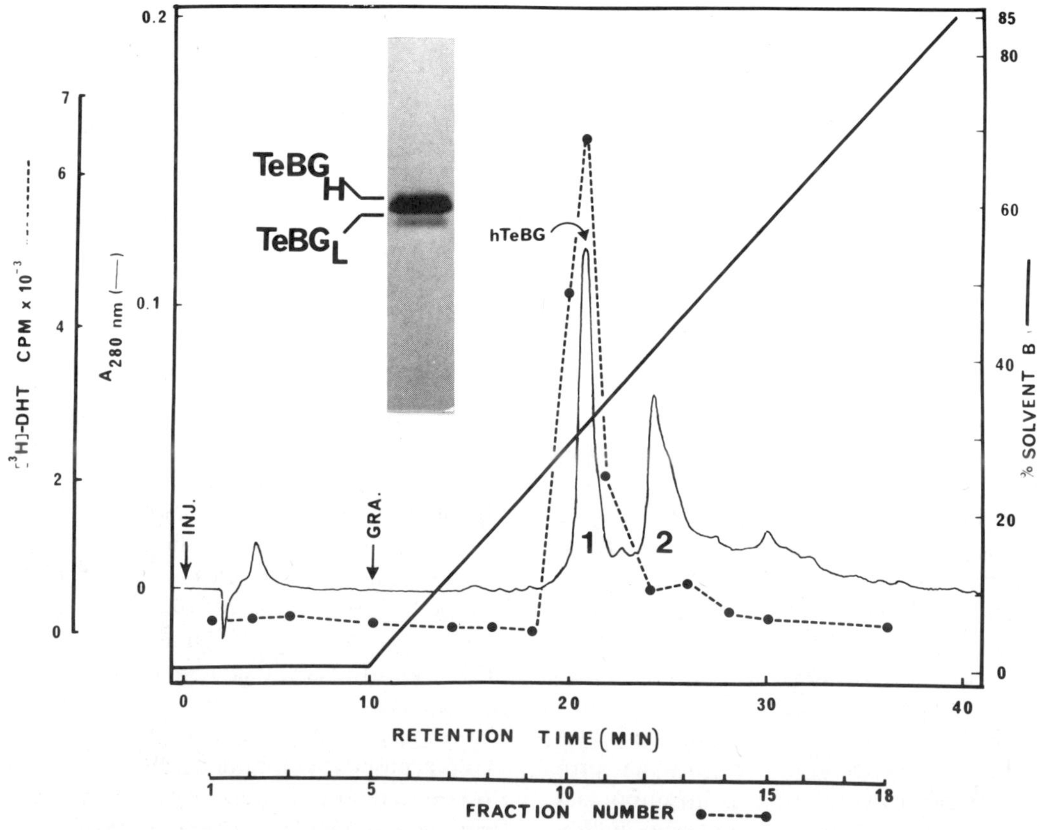

FIG. 2. Anion-exchange HPLC of partially purified hTeBG after affinity chromatography. INJ indicates where sample was loaded, GRA indicates beginning of gradient. The insert is a silver-stained SDS-polyacrylamide gel of the hTeBG purified by HPLC. The H and L indicate the relative mobility of $hTeBG_H$ and $hTeBG_L$. (Adapted from ref. 108).

and hTeBG, both proteins were purified, from testicular extracts and serum, respectively, by sequential androgen affinity and high-performance liquid chromatography. The two forms of hABP were resolved on Con A-Sepharose. Form I hABP, like hTeBG, possesses heavy (H) and light (L) protomers after fractionation by SDS-PAGE (Fig. 5). The relative molecular weights of the individual protomers are: Form I $hABP_H$ > Form I $hABP_L \cong hTeBG_H > hTeBG_L$. The relative amounts of each protomer in both proteins also differ: hABP has more of the L component, whereas hTeBG has more of the H component. Peptide maps prepared from the H and L protomers of the two proteins suggest that they are similar but not identical (118). hTeBG and hABP photolabeled with $[^3H]$-Δ^6-testosterone both have a portion of the steroid-binding site on the H and L protomers (Fig. 5). Furthermore, the distribution of protomers seen with affinity labeling is identical to that observed by silver staining of the purified protein. These observations indicate that both the H and L protomers of the purified protein are components of native hABP. With the information available to date, it is not possible to know whether H:L in highly purified Form I hABP is the same (i.e., 2:3) as that secreted by Sertoli cells.

Form II hABP is similar to hTeBG with regard to Con A binding (80); on SDS-polyacrylamide gels, it migrates as a heterogeneous band with an average molecular weight greater than that of hTeBG (Fig. 5) (118). The peptide maps generated by Form II hABP are essentially the same as those of hTeBG when the peptide fragments are visualized by immunoblots using monospecific hTeBG antiserum, but slightly different from hTeBG when visualized by silver staining or lectin-blotting using Con A (118). Steroid-binding assays and an hTeBG ra-

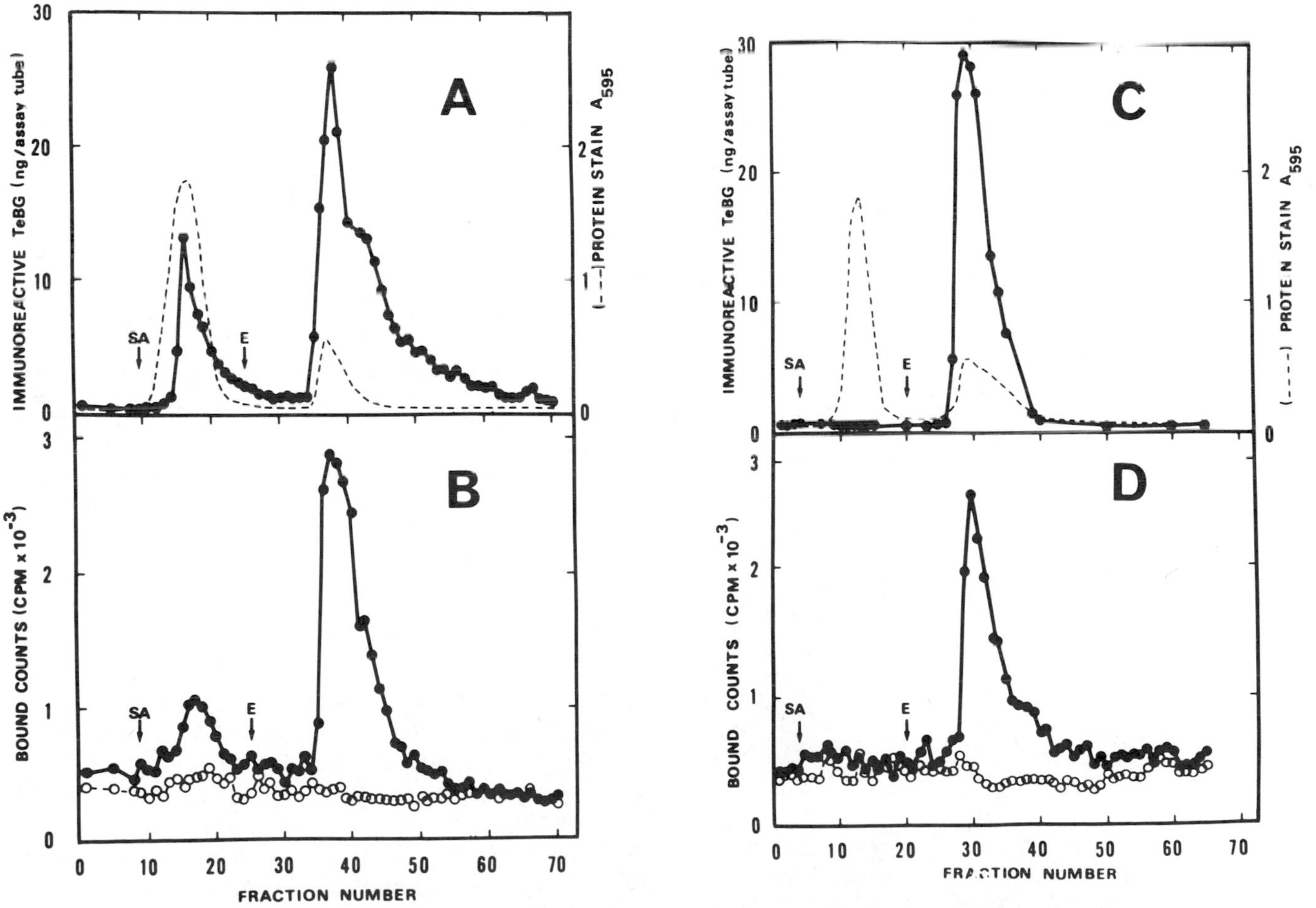

FIG. 3. Con A-Sepharose affinity chromatography of human testicular cytosol (**A,B**) and serum from a normal man (**C,D**). In A and C, the concentration of immunoreactive hTeBG-like material was measured by radioimmunoassay using an aliquot from each fraction; total protein was also estimated by dye binding. In B and D, an aliquot from each fraction was assayed for steroid binding by incubation with $[^3H]$DHT in the absence (●) or presence (○) of 2000-fold excess of nonradioactive DHT. SA indicates where sample was applied; E indicates elution of glycoproteins bound to Con A using methylglucoside. It is of note that human testicular cytosol contains two peaks showing immunoreactivity to hTeBG antiserum and binding, whereas human serum contains only one. (Adapted from ref. 80).

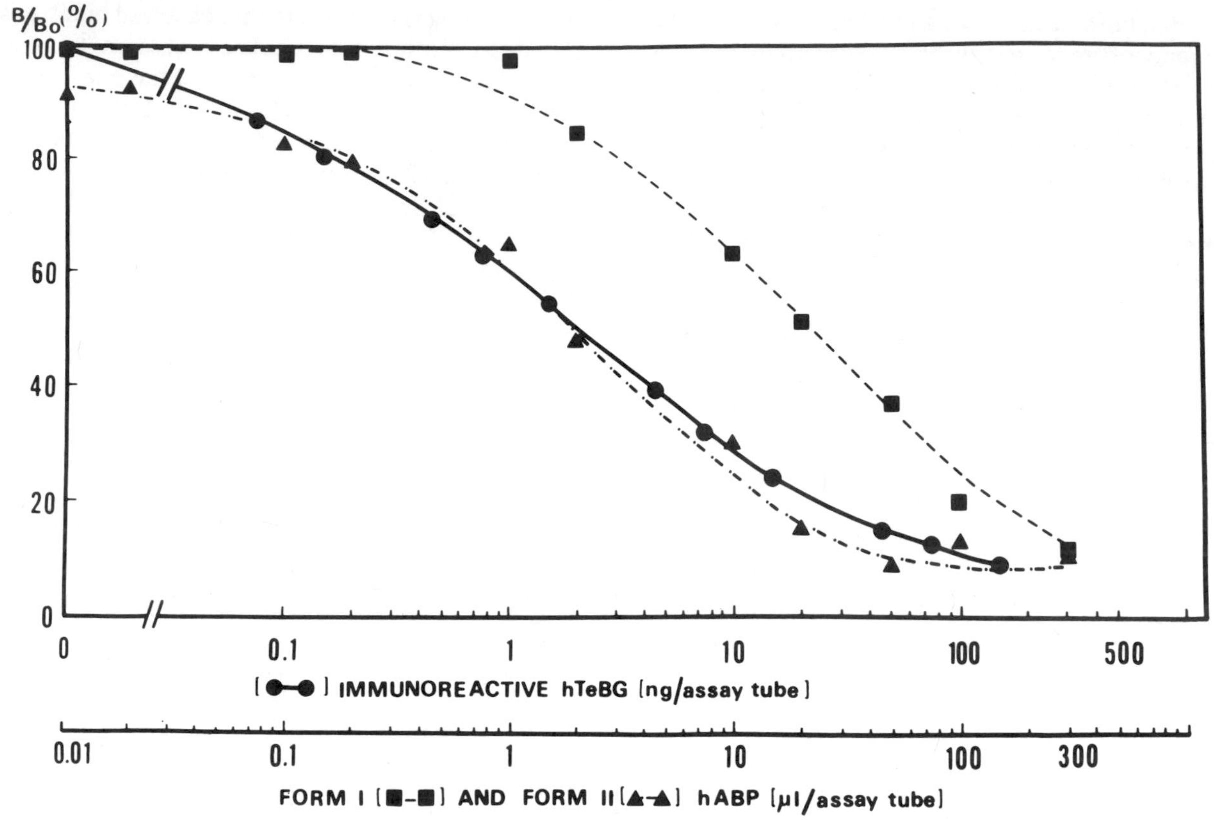

FIG. 4. Competition of [^{125}I]hTeBG binding to hTeBG antiserum by Form I and Form II hABP derived from human testicular extracts fractionated on Con A-Sepharose columns and by hTeBG from a pool of human pregnancy sera. The abscissa is the log dose of competitor. The ordinate is expressed as B/B_0, where B and B_0 are counts bound in the presence and absence of unlabeled competitor, respectively. (Adapted from ref. 80.)

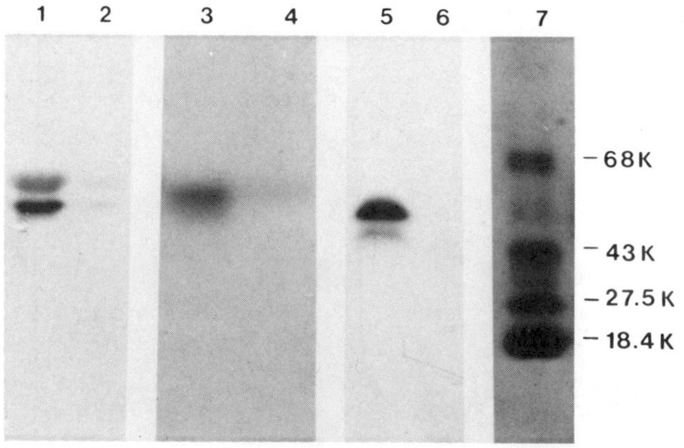

FIG. 5. SDS-polyacrylamide gel electrophoresis of photolabeled hABP and hTeBG. Highly purified Form I hABP (lanes 1 and 2), Form II hABP (lanes 3 and 4), and hTeBG (lanes 5 and 6) were photolyzed in the presence of Δ^6-[^{3}H]testosterone with or without nonradioactive DHT. After photolysis, samples were fractionated on an SDS-polyacrylamide slab gel, and the radioactive components were demonstrated by fluorography. Lanes 1, 3, and 5 indicate proteins photolyzed in the absence of competitor; lanes 2, 4, and 6 indicate samples that were photolyzed in the presence of competitor. Lane 7 is ^{14}C-labeled molecular-weight standards. (Adapted from ref. 118.)

dioimmunoassay demonstrated that both proteins have similar binding sites and shared immunodeterminants. The demonstration that the isoforms of hABP are distinct from hTeBG provides hope that both of these proteins may eventually be quantified in biological fluids. However, the ability to distinguish how these isoforms differ from one another and from hTeBG must await their primary sequence analysis.

ABP in Other Species. In addition to being present in rat, rabbit, and human testes, ABPs are present in guinea-pig (77), monkey, and ovine testes. Since hTeBG shares immunodeterminants with monkey steroid-binding proteins (112,119,120), antiserum against this hTeBG can be used for studies in primates (120). Monkey ABP (mABP), like hABP, resolves into two forms on Con A chromatography, namely, two protomers of molecular weight (MW) 48,000 and 46,000, which are present in nonequivalent amounts. Purified ovine ABP differs from ovine TeBG in much the same way as rbABP differs from rbTeBG (C. Y. Cheng and C. W. Bardin, *unpublished observations*).

It has not been possible to detect androgen-binding activity in the reproductive tract of porcine and murine species using assays that could easily detect such binding sites in rat tissues. These observations raise some doubts as to the necessity for ABP in normal reproduction. It was of interest, therefore, to find immunostainable ABP-like activity (using anti-rABP) in mouse Sertoli cells, neural tissue, and epithelia of rete testis, efferent ductules, proximal caput epididymis, and vas deferens (S. D. Tsong, *unpublished observations*). In contrast, other cells in these tissues, as well as in 10 other control organs, were immunonegative. These observations suggest that there is a protein in the mouse that does not have a steroid-binding site detectable by conventional assays, but contains immunodeterminants similar to those of rABP. Since the tissue and cellular distribution of the immunostainable material in the mouse is exactly the same as the distribution of rABP in rat tissues using the same antisera, these observations suggest that the tissue distribution of this ABP-like immunoreactive protein in the mouse may not be dependent on the presence of a high-affinity testosterone-binding site. Whether similar ABP immunostainable activity exists in the same tissue of other species without steroid-binding sites remains to be established.

Functions of ABP. Although it is 10 and 20 years since the identification of rABP and hTeBG, respectively, their physiologic function is still not completely understood. It was once thought that ABP, like TeBG, could not be important because these proteins were not found in all species (2,83). Such a postulate was acceptable as long as it was believed that they served only as extracellular steroid transport proteins. Several observations suggest, however, that steroid-binding proteins are not just curiosities of evolution. First, ABP and TeBG have been found in several species that were originally thought not to have such proteins. Second, the conservation of a specific steroid-binding site for androgens and estrogens through philogeny suggests a selective advantage. Finally, it has become increasingly clear that ABP and TeBG are both present in cells other than those in which they are synthesized. For example, ABP and TeBG are localized immunocytochemically in selected cells that respond to, or metabolize, androgens. These observations suggest there may be a specific mechanism for transport of these proteins into such cells. Moreover, a specific saturable binding site for hTeBG has recently been demonstrated on prostatic cells (121). A similar binding site for rABP has also been postulated to occur on cells of the proximal caput epididymis, where the intracellular concentration of this protein is high (122).

The physiologic roles postulated for ABP have included: (a) a carrier of testosterone within the Sertoli cells; (b) a carrier to maintain high concentrations of androgens in seminiferous tubules and epididymides; and (c) a transporter of testosterone from the testis into the epididymis. Although data to support these functions are limited, they all are consistent with the steroid-binding activity exhibited by ABP (123,124). If binding of steroids by ABP is relevant, then this protein may influence androgen action or metabolism, particularly in the caput epididymis, where ABP is concentrated. This speculation is supported by studies indicating that the androgen concentrations in blood are not sufficient to maintain the function of this region once the entry of testicular androgens and proteins is limited by ligation of the efferent ductules (for a review see ref. 3). However, if ABP is the product of Sertoli cells that is important for the functioning of the caput epithelium, then the finding of immunoreactive ABP without demonstrable binding activity in the mouse questions whether all the functions postulated for this protein are related to its steroid-binding activity. In contrast to these speculations, it is clear that the Sertoli cells of many species produce ABP, presumably to serve the same function in the reproductive tract as TeBG serves in the systemic circulation.

Metal-Binding Proteins

As noted above, several investigators have demonstrated that Sertoli cells synthesize and secrete iron- and copper-transport proteins (10,12,67). These proteins have been called *testicular transferrin* and *ceruloplasmin,* respectively. The presence of both of these proteins in tubular fluid suggests a mechanism by which iron and copper can be transported to germ cells in the adluminal compartment (125).

A comparison of highly purified testicular transferrin to its homolog in serum using amino acid analysis and tryptic peptide patterns indicates that the only apparent difference between these two proteins is their carbohydrate content (11). This suggests that testicular and serum transferrin are the products of the same gene which have differential patterns of post-translational processing.

When serum-free culture media were developed for the growth of testicular cells, it was shown that Sertoli cells required transferrin for growth (126). It was postulated that this protein might serve as a specific mitogen for this cell type, independent of its ability to transport iron. Results of studies investigating this possibility demonstrate that in the absence of iron, transferrin has no growth-promoting activity (127). The proposed function of this protein on testicular cells is, therefore, to transport iron. It has been postulated that Sertoli cells synthesize and secrete this protein into the seminiferous tubular lumen to provide a mechanism for transport of Fe^{3+} to developing germ cells (10). The demonstration of transferrin's specific binding to spermatocytes (128) and of transferrin receptors on spermatids (M. Serio et al., *personal communication*) is consistent with this hypothesis.

Transferrin production by Sertoli cell cultures was stimulated by FSH, testosterone, retinol, and retinoic acid treatment (129). However, the effects of FSH on transferrin production by Sertoli cell-enriched cultures have not been routinely reproduced by other laboratories, probably because the concentration of some other factor(s) in the medium is critical for FSH action (24,127).

Thorbecke (130) surveyed several tissues with transferrin antiserum and observed that this protein is synthesized by both the testis and the ovary. Studies on seminal fluid of normal and vasectomized men suggest that more than 80% of seminal transferrin comes from the testes (or epididymides) (131), whereas seminal ceruloplasmin is from another part of the reproductive tract. More importantly, these studies show that seminal transferrin is a reliable index of seminiferous tubular function because levels of this protein are lower in patients with oligo- and azoospermia (131,132). These observations are important since they demonstrate that at least one Sertoli cell protein can pass through the epididymis and can be measured in semen. This is strikingly different from ABP that is quantitatively removed by the reproductive tract.

Clusterin

Fritz et al. (18) reported the presence of a macromolecule in ram rete testis fluid which elicited "clustering" of Sertoli cells from immature rats, TM_4 Sertoli cells, and erythrocytes of several species. Purified clusterin from ram rete testis fluid is a dimeric glycoprotein containing 36% carbohydrate (19,133). The protein is synthesized and secreted by Sertoli cells (19). The native dimer (MW 80,000) consists of two monomers of MW 40,000, each with different *N*-terminal amino acid sequences (C. Y. Cheng and C. W. Bardin, *unpublished observations*).

Recently, a glycoprotein that is responsive to FSH and testosterone was identified in primary Sertoli cell-enriched cultures prepared from rat testes (24), partially purified using sequential high-performance liquid chromatography (HPLC) columns, and designated CMB-21 (C. Y. Cheng and C. W. Bardin, *unpublished observations*). CMB-21 is a dimer of MW 90,000 consisting of two monomers of MW 45,000 with identical electrophoretic mobilities. A monospecific antiserum against this protein cross-reacts with ram clusterin and with a protein of similar size found in media from mouse Sertoli cell-enriched cultures (C. Y. Cheng and C. W. Bardin, *unpublished observations*). These observations suggest that the Sertoli cell protein, clusterin, is not limited to the ovine species.

Immunocytochemical studies using monoclonal antibodies against ram clusterin, in combination with indirect immunofluorescence microscopy, indicated that this protein is concentrated in the adluminal region of the seminiferous epithelium and in the epithelial cells of the rete testis and caput epididymides (20). The physiologic function of clusterin is unknown; however, it may act to facilitate cell-cell interactions (18). In this regard, immunoassayable clusterin has also been identified in the blood of rams, suggesting that it could have some actions outside the reproductive tract (C. Y. Cheng, J. P. Mather, and C. W. Bardin, *unpublished observations*).

Testicular Plasminogen Activators

The presence of serine proteases, plasminogen activators (PA), in Sertoli cell-enriched cultures was first reported in 1977 (16). The activity of this enzyme is stimulated by FSH or dibutyryl cAMP in the medium. It was proposed that PAs are involved in tissue restructuring and cell migration processes in normal tissues. In the reproductive tissue, PA may play a role in facilitating either the release of mature spermatids by Sertoli cells or the migration of germ cells (mainly preleptotene spermatocytes) from the basal compartment to the adluminal compartment of the seminiferous tubule by opening the occluding inter-Sertoli cell junctions, or both. The enzyme might also participate in remodeling the seminiferous epithelium (17,134,135).

More recent studies indicate that the secretion of PA is dependent on the stage of the seminiferous epithelium cycle (136,137). Secreted PA is of the urokinase type, which predominates in stages VII and VIII of the seminiferous epithelium cycle, whereas tissue-type PA is maximal in stages IX to XII of the cycle. Immunohistochemical analysis using specific antibodies revealed that urokinase-type PA is localized in Sertoli cells in stages VII and VIII; and tissue-type PA is in pachytene and diakinetic primary spermatocytes in stages VII to XIII. These studies suggest that the cyclic secretion of PA is related to the stages of the spermatogenic cycle. Thus, they provide insights into the relationship between the tissue-restructuring processes, such as movement of the preleptotene primary spermatocytes from basal lamina (134) and release of the spermatids from the seminiferous epithelium (138).

H-Y Antigen

H-Y antigen is a male-specific protein that binds to receptors on Sertoli cells of the primordial gonad. Specific receptors for H-Y antigen are found on testicular and ovarian cells but not on cells of extragonadal tissues (139,140). The coupling of H-Y antigen and its receptor is believed to elicit the formation of the testicular cords (141–143). There are two reports indicating that Sertoli cells secrete H-Y antigen. It has been shown that in Sertoli cell culture medium there is a product, similar to the H-Y antigen, which neutralizes the cytotoxicity of anti-

H-Y serum against rat-tail epidermal cells (142). In another study, a monoclonal antibody developed against H-Y antigen shows that medium from both primary Sertoli cell-enriched cultures and TM_4 (a mouse Sertoli cell line) contain H-Y antigen (15). These observations, however, were not confirmed by another laboratory, where radiolabeled proteins secreted by rat Sertoli cells in primary culture were examined for specific interactions with polyclonal and monoclonal antibodies directed against serologically detectable H-Y antigen. It is of note that none of the Sertoli cell secretory proteins reacted specifically with H-Y antibodies as determined by immunoprecipitation (144). The reason for the discrepancies between these independent observations remains to be elucidated.

Growth Factors

It was first shown that mouse testes contain a potent mitogen that induces DNA synthesis and cell division in cultures of confluent, quiescent BALB/c 3T3 cells (5,7,145). This mitogen apparently originates from Sertoli cells because this component of the seminiferous epithelium from the prepubertal testis exhibits substantially higher levels of mitogenic activity than do components of other cell types (5). This growth factor is present in the seminiferous epithelium of several mammalian species, including rat, guinea pig, and calf (6). The partially purified growth factor has an MW of 15,700 and a pI between 4.8 and 5.8 (6). The physiologic function of this protein is not yet known; however, it is presumably involved in the regulation of cell proliferation in developing and adult testes (146).

An independent line of research showed that the fibroblast growth factor (FGF) originally isolated from pituitary fractions is a potent stimulator of ovarian cells in culture (147). Similar growth factors can be purified from a wide variety of tissues using heparin-Sepharose affinity chromatography (147,148). These growth factors have similar molecular weights and have relative affinities for heparin-Sepharose. Based on their isoelectric points, it appears that the majority of these endothelial cell mitogens fall into two general classes, namely, acidic and basic FGFs. Both of these peptides will stimulate proliferation of multiple endothelial cell types and both are potent angiogenic agents. Basic FGF is present in pituitary, brain, adrenal, retina, corpus luteum, and kidney, whereas acidic FGF is present in brain, retina, and testes. The cellular localization of FGF in the testis has not yet been established (149).

Recent completion of the amino acid sequences of both basic and acidic FGF has allowed comparison with each other, as well as with other potentially related proteins. Based on amino and carboxyl terminal sequences, there is homology between selected regions of interleukin I and the FGFs. This homology, however, is far less than between the two forms of FGF. For example, interleukin I has approximately 25% and 27% homology with bovine basic and acidic FGF, respectively. By contrast, there is a 53% homology between basic and acidic FGF, and up to 42 of the remaining 66 residues involve nucleotide substitution where a single base change could result in amino acid replacement (149–151). How FGF in the testis relates to the Sertoli cell growth factor of the same MW described above remains to be established.

Another growth factor that has been identified in Sertoli cell-enriched cultures is somatomedin C (9). Studies performed on ovarian cells indicate that this growth factor acts synergistically with FSH (152). It is highly likely that this factor has a similar effect on Sertoli cells. Epidermal growth factor has also been identified in testicular extracts and is known to bind to multiple testicular cells (153). Its site of origin is not known.

Testibumin

During a search for hormonally responsive products in media from Sertoli cell-enriched cultures, a protein that responds synergistically to FSH and testosterone was identified and designated *CMB-1* (154). Structural and immunological analyses, including *N*-terminal sequence determination and immunoblots, indicate that CMB-1 is related to albumin and alpha-fetoprotein (AFP) (25). Furthermore, CMB-1 is highly concentrated in the testicular and epididymal compartments in adult rats. In view of its localization and its similarity to albumin and AFP, we postulate that this may be the albumin homolog of the adluminal compartment of the testis and have called it *testibumin.* The fact that this protein is also found in the blood of adult female rats indicates that, unlike rABP, this protein is not synthesized exclusively in the testis.

Identification and Isolation of Other Sertoli Cell Proteins

As noted above, Sertoli cell products have been, and will continue to be, used as probes for studying Sertoli cells and their interactions with the multiple-germ cell types in the adluminal and basal compartments of the seminiferous tubules. The isolation of these proteins has been difficult because, in many instances, the procedures used to identify them, including one- or two-dimensional gel electrophoresis (21,67,155), have not been useful in subsequent purification as a result of their limited loading capacities. In addition, the use of radioac-

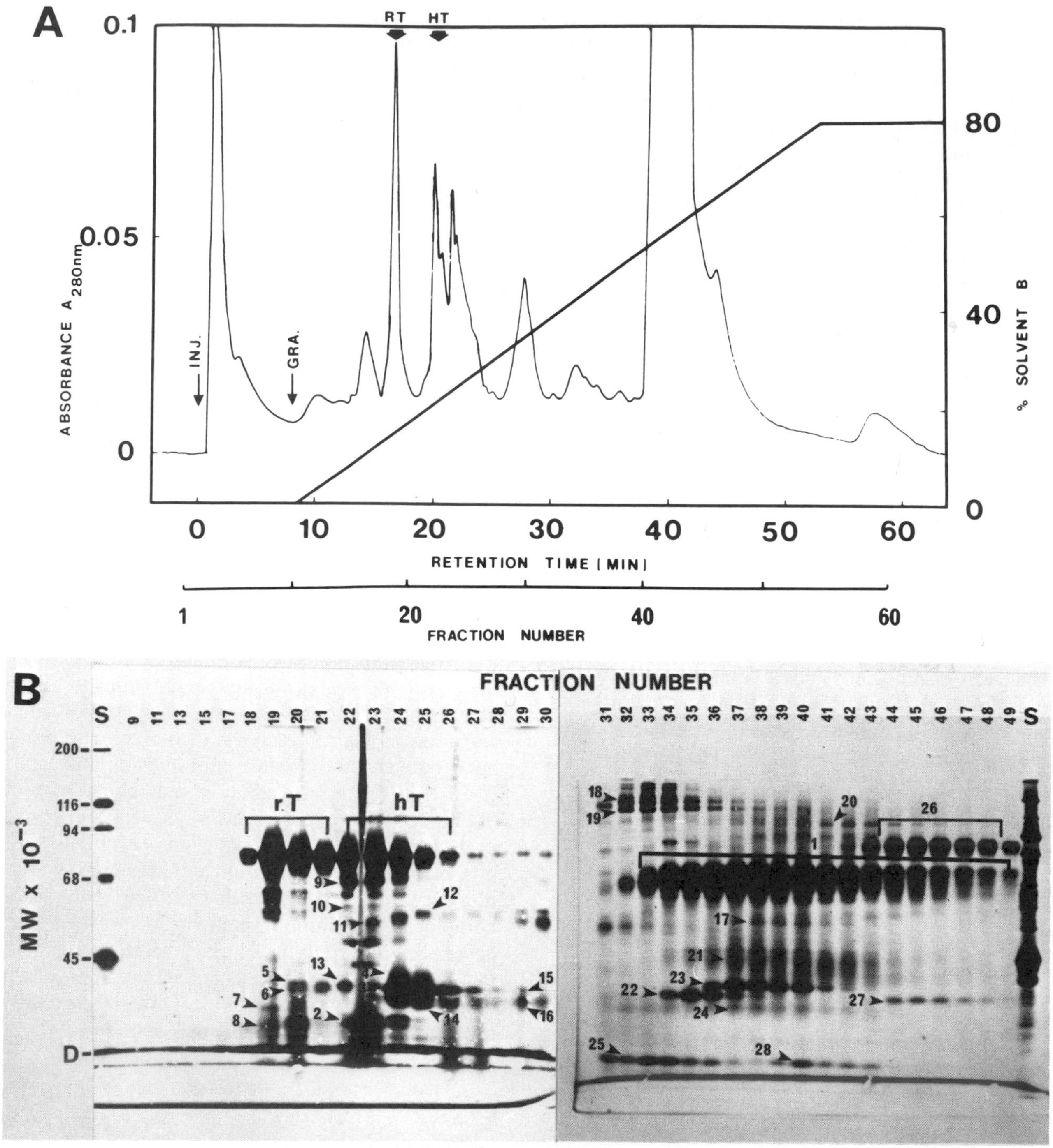

FIG. 6. Fractionation and identification of total secreted proteins, contained in Sertoli cell-enriched culture medium. **A:** Proteins in Sertoli cell-enriched culture medium. Spent medium obtained from Sertoli cells grown in the presence of FSH (300 ng/ml) and testosterone (2×10^{-7} M) was resolved by anion-exchange HPLC. After injection (INJ.) a gradient (GRA.) of 0–80% solvent B (20 mM Tris, 600 mM NaCl, pH 7.4 at 22°C) was applied to the column. Fractions were collected and proteins were monitored by UV absorbance at 280 nm. A total of 15 major protein peaks were resolved. **B:** Polyacrylamide gel electrophoresis of total proteins contained in the fractions resolved by HPLC as shown in A. The numbers indicate the tentative names for these Sertoli cell proteins. (Adapted from ref. 24.)

tive amino acids to identify Sertoli cell proteins may confound a subsequent purification strategy because the intensity of labeling does not necessarily indicate which of the proteins in the medium are the major secretory products of Sertoli cells. This problem may be particularly pertinent in products having rapid turnover rates or a large number of the radiolabeled amino acid residues.

The recent application of newly developed HPLC columns to the rapid isolation of TeBGs from serum of human, rabbit, bull (156), and ram (C. Y. Cheng, *unpublished observations*) and of ABP from human testes (108) encouraged us to take a similar approach for the identification and isolation of major Sertoli cell secretory products. The first two steps of this procedure, anion-exchange HPLC and SDS-PAGE, applied to media from Sertoli cell-enriched cultures, are illustrated in Fig. 6. In such media there are more than 30 major acidic proteins (Fig. 6), which have been termed *CMB proteins* (24). When culture media are prepared from Sertoli cells grown with testosterone, FSH, or both hormones, these proteins are classified as those responding (a) to neither hormone, (b) primarily to testosterone, (c) primarily to FSH, or (d) to both hormones (24). It is now possible to isolate many of these proteins from 1 to 2 liters of medium using a variety of HPLC columns (25). It is of note that Sertoli cell-enriched cultures are likely to contain small amounts of peritubular cells and germ cells that can contribute directly or indirectly to the secreted proteins (157,158). Thus, proteins in the Sertoli cell media could be derived from peritubular and residual germ cells. In this regard, Sertoli cells do not secrete fibronectin or Type I collagen into the medium when maintained for up to 6 days under serum-free conditions. By contrast, peritubular cells in culture secrete both of these proteins, and, when co-cultured with Sertoli cells, the secretion of both proteins is enhanced (159). Using a monospecific fibronectin antiserum, no fibronectinlike macromolecules were present by Western blotting in the Sertoli cell-enriched cultures used for the isolation of CMB proteins (C. Y. Cheng and C. W. Bardin, *unpublished observations*). This suggests that most of the CMB proteins are of Sertoli cell origin. Nonetheless, the origins of CMB proteins must be established with more direct methods following purification, assay development, and sequence analysis. The characterization of such proteins should show homology with Sertoli secretory products that have been identified by others (21,22,67,155, 160–162).

Secretion of Sertoli Cell Hormones

Although many of the proteins and peptides produced by Sertoli cells have autocrine and paracrine effects on the testis, a few of these products are secreted into the blood and act as endocrine mediators on other tissues.

Inhibin

The existence of water-soluble substances of gonadal origin that selectively suppress FSH secretion has been suspected for more than five decades (163). The quest to chemically characterize these molecules, referred to as *inhibin,* proceeded slowly until 1985 (4,164). In the past few years, several investigators have isolated inhibinlike molecules from a variety of sources. Primary structures of a 31-peptide and 94-peptide with inhibinlike activities were reported by Ramasharma et al. (165) and Seidah et al. (166). These peptides were isolated from human seminal plasma. Subsequently, two additional peptides containing 52 and 92 amino acids were also reported (167). Studies using the synthetic 31-peptide demonstrated that it did not have the properties expected of inhibin, since it did not suppress the plasma levels of FSH in castrated rats (168). Robertson and colleagues reported on the isolation of inhibin, from bovine follicular fluid, that had an apparent MW of 56,000. This protein was characterized by two peptide chains of 14,000 and 46,000 MW connected by disulfide bonds (169). Inhibin from porcine follicular fluid was also isolated, but showed an apparent MW of 32,000 (150,170). This peptide consisted of dissimilar polypeptide subunits of 18,000 (α-inhibin) and 14,000 (β-inhibin) MW linked by disulfide bonds (168). A similar protein has also been isolated from ram rete testis fluid. All the preparations purified from ovarian and testicular fluids are several hundredfold more potent than any of the peptides isolated from seminal plasma.

Recently, the *N*-terminal amino acid sequence of α- and β-inhibin was determined, and the data were used to identify cloned complementary DNAs corresponding to the mRNA for pro-inhibin α and β (150,171,172). The complete amino acid sequences of these subunits were predicted from their nucleotide sequences, and it was found that β-inhibin shares a high homology with transforming growth factor β. It is of interest that molecules regulating reproduction and cell growth appear to be related. A more complete description of the history and biological activities of inhibin is given in Chapter 15 of this volume.

Steroids

In the 1930s, testosterone was first isolated from testicular tissue (173); however, it was not until the 1950s that *in vitro* studies using radiolabeled steroid precursors demonstrated that testicular tissue is capable of *de novo* synthesis of testosterone (174,175). *In vitro* studies showed that Leydig cells are responsible for the synthesis of most, if not all, of the androgens in the testis. This topic has been reviewed previously (176) and is also reviewed in another chapter in this volume.

The possibility that Sertoli cells are also involved in steroid biosynthesis has been raised by several observations over the years. One line of evidence is that tumors of Sertoli cell origin secrete steroids (177). In addition, electron microscopic studies show that Sertoli cells possess cytoplasmic organelles typical of steroid-secreting endocrine glands, including extensive smooth endoplasmic reticulum and cholesterol-containing lipid droplets (35). The ability to prepare various testicular cells for *in vitro* studies shows the extent to which various testicular cells are capable of secreting and metabolizing steroids (28,29,178). For example, isolated Sertoli cells exhibit 17β-hydroxysteroid oxidoreductase, 17α-hydroxylase, C17–C20 lyase, and 20α-hydroxysteroid oxidoreductase activities (179–182). In addition, Sertoli cell-enriched cultures from adult rats metabolize progesterone to testosterone, androstenedione, and 3α-hydroxy-5α-androstan-17-one (183). Primary Sertoli cell-enriched cultures from 10- to 20-day-old rats metabolize androstenedione to testosterone, dihydrotestosterone (DHT), and 5α-androstane-3α,17β-diol. The observation that these metabolic conversions are stimulated by FSH suggests that they occur in Sertoli cells rather than in another cell type present in the cultures. In addition, they are age-dependent because the conversion rate is higher in Sertoli cells cultured from 10- to 20-day-old rats than from rats after 20 days of age. This age-dependent pattern is the reverse of that seen in Leydig cells (180,182). Based on these studies it seems unlikely that Sertoli cells contribute significantly to the androgen pool in the blood of adult animals. However, it is possible that some of the steroids produced by Sertoli cells are important for the function of the seminiferous tubule, rete testis, or epididymis.

Following the demonstration that the prostate and seminal vesicles convert testosterone to DHT and the suggestion that the latter steroid may be the biologically active androgen in the male reproductive tract, many investigators measured the formation of DHT by testes (184–186). 5α-Reductase is higher in testes from younger animals and is stimulated by FSH and decreased by LH (187,188). Spermatocytes and Sertoli cells have a greater 5α-reductase activity than do spermatids, but there is very little of this enzyme in Leydig cells. In spermatocytes, the major 5α-reductase product of testosterone is DHT; however, in Sertoli cells, testosterone can be further metabolized to 5α-androstane-3α,17β-diol. In cells from intact testes, the formation of both 3α- and 3β-diol increases until puberty and then declines (189). Even though the testis shows 5α-reductase activity, it is important to compare its *in vivo* efficiency with that of the prostate and seminal vesicle. In prostate and seminal vesicle, the ratio of 5α-reduced metabolites to testosterone is 7:1 whereas in the testis it was 1:2 (190). These observations indicate that the pattern of testosterone metabolism in the seminiferous tubule is very different than that found in the accessory sex organs. Perfusion of the male reproductive tract with [^{3}H]testosterone indicates that dihydrotestosterone, the major androgen, binds to nuclear receptors in epididymis, prostate, and seminal vesicle, whereas testosterone is the major nuclear androgen in the testis (191). Taken together, these observations indicate that dihydrotestosterone is the major active androgen in the accessory sex organs, whereas in the mature testis it is testosterone.

Although Sertoli cell testosterone and androstenedione are not major components of the blood androgen pool, they are important substrates for estradiol and estrone produced in the seminiferous tubular epithelium of the developing animal. Aromatase is highest in young animals and is highly responsive to FSH (192,193). The estradiol production of cultured Sertoli cells in response to FSH has been used as a bioassay for this hormone (194). In the adult human, on whom the most extensive studies have been done, only a small fraction of the estradiol in blood is secreted by the testes; most of this steroid is derived from testosterone in extragonadal tissues. However, in patients with testicular disorders associated with elevated FSH levels, up to 40% of estradiol in blood is of testicular (and possibly of Sertoli cell) origin (195).

HUMORAL REGULATION OF SERTOLI CELL FUNCTION

The major hormonal regulators of the seminiferous epithelium *in vivo* are testosterone and FSH. From *in vitro* studies it is clear that the Sertoli cell is the principal site of action of these hormones and that the regulation of Sertoli cell function is more complex than could be appreciated from *in vivo* studies. The ability to maintain Sertoli cells under serum-free conditions permitted careful definition of the multiple hormones, growth factors, vitamins, metal transport proteins, and attachment factors that are required to maintain growth, protein secretion, and specific morphological features. Furthermore, various combinations of these humoral factors result in different patterns of growth and differentiated function of Sertoli cells *in vitro*. In addition, various cells of the testis regulate Sertoli cells either through direct contact or by modulating the environment of this cell through paracrine factors. These observations, coupled with those described above, indicate that the internal environment of the testis is controlled by Sertoli cells, whose function is, in turn, regulated by multiple humoral and cellular factors. The following is a compilation of some of the factors that have been shown to affect Sertoli cell function.

Polypeptide Hormones

FSH

FSH produces hypertrophy and changes in nuclear morphology of Sertoli cells when administered to hypophysectomized rats (196). In addition, FSH receptors are present on Sertoli cells, which constitute the major site of FSH binding in the testis (197–199). The actions of FSH on diverse functions such as energy metabolism, protein secretion, cell shape, and cell division are mediated via several second messengers, including cAMP and Ca^{2+}.

FSH receptor. Although the FSH receptor is located predominantly on Sertoli cells, recent observations suggest that some binding sites for this hormone may also be located on macrophages in the interstitium of the testis (200,201). The membrane-bound FSH receptor isolated from testis meets the requirements of a physiologically relevant receptor in that the binding of hormone results in activation of adenylate cyclase. This receptor can be detergent solubilized, and a variety of studies suggest that this represents the same molecular form as that present in the membrane. In addition, a cytoplasmic (buffer-soluble) FSH-binding component can be prepared from testes in the absence of detergent (202). The origin of the buffer-soluble binding component is not clear. However, FSH interacts with both forms of receptor in seemingly identical ways. Treatment with FSH produces a decline in the membrane receptor concentration which is coincident with an increase in the buffer-soluble component, suggesting that the latter may be derived from the membrane-bound form (203). It is, therefore, entirely possible that the FSH receptorlike material in cytoplasm is formed as a consequence of receptor processing or recycling. Until the membrane and cytoplasmic FSH-binding forms can be purified, their homologies cannot be confirmed.

Even though the receptor has not been purified to homogeneity, a considerable amount is known about its structure. It is of note that receptors for many peptides and protein hormones are glycoproteins. For example, receptors for growth hormone, insulin, epidermal growth factor, prolactin, TSH, and LH bind to concanavalin A (202). It is surprising, therefore, to find that the solubilized FSH receptor does not bind to this lectin. Evidence for the glycoprotein nature of the FSH receptor is derived from studies using neuraminidase. Removal of sialic acid from the receptor results in increased binding of [^{125}I]FSH which is secondary to a fivefold increase in binding affinity. The role of receptor-associated carbohydrates in hormone recognition and promotion of postbinding effects can be more clearly delineated once the structure of the receptor is known and mutations are produced with selected deletions of specific carbohydrates.

Phospholipids are believed to be components of a number of membrane receptors. Incubation of testicular membranes with phospholipase markedly reduces the specific binding of FSH to membrane-bound receptors. Treatment with this enzyme did not, however, reduce FSH binding to the detergent-solubilized receptor. These results suggest that phospholipids are important in maintaining the receptor in a conformation necessary for FSH binding when it is in the membrane (202).

The MW of the native FSH receptor has been estimated to be approximately 146,000 (204). Studies using cross-linking and photoaffinity-labeling reagents suggest that the FSH receptor may be multimeric, containing at least one 48,000-MW subunit plus other nonidentical subunits (204,205). Similar results have also been obtained for the LH receptor (206). Another interpretation of the presence of multiple nonidentical subunits is that they are produced by limited proteolysis during isolation of the cells or receptor. Such a possibility is suggested by recent studies showing only a single receptor subunit with an MW of 89,000 in the testis and in the ovary when protease inhibitors are used (207).

Large doses of FSH are known to induce the loss of FSH receptors from Sertoli cells both *in vivo* and *in vitro* (208,209). Although the exact mechanism by which FSH mediates this effect on its receptors is not established in detail, it is assumed, based on the large amount of data available on other hormones, that this occurs through receptor-mediated endocytosis. Under such conditions, virtually 100% of receptors are occupied as a result of excess hormone, thus the endocytotic route predominates and most of the surface receptor is depleted. If, however, cells are incubated with an amount of FSH to occupy only 35% of the available receptors, then only 8% of receptors are lost. If the same proportion of receptors are lost following the small and the large doses of FSH, then these observations are consistent with considerable receptor turnover and/or recycling (202). Studies using radioactive FSH indicate that much of the specifically bound hormone is removed from the cell surface within 15 min; following internalization, it is degraded to its component amino acids. Studies with inhibitors suggest that this latter process occurs in lysosomes (210). Receptors for other hormones have similar mechanisms of internalization, degradation, and repletion.

The interaction of FSH with its receptors is influenced by a wide variety of factors. Binding of FSH to membrane-bound receptor is stimulated by Mn^{2+}, Mg^{2+}, or Ca^{2+} and inhibited by Co^{2+} or Ni^{2+}. Binding is also inhibited by monovalent ions (211); bacitracin, polyamines (212), and low-MW factor(s) in seminal plasma (213) or serum (214). In the testes of several species, there are also factors with an MW of 10,000 to 33,000 which inhibit FSH binding to its receptor (215,216). The roles of all the above agents on receptor function and biological activity of FSH *in vivo* remain to be established.

Mediators of FSH Action. It is well established that some of the actions of FSH are mediated via the adenylate cyclase-protein kinase system. FSH results in an increase of cAMP (217–222), and either cAMP or substances that elevate cAMP (i.e., cholera toxin) can mimic some of the actions of FSH. In addition to increasing the synthesis of cAMP, FSH also affects various components of this system such as phosphodiesterase and protein kinase inhibitor levels as well as protein phosphorylation per se (223–228).

Following the binding reaction, FSH stimulates adenylate cyclase activity (220). This results in an increase in the intracellular cAMP concentration (217), which, in turn, activates protein kinase (220,229). The phosphorylation of proteins is involved in stimulation and the cascade of subsequent events in the Sertoli cell which ultimately lead to altered function. The observations that FSH stimulates both RNA (230–234) and protein synthesis in the Sertoli cell (235–237) suggested that this hormone affects a number of specific differentiated functions by mechanisms other than modifying the activities of existing protein.

In addition to activating a variety of cellular functions, protein hormones also produce adaptive changes that tend to reduce the response of the cell to further stimulation. This is a general phenomenon that has been observed in many cell types (238–240). Refractoriness to continued hormonal stimulation is usually the result of receptor loss, impaired accumulation of the second messenger, cAMP, and/or alteration of other regulatory mechanisms. FSH-induced refractoriness of Sertoli cells is associated with a decreased number of FSH receptors (208,241), a reduced adenylate cyclase activity (242, 243), and a large stimulation of high-affinity cAMP phosphodiesterase, both *in vivo* and *in vitro* (226,227, 244). When refractory cells are treated with phosphodiesterase inhibitors, methyl-isobutyl-xanthine, or the nonxanthine phosphodiesterase inhibitor, RO20-1724, the FSH response returns to normal. Treatment of Sertoli cells with FSH also produces an impaired response to a secondary incubation with isoproterenol, cholera toxin, or forskolin. The responses of these compounds are also restored to normal in the presence of phosphodiesterase inhibitors. From these studies it is concluded that even though FSH treatment produces FSH-receptor down regulation and a desensitization of adenylate cyclase, these events are not sufficient to decrease the FSH response. The refractory state can be fully expressed only when adenylate cyclase desensitization is associated with the stimulation of high-affinity cAMP phosphodiesterase. These two regulatory mechanisms cooperate to decrease the intercellular cAMP level, which consequently blunts the subsequent actions of FSH (245).

The intercellular events mediated by peptide hormones are also regulated by calcium. Calmodulin can be thought of as the primary receptor for calcium in much the same way as the regulatory subunits of cAMP-dependent protein kinase are the predominant cAMP receptors in eukaryotic cells (246,247). The interaction of calcium with calmodulin causes a conformational change in this protein so that it can interact with a variety of enzymes to alter their activities (248,249). In some instances, the effects of calcium are antagonistic to those of cAMP, but there are examples of additive or synergistic effects of these intercellular mediators.

In Sertoli cells, widely divergent cellular processes are regulated by common phosphorylation-dephosphorylation reactions, as is the case in other cells. For example, in Sertoli cells, reactions that regulate energy generation involve glycogen synthetase, phosphorylase kinase, and phosphorylase. FSH markedly alters phosphorylase activity, leading to glycogen breakdown and energy production (250). The phosphorylase in these cells is activated by increased concentrations of either cAMP or calcium. The mechanism involves conversion of inactive phosphorylase-b to active phosphorylase-a by phosphorylation. The converting enzyme, phosphorylase kinase, is also activated by phosphorylation. In Sertoli cells, the phosphorylation occurs via the catalytic subunit of cAMP-dependent protein kinase in response to FSH-induced cAMP accumulation. In addition, increases in intercellular calcium also stimulate phosphorylase kinase. In addition to energy generation, calcium effects mediated via calmodulin are believed to affect functions as divergent as cell motility, protein secretion, and cell proliferation (251).

Effects of FSH on Differentiated Function. The hormonal control of protein secretion by Sertoli cells has been studied by many laboratories. Because rABP was the first specific Sertoli cell protein for which there was a specific immunoassay, it was extensively studied both *in vivo* and *in vitro.* Many studies confirm that rABP levels are increased by chronic FSH treatment both *in vivo* and *in vitro* (62,178,252). The acute effects of this hormone *in vivo* are somewhat more controversial. Tindall and Means (253) showed rapid increases in rABP within 2 hr following FSH treatment. These investigators suggested that this was attributed to the presence of LH contamination, which caused increased testicular testosterone levels. The increased testosterone levels, in turn, had a protective effect on rABP steroid-binding activity, resulting in increased amounts of measurable rABP. This line of reasoning is supported by the observation that enhanced recovery of rABP could be mimicked by the addition of calcium, testosterone, glycerol, or *p*-chloro-mercurophenylsulfonate to the homogenization medium. It was concluded that the rapid effects of FSH were not due to increased synthesis of rABP, but rather to better recovery of androgen-binding activity from testicular extracts. These conclusions are in contrast to those of Kotite et al. (254), who observed that FSH produced a rapid increase in rABP even when steps were taken to ensure maximum stabilization of rABP with glycerol and testosterone. This apparent dilemma has not been resolved. It is of note that it takes many hours before the *in vitro* effects of FSH on rABP accumulation in the culture medium can be observed (255).

In addition to rABP, the secretion of a number of other proteins is affected by FSH: this includes (a) several secretory proteins with unknown function (24,256), (b) plasminogen activator (16,257,258), and (c) the iron-carrier protein, transferrin (127,129,259). However, it is of note that FSH does not have a general effect on the secretion of all Sertoli cell products, since several secreted proteins are unaffected by treatment with this hormone (24).

The secretion of a Sertoli cell product, functionally identified as a *Leydig cell stimulatory factor* (LCSF), has also been shown to be increased *in vitro* by FSH (260,261). This factor has been shown to be a heat-labile, nondialyzable substance that stimulates steroidogenesis in Leydig cells and may be a paracrine substance that is a communication link between the Sertoli and Leydig cells (260,262,263). The existence of such a paracrine system is supported by several lines of evidence that are presented in more detail below.

In addition to protein secretion, several other aspects of Sertoli cell metabolism are regulated by FSH. There are changes in lipids in Sertoli cells that result from hypophysectomy, suggesting that FSH and/or testosterone influence lipid metabolism in this cell; however, the exact nature of the effect is not well established. Sertoli cell cholesterol esterase activity is also modulated by FSH. Two forms of cholesterol esterase are present in the testis: One is a heat-labile enzyme, found exclusively in the Sertoli cell, that increases 20-fold in response to FSH treatment of hypophysectomized rats; the other form is a heat-stable species that is located in Sertoli and Leydig cells and is increased by both LH and FSH. The role of this enzyme in the physiology of these cells is not known (264).

As noted above, FSH influences Sertoli cell energy metabolism. This includes the stimulation of glucose uptake (265), lactate production (266), and the activity of glycogen phosphorylase (250). Because it has been shown that germ cells depend heavily on lactate as an energy source (267) this mobilization of energy resources and the concomitant increase in lactate and pyruvate secretion may play a role in their nourishment.

In addition to affecting Sertoli cell secretory proteins FSH also increases the synthesis of cell surface glycoproteins (268), which appear to be involved with one another in the interaction of Sertoli cells. FSH-induced cell-cell associations *in vitro* are blocked by specific lectins, inhibitors of protein synthesis, inhibitors of RNA synthesis, and cell surface modification (268,269). These results are consistent with the thesis that FSH increases the production of cell surface glycoproteins, which, in turn, serve as cell adhesion molecules.

Effects of FSH on Cell Division. In addition to its influence on differentiated function, FSH has a profound affect on the proliferation of Sertoli cells both in the pre- and postnatal period. Exogenous FSH stimulates thymidine incorporation into the DNA of Sertoli cells in fetal rats denied endogenous FSH by hypophysectomy (270). In addition, this hormone also regulates Sertoli cell proliferation in the neonate (271). Prior to 20 days of age in the rat, FSH increases DNA synthesis and mitotic activity (272,273). This response diminishes with increasing age and is not present in the adult. Indeed, this apparent change in FSH responsiveness of the Sertoli cells is observed with other endpoints as well (223,274,275) and may be a reflection of Sertoli cell differentiation prior to and during puberty. A more extensive discussion of Sertoli cell division is presented below with information about testicular hypertrophy.

Insulin and Insulinlike Growth Factors

Although other polypeptide hormones such as insulin are not as extensively studied as FSH, they are known to play essential roles in regulating Sertoli cell function. Insulin is considered to be an essential factor for growth of these cells in serum-free medium, where it has effects on multiple metabolic parameters (28,276). Insulin appears to have an effect on uptake and incorporation of labeled orthophosphate into free nucleotide pools, which, in turn, is manifested by an increased rate of label incorporation into poly $(A)^+$ RNA (277). Moreover, it has been shown to increase thymidine incorporation into DNA, leucine incorporation into protein, lactate production (278), and hexose uptake (279). With regard to its effects on specific differentiated function in Sertoli cells, insulin has been shown to be essential for the secretion of both transferrin and rABP (276). All of the effects of insulin on Sertoli cells are observed *in vitro* at micromolar concentrations even though most of the actions that are thought to be mediated via the insulin receptor are believed to be maximally stimulated by nanomolar quantities of this hormone. Insulinlike effects are also observed with nanomolar concentrations of insulinlike growth factor I (DNA synthesis and hexose uptake) and insulinlike growth factor II (DNA and protein synthesis as well as lactate production) (278,279). It is, therefore, possible that many, if not all, of these responses of Sertoli cells to insulin may result from the binding of this hormone to insulinlike growth receptors. An alternative explanation for the requirement for supraphysiological amounts of insulin is that Sertoli cells produce insulinase *in vitro* which is particularly active in serum-free medium.

Glucagon. Another polypeptide hormone known to have an affect on the Sertoli cell is glucagon (280). This hormone increases cAMP levels and has a magnitude and kinetic response similar to that of FSH. One of the consequences of glucagon stimulation is an increase in the rate of testosterone aromatization, a response also produced by other substances, including FSH, that stimulate cAMP production by Sertoli cells (280).

Calcitonin. Receptors for calcitonin are present in membrane fractions of testes, and autoradiographic studies show these binding sites are located primarily on Leydig cells (281,282); however, examination of published autoradiographs suggests that binding sites for calcitonin are also present in seminiferous tubules, possibly on Sertoli cells. Although the physiologic functions of calcitonin receptors on testicular cells are not known, this hormone regulates (a) cAMP accumulation in the TM_4 Sertoli cell line and (b) rABP secretion by primary Sertoli cells (283). In addition, this peptide increases the total concentration of both androgen and estrogen receptors in TM_4 cells (283). The observation that 8-bromo-cAMP decreases androgen and estrogen receptor concentrations suggests that the calcitonin effect is not mediated by cAMP. The fact that calcitonin-induced increases in receptor levels can be reversed by lowering extracellular calcium concentrations suggests that the effects of calcitonin might be modulated by this cation. The effects of calcium channel blockers and calcium ionophores are consistent with this hypothesis (283). Thus, part of the effects of calcitonin on Sertoli cell function are mediated by cAMP and others by changes in intracellular calcium.

Pro-Opiomelanocortin (POMC)-Derived Peptides. Peptides derived from the hormone precursor POMC, including ACTH, α-MSH, and β-endorphin, have a variety of effects on Sertoli cells (284,285). This conclusion was reached after the demonstration of the presence of POMC-derived peptides in the male reproductive tract (286,287). In the testis, immunostainable β-endorphin and ACTH-like substances are in the cytoplasm of Leydig cells (288,289), suggesting that POMC-derived peptides are synthesized in this cell type. This postulate is supported by the demonstration of POMC mRNA in Leydig cells (290–292). The low concentrations of secreted peptides suggest that they might have autocrine and/or paracrine functions within the testis rather than effects via the general circulation (288).

Following the demonstration that all peptides with MSH-like activity, including ACTH, stimulate adenylate cyclase activity in the Sertoli cell (284,293,294), a detailed study was performed to determine the effects of α-MSH and des-acetyl-α-MSH on Sertoli cell function *in vitro* (295). Both peptides stimulate cAMP secretion and aromatase activity in primary Sertoli cell cultures when incubated in the presence of a phosphodiesterase inhibitor, FSH, or forskolin. Both peptides shift the FSH dose-response curve to the left, thus making the cells more sensitive to this gonadotropin. Furthermore, the apparent potencies of α-MSH and its desacetyl derivative are similar when measured on Sertoli cells. In this regard, it is well known that *N*-acetylation has an important effect on the biological activities of POMC-derived peptides in the central nervous system. For example, in several behavioral actions such as arousal and expressive grooming, α-MSH is much more potent than des-acetyl-α-MSH (296,297). By contrast, only the des-acetylated form is able to block opiate analgesia and opiate receptor binding (298). In addition, the activity of α-MSH on melanosome dispersion in melanocytes of *Rana pipiens* is also influenced by *N*-acetylation because α-MSH is much more active than des-acetyl-α-MSH (299). In view of these observations, it is surprising that these peptides are equipotent in their actions on Sertoli cells (295).

To search for possible effects of β-endorphin on the testis, an investigation of its influence on testis growth in young animals was undertaken. Potent opiate antagonists, nalmefene or naloxone, injected intratesticularly in neonatal rats increased the compensatory hypertrophy following unilateral castration (300–302). Naloxone and β-endorphin antiserum increase Sertoli cell division in explants of neonatal testis (303). Treatment of hemicastrate male rats with the opiate antagonists was also associated with a marked rise in rABP secretion (284,302). The increase in testicular size and rABP secretion following antagonist administration is consistent with the hypothesis that β-endorphin or other endogenous opiates inhibit Sertoli cell growth and secretion during early testicular development and are antagonistic to gonadotropins during this time period. Recent studies have demonstrated the presence of receptors for β-endorphin on Sertoli cells (304). It is of note that other opiates in addition to β-endorphin are present in testes based on the results of peptide isolation and the presence of proenkephalin and prodynorphin mRNA (305).

Taken together, the results from *in vivo* and *in vitro* experiments suggest that peptides derived from various portions of the POMC molecule have differential effects on Sertoli cells. For example, ACTH stimulates proliferation and both ACTH and MSH-like peptides increase cAMP production by primary Sertoli cells and Sertoli cell lines. By contrast, β-endorphin or another endogenous opiate inhibits Sertoli cell proliferation and secretion of specific proteins. Opposing effects of different POMC-derived peptides in other tissues are also known. For example, ACTH-like peptides and β-endorphin have opposing effects on different types of behavior. β-Endorphin is a potent inhibitor of the lordosis response in rats, whereas α-MSH facilitates female sexual behavior (306). The interesting question raised by these observations is how two peptides, which can be produced in equimolar amounts from the same precursor, regulate opposite biological responses. The answer to this question is not known for any tissue where POMC is synthesized, but several possibilities may exist. First, there may be selective processing of POMC, as is the case for ACTH in anterior pituitary and α-MSH in intermediate pituitary. Second, the activity of a peptide can be altered by *N*-acetylation, as occurs for MSH and β-endorphin in the intermediate pituitary. Finally, there may be rapid turnover of a peptide from one portion of POMC by a locally produced protease which would allow a peptide from another part of the molecule to dominate (307). Thus, the biological consequences of POMC synthesis in the testis will depend not only on the amount of the precursor that is made but also on which of its component peptides are present in biologically active form. The autocrine effects of POMC-derived peptides on Leydig cells are reviewed elsewhere (308).

Steroid Hormones

A number of steroid hormones are known (or believed) to affect Sertoli cells because of either demonstrated effects or the presence of specific steroid receptors. The most extensively studied steroid is testosterone. In addition, other molecules, including estrogens, progestins, and glucocorticoids, also have effects on these cells. *In vitro* experiments permit detailed studies of the action of steroid hormones on Sertoli cells which are difficult to achieve with *in vivo* experiments.

Androgens

Sertoli cells have typical androgen receptors (309,310) that mediate the effects of testosterone. Some of the effects of this steroid mimic those of FSH. This can be observed on the secretion of selected proteins (24) and on the maintenance of spermatogenesis after hypophysectomy. In addition, some of the actions of testosterone appear to oppose those of FSH. For example, androgens inhibit FSH-induced "rounding up" of Sertoli cells in culture, presumably by enhancing actin organization, whereas FSH stimulates disorganization (311). In addition, testosterone inhibits FSH induced inhibin secretion (P. Morris, *unpublished observations*). There are also morphological changes in Sertoli cells deprived of androgens. These include alteration in nuclear and mitochondrial morphology, increase in the amount of lipid droplets, and decreases in smooth endoplasmic reticulum (312).

Testosterone also has a general effect on transcriptional activity (232). The addition of this hormone to Sertoli cells in culture produces a rapid but transient (15 min) increase in RNA polymerase II activity followed by a further and more prolonged increase 3 to 6 hr later. This is in contrast to the response to FSH which increases polymerase, I, II, and III over a longer time period (232,233).

The effects of androgens on more terminally differentiated functions have also been studied using rABP as an endpoint both *in vivo* (313,314) and *in vitro* (255,315,316). Rat Sertoli cells cultured in serum-free medium survive longer and secrete more rABP when cultured with physiological concentrations of testosterone (255,317).

The *in vivo* effects of testosterone are dependent upon the stage of differentiation of the seminiferous epithelium. In immature long-term hypophysectomized animals, testicular but not epididymal levels of rABP increase following androgen treatment (91). This is consistent with the *in vitro* data outlined above. In mature animals, there is a slow decrease in testicular and epididymal rABP levels following hypophysectomy that can be prevented by the administration of androgen (318). If the testis is allowed to fully regress, subsequent androgen administration will increase rABP levels in the blood and testis but not in the epididymis (319). In this latter instance, FSH is required in order to facilitate secretion of rABP into the tubular lumen as well as facilitate its transport to the epididymis. These different effects of testosterone on the Sertoli cells of newly hypophysectomized and on fully regressed hypophysectomized animals are likely to be a function of the differentiated state of this cell. If Sertoli cells are fully differentiated, their function can be maintained by testosterone alone, whereas the acquisition of the differentiated state typical of intact adults occurs in response to FSH. Other explanations for these findings are also possible. For example, little is known about the *in situ* degradation of rABP during testicular regression and about the effects of testosterone on this process. It is, therefore, not known whether testosterone affects degradation as well as synthesis of rABP under these experimental conditions. It is possible that some effects of testosterone on maintaining the differentiated state may be to slow the turnover of rABP and other proteins as it is known to do in other organs (320).

Studies by Tsutsui and Ishii (321,322) suggest that, in some species, androgens play a role in regulating the number of FSH receptors. Testosterone administration to birds during photoperiod-induced testicular regression results in an increase in the density of FSH receptors. This response could also be observed with the administration of FSH, but combined treatment with both hormones caused a greater increase in these receptors. These authors suggest that testosterone and FSH act synergistically to induce FSH-receptor synthesis.

Finally, it should be noted that part of the effects of testosterone on Sertoli cells appear to be mediated by the action of this steroid on testicular myoid cells. An androgen-dependent product from these cells has marked effects on several Sertoli cell functions (157,158). These observations are perhaps similar to those in prostate, where mesenchyme cells appear to mediate most, if not all, of the actions of testosterone on the epithelium (323,324).

Estrogens

As noted above, Sertoli cells produce estradiol, which is under the influence of FSH. The observation that Sertoli cell lines have estrogen receptors and are growth inhibited by low levels of estradiol suggested that these cells might also respond to this class of hormones (31). Interestingly, estrogen receptors are present at or below the level of detection (12 ± 3 fmole/mg protein) in newly isolated Sertoli cells. However, following 15 days of culture, estrogen receptors rise to 50 ± 5 fmole/mg protein (325). The appearance of estrogen receptors in primary Sertoli cells with increasing time in culture suggests that these cells are capable of producing receptors even though they are undetectable in freshly isolated cells. There are many reasons why estrogen receptors may not be measurable in newly isolated Sertoli cells. One possibility is that these receptors are present in only a limited number of Sertoli cells along the length of the tubule as a result of interaction with germ cells of a specific stage of the cycle. The fact that estrogen receptors are not detectable in segments of tubules isolated and pooled according to stage of spermatogenic cycle argues against this possibility (326). An alternative possibility is that estrogen receptors are uniformly suppressed in all Sertoli cells by some testicular product(s). One candidate for such an agent is estradiol per se, since it is locally produced and causes translocation of receptors to the nucleus so that the content available in the cytoplasm at any one time is low. On the other hand, testosterone decreases estrogen receptors in a Sertoli cell line, suggesting that androgens may regulate this class of receptors in the seminiferous epithelium (325).

Other Steroid Hormones

There are limited studies on the effects of steroids other than androgens and estrogens on Sertoli cells. Both hydrocortisone and progesterone can be shown to increase ABP secretion *in vitro* (255). Progesterone also increases RNA polymerase II in Sertoli-enriched cultures, and Wagle et al. (327) suggested that these responses may be mediated through the androgen receptor.

Vitamins

Deficiencies of certain vitamins reduce fertility in male rats. Although reduced fertility in such animals could result from the systemic effects of the deficient states, the finding that at least two vitamins influence Sertoli cell function *in vitro* and that another has receptors in Sertoli cells suggests that these agents might directly influence testicular function.

Vitamin A

Vitamin A (retinol) is a lipid soluble vitamin known to be important in vision and fertility. Male animals made deficient in this vitamin cease production of spermatozoa, and several markers of Sertoli cell function also change. The production of at least two secretory proteins by Sertoli cells *in vitro* is influenced by retinol. This includes the increased secretion of transferrin in the presence of either retinol or retinoic acid (127,129). In addition, rABP is also influenced similarly by this vitamin (127,255,276). There is one report indicating that vitamin A also lowers uridine pools in Sertoli cells (328) but does not change either total protein synthesis or growth rate.

Retinoids exert their actions via an intracellular binding protein much like the classic steroid hormone receptor. Vitamin A is concentrated by Sertoli cells (329); in addition, these cells contain an intracellular retinol-binding protein (13). This receptor has the same physical characteristics as the cellular retinol-binding protein found in the liver but is distinct from the cellular retinoic acid-binding protein found in germ cells (330). The amount of this cellular retinol-binding protein in the Sertoli cells is influenced by both FSH (13) and germ cell association (330).

Vitamin E

Another lipoidal vitamin that affects Sertoli cells is vitamin E. This substance appears to have no effect on transferrin production by Sertoli cells, but it does influence rABP secretion (127). In addition, vitamin E influences both plating efficiency and multiplication of immature Sertoli cells in culture (127).

Vitamin D

There are few studies on the effects of vitamin D_3 and its analogs on Sertoli cell function either *in vivo* or *in vitro*. There is, however, a high-affinity low-capacity receptor for this steroid. There is little or no vitamin D_3 receptor in testes from prepubertal rats, but there is a progressive increase as animals mature (331). Several studies suggest that these receptors are localized in a nongerminal component of seminiferous tubules, probably Sertoli cells (332). These findings support the postulate that the Sertoli cell is a site of action for vitamin D_3, but do not explain its role in testicular biology.

Cell Matrix and Attachment Factors

One of the more significant advances in cell biology in recent years has been the elucidation of how the insoluble extracellular matrix (ECM) which comprises the basal lamina influences the differentiated function of epithelial cells. This subject has been reviewed in detail by several groups of investigators (333–336). When Sertoli cells are grown *in vitro* on plastic, they form a flattened and well-spread monolayer. By contrast, the same cells grown on plastic covered by peritubular myoid cells (which produce ECM) (337), testicular extracellular matrix (338), or extracellular matrix derived from a tumor (339) attain a more cuboidal shape and spread more slowly. These morphological characteristics more closely resemble those of Sertoli cells *in vivo* (Fig. 7). Other characteristics of Sertoli cells grown on ECM are the formation of typical basolateral junctional complexes (338,339) and a decrease in the rate of DNA synthesis. These are also characteristics of Sertoli cells as they mature *in vivo* (273,339).

The effects of ECM on various differentiated functions revealed that the basal secretion of several proteins is enhanced when cells are grown on this substance. These include the well-established markers such as ABP and transferrin, as well as type-1 collagen. Furthermore, there is a substantial increase in total protein secretion (339). In addition to improving the basal secretion of proteins, ECM of all types markedly increases the response of Sertoli cells to FSH. The ECM formed by myoid cells had the most pronounced effect when compared to matrix components (337).

One poorly understood function of differentiated Sertoli cells is their ability to support the growth of germ cells. When Sertoli cells and their accompanying germ cells are plated on plastic surfaces, the germ cells degenerate over a period of several days. When comparable cultures are grown on ECM, viable germinal elements are retained in the Sertoli cell monolayer, but do not show signs of further development (339). These observations suggest that ECM contributes to Sertoli cell differentiation so as to allow them to maintain one component of Sertoli cell/germ cell interaction; however, contact alone is not sufficient to support further maturation. Germ cells can mature in culture in defined medium when a tubular segment is grown with intact basal lamina (ECM) and myoid cells (340).

One exciting observation is the demonstration that mixed Sertoli and germ cell cultures from 10-day-old rat testes are capable of reassociating into structures that resemble seminiferous tubules when grown on thick ECM layers. These cords of Sertoli cells are organized with spermatogonia embedded on their outer surfaces; junctional complexes form between adjacent Sertoli cells, and the interior of these cords becomes inaccessible to large molecules. With further time in culture, cells with morphological characteristics of late pachytene spermatocytes appear within the tubules (339). These results

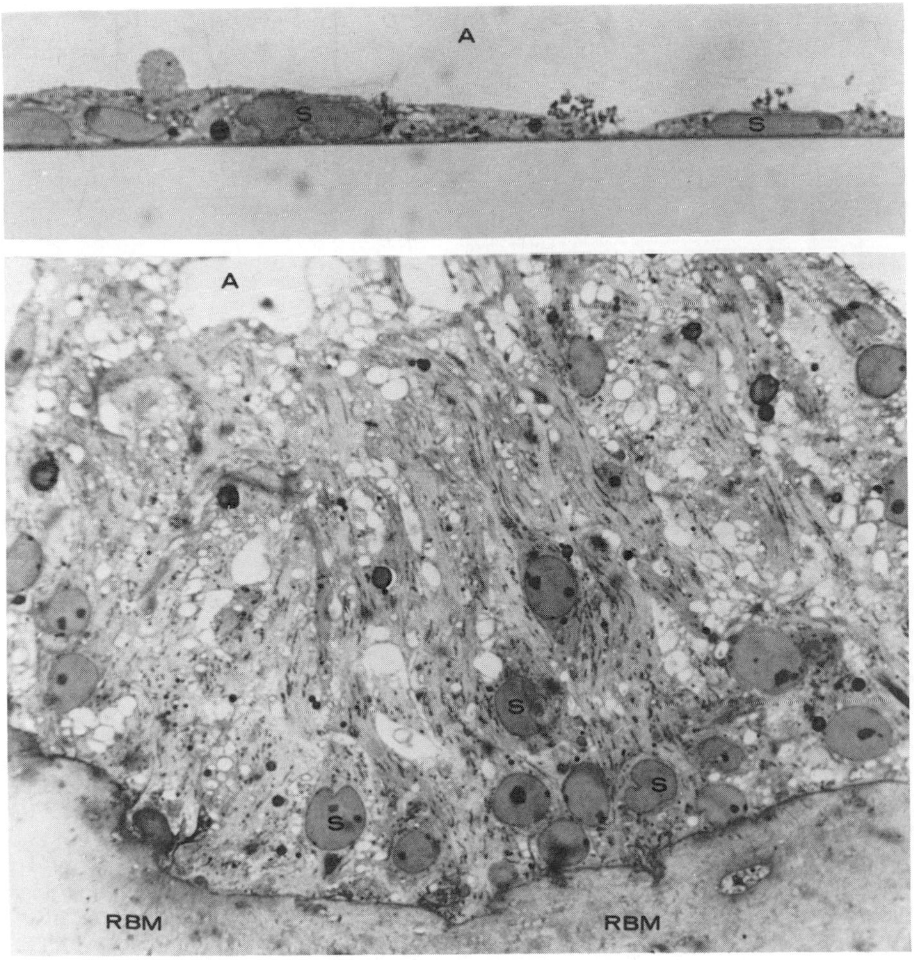

FIG. 7. Light micrographs (×780) of Sertoli cells grown in serum-free media in the presence of various substrata. **Top:** Cells on plastic appear as low squamous cells with flattened nuclei. **Bottom:** Sertoli cells on reconstituted basement membrane (RBM) from the ETS tumor form tall monolayers with extensive cytoplasmic stalks. Sertoli cell nuclei (S) and apical surface (A) are indicated. (From ref. 339.)

suggest that under appropriate conditions the native ability of Sertoli cells to form tubules occurs, thus producing an isolated environment that will allow the development of germ cells.

THE CELLULAR REGULATION OF SERTOLI CELLS

In addition to the effects of various humoral factors, Sertoli cells are also dramatically altered by the cells that surround them. These include germ, myoid, and Leydig cells. In some instances, these interactions require direct contact between cells, whereas other interactions depend upon paracrine factors. In many instances, the type of factor that mediates such interactions is not known.

Germ Cell/Sertoli Cell Interactions

The ability to examine Sertoli cell/germ cell interaction is based upon the observation that germ cells are not randomly distributed along the length of the seminiferous epithelium but are strictly arranged in defined cell associations or stages. The most commonly used classification of germ cell associations makes use of the "steps of spermatogenesis," as seen in sections stained with periodic acid-Schiff reagent (138). In the rat, there are 14 morphologic stages, and each stage has a constant duration. The succession of different stages in time at a given point in the tubular epithelium is called the *spermatogenic cycle.* For each species, the duration of the cycle is constant and can be thought of as a biological clock for that species. In the rat, the complete cycle of stages lasts 12 days. Thus, at any site along the seminiferous tubule, the germ cells associated with a group of Sertoli cells are morphologically distinct from those associated with an adjacent group of Sertoli cells just a few millimeters away (Fig. 8) (32).

Sertoli cell morphology also varies along the length of the seminiferous tubule in conjunction with the changes in germ cells. These include changes in nuclear morphology, the quantity of cytoplasmic lipid, and the variation of the number of enzymes, as analyzed by histochemistry (138,341,342). These changes in Sertoli cells are coordinated with the spermatogenic cycle.

The different stages of the spermatogenic cycle in adjacent segments of the seminiferous tubular epithelium can be demonstrated by transillumination in freshly isolated, unstained, seminiferous tubules (Fig. 8) (343). Based on light transmission, tubular segments representing different stages can be isolated and studied *in vitro.* Using these segments, it is possible to demonstrate that many aspects of Sertoli cell function vary along the length of the tubule in concert with the stage of the cycle (32). For example, maximal FSH binding to receptors occurs on Sertoli cells in Stage I, whereas the maximal

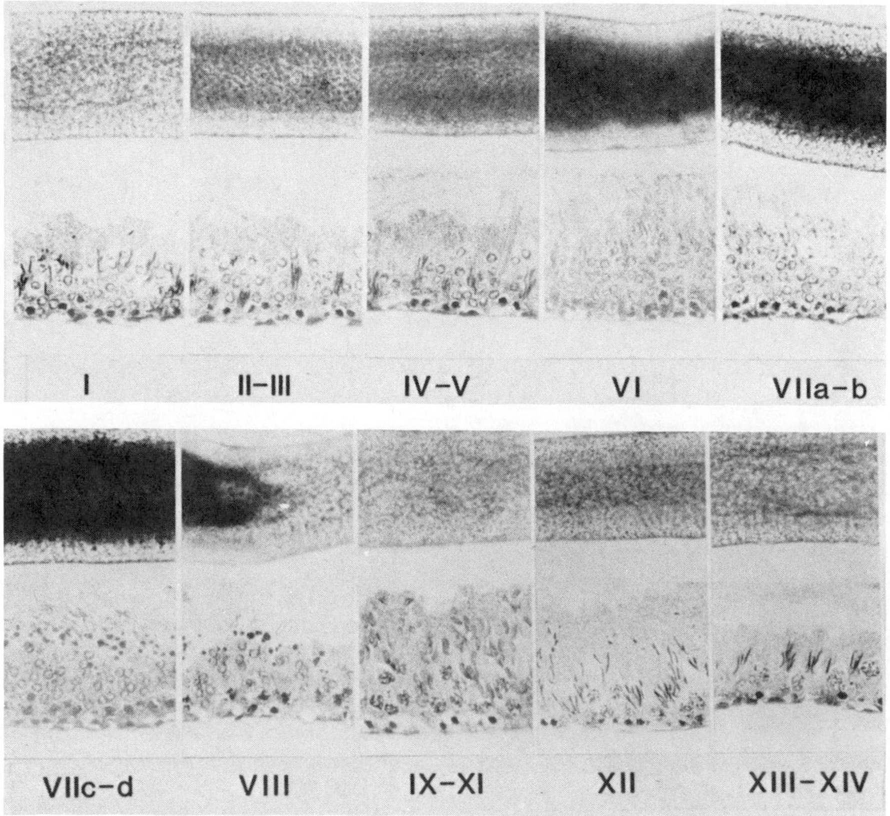

FIG. 8. Transillumination pattern of freshly isolated rat seminiferous tubule related to the stage of the cycle of the seminiferous tubule epithelium. The roman numerals indicate the stages of the cycle as defined by the fixed stained sections along the lower portion of the figure. These are correlated with the transillumination of the unfixed tubules in the upper portion of the figure. (From ref. 32.)

FSH-stimulated cAMP production occurs in stages I to III and cAMP phosphodiesterase is highest in stages VI and VII (32). In addition to the cyclic changes in constitutive Sertoli cell proteins, the secretion of a number of products by these cells is also enhanced during specific stages of the germ cell cycle (Fig. 9). For example, plasminogen activator is specifically secreted only in stages VII and VIII of the cycle (344). As noted above, this enzyme is believed to play a role in the release of maturing spermatids from the seminiferous tubular epithelium at stage VIII. Also at stage VIII, primary spermatocytes move from the basal compartment of the seminiferous tubular epithelium, through the junctional complexes between adjacent Sertoli cells, into the adluminal compartment. This process is also thought to involve plasminogen activator secreted by Sertoli cells. Androgen-binding protein is also secreted in a cyclic manner with a peak at stages IX to XI (318,345). The cyclic secretion of many other Sertoli cell products is known from *in vitro* studies using tubular segments isolated by the transillumination technique. Results of these studies indicate that both the morphology and the biological functions of Sertoli cells cycle with the germinal components of the seminiferous tubular epithelium. Existing information suggests that germ and Sertoli cells are the minimal elements required to form the biological clock in the seminiferous tubule (21).

Myoid Cell/Sertoli Cell Interactions

In addition to the germ cell/Sertoli cell interaction, myoid cells also interact with Sertoli cells and influence their behavior. As noted above, a factor elicited by these cells influences the secretion of specific proteins (157,158,259) by Sertoli cells *in vitro.* The secretion of rABP and transferrin, but not plasminogen activator, are stimulated. In addition, it appears not to be a mitogenic factor (158). The induction of this putative paracrine factor by peritubular myoid cells is stimulated by androgens but not estrogens (157). This observation raises the question as to whether the testosterone effects on Sertoli cells are direct; they might be indirect through testosterone's action on peritubular myoid production of this factor (157,158,346).

The effects of myoid cell interaction with Sertoli cells are not confined to secreted proteins. Several enzymes (i.e., lactic dehydrogenase, succinic dehydrogenase,

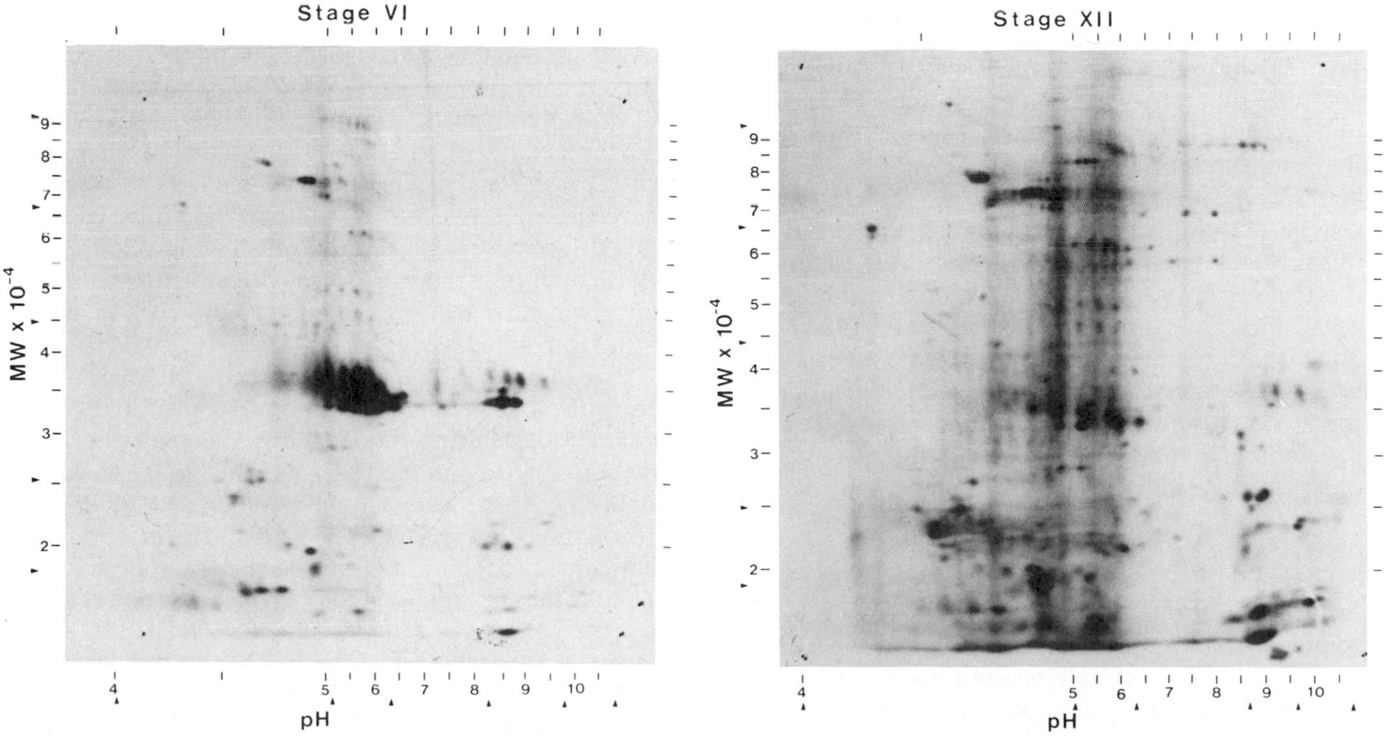

FIG. 9. Two-dimensional gel of electrophoresis of total ^{35}S-labeled secreted proteins at stage VI and stage XII of the cycle of the seminiferous tubular epithelium. Radiolabeled proteins were detected by fluorography. The position of the standards of each gel are indicated by the arrows next to the scales. The spots shown are believed to be proteins of Sertoli cell origin, because the segments were incubated in the absence of myoid cells. The pattern of secretion is reminiscent of those from two separate organs rather than from the same cells a few millimeters apart along the length of the seminiferous tubule. (From ref. 21.)

glucose-6-phosphate dehydrogenase, and nonspecific esterases) are maintained in Sertoli cells only when they are co-cultured with peritubular cells (347). In addition, there appears to be interaction between these two cell types with regard to the production and/or deposition of ECM (159,348). The presence of this ECM enhances plating efficiency and viability and accounts for the unique morphological characteristics seen in such cocultures (346,348). Finally, myoid cells can modulate the cyclic secretion of Sertoli cell proteins that are entrained by the spermatogenic cycle. As noted above, rABP secretion is maximal at stages IX to XI. The peak secretion occurs at the same stages whether myoid cells are present or not. However, in the presence of myoid cells, rABP secretion is three to five times higher than in the absence of these cells (59). We conclude that myoid cells act as an amplifier of the clock created by the Sertoli cell/germ cell unit.

Leydig Cell/Sertoli Cell Interactions

Cellular interactions of Sertoli cells also affect Leydig cells, either directly or in their link between germ cells and myoid cells. Paracrine factors rather than cell-cell contacts are believed to be the important means of communication between Leydig cells and the seminiferous tubule (349). Leydig cells show a cyclic variation in size which is dependent on the stage of tubules adjacent to them (350). In this case, the cells adjacent to stages VII and VIII tubules are larger than those associated with other stages. These observations are further enhanced by the demonstration that rat (260,351) and pig (352,353) Sertoli cells secrete a product that can stimulate Leydig cell steroid production. Furthermore, the secretion of this factor is enhanced by FSH. Thus, it is tempting to speculate that there is a substance produced by Sertoli cells which is regulated by endocrine (FSH) and paracrine factors (germinal cell associations) and communicates with the adjacent Leydig cells to modulate the local production of testosterone. Inhibin is one possible candidate for such a substance, since its production by Sertoli cells is stimulated by FSH and it, in turn, stimulates steroidogenesis in Leydig cells (C. W. Bardin, *unpublished observations*).

In summary, it appears that Sertoli cell functions are controlled not only by humoral factors but also by a complex paracrine system that modulates this cell's responses and modifies its functions in a manner dependent on cell-cell interactions between Sertoli cells, germ cells, Leydig cells, and myoid cells.

THE SERTOLI CELL *IN VIVO*

The multiple factors implicated in control of Sertoli cell function are derived not only from the different cell types within the testis, but also from the circulation and possibly the nervous system. This complexity of control mechanisms, coupled with the implicit heterogeneity of the Sertoli cell population arising from the cycle of the seminiferous epithelium, cannot, as yet, be replicated for *in vitro* studies. Thus, there is impetus for studies of Sertoli cell function in the intact animal to complement the *in vitro* approach. The areas where significant advances have been made in recent years include: Sertoli cell differentiation; Sertoli cell proliferation; and the bidirectional release of Sertoli cell products in naturally occurring and experimentally induced pathophysiologic states.

Sertoli Cell Differentiation and Proliferation

The differentiation of Sertoli cells *in utero* and their subsequent proliferation during fetal and neonatal life are complex events involving presently unknown signals for the initiation of differentiation from within the testis as well as humoral factors from extratesticular sites. In the normal animal, this sequence of events results in the complement of mature Sertoli cells required to support spermatogenesis and fertility. Although there are, at present, several clearly identifiable factors modulating this progression, it appears that, once initiated, the process continues in an orderly fashion and is completed prior to puberty. In the rat, this occurs over a period of about 30 days of fetal and neonatal life. During this period a number of events are characterized by the appearance of clear markers that provide convenient indices for investigating the factors involved in modulating this developmental process. Recent morphological studies describe the developmental aspects of Sertoli cell ultrastructure in the rat (354), mouse (355), pig (356), and human (357). Specific reference to those aspects of ultrastructure development which have direct bearing on Sertoli cell function *in vivo* are noted below.

In mammals, the appearance of the primordial Sertoli cell is the first identifiable event in testicular differentiation. Early histological studies of the differentiating fetal rat testis (358), confirmed later by careful ultrastructural studies (359), indicate that these cells appear on day 13 post-fertilization and then aggregate and form seminiferous cords the following day. The signal responsible for eliciting the appearance of the primordial Sertoli cell has not been identified but presumably is related to gene products, encoded on the Y chromosome, that signal the bipotential fetal gonad to develop into a testis. The initial appearance of the differentiating Sertoli cell and subsequent organogenesis, that is, aggregation and formation of seminiferous cords, are apparently regulated independently, since early organogenesis is inhibited by factors present in fetal calf serum while morphologically distinct Sertoli cells are maintained (360,361).

Following the initial appearance of distinct Sertoli cells and the early stages of organogenesis, there is a period of rapid proliferation. In the rat this begins in fetal life, continues during early neonatal life, and is complete before closure of the blood-testis barrier (271,362). Since the Sertoli cell population in the adult animal is determined during this period, any disruption of the proliferative process will have a profound effect by reducing the ultimate Sertoli cell population, which will, in turn, influence testicular size of the adult animal. Recent studies confirm that inhibition of Sertoli cell proliferation in neonatal rats causes a decreased Sertoli cell population in the adult animal, with a commensurate decrease in germinal elements (363).

A number of investigators have studied this critical period in Sertoli cell development. Short-term uptake (2 hr) of [^{3}H]thymidine indicates that an appreciable fraction of Sertoli cells (~15%) are undergoing replication as early as day 16 post-conception (pc) (271). This fraction increases steadily to reach a peak value of about 27% on day 20 pc and then decreases monotonically to reach undetectable levels by day 21 post-partum. Thus, in the rat, maximum rates of Sertoli cell proliferation occur during fetal life. The cessation of Sertoli cell proliferation prior to puberty also occurs in other species. Studies of [^{3}H]thymidine uptake by Sertoli cell nuclei suggest that proliferation ceases by day 12 postpartum in the mouse (364) and does not occur in the post pubertal monkey (365). Histometric studies of the developing testis in the human indicated that a relatively constant Sertoli cell population may be achieved by as early as 3 years of age (366).

Based on proliferation rates found for Sertoli cells in the rat, it would appear that factors influencing this process in fetal animals have the greatest potential for affecting testicular function in adults, whereas events during late neonatal and prepubertal life may have a less dramatic affect on the adult Sertoli cell population.

Since FSH and androgens have long been considered to be of primary importance in regulation of Sertoli cell function *in vivo,* both in immature and adult animals, it is reasonable to expect them also to play a role in Sertoli cell function in the fetal animal. Recent studies employing *in utero* neutralization of FSH as well as ablation of the fetal pituitary by decapitation suggest that FSH is a major factor in controlling expansion of the Sertoli cell population in fetal rats (270). In addition, Sertoli cells from fetuses deprived of endogenous FSH are responsive to both FSH and cyclic nucleotides *in vitro,* and these agents can restore rates of Sertoli cell proliferation to those found in intact animals. Ablation studies performed in the fetal pig show that Sertoli cell ultrastructure develops normally, even in the absence of the fetal pituitary (356). These findings are consistent with the notion that a pattern for development of Sertoli cells is laid down early in fetal life and proceeds according to this intrinsic pattern.

The observation that FSH is essential for initiating spermatogenesis in immature animals, an event occurring near the end of the proliferative phase of Sertoli cell development, suggests the continued influence of FSH on Sertoli cells during this period (367). Studies using antibodies to neutralize FSH and LH in immature animals pointed out the importance of FSH to the normal developmental process (368). Further discussions of the *in vivo* effects of FSH as well as other modulating factors during the proliferative period are presented at several points later in this review.

Since FSH action on the Sertoli cell is dependent on its binding to surface receptors, the strong influence of this hormone on proliferation, as well as its continued action during prepubertal life, implies the existence of an adequate receptor population. Autoradiographic studies showing that Sertoli cells have most of the FSH-binding sites in the testis (369) are supported by binding studies using enriched Sertoli cell preparations and highly purified Leydig cells as negative controls (193). FSH binding is detectable in fetal rat testes shortly after the appearance of differentiated Sertoli cells (370). Thereafter, total testicular receptor content rises slowly until about 19 days pc, when there is a dramatic increase concomitant with the rapid rise in testis weight during the period of maximal Sertoli cell proliferation (271). Following birth, FSH binding per testis continues to increase, although there are conflicting data regarding the duration of the increase. One study shows a 10-fold increase, leading to a plateau on day 15, and then constant levels until at least day 60 of age (371), whereas other studies indicate a steady increase until well past puberty (372). Studies in the sheep (373) and mouse (372) also show that steady increases in total testicular FSH receptors continue through puberty. Experiments using isolated Sertoli cells confirm the early increase in FSH receptors, but do not resolve the question regarding FSH receptor numbers in nonproliferating Sertoli cells because the studies were not continued beyond 15 days of age (193). The attainment of a constant level of binding at about day 15, concomitant with cessation of Sertoli cell proliferation, would be consistent with a constant number of FSH receptors per Sertoli cell from day 15 through puberty, whereas continuously increasing FSH binding per testis would imply increasing numbers of FSH receptors per Sertoli cell during this period. Regardless of this problem, it appears that the number of FSH receptors per Sertoli cell does not change dramatically during the proliferative period, since the increase in total receptor content roughly parallels testicular growth during this time when the Sertoli cell is the dominant cell type in the testes.

During the period of rapid cell proliferation, Sertoli cells must begin to acquire the machinery required to support spermatogenesis in the mature animal. These changes include ultrastructural development of organelles and acquisition of metabolic and synthetic activities characteristic of the mature cell. Some of the morphological properties and expressed functions of these cells are held in common with other cell types in the animal, whereas others are unique to Sertoli cells. Although these general properties are important indices of Sertoli cell function, they can be used only when it can be verified that the responses originate in the Sertoli cell. Several of the secretory proteins synthesized by the Sertoli cell have been enumerated in previous sections of this review, as has their usefulness for *in vitro* studies of cell regulation. However, it is the Sertoli cell specific properties that provide the most convenient markers for the study of Sertoli cell function *in vivo.*

Concomitant with the morphological changes marking the differentiation of Sertoli cells *in utero* is the appearance of distinct Sertoli cell products. Of the known Sertoli cell proteins, the first to appear is anti-Müllerian hormone (AMH), or Müllerian duct inhibiting factor (MIF), the product responsible for causing regression of the Müllerian ducts in male fetuses (374). In addition to producing regression of normal fetal tissue, AMH also produces regression of carcinomas both *in vitro* (375–377) and *in vivo* (378). The appearance of AMH in the testis is associated with differentiating seminiferous cords in both fetal calves (379) and rats (380). Although cross-species bioreactivity provides a means for assay of bovine (381) and porcine (382) AMH using rat Müllerian ducts as target organs, there are species differences in molecular structure as evidenced by the inability of antibodies directed toward bovine AMH to cross-react with chicken, pig, mouse, rat, or human AMH (379,383). The expression of AMH in fetal rats occurs shortly after Sertoli cell differentiation and is not dependent on testicular organogenesis (380). Precise timing for the onset of AMH synthesis in the fetal rat awaits the development of sensitive species-specific probes. It has been shown that porcine (384) and bovine (379) Sertoli cells continue to secrete AMH during the postnatal period. AMH secretion drops sharply before any histological markers of puberty, including formation of the blood-testis barrier, are seen in the pig (384), and AMH levels drop to near the limit of detection in testes of 3-month-old calves (379).

One of the most striking morphologically and physiologically important features of Sertoli cells to develop in the prepubertal rat is the formation of Sertoli-Sertoli junctional complexes, which form an important part of the blood-testis barrier.

Although investigators have described several factors that can modulate formation of Sertoli-Sertoli junctional complexes, this process appears to proceed according to a predetermined pattern in much the same manner as seen in the proliferative phase. In normal rats the formation of the blood-testis barrier begins at about day 15 post-partum, just as Sertoli cell proliferation declines, and is completed between days 16 and 19. Junctional complexes do not form synchronously along the length of the developing seminiferous tubule, but rather seem to reflect the stage of spermatogenesis of the associated germ cells (385). Thus, although formation of the blood-testis barrier is modulated by germ cells, it is not dependent on their presence, since testes depleted of germinal elements by *in utero* irradiation still form junctional complexes (386,387). Although the junctional complexes in these Sertoli cell-enriched (SCE) testes appear about 10 days later than normal, they exclude electron opaque tracers and allow the formation of patent tubules capable of directing Sertoli cell secretory products to the epididymis. Competent blood-testis barriers also are formed in testes of several other animals with impaired fertility (367,388–390). The time of barrier formation seems also to be delayed in some of these animals.

Of the many Sertoli cell products characterized to date, androgen-binding protein remains the best marker of this cell *in vivo.* Measurement of this protein provides a useful index of Sertoli cell function during neonatal development and at puberty. However, studies in fetal rats are complicated by immunoreactive rABP-like material in the serum from fetuses of both sexes (2). This latter protein is produced by the fetal liver (391); synthesis by the liver commences prior to testicular differentiation, peaks at about 17 days pc, and then declines rapidly to undetectable levels prior to birth (Fig. 10) (92). This is associated with a decline of the levels of this protein in serum (Fig. 11). As noted above in the section on Sertoli cell proteins, this product of the fetal liver is believed to be the serum protein TeBG, which is present in adult animals of other species, but not in the adult rat.

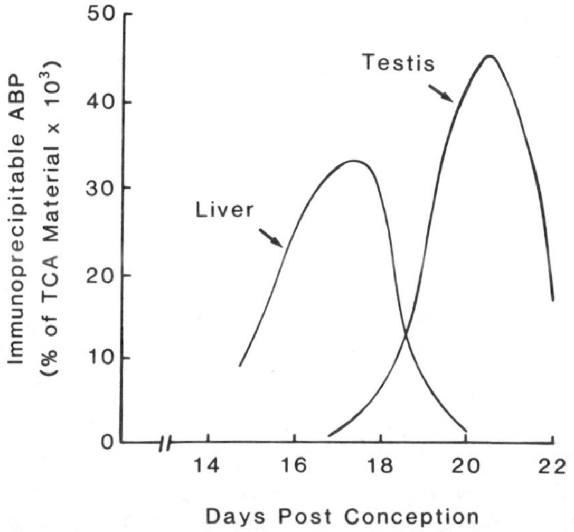

FIG. 10. Synthesis of immunoprecipitable ABP by liver and testes of fetal rats. Tissue minces of liver and testes, obtained from fetal rats at several times post-conception, were incubated for 17 hr in tissue culture medium supplemented with [^{35}S]methionine. Media were collected and centrifuged, and the ABP in the supernatants was immunoprecipitated with rabbit anti-rat ABP. Results are expressed as percentage of total TCA precipitable counts. (Adapted from ref. 392.)

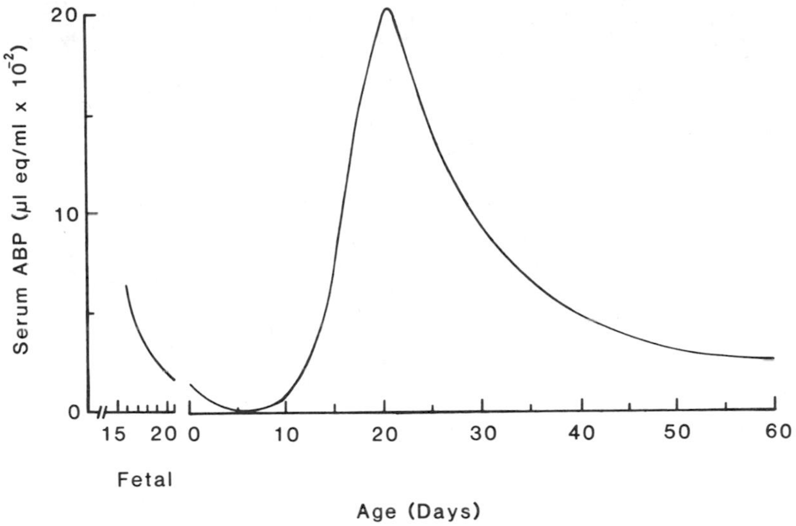

FIG. 11. Serum ABP levels in rats from 16 days post-conception to 60 days of age. Data are expressed as microliter equivalents (μl eq) of a standard rat epididymal cytosol measured in each assay (393). 1 μl eq, when measured by steady state polyacrylamide gel electrophoresis (72), is equivalent to 9.8 ± 0.9-fmole binding sites. Data are a composite from several studies: fetal and neonatal data (92), days 10–60 (388–390).

Synthesis of rABP by the fetal testis is first detectable on day 18 pc, the time at which high synthetic rates are also observed in the liver (Fig. 10). Production of rABP by the testis increases rapidly, reaching a maximum at about day 21 pc, and then declines quickly before birth (392). Synthesis of rABP by the fetal testis corresponds to the time of maximum Sertoli cell proliferation (271) and the onset of the dramatic increase in total testicular FSH receptor levels (370). Except for this short burst of secretory activity late in fetal life, the Sertoli cell appears to be relatively quiescent during the remainder of the proliferative phase of development. Because of its small size, the fetal testis presumably contributes very little to rABP in blood at this time.

For the first few days following birth, immunoreactive rABP levels in blood are similar in both sexes and continue to decrease. This immunoreactive material is presumably the residual from the protein produced by the liver prior to birth, since the testes are quiescent with regard to rABP production during this period (Fig. 11). By day 4 postpartum, evidence for renewed synthetic activity by the Sertoli cell is marked by increasing levels of rABP in the blood of male rats, whereas those in females continue to decrease and reach undetectable levels by day 5 (92). During this time, and prior to formation of Sertoli-Sertoli junctional complexes, the entire surface of the Sertoli cell is in communication with the extracellular compartment. As a consequence, secretory products of Sertoli cells are released directly into the extracellular compartment and can presumably pass readily into blood. Thus, rABP levels in blood provide an index of the relative synthetic and secretory activity of the Sertoli cell over this time period. From days 4 through 10, serum rABP levels are maintained at a steady low level and then begin to rise slowly (Fig. 11). Then, at about the time Sertoli cell proliferation stops, serum rABP dramatically rises, increasing over 10-fold between days 12 and 20 (66). Testicular rABP concentration also shows a dramatic rise over this time period as a result of (a) increased synthesis and (b) retention following formation of the junctional complexes (Fig. 12, bottom panel) (388). Sometime between days 17 and 25 (the exact time depends on the animal strain or experimental manipulation), serum rABP levels peak and then begin to drop once the patent tubules form and direct the bulk of ABP to the epididymis. Prior to this time, low but detectable levels of rABP are in the epididymis (388). Nonetheless, the appearance of rABP, as measured by steroid binding, or the abrupt increase in immunoassayable rABP in the epididymis serves as a marker for formation of a patent tubule (386). Unlike serum rABP, testicular and epididymal ABP content continue to increase after day 25, then plateau at adult levels by day 60 (Fig. 12, top panel) (388,390).

Although it was known for several years that the testis was capable of synthesizing estrogen, there were conflicting views regarding the role of Sertoli cells in this process (394–397). It is now clear that in the immature rat, Sertoli cells express FSH-dependent aromatase activity (192,193). In the mature animal, aromatase activity in Sertoli cells declines as they become relatively refractory to the action of FSH, whereas Leydig cells are the major site of estrogen synthesis in the adult (193). The physiological importance of aromatization by Sertoli cells in the immature animal has yet to be determined.

The Control of Testicular Size

Morphometric analysis of the adult rat testis shows the seminiferous tubule to comprise over 80% of testicular volume (398). Thus, the more important contributors to

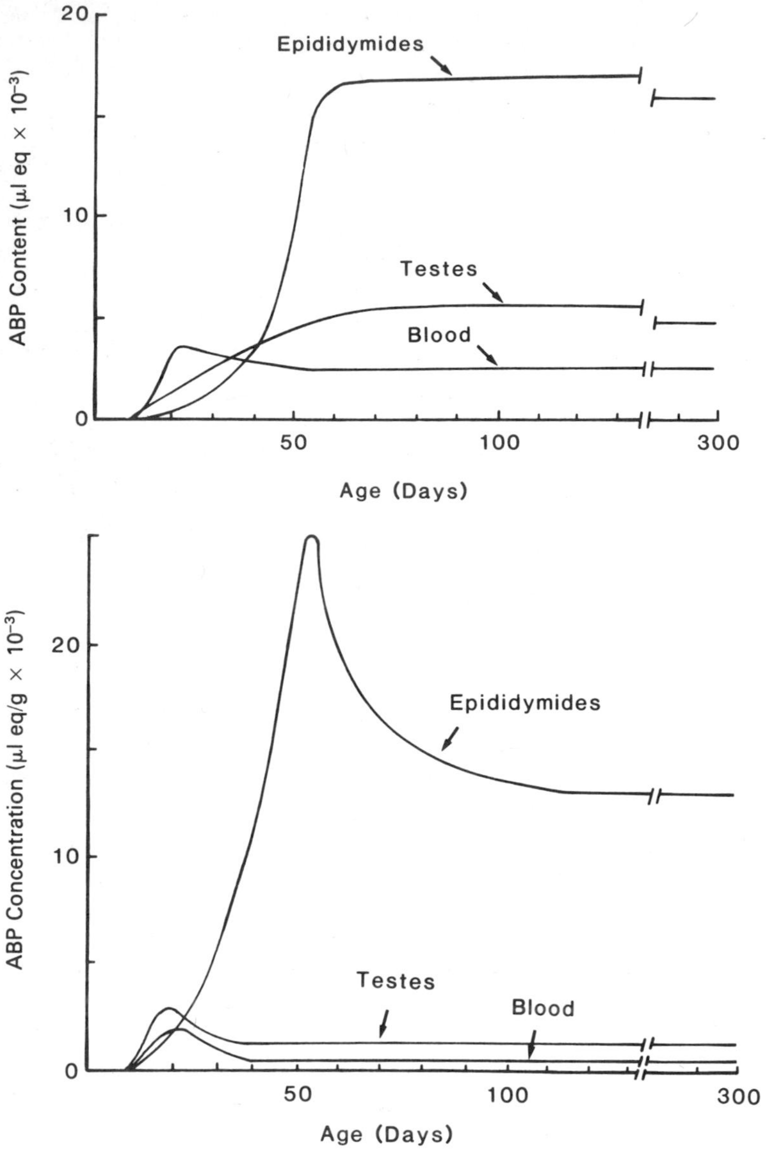

FIG. 12. Distribution of ABP in rat testes, epididymides and blood. **Top panel:** Total rABP content per organ pair or in the vascular compartment, expressed as μl eq (see legend of Fig. 11 for details). **Bottom panel:** rABP concentration in testes, epididymides, and blood. Tissue concentration is expressed as μl eq per g tissue (wet weight); serum concentration is expressed as μl eq per ml. Data are a composite of data from several studies (388–390).

determination of adult testis size are Sertoli and germ cell populations. The highly irregular shape of the Sertoli cell relative to the germ cell makes it difficult to provide a quantitative measurement of the volume density of the former cell (399). However, careful measurement of the numerical density of both these cell types shows the ratio of germ cells to Sertoli cells to be about 16:1, with the distribution of cell types staying relatively constant throughout the cycle of the seminiferous epithelium (400). The ratio of volume density of germ cells to Sertoli cells is somewhat less than this figure because the germinal elements are smaller than Sertoli cells. A quantitative estimate based on comparison of testis weights of normal adult animals and of those in which germ cells were depleted by *in utero* irradiation (the SCE animal) puts this ratio at about 5:1 (386). This estimate does not take into consideration the possibility that Sertoli cells in these animals may not have the same volume as those in normal animals. A second estimation of this latter ratio can be made using the Sertoli cell volume of 6,012 μm^3 (derived from a completely reconstructed rat Sertoli cell) (401), the estimate of 22×10^6 Sertoli cells per adult testis, and the observation that the epithelium comprises 80% of the cross-sectional area of the seminiferous tubule (400). This yields a 10:1 ratio of volume density of germ cells to Sertoli cells. These calculations provide crude estimates at best and point to some of the problems that must be overcome if the quantitative aspects of testicular growth are to be understood. The most formidable problem is related to the complex structure of the Sertoli cell and the attendant problem of providing easily accessible number and volume densities of this cell type, as well as others in the testis, under a variety of experimental conditions. The effort involved in the elegant reconstructions of a single Sertoli cell in the rat (399,401,402), and more recently the monkey (403), emphasizes this point.

In spite of the difficulty in providing detailed quantitative measurement of the individual testicular cell types, it is still possible to approach the study of testis growth by other means. One approach is to focus on events occurring in the perinatal period, since this is a period of rapid Sertoli cell proliferation and testis growth. Factors affecting Sertoli cell proliferation, either positively or negatively, have a large potential for influencing testicular function in the adult animal. This notion is supported by the observation that, in the mouse, once Sertoli cell proliferation stops there is a constant numerical relationship between Sertoli cells and germ cells (364). This implies that the germ cell population in the adult animal is dependent on the number of Sertoli cells. The decision to study factors that influence Sertoli cell number during the neonatal period is bolstered by the observation that agents influencing this parameter during this period have permanent effects on testicular size in the adult animal, whereas the same treatments may be ineffectual or transitory when performed after puberty. Hemicastration and LH-releasing hormone (LHRH) antiserum are examples of such treatments that increase and decrease testicular size, respectively (388,404).

The fact that there is compensatory increase in weight by the testis remaining after hemicastration of prepubertal animals has been known for over 90 years (405). For a complete bibliography, see ref. 404. The weight increase has been fairly consistently referred to as *compensatory hypertrophy,* but there is evidence for both hypertrophy and hyperplasia. Compensatory increase in testicular size occurs only in rats hemicastrated before puberty, and the relative increase over that of a testis from an intact animal persists in the adult (404). The earlier the hemicastration is performed, the more pronounced its effect on testicular weight (404), an observation consistent with the finding that Sertoli cell proliferation after birth is programmed to continuously decrease, and thus there is presumably less time for the Sertoli cell population to respond before cell division is no longer possible (271). In rats hemicastrated on day 3, it is possible to see increased Sertoli cell proliferation, as measured by [^{3}H]-thymidine incorporation into nuclei, as soon as 8 hr following surgery; however, this is not manifested as a significant weight increase until day 1 after surgery (406). In such animals, increasing Sertoli cell proliferation is observed for at least 4 days following hemicastration; however, 1 week following surgery, Sertoli cells in hemicastrated and intact animals showed comparable labeling, which became undetectable by 3 weeks following surgery. Thus, although the Sertoli cells in the testis remaining after hemicastration respond by increasing their proliferative rate relative to intact animals, the duration of the proliferative phase is not affected. This is consistent with the concept, noted earlier, that the temporal events influencing Sertoli cell development unfold according to a predetermined pattern, although the responses at a given time are subject to modulation. Increased Sertoli cell proliferation in the hemicastrated animal implies that a portion of the testis weight gain is attributable to Sertoli cell hyperplasia.

As noted before, FSH is implicated as a major factor in regulation of Sertoli cell proliferation. The hyperplasia noted following hemicastration in rats is associated with a doubling of serum FSH levels within 4 to 5 days of surgery (404,406) that is maintained throughout the proliferative phase (404). Similar studies in the hemicastrated lamb show serum FSH levels three to four times those found in intact animals (407,408). Serum FSH in hemicastrated lambs also remains elevated for several weeks and then returns, before lumen formation, to values found in intact animals. In addition to augmented cell division, Sertoli cells in these animals also show an increase in their cytoplasm (408), an observation consistent with both hypertropic and hyperplastic responses to hemicastration in some species. In contrast to serum FSH, LH levels in hemicastrated animals are either unaffected (406,407) or elevated only transiently (408). Whether this differential response in gonadotropin release is due to reduced inhibin levels secondary to the reduced Sertoli cell component in hemicastrated animals or due, instead, to other modulatory factors is not presently known. The fact that testis weight gain in hemicastrated rats can be inhibited by administration of testicular extracts, presumably containing inhibin, would be consistent with the former possibility (409).

The increased division of Sertoli cells seen in hemicastrated rats (406) and sheep (408) implies that Sertoli cell hypertrophy is an important factor in the increase in testicular weight observed immediately after surgery in these animals. This is supported by studies on animals with SCE testes in which hemicastration produced the same relative growth found in normal hemicastrates of the same age (404). Since animals with SCE testes are essentially devoid of germ cells, we can also conclude that the bulk of Sertoli cell hypertrophy is mediated by nongerminal elements.

Evidence presented thus far indicates that the FSH-provoked Sertoli cell proliferation in response to hemicastration in young animals is the major influence on testicular development at this time. In contrast, testosterone, a hormone known to be important for maintenance of spermatogenesis in the adult animal, plays an inhibitory role in this process. That is, the administration of testosterone to hemicastrated animals prevents the compensatory increase in testis weight (409). Studies using [^{3}H]thymidine as an index of Sertoli cell division indicate that this is due to suppression of Sertoli cell proliferation in the remaining testis (406). In addition, there is short-term suppression of Sertoli cell proliferation in intact animals that were administered testosterone. Whether testosterone has a direct effect on the Sertoli cell or is acting indirectly, perhaps via negative feedback on FSH levels, is not known.

The growth of the testes following hemicastration is in contrast to arrested or incomplete testicular development associated with hypogonadotropic hypogonadism, an inherited condition in humans (410) and other species, which is believed to be due, in most instances, to a deficiency of LHRH. In such animals, testicular size is reduced and spermatogenesis is incomplete, as expected, as a result of LH and FSH deficiency. Interestingly, testicular size increases but is never restored to normal when men with severe hypogonadotropic hypogonadism are treated for many months with FSH and hCG to restore spermatogenesis. Similarly, hypogonadotropic mice show an increase in testicular size to only 50% of normal following restoration of LH and FSH secretion by brain transplants, even though spermatogenesis was restored (292). It was suspected that the reason why testicular size was not restored following treatment for hypogonadotropism was that adequate replacement therapy was never achieved. Studies on transient hypogonadotropism provide an alternative explanation for these observations.

Transient hypogonadotropism can be produced in adult and immature animals by passive immunization with antiserum to LHRH (LHRH-AS) (for additional references see ref. 92). Male rats passively immunized at 5 days of age with a single injection of LHRH-AS have small testes and reduced fertility as adults despite normal serum concentrations of gonadotropins and testosterone (411,412). The LHRH-AS treatment results in a transient decrease of FSH, LH, and androgen levels during the period of Sertoli cell proliferation. This is associated with decreased testicular weights from day 10 onward to adult life (Fig. 13). In addition, altered Sertoli cell function is also apparent. There is a delay of 5 days in the peaks of serum and testicular rABP concentrations, suggesting that closure of the blood-testis barrier may also be retarded in animals treated with LHRH-AS. This was corroborated by a similar delay in the increase of epididymal rABP concentrations. A second effect is the decrease in secretory activity of Sertoli cells, which is reflected in reduced testicular, epididymal, and serum ABP levels from day 10 on. Testicular rABP and LH/hCG receptor content are commensurate with testis weight at all time points, a finding consistent with the fact that Sertoli and Leydig cell compartments are equally affected by LHRH-AS treatment. By contrast, at all ages, the cross sections of seminiferous tubules in animals that received LHRH-AS are normal, and spermatogenesis develops at the expected time (92). Since the seminiferous tubules appear to have a normal complement of germ cells when viewed in cross section, the most likely explanation for the marked reduction in testes size is that the length of

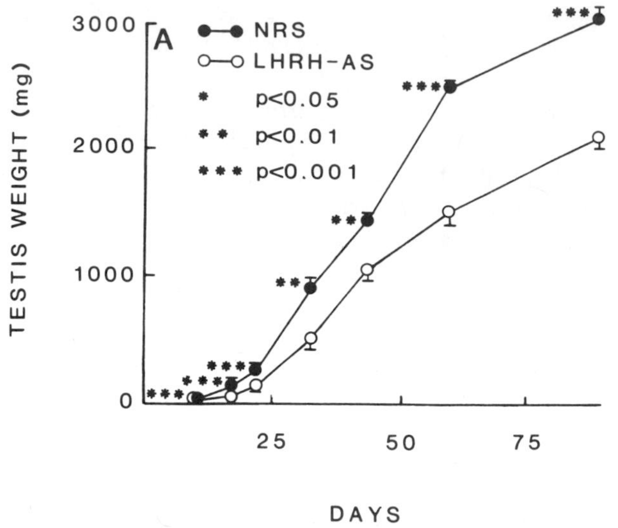

FIG. 13. Testis weight (organ pairs) in animals treated at 5 days of age with LHRH-AS or NRS. Values expressed as means ± SEM. (Data from ref. 388.)

the tubules is foreshortened by a decrease in the Sertoli cell number, which is accompanied by a parallel decrease in germ cells. Since FSH plays a central role in Sertoli cell proliferation, one possible explanation for the decreased testis size in animals treated with LHRH-AS would be the lack of adequate FSH to support the normal proliferative phase which occurs prior to puberty. Thereafter, the testes were unable to show a proliferative response to normal gonadotropin levels, which returned after the Sertoli cell proliferative phase was complete. This suggests a physiological basis for the inability of testes in adult mice and humans with hypogonadotropic hypogonadism to respond to seemingly adequate gonadotropin treatment with an increase to normal testicular size.

Following neonatal hemicastration, testis size is permanently increased, probably because of the FSH-provoked proliferative response of Sertoli cells in the remaining testis; after LHRH-AS administration, testis size permanently decreases, possibly as a result of inadequate FSH during the proliferative phase. Since these two treatments produce opposite effects on adult testes, they were combined in a 2^2 factorial design to investigate whether they operate through a common factor. LHRH-AS treatment was found to decrease testis weights in both intact and hemicastrated animals, and there was an increase in testis size in response to hemicastration in both LHRH-AS-treated and control animals. Analysis of variance failed to show any interactive terms between the two treatments (413), a finding consistent with both affecting a common regulatory system. Whether these two treatments result in different distributions in cell volume and number density of the various cell types comprising the adult testis is not known. Resolution of this question requires a detailed morphometric study of the testes from these animals, a rather formidable undertaking. Although there is compelling evidence that FSH is the primary mediator of Sertoli cell proliferation, it is clear that factors other than FSH are important in determinating testis size in the adult animal. These include the complex interaction of the various cell types within the testis, mediated by paracrine function as well as by cell-cell contact.

The identification of β-endorphin-related and other peptides derived from pro-opiomelanocortin (POMC) in the male reproductive tract (286), and specifically in Leydig cells of hypophysectomized rats (287,288), suggested that opiatelike molecules were produced within the testis and, thus, could have direct action on testicular function. The presence of immunoreactive β-endorphin in testicular interstitial fluid, at levels severalfold higher than in peripheral blood, and the ability of hCG and LHRH analogs to modulate its levels in interstitial fluid (414) strongly support this hypothesis. Furthermore, the observation that Sertoli cells isolated from adult testes possess opiate receptors, coupled with the ability of naloxone to block the suppression of rABP synthesis by [D-Ala^2]-β-endorphin in Sertoli cells isolated from 18-day-old animals (304), are consistent with the direct action of opiates on the Sertoli cell.

Several lines of evidence suggest that testicular opiates may regulate Sertoli cell proliferation. A single intratesticular injection of opiate antagonist on day 5 was found to enhance testis weight gain and to promote testicular differentiation, which was evident in both hemicastrated and intact animals 5 to 6 days later (300); however, the effect of enhanced weight gain did not persist in hemicastrated animals (302). The inability to affect testis size by systemic administration of these antagonists, at dosages found to cause maximal weight gain by intratesticular delivery (302), supports the concept of a localized function for intratesticular opiates. Decreased serum testosterone levels (300) and tetosterone production (302) in animals treated with opiate antagonist suggest that intratesticular opiates also facilitate testosterone secretion by Leydig cells, whereas increased serum rABP levels in the same animals suggests that intratesticular opiates may exert a direct suppressive effect on Sertoli cell function. The correlation of decreased androgen levels and enhanced testicular weight gain in young hemicastrated animals treated with opiate antagonists may be related to consistent findings that administration of testosterone to young hemicastrated animals suppresses Sertoli cell proliferation and testis weight gain (406). Studies indicating that β-endorphin inhibits Sertoli cell proliferation in fetal (415) and in neonatal animals (303), when Sertoli cell proliferation is at a maximum (271), imply paracrine communication between Leydig and Sertoli cells. Whether the effect on Sertoli cells is a result of the direct action of intratesticular opiates or is the consequence of their action on Leydig cells remains to be elucidated.

The studies on testicular growth during fetal and neonatal life suggest that there are both positive and negative regulators of this process. FSH and possibly other agents that increase Sertoli cell cAMP production, such as β-adrenergic agonists and peptides with MSH activity, stimulate, whereas β-endorphin and other intratesticular opiates inhibit, Sertoli cell growth. Since total sperm production by a testis is limited by the number of Sertoli cells, the regulatory mechanisms that modulate Sertoli cell division are, in turn, determinants of testicular size and sperm output.

Bidirectional Secretion of Sertoli Cell Products into Seminiferous Tubules and Blood

Bidirectional Secretion by Normal Seminiferous Tubules

As outlined previously, in adult rats the majority of rABP is secreted into the lumen of the seminiferous tubule and subsequently transported, along with spermatozoa, to the epididymis via the rete testis and efferent ductules. In the epididymis a portion of rABP is taken up by the initial segment of the caput (63,64), and the remainder disappears during its passage through the epididymis (68), with minimal amounts being detectable in the vas deferens (416). Direct measurements of luminal fluid obtained by micropuncture from various points in the reproductive tract indicate that more than 95% of rABP is lost between the rete testis and cauda epididymis (43).

In the rat, extracellular proteins capable of binding androgens were considered to be confined to the reproductive tract because no specific binding activity could be found in serum (83). However, the development of a sensitive radioimmunoassay led to the discovery of rABP in the blood of mature male rats (74). Although serum rABP concentration is low compared to testicular and epididymal tissue concentrations, in the adult rat the total rABP content of the vascular compartment is equivalent to half the testicular content and accounts for an appreciable fraction of daily rABP production (Fig. 12). Evidence suggesting that proteins as large as rABP cannot pass from the lumen of the reproductive tract into blood, and the observation that several factors have differential effects on the rABP content of the testicular, epididymal, and blood compartments, gave rise to the concept of bidirectional release of this protein from the Sertoli cell (66). The major route of release is into the lumen of the seminiferous tubule, with subsequent transport to the epididymis; the minor route is from the basal aspect of the Sertoli cell into the interstitial space of the testis, with subsequent passage through the lymphatics to the vascular compartment. The decreasing gradient of rABP levels from the lumen of the seminiferous tubule to interstitial fluid, to peripheral blood, is consistent with this hypothesis (43). Calculations based on rABP pool sizes and half-lives in blood and epididymis of normal adult animals indicate that of the daily ABP production by the testes, 80% is transported to the epididymides and 20% is released into blood (66). More recent measurements permitting refinement of the values on which these calculations are based indicate no substantial changes in the conclusions drawn from the earlier studies (G. L. Gunsalus, *unpublished results*). An alternative calculation based on direct measurements of rABP levels in seminiferous tubular and interstitial fluid, as well as on flow rates of testicular lymph and of rete testis fluid to the efferent ducts, estimates rABP secretion to be 67% intratubular and 33% extratubular (43).

Several lines of evidence support the concept for basal release of Sertoli cell secretory proteins. As discussed briefly in a previous section of this review, the Sertoli-Sertoli junctional complexes separate the seminiferous tubule into the exterior and interior compartments (36,417). The inability of electron-opaque molecules (418) as well as proteins (419) and hormones (420), found normally in the blood, to move from the basal compartment past the Sertoli-Sertoli tight junctions and into the adluminal compartment implies that passage in the direction opposite the adluminal compartment would also be restricted. Indeed, the ability of the tight junctions in the seminiferous tubule and rete testis to withstand increased intraluminal pressure generated by efferent duct ligation and to restrict fluid loss from the lumen attests to the physical integrity of the barrier. A number of studies, in one or more species, have confirmed that, after ligation, tight junctions are maintained in both seminiferous tubules and rete testis under this condition (421–425). Although the tight junctions in the rest of the reproductive tract are not as extensively developed as in the testis, they are sufficient to maintain patent tubules and to prevent escape of luminal contents into the blood. Studies to determine whether rABP could escape from the epididymis and thus be an additional source of blood rABP showed that this pathway could, at best, contribute minimally (416). This also confirmed earlier studies (68) that indicated the epididymis to be the major site of ABP degradation. The site of blood ABP degradation is not known, but, by analogy to other serum glycoproteins, is presumed to be the liver (426).

The distribution and levels of rABP in the rat change dramatically between the appearance of Sertoli cells in the fetus and the achievement of sexual maturity in the adult. Over this time period, rABP levels in the various compartments correlate with several important events in the developmental process. In a previous section we described the distribution of rABP during the time of Sertoli cell proliferation (late fetal life to 15 days postpartum) and the temporal correlations with formation of the blood-testis barrier and arrival of mature spermatozoa in the epididymis (refer to Figs. 11 and 12). After 60 days of age, when the animal reaches full reproductive potential, rABP levels in the testes, epididymides, and serum achieve a steady state that is maintained throughout adult life. In the adult animal, the relative rABP contents are 2:6:1 (testes:epididymides:serum). In animals affected by genetic abnormalities, hormonal treatment, or surgical manipulation, the distribution of rABP is altered dramatically. Thus, it is possible to determine the factors that regulate the bidirectional release of Sertoli cell products. There are *in vitro* and *in vivo* studies that suggest bidirectional secretion of Sertoli cell transferrin and testibumin, respectively (25,34), but these proteins are not as useful as rABP because they are synthesized by extragonadal cells.

Bidirectional ABP Release by Abnormal Tubules

Animals homozygous for the *grc* complex or heterozygous for *Hre* have severe germ cell depletion and are infertile, as are rats depleted of germ cells by *in utero* X-irradiation (SCE testes). Although animals with both genetic defects have small testes, they are not genetically related to each other (427). These unrelated genes were both associated with markedly reduced rABP content of the testes and epididymides (389,390). By contrast, the serum rABP concentrations were normal or near normal in both groups at all ages. These observations are compatible with the hypothesis that both *grc* and *Hre* influence the secretion of rABP from the apical portion of Sertoli cells and its subsequent transport to the epididymis, but have little or no effect upon rABP secretion from the base of Sertoli cells into blood. Animals with SCE testes have patterns of rABP secretion similar to those shown by animals carrying the *grc* and *Hre* genes (390). It is possible, therefore, that abnormal ABP secretion into the tubular lumen of these animals is secondary to germ cell depletion, a feature common to *grc/grc, Hre/+*, and X-ray-treated rats.

The very low epididymal rABP content but normal serum rABP levels seen in animals with germ cell depletion implies that little of the blood rABP is derived from the epididymis, an observation consistent with the testicular origin of blood rABP. This hypothesis was further supported by data from a whole-body kinetic study performed to determine rABP half-life ($t_{1/2}$) and metabolic clearance rate using endogenous and exogenous protein (416). In studies performed using both intact rats and animals with testes removed but epididymides intact, it was possible to conclude that under androgen deprivation the epididymides are capable of releasing substantial amounts of rABP into the blood, but that the epididymides of normal animals contribute little, if any, rABP to the vascular compartment. These studies are consistent with the hypothesis that the testes release rABP directly into the lymph and/or blood. This is also confirmed by measurements of rABP in samples obtained from the testis by micropuncture that show that the concentration of rABP in the interstitial fluid is eight times higher than that present in thoracic duct lymph and four times higher than that in serum (428).

Several other studies provided corroborating evidence for differential control of the bidirectional release of rABP from the testis. For example, the ability to increase the release of rABP into blood, independent of that to the epididymides, by administration of medroxyprogesterone acetate (MPA) (but not potent androgens) (429) or the antispermatogenic compound, tolnidamine (430), is consistent with this concept. Knowledge about factors that alter bidirectional secretion of rABP provides insight into *in vivo* and *in vitro* approaches that can be used to examine intracellular sorting of Sertoli cell products between the basal and adluminal compartments. In addition, measurements of rABP and other Sertoli cell proteins in the blood and reproductive tract provide a means of studying the pathophysiology of the seminiferous tubule.

The Functional Basis for Bidirectional Secretion

Since the bidirectional secretion of Sertoli cells has been studied using rABP as an indicator, it is appropriate to determine whether there are structural features of this protein that favor secretion into the adluminal, rather than the basal, compartment. rABP can be fractionated into two forms by concanavalin A-Sepharose (Con A) chromatography: Form I, which does not bind, and Form II, which does. The ratio of the two forms of rABP is 1:1 in blood and cytosols prepared from the testes and epididymides of young rats before closure of the blood-testis barrier. After maturity, there is a fivefold decrease in the amount of Form I rABP relative to Form II secreted into the blood (i.e., a ratio of 1:5) (89). These observations led to a study of the heterogeneity of rABP in samples collected by micropuncture from the testes of adult rats; the ratio of Form I to Form II rABP was approximately 1:1 in seminiferous tubular and rete testis fluids. By contrast, this ratio was approximately 1:5 in interstitial fluid. These results indicate that Form I rABP is secreted preferentially into the adluminal compartment of the seminiferous tubule rather than into the interstitial fluid in the mature rat and suggest that partitioning of rABP between the basal and adluminal compartments may depend, in part, on its carbohydrate composition (428). These observations provide the first insight into a possible mechanism for how differential partitioning of rABP into blood and tubular fluid might occur. It is also possible that other structural features of rABP could contribute to this process, as is the case for proteins in other bipolar cells.

If a structural feature of rABP can account for differential secretion of this protein into basal and adluminal compartments of the normal adult animals, then this same mechanism could also explain changes in secretion during maturation or hormonal treatment. For example, there is a peak in the serum rABP between 20 and 25 days of age in developing rats. The rapid decline in the blood levels of this protein after the peak has been associated with formation of the blood-testis barrier (Fig. 11). There may be, however, a discrepancy between the formation of the barrier at age 19 days and the beginning of the decline in serum levels, at least in some strains of rats. One explanation is that different strains have a 4- to 5-day variation in the time of blood-testis barrier closure. An alternate possibility is that the sorting mechanism for this protein has not yet matured, resulting in continued secretion of rABP into blood after formation of the barrier. One test of this hypothesis is provided by measurement of serum testibumin over this time period. Serum levels of this protein do not rise or fall before or after day 25. This suggests that formation of the blood-testis barrier per se may not be responsible for the decline of serum rABP during puberty. At this point, such a possibility remains to be established because testibumin is synthesized by extragonadal cells in the rat; thus, a rise and fall in testicular secretion into blood may not have been detected if the contribution of extratesticular sources were large relative to that from the testes (25). Either closure of the barrier or maturation of a sorting process for ABP could also explain why secretion of form I rbABP does not occur past 24 weeks of age in rabbits (341).

The Study of Sertoli Cell Function in Humans

It is presumed that Sertoli cells in human testes are bipolar, as they appear to be in the rat. If an appropriate group of unique testicular proteins can be identified that are secreted into blood as well as the seminiferous tubular lumen, then Sertoli cell (and therefore tubular) function in humans can be studied in much the same way as in other bipolar cells, for example, hepatocytes. Deranged liver function can be monitored by measurement of hepatic products that partition abnormally between blood and bile ducts. It is hoped that, in the future, abnormalities of testicular function can be assessed by detecting deranged secretion of Sertoli cell proteins. At present, the only such test that is believed to be an index of Sertoli cell function in humans is semen transferrin (131).

REFERENCES

1. Hansson V, Ritzén EM, French FS, Nayfeh SN. Androgen transport and receptor mechanisms in testis and epididymis. In: *Handbook of Physiology, Section 7: Endocrinology, Volume V: Male Reproductive System,* edited by Hamilton DW and Greep RO, Washington, D.C.: American Physiological Society; 1975: 173–201
2. Bardin CW, Musto N, Gunsalus G, Kotite N, Cheng S-L, Larrea F, Becker R. Extracellular androgen binding proteins. *Annu. Rev. Physiol.* 1981;43:189–198.
3. Ritzén EM, Hansson V, French FS. The Sertoli cell. In: *The Testis,* edited by Burger H and de Kretser D, New York: Raven Press; 1981:171–197.
4. de Jong FH, Robertson DM. Inhibin: 1985 Update on action and purification. *Mol. Cell. Endocrinol.* 1985;42:95–103.
5. Feig LA, Bellve AR, Erickson NH, Klagsbrun M. Sertoli cells contain a mitogenic poly peptide. *Proc. Natl. Acad. Sci. USA,* 1980;77:4774–4778.
6. Feig LA, Klagsbrun M, Bellve AR. Mitogenic polypeptide of the mammalian seminiferous epithelium: Biochemical characterization and partial purification. *J. Cell Biol.,* 1983;97:1435–1443.
7. Brown KD, Blakeley DM, Henville A, Setchell BP. Rete testis fluid contains a growth factor for cultured fibroblasts. *Biochem. Biophys. Res. Commun.,* 1982;105:391–397.
8. Holmes SD, Spotts G, Smith RG. Rat Sertoli cells secrete a growth factor that blocks epidermal growth factor (EGF) binding to its receptor. *J. Biol. Chem.* 1986;261:4076–4080.
9. Hall K, Ritzén EM, Johnsonbaugh RE, Parvinen M. Secretion of somatomedin-like compound from Sertoli cells *in vitro.* In: *Insulin-Like Growth Factors/Somatomedins,* edited by Spencer EM, New York: Walter de Gruyter; 1983:611–614.
10. Skinner MK, Griswold MD. Sertoli cells synthesize and secrete transferrin-like protein. *J. Biol. Chem.* 1980;255:9523–9525.
11. Skinner MK, Cosand WL, Griswold MD. Purification and characterization of testicular transferrin secreted by rat Sertoli cells. *Biochem. J.,* 1984;218:313–320.
12. Skinner MK, Griswold MD. Sertoli cells synthesize and secrete a ceruloplasmin-like protein. *Biol. Reprod.* 1983;28:1225–1230.
13. Huggenvik J, Griswold MD. Retinol binding protein in rat testicular cells. *J. Reprod. Fertil.* 1981;61:403–408.
14. Carson DD, Rosenberg LI, Blaner WS, Kato M, Lennarz WJ. Synthesis and secretion of a novel binding protein for retinol by a cell line derived from Sertoli cells. *J. Biol. Chem.* 1984;209: 3117–3123.
15. Brunner M, Moreira-Filho CA, Wachtel G, Wachtel S. Secretion of H-Y antigen. *Cell* 1984;37:615–620.
16. Lacroix M, Smith FE, Fritz IB. Secretion of plasminogen activator by Sertoli cell enriched cultures. *Mol. Cell. Endocrinol.* 1977;9:227–236.
17. Vihko KK, Suominen JJO, Parvinen M. Cellular regulation of plasminogen activator secretion during spermatogenesis. *Biol. Reprod.* 1984;31:383–390.
18. Fritz IB, Burdzy K, Setchell B, Blaschuk O. Ram rete testis fluid contains a protein clusterin which influences cell-cell interactions *in vitro. Biol. Reprod.* 1983;28:1173–1188.
19. Blaschuk OW, Fritz IB. Isoelectric forms of clusterin isolated from rate rete testis fluid and from secretions of primary cultures of ram and rat Sertoli cell enriched preparations. *Can. J. Biochem. Cell Biol.* 1984;62:456–461.
20. Tung PS, Fritz IB. Immunolocalization of clusterin in the ram testis, rete testis, and excurrent ducts. *Biol. Reprod.* 1985;33: 177–186.
21. Wright WW, Parvinen M, Musto NA, Gunsalus GL, Phillips DM, Mather JP, Bardin CW. Identification of stage-specific proteins synthesized by rat seminiferous tubules. *Biol. Reprod.* 1983;29:257–270.
22. Sylvester SR, Skinner MK, Griswold MD. A sulfated glycoprotein synthesized by Sertoli cells and by epididymal cells is a component of the sperm membrane. *Biol. Reprod.* 1984;31: 1087–1102.
23. DePhilip RM, Kierszenbaum AL. Hormonal regulation of protein synthesis, secretion and phosphorylation in cultured rat Sertoli cells. *Proc. Natl. Acad. Sci. USA* 1982;79:6551–6555.
24. Cheng CY, Mather JP, Byer AL, Bardin CW. Identification of hormonally responsive proteins in primary Sertoli cell culture medium by high performance liquid chromatography. *Endocrinology* 1986;118:480–488.
25. Cheng CY, Bardin CW. Rat testicular testibumin is a glycoprotein responsive to FSH and testosterone that shares immunodeterminants with albumin. *Biochemistry* 1986;25:5276–5288.
26. Cheng CY. A FSH and testosterone (T) responsive glycoprotein isolated from rat primary Sertoli cell-enriched cultures (SCCM) shares immunodeterminants with ram clusterin. *The Endocrine Society 68th Annual Meeting, June 25–27, 1986* (abstract 238).
27. Cheng CY, Grima JG, Bardin CW. Identification, purification and characterization of two testosterone (T) responsive glycoproteins from rat primary Sertoli cell culture medium (SCCM). *J. Cell Biol.* 1985;101:371a (abstract 1406).
28. Mather JP, Sato GH. The use of hormone-supplemented serum-free media in primary cultures. *Exp. Cell Res.* 1979;124: 215–222.
29. Mather JP. Establishment and characterization of two distinct mouse testicular epithelial cell lines. *Biol. Reprod.* 1980;23: 243–252.
30. Galdieri M, Ziparo E, Palombi F, Russo MA, Stefanini M. Sertoli cell cultures: A new model for the study of somatic germ cell interactions. *J. Androl.* 1981;2:249–254.
31. Mather JP, Zhuang L-Z, Perez-Infante V, Phillips DM. Culture of testicular cells in hormone-supplemented serum-free medium. In: *The Cell Biology of the Testis, Vol. 383,* edited by Bardin CW and Sherins RJ, New York: New York Academy of Sciences; 1982: 44–68.
32. Parvinen M. Regulation of the seminiferous epithelium. *Endocr. Rev.* 1982;3:404–417.
33. Byers SW, Hadley MA, Djakiew D, Dym M. Growth and characterization of polarized monolayers of epididymal epithelial cells and Sertoli cells in dual environment culture chambers. *J. Androl.* 1986;7:59–68.
34. Janecki A, Steinberger A. Polarized Sertoli cell function in a new two-component culture system. *J. Androl.* 1986;7:69–71.
35. Fawcett DW. Ultrastructure and function of the Sertoli cell. In: *Handbook of Physiology, Section 7: Endocrinology, Volume V: Male Reproductive System,* edited by Hamilton DW and Greep RO, Washington, D.C: American Physiological Society; 1975:21–55.
36. Setchell BP. *The Mammalian Testis,* Ithaca, New York: Cornell University Press; 1978.
37. Nicander L. An electron microscopical study of cell contacts in the seminiferous tubules of some mammals. *Z. Zellforsch. Mikrosk. Anat.* 1967;83:375–397.
38. Dym M, Fawcett DW. The blood-testis barrier in the rat and the physiological compartmentation of the seminiferous epithelium. *Biol. Reprod.* 1970;3:308–326.
39. Dym M. The fine structure of the monkey macaca Sertoli cell and its role in maintaining the blood-testis barrier. *Anat. Rec.* 1973;175:639–656.
40. Russell LD. The blood testis barrier and its formation relative to spermatocyte maturation in the adult rat: A lanthanum tracer study. *Anat. Rec.* 1978;190:99–112.
41. Mufly KE, Turner TT, Brown M, Hall PF. Contents of K^+ and Na^+ in seminiferous tubule and rete testis fluids from Sertoli cell-enriched testes. *Biol. Reprod.* 1985;33:1245–1251.
42. Johnson MH, Setchell BP. Protein and immunoglobin content in rete testis fluid of rams. *J. Reprod. Fertil.* 1968;17:403–406.
43. Turner TT, Jones CE, Howards SS, Ewing LL, Zegeye B, Gunsalus GL. On the androgen microenvironment of maturing spermatozoa. *Endocrinology* 1984;115:1925–1932.
44. Voglmayr JK, Scott TW, Setchell BP, Waites GMH. Metabolism of testicular spermatozoa and characteristics of testicular fluid collected from the conscious ram. *J. Reprod. Fertil.* 1967;14: 87–99.
45. Voglmayr JK, Larsen LH, White IG. Metabolism of spermatozoa and composition of fluid collected from the rete testis of living bulls. *J. Reprod. Fertil.* 1970;21:449–460.
46. Tuck RR, Setchell BP, Waites GMH, Young JA. The composi-

tion of fluid collected by micropuncture and catheterization from the seminiferous tubules and rete testis of rats. *Eur. J. Physiol. (Pflugers Arch.)* 1970;129:225–243.
47. Waites GMH, Einer-Jensen N. Collection and analysis of rete testis fluid from macaque monkeys. *J. Reprod. Fertil.* 1974;41: 505–508.
48. Free MJ, Jaffee RA. Collection of rete testis fluid from rats without previous efferent duct ligation. *Biol. Reprod.* 1979;20: 269–274.
49. Setchell BP. The secretion of fluid by the testis of rats, rams and goats with some observations on the effect of age, cryptorchidism and hypophysectomy. *J. Reprod. Fertil.* 1970;23:79–85.
50. Setchell BP, Duggan MC, Evans RW. The effect of gonadotropins on fluid secretion and sperm production by the rat and hamster testis. *J. Endocrinol.* 1973;56:27–36.
51. Setchell BP. Do the Sertoli cells secrete the rete testis fluid? *J. Reprod. Fertil.* 1969;19:391–392.
52. Tuck RR. "An investigation of the fluid secreted by the seminiferous tubules and the rete testis of the rat." BSc. (Med.) thesis, Sydney: University of Sydney; 1969.
53. Levine N, Marsh DJ. Micropuncture study of the fluid composition of 'Sertoli cell-only' seminiferous tubules in rats. *J. Reprod. Fertil.* 1975;43:547–550.
54. Linzell JL, Setchell BP. Metabolism, sperm and fluid production of the isolated perfused testis of the sheep and goat. *J. Physiol.* 1969;201:129–143.
55. Setchell BP, Voglmayr JK, Hinks NT. The effect of local heating on the flow and composition of rete testis fluid in the conscious ram. *J. Reprod. Fertil.* 1971;24:81–89.
56. Ribbert H. Die abscheidung intravenos injizierten gelosten Karmins in den Geweben. *Z. Allgem. Physiol.* 1904;4:201–214.
57. Bouffard G. Injection des couleurs de benzidine aux animaux normaux. *Ann. Inst. Pasteur* 1906;20:539–546.
58. Mostov KE, Simister NE. Transcytosis. *Cell* 1985;43:389–390.
59. Mather JP, Gunsalus GL, Musto NA, Cheng CY, Parvinen M, Wright W, Perez-Infante V, Margioris A, Liotta A, Becker R, Krieger DT, Bardin CW. The hormonal and cellular control of Sertoli cell secretion. *J. Steroid Biochem.* 1983;19:41–51.
60. Hansson V, Tveter KJ. Uptake and binding *in vivo* of ^{3}H-labelled androgen in the rat epididymal and ductus deferens. *Acta Endocrinol.* 1971;66:745–755.
61. Ritzén EM, Nayfeh SN, French FS, Dobbins MC. Demonstration of androgen binding components in rat epididymis cytosol and comparison with binding components in prostate and other tissues. *Endocrinology* 1971;89:143–151.
62. Vernon RG, Kopec B, Fritz IB. Observations on the binding of androgens by rat testis seminiferous tubules and testis extracts. *Mol. Cell. Endocrinol.* 1974;1:167–187.
63. Pelliniemi LJ, Dym M, Gunsalus GL, Musto NA, Bardin CW, Fawcett DW. Immunocytochemical localization of androgen binding protein in the male rat reproductive tract. *Endocrinology* 1981;108:925–931.
64. Attramadal A, Bardin CW, Gunsalus GL, Musto NA, Hansson V. Immunocytochemical localization of androgen binding protein in rat Sertoli and epididymal cells. *Biol. Reprod.* 1981;25: 983–988.
65. Musto N, Gunsalus G, Cheng CY, Tsong SD, Goldstein M, Phillips D, Bardin CW. Identification of androgen-binding proteins and their localization in the testis and male reproductive tract. In: *Recent Advances in Male Reproduction: Molecular Basis and Clinical Implications,* edited by D'Agata R, Lipsett MB, Polosa P, and van der Molen HJ, New York: Raven Press; 1983:37–45.
66. Gunsalus GL, Musto NA, Bardin CW. Bidirectional release of a Sertoli cell product, androgen binding protein, into the blood and seminiferous tubule. In: *Testicular Development, Structure and Function,* edited by Steinberger A and Steinberger E, New York: Raven Press; 1980:291–297.
67. Wright WW, Musto NA, Mather JP, Bardin CW. Sertoli cells secrete both testis-specific and serum proteins. *Proc. Natl. Acad. Sci. USA* 1981;78:7565–7569.
68. French FS, Ritzén EM. A high affinity androgen binding protein (ABP) in rat testis: Evidence for secretion into efferent duct fluid and absorption by epididymis. *Endocrinology* 1973;93:88–95.
69. Hagenas L, Ritzén EM, Ploen L, Hansson V, French FS, Nayfeh SN. Sertoli cell origin of testicular androgen binding protein. *Mol. Cell. Endocrinol.* 1975;2:339–350.
70. Sanborn BM, Elkington JSH, Steinberger A, Steinberger E. Androgen binding in the testis: *In vivo* production of androgen binding protein (ABP) by Sertoli cell cultures and measurement of nuclear bound androgen by a nuclear exchange assay. In: *Hormonal Regulation of Spermatogenesis,* edited by French FS, Hansson V, Ritzén EM, and Nayfeh SN, New York: Plenum Press; 1975:293–309.
71. Fritz IB, Rommerts FG, Louis BG, Dorrington JH. Regulation by follicle stimulating hormone and dibutyryl cyclic AMP of the formation of androgen-binding protein in Sertoli cell-enriched cultures. *J. Reprod. Fertil.* 1976;46:17–24.
72. Ritzén EM, French FS, Weddington SC, Nayfeh SN, Hansson V. Steroid binding in polyacrylamide gels: Quantitation at steady state conditions. *J. Biol. Chem.* 1974;249:6597–6604.
73. Musto NA, Bardin CW. Decreased levels of androgen binding protein in the reproductive tract of the restricted (H^{re}) rat. *Steroids* 1976;28:1–11.
74. Gunsalus GL, Musto NA, Bardin CW. Immunoassay of androgen binding protein in blood: A new approach for the study of the seminiferous tubule. *Science* 1978;200:65–66.
75. Taylor CA, Smith HE, Danzo BJ. Photoaffinity labeling of rat androgen binding protein. *Proc. Natl. Acad. Sci. USA* 1980; 234–238.
76. Danzo BJ, Taylor CA Jr, Eller BC. Some physiochemical characteristics of photoaffinity-labeled rabbit androgen-binding protein. *Endocrinology* 1982;111:1270–1277.
77. Danzo BJ, Dunn JC, Davies J. The presence of androgen-binding protein in the guinea-pig testis, epididymis and epididymal fluid. *Mol. Cell. Endocrinol.* 1982;28:513–527.
78. Weddington SC, Brandtzaeg P, Hansson V, French FS, Petrusz P, Nayfeh SN, Ritzén EM. Immunological cross reactivity between testicular androgen-binding protein and serum testosterone-binding globulin. *Nature* 1975;258:257.
79. Musto NA, Larrea F, Cheng S-L, Kotite N, Gunsalus GL, Bardin CW. Extracellular androgen binding proteins: Species comparison and structure-function relationships. *Ann. N.Y. Acad. Sci.* 1982;383:343–359.
80. Cheng CY, Frick J, Gunsalus GL, Musto NA, Bardin CW. Human testicular androgen binding protein shares immunodeterminants with serum testosterone-estradiol-binding globulin. *Endocrinology* 1984;114:1395–1401.
81. Kotite NJ, Cheng S-L, Musto NA, Gunsalus GL. Comparison of rabbit epididymal androgen binding protein and serum testosterone estradiol binding globulin. II. Immunological properties. *J. Steroid. Biochem.* 1986;25:171–176.
82. Musto NA, Gunsalus GL, Miljkovic M, Bardin CW. A novel affinity column for isolation of androgen binding protein from rat epididymis. *Endocr. Res. Commun.* 1977;4:147–157.
83. Corvol P, Bardin CW. Species distribution of testosterone binding globulin. *Biol. Reprod.* 1973;8:277–282.
84. Musto NA, Gunsalus GL, Bardin CW. Purification and characterization of androgen binding protein from the rat epididymis. *Biochemistry* 1980;19:2853–2860.
85. Larrea F, Musto NA, Gunsalus GL, Mather JP, Bardin CW. Origin of the heavy and light protomers of androgen-binding protein from the rat testis. *J. Biol. Chem.* 1981;256:12566–12573.
86. Larrea F, Musto NA, Gunsalus GL, Bardin CW. The microheterogeneity of rat androgen binding protein from the testis, rete testis fluid, and epididymis as demonstrated by immunoelectrophoresis and photoaffinity labeling. *Endocrinology* 1981;109: 1212–1220.
87. Joseph DR, Hall SH, French FS. Identification of complementary DNA clones that encode rat androgen binding protein. *J. Androl.* 1985;6:392–395.
88. Hansson V. Heterogeneity in end-terminal sugars of rabbit and rat androgen binding protein (ABP). *J. Androl.* 1981;4:220.
89. Cheng CY, Gunsalus GL, Musto NA, Bardin CW. The heterogeneity of rat androgen binding protein (rABP) in serum differs from that in testis and epididymis: Evidence for differential secretion. *Endocrinology* 1984;114:1386–1394.
90. Suzuki Y, Ito M, Sinohara H. Isolation and characterization of

sex-steroid-binding protein from rat and rabbit plasma. *J. Biochem.* 1981;89:231–236.

91. Gunsalus GL, Musto NA, Bardin CW. Factors affecting blood levels of androgen binding protein in the rat. *Int. J. Androl. (Suppl.)* 1978;2:482–493.
92. Gunsalus GL, Carreau S, Vogel DL, Musto NA, Bardin CW. Use of androgen binding protein to monitor development of the seminiferous epithelium. In: *Sexual Differentiation: Basic and Clinical Aspects,* edited by Serio M, Motta M, Zanisi M, Martini L, New York: Raven Press; 1984:53–64.
93. Carreau S, Musto NA, Bercu BB, Bardin CW, Gunsalus GL. L'Androgen binding protein, un marqueur de la fonction Sertolienne chez le rat (The androgen binding protein as an index of the rat Sertoli cell function). In: *Recent Progress in Cellular Endocrinology of the Testis, Proceedings of the 3rd European Workshop on the Testis,* INSERM. 1985;123:157–162.
94. Cheng S-L, Musto NA. Purification and characterization of androgen binding protein from rabbit epididymis. *Biochemistry* 1982;21:2400–2405.
95. Kotite NJ, Musto NA. Subunit structure of rabbit testosterone estradiol-binding globulin. *J. Biol. Chem.* 1982;257:5118–5124.
96. Danzo BJ, Taylor CA Jr, Eller BC. Some physicochemical characteristics of photoaffinity-labeled rabbit testosterone-binding globulin. *Endocrinology* 1982;111:1278–1285.
97. Cheng S-L, Wright WW, Musto NA, Gunsalus GL, Bardin CW. Testicular proteins which can be used to study seminiferous tubular function: A study of ABP and other testis-specific markers. In: *Physiopathology of Hypophysial Disturbances and Diseases of Reproduction,* edited by de Micola A, Blaquier J and Soto RJ, New York: Alan R. Liss; 1982:193–216.
98. David GFX, Koehler JK, Brown JA, Petra PH, Farr AG. Light and electron microscopic studies on the localization of steroid-binding protein (SBP) in rabbit spermatozoa. *Biol. Reprod.* 1985;33:503–514.
99. Mercier C, Alfsen A, Baulieu EE. A testosterone binding globulin. In: *Proceedings of the Second Symposium on the Steroid Hormones, International Congress Series 101,* Amsterdam: Excerpta Medica Foundation; 1966:212.
100. Rosenbaum W, Christy NP, Kelly WG. Electrophoretic evidence for the presence of an estrogen-binding β-protein in human plasma. *J. Clin. Endocrinol.* 1966;26:1399–1403.
101. Siiteri PK, Murai JT, Hammond GL, Nisker JA, Raymoure WJ, Kuhn RW. The serum transport of steroid hormones. In: *Recent Progress in Hormone Research,* New York: Academic Press; 1982;38:457–510.
102. Rosner W, Smith RN. Isolation and characterization of the testosterone-estradiol-binding globulin from human plasma. Use of a novel affinity column. *Biochemistry* 1975;14:4813–4820.
103. Mickelson KE, Petra PH. Purification of the sex steroid binding protein from human serum. *Biochemistry* 1975;14:957–963.
104. Mercier-Bodard C, Renoir JM, Baulieu EE. Further characterization and immunological studies of human sex steroid binding plasma protein. *J. Steroid Biochem.* 1979;11:253–259.
105. Iqbal MJ, Johnson MW. Purification and characterization of human sex hormone binding globulin. *J. Steroid Biochem.* 1979;10:535–540.
106. Fernlund P, Laurell CB. A simple two-step procedure for the simultaneous isolation of corticosteroid binding globulin and sex hormone binding globulin from human serum by chromatography on cortisol-Sepharose and phenyl-Sepharose. *J. Steroid Biochem.* 1981;14:545–552.
107. Cheng CY, Musto NA, Gunsalus GL, Bardin CW. Demonstration of heavy and light protomers of human testosterone-estradiol-binding globulin. *J. Steroid Biochem.* 1983;19:1379–1389.
108. Cheng CY, Musto NA, Gunsalus GL, Bardin CW. The role of the carbohydrate moiety on the size heterogeneity and immunologic determinants of human testosterone-estradiol binding globulin. *J. Steroid Biochem.* 1985;22:127–134.
109. Petra PH, Stanczyk FZ, Senear DF, Namkung PC, Novy MJ, Ross JBA, Turner E, Brown JA. Current status of the molecular structure and function of the plasma sex steroid binding protein (SBP). *J. Steroid Biochem.* 1983;19:699–706.
110. Khan MS, Ehrlich P, Birkens S, Rosner W. Size isomers of testosterone-estradiol-binding globulin exist in the plasma of individual men and women. *Steroids* 1985;45:463–472.
111. Khan MS. Radioimmunoassay for human testosterone-estradiol binding globulin. *J. Clin. Endocrinol.* 1982;54:705–710.
112. Cheng CY, Bardin CW, Musto NA, Gunsalus GL, Cheng S-L, Ganguly M. Radioimmunoassay of testosterone-estradiol-binding globulin in humans: A reassessment of normal values. *J. Clin. Endocrinol. Metab.* 1983;56:68–75.
113. Vigersky RA, Loriaux DL, Howard SS, Hodgen GB, Lipsett MB, Chrambach A. Androgen binding protein of testis, epididymis and plasma in man and monkeys. *J. Clin. Invest.* 1976;58:1061–1068.
114. Lipshultz LI, Tsai YH, Sanborn BM, Steinberger E. Androgen-binding activity in the human testis and epididymis. *Fertil. Steril.* 1977;28:947–951.
115. Purvis K, Calandra R, Sander S, Hansson V. Androgen binding proteins and androgen levels in the human testis and epididymis. *Int. J. Androl.* 1978;1:531–548.
116. Burke WR, Aten RF, Eisenfeld AJ, Lytton B. Androgen binding in human testis. *J. Urol.* 1977;118:52–57.
117. Hsu A-F, Troen P. An androgen binding protein in the testicular cytosol of human testis. Comparison with human plasma testosterone-estrogen binding globulin. *J. Clin. Invest.* 1978;61:1611–1619.
118. Cheng CY, Musto NA, Gunsalus GL, Frick J, Bardin CW. There are two forms of androgen binding protein in human testes: Comparison of their protomeric variants with serum testosterone-estradiol-binding globulin. *J. Biol. Chem.* 1985;260:5631–5640.
119. Waheed A, Winter SJ, Farrow GM, Oshima H, Troen P. Studies of the human testis. XIX. Preparation of an antibody to human testosterone-oestradiol-binding globulin and its application to the study of testicular androgen-binding protein. *Acta Endocrinol.* 1985;108:284–288.
120. Keeping HS, Winters SJ, Troen P. Identification of androgen-binding protein from testis cytosol and Sertoli cell culture medium of the cynomolgus monkey, *Macaca fascicularis. Endocrinology* 1985;117:1521–1529.
121. Hryb DJ, Khan SM, Rosner R. Testosterone-estradiol-binding globulin binds to human prostatic cell membranes. *Biochem. Biophys. Res. Commun.* 1985;128:432–440.
122. Byers SW, Musto NA, Dym M. Culture of ciliated and nonciliated cells from rat ductuli efferentes. *J. Androl.* 1985;6:271–278.
123. Lobl TJ. Androgen transport proteins: Physical properties, hormonal regulation, and possible mechanism of TeBG and ABP action. *Arch. Androl.* 1981;7:133–151.
124. Campo S, Pellizzari E, Cigorraga S, Monteagudo C, Nicolau G. Androgen binding to subcellular particles of rat testis. *J. Steroid Biochem.* 1982;17:165–173.
125. Mather JP. Ceruloplasmin, a copper-transport protein, can act as a growth promoter for some cell lines in serum-free medium. *In Vitro,* 1982;18:990–996.
126. Perez-Infante V, Mather JP. The role of transferrin in the growth of testicular cell lines in serum-free medium. *Exp. Cell Res.* 1982;142:325–332.
127. Perez-Infante V, Bardin CW, Gunsalus GL, Musto NA, Rich KA, Mather JP. Differential regulation of testicular transferrin and androgen-binding protein in primary cultures of rat Sertoli cells. *Endocrinology* 1986;118:383–392.
128. Holmes SD, Bucci LR, Lipshultz LI, Smith RG. Transferrin binds specifically to pachytene spermatocytes. *Endocrinology* 1983;113:1916–1918.
129. Skinner MK, Griswold MD. Secretion of testicular transferrin by cultured Sertoli cells is regulated by hormones and retinoids. *Biol. Reprod.* 1982;27:211–222.
130. Thorbecke CJ, Liem HH, Knight S, Cox K, Muller-Eberlard U. Sites of formation of the serum proteins, transferrin and hemopexin. *J. Clin. Invest.* 1973;32:725–731.
131. Holmes SD, Lipshultz LI, Smith RG. Transferrin and gonadal dysfunction in man. *Fertil. Steril.* 1982;38:600–604.
132. Orlando C, Caldini AL, Barni T, Wood WG, Strasburger CJ. Ceruloplasmin and transferrin in human seminal plasma: Are they an index of seminiferous tubular function. *Fertil. Steril.* 1985;43:280–284.
133. Blaschuk O, Burdzy K, Fritz IB. Purification and characteriza-

tion of a cell-aggregating factor (clusterin), the major glycoprotein in ram rete testis fluid. *J. Biol. Chem.* 1983;258:7714–7720.
134. Russell L. Movement of spermatocytes from the basal to the adluminal compartment of the rat testis. *Am. J. Anat.* 1977;148: 313–328.
135. Russell LD. Sertoli germ cell interrelations: a review. *Gamete Res.* 1980;3:179–202.
136. Vihko KK, Kristensen P, Toppari J, Saksela O, Dano K, Parvinen M. The function of plasminogen activator in the seminiferous epithelium. *J. Cell Biol.* 1985;101:367a (abstract 1392).
137. Toppari J, Vihko KK, Rasanen KGE, Eerola E, Parvinen M. Regulation of stages VI and VIII of the rat seminiferous epithelial cycle *in vitro*. *J. Endocrinol.* 1986;108:417–422.
138. Leblond CP, Clermont Y. Definition of the stages of the cycle of the seminiferous epithelium in the rat. *Ann. NY Acad. Sci. USA* 1952;55:548–573.
139. Ohno S, Nagai Y, Ciccarese S, Iwata H. Testis-organizing H-Y antigen and the primary sex determining mechanism of mammals. *Recent Prog. Horm. Res.* 1979;35:449–478.
140. Muller U, Wolf U, Siebers JW, Gunther E. Evidence for a gonad-specific receptor for H-Y antigen: Binding of exogenous H-Y antigen to gonadal cells is independent of β2-microglobulin. *Cell* 1979;17:331–335.
141. Ciccarese S, Ohno S. 2 plasma membrane antigens of testicular Sertoli cells and h-2 restricted vs unrestricted lysis by female thymus derived cells. *Cell* 1978;13:643–650.
142. Zenzes MT, Wolf U, Gunther E, Engel W. Studies on the function of H-Y antigen: Dissociation and reorganization experiments on rat gonadal tissue. *Cytogenet. Cell Genet.* 1978;20: 365–372.
143. Wachtel SS. *H-Y Antigen and the Biology of Sex Determination*, New York: Grune and Stratton; 1983.
144. Gore-Langton RE, Tung PS, Fritz IB. The absence of specific interactions of Sertoli cell secreted proteins with antibodies directed against h-y antigen. *Cell* 1983;32:289–302.
145. Braunhut SJ, Rufo GA Jr, Ernisse BJ, Bellve AR. The seminiferous growth factor (SGF) stimulates the proliferation of transformed mouse Sertoli cells (TM_4) in a serum-free medium. *J. Cell Biol.* 1985;101:372a (abstract 1408).
146. Bellve AR, Feig LA. Cell proliferation in the mammalian testis: Biology of the seminiferous growth factor (SGF). *Recent Prog. Horm. Res.* 1984;40:531–567.
147. Esch F, Baird A, Ling N, Ueno N, Hill F, Denoroy L, Klepper R, Gospodarowicz D, Böhlen P, Guillemin R. Primary structure of bovine pituitary basic fibroblast growth factor (FGF) and comparison with the amino-terminal sequence of bovine brain acidic FGF. *Proc. Natl. Acad. Sci. USA* 1985;82:6507–6511.
148. Gospodarowicz D, Baird A, Cheng J, Lui GM, Esch F, Böhlen P. Isolation of fibroblast growth factor from bovine adrenal gland: Physiochemical and biological characterization. *Endocrinology* 1986;118:82–90.
149. Böhlen P, Esch F, Baird A, Gospodarowicz D. Acidic fibroblast growth factor (FGF) from bovine brain: Amino-terminal sequence and comparison with basic FGF. *EMBO* 1985;4:1951–1956.
150. Ling N, Ying S-Y, Ueno N, Esch F, Denoroy L, Guillemin R. Isolation and partial characterization of a M_r 32,000 protein with inhibin activity from porcine follicular fluid. *Proc. Natl. Acad. Sci. USA* 1985;82:7217–7221.
151. Esch F, Ueno N, Baird A, Hill F, Denoroy L, Ling N, Gospodarowicz D, Guillemin R. Primary structure of bovine brain acidic fibroblast growth factor (FGF). *Biochem. Biophys. Res. Commun.* 1985;133:554–562.
152. Adashi EY, Resnick CE, Svoboda ME, Van Wyk JJ. Somatomedin-C as an amplifier of follicle-stimulating hormone action: Enhanced accumulation of adenosine 3′,5′-monophosphate. *Endocrinology* 1986;118:149–155.
153. Elson SD, Browne CA, Thorburn GD. Identification of epidermal growth factor-like activity in human male reproductive tissue and fluids. *J. Clin. Endocrinol. Metab.* 1984;58:589–594.
154. Cheng CY, Grima J, Lee WM, Bardin CW. The distribution of rat testibumin in the male reproductive tract. *Biol. Reprod. (in press).*
155. Kissinger C, Skinner MK, Griswold MD. Analysis of Sertoli cell-secreted proteins by 2 dimensional gel electrophoresis. *Biol. Reprod.* 1982;27:233–240.
156. Cheng CY, Bardin CW, Nagendranath N, Escobar N, Han AC, Musto NA, Gunsalus GL. Purification of testosterone-estradiol-binding globulins from mammalian sera by anion-exchange high-performance liquid chromatography. *Int. J. Androl.* 1985;8: 1–12.
157. Skinner MK, Fritz IB. Testicular peritubular cells secrete a protein under androgen control that modulates Sertoli cell functions. *Proc. Natl. Acad. Sci. USA* 1985;82:114–118.
158. Skinner MK, Fritz IB. Androgen stimulation of Sertoli cell function is enhanced by peritubular cells. *Mol. Cell. Endocrinol.* 1985;40:115–122.
159. Skinner MK, Tung PS, Fritz IB. Cooperativity between Sertoli cells and testicular peritubular cells in the production and deposition of extracellular matrix components. *J. Cell Biol.* 1985;100: 1941–1947.
160. Spruill WA, Steiner AL, Tres LL, Kierszenbaum AL. FSH dependent phosphorylation of vimentin in cultures of rat Sertoli cells. *Proc. Natl. Acad. Sci. USA* 1983;80:993–997.
161. Perrard MH, Saez JM, Dazord A. FSH stimulation of cytosolic protein synthesis in cultured pig Sertoli cells. *J. Steroid Biochem.* 1985;22:281–284.
162. Perrard-Sapori MH, Saez JM, Dazord A. Hormonal regulation of proteins secreted by cultured pig Sertoli cells: Characterization by two-dimensional polyacrylamide gel electrophoresis. *Mol. Cell. Endocrinol.* 1985;43:189–197.
163. McCullagh DD. Dual endocrine activity of the testis. *Science* 1932;76:19–20.
164. Channing CP, Gordon WL, Liu VK, Ward DN. Minireview: Physiology and biochemistry of ovarian inhibin. *Biol. Med.* 1985;178:339–361.
165. Ramasharma K, Sairam MR, Seidah NG, Chirtien M, Manjunath P, Schiller PW, Yamashiro D, Li CH. Isolation, structure and synthesis of a human seminal plasma peptide with inhibin-like activity. *Science* 1984;223:1199–1202.
166. Seidah NG, Ramasharma K, Sairam MR, Chretien M. Partial amino acid sequence of a human seminal plasma peptide with inhibin-like activity. *FEBS Lett.* 1984;167:98–102.
167. Li CH, Hammonds RG, Ramasharma K, Chung D. Human seminal α-inhibins: Isolation, characterization, and structure. *Proc. Natl. Acad. Sci. USA* 1985;82:4041–4044.
168. Rivier J, McClintock R, Vaughan J, Yamamoto G, Anderson H, Spiess J, Vale W, Voglmayr J, Cheng CY, Bardin CW. Partial purification of inhibin from ovine rete testis fluid. In: *Male Contraception: Advances and Future Prospects,* edited by Zatuchni G, Goldsmith A, and Sciarra J, Philadelphia: Harper and Row; 1986:401–407.
169. Robertson DM, Foulds LM, Leversha L, Moran FJ, Hearn MTW, Burger HG, Wettenhall REH and de Kretser DMV. Isolation of inhibin from bovine follicular fluid. *Biochem. Biophys. Res. Commun.* 1985;126:220–226.
170. Miyamoto K, Hasegawa Y, Fukuda M, Nomura M, Igarashi M, Kangawa K, Matsuo A. Isolation of porcine follicular fluid inhibin of 32K daltons. *Biochem. Biophys. Res. Commun.* 1985;128: 396–403.
171. Mason AJ, Hayflick JS, Ling N, Esch F, Ueno N, Ying S-Y, Guillemin R, Niall H, Seeburg PH. Complementary DNA sequences of ovarian follicular fluid inhibin show precursor structure and homology with transforming growth factor-β. *Nature* 1985;318:659–663.
172. Mason AJ, Niall HD, Seeburg PH. Structure of two human ovarian inhibins. *Biochem. Biophys. Res. Commun.* 1986;135: 957–964.
173. David K, Dingemanse E, Freud J, Laqueur E. Uber krystallinisches mannliches Hormon aus Hoden (Testosteron), Wirksamer als aus Harn oder aus Cholesterin bereitetes Androsteron. *Z. Physiol. Chem.* 1935;233:281–282.
174. Srere PA, Chaikoff IL, Treitman SS, Burstein LS. The extrahepatic synthesis of cholesterol. *J. Biol. Chem.* 1950;182:629–634.
175. Brady RO. Biosynthesis of radioactive testosterone *in vitro*. *J. Biol. Chem.* 1951;193:145–148.
176. Steinberger E, Steinberger A, Ficher M. Study of spermatogenesis

and steroid metabolism in cultures of mammalian testes. *Recent Prog. Horm. Res.* 1970;26:547–588.
177. Huggins C, Moulder PV. Estrogen production by Sertoli cell tumors of the testes. *Cancer Res.* 1945;5:510–514.
178. Steinberger A, Elkington JSH, Sanborn BM, Steinberger E, Heindel J, Lindsey JN. Culture of FSH response of Sertoli cells isolated from sexually mature rat testes. In: *Hormonal Regulation of Spermatogenesis,* edited by French FS, Hansson V, Ritzén EM, and Nayfeh SN, New York: Plenum Press; 1975:398–411.
179. Oshima HD, Fan DF, Troen P. Studies of the human testis. V. Properties of Δ^5-3β- and 17β-hydroxysteroid dehydrogenase in the biosynthesis of testosterone from dehydroepiandrosterone. *J. Clin. Endocrinol. Metab.* 1975;40:573–581.
180. Welsh MJ, Wiebe JP. Sertoli cells from immature rats: *in vitro* stimulation of steroid metabolism by follicle stimulating hormone. *Biochem. Biophys. Res. Commun.* 1976;69:936–941.
181. Tcholakian RK, Steinberger A. Progesterone metabolism by cultured Sertoli cells. *Endocrinology* 1979;103:1335–1343.
182. Welsh MJ, Wiebe JP. Sertoli cell capacity to metabolize C-19 steroids: Variation with age and the effect of follicle stimulating hormone. *Endocrinology* 1978;103:838–844.
183. Tcholakian RK, Steinberger A. *In vitro* metabolism of testosterone by cultured Sertoli cells and the effect of FSH. *Steroids* 1979;33:495–526.
184. Yamada M, Yasue S, Matsumoto K. Formation of 5α-reduced products from testosterone *in vitro* by germ cells from immature rats. *Acta Endocrinol. (Copenh.)* 1972;71:383–400.
185. Payne AH, Kawano A, Jaffe RB. Formation of dihydrotestosterone and other 5α-reduced metabolites by isolated seminiferous tubules and suspension of interstitial cells in a human testis. *J. Clin. Endocrinol. Metab.* 1973;37:448–453.
186. Wiebe JP, Tilbe KS, Buckingham KD. An analysis of the metabolites of progesterone produced by isolated Sertoli cells at the onset of gametogenesis. *Steroids* 1980;35:561–578.
187. Folman Y, Sowell JG, Eik-Nes KB. Presence and formation of 5α-dihydrotestosterone in rat testes *in vivo* and *in vitro. Endocrinology* 1972;91:702–709.
188. Dorrington JH, Fritz IB. Cellular localization of 5-alpha reductase and 3-alpha hydroxy steroid dehydrogenase in the seminiferous tubule of the rat testis. *Endocrinology* 1975;96:879–889.
189. Cochran RC, Schuetz AW, Ewing LL. Age-related changes in conversion of 5α-androstan-17β-ol-3-one to 5α-androstane-3α,17β-diol and 5α-androstane-3β,17β-diol by rat testicular cells *in vitro. J. Reprod. Fertil.* 1979;57:143–147.
190. Kasai H, Mizutani S, Matsumoto K. Detection of [^{3}H]5α-androstane-3α, 17β-diol and [^{3}H]17β-hydroxy-5α-androstan-3-one in mouse testes following administration of [^{3}H]testosterone. *Acta Endocrinol.* 1973;74:177–185.
191. Baker HWG, Bailey DJ, Feil PD, Jefferson LS, Santen RJ, Bardin CW. Nuclear accumulation of androgens in perfused rat accessory sex organs and testes. *Endocrinology* 1977;100:709–721.
192. Suarez-Quian CA, Dym M, Makris A, Brumbaugh J, Ryan KJ, Canick JA. Estrogen synthesis by immature rat Sertoli cells *in vitro. J. Androl.* 1983;4:203–209.
193. Tsai-Morris C-H, Aquilano DR, Dufau ML. Cellular localization of rat testicular aromatase activity during development. *Endocrinology* 1985;116:38–46.
194. Ritzen EM, Van Damme MP, Froysa B, Reuter C, De La Torre B, Diczfalusy E. Identification of estradiol produced by Sertoli cell enriched cultures during incubation with testosterone. *J. Steroid Biochem.* 1981;14:533–536.
195. Siiteri PK, MacDonald PC. Role of extraglandular estrogen in human endocrinology. In: *Handbook of Physiology: Endocrinology, Section 7, Vol. 11,* edited by Greep RO and Astwood EB, Washington, D.C.: American Physiological Society; 1973: 615–629.
196. Murphy HD. Sertoli cell stimulation following intratesticular injection of FSH in the hypophysectomized rat. *Proc. Soc. Exp. Biol. Med.* 1965;118:1202–1205.
197. Means AR, Vaitukaitis J. Peptide hormone "receptors": Specific binding of ^{3}H-FSH T_4 testis. *Endocrinology* 1972;90:39–46.
198. Bhalla VK, Reichert LE. Properties of follicle-stimulating hormone-receptor interaction. *J. Biol. Chem.* 1974;249:43–51.
199. Steinberger E, Chowdhury M. Control of pituitary FSH in male rats. *Acta Endocrinol. (Copenh.)* 1974;76:235–241.
200. Yee JB, Hutson JC. Testicular macrophages: Isolation, characterization and hormonal responsiveness. *Biol. Reprod.* 1983;29: 1319–1326.
201. Yee JB, Hutson JC. *In vivo* effects of follicle-stimulating hormone on testicular macrophages. *Biol. Reprod.* 1985;32: 880–883.
202. Reichert LE Jr, Andersen TT, Dias JA, Fletcher PW, Sluss PM, O'Neill WC, Smith RA. Studies on the molecular biology of the interaction of follicle-stimulating hormone with receptors from testis. In: *Hormone Receptors in Growth and Reproduction,* edited by Saxena BB et al. New York: Raven Press; 1984.
203. Dias JA, Reichert LE Jr. Characterization of a follicle-binding component prepared from immature bovine testis in the absence of detergent. *J. Biol. Chem.* 1982;257:613–620.
204. Branca AA, Sluss PM, Smith RA, Reichert LE Jr. The subunit structure of the follitropin receptor: Chemical cross-linking of the solubilized follitropin receptor complex. *J. Biol. Chem.* 1985; 260:9988–9993.
205. Smith RA, Branca AA, Reichert LE Jr. The subunit structure of the follitropin (FSH) receptor: Photoaffinity labeling of the membrane-bound receptor follitropin complex *in situ. J. Biol. Chem.* 1985;260:14297–14303.
206. Dattatreyamurty B, Rathnam P, Saxena BB. Isolation of the luteinizing hormone-chorionic gonadotropin receptor in high yield from bovine corpora lutea. *J. Biol. Chem.* 1983;258:3140–3158.
207. Ascoli M, Segaloff DL. Effects of 'collagenase' on the structure of the lutropin/choriogonadotropin (LH/CG) receptor. *J. Biol. Chem.* 1986;261:3807–3815.
208. Francis GL, Brown TJ, Bercu BB. Regulation by homologous hormone exposure. *Biol. Reprod.* 1981;24:995–961.
209. Francis GL, Triche TJ, Brown TJ, Brown HC, Bercu BB. *In vitro* gonadotropin stimulation of bovine Sertoli cell ornithine decarboxylase EC-4.1.1.17 activity. *J. Androl.* 1981;2:312–320.
210. Fletcher PW, Reichert LE Jr. Cellular processing of follicle-stimulating hormone by Sertoli cells in serum-free culture. *Mol. Cell. Endocrinol.* 1984;34:39–50.
211. Andersen TT, Reichert LE Jr. Correlation of β coefficient of viscosity for monovalent salts with effects on binding of human follitropin to receptor. *Mol. Cell. Endocrinol.* 1984;35:41–46.
212. Dias JA, Treble DH, Reichert LE. Effect of bacitracin and polyamines on follicle-stimulating hormone binding to membrane-bound and detergent-solubilized bovine calf testis receptor. *Endocrinology* 1983;113:2029–2034.
213. Dias JA, Treble DH, Bennett AH, Reichert LE Jr. Follicle-stimulating hormone receptor binding inhibitors in human seminal plasma. *J. Androl.* 1981;5:259–268.
214. Sanzo MA, Reichert LE Jr. Gonadotropin receptor binding regulators in serum: Characterization and separation of follitropin binding inhibitor and lutropin binding stimulator. *J. Biol. Chem.* 1982;257:6033–6040.
215. Papkoff H, Niswender GD, Murthy HMS, Wiebe JP. Properties of an ovine testicular peptide that inhibits the binding of FSH to gonadal tissues. *Endocrinology* 1983;112:267.
216. Dias JA, Reichert LE Jr. Evidence for a high molecular weight follicle-stimulating hormone binding inhibitor in bovine testis. *Biol. Reprod.* 1984;31:975–983.
217. Murad F, Strauch BS, Vaughn M. The effect of gonadotrophins on testicular adenylate cyclase. *Biochim. Biophys. Acta* 1969;177: 591–598.
218. Kuehl F, Patanelli DJ, Humes JL, Tarnoff J. Testicular adenylate cyclase: Stimulation by the pituitary gonadotrophins. *Biol. Reprod.* 1970;2:153–163.
219. Dorrington JH, Vernon RG, Fritz IB. The effect of gonadotrophins on the 3′,5′-AMP levels of seminiferous tubules. *Biochem. Biophys. Res. Commun.* 1972;46:1523–1528.
220. Means AR. Early effects of FSH upon testicular metabolism. *Adv. Exp. Med. Biol.* 1973;36:431.
221. Dorrington JH, Fritz IB. Effects of gonadotrophins on cyclic AMP production by isolated seminiferous tubules and interstitial cell preparations. *Endocrinology* 1974;94:395–403.
222. Heindel JJ, Rothenberg R, Robinson GA, Steinberger A. LH and

FSH stimulation of cyclic AMP in specific cell types isolated from the testes. *J. Cyclic Nucleotide Res.* 1975;1:69–79.
223. Means AR. Biochemical effects of follicle-stimulating hormone on the testis. In: *Handbook of Physiology, Vol. V,* edited by Greep RO, Washington, D.C.: American Physiological Society; 1975:203–218.
224. Beale EG, Dedman JR, Means AR. Isolation and regulation of the protein kinase inhibitor and the calcium dependent cyclic nucleotide phosphodiesterase regulator in the Sertoli cell enriched testis. *Endocrinology* 1977;101:1621–1634.
225. Beale EG, Dedman JR, Means AR. Isolation and characterization of a protein from rat testis which inhibits cyclic AMP dependent protein kinase EC-2.7.1.37 and phosphodiesterase. *J. Biol. Chem.* 1977;252:6322–6327.
226. Conti M, Geremia R, Adamo S, Stefanini M. Regulation of Sertoli cell cyclic adenosine 3′:5′-monophosphate phosphodiesterase activity by follicle stimulating hormone and dibutyryl cyclic AMP. *Biochem. Biophys. Res. Commun.* 1981;98:1044–1050.
227. Conti M, Toscano MV, Geremia R, Stefanini M. Follicle-stimulating hormone regulates *in vivo* testicular phosphodiesterase. *Mol. Cell. Endocrinol.* 1983;29:79–90.
228. Ireland ME, Rosenblum BB, Welsh MJ. Two-dimensional gel analysis of Sertoli cell protein phosphorylation: Effect of short term exposure to follicle-stimulating hormone. *Endocrinology* 1986;118:526–532.
229. Means AR, MacDougall E, Soderling T, Corbin JD. Testicular adenosine 3′:5′-monophosphate-dependent protein kinase. *J. Biol. Chem.* 1974;249:1231–1238.
230. Means AR. Concerning the mechanism of FSH action: Rapid stimulation of testicular synthesis of nuclear RNA. *Endocrinology* 1971;89:981–989.
231. Means AR, Tindall DJ. FSH-induction of androgen binding protein in testis of Sertoli cell-only rats. In: *Hormonal Regulation of Spermatogenesis,* edited by French FS, Hansson V, Nayfeh SH, and Ritzén M, New York: Plenum; 1975:383–398.
232. Lamb DJ, Lee AL, Steinberger A, Sanborn BM. Correlation between androgen binding and stimulation of nuclear RNA polymerase II activity in cultured Sertoli cells. In: *Cell Biology of the Testis,* edited by Bardin CW and Sherins RJ, New York: New York Academy of Science; 1982;383:470–471.
233. Lamb DJ, Tsai Y-H, Steinberger A, Sanborn BM. Sertoli cell nuclear transcriptional activity. Stimulation by follicle stimulating hormone and testosterone *in vitro. Endocrinology* 1981;108:1020–1026.
234. Lamb DJ, Wagle JR, Tsai YH, Lee AL, Steinberger A, Sanborn BM. Specificity and nature of the rapid steroid stimulated increase in Sertoli cell nuclear RNA polymerase activity. *J. Steroid Biochem.* 1982;16:653–660.
235. Means AR, Hall PF. Effect of FSH on protein biosynthesis in testis of the immature rat. *Endocrinology* 1967;81:1151–1160.
236. Abney TO, Skipper JK, Williams WL. Gonadotropin stimulation of rat testicular protein synthesis. Polysome isolation and activity in a cell-free system. *Biochemistry* 1974;13:3956–3961.
237. Dorrington JH, Roller NF, Fritz IB. Effects of follicle-stimulating hormone on cultures of Sertoli cell preparations. *Mol. Cell. Endocrinol.* 1975;3:57–70.
238. Terasaki WL, Brooker G, de Vellis J, Inglish D, Hsu C, Moylan RD. Involvement of cyclic AMP and protein synthesis in catecholamine refractoriness. In: *Advances in Cyclic Nucleotide Research,* edited by George WJ and Ignarro LJ. New York: Raven Press; 1978.
239. Catt KT, Harwood JP, Aquilera G, Dufau ML. Hormonal regulation of peptide receptors and target cell response. *Nature* 1979;280:109–116.
240. Harden T. Agonist-induced desensitization of the β-adrenergic receptor-linked adenylate cyclase. *Pharmacol. Rev.* 1983;35:5.
241. O'Shaughnessy PJ. FSH receptor autoregulation and cyclic AMP production in the immature rat testis. *Biol. Reprod.* 1980;23:810.
242. Conti M, Toscano MV, Petrelli L, Geremia R, Stefanini M. Involvement of phosphodiesterase in the refractoriness of the Sertoli cell. *Endocrinology* 1983;113:1845–1853.
243. Attramadal H, Le Gac F, Jahnsen T, Hansson V. β-Adrenergic regulation of Sertoli cell adenylate cyclase: Desensitization by homologous hormone. *Mol. Cell. Endocrinol.* 1984;34:1–6.
244. Verhoeven G, Cailleau J, De Moor P. Hormonal control of phosphodiesterase activity in cultured rat Sertoli cells. *Mol. Cell. Endocrinol.* 1981;24:41–52.
245. Conti M, Monaco L, Geremia R, Stefanini M. Effect of phosphodiesterase inhibitors on Sertoli cell refractoriness: Reversal of the impaired androgen aromatization. *Endocrinology* 1986;118:901–908.
246. Means AR. Calmodulin: Properties, intracellular localization and multiple roles in cell regulation. *Recent Prog. Horm. Res.* 1981;37:333–368.
247. Means AR, Tash JS, Chafouleas JG. Physiological implications of the presence, distribution, and regulation of calmodulin in eukaryotic cells. *Physiol. Rev.* 1982;62:1–38.
248. LaPorte DC, Wierman BM, Storm DR. Calcium-induced exposure of a hydrophobic surface on calmodulin. *Biochemistry* 1980;19:3814–3819.
249. Tanaka T, Hidaka H. Hydrophobic regions function in calmodulin enzyme(s) interactions. *J. Biol. Chem.* 1980;255:11078–11080.
250. Slaughter GR, Means AR. FSH activation of glycogen phosphorylase in the Sertoli cell enriched rat testis. *Endocrinology* 1983;113:1476–1485.
251. Means AR, Slaughter GR, Putkey JA. Postreceptor signal transduction by cyclic adenosine monophosphate and the Ca^{2+}-calmodulin complex. *J. Cell Biol.* 1984;99:226s–231s.
252. Hansson V, Reusch E, Trygstad O, Torgersen O, French FS, Ritzén EM. FSH stimulation of androgen binding protein (ABP). *Nature (New Biol.)* 1973;246:56–59.
253. Tindall DJ, Means AR. Concerning the hormonal regulation of androgen binding protein in rat testis. *Endocrinology* 1976;99:809–818.
254. Kotite NJ, Nayfeh SN, French FS. Follicle stimulating hormone and androgen regulation of Sertoli cell function in the immature rat. *Biol. Reprod.* 1978;18:65–73.
255. Rich KA, Bardin CW, Gunsalus GL, Mather JP. Age-dependent pattern of androgen binding protein (ABP) secretion from rat Sertoli cells in primary culture. *Endocrinology* 1983;113:2284–2293.
256. Wilson RM, Griswold MCD. Secreted proteins from rat Sertoli cells. *Exp. Cell Res.* 1979;123:127–135.
257. Lacroix M, Fritz IB. Control of synthesis and secretion of plasminogen activator by rat Sertoli cells in culture. *Mol. Cell. Endocrinol.* 1982;26:247–258.
258. Fritz IB, Karmally K. Hormonal influences on formation of plasminogen activator by cultured testis tubule segments at defined stages of the cycle of the seminiferous epithelium. *Can. J. Biochem. Cell Biol.* 1983;61:553–560.
259. Holmes SD, Lipshultz LI, Smith RG. Regulation of transferrin secretion by human Sertoli cells cultured in the presence or absence of human peritubular cells. *J. Clin. Endocrinol. Metab.* 1984;59:1058–1062.
260. Verhoeven G, Cailleau J. A factor in spent media from Sertoli cell-enriched cultures that stimulates steroidogenesis in leydig cells. *Mol. Cell. Endocrinol.* 1985;40:57–68.
261. Benahmed M, Reventos J, Tabone E, Saez JM. Cultured Sertoli cell-mediated FSH stimulatory effect on Leydig cell steroidogenesis. *Am. J. Physiol.* 1985;248:E176–E181.
262. Sharpe RM, Bartlett JMS. Stimulation of Leydig cell function by a polypeptide present in testicular interstitial fluid. *Med. Biol.* 1985;63:245–250.
263. Saez JM, Tabone E, Perrard-Sapori MH, Rivarola MA. Paracrine role of Sertoli cells. *Med. Biol.* 1985;63:225–236.
264. Durham LA, III, Grogan WM. Characterization of multiple forms of cholesteryl ester hydrolase EC-3.1.1.13 in the rat testis. *J. Biol. Chem.* 1984;259:7433–7438.
265. Hall PF, Mita M. Influence of FSH on glucose transport by cultured Sertoli cells. *Biol. Reprod.* 1984;31:863–869.
266. Mita M, Price JM, Hall PF. Stimulation by FSH of synthesis of lactate by Sertoli cells from rat testis. *Endocrinology* 1982;110:1535–1541.
267. Mita M, Hall PF. Metabolism of round spermatids from rats lactate as the preferred substrate. *Biol. Reprod.* 1982;26:445–455.

268. Marzowski J, Sylvester SR, Gilmont RR, Griswold MD. Isolation and characterization of Sertoli cell plasma membranes and associated plasminogen activator activity. *Biol. Reprod.* 1985;32: 1237–1246.
269. Bordy MJ, Berger S, Desjardins C, Davis JC. Active cell aggregation by immature rat Sertoli cells in primary culture: a role for cell surface glyco proteins. *J. Cell. Physiol.* 1979;99:175–182.
270. Orth JM. The role of FSH in controlling Sertoli cell proliferation in testes of fetal rats. *Endocrinology* 1984;115:1248–1255.
271. Orth JM. Proliferation of Sertoli cells in fetal and post natal rats: A quantitative autoradiographic study. *Anat. Rec.* 1982;203: 485–492.
272. Griswold MD, Mably ER, Fritz IB. Follicle stimulating hormone stimulation of DNA synthesis in Sertoli cells in culture. *Mol. Cell. Endocrinol.* 1976;4:139–149.
273. Griswold MD, Solari A, Tung PS, Fritz IB. Stimulation by follicle-stimulating hormone of DNA synthesis and of mitosis in cultured Sertoli cells prepared from testes of immature rats. *Mol. Cell. Endocrinol.* 1977;7:151–165.
274. Fakunding JL, Tindall DJ, Dedman JR, Mena CR, Means AR. Biochemical actions of follicle stimulating hormone in the Sertoli cell of the rat testis. *Endocrinology* 1976;98:392–402.
275. Means AR. Mechanisms of action of follicle-stimulating hormone (FSH). In: *The Testis, Vol. IV,* edited by Johnson AD and Gomes WR, New York: Academic Press; 1977:163–188.
276. Karl AF, Griswold MD. Actions of insulin and vitamin A on Sertoli cells. *Biochem. J.* 1980;186:1001–1004.
277. Griswold MD, Merryweather J. Insulin stimulates the incorporation of inorganic phosphorus-32 into RNA in cultured Sertoli cells. *Endocrinology* 1982;111:661–667.
278. Borland K, Mita M, Oppenheimer CL, Blinderman LA, Massague J, Hall PF, Czech MP. The actions of insulin-like growth factors I and II on cultured Sertoli cells. *Endocrinology* 1984;114:240–246.
279. Mita M, Borland K, Price JM, Hall PF. The influence of insulin and insulin-like growth factor-I on hexose transport by Sertoli cells. *Endocrinology* 1985;116:987–992.
280. Eikvar L, Levy FO, Attramadal H, Jutte NHPM, Froysa A, Tvermyr SM, Hansson V. Glucagon-stimulated cyclic AMP production and formation of estradiol in Sertoli cell cultures from immature rats. *Mol. Cell. Endocrinol.* 1985;39:107–114.
281. Chausmer A, Stuart C, Stevens M. Identification of testicular cell plasma membrane receptors for calcitonin. *J. Lab. Clin. Med.* 1980;96:933.
282. Chausmer AB, Stevens MD, Severn C. Autoradiographic evidence for a calcitonin receptor on testicular Leydig cells. *Science* 1982;216:735.
283. Nakhla AM, Mather JP, Jänne OA, Bardin CW. The action of calcitonin on cultured testicular cells. II. Changes in androgen binding protein secretion and sex steroid receptor concentrations in Sertoli cells. *J. Androl. (submitted for publication.)*
284. Bardin CW, Shaha C, Mather J, Salomon Y, Margioris AN, Liotta AS, Gerendai I, Chen C-L, Krieger DT. Identification and possible function of pro-opiomelanocortin-derived peptides in the testis. *Ann. NY Acad. Sci.* 1984;438:346–364.
285. Krieger DT, Margioris AN, Liotta AS, Shaha C, Gerendai I, Pintar J, Bardin CW. Pro-opiomelanocortin (POMC)-derived peptides in the rodent male reproductive tract. In: *Opioid Modulation of Endocrine Function,* edited by Delitala G, Motta M and Serio M, New York: Raven Press; 1984:223–235.
286. Sharpe B, Pekary AE, Meyer NV, Hersham JM. β-Endorphin in male rat reproductive organs. *Biochem. Biophys. Res. Commun.* 1980;95:618–623.
287. Tsong SD, Phillips DM, Halmi N, Krieger D, Bardin CW. β-Endophin is present in the male reproductive tract of five species. *Biol. Reprod.* 1982;27:755–764.
288. Tsong S-D, Phillips DM, Bardin CW, Halmi N, Liotta AJ, Margioris A, Krieger DT. ACTH and β-endorphin related peptides are present in multiple sites in the reproductive tract of the rat. *Endocrinology* 1982;110:2204–2206.
289. Shaha C, Liotta AS, Krieger DT, Bardin CW. The ontogeny of immunoreactive β-endorphin in the fetal, neonatal, and pubertal testes from mouse and hamster. *Endocrinology* 1984;114:1584–1591.
290. Chen C-L, Mather JP, Morris PL, Bardin CW. Expression of pro-opiomelanocortin-like gene in the testis and epididymis. *Proc. Natl. Acad. Sci. USA* 1984;81:5672–5675.
291. Melner MH, Puett D. Evidence for the synthesis of multiple pro-opiomelanocortin-like precursors in murine Leydig tumor cells. *Arch. Biochem. Biophys.* 1984;232:197–201.
292. Pintar JE, Schachter B, Herman AB, Durgerian S, Krieger DT. Characterization and localization of pro-opiomelanocortin mRNA in the adult rat. *Science* 1984;225:632.
293. Shaha C, Boitani C, Hahn EF, Gerendai I, Mather J, Margioris AN, Liotta AS, Chen C-L, Krieger DT, Bardin CW. The presence and possible function of pro-opiomelanocortin-derived peptides in the testis and ovary. In: *Opioid Peptides in Periphery,* edited by Fraioli F, Isidori A, and Mazzetti M, Amsterdam: Elsevier; 1984:53–59.
294. Mather J, Bardin CW, Byer A, Salomon Y. Modulation of adenylate cyclase activity in Sertoli cells *in vitro.* In: *Recent Progress in Cellular Endocrinology of the Testis, Vol. 122,* edited by Saez JM, Forest MG, Dazord A, and Bertrand J, Paris: INSERM; 1985:183–186.
295. Boitani C, Mather JP, Bardin CW. Stimulation of cAMP production in rat Sertoli cells by α-MSH and des-acetyl α-MSH. *Endocrinology* 1986;118:1513–1518.
296. O'Donohue TL, Handelmann TL, Chaconas T, Miller RL, Jacobowitz DM. Evidence that *N*-acetylation regulates the behavioral activity of MSH in the rat and human central nervous system. *Peptides* 1981;2:333.
297. O'Donohue TL, Handelmann GE, Miller RL, Jacobowitz DM. *N*-Acetylation regulates the behavioral activity of α-melanotropin in a multineurotransmitter neuron. *Science* 1982;215:1125.
298. Akil H, Hewlitt H, Barchas JD, Ki CH. Binding of ^{3}H-β-endorphin to rat brain membranes: Characterization of opiate properties and interaction with ACTH. *Eur. J. Pharmacol.* 1980;64:1.
299. McCormack AM, Carter RJ, Thody AJ, Shuster S. Des-acetyl-α-MSH and α-MSH act as partial agonists to MSH on the Anolis melanophore. *Peptides* 1982;3:13.
300. Gerendai I, Nemeskéri A, Csernus V. Naloxone has a local effect on the testis of immature rats. *Andrologia* 1983;15:398–403.
301. Chen C-LC, Margioris AN, Liotta AS, Morris PL, Boitani C, Mather JP, Krieger DT, Bardin CW. Pro-opiomelanocortin-derived peptides of Leydig cell origin may be modulators of testicular function. In: *Gonadal Proteins and Peptides and Their Biological Significance,* edited by Sairam MR and Atkinson LE, Singapore: World Scientific; 1984:339–352.
302. Gerendai I, Shaha C, Gunsalus GL, Bardin CW. The effects of opioid receptor antagonists suggest that testicular opiates regulate Sertoli and Leydig cell function in the neonatal rat. *Endocrinology* 1986;118:2039–2044.
303. Orth J. FSH-induced Sertoli cell proliferation in the developing rat is modified by β-endorphin produced in the testis. *Endocrinology* 1986;119:1876–1878.
304. Fabbri A, Tsai-Morris CH, Luna S, Fraioli F, Dufau ML. Opiate receptors are present in the rat testis. Identification and localization in Sertoli cells. *Endocrinology* 1985;117:2544–2546.
305. Kilpatrick DL, Rosenthal JL. The proenkephalin gene is widely expressed within the male and female reproductive systems of the rat and hamster. *Endocrinology* 1986;119:370–374.
306. Thody AT, Wilson CA, Everard D. α-Melanocyte stimulating hormone stimulates sexual behaviour in the female rat. *Psychopharmacology* 1981;74:153.
307. Krieger DT, Liotta AS, Brownstein MJ, Zimmerman EA. ACTH, β-lipotropin, and related peptides in brain, pituitary, and blood. *Recent Prog. Horm. Res.* 1980;36:277–344.
308. Chen C-L, Mather JP, Morris PL, Bardin CW. Expression of Pro-opiomelanocortin-like gene in the testis and Leydig cell lines. In: *Hormone Action and Testicular Function, Vol. 438,* edited by Catt KJ and Dufau ML, New York: Annals of the New York Academy of Science; 1985:659–662.
309. Tindall DJ, Miller DA, Means AR. Characterization of androgen receptor in Sertoli cell enriched testis. *Endocrinology* 1977; 101:13–23.
310. Sanborn BM, Steinberger A, Tcholakian RK, Steinberger E. Direct measurement of androgen receptors in cultured Sertoli cells. *Steroids* 1977;29:493–502.

311. Chevalier M, Dufaure J-P. Effect of FSH testosterone and calcium on Sertoli cell micro filaments in the immature pig testis. *Biol. Cell* 1981;41:105–112.
312. Dym M, Raj HGM. Response of adult rat Sertoli cells and Leydig cells to depletion of luteinizing hormone and testosterone. *Biol. Reprod.* 1977;17:676–696.
313. Elkington JS, Sanborn BM, Steinberger E. The effect of testosterone propionate on the concentration of testicular and epididymal androgen binding activity in hypophysectomized rat. *Mol. Cell. Endocrinol.* 1975;2:157–170.
314. Weddington SC, Hansson V, Purvis K, Varaas T, Verjans HL, Eik-Nes KB, Ryan WH, French FS, Ritzén EM. Biphasic effect of testosterone propionate on Sertoli cell secretory function. *Mol. Cell. Endocrinol.* 1976;5:137–145.
315. Louis BG, Fritz IB. Stimulation by androgens of the production of androgen binding protein by cultured Sertoli cells. *Mol. Cell. Endocrinol.* 1977;7:9–16.
316. Louis BG, Fritz IB. Follicle stimulating hormone and testosterone independently increase the production of androgen binding protein by Sertoli cells in culture. *Endocrinology* 1979;104: 454–461.
317. Louis BG, Fritz IB. Regulation by testosterone and follicle stimulating hormone of androgen binding protein production by Sertoli cells in culture. *Proc. Can. Fed. Biol. Soc.* 1976;19:148.
318. Gunsalus GL, Larrea F, Musto NA, Becker RR, Mather JP, Bardin CW. Androgen binding protein as a marker for Sertoli cell function. *J. Steroid Biochem.* 1981;15:99–106.
319. Elkington JSH, Sanborn BM, Martin MW, Chowdhury AK, Steinberger E. Effect of testosterone propionate on ABP levels in rats hypophysectomized at different ages using individual sampling. *Mol. Cell. Endocrinol.* 1977;203–209.
320. Isomaa VV, Pajunen AEI, Bardin CW, Jänne OA. Ornithine decarboxylase in mouse kidney. Purification, characterization and radioimmunological determination of the enzyme protein. *J. Biol. Chem.* 1983;258:6735–6740.
321. Tsutsui K, Ishii S. Effects of follicle stimulating hormone and testosterone on receptors of follicle stimulating hormone in the testis of the immature Japanese quail. *Gen. Comp. Endocrinol.* 1978;36:297–305.
322. Tsutsui K, Ishii S. Hormonal regulation of follicle stimulating hormone receptors in the testes of Japanese quail. *J. Endocrinol.* 1980;85:511–518.
323. Cunha GR, Chung LWK, Shannon JM, Taguchi O, Fujii H. Hormone induced morphogenesis and growth: Role of mesenchymal-epithelial interactions. In: *Recent Prog. Horm. Res.* 1983;39: 559–598.
324. Cunha GR, Bigsby RM, Cooke PS, Sugimura Y. Stromal-epithelial interactions in adult organs. *Cell Differ.* 1985;17: 137–148.
325. Nakhla AM, Mather JP, Jänne OA, Bardin CW. Estrogen and androgen receptors in Sertoli, Leydig, myoid, and epithelial cells: Effects of time in culture and cell density. *Endocrinology* 1984;115:121–128.
326. Isomaa V, Parvinen M, Jänne OA, Bardin CW. Nuclear androgen receptors in different stages of the seminiferous epithelial cycle and the interstitial tissue of rat testis. *Endocrinology* 1985;116:132–136.
327. Wagle JR, Steinberger A, Sanborn BM. Interaction of progestins with Sertoli cell androgen receptors. *J. Steroid Biochem.* 1983;18:253–256.
328. Carson DD, Lennarz WJ. Vitamin A deprivation selectively lowers uridine nucleotide pools in cultured Sertoli cells. *J. Biol. Chem.* 1983;258:1632–1636.
329. Rajguru SU, Kang Y-H, Ahluwalia BS. Localization of retinol vitamin A in rat testes. *J. Nutr.* 1982;112:1881–1891.
330. Porter SB, Ong DE, Chytil F, Orgebin-Crist M-C. Localization of cellular retinol-binding protein and cellular retinoic-acid-binding protein in the rat testis and epididymis. *J. Androl.* 1985;6: 197–212.
331. Levy FO, Eikvar L, Jutte NHPM, Cervenka J, Yoganathan T, Hansson V. Appearance of the rat testicular receptor for calcitriol 1,25-dihydroxyvitamin d-3 during development. *J. Steroid Biochem.* 1985;23:51–56.
332. Merke J, Huegel U, Ritz E. Nuclear testicular 1,25-dihydroxyvitamin d-3 receptors in Sertoli cells and seminiferous tubules of adult rodents. *Biochem. Biophys. Res. Commun.* 1985;127: 303–309.
333. Kleinman HK, Klebe RJ, Martin GR. Role of collagenous matrices in the adhesion and growth of cells. *J. Cell Biol.* 1981;88: 473–485.
334. Gospodarowicz DJ. Extracellular matrices and the control of cell proliferation and differentiation *in vitro.* In: *New Approaches to the Study of Benign Prostatic Hyperplasia,* edited by Kimball FA, Buhl AE, and Carter DB, New York: Alan R. Liss; 1984:103–128.
335. Hay ED. (1984): Cell-matrix interaction in the embryo: Cell shape, cell surface, cell skeletons, and their role in differentiation. In: *The Role of the Extracellular Matrix in Development,* edited by. Trelstad RL, pp. 1–31. Alan R. Liss, New York.
336. Reid LM, Jefferson DM. Cell culture studies using extracts of extracellular matrix to study growth and differentiation in mammalian cells. In: *Mammalian Cell Culture,* edited by Mather JP. New York: Plenum; 1984.
337. Mather JP, Wolpe SD, Gunsalus GL, Bardin CW, Phillips DM. Effect of purified and cell-produced extracellular matrix components on Sertoli cell function. In: *Hormone Action and Testicular Function, Vol. 438,* edited by Catt KJ and Dufau ML, New York: Annals of the New York Academy of Science; 1985: 572–575.
338. Tung PS, Fritz IB. Extracellular matrix promotes rat Sertoli cell histotypic expression *in vitro. Biol. Reprod.* 1984;30:213–230.
339. Hadley MA, Byers SW, Suarez-Quian CA, Kleinman HK, Dym M. Extracellular matrix regulates Sertoli cell differentiation, testicular cord formation, and germ cell development *in vitro. J. Cell Biol.* 1985;101:1511–1522.
340. Parvinen M, Wright WW, Phillips DM, Mather JP, Musto NA, Bardin CW. Spermatogenesis *in vitro:* Completion of meiosis and early spermiogenesis. *Endocrinology* 1983;112:1150–1152.
341. Lacy D. Light and electron microscopy and its use in the study of factors influencing spermatogenesis in the rat. *J. Microsc. Soc.* 1960;79:209.
342. Hilscher B, Passia D, Hilscher W. Kinetics of the enzymatic pattern in the testis. I. Stage dependence of enzymatic activity and its relation to cellular interactions in the testis of the Wistar rat. *Andrologia* 1979;11:169–181.
343. Parvinen M, Vanha-Perttula T. Identification and enzyme quantitation of the stages of the seminiferous epithelial wave in the rat. *Anat. Rec.* 1972;174:435–450.
344. Lacroix M, Parvinen M, Fritz IB. Localization of testicular plasminogen activator in discrete portions T stages VII and VIII of the seminiferous tubule. *Biol. Reprod.* 1981;25:143–146.
345. Ritzen EM, Boitani C, Parvinen M, French FC, Feldman M. Stage dependent secretion of androgen binding protein by rat seminiferous tubules. *Mol. Cell. Endocrinol.* 1982;25:25–34.
346. Tung PS, Fritz IB. Interactions of Sertoli cells with myoid cells *in vitro. Biol. Reprod.* 1980;23:207–218.
347. Cameron DF, Syndle E. Selected enzyme histochemistry of Sertoli cells. 2. Adult rat Sertoli cells in co-culture with peritubular fibroblasts. *Andrologia* 1985;17:185–193.
348. Cameron DF, Markwald RR. Structural response of adult rat Sertoli cells to peri tubular fibroblasts *in vitro. Am. J. Anat.* 1981;160:343–358.
349. Parvinen M, Ruokonen A. Endogenous steroids in the rat seminiferous tubules. Comparison of the stages of the epithelial cycle isolated by transillumination-assisted microdissection. *J. Androl.* 1982;3:211–220.
350. Bergh A. Paracrine regulation of Leydig cells by the seminiferous tubules. *Int. J. Androl.* 1983;6:57–65.
351. Sharpe RM, Fraser HM, Cooper I, Rommerts FFG. Sertoli-Leydig cell communication via a luteinizing hormone releasing hormone like factor. *Nature* 1981;209:785–787.
352. Reventos J, Benahmed M, Tabone E, Saez JM. Modulation of Leydig cell functions by Sertoli cells: *in vitro* studies. *C. R. Acad. Sci. III* 1983;296:123–126.
353. Tabone E, Benahmed M, Reventos J, Saez JM. Interactions between immature porcine Leydig and Sertoli cells *in vitro:* An ultrastructural and biochemical study. *Cell Tissue Res.* 1984;237: 357–362.

354. Hatier R, Grignon G. Ultrastructural study of Sertoli cells in rat seminiferous tubules during intra uterine life and post natal period. *Anat. Embryol.* 1980;160:11–28.
355. Almond DG, Singh RP. Development of the Sertoli cell in the fetal mouse. *Acta Anat.* 1980;106:276–280.
356. Van Vorstenbosch CJAHV, Spek E, Colenbrander B, Wensing CJG. Sertoli cell development of pig testis in the fetal and neonatal period. *Biol. Reprod.* 1984;31:565–578.
357. Nistal M, Paniagua R. Post natal development of human Sertoli cells. *Z. Mikrosk. Anat. Forsch.* 1983;97:739–752.
358. Jost A. Preliminary data on the initial stages of testicular differentiation in the rat. *Arch. Anat. Microsc. Morphol. Exp.* 1972;61: 415–437.
359. Magre S, Jost A. The initial phases of testicular organogenesis in the rat: an electron microscopic study. *Arch. Anat. Microsc. Morphol. Exp.* 1980;69:297–318.
360. Agelopoulou R, Magre S, Patsavoudi E, Jost A. Initial phases of the rat testis differentiation *in vitro*. *J. Embryol. Exp. Morphol.* 1984;83:15–32.
361. Jost A, Magre S. Testicular development phases and dual hormonal control of sexual organogenesis. In: Serio M, Motta M, Zanisi M, and Martini L. *Sexual Differentiation: Basic and Clinical Aspects, Vol. 11.* New York: Raven Press; 1984;1–16.
362. Steinberger A, Steinberger E. Replication pattern of Sertoli cells in maturing rat testis *in vivo* and in organ culture. *Biol. Reprod.* 1971;84:84–94.
363. Orth JM. Effect of Sertoli cell depletion during neonatal life on spermatid production in adults. *Anat. Rec.* 1985;211:144A (abstract).
364. Kluin PM, Kramer MF, De Rooij DG. Proliferation of spermatogonia and Sertoli cells in maturing mice. *Anat. Embryol.* 1984;169:73–78.
365. Kluin PM, Kramer MF, De Rooij DG. Testicular development in macaca-irus after birth. *Int. J. Androl.* 1983;6:25–43.
366. Nistal M, Abaureea MA, Paniagua R. Morphological and histometric study on the human Sertoli cell from birth to the onset of puberty. *J. Anat.* 1982;134:351–363.
367. Chemes HE, Dym M, Raj HGM. The role of gonadotropins and testosterone on initiation of spermatogenesis in the immature rat. *Biol. Reprod.* 1979;21:241–249.
368. Chemes HF, Dym M, Raj HGM. Hormonal regulation of Sertoli cell differentiation. *Biol. Reprod.* 1979;21:251–262.
369. Orth J, Christensen AK. Localization of iodine-125 labeled follicle stimulating hormone in the testes of hypophysectomized rats by auto radiography at the light microscope and electron microscope levels. *Endocrinology* 1977;101:262–278.
370. Warren DW, Huhtaniemi IT, Tapanainen J, Dufau ML, Catt KJ. Ontogeny of gonadotropin receptors in the fetal and neonatal rat testis. *Endocrinology* 1984;114:470–476.
371. Means AR, Fakunding JL, Huckins C, Tindall DJ, Vitale R. Follicle-stimulating hormone, the Sertoli cell, and spermatogenesis. *Recent Prog. Horm. Res.* 1976;32:477–528.
372. Tsutsui K, Shimizu A, Kawamoto K, Kawashima S. Developmental changes in binding of follicle-stimulating hormone (FSH) to testicular preparations of mice and the effects of hypophysectomy and administration of FSH on the binding. *Endocrinology* 1985;117:2534–2543.
373. Barenton B, Hochereau-De Reviers MT, Perreau C, Saumande J. Changes in testicular gonadotropin receptors and steroid content through postnatal development until puberty in the lamb. *Endocrinology* 1983;112:1447–1453.
374. Tran D, Meusy-Dessolle N, Josso N. Anti-muellerian hormone is a functional marker of fetal Sertoli cells. *Nature* 1977;269: 411–412.
375. Donahoe PK, Swann DA, Hayashi A, Sullivan MD. Mullerian duct regression in the embryo correlated with cytotoxic activity against a human ovarian cancer. *Science* 1979;205:913.
376. Fuller A, Guy S, Donahoe P. Mullerian inhibiting substance inhibits colony growth of a human ovarian carcinoma cell line. *J. Clin. Endocrinol. Metab.* 1982;54:1051–1055.
377. Fuller AF, Krane IM, Budzik GP, Donahoe PK. Mullerian inhibiting substance reduction of colony growth of human gynecologic cancers in a stem cell assay. *Gynecol. Oncol.* 1985;2:135.
378. Donahoe P, Fuller A, Scully R, Guy S. Mullerian inhibiting substance inhibits growth of a human ovarian cancer in nude mice. *Am. Surg.* 1981;194:472.
379. Tran D, Josso N. Localization of antimuellerian hormone in the rough endoplasmic reticulum of the developing bovine Sertoli cell using immunocytochemistry with a monoclonal antibody. *Endocrinology* 1982;111:1562–1567.
380. Magre S, Jost A. Dissociation between testicular organogenesis and endocrine cytodifferentiation of Sertoli cells. *Proc. Natl. Acad. Sci. USA* 1984;81:7831–7834.
381. Blanchard M-G, Josso N. Source of the anti-muellerian hormone synthesized by the fetal testis: Muellerian inhibiting activity of fetal bovine Sertoli cells in tissue culture. *Pediatr. Res.* 1974;8:968–971.
382. Josso N, Picard JY, Dacheaux JL, Courot M. Detection of anti-Müllerian activity in boar rete testis fluid. *J. Reprod. Fertil.* 1979;57:397–403.
383. Necklaws EC, LaQuaglia MP, MacLaughlin D, Hudson P, Mudgett-Hunter M, Donahoe PK. Detection of mullerian inhibiting substance in biological samples by a solid phase sandwich radioimmunoassay. *Endocrinology* 1986;118:791–796.
384. Tran D, Meusy-Dessolle N, Josso N. Waning of anti-muellerian activity: An early sign of Sertoli cell maturation in the developing pig. *Biol. Reprod.* 1981;24:923–932.
385. Bergmann M, Dierichs R. Post natal formation of the blood testis barrier in the rat with special reference to the initiation of meiosis. *Anat. Embryol.* 1983;168:269–276.
386. Tindall DJ, Vitale R, Means AR. Androgen binding protein as a biochemical marker of formation of the blood testis barrier. *Endocrinology* 1975;97:636–648.
387. Hatier R, Grignon G, Touati F. Ultrastructural study of seminiferous tubules in the rat after pre natal irradiation. *Anat. Embryol.* 1982;165:425–436.
388. Vogel DL, Gunsalus GL, Bercu BB, Musto NA, Bardin CW. Sertoli cell maturation is impaired by neonatal passive immunization with antiserum to luteinizing hormone-releasing hormone. *Endocrinology* 1983;112:1115–1121.
389. Gunsalus GL, Musto NA, Bardin CW, Kunz HW, Gill TJ III. Rats homozygous for the *grc* complex have defective transport of androgen binding protein to the epididymis, but normal secretion into the blood. *Biol. Reprod.* 1985;33:1057–1063.
390. Gunsalus GL, Musto NA, Becker RR, Bardin CW. (1986): The bidirectional secretion of androgen binding protein in rats with germ cell depletion secondary to the H^{re} gene and prenatal x-ray. *Endocrinology (in press).*
391. Carreau S, Musto NA, Gunsalus GL. In fetal rats androgen binding protein (ABP) is synthesized by liver and testis. *Endocrinology* 1983;112:238 (abstract).
392. Carreau S, Gunsalus GL, Musto NA, Bardin CW. Sertoli rat androgen-binding protein is synthesized by liver and testis. *Endocrinology (submitted for publication).*
393. Gunsalus GL, De Besi L, Musto NA, Bardin CW. Measurement of rat androgen-binding protein (rABP) by steroid binding, radioimmunoassay (RIA), and enzyme linked immunosorbent assay (ELISA). In: *Binding Proteins of Steroid Hormones,* INSERM, Paris, 1986;149:227–236.
394. Dorrington JH, Fritz IB, Armstrong DT. Site at which follicle stimulating hormone regulates estradiol 17-β biosynthesis in Sertoli cell preparations in culture. *Mol. Cell. Endocrinol.* 1976;6: 117–122.
395. Steinberger E, Tcholakian RK, Steinberger A. Steroidogenesis in testicular cells. *J. Steroid Biochem.* 1979;11:185–192.
396. Canick JA, Makris A, Gunsalus GL, Ryan KJ. Testicular aromatization in immature rats: Localization and stimulation after gonadotropin administration *in vivo*. *Endocrinology* 1979;104: 285–288.
397. Gore-Langton R, Mckeracher H, Dorrington J. An alternative method for the study of follicle stimulating hormone effects on aromatase activity in Sertoli cell cultures. *Endocrinology* 1980;107:464–471.
398. Mori H, Christensen AK. Morphometric analysis of Leydig cells in the normal rat. *J. Cell Biol.* 1980;84:340–354.
399. Wong V, Russell LD. Three-dimensional reconstruction of a rat

stage V Sertoli cell. I. Methods, basic configuration, and dimensions. *Am. J. Anat.* 1983;167:143–162.

400. Wing T-Y, Christensen AK. Morphometric studies on rat seminiferous tubules. *Am. J. Anat.* 1982;165:13–26.
401. Weber JE, Russell LD, Wong V, Peterson RN. Three-dimensional reconstruction of a rat stage V Sertoli cell. II. Morphometry of Sertoli-Sertoli and Sertoli germ cell relationships. *Am. J. Anat.* 1983;167:163–180.
402. Russell LD, Tallon-Doran M, Weber JE, Wong V, Peterson RN. Three-dimensional reconstruction of a rat stage V Sertoli cell. III. A study of specific cellular relationships. *Am. J. Anat.* 1983;167:181–192.
403. Gardner R, Weber JE, Russell LD. Morphometric analysis of a reconstructed stage V monkey Sertoli cell. *J. Androl.* 1985;6:66-P (abstract).
404. Cunningham GR, Tindall DJ, Huckins C, Means AR. Mechanisms for the testicular hypertrophy which follows hemicastration. *Endocrinology* 1978;102:16–22.
405. Ribbert H. Ueber die compensatorische Hypertrophie der Geschlechtsdrusen. *Virchows Arch.* 1890;120:247.
406. Orth JM, Higginbotham CA, Salisbury RL. Hemicastration causes and testosterone prevents enhanced uptake of tritium labeled thymidine by Sertoli cells in testes of immature rats. *Biol. Reprod.* 1984;30:263–270.
407. Walton JS, Evins JD, Hillard MA, Waites GMH. Follicle stimulating hormone release in hemicastrated prepubertal rams and its relationship to testicular development. *J. Endocrinol.* 1980;84:141–152.
408. Waites GMH, Wenstrom JC, Crabo BG, Hamilton DW. Rapid compensatory hypertrophy of the lamb testis after neonatal hemiorchiectomy: Endocrine and light microscopic morphometric analyses. *Endocrinology* 1983;112:2159–2167.
409. Hochereau-De Reviers M-T, De Reviers M. Inhibition de la croissance compensatrice du testicule restant chez le Raton Hemicastre par de la testosterone ou des extraits aqueux de testicule de Rat adulte. *C. R. Acad. Sci. (Paris)* 1978;287:1015–1018.
410. Santen RJ, Paulsen CA. Hypogonadotropic eunuchoidism. I. Clinical study of the mode of inheritance. *J. Clin. Endocrinol. Metab.* 1973;36:47–53.
411. Bercu BB, Jackson IMD, Sawin CT, Safaii H, Reichlin S. Permanent impairment of testicular development after transient immunological blockade of endogenous luteinizing hormone releasing hormone in the neonatal rat. *Endocrinology* 1977;101:1871.
412. Bercu BB, Jackson IMD. Response of adult male rats to LHRH after neonatal immunization with antiserum to LHRH. *J. Reprod. Fertil.* 1980;59:501–507.
413. Carreau S, Bercu BB, Musto NA, Bardin CW, Gunsalus GL. Rat Sertoli cell maturation: Effects of neonatal hemicastration and LHRH antiserum treatment. *Endocrinology (submitted for publication).*
414. Valenca MC, Negro-Vilar N. Proopiomelanocortin-derived peptides in testicular interstitial fluid: Characterization and changes in secretion after human chorionic gonadotropin or luteinizing hormone-releasing hormone analog treatment. *Endocrinology* 1986;118:32–37.
415. Orth JM. Evidence that β-endorphin inhibits Sertoli cell proliferation in fetal rats. In: *7th International Congress of Endocrinology, Quebec, Canada,* Amsterdam (abstract 1902): Excerpta Medica; 1984:1211.
416. Becker RR, Gunsalus GL, Musto NA, Bardin CW. The epididymis contributes minimally to serum androgen binding protein in the rat: A whole body kinetic study. *Endocrinology* 1984;114:2354–2360.
417. Setchell BP, Waites GMH. The blood-testis barrier. In: *Handbook of Physiology, Section 7: Endocrinology, Volume V: Male Reproductive System,* edited by Hamilton DW and Greep RO, Washington D.C.: American Physiological Society; 1975:143.
418. Dym M. The mammalian rete testis-A morphological examination. *Anat. Rec.* 1976;186:493–520.
419. Christensen AK, Komorowski TE, Wilson B, Ma S-F, Stevens RW III. The distribution of serum albumin in the rat testis studied by electron microscope immunocytochemistry on ultrathin frozen sections. *Endocrinology* 1985;116:1983–1996.
420. Setchell BP, Hinton BT, Jacks F, Davies RV. The restricted penetration of iodinated FSH and LH into the seminiferous tubules of the rat testis. *Mol. Cell. Endocrinol.* 1976;6:59.
421. Ross MH. Sertoli Sertoli junctions and Sertoli spermatid junctions after efferent ductule ligation and lanthanum treatment. *Am. J. Anat.* 1977;148:49–56.
422. Osman DI, Ploen L. The terminal segment of the seminiferous tubules and the blood testis barrier before and after efferent ductule ligation in the rat. *Int. J. Androl.* 1978;1:235–249.
423. Nykanen M, Kormano M. Early effects of efferent duct ligation on the rat rete testis. *Int. J. Androl.* 1978;1:225–234.
424. Osman DI. A comparative ultrastructural study on typical and modified Sertoli cells before and after ligation of the efferent ductules in the rabbit. *Anat. Histol. Embryol.* 1979;8:114–123.
425. Anton E. Preservation of the rat blood testis barrier after ligation of the ductuli efferentes as demonstrated by intra-arterial perfusion with peroxidase. *J. Reprod. Fertil.* 1982;66:227–230.
426. Ashwell G, Morell AG. The role of surface carbohydrates in the hepatic recognition and transport of circulating glycoproteins. In: *Advances in Enzymology, Vol. 41,* edited by Meister A, New York: John Wiley & Sons; 1974:99–128.
427. Gill TJ IV, Gill TJ III, Kunz HW, Musto NA, Bardin CW. Genetic and morphometric studies of the heterogeneity in the testicular defect of the H^{re} rat and the interaction between the H^{re} and grc genes. *Biol. Reprod.* 1984;31:595–603.
428. Cheng CY, Gunsalus GL, Morris ID, Turner TT, Bardin CW. The heterogeneity of rat androgen binding protein (rABP) in the vascular compartment differs from that in the testicular tubular lumen: Further evidence for bidirectional secretion of rABP. *J. Androl.* 1986;7:175–179.
429. Lobl TJ, Musto NA, Gunsalus GL, Bardin CW. Medroxyprogesterone acetate has opposite effects on the androgen binding protein concentrations in serum and epididymis. *Biol. Reprod.* 1983;29:697–712.
430. Spitz IM, Gunsalus GL, Mather JP, Thau R, Bardin CW. The effects of the indazole carboxylic acid derivative, tolnidamine, on testicular function. I. Early changes in androgen binding protein secretion in the rat. *J. Androl.* 1985;6:171–178.
431. Escobar N, Musto NA. Assessing Sertoli cell function in the rabbit by measurement of serum androgen-binding protein. In: *7th International Congress of Endocrinology, Quebec, Canada,* Amsterdam (abstract 766): Excerpta Medica; 1984:643.

The Physiology of Reproduction, Second Edition,
edited by E. Knobil and J.D. Neill,
Raven Press, Ltd., New York © 1994.

CHAPTER 21

Testicular Steroid Synthesis: Organization and Regulation

Peter F. Hall

The function of the Leydig cells of the testis is to secrete androgens in a regulated fashion. The principal regulating mechanism consists of the secretion of pulses of luteinizing hormone (LH) by the adenohypophysis (1). Androgens are responsible for the development and maintenance of the internal and external genitalia, the appearance of the secondary sexual characteristics, the development of the musculoskeletal system, feedback inhibition of the hypothalamus-pituitary, and stimulation of spermatogenesis. In addition, androgens stimulate a variety of other tissues including the skin and the kidneys. To a considerable extent, the difference between male and female mammalian organisms with respect to androgens is one of degree, so that male appearances can be induced in females by the administration of androgens.

Department of Endocrinology, Prince of Wales Hospital, Randwick, Sydney, N.S.W. 2031 Australia

The principal steroids secreted by the testis are androgens, and testosterone is by far the most important androgen because of its potency. Androstenedione and dehydroepiandrosterone are also secreted by the testis and show lesser degrees of androgenicity (2).

SOURCE OF TESTICULAR ANDROGENS

Without doubt, almost all testicular androgens are formed and secreted by the Leydig cells (2,3). Some steroidogenic enzymes are found within the seminiferous tubule (4).

It has been proposed that the seminiferous tubule can convert cholesterol to pregnenolone and is therefore capable of synthesizing androgens. Hall et al. (4) found no detectable production of [^{3}H]pregnenolone when seminiferous tubules of the rat were incubated with [7α-^{3}H]cholesterol. This failure could not be attributed to failure of the substrate to enter the germ cells or fibroblasts, first because cholesterol enters most cells freely, so that [^{3}H]cholesterol would be expected to label intracellular cholesterol by exchange, if not by net uptake (5). Second, homogenate of seminiferous tubules incubated with [^{3}H]cholesterol does not produce detectable [^{3}H]-pregnenolone or [^{3}H]androgens (6). On the one hand, it is never possible to say that there has been *no* conversion of one substance to another, only less than the minimal amount detected by the methods used. On the other hand, it is always difficult to exclude some contamination of seminiferous tubules by Leydig cells, and vice versa. The problem is best considered functionally. There is no evidence that the seminiferous tubules can make a physiologically detectable contribution to androgen production, and there is no evidence that the seminiferous tubules can maintain spermatogenesis by their own production of androgens.

In addition to the secretion of androgens, the testis also produces small amounts of estrogens (7,8). Indirect evidence points to the Leydig cell as the source of such estrogens (9,10), although the Sertoli cell also contributes (7,11,12).

It should be added that an important part of plasma estrogen in the male comes from extratesticular conversion of nonestrogenic steroids (13).

SYNTHESIS OF ANDROGENS BY LEYDIG CELLS

The synthesis of steroid hormones requires a substrate, that is, a source of the steroid ring system, a series of enzymes and cofactors that together constitute the biosynthetic pathway and a source of energy.

The Substrate

The immediate source of the steroid ring system used for the synthesis of steroid hormones consists of depots of cholesterol in the cytoplasm (14). Stores of cholesterol are to be seen in Leydig cells of various species in the form of conspicuous lipid droplets in the cytoplasm (15). Much work has been performed to determine whether this cholesterol is made in Leydig cells or brought from plasma in lipoproteins. It is clear that both sources are used (6,16). To determine the relative importance of these two sources of cholesterol, Chaikoff and coworkers (17,18) studied the equilibration of plasma [^{14}C]-cholesterol with testicular cholesterol and testosterone. They found that plasma cholesterol contributes no more than 13% to the total production of androgens in the guinea pig (17) and 40% in rat (18).

Evidently the testis makes an important contribution to the steroidogenic cholesterol. When slices of testis are incubated *in vitro* with [^{14}C]acetate, the label is readily incorporated into testosterone in rabbit (19) but not demonstrably in rat (20). Unfortunately, the testis is complex in structure, and Leydig cells constitute no more than a small part of the organ. This limits the experimental approaches that can be used to answer such questions. Cultured Leydig cells offer a useful system for such studies. Clearly, the contribution of plasma cholesterol varies from species to species and is different in the adrenal (21). Future studies must evaluate each system individually. The relevant methods are now available (21); in the meantime, it must be concluded that steroidogenic cholesterol comes from both plasma and local production in the Leydig cell.

The contribution of plasma cholesterol to the synthesis of steroid hormones comes from lipoproteins. Leydig tumor cells (MA-10) use low-density lipoprotein (LDL) as a source of steroidogenic cholesterol (22). The so-called classical pathway from LDL receptor to lysosomes to cholesterol depots is employed in these (22), as in other cells that import LDL from plasma (5). During stimulation by human chorionic gonadotropin (hCG), more than half of the steroidogenic cholesterol comes from LDL, and cholesterol stores are depleted within 4 h (22).

The pathway in these cells is unusual in that cholesterol from LDL does not inhibit the synthesis of cholesterol from acetate (5,22). On the other hand, rat testis has been shown to possess specific receptors for high-density lipoprotein (HDL) (23), so this form of lipoprotein may be important as a source of cholesterol for steroid synthesis, as in rat adrenal (24).

The lipid droplets of Leydig cells are depleted during times of increased synthesis of androgens (15), in keeping with the well-accepted idea that the stored cholesterol is used for the synthesis of these hormones. The testis possesses a cholesterol ester hydrolase that is stimulated by hCG (25). Presumably, this enzyme serves to mobilize cholesterol for steroid synthesis, as in the adrenal (26). From there on, no details are known concerning the steroid synthetic pathway in Leydig cells until cholesterol appears in the inner mitochondrial membrane, where the pathway continues with the conversion of cholesterol to pregnenolone. The adrenal cortex has been studied more intensely in this respect. Here, the cholesterol from LDL is reesterfied for storage, and when cholesterol ester hydrolase releases free cholesterol, this substrate binds to sterol carrier protein (SCP_2), which accompanies it to mitochondria (21). This, or another protein, takes the cholesterol to the inner mitochondrial membrane (21,27). It is also clear that reesterification of cholesterol for storage involves different fatty acids from those esterified to the cholesterol of LDL (21). Only future studies will reveal how closely the handling of cholesterol in Leydig cells resembles that in the adrenal. It seems reasonable to proceed with this discussion on the assumption that the two cells handle steroidogenic cholesterol in essentially the same way, provided the extent of this assumption is not overlooked.

The Pathway

The synthesis of androgens involves the conversion of cholesterol to testosterone:

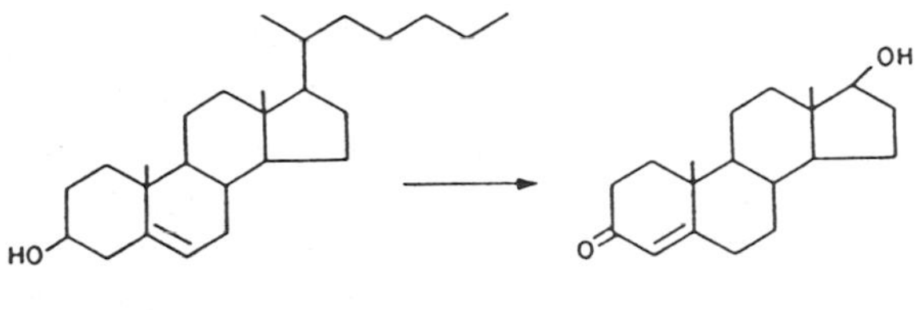

The enzymatic reactions required for this conversion are as listed in Table 1.

Hydroxylation and lyase activities require cytochromes P-450 (28). Dehydrogenation requires typical pyridine nucleotide dehydrogenases, and an isomerase moves the double bond to the more stable α,β-unsaturated ketone (16).

The pathway begins with the conversion of cholesterol to pregnenolone (C_{27} side-chain cleavage), which takes place in mitochondria. Pregnenolone is converted to testosterone by microsomal enzymes. Before discussing the individual enzymes involved, we must consider the general properties of cytochromes P-450, since two of these enzymes catalyze key reactions in the pathway to androgens, i.e., C_{27} side-chain cleavage (29) and C_{21} side-chain cleavage (30).

Cytochromes P-450

The remarkable family of enzymes known as cytochromes P-450 is widely distributed in nature, where they are best known as enzymes for the disposal of lipophilic substrates by rendering these substances more soluble in water as the result of hydroxylation. The prototype for reactions catalyzed by these enzymes in the presence of $^{18}O_2$ can be summarized as follows (31):

$$R—H + NADPH + H^+ + {}^{18}O_2 \xrightarrow{[P\text{-}450]} R\text{-}{}^{18}OH + H_2{}^{18}O + NADP^+$$

This statement of the reaction indicates a number of important features of hydroxylation of substrates (RH) catalyzed by these enzymes. The enzyme uses atmospheric or molecular oxygen, one atom of which is attached to the substrate in a hydroxyl group, while the second is reduced to water. This type of oxidation is referred to as monooxygenation, since only one atom of oxygen appears in the product. The hydroxyl group in the product replaces a hydrogen in the substrate, so the product is more soluble in water than the substrate. This change facilitates the removal of the product from the body, because the more soluble product can be filtered by the kidney and because it is less able to dissolve in cell membranes to enter cells than the more lipophilic substrate. This mechanism provides a major defence against xenobiotics and drugs that are frequently lipophilic (32). In addition, the body uses this mechanism to remove such lipophilic substrates as steroids and prostaglandins that are no longer required by the body; these substances are referred to as endogenous substrates to distinguish them from xenobiotics (exogenous substrates) (33). The reactions to be considered here fall into another category, in which the changes produced in the substrate provide those features of the steroid hormones that are recognized by receptors and other intracellular molecules and that therefore enable the steroids to act as hormones.

The equation also shows the characteristic stoichiometry of monooxygenation, i.e., NADPH:O_2:RH of 1:1:1 (31,34). The above statement does not show the electron carriers used to convey electrons from reduced pyridine nucleotide to P-450. Microsomal cytochromes P-450 use a single flavoprotein reductase to discharge this function (35), whereas mitochondrial P-450 uses two carriers—a flavoprotein reductase and an iron-sulfur protein (36). The iron sulfur proteins are referred to by the suffix *-oxin,* e.g., andrenodoxin for the adrenal protein, and presumably testodoxin will be used for the testicular enzyme, which has not been studied in detail. The reductase proteins are referred to as adrenodoxin reductase, etc. It will be pointed out that the steroidogenic cytochromes P-450 are capable of reactions other than simple hydoxylation, e.g., cleavage of C—C bonds.

Cytochromes P-450 are heme proteins: each molecule of protein contains a heme moiety that is not covalently bound to the protein but lies in a hydrophobic crevice. It turns out that all cytochromes P-450 show a number of important structural features, so it is useful to discuss

TABLE 1. *Enzymatic reactions required for the conversion of cholesterol to testosterone*

Activity	C atom
Hydroxylation	17,20,22
Dehydrogenation	3β, 17β
Isomerization	$\Delta^{4,5}$
C-C cleavage (lyase)	20,22 and 17,20

this group of enzymes as a whole. The iron of the heme has the potential to engage in six bonds, of which four are of necessity made to the four pyrrole nitrogens of the heme; in P-450 one is to a cysteine in the protein. The four bonds with nitrogen lie in the plane of the pyrrole ring system, and the fifth and sixth bonds are at right angles to this plane and are thus called axial. The fifth bond takes the form of a thiolate bond with the sulfur of cysteine (37,38). The nature of the sixth ligand is uncertain. Finally, it should be pointed out that the iron may be hexacoordinate or pentacoordinate (six or five bonds). The pentacoordinate iron is displaced from the plane of the ring, and the electrons of the d orbital of the iron are arranged so as to give the so-called high-spin form of this atom, in contrast to the low-spin hexacoordinate form in which the iron lies in the plane of the heme ring system.

The conjugated double-bond system of heme gives rise to a striking property on absorption spectroscopy, namely, a conspicuous peak at approximately 420 nm, the so-called Soret peak. The intensity and position of the Soret peak are influenced by the protein moiety of the heme proteins. In the absence of bound substrate, the heme moiety has a low-spin, hexacoordinate iron with a Soret peak in the vicinity of 420 nm. When substrate binds to P-450, the accompanying conformational change results in the formation of pentacoordinate high-spin iron displaced from the plane of the heme ring system. These changes are accompanied by a shift in the Soret peak to approximately 390 nm, the so-called substrate-induced spectral shift:

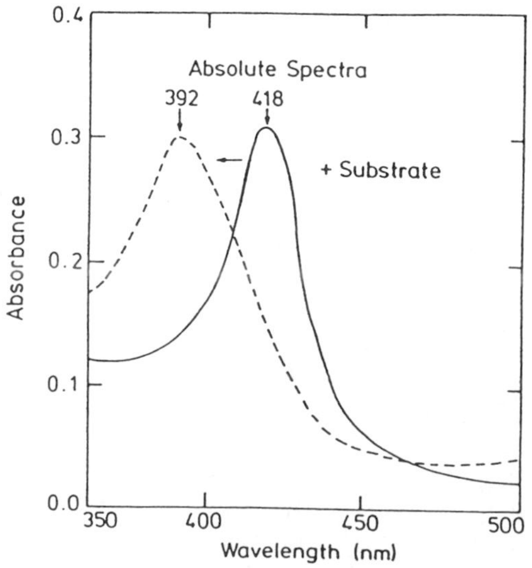

This shift is of great practical significance, because it can be measured by difference, i.e., substrate-induced difference spectroscopy. The spectrophomometer is set to subtract the absorbance of enzyme plus solvent (reference cuvette) from that of enzyme plus substrate (sample cuvette). The high-spin form (ES) gives a positive peak at 390 nm, and the low-spin form (no substrate) gives a negative peak, or trough, at 420 nm, because the absorbance in the reference cuvette is subtracted from that in the sample cuvette. The peak plus trough (A 390–420 nm) is proportional to the amount of enzyme present in the form of ES, as illustrated below:

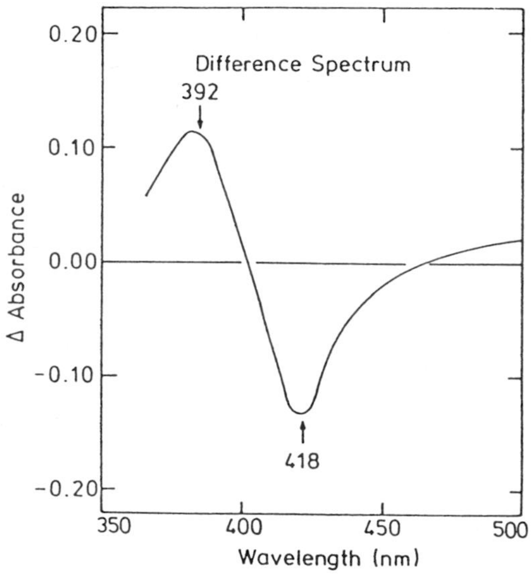

This provides a simple, rapid, direct, and nondestructive method of measuring binding as a function of substrate concentration. This difference spectrum (peak at 390 nm and trough at 420 nm) is referred to as a type 1 spectrum.

In the low-spin form of iron, all the *d* orbital electrons are of the low-energy form called t_{2g}, and there is one unpaired electron.

In short-hand nomenclature, this is referred to as 1/2. In the high-spin form of iron, all five electrons of the *d* orbitals are unpaired, and two have the high-energy form, e.g., in short-hand nomenclature, this is referred to as 5/2. These spectral properties of P-450 are summarized in Table 2 (37–39).

We must consider one further spectral property that is also of practical importance since it is used to identify and measure all cytochromes P-450. Reduced heme proteins bind CO as the sixth ligand, and this shifts the Soret peak. The oxidized form does not bind CO. In most heme proteins the shift amounts to no more than a few nanometers. With P-450, the shift is unusually extensive (420–450 nm). The spectrum can be examined by difference: reduced P-450-CO minus oxidized P-450 plus CO (40). In addition to giving P-450 its name (pigment 450), this spectral property provides an accurate method for measuring P-450:

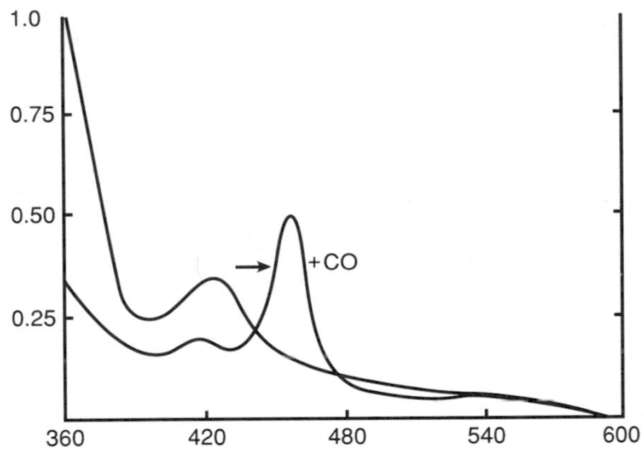

An important feature of all cytochromes P-450 is the so-called P-450 cycle, by which the enzyme becomes reduced so that it can carry out its alloted function. The reduced (Fe^{2+}) enzyme must be reoxidized in readiness for the next cycle.

TABLE 2. *Spectral properties of P-450*

Substrate	Coordination valence	Spin state	*d* electrons	Soret band (nm)
Absent	6	Low	1/2	420
Bound	5	High	5/2	390

Since P-450 is reduced to the ferrous form by electrons from NADPH and reoxidized during catalytic activity, the enzyme must undergo cycles of oxidation and reduction. For descriptive purposes each cycle can be considered in five steps, although the steps flow rapidly into one another, and the last step is itself made up of several steps (37,38,41).

Step 1. Binding the substrate:

$$Fe^{3+} + RH + e \rightarrow Fe^{2+} - RH$$

where P-450 is represented by Fe. This step has two important consequences. First, it is associated with a conformational change that displaces the iron from the plane of the ring and produces the high-spin form of heme iron with a type 1 spectral shift. Second, binding of substrate promotes the passage of one electron (the so-called first electron) from adrenodoxin to the enzyme substrate complex.

Step 2. Reduction of the enzyme-substrate complex by the first electron:

$$Fe^{3+} - RH + e \rightarrow Fe^{2+} - RH$$

Step 3. Binding of oxygen. The reduced enzyme-substrate complex binds oxygen:

$$Fe^{2+} - RH + O_2 \rightarrow Fe^{2+} - \underset{\displaystyle O_2}{\overset{|}{RH}}$$

Step 4. Activation of bound oxygen by a second electron. The second electron activates oxygen bound to iron as the result of rearrangement of electrons:

$$\underset{\displaystyle O_2}{\overset{|}{Fe^{2+}}} - RH + e + H^+ \rightarrow \underset{\displaystyle O_2^{2-}}{\overset{|}{Fe^{3+}}} - RH + OH^-$$

Step 5. Hydroxylation of substrate. This complex step results in the formation of the hydroxylated product:

$$\underset{\displaystyle O_2^{2-}}{\overset{|}{Fe^{3+}}} - RH \rightarrow Fe^{3+} + ROH$$

The hydroxyl group of the product produces repulsive forces at the hydrophobic active site of the enzyme, which facilitates removal of the product. The enzyme is now ready to start the cycle again:

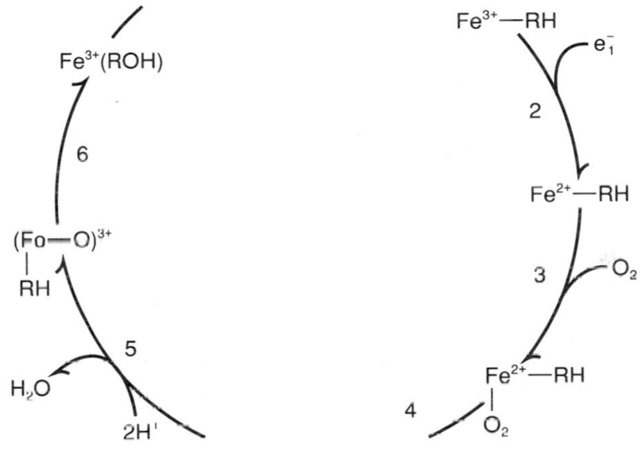

We can now consider the individual enzymes of the steroidogenic pathway beginning with the cytochromes P-450.

C_{27} Side-Chain Cleavage

The conversion of cholesterol to pregnenolone is catalyzed by a mitochondrial cytochrome P-450 in three steps: (see top of next page). The classical hydroxylase activity of P-450 is used in the first two steps, and the intervening C—C bond is cleaved to give two oxygenated products. This enzyme was the first cytochrome P-450 to be purified. It was isolated from mitochondria of bovine adrenal cortex using conventional chromatographic procedures (29,42,43). A variety of other methods have been used subsequently (44–47). Since the enzyme was shown to be homogeneous by gel electropho-

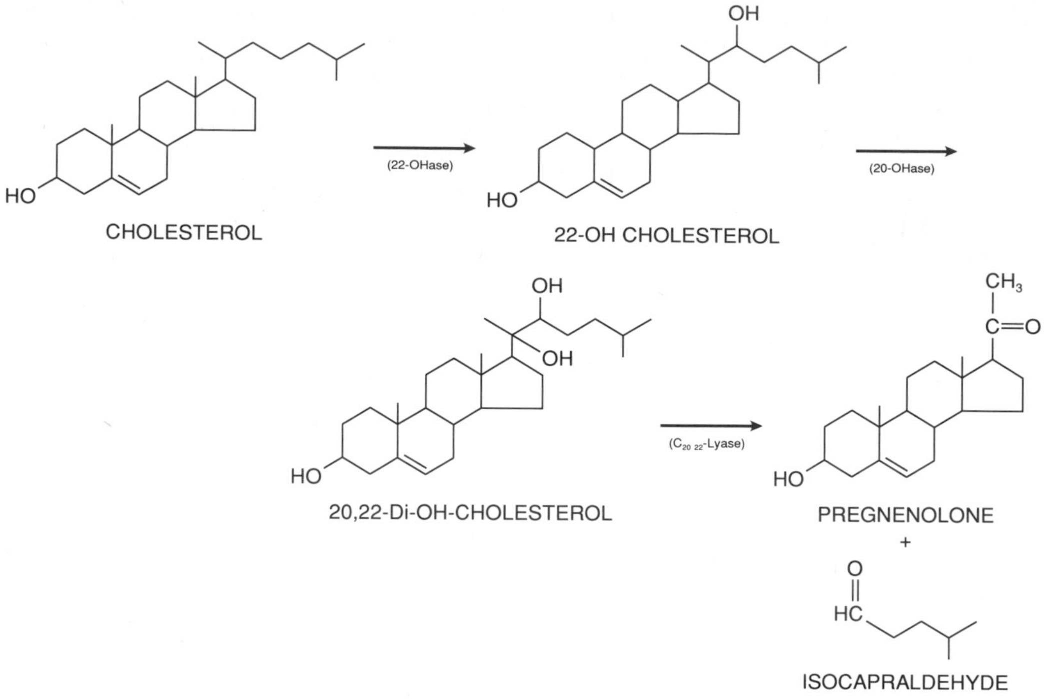

resis and by double diffusion with an antibody raised against the pure enzyme showing the line of identity, as well as by immunoelectrophoresis (29,43), we must conclude that all three steps in the above reaction are catalyzed by a single protein. The enzyme shows a single NH_2 terminal amino acid (namely, glutamate) (43). Moreover, when the substrate used is [^{14}C]cholesterol, virtually all the disappearing cholesterol can be accounted for as [^{14}C]pregnenolone plus unused substrate (48,49). The existence of the two intermediates was demonstrated first by showing that the intermediates are rapidly converted to pregnenolone and later by the work of Burstein and Gut (50) in which the kinetics of the conversion were studied using large-scale preparations of a crude enzyme system.

The next question to be raised was whether there is more than one active site on the enzyme. Kinetic and binding studies by Duque et al. (51) are consistent with a single binding site. Since the cleavage of a C—C bond is unusual for cytochrome P-450, it was important to demonstrate that the heme moiety of P-450 is involved in the last step of the conversion. This was accomplished by means of a photochemical action spectrum, which showed that CO inhibits the conversion of the dihydroxycholesterol to pregnenolone and that this inhibition is specifically reversed by light of wavelength 450 nm (52). This finding unequivocally established the involvement of the heme moiety in a classical P-450-catalyzed reaction. This conclusion was supported by measurement of the stoichiometry of the overall reaction and that of the individual steps. The overall action shows the following stoichiometry (53):

$$C_{27}H_{46}O + 3O_2 + 3\ NADPH + 3H^+ \rightarrow C_{21}H_{32}O_2 + C_6H_{12}O + 4H_2O$$

The stoichiometry of each step was found to be that of monooxygenation, i.e., 1 NADPH + 1H^+ + 1O_2 + 1 mole of substrate (31,53).

Evidently the cleavage of the C_{20}—C_{22} bond involves a typical monooxygenation using the heme group of P-450. This finding established, for the first time, such C—C cleavage as a reaction catalyzed by P-450. A detailed study of the binding of substrate, intermediates, and product to the pure enzyme using electron spin resonance and absorption spectroscopy revealed a single binding site for each of these steroids (54). The values for the respective dissociation constants are shown as follows in Table 3:

TABLE 3. *Dissociation constants for three steroids*

Steroid	K_d (nM)
22R-OH cholesterol	4.9
20R, 22R-diOH cholesterol	81.0
Pregnenolone	2,900.0

Moreover, 22R-OH cholesterol shows a dissociation frequency of 5S^{-1}. It is therefore apparent that the two intermediates are tightly bound and that the product dissociates readily. It is also clear why the intermediates are so difficult to isolate: they are tightly bound to the enzyme, and one intermediate is rapidly converted to the next. The intermediates are therefore only present bound to the enzyme, i.e., virtually no free intermediates exist. It was for this reason that Burstein and Gut (50) were forced to use large amounts of enzyme to recover measurable amounts of intermediates (50). Unfortunately, the insolubility of cholesterol has made it impossible to obtain reliable values for Kd of this substrate.

Evidently the catalytic cycle of P-450 is modified for side-chain cleavage in such a way that a second cycle begins with the product of the first cycle still at the active site, and the same is true for the third cycle. When the third cycle is complete, the product (pregnenolone) dissociates from the active site, and the whole process starts again with the binding of cholesterol.

It should be pointed out that when pregnenolone is added to the pure C_{27} side-chain cleavage P-450, a spectral shift occurs that is the inverse of the usual shift produced by substrates, i.e., peak at 420 and trough at 390 nm, instead of vice versa (55). This shift (called inverse type 1) results from the binding of pregnenolone to a site that differs from the active site (54–56). This binding is responsible for inhibition of the side-chain cleavage of cholesterol by pregnenolone (48).

In aqueous media, the C_{27} side-chain cleavage enzyme associates into oligomeric forms—tetramers, octomers, and hexadecamers (42). When the enzyme was centrifuged through buffered sucrose containing adrenodoxin, adrenodoxin reductase, cholesterol, and NADPH, it was found that only the hexadecamer form (16 subunits, MW 850,000) is enzymatically active (57). The nature of the active form in the inner mitochondrial membrane is unknown.

C_{21} Side-Chain Cleavage

The conversion of C_{21} steroids to C_{19} steroids proceeds in two steps: 17α-hydroxylation and $C_{17,20}$-lyase:

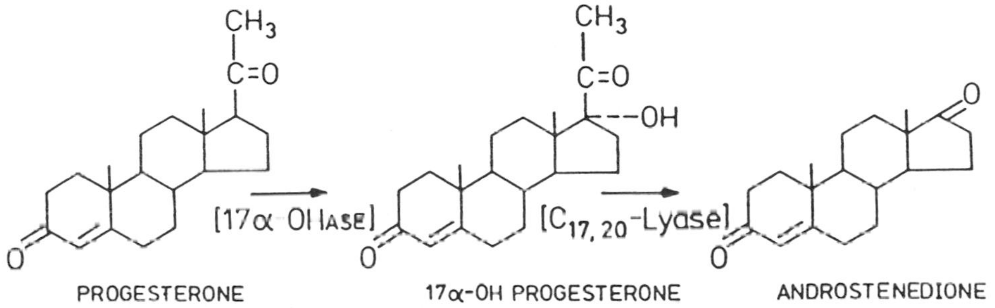

In view of the mechanism of C_{27} side-chain cleavage just described, it might have been predicted that a single cytochrome P-450 is responsible for catalyzing both reactions. However, because the adrenal cortex synthesizes the 17α-hydroxy-C_{21} steroid cortisol, it seemed clear that 17α-hydroxylation can proceed without $C_{17,20}$-lyase activity. This pointed to two separate enzymes, and some indirect evidence seemed to support this view (58).

The next question to arise was whether there is one active site or two to catalyze the two steps in C_{21} side-chain cleavage. Studies with inhibition by antibody to the pure enzyme and competitive inhibition by two synthetic inhibitors, together with substrate-induced difference spectra and equilibrium dialysis, all support the idea of a single active site (59,60,66,67). An additional line of evidence proved important in support of the concept of a single active site. The enzyme was subjected to affinity alkylation by 17α-bromoacetoxyprogesterone. This substrate analogue binds covalently to a specific cysteine residue:

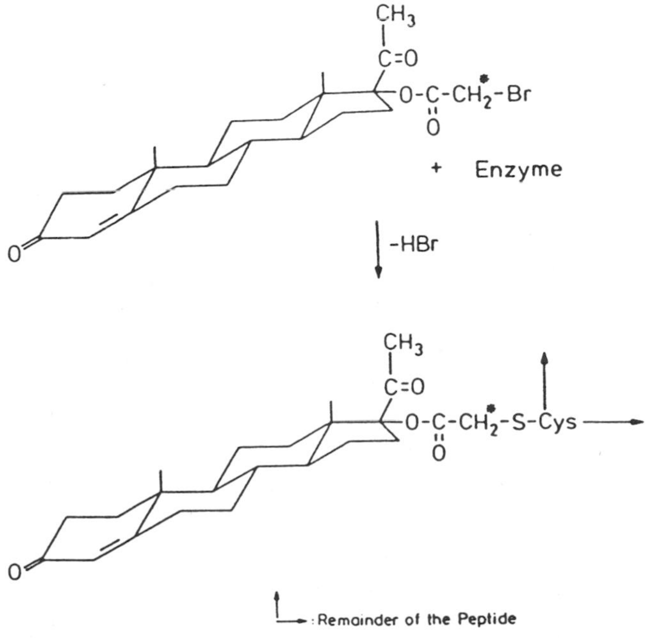

However, when the testicular enzyme was purified to homogeneity, it was found that one enzyme catalyzes both reactions (59,60). The enzyme is microsomal, but otherwise it resembles the C_{27} side-chain cleavage enzyme to such an extent that they have been mistaken during purification (61). Evidence for homogeneity of the enzyme rests on gel electrophoresis, double diffusion, and immunoelectrophoresis with antibodies raised against the pure enzyme and extensive sequence determination with a single amino acid at each position in the molecule (59,60). Incidentally, the difference between the testicular and adrenal enzymes provides a most unexpected result. The two enzymes are very similar (not quite identical) in almost every way (62,63). Binding and kinetic constants for the substrates are almost the same for both enzymes. The difference must lie in the microsomes, because in adrenal microsomes very little lyase activity is seen, yet the pure enzyme shows the same lyase activity as the pure testicular enzyme (62). This provides an intriguing example of microsomal regulation. One factor that promotes lyase activity is P-450 reductase, which is present in greater concentration in the microsomes of testis than in those of adrenal (64). In addition, cytochrome b_5 increases activity of lyase relative to hydroxylase, and testicular microsomes contain more cytochrome b_5 per milligram of protein than do adrenal microsomes (64,65). However, there may be additional factors involved in microsomal regulation.

The process of affinity alkylation inactivates the enzyme. Inactivation proceeds by a first-order process that shows the same value of $t_{1/2}$ for both enzyme activities (hydroxylase and lyase) (67). Moreover, both substrates (progesterone and 17α-hydroxyprogesterone) protect both activities against inactivation (67). In other words, the substrate analogue and both substrates compete for a single active site (67).

The concept of one active site was confirmed by two additional observations. First, the $C_{17,20}$-lyase activity was shown to involve the heme moiety of the enzyme in a typical P-450 catalyzed reaction (68). Second, there is one heme group per peptide moiety. If heme is required for both reactions, it means that there is one active site or two overlapping sites both of which include the heme moiety.

Evidently, these two systems for C—C cleavage (C_{27} and C_{21}) use similar mechanisms. However, two important differences are seen between these enzymes: namely, the C_{27} system is mitochondrial whereas the C_{21} system is microsomal, and the C_{27} systems require three steps whereas the C_{21} substrate is already oxygenated at C_{20}, so only two steps are necessary.

Dehydrogenase-Isomerase

The A and B rings of pregnenolone are converted to the Δ^4-3-keto structure by a microsomal enzyme system that has not been purified to homogeneity:

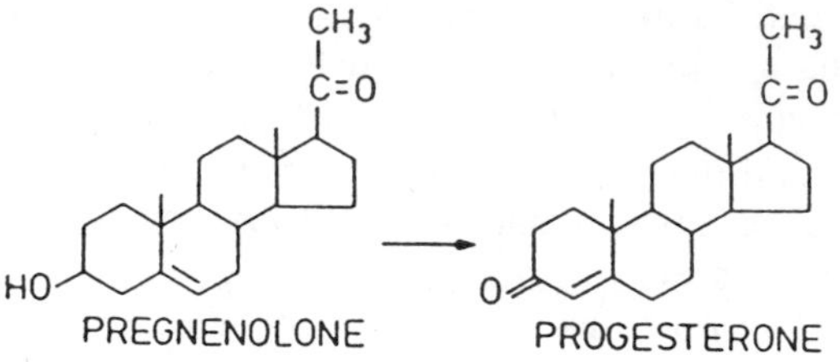

The enzyme has been purified from rat adrenal and shows an MW of 46,800. The intermediate Δ^5-3-ketosteroid was identified, and both activities were found in a single protein (69). The corresponding enzyme has also been reported from rat testis (70). It was found that the dehydrogenase and isomerase activities require NAD^+, but the former activity does not change the redox state of the cofactor required as an activator for the enzyme (70). The enzyme from human placenta is a tetramer of MW 70,800 with monomers of 19,000 (71). The enzyme is found in a number of tissues not usually associated with steroid synthesis, e.g., liver and prostate (72). There may be a single, active site for this enzyme, but if this is so the two activities probably involve different amino acid side-chains because the dehydrogenase and isomerase functions show pH optima of 9.8 and 7.5, respectively (73).

17β-Hydroxysteroid Dehydrogenase

The microsomal enzyme 17β-hydroxysteroid dehydrogenase catalyzes the interconversion of androstenedione and testosterone with the aid of NAD^+:

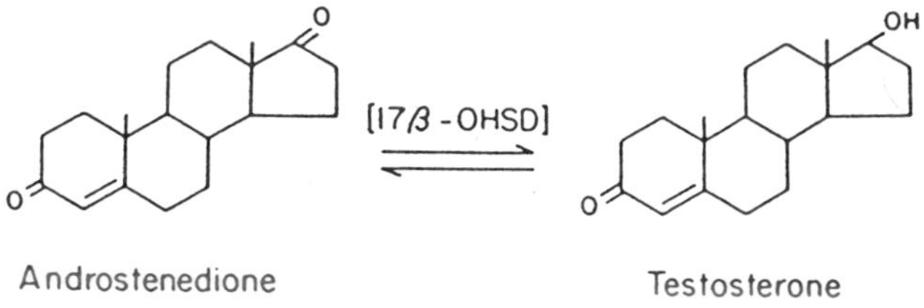

OHSD: HYDROXYSTEROID DEHYDROGENASE

The enzyme shows the unusual property of product activation, i.e., testosterone promotes the formation of testosterone from androstenedione, and androstenedione does the same from testosterone (74). The reaction catalyzed is freely reversible, and the enzyme possesses two active sites (75). These remarkable properties suggest that the activity of the enzyme may be greatly influenced by the available concentrations of the two substrates and by the rate of removal of the products of the reaction. Special methods may be required to understand the regulation of this enzyme *in vivo*. The activity of the enzyme in the microsome is greatly decreased by the action of phospholipase C, indicating a stabilizing action of lipids on the enzyme (76). In addition, there appears to be a keto-reductase distinct from the dehydrogenase and a separate enzyme within the seminiferous tubule, i.e., apart from that in Leydig cells (77). The details of the kinetics of this complex enzyme have been reviewed (78).

The Energy

Reactions catalyzed by cytochromes P-450 use NADPH. Energy is also presumably required for movement of substrate and intermediates through the cell, but the nature of these processes is not sufficiently understood to describe the sources of the energy required.

Organization of the Steroidogenic Pathway in the Cell

In discussing the performance of this pathway in the cell, it is important to consider the relationship between the mitochondrial and microsomal compartments, which is illustrated as follows:

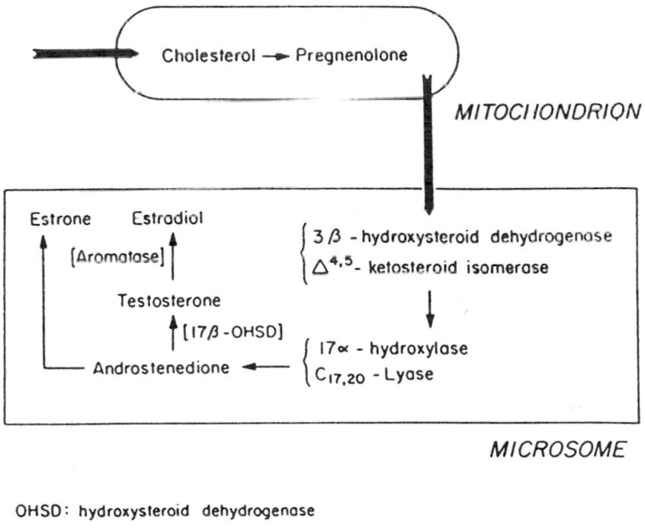

It is clear that the pathway begins in the mitochondrion and that pregnenolone is transferred to microsomes to complete the synthesis of androgens.

Steroidogenic Inner Mitochondrial Membrane

The side-chain cleavage enzyme system is found only in the inner mitochondrial membrane, and immunoelectron microscopy with colloidal gold (79) showed that, at least in the adrenal cortex, all mitochondria contain the enzyme, and within each organelle the distribution is random (80). To study the enzyme in an environment that more closely resembles the mitochondrial membrane, it was incorporated into lipid vesicles prepared from an equimolar mixture of phosophatidylcholine and phosphatidylethanolamine with and without cholesterol (81). The entire side-chain cleavage system (adrenodoxin reductase, adrenodoxin, and P-450) can be incorporated into lipid vesicles so that on addition of NADPH, production of pregnenolone occurs. The enzyme is converted to the high-spin form and shows a great reduction of K_m for cholesterol (81). The reconstituted side-chain cleavage system in lipid vesicles was studied in greater detail by Seybert et al. (82,83). These workers showed that P-450 in one vesicle does not use cholesterol incorporated into a different vesicle and that the binding site on P-450 for cholesterol is associated with the hydrophobic region of the bilayer, whereas the binding site on P-450 for adrenoxdoxin is on the surface of the vesicle facing the external water phase (82,83). The same group went on to show that adrenodoxin shuttles between the reductase and P-450 as follows. Oxidized adrenodoxin binds to reduced reductase, and, after transfer of one electron, the reduced adrenodoxin shows low affinity for the oxidized reductase and now binds to P-450 (84,85). Adrenodoxin and P-450 are present in approximately equimolar amounts in the inner mitochondrial membrane, and reductase is present at a lower concentration (86).

As a result of the dissociation and reassociation of adrenodoxin and reductase, one molecule of reductase can serve numerous molecules of adrenodoxin and, hence, P-450 (84,85). Presumably, this mechanism explains the ability of the system to function *in vivo* with a low concentration of reductase. It is not clear at present whether this adrenodoxin shuttle regulates the rate of side-chain cleavage *in vivo* (86).

Steroidogenic Endoplasmic Reticulum

Less work has been performed with the organization of the endoplasmic reticulum than with the inner mitochondrial membrane. However, the homogeneous enzymes are available, and the same methods can be used. We can consider three problems associated with the microsomal system that have been investigated experimentally.

Sequence of Reactions

Since the product of C_{21} side-chain cleavage is adrostenedione, the 17β-hydroxysteroid dehydrogenase must catalyze the last reaction in the pathway. If we consider the conversion of pregnenolone to androstenedione, and if we keep in mind that both C_{21} side-chain cleavage P-450 and dehydrogenase-isomerase are single enzymes, we can see that there are two possible pathways for this conversion, depending on which enzyme acts first:

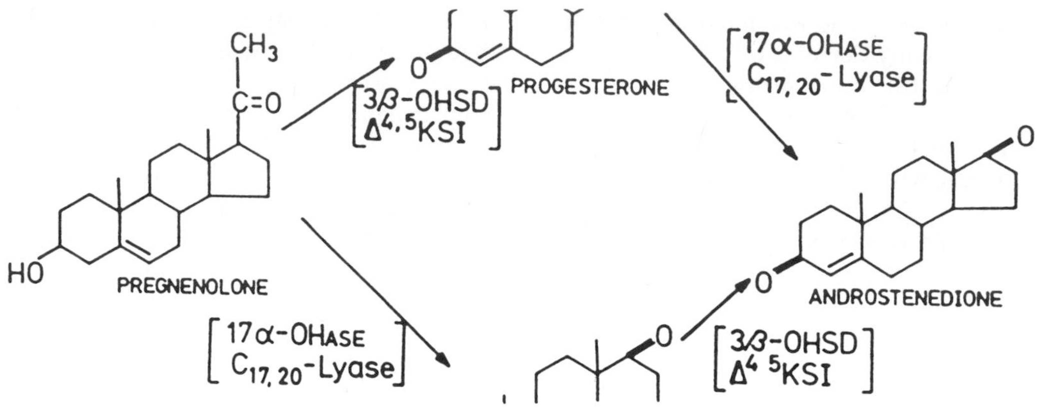

The "upper" pathway is referred to as the progesterone, or Δ^4, pathway, in contrast to the "lower pathway," referred to as the Δ^5, or dehydroepiandrosterone pathway. The choice of pathways is not random. For example, the rat uses the Δ^4 pathway largely if not exclusively (73). Pigs (87), rabbits, and dogs (88) use the Δ^5 pathway to varying degrees. In theory, regulation of the choice of pathway could arise either as the result of the properties of the enzymes or by their arrangement within the membrane. If, for example, the C_{21} side-chain cleavage enzyme has a higher affinity for pregnenolone than for progesterone, the Δ^5 pathway would prevail.

Similar considerations apply to the dehydrogenase-isomerase. The only evidence we have at present is consistent with that view, because the porcine C_{21} side-chain cleavage enzyme shows a considerably higher affinity for pregnenolone and 17α-hydroxypregnenolone than for the corresponding Δ^4 compounds (66). This affinity may help to explain the fact that, in pig testes, the Δ^5 pathway is extensively used (87). Clearly, much more information is needed before we can conclude that the sum of the properties of the individual enzymes accounts for the properties of the endoplasmic reticulum.

The alternative possibility is that the enzymes are arranged in a specific order and that pregnenolone enters the microsome at certain preferred points—entry ports established by the presence (for example) of a pregnenolone-binding protein. Preliminary evidence suggests that such a protein exists (28). The location of the binding protein relative to the two steroidogenic enzymes could influence the sequence of the reactions involved in the conversion of pregnenolone to androstenedione. There is no evidence for this concept, but recent advances in immunoelectron microscopy (79) and methods for chemical cross-linking of membrane proteins (89–91) make it possible to approach this question.

Location of Enzymes in the Lipid Bilayer

The endoplasmic reticulum *in situ* shows an external or cytoplasmic surface and an internal surface. When cells are disrupted by homogenization, fragments of endoplasmic reticulum form vesicles that are called right side out if the cytoplasmic surface remains outside and inside out if not. Membrane proteins may be associated with the bilayer by powerful hydrophobic forces that result in location of the protein buried in the interior of the bilayer or by a mixture of hydrophobic and hydrophilic forces, in which case the proteins may be predominantly disposed on one or the other side of the membrane, or the protein may cross the membrane several times. Proteins may also be associated loosely with the surface of the membrane by hydrophilic forces; such proteins are, to a greater or lesser degree, removed during washing of the microsomes.

Since many enzymes cannot penetrate a lipid bilayer, proteolytic enzymes and phospholipases can be used to determine whether the proteins in the membrane are accessible to these enzymes. Proteolytic enzymes can be used to demonstrate that a particular protein can be attacked from one surface or another, or whether it is buried in the bilayer and, hence, inaccessible to water-soluble proteolytic enzymes. Phospholipases can be used to show whether the enzyme in the microsomal membrane requires phospholipids for activity. It is then important to know whether the vesicles are right side out or not in order to relate these findings to the situation in the cell. This is usually easy with rough endoplasmic reticulum because ribosomes bind to the cytoplasmic surface of the membrane. It is generally assumed that the vesicles routinely produced from smooth endoplasmic reticulum are right side out, but this should be confirmed for each organ. It is likely that such questions will be successfully approached by immunoelectron microscopy, using second antibodies conjugated to gold particles (79).

Phospholipases A and C and trypsin were found by Samuels et al. (78) to exert the following effects on testicular microsomes:

TABLE 4. *Effects of phospholipase and trypsin on testicular microsomes*

	Pregnenolone binding	3β-OHSD	Hydroxylase/ lyase activity
Phospholipase	↓	↓↓↓	No change
Trypsin	↓↓↓	↓↓↓	↓↓↓

OHSD, hydroxsteroid dehydrogenase.

Since it has been shown that, in hepatic microsomes, cytochrome P-450 is on the inside of microsomes (92), these results were taken to mean that hydroxylase/lyase activity is inhibited because the reductase is located on the outside of the microsome, and trypsin inhibits the activity of P-450 by interfering with electron transport (reductase activity) rather than by acting on P-450 itself. The activity of the dehydrogenase-isomerase apparently depends on the presence of phospholipid. Pregnenolone binding depends on a protein that faces the external (cytoplasmic) surface of the microsome (94).

These findings should be considered in the light of earlier observations by Samuels et al. (78) showing that microsomal P-450 acts on intramembrane steroid substrate, whereas the dehydrogenase-isomerase acts on substrate from the surrounding water phase. These observations are summarized in diagramatic form:

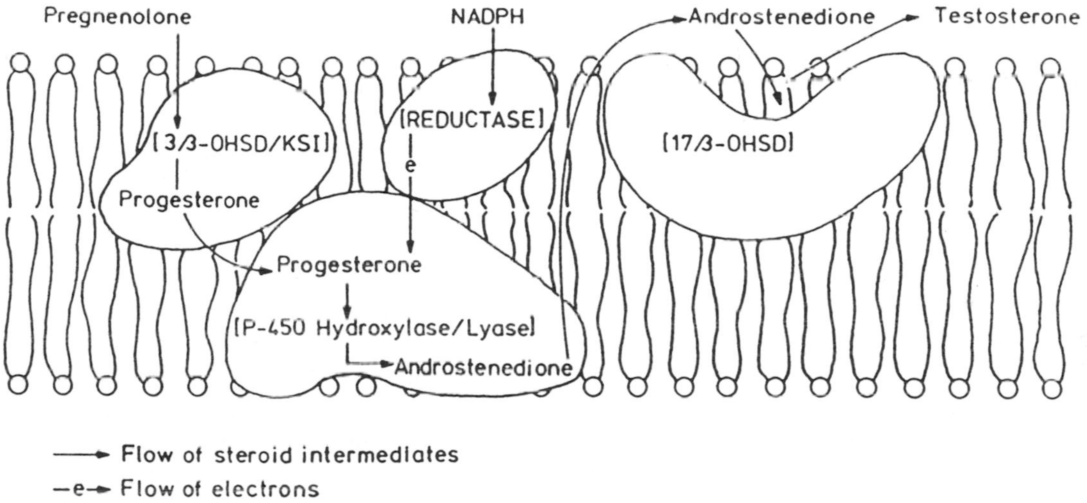

The diagram presents a schematic illustration of the findings of Samuels and colleagues (78). No doubt it will require repeated revision as more information becomes available.

Samuels et al. (93,94) also showed that when testicular microsomes are incubated with [^{3}H]progesterone and 17α-hydroxy-[^{14}C]progesterone, the resulting androstenedione shows a higher ratio of [^{3}H]:[^{14}C] than the original mixture of substrates. This finding suggested that the access of progesterone to the active site of the hydroxylase/lyase is greater than that of 17α-hydroxyprogesterone. These workers also showed that the partition ratio of progesterone from water to microsomes was greater than that of the 17α-hydroxysteroid (93,94). We now know that the two steroids show the same affinity for the single active site on pure C_{21} side-chain cleavage P-450 (60,66) and that 17α-hydroxyprogesterone in the water phase exchanges freely with 17α-hydroxyprogesterone generated by the enzyme from progesterone (95).

It would seem, therefore, that the difference between the two substrates lies in their respective rates of entry into the lipid bilayer. This presents us with a problem. We would expect progesterone to be formed from pregnenolone by P-450 in the lipid bilayer. There would seem to be no reason for progesterone to leave the membrane only to return. Moreover, it was pointed out above that the hydroxylase/lyase allows immediate exchange between the intermediate 17α-hydroxyprogesterone generated by the enzyme and exogenous 17α-hydroxyprogesterone added to the surrounding water phase (95). We clearly cannot interpret these findings without more information. There may be proteins in the microsome that influence the affinity of the substrate for the hydroxylase/lyase. Although these studies have exposed rather than resolved the problems, such approaches provide our first insight into the organization of the steroidogenic microsome.

Influence of the Microsomal Environment

A comparison between the 17α-hydroxylase of adrenal microsomes and the hydroxylase/lyase of testicular microsomes proves instructive. As mentioned above, when progesterone is incubated with adrenal microsomes, only products of 17α-hydroxylation are found; no C_{19} steroids are isolated (62). On the other hand, testicular microsomes produce a mixture of steroids in which C_{19} steroids predominate (96). However, when the two enzymes are purified, they are indistinguishable, and both produce large amounts of C_{19} steroids (62,63). Clearly, the microsomal environment influences the behavior of the adrenal enzyme. Since the two enzymes behave in the same way when they are incorporated in liposomes prepared from lipids extracted from either adrenal or testicular microsomes, the difference cannot be attributed to the microsomal lipids (64). Testicular microsomes contain four times as much reductase relative to P-450 as adrenal microsomes, and addition of exogenous reductase to adrenal microsomes increases lyase activity (64). In addition, it was observed that cytochrome b_5 increases lyase activity relative to hydroxylase in both adrenal and testicular microsomes (64,65). Although it is generally believed that the rate of reduction of P-450 is not rate-limiting for the actions of cytochromes P-450, lyase is at a disadvantage relative to hydroxylase, because a second turn of the P-450 cycle (and therefore a second input from reductase) is required. Agents that facilitate reduction of P-450 evidently favor lyase activity (64).

Hepatic microsomes are known to contain much more P-450 than reductase (97). Attempts have been made to determine whether one molecule of reductase remains in a fixed cluster with many molecules of P-450 all served by the one molecule of reductase, or whether P-450 can diffuse rapidly within the microsomal membrane so that each P-450 binds transiently to various reductase molecules in a random manner. Most available evidence concerning the mobility of proteins in membranes comes from studies with the more accessible plasma membrane in which proteins, even though restrained by attachment to the cytoskeleton, are sufficiently mobile to make the idea of a permanent cluster of molecules unthinkable (98). The concept has been extended, with less confidence, to mitochondrial membranes (99). If clusters of protein are possible in microsomal membranes, as the result of low mobility of proteins, these membranes must differ considerably from other cellular membranes. The relatively high content of protein in microsomal membranes would be a possible factor in accounting for such differences. Studies showing a break in the Arrhenius plots of microsomal membranes (activity versus 1/T) have been interpreted to favor the concept of a cluster of P-450 molecules associated with each molecule of reductase (100). On the other hand, spectroscopic studies suggest a high mobility of P-450 in microsomal membranes, so that interaction with reductase may not require a long-lived complex (101). It has also been suggested that P-450 may not be active as a monomer but rather in the form of molecular aggregates (101). Similar studies need to be performed in the steroidogenic microsomes, where the number of molecules of P-450 is much closer to the number of molecules of reductase (unpublished data).

REGULATION OF ANDROGEN SYNTHESIS BY LUTEINIZING HORMONE

In hypophysectomized animals, the synthesis of androgens by the testis proceeds at a greatly reduced rate (102). The pituitary owes its ability to stimulate the synthesis of androgens to the synthesis and secretion of LH. This hormone provides the most important physiological regulation of the production of androgens by the testis (1,103,104).

Within recent years, it has become clear that most (perhaps all) cells use a limited number of molecular mechanisms, all of which eventually involve proteins. When any cell responds to a stimulus, it does so by changing its proteins—either synthesizing new proteins, phosphorylating, or otherwise modifying existing proteins or both. Two major messengers have been discovered to convert blood-borne stimuli into cellular responses, namely, cyclic AMP and Ca^{2+}. These are the fundamental mechanisms used by cells to respond to various stimuli. The nature of the stimuli and the responses vary greatly from one cell type to another, but the underlying mechanisms are similar. These messengers, and the changes they produce in intracellular proteins, modify the functions of the various components of the cell, which in turn provide the response to the original stimulus: the plasma membrane transduces stimuli and provides second messengers; the cytoskeleton organizes the compartments and surfaces of the cell, modifies its shape, and provides direction (i.e., vectors for movements inside the cell); the endoplasmic reticulum synthesizes proteins (rough) and steroids (smooth); the mitochondria provide energy; and the nucleus determines the nature and number of proteins synthesized by the cell.

With these mechanisms and these cellular components, luteinizing hormone (LH) stimulates the synthesis of testosterone by Leydig cells. We will now consider how this comes about. To do this, reference must be made to some studies that have been performed with adrenocorticotropic hormone (ACTH) and adrenal cells. It was pointed out above that studies with the adrenal cortex have proceeded more rapidly than those with the testis, largely for technical reasons. It is time that this disparity was put right; in the meantime, cautious extrapolation from studies with the adrenal will make the testicular system more readily interpretable.

Site of Action of Luteinizing Hormone

Early experiments with LH showed that stimulation of steroidogenesis by this hormone occurs in the steroidogenic pathway after cholesterol but before pregnenolone; in short, it appeared that the side-chain cleavage of cholesterol is stimulated by LH (14,105–107). When these experiments were performed, nothing was known about intracellular transport as a biological phenomenon. Although it was known that cholesterol is stored in cytoplasmic droplets and that the side-chain cleavage reaction occurs in mitochondria, little thought was given to the mechanism by which the enzyme is supplied with cholesterol. When Garren et al. (108) observed that the action of ACTH is inhibited by cycloheximide at a step before side-chain cleavage of cholesterol, these workers proposed that ACTH stimulates the transport of cholesterol to mitochondria. This was confirmed directly by other studies (109,110).

When preparations of Leydig cells from rat testes became available (111), this idea was tested with the response to LH. It was found that this hormone, like ACTH, stimulates the transport of cholesterol to the inner mitochondrial membrane (112). On the other hand, the rate of conversion of cholesterol to pregnenolone by isolated mitochondra from Leydig cells incubated with and without LH is the same (112). At this point, it is important to consider the state of mitochondria in such experiments. It is difficult to prepare aerobic mitochondria unless special care is taken (113). If mitochondria become anaerobic, side-chain cleavage is inhibited, because this reaction requires oxygen (53), and cholesterol accumulates in the mitochondria (113).

When such mitochondria are incubated, they show a burst of synthesis of pregnenolone that is greater in mitochondria from cells incubated with LH, because these mitochondria are loaded with cholesterol (112). This point is crucial to the interpretation of such experiments, because the findings distinguish between an effect of LH on cholesterol transport, as opposed to an effect on the side-chain cleavage system per se (114). The problem has been more intensively studied in the adrenal, where it is now clear that the trophic hormone acts on cholesterol transport to the mitochondrial side-chain cleavage P-450 (114). Studies have not so far been reported with inner and outer mitochondrial membranes from Leydig cells to determine whether or not LH also stimulates the movement of cholesterol from the outer to the inner mitochondrial membrane, but it is clear that ACTH stimulates transport both to and within mitochondria (114). It seems likely that LH does the same.

Role of Cyclic AMP

It has long been known that cyclic AMP accelerates the synthesis of androgens by Leydig cells (115) and that LH increases the levels of cyclic AMP in these cells (116–118). In view of the extensive evidence that cyclic AMP mediates the actions of various hormones, it has been concluded that the responses of Leydig cells to LH and hCG result from increased production of cyclic AMP as the result of the binding of LH to its receptor. Cyclic AMP in turn phosphorylates a number of proteins, which presumably acquire different properties in the phosphorylated form. These different properties directly or indirectly lead to increased synthesis of androgens. There is no reason to doubt that this chain of events is the consequence of LH binding and the cause of increased production of androgens. The question has been raised as to whether or not cyclic AMP is the only mediator of the action of LH. To act in this way, cyclic AMP must stimulate cyclic AMP-dependent protein kinase (protein kinase A). It must then be asked whether kinase A, in turn, is the only mediator of the action of cyclic AMP and hence that of LH. In the adrenal cortex this question was approached by Schimmer (117), who studied a series of Y-1 adrenal cells in which protein kinase A had undergone various mutations. It was shown that deficiency of protein kinase A is associated with defective response to ACTH (117). These studies show that normal kinase activity is necessary for a normal response to ACTH. If the same is true for LH and Leydig cells, it could be concluded that the kinase (and hence cyclic AMP) is an obligatory messenger in the response to LH. It should be added that in the studies of Schimmer, small responses to ACTH were always seen and the kinase activity was never entirely eliminated (117). The possibility of a minor pathway not involving the kinase cannot be excluded.

Much has been written to justify this obligatory role of cyclic AMP and hence kinase A, by pointing to the sensitivity of present methods of measuring this nucleotide. It is argued that compartmentation of cell contents is a theoretical abstraction and, in any case, however small the responding compartment, it will be revealed by methods of measuring cyclic AMP that are sufficiently sensitive. To the first of these comments one must say that a cell in which cyclic AMP is randomly distributed is hard to imagine since such a cell would respond to all stimuli acting via cyclic AMP with increase in cyclic AMP throughout the cell. In such a cell there could be no more than one response to all agents that cause increase in the production of cyclic AMP. The involvement of cyclic AMP in so many cellular activities makes it unlikely that any cell could function with an all-or-none response to this agent. Moreover, positive evidence of inhomogeneity of cellular cyclic AMP has been reported. For example, to explain the absence of increased total concentrations of cyclic AMP in Leydig cells treated with low doses of LH that increase steroid production, Dufau and Catt (119) showed that under these conditions the number of molecules of regulatory subunit (R) bound to cyclic AMP increases at the expense of free molecules of R (i.e., no bound cyclic AMP). The results are compatible with an obligatory role for cyclic AMP in the response to LH (119).

Further evidence to support this idea was presented by Moger (120), who showed that endogenous cyclic AMP in Leydig cells binds preferentially to type I protein kinase, although both the I and II forms of the kinase are capable of stimulating steroid synthesis. Clearly, the endogenous nucleotide is not randomly distributed. Again, Pereia et al. (121) showed that at low concentrations of LH—conditions under which correlation between the concentration of cellular cyclic AMP and steroid synthesis is poor—a specific inhibitor of cyclic AMP, namely (Rp)-cAMPs, still decreases the steroidogenic response to LH. It follows that even if cyclic AMP is not the only second messenger for LH, it is still a necessary component in the response to that hormone. This is true even at low concentrations of LH.

The process of attempting to exclude all other second messengers proves less convincing than positive evidence for the existence of another messenger. Ca^{2+} has been the most successful alternative so far. The role of Ca^{2+} in the response to LH is discussed below. Here it should be mentioned that several groups have shown that Ca^{2+} stimulates synthesis of androgens by a mechanism involving Cl^- channels (122,123). This response does not appear to involve cyclic AMP. It would seem therefore that cyclic AMP is compartmentally distributed in the cell and is an important (probably essential) ingredient in the steroidogenic response to LH. Ca^{2+} can also stimulate the synthesis of androgens. The challenge now remains to determine the physiological conditions under which each of these second messengers acts on steroid synthesis.

Role of Protein Synthesis

In 1962, it was discovered that the steroidogenic response to LH is inhibited by puromycin (19). It was subsequently shown that LH increases incorporation of labeled amino acids into the total protein of Leydig cells (124). A detailed study by Janszen et al. (125) revealed increased synthesis of two proteins in Leydig cells produced by LH. One of these proteins (21K) appears 2 hours after addition of LH and shows a half-life greater than 30 minutes (125). The second protein (33K) has a short half-life (11 minutes). In both cases, the effect of LH on these proteins may be indirect. The authors propose that 33K may be an inactive precurser of short half-life that is activated in the presence of LH (125). The roles of these proteins in the response to LH deserve further study.

Further progress has been made in elucidating the roles of several proteins in trophic stimulation by ACTH of adrenal cells. A 30K protein of considerable interest was identified by Epstein and Orme-Johnson (126–128) in mitochondria of adrenal, Leydig, and corpus luteal cells. The synthesis of the protein is accelerated by the appropriate trophic hormone (ACTH or LH). This protein begins as 37K and gives rise to a 32K and finally to a 30K protein (126). The 30K form is phosphorylated and turns over relatively slowly (126). These features of 30K suggest that it plays an important role in the response to LH. Clearly the protein in one or more of its various forms or sizes must be isolated and its properties studied directly.

Adrenal and Leydig cells contain a so-called sterol carrier protein (SCP-2) that increases the synthesis of pregnenolone when added to isolated mitochondria. SCP-2 is believed to promote transport of cholesterol from outer to inner mitochondrial membrane, but it does not load cholesterol into the active site of the enzyme P450scc (129,130). It is difficult to understand how SCP-2 stimulates side-chain cleavage if the protein does not increase the amount of cholesterol bound to P450scc since loading of the enzyme appears to limit the rate of side-chain cleavage (114). It has also been found that the concentration of SCP-2 in the inner membrane is correlated with the concentration of cholesterol in that membrane (131). Although ACTH stimulates synthesis of SCP-2, the response is relatively slow, suggesting a trophic action rather than an acute metabolic effect (132). Nevertheless, it is still possible that SCP-2 is important in the regulation of steroid synthesis. Although most of this work has been performed in adrenal cells, it is likely that the same findings apply to Leydig cells.

A protein called sterol activating protein (SAP) of MW 2,200 was isolated from adrenal cells (133), and a similar protein was found in Leydig and ovarian cells (134,135). These proteins show an amino acid sequence that closely resembles the carboxy terminus of a heat shock protein. The synthesis of this protein is stimulated by ACTH or LH, and this effect is inhibited by cycloheximide. This protein may be formed by co-translational cleavage of a larger precursor protein—possibly the heat shock protein called glucose-regulated protein (GRP78). The co-translational cleavage would account for inhibition of synthesis of SAP by cycloheximide (132). SAP does not itself bind cholesterol but appears to promote binding of cholesterol to P450scc (132). This protein might play an important role in the response to LH.

A protein of MW approximately 9,000 was isolated from bovine adrenal cortex, using an assay based on stimulation of side-chain cleavage in isolated adrenal mitochondria, by Yanagibashi and colleagues (136,137). It was found to be identical with endozepine, already well known in the central nervous system as a form of endogenous valium, i.e., an anxiolytic agent. However, the two carboxy-terminal amino acids were not present in the adrenal form of endozepine. The protein was referred to as des-(gly-ile)-endozepine. It stimulates the transport of cholesterol from outer to inner mitochondrial membrane when added to the two membranes incubated together (136). In addition, endozepine promotes loading of P450scc with substrate (cholesterol) (136). The protein also exerts this effect when added to the inner membrane *in vitro* (136). This observation means that endozepine can act on whatever cholesterol is present in the inner membrane so that the effect of the protein on transport of cholesterol from outer to inner membrane is not necessary for the effect on inner membrane. In addition, endozepine accelerates reduction of P-450 when added to the pure enzyme in a reconstituted system that includes adrenodoxin reductase, adrenodoxin, and NADPH (138). It will be recalled that binding of substrate to P-450 promotes the passage of the first electron from NADPH. It seems likely that the increased binding of cholesterol by endozepine may cause increase in the rate of reduction of P450scc and hence acceleration of side-chain cleavage (138). Since the synthesis of endozepine is accelerated by ACTH, this protein may be one of the newly synthesized proteins that mediate the steroidogenic action of ACTH. Endozepine, as well as des-endozepine, has been isolated from Leydig cells, so the conclusions concerning endozepine probably apply to Leydig cells (unpublished data). It is inferred that, as in the nervous system, the full molecule, i.e., endozepine itself rather than des-endozepine, is the active form of the molecule. Finally, it has been proposed that the first of the responses to endozepine (increased transport of cholesterol from outer to inner mitochondrial membrane) may result from the action of a mitochondrial outer membrane receptor for benzodiazepines to which it is proposed that endozepine binds (138a).

Each of these proteins can lay claim to a role in the response of adrenal and Leydig cells to trophic stimulation. Whether one is the prime mover or whether all are directly involved remains to be seen. Meanwhile, it has been shown that GTP stimulates the synthesis of pregnenolone by isolated adrenocortical mitochondria (139). It has been proposed that GTP promotes intramitochondrial transport of cholesterol (139). The GTP must be hydrolyzed to act in this way, and the response is specific for the guanosine nucleotide. Although the effect of GTP has not been analyzed in Leydig cell mitochondria, this nucleotide is a candidate for a role in the response to trophic stimulation in addition to the proteins discussed above. How these various agents act in regulating side-chain cleavage is entirely unclear at present.

Role of Ca^{2+}

Since most biological processes require Ca^{2+}, at least as a permissive agent, and since the steroidogenic response to ACTH requires Ca^{2+} (140), it is likely that the action of LH on Leydig cells also requires this cation. So far, the nature of the involvement of Ca^{2+} in response to LH has not been clarified. However, it was found that trifluoperazine inhibits the steroidogenic action of LH (141). Moreover, when calmodulin is injected into Leydig cells by means of liposomes, the protein accelerates the synthesis of testosterone (141), and this acceleration is accompanied by increased transport of cholesterol to the inner mitochondrial membrane (141). Injection of Ca^{2+} alone is without effect, and the action of calmodulin is enhanced if it is first saturated with Ca^{2+} (141). These studies were interpreted to mean that in the unstimulated cell, insufficient Ca^{2+}-calmodulin is present in those regions of the cell at which the complex is required to accelerate steroid synthesis. The injected Ca^{2+}-calmodulin floods the cell and increases the concentration of this complex in various parts of the cell including those places in which it is required for increased steroid synthesis. This finding suggests that LH may cause redistribution of calmodulin, and this redistribution plays an important part in the stimulation of the synthesis of androgens by LH. Such an idea would be in keeping with observations made with luteinizing hormone-releasing hormone (LHRH), which causes redistribution of calmodulin in pituitary cells (142). Further studies are needed to characterize such redistribution of endogenous calmodulin.

Apart from this action of Ca^{2+}-calmodulin, Ca^{2+} may be involved elsewhere in the regulation of steroidogenesis. For example, Ca^{2+} is required for interaction of ACTH with its receptor (143). This effect of Ca^{2+} involves coupling of the receptor to the protein Gs, and this action requires calmodulin (144). Ca^{2+} also enters adrenal cells through voltage-dependent channels and can in this way stimulate steroid synthesis without increase in cellular cyclic AMP (144,145). It will be important to demonstrate whether or not these actions of Ca^{2+}-calmodulin apply to the Leydig cell.

Role of Phosphorylation

Since cyclic AMP serves as a second messenger for LH and since the only known mechanism of action of cyclic AMP is to phosphorylate proteins (146), it follows that LH should promote phosphorylation of Leydig cell proteins. Indeed, Cooke et al. (147) found that LH produces phosphorylation of three Leydig cell proteins, identified as 14K, 57K, and 78K. The extent of phosphorylation of these proteins showed some correlation with the steroidogenic response to LH (147). Some relevant information on the role of phosphorylation in the action of LH comes from studies in the ovary. Special attention has been paid to mitochondrial proteins because of the importance of the side-chain cleavage of cholesterol in that organelle. LH stimulates phosphorylation of two mitochondrial proteins in ovarian follicles, but the relationship of these changes to steroidogenesis is not clear (148). Studies by Inaba and Wiest (149) showed that the mitochondrial membrane prevents protein kinase A from stimulating the side-chain cleavage of cholesterol. However, disruption of the mitochondrial membrane by Ca^{2+} allows the protein kinase to stimulate side-chain cleavage of cholesterol—possibly by facilitating access of cholesterol to the enzyme (149).

In addition to the role of protein kinase A in the response to LH, phorbol esters stimulate the phosphorylation of Leydig cell proteins and also increase the synthesis of androgens by these cells (150,151). The problem in understanding the role of phosphorylation of proteins in this and other biological responses lies not so much in cataloguing the nature and number of responding proteins but rather in defining the changes in the functions of these proteins when phosphorylated. This is the next step that must be undertaken in the case of LH.

Role of Phospholipids

The discovery that phosphatidylinositol is rapidly formed and degraded in a cyclic process occurring in most cells has revolutionized current ideas on metabolic regulation. The breakdown of phosphatidylinositol can be visualized as a cycle:

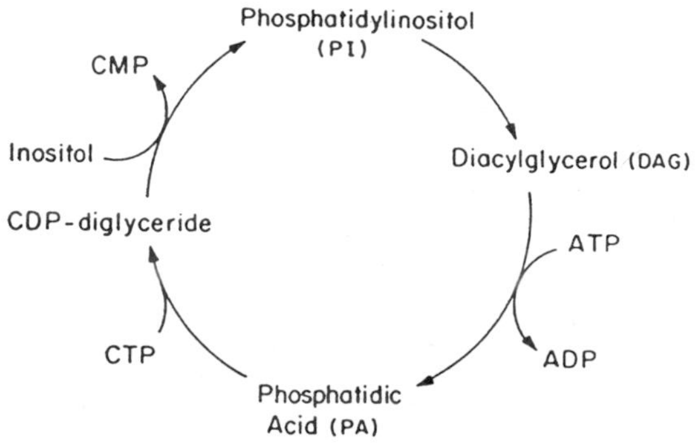

Phosphatidylinositol is, in turn, degraded to inositol triphosphate by phospholipase C, and this triphosphate is a powerful Ca^{2+} ionophore. The second important product of the cycle is diacylglycerol, which activates the Ca^{2+}/phospholipid-dependent protein kinase commonly called PKC. Clearly the cycle provides both of the cofactors required for the activation of PKC. In addition, intracellular Ca^{2+} will be increased or redistributed or both (152,153). In view of the far-reaching metabolic effects of Ca^{2+}, it is obvious that phospholipase C is capable of greatly influencing cell metabolism. There is no doubt that these processes are of major importance in many cells. However, it would appear that although PKC may be involved in the regulation of steroidogenesis, unlike cyclic AMP, it does not appear to play a direct role in this process. It has been suggested that some cells and some regulatory systems are dependent on cyclic AMP and others on Ca^{2+}, although such complete separation between these two second messengers may not always turn out to be hard and fast. If the role of PKC in the response to LH is uncertain, the significance of the phosphoinositide cycle in Leydig cells remains even more uncertain. The classical phospholipase C response with breakdown of phosphatidylinositol and increased cellular Ca^{2+} does not occur in adrenal cells in response to ACTH (154).

It has been proposed that in steroidogenic and some other cells, the phosphatidylinositol cycle serves a different function. LH and ACTH were reported to stimulate the synthesis of phosphatidic acid from sources outside the above cycle (155–157). Increase in the cellular concentration of phosphatidic acid would be expected to increase the amounts of the phosphoinositides including phosphorylated phosphoinositides (called phosphatidylphosphoinositides) (157), which can influence the activity of mitochondria in these cells by a direct action that results in the increased production of pregnenolone and hence increased synthesis of steroid hormones (155–157). So far direct evidence for this interesting proposal has not been presented. This will require correlation of the concentrations of specific phosphatidylphosphoinositides with the rate of side-chain cleavage. Such an action would constitute a major departure from the established metabolic roles of the phosphatidylinositol cycle (152,153).

Role of Gene Expression

It is now clear that a major role in determining the amounts of specific proteins in cells is played by the regulation of gene expression. Existing mRNA can be translated more rapidly or it can be rendered more stable, but the amount of a protein in a cell is frequently determined by the rate of transcription of the relevant gene. Such transcription can be involved in acute metabolic regulation as well as in long-term responses. As discussed above, the steroidogenic response to LH requires new proteins. This acute response is inhibited by actinomycin D, so that new mRNA is presumably required for the synthesis of these proteins (158). It is now clear that LH increases the amounts of at least some steroidogenic enzymes over a longer time scale than the acute increase in steroid synthesis that occurs in the acute response to LH. This should be contrasted with the rapid responses seen with the other proteins that are discussed above.

The study of these processes is commonly called molecular biology, although biology can be studied in molecular terms without necessarily considering gene transcription. Nevertheless, we are concerned here with the transcription of DNA to RNA in connection with the action of LH. This involves demonstrating increased production of molecules of specific RNA. This is achieved by preparing a specific labeled (usually radioactive) DNA probe that is added to total cell RNA to detect a specific species of mRNA complementary to the specific probe—a procedure called Northern blotting. This in turn commonly follows isolation of the gene in question (usually called cloning). Methods are available to work backwards from an antibody to a protein and from the protein to a degenerate DNA probe. Knowing a relatively short amino acid sequence, it is possible to construct a DNA probe based upon the possible codons corresponding to this sequence (degenerate probe). Alternatively, an antibody to the protein makes it possible to identify the relevant DNA.

The isolated gene is characterized in order to demonstrate size, introns and exons, and DNA at either end of the gene that is not transcribed (5′ and 3′ ends). In addition to this genomic DNA, it is usual to prepare complementary DNA (cDNA) by reversing the process of transcription (RNA → DNA) using a viral enzyme called reverse transcriptase. DNA is much more stable than RNA, and cDNA has the great virtue of not containing introns and other DNA that is not transcribed since it is complementary to mRNA as opposed to the gene itself. The important approaches to regulation of transcription are twofold. Untranscribed DNA (usually 5′ upstream) is attached to a gene not present in the cell under investigation (reporter gene), and this so-called DNA construct is transfected into the cells of interest, e.g., Leydig cells. The effects of various agents (e.g., LH or cyclic AMP) on the expression of the reporter gene are studied by measuring either the RNA or the protein corresponding to the reporter gene. In this way it is possible to determine which sequences of untranscribed DNA are responsible for promoting the transcription of the reporter gene and by inference the corresponding endogenous gene. It is an assumption of the method that the untranscribed DNA promotes transcription of the reporter gene in the same way and in response to the same stimuli as the same (5′) DNA regulates transcription of the endogenous gene of interest from which this DNA was prepared.

These studies will define the start site of transcription (referred to as nucleotide + 1) and can be expected to define those sequences of DNA that enable the gene to be expressed. The sequences are referred to as elements, and the regulation of expression of genes by sequences or elements of untranscribed DNA is referred to as cis regulation, in contrast to trans regulation, to be discussed below. Among the elements involved in cis regulation two common (perhaps universal) types of regulation are recognized. Firstly, sequences around the start site of transcription (usually within −100 to +1) are involved in establishing correct binding of the necessary proteins (transcription factors, as they are called) to the DNA and to RNA polymerase to secure the correct start site. These elements are thought to permit basal levels of transcription of the gene in question and are referred to as promoters. Further upstream it is possible to recognize positive and negative elements that influence the basal rate of expression established by the promoter. Positive upstream elements beyond the promoter (usually beyond −100) are referred to as enhancers. Enhancers may be involved in expressing regulatory influences exerted by intracellular messengers such as cyclic AMP. By means of studies of upstream DNA it is possible to establish cis regulation exterted not only by the upstream DNA but also by intracellular messengers.

The second thrust of studies concerning the regulation of transcription consists of a search for specific nuclear proteins that are capable of binding to specific elements of DNA. Such binding influences the regulatory activities of positive (enhancers) and negative (suppressors) upstream sequences. This form of regulation by way of nuclear proteins is called trans regulation.

Finally, it should be added that since all the DNA of all the cells of an organism is the same, one could reasonably expect that the role of untranscribed DNA of a given gene in regulating transcription of that gene is likely to be the same in different organs that express the gene under the influence of the same or even perhaps different stimuli. This means that studies of the regulation of a steroidogenic gene are frequently made indiscriminately in the cell familiar to the laboratory in question, so that in what follows we will frequently need to turn to studies performed in the adrenal and the ovary to learn what is believed to occur in all steroidogenic cells. Unfortunately, this logical expectation is not always realized. Finally, because transformed cells (so-called cell lines) are easier to work with than primary cultures of the corresponding normal cells, we will find it necessary to discuss studies performed in such mutant cells. Because the nature and number of mutations in a given cell line are not known, the results may be misleading. We can now turn to individual steroidogenic enzymes.

Cytochrome P450scc

Measurement of the amounts of P450scc in rat Leydig cells by immunoprecipitation reveal that LH causes increased synthesis of this enzyme (159). Similar findings have been made in Leydig cells from immature pigs (160) and in ovarian cells (161,162). However, the use of cycloheximide in studying this effect of cyclic AMP and LH has given conflicting results. The inhibitor decreases the response to cyclic AMP in bovine adrenocortical cells (163) and in JEG-3 choriocarcinoma cells (164) but not in human granulosa cells (165) or in mouse Leydig cells (166). If we consider that cycloheximide is a specific inhibitor of protein synthesis, we must assume that LH and its second messenger (cyclic AMP) promote synthesis of P450scc in adrenal but not in Leydig cells or granulosa cells. It would be concluded that in adrenal cells cyclic AMP promotes synthesis of a protein that binds to regulatory DNA and increases transcription of the P-450scc gene, which is called CYPIIA. In Leydig and granulosa cells, on the other hand, it could reasonably be concluded that cyclic AMP promotes phosphorylation of a protein (perhaps a nuclear protein) that is capable of binding to a specific sequence in the regulatory DNA of CYPIIA. The phosphorylation of the protein would alter its function in such a way as to promote binding to specific DNA. However, neither of these effects of cyclic AMP (synthesis of new protein and phosphorylation) has so far been directly demonstrated in the relevant steroidogenic cells. The striking difference between adrenal and Leydig cells in the regulation of transcription of CYPIIA is out of keeping with the general similarity seen in other aspects of the regulation of steroid synthesis in the two cell types. These apparent inconsistencies will be clarified when the regulation of gene expression is better understood. How cyclic AMP acts in promoting synthesis of P450scc is therefore not understood and may differ in different types of steroidogenic cells. It is, however, clear that the cyclic nucleotide stimulates transcription of CYPIIA since treatment of cultured adrenal cells with the nucleotide results in increased levels of the specific mRNA for P450scc (167). It should be noted that it is not clear whether or not the effect of cyclic AMP on transcription requires the action of protein kinase A. The effect on transcription may turn out to be an exception to the general rule.

Examination of the cDNA for CYPIIA reveals a larger or preform of the protein in which it is extended at the NH_2 terminus by 39 amino acids (168,169). This extension or signal peptide serves to permit recognition and internalization into mitochondria. Once inside this organelle, the signal peptide is removed by specific proteolysis to give the mature form of P450scc.

Attempts to define those regions of upstream DNA that are necessary for the basal expression of CYPIIA have proved disappointing and confusing. Basal expression of the human, mouse, and bovine genes has been examined in Y-1 mouse adrenal cells. Each of these genes appears to require one or more quite different upstream sequences for expression. The differences involve not only differences in the sequence of bases in these regulatory elements but also differences in distance of these sequences from the start site of transcription (+1). Since a major problem for RNA polymerase is to secure the correct starting base (+1), the arrangement of the relevant regulatory sequences relative to +1 is critical. Although distant sequences can fold over to approach the RNA polymerase bound in the region of +1, the differences noted above between the three species would suggest radically different arrangements for assembling the complex of proteins required for transcription (170). Such differences are surprising when we consider how highly conserved the genes themselves are known to be. At least two important possibilities may account for these differences, namely, these studies were all performed in a mouse cell line (Y-1) and also the chromosomal structure may be important in gene expression; the construct introduced from outside a given cell may not accurately reflect what happens with the endogenous gene within its chromosome.

When the upstream region of CYPIIA from the same three species (human, bovine, and mouse) was examined with expression vectors to determine sequences that are necessary for the stimulating effect of cyclic AMP on expression of the gene, the results are as confusing as those just discussed for basal transcription. Many genes the transcription of which is stimulated by cyclic AMP show an upstream sequence of CGTCA that is called cyclic AMP responsive element (CRE). In human CYPIIA three upstream sequences that are necessary for the action of cyclic AMP on expression of the gene have been defined. Although the three sequences are very different from each other, they all include a sequence that contains four of the five bases in the CRE (171). On the other hand, the bovine gene requires the sequence −183/−83 to permit stimulation by cyclic AMP; this sequence shows no evidence of a CRE (172). The mouse gene shows two sequences required for the cyclic AMP response, namely −424/−327 and −219/−77 (173). Neither of these sequences shows homology to those of the other two species and neither contains a CRE (170–172). It is of interest, however, that the mouse gene contains two elements at −70 and −40 that closely resemble upstream DNA of the gene for steroid 21-hydroxylase where these sequences are involved in the regulation of expression of this gene (173). When −1500/+28 of the mouse gene was used in an expression vector in Y-1 cells and in cells of the MA-10 Leydig cell line, expression of the reporter gene was much lower in MA-10 than in Y-1 cells (173). Clearly the host cell is important and additional unknown factors may be necessary for normal expression of the gene in the two mutant cells. It seems strange that such a highly conserved gene shows such differences in the DNA sequences necessary for the effect of cyclic AMP on expression of this gene-differences not only in sequence but also in location upstream relative to +1.

The action of nuclear proteins on upstream DNA is usually studied either by the effect of protein on the migration of DNA in an agarose gel (gel retardation) or by protection of the DNA by specifically bound nuclear protein from digestion by DNase (footprinting). These methods have been applied to the study of expression of CYPIIA in the human (171) and mouse (173) genes. Nuclear proteins have been shown to bind specifically to the CRE elements described above (171,173). These include proteins that bind to the two motifs seen in upstream DNA of 21-hydroxylase (a gene not expressed in Leydig cells) (see above) and others that bind to a sequence near −120 (173). It is clear that much work remains to be done before it will be possible to present a clear account of regulation of expression of CYPIIA. However, these fragments of information must be part of a larger picture that is likely to be clarified by future experiments in which all the regulatory elements of CYPIIA in at least the above three species will be clarified.

Cytochrome P-450 C21scc (P-450 17)

LH and cyclic AMP increase amounts of the mRNA for this gene in rat Leydig cells (174). In adrenocortical cells ACTH increases the synthesis of the enzyme (175). The relevant gene is called CYP17. Expression vectors containing 5′ upstream DNA from bovine CYP17 were used to identify two elements that separately respond to cyclic AMP when the vectors are transfected into Y-1 cells (176). These two DNA sequences are situated at −243/−225 and at −80/−40. The two elements show no homology one to the other. In addition, a CRE is seen at −425. In the human gene the same CRE-like sequence is seen at −434 (177). When the response to −243/−225 from the bovine gene was studied in Y-1 cells, cyclic AMP was found to cause a rapid response that is not inhibited by cycloheximide (176). When the effect of cyclic AMP is studied in normal bovine adrenocortical cells, the response is slow but is inhibited by cycloheximide (178). Interpretation of these findings is complicated by the fact that the endogenous gene is not expressed in Y-1 cells. Clearly, the expression vector, at least in this case, is not providing a complete system capable of reflecting regulation of the gene in the intact cell.

A start has been made with the study of nuclear proteins in Y-1 cells. The sequence −243/−225 (which includes a CRE-like motif) specifically binds a protein of MW 47,000 that was found in nuclear extracts of Y-1 cells treated with ACTH. Moreover, a 47,000-MW protein from these cells (presumably the same protein) also binds a perfect synthetic CRE (179). These findings are encouraging but must be interpreted with caution because CYP17 is not normally expressed in Y-1 cells with or without cyclic AMP. Nevertheless, identification of a protein made under the influence of cyclic AMP that binds an upstream CRE will surely prove important.

3β-Hydroxysteroid Dehydrogenase-Isomerase

It was pointed out above that these two reactions are catalyzed by a single protein. The final proof of this assertion came from studies in which the gene was expressed in COS-1 cells. The resulting protein was found to catalyze both reactions (180). Some studies have been reported on the expression of the relevant gene. Basal levels of expression are high in Leydig cells, but maximal expression requires cyclic AMP (181). Cortisol and testosterone inhibit this expression (182).

17β-Hydroxysteroid Dehydrogenase

Two genes in tandem (I and II) corresponding to this enzyme have been isolated (183). Gene II gives rise to the so-called estrogenic enzyme, which converts estrone to estradiol and vice versa (183). It has been proposed that gene I is responsible for the androgenic form that converts androstenedione to testosterone (183,184).

ROLES OF COMPONENTS OF THE LEYDIG CELL

In the previous sections of this chapter, we have considered the molecular mechanisms that the Leydig cell uses in the synthesis of androgens. We must now turn to the morphology of the cell and the activities of those subcellular components of the cell in which these mechanisms are employed. The Leydig cell itself varies in appearance from species to species, although the functional significance of these variations is unclear. A detailed comparative approach to the morphology of the Leydig cell may prove rewarding. In the meantime, we will consider the human Leydig cell, because it has been thoroughly studied by Christensen (15), who has pointed out that the cell is typical of Leydig cells in general. The Leydig cell is polygonal and has a diameter of 15 to 20 μm. The surface area of the human Leydig cell has been estimated to be 800 μm^2 (15).

Plasma Membrane

The plasma membrane is not unusual in appearance. In places it shows well-developed microvilli (15). This membrane contains the LH receptor coupled to adenylate cyclase.

LH Receptor–Adenylate Cyclase

Each Leydig cell in the rat contains approximately 20,000 receptors, and the testis can bind about 1 pmole LH/g wet weight (185). The receptor can bind both LH and hCG, so that it is known as the LH/hCG receptor. For the sake of brevity, these receptors will be referred to here as LH receptors. The receptor has been partly purified and found to be a glycoprotein of MW 190,000 made up of two identical subunits of MW 90,000 (185). Attempts to remove all bound phospholipid result in loss of binding activity (185). The Leydig cell is said to show spare receptors, because maximal steroidogenesis can be obtained at concentrations of LH that are sufficient to occupy only a fraction of the total number of available LH receptors (186).

The LH receptor is coupled to adenylate cyclase, and, as in other cells, the cyclase contains GTP-binding or G proteins. Binding of GTP to the stimulatory G protein (Gs) results in activation of the cyclase, and activation is terminated by hydrolysis of GTP. An analogous inhibitory G protein (Gi) is also present in the adenylate cyclase complex. The process of activation can be studied with Gpp (NH)p, an analogue of GTP that is not hydrolyzed (187). Since the amount of Gpp (NH)p bound to Leydig cell membranes (pmoles/mg protein) exceeds the number of LH receptors, it is concluded that one occupied receptor can activate many GTP-binding sites, which results in a 20-fold amplification of the binding of LH (188). Moreover, binding of LH to its receptor results in phosphorylation of several membrane proteins, including one of MW 44,000. It has been suggested that this protein may be Gs (189).

Downregulation and Desensitization

When a single injection of LH or hCG is administered to a rat, a second injection produces a response that is quantitatively different from the first injection. Usually, the second injection produces a smaller response than the first (187). Since the administration of LH to a rat in any dose is unphysiological, the significance of the changes to be described is uncertain. Moreover, the field has been burdened with inappropriate colloquialisms that are not always adequately defined. It is common practice to refer to the diminished response to a second injection as downregulation, if the full extent seen with the first response can be obtained with cyclic AMP, that is, if the limitation set on the second response results from a change in the LH receptor.

The confusion in nomenclature has been compounded with the terms homologous and heterologous downregulation, which refer respectively to altered responses produced by the same stimulating agent (e.g., LH and hCG) or different agents (e.g., LH and forskolin). When the lesser second response cannot be corrected by cyclic AMP, the unfortunate term desensitization is used. This leaves an undefined group of responses in which the diminished second response results from changes in the cyclase itself. Under some conditions, which have not been fully studied, upregulation, with the second response greater than the first, may be seen (190). This situation will not be discussed here.

The following changes have been reported in Leydig cells after an injection of LH: (a) decrease in number, but not affinity, of LH receptors (191,192); (b) regulated proteolysis of the receptor resulting from exposure of a peptide bond on binding ligand (192a); (c) alterations in the coupling and function of the cyclase (193,194); (d) depletion of substrate (195,196); (e) changes in the steroidogenic pathway at C_{21} side-chain cleavage (hydroxylase/lyase) (197,198) and, with larger doses, a decrease in C_{27} side-chain cleavage (199,200).

Decrease in Number of Receptors

The term downregulation refers to a decrease in the number of receptors on the surface of the Leydig cell following an injection of LH. It appears that the receptors are internalized but not degraded (191,192). Presumably, the fate of occupied receptors includes internalization, dissociation of LH, and a regulated return of the free receptors to the surface of the cell. This cycle of receptors, from cell surface to the interior of the cell and back to the surface, has been studied intensely in other systems, and the findings have been reviewed (197,198). The binding of ligand (LH) to receptor influences the distribution of the receptor in the plasma membrane in such a way as to encourage internalization via coated vesicles. In the lysosome, the ligand is released and follows its own fate, which may be degradation (201,202). The receptor may be sorted in the Golgi apparatus and returned to the plasma membrane to function once again as a free receptor. The LH receptor acts in this respect like other receptors, and perhaps downregulation should be seen in this light—as part of the normal cellular processing of receptors. It has been proposed that downregulation may serve to limit the response to pulses of LH—one pulse could deplete receptors before later pulses appear (203). We are a long way from the sort of evidence necessary to discuss the physiological importance of the phenomenon of downregulation, which has, however, prompted important research on the intracellular movement of receptors.

Proteolysis of Receptor

Proteolysis is well-known with other receptors and has been described for LH (192a).

Alterations in Adenylate Cyclase

Studies with forskolin and cholera toxin, which stimulate adenylate cyclase, suggest that homologous and heterologous downregulation result respectively from lesions before and after Gs in the process of activation of adenylate cyclase (204). Again, the physiological relevance of the findings is uncertain. It is also unclear whether these lesions are better referred to as downregulation or desensitization.

Desensitization

Before reviewing the phenomena associated with desensitization, it is well to consider how far removed our best cell culture systems are from providing physiological conditions, because one of the most important contributions to come from the study of desensitization is the emphasis these investigations have given to the importance of the details of cell culture. Present systems of cell culture frequently use serum, almost always induce oxygen toxicity in the cells, and do not provide a regulated circulation of fresh medium. While serum-free medium is becoming commonplace, such media are still far removed from normal interstitial fluid, and perfusion is but a beginning of attempts to mimic circulatory conditions *in vivo*. The worst and least generally understood problem is that of oxygen toxicity. It is still necessary to point out that oxygen is highly toxic and that 20% O_2 is well above physiological levels for individual cells. Manufacturers of tissue culture apparatus have been slow to take up this challenge. We will see that availability of substrate and adverse effects of high O_2 tension may be important in desensitization.

Supply of Cholesterol

It is clear that in some experimental studies, desensitization can be relieved by addition of LDL to cultured Leydig cells (195,196). The first injection of LH causes sufficient stimulation of steroid synthesis to produce depletion of cholesterol. What is not clear is whether such depletion occurs *in vivo* under physiological circumstances.

Inhibition of the Steroidogenic Pathway

When the individual steps in the biosynthetic pathway to testosterone are examined in desensitized Leydig cells, C_{21} side-chain cleavage is seen to be depressed (197,198), and with higher doses of LH at the first injection, side-chain cleavage of cholesterol (C_{27}) may be inhibited (199,200). It is no coincidence that these reactions are both catalyzed by cytochromes P-450. It will be recalled that binding of substrate to P-450 promotes the flow of the first electron to the cytochrome and that this is followed by activation of oxygen. The active oxygen is used to hydroxylate the substrate. Some steroids (e.g., the products of reactions catalyzed by P-450) can bind to the active site of P-450 but cannot be hydroxylated, for example, they may already be hydroxylated at the only accessible C atom. Such steroids are called pseudosubstrates. The binding of the pseudosubstrate will promote the activation of oxygen, and the active oxygen cannot be used for hydroxylation. Active oxygen can exist in a variety of forms, e.g., peroxide, hydroxyl radical, superoxide, etc. These forms of oxygen can attack heme and inactive P-450 (205,206). Given the high oxygen tensions present in cell cultures, the question of active oxygen could be important in the inactivation of the two steroidogenic cytochromes P-450 involved in the synthesis of androgens. The topic of active oxygen has been extensively reviewed (205–207). Moreover, Quinn and Payne (197) have shown that at low oxygen tension (1%), inhibition of P-450 during desensitization to LH is greatly diminished. It will be necessary to study the effects of more physiological conditions of oxygen tension between 1% and 20% before these findings can be fully interpreted.

Synthesis of Estrogen

Yet another factor in the mechanism of desensitization appears to be the synthesis of estrogens by the Leydig cell. Desensitization can be diminished by treating Leydig cells with antiestrogen (tamifoxen) (208). There are at least two ways in which estrogens can inhibit C_{21} side-chain cleavage. First, estradiol causes inhibition of the enzyme itself (209), and second, estradiol promotes synthesis of a protein (24K) that can inhibit both C_{21} and C_{27} side-chain cleavage (210). The nature of this protein and the mechanism of inhibition are likely to be important. It is proposed that the first injection of LH increases the synthesis of estrogens as well as that of androgens by the Leydig cell, and the estrogen inhibits the response to the second injection by one or both of the above mechanisms (211).

Endoplasmic Reticulum

The most conspicuous feature of the Leydig cell is an extensive endoplasmic reticulum (ER), most of which is smooth. The smooth ER is generally believed to be related to the synthesis of steroids. It has been proposed that the development of smooth ER is specifically related to the synthesis of cholesterol, which is consistent with the idea that, at least in some species, the Leydig cell makes much of its own steroidogenic cholesterol. The smooth ER forms a network of tubules 80 to 120 nm in diameter, with an estimated surface area of 4,000 μm^2 (15). This enormous surface is used by the membrane-bound enzymes that synthesize cholesterol and steroid hormones. In addition, the Leydig cell contains rough ER with ribosomes. The rough ER interconnects with the smooth ER (15) and must be responsible for the synthesis of the proteins required for the response of Leydig cells to LH.

Cytoplasm

The most striking feature of Leydig cell cytoplasm is the presence of lipid droplets, which are bounded by a membrane of 5 nm in width. This cannot be a typical bilayer structure, since the width of such a structure is approximately 7.5 nm (15). Presumably, cholesterol can pass freely through this membrane. Histochemical studies show that the droplets consist chiefly of cholesterol and neutral fats (212). In view of what is known of adrenal lipid stores, it seems reasonable to conclude that the droplets contain stores of cholesterol ester to be used in steroid synthesis. Christensen (15) has pointed out that the content of lipid droplets varies greatly from cell to cell in one testis, and, since LH causes depletion of lipid droplets, these variations may reflect cycles of synthetic activity (15). This is a point of some importance in interpreting biochemical studies in which we may be examining the activity of a small number of cells at any one time in a given population, since many of the cells may not be in a phase of activity.

The functional contributions of the cytoplasm include the synthesis of new proteins, the storage of cholesterol, and the mobilization of this substrate. Mobilization includes cleavage of stored esters by cholesterol ester hydrolase and, presumably, binding to a carrier protein. It is also impossible to ignore the crystals of Reinke that are seen in the cytoplasm of human Leydig cells but in no other species. These functional structures consist largely of protein, but their functional significance remains obscure (15).

Mitochondria

In view of the importance of mitochondria in the synthesis of steroid hormones, it is disappointing that we learn so little from the morphology of those of the Leydig cell. These organelles vary considerably from species to species, but in all cases so far examined, some tubular, some lamellar, and some intermediate forms of cristae are seen (15). The mitochondria are responsible for the conversion of cholesterol to pregnenolone and for the transport of the cholesterol to the inner membrane (213,214). Mention has already been made of an 8.2K protein (endozepine) that may regulate this process (136). It is important that similar studies be performed with Leydig cells.

Cytoskeleton

Unfortunately, a systematic description of the cytoskeleton of the Leydig cell has not been reported, but the usual cytoskeletal elements are present in this cell (15). Although the full functional significance of the cytoskeleton in the economy of the cell is not known, some important functions deserve mention. The cytoskeleton provides surfaces and compartments within the cell that are responsible for the inhomogeneity of the cytoplasm (215). This inhomogeneity arises from subdivisions created by microtubules and perhaps by finer trabecular structures (216,217). Within the compartments, enzymatic activity takes place in bound water associated with the surfaces of the cytoskeleton (218). It is significant that the enzymes of glycolysis are associated with microtubules (219). In addition, the shape of the cell is determined by intermediate filaments (220). The presence of actin in microfilaments suggests the possibility of contractile activity that may be used for intracellular movements. The subject has been reviewed elsewhere (221). The steroidogenic response of Leydig cells to LH is inhibited by antiactin injected into Leydig cells by fusion with liposomes (112). The inhibitory action of antiactin arises from inhibition of the transport of cholesterol to mitochondria (112). When these findings are considered in relation to the more detailed studies in the adrenal (222–224), we are left to conclude that LH requires a pool of G actin available for polymerization, and this, in turn, results in increased transport of cholesterol to mitochondria. This effect of LH is not inhibited by cycloheximide and does not, therefore, require newly synthesized proteins (unpublished data). The mechanism by which actin is involved in cholesterol transport is not known. Microfilaments may promote bulk movement within the cytoplasm, they may provide direction and shortening, or they may construct new compartments within the cytoplasm that may constrain the movement of cholesterol in such a way as to increase the efficiency of the transfer of this substrate to mitochondria. These and other possibilities must be explored by new methods that can be used in the living cell, including video-intensified Nomarski optics (225).

In exploring the role of the cytoskeleton in cholesterol transport, extracts of adrenal cells were made with buffered media that progressively remove membranes, microtubules, microfilaments, and all organelles except lipid droplets, which remain tightly bound to the intermediate filaments (226,227). It was also found that mitochondria are attached to intermediate filaments (228). The fact that the source and the endpoint for transport of cholesterol in steroidogenic cells (i.e., droplets and mitochondria) are both tethered to intermediate filaments suggests that these filaments may play an important part in the directed transport of this substrate from the site of storage to the steroidogenic pathway (228). It is also interesting that in fibroblasts ATP has been shown to collapse intermediate filaments by a mechanism based on actomyosin (229). Such a mechanism could account for the roles of both microfilaments and intermediate filaments in the rate-limiting step of cholesterol transport to mitochondria.

CONCLUSIONS

The synthesis of androgens in Leydig cells begins with the mobilization of cholesterol from depots of cholesterol esters in lipid droplets within the cytoplasm. The cholesterol is taken to the inner mitochondrial membrane in which it is converted to pregnenolone by C_{27} side-chain cleavage P-450. These events appear to include the slow step or steps in the steroidogenic pathway. Side-chain cleavage involves shuttling of adrenodoxin to and fro between adrenodoxin reductase and P-450. The pregnenolone so formed moves to the microsomal compartment, in which it is attacked by membrane-bound enzymes including the C_{21} side-chain cleavage P-450, which converts the 21-carbon steroid to a 19-carbon androgen, androstenedione, or dehydroepiandrosterone, depending on whether the Δ^4 or Δ^5 pathway is used. Androstenedione is converted to the principal androgen, testosterone, by 17β-hydroxysteroid dehyrogenase.

The microsomal enzymes are organized in a specific arrangement in which some of the active sites are further removed from the aqueous surroundings of the microsomes than others. The two steroidogenic cytochromes P-450, especially the microsomal C_{21} side-chain cleavage system, are susceptible to degradation by various forms of active oxygen.

This pathway is chiefly regulated by pulses of LH from the pituitary. LH binds to a specific surface receptor, and binding activates a stimulatory GTP-binding protein (G protein), which in turn stimulates neighboring adenylate cyclase. The resulting increase in cyclic AMP is probably responsible for all of the ensuing changes; if other second messengers exist, they have not been unequivocally identified at this time. The increased levels of cyclic AMP trigger a second response—it appears that the only action of cyclic AMP is to phosphorylate proteins via protein kinase A. One protein affected by this form of posttranslational modification is cholesterol ester hydrolase, which becomes active (or more active) on phosphorylation. The active hydrolase releases free cholesterol, which is conveyed to the mitochondrion by a mechanism that involves microfilaments. To this point, the synthesis of new protein is not required—LH achieves these responses with the existing Leydig cell proteins.

As a result of the action(s) of one or more proteins synthesized at accelerated rates under the influence of LH, cholesterol is transported to the inner mitochondrial membrane, where C_{27} side-chain cleavage takes place. The two processes of transport to and within the mitochondria appear to be points at which LH accelerates steroid synthesis. There may be, in addition, stimulation of the side-chain cleavage reaction itself.

Pregnenolone, formed as the result of C_{27} side-chain cleavage, proceeds to the microsomal system in which the remaining steps of the pathway take place. These reactions proceed more rapidly than the delivery of cholesterol to the C_{27} side-chain cleavage enzyme. However, the microsomal contribution to steroid synthesis is not without regulation. The degree to which the lyase activity of C_{21} side-chain cleavage is expressed, the relative activities of the Δ^4 and Δ^5 pathways, and the presence of pregnenolone-binding protein are examples of regulation in the microsomal compartment.

The expression of genes connected with steroid synthesis, including the four steroidogenic enzymes, is regulated by LH and cyclic AMP. This regulation takes place in a slower time frame than that of the acute synthesis of androgens in response to LH. Such changes in gene expression may represent trophic or maintenance effects or they may be important in circadian and other slower responses.

The most pressing challenge in our attempts to understand the mechanism of action of LH appears to involve assignment of functions to bands or spots on polyacrylamide gels and autoradiograms—bands or spots corresponding to proteins that change in amount and/or are subjected to posttranslational modification in response to LH.

ACKNOWLEDGMENTS

The author is extremely grateful to Ms. Vanessa Williamson for patience and skill in preparing the manuscript.

REFERENCES

1. Dufau ML, Veldhuis J, Fraioli F, Johnson MH, Catt KJ. Mode of bioactive LH secretion in man. *J Clin Endocrinol Metab* 1983;57:993–1003.
2. Eik-Nes KB, Hall PF. Secretion of steroid hormones in vivo. *Vitam Horm* 1965;23:153–181.
3. Christensen AK, Mason NR. Comparative ability of seminiferous tubules and interstitial tissue of rat testes to synthesize androgens from progesterone-4-^{14}C *in vitro. Endocrinology* 1965;76: 646–650.
4. Hall PF, Irby DC, De Kretser DM. Conversion of cholesterol to androgens by rat testes: comparison of interstitial cells and seminiferous tubules. *Endocrinology* 1969;84:488–492.
5. Brown MS, Goldstein JL. Receptor-mediated control of cholesterol metabolism. *Science* 1976;191:150–154.
6. Hall PF. Testicular hormones: synthesis and control. In: De Groot LJ, Cahill GF, Martini L et al., eds. *Endocrinology.* Vol. 3. New York: Grune & Stratton, 1979;1511–1519.
7. Dorrington JH, Armstrong DT. FSH stimulates estadiol-17β0 synthesis in cultured Sertoli cells. *Proc Natl Acad Sci USA* 1975;72:2677–2681.
8. Nyman MA, Geiger J, Goldzieher JW. Biosynthesis of estrogen by the perfused stallion testis. *J Biol Chem* 1959;234:16–21.
9. De Jong FH, Hey AH, Van der Molen HJ. Estradiol and testosterone in rat testis tissue: Localization and production *in vitro. J Endocrinol* 1974;60:409–416.
10. Tcholakian RK, Steinberger A. *In vitro* metabolism of testosterone by Sertoli cells and interstitial cells. In: Steinberger A, Steinberger E, eds. *Testicular development, structure and function.* New York: Raven Press, 1979;177–193.
11. Ritzen EM, Van Damme MP, Froysa B, Reuter C, De La Torre

B, Dicafalusy E. Identification of estradiol produced by Sertoli cell-enriched cultures. *J Steroid Biochem* 1981;14:533–537.
12. Camick JA, Makris A, Gunsalus GL, Ryan KJ. Testicular aromatization in immature rats. *Endocrinology* 1979;104:285–289.
13. Fishman LM, Safarty GA, Wilson H, Lipsett MB. The role of the testis in oestrogen production. *Ciba Found Colloq Endocrinol* 1967;16:156–161.
14. Hall PF. The effect of interstitial cell-stimulating hormone on the biosynthesis of testicular cholesterol from acetate-1-C^{14}. *Biochemistry* 1963;2:1232–1236.
15. Christensen AK. Leydig cells. In: Greep RO, Astwood EB, eds. *Handbook of physiology.* Sect. 7, Vol. V. Washington: American Physiological Society, 1975;21–55.
16. Hall PF. Endocrinology of the testis. In: Johnson AD, Gomez WR, van Denmark VL, eds. *Testicular physiology and biochemistry.* Vol. II. New York: Academic Press, 1970;1.
17. Werbin H, Chaikoff IL. Utilization of adrenal gland cholesterol for the synthesis of cortisol. *Arch Biochem Phys* 1961;19: 833–838.
18. Morris MD, Chaikoff IL. The origin of cholesterol in liver, adrenal gland and testis of the rat. *J Biol Chem* 1959;234:1095–1099.
19. Hall PF, Eik-Nes KB. The action of gonadotropic hormones upon rabbit testis *in vitro*. *Biochim Biophys Acta* 1962;63: 411–419.
20. Sandler R, Hall PF. The response of rat testis to interstitial cell-stimulating hormone *in vitro*. *Comp Biochem Physiol* 1966;19:833–840.
21. Vahouny GV, Chanderbhan R, Noland BJ, Scallen TJ. Cholesterol ester hydrolase and sterol carrier proteins. *Endocrinol Res* 1985;10:473–489.
22. Freeman DA, Ascoli M. The LDL pathway of cultured Leydig tumor cells. *Biochim Biophys Acta* 1983;754:72–76.
23. Chen YI, Kraemer F, Reaven GM. Identification of specific HDL-binding sites in rat testis. *J Biol Chem* 1980;255: 9162–9169.
24. Gwynne JT, Hess B, Hughes T, Rountree R, Mahaggee D. The role of high density liproproteins in adrenal steroidogenesis. *Endocrinol Res* 1985;10:411–429.
25. Albert DH, Ascoli M, Puett D, Coniglio JG. Lipid composition and gonadotropin-mediated lipid metabolism of the M5480 murine Leydig cell tumor. *J Lipid Res* 1980;21:862–865.
26. Naghshineh S, Treadwell CR, Gallo LH, Vahouny GV. Protein-kinase mediated phosphorylation of purified ester hydrolase from bovine adrenal cortex. *J Lipid Res* 1978;19:561–567.
27. Conneely OM, Headon DR, Olson CD, Ungar F, Dempsey ME. Intramitochondrial movement of cholesterol carrier protein with cholesterol in response to corticotropin. *Proc Natl Acad Sci USA* 1984;81:2970–2974.
28. Hall PF. Cellular organization for steroidogenesis. *Int Rev Cytol* 1984;86:53–92.
29. Shikita M, Hall PF. Cytochrome P-450 from bovine adrenocortical mitochondria: an enzyme for the side-chain cleavage of cholesterol. I. Purification and properties. *J Biol Chem* 1973;248: 5598–5606.
30. Nakajiin S, Hall PF. Microsomal cytochrome P-450 from neonatal pig testis: purification and properties of a C_{21} steroid side-chain cleavage (17α-hydroxylase and $C_{17,20}$-lyase). *J Biol Chem* 1981;256:3871–3878.
31. Mason HS. Mechanisms of oxygen metabolism. *Science* 1957;125:1185–1189.
32. Bresnick E. The molecular biology of the induction of the hepatic mixed function oxidase. In: Schenkman JB, Kupfer D, eds. *Hepatic cytochrome P450 monooxygenase system.* New York: Pergamon Press, 1980;191–224.
33. Hall PF. Microsomal metabolism of endogenous substrates: chairman's introduction. In: Sato R, Kato R, eds. *Microsomal metabolism of endogenous substrates.* Fifth International Symposium on Microsomes, Drug Oxidations and Drug Toxicity. Tokyo: Japan Societies Press, New York: Wiley Interscience, 1982.
34. Hayaishi O. Oxygenases: history and scope. In: *Oxygenases.* New York: Academic Press, 1962;1–22.
35. Masters BSS, Okita RT. The history, properties and function of NADPH-cytochrome P-450 reductase. In: Schenkman JB, Kupfer D, eds. *Hepatic cytochrome P-450 monooxygenase system.* New York: Pergamon Press, 1982;343–361.
36. Omura T, Sanders E, Estabrook RW, Cooper DY, Rosenthal O. Isolation from adrenal cortex of a nonheme iron protein and a flavoprotein as a TPNH-cytochrome P-450 reductase. *Arch Biochem Biophys* 1966;117:660–671.
37. Ullrich V. Cytochrome P-450 and biological hydroxylation reactions. *Top Curr Chem* 1979;83:68–115.
38. White RE, Coon MJ. Oxygen activation by cytochrome P-450. *Annu Rev Biochem* 1980;49:315–349.
39. Rein H, Ristan O. The importance of the high spin-low spin equilibrium existing in the cytochrome P450 for the enzyme mechanism. *Pharmazie* 1978;33:325–338.
40. Omura T, Sato R. The carbon monoxide-binding pigment of liver microsomes. *J Biol Chem* 1964;239:2370–2376.
41. Gunsalus IC, Meeks JR, Lipscomb JD, De Brunner P, Munck E. Bacterial monooxygenase—the P450 cytochrome system. In: Hayaishi O, ed. *Molecular mechanisms of oxygen activation.* New York: Academic Press, 1974;559–572.
42. Shikita M, Hall PF. Cytochrome P-450 from bovine adrenocortical mitochondria: an enzyme for the side-chain cleavage of cholesterol. II. Subunit structure. *J Biol Chem* 1973;248:5605–5610.
43. Watanuki M, Granger GA, Hall PF. Cytochrome P-450 from bovine adrenocortical mitochondria: immunochemical properties and purity. *J Biol Chem* 1978;253:2927–2934.
44. Tilley BE, Watanuki M, Hall PF. Preparation and properties of side-chain cleavage cytochrome P-450 from bovine adrenal cortex by affinity chromatography with pregnenolone as ligand. *Biochem Biophys Acta* 1977;493:260–269.
45. Takemori S, Sato H, Gomi T, Suhara K, Katagiri M. Purification and properties of cytochrome P-450 11β from adrenal mitochondria. *Biochem Biophys Res Commun* 1975;67:1151–1155.
46. Ramseyer J, Harding BW. Solubilization of adrenal cortical cytochrome P-450 which cleaves the cholesterol side-chain. *Biochem Biophys Acta* 1973;315:306–313.
47. Wang HP, Kimura T. Purification of adrenal cortex mitochondrial cytochrome P-450 specific for cholesterol side-chain cleavage activity. *J Biol Chem* 1977;251:6068–6074.
48. Koritz SB, Hall PF. Feedback inhibition by pregnenolone: a possible mechanism. *Biochim Biophys Acta* 1964;92:215–218.
49. Hall PF, Kortiz SB. Inhibition of the biosynthesis of pregnenolone by 20α-hydroxycholesterol. *Biochim Biophys Acta* 1964;93:441–445.
50. Burstein S, Gut M. Intermediates in the conversion of cholesterol to pregnenolone. *Steroids* 1976;38:115–129.
51. Duque C, Morisaki M, Ikekawa N, Shikita M. The enzyme activity of bovine adrenocortical cytochrome P450 producing pregnenolone from cholesterol. *Biochem Biophys Res Commun* 1978;82:179–185.
52. Hall PF, Lee Lewes J, Lipson ED. The role of mitochondrial cytochrome P450 from bovine adrenal cortex in side chain cleavage of 20S, 22R-dihydroxycholesterol. *J Biol Chem* 1975;250: 2283–2290.
53. Shikita M, Hall PF. The stoichiometry of the conversion of cholesterol and hydroxycholesterols to pregnenolone (3β-hydroxypregn-5-en-20-one) catalyzed by adrenal cytochrome P-450. *Proc Natl Acad Sci USA* 1974;71:1441–1446.
54. Orme-Johnson NR, Light DR, White-Stevens RW, Orme-Johnson WH. Steroid-binding properties of beef adrenal cortical cytochrome P450 which catalyzes conversion of cholesterol to pregnenolone. *J Biol Chem* 1979;254:2103–2109.
55. Young DG, Holroyd JD, Hall PF. Enzymatic and spectral properties of solubilized cytochrome P-450 from bovine adrenocortical mitochondria. *Biochem Biophys Res Commun* 1970;38: 184–188.
56. Kido T, Arakawa M, Kimura T. Adrenal cortex mitochondrial cytochrome P-450 specific to cholesterol side chain cleavage reaction. *J Biol Chem* 1979;254:8377–8384.
57. Tagaki Y, Shikita M, Hall PF. The active form of cytochrome P-450 from bovine adrenocortical mitochondria. *J Biol Chem* 1975;250:845–851.
58. Betz G, Tsai P, Weakley R. Heterogeneity of cytochrome P-450 in rat testis microsomes. *J Biol Chem* 1976;251:2839–2846.
59. Nakajin S, Hall PF. Microsomal cytochrome P-450 from neonatal pig testis: purification and properties of a C_{21} steroid side-chain cleavage system (17α-hydroxylase and $C_{17.20}$ lyase). *J Biol Chem* 1981;256:3871–3878.

60. Nakajiin S, Shively J, Yuan PM, Hall PF. Microsomal cytochrome P-450 from neonatal pig testis: two enzymatic activities (17α-hydroxylase and $C_{17,20}$-lyase) associated with one protein. *Biochemistry* 1981;20:4037–4045.
61. Bumpus JA, Dus KM. Bovine adrenocortical microsomal hemeproteins P450 C_{17} and P450 C_{21}. *J Biol Chem* 1982;257: 12696–12703.
62. Nakajiin S, Shinoda M, Hall PF. Purification and properties of 17α-hydroxylase from microsomes of pig adrenal: a second C_{21} side-chain cleavage system. *Biochem Biophys Res Commun* 1983;111:512–516.
63. Nakajiin S, Shinoda M, Hanui M, Shively JE, Hall PF. The C_{21} steroid side-chain cleavage enzyme from porcine adrenal microsomes: purification and characterization of the 17α-hydroxylase-$C_{17,20}$-lase cytochrome P450. *J Biol Chem* 1984;259:3971–3978.
64. Yanagabashi K, Hall PF. Role of electron transport in the regulation of lyase activity of C_{21} side-chain cleavage P-450 from porcine adrenal and testicular microsomes. *J Biol Chem* 1987;261:8429–8433.
65. Onoda M, Hall PF. Cytochrome b_5 stimulates purified testicular microsomal cytochrome P450 (C_{21} side chain cleavage). *Biochem Biophys Res Commun* 1982;108:454–458.
66. Nakajiin S, Hall PF, Onoda M. Testicular microsomal cytochrome P-450 for C_{21} steroid side-chain cleavage; spectral and binding studies. *J Biol Chem* 1981;256:6134–6141.
67. Onada M, Haniu M, Yanagabashi K, Sweet, Shively JE, Hall PF. Affinity alkylation of the active site of C_{21} side-chain cleavage P-450: unique cysteine residue alkylated by 17β-bromoacetoxyprogesterone. *Biochemistry* 1987;26:657–662.
68. Nakajiin S, Hall PF. Side-chain cleavage of C_{21} steroids by testicular microsomal cytochrome P-450 (17α-hydroxylase/lyase): involvement of heme. *J Steroid Biochem* 1983;19:1345–1348.
69. Ishii-Ohba H, Saiki N, Inano H, Takemori B. Purification and characterization of rat adrenal 3β-hydroxysteroid dehydrogenase with steroid 5-ene-4-ene-isomerase. *J Steroid Biochem* 1986;24:753–760.
70. Ishii-Ohba H, Saiki N, Inano H, Takemori B. Purification and properties of testicular 3β-hydroxysteroid dehydrogenase and 5-ene-4-ene-isomerase. *J Steroid Biochem* 1986;25:255–260.
71. Thomas JL, Ebenezer T, Berko A, Faustino A, Myers RP, Strickler RC. Human placental 3β-hydroxy-5-ene-steroid dehydrogenase and steroid 5-4-ene-isomerase: purification and inhibition by product steroids. *J Steroid Biochem* 1988;31:785–796.
72. Lorence MC, Murry BA, Trant JM, Mason JI. Human 3β-hydroxysteroid dehydrogenase/isomerase: expression in nonsteroid organic cells of a protein showing both activities. *Endocrinology* 1990;126:2493–2498.
73. Thomas JL, Myers RP, Strickler RC. Human placental 3β-hydroxy-5-ene-steroid dehydrogenase and steroid-5-4-ene-isomerase: purification and characterization of mitochondrial microsomal enzymes. *J Steroid Biochem* 1989;33:209–217.
74. Oshima H, Ochi AI. On testicular 17β-hydroxysteroid oxidoreductase: product activation. *Biochim Biophys Acta* 1973;306: 227–235.
75. Bogovich K, Payne AH. Purification of rat testicular microsomal 17β-ketosteroid reductase. *J Biol Chem* 1980;255:5552–5558.
76. Murano EP, Payne AH. Distinct testicular 17β-ketosteroid reductases, one in interstitial tissue and one in seminiferous tubules. *Biophys Acta* 1976;450:89–95.
77. Ohba H, Inano H, Tamaoki B. Kinetic mechanism of porcine testicular 17β-hydroxysteroid dehydrogenase. *J Steroid Biochem* 1982;17:381–389.
78. Samuels LT, Bussman L, Matsumoto K, Huseby RA. Organization of androgen biosynthesis in the testis. *J Steroid Biochem* 1975;6:291–301.
79. Bendayan M. Protein A-gold electron microscopic immunocytochemistry: methods, applications and limitations. *J Electron Microsc* 1984;1:243–250.
80. Guezse HJ, Slot JW, Yanagibashi K, McCracken JA, Hall PF. Immunoelectron microscopy of cytochromes P450 in porcine adrenal cortex: two enzymes (11β-hydroxylase and side-chain cleavage) are co-localized in the same mitochondria. *Histochemistry* 1987;86:551–559.
81. Hall PF, Watanuki M, Hamkalo BA. Adrenocortical cytochrome P-450 side-chain cleavage: preparation of membrane-bound side-chain cleavage system from purified components. *J Biol Chem* 1979;254:547–553.
82. Seybert DW, Lancaster JR, Lambert JD, Kamin H. Participation of the membrane in the side-chain cleavage of cholesterol. *J Biol Chem* 1979;254:12088–12093.
83. Seybert DW, Lambeth JD, Kamin H. The participation of a second molecule of adrenodoxin in cytochrome P-450 catalyzed 11β-hydroxylation. *J Biol Chem* 1978;253:8355–8361.
84. Lambeth JD, Seybert DW, Kamin H. Ionic effects on adrenal steroidogenic electron transport. *J Biol Chem* 1979;254: 7255–7261.
85. Lambeth JD, Seybert DW, Kamin H. Phospholipid vesicle-reconstituted cytochrome P450 SCC. *J Biol Chem* 1980;255: 138–145.
86. Kimura T, Parcells JH, Wang H. Purification of adrenodoxin, adrenodoxin reductase and cytochrome P-450 from adrenal cortex. *Methods Enzymol* 1978;LII:132–151.
87. Ruokenen A, Vihko R. Concentrations of unconjugated and sulfated neutral sterols in boar testis. *J Steroid Biochem* 1974;5:33–39.
88. Hall PF, Sozer CC, Eik-Nes KB. Formation of dehydroepiandrosterone during *in vivo* and *in vitro* biosynthesis of testosterone by testicular tissue. *Endocrinology* 1964;74:35–43.
89. Baskin LS, Yang S. Cross-linking studies of the protein topography of rat liver microsomes. *Biochem Biophys Acta* 1982;684:263–270.
90. Nisimoto Y, Lambeth JD. NADPH-cytochrome P-450 reductase-cytochrome b_5 interactions: crosslinking of the phospholipid vesicle-associated proteins by a water-soluble carbodiimide. *Arch Biochem Biophys* 1985;241:386–395.
91. Lambeth JD, Green LM, Millett F. Adrenodoxin interaction with adrenodoxin reductase and cytochrome P-450 SCC. *J Biol Chem* 1984;259:10025–10031.
92. Welton AF, Aust SD. The effects of 3-methylcholanthrene on the structure of the rat liver endoplasmic reticulum. *Biochim Biophys Acta* 1974;373:197–205.
93. Samuels LT, Matsumoto K. Localization of enzymes involved in testosterone biosynthesis in mouse testis. *Endocrinology* 1974;94:55–61.
94. Matsumoto K, Samuels LT. Influence of steroid distribution between microsomes and soluble fraction on steroid metabolism by microsomal enzymes. *Endocrinology* 1969;85:402–409.
95. Nakajiin S, Hall PF. Side-chain cleavage of C_{21} steroids to C_{19} steroids by testicular microsomal cytochrome P-450: 17α-hydroxy-C_{21} steroids as obligatory intermediates. *J Steroid Biochem* 1981;14:1249–1255.
96. Tamaoki B, Shikita M. Biosynthesis of steroids in testicular tissue *in vitro*. In: Pincus G, Tait J, Nakamo T, eds. *Steroid dynamics*. New York: Academic Press, 1966;493.
97. Estabrook RW, Frankle MR, Cohen B, Shigamatzu A, Hildebrandt AG. Influence of hepatic microsomal mixed function oxidation on cellular metabolism. *Metabolism* 1971;20:187–198.
98. Wu ES, Tank DW, Webb WW. Unconstrained lateral diffusion of ConA receptors in bulbous lymphocytes. *Proc Natl Acad Sci USA* 1982;79:4962–4966.
99. Hochman JH, Schindler M, Lee JG, Ferguson-Miller S. Lateral mobility of cytochrome c in intact mitochondrial membranes as determined by fluorescence redistribution after photobleaching. *Proc Natl Acad Sci USA* 1982;79:6866–6870.
100. Peterson JA, Ebel RE, O'Keefe DH, Matsubara T, Estrabrook RW. Temperature dependence of cytochrome P450 reduction. *J Biol Chem* 1976;251:4010–4016.
101. Dean WL, Gray RD. Relationship between state of aggregation and catalytic activity of P450 LM_2 and P450 reductase. *J Biol Chem* 1983;257:14679–14686.
102. Li CH, Evans HM. Chemistry of anterior pituitary hormones. In: Pincus G, Thimann K, eds. *The hormones*. Vol. 1. New York: Academic Press, 1948;631.
103. Hall PF, Eik-Nes KB. The action of gonadotropic hormones upon rabbit testis *in vitro*. *Biochim Biophys Acta* 1962;63: 411–419.
104. Hall PF, Eik-Nes KB. The influence of gonadotropins in vivo upon the biosynthesis of androgens by homogenate of rat testis. *Biochem Biophys Acta* 1963;71:438–447.
105. Hall PF. On the stimulation of testicular steroidogenesis in the

rabbit by interstitial cell-stimulating hormone. *Endocrinology* 1966;78:690–697.
106. Hall PF, Young DG. Site of action of trophic hormones upon the biosynthetic pathways to steroid hormones. *Endocrinology* 1968;82:559–565.
107. Mori M, Marsh JM. The site of LH stimulation of steroidogenesis in mitochondria of the rat corpus luteum. *J Biol Chem* 1982;257:6178–6185.
108. Garren LD, Ney RH, Davis WW. Studies on the role of protein synthesis in the regulation of corticosterone production by ACTH *in vivo*. *Proc Natl Acad Sci USA* 1965;53:1443–1447.
109. Hall PF, Charpponnier C, Nakamura M, Gabbiani G. The role of microfilaments in the response of adrenal tumor cells to adrenocorticotropic hormone. *J Biol Chem* 1979;254:9080–9084.
110. Crivello JF, Jefcoate CR. Intramitochondrial movement of cholesterol in rat adrenal cells. *J Biol Chem* 1980;255:8144–8149.
111. Dufau ML, Catt KJ. Gondaotropic stimulation of interstitial cell functions of the rat testis in vitro. In: Hardman JG, O'Malley BW, eds. *Methods in enzymology XXXIX*. New York: Academic Press, 1975;252–257.
112. Hall PF, Charpponnier C, Nakamura M, Gabbiani G. The role of microfilaments in the response of Leydig cells to luteinizing hormone. *J Steroid Biochem* 1979;11:1361–1369.
113. Bell JJ, Harding B. The acute action of ACTH on adrenal steroidogenesis. *Biochim Biophys Acta* 1984;348:285–292.
114. Hall PF. Trophic stimulation of steroidogenesis: in search of the elusive trigger. In: Greep RO, ed. *Recent progress in hormone research*. Vol. 41. Laurentian Hormone Conference New York: Academic Press, 1985;1–39.
115. Sandler R, Hall PF. The influence of age upon the response of rat testis to intestitial cell-stimulating hormone *in vitro*. *Biochem Biophys Acta* 1968;164:445–451.
116. Marsh JM. The role of cyclic AMP in gonadal steroidogenesis. *Biol Reprod* 1976;14:30–55.
117. Schimmer BP. Cyclic nucleotides in hormonal regulation of adrenocortical function. *Adv Cyclic Nucleotide Res* 1980;13:181–198.
118. Moyle WR, Kong YC, Ramachandran J. Steroidogenesis and cyclic AMP accumulation in rat adrenal cells. *J Biol Chem* 1973;248:2409–2417.
119. Dufau ML, Baukal AJ, Catt KJ. Intermediate role of cyclic AMP and protein kinase during gonadotropin-induced steroidogenesis in Leydig cells. *Proc Natl Acad Sci USA* 1977;74:3419–3423.
120. Moger WH. Evidence for compartmentation of C'AMP-dependent protein kinase in rat Leydig cells. *Endocrinology* 1991;128:1414–1418.
121. Pereira ME, Segaloff DL, Ascoli M, Eckstein F. Inhibition of gonadotropin-activated steroidogenesis in cultured Leydig tumour cells by the Rp diastereoisomer of adenosine-3'5'-cyclic phosphothioate. *J Biol Chem* 1987;262:6093–6100.
122. Duchatelle P, Joffre M. Ca^{2+}-dependent-chloride and potassium currents in rat Leydig cells. *FEBS Lett* 1987;217:335–339.
123. Choi MSK, Cooke BA. Evidence for two independent pathways in the stimulation of steroidogenesis by LH. *FEBS Lett* 1990;261:402–404.
124. Irby DC, Hall PF. Stimulation by ICSH of protein biosynthesis in isolated Leydig cells from hypophysectomized rats. *Endocrinology* 1971;89:1367–1374.
125. Janszen FHA, Cooke BA, Van der Molen HJ. Specific protein synthesis in isolated rat Leydig cells. Influence of LH and cycloheximide. *Biochem J* 1977;162:341–346.
126. Epstein LF, Orme-Johnson NR. Regulation of steroid hormone biosynthesis. Identification of precursors of a phosphoprotein targeted to the mitochondrion in stimulated rat adrenal cortex cells. *J Biol Chem* 1991;266:19739–19745.
127. Pon LA, Epstein LF, Orme-Johnson NR. Protein synthesis requirement for acute ACTH stimulation of adrenal corticosteroidogenesis. *Endocr Res* 1986;12:429–446.
128. Pon LA, Orme-Johnson NR. Acute stimulation of steroidogenesis in corpus luteum and adrenal cortex by peptide hormones. *J Biol Chem* 1986;261:6594–6599.
129. Chanderbahn R, Noland BJ, Scallen TJ, Vahouny GV. Sterol carrier protein 2. Delivery of cholesterol from adrenal lipid droplets to mitochondria for pregnenolone synthesis. *J Biol Chem* 1982;257:8928–8935.
130. Vahouny GV, Chanderbahn R, Nolan BJ, et al. Sterol carrier protein 2. Identification of adrenal SCP and site of action for mitochondrial cholesterol utilization. *J Biol Chem* 1983;258: 11731–11737.
131. Conneely OM, Headon DR, Olson ED, Ungar F, Dempsey ME. Intramitochondrial movement of adrenal sterol carrier protein with cholesterol in response to corticotropin. *Proc Natl Acad Sci USA* 1984;81:2970–2976.
132. Pederson RC. Polypeptide activators of cholesterol side-chain cleavage. *Endocr Res* 1984;10:533–561.
133. Pedersen RC, Brownie AC. Cholesterol side-chain cleavage in the rat adrenal cortex: isolation of a cycloheximide sensitive activator protein. *Proc Natl Acad Sci USA* 1983;80:1882–1886.
134. Pederson RC. Steroidogenesis activator polypeptide (SAP) in rat ovary and testis. *J Steroid Biochem* 1987;27:731–735.
135. Pedersen RC, Brownie AC. Steroidogenesis-activator polypeptide isolated from a Leydig cell tumor. *Science* 1987;236: 188–190.
136. Yanagibashi K, Ohno Y, Kawamura M, Hall PF. The regulation of intracellular transport of cholesterol in bovine adrenal cells. Purification of a novel protein. *Endocrinology* 1988;123: 2075–2082.
137. Besman MJ, Yanagibashi K, Lee TD, Kawamura M, Hall PF, Shively JE. Identification of des-(Gly-Ile)-endozepine as an effector of corticoprotein-dependent adrenal steroidogenesis: stimulation of cholesterol delivery is mediated by the peripheral benzodiazepine receptor. *Proc Natl Acad Sci USA* 1989;86:4897–4901.
138. Brown AS, Hall PF. Stimulation by endozepine of the side-chain cleavage of cholesterol in a reconstituted enzyme system. *Biochem Biophys Res Commun* 1991;180:609–614.
138a. Papadopoulos V, Mukhin AG, Cost E, Krueger KE. Peripheral type benzodiazepine receptor is functionally linked to Leydig cell steroidogenesis. *J Biol Chem* 1990;265:3772–3779.
139. Xu X, Xu T, Roberston DG, Lambeth JD. GTP stimulates pregnenolone generation in isolated rat adrenal mitochondria. *J Biol Chem* 1989;264:17674–17680.
140. Birmingham MK, Elliot FH, Valere PHL. The need for the presence of Ca^{2+} for the stimulation *in vitro* of rat adrenal glands by ACTH. *Endocrinology* 1953;53:687–693.
141. Hall PF, Osawa S, Mrotek JJ. Influence of calmodulin on steroid synthesis in Leydig cells from rat testis. *Endocrinology* 1981;109:1677–1684.
142. Conn PM, Chafouleas JG, Rogers D, Means AR. Gonadotropin releasing hormone stimulates calmodulin redistribution in rat pituitary. *Nature* 1981;292:264–266.
143. Cheitlin R, Buckley DI, Ramachandran J. The role of extracellular calcium in corticotropin stimulated steroidogenesis. *J Biol Chem* 1985;260:5327–5334.
144. Widmaier EP, Papadopoulos V, Hall PF. The role of calmodulin in the responses to adrenocorticotropin of plasma membranes from adrenal cells. *Endocrinology* 1990;126:2465–2473.
145. Yanagibashi K, Kawamura M, Hall PF. Voltage-dependent Ca^{2+} channels are involved in regulation of steroid synthesis by bovine but not rat fasciculata cells. *Endocrinology* 1990;126:311–318.
146. Kuo JF, Greengard P. Cyclic nucleotide-dependent kinase: widespread occurrence of cyclic AMP-dependent protein kinase. *Proc Natl Acad Sci USA* 1969;64:1349–1353.
147. Cooke BA, Lindh ML, Janzen FHA. Effect of lutropin on phosphorylation of endogenous proteins in testis Leydig cells. *Biochem J* 1977;168:43–48.
148. Neymark MA, Bieszczad RR, Dimino MJ. Phosphorylation of mitochondrial proteins in isolated porcine follicles after treatment with LH. *Endocrinology* 1984;114:588–595.
149. Inaba T, Wiest WG. Protein kinase stimulation of steroidogenesis in rat luteal cell mitochondria. *Endocrinology* 1985;117: 315–322.
150. Lin T. The role of Ca^{2+}/phospholipid-dependent protein kinase in Leydig cell steroidogenesis. *Endocrinology* 1985;117:119–126.
151. Moger WH. Stimulation and inhibition of Leydig cell steroidogenesis by the phorbol ester 12-0-tetradecanoylphorbol-13-acetate. *Life Sci* 1985;37:869–874.
152. Berridge MJ, Dawson RMC, Downes CPP, Heslop JP, Irvine RF. Changes in levels of inositol phosphates after agonist-dependent hydrolysis of membrane phosphoinositide. *Biochem J* 1983;212: 473–479.
153. Burgess GM, Godfrey PP, McKinney JS, Berridge MJ, Irvine

RR, Putney JW. The second messenger linking receptor activation to internal Ca release in liver. *Nature* 1984;309:63–65.
154. Iida S, Widmaier E, Hall PF. The phosphoinositide-Ca^{2+} hypothesis does not apply to the steroidogenic action of ACTH. *Biochem J* 1986;236:53–61.
155. Lowitt S, Farese RV, Sabir MA, Root AW. Rat Leydig cell phospholipid content is increased by LH and 8-bromo-cyclic AMP. *Endocrinology* 1982;111:1415–1422.
156. Farese RV, Sabir MA, Larson RE, Trudeau W, III. Further observations on the increases in phospholipids after stimulation by ACTH, cyclic AMP and insulin. *Cell Calcium* 1983;4:195–203.
157. Farese RV. Phospholipids as intermediaries in hormone action. *Mol Cell Endocrinol* 1984;35:1–24.
158. Mendelson O, Dufau M, Katt K. Dependence of gonadotropin-induced steroidogenesis upon RNA and protein synthesis in the interstitial cells of the rat testis. *Biochem Biophys Acta* 1975;411:222–230.
159. Anderson CM, Mendelson CR. Regulation of steroidogenesis in rat Leydig cells in culture. *Arch Biochem Biophys* 1985;238: 378–387.
160. Mason JI, MacDonald AA, Laptook A. The activity and biosynthesis of cholesterol side-chain cleavage enzyme in cultured immature pig testis cells. *Biochim Biophys Acta* 1984;795:504–512.
161. Goldring NB, Durica JM, Lifka J, et al. Cholesterol side-chain cleavage P450 messenger ribonucleic acid: evidence for hormonal regulation in rat ovarian follicles and constitutive expression in corpora lutea. *Endocrinology* 1987;120:1942–1950.
162. Voutilainen R, Miller WL. Coordinate tropic hormone regulation of mRNAs for insulin-like growth factor II and the cholesterol side-chain cleavage enzyme P450scc, in human steroidogenic tissues. *Proc Natl Acad Sci USA* 1987;84:1590–1594.
163. John ME, John MC, Boggaram V, Simpson ER, Waterman MR. Transcriptional regulation of steroid hydroxylase genes by corticotropin. *Proc Natl Acad Sci USA* 1986;83:4715–4719.
164. Picardo-Leonard J, Voutilainen R, Kao L, Chung B, Strauss JF, III, Miller WL. Human adrenodoxin: cloning of three cDNAs and cycloheximide enhancement in JEG-3 cells. *J Biol Chem* 1988;263:3240–3244.
165. Golos TG, Miller WL, Strauss JE III. Human chorionic gonadotropin and 8-bromo cyclic adenosine monophosphate promote an acute increase in cytochrome P450scc and adrenodoxin messenger RNAs in cultured human granulosa cells by a cycloheximide-insensitive mechanism. *J Clin Invest* 1988;80: 896–899.
166. Mellon SH, Vaisse C. cAMP regulates P-450scc gene expression by a cycloheximide insensitive mechanism in cultured mouse Leydig MA-10 cells. *Proc Natl Acad Sci USA* 1989;86: 7775–7779.
167. John ME, John MC, Boggaram V, Simpson ER, Waterman MR. Transcriptional regulation of steroid hydroxylase genes by corticotropin. *Proc Natl Acad Sci USA* 1986;83:4715–4719.
168. Kumamoto T, Morohashi K, Ito A, Omura T. Site-directed mutagenesis of basic amino acid residues in the extension peptide of P-450(SCC) precursor: effects on the import of the precursor into mitochondria. *J Biochem* 1987;102:833–838.
169. Kumamoto T, Morohashi K, Ito A, Omura T. Critical region in the extension peptide for the import of cytochrome P-450 (SCC) precursor into mitochondria. *J Biochem* 1989;105:72–78.
170. Johnson FF, McKnight SL. Eukaryotic transcriptional regulatory proteins. *Annu Rev Biochem* 1989;58:799–839.
171. Inoue H, Watanabe N, Hiyashi Y, Fujii-Kuriyama Y. Structures of regulatory regions in the human cytochrome P450scc (desmolase) gene. *Eur J Biochem* 1991;195:563–569.
172. Ahlgren R, Simpson RR, Waterman MR, Lund J. Characterization of the promoter/regulatory region of bovine CYP11A (P_{450}scc) gene. *J Biol Chem* 1990;265:3313–3319.
173. Rice DA, Kirkman MS, Aitken LD, Mouw AR, Schimmer BP, Parker KL. Analysis of the promoter region of the gene encoding mouse cholesterol side-chain cleavage enzyme. *J Biol Chem* 1990;265:11713–11720.
174. Nishihara M, Winters CA, Buzko E, Waterman MR, Dufau ML. Hormonal regulation of rat Leydig cell cytochrome P45017α mRNA levels. *Biochem Biophys Res Commun* 1988;154: 151–158.
175. McCarthy JL, Waterman MR. Co-induction of 17α-hydroxylase and C-17,20-lyase activities in primary cultures of bovine adrenocortical cells in response to ACTH treatment. *J Steroid Biochem* 1983;29:307–312.
176. Lund J, Ahlgren R, Wu D, Kagimoto M, Simpson ER, Waterman MR. Transcriptional regulation of the bovine CYP17 (P-45017α) gene. *J Biol Chem* 1990;265:3304–3312.
177. Picado-Leonard J, Miller WL. Cloning and sequence of the human gene for P450CYP17 (17α-hydroxylase/17.20 lyase). *DNA* 1987;6:439–448.
178. Zuber MX, John ME, Okamura T, Simpson E, Waterman MR. Bovine adrenocortical P-450 17α. Regulation of gene expression by ACTH. *J Biol Chem* 1986;261:2475–2482.
179. Zanger UM, Lund J, Simpson ER, Waterman MR. Activation of transcription in cell-free extracts by a novel cAMP-responsive sequence from the bovine CYP17 gene. *J Biol Chem* 1991;266:11417–11420.
180. Zhao H, Simard J, Labrie C, et al. Molecular cloning, cDNA structure and predicted amino acid sequence of bovine 3β-hydroxy-5-ene steroid dehydrogenase/isomerase. *FEBS Lett* 1989;259:153–157.
181. Chedrese PJ, Luu-Thé V, Labrie F, Juros AV, Murphy BD. Evidence for the regulation of 3β-hydroxysteroid dehydrogenase mRNA by hCG. *Endocrinology* 1990;126:2228–2230.
182. Payne AH, Sha L. Multiple mechanisms for regulation of 3β-hydroxysteroid dehydrogenase/isomerase, 17α-hydroxylase/lyase and side-chain cleavage P450 mRNA levels in primary cultures of mouse Leydig cells. *Endocrinology* 1991;129:1429–1435.
183. Luu-Thé V, Labrie C, Zhao F, et al. Characterization of cDNAs for human estradiol 17β-dehydrogenase. *Mol Endocrinol* 1989;3:1301–1309.
184. Tremblay Y, Ringler GE, Morel Y, et al. Regulation of the gene for estrogenic 17-ketosteroid reductase lying on chromosome 17cen-q25. *J Biol Chem* 1989;264:20458–20462.
185. Aubry M, Collu R, Ducharme JR, Crine P. Biosynthesis of a putative gonadotropin receptor component by rat Leydig cells. *Endocrinology* 1982;111:2129.
186. Dufau ML, Horner KA, Hayashi K, Tsuruhara T, Conn PM, Catt KJ. Actions of choleragen and gonadotropin in isolated Leydig cells. *J Biol Chem* 1978;253;3721–3729.
187. Dufau ML, Baukal AJ, Catt KJ. Hormone-induced guanyl nucleotide binding and activation of adenylate kinase in the Leydig cell. *Proc Natl Acad Sci USA* 1980;77:5837–5841.
188. Dufau ML, Winters CA, Hattori M, et al. Hormonal regulation of androgen production by the Leydig cell. *J Steroid Biochem* 1984;20:161–171.
189. Dufau ML, Baukal AJ, Winters CA, Catt KJ. Guanyl nucleotide-induced phosphorylation of Leydig cell membrane protein. *Endocrinology* 1982;110:256–262.
190. Barano JL, Dufau ML. Gonadotropin-induced changes in the LH receptors of cultured Leydig cells; evidence for up-regulation *in vitro*. *J Biol Chem* 1983;258:7322–7326.
191. Freeman DA, Ascoli M. Desensitization to gonadotropin receptors. *Proc Natl Acad Sci USA* 1981;75:6309–6313.
192. Freeman DA, Ascoli M. Desensitization of steroidogenesis in cultured Leydig tumour cells: role of cholesterol. *Proc Natl Acad Sci USA* 1982;79:7796–7801.
192a. West AP, Cooke BA. Regulation of the function of LH receptors at the plasma membrane is different in rat and mouse Leydig cells. *Endocrinology* 1991;128:363–370.
193. Ezra E, Salomon Y. Mechanism of desensitization of adenylate cyclase by lutropin. *J Biol Chem* 1980;255:653–659.
194. Rebois RV, Fishman PH. Down-regulation of gonadotropin receptors in a murine Leydig cell tumour. *J Biol Chem* 1984;259:3096–3102.
195. Quinn PG, Dombrausky LJ, Chen YDI, Payne AH. Serum lipoproteins increase in testosterone production in hCG-desensitized Leydig cells. *Endocrinology* 1981;109:1790–1798.
196. Charreau EH, Calvo JC, Nozu K, Pignataro O, Catt KJ, Dufau ML. Hormonal modulation of HMG CoA reductase in desensitized Leydig cells. *J Biol Chem* 1981;256:12719–12725.
197. Quinn PG, Payne AH. Steroid product-induced, oxygen-mediated damage of microsomal cytochrome P450 enzymes in Leydig cell cultures. *J Biol Chem* 1985;260:2092–2097.
198. Chasalow F, Marr H, Haour F, Saez JM. Testicular steroidogene-

sis after hCG desensitization in rats. *J Biol Chem* 1979;254: 5613–5618.
199. Cigorraga SB, Dufau ML, Catt KJ. Regulation of LH receptors and steroidogenesis in gonadotropin-desensitized Leydig cells. *J Biol Chem* 1978;253:4297–4302.
200. Catt KJ, Harwood JP, Clayton RN, et al. Regulation of peptide hormone receptors and gonadal steroidogenesis. *Recent Prog Horm Res* 1980;36:557–576.
201. Tycko B, Keith CH, Maxfield FR. Rapid acidification of endocytic vesicles containing asialoglycoprotein in cells of a human hepatoma line. *J Cell Biol* 1983;97:1762–1767.
202. Steinman RM, Mellman IS, Muller WA, Cohn ZA. Endocytosis and the recycling of plasma membrane. *J Cell Biol* 1983;96:1–7.
203. Guillou F, Martinat N, Combarnous Y. Rapid *in vitro* desensitization in rat Leydig cells by subactive concentrations of porcine LH. *FEBS Lett* 1985;184:6–10.
204. Dix CJ, Haberfield D, Cooke BA. Characterization of the homologous and heterologous desensitization of rat Leydig-tumour-cell adenylate cyclase. *J Biochem* 1984;220:803–810.
205. Hornsby PJ, Crivello JF. The role of lipid peroxidation and biological antioxidents in the function of the adrenal cortex. Part 1. *Mol Cell Endocrinol* 1983;30:1–22.
206. Hornsby PJ, Crivello JF. The role of lipid peroxidation and biological antioxidents in the function of the adrenal cortex. Part 2. *Mol Cell Endocrinol* 1983;30:123–142.
207. Crivello JF, Hornsby PJ, Gill GN. Metyrapone and antioxidants are required to maintain aldosterone synthesis by cultured bovine adrenocortical zona glomerulosa cells. *Endocrinology* 1982;111: 469–475.
208. Nozu K, Dufau ML, Catt KJ. Estradiol-receptor mediated regulation of steroidogenesis in gonadotropin-desensitized Leydig cells. *J Biol Chem* 1981;256:1915–1922.
209. Onoda M, Hall PF. Inhibition of testicular microsomal cytochrome P450 (17α-hydroxylase-$C_{17,20}$-lase) by estogens. *Endocrinology* 1981;109:763–767.
210. Nozu K, Dehejia A, Zawistowich L, Catt KJ, Dufau ML. Gonadotropin-induced receptor regulation in cultured Leydig cells. *J Biol Chem* 1981;256:12875–12882.
211. Nozu K, Dehejia A, Zawistowich L, Catt KJ, Dufau ML. Gonadotropin-induced desensitization of Leydig cells *in vivo* and *in vitro*. *Ann NY Acad Sci* 1982;383:230–242.
212. Johnson AD. Testicular lipids. In: Johnson AD, Gomes NL, Van Denmark NL, eds. *The testis.* Vol. 2. New York: Academic Press, 1979;193–217.
213. Ohno Y, Yanagibashi K, Yonezawa Y, Ishiwatari S, Matsuba M. Effect of ACTH, cycloheximide and aminoglutethimide on the content of cholesterol in the outer and inner mitochondrial membrane of rat adrenal cortex. *Endocrinol Jpn* 1983;30:335–344.
214. Privalle CT, Crivello JF, Jefcoate CR. Regulation of intramitochondrial cholesterol side-chain cleavage P450 in rat adrenal gland. *Proc Natl Acad Sci USA* 1983;80:702–706.
215. Clegg JS. Interrelationships between water and cell metabolism in Artemia cysts. *Cold Spring Harbor Symp Quant Biol* 1982;46:23–38.
216. Wolosewick JJ, Porter KR. Microtrabecular lattice of the cytoplasmic ground substance. Artifact or reality. *J Cell Biol* 1979;82:114–139.
217. Gershon ND, Porter KR, Trus BL. The cytoplasmic matrix: its volume and surface area; the diffusion of molecules through it. *Proc Natl Acad Sci USA* 1985;82:5030–5034.
218. Clegg JS. Properties and metabolism of the aqueous cytoplasm and its boundaries. *Am J Physiol* 1984;246:R133–141.
219. Ottaway JH, Mowbray J. The role of compartmentation in the regulation of glycolysis. *Curr Top Cell Regul* 1977;12:108–149.
220. Lazarides E. Intermediate filaments as mechanical integrates of cellular space. *Nature* 1980;283:249–253.
221. Hall PF. The role of cytoskeleton in hormone action. *Can J Biochem Cell Biol* 1984;62:653–674.
222. Hall PF. The role of the cytoskeleton in endocrine function. In: Conn MP, ed. *Cellular regulation of secretion and release.* New York: Academic Press, 1982;195–221.
223. Hall PF. The role of the cytoskeleton in the responses of target cells to hormones. In: McKerns KW, Aakvaag A, Hanson V, eds. *Regulation of target cell responsiveness.* Vol. 1. New York: Plenum, 1984;205–227.
224. Osawa S, Betz G, Hall PF. The role of actin in the responses of adrenal cells to ACTH and cyclic AMP: inhibition by DNase I. *J Cell Biol* 1984;99:1335–1342.
225. Allen RD, Travis JL, Allen NS, Yilmaz H. Video-enhanced contrast polarization (AVEC-POL) microscopy. *Cell Motil* 1981;1:275–290.
226. Almahbobi G, Hall PF. The role of intermediate filaments in adrenal steroidogenesis. *J Cell Sci* 1990;97:679–687.
227. Almahbobi G, Williams LJ, Hall PF. Attachment of steroidogenic lipid droplets to intermediate filaments in adrenal cells. *J Cell Sci* 1992;101:383–393.
228. Almahbobi G, Williams LJ, Hall PF. Attachment of mitochondria to intermediate filaments in adrenal cells. *Exp Cell Res* 1992;200:361–369.
229. Tint LS, Hollenbeck PJ, Berkhovsky AB, Surgucheva LG, Bershadsky AD. Evidence that intermediate filament reorganization is induced by ATP-dependent contraction of the actomyosin cortex in permeabilized fibroblasts. *J Cell Sci* 1991;98:375–384.

The Physiology of Reproduction, Second Edition,
edited by E. Knobil and J.D. Neill,
Raven Press, Ltd., New York © 1994.

CHAPTER 22

Regulation of Spermatogenesis

Richard M. Sharpe

INTRODUCTION AND HISTORICAL ASPECTS

Spermatogenesis is one of the keys to the future because without the successful production of astronomical numbers of competent spermatozoa daily we are infertile as a species and are thus incapable of passing on our genes. We appear to be all too successful in this respect, though the recent report (1) that the sperm counts of men in the Western World have declined by approximately half in the past 50 years, should give us pause for thought. Whether this decrease is real or not (2–4), it has served to highlight our woeful ignorance about how spermatozoa are made and what factors affect or regulate this process. This chapter explores the little that we do know about the regulation of spermatogenesis. But before diving into this information it is appropriate to begin by considering our progress in understanding from a historical perspective, as it provides considerable food for thought.

MRC Reproductive Biology Unit, Centre for Reproductive Biology, Edinburgh EH3 9EW, UK

We now have at our disposal far more "facts" about spermatogenesis than were available 20 years ago and incalculably more than were available to the scientific pioneers of earlier centuries. Unfortunately, our understanding of the regulation of spermatogenesis has not increased in proportion to the "facts" over this time period. To understand why let me remind the reader briefly of some historical "facts."

The existence of seminiferous tubules and their essential role in male fertility was established over three centuries ago (5), as was the presence of spermatozoa in semen by van Leeuwenhoek (6). The endocrine effects of testosterone have been known about for half of this time period (7) and, arguably, for a few thousand years earlier in one form or another (8). Testosterone was first purified more than 60 years ago (9), and our knowledge of the essential role of the pituitary gland in maintaining spermatogenesis derives from around the same time period (10,11), as does our understanding that exogenous testosterone could to some extent substitute for the pituitary gland (12,13). Moreover, we have known for more than 60 years that two pituitary hormones (FSH and

LH) with separate sites of action in the testis are involved in the control of spermatogenesis (14), and we have been aware for more than half a century that age is an important factor in determining the response of the testis to these hormones (15,16). Indeed, it was worked out by Ludwig (16) more than 40 years ago that low doses of testosterone propionate (TP) suppressed, whereas higher doses maintained, spermatogenesis. Not only this, he showed how low doses of TP suppressed pituitary gonadotropic bioactivity, whereas higher doses supported spermatogenesis directly. The latter was based on his observation that implantation of pellets containing different doses of testosterone into the rat testis resulted in dose-dependent stimulation of spermatogenesis, but only in the vicinity of the implants.

These early pioneers had no gene probes or purified growth factors—they did not even have radioimmunoassays with which to measure hormone levels; yet they were not much further away from understanding broadly *how* spermatogenesis is regulated than we are now. Why? There is probably no easy answer, but there is one important difference between then and now. Then, the researchers' model was the whole animal, whereas today it is often an isolated cell or cell line. The latter have an important role to play in advancing our understanding, but they should never be our front line. Logic dictates that we first understand how a process works in vivo before we attempt to unravel how it is effected at the cellular or subcellular level. In practice it appears that many researchers work the other way around. We know now that a Sertoli cell isolated from its normal complement of germ cells looks different and functions differently (17); indeed, in many instances the functions of the "normal" Sertoli cell (i.e., in association with its germ cells) are not even detectable when these cells are isolated. The fact that responsiveness to testosterone is one such example (discussed later) serves to highlight the importance of the problem.

The objective of this chapter is not, however, to indulge in scientific chastisement or to lament what could or should have been. My reason for raising these points at the beginning is, first, so that the reader may keep them in mind whilst reading this chapter. Second, my hope is that we may all learn from the scientific shortcomings of the recent past as applied to studying the regulation of spermatogenesis and that, as a consequence, we will change our experimental approaches.

This chapter reviews what is known about the regulation of spermatogenesis and attempts to formulate this into mechanisms and pathways. Wherever possible, I have tried to "judge" the merits of the data and to point out shortcomings (as I see them). My ideas on how FSH and testosterone regulate spermatogenesis are offered as points of focus for further research rather than as a definitive account of the way things work. My hope is that the reader (with stamina) will not come away thinking "so that's how it works" but more "that cannot be right and I've thought of just the way to test it."

SCOPE OF THIS CHAPTER

The primary aim of this chapter is to give an in-depth and wide-ranging review of what is known currently about the hormonal regulation of spermatogenesis in mammals. It is therefore inevitable that the emphasis is very much on the roles of testosterone and FSH in controlling spermatogenesis. Although the process and organization of spermatogenesis are covered, my approach has been to provide only the information the reader requires to understand the key events and phases of this process in different species and at what points regulation is possible or occurs. I have adopted a similar approach with respect to the role of specific factors in the process of spermatogenesis. There is a burgeoning literature on the expression of various genes or gene products in one or more cell types of the seminiferous tubule, but in most instances we cannot even guess at their specific roles, let alone say what part (if any) they might play in the overall process of spermatogenesis. At this stage in our understanding (or lack of it!), I see no point in listing all of this data, and instead I refer the reader to a number of detailed reviews that contain such information (17–25).

I have also not dealt to any extent with events that lie outside of the seminiferous tubule. In particular, I have not discussed the intimate and closely regulated relationship between the seminiferous tubules and the Leydig cells, with the one obvious exception being the effects of testosterone itself on spermatogenesis. This exclusion does not mean that I consider dialogue between the seminiferous tubules and Leydig cells to be unimportant. Indeed, such interactions are at the heart of the normal functioning of the testis, and I urge the reader to keep this firmly in mind. It is really impossible to consider the regulation of spermatogenesis as if it were an autonomous event occurring within the seminiferous tubules. It is the culmination of "building" events during fetal and neonatal life and of activation by the brain during puberty so that, in adulthood, the beautifully organized process of spermatogenesis can occur via a complex series of cell–cell interactions that involves all of the testicular cell types (including the vasculature) all of the time (see refs. 17,26).

It is potentially dangerous to dissect out any part of this process and then discuss it in isolation from its normal environment, though at the practical, experimental level this is what we have spent most of our research effort in doing (and I would argue that this investment has not yielded value for money). We know that there is a multifactorial dialogue between the seminiferous tubules and the neighboring Leydig cells and Leydig precursor cells to regulate their numbers, structure, and function; moreover, we know that this dialogue changes according to events within the seminiferous tubule, e.g., during puberty or after germ cell depletion (reviewed in refs. 17,27). I would therefore urge the committed reader to consult this information also in order that he or she may gain a more accurate impression of the whole picture of normal testicular function.

In the past, the hormonal regulation of spermatogenesis has been discussed in terms of the steps in development that are FSH or testosterone dependent (e.g., 28). I have approached the problem in a different way by considering the stages of the cycle of the seminiferous epithelium (or, as I will term it, the stages of the spermatogenic cycle) at which there is hormonal regulation. Each stage in fact encompasses several different steps in development of the germ cells (see below). My reason for adopting this approach is simply that this appears to be the way in which hormones regulate spermatogenesis. It also has the distinct advantage that it forces the reader to consider spermatogenesis as a whole, not as a series of steps that can be viewed in isolation from one another. It is becoming increasingly evident that the function of a Sertoli cell at a particular stage of the spermatogenic cycle is determined by its complement of germ cells (17–19). As the various germ cell classes are removed, the functions of the Sertoli cell change, and this appears to be equally true for hormone-dependent regulatory events, as this chapter will demonstrate.

It is therefore by no means certain that the effects of FSH or testosterone on the Sertoli cell to regulate, for example, spermatogonial replication will be the same when just Sertoli cells and spermatogonia are present as they will be when a full complement of other germ cell classes is also present. Indeed, the available information suggests that puberty is very much a "learning" process for the Sertoli cell as its expanding germ cell population programs its functions in an increasingly efficient way (see refs. 17,29). In addition, the germ cell type that regulates specific functions of the Sertoli cell may also change during puberty as the vanguard of "new" germ cell types appears (see refs. 17,20–22,30). I mention these facts at this stage in my review to highlight that what regulates spermatogenesis in the normally functioning adult testis may not be the same as during puberty or during the reinitiation of spermatogenesis after its regression. The emphasis of this chapter is on delineating the regulation of spermatogenesis in the fully developed, normally functioning testis, as I consider that our priority is to understand these events before we attempt to define how they change in pathological situations.

The vast majority of available information on the organization and regulation of spermatogenesis derives from studies in the laboratory rat. From necessity, I have therefore built this chapter around what is known for the rat. I have, however, discussed in detail how this information relates to other species, giving particular emphasis to man. The process of spermatogenesis is remarkably similar between different mammals (even between different vertebrate classes) (31,32), and it is highly likely that many of the key regulatory events are conserved between species. Certainly, we know that testosterone is the primary driving force for spermatogenesis in the adult testis of all mammals for which we have information (see below). Nevertheless, it must be kept firmly in mind that the regulatory events described for the rat may not be applicable in a wholesale fashion to man or other mammals. Indeed, it is certain that there will be differences in the "detail" of regulatory events as has been described elsewhere in this book for other reproductive control systems.

The other factors I have used to focus this chapter are the seemingly never-ending arguments about (a) what is the normal level of testosterone in the testis, and how much of this level is needed for the support of full spermatogenesis (33–35), and (b) is FSH essential for spermatogenesis in the adult, and does this vary from species to species (36)? These are old, and some would say extremely boring, arguments that have echoed down the years and appear to have defied a widely accepted explanation. My hope is that by considering the various aspects of each argument within the context of this in-depth review, I will at least provide a common point on which future research can focus even if I do not succeed in finally resolving the arguments to everybody's satisfaction.

ORGANIZATION OF SPERMATOGENESIS

The general organization of spermatogenesis is essentially the same in all mammals and can be divided into phases of development through which all germ cells pass sequentially over time (Fig. 1). The initial phase is the proliferative or spermatogonial phase during which the large numbers of spermatozoa produced by most mammals (41) are determined. An initial division of stem-cell spermatogonia (termed A_o in the rat and A_d in man) gives rise to two daughter cells, one of which then enters the process of spermatogenesis while the other remains as a stem cell. There are then further sequential mitotic divisions of which there are six in the rat (42) and two (37,43) or perhaps more (44) in man (this is discussed more fully below). Each of these mitoses occurs at a precisely timed point of development at a particular stage (Fig. 1), and the final mitotic division of B-spermatogonia gives rise to daughter cells that then enter a lengthy meiotic phase as preleptotene spermatocytes. The latter cells become assimilated into the "adluminal"

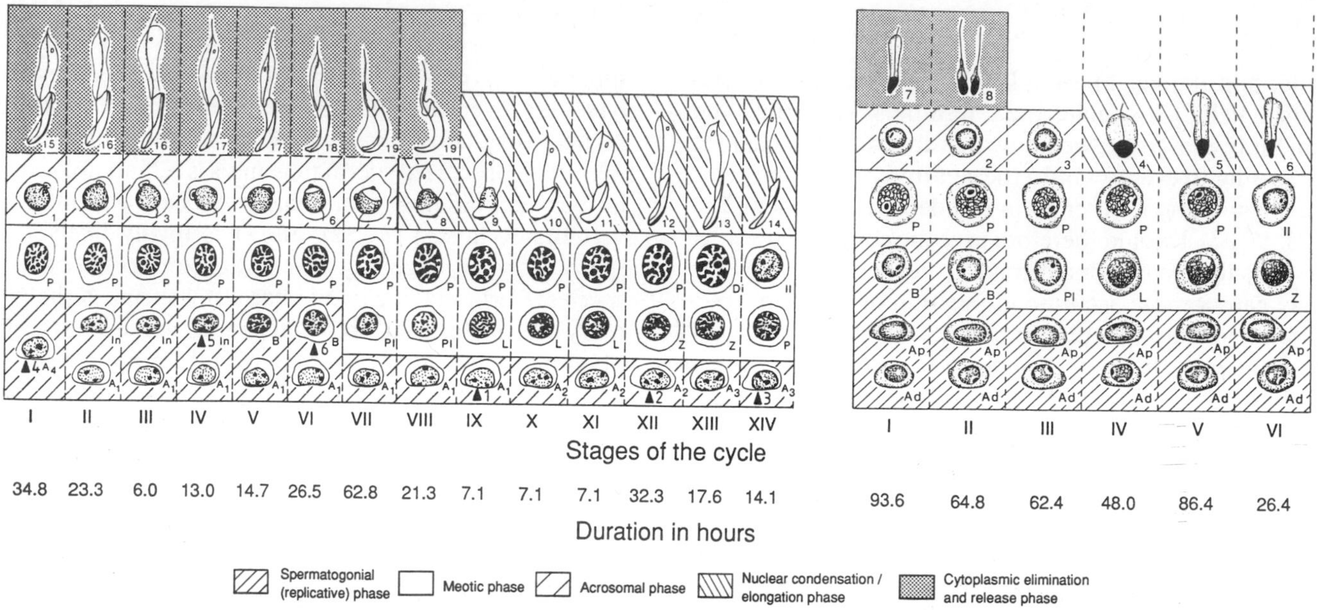

FIG. 1. Germ cell associations at the different stages of the spermatogenic cycle in the rat and man. Each *vertical column* or *stage* describes the fixed complement of germ cells associated with Sertoli cells at that particular stage, with the lumen of the tubule to the top and the basement membrane to the bottom of the diagram. Each stage lasts for a fixed period of time (*bottom*) at the end of which each germ cell type within that stage will have developed into a germ cell characteristic of the following stage; e.g., at the end of 34.8 hours a step 1 spermatid in the rat (stage I) will have developed into a step 2 spermatid characteristic of stage II. When germ cells reach the final stage of the cycle (stage XIV in the rat, stage VI in man), they progress to stage I again; e.g., a secondary spermatocyte in the third layer of germ cells at stage XIV in the rat gives rise to daughter step 1 spermatids at stage I. To follow the development of a single germ cell, scan from left to right, starting at stage I, and move up a row each time you return to stage I after the completion of one passage through the cycle. Although the total duration of the cycle is the sum of the durations of the different stages, the duration of the complete process of spermatogenesis is far longer because each germ cell passes through the cycle $4\frac{1}{2}$ (rat) or $5\frac{1}{2}$ (human) times before its eventual release as a spermatozoon at stage VIII (rat) or stage II (human). The complete process of spermatogenesis can be divided into phases based on the major developmental event(s) that occurs. Thus, there is an initial spermatogonial phase (**A**) (*arrowheads* show when sequential mitoses occur), at the completion of which the B-spermatogonia (**B**) enter the meiotic phase as preleptotene spermatocytes (**Pl**) and then develop through leptotene (**L**), zygotene (**Z**), and pachytene (**P**) primary spermatocyte stages before the final meiotic division (**II**, secondary spermatocyte), during which each spermatocyte gives rise to four haploid round (step **1**) spermatids, which enter the first of three phases of spermiogenesis (acrosomal phase), during which the acrosome develops. Then follows the phase of nuclear condensation and elongation, during which most of the structures of the tail are formed. The final phase of spermatid development involves elimination of remaining cytoplasm and release of the spermatid from the apex of the Sertoli cell (it is called a spermatozoon upon release). The overall process of spermiogenesis, which encompasses these three phases, involves sequential steps of which there are 19 in the rat and 8 in man; hence, the spermatids are numbered 1 to 19 in the rat and 1 to 8 in the human (it is more normal in the human to refer to spermatid development in a different way [37], but this only adds to confusion when comparing across species). *Important points to note:* (a) The division into stages represents a convenient classification, devised by man, based on morphological changes that can be distinguished—it relies mainly on development of the spermatids, especially of their acrosome in the rat (37,38). The number of stages is therefore arbitrary, and the reader should remember that, in reality, there is a continuous gradation between stages (see also Table 1). (b) Because the number of stages that can be distinguished in man is fewer than in the rat, the division of the phases of spermiogenesis is a little more arbitrary than in the rat; e.g., nuclear condensation is initiated late in stage III (in step 3 spermatids) rather than precisely at the beginning of stage IV (in step 4 spermatids) as shown. (c) These pictorial "roadmaps" of spermatogenesis do not illustrate numerical differences in the different germ cell types, which change considerably because of the mitotic and meiotic divisions (see Fig. 2). Nor do they indicate that the position of the elongate spermatids (steps 14–19 in the rat; steps 6–8 in man) is not always around the edge of the lumen but changes according to the stage. (d) Because of the presence of tight junctions between adjacent Sertoli cells (the so-called blood-testis barrier), each stage is also divided vertically (not shown on the diagrams) into basal and adluminal compartments (see Fig. 2). The latter contains all of the germ cells other than spermatogonia, though preleptotene spermatocytes (**Pl**) represent the step at which germ cells pass from the basal to the adluminal compartment (45,46). The spermatogonia (**A** and **B** in rat; **Ad, Ap,** and **B** in man) always form a single layer adjacent to the basement membrane and occupy the basal compartment beneath the Sertoli cells (see Fig. 2). The diagrams above have been adapted from various sources (37–40,44).

compartment of the seminiferous tubule by the formation of tight junctions (inter-Sertoli cell junctions) below them (45,46). All other meiotic and postmeiotic germ cells reside in the adluminal compartment (i.e., sequestered behind the tight junctions), whereas the spermatogonia all reside outside of this barrier in the "basal" compartment (Fig. 2). The germ cells in the adluminal compartment are thus isolated and do not have direct access to nutrients, hormones, etc. derived from the bloodstream and interstitial fluid; they are therefore dependent on the Sertoli cells for providing all such requirements (see ref. 47).

The meiotic phase involves DNA synthesis in preleptotene spermatocytes (48), RNA synthesis in pachytene spermatocytes (especially in mid- to late-stage pachytene spermatocytes, i.e., at stages VII–VIII in the rat, stages III–IV in man) (49–51), and the completion of meiosis (stage XIV in rat; stage VI in man), during which there is a reduction division and a mitotic division such that, theoretically, every pachytene spermatocyte gives rise to four haploid spermatids. However, meiosis is a point in the process of spermatogenesis when degeneration of some of the meiotic germ cells always occurs (52), and, for reasons we do not understand, such degeneration is particularly prevalent in man (discussed below). As there is no further mitotic division, the number of daughter spermatids that emerge from the completion of meiosis represents the number of spermatozoa that will eventually be released from the Sertoli cell assuming that there is no subsequent cell degeneration.

Spermiogenesis is the term used to describe the remarkable process whereby each round spermatid differentiates into a spermatozoon, which is quite different from any other cell type in the body. It has a compact head, which varies in shape between species (see Eddy, Chapter 2, *this volume*), and within which the nuclear DNA is compacted and inactive (53). On the anterior surface of the head is the acrosome, a store of enzymes that will aid the spermatozoon to penetrate the investments of the oocyte and its zona pellucida (see Yanagimachi, Chapter 5, *this volume*). Most of the spermatozoon is made up of a tail containing abundant mitochondria, but otherwise the spermatozoon is remarkable in that it lacks virtually all cytoplasm and thus all cytoplasmic organelles.

For convenience I have separated the process of spermiogenesis into three separate phases according to the major event(s) the spermatid is undergoing (Fig. 1). However, the reader should recognize that the demarcation between these phases is not as sharp as is shown and that initiation and completion of the major morphological changes to the spermatid overlap one another. For exam-

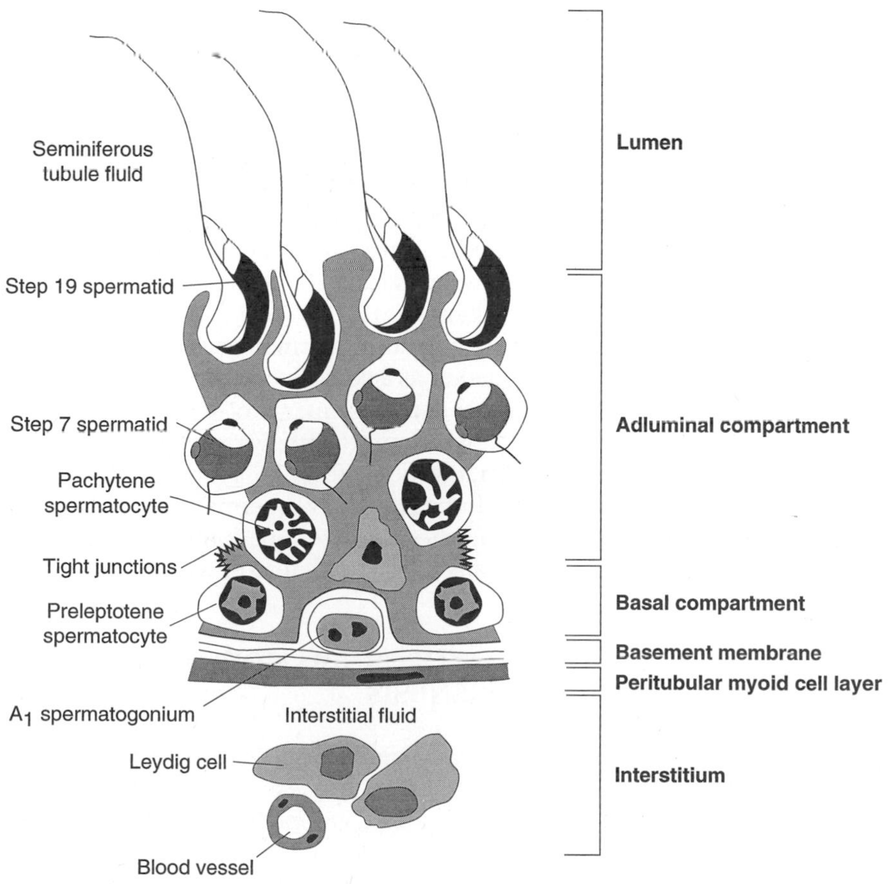

FIG. 2. Schematic two-dimensional illustration of a Sertoli cell and its associated germ cells at stage VII of the spermatogenic cycle in the rat, showing the division of the cell into basal and adluminal compartments. Note that the relative proportions of the different germ cell types are not accurate.

ple, although the acrosomal phase is shown, in the rat, as occurring during spermatid steps 1 to 7 (i.e., during stages I–VII), the acrosome continues to develop and change its shape and position after stage VII; indeed, the 14 stages of the spermatogenic cycle are defined in terms of the acrosomal development of the early spermatids (38).

The second phase of spermatid development involves two main events, elongation of the spermatid and nuclear condensation. During nuclear condensation, histones within the nuclear chromatin are replaced by transition proteins, which are then in turn replaced by protamines (54), thus converting the nucleosome type of chromatin organization into smooth compact chromatin fibers that can be packaged in parallel arrays, i.e., in a condensed form (53). The net result of these changes is to convert a transcriptionally active nucleus into the compact and transcriptionally inactive nucleus characteristic of the spermatozoon (54). In terms of the regulation of spermatogenesis and ongoing spermatid development, the major implication of nuclear condensation is that transcription of genes ceases in the rat in step 8 spermatids (during late step 3 in man). Therefore, all of the mRNAs that code for proteins required during the period of spermiogenesis beyond step 8 must be transcribed in earlier steps (54). As a result, many unusual long-lived mRNAs are made during spermatogenesis, and some may be made as early as midpachytene, when RNA synthesis is maximal (50,54). A simple example involves the genes coding for the transition proteins (TP), which play a role in nuclear condensation. In the rat there are two transition proteins, TP-1 and TP-2, and their mRNAs first appear in step 7 spermatids, and the level of detectable mRNA then becomes maximal during steps 8 to 13 before disappearing (55–57). Polysomal analysis (58), high-resolution in situ hybridization (57), and immunocytochemical localization of the protein products (55) all suggest that the mRNAs for TP-1 and TP-2 are transcribed some time before they are translated and that, prior to translation, they exist in a highly stabilized and inactive form (59), perhaps sequestered in the chromatoid body (57). Although the mRNA for these two proteins first becomes detectable in step 7 spermatids, it is possible that the mRNA is synthesized some time before this step but that it cannot be detected (i.e., hybridized to) because of its method of storage, configuration, etc.

Elongation of the spermatids is initiated at about the same time as nuclear condensation but continues up until step 14 or 15 in the rat. This period is characterized by elongation of the flagellum (a short flagellum is present from step 1) and accumulation of the associated mitochondria; however, little is known about the control of these events. Associated with spermatid elongation there is a progressive reduction in cytoplasmic volume between steps 8 and 14 that is accomplished mainly by the elimination of water (60,61). The latter continues throughout the remaining phase of spermiogenesis, i.e., during spermatid steps 15 to 19, and is thought to be accomplished primarily via specialized structures, tubulobulbar complexes, which form between the Sertoli cell and the head region of the spermatid (62,63); as these structures appear to be present in all mammals so far examined (60,63), it is presumed that the methods used to eliminate spermatid cytoplasm are highly conserved.

The morphologically mature spermatid rids itself of its remaining cytoplasm at the time of its release from the Sertoli cell. This cytoplasm is termed the residual body and is phagocytosed by the Sertoli cell and pulled down through the epithelium to the base of the Sertoli cell, where it is degraded lysosomally (46,64). Historically, residual bodies were suggested as a means by which the released spermatozoa exercised regulatory effects on the Sertoli cell in the rat to time various events such as the first mitosis of A_1 spermatogonia (stage IX), entry of spermatocytes into meiotic prophase, and the changes in spermatids described above (31,65). These possibilities have been reawakened in recent years (20–22) following the demonstration that the elongated spermatids that are about to be released can exert important effects on a range of Sertoli cell functions such as the secretion of seminiferous tubule fluid (66,67), androgen-binding protein (ABP) (68,69), and inhibin (30). Moreover, the addition of residual bodies to isolated Sertoli cells in vitro is able to induce various functional changes in the Sertoli cells, notably increased secretion of interleukin 1 (70).

Having shed its residual cytoplasm the spermatid is released from the apex of the Sertoli cell (at stage VIII in the rat, stage II in man). The mechanism of release is not fully understood but may involve detachment of the tubulobulbar complexes from the head of the spermatid as well as other changes (61,71). Spermiation is one of the most important aspects of spermatogenesis, as it is easily perturbed, whether as a consequence of inadequate hormonal support or as a consequence of exposure to chemicals, heat, etc., which exert an adverse effect on the process of spermatogenesis (61,71). However, it is not known how impairment of spermatogenesis causes problems with sperm release. Spermatids that are not released normally are phagocytosed by the Sertoli cells.

FUNCTIONAL ORGANIZATION OF SPERMATOGENESIS

Why is spermatogenesis organized such that four or five layers of germ cells that are at vastly different stages of their development are grouped into cellular associations or stages? As this organization appears to be conserved among mammals (Table 1), it is clearly a fundamentally important aspect of spermatogenesis. Current thinking (17–19) is that within each stage the Sertoli cells function somewhat differently, their functions changing according to the germ cell complement (i.e., the sum of the different types of germ cells) with which they are associated. As the germ cell complement changes with time (remember that each germ cell is maturing and developing inexorably), so does their feedback to the Sertoli cells, and hence the function of the latter changes in accordance with the requirements of its associated germ cells. This represents a broad, general interpretation of a limited amount of data, but it represents a plausible working hypothesis.

What should be remembered is that it does not mean that every germ cell type present within a stage has the same or similar requirements, as this is clearly not the case. For example, at stage VIII in the rat (Fig. 1) the step 19 spermatids are awaiting release, the step 8 spermatids are just commencing nuclear condensation and elongation, the pachytene spermatocytes are synthesizing RNA, and the preleptotene spermatocytes are synthesizing DNA and are being translocated from the basal to the adluminal compartment. Clearly, no one signal is likely to effect these different changes, and it seems likely that, within the cell association at any one stage, each germ cell type "selfishly" controls aspects of Sertoli cell function that are important for its own development (17). However, it is also likely that the function of the Sertoli cells at any one stage is not determined simply by the sum of the feedback signals from the different germ cell types; e.g., certain functions might be triggered only by the presence of two different germ cell types. What does seem inherently certain is that the functions of the Sertoli cell at any one stage will be compatible with the onward development of each of the associated germ cell types.

It has been established for many years that the structure and function of the Sertoli cells change according to the stage of the spermatogenic cycle (18,19,64,103), and there are undoubtedly other cyclical aspects of Sertoli cell function of which we are currently unaware. It is not my intention to discuss each of the known cyclical changes in the Sertoli cells except for those that are relevant to the roles of FSH and testosterone in regulating spermatogenesis. I will also cover the general principles and implications of cyclical changes in function at the different stages of the cycle (see below). For details that are not covered in these sections, the reader is referred to the reviews cited above.

One of the obstacles to understanding spermatogenesis is the inability to place this thinking on the functional significance of the stages within the overall process of spermatogenesis. I will therefore endeavor to give an explanation by analogy that explains the organization as I see it. Imagine that spermatogenesis is like a car produc-

TABLE 1. *Some of the basic characteristics of the organization and kinetics of spermatogenesis in a range of mammals*

Species	Duration of spermatogenic cycle (days)	Stages of the spermatogenic cycle: Classification[a]	Stages of the spermatogenic cycle: Arrangement	Duration of spermatogenesis (days)	References
Rat	12.5–13.3	14	Segmental	51.6–53.2	38,72–75
Mouse	8.6	12	Segmental	35	76,77
Hamster	8.7–9.0	13	Segmental	35–36	77–79
Rabbit	10.3	8	Segmental	48	80,81
Guinea pig	8.5	12	Segmental	33.8	82,83
Dog	13.6	8	Segmental	54.4	84
Coyote	13.6	8	Segmental	54	85
Blue fox	12	8	Segmental	48	86
Opossum	Not known	12	Segmental	Not known	102
Ram	10.4	8	Segmental	49	78,87
Boar	8.6	8	Segmental	34.4	78,88
Stallion	12.2	8	Segmental	49	78,89,90
Bull	13.5	12	Segmental	54	87,91
Baboon	10.2	12	Helical[b]	57	92–94
M. arctoides	10.5	12	Segmental	44	95
M. fascicularis	10.5	12	Segmental/helical	42	96,97
M. mulatta	10.5	12	Segmental	44	98,99
Man	16	6	Helical	74–76	37,40,100,101

[a] Note that differences between species in the number of stages are arbitrary and reflect the ability of morphologists to identify distinguishable changes in the appearance of cells within a stage rather than an inherent difference in the organization or kinetics of spermatogenesis.

[b] Note that most primates have a segmental arrangement of the stages, whereas man, the olive baboon (93,100,101), and possibly the orang-utang (97) have a helical arrangement. The cynomolgus macaque may exhibit an intermediate pattern in which both segmental and helical arrangements may occur (97).

tion line on which germ cells are "assembled." Instead of one continuous conveyor belt, as occurs on car production lines, spermatogenesis has five (rat) or six (human) parallel conveyor belts that run the length of the factory (i.e., the horizontal rows in Fig. 1); each conveyor belt runs at exactly the same speed. When a germ cell reaches the end of each of these conveyor belts it is transported back to the start of the next conveyor belt, except that the final conveyor belt passes out of the factory, where it releases the finished product, the spermatozoon. Now imagine that within this factory there are workshops that traverse its width and that in the rat there are 14 such workshops (six in man); i.e., each stage of the cycle is equivalent to a workshop. Remember that each of the conveyor belts passes through each of the workshops. Let us consider that, for example, workshop III is the painting workshop. When a car is being manufactured, it is not assembled completely and then spray-painted, because some parts that need to be painted would be inaccessible, and others (e.g., windshield, headlamps) would need to be masked. Therefore, painting is done at several different points of assembly, and it is most convenient (and probably more efficient) if all of this is grouped together in one workshop so as to make the most efficient use of the special machinery and facilities required for spray-painting and to cause minimum disruption to events that are due to occur in workshops both before and after painting. Thus, in spermatogenesis in the rat we have to imagine that the developmental equivalent of spray-painting occurs in workshop III (stage III) and that each of the germ cells on each of the conveyor belts either requires painting as it passes through this workshop or would not be affected adversely by the other germ cell types being painted. It is presumed that evolution has placed these particular germ cells in association at stage III because they have the most similar or most compatible requirements.

The analogy with a car production line is quite a useful way of trying to understand spermatogenesis, as it also makes sense of why each of the conveyor belts is always fully loaded—to ensure that sperm production is maximized by making the most efficient use of limited space. Unfortunately, the analogy does not allow easy incorporation of the fact that the number of germ cells on any one part of the conveyor belt is not constant (as it is with cars) because of multiplication, mainly on the first and second conveyor belts (Fig. 1). However, the reader should remember that when these cell divisions occur, the "daughter" cells all remain connected by cytoplasmic bridges, and this clone of cells then literally goes through the process of spermatogenesis hand in hand until late in spermiogenesis (45). In terms of the analogy, the reader should therefore imagine that one cell starts along the conveyor belt but that its numbers double at each mitosis (Fig. 1) and that the resultant group of interconnected cells then travel together on the conveyor belt to the next workshop.

Now back to reality and one important fact: in spermatogenesis there are no conveyor belts, and germ cells do not move (at least not laterally). Instead, it is time that changes, and with time the germ cells develop (at fixed rates so that the cell associations remain constant) and tell the Sertoli cells to change the workshop from III to IV. However, despite this complication I urge the reader to think in terms of conveyor belts and workshops as we progress through this chapter, as it is probably the most straightforward way we have at present of trying to make sense of the complicated workings of spermatogenesis. It is particularly useful for understanding how we think hormones regulate the process of spermatogenesis, and I will use the car production analogy again to do this (see sections on testosterone and FSH).

DETERMINANTS OF SPERM OUTPUT DURING SPERMATOGENESIS

There are several key factors that determine the number of spermatozoa produced, and modulation of these factors clearly has important implications in terms of the regulation of spermatogenesis. The first, and possibly the least well recognized, determinant of sperm output is the number of Sertoli cells each testis contains.

Regulation of Sertoli Cell Numbers

It is well documented that each Sertoli cell can support only a finite number of germ cells through their development into spermatozoa (104–106); indeed, common sense tells us that this must be the case. The consequence is that the number of Sertoli cells per testis determines the theoretical maximum or ceiling of sperm output. Thus, inhibition of Sertoli cell replication neonatally in rats results in fewer Sertoli cells and hence reduced sperm output and testicular weight in adulthood (107). Moreover, prolongation of the period during which Sertoli cells replicate, achieved by the induction of transient hypothyrodism, results in exactly the opposite change, namely, an increased number of Sertoli cells, increased sperm output, and increased testicular weight (108–113). These changes are not minor—testicular weight and sperm output can be increased by as much as 80%. It is important to emphasize that these experimentally induced changes in Sertoli cell number have no effect on spermatogenesis or on the quality of the spermatozoa produced, just on the numbers of spermatozoa produced.

These changes in Sertoli cell numbers can be induced because Sertoli cell replication in the rat largely ceases at around postnatal day 14 or 15, having commenced on day 19 or 20 of fetal life (114–121). Cessation of Sertoli cell replication occurs at the time of formation of the inter-Sertoli-cell junctions and lumen formation and is associated with various functional (122–124) and morphological (122,125) changes to the Sertoli cells, which together are termed "maturation." Both Sertoli cell replication and their "maturation" appear to be hormonally regulated or at least hormonally modulable effects.

It is clear that, in the rat, FSH is probably the most important regulator of Sertoli cell replication during fetal and neonatal life as judged by the reduction in Sertoli cell numbers induced by suppression of FSH levels (126,127) and the reversal of this effect by the administration of FSH (118,120,121,128–130). Although it is clear from these and other (131) studies that the rate of Sertoli cell replication can be increased by the administration of FSH to neonatal rats, the increase in Sertoli cell number induced by neonatal hypothyroidism is associated with reduced rather than increased FSH levels both prepubertally and in adulthood (132). Instead, neonatal hypothyroidism appears to work by delaying "maturation" of the Sertoli cells and thus prolonging the period of Sertoli cell replication (see Fig. 3). It is not entirely clear why this happens, though it is well established that Sertoli cells from rats of this age possess receptors for triidothyronine (133,134), and Sertoli cells isolated from immature rats that have been hypothyroid since birth show delayed changes in maturation of various aspects of their morphology and function, such as the secretion of estradiol and ABP (135,136). Moreover, addition of triidothyronine to isolated Sertoli cells is able to stimulate various functions typical of the "mature" Sertoli cell such as the secretion of ABP (135,137,138). It seems likely that these results indicate a fundamental interlinking between control of the onset of puberty and thyroid gland function (139). It is unknown whether these observations have relevance to all species, but, in the human, untreated juvenile hypothyroidism is associated with marked and precocious testicular enlargement, precocious puberty, and delayed maturation (140–142), and although it is not known whether Sertoli cell number is increased, these findings are consistent with this having occurred. More recently, a cDNA for a novel thyroid hormone receptor has been isolated from a human testis cDNA library (143). In more general terms, the discovery that thyroid hormone can increase levels of the mRNA for a transmembrane glucose transporter (GLUT 1) and, like FSH (144), can stimulate glucose transport into isolated Sertoli cells from the immature rat (145) perhaps indicates that thyroid hormone simply up-regulates the general metabolic activity of the Sertoli cell, which is surely a prerequisite for the expansion of spermatogenesis.

Thyroid hormone and FSH are probably not the only factors that may modulate Sertoli cell replication. The observation that the growth-hormone-deficient rat has qualitatively normal spermatogenesis but smaller testes (146) could indicate a role for growth hormone in Sertoli cell replication, and evidence from the boar (147) supports this possibility. At the local level, there is good evidence for the rat that β-endorphin produced by the fetal Leydig cells (148) binds to opiate receptors on the Sertoli cells (149) and inhibits their multiplication (150–151a). These findings are of interest because the studies described above for the neonatal hypothyroid rat and for compensatory testicular hypertrophy following neonatal hemicastration all demonstrate that the number of Leydig cells changes in proportion to the number of Sertoli cells, and it is well established that FSH can regulate Leydig cell development via effects on the Sertoli cells (see below and ref. 17). In this context, production of β-endorphin could represent a local feedback mechanism by which the Leydig cells aid in locally determining Sertoli cell numbers. Even more intriguing is the recent demonstration that targeted deletion of the α-inhibin gene in transgenic mice results in a 100% incidence of gonadal (stromal) tumors in pubertal or adult life (152), implying that inhibin derived from the Sertoli cells may exert a negative autocrine effect on Sertoli cell replication. It may therefore be more than coincidence that intratesticular inhibin levels are very high at around the time of Sertoli cell replication in the rat (0–15 days postnatally) and then decline exponentially beyond this time (see "Inhibin," below).

Regulation of Sertoli cell numbers appears to be the main determinant of ultimate testicular size between species (46,105), within strains of the same species (153), and between individuals of the same strain (154). As has been indicated already, Sertoli cell replication in the rat ceases at around day 15, or, if it continues after this time (117), it is of minor significance. A similar time span applies to Sertoli cell replication in the mouse (155,156) and the rabbit (157), whereas in the sheep (158), the boar (147,159), and the bull (154,160), it probably extends to 6 to 10 weeks postnatally. However, the available (though more limited) evidence for cynomolgus monkeys (161) and for man (162) suggests that Sertoli cell replication may continue throughout the prepubertal period (see Fig. 3). Nevertheless, even in these species Sertoli cell replication during the fetal and neonatal period is clearly considerable and, as in the rat, is probably under the predominant control of FSH (162–165). In seasonal breeders, the majority of evidence suggests that Sertoli cell number in the adult remains constant in the breeding and nonbreeding seasons (ram, 166–168; hamster, 169; stallion, 170), though there is evidence to the contrary for the stallion (171,172) and the red deer (173). The limited period during which Sertoli cells multiply in most species explains why unilateral orchidectomy only results in compensatory hypertrophy of the contralateral testis (rat, 128,174; ram, lamb, 175,176; boar, 147,159;

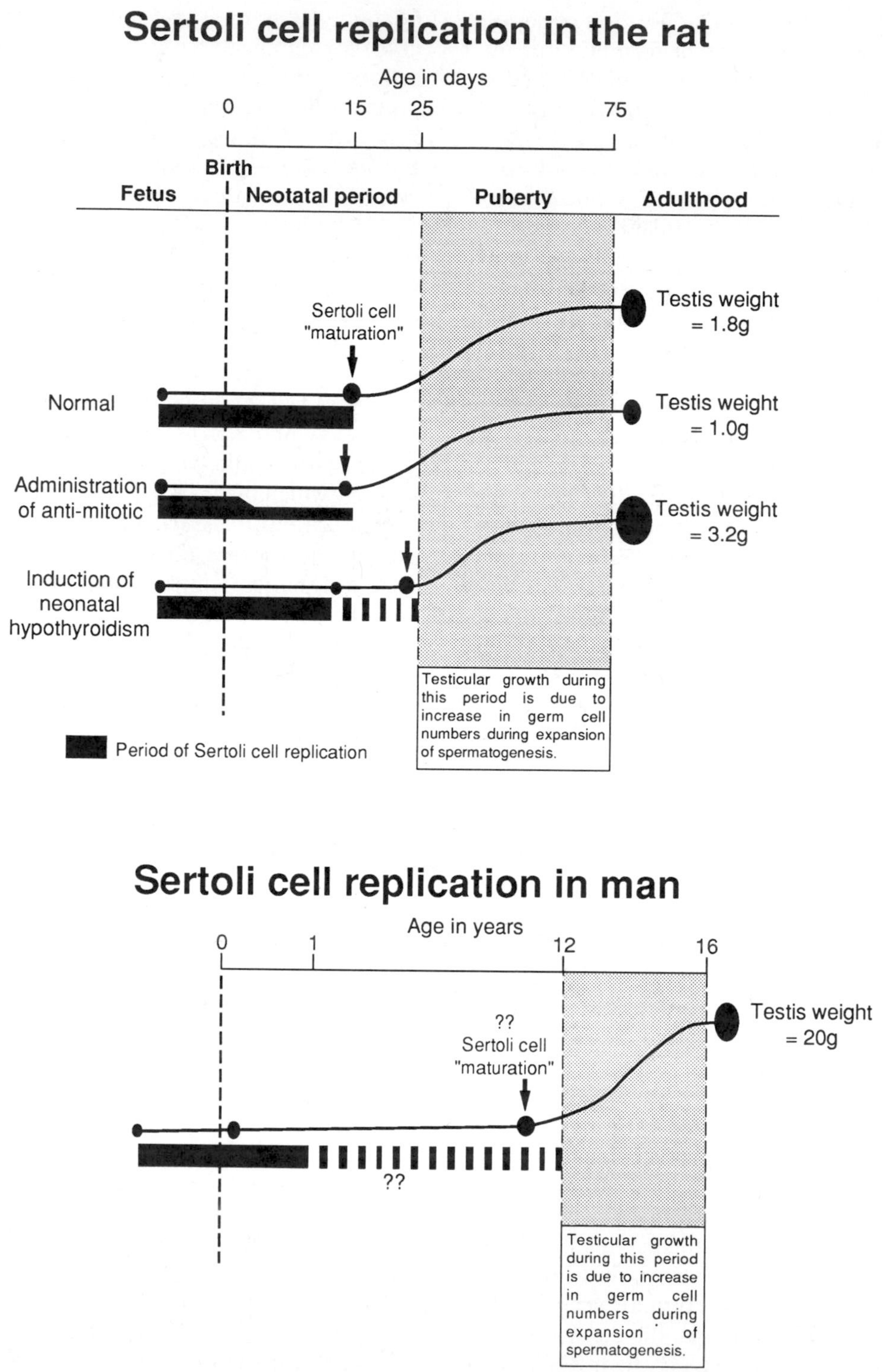

FIG. 3. The timing and duration of the period of Sertoli cell replication in relation to puberty in the rat and man. Also illustrated are the consequences of experimental inhibition of Sertoli cell replication by administration of an antimitotic drug or prolongation of the period of Sertoli cell replication by the induction of neonatal hypothyroidism in rats. Note that although the bulk of the weight of the adult testis is that of germ cells, the number of germ cells per testis (and hence testicular size) is determined by the number of Sertoli cells. There is uncertainty about the duration of Sertoli cell replication in some instances, and this is indicated by the *broken horizontal bar*.

bull, 160) if the orchidectomy is performed during the period of active Sertoli replication (see Fig. 3). In instances when compensatory hypertrophy occurs, it is accompanied by raised blood levels of FSH, and prevention of this increase blocks the compensatory hypertrophy of the remaining testis (178). In species such as man, when the period of Sertoli cell replication may be protracted (162), it is theoretically possible that compensatory hypertrophy of the contralateral testis after hemiorchidectomy could occur throughout this period; although there is some evidence that this does occur (177), it is not known to what extent the compensatory hypertrophy occurs.

Because Sertoli cell number is so important in determining the ultimate "ceiling" of sperm output, the intriguing question is whether variations in Sertoli cell number in man are responsible to any extent for the wide variations in sperm count in normal (or infertile) men and the reported ethnic differences in testicular size (179). Quantification of Sertoli cell numbers in adult men (162,180) has certainly revealed a wide variation (25×10^6 to 900×10^6 per testis), but with a strong positive correlation between Sertoli cell number and sperm production; similar data exist for the bull (154,160). Other evidence derives from hypogonadotropic men who, because of subnormal FSH levels, would be expected to have reduced Sertoli cell numbers. When such men are treated with human chorionic gonadotrophin, its success (in terms of the sperm count achieved) is determined by initial testicular size (181,182), which, in turn, would be expected to be related directly to Sertoli cell number. At the more general level, a persuasive case can be made for the reported drop in sperm counts in men over the past half-century (1) being a consequence of reduced Sertoli cell number (3,4), though there is no direct evidence that this is the case.

The Efficiency of Spermatogenesis

Although Sertoli cell number is an important determinant of the maximum achievable sperm output, another key factor is the efficiency of spermatogenesis. Put more simply, how many germ cells can each Sertoli cell shepherd through development into spermatozoa? As will be clear from Table 2, there appear to be large differences in this figure between species, with man placed firmly at the bottom of the league with the most inefficient spermatogenesis, whether measured simply by the daily sperm production (DSP) per gram of testis (41) or more definitively by the elongate spermatid : Sertoli cell ratio (97,104). Of the nonhuman primates that have been investigated, the rhesus monkey shows vastly superior efficiency of spermatogenesis compared to man, whereas the orang-utang and cynomologus monkey are somewhat intermediate. Of particular interest is that there appears to be considerable variation between individuals in the elongate spermatid : Sertoli cell (ES : SC) ratio in

TABLE 2. *Comparative efficiency of spermatogenesis in a number of mammals using either the elongate spermatid: Sertoli cell ratio or the rate of daily sperm production (DSP) per gram of testis*

	Efficiency of spermatogenesis			
Species	Number of elongate spermatids per Sertoli cell	DSP per gram of testis (10^6/g)	Paired testis weight (g)	Total DSP (10^9/both testes)
Rabbit	12.2 ± 2.0[a]	25	6.4	0.16
Hamster	10.8 ± 1.4	24	3	0.07
Rat	10.3 ± 1.6[b]	24	3.7	0.09
Rhesus monkey	—	23	49	1.1
Boar	—	23	720	16.2
Ram	—	21	500	9.5
Stallion	[11.5 ± 1.0][c]	16	340	5.3
Bull (Charolais)	—	13	775	8.9
Cynomolgus monkey	8.2 ± 3.6[d]	—	—	—
Orang-utang	5.7 ± 2.3[e]	—	—	—
Human	3.9 ± 0.5[f]	4.4	34	0.13[g]

The data in the table have been adapted from several sources (41,97,104).
[a] Another study put the number of round spermatids per Sertoli cell at approximately 10 (80).
[b] Another study gives a figure of 8.4 (183).
[c] Number of round spermatids per Sertoli cell (184).
[d] Other data based on testicular biopsies yielded values of 4.7–6.6 round spermatids or elongate spermatids per Sertoli cell (185,186).
[e] Data are from only one animal.
[f] Other studies in man put the number of round spermatids per Sertoli cell at 2 to 4 (43,187,188).
[g] This is an average figure. It may range from 0.02 to 0.27 × 10^9/day (180).

cynomologus monkeys: of the three animals that have been assessed in two separate studies, the ES : SC ratio was 5.9 (104), 6.4, and 12.5 (97). This variation perhaps gives clues to the cause of the marked differences in spermatogenic efficiency between species, as cynomologus monkeys appear to exhibit a mixture of segmental and helical arrangements of the stages of the spermatogenic cycle (see Figs. 4 and 5) with the helical arrangement associated with inefficiency (97). This thinking would fit well with what is observed in the rhesus monkey and the other species cited, all of which have high efficiency of spermatogenesis associated with a segmental arrangement of the stages of the spermatogenic cycle. In this respect it is of interest that the stallion, which has appreciably less efficient spermatogenesis than many of the animals listed in Table 2, is sometimes cited as having some "irregularities" in the spatial organization of stages (41), perhaps also indicating some mixing of segmental and helical arrangements. The Japanese quail also has a helical arrangement of stages (189), though the efficiency of spermatogenesis is not known.

Based on the above evidence it is tempting to suggest that the helical arrangement of stages is the *cause* of the inefficiency of spermatogenesis in man. From all of the other evidence discussed in this chapter it is clear that what distinguishes one stage from another is not just the differences in morphological appearance but also dramatic differences in function, especially in the secretory function of the Sertoli cells (18,19,190). It is generally accepted that the latter functional changes vary the local milieu of the germ cells according to their requirements (17). Clearly, a long stretch of seminiferous tubule at one stage is likely to maintain a more homogeneous (better?) environment than is a stretch of tubule in which the stages are mixed because of their helical arrangement (see Fig. 4). However, it is equally possible that it is not the helical arrangement of stages that causes the inefficiency of spermatogenesis but rather that inefficiency in spermatogenesis leads to a helical arrangement (97). Based on the available data it is not really possible to say which of these two possible interpretations is more likely, though consideration of other aspects of spermatogenesis in man might just favor the second interpretation. Thus, in man there appear to be only three spermatogonial divisions (there may be more—see ref. 44) as opposed to five or six in the rat (Fig. 1), mouse, hamster, rabbit, bull, ram, rhesus monkey, stumptailed macaque, and cynomologus monkey (see references in Table 1). Therefore one possible reason for the low efficiency of spermatogenesis in man is that the supply of B-spermatogonia ready to enter meiosis may be more limited than in other species (see also below).

Not all preleptotene spermatocytes that enter meiosis complete development into spermatids and are then released as spermatozoa. Some degenerate during meiosis or, more rarely, during spermiogenesis, and the most crit-

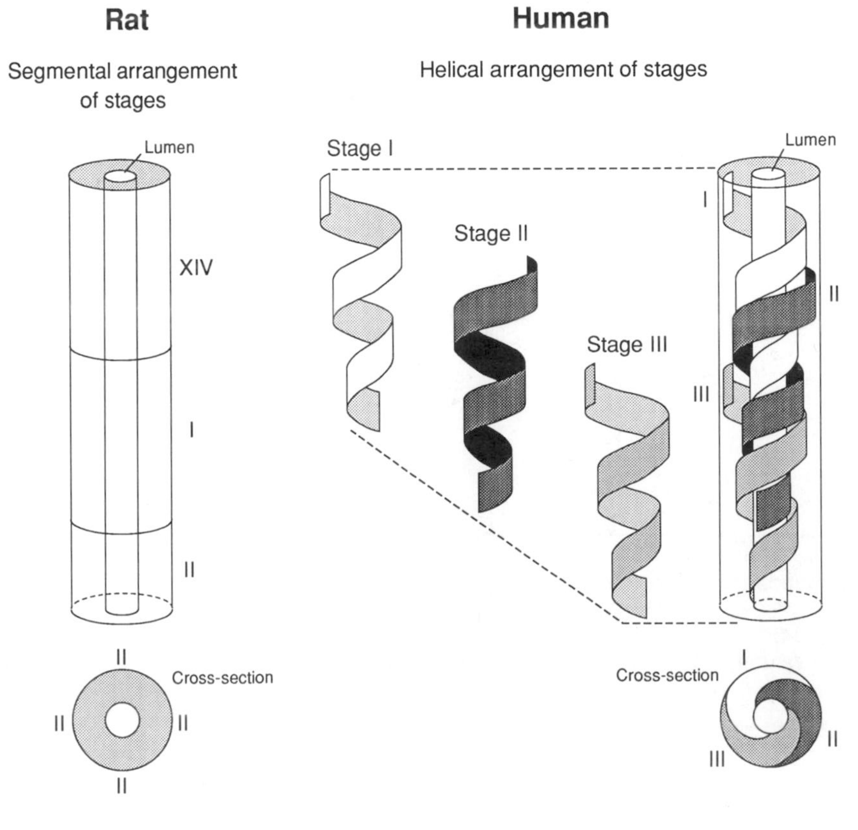

FIG. 4. Diagrammatic illustration of the different spatial organization of the stages of the spermatogenic cycle along a short length of seminiferous tubule in the rat and human. The latter is based on the observations of Schulze and colleagues (100,101).

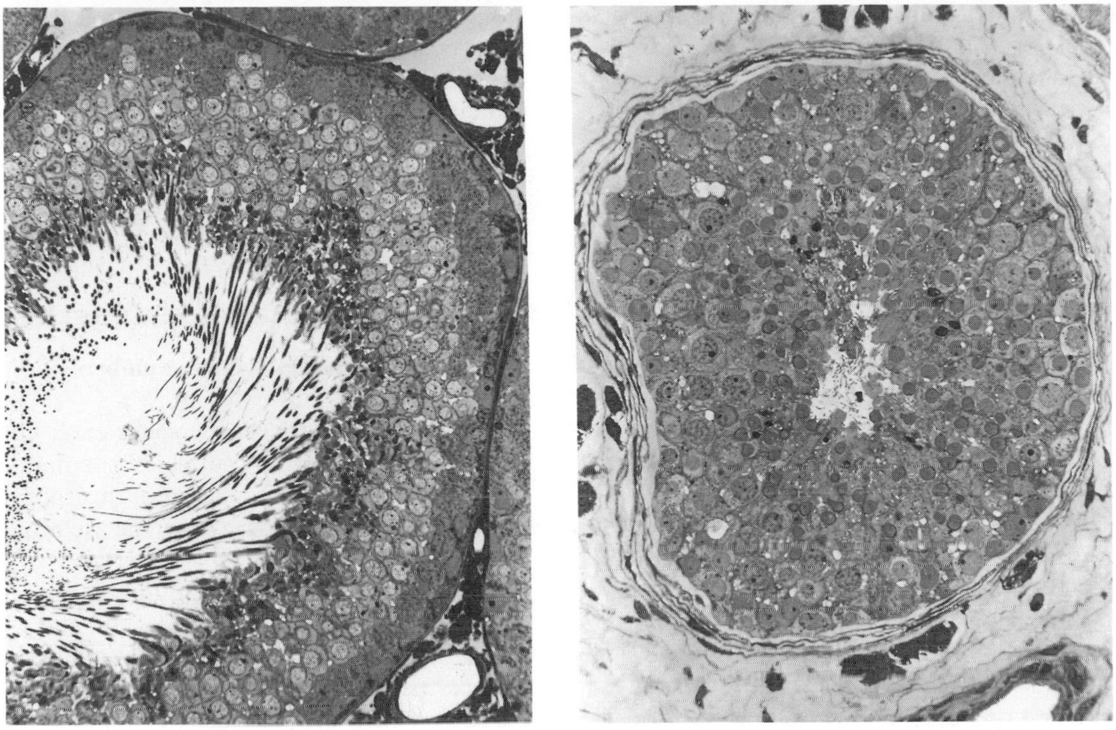

FIG. 5. Photomicrographs of cross sections of a seminiferous tubule from a normal adult rat (**left**) and a normal adult man (**right**). Note that the epithelium of the rat tubule cross section is homogeneous (all at late stage VII/early stage VIII), whereas that for the human contains a mixture of stages. Refer also to Figs. 1 and 4. (Photomicrographs were kindly supplied by Professor Jeffrey Kerr, Monash University.)

ical time for this to happen is during metaphase at the end of meiosis (stage XIV in rat, stage VI in man; see Fig. 1). Germ cell degeneration in metaphase is a feature common to most mammals (52,78). In the rat, such degenerating cells are seen frequently in cross sections of seminiferous tubules at stages XIV and early I of the spermatogenic cycle (29,191,192), though on average there is only one degenerating cell per two stage XIV/I tubules. It is this cell loss during the final stages of meiosis that leads to a reduction in the ratio of spermatids to pachytene spermatocyte below the expected ratio of 4 : 1; i.e., each pachytene spermatocyte that completes meiosis should give rise to four daughter spermatids. In the normal adult rat there is a shortfall of 4% to 6% in this yield (26,29,191), and this shortfall is also very low in the dog (84) and in the ram in the breeding season (166,193). In stark contrast, the calculated shortfall in man is 39% (187,194–198), and it appears to worsen with age (199,200). Interestingly, in the bull the loss of germ cells during the two divisions of meiosis is in excess of 20% (91,201), and, of the nonprimate species listed in Table 2, the bull has the most inefficient spermatogenesis. However, the rabbit, which boasts the most efficient spermatogenesis (Table 2), also appears to have a 24% shortfall in the number of round spermatids resulting from the meiotic divisions, though this may be an overestimate (80).

It is presumed that the degeneration of germ cells during meiosis represents some sort of selection process that prevents aberrant cells (especially those with chromosomal aberrations) from progressing further through spermatogenesis (52). This selection process may not be that effective in man, as it has been suggested that faulty meiotic divisions are one of the causes of the high percentage of morphologically abnormal spermatozoa in the ejaculate of normal (and infertile) men (202). However, it is not known what causes or controls degeneration of meiotic spermatocytes, although one study in rats has shown that active immunization against oxytocin or removal of the Leydig cells (the testicular source of oxytocin in the rat) and replacement of testosterone exogenously results in a three- to fourfold increase in the number of degenerating metaphase spermatocytes at stages XIV–I (191). The physiological significance of this finding is unknown, though recent evidence suggests that oxytocin in the rat testis may somehow alter testosterone metabolism or utilization (203a). As is detailed later in this chapter, testosterone insufficiency can lead to increased germ cell degeneration and less efficient spermatogenesis, so subtle deficiencies in androgen levels or action within the testis are other possible contributory factors.

Germ cell degeneration is not restricted to the maturation divisions during meiosis. It also occurs commonly in spermatogonia during mitotic division and may affect clusters (clones) of cells (52). This explains why, in the adult rat, the incidence of degenerating cells is stage dependent, the stages at which degeneration occurs coinciding mainly with those at which mitotic (or meiotic) divisions occur (192). Clearly, the degeneration of spermatogonia has major potential implications in terms of affecting sperm output as all of the potential progeny from that cell are lost. If a spermatogonium degenerates that would otherwise have undergone a further four or five mitotic divisions, it can be appreciated how large an effect this could have. Even in the rat, the available evidence suggests that cell loss in the spermatogonial stages probably exceeds 75% (42,52). This implies that germ cell degeneration is an integral and important part of normal spermatogenesis. Indeed, as all of the available evidence suggests that each Sertoli cell can only shepherd a limited number of germ cells through meiotic and postmeiotic development (Table 2), it might be presumed that, under normal circumstances, the supply of spermatogonia was not a limiting factor; i.e., more than enough B-spermatogonia will always be available to enter meiosis. This proves to be true of some, but not all, species (see below).

Finally, brief mention should be made of germ cell degeneration during phases of spermatogenesis other than meiosis and the spermatogonial phase. In the adult rat, degeneration of spermatids during nuclear condensation can occur (52), although calculations suggest that the rate of cell loss during spermiogenesis must be trivial compared to that which occurs during meiosis (29,191). However, the situation is radically different during puberty, when the first wave of spermatogenesis is developing. During this period in the rat, germ cell degeneration is relatively common and occurs at many different stages, though with a peak at the androgen-dependent stages, VII–VIII (29). It is likely that this apparent inefficiency is related to the "inexperience" of the Sertoli cell in adjusting its functions to the requirements of the new types of germ cells that appear in succession, although there might also be suboptimal hormonal support at this time (29) or inadequate production of seminiferous tubule fluid (see below). Presumably the functions of the Sertoli cell become increasingly better programmed as fewer and fewer germ cells degenerate so that eventually the highly efficient spermatogenesis characteristic of the adult is attained and then subsequently maintained (see below and refs. 17,22,205). The reverse situation occurs during involution of the testis during the nonbreeding season in seasonal animals. In this instance there is widespread degeneration of many different types of germ cells, especially during the initial period of involution (206–208). This presumably reflects a generalized decline in metabolic/nutritional support for the various classes of germ cells by the Sertoli cells as a consequence of the withdrawal of pituitary gonadotropic support and reduced testosterone levels. In those species in which low levels of spermatogenesis may continue during the nonbreeding season, morphological abnormalities in the resultant spermatozoa are commonplace (209). When spermatogenesis is reinitiated in the breeding season, germ cell degeneration declines, and each Sertoli cell is able to support the development of more postmeiotic germ cells than in the nonbreeding season, at least in the stallion (170) and red deer (173).

Regulation of Spermatogonial Numbers

As the number of spermatocytes entering meiosis is clearly dependent on the supply of spermatogonia, it is readily apparent that regulation of this supply is potentially important in determining the yield of spermatozoa. There is still considerable uncertainty about the extent to which spermatogonial numbers are regulated, at what steps this regulation might occur, and what are the regulatory factors involved; there also appear to be differences between rodents and primates (210). Perhaps the biggest difference between rodents and primates is in regulation of the supply of differentiating spermatogonia (see Fig. 6; A_1–A_4, In- and B-spermatogonia for the rat; just B-spermatogonia in the human). In rodents such as the rat, mouse, and hamster the number of early differentiating spermatogonia (A_1, A_2, A_3, A_4) is controlled locally by density-dependent degeneration; i.e., only a fixed number of spermatogonia develop into B-spermatogonia, and the excess cells degenerate (211–213). Essentially what this means is that an excess of A-type spermatogonia are produced, and the surplus degenerate (Fig. 6). Studies in the hamster in which spermatogonial numbers were manipulated experimentally demonstrated that the degree of degeneration of A-spermatogonia was dictated simply by their numerical density (213). Presumably this is one way in which the number of germ cells entering meiosis is tailored to the number that the Sertoli cell can support (see above). There is also some evidence that the early differentiation of A_1-spermatogonia may be hormonally controlled (probably by testosterone) in rodents (28,214) and rams (166).

Regulation of the supply of differentiating spermatogonia in primates, including man, appears to differ from that in rodents in that there is no surplus of cells and thus no density-dependent degeneration (78,95,98,210); this appears to be simply a consequence of a much lower rate of division of the undifferentiated spermatogonia. One result is that, unlike in rodents, the number of B-spermatogonia available to enter meiosis may not be maximal. Indeed, administration of FSH to adult cynomologus (186) or rhesus (215) monkeys is able to increase the number of B-spermatogonia, spermatocytes, and spermatids substantially over the ensuing week or

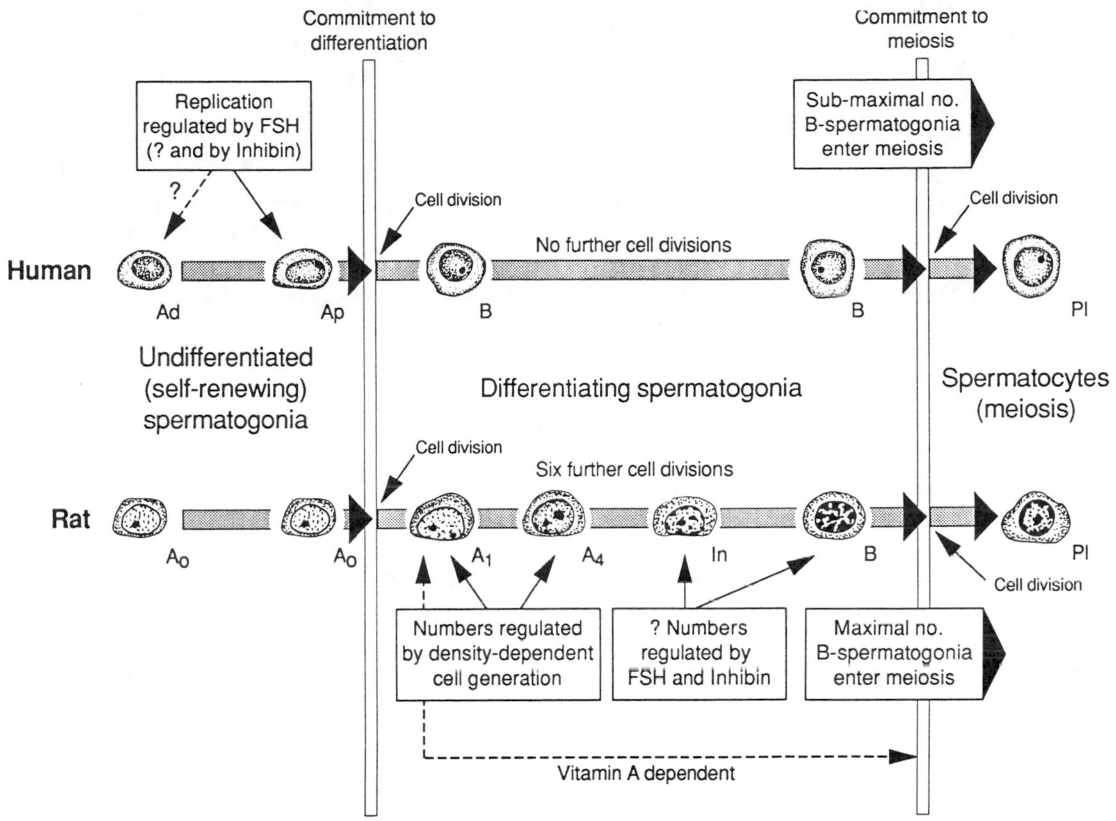

FIG. 6. Regulatory factors involved in the control of spermatogonial replication and differentiation in the human and the rat and the consequences for the number of B-spermatogonia that are available to enter meiosis as preleptotene spermatocytes (Pl). Most nonprimates follow a similar pattern to the rat, whereas most primates follow a similar scheme to the human except that there are usually further divisions of the differentiating spermatogonia as occurs in the rat. Further details are given in the text and references in Table 1. The illustrated scheme is based on that proposed by de Rooij et al. (210).

two of treatment; data for immature rhesus monkeys are indicative of similar effects of FSH (216). This stimulatory effect of FSH is mediated by an increase in numbers of Ap, but not of Ad, spermatogonia (Fig. 6). This finding is of considerable potential importance for a number of reasons. First, it probably explains to a large extent the well-described difference in response of primates and rodents to the withdrawal of FSH (discussed later in this chapter). It probably also explains why FSH administration to intact immature or adult rats is without discernible effect on spermatogenesis, a finding that has always been interpreted as evidence that the rat is stimulated maximally by endogenous FSH (217,218). Second, and of far more clinical significance, the stimulatory effects of FSH on germ cell numbers in monkeys suggest that the number of germ cells entering meiosis in primates (and perhaps especially in man) is actually less than the Sertoli cell can support. If this is true for man, then it implies that FSH administration may be able to improve spermatogenesis in some men, e.g., oligozoospermic men with reduced bioactivity of their FSH in blood (218a). There is some evidence that administration of clomiphene citrate to normal men (to increase FSH and LH levels) can increase sperm output in some men at some doses (e.g., ref. 219), but clinical use of this drug in infertile men has not been successful (220). However, there is one recent report showing that administration of recombinant human FSH to subfertile men is able to increase the fertilizing ability of their spermatozoa during in vitro fertilization, although the FSH treatment did not alter sperm counts (221). This could have been because the treatment did not extend beyond 3 months, thus giving insufficient time for an effect of FSH on spermatogonial stem cell renewal to become manifest as a change in sperm output (4 to 5 months of treatment is probably required). Alternatively, the observed effect may result from FSH-induced changes in Sertoli cell function (described later) rather than effects on spermatogonial replication, as there is other evidence in normal men that suppression of blood FSH to very low levels does not result in much, if any, decrease in sperm counts provided that adequate levels of testosterone are maintained by hCG administration (222); nor do low FSH levels prevent reinitiation of spermatogenesis by hCG in normal adult men (223). Furthermore, during aging in man there is a reduction in the number of Ap spermatogonia (224) despite the generally increased FSH levels.

Although adult rodents and primates may differ in their spermatogonial response to FSH, it appears that during puberty or after recovery of spermatogenesis following its regression, FSH may play a role also in rodents either in regulating the replication of differentiated spermatogonia or in reducing the number of these cells that degenerate (29,225–228). The reported effects of hypophysectomy in reducing the numbers of differentiated spermatogonia in the rat (229) and the ram (230) are also consistent with this view. Data from seasonally breeding species also suggest that spermatogonial numbers are reduced when gonadotropin levels fall (208), though it is not possible to identify the lack of FSH as the definitive causal factor. The type of spermatogonia affected in this situation may also differ between species. For example, in the ram the numbers of both nondifferentiating and differentiating spermatogonia are reduced in the nonbreeding season (231), whereas in the red deer only the number of differentiating spermatogonia is reduced, and the number of nondifferentiating spermatogonia is actually increased (173). Reinitiation of spermatogenesis in the breeding season, which is primarily an FSH-driven event (208,232), presumably involves the reversal of these trends as well as improvements in the number of germ cells successfully completing meiosis (233).

Data for the rat suggest that there are other intriguing aspects to the involvement of FSH in possibly regulating the supply of differentiated spermatogonia available to enter meiosis. First, the effects of FSH on the Sertoli cell in the adult testis are stage dependent. Levels of the FSH receptor (234) and its mRNA (235) are highest at stages XIV and I (the time of division of A_3- and A_4-spermatogonia, respectively), but more importantly the response of the Sertoli cell to FSH stimulation, in terms of cAMP production, is dramatically higher at stages XIV–VI and at a nadir at stages VII–VIII (19,236,237). Stages XIV–VI encompass the last four mitotic divisions of the differentiating spermatogonia (see Fig. 1) leading up to their entry into meiosis at stage VII. These changes in FSH responsiveness of the Sertoli cell are consistent with the suggested role of FSH in regulating the survival of differentiated spermatogonia. However, FSH is probably not the only factor that modulates the number of spermatogonia about to enter meiosis (238), and it must also be remembered that adult rat seminiferous tubules respond very poorly to FSH stimulation (239,240); this implies that at least the FSH-driven processes that regulate the division and survival of differentiating spermatogonia in the normal adult rat are maximally stimulated. When these processes go wrong, sterility results (241).

Inhibin

Usually where there is a stimulatory biological process there is also a counterbalancing inhibitory process, and data are beginning to emerge to suggest that the Sertoli-cell-secreted protein inhibin might negatively regulate the supply of differentiating spermatogonia (242). Inhibin is a glycoprotein heterodimer consisting of an α and one of two types of β subunit covalently linked (see Vale, Chapter 17, *this volume*) and is secreted by the Sertoli cell under FSH stimulation; it can, under certain circumstances (e.g., in early puberty), negatively regulate the secretion of FSH from the pituitary gland in the male (243,244). In the adult, it appears that testosterone is more important in this respect. Inhibin is secreted bidirectionally by the Sertoli cell, i.e., into seminiferous tubule fluid (STF) and, from the base of the Sertoli cell, into testicular interstitial fluid (IF) (17,245). The latter would have access to the spermatogonia that lie underneath the base of the Sertoli cell, whereas that secreted apically into STF would not. An intriguing finding, therefore, is that the secretion of inhibin via the base of the Sertoli cell into IF declines exponentially during puberty and testicular growth in the rat (246–248) (Fig. 7), i.e.,

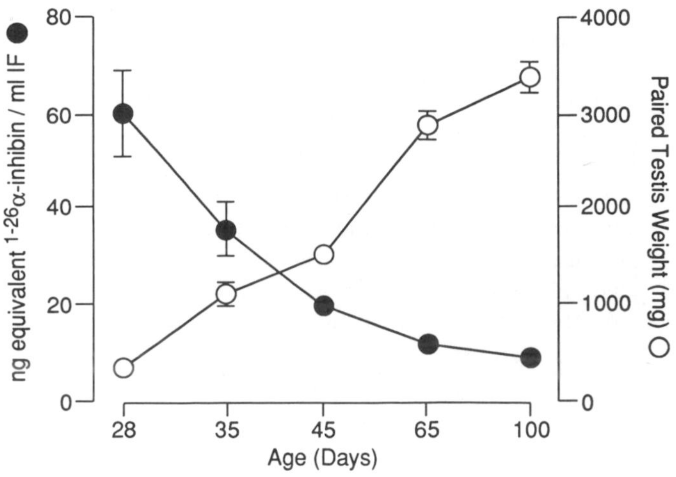

FIG. 7. Maturational decrease in the levels of inhibin in testicular interstitial fluid in the rat and its relationship to the expansion of spermatogenesis as indicated by testicular weight. (Reproduced with permission from Maddocks and Sharpe, ref. 248.)

during the period when there is a progressive expansion in germ cell numbers and in the efficiency of spermatogenesis (29) (see also below). Indeed, the inhibin destined for the pituitary gland derives predominantly from that secreted into STF in the adult (but not in the immature) rat (248–250), implying that this function (i.e., feedback regulation of FSH) is kept separate from any local effects on spermatogonia.

When semipurified inhibin or inhibin-containing preparations were injected intratesticularly into mice or hamsters, they reduced substantially the numbers of differentiated spermatogonia entering meiosis (242). As these studies involved the injection of very high levels of inhibin, the physiological significance of these findings might be a little in doubt, although the levels of inhibin in IF in the rat are quite high (Fig. 7), and inhibin-A appears to bind to spermatogonia as well as to other germ cell types (251). The α subunit of inhibin, or extended forms of the α-subunit, can also be secreted by Leydig cells into IF in both the rat (252,253) and man (254), but it is unknown whether this might have an effect on spermatogonia; it does not seem to contribute appreciably to the "inhibin" levels in IF in the adult rat (255). Support for the possible role of inhibin in antagonizing the stimulatory effects of FSH on the survival of differentiating spermatogonia comes from analysis of the stage-dependent expression of the mRNA for the α subunit (256,257). As only the Sertoli cell appears to make the β subunits of inhibin in the adult rat testis (258,259), it appears that only the Sertoli cell can produce bioactive, heterodimeric inhibin. Therefore, in the absence of any evidence (as yet) for effects of free α subunit on spermatogonial numbers, the present conclusion would be that, via FSH and inhibin, the Sertoli cell in the adult rodent may regulate the numbers of B-spermatogonia available for entry into meiosis (Fig. 6). This modulatory pathway may be of less significance in man and primates, as they appear to regulate the supply of B-spermatogonia in a rather different way from rodents and ungulates (Fig. 6) though perhaps inhibin will prove to be a negative regulator of stem cell renewal in primates.

Finally, a piece of speculation relating to inhibin. Secretion of bioactive inhibin by seminiferous tubules in the adult rat is modulated by the most mature germ cell types, the elongate spermatids (30). When these cells are depleted experimentally from the seminiferous epithelium, FSH levels in blood increase (30,66,68,69,260) as the levels of inhibin in blood decrease (30). Could this represent a long-term (i.e., the duration of spermatogenesis) mechanism by which the numbers of spermatozoa about to be released regulate the number of differentiated spermatogonia entering meiosis? The need for such a mechanism seems considerable. Moreover, this would have general application to rodents and primates, as the net result of reduced inhibin levels in blood would be an increase in blood FSH levels, which then increased the number of differentiated spermatogonia by either modulating stem cell multiplication (primates) or the survival of differentiating spermatogonia (other species).

The critical factor determining the supply of germ cells in man is the number of undifferentiated or self-renewing (Ap) stem spermatogonia, as the progeny of these cells will only undergo two further divisions before entry into meiosis, compared to six further cell divisions in most other species including the rat, mouse, hamster, ram, and stallion (Fig. 6; Table 2). In nonhuman primates, the difference from these other species is not so great as the B-type spermatogonia undergo replication (typically four mitotic divisions) in addition to the cell division leading to their formation (Ap → B; Fig. 6). Therefore, although sperm output in primates as a group may be more dependent than that in nonprimate species on the replication of stem cell spermatogonia, man appears particularly dependent because of the paucity of subsequent mitoses that these cells will undergo before entry into meiosis (Fig. 6). Considering as well the inefficiency of the meiotic and postmeiotic steps of spermatogenesis in man, it is perhaps not surprising that our daily sperm output is only marginally higher than that in the rat despite having eightfold larger testes (Table 2).

Replication of the undifferentiated spermatogonia is generally reckoned to be Sertoli cell modulated irrespective of whether this is FSH stimulable or not (210). Unfortunately, we have little idea of the factors involved in these steps or indeed the factors involved in either triggering or allowing the subsequent mitoses of the differentiating spermatogonia. This is not to imply that there is any shortage of candidates because, in addition to inhibin, which has already been discussed, virtually every known growth or transforming factor or oncogene product has been identified as being present in one or more cell types of the testis (24,25,124,261,262). Unfortunately, there is little information that permits any of these growth factors to be assigned particular roles in spermatogonial replication. I will just consider four factors in detail, as on present evidence they appear to be the most promising in terms of the regulation of spermatogonial development.

Vitamin A

It has been established for many years that adequate dietary intake of vitamin A is essential for normal spermatogenesis (263), and depletion of vitamin A in adult rats leads to the failure of spermatogenesis and disappearance from the seminiferous epithelium of all germ cell types except for A_0 (stem) spermatogonia, A_1 (differentiating) spermatogonia, and a few preleptotene spermatocytes (264–268); the spermatogonial types A_2, A_3, A_4, In, and B are completely absent (see Figs. 1 and 6). As no mitoses of the residual A_1 spermatogonia are observed in vitamin A-deficient animals, the presumption is that the A_1 spermatogonia are arrested at stage VIII of the spermatogenic cycle (Fig. 1) and that vitamin A is essential for the first division of the differentiating spermatogonia at stage IX ($A_1 \rightarrow A_2$) and perhaps for the subsequent further mitoses of the A- and B-type spermatogonia (266–268). When vitamin-A-deficient rats or mice are then supplemented with retinol, the remaining A_1 spermatogonia divide synchronously, and spermatogenesis is reinitiated from these cells (not from the few preleptotene spermatocytes) (75,266,269–273). The most remarkable feature of this reinitiation is that all of the seminiferous tubules begin redevelopment at more or less the same time with the result that the testis contains seminiferous tubules only at three or four stages of the spermatogenic cycle rather than 14 as normal. This consequence has been exploited for study of the role of stage-dependent changes in spermatogenesis (e.g., refs. 266,274–276).

What is not clear is whether the effects of vitamin A on spermatogonial division represent a specific effect directly on the spermatogonia (i.e., is vitamin A essential for A_1 spermatogonia to divide) or whether the arrested development of the A_1 spermatogonia is a secondary consequence of altered Sertoli cell function because of the lack of effect of vitamin A on the Sertoli cells (268). The marked degeneration of postmeiotic germ cells that accompanies vitamin A depletion (265,266) probably suggests that impaired Sertoli cell function is an important factor. The biochemistry of vitamin A metabolism and action is fairly complex but involves two intracellular binding proteins, cellular retinol binding protein (CRBP) and cellular retinoic acid binding protein (CRABP), as well as a variety of retinoic acid receptors and related (retinoid-X) receptors (268); this is a subject that is still evolving. CRBP appears to localize exclusively to Sertoli cells, whereas CRABP localizes preferentially to pachytene spermatocytes and spermatids (277,278) and, in lower amounts, probably to spermatogonia (277,279). However, there is no universal agreement about the latter findings (278,280). There is no definitive evidence that spermatogonia contain retinoic acid receptors, though the various subtypes of receptors are otherwise distributed in Sertoli cells and germ cells (268). A fuller account of vitamin A and spermatogenesis can be found in the last cited review.

c-*kit*

This is a proto-oncogene involved in, among other things, hemopoiesis. Mutation in the c-*kit* gene leads to nondevelopment of primordial germ cells in mutant mice (281), but, more interestingly, c-*kit* mRNA is also expressed in spermatogonia postnatally (282,283). Intravenous or intraperitoneal administration of a monoclonal antibody to c-*kit* to adult or prepubertal mice causes depletion of differentiating spermatogonia in the ensuing 36 hours but has no effect on the nondifferentiating spermatogonia or spermatocytes (283). These authors speculate that postnatal expression of c-*kit* is a function of spermatogonial differentiation, and the presumption would be that the ligand for c-*kit* derived from the Sertoli cell. This looks to be the case, as the protein coded for by the *steel* gene has been identified as the ligand for the c-*kit* receptor (see ref. 262), and this gene is expressed in Sertoli cells of the adult mouse (284,285) and *steel* factor can stimulate proliferation of primordial germ cells in vitro (286–289).

Interleukin-1

An interleukin-1 (IL-1)-like factor has been shown to be produced by seminiferous tubules from both the rat (290) and man (291), and the evidence suggests that it probably originated from the Sertoli cells (292). The latter has now been shown definitively, and the factor is probably IL-1α (293). In the rat, secretion of IL-1 by the seminiferous tubules increases during sexual maturation (292), varies according to the stage of the spermatogenic cycle, and appears to correlate with increased DNA synthesis by differentiating spermatogonia at the relevant stages of the spermatogenic cycle (48,294). There is evidence that intratesticular injection of recombinant IL-1α into hypophysectomized rats can induce a small increase in uptake of [^{3}H]thymidine by spermatogonia (295), but the data are not impressive. Of far more interest is the demonstration that phagocytosis of residual bodies or cytoplasm from elongate spermatids, or even the phagocytosis of latex beads, induces secretion of IL-1 by rat Sertoli cells *in vitro* (70). These data have been interpreted (20–22) as evidence that, in the normal spermatogenic cycle of the rat, phagocytosis of the residual bodies at stage VIII and their lysosomal digestion at stage IX trigger production of IL-1, which, in turn, stimulates the first division of the differentiated (type A_1) spermatogonia (see Fig. 1). The secretion of IL-6 by Sertoli cells in response to autocrine effects of IL-1 might also be involved in this cascade (21,296). This linking together of the final (spermatid release) and initial events of spermatogenesis in the rat is very appealing and has already been discussed with respect to inhibin.

Activin

One study (297) has shown that addition of activin-A to cocultures of germ cells and Sertoli cells from immature rats increases DNA synthesis and multiplication of spermatogonia; inhibin-A had no effect. Although there is as yet no evidence that activin plays such a role *in vivo*, this single observation is of interest because activin is a member of the inhibin family of peptides. Activin is a homodimer of the β subunits of inhibin (244) and has considerable homology with the β-transforming growth factors, which are also produced within the seminiferous tubule (124). The Sertoli cell expresses mRNA for the β-subunits of inhibin (256,298) and therefore can make activin (299). However, recent data on localization of mRNA for the activin receptor (298,300a) and studies on the localization (253) or binding of activin-A to isolated germ cells (251) suggest strongly that step-1 to -5 spermatids and pachytene and secondary spermatocytes are the main targets for activin in the adult rat seminiferous tubule.

There is a considerable amount of data, which I have not discussed, that could be interpreted as evidence for a role of this or that growth factor in the regulation of spermatogonial replication and development. I have not discussed these because, at the present time, there are insufficient data to enable anything other than a speculative assessment of their possible roles (24,25,262,274, 300). However, if we are to look for likely regulators of spermatogonial development, then perhaps we should take note of developments in hemopoiesis, a field considerably in advance of spermatogenesis in terms of understanding of the roles of individual growth and differentiation-regulating factors. Already we have evidence, as discussed above, that factors involved in hemopoiesis such as vitamin A, activin, *c-kit*, and IL-1 may be involved in spermatogonial development. Further support comes from preliminary evidence that leukemia inhibitory factor can stimulate proliferation of primordial germ cells *in vitro* (289) and the demonstration that the erythroid transcription factor GATA-1 is transcribed in spermatogonia of the mouse testis (301). The latter factor plays a key role in the regulation of genes in hemopoietic cell lineages. It would not be too much of a surprise if spermatogenesis proved to be a modified version of hemopoiesis with many of the same regulatory pathways and factors involved.

Initiation and Reinitiation of Spermatogenesis

Spermatogenesis is initiated at the time of puberty as a consequence of increased secretion of FSH and, to a lesser extent initially, LH (see Ward, Chapter 32; ref. 302). Before this time, events will already have taken place that prepare the ground for the onset of spermatogenesis, including testicular descent (303), masculinization of the reproductive tract (304), multiplication of Sertoli cells (discussed earlier), and multiplication of the early germ cells (prespermatogonia) (305). Most of these events occur during fetal or early neonatal life and then await puberty. This may not occur for another 11 to 13 years (human) or may have been initiated almost immediately (rat), but in either instance similar events are involved. For many of these we have only a sketchy idea of the precise mechanisms responsible, though there is general agreement that FSH is one of the prime factors. At this time (it may be over many months, as in man) FSH (and perhaps testosterone) stimulate considerable changes in Sertoli cell structure and function, and it is presumably these changes that allow spermatogenesis to be initiated. A detailed, up-to-date review of these changes is available (122), so I will provide only an outline of the important events and how they may be regulated.

Sertoli Cell Barrier and Lumen Formation

Probably one of the earliest events to occur in puberty is the proliferation of spermatogonia, and it is presumed that this is under the control of the Sertoli cell (306); there may also be selective degeneration of germ cells at this time, with just those located around the periphery of the seminiferous cords surviving (307). As the spermatogonia proliferate and differentiate, they approach meiosis, and it is with the approach of the first germ cells to meiosis that the most dramatic structural changes occur. These involve the formation of tight junctions between adjacent Sertoli cells so as to form two compartments (see Fig. 2) and, more or less coincident with this change, the appearance of a lumen, reflecting the secretion of seminiferous tubule fluid (STF) by the Sertoli cell (29,203). Formation of this so-called blood–testis barrier occurs at different ages in different species, depending on the timing of puberty, varying from 15 to 18 days in the rat (203,308) to 24 to 28 weeks in the bull (309,310) and 11 to 14 years in the human (311,312). It is widely accepted that this barrier is essential for the progression of germ cells through meiosis and spermiogenesis, presumably because the adluminal compartment has a substantially different ionic and protein composition than the basal compartment, and it affords a barrier between the "foreign" haploid germ cells and the body's immune system (39,313). However, there are certain situations such as during the seasonal development and recrudescence of spermatogenesis in the mink (314) when these arguments do not fit the facts. At several places in this chapter, it is emphasized how vitally important the production of STF appears to be, presumably because it represents the main route via which nutrients and messages are delivered to the huge mass of germ cells in the adluminal compartment (313).

What controls these initial events? Unfortunately our information on this subject is extremely sketchy, but obviously the key is the changing function of the Sertoli cells. The astute reader will have realized that, in the rat, cessation of Sertoli replication (discussed above) and formation of the inter-Sertoli-cell tight junctions are more or less coincident. Moreover, other dramatic changes happen to the rat Sertoli cell at this time. Its nuclear and cytoplasmic morphology change (122,311,315), it increases considerably in size (122,316), and it down-regulates functions that have been predominant in the fetal/neonatal period such as the secretion of estrogens (317,318) and Müllerian-inhibiting substance (123,319, 320) and up-regulates functions that are going to predominate in the adult testis such as the secretion of STF (203) and androgen-binding protein (240,321,322). All of these changes are collectively termed *maturation* of the Sertoli cells, though it should be remembered that maturation occurs progressively over a period of time but is probably at its most abrupt in early-maturing species such as the rat and mouse (122).

The Switch from FSH to Testosterone Responsiveness

There are also other important changes at this time in what regulates the functions of the Sertoli cell. In species for which information is available (most is from the rat), maturation of the Sertoli cells involves a progressive switch from being mainly FSH-modulated to be mainly testosterone-modulated. This is evident from the age-dependent decline in responsiveness of the Sertoli cell to FSH in terms of the secretion of cAMP, protein, transferrin, estrogen, ABP, inhibin, and STF (68,217,321, 323–336a). Although the blood levels of FSH fall quite markedly during early puberty in the rat (218,247,248, 337), the changing responsiveness of the Sertoli cell is not related directly to this or to any reduction in the number of FSH receptors (240,338). Instead it appears to result from increased activity of cAMP phosphodiesterase activity (240). However, in the adult rat, the effects of FSH and phosphodiesterase activity vary according to the stage of the spermatogenic cycle (19).

The maturational changes in FSH responsiveness of the Sertoli cell are not caused by the fall in blood levels of FSH, and the other obvious causal factor is the expanding population of germ cells. This, indeed, appears to be the case. Addition of mixed germ cells or enriched preparations of pachytene spermatocytes or round spermatids to Sertoli cells in culture reduces responsiveness of the Sertoli cells to FSH in a more or less dose-dependent manner (21,323,326). So does it follow that all of the maturational events in the Sertoli cell described above are simply a consequence of the appearance of an increase in numbers of germ cells? The answer is No. Formation of the inter-Sertoli-cell tight junctions in the rat still occurs in the absence of germ cells (destroyed by X-irradiation in utero), although their formation is delayed until about 30 days of age as opposed to the normal 15 to 18 days of age (217,250). Instead, the available evidence suggests that their formation is at least partly dependent on adequate FSH stimulation (239,339,340,340a), and initiation and completion of the first wave of spermatogenesis are in turn dependent on this event. However, in light of the results discussed in the preceding section, it seems likely that factors other than FSH (e.g., thyroid hormone, growth hormone, testicular opiates) may be involved in maturational changes in the Sertoli cell that are a prerequisite for the expansion of spermatogenesis. Nevertheless, FSH is clearly the major factor in *initiating* expansion of spermatogenesis, and, though the precise pathways involved are not clear, there is a substantial literature describing a multiplicity of effects of FSH on various metabolic aspects of Sertoli cell function (341,342) and on spermatogonial multiplication and/or development as described above. This is also evident from studies in which FSH has been immunoneutralized in vivo in immature rats (125,339). However, care should be taken in interpreting the latter results, as the period of FSH suppression included the first two postnatal weeks, which, in rats, will have impaired Sertoli cell multiplication and thus reduced testicular size and germ cell numbers per testis (see above).

As the responsiveness of the Sertoli cell to FSH declines during early puberty, its responsiveness to testosterone increases, based on its effects on the secretion of STF (332,333,343), ABP (321,335), and androgen-regulated proteins (190,329). These changes may result partly from an increase in the levels of androgen receptor in the Sertoli cells (344,345), which may be induced by FSH (346–349) but also appears to be induced by the presence of particular types of germ cells (329,350). As discussed later in this chapter, the pubertal increase in secretion of ABP (321,322) may also be of importance in switching control of spermatogenesis from FSH to testosterone. This switch in hormone dependence of Sertoli cell function presumably also explains why in the adult rat it appears to be testosterone that is the major regulator of FSH secretion, whereas in the prepubertal rat (up to ~20 days of age) it is inhibin secreted by the Sertoli cells (351,352).

Regulation of Leydig Cell Development by FSH

As a preparation for the "switch" from FSH to testosterone dependence of spermatogenesis, FSH also appears to play an important role in regulating development of the appropriate number of Leydig cells in order that high levels of testosterone can be produced when required (17). This coordinating effect of FSH operates via the Sertoli cell, although there is as yet no definitive evidence of the growth regulatory factors involved (17,27). Data on the effects of FSH on Leydig cell development have come from studies both *in vivo* and *in vitro,* and both show complementary effects.

The most extensive evidence derives from studies involving the administration of FSH to hypophysectomized immature rats (~20–30 days of age). As a consequence of this treatment, testicular weight increases (relative to hypophysectomized controls) reflecting an increase in germ cell numbers. However, this treatment also induces an increase in the number of LH receptors and in the capacity of the testis to secrete testosterone *in vivo* or *in vitro* in response to LH stimulation (218,353–358); similar changes have been observed in isolated Leydig cells from FSH-treated hypophysectomized rats (359,360). More recently, comparable effects of FSH on Leydig cell development and responsiveness have been described in the hypogonadal mouse (361) as well as in hypophysectomized or photoperiod-inhibited hamsters (362). Moreover, the effects of FSH in immature hypophysectomized rats described above have been repeated recently using recombinant FSH (363). It is emphasized that in all of these studies, the FSH treatment did not affect testosterone secretion to any perceptible degree; what it did was to increase the capacity of the Leydig cells, and of the testis as a whole, to respond to LH stimulation. The FSH treatment increases Leydig cell size and number (360,364) and appears to induce the differentiation of Leydig cells that are morphologically (360,365) and functionally (361,366) adult in type. In contrast to these findings, administration of comparable doses of FSH to intact immature rats older than 18 days of age has no detectable effects on the Leydig cells (217,218, 367), presumably indicating that at this time in the rat all FSH-regulated events are activated maximally and/or FSH responsiveness has largely been lost (see above). These experimental findings fit well with the high FSH levels (218,337,351,352) during the period of pubertal increase in Leydig cell numbers in the developing rat (338,368,369).

FSH probably plays a similar role in controlling seasonal development or redevelopment of the Leydig cells in seasonally breeding animals. FSH levels can increase within 3 days of transfer to a stimulatory photoperiod (232,370), and the protracted increase in blood levels of FSH that then ensues precedes the return of full Leydig cell numbers and function in most species that have been studied (166,168,173,208,371–374). However, in the hamster (375,376), though not in the sheep (377), prolactin may also play an important role in regulating seasonal changes in responsiveness of the Leydig cells to LH by altering the number of LH receptors; in nonseasonal rodents such as the rat, prolactin may have similar effects on LH receptor numbers (378).

In the human there is also evidence for a role of FSH in regulating development of the adult Leydig cell population, though it is all indirect. FSH levels increase during early puberty in boys, though LH levels also increase at around the same time (302), and, in cryptorchid boys, testosterone levels both before and after treatment with hCG have been shown to correlate with the basal levels of FSH, not LH (379). In hypophysectomized or hypogonadotropic men (who are endocrinologically prepubertal), pretreatment with human menopausal gonadotropin (which contains FSH and LH bioactivity) before hCG treatment induces Leydig cell differentiation (380) and initiates spermatogenesis (381,382).

In vitro evidence, though more limited, has provided strong support for the *in vivo* observations described above. Culture medium conditioned by Sertoli cells from immature 19-day-old rats is able to stimulate incorporation of [^{3}H]thymidine into purified Leydig cells from both immature and adult rats, though the effect is highest with Leydig cells from 26-day-old rats (383). This is also the age of highest basal DNA synthesis by isolated Leydig cells (383) and by Leydig cells *in vivo* (369,384) and coincides with the period of peak increase in Leydig cell numbers (368,384) and highest FSH levels, as noted above. Production of the Leydig cell mitogenic activity by immature rat Sertoli cells *in vitro* (383) is dependent on the presence of FSH and testosterone in the culture medium; hCG has no effect. Therefore, Sertoli-cell-mediated effects of FSH on Leydig cell replication and also on replication and/or differentiation of Leydig precursor cells (23,360,364) probably regulate the pubertal increase in Leydig cell numbers in the rat. FSH may also control the cellular morphology of these developing Leydig cells. Coculture of Sertoli and Leydig cells from the testes of immature pigs has been shown to increase both the LH-stimulated testosterone response and the volume of smooth endoplasmic reticulum (SER) in the Leydig cells, an effect that is FSH but not LH stimulable (385,386). This is a finding of particular significance because the volume of SER clearly determines the capacity of the Leydig cell to secrete testosterone (387), and several pieces of *in vivo* evidence have shown that the seminiferous tubules are able to regulate the SER content of neighboring Leydig cells (see ref. 17).

The Role of Seminiferous Tubule Fluid

During the period in the rat when Sertoli cell function is transitional between being predominantly FSH regulated (<20 days of age) to being predominantly testosterone regulated (>40 days of age) it appears that either FSH or testosterone may support spermatogenesis. Thus, in rats hypophysectomized at the age of 29 days, administration of either FSH or LH or the two hormones together over the next 3 days is able to maintain normal germ cell numbers and largely (FSH or LH alone) or completely (FSH + LH) prevent the hypophysectomy-induced increase in number of degenerating germ cells (Fig. 8). The latter parameter is probably the most sensitive index of the maintenance of spermatogenesis, and it has already been remarked that a progressive decrease in the incidence of degenerating germ cells is one of the hallmarks of puberty (29). One of

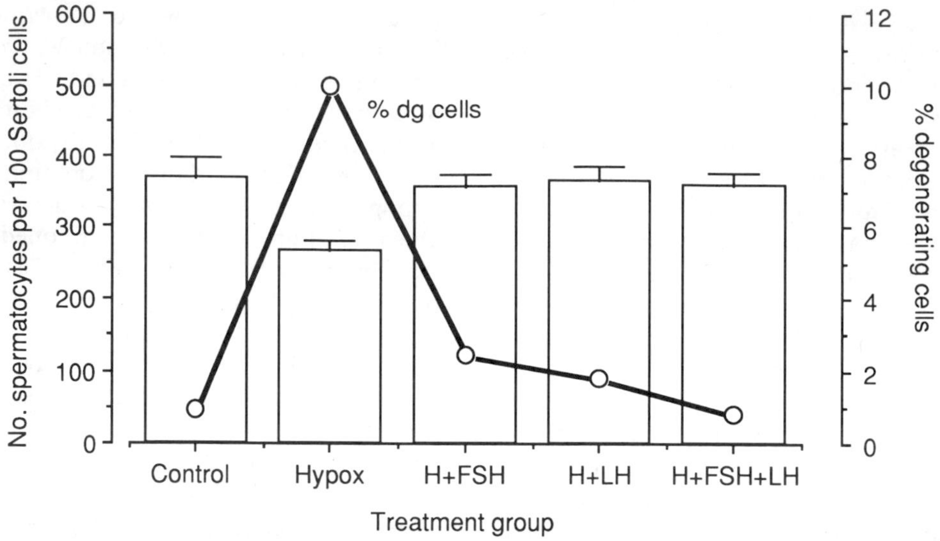

FIG. 8. Effect of hypophysectomy (*Hypox* or *H*) of 29-day-old male rats with or without gonadotropin replacement on the number of spermatocytes (means ± SEM) per 100 Sertoli cells and the percentage of total germ cell numbers that were degenerating (dg) three days later. Gonadotropin treatment (13 mg oLH-S19, 60 mg oFSH-S11) was administered every 12 hours. Note the greater sensitivity of degenerating germ cells compared with spermatocyte numbers as a measure of the degree of maintenance of spermatogenesis. (The diagram is based on data adapted from Russell et al., ref. 29).

the factors responsible for this may be the progressive increase in production of STF, based on lumen size and direct measurement of STF (203,388) (see Fig. 9). Quite clearly the production of STF appears to parallel the increase in germ cell numbers and to show a mirror-image relationship with the proportion of degenerating germ cells (Fig. 9). The production of STF is first detectable at the time of formation of the tight junctions, as manifest by the appearance of a lumen (203), but it seems likely that STF production may be a constitutive feature of the Sertoli cell and may therefore occur before lumen formation—we simply have no method of detecting it. Certainly, part of the reason for the maturational increase in lumen size and STF production is improved efficiency of

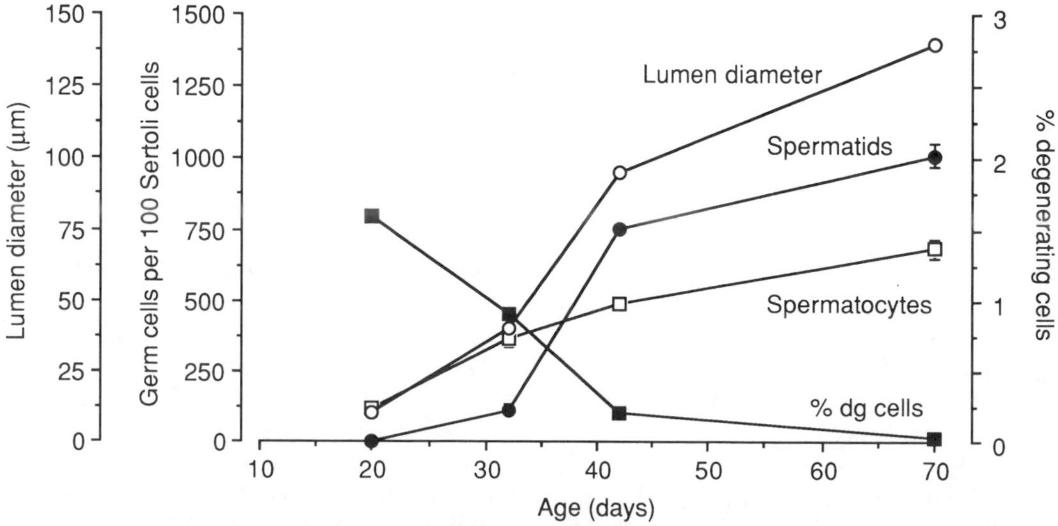

FIG. 9. Relationship between the production of seminiferous tubule fluid (as indicated by lumen diameter) and the increase in numbers of spermatocytes and spermatids (means ± SEM) per 100 Sertoli cells during the expansion of spermatogenesis throughout puberty in the rat. Note the reciprocal relationship between the increase in lumen diameter and the number of degenerating germ cells expressed as a percentage of total germ cell numbers. (The diagram is based on data adapted from a number of studies by Russell et al., refs. 29, 203, and 204.)

the occluding inter-Sertoli-cell tight junctions (245,389); i.e., less STF escapes via the junctions into the interstitium. However, the increasing testosterone levels during puberty (see Plant, Chapter 43, *this volume*) and the appearance of elongate spermatids (66,67) probably also play a part in promoting increased production of STF.

Evidence from seasonal species also suggests that there is a clear relationship between the production of STF and the initiation and expansion of spermatogenesis during the breeding season, based on measurements of rete testis fluid (390), and the reverse is true during "seasonal" regression of the testis induced by exposure of hamsters to an inhibitory photoperiod (391) (Fig. 10). In all of these situations it can of course be argued that STF production is simply reflecting the overall level of activity of the Sertoli cell, and this is probably the case to some extent. Nevertheless, STF production appears to be the first factor to change in many situations, notably after testosterone withdrawal (described later), and, because it probably represents the major route by which all nutrients are delivered to the developing germ cells, it perhaps demands that we focus more of our attention on this underresearched product of the Sertoli cell (392, 393). The fact that it cannot be measured *in vitro* probably explains why it has received relatively little attention.

Hormones and Initiation/Reinitiation of Spermatogenesis

I have emphasized the potential importance of STF production because it probably helps to illustrate some of the overlap between the effects of FSH and testosterone during the initiation and maintenance of spermatogenesis or during the reinitiation of spermatogenesis after its seasonal or experimentally induced regression. In many situations, testosterone alone can induce qualitatively complete spermatogenesis without prior or concomitant exposure to FSH. This has been shown in hypophysectomized (394–397) or GnRH-immunized (398) adult rats and in stalk-sectioned (399) or hypophysectomized adult monkeys (185) in which testicular regression had been allowed to occur over at least 4 weeks. Moreover, in normal adult men with suppressed FSH levels and testicular regression induced over a 9-month period, treatment with hCG induced qualitatively normal spermatogenesis in the presence of minimal FSH levels (223). Similarly, spermatogenesis can be induced by testosterone alone in intact immature monkeys (400) and in prepubertal boys with Leydig cell tumors (401,402) or "familial testotoxicosis" (403–405). Rather surprisingly, testosterone administration to immature rats appears to be unable to induce complete spermatogenesis (227). Bearing in mind the differences between rodents and primates in FSH dependence of spermatogonial multiplication discussed earlier (Fig. 6), these findings on the induction of spermatogenesis appear contradictory. However, there are two important points to note. First, studies involving the administration of testosterone to neonatal rats to induce spermatogenesis invade the period of (FSH-dependent) Sertoli cell replication (0–15 days; see Fig. 3), and this is almost certain to have confounding effects. Second, although complete spermatogenesis can be induced by testosterone in immature monkeys, the testicular weights achieved are only 10% of normal adult levels (400), implying that this

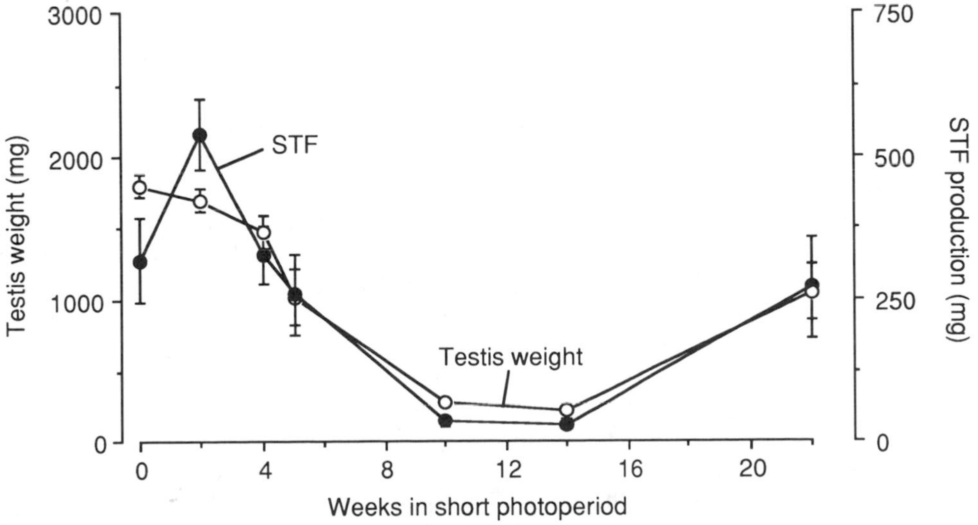

FIG. 10. Relationship between the secretion of seminiferous tubule fluid (STF) and testicular weight during photoperiod-induced testicular regression in the seasonally breeding hamster. STF was measured by the efferent duct ligation method. (Data have been redrawn with permission from Bartke et al., ref. 391.)

is an extremely unphysiological situation and probably also indicating that Sertoli cell number has been reduced.

It therefore seems likely that the ability of testosterone to initiate or reinitiate spermatogenesis in mammals will vary because of a variety of factors that will differ according to age, species, and probably the degree of regression of spermatogenesis. This is not to imply that testosterone does not have a role to play early on in spermatogenesis, as there is reasonable evidence that this may be the case in some species (28,166,193). However, most such data have been obtained under experimental conditions that have no physiological counterpart, and this makes it difficult to assess its relevance. The exception is in the study of the seasonal reinitiation of spermatogenesis in seasonal breeders, though it does not necessarily follow that such findings can be extrapolated to nonseasonal species such as man. It has already been remarked that seasonal mammals show wide variation between species and between strains in the degree of regression of spermatogenesis during the nonbreeding season, and this is partly related to the latitude at which they have evolved or become adapted (208). However, it may also reflect inherent differences in how spermatogonial replication and development are controlled; for example, in the absence of FSH, spermatogonial development in rodents would probably arrest at a later step than in a primate (Fig. 6). As a result, some species (e.g., field mouse, mole, stoat, and red squirrel) show regression of spermatogenesis back to just spermatogonia, other species (e.g., most deer, red fox, weasel, and hare) show severe regression, though with some germ cells still entering (but not completing) meiosis, and still other species (e.g., sheep, badger, hedgehog, wild rabbit) show complete spermatogenesis ("seasonal oligospermia") (208).

Reinitiation of spermatogenesis in a seasonal breeding animal is often likened to seasonal puberty, and for a species that regresses spermatogenesis back to early spermatogonial stages, this is probably true. The only difference is that the number of Sertoli cells has already been fixed, though there are exceptions to this rule (171,173).

Judging by the pattern of change in blood hormone levels it is FSH alone, or together with LH, that reinitiates spermatogenesis in most seasonal species, ranging from the hamster (232,362,406,407) to the ram (166,208). Although testosterone also clearly has an indispensable role in maintaining (and perhaps in initiating) spermatogenesis in seasonal mammals, its role may be somewhat more restricted than in a nonseasonal species. Testosterone also controls reproductive behavior in seasonal animals, and because this behavior is not usually expressed until spermatozoa are available for ejaculation (i.e., spermatogenesis is complete), it may be that the switch from FSH to testosterone dependence of Sertoli cell function may occur later than in a nonseasonal animal such as the laboratory rat. Alternatively, the switch may not be as complete, so that a greater degree of FSH dependence persists in a seasonal than in a nonseasonal species. This might explain, for example, why spermatogenesis is apparently maintained so poorly by very high levels of testosterone in hypophysectomized rams (discussed later).

Overlap in the Roles of FSH and Testosterone

Irrespective of whether a mammal is seasonal or not, perhaps the easiest general concept to advance for the hormonal regulation of spermatogenesis is that FSH and testosterone appear to control many of the same basic metabolic functions of the Sertoli cell that are essential for normal spermatogenesis. Usually during puberty or in the later stages of seasonal development of spermatogenesis there is a switch from FSH to testosterone dependence, perhaps related to changes in the number of androgen receptors, the secretion of ABP, or the appearance of a particular germ cell type. The overlap in functions controlled by FSH and testosterone (LH) probably explains why in many species either hormone alone can maintain qualitatively complete spermatogenesis, though the quantitative extent to which this can be achieved is probably determined by what other, nonoverlapping, roles FSH and testosterone (LH) may have.

If this generalized concept is true, why can an animal not use just FSH or just testosterone to initiate and maintain spermatogenesis? The answer is that two separate controlling systems are required so that developmental and behavioral maturation can be divorced from spermatogenesis during the lengthy process of its initiation and expansion (i.e., FSH-modulated phase) but linked closely to spermatogenesis when it is fully established and mature gametes are available to pass on the animals genes (i.e., testosterone-modulated phase). The case for this dual control system has already been mentioned with regard to seasonally breeding animals, but the need is as great in a nonseasonal animal such as man. If testosterone initiated spermatogenesis in man, then its wide range of peripheral effects would also occur. There would be precocious development of secondary sexual characteristics and genital development, and although these would perhaps be the most incongruous consequence, the premature and final cessation of long bone growth would probably be the most limiting in the long term. There is a wealth of data in the medical literature that demonstrate the devastating impact that premature activation of testosterone secretion can have in boys as a consequence of a range of metabolic or neoplastic disorders (408) (see Coffey, Chapter 25, *this volume*).

Armed with these concepts the reader should be ready to do battle with the data on hormonal regulation of the maintenance of spermatogenesis. And armed the reader probably needs to be, for there have been many battles down the years as to the level of testosterone required to maintain spermatogenesis and whether FSH is or is not required. Indeed, these battles go on. I have tackled the subject with a view to separating the opposing armies of thought and identifying the causes of the disagreement and how these can perhaps be resolved.

HORMONAL REGULATION OF SPERMATOGENESIS

Having dealt with the hormonal effects on the development of Sertoli cell numbers and spermatogenesis, we now move on to consider the role of hormones in the maintenance of spermatogenesis. Again, as in development, it is the same two hormones, FSH and testosterone, that dominate the scene, except that it is testosterone that now has the predominant role. For this reason it will be discussed first. But before I do so, I present a few cautionary words about the animal models that have been used to explore the hormonal regulation of spermatogenesis. Hypophysectomy has been probably the most widely used approach, and everybody admits to the "unknown" consequences for spermatogenesis that result from the removal of pituitary hormones other than the gonadotropins. Not so well appreciated is that, after hypophysectomy, a significant level of Leydig cell testosterone secretion persists, which blurs the picture in studies of testosterone withdrawal and replacement (see below).

This deficit has been overcome by the introduction of a new model system, the ethane dimethane sulfonate (EDS)-treated adult rat. A single intraperitoneal injection of EDS results in destruction of all of the Leydig cells within 36 hours, and these only regenerate some 2 to 6 weeks later if LH and FSH levels are not suppressed (26,409–413). This model has many advantages over the hypophysectomized rat in that the destruction of the Leydig cells is highly selective—or is it? EDS is an alkylating agent and could therefore have effects other than those on the Leydig cells, although it does appear to be relatively nontoxic and to have no direct effect on proliferating germ cells and hemopoiesis (414,415). It certainly has fairly obvious adverse effects on the epydidymis (191,416,417), and, at high levels, it can cause impairment of certain aspects of Sertoli cell function *in vitro* (418) and possibly *in vivo* (419). However, it is equally clear that when testosterone is administered at an appropriately high dose (see below) to EDS-treated rats, then all of the adverse morphological changes to the testis induced by EDS are prevented (except the loss of Leydig cells) (26), and if two successive doses of EDS are administered several days apart, the second dose has no discernible additional effect on testicular morphology (420); i.e., all of the changes observed are caused by the loss of Leydig cells (and testosterone) induced by the first injection of EDS. This implies that the side-effects of EDS are not a major confounding factor, though all who use this compound should not forget that, under particular experimental circumstances, they may be of importance (419).

Irrespective of the model system used, time is the other important factor. Studies of the roles of testosterone and FSH should really cover a lengthy experimental period so that at least the duration of the process of spermatogenesis (see Table 1) is covered. Deficiencies in the support of spermatogenesis that are not obvious after 2 weeks of treatment will become obvious by 8 to 10 weeks. This is particularly true when suboptimal replacement doses of testosterone are administered to hypophysectomized or EDS-treated rats (421–423), as this **delays** (but does not prevent) regression of the seminiferous epithelium and can lead to misinterpretation of the degree of maintenance of spermatogenesis. Indeed, most studies involving FSH administration to hypophysectomized rats have been for only 2 to 4 weeks, usually because of limitations in the supply of FSH, so the data should be viewed with a degree of circumspection.

A final word on models. The vast majority of studies have used the laboratory rat, and although much of these data do appear to be applicable in general terms to most other mammals that have been studied, the reader must keep in mind that there are also differences; e.g., the regulation of spermatogonial development is different from that in primates (see Fig. 6). The latter is really only a difference in detail, but it does have quite major consequences, especially for the human. There may be other such differences of which we are currently unaware.

The Role of Testosterone

There is general agreement that testosterone is essential for the maintenance of normal spermatogenesis and fertility in all male mammals that have been investigated. Despite our certainty on this aspect, there remain important areas of doubt, dispute, and ignorance relating to testosterone action on spermatogenesis. These can be categorized into three principal areas: (1) dispute about whether testosterone alone can maintain ***quantitatively*** normal spermatogenesis, (2) dispute about what level of testosterone is required to maintain maximum (i.e., normal) spermatogenesis and how this figure relates to the levels of testosterone found in the normal testis, and (3) ignorance of how testosterone plays its all-important role in spermatogenesis. Of these three, the last is by far the most important to address, yet it is remarkable that far more research effort has been directed at the first two areas of concern without really advancing our understanding of **how** testosterone supports spermatogenesis. I hope that this review of the literature will finally lay to rest the disputes over "how much testosterone is required for normal spermatogenesis" and point us firmly in the directions we need to go if we are to answer the more important question regarding *how* testosterone works.

The way that I have chosen to do this is to first address the question relating to normal testosterone levels in the testis, as it is this that dictates the accuracy of our estimates of how much testosterone is really needed to support spermatogenesis. Then I will review the main studies in the literature that have administered testosterone to hypophysectomized or intact rats and list these according to the mean level of testosterone that was achieved. This figure can then be compared readily with the normal values, which will have already been discussed, and the degree of maintenance of spermatogenesis assessed by reference to testicular weight. This can then be used as a reference point for studies involving the administration of testosterone to other species including man.

The Level of Testosterone Within the Testis

The reader new to this area may be puzzled as to why there should be problems or disputes relating to determination of testicular testosterone levels. Simple techniques for the collection of testicular interstitial fluid (IF) from rats have been devised (424,425) and applied widely in a range of experimental situations (see references below), and this gives the opportunity to determine the level of testosterone in the fluid that actually bathes the outside of the seminiferous tubules. Such studies have shown that, in untreated controls, testosterone levels in IF are in the range 60 to 400 ng/ml (the levels vary considerably between animals and between studies), which is not dissimilar to the values (150 ng/ml) reported for IF collected by micropuncture from anesthetized rats (426). The problem emerges when we consider what values are reported for the level of testosterone in testicular venous (TV) blood, i.e., samples of blood collected from veins on the surface of the testis and that contain blood that has just perfused through the testicular interstitium. These TV samples should not be confused with samples collected from the spermatic cord (I shall refer to these as spermatic venous blood), because it will become apparent (below) that testosterone levels in these two samples are consistently different. The TV blood collected from the testes of adult rats contains 25 to 100 ng/ml testosterone as determined by a number of different authors using slightly different approaches (e.g., refs. 248,393,422,425,427–433), and similar or higher values are found in other species, with man having particularly high levels (see below).

Although the values for TV levels of testosterone in the rat overlap with those for testicular IF, the important fact is that when IF and TV levels of testosterone are measured in the same animal or from the same testes, the levels of testosterone in IF are consistently and significantly higher than those in TV, the difference usually being of the order of two- to threefold or more (248,422,425,429,432). This could mean that mechanisms exist that maintain higher levels of testosterone in IF and limit its diffusion or transfer into the bloodstream. Certainly, in the rat, androgen-binding protein (ABP) is secreted into IF by the Sertoli cells in fairly high amounts (245), and albumin is present in IF at levels similar to those in serum (430,431,442), and both of these proteins will bind testosterone. If this is the explanation, then it would be expected that a relatively constant gradient of testosterone levels would be maintained from IF to TV blood. This proves to be the case in situations in which the Leydig cells are functioning normally or are stimulated by hCG (248,429,432) but is not the case when Leydig cell steroidogenesis is blocked **acutely** using aminoglutethimide (431,432). In the latter instance, the levels of testosterone in IF and TV blood are exactly comparable (both are lower than normal) (see Fig. 11), yet the levels of ABP and albumin do not change, and it would have been predicted that, if anything, the ratio of testosterone in IF to TV blood would have increased if mechanisms existed to "preserve" intratesticular levels of testosterone.

The alternative explanation for the "discrepancy" between IF and TV levels of testosterone in the control situation is that the levels measured in IF are artifactually high. The first suspicion that this could be the case came from a study in which a push–pull cannula was inserted into the testicular interstitium of anesthetized rats and the IF sampled (430). This method yielded values of around 25 ng/ml in IF which were a little lower than the levels of testosterone found in TV blood from the same animals. There remain doubts about whether this method of sampling IF is absolutely accurate, but a number of different approaches in which IF has been collected by easier drip methods have supported its conclusions. As mentioned above, when the process of steroidogenesis is inhibited acutely by administration of aminoglutethimide, then the IF and TV levels of testosterone are comparable (248,431,432). Similarly, when endogenous levels of testosterone are suppressed because of exogenous testosterone administration (i.e., the majority of testosterone in the blood and in the testis is derived from the subcutaneous injection/implant site), then the levels of testosterone in TV blood and IF become far more comparable (430). Indeed, in instances when testosterone is administered exogenously to rats lacking Leydig cells, the levels of testosterone in IF and **peripheral** venous (PV) blood are comparable (35,191) because testosterone levels in PV blood are the sole determinant of the levels in IF. However, if the Leydig cells are intact, then the levels of testosterone in IF in testosterone-treated rats still tend to be a little higher than in TV

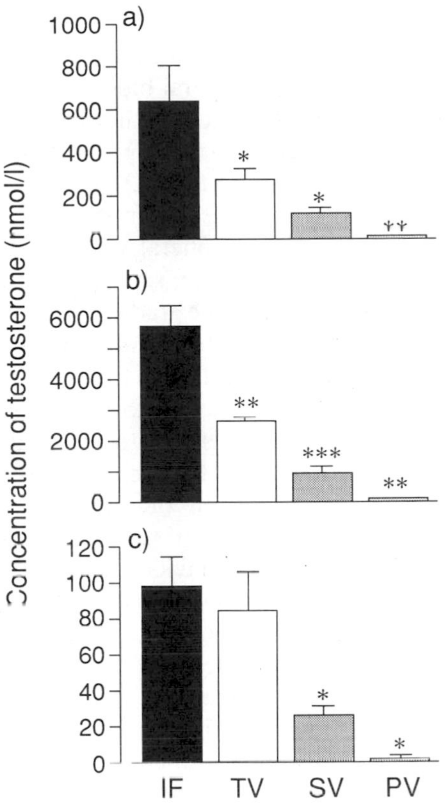

FIG. 11. Levels of testosterone in testicular interstitial fluid (IF) and in testicular venous (TV), spermatic venous (SV), and peripheral venous (PV) blood from (**A**) control rats or rats treated 8 hours previously with (**B**) hCG or (**C**) aminoglutethiomide (administered every 4 hours). Note the difference in scale for each of the graphs. Note also that the difference in testosterone levels between IF and TV samples disappears when Leydig cell steroidogenesis is inhibited by aminoglutethimide, whereas the relative differences in testosterone levels between TV and SV blood and between SV and PV blood remain more or less the same. Values are means ± SEM (n = 5 or 6 per group). *$p < 0.05$, **$p < 0.01$, ***$p < 0.001$ compared with values for the immediately preceding column (paired t test). (Reproduced with permission from Maddocks and Sharpe, ref. 432.)

blood (35,191) though this difference is nowhere near as large as in untreated control rats. What all of these findings demonstrate is that when **active** Leydig cell steroidogenesis is occurring, the relative level of testosterone in IF is higher than that in TV blood, whereas when steroidogenesis is suppressed or the Leydig cells are removed, then the level of testosterone in IF and TV blood are comparable. There is a simple and likely explanation for this difference.

It is an accepted fact that Leydig cells do not store testosterone but rapidly secrete all that is manufactured (444,445). The secreted testosterone first enters IF and may then diffuse (or perhaps be transported) into the seminiferous tubules or into the bloodstream. The amount of testosterone leaving the testis in blood is clearly determined by blood flow (446), and it is obvious that cessation of blood flow will prevent any further testosterone from leaving the testis. When a testis is removed from a rat at autopsy for "drip" collection of IF, its blood supply is severed, and even though the testis may be placed rapidly in ice, any testosterone that is still synthesized and secreted will accumulate in IF and testicular tissue, as there is no route out. As a consequence, if a whole testis is removed rapidly after clamping its blood supply and is frozen immediately in liquid nitrogen and then extracted, it has approximately half the testosterone content of the contralateral testis that is cooled in ice before extraction (35).

However, even this approach to "accurately measuring intratesticular testosterone" has a flaw in that it also homogenizes the Leydig cells and any testosterone they contain. Although Leydig cells do not store testosterone, it is obvious that ongoing steroidogenesis will leave testosterone that was "in transit," trapped in the cell, and extracts of Leydig cells do contain appreciable amounts of testosterone (444,445). Therefore, it is not just studies in which IF has been collected that have this problem but all studies in which intratesticular testosterone has been measured (33). As described below, many of the studies in which testosterone has been administered to hypophysectomized or intact rats in order to assess the level of intratesticular testosterone required for maintenance of spermatogenesis have reportedly maintained various degrees of spermatogenesis with intratesticular levels of testosterone <10% of that in controls. However, the figure of <10% must be viewed with suspicion for the following reasons. In each experiment, the control testes containing active Leydig cells will contain more testosterone and manufacture and secrete more testosterone in the period after severing of the blood supply and freezing/cooling, than will the testes from the experimental group. The latter will consist of either hypophysectomized rats (lacking LH) or intact rats in which LH has been suppressed by exogenous testosterone administration and/or other means (e.g., GnRH immunization); the endogenous Leydig cells are very inactive compared with the controls, and therefore the artifactual accumulation of testosterone in the testis after its isolation will be **proportionately** far less than in the control situation (33).

At this point, the reader may have become irritated by what appears to be a rather detailed dissection of something rather trivial—does it really matter what the intratesticular level of testosterone is? The answer is yes, it does matter if we are to make a rational assessment of the relative importance of testosterone in maintaining spermatogenesis, because very disparate claims have been made by various authors based on studies in which widely different levels of testosterone have been achieved. It is therefore vital to ascertain what the real level of testosterone is within the normal adult testis and, most importantly of all, to identify how this real value can be most accurately determined.

The arguments and interpretation voiced above have been contested (e.g., ref. 422), but the evidence on which this is based is subject to the same flaws as described above (i.e., measurements are made in intact rats with varying, but incomplete, suppression of endogenous Leydig cell function). When LH secretion in adult rats is abolished by hypophysectomy or is suppressed by administration of GnRH agonists or antagonists or exogenous testosterone or antisera to LH, there is the mistaken assumption that testosterone secretion by the Leydig cells is abolished. In fact, though the Leydig cells become atrophic very rapidly after LH suppression (447), they continue to secrete **small** but significant amounts of testosterone even after the prolonged and complete absence of LH. Numerous studies in the literature attest unwittingly to this situation (397,429,443,448). For example, in two separate studies of hypophysectomized adult rats at 21 (429) or 26 (443) days after hypophysectomy, levels of testosterone in IF were reported to be around 3 ng/ml, a value far far lower (<5%) than even the most accurate assessment of "normal." Yet this value of 3 ng/ml is more than ten times higher than the level of testosterone in peripheral blood in the same rats (~0.3 ng/ml) and is similar to the levels found in peripheral blood of normal adult rats. So, the Leydig cells do continue to secrete some testosterone, even in the absence of LH.

The significance of this low level of testosterone secretion within the testis has been highlighted by studies in which the Leydig cells have been destroyed using EDS. Thus, administration of EDS to hypophysectomized adult rats causes major loss of germ cells and more than halves testicular weight (228 mg) 3 weeks later, when compared with hypophysectomized controls (474 mg), an effect that is reversed by testosterone administration (449; see also ref. 450), and comparable changes are observed in GnRH-antagonist-treated rats when an antiandrogen (flutamide) is coadministered (451). In EDS-treated, hypophysectomized, or intact rats the testosterone levels in IF (and blood) are reduced to <0.2 ng/ml within 3 to 4 days of EDS administration (412,443,449), a level that is at least tenfold lower than that found in long-term hypophysectomized rats (429,443).

Convincing though they are, the above arguments cannot completely rule out the possibility that levels of testosterone within IF in the testis are somehow maintained at a level that is higher than that in TV blood. However, if this is the case, then nobody has yet provided any explanation for how this gradient is maintained or has explained why this gradient disappears when Leydig cell steroidogenesis is suppressed acutely or when the Leydig cells are destroyed and the intratesticular levels of testosterone are restored by exogenous administration (see above). It therefore seems prudent to view reported levels of testosterone in whole testes or IF as likely to be overestimates of the level under physiological conditions *in situ*, in which case, how should intratesticular levels of testosterone be assessed, or how can they be inferred from other measurements?

Measurement of the peripheral blood levels of testosterone gives some insight into whether the Leydig cells are functioning normally but really gives little clue as to the likely levels within the testis (433). Consideration of the levels of testosterone in testicular venous (TV), spermatic venous (SV), and peripheral venous (PV) blood from four species including man serves to illustrate this point (Fig. 12). In all species the gradient from TV to PV blood is massive, ranging from about 40-fold in the rat and macaque monkey to 250-fold in man. Perhaps more important is the observation that there is no constant relationship between the levels of testosterone in TV and PV blood (432,433), so the latter cannot be used to infer the level in TV blood. Based on the arguments expounded above, measurement of the levels of testosterone in TV blood probably provides the most accurate measure of testosterone levels within the testis (432,433), so the simple conclusion is that PV blood cannot be used to assess the intratesticular level of testosterone under normal circumstances. An example will serve to emphasize this point. When TV and PV levels of testosterone are evaluated in adult rats in which testicular size is reduced because of absence of germ cells induced by X-irradiation in utero, then the level of testosterone in PV blood is <10% of that in controls, whereas the level in TV blood (and IF) is more than four times higher than that in controls (250). This difference is simply a consequence of the grossly smaller testes in the X-irradiated animals (~300 mg) compared with the controls (~1600 mg), because testicular size largely dictates testicular blood flow (446). Thus, the smaller the testis, the lower is the rate of blood flow, and consequently the higher will be the level of testosterone in blood leaving the testis, assuming that the Leydig cells are functioning normally. Similar discrepancies can be demonstrated in other situations (446) or can be inferred to occur from marked discrepancies between intratesticular and PV levels of testosterone, e.g., after hypophysectomy (429,448), when compared with appropriate controls. Indeed, our own unpublished studies (R. M. Sharpe, S. Maddocks, and T. B. Hargreave, *unpublished data*) of azoospermic men at the time of testicular biopsy again suggest that in men with abnormally small testes, the level of testosterone in TV blood is approximately twice that of the (already) very high level found in controls, i.e., men undergoing vasectomy reversals (433) (see Fig. 12).

It is therefore fairly obvious that, under normal conditions, the PV level of testosterone is not a reliable guide to the intratesticular level of testosterone, and this is especially true for man in whom the gradient from TV to PV blood is so large. Other than PV blood, SV blood is probably the most commonly collected blood sample and in

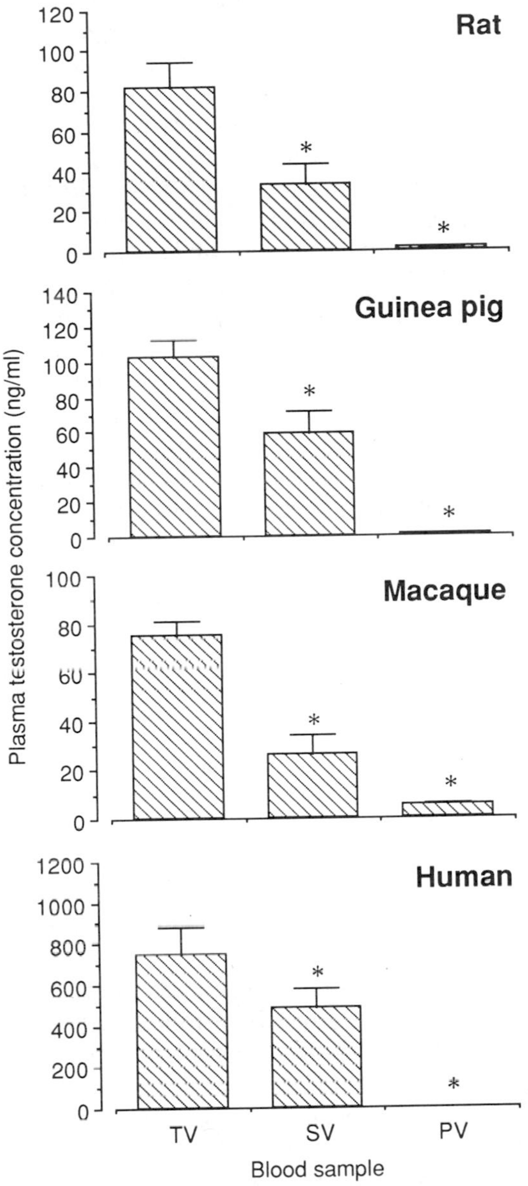

FIG. 12. Comparison of the levels of testosterone in testicular venous (TV), spermatic venous (SV), and peripheral venous (PV) blood in normal adult rats, guinea pigs, stumptailed macaques, and men (means ± SEM, n = 3–10) collected under general anaesthesia. Note the substantial decrease in testosterone levels between TV and SV samples and the even larger decrease following dilution of SV blood in the peripheral circulation (PV). *Asterisks* indicate a significant difference ($p < 0.05$) from the corresponding testosterone level in TV blood. Note the difference in scale on the left for the human samples, which were collected from ten young men undergoing vasectomy reversal; comparable levels have been reported in hypogonadal men (434). The values shown for SV blood from the men in the illustrated figure are similar to the range of values (310–740 ng/ml) reported elsewhere in the literature for normal young men (401,435–437). It should be kept in mind that in both animals (438,439) and man (440), anesthesia can reduce the blood levels of testosterone. On the other hand, it is also possible that general anesthesia could reduce testicular blood flow (441), and this might lead to an artificially high level of testosterone in TV and SV samples (see text). (Data adapted with permission from Maddocks et al., ref. 433.)

the past has been thought to provide a more accurate indication of the intratesticular level of testosterone. In man, the SV level of testosterone is some 60- to 170-fold greater than the level in PV blood (Fig. 12); in the conscious ram the difference is about 30-fold (392,439, 452); and in the rat it is approximately the same (425, 432,433). However, in situations where TV and SV blood have been collected from the same animals/persons the level of testosterone in SV blood is **always** some 50% to 100% lower than in the corresponding sample of TV blood (Figs. 11 and 12). This has been shown to occur in rats, guinea pigs, sheep, pigs, monkeys, and man (433,453). The basis for this consistent decrease in testosterone levels as blood passes from the testis up the spermatic cord is the presence of arteriovenous anastomoses or shunts between the testicular artery and the spermatic veins within the pampiniform plexus (453–456). Approximately 50% to 60% of incoming arterial blood is shunted across these arteriovenous (A-V) anastomoses such that outgoing venous blood is effectively diluted by this arterial blood, and hence the drop in testosterone levels. Transfer of testosterone from outgoing venous blood to incoming arterial blood also does occur (432,441,457), but this accounts for only a tiny proportion of the reduction in testosterone levels that occurs between TV and SV blood. The available evidence suggests that the A-V anastomoses in the spermatic cord may be opened or closed preferentially (453), and this could have significance in clinical conditions such as varicocele. However, one more obvious consequence is that the ratio of the testosterone level in TV : SV blood is unlikely to be constant (it is extremely variable; see ref. 433), and therefore measurement of the testosterone level in SV blood will not provide an **accurate** estimate of the level within the testis.

Based on the above discussion it is likely that measurement of testosterone levels in TV blood provides the most accurate estimate of the **minimum** level present in IF surrounding the tubules, and in the rat these levels range from 25 to 100 ng/ml as detailed above. It could be argued that the levels of testosterone measured in seminiferous tubule fluid (STF), or perhaps in rete testis fluid (RTF), are more appropriate in terms of the regulation of spermatogenesis. Testosterone levels in STF from rats have been measured after collection by micropuncture from anesthetized animals (426,457) or post-mortem by a homogenization method that apparently gives comparable results to micropuncture studies (397,425,458, 459); these methods have yielded values of 80 to 90 and 50 to 62 ng/ml, respectively. In both types of study, the levels of testosterone in RTF (collected by micropuncture after efferent duct ligation) were found to be somewhat lower (33–35 and 18 ng/ml, respectively), and other data in the literature give values of around 20 to 40 ng/ml (439,447). There may be physiological reasons for lower levels of testosterone in RTF than in STF (e.g., utilization of testosterone, very low albumin levels; see refs. 392,393,538). Alternatively, it may be that the problems described above for the potential overestimation of testosterone levels in IF may apply more to STF than to RTF. Curiously, in every study in which IF and STF levels of testosterone have been measured concurrently in adult rats, either by micropuncture or postmortem collection, testosterone levels reported for IF have been some 50% higher than the levels in STF (425,426, 429). This perhaps suggests that testosterone levels measured in STF are more accurate than those reported for IF, and this could perhaps be related to the way in which STF is collected in most of the studies (425).

The adult rat is the animal that has been used most widely to evaluate the role of testosterone in spermatogenesis. Based on the arguments and analysis above, testosterone levels within the normal adult rat testis would be placed somewhere in the region of 25 to 100 ng/ml, with the majority of evidence favoring 25 to 50 ng/ml. These figures should be kept prominently in mind as we move now to review those studies that have sought to establish the minimum level of testosterone required for quantitative maintenance of spermatogenesis in the rat and/or to establish whether testosterone alone can maintain quantitatively normal spermatogenesis. As will become apparent, relatively few of the studies that have attempted to address these questions have restored intratesticular testosterone levels to within the "normal range" identified above.

Effects of Testosterone on Spermatogenesis in Rats

In describing the role of testosterone in spermatogenesis, the main aim of this section is to address the questions raised earlier, namely, can testosterone **alone** maintain quantitatively normal spermatogenesis, and, if so, what level of testosterone is required to achieve this? This task is not straightforward, as a variety of experimental approaches in different species have been tried. The majority of these studies have used the intact or hypophysectomized rat, and it is therefore easiest to consider these results before discussing whether they have general relevance to studies in other species. Some of the studies in rats have been excluded from consideration here because they have involved administration of testosterone for less than 2 weeks, a period that does not enable satisfactory distinction between true maintenance of spermatogenesis and delayed regression (see above). Indeed, studies that have administered testosterone for less than 7 weeks to rats should be viewed circumspectly for the same reasons (see Table 3), as the period of treatment will not have encompassed the duration of the process of spermatogenesis.

Studies in hypophysectomized rats have been distinguished from those using rats with an intact pituitary gland in order that the possible requirements of gonadotropic or nongonadotropic pituitary hormones for the support of spermatogenesis can be highlighted (see also below). Finally, and probably most importantly, I have tried to distill a considerable body of information into something meaningful by tabulating the data (Table 3) and listing them according to the level of testosterone achieved. From the lengthy discussions in the preceding section the reader should appreciate the reasons for organizing the data in this way. It will be evident that I have used the peripheral blood level of testosterone for this purpose and **not** the intratesticular level. There are two main reasons for this. First, many of the studies have not reported intratesticular levels of testosterone, and those that did measured testosterone levels in IF, STF, or whole testis; for the reasons discussed in the preceding section such values may be overestimates of the real testosterone level, and it is also not really possible to equate these different measurements with confidence. Second, because all of the studies quoted in Table 3 administered testosterone by subcutaneous implant or injection, the level of testosterone achieved within the testis will have been determined largely or completely by the level in peripheral blood; the only caveat to this statement is that in the studies in intact or hypophysectomized rats with intact Leydig cells (i.e., not treated with EDS), it is likely that their intratesticular level of testosterone will be a little higher than the value reported for peripheral blood because of continued low-level secretion of testosterone by the Leydig cells. Where such measurements have been made, they all support this contention (422,423, 429,459,462,469,472).

Although I have emphasized earlier that the low-level production of testosterone by atrophic Leydig cells in such circumstance can have considerable biological effects (449), these should be seen in perspective. In studies in which very low levels of testosterone have been administered to rats (e.g., implants of ≤2 cm or injections of 0.1 mg testosterone propionate), residual testosterone production by the Leydig cells will undoubtedly make a significant contribution to intratesticular levels. In contrast, in situations in which very high levels of testosterone have been administered (e.g., >20 cm implants), the contribution from the Leydig cells will probably be proportionately less important. For this reason, and also because, physiologically, intratesticular levels of testosterone are normally high (25–100 ng/ml), I have only included data in Table 3 for the maximum implant size/dose of testosterone administered in each of the cited studies. Where lower doses of testosterone were administered, they maintained testicular weight at a lower level than that shown in Table 3, the exception being when very low doses were administered to intact rats that failed to suppress endogenous gonadotropin and testosterone production (238,467,469–471).

In Table 3, the degree of quantitative maintenance of spermatogenesis has been inferred simply from testicular

TABLE 3. *Compilation of data from the main studies in the literature that have attempted to maintain normal testicular weight (? = quantitative maintenance of spermatogenesis) by administration of testosterone (T) or testosterone derivatives (TP, TC, Te) to hypophysectomized or intact adult rats*[1]

Experimental approach/No.	Method of testosterone administration and dose	Duration of treatment weeks	Serum level of testosterone achieved (ng/ml)	Percentage maintenance of testicular weight	Reference
Hypophysectomized rats					
1	T-implant, 24 cm	7–9	35.8	66%*	(460)
2	T-implant, 20 cm	7	18.0	60%	(343)
3	*T-implant, 22 cm*	*4*	*17.7*	*77%*	*(461)*
4[a]	T-implant, 24 cm	12	14.0[e]	65%	(423)
5	T-implant, 10 cm	13	11.0	57%	(422)
6	T-implant, 10 cm	13	10.3	51%	(462)
7	*Injection, 1 mg TP/day*	*4*	*4.8*	*69%*	*(463)*
8	*T-implant, 1.5 cm*	*2*	*4.0*	*54%*	*(464)*
9	*Injection, 0.2 mg TP/day*	*4*	*[161.9][b]*	*74%*	*(465)*
10	*Injection, 1 mg DHT/day*	*4*	*n·m*	*73%*	*(466)*
Intact rats					
EDS-treated	*Injection, 25 mg Te/3 days*[c]	*3*	*76*	*98%*	*(35)*
EDS-treated	Injection, 10 mg TE/3 days[c]	10	51	99%*	(191)
Untreated	TP-implant, 20 cm	8	46.0	98%	(467)
Untreated	T-implant, 50 cm	8	45.0	82%	(238)
Untreated	T-implant, 20 cm	8	26.0	86%	(467)
GnRH immunized	T-implant, 24 cm	8	24.0[d]	93%	(459)
Untreated	TC-implant, 20 cm	8	20.0	93%	(467)
Untreated	*T-implant, 15 cm*	*4*	*18.3*	*92%*	*(468)*
Untreated	*T-implant, 20 cm*	*7*	*16.5*	*70%*	*(343)*
GnRH antag. treated	*T-implant, 15 cm*	*4*	*13.2*	*94%*	*(468)*
Untreated	T-implant, 40 cm	8	*12.3*[f]	84%	*(469)*
Untreated	T-implant, 12 cm	12	7.8	67%	(470)
Untreated	T-implant, 10 cm	13	7.5	80%	(462)
Untreated	T-implant, 5 cm	10	7.2	60%	(471)
Untreated	*Injection, 0.1 mgTP/g/day*	$5\frac{1}{2}$	*4.0*	*87%*	*(472)*

[a] Delay of 4 days after hypophysectomy before initiation of testosterone treatment.
[b] Value must be erroneous.
[c] Administration by injection every third day.
[d] Testosterone level in seminiferous tubule fluid (STF) not serum; based on other studies by the same authors this value is probably a littler higher than the testosterone level in serum (see footnotes, e, f).
[e] In the same animals, the reported level of testosterone in STF was 24 ng/ml.
[f] In the same animals, the reported level of testosterone in STF was 23 ng/ml.
* Rats were fertile at the end of treatment. TP, testosterone propionate. TC, testosterone cypionate. Te, mixture of long-acting testoterone esters. DHT, 5α-dihydrotestosterone. n.m., not measured.
[1] Note that for each of the studies cited only data for the highest dose of testosterone/length of implant has been included and results have been listed in descending order based on the reported blood levels of testosterone achieved. Data has not been included from studies in which testicular regression had been allowed to occur after hypophysectomy etc: before initiation of testosterone treatment, nor has data from studies in which other hormones (e.g. FSH) have been administered together with testosterone. Studies listed in italics are those in which testosterone administration was for a period too short to permit reliable assessment of the ability of testosterone to maintain testicular weight (i.e. a period less than the duration of spermatogenesis).

weight. Although this may seem a very crude index, it is the one measured parameter that is common to all of the studies and for which there is likely to be very little between-laboratory error. Otherwise, a wide variety of endpoints of the maintenance of spermatogenesis have been used in various studies, many involving fixation of the testis. These include germ cell counts in seminiferous tubule cross sections, either at various stages of the spermatogenic cycle (395,473) or specifically at stage VII of the cycle (see below) (35,191,396,397,458,463,467), enumeration of the number of homogenization-resistant spermatids per testis (398,419,422,423,459,461,469, 470,474), measurement of seminiferous tubule diameter (35,191,204,462,475), counts of the number of degenerating germ cells in stage VII tubule cross sections (35,191,229,447,476), evaluation of spermatogonial numbers (238,471), or qualitative assessment of spermatogenesis from histology (421,466,472).

Various arguments could be put forward in support of a number of these endpoints, but none of them would enable a reliable comparison to be made between the **effectiveness** of treatments in **all** of the different studies with regard to the quantitative maintenance of spermatogenesis. In contrast, testicular weight does allow such a comparison to be made. Moreover, there are several distinct advantages to using this endpoint. First, it does not rely on the quality of fixation of testicular tissue as do many of the endpoints listed above; most laboratories that use perfusion-fixed testes for their analyses have misgivings about the use of immersion-fixed tissue, as the latter can induce many artifacts and hide subtle adverse changes (477–480). Second, because the available evidence now suggests strongly that testosterone acts only at around stage VII of the spermatogenic cycle in the rat (see below), it may be that measurements that do not involve analysis of this stage will miss relatively minor observations that are restricted to this stage, e.g., small numbers of degenerating germ cells (35,191,204,475, 476). In contrast, testicular weight effectively "sums" all abnormal changes within the testis.

A strong argument can be advanced for the measurement of homogenization-resistant elongate spermatids as a measure of daily sperm production (DSP) in the testis (197,481). Not only are these the final product of spermatogenesis, but they also come from a large number of the stages of the spermatogenic cycle (including stage VII). In general, testicular weight and the DSP give extremely comparable results, and there is no question that, when spermatogenesis is not maintained quantitatively (as evaluated by a variety of methods), neither is the DSP, and neither is testicular weight (398,422,423, 469,470,474). However, there are a number of studies (398,459,461,469,474) in intact rats bearing 20- to 40-cm testosterone implants that demonstrate **quantitative** maintenance or restoration of the DSP (i.e., no difference from vehicle-treated controls) but subnormal testicular weights (77–93% of controls); other studies also show that maintenance of DSP may exceed maintenance of testicular weight (422,470). These findings are puzzling because virtually every other piece of evidence suggests that subnormal testicular weights are associated with abnormalities of spermatogenesis. A possible explanation is that measurement of the DSP by homogenization of the testis overestimates the true DSP (104,481). For example, it is known that testosterone withdrawal leads to abnormal retention (and subsequent phagocytosis) of step 19 spermatids at stages IX–XII or later (412, 447,476,482). These spermatids would be "measured" in the DSP assessment based on homogenization but would in fact never be released. It is a well-recognized fact that abnormal retention or failed release of step 19 spermatids beyond stage VIII is one of the earliest and most subtle abnormal changes associated with damage to spermatogenesis induced by a wide variety of experimental approaches (61,71,478,483).

It is therefore possible that in studies in which the DSP is maintained but testicular weight is below normal, there are still subtle abnormalities of spermatogenesis such as retained step 19 spermatids. No such changes have been reported in the various studies, but they are easy to overlook, and it would be reassuring if this possibility could be checked properly and a definitive answer provided. As well as direct evidence that measurement of the DSP by homogenization may overestimate the number of spermatozoa that are released (104), there is also indirect evidence. Thus, studies in intact rats have demonstrated 98% to 99% maintenance of testicular weight (i.e., indistinguishable from controls) using either implants of testosterone propionate (467) or injections of testosterone esters every third day (191) (see Table 3), and the latter study also reported approximately 10% **lower** sperm numbers in the cauda epididymis of the testosterone-treated rats than in controls. Comparable findings (9% decrease in sperm counts) have been reported in rabbits bearing 26-cm testosterone implants for 9 weeks and that maintained testicular weight at 96% of control levels (484). In the latter study, the testosterone implant maintained blood levels in the rabbits at 40 ng/ml, and in the two studies in intact rats in which testicular weights were maintained at 98% to 99% of control levels (191,467) blood levels of testosterone were 46 and 51 ng/ml, values that are noticeably higher than any of those reported in other studies except for 45 ng/ml in rats bearing 50-cm testosterone implants (238). In contrast to the aforementioned studies, the latter study only demonstrated 82% maintenance of testicular weight, though it is of interest that the controls exhibited an unusually large mean testicular weight (2150 mg).

These differences between studies make it difficult to draw definitive conclusions, but perhaps it should be accepted that true quantitative maintenance of spermatogenesis requires demonstration of normal testicular weight (consistently 90% of control levels is *not* normal) ***plus*** demonstration of normal DSP (or sperm number in the epididymis). In this regard, it should be noted that though Berndston et al. (467) reported 98% maintenance of testicular weight with implants of testosterone propionate, compared with 86% for implants of testosterone, the latter was more effective at maintaining germ cell counts in stage VII seminiferous tubules; indeed, germ cell counts were reportedly reduced by around 20% at stage VII in the animals with 98% maintenance of testicular weight, findings decidedly at odds with one another. However, another study disagrees in showing quantitative maintenance of testicular weight and germ cell counts at stage VII following administration of testosterone for 10 weeks to EDS-treated rats (191).

The reader may consider that the above arguments are "much ado about nothing" and that 90% maintenance of testicular weight and sperm output during long-term testosterone administration to rats is close enough to the controls. However, this loses sight of the important dose–response relationship between testosterone levels within the testis and the degree of quantitative maintenance of spermatogenesis as discussed earlier. It is beyond dispute that full (i.e., qualitatively normal) spermatogenesis can be maintained with remarkably low levels of testosterone (33,394,399,460), but it may be equally true that the difference between 90% and 100% quantitative maintenance of spermatogenesis in the rat is simply a consequence of differences in testosterone levels. This is obviously of fundamental importance when it comes to answering the question, How much testosterone is required to support spermatogenesis? Unfortunately, it is not feasible to provide a definitive answer to this question based on current data. However, there are simple ways to resolve this matter, and they depend on applying the most sensitive index of testosterone insufficiency. This involves counting the number of degenerating germ cells in seminiferous tubules at stage VII of the spermatogenic cycle. In the normal **adult** rat, degenerating germ cells are observed only very rarely at stage VII, perhaps one degenerating cell every 100 to 150 stage VII cross sections (29,35,192,482); this level of germ cell degeneration is appreciably lower than that observed at many other stages (192), when it is often associated with mitotic or meiotic divisions (29,52). It should also be remembered that the situation during puberty is very different, as more widespread germ cell degeneration is a normal phenomenon (see Fig. 9).

When testosterone is withdrawn from adult rats by hypophysectomy (475,476), immunoneutralization of LH (447), administration of antiandrogens (477), or destruction of the Leydig cells using EDS (26,190,412, 482), the earliest morphological change (at about 3–5 days after treatment) is the appearance of occasional degenerating germ cells at stage VII. These changes are restricted initially to stage VII (see below) and are prevented completely by administering testosterone in **high** doses (26,35,190,482) or by the administration of LH (476,477). However, the degree to which the increased germ cell degeneration at stage VII is reversed is related to the dose of testosterone administered, and doses of testosterone that maintain testicular weight at 92% of that in controls do not completely prevent germ cell degeneration at stage VII (35); this occurred despite a testosterone level of around 25 ng/ml in blood and IF (compare with Table 3). This observation, combined with other evidence (discussed below) that demonstrates that testosterone acts specifically at around stage VII of the spermatogenic cycle, suggests that detection of degenerating germ cells at this stage is the most **sensitive** index of testosterone insufficiency (29; see also Fig. 8). None of the studies that have enumerated the DSP by homogenization have reported counts of degenerating germ cells at stage VII, and it would appear to be an important (and easy) matter to address in future studies.

It will already be clear that there are obstacles to pinpointing the relative importance of testosterone (and its level) required to maintain quantitatively normal spermatogenesis in the rat. Nevertheless, perusal of Table 3 makes two facts clear. First, the administration of testosterone is far more effective at maintaining testicular weight (i.e., spermatogenesis) in animals with an intact pituitary gland than in hypophysectomized rats. Second, in intact rats the highest levels of testosterone achieved are associated with the best maintenance of testicular weight, and the lowest levels of testosterone with the poorest maintenance of testicular weight. The latter observations may have relevance to the findings in hypophysectomized rats because, with the exception of study 1 (460), the levels of testosterone in blood achieved by exogenous administration bear poor comparison with many of the studies in intact rats. Indeed, even the level of 35.8 ng/ml reported in study 1 looks suspiciously high when placed alongside other values for comparable-length testosterone implants (e.g., 14 ng/ml in study 4), as, overall, equivalent-sized implants seem to produce equivalent testosterone levels in intact and hypophysectomized rats. Clearly, a study in which higher blood levels of testosterone are achieved (e.g., >40 ng/ml) in hypophysectomized rats would go a long way toward identifying whether or not there is an inherent difference in the ability of testosterone to maintain spermatogenesis in rats with or without an intact pituitary gland.

The most obvious difference between hypophysectomized and intact rats is that the latter still have the capacity to secrete FSH and/or LH. The role of FSH in spermatogenesis is discussed more fully below, but it is appropriate to make some observations on FSH (and LH) at this point. All of the studies listed in intact rats in which blood levels of LH have been measured are unanimous in showing that testosterone administration, even at doses far lower than those listed in Table 3, suppresses the secretion of LH to virtually undetectable levels. Based on this evidence, it therefore seems relatively unlikely that the better maintenance of spermatogenesis by exogenous testosterone in intact rats is a consequence of higher endogenous production of testosterone by Leydig cells as a result of LH stimulation. Measurement of testosterone levels in STF from intact and hypophysectomized rats bearing the same size testosterone implant support this view (423,469,474), though similar measurements for testicular IF show consistently higher values in intact than in hypophysectomized rats bearing the same size testosterone implants (422,462). Both sets of studies agree in showing higher levels of testosterone in STF or IF than in peripheral blood samples from the same animals.

As FSH clearly has supportive effects on spermatogenesis (see below), the presence of this hormone in intact, but not in hypophysectomized, rats would provide a ready explanation for the different effectiveness of testosterone in the two situations. However, the studies listed in Table 3 do not provide unequivocal support for this possibility. The most definitive evidence comes from a study in which rats were actively immunized against GnRH and given testosterone implants (459). Despite the fact that GnRH immunization reduced FSH (and LH) to undetectable levels in blood, 24-cm implants of testosterone maintained testicular weight and DSP at >90% of control levels after 8 weeks, a degree of maintenance far better than any of the studies in hypophysectomized rats and considerably better than the equivalent degree of maintenance (65%) reported in hypophysectomized rats by the same authors (423). The other studies are less clear-cut in this respect. For example, Sun et al. (462) also reported 80% maintenance of testicular weight in intact rats bearing 10-cm testosterone implants for 13 weeks and only 51% to 57% maintenance in equivalent studies in hypophysectomized rats (422,462). However, in their studies in intact rats these authors reported that, although testosterone implants lowered FSH levels in blood, this suppression was only partial—indeed, it appears from their studies that larger testosterone implants suppress FSH secretion less effectively than do smaller implants. Other studies using testosterone implants have reported little if any effect of even large implants on FSH levels in intact rats (470,474); some report partial and perhaps testosterone dose-dependent suppression of FSH (238,469), and others report virtually complete suppression (467). Where testosterone esters have been administered to intact rats by injection in low or high doses, suppression of FSH levels into the range found in hypophysectomized rats has been reported (35,191), and studies in man involving comparable treatment with low doses of testosterone esters have reported identical findings (222,485–488). In complete contrast, in intact rats administered a GnRH antagonist to lower FSH levels into the nondetectable range, administration of testosterone by implant or injection returned FSH levels into the normal control range (468,489).

It is impossible to make complete sense of these disparate findings, and the picture is all the more puzzling in that the majority of the studies in rats have used the same assay kit for measuring FSH levels. However, it can probably still be concluded with some confidence that the better maintenance of spermatogenesis by testosterone in intact as opposed to hypophysectomized rats (Table 3) is **not** accountable for by FSH. This is discussed further below in relation to the effects of exogenous FSH administration.

Hypophysectomy also deprives the animal of nongonadotropic pituitary hormones, and it could be argued that it is the absence of these hormones that results in testosterone failing to maintain spermatogenesis as effectively as in rats with an intact pituitary gland. This possibility cannot be dismissed, though there are not particularly strong supportive data. As discussed below, the administration of prolactin has been shown to have stimulatory effects on testicular weight in hypophysectomized rats, and insulin and thyroid-stimulating hormone (TSH) can also exert effects under certain circumstances (discussed elsewhere in this chapter). However, there are insufficient data to enable rational assessment of the relevance of these findings to the differences in maintenance of spermatogenesis between hypophysectomized and intact rats (Table 3). Indeed, the first priority should be to administer higher doses/implants of testosterone to hypophysectomized rats (to give blood levels of ≥40 ng/ml) with or without concomitant FSH administration to ascertain whether a comparable degree of spermatogenesis can be maintained to that in the intact rat.

Intratesticular Factors and Testosterone Support of Spermatogenesis: Role of Estrogens

It is perhaps also appropriate at this stage to discuss whether there might be other **intratesticular** factors that differ between intact and hypophysectomized rats and that might contribute to the apparently different effects of testosterone on spermatogenesis in these two groups (Table 3). Surprisingly, there is good evidence for such a difference, though its relevance is difficult to assess. A number of studies have shown that administration of GnRH agonists to intact rats leads, within 3 days, to drastic impairment of spermatogenesis and a 20% drop in testicular weight (490) and that longer periods of treatment lead not only to widespread disruption of spermatogenesis but also to the appearance of tubules devoid of both Sertoli cells and germ cells (490–494); spermatogenesis in the latter tubules does not recover 16 weeks after cessation of treatment (492). Remarkably, these adverse effects do not occur in GnRH agonist-treated hypophysectomized rats (490,492,495), though comparable changes can be induced by the administration of relatively high doses of LH, and the disruptive effects of this treatment are exacerbated by coadministration of a GnRH agonist (496). Therefore, the key factor in inducing this pronounced disruption of spermatogenesis is exposure of the testis to high (abnormally high?) levels of LH. Indeed, the administration of hCG + PMSG for 1 to 2 weeks to intact adult rats also causes gross disruption of spermatogenesis (490), and, more remarkably, within 12 hours of administration of a single dose of hCG focal disruption of spermatogenesis is evident (497,498); it is stage-dependent (498) and can be exacerbated by activation of the intratesticular macrophages (498).

A number of pieces of information demonstrate that the adverse effects of LH/GnRH agonists on spermatogenesis are not related to effects on intratesticular testosterone. First, the effects occur earlier (12–24 hours) (497,498) than the earliest detectable adverse changes following testosterone withdrawal (72 hours; discussed later) and are associated with normal or raised intratesticular levels of testosterone (496,498). Moreover, different stages of spermatogenesis are affected adversely by hCG/LH-administration (498) than are affected by testosterone withdrawal (482), and administration of testosterone propionate to GnRH agonist-treated intact rats is unable to prevent the focal tubular atrophy induced by the GnRH agonist (490,492).

Possible explanations for these rather paradoxical adverse effects of LH/hCG on spermatogenesis in the rat have been discussed, including focal ischemia (499) or inflammatory changes (498). However, neither of these possibilities really stands close scrutiny (498). A further possibility is that estrogens are involved based on a recent finding (419) that showed that coadministration of implants of testosterone and estradiol to EDS-treated rats (i.e., lacking mature Leydig cells) caused marked atrophy of the seminiferous tubules, the degree of atrophy being related dose-dependently to the amount of testosterone administered. It is emphasized that the tubular atrophy induced in this instance is unrelated to the administration of EDS, as it is clear from other studies that administration of testosterone alone dose-dependently supports spermatogenesis in EDS-treated rats (26,35,191), and administration of EDS alone (i.e., without testosterone replacement) results subsequently in only a small incidence of tubular atrophy (412,419).

There are many reports in the literature that demonstrate that the administration of estrogens to adult rats is able to induce impairment of spermatogenesis and sperm output (470,500–502). These changes have usually been explicable on the basis of impaired LH (and/or FSH) secretion and consequent changes in intratesticular testosterone (470,502,503), though other findings in hypophysectomized rats (504,505) or in rams (505a) have suggested intratesticular effects, including inhibition of Leydig cell steroidogenesis.

Can the findings on the induction of tubule atrophy by estradiol implants in animals lacking adult Leydig cells (419) be linked to the observations of the adverse effects of LH/hCG on spermatogenesis discussed above? The answer is probably yes, because in the adult rat testis it is the Leydig cells that are the sole source of estradiol, and it is established that overstimulation of the Leydig cells with high levels of LH or hCG leads to increased estradiol secretion (445; reviewed in ref. 378). Therefore, the seminiferous tubule atrophy induced in intact rats by GnRH agonists or in hypophysectomized and intact rats by LH/hCG may well be mediated by elevation of the intratesticular levels of estradiol. If this interpretation is correct, how does it occur?

Unfortunately, we have little idea as to how estrogens could locally impair spermatogenesis in the rat, as there is no evidence for direct effects on the seminiferous epithelium. Impairment of testosterone production by effects of estrogens on the cytoplasmic steroidogenic enzymes of the Leydig cells is demonstrable within a few days of estrogen administration to hypophysectomized rats (505), but these could not account for the marked tubular atrophy induced by estrogens (+ testosterone) in adult rats lacking Leydig cells (419). There is recent evidence that suggests that estrogens can prevent proliferation of Leydig precursor cells (506), and this may represent a normal intratesticular mechanism whereby adult Leydig cells negatively regulate the number of their developing precursor cells in the medium term (23). However, unless the Leydig precursor cells are assumed normally to exhibit an important influence on the seminiferous epithelium (and there is no evidence to support this), it is not immediately apparent how an effect of estrogens on Leydig precursor cell proliferation could lead to the rapid (within 12–24 hours) and pronounced adverse effects of LH/hCG or GnRH agonists on spermatogenesis in rats.

It is also uncertain whether this is a line of inquiry that should be pursued, for although administration of GnRH agonists by injection or implants can suppress spermatogenesis in a number of species including the dog (507,508), baboon (509), rhesus monkey (510–512), and man (513,514), this suppression appears to be a consequence of lowered LH and FSH secretion. Certainly, in all instances in which recovery of spermatogenesis has been checked following cessation of GnRH agonist treatment, it appears to be complete (508–510,512,515), with no evidence of the presumably irreversible focal degeneration of seminiferous tubules induced by GnRH agonist administration to intact rats (490,492). The latter may thus be a feature unique to the rat and is perhaps related to the presence of GnRH receptors on Leydig cells in the testis (27,496). However, there is an old report (516) showing that prolonged hCG administration to men can cause seminiferous tubule damage in association with increased levels of estradiol, and a more recent study in oligoasthenospermic men could be interpreted as supporting these observations (517). Another study (518) has suggested that suppression of endogenous estrogen production in oligospermic men can improve sperm numbers in the ejaculate. In contrast, studies involving prolonged administration of either hCG (222,487) or LH (486) to normal men have reported full recovery of normal sperm output following treatment, even when there was clear evidence for raised estrogen levels during gonadotropin treatment (487). Similar studies in infertile men, most of whom were oligospermic or oligoasthenospermic, have also failed to demonstrate any consistent evidence for impairment of spermatogenesis induced by prolonged administration of hCG (519–526).

The Role of Testosterone in Control of Spermatogenesis in Man and Other Mammals

The aim of this section is to address whether the findings described above for the rat can be applied to man and other mammals. The general answer is Yes, although this should be qualified by stating that, for man at least, the amount of information on which this answer is based is strictly limited; moreover, much of this information is rather indirect. What is completely clear is that spermatogenesis in man and other mammals is absolutely dependent on "high" intratesticular levels of testosterone, as in the rat (for the moment, the term "high" should be construed as meaning substantially higher than the levels in peripheral blood). Thus, when testosterone is administered exogenously in doses that maintain normal blood levels of this steroid or increase it by two- to threefold, then spermatogenesis is suppressed progressively over the next 6 to 20 weeks. This has been demonstrated in rabbits (484), rams (527), rhesus monkeys (186,502,528,529), and man (222,485,486,530–532,539). In most of these instances the suppression of spermatogenesis was inferred by changes in testicular volume and/or quantitation of spermatozoa in the ejaculate, but earlier studies in men in which testicular biopsies were taken (530,533,539) have confirmed that spermatogenesis is suppressed by administration of low doses of testosterone, and comparable data were found in the rhesus monkey (186,538), ram (527), and rabbit (484). In man, blockade of androgen action in the testis by administration of 200 mg/day cyproterone acetate for 16 to 20 weeks also results in gross impairment of spermatogenesis and associated oligospermia (534).

It also appears that, as in the rat, the intratesticular levels of testosterone in man and other mammals need to be at a high level if quantitatively normal spermatogenesis and/or sperm output are to be maintained. Although direct measurement of testosterone levels (i.e., in homogenates of testicular tissue) has been undertaken in the ram (200 ng/g; ref. 163), monkeys (200 ng/g; ref. 399), and man (>500 ng/g; refs. 436,440,530,535), these are likely to be overestimates of the physiological level in situ for the same reasons that have been given for the rat (above). In the latter, it was argued that TV levels of testosterone were likely to be the most accurate guide to levels within the testis, and in the one study in normal men in which these have been measured (433) the TV level of testosterone varied from 500 to 1200 ng/ml, an order of magnitude higher than values reported for comparable samples from the rat (see Fig. 12); an earlier study of hypogonadal men (434) in which a testicular vein was cannulated reported similarly high values ranging up to 1030 ng/ml. These very high levels of testosterone are not erroneous because many studies in the literature report levels of testosterone in SV blood in man of 310 to 740 ng/ml (401,435–437), and these are clearly lower than those in TV blood (see Fig. 12). Nonhuman mammals (guinea pig, ram, stumptailed macaque) appear much more similar to the rat in terms of their testosterone levels in TV or SV blood or in STF or RTF (433,439,452,527). Based on these measurements it would therefore be reasonable to conclude that, in other mammals, intratesticular testosterone would need to be at levels as high as in studies in the rat (see Table 3) to maintain quantitatively normal spermatogenesis; arguably, in man, this level could be considerably higher still. With the latter in mind, it is not surprising that studies in normal men in which testosterone has been administered to achieve levels in peripheral blood of 8 to 19 ng/ml (i.e., <4% of the levels in TV blood) have all reported massive suppression of spermatogenesis (Table 4); indeed, the primary objective of these (and other) studies involving testosterone administration to man has been to suppress spermatogenesis (529). It seems highly unlikely that doses of testosterone that are high enough to achieve >50% of TV testosterone levels (i.e., >250 ng/ml) will ever be administered clinically to normal men because of ethical and safety considerations (529,536). Historically, these sorts of levels may have been achieved in one study in which "an exceptionally well-developed" oligospermic 30-year-old man was administered doses of testosterone propionate ranging from 250 to 1000 mg per day (537). This treatment was reportedly without side effects or effects on spermatogenesis (as judged by biopsy), though the duration of treatment (4–11 days) and follow-up were really inadequate in this respect. Nowadays, this sort of study would have lawyers reaching for their calculators!

The majority of studies involving testosterone administration to nonhuman primates have also aimed to suppress rather than maintain spermatogenesis as part of a program of development of new male contraceptive strategies (529). Nevertheless, those studies that have achieved reasonably high levels of testosterone by exogenous administration have produced results comparable to those in the rat (compare Tables 3 and 4). Thus, a serum testosterone level of around 16.5 ng/ml was unable to maintain quantitatively normal spermatogenesis in intact rhesus monkeys though it did maintain qualitatively complete spermatogenesis (538). Again, in hypophysectomized cynomolgus monkeys, achievement of a level of testosterone (46 ng/ml) close to the likely intratesticular level failed by a wide margin to maintain quantitatively normal spermatogenesis (Table 4), a finding remarkably similar to that in hypophysectomized rats (Table 3).

Studies involving testosterone administration to rams have generally achieved much higher levels of testosterone than in man and monkeys, though they have been singularly unsuccessful in maintaining normal spermatogenesis or sperm output (Table 4). In some instances, the blood levels of testosterone quoted may be erroneously

TABLE 4. *Effects of testosterone on spermatogenesis in various mammals*

Species	Method of testosterone administration and dose	Duration of treatment (weeks)	Serum level of testosterone achieved (ng/ml)	Endpoint of spermatogenesis	Percentage maintenance of spermatogenesis	Reference
Man	Injection 50 mg TP/day	10–25	19.0[a]	Sperm count	reduced	530
	Injection 300 mg TE/week	24	15.0[b]	Sperm count	3%	488
	Injection 250 mg TE/week	21	8–10	Sperm count	4%	539
Cynomologous monkey (hypophysectomized)	T implant 100 cm	13	46.0	Germ cell counts[c] Testis weight	50% 60%	185
Rhesus monkey	TP implant (330 μg/kg per day)	10	16.5	Sperm count Testis weight	38% 60%	538
Ram	Injection 500 mg/day	10	100.0[d]	DSP Testis weight	33% 60%	527
Ram	T implants (×20)	10	28.0[e]	DSP Testis weight	<5% 25%	527
Ram (hypophysectomized)	T injection 2000 mg/day	2–6	316.0[f]	Testis weight	100%[f]	230 540
Rabbit	T implant 26 cm	9	40.0	DSP Testis weight	91% 96%	484

Compilation of data from the main studies in the literature that have assessed the effects on spermatogenesis of large doses of testosterone administered to normal adult men, to intact or hypophysectomized adult monkeys and rams (during their breeding season), or to rabbits. Note that for each of the studies cited, only data for the highest dose of testosterone or length of implant have been included. Data have not been included from immature animals or animals in which testicular regression had been induced (e.g., by hypophysectomy several weeks earlier) prior to initiation of testosterone treatment. Compare with comparable data for the rat listed in Table 3.

[a] Study reported that intratesticular levels of testosterone were reduced by >95%, compared with levels measured in pretreatment biopsies.

[b] Several earlier studies from this group in which lower doses of TE were administered have not been included in the Table (see text).

[c] In seminiferous tubule cross sections from testicular biopsies.

[d] Testosterone level is suspiciously high: in the same animals testosterone levels in RTF were 12.7 ng/ml, which was only 40% of the levels found in controls.

[e] Testosterone levels in RTF from the same animals were 6.6 ng/ml (20% of control levels).

[f] Data are for rams treated for 2 weeks from ref. 230. The study of Courtens and Courot (540) did not report testicular weight but said that subnormal numbers of spermatozoa were produced, and many of these were abnormal. TP, testosterone propionate; DSP, daily sperm production derived by measurement of homogenization-resistant spermatids in testicular tissue.

high (e.g., 100 ng/ml quoted in ref. 527, whereas levels in RTF in the same animals were eightfold lower), and in other studies the failure to maintain qualitatively or quantitatively normal spermatogenesis (230,540) could be related to the fact that the animals had been hypophysectomized. However, even in studies in which blood testosterone levels in intact rams were maintained at 28 ng/ml, testicular weight and DSP were <25% of control levels (527). In the intact rat, this level of testosterone would probably have maintained spermatogenesis at >80% of control levels (Table 3). However, normal testicular weight was maintained in hypophysectomized rams for 2 weeks when blood levels of testosterone were reportedly 316 ng/ml (230), though at 3 to 6 weeks testicular weight was reduced, and spermatogenesis was abnormal (193,540). Based on these observations, it would have to be concluded either that rams (in their breeding season) have a requirement for particularly high levels of testosterone for quantitative maintenance of spermatogenesis or that the requirement for FSH is far greater in this species than it is in the rat. The former possibility seems untenable in view of the likely similarity in intratesticular testosterone levels in the rat and ram (see above), and the second possibility is discussed later in this chapter.

In contrast to findings in the ram, the only study in which testosterone was administered at high levels to intact rabbits for 10 weeks produced virtually the same effects as in the rat, i.e., >90% maintenance of testicular weight and DSP with a testosterone level of 40 ng/ml (compare Tables 3 and 4).

With the exception of findings in the ram, it could therefore be concluded that the data on testosterone and spermatogenesis in mammals other than the rat are comparable to the detailed findings in this species. However, it is emphasized that studies that would permit a truly accurate comparison (e.g., administration of testosterone in doses high enough to achieve >40 ng/ml) have not been undertaken in **intact** monkeys and men, and without such information it is prudent to keep an open mind.

Testosterone and Male Infertility

The question of most immediate clinical significance is whether there is a subgroup of infertile men who have a deficiency in intratesticular testosterone; i.e., their testosterone level is not sufficient to maintain spermatogenesis at its maximum possible level. Data based on testosterone levels can be cited to support this possibility (435,541–547), but it should be viewed with caution, as these studies have used either the PV blood level of testosterone or the level in biopsied testicular tissue as their guide, and both of these are likely to be an inaccurate reflection of the true intratesticular testosterone level (discussed above). Nevertheless, it is beyond dispute that there is a small subgroup of phenotypically normal young men in whom "androgen insensitivity" is demonstrable (548–550) and who exhibit raised blood levels of LH and testosterone (implying androgen resistance) in association with severe oligozoospermia (544,548,551–553,553a) or even normospermia (554). A proportion of these men may be androgen resistant because of conservative mutations in the gene coding for the androgen receptor (548,551,555), though at present definitive evidence to support this possibility is lacking. However, it is also possible that a proportion of these patients may be infertile because of deficiencies in the intratesticular level of testosterone resulting from Leydig cell abnormalities. There is evidence to support this possibility (541–543,546,547,556,557), but it is indirect.

A number of studies down the years have claimed that administration of hCG to infertile men or men with oligozoospermia and/or asthenospermia improves sperm numbers and/or motility, either during treatment or following cessation of treatment (519–526). However, other studies have found no such effect (517), and properly controlled trials of the effectiveness of hCG treatment have yielded negative results (220,526). This could be because patients with definitive evidence of "androgen resistance" have not been selected for study (558), although because these patients already have raised blood levels of LH (544,548), the prospects of hCG treatment having a positive effect must be considered slim. Administration of very high doses of testosterone to such men (i.e., to achieve probable intratesticular levels of >40 and preferably >300 ng/ml) would go a long way toward resolving this problem definitively, but it seems highly unlikely that such a study will ever take place.

There is other, indirect, evidence that can be interpreted as suggesting that inadequate production of testosterone leads to increased germ cell degeneration during spermatogenesis, which in turn leads to a reduction in daily sperm production during aging in some men. It is generally recognized that such men have reduced numbers of Leydig cells (559), reduced levels of total and free testosterone in blood (560–562), and loss of circadian rhythmicity in their testosterone levels (563). These changes are associated with falling daily sperm production (187,199,200) as a consequence of increased germ cell degeneration late in meiosis (198,200); these changes are associated with an increase in the blood levels of FSH (200). Based on the data discussed above for the rat, it could be speculated that the increased germ cell degeneration was simply a manifestation of decreased efficiency of spermatogenesis because of suboptimal testosterone levels and that the latter would also lead to reduced production of STF. If in man, STF provides the main vehicle and route via which inhibin from the Sertoli cell reaches the peripheral bloodstream, as it does in the adult rat (17,248,432,433), then decreased secretion of STF and inhibin would lead to an increase in blood levels of FSH. Certainly in the rat it is clear that reduced production of STF and raised FSH levels go hand in hand, and both are associated with changing numbers of elongate spermatids (66,67), which in turn regulate inhibin secretion and exit from the testis (30,250).

The important question is whether the possible association of these age-related changes to declining testosterone levels has relevance to younger subfertile men. As detailed earlier, humans have the most inefficient spermatogenesis of any mammal so far investigated, and one important reason for this is a "naturally" high level of germ cell degeneration during meiosis, especially in late pachytene and in diakinesis (187,194–196,200); it is the latter that appears to worsen with aging (200). Pachytene spermatocytes at stages VII–VIII of the spermatogenic cycle (the androgen-dependent stages) are the first germ cells to degenerate following testosterone withdrawal in the rat (35,190,475,476,482), and during supplementation of EDS-treated rats with suboptimal doses of testosterone, it is mainly the pachytene spermatocytes that continue to degenerate in abnormal numbers (26,35).

A number of pieces of evidence imply that there may be a similar sensitivity of these germ cells to ambient testosterone levels and/or action in human spermatogenesis. For example, patients with suspected mild androgen insensitivity (i.e., raised blood levels of LH **and** testosterone, slow beard growth, etc.) and/or 5α-reductase deficiency often display arrest of germ cell development at mid- to late pachytene (548,551,564). Because such arrest is also a feature of a proportion of azoospermic men (565,566), it remains possible that mild insufficiency in androgen production or action could be a contributory factor to low sperm output in some men (567,568).

The Mechanisms by Which Testosterone Supports Spermatogenesis

As was indicated at the beginning of this chapter, probably one of the most remarkable aspects of the regulation of spermatogenesis is that we still have little idea how testosterone exerts its supportive effects on this process despite the fact that these effects are clearly all-important. This now shows signs of changing, but in reviewing what we know now, I think it is important first to highlight the obstacles that we have inadvertently placed in the way of developing such understanding over the past 20 or so years. This is done most easily by considering some curious facts about testosterone action and spermatogenesis, most of which have been known for a long time and that really should have alerted us to the possibility that all was not straightforward.

The first fact is that testosterone or dihydrotestosterone acts via the androgen receptor, one of the members of the steroid family of receptors (569–571), which is coded for by a single copy gene on the X chromosome (572). Androgen receptors within the testis of the rat are confined to the Leydig cells, peritubular cells, and Sertoli cells (573–576), but very recent studies have shown that they are also present in the muscular layer of most arteries within the rat testis (576,577). What is clear from these and other (578,579) studies is that androgen receptors are not present in germ cells and are not required in germ cells for their normal development (580). Evidence has been presented for the presence of androgen receptors in germ cells (581–584), but these data are generally considered to be inaccurate because of the methods used. It is, however, possible that the latter studies were detecting some form of androgen-binding moiety other than the androgen receptor, and this is discussed further below. Therefore, the vast majority of the available data suggest that the mechanisms by which testosterone supports the development of germ cells are indirect and presumably occur via the Sertoli (576) or peritubular myoid cells (24,585) of the seminiferous tubule.

A further important finding concerning the androgen receptor in the rat testis is that levels of this receptor in the Sertoli cell increase quite markedly from 10 to 20 days to 35 or 60 days of age (344,345,384,576), implying that the role of testosterone in regulating the Sertoli cell in the pubertal and adult rat testis is more important than in the prepubertal testis. Indeed, this finding fits very well with the little that is known about the functional effects of testosterone on the rat testis. For example, in the adult rat the production of seminiferous tubule fluid (STF) is under the control of testosterone rather than FSH (333,343,586), whereas the converse is true for the immature rat (332). The same probably holds true for the production of ABP (321,335). Indeed, there is abundant evidence that, in the immature rat, the Sertoli cell is primarily FSH rather than testosterone driven and that the responsiveness of the Sertoli cell to FSH declines dramatically during puberty and into adulthood as detailed earlier. It is therefore all the more remarkable that the majority of studies that have tried to assess how testosterone controls spermatogenesis via the Sertoli cell have utilized Sertoli cells isolated from immature rats (15–20 days of age), a singularly inappropriate starting point.

The second curious fact about testosterone and spermatogenesis stems from observations in the 1970s and 1980s that demonstrated that testosterone withdrawal led (initially at least) not to wholesale degeneration of germ cells but to germ cell degeneration just at stages VII–VIII of the rat spermatogenic cycle (447,476,477, 587,588). These findings, coupled with the growing awareness of stage-dependent changes in Sertoli cell function (103), should have alerted us to the possibility that testosterone did not affect the whole process of spermatogenesis but, instead, acted only at one or two stages of the spermatogenic cycle. Anyone who thinks that this concept is a recent development in our thinking should read the older literature (28), where it is prominently voiced. The critically important aspect about stage-dependent changes in Sertoli cell function is that they are germ cell modulated; i.e., the cyclical changes in Sertoli cell function are determined by the complement of germ cells associated with the Sertoli cell; again, there is nothing new in this sort of reasoning, although today we have many more examples of this germ cell modulation of Sertoli cell function than 20 years ago (17,19,103). Therefore, what the available information was shouting out was that the mechanisms by which testosterone controlled spermatogenesis via the Sertoli cell were likely to be manifest only in the presence of an appropriate complement of germ cells. The choice of isolated Sertoli cells from immature rats to investigate such effects again seems wholly inappropriate.

Finally, we come to another curious fact about testosterone and spermatogenesis that has particular relevance to us today because it is perhaps our current blind spot, namely, the levels of testosterone required to support spermatogenesis. This is a subject we have already dealt with in depth, including the various arguments about just what level of testosterone is required for the quantitative maintenance of normal spermatogenesis. As was concluded earlier, there is unanimity in recognizing that testosterone levels within the testis have to be high to support spermatogenesis—in my opinion, 40 ng/ml at least in the rat, but everyone would accept at least 20 ng/ml. But why? If the testosterone support for spermatogenesis is mediated via androgen receptors, then all of these receptors will be occupied at levels of testosterone of 1 ng/ml or less based on known kinetics (569,589–591)—this is certainly the case for androgen receptors in peripheral target tissues (571,589,590), and as there is only one androgen receptor (572), the presumption must be that the same holds true for the testis. It cannot even be argued that the number of androgen receptors in seminiferous tubules changes according to the different stages of the spermatogenic cycle, as there is relatively little difference between the stages (275,592), and levels of testosterone in (270,593) or around (17) the tubules also probably do not differ greatly.

It therefore remains a mystery why testosterone levels in the testis need to be so high to support spermatogenesis. But it does indicate that there is some important aspect of androgen action on the seminiferous tubule of which we are unaware. There are perhaps three distinct possibilities, which are not mutually exclusive. The first centers around growing understanding of how steroids interact with their receptors to alter gene transcription. These suggest that a variety of cofactors are required to enable steroid-dependent gene transcription to occur and that these cofactors can dramatically alter the dose–response relationship (571,590,594; reviewed in ref. 595). In the context of spermatogenesis it can be envisaged that the presence of the different germ cell types might be the triggers for various cofactors, which then enable androgen bound to its receptor to activate gene transcription in the Sertoli cells. This model would fit well with recent findings on the biochemistry of androgen action on the seminiferous tubule, as described below. However, although this would explain the stage specificity of androgen action, it would still not provide a straightforward explanation for why intratesticular levels of testosterone have to be so high to support spermatogenesis. Therefore, the second possibility relates to the type of androgen interacting with the androgen receptor in the Sertoli and peritubular cells.

In most androgen-responsive tissues testosterone is first converted to 5α-dihydrotestosterone (DHT) by the enzyme 5α-reductase (596). Although testosterone and DHT have similar affinity for the androgen receptor, DHT forms a more stable complex and hence is about an order of magnitude more potent at concentrations of steroid (~0.6 ng/ml) that saturate the receptor (589). However, if the concentration of testosterone is increased about tenfold (6–7 ng/ml), it is then just as potent as DHT (589). Could it be that testosterone is not converted to DHT in the testis and that this explains why such high intratesticular levels of testosterone are needed to support spermatogenesis? Several pieces of information demonstrate that this is almost certainly not the case. Thus, the concentrations of testosterone (6–7 ng/ml) needed to stabilize the androgen–steroid receptor complex are still far lower than those needed to support spermatogenesis, as described above. It is also quite clear that testosterone can be converted to DHT within the testis of both rat and man, and although there may be changes in activity of 5α-reductase during pubertal development (597–600), the levels of DHT in spermatic vein blood from adult men are far higher than those in peripheral blood (601), indicating that 5α-reduction of testosterone still occurs in the normal adult testis. Data from the adult rat support this view (see ref. 203a). Finally, data from individuals with 5α-reductase deficiency indicate that spermatogenesis is impaired or arrested (552,564), though as this condition may also adversely affect testicular descent, it is difficult to be certain that the abnormalities in spermatogenesis are solely a consequence of the 5α-reductase deficiency.

Based on the available evidence it therefore seems unlikely that an unusual pattern of androgen metabolism within the testis can explain the requirement for high intratesticular levels of testosterone. The final possibility is that testosterone does not act only via the androgen receptor to support spermatogenesis but also by other pathways (e.g., membrane effects or via androgen-binding protein) that require higher testosterone levels. This is discussed further below.

Current Understanding of Testosterone Action

In view of the concentration of research effort on isolated Sertoli cells from immature rats, we should perhaps not be surprised that few effects of testosterone have been identified. It has been recognized for many years that testosterone can stimulate the secretion of androgen-binding protein (ABP) by the Sertoli cell both *in vivo* and *in vitro* and in the presence or absence of FSH (217,334,602). Testosterone can have small effects on overall protein secretion by Sertoli cells (336), which are perhaps related to effects on RNA polymerase II (603), but other studies have identified specific (but low-abundance) proteins the secretion of which is testosterone modulated in culture (604–607). However, overall, there is a remarkable lack of evidence for effects of testosterone on Sertoli cell function, but, as has been stressed already, this is probably because of the use of an inappropriate model for addressing this problem. The studies cited above have exclusively used isolated Sertoli cells (i.e., the germ cells have been removed) from either immature (~20 days of age) rats or from older rats (40 days or older) that had been hypophysectomized several weeks beforehand (to induce degeneration and hence removal of the germ cells). There is no question that the function of the Sertoli cells changes ("matures") with age, even in the absence of germ cells, but it is equally evident that the response of the Sertoli cells to germ cells also changes with age (17,20,21,23,323,326,327). It is therefore unlikely that the use of Sertoli cells from older animals will enable the identification of testosterone-regulated Sertoli cell proteins involved in spermatogenesis if the Sertoli cells are isolated from their normal germ cell complement.

Reasoning as above led us to adopt a different approach toward identifying how testosterone regulates spermatogenesis based on the use of isolated seminiferous tubules with a normal germ cell complement but deprived acutely of **all** testosterone by the EDS-induced destruction of the Leydig cells (26,190,482). Such studies showed that, in association with the appearance of a small number of degenerating germ cells at stage VII of the spermatogenic cycle, which is the first biological manifestation of androgen insufficiency (26,35,190,476,477,482), there was a marked decrease in total protein secretion (based on [^{35}S]methionine incorporation) by isolated seminiferous tubules at stages VI–VIII of the spermatogenic cycle following acute testosterone withdrawal (Fig. 12). This decrease was specific for stages VI–VIII, as seminiferous tubules at stages before or after VI–VIII from the same animals showed no change in protein secretion (Fig. 12), and, moreover, the incorporation of [^{35}S]methionine into intracellular proteins was unaffected at any of the stages (190,608). It was then realized that testosterone withdrawal had not in fact reduced protein secretion by seminiferous tubules at stages VI–VIII but had **prevented** the normal twofold increase in protein secretion that occurs at these stages (Fig. 13). Administration of exogenous testosterone to EDS-treated rats at a dose sufficient to achieve testosterone levels of ~40 ng/ml was able to restore the normal stage-dependent pattern of protein secretion (Fig. 13) and prevent the appearance of degenerating germ cells (190).

This stage-dependent pattern of ST-protein secretion fits well with a previous report of stage-dependent changes in RNA synthesis by ST (609) and its possible regulation by testosterone (610), findings that appear to have been generally ignored. Analysis of the radiolabeled proteins secreted by isolated seminiferous tubules at different stages from the various treatment groups described above has identified seven putative androgen-regulated proteins (ARPs), the secretion of which is largely stage dependent (i.e., restricted to stages VI–VIII) as well as being testosterone dependent (Fig. 14) (190). The cellular source of these proteins is, of course, difficult to delineate when intact seminiferous tubules are used, but a variety of approaches suggest that the different ARPs probably derive from Sertoli cells (ARP-3, ARP-4, ARP-5), peritubular cells (ARP-6, ARP-7), and round spermatids (ARP-1, ARP-2) (190,350,608).

What the findings illustrated in Figs. 13 and 14 demonstrate is that testosterone does indeed have major general (i.e., overall protein secretion) and specific (i.e., on the ARPs) effects on cells within the seminiferous tubule of adult rats and that these effects are highly stage specific. Moreover, the stages within which testosterone has its effects include stage VII, which is the first stage to show morphological signs of testosterone withdrawal following experimental manipulation, as has been discussed already. This stage specificity implies that germ cells are somehow involved in programming the response to testosterone of the androgen target cells with which they are associated (i.e., the Sertoli cells), as the germ cell complement is really the only factor that differs from stage to stage (17,19). This presumption has been shown to be true by assessing the effect of depletion of each of the germ cell types at stages VI–VIII on the normal androgen-dependent changes (350,608). These studies have shown that depletion of **either** pachytene spermatocytes, round spermatids, or elongate spermatids from seminiferous tubules at stages VI–VIII largely prevents the normal stage-dependent increase in total protein secretion as well as affecting secretion of the ARPs. Indeed, if both pachytene spermatocytes and round spermatids are depleted from seminiferous tubules at stages VI–VIII, then most of the androgen-dependent changes are abolished completely (C. McKinnell and R. M. Sharpe, *unpublished data*). Moreover, if seminiferous tubules or Sertoli cells are isolated from young rats aged 28 days, then none of the ARPs are detectable secretory products (329). All of these findings are consistent and demonstrate that a normal germ cell complement is a prerequisite for testosterone to exert its normal stage-dependent effects on protein secretion by the cells of the seminiferous epithelium.

It remains largely unknown how germ cells are able to regulate responsiveness of the Sertoli cell to testosterone, although it can presumably occur via specialized junctional interactions between the germ and Sertoli cells (23,46) and/or by the secretion of soluble factors. With respect to the latter, the germ cells of the mouse and rat testis have been shown to produce nerve growth factor (NGF) (611), low-affinity receptors for NGF have been

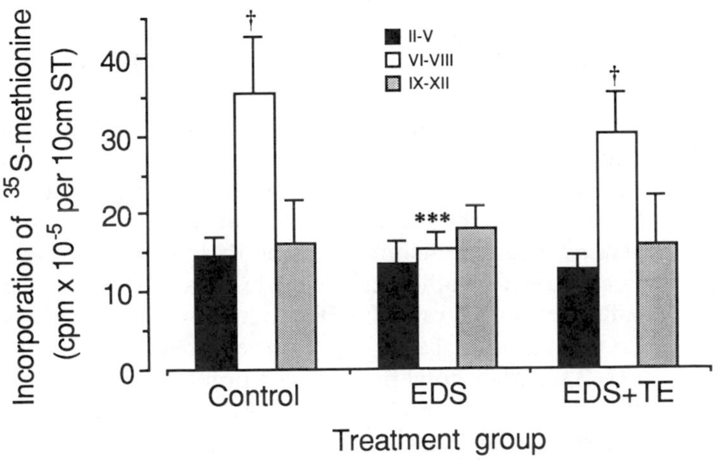

FIG. 13. Regulation by testosterone of stage-dependent differences in total protein secretion (means ± SD) in vitro over 24 hours by seminiferous tubules isolated at stages II–V, VI–VIII, or IX–XII from control rats, rats treated 4 days earlier with ethane dimethane sulfonate (EDS) or treated with EDS and supplemented with high doses of testosterone (EDS + TE). $^{\dagger}p < 0.001$ compared with stages II–V and IX–XII from the same group. $^{***}p < 0.001$ compared with ST at stages VI–VIII in the other two groups. (Reproduced with permission from Sharpe et al., ref. 190.)

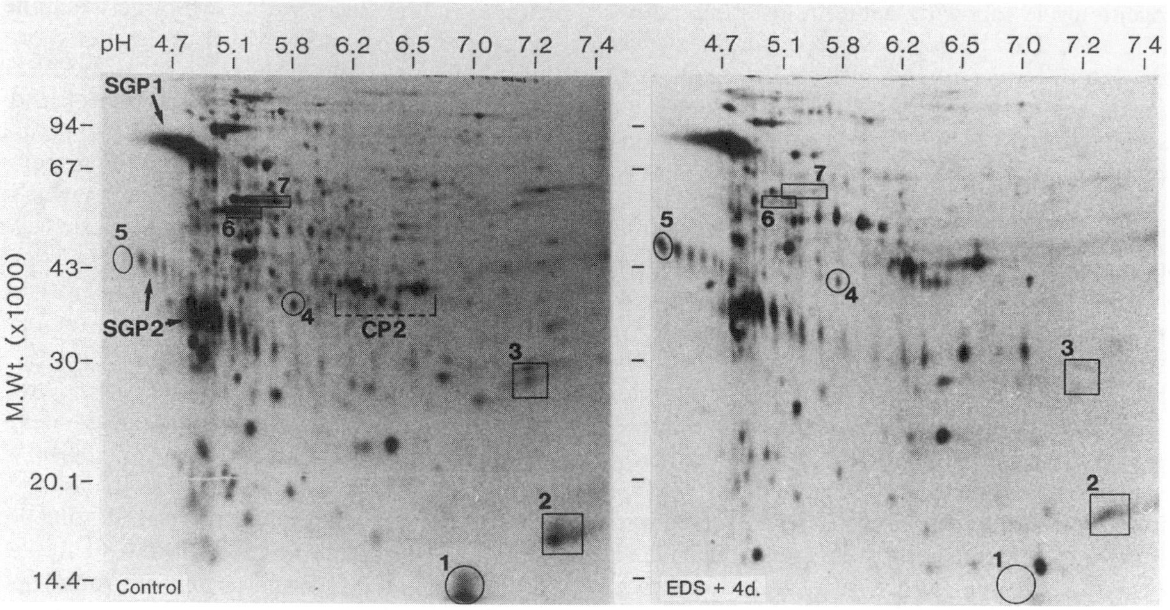

FIG. 14. Identification, using two-dimensional SDS-PAGE, of putative androgen-regulated proteins (ARPs) secreted *in vitro* over 24 hours by seminiferous tubules (ST) at stages VI–VIII of the spermatogenic cycle that had been isolated from control rats (**left**) or from rats in which testosterone withdrawal had been induced by treatment with ethane dimethane sulfonate (EDS); ST were cultured in the presence of ^{35}S-labeled methionine. Seven ARPs are indicated, one of which (ARP-5) is regulated negatively by testosterone and the others regulated positively by testosterone. The ARPs are secreted predominantly at stages VI–VIII of the spermatogenic cycle, and their secretion in EDS-treated rats is restored by testosterone administration (190,350,608). The three major Sertoli cell-secreted proteins, sulfated glycoprotein-1 (SGP-1), sulfated glycoprotein-2 (SGP-2), and cyclic protein-2 (CP2), are also indicated for reference. Gels were loaded with equal counts of radiolabeled proteins.

localized to Sertoli cells at stages VII–VIII of the spermatogenic cycle, and the mRNA for the receptor is apparently regulated negatively by testosterone (612). A role for NGF in the onset of meiosis (DNA synthesis in preleptotene spermatocytes) has been proposed (613), and recent data suggest that NGF production by the germ cells may modulate levels of mRNA for ABP in the Sertoli cell (614). These findings are of obvious potential significance, but far more detailed assessment is required to establish the importance of these observations. Many such factors have been identified in the testis at one time or another, but establishment of their physiological role (if any) has proved extremely problematical (17,23, 24,300).

As yet, the identity and function of the ARPs secreted by seminiferous tubules at stages VI–VIII has not been established. However, perhaps the most intriguing effect of testosterone is the "up-regulation" of protein secretion at stages VI–VIII (Fig. 13). It appears to be a fairly general effect, with the secretion of most proteins being increased, irrespective of their cellular source. The volume of rough endoplasmic reticulum is known to increase substantially in Sertoli cells at stages VII–VIII of the spermatogenic cycle (615,616), and this could be related to the increased secretion of Sertoli cell proteins. It is perhaps more likely that testosterone is exerting an effect on total protein secretion via some other route, e.g., by increasing the stability of mRNAs, by increasing the efficiency of peptide elongation, or by increasing the transcription of genes regulating the packaging and secretion of proteins. As yet there is no information available that would enable these various possibilities to be assessed. However, there is one other possibility that merits serious consideration—seminiferous tubule fluid (STF) production. The secretion of STF is androgen regulated in the adult rat testis (333,343,586), and it could be envisaged that the secretion of STF and proteins could be interconnected (17).

Other indirect evidence supports the notion that the production of STF is greatest at stages VII–VIII (the androgen-dependent stages) based on the large increase in diameter of the lumen of the seminiferous tubule that occurs specifically at these stages of the spermatogenic cycle (67,183,615). This increase in lumen diameter is dependent on the presence of elongate spermatids in the seminiferous epithelium (67), and these germ cells have been shown in other studies to exert a strong positive influence on the rate of STF production (66) as well as on the secretion of a variety of proteins by the Sertoli cell (21–23) and on total protein secretion by isolated seminiferous tubules (350). Indeed, STF production clearly decreases after testosterone withdrawal. For example, direct measurement using the efferent duct ligation method has shown that STF production is reduced by nearly half at 7 days after EDS treatment (617), and in rats 6 days after hypophysectomy, a comparable decrease was inferred from reduction in diameter of the seminiferous tubule lumen at stage VII (204). However, we have been unable to show any significant decrease in STF production at 4 days after EDS-induced testosterone withdrawal using the efferent duct ligation method (S. Maddocks and R. M. Sharpe, *unpublished data*), a time at which protein secretion by isolated seminiferous tubules at stages VI–VIII of the spermatogenic cycle is suppressed maximally (190). Nevertheless, it still seems a distinct possibility that the overall secretion of proteins and STF at stages VII–VIII is somehow linked, in view of the clear testosterone dependence of both of these phenomena at just these particular stages. In this respect it is also of interest that, in man, the volume of the seminiferous tubule lumen is correlated with the volume of dark but not light Leydig cells (618), also implying a relationship between testosterone and STF production.

One recent study (619) has shown that, in the 4 to 8 days following testosterone withdrawal in rats by either EDS or hypophysectomy, there is the appearance of a ring of small basally situated vacuoles in the seminiferous epithelium specifically in tubules at stages VII–VIII of the spermatogenic cycle. (Fig. 15) (see also ref. 475). Ultrastructural analysis has shown these vacuoles to be multiple focal dilatations of the inter-Sertoli-cell tight junctions, and it is suggested that the vacuoles arise because of inappropriate secretion of STF into the clefts of the tight junctions. These changes were clearly related to testosterone withdrawal as opposed to degeneration of germ cells, as comparable changes occurred in rats lacking germ cells and in which testosterone withdrawal was then induced. Small groups of basally situated intercellular vacuoles are also evident in men treated with the antiandrogen cyproterone acetate (312), and similar vacuoles may be present in the testes of some infertile men with pronounced germ cell loss (620,621), though it is not known whether this might reflect deficiencies in testosterone action.

Another important site of testosterone action within the testis is on the vasculature. Androgen receptors are present on the muscular layer of small arteries in the rat testis (577), and these are presumably responsible for mediating effects of testosterone on vasomotion (rhythmic variations in testicular blood flow in arterioles) (622). Vasomotion is thought to be a mechanism by which the movement of fluids is effected from the vasculature to the interstitial space, and it is of considerable interest that both the volume of testicular interstitial fluid (26,623) and vasomotion (624,625), as well as overall testicular blood flow (624), are all regulated acutely by testosterone. In addition, the germ cells exert an important modulatory effect on all of these phenomena (625,626), presumably via effects on the Sertoli cells. Curiously, it appears to be the elongate spermatids that exert the most marked effect on testicular haemodynamics, and it is these same germ cells that regulate the production of STF by the Sertoli cell, another androgen-dependent event (discussed above). Other relevant information is that vasomotion is not present in the testes of 20-day-old rats (627) despite the presence of sufficient intratesticular levels of testosterone, and permeability of the testicular vasculature also changes during puberty (389), evidence that again probably argues for an essential modulatory or inductive effect by the germ cells.

Despite their similarity in temporal sensitivity and germ cell dependence, the effects of testosterone on vasomotion and spermatogenesis differ in one important aspect: Far lower levels of testosterone are required to maintain vasomotion (625). Indeed, normal peripheral blood levels of testosterone will maintain vasomotion in contrast to the much higher levels required to maintain spermatogenesis, as discussed earlier; however, this is only true provided that a normal germ cell complement is present (625). The significance of these findings showing that blood flow, vasomotion, interstitial fluid volume, and STF production are all androgen dependent should not be underestimated. Blood flow to the testis is probably one of the most important factors in terms of the metabolic constraints that subnormal blood flow would impose (392,628). Indeed, it is quite clear that testicular size and blood flow go hand in hand (629,630), though it is not always entirely clear which is determining which. Clearly, abnormalities in any aspect of blood flow and fluid dynamics of the testis could have considerable consequences for spermatogenesis. Whether such defects might be involved in the etiology of infertility in the human male is unknown, but histological abnormalities of the vasculature in the testis associated with focal seminiferous tubule damage have been reported in connection with varicocele, aging, etc. (631–635). A summary of the known testosterone-modulated events in the normal adult rat testis is given in Table 5. This makes clear that testosterone appears to control all of the aspects of testicular function that involve the transport of nutrients, etc., to the testis, from the vasculature to the interstitium and thence from the Sertoli cell to the germ cells.

There are no specific data from man or other mammals on the mechanisms by which testosterone supports spermatogenesis in the adult testis, so it is not possible to assess meaningfully whether the data described above for the rat have general relevance to other species. However, in view of the remarkable similarities in organization of the process of spermatogenesis in mammals (32) and the fundamental aspects of testicular function that are regulated by testosterone in the rat, it seems likely that the effects of testosterone on spermatogenesis will be highly conserved between species.

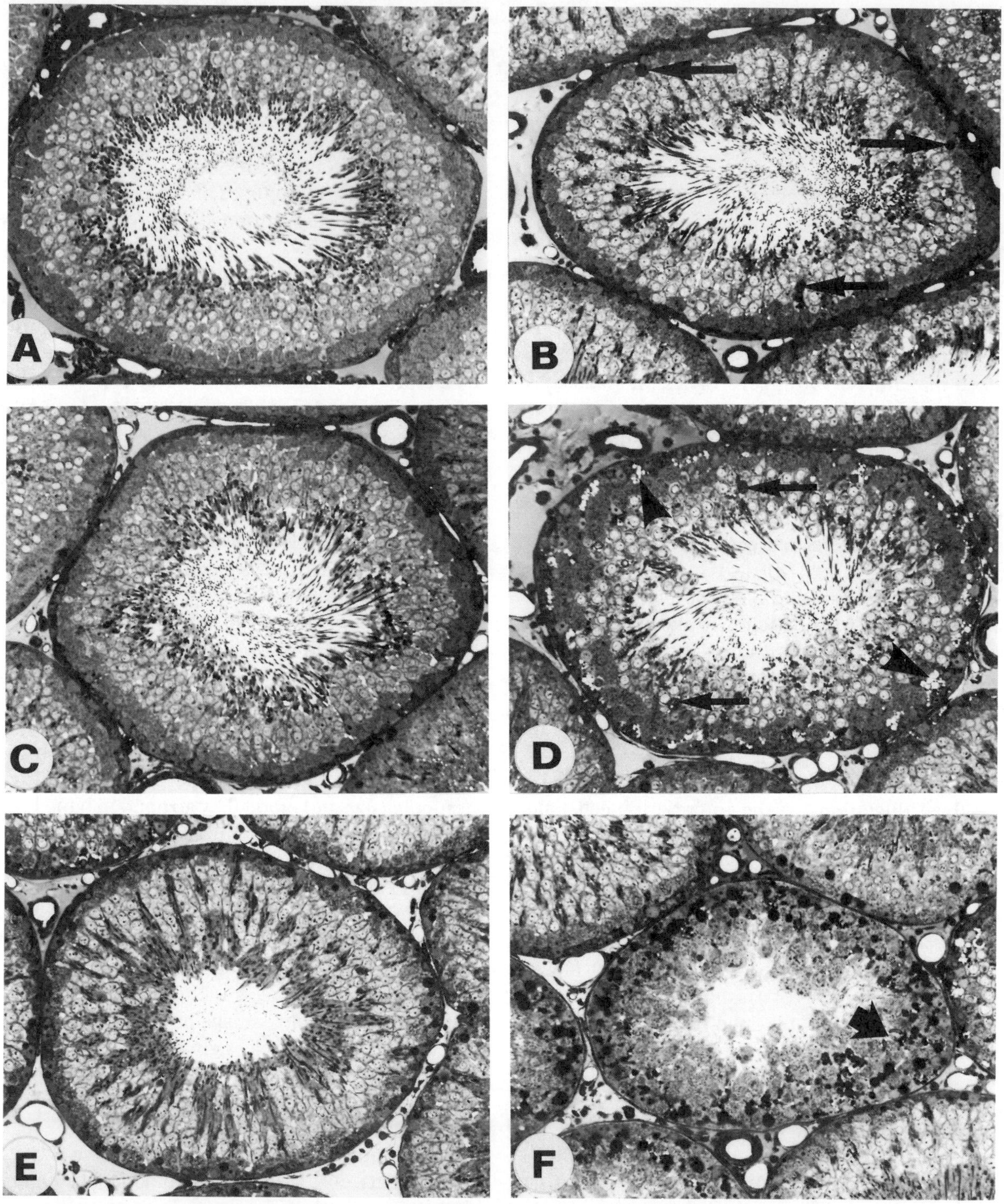

FIG. 15. Temporal and stage-dependent effects of testosterone withdrawal on spermatogenesis in the adult rat, induced by administration of ethane dimethane sulfonate (EDS). **A:** Stage VII in a normal rat. Note that no degenerating germ cells or vacuoles are evident in the epithelium. **B:** Stage VII in a rat 6 days after EDS treatment illustrating the presence of three degenerating germ cells (*arrows*). Note, however, that the majority of germ cells appear normal. **C:** Stage VII in a rat 6 days after EDS + testosterone (TE) treatment (25 mg testosterone esters every 3 days) to illustrate that the TE prevents the appearance of degenerating germ cells. **D:** Stage VII in a rat 8 days after EDS-treatment. Note the appearance of a ring of small vacuole clusters (arrowheads) in the vicinity of the inter-Sertoli cell tight junctions. Note also that degenerating germ cells are still evident (*arrows*), although the majority of germ cells are still present and appear normal. **E:** Stage IV in a rat 8 days after EDS treatment, illustrating a completely normal appearance. **F:** Stage XII in a rat 8 days after EDS-treatment illustrating gross impairment of spermatogenesis at this stage. Note the loss of all but two of the step 12 spermatids (*large arrow*) and the abnormal accumulation of darkly staining lipid droplets resulting from germ cell degeneration. Note that in panels **B** to **F** no Leydig cells are evident in the interstitium. For further details and references see the text.

TABLE 5. *Stage specificity of testosterone effects on the adult rat testis*[a]

Parameter[b]	Stage specificity	References
Testosterone-responsive parameters of seminiferous tubule (ST) function		
Lumen diameter	Maximal at VII–VIII	67,183,204,615
STF production	Unknown (?maximal at VII–VIII)	33,343,586
ST protein secretion	Maximal at VI–VIII	190,329,350,608
Secretion of ARP's	Maximal at VI–VIII	190,350,608
Secretion of ABP	Maximal at VII–VIII	321,335,668
Effects of acute (days 3–7) testosterone withdrawal		
Decrease in lumen size	Occurs at VII–VIII (unknown for other stages)	204
Decrease in STF production	? Decreased at VII (unknown for other stages)	204,333,343
Vacuolation of tight junctions	Mainly VII–VIII	619
Decrease in ST protein secretion	Only at VI–VIII	190,350,608
Decrease in secretion of ARP's	Only at VI–VIII	190,350,608
Degenerating germ cells	Appear first at VII–VIII (then spread sequentially to following stages)	35,190,191,475, 476,482
Decrease in blood flow/vasomotion	—	624,625
Decrease in IF volume	—	26,190,623

[a] Summary of the major known effects of testosterone on the adult rat testis and their stage-specificity, based on testosterone-responsive parameters and the effects of acute testosterone withdrawal. Note that most of the parameters in the table are also germ cell-modulated phenomena, especially by elongate (step 19) spermatids (66–69,260,350,625,626)].

[b] STF, seminiferous tubule fluid; ARPs, androgen-regulated proteins; ABP, androgen-binding protein; IF, interstitial fluid.

Failure of Spermatogenesis Following Testosterone Withdrawal

Additional insight into how testosterone controls spermatogenesis might be gained by detailed analysis of exactly how the process fails following testosterone withdrawal. Surprisingly, this has received remarkably little attention, with most studies having concentrated on either the short-term (<6 days) or longer-term (>28 days) effects of testosterone withdrawal; only one recent study (482) has attempted a longitudinal analysis, and then only covering the first 8 days of testosterone withdrawal. It is particularly important to have such a longitudinal analysis because the degeneration and loss of germ cells that follow testosterone withdrawal become progressively more pronounced with time (204,412,482), and this loss will clearly induce other, secondary changes in Sertoli cell structure and function that are not related **directly** to the mechanisms of testosterone action (17,23,190,204).

Detailed morphometric analysis of the structure of Sertoli cells at stage VII in the rat at either 6 or 28 days after hypophysectomy revealed virtually no significant changes at 6 days despite a 28% reduction in testicular weight and the presence of some degenerating germ cells (204); the reduction in testicular weight was attributed to altered production of STF, as discussed above. Therefore, at a time when, biochemically, Sertoli cell function is clearly disturbed in a major way (see above), with consequent degeneration/loss of a small percentage of germ cells, the ultrastructure of the Sertoli cell remains virtually normal (see Fig. 15). In contrast, by day 28 after hypophysectomy, when testicular weight had decreased by 75%, virtually every parameter of Sertoli cell structure was altered drastically (204). However, as these authors pointed out, it is almost certain that these adverse changes are a consequence of germ cell loss rather than testosterone withdrawal per se.

In the rat, seminiferous tubules at stage VII of the spermatogenic cycle are the first to show signs of testosterone withdrawal in terms of the appearance of degenerating germ cells (26,190,476,482), and it has been argued above that all of the available evidence suggests that testosterone exerts its supportive effect on spermatogenesis via effects at stage VII and perhaps stage VIII of the spermatogenic cycle. Therefore, the obvious prediction would be that, following testosterone withdrawal, there would be a progressive increase with time in the number of degenerating germ cells at stages VII–VIII and that spermatogenesis would fail because of the inability of germ cells to pass successfully through this "window" or "gate," leading to progressive maturation depletion of germ cells. In fact, this is not what happens. The number of degenerating germ cells at stage VII does increase progressively from day 4 to day 8 after testosterone withdrawal induced by EDS (Fig. 16), but the number of germ cells thus affected is still only a small proportion of those present in the epithelium (Fig. 15). However, what does happen with increasing time of testosterone withdrawal is the appearance of degenerating germ cells at the stages following VII and VIII, and there is a rapid and progressive increase in their numbers, such that by day 8 the number of degenerating germ cells at stages X and XI far exceeds that at stage VII (Fig. 16). Indeed, >80% of the elongating (step 10–12) spermatids are either absent or degenerating by day 8 (Fig. 15), and the current conclusion is that spermatogenesis fails because of the degeneration of germ cells in the stages **following** VII–VIII (482). Remarkably, whilst all of this germ cell degeneration is occurring, seminiferous tubules in the first half of the spermatogenic cycle exhibit normal morphology, a normal germ cell complement, and virtually no degenerating germ cells (Figs. 15 and 16).

Do these observations mean that testosterone is exerting effects at stages of the spermatogenic cycle other than VII–VIII? The answer is almost certainly No. Careful inspection of the time course of appearance of degenerating germ cells at stages IX–XIV (Fig. 17) reveals why. Calculation of the time taken for germ cells to pass through stage VII (without testosterone support) and to reach a subsequent stage coincides with the time of appearance of degenerating germ cells at these later stages —in other words, germ cells degenerate at stage XI as a delayed consequence of testosterone not acting as normal at stage VII. Perhaps the easiest way to imagine this is to think again about the concept of a car production line that was introduced at the start of this chapter. As the car (i.e., germ cell) passes through workshop VII various changes are made to it under the influence of testosterone; e.g., the car has its doors fitted. When the car reaches workshop XI it is due to have the windows fitted into the doors, and in workshop XII they fit the door handles. If the door has not been fitted to the car in workshop VII, because of the absence of testosterone, then these subsequent events cannot occur in workshops XI and XII. The deficient cars are therefore scrapped when they reach these workshops, or in the case of germ cells, they are phagocytosed by the Sertoli cells.

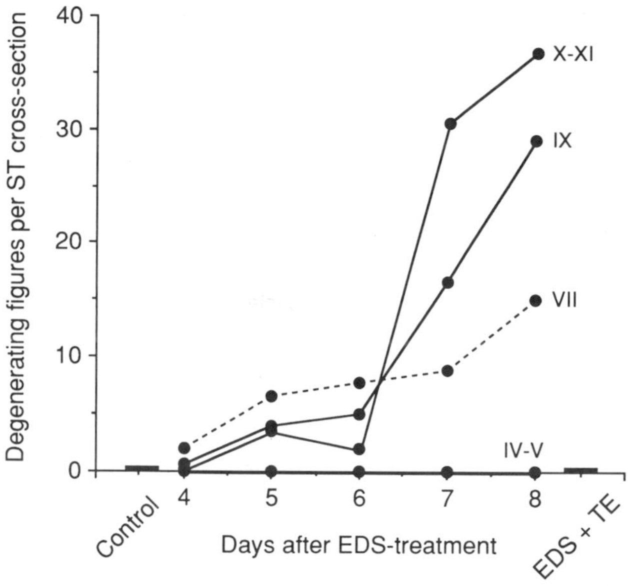

FIG. 16. Stage-dependent changes in the number of degenerating germ cells per seminiferous tubule (ST) cross section in control rats, rats treated 4 to 8 days earlier with ethane dimethane sulfonate (EDS), or rats treated 6 days earlier with EDS and supplemented every 3 days with 25 mg testosterone esters (EDS + TE); the latter treatment maintained normal testicular weight and tubule diameter (35). Note that degenerating germ cells are first evident at stage VII but appear progressively with time after EDS treatment in the stages following stage VII; stages IV–V are unaffected. Treatment with TE prevents the appearance of degenerating germ cells at all of the stages shown. It should be keep in mind that although degenerating germ cells probably provide the most sensitive index of testosterone withdrawal, this measure does not take into account germ cells that have degenerated earlier and been phagocytosed. Thus, at 8 days after EDS treatment, many of the germ cells at stages XI–XII (especially the elongating spermatids) have already disappeared (see Fig. 15). (This figure is based on data from Kerr et al., ref. 482, and *error bars* have been omitted for the sake of clarity.)

This interpretation presupposes that stages VII–VIII are workshops rather than "gates," as the majority of germ cells entering stages VII and VIII are able to pass through irrespective of the presence or absence of testosterone; i.e., there is no gate "shut" in the absence of testosterone. However, it must be remembered that as more and more germ cells degenerate in stages VII–XIV, including early and later spermatocytes (475), then fewer germ cells will pass through into stages I–VI and eventually through again to stage VII. Thus, it can be envisaged how spermatogenesis gradually and progressively winds down. It may well be, also, that this gradual attrition of germ cells at the various stages, including stage VII, will lead to secondary abnormal changes in Sertoli cell function, as there is abundant evidence for such effects (17,21–23). In their turn, these changes may result in inadequate support for the germ cells still present at that stage, thus predisposing them to degenerate then or at a later stage. Although there is no direct evidence that this chain of abnormal events occurs, it is a likely scenario based on several pieces of indirect information.

First, in man and other primates administered low-dose testosterone or other treatment to induce azoospermia, suppression of sperm production is not sudden but involves a progressive decrease with time in sperm output (186,529,636,637). Second, in seasonally breeding animals such as the hamster, sheep, and deer, it is clear that at the end of the breeding season the withdrawal of pituitary hormone (LH, FSH, and prolactin) support leads to slow but progressive winding down of spermatogenesis (168,173,406,407; reviewed in ref. 208); indeed, in the nonbreeding season complete spermatogenesis may still occur in some species, but it is always inefficient and low-key, whereas in other species virtually all germ cells other than spermatogonia disappear (168,184,638,639; reviewed in ref. 208). Similarly, during puberty in the laboratory rat the most mature germ cells present at any particular time show widespread de-

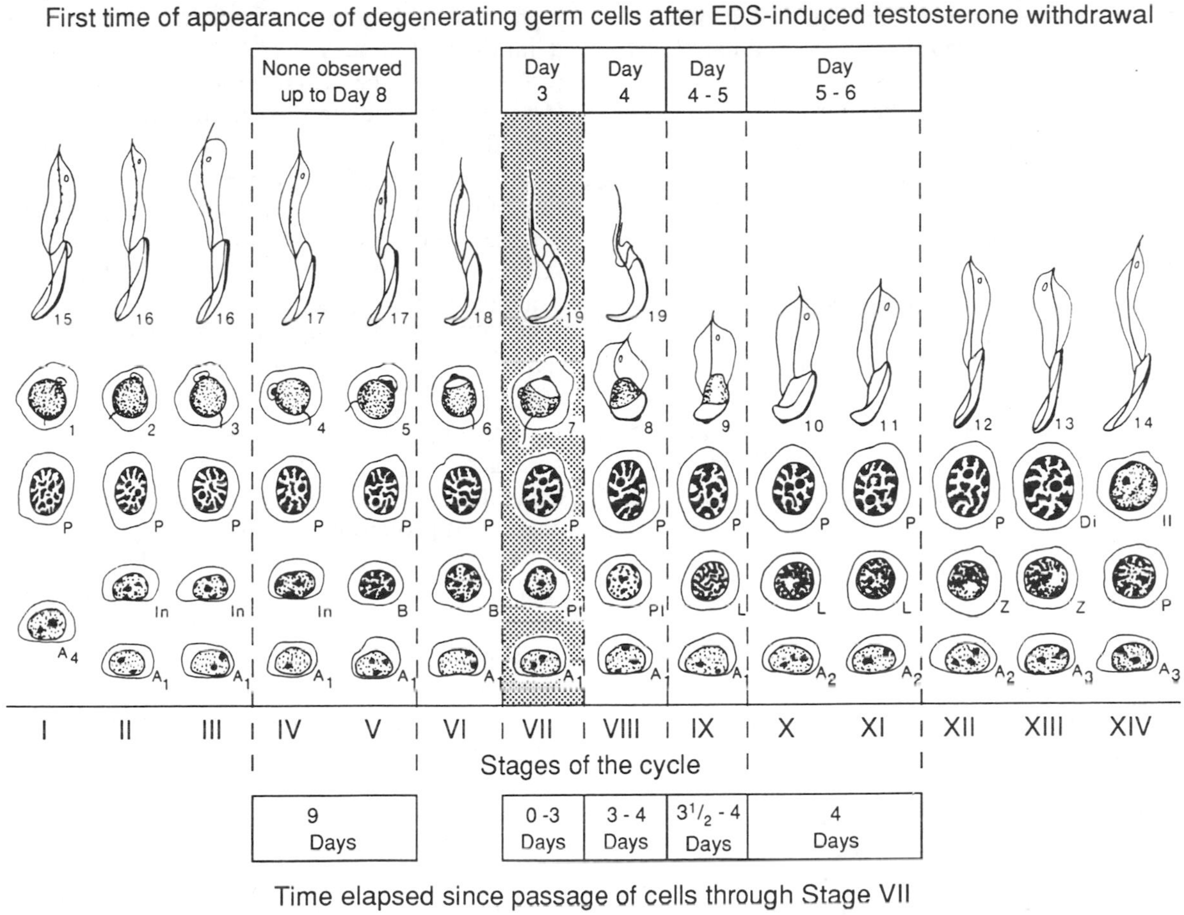

FIG. 17. Temporal appearance of abnormally degenerating germ cells following EDS-induced testosterone withdrawal in adult rats, shown in relation to the stages of the spermatogenic cycle. Note that, following EDS-induced destruction of the Leydig cells, testosterone levels take 24–30 hours to decline to <10% of control levels (412), and this probably accounts for the difference in timing between the first appearance of degenerating germ cells (*top time scale*) and the time elapsed since passage of these cells through stage VII (*bottom time scale*). Note also that, following EDS-induced testosterone withdrawal, the effects on androgen-dependent protein secretion by seminiferous tubules at stages VI–VIII are first evident on day 3 but are not maximal until day 4 after EDS treatment (190); this may account for the progressive increase with time in the numbers of degenerating germ cells evident at the different stages (Fig. 16).

generation (29), presumably because the required functions of the Sertoli cell are not yet working optimally. The latter presumably improve progressively with increase in the germ cell complement (21–23) so that the process "winds up" progressively to its maximum. Probably the best overall description of these changes is the **efficiency** of spermatogenesis. This has more than theoretical relevance. As was discussed earlier, qualitatively complete spermatogenesis can be maintained by subnormal levels of testosterone in a number of species, but quantitative maintenance requires normal (i.e., higher) levels of testosterone. The difference between these two situations is presumably one of efficiency. With high levels of testosterone, Sertoli cell function is maintained at normal levels, which allows the full normal complement of germ cells to develop successfully, whereas lower levels of testosterone will lead to suboptimal Sertoli cell function such that only a proportion of the germ cells present are able to complete their development successfully. The presence of a normal germ cell complement under optimal conditions of hormonal support may also have a "reinforcing effect" on Sertoli cell function, and this may be reduced dose-dependently (dose meaning the number of germ cells) when subnormal numbers of germ cells are present (21,22). Similar arguments probably apply to FSH (see below) except the effects of this hormone are manifest at different stages from those of testosterone. It is also likely that differences between species in the degree of shutdown of hormonal support for spermatogenesis in the nonbreeding season may partly explain differences in the degree of suppression of spermatogenesis (208).

It must also be kept in mind that even though qualitatively complete spermatogenesis can be maintained by suboptimal levels of intratesticular testosterone, this does not necessarily mean that the spermatozoa that develop under such conditions are normal. This has not been the subject of extensive studies, but evidence from the rat (640) and ram (540) suggest that many of the spermatozoa produced under these conditions may have morphological (especially nuclear) defects, though the evidence from functional studies is more equivocal (641). Data for man are equally ambiguous; ejaculated spermatozoa from men in whom severe oligospermia had been induced by testosterone enanthate (for contraceptive purposes) showed subnormal penetration of hamster oocytes *in vitro* (488,642), yet in some instances such men were still able to initiate pregnancies in their partners (643).

Alternative Methods of Testosterone Support for Spermatogenesis

Current dogma assumes that testosterone supports spermatogenesis (i.e., germ cell development) indirectly via the peritubular and Sertoli cells, as these are the only cells in the seminiferous tubule that possess androgen receptors (575,576,579). This assumption does not fit well with what is known about testosterone levels in the testis (see above) (591,596), and, on conceptual grounds, it could be argued that it is rather nonsensical for testosterone **not** to act directly on the germ cells. Evidence is beginning to emerge (591,596,644,645) that demands that we give this possibility more serious consideration. In the past, there has been intense debate about whether or not germ cells possess androgen receptors (646–649), though the clear consensus now is that they do not (579,591,648). However, attention has now switched to deciding whether testosterone might also act via androgen-receptor-independent mechanisms, either via interactions directly with the cell membrane of germ cells (or Sertoli cells), which then alter events such as calcium uptake (591,596,645), or via membrane receptors for androgen-binding protein (ABP) (591,644). There is as yet no direct evidence for the former in the testis, but there is growing evidence for a role for ABP.

ABP has been known for a long time and, like sex hormone-binding globulin (SHBG), its counterpart in peripheral blood in man, was generally thought to play a role in "buffering" the supply of testosterone or in transporting this steroid to the head of the epididymis (240,367,650,651). In addition there was some evidence that ABP could bind reversibly to a testicular protein (652) or to germ cells (653,654), and there was immunohistochemical evidence that SHBG might be taken up or localized in particular tissues of monkeys including the testis (655). More recent evidence suggests strongly that high-affinity binding sites for SHBG/ABP are present in a number of tissues (644,656) including the prostate (657–659) and testicular germ cells from both the rat (660) and monkey (661). On the basis of studies in the prostate and prostatic cell lines it appears that the ABP receptor is coupled to adenylate cyclase and that interaction of ABP with its receptor and activation of adenylate cyclase are modulated by the binding of steroid to the ABP (644,656,658,659,662,663). No evidence is yet available as to whether the same cascade exists in germ cells, although they endocytose ABP via coated pits (661) as happens with other membrane receptors, and the germ cells clearly possess adenylate cyclase and a variety of modulators of cAMP production (19,236,664) and action (665,666) as well as exhibiting stage-dependent differences in expression of cyclic AMP-dependent protein kinases (667).

At present we do not know the physiological significance of these findings, but there is indirect evidence that suggests that ABP could be of fundamental importance. To begin with, in the rat, ABP is secreted in substantially higher amounts by seminiferous tubules at stages VII–VIII of the spermatogenic cycle than at stages XIV–VI (668), and measurement of the mRNA levels for ABP also fits this picture (275). Thus, the secretion of ABP is highest at the androgen-dependent stages (see above and Table 5). There is also evidence that links the production rate of ABP to the rate of sperm production and/or their fertilizing ability in rats (650,669–671) and hamsters (672). However, there are a number of other possible explanations for the latter association, including the regulation by elongate spermatids (spermatozoa) of ABP production (66,68,69,260,673) and the secretion of STF (66,67). However, the fact that both of these secretory processes are apparently maximal at stages VII–VIII (see above) and both are at least under some degree of control by testosterone (333,343,367,650) perhaps suggests that they are associated for a reason rather than by accident.

ABP is produced in the testes of a number of species in addition to the rat, including the hamster (672), guinea pig (672), rabbit (675), ram (676,731), bull (650), cynomolgus monkey (677,678), and man (679–681). ABP and SHBG are coded for by the same gene (682–684), and screening of a human testicular cDNA library using a cDNA for SHBG identified that, in addition to the presence of an mRNA for SHBG/ABP, there were two other mRNAs derived by alternative splicing (651); the function of the proteins coded for by these mRNAs is unknown. Important changes take place developmentally in the production of ABP (240,321), and data for the rat (322) and monkey (678), suggest that intratesticular levels of ABP increase during puberty and into adulthood. ABP is secreted bidirectionally by the Sertoli cell (245), and this changes progressively during puberty (17,245,246); a different pattern is observed for the blood levels of ABP in the rat compared to testicular levels, as ABP levels in plasma decline progressively from about 15–20 days of age onwards (247,322,685). All of these data on testicular ABP are consistent with it having a role in spermatogenesis, though on present evidence this is only a possibility. However, it could be envisaged that transport of testosterone to the germ cells bound to ABP or the interaction of testosterone with ABP in the vicinity of germ cells could play a role in germ cell development, and such effects would probably be stage dependent (see Fig. 18). It will be an important task for researchers in this area to put this idea to the test by providing definitive evidence as to whether or not ABP plays an essential role in spermatogenesis.

The Role of FSH in the Adult

Similar to the story of intratesticular levels, there have been many arguments over the past 20 years as to whether FSH is or is not required for full normal spermatogenesis in the adult male (36). It seems likely that much of the disagreement can now be resolved, but it is probably informative to restate the principal findings that have contributed to the debate about the role of FSH in the adult male.

The first centers on a major difference between rodents and nonhuman primates in their response to suppression of FSH levels. Active or passive immunoneutralization of endogenous FSH using antibodies to FSH or its β subunit has little or no impact on spermatogenesis in rats (686,687), whereas in nonhuman primates it results in considerable (though generally incomplete) suppression of spermatogenesis and sperm output (688–693,733). In normal men in whom endogenous FSH levels are grossly suppressed, testosterone alone (via hCG injection) is able to stimulate qualitatively normal sperm production, but, quantitatively, sperm output is subnormal (223) but can be returned to within the control range by the coadministration of FSH (487). Based on what we know now, this radically different response between primates and rats can probably be explained by FSH-dependent differences in the regulation of spermatogonial stem cell divisions (as discussed earlier in this chapter). Indeed, in the adult rat the available evidence suggests that FSH may have only a minor role to play in regulating the number of B-spermatogonia available for entry into meiosis, although in view of this role, it might still be anticipated that suppression of FSH levels would have some negative impact on sperm output. Careful inspection of the data suggests that there is such a decrease. Passive immunization of adult rats against FSH results in about a 10% decrease in testicular weight, germ cell numbers, and sperm output (686,687). Suppression of endogenous FSH secretion either by injecting high doses of testosterone (191) or by active immunization against GnRH (459) also results in a similar shortfall in

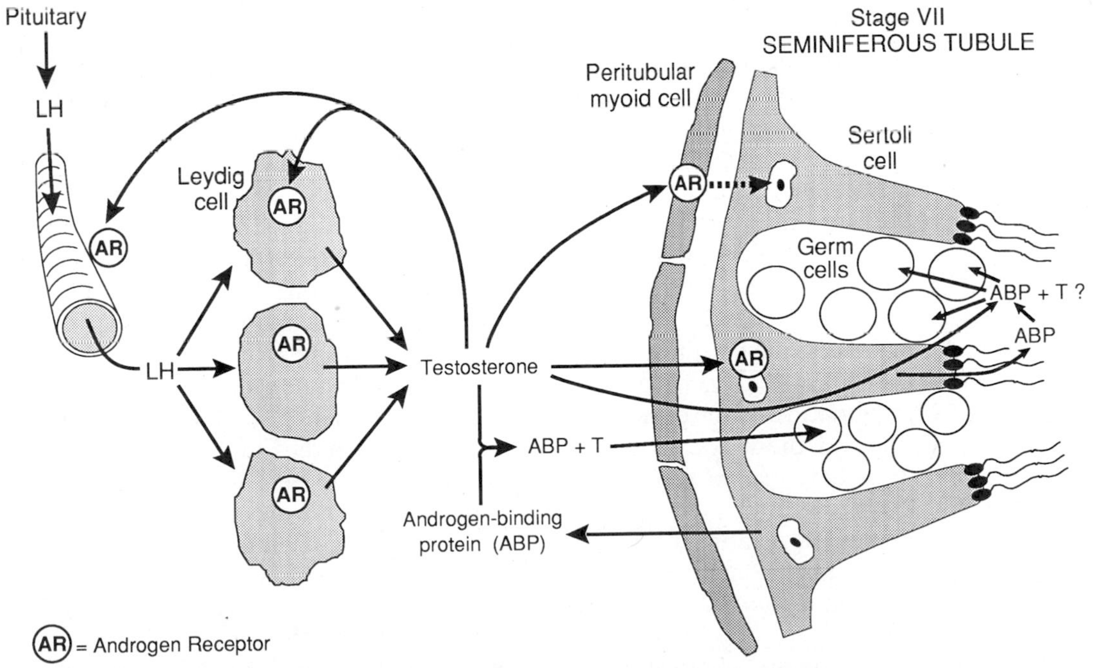

FIG. 18. Schematic diagram illustrating the possible sites of testosterone (T) action in the rat testis based on the distribution of androgen receptors and the secretion of androgen-binding protein by Sertoli cells in a stage VII seminiferous tubule. Note that ABP is secreted from the Sertoli cell into both seminiferous tubule fluid around the germ cells and, via the base of the Sertoli cell, into interstitial fluid around the Leydig cells.

sperm output despite the maintenance of high intratesticular levels of testosterone, and similar data exist for the rabbit (484).

Therefore, the differences between rats and primates in their response to FSH suppression appears to be explicable by the different effects of this hormone during the spermatogonial phase. Despite this difference, testosterone (or hCG) alone can maintain qualitatively complete spermatogenesis in the rat (see Table 3), man (484,486), and monkeys (185), though there may be some exceptions to the latter (690). It has also not been tested whether administration of particularly high levels of testosterone to monkeys or to man with suppressed FSH levels might override their dependence on FSH and maintain spermatogenesis quantitatively (36); however, the logical expectation would be that this would not work.

The other experimental situation that has been touted widely as evidence for the FSH dependence of spermatogenesis in the adult is the effect of hypophysectomy. However, in this situation data for rodents and primates are remarkably similar (Tables 3 and 4), which is rather incongruous considering their rather different responses to the selective suppression of FSH outlined above. In all species of mammals that have been investigated, hypophysectomy results in regression of spermatogenesis over the ensuing 3 to 6 weeks, and though the administration of testosterone is able to maintain qualitatively complete spermatogenesis in most hypophysectomized animals, not even in the rat is spermatogenesis maintained quantitatively (see Tables 3 and 4 and associated discussion). This statement should be qualified by reiterating that doses of testosterone that would restore normal intratesticular levels of this steroid have not been administered in most studies using hypophysectomized animals. Nevertheless, where comparable doses of testosterone have been administered to hypophysectomized and intact animals (mainly rats), spermatogenesis is always maintained better in the intact animals (Tables 3 and 4). Although this could reflect differences in FSH levels, this suggestion does not stand up to scrutiny. First, many (but not all) of the studies involving the administration of testosterone or hCG to intact animals (26,35,191,467) or men (222,485–487,694) reported very low or nondetectable FSH levels. Second, and more convincingly, when the secretion of FSH (and LH) is suppressed selectively in adult rats by active immunization against GnRH, spermatogenesis is maintained more effectively by testosterone implants than it is in hypophysectomized rats by comparable sized implants (423,459) (see Table 3).

There are many studies involving the administration of FSH, with or without LH or testosterone, to hypophysectomized adult rats. These show that FSH, on its own, cannot support qualitatively complete spermatogenesis for anything other than a brief period of time (28,449,451,476,695–697), whereas administration of FSH together with LH or testosterone augments the supportive effects of LH or testosterone on spermatogenesis (28,331,395,449,464,697,698). Data obtained for the ram (193), for the cynomolgus monkey (734), and for man (381,694) are in broad agreement with these findings in the rat. However, there are a number of drawbacks to most of these studies that render their interpretation less than straightforward. Many of the older studies used FSH preparations (or PMSG) that were contaminated significantly by small amounts of LH; this could stimulate low levels of testosterone production, which would synergize (see below) with the FSH to support spermatogenesis. This would cast some doubt on findings involving FSH treatment alone. Now that highly pure FSH preparations and recombinant FSH are available, this problem can be avoided, and, reassuringly, highly pure FSH does appear to have similar supportive effects on spermatogenesis in hypophysectomized rats as in older studies (464). Or does it? There are two further related problems that also affect interpretation of these findings, and both have been touched on earlier in this chapter. The first is the presence of Leydig cells in hypophysectomized rats and their continued secretion of testosterone in low but significant amounts for many weeks after hypophysectomy in the absence of LH (397,429,443). This testosterone undoubtedly has a significant influence in maintaining some degree of spermatogenesis because when the Leydig cells are destroyed with EDS (449), or when action of the testosterone is blocked in GnRH antagonist-treated rats with an antiandrogen (451), there is a marked drop in testicular weight and impairment of spermatogenesis. However, even in both of these situations FSH is still able to exert a stimulatory effect on spermatogenesis. The second problem is related and involves the well-described effects of FSH in stimulating Leydig cell development and differentiation, discussed in detail earlier in this chapter. Clearly such an effect can be of considerable importance in interpreting the observed effects of FSH on spermatogenesis, especially when the FSH is coadministered with LH or is contaminated with low levels of LH.

The consequences of the above arguments are that many of the studies in animals other than the rat, in which either impure FSH (or PMSG) was administered or in which the Leydig cells remained intact (this applies to every study), need to be interpreted with the above facts in mind. This includes all of the data for man (222,381,485). In physiological terms these concerns are almost certainly irrelevant, as the normal adult testis is rarely, if ever, exposed to FSH in the absence of LH, and Leydig cells are present in one form or another throughout all but the early stages of fetal life. However, the concerns are of relevance to the interpretation of past findings and, indeed, to the resolution of long-standing arguments about the importance of FSH in normal spermatogenesis.

Another problem that affects interpretation of the data for FSH is the duration of its administration. In the vast majority of the studies cited, FSH has been administered for only 2 or 3 weeks, far less than the duration of the process of spermatogenesis. As with the administration of suboptimal doses of testosterone, the effects of FSH over this short time period are likely to be exaggerated because, in effect, FSH administration has delayed or slowed down the regression of spermatogenesis caused by testosterone withdrawal. This has been demonstrated most clearly, but in different ways, in recent studies in rats (451) and GnRH-antagonist-treated cynomolgus monkeys (734). The latter study showed simply that as the duration of treatment with a highly pure preparation of FSH increased from 0 to 8 weeks, the number of meiotic and postmeiotic germ cells **declined** progressively. The second study involved administration of the same FSH preparation for only 2 weeks to GnRH-antagonist-treated rats (451). Although this treatment maintained near-normal numbers of germ cells at stage VII of the spermatogenic cycle, testicular weight was reduced, and the number of degenerating germ cells was increased; the latter in particular has been argued earlier as being the most sensitive index of suboptimal support of spermatogenesis. Indeed, in this study, blockade of androgen action by flutamide in FSH-treated rats largely wiped out all of the apparent supportive effects of FSH on germ cell counts, implying that even these apparent effects of FSH were mediated by effects on the Leydig cells via the mechanisms outlined above.

Interactions Between FSH and Testosterone

Experiments that would definitively identify the importance of FSH relative to testosterone in supporting spermatogenesis have not been done. Ideally, a range of doses of testosterone should be administered for 8 to 12 weeks with or without purified FSH to GnRH-antagonist-treated adult animals. In this way it could be evaluated whether spermatogenesis could be maintained **quantitatively** by lower doses of testosterone in the presence of FSH than could be achieved in the absence of FSH. At present we know that in intact adult rats, spermatogenesis can be maintained for long periods at >95% of normal levels with high doses of testosterone in the near absence of FSH (26,191) (see Table 3). However, this does not prove that FSH is not important, as these studies did not evaluate whether **lower** doses of testosterone would have maintained spermatogenesis just as effectively as a higher dose if FSH were present. Two recent studies in hypophysectomized adult rats (449,464) provide evidence that supports this possibility, though neither study extended beyond 3 weeks, and both also had one or more of the other limitations described above. Both studies showed clearly that combined treatment with FSH and a relatively low dose of testosterone supported spermatogenesis far better than did either treatment alone; in one study the FSH was a highly purified preparation (464), whereas in the other study the animals lacked Leydig cells (449). The latter study also quantified the effects of the various treatments at different stages of the spermatogenic cycle. This showed that the effect of FSH was manifest up to stage VI of the spermatogenic cycle, whereas progression of the meiotic and postmeiotic germ cells beyond stage VI was largely dependent on the presence of testosterone, in keeping with more detailed findings that were described earlier (see Fig. 17). These findings are consistent with a wide range of other data from hypophysectomized or GnRH-antagonist-treated rats treated with FSH ± LH or testosterone (28,73,451,462,472,695,698). The data on the stage specificity of FSH action in spermatogenesis are also consistent with the stage-dependent expression of FSH receptors (234,235,699) and FSH responsiveness of the Sertoli cell in the adult rat (236,237,699,700).

A summary diagram that puts together the above data on FSH action in the adult rat with that which was elucidated earlier for testosterone is illustrated in Fig. 19. It remains unknown to what extent this scheme might apply to other species, although, in view of the fact that spermatogenesis is regulated primarily by testosterone and FSH in all mammalian species that we know of, it is likely that the principles of the scheme may apply to most species (193,362,487), even if the detail does not. In this respect it should be kept in mind that one of the important effects of FSH in primates is on the replication of spermatogonial stem cells, as discussed earlier, an effect that is not represented in Fig. 19, as it does not occur in the rat. However, what Fig. 19 should make clear is how FSH and testosterone can have synergistic effects on spermatogenesis; i.e., FSH increases the availability of germ cells at four different steps of development (B-spermatogonia, pachytene spermatocytes, step 6 spermatids, step 18 spermatids) for entry into the androgen-dependent phase (stages VII–VIII). Under the influence of testosterone, these cells safely negotiate this and the subsequent stages (IX–XIV) (or in the case of the step 19 spermatids are released) so that most of these germ cells reach stage XIV and then pass into their next phase of FSH dependence, and so on. This sort of scheme also has appeal in explaining seasonal regression of spermatogenesis and its variability between species (208), with the degree of FSH and testosterone withdrawal determining both the degree of regression and the step(s) at which spermatogenic arrest does or does not occur.

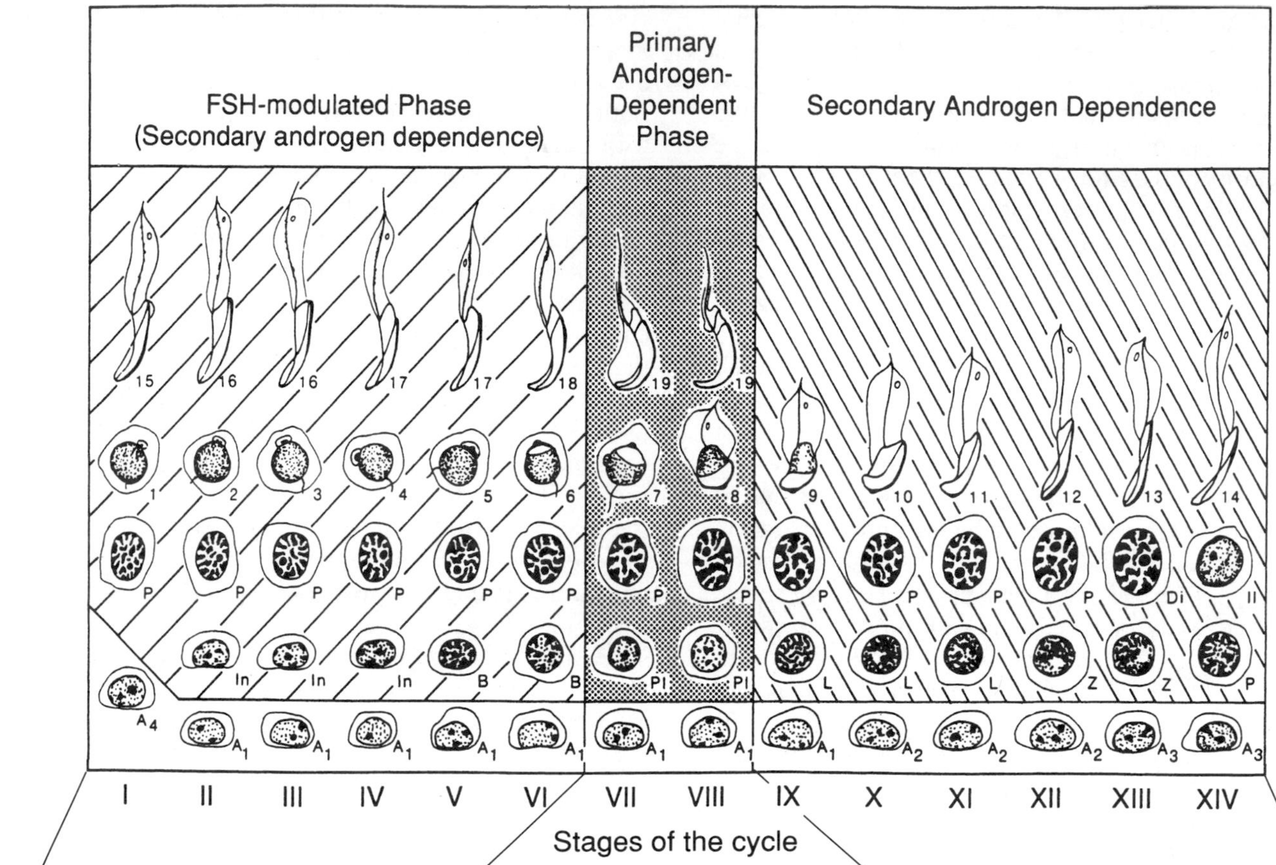

• Some of the events in these stages are probably FSH-modulated rather than being *absolutely* FSH dependent in the rat, though this may vary between species.
• FSH may regulate the number of B-spermatogonia that enter meiosis and can support limited development of spermatids up to step 6.
• Successful passage of nonspermatogonial germ cells through these stages is largely dependent on their having undergone androgen-regulated changes during their last passage through stages VII–VIII.
• FSH receptor numbers and especially FSH responsiveness of the Sertoli cells are high during these stages.

• Each of the non-spermatogonial germ cells undergoes changes in structure and/or function that are androgen regulated. These changes are *essential* prerequisites for other programmed changes that are due to happen in stages IX–XIV and to a lesser extent in stages I–VI.
• Possible programmed events affected are:
PL, DNA synthesis, translocation; *P,* RNA synthesis, completion of meiosis; *step 7–8,* nuclear condensation, elongation; *step 19,* final cytoplasmic elimination (RB formation), release from the Sertoli cell.

• Changes to the non-spermatogonial germ cells during these stages are dependent on prior androgen-regulated changes during their last passage through stages VII–VIII.
• Particularly vulnerable are the step 9–14 spermatids and the meiotically dividing spermatocytes at stage XIV.

FIG. 19. Summary diagram illustrating the probable stage dependence of the effects of FSH and testosterone on spermatogenesis in the adult rat.

It is implicit in this scheme that it is the changing germ cell complement from stage to stage that determines the alterations in hormonal responsiveness of the Sertoli cells (or of the germ cells or peritubular cells), and all of the available evidence supports this contention (17,19). Furthermore, this imposition of stage-dependent hormonal control on the spermatogenic cycle should not be viewed as indicating that every function of the Sertoli cells within stages I–VI is different from that in stages VII–VIII and from stages IX–XIV, because this is clearly not the case. Some functions of the Sertoli cell (e.g., the secretion of SGP-1 and SGP-2) remain more or less constant throughout the different stages and appear to be under little or no influence of age (329,701) or hormonal status or the germ cell complement (190,397,458,608). Other functions of the Sertoli cell, such as the secretion of cyclic protein-2 (CP-2), straddle the FSH- and androgen-dependent phases, as expression of the CP-2 gene and secretion of the protein product occur in stages IV–VII of the spermatogenic cycle (701–704).

The synergistic effects of FSH and testosterone on spermatogenesis can probably be explained by the scheme depicted in Fig. 18 without the need for any biochemical changes, e.g., FSH induction of responsiveness to testosterone. However, the latter possibility should not be excluded. In cultures of Sertoli cells from immature rats, exposure to FSH can increase levels of the mRNA for the androgen receptor and levels of the receptor itself (346–349). It is unknown whether this finding has any relevance to the adult, as there are no major stage-specific differences in the level of androgen receptors in isolated seminiferous tubules (275,592) that can account for the altered androgen responsiveness of stages VII–VIII (190), although there are older reports (705,706) that suggested that FSH was able to increase uptake of testosterone by adult rat seminiferous tubules *in vivo* and *in vitro*. As discussed earlier in this chapter, there are also a range of basic key functions of the Sertoli cell, such as the secretion of STF and proteins such as ABP, that switch during puberty from being predominantly FSH regulated to being predominantly testosterone regulated, so it may yet prove that, in the adult, both hormones together might regulate these functions more effectively than does testosterone on its own. Effects of FSH on the number or size of Leydig cells, as discussed earlier, should also be kept in mind when considering synergism between FSH and LH (or testosterone).

Brief mention should be made about the reinitiation of spermatogenesis in the adult under experimental conditions. This topic has been dealt with earlier in this chapter, especially in relation to seasonal breeding. However, in the context of the scheme presented in Fig. 19, a little more discussion is probably relevant. The available evidence for the rat (396–398,474), the rabbit (484), monkeys (185,186,707), and man (28,223,486) is that once spermatogenesis has regressed (as a result of hypophysectomy, GnRH antagonist administration, or steroid-induced suppression of gonadotropin secretion), it can be reinitiated by testosterone (or LH/hCG) alone, but never as effectively as if the testosterone (or LH/hCG) had been administered immediately to prevent regression of spermatogenesis. After regression of spermatogenesis, administration of FSH (or hMG) or elevation of endogenous FSH levels before or concomitant with the administration of testosterone (or LH/hCG) appears to be able to restore spermatogenesis more effectively than administration of the testosterone (or LH/hCG) alone (28,223,395,468,474,487,732). Data from hypogonadotropic men treated with various gonadotropin preparations alone or together (381,382, 708,709) are in general agreement with these findings, although in these men it is initiation rather than reinitiation of spermatogenesis that is involved, and there may be differences between these two situations (see below and ref. 694).

What the above data may mean is that once most of the layers of different germ cell types at each stage have been lost, programming of Sertoli cell functions is altered to the extent that, for example in the rat, germ cell survival during passage through stages I–VI becomes far more dependent on hormonal (FSH) stimulation than is the case when complete spermatogenesis is up and running. Consistent with this interpretation, our own unpublished evidence is that when two layers of germ cells are depleted from a tubule, there are dramatic changes in Sertoli cell secretory function that are not evident when either layer of germ cells is depleted on its own. Therefore, when full normal spermatogenesis is established, essential supporting functions of the Sertoli cell that are both hormonally and germ-cell regulated (secretion of STF, ABP, total protein, inhibin, etc., as discussed earlier) may be less critically hormone dependent than when these functions have to be initiated from scratch (when most germ cells are not present). Data from both normal and hypogonadotropic men fully support this interpretation (694), although in man and other primates the ability of FSH to increase replication of the self-renewing spermatogonia could be a critically important factor.

The Role of Other Hormones

From the preceding discussions it should be apparent to the reader that FSH and LH (working via stimulation of testosterone) are the major and almost exclusive regulators of spermatogenesis, and, apart from prolactin, there is very little direct evidence that other hormones play any important modulatory roles in the adult. The situation may be somewhat different during prepuberty and puberty, when general metabolic factors such as thyroid hormone and growth hormone may have effects on testicular development, especially on Sertoli cell replication. These have been discussed already. However, it must be presumed that these hormones also exert basic supportive effects on cell metabolism (primarily of the Sertoli cell) in the adult testis, so their importance cannot be dismissed, although this is more likely to be of significance in disease states involving gross changes in the level of these hormones.

Prolactin

Brief mention has already been made of the role that prolactin may play, especially in seasonally breeding animals (208,407,710,711), where it may act as one of the seasonal cues for switching reproductive activity on or off. These effects of prolactin, and the consequent changes in spermatogenesis, are caused primarily by altered secretion of gondadotropins by the pituitary gland (see Chapter 27–35, *this volume*), although in species such as the hamster (375,376) and rat (378), prolactin can also exert modulatory effects on the number of Leydig cell LH receptors. In general, the effect of prolactin is to increase the number of LH receptors and hence increase sensitivity of the Leydig cells to LH stimulation. Hyperprolactinemia is commonly associated with infertility in both females (Weiner et al., Chapter 29, *this volume*) and males (712,713) and usually results from a prolactin-secreting tumor. In hyperprolactinemic men there are abnormalities of spermatogenesis, which can be severe, (714,715), but these appear to be a consequence of reduced LH secretion and hence reduced testosterone levels (712,716); as a consequence, most of the men are also impotent. Normal testicular size, function, and sperm output usually resume when prolactin levels are normalized by treatment (716). Therefore, the available data indicate that irrespective of whether the effects oı prolactin on spermatogenesis in man and animals involve testicular (Leydig cells) or central (pituitary gland) effects, all of the changes in spermatogenesis appear to be a consequence of altered testosterone secretion.

Oxytocin

Oxytocin is produced at various points along the male reproductive tract, including the testis, as well as by the posterior pituitary gland (726). The available evidence suggests that oxytocin is produced by the Leydig cells and that its secretion exerts a paracrine influence on contractility of the peritubular myoid cells in the rat and mouse (717,718). However, destruction and removal of all of the Leydig cells from the adult rat testis using EDS, which clearly results in the loss of oxytocin (719), has very little if any effect on spermatogenesis **provided** that high intratesticular levels of testosterone are maintained by exogenous administration (191). However, what the latter study did observe was that there was a two- to threefold increase in the number of degenerating meiotic spermatocytes at stages XIV–I; this appeared to be related to the absence of oxytocin, as active immunization of adult rats against oxytocin caused a similar change. The physiological significance of these observations is unknown, but, as discussed earlier (see "Efficiency of Spermatogenesis"), germ cell degeneration during meiosis is a universal feature of mammalian spermatogenesis and is particularly prevalent in the human. A more recent study (203a) has shown quite dramatic changes in intratesticular and blood levels of testosterone (decreased) and DHT (increased) in rats with intratesticular oxytocin implants, though there were, surprisingly, no effects on spermatogenesis. These findings suggest that the role of oxytocin in testicular function merits closer scrutiny.

Insulin

The Sertoli cells control the environment of all non-spermatogonial germ cells, and one of the key requirements is energy, which the Sertoli cell provides primarily in the form of lactate and pyruvate rather than glucose (720,721), and this may be under the control of FSH, at least in the immature rat (722). Glucose appears to have detrimental effects on germ cells (723). Because insulin plays an important role in regulating glucose uptake and metabolism by all cells, including Sertoli cells (724,725), gross abnormalities in insulin production, as occur in diabetes, could have adverse effects on spermatogenesis. There are reports of such adverse effects in men with diabetes, though there are also reports that diabetes can be without any discernible effect on spermatogenesis and fertility (735). Experimentally induced diabetes in rodents results in abnormalities of spermatogenesis (727,728), though as in man it remains undecided whether these adverse changes are a consequence of altered gonadotropin secretion or altered glucose uptake/metabolism by the Sertoli cells.

CONCLUDING REMARKS

I began this chapter by urging that we redirect our research on spermatogenesis because of the relatively poor progress in our understanding when viewed from a historical perspective. Many many pages later, the reader may have forgotten my introduction and be thinking that we are at least beginning to get some idea of how spermatogenesis is regulated. In my opinion the emphasis should be on *beginning* because it does not take much digging to realize that our understanding is woefully superficial. We still do not know **how** FSH and, in particular, testosterone actually regulate spermatogenesis at the cellular and cell–cell level. Yet, remarkably, this is the area of biomedicine in which there has been an explosion of information in the past two decades. Unfortunately, it has been an explosion that has had little impact on our understanding. Why? The answer is simple: we have studied cellular regulation out of context, with the result that the information obtained cannot be fitted in confidently to any physiological picture or scheme that we might devise to explain the regulation of spermatogenesis. Indeed, there are probably readers who are grossly disappointed that I have not dissected apart the many different findings on this or that factor and the regulation of its production by immature rat Sertoli cells. This omission is deliberate—I simply do not know where to fit the information. For some of it I do not even feel confident that it will ever fit into any physiological scheme. These are hard words, and I know that they will not make agreeable reading to everyone, but if it forces the reader to prove me wrong then it will have been worthwhile, for I see no way that he or she can do it without starting at the whole-animal level rather than at the cellular level.

I am not calling for an end to *in vitro* work or to work on isolated cells; I am asking that we use these valuable approaches at the right time. The first task is to identify the physiological mechanism of interest and then to devise a way that this can be studied **within** that physiological context. Knowing that FSH has a role in spermatogenesis does not mean that once the Sertoli cell is isolated from the testis and from **all** of its neighboring cells, its FSH-responsive functions that occur during normal spermatogenesis will be preserved; indeed, the available evidence says that it will not. However, if it can be proved that this or that function is maintained in a physiological way **after** isolation, **then** isolated cells are both the most convenient and the most logical research approach to employ. But this is not the way that we do it. Instead, we identify some novel function of the isolated cell and **then** begin the task of fitting this into the physiological picture. This would not be unreasonable if our picture were a jigsaw with only 30 pieces to it, but we do not know how many pieces there are in the picture of spermatogenesis (though we would guess many hundred), and we do not even known that a "piece" of data obtained in the way just described will actually fit into the picture—its shape may change when it is placed alongside a neighboring piece.

We must also be more aware of studying hormonal effects out of context. The majority of studies that have endeavored to assess the roles of FSH and testosterone in spermatogenesis have studied them in isolation from each other or in situations in which physiological levels of both are not maintained. We cannot be at all confident that the results obtained under these conditions reflect the physiological situation. When nature has taken so many millenia to fashion spermatogenesis, we can be sure that multiple feedback, compensatory, and backup systems will be in place ready to operate under certain circumstances in an effort to maintain spermatogenesis. These may be activated under experimental conditions and obscure our understanding of the normal, physiological situation.

But what of the future? Despite what I have said above, I feel strongly that we are on the verge of a new understanding of spermatogenesis, and this breakthrough comes from the unlikely source of molecular biology. I say unlikely because molecular biology is really concerned with subcellular aspects of cell regulation, a focus that is potentially far worse than isolated cells in view of its "distance" from the testis as a functioning organ. However, it is *in situ* hybridization that is once again forcing researchers to look at the testis as a whole and, in so doing, to realize the beautiful, if complex, organization and control of spermatogenesis. This is an area that is about to take off, especially now that methods have been developed for *in situ* hybridization studies on the testis that preserve good morphology and permit **accurate** cellular, and even subcellular, localization of mRNAs (729). The amount of information gained from such studies (basic morphology, cellular sites of expression, stage dependency of gene expression, and, if prior treatments are applied, the hormonal regulation of gene expression and morphology) is far in advance of any other single research technique and yet involves a basically physiological approach. There is only one word of caution—detection of an mRNA does not necessarily mean that there is a protein product, a warning that appears to have particular relevance to the testis (730). However, as a front line, physiological approach, *in situ* hybridization studies are likely to initiate a quantum leap in our understanding of the regulation of spermatogenesis in the next 5 years.

In writing this chapter, one factor has cropped up time and time again and has forced me to recognize for the first time its potential importance—seminiferous tubule fluid (STF). Many readers, like myself, will have viewed STF primarily as a means of transporting spermatozoa, inhibin, ABP, etc., out of the testis. Although these functions are indisputable (see also Setchell, Chapter 20, *this volume*), I am now persuaded by the data that STF is perhaps the single most important factor in the regulation and maintenance of spermatogenesis. I will not reiterate the data on which this is based except to say that in virtually every situation in which spermatogenesis changes, whether during puberty, during seasonal regression of the testis, or in the failure of spermatogenesis after the withdrawal of testosterone, it is the secretion of STF that changes first. Maybe STF is just a transport medium, but nearly every messenger protein, nutrient, energy source, etc., has to be transported to the germ cells from the Sertoli cells, and STF is the major route via which this can occur (see Setchell, Chapter 20, *this volume*). It merits a lot more attention, and it is surely not a coincidence that such studies will have to be *in vivo* because STF production cannot yet be measured *in vitro*. This seems a particularly appropriate note on which to conclude this chapter.

ACKNOWLEDGMENTS

I thank my family, colleagues, and friends for their unstinting support while I was writing this chapter and, more importantly, for the data, ideas, discussions, and inspirations that provided the essential background for the concepts I have proposed. I thank Ted Pinner for preparing the figures and Mike Millar for help with the photomicrographs. Last, but certainly not least, I thank Madeleine Stevenson and Sandie Harley for their speed, skill, and perseverance with typing this chapter.

REFERENCES

1. Carlsen E, Giwercman A, Keiding N, Skakkebaek NE. Evidence for decreasing quality of semen during past 50 years. *Br Med J* 1992;305:609–613.
2. Giwercmann A, Skakkebaek NE. The human testis—an organ at risk? *Int J Androl* 1992;15:373–375.
3. Sharpe RM. Declining sperm counts in men—is there an endocrine cause? *J Endocrinol* 1993;136:357–360.
4. Sharpe RM, Skakkebaek NE. Are oestrogens involved in falling sperm counts and disorders of the reproductive tract? *Lancet* 1993;341:1392–1395.
5. de Graff R. On the human reproductive organs (1668). Translated by Jocelyn HD, Setchell BP (1972). *J Reprod Fertil Suppl* 17;1–122.
6. Bodemer C. The microscope in early embryological investigation. *Gynecol Invest* 1973;4:188–209.
7. Berthold AA. Transplantation der Hoden. *Arch Anat Physiol Wiss Med* 1849;16:42–46.
8. Bremner WJ. Historical aspects of the study of the testis. In: Burger H, de Kretser DM, eds. *The testis.* New York: Raven Press; 1981:1–5.
9. Butenandt A. Uber die chimische Untersuchung der Sexual hormone. *Z Angew Chem* 1931;44:905–911.
10. Smith PE. Maintenance and restoration of spermatogenesis in hypophysectomized rhesus monkeys by androgen administration. *Yale J Biol Med* 1944;17:283–287.
11. Smith PE. Hypophysectomy and a replacement therapy in the rat. *Am J Anat* 1930;45:205–256.
12. Walsh EL, Cuyler WK, McCullagh DR. Physiologic maintenance of male sex glands; effect of androtin on hypophysectomized rats. *Am J Physiol* 1934;107:508–512.
13. Nelson WO, Merckel CE. Maintenance of spermatogenesis in hypophysectomized mice with androgenic substances. *Proc Soc Exp Biol Med* 1938;38:737–740.
14. Greep RO, Fevold HL. The spermatogenic and secretory function of the gonads of hypophysectomized adult rats treated with pituitary FSH and LH. *Endocrinology* 1937;21:611–618.
15. Cutuly E, Cutuly EC. Observations on spermatogenesis in rats. *Endocrinology* 1940;26:503–507.
16. Ludwig DG. The effect of androgen on spermatogenesis. *Endocrinology* 1950;46:453–481.
17. Sharpe RM. Experimental evidence for Sertoli–germ cell and Sertoli–Leydig cell interactions. In: Russell LD, Griswold MD, eds. *The Sertoli cell.* Clearwater, Florida: Cache River Press; 1993:391–418.
18. Parvinen M, Vihko KK, Toppari J. Cell interactions during the seminiferous epithelial cycle. *Int Rev Cytol* 1986;104:105–119.
19. Parvinen M. Cyclic function of Sertoli cells. In: Russel LD, Griswold MD, eds. *The Sertoli cell.* Clearwater, Florida: Cache River Press; 1993:331–347.
20. Jégou B. Spermatids are regulators of Sertoli cell function. *Ann NY Acad Sci* 1991;637:340–353.
21. Jégou B. The Sertoli-germ cell communication network in mammals. *Int Rev Cytol* 1993; [*in press*].
22. Jégou B, Syed V, Sourdaine P. The dialogue between late spermatids and Sertoli cells: A century of research. In: Nieschlag E, Habenicht UF eds. *Spermatogenesis, fertilization, contraception.* Berlin: Springer-Verlag 1992;57–95.
23. Jégou B, Sharpe RM. Paracrine mechanisms in testicular control In: de Kretser DM, ed. *The Molecular Biology of the Male Reproductive System.* Academic Press, 1993;271–310.
24. Skinner MK. Cell–cell interactions in the testis. *Endocrine Rev* 1991;12:45–77.
25. Skinner MK. Secretion of growth factors and other regulatory factors. In: Russell LD, Griswold MD, ed. *The Sertoli cell.* Clearwater, Florida: Cache River Press; 1993:237–247.
26. Sharpe RM, Maddocks S, Kerr JB. Cell–cell interactions in the control of spermatogenesis as studied using Leydig cell destruction and testosterone replacement. *Am J Anat* 1990;188:3–20.
27. Sharpe RM. Intratesticular control of steroidogenesis. *Clin Endocrinol* 1990;33:787–807.
28. Steinberger E. Hormonal control of mammalian spermatogenesis. *Physiol Rev* 1971;51:1–23.
29. Russell LD, Alger LE, Nequin LG. Hormonal control of pubertal spermatogenesis. *Endocrinology* 1987;120:1615–1632.
30. Allenby G, Foster PMD, Sharpe RM. Evidence that secretion of immunoactive inhibin by seminiferous tubules from the adult rat testis is regulated by specific germ cell types: Correlation between *in vivo* and *in vitro* studies. *Endocrinology* 1991;128:467–476.
31. Roosen-Runge EC. Kinetics of spermatogenesis in mammals. *Ann NY Acad Sci* 1952;55:574–584.
32. Roosen-Runge EC. *The process of spermatogenesis in animals.* Cambridge: Cambridge University Press; 1977.
33. Sharpe RM. Testosterone and spermatogenesis. *J Endocrinol* 1987;113:1–2.
34. Rommerts FFG. How much androgen is required for maintenance of spermatogenesis? *J Endocrinol* 1988;116:7–9.
35. Sharpe RM, Donachie K, Cooper I. Re-evaluation of the intratesticular level of testosterone required for quantitative maintenance of spermatogenesis in the rat. *J Endocrinol* 1988; 117:19–26.
36. Sharpe RM. Follicle-stimulating hormone and spermatogenesis in the adult male. *J Endocrinol* 1989;121:405–407.
37. Clermont Y. The cycle of the seminiferous epithelium in man. *Am J Anat* 1963;112:35–51.
38. Leblond CP, Clermont Y. Definition of the stages of the cycle of the seminiferous epithelium in the rat. *Ann NY Acad Sci* 1952;55:548–573.
39. Dym M, Clermont Y. Role of spermatogonia in the repair of the seminiferous epithelium following X-irradiation of the rat testis. *Am J Anat* 1970;128:265–282.
40. Heller CG, Clermont Y. Kinetics of the germinal epithelium in man. *Recent Prog Horm Res* 1964;20:545–575.
41. Amann RP. A critical review of methods for evaluation of spermatogenesis from seminal characteristics. *J Androl* 1981; 2:37–58.
42. Clermont Y. Quantitative analysis of spermatogenesis of the rat: A revised model for the renewal of spermatogonia. *Am J Anat* 1962;111:111–129.
43. Paniagua R, Codesal J, Nistal M, Rodriguez MC, Santamaria L. Quantification of cell types throughout the cycle of the human seminiferous epithelium and their DNA content. *Anat Embryol* 1987;176:225–230.
44. Kerr JB. The cytology of the human testis. In: Burger H, de Kretser DM, eds. *The testis,* 2nd ed. New York: Raven Press; 1989:197–229.
45. Russell LD. Sertoli-germ cell interrelations—a review. *Gamete Res* 1980;3:179–202.
46. Russell LD. Morphological and functional evidence for Sertoli-germ cell relationships. In: Russel LD, Griswold MD. *The Sertoli cell.* Clearwater, Florida: Cache River Press; 1993:365–390.
47. Russell LD, Griswold MD (eds.). *The Sertoli cell.* Clearwater, Florida: Cache River Press; 1993.
48. Parvinen M, Soder O, Mali P, Froysa B, Ritzen EM. In vitro stimulation of stage-specific deoxyribonucleic acid synthesis in rat seminiferous tubule segments by Interleukin-1α. *Endocrinology* 1991;129:1614–1620.
49. Monesi V. Synthetic activities during spermatogenesis in the mouse, RNA and protein. *Exp Cell Res* 1965;39:197–224.
50. Monesi V, Geremia R, D'Agostino, Boitani C. Biochemistry of male germ cell differentiation in mammals: RNA synthesis in meiotic and postmeiotic cells. *Curr Top Dev Biol* 1978;12:11–36.
51. Tres LL, Kierszenbaum AL. Premeiotic and meiotic prophase RNA synthesis in human testes. In: Troen P, Nankin HR, ed. *The testis in normal and infertile men.* New York: Raven Press; 1977:9–23.
52. Roosen-Runge EC. Germinal cell loss in normal metazoan spermatogenesis. *J Reprod Fertil* 1973;35:339–348.
53. Ward SW, Coffey DS. DNA packaging and organization in mammalian spermatozoa: Comparison with somatic cells. *Biol Reprod* 1991;44:569–574.

54. Hecht NB. Regulation of 'haploid expressed genes' in male germ cells. *J Reprod Fertil* 1990;88:679–693.
55. Heidaran MA, Showman RM, Kistler WS. A cytochemical study of the transcriptional and translational regulation of nuclear transition protein (TP-1), a major chromosomal protein of mammalian spermatids. *J Cell Biol* 1988;106:1427–1433.
56. Mali P, Kaipia A, Kangasniemi M, et al. Stage-specific expression of nucleoprotein mRNA's during rat and mouse spermiogenesis. *Reprod Fertil Dev* 1989;1:369–382.
57. Saunders PTK, Millar MR, Maguire SM, Sharpe RM. Stage-specific expression of rat transition protein-2 mRNA and possible localization to the chromatoid body of step 7 spermatids by in situ hybridization using a nonradioactive riboprobe. *Mol Reprod Dev* 1992;33:385–391.
58. Kleene KC. Poly (A) shortening accompanies the activation of translation of five mRNA's during spermiogenesis in the mouse. *Development* 1989;106:367–373.
59. Yelick PC, Kwon Y, Flynn JF, Borzorgzadeh A, Kleene KC, Hecht NB. Mouse transition protein 1 is translationally regulated during the post-meiotic stages of spermatogenesis. *Mol Reprod Dev* 1989;1:193–200.
60. Sprando RL, Russell LD. Comparative study of cytoplasmic elimination in spermatids of selected mammalian species. *Am J Anat* 1987;178:72–80.
61. Russell LD. Role in spermiation. In: Russell LD, Griswold MD, eds. *The Sertoli cell.* Clearwater, Florida: Cache River Press; 1993:269–303.
62. Russell LD. Spermatid–Sertoli tubulobulbar complexes as devices for elimination of cytoplasm from the head region of late spermatids of the rat. *Anat Rec* 1979;194:233–246.
63. Russell LD, Malone JP. A study of Sertoli-spermatid tubulobulbar complexes in selected mammals. *Tissue Cell* 1980; 12:263–285.
64. Morales C, Clermont Y. Structural changes of the Sertoli cell during the cycle of the seminiferous epithelium. In: Russell LD, Griswold MD, ed. *The Sertoli cell,* Clearwater, Florida: Cache River Press; 1993:306–329.
65. Regaud C. Etudes de la structure des tubes séminiféres et sur la spermatogénése chez les mammiféres. *Arch Anat Microscop Morphol Exp* 1901;4:101–156, 231–380.
66. Jégou B, Laws AO, De Kretser DM. Changes in testicular function induced by short-term exposure of the rat testis to heat; further evidence for interaction of germ cells, Sertoli cells and Leydig cells. *Int J Androl* 1984;7:244–257.
67. Sharpe RM. Possible role of elongated spermatids in control of stage-dependent changes in the diameter of the lumen of the rat seminiferous tubule. *J Androl* 1989;10:304–310.
68. Pineau C, Velez de la Calle JF, Pinon-Lataillade G, Jégou B. Assessment of testicular function after acute and chronic irradiation: Further evidence for an influence of late spermatids on Sertoli cell function in the adult rat. *Endocrinology* 1989; 124:2720–2728.
69. Pinon-Lataillade G, Velez de la Calle JF, Viguier-Martinez MC, et al. Influence of germ cells upon Sertoli cells during continuous low-dose rate γ-irradiation of adult rats. *Mol Cell Endocrinol* 1988;58:51–63.
70. Gerard N, Syed V, Jégou B. Lipopolysaccharide, latex beads and residual bodies are potent activators of Sertoli cell interleukin-1α production. *Biochem Biophys Res Commun* 1992;185:154–161.
71. Russell LD. The perils of sperm release—"Let my children go." *Int J Androl* 1991;14:317–311.
72. Perey B, Clermont Y, Leblond CP. The wave of the seminiferous epithelium in the rat. *Am J Anat* 1961;108:47–77.
73. Clermont Y, Harvey SC. Duration of the cycle of the seminiferous epithelium in normal, hypophysectomized and hypophysectomized-hormone treated albino rats. *Endocrinology* 1965; 76:80–89.
74. Huckins C. Duration of spermatogenesis in pre- and postpubertal Wistar rats. *Anat Rec* 1965;151:364.
75. van Beek MEAB, Meistrich ML. A method for quantifying synchrony in testes of rats treated with vitamin A deprivation and readministration. *Biol Reprod* 1990;42:424–431.
76. Oakberg EF. Duration of spermatogenesis in the mouse and timing of stages of the cycle of the seminiferous epithelium. *Am J Anat* 1956;99:507–516.
77. Clermont Y, Trott M. Duration of the cycle of the seminiferous epithelium in the mouse and hamster determined by means of ^{3}H-thymidine and radioautography. *Fertil Steril* 1969;20: 805–817.
78. Clermont Y. Kinetics of spermatogenesis in mammals: Seminiferous epithelium cycle and spermatogonial renewal. *Physiol Rev* 1972;52:198–236.
79. De Rooij DG. Stem cell renewal and duration of the spermatogonial cycle in the golden hamster. *Z Zellforsch* 1968; 89:133–136.
80. Swierstra EE, Foote RH. Cytology and kinetics of spermatogenesis in the rabbit. *J Reprod Fertil* 1963;5:309–322.
81. Orgebin-Crist MC. Passage of spermatozoa labelled with thymidine-^{3}H through the ductus epididymis of the rabbit. *J Reprod Fertil* 1965;10:241–251.
82. Clermont Y. Cycle of the seminiferous epithelium of the guinea pig. A method for identification of the stages. *Fertil Steril* 1960;11:563–573.
83. Noller DW, Flickinger CJ, Howards SS. Duration of the cycle of the seminiferous epithelium in the guinea pig determined by tritiated thymidine autoradiography. *Biol Reprod* 1977;17: 532–534.
84. Foote RH, Swierstra EE, Hunt WL. Spermatogenesis in the dog. *Anat Rec* 1972;173:341–352.
85. Kennelly JJ. Coyote reproduction I. The duration of the spermatogenic cycle and epididymal sperm transport. *J Reprod Fertil* 1972;31:163–175.
86. Bergh KA, Clausen OPF, Huitfeldt HS. The spermatogenic cycle in the blue fox (*Alopex iagopus*): Relative frequency and absolute duration of the different stages. *Int J Androl* 1990;13:315–326.
87. Hocherau MT, Courot M, Ortavant R. Marquage des cellules germinales du belier et du taureau per injection de thymidine tritiee dans l'artere spermatique. *Ann Biol Anim Biochem Biophys* 1964;2:157–159.
88. Swierstra EE. Cytology and duration of the cycle of the seminiferous epithelium of the boar: Duration of spermatozoan transit through the epididymis. *Anat Rec* 1968;161:171–185.
89. Amann RP. Spermatogenesis in the stallion: a review. *J Equine Vet Sci* 1981;1:131–139.
90. Swierstra EE, Gebauer MR, Pickett BW. Reproductive physiology of the stallion. I. Spermatogenesis and testis composition. *J Reprod Fertil* 1974;40:113–123.
91. Berndtson WE, Desjardins C. The cycle of the seminiferous epithelium and spermatogenesis in the bovine testis. *Am J Anat* 1974;140:167–180.
92. Barr AB. Timing of spermatogenesis in four nonhuman primate species. *Fertil Steril* 1973;24:381–389.
93. Chowdhury AK, Steinberger E. A study of germ cell morphology and duration of spermatogenic cycle in the baboon, *Papio anubis*. *Anat Rec* 1976;185:155–169.
94. Chowdhury AK, Marshall G. Irregular pattern of spermatogenesis in the baboon (*Papio anubis*) and its possible mechanism. In: Steinberger A, Steinberger E, eds. *Testicular development, structure and function.* New York: Raven Press; 1980:129–137.
95. Clermont Y, Antar M. Duration of the cycle of the seminiferous epithelium and spermatogonial renewal in the monkey *Macaca arctoides*. *Am J Anat* 1973;136:153–166.
96. Fouquet JP, Dadoune JP. Renewal of spermatogonia in the monkey (*Macaca fascilcularis*). *Biol Reprod* 1986;35:199–207.
97. Schulze W, Salzbrunn A. Spatial and quantitative aspects of spermatogenic tissue in primates. In: Neischlag E, Habenicht, U-F, eds. *Spermatogenesis, fertilization, contraception.* Berlin: Springer-Verlag; 1992:267–283.
98. Clermont Y, Lebond CP. Differentiation and renewal of spermatogonia in the monkey, *Macacus rhesus*. *Am J Anat* 1959; 104:237–273.
99. De Rooij DG, Van Alphen MMA, Van De Kant HJG. Duration of the cycle of the seminiferous epithelium and its stages in the rhesus monkey (*Macaca mulatta*). *Biol Reprod* 1986;35: 587–591.
100. Schulze W, Rehder U. Organization and morphogenesis of the human seminiferous epithelium. *Cell Tissue Res* 1984; 237:395–407.
101. Schulze W, Riemer M, Rehder U, Hohne KH. Computer-aided three-dimensional reconstructions of the arrangement of primary

spermatocytes in human seminiferous tubules. *Cell Tissue Res* 1986;244:1–8.
102. Orsi AM, Ferreira AL. Definition of the stages of the cycle of the seminiferous epithelium of the opossum (*Didelphis azarae,* Temminck, 1825). *Acta Anat* 1978;100:153–160.
103. Parvinen M. Regulation of the seminiferous epithelium. *Endocrine Rev* 1982;3:405–417.
104. Russell LD, Peterson RN. Determination of the elongate spermatid–Sertoli cell ratio in various mammals. *J Reprod Fertil* 1984;70:635–641.
105. Russell LD, Ren HP, Sinha Hikim S, Schulze W, Sinha Hikim AP. A comparison study in twelve mammalian species with respect to key morphometric parameters related to volume densities and volumes of selected testis components. *Am J Anat* 1990;188:21–30.
106. Berndtson WE, Thompson TL. Changing relationships between testis size, Sertoli cell number and spermatogenesis in Sprague-Dawley rats. *J Androl* 1990;11:429–435.
107. Orth JM, Gunsalus GM, Lamperti AA. Evidence from Sertoli cell-depleted rats indicates that spermatid numbers in adults depends on numbers of Sertoli cells produced during perinatal development. *Endocrinology* 1988;122:787–794.
108. Cooke PS, Hess RA, Porcelli J, Meisami E. Increased sperm production in adult rats after transient neonatal hypothyroidism. *Endocrinology* 1991;129:244–248.
109. Cooke PS, Meisami E. Early hypothyroidism in rats causes increased adult testis and reproductive organ size but does not change testosterone levels. *Endocrinology* 1991;129:237–243.
110. Cooke PS. Thyroid hormones and testis development: A model system for increasing testis growth and sperm production. *Ann NY Acad Sci* 1991;637:122–132.
111. Cooke S, Porcelli J, Hess RA. Induction of increased testis growth and sperm production in adult rats by neonatal administration of the goitrogen propylthiouracil (PTU): The critical period. *Biol Reprod* 1992;46:146–154.
112. Meisami E, Sendera TJ, Clay LB. Paradoxical hypertrophy and plasticity of the testis in rats recovering from early thyroid deficiency: A growth study including effects of age and duration of hypothyroidism. *J Endocrinol* 1992;135:495–505.
113. van Haaster LH, De Jong FH, Docter R, De Rooij DG. The effect of hypothyroidism on Sertoli cell proliferation and differentiation and hormone levels during teticular development in the rat. *Endocrinology* 1992;131:1574–1576.
114. Clermont Y, Perey B. Quantitative study of the cell population of the seminiferous tubules in immature rats. *Am J Anat* 1957;100:241–267.
115. Steinberger A, Steinberger E. Replication pattern of Sertoli cells in maturing rat testis *in vivo* and in organ culture. *Biol Reprod* 1971;4:84–87.
116. Steinberger A, Steinberger E. The Sertoli cells. In: Johnson AD, Gomes WR, eds. *The testis.* New York: Academic Press; 1977:371–399.
117. Nagy F. Cell division kinetics and DNA synthesis in the immature Sertoli cells of the rat testis. *J Reprod Fertil* 1972; 28:389–395.
118. Griswold MD, Solari A, Tung PS, Fritz IB. Stimulation by FSH of DNA synthesis and of mitosis in cultured Sertoli cells prepared from testes of immature rats. *Mol Cell Endocrinol* 1977; 7:151–165.
119. Orth JM. Proliferation of Sertoli cells in fetal and postnatal rats: A quantitative autoradiographic study. *Anat Rec* 1982; 203:485–492.
120. Orth JM. The role of FSH in controlling Sertoli cell proliferation in testes of fetal rats. *Endocrinology* 1984;115:1248–1255.
121. Almiron I, Chemes H. Spermatogenic onset. II. FSH modulates mitotic activity of germ and Sertoli cells in immature rats. *Int J Androl* 1988;11:235–246.
122. Gondos B, Berndtson WE. Postnatal and pubertal development. In: Russell LD, Griswold MD, eds. *The Sertoli cell.* Clearwater, Florida: Cache River Press; 1993:115–153.
123. Hirobe S, He W-W, Lee MM, Donahoe PK. Mullerian inhibiting substance mRNA expression in granulosa and Sertoli cells coincides with their mitotic activity. *Endocrinology* 1992; 131:854–862.
124. Teerds KJ, Dorrington JH. Localization of transforming growth factor β_1, and β_2 during testicular development in the rat. *Biol Reprod* 1993;48:40–45.
125. Chemes HE, Dym M, Raj HGM. Hormonal regulation of Sertoli cell differentiation. *Biol Reprod* 1979;21:251–262.
126. Huhtaniemi IT, Nevo N, Amsterdam A, Naor Z. Effect of postnatal treatment with a gonadotropin-releasing hormone antagonist on sexual maturation of male rats. *Biol Reprod* 1986; 35:501–509.
127. van Den Dungen HM, van Dieten JAMJ, van Rees GP, Shoemaker J. Testicular weight, tubular diameter and number of Sertoli cells in rats are decreased after early prepubertal administration of an LHRH antagonist: the quality of spermatozoa is not impaired. *Life Sci* 1990;46:1081–1089.
128. Orth JM, Higginbotham CA, Salisbury RL. Hemicastration causes and testosterone prevents enhanced uptake of ^{3}H-thymidine by Sertoli cells in testes of immature rats. *Biol Reprod* 1984;30:263–270.
129. Feigelson M. Suppression of testicular maturation and fertility following androgen administration to neonatal male rats. *Biol Reprod* 1986;35:1321–1332.
130. Gernelo P, Pinilla L, Gaytan F, Aguilar E. Pituitary-testis function in rats treated neonatally with a gonadotrophin-releasing hormone agonist: Short- and long-term effects. *J Endocrinol* 1992;134:269–277.
131. Ultee-Van Gessel AM, Timmerman MA, De Jong FH. Effects of treatment of neonatal rats with highly purified FSH alone and in combination with LH on testicular function and endogenous hormone levels at various ages. *J Endocrinol* 1988;116:413–420.
132. Kirkby JD, Jetton AE, Cooke PS. Developmental hormonal profiles accompanying the neonatal hypothyroidism-induced increase in adult testicular size and sperm production in the rat. *Endocrinology* 1992;131:559–565.
133. Palmero S, Maggiani S, Fugassa E. Nuclear triidothyronine receptors in rat Sertoli cells. *Mol Cell Endocrinol* 1988;58:253–256.
134. Ontogenesis of the nuclear 3,5,3′-triidothyronine receptor in the rat testis. *Endocrinology* 1990;12:2521–2526.
135. Palmero S, de Marchis M, Gallo G, Fugassa E. Thyroid hormone affects the development of Sertoli cell function in the rat. *J Endocrinol* 1989;123:105–111.
136. Francavilla S, Cordeschi G, Properzi G. Effect of thyroid hormone on the pre- and post-natal development of the rat testis. *J Endocrinol* 1991;129:35–42.
137. Fugassa E, Palmero S, Gallo G. Triidothyronine decreases the production of androgen-binding protein by rat Sertoli cells. *Biochem Biophys Res Commun* 1987;147:241–247.
138. Beraldi E, Pezzi V, Salerno M. Influence of thyroid hormone on androgen metabolism in peripubertal rat Sertoli cells. *J Endocrinol* 1993; [*in press*].
139. Longcope C. The male and female reproductive systems. In: Ingbar SH, Braverman LE, eds. *Thyroid.* Philadelphia: Lippincott; 1986:920–1199.
140. De la Balze FA, Arrillaga F, Mancini RE, Janches M, Davidson OW, Gurtman AI. Male hypogonadism in hypothyroidism: A study of six cases. *J Clin Endocrinol Metab* 1962;22:212–222.
141. Franks RC, Stempfel RS. Juvenile hypothyroidism and precocious testicular maturation. *J Clin Endocrinol Metab* 1963;23:805–810.
142. Laron Z, Karp M, Dolberg L. Juvenile hypothyroidism with testicular enlargement. *Acta Paediatr* 1970;59:317–322.
143. Benbrook D, Pfahl M. A novel thyroid hormone receptor encoded by a cDNA clone from a human testis library. *Science* 1987;238:788–791.
144. Hall PF, Mita M. Influence of FSH on glucose transport by cultured Sertoli cells. *Biol Reprod* 1984;31:863–869.
145. Ulisse S, Jannini EA, Pepe M, de Matteis S, D'Armiento M. Thyroid hormone stimulates glucose transport and GLUT1 mRNA in rat Sertoli cells. *Mol Cell Endocrinol* 1992;87:131–137.
146. Bartlett JMS, Charlton HM, Robinson ICAF, Nieschlag E. Pubertal development and testicular function in the male growth hormone-deficient rat. *J Endocrinol* 1990;126:193–201.
147. Kosco MS, Bolt DJ, Wheaton JE, Loseth KJ, Crabo BG. Endocrine responses in relation to compensatory testicular growth after neonatal hemicastration in boars. *Biol Reprod* 1987; 36:1177–1185.
148. Fabbri A, Knox G, Buczko E, Dufau ML. β-Endorphin produc-

tion by the fetal Leydig cell: regulation and implications for paracrine control of Sertoli cell function. *Endocrinology* 1988; 122:749–755.
149. Fabbri A, Tsai-Morris CH, Luna S, Fraioli F, Dufau ML. Opiate receptors are present in the rat testis. Identification and localization in Sertoli cells. *Endocrinology* 1985;117:2544–2546.
150. Gerendai I, Chandrima S, Gunsalus GL, Bardin CW. The effects of opioid receptor antagonists suggest that testicular opiates regulate Sertoli and Leydig cell function in the neonatal rat. *Endocrinology* 1986;118:2039–2044.
151. Orth JM. FSH-induced Sertoli cell proliferation in the developing rat is modified by β-endorphin produced in the testis. *Endocrinology* 1986;119:1876–1878.
151a. Orth JM, Boehm R. Endorphin suppresses FSH-stimulated proliferation of isolated neonatal Sertoli cells by a pertussis toxin-sensitive mechanism. *Anat Rec* 1990;226:320–327.
152. Matzuk MM, Finegold MJ, Su J-G, Hsueh AJW, Bradley A. α-inhibin is a tumour-suppressor gene with gonadal specificity in mice. *Nature* 1992;360:313–319.
153. Chubb C. Genes regulating testis size. *Biol Reprod* 1992; 47:29–36.
154. Berndtson WE, Igboeli G, Parker WG. The numbers of Sertoli cells in mature Holstein bulls and their relationship to quantitative aspects of spermatogenesis. *Biol Reprod* 1987;37:60–67.
155. Kluin PM, Kramer MR, De Rooij DG. Proliferation of spermatogonia and Sertoli cells in maturing mice. *Anat Embryol* 1984;169:73–78.
156. Vergouwen RPFA, Jacobs SGPM, Huiskamp R, Davids JAG, de Rooij DG. Proliferative activity of gonocytes, Sertoli cells and interstitial cells during testicular development in mice. *J Reprod Fertil* 1991;93:233–243.
157. Sun EL, Gondos B. Proliferative activity in the rabbit testis during postnatal development. In: Byskov AG, Peters H, eds. *Development and function of reproductive organs.* Amsterdam: Excerpta Medica; 1981:140–148.
158. de Reviers M, Hocherau de Reviers MT, Blanc MR. Control of Sertoli and germ cell populations in the cock and sheep testes. *Reprod Nutr Dev* 1980;20:241–249.
159. Kosco MS, Loseth KJ, Crabo BG. Development of the seminiferous tubules after neonatal hemicastration in the boar. *J Reprod Fertil* 1989;87:1–11.
160. Berndtson WE, Igboeli G, Pickett BW. Relationship of absolute numbers of Sertoli cells to testicular size and spermatogenesis in young beef bulls. *J Anim Sci* 1987;64:241–246.
161. Kluin PM, Kramer MF, de Rooij DG. Testicular development in *Macaca irus* after birth. *Int J Androl* 1983;6:25–43.
162. Cortes D, Müller J, Skakkebaek NE. Proliferation of Sertoli cells during development of the human testis assessed by stereological methods. *Int J Androl* 1987;10:589–596.
163. Gulyas BJ, Tullner WW, Hodgen GD. Fetal or maternal hypophysectomy in rhesus monkeys (*Macaca mulatta*): Effects on the development of testes and other endocrine organs. *Biol Reprod* 1977;17:650–660.
164. Nistal M, Abaurrea MA, Paniagua R. Morphological and histometric study on the human Sertoli cell from birth to the onset of puberty. *J Anat* 1982;14:351–363.
165. Mann DR, Gould KG, Collins DC, Wallen K. Blockade of neonatal activation of the pituitary-testicular axis: effect on peripubertal LH and testosterone secretion and on testicular development in male monkeys. *J Clin Endocrinol Metab* 1989;68:600–607.
166. Courot M, Ortavant R. Endocrine control of spermatogenesis in the ram. *J Reprod Fertil* 1981;Suppl 30:47–60.
167. Barenton B, Pelletier J. Seasonal changes in testicular gonadotropin receptors and steroid content in the ram. *Endocrinology* 1983;112:1441–1446.
168. Hocherau-de-Reviers MT, Perreau C, Lincoln GA. Photoperiodic variations of somatic and germ cell populations in the Soay ram testis. *J Reprod Fertil* 1985;74:329–334.
169. Sinha Hikim AP, Bartke A, Russell LD. Morphometric studies on hamster testes in gonadally active and inactive states: light microscope findings. *Biol Reprod* 1988;39:1225–1237.
170. Jones LS, Berndtson WE. A quantitative study of Sertoli cell and germ cell populations as related to sexual development and aging in the stallion. *Biol Reprod* 1986;35:138–148.
171. Johnson L, Nguyen HB. Annual cycle of the Sertoli cell population in adult stallions. *J Reprod Fertil* 1986;76:311–316.
172. Johnson A, Varner DD, Tatum ME, Scrutchfield W. Season but not age affects Sertoli cell number in adult stallions. *Biol Reprod* 1991;45:404–410.
173. Hocherau-de-Reviers MT, Lincoln GA. Seasonal variations in the histology of the testis of the red deer, *Cervus elaphus*. *J Reprod Fertil* 1978;54:209–213.
174. Ultee-van Gessel AM, Leemborg FG, de Jong FH, van der Molen HJ. Influence of neonatal hemicastration on in-vitro secretion of inhibin, gonadotrophins and testicular steroids in male rats. *J Endocrinol* 1985;106:259–265.
175. Waites GMH, Wenstrom JC, Crabo BG, Hamilton DW. Rapid compensatory hypertrophy of the lamb testis after neonatal hemiorchidectomy: Endocrine and light microscopical morphometric analyses. *Endocrinology* 1983;112:2159–2167.
176. Walton JS, Evins JD, Hillard MA, Waites GMH. Follicle-stimulating hormone release in hemicastrated prepubertal rams and its relationship to testicular development. *J Endocrinol* 1980; 84:141–152.
177. Laron Z, Zilka E. Compensatory hypertrophy of testicle in unilateral cryptorchidism. *J Clin Endocrinol Metab* 1969;29: 1409–1413.
178. Jenkins N, Waites GMH. Effects of hemicastration at various ages and of oestradiol-17β on plasma concentrations of gonadotrophins and androgens, testicular growth and interstitial cell responses in prepubertal lambs. *J Reprod Fertil* 1983;67:325–334.
179. Mittwoch U. Ethnic differences in testis size: A possible link with the cytogenetics of true hermaphroditism. *Hum Reprod* 1988;3:445–449.
180. Johnson L, Zane RS, Petty CS, Neaves WB. Quantification of the human Sertoli cell population: its distribution, relation to germ cell numbers and age-related decline. *Biol Reprod* 1984; 31:785–795.
181. Burris AS, Rodbard HW, Winters SJ, Sherins RJ. Gonadotropin therapy in men with isolated hypogonadotropic hypogonadism: The response to hCG is predicted by initial testicular size. *J Clin Endocrinol Metab* 1988;66:1144–1151.
182. Vicari E, Mongioi A, Calogero AE. Therapy with hCG alone induces spermatogenesis in men with isolated hypogonadotrophic hypogonadism—long term follow-up. *Int J Androl* 1992; 15:320–329.
183. Wing T-Y, Christensen AK. Morphometric studies on rat seminiferous tubules. *Am J Anat* 1982;165:13–25.
184. Johnson L. Increased daily sperm production in the breeding season of stallions is explained by an elevated population of spermatogonia. *Biol Reprod* 1985;32:1181–1190.
185. Marshall GR, Jockenhovel F, Ludecke D, Nieschlag E. Maintenance of complete but quantitatively reduced spermatogenesis in hypophysectomized monkeys by testosterone alone. *Acta Endocrinol* 1986;113:424–431.
186. Weinbauer GF, Nieschlag E. Peptide and steroid regulation of spermatogenesis in primates. *Ann NY Acad Sci* 1991; 637:107–121.
187. Johnson K, Petty CS, Porter JC, Neaves WB. Germ cell degeneration during postprophase of meiosis and serum concentrations of gonadotropins in young adult and older adult men. *Biol Reprod* 1984;31:770–784.
188. Skakkebaek NE, Hulten M, Jacobsen P, Mikkelsen M. Quantification of human seminiferous epithelium. II. Histological studies in eight 47,XYY men. *J Reprod Fertil* 1973;32:391–401.
189. Lin M, Jones RC. Spatial arrangement of the stages of the cycle of the seminiferous epithelium in the Japanese quail, *Coturnix coturnix japonica*. *J Reprod Fertil* 1990;90:361–367.
190. Sharpe RM, Maddocks S, Millar M, Saunders PTK, Kerr JB, McKinnell C. Testosterone and spermatogenesis: Identification of stage-dependent, androgen-regulated proteins secreted by adult rat seminiferous tubules. *J Androl* 1992;13:172–184.
191. Sharpe RM, Fraser HM, Ratnasooriya WD. Assessment of the role of Leydig cell products other than testosterone in spermatogenesis and fertility in adult rats. *Int J Androl* 1988;11:507–523.
192. Kerr JB. Spontaneous degeneration of germ cells in normal rat restis: assessment of cell types and frequency during the spermatogenic cycle. *J Reprod Fertil* 1992;95:825–830.
193. Courot M, Hocherau de Reviers MT, Monet-Kuntz C, et al. En-

docrinology of spermatogenesis in the hypophysectomized ram. *J Reprod Fertil* 1979;Suppl 26:165–173.
194. Barr AB, Moore DJ, Paulsen CA. Germinal cell loss during human spermatogenesis. *J Reprod Fertil* 1971;25:75–80.
195. Johnson L, Nguyen HB, Petty C, Neaves WB. Quantification of human spermatogenesis: germ cell degeneration during spermatocytogenesis and meiosis in testes from younger and older adult men. *Biol Reprod* 1980;37:739–747.
196. Johnson L, Khaturvedi PK, Williams JD. Missing generations of spermatocytes and spermatids in seminiferous epithelium contribute to low efficiency of spermatogenesis in humans. *Biol Reprod* 1992;47:1091–1098.
197. Johnson L, Petty CS, Neaves WB. A comparative study of daily sperm production and testicular composition in humans and rats. *Biol Reprod* 1980;22:1233–1243.
198. Johnson L, Petty CS, Neaves WB. Further quantification of human spermatogenesis: germ cell loss during postprophase of meiosis and its relationship to daily sperm production. *Biol Reprod* 1983;29:207–215.
199. Johnson L. Spermatogenesis and ageing in the human. *J Androl* 1986;7:331–354.
200. Johnson L, Grumbles JS, Bagheri A, Petty CS. Increased germ cell degeneration during postprophase of meiosis is related to increased serum FSH concentrations and reduced daily sperm production in aged men. *Biol Reprod* 1990;42:281–287.
201. Attal J, Courot M. Développement testiculaire et établissment de la spermatogenése chez le taureau. *Ann Biol Anim Biochem Biophys* 1963;3:219–241.
202. Skakkebaek NE, Bryant JI, Philip J. Studies on meiotic chromosomes in infertile men and controls with normal karyotypes. *J Reprod Fertil* 1973;35:23–34.
203. Russell LD, Bartke A, Gosh JC. Postnatal development of the Sertoli cell barrier, tubular lumen and cytoskeleton of Sertoli and myoid cells in the rat, and their relationship to tubular fluid secretion and flow. *Am J Anat* 1989;184:179–189.
203a. Nicholson HD, Guldenaar SEF, Boer GJ, Pickering BT. Testicular oxytocin: Effects of intratesticular oxytocin in the rat. *J Endocrinol* 1991;130:231–238.
204. Ghosh S, Bartke A, Grasso P, Reichert LE Jr, Russell LD. Structural manifestations of the rat Sertoli cell to hypophysectomy: A correlative morphometric and endocrine study. *Endocrinology* 1992;131:485–497.
205. Zhengwel Y, Wreford NG, De Kretser DM. A quantitative study of spermatogenesis in the developing rat testis. *Biol Reprod* 1990;43:629–635.
206. Hodgson TM, Irby DC, Kerr JB, De Kretser DM. Studies of the structure and function of the Sertoli cell in a seasonally breeding rodent. *Biol Reprod* 1979;21:1091–1098.
207. Mortimer D, Lincoln GA. Ultrastructural study of regressed and activated testes from Soay rams. *J Reprod Fertil* 1982; 64:437–442.
208. Lincoln GA. Seasonal aspects of testicular function. In: Burger H, de Kretser DM, eds. *The testis,* 2nd ed. New York: Raven Press; 1989:329–385.
209. Mickelsen WD, Paisley LG, Dahmen JJ. The effect of season on scrotal circumference and sperm motility and morphology in rams. *Theriogenology* 1981;16:45–51.
210. De Rooij DG, Van Dissel-Emiliani FMF, Van Pelt AMM. Regulation of spermatogonial proliferation. *Ann NY Acad Sci* 1989;564:140–153.
211. Huckins C. The morphology and kinetics of spermatogonial degeneration in adult rats: An analysis using a simplified classification of the germinal epithelium. *Anat Rec* 1978;190:905–926.
212. Huckins C, Oakberg EF. Morphological and quantitative analysis of spermatogonia in mouse testes using whole mounted seminiferous tubules I. The normal testes. *Anat Rec* 1978;192:519–528.
213. De Rooij DG, Lok D. The regulation of the density of spermatogonia in the seminiferous epithelium of the Chinese hamster. II. Differentiating spermatogonia. *Anat Rec* 1987;217:131–136.
214. Viguier-Martinez MC, Hocherau-de Reviers MT. Comparative action of cyproterone and cyproterone acetate on pituitary and plasma gonadotrophin levels, the male genital tract and spermatogenesis in the growing rat. *Ann Biol Anim Biochem Biophys* 1977;117:1069–1076.
215. van Alphen MMA, van de Kant HJG, de Rooij DG. Follicle-stimulating hormone stimulates spermatogenesis in the adult monkey. *Endocrinology* 1988;123:1449–1455.
216. Arslan M, Weinbauer GF, Schlatt S, Shahab M, Nieschlag E. FSH and testosterone, alone or in combination, initiate testicular growth and increase the number of spermatogonia and Sertoli cells in a juvenile non-human primate (*Macaca mulatta*). *J Endocrinol* 1992;136:235–243.
217. Means AR, Fakunding JL, Huckins C, Tindall DJ, Vitale R. Follicle-stimulating hormone, the Sertoli cell and spermatogenesis. *Recent Prog Horm Res* 1976;32:477–527.
218. Odell WD, Swerdloff RS. Etiologies of sexual maturation. A model system based on the sexually maturing rat. *Recent Prog Horm Res* 1976;32:245–288.
218a. Wang C, Dahl KD, Leung A, Chan SYW, Hsueh AJW. Serum bioactive FSH in men with idiopathic azoospermia and oligospermia. *J Clin Endocrinol Metab* 1987;65:629–633.
219. Heller CG, Rowley MJ, Heller GV. Clomiphene citrate: A correlation of its effect on sperm concentration and morphology, total gonadotropins, ICSH, estrogen and testosterone excretion, and testicular cytology in normal men. *J Clin Endocrinol Metab* 1969;29:638–649.
220. Baker HWG. Clinical evaluation and management of testicular disorders in the adult. In: Burger H, de Kretser DM, eds. *The testis,* 2nd edition. New York: Raven Press, 1989:419–440.
221. Acosta AA, Khalifa E, Oehningers S. Pure FSH has a role in the treatment of severe male infertility by assisted reproduction: Norfolk's total experience. *Hum Reprod* 1992;7:1067–1072.
222. Bremner WJ, Matsumoto AM, Sussman AM, Paulsen CA. Follicle-stimulating hormone and human spermatogenesis. *J Clin Invest* 1981;68:1044–1052.
223. Matsumoto AM, Bremner WJ. Stimulation of sperm production by human chorionic gonadotropin after prolonged gonadotropin suppression in normal men. *J Androl* 1985;6:137–143.
224. Nistal M, Codesal J, Paniagua R, Santamaria L. Decrease in the number of human Ap and Ad spermatogonia and in the Ap/Ad ratio with advancing age. *J Androl* 1987;8:64–68.
225. Mills NC, Means AR. Sorbitol dehydrogenase of rat testis: Changes of activity during development, after hypophysectomy and following gonadotropic hormone administration. *Endocrinology* 1972;91:147–156.
226. Eshkol A, Lunenfeld B. Use of antisera to gonadotrophins in reproduction. In: Nieschlag E, ed. *Immunization with hormones in reproductive research.* Amsterdam: North Holland; 1975: 55–71.
227. Chemes HE, Dym M, Raj HGM. The role of gonadotropins and testosterone on initiation of spermatogenesis in the immature rat. *Biol Reprod* 1979;21:241–249.
228. Haneji T, Maekawa M, Nishimune Y. Vitamin A and FSH synergistically induce differentiation of type A spermatogonia in adult male mouse cryptorchid testes *in vitro. Endocrinology* 1984; 114:801–805.
229. Clermont Y, Morgentaler H. Quantitative study of spermatogenesis in the hypophysectomized rat. *Endocrinology* 1955; 57:369–382.
230. Monet-Kuntz C, Terqui M, Locatelli A, Hocherau-de Reviers MT, Courot M. Effects de la supplementation en testosterone sur la spermatogenèse de bélièrs hypophysectomisés. *C R Hebd Seanc Acad Sci Paris D* 1976;283:1763–1766.
231. Hocherau-De-Reviers MT, Loir M, Pelletier J. Seasonal variation in the response of the testis and LH levels to hemicastration of adult rams. *J Reprod Fertil* 1976;46:203–209.
232. Milette JJ, Schwartz NB, Turek FW. The importance of FSH in the initiation of testicular growth in the photostimulated Djungarian hamster. *Endocrinology* 1988;122:1060–1066.
233. Johnson L. Seasonal differences in equine spermatocytogenesis. *Biol Reprod* 1991;44:284–291.
234. Kangasniemi M, Kaipia A, Toppari J, Perheentupa A, Huhtaniemi I, Parvinen M. Cellular regulation of FSH binding in rat seminiferous tubules. *J Androl* 1990;11:336–343.
235. Heckert LL, Griswold MD. Expression of follicle-stimulating hormone receptor mRNA in rat testes and Sertoli cells. *Mol Endocrinol* 1991;5:670–677.
236. Kangasniemi M, Kaipia A, Mali P, Toppari J, Huhtaniemi I,

Parvinen M. Modulation of basal and FSH-stimulated cyclic AMP production in rat seminiferous tubules staged by an improved transillumination technique. *Anat Rec* 1990;227:62–70.
237. Kangasniemi M, Kaipia A, Toppari J, Mali P, Huhtaniemi IP, Parvinen M. Cellular regulation of basal and FSH-stimulated cyclic AMP production in irradiated rat testes. *Anat Rec* 1990;227:32–36.
238. Huang HFS, Neischlag E. Suppression of the intratesticular testosterone is associated with quantitative changes in spermatogonial populations in intact adult rats. *Endocrinology* 1986; 118:619–627.
239. Fritz IB. Sites of action of androgens and FSH on cells of the seminiferous tubule. In: Litwack G, ed. *Biochemical actions of hormones,* New York: Academic Press; 1978:249–281.
240. Ritzen EM, Hansson V, French FS. The Sertoli cell. In: Burger H, de Kretser DM, eds. *The testis,* 2nd ed. New York: Raven Press; 1989:269–302.
241. Beamer WG, Cunliffe-Beamer TL, Shultz KL, Langley SH, Roderick TH. Junvenile spermatogonial depletion (jsd): A genetic defect of germ cell proliferation of male mice. *Biol Reprod* 1988;38:899–908.
242. Van Dissel-Emiliani FM, Grootenhuis AJ, De Jong FH, De Rooij DG. Inhibin reduces spermatogonial numbers in testes of adult mice and Chinese hamsters. *Endocrinology* 1989;125:1899–1903.
243. De Jong FH. Inhibin. *Physiol Rev* 1988;68:555–607.
244. McLachlan RI, Robertson DM, De Kretser DM, Burger HG. Advances in the physiology of inhibin and inhibin-related peptides. *Clin Endocrinol* 1988;29:77 112.
245. Sharpe RM. Bidirectional secretion by the Sertoli cell. *Int J Androl* 1988;11:87–91.
246. Sharpe RM, Bartlett JMS. Changes in the secretion of ABP into testicular interstitial fluid with age and in situations of impaired spermatogenesis. *Int J Androl* 1987;10:701–710.
247. Sharpe RM, Swanston IA, Cooper I, Tsonis CG, McNeilly AS. Factors affecting the secretion of immunoactive inhibin into testicular interstitial fluid in rats. *J Endocrinol* 1988;119:315–326.
248. Maddocks S, Sharpe RM. The effects of sexual maturation and altered steroid synthesis on the production and route of secretion of inhibin-α from the rat testis. *Endocrinology* 1990; 126:1541–1550.
249. Maddocks S, Sharpe RM. The route of secretion of inhibin from the rat testis. *J Endocrinol* 1989;120:R5–R8.
250. Maddocks S, Kerr JB, Allenby G, Sharpe RM. Evaluation of the role of germ cells in regulating the route of secretion of immunoactive inhibin from the rat testis. *J Endocrinol* 1992; 132:439–448.
251. Woodruff TK, Borree J, Attie KM, Cox ET, Rice GC, Mather JP. Stage-specific binding of inhibin and activin to subpopulations of rat germ cells. *Endocrinology* 1992;130:821–837.
252. Risbridger GP, Clements J, Robertson DM, et al. Immuno- and bioactive inhibin and inhibin α subunit expression in rat Leydig cell cultures. *Mol Cell Endocrinol* 1989;66:119–122.
253. Shaha C, Morris PL, Chen CLC, Vale W, Bardin CW. Immunostainable inhibin subunits are in multiple types of testicular cells. *Endocrinology* 1989;125:1941–1950.
254. Bergh A, Cajander S. Immunohistochemical localization of inhibin-α in the testes of normal men and in men with testicular disorders. *Int J Androl* 1990;13:463–469.
255. Maddocks S, Sharpe RM. Assessment of the contribution of Leydig cells to the secretion of inhibin by the rat testis. *Molec Cell Endocrinol* 1989;67:113–118.
256. Bhasin S, Krummen LA, Swerdloff RS, et al. Stage dependent expression of inhibin α and β-B subunits during the cycle of the rat seminiferous epithelium. *Endocrinology* 1989;124:987–991.
257. Kaipia A, Parvinen M, Shimasaki S, Ling N, Toppari J. Stage-specific cellular regulation of inhibin α-subunit mRNA expression in the rat seminiferous epithelium. *Mol Cell Endocrinol* 1991;82:165–173.
258. Roberts V, Meunier H, Sawchenko PE, Vale W. Differential production and regulation of inhibin subunits in rat testicular cell types. *Endocrinology* 1989;125:2350–2359.
259. De Winter JP, Timmerman MA, Vanderstichele HMJ, et al. Testicular Leydig cells in vitro secrete only inhibin α-subunits, whereas Leydig cell tumours can secrete bioactive inhibin. *Mol Cell Endocrinol* 1992;83:105–115.
260. Bartlett JMS, Kerr JB, Sharpe RM. The selective removal of pachytene spermatocytes using methoxy acetic acid as an approach to the study in-vivo of paracrine interactions in the testis. *J Androl* 1988;9:31–40.
261. Bellvé AR, Zheng W. Growth factors as autocrine and paracrine modulators of male gonadal functions. *J Reprod Fertil* 1989;85:771–793.
262. Wolgemuth DJ, Don J, Chapman DL, Winer MA. Expression of proto-oncogenes and protein kinases in the testis. In: Nieschlag E, Habenicht U-F, eds. *Spermatogenesis, fertilization, contraception,* Berlin: Springer-Verlag; 1992:201–224.
263. Thompson JN, Howell JMC, Pitt GAJ. Vitamin A and reproduction in rats. *Proc R Soc [Biol]* 1964;159:510–535.
264. Mitranon V, Sobhon P, Tosukhowong P, Chindaduangrat W. Cytological changes in the testes of vitamin A-deficient rats. I. Quantitation of germinal cells in the seminiferous tubules. *Acta Anat* 1979;103:159–168.
265. Unni E, Rao MR. Histological and ultrastructural studies on the effect of vitamin A depletion and subsequent repletion with vitamin A on germ cells and Sertoli cells in the rat testis. *Indian J Exp Biol* 1983;21:180–192.
266. Griswold MD, Bishop PD, Kim KH, Ren P, Siiteri KE, Morales C. Function of vitamin A in normal and synchronized seminiferous tubules. *Ann NY Acad Sci* 1989;564:154–172.
267. Ismail N, Morales C, Clermont Y. Role of spermatogonia in the stage-synchronization of the seminiferous epithelium in vitamin A-deficient rats. *Am J Anat* 1990;188:57–63.
268. Kim KH, Wang ZO. Action of vitamin A on the testis: role of the Sertoli cell. In: Russell LD, Griswold MD, eds. *The Sertoli cell.* Clearwater, Florida: Cache River Press; 1993:515–535.
269. Morales CR, Griswold MD. Retinol-induced stage synchronization in seminiferous tubules of the rat. *Endocrinology* 1987; 121:432–434.
270. Bartlett JMS, Weinbauer GF, Nieschlag E. Stability of spermatogenic synchronization achieved by depletion and restoration of vitamin A in rats. *Biol Reprod* 1990;42:603–612.
271. van Beek MEAB, Meistrich ML. Stage-synchronized seminiferous epithelium in rats after manipulation of retinol levels. *Biol Reprod* 1991;45:235–244.
272. van Pelt AMM, De Rooij DG. Synchronization of the seminiferous epithelium after vitamin A replacement in vitamin A-deficient mice. *Biol Reprod* 1990;43:363–367.
273. Siiteri JE, Karl AF, Linder CC, Griswold MD. Testicular synchrony: Evaluation and analysis of different protocols. *Biol Reprod* 1991;46:284–289.
274. Bartlett JMS, Weinbauer GF, Nieschlag E. Quantitative analysis of germ cell numbers and relation to intratesticular testosterone following vitamin A-induced synchronization of spermatogenesis in the rat. *J Endocrinol* 1989;123:403–412.
275. Linder C, Heckert L, Roberts K, Kim KH, Griswold MD. Expression of receptors during the cycle of the seminiferous epithelium. *Ann NY Acad Sci* 1991;637:313–321.
276. Unni E, Rao MR. Androgen binding protein levels and FSH binding to testicular membranes in vitamin A deficient rats and during subsequent replenishment with vitamin A. *J Steroid Biochem* 1986;25:579–583.
277. Blaner WAS, Galdieri M, Goodman DS. Distribution and levels of cellular retinol- and cellular retinoic acid-binding protein in various types of rat testis cells. *Biol Reprod* 1987;36:130–137.
278. Porter SB, Ong DE, Chytil F, Orgebin-Crist M-C. Localization of cellular retinol-binding protein and cellular retinoic acid-binding protein in the rat testis and epididymis. *J Androl* 1985;6:197–212.
279. Eriksson U, Hansson E, Nordlinder H, Busch C, Sundelin J, Peterson PA. Quantitation and tissue localization of the cellular retinoic acid-binding protein. *J Cell Physiol* 1987;133:482–490.
280. Kato M, Sung WK, Kato K, Goodman DS. Immunohistochemical studies on the localization of cellular retinol-binding protein in rat testis and epididymis. *Biol Reprod* 1985;32:173–189.
281. Russell ES. Heriditary anemias of the mouse: a review for geneticists. *Adv Genetics* 1979;20:357–459.
282. Manova K, Nocka K, Besmer P, Bachvarova RF. Gonadal ex-

pression of c-*kit* encoded at the *W* locus of the mouse. *Development* 1990;110:1057–1069.
283. Yoshinaga K, Nishikawa S, Ogawa M, et al. Role of c-*kit* in mouse spermatogenesis: identification of spermatogonia as a specific site of c-*kit* expression and function. *Development* 1991;113:689–699.
284. Rossi P, Albanesi C, Grimaldi P, Geremia R. Expression of the mRNA for the ligand of c-*kit* in mouse Sertoli cells. *Biochem Biophys Res Commun* 1991;176:910–914.
285. Tajima Y, Onoue H, Kitamura Y, Nishimune Y. Biologically active kit ligand growth factor is produced by mouse Sertoli cells and is defective in Sid mutant mice. *Development* 1991; 113:1031–1035.
286. Rossi P, Mavrail G, Albanesi C, Charlesworth A, Geremia R, Sorrentino V. A novel c-*kit* transcript potentially encoding a truncated receptor originates within a kit gene intron in mouse spermatids. *Dev Biol* 1992;152:203–207.
287. Dolci S, Williams DE, Ernst MK, et al. Requirement for mast cell growth factor for primordial germ cell survival in culture. *Nature* 1991;352:809–811.
288. Godin I, Deed R, Cooke J, Zsebo K, Dexter M, Wylie CC. Effects of the *steel* gene product on mouse primordial germ cells in culture. *Nature* 1991;352:807–809.
289. Matsui Y, Toksoz D, Nishikawa S, et al. Effect of *Steel* factor and leukaemia inhibitory factor on murine primordial germ cells in culture. *Nature* 1991;353:750–752.
290. Khan SA, Soder O, Syed V, Gustafsson K, Lindh M, Ritzen EM. The rat testis produces large amounts of an interleukin-1-like factor. *Int J Androl* 1987;10:495–503.
291. Khan SA, Schmidt K, Hallin P, Di Pauli R, De Geyter Ch, Nieschlag E. Human testis cytosol and ovarian follicular fluid contain high amounts of interleukin-1-like factor(s). *Mol Cell Endocrinol* 1988;58:221–230.
292. Syed V, Soder O, Arver S, Lindh M, Khan S, Ritzen EM. Ontogeny and cellular origin of an interleukin-1-like factor in the reproductive tract of the male rat. *Int J Androl* 1988;11:437–447.
293. Gerard N, Syed V, Bardin CW, Genetet N, Jégou B. Sertoli cells are the site of interleukin-1α synthesis in the rat. *Mol Cell Endocrinol* 1991;82:R13–R16.
294. Soder O, Syed V, Callard GV, et al. Production and secretion of an interleukin-1-like factor is stage-dependent and correlates with spermatogonial DNA synthesis in the rat seminiferous epithelium. *Int J Androl* 1991;14:223–231.
295. Pollanen P, Soder O, Parvinen M. Interleukin-1α stimulation of spermatogonial proliferation *in vivo*. *Reprod Fertil Dev* 1989;1:85–87.
296. Syed V, Gérard N, Kaipia A, Bardin CW, Parvinen M, Jégou B. Identification, ontogeny and regulation of an interleukin-6-like (IL-6) factor in the rat testis. *Endocrinology* 1993;132:293–299.
297. Mather JP, Attie KM, Woodruff TK, Rice GC, Phillips DM. Activin stimulates spermatogonial proliferation in germ-Sertoli cell cocultures from immature rat testis. *Endocrinology* 1990;127:3206–3214.
298. Kaipia A, Penttila T-J, Shimasaki S, Ling N, Parvinen M, Toppari J. Expression of inhibin β_A and β_B, follistatin and activin A receptor messenger ribonucleic acids in the rat seminiferous epithelium. *Endocrinology* 1992;131:2703–2710.
299. Grootenhuis AJ, Steenbergen J, Timmerman MA. Inhibin and activin-like activity in fluids from male and female gonads: Different molecular weight forms and bioactivity/immunoactivity. *J Endocrinol* 1989;122:293–301.
300. Mather JP, Krummen LA. Inhibin, activin and growth factors: paracrine regulators of testicular function. In: Nieschlag E, Habenicht U-F, eds. *Spermatogenesis, fertilization, contraception.* Berlin: Springer-Verlag; 1992:169–200.
300a. De Winter JP, Themmen APN, Hoogerbrugge JW, Klaij IA, Grootegoed JA, De Jong FH. Activin receptor mRNA expression in rat testicular cell types. *Mol Cell Endocrinol* 1992;83:R1–R8.
301. Ito E, Toki T, Ishihara H, et al. Erthyroid transcription factor GATA-1 is abundantly transcribed in mouse testis. *Nature* 1993;362:466–468.
302. Ojeda SR, Andrews WW, Advis JP, White SS. Recent advances in the endocrinology of puberty. *Endocrine Rev* 1980;1: 228–257.
303. Hutson JM, Williams MPL, Fallat ME, Attah A. Testicular descent: New insights into its hormonal control. *Oxford Rev Reprod Biol* 1990;12:1–56.
304. Forest MG. Development of the male reproductive tract. In: de vere White R, ed. *Aspects of male infertility* Baltimore: Williams & Wilkins; 1982:1–60.
305. Wartenberg H. Differentiation and development of the testes. In: Burger H, de Kretser DM. *The testis,* 2nd ed. New York: Raven Press; 1989:67–118.
306. Gondos B, Renston RH, Conner LA. Ultrastructure of germ cells and Sertoli cells in the postnatal rabbit testis. *Am J Anat* 1993;136:427–440.
307. Gondos B, Byskov AG. Germ cell kinetics in the neonatal rabbit testis. *Cell Tissue Res* 1981;215:143–151.
308. Dym M, Fawcett DW. The blood–testis barrier in the rat and the physiological compartmentation of the seminiferous epithelium. *Biol Reprod* 1970;3:308–326.
309. Curtis SK, Amann RP. Testicular development and establishment of spermatogenesis in Holstein bulls. *J Anim Sci* 1981;53:1645–1657.
310. Sinoratz F, Amselgruber W. Postnatal development of bovine Sertoli cells. *Anat Embryol* 1986;174:413–423.
311. Nistal M, Paniagua R. The postnatal development of the human Sertoli cells. *Z Mikrosk-Anat Forsch* 1983;5:739–752.
312. Schulze C. Sertoli cells and Leydig cells in man. *Adv Anat Embryol Cell Biol* 1984;88:1–104.
313. Hinton BT, Setchell BP. Fluid secretion and movement. In: Russell LD, Griswold MD eds. *The Sertoli cell.* Clearwater, Florida: Cache River Press; 1993:249–267.
314. Pelletier G. Cyclic formation and decay of the blood–testis barrier in the mink (*Mustel vison*), a seasonal breeder. *Am J Anat* 1986;175:91–117.
315. Ramos AM, Dym M. Ultrastructural differentiation of rat Sertoli cells. *Biol Reprod* 1979;21:909–922.
316. Kelly CW, Janecki A, Steinberger A, Russell LD. Structural characteristics of immature rat Sertoli cells *in vivo* and *in vitro. Am J Anat* 1991;192:183–193.
317. Pomerantz D. Effects of *in-vivo* gonadotropin treatment on estrogen levels in the testis of the immature rat. *Biol Reprod* 1979;21:1247–1255.
318. Rosselli M, Skinner MK. Developmental regulation of Sertoli cell aromatase activity and plasminogen activator production by hormones, retinoids and the testicular paracrine factor, PModS. *Biol Reprod* 1992;46:586–594.
319. Josso N, Picard J-Y. Anti-mullerian hormone. *Physiol Rev* 1986;66:1038–1090.
320. Kuroda T, Lee MM, Haqq CM, Powell DM, Manganaro TF, Donahoe PK. Mullerian inhibiting substance ontogeny and its modulation by FSH in the rat testis. *Endocrinology* 1990;127:1825–1832.
321. Rich KA, Bardin CW, Gunsalus GL, Mather JP. Age-dependent pattern of ABP secretion from rat Sertoli cells in primary culture. *Endocrinology* 1983;113:2284–2293.
322. Danzo BJ, Eller BC. The ontogeny of biologically active androgen-binding protein in rat plasma, testis and epididymis. *Endocrinology* 1985;117:1380–1387.
323. Le Magueresse B, Jégou B. *In vitro* effects of germ cells on the secretory activity of Sertoli cells recovered from rats of different ages. *Endocrinology* 1988;122:1672–1680.
324. Le Magueresse B, Jégou B. Paracrine control of immature Sertoli cells by adult germ cells in the rat (an *in-vitro* study). Cell–cell interactions within the testis. *Mol Cell Endocrinol* 1988; 58:65–72.
325. Le Magueresse B, Le Gac F, Loir M, Jégou B. Stimulation of rat Sertoli cell secretory activity *in-vitro* by germ cells and residual bodies. *J Reprod Fertil* 1986;77:489–498.
326. Castellon E, Janecki A, Steinberger A. Age-dependent Sertoli cell responsiveness to germ cells *in vitro. Int J Androl* 1989;12:439–450.
327. Castellon E, Janecki A, Steinberger A. Influence of germ cells on Sertoli cell secretory activity in direct and indirect co-culture with Sertoli cells from rats of different ages. *Mol Cell Endocrinol* 1989;64:169–178.
328. Ritzen EM, Hagenas L, Ploen L, French FS, Hansson V. *In vitro*

synthesis of rat testicular androgen-binding protein (ABP). *Mol Cell Endocrinol* 1977;8:335–346.
329. McLaren TT, Foster PMD, Sharpe RM. Effect of age on seminiferous tubule protein secretion and the adverse effects of testicular toxicants in the rat. *Int J Androl* 1993; [*in press*].
330. Purvis K, Hansson V. Hormonal regulation of spermatogenesis: regulation of target cell response. *Int J Androl* 1981;3:85–125.
331. Hugly S, Roberts K, Griswold MD. Transferrin and sulfated glycoprotein-2 messenger ribonucleic acid levels in the testis and isolated Sertoli cells of hypophysectomized rats. *Endocrinology* 1988;122:1390–1396.
332. Jégou B, Le Gac F, De Kretser DM. Seminiferous tubule fluid and interstitial fluid production. I. Effects of age and hormonal regulation in immature rats. *Biol Reprod* 1982;27:590–595.
333. Jégou B, Le Gac F, Irby DC, De Kretser DM. Studies on seminiferous tubule fluid production in the adult rat: effect of hypophysectomy and treatment with FSH, LH and testosterone. *Int J Androl* 1983;6:249–260.
334. Tindall DJ, Rowley DR, Murthy L, Lipshultz LI, Chang CH. Structure and biochemistry of the Sertoli cell. *Int Rev Cytol* 1985;94:127–149.
335. Danzo BJ, Pavlou SN, Anthony HL. Hormonal regulation of androgen-binding protein in the rat. *Endocrinology* 1990; 127:2829–2838.
336. Sanborn BM, Wagle JR, Steinberger A, Greer-Emmert D. Maturational and hormonal influences on Sertoli cell function. *Endocrinology* 1986;118:1700–1709.
336a. Steinberger A, Hintz M, Heindel JJ. Changes in cyclic AMP responses to FSH in isolated rat Sertoli cells during sexual maturation. *Biol Reprod* 1978;19:566–572.
337. Ketelslegers JM, Hetzel WD, Sherins RJ, Catt KJ. Developmental changes in testicular gonadotrophin receptors, plasma gonadotropins and plasma testosterone in the rat. *Endocrinology* 1978;103:212–222.
338. Bortolussi M, Zanchetta R, Belvedere P, Colombo L. Sertoli and Leydig cell numbers and gonadotropin receptors in rat testis from birth to puberty. *Cell Tissue Res* 1990;260:185–191.
339. Madhwa Raj HG, Dym M. The effects of selective withdrawal of FSH or LH on spermatogenesis in the immature rat. *Biol Reprod* 1976;14:489–494.
340. Solari AJ, Fritz IB. The ultrastructure of immature Sertoli cells. Maturation-like changes during culture and the maintenance of mitotic potentiality. *Biol Reprod* 1978;18:329–345.
340a. Posalaky Z, Meyer R, McGinley D. The effects of FSH on Sertoli cell junctions *in vitro:* A freeze-fracture study. *J Ultrastruct Res* 1981;74:241–254.
341. Means AR, Dedman JR, Tash JS, Tindall DJ, Van Sickel M, Welsh MJ. Regulation of the testis Sertoli cell by follicle-stimulating hormone. *Annu Rev Physiol* 1980;42:59–70.
342. Griswold MD. Actions of FSH on mammalian Sertoli cells. In: Russell LD, Griswold MD, eds. *The Sertoli cell.* Clearwater, Florida: Cache River Press; 1993:493–508.
343. Au CL, Irby DC, Robertson DM, De Kretser DM. Effects of testosterone on testicular inhibin and fluid production in intact and hypophysectomized adult rats. *J Reprod Fertil* 1986; 76:257–266.
344. Buzek SW, Caston LA, Sanborn BM. Evidence for age-dependent changes in Sertoli cell androgen receptor concentration. *J Androl* 1987;8:83–90.
345. Buzek SW, Sanborn BM. Increase in testicular androgen receptor during sexual maturation in the rat. *Biol Reprod* 1988;39:39–49.
346. Verhoeven G, Caillaeu J. Follicle-stimulating hormone and androgens increase the concentration of the androgen receptor in Sertoli cells. *Endocrinology* 1988;122:1541–1550.
347. Blok LJ, Mackenbach P, Trapman J, Themmen APN, Brinkmann AO, Grooteogoed JA. Follicle-stimulating hormone regulates androgen receptor mRNA in Sertoli cells. *Mol Cell Endocrinol* 1989;63:267–271.
348. Blok LJ, Hoogerbrugge JW, Themmen APN, Baarends WM, Post M, Grootegoed JA. Transient down-regulation of androgen receptor mRNA expression in Sertoli cells by FSH is followed by up-regulation of androgen receptor mRNA and protein. *Endocrinology* 1992;131:1343–1349.
349. Sanborn BM, Caston LA, Chang C, et al. Regulation of androgen receptor mRNA in rat Sertoli cells and peritublar cells. *Biol Reprod* 1991;45:634–641.
350. McKinnell C, Sharpe RM. The role of specific germ cell types in modulation of the secretion of androgen-regulated proteins (ARP's) by stage VI-VIII seminiferous tubules from the adult rat. *Mol Cell Endocrinol* 1992;83:219–231.
351. Culler MD, Negro-Vilar A. Passive immunoneutralization of endogenous inhibin: Sex-related differences in the role of inhibin during development. *Mol Cell Endocrinol* 1988;58:263–272.
352. Rivier C, Cajander S, Vaughan J, Hsueh AJW, Vale W. Age-dependent changes in physiological action, content and immunostaining of inhibin in male rats. *Endocrinology* 1988; 123:120–126.
353. Odell WD, Swerdloff RS, Jacobs HS, Hescox MA. FSH induction of sensitivity to LH: One cause of sexual maturation in the male rat. *Endocrinology* 1973;92:160–165.
354. Odell WD, Swerdloff RS. The role of testicular sensitivity to gonadotropins in sexual maturation of the male rat. *J Steroids Biochem* 1975;6:853–857.
355. Chen YDI, Payne AH, Kelch RP. FSH stimulation of Leydig cell function in the hypophysectomized immature rat. *Proc Soc Exp Biol Med* 1976;153:473–475.
356. Chen YDI, Shaw MJ, Payne AH. Steroid and FSH action on LH receptors and LH-sensitive testicular responsiveness during sexual maturation of the rat. *Mol Cell Endocrinol* 1977;8:291–299.
357. Hsueh AJW, Dufau ML, Catt KJ. Direct inhibitory effect of estrogen on Leydig cell function of hypophysectomized rats. *Endocrinology* 1978;103:1096–1102.
358. Selin LK, Moger WH. The effect of FSH on LH induced testosterone secretion in the immature hypophysectomized male rat. *Endocrine Res Commun* 1977;4:171–182.
359. van Beurden WMO, Roodnat B, de Jong FH, Mulder E, van der Molen HJ. Hormonal regulation of LH stimulation of testosterone production in isolated Leydig cells of immature rats: The effect of hypophysectomy, FSH and estradiol-17β. *Steroids* 1976;28:847–866.
360. Kerr JB, Sharpe RM. FSH induction of Leydig cell maturation. *Endocrinology* 1985;116:2592–2604.
361. O'Shaughnessy PJ, Bennett MK, Scott IS, Charlton HM. Effects of FSH on Leydig cell morphology and function in the hypogonadal mouse. *J Endocrinol* 1992;135:517–525.
362. Niklowitz P, Khan S, Bergmann M, Hoffmann K, Nieschlag E. Differential effects of FSH and LH on Leydig cell function and restoration of spermatogenesis in hypophysectomized and photoinhibited Djungarian hamsters (*Phodopus sungorus*). *Biol Reprod* 1989;41:871–880.
363. Vihko KK, Lapolt PS, Mishimor K, Hsueh AJW. Stimulatory effects of recombinant FSH on Leydig cell function and spermatogenesis in immature hypophysectomized rats. *Endocrinology* 1991;129:1926–1932.
364. Teerds KJ, Closset J, Rommerts FFG, de Rooij DG, Stocco DM. Colenbrander B< Wensing CJG, Hennen G. Effects of pure FSH and LH preparations on the number and function of Leydig cells in immature hypophysectomized rats. *J Endocrinol* 1989; 120:97–106.
365. Kerr JB, Sharpe RM. Stimulatory effect of FSH on rat Leydig cells. A morphometric and ultrastructural study. *Cell Tissue Res* 1985;239:405–415.
366. Murono EP, Payne AH. Testicular maturation in the rat. *In vivo* effect of gonadotropins on steroidogenic enzymes in the hypophysectomized immature rat. *Biol Reprod* 1979;20:911–918.
367. Hansson V, Calandra R, Purvis K, Ritzen EM, French FS. Hormonal regulation of spermatogenesis. *Vit Horm* 1976;34: 187–214.
368. Knorr DW, Vaha-Perttula T, Lipsett MB. Structure and function of the rat testis through pubescence. *Endocrinology* 1970; 86:1298–1304.
369. Hardy MP, Zirkin BR, Ewing LL. Kinetic studies on the development of the adult population of Leydig cells in the testes of the pubertal rat. *Endocrinology* 1989;124:762–770.
370. Matt KS, Stetson MH. Hypothalamic–pituitary–gonadal interactions during spontaneous testicular recrudescence in the golden hamster, (*Mesocricetus auratus*). *Biol Reprod* 1979;20:739–746.
371. Sinha Hikim AP, Amador AG, Bartke A, Russell LD. Structural/

function relationships in active and inactive hamster Leydig cells: A correlative morphometric and endocrine study. *Endocrinology* 1989;125:1844–1856.
372. Sinha Hikim AP, Bartke A, Russell LD. The seasonally breeding hamster as a model to study structure-function relationships in the testis. *Tissue Cell* 1988;20:63–78.
373. Christensen AK. Leydig cells. In: Hamilton DW, Greep RO, eds. *Handbook of physiology, vol V.* Washington DC: American Physiological Society; 1975:57–94.
374. Johnson L, Neaves WB. Age-related changes in the Leydig cell population, seminiferous tubules and sperm production in stallions. *Biol Reprod.* 1981;24:703–712.
375. Bex FJ, Bartke A. Testicular LH-binding in the hamster: modification by photoperiod and prolactin. *Endocrinology* 1977; 100:1223–1226.
376. Bex F, Bartke A, Goldman BD, Dalterio S. Prolactin, growth hormone, luteinizing hormone receptors and seasonal changes in testicular activity in the golden hamster. *Endocrinology* 1978;103:2069–2080.
377. Barenton B, Pelletier J. Prolactin, testicular growth and LH-receptors in the ram following light and 2-Br-α-ergocryptine treatments. *Biol Reprod* 1980;22:781–790.
378. Sharpe RM. The hormonal regulation of the Leydig cell. In: Finn CA, ed. *Oxford reviews of reproductive biology.* Oxford: Oxford University Press; 1982:241–317.
379. Sizonenko PC, Cuendet A, Paunier L. FSH. I. Evidence for its mediating role on testosterone secretion in cryptorchidism. *J Clin Endocrinol Metab* 1973;37:68–73.
380. Nistal M, Paniagua R. Leydig cell differentiation induced by stimulation with HCG and HMG in two patients with hypogonadotropic hypogonadism. *Andrologia* 1979;11:211–222.
381. Mancini RE. Effect of different types of gonadotrophins on the induction and restoration of spermatogenesis in the human testis. *Acta Eur Fertil* 1969;1:401–429.
382. Johnsen SG. Maintenance of spermatogenesis induced by HMG treatment by means of continuous HCG treatment in hypogonadotrophic men. *Acta Endocrinol* 1978;89:763–769.
383. Ojeifo JO, Byers SW, Papadopoulos V, Dym M. Sertoli cell-secreted protein(s) stimulates DNA synthesis in purified rat Leydig cells *in-vitro. J Reprod Fertil* 1990;90:93–108.
384. Hardy MP, Gelber SJ, Zhou Z, et al. Hormonal control of Leydig cell differentiation. *Ann NY Acad Sci* 1991;637:152–163.
385. Benhamed M, Tabone E, Reventos J, Saez JM. Role of Sertoli cells in Leydig cell function. *INSERM Coll* 1984;123:363–385.
386. Tabone E, Benahmed M, Reventos J, Saez JM. Interactions between immature porcine Leydig and Sertoli cells *in vitro.* An ultrastructural and biochemical study. *Cell Tissue Res* 1984; 237:357–362.
387. Ewing LL, Zirkin B. Leydig cell structure and steroidogenic function. *Recent Prog Horm Res* 1983;39:599–635.
388. Setchell BP. The secretion of fluid by the testes of rats, rams and goats with some observations on the effect of age, cryptorchidism and hypophysectomy. *J Reprod Fertil* 1970;23:79–85.
389. Setchell BP, Pollanen P, Zupp JL. Development of the blood–testis barrier and changes in vascular permeability at puberty in rats. *Int J Androl* 1988;11:225–233.
390. Dacheux JL, Pisselet C, Blanc MR, Hocherau De Reviers MT, Courot M. Seasonal variations in rete testis fluid secretion and sperm production in different breeds of ram. *J Reprod Fertil* 1981;61:363–371.
391. Bartke A, Amador AG, Chandrashekar V, Klemcke HG. Seasonal differences in testicular receptors and steroidogenesis. *J Steroid Biochem* 1987;27:581–587.
392. Setchell BP. *The mammalian testis.* London: Paul Elek; 1978.
393. Setchell BP. The functional significance of the blood–testis barrier. *J Androl* 1980;1:3–10.
394. Boccabella AV. Reinitiation and restoration of spermatogenesis with testosterone propionate and other hormones after long-term and post-hypophysectomy regression period. *Endocrinology* 1963;72:787–798.
395. Elkington JSH, Blackshaw AW. Studies on testicular function. I. Quantitative effects of FSH, LH, testosterone and dihydrotestosterone on restoration and maintenance of spermatogenesis in the hypophysectomized rat. *Aust J Biol Sci* 1974;27:47–57.
396. Huang HFS, Marshall GR, Rosenberg R, Nieschlag E. Restoration of spermatogenesis by high levels of testosterone in hypophysectomized rats after long-term regression. *Acta Endocrinol* 1987;116:433–444.
397. Roberts KP, Awoniyi CA, Santulli R, Zirkin BR. Regulation of Sertoli cell tansferrin and sulfated glycoprotein-2 mRNA levels during the restoration of spermatogenesis in the adult hypophysectomized rat. *Endocrinology* 1991;129:3417–3423.
398. Awoniyi CA, Santulli R, Chandrashekar V, Schanbacher BD, Zirkin BR. Quantitative restoration of advanced spermatogenic cells in adult male rats made azoospermic by active immunization against LH or GnRH. *Endocrinology* 1989;125:1303–1309.
399. Marshall GR, Wickings EJ, Ludecke DK, Nieschlag E. Stimulation of spermatogenesis in stalk-sectioned rhesus monkeys by testosterone alone. *J Clin Endocrinol Metab* 1984;57:152–159.
400. Marshall GR, Wickings EJ, Nieschlag E. Testosterone can initiate spermatogenesis in an immature nonhuman primate, *Macaca fascicularis. Endocrinology* 1984;114:2228–2233.
401. Steinberger E, Root A, Ficher M, Smith KD. The role of androgens in the initiation of spermatogenesis in man. *J Clin Endocrinol Metab* 1973;37:746–751.
402. Chemes HE, Pasqualini T, Rivarola MA, Bergada C. Is testosterone involved in the initiation of spermatogenesis in humans? A clinicopathological presentation and physiological consideration in four patients with Leydig cell tumours of the testis or secondary Leydig cell hyperplasia. *Int J Androl* 1982;5:229–245.
403. Rosenthal SM, Grumbach MM, Kaplan SL. Gonadotrophin-independent familial sexual precocity with premature Leydig and germinal cell maturation (familial testotoxicosis): Effects of a potent LHRH agonist and medroxyprogesterone acetate therapy in four cases. *J Clin Endocrinol Metab* 1983;57:571–579.
404. Reiter EO, Brown RS, Longcope C, Beitins IZ. Male-limited familial precocious puberty in three generations: apparent Leydig cell autonomy and elevated glycoprotein hormone alpha subunit. *N Engl J Med* 1986;311:515–519.
405. Holland FJ, Fishman L, Bailey JD, Fazekas ATA. Ketoconazole in the management of precocious puberty not responsive to LHRH-analogue therapy. *N Engl J Med* 1985;312:1023–1028.
406. Berndtson WE, Desjardins C. Circulating LH and FSH levels and testicular function in hamsters during light deprivation and subsequent photoperiodic stimulation. *Endocrinology* 1974;95: 195–205.
407. Bartke A, Sinha Hikim AP, Russell LD. Sertoli cell structure and function in seasonally breeding mammals. In: Russell LD, Griswold MD, eds. *The Sertoli cell.* Clearwater, Florida: Cache River Press; 1993:349–364.
408. Kulin HE. Disorders of sexual maturation: delayed adolescence and precocious puberty. In: de Groot LJ, ed. *Endocrinology,* 2nd ed., vol 3. Philadelphia: WB Saunders, 1989:1873–1899.
409. Kerr JB, Donachie K, Rommerts FFG. Selective destruction and regeneration of rat Leydig cells *in-vivo.* A new method for the study of seminiferous tubular–interstitial tissue interaction. *Cell Tissue Res* 1985;242:145–156.
410. Molenaar R, de Rooij DG, Rommerts FFG, van der Molen HJ. Repopulation of Leydig cells in mature rats after selective destruction of the existent Leydig cells with ethylene dimethane sulfonate is dependent on LH and not FSH. *Endocrinology* 1986;118:2546–2554.
411. Morris ID, Philips DM, Bardin CW. Ethylene dimethanesulfonate destroys Leydig cells in the rat testis. *Endocrinology* 1986;118:709–719.
412. Bartlett JMS, Kerr JB, Sharpe RM. The effect of selective destruction and regeneration of rat Leydig cells on the intratesticular distribution of testosterone and morphology of the seminiferous epithelium. *J Androl* 1986;7:240–253.
413. Jackson AE, O'Leary PC, Ayers MM, de Kretser DM. The effects of ethylene dimethane sulphonate (EDS) on rat Leydig cells: Evidence to support a connective tissue origin of Leydig cells. *Biol Reprod* 1986;35:425–437.
414. Dunn DR, Elson LA. The effect of a homologous series of dimethane sulphonylalkanes on haemopoietic colony forming units in the rat. *Chem-Biol Interact* 1970;2:273–280.
415. Jackson CM, Jackson H. Comparative protective actions of gonadotrophins and testosterone against the antispermatogenic action of ethane dimethanesulphonate. *J Reprod Fertil* 1984;71:393–401.

416. Cooper ERA, Jackson H. Chemically induced sperm retention cysts in the rat. *J Reprod Fertil* 1973;34:445–449.
417. Klinefelter GR, Roberts NL, Suarez JD. Direct effects of ethane dimethanesulphonate on epididymal function in adult rats: An *in-vitro* demonstration. *J Androl* 1992;13:409–421.
418. Verhoeven G, Cailleau J, Morris ID. Inhibitory effects of alkane sulphonates on the function of immature rat Leydig, Sertoli and peritubular cells cultured *in-vitro. J Mol Endocrinol* 1989; 2:145–155.
419. Sprando RL, Santulli R, Awoniyi CA, Ewing LL, Zirkin BR. Does ethane 1,2-dimethanesulphonate (EDS) have a direct cytotoxic effect on the seminiferous epithelium of the rat testis? *J Androl* 1990;11:344–352.
420. Morris ID. Leydig cell resistance to the cytotoxic effect of ethylene dimethanesulphonate in the adult rat testis. *J Endocrinol* 1985;105:311–316.
421. Ahmad N, Haltmeyer GC, Eik-Nes KB. Maintenance of spermatogenesis in rats with intratesticular implants containing testosterone or dihydrotestosterone (DHT). *Biol Reprod* 1973; 8:411–419.
422. Sun Y-T, Irby DC, Robertson DM, de Kretser DM. The effects of exogenously administered testosterone on spermatogenesis in intact and hypophysectomized rats. *Endocrinology* 1989;125: 1000–1010.
423. Santulli R, Sprando RL, Awoniyi CA, Ewing LL, Zirkin RB. To what extent can spermatogenesis be maintained in the hypophysectomized adult rat testis with exogenously administered testosterone. *Endocrinology* 1990;126:95–102.
424. Sharpe RM. Gonadotrophin-induced accumulation of interstitial fluid in the rat testis. *J Reprod Fertil* 1979;55:365–371.
425. Turner TT, Jones CE, Howards SS, Ewing LL, Zegeye B, Gunsalus GL. On the androgen microenvironment of maturing spermatozoa. *Endocrinology* 1984;115:1925–1932.
426. Comhaire FH, Vermeulen A. Testosterone concentration in the fluids of seminiferous tubules, the interstitium and the rete testis of the rat. *J Endocrinol* 1976;70:229–235.
427. Suzuki K, Eto T. Androgens in testicular venous blood in the adult rat. *Endocrinol Jpn* 1962;9:277–283.
428. Nishihara M, Takahashi M. Effects of active immunization against estradiol-17β on luteinizing hormone and testosterone in male rats. *Biol Reprod* 1983;29:1092–1094.
429. Turner TT, Ewing LL, Jones CE, Howards SS, Zegeye B. Androgens in various fluid compartments of the rat testis and epididymis after hypophysectomy and gonadotropin supplementation. *J Androl* 1985;6:353–358.
430. Maddocks S, Setchell BP. The composition of extracellular interstitial fluid collected with a push-pull cannula from the testes of adult rats. *J Physiol (Lond)* 1988;407:304–312.
431. Maddocks S, Setchell BP. Testosterone concentrations in testicular interstitial fluid collected with a push–pull cannula or by drip-collection from adult rats given testosterone or aminoglutethimide. *J Endocrinol* 1989;121:303–309.
432. Maddocks S, Sharpe RM. Dynamics of testosterone secretion by the rat testis: Implications for measurement of the intratesticular levels of testosterone. *J Endocrinol* 1989;122:323–329.
433. Maddocks S, Hargreave TB, Reddie K, Fraser HM, Kerr JB, Sharpe RM. Intratesticular hormone levels and the route of secretion of hormones from the testis of the rat, guinea pig, monkey and human. *Int J Androl [in press]*.
434. Jeffcoate SL, Brooks RV, Lim NY, London DR, Prunty FTG, Spathis GS. Androgen production in hypogonadal men. *J Endocrinol* 1967;37:401–411.
435. de la Torre B, Noren S, Hedman M, Diczfalusy E. Studies on the relationship between sperm count and steroid levels in the spermatic and cubital veins of patients with varicocele. *Int J Androl* 1978;1:297–307.
436. Ishida H, Tashiro H, Watanabe M, et al. Measurement of inhibin concentrations in men: study of changes after castration and comparison with androgen levels in testicular tissue, spermatic venous blood and peripheral venous blood. *J Clin Endocrinol Metab* 1990;70:1019–1022.
437. Winters SJ. Inhibin is secreted together with testosterone by the human testis. *J Clin Endocrinol Metab* 1990;70:548–550.
438. Bardin CW, Peterson RE. Studies on androgen production by the rat: Testosterone and androstenedione content of blood. *Endocrinology* 1967;80:38–44.
439. Cooper TG, Waites GMH. Testosterone in rete testis fluid and blood of rams and rats. *J Endocrinol* 1974;62:619–629.
440. Hirsh AV, Tyler JPP, Landon G, et al. Testicular testosterone concentration, interstitial cell density and spermatogenesis in infertile men. *Int J Androl* 1981;4:409–420.
441. Free MJ. Blood supply to the testis and its role in local exchange and transport of hormones. In: Johnson AD, Gomes WR, eds. *The testis*. New York: Academic Press; 1977:39–90.
442. Sharpe RM. Gonadotrophin-induced accumulation of interstitial fluid in the rat testis. *J Reprod Fertil* 1979;55:365–371.
443. Sharpe RM, Bartlett JMS. Stimulation of Leydig cell function by a polypeptide present in testicular interstitial fluid. *Med Biol* 1985;63:245–250.
444. Cooke BA, De Jong FH, Van Der Molen HJ, Rommerts FFG. Endogenous testosterone concentrations in rat testis interstitial tissue and seminiferous tubules during in vitro incubation. *Nature [New Biol]* 1972;237:255–256.
445. De Jong FH, Hey AG, van der Molen HJ. Oestradiol-17β and testosterone in rat testis tissue: effect of gonadotrophins, localization and production in vitro. *J Endocrinol* 1974;60:409–419.
446. Galil KAA, Setchell BP. Effect of local heating of the testes on the concentration of testosterone in jugular and testicular venous blood of rats and on testosterone production *in vitro*. *Int J Androl* 1987;11:61–72.
447. Dym M, Madhwa Raj HG. Response of adult Sertoli rat cells and Leydig cells to depletion of luteinizing hormone and testosterone. *Biol Reprod* 1977;17:676–696.
448. Harris ME, Bartke A. Concentration of testosterone in testis fluid of the rat. *Endocrinology* 1974;95:701–706.
449. Kerr JB, Maddocks S, Sharpe RM. Testosterone and FSH have independent, synergistic and stage-dependent effects upon spermatogenesis in the rat testis. *Cell Tissue Res* 1992;268: 179–189.
450. Teerds KJ, De Rooij DK, Rommerts FFG, Wensing CJG. The regulation of the proliferation and differentiation of Leydig cell precursor cells after EDS administration or daily hCG treatment. *J Androl* 1988;9:343–351.
451. Chandolia RK, Weinbauer GF, Fingscheidt U, Bartlett JMS, Nieschlag E. Effects of flutamide on testicular involution induced by an antagonist of gonadotrophin-releasing hormone and on stimulation of spermatogenesis by FSH in rats. *J Reprod Fertil* 1991;93:313–323.
452. Voglmayr JK, Roberson C, Musto NA. Comparison of androgen levels in ram rete testis fluid, testicular lymph and spermatic venous blood plasma: evidence for a regulatory mechanism in the seminiferous tubules. *Biol Reprod* 1980;23:29–39.
453. Noordhuizen-Stassen EN, Charbon GA, de Jong FH, Wensing CJG. Functional arterio-venous anastomoses between the testicular artery and the pampiniform plexus in the spermatic cord of rams. *J Reprod Fertil* 1985;75:193–201.
454. Wensing CJG, Djikstra G. The morphological relation between the testicular artery and the pampiniform plexus in the spermatic cord. *Acta Morphol Neer Scand* 1981;19:162.
455. Wensing CJG, Djikstra G, Frankenhuis MT. The intricate morphological relations between the testicular artery and pampiniform plexus. *Int J Androl Suppl* 1981;4:77–78.
456. Hees H, Leiser R, Kohlter T, Wrobel KH. Vascular morphology of the bovine spermatic cord and testis. *Cell Tissue Res* 1984;237:31–38.
457. Bayard F, Boulard PY, Huc A, Pontonnier F. Arterio-venous transfer of testosterone in the spermatic cord of man. *J Clin Endocrinol Metab* 1975;40:345–346.
458. Roberts KP, Santulli R, Seiden J, Zirkin BR. The effect of testosterone withdrawal and subsequent germ cell depletion on transferrin and sulfated glycoprotein-2 mRNA levels in the adult rat testis. *Biol Reprod* 1992;47:92–96.
459. Awoniyi CA, Zirkin BR, Chandrashekar V, Schlaff WD. Exogenously administered testosterone maintains spermatogenesis quantitatively in adult rats actively immunized against GnRH. *Endocrinology* 1992;130:3283–3288.
460. Buhl AE, Cornette JC, Kirkton KT, Yuan Y-D. Hypophysectomized male rats treated with polydimethylsiloxane capsules containing testosterone: Effects on spermatogenesis, fertility and re-

productive tract concentrations of androgens. *Biol Reprod* 1982;27:183–188.
461. Robaire B, Zirkin BR. Hypophysectomy and simultaneous testosterone replacement: effects on male rat reproductive tract and epididymal Δ^4-5α-reductase and 3α-hydroxysteroid dehydrogenase. *Endocrinology* 1981;109:1225–1233.
462. Sun Y-T, Wreford NG, Robertson DM, de Kretser DM. Quantitative cytological studies of spermatogenesis in intact and hypophysectomized rats: Identification of androgen-dependent stages. *Endocrinology* 1990;127:1215–1223.
463. Chowdhury AK, Tcholakian RK. Effects of various doses of testosterone propionate on intratesticular and plasma testosterone levels and maintenance of spermatogenesis in adult hypophysectomized rats. *Steroids* 1979;34:151–162.
464. Bartlett JMS, Weinbauer GF, Nieschlag E. Differential effects of FSH and testosterone on the maintenance of spermatogenesis in the adult hypophysectomized rat. *J Endocrinol* 1989;121:49–58.
465. Collins PM, Tsang WN. A quantitative assessment of the gametogenic and androgenic properties of testicular steroids in hypophysectomized rats. *J Reprod Fertil* 1985;75:285–292.
466. Ahmad N, Haltmeyer GC, Eik-Nes KB. Maintenance of spermatogenesis with testosterone or dihydrotestosterone in hypophysectomized rats. *J Reprod Fertil* 1975;44:103–107.
467. Berndtson WE, Desjardins C, Ewing LL. Inhibition and maintenance of spermatogenesis in rats implanted with polydimethylsiloxane capsules containing various androgens. *J Endocrinol* 1974;62:125–135.
468. Rea MA, Marshall GR, Weinbauer GF, Nieschlag E. Testosterone maintains pituitary and serum FSH and spermatogenesis in gonadotrophin-releasing hormone antagonist-suppressed rats. *J Endocrinol* 1986;108:101–107.
469. Zirkin BR, Santulli R, Awoniyi CA, Ewing LL. Maintenance of advanced spermatogenic cells in the adult rat testis: quantitative relationship to testosterone concentration within the testis. *Endocrinology* 1989;124:3043–3049.
470. Robaire B, Ewing LL, Irby DC, Desjardins C. Interactions of testosterone and estradiol-17β on the reproductive tract of the male rat. *Biol Reprod* 1979;21:455–463.
471. Huang HFS, Boccabella AV. Dissociation of qualitative and quantitative effects of the suppression of testicular testosterone upon spermatogenesis. *Acta Endocrinol* 1988;118:209–217.
472. Cunningham GR, Huckins C. Persistence of complete spermatogenesis in the presence of low intratesticular concentrations of testosterone. *Endocrinology* 1979;105:177–186.
473. Chowdhury AK. Dependence of testicular germ cells on hormones: A quantitative study in hypophysectomized testosterone-treated rats. *J Endocrinol* 1979;82:331–340.
474. Awoniyi CA, Sprando RL, Santulli R, Chandrashekar V, Ewing LL, Zirkin BR. Restoration of spermatogenesis by exogenously administered testosterone in rats made azoospermic by hypophysectomy or withdrawal of luteinizing hormone alone. *Endocrinology* 1990;127:177–184.
475. Ghosh S, Sinha-Hikim AP, Russell LD. Further observations of stage-specific effects seen after short-term hypophysectomy in the rat. *Tissue Cell* 1991;23:613–630.
476. Russell LD, Clermont Y. Degeneration of germ cells in normal, hypophysectomized and hormone treated hypophysectomized rats. *Anat Rec* 1977;187:347–366.
477. Russell LD, Malone JP, Karpas SL. Morphological pattern elicited by agents affecting spermatogenesis by disruption of its hormonal stimulation. *Tissue Cell* 1981;13:369–380.
478. Russell LD, Ettlin RA, Sinha Hikim AP, Clegg ED. *Histological and histopathological evaluation of the testis.* Clearwater, Florida: Cache River Press; 1990.
479. Hess RA. Quantitative and qualitative characteristics of the stages and transitions in the cycle of the rat seminiferous epithelium: Light microscopic observations of perfusion-fixed and plastic-embedded testes. *Biol Reprod* 1990;43:525–542.
480. Linder RE, Strader LF, Slott VL, Suarez JD. Endpoints of spermatotoxicity in the rat after short duration exposures to fourteen reproductive toxicants. *Reprod Toxicol* 1992;6:491–505.
481. Johnson L, Petty CS, Neaves WB. The relationship of biopsy evaluations and testicular measurements to overall daily sperm production in human testes. *Fertil Steril* 1980;32:36–40.
482. Kerr JB, Millar M, Maddocks S, Sharpe RM. Stage-dependent changes in spermatogenesis and Sertoli cells in relation to the onset of spermatogenic failure following withdrawal of testosterone. *Anat Rec* 1993;235:547–559.
483. Boekelheide K. Sertoli cell toxicants. In: Russell LD, Griswold MD, eds. *The Sertoli cell.* Clearwater, Florida: Cache River Press; 1993:552–575.
484. Desjardins C, Ewing LL, Irby DC. Response of the rabbit seminiferous epithelium to testosterone administered via polydimethylsiloxane. *Endocrinology* 1973;93:450–460.
485. Matsumoto AM, Karpas AE, Paulsen CA, Bremner WJ. Reinitiation of sperm production in gonadotropin-suppressed normal men by administration of follicle-stimulating hormone. *J Clin Invest* 1983;72:1005–1015.
486. Matsumoto AM, Paulsen CA, Bremner WJ. Stimulation of sperm production by human luteinizing hormone in gonadotropin-suppressed normal men. *J Clin Endocrinol Metab* 1984;55:882–887.
487. Matsumoto AM, Karpas AE, Bremner WJ. Chronic hCG administration in normal men: Evidence that FSH is necessary for the maintenance of quantitatively normal spermatogenesis in man. *J Clin Endocrinol Metab* 1986;62:1184–1192.
488. Matsumoto AM. Is high dosage testosterone an effective male contraceptive agent? *Fertil Steril* 1990;50:324–328.
489. Bhasin S, Fielder TJ, Swerdloff RS. Testosterone selectively increases serum FSH but not LH in GnRH antagonist-treated male rats: Evidence for differential regulation of LH and FSH secretion. *Biol Reprod* 1987;37:55–59.
490. Rivier C, Rivier J, Vale W. Chronic effects of [D-Trp^6, Pro^9-NET] luteinizing hormone-releasing factor on reproductive processes in the male rat. *Endocrinology* 1979;105:1191–1201.
491. Labrie F, Belanger A, Cusan I, et al. Antifertility effects of LHRH agonists in the male. *J Androl* 1980;1:209–228.
492. Pelletier G, Cusan GL, Belanger A, Seguin C, Kelly PA, Labrie F. Further studies on the inhibitory effect of [D-Ala^6, des-Gly-NH_2^{10}] LHRH ethylamide on spermatogenesis and steroidogenesis in the rat: reversibility and effect of androgen administration. *J Androl* 1980;1:171–181.
493. Vickery B, McRae GI, Bergstrom K, Briones W, Worden A, Seidenberg R. Inability of long-term administration of D-Nal(2)6-LHRH to abolish fertility in male rats. *J Androl* 1983;4:283–291.
494. Lefebvre FA, Belanger A, Pelletier G, Labrie F. Recovery of gonadal functions in the adult male rat following cessation of five-month daily treatment with an LHRH agonist. *J Androl* 1984;5:181–192.
495. Labrie F, Cusan L, Sequin C, et al. Antifertility effects of LHRH agonists in the male rat and inhibition of testicular steroidogenesis in man. *Int J Fertil* 1980;25:157–170.
496. Kerr JB, Sharpe RM. Effects and interaction of LH and LHRH agonist on testicular morphology and function in hypophysectomized rats. *J Reprod Fertil* 1986;76:175–192.
497. Kerr JB, Sharpe RM. Focal disruption of spermatogenesis in the testis of adult rats after a single administration of hCG. *Cell Tissue Res* 1989;257:163–169.
498. Kerr JB, Sharpe RM. Macrophage activation enhances the hCG-induced disruption of spermatogenesis in the rat. *J Endocrinol* 1989;121:285–292.
499. Van Vliet J, Rommerts FFG, De Rooij DG, Buwalda G, Wensing CJG. Reduction of testicular blood flow and focal degeneration of tissue in the rat after administration of hCG. *J Endocrinol* 1988;117:51–57.
500. Verjans HL, De Jong FH, Cooke BA, Van Der Molen HJ, Eik-Nes KB. Effects of estradiol benzoate on pituitary and testis function in normal adult male rats. *Acta Endocrinol [Kbh]* 1974;77:636–642.
501. Steinberger E, Duckett GE. The effect of estrogen or testosterone on the initiation and maintenance of spermatogenesis in the rat. *Endocrinology* 1965;76:1184–1189.
502. Ewing LL, Desjardins C, Irby DC, Robaire B. Synergistic interaction of testosterone and oestradiol inhibits spermatogenesis in rats. *Nature* 1977;269:409–411.
503. Van Beurden WMO, Mulder E, De Jong FH, van der Molen HJ. The effect of estrogens on luteinizing hormone plasma levels and

on testosterone production in intact and hypophysectomized rats. *Endocrinology* 1977;101:342–349.
504. Sivelle PC, McNeilly AS, Collins PM. A comparison of the effectiveness of FSH, LH and prolactin in the reinitiation of testicular function of hypophysectomized and estrogen-treated rats. *Biol Reprod* 1978;18:878–885.
505. Kalla NR, Nisula BC, Menard R, Loriaux DL. The effect of estradiol on testicular testosterone biosynthesis. *Endocrinology* 1980;106:35–39.
505a. Sanford L. Evidence that estrogen regulation of testosterone secretion in adult rams is mediated by both indirect (gonadotropin dependent) and direct (gonadotropin independent) means. *J Androl* 1985;6:306–314.
506. Abney TO, Myers RB. 17β-Estradiol inhibition of Leydig cell regeneration in the ethane dimethylsulfonate-treated mature rat. *J Androl* 1991;12:295–304.
507. Tremblay Y, Belanger A. Reversible inhibition of gonadal functions by a potent gonadotropin-releasing hormone agonist in adult dogs. *Contraception* 1984;30:483–497.
508. Vickery BH, McRae GI, Briones W, et al. Effects of an LHRH analog upon sexual function in male dogs. Suppression, reversibility and effect of testosterone replacement. *J Androl* 1984;5:28–42.
509. Vickery BH, McRae GI. Responses of the males of different laboratory species to continuous administraiton of an LHRH agonist. *J Androl* 1980;1:62.
510. Akhtar FB, Marshall GR, Wickings EJ, Nieschlag E. Reversible induction of azoospermia in rhesus monkeys by constant infusion of a GnRH agonist using osmotic minipumps. *J Clin Endocrinol Metab* 1983;56:534–540.
511. Mann DR, Gould KG, Smith MM, Duffy T, Collins DC. Influence of simultaneous gonadotropin-releasing hormone agonist and testosterone treatment on spermatogenesis and potential fertilizing capacity in male monkeys. *J Clin Endocrinol Metab* 1987;65:1215–1224.
512. Sundaram K, Keizer-Zucker A, Thau RB, Bardin CW. Reversal of testicular function after prolonged suppression with an LHRH agonist in rhesus monkeys. *J Androl* 1987;8:103–107.
513. Schurmeyer TH, Knuth UA, Fresichem CW, Sandow J, Akhtar FB, Nieschlag E. Suppression of pituitary and testicular function in normal men by constant GnRH agonist infusion. *J Clin Endocrinol Metab* 1984;59:19–24.
514. Swerdloff RS, Steiner BS, Bhasin S. Gonadotropin releasing hormone (GnRH) agonists in male contraception. *Med Biol* 1985;63:218–224.
515. Weinbauer GF, Respondek M, Themann H, Nieschlage E. Reversibility of long-term effects of GnRH agonist administration on testicular histology and sperm production in the nonhuman primate. *J Androl* 1987;8:319–329.
516. Maddock WO, Nelson WO. The effects of chorionic gonadotropin in adult men: increased estrogen and 17-ketosteroid excretion, gynecomastia, Leydig cell stimulation and seminiferous tubule damage. *J Clin Endocrinol Metab* 1952;12:985–1007.
517. Margalioth EJ, Laufer N, Persistz E, Gaulayev B, Shemesh A, Schenker JG. Treatment of oligoasthenospermia with human chorionic gonadotropin: Hormonal profiles and results. *Fertil Steril* 1983;39:841–844.
518. Vigersky RA, Glass AR. Effects of Δ^1-testolactone on the pituitary–testicular axis in oligospermic men. *J Clin Endocrinol Metab* 1981;52:987–902.
519. Dorner G, Moch G, Zabel H. The "overproduction effect" of the testes after cessation of human chorionic gonadotropin administration in men with oligoasthenospermia. *Fertil Steril* 1960;11:457–464.
520. Glass SJ, Holland HM. Treatment of oligospermia with large doses of human chorionic gonadotropin: A preliminary report. *Fertil Steril* 1963;14:500–506.
521. Futterweit W, Sobrero AJ. Treatment of normogonadotropic oligospermia with large doses of chorionic gonadotropin. *Fertil Steril* 1968;19:971–976.
522. Misurale F, Cagnazzo G, Storage A. Asthenospermia and its treatment with hCG. *Fertil Steril* 1969;20:650–653.
523. Szollosi J, Apro G, Falkay G, Sas M. Choriogonin treatment of patients with pathospermia. *Int Urol Nephrol* 1978;10:65–71.
524. Homonnai ST, Peled M, Paz GF. Changes in semen quality and fertility in response to endocrine treatment of subfertile men. *Gynecol Obstet Invest* 1978;9:244–251.
525. Chehval MJ, Mehan DJ. Chorionic gonadotropins in the treatment of the subfertile male. *Fertil Steril* 1979;31:666–668.
526. Knuth UA, Honigl W, Bals-Pratsch M, Schleicher G, Nieschlag E. Treatment of severe oligospermia with hCG/hMG: A placebo-controlled, double blind trial. *J Clin Endocrinol Metab* 1987;65:1081–1087.
527. Schanbacher BD. Dose-dependent inhibition of spermatogenesis in mature rams with exogenous testosterone. *Int J Androl* 1980;3:563–573.
528. Weinbauer GF, Gockeler E, Nieschlag E. Testosterone prevents complete suppression of spermatogenesis in the GnRH antagonist-treated nonhuman primate (*Macaca fascicularis*). *J Clin Endocrinol Metab* 1988;67:284–290.
529. Nieschlag E, Behre HM, Weinbauer GF. Hormonal male contraception: a real chance? In: Nieschlag E, Habenicht U-F, eds. *Spermatogenesis, fertilization, contraception.* Berlin: Springer-Verlag; 1992:477–502.
530. Morse HC, Horike N, Rowley MJ, Heller CG. Testosterone concentrations in testes of normal men: effects of testosterone propionate administration. *J Clin Endocrinol Metab* 1973;37:882–886.
531. Schurmeyer T, Knuth UA, Belkien L, Neischlag E. Reversible azoospermia induced by the anabolic steroid 19-nortestosterone. *Lancet* 1984;1:417–420.
532. Swerdloff RS, Palacios A, McClure D. Suppression of human spermatogenesis by depot androgen: Potential for male contraception. *J Steroid Biochem* 1979;11:663–670.
533. Barham SS, Berlin JD. Fine structure and cytochemistry of testicular cells in men treated with testosterone propionate. *Cell Tissue Res* 1974;148:159–182.
534. Morse HC, Leach DR, Rowley MJ, Heller CG. Effect of cyproterone acetate on sperm concentration, seminal fluid volume, testicular cytology and levels of plasma and urinary ICSH, FSH and testosterone in normal men. *J Reprod Fertil* 1973;32:365–378.
535. Purvis K, Calandra R, Sander S, Hansson V. Androgen binding proteins and androgen levels in the human testis and epididymis. *Int J Androl* 1978;1:531–548.
536. Bardin CW, Swerdloff RS, Santen RJ. Androgens: Risks and benefits. *J Clin Endocrinol Metab* 1992;73:4–7.
537. Hotchkiss RS. Effects of massive doses of testosterone propionate upon spermatogenesis. *J Clin Endocrinol Metabl* 1944;4:117–120.
538. Setchell BP, Davies RV, Gladwell RT, et al. The movement of fluid in the seminiferous tubule and rete testis. *Ann Biol Anim Biochem Biophys* 1978;18:623–632.
539. Mauss J, Borsch G, Bormacher K, Richter E, Leyandecker C, Nocke W. Effect of long-term testosterone oenanthate administration on male reproductive function: clinical evaluation, serum FSH, LH, testosterone and seminal fluid analysis in normal men. *Acta Endocrinol (Kbh)* 1975;78:373–384.
540. Courtens JL, Courot M. Acrosomal and nuclear morphogenesis in ram spermatids: an experimental study of hypophysectomized and testosterone supplemented animals. *Anat Rec* 1980;197:143–152.
541. Booth JD, Merriam GR, Clark RV, Loriaux DL, Sherins RJ. Evidence for Leydig cell dysfunction in infertile men with a selective increase in plasma FSH. *J Clin Endocrinol Metab* 1987;64:1194–1201.
542. Dony JMJ, Smals AGH, Rolland R, Rauser BCJ, Thomas CMG. Differential effect of LHRH infusion on testicular steroids in normal men and patients with idiopathic oligospermia. *Fertil Steril* 1984;42:274–280.
543. Morrow AF, Baker HWG, Burger HG. Different testosterone and LH relationships in infertile men. *J Androl* 1986;7:310–315.
544. Glass AR, Vigersky RA. Leydig cell function in idiopathic oligospermia. *Fertil Steril* 1980;34:144–148.
545. Ruder HJ, Loriaux DL, Sherins RJ, Lipsett MB. Leydig cell function in men with disorders of spermatogenesis. *J Clin Endocrinol Metab* 1974;30:244–247.
546. Rodriguez-Rigau LJ, Weiss DB, Zukerman Z, Grotjan He, Smith KD, Steinberger E. A possible mechanism for the detrimental

effect of varicocele on testicular function in man. *Fertil Steril* 1978;30:577–585.
547. Rodriguez-Rigau LJ, Smith KD, Steinberger E. A possible relation between elevated FSH levels and Leydig cell dysfunction in azoospermic and oligospermic men. *J Androl* 1980;1:127–132.
548. Aiman J, Griffin JE, Gazak JM, Wilson JD, MacDonald PC. Androgen insensitivity as a cause of infertility in otherwise normal men. *N Engl J Med* 1979;300:223–229.
549. Griffin JE. Androgen resistance—the clinical and molecular spectrum. *N Engl J Med* 1992;326:611–618.
550. Wilson JD. Syndromes of androgen resistance. *Biol Reprod* 1992;46:168–173.
551. Migeon CJ, Brown TR, Lanes R, Palacios A, Amrhein JA, Schoen EJ. A clinical syndrome of mild androgen insensitivity. *J Clin Endocrinol Metab* 1984;59:672–678.
552. Jukier J, Kaufman M, Pinsky L, Peterson RE. Partial androgen resistance associated with secondary 5α-reductase deficiency: Identification of a novel qualitative androgen receptor defect and clinical implications. *J Clin Endocrinol Metab* 1984;59:679–688.
553. Schulster A, Ross L, Scommegna A. Frequency of androgen insensitivity in infertile phenotypically normal men. *J Urol* 1983;130:699–701.
553a. Giagulli VA, Vermeulen A. Leydig cell function in infertile men with idiopathic oligospermic infertility. *J Clin Endocrinol Metab* 1988;66:62–67.
554. Larrea F, Benavides G, Scaglia H, et al. Gynecomastia as a familial in complete male pseudohermaphroditism type I: A limited androgen resistance syndrome. *J Clin Endocrinol Metab* 1978;46:961–970.
555. McPhaul MJ, Marcelli M, Zoppi S, Griffin JE, Wilson JD. Genetic basis of endocrine disease. 4. The spectrum of mutations in the androgen receptor gene that causes androgen resistance. *J Clin Endocrinol Metab* 1993;76:17–23.
556. de Kretser DM, Burger HG, Fortune D, et al. Hormonal, histological and chromosomal studies in adult males with testicular disorders. *J Clin Endocrinol Metab* 1972;35:392–401.
557. Yoshida K-I, Lanasa JA, Takahashi J, Winters SJ, Oshima H, Troen P. Studies of the human testis. XVI. Evaluation of multiple indexes of testicular function in relation to advanced age, idiopathic oligospermia or varicocele. *Fertil Steril* 1982;38:712–720.
558. Paulson RJ, Bernstein GS, Marrs RP, Lobo RA. Idiopathic oligospermia and peripheral androgen metabolism. *Fertil Steril* 1986;46:480–483.
559. Neaves WB, Johnson L, Porter JT, Parker CR Jr, Petty CS. Leydig cell numbers, daily sperm production and serum gonadotropin levels in ageing men. *J Clin Endocrinol Metab* 1984;59:756–763.
560. Baker HWG, Hudson B. Changes in the pituitary-testicular axis with age. In: de Kretser DM, Burger HG, Hudson B, eds. *Monographs on endocrinology, vol 25.* Berlin: Springer-Verlag; 1983:711–784.
561. Paniagua R, Martin A, Nistal M, Amat P. Testicular involution in elderly men: Comparison of histologic quantitative studies with hormone patterns. *Fert Steril* 1987;47:671–679.
562. Vermeulen A. Androgens in the ageing male. *J Clin Endocrinol Metab* 1991;73:221–224.
563. Bremner WJ, Vitiello MV, Prinz PN. Loss of circadian rhythmicity in blood testosterone levels with ageing in normal men. *J Clin Endocrinol Metab* 1983;56:1278–1281.
564. Johnson L, George FW, Neaves WB. Characterization of the testicular abnormality in 5α-reductase deficiency. *J Clin Endocrinol Metab* 1986;63:1091–1099.
565. Kula K, Rodriguez-Rigau LJ, Wlodarczyk WP. Three principal types of spermatogenic activity in man as determined by quantitative analysis of the seminiferous epithelium: Partial meiotic spermatogenic arrest is associated with accumulation of spermatocytes. In: Frajese G, et al., eds. *Oligospermia: Recent progress in andrology.* New York: Raven Press; 1981:55–64.
566. Müller J, Skakkebaek NE. Quantitative assessment of the seminiferous epithelium in male infertility. In: Santen RJ, Swerdloff RS, eds. *Male reproductive dysfunction.* New York: Marcel Dekker; 1986:321–330.
567. Brown T. Male pseudohermaphroditism: Defects in androgen-dependent target tissues. *Sem Reprod Endocrinol* 1987;5: 243–260.
568. Steinberger E, Weidman ER. Abnormalities of spermatogenesis in the human testis. *Sem Reprod Endocrinol* 1988;6:309–321.
569. Yamamoto KR. Steroid receptor regulated transcription of specific genes and gene networks. *Annu Rev Genet* 1985;19:209–252.
570. Parker MG. Mechanisms of action of steroid receptors in the regulation of gene transcription. *J Reprod Fertil* 1990; 88:717–720.
571. Parker MG. *Nuclear hormone receptors.* New York: Academic Press; 1991.
572. Lubahn DB, Joseph DR, Sullivan PM, Willard HF, French FS, Wilson EM. Cloning of human androgen receptor complementary DNA and localization to the x-chromosome. *Science* 1988;240:327–330.
573. Sanborn BM, Steinberger A, Tcholakian RK, Steinberger E. Direct measurement of androgen receptors in cultured Sertoli cells. *Steroids* 1977;29:493–502.
574. Tindall DJ, Miller A, Means AR. Characterization of androgen receptor in Sertoli cell-enriched testis. *Endocrinology* 1977; 101:13–23.
575. Sar M, Lubahn DB, French FS, Wilson EM. Immunohistochemical localisation of the androgen receptor in rat and human tissues. *Endocrinology* 1990;127:3180–3186.
576. Sar M, Hall SH, Wilson EM, French FS. Androgen regulation of Sertoli cells. In: Russell LD, Griswold MD, eds. *The Sertoli cell.* Clearwater, Florida: Cache River Press; 1993:509–516.
577. Bergh A, Damber JE. Immunohistochemical demonstration of androgen receptors on testicular blood vessels. *Int J Androl* 1992;15:425–434.
578. Anthony CK, Kovacs WJ, Skinner MK. Analysis of the androgen receptor in isolated testicular cell types with a microassay that uses an affinity ligand. *Endocrinology* 1989;125:2628–2635.
579. Grootegoed JA, Peters MJ, Mulder E, Rommerts FFG, Van Der Molen HJ. Absence of a nuclear androgen receptor in isolated germinal cells of rat testis. *Mol Cell Endocrinol* 1977;9:159–167.
580. Lyon MF, Glenister PH, Lamoreux ML. Normal spermatozoa from androgen-resistant germ cells of chimaeric mice and the role of androgen in spermatogenesis. *Nature* 1975;258:620–622.
581. Galena HJ, Pillai AK, Terner C. Progesterone and androgen receptors in nonflagellate germ cells of the rat testis. *J Endocrinol* 1974;63:223–237.
582. Sanborn BM, Steinberger A, Meistrich ML, Steinberger E. Androgen binding sites in testis cell fractions as measured by a nuclear exchange assay. *J Steroid Biochem* 1975;6:1459–1465.
583. Tsai YK, Sanborn BM, Steinberger A, Steinberger E. The interaction of testicular androgen-receptor complex with rat germ cell and Sertoli cell chromatin. *Biochem Biophys Res Commun* 1977;75:366–372.
584. Wright WW, Frankel AI. An androgen receptor in the nuclei of late spermatids in testes of male rats. *Endocrinology* 1980;107:314–317.
585. Skinner MK. Sertoli cell-peritubular myoid cell interactions In: Russell LD, Griswold MD, eds. *The Sertoli cell.* Clearwater, Florida: Cache River Press; 1993:493–508.
586. Free MJ, Jaffe RA, Morford DE. Sperm transport through the rete testis in anaesthetized rats: Role of the testicular capsule and effect of gonadotropins and prostaglandins. *Biol Reprod* 1980;2:1073–1078.
587. Flickinger CJ. Effects of clomiphene on the structure of the testis, epididymis and sex accessory glands of the rat. *Am J Anat* 1977;149:533–562.
588. Flickinger CJ. The influence of progestin and androgen on the fine structure of the male reproductive tract of the rat. I. General effects and observations on the testis. *Anat Rec* 1977;187: 405–430.
589. Grino PB, Griffin JE, Wilson JD. Testosterone at high concentrations interacts with the human androgen receptor similarly to dihydrotestosterone. *Endocrinology* 1990;126:1165–1172.
590. Landers JP, Spelsberg TC. Updates and new models for steroid hormone action. *Ann NY Acad Sci* 1991;637:26–55.
591. Rommerts FFG. Cell surface action of steroids: a complementary

mechanism for regulation of spermatogenesis? In: Neischlag E, Habenicht UF, eds. *Spermatogenesis, fertilization, contraception.* Berlin: Springer-Verlag; 1992:1–19.
592. Isomaa V, Parvinen M, Janne OA, Bardin CW. Nuclear androgen receptors in different stages of the seminiferous epithelial cycle and the interstitial tissue of rat testis. *Endocrinology* 1985;116:132–137.
593. Parvinen M, Huhtaniemi I. Testosterone micromilieu in staged rat seminiferous tubules. *J Steroid Biochem* 1990;36:377–381.
594. Smith DF, Toft DO. Steroid receptors and their associated proteins. *Mol Endocrinol* 1993;7:4–11.
595. Simons SS, Oshima H, Szapary D. Higher levels of control: Modulation of steroid hormone-regulated gene transcription. *Mol Endocrinol* 1992;6:995–1002.
596. Sheridan PJ. Can a single androgen receptor fit the bill? *Mol Cell Endocrinol* 1991;76:C39–C45.
597. Matsumoto K, Yamada M. 5α-Reduction of testosterone *in-vitro* by rat seminiferous tubules and whole testes at different stages of development. *Endocrinology* 1973;93:253–255.
598. Rivarola MA, Podesta EJ, Chemes HE, Aguilar D. *In vitro* metabolism of testosterone by whole human testis, isolated seminiferous tubules and interstitial tissue. *J Clin Endocrinol Metab* 1973;37:454–460.
599. Rivarola MA, Podesta EJ, Chemes HE, Calandra RS. Androgen metabolism and concentration in the seminiferous tubules at different stages of development. *J Steroid Biochem* 1975;6:365–369.
600. Nayfeh SN, Coffey JC, Hansson V, French FS. Maturational changes in testicular steroidogenesis: Hormonal regulation of 5α-reductase. *J Steroid Biochem* 1975;6:329–355.
601. Pazzagli M, Borrelli D, Forti G, Serio M. Dihydrotestosterone in human spermatic venous plasma. *Acta Endocrinol (Kbh)* 1974;76:388–391.
602. Louis BG, Fritz IB. Stimulation by androgens of the production of androgen binding protein by cultured Sertoli cells. *Mol Cell Endocrinol* 1977;7:9–16.
603. Lamb DJ, Tsai YH, Steinberger A, Sanborn BM. Sertoli cell nuclear transcriptional activity: Stimulation by follicle-stimulating hormone and testosterone *in vitro*. *Endocrinology* 1981; 108:1020–1026.
604. Cheng YC, Mather JP, Byer AL, Bardin CW. Identification of hormonally responsive proteins in primary Sertoli cell culture medium by anion-exchange high performance liquid chromatography. *Endocrinology* 1986;118:480–489.
605. Cheng YC, Bardin CW. Identification of two testosterone responsive testicular proteins in Sertoli cell enriched culture medium whose secretion is suppressed by cells of the intact seminiferous tubule. *J Biol Chem* 1987;262:12768–12775.
606. Mills NC. Androgen effects on Sertoli cells. *Int J Androl* 1990;13:123–134.
607. Roberts K, Griswold MD. Testosterone induction of cellular proteins in cultured Sertoli cells from hypophysectomized rats and rats of different ages. *Endocrinology* 1989;125:1174–1179.
608. Sharpe RM, Millar M, McKinnell C. Relative roles of testosterone and the germ cell complement in determining stage-dependent changes in protein secretion by isolated rat seminiferous tubules. *Int J Androl* 1993;16:71–81.
609. Soderstrom KO, Parvinen M. RNA synthesis in different stages of rat seminiferous epithelial cycle. *Mol Cell Endocrinol* 1976;5:181–189.
610. Parvinen M, Soderstrom KO. Effects of FSH and testosterone on RNA synthesis in different stages of rat spermatogenesis. *J Steroid Biochem* 1976;7:1021–1023.
611. Ayer-Le Lievre C, Olson L, Ebendal T, Hallbrook F, Persson H. Nerve growth factor mRNA and protein in the testis and epididymis of mouse and rat. *Proc Natl Acad Sci* 1988;85:2628–2632.
612. Persson H, Ayer-Le Lievre C, Soder O, et al. Expression of β-nerve growth factor receptor mRNA in Sertoli cells downregulated by testosterone. *Science* 1990;247:707–707.
613. Parvinen M, Pelto-Huikko M, Soder O, et al. Expression of β-nerve growth factor and its receptor in rat seminiferous epithelium: Specific function at the onset of meiosis. *J Cell Biol* 1992;117:629–641.
614. Lonnerberg P, Soder O, Parvinen M, Ritzen EM, Persson H. β-nerve growth factor influences the expression of ABP messenger ribonucleic acid in the rat testis. *Biol Reprod* 1992;47:381–388.
615. Kerr JB. A light microscopic and morphometric analysis of the Sertoli cell during the spermatogenic cycle of the rat. *Anat Embryol* 1988;179:191–203.
616. Ueno H, Mori H. Morphometrical analysis of Sertoli cell ultrastructure during the seminiferous epithelial cycle in rats. *Biol Reprod* 1990;43:769–776.
617. O'Leary PC, Jackson AE, Irby DC, De Kretser DM. Effects of ethane dimethane sulphonate (EDS) on seminiferous tubule function in rats. *Int J Androl* 1987;10:625–634.
618. Qureshi SJ, Sharpe RM. Evaluation of possible determinants and consequences of Leydig cell heterogeneity in man. *Int J Androl* [*in press*].
619. Kerr JB, Savage GN, Millar M, Sharpe RM. Response of the seminiferous epithelium of the rat testis to withdrawal of androgen: Evidence for direct effects upon inter-Sertoli cell tight junctions. *Cell Tissue Res* [*in press*].
620. Chemes HE, Dym M, Fawcett DW, Javadpour N, Sherins RJ. Pathophysiological observations of Sertoli cells in patients with germinal aplasia or severe germ cell depletion. Ultrastructural findings and hormone levels. *Biol Reprod* 1977;17:108–123.
621. De Kretser DM, Kerr JB, Paulsen CA. Evaluation of the ultrastructural changes in the human Sertoli cell in testicular disorders and the relationship of the changes to the levels of serum FSH. *Int J Androl* 1981;4:129–144.
622. Bergh A, Damber J-E, Widmark A. Hormonal control of testicular blood flow, microcirculation and vascular permeability. In: Cooke BA, Sharpe RM, eds. *The molecular and cellular endocrinology of the testis.* New York: Raven Press; 1988:122–134.
623. Maddocks S, Sharpe RM. Interstitial fluid volume in the rat testis—androgen dependent regulation by the seminiferous tubules. *J Endocrinol* 1989;120:215–222.
624. Damber JE, Maddocks S, Widmark A, Bergh A. Testicular blood flow and vasomotion can be maintained by testosterone in Leydig cell-depleted rats. *Int J Androl* 1992;15:385–393.
625. Collin O, Bergh A, Damber J-E, Widmark A. Control of testicular vasomotion by testosterone and tubular factors in rats. *J Reprod Fertil* 1993;97:115–121.
626. Sharpe RM, Bartlett JMS, Allenby G. Evidence for the control of testicular interstitial fluid volume in the rat testis by specific germ cell types. *J Endocrinol* 1991;128:359–367.
627. Damber J-E, Bergh A, Widmark A. Age-related differences in testicular microcirculation. *Int J Androl* 1990;13:197–206.
628. Setchell BP. Local control of testicular fluids. *Reprod Fertil Dev* 1990;2:291–309.
629. Setchell BP, Galil KAA. Limitations imposed by testicular blood flow on the function of Leydig cells in rats *in-vivo*. *Austr J Biol Sci* 1983;36:285–294.
630. Wang J, Galil KAA, Setchell BP. Changes in testicular blood flow and testosterone production during aspermatogenesis after irradiation. *J Endocrinol* 1983;98:35–46.
631. Sasano N, Ichijo S. Vascular patterns of the human testis with special reference to its senile changes. *Tohoku J Exp Med* 1969;99:269–280.
632. Suoranta H. Changes in the small blood vessels of the adult human testis in relation to age and to some pathological conditions. *Virchows Arch* 1971;352:165–181.
633. Spera G, Alei G, Coia L. Histological lesions in the testis of infertile men with varicocele. *Arch Androl* 1979;2:335–339.
634. Hatakeyama S, Takizawa T, Kawahara Y. Focal atrophy of the seminiferous tubules in the human testis. *Acta Pathol Jpn* 1979;29:901–910.
635. Regadera J, Nistal M, Paniagua R. Testis, epididymis and spermatic cord in elderly men. Correlation of angiographic and histologic studies with systemic arterioslerosis. *Arch Pathol Lab Med* 1985;109:663–667.
636. Wu FCW. Male contraception—current status and future prospects. *Clin Endocrinol* 1988;29:443–465.
637. WHO Task Force on Methods for the Regulation of Male Fertility. Contraceptive efficacy of testosterone-induced azoospermia in normal men. *Lancet* 1990;336:955–959.

638. Ortavant R. Action de la durée de eclairment sur les processes spermatogénétiques chez le bélier. *CR Soc Biol (Paris)* 1956;150:471–474.
639. Millar RP, Glover TD. Seasonal changes in the reproductive tract of the male rock hyrax, *Procavia capensis. J Reprod Fertil* 1970;23:497–499.
640. Huang HFS, Nieschlag E. Alteration of free sulphydryl content of rat sperm heads by suppression of intratesticular testosterone. *J Reprod Fertil* 1986;70:31–38.
641. Robaire B, Smith S, Hales BF. Suppression of spermatogenesis by testosterone in adult male rats: Effect on fertility, pregnancy outcome and progeny. *Biol Reprod* 1984;31:221–230.
642. Wu FCW, Aitken RJ. Suppression of sperm function by depot medroxyprogesterone acetate and testosterone enanthate in steroid male contraception. *Fertil Steril* 1989;51:691–697.
643. Wallace EM, Aitken RJ, Wu FCW. Residual sperm function in oligozoospermia induced by testosterone enanthate administered as a potential male contraceptive. *Int J Androl* 1992;15:416–424.
644. Rosner W. The functions of corticosteroid-binding globulin and sex hormone-binding globulin: Recent advances. *Endocrinol Rev* 1990;11:80–91.
645. Nemere I, Norman AW. Steroid hormone actions at the plasma membrane: induced calcium uptake and exocytotic events. *Mol Cell Endocrinol* 1991;80:C165–C169.
646. Ericsson RI, Cornette JC, Buttala DA. Binding of sex steroids to rabbit sperm. *Acta Endocrinol* 1967;56:424–432.
647. Cheng CY, Boetcher B, Rose RJ, Kay DJ, Tinnenberg HR. The binding of sex steroids to human spermatozoa. An autoradiographic study. *Int J Androl* 1981;4:1–17.
648. Frankel AI, Chapman JC, Wright WW. The equivocal presence of nuclear androgen-binding proteins in mammalian spermatids and spermatozoa. *J Steroid Biochem* 1989;33:71–79.
649. Wright WW, Frankel AI. Characterization of the androgen receptor in nuclei of seminiferous tubules of the mature male rat based upon radioimmunoassay of endogenous levels of bound testosterone. *Endocrinology* 1979;104:1580–1587.
650. Hansson V, Ritzen EM, French FS, Nayfeh SN. Androgen transport and receptor mechanisms in testis and epididymis. In: Hamilton D, Greep RO, eds. *Handbook of physiology,* Sec 7. Baltimore: Williams & Wilkins; 1975:173–201.
651. Hammond GL, Underhill DA, Rykse HM, Smith CL. The human sex hormone-binding globulin gene contains exons for androgen-binding protein and two other testicular messengers. *Mol Endocrinol* 1989;3:1869–1876.
652. Rommerts FFG, Kruger BCH, Grootegoed JA, Van der Molen HJ. Reversible interaction between androgen binding protein and testicular macromolecules causing inhibition of androgen binding activity. *Steroids* 1979;33:659–673.
653. David GFX, Koehler JK, Brown JA, Petra PH, Farr AG. Light and electron microscopic studies on the localization of steroid-binding protein (SBP) in rabbit spermatozoa. *Biol Reprod* 1985;33:503–514.
654. Steinberger A, Dighe RR, Diaz J. Testicular peptides and their endocrine and paracrine functions. *Arch Biol Med Exp* 1984;17:267–271.
655. Bordin S, Petra PH. Immunochemical localization of the sex steroid-binding protein of plasma in tissues of the adult monkey *Macaca nemestrina. Proc Natl Acad Sci USA* 1980;77: 5678–5682.
656. Rosner W, Hryb DJ, Khan MS, Nakhla AM, Romas NA. Sex hormone-binding globulin. Binding to cell membranes and generation of a second messenger. *J Androl* 1992;13:101–106.
657. Hryb DJ, Khan MS, Rosner W. Testosterone-estradiol-binding globulin binds to human prostatic cell membranes. *Biochem Biophys Res Commun* 1985;128:432–440.
658. Hryb DJ, Khan MS, Romas NA, Rosner W. Solubilization and partial characterization of the sex hormone-binding globulin receptor from human prostate. *J Biol Chem* 1989;264:5378–5383.
659. Hryb DJ, Khan MS, Romas NA, Rosner W. The control of the interaction of SHBG with its receptor by steroid hormones. *J Biol Chem* 1990;265:6048–6054.
660. Porto CS, Abreu LC, Gunsalus GL, Bardin CW. Binding of sex-hormone-binding globulin (SHBG) to testicular membranes and solubilized receptors. *Mol Cell Endocrinol* 1992;89:33–38.
661. Gerard A, Nya AE, Egloff M, Domingo M, Degrelle H, Gerard H. Endocytosis of human sex steroid-binding protein in monkey germ cells. *Ann NY Acad Sci* 1991;637:258–276.
662. Damassa DA, Lin TM, Sonnenschein C, Soto AM. Biological effects of sex hormone-binding globulin on androgen-induced proliferation and androgen metabolism in LNCaP prostate cells. *Endocrinology* 1991;129:75–84.
663. Nakhla AM, Khan MS, Rosner W. Biologically active steroids activate receptor-bound sex hormone-binding globulin to cause LNCaP cells to accumulate adenosine 3′,5′-monophosphate. *J Clin Endocrinol Metab* 1990;71:398–404.
664. Welch JE, Swinnen JV, O'Brien DA, Eddy EM, Conti M. Unique adenosine 3′,5′ cyclic monophosphate phosphodiesterase messenger ribonucleic acids in rat spermatogenic cells: Evidence for differential gene expression during spermatogenesis. *Biol Reprod* 1992;46:1027–1033.
665. Waeber G, Meyer TE, Lesieur M, Hermann HL, Gerard N, Habener JF. Developmental stage-specific expression of cyclic adenosine 3′,5′-monophosphate response element binding protein CREB during spermatogenesis involves alternative exon splicing. *Mol Endocrinol* 1991;5:1418–1430.
666. Waeber G, Habener JF. Novel testis germ cell-specific transcript of the CREB gene contains an alternatively spliced exon with multiple in-frame stop codons. *Endocrinology* 1992;131: 2010–2015.
667. Lonnerberg P, Parvinen M, Jahnsen T, Hansson V, Persson H. Stage- and cell-specific expression of cyclic adenosine 3′,5′-monophosphate-dependent protein kinases in rat seminiferous epithelium. *Biol Reprod* 1992;46:1057–1068.
668. Ritzen EM, Boitani C, Parvinen M, French FS, Feldman M. Stage-dependent secretion of ABP by rat seminiferous tubules. *Mol Cell Endocrinol* 1982;25:25–34.
669. Anthony CT, Danzo BJ, Orgebin-Crist MC. Investigations on the relationship between sperm fertilizing ability and androgen-binding protein in the restricted rat. *Endocrinology* 1984; 114:1413–1418.
670. Anthony CT, Danzo BJ, Orgebin-Crist MC. Investigations on the relationship between sperm fertilizing ability and androgen-binding protein in the hypophysectomized, pregnenolone-injected rat. *Endocrinology* 1984;114:1419–1425.
671. Huang HFS, Pogach L, Giglio W, Nathan E, Seebode J. GnRH-A induced arrest of spermiogenesis in rats is associated with altered ABP distribution in the testis and epididymis. *J Androl* 1992;13:153–159.
672. Holland MK, Rogers BJ, Orgebin-Crist M-C, Danzo BJ. Effects of photoperiod on androgen-binding protein and sperm fertilizing ability in the hamster. *J Reprod Fertil* 1987;81:99–112.
673. Morris ID, Bardin CW, Musto NA, Thau RB, Gunsalus GL. Evidence suggesting that germ cells influence the bidirectional secretion of androgen binding protein by the seminiferous epithelium demonstrated by selective impairment of spermatogenesis with busulphan. *Int J Androl* 1987;10:691–700.
674. Danzo BJ, Dunn JC, Davies J. The presence of androgen binding protein in the guinea pig testis, epididymis and epididymal fluid. *Mol Cell Endocrinol* 1982;28:512–527.
675. Ritzen EM, French FS. Demonstration of an androgen-binding protein (ABP) in rabbit testis: secretion in efferent duct fluid and passage into epididymis. *J Steroid Biochem* 1974;5:151–154.
676. Jégou B, Dacheux LJ, Terqui M, Garnier DH, Courot M. Studies on the androgen binding protein in rete testis fluid of the ram and its regulation by sexual season. *Mol Cell Endocrinol* 1978;9:335–346.
677. Keeping HS, Winter SH, Troen P. Identification of androgen-binding protein from testis cytosol and Sertoli cell culture medium of the cynomolgus monkey, *Macaca fascicularis. Endocrinology* 1985;117:1521–1529.
678. Keeping HS, Winters SJ, Attardi B, Troen P. Developmental changes in testicular inhibin and androgen-binding protein during sexual maturation in the cynomolgus monkey, *Macaca fascicularis. Endocrinology* 1990;126:2858–2867.
679. Cheng CY, Frick J, Gunsalus GL, Musto NA, Bardin CW. Human testicular ABP shares immunodeterminants with serum testosterone-estradiol binding globulin. *Endocrinology* 1984; 114:1395–1401.

680. Cheng CY, Musto NA, Gunsalus GL, Frick J, Bardin CW. There are two forms of androgen binding protein in human testes. *J Biol Chem* 1985;260:5631–5640.
681. Hsu AF, Troen P. An androgen binding protein in the testicular cytosol of human testis. Comparison with human plasma testosterone-estrogen binding globulin. *J Clin Invest* 1988; 58:1611–1619.
682. Joseph DR, Hall SH, French FS. Rat androgen-binding protein: Evidence for identical subunits and amino acid sequence homology with human sex hormone-binding globulin. *Proc Natl Acad Sci USA* 1987;84:4339–4343.
683. Joseph DR, Hall SH, Conti M, French FS. The gene structure of rat androgen-binding protein: Identification of potential regulatory deoxyribonucleic acid elements of a follicle-stimulating hormone regulated protein. *Mol Endocrinol* 1988;2:3–13.
684. Reventos J, Hammond GL, Crozat A, et al. Hormonal regulation of rat androgen-binding protein (ABP) messenger ribonucleic acid and homology of human testosterone–estradiol-binding globulin and ABP complementary deoxyribonucleic acids. *Mol Endocrinol* 1988;2:125–132.
685. Nazian SJ. Concentrations of free testosterone, total testosterone and androgen-binding protein in the peripheral serum of male rats during sexual maturation. *J Androl* 1986;7:49–54.
686. Davies RV, Main SJ, Laurie MS, Setchell BP. The effects of long-term administration of either a crude inhibin preparation or an antiserum to FSH on serum hormone levels, testicular function and fertility of adult male rats. *J Reprod Fertil* 1979;26:183–191.
687. Dym M, Raj HGM, Lin YC, et al. Is FSH required for maintenance of spermatogenesis in adult rats? *J Reprod Fertil* 1979;26:175–181.
688. Wickings EJ, Nieschlag E. Suppression of spermatogenesis over two years in rhesus monkeys actively immunized with follicle-stimulating hormone. *Fertil Steril* 1980;34:269–274.
689. Wickings EJ, Usadel KH, Dathe G, Nieschlag E. The role of follicle-stimulating hormone in testicular function of the mature rhesus monkey. *Acta Endocrinol* 1980;95:117–128.
690. Moudgal NR. A need for FSH in maintaining fertility of adult subhuman primates. *Arch Androl* 1981;7:117–125.
691. Neischlag E, Wickings EJ. Immunological neutralization of FSH as an approach to male fertility control. *Int J Androl* 1982;5:18–26.
692. Srinath BR, Wickings EJ, Witting C, Nieschlag E. Active immunization with follicle-stimulating hormone for fertility control: A $4\frac{1}{2}$ year study in male rhesus monkeys. *Fert Steril* 1983;40:110–117.
693. Raj HGM, Murty GSRC, Sairam MR, Tabert LM. Control of spermatogenesis in primates: Effects of active immunization against FSH in the monkey. *Int J Androl* 1982;5:27–33.
694. Matsumoto AM. Hormonal control of spermatogenesis. In: Burger H, de Kretser DM, eds. *The testis,* 2nd ed. New York: Raven Press; 1989:181–196.
695. Clermont Y, Harvey SC. Effects of hormones on spermatogenesis in the rat. *CIBA Found Colloq Endocrinol* 1967;16:173–189.
696. Woods MC, Simpson ME. Pituitary control of the testis of the hypophysectomized rat. *Endocrinology* 1961;69:91–125.
697. Toppari J, Tsutsumi I, Bishop PC. Flow cytometric quantification of rat spermatogenic cells after hypophysectomy and gonadotropin treatment. *Biol Reprod* 1989;40:623–634.
698. Vernon RG, Go VLW, Fritz IB. Hormonal requirements of the different cycles of the seminiferous epithelium during reinitiation of spermatogenesis in long-term hypophysectomized rats. *J Reprod Fertil* 1975;42:77–94.
699. Parvinen M, Marana R, Robertson DM, Hansson V, Ritzen EM. Functional cycle of rat Sertoli cells: Differential binding and action of FSH at various stages of the spermatogenic cycle. In: Steinberger A, Steinberger E, eds. *Testicular development, structure and function.* New York: Raven Press; 1980:425–432.
700. Huhtaniemi I, Nikula H, Parvinen M. Pertussis toxin enhances FSH-stimulated cAMP production in rat seminiferous tubules in a stage-dependent manner. *Mol Cell Endocrinol* 1989;62:89–94.
701. Zabludoff SD, Karzai AW, Wright WW. Germ cell-Sertoli cell interactions. The effect of testicular maturation on the synthesis of cyclic protein-2 by rat Sertoli cells. *Biol Reprod* 1990;43:25–33.
702. Wright WW, Parvinen M, Musto NA, et al. Identification of stage-specific proteins synthesized by rat seminiferous tubules. *Biol Reprod* 1983;29:257–270.
703. Wright WW. Germ cell-Sertoli cell interactions: analysis of the biosynthesis and secretion of cyclic protein-2. *Dev Biol* 1988;130:45–56.
704. Maguire SM, Millar MR, Sharpe RM, Saunders PTK. Stage-dependent expression of mRNA for cyclic protein 2 during spermatogenesis is modulated by elongate spermatids. *Mol Cell Endocrinol* 1993;94:79–88.
705. Seilicovich A, Rosner JM. Effect of FSH on the *in vivo* uptake of ^{3}H-testosterone by rat seminiferous tubules. *Steroids Lipids Res* 1972;3:214–219.
706. Seilicovitch A, Perez Bedes GD, Monastirsky R, Gonzalez N, Rosner JM. Effect of FSH on the *in-vitro* uptake of ^{3}H-testosterone by the cultured seminiferous tubule. *Steroids Lipids Res* 1973;4:224–234.
707. Smith PE. The disabilities caused by hypophysectomy and their repair. *JAMA* 1927;88:158–161.
708. Finkel DM, Philips JI, Snyder PJ. Stimulation of spermatogenesis by gonadotropins in men with hypogonadotropic hypogonadism. *N Engl J Med* 1985;313:651–655.
709. D'Agata R, Heindel JJ, Vicari E, Aliffi A, Gulizia S, Polosa P. hCG-induced maturation of the seminiferous epithelium in hypogonadotropic men. *Horm Res* 1984;19:23–32.
710. Bartke A, Hogan MP, Cutty GB. Effects of hCG, prolactin and bromocriptine on photoperiod-induced testicular regression and recrudescence in golden hamsters. *J Androl* 1980;1:115–123.
711. Bartke A. Male hamster endocrinology. In: Siegel HI, eds. *The hamster: Reproduction and behavior.* New York: Plenum Press; 1985:73–98.
712. Carter JN, Tyson JE, Tolis G, Van Vliet S, Faiman C, Frieson HG. Prolactin-secreting tumors and hypogonadism in 22 men. *N Engl J Med* 1978;299:847–852.
713. Segal S, Yaffe H, Laufer N, Ben-David M. Male hyperprolactinaemia: Effects on fertility. *Fertil Steril* 1979;32:556–561.
714. Jequier AM, Crich J, Ansell ID. Clinical findings and testicular histology in three hyperprolactineamic infertile men. *Fertil Steril* 1979;31:525–530.
715. Cameron DF, Murray FT, Drylie DD. Ultrastructural lesions in testes from hyperprolactinaemic men. *J Androl* 1984;5:283–293.
716. Murray FT, Cameron DF, Ketchum C. Return of gonadal function in men with prolactin-secreting pituitary tumors. *J Clin Endocrinol Metab* 1984;59:79–85.
717. Worley RTS, Nicholson HD, Pickering BT. Testicular oxytocin: an initiator of seminiferous tubule movement? In: Saez JM, Forest MG, Dazord A, Bertrand J, eds. *INSERM Coll* 1985;Vol 123:205–212.
718. Nicholson HD, Worley RTS, Charlton HM, Pickering BT. LH and testosterone cause the development of seminiferous tubule contractile activity and the appearance of testicular oxytocin in hypogonadal mice. *J Endocrinol* 1986;110:159–167.
719. Nicholson HD, Worley RTS, Guldenaar SEF, Pickering BT. Ethan-1,2-dimethane sulphonate reduces testicular oxytocin content and seminiferous tubule movements in the rat. *J Endocrinol* 1987;112:311–316.
720. Grootegoed JA, Jansen R, Van Der Molen HJ. The role of glucose, pyruvate and lactate in ATP production by rat spermatocytes and spermatids. *Biochim Biophys Acta* 1984;767:248–256.
721. Griswold MD. Unique aspects of the biochemistry and metabolism of Sertoli cells. In: Russell LD, Griswold MD, eds. *The Sertoli cell,* Clearwater, Florida: Cache River Press; 1993:485–492.
722. Jutte NHPM, Janse R, Grootegoed JA, Rommerts FFG, Van Der Molen HJ. FSH stimulation of the production of pyruvate and lactate by rat Sertoli cells may be involved in hormonal regulation of spermatogenesis. *J Reprod Fertil* 1983;68:219–226.
723. Grootegoed JA, Jansen R, Van Der Molen HJ. Effect of glucose on ATP dephosphorylation in rat spermatids. *J Reprod Fertil* 1986;77:99–107.
724. Oonk RB, Grootegoed JA, Van Der Molen HJ. Comparison of the effects of insulin and follitropin on glucose metabolism by Sertoli cells from immature rats. *Mol Cell Endocrinol* 1985;42:39–48.
725. Oonk RB, Grootegoed JA. Identification of insulin receptors on rat Sertoli cells. *Mol Cell Endocrinol* 1987;49:51–62.

726. Wathes DC. Possible actions of gonadal oxytocin and vasopressin. *J Reprod Fertil* 1984;71:315–345.
727. Schoffling K, Federlin K, Schmitt M, Pfeiffer EF. Histometric investigations on the testicular tissue of rats with alloxan diabetes and Chinese hamsters with spontaneous diabetes. *Acta Endocrinol* 1976;54:335–346.
728. Foglia VG, Rosner JM, Cattaneo De Peralta Ramos M, Lema BE. Sexual disturbances in the male diabetic rat. *Horm Met Res* 1969;1:72–77.
729. Millar M, Sharpe RM, Maguire SM, Saunders PTK. Cellular localisation of messenger RNAs in rat testis: Application of digoxigenin-labelled probes to embedded tissue. *Cell Tissue Res* [*in press*].
730. Ivell R. All that glisters is not gold: Common testis gene transcripts are not always what they seem. *Int J Androl* 1992;15:85–92.
731. Carreau S, Drosdowsky MA, Pisselet C, Courot M. Hormonal regulation of androgen-binding protein in lamb testes. *J Endocrinol* 1980;85:443–448.
732. Matsumoto AM, Bremner WJ. Endocrinology of the hypothalamic–pituitary–testicular axis with particular reference to the hormonal control of spermatogenesis. *Baillieres Clin Endocrinol Metab* 1987;1:71–87.
733. Nieschlag E, Usadel KH, Wicking EJ, Kley HK, Wuttke W. Effects of active immunization with steroids on endocrine and reproductive functions in male animals. In: Nieschlag E, ed. *Immunization with hormones in reproduction research.* Amsterdam: North Holland; 1975:155–172.
734. Weinbauer GF, Behre HM, Fingscheidt U, Nieschlag E. Human FSH exerts a stimulatory effect on spermatogenesis, testicular size and serum inhibin levels in the GnRH antagonist-treated nonhuman primate (*Macaca fascicularis*). *Endocrinology* 1991;129:1831–1839.
735. Rodriguez-Rigau LJ. Diabetes and male reproductive function. *J Androl* 1980;1:105–110.

The Physiology of Reproduction, Second Edition,
edited by E. Knobil and J.D. Neill,
Raven Press, Ltd., New York © 1994.

CHAPTER 23

The Male Sex Accessory Tissues

Structure, Androgen Action, and Physiology

Markham C. Luke and Donald S. Coffey

GENERAL OVERVIEW

Male sex accessory tissues such as the prostate, seminal vesicles, ampullary, and bulbourethral (Cowper's) glands (see Fig. 1) play an important role in reproductive function. As an overview, we will examine some of the frontier research in this area as exemplified by the following examples.

Department of Urology, The Johns Hopkins University, School of Medicine, Baltimore, Maryland 21287

Evolutionary Variation

Great variation among species is observed in the anatomy, biology, and function of the sex accessory tissues.

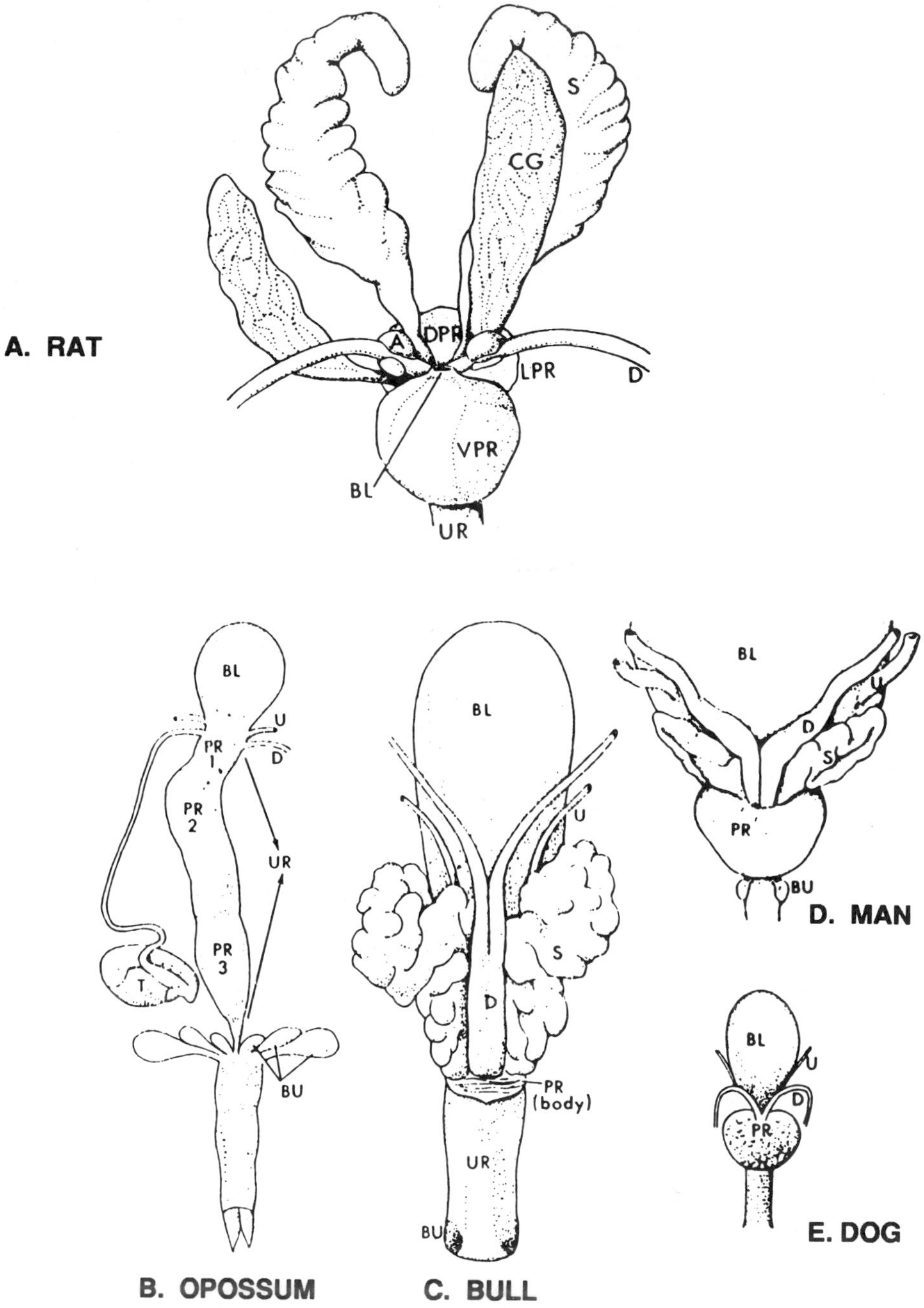

FIG. 1. Comparative anatomy of sex accessory tissue: **(A)** rat; **(B)** opossum; **(C)** bull; **(D)** man; **(E)** dog. *BL,* bladder (which was removed in the rat schematic); *BU,* bulbourethral gland; *D,* ductus deferens; *DPR,* dorsal prostate; *LPR,* lateral prostate; *PR,* prostate; *S,* seminal vesicle; *T,* testis; *U,* ureter; *UR,* urethra; *VPR,* ventral prostate. Adapted from Price (1).

For example, the seminal vesicles are large and prominent in the human and rat, but are not present in the cat and dog. Although the presence of the prostate is universal in mammals, among species, it is marked by considerable variation in anatomy, biochemistry, and pathology. For example, the rat prostate is characterized by distinct and separate anatomical lobes such as the dorsal, ventral, and lateral, each with separate functions, while in the human and dog, these corresponding anatomical lobes are not apparent but may exist only as zones in what anatomically appears to be a single uniform prostate. The sex accessory tissues also produce secretions that form the ejaculate volume, and even this varies dramatically. For example, the volume of boar ejaculate is approximately 250 ml; stallion, 70 ml; dog, 9 ml; bull, 4 ml; human, 3 ml; and ram, only 1 ml. The human ejaculate clots and then lyses, whereas in many rodents, a solid copulatory plug is ejaculated. Not only is there a vast variation in anatomical features and in secretion volumes, but this variation is also reflected in the biochemical composition of the glandular secretions and combined ejaculate. In the human ejaculate, the major anion is citrate ion (4 mg/ml), while in the dog seminal plasma, it is chloride ion.

In summary, in mammals, no other organ has such anatomical and biochemical diversity as the sex accessory tissues. If known, the evolutionary and physiological reasons for this large variation might shed insight into the functions of these glands because it is difficult to understand why such changes should be limited to sex accessory tissues. It might be suggested that the great diversity of environments and reproductive habits of mammals regulates different sex accessory functions to protect their genitourinary tracts from invasion by pathogens of external insult. Much speculation will always be generated until firm evidence is forthcoming to explain these large biological differences.

The Sex Accessory Tissue and Secretions

At present, the only firm insight we have about the specific biological functions of the sex accessory tissues such as the prostate, seminal vesicles, and bulbourethral (Cowper's glands) is that they provide the bulk of the volume of the ejaculate. The secretions of these glands constitute most of the volume and chemical composition of the seminal plasma; fluids from other parts of the male reproductive tract, such as the testes and epididymes, comprise less than 1% of the total semen volume. These sex accessory tissues produce high concentrations of many important biological substances, such as prostaglandins (200 μg/ml), spermine (3 mg/ml), fructose (2 mg/ml), citric acid (4 mg/ml), and extremely high concentrations of zinc (150 μg/ml), proteins (40 mg/ml), and specific enzymes such as immunoglobulins, proteases, esterases, and phosphatase. At present, we have only limited knowledge of the physiological functions of many of these secretory products in the seminal plasma, with the exception of some roles in the clotting and lysing processes that occur with seminal plasma. Some investigators even question the necessity for these sex accessory secretions in the fertilization process, since, in some mammals, it has been observed that sperm removed from the epididymis are capable of fertilizing the ovum; therefore, the sperm are capable of fertilization without ever having made contact with the secretions of the prostate or seminal vesicles. In addition, the surgical removal of some lobes of the rodent prostate or seminal vesicles (but not both) does not abolish male fertility (2). Although the seminal plasma may not contain factors that are absolutely essential for fertilization, the secretions may nevertheless optimize conditions for fertilization by providing a buffer effect or by increasing sperm motility and survival, and by enhancing transport in both the male and female reproductive tracts. It is suggested that the high concentrations of sugars, such as fructose, and lipids in the seminal plasma may provide nutrients or beneficial substrates to the sperm. The seminal plasma may therefore extend viability and decrease environmental shock to the sperm. A role for the sex accessory secretions in male infertility has long been suspected, but, at present, no single factor has been implicated clearly (3).

It remains to be resolved what biological materials, and drugs can be transported from the serum into the seminal plasma. Our knowledge of the mechanisms and types of transport of ions, drugs, and natural products in and out of the secretions of the sex accessory tissues is very sparse (4).

The prostate may itself serve with other sex accessory tissues in forming secretions that protect the lower urinary tract and reproductive system from the insults of pathogens that may invade via the urethra. These sex accessory glands are well positioned to block or intercept pathogens by secreting potent biological substances, such as metal ions like zinc or spermine, and proteases like lysozymes, as well as secretory immunoglobulins. The mechanical washing of the urethra by these secretions, thereby establishing a milieu hostile to invading pathogens, may be one of the primary functions of the sex accessory tissues and may account for why these glands have such a large variability in structure and composition among species. Of all the organs in evolution, the sex accessory organs vary the most; for example, the seminal vesicles are large in the human, European rabbit, rat, and hamster, but are absent from the dog, cat, cottontail rabbit, bear, and aquatic mammals. Is this evolutionary selection of a wide range of sex accessory tissue structure and function among species required because of variations in environmental factors or pathogens, or were they selected for roles in reproductive behavior? In some species the size and function of the sex accessory tissues are seasonally regulated to coincide with periods of rutting and thus may suggest their primary role in reproductive behavior or fertilization.

Infections and the Role of Sex Accessory Tissues in the Transmission of AIDS

Of great current importance is the mechanism of transport of pathogens such as the HIV-1 virus into human semen. The ejaculate is one of the major routes of sexual transmission of these viruses, but we know little about how they enter the semen, whether in free virus form (5) or carried within cells that appear in the ejaculate (6–9). If the virus enters the semen distally from the testes or epididymes, then vasectomy would stop transmission of AIDS through the ejaculate (10). The prostate is one of the leading organs in the male for other types of infections and inflammatory processes producing both acute and chronic bacterial prostatitis and the more common nonbacterial prostatitis that is of unknown origin. The influx of lymphocytes and inflammatory cells into the prostate and their presence in semen is still a mystery, since these cells can be present in both normal heterosexual males and apparently asymptomatic homosexual men who are either HIV sera-positive or -negative (7). Since these lymphocytes and inflammatory cells in the ejaculate can carry the HIV virus as a major route of sexual transmission of AIDS in heterosexuals and homosexuals, then it is obviously of great medical and social importance to understand these mechanisms and the role that the prostate and seminal vesicles play in pathogen transmission (11).

Mechanism of Androgen Action

Recently, much has been learned about the mechanism of androgen action on both the systemic and molecular level, but work remains in identifying the exact role of the androgens and the androgen receptor in the development of the organs. Advances made in the androgen receptor field include the cloning and sequencing of the receptor, the expression of the receptor in a variety of mammalian and nonmammalian cells, and the identification of androgen DNA response elements in the control regions of various genes.

Work remains to be done regarding the nature of tissue specificity of androgen action.

Why are some genes turned on in the prostate and not in the seminal vesicle?
What prevents cross-talk between androgen, progesterone, and glucocorticoid receptors if their DNA response elements are of similar sequences?
What is the role of other nuclear and cytoplasmic proteins and their interaction with androgen receptors?
What interplay exists between other signal transduction pathways and that of androgen action?

These questions currently are being addressed by researchers.

Pathology of the Prostate and Seminal Vesicles

The medical problems caused by the prostate gland are increasing (12), and their full magnitude and impact have only recently been established (13). Much of the physiology, biochemistry, and molecular biology of the prostate remains to be elucidated and yet new understanding of basic anatomy (14) has already led to important surgical considerations; and the identification of prostatic-specific antigen (15), and its presence in the sera of prostatic cancer patients (16–18) has proven to be a most useful marker for clinical monitoring (18–22).

Surprisingly, all of these abnormalities of prostate growth, including benign prostatic hypertrophy and prostate cancer, are common only to humans and dogs. It is still a mystery as to why other species such as bulls, horses, cats, and rodents are essentially free of abnormal growth of the prostate, since these animals share much of our environment. In fact, it is not understood why in humans the prostate gland should be the only common site within the sex accessory tissues for these diseases. For example, the seminal vesicles are almost devoid of abnormal growth such as benign or malignant hyperplasia. On first examination, it would appear that because of proximity, both the prostate and seminal vesicles might receive essentially the same endogenous bloodborne hormones and might be subjected to the same pathological insults by carcinogens and pathogens. Some believe the difference in disease in the two glands could be due to differences in the embryonic origins: the prostate arising from the urogenital sinus and the seminal vesicles from the wolffian ducts. Whether the marked difference between the pathology of the prostate and seminal vesicles resides in intrinsic factors within the gland, or with extrinsic environmental or pathological factors, must obviously await further study.

In summary, the purpose of this overview is to bring the reader's attention to some important problems about the sex accessory tissues and to challenge them to the importance of further studies of the sex accessory tissue. These are not only critical questions for reproduction and evolution, but also are central to important medical and social problems. The remainder of this chapter will provide the reader with a basic review that assists in the assessment of our present progress, and of areas that need further investigation.

ORGANIZATION AND CELL BIOLOGY OF SEX ACCESSORY TISSUES

Embryonic Development

Aumuller (26) has provided a detailed review of the embryology, histology, and endocrinological aspects of the development of both the prostate and seminal vesicles. These glands are very different with regard to their embryonic origin and the type of steroid that induces their developmental growth. The wolffian ducts develop into the seminal vesicles, epididymis, vas deferens, ampulla, and ejaculatory duct, and the developmental growth of this group of glands is stimulated by fetal testosterone and not dihydrotestosterone. The growth of these wolffian-derived sex accessory glands is primarily completed by the thirteenth week. In contrast, the prostate first appears and starts its development from the urogenital sinus during the third month of fetal growth, and development is directed primarily by dihydrotestosterone that is produced from the metabolic conversion of fetal testosterone through the action of the enzyme 5α-reductase that is located within the urogenital sinus. Five epithelial buds form in a paired manner on the posterior side of the urogenital sinus on both sides of the verumontanum, and they then invade the mesenchyme to form the prostate. The top pairs of buds form the inner zone of the prostate and appear to be of mesoderm origin, while the lower buds form the outer zone of the prostate and appear to be of endoderm origin. This is of potential importance, since the inner zone will give tissue of benign prostatic hyperplasia origin, while the outer zone contains the primary origin of cancer. These two zones of the prostate develop as concentric circles around the urethra. The long, branched ducts on the outside form the thick outer layer of the true prostate gland. The center portion that contains the mucosal and submucosal gland and the ejaculatory ducts, as well as the small remnants of the Müllerian duct, the utriculum prostaticus, which forms the small prostatic utricle. The prostate is well differentiated by the fourth month.

There has been much debate and divergent views on the development of the zones of the prostate. This has been reviewed in detail by McNeal (27) and in an in-depth historical review by Aumuller (26). The full embryology of the prostate in relation to its zones still requires modern biological and molecular techniques for a precise definition.

The prostate forms acini and collecting ducts that branch into the urethra and may be visualized as similar to a small tree with the growth occurring primarily on the tips as the ducts extend and branch during development. This clear indication that dynamic growth processes occur along a budding and branching system was developed from studies on the mouse prostate (28).

During the development of the prostate from the urogenital sinus, there is a close reciprocal interaction between the stromal and epithelial tissue components. Dihydrotestosterone (DHT) is produced from testosterone by both the epithelium and the mesenchyme; however, the epithelium appears to make much larger amounts of DHT. In contrast, the stromal cells appear to contain larger amounts of androgen receptor and Cunha and colleagues (29) believe that during development it is exclusive to the mesenchyme. It is visualized that a reciprocal action occurs in that DHT is formed in the epithelial cells and diffuses to the DHT receptor in the stromal nuclei of the mesenchymal cells that then produce an unknown inductive factor that drives the morphogenesis of the epithelial cells. This is thought to be accomplished in part by the DHT induction of specific soluble growth factors and alterations in the insoluble extracellular matrix components binding the stromal and epithelial cells. Resolving the exact growth factors in these temporal developments will be an important research frontier. In the development of other organs it is apparent that growth factors are of a multifunctional nature and can be either a stimulator or an inhibitor of growth, depending upon their dose combinations and sequence of presentation to target cells. For example, the interaction and combination of epidermal growth factor with transforming growth factor β and insulinlike growth factor, as well as gonadotropins, have all been shown to affect the differentiation of other types of reproductive cells and it is expected that similar roles will soon be elucidated for prostate cells (30). Growth factors will be discussed later, but it is important to note that the Müllerian inhibiting substance (MIS) that is expressed early in gonadal differentiation of the male causes the regression of the Müllerian duct as a prerequisite for virilization in the male (31). The requirement for MIS in human male development is well established; the human gene has been isolated, the primary amino acid sequence of MIS has been determined, and it now appears that it is closely related to a family of proteins that includes transforming growth factor β, which is a very potent inhibitor of growth and function of a wide variety of cell types.

The temporal events that are involved in the development of the male reproductive tract and the involvement of both steroids and growth hormones is of fundamental importance in developmental biology, but also may be of great interest in pathology of the prostate. It has been proposed by McNeal (32) that benign prostatic hyperplasia may be caused by an adult reawakening of dormant embryonic growth potential of the adult stroma and that the proliferation of the stromal elements in the periurethral region of the human prostate can stimulate the ingrowth of epithelial cells to produce a benign growth. Animal models have been made by constructing sandwiches of chimeric tissue implants composed of embryonic urogenital mesenchyme and adult prostate tissues, and it does appear that in these models the fetal mesenchyme can drive both the differentiation and growth of adult urogenital cells (29,33–40). The role of steroids and growth factors in the development of the male urogenital tract has recently been reviewed (33).

Postnatal Development and Hormone Imprinting of Growth

At birth, the majority of the acini are lined with squamous epithelium metaplasia and scattered secretory activity and cyst formation (26,41). This stimulation is believed to be under the control of residual maternal steroids such as estrogens, and there is a postnatal involution phase that occurs over the first 5 months following birth. Large transient surges of serum levels of androgen, estrogen, and progesterone normally occur very early in life both in rats and in humans. In the human male neonate a surge in testosterone is observed that peaks between 2 and 3 months of age, and during this period, blood testosterone levels rise to 60 times that of normal prepubertal levels and reach the adult range of about 400 ng/dl (42,43). Serum estradiol levels are very high at birth in both humans and rats but fall to very low levels in the first few days after birth; there is a subsequent transient surge prepubertally in the rat but not in the human. The progesterone level is high at birth in humans, which is believed to be the result of placental progesterone production. There is a second transient progesterone surge that occurs in humans at approximately

2 months of age (42). Studies in the rat have shown that neonatal and prepubertal steroids are of critical importance in setting the long-term growth regulation of the prostate that can occur later in life when the organ is subjected to testosterone stimulation (44–52). The ability of neonatal and prepubertal steroids to imprint the prostate has been established as a critical factor in these animal studies but has not been determined for the human prostate. It is important to note that there are critical differences in the postnatal development of the male reproductive trace between human and rodents, but the correlation of these prepubertal surges in both the rat and human in steroid blood levels might indicate that similar imprinting can be expected in the human. Naslund and Coffey (51,52) have proposed that neonatal imprinting may be an important factor in setting the response of the prostate in later adult life and could have implications for benign prostatic hyperplasia. Higgins and associates (53) have shown that differentiation of the rat prostate as determined by DNA methylation of specific genes in the seminal vesicles and ventral prostate is determined by similar types of imprinting phenomena, and this may provide the molecular mechanism for these effects.

Structure of the Prostate and Seminal Vesicle Glands

Overview of the Sex Accessory Glands

The prostate contains a number of individual glands composed of from 30 to 50 lobules, which then form 15 to 30 secretory ducts that open into the urethra lateral to the colliculus seminalis (26,54). The term "lobes" for prostate organization has given way to the discussion of zones (55,56). The prostate shape is most often said to be analogous to a horse chestnut with the length of the anterior aspect being between 3 and 4 cm and its width between 3.5 and 5 cm. A normal adult human prostate weighs approximately 20 ± 6 g (57) and lies immediately below the base of the bladder surrounding the proximal portion of the urethra. The gland is located behind the inferior part of the symphysis pubis and rests directly above the urogenital diaphragm and in front of the rectal ampulla. The gland is composed of alveoli that are lined with tall columnar secretory epithelial cells. The acini of these alveoli drain, by a system of branching ducts and tubules, into the floor and lateral surfaces of the posterior urethra. The alveoli and ducts are embedded within a stroma of fibromuscular tissue.

The weight of the seminal vesicles is 8–9 g in the human and develops as paired pouches (capacity, 4.5 ml each) forming from the vas deferens. The glands are 4 to 5 cm in length and are located directly on the posterior side of the bladder and adjacent to the rectum. The glands are composed of tubular alveoli containing viscous secretions, and the ducts can be highly variable from a simple tube to the more common short main ducts with clusters of large side-ducts. The seminal vesicles were so named because it was erroneously believed that they stored semen and sperm. Their secretions contribute to semen, but they do not store secretions made elsewhere. The ampulla at the distal end of the vas deferens does store sperm, and the seminal vesicles join the ampulla to form the beginning of the ejaculatory ducts. The ejaculatory ducts pass through the prostate and finally terminate below the utricle within the prostate urethra at the verumontanum. Aumuller and Riva (58) have written a recent review on seminal vesicle anatomy and function.

The bulbourethral, or Cowper's gland, is a paired, pea-sized, typically mucous compound tubular gland located directly below the prostate within the urogenital sinus. This gland was named after its founder William Cowper, who described it in 1698. It is variable in evolution, being a very large gland in the squirrel and boar, but absent from the dog. The glands empty into the urethra, and the function and composition of their secretions are poorly understood but contain high concentrations of sialic acid. Very small urethral glands, termed glands of Littre, line the penile urethra. It is believed that the Cowper and Littre glands lubricate the urethra, facilitating intromission. All of these sex accessory tissues depend on androgens for development, growth, and maintenance of their size and secretory products and contribute to the composition of the seminal plasma of the ejaculate.

Prostate Anatomy

For many years the prostate was believed to have a lobular structure. Prior to 1906, when Home described the middle lobe, the prostate was generally considered to be composed of two lateral lobes (59). For the next century the importance of the two or three lobes of the prostate was debated widely. However, in 1912 Lowsley proposed the existence of five prostatic lobes based upon embryologic findings: two lateral lobes, a posterior lobe, and the middle lobe; an anterior lobe, which was present in fetal material, atrophied and disappeared by the time of birth. This concept was adopted widely for the next 50 years. It is difficult to understand why this theory remained unchallenged over this period of time. Franks (60) has emphasized that these divisions were only identifiable in the embryo, and from the last months of gestation into postnatal life no divisions into separate glands was possible. Furthermore, LeDuc (59) was unable to demonstrate a posterior row of prostatic ducts, thus seriously challenging the existence of the posterior lobe of the prostate, which was given such anatomical prominence by Lowsley. In retrospect, this old concept most likely arose from confusion between the anatomy of the truly normal prostate and the prostate affected by hyperplastic changes. Urological surgeons frequently refer to midline and laterally projecting nodules of benign prostatic hyperplasia as middle and lateral lobes, respectively. However, these "lobes" are not reference points of normal anatomy but exist only in glands with benign prostatic hyperplasia.

Today the concept of a lobular structure has been replaced by a concept based on concentric zones. Many authors have suggested that the prostate could be separated into at least two independent structures: an inner and outer zone (60–62). In more recent years the morphology of the prostate has come under intense study by several talented investigators (27,55,56,63–67). Of these, McNeal's work appears to be the most widely accepted. A historical and comparative analysis of McNeal's terminology to the contributions of others has been made (27,68). Rather than dividing the prostate into arbitrary lobes, McNeal has identified zones that appear to have morphological, functional, and pathological significance. To understand his descriptions of the prostate it is important to recognize that the prostatic urethra is not a straight tube. Rather, at the midpoint of the prostatic urethra between the apex of the prostate and the bladder neck (i.e., at the upper end of the verumontanum) the posterior wall of the urethral is kinked anteriorly in such a way that the entire proximal urethra is angled 35 degrees anterior to the course of the distal urethral segment (Fig. 2). Previously, many investigators used transverse sections of the prostate taken at the level of the verumontanum for their studies. However, McNeal (63) has emphasized the need for planes other than conventional transverse sections to demonstrate differences between one part of the prostate and the other. Using sagittal, coronal, and oblique coronal sections he has divided the prostate into four distinct zones. Each zone makes contact with a specific portion of the prostatic urethra, which can be taken as the primary anatomical landmark for defining them (Fig. 2). The subsequent descriptions of these zones are taken directly from McNeal's many contributions (27,55,56,63–65).

Anterior Fibromuscular Stroma

The anterior fibromuscular stroma is a thick sheet of connective tissue that covers the entire anterior surface of the prostate. It is a continuous sheet of smooth muscle that surrounds the urethra proximally at the bladder neck where it merges with the internal sphincter and detrusor muscle from which it originates. Near the apex, the smooth muscle merges with transverse loops of striated muscle, which represent a proximal extension of the external sphincter, thus forming an incomplete sphincter along the anterior aspect of the distal urethral segment. The anterior fibromuscular stroma comprises up to one-third of the total bulk of the prostate. It is entirely lacking in glandular elements.

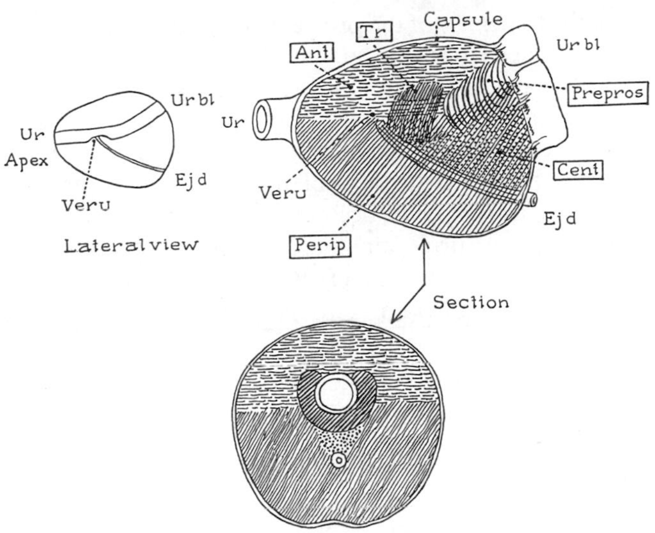

FIG. 2. Diagrammatic representation of prostatic anatomy as described by McNeal (see text). **Upper left,** Path of the urethra (*Ur*) as it courses from the apex of the prostate to the bladder (*bl*). **Upper right,** Sagittal view illustrating the four zones of the prostate and their relationship to the ejaculatory ducts (*Ejd*). anterior fibromuscular stroma (*Ant*); peripheral zone (*Perip*); central zone (*Cent*); preprostatic tissue (*Prepros*); and transition zone (*Tr*). **Bottom,** Relationship of the zones in a transverse section. *Veru,* verumontanum. From *Campbell's Urology,* 6th ed. P. C. Walsh et al., eds. Philadelphia: W. B. Saunders, 1992.

Peripheral Zone

The peripheral zone is the largest anatomical subdivision of the prostate. It is a flat disk of secretory tissue whose ducts branch out laterally from either side of the distal urethra. Laterally, some of the terminal ducts curve anteriorly to form a shallow cup around the striated sphincter and then anchor into the lateral extent of the anterior fibromuscular stroma. This zone contains 75% of the total glandular tissue of the prostate. In this region, almost all carcinomas arise. Furthermore, this is the tissue sampled in most random biopsies of the prostate.

Central Zone

The central zone is the smaller of the two subdivisions of functioning glandular prostate making up about 25% of its mass. It contacts the urethra only at the upper end of the verumontanum where its duct orifices open in a tight circle immediately around the ejaculatory duct orifices. The ducts branch laterally to form a flat wedge of glandular tissue with its apex at the verumontanum and its base at the base of the prostate posterior to the bladder neck. The central zone surrounds the ejaculatory ducts completing the proximal quadrant of glandular tissue above and behind the verumontanum. McNeal distinguishes the central from the peripheral zone based on differences in architecture of the glands and cytologic detail. He feels that the architecture and histological features of the central zone closely resemble those of the seminal vesicle, suggesting that the central zone could be of wolffian duct origin. This possibility correlates with the uncommon occurrence of carcinoma in both the seminal vesicle and central zone.

Preprostatic Tissues

The preprostatic tissues, which surround the anteriorly displaced urethra proximal to the upper end of the verumontanum, is the smallest of the four regions and the most complex in its arrangement of both glandular and nonglandular elements. This term has been applied to this zone because of its sphincteric function at the time of ejaculation to prevent the reflux of seminal fluid into the bladder. Its main components is a cylindrical smooth muscle sphincter surrounding the entire preprostatic urethra. Inside this cylinder of smooth muscle are the tiny periurethral glands, which constitute less than 1% of the mass of the glandular prostate. They do not possess their own periglandular musculature and are confined in their extent to the immediate periurethral stroma. Because the smooth muscle cylinder limits the expansion of the glands laterally away from the urethra, these glands grow proximally toward the bladder neck. However, at the distal margin of the smooth muscle sphincter some ducts escape below the most distal rings of the smooth muscle sleeve thus enabling them to develop outside its confines.

Transition Zone

The *transition zone* is a small group of ducts, arising at a single point at the junction of the proximal and distal urethral segments. The ducts in this region, which comprise less than 5% of the mass of the normal glandular prostate, demonstrate more branching and acinar proliferation than the other periurethral ducts. Though insignificant in size and functional importance, the transition zone and the other periurethral glands are the exclusive site of origin of benign prostatic hyperplasia.

Prostate Cell Types

Epithelial Cells

A summary of the tissue elements and organization of the prostate are listed in Table 1. The prostatic epithelium in the human is composed of three major cell types: the secretory epithelial cells, the basal cells, and the neuroendocrine cells. In most glands with cell-renewing populations there is a steady-state flow of cells from reserve quiescent stem cells to a more rapidly dividing transient proliferating population that finally proceeds to the formation of the fully mature nondividing terminally differentiated secretory cells that are then programmed to senesce and die off. It is still unclear how this generalized scheme functions in the normal and hyperplastic prostate (69). In the prostate the most common tall (12–10 μm) columnar secretory epithelial cells are terminally differentiated and are easily distinguished by their morphology and abundant secretory granules and enzymes that stain abundantly with prostatic specific antigen, acid phosphatase, and other enzymes such as leucine aminopeptidase. These tall columnar secretory cells appear like rows of a picket fence resting next to each other connected by cell adhesion molecules and with their base attached to a basement membrane through integrin receptors. The nucleus is at the base just below a clear zone (2–8 μm) of abundant Golgi apparatus and the upper cellular periphery is rich in secretory granules and enzymes. The apical plasma membrane facing the lumen possesses a microvilli and secretions move out into the open collecting spaces of the acinus. These epithelial cells ring the periphery of the acinus and produce secretions into the acini that drain into the ducts that connect to the urethra. In androgen ablation the typical secretory cells decrease by 90% in total numbers, become cuboidal, and shrink by 80% in cell volume and 60% in cell height (70). Kastendieck (71) suggested more than three types and identified five different prostatic epithelial cell types: type I, the basal cell, type II, the immature nonsecretory glandular cell, type III, the mature secretory glandular cell, type IV, the nonsecreting predegenerative glandular cell, and type V, the degenerating glandular cell.

Basal/Stem Cells

In comparison to the secretory epithelial cells, the basal cells are much smaller and less abundant in number and are present in less than 10% the number. These small cells are not columnar, are more round with little cytoplasm and large irregular-shaped nuclei. They are less differentiated and almost devoid of secretory products such as acid phosphatase. These basal cells are always resting on the basement membrane and appear wedged between the bases of adjacent tall columnar epithelial cells. The plasma membrane is rich in ATPase, suggesting that these cells may be involved in active transport. These basal cells are rich in 5-nm tonofilaments and stain brightly with fluorescent antibodies to keratin (72). It was mistakenly believed that these cells were myo-

TABLE 1. *Summary of the anatomy and cell biology of the prostate gland*

Components	Properties
Development	
Seminal vesicles	From wolffian ducts via testosterone stimulation
Prostate	From urogenital sinus via DHT stimulation
Prostate zones	
Anterior fibromuscular	30% of prostate mass, no glandular elements, smooth muscle
Peripheral	Largest zone, 75% of prostate glandular elements, site of carcinomas
Central	25% of prostate glandular elements, surrounds ejaculatory ducts, may be of wolffian duct origin, seminal vesicle-like
Preprostatic	Smallest, surround upper urethra, complex, sphincter
Transition	5% of prostate glandular elements, site of BPH
Epithelial cells	
Basal	Small undifferentiated, keratin-rich (type 4, 5, 6) pluripotent cells, less than 10% of epithelial cell number
Transient proliferating	Incorporate thymidine
Columnar secretory	Terminal differentiated, nondividing, rich in acid phosphatase and PSA; 20 μm tall, most abundant cell, keratin types 8, 18, 19
Neuroendocrine	Serotonin-rich, APUD type
Stroma cells	
Smooth muscle	Actin-rich
Fibroblast	Vimentin-rich and associated with fibronectin
Endothelial	Associated with fibronectin, alkaline phosphatase-positive
Tissue matrix	
Extracellular	
Basement membrane	Type IV collagen meshwork, laminin-rich, fibronectin
Connective tissue	Type I and type II fibrillar collagen, elastin
Glycosaminoglycans	Sulfates of dermatan, chondroitin, and heparan; hyaluronic acid
Cytomatrix	Tubulin, actin, and intermediate filaments of keratin
Nuclear matrix	DNA tight-binding proteins, RNA, and residual nuclear proteins

From *Campbell's Urology*, 6th ed. P. C. Walsh et al., eds. Philadelphia: W. B. Saunders, 1992.

APUD, amine precursor uptake decarboxylase cell; DHT, dihydrotestosterone; BPH, benign prostatic hyperplasia; PSA, prostate-specific antigen.

epithelial (60), but this may not be the case, since they are not rich in actin or myosin. It is believed that these undifferentiated basal cells give rise to secretory epithelial cells and as such function as a type of stem cell (73). Evans and Chandler (74) used pulse chase DNA-labeling experiments to challenge the concept of the basal cell as a stem cell for secretory epithelial cells. Basal cell proliferation has been measured in relation to benign prostatic hyperplasia (75). The importance of understanding the biology of these basal cells is realized because of the growing evidence that many neoplasias, both benign and malignant, really represent stem cell diseases. The stem cell concept of normal and abnormal growth has been reviewed by Isaacs and Coffey (69).

The proper identification in the prostate of stem cells and the transient proliferating cells has not been realized. Indeed, there may be several types of stem cells as well as several types of secretory cells. Functional and immunological markers are needed to answer these questions. Lectins as cell markers have been used to identify some types of basal and secretory cells (76). Merk and coworkers (77) have presented evidence that canine prostatic epithelial cells have a pluripotentiality of response and can change their keratin pattern, secretory granules, and phenotype base on treatment with estrogens and/or androgens.

Neuroendocrine Cells

There are also significant populations of neuroendocrine cells that reside among the more abundant secretory epithelium in the normal prostate gland. These cells are found in the epithelium of the acini and in ducts of all parts of the gland, as well as in the urothelium of the prostatic urethral mucosa (78–80). The distribution, morphology and secretory products of these cells have been studied in both normal and benign prostatic hyperplasia tissues (81,82). There are three types of prostate neuroendocrine cells with the major type containing both serotonin (5-hydroxytryptamine, 5-HT) and thyroid-stimulating hormone. The two minor cell types contain calcitonin and somatostatin (78). Neuroendocrine cells—also termed APUD (amine precursor uptake decarboxylase) cells—carry out their regulatory activity by the secretion of hormonal polypeptides or biogenic amines such as serotonin, which is a common marker for these cells. High pressure liquid chromatography measurements have shown that normal human prostate tissue contains approximately 1,400 ng of serotonin/g of tissue and this would certainly emphasize the importance of these cells (80). It is most probable that these neuroendocrine cells may be involved in the regulation of prostatic secretory activity and cell growth. Chung and his coworkers (83) have shown that the rat ventral prostate growth can be uncoupled from secretory function by transplanting the ventral prostate subcutaneously and that the synthesis of prostatin, a secretory protein, can be restored by a β-agonist treatment using L-isoproterenol, thus suggesting β-adrenergic receptors in the regulation of prostatic epithelial cells. They also demonstrated that norepinephrine has a direct mitogenic effect on cultured prostatic stromal cells. They demonstrated that norepinephrine and 5-hydroxytryptamine was greatly increased in the prostate of castrated animals and that the level of the biogenic amine was regulated reversibly by androgens (38,83,84).

Higgins and Gosling (85) have studied the structure and intrinsic innervation of the normal human prostate and have observed acetylcholine esterase nerves associated with smooth muscle in both the peripheral and central parts of the prostate. In addition, they have shown that the majority of the acini in the peripheral and central regions possess a rich plexus of autonomic nerves and that vasoactive intestinal peptide (VIP)-positive nerve fibers were found in relation to the epithelial lining acini in the central and peripheral regions of the gland. They concluded that an autonomic innervation of peripheral and central regions of the gland were indistinguishable and they were unable to morphologically find a distinct transitional zone. In contrast, Reese and colleagues (86) have found plasminogen activator as a mark for functional zones within the human prostate gland.

Lepor and Kuhar (87) characterized and studied the location of the muscarinic cholinergic receptor in human prostate tissue and localized it to the epithelial cells which is consistent with the neuropharmacology of muscarinic cholinergic agonist having a marked effect on increasing prostatic secretion. In addition, the alpha, adrenergic receptor has also been studied in the human prostate. This is of great clinical importance because of the use of selected alpha, adrenergic antagonists to alleviate bladder outlet obstruction secondary to benign prostatic hyperplasia (88–90).

The Stroma and Tissue Matrix

The epithelial cells rest upon the basement lamina or membrane that is about 100 nm thick and surrounds the acini. The basement membrane is not a membrane, but a complex structure containing collagen types IV and V, glycosoaminoglycans, complex polysaccharides, and glycolipids. This forms an interface to the stromal compartment that consists of a structural extracellular matrix, ground substance, and a variety of stromal cells including the fibroblasts, capillary and lymphatic endothelial cells, smooth muscle cells, neuroendocrine cells, and axons (91,92). The smooth muscle cells are clustered around the acinar structure and the capsule and are believed to be involved in the mechanical expression of ejaculate fluid under neural stimulation. These smooth muscle cells change their morphology in association with BPH in the plasma reticulum and Golgi apparatus appear to be enlarged as measured by morphometric techniques (93). They hypothesize that under hormonal stimulation, the smooth muscle is stimulated, producing collagen which forms part of the extracellular matrix and enhances epithelial growth by a stromal-epithelial type of interaction (see later discussion).

A tissue matrix system is defined as a biological scaffolding or residual skeleton structure that organizes and locates cells and their polarity and interactions within the organ (94). The tissue matrix system forms an interacting three-dimensional framework and is one of the most active areas of modern cell biology and involves the interaction of the matrix components including the extracellular matrix, cytoskeleton and nuclear matrix. The epithelial cell rests upon the basement membrane that is connected by an extracellular matrix to the stromal cells. It is believed that structural phase shifts and communication through these matrix elements may play a central role in controlling prostatic development and function of the prostate and in transmitting structural signals from the cell periphery to the DNA, and thus play a central role in regulating chromatin structure and gene expression (94). All mammalian cells are composed of a cytomatrix or cytoskeleton network that is formed from a network of microtubules of 20 nm (tubulins), microfilaments of 6 nm (actins), and intermediate filaments of 10 nm (keratin, desmin, vimentin). Tubulin is ubiquitous in all cells as a microtubular structure that appears to anchor many cellular structures and is a critical factor in determining the shape of the cell. The microfilaments are composed primarily of actin, one of the major proteins in all cells. Actin has the ability to polymerize and depolymerize and as such, makes one of the important structural chemomechanical systems when it interacts with myosin within the cell. The cytomatrix composed of these filaments is involved in a central way with transport of particles and components within the cell and with cell motility.

There are several types of intermediate filaments of the cytomatrix that are extremely important because they vary in type and composition with differentiation and appear to define the various cell types within the body. For example, one of the intermediate filaments called desmin is a central component of all muscle cells, while the intermediate filament vimentin is found in all fibroblasts. The intermediate filaments made of keratins are universal as major components of the cytomatrix of all epithelial cells. There is usually just one type of vimentin and desmin in the fibroblast or muscle cells. In contrast, in the epithelial cells the keratins represent over 20 different molecular types that vary with the state of cellular differentiation and the types of epithelial cells ranging from stratified squamous to simple epithelial cells. Keratins can change in prostate epithelial cells with pathology or hormone action (72,77,95–98). Of particular interest is the combination of cytoskeletal studies with steroid receptor and secretory function that has been carried out on the human prostate, comparing the keratin patterns in the epithelium of the prepubertal and pubertal prostate with those found in benign prostatic hyperplasia and prostatic adenocarcinoma (99).

The cytomatrix (cytoplasmic skeleton) just described terminates in the center of the cell by direct attachment to the nuclear matrix (Fig. 3). The prostatic epithelial cell therefore has direct structural linkage via the matrix systems from the DNA to the plasma membrane. The cytomatrix then makes direct contact to the basement membrane and extracellular matrix and ground substance of the stroma. This entire interlocking tissue scaffolding or superstructure is termed the *tissue matrix* (94) and may have dynamic properties in ordering biological processes and the transport of secretion from the sex accessory tissues.

Understanding the biological components of the tissue matrix system within sex accessory tissues is of paramount importance (see review in ref. 94). The epithelial cell is anchored to the basement membrane or basement lamina by an extracellular matrix protein called laminin. The laminin proteins are glycoproteins of the extracellular matrix that mediate attachment of cells to the collagen IV of the basement membrane. Laminin is produced by epithelial cells, but not by fibroblasts, and is a large molecule with molecular domains that interact with the type IV collagen of the basement membrane and integrin type of receptors within the cell surface glycocalyx of the epithelial cell. Laminin surrounds the basement membrane of prostate acinar epithelial cells, capillaries, smooth muscle and nerve fibers, but not lymphatics, lymphocytes, or fibroblast, and the laminin distribution was disrupted in higher grade prostate neoplasias (100).

A second type of important prostatic glycoprotein that is involved in cell adherence to the extracellular matrix is fibronectin that also binds to the family of cell integrin-type receptors. Fibronectin is secreted primarily by prostatic fibroblasts and forms an adhesive material that makes a binding interface of mesenchymal and epithelial cells to various types of collagen and proteoglycans of the extracellular matrix. There are several types of fibronectin and they have been proposed to play a key role in morphogenesis and control of cell growth.

The connective tissue of the prostate is primarily collagen of types I and III, which form the interstitial collagen (101), while types IV and V are found primarily in the basement membrane woven through the stroma and connective tissue of the extracellular matrix in a complex network of glycosaminoglycans and complex polysaccharides. Glycosaminoglycans are large negatively charged polymers (polyanions) that have proven to be critical factors in the signaling of extracellular matrix events in many different tissues (102). These latter polysaccharide polymers have long been proposed to play an important role in prostate growth (103), and DeKlerk (104) has isolated and quantitated these important glycosaminoglycans from the normal and benign human prostates and reports that dermatan sulfate is the predominant (40%) glycosaminoglycans followed by hepa-

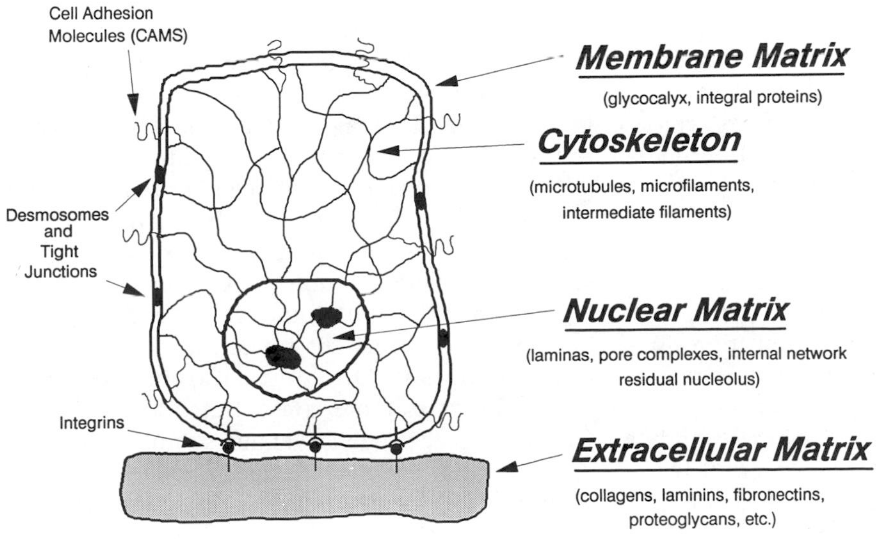

FIG. 3. The tissue matrix system. A superstructure scaffold network connects the extracellular matrix components to the integrin receptors that extend through the plasma membrane and connect directly to the cytomatrix structures. The cytomatrix couples directly to the nuclear matrix, which attaches and organizes the DNA. The cell adhesion molecules (*CAMs*) and desmosomes connect neighboring cells. From Getzenberg et al. (94).

rin (20%), chondroitin (16%), and hyaluronic acid (20%). Fetal prostates are devoid of dermatan and chondroitin sulfate increases with benign prostatic hyperplasia. Chan and Wong (105,106) have studied the histochemical distribution in the guinea pig lateral prostate and have identified three different types of proteoglycan fibers in different tissue compartments. It will be of interest to determine the role of glycosaminoglycans in sex accessory tissue function. It has been shown that synthesis of proteoglycans can be regulated in the rat prostate by androgens (107,108).

In the near future one of the most active areas of unraveling the control of sex accessory tissue function will revolve around a clearer understanding of the interactions of these complex tissue matrix components. At present, there have been several important studies (29,36,104, 109) that all point to the importance of these structural elements. Of particular importance are the studies that have shown the localization of keratins, laminin, fibronectin and actin within the various cell types of the prostate, and the studies of Bartch and colleagues (101), and Thornton and colleagues (109) on the collagens of the prostate (91).

ENDOCRINE CONTROL OF SEX ACCESSORY TISSUE

Endocrine Overview

The prostate, like other sex accessory tissues, is stimulated to grow and is maintained in size and secretory function by the continued presence of serum testosterone, which is a prohormone and must be converted by metabolism within the prostate into dihydrotestosterone. It is important to realize that testosterone is synthesized originally from the precursor of progesterone by reversible reactions; however, when testosterone forms estrogens or dihydrotestosterone, it is by irreversible reactions. All of these steroids are believed to have strong effects on different cells and tissues in the body, ranging from differentiation and neonatal imprinting, through puberty and into adult maintenance and later senescence (Fig. 5). Therefore, androgen ablation or androgen treatment have a wide variety of physiological effects that must be taken into consideration. The effect of the endocrine glands on the prostate is depicted in Fig. 4. The hypothalamus releases a small protein with only 10 amino acids (decapeptide) called the luteinizing hormone releasing hormone (LHRH) or the gonadotropin releasing hormone (GnRH). Under the stimulation of LHRH, the pituitary releases the luteinizing hormone (LH) that is transported to the testes and acts directly on the Leydig cells to stimulate the steroid synthesis and release of testosterone that becomes the major serum androgen capable of stimulating prostatic growth. Most of the estrogen in the male is also derived from peripheral conversion of testosterone to estrogens through an enzymatic aromatization reaction. Therapeutic estrogens, such as diethylstilbestrol, do not primarily block androgen action by direct effects on the prostate, but indirectly through blocking pituitary function by decreasing LH release that reduces the serum signal for testicular testosterone production; therefore, estrogen acts as an effective "chemical castration." Other androgens capable of stimulating prostate growth include adrenal androgens formed from androstenedione; however, this is not a major pathway, since, in both animals and humans, castration leads to almost complete involution of the prostate, therefore adrenal androgens are insufficient to stimulate any meaningful growth of the prostate. Only when the adrenals are stimulated by excess adrenocorticotropic hormone (ACTH) or are overactive do they have any significant effect in stimulating prostatic growth. The role of adrenal androgens is minor, but this is a very controversial issue and has led to the total androgen blockade concept of claiming additional control of prostate cancer by eliminating adrenal androgens or their function. This is the concept of using LHRH analogs in combination with antiandrogens like flutamide to theoretically block residual androgen stimulation from the adrenal gland.

Prolactin has often been postulated to enhance androgen-induced growth; however, several decades of study have failed to indicate the mechanism of this action, but it does not appear at present to be a major means of regulating normal prostatic growth. Prolactin is believed to enhance the uptake of androgens into the prostate and to affect the synthesis of citric acid.

The following section reviews endocrine factors released by other organs, their synthesis, serum levels, and transport to the prostate.

Androgen Production by the Testes

Since the testes produce the major serum androgen supporting prostate and sex accessory tissue growth, it is important to briefly review this function. In the normal human male, the major circulating serum androgen is testosterone, which is almost exclusively (more than 95%) of testicular origin. Under normal physiological conditions the Leydig cells of the testis are the major source of the testicular androgens. The Leydig cells are stimulated by the gonadotropins (primarily the luteinizing hormone (LH) to synthesize testosterone from acetate and cholesterol. The spermatic vein concentration of testosterone is 40 to 50 μg/100 ml and is approximately 75 times more concentrated than the level detected in the peripheral venous serum (110), which is approximately 600 ng of testosterone/100 ml. Other androgens also leave the testes by the spermatic vein, and

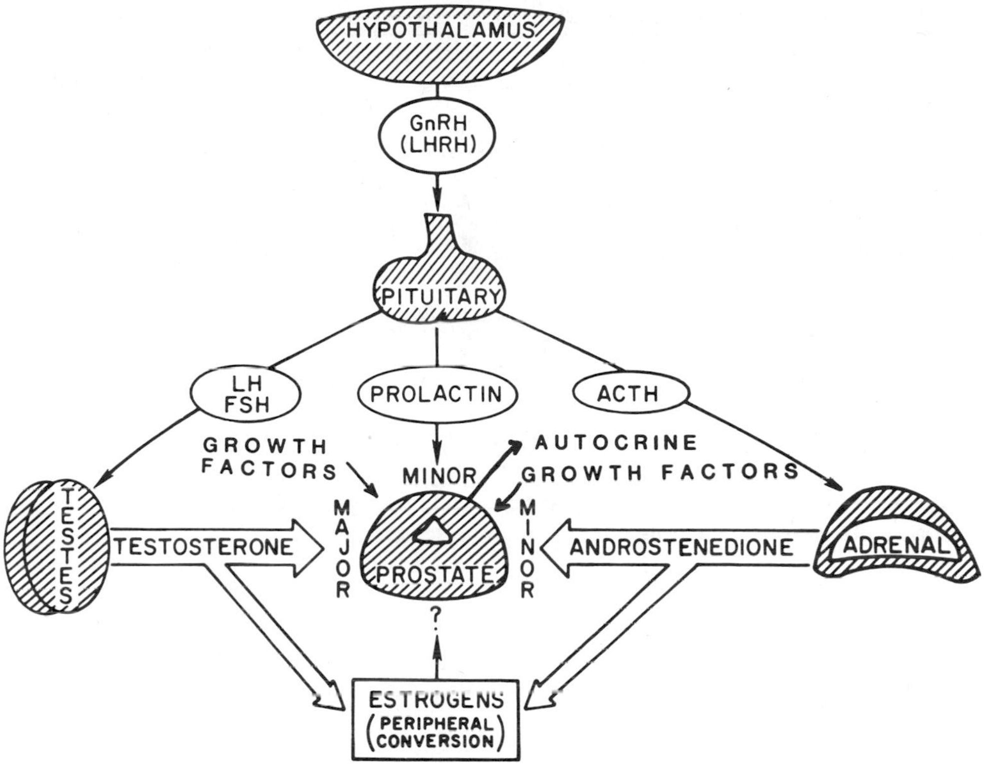

FIG. 4. A schematic of factors affecting the growth of the prostate. *GRH,* gonadotropin-releasing hormone; *LH,* luteinizing hormone; *FSH,* follicle-stimulating hormone; *ACTH,* adrenocorticotropic hormone; growth factors are present in the serum; autocrine growth factors are protein factors released within the prostate that function either by autocrine or paracrine mechanisms. The schematic indicates that prolactin and the adrenal glands have only minor effects on prostate growth, whereas the effects of estrogens are still not established. Adapted from *Campbell's Urology,* 5th ed. P. C. Walsh et al., eds. Philadelphia: W. B. Saunders, 1985.

these include androstanediol, androstenedione (3 μg/100 ml), dehydroepiandrosterone (7 μg/100 ml), and dihydrotestosterone (0.4 μg/100 ml); therefore, the concentrations of these androgens are much lower in the spermatic vein than those of testosterone, with all being less than 15% of that of testosterone.

The total testosterone that enters the plasma is referred to as the testosterone blood production rate and is 6 to 7 mg/day in the human. Although other steroids, such as androstenedione from the adrenals, can be converted by peripheral metabolism to testosterone, they probably account for less than 5% of the overall production of plasma testosterone. The mean metabolic clearance rate for testosterone is around 1,000 liters per 24 hours and results in a plasma half-life of only 10–20 minutes.

The average testosterone concentration in the adult human male plasma is approximately 611 ng/100 ml ± 186 with a normal range of 300 to 1,000 that is equal to 10.4–34.7 nmol/L in SI units (Table 2). Serum testosterone levels are not remarkably related to age between 25 and 70 years, although it does decline gradually to approximately 500 ng/100 ml after 70 years of age. It is recognized that plasma concentrations of testosterone can vary widely in an individual in any one day and may reflect both episodic and diurnal variations in the production rate.

Only 2% of the total serum testosterone is not protein-bound—called free testosterone—and it is at a concentration of approximately 15 ng/100 ml or less than 1 nM. It is only this free testosterone that is available for prostate uptake for metabolism to dihydrotestosterone or uptake by the liver and intestines primarily to form 17-ketosteroids. Metabolic androgen such as 17-ketosteroids are then secreted into the urine as final water-soluble conjugates with either sulfuric acid or glucuronic acid. The total 17-ketosteroids in the urine in adult males is from 4 to 25 mg/24 h and is not an accurate index of testosterone production, since other steroids from the adrenals as well as nonandrogenic steroids can be metabolized to 17-ketosteroids. Only small (25 to 160 μg/day) amounts of testosterone enter the urine without metabolism, and this urinary testosterone represents less than 2% of the daily testosterone production (Fig. 5).

Although testosterone is the primary plasma androgen inducing growth of the prostate gland and other sex acces-

TABLE 2. *Average plasma levels of sex steroids in healthy human males*

Steroid (common name)	Plasma concentration ng/100 ml	Plasma concentration Relative molarity	Daily blood production rate (mg/day)	Relative androgenicity rat VP assay[a]
Testosterone	611 ± 186	100	6.6 ± 0.5	100
Dihydrotesterone (DHT)	56 ± 20	9	0.3 ± 0.06	181
5α-Androstane-3α,17β-diol (3α-androstanediol)	14 ± 4	2	0.2 ± 0.03	126
5α-Androstane-3β,17β-diol (3β-androstanediol)	<2	<0.3		18
Androstenediol	161 ± 52	26		0.21
Androsterone	54 ± 32	9	0.28	53
Androstenedione	150 ± 54	25	1.4	39
Dehydroepiandrosterone (DHEA)	501 ± 98	81	29	15
Dehydroepiandrosterone sulfate (DHEAS)	135,925 ± 48,000	17,619		<1
Progesterone	30	4.5	0.75	
17β-Estradiol (E_2)	2.5 ± 0.8	0.4	0.045	
Estrone	4.6	0.8		

Adapted from *Campbell's Urology,* 5th ed. P. C. Walsh et al., eds. Philadelphia: W. B. Saunders, 1985.
[a] VP assay, ventral prostate growth in castrated rat.

sory tissues, it appears to function as a prohormone in that the active form of the androgen in the prostate is not testosterone but a more androgenic metabolite, *dihydrotestosterone* (DHT) (111–116) (Fig. 6). The formation of dihydrotestosterone involves the reduction of the double bond in the A ring of testosterone through the enzymatic action of the enzyme 5α-reductase (Fig. 6). This conversion can take place directly in the prostate and seminal vesicles or in peripheral tissues such as the liver. Dihydrotestosterone concentration in the plasma of normal men is very low, 56 ± 20 ng/100 ml, in comparison to testosterone, which is 11-fold higher at approximately 611 ng/100 ml (see Table 2).

In summary, although dihydrotestosterone is a potent androgen (1.5 to 2.5 times as potent as testosterone in most bioassay systems), its low plasma concentration and tight binding to plasma proteins diminishes its direct importance as a circulating androgen affecting prostate and seminal vesicle growth. In contrast, dihydrotestosterone is of paramount importance for growth within the

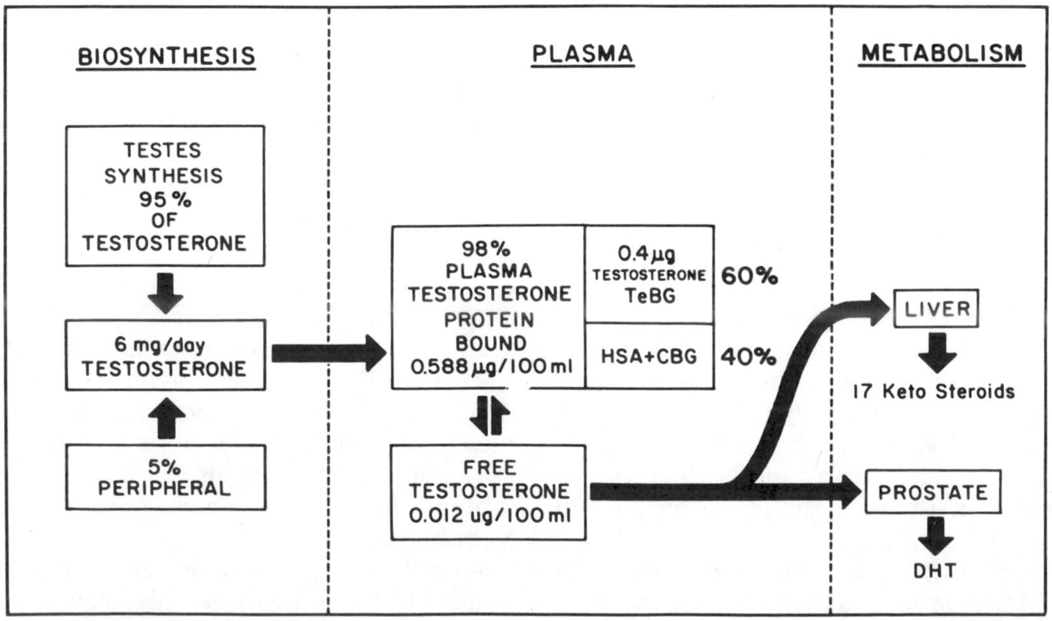

FIG. 5. The biosynthesis, plasma concentrations, and metabolism of testosterone. **Left:** Indicates the daily production of 6 mg/day of testosterone that is formed, 95% by the testes and 5% by peripheral synthesis. This testosterone enters the plasma, where it is present at a circulating level of 600 ng/100 ml. This is equivalent to 0.6 μg/dl. About 98% of serum testosterone is bound to plasma proteins. Free testosterone enters the liver and prostate for further metabolism to 17-ketosteroids and dihydrotestosterone (DHT), respectively.

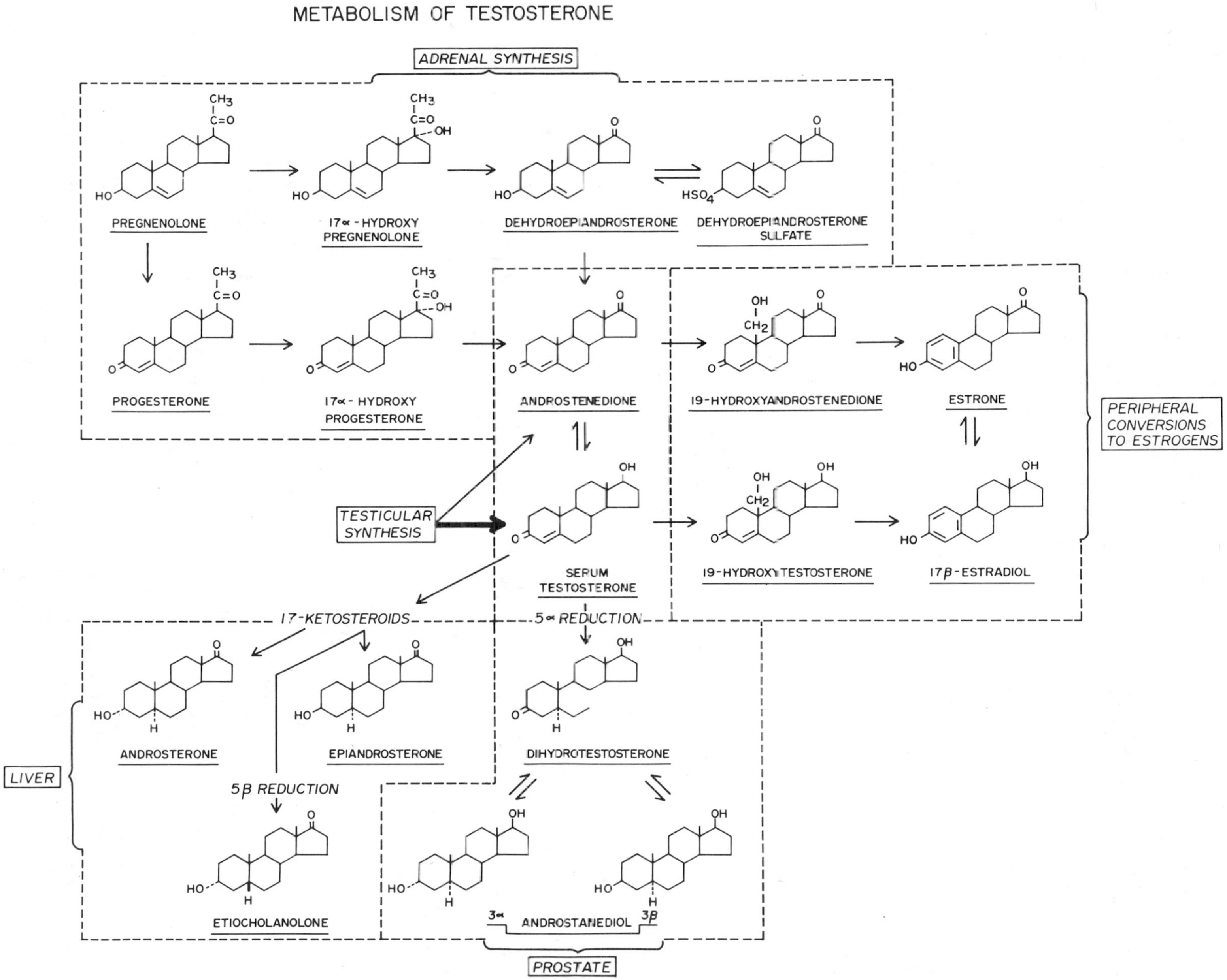

FIG. 6. The metabolism of testosterone in various organs and compartments. The adrenal gland contributes to androgens primarily through androstenedione. Both adrostenedione and serum testosterone are converted to estrogens by peripheral aromatase reactions. Serum testosterone enters the prostate gland, where it is metabolized to the androgens dihydrotestosterone 3α-androstanediol, or 3β-androstanediol. Testosterone enters the liver, where it is converted to the 17-ketosteroids.

prostate, where it is formed from testosterone. Dihydrotestosterone is the major form of androgen found within the prostate gland (5 ng/g tissue wet weight) and is fivefold higher than testosterone, that is, at approximately 1 ng/g. In the prostate, dihydrotestosterone binds to specific androgen receptors within the nucleus where approximately 100,000 DHT molecules reside per nucleus.

In summary, DHT becomes the major androgen regulating the cellular events of growth, differentiation, and function in the prostate.

The normal plasma levels of some important steroids are summarized in Table 4. These values are derived as averages and can fluctuate with stress, hospitalization, and environmental changes.

Adrenal Androgens

There is evidence that hyperstimulation of the adrenal cortex can cause the overproduction of adrenal steroids, which can stimulate the growth of the prostate gland. For example, in humans, abnormal virilism has been observed in immature males with hyperfunction of the adrenal cortex resulting from neoplasia or hyperplasia of the adrenal gland. In rodents, overstimulation of the adrenals can also induce limited prostate growth even in the absence of testicular androgens. For example, administration of exogenous ACTH to castrated animals does significantly increase the growth of sex accessory tissue (117–119).

The effect of normal levels of adrenal androgens on the prostate in noncastrated humans and adult male rats may not be significant because adrenalectomy has very little effect on prostate size, DNA, or morphology of the sex accessory tissue (120,121). Furthermore, following castration in animals, the prostate diminishes to a very small size (90 percent reduction in cell mass) without concomitant adrenalectomy. Finally, the small involuted ventral prostate in the castrated rat cannot be significantly reduced further by performing additional adrenalectomy or hypophysectomy (122). In rats that are castrated, the DHT level in the prostatic tissue is approximately 20% of that in normal intact animals. Adrenalectomy lowers the DHT to nondetectable levels without further diminution in prostate growth. This indicates that a threshold level of DHT is required in the prostate to stimulate growth and the castrate level is below this threshold. It has also been concluded similarly that the prostate of man does not restore itself following castration, indicating that adrenal androgens are insufficient to compensate for the loss of testicular function. Quantitative morphometry of the human prostate (120) also confirms that the adrenal gland has little effect on the normal prostate.

The adrenal steroids, dehydroepiandrosterone, and the conjugate dehydroepiandrosterone sulfate, as well as androstenedione, are androgens synthesized from acetate and cholesterol (Fig. 6), which are secreted by the normal human adrenal glands. Essentially all of the dehydroepiandrosterone in the male plasma is of adrenal cortex origin, and the production rate in man is 10 to 30 mg/day. Less than 1% of the total testosterone in the plasma is derived from dehydroepiandrosterone (123,124).

The prostate and seminal vesicles of the rat and the human prostate can slowly hydrolyze dehydroepiandrosterone sulfate (DHEAS) to free steroids through a prostate sulfatase enzymatic activity, but the degree of 5α-conversion is low, thereby explaining why DHEAS is not a very potent androgen.

A second adrenal androgen is androstenedione, and the plasma concentration in adult males is approximately 150 ± 54 ng/100 ml (Table 4). The blood production rate of androstenedione in human males is about 2–6 mg/day, with approximately 20% of the androstenedione being generated by peripheral metabolism of other steroids. Androstenedione cannot be converted directly to DHT and therefore is a weak androgen. An important role for androstenedione in the male may be its peripheral conversion to estrogens through the aromatase reaction (see Fig. 6).

The adrenal gland also produces C 21 steroids (e.g., progesterone). The plasma production rate at 0.75 mg/day is low, producing a low plasma progesterone concentration of 30 ng/100 ml. Although progesterone is weakly androgenic, it does not exert a significant effect on the prostate at the low concentrations present in normal male plasma.

In summary, under normal conditions the adrenals do not support significant growth of prostatic tissue.

Estrogens in the Male

Only small amounts of estrogen are produced directly by the testes. Approximately 75% to 90% of the estrogens in the plasma of young healthy human males is derived from the peripheral conversion of androstenedione and testosterone to estrone and estradiol via the aromatase reaction (Fig. 6) (123,124). The androgenic C19 steroids (testosterone and androstenedione) are converted to the estrogenic C18 steroids first by removing the 19-methyl group and subsequently the formation of an aromatic or phenolic steroid A ring (aromatase reaction), present in both estradiol and estrone. Estradiol is formed from testosterone and estrone from androstenedione; these two estrogens are then interconvertible. The daily production of estradiol in the human male is about 40 to 50 μg, and only 5 to 10 μg (10% to 25%) can be accounted for by direct testicular secretion. The dynamics of the synthesis of estrogens in human males have been quantitated by Siiteri and MacDonald (125), who showed that of the 7.0

mg of testosterone produced in man each day, only 0.35% was converted directly to estradiol, forming 24 μg/day. Of the 2.5 mg of androstenedione produced per day, 1.7% was converted to estrone, producing 42 μg/day. The interconversion of estrone and estradiol yielded a final total peripheral production of approximately 40 μg of estradiol/day. The exact location in the periphery where estrogen production occurs has not been elucidated on a quantitative basis, but it is believed that most of the daily production may involve adipose tissue. The small amount of estrogens secreted directly from the testes may originate in part from the Sertoli cells, since in culture these cells respond to FSH stimulation by producing small amounts of estradiol (126); in the adult rat the Leydig cell may be the source of estradiol.

Men over 50 years of age may have an increase in total plasma estradiol levels of approximately 50%, with minimal change (less than 10%) in the free estradiol levels because of increases in binding of the estradiol by elevated serum testosterone-estrogen-binding globulin (TeBG) levels, which are also age-related (127). The result of an age-related decrease in the plasma free testosterone level while the free estradiol level is maintained produces a 40% increase in the ratio of free estradiol/free testosterone (127,128). It is apparent that the availability of estrogens and androgens in the serum is regulated not only by their total level but by the free level (i.e., unbound). Since the steroid binding proteins in the serum can regulate the free levels, it is important to understand how they function.

Androgen Binding Proteins in the Plasma

The great bulk of serum steroids do not circulate free in males but are reversibly bound to a variety of serum proteins. Less than 2% of the total testosterone in human plasma is free or unbound and the remaining 98% is bound to several different types of plasma proteins (Fig. 5). The plasma proteins that bind steroids include human serum albumin, testosterone-estrogen-binding globulin (denoted TeBG or SBG, steroid-binding globulin), corticosteroid-binding globulin (CBG, also termed transcortin), progesterone-binding globulin (PBG), and, to a lesser extent, the alpha-acid glycoprotein (AAG). The total amount of testosterone bound to PBG and AAG is not large and is usually ignored.

The regulation of the amount of androgen that is free is an important physiological variable and varies in different species. The total amount of steroid bound depends on two factors: (1) the *affinity* of the steroid to bind to a specific protein, and (2) the *capacity,* which is the maximal potential binding when all of a binding protein is saturated with bound steroid; the capacity is governed by the amount of binding protein in the plasma. Serum albumin has a relatively low affinity for testosterone, but because albumin is at high concentration in the plasma, it can bind appreciable quantities of testosterone. Therefore, albumin is termed a low affinity, high capacity binding protein. In contrast, steroid-binding globulin (SBG or TeBG), which has been isolated from plasma, has a high affinity for binding steroids, but the protein is present in relatively low concentrations; however, the plasma molarity of each binding protein exceeds the plasma molarity for total testosterone concentration. The majority of testosterone bound to plasma protein is associated with TeBG. For example, Vermeulen (1973) has calculated that in the normal human male, 57% of testosterone in the plasma is bound to TeBG and 40% is bound to human serum albumin. Less than 1% is bound to CBG, and only 2% of the total testosterone is free (see Fig. 5). The normal plasma free testosterone level is therefore 12.1 ± 3.7 ng/100 ml or 0.42 nM; this non-protein-bound "free testosterone" is available to diffuse into the sex accessory tissue and into liver cells for metabolism. In addition, a large percentage of the TeBG is saturated, whereas only a small fraction of the total capacity of CBG and albumin is utilized under normal conditions. As testosterone levels increase in the plasma, the order of increasing saturation of the plasma proteins proceeds from TeBG to CBG to albumin. Therefore the binding of androgen is a dynamic equilibrium between various serum proteins.

The total plasma levels of TeBG can be altered by hormone therapy. Administration of testosterone decreases TeBG levels in the plasma, while estrogen therapy stimulates TeBG levels (128–130). Estrogen also competes with testosterone for binding to TeBG, but estrogen has only one-third the binding affinity of testosterone. Therefore, administration of small amounts of estrogen increases the total concentration of TeBG, and this effectively increases the binding of testosterone and thus lowers the free testosterone plasma concentration.

Therefore, since free testosterone enters sex accessory tissue, the binding of testosterone to plasma proteins would inhibit the uptake into the prostate (131). It is apparent that androgenic activity is regulated in part by the extent of binding of an androgen to the steroid-binding proteins in the plasma. Indeed, Anderson and colleagues (132) have postulated that altered testosterone binding to plasma proteins might produce amplified changes in free estrogen and androgen levels, and this could be an important factor in inducing gynecomastia and impotence.

The plasma concentration is inversely related to the rate of testosterone metabolism (metabolic clearance rate [MCR]); this is obvious because free testosterone is the form metabolized by the liver. In addition, estrogen therapy increases the level of TeBG and lowers the metabolic clearance rate of testosterone. This may be explained by the fact that estrogen treatment increases the amount of TeBG and thus the percentage of plasma testosterone that is protein bound; therefore, there is a reduction in the amount of free testosterone in the plasma that is available either to the liver for metabolism or to the prostate for androgenic stimulation.

TeBG has more recently been found to be a plasma glycoprotein that binds to receptor sites on plasma membranes with the unusual kinetics of having slow on and off rates. Steroid binding and membrane binding functions have an allosteric relationship with binding of TeBG to membrane inhibiting the binding to steroids. Additional work appears to indicate that membrane bound TeBG may activate adenylate cyclase and its concommitant increase in cyclic AMP on steroid binding. A recent review discusses the most recent research on TeBG (133).

Prolactin

Exogenous androgens can restore 80% of the normal adult prostate size in hypophysectomized rats. To obtain full restoration with androgens in these hypophysectomized rats, supplements of exogenous prolactin are required (134). This early observation has been confirmed in numerous animal experiments, in which prolactin was shown to be synergistic with androgens on prostate growth (135). In addition, prolactin increases zinc uptake in the tissue (136), alters androgen uptake and metabolism (137), and regulates citric acid and fructose levels. Prolactin receptors have been identified in prostatic tissue (138). Prolactin has a permissive effect on the growth of the lateral prostate of the rat and this may be associated with increased nuclear androgen levels (135,139).

It is of interest that some cellular growth factors have homology with prolactin. Indeed, Lee and colleagues (140) have suggested that prolactin may enhance rat lateral prostate growth by an androgen-independent pathway since hyperprolactin levels caused a decrease in the DHT levels in the lateral prostate while increasing growth. It is well known that the prostate contains an abundance of prolactin receptors (141). The direct action of prolactin on prostate epithelial cells has also been suggested through tissue and organ culture experiments (142).

The aforementioned evidence that prolactin affects prostatic growth in animals has led to much speculation about a similar role in humans. Prolactin levels in human blood are elevated with estrogens, some tranquilizing drugs, and stress, and can be decreased by L-dopa and ergot derivatives. With improved assays, the levels are being monitored in patients of advanced age and in those with benign prostatic hyperplasia, but no clear correlation of cause of prostate pathology and prolactin effect is yet apparent (143).

Insulin

Other circulating endocrine factors have been reported to affect sex accessory tissue growth. For example, insulin has been reported to have synergistic or permissive effects on prostatic growth, but these data have been obtained previously in rodents and often in tissue or organ culture (142,144). Sufrin and Prutkin (145) have demonstrated that diabetic castrated rats have a diminished response to exogenous androgens that can be restored with supplements of insulin, and these findings support the earlier conclusions of Calame and Lostroh (146) and Lostroh (147), who found that insulin was required for androgen response of the mouse prostate in organ culture. There is little information on the possible role of insulin in the growth of the human prostate. Recent focus on insulinlike growth factors in many tissues and cell types leaves open the importance of these factors on the growth of sex accessory tissue.

CELLULAR AND MOLECULAR REGULATION OF PROSTATIC GROWTH BY HORMONES AND GROWTH FACTORS

Overview

It now appears that there are many levels of cell regulation that include hormone action and direct cell-cell communication and growth factors and these are also at the research forefront of biological regulation of sex accessory tissue. These types of growth control are usually accomplished by several generalized systems, and they include the following:

1. *Endocrine factors* or long-range signals arriving at the prostate by serum transport of hormone originating from the secretions of distant organs; this would include serum hormonelike steroids such as testosterone, estrogens and serum polypeptide hormones like prolactin, and insulin as discussed above
2. *Neuroendocrine* signals originating from neural stimulation such as 5-hydroxytryptamine, acetylcholine, and norepinephrine
3. *Paracrine factors* or soluble tissue growth factors that stimulate or inhibit (chalones) growth that are elaborated over short ranges between neighboring cells within the prostate tissue compartment such as β-fibroblast growth factor, epidermal growth factor, etc.
4. *Autocrine factors* are soluble growth factors that are released by a cell and then feed back on the same cell to regulate growth or function such as autocrine motility factor
5. *Intracrine factors,* autocrine factors that are not released but work inside the cell
6. *Extracellular matrix factors* that are insoluble tissue

matrix systems and make direct and coupled contact by being attached through integrins and adhesions molecules to the basal membrane and the extracellular matrix components that include the glycosaminoglycans such as heparan sulfate, etc. (94)

7. *Cell-cell interactions* of the epithelial or stromal cells occurring through tight membrane junctions on intramembrane proteins such as the cell adhesion molecules, like uvomorulin that couple neighboring cells.

Of these seven growth control systems, the first studied on the prostate was the endocrine effects of androgenic steroid in the regulation of prostatic growth via changes in serum testosterone levels and steroid receptor interactions. However, recently rapid progress has been made in the understanding of the other systems, particularly the growth factors. At present, structural elements in cellular control involving the tissue matrix are being developed. We first review these mechanisms, starting with androgen action at the prostate cell level beginning with the arrival of testosterone.

Androgen Action at the Cellular Level

Testosterone in the serum arrives at the prostate bound to albumin and to the steroid binding globulins as depicted in Fig. 7. Only the free testosterone enters the prostate cell by diffusion where it is then subjected to a variety of steroid metabolic steps that appear to regulate the activity, and, finally, inactivation of the steroid hormone. The temporal sequence of intracellular events are depicted in Fig. 7 and include

1. Cellular uptake of testosterone.
2. Testosterone converted to DHT by metabolism of 5α-reductase.
3. DHT or testosterone binding to specific androgen receptors in the nucleus
4. Activation of the steroid receptor in the nucleus by conformational change and phosphorylation and the binding of the receptor to DNA androgen response elements (AREs) that are short specific sequences of DNA, and by binding of the receptor to tissue-specific proteins of the nuclear matrix.
5. Receptor-induced changes in DNA loop topology and chromatin structure.
6. The receptor acts as a transcription factor and when bound to the DNA and matrix in proximity to androgen target genes regulates the RNA polymerase transcription of the DNA into messenger RNA (mRNA).
7. The transcribed message (mRNA) is very large and contains introns, exons, and a poly A tail. Only the exon portion will be retained in the final message. The trimming and processing of the mRNA is accomplished on the nuclear matrix as it is transported through the nucleus and out through the nuclear pore complex, it is possible that androgen receptors may play a role in stabilization of the messenger RNA, but no definitive evidence has been shown yet.
8. The stabilized mRNA is transported into the cytoplasmic compartment to be translated at the ribosome into protein.
9. The transportation of the proteins to specific cellular sites and its subsequent posttranslational modification.
10. The storage of the protein in secretory granules poised for secretion into the lumen on neurological command during the process of ejaculation.

The epithelial cell is the primary unit in secretion but specific genes are also activated in the stromal cells, and these events are also regulated by testosterone, estrogens, and growth factors in a similar chain of events, as just discussed. Not all cells respond the same to androgens or estrogens. For simplicity, these steps will be discussed in relation to the epithelial cells because differences between the cell types are important but have not yet been resolved. Androgens and estrogens, both together, and separately, can affect prostate cells through the interaction with receptors and it appears that estrogens might have their primary effect on the stromal cells. We will now discuss these aforementioned events in androgen action within the prostate in more detail and at the molecular level.

5α-Reductase and Androgen Metabolism Within the Prostate

After the free testosterone in the plasma has entered the prostatic cells through diffusion, it is rapidly metabolized to other steroids by a series of prostatic enzymes (148–152). Over 90% of the testosterone is *irreversibly* converted to the main prostatic androgen, dihydrotestosterone (DHT) (see Fig. 8) through the action of NADPH and the enzyme 5α-reductase (EC 1.3.99.5) located on the endoplasmic reticulum and on the nuclear membrane. The enzyme 5α-reductase reduces the unsaturated bond in testosterone between the 4 and 5 positions to form the 5α-reduced product DHT. The K_m for testosterone is 8.3 nM and the serum level of testosterone is only in the range of 0.5–3.0 nM, indicating that the enzyme cannot be saturated, since the testosterone substrate would be less than the K_m value (152). 5α-Reductase can also convert androstenedione or progesterone to the 5α-reduced form.

Bruchovsky and Dunstan-Adams (152) have reported a 10-fold increase in the maximal velocity, V_{max}, which indicates an activity showing 262 pmol of DHT formed/

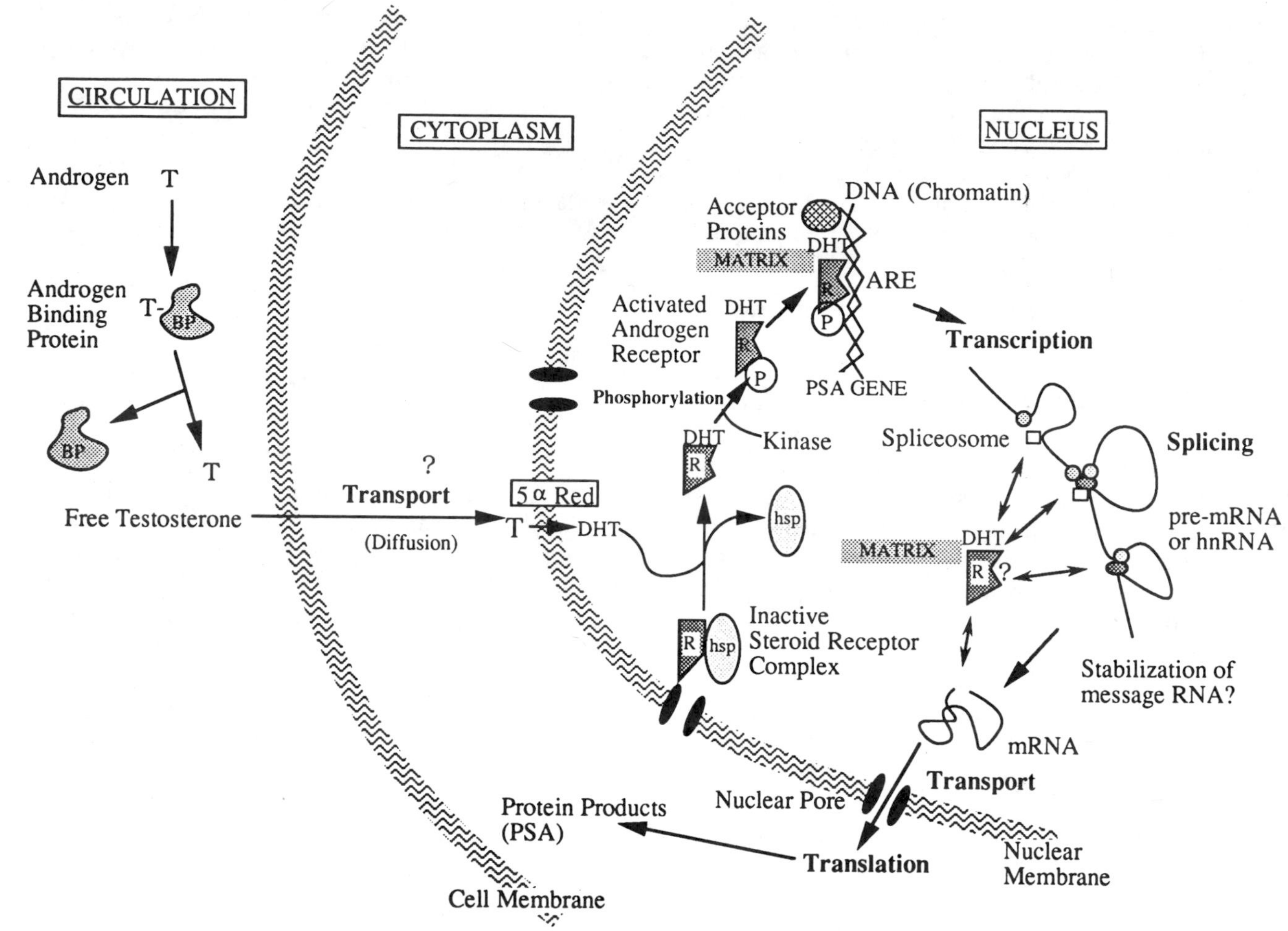

FIG. 7. Mechanism of androgen action in a prostate cell. Target tissue action of androgens in prostate begins with the transport of testosterone to the site of action via the circulation. Current thought suggests that the steroid is transported across the cell membrane at the target cell via passive diffusion. The testosterone is metabolized to dihydrotestosterone which specifically activates androgen receptor. The androgen receptor dissociates from heat shock protein, is phosphorylated and allowed to interact with its DNA hormone response element. The androgen receptor may also interact with various nuclear acceptor proteins which may modulate its transcription activating function. The targeted gene is transcribed and the messenger RNA is processed by splicing. It is still debated as to whether androgen receptor has any effect on splicing, message transport, or mRNA stability. The mRNA is then translated in the cytoplasm by ribosomal complexes to yield protein products, in this case the prostate-specific antigen (PSA) protein. T, testosterone; BP, steroid hormone binding protein; DHT, dihydrotestosterone; R, androgen receptor; hsp, heat shock protein; ARE, androgen response element.

30 min/mg protein from testosterone when measured in the stroma and less than 10% of that amount with a V_{max} of 19 for the epithelium. The stromal K_m was 76 nM and the epithelial 13. It is unknown why these values are different between normal, benign prostatic hyperplasia, and cancer, but it is intriguing that there may be alterations occurring in the enzyme or in its regulatory mechanism.

The human and rat 5α-reductase genes have been cloned and expressed (153). The enzyme is a hydrophobic protein of 259 amino acids with a molecular weight of 29,462. The rat and human 5α-reductase have a 60% homology. The 5α-reductase inhibitor 4-azasteroids demonstrated marked differences in their ability to inhibit the human and rat steroid 5α-reductase with it being far more inhibitory on the rat enzyme. The 4-azasteroids of importance are MK-906, finasteride, or Proscar [17β-(*N*-*t*-butyl)carbamyl-4-aza-5α-androst-1-en-3-one] and a related compound called 4MA. These inhibitors work as competitive inhibitors for 5α-reductase. The enzyme is primarily present in the prostate, other sex accessory tissues, liver, and adrenal glands.

5α-Reductase is of great importance because the product DHT is important in the differentiation of the prostate during fetal development, and mutations in 5α-

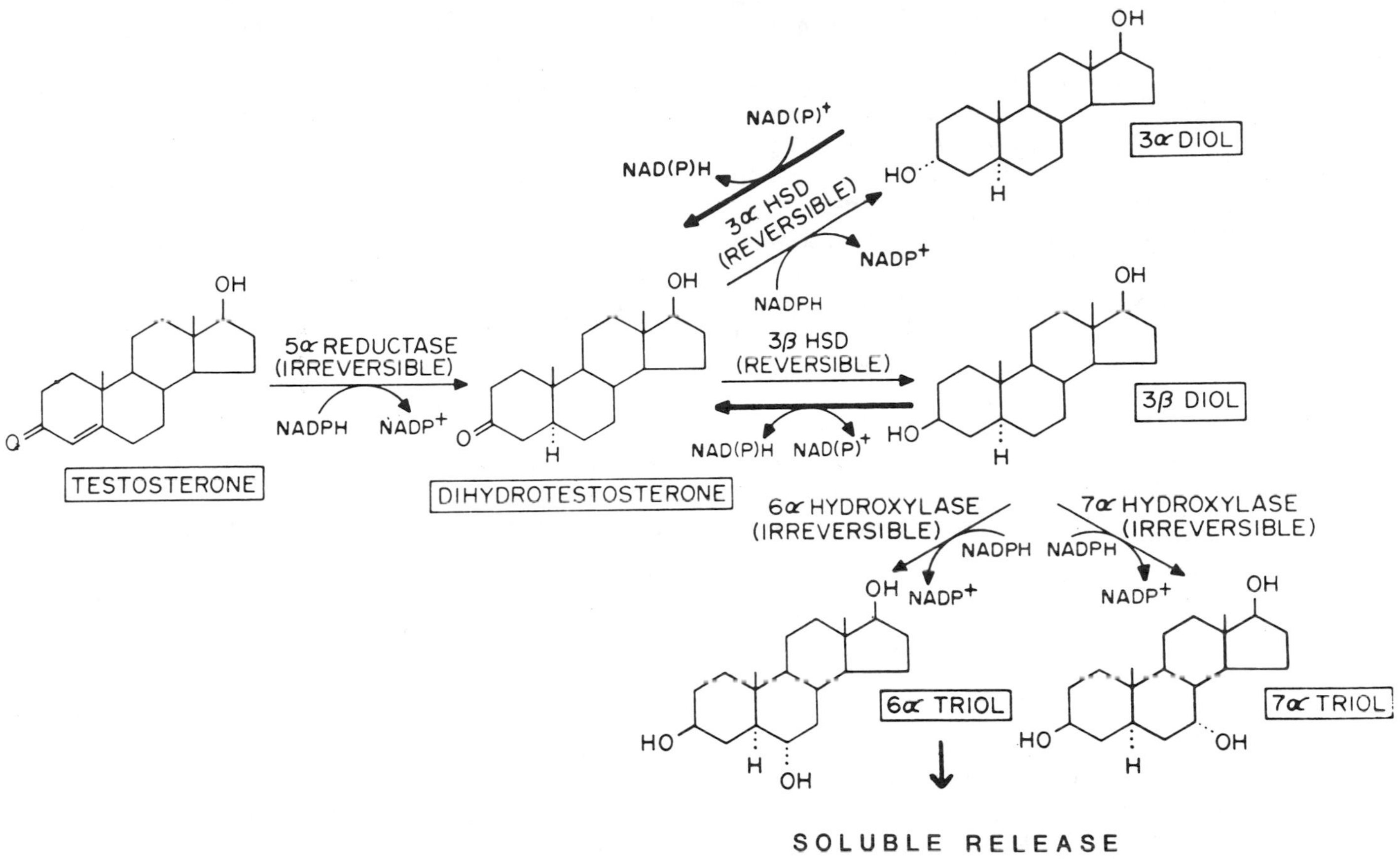

FIG. 8. The metabolic pathways of testosterone within the prostate. Testosterone is irreversibly converted to DHT, which is then reversibly converted to 3α-diol or 3β-diol. The diols are hydroxylated in either the 6α or 7α position in an irreversible manner, thus forming a triol. The triols are highly soluble and are released from the prostate in an inactive form.

reductase give rise to a rare form of pseudohermaphroditism. In prostate physiology expression of the 5α-reductase gene is regulated by androgens in both the prostate and liver. It is also believed that the 5α-reductase is involved in male pattern baldness, acne, and hirsutism, as well as often postulated to be involved in benign prostatic hyperplasia. A 5α-reductase inhibitor, MK-906 (finasteride, Proscar), a 4-azasteroid is now being used in the pharmacological management of benign prostatic hyperplasia. The use of 5α-reductase inhibitors in the therapy of BPH has recently been reviewed (154,155).

After the DHT is formed from testosterone in the prostate, it is then subjected to a series of reversible metabolic reactions to form 3α-diol (5α-androstane 3α,17β-diol) and 3β-diol (5α-androstane 3β,17β-diol) (see Fig. 8). The enzymes that perform this transformation of DHT are 3α- or 3β-hydroxysteroid oxidoreductases (3α-HSOR or 3β-HSOR). These enzymes utilize NADP as a cofactor but in contrast, to 5α-reductase, they can also utilize NAD. The equilibrium for the metabolism of DHT favors the formation of DHT, that is the oxidation of the 3-hydroxy group of 3α- and 3β-diol to the 3-ketone that is present in DHT. It is known that administering 3α-diol to an animal is a strong androgen through its rapid conversion to the effective DHT. On the other hand, 3β-diol is not very effective as an androgen because it is rapidly and irreversibly converted to the triol form by hydroxylation in the 6α- or 7α-position (see Fig. 8). The triols are dead end products of testosterone metabolism and are very water-soluble and inactive as androgens and cannot reform DHT. Steroids also can form glucuronide or sulfate conjugates and be secreted in a more soluble form.

In summary, testosterone is irreversibly metabolized to DHT that is in equilibrium with other reduced steroids primarily through oxidation and reduction at the 3-position. The steroids are inactivated by being irreversibly hydroxylated to the inactive triols.

Estrogens and Estrogen/Androgen Synergism

Estrogens do not block androgen-induced growth of the prostate cell but, on the contrary, may even synergize androgen effects. This has been well documented in the canine prostate first by Walsh and Wilson (156) and subsequently DeKlerk coworkers (157), Tunn coworkers (158), and Juniewicz et al. (159). In the aforementioned studies the simultaneous administration of estradiol to castrate dogs receiving 5α-androstane metabolites such as DHT or 3α-diol produced a 2- to 4-fold enhancement in the size of the prostate that was due to an increase in total cell number and was a true glandular hyperplasia. The mechanism of the androgen-estrogen synergism on prostate growth is not understood, however, it has been shown that estrogens increase the androgen nuclear receptor content in the prostate cell which might be an important factor in this phenomenon (160). Estrogen combined with DHT also induces other changes such as increase in steroid metabolism towards DHT formation, collagen formation and alteration in cell death modification. These changes have been summarized by Coffey and Walsh in relation to benign prostatic hyperplasia (161).

The synergism of estrogens on androgen-induced growth in the dog prostate is observed only with the 5α-reduced androgens such as dihydrotestosterone or 3α-diol and is not observed when testosterone is administered (156,157,162). In addition, this synergism with androgens and estrogens in the dog does not occur in the rat prostate (163). Whether this species difference is due to the fact that the rat does not develop benign prostatic hyperplasia, and the dog does, is a matter of conjecture.

Estrogens are capable, either directly or indirectly, of stimulating the stromal elements of the prostate. These studies have been carried out in animal models such as the monkey (164) and the guinea pig (165–168). Young males receiving androgen blockade with antiandrogens combined with estrogen therapy did not have enlarged prostates, but their stromal elements were markedly enhanced while the epithelial component involuted (169). In human BPH nuclei, total assayed estrogens in stromal nuclei (58 fmoles/mg of DNA) are five times higher than those found in epithelial nuclei (9 fmoles/mg of DNA) (170). It is unknown what this large amount of estrogen is bound to in the nucleus.

The distribution of estrogen receptors and binding in the prostate is heterogeneous but it is clear that stroma is a major target for these estrogens (171–175). It is still uncertain whether the very modest amounts of estrogen receptor in the prostate (173,176) can account for any of the pathological growths that occur in the prostate. Of great interest will be the localization of estrogen receptors in specific cellular compartments of the prostate, particularly with regard to their role in stem cell growth, cell death and the secretion of extracellular matrix components such as collagen. It is also still not clear whether the prostate can make any significant amount of estrogens and whether antiestrogens would be an effective treatment for abnormal prostate growth (164,165,177, 178). It is apparent that estrogens do imprint the prostate growth and their role in development may be of paramount importance (51,52). Estrogens can cause a florid squamous cell metaplasia in prostatic growth that can be offset by androgens (157,159). How this is regulated by stem cells is of paramount importance for the role of estrogen in abnormal growth (73,157). Estrogens may have other actions including affecting prostatic secretion and water and electrolyte transport (151), as well as the potential for affecting urethral musculature and its neurological control (179).

Steroid Receptors

In almost all cells in the body, steroids can enter the nucleus, but only a few cells can retain this steroid within their nucleus for any length of time. The cells that retain the steroid have receptors that are specific and can activate specific androgen-sensitive genes within the nucleus to increase the expression of certain protein products that are under steroid control. Earlier, many investigators focused their attention on the cytoplasmic receptor instead of the nuclear compartment where the androgen action is believed to occur. In fact, the cytoplasmic receptor appears to be an extraction artifact and most receptors may actually reside within the nucleus. For years it was believed that steroids get into the cell and bind specific cytoplasmic receptors and then by a temperature sensitive step, these cytoplasmic receptors are activated and then translocated into the nucleus where they bind to a mysterious nuclear acceptor. The androgen receptor's affinity for the nuclear acceptor site to which it binds in the nucleus, which is probably a compilation of binding to specific sequences on DNA and to the nuclear matrix, is strongly regulated by the presence of the androgen ligand bound to the receptor. When androgens are not present the receptor decreases its affinity for nuclear binding and can be easily removed, and indeed, under castrate conditions, some receptors may leak out into the cytoplasm (180). Immunohistochemical technique indicate that the nucleus is the primary place in which the receptor resides.

The prostate and seminal vesicles contain steroid specific and high affinity (10^{-9} to 10^{-10} M K_d) saturable (100–1,000 fmol of receptor/mg DNA equivalents of tissue) androgen receptors. There are 5,000 to 20,000 molecules of these receptors per cell. It is believed that the androgen receptors in the nucleus bind to specific nuclear acceptors that include chromatin, DNA, and the nuclear matrix. The properties and hormonal regulation of androgen receptors, as well as their uses, have been reviewed in detail (181).

The cloning of the human androgen receptor and its expression was a hallmark in the study of the mechanism of hormone action (182–184). This has led to the study of the sequence of the gene and its protein product and how this is altered in inherited androgen insensitivity syndromes as well as receptor function (183–188). This powerful new technique is providing the resolution to many questions of andrology (189–191).

Molecular Biology of Androgen Receptor Action

Overview of Steroid Receptors

Steroids play an important role in the control of gene expression directly at the nuclear level by binding to steroid receptors. Once activated, these steroid receptors act as controllers of gene transcription by binding to DNA at specific sequences termed hormone response elements or HREs. Additionally, in the DNA-depleted nuclear matrix, evidence suggests that steroid receptors are bound in a hormone and target tissue specific manner to a non-DNA acceptor (192–194). However, the mechanism and exact nature of such interactions remain unresolved.

The androgen receptor binds the male sex steroids, testosterone and dihydrotestosterone, and regulates many of the genes necessary for male sex differentiation and development. It is a member of the large superfamily of ligand-activated transcription factors termed the nuclear hormone receptors (Fig. 9). The members of the superfamily include the steroid hormone receptors (estrogen, progesterone, androgen, glucocorticoid, mineralocorticoid, vitamin D, ecdysteroid), thyroid hormone receptors, and retinoid receptors. Over 30 members of the receptor family have been identified, including a number of "orphan" receptors, whose ligands have not yet been found.

Nuclear Hormone Receptor Domains

Many of the nuclear hormone receptors have been sequenced and the structural domains of these receptors have been correlated with their functions (195). These nuclear receptors have each been shown to have at least three major structural domains that are involved in binding to DNA, hormone, and nuclear proteins (Fig. 9).

DNA-Binding Domain

All of the nuclear hormone receptors have a 66 to 68 amino acid *DNA-binding domain* (C domain) which contains two looped nonhomologous zinc fingers. The zinc atom in each finger is coordinated tetrahedrally to cysteine residues. The region between the two zinc fingers contain amino acids that can discriminate between the DNA sequences of the respective DNA response elements to which these nuclear hormone receptors may bind. In fact, it has been proposed that a region of three discriminatory amino acids in the DNA binding domain could serve as the locus for the subclassification of the nuclear hormone receptors (196). The structural interaction of the DNA binding domain fragment from glucocorticoid receptor with bound DNA has been solved using two-dimensional nuclear magnetic resonance (2D-NMR) and confirms direct interactions of the amino acids with the DNA response element (197).

The DNA binding domain is thought to be transcriptionally active in the absence of the hormone binding region, though to a lesser extent than with the intact receptor with bound ligand. A good example of this is the v-erbA oncogene, which is essentially a differentially spliced thyroid hormone receptor with a modified C-terminal domain. This oncogene product is transcriptionally active in the absence of an active thyroid ligand binding domain.

Hormone- or Ligand-Binding Region

The *hormone or ligand binding region* (domain E) of the nuclear receptors is approximately 210 amino acids in length at the carboxyl-terminal of the receptor and determines ligand specificity. Ligand binding induces a conformational change which transforms the nuclear receptor enabling transcriptional activation. The steroid binding region of the androgen receptor is well conserved across different species.

Hinge Domain

Between the DNA-binding domain and the hormone binding domain is a region known as the *hinge domain* (domain D). This region contains a putative nuclear localization peptide sequence (198,199).

Amino-Terminal Regulatory Domain

The *amino-terminal regulatory domain* (A/B domains) of the nuclear hormone receptors is the most variable region. The function of the amino terminal region has not yet been well defined. In steroid receptors, this region appears to be responsible for a ligand-independent transactivation function. The multiple stretches of polyamino acids contained within this amino-terminal domain of androgen receptors include polyproline, polyglycine, polyglutamine, and polyalanine, and their functions are yet to be determined. Additionally, some of the nuclear hormone receptors have a carboxyl-terminal regulatory domain whose function is not yet entirely defined.

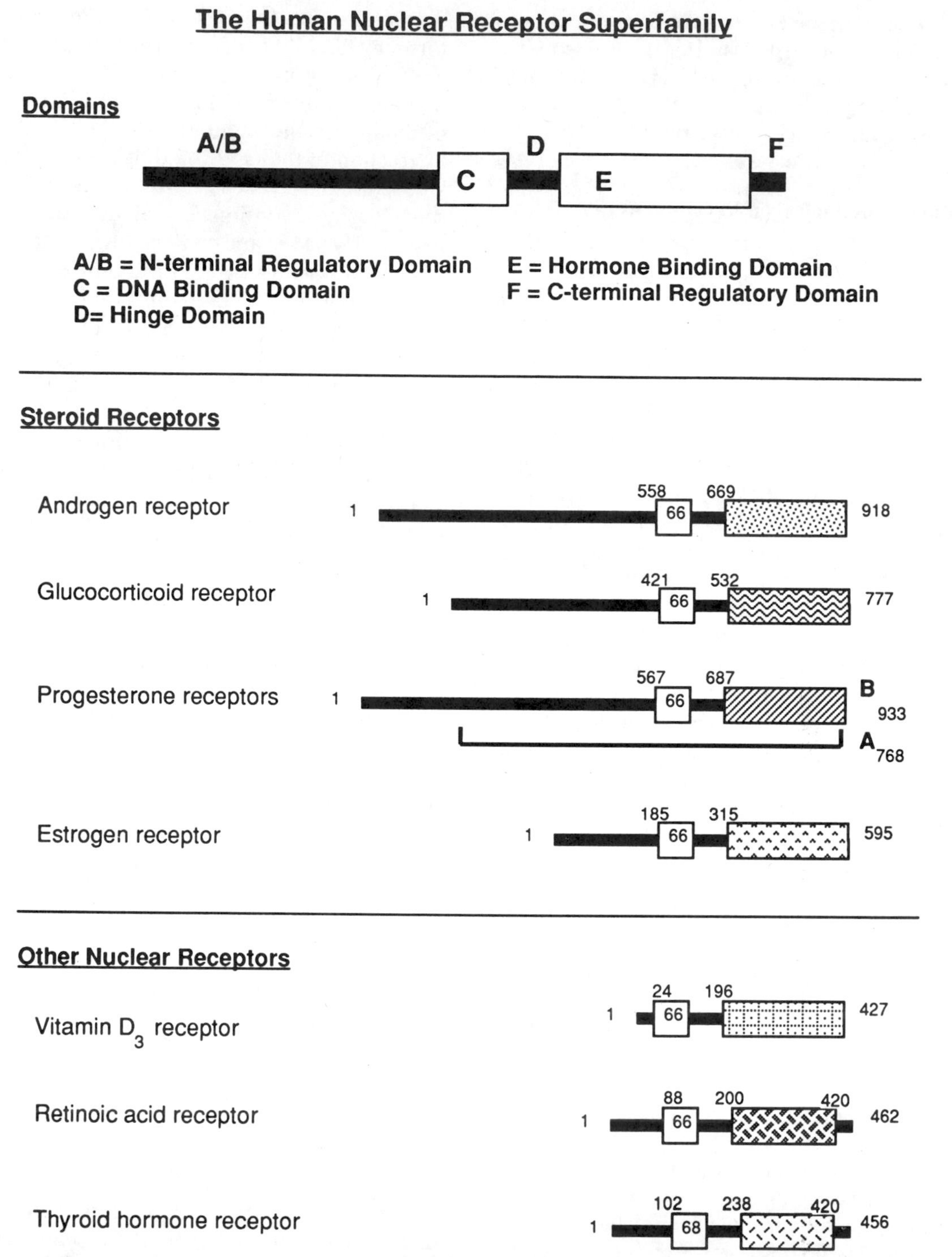

FIG. 9. The human nuclear receptor superfamily. The steroid receptors are members of the nuclear hormone receptor superfamily. The receptor peptide sequence can be divided into functional domains. The steroid receptors have four major functional domains while some of the other nuclear receptors also have an additional carboxyl-terminal regulatory domain. The comparative peptide lengths of the receptors are shown with the lengths of the various homologous domains. Progesterone receptor A is a shorter splice variant of the type B receptor.

Structure of Human Androgen Receptor

The human androgen receptor has been cloned and sequenced (182,184). The receptor has been localized to the X-chromosome between the centromere and q13 in humans. It is currently believed that there is only a single androgen receptor protein coded for by the human genome. The exon-intron structure and the promoter region of androgen receptor have been determined. Figure 10 shows the exon structure of the gene for the human androgen receptor, and the unique restriction map of the receptor cDNA. The human androgen receptor has its coding information separated over eight exons (183). The N-terminal domain is encoded by the large first exon, the two zinc fingers of the DNA-binding domain are separately encoded by exons 2 and 3. Finally, exons 4 through 8 encode the ligand-binding domain. Exons are that part of the DNA coding sections of the gene that have the final information that will be transcribed into message RNA and then subsequently translated into protein amino acid sequences. They are called exons because this information will exit the nucleus. The exon sections are separated in the gene by intervening introns which will also be translated into mRNA but will be subsequently deleted out of the final message by splicing that occurs in the nucleus. The exon and intron DNA makes a large gene for the androgen receptor that spans a minimum of 54 kilobases (kb) (185). Only the information contained in the 8 exons will be translated into the receptor. This is very similar to the organization of many other steroid receptors that also contain information from 8 exons, such as the progesterone and estrogen receptor. The large androgen receptor gene (54 kb) of DNA is translated into a message of RNA (mRNA) that is only 17% as large as the gene, being only 9.6 kb and this contains an added tail of poly(A) RNA that will aid in translation (200). This messenger RNA is then translated into a hormone receptor protein of approximately 110,000 MW that contains 917 amino acids. In summary, the gene for making the androgen receptor is very large at 54 kb, but only 17% of these nucleotide bases will actually form message. The other 83% of the gene is used for regulatory control and represents sites that are binding to protein to control its translation into RNA. Only a small fraction of the messenger RNA will actually be translated into protein and this portion represents the 2,751 base pair located in the 8 exons. Therefore, the final protein is only 5% of the genetic information in the gene and the only 95% is involved in processing and regulation (Fig. 11).

The structure and functional domain organization of the androgen receptor protein resembles that of the other steroid receptors (Fig. 9). Phylogenetically, it is most closely related to the progesterone, glucocorticoid, and mineralocorticoid receptors upon examination and comparison of its peptide sequence (201,202). Figure 12 shows a schematic representation of the androgen receptor protein with its structural domains.

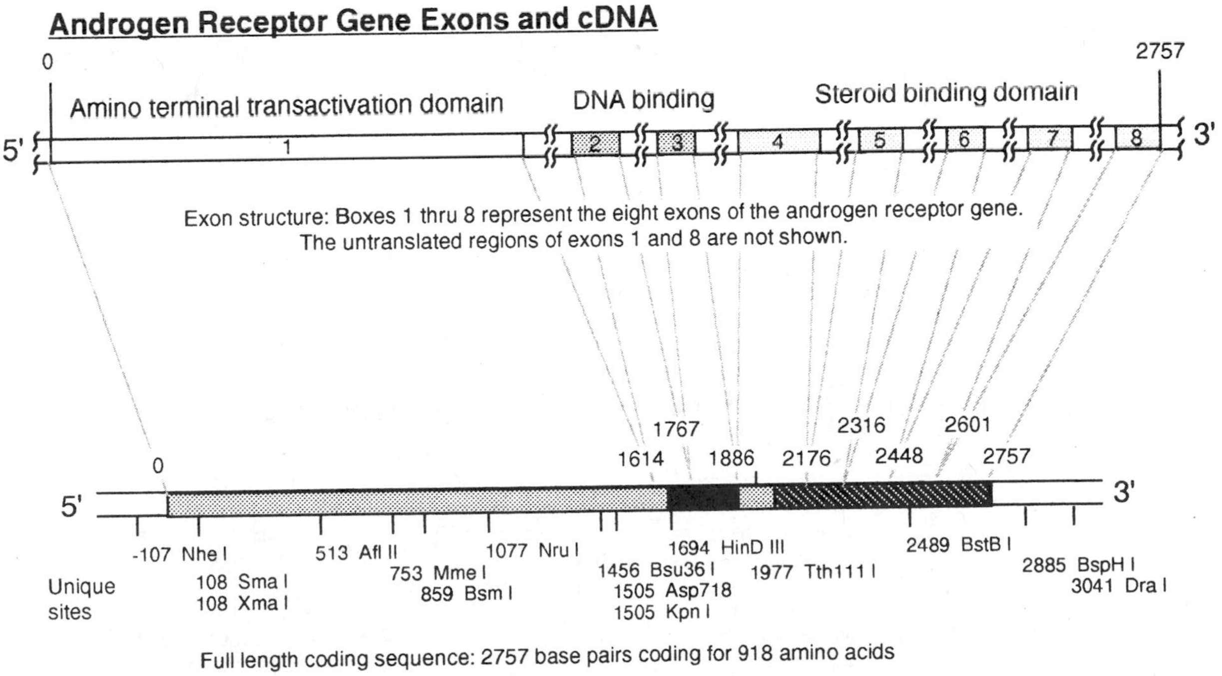

FIG. 10. Androgen receptor functional domains. The androgen receptor, like other steroid receptors, have four major functional domains. The N-terminal regulatory domain, the DNA-binding domain, the hinge domain, and the steroid-binding domain.

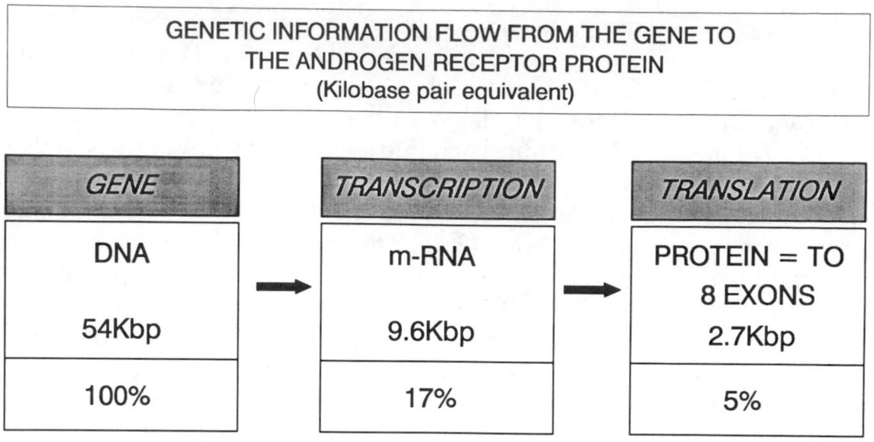

FIG. 11. About 95% of genetic information is not translated into protein. Information located in the gene for the androgen receptor is reduced during formation of the final receptor message. The gene contains 54,000 base pairs of nucleotides. This vast amount of information is used for regulation, with only 5% reaching the final message of eight exons that will be translated into the receptor protein.

The DNA binding domain of the androgen receptor contains 72 amino acids that are rich in cysteine and have the sequence that indicates that they form several small loops of protein of 12–13 amino acid sequences that are anchored at their base by complexing with zinc molecules. These small finger loops are referred to as "zinc fingers" and are commonly found in all types of steroid receptors and many other types of transcription activating factors. These fingers on the receptor that bind directly to the DNA must recognize specific sequences in what is called a hormone responsive element (HRE); this will instruct the gene to be androgen activated. This DNA binding domain of fingers in the steroid receptor molecule is highly conserved. Therefore, there is a high evolutionary conservation of amino acid sequence homology in this DNA binding domain between all classes of steroid receptors. In this region there is a 79% homology to the progesterone receptor, 76% with the glucocorticoid receptor and 56% with the estrogen receptor (188). Androgen receptor is most homologous with the proges-

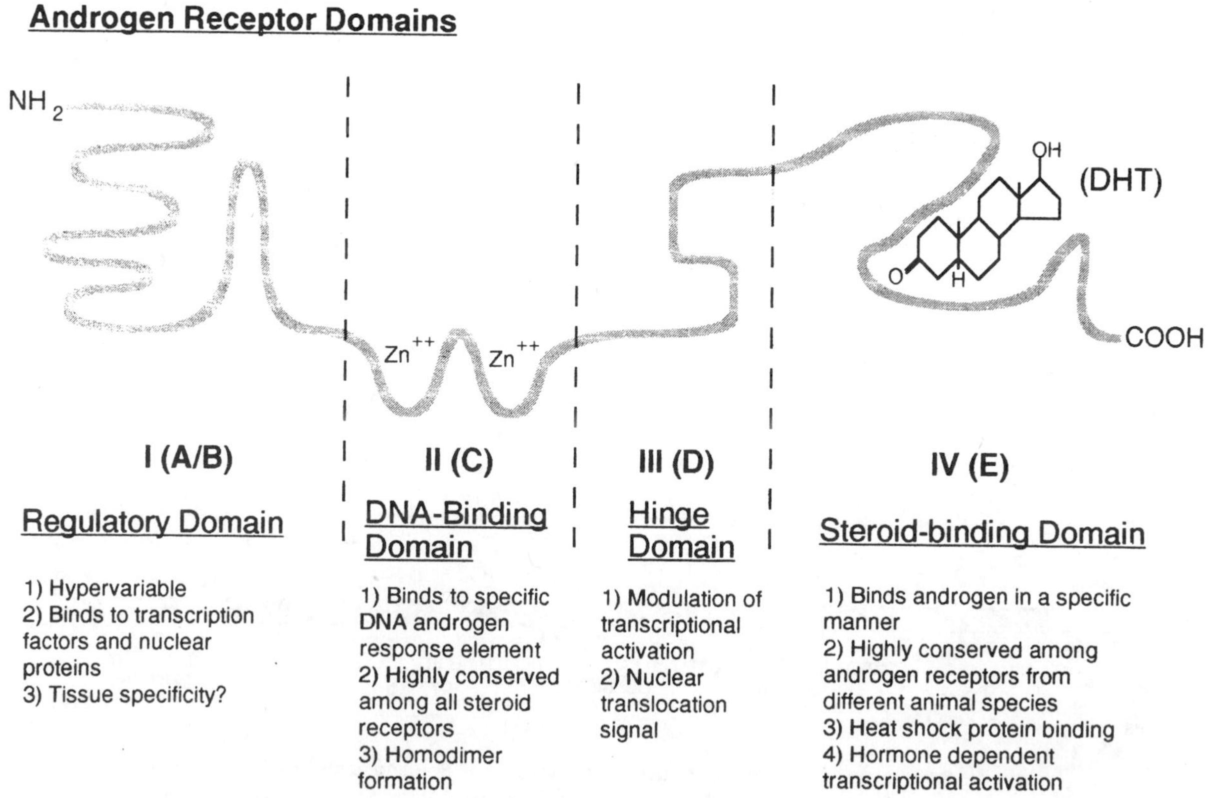

FIG. 12. Androgen receptor gene exons and cDNA. The exon structure for the human androgen receptor is shown. Boxes 1 thru 8 represent the eight exons of the androgen receptor gene. The untranslated regions of exons 1 and 8 are not shown. The base pairs where the splice junctions occur are indicated. The cDNA is shown with selected unique restriction enzyme sites.

terone receptor. Mutations of amino acids in this area of the androgen receptor can make the receptor unable to activate androgen-sensitive genes (203).

The receptor must have steroid specificity and the androgen binding domain is on the carboxylic acid or C-terminal end of the receptor. It is believed that binding of either dihydrotestosterone or testosterone to this region changes the conformation of the protein and this permits the receptor to act as a transcription factor by increased binding to target genes, a general process called "transactivation." If certain activations or deletions occur in this C-terminal portion of the molecule, it is able to constitutively activate target genes and transactivate even in the absence of steroids (185). Marcelli and his colleagues (185) observed that mutations in the androgen receptor at amino acids 587 or 794 are inactive in the assay for androgen binding and for transcriptional activation, however, the removal of amino acids from 708 to the carboxyl end at 917 leads to the synthesis of a receptor protein that does not bind the androgen receptor, but is still constitutively active in functional assays as a transactivating factor without needing androgens. This may have profound implications on how prostate cancer may become androgen-insensitive and continue to grow in the absence of androgens by producing a steroid receptor that functions without a steroid.

Androgen Response Elements and Gene Expression

A typical gene in the open regions of DNA appear to be composed of two major areas: the *structural* region which is going to be transcribed and become part of the message RNA, and adjacent to this and upstream towards the 5′ end is a large *regulatory* region of DNA that contains the control sites for the activation of this gene. The structural area is called the coding region of the gene and, starting at its 5′ end, where it will initiate transcription, the nucleotide bases are numbered as +1 and increase as they move to the right (downstream) into the gene and toward the 3′ end. Moving away from the gene and to the left of the initiation site and upstream in the 5′ direction, the nucleotide bases are numbered from right to left starting with −1 and increasing in negative value as one moves to the left of the gene. The regulatory region is divided into a *promoter element* that is present in all genes. This promoter element specifies the site to which RNA polymerase II will attach to the DNA and will determine the accuracy point for the initiation of transcription. The RNA polymerase will copy or transcribe the DNA code into mRNA, a process termed transcription. This promoter area was originally referred to as the Goldberg-Hogness box and has a consensus sequence of TATAAAAG. The RNA polymerase II enzyme binds to this TATA box as one of the initial steps in transcription. Further upstream from the TATA box lie some of the DNA regulatory promoter elements to which a variety of DNA binding proteins such as transcription factors and steroid receptors can bind and either enhance or inhibit transcription, perhaps by affecting RNA polymerase II transcription complex formation.

Once the DNA is transcribed into messenger RNA, a series of adenine units are added to the end (called the poly(A) tail) and then the messenger RNA is cut and spliced on small nuclear particles (called splicesomes) located on the nuclear matrix, and this splicing removes the intron portion of the message. The final messenger RNA is shipped out of the nucleus, believed to occur on the structural components of the nuclear matrix, and passes through the pore complexes of the nucleus and out to the ribosomes where the mRNA is then translated into protein product, a step termed "translation." The proteins have specific amino acid sequences that instruct the cell where to ship the protein in relation to secretory granules or to the membrane area. The protein can also be modified after translation by the subsequent addition of carbohydrates, such as sugars, to become glycoproteins or be phosphorylated by enzymes called kinases; this is termed "posttranslational modification." Under appropriate signals, such as neurological control, secretory proteins can then be excreted into the lumen of the prostate. This is a process that occurs when secretory proteins of the prostate and seminal vesicles are formed into the ejaculate.

Hormone response elements (HREs) are the nucleotide sequences recognized by the steroid hormone receptors and are responsible in part for their gene regulatory activity. These sequences are usually palindromic in nature with two unequal half-sites separated by a spacer of a few nucleotides. The nuclear receptor superfamily can be divided in to subgroups according to the structure of their DNA binding domains. Likewise, the hormone response elements can be similarly divided, e.g. the glucocorticoid/progesterone response element (GRE/PRE) subgroup, which has a half-site consensus sequence of TGTTCT, and the estrogen response element (ERE) subgroup, whose prototype half-site sequence is TGACC. The HREs to which androgen receptors have been shown to bind belong to the GRE/PRE subgroup. A consensus sequence for the androgen response element (ARE) has been determined using a DNA-binding site selection assay with an androgen receptor fusion protein to be GG(A/T)ACAnnnTGTTCT (204). Among the identified AREs there exists some degree of sequence variation (Table 3). The only identified human ARE to date is that for the prostate specific antigen.

Glucocorticoid receptor and progesterone receptor binding sequences, such as those found in the mouse mammary tumor virus (MMTV) promoter region, can bind androgen receptors and have been used to confer androgen responsiveness to reporter genes (205). Moreover, additional androgen response elements have been identified within the last few years for various genes that are responsive to androgen action (Table 3). The androgen regulated rat secretory protein C3 or prostatein has an ARE within its first intronic element which has been shown to function as an androgen responsive promoter (206). This particular androgen response element demonstrates that some of the hormone response elements may not be located in the classical promoter region upstream of a gene's first exon, but rather elsewhere in the gene. Additional androgen regulated rodent proteins have been found, and include the rat amino-transferase and probasin protein, as well as, the mouse sex-limited protein and ornithine decarboxylase (207–210). In humans the prostate specific antigen (PSA) is a major protein in the male ejaculate that is androgen regulated. An androgen regulatory element has been found upstream of the genes first exon in the promoter region (211).

Androgen Receptor Nuclear Translocation

Androgen receptors, like other steroid receptors, exert their function primarily in the cell nucleus. How do these receptors transit to their sites of action within the nucleus? According to their 1974 book, King and Mainwaring (212) asserted that nuclear translocation of the activated steroid receptor was the sine qua non of any discussion of steroid hormone action. Currently, the importance of nuclear translocation as a limiting step in steroid action has become less defined. Controversy now exists over the initial location of the inactive steroid receptor and the site of steroid ligand binding. Previous work had localized steroid receptors to the cytosolic portion of cells when they were fractionated. However, the methods of extraction may have resulted in the artifactual presence of steroid receptor. Much of the current localization work has been done in cultured cells, which has resulted in different findings depending on cell and steroid receptor type.

Estrogen and progesterone receptors have been localized by indirect immunofluorescence to the nucleus of cells even in the absence of ligand (213–216). Unliganded glucocorticoid receptors are usually found in the cytoplasm (217–219). However, in the stably transfected WCL2 Chinese hamster ovary cell line the glucocorticoid receptor is located in the nucleus even in the absence of hormone (220). Without their steroid ligand, androgen receptors in transiently transfected COS cells, a monkey kidney cell line, are found in a punctate perinuclear distribution in the cytoplasm (221). Addition of androgen results in strong nuclear immunostaining. In the absence of hormone, all steroid receptors can be recovered in the cytosolic fraction upon cell rupture, indicating ligand-free receptors are loosely bound in the nucleus.

Currently it is thought that signal peptide sequences direct proteins to their respective cellular compartments. Nuclear proteins are thought to be transported to the nucleus across the nuclear pore complex via a nuclear signal binding protein. Evidence exists for nuclear localization signals (NLSs) in nuclear proteins, the prototype of which is that for SV40 large T antigen which contains a single stretch of basic amino acids, PKKKRKV. Various other basic sequences have also been implicated in nuclear localization signaling. Proteins which lack NLSs may be imported to the nucleus by "piggybacking" onto a NLS-containing protein. It has been demonstrated that an analogous sequence is present in steroid receptors and is required for their nuclear translocation (198). It is currently thought that the mechanism of regulation of the nuclear import of steroid receptors involves the unmasking of a NLS. This putative nuclear translocation signal is located in proximity to the second zinc

TABLE 3. *Androgen-responsive elements*

Gene promoter	Species	ARE binding site sequence	Reference
MMTV-LTR promoter	Mouse Virus	GTTACAaacTGTTCT GGTATCaaaTGTTCT AGCTCTtagTGTTCT ATTTTCctaTGTTCT	Darbre et al., 1986
C3(I) gene first intron	Rat	AGTACCtgaTGTTCT	Claessens et al. (206)
Tyrosine aminotransferase	Rat	TGTACAggaTGTTCT	Denison et al. (202)
Sex-limited protein (SLP)	Mouse	AGAACAggcTGTTTC	Loreni et al. (209)
Prostate-specific antigen	Human	AGAACAgcaAGTGCT	Reigman et al. (211)
Ornithine decarboxylase	Mouse	AGTACCactTGTTCT	Crozat et al. (210)
Probasin promoter	Rat	ATAGCAtctTGTTCT	Rennie et al. (208)
ARE consensus		GG(A/T)ACAnnnTGTTCT	Roche et al. (204)
GRE/PRE consensus		GGTACAnnnTGTTCT	Beato et al., 1989

MMTV, mouse mammary tumor virus.

binding finger in the hinge region between the DNA binding and ligand binding domains. In the androgen receptor this sequence is [628]RKLKKLGN. However, some recent work with androgen receptor nuclear localization seems to indicate that this one putative nuclear signal peptide is not sufficient by itself for translocation (222). Additional nuclear localization signals may exist in the steroid receptor protein, one of which has been localized to the steroid binding domain, but not yet isolated (223). Multiple nuclear localization signals have been shown to be either hormone dependent or independent in both estrogen and progesterone receptors (224). Recent data appear to point towards receptor phosphorylation upon activation as being an important mechanism in the nuclear translocation of steroid receptors. Both serine and tyrosine residues have been found to be phosphorylated in other steroid receptors (reviewed in ref. 225). In a mammalian cell system, expressed progesterone receptors can be found localized to the nucleus in the absence of progesterone ligand when the cells are treated with okadaic acid, a phosphatase inhibitor (226).

Molecular Regulation of Androgen Receptor Action

It is of interest that not only is androgen receptor capable of activating specific target genes, but is also capable of autoactivating its own gene that makes the androgen receptor. Frequently as the tissue levels of androgen increase, the messenger RNA levels for the androgen receptor decrease, but mysteriously the levels of androgen receptor still remain high in the tissues. This mechanism of autoregulation of the receptor gene and the receptor stability and turnover in tissue needs to be resolved.

The binding of steroids to the receptor is important. The dissociation constant for the androgen receptor, the K_d, is 0.2–4 nM and it is important to determine whether this affinity for steroid can be modulated by modification of the receptor. Androgen receptors, like all steroid receptors, are known to bind to heat-shock proteins that are ubiquitous and are believed to be involved in sequestering the receptor. In addition, many steroid receptors are regulated by the level of phosphorylation of tyrosine or serine residues on the receptor. Recently it has been shown that the androgen receptor can be phosphorylated in the rat ventral prostate and it has been reported to occur through a nuclear cAMP-independent protein kinase (227). It has been suggested that the rich acid phosphatases in the prostate may be acting on phosphotyrosyl residues of the androgen receptor, thus playing a role in dephosphorylation and inactivation of androgen receptors (228).

What produces the tissue specificity in receptor action? Two cell types in different tissues from the same animal can contain the same androgen receptors present in their nuclei but a cell in one tissue type will respond to the receptor by making one type of androgen-induced protein while another cell in a different tissue will produce a second type of androgen-induced protein. For example, in the rat, the ventral prostate and the seminal vesicles both have androgen receptors and in the presence of dihydrotestosterone they bind to the same genome (DNA) in their nuclei; however, the prostate makes a different pattern of androgen-controlled gene expression of secretory proteins from the secretory proteins induced by androgen in the seminal vesicles. How two cells with the same DNA respond to the same receptor in a totally different manner remains a mystery. Is it because the receptors are different in these two tissues in some subtle way or that certain DNA sequences have been slightly modified by methylation or changes in topology or chromatin structure? This is one of the major frontiers of endocrine molecular biology.

Part of the tissue and gene specificity in the recognition of receptors and DNA may depend on the organization of the DNA within different nuclei (94). The steroid receptor complex can only interact with genes that are in regions that are "open" or in the transcriptionally active form, which means that they are susceptible to digestion by incubation with the enzyme DNase I. This indicates that the DNA in this region is in an accessible form to the DNase enzyme. Studies show that these open regions of chromatin with altered conformation extend up to 100,000 base pairs in length, or more than 10-fold the size of a gene which usually ranges from 1,000 to 10,000 base pairs. It is unknown how such a large range of DNA is altered in conformation, but it may be through binding to structures like the nuclear matrix which can order large loop domains in the region of 60,000–120,000 base pairs.

We now turn our attention to the structure of the nucleus where the genetic information of the genes, the androgen receptor interactions and the messenger RNA processing occur and are integrated. This is within a highly ordered structure of the nucleus that is determined by a residual scaffolding framework, called the nuclear matrix, that provides three-dimensional organization to both the nucleus and the DNA.

The Role of the Nuclear Matrix in Androgen Action

The DNA may be similar in every cell of different tissues in the body but it appears to be organized in a different three-dimensional array in these different cell types. This spatial organization of DNA appears to be determined by nuclear architecture and structure dictated by the scaffolding element termed the nuclear matrix. Therefore, more may be required than just a steroid receptor and a DNA sequence with an ARE to determine the high tissue specificity of androgen hormone action. It may require regulation of DNA conformation and three-dimensional structure. It is known that there are great regions of at least 100 kb of DNA that are larger than many genes that are in an open conformation and this varies between cells with the same genome. There is strong evidence to believe that structural components of the nucleus may organize the DNA into different topological constraints that permit specific steroid receptor interactions themselves. It is also believed that these structural modifications of topology of DNA may be an integral part of differentiation. The nuclear matrix has been proposed to be an important structural element in this type of DNA organization (94). The nuclear matrix is an important site that binds hormone receptor complexes and organizes the location of active genes that can be expressed by the action of the steroid receptor. The matrix facilitates the location of target genes, and their conformation, and facilitates their cointeraction with steroid receptors. For this reason, we will review the properties and describe the nuclear matrix structure.

Barrack and Coffey (229,230) first showed that the nuclear matrix is a major target for androgen and estrogen receptor binding. Because the matrix has been implicated in many important nuclear events it would provide an ideal target for androgen action. The matrix also organizes DNA and alterations in chromatin structure are known to be affected by hormonal action.

The nuclear matrix has been defined as the dynamic structural subcomponent of the nucleus that directs the functional organization of DNA into loop domains and provides sites for the specific control of nucleic acids (94,231). Conceptually, it can be viewed as the nuclear equivalent to the cytomatrix or cytoskeleton. The nuclear matrix contains residual nuclear elements, including the pore-complex-lamina, the residual nucleolus, and an internal ribonucleoprotein particle (RNP) network attached to a dynamic fibrous protein mesh (232). The nuclear matrix may be isolated by sequential extractions employing nonionic detergent, brief digestion with DNase I, and a hypertonic salt buffer wash. The residual nuclear matrix structures represent only 15% or less of the original total nuclear mass. Over 98% of the DNA, 70% of the RNA, and 90% of the nuclear proteins have been extracted and the remaining structure is essentially devoid of histones and lipids.

The nuclear matrix has been implicated as an important structural component in a wide variety of important biological functions. The nuclear matrix serves an important role in DNA organization. There are approximately 50,000 DNA loop-domains in a nucleus, each containing about 60 kbp of DNA and these loops are attached at their bases to the nuclear matrix (233,234). This loop organization is maintained during interphase and throughout metaphase (231). Topoisomerase II, an enzyme which modulates DNA twisting and topology, is associated with the nuclear matrix and the mitotic chromosome scaffold. Hormones are known to activate genes and alter DNA structure. Many studies with a wide variety of systems have demonstrated that active genes are associated with the nuclear matrix while transcriptionally inactive genes are not in close proximity to the matrix. This location of active genes on the matrix provides evidence that the matrix plays an important organizing role in differentiation, placing genes in different configuration.

Androgens can activate DNA synthesis and cell replication in target tissues. The nuclear matrix also serves an important role in DNA replication. The matrix contains fixed sites for DNA synthesis (233) located at the base of the DNA loop. During DNA synthesis, the DNA loop domains are reeled down through the attached replicating complex that are fixed on the matrix. Therefore, the DNA replication fork, DNA polymerase, and newly replicated DNA have been shown to be associated with the nuclear matrix. It is easy to visualize how hormone action and alteration in the nuclear matrix structures could impinge on the androgen regulation of DNA synthesis and growth in a prostate cell (See Fig. 13).

The nuclear matrix is also associated with mRNA synthesis during transcription. Transcriptional complexes have been identified on the nuclear matrix. O'Malley and his colleagues (235) observed that over 95% of the unprocessed mRNA precursor for ovalbumin was associated with nuclear matrix of the chick oviduct. When the intron portions of the RNA were spliced out the mature mRNA was released from the nuclear matrix. This led them to suggest that the nuclear matrix was involved in RNA processing. Marriman and van Venrooij (236) have reported that all RNA cleavage products and RNA processing intermediates are firmly bound to nuclear matrix. Once again, alterations in nuclear matrix structures with steroid receptor interactions could alter important steps in transcription and RNA processing. The nuclear matrix contains the attachment sites for the small nuclear ribonucleoprotein particles (snRNP) that are part of the nuclear splicesome system that is central to the nuclear processing of RNA to the final mRNA that is transported out to the cytoplasm to be translated.

In summary, the nuclear matrix is an important modulator of nuclear regulation and is an ideal target for hormonal regulation. Indeed, the nuclear matrix is a major site of steroid hormone receptor binding (176,192,230, 237–239). In the prostate, over 60% of all nuclear androgen receptors are associated with the nuclear matrix (230). The matrix is also a target for many other types of regulatory interactions including the nuclear products of oncogenes and viral proteins that can also induce growth regulation similar to hormone induced growth. For example, the nuclear matrix is reported to be a cellular target for the retrovirus myc oncogene protein, and the adenovirus E1A transforming protein, as well as the poly-

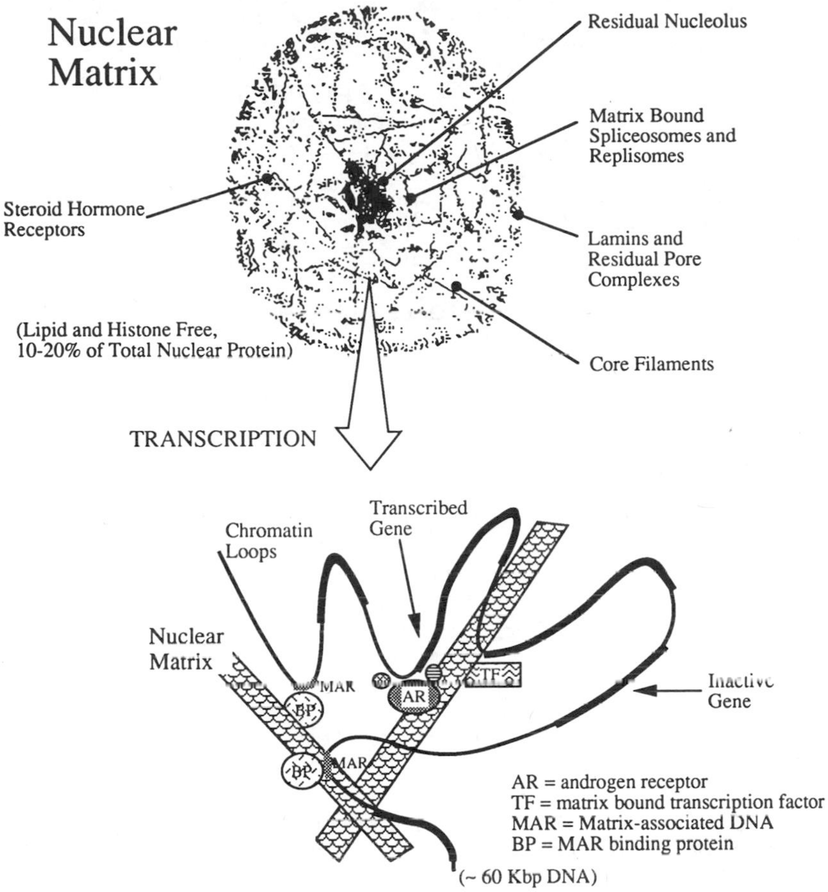

FIG. 13. Model of transcription on the nuclear matrix. Among the functional and structural components of the nuclear matrix are the proteins that organize DNA into 60 kbp loop domains. A 60 kbp loop is depicted in this model as being bound at the bases by matrix associated region (MAR) DNA binding proteins. Additionally, binding of specific DNA sequences to various transcription factors, including the binding of AREs to androgen receptor can lead to the formation of minor loops which regulate transcription of genes on those loops. This interaction can be modulated by additional accessory acceptor proteins. Additional transcription factors may also work in a similar way. Inactive genes have been shown previously not to be associated with the nuclear matrix.

oma large T antigen. All of these transformation proteins that bind to the nucleus are believed to be early molecular events in carcinogenesis or transformation. Therefore, the observation that androgen receptors interact with the matrix has precedence with the matrix as a common target in factors that regulate cell structure and function. For a more detailed review of the matrix in hormone action, see the review of Getzenberg and colleagues (94), and for the role in cancer, see Pienta and colleagues (240).

Stromal-Epithelial Interactions

The non-cellular stroma and connective tissue of the prostate comprise what is termed the ground substance and extracellular matrix and was first proposed by Arcadi (103) to play an important role in prostate function and pathology. The extracellular matrix has long been recognized as one of the important inductive components during normal development of many different types of cells (102,241,242). The extracellular matrix is far more than a supporting scaffolding for cells because it has been shown to play a central role in development and the control of cellular function (102). It now appears that the extracellular matrix is just one of the three major matrix systems that interact and form the overall tissue matrix system of the prostate (94,243).

There has been increasing interest in the role of stromal tissue elements in inducing the growth of the sex accessory tissue since the early suggestions of Franks in 1970 that epithelial cells require stroma for their growth; in addition, the classic experiments of Cunha and colleagues (29,34), Chung and Cunha (35), and Biller and colleagues (244) have clearly shown the direct importance of the embryonic mesenchyme in the induction of the differentiation of the normal prostatic epithelial cells (see discussion in earlier section). McNeal proposed that in BPH the stroma may be reactivated in adult life to an embryonic state, thus stimulating abnormal growth; this concept has generated a great deal of interest and effort to understand these tissue components of the prostate. To test whether adult prostate cells could be stimulated by embryonic factors, Chung and coworkers (37,39) transplanted a fetal urogenital sinus into an adult rat prostate and induced a large hyperplastic overgrowth of adult prostatic tissue apparently stimulated by the presence of the factors from the fetal tissue. It is unknown whether direct contact with an insoluble embryonic extracellular matrix and/or soluble diffusible growth factor(s) and steroids are responsible for these observations. Figure 14 is a schematic of pathways of coupling

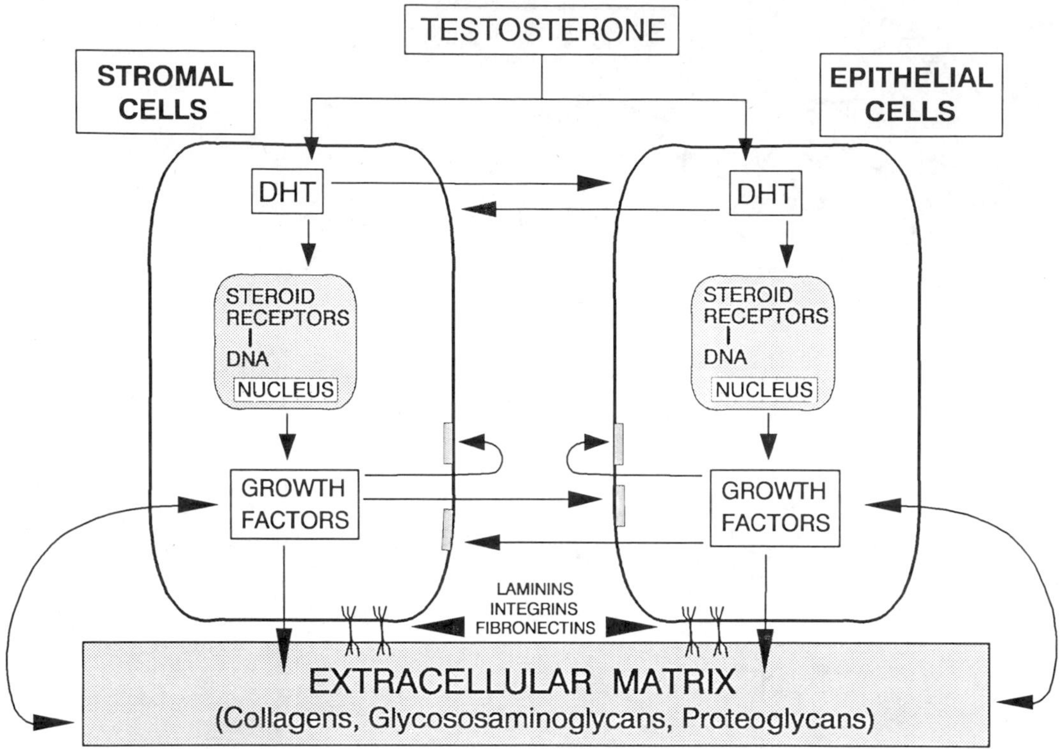

FIG. 14. Types of stromal-epithelial interactions in information transfer and regulation within the prostate. Testosterone and growth factors interact on and between stromal and epithelial cells. The formation of dihydrotestosterone (*DHT*), the production of growth factors, and extracellular matrix components regulate stromal-epithelial interactions.

stromal-epithelial interactions involving both soluble (growth factors and steroids) and insoluble (extracellular matrix and integrin) interactions.

Cell-matrix interactions can also limit growth. Muntzing (245) proposed that collagen of the prostate might limit prostate growth. Mariotti and Mawhinney (246) and Thornton and associates (109) have provided evidence that collagen synthesis and degradation can be important events in accompanying limitations on prostatic growth in animals. At present, a clear cause and effect of collagen on normal prostate growth and function has not been fully established, but several types of collagens are critical components of the extracellular matrix. The extracellular matrix is becoming a major target for understanding how the phenotype of a cells is regulated. Membrane receptors on the cell surface extend out through the plasma membrane and form a bridge directly connecting the cell skeleton with proteins on the extracellular matrix. These transmembrane receptors are called *integrins* and are made up of two subunits termed alpha and beta. These integrins serve to externally contact the extracellular matrix as receptors for fibronectin and laminin, as well as glycosoaminoglycans in the proteoglycans of the extracellular matrix. The integrin receptor domains inside the cell compartment serve as focal points for determining the structure and organization of the cytoskeleton. In addition, other types of transmembrane receptors also extend through the cell to make direct contact with the neighboring cell by recognizing similar receptors and forming hormone-dimer bonds. This permits direct cell-cell interaction; these receptors to neighboring cells are called cell adhesion molecules and require calcium for their action. One type of cell adhesion molecule of growing importance, uvomorulin, appears to bind many types of epithelial cells together, including the prostate. These interlocking matrix systems interact to form a structural network extending externally from cell-cell contact and extracellular matrix interactions, internally to cytoskeleton organization and centrally, terminating by contact with the nuclear matrix and DNA. The interactions of the tissue matrix regulate many aspects of DNA functions that are involved in growth and differentiation, and the study of this system is at the forefront of molecular endocrinology. These types of tissue matrix interactions are essential to the understanding of stromal-epithelial interactions because they form direct structural linkages and communications between the stroma and epithelial nuclear DNA.

Elements of the stroma and tissue matrix can be isolated as a *biomatrix;* when this is used as a substratum for epithelial growth in tissue culture, it regulates the growth and function of the prostate epithelial cells (72).

Canine prostatic epithelial cells will grow rapidly as primary outgrowth on plastic and do not require stromal elements, however, when these cells are growing on prostatic biomatrix they reduce their growth and maintain their morphology and secretory ability and more closely approximate that occurring *in vivo* (72). This indicates that the stromal elements act as a braking system for growth and therefore limit proliferation and maintain the state of functional differentiation and secretion. Indeed, in normal prostate and in benign prostatic hyperplasia where there is stromal-epithelial interactions, there is usually very little growth and mitotic figures are rare. Removing cells from this normal state and placing them on plastic removes the brake and permits the epithelial cells to grow. The extent of disruption in these braking systems in benign prostatic hyperplasia and cancer is a developing area of tumor biology.

Cancer cells can migrate out of the prostate and are capable of growing elsewhere in the body as metastatic lesions and, therefore, either can use stromal elements from other tissues to support their growth or are free of stromal cell restraints, possibly because of autocrine factors. Chung and his colleagues (247) have shown that the development and establishment of transplanted cancer cells is dependent upon their transplantation with collagen and either live or dead fibroblasts.

In summary, different components of matrix interactions can either have an inhibitory role in negative regulation of normal prostate growth and/or a positive role in establishing tumor growth. There have been many hypotheses concerning the mechanism of these epithelial-stromal interactions, but they have yet to be fully resolved (94,245,248).

The discussion until this point has concerned primarily insoluble elements in inducing stromal-epithelial interactions, but soluble hormones such as steroids and growth factors, are also important. The prostatic stroma does contain steroid receptors and does respond to both androgens and estrogens (see earlier discussion), and the stroma has an androgen metabolizing ability to form dihydrotestosterone almost equal to that of the epithelium. Steroids can alter the formation of collagen and other extracellular matrix components.

Prostatic Growth Factors and Growth Suppressors

Since the normal adult prostate is not growing rapidly or increasing in size, one would not anticipate an abundance of active growth factors in the normal prostate. However, this is a paradox because many adult tissues, not rapidly growing like the prostate, still have high levels of growth factors that can be demonstrated by extracting the tissues and showing that they contain soluble factors that can stimulate *in vitro* fibroblast growth.

It has been proposed that many of these prostate growth factors may not be active because they are sequestered by binding to components of the extracellular matrix, such as heparan or heparin sulfates that are part of the glycosaminoglycans. Indeed, it is known that heparin binding to growth factors is one of the most efficient ways to remove and purify many growth factors such as those in the basic fibroblast growth factor family. If the prostate growth factors are sequestered at the extracellular matrix, it would be important to know what mechanisms are involved in their binding and in their release. Therefore, the simple measuring of total growth factor levels in the prostate is, in itself, not sufficient to define their actual biological activity in the prostate. In all types of growth, it now appears that there is a balance between factors that activate growth and factors which suppress these growth promoting factors. These latter inhibitory or braking elements have been termed "suppressor." In this regard, the extracellular matrix could be termed a "suppressor element" in regard to its ability to sequester growth factors. In addition, extracellular matrix interactions with cells can determine or direct the response of a cell to a mitogen like a growth factor.

Both stromal and epithelial cells themselves can synthesize and respond to growth factors in a reciprocal and interactive manner (Fig. 14). Many of these growth factors appear to be under hormonal regulation, particularly in response to androgens, estrogens, and other endocrine factors. Androgens and growth factors can also stimulate the synthesis and degradation of extracellular matrix components that can alter a cell's response to steroids and growth factors. Therefore, the interactions of steroids, growth factors and the extracellular matrix with the cell is reciprocal and dynamic and can have either positive or negative effects in regulating cell growth.

The combination of steroid hormones and different growth factors and their temporal sequence on different cells of the prostate at various times of development will be complex, and it is certainly too early to conclude mechanisms, but it will be an important area in understanding the biology and pathology of the prostate. In this regard, the effects and mechanism of growth factors on any cell is complicated. Not all steps are realized with each growth factor, but they are usually modifications of the generalized scheme and pathways and involve four phases of regulation: synthesis, secretion, target cell interactions, and effects. The cell is signaled to produce synthesis of a growth factor by environmental signals that include cell-cell-extracellular matrix communications and hormonal levels. The genes for making the growth factors are activated making messenger RNAs which can be processed to various forms which are then translated, usually to an inactive or progrowth factor form. Proteolysis activates the growth factor which then can either work internally in the cell (intracrine), or be secreted extracellularly to serve as soluble signals either to its own cell in which it was synthesized (autocrine), or to stimulate a nearby cell (paracrine). After being secreted, the growth factor can be sequestered by binding to the extracellular matrix, but upon release, is capable of binding to specific growth factor receptors that reside on the plasma membrane of the target cell. The degree of occupancy of these membrane growth factor receptors activates a series of second messenger signals that involve either protein kinases, membrane phospholipases, or G protein pathways. The early result of binding to the receptor is the activation of one of these three general types of enzymes that phosphorylate proteins that are called kinases. These kinases are: tyrosine kinase, cAMP protein kinase A, or protein kinase C and they are either part of the growth factor receptor itself or are located adjacent to the receptor in the plasma membrane. The growth factor-induced activation of these kinases and second messengers cause a cascade of phosphorylation of specific target regulatory proteins and often the subsequent release of calcium ions from the mitochondria and endoplasmic reticulum. Usually in concert, this cascade brings about the final signal to the nucleus to turn on the expression of specific growth factor-activated genes or to induce DNA synthesis and cell replication. Overall growth is always a net balance between the rate of cell replication and the rate of cell death and growth factors can either stimulate or suppress growth through affecting this balance.

Fibroblast Growth Factor

The same growth factors often received a wide variety of names as they were first isolated from different tissues and this has caused much confusion. For example, basic fibroblast growth factor (bFGF) is the same, or very similar to, prostate growth factor, osteoblastic growth factor, a form of tumor angiogenesis factor, endothelial growth factor, uterine growth factor, seminiferous growth factor, and keratinocyte growth factor just to name a few. Fibroblast growth factors can be isolated from many tissues and come from cells of embryonic mesoderm or neuroectoderm origin. They can also be found in a wide variety of tumors and are produced by many cells in culture. In 1979, Jacobs and colleagues (249–251) identified a prostatic growth factor which they were able to show was a mitogenic factor present in human prostatic extracts.

There are 7 related genes that code for a family of related fibroblast growth factor; for specific details consult the review of Goldfarb (252). In general, there are two major types, both basic and acidic forms of the growth factor, but the acidic form is found primarily in neural tissue such as the brain and hypothalamus, and the basic form (bFGF) may be more important in the prostate. Both of these growth factors bind very tightly to heparin and are sometimes referred to as heparin binding growth factors. FGF is very mitogenic for mesoderm-derived cells and will stimulate capillary growth; it is often therefore termed the "tumor angiogenesis factor" and may be involved in neovascularization in any rapidly growing or developing tissue. The acid and basic FGFs have a 55% amino acid sequence homology. The gene for basic FGF codes for a precursor form of 155 amino acids, and if the protein is kept at neutral pH in the presence of protease inhibitors, 154 amino acid units can be isolated from the prostate (251), but the usual form isolated is often 146 amino acids. The ability of the prostate to manufacture its own growth factors, such as basic fibroblast growth factor (253) and TGFβ2 (254), and the changes of these levels with pathological growth such as BPH and cancer is obviously of great interest (255).

Oncogenes are genes that are abberant in expression or form in cancer cells. One of the oncogenes, termed "int-2", is a gene very similar to fibroblast growth factor but is larger, containing 239 amino acids. It has now been possible to clone this gene and to place it into germ cells that upon fertilization, produce a mouse which can overexpress the int-2 gene. These transgenic mice produce high levels of int-2 product causing epithelial overgrowth as the mice develop. In females, this overproduction produces a mammary gland hyperplasia, and in the male it produces a dramatic prostatic epithelial hyperplasia, but the stromal components do not produce a fibromuscular hyperplasia (256). Int-2 is expressed in normal cells of other tissues during embryogenesis but is usually not found in adult tissues. Whether the re-expression of int-2 or a similar growth factor gene occurs as an embryonic "re-awakening" in human BPH needs to be determined.

The molecular weight of the membrane receptor that binds basic fibroblast growth factor is approximately 100,000 and extends through the membrane with the cytoplasmic domain having a tyrosine kinase function which permits the receptor to function as an enzyme phosphorylating tyrosine protein residues.

In summary, the fibroblast growth factors are broad spectrum mitogens and in addition, can stimulate angiogenesis. Since they also induce the expression of plasminogen activator, it has been suggested that they have the properties to support tumor growth and enhance its ability to invade, but this has yet not been established. It seems a paradox that normal adult prostate tissue that is not growing still contains remarkably high concentrations of these growth factors; this may be because the growth factor is sequestered, inactivated or incapable of function because of receptor limitations.

Epidermal Growth Factor

Urogastrone, a growth factor which is a polypeptide of 53 amino acids was first found in the urine and is now known to be similar to mouse epidermal growth factor (EGF) (mol. wt. 16,000). EGF is present in high concentration (272 ng/ml) in human ejaculate and is produced in the prostate.

High levels of fibroblast growth factor (bFGF) are found in all prostates, but epidermal growth factor level is usually much lower. This has led Store and associates (257) to conclude that EGF is not the major growth factor in the human prostate; indeed, messenger RNA for EGF has been difficult to detect in normal or abnormal growth of the human prostate (254). It has been reported that epidermal growth factor related mitogen with a slightly higher molecular weight than EGF is present in the dorsal prostate of the rat (258). It has also been reported that the prostatic epidermal growth factor receptor can be regulated by androgens in the prostate (259).

There is still much conflict over the role of epidermal growth factor in the human prostate because prostate cancer cells in culture (LNCaP) do have significant levels of EGF that is 100 times the TGF-α level when measured intracellularly (260). Morris and Dodd (261) have measured the level of EGF and its receptor EGF-R in the human prostate and have shown the highest levels in prostate cancer tissues, thus emphasizing the potential importance of EGF in cancer.

The epidermal growth factor receptor extends through the plasma membrane, has a molecular weight of 170,000 and, like basic fibroblast growth factor, the receptor is an enzyme tyrosine kinase.

Transforming Growth Factor α

The transforming growth factors (TGF) were named because of their ability to promote cell colony formation in suspension cultures and it therefore was an operational definition. TGF-α is made as a precursor of 160 amino acids and is processed to 50 amino acids with a molecular weight of 5,600. TGFα is structurally similar to EGF and is believed to bring about most of its effects by interacting with the EGF receptor. TGFα has been shown to stimulate the growth of human prostate cancers in culture (262). TGFα is present in breast cancer and is thought to be an autocrine growth factor stimulated by estrogen treatment. Transgenic mice that overexpress TGFα produce both mammary cancers and, in males, an epithelial hyperplasia in the mouse prostate lobe called the coagulating gland (263).

Transforming Growth Factor β

Transforming growth factor β is not related to transforming growth factor α, and the similarity in names causes confusion. There are two genes for TGFβ, termed 1 and 2, and they have a 70% homology. There are three combinations possible between these two genes when a dimer is formed. TGFβ is made as a precursor of 391 amino acids that is inactive in a latent form and it can be activated by proteolysis, such as plasminogen activator, or by acid to produce a 25,000 M.W. growth factor of 1 monomers each with 112 amino acids. Although both TGFβ1 and 2 are expressed in prostate tissue, TGFβ2 has been shown to be significantly increased in expression in BPH as compared to the normal prostate, while TGFβ1 was not (254). TGFβ is of paramount interest because it may function as a braking system in negatively regulated epithelial cell growth while being a positive factor in stimulating stromal cell growth. These generalizations may be changed in cancers or benign prostatic hyperplasia tissues where the epithelial cells have changed their response to TGFβ. This may be mediated by changes in the function of the receptors or TGFβ and at present there are three of these receptors that have been identified and they appear to function through G proteins activating cAMP pathways. The down regulation of these receptors could release the brake on epithelial growth. This is a complex area because alternate splicing of the messenger RNA for TGFβ and its multiple forms due to the combinations of these dimers, as well as the multiple receptor action, attest to the complexity of this important growth factor systems. In addition, TGFβ is also an angiogenesis factor and can regulate neovascularization that is essential to tumor growth. It has recently been reported by Steiner and Barrack (255) that overexpression of TGFβ1 enhances tumor growth in vivo.

Two other growth factors related to the TGFβ family are Müllerian inhibitory substance, which is a 14,000 MW protein that causes regression in the mullerian ducts, and inhibin, a peptide involved in feedback control of follicle-stimulating hormone, FSH. Inhibin has been reported to be present in the human prostate and seminal plasma and is synthesized in the rat ventral prostate under hormonal control (264,265).

Insulinlike Growth Factors I and II (Somatomedin)

Insulinlike substances have also been detected in the prostate (266). Insulinlike growth factors, termed somatomedin, are in two closely related forms, type I and type II, and are 75,000 M.W. single-chain polypeptides that share sequence homology with human pro-insulin. These growth hormones can be found in circulating blood and therefore are endocrine factors, as well as in their production in target tissue and therefore are growth factors. These growth factors bind to receptors on the cell membrane that are similar to the insulin receptor consisting of 2 alpha chains and 2 beta chains. This receptor has a tyrosine kinase activity. IGF-1 is locally produced in connective tissue such as the chondrocyte and has an anabolic effect on bone formation through the stimulation of osteoblasts. Many growth factors affect the synthesis of other growth factors and TGFβ-1 has the ability to strongly stimulate the production of IGF-1 in bone and cartilage. Of interest, has been the observation that IGF-2 and cathepsin-D both have a common type of receptor on breast cancer cells that involves a mannose-6-phosphate receptor and may indicate the importance of proteolytic enzymes to function also as growth factors. High cathepsin-D levels are seen in breast cancer and in the involuting prostate following androgen withdrawal.

Platelet-Derived Growth Factor

PDGF is expressed in many tissues and found in the urine, although it is primarily derived from platelets, and is expressed by the c-sis oncogene. PDGF has a strong mitogenic effect on connective tissue cells and makes cells competent to respond to other growth factors. It has been shown to be expressed in prostate tumor models and cells in culture (267,268), but has not received as much attention as has the basic fibroblast growth factor.

Other Types of Prostate Growth Factors

Other identified growth factors that are claimed to originate in the prostate but as yet there is no proven growth factor that is unique to the prostate that could be termed a true prostate-specific structure that does not exist in other tissues. It is possible that growth factors may be altered in processing so as to produce increased specificity for an organ, but this is not established. Crabb and coworkers (269) have reported the complete primary structure of a prostate epithelial growth factor that they have termed prostatropin. Much work will be required to demonstrate that any growth factor is found only in the prostate and to eliminate the possible contamination of other known growth factors. Proteases in the prostate can also clip and modify known growth factors to produce altered forms.

Other growth factors, such as insulin, that originate in distant organs and are transported by the blood are usually termed "endocrine" and not growth factors; however, this is only a matter of classification and does not diminish their importance. For example, prolactin has been shown to have an effect on the increase in DNA synthesis and isolated human BPH tissue (270). Receptors for many pituitary factors, including prolactin, LHRH, growth hormone, somatostatin, and thyroid-stimulating hormone have been sporadically reported in the prostate, but most of the attention has focused on the prolactin and LHRH receptors (271,272). It is still unclear how these endocrine and pituitary factors might act as growth hormones in direct interaction on the prostate cells.

Grayhack and his colleagues (273) have long proposed that there is a second factor released by the testes other than testosterone that may be involved in prostatic growth in both the rat and dog, but this factor has not been isolated and characterized.

The Regulation of Prostate Growth: Balance of Cell Replication and Cell Death

There is little doubt that most tissues are susceptible to stimulation by growth factors or by inhibition of growth by growth factors and poorly defined tissue chalones, and the action of these positive and negative growth factors are in a dynamic balance. The net balance between the rate of cell growth and cell death maintains the steady state size of the prostate; it appears to be under hormonal and growth factor control, and is age-dependent. Resolving the mechanisms which control this normal growth balance is most crucial to understanding the imbalance that occurs in tumor growth.

For cells to grow they must first undergo DNA synthesis and this can be determined on human prostatic tissue by the incorporation of precursors into the DNA, such as thymidine (274), iododeoxyuridine (275), or bromodeoxyuridine (276). Other markers include antibodies against nuclear proteins associated with proliferation, such as KI-67, histones, topoisomerase enzymes, or counting mitotic indices have all been used to detect the proliferation of DNA in prostate cells. These techniques have been very helpful in working out the temporal sequence of events that occur in the growth of the prostate under hormonal stimulation in animal models (70,277–284). Castration causes a 90% loss in the total number of prostatic epithelial cells and a slower, but less complete, reduction of approximately 40% in the number of stromal cells. In castrates, following androgen treatment, there is a delay of 1 day before the onset of DNA synthesis, which reaches a maximum rate at 2–3 days and then subsides to normal levels even in the continued presence of androgen stimulation (277,278). It is unknown why the rapid synthesis of DNA stops after the gland is restored to its full size. Buttyan and his colleagues (285) have studied the sequence that occur following testosterone repletion that precede the onset of DNA synthesis. They demonstrated that the oncogene c-fos showed the earliest transient rise, increasing threefold within 1 hour, followed by an increase in ras oncogenes within 2 hours, followed by the transient transcription of both myc and myb within 6 to 8 hours. This is typical of many other tissues that are stimulated to grow where similar transient rises in oncogenes precede the onset of DNA synthesis.

Many oncogenes are expressed during growth and development and it has been proposed that mutated oncogenes, or aberrant forms, may be at the heart of genetic expression in cancer. At present, the ras oncogene is the most common oncogene mutated in many human solid tumors, but it does not have a high instance in human prostate cancer. Deletion of genetic materials has been shown to release the brake that holds tissues and growth in check. This genetic material has been termed "suppressor" genes which means that their absence induces growth and so far, the only one implicated in prostatic tissues in culture has been the retinoblastoma gene (286). This will obviously be an active area of pursuit in the future as allelotyping identifies specific areas of deletion in human prostate cancer.

It was long believed that cell death following androgen withdrawal was simply the reduction of an important biological factor required to maintain the life of the cell. Recent studies have shown that this involution is an active process rather than passive. For example, Lee, Grayhack and associates (287–289) reported that if protein or RNA synthesis is blocked following castration, the rate of prostate gland involution was markedly reduced. This suggested that specific proteins might be expressed to produce active cell death following androgen deprivation. This process is reminiscent of the system that occurs in bacteria where bactericidal death requires the synthesis of over a dozen specific proteins required to kill the bacteria, and it now appears that a similar process of specific protein synthesis required for involution following androgen withdrawal occurs in the prostate. This process is termed "programmed cell death."

There are a series of proteins that are induced following castration in the prostate and the most actively studied is trpm-2 (Tenniswood and colleagues; 290). This has been aided by the characterization and cloning of this gene (291,292). This trpm-2 protein was dramatically increased 48 hours following castration and has proven to be one of the most reliable indicators of epithelial cell involution in the prostate. It is still not certain what the role of trpm-2 is in cell death, or if it is merely a secondary marker associated with, but not causing, involution. Trpm-2 has been shown to be similar to clusterin, a sulfated glycoprotein-2 normally found in Sertoli cells and present in human seminal plasma, and is suggested to be important in fertility (293).

Proteolytic enzymes, such as cathepsin D, are activated during castration-induced involution in the rat prostate (294,295). Plasminogen activators are also increased following castration (296) and three forms are increased following castration in the prostate epithelial cells (297).

Several groups have studied the appearance of two-dimensional protein patterns that were altered by castration or androgen treatment (140,298,299). The colleagues of Liao (300) have shown that specific messages and products are required to be synthesized in the prostate during the process of involution. Saltzman (300) has shown that androgen withdrawal causes the production of a 29,000 MW protein and its messenger RNA during the involution of the rat ventral prostate. Chang and colleagues (301) have shown that glutathione *S*-transferase is induced following castration; this is an enzyme located at the cell nucleus that appears to be a DNA binding protein.

As a cell undergoes programmed cell death, dramatic changes are seen in the nucleus with a clear zone forming in the perinuclear area (302). This process, termed apoptosis, has been shown to be a major pathway in prostatic involution (283,303–307).

Isaacs and his colleagues (283,306,307) have shown that a calcium influx activates a calcium-dependent DNase that causes fragmentation of the DNA molecule that is an early event in programmed cell death. The timing of these events has been studied (283) and the role of cell calcium levels has become paramount (307,308). Buttyan and colleagues (309) have studied the cascade of induction of a series of oncogenes and heat-shock proteins that follows castration and precedes cell loss.

Kyprianou and Isaacs (306) have reported that there is an increase in TGFβ receptors during castration and this may regulate cell death. Barrack and Berry (310) have studied DNA synthesis in canine prostates induced to massive growth by the combination of androgens and estrogens, and have shown that there is a decrease in the amount of DNA synthesis per unit amount of DNA required to maintain a large gland when 5α-reduced androgens and estrogens are given simultaneously. This has led them to suggest that estrogens are decreasing the rate of cell death in the prostate in the presence of 5α-reduced androgens and not an increase in proliferation. What determines the setpoint for determining the level of cells in the prostate and their rates of growth and death is of paramount importance in understanding BPH and prostate cancer.

FUNCTIONS OF THE CONSTITUENTS SEX ACCESSORY GLAND SECRETIONS

The average volume of the normal human ejaculate is approximately 3 ml, ranging from 2 to 6 ml and is composed of two components, spermatozoa and the seminal plasma. The spermatozoa are present in the range of 100 million per milliliter, but the volume of the spermatozoa component is insignificant in the volume of the total ejaculate (less than 1 per cent). The seminal plasma is formed primarily from the secretions of the sex accessory tissues, which include the epididymis, vas deferens, ampullae, seminal vesicles, prostate, Cowper's (bulbourethral) gland, and glands of Littre. In an average ejaculate volume of 3 ml, the major contribution to the volume of the seminal plasma comes from the seminal vesicles, 1.5 to 2 ml; from the prostate, 0.5 ml; and from Cowper's gland and glands of Littre, 0.1 to 0.2 ml. During ejaculation the secretions of these glands are released in a sequential manner (311–313).

The first fractions of the human ejaculate are rich in sperm and components from the prostatic secretion such as citric acid. The concentration of fructose represents a major secretory product from the seminal vesicles and is elevated in the later fractions of the ejaculate. The overall chemical composition of prostatic secretions and the normal human seminal plasma has been studied by many laboratories and the results have been summarized in excellent reviews (314–316).

In relation to other body fluids, the seminal plasma is unusual because of its very high concentrations of potassium, zinc, citric acid, fructose, phosphorylcholine, spermine, free amino acids, prostaglandins, and enzymes, most notably acid phosphatase, diamine oxidase, beta-glucuronidase, lactic dehydrogenase, alpha-amylase, prostatic specific antigens, and seminal proteinases, and much of this originates from the prostate (see Table 4).

Citric Acid

Tremendous amounts of citric acid are formed by the prostate that is almost 100 time higher than that seen in other soft tissues. For example, the prostate tissue contains approximately 30,000 nmol/g, while other tissues are in the range of 150–450 and the concentration of citrate in the ejaculate is 500–1,000 times higher than in the plasma. The prostate secretory epithelial cells have a very special metabolic ability to form citrate from aspartic acid and glucose and this results partly from the inability of the mitochondria of the prostate cells to readily oxidize citrate once it is formed; therefore, the rate of citrate synthesis far exceeds the rate of citrate oxidation (317).

One of the major anions in the human seminal plasma is citrate (mean, 376 mg/100 ml) in the range of 20 mM or 60 mEq/L. This is compared to the chloride ion (155 mg/100 ml) at 40 mM. Citrate is a potent binder of metal ions, and the seminal plasma concentration of citrate, 20 mM, is comparable to that of the total divalent metals at 13.6 mM (calcium 7 mM; magnesium, 4.5 mM; zinc, 2.1 mM). Citric acid is localized in different sex accessory tissues according to species; however, in the human the prostate is the major source for citric acid that is present in the semen. Prostatic secretions approximate 15.8 mg/ml (316) and the values for seminal vesicle citric acid secretions were almost 100-fold less, being only 0.2 mg/ml.

Fructose

The source of fructose in human seminal plasma is the seminal vesicles (315). Patients with congenital absence of the seminal vesicles have an associated absence of fructose in their ejaculates (318). The seminal vesicle secretion contains smaller amounts of other free sugars such as glucose, sorbitol, ribose, and fucose, and these sugars usually amount to less than 10 mg/100 ml. In comparison, the concentration of the reducing sugar, fructose, is approximately 300 mg/100 ml in human seminal secretion and has a level of 200 mg/100 ml in seminal plasma. Fructose levels are under androgenic regulation, but many factors such as storage, frequency of ejaculation, blood glucose levels, and nutritional status can also affect the seminal plasma concentration (315); these considerations may account for the wide variations encountered in different semen samples from the same patient. Furthermore, plasma levels of androgens do not always correlate with seminal plasma fructose levels, therefore these levels are not a reliable index of the androgenic state of the subject.

The source of fructose in seminal vesicles appears to proceed from glucose by aldose reduction to sorbitol and a subsequent ketone reduction to form fructose. The fructose of the seminal plasma appears to provide an anaerobic and aerobic source of energy for the spermatozoa (315). The cervical mucus has high concentrations of glucose and very low levels of fructose, and the sperm are capable of utilizing both types of sugars.

TABLE 4. *Predominant proteins secreted by the prostate gland*

Protein	Mol. wt. (kDa)	Isoelectric point (pi)	Prostatic fluid (mg/ml)	Seminal plasma (mg/ml)	Activity
Prostatic acid phosphatase (PAP)	102–106 (dimer)	3.8–5.0	2–5	0.3–1.0	Phosphotyrosyl protein phosphatase
Prostate-specific antigen (PSA); gamma-seminoprotein (γ-SM)	33–36	6.9	3	0.7	Kallikrein, serine protease, arginine esterase
Prostate-specific protein (PSP-94); β-microseminoprotein (β-MSP); β-inhibin	10.7–16	—	—	0.6–0.9	Also in epithelial cells of antrum of stomach

Polyamines

Polyamines are the most basic and positively charged small organic molecules in nature. They occur ubiquitously in tissues at very high concentrations and are believed to be involved in diverse physiological processes that share a close relationship to cell proliferation and growth. Indeed, polyamines can serve as growth factors for cultured mammalian cells and bacteria, as well as inhibitors of enzymes that include protein kinases. The role of polyamines at a molecular level still eludes science but they are potent biological compounds and are at very high levels in the ejaculate. Spermine levels in the normal human seminal plasma range from 50 to 350 mg/100 ml and originate primarily from the prostate gland; which is the richest source of spermine in the body. Spermine [NH_2—$(CH_2)_3$—NH—$(CH_2)_4$—$(CH_2)_4$—NH—$(CH_2)_3$—NH_2] is a very basic aliphatic polyamine, and because of its four positive charges binds strongly to acidic or negatively charged molecules such as phosphate ions, nucleic acid, or phospholipids. When semen is allowed to stand at room temperature, acid phosphatase enzymatically hydrolyzes seminal phosphorylcholine to form free inorganic phosphate ions, which then interact with the positively charged spermine and precipitate as large translucent salt crystals of spermine phosphate. Polyamines can also form amide bonds and make their covalent addition to protein carboxylic groups (319,320), and this modification may be involved in regulatory function. There has been much interest in spermine and other related polyamines such as spermidine and putrescine because of the rapid and dramatic changes in levels and ratios associated with many types of cells that have been induced into growth. Williams-Ashman and his colleagues (319,321,322) have investigated in detail the biosynthesis and regulation of polyamines in the male reproductive tract and have characterized the enzymatic reactions that progress from ornithine to putrescine to spermidine to spermine. The polyamines are oxidized enzymatically by diamine oxidase (present in the seminal plasma) to form very reactive aldehyde compounds that can be toxic to both sperm and bacteria (320). The formation of these aldehyde products produces the characteristic odor of semen. It is also possible that these aldehydes or polyamines themselves may protect the genitourinary tract from infective agents. Relationships between spermine levels in seminal plasma and sperm count and motility have also been suggested (323–325).

Phosphorylcholine

Other positively charged amines are at high concentrations in the ejaculate, including choline and phosphorylcholine which are usually found as components of lipid or as lipotropic factors.

The semen of mammals is very rich in choline [(CH3)3—N+—(CH2)2—OH]. In man, phosphorylcholine predominates, while in most other species much higher levels of α-glycerylphosphorylcholine are present, often exceeding 1 g/100 ml of seminal plasma. Seligman and associates (326) have demonstrated that phosphorylcholine is a highly specific substrate for prostatic acid phosphatase, which is also very active in seminal plasma. The result of this enzymatic activity is the rapid formation of free choline in the first ejaculate. In contrast, α-glycerylphosphorylcholine is secreted primarily in the epididymis and is not readily hydrolyzed by acid phosphatase. For these reasons, Mann and Mann (315) have suggested that the level of α-glycerylphosphorylcholine can be used as an index for assessing the contribution of the epididymal secretion to the ejaculate. The secretion from the epididymis is also under androgenic control. The function of these choline compounds is unknown; it appears that they are not metabolized by spermatozoa nor do they affect the respiration of the sperm.

Prostaglandins

The richest sources of prostaglandins in the human are the seminal vesicles. Prostaglandins are present in seminal plasma at a concentration of approximately 100 to 300 μg/ml. Injected seminal plasma produces strong pharmacological effects, producing both stimulatory and depressor effects on smooth muscle. Von Euler (327) proposed the name prostaglandins for the active components in seminal plasma in the belief that they originated from the prostate gland but Eliasson (328) established that the primary source of prostaglandin was the seminal vesicles, not the prostate; however, the original name has survived to date. Prostaglandins have a wide distribution in mammalian tissues but at much lower concentrations than found in the seminal vesicles. There are 15 different prostaglandins present in human semen, and they are all 20-carbon hydroxy fatty acids with a cyclopentane ring with two side chains; as such they are derivatives of prostanoic acid. The 15 types of prostaglandins are divided into four major groups, designated A, B, E and F according to the structure of the five-membered cyclopentane ring, and each of these groups is further subdivided according to the position and number of double bonds in the side chain (therefore, PGE3 indicates prostaglandins of E type with three double bonds in the side chain). The E group of prostaglandins is the major component in the male reproductive tract, while the F predominates in the female system. Fuchs and Chantharaski (329) have summarized the reported levels of human seminal plasma prostaglandins and report the following mean values (μg/ml): PGE1, 20; PGE2, 15; (PGE1 + E2)-19 OH, 100; PGA1 + A2, 9; (PGA1 + A2)-19 OH1, 31; PGB1 + B2, 18; (PGB1 + B2)-19 OH, 13; PGF1a, 3; and PGF2a, 4. These compounds are very potent pharmacologic agents that have been implicated in a wide variety of biologic events in the male, including erection, ejaculation, sperm motility and transport, as well as testicular and penile contractions. In addition, prostaglandins from seminal fluid deposited in the vagina have been reported to affect cervical mucus, vaginal secretion, and sperm transport in the female genital tract.

Cholesterol and Lipids

Scott (330) reported that human seminal plasma contained 185 mg/100 ml of total lipids, 103 mg/100 ml of cholesterol, and 83 mg/100 ml of phospholipids. In comparison, human prostatic secretion contained: total lipids, 186 mg/100 ml; cholesterol, 80 mg/100 ml; and phospholipids, 180 mg/100 ml. The lipids of semen have been further described (331), and the phospholipids of the seminal plasma are composed of 44% sphingomyelin, 12.3 percent ethanolamine plasmalogen, and 11.2% phosphatidylserine (332).

The reported levels of cholesterol in seminal plasma have varied considerably from 11 to 103 mg/100 ml (326,328,330). White and colleagues (331) believe that the ratio of cholesterol to phospholipid in the seminal plasma stabilizes the sperm against temperature and environmental shock.

Zinc

The high level of zinc in human seminal plasma (140 μg/ml) appears to originate primarily from secretions of the prostate gland (488 ± 18 μg/ml) that has the highest concentration of zinc (50 mg/100 g dry weight) of any organ. Mackenzie and colleagues (333) reported that human seminal plasma contained 310 mg of zinc/100 gm dry weight and that spermatozoa contained 200 mg/100 g dry weight. In comparison, prostatic secretions from 8 normal subjects had 720 mg zinc/100 g dry weight. Many of the early experiments and concepts related to zinc in the reproductive tract have been reviewed in detail by Byar (334). Zinc levels are elevated or stable in BPH, while there is a marked decrease in zinc content associated with prostatic adenocarcinoma. The localization of zinc-65 in the human prostate by radioautography appears to be within the epithelial cells; however, in the lateral prostate of the rat, large quantities of zinc were also associated with the stroma and particularly with the basal membrane and the elastin protein component (335). Oral intake of zinc does not alter zinc levels in prostatic fluid.

Many physiologic roles have been postulated for zinc since the classic studies of Gunn and Gould (336,337), who correlated endocrine effects on zinc uptake and concentration in the prostate of the rodent. There are many important zinc-containing metalloenzymes, but the concentration of zinc in the prostate probably exceeds that present in zinc-associated enzymes. Zinc is known to bind many proteins. Johnson and coworkers (338) characterized zinc-binding protein in the prostatic secretion of the dog that contained only eight types of amino acids upon hydrolysis. Heathcote and Washington (339) described a zinc-binding protein in human BPH that was rich in histidine and alanine. There have been other studies on zinc-binding proteins from the prostate (340,341), and additional information on these interesting proteins is needed.

An important role for zinc in the prostatic secretion has been suggested in the studies of Fair and Wehner (340), who suggest the direct role of zinc as a prostatic antibacterial factor. In the study of 36 normal men free from bacterial prostatic infections, the mean value of zinc in the prostatic secretion was approximately 350 μg/ml, with a wide range of 150 to 1,000. In comparison, the prostatic fluid obtained from 61 specimens collected from 15 patients with documented chronic bacterial prostatitis had over an 80% reduction and averaged only 50 μg/ml, with a range of 0 to 139. The authors proposed a lower limit of normal at 150 μg/ml. In addition, *in vitro* studies of free zinc ions at concentrations normally found in prostatic fluid have confirmed the bactericidal activity of zinc against a variety of gram-positive and gram-negative bacteria.

However, a considerable portion of the zinc in the prostate appears to be bound to unique proteins, such as metallothionein, and it is not certain how this might alter the biologic properties of zinc.

Prostatic Secretory Proteins

The protein secretions of the sex accessory tissues have been reviewed by Aumuller and Seitz (314). There have been several studies to identify high resolution two-dimensional electrophoresis profiles of major secretory protein markers from human ejaculate, seminal plasma and prostatic secretions (342–347). There are three major proteins secreted by the human prostate gland (314,347) (see Table 4):

1. Prostate-specific antigen (PSA) (also called seminin, or gamma-seminoprotein)
2. Prostatic acid phosphatase (PAP)
3. Prostatic specific protein (PSP-94) (also termed β-microseminoprotein, β-MSP, or β-inhibin

These three major proteins stain immuno-histochemically as a group in the epithelial cells of the prostate (348).

Prostate Specific Antigen

Prostatic-specific antigen (PSA) was the result of a search of the ejaculate and prostate to find specific proteins. In 1971, Japanese researchers isolated from the seminal plasma a protein that proved to be antigenically specific for the semen and reported its chemical and physical characteristics; they termed it gamma-seminoprotein (349). Later, in 1973, Lee and Beating also isolated this protein from human seminal plasma. Five years later in 1978, in an attempt to develop a forensic marker for semen identification, Sensibar (299) purified this protein from the seminal plasma. These seminal proteins called, gamma-seminoproteins, have now been shown to be the same as PSA (348). They reported the same proteolytic activity, site of glycosylation, the same molecular weight and that they have identical immunohistochemical characteristics as well as similar serum characteristics.

The first identification of gamma-seminoprotein as a prostatic-specific antigen (PSA) was the result of the important studies reported in 1979 by Wang. Wang and colleagues (15) reported this human prostate-specific antigen (PSA) that has proven to be a very important marker of prostate pathology. PSA is a glycoprotein of 33,000 MW that contains 7% carbohydrate (350), and is detected only in the epithelial cells of the prostate. PSA in the serum was demonstrated to be clinically important assay for the monitoring of prostate cancer (17,18). For a detailed description of the use of prostatic-specific antigen and the limitations, both clinically and in the laboratory medicine analysis, consult the book reporting a major comprehensive meeting on this topic (23).

Watt and colleagues (350) have made an extensive study of PSA and have reported the complete amino acid sequence. The single polypeptide chain contains 240 amino acids and an O-linked carbohydrate side chain attached to serine. Lundwall and Lilja (349) have cloned the cDNA that encodes the PSA gene. Their study indicates that the messenger RNA in the prostate is 1.5 kb.

Prostatic specific antigen is a serine protease and an esterase with both chymotrypsin-like and trypsin-like activity. The sequence of the protein is similar to the kallikreins that are important proteolytic enzymes involved in cell regulatory mechanism (350,352). Lilja (352) reported that the structural protein (semenogelin) of the seminal coagulum that causes the ejaculate to clot, and is the predominant seminal vesicle secreted protein, might be the physiological substrate for prostatic-specific antigen. One of the possible biological roles of PSA would be to lyse the ejaculate clot, but it is unknown why this clotting and lysing mechanism is important to the reproductive process.

Prostatic Acid Phosphatase

Acid phosphatase activity is about 200 times more abundant in prostate tissue than in any other tissue and is the source of the high levels of acid phosphatase in the ejaculate. Phosphatase enzymes hydrolyze many types of organic monophosphate esters to yield inorganic phosphate ions and alcohol. Many phosphatase enzymes exhibit optimal activity *in vitro* in the acid (pH 4 to 6) or alkaline (pH 8 to 11) ranges and thus are classified broadly as either acid or alkaline phosphatase. Both types of phosphatase appear to be ubiquitous in animal tissues.

Acid phosphatase activity may be further defined by factors that inhibit its enzymatic activity. For example, erythrocyte acid phosphatase is particularly sensitive to inhibition of 0.5 percent formaldehyde or copper ions (0.2 mM), while prostatic acid phosphatase activity is far more sensitive to inhibition by fluoride ions (1 mM) or L-tartrate (1 mM).

Osteoclasts are also a rich source of acid phosphatase that is tartrate insensitive, and this fact is useful because of the minor elevation in serum acid phosphatase levels that accompany Paget's disease, osteoporosis, nonprostatic bone metastasis, and other conditions of increased bone resorption.

All acid phosphatases hydrolyze a wide range of natural and synthetic phosphomonoesters, and this has provided a wide variety of assay systems and the expression of many different units of activity. These synthetic substrates include, in part: phenylphosphate (353); phenolphthalein phosphate; paranitrophenyl phosphate, also called Sigma 104; and thymolphthalein phosphate (354). The specificity of these substrates varies with the type and source of acid phosphatase; it appears that thymolphthalein phosphate may be the most specific substrate for assaying serum levels of prostatic acid phosphatase but now specific antibodies are available for immunoassays. Interest in assays for acid phosphatase in serum as a measure of prostatic cancer metastasis has decreased with the availability of the more sensitive and specific prostatic specific antigen (PSA) assay. The natural substrate for prostatic acid phosphatase may be phosphorylcholine phosphate, which is rapidly hydrolyzed in the semen (355). The biologic functions of this enzyme and its reactions are not known but it is of interest that prostatic acid phosphatase can hydrolyze protein tyrosine phosphate esters, which are natural products of many oncogene protein tyrosine kinases (356,357). It is unknown whether acid phosphatase is a regulatory factor in controlling the tyrosyl protein kinase systems that are so essential as signalling mechanisms in growth factor function.

Many tissues contain several forms of acid phosphatase that can be separated by subfractionation of the tissue and may be associated primarily with either the lysosomes, secretions, or particular membrane fractions. Electrophoresis of prostate tissue extracts revealed 13 bands of activity that might be multiple forms of a common enzyme in various states of being processed for secretion because removal of sialic acid residues from the glycoprotein enzyme converted many of these bands to only 1 or 2 entities.

Human prostatic acid phosphatase is a glycoprotein dimer of molecular weight 102,000 and contains about 7% by weight of carbohydrate, which is composed of 15 residues per mole of neutral sugars (fucose, galactose, and mannose); 6 residues per mole of sialic acid; and 13 residues of *N*-acetylglucosamine (358). The protein can be dissociated into two subunits of 50,000 m.w.. In summary, many secretory proteins and enzymes are glycosylated after they have been synthesized, and it appears that this accounts for some of the isoenzyme patterns of prostatic acid phosphatase. The secretory enzyme is probably the major form in the prostate, and the lysosomal acid phosphatase form may be similar in properties to the acid phosphatase found in other tissue lysosomes. The genes for these two acid phosphatases are located on different chromosomes.

The activity of the purified human enzyme is 723 U/mg with α-napthyl phosphate, and the seminal plasma contains 0.3–1 g/L or 177–760 U/ml. The high enzymatic activity of prostatic acid phosphatase is not characteristic of accessory tissues in many other species; the level is 1,000 times higher per gram tissue in the human prostate than in the rat prostate.

Prostatic Specific Protein 94, β-Microseminoprotein, and β-Inhibin

A major 16-kDa molecular weight protein has been found in prostatic secretions that contains 94 amino acids and has been termed PSP 94. This protein had previously been designated as β-inhibin and also as β-microseminoprotein (359,360). Transcripts of messenger RNA for this protein have also been identified in nongenital tissues (359). It remains to be determined how useful PSP 94 will be in diagnosing or monitoring prostate cancer.

Zn-α_2-Glycoprotein

Lin and Clinton (356) identified a 40 kDa glycoprotein which they had purified from seminal plasma that is similar to Zn-α_2 glycoprotein isolated from blood plasma. It receives its name from its ability to be precipitated by zinc acetate It is present in the kidney and other biological fluids and its function is unknown.

Leucine Aminopeptidase

Aminopeptidases hydrolyze the *N*-terminal amino acid from small polypeptides. Leucine aminopeptidases are particularly active against the substrate L-leucylglycine, and some of these enzymes are referred to as arylamidases because the optimal substrate is L-leucyl-β-naphthylamine. The human prostate is rich in the latter arylamidase type of leucine aminopeptidase with an activity in prostatic fluid of 30,000 units/ml. Mattila (361) demonstrated two forms of the enzyme in human prostatic tissue (molecular weights 107,000 and 305,000), only one of which was similar to that of the kidney. The kidney is one of the richest sources of leucine aminopeptidases, but at present, the tissue-specific nature of any of these isoenzymes has not been established.

Leucine aminopeptidase is a product of the epithelial cells of the prostate (362) and is secreted into the lumen of the acini (363).

Lactic Dehydrogenase

The isoenzyme ratios of lactic dehydrogenases (LDH) in human semen may be altered in a patient with prostatic cancer (364). Lactic dehydrogenase (150,000 MW) is composed of four subunits (each of 35,000 molecular weight) of only two different types of proteins, denoted M and H. The LDH of muscle has four M units and that of heart has four H units. Five isoenzymes of LDH can be found in tissues with a four subunit composition as follows: LDH I, MMMM; LDH II, MMMH; LDH III, MMHH; LDH IV, MHHH; and LDH V, HHHH). The M and H subunits appear to be the same in all tissues, but the amounts of LDH I to V can vary. Denis and Prout (365) observed increased levels of LDH IV and V in prostatic cancer tissue. Several investigators have observed elevated ratios of LDH V/LDH I in human prostatic cancer (364,366–368).

Immunoglobulins, C3 Complement and Transferrin

There are many reports establishing the presence of immunoglobulins in human seminal plasma. It is possible to measure levels of IgG from 7 to 22 mg/100 ml and IgA from 0 to 6 mg/100 ml; however, IgM is very low and often not detected (369). The complete source of these antibodies is not known, although they are found in expressed prostatic fluid (370) and may be related to infections (371,372). They are usually found at lower levels in seminal plasma than in blood, but the possibility of diffusion across the "blood-seminal plasma barrier" has not been eliminated (see discussion in ref. 369). Expressed prostatic fluid contains considerable amounts of the C_3 component of complement, being present at 1.82 mg/100 ml and this increases almost 10-fold in fluid collected from patients with prostatic adenocarcinoma to levels of 16.9 mg/100 ml (373). Prostatitis and BPH only increase the level approximately twofold. In the same manner, a protein-carrying iron, termed transferrin, is increased in a similar manner going from normal levels of prostatic fluid of 5.3 mg% to 42.4 mg% in prostatic carcinoma (373). The function of these serum proteins in the secretion of prostatic fluid remains to be resolved.

Seminal Vesicle Secretory Proteins: Semenogelin

Williams-Ashman (374) presented a classical review on the regulatory features of the seminal vesicles development and function. The secretory proteins of the seminal vesicles are major proteins and enzymes involved in the rapid clotting of the ejaculate. The major clotting protein has been termed semenogelin (375), which has been shown to be the seminal vesicle specific antigen. These clotted proteins from the seminal vesicle serve as substrates for PSA from the prostate that enzymatically lyse the clot through its protease activity (342,352). Beyond the coagulation reaction, we are not certain what role these seminal vesicle proteins play, but their effect on fertility and uterine sperm motility have been studied in the mouse (2). A more current review is that by Aumuller and Riva (58).

Coagulation and Liquefaction of Semen

Within 5 min following ejaculation, human semen coagulates into a semi-solid gel and upon further standing for a 5 to 20 minute period, the clot spontaneously liquefies to form a viscous liquid (313,373,374). Calcium-binding substances such as sodium citrate and heparin do not inhibit the coagulation process, nor are prothrombin, fibrinogen, or factor XII required, since they are absent in seminal plasma. The seminal clot is formed of fibers 0.15 to 10 nm in width, and its morphology differs from that of a blood fibrin clot (315,376,377). Factors affecting blood coagulation do not regulate semen viscosity (378). From these observations and others, it appears that the coagulation of human semen is different from that of blood.

Examination of split human ejaculates indicates that the first fraction, originating primarily from Cowper's gland and the prostate, contains the liquefaction factors, and the final fraction of the ejaculate is enriched in seminal vesicle secretions, and is responsible for the coagulation of the ejaculate (375).

It has long been known that prostatic fluid has a dramatic fibrinolytic-like activity and that 2 ml of this secretion can liquefy 100 ml of clotted blood in 18 hr at 37°C (315,376). The factors involved in such proteolytic activity in semen have been resolved (312,315,375–377,379,380). Two types of seminal plasma proteolytic enzymes appear to be major factors in the liquefaction process-plasminogen activators and PSA prostatic specific antigen (seminin).

Two plasminogen activators have been isolated from seminal plasma; they have molecular weights of 70,000 and 74,000 and appear to be related to urokinase (381). It is believed that the plasminogen activators originate from the prostatic secretions.

Seminin is an early term for what is now prostatic specific antigen, a proteolytic enzyme (molecular weight 30,000) that appears in the first fraction of split ejaculates and therefore originates from the prostate gland (312,313,379,381–383).

The seminal plasma contains a variety of other proteolytic enzymes, including pepsinogen, lysozyme, alpha-amylase, and hyaluronidase. In addition, human semen inhibits the activity of the proteolytic enzyme trypsin, and this is due to the presence in the seminal plasma of such proteinase inhibitors as alpha 1-antitrypsin and alpha 1-antichymotrypsin. Coagulation and liquefaction vary in different species. For example, the semen of the bull or dog does not coagulate, while the semen of rodents such as the rat and guinea pig ejaculate a firm pellet that does not appear to liquefy (313,377). In rodents, the plugs form through the action of an enzyme called vesiculase, which comes from the anterior lobe of the prostate and reacts with seminal vesicle secretions. Because of this action, the anterior lobe of the rodent prostate is also called the coagulating gland. Vesiculase is not identical with thrombin, since it does not coagulate fibrinogen nor does thrombin clot the secretions of the seminal vesicles. Williams-Ashman and colleagues (384) have established that vesiculase has transamidase activity, catalyzing the formation of gamma-glutamyl-ϵ-lysine crosslinks in a clottable protein derived from the seminal vesicles. This seminal vesicle protein which serves as a substrate for vesiculase, is a very basic substance with a molecular weight of 17,900.

In summary, it appears that seminal plasma coagulation and liquefaction is under enzymatic control, but the biologic purpose of this process has not been resolved. Enzymes and proteins of the seminal vesicles and prostate glands are involved in this system. There have been reports that some infertile men may have impairment of the liquefaction process (385,388).

Seminal Plasma Analysis, Fertility

There have been several reviews related to semen analysis and fertility (3,385,386,389,390). Parson and Lipshultz (3) have suggested that there is evidence of antisperm antibodies, primarily the IgG and secretory IgA classes, that can impair sperm motility, possibly, sperm-egg fusion and possibly important factors in infertility, and they suggest the possibility of testing immunosuppressive treatment to block this impairment. Eliasson (386) emphasizes that decreased secretory function of the accessory genital glands is a common finding in men with acute and chronic infection or inflammation of the prostate or seminal vesicles, and further states that a decreased secretory capacity of the male sex accessory glands is not in itself a factor in infertility. Chemical alterations in the seminal plasma, however, may indicate abnormalities. Since seminal fructose is a secretory product of the seminal vesicles, it is often used as an index of the function of this gland. Fructose is absent from the semen in three conditions (385):

1. Azoospermic males with congenital bilateral absence of the vas deferens and seminal vesicles (Embryologically, the seminal vesicles and vas deferens develop from the Wolffian ducts; therefore, when the vas deferens is absent in development, so are the seminal vesicles, no fructose is present in the semen, and the ejaculate also does not coagulate.)
2. Obstruction of both ejaculatory ducts
3. The presence of retrograde ejaculation

Fructose analysis of the semen is a simple test and should be performed routinely in every case of azoospermia (385). For additional details on obstructive occlusions in the reproductive tract and diagnostic approaches, see the review of Marina and colleagues (391).

Prostatic Secretions and Drug Transport

Aumuller and Seitz (314) have reviewed the secretory mechanism for the sex accessory tissues. Isaacs (392) has also reviewed the concepts related to the fluid and drug transport properties of the prostate and seminal vesicles. He has compared the composition and volume of prostatic secretion under basal stimulation and under neurological stimulation during ejaculation or pilocarpine stimulation. He calculates that under neurological stimulation an increase of 205-fold in the total potassium, chloride, and sodium output over the basal secretory rate, and has shown that the prostate is capable of secreting 5 times its total content of sodium and chloride during this active secretion. This obviously shows the tremendous transport powers of this system. Smith and his colleagues (267) have studied the transepithelial voltage changes during prostatic secretion in the dog and have concluded that sodium may move passively through the plasma in the prostatic fluid during ejaculation but that the movement of potassium and chloride ions involves active transcellular transport.

Only a few compounds are capable of entering the semen by simple diffusion, including ethanol, iodine, and a few antibiotics. Drugs entering prostatic secretions have been of interest because of the prevalence of prostatitis and the need for new modalities of chemotherapy. Earlier, Stamey and his colleagues (393,394), have made extensive studies of the ability of chemotherapeutic agents to concentrate in the prostatic fluid of humans and dogs and many other laboratories have also contributed to this knowledge (395–398). Few drugs reach concentrations in the prostatic secretion that approach or surpass their concentrations in blood, but some exceptions are the basic macrolides, erythromycin and oleandomycin; sulfonamides; chloramphenicol; tetracycline; clindamycin, and trimethoprim (see ref. 399 for a review). In general, these drugs are assumed to pass across the membrane by nonionic diffusion, possibly by lipid solubility through the membrane; when they reach the more acidic prostatic fluid, they are protonated and acquire a more positive charge, thus the charged drugs become relatively trapped within the prostatic secretions. Several factors are critical, including the pK' of the drug and the pH of the prostatic secretions, as well as the drug binding to proteins in each compartment. Basic drugs would be more positively charged in acidic prostatic fluid than in blood. Slight changes in pH can have large effects on this nonionic diffusion. Samples of prostatic secretions from humans varied widely in pH from 6 to 8 with a mean value of 6.6; however, with prostatic inflammation the pH tended to be 7 or greater (400). It should be realized that, although prostatic secretions are slightly acidic, the pH of freshly ejaculated human semen is slightly alkaline (pH 7.3 to 7.7); on standing, semen first becomes more alkaline with the loss of carbon dioxide and then later acidic owing to accumulation of lactic acid.

Drugs may be developed in the future that are transported into the prostate as therapeutic agents, chemoprotectors, or as a route to the semen to regulate fertility; however, more must be learned about the fundamental transport system in and out of the male reproductive tract before such an approach is feasible.

REFERENCES

1. Price D. Comparative aspects of development and structure in the prostate. *Natl Cancer Inst Monogr* 1962;12:2.
2. Pietz B, Olds-Clark EP. Effect of seminal vesicle removal on fertility and uterine sperm motility in the house mouse. *Biol Reprod* 1988;35:608–17.

3. Parson SJ, Lipshultz LI. The effects of prostatic secretions on male fertility. In: Fitzpatrick JM, Krane RJ, eds. *The prostate.* New York: Churchill Livingston; 1989:53–9.
4. Smith ER, Hagopian M. Uptake in secretion of carcinogenic chemicals by the dog and rat prostate. In: Murphy GP, Sandberg AA, Karr JP, eds. *The prostate cell: structure and function,* Part B. New York: Alan Liss; 1981:131–63.
5. Borzy MS, Connell RS, Kiessling AA. Detection of human immunodeficiency virus in cell-free seminal fluid. *J AIDS* 1989;1:1–6.
6. Meltzer MS, Gendelman HE. Mononuclear phagocytes as targets, tissue reservoirs, and immunoregulatory cells in human immunodeficiency virus disease. *Curr Top Microbiol Immunol* 1992;181:239–63.
7. Anderson DJ, Wolff H, Pudney J, Wenhao Z, Martinez A, Mayer K. Presence of HIV in semen. In: Alexander NJ, Gabelnick HL, Spiler JM, eds. *Heterosexual transmission of AIDS.* New York: Alan R Liss; 1990:167–80.
8. Anderson DJ, Hill JA. CD4 (T4+) lymphocytes in semen of healthy heterosexual men: implication for the transmission of AIDS. *Fertil Steril* 1983;48:703.
9. Anderson DJ, Yunis EJ. "Trojan horse" leukocytes in acquired immunodeficiency syndrome (AIDS). *N Engl J Med* 1983; 309:984.
10. Dym M, Orenstein J. Structure of the male reproductive tract in AIDS patients: In: Alexander NJ, Gabelnick HL, Spieler JM, eds. *Heterosexual transmission of AIDS.* Wiley-Liss; New York: 1990:181–96.
11. Wolff H, Anderson DJ. Male genital tract inflammation is associated with increased numbers of potential human immunodeficiency virus host cells in semen. *Andrologia* 1988;20:404–5.
12. Carter HB, Coffey DS. The prostate: an increasing medical problem. *Prostate* 1990;16:39–48.
13. National Kidney and Urological Disease Advisory Board. *Long-range plan window on the 21st century.* National Institutes of Health Publ. 90-583. Bethesda, MD: US Department of Health & Human Services; 1990.
14. Walsh PC. Techniques for radical retropubic prostatectomy with preservation of sexual function: an anatomical approach. In: Skinner DJ, Lieskovsky G, eds. *Diagnosis and management of genitourinary cancer.* Philadelphia: WB Saunders; 1988:735–78.
15. Wang MC, Valenzuela LA, Murphy GP, Chu TM. Purification of a human prostate specific antigen. *Invest Urol* 1979;17: 159–63.
16. Papsidero LD, Wang MC, Valenzuela LA, Murphy GP, Chu TM. A prostate antigen in sera of prostatic cancer patients. *Cancer Res* 1980;40:2428–32.
17. Kuriyama M, Wang MC, Papsidero LD, et al. Quantitation of prostatic specific antigen in serum by a sensitive enzyme immunoassay. *Cancer Res* 1980;40:4658–62.
18. Kuriyama M, Wang MC, Lee CL, et al. Use of human prostate-specific antigen in monitoring prostate cancer. *Cancer Res* 1981;41:3874–6.
19. Killian CS, Yang N, Emrich JL, et al. Prognostic importance of prostate-specific antigen for monitoring patients with stages B2 to D1 prostate cancer. *Cancer Res* 1985;45:886–91.
20. Stamey TA, Wang N, Hay AR, et al. Prostate-specific antigen as a serum marker for adenocarcinoma of the prostate. *N Engl J Med* 1987;317:909–16.
21. Chan DW, Bruzek DJ, Oesterling JE, et al. Prostate-specific antigen as a marker of prostatic cancer: a monoclonal and a polyclonal immunoassay compared. *Clin Chem* 1987;33:1916–20.
22. Oesterling JE. Prostate specific antigen: a critical assessment of the most useful tumor marker for adenocarcinoma of the prostate. *J Urol* 1991;145:907–23.
23. Catalona WJ, Coffey DS, Karr JP. In: *Clinical aspects of prostate cancer: assessment of new diagnostic and management procedures.* New York: Elsevier; 1989.
24. Coffey DS, Resnick MI, Dorr FA, Karr JP. *A multidisciplinary analysis of controversies in the management of prostate cancer.* New York: Plenum; 1988.
25. Carter BS, Carter HB, Isaacs JT. Epidemiologic evidence regarding predisposing factors to prostate cancer. *Prostate* 1990;16: 187–97.
26. Aumuller G. In: *Prostate gland and seminal vesicles.* Berlin: Springer-Verlag; 1979.
27. McNeal JE. Anatomy of the prostate: an historical survey of divergent views. *Prostate* 1980;1:3.
28. Sugimura Y, Cunha GR, Donjacour AA, Bigsby RM, Brody JR. Whole mount autoradiography studies of DNA synthetic activity during postnatal development and androgen-induced regeneration in the mouse prostate. *Biol Reprod* 1986;34:985.
29. Cunha GR, Chung LWK, Shannon JM, Toguchi O, Fujii H. Hormonal induced morphogenesis and growth: role of the mesenchymal-epithelial interactions. *Recent Prog in Horm Res* 1983;39:559.
30. Bendell JL, Dorrington JH. Epidermal growth factor influences growth and differentiation of rat granulosa cells. *Endocrinology* 1990;127:533–40.
31. Jost A. Hormonal factors in development of the fetus. *Cold Spring Harbor Symp Quant Biol* 1954;19:167.
32. McNeal JE. Origin and evolution of benign prostatic enlargement. *Invest Urol* 1978;15:340–5.
33. Cunha GR, Alarid ET, Turner T, Donjacour AA, Boutin EL, Foster BA. Normal and abnormal development of the male urogenital tract. Role of androgens, mesenchymal-epithelial interactions, and growth factors. *J Androl* 1992;13:465–75.
34. Cunha GR, Fujii H, Neubauer BL, Shannon JM, Sawyer L, Reese BA. Epithelial-mesenchymal interactions in prostatic development: I. Morphological observations of prostatic induction by urogenital sinus mesenchyma in epithelium of the adult rodent urinary bladder. *J Cell Biol* 1983;96:1662–70.
35. Chung LWK, Cunha GR. Stromal-epithelial interactions: II. Regulation of prostatic growth by embryonic urogenital sinus mesenchyme. *Prostate* 1983;4:503.
36. Chung LWK, Matsuura J, Rocco AK, Thompson TC, Miller GJ, Runner MN. A new mouse model for prostatic hyperplasia: Induction of adult prostatic overgrowth of fetal urogenital sinus implants. In: Kimball FA, Buhl AE, Carter DB, eds. *New approaches to the study of benign prostatic hyperplasia.* New York: Alan Liss; 1984:291.
37. Chung LWK, Matsuura J, Rocco AK, Thompson TC, Miller GJ, Runner MN. Tissue interactions in prostatic growth: a new mouse model for prostatic hyperplasia. *Ann NY Acad Sci* 1984;438:394–404.
38. Chung LWK, Thompson TC, Chao H, Bell C, Ruth JA. Catecholamines are involved in stromal-epithelial interactions in the rat ventral prostate gland. In: Rodgers CH, Coffey DS, Cunha G, Grayhack JT, Hinman F, Horton R, eds. *Benign prostatic hyperplasia,* vol. 2. National Institutes of Health Publ. 87-2881. Bethesda, MD: US Department of Health & Human Services; 1987:27–33.
39. Chung LWK, Matsuura J, Runner MR. Tissue interactions and prostatic growth: I. Induction of adult mouse prostatic hyperplasia by fetal urogenital sinus implants. *Biol Reprod* 1984; 31:155–63.
40. Thompson TC, Chung LWK. Regulation of overgrowth and expression of prostatic binding protein in rat chimeric prostate gland. *Endocrinology* 1986;118:2437–44.
41. Andrews GS. The histology of the human fetal and prepubertal prostate. *J Anat* 1951;85:44–54.
42. Forest MG. Plasma androgens (testosterone and 4-androstenedione) and 17-hydroxyprogesterone in the prenatal, prepubertal and peripubertal periods in the human and the rat: differences between species. *J Steroid Biochem* 1979;11:543–8.
43. Pang S, Levine L, Chow D, Sagiani F, Saenger P, New M. Dihydrotestosterone and its relationship to testosterone in infancy and childhood. *J Clin Endocrinol Metab* 1979;48:821–6.
44. Kincl FA, Folch Pi AF, Herrera Lasso LH. The effect of estradiol benzoate treatment in the newborn male rat. *Endocrinology* 1963;72:966–8.
45. Swanson HE, Vanderwer FF, Werff ten Bosch JJ van der. Sex differences in growth of rats and their modification by a single injection of testosterone propionate shortly after birth. *J Endocrinol* 1963;26:197–207.
46. Morrison RL, Johnson DC. The effects of androgenation in male rats castrated at birth. *J Endocrinol* 1966;34:117–23.

47. Bronson FH, Whisett MJ, Hamilton TH. Responsiveness of accessory glands of adult mice to testosterone: priming with neonatal injections. *Endocrinology* 1972;90:10–6.
48. Rajfer J, Coffey DS. Sex steroid imprinting of the immature prostate: Long term effects. *Invest Urol* 1979;16:186.
49. Rajfer J, Coffey DS. Effects of neonatal steroids on male sex tissues. *Invest Urol* 1979;17:3.
50. Chung LWK, McFadden DK. Sex steroid imprinting and prostatic growth. *Invest Urol* 1980;17:337.
51. Naslund MJ, Coffey DS. The differential effects of neonatal androgens, estrogens and progesterones on adult rat prostate growth. *J Urol* 1986;136:1126–40.
52. Naslund MJ, Coffey DS. The hormonal imprinting of the prostate and the regulation of stem cells in prostatic growth. In: Rodgers CH, Coffey DS, Cunha G, Grayhack JT, Hinman F Jr, Horton R, eds. *Benign prostatic hyperplasia,* vol. 2. NIH Publication No. 87-2881. Bethesda, MD: US Department of Health & Human Services; 1987:73–83.
53. Higgins SJ, Smith SE, Wilson J. Development of secretory protein synthesis in the seminal vesicle and ventral prostate of the male rat. *Mol Cell Endocrinol* 1982;27:55–65.
54. Narbaitz R. Embryology, anatomy and histology of the male accessory glands. *In:* Brandes D, ed. *Male accessory sex organs: structure and function in mammals.* New York: Academic Press; 1974:3–17.
55. McNeal JE. Normal histology of the prostate. *Am J Surg Pathol* 1988;12:619.
56. McNeal JE. Pathology of benign prostatic hyperplasia. *Urol Clin North Am* 1990;17:477–86.
57. Berry SJ, Coffey DS, Walsh PC, Ewing LL. The development of human benign prostatic hyperplasia with age. *J Urol* 1984;132:474–9.
58. Aumuller G, Riva A. Morphology and functions of the human seminal vesicle. *Andrologia* 1992;24:183–96.
59. LeDuc IE. The anatomy of the prostate and the pathology of early benign prostatic hypertrophy. *J Urol* 1939;42:1217.
60. Franks LM. Benign nodular hyperplasia of the prostate: a review. *Ann R Coll Surgeons* 1954;14:92.
61. Young HH. *Young's practice of urology,* vol. 1. Philadelphia: WB Saunders; 1926:419.
62. Huggins C, Webster WO. Duality of human prostate in response to estrogen. *J Urol* 1948;59:258.
63. McNeal JE. Regional morphology and pathology of the prostate. *Am J Clin Pathol* 1968;49:347.
64. McNeal JE. Developmental and comparative anatomy of the prostate. In: Grayhack JT, Wilson JD, Scherbenske, eds. *Benign prostatic hyperplasia.* Proceedings of a workshop sponsored by the Kidney Disease and Urology Program of the NIAMDD. Washington, DC: US Government Printing Office; 1976:1–6.
65. McNeal JE. The zonal anatomy of the prostate. *Prostate* 1981;1:35.
66. Tisell LE, Salander H. The lobes of the human prostate. *Scand J Urol Nephrol* 1975;9:185.
67. Blacklock NJ, Bouskill K. The zonal anatomy of the prostate in man and the rhesus monkey. *Urol Res* 1977;5:163.
68. Villers A, Steg A, Boccon-Gibod L. Anatomy of the prostate: review of the different models. *Eur Urol* 1991;20:261–8.
69. Isaacs JT, Coffey DS. Etiology and disease processes of benign prostatic hyperplasia. *Prostate* 1989;2(Suppl):33–50.
70. DeKlerk DP, Heston WDW, Coffey DS. Studies on the role of macromolecular synthesis in the growth of the prostate. In: Grayhack JT, Wilson JD, Scherbenske MJ, eds. *Benign prostatic hyperplasia.* Proceedings of a workshop sponsored by the Kidney Disease and Urology Program of the NIAMDD. Washington, DC: US Government Printing Office; 1976:43–51.
71. Kastendieck H. Ultrastrukturpathologie der menschlichen Prostatadruse: Cyto- und Histomorphogeneses von Atrophie, Hyperplasie, Metaplasie, Dysplasie und Carcinom. *Veroeff Pathol* 1977;106.
72. Isaacs WB. *Structural and functional components in normal and hyperplastic prostate.* [Doctoral dissertation]. Department of Pharmacology, Baltimore: The Johns Hopkins University School of Medicine, 1984.
73. Merk FB, Ofner P, Kwan PWL, Leav I, Vena RL. Ultrastructural and biochemical expression of divergent differentiation in prostates of castrated dogs treated with estrogens and androgens. *Lab Invest* 1982;47:437.
74. Evans GS, Chandler JA. Cell proliferation studies in the rat prostate: II. The effects of castration and androgen-induced regeneration upon basal and secretory cell proliferation. *Prostate* 1987;11:339–51.
75. Dermer GB. Basal cell proliferation in benign prostatic hyperplasia. *Cancer* 1978;41:1857–62.
76. Sinowatz F, Gabius HJ, Hellmann KP, Amselgruber W, Schneider MR. Expression of endogenous receptor for neoglycoproteins in Dunning R-3327 rat prostatic carcinoma. *Prostate* 1990;16:173–84.
77. Merk FB, Warhol MJ, Kwan P, et al. Multiple phenotypes of prostatic glandular cells in castrated dogs after individual or combined treatment with androgens and estrogens. *Lab Invest* 1986;54:442–56.
78. Abrahmsson PA, Lilija H. Partial characterization of a thyroid-stimulating hormone-like peptide in neuroendocrine cells of the human prostate gland. *Prostate* 1989;14:71–81.
79. Abrahmsson PA, Wadstrom LB, Alumets J, Falkmer S, Grameliu L. Peptide hormone-serotonin-immunoreactive cells in normal and hyperplastic prostate glands. *Pathol Res Pract* 1986;181:675–83.
80. Davis NS. Determination of serotonin and 5-hydroxyendolacetic acid in guinea pig and human prostate using HPLC. *Prostate* 1987;11:353–60.
81. diSant-Agnese PA, deMesy-Jensen KL, Churukien CJ, Agarwall MM. Human prostatic endocrine-paracrine (APUD) cells: distribution analysis for the comparison of serotonin and neuron-specific amylase immunoreactivity in silver stains. *Arch Pathol Lab Med* 1985;109:607–12.
82. diSant-Agnese PA, deMesy-Jensen KL. Endocrine-paracrine cells of the prostate and prostatic urethra: an ultrastructural study. *Hum Pathol* 1984;15:1034–41.
83. Guthrie PD, Freeman MR, Liao S, Chung LWK. Regulation of gene expression in rat prostate by androgen and β-adrenergic receptor pathways. *Mol Endocrinol* 1990;4:1343–53.
84. Thompson TC, Zhau H, Chung LWK. Catecholamines are involved in the growth and expansion of prostatic binding protein by the rat ventral prostatic tissue. *Prog Clin Biol Res* 1987;239:239–48.
85. Higgins JRA, Gosling JA. Studies of the structure and intrinsic innervation of the normal human prostate. *Prostate* 1989; 2(Suppl):5–16.
86. Reese JH, McNeil JE, Redwine EA, Samloff IN, Stamey TA, Freiha FS. Tissue type plasminogen activator as a marker for functional zones, within the human prostate gland. *Prostate* 1988;12:47–53.
87. Lepor H, Kuhar MJ. Characterization and localization of the muscarinic cholinergic receptor in human prostate tissue. *J Urol* 1984;132:397–402.
88. Lepor H, Shapiro E. Characterization of the alpha-1 adrenergic receptor in human benign prostatic hyperplasia. *J Urol* 1984;132:1226–9.
89. Lepor H, Shapiro E, Gup DI, Baumann M. Laboratory assessment of terazosin and alpha1 blockade in prostatic hyperplasia. *Urology* 1988;32(Suppl):21.
90. Lepor H. Role of long-acting selective $\alpha 1$ blocker in the treatment of benign prostatic hyperplasia. *Urol Clin North Am* 1990;17:651–9.
91. Mawhinney M. The extracellular matrix and cellular proliferation in etiology of benign prostatic hyperplasia. In: Ackermann R, Schroeder FA, eds. *Prostatic hyperplasia: new developments in biosciences V.* 1989;55–62.
92. Aumuller G. Morphology and endocrine aspects of prostatic function. *Prostate* 1983;4:195.
93. Rohr HP, Bartsch G. Human benign prostatic hyperplasia: a stromal disease? *Urology* 1980;16:625–33.
94. Getzenberg RH, Pienta KJ, Coffey DS. The tissue matrix: cell dynamics and hormone action. *Endocr Rev* 1990;11:399–416.
95. Ellis DW, Leffer S, Davies J, Meek NG. Multiple immunoperoxidase markers in benign prostatic hyperplasia and adenocarcinoma of the prostate. *Am J Clin Pathol* 1984;81:279–84.

96. Purnell DM, Heathfield BM, Trump BF. Immunocytochemical evaluation of human prostatic carcinomas for carcinoembryonic antigen, nonspecific cross-reactivating antigen, beta chorionic gonadotropins and prostate-specific antigen. *Cancer Res* 1984; 44:285–92.
97. Achtstatter TH, Moll R, Moore B, Franke WW. Cytokeratin polypeptide patterns of different epithelial cells from human male urogenital tract: immunofluorescence and gel electrophoretic studies. *J Histochem Cytochem* 1985;33:415–26.
98. Brawer MK, Peehl DM, Stamey T, Bostwick DG. Keratin immunoreactivity in the benign and neoplastic human prostate. *Cancer Res* 1985;45:3663–7.
99. Warner TN, Dohm G. Immunohistochemistry of the prostate and diverse prostate carcinomas. In: Krieg K, Senge Th, eds. *New aspects in the regulation of prostatic function.* Cansteiner Colloquium, Schloss Canstein. München: Zuckschwerdt; 1989: 69–81.
100. Sinha AA, Gleason DF, Wilson MJ, et al. Immunohistochemical localization of laminin in basement membranes of normal, hyperplastic and neoplastic human prostate. *Prostate* 1989;15: 299–313.
101. Bartsch G, Brungger A, Schweikert U, et al. The importance of stromal tissue in benign prostatic hyperplasia: morphological, immunofluorescence and endocrinological investigations. In: Kimball FA, Buhl AE, Carter DB, eds. *New approaches to the study of benign prostatic hyperplasia.* New York: Alan Liss; 1984:179.
102. Hay ED, ed. *The cell biology of the extracellular matrix.* New York: Plenum, 1981.
103. Arcadi JA. Role of ground substance in atrophy of normal and malignant prostatic tissue following estrogen administration in orchiectomy. *J Clin Endocrinol Metab* 1954;14:1113.
104. DeKlerk DP. Glycosoaminoglycans of benign prostatic hyperplasia. *Prostate* 1983;4:73.
105. Chan L, Wong YC. Cytochemical characterization of cuprolinic blue stain proteoglycans in the epithelial-stromal interface of the guinea pig lateral prostate. *Prostate* 1989;14:133–45.
106. Chan L, Wong YC. Ultrastructural localization of proteoglycans by cationic dyes in the epithelial-stromal interface of the guinea pig lateral prostate. *Prostate* 1989;14:147–62.
107. Hiler L. *The effects of hormones on the proteoglycans of the rat prostate.* [Doctoral dissertation]. Baltimore: Department of Pathology, University of Maryland Medical School, 1987.
108. Kofoed JA, Tumilasci OR, Curbelo HM, Fernandez-Lemos SM, Arias NH, Houssay AB. Effect of castration of androgens upon prostatic proteoglycans in rats. *Prostate* 1990;16:93–102.
109. Thornton MO, Frederickson R, Matal J, Mawhinney M. Preliminary studies on the relationship between collagen and the growth of the male accessory sex organ epithelial cells. In: Kimball FA, Buehl AE, Carter DP, eds. *New approaches to the study of benign prostatic hyperplasia,* New York: Alan Liss; 1984:143.
110. Hammond GL. Endogenous steroid levels in the human prostate from birth to old age: a comparison of normal and diseased states. *J Endocrinol* 1978;78:7.
111. Bruchovsky N, Wilson JD. The conversion of testosterone to 5α-androstan-17β-ol-3-one by rat prostate in vivo and in vitro. *J Biol Chem* 1968;243:2012.
112. Bruchovsky N, Wilson JD. The intranuclear binding of testosterone and 5α-androstan-17β-ol-3-one by rat prostate. *J Biol Chem* 1968;243:5953.
113. Anderson KM, Liao S. Selective retention of dihydrotestosterone by prostatic nuclei. *Nature* 1968;219:277.
114. Shimazaki J, Kurihara H, Ito Y, Shida K. Metabolism of testosterone in prostate: separation of prostatic 17b-ol-dehydrogenase and 5α-reductase. *Gunma J Med Sci* 1965;14:326.
115. Shimazaki J, Kurihara H, Ito Y, Shida K. Testosterone metabolism in prostate: formation of androstane-17b-ol-3-one and androst-4-ene-3,17a-dione, and inhibitory effect of natural and synthetic estrogens. *Gunma J Med Sci* 1965;14:313.
116. Farnsworth WE, Brown JR. Testosterone metabolism in the prostate. In: Vollmer EP, ed. Biology of the prostate and related tissues. *Natl Cancer Inst Monogr* 1963;12:323–9.
117. Walsh PC, Gittes RF. Inhibition of extratesticular stimuli to prostatic growth in the castrate rat by antiandrogens. *Endocrinology* 1970;87:624.
118. Tisell LE. Effect of cortisone on the growth of the ventral prostate, the dorsolateral prostate, the coagulating gland and the seminal vesicles in castrated adrenalectomized and in castrated nonadrenalectomized rats. *Acta Endocrinol* 1970;64:637.
119. Tullner WW. Hormonal factors in the adrenal dependent growth of the rat ventral prostate. In: Vollmer EP, ed. Biology of the prostate and related tissues. *Natl Cancer Inst Monogr* 1963;12:211.
120. Oesterling JE, Epstein JI, Walsh PC. The inability of adrenal androgens to stimulate the adult prostate: an autopsy evaluation of men with hypogonadotropic hypogonadism and panhypopituitarism. *J Urol* 1986;136:103–4.
121. Mobbs BJ, Johnson LE, Connolly JG. Influence of the adrenal gland on prostatic activity in adult rats. *J Endocrinol* 1973;59:335.
122. Kyprianou N, Isaacs JT. Significance of measurable androgen levels in the rat ventral prostate following castration. *Prostate* 1987;10:313–24.
123. Horton RJ. Androgen hormones and prehormones in young and elderly men. In: Grayhack JT, Wilson JD, Scherbenske MJ, eds. *Benign prostatic hyperplasia.* Proceedings of a workshop sponsored by the Kidney Disease and Urology Program of the NIAMDD. Washington, DC: US Government Printing Office; 1976:183–8.
124. MacDonald PC. Origin of Estrogen in Men. In Grayhack JT, Wilson JD, Scherbenske MJ, eds. *Benign prostatic hyperplasia.* Proceedings of a workshop sponsored by the Kidney Disease and Urology Program of the NIAMDD, Feb 20–21, 1975. Washington, DC: US Government Printing Office; 1976:191–2.
125. Siiteri PK, MacDonald PC. Role of extraglandular estrogen in human endocrinology. *Handb Physiol* 1973;2:615–29.
126. Dorrington JH, Armstrong DT. Follicle stimulating hormone stimulates estradiol-17β synthesis in cultured Sertoli cells. *Proc Natl Acad Sci USA* 1975;72:2677.
127. Vermeulen A. Testicular hormonal secretion and aging in males. In: Grayhack JT, Wilson JD, Scherbenske MJ, eds. *Benign prostatic hyperplasia.* Proceedings of a workshop sponsored by the Kidney Disease and Urology Program of the NIAMDD, Feb. 20–21, 1975. Washington, DC: US Government Printing Office; 1976:177.
128. Vermeulen A, Verdonck L, Van der Straeten M, Orie N. Capacity of the TeBG in human plasma and influence of specific binding of testosterone on its metabolic clearance rate. *J Clin Endocrinol* 1969;29:1470.
129. Burton RM, Westphal U. Steroid hormone binding proteins in blood plasma. *Metabolism* 1972;21:253.
130. Forest MG, Rivarola MA, Migeon CJ. Percentage binding of testosterone, androstenedione and dehydroisoandrosterone in human plasma. *Steroids* 1968;12:323.
131. Lasnitzki I, Franklin HR. The influence of serum on uptake, conversion and action of testosterone in rat prostate glands in organ culture. *J Endocrinol* 1972;54:333.
132. Anderson DC, Marshall JC, Galuao-Teles A, et al. Gynaecomastia and impotence associated with testosterone binding. *Proc R Soc Med* 1972;65:787.
133. Rosner W, Hryb DJ, Khan MS, Hakhla AM, Romas NA. Sex hormone-binding globulin: anatomy and physiology of a new regulatory system. *J Steroid Biochem Mol Biol* 1991;40:813–20.
134. Grayhack JT, Bunce PL, Kearns JW, Scott WW. Influence of the pituitary on prostatic response to androgen in the rat. *Bull Johns Hopkins Hosp* 1955;96:154.
135. Assimos D, Smith C, Lee C, Grayhack JT. Action of prolactin in regressing prostate: independent of action mediated by androgen receptors. *Prostate* 1984;5:589–95.
136. Moger WH, Geschwind LL. The action of prolactin on the sex accessory glands of the male rat. *Proc Soc Exp Biol Med* 1972;141:101.
137. Lloyd JW, Thomas JA, Mawhinney MG. A difference in the in vitro accumulation and metabolism by the rat prostate gland with prolactin. *Steroids* 1973;22:473.
138. Aragona C, Friesen HG. Specific prolactin binding sites in the prostate and testis of rat. *Endocrinology* 1975;97:677.
139. Manandhar MSP, Thomas JA. Effect of prolactin on the metabo-

lism of androgens by the rat ventral prostate. *Invest Urol* 1976;14:20.
140. Lee C, Hopkins D, Holland JM. Reduction in prostatic concentration of endogenous dihydrotestosterone in rats by hyperprolactinemia. *Prostate* 1985;6:361–367.
141. Witorsch RJ, Smith JP. Evidence for androgen-independent intracellular binding of prolactin in the rat ventral prostate gland. *Endocrinology* 1977;101:929–938.
142. McKeehan WL, Adams PS, Rosser MP. Direct mitogenic effects of insulin, epidermal growth factor, glucocorticoid, cholera toxin, unknown pituitary factors and possibly prolactin, but not androgens, on normal rat prostate epithelial cells in serum-free primary cell culture. *Cancer Res* 1984;44:1998–2010.
143. Birkoff JD, Lattimer JK, Frantz AG. Role of prolactin in benign prostatic hyperplasia. *Urology* 1974;4:557.
144. Angervall L, Hesselsjo R, Nilsson S, Tissel LE. Action of testosterone on ventral prostate, dorsolateral prostate, coagulating glands, and seminal vesicles of castrated alloxan-diabetic rats. *Diabetologia* 1967;3:395.
145. Sufrin G, Prutkin L. Experimental diabetes and the response of the sex accessory organs on the castrate male rat to testosterone propionate. *Invest Urol* 1974;11:361.
146. Calame SS, Lostroh AJ. Effect of insulin and lack of effect of testosterone on the protein of ventral prostate from castrate mice maintained as organ cultures. *Endocrinology* 1964;75:451.
147. Lostroh AJ. Effect of testosterone and insulin in vitro on maintenance and repair of the secretory epithelium of the mouse prostate. *Endocrinology* 1971;88:500.
148. Isaacs JT, Coffey DS. Changes in dihydrotestosterone metabolism associated with the development of canine benign prostatic hyperplasia. *Endocrinology* 1981;108:445.
149. Isaacs JT, Coffey DS. Androgen metabolism of the prostate: new concepts related to normal and abnormal growth. In: Everett JE, Altwein G, Bartsch G, Jacoby GH, eds. *Antihormones: Bedeutung in der Urologie.* Munchen: Zuckschwerdt; 1981.
150. Isaacs JT, Berry SJ. Changes in dihydrotestosterone metabolism in development of benign prostatic hyperplasia in the aging beagle. *J Steroid Biochem* 1983;18:749–757.
151. Isaacs JT, Brendler CB, Walsh PC. Changes in the metabolism of dihydrotestosterone in the hyperplastic human prostate. *J Clin Endocrinol Metab* 1983;56:139–146.
152. Bruchovsky N, Dunstan-Adams E. Regulation of 5α-reductase activity in stroma and epithelium of human prostate. In: Bruchovsky N, et al., eds. *Regulation of androgen action.* Proceedings of an International Symposium. Berlin: Congressdruck R. Bruckner; 1985:31–34.
153. Anderson S, Russell DW. Structural and biochemical properties of cloned and expressed human and rat steroid 5α-reductases. *Proc Natl Acad Sci USA* 1990;87:3640–3644.
154. Stoner E. The clinical development of a 5-alpha-reductase inhibitor, finasteride. *J Steroid Biochem Mol Biol* 1990;37:375–378.
155. Steiner JF. Finasteride: a 5-alpha-reductase inhibitor. *Clin Pharmacol* 1993;12:15–23.
156. Walsh PC, Wilson JD. The induction of prostatic hypertrophy in the dog with androstanediol. *J Clin Invest* 1976;57:1093.
157. DeKlerk DP, Coffey DS, Ewing LL, et al. Comparison of spontaneously and experimentally induced canine prostatic hyperplasia. *J Clin Invest* 1979;64:842.
158. Tunn S, Senge Th, Schenck B, Neumann F. Biochemical and histological studies on prostates in castrated dogs after treatment with androstanediol, estradiol and cyproterone acetate. *Acta Endocrinol* 1979;91:373–384.
159. Juniewicz PE, Lemp BM, Barbolt TA, Labrie TK, Batzold FH, Reel JR. Dose-dependent hormonal induction of benign prostatic hyperplasia (BPH) in castrated dogs. *Prostate* 1989;14: 341–352.
160. Trachtenberg J, Hicks LL, Walsh PC. Methods for the determination of androgen receptor concentration in human prostatic tissue. *Invest Urol* 1981;18:349.
161. Coffey DS, Walsh PC. Clinical and experimental studies in benign prostatic hyperplasia. *Urol Clin North Am* 17, pp. 461–476.
162. Moore RJ, Gazak JM, Quebbeman JF, Wilson JD. Concentration of dihydrotestosterone in 3a-androstanediol in naturally occurring and androgen induced prostatic hyperplasia in the dog. *J Clin Invest* 1979;64:1003.
163. Ehrlichman RJ, Isaacs JT, Coffey DS. Differences in the effects of estradiol on dihydrotestosterone-induced growth of the castrate rat and dog. *Invest Urol* 1981;18:466–470.
164. Habenicht U-F, El Etreby MF. The periurethral zone of the prostate of the cynomologus monkey is the most sensitive prostate part for an estrogenic stimulus. *Prostate* 1988;13:305–316.
165. Neubauer B, Bisser T, Jones CD, et al. Antagonism of androgen and estrogen effects in the guinea pig seminal vesicle, epithelium and fibromuscular stroma by keoxifene (LY 156758). *Prostate* 1989;15:273–286.
166. Mawhinney MG, Neubauer BL. Action of estrogens in the male. *Invest Urol* 1979;16:409–420.
167. Mariotti J, Mawhinney MG. Androgenic regulation of estrogenic action on accessory sex organ smooth muscle. *J Urol* 1983;129:180–185.
168. Goodwin WE, Cummings RH. Squamous metaplasia of the verumontanum with obstruction due to hypertrophy: long term effects of estrogen on the prostate in aging male to female transsexuals. *J Urol* 1984;131:553–554.
169. deVoogt HJ, Rao BR, Geldof AA, Gooren LJG, Bauman FG. Androgen action blockade does not result in reduction in size but changes the histology of the normal human prostate. *Prostate* 1987;11:305–311.
170. Kozak I, Bartsch W, Krieg M, Voigt K. Nuclei stroma: Site of highest estrogen concentration in human benign prostatic hyperplasia. *Prostate* 1982;3:433–438.
171. Schulze H, Barrack ER. The immunocytochemical localization of estrogen receptors in the normal male and female canine urinary tract and prostate. *Endocrinology* 1987;121:1773–1783.
172. Schulze H, Barrack ER. The immunocytochemical localization of estrogen receptors in spontaneous and experimentally induced canine prostatic hyperplasia. *Prostate* 1987;11:145–162.
173. Mobbs BJ, Johnson LE, Liu Y. The quantitation of cytosolic and nuclear estrogen and progesterone receptors in benign, untreated and treated malignant human prostatic tissue by radioligand binding and enzyme immunoassays. *Prostate* 1990;16:235–244.
174. Eaton CL, Hamilton TC, Kenvyn K, Pierrepoint CG. Studies of androgen and estrogen binding in normal canine prostatic tissue and epithelial stromal cell lines derived from the canine prostate. *Prostate* 1985;7:377.
175. Krieg M, Klotzl G, Kaufmann J, Voigt KD. Stroma of human benign prostatic hyperplasia: Preferential tissues for androgen metabolism and estrogen binding. *Acta Endocrinol* 1981;96: 422–432.
176. Donnelly BJ, Lakey WH, McBlain WA. Estrogen receptors in human benign prostatic hyperplasia. *J Urol* 1983;130:183.
177. Stone NN, Fair WR, Fishman J. Estrogen formation in human prostatic tissue from patients with and without benign prostatic hyperplasia. *Prostate* 1986;9:311.
178. Oesterling JE, Juniewicz PE, Walters JR, et al. Aromatase inhibition in the dog: II. Effects of growth, function and pathology of the prostate. *J Urol* 1988;139:832–839.
179. Schreiter F, Fuchs P, Stockamp K. Estrogenic sensitivity of α-receptors in the urethra musculature. *Urol Int* 1976;31:13.
180. Husmann DA, Wilson CM, McPhaul MJ, Tilley WD, Wilson JD. Anti-peptide antibodies to two distinct regions of the androgen receptor localize the receptor protein to the nuclei of target cells in the rat and human prostate. *Endocrinology* 1990;126: 2359–23568.
181. Barrack ER, Tindall DJ. A critical evaluation of the use of androgen receptor assays to predict the androgen responsiveness of prostate cancer. In: Coffey DS, et al., eds. *Current concepts and approaches to the study of prostate cancer.* New York: Alan R. Liss; 1987:155–187.
182. Chang C, Kokontis J, Liao S. Molecular cloning of human and rat complementary DNA in coding androgen receptors. *Science* 1988;240:324–326.
183. Lubahn DB, Josephs DR, Sullivan PM, Willard HF, French FS, Wilson AM. Cloning of the human androgen receptor complementary DNA and localization to the X chromosome. *Science* 1988;240:327–330.

184. Lubahn DB, Josephs DR, Sar M, et al. The human androgen receptor: complementary deoxyribonucleic acid cloning sequence analysis and gene expression in prostate. *Mol Endocrinol* 1988;2:1265–1275.
185. Marcelli M, Tilley WD, Wilson CM, Griffin JE, Wilson JD, McPhaul MF. Definition of the human androgen receptor gene structure permits the identification of mutations that cause androgen resistance: premature termination of the receptor protein at amino acid residue 588 causes complete androgen resistance. *Mol Endocrinol* 1990;4:1105–1116.
186. Kuiper GGJM, Faber PW, van Rooij HCG, van der Korput JAGM, et al. Structural organization of the human androgen receptor gene. *J Mol Endocrinol* 1989;2:R1–R4.
187. Tilley WD, Marcelli M, Wilson JD, McPhaul MJ. Characterization and expression of cDNA encoding the human androgen receptor. *Proc Natl Acad Sci USA* 1989;86:327–331.
188. Chang C, Kokontis J, Liao S. Structural analysis of the complementary DNA in amino acid sequence of human and rat androgen receptor. *Proc Natl Acad Sci USA* 1988;85:7211–7215.
189. Tilley WD, Marcelli M, McPhaul MJ. Recent studies of the androgen receptor: new insights into old questions. *Mol Cell Endocrinol* 1990;68:C7–C10.
190. Brown TR, Lubahn DB, Wilson EM, Josephs DR, French FW, Migeon CJ. Deletion of the steroid-binding domain of the human androgen receptor gene in one family with complete androgen insensitivity syndrome: evidence for further genetic heterogeneity in this syndrome. *Proc Natl Acad Sci USA* 1988;85: 8151–8155.
191. Newmark JR, Hardy DO, Tonb DC, et al. Androgen receptor gene mutation in human prostate cancer. *Proc Natl Acad Sci USA* 1992;89:6319–6323.
192. Barrack ER. Steroid hormone receptor localization in the nuclear matrix: interaction with acceptor sites. *J Steroid Biochem* 1987;27:115.
193. Spelsberg TC, Ruh T, Ruh M, et al. Nuclear acceptor sites for steroid hormone receptors: Comparisons of steroids and antisteroids. *J Steroid Biochem* 1988;31:579–592.
194. Darling DS, Beebe JS, Burnside J, Winslow ER, Chin WW. 3,5,3′-Triiodothyronine (T#) receptor-auxiliary protein (TRAP) binds DNA and forms heterodimers with the T3 receptor. *Mol Endocrinol* 1991;5:73–74.
195. Parker MG, ed. *Nuclear hormone receptors: molecular mechanisms, cellular functions, clinical abnormalities.* London: Academic Press; 1991.
196. Forman BM, Samuels HH. Interactions among a subfamily of nuclear hormone receptors: the regulatory zipper model. *Mol Endocrinol* 1990;4:1293–1301.
197. Härd T, Kellenbach E, Boelens R, et al. Solution structure of the glucocorticoid receptor DNA-binding domain. *Science* 1990; 249:157–160.
198. Guiochon-Mantel A, Loosfelt H, Lescop P, et al. Mechanisms of nuclear translocation of the progesterone receptor: evidence for interaction between monomers. *Cell* 1989;57:1147–1154.
199. Simental JA, Sar M, Lane MV, French FS, Wilson EM. Transcriptional activation and nuclear targeting signals of the human androgen receptor. *J Biol Chem* 1991;266:510–518.
200. Trapman J, Klaassen P, Kuiper GGJM, et al. Cloning, structure and expression of a cDNA encoding the human androgen receptor. *Biochem Biophys Res Commun* 1988;153:241–248.
201. Laudet V, Hänni C, Coll J, Catzeflis F, Stéhelin D. Evolution of the nuclear receptor gene superfamily. *EMBO J* 1992;11: 1003–13.
202. Amero SA, Kretsinger RH, Moncrief ND, Yamamoto KR, Pearson WR. The origin of nuclear receptor proteins: a single precursor distinct from other transcription factors. *Mol Endocrinol* 1992;6:3–7.
203. Govindan MV. Specific regions in hormone binding domains is essential for hormone binding and trans-activation by human androgen receptor. *Mol Endocrinol* 1990;4:417–427.
204. Roche PJ, Hoare SA, Parker MG. A consensus DNA-binding site for the androgen receptor. *Mol Endocrinol* 1992;6:2229–2235.
205. Ham J, Thomson A, Needham M, Webb P, Parker M. Characterization of response elements for androgens, glucocorticoids, and progestins in mouse, mammary tumour virus. *Nucl Acids Res* 1988;16:5263–5267.
206. Claessens F, Celis L, Peeters B, Heyns W, Verhoeven G, Rombauts W. Functional characterization of an androgen response element in the first intron of the C3(1) gene of prostatic binding protein. *Biochem Biophys Res Commun* 1989;164:833–840.
207. Denison SH, Sands A, Tindall DJ. A tyrosine aminotransferase glucocorticoid response element also mediates androgen enhancement of gene expression. *Endocrinology* 1989;124:1091–1093.
208. Rennie PS, Bruchovsky N, Leco KJ, et al. Characterization of two cis-acting DNA elements involved in the androgen regulation of the probasin gene. *Mol Endocrinol* 1993;7:23–36.
209. Loreni F, Stavenhagen J, Kalff M, Robins DM. A complex androgen-responsive enhancer resides 2 kilobases upstream of the mouse Slp gene. *Mol Cell Biol* 1988;8:2350–2360.
210. Crozat A, Palvimo JJ, Julkunen M, Janne OA. Comparison of androgen regulation of ornithine decarboxylase and S-adenosylmethionine decarboxylase gene expression in rodent kidney and accessory sex organs. *Endocrinology* 1992;130: 1131–1144.
211. Riegman PHJ, Vlietstra RJ, van der Korput JAGM, Brinkmann AO, Trapman J. The promoter of the prostate specific antigen gene contains a functional androgen responsive element. *Mol Endocrinol* 1991;5:1921–1930.
212. King RJB, Mainwaring WIP. *Steroid-cell interactions.* Baltimore: University Park Press; 1974.
213. King WJ, Greene GL. Monoclonal antibodies localize oestrogen receptor in the nuclei of target cells. *Nature* 1984;307:745–747.
214. Welshons WV, Lieberman ME, Gorski J. Nuclear localization of unoccupied oestrogen receptors. *Nature* 1984;307:747–749.
215. Perrot-Applanat M, Logeat F, Groyer-Picard MT, Milgrom E. Immunocytochemical study of mammalian progesterone receptor using monoclonal antibodies. *Endocrinology* 1985;116: 1473–1484.
216. Gasc JM, Renoir JM, Faber LE, Delahaye F, Baulieu EE. Nuclear localization of two steroid receptor-associated proteins, hsp90 and p59. *Exp Cell Res* 1989;181:492–504.
217. Antakly T, Eisen HJ. Immunocytochemical localization of glucocorticoid receptor in target cells. *Endocrinology* 1984;115: 1984–1989.
218. Wikström A-C, Bakke O, Okret S, Brönnegård M, Gustafsson J-A. Intracellular localization of the glucocorticoid receptor: evidence for cytoplasmic and nuclear localization. *Endocrinology* 1987;120:1232–1242.
219. Qi M, Hamilton BJ, DeFranco D. v-mos oncoproteins affect the nuclear retention and reutilization of glucocorticoid receptors. *Mol Endocrinol* 1989;3:1279–1288.
220. Sanchez ER, Hirst M, Scherrer LC, Hormone-free mouse glucocorticoid receptors overexpressed in Chinese hamster ovary cells are localized to the nucleus and are associated with both hsp70 and hsp90. *J Biol Chem* 1990;265:20123–20130.
221. Kemppainen JA, Lane MC, Sar M, Wilson EM. Androgen receptor phosphorylation, turnover, nuclear transport, and transcriptional activation. *J Biol Chem* 1992;267:968–974.
222. Simental JA, Zhou ZX, Vilchis F, Sar M, Wilson EM. A bipartite nuclear targeting signal spanning the DNA binding and hinge regions of the human androgen receptor. *Proceedings of the 74th Annual Meeting of the Endocrine Society, San Antonio, TX;* 1992:127 [Abstract].
223. Picard D, Yamamoto KR. Two signals mediate hormone-dependent nuclear localization of the glucocorticoid receptor. *EMBO J* 1987;6:3333–3340.
224. Ylikomi T, Bocquel MT, Berry M, Gronemeyer H, Chambon P. Cooperation of proto-signals for nuclear accumulation of estrogen and progesterone receptors. *EMBO J* 1992;11:3681–3694.
225. Landers JP, Spelsberg TC. New concepts in steroid hormone action: transcription factors, proto-oncogenes, and the cascade model for steroid regulation of gene expression. *Crit Rev Euk Gene Exp* 1992;2:19–63.
226. Beck CA, Weigel NL, Edwards DP. Effects of hormone and cellular modulators of protein phosphorylation on transcriptional activity, DNA binding, and phosphorylation of human progesterone receptors. *Mol Endocrinol* 1992;6:607–620.

227. Goueli SA, Holtzman JL, Ahmed K. Phosphorylation of the androgen receptor by a nuclear cAMP-independent protein kinase. *Biochem Biophys Res Commun* 1984;123:778–784.
228. Goldsteyn EJ, Graham JS, Goren HJ, LeFebvre YA. Phosphorylation status of the nuclear cytosolic androgen receptors in the rat ventral prostate. *Prostate* 1989;14:91–101.
229. Barrack ER, Coffey DS. Specific binding of estrogens and androgens to the nuclear matrix of sex hormone responsive tissue. *J Biol Chem* 1980;255:7265.
230. Barrack ER, Coffey DS. Biological properties of the nuclear matrix: steroid hormone binding. *Recent Prog Hormone Res* 1982;38:133.
231. Nelson WG, Pienta KJ, Barrack ER, Coffey DS. The role of the nuclear matrix in the organization and function of DNA. *Ann Rev Biophys Biophys Chem* 1986;15:457–475.
232. Berezney R, Coffey DS. Nuclear matrix: isolation and characterization of a framework structure from rat liver nuclei. *J Cell Biol* 1977;73:616–637.
233. Pardoll DM, Vogelstein B, Coffey DS. A fixed site of DNA replication in eukaryotic cells. *Cell* 1980;19:527–536.
234. Vogelstein B, Pardoll DM, Coffey DS. Supercoiled loops in eukaryotic DNA replication. *Cell* 1980;22:79–85.
235. Ciejek EM, Nordstrom JL, Tsai M, O'Malley BW. Ribonucleic acid precursors are associated with the chick oviduct nuclear matrix. *Biochemistry* 1982;21:4945–4953.
236. Marriman EC, van Venrooij WJ. The nuclear matrix and RNA processing: use of human antibodies. In: Schmuckler EG, Claussen GA, eds. *Nuclear envelope structure and RNA maturation.* New York: Alan R. Liss; 1985:315–319.
237. Metzger DA, Korach KS. Cell-free interactions of the estrogen receptor with mouse uterine nuclear matrix: evidence of saturability, specificity and resistance to KCl extraction. *Endocrinology* 1990;162:2190.
238. Alexander RB, Greene GL, Barrack ER. Estrogen receptors in the nuclear matrix: direct demonstration using monoclonal antireceptor antibodies. *Endocrinology* 1987;120:1851.
239. Wilson EM, Colvard DS. Factors that influence interaction of the androgen receptor with nuclei and nuclear matrix. *Ann NY Acad Sci* 1984;438:85.
240. Pienta KJ, Partin AW, Coffey DS. Cancer as a disease of DNA organization and dynamic cell structure. *Cancer Res.* 1989;49:2525–2532.
241. Bissel MJ, Hall HG, Perry G. How does the extracellular matrix direct gene expression? *J Theor Biol* 1982;99:31.
242. Grobstein C. The developmental role of the intracellular matrix: A retrospective and prospective. In: Slavkin HC, Greulich RC, eds. *Extracellular matrix influence on gene expression.* New York: Academic Press; 1975:9–16.
243. Isaacs JT, Barrack ER, Isaacs WB, Coffey DS. The relationship of cellular structure and function: the matrix system. In: Murphy GP, Sandberg AA, Karr JP, eds. *The prostate cell structure and function,* part A. New York: Alan Liss; 1981:1.
244. Biller GH, Runner MN, Chung LWK. Tissue interactions in prostatic growth: morphological-biochemical characterization of adult mouse prostatic hyperplasia induced by fetal urogenital sinus implants. *Prostate* 1985;6:241–253.
245. Muntzing J. Androgen and collagen as growth regulators of the rat ventral prostate. *Prostate* 1980;1:71.
246. Mariotti J, Mawhinney MG. Hormonal control of accessory sex organ fibromuscular stroma. *Prostate* 1981;2:397.
247. Chung LWK, Chang SM, Bell C. Coinoculation of tumorigenic rat prostate mesenchymal cells with nontumorigenic epithelial cells results in the development of carcinosarcoma in syngeneic and athymic animals. *Int J Cancer* 1989;43:1129.
248. Tenniswood M. Role of epithelial-stromal interactions in the control of gene expression in the prostate: an hypothesis. *Prostate* 1986;9:375–385.
249. Jacobs SC, Pikna D, Lawson RK. Prostatic osteoblastic factor. *Invest Urol* 1979;17:195.
250. Jacobs SC, Lawson RK. Mitogenic factors in human prostate extracts. *Urology* 1980;16:488–491.
251. Lawson RK, Storey MT, Jacobs SC, Begun FP. Growth factors in benign prostatic hyperplasia. In: Ackermann R, Schroeder, FH, eds. *Prostatic hyperplasia: etiology, surgical and conservative management;* 1989:73–80.
252. Goldfarb M. The fibroblast growth factor family. *Cell Growth Differentiation* 1990;1:439–445.
253. Mydlo JK, Bulbul MA, Richon VM, Heston WDW, Fair WR. Heparin binding growth factors isolated from human prostatic extracts. *Prostate* 1988;12:343–355.
254. Mori H, Maki M, Oishi K, et al. Increased expression of genes for basic fibroblast growth factor: a transforming growth factor type $\beta 2$ in human benign prostatic hyperplasia. *Prostate* 1990;16:71–80.
255. Steiner MS, Barrack ER. Transforming growth factor-B, overproduction in prostate cancer: effects on growth in vivo and in vitro. *Mol Endocrinol* 1992;6:15–25.
256. Muller WJ, Lee FS, Dickson C, Peters G, Pattengale P, Leder P. The int-2 gene product acts as an epithelial growth factor in transgenic mice. *EMBO J* 1990;9:909–913.
257. Storey MT, Jacobs SC, Lawson RK. Epidermal growth factor is not the major growth-promoting agent in extracts of prostatic tissues. *J Urol* 1983;130:175.
258. Nishi N, Matuo Y, Wada F. Partial purification and of the major type of rat prostatic growth factor: characterization as an epidermal growth factor related mitogen. *Prostate* 1988;13:209–220.
259. Traish AM, Wotiz HH. Prostatic epidermal growth factor receptors and their regulation by androgens. *Endocrinology* 1987;121:1461–1467.
260. Connolly JM, Rose DP. Production of epidermal growth factor and transforming growth factor-α by the androgen responsive LNCaP human prostate cancer cell lines. *Prostate* 1990;16:209–218.
261. Morris GL, Dodd JG. Epidermal growth factor receptor: mRNA levels in human prostatic tumors and cell lines. *J Urol* 1990;143:1272–1274.
262. Wilding G, Valvaerius E, Knabbe C, Gelman EP. The role of transforming growth factor α in human prostate cancer cell growth. *Prostate* 1989;15:1–2.
263. Jhappan C, Stahle C, Harkins R, Fauston R, Smith GA, Merlino GT. TGFα overexpression in transgenic mice induces liver neoplasia and abnormal development of the mammary gland and pancreas. *Cell* 1990;61:1137–1146.
264. Sathe VA, Sheth AR, Sheth NA. Biosynthesis of immunoreactive inhibin-like material (IR-ILM) by rat prostate. *Prostate* 1986;8:401–408.
265. Sheth AR, Pan SE, Vaze AY, Geller J, Albert J. Inhibin in the human prostate. *Arch Androl* 1981;6:317–321.
266. Stahler MS, Pansky B, Budd GC. Immunocytochemical demonstration of insulin or insulin-like immunoreactivity in the rat prostate gland. *Prostate* 1988;13:189–198.
267. Smith RG, Syms AJ, Nag A, Lerner S, Norris JS. Mechanisms of the glucocorticoid regulation and growth of the androgen-sensitive prostate-derived R3327 H-G8-A1 tumor cells. *J Biol Chem* 1985;260:12454–12463.
268. Rijnders AWM, van der Korput JAGM, van Stenbrugge GJ, Romijn TC, Trapman J. Expression of cellular oncogenes in human prostatic carcinoma cell lines. *Biochem Biophys Res Commun* 1985;132:548–54.
269. Crabb JW, Armes LG, Carr SA, et al. Complete primary structure of prostatropin, a prostate epithelial cell growth factor. *Biochemistry* 1986;225:4988–93.
270. Launoit Y, Kiss R, Jossa V, et al. The influence of dihydrotestosterone, testosterone, estradiol, progesterone or prolactin on the cell kinetics of human hyperplastic prostatic tissue in organ culture. *Prostate* 1988;13:143–53.
271. Kadar T, Redding TW, Ben-David M, Schally AV. Receptors for prolactin, somatostatin and lutenizing hormone-releasing hormone (LH-RH) on experimental prostate cancer after treatment with analogs of LH-RH and somatostatin: decrease in prolactin binding sites. *Proc Natl Acad Sci USA* 1988;85:890–4.
272. Kadar T, Ben-David M, Pontes EJ, Fekete M, Schally AV. Prolactin and leutenizing hormone-releasing hormone receptors in human benign prostatic hyperplasia and prostate cancer. *Prostate* 1988;12:299–307.
273. Dalton DP, Lee C, Huprikar S, Grayhack JT. Nonandrogenic

role of testes in ventral prostate growth in rats. *Prostate* 1990;16:225–233.
274. Meyer JS, Sufrin G, Martin SA. Proliferative activity of benign human prostate, prostatic adenocarcinoma and seminal vesicles evaluated by thymidine labeling. *J Urol* 1982;128:1353–6.
275. Masters JRW, O'Donoghue EPN. Human benign prostatic hyperplasia in organ culture: studies on iododeoxyuridine uptake. *Prostate* 1983;4:167–78.
276. Nemoto R, Hattori K, Uchida K, et al. S-phase fraction of human prostate adenocarcinoma studied with in vivo bromodeoxyuridine labeling. *Cancer* 1990;66:509–14.
277. Coffey DS, Shimazaki J, Williams-Ashman HG. Polymerization of deoxyribonucleotides in relation to androgen-induced prostatic growth. *Arch Biochem Biophys* 1968;124:184–98.
278. Sufrin G, Coffey DS. A new model for studying the effects of drugs on prostatic growth: I. Antiandrogens in DNA synthesis. *Invest Urol* 1973;11:45–54.
279. Lesser B, Bruchovsky N. The effects of testosterone, 5α-dihydrotestosterone and adenosine 3′,5′ monophosphate on cell proliferation and differentiation in rat prostate. *Biochem Biophys Acta* 1973;308:426–37.
280. English HF, Drago JR, Santen RJ. Cellular response to androgen depletion and repletion in the rat ventral prostate: autoradiography and morphometric analysis. *Prostate* 1985;7:41–51.
281. English HF, Santen RJ, Isaacs JT. Response of glandular vs. basal rat ventral prostatic epithelial cells to androgen withdrawal and replacement. *Prostate* 1987;11:229–42.
282. English HF, Kloszewski ED, Valentine EG, Santen RJ. Proliferative response of the Dunning R3327-H experimental model of prostatic adenocarcinoma to conditions of androgen depletion and repletion. *Cancer Res* 1986;46:839–44.
283. English HF, Kyprianou N, Isaacs JT. Relationship between DNA fragmentation and apoptosis in programmed cell death in the rat prostate following castration. *Prostate* 1989;15:233–250.
284. Humphries JE, Isaacs JT. Unusual androgen sensitivity of the androgen-independent Dunning R3327-G rat prostatic adenocarcinoma: androgen effects on tumor cell loss. *Cancer Res* 1982;41:3148–56.
285. Katz A, Wise G, Olsson C, Benson M, Buttyan R. A map of molecular events during the early phase of prostate growth. *J Urol* [Abstract 380]. 1989.
286. Bookstein R, Shew JY, Chen PL, Scully P, Lee WH. Suppression of tumorigenicity of human prostate carcinoma cells by replacing a mutated RB gene. *Science* 1990;247:712–5.
287. Stanisic T, Sadlowski R, Lee C, Grayhack JT. Partial inhibition of castration-induced ventral prostate regression with actinomycin D and cyclohexamide. *Invest Urol* 1978;16:15–18.
288. Engels G, Lee C, Grayhack JT. Acid ribonuclease in rat prostate during castration-induced involution. *Biol Reprod* 1980;22:827–831.
289. Lee C, Tsai Y, Harrison H, Sensiber J. Proteins of the rat prostate: I. Preliminary characterization by 2-dimensional electrophoresis. *Prostate* 1985;7:171–182.
290. Montpetit ML, Lawless KR, Tenniswood M. Androgen repressed messages in the rat ventral prostate. *Prostate* 1986;8:25–36.
291. Leger JG, Montpetit ML, Tenniswood M. Characterization and cloning of androgen repressed messenger RNase from rat ventral prostate. *Biochem Biophys Res Commun* 1987;147:196–203.
292. Leger JG, Guellec RL, Tenniswood M. Treatment with antiandrogens induces an androgen-repressed gene in the rat ventral prostate. *Prostate* 1980;13:131–142.
293. O'Bryan MK, Baker HWG, Saunders JR, et al. Human seminal clusterin (SP-40, 40). *J Clin Invest* 1990;85:1477–1486.
294. Tanabe E, Lee C, Grayhack JT. Activities of cathepsin D in rat prostate during castration-induced involution. *J Urol* 1982; 127:826–828.
295. Sensibar JA, Liu X, Patai B, Alger B, Lee C. Characterization of castration-induced cell death in the rat prostate by immunohistochemical localization of cathepsin D. *Prostate* 1990;16:263–276.
296. Rennie PS, Bouffard R, Bruchovsky N, Chang H. Increased activity of plasminogen activators during involution of the rat ventral prostate. *Biochem J* 1984;221:171–278.
297. Andreasen PA, Kristensen P, Lund LR, Dano K. Urokinase-type plasminogen activator is increased in the involuting ventral prostate of castrated rats. *Endocrinology* 1990;126:2567–2577.
298. Anderson KM, Baranowski J, Ekonomous SG, Rubenstein M. A qualitative analysis of acetic proteins associated with regressing, growing or dividing rat ventral prostate cells. *Prostate* 1983;4:151–166.
299. Lee C, Sensibar J. Proteins of the rat prostate: II. Synthesis of new proteins in the ventral lobe during castration-induced regression. *J Urol* 1987;138:903–908.
300. Saltzman AG, Hiipakka ARA, Chang C, Liao S. Androgen repression of the production of a 29-kilodalton protein and its mRNA in the rat ventral prostate. *J Biol Chem* 1987;262: 432–437.
301. Chang GC, Saltzman AG, Sorensen MS, Hiipakka RA, Liao S. Identification of a glutathione *S*-transferase Yb1 mRNA as an androgen-repressed mRNA by cDNA cloning and sequence analysis. *J Biol Chem* 1987;262:11901–11903.
302. Wyllie AH, Kerr JFR, Currie AR. Cell death: the significance of apoptosis. *Int Rev Cytol* 1986;68:251–306.
303. Kerr JFR, Searle J. Deletion of cells by apoptosis during castration-induced involution of the rat prostate. *Virchows Arch Cell Pathol* 1973;13:87–102.
304. Dahl E, Kjaerheim A. The ultrastructure of the accessory sex organs of male rats: II. Post-castration involution of the ventral, lateral and dorsal prostate. *Z Zellforsh Mikrosk Anat* 1973;144:167–170.
305. Sanford ML, Searle JW, Kerr JFR. Successive waves of apoptosis in the rat prostate after repeated withdrawal of testosterone stimulation. *Pathology* 1984;16:406–410.
306. Kyprianou N, Isaacs JT. Activation of programmed cell death in the rat ventral prostate after castration. *Endocrinology* 1988;122:552–62.
307. Kyprianou N, English HF, Isaacs JT. Activation of calcium-magnesium dependent endonuclease as an early event in castration-induced prostate cell death. *Prostate* 1988;13: 103–117.
308. Connor J, Sawczuk IS, Benson MC, et al. Calcium channel antagonists delay regression of androgen-dependent tissues and suppress gene activity associated with cell death. *Prostate* 1988;13:119–130.
309. Buttyan R, Zacker Z, Lochshin R, Wolgemuth D. Cascade induction of c-fos, c-myc and heat-shock 70k transcript during regression of the rat ventral prostate gland. *Mol Endocrinol* 1988;2:650–657.
310. Barrack ER, Berry SJ. DNA synthesis in the canine prostate: Effects of androgen and estrogen treatment. *Prostate* 1987;10: 45–56.
311. Amelar RD, Hotchkiss RS. The split ejaculate: its uses in the management of male infertility. *Fertil Steril* 1965;16:46.
312. Tauber PF, Zaneveld LJD, Propping D, Schumacher GFB. Components of human split ejaculates: II. Enzymes and proteinase inhibitors. *J Reprod Fertil* 1976;46:165.
313. Tauber PF, Zaneveld LJD, Propping D, Schumacher GFB. Components of human split ejaculate. *J Reprod Fertil* 1975;43:249.
314. Aumuller G, Seitz J. Protein secretion and secretory processes in male sex accessory glands. *Int Rev Cytol* 1990;121:127–231.
315. Mann T, Mann CL. *Male reproductive function and semen.* New York: Springer-Verlag; 1981.
316. Zaneveld LJD, Tauber PF. Contributions of prostatic fluid components to the ejaculate. In: Murphy GP, Sandberg AA, Karr JP, eds. *The prostate: cell structure and function,* part A. New York: Alan R. Liss; 1981:265.
317. Costello LC, Franklin RB. Prostate epithelial utilize glucose and aspartate as a carbon source for net citrate production. *Prostate* 1989;15:335–342.
318. Phadke AM, Samant NR, Deval SP. Significance of seminal fructose studies in male fertility. *Fertil Steril* 1973:24:894.
319. Williams-Ashman HG, Corti A, Sheth AR. Formation and functions of aliphatic polyamines in the prostate gland and its secretions. In: Goland M, ed. *Normal and abnormal growth of the prostate.* Springfield, IL: Charles C Thomas; 1975:222.

320. Falk JE, Park MH, Chung SI, et al. Polyamines as physiological substrates for transglutaminases. *J Biol Chem* 1980;255:3695.
321. Williams-Ashman HG, Janne J, Coppoc GC, Geroch ME, Schenone A. New aspects of polyamine biosynthesis in eukaryotic organisms. *Adv Enzyme Regul* 1972;10:225.
322. Williams-Ashman HG, Pegg AE, Lockwood DH. Mechanisms and regulation of polyamine and putrescine biosynthesis in male genital glands and other tissues of mammals. *Adv Enzyme Regul* 1969;7:291.
323. Fair WR, Parrish RT. Antibacterial substance in prostatic fluid. In: Murphy GP, Sandberg AA, Karr JP, eds. *The prostate: cell structure and function,* part A. New York: Alan R. Liss; 1981:247–264.
324. Fair WR, Couch J, Wehner N. The purification and assay of the prostatic antibacterial factor (PAF). *Biochem Med* 1973;8:329.
325. Stamey TA, Fair WR, Timothy MM, et al. Antibacterial nature of prostatic fluid. *Nature* 1968;218:444.
326. Seligman AM, et al. Design of spindle poisons activated specifically by prostatic acid phosphatase (PAP) and new methods for PAP cytochemistry. *Cancer Chemother Rep* 59:233.
327. von Euler US. Zur Kenntnis der pharmakologischen Wirkungen von Natirsekreten und Extrackten männlicher accessorischer Geschlechtsdrusen. *Arch Pathol Pharmakol* 1934;175:78.
328. Eliasson R. Studies on prostaglandins: occurrence formation and biological actions. *Acta Physiol Scand* 1959;158 Suppl 46:1.
329. Fuchs AR, Chantharaski U. Prostaglandins and male fertility. In: Hafez ESE, ed. *Human semen and fertility regulation in men.* St. Louis: CV Mosby; 1976.
330. Scott WW. The lipids of the prostatic fluid, seminal plasma and enlarged prostate gland of man. *J Urol* 1945;53:712.
331. White IG, Darin-Bennett A, Poulos A. Lipids of human semen. In: Hafez ESE, ed. *Human semen and fertility regulation in men.* St. Louis: CV Mosby; 1976.
332. Poulos A, White LG. Phospholipids of human spermatozoa and seminal plasma. *J Reprod Fertil* 1973;35:265.
333. Mackenzie AR, Hall T, Whitmore WF, Jr. Zinc content of expressed human prostatic fluid. *Nature* 1962;193:72.
334. Byar DP. Zinc in male sex accessory organs: distribution and hormonal response. In: Brandes D, ed. *Male sex accessory organs: structure and function in mammals.* New York: Academic Press; 1974:161–71.
335. Chandler JA, Timms BG, Morton MS. Subcellular distribution of zinc in rat prostate studied by x-ray microanalysis: I. Normal prostate. *Histochem J* 1977;9:103.
336. Gunn SA, Gould TC. The relative importance of androgen and estrogen in the selective uptake of Zn by the dorsolateral prostate of the rat. *Endocrinology* 1956;58:443.
337. Gunn SA, Gould TC, Anderson WA. The effect of growth hormone and prolactin preparations on the control by interstitial cell-stimulating hormone of uptake of 65-Zn by the rat dorsolateral prostate. *J Endocrinol* 1965;32:205.
338. Johnson L, Wickstrom S, Nylander G. The vehicle of zinc in the prostatic secretion of dog. *Scand J Urol Nephrol* 1969;3:9–11.
339. Heathcote JG, Washington RJ. Analysis of the zinc-binding protein derived from the human benign hypertrophic prostate. *J Endocrinol* 1973;58:421.
340. Fair WR, Wehner N. The prostatic antibacterial factor: identity and significance. In: Marberger H, et al, eds. *Prostatic disease,* vol. 6. New York: Alan R. Liss; 1976.
341. Reed MJ, Stitch SR. The uptake of testosterone and zinc in vitro by the human benign hypertrophic prostate. *J Endocrinol* 1973;58:405.
342. Aumuller G, Seitz J, Lilja H, Abrahamsson TA, Vonderkammer H, Scheit KH. Species-specificity and organ-specificity of secretory proteins derived from human prostate and seminal vesicle. *Prostate* 1990;17:31–40.
343. Frenette G, Dube JY, Lazure C, Paradis G, Chretien M, Tremblay RR. The major 40-kDa glycoprotein in human prostatic fluid is identical to Zn-α2-glycoprotein. *Prostate* 1987;11:257–270.
344. Tsai YC, Harrison HH, Lee C, et al. Systematic characterization of human prostatic proteins with 2-dimensional electrophoresis. *Clin Chem* 1984;30:2026.
345. Rui H, Mevag B, Purvis K. Two-dimensional electrophoresis of proteins in various fractions of human split ejaculate. *J Androl* 1984;7:509–520.
346. Carter DB, Resnick MI. High resolution analysis of human prostatic fluid by 2-dimensional electrophoresis. *Prostate* 1982;3:27–31.
347. Edwards JE, Pollaksen SL, Anderson NG. Proteins of human semen: I. Two-dimensional mapping of human seminal plasma. *Clin Chem* 1981;27:135–144.
348. Lilja H, Abrahamson PA. Three predominant proteins secreted by the human prostate gland. *Prostate* 1988;12:29–38.
349. Hara M, Inove T, Fukuyama T. Some physico-chemical characteristics of gamma seminoprotein, an antigenic component specific for human seminal plasma-antigenic component specific for human seminal plasma. *Nippon Hoigaka Zasshi* 1971;25:322–324.
350. Watt KWK, Lee PJ, Tinkulu TM, et al. Human prostatic specific antigen: structural and functional similarities with serum proteases. *Proc Natl Acad Sci USA* 1986;83:3166–3170.
351. Lundwall A, Lilja H. Molecular cloning in human prostatic specific antigen cDNA. *FEBS Lett* 1977;214:317–322.
352. Lilja H. A kallikrein-like serum protease in prostatic fluid cleaves the predominant seminal vesicle protein. *J Clin Invest* 1985;76:1899–1903.
353. Gutman AB, Gutman EB. An acid phosphatase occurring in serum of patients with metastasizing carcinoma of the prostate gland. *J Clin Invest* 1938;17:473.
354. Roy AV, et al. Sodium thymolphthalein monophosphate: a new acid phosphatase substrate with greater specificity for the prostatic enzyme in serum. *Clin Chem* 1971;17:1093.
355. Seligman AM, et al. The colorimetric determination of phosphatases in human serum. *J Biol Chem* 1951;190:7.
356. Lin MF, Clinton GM. Human prostatic acid phosphatase has phosphotyrosyl protein-phosphatase activity. *Biochem J* 1986;235:351–357.
357. Li HC, Chernoff J, Chen LB, Kirschonbaum A. A phosphotyrosyl-protein phosphatase activity associated with acid phosphatase from human prostate gland. *Eur J Biochem* 1984;138:45–51.
358. Chu TM, Wang MC, Kuciel L, Valenzuela L, Murphy GP. Enzyme markers in human prostatic carcinoma. *Cancer Treat Rep* 1977;61:193.
359. Ulvsback M, Lindstrom C, Weiber H, Abrahamsson TA, Lilja H, Lundwall A. Molecular cloning of a small prostate protein, known as β-microsemenoprotein, PSP 90 or β-inhibin, and demonstration of transcripts in non-genital tissues. *Biochem Biophys Res Commun* 1989;164:1310–1315.
360. Dube JY, Frenette G, Paquin R, et al. Isolation from human seminal plasma of an abundant 16 kDa protein originating from the prostate: Its identification to a 94 residue peptide originally described as β-inhibin. *J Androl* 1987;8:182–189.
361. Mattila S. Further studies on the prostatic tissue antigens. Separation of two molecular forms of aminopeptidase. *Invest Urol* 1969;7:1.
362. Niemi M, Harkonen M, Larmi TKL. Enzymic histochemistry of human prostate. *Arch Pathol* 1963;75:528.
363. Kirchheim D, Byorkey F, Brandes D, Scott WW. Histochemistry of the normal hyperplastic and neoplastic human prostate gland. *Invest Urol* 1964;4:403.
364. Oliver JA, et al. LDH isoenzymes in benign and malignant prostate tissue: the LDH/VI ratio as an index of malignancy. *Cancer* 1970;25:863.
365. Denis LJ, Prout GR Jr. Lactic dehydrogenase in prostatic cancer. *Invest Urol* 1963;1:101.
366. Grayhack JT, Wendel EF, Lee C, Oliver L, Choen E. Lactate dehydrogenase isoenzymes in human prostatic fluid: an aid in recognition of malignancy. *J Urol* 1977;118:204.
367. Elhilali MM, et al. Lactate dehydrogenase isoenzymes in hyperplasia and carcinoma of the prostate: a clinical study. *J Urol* 1968;98:686.
368. Flocks RH, Schmidt JD. Lactate dehydrogenase isoenzyme patterns of prostatic cancer and hyperplasia. *J Surg Oncol* 1972;4:161.
369. Friberg J, Tilly-Friberg I. Antibodies in human seminal fluid. In:

Hafez ESE, ed. *Human semen and fertility regulation in men.* St. Louis: CV Mosby; 1976.
370. Grayhack JT, Wendel EF, Oliver L, et al. Analysis of specific proteins in prostatic fluid for detecting prostatic malignancy. *J Urol* 1979;121:295.
371. Fowler JE Jr, Mariano M. Immunologic response of the prostate to bacteriuria and bacterial prostatitis: II. Antigen-specific immunoglobulins in prostatic fluid. *J Urol* 1982;128:165.
372. Fowler JE Jr, Kaiser DL, Mariano M. Immunologic response of the prostate to bacteriuria and bacterial prostatitis: I. Immunoglobulin concentrations in prostatic fluid. *J Urol* 1982;128:158.
373. Grayhack JT, Lee C. Evaluation of prostatic fluid and prostatic pathology. In: Murphy GP, Sandberg AA, Karr JP, eds. *The prostate: cell structure and function,* part A. New York: Alan R. Liss; 1981:231.
374. Williams-Ashman HG. Regulatory features of the seminal vesicle development and function. *Curr Top Cell Regul* 1983;22: 201–275.
375. Lilja H, Oldbring J, Rannevik G, Laurell CB. Seminal-secreted proteins and their reactions during gelation and liquefaction of human semen. *J Clin Invest* 1987;80:281–285.
376. Huggins C, Neal W. Coagulation and liquefaction of semen: proteolytic enzymes and citrate in prostatic fluid. *J Exp Med* 1942;7:527.
377. Tauber PF, Zaneveld LJD. Coagulation and liquefaction of human semen. In: Hafez ESE, ed. *Human semen and fertility regulation in men.* St. Louis: CV Mosby; 1976.
378. Amelar RD. Coagulation, liquefaction and viscosity of human semen. *J Urol* 1962;87:187.
379. Syner FN, Moghissi KS, Yanez J. Isolation of a factor from normal human semen that accelerates dissolution of abnormally liquefying semen. *Fertil Steril* 1975;26:1064.
380. Zaneveld LJD, Chatterton RT. *Biochemistry of mammalian reproduction.* New York: Wiley; 1982.
381. Propping D, Tauber PF, Zaneveld LJD, Schumacher GFB. Purification and characterization of two plasminogen activators from human seminal plasma. *Fed Proc* 1974;33:289.
382. Fritz H, Arnhold M, Forg-Brey B, Zaneveld LJD, Schumacher GFB. Verhalten der chymotrypsin-ahnlichen Proteinase aus Humansperma gegenuber Protein-Proteinase-Inhibitoren. *Hoppe-Seylers Z Physiol Chem* 1972;353:1651.
383. Lundquist F, Thorsteinsson T, Buus O. Purification and properties of some enzymes in human seminal plasma. *Biochem J* 1955;56:69.
384. Williams-Ashman HG, Wilson J, Beil R, et al. Transglutaminase reactions associated with the rat semen clotting system. *Biochem Biophys Res Commun* 1977;79:1192.
385. Amelar RD, Dubin L. Semen analysis. In: *Male infertility.* Philadelphia: WB Saunders; 1977.
386. Eliasson R. Parameters of male infertility. In: Hafez ESE, Evans TN, eds. *Human reproductive conception and contraception.* New York: Harper & Row; 1973.
387. Bunge RG. Some observations on the male ejaculate. *Fertil Steril* 1970;21:639.
388. Bunge RG, Sherman JK. Liquefaction of human semen by α-amylase. *Fertil Steril* 1954;5:353.
389. Freund M, Peterson RN. Semen evaluation and fertility. In: Hafez ESE, ed. *Human semen and fertility regulation in men.* St. Louis: CV Mosby; 1976.
390. Walsh PC, Amelar R. Embryology, anatomy and physiology of the male reproductive system. In: Amelar R, et al, eds. *Male infertility.* Philadelphia: WB Saunders; 1977.
391. Marina S, Pomerlo JM, Zungri ER. Occlusions in the male reproductive tract: diagnostic radiology. In: Hafez ESE, ed. *Human semen and fertility regulation in men.* St. Louis: CV Mosby; 1976.
392. Isaacs JT. Prostatic structure and function in relation to the etiology of prostate cancer. *Prostate* 1983;4:351.
393. Hessl JM, Stamey TA. The passage of tetracyclines across epithelial membranes with special reference to prostatic epithelium. *J Urol* 1971;106:253.
394. Stamey TA, Bushby SRM, Bragonje J. The concentration of trimethoprim in prostatic fluid: nonionic diffusion or active transport? *J Infect Dis* 1973;128 Suppl:686.
395. Fowle ASE, Bye A. Concentrations of trimethoprim and sulfamethoxazole in human prostatic fluid. In: Hejzlar M, ed. *Advances in antimicrobial and antineoplastic chemotherapy.* Munich: Urban & Schwarzenberg; 1972:1289.
396. Madsen PO, Wolf H, Barquin OP, Rhodes P. The nitrofurantoin concentration in prostatic fluid of humans and dogs. *J Urol* 1968;100:54.
397. Madsen PO, Kjaert B, Baumueller A, Mellin HE. Antimicrobial agents in prostatic fluid and tissue. *Infection* 1976;4(Suppl 2):154.
398. Madsen PO, Baumueller A, Hoyne U. Experimental models for determination of antimicrobials in prostatic tissue, interstitial fluid and secretion. *Scand J Infect Dis* 1978;14(Suppl):145.
399. Reeves DS. Pharmacology of the prostate. In: Chisolm GD, Williams DI, eds. *Scientific foundations of urology,* 2nd ed. London: Heineman Medical Books; 1982:514–520.
400. White MA. Changes in pH of expressed prostatic secretion during the course of prostatitis. *Proc R Soc Med* 1975;68:511.

The Physiology of Reproduction, Second Edition,
edited by E. Knobil and J.D. Neill,
Raven Press, Ltd., New York © 1994.

CHAPTER 24

Male Sexual Function: Erection, Emission, and Ejaculation

George S. Benson

Our knowledge of the physiologic mechanisms that control male sexual function is rapidly expanding. The development of successful therapy for impotence, both surgical and pharmacological, in the past decade has been primarily responsible for stimulating the considerable research effort presently being undertaken to understand better both the normal physiology of penile erection and the pathophysiology of disease states leading to sexual dysfunction. Although significant progress has been made, many basic questions remain unanswered.

Three components of male sexual function will be discussed in this chapter: erection, emission, and ejaculation. Erection is defined as penile rigidity or tumescence. What is generally referred to as the "ejaculatory process" is, in fact, two distinct events: emission and ejaculation. Emission, by definition, is the deposition of seminal fluid components from the vasa deferentia, seminal vesicles, and prostate gland into the posterior urethra, while ejaculation refers to the passage of seminal fluid through the urethra and its expulsion from the urethral meatus (1).

Department of Surgery, Division of Urology, The University of Texas Medical School at Houston, Houston, Texas 77030

ERECTION

Our understanding of the mechanisms involved in the production of penile erection remains incomplete. Much of our data are derived from clinical observation and are subjective. Recently, however, several new approaches to obtaining objective data in man have been developed and have been instrumental in redirecting our thinking and correcting widely accepted misconceptions. The lack of a universally accepted animal model for penile erection has also hampered research efforts in the past, but recent *in vivo* data obtained in the dog and monkey have nevertheless clarified much of our misunderstanding.

Penile Anatomy

Unlike several animal species, the human does not possess an os penis (like the canine) or a retractor penis muscle (multiple animal species) (2–4). Anatomic and physiologic data obtained from much animal work to explain the complex events responsible for human penile erection are therefore suspect. In the human, erectile tissue is contained within three corporal bodies, two dorsally positioned corpora cavernosa and a ventrally positioned corpus spongiosum that also contains the urethra (Fig. 1). Each of the three corpora is surrounded by a thick layer of fibrous tissue (tunica albugenia), which separates the corpora from each other. Buck's fascia lies superficial to the tunica albugenia and surrounds all three corporal bodies.

Following the realization that the erectile tissue of the corpora acts not only as a reservoir for blood, but also plays an active role in the development of erection, this tissue has been the subject of much recent anatomic, physiologic, and pharmacologic investigation. Anatomically, the erectile tissue of both the corpora cavernosa and corpus spongiosum is composed of numerous cavernous spaces separated by trabeculae. The trabeculae are composed not only of fibroblasts, collagen, and elastic fibers, but also of significant amounts of smooth muscle. Endothelial cells, which resemble those found in blood vessels, cover the surfaces of the trabeculae. In general, the corpus spongiosum differs from the corpus cavernosum in that the spongiosum contains larger cavernous spaces and the trabeculae are smaller and contain fewer smooth muscle cells (5).

Penile Vasculature

It has long been recognized that penile erection is primarily a vascular event. The basis for increasing penile blood flow (and pressure) is, however, incompletely understood.

Arterial Supply

In the human, penile arterial blood supply is derived from the pudendal arteries, which are branches of the internal iliac (hypogastric) arteries (Fig. 2). Each of the paired internal pudendal arteries supplies two arteries to the corpus spongiosum: (a) a bulbar branch, which supplies the proximal corpus spongiosum, and (b) the urethral artery, which courses from the perineum to the glans penis. Prior to entering the crus of the penis, the internal pudendal artery divides into two terminal branches, the deep penile and the dorsal penile artery.

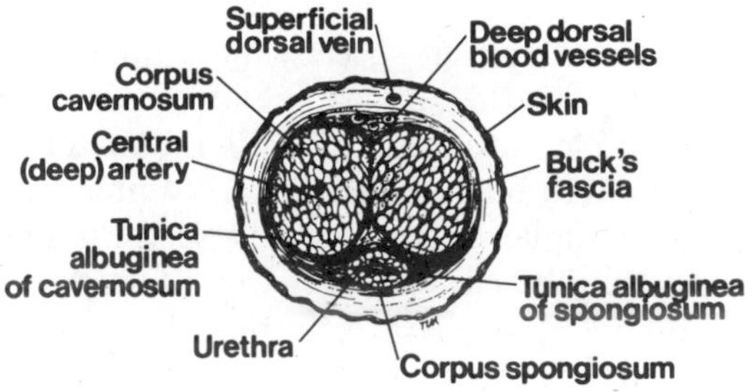

FIG. 1. Cross-sectional anatomy of human penis.

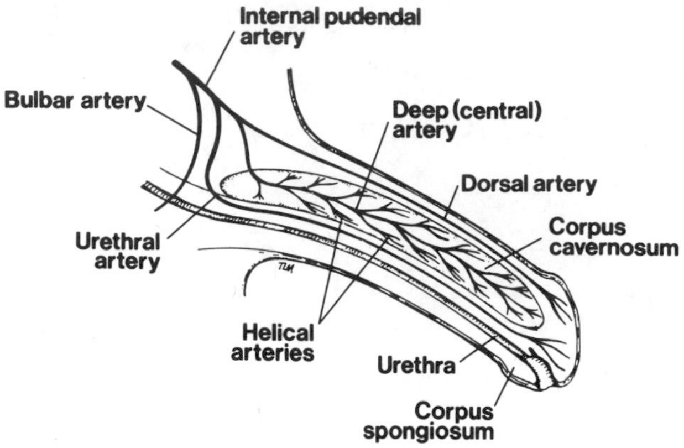

FIG. 2. Arterial blood supply to the human penis.

The dorsal penile artery anatomically does not enter the corpora cavernosa. It courses distally between the tunica albuginea of the corpora cavernosa and Buck's fascia. Each of the paired deep arteries enters the crus of the penis in the perineum and then courses distally through each corpus cavernosum as the central (deep) artery. The central arteries supply nutrient vessels to the corpora cavernosa and numerous small vessels (helical arteries), which further divide into end-arteries as they open directly into the cavernous spaces (6). In the human, the central artery also sends anastomotic branches to the opposite corpus cavernosum; the result of these anastomoses is that the two human corpora cavernosa act as one functional unit (7,8). In the dog, however, such anastomoses do not exist, and the two corpora are capable of functioning independently (9). Although it would appear that the arterial supply to the corpora cavernosa is derived solely from the deep arteries, numerous anastomotic channels interconnect all arteries of the penis. In addition, "shunt arteries," which connect the central arteries in the corpora cavernosa with arteries in the corpus spongiosum, have been described (10). The significance of these arterial interconnections and, specifically, their role in the production of penile erection is not understood.

Venous Drainage

The venous drainage of the penis is anatomically more complex than the arterial supply. Although numerous anastomotic interconnections exist in the penile venous system, at least four major components have been identified (11,12). The superficial dorsal vein is formed by the confluence of multiple superficial veins and lies subcutaneously superficial to Buck's fascia. Bulbar and urethral veins provide drainage for the proximal corpus spongiosum. The major venous systems draining the primary erectile bodies, the corpora cavernosa, are the deep dorsal veins and the deep veins (crural and cavernous).

The deep dorsal vein receives veins from the glans penis as well as emissary and circumflex veins from the corpora cavernosa. These anastomosing vessels, as well as the deep dorsal vein itself, course between the tunica albuginea of the corpora and Buck's fascia. The cavernous and crural veins exit the corpora cavernosa proximally in the area of the penile crura and drain into the internal pudendal venous system. The distal and mid-corpora cavernosa drain into the deep dorsal veins and the proximal corpora drain into the cavernous and crural veins (12).

The anatomy and significance of the venous drainage of the penis requires much further investigation. For years, the venous drainage systems were thought to contribute minimally, if at all, to the physiology of normal erection. The differences in venous drainage between the corpora cavernosa and the corpus spongiosum/glans penis were appreciated and formed the basis for "shunting" operations (cavernosum-spongiosum and cavernosum-glans penis shunts) used to divert blood from the corpora cavernosa in patients with priapism. Recently, however, the importance of increased corporal outflow resistance in attaining normal erection has been demonstrated in animals (9), and impotence secondary to "venous leakage" has been observed clinically (13). These data and their significance will be discussed subsequently.

Penile Innervation

The penis is innervated by both divisions of the autonomic nervous system (sympathetic and parasympathetic) as well as by the somatic nervous system (Fig. 3). The innervation of the penis and its vasculature is complex and controversial.

The penis, and presumably its vasculature, receives its autonomic innervation from the pelvic plexus. In man, this ganglionic plexus is located retroperitoneally near the rectum (14). The pelvic plexus receives autonomic nerve input from both the sympathetic and parasympathetic systems. Sympathetic nerves originate in the low thoracic and upper lumbar regions of the spinal cord and course retroperitoneally to condense into the superior hypogastric plexus (presacral nerve) located just inferior to the aortic bifurcation. Nerve fibers leave the superior hypogastric plexus as the paired hypogastric nerves, which fuse distally and then enter the pelvic (inferior hypogastric) plexus (15). The parasympathetic contribution to the pelvic plexus is derived from nerves whose cell bodies are located in the sacral (S_{2-4}) spinal cord. Parasympathetic fibers fuse to form the pelvic nerve, which courses in the endopelvic fascia prior to reaching the pelvic plexus (14).

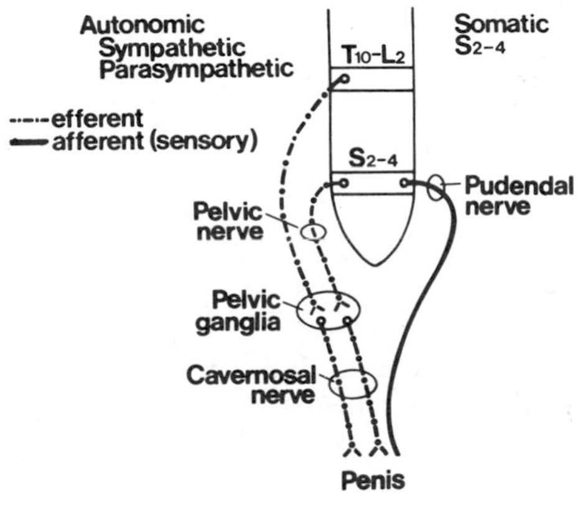

FIG. 3. Innervation of the human penis.

Anatomically, it is extremely difficult to trace nerve fibers leaving the pelvic plexus and more difficult (if not impossible) to determine the origin of specific nerve fibers leaving the pelvic plexus. Nerve fibers leaving the pelvic plexus innervate not only the penis, but also other pelvic viscera including the urinary bladder, prostate, and rectum. Significant recent anatomic studies have clarified the gross anatomy of the autonomic nerves that supply the corpora cavernosa. These cavernosal nerves leave the pelvic plexus, course between the rectum and urethra, enter the urogenital diaphragm in proximity to the muscular wall of the urethra, and finally enter the dorsal medial aspect of the corpora cavernosa. These nerves presumably innervate the smooth musculature and vasculature located within the corpora cavernosa (14).

The somatic innervation to the penis is carried via the pudendal nerve; periurethral striated muscles as well as the sensory innervation of the penis are supplied by this system. The pudendal nerve, like the parasympathetic autonomic fibers, arises from the sacral (S_{2-4}) spinal cord. The pudendal nerve accompanies the internal pudendal blood vessels along the lateral wall of the ischiorectal fossa (14). Penile sensation is carried in the dorsal nerve of the penis, a branch of the pudendal nerve.

Histochemical techniques have been utilized to study the autonomic innervation of the smooth musculature of the corpora cavernosa and the penile vasculature. Adrenergic nerves, whose neurotransmitter is by definition a catecholamine, have been studied by histofluorescent techniques. Initial studies in man described a sparse adrenergic innervation to the smooth muscle of the corpora (16); subsequent investigation demonstrated a considerable adrenergic innervation (5).

Adrenergic nerves can be identified coursing through trabeculae of the corpora cavernosa and approaching the walls of the cavernous spaces. In addition, the blood vessels within the corpora contain dense aggregations of nerve varicosities in the outer tunic (17,18). Adrenergic nerves are also found in the corpus spongiosum. Unlike the corpora cavernosa, however, the density of innervation in the spongiosum is sparse. Electron microscopic evaluation of the corpora is consistent with the light microscopic data; nerves containing small (400–600 Å), electron-dense vesicles that are considered to be adrenergic have been identified (18).

Cholinergic nerves, whose neurotransmitter by definition is acetylcholine, have also been anatomically identified. Although acetylcholinesterase staining may not be specific for only cholinergic neurons (19), this technique has classically been utilized to demonstrate cholinergic innervation. Although cholinergic (acetylcholinesterase-positive) nerves have been found in the trabeculae of the corpora cavernosa, their density is controversial. Like the adrenergic innervation, the corpora cavernosa contains more cholinergic nerves than the corpus spongiosum, and cholinergic nerves are found in the outer tunic of most penile arterioles (18) (Fig. 4).

Neuropharmacologically, penile erection does not appear to be entirely dependent upon classic adrenergic and cholinergic mechanisms. This will be discussed below. Anatomically, nerves containing other putative neurotransmitters have been described in penile tissue from animals and man. Vasoactive intestinal polypeptide (VIP) has been identified at both the light and electron microscopic levels utilizing histochemical techniques (20–22). Electron microscopically, in addition to VIP-immunopositive vesicles, a variety of large vesicles that are not VIP positive have also been seen and are hypothesized to contain other peptides that may act as neurotransmitters (22). Substance P, somatostatin, and neuropeptide Y (NPY) have been demonstrated in nerves within the penis with radioimmunoassay and immunocytochemistry (21). Neuropeptide Y has been colocalized with norepinephrine in the same nerve terminal in perivascular nerve fibers and with VIP in penile cavernous tissue of green monkeys (23–25).

Hemodynamic Aspects

Penile erection is clearly dependent upon vascular events. The importance of increased arterial flow was demonstrated experimentally by Semans and Langworthy (26) in their classic experiments in cats. Aortic occlusion prevented the development of penile erection produced by sacral nerve root stimulation. Furthermore, after an erection had been produced by nerve stimulation, aortic occlusion resulted in prompt detumescence. The importance of arterial flow was recognized clinically by Leriche and Morel (27). Patients with aortoiliac occlusive vascular disease were recognized to suffer from not only intermittent claudication of the lower extremities, but also from impotence.

Although general agreement exists concerning the importance of increased arterial blood flow in the production and maintenance of erection, the role of the venous drainage system, despite extensive investigation, is still controversial. In 1967, Dorr and Brody (28) extensively studied the hemodynamic aspects of erection in the canine. With erection produced by pelvic nerve stimulation, these investigators demonstrated that dorsal artery perfusion pressure fell while venous pressure rose. Blood flow through not only the dorsal artery, but also the dorsal vein, markedly increased. To ascertain whether a venous occlusive mechanism was, at least in part, responsible for the production and maintenance of erection, pressures were measured at multiple venous sites from the corpora cavernosa distally to the internal pudendal vein proximally. No venous pressure gradient could be found, and these investigators concluded that increased arterial inflow was of primary importance in the produc-

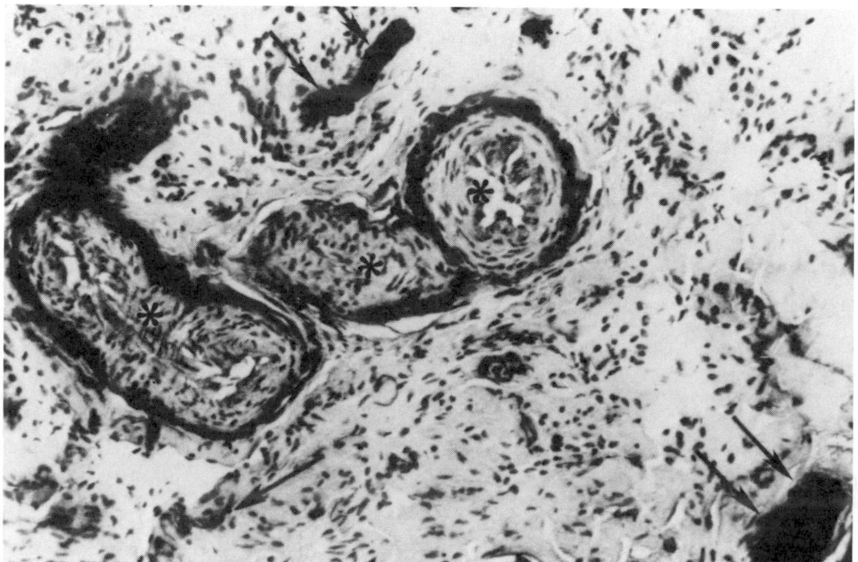

FIG. 4. Acetylcholinesterase-positive fibers in corpus cavernosum in the outer tunic of tortuous arteriole (*asterisks*). Nerve bundles containing acetylcholinesterase are also seen (*arrows*). ×180. From ref 8, with permission.

tion of erection and that increased venous outflow resistance was of little, if any, significance.

In other animal experiments performed in several species, however, data exist that do implicate the obstruction of venous flow from the penis as being mechanistically important in the production of erection. In dogs, the highest recorded pressures in the corpora cavernosa occur during intromission and coincide with electromyographically demonstrable contraction of the ischiocavernosus muscle (29). A plausible explanation for this observation is that skeletal muscle contraction produces compression and, therefore, blockade of venous flow. An equally plausible explanation, however, is that the skeletal muscle is simply compressing the corpora cavernosa in an already erect, high-pressure, state. In goats, bulls, and stallions, anesthesia of the ischiocavernosus muscles prevents these animals from copulating because of their inability to achieve erection (30). In man, however, the importance of striated perineal muscle activity in the production of erection appears to be insignificant. Human erection can occur with no increase in electromyographic activity of the bulbocavernosus, deep transverse perineal, or urethral sphincter muscles (31).

In the early 1980s, xenon washout techniques were utilized to study hemodynamic changes in penile erection in man. This technique appeared ideal to resolve the question of whether increased venous resistance significantly contributes to the production of penile erection. Blood flow through the corpora cavernosa in the flaccid state is minimal. If Xe^{133} were to be injected into the corpora cavernosa and penile erection produced by visual sexual stimulation, the rate of Xe^{133} washout in the flaccid and erect states should determine whether venous flow was increased or decreased with erection. Xe^{133} washout techniques have been utilized by two groups of investigators with remarkably conflicting results. Shirai and Ishii (32) reported an increase in the washout of Xe^{133}, therefore concluding that venous flow increases with erection and that no increase in venous vascular resistance thus occurs. Utilizing similar techniques, however, Wagner (33) found that the rate of washout of Xe^{133} decreased with erection. Wagner concluded that decreased venous flow and therefore increased resistance was an important physiologic event occurring with erection.

Recently, more sophisticated animal experimentation and clinical laboratory techniques have emerged; these data in general support the necessity for increased venous resistance in the production and maintenance of erection. In the canine model, Lue et al. (9) determined that with electrical stimulation of the cavernosal nerve arterial flow through the internal pudendal artery increased by 250%. With erection, pressure within the corpora cavernosa is approximately 10 mmHg below the systolic arterial blood pressure, and blood flow into and out of the corpora cavernosa, although present, is markedly reduced. Utilizing a technique of saline infusion into the corpora with the aorta clamped, an initial drop in cavernosal pressure as well as decreased venous flow was observed during erection produced by cavernosal nerve stimulation. Thus, these investigators conclude that erection is the result of increased arterial inflow, active relaxation of the smooth muscle of the trabeculae of the corpora cavernosa, and active increase in venous outflow resistance. The mechanism responsible for the increase in venous outflow resistance is unclear, but is probably secondary to relaxation of the trabeculae of the corpora cavernosa and increased intracavernosal pressure rather than to active constriction of veins and venules *per se*. Venous compression appears to occur within the corpora cavernosa, between the expanding sinusoidal wall and the noncompliant tunica albuginea during full erection (34).

Clinical studies utilizing cavernosography also support the concept of increased venous resistance. When an erection is produced pharmacologically in man, contrast agents infused into the corpora cavernosa can be radiologically observed to remain in the corpora cavernosa; venous drainage systems of the penis are not normally visualized. In fact, a new etiology for impotence, "venous leak" impotence, has been proposed (35). The pathological event in these patients is probably dysfunction of the smooth muscle of the corpora cavernosa rather than dysfunction of the veins themselves; this new concept will be discussed in further detail in the section on neuropharmacology. Although the controversy concerning the importance of increased venous resistance in the production of penile erection remains unresolved, current evidence supports the concept that both increased arterial inflow and decreased venous outflow contribute to normal erectile physiology.

An equally controversial area concerns the mechanism(s) by which blood is shunted into the penis during the development of erection. In the flaccid state, blood flow through the corpora cavernosa is low. With erection, the cavernous spaces are dilated and filled with blood and the pressure within the corpora cavernosa increases. For years, extremely complex shunt mechanisms were believed to be responsible for increasing blood flow within the corpora cavernosa. In 1939, Deysach (8) hypothesized that "venous sluices" opened and closed and produced erection by altering venous outflow resistance. In 1952, Conti (36), in an anatomic study performed on cadavers, described "polsters," columns of smooth muscle within the intima of penile arteries and veins. Conti proposed that relaxation and contraction of "polsters" could divert blood into and away from the corpora cavernosa and thereby control erection and detumescence. Conti's "polster theory" was widely accepted until evidence was presented that "polsters" are not specialized anatomic structures, but rather atherosclerotic changes in penile blood vessels (37,38). In addition, no innervation to these structures has ever been identified.

Recently, another "shunt theory" has been proposed based on "shunt arteries" (10). According to this hypothesis, the helicine arteries that supply the corpora cavernosa are constricted during detumescence, and blood is diverted to the corpus spongiosum through "shunt arteries." With appropriate stimuli for erection, "shunt arteries" constrict, the helicine arteries dilate, and the net result is that blood flow is increased to the corpora cavernosa. All theories concerning specialized structures that shunt blood away from the corpora in detumescence and into the corpora with erection are speculative. No physiologic data exist to support such mechanisms. In all probability, dilation of the arterial supply to the penis, the helicine arteries, and the trabeculae of the corpora cavernosa are all that is required to shunt blood into the corpora cavernosa.

Neurophysiology

The fact that penile erection is under neurologic control cannot be disputed; the neural pathways involved and the neurophysiologic events responsible for penile erection have been studied since the mid-nineteenth century. The importance of the pelvic parasympathetic nerve was first recognized by the classic observations of Eckhard (39). In the canine, stimulation of these nerves ("nervi erigentes") resulted in penile erection; stimulation of the hypogastric nerve (a sympathetic nerve) did not produce erection.

Similar, but refined, experiments were performed by Muller (40) in the dog and Root and Bard (41) in the cat. The results of these two classic experiments are similar. Two types of stimuli are capable of producing penile erection in these species: (a) tactile genital stimulation, and (b) psychogenic stimulation through proximity to a bitch in heat or cat in estrous. When the entire sacral and most of the lumbar spinal cord is surgically excised, these animals no longer develop erection with genital stimulation. These animals are, however, still capable of developing psychogenic erections. In Root and Bard's study, when cats, in addition to having the lumbosacral spinal cord ablated, also underwent spinal cord transection between T_{11} and T_{12} or T_{13} and L_1, no erectile activity could be seen with either tactile or psychogenic stimuli. In addition, in those animals that had undergone lumbosacral ablation, removal of the hypogastric nerves also resulted in cessation of psychogenically stimulated erection. With the lumbosacral cord intact, however, resection of the hypogastric nerves or inferior mesenteric ganglion had no effect on erections produced by either tactile or psychic stimuli. The results of these studies can be summarized as follows. In the dog and cat, two peripheral neural pathways are capable of producing penile erection. The lumbosacral portion of the spinal cord appears capable of mediating erection by both tactile and psychic stimuli, and the lower thoracic cord and peripheral sympathetic nerves appear capable of mediating erection secondary to psychic stimuli.

Other animal data exist, however, that do not support such relatively simplistic neurologic control mechanisms. In all animal studies performed in the dog, cat, and rabbit, parasympathetic nerve or nerve root stimulation produces erection. Results obtained with sympathetic nerve stimulation have not been so consistent. With hypogastric nerve stimulation, Eckhard (39) reported erection in rabbits, but not in dogs. Other investigators have indicated that hypogastric nerve stimulation in the canine results in a slight increase in penile volume (42). In the feline, Semans and Langworthy (26) did not find penile erection with hypogastric nerve stimulation; in fact, stimulation of these sympathetic nerves produced contraction of penile arteries and actually caused an erect penis to become flaccid. In animal experimentation, therefore, parasympathetic nerve stimulation consistently results in penile erection. Although the sympathetic nervous system may be capable of mediating psychogenic erection, experimental evidence supporting this concept is not conclusive.

Available human data, although scant, are in general consistent with the results of animal experimentation. However, two major flaws exist in most studies in man. First, the completeness of the neurologic lesion can rarely be accurately defined by clinical testing. Second, much of the data is retrospective and has been obtained by interview technique. Few, if any, studies are available that are convincing, because of the lack of objective clinical data pertaining to potency in the presence of neurologic injury or neurologic disease.

The largest series of patients dealing with sexual function in spinal cord injured patients was published by Bors and Comarr (43). No patient with a complete lower motor neuron lesion achieved an erection with genital stimulation. Twenty-four percent of these patients, however, reported penile erection with psychogenic stimulation. Most patients with spinal cord lesions above the level of the sacral spinal cord did report erections with genital tactile stimulation. Patients with spinal cord injuries above the level of the sacral spinal cord also reported erections with psychic stimulation; the percentage of patients achieving psychogenic erection, however, depended on the level of the injury. Psychogenic erections were reported by 4% with cervical lesions; 0% with thoracic, T_1–T_6 lesions; 8% with thoracic, T_7–T_{12} lesions; and 56% with lumbar lesions. These human data are, in general, consistent with the previously described animal data. In man, penile erection produced by tactile genital stimulation appears to be dependent upon an intact sacral spinal reflex arc. The sympathetic nervous system does appear, at least in some patients, to be capable of mediating psychogenic erection through pathways that connect the cerebral cortex, thoracolumbar spinal cord, and peripheral sympathetic pathways to the penis and its vasculature.

In man, as in animal studies, the importance of the parasympathetic nervous system in erectile physiology appears clear. Clinical data relating to importance of the sympathetic innervation of the penis are obtained from young male patients undergoing retroperitoneal lymph node dissection for testis cancer. In these patients, the periaortic sympathetic chain as well as the entire sympathetic innervation to the pelvis is removed from the level of the renal vein to the aortic bifurcation. These patients almost uniformly develop symptoms referable to peripheral sympathetic denervation (lack of seminal fluid emission or retrograde ejaculation), but they do not experience impotence (44,45). Sympathetic innervation, therefore, does not appear to be necessary for the development of erection from tactile or psychogenic stimulation in man. In some patients with sacral spinal cord lesions, the sympathetic nervous system may be responsible for psychogenically induced erections. The overall importance of the sympathetic nervous system in the neurologically normal patient requires better definition.

Supraspinal neurologic control of penile erection undoubtedly is of major importance. Psychogenic impotence is a well-recognized clinical phenomenon. Our understanding of the specific significant central neural pathways is limited. Some animal data exist that describe the results of central nervous system ablation and stimulation experiments. Human data are scarce and are based primarily on isolated case reports of patients with central nervous system diseases or patients following ablative neurosurgical procedures.

Experimentally, the importance of the supraspinal nervous system in regulating penile erection was emphasized by Kluver and Bucy (46). These investigators reported hypersexual behavior in monkeys following removal of both temporal lobes including the uncus and part of the hippocampus. Even under nonstimulated conditions, these monkeys exhibited frequent penile erections. Other experiments utilizing stereotaxic electrical stimulation of various parts of the brain, particularly the limbic system, have demonstrated that the supraspinal central nervous system is capable of mediating penile erection (47–49). Cortical lesions in man are also associated with impotence (50,51).

Neuropharmacology

A significant amount of recent research has concentrated on the peripheral neuropharmacology of penile erection. Man has been searching for an effective aphrodisiac for centuries; recent reports of possibly effective oral therapy for impotence have emphasized the importance of better definition of the end-organ neuropharmacology (52). In addition, effective intracorporal injection therapy has emerged and will be subsequently discussed. Despite concentrated research efforts, the identification of the neurotransmitter(s) responsible for the production of penile erection remains elusive.

As previously discussed, in animals and man, the parasympathetic nervous system (specifically the pelvic nerve) is the primary neural pathway responsible for mediating penile erection. Since the parasympathetic nervous system has been classically thought to be composed of cholinergic neurons, acetylcholine would appear to be the logical candidate for the neurotransmitter responsible for penile erection. Acetylcholine should, therefore, dilate penile blood vessels and relax the smooth muscle of the corpora cavernosa.

Available experimental data, however, do not support the fact that acetylcholine is the primary neurotransmitter, or the only neurotransmitter, responsible for penile erection (17). In animals, erection produced by pelvic nerve stimulation can be prevented by pretreatment with the ganglionic blocking agent hexamethonium, but not by pretreatment with atropine (28,53). Available studies in man also support the concept that penile erection is at least partially atropine resistant (54). If acetylcholine is the neurotransmitter responsible for penile erection, infusion of this agent should produce erection. In animal models, however, penile erection does not follow the intravascular injection of acetylcholine (28,55). Furthermore, corporal smooth muscle relaxation is thought to be of primary importance in producing erection, and, in *in vitro* experiments, strips of corporal smooth muscle respond minimally, if at all, to acetylcholine stimulation (5). Relevant criticisms of these experiments have been forwarded, including the possibility that acetylcholine infused intravascularly may be hydrolyzed before it reaches the smooth muscle receptor and that, in these experimental situations, acetylcholine and atropine do not reach the vascular and corporal receptors. An alternative explanation is that penile erection is not a cholinergically (or exclusively cholinergically) mediated event.

If acetylcholine is not the neurotransmitter responsible for penile arterial dilation and corporal smooth muscle relaxation, could a catecholamine be responsible for the physiologic events leading to penile erection? Adrenergic neurons are carried in the pelvic parasympathetic nerves of rats and cats (56,57), and this could conceivably also be true in man. Stimulation of the pelvic parasympathetic nerve could perhaps, therefore, activate adrenergic as well as cholinergic neurons. As previously discussed, the penile vasculature and corporal smooth muscle are anatomically richly supplied by adrenergic neurons, and high norepinephrine levels in the corpora cavernosa have been demonstrated (58). In addition, in man, radioligand binding studies have demonstrated high α-adrenergic receptor density in corporal preparations (59).

In the cat, the intravenous infusion of the β-adrenergic agonist salbutamol and the α-adrenergic blocker phenoxybenzamine produces penile erection (55). In addition, isolated strips of human corpora cavernosa relax when exposed to isoproterenol and salbutamol (60). β-adrenergic stimulation or α-adrenergic blockade would appear, therefore, to promote erection. Stimulation of isolated human corporal strips with norepinephrine, however, results in contraction; this contractile response can be blocked by pretreating the strips with phentolamine (5). The infusion of norepinephrine in the dog (28) and cat (55) does not cause erection. Epinephrine infusion, in fact, causes contraction of canine penile arteries (61). The oral administration of large doses of α- and β-adrenergic antagonists (phenoxybenzamine and propranolol) has no effect on erections produced by mechanical or visual sexual stimulation in man (54). The evidence concerning the possibility that a catecholamine is the neurotransmitter responsible for erection appears to favor the conclusion that adrenergic stimulation promotes penile detumescence (vascular constriction and corporal contraction) rather than penile erection (62). Further, more convincing, evidence is presented below in the discussion of the intracorporal injection of vasoactive agents.

Thus, the neuropharmacology of penile erection cannot be totally explained by classic adrenergic and cholinergic mechanisms (17). Numerous putative nonadrenergic, noncholinergic neurotransmitters have been neuropharmacologically investigated. Available evidence indicates that prostaglandins (PGE_1, PGE_2, and $PGF_{2\alpha}$), bradykinin, 5-hydroxytryptamine, histamine, and several amino acids are not the neurotransmitters responsible for the vascular and corporal smooth muscle relaxation necessary for the production of penile erection (3,4). Adenosine triphosphate (ATP, a putative purinergic neurotransmitter) has not been physiologically linked to the erectile process.

The search for a nonadrenergic, noncholinergic mechanism to explain the neuropharmacology of penile erection has in recent years been concentrated on possible peptidergic mechanisms. The polypeptide that has been most extensively investigated is VIP. As previously discussed, nerves containing VIP have been anatomically demonstrated in the trabeculae of the corpora cavernosa and in the outer tunic of penile blood vessels at both the light and electron microscopic levels. It not only causes vasodilation (63,64), but also has been demonstrated *in vitro* to cause relaxation of strips of rabbit, cat, monkey, and human corpora cavernosa (21,22,65,66). Other animal experiments have yielded conflicting results. In *in vitro* experiments, VIP has been reported to have little or no effect on the corpora cavernosa urethra of the rabbit, guinea pig, dog, or cat. In addition, VIP stimulation also did not produce relaxation of penile blood vessels in the bull (67). In strips of human corpora cavernosa, VIP exerts no effect unless the strips have been previously contracted via norepinephrine stimulation. After norepinephrine stimulation, a weak relaxant effect is noted (22).

A major reason for the interest in a peptidergic mechanism being responsible for penile erection deals with the issue of atropine resistance. As previously discussed, atropine does not completely block the erectile response elicited by pelvic nerve stimulation. A similar situation has been shown to occur in the cat submandibular gland. Specifically, the vasodilation seen with nerve stimulation in this organ is also atropine resistant. VIP has been demonstrated to be responsible for the atropine-resistant vasodilation; both VIP and acetylcholine are present in the same neuron, and both are released with nerve stimulation (68). If similar mechanisms exist in the penis, many basic questions concerning the neuropharmacology of erection could be answered.

A breakthrough in our understanding of the neuropharmacology and neurophysiology of erection occurred with the description of the intracorporal injection of vasoactive agents. In 1982, Virag et al. (69) reported that papaverine injected directly into the corpora cavernosa caused penile erection. This agent produces smooth muscle relaxation by direct action(s) on the smooth muscle cell and does not act through neuroreceptors. Brindley's (70) observation that the intracorporal injection of phenoxybenzamine (an α-adrenergic blocking agent) also results in penile erection in man clarified the situation further. As previously discussed, norepinephrine causes the smooth muscle of the corpora cavernosa to contract; this effect is α-adrenergic receptor mediated and is prevented by the α-adrenergic blocking agents phenoxybenzamine and phentolamine. Although both of these agents probably also increase arterial blood flow into the penis, the importance of relaxation of the trabeculae of the corpora cavernosa in initiating and maintaining penile erection is now appreciated. A variety of other agents, including imipramine and verapamil (a calcium channel blocker), also produce erection when they are injected intracorporally (71). Since agents that cause smooth muscle relaxation produce erection, pharmacologic agents that cause the corporal smooth muscle to contract should produce detumescence. Norepinephrine, the postganglionic sympathetic neurotransmitter, causes both penile vasoconstriction and contraction of the corporal smooth muscle. The sympathetic nervous system, therefore, appears to be responsible for penile detumescence. The use of intracorporal injection is not only an important research method, but is also a valuable diagnostic and therapeutic modality in the patient with impotence. This will be discussed below.

The recent recognition of the importance of endothelium-derived relaxation factor (EDRF) in the physiology of vascular smooth muscle relaxation has led to new insights into the mechanisms responsible for penile erection. This endothelium-dependent relaxation appears to be mediated by nitric oxide (72). In strips of corporal smooth muscle from rabbit and man, nitric oxide causes relaxation that is similar to that produced by electrical field stimulation. This relaxation occurs in the presence of guanethidine and atropine in the bathing media and is therefore thought to be mediated by nonadrenergic, noncholinergic neurons (73). Acetylcholine is also capable of causing endothelium-dependent relaxation by mechanisms that appear to involve nitric oxide (74). The relaxation produced by nitric oxide is mediated through increased intracellular levels of cyclic GMP. Relaxant responses to nitric oxide are enhanced by pretreating the smooth muscle strips with a cyclic GMP phosphodiesterase inhibitor (73). These observations support the hypothesis that stimulation of nonadrenergic, noncholinergic neurons in the corpus cavernosum stimulates the endogenous formation of nitric oxide in either the neurons, smooth muscle, or endothelial cells. Nitric oxide then causes smooth muscle relaxation through a cyclic GMP mechanism.

Although significant advances have been made in clarifying the neuropharmacology of the peripheral nervous system as it relates to erection, our knowledge of central nervous system mechanisms is limited. Serotonin has been demonstrated to inhibit and dopamine to stimulate male sexual activity in the rat (75). In male patients with Parkinson's disease treated with L-dopa, increased sexual activity has been reported (76,77). Trazodone, an antidepressant used commonly clinically, is associated with the occurrence of priapism (78). Trazodone is thought to act primarily by blocking the reuptake of serotonin into nerve terminals. In addition, chlorophenylpiperazine, a metabolite of trazodone, causes erection in monkeys when this agent is injected intravenously (79,80).

Clinical Importance of Recent Basic Science Advances

The description of acceptable penile prostheses in the mid-1970s (81,82) not only popularized the evaluation and treatment of impotence, but also emphasized how little was actually known about the basic physiology of erection. Recent research has clarified the fact that the two major events responsible for penile erection are increased arterial flow to the penis and relaxation of the smooth muscle of the trabeculae, which allows blood to be shunted into the corpora cavernosa. As previously discussed, increased venous outflow resistance also occurs, not by active constriction of the venous outflow, but by passive occlusion caused by increased intracorporal pressure.

Although erectile difficulty secondary to atherosclerotic disease has been recognized for years (27), the standardization of techniques to measure penile blood flow has significantly clarified our understanding of the importance of arterial flow in several disease processes. Until relatively recently, the penile arterial supply was routinely evaluated by measuring the penile blood pressure with a Doppler stethoscope and a pneumatic cuff (83). The accuracy of this noninvasive study has recently been questioned. The conventional Doppler spreads a wide ultrasound wave, and the operator cannot be sure which artery (dorsal, cavernosal, or urethral) is being evaluated. In addition, this study has been performed with the penis in thc flaccid statc, and the significance of the results is in question.

Currently, the study of choice to evaluate the penile arterial supply is either duplex Doppler or color Doppler evaluation. Individual arteries can be visualized, their diameters measured, and velocity of blood flow determined (84). The measurements are made with the penis in both the flaccid and the erect state. Erection is produced by the intracorporal injection of vasoactive drugs; this is discussed below. An increase in mean arterial diameter of more than 75% of the flaccid value and a mean peak flow velocity of greater than 25 cm/sec after intracorporal drug injection are considered normal values (85). The use of objective measurements of penile arterial flow has allowed description of several clinical entities. For example, patients who initially develop a good erection and then experience difficulty maintaining it during intercourse may demonstrate the "external iliac" or "pelvic steal" syndrome (86,87). In these patients, with exercise, blood is shunted from the pelvis to the buttocks and legs.

Impotence in patients who have undergone successful renal transplantation may also be secondary to vascular factors. In renal transplantation, the internal iliac (hypogastric) artery is often transected and used in an end-to-end anastomosis to the transplant renal artery. If a second transplant is performed utilizing the opposite internal iliac artery in a similar fashion, impotence secondary to decreased arterial flow to the penis is likely to occur (88). Second renal transplants can be performed by an end-to-side technique on the external iliac or common iliac artery and penile blood flow preserved.

Although much experimental information concerning the neuroanatomy and neurophysiology of erection has been recently generated, clinical studies to assess the integrity of sensory and motor pathways are less than adequate. The integrity of neural pathways can be ascertained by measuring evoked potentials. The sacral evoked potential (sacral latency time) is performed by stimulating penile skin and recording from a needle electrode placed in the bulbocavernosus muscle (89). The time from stimulation to the first electrical response in the bulbocavernosus muscle is measured and is the sacral latency time. The neural reflex controlling penile erection consists of pudendal afferent (sensory) fibers and parasympathetic efferent (motor) fibers. The sensory portion of the sacral reflex that governs erection and the sensory portion of the reflex that is measured by sacral evoked potential testing are, therefore, identical. This sensory portion of the reflex arc can also be evaluated by measuring dorsal penile nerve conduction velocity (90). The efferent part of the reflex that controls erection is, however, different from the efferent innervation, which is measured by sacral evoked potential testing. This study measures pudendal sensory afferent and pudendal (somatic) motor efferent nerves. At present, no methodology exists that can directly measure the efferent (parasympathetic) portion of the reflex controlling erection. Measurement of sacral latency times provides some information concerning reflex activity through the sacral spinal cord, but does not directly test efferent penile innervation.

Neurologic testing of central nervous system pathways that control erection is even less precise. Genitocerebral evoked potentials can be measured; the penis is stimulated as in the sacral evoked response examination, and recordings are taken from electroencephalographic leads placed on the scalp (91). The clinical significance of such studies is not yet clear. Methods to evaluate penile innervation clinically and directly are needed.

The recent description of the anatomy of the corporal nerves in man has allowed the technique of several surgical procedures to be modified. Previously, most patients undergoing radical prostatectomy for prostate cancer experienced postoperative impotence. Following the precise anatomic description of the cavernosal nerves, Walsh and Mostwin (92) concluded that impotence in these patients results from injury to the autonomic innervation during transection of the prostatic apex and the urethra, or during division of the lateral pelvic fascia and lateral pedicle. After modification of the surgical technique to preserve these nerves, 86% of patients who have undergone radical prostatectomy are potent 1 year after surgery.

Recent advances in our understanding of erectile neuropharmacology have already become clinically useful. The intracorporal injection of various drugs causes penile erection. In man, the injection of papaverine alone and papaverine combined with phentolamine has been utilized both diagnostically and therapeutically (84,93). Currently, PGE_1 alone or PGE_1 in combination with low doses of papaverine and phentolamine are the most commonly utilized drugs for intracorporal injection (94,95). These injection techniques have improved the accuracy of the diagnostic evaluation of both the penile arterial supply and venous drainage. Pressure responses to drug injection and the physiologic measurements of blood flow under various test situations can be measured. Both arterial and venous channels can be visualized in both the tumescent and flaccid states. These techniques, however, require further standardization, and determination of normal values in potent men of all ages is needed. Intracorporal injection therapy for impotence has reportedly been successful in large numbers of patients (93,94,96). Self-injection with PGE_1 and combinations of papaverine and phentolamine is thought to be relatively free of side effects (96); the long-term effects of such therapy in man, however, is not known.

A significant complication of the intracorporal injection of drugs that produce erection is priapism (97). In the past, priapism has been treated primarily by surgical procedures that shunt blood out of the corpora cavernosa and into either the saphenous vein, glans penis, or corpus spongiosum (98,99). By applying new knowledge of the neuropharmacology of the penis, it is now possible to treat some patients with priapism by pharmacologic methods. Laboratory studies have demonstrated that catecholamines cause the smooth muscle of the corpora to contract and constrict penile arteries. Since erection is produced by corporal dilation and vasodilation, the intracorporal injection of catecholamines into an already erect penis should, theoretically, produce detumescence. This, in fact, is the case, and some patients with priapism, particularly those patients whose priapism is secondary to the prolonged effects of intracorporally injected drugs, can be successfully treated by the intracavernous injection of α-adrenergic agonists such as norepinephrine and phenylephrine (97,100).

The ultimate goal of pharmacologic therapy of impotence is the discovery and development of a drug that can be taken orally and that would reproducibly result in the development of penile erection. Various agents have been utilized for this purpose in the past; none have yielded satisfactory results. Testosterone therapy in impotent patients with normal serum testosterone levels is no more efficacious than a placebo (101). Recently, renewed interest in yohimbine has emerged. For many years this agent was considered an aphrodisiac and, in combination with testosterone and nux vomica extract, was widely used for the therapy of impotence in the 1960s. Clinical trials with yohimbine have again emerged. Morales et al. (52) initially reported that 6 of 23 patients treated with this drug note the reappearance of full, sustained erections. Further controlled studies, however, did not show that yohimbine was statistically more efficacious than a placebo (102).

An equally important pharmacologic question concerns the incidence and mechanisms by which many commonly used drugs cause erectile dysfunction. Medication may be the single most common cause of impotence in the United States. Objective evidence is so limited, however, that very few conclusions can be reached. Virtually every class of drugs has been implicated as being causally related to impotence; the theoretical mechanisms for these adverse drug effects include central nervous system sedation or depression, drug-related hyperprolactinemia, direct antiandrogen effects, and anticholinergic or antiadrenergic effects (103). An example of the complexity of drug effects on erectile function is cimetidine, a histamine (H_2) receptor antagonist widely used in the treatment of duodenal ulcer disease. This agent has been associated with diminished libido and impotence in up to 50% of male patients (104). The mechanisms, however, by which cimetidine causes impotence are unclear. Cimetidine has been associated with elevated prolactin levels and gynecomastia (105, 106). In addition, peripheral H_2 receptor blockage in corporal smooth muscle may also be responsible (107). The pharmacologic central effects of most medications are unknown. Few, if any, well-controlled studies exist that have utilized objective parameters to evaluate the adverse effects of most commonly used medications on penile erection.

In summary, a significant amount of new basic laboratory information concerning the physiology of erection has been obtained during the past decade. Much of this information has been directly applicable to clinical practice. Many important questions remain unanswered. Which neurotransmitter(s) control vascular dilatation and corporal smooth muscle relaxation? What role does the sympathetic nervous system play in man? What are the mechanisms by which the central nervous system controls erection? What are the mechanisms by which commonly prescribed drugs adversely affect erection? In contrast to a decade ago, a significant number of laboratories are now currently involved in basic science and clinical research in the areas of penile erection and impotence. Answers to many questions concerning male erectile dysfunction should be available in the near future.

EMISSION AND EJACULATION

In recent years, research in the area of erectile dysfunction has produced a significant amount of new clinical information. The study of erectile dysfunction is at present receiving much attention primarily because of the high incidence of impotence and public awareness that satisfactory therapy exists. Fewer patients experience primary disorders of emission and ejaculation. The physiology of these events is understood to some extent, and treatment is available for some patients with disorders of seminal fluid emission and ejaculation. Emission, the deposition of seminal fluid into the posterior urethra, is dependent upon the integrity of the vasa deferentia, seminal vesicles, prostate gland, and bladder neck. Ejaculation is dependent primarily upon the function of the striated perineal musculature.

Anatomy

Spermatozoa are transported from the testes and epididymides to the posterior urethra by the vasa deferentia. The tubular vas deferens is approximately 35 cm long in the human adult. It extends from the tail of the epididymis to the region of the verumontanum in the posterior urethra. (Fig. 5) The vas deferens joins the duct of the seminal vesicle to form the ejaculatory duct. Anatomically, the vas deferens in man can be divided into five parts: (a) the sheathless epididymal portion contained within the tunica vaginalis, (b) the scrotal portion, (c) the inguinal portion, (d) the retroperitoneal portion, and (e) the ampulla.

Embryologically, the vas deferens is derived from the Wolffian ductal system. On physical examination, the vas deferens is easily palpable as a thick, cordlike structure in the scrotum. The vas is not present in patients with cystic fibrosis and in some patients with renal agenesis. Histologically, the thick wall of the vas surrounds a very narrow lumen (approximately 0.05 cm). The wall is composed of three layers: (a) a mucosal layer; (b) a thick muscular layer consisting of inner longitudinal, middle circular, and outer longitudinal layers; and (c) an adventitial layer composed of a sheath of connective tissue containing numerous small blood vessels and nerves (108).

At the time of seminal fluid emission and ejaculation, the bladder neck closes to prevent the retrograde ejaculation of seminal fluid into the bladder (109). The anatomy of the bladder neck is controversial, and the anatomic basis for bladder neck closure in preventing not only retrograde ejaculation, but also urinary incontinence is unclear. Most investigators agree that no anatomic sphincter consisting of circular smooth muscle fibers exists in the area of the bladder outlet (110,111). A physiologic sphincter, however, does exist. The bladder neck probably remains collapsed because of tension created by the large amount of elastic tissue in this area as well as smooth muscle contraction under α-adrenergic control (112). Following transurethral resection of the

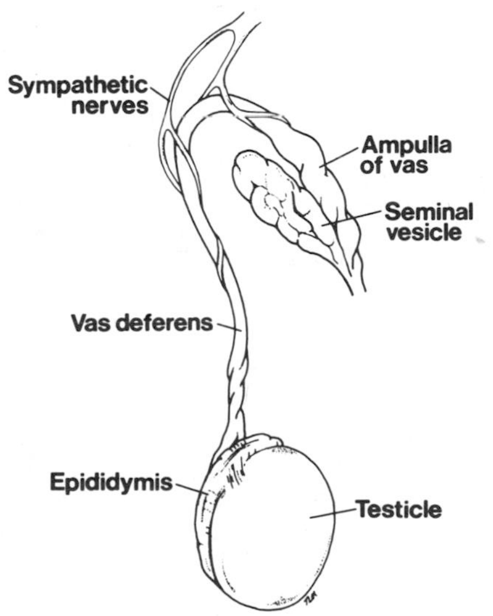

FIG. 5. Anatomy of the human vas deferens.

prostate, the bladder neck closure mechanism is destroyed. Patients remain continent because of a second, more distal, continence mechanism that is present in the region of the membranous urethra (113) (Fig. 6). Most patients who have undergone transurethral resection of the prostate, however, do experience retrograde ejaculation.

Following emission, the seminal fluid that has been deposited in the posterior urethra is expelled out the urethral meatus by the process of ejaculation. Clonic contractions of the perineal striated musculature, primarily the bulbocavernosus and ischiocavernosus muscles, are responsible for this event (114). The bulbocavernosus muscle takes its origin from the central tendon, encircles the corpus spongiosum, and inserts into the corpus cavernosum. The ischiocavernosus muscle arises from the inner surface of the ischial tuberosity and inserts into the penile crura. In man, the experience of orgasm occurs simultaneously with the clonic contractions of these striated muscles during ejaculation (31).

Neuroanatomy of the Vas Deferens, Bladder Neck, and Perineal Musculature

The vas deferens and bladder neck, like the penis, are supplied by nerves from the pelvic plexus. For reasons that will be subsequently discussed, the innervation to these organs is thought to be primarily sympathetic in origin. In man, the cell bodies of the sympathetic neurons are located in the lateral columns of gray matter in the thoracic and upper lumbar segments of the spinal

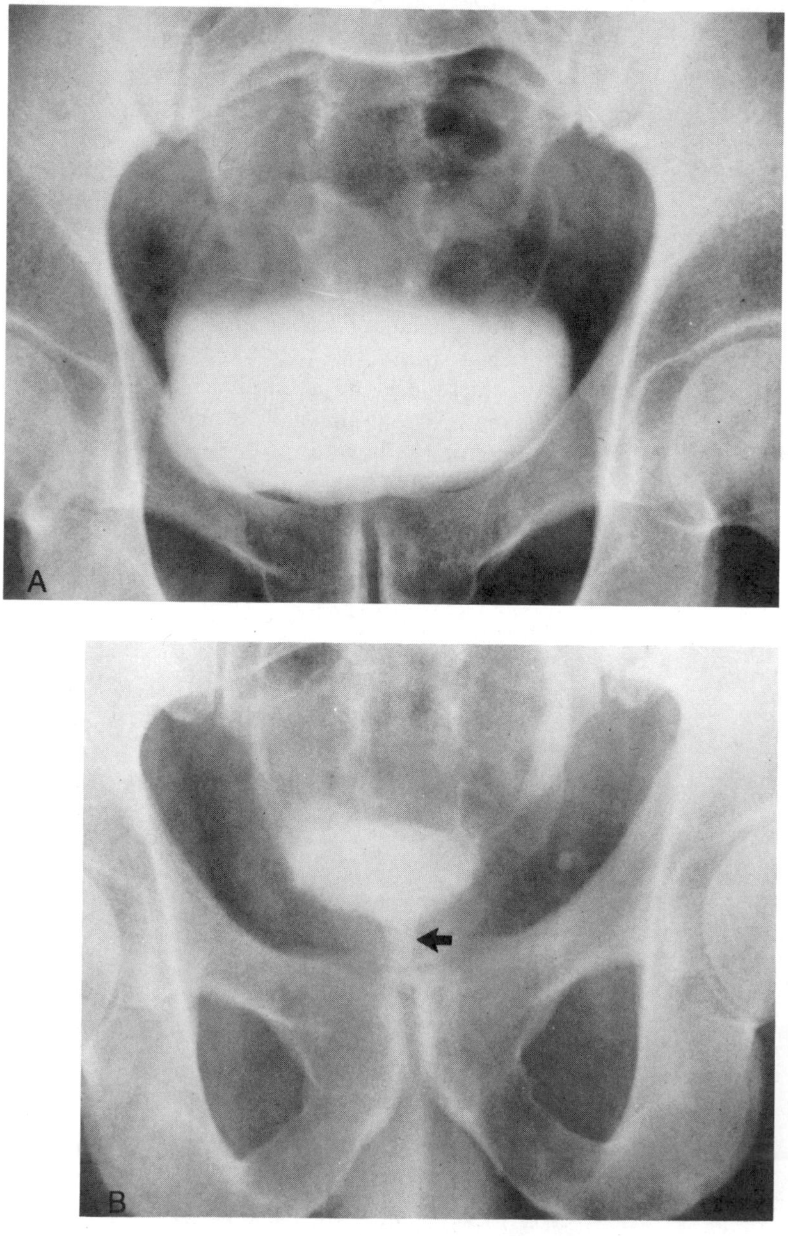

FIG. 6. Cystogram before (**A**) and after (**B**) transurethral resection of prostate (TURP). Note that contrast in A is contained within bladder by competent bladder neck. After TURP, contrast is seen past the area of the bladder neck in the region of the prostatic urethra (*arrow*).

cord. Sympathetic nerve fibers exit the spinal cord via the ventral roots. These preganglionic sympathetic fibers synapse with either (a) paravertebral sympathetic chain ganglia, (b) abdominal or pelvic plexuses, or (c) ganglia located near or in the end organ. The anatomy of the abdominal and pelvic sympathetic nervous system is complex and variable, and its nomenclature is poorly standardized. Peripheral sympathetic nerves are extremely difficult to trace anatomically, and individual variability of even the paravertebral sympathetic chain is marked. Pick and Sheehan (115) carefully dissected the paravertebral sympathetic chain in 25 cadavers. They found the first lumbar ganglion to be independent in 11, fused with other ganglia in 10, and separated into two parts in 2. The second lumbar ganglion was absent in 2, independent in 12, fused in 7, and split in four.

Sympathetic nerve fibers exiting the thoracolumbar spinal cord synapse in all of the abdominal and pelvic plexuses (celiac, superior mesenteric, aortic, inferior mesenteric, superior hypogastric, inferior hypogastric, and pelvic). In man, the paired hypogastric nerves exit the superior hypogastric ganglion, which is also called the presacral nerve (15). The superior hypogastric ganglion anatomically extends from approximately the fourth lumbar to the first sacral vertebra. The pelvic plexus is located retroperitoneally beside the rectum and receives input from both the sympathetic and parasympathetic nervous systems. Autonomic nerves leaving the pelvic plexus supply the penis, prostate, seminal vesicle, vas deferens, and bladder (Fig. 7).

The perineal striated musculature (including the bulbocavernosus and ischiocavernosus muscles) is innervated by the pudendal nerve. The pudendal nerve is a somatic nerve that emanates from the sacral spinal cord (S_{2-4}). Peripherally, the pudendal nerve does not enter

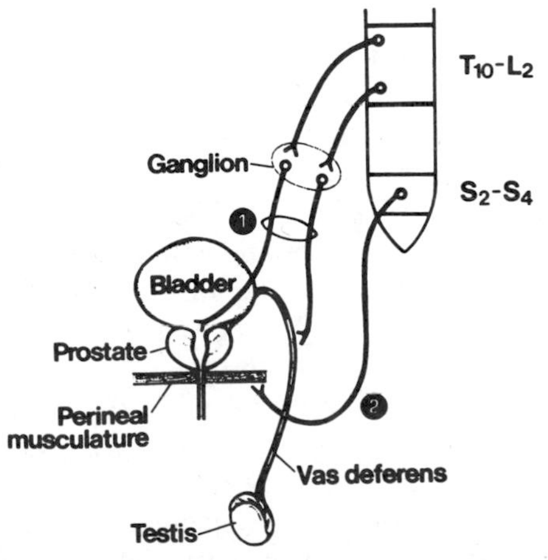

FIG. 7. Innervation of bladder neck, vas deferens, and perineal striated musculature: (*1*) sympathetic innervation to bladder neck and vas deferens; (2) somatic innervation to striated perineal musculature.

the pelvic plexus, but exits the pelvis through the greater sciatic foramen, crosses the spine of the ischium, and reenters the pelvis through the lesser sciatic foramen (14).

Striated muscle fibers can be seen histologically periurethrally as far cephalad as the area of the bladder neck (116). Anatomic evidence has been presented that this periurethral striated musculature is composed of two distinct types of muscle fibers, fast twitch and slow twitch (117). Evidence has also been presented that this periurethral striated musculature is innervated not by the pudendal (somatic) nerve, but by autonomic fibers from the pelvic plexus (118). In addition, Elbadawi and Shenk (119) have reported finding a "triple innervation" (somatic, adrenergic, and cholinergic) to the periurethral striated musculature. Other studies, however, have failed to demonstrate an autonomic innervation to this striated musculature (120,121). At present, most anatomic evidence supports the concept that the innervation of the musculature responsible for ejaculation is somatic and not autonomic (Fig. 7).

Microscopically, utilizing histofluorescent techniques, the vas deferens in animals (cat, rat, dog, and monkey) as well as man is heavily innervated by adrenergic nerves (122). High concentrations of norepinephrine determined by fluorimetric techniques have also been demonstrated (123). The inguinal portion of the vas deferens appears to be more densely adrenergically innervated and to possess a higher norepinephrine content than that portion of the vas nearer the testicle (124). Electron microscopic studies relating to the adrenergic innervation of the vas deferens are consistent with the light microscopic data. Nerve varicosities containing small (400–600 Å), dense-core vesicles have been identified. Utilizing a glutaraldehyde-dichromate technique, these small vesicles have been shown to contain catecholamine (125).

Although, anatomically, the primary innervation to the vas appears to be adrenergic, other types of nerve fibers have been demonstrated. A sparse cholinergic component was observed by Baumgarten et al. (124). Recent light and electron microscopic studies have confirmed the presence of a cholinergic innervation and also demonstrated a peptidergic innervation. Presumptive cholinergic vesicles (400–600 Å small clear vesicles) are present in the vas (125). Close beneath the basement membrane of the epithelium VIP immunoreactive nerve fibers have been seen, but only occasionally in the smooth musculature of the vas. In addition, avian pancreatic polypeptide immunoreactive nerves are particularly dense in the muscular coat of the vas deferens, and somatostatin has been demonstrated to be present in the vas by radioimmunoassay (21). The physiologic significance of the peptidergic innervation is unclear.

Morphologically, in animal models, the bladder base is richly innervated by both adrenergic and cholinergic nerves. In the dog, the bladder base contains a much denser adrenergic innervation than does the bladder body (112). Human data are, in general, consistent with those obtained in animals. Acetylcholinesterase-positive (presumptive cholinergic) and histofluorescent (adrenergic) nerve fibers are reported to be numerous in the trigone and less dense in the anterior bladder base in both males and females (126). Gosling et al. (127), however, have reported a sexual difference and describes a dense adrenergic innervation throughout the bladder base in the male and a sparse adrenergic innervation in this area in the female. In considering the neuroanatomic basis for bladder neck closure during emission and ejaculation, however, there is general agreement that, in the male, this region possesses a significant adrenergic innervation.

Neurophysiology and Neuropharmacology

Electrical stimulation of either the superior hypogastric ganglion (presacral nerve) or the hypogastric nerves in man results in contraction of the bladder neck, prostatic musculature, seminal vesicles, and ejaculatory ducts (15). Similar results have been obtained from experiments in the cat (26). The exact spinal cord level from which these sympathetic nerves originate is difficult to ascertain because of the previously discussed marked anatomic variability.

The neuropharmacology of the vas deferens in several animal species has been extensively studied. Although the importance of the sympathetic nervous system and adrenergic innervation to the vas is well recognized, evidence has accumulated indicating that nonadrenergic neurotransmission may be responsible for part of the contraction of the vas deferens in several animal species including the guinea pig and the rat (128–130). In man, however, norepinephrine is most probably the only significant neurotransmitter responsible for vasal contraction. Norepinephrine causes a marked contractile response in *in vitro* preparations of the human vas deferens. These norepinephrine-induced contractions can be blocked by phentolamine, phenoxybenzamine, and prazosin (131–133). The smooth muscle of the vas deferens exhibits spontaneous motility unless it has been exposed to local anesthetic agents. Local anesthetics also inhibit the response of the vas to norepinephrine stimulation. Other pharmacologic agents (acetylcholine, isoproterenol, histamine, and serotonin) exert little or no effect on the human vas deferens (134). In summary, in man the primary neurologic control of the contractility of the vas deferens is the sympathetic nervous system; adrenergic nerves release norepinephrine, which acts via stimulation of α_1-adrenergic receptors.

Strips of muscle from the bladder base (bladder neck) also contract when stimulated *in vitro* with norepinephrine. Like the vas deferens, these contractile responses are blocked by pretreating the tissue with α-adrenergic antagonists (135). On the other hand, strips of bladder body, that part of the bladder circumferentially above the level of the ureteral orifices, respond to adrenergic stimulation by norepinephrine with β-adrenergic receptor-mediated relaxation (112). Radioligand binding studies in animals have shown that α-adrenergic receptors outnumber β-adrenergic receptors in the bladder base (bladder neck). β-Adrenergic receptors outnumber α-adrenergic receptors in the bladder body (136). It therefore appears that increased sympathetic (adrenergic) nerve activity causes both contraction of the vas deferens (emission) and closure of the bladder neck to prevent retrograde ejaculation.

The neurophysiology and neuropharmacology of ejaculation is less well understood. In man, ejaculation is associated with rhythmic contractions of the periurethral and anal sphincter muscles (114,137). Some animal data concerning central nervous system control of emission and ejaculation have been generated. Seminal fluid emission in rats occurs after stimulation of parts of the hypothalamus (138), and ejaculation in monkeys has been produced by stimulating the preoptic area (139). In man, both erection and ejaculation have occurred following the intrathecal injection of Prostigmin, a drug that blocks cholinesterase (140). This technique has been utilized clinically to obtain semen in patients with neurologic injury. Its usefulness is limited by the fact that significant hypertension commonly occurs. The physiologic and pharmacologic bases for the central nervous system actions of this drug are not known.

Conclusions and Clinical Correlation

Clinical observation has significantly contributed to our understanding of the basic physiologic mechanisms involved in emission and ejaculation. Following retroperitoneal lymph node dissection (RLND) for testicular cancer, many patients report that, although penile erection and orgasm are unchanged postoperatively, they experience a "dry ejaculate" or "shoot blanks." An extensive retroperitoneal dissection, RLND includes removal of the sympathetic nerves and ganglia lying on the aorta and vena cava as well as the paravertebral ganglia. For years the "dry ejaculate" was thought to be secondary to retrograde ejaculation of seminal fluid into the bladder; the extensive "sympathectomy" had presumably rendered the bladder unable to close during emission and ejaculation. Further study of these patients revealed that this explanation for the "dry ejaculate" was incomplete. Examination of postmasturbation bladder washings in these patients failed to demonstrate any sperm or fructose (44,45). The most reasonable explanation for the occurrence of a "dry ejaculate" following RLND is not retrograde ejaculation, but rather the absence of seminal fluid emission. Although lack of emission is the most common cause of sexual dysfunction following RLND, some patients do exhibit retrograde ejaculation. The etiology of these disorders appears to be interruption of the sympathetic innervation of the vas deferens and/or bladder neck.

Except for the previously mentioned attempts to produce emission and ejaculation with the intrathecal administration of Prostigmin, efforts to manipulate these processes pharmacologically are directed at the end organ. No specific therapy for disturbances of ejaculation *per se* are available. Attempts to alter ejaculation pharmacologically are actually directed toward seminal fluid emission and bladder neck closure.

Since seminal fluid emission and bladder neck closure are controlled by sympathetic innervation acting through α-adrenergic receptors, rational drug therapy directed toward correcting vas deferens and bladder neck dysfunction is at least theoretically possible. The sequence of events at the adrenergic nerve terminal is depicted in Fig. 8. With adrenergic nerve stimulation, norepinephrine is released from the nerve terminal and then interacts with α_1-adrenergic receptors located on the smooth muscle membrane. Norepinephrine reuptake into the nerve terminal as well as degradation by monamine oxidase and catechol-O-methyl-transferase then occurs. In addition, norepinephrine interacts with presynaptic α_2-adrenergic receptors on the nerve terminal in a "negative-feedback" fashion whereby stimulation of the α_2-receptors decreases the amount of norepinephrine released by the nerve terminal. Pharmacologic agents are available that can influence several of these events at the nerve terminal.

A number of adrenergic receptor agonists have been used clinically to stimulate contraction of the vas deferens, prostate, seminal vesicle, and bladder neck. Ephedrine sulfate directly stimulates both α- and β-adrenergic receptors and also causes norepinephrine to be released from nerve terminals. Prolonged usage of this drug results in tachyphylaxis, probably because of depletion of norepinephrine in the nerve terminal (141). Pseudoephedrine hydrochloride (a stereoisomer of ephedrine) exerts similar pharmacologic effects. Phenylpropanolamine hydrochloride, an ingredient in many commonly used nasal decongestants, also directly stimulates α-adrenergic receptors. These agents have been used to treat patients with both urinary incontinence and lack of seminal fluid emission and retrograde ejaculation (142).

Imipramine, a tricyclic antidepressant, has also been clinically utilized to treat disorders of emission (143). Imipramine probably potentiates peripheral adrenergic activity by blocking the reuptake of norepinephrine into the nerve terminal. This "cocainelike" effect occurs in the central nervous system; the peripheral effects on this drug are less clear. Imipramine does possess both anticholinergic and direct smooth muscle depressant properties (144,145). It is not known whether the clinical benefits of this drug on the urogenital tract are primarily from central or peripheral nervous system effects.

Clinical disorders of emission and ejaculation can be broadly categorized into four groups: (a) anatomic (e.g., secondary to transurethral resection of the prostate or Y-V plasty of the bladder neck); (b) neuropathic (e.g., secondary to diabetes or RLND); (c) psychogenic ("ejaculatory incompetence"); or (d) idiopathic (142). Exogenous drugs possessing α-adrenergic blocking properties, e.g., phenoxybenzamine, can also result in failure of seminal fluid emission and/or retrograde ejaculation. Surgical and medical management of patients with "ejaculatory dysfunction" is improving. The use of electroejaculation techniques utilizing rectal probes is being advocated, particularly in patients with neurologic deficits (146). Major breakthroughs, however, await a better understanding of the physiologic, particularly central nervous system, mechanisms involved.

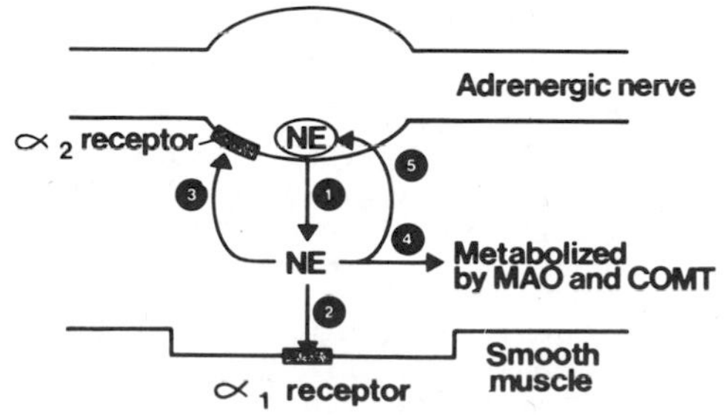

FIG 8. Physiologic events at adrenergic nerve terminal: *(1)* with nerve stimulation, norepinephrine is released from the nerve terminal; *(2)* norepinephrine stimulates α_1-adrenergic receptors on smooth muscle membrane; *(3)* norepinephrine also stimulates presynaptic α_2-receptors; *(4)* norepinephrine is degraded by monamine oxidase and catechol-O-methyl-transferase; *(5)* remaining norepinephrine undergoes reuptake into the nerve terminal.

REFERENCES

1. Benson GS, Lipshultz LI, McConnell JA. Mechanisms of human erection, emission, and ejaculation: current clinical concepts. In: vonEschenbach AC, Rodrigues DB, eds. *Sexual rehabilitation of the urologic cancer patient.* Boston: GK Hall, 1981;54–68.
2. Benson GS. Mechanisms of penile erection. *Invest Urol* 1981;19:65–69.
3. Klinge E, Sjostrand NO. Contraction and relaxation of the retractor penis muscle and the penile artery of the bull. *Acta Physiol Scand (Suppl)* 1974;420:1–88.
4. Klinge E, Sjostrand NO. Comparative study of some isolated mammalian smooth muscle effectors of penile erection. *Acta Physiol Scand* 1977;100:354–367.
5. Benson GS, McConnell JA, Lipshultz LI, Corriere JN, Jr, Wood J. Neuromorphology and neuropharmacology of the human penis. *J Clin Invest* 1980;65:506–513.
6. Newman HF, Northrup JD. Mechanism of human penile erection: an overview. *Urology* 1981;17:399–408.
7. Reiss HF, Northrup HF, Zorgniotti A. Artificial erection by perfusion of penile arteries. *Urology* 1982;20:284–288.

8. Deysach LJ. The comparative morphology of the erectile tissue of the penis with especial emphasis on the probable mechanism of erection. *Am J Anat* 1939;64:111–131.
9. Lue TF, Takamura T, Umraiya M, Schmidt RA, Tanagho EA. Hemodynamics of canine corpora cavernosa during erection. *Urology* 1984;24:347–352.
10. Wagner G, Bro-Rasmussen F, Willis EA, Neilsen MH. New theory on the mechanism of erection involving hitherto undescribed vessels. *Lancet* 1982;1:416–418.
11. Van Arsdalen HN, Malloy TR, Wein AJ. Erectile physiology, dysfunction and evaluation. Part 1: Physiology of erection. In: Stamey TA, ed. *1983 Monographs in urology.* Princeton: Custom Publishing Services, 1983;137.
12. Lue TF, Tanagho EA. Hemodynamics of erection. In: Tanagho EA, Lue TF, McClure RD, eds. *Contemporary management of impotence and infertility.* Baltimore: Williams & Wilkins, 1988;28–38.
13. Wespes E, Schulman CC. Venous leakage: surgical treatment of a curable cause of impotence. *J Urol* 1985;133:796–798.
14. Walsh PC, Donker PJ. Impotence following radical prostatectomy: insight into etiology and prevention. *J Urol* 1982;128: 492–497.
15. Learmonth JR. A contribution to the neurophysiology of the urinary bladder in man. *Brain* 1931;54:147–176.
16. Shirai M, Sasaki K, Rikimaru A. Histochemical investigation on the distribution of adrenergic and cholinergic nerves in the human penis. *Tohoku J Med* 1972;107:403–404.
17. Benson GS. Penile erection: in search of a neurotransmitter. *World J Urol* 1983;1:209–212.
18. McConnell JA, Benson GS. Innervation of human penile blood vessels. *Neurourol Urodyn* 1982;1:199–210.
19. Chubb IW, Hodgson AJ, White GH. Acetylcholinesterase hydrolyzes substance P. *Neuroscience* 1980;5:2065–2072.
20. Polak JM, Gu J, Mina S, Bloom SR. Vipergic nerves in the penis. *Lancet* 1981;2:217–219.
21. Gu J, Polak JM, Probert L, et al. Peptidergic innervation of the human male genital tract. *J Urol* 1983;130:386–391.
22. Steers WD, McConnell JA, Benson GS. Anatomical localization and some pharmacologic effects of vasoactive intestinal polypeptide in human and monkey corpus cavernosum. *J Urol* 1984;132:1048–1053.
23. Kirkeby HJ, Jorgensen JC, Ottesen B. Neuropeptide Y (NPY) in human penile corpus cavernosum tissue and circumflex veins—occurrence and in vitro effects. *J Urol* 1991;145:605–609.
24. Ekblad E, Edvinsson L, Wahlestedt C, Udman R, Hakanson R, Sundler F. Neuropeptide Y coexists and cooperates with noradrenaline in perivascular nerve fibers. *Regul Pept* 1984;8: 225–235.
25. Schmalbruch H, Wagner G. Vasoactive intestinal polypeptide (VIP)- and neuropeptide Y (NPY)-containing nerve fibers in the penile cavernous tissue of green monkeys (*Cercopithecus aethiops*). *Cell Tissue Res* 1989;256:529–541.
26. Semans JH, Langworthy OR. Observations on the neurourophysiology of sexual function in the male cat. *J Urol* 1939;40: 836–846.
27. Leriche R, Morel A. Syndrome of thrombotic obliteration of the aortic bifurcation. *Ann Surg* 1948;127:193–206.
28. Dorr LD, Brody MJ. Hemodynamic mechanism of erection in the canine penis. *Am J Physiol* 1967;213:1526–1531.
29. Purohit RC, Beckett SD. Penile pressures and muscle activity associated with erection and ejaculation in the dog. *Am J Physiol* 1976;231:1343–1348.
30. Beckett SD, Hudson RS, Walker DF, Vachon RI, Reynolds TM. Corpus cavernosum penis pressure and external penile muscle activity during erection in the goat. *Biol Reprod* 1972;7:359–364.
31. Kollberg S, Peterson I, Stener I. Preliminary results of an electromyographic study of ejaculation. *Acta Chir Scand* 1962;123: 478–483.
32. Shirai M, Ishii N. Hemodynamics of erection in man. *Arch Androl* 1981;6:27–32.
33. Wagner G. Erection, physiology and endocrinology. In: Wagner G, Green R, eds. *Impotence.* New York: Plenum Press, 1981;29–30.
34. Lue TF, Tanagho EA. Functional anatomy and mechanism of penile erection. In: Tanagho EA, Lue TF, McClure RD, eds. *Contemporary management of impotence and infertility.* Baltimore: Williams & Wilkins, 1988;39–54.
35. Lue TF, Hricak H, Schmidt RA, Tanago EA. Functional evaluation of penile veins by cavernosography in papaverine-induced erection. *J Urol* 1986;135:479–482.
36. Conti G. L'erection du penis humain et ses bases morphologico-vascularies. *Acta Anat (Basel)* 1952;14:217–262.
37. Benson GS, McConnell JA, Schmidt WA. Penile "polsters": functional structures or atherosclerotic changes? *J Urol* 1981; 125:800–803.
38. McConnell JA, Benson GS, Schmidt WA. The vasculature of the human penis: a reexamination of the morphological basis for the polster theory of erection. *Anat Rec* 1982;203:475–484.
39. Eckhard C (ed). Untersuchungen uber die Erection das Penis beim hunde. *Beitrage zur Anatomie und Physiologie* 1863;3: 123–166.
40. Muller LR. Klinische and experimentelle Studien uber die Innervation der Blase, des Mastdarms, und des Genitalapparates. *Deutsch Z Nervenheilk* 1902;21:86–154.
41. Root WAS, Bard P. The mediation of feline erection through sympathetic pathways with some remarks on sexual behavior after deafferentiation of the genitalia. *Am J Physiol* 1947; 151:80–90.
42. Bacq ZM. Recherches sur la physiologie et la pharmacologie du systéme nerveux anatonome: XII. Nature cholinergique et adrenergique des diverses innervations vasomotrices du penis chez le chien. *Arch Int Physiol* 1934;40:311–321.
43. Bors E, Comarr AE. Neurologic disturbances of sexual function with special reference to 529 patients with spinal cord injury. *Urol Survey* 1960;10:191–222.
44. Kedia KR, Markland C, Fraley EE. Sexual function following high retroperitoneal lymphadenectomy. *J Urol* 1975;114: 237–239.
45. Kom C, Mulholland SG, Edson M. Etiology of infertility after retroperitoneal lymphadenectomy. *J Urol* 1971;105:528–530.
46. Kluver H, Bucy PC. Preliminary analysis of functions of the temporal lobes in monkeys. *Arch Neurol Psychiatry* 1939;42: 979–1000.
47. Dua S, MacLean PD. Localization for penile erection in medial frontal lobe. *Am J Physiol* 1964;207:1425–1434.
48. MacLean PD. The limbic system ("visceral brain") in relation to central gray and reticulum of the brain stem. Evidence of interdependence in emotional processes. *Psychosom Med* 1955;17: 355–366.
49. MacLean PD, Ploog DW. Cerebral representation of penile erection. *J Neurophysiol* 1962;25:29–55.
50. Hierons R, Saunders M. Impotence in patients with temporal-lobe lesions. *Lancet* 1966;2:761–763.
51. Meyers R. Three cases of myoclonus alleviated by bilateral ansotomy, with a note on postoperative alibido and impotence. *J Neurosurg* 1962;19:71–81.
52. Morales A, Surridge DHC, Marshall PG, Fenemore J. Nonhormonal pharmacological treatment of organic impotence. *J Urol* 1982;128:45–47.
53. Henderson VE, Roepke MH. On the mechanism of erection. *Am J Physiol* 1933;106:441–448.
54. Wagner G, Brindley GS. The effect of atropine, alpha and beta blockers on human penile erection: a controlled pilot study. In: Zorgniotti A, Rossi J, eds. *Vasculogenic impotence. International symposium on corporal revascularization.* Springfield, IL: Charles C Thomas, 1980;77–81.
55. Domer FR, Wessler G, Brown RL, Charles HC. Involvement of the sympathetic nervous system in the urinary bladder internal sphincter and in penile erection in the anesthetized cat. *Invest Urol* 1978;15:404–407.
56. Alm P, Elmer M. Adrenergic and cholinergic innervation of the rat urinary bladder. *Acta Physiol Scand* 1975;94:36–45.
57. Sundin T, Dahlstrom A. The sympathetic innervation of the urinary bladder and urethra in the normal state and after parasympathetic denervation at the spinal root level: an experimental study in cats. *Scand J Urol Nephrol* 1973;7:131–149.
58. Melman A, Henry D. The possible role of the catecholamines of the corpora in penile erection. *J Urol* 1979;121:419–421.

59. Levin RM, Wein AJ. Adrenergic alpha receptors outnumber beta receptors in human penile corpus cavernosum. *Invest Urol* 1980;18:225–226.
60. Adaikan PG, Karim SMM. Adrenoreceptors in the human penis. *J Auton Pharmacol* 1981;1:199–203.
61. Elliott TR. The action of adrenalin. *J Physiol (Lond)* 1905; 32:401–467.
62. Diedrichs W, Stief CG, Lue TF, Tanagho EA. Sympathetic inhibition of papaverine induced erection. *J Urol* 1991;146:195–198.
63. Said SI, Rosenberg RN. Vasoactive intestinal polypeptide: abundant immunoreactivity in neural cell lines and normal nervous tissue. *Science* 1976;192:907–908.
64. Uddman R, Alumets J, Efvinsson L, Hakanson R, Sundler F. VIP nerve fibers around peripheral vessels. *Acta Physiol Scand* 1981;112:65–70.
65. Willis E, Ottesen B, Wagner G, Sundler R, Fahrenkrug J. Vasoactive intestinal polypeptide (VIP) as a possible neurotransmitter involved in penile erection. *Acta Physiol Scand* 1981;113: 545–547.
66. Larsson LI, Fahrenkrug J, Schaffalitzky de Muckadell OB. Occurrence of nerves containing vasoactive intestinal polypeptide immunoactivity in the male genital tract. *Life Sci* 1977;21:503–508.
67. Sjostrand NO, Klinge E, Himberg JJ. Effects of VIP and other putative neurotransmitters on smooth muscle effectors of penile erection. *Acta Physiol Scand* 1981;113:403–405.
68. Lundberg JM, Anggard A, Fahrenkrug J, Hokfelt T, Mutt V. Vasoactive intestinal polypeptide in cholinergic neurons of exocrine glands: functional significance of coexisting transmitters for vasodilation and secretion. *Proc Natl Acad Sci USA* 1980;77: 1651–1655.
69. Virag R, Frydman D, Legman M, Virag H. Intravenous injection of papaverine as a diagnostic and therapeutic method in erectile failure. *Angiology* 1984;35:79–87.
70. Brindley GS. Cavernosal alpha blockade: a new technique for investigating and treating penile impotence. *Br J Psychiatry* 1983;143:332–337.
71. Brindley GS. Pilot experiments on the actions of drugs injected into the human corpus cavernosum penis. *Br J Pharmacol* 1986;87:495–501.
72. Kim N, Azadzoi KM, Goldstein I, Saenz de Tejada I. A nitric oxide-like factor mediates nonadrenergic-noncholinergic neurogenic relaxation of penile corpus cavernosum smooth muscle. *J Clin Invest* 1991;88:112–118.
73. Bush PA, Aronson WJ, Buga GM, Rajfer J, Ignarro LJ. Nitric oxide is a potent relaxant of human and rabbit corpus cavernosum. *J Urol* 1992;147:1650–1655.
74. Saenz de Tejada I, Goldstein I, Azadzoi K, Krane RJ, Cohen RA. Impaired neurogenic and endothelium-mediated relaxation of penile smooth muscle from diabetic men with impotence. *N Engl J Med* 1989;320:1025–1030.
75. Gessa GL, Tagliamonte A. Role of brain monoamines in male sexual behavior. *Life Sci* 1974;14:425–436.
76. Barbeau A. L-dopa therapy in Parkinson's disease: a critical review of nine years' experience. *Can Med Assoc J* 1969;101: 791–799.
77. Jenkins RB, Groh RH. Mental symptoms in parkinsonian patients treated with L-dopa. *Lancet* 1970;2:177–179.
78. Priapism with trazodone. *Med Lett* 1984;26:35.
79. Caccia S, Ballabio M, Samanin R, Zanini MG, Garattini S. ( )-*m*-Chlorophenylpiperazine, a central 5-hydroxytryptamine agonist, is a metabolite of trazodone. *J Pharm Pharmacol* 1981;33: 477–478.
80. Aloi JA, Insel TR, Mueller EA, Murphy DL. Neuroendocrine and behavioral effects of *m*-chlorophenylpiperazine administration in rhesus monkeys. *Life Sci* 1984;34:1325–1331.
81. Scott FB, Bradley WE, Timm GW. Management of erectile impotence: use of implantable inflatable prosthesis. *Urology* 1973;2:80–82.
82. Small MP, Carrion HM, Gordon JA. Small-Carrion penile prosthesis: new implant for management of impotence. *Urology* 1975;5:479–486.
83. Gewertz BL, Sarins CK. Vasculogenic impotence. In: Seagraves RT, Schoenberg HW, eds. *Diagnosis and treatment of erectile disturbances: a guide for clinicians.* New York: Plenum Press, 1985;105–113.
84. Lue TF, Hricak H, Marick KW, Tanagho EA. Vasculogenic impotence evaluated by high-resolution ultrasonography and pulsed Doppler spectrum analysis. *Radiology* 1985;155:777–781.
85. Lue TF, Hricak H, Marich KW, Tanagho EA. Evaluation of arteriogenic impotence with intracorporal injection of papaverine and the duplex ultrasound scanner. *Semin Urol* 1985;3:21–26.
86. Michal V, Kramar R, Pospichal J. External iliac "steal syndrome." *J Cardiovasc Surg* 1978;19:355–357.
87. Goldstein I, Siroky MB, Nath RL, McMillian TN, Menzoian JO, Krane RJ. Vasculogenic impotence; role of the pelvic steal test. *J Urol* 1982;128:300–306.
88. Gittes RF, Waters WB. Sexual impotence: the overlooked complication of a second renal transplant. *J Urol* 1979;121:719–720.
89. Krane RJ, Siroky MB. Studies on sacral evoked potentials. *J Urol* 1980;124:872–876.
90. Gerstenberg TC, Bradley WE. Nerve conduction velocity measurement of dorsal nerve of penis in normal and impotent males. *Urology* 1983;21:90–92.
91. Haldeman S, Bradley WE, Bhatia NN. Pudendal evoked responses. *Arch Neurol* 1982;39:280–283.
92. Walsh PC, Mostwin JL. Radical prostatectomy and cystoprostatectomy with preservation of potency. Results utilizing a new nerve sparing technique. *Br J Urol* 1984;56:694–697.
93. Sidi AA, Cameron JS, Duffy LM, Lange PH. Intracavernous drug-induced erections in management of male erectile dysfunction: experience with 100 patients. *J Urol* 1986;135:704–706.
94. Stackl W, Hasun R, Marberger M. Intracavernous injection of prostaglandin E_1 in impotent men. *J Urol* 1988;140:66–68.
95. Bennett AH, Carpenter AJ, Barada JH. An improved vasoactive drug combination for a pharmacological erection program. *J Urol* 1991;146:1564–1565.
96. Zorgniotti AW, Lefleur RS. Autoinjection of the corpus cavernosum with a vasoactive drug combination for vasculogenic impotence. *J Urol* 1985;133:39–41.
97. Lue TF, Hellstrom WJG, McAninch JW, Tanagho EA. Priapism: a refined approach to diagnosis and treatment. *J Urol* 1986;136:104–108.
98. Grayhack JT, McCullough W, O'Conor VJ Jr, Trippel O. Venous bypass to control priapism. *Invest Urol* 1964;1:509–513.
99. Winter CC. Cure of idiopathic priapism: new procedure for creating fistula between glans penis and corpora cavernosa. *Urology* 1976;8:389–391.
100. Walther PJ, Meyer AF, Woodworth BE. Intraoperative management of penile erection with intracorporeal phenylephrine during endoscopic surgery. *J Urol* 1987;137:738–739.
101. Benkert O, Witt W, Adam W, Leitz A. Effects of testosterone undecanoate on sexual potency and the hypothalamic-pituitary-gonadal-axis of impotent males. *Arch Sex Behav* 1979;8: 471–479.
102. Morales A, Condra M, Owen JA, Surridge DH, Fenemore J, Harris C. Is yohimbine effective in the treatment of organic impotence? Results of a controlled trial. *J Urol* 1987;137:1168–1172.
103. Horowitz JD, Gobel AJ. Drugs and impaired male sexual function. *Drugs* 1979;18:206–217.
104. Jensen RT, Collen MJ, Pandol SJ, et al. Cimetidine-induced impotence and breast changes in patients with gastric hypersecretory states. *N Engl J Med* 1983;308:883–887.
105. Hall WH. Breast changes in males on cimetidine. *N Engl J Med* 1976;295:841.
106. Carlson HE, Ippoliti AF. Cimetidine, an H_2-antihistamine, stimulates prolactin secretion in man. *J Clin Endocrinol Metab* 1977;45:367–370.
107. Adaikan PG, Karim SMM. Male sexual dysfunction during treatment with cimetidine [Letter]. *Br Med J* 1979;1:1282.
108. Hackett RE, Waterhouse K. Vasectomy—reviewed. *Am J Obstet Gynecol* 1973;116:438–455.
109. Koraitim M, Schafer W, Melchior H, Lutzeyer W. Dynamic activity of bladder neck and external sphincter in ejaculation. *Urology* 1977;10:130–132.
110. Woodburne RG. Anatomy of the bladder and bladder outlet. *J Urol* 1968;100:474–487.

111. Tanagho EA, Smith DR. The anatomy and function of the bladder neck. *Br J Urol* 1966;38:54–71.
112. Raezer DM, Wein AJ, Jacobowitz D, Corriere JN, Jr. Autonomic innervation of canine urinary bladder: cholinergic and adrenergic contributions and interaction of sympathetic and parasympathetic nervous systems in bladder function. *Urology* 1973; 2:211–221.
113. Turner-Warwick R, Whiteside CG, Arnold EP, et al. A urodynamic view of prostatic obstruction and the results of prostatectomy. *Br J Urol* 1973;45:631–645.
114. Peterson I, Stener I. An electromyographic study of the striated urethral sphincter, the striated anal sphincter, and the levator ani muscle during ejaculation. *Electromyography* 1970;1:23–44.
115. Pick J, Sheehan D. Sympathetic rami in man. *J Anat (Lond)* 1946;80:12–20.
116. Wesson MB. Anatomical, embryological, and physiological studies of the trigone and neck of the bladder. *J Urol* 1920;4:279–307.
117. Gosling JA, Dixon JS, Critchley HOD, Thompson SA. A comparative study of the human external sphincter and periurethral levator ani muscles. *Br J Urol* 1981;53:35–41.
118. Donker DJ, Droes JTPM, Van Ulden BM. Anatomy of the musculature and innervation of the bladder and urethra. In: Williams DE, Chisholm GD, eds. *Scientific foundations of urology.* Vol. 2. Chicago: Year Book Medical Publishers, 1976;32–39.
119. Elbadawi A, Schenk EA. A new theory of the innervation of the bladder musculature. Part 4. Innervation of vesicourethral junction and external urethral sphincter. *J Urol* 1974;111:613–615.
120. Wein AJ, Benson GS, Jacobowitz D. Lack of evidence for adrenergic innervation of the external urethral sphincter. *J Urol* 1979;121:324–326.
121. Lincoln J, Crowe R, Bokor J, Light JK, Chilton CP, Burnstock G. Adrenergic and cholinergic innervation of the smooth and striated muscle components of the urethra from patients with spinal cord injury. *J Urol* 1986;135:402–408.
122. McConnell JA, Benson GS, Wood JG. Autonomic innervation of the urogenital system: adrenergic and cholinergic elements. *Brain Res Bull* 1982;9:679–694.
123. Baumgarten HG, Falck B, Holstein AF, Owman C, Owman T. Adrenergic innervation of the human testis, epididymis, ductus deferens, and prostate: a fluorescence microscopic and fluorimetric study. *Z Zellforsch* 1968;90:81–85.
124. Baumgarten HG, Holstein AF, Rosengren E. Arrangement, ultrastructure, and adrenergic innervation of smooth musculature of the ductuli efferentes, ductus epididymis, and ductus deferens of man. *Z Zellforsch* 1971;120:37–79.
125. McConnell JA, Benson GS, Wood J. Distribution of autonomic fibers to pelvic/perineal viscera of the human male. *Anat Rec* 1978;190:475.
126. Ek A, Alm P, Andersson KE, Persson CGA. Adrenergic and cholinergic nerves of the human urethra and urinary bladder. A histochemical study. *Acta Physiol Scand* 1977;99:345–352.
127. Gosling JA, Dixon JS, Lendon RG. The autonomic innervation of the human male and female bladder neck and proximal urethra. *J Urol* 1977;118:302–305.
128. Ambache N, Aboo Zar M. Evidence against adrenergic motor transmission in the guinea-pig vas deferens. *J Physiol* 1971; 216:359–389.
129. Jenkins DA, Marshall I, Nasmyth PA. Is noradrenaline the motor transmitter in the mouse vas deferens? *J Physiol* 1976;254: 49P–50P.
130. McGrath JC. Adrenergic and "non-adrenergic" components in the contractile response of the vas deferens to a single indirect stimulus. *J Physiol* 1978;283:23–39.
131. Anton PG, McGrath JC. Further evidence for adrenergic transmission in the human vas deferens. *J Physiol* 1977;273:45–55.
132. Birmingham AT. The human isolated vas deferens: its response to electrical stimulation and to drugs. *Br J Pharmacol* 1968;34:692P–693P.
133. Hedlund H, Andersson KE, Larson B. Effect of drugs interacting with adrenoceptors and muscarinic receptors in the epididymal and prostatic parts of the isolated human vas deferens. *J Auton Pharmacol* 1985;5:261–270.
134. McLeod DG, Reynolds DG, Demaree GE. Some pharmacologic characteristics of the human vas deferens. *Invest Urol* 1973; 10:338–341.
135. Benson GS, Wein AJ, Raezer DM, Corriere JN, Jr. Adrenergic and cholinergic stimulation and blockade of the human bladder base. *J Urol* 1976;116:174–175.
136. Levin RM, Wein AJ. Distribution and function of adrenergic receptors in the urinary bladder of the rabbit. *Mol Pharmacol* 1979;16:441–448.
137. Mitsuya H, Asai J, Suyama K, Ushida T, Hosoe K. Application of x-ray cinematography in urology: I. Mechanism of ejaculation. *J Urol* 1960;83:86–92.
138. Herberg LJ. A hypothalamic mechanism causing seminal ejaculation. *Nature* 1963;198:219–220.
139. Robinson BW, Mishkin M. Ejaculation evoked by stimulation of the preoptic area in monkey. *Physiol Behav* 1966;1:269–272.
140. Guttmann L, Walsh JJ. Prostigmin assessment test of fertility in spinal man. *Paraplegia* 1971;9:39–51.
141. Innes IR, Nickerson M. Norephinephrine, epinephrine and the sympathomimetic amines. In: Goodman LS, Gilman A, eds. *The pharmacological basis of therapeutics.* New York: Macmillan, 1975;477.
142. Lipshultz LI, McConnell JA, Benson GS. Current concepts of the mechanisms of ejaculation. *J Reprod Med* 1981;26:499–507.
143. Kelly ME, Needle MA. Imipramine for aspermia after lymphadenectomy. *Urology* 1979;13:414–415.
144. Benson GS, Sarshik SA, Raezer DM, Wein AJ. Bladder muscle contractility: comparative effects and mechanisms of action of atropine, propantheline, flavoxate, and imipramine. *Urology* 1977;9:31–35.
145. Gregory JG, Wein AJ, Schoenberg HW. A comparison of the action of tofranil and probanthine on the urinary bladder. *Invest Urol* 1974;12:233–235.
146. Bennett CJ, Seager SW, Vasher VA, McGuire EJ. Sexual dysfunction and electroejaculation in men with spinal cord injury: review. *J Urol* 1988;139:453–457.

The Pituitary and the Hypothalamus

The Physiology of Reproduction, Second Edition,
edited by E. Knobil and J.D. Neill,
Raven Press, Ltd., New York © 1994.

CHAPTER 25

Pituitary and Hypothalamus: Perspectives and Overview[1]

John W. Everett

Nearly all our knowledge on the hypothalamic-pituitary system has been gathered during the 20th century, building on fragmentary notions from earlier times. Galen regarded the pituitary as a sump for waste products (phlegm = *pituita*) derived in the brain from distillation of "animal spirit." Supposedly the phlegm would then filter through openings in the ethmoid bone into the nasal passages. That notion held without question until 1655, when Conrad Victor Schneider of Wittenburg concluded, on anatomical grounds, that the openings in the cribriform plate of the ethmoid bone are for the olfactory nerves and that fluids cannot pass from the cranial cavity into the nose (1). Richard Lower of Oxford confirmed this in 1670 with a case of hydrocephalus and a series of experiments in cadavers. Although intraventricular fluid was greatly increased after injection of water into the jugular veins, no fluid appeared in the nasal cavities. Lower envisioned substances to be conducted from the ventricles through the infundibulum to the pituitary, there to be "distilled" into the blood stream (1).

Recognition of the dual embryonic origin of the pituitary from the diencephalon and the buccal epithelium awaited disclosure in 1838 by Martin Heinrich Rathke (2) of Königsberg, an embryologist noted for discovering the embryonic gill slits and gill arches. Rathke described a dorsal outpocketing from the roof of the stomodeum extending to meet a ventral process from the diencephalic floor. Knowledge of the histological structure of the respective components was many years in the future, however. In the same year as Rathke's report, the cell theory was proposed for plants by Schleiden and extended the following year by Schwann to include animals. Methods for fixing tissues were in use, but histology did not come into its own until the latter part of the 19th century. Staining with hematoxylin (Waldeyer) and aniline dyes (Beneke) was described in 1863, and the microtome was introduced by His in 1870. Although the distinction between glands with and without ducts was apparent by older methods, the identification of ductless glands structurally specialized for internal secretion required the microscopic observations made possible by these procedures and by improved lens systems.

Claude Bernard first conceptualized "internal secretion," noting that all tissues and organs influence the

Department of Neurobiology, Duke University School of Medicine, Durham, North Carolina 27710 (Deceased)

[1] This chapter reprinted from *The Physiology of Reproduction*, edited by E. Knobil and J. D. Neill. Raven Press, Ltd., New York © 1988.

body as a whole by discharging substances into the blood (3). The idea was extended by Brown-Séquard and d'Arsonval with the view that internal secretions serve to coordinate body functions (3). The concept of control of specific target tissues by circulating messengers ("hormones") was stated by Bayliss and Starling in their Croonian Lecture (4) that reported their discovery of secretin.

Although histology of the pituitary complex (Table 1) clearly showed the glandular features of the pars distalis, the neural lobe did not appear to be a secretory organ. Silver-staining methods devised by Golgi and modified by Ramón y Cajal disclosed a rich content of nerve fibers in the neural lobe that Cajal (5) judged to be sensory fibers with terminals in the surrounding epithelium of the pars intermedia. Camus and Roussy (6), on the other hand, considered the neural lobe to be merely a "fragment nerveux atrophié." Bailey and Bremer (7), as late as 1921, agreed, after observing that experimental removal of the neural lobe had no evident effect. They interpreted pituitrin as nothing more than a "pharmacologically interesting extract." They also noted, with respect to the pars distalis, that in spite of its obviously glandular structure there was "little actual knowledge of its functional significance." Nonetheless, Evans and Long (8) had already produced gigantism in rats by long-term daily treatment with extracts of beef anterior pituitary (AP).

In retrospect, the functional relationship between the pars distalis and body growth is apparent in clinical reports beginning in 1864. The syndrome of acromegaly described by Pierre Marie was shown by Minkowski to be accompanied consistently by the presence of a pituitary tumor (9). Unfortunately, he wrongly assumed that a tumor must represent loss of function and, hence, that the syndrome must be due to impaired pituitary activity. That notion persisted into the 20th century and led to various attempts at experimental hypophysectomy. Most notable of these attempts were reported by Paulesco (9), Cushing and associates (10–12), and Aschner (13,14). Because Paulesco had been unable to obtain survival of hypophysectomized dogs for more than a few days, the concept at first arose that the pituitary is essential for life. There were also arguments about complications from possible damage to the hypothalamus. However, Aschner, operating on puppies, obtained survival for several months in the total absence of the hypophysis and without damage to the brain. The puppies failed to grow. It was by no means clear, however, that this failure represented specific loss of a particular hormone, for there were metabolic defects in the cachectic animals, and the thyroids and adrenal cortex were obviously impaired. Impairment of the reproductive organs could similarly have been due to the general debility. Questions of specificity also applied to the early AP extracts alleged to contain growth hormone. The sorting out of the specific trophic hormones present in the gland and their eventual purification were to occupy investigators for many years to come.

Several other lines of evidence stand in the background of present awareness of the central position of the hypothalamic-pituitary apparatus in regulating gonadal functions. Seasonal influences of the environment on animal reproduction in temperate zones have been well known from time immemorial (15,16). Especially noteworthy is the fact that in some species ovulation and corpus luteum formation require the stimulus of copulation. This was demonstrated in domestic rabbits by both Haighton (17) and Cruikshank (18) in presentations to the Royal Society of London in 1797, confirmed later by Barry (19), Heape (20), and many others. By mating rabbits after cutting the fallopian tubes, Haighton showed that the effect could not be due to contact of the semen with the ovary. Provoked ovulation was later described in ferrets (21) and domestic cats (22). Numerous other species have been added in recent years (1).

Retroactive influence of the gonads on the AP was recognized by Fichera (23), who reported that in several species gonadectomy was followed by AP enlargement and, in the rat, by the occurrence of many enlarged, vacuolated cells having a signet-ring appearance. Such "castration cells" were identified by Addison (24) as belonging to the basophil cell class. Other phenomena now recognized as reflecting the influence of the gonads on the AP were the suppression of estrous and menstrual cycles during pregnancy and the prompt return of cycles after removal of corpora lutea (25). The tendency for lactation to suppress cycles, likewise a hypothalamic-pituitary effect, was well known from early times.

The period from 1916 to 1926 was marked by a series of discoveries fundamental for modern endocrinology and reproductive biology. Development of the vaginal

TABLE 1. *Terminology of the subdivisions of the hypophysis*

Neurohypophysis	Median eminence	Infundibulum
	Infundibular stem	
	Neural lobe (infundibular process)	Posterior lobe
Adenohypophysis (glandular lobe)	Pars intermedia	
	Pars tuberalis	Anterior lobe (AP)
	Pars distalis	

smear method by Stockard and Papanicolaou (26) to reveal the estrous cycle of the guinea pig was a breakthrough that led eventually to the isolation and synthesis of the estrogens. The method was soon applied to the rat by Long and Evans (27), and to the mouse by Edgar Allen (28). Allen and Doisy (28a) and Allen et al. (29) soon reported that oily extracts of porcine follicular fluid when injected into spayed mice brought about full cornification of the vagina; the Allen-Doisy test became a basic procedure for the biochemical studies that followed.

Procedures for hypophysectomy received continuing attention. Both Allen (30,31) and Smith (32) investigated effects of hypophysectomy (removal of Rathke's pouch) in amphibian larvae, noting atrophy of the adrenals and thyroids and failure to metamorphose. Smith and Smith (33,34) counteracted these losses by intraperitoneal administration of bovine AP material. Smith (35–37) subsequently devised the parapharyngeal technique for pituitary ablation in rats, a breakthrough that enabled isolation, purification, and chemical characterization of the various AP hormones. Smith and Engle (38) promptly demonstrated maintenance and repair of gonads by repeated intramuscular implants of fresh AP tissue in hypophysectomized rats.

No less important was the classic monograph by Long and Evans (27) detailing many aspects of reproduction in the rat. The usual length of the estrous cycles was shown to be either 4 or 5 days, not 10 days or longer, as most earlier reports had indicated. Stages of the vaginal cycle were defined and correlated with events in the ovary, reproductive tract, and mammary glands. Pseudopregnancy was described and named as the result of infertile copulation or mechanical stimulation of the cervix. The production of deciduomata by uterine trauma was described, and the importance of the critical timing of traumatization was noted. Since pseudopregnancy occurred readily in animals whose ovaries had been transplanted, it did not involve the ovarian innervation. In the correlated investigation by Evans and Long (8) of the effects of prolonged daily intraperitoneal administration of bovine AP substance, in addition to gigantism the females showed marked enlargement of the ovaries with masses of corpora lutea, together with suppression of estrous cycles. Here was the first demonstration of the presence of both growth-promoting and gonad-stimulating substances in the anterior lobe.

Evans et al. (39,40) succeeded in separating fractions of AP extracts having these respective activities. Separation of thyroid-stimulating and gonadotropic fractions was achieved by Greep (41). Eventually, by the late 1930s the existence of six AP hormones had been established: hormones controlling body growth, the gonads, mammary glands, thyroids, and adrenal cortex. The advances toward their eventual isolation and determination of their chemical structures required progressive sophistication of *in vitro* techniques. This was accompanied by progressive refinement of definitions of the biological actions of the respective hormones.

In the case of the gonadotropins, progress was delayed from time to time by certain faulty assumptions, sometimes engendered by impurities in the substances administered. The existence of two gonadotropic principles was first proposed by Zondek (42,43), who had obtained a follicle-stimulating material (Prolan A) from the urine of ovariectomized or postmenopausal women and a luteinizing material (Prolan B) from human pregnancy urine. He assumed both to be secreted by the AP. Although Prolan B was later shown to originate from the placenta (44–47), the idea of a separate luteinizer led to intensive search for distinct pituitary principles having potencies resembling the two Prolans. The dual hormone concept was championed by Fevold, Hisaw, and associates in Wisconsin. Fevold et al. (48) were first to succeed in separating the respective fractions from pyridine extracts. Details of the efforts leading to eventual isolation and determination of the chemical structure of follicle-stimulating hormone (FSH) and luteinizing hormone (LH) have been admirably reviewed by Greep (49). A major misapprehension not emphasized was the early failure to distinguish formation, *per se,* of corpora lutea (luteinization) and maintenance of their function (luteotropic action). In rats and mice the principal luteotropin is prolactin, a fact unknown until demonstrated in 1941 by Astwood (50) and Evans et al. (51).

Prolactin research stems from an observation by Stricker and Grueter (52,53) after induction of ovulation in rabbits by administration of AP extract. In rabbits that received the material for several days after ovulation the mammary glands were distended with milk. The effect was confirmed by Corner (54), who also obtained it in ovariectomized estrous rabbits. Evans and Simpson (55) saw mammary glands distended with milk in rats that had received an AP extract for 20 to 30 days. A series of studies by Riddle and associates (56–59) between 1931 and 1935 disclosed that, in the pigeon and ring-dove, secretion of crop milk was governed by the AP and that the same hormone, which they named prolactin, caused milk secretion in mammals. It suppressed gonadal function by inhibiting FSH secretion. In both mice and rats, daily treatment interrupted estrous cycles for approximately 2 weeks (60,61). Although Lahr and Riddle (61) saw large corpora lutea, demonstration of the luteotropic action of prolactin was 5 years in the future, as noted above. The growth-promoting power of prolactin was shown in hypophysectomized pigeons, as for years Riddle, Bates, and others questioned "the concept of a growth hormone as an individual entity." The disagreement was finally resolved by Bates et al. (62) through use of highly purified AP hormones. Optimal metabolic effects were obtained in hypophysectomized pigeons by giving a combination of ovine prolactin, bovine growth hormone, thyroxine, and prednisone.

ANTERIOR PITUITARY CYTOLOGY

From the very beginning of microscopic observation of the pituitary, considerable variation was evident in size, shape, and granule content of pars distalis cells. Application of dyes disclosed coloration differences as well. Schönemann (63) is credited with having made the original distinction among basophils ("cyanophils"), acidophils ("eosinophils"), and "chromophobes" as seen in human pituitaries stained with alum hematoxylin and eosin. Holmes and Ball (64) present a useful summary of the complex story of efforts in this century to subdivide these classes and to relate the subclasses to particular hormones and functional states. Underlying these efforts was the developing knowledge of the number of AP hormones, coupled with the feeling that the number of cell types ought to correspond.

Early confusion arose from the finding that in most animals other than humans the basophil cells cannot be stained by hematoxylin. Staining of ergastoplasm by basic dyes like toluidin blue added further confusion. The use of the multiple acid dyes introduced by Mallory (65) produced an array of tinctorial cell types. Modifications of the Mallory procedure were especially useful in some species and appeared to distinguish cells with granules containing simple proteins from cells having granules of glycoprotein. Application of the McManus (66) periodic acid (PAS) histochemical method provided a generally useful distinction between "serous" cells (67) and "mucoid" cells (68). The latter types are those producing FSH, LH, melanocyte-stimulating hormone (MSH), and thyroid-stimulating hormone (TSH), all of which are glycoproteins.

The eventual availability of highly purified AP hormones and antibodies and the advent of immunocytochemical methods (69) in both light microscopy and electron microscopy have led far in recent years toward the ideal of a functional classification. The older terminologies have given way largely to the naming of cells according to the hormone produced, whenever known. Some problems remain, as when a gonadotropic cell contains granules that react with both FSH and LH antibodies. Special difficulties attend the localization of adrenocorticotropic hormone (ACTH), MSH, and the related peptides, several of which may be contained within a parent molecule in some cells (70).

Pituitary histology and cytology have moved hand-in-hand with progress in pituitary physiology and biochemistry. Regional variations of cell types in the bovine AP made it possible for Smith and Smith (33) to distinguish the selective growth-promoting power of the acidophilic lateral portions from the thyrotropic power of the anteromedial portion containing basophils and chromophobes. Enlargement of AP and castration cell formation after gonadectomy provided means for testing the feedback actions of gonadal hormones. The lack of castration cells in rat AP transplants to sites away from the brain was an early sign of the importance of the brain in regulating AP secretions (71).

EVIDENCE FOR NEURAL CONTROL OF PARS DISTALIS SECRETION

Frölich's (72) original description of the syndrome termed urogenital dystrophy was the start of prolonged controversy about the respective roles of damage to the hypothalamus or the pituitary gland in causing the disease. An intracranial cystic tumor thought to be a craniopharyngioma was surgically drained, after which there was satisfactory recovery. Eventually, following experimental studies by Camus and Roussy (6), Bailey and Bremer (7), Smith (36), and Hetherington and Ranson (73–75), it became clear that both obesity and genital atrophy can result from injury to the hypothalamus without direct involvement of the AP. Among 60 clinical cases of hypothalamic pathology assembled by Bauer (76), 43 manifested either hypogonadism or sexual precocity, five showing obesity. Precocity was commonly associated with basal tuberal lesions, while hypogonadism accompanied lesions located more rostrally.

Smith's observations of the effects of hypothalamic damage were made as he developed his method for parapharyngeal hypophysectomy (36). One attempt to ablate the gland was to inject chromic acid into the pituitary capsule, with the result that some of the acid passed beyond and damaged the brain. He then found that selective damage to the hypothalamus itself produced genital atrophy and obesity. Soon afterward Grafe and Grünthal (77) reported similar results. During the following 25 years, paralleling the progressive purification of the several AP secretions and determination of their actions, there was growing interest in the possible control of these secretions by the nervous system. Although the Moore and Price hypothesis (78) of pituitary-gonad reciprocity did not seem to take the nervous system into account, the authors recognized the modifying influences of environmental factors.

There was also strong implication of neural participation in the special case of the coitally induced ovulation in rabbits. Fee and Parkes (79,80) demonstrated two important features of that process; since the hypophysis must remain in place for only an hour after copulation, the necessary release of hormone must be relatively acute, and since anesthesia of the vagina prevented the ovulation, the nervous system must be directly involved. Participation of the brain was more directly indicated by Marshall and Verney (81), who obtained ovulation in estrous rabbits by passing an electric current through the head. With greater precision, Harris (82) and Haterius and Derbyshire (83) produced the same effect by local stimulation of the hypothalamus. The importance of the pituitary stalk to complete the reflex connection to the pars distalis was shown by Westman and Jacobsohn (84). Ovulation failed when the stalk had been cut and a metal foil barrier placed between the hypothalamus and pituitary gland, supposedly interrupting neural connections. The result also seemed to eliminate participation of autonomic fibers directly innervating the pars distalis.

Several workers had described autonomic fibers within the pars distalis parenchyma. However, a careful study by Rasmussen (85) of the pituitaries of human, rat, guinea pig, rabbit, dog, cat, and monkey led him to conclude that the only nerve fibers present in the AP must be vasomotor. Many parts of the gland were free of nerves. This view has been widely corroborated.

Meanwhile, the concept of a "sexual center" in the hypothalamus arose from the studies in rats by Hohlweg and associates (71,86), confirmed and amplified by Westman and Jacobsohn (87–89). As noted above, Hohlweg and Junkmann (71) saw that gonadectomy failed to produce castration cells in hypophyses that had been transplanted to a site away from the brain. Searching for effects of estrogen on the AP, Hohlweg and Chamorro (86) discovered that a single injection of estradiol benzoate into prepubertal rats induced formation of a set of corpora lutea within 7 days, presumptive evidence of increased LH secretion and ovulation. Luteinization was prevented by hypophysectomy 2 days after injection, but not at 4 days. Westman and Jacobsohn (87–89), after confirming the Hohlweg effect, examined the results of stalk section and insertion of a barrier of metal foil. Stalk section less than $2\frac{1}{2}$ days after estrogen injection prevented luteinization, but not when performed later on. As in the rabbit reflex, the estrogen stimulus was thought to operate through an essential neural link from the hypothalamus. The pituitary portal vessels were not yet generally recognized.

Pituitary Portal Vessels

Prominent vessels on the pituitary stalk were first well described by Pietsch (90) and Popa and Fielding (91,92). The latter authors described them as *portal vessels connecting capillary beds in the median eminence and pars distalis.* Erroneously, they concurred with Pietsch that blood moves "upward" from the gland toward the brain. That conclusion was based partly on the experimental observation in rabbits that when a clamp was placed on the stalk the vessels distended below the clamp. Unknown at the time was the fact that rabbits, unlike most mammals, have a direct arterial supply to the pars distals.

Evidence for "downward" flow in the portal vessels was first reported by Houssay et al. (93) from direct microscopic observation of the exposed vessels in South American toads. Furthermore, lesioning of the infundibulum caused infarction of the pars distalis. On histologic grounds, Wislocki and King (94) and Wislocki (95) reached the conclusion that the primary capillary bed occupies the median eminence and the infundibular stem, whence blood is transported by the portal vessels to the secondary capillaries in the pars distalis. They further recognized the median eminence as a part of the neurohypophysis, not of the hypothalamus. Direct observation of downward blood flow was later reported in several species [amphibia: Green (96); duck: Benoit and Assenmacher (97); rat: Green and Harris (98,99) and others; mouse: Worthington (100,101); dog and cat: Török (102,103); baboon and monkey: Daniel (104)]. Although the possibility of some recurrent flow was indicated recently (105–107), the present view is that the principal flow is downward, transmitting hypophysiotropic agents to the AP.

Considerable territorial specificity exists in the origins of the various portal vessels from the primary capillaries and distributions of the secondary capillaries within the pars distalis. After stalk sectioning in the rat, sheep, goat, monkey, and human the extent of the infarcted area in the AP depends on the number and location of portal vessels interrupted (108). Daniel (104) proposed that the territorial specificity may explain the regional variation of cell types. An experimental basis for such a view was shown by Pasteels (109). In the amphibian *Pleurodeles waltlii,* he removed the hypophysis and reimplanted it in the original location, but inverted and rotated 180°. The cytology of the gland became regionally reversed in accord with the relationship to the portal circulation. A contrary view has been expressed by Porter et al. (110) after they found in rats that when the portal vessels were exposed and a colored fluid was injected into a single vessel through a microcannula, the distribution of the dye in the AP was greatly varied, sometimes reaching the entire gland. One may suggest, however, that under physiological conditions of balanced pressure territorial specificity would be maintained.

Neurohumoral Regulation

The concept of neurohumoral control of the pars distalis can be traced back to a paper by Hinsey and Markee (111). Failing to prevent postcoital ovulation in rabbits by severing the cervical sympathetic trunks, they suggested that the reflex involves a humoral link, transmitting some substance from the "posterior lobe" to the pars distalis. After Wislocki and King (94) presented their strong evidence for downward movement of blood in the portal vessels, there was speculation that these channels might constitute the humoral pathway (see ref. 112 and accompanying discussions). Resistance to the idea continued for a while, partly because in avian and cetacean forms a heavy connective tissue septum separates the neural lobe from the pars distalis. However, it has been fully demonstrated that in such cases a "porto-tuberal tract" transmits the portal vessels rostral to that septum (97,113). Green (114) concluded from his comparative study that the pituitary portal vessels or their equivalent are a constant feature of all vertebrates.

Green and Harris (98), reversing Harris' earlier view (82), presented several strong arguments in favor of the humoral transmission via the portal vessels. They proposed that the variable effects others had encountered from cutting the stalk may have resulted from ability of the vessels to regenerate. Harris (115) conclusively demonstrated in stalk-sectioned rats that recovery of reproductive function was directly proportional to the extent of portal vessel regeneration. Regeneration was also demonstrated in monkeys (116) and rabbits (117). Thus, to interrupt fully hypothalamic influence on the AP by stalk section, an impermeable barrier is mandatory.

These findings seemed to explain the restoration of function in the pars distalis grafts that Greep (118) placed in the original site after hypophysectomy. Yet there remained some uncertainty, since it would be difficult to distinguish remnants of the gland left *in situ.* To avoid this, Harris and Jacobsohn (119) modified the experiment with a dual operation, hypophysectomizing female rats by the parapharyngeal route and implanting pars distalis tissue by the transtemporal approach to a location beneath the median eminence. Donors of the grafts were either several of the subjects' own male or female young, adult females, or adult males. Control subjects received the grafts under the temporal lobe. Estrous cycles returned in all rats bearing infantile grafts under the median eminence, often within a week. Several became pregnant and delivered normal young. Adrenals and thyroids were histologically normal. Significantly, similar results appeared in the few subjects bearing adult male grafts, one having a successful pregnancy. No traces of AP tissue were microscopically detectable in the original sites. These highly significant findings were confirmed and supplemented by Nikitovitch-Winer and Everett (120,121) in a two-stage experiment. The pars distalis of adult female rats was first autografted to the renal capsule where capacity for secretion of FSH, LH, ACTH, and TSH was largely lost. Several weeks later, the graft was retransplanted by the transtemporal route beneath the median eminence. Controls either received the graft under the temporal lobe or were left with the graft on the kidney. Estrous cycles reappeared in most rats having grafts revascularized from the median eminence, and in many cases the animals became pregnant when mated. Secretion of ACTH and TSH appeared to be moderately restored, whereas the control grafts continued to secrete mostly prolactin. Grafts under the median eminence contained many large gonadotrophs and thyrotrophs, which were absent from the controls. Thus, in spite of the double surgical insult with considerable loss of tissue due to infarction at each operation, the gland could rapidly renew its several trophic secretions once it received blood from the median eminence. Smith (122,123) contributed a further confirmatory variation of Greep's experiment. In both male and female rats, months after hypophysectomy he introduced homografts of pars distalis tissue near the median eminence through the reopened pituitary capsules. Fertility was restored along with significantly improved thyrotropic and adrenotropic functions. During the long intervals after hypophysectomy the typical apituitary syndrome had shown the essential completeness of that operation. Since hypophysectomy was performed in young subjects around 40 days of age, the return of somatotropin secretion was demonstrable after the grafts were introduced.

Thus it became fully evident that the hypophysial portal circulation is essential for stimulating the pars distalis to secrete FSH, LH, TSH, ACTH, and somatotropin (GH, STH). Although Green and Harris (98) had suggested that there might be separate transmitter agents, excitatory or inhibitory, controlling these respective secretions, there were alternative possibilities (124). A single agent might act permissively or its different concentrations in the portal blood might selectively influence particular secretions. Nevertheless, the territorial variations in cell types argued strongly for multiple stimulative factors. Saffran et al. (125) coined the term *releasing factor* and the acronym RF.

Although inhibitory neural action on the pars intermedia was known, the first evidence of inhibitory neurohumoral control of a pars distalis secretion emerged in experiments involving autotransplantation of the gland to the renal capsule (126,127). When the operation was performed in female rats on the day after ovulation, the newly forming corpora lutea were activated and continued to secrete progesterone for weeks or months until the experiment concluded. Since the principal luteotropin in rats is prolactin, the results demonstrated enhancement of prolactin secretion by removal of the pars distalis from hypothalamic influence. Although not recognized at the time, this effect had previously been obtained by Westman and Jacobsohn (89) after separating the gland from the hypothalamus by stalk section and placement of an impermeable barrier; they interpreted the result as being due to stimulation of the cervix. Desclin (128) also had evidence of prolactin secretion by transplanted pars distalis, but thought it due to the direct stimulative effect of treatment with estrogen. Nikitovitch-Winer (129) repeated the stalk-sectioning experiment of Westman and Jacobsohn, but omitting the cervical stimulation showed clearly that the enhanced prolactin secretion must be due to removal from hypothalamic inhibition. *In vitro* organ cultures and tissue cultures of pars distalis from several mammals show autonomous secretion of prolactin, increasing with time, while other secretions diminish (130–134). Addition of hypothalamic tissue or extract to the cultures reduces prolactin output, extracts of cerebral cortex having no such effect.

Hypothalamic Hormones

Several different releasing (and inhibiting) factors are recognized today as hypothalamic hormones transmitted to the pars distalis via the portal vessels, each factor having more or less selective action on pituitary secretions. The agents of primary importance for reproduction include first and foremost the luteinizing hormone-releasing hormone LHRH (or GnRH, since it stimulates both FSH and LH secretion). Thyroid-releasing hormone (TRH), the releasing agent for the thyroid-stimulating hormone, has the added capacity for stimulating prolactin secretion. The chemical structures of both LHRH, a decapeptide, and TRH, a tripeptide, are known, and both are available in synthetic form. The remarkable story of the elucidation of their chemistry and synthesis has been fully told by Wade (135). Prolactin-inhibiting factor (PIF), remains to be fully characterized. Dopamine, a potent inhibitor (136), appears in the arcuate nuclei-median eminence and portal vessels (137), but may not be the only inhibiting agent.

Hypothalamic-Pituitary Control of Ovulation

Pharmacologic Blockade

In rabbits, the sequence of events provoked by the copulatory stimulus and culminating in ovulation begins with a very brief triggering period during which the process can be blocked by the intravenous injection of certain drugs (138–140). The α-adrenergic blockers Dibenamine or a congener SKF-501, when injected intravenously within 1 minute after coitus, prevented ovulation in 80% of the subjects. Atropine sulphate or another cholinergic blocker, Banthine, also blocked, but they had to be injected more rapidly still, indicating that a cholinergic mechanism precedes the adrenergic trigger. This was further indicated when ovulation was induced by injecting a high dose of Adrenaline (Parke-Davis) into estrous rabbits protected from the lethal effects by atropine. The initial postulate that the neurohumoral transmitter carried to the pars distalis by the portal vessels is a catecholamine was later abandoned. Sawyer (141) determined that ovulation could be induced in rabbits by intraventricular injection of either epinephrine or norepinephrine (see also ref. 142). Thus, both the cholinergic and adrenergic links in the rabbit ovulatory reflex are central neural processes, completed within a very few minutes *post coitum*. Although no means has been devised for sampling the portal blood content after the mating stimulus, indirect evidence indicates that LHRH rises rapidly during the first hour, and then remains high for several hours (143). The LHRH rise is thought to slightly precede the LH surge, which peaks at 60 to 90 minutes, remains high for approximately an hour, and then declines (143–146). The prolonged high level of LHRH recalls a report by Westman (147), who placed clamps on the pituitary stalks of estrous rabbits, mated them, and removed the clamps 50 to 60 minutes later; ovulation followed unless the pituitaries were also removed. A related observation by Westman and Jacobsohn (84) was that, while hypophysectomy 30 minutes *post coitum* prevented ovulation, exsanguination and replacement with blood from another rabbit at that time allowed ovulation to take place. It failed, however, if exsanguination and replacement were delayed until 75 to 90 minutes *post coitum*. In the first instance, the continuing LH surge surely added enough for ovulation, whereas in the latter case any added LH was inadequate.

Reflex Ovulators

During the interval between the LH surge and ovulation, in both reflex ovulators and spontaneous ovulators, certain maturation changes take place in the Graafian follicles and ova: follicular hyperemia and swelling, appearance of "secondary liquor," dispersal of cells in the cumulus oophorus, formation of a prominent corona, production of the first polar body (typically), and formation of the second polar division spindle. In retrospect, the relatively brief preovulatory spurt of follicle enlargement described in the guinea pig by Dempsey (148) was an early indication of a spontaneous abrupt increase of gonadotropin secretion.

Spontaneous Ovulators

Clear demonstration of acute timing of a preovulatory gonadotropin surge in the spontaneously ovulating rat was presented in a series of studies by Everett, Sawyer, and associates (149–155) employing a number of drugs including those that blocked the rabbit reflex. In addition to Dibenamine and atropine, drugs effective in rats included several barbiturates, chlorpromazine, reserpine, morphine, and urethane. Their use defined a "critical period" of 2 to 3 hours on the afternoon of proestrus, beginning predictably at approximately 1400 hours. Analysis by injecting atropine sulphate or pentobarbital or by hypophysectomy at progressively later times during the critical period indicated temporal variation in the beginning of LH release among different individuals (156–158). Hormone release could be interrupted while in progress as readily by the drugs as by hypophysectomy. Hence, although an atropine-sensitive mechanism controls the spontaneous surge in rats, the action is essential throughout the surge, not a brief trigger, as in the rabbit reflex. The analysis also indicated that the time needed to release the minimal ovulation quota of LH in rats is approximately 30 minutes. There were indications that the normal surge continues much longer, however. Modern data from radioimmunoassay confirm this finding and show that the full amount of LH released is far greater than the minimum quota. The surge begins during the critical period, but reaches peak level later, remaining high for 2 to 3 hours and returning to baseline typically by 1800 to 1900 hours (159). It is provoked by a rise of LHRH in the pituitary-portal blood (160).

The occurrence of acute preovulatory surges of LH and FSH is now recognized as universal among spontaneous and reflex ovulators alike. The duration of the surges tends to be considerably longer in larger mammals; in the human female and other large primates it exceeds 24 hours.

The use of barbiturates for blocking spontaneous ovulation in rats led to three discoveries: (a) circadian periodicity of the neural stimulus for release of the LH surge; (b) "delayed pseudopregnancy"; and (c) the fact that rats pharmacologically blocked from ovulating spontaneously can nevertheless be made to release an ovulatory surge of LH by stimulating the brain.

Circadian Periodicity of the Luteinizing Hormone Surge Mechanism

Rats that were blocked with pentobarbital on the proestrus afternoon presented a similar critical period on the next day; if they were blocked at that time, the critical period was repeated on the third afternoon (152). Blockade for 3 days produced an anovulatory cycle, followed by a short diestrus and return of cyclic ovulation. Thus, circadian rhythmicity was clearly evident. This had been implied by the 24-hour advance of ovulation through treatment of rats with progesterone (161), by the fact that this advance could be blocked pharmacologically on the preceding afternoon (151), and by the temporal dependency of the LH surge on regularity of environmental lighting (162). As noted later (*this chapter*), although the close relationship of the spontaneous ovulatory surge of LH to time of day has been amply demonstrated in rats and hamsters, this feature appears to be limited to the small polyestrous rodents.

Delayed Pseudopregnancy

A serendipitous finding occurred during experiments that were intended to search for reflex ovulation in rats blocked with pentobarbital (163,164). They were caged with fertile bucks overnight, and proof of copulation was shown next morning by presence of vaginal plugs and spermatozoa. A few had ovulated, but when similarly treated rats were blocked again on the second afternoon, the usual result was early follicular atresia, a short diestrus of 2 to 3 days, then a new proestrus and estrus with spontaneous ovulation, followed by pseudopregnancy of normal duration. The influence of the copulatory stimulus had been retained for over a week, supposedly through some functional change in the central nervous system. Such a long-delayed effect could not be obtained by stimulating the cervix, but shorter delay had been shown by Greep and Hisaw (165) when cervical stimulation during late diestrus caused pseudopregnancy beginning 2 days later, after completion of the cycle. Quinn and Everett (166) produced delayed pseudopregnancy by electrically stimulating the dorsomedial-ventromedial hypothalamus, a stimulation site not conducive to ovulation. As with genital stimulation, there was a quantitative effect, depending in this case on duration of the stimulus: 10-minute stimulation was adequate for short-term delay, but 30-minute stimulation was needed for long-term delay. This was confirmed by Beach et al. (167,168), who also recorded twice-daily surges of prolactin secretion during the long-delay interval. It is known, however, that these surges during the interval are not essential to the subsequent pseudopregnancy (169). The mnemonic influence of genital or hypothalamic stimulation suggests a protracted change in brain chemistry somehow expressed in the prolactin surges.

Brain Stimulation of Gonadotropin in Rats

In spite of the strong indirect evidence that the central nervous system controls spontaneous as well as reflex ovulation, until 1957 there were no reports of gonadotropin release induced in spontaneous ovulators by brain stimulation. In that year, Anand et al. (170) appear to have had some success from daily hypothalamic stimulation of monkeys early in their menstrual cycles. Bunn and Everett (171), using rats in constant estrus under continuous illumination, consistently induced ovulation and luteinization by electrical stimulation of the amygdala and, in one case, the lateral septum. Critchlow (172) discovered that rats blocked during the proestrus critical period with pentobarbital can be ovulated by stimulating the medial basal tuber (MBT) close to the median eminence. Such pharmacologically blocked rats have become favorite experimental subjects for artificial stimulation of gonadotropin release.

Attempts in the writer's laboratory to repeat Critchlow's work led to the demonstration that the medial preoptic area (MPOA) is an especially useful stimulation site. In contrast to the MBT, electrode placement in the MPOA is much less restricted. Everett and Radford (173) encountered the fact that passage of anodic direct current or anodic pulse trains through electrodes containing iron will produce an irritative focal lesion. Such an *electrochemical stimulus* in the MPOA or anterior hypothalamus can induce ovulation, its effectiveness being determined by the amount of iron deposited. A dose-response relationship between size of the electrochemical (EC) focus and the amount of LH released has been well documented, initially by its ovulatory effectiveness (174–177), and later by radioimmunoassay of the LH surge. Large bilateral EC foci involving most of the MPOA may produce enough gonadotropin within 30 minutes for full ovulation, as shown by hypophysectomy at that time (174). The amount of LH in the complete surge produced by the large bilateral stimulus reportedly resembles the normal proestrous surge in magnitude and duration (176).

Electrochemical stimulation is especially useful because of the very short time required for the passage of current (<60 seconds) and the long period of the stimulative action. Plasma LH typically rises slowly at first, then rapidly to reach peak concentration at 90 to 120 minutes, falling gradually thereafter. The stimulative processes near the EC lesion are poorly understood, but increased electrical activity in zones 0.4 to 0.8 mm from center of EC lesions has been reported (178). Spiking activity has also been observed 1 mm behind the MPOA, rising sharply after some 15 minutes and continuing for several hours (179). Although on the day after stimulation the EC lesion consists of a coagulated core of damaged tissue surrounded by an extensive halo devoid of nerve cells and fibers, on the preceding day soon after the passage of current, the region of the eventual halo shows no apparent neuronal damage. It is likely that this outlying region is the site of the increased neural activity. Although there has been some controversy over the possibility that EC lesions act by disinhibition rather than by direct neuronal excitation (180,181), the weight of evidence favors the latter alternative. After Hillarp et al. (182) placed electrolytic lesions with nichrome electrodes in the lateral preoptic areas of male rats there were pronounced behavioral manifestations for as long as 6 hours. Recent investigations by Willmore et al. (183,184) of the effects of ferrous ions introduced into the cerebral cortex indicate that the resulting epileptiform focus is produced by transient formation of free radical oxygen, hydroxyl radicals, and peroxides, causing neural lipid peroxidation.

A major limitation of electrochemical stimulation, aside from uncertainties about how it acts, is that a bulk of tissue is destroyed. That precludes repeated stimulation at the same site and may eliminate neurons important for effective stimulation elsewhere. When EC stimulation is applied near the median eminence, the damage itself may confound the experiment nonspecifically by emptying LHRH into the portal vessels. Knife cuts across the basal tuber (185) or radiofrequency lesions in the arcuate nucleus-median eminence (186) can cause release of an ovulatory quantity of LH. A further limitation of EC stimulation is that the duration of stimulation cannot be controlled.

Such problems are avoided by *electrical stimulation*, especially with platinum electrodes and nonlesioning current, such as matched biphasic pulse pairs. As with EC stimulation, electrical stimulation can induce ovulation in rats under blockade with pentobarbital (and several other drugs), except that it must continue much longer. The amount of LH released and the proportionate numbers of rats ovulating vary with microamperage of the pulses, overall duration of the stimulus, pulse frequency, and other features (187–192). The amount of LH released in a given time by MPOA electrical stimulation is less than expected after EC stimulation, perhaps because of involvement of fewer components of the preoptic-tuberal neuronal system, judged to be diffuse at that level (187–189). Where that system converges upon the arcuate nucleus-median eminence (ARC-ME), electrical stimulation consistently produces more LH than stimulation of the MPOA (174).

Curvilinear Pattern of Ovulatory Gonadotropin Surges

Comparison of the patterns of LH secretion induced by MPOA and ARC-ME stimulations (189) presents a distinct curvilinear parallel, with relatively slow increase during the first 30 to 60 minutes, followed by rapid increase thereafter. The greater amount of LH discharged during the second hour corresponds to the great excess commonly produced in the spontaneous proestrus surge and undoubtedly reflects the self-priming action of LHRH on the pars distalis (193–195). Aiyer et al. (193) disclosed that if two identical amounts of LHRH were injected intravenously 1 hour apart, plasma LH rose sixfold after the second injection. Comparable priming occurred *in vitro* (195). Fink et al. (194) noted a similar response pattern when the MPOA was electrically stimulated with two 15-minute pulse trains at a 45-minute interval. Grieg and Weisz (196) calculated that only approximately 15% of the normal surge is needed for ovulation. This conforms with the minimal ovulation quota released in the first 20 to 40 minutes as estimated from the results of hypophysectomy or atropine block during the critical period (156,157).

The curvilinear pattern of the ovulatory surge of LH (and FSH) is apparent in other species, both reflex ovulators and spontaneous ovulators, provided that frequent blood samples are assayed. Note, for example, the characteristic surges at midcycle in rhesus monkeys shown by Weick et al. (197). From beginning to end, the LH surge in monkeys lasts for 48 hours, but how much of this constitutes the minimal ovulation quota? That information is available only for the rat and, from the pioneer hypophysectomy experiments of Fee and Parkes (79,80) and others (198), for rabbits. While the quota is released within 60 minutes *post coitum* in rabbits, peak levels of plasma LH may be reached later and are said to continue for 1 or 2 hours longer (199). The function of the great excess is not understood, although one effect was noted in rats (156). After hypophysectomy or atropine blockade during the critical period, rats that had ovulated by the next morning characteristically lacked the depletion of cholesterol from the interstitial tissue normally shown at that time.

ACTIONS OF GONADAL SECRETIONS ON PITUITARY SECRETION

Functional mammalian corpora lutea suppress estrous cycles and ovulation. This view, expressed by Beard late in the 19th century (200), was supported experimentally by Loeb (201), who noted the early return of estrus and ovulation in guinea pigs after removal of corpora lutea during pregnancy or during the luteal phase of the cycle. Luteectomy in the pregnant goat (202) and cow (203) had the same effect. After confirming Loeb's finding in cyclic guinea pigs (204), Papanicolaou (205) determined that administration of a lipid extract of corpora lutea had the same inhibitory action as the active luteal tissue. Similar findings were reported for the mouse (206) and the rat (207). Once progesterone became available, its daily administration gave the same result (208,209). According to Kennedy (210) and Mahnert (211) corpus luteum extracts prevented ovulation in rabbits if injected before coitus: that effect was later shown by Makepeace et al. (212) with pure progesterone. Mahnert, in fact, speculated on the possibility of female sterilization with luteal extracts, apparently the first expression of an idea that would emerge 30 years later as a primary means of population control, the Pincus Pill. Inhibition of gonadotropic potency of the AP by gonadal hormones was the basis for the Moore and Price (213) hypothesis of pituitary-gonadal reciprocity. The idea of negative feedback control was so firmly entrenched by the early 1930s that the equally important stimulative actions were slow to emerge.

The first indication of a positive stimulative influence of estrogen lay in its induction of early puberty (214). As mentioned earlier, Hohlweg and Chamorro (86) induced corpus luteum formation in prepubertal rats by treating them with estradiol benzoate, a result that could be prevented by hypophysectomy 2 days later. Confirming this finding, Westman and Jacobsohn (87–89) noted that the effect could also be prevented by pituitary stalk section. In adult rats, Hohlweg (215) observed that daily, month-long injections of estrogen resulted in great enlargement of the corpora lutea, an effect that can now be ascribed to the luteotropic action of prolactin. Although he states (216) that he observed estrogen-induced ovulation in adult rats, I am not aware of a published record.

Induction of ovulation by estrogen treatment of adult mammals was first recorded by Hammond et al. (217) for anestrous ewes and confirmed by Hammond (218) and Casida (219). Everett (220) reported that in rats having regular 5-day cycles ovulation was advanced 24 hours by administering estradiol benzoate or implanting an estradiol crystal on the second day of diestrus. In pregnant (221) or pseudopregnant rats (222), treatment with estradiol benzoate on day 4 or 5 of vaginal leukocytosis resulted in renewed ovulation and formation of new corpora lutea. These stimulative effects in the rat were subject to pharmacologic blockade with either atropine or Dibenamine (222,223).

The first indication that progesterone has a positive as well as a negative influence on gonadotropin secretion arose from Everett's observation that in rats persistently presenting spontaneous vaginal estrus and polycystic ovaries, ovulation could be induced by certain progesterone treatments. It was known that in normal rats the minimal daily subcutaneous dose for suppressing estrous cycles is 1.5 mg in oil. This was confirmed in the persistent-estrous rats, but daily injection of smaller amounts induced sequences of ovulatory cycles (224). Further study showed progesterone to be primarily important each time that the animal returned to proestrus-estrus, whereupon a single injection of 0.5 mg or more consistently induced ovulation (225). The positive action was next demonstrated in normal rats having 5-day cycles. Progesterone injection on diestrus day 3 induced 24-hour advancement of ovulation. As with advancement by estrogen, the progesterone effect was subject to pharmacologic blockade (226).

Biphasic Action of Progesterone: Interaction with Estrogen

There is an obvious interaction between progesterone and estrogen to produce the positive influence on gonadotropin secretion. In most such cases, progesterone acts acutely against a background of elevated estrogen. The action is biphasic (220): stimulation during the first several hours, followed by inhibition. Daily administration thereafter of a large amount of progesterone will suppress the next cyclic proestrus day-to-day until after treatment stops, thus reproducing the effect of functional corpora lutea. For example, injection for 2 days on diestrus days 1 and 2 of the rat cycle extends the normal diestrus exactly 2 days, proestrus occurring 3 days thereafter. However, omission of one daily injection allows the next injection of progesterone to exert its stimulative effect.

The timing of a progesterone injection on the day of proestrus is critical for determining whether it will stimulate or inhibit an ovulatory LH surge (227–229). Injection at 0200 hours will inhibit ovulation (227), whereas injection between 0900 and 1200 hours will produce an ovulatory surge of hormone in advance of the normal critical period (227–229). Comparable temporal relationships are seen in estrogen-primed ovariectomized rats (230). Progesterone's biphasic influence is well documented in the rabbit also (231), where for a few hours it enhances but later inhibits the coital ovulation reflex. Correlated biphasic effects were recorded (232) on behavior and on thresholds for the EEG afterreactions to electrical stimulation of the hypothalamus or the rhinencephalon.

In the special case of ovulation induced in pregnant or pseudopregnant rats by estrogen administration, progesterone serves as a background for the stimulative action of acutely rising estrogen. It is of some interest that the induced gonadotropin release occurs during an afternoon critical period like that in proestrus (222). The progesterone produced by the corpora lutea does not apparently advance the time of release under these circumstances.

Episodic Gonadotropin Release

Gonadectomized animals of either sex are valuable subjects in these inquiries. The finding of highly variable plasma levels of LH in ovarectomized rhesus monkeys led to the first demonstration that gonadotropins tend to be released in pulsatile fashion (233). Pulsatile (episodic, ultradian) release is now recognized as a general phenomenon of AP physiology in many species, including humans (234–237). The concentrations of circulating gonadotropins are known to depend on the frequency and amplitude of LHRH pulses discharged into the pituitary portal vessels; these, in turn, depend upon the endocrine status. The extensive studies of rhesus monkeys by Knobil and associates (236) show that while continuous infusion of LHRH fails to release LH, pulsatile infusion is effective, optimal results being obtained with a pulse frequency of 1/hr. In rats, while continuous infusion of LHRH will stimulate LH release (237), pulsatile infusion is nevertheless more effective (238). Castration of either sex increases the magnitude of episodic LHRH release, resulting in a rise of circulating gonadotropins (239–243). Replacement with gonadal steroids reduces the pulse frequency of LH at first, thus depressing plasma LH and FSH, but prolonged exposure to estrogen in gonadectomized females reverses the inhibition. There are correlated changes in electrical activity in the medial basal hypothalamus. Dufy et al. (244) recorded pronounced pulsatile multiunit events in the arcuate nuclei of ovariectomized monkeys immediately preceding each LH pulse.

Since LHRH promotes secretion of both LH and FSH, and no specific FSH releaser has been identified, the means for differential regulation of these two secretions has been a mystery. A suggestion of an answer comes from observations that the LH/FSH ratios are influenced by changes in the LHRH pulse frequency (239,243), LH secretion being favored by higher frequencies and FSH by lower frequencies. Controls of the respective gonadotropins may thus be served entirely by the one neurohumor. (There is some evidence that certain regions of the hypothalamus contain a specific releaser for FSH, and the search for such an agent continues.)

Steroids and the Phasic Release of Gonadotropins

Whereas the episodic discharge of LH appears to be universally determined by hypothalamic signals mediated by LHRH, the relative involvement of the hypothalamus and the AP itself in the phasic (preovulatory) surge of gonadotropins varies greatly from species to species. In the rat, mouse, and hamster, whose reproductive processes are closely attuned to the photoperiod, the hypothalamus has the leading role. Under the influence of the gonadal steroids there is a rapid increase of LHRH content in the medial basal hypothalamus just before the critical afternoon period of proestrus (245). Multiple pulses of LHRH in the portal blood follow, accompanied by increased frequency of pulsatile LH release, at intervals of 16 to 25 seconds (246). The magnitude of these LH pulses is governed initially by the responsiveness of the AP after being primed by estrogen. As the plasma LH concentration rises, the responsiveness is enhanced, partly by the self-priming action of LHRH and probably also by the increased exposure of the gonadotrophs to progesterone. Whether progesterone or some other progestin is active at the very start of the surge has long been debated.

At the other extreme from the rat is the rhesus monkey, in which the role of the hypothalamus is judged to be more permissive and the timing of the LH surge is determined directly by the response of the AP to the rising tide of estrogen (236,247). Knobil et al. (248) have shown that in female monkeys bearing long-term lesions of the arcuate nuclei, the month-long infusion of the LHRH pulses once per hour sustained complete menstrual cycles. In long-term ovariectomized females having similar hypothalamic lesions and similarly treated with LHRH, administration of estrogen invoked LH surges. No relationship to the time of day was evident in such responses. Nevertheless, the amount of LHRH in the portal blood does vary in the rhesus monkey, being relatively high during the estrogen-induced LH surge (249). A modulating, though nonessential, influence of the hypothalamus has been suggested (247), and others have proposed a specific hypothalamic message (250).

The guinea pig is intermediate between the rat and monkey, such that in ovariectomized subjects the time of an LH surge induced by estrogen depends not only on the time of injection, but also on the time of day and dosage (251,252); the surge is larger in the dark than in the light phase of the daily rhythm. In intact animals, spontaneous surges are also more frequent in the dark phase. Furthermore, unlike the rat and hamster, the ovariectomized guinea pig receiving estrogen fails to present repeated daily surges of LH.

The ovariectomized rat, chronically supplied with estrogen, either by repeated injection of estradiol benzoate (253) or by implanted Silastic capsules containing estradiol (254,255), displays daily proestrus-like surges of LH secretion, confirming that there is an innate circadian periodicity in the control mechanism in this species. When progesterone is introduced into such a preparation early in the day, the amount of LH released is enhanced, but release on the days following is diminished or prevented (230,256). Both effects are dose dependent (257).

The female hamster presents interesting variations on the circadian manifestations displayed by the rat (258–260). During the anestrus induced by short photoperiods, when estrogen levels are low and progesterone is high, there are daily afternoon surges of LH (261,262). Estrogen treatment of long-day subjects intensifies the surges at first, but later suppresses them; that inhibition is hastened by progesterone.

Investigation of the positive and negative actions of the sex steroids on the hypothalamic-pituitary complex proceeds apace, resulting already in a voluminous literature that defies balanced analysis. A recent review (245) addressed selectively to the control of LH secretion in the laboratory rat cites over 400 articles, of which over 300 were published during the last decade. The broad perspective embraces similarities and differences among species, sex differences, developmental aspects, changes during pregnancy, and the influences of old age. There are concerns with anatomy of the LHRH nerve cells and fibers and their physical connections with steroid-concentrating neurons and other neural systems. Much interest focuses on the influence of the steroids on hypothalamic neurochemistry and on the participation of several neurotransmitters and hypothalamic enzymes that affect LHRH synthesis, transport, and release.

Nonsteroid Gonadal Feedback

The participation of nonsteroidal gonadal secretions in modulating the pars distalis responses to LHRH assumes increasing significance for the differential regulation of FSH and LH synthesis and discharge. Such material obtained from ovarian follicular fluid or testis extracts (inhibin, folliculostatin, gonadostatin) selectively inhibits FSH secretion *in vivo* and *in vitro* (263,264). On the other hand, inhibin is said to enhance the secretion *in vitro* of LH in response to LHRH, adding to the stimulative action of estradiol (265).

CONCLUSIONS

This chapter focuses primarily on background studies of the regulation of gonadotropin and prolactin secretion in adult female mammals. Little or no attention is given to a number of important subjects such as the pars intermedia and the classical neurosecretory system terminating in the neural lobe. Present knowledge of the mammalian hypothalamo-pars distalis apparatus is necessarily limited to a few readily available species. For the vast majority, distributed through more than 900 genera, the details of reproductive physiology are poorly known and for practical reasons will probably remain so. One can only assume that the range of specializations recognized among familiar species is representative. Each has contributed importantly in its own way. Thus, as principal representative of the reflex ovulators, the rabbit gave the first clues to the importance of the central nervous system and the hypothalamic-pars distalis connection for the ovulation process. The guinea pig gave the initial evidence that the corpora lutea suppress ovulation. The mouse, through the Allen-Doisy test, was influential in the purification and synthesis of estrogens. The rat, through the technique of hypophysectomy, greatly facilitated the isolation and purification of the several pars distalis hormones. From the rat also came the first proof of the regenerative capacity of the pituitary portal vessels and demonstration of the importance of the vascular supply to the gland from the median eminence, as well as the evidence for neurohumoral inhibition of prolactin secretion. The ovulation-blocking action of certain drugs in rabbits and rats gave the first clear evidence for an acute preovulatory surge of gonadotropins in spontaneous ovulators. The predictable time of this surge in rats, its dependence on the lighting rhythm, and failure of the surge in old rats led to disclosure of the biphasic action of progesterone and its interaction with estrogen in promoting the surge. Blockage of the surge pharmacologically or by exposure to continuous lighting fostered various studies of the central neural apparatus controlling spontaneous ovulation. Critical comparisons among rats, hamsters, guinea pigs, sheep, and monkeys, facilitated by radioimmunoassay and other modern techniques, have yielded interpretations that seem generally applicable to human subjects, a major goal of all research in reproductive biology.

ACKNOWLEDGMENTS

This research was supported in part by grants from the Research Council of Duke University and, since 1957, from the National Science Foundation. The author is also grateful to John Graves for typing the manuscript.

REFERENCES

1. Harris GW. Humours and hormones, the Sir Henry Dale lecture for 1971. *J Endocrinol* 1972;53:ii–xxii.
2. Rathke MH. Uber die Entstehung der Glandula pituitaria. *Arch Anat Physiol Wiss Med* 1838;482–485. Cited by Medvei VC. *A history of endocrinology.* Boston: MTP Press, 1982.
3. Bayliss WM. *Principles of general physiology.* London: Longmans, Green, 1915.
4. Bayliss WM, Starling EH. The chemical regulation of the secretory process. *Proc R Soc Lond (Biol)* 1904;73:310–322.
5. Ramón y Cajal S. Algunas contribuciónes conociamento de los ganglios del encéfale. *Anal Soc Espan Hist Nat* 1894;23:214–215.
6. Camus J, Roussy G. Experimental researches on the pituitary body. Diabetes insipidus, glycosuria, and those dystrophies considered as hypophysial in origin. *Endocrinology* 1920;4:507–522.
7. Bailey P, Bremer F. Experimental diabetes insipidus. *Arch Intern Med* 1921;28:773–803.
8. Evans HM, Long JA. Effect of anterior lobe of hypophysis administered intraperitoneally upon growth, maturity, and oestrous cycles in the rat. *Anat Rec* 1921;21:61 (abstract).
9. Anderson E. Earlier ideas of hypothalamic function, including irrelevant concepts. In: Haymaker W, Anderson E, Nauta WJH, eds. *The hypothalamus.* Springfield, IL: Charles C Thomas, 1969;1–12.
10. Cushing H. The hypophysis cerebri: chemical aspects of hyperpituitarism and hypopituitarism. *JAMA* 1909;53:249–255.
11. Crowe SJ, Cushing H, Homans J. Experimental hypophysectomy. *Bull Johns Hopkins Hosp* 1910;21:127–169.
12. Cushing H. *The pituitary and its disorders.* Philadelphia: JB Lippincott, 1912.
13. Aschner B. Demonstration von Hunden nach Extirpation der Hypophyse. *Wien Klin Wochenschr* 1909;22:1730–1732.
14. Aschner B. Ueber die Function der Hypophyse. *Pflugers Arch Ges Physiol* 1912;146:1–147.
15. Marshall FHA. Sexual periodicity and the causes which determine it. The Croonian lecture. *Philos Trans R Soc Lond (Biol)* 1936;226:423–456.
16. Marshall FHA. Exteroceptive factors in sexual periodicity. *Biol Rev* 1942;17:68–90.
17. Haighton J. An experimental study concerning animal impregnation. *Philos Trans R Soc* 1797;87:157–196.
18. Cruikshank W. Experiments in which, on the third day after impregnation, the ova of rabbits were found in the Fallopian tubes; and on the fourth day after impregnation in the uterus itself; with the first appearance of the foetus. *Philos Trans R Soc* 1797;87:197–214.
19. Barry M. Researches in embryology. *Philos Trans R Soc* 1839;129:307–380.
20. Heape W. Ovulation and degeneration of ova in rabbit. *Proc R Soc Lond (Biol)* 1905;76:266–268.
21. Marshall FHA. The oestrous cycle of the common ferret. *Q J Microsc Sci* 1904;48:323–345.
22. Longley WH. Maturation of the egg and ovulation in the domestic cat. *Am J Anat* 1911;12:139–172.
23. Fichera G. Sur l'hypertrophie de la gland pituitaire consecutive à la castration. *Arch Ital Biol* 1905;43:405–426.
24. Addison WHF. The cell changes of the hypophysis of the albino rat after castration. *J Comp Neurol* 1917;28:441–461.
25. Loeb L. Über die Bedeutung des Corpus luteum für die Periodizität des sexuellen Zyklus beim weiblichen Säugetier-organismus. *Dtsch Med Wochenschr* 1911;37:17–21.
26. Stockard CR, Papanicolaou GN. The existence of a typical oestrous cycle in the guinea pig—with a study of its histological and physiological changes. *Am J Anat* 1917;22:225–283.
27. Long JA, Evans HM. The oestrous cycle in the rat and its associated phenomena. *Mem Univ Calif* 1922;6:1–111.
28. Allen E. The oestrous cycle in the mouse. *Am J Anat* 1922;30:297–371.

28a. Allen E, Doisy EA. An ovarian hormone; a preliminary report on its localization, extraction and partial purification, and action in test animals. *JAMA* 1923;81:819–821.

29. Allen E, Pratt JP, Doisy EA. The ovarian follicular hormone. Its distribution in human genital tissues. *JAMA* 1925;85:399–405.
30. Allen BM. The results of extirpation of the anterior lobe of the hypophysis and of the thyroid of *Rana pipiens* larvae. *Science* 1916;44:755–757.
31. Allen BM. Experiments in the transplantation of the hypophysis of adult *Rana pipiens* to tadpoles. *Science* 1920;52:274–276.
32. Smith PE. The effect of hypophysectomy in the early embryo upon growth and development of the frog. *Anat Rec* 1916;11:57–64.
33. Smith PE, Smith IP. The effect of intraperitoneal injection of fresh anterior lobe substance in hypophysectomized tadpoles. *Anat Rec* 1922;23:38–39.
34. Smith PE, Smith IP. The repair and activation of the thyroid in the hypophysectomized tadpole by the parenteral administration of fresh anterior lobe of the bovine hypophysis. *J Med Res* 1922;43:267–283.
35. Smith PE. Ablation and transplantation of the hypophysis in the rat. *Anat Rec* 1926;32:221 (abstract).
36. Smith PE. The disabilities caused by hypophysectomy and their repair. *JAMA* 1927;88:158–161.
37. Smith PE. Hypophysectomy and replacement therapy in the rat. *Am J Anat* 1930;45:205–274.
38. Smith PE, Engle ET. Experimental evidence regarding the role of the anterior pituitary in the development and regulation of the genital system. *Am J Anat* 1927;40:159–217.
39. Evans HM, Meyer K, Simpson ME. The growth and gonad-stimulating hormones of the anterior hypophysis. *Mem Univ Calif* 1933;11:67–229.
40. Evans HM, Pencharz RI, Meyer K, Simpson ME. The growth and gonad-stimulating hormones of the anterior hypophysis. *Mem Univ Calif* 1933;11:315–334.
41. Greep RO. Separation of a thyrotropic from the gonadotropic substances of the pituitary. *Am J Physiol* 1935;110:692–699.
42. Zondek B. Über die Hormone des Hypophysenvorderlappens. I. Wachstumshormon, Follikelreifungshormon (Prolan A), Luteinisierungshormon (Prolan B), Stoffwechselhormon. *Klin Wochenschr* 1930;9:245–248.
43. Zondek B. Über die Hormone des Hypophysenvorderlappens. II. Follikelreifungshormon Prolan A-Klamakterium-Kastration. *Klin Wochenschr* 1930;9:393–396.
44. Reichert FL, Pencharz RI, Simpson ME, Meyer K, Evans HM. Relative ineffectiveness of Prolan in hypophysectomized animals. *Am J Physiol* 1932;100:157–161.
45. Leonard SM, Smith PE. Responses of the reproductive system of hypophysectomized rats to injections of pregnancy-urine extracts. II. The female. *Anat Rec* 1934;58:175–200.
46. Gey GO, Seegar GE, Hellman LM. The production of gonadotropic substance (Prolan) by placental cells in tissue culture. *Science* 1938;88:306–307.
47. Jones GES, Gey GO, Cey MK. Hormone production by placental cells maintained in continuous culture. *Bull Johns Hopkins Hosp* 1943;72:26–38.
48. Fevold HL, Hisaw FL, Leonard SL. The gonad-stimulating and the luteinizing hormones of the anterior lobe of the hypophysis. *Am J Physiol* 1931;97:291–301.
49. Greep RO. History of research on anterior hypophysial hormones. In: *Handbook of Physiology, Section 7, Endocrinology,* Vol. IV, part 2. Washington, DC: American Physiological Society, 1974;1–27.
50. Astwood EB. The regulation of corpus luteum function by hypophysial luteotropin. *Endocrinology* 1941;28:309–320.
51. Evans HM, Simpson ME, Lyons WR, Turpeinen K. Anterior pituitary hormones which favor production of traumatic uterine placentoma. *Endocrinology* 1941;28:933–945.
52. Stricker P, Grueter F. Action du lobe antérieur de l'hypophyse sur la montée laiteuse. *C R Soc Biol (Paris)* 1928;99:1978–1980.
53. Stricker P, Grueter F. Fonctions du lobe antérieur de l'hypophyse: influence des extraits du lobe antérieur sur l'appareil génitale de la lapine et sur la montée laiteuse. *Presse Med* 1929;37:1268–1271.

54. Corner GW. The hormonal control of lactation. I. Noneffect of the corpus luteum. II. Positive action of extracts of the hypophysis. *Am J Physiol* 1930;95:43–55.
55. Evans HM, Simpson ME. Hyperplasia of the mammary apparatus of adult virgin females induced by anterior hypophyseal hormones. *Proc Soc Exp Biol Med* 1929;26:598.
56. Riddle O. Physiological responses to prolactin. *Cold Spring Harbor Symp Quant Biol* 1937;5:218–228.
57. Riddle O. Prolactin. *Assoc Res Nerv Mental Dis* 1938;17: 287–297.
58. Riddle O, Braucher PF. Studies on the physiology of reproduction in birds. XXX. Control of the special secretion of the crop gland in pigeons by an anterior pituitary hormone. *Am J Physiol* 1931;97:617–625.
59. Riddle O, Bates RW, Dykshorn SW. The preparation, identification and assay of prolactin—a hormone of the anterior pituitary. *Am J Physiol* 1933;105:191–216.
60. Dresl L. The effect of prolactin on the estrus cycle of nonparous mice. *Science* 1935;82:173.
61. Lahr L, Riddle O. Temporary suppression of estrous cycles in the rat by prolactin. *Proc Soc Exp Biol Med* 1936;34:880–893.
62. Bates RW, Miller RA, Garrison MM. Evidence in the hypophysectomized pigeon of a synergism among prolactin, growth hormone, thyroxine and prednisone upon weight of the body, digestive tract, kidney and fat stores. *Endocrinology* 1962;71:345–360.
63. Schönemann A. Hypophysis und Thyroidea. *Virchows Arch (Pathol Anat)* 1892;129:310–336.
64. Holmes RL, Ball JN. *The pituitary gland—a comparative account.* Cambridge: Cambridge University Press, 1974.
65. Mallory FB. A contribution to staining methods. *J Exp Med* 1900;5:15–20.
66. McManus JFA. Histological demonstration of mucin after periodic acid. *Nature* 1946;158:202.
67. Herlant M. Étude critique de deux techniques nouvelles destinées à mettre en evidence les différentes catégories cellulaires présente dans la glands pituitaire. *Bull Microsc Appl* 1960;10:37–44.
68. Pearse AGE. Cytological and cyto-chemical investigations on the foetal and adult hypophysis in various physiological and pathological states. *J Pathol Bacteriol* 1953;65:355–370.
69. Coons AH. Histochemistry with labelled antibody. *Int Rev Cytol* 1956;5:1–23.
70. Halmi NS, Krieger D. Immunocytochemistry of ACTH-related peptides in the hypophysis. In: Bhatnagar AS, ed. *The anterior pituitary gland.* New York: Raven Press, 1983;1–15.
71. Hohlweg W, Junkmann K. Die hormonal-nervöse Regulierung der Funktion des Hypophysenvorderlappens. *Klin Wochenschr* 1932;11:321–323.
72. Fröhlich A. Ein Fall von Tumor der Hypophysis cerebri ohne Akromegalie. *Wien Klin Rundschau* 1901;15:883–886; 906–908.
73. Hetherington AW, Ranson SW. Experimental hypothalamico-hypophyseal obesity in the rat. *Proc Soc Exp Biol Med* 1939;41:465–466.
74. Hetherington AW, Ranson SW. Hypothalamic lesions and adiposity in the rat. *Anat Rec* 1940;78:149–172.
75. Hetherington AW, Ranson SW. The relation of various hypothalamic lesions to adiposity in the rat. *J Comp Neurol* 1942;76:475–499.
76. Bauer HG. Endocrine and other clinical manifestations of hypothalamic disease. *J Clin Endocrinol* 1954;14:13–31.
77. Grafe E, Grünthal E. Über isolierte Beinflussung des Gesamtstoffwechsels vom Zwischenhirn aus. *Klin Wochenschr* 1929;8:1013–1016.
78. Moore CR, Price D. Gonad hormone functions and the reciprocal influence between gonads and hypophysis with its bearing on the problem of sex-hormone antogonisms. *Am J Anat* 1932; 50:13–71.
79. Fee AR, Parkes AS. The relation of the anterior pituitary body to ovulation in the rabbit. *J Physiol (Lond)* 1929;67:383–388.
80. Fee AR, Parkes AS. Effects of vaginal anesthesia on ovulation in the rabbit. *J Physiol (Lond)* 1930;70:385–388.
81. Marshall FHA, Verney EB. The occurrence of ovulation and pseudopregnancy in the rabbit, as a result of central nervous stimulation. *J Physiol (Lond)* 1936;86:327–336.
82. Harris GW. The induction of ovulation in the rabbit by electrical stimulation of the hypothalamo-hypophysial mechanism. *Proc R Soc Lond (Biol)* 1937;122:374–394.
83. Haterius HO, Derbyshire AJ Jr. Ovulation in the rabbit upon stimulation of the hypothalamus. *Am J Physiol* 1937;119: 329–330.
84. Westman A, Jacobsohn D. Experimentelle Untersuchungen über die Bedeutung des Hypophysen-Zwischenhirnsystems für die Produktion gonadotroper Hormone des Hypophysenvorderlappens. *Acta Obstet Gynecol Scand* 1937;17:235–265.
85. Rasmussen AT. Innervation of the hypophysis. *Endocrinology* 1938;23:263–278.
86. Hohlweg W, Chamorro A. Über die luteinisierende Wirkung des Follikelhormons durch Beinflussung der endogenen Hypophysenvorderlappensekretion. *Klin Wochenschr* 1937;16:196–197.
87. Westman A, Jacobsohn D. Endokrinologische Untersuchungen an Ratten mit durchtrenntem Hypophysenstiel. I. Hypophysenveränderungen nach Kastration und nach Oestrinbehandlungen. *Acta Obstet Gynecol Scand* 1938;18:99–108.
88. Westman A, Jacobsohn D. Endokrinologische Untersuchungen an Ratten mit durchtrenntem Hypophysenstiel. III. Über die luteinisierende Wirkung des Follikelhormons. *Acta Obstet Gynecol Scand* 1938;18:115–123.
89. Westman A, Jacobsohn D. Endokrinologische Untersuchungen an Ratten mit durchtrenntem Hypophysenstiel. VI. Produktion und Abgabe der gonadotropen Hormone. *Acta Pathol Microbiol Scand* 1938;15:445–453.
90. Pietsch K. Aufbau und Entwicklung der Pars tuberalis des menschlichen Hirnanhangs in ihren Beziehung zu den übrigen Hypophysenteilen. *Z Mikrosk Anat Forsch* 1930;22:227–257.
91. Popa GT, Fielding U. A portal circulation from the pituitary to the hypothalamic region. *J Anat (Lond)* 1930;65:88–91.
92. Popa GT, Fielding U. Hypophysio-portal vessels and their colloid accompaniment. *J Anat (Lond)* 1933;67:227–232.
93. Houssay BA, Biosotti A, Sammartino R. Modificationes fonctionelles de l'hypophyse après les lésions infundibulotubériennes chez le crapaud. *C R Soc Biol (Paris)* 1935;120:725–727.
94. Wislocki GB, King LS. The permeability of the hypophysis and the hypothalamus to vital dyes, with a study of the hypophysial vascular supply. *Am J Anat* 1936;58:421–472.
95. Wislocki GB. The vascular supply of the hypophysis cerebri of the rhesus monkey and man. *Res Publ Assoc Nerv Ment Dis* 1938;17:48–68.
96. Green JD. Vessels and nerves of the amphibian hypophysis: a study of the living circulation and of the histology of the hypophysial vessels and nerves. *Anat Rec* 1947;99:21–54.
97. Benoit J, Assenmacher I. Le controle hypothalamique de l'activité préhypophysaire gonadotrope. *J Physiol (Paris)* 1955; 47:427–567.
98. Green JD, Harris GW. The neurovascular link between the neurohypophysis and adenohypophysis. *J Endocrinol* 1947; 5:136–146.
99. Green JD, Harris GW. Observations of the hypophysial portal vessels of the living rat. *J Physiol (Lond)* 1949;108:359–361.
100. Worthington WC Jr. Some observations on the hypophyseal portal system in the living mouse. *Bull Johns Hopkins Hosp* 1955;97:343–357.
101. Worthington WC Jr. Vascular responses in the pituitary stalk. *Endocrinology* 1960;66:19–31.
102. Török B. Lebendbeobachtung des Hypophysenkreislaufes an Hunden. *Acta Morphol Hung* 1954;4:83–89.
103. Török B. Neue Angaben zum Blutkreislauf der Hypophyse. *Anat Anz* 1962:109(Suppl.):622–629.
104. Daniel PM. The anatomy of the hypothalamus and pituitary gland. In: Martini L, Ganong WF, eds. *Neuroendocrinology,* Vol. 1. New York: Academic Press, 1966;15–80.
105. Page RB, Bergland RM. The neurophysial capillary bed. I. Anatomy and arterial supply. *Am J Anat* 1977;148:345–358.
106. Bergland RM, Page RB. Can the pituitary secrete directly to the brain? (Affirmative anatomical evidence). *Endocrinology* 1978; 102:1325–1338.
107. Oliver C, Mical RS, Porter JC. Hypothalamic-pituitary vasculature: evidence for retrograde blood flow in the pituitary stalk. *Endocrinology* 1977;101:598–604.
108. Daniel PM, Prichard MML. Studies of the hypothalamus and the

pituitary gland with special reference to the effects of transection of the pituitary stalk. *Acta Endocrinol* 1975;80(Suppl. 201): 1–216.
109. Pasteels JL. Étude expérimentale des différentes catégories d'éléments chromophiles de l'hypophyse adulte de *Pleurodeles waltlii* et de leur controle par l'hypothalamus. *Arch Biol (Paris)* 1960;71:409–471.
110. Porter JC, Kamberi IA, Grazia YA. Pituitary blood flow and portal vessels. In: Martini L, Ganong WF, eds. *Frontiers in neuroendocrinology.* New York: Oxford University Press. 1971; 145–175.
111. Hinsey JC, Markee JE. Pregnancy following bilateral section of the cervical sympathetic trunks in the rabbits. *Proc Soc Exp Biol Med* 1933;31:270–271.
112. Hinsey JC. The relationship of the nervous system to ovulation and other phenomena of the female reproductive tract. *Cold Spring Harbor Symp Quant Biol* 1937;5:269–279.
113. Wingstrand KG. Comparative anatomy and evolution of the hypophysis. In: Harris GW, Donovan BT, eds. *The pituitary gland,* Vol. 1. London: Butterworths, 1966;58–126.
114. Green JD. The comparative anatomy of the hypophysis, with special reference to its blood supply and innervation. *Am J Anat* 1951;88:225–312.
115. Harris GW. Oestrous rhythm, pseudopregnancy and the pituitary stalk in the rat. *J Physiol (Lond)* 1950;111:347–360.
116. Harris GW, Johnson RT. Regeneration of the hypophysial portal vessels after section of the hypophysial stalk, in the monkey *Macaca rhesus. Nature* 1950;165:819–820.
117. Jacobsohn D. Regeneration of hypophysial portal vessels and grafts of anterior pituitary glands in rabbits. *Acta Endocrinol (Copenh)* 1954;17:187–197.
118. Greep RO. Functional pituitary grafts in rats. *Proc Soc Exp Biol Med* 1936;34:754–755.
119. Harris GW, Jacobsohn D. Functional grafts of the anterior pituitary gland. *Proc R Soc Lond (Biol)* 1952;139:263–276.
120. Nikitovitch-Winer M, Everett JW. Functional restitution of pituitary grafts re-transplanted from kidney to median eminence. *Endocrinology* 1958;63:916–930.
121. Nikitovitch-Winer M, Everett JW. Histo-cytologic changes in grafts of rat pituitary on the kidney and upon retransplantation under the diencephalon. *Endocrinology* 1959;65:357–368.
122. Smith PE. Postponed homotransplants of the hypophysis into the region of the median eminence in hypophysectomized male rats. *Endocrinology* 1961;68:130–143.
123. Smith PE. Postponed pituitary homotransplants into the region of the hypophysial portal circulation in hypophysectomized female rats. *Endocrinology* 1963;73:793–806.
124. Harris GW. *Neural control of the pituitary gland.* London: Arnold, 1955.
125. Saffran M, Schally AV, Benfry BG. Stimulation of the release of corticotropin from the adenohypophysis by a neurohypophysial factor. *Endocrinology* 1955;57:439–444.
126. Everett JW. Luteotrophic function of autografts of the rat hypophysis. *Endocrinology* 1954;54:685–690.
127. Everett JW. Functional corpora lutea maintained for months by autografts of rat hypophyses. *Endocrinology* 1956;58:786–796.
128. Desclin L. A propos du méchanisme d'action des oestro-gènes sur le lobe antérieur de l'hypophyse chez le rat. *Ann Endocrinol* 1950;11:656–659.
129. Nikitovitch-Winer MB. Effect of hypophysial stalk transection on luteotropic hormone secretion in the rat. *Endocrinology* 1965;77:658–666.
130. Nicoll CS, Meites J. Prolactin secretion *in vitro:* comparative aspects. *Nature* 1962;195:606–607.
131. Nicoll CS. Neural regulation of adenohypophysial prolactin secretion in tetrapods: indications from *in vitro* studies. *J Exp Zool* 1965;158:203–210.
132. Meites J. Control of prolactin secretion. *Arch Anat Microsc Morphol Exp* 1967;56(Suppl.):516–529.
133. Pasteels JL. Sécrétion de prolactine par l'hypophyse en culture de tissues. *C R Acad Sci (Paris)* 1961;253:2140–2142.
134. Pasteels JL. Premiers résultats de culture combinée *in vitro* d'hypophyis et d'hypothalamus dans le but d'en apprécier la sécrétion de prolactine. *C R Acad Sci (Paris)* 1961;253:3074–3075.
135. Wade N. *The Nobel duel.* New York: Anchor Press/Doubleday, 1981.
136. MacLeod RM. Regulation of prolactin secretion. In: Martini L, Ganong WF, eds. *Frontiers in neuroendocrinology.* New York: Raven Press, 1976;169–194.
137. Ben-Jonathan N, Oliver C, Weiner HJ, Mical RS, Porter JC. Dopamine in hypophysial portal plasma of the rat during the estrous cycle and throughout pregnancy. *Endocrinology* 1977; 100:452–458.
138. Sawyer CH, Markee JE, Hollinshead WH. Inhibition of ovulation in the rabbit by the adrenergic-blocking agent Dibenamine. *Endocrinology* 1947;41:395–402.
139. Markee JE, Sawyer CH, Hollinshead WH. Adrenergic control of the release of luteinizing hormone from the hypophysis of the rabbit. *Recent Prog Horm Res* 1948;2:117–151.
140. Sawyer CH, Markee JE, Townsend BF. Cholinergic and adrenergic components in the neurohumoral control of the release of LH in the rabbit. *Endocrinology* 1949;44:18–37.
141. Sawyer CH. Stimulation of ovulation in the rabbit by the intraventricular injection of epinephrine or norepinephrine. *Anat Rec* 1952;112:385 (abstract).
142. Sawyer CH. The Seventh Stevenson Lecture. Brain amines and pituitary gonadotrophin secretion. *Can J Physiol Pharmacol* 1979;57:667–680.
143. Tsou RC, Dailey RA, McLanahan CS, Parent AD, Tindall GT, Neill JD. Luteinizing hormone releasing hormone (LHRH) levels in pituitary stalk plasma during the preovulatory gonadotropin surge of rabbits. *Endocrinology* 1977;101:534–539.
144. Dufy-Barbe L, Franchimont P, Faure JMA. Time courses of LH and FSH release in the female rabbit. *Endocrinology* 1973; 92:1318–1321.
145. Kanematsu S, Scaramuzzi RJ, Hilliard J, Sawyer CH. Patterns of ovulation-inducing LH release following coitus, electrical stimulation and exogenous LH-RH in the rabbit. *Endocrinology* 1974;95:247–252.
146. Goodman AL, Neill JD. Ovarian regulation of postcoital gonadotropin release in the rabbit: reexamination of a functional role for 20α dihydro-progesterone. *Endocrinology* 1976;99:852–860.
147. Westman A. Der Einfluss des Hypophysenzwishchenhirnsystems auf die Sexualfunktionen. *Schweiz Med Wochenschr* 1942; 72:113–116.
148. Dempsey EW. Follicular growth rate and ovulation after various experimental procedures in the guinea pig. *Am J Physiol* 1937;120:126–132.
149. Everett JW, Sawyer CH, Markee JE. A neurogenic timing factor in control of the ovulating discharge of luteinizing hormone in the cyclic rat. *Endocrinology* 1949;44:234–250.
150. Sawyer CH, Everett JW, Markee JE. A neural factor in the mechanism by which estrogen induces the release of luteinizing hormone in the rat. *Endocrinology* 1949;44:218–233.
151. Everett JW, Sawyer CH. A neural timing factor in the mechanism by which progesterone advances ovulation in the cyclic rat. *Endocrinology* 1949;45:581–595.
152. Everett JW, Sawyer CH. A 24-hour periodicity in the "LH-release apparatus" of female rats, disclosed by barbiturate sedation. *Endocrinology* 1950;47:198–218.
153. Barraclough CA, Sawyer CH. Inhibition of the release of pituitary ovulatory hormone in the rat by morphine. *Endocrinology* 1955;57:329–337.
154. Barraclough CA, Sawyer CH. Blockade of the release of pituitary ovulating hormone in the rat by chlorpromazine and reserpine: possible mechanisms of action. *Endocrinology* 1957;61:341–351.
155. Blake CA, Sawyer CH. Ovulation blocking actions of urethane in the rat. *Endocrinology* 1972;91:87–94.
156. Everett JW, Sawyer CH. Estimated duration of the spontaneous activation which causes release of ovulating hormone from the rat hypophysis. *Endocrinology* 1953;52:83–92.
157. Everett JW. The time of release of ovulating hormone from the rat hypophysis. *Endocrinology* 1956;59:580–585.
158. Everett JW, Tejasen T. Time factor in ovulation blockade in rats under differing lighting conditions. *Endocrinology* 1967; 80:790–792.
159. Blake CA. A detailed characterization of the proestrous luteinizing hormone surge. *Endocrinology* 1976;98:445–450.

160. Sarkar DK, Chiappa SA, Fink G, Sherwood NM. Gonadotropin-releasing hormone surge in pro-oestrous rats. *Nature* 1976; 264:461–463.
161. Everett JW. Progesterone and estrogen in the experimental control of ovulation time and other features of the estrous cycle in the rat. *Endocrinology* 1948;43:389–405.
162. Everett JW. Photoregulation of the ovarian cycle in the rat. In: Benoit J, Assenmacher I, eds. *La photoregulation de la reproduction chez les oiseaux et les mammiféres.* Paris: C.N.R.S., 1970;387–403.
163. Everett JW. Presumptive hypothalamic control of spontaneous ovulation. *Ciba Found Coll Endocrinol* 1952;4:167–178.
164. Everett JW. Provoked ovulation or long-delayed pseudopregnancy from coital stimuli in barbiturate-blocked rats. *Endocrinology* 1967;80:145–154.
165. Greep RO, Hisaw FL. Pseudopregnancies from electrical stimulation of the cervix in the diestrum. *Proc Soc Exp Biol Med* 1938;39:359–360.
166. Quinn DL, Everett JW. Delayed pseudopregnancy induced by selective hypothalamic stimulation. *Endocrinology* 1967; 80:155–162.
167. Beach JE, Tyrey L, Everett JW. Serum prolactin and LH in early phases of delayed versus direct pseudopregnancy in the rat. *Endocrinology* 1975;96:1241–1246.
168. Beach JE, Tyrey L, Everett JW. Prolactin secretion preceding delayed pseudopregnancy in rats after electrical stimulation of the hypothalamus. *Endocrinology* 1978;103:2247–2251.
169. de Greef WJ, Zeilmaker GH. Prolactin and delayed pseudopregnancy in the rat. *Endocrinology* 1976;98:305–310.
170. Anand BK, Malkani PK, Dua S. Effect of electrical stimulation of the hypothalamus on menstrual cycle in monkey. *Indian J Med Res* 1957;45:499–502.
171. Bunn JP, Everett JW. Ovulation in persistent-estrous rats after electrical stimulation of the brain. *Proc Soc Exp Biol Med* 1957;96:369–371.
172. Critchlow V. Ovulation induced by hypothalamic stimulation in the anesthetized rat. *Am J Physiol* 1958;195:171–174.
173. Everett JW, Radford HM. Irritative deposits from stainless steel electrodes in the preoptic rat brain causing release of pituitary gonadotropin. *Proc Soc Exp Biol Med* 1961;108:604–609.
174. Everett JW. Preoptic stimulative lesions and ovulation in the rat: "thresholds" and LH-release time in late diestrus and proestrus. In: Bajusz E, Jasmin G, eds. *Major problems in neuroendocrinology.* Basel: Karger, 1964;346–366.
175. Everett JW, Krey LC, Tyrey L. The quantitative relationship between electrochemical preoptic stimulation and LH release in proestrous *versus* late diestrous rats. *Endocrinology* 1973; 93:947–953.
176. Turgeon J, Barraclough GA. Temporal patterns of LH release following graded preoptic electrochemical stimulation in proestrous rats. *Endocrinology* 1973;92:755–761.
177. Velasco ME, Rothchild I. Factors influencing the secretion of luteinizing hormone and ovulation in response to electrochemical stimulation of the preoptic area in rats. *J Endocrinol* 1973;58:163–176.
178. Colombo JA, Whitmoyer DI, Sawyer CH. Local changes in multiple unit activity induced by electrochemical means in preoptic and hypothalamic areas in the female rat. *Brain Res* 1974;71:1175–1183.
179. van der Schoot P, Lincoln DW, Clark JS. Activation of hypothalamic neuronal activity by electrolytic deposition of iron into the preoptic area. *J Endocrinol* 1978;79:107–120.
180. Dyer RG, Burnet F. Effects of ferrous ions on preoptic area neurons and luteinizing hormone secretion in the rat. *J Endocrinol* 1976;69:247–254.
181. Dyball RE, Dyer RG, MacLeod NK, Wright RJ, Yates JO. Effects of ferrous ions on secretion from incubated nerve terminals. *J Endocrinol* 1976;72:73P.
182. Hillarp NA, Olivecrona H, Silferskiöld W. Evidence for the participation of the preoptic area in male mating behaviour. *Experientia* 1954;10:224–225.
183. Willmore LJ, Hurd RW, Sypert GW. Epileptiform activity initiated by pial iontophoresis of ferrous and ferric chloride on rat cerebral cortex. *Brain Res* 1978;152:406–410.
184. Willmore LJ, Hiramatsu M, Kochi H, Mori A. Formation of superoxide radicals after $FeCl_3$ injection into rat isocortex. *Brain Res* 1983;277:393–396.
185. Tejasen T, Everett JW. Surgical analysis of the preoptico-tuberal pathway controlling ovulatory release of gonadotropins in the rat. *Endocrinology* 1967;81:1387–1396.
186. Everett JW, Tyrey L. Induction of LH release and ovulation in rats by radiofrequency lesions of the medial basal tuber cinereum. *Anat Rec* 1977;187:575 (abstract).
187. Everett JW, Quinn DL, Tyrey L. Comparative effectiveness of preoptic and tuberal stimulation for luteinizing hormone release and ovulation in two strains of rats. *Endocrinology* 1976; 98:1302–1308.
188. Gosden RG, Everett JW, Tyrey L. Luteinizing hormone requirement for ovulation in the pentobarbital-treated proestrous rat. *Endocrinology* 1976;99:1046–1053.
189. Everett JW, Tyrey L. Comparative increments of circulating luteinizing hormone in rats with increasing duration of electrical stimulation in medial preoptic or medial basal tuberal sites. *Endocrinology* 1981;109:691–696.
190. Fink G, Jamieson MG. Immunoreactive luteinizing hormone releasing factor in rat pituitary stalk blood: effects of electrical stimulation of the medial preoptic area. *J Endocrinol* 1976;68:71–87.
191. Cramer OM, Barraclough CA. Effect of electrical stimulation of the preoptic area on plasma LH concentrations in proestrous rats. *Endocrinology* 1971;88:1175–1183.
192. Everett JW, Tyrey L. Similarity of luteinizing hormone surges induced by medial preoptic stimulation in female rats blocked with pentobarbital, morphine, chlorpromazine, or atropine. *Endocrinology* 1982;111:1979–1985.
193. Aiyer MS, Chiappa SA, Fink G. A priming effect of luteinizing hormone releasing factor on the anterior pituitary gland in the female rat. *J Endocrinol* 1974;62:573–588.
194. Fink G, Chiappa SA, Aiyer MS. Priming effect of luteinizing hormone releasing factor elicited by preoptic stimulation and by intravenous infusion and multiple injections of the synthetic peptide. *J Endocrinol* 1976;69:359–372.
195. Pickering AJMC, Fink G. Priming effect of luteinizing hormone releasing factor *in vitro:* role of protein synthesis contractile elements, Ca^{++} and cyclic AMP. *J Endocrinol* 1979;81:223–234.
196. Grieg F, Weisz J. Preovulatory levels of luteinizing hormone, the critical period and ovulation in rats. *J Endocrinol* 1973; 57:235–245.
197. Weick RF, Dierschke DJ, Karsch FJ, Butler WR, Hotchkiss J, Knobil E. Periovulatory time courses of circulating gonadotropic and ovarian hormones in the rhesus monkey. *Endocrinology* 1973;93:1140–1147.
198. Westman A, Jacobsohn D. Über Ovarialveränderungen beim Kaninchen nach Hypophysektomie. *Acta Obstet Gynecol Scand* 1936;16:483–508.
199. Hilliard J, Haywood JN, Sawyer CH. Postcoital patterns of secretion of pituitary gonadotropin and ovarian progestin in the rabbit. *Endocrinology* 1964;75:957–963.
200. Beard J. The rhythm of reproduction in animals. *Anat Anz* 1898;14:97–102.
201. Loeb L. Über die Bedeutung des Corpus luteum für die Periodizität des sexuellen Zyklus beim weiblichen Säugetierorganismus. *Dtsch Med Wochenschr* 1911;37:17–21.
202. Drummond-Robinson G, Asdell SA. The relation between the corpus luteum and the mammary gland. *J Physiol (Lond)* 1926;61:608–614.
203. Hammond J. *The physiology of reproduction in the cow.* Cambridge: Cambridge University Press, 1927.
204. Papanicolaou GN. Effect of removal of corpora lutea and ripe follicles on oestrous periodicity in guinea pigs. *Anat Rec* 1920;19:251 (abstract).
205. Papanicolaou GN. A specific inhibitory hormone of the corpus luteum. *JAMA* 1926;86:1422–1424.
206. Parkes AS, Bellerby CW. Studies on the internal secretion of the ovary. V. The oestrus-inhibiting function of the corpus luteum. *J Physiol (Lond)* 1928;64:233–245.
207. Gley P. Sur l'inhibition de l'ovulation par le corps jaune. *C R Soc Biol (Paris)* 1928;98:504–505.
208. Selye H, Browne JSL, Collip JB. Effects of large doses of progesterone in the female rat. *Proc Soc Exp Biol Med* 1936; 34:472–474.

209. Dempsey EW. Follicular growth rate and ovulation after various experimental procedures in the guinea pig. *Am J Physiol* 1937;120:126–132.
210. Kennedy WP. Corpus luteum extracts and ovulation in the rabbit. *Q J Exp Physiol* 1925;15:103–112.
211. Mahnert A. Weitere Untersuchungen über die Beziehungen zwischen Hypophysenvorderlappen und Ovarium. Zugleich ein Beitrag zur Frage der hormonalen Sterilisierung. *Zentralbl Gynaekol* 1930;54:2883–2887.
212. Makepeace AW, Weinstein GL, Friedman MH. The effect of progestin and progesterone on ovulation in the rabbit. *Am J Physiol* 1937;119:512–516.
213. Moore CR, Price D. Gonad hormone functions and the reciprocal influence between gonads and hypophysis. *Am J Anat* 1932;50:13–72.
214. Engle ET. The pituitary gonadal relationship and the problem of precocious sexual maturity. *Endocrinology* 1931;15:405–420.
215. Hohlweg W. Veränderungen des Hypophysenvorderlappens und des Ovariums nach Behandlungen mit grossen Dosen von Follikelhormonen. *Klin Wochenschr* 1934;13:92–95.
216. Hohlweg W. The regulatory centers of endocrine glands in the hypothalamus. In: Meites J, Donovan B, McCann SM, eds. *Pioneers in neuroendocrinology,* Vol. 1. New York: Plenum Press, 1975;161–172.
217. Hammond J Jr, Hammond J, Parkes AS. Hormonal augmentation of fertility in sheep. I. Induction of ovulation, superovulation, and heat in sheep. *J Agric Sci* 1942;32:308–323.
218. Hammond J Jr. Induced ovulation and heat in anestrous sheep. *J Endocrinol* 1945;4:169–180.
219. Casida LE. Induction of ovulation and subsequent fertility in domestic animals. In: Engle ET, ed. *The problem of fertility.* Princeton: Princeton University Press, 1946;49–59.
220. Everett JW. Progesterone and estrogen in the experimental control of ovulation time and other features of the estrous cycle in the rat. *Endocrinology* 1948;43:389–405.
221. Everett JW. Hormonal factors responsible for deposition of cholesterol in the corpus luteum of the rat. *Endocrinology* 1947;41:364–377.
222. Everett JW, Nichols DC. The timing of ovulatory release of gonadotropin induced by estrogen in pseudopregnant and diestrous cyclic rats. *Anat Rec* 1968;160:346 (abstract).
223. Everett JW, Sawyer CH, Markee JE. A neurogenic timing factor in control of the ovulatory discharge of luteinizing hormone in the cyclic rat. *Endocrinology* 1949;44:234–250.
224. Everett JW. The restoration of ovulatory cycles and corpus luteum formation in persistent-estrous rats by progesterone. *Endocrinology* 1940;27:681–686.
225. Everett JW. Further studies on the relationship of progesterone to ovulation and luteinization in the persistent-estrous rat. *Endocrinology* 1943;32:285–292.
226. Everett JW, Sawyer CH. A neural timing factor in the mechanism by which progesterone advances ovulation in the cyclic rat. *Endocrinology* 1949;45:581–595.
227. Zeilmaker GH. The biphasic effect of progesterone on ovulation in the rat. *Acta Endocrinol* 1966;51:461–468.
228. Everett JW. Effects of estrogen-progesterone synergy on thresholds and timing of the "LH-release apparatus" of the female rat. *Anat Rec* 1951;109:291 (abstract).
229. Redmond WC. Ovulatory response to brain stimulation or exogenous luteinizing hormone in progesterone-treated rats. *Endocrinology* 1968;83:1013–1022.
230. Caligaris L, Astrada JJ, Taleisnik S. Biphasic effect of progesterone on the release of gonadotropin in rats. *Endocrinology* 1971;89:331–337.
231. Sawyer CH, Everett JW. Stimulatory and inhibitory effects of progesterone on the release of pituitary ovulatory hormone in the rabbit. *Endocrinology* 1959;65:644–651.
232. Kawakami M, Sawyer CH. Neuroendocrine correlates of changes in brain activity thresholds by sex steroids and pituitary hormones. *Endocrinology* 1959;65:652–668.
233. Dierschke DJ, Bhattacharya AN, Atkinson LE, Knobil E. Circhoral oscillations of plasma LH levels in the ovariectomized monkey. *Endocrinology* 1970;87:850–853.
234. Brinkley HJ. Endocrine signaling and female reproduction. *Biol Reprod* 1981;24:22–43.
235. Knobil E. Patterns of hypophysiotropic signals and gonadotropin secretions in the rhesus monkey. *Biol Reprod* 1981;24:44–49.
236. Knobil E. The neuroendocrine control of the menstrual cycle. *Recent Prog Horm Res* 1980;36:53–88.
237. Blake CA. Simulation of the proestrous luteinizing hormone (LH) surge after infusion of LH-releasing hormone in phenobarbital-blocked rats. *Endocrinology* 1976;98:451–460.
238. Weick RF. The pulsatile nature of luteinizing hormone secretion. *Can J Physiol Pharmacol* 1981;59:779–785.
239. Wise PM, Rance N, Barr GD, Barraclough CA. Further evidence that luteinizing hormone-releasing hormone also is follicle-stimulating hormone-releasing hormone. *Endocrinology* 1979; 104:940–947.
240. Carmel PW, Araki S, Ferin M. Pituitary stalk portal blood collection in rhesus monkeys: evidence for pulsatile release of gonadotropin-releasing hormone. *Endocrinology* 1976;99:243–248.
241. Nett TM, Akbar AM, Niswender GD. Serum levels of luteinizing hormone and gonadotropin-releasing hormone in cycling, castrated and anestrous ewes. *Endocrinology* 1974;94:713–718.
242. Savoy-Moore RT, Schwartz NB. Differential control of FSH and LH secretion. In Greep RO, ed. *Reproductive physiology III, International review of physiology,* Vol. 22. Baltimore: University Park Press, 1980;203–248.
243. Wildt L, Häusler A, Marshall G, et al. Frequency and amplitude of gonadotropin-releasing hormone stimulation and gonadotropin secretion in the rhesus monkey. *Endocrinology* 1981; 109:376–385.
244. Dufy B, Dufy-Barbe L, Vincent JD, Knobil E. Étude électrophysiologique des neurones hypothalamiques et régulation gonadotrope chez de singe rhesus. *J Physiol (Paris)* 1979;75:105–108.
245. Kalra SP. Neural circuitry involved in the control of LHRH secretion: a model for preovulatory LH release. In: Ganong WF, Martini L, eds. *Frontiers in neuroendocrinology.* New York: Raven Press, 1986;203–246.
246. Gallo RV. Pulsatile LH release during the ovulatory LH surge on proestrus in the rat. *Biol Reprod* 1981;24:100–104.
247. Cogen PH, Antunes JL, Louis KM, Dyrenfurth I, Ferin M. The effects of anterior hypothalamic disconnection on gonadotropin secretion in the female rhesus monkey. *Endocrinology* 1980; 107:677–683.
248. Knobil E, Plant TM, Wildt L, Belchetz PE, Marshall G. Control of the rhesus monkey menstrual cycle: permissive role of hypothalamic gonadotropin-releasing hormone. *Science* 1980; 207:1371–1373.
249. Neill JD, Patton JM, Dailey RA, Tsou RC, Tindall GT. Luteinizing hormone releasing hormone (LHRH) in pituitary stalk blood of rhesus monkeys: relationship to level of LH release. *Endocrinology* 1977;101:430–434.
250. Norman RL, Gliessman P, Lindstrom SA, Hill J, Spies HG. Reinitiation of ovulatory cycles in pituitary stalk-sectioned rhesus monkeys: evidence for a specific hypothalamic message for the preovulatory release of luteinizing hormone. *Endocrinology* 1982;111:1874–1882.
251. Terasawa E, Rodriguez JS, Bridson WE, Wiegand SJ. Factors influencing the positive feedback action of estrogen upon the luteinizing hormone surge in the ovariectomized guinea pig. *Endocrinology* 1979;104:680–686.
252. Terasawa E, King MK, Wiegand SJ, Bridson WE, Goy RW. Barbiturate anesthesia blocks the positive feedback effect of progesterone, but not of estrogen, on luteinizing hormone release in ovariectomized guinea pigs. *Endocrinology* 1979;104:687–692.
253. Caligaris L, Astrada JJ, Taleisnik S. Release of luteinizing hormone induced by estrogen injection into ovariectomized rats. *Endocrinology* 1971;88:810–815.
254. Legan SJ, Coon GA, Karsch FJ. Role of estrogen as initiator of daily LH surges in the ovariectomized rat. *Endocrinology* 1975;96:50–56.
255. Wise PM, Camp-Grossman P, Barraclough CA. Effects of estradiol and progesterone on plasma gonadotropins, prolactin, and LHRH in specific brain areas of ovariectomized rats. *Biol Reprod* 1981;24:820–830.
256. Banks JA, Freeman ME. The temporal requirement of progester-

one on proestrus for extinction of the estrogen-induced daily signal controlling luteinizing hormone release in the rat. *Endocrinology* 1978;102:426–432.
257. DePaolo LV, Barraclough CA. Dose-dependent effects of progesterone on the facilitation and inhibition of spontaneous gonadotropin surges in estrogen treated ovariectomized rats. *Biol Reprod* 1979;21:1015–1023.
258. Norman RL, Blake CA, Sawyer CH. Estrogen-dependent twenty-four-hour periodicity in pituitary LH release in the female hamster. *Endocrinology* 1973;93:965–970.
259. Norman RL, Spies HG. Neural control of the estrogen-dependent twenty-four-hour periodicity of LH release in the golden hamster. *Endocrinology* 1974;95:1367–1372.
260. Stetson MH, Watson-Whitmyre M, Matt KS. Cyclic gonadotropin release in the presence and absence of estrogenic feedback in ovariectomized golden hamsters. *Biol Reprod* 1978;19:40–50.
261. Seegal RF, Goldman BD. Effects of photoperiod on cyclicity and serum gonadotropins in the Syrian hamster. *Biol Reprod* 1975;12:223–231.
262. Bridges RD, Goldman BD. Diurnal rhythms in gonadotropins and progesterone in lactating and photoperiod induced acyclic hamsters. *Biol Reprod* 1975;13:617–622.
263. Schwartz NB. Role of ovarian inhibin (folliculostatin) in regulating FSH secretion in the female rat. In: Channing CP, Segal SJ, eds. *Intraovarian control mechanisms.* New York: Plenum Press, 1982;15–36.
264. Thomas CL Jr, Nikitovitch-Winer MB. Complete suppression of plasma follicle-stimulating hormone in castrated male and female rats during continuous administration of porcine follicular fluid. *Biol Reprod* 1984;30:427–433.
265. Miller WL, Huang ESR. Secretion of ovine luteinizing hormone *in vitro:* differential positive control by 17β-estradiol and a preparation of porcine ovarian inhibin. *Endocrinology* 1985; 117:907–911.

The Physiology of Reproduction, Second Edition,
edited by E. Knobil and J.D. Neill,
Raven Press, Ltd., New York © 1994.

CHAPTER 26

The Anatomy of the Hypothalamo-Hypophysial Complex

Robert B. Page

INTRODUCTION

Consider the pituitary gland as did Harvey Cushing almost 80 years ago (1). The pituitary gland that Cushing (1) saw differed from that seen by others. It was described by a dictionary of the time as "a small bilobed body of unknown function attached to the infundibulum at the base of the brain" (2). Common wisdom of the day held it to be a vestigial organ. He saw a structure composed of neural and epithelial elements lying in the sella turcica in the base of the skull. He realized that the epithelial component developed from an oral pouch that was derived from the ectoderm of the primitive mouth and not from the endoderm of the primitive foregut, as initially proposed by Rathke (3). He further realized that the epithelial portion, the anterior lobe, was organized in a glandular pattern (4,5) and that its cells could be differentiated into chromophobes and chromophiles on the basis of their staining affinity for hematoxylin and eosin dyes (1). He observed that the anterior lobe of the gland was very vascular and that its glandular cells assumed an intimate relationship with its sinusoids. His understanding of the blood supply to the pituitary was based on the studies of Dandy and Goetsh (6), who had described an arterial supply to the canine anterior lobe that arose from the vessels of the circle of Willis and coursed centripetally over the tuber cinereum to supply it at its junction with the anterior lobe. These authors (6) described the venous drainage of the anterior lobe to be directed toward the base of the brain. Based on the writings of Claude Bernard (1853) and of Brown-Sequard (1856), who had proposed that one cell could secrete "on its own account certain products or special ferments which influence all other cells of the body by a mechanism other than the central nervous system," and on his experience with patients suffering from acromegaly (7), Cushing (1) came to believe that the anterior lobe of the pituitary body was a gland of internal secretion and that a tumor of this apparently insignificant organ might cause profound changes in body habitus and metabolism because it released its secretions into the bloodstream in excessive amounts.

Cushing recognized that acromegaly was not the uniform result of any tumor of the anterior lobe of the pituitary. Some patients with pituitary tumors developed adiposal-genital dystrophy and died (8). To test the hypothesis that this syndrome might be due to destruction

Department of Surgery, Pennsylvania State College of Medicine, Hershey, Pennsylvania 17033 of the gland with a consequent reduction or cessation of its secretions, he began a series of ablative experiments on dogs in the newly established Hunterian Laboratory at the Johns Hopkins Hospital (9). He was able to demonstrate that the anterior lobe was necessary to support the structure and function of the gonads, adrenals, and thyroid, to support the normal growth of the young animal, and to support even life itself. The injection or ingestion of pituitary extracts did not reverse the effect of hypophysectomy. His attempt to reverse the deficits produced by hypophysectomy by transplanting the pituitary gland (to the rectus sheath, to bone marrow, or to brain) met with only limited success (10). He was able to establish that, in cases of partial ablation of the gland, the transplant seemed to support the dog (which otherwise would have died) until the remaining fragments could recover and hypertrophy. Although it was not until some 20 years later that P. E. Smith (11) was able to reverse all the deficits caused by hypophysectomy in rats by the injection of pituitary extract, Cushing (1) in 1912 clearly saw the anterior lobe of the pituitary as a ductless gland that synthesized hormones and secreted them into the bloodstream, which carried them toward the brain. These secretions of the anterior lobe of the pituitary gland supported the function of the other ductless glands and permitted normal body growth.

In 1912, Cushing (1) realized that most of the posterior lobe (the neural portion of the pituitary gland) was derived from the brain (3), but he included the pars intermedia with the neural lobe under the rubric of the "posterior lobe." In his morphological studies he saw "colloid" in the posterior lobe as had Herring (4) when he examined the posterior lobe histologically (1) (Fig. 1). He proposed, on the basis of the analogy with the thyroid, that colloid, now called *Herring bodies,* was a secretion of the posterior lobe; but he believed it was a secretion of the pars intermedia, not of the pars nervosa. The pars nervosa (along with the cervical sympathetics) served to innervate the pars intermedia (1,12). His visualization of colloid on microscopic examination within the pars intermedia, the neural lobe, beneath the ependyma of the diencephalic floor, and apparently bursting into the third ventricle on microscopic examination convinced him that the posterior lobe secreted directly to the brain (13). The paucity of blood vessels in the posterior lobe (6) reinforced his belief that the secretions of the neural lobe entered the third ventricle, not the circulation.

To determine the function of the posterior lobe, he performed hypophysectomies, selective ablation of the anterior or posterior lobes, or selective stimulations of these regions of the pituitary gland in dogs. On the basis of these experiments, Cushing proposed that the posterior lobe secretions caused a fall in glucose tolerance (glucosuria), whereas their absence resulted in a rise in glucose tolerance (14). This surmise was strengthened by

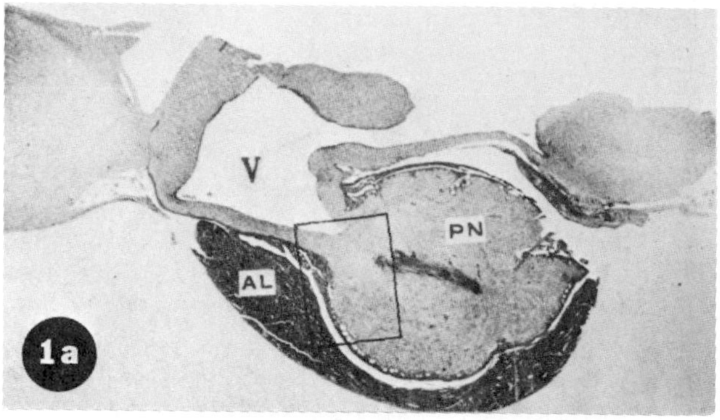

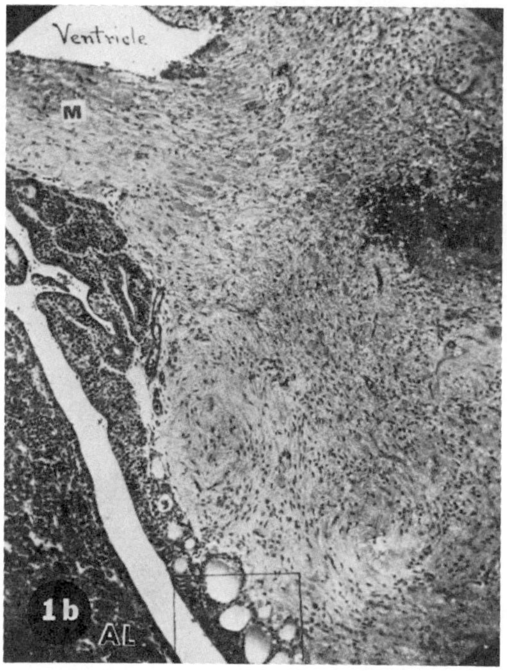

FIG. 1. A: Midsagittal section of canine pituitary gland. Note layer of colloid globules arising from the epithelial investment of the par nervosa (*PN*). Anterior lobe (*AL*) is separated from posterior lobe by cleft. *V,* third ventricle. **B:** Enlargement of squared-off area in Fig. **A.** Anterior lobe (*AL*) is separated by cleft from investment of pars nervosa containing colloid masses. (From ref. 1, with permission.)

his finding that stimulation of the pars nervosa or of the superior cervical ganglion, both of which structures he envisioned as innervating the intermediate lobe (1,12), caused glucosuria (15). He was aware that a vasopressor effect of posterior lobe extract had been reported (16,17) as had an oxytotic effect (18). He accepted these observations as true but thought these roles were subordinate to the role of the posterior lobe in glucose metabolism. He did not accept the proposal that the posterior lobe secreted an antidiuretic substance. As late as 1930 he stated "too much attention has been paid to the symptoms of thirst and polyuria, and too little to the symptoms of the opposite of these, oliguria having been observed not infrequently as a sequel of our early (1908–1910) canine hypophysectomies" (2). In 1912,

Cushing (1) saw the posterior lobe as a gland (the pars intermedia) that was innervated principally by the pars nervosa. Hormones synthesized in the pars intermedia were carried through the pars nervosa to the third ventricle and functioned to regulate glucose metabolism, vascular tone, and uterine contractions.

In the intervening years from 1912 to 1930, when he delivered the Lister Memorial Lecture (2), Cushing clung to these two tenets: that the anterior lobe released its secretions into blood vessels draining toward the brain and that the posterior lobe released its secretions into the third ventricle. The discovery of a portal system in the pituitary gland by Popa and Fielding (19,20) did not alter his convictions, which were based on his concept that the anterior and posterior lobes each received an independent blood supply and the posterior lobe drained to the cavernous sinus (6). A portal system supplied a route to Cushing by which anterior pituitary secretions could be delivered to the brain prior to being delivered to the remainder of the body (21). He continued to believe that the posterior lobe was a special brain gland whose secretory cells in the pars intermedia were innervated by the pars nervosa and that it released its secretions into the brain's ventricular system (22).

In those intervening years he had become aware that in some unknown fashion the hypothalamus and the pituitary gland are inextricably joined. The accepted belief at the time was that the secretions of the posterior lobe were synthesized there in glial cells of the pars nervosa (23,24), in epithelial cells of the pars intermedia (22), or in glandular cells in the neural lobe (25) (for review, see ref. 26). As early as 1912, Cushing had been aware of the report of Cajal (1894) describing a neural tract that originated in the hypothalamus and ended in the neural lobe. He cited reports of Greving (1926) and of Pines (1928) describing a fiber tract passing from the supraoptic nuclei (SON) and paraventricular nuclei (PVN) to the neural lobe, but he persisted in thinking this tract innervated the pars intermedia (2). The true function of the supraoptico-hypophysial tract remained unsuspected (27,28). He acknowledged that diabetes insipidus could be caused by making tuberal lesions in rats that interrupted the supraoptico-hypophysial tract and could be cured by giving the rats posterior lobe extract; but he did not accept the significance of this observation. Although he misunderstood the means by which the hypothalamus regulated posterior lobe function, he realized that "it is highly improbable that two corresponding effects should be produced, the one by a hypothalamic lesion, the other by removing the source of chemical messages, in the absence of any functional interaction" (2).

Cushing also noted that the brain apparently controlled certain aspects of anterior lobe function—such as ovulation in the rabbit because it regularly follows 10 hours after copulation in that species and hence resembles a reflex act. He became further aware of the role of the diencephalon in regulating sympathetic tone, alertness, body temperature, body habitus, and sexual function from caring for patients with tumors that invaded the third ventricle and hypothalamus such as gliomas of the optic chiasm and craniopharyngiomas but that spared the pituitary gland. Their occurrence brought home to Cushing the realization that there is an "interdependence of the diencephalon and the pituitary body." He explained this interdependence in the following manner. Nerves in the diencephalon projecting to the pituitary gland through the supraoptico-hypophysial tract stimulate the release of substances from the pars intermedia in the posterior lobe, which are transported directly into the third ventricle from which site they influence neural centers in its walls. Discharge from these diencephalic centers activates sympathetic mechanisms that result in the stimulation of the glandular cells in the anterior lobe by way of the cervical sympathetic plexus. In his picture the peripheral sympathetic nervous system was the final common pathway to the epithelial cells of the anterior lobe of the pituitary and to the epithelial cells of the adrenal medulla, as well as to the smooth muscle cells of the intestines and the blood vessels (2). His belief that the diencephalon coordinated the functions of the anterior pituitary gland and the sympathetic nervous system passed into the background as forces marshalled that would undo many of his concepts and change the way investigators see the pituitary gland.

To see the gland as most see it today, it is necessary to start with a consideration of the work of Wislocki and King (29). Published 6 years after Cushing's last public lecture on the pituitary gland, their work challenged several of his basic concepts. They stressed the observation that the pituitary gland and viscera stained after the intravascular injection of acid vital dyes into monkeys, cats, and rabbits, whereas the brain (with the exception of the choroid plexus and several small regions surrounding the third ventricle and the area postrema of the fourth ventricle) did not. The contents of the third ventricle were not stained following the intravascular injection with acid dyes even when the neural lobe was heavily stained. They thus demonstrated that substances could enter, and presumably leave, the neural portion of the hypophysis by vascular routes but that it was unlikely that substances in the neurohypophysis were discharged into the third ventricle. Wislocki and King (29) also studied the vascular anatomy of the pituitary. They made intravascular injections of monkeys, rabbits, and rats with India ink and examined either serial sections of the injected gland or whole mounts after clearing the tissue. They concluded that they could not corroborate the observations of Popa and Fielding (19,20) that a large artery arising from each supraclinoid carotid artery supplies the pars distalis and that large venuoles connect the pars distalis to the hypothalamus. Their report erased a picture of the pituitary gland that had been held for almost 30 years. Neither the neural or the glandular portion of the pituitary could discharge its contents directly to the brain. A new concept had to be erected.

Wislocki and King (29) provided the basis for it. First, they noted that the eminentia saccularis (the median eminence of the tuber cinereum or the infundibulum) was stained, as were the anterior and posterior lobes, after the intravascular injection of acid dyes, whereas the tuber cinereum was not. They proposed that the median eminence should, as a consequence of this similarity with the pituitary gland, be classified as part of it. In this schema, based on the observation that the hypophysis lacks a blood-brain barrier, the neurohypophysis is composed of the infundibulum (median eminence, eminentia saccularis), infundibular stem, and infundibular process (neural lobe). The adenohypophysis is composed of the pars tuberalis (applied to the infundibulum and infundibular stem), the pars intermedia (applied to the infundibular stem and infundibular process), and the pars distalis (anterior lobe) (29,30). This classification recognizes that the pituitary gland lies not only within the sella turcica (the lower infundibular stem and infundibular process with the pars intermedia and the pars distalis) but also in the subarachnoid space and applied to the base of the brain (the median eminence and upper infundibular stem with the pars tuberalis). Wislocki and King (29) observed, after the intravascular injection of vital dyes, that the boundary of the stained pituitary gland with the unstained hypothalamus lay at the level of the tuberoinfundibular sulcus. This sulcus, which separates the tuber cinereum of the hypothalamus from the infundibulum, not the diaphragm sella, forms the rostral boundary of the pituitary gland (Fig. 2).

Second, they correctly surmised the direction of blood flow in the portal system and suggested its role in control of anterior pituitary function. They described superior hypophysial arteries in the monkey that arose from the supraclinoid internal carotid arteries and the vessels of the circle of Willis. These vessels approached the eminentia saccularis (median eminence) and pituitary stalk (pars tuberalis and infundibular stem) and the rostral pole of the pars distalis. The superior hypophysial arteries bifurcated, sending one branch to the pars distalis and one branch to the infundibular stem and median eminence. The capillary bed in the median eminence and upper part of the infundibular stem was fed by the superior hypophysial arteries. It was drained by portal vessels that discharged their contents into a secondary capillary bed in the pars distalis. The pars distalis in turn drained by lateral hypophysial veins into the adjacent cavernous sinuses. The pars distalis, according to the account of Wislocki and King (29), resembled the liver, receiving both an arterial and a venous blood supply. They surmised that the direction of blood flow through the portal vessels had to be from the median eminence to the pars

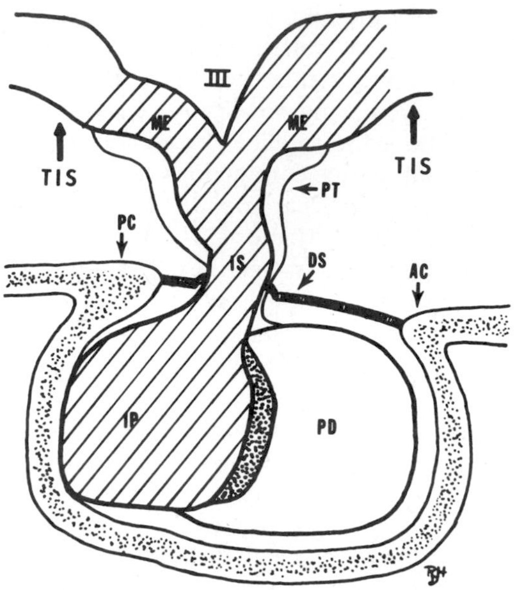

FIG. 2. Midsagittal section of the human pituitary gland. The neurohypophysis (*hatching*) consists of the median eminence (*ME*) (or infundibulum), infundibular stem (*IS*), and infundibular process (*IP*) (neural lobe). The adenohypophysis consists of the pars tuberalis (*PT*), which is applied to the ME and IS and lies in the subarachnoid space above the diaphragm sella (*DS*) and the pars distalis (*PD*), which lies within the sella turcica beneath the DS. The region corresponding to the pars intermedia of other forms is indicated by the *stippled area* between the PD and the IP. *AC*, anterior clinoid; *PC*, posterior clinoid; *III*, third ventricle; *TIS*, tuberoinfundibular sulcus. (From ref. 1066, with permission.)

distalis, as they could demonstrate no significant outflow routes from the median eminence to the vessels at the base of the brain. The only apparent outflow was from the median eminence to the pars distalis, which could in turn drain to the adjacent cavernous sinuses through lateral hypophysial veins (Fig. 3).

Third, they saw the circulation of the neural lobe as isolated from that of the portal system. They described the origin and course of the inferior hypophysial arteries from the intracavernous segment of the carotid arteries to the infundibular process and the paired venous structures (inferior hypophysial veins) that drained it. The function of the neural lobe had been clarified by 1936. In 1924, Starling and Verney (31) had reported that posterior lobe extract corrected diabetes insipidus, reduced urinary flow, and raised urinary solute concentration. The posterior (neural) lobe was also recognized to regulate urine flow and blood pressure (16) and to stimulate uterine contractions (18). Its structure was also clear. The neural lobe contained axons and terminals of the supraoptico-hypophysial tract, specialized glial cells called *pituicytes,* and blood vessels (27,28). With the demonstration by Ingram and his co-workers (32–34) that lesions of the supraoptico-hypophysial tract caused diabetes insipidus, atrophy of the neural lobe, and de-

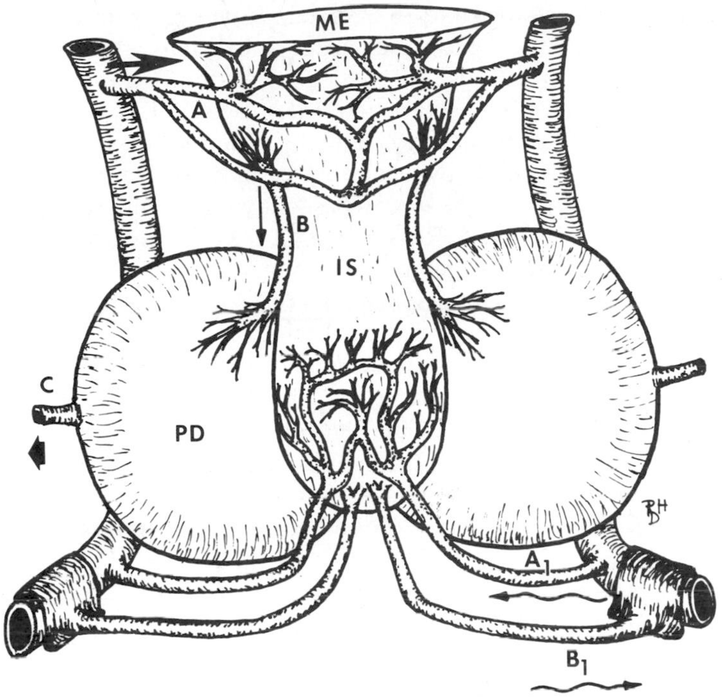

FIG. 3. Classic schema of pituitary blood flow proposed by Wislocki and King (29). Blood enters the median eminence (*ME*) at point A through superior hypophysial arteries (*large arrow*). It passes through the ME primary capillary plexus in the pars distalis (*PD*). From the PD, blood drains through lateral hypophysial veins (*C*) to the cavernous sinus (*arrowhead*). Blood enters the neural lobe through inferior hypophysial arteries (A_1). It drains from the neural lobe through inferior hypophysial veins (B_1). *IS*, infundibular stem. (From ref. 626, with permission.)

generation of cell bodies in the supraoptic nucleus, it became apparent that the supraoptico-hypophysial tract regulated in some unknown manner the release of hormones from the neural lobe.

Ernest and Berte Scharrer provided the answer to this puzzle explaining how the brain regulates not only neural lobe function (35,36) but by extension of their ideas how the brain also regulates adenohypophysial function. The concept of neurosecretion, first promulgated by E. Scharrer, received support from the observations of Palay (37), who found the presence of a colloid material, stainable with silver or Masson's trichrome technique, that was unique to the preoptico-hypophysial tract of the goldfish (a tract analogous to the supraoptico-hypophysial tract of mammals). Bargmann and Hild (38) found that the chrome-alumhematoxylin technique of Gomori selectively stained neurosecretory (colloid) material within the supraoptico-hypophysial tract, as it selectively stained secretory material in the islet cells of the pancreas. On the basis of the finding of stainable neurosecretory material in the cell bodies of large cells in the supraoptic nucleus and of finding this material in the axons of these cells and in their terminals in the neural lobe, Bargmann and Scharrer (39) proposed that hormones released from the posterior lobe of the pituitary were not synthesized there. They were synthesized in the supraoptic nucleus of the hypothalamus, transported down their axons to their terminals in the posterior lobe, and released from these terminals into the bloodstream. Cushing had seen stainable (colloid) material in the neural lobe and proposed on the basis of analogy with the thyroid that it was a secretion of the pars intermedia in the posterior lobe. Because he saw few vessels in the posterior lobe and because he saw colloid bursting into the third ventricle, he came to believe that the neural lobe secreted to the brain. Scharrer saw the same material within nerves lying in the hypothalamus and in their terminals in the neural lobe. Based on the analogy with the neurosecretory system of insects and the knowledge that the neural lobe lacked a blood-brain barrier but possessed direct venous connections to the cavernous sinuses, he proposed the (correct) mechanism by which the brain controls pituitary function. He saw that secretions of the neural lobe were made in the hypothalamus, transported to the neural lobe, and were released into the circulation. Each looked at the pituitary and saw a different organ.

Scharrer (40–42) broadened the scope of his histological observations, but it was the biochemical and physiological investigations of others that confirmed his seminal concept. The neural lobe hormone responsible for uterine contraction and for milk injection was identified as oxytocin (43,44). The neural lobe hormone responsible for antidiuresis was identified as vasopressin (45–47). They were found not only in the neural lobe of the pituitary but also in the hypothalamic supraoptic (and paraventricular) nuclei (48). Subsequent anatomical and physiological studies have demonstrated that oxytocin and vasopressin are synthesized in separate neuronal cell bodies lying in the supraoptic and paraventricular nuclei, are transported down the axons of the supraoptico-hypophysial tract to their axon terminals in the neural lobe, and are released into the systemic circulation in response to appropriate stimulation (49–64).

Harris (65) pursued the observation that in the rabbit ovulation reflexly follows copulation. He induced ovulation by stimulation of the hypothalamus but not the pituitary. The mechanism could not be a direct neural innervation of glandular cells, as the pars distalis lacked nerves other than those terminating on vessels (66). In 1947, Green and Harris (67) proposed that there was a neurovascular link between axons terminating in the median eminence and glandular cells in the pars distalis. This link was provided by the portal vessels on the anterior surface of the pituitary stalk. Green and Harris supported their proposal with the following observations: (a) Nerves terminating in the median eminence and upper infundibular stem are in close contact with capillaries that drain into portal vessels (67,68), (b) blood flowed through portal vessels of living animals (frog and rats) from the median eminence to the pars distalis (69,70), (c) stimulation of the hypothalamus caused ovulation in the anesthetized (65) and unanesthetized rabbit (71), (d) stalk section disrupted trophic function of gland and disrupted estrous cycles but trophic function and estrous cycles returned if portal vessels were permitted to regenerate (72–74), and (e) functional grafting of the excised pituitary gland only occurred if the excised portion was replaced beneath the median eminence and the portal vessels were permitted to regenerate (75,76). In monographs published in 1948 and 1955, Harris (21,77) summarized the extant evidence that the anterior pituitary is regulated by the brain.

The findings of Green and Harris gained more significance when it was appreciated that a portal vascular system characteristically links the median eminence with the pars distalis in vertebrates (66,78–80), including humans (81–83). Although Harris (84) reported that there was an independent arterial supply to the pars distalis of the rabbit (in addition to the portal [venous] supply), Green (66) could not identify a separate arterial supply to the pars distalis in 76 other species. Reexamination of the vascular supply of the rabbit pituitary employing scanning electron microscopy of vascular casts (85) failed to confirm Harris's findings. Contrary to Wislocki's belief (29,86–89), the pars distalis does not appear to have a dual blood supply as does the liver. It appears to be bathed entirely by blood that has passed through the neurohypophysis.

Stalk section experiments strengthened the case for a neurovascular link and further weakened the case for a separate arterial supply to the pars distalis. Such sections divided the supraoptico-hypophysial tract, which linked cells of the supraoptic nucleus with their terminals in the neural lobe, and the portal vessels, which linked terminals in the median eminence with glandular cells in the pars distalis. Stalk section transiently disrupts neural lobe function until regeneration of divided axons, or establishment of new neurohemal contacts, can occur (90–94). With interruption of the portal vessels, the pars distalis atrophies, but the degree of atrophy depends on the species studied and on the extent to which channels from the neural lobe to the adjacent pars distalis are available (95–99). Estrous cycles are abolished (73), and trophic anterior pituitary function is destroyed (74,75,93).

Halasz sought to evaluate the neural influences on pituitary function by separating the pituitary gland with its attachment to the medial basilar hypothalamus from the rest of the brain. Reasoning that the only portion of the brain that could support a pituitary transplant lay in the region of the tuber cinereum (76,100,101), he and Pupp set out to study this hypophysiotropic area (102). They were able to isolate this region, which included the infundibulum and entire pituitary gland as well as the arcuate nuclei, a portion of the ventromedial nucleus, the periventricular nuclei, the ventral premammillary, the median mammillary nuclei, and the retrochiasmatic area from the remainder of the brain. All neural input into the hypophysiotropic area was interrupted. However, neural output to the median eminence from the arcuate nucleus (the tuberoinfundibular tract) (103) was spared (102). Isolation of the hypophysiotropic area and the pituitary gland from the brain produced (in the rat) a different picture than did isolation of the pars distalis from the median eminence by stalk section. Trophic pituitary function was not seriously disturbed (102). Basal thyroid function, adrenal output of corticosteroids, and testicular sperm production were maintained. The histological picture of the thyroid, adrenals, and testis was not markedly altered, and compensatory hypertrophy of the remaining adrenal gland occurred after unilateral adrenalectomy (104–108). Modulating neural influences on pituitary function were disrupted, however, as the estrous cycle was abolished and an increased secretion of adrenal corticosteroids in response to stress did not occur (see ref. 107, for summary). These observations focused attention on the hypophysiotropic area, now defined as comprising the periventricular nuclear groups in the hypothalamus, and particularly upon the median eminence, as the focal point of converging neural systems for the humoral relay of information from the brain to the anterior pituitary gland.

The median eminence was found to contain substances that were capable of stimulating or inhibiting the release of anterior pituitary hormones (109,110). Saffran and Schally (111) and Guillemin and Rosenberg (112) incubated pituitary tissue with hypothalamic tissue *in vitro* and were able to demonstrate support of adrenocorticotropin (ACTH) production using bioassay techniques. Further studies employing such *in vitro* assays revealed hypothalamic factors capable of stimulating ACTH (113,114), thyroid-stimulating hormone (TSH) (115), growth hormone (GH) (116), and luteinizing hormone (LH) (117) release from incubated pituitary glands. Prolactin (PRL) production from anterior pituitary cells was inhibited by incubation with hypothalamic tissue (118–121). Anterior pituitary hormone release of ACTH (122,123), TSH (124), GH (125), follicle-stimulating hormone (FSH) (126,127), and LH (128,129) *in vivo* could also be stimulated by injection of hypothalamic extracts.

Porter et al. (130,131) developed a technique for perfusion of and sampling from the long portal vessels on the anterior surface of the rat's pituitary stalk. Perfusion of the long portal vessels with hypothalamic extract stimulated FSH and LH release from the anterior pituitary (132,133). Thyroid-stimulating hormone release was also stimulated by infusion of hypothalamic extracts into portal vessels (134). Gonadotropin-releasing activity (135) has been found in portal blood collected from the severed pituitary stalk; and GH-releasing activity, TSH-releasing activity (136), and gonadotropin-releasing activity (133) have been found in blood sampled by cannulation of portal vessels.

The chemical composition of thyrotropin-releasing hormone (TRH) was the first of the hypothalamic-releasing hormones to be discovered (137–139). Thyroid-stimulating hormone was released from the anterior pituitary following the infusion of thyrotropin-releasing hormone (TRH) into a portal vessel on the surface of the rat pituitary stalk (140). Subsequently the structures of gonadotropic-releasing hormone (GnRH) (141–143), corticotropin-releasing factor (CRF) (144, 145), somatostatin (SRIF) (146), and growth hormone-releasing hormone (GRH) (147–150) have been elucidated. There is an increasing body of evidence supporting the role of dopamine as a PRL-inhibiting factor (151–158). The chemical characterization of hypothalamic hypophysiotropic hormones has permitted their localization within hypothalamic neurons by immunohistochemical techniques (159,160). The pattern revealed by their localization is one of convergence of axons containing peptide hormones (peptidergic neurons) upon the median eminence from diverse medial preoptic (MPOA) and hypothalamic periventricular loci (161,162).

Immunohistochemistry, when combined with transmission electron microscopy, permitted the subcellular localization of hypothalamic hormones (163,164). Gonadotropic-releasing hormone–containing cells were believed by early investigators to originate in the hypothalamus and terminate in the median eminence of the rat. In the median eminence, GnRH was localized in granular vesicles in axon terminals (165) that lay in the perivascular space of median eminence capillaries. In cell bodies in the hypothalamus, GnRH was identified in granular vesicles associated with the Golgi apparatus. On the basis of morphological evidence, it was proposed that GnRH is synthesized on polysomes in the cell body, packaged into dense-cored vesicles in the Golgi apparatus, and transported with vesicles down the axon by axoplasmic flow to be stored within axon terminals and released upon appropriate stimulation (163,164,166,167). The process of the synthesis of a hypothalamic-releasing (or -inhibiting) hormone in cell bodies lying in diverse hypothalamic nuclei and their delivery to and their release from neural terminals in the median eminence was generally held to be analogous to the synthesis of vasopressin or oxytocin in cell bodies lying in the supraoptic nuclei and their delivery to and release from axon terminals in the neural lobe.

Cushing (1) saw an organ composed of a neural and an epithelial portion lying in the sella turcica. His pars anterior released its secretions under regulation of the peripheral sympathetic system into veins that carried them to the brain and then to distant glands that they supported. His posterior lobe released its secretions, which were synthesized in the pars intermedia, under the regulation of the supraoptico-hypophysial tract. They were carried through the neural lobe to the third ventricle, which they entered to influence periventricular hypothalamic centers. These in turn regulated the sympathetic system, which controlled the tone of smooth muscle in the intestines and arteries, regulated adrenal medullary function, and controlled the function of the anterior lobe of the pituitary. Some 80 years later we see a different organ—one that has a neural and an epithelial region. The rostral end of the neural region lies on the base of the brain and is the site where secretions manufactured outside the pituitary and behind the blood-brain barrier in the hypothalamus are released from nerve terminals and are carried by restricted portal routes to the epithelial portion of the pituitary gland (pars distalis within the sella turcica) to regulate its function. The caudal region of the neural portion lies within the sella turcica and is the site where secretions (synthesized in the hypothalamus) are released from terminals of the supraoptico-hypophysial tract and are carried by systemic routes to regulate the function of the kidneys, breast, and uterus. The means by which the brain controls pituitary function are now well understood.

In the past 10 years, Cushing's concept that the pituitary gland and the autonomic nervous system were inextricably linked through the diencephalon has received considerable attention. Not only do the periventricular nuclear groups of the hypothalamus and the MPOA house cells that project to the median eminence to regulate pituitary function, they also house neurons that project to the intermediolateral cell column of the spinal cord and to brainstem visceral efferent nuclei to regulate autonomic function (168). The objective of this chapter is to explore, in further detail, (a) the structures employed by the brain to control pituitary function and (b) the organization employed by the diencephalon to coordinate endocrine and neural responses to changes in the internal milieu and external environment.

THE ADENOHYPOPHYSIS

Epithelial Cells of the Adenohypophysis

Epithelial cells and smooth muscle cells are the motor elements of the neuroendocrine and autonomic nervous

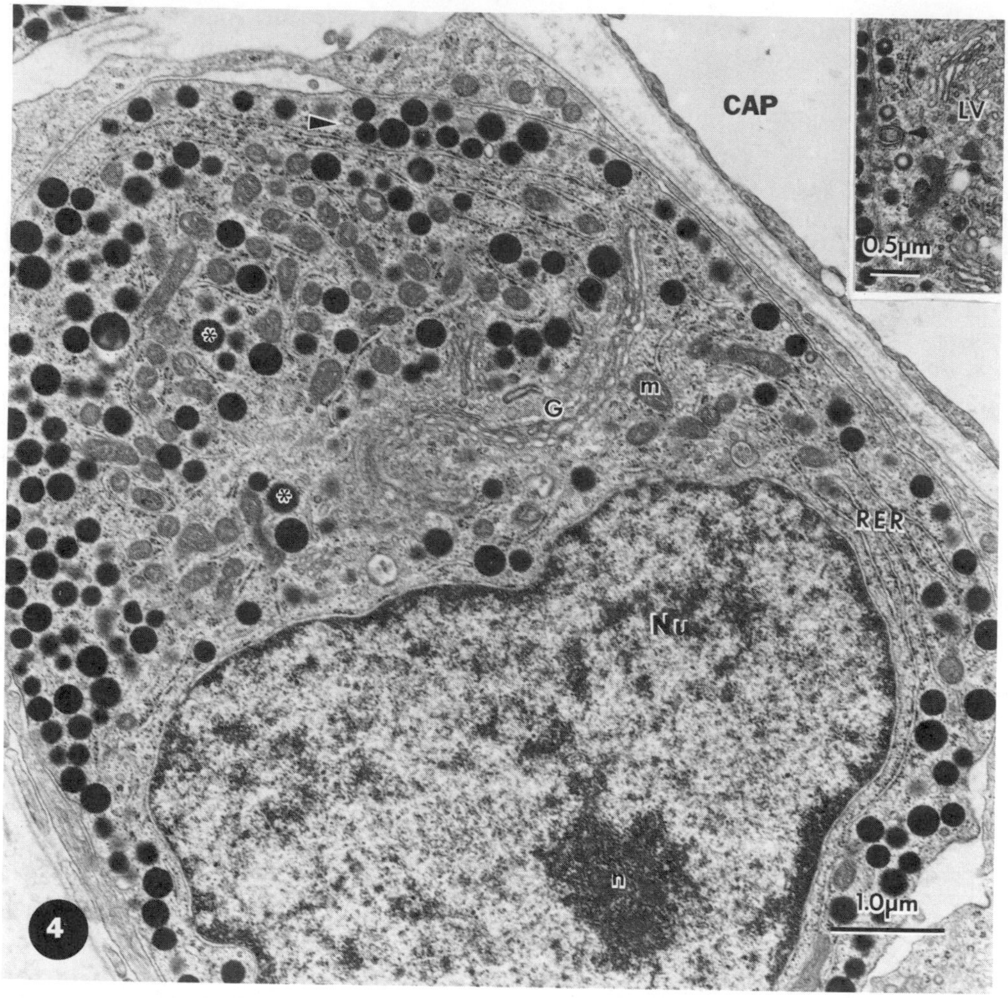

FIG. 4. A: Transmission electron micrograph of a rabbit pars distalis epithelial cells. The large nucleus (*Nu*) contains a single nucleolus (*n*). Nuclear chromatin is homogeneously dispersed except at the nuclear membrane, where it is aggregated. The cytoplasm contains many electron-dense granules (*). Mitochondria (*m*) are abundant. The rough endoplasmic reticulum (*RER*) is plentiful. The Golgi apparatus (*G*) is found close to the nucleus. The cis border faces the nucleus. The trans (concave) border is associated with dense granules of varying size. A coated vesicle is indicated by the *small arrowhead.* Note fenestra in capillary endothelial tube. *CAP,* capillary. **Inset:** Extrusion of granule with formation of omega figure at *arrowhead.* Both dense granules and coated vesicles are present at cell plasmalemma. *LV,* lucent vesicles. **B:** Transmission electron micrograph of a rat pars tuberalis cell. Many mitochondria and glycogen granules are present in the cytoplasm. Secretory granules are designated by *small white arrowheads* and are aggregated at the vascular pole of the cell. Lysosomes are not seen in this pars tuberalis specific cell. A cilium is seen in an adjacent follicular cell (*black arrowhead*).

systems, which arise in the diencephalon. The epithelial cells of the neuroendocrine system are found in the adenohypophysis, the glandular portion of the pituitary body at the base of the brain. These epithelial cells carry out their role as effector elements of the neuroendocrine system by synthesizing peptide hormones and secreting them into nearby capillaries (Fig. 4A). They are round to polygonal in shape and are characterized by the presence of electron-dense granules, lucent vesicles, rough endoplasmic reticulum, and a Golgi apparatus in their cytoplasm. The electron-dense granules are round to ovoid in shape and range from about 100 to 700 nm in diameter, depending on the type of the cell, its age, and its functional state. They are the site of storage of pituitary hormones (169–171).

The Golgi apparatus in these cells is prominent and composed of a half-moon-shaped system of stacked parallel cisternae. The cis face of the Golgi apparatus is the convex surface, which faces the rough endoplasmic reticulum. The trans face is the concave surface, which faces the plasmalemma. Platelike cisternae are closely associated with the trans elements of the Golgi (172) and are analogous to the GERL apparatus described in dorsal root ganglia (173,174). Cytochemical staining tech-

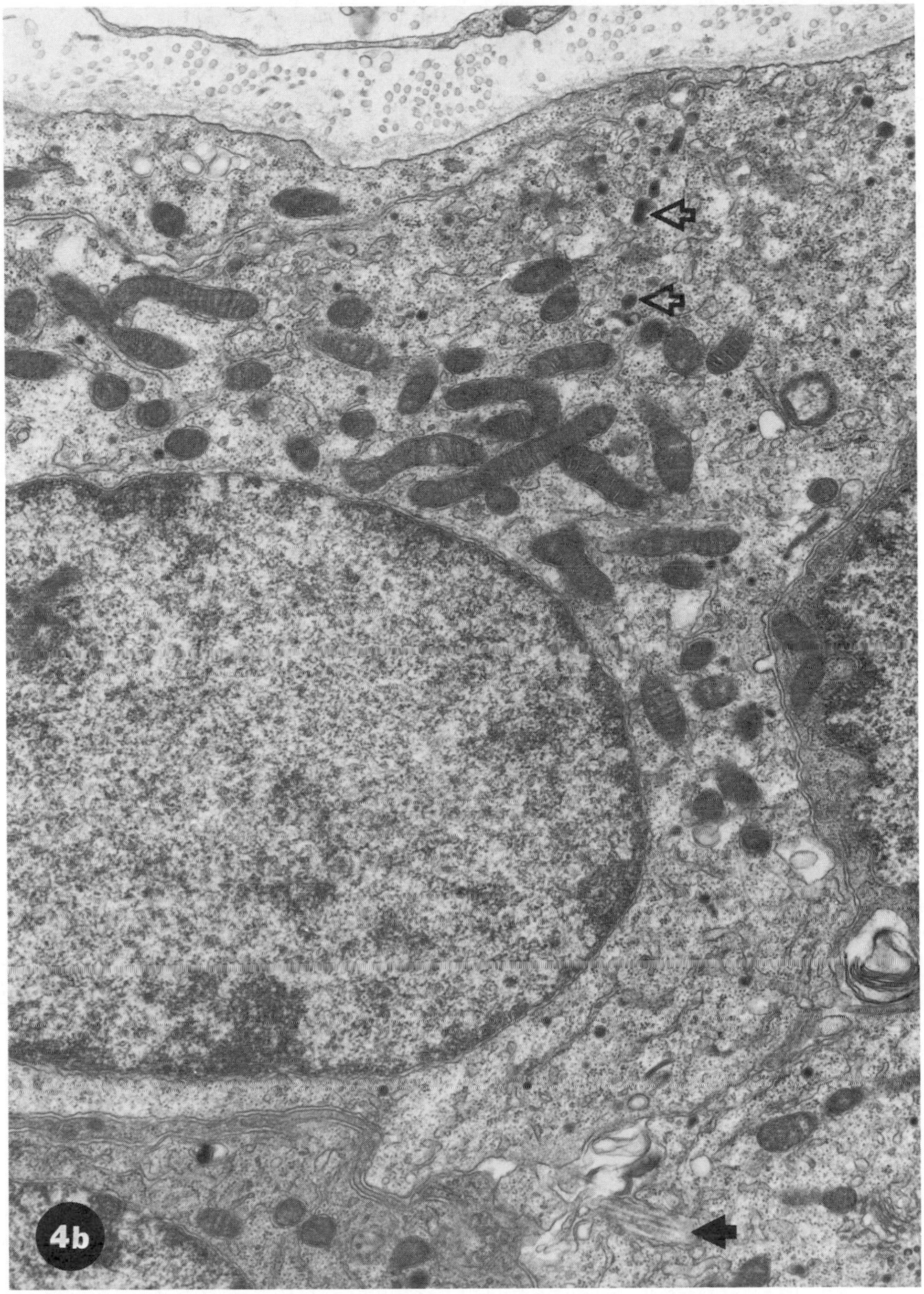

FIG. 4. *Continued.*

niques revealed specific enzymes localized to specific membranes of the Golgi stack (see ref. 175, for review). With fractionation of the Golgi membranes phosphorylation was demonstrated in the cis region, glycosolation in the middle region, and addition of siliac acid or galactoside residue in the trans region (172). These experiments support the earlier cytochemical observations. In the most trans region, often called the *GERL,* acid phosphatase has been demonstrated (174). The existing evidence demonstrates that enzymatic functions in the Golgi apparatus are compartmentalized.

The electron-lucent vesicles in the region of the cis face are about 40 nm in diameter. They lie between the rough endoplasmic reticulum and the Golgi apparatus and are believed to "shuttle" nascent proteins from the former to the latter. Farquhar and Wellings (176) first presented transmission electron microscopic (TEM) evidence that suggested that hormones were packaged into secretory granules within the Golgi apparatus. Electron micrographs revealed small vesicles surrounded by membranes budding from the end of the Golgi lamellae. They progressively enlarged as they became increasingly displaced from the Golgi (176,177).

Pulse labeling experiments employing labeled amino acids revealed a path from rough endoplasmic reticulum via lucent vesicles to the Golgi apparatus and then to secretory granules (178–181). Further biochemical evidence suggested that at least two pituitary hormones (GH and PRL) are assembled on polyribosomes as prohormones with an excess 27 amino acids at the amino terminus. This segment serves as a signal sequence to permit passage of the hormone being assembled from the polysome through the membranous lamellae of the rough endoplasmic reticulum into its channels (182,183). Membrane, pinched off from the channels of the endoplasmic reticulum, is believed to form the lucent vesicles that transport the protein to the Golgi apparatus for packaging into secretory granules (or alternatively to the plasmalemma for discharge under conditions of maximal stimulation). The Golgi apparatus is compartmentally organized, and processing occurs in a cis to trans sequence (172). The proteins pass sequentially through channels in the Golgi from stack to stack by vesicular transport and during that transport undergo a series of modifications. In addition to the packaging of hormone and to their modification by phosphorylation, glycosylation, or sialation (172,184, 185) posttranslational modification of prohormones by enzymatic cleavage of peptide bonds begins (186).

The large electron-dense granules are usually aggregated near the concave trans face, as well as dispersed throughout the cytoplasm. Membrane for the formation of secretory granules is provided by recycling the membrane of secretory granules after exocytosis (187). The site of formation of large secretory granules has been found to be the outermost trans elements of the Golgi (188). Cationic ferritin, endocytosed from the cell's surface by lucent coated vesicles, was carried to the trans face of the Golgi. The marker membrane was observed to fuse with nascent secretory granules budding from the Golgi apparatus, thus providing material for their enlargement. This region is characterized by the presence of plate-like cisternae (173) and stains with acid phosphatase. Novikoff et al. (174) attributed the function of lysosome formation to the GERL region because of the localization of acid phosphatase to it. It now appears that its function is more complex and that it is the site of both secretory granule and lysosome formation.

With stimulation of adenohypophysial cells (such as stimulation of lactotrophs by suckling or stimulation of somatotropes with GRH), the rough endoplasmic reticulum became more pronounced, vesicles increased in number, and the granules discharged their contents by exocytosis (189,190). Transmission electron microscopy examination of ultrathin sections and of freeze-fractured material demonstrated migration of secretory granules to the cell periphery and fusion of the granular and plasma membranes (191). Actin filaments and microtubules have both been implicated in the migration of secretory granules to the periphery of the cell (192). Omega figures (Ω) formed with discharge of hormone into the extracellular space (193). Membrane retrieval was demonstrated with internalization of membrane at the exocytotic site and its migration as coated vesicles to the trans Golgi region (187,188). Exocytotic events have been quantified by electron microscopy after preparation of stimulated somatotropes by freezing techniques before and after stimulation of somatotropes with GRH. The number of exocytotic events paralleled the amount of growth hormone released (194). Although it appears that exocytosis is the primary mechanism for release of peptide hormones from pituitary cells, debate persists as to whether the only pathway employed in the synthesis and release of protein is from rough endoplasmic reticulum to vesicles to Golgi to granules to discharge at the plasma membrane (184) or whether, under conditions of prolonged stimulation, the formation of secretory granules may be short circuited and newly synthesized peptide hormone released from cytoplasmic sites such as the channels of the endoplasmic reticulum (Fig. 5) (195,196).

The release of protein hormones from adenohypophysial cells is in part regulated by the secretions from distant sites that are carried to the glandular pituitary via the systemic circulation. Secretions of the target organs of the pituitary (the adrenal cortex, the gonads, or the thyroid) regulate anterior pituitary function through feedback loops. In addition, catecholamines secreted from the adrenal medulla (197) and cytokines (198–200) released from multiple sites can regulate the function of adenohypophysial cells. The release of hormones is also regulated by peptide secretions of nerves that terminate in the neurohypophysis. These hypothalamic releasing and inhibiting hormones are carried to the adenohypophysial cells through a restricted portal circulation. There is ample evidence that peptide hypothalamic hypophysiotropic releasing hormones cause degranulation of target adenohypophysial cells with consequent hormone release (201–205). Hypothalamic releasing hormones, catecholamines, and cytokines interact with receptors at the cell surface. The transduction of receptor binding at the cell's surface to hormone release at the cell surface is mediated by second messenger systems. G proteins, cyclic AMP, calcium, and phosphatidylinositol have each been implicated as the second messengers mediating exocytosis and are the subjects of more in-depth discussion in later chapters.

Development of the Adenohypophysis

The adenohypophysis arises from the ectodermal tissue of the primitive mouth (3,206,207). The pouch of

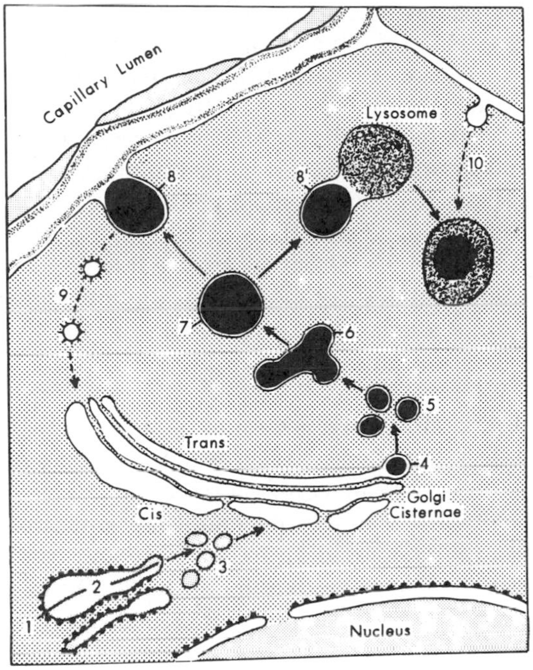

FIG. 5. The intracellular traffic that takes place in connection with the synthesis, packaging, and secretion of prolactin, as documented by work from many laboratories. Protein is synthesized on ribosomes (*1*), segregated into rough endoplasmic reticulum (2), and transported by small vesicles (*3*) to the Golgi complex; then it passes through the Golgi complex and is concentrated into small granules on the trans side of the stack (*4*). Several of these aggregate (*5* and *6*) to form the mature secretory granule (*7*). During active secretion, the latter fuses with the cell membrane by exocytosis (*8*), its content is discharged into the perivascular spaces, and the granule membrane recycles back to the Golgi cisternae (*9*). When secretory activity is suppressed and the cell must dispose of excess stored hormone, some granules fuse with lysosomes (*8'*) and their content is degraded. Besides these routes, an endocytic pathway from the cell surface to lysosomes has been demonstrated. (From ref. 1068, with permission.)

Rathke, which evaginates from the stomadeum, migrates dorsally. The floor of the diencephalon, the saccus infundibuli, migrates ventrally. This hollow diverticulum of brain is made up of a ventral (pituitary) and dorsal (saccular) wall. Caudally, these walls fuse to form the lower infundibular stem and infundibular process. As the pouch of Rathke migrates dorsally its aboral (posterior) wall becomes apposed to the caudal region of the saccus infundibuli (the presumptive lower infundibular stem and infundibular process). It will become the pars intermedia. In the account of Herring (3), the anterior, oral wall of Rathke's pouch grows massively, whereas the posterior, aboral wall does not. Hence the pars intermedia (aboral lobe) remains a thin band of glandular tissue separated from the expanded pars anterior (oral lobe) by Rathke's cleft except at the apex of the pouch, where the oral and aboral walls are united. Wingstrand (79) agrees that the aboral wall becomes apposed to the lower infundibular stem and infundibular process to form the pars intermedia. However, he proposes that the aboral wall of Rathke's pouch enlarges to form most of the pars distalis. The rostral region of the ventral diencephalic floor develops into the median eminence or infundibulum. The oral wall (anterior lobe) makes contact with the presumptive median eminence and becomes the site where portal connections between the median eminence and the pars distalis develop. From the anterior lobe two lateral buds develop that enlarge. These lateral lobes migrate cranially to approach the rostral portion of the ventral (or pituitary) surface of the evaginating saccus infundibuli. They become applied to it, fuse together, and develop into the pars tuberalis, which lies on the surface of the pars intermedia and the external and posterior regions of the infundibular stem and the zona tuberalis of the pars distalis, which is continuous with the pars tuberalis and lies on the anterior surface of the infundibular stem (Fig. 6).

Takor and Pearse (208) proposed that the entire hypophysis (neural and glandular) is of neuroectodermal origin. They reported that the ventral neural ridge of the white leghorn chick embryo is the origin of both pituitary components. As some adenohypophysial cells demonstrate amine precursor uptake and decarboxylation (APUD) activity and as such cells are held to be of neural origin, their theory is consistent. However, immunohistochemical staining of pars distalis cells for neurofilament protein is negative (209), and hence their neural origin is unlikely.

The adenohypophysis is applied to the neurohypophysis in all chordates. The pars tuberalis is applied to the median eminence (the infundibulum) and the upper infundibular stem, and the pars intermedia is applied to

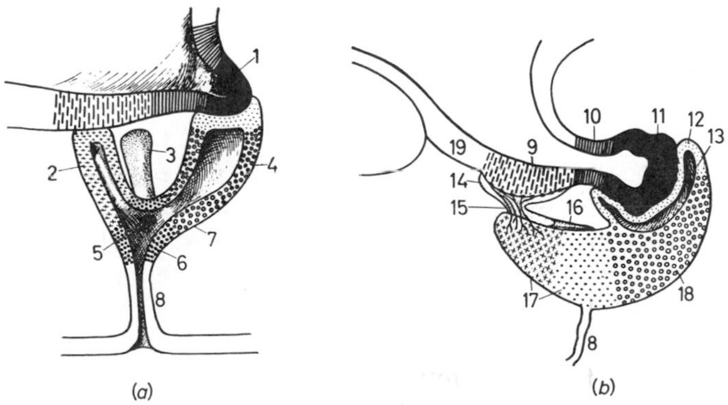

FIG. 6. Diagrams showing the structure of a generalized amniote pituitary (**B**) and its embryonic origin (**A**) as seen particularly in reptiles. *1,* Saccus infundibuli; *2,* anterior process; *3,* lateral lobe; *4,* aboral lobe; *5,* opening of the lateral lobe cavity; *6,* oral lobe, *7,* constriction of Rathke's pouch; *8,* epithelial stalk, *9,* median eminence; *10,* infundibular stem; *11,* neural lobe; *12,* pars intermedia; *13,* hypophysial cleft; *14,* juxtaneural pars tuberalis; *15,* portotuberal tract; *16,* pars tuberalis interna; *17,* cephalic lobe of the pars distalis; *18,* caudal lobe of the pars distalis; *19,* pars oralis tuberis. (From ref. 79, with permission.)

the lower infundibular stem and infundibular process (78). There is considerable variation in the development of the neurohypophysis and in the relationship of the neurointermediate lobe to the pars distalis among classes of animals. For example, in fishes and in some birds, the saccus vasculosus is well developed. In birds, the intermediate lobe does not develop, and the neural lobe is separated from the pars distalis by connective tissue, in some cases even by bone, of variable thickness. Neither neural nor vascular structures cross between the pars distalis and the infundibular process in birds. Furthermore, there is some dispute as to whether the pouch of Rathke is the analogue of the pituitary in all classes of vertebrates. Some feel that the pituitary may arise from Hatschek's pit in cyclostomes or from the nasal placode or dorsal lip in other lower species (79,80,210).

Even among mammals, species differences (e.g., the degree of persistence of Rathke's cleft or amount of coaptation of the saccular and ventral surfaces of the saccus infundibuli and hence the depth of the infundibular recess) will exist. Nevertheless, the apposition of glandular tissue to the rostral region of the evolving neurohypophysis with the consequent trapping of an interposed layer of vascular mesenchyme that will supply both the glandular and neural tissue at the base of the brain is a common characteristic of the (fetal) pituitary body in vertebrates (79). The pouch of Rathke develops into the adenohypophysis, which consists of a pars tuberalis applied to the median eminence at the base of the brain, a pars intermedia applied to the neural lobe (infundibular process) within the sella turcica, and a pars distalis that lies in the sella turcica separated from the neurohypophysis.

Organization of the Adenohypophysis

Pars Distalis

Upon the completion of its development, the pars distalis is comprised of epithelial cells, a connective tissue stroma, and many capillaries. Nerves do not terminate on or near pars distalis cells (78). There is no blood-brain barrier in the adenohypophysis (29,211). The capillaries in the adenohypophysis are not sinusoids (as believed by early investigators), because there are no phagocytic elements or large gaps in their walls. The capillaries of the adenohypophysis are fenestrated. Interposed between the epithelial cells and the fenestrated capillary tubes is a double basement membrane that on occasion is widely split with the space between the basal lamina containing connective tissue elements (212). The epithelial cells are arranged in cords (4,5). Both secretory cells (containing cytoplasmic secretory granules) and nonsecretory cells (lacking cytoplasmic granules) are present, but secretory cells predominate. Adjacent granulated cells are united by desmosomes. The nonsecretory cells are called *folliculostellate* cells. These stellate-shaped cells have long cytoplasmic processes that extend between neighboring granulated cells. Although it was initially claimed that adjacent epithelial cells are united by desmosomes and gap junctions (213,214), subsequent studies have demonstrated that gap junctions are present only between folliculostellate cells and granulated cells (215). Soji and Herbert (215), on the basis of freeze-fracture electron microscopic studies, proposed that the folliculostellate cells form a scaffold that serves as a syncytium to permit rapid communication between cells that lack innervation.

This anatomical organization of capillaries and cords of secretory epithelial cells has the obvious consequence that hormones released into the extracellular space of the adenohypophysis from any epithelial cell can reach nearby capillaries by diffusion or bulk flow and enter them through fenestrations in their endothelial tubes (Fig. 7). However, three other consequences can also be foreseen: (a) hormones can as easily reach adenohypophysial cells from the brain or from distant glands such as the thyroid, gonads, adrenal cortex or adrenal medulla; (b) hormones released by one epithelial cell are free to interact with neighboring cells that contain appropriate receptors in their cell membranes (216); and (c) intercellular communication between secretory cells is possible by electrotonic means through mutual connections with folliculostellate via gap junctions (213,215,217). The anatomy of the pars distalis permits hormonal, paracrine, and electrotonic communication.

The structure of eight hormones secreted by the adenohypophysis has been identified. Although species differences occur frequently, TSH, FSH, LH (218), PRL (219–223), GH (224,225), ACTH (226–228), melanocyte-stimulating hormones (MSH) (229–234), and β-endorphin (β-END) (235–239) have been isolated from several species and sequenced. That each hormone secreted by the pituitary gland is synthesized in and released from a functionally specific group of cells (i.e., TSH by thyrotropes, ACTH by corticotropes, and so forth) has long been postulated. This hypothesis was initially explored by attempting to correlate clinical syndromes produced by pituitary tumors with pituitary histology. Subsequent attempts have employed histochemistry (240), immunohistochemistry (241), TEM (242), and radioautographic localization of messenger RNA by light microscopic examination of histological sections after in situ hybridization (243); however, to date, not every pituitary hormone has been housed in its own unique cell.

The attempt to relate structure to function began with light microscopic examination of stained pituitary sections, which revealed glandular cells with unstained cytoplasm (chromophobes) and glandular cells with stained cytoplasm (chromophiles). Those chromophiles

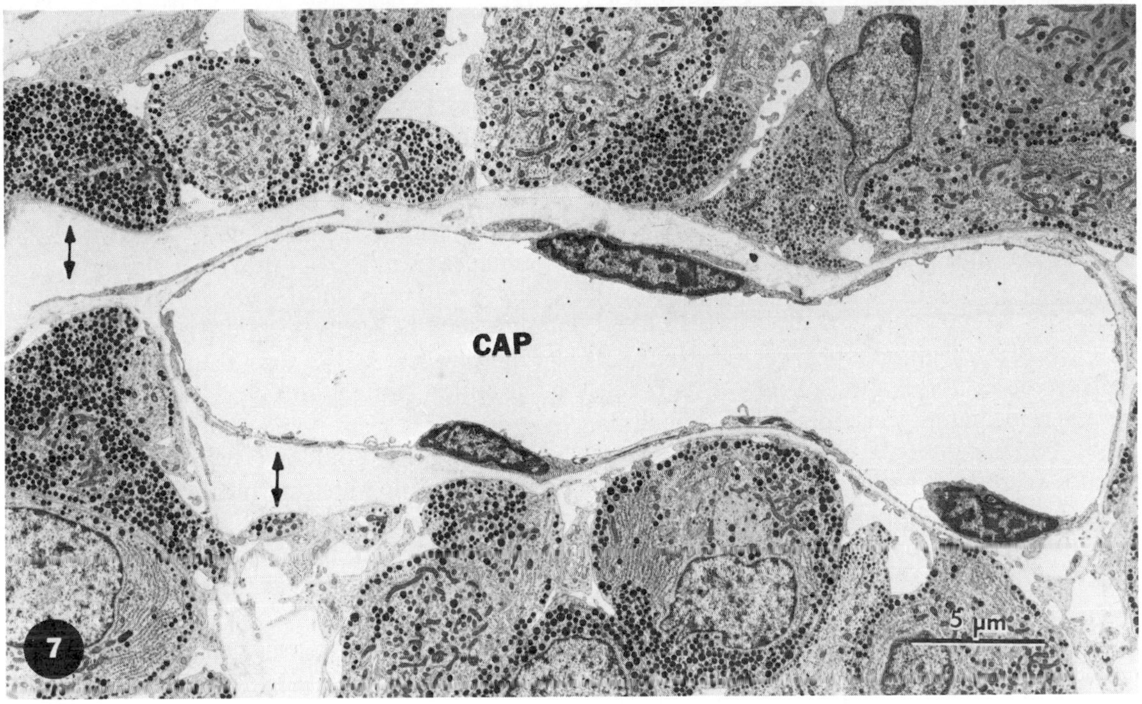

FIG. 7. Transmission electron micrograph of rabbit pars distalis. A fenestrated capillary (*CAP*) is surrounded by a double basement membrane (*arrows*) that defines the perivascular space upon which epithelial cells abut. Note occasional wide expansions of the perivascular space (↕) on which cell processes of connective tissue elements are seen. Glandular epithelial cells, identified by the presence of secretory granules, are closely related to the perivascular space and closely apposed to each other.

that stained with acid dyes were called *acidophils* (eosinophiles), whereas those that stained with basic dyes were called *basophils*. The human male gland was reported to be composed of 52% chromophobes, 37% acidophils, and 11% basophils (244). In females the proportions differed in different stages of the menstrual cycle and with pregnancy (245). Acidophils lay in the lateral wings of the human pars distalis and basophils in the central (mucoid) wedge (244). It was recognized early that the staining of chromophiles was due to the staining of granules in their cytoplasm (246,247). The belief that these granules represented a stored source of hormone was based on the observed depletion of granules following castration, thyroidectomy, or adrenalectomy of experimental animals, and this has been subsequently substantiated (169–171). Cushing (248,249) had noted a preponderance of acidophils in the pituitary tumors associated with acromegaly, and he proposed that the substance responsible for excess growth in these individuals was released from these cells. His finding of a predominance of basophils in tumors associated with bilateral adrenal cortical hyperplasia (subsequently called *Cushing's disease*) convinced him that the hormone responsible for the support of the adrenal glands (ACTH) was made in and released from basophils (250).

This picture became muddied when it was found that the number of acidophils increased in female animals at the time of parturition and that this increase was maintained during lactation (247). It was not known if acidophils secrete two hormones (one to support lactation and one to support growth) or just one. In addition, changes in the morphology of both acidophils and basophils occurred during the estrous cycle, during pregnancy, and following castration (for review, see ref. 247). Furthermore, thyroidectomy produced a decrease in the number of acidophils as well as a degranulation of basophils while adrenalectomy also produced degranulation of basophils. To clarify the situation, more histochemical techniques were employed based on modifications of the use of an acid dye such as eosin or orange G to stain acidophiles and of the periodic acid-Schiff (PAS) reaction to stain basophils. The result was a chaotic picture adding little to knowledge of the problem at hand—the localization of specific hormones within specific cell types as defined by histochemical staining. Confusion arose because of the vagaries of staining by different lots of analine dyes, the lack of knowledge of the chemical reaction between the dye and the cellular or hormone elements, species differences in staining patterns, and the use of the same terminology to describe cells stained by different dyes and thus of different appearance. The subject is reviewed in detail by Romeis (251), Pearse (252), Herlant (253), Pearse and Noorden (240), and Purves (254). From light microscopic examinations of stained sections, the following firm conclusions were reached: (a) hormones are stored in granules in pituitary epithelial cells; (b) the hormone (or hormones) responsible for growth and lactation are found in eosinophils; (c) these eosinophils are localized predominantly in the lateral wings of the gland (244,255); (d) basophilic cells can be thyrotropic, gonadotrophic, or adrenocorticotrophic, and they lie predominantly in the middle of the gland (240,244,253–255); and (e) the positive PAS reaction that characterizes basophils indicates glycosolation of the protein hormone molecule in these cells (240,252).

The nature of the chromophobes was resolved with electron microscopy. Observation of pars distalis cells with TEM revealed that all the epithelial cells, with the exception of folliculostellate cells, contain electron-dense granules in their cytoplasm (189,242,256). The granules seen in TEM studies of the cytoplasm of chromophobes were too small, or too few, to be observed by light microscopy. Hence the large population of chromophobes, about 50%, observed by light microscopy in the human gland could not represent a population of uncommitted cells (246,247).

The eosinophils were divided by light microscopists into two groups (α cells and η [or ϵ] cells) (251): orangeophils and carminophils (253). The color of the granules differed with the stain employed and the species studied, but appropriate techniques revealed one type of acidophil that is found predominantly in the lateral wings of the pars distalis and does not vary with pregnancy and a second type that also lies in the lateral wings and becomes much more frequent at the time of pregnancy and parturition (254,256). Purves and Greisbach (257) described two classes of acidophils in rats. Acidophils found on the interior of cell cords became degranulated after castration or estrogen therapy and were believed to be lactotrophs. Columnar acidophils arranged radially about capillaries became prominent following castration or estrogen therapy, but became degranulated after thyroidectomy and were classified as somatotropes.

On electron microscopic examination somatotropes were described by Farquhar and Rinehart (258) as containing secretory granules of about 350 nm in their cytoplasm that lined up along the plasmalemma in a single row. Interestingly these cells became more prominent after castration (258) and less prominent (degranulated) after thyroidectomy (259). The somatotrope in the rat pituitary is described by Kurosumi (242) as a round, oval, or polygonal cell with distinctive short clubbed mitochondria and round dense secretory granules with a maximum diameter of 350 nm. Injection of a stalk median eminence extract rich in GRF activity results in rapid degranulation of these cells (201).

The use of immunoelectron microscopy (241) further strengthened the argument that growth hormone is produced by a functionally specific line of cells and is stored within cytoplasmic secretory granules (256,260–262). However, it cast doubt upon the concept that all the somatotropes can be recognized solely by the size and shape of their secretory granules. Kurosumi and Tosaka (263) have described three morphological appearances of somatotropes identified by immunogold electron microscopy. Type I cells contained granules of ~350 nm in diameter and corresponds to the cells described by Farquhar and Rinehart (258). Type II cells contained smaller granules, but these were larger than those found in type III cells, which were ~100 nm in diameter. In the late fetal stages, type III cells predominated among somatotropes. As the animals matured the frequency distribution shifted, and type I cells became the most frequent. They proposed that type I cells were mature somatotropes and that type III cells were immature. Type II cells were intermediate (263). The morphology of somatotropes is thus variable and depends, among other things, on their maturity.

The presumptive lactotrope was believed by Farquhar and Rinehart (258,259) to contain elliptical rather than round secretory vesicles that were as large as 600 to 900 mm in their longest diameter. Such cells became degranulated and developed large laminar areas of rough endoplasmic reticulum under the stimulus of suckling (189). Similar cells were identified by Kurosumi (242) as lactotrophs. Nakane (260,261) localized immunoreactive PRL within these granules. When immunohistochemistry was combined with electron microscopy the picture became more complex. The ultrastructural characteristics of cells that were immunostained for PRL were not uniform. Granule size varied from ~150 to ~600 nm in diameter. The prominence of the Golgi apparatus, the degrees of dilation of the cisternae of the endoplasmic reticulum, the prominence of the nucleolus, and the shape of the nucleus also varied among cells that were immunostained for PRL. Several classifications of lactotropes (as defined by immunohistochemistry) based principally on granule size and shape were made (see ref. 264 for review). Kurosumi et al. (265) classified lactotropes into three types. Type I is a crescent-shaped cell with an eccentric, oval nucleus. The Golgi and rough endoplasmic reticulum are well developed. Most of the mitochondria are perinuclear in location. Granules are large (~500 nm) and are mostly arranged along the periphery. Type II is polygonal or elongated in shape. The nucleus is kidney shaped. Some lysosomes contain secretory granules that stain for PRL. These cells are usually more granulated than type I, and the granules are smaller (~150 to 250 nm). Type III cells are small and polygonal. A few small secretory granules (~100 nm) are present in the cytoplasm. In adult males, type I cells comprised 46% of the lactotropes, type II cells comprised 48%, and type III cells comprised 6%. In perinatal rats, type III cells made up 83% of the total lactotrope population. In female rats, the type I cell comprised 91% of the lactotropes. Lactotrope morphology varied in females with the state of the estrous cycle (265) and in males with age (266).

Growth hormone and PRL are thus present in functionally distinct cell lines that are best differentiated by immunohistochemistry to identify the protein stored in their granules or by hybrid histochemistry to identify the nature of their messenger RNA (267,268). The ultrastructural morphology of the lactotropes varies with age, hormonal milieu, and function and will be the subject of an in-depth discussion in a later chapter.

Basophils may be thyrotropes, gonadotropes, or corticotropes. Thyrotropes and gonadotropes aggregate in the central region of the pars distalis: the mucoid wedge—so named because its cells contain glycoproteins. Corticotropes aggregate in the anterior portion of the mucoid wedge. The mucoid wedge occupies the zona tuberalis, which, according to Wingstrand (79), with the pars tuberalis arises from the oral lobe of Rathke's pouch. On the bases of their reaction with such stains as Alcian Blue, Aldehyde Fuchsin, and Resorcin Fuchsin and on their staining characteristics with such dyes following oxidation with potassium permanganate, PAS positive cells have been subclassified into FSH-, LH-, TSH-, and ACTH-containing cells (240,251–254,256). Such schemes are complex, with patterns of staining that vary from species to species, and they have never gained wide acceptance. Differentiation of cell types now relies principally on immunohistochemistry at the light and electron microscopic levels.

Thyroid-stimulating hormone is a glycoprotein that contains two chains, designated α and β. TSH containing cells thus stain with PAS (254,269,270). The α-chain is common to TSH, LH and FSH, and the β-chain is specific for TSH (218,271). Small angular cells in the rat's pituitary gland, which contain granules with a maximal diameter of 140 nm, were found on TEM examination by Farquhar and Rinehart (259) to exhibit a depletion of cytoplasmic dense granules and a marked increase in the number of lucent cytoplasmic vesicles following thyroidectomy and were thus identified as thyrotropes. Kawarai (272) published similar findings. Using antibodies to TSH, preabsorbed with β-human chorionic gonadotropin and without cross reaction with FSH or LH, Baker et al. (271) were able to localize immunoreactive TSH to cells in the rat pituitary that corresponded to the thyroidectomy cells described by Farquhar and Rinehart (259). Moriarity and Tobin (273,274) employed antibodies to the β-chain of TSH and obtained similar results. Immunohistochemically identified thyrotropes in human pituitaries resemble those described in the rat (275). The morphology of thyrotropes in the rat also varies with the state of development (276). In adult rats, angular cells resembling those described by Farquhar and Rinehart (259), with cytoplasmic granules ranging between 120 to 180 nm, predominated. In neonatal rats, thyrotropes identified by immunoelectron microscopy contained few granules of 50 to 100 nm in diameter. By 20 days postpartum, almost 70% of the thyrotropes were intermediate in type, containing granules 80 to 120 nm in diameter. By 60 days, ~70% were mature in appearance.

Follicle-stimulating hormone and LH are also glycoproteins that contain an α-chain common to TSH, FSH and LH and a β-chain specific for each gonadotropin (218). PAS staining pituitary cells that become hyalinized following castration are termed *signet ring* or *castration cells* and are presumed to be gonadotropes. Farquhar and Rinehart (258) described two types of castration cell in the rat based on their TEM observations. The first appeared soon after castration and contained ovoid cytoplasmic vesicles. The second did not appear until later and contained irregularly shaped vesicles separated by cytoplasmic strands. It was described as resembling a filigree. The authors proposed that the former cells were *FSH producers* and the latter were *LH producers*. Kurosumi and Oota (277) proposed that FSH gonadotropes are large and round with two populations of granules in their cytoplasm one of 200 nm diameter and the second as large as 700 nm in diameter. LH gonadotropes were described as smaller than FSH gonadotropes and frequently located along blood vessels (a site presumptively not occupied by FSH gonadotropes). Luteinizing hormone gonadotropes were said to be polygonal with secretory vesicles measuring 250 nm situated at the periphery of the cell. In contrast to the FSH cell, the LH cell was said to have a small Golgi apparatus with little development of the rough endoplasmic reticulum. However, Moriarity (278) demonstrated the presence of immunoreactive LH-β in each of these cell types. Immunoreactive FSH and LH have been localized in the same cells in the human pituitary (279). In male rats, 80% of gonadotropes contained both FSH and LH, 10% contained only LH, and 10% contained only FSH (280). Childs et al. (281) also have employed in situ hybridization techniques along with immunoelectron microscopy to study gonadotropes in normal and castrated male rats. In 80% of gonadotropes that contained FSH in secretory granules, LH mRNA was found in the cytoplasm.

The usual appearance of a gonadotrope was of a large ovoid or polyhedral cell. The nucleus was spherical, and the Golgi was prominent. The rough endoplasmic reticulum was abundant. Gonadotropes were divided into types, depending on granule size: type I harbored two granule sizes (200 to 250 and 450 to 700 nm); type II contained only the smaller granules. Lloyd and Childs (282) were able to separate gonadotropes into two populations (of large and small cells) on the basis of density centrifugation. Large cells tended to be multihormonal, and small cells tended to be monohormonal. Whether there is a correlation between large cells and type I cells and small cells and type II cells has yet to be determined. The ultrastructure of the gonadotrope is thus not predictive of the gonadotropic hormone(s) it contains (283,284). Gonadotropes may assume one of several appearances upon TEM examination. Their ultrastructural appearance varies as a function of the (estrous) cycle or cellular activity (synthesis, storage, or release of hormone[s]) (265). This topic is discussed in detail in a subsequent chapter.

Basophils (thyrotropes and gonadotropes) aggregate in the central portion of the pars distalis, (i.e., the *mucoid wedge* [so called because its cells contain glycoproteins]). The wedge occupies the zona tuberalis, which, with the pars tuberalis, arises from the oral lobe of Rathke's pouch (79). ACTH is not a glycoprotein in humans (285). It is a single-chain protein hormone 39 amino acids in length. However, in rats and mice, both glycosylated and nonglycosylated forms of ACTH 1-39 have been identified (286). ACTH-containing cells have been described as basophilic, as well as acidophilic, amphophilic, and chromophobic (see refs. 253,254,256, and 262 for reviews). In the human, ACTH cells are described by Baker (256) as intensely basophilic. His description of ACTH containing basophilic cells is consistent with the finding of basophils in adenomas of the human pituitary that secrete ACTH and cause Cushing's disease (250). The source of the positive reaction obtained with PAS staining of human corticotropes has in the past been attributed to glycolipids (such as phosphatidylinositol), glycoproteins, or mucoproteins in the secretory granules or in their membranes (240,252,256). Proopiomelanocortin (POMC) (285,287), the 31K prohormone from which ACTH and MSH are derived, is glycosylated; and POMC, not ACTH, may be the source of PAS positivity in corticotropes that contain the nonglycosylated form of ACTH in their granules (262).

The TEM description of corticotropes was at first based on the description of cells that showed signs of increased protein secretion following adrenalectomy. Adrenalectomy cells were described as large, irregular in outline, and with a tendency "to insinuate cytoplasmic projections between neighboring cells in the direction of sinusoids" (288). Their cytoplasm contained many vesicles, and their granules measured 200 nm on average. Following the administration of cortisol to normal rats, dense granules accumulated in the cytoplasm in large angular cells believed to be corticotropes. Following the administration of cortisol to adrenalectomized rats, an increase in the number of cytoplasmic granules was accompanied by a decrease in the number of cytoplasmic vesicles that are found in adrenalectomy cells of untreated animals (289,290). Employing an antibody to 17-39 or 25-39 ACTH, Moriarity and Halmi (291) were able to localize immunoreactive ACTH within granules in the cytoplasm of angular cells with long processes insinuated between neighboring and with granules of about 200 nm in diameter—cells that resembled those described by Siperstein and colleagues (288–290).

The adult human, unlike the rat, lacks a pars intermedia, and thus corticotropes and melanotropes are present in the pars distalis. However, identification of each cell type by immunohistochemistry may be difficult. α-MSH shares a common sequence of amino acids with ACTH (1-13), and β-MSH shares a common sequence with ACTH (4-10) (226–235). Furthermore, ACTH, α-MSH, β-lipotropin (β-LPH), and β-END are all derived from the same 31 kD parent hormone by enzymatic cleavage of peptide bonds (285,291–294). In the rat, pars distalis corticotropes process this parent hormone principally to ACTH, β-LPH and β-END, whereas pars intermedia melanotropes further process (a) ACTH to α-MSH and corticotropin-like intermediate peptide (CLIP) and (b) β-LPH to β-END and α-lipotropin (which in turn can be processed to β-MSH) (285,294). Immunohistochemical studies to localize these hormones must be done with particular care, because binding of the antibody to one sequence of amino acids may stain several protein hormones. For example, an antibody to ACTH 4-9 may stain ACTH, α-MSH, β-MSH, and POMC, and antibodies to β-LPH may react with β-END as well as with the 31 kD prohormone.

Immunohistochemical study of the human pars distalis with antibody against ACTH 17-39 demonstrates ACTH-containing cells in the pars distalis that are basophilic (PAS positive) (295). The same cells also react with antibody against β-MSH (296), but this reaction may reflect LPH rather than β-MSH activity (297). β-Lipoprotein has been localized in the same secretory granules of corticotropes in the pars distalis as has ACTH by electron microscopic examination of human, monkey, ox, pig, and rat pituitaries (298). It also appears that ACTH and β-LPH (or β-END) are found in the same granules of corticotropes in the rat pars distalis (299).

Corticotropes in the rat's pars distalis rarely stain for melanotropin (300). Kurosumi et al. (301) employed immunogold labeling of POMC cells in the rat's pars distalis to identify putative corticotropes in fetal, neonatal, and adult rats. They found that in fetal pituitaries POMC-containing cells were polygonal and characterized by the presence of many mitochondria about the nucleus. The mitochondria were "thread-like," and sometimes bifurcated. Secretory granules were small. With advancing development the cell type became scarce and was replaced by angular cells with an average granular diameter of $\sim$100 nm and then by cells with larger granules (average $\sim$140 nm with a maximum diameter of 200 nm). The granule size of POMC-containing cells was a function of the maturity of the animal, as was the granule size of somatotropes, lactotropes, thyrotropes, and gonadotropes.

Colocalization of hormones from apparently different cell lines within a single cell type has recently been reported. Double-label immunogold immunohistochemistry of the rat pituitary has revealed a small number of cells in which GH and PRL are costored in the same secretory granules (302). These mammosomatotropes do not resemble either lactotropes or somatotropes but contain small secretory granules (50 to 100 nm in diameter). Mammosomatotropes have also been reported in the cow and human pituitary gland (275,303). The presence of somatotropes (identified by immunoelectron microscopic techniques) that contain TSH mRNA (identified by in situ hybridization) has been described in rats made hypothyroid by propylthiouracil treatment (304). This finding could not be confirmed in rat pituitaries following surgical ablation of the thyroid (305). Whether transdifferentiation of pituitary cells occurs is a matter of investigation.

The concept a pleuripotential stem cell that can be recruited into a population of secreting adenohypophysial cells upon appropriate stimulation has recently gained considerable support from the laboratory of Dr. Childs. Wu and Childs (306) observed that the number of cells containing POMC mRNA in the dissociated anterior pituitary gland was increased after 15 minutes of cold stress. Sasaki et al. (307) also found an increased number of corticotropes (as identified by immunohistochemistry) and an increased number of cells binding biotinylated CRF. Dual immunohistochemical studies done under nonstimulated conditions have revealed a small number of adenohypophysial cells that costore ACTH and TSH (307). Upon appropriate stimulation, such as cold stress, these cells, increased in number, add significantly to the population of actively secreting corticotropes and thyrotropes (307).

In addition to the granulated cells described above, the pars distalis contains a stellate-shaped nongranulated cell—the folliculostellate cell. These angular epithelial cells contain a few secretory granules in their cytoplasm. Microfilaments, lysosomes, and lipid bodies are plentiful. They are frequently joined by junctional complexes to each other to create a follicle with a central lumen (308). Microvilli and cilia protrude from the folliculostellate cell membrane lining the lumen, which contains colloid (275). They make contact with adjacent secretory cells through gap junctions. These cells are characterized by the presence of the immunoreactive S-100 neuronal protein in their cytoplasm (194,309). In addition, fibronectin has been immunohistochemically demonstrated in the cytoplasm of these cells (310). The role of these cells has not firmly been established, but a role in intercellular communication or phagocytosis has been postulated (215,308). Recent immunohistochemical studies demonstrated that folliculostellate cells can synthesize interleukin-6 (311,312)—a cytokine capable of stimulating ACTH release from corticotropes (313,314).

The pars distalis contains somatotropes, lactotropes, thyrotropes, gonadotropes, corticomelanotropes, and folliculostellate cells. In addition, it appears to contain pleuripotential cells that can contribute to a population of secreting cells upon appropriate stimulation. Ultrastructural morphology of these cells alone is not a very good indicator of their function, because the ultrastructure is not constant with time or with circumstance. The morphology of a given clone depends on its age, its state of function, and its hormonal milieu. Furthermore, some clones contain more than one hormone (e.g., gonadotropes, corticomelanotropes, and pleuripotential cells). The epithelial cells of the pars distalis are not innervated. In some cases they are regulated by feedback mechanisms and/or by the interaction of catecholamines with receptors on their cell surfaces. In some cases they are regulated by their interaction with cytokines. In all cases they are regulated by hypothalamic releasing and inhibiting hormones that are released from nerve endings in the neurohypophysis and that, through restricted portal routes, reach receptors on the surface of the epithelial cells of the adenohypophysis.

Pars Intermedia

The pars intermedia is prominent in many species, including the rat, but is lacking in others such as birds or humans with the exception of the pregnant human female and the human fetus. Although neither α-MSH nor β-MSH is a glycoprotein, pars intermedia cells have long been recognized as intensely basophilic and as the source of a hormone that regulates skin color in amphibians (315). As in corticomelanotropes in the pars distalis, the source of this PAS positivity may be the presence of proopiomelanocortin, a glycosylated protein, in the storage granules of pars intermedia cells.

The (rat) pars intermedia was found to be lobulated. Capillaries separated adjacent lobules, but are sparse. The cells, with the exception of those that line the lumen of the hypophysial cleft, were polygonal. Light and dark cells have been distinguished by light microscopy (on the basis of their staining affinity for PAS) and by TEM. There were more light cells than dark ones. Light cells had large ovoid nuclei. Their cytoplasm contained many clear vesicles that were round and measured 200 to 300 nm. Round, dense granules measuring 200 to 300 nm in diameter lay in the Golgi region, which was well developed and lies near the nucleus. Dark cells were irregular in outline and contained lobulated nuclei. The cytoplasm contained closely packed particles measuring 20 nm in diameter, which gave the cells their dark appearance. The endoplasmic reticulum was well developed, but vesicles are scant (316).

α-Melanocyte-stimulating hormone is localized in pars intermedia cells of the human fetus and in the pregnant human female (317). Both light and dark cells in the pars intermedia of the rat contain immunoreactive β-melanotropin (318). In cows, pigs, rabbits, and rats immunoreactive ACTH 17-39 was found in pars intermedia cells (319), although the concentration of ACTH is believed to be much less than β-MSH in these cells (300). Moriarity and Halmi (320) localized immunoreactive ACTH 17-39 to granules of dark and light cells, and subsequently Moriarity and Garner (297) found that the granules in corticomelanotropes in the rat intermediate lobe immunostained for both ACTH 17-39 and β-MSH. Similar findings have been reported in the mouse (318). β-Melanocyte-stimulating hormone staining may also have indicated the presence of β-LPH, as the entire sequence of β-MSH is found in β-LPH.

The pars intermedia is less well vascularized than the pars distalis (321). In the rat's pars intermedia, capillaries join with the capillaries of the pars distalis to form a portal system within the adenohypophysis (321). The extracellular space is well developed and communicates with the hypophysial cleft and the extracellular space of the adjacent infundibular process (neural lobe) and pars distalis (322). These vascular arrangements provide mechanisms to deliver the products of the pars intermedia to the neural lobe and pars distalis or alternatively to deliver secretions from the neural lobe and pars distalis to the pars intermedia. The side chain of oxytocin, pro-leu-gly-NH_2, has been proposed as a melanocyte-hormone-inhibiting factor (323) and can reach melanotropes from the extracellular spaces of the neural lobe. Corticotropin-releasing factor, which releases melanotropin from pars intermedia cells as well as corticotropin from pars distalis corticotropes (324,325), can reach melanotropes from the extracellular spaces of the pars distalis. The vascular architecture of the pars intermedia probably plays an important role in the regulation of its function.

Axons terminate in the pars intermedia and make synaptoid contact with its epithelial cells (316,326), and hence pars intermedia cells can be regulated by direct neural contact. β-Adrenergic receptors have been demonstrated on melanotropes, and β-adrenergic agonists stimulated the release of α-MSH (327,328). Early evidence for the presence of a (nor)adrenergic input to the neurointermediate lobe of the rat was obtained by microspectrofluorometric analysis of the neurointermediate lobe following formaldehyde fixation and exposure to hydrochloric acid vapors. The shifts in emission wavelength (and hence in color) were specific for dopamine and norepinephrine. Both dopaminergic and norepinergic terminals were demonstrated in the pars intermedia (329). A direct innervation of melanocytes by noradrenergic or adrenergic systems arising in the brainstem was proposed on the basis of early ultrastructural studies (330), but a more recent immunohistochemical study failed to demonstrate immunoreactive dopamine β-hydroxylase in the pars intermedia (331).

Serotonergic fibers have been shown to terminate in the rat's pars intermedia (332) and putatively to stimulate MSH release. Immunoreactive dopaminergic (333) terminals have been demonstrated in the pars intermedia of the rat and cat (333,334). Dopamine has been shown to inhibit the release of POMC-derived products from dispersed pars intermedia cells and from the incubated neurointermediate lobe (334). GABAergic (335–338) fibers also terminated in the pars intermedia and made synaptoid contact with pars intermedia cells (339). They (presumably) also inhibit MSH release from melanotropes. Immunoreactive GABA and immunoreactive TH have been colocalized in the same terminals in the pars intermedia of the rat (340). Dopamine has also been reported to be costored with serotonin in terminals innervating melanotropes (341), as has colocalization of GABA and dopamine (342). Saland et al. (341) suggest that all three neurotransmitters may be costored together in one terminal type. GABA and dopamine are not costored in the pars intermedia of the rabbit or hare (342). Immunohistochemical studies have demonstrated immunoreactive serotonergic fibers innervating pars intermedia cells in the rat (332). In this species pro-leu-gly-NH_2 may reach melanotropes directly by synaptoid contact between oxytocinergic fibers and melanotropes in the pars intermedia (323). The epithelial cells of the pars intermedia can thus be regulated by three different mechanisms—long portal routes from the median eminence via the pars distalis, "short" portal routes from the neural lobe, and synaptoid contact.

Pars Tuberalis

The pars tuberalis as described is comprised of glandular epithelial cells arranged in cords and containing dense cytoplasmic granules. Pars tuberalis specific cells, "invasive cells," and follicular cells reside there (343). Pars tuberalis specific cells are spheroid in shape and are characterized by the presence of only a few secretory granules located at the vascular pole of the cell. These granules are generally smaller than those found in pars distalis cell. In the adult rat they range from 120 to 150 nm. A large number of lysosomes may be found in these cells. They typically consist of a dense core with a cup-like extension. Varying numbers of glycogen granules are present in the cytoplasm and are a distinguishing characteristic of pars tuberalis specific cells (Fig. 4B). Invasive cells appear to be gonadotropes that have migrated into the pars tuberalis from the pars distalis. Follicular cells, in the human fetal pituitary, had irregular heterochromatic nuclei, no secretory granules, and long processes that extended between secretory cells. At times they aggregated to form typical follicles. At their cell surface, the follicle is lined with microvilli and cilia (343). In addition, connective tissue elements are present, as are many (fenestrated) capillaries. Occasionally, an axon terminal is found adjacent to a glandular epithelial cell (344).

The glandular epithelial cells in several species have been characterized by immunohistochemistry that revealed cells that stain with antibodies to TSH and GnRH. The nature of the cells that react with anti-TSH is open to question, however, as only faint staining of pars tuberalis specific cells occurs. Gonadotropes have been localized within the pars tuberalis of the rat (345) and in the pars tuberalis of the monkey (*Macacca mulatta*) (346,347). Girod et al. (347) reported localization of β-LH in scattered cells of the pars tuberalis in *Macacca irus*. With hypophysectomy of rats, there was an increase in the number and size of immunoreactive gonadotropes and an increase in gonadotropin hormone production (348).

The function of the pars tuberalis is unknown. It has recently been found that the pars tuberalis is rich in melatonin receptors, and there is suggestive evidence that these receptors are found in pars tuberalis specific cells (349). Their morphology, in some species, varied with photoperiod and not with functional changes in endocrine organs that are targets of the pituitary. Wittokski et al. (349) postulated that the pars tuberalis modulates pars distalis function by secreting an as yet uncharacterized peptide from pars tuberalis specific cells in response to melatonin secreted by the pineal gland. This postulated hormone is carried to the pars distalis by vascular routes. Nakazawa et al. (350) also posit a short loop feedback role for the pars tuberalis. Incubation of median eminence–pars tuberalis fragments with GnRH stimulated the release of LH into the medium. Incubation of the median eminence–pars tuberalis fragments in the presence of LH decreased the release of GnRH into the medium while incubation with an antibody to LH caused an increase in the amount of GnRH released. They found that incubation of the median eminence and pars tuberalis in the presence of melatonin increased the release of GnRH into the medium. The increase in GnRH release was blocked by the coincubation of LH with the melatonin. The authors proposed that melatonin suppressed LH release from pars tuberalis gonadotropes and that this local decrease in LH stimulated the increased release of GnRH from terminals in the median eminence by releasing the terminals from (short loop) feedback inhibition.

THE NEUROHYPOPHYSIS

Nerve Terminals of the Neurohypophysis

Nerve terminals in the neurohypophysis release hormones (employed by other terminals to perform other tasks) into blood vessels to be carried to the adenohypophysis or to distant target organs to regulate their function. The neurohypophysis is composed of the median eminence (the infundibulum), the infundibular stem, and the neural lobe (infundibular process) (30). The terminals there can be viewed as the terminals of the segmental motor neurons of the neuroendocrine system.

Three basic types of terminals can be recognized by TEM. The first is found predominantly in the neural lobe and in the rat measures 1.5 to 7.0 μm in diameter. These terminals of the magnocellular supraoptico-hypophysial tract contain mitochondria, large dense-cored vesicles that measure 180 nm on average, and small lucent synaptic vesicles of 50 nm average diameter. The second type of terminal lies predominantly in the median eminence. These terminals of the parvicellular tuberohypophysial tract are smaller, measuring 0.3 to 1.4 μm in the rat. They contain mitochondria, large granular vesicles measuring 90 nm on average, and small lucent vesicles about 50 nm in diameter. The third type of terminal is the same size as the second but contains only lucent vesicles measuring about 50 nm in diameter (351). In the rabbit, terminals of the supraoptico-hypophysial tract contain large dense-cored vesicles that are 250 to 300 nm in diameter, as well as small lucent vesicles with an average diameter of 50 nm. In the rabbit's median eminence, some axon terminals contain large granular vesicles that average 120 nm in diameter and small lucent vesicles, whereas others contain only small lucent vesicles with an average diameter of 50 nm (352,353). Similar observations have been made by others in the rat (354,355) and in the human (356,357), and even in submammalian species, for example, the toad (358,359). However, the number of groups into which the terminals are classified by the authors, based on the size of their vesicles, varies with the author and with the species (Fig. 8).

Magnocellular neurons that originate in the hypothalamic supraoptic and paraventricular nuclei course through the hypothalamus as the supraoptico-hypophysial tract and terminate in the neural lobe (33,34,360–362). This magnocellular neurosecretory system has been classified as peptidergic, as it synthesizes, stores, and secretes oxytocin and vasopressin with their associated neurophysins (I and II, respectively) (62,363). These hormones are stored in the dense-cored vesicles in terminals of the supraoptico-hypophysial tract (63). Oxytocin and vasopressin have been isolated from bovine dense-cored vesicles (364). Vasopressin and neurophysin have been localized in terminals of the supraoptico-hypophysial tract of the guinea pig by combining TEM and immunohistochemical techniques (365). The large dense-cored vesicles containing peptide hormones are transported from nuclei in the hypothalamus by axoplasmic flow to terminals in the neural lobe (55,58).

The contents of the dense-cored vesicles are released from the nerve terminal by exocytosis (366). Transmission electron microscopy of thin sections (366,367) and of freeze-fracture preparations (368) demonstrated fusion of the dense-cored vesicles with the terminal membrane and then the formation of omega figures with opening of the membrane at the fusion site and release of

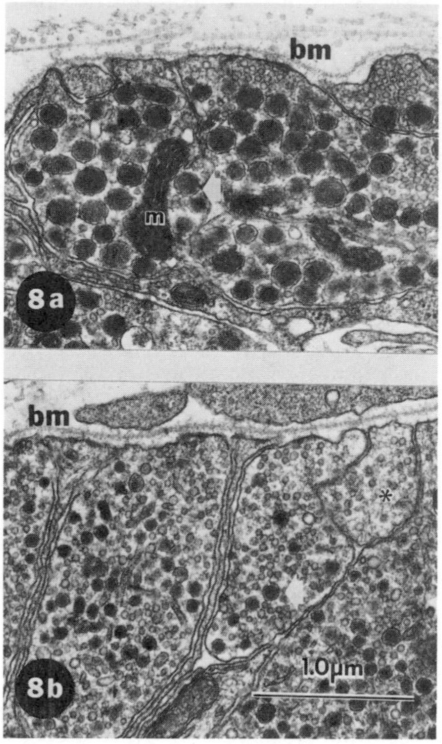

FIG. 8. Transmission electron micrograph of neural terminals in the rat neurohypophysis. **A:** Neural lobe. Large dense-cored vesicles (*white arrowhead*) and small lucent vesicles fill neural terminals. *bm,* Basement membrane; *m,* mitochondria. **B:** Median eminence. Smaller terminals contain large granular vesicles (*white arrowhead*) and lucent vesicles. One terminal (*) contains only lucent vesicles. Dense-cored vesicles (Fig. A) are larger than large granular vesicles (Fig. B). Lucent vesicles in Fig. A resemble those in Fig. B.

the contents of the vesicles. Calculations based on the estimated hormone content of a single vesicle and the decrease in the number of dense-cored vesicles in terminals following stimulation suggested that all the hormone released can be accounted for by this mechanism (369).

Large dense-cored vesicles in the terminals of the supraoptico-hypophysial tract of a single specimen are not always uniform in appearance when viewed by TEM (351,356,370–374). Frequently large vacuoles devoid of osmophilic material are found. Following the injection of histamine (370) or following ether treatment (371), the number of large dense-cored vesicles was reported to decrease and the number of large empty vacuoles to increase. Such observations led to the concept that hormone release from magnocellular terminals was due to escape of hormone through the membranes of dense-cored vesicles into the axoplasm, leaving behind an empty vacuole, and then escape from the axoplasm of the nerve terminal into the extracellular space. Thus hormone was released through a process of molecular dispersion. This theory is at odds with the concept that hormones are secreted from nerve terminals by exocytotic release from dense-cored vesicles at the plasmalemma. Douglas et al. (366) stated that, with optimal fixative techniques, empty vacuoles were few in number and believed them to be a fixation artifact. He reported that with stimulation the number of large empty vacuoles remained unchanged but the number of small "synaptic" vesicles increased.

The role of these small "synaptic" vesicles in large axon terminals of the supraoptico-hypophysial tract has been debated. Douglas et al. (366) proposed that these clear vesicles about 50 nm in diameter, were involved in membrane retrieval, because they observed that the vesicles, increased in number after stimulation as the number of large secretory granules decreased. Morris and Nordmann (369) disputed the observation of Douglas et al. (366) that the number of microvesicles was increased after stimulation. They found that the number of large empty vacuoles (not small lucent vesicles) to be increased after stimulation. They proposed that the vacuoles were retrieved neurosecretory granules that had been emptied by exocytosis. On the basis of experiments that demonstrated ATP-dependent Ca^{2+} binding in microvesicles, Nordmann and Chevallier (375) and Shaw and Morris (376) proposed that small lucent vesicles are involved in calcium homeostasis within the nerve terminal. Broadwell et al. (377) presented evidence, based on transmission electron microscopic observations of endocytosis of wheat germ agglutinin by terminals of the supraoptico-hypophysial tract, that microvesicles as well as vacuoles participate in the neurosecretory process by endocytosis and recycling of the membrane of neurohypophysial terminals.

The nature of the microvesicles has become clarified with the observation that their membranes have been found to contain synapsin, synaptophysin, and protein III. These proteins were not found associated with the membrane of secretory granules (378). Meeker et al. (379,380) have presented convincing evidence that glutamate is present as a neurotransmitter in microvesicles of the terminals in the neural lobe. The microvesicles in neurosecretory neuron terminals thus serve the same role that they do in axon terminals at synapses. They house and release neurotransmitters. The previous investigations cited demonstrated that following exocytosis secretory granules appear empty and that membrane recycling, as indicated by labeling of the membranes with wheat germ agglutinin occurs in the life cycles of the both secretory granules and microvesicles.

Axon terminals of parvicellular neurons contain granular vesicles measuring about 90 nm (in the rat) and small lucent vesicles. They have been until recently classified as aminergic or peptidergic (381–383). The colocalization of amines and peptides within the same neurosecretory neuron is now recognized as commonplace (384) and makes this method of classification less useful than it previously seemed to be. The localization of peptides and amines within separate organelles at the neurosecretory neuron's terminal has not been completely accomplished. TRH (385,386), SRIF (387,388), and GnRH (389) have been localized by immunohistochemical techniques to large granular vesicles in the terminals of parvicellular systems. Exocytosis characterized by fusion of the large granular vesicles with the terminal membrane and release of their granular material has been demonstrated (390–392).

The role of small lucent vesicles in parvicellular neurosecretory systems remains elusive, although a preponderance of evidence suggests that they house neurotransmitters. Ajika (393) employed antibodies to LHRH and to tyrosine hydroxylase to identify LHRH and dopamine-containing cells in the same sections, and LHRH was preferentially localized over large granular vesicles. Tyrosine hydroxylase was localized over small lucent vesicles of different cells. Small lucent vesicles in GnRH-containing cells did not stain. A similar study localized TRH by immunohistochemistry and monoamines by autoradiography (after injection with tritiated monoamines) and demonstrated similar findings (394). Although uptake of the false neurotransmitter 5-hydroxydopamine occurred in both the large granular and the small lucent vesicles (353,382,395–397), immunohistochemical techniques employing antibodies against specific enzymes in the biosynthetic pathway of amines localized them to lucent microvesicles in terminals (382,397–400). Autoradiographic techniques have also localized amines to small lucent vesicles (257,258).

Terminals containing only small lucent vesicles are also found on TEM examination of the neurohypophysis after aldehyde fixation (353). While some of these neurons may be aminergic, systems containing other neurotransmitters such as ACh and GABA terminate in the neurohypophysis (335–337,401). The full spectrum of neurotransmitters and neurohormones and their subcellular localizations in terminals of the neurohypophysis remain to be discovered.

Nerve terminals in the neurohypophysis are organized to release their contents into the perivascular space of fenestrated capillaries and not into a synaptic cleft between neuronal elements. Although terminals in the hypothalamus and other regions of the brain may contain peptides or amines, the distribution of vesicles within their terminals differs from that in the terminals in the neurohypophysis. In brain regions organized for neurotransmission, lucent synaptic vessels are often aggregated within terminals near a presynaptic thickening of the terminal membrane that borders a synaptic cleft. In the cerebrum, presynaptic TRH neurons are characterized by the presence of small lucent vesicles aggregated near the thickening of the presynaptic terminals, whereas the large granular vesicles are randomly distributed throughout the terminal (385). In the neurohypophysis this organizational pattern is seldom seen. The axon terminals are remarkably free of synaptic specializations, and synapses are not frequently found on TEM examination. Both large and small vesicles are randomly distributed within the axon terminals. Thickening of an axon terminal, when present, occurs at its free surface facing the outer basal lamina and the perivascular space. The neural systems in the neurohypophysis are not organized for neurotransmission but are organized for neurosecretion and release the contents of their vesicles into the extracellular space of the neurohypophysis or the perivascular space of its fenestrated capillaries. The termination of a secretory neuron near a blood vessel without an interposed blood-brain barrier constitutes the fundamental organizational pattern of the neurohypophysis.

Development of the Neurohypophysis

The saccus infundibuli is discernible on the 15th day of gestation in the fetal rat (402). At that time the floor of the third ventricle is made up only of six to ten layers of round or oval cells. The presumptive infundibular process is an oval mass of cells with its long axis directed perpendicular (not parallel, as in the adult case) to the floor of the diencephalon. The aboral wall of Rathke's pouch has become apposed to the presumptive neural lobe, and the oral wall has become apposed to the presumptive median eminence by this time. However, it is unlikely that migration of Rathke's pouch was induced by the presence of neurosecretory terminals, as none are present in the saccus infundibuli at this time (402,403). The capillaries, entrapped between the anterior (oral) wall of Rathke's pouch and the presumptive median eminence, display only a few fenestrations, but pinocytotic vesicles are present in their endothelial cells. Ependymal terminals, not neural terminals, lie in the perivascular space of this developing tuberal (mantle) plexus.

On the 16th fetal day, neuronal processes can be clearly identified in the ventral region of the developing median eminence in the rat. These neurites contain only a few electron-dense granules and neurotubules, and hence their site of origin in the hypothalamus cannot be deduced (402). They are oriented parallel to the ventral (oral) surface of the median eminence and lie between extended processes of ependymal cells (tanycytes) that stretch between the ventricular surface and the external surface of the median eminence. The nuclei of these stretched ependymal cells are indistinguishable from the nuclei of the primitive matrix cells found in abundance in the median eminence on day 15.

During the next two days (days 17 and 18) in the fetal life of the rat, the median eminence thickens as more axons enter it. The stretched ependymal cells lengthen in response to the thickening of the median eminence. The number of fenestra increases and the number of pinocytotic vesicles decreases in the endothelial tubes of the tuberal plexus at this time. Surface vascular connections are established by this plexus between the developing median eminence and the pars distalis. In the adenohypophysis mitotic figures are frequently found, and the Golgi apparatus becomes prominent in many of the developing glandular epithelial cells. Nerve fibers arrive in the neural lobe on the 17th day of gestation, one day after they were first demonstrated in the median eminence.

Neurohemal contact can first be detected by TEM in the rat and in the mouse median eminence 2 to 3 days before birth. Abundant numbers of large granular and small clear vesicles and of mitochondria are found within the enlarged neural terminals that have displaced ependymal terminals and lie next to the outer basal lamina in the perivascular space of fenestrated capillaries near the surface of the median eminence (402,404–406). Concurrently, dense-cored granules first appear in the cytoplasm of adenohypophysial cells (402). Immunoreactive GnRH-, SRIF-, and CRF-containing terminals are first identified in the rat median eminence on the 19th fetal day by TEM examination of immunostained material (405–407). Setalo et al. (408) could not detect immunoreactive GnRH in the median eminence of the rat with light microscopic techniques until the day of birth. However, TEM examination has demonstrated immunoreactive GnRH-containing fibers in the median eminence when light microscopic examination of immunostained sections failed (405). Similar findings are reported in mice in which immunoreactive GnRH was first detected in the median eminence 3 days prior to birth, on day 17 of gestation (409). Both neurohemal contact in the median eminence and the presence of immunoreactive LH in adenohypophysial cells could first be demonstrated on that day (403,410). The functional significance of these observations for the rodent fetus was questioned by Monroe and Paull (406), who demonstrated that neurohemal contact, although begun, was not "well established" until the day of birth. Freeze-fracture studies first demonstrated configurations suggesting exocytosis from nerve terminals on the third postnatal day. However, the number of adequate preparations from earlier time periods was limited, and exocytosis may have been initiated at an earlier stage (411). In the light of these limited and sometimes conflicting observations, it is not clear when the pituitary gland of the rat is first able to function.

The epithelium lining the saccus infundibuli also changes markedly with development. The infundibular recess in the rat brain is slit-like on the 15th and 16th days of gestation when viewed in coronal section. The ependymal cells of the saccus infundibulae are several layers thick and cannot be distinguished from the matrix cells. The floor of the ventricle is formed by round cells and by cells with apical processes, ovoid perikarya, and basal processes (412). The apical processes of these tanycytes line the ventricular surface and are bathed by ventricular fluid. Their basal processes abut the outer basal lamina and lie in the perivascular space of capillaries of the tuberal plexus, which are interposed between the rostral region of the saccus infundibuli and the oral lobe of Rathke's pouch. The tanycytes demonstrate polarity with the Golgi apparatus and mitochondria gathered in the apical process of each cell between the nucleus and the ventricular surface. The rough endoplasmic reticulum and ribosomes are poorly developed.

Between the 16th and 18th days, the number of these cells (relative to the thickness of the median eminence) decreases with the ingrowth of axons from the hypothalamus. The median eminence becomes thicker and the floor of the infundibular recess widens, increasing its ventricular surface. The apical processes of tanycytes shorten, bringing the nuclei closer to the surface. A second type of ependymal cell, which is cuboidal and without apical or basal processes, appears in the expanding epithelial lining. The number and types of organelles in the cytoplasm of the tanycytes (mitochondria, polysomes, lipid bodies, lysosomes, and laminated dense bodies) increases until in cross section the cells come to resemble those seen in adult animals (404). Gap junctions between ependymal cells are numerous on day 17, while the development of tight junctions is rudimentary. Tight junctions between ependymal cells of the ventricular floor in the infundibular recess are not mature until birth (413). The surface of the floor of the third ventricle remains flat, without microvilli or apical blebs throughout gestation. The specializations at the ventricular surface that are characteristic of some tanycytes in the adult median eminence do not appear until after birth.

By the 18th day of gestation, 3 days before birth, the thickness of the median eminence has attained one-half the thickness of the adult rat. Further differentiation of the median eminence will occur prior to and after birth, and the median eminence will not assume its adult morphology for several weeks (402–404,414,415). However, in the rat by the 18th day of gestation, the basic organizational pattern of the adult neurohypophysis has been established. The neurohypophysis has differentiated into an infundibular process (neural lobe), an infundibular stem, and an infundibulum (median eminence). Neurohemal contact has been initiated. The median eminence has further differentiated into an ependymal zone, an internal layer defined by the presence of the supraoptico-hypophysial tract, and an external layer of small axons and terminals (Fig. 9) (416–418).

Organization of the Neurohypophysis

Infundibular Process

The principal elements of the neural lobe as ascertained by light microscopy are nerve terminals, glial cells called *pituicytes,* and capillaries (27). Transmission electron microscopic studies of the neural lobe have been

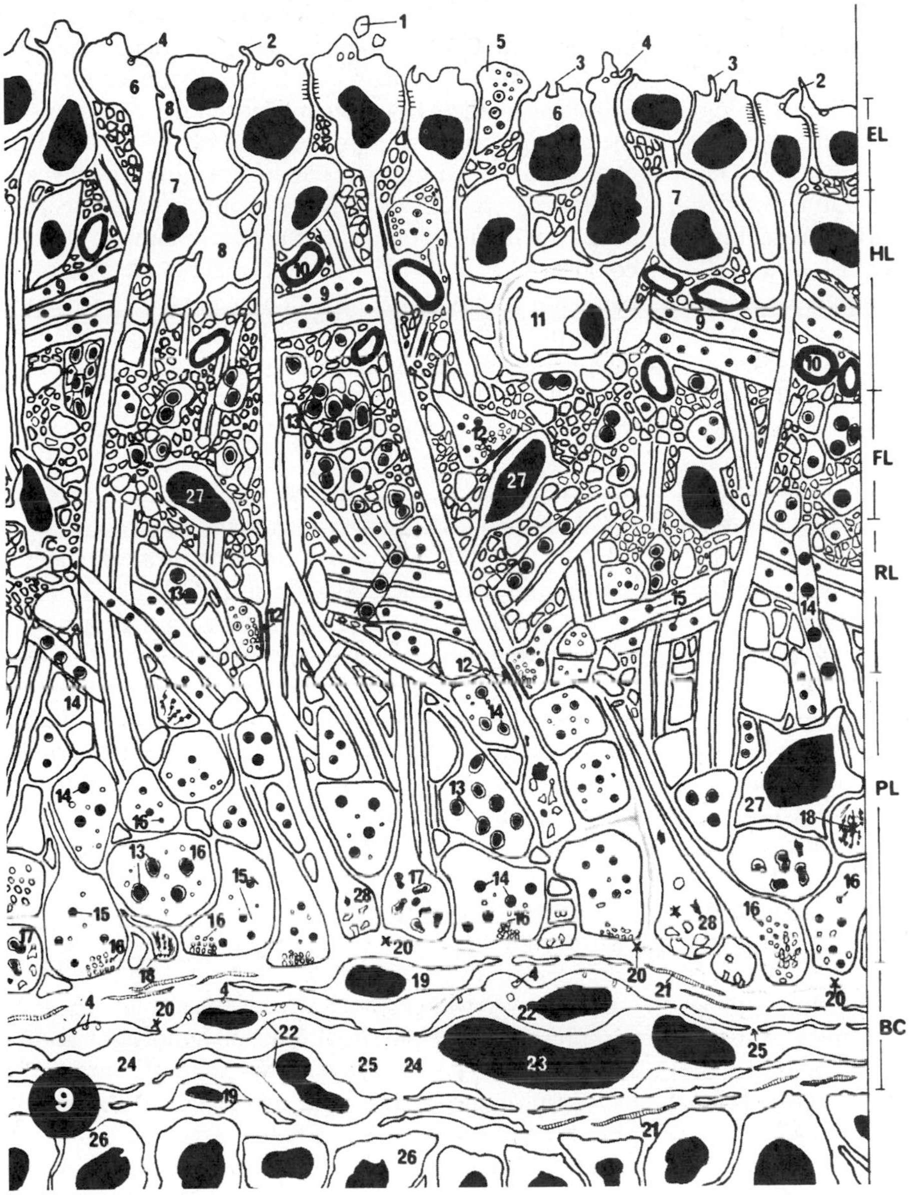

FIG. 9. Diagram of the fine structure of the rat median eminence. *BC*, capillaries of the primary plexus; *EL*, ependymal layer; *FL*, fiber layer; *HL*, hypendymal layer; *PL*, palisade layer; *RL*, reticular layer. *1*, Cytoplasmic masses released from ependymal cells into the third ventricle; *2*, marginal fold; *3*, finger-like microvilli; *4*, pinocytotic vesicles; *5*, monoaminergic axon terminals protruding into the third ventricle; *6*, ependymal cell; *7*, hypendymal cell; *8*, intercellular cavity; *9*, commissure of monoaminergic axons; *10*, myelinated axon; *11*, capillaries (note thin pericapillary space; *12*, synaptoid contact; *13*, large granule; *14*, intermediate granule; *17*, *18*, two types of unidentified processes; *19*, fibroblast; *20*, basement membranes; *21*, collagen fiber; *22*, endothelial cell; *23*, red cell; *24*, capillary lumen; *25*, fenestration; *26*, pars tuberalis cell; *27*, glial cell; *28*, terminal of ependymal, hypendymal, or glial process. (From ref. 416, with permission.)

performed in the rat (351,370), mouse (419), rabbit (371), and human (356,357), as well as in submammalian species (373). A basic picture of nerve terminals in the perivascular space of fenestrated capillaries is maintained, and differences between mammalian species at the ultrastructural level are not marked. The axons of the supraoptico-hypophysial tract in the neural lobe are not uniform in diameter. Discrete swellings along the course of these axons give them a varicose appearance. Swellings contain dense-cored vesicles but not lucent vesicles, a feature that helps to differentiate them from terminals. Large swellings, filled with dense-cored vesicles, are called *Herring bodies.* Pulse labeling experiments suggest that newly synthesized hormone is first transported in dense-cored vesicles to terminals, but subsequently the hormone is transported to the axon swellings if the hormone newly arrived at the axon terminal is not released (420).

Swellings have been viewed traditionally as a site for storage of hormones. More recently, Tweedle et al. (421) made three-dimensional reconstructions of axons, axonal swellings, and axon terminals and neighboring terminals. Individual axons made multiple contacts with a target capillary through axonal swellings before ending in a terminal. The authors proposed that, with brief stimulation, hormone is only released from large dense-cored vesicles in the terminals, but, with more prolonged stimulation, hormone release also occurs from the large dense-cored vesicles in the axonal swellings.

Most of the terminals in the neural lobe are large and contain dense-cored and lucent vesicles (373). Under resting conditions, oxytocin (OT) and vasopressin

(AVP) are stored in the large dense-cored vesicles in separate terminals of the supraoptico-hypophysial tract (422). In the rat, AVP-containing fibers are congregated centrally in the neural lobe, whereas OT-containing fibers lie peripherally (423). Somewhat surprisingly, in situ hybridization experiments have demonstrated OT mRNA in dense-cored granules in axons and terminals of the supraoptico-hypophysial tract (424). Stalk section abolished the signal confirming the conclusion the OT mRNA was present in the terminals and not in the pituicytes (425). The dogma that AVP and OT are always to be found in separate terminals and hence synthesized in separate cell populations has recently been challenged with the demonstration that both hormones can be found in the same in terminal (in the same dense-core vesicle) under conditions of chronic stimulation such as lactation (426).

Opioid peptides have been demonstrated in the neural lobe. However, the nature of the opioid peptides in the terminals in the neural lobe has been a matter of debate. Methionine (met) and leucine (leu)-enkephalin (ENK) were isolated from the rat neural lobe, and immunohistochemical light microscopic studies demonstrated immunoreactive leu-ENK in varicose fibers in the neural lobe. Their cell bodies in the paraventricular and supraoptic nuclei were reported to have the characteristics of magnocellular neurons (427). Zamir (428) concluded on the basis of lesioning experiments that met- and leu-ENK have different cells of origin and that separate populations of magnocellular neurons contribute to the met- and leu-ENK content of the posterior pituitary. Martin and Voigt (429) presented light microscopic studies that suggested (from examination of serial sections) that met-ENK is colocalized with OT and leu-ENK is colocalized with AVP. Martin et al. (430) subsequently reported colocalization of immunoreactive OT and met-ENK in dense-cored vesicles within magnocellular terminals. Met-enkephalin, proenkephalin, and OT have been localized by immunohistochemistry within the same magnocellular neurons in the bovine hypothalamus (431). Leu-enkephalin was colocalized in dense-cored vesicles with immunoreactive AVP, but, because staining was enhanced by trypsin pretreatment, the leu-ENK was believed to be incorporated into a larger prohormone. Because α-neoendorphin and dynorphin have also been colocalized with AVP and because the sequence of leu-ENK is found at the N terminus of these peptides, the antigenic sequence of leu-ENK demonstrated in the AVP-containing terminals was subsequently believed to be contained within these larger molecules (430). This conclusion is strengthened by the observation that the products of proenkephalin processing are not found in AVP-containing neurons, but dynorphin-A-(1-8) and the other products of preprodynorphin processing (including leu-ENK) are colocalized with AVP in terminals in the rat neural lobe (432).

Whether met-ENK is colocalized in magnocellular neurons with OT or is found in terminals of parvicellular neurons has been a matter of debate. Evidence for colocalization with OT within magnocellular terminals in the neural lobe has already been presented. VanLeeuwen et al. (433) have reported that enkephalins are localized in granular vesicles of about 120 nm in diameter and hence not in the terminals of magnocellular neurons that contain AVP or OT. These terminals made synaptoid contact with pituicytes. Merchenthaler et al. (434) could not demonstrate met-ENK in OT-containing magnocellular neurons in the SON or PVN or in large axons in the internal zone of the median eminence. Opiate systems terminating in the neural lobe are believed to play an inhibitory role in the regulation of AVP and OT secretion (435,436).

Other peptides have also been found to be colocalized with AVP or OT. Neurons containing immunoreactive gastrin-like and cholecystokinin (CCK)-like peptide have been demonstrated to arise in the paraventricular and supraoptic nuclei and to terminate in the neural lobe of the rat (437). Based on light microscopic examination of immunostained sections of the rat hypothalamus, Kiss et al. (438) concluded that immunoreactive cholecystokinin is colocalized with oxytocin. Galanin (GAL) has been demonstrated by immunohistochemical techniques to be colocalized with OT (439) and with AVP (440). In addition, immunoreactive substance P is present in terminals in the mouse neural lobe in the same distribution as AVP-containing terminals (441,442). Large terminals of the magnocellular system could thus contain AVP with its associated neurophysin II (443), vasopressin, neurophysin II, and/or dynorphin and/or substance P; OT with its associated neurophysin I (443); oxytocin, neurophysin I, and met-ENK or OT, neurophysin I and gastrin-like, CCK-like peptide.

Parvicellular terminals in the neural lobe contain large granular and small lucent vesicles (373). Thyrotropin-releasing hormone-containing fibers are abundant in the rat neural lobe (444). Somatostatin-containing fibers are also present in the rat neural lobe but in fewer numbers (423,445). The axons of the dopaminergic tuberohypophysial tract terminate in the neural lobe (446–448) in close proximity to AVP terminals (449). Colocalization of immunoreactive serotonin within immunoreactive tyrosine hydroxylase (TH) terminals has been demonstrated (341). Immunoreactive GABA-containing terminals have been demonstrated in the neural lobe by light microscopy (335–337). Immunohistochemical studies at the ultrastructural level have demonstrated immunoreactive GABA within clear microvesicles but also within large granular vesicles of parvicellular terminals (450–452). Colocalization with immunoreactive TH has been demonstrated by immunohistochemistry (340,342). Thus dopamine, serotonin, and GABA are colocalized within some parvicellular terminals in the neural lobe.

Norepinephrine has been isolated in the neurointermediate lobe of the rat pituitary. The concentration of norepinephrine decreased by only ~30% with bilateral superior cervical ganglionectomy (453). It decreased by ~70% following stalk section (449). A recent study has reported the presence of immunoreactive dopamine β-hydroxylase (DBH) in terminals in the neural lobe (331). A retrograde transport study employing injection of horseradish peroxidase (HRP) into the neural lobe of the rat demonstrated HRP-containing neurons in the dorsal vagal nucleus of the medulla (454). The presence of a central noradrenergic system that terminates in the neural lobe seems to be well accepted, but the details of its terminus, or even of its origins, are not firmly established.

Both dopamine and GABA are inhibitory to the release of neurohormones in the neural lobe. Incubation of isolated neurointermediate lobes in medium containing dopamine reduced the release of milk ejecting factor into the media (455). The amount of OT released from incubated neurointermediate lobes was increased when incubated with α-methyltyrosine (456). Dopamine agonists suppressed the release of AVP from incubated neurointermediate lobes that had been electrically stimulated (457). Dynorphin, coreleased with AVP, is posited to suppress release of OT from neighboring terminals in a paracrine fashion. This postulate is based on the observation that the administration of naloxone to dehydrated or stressed rats increased the plasma levels of oxytocin (435). *In vitro* study of the release of oxytocin and vasopressin from incubated neurointermediate lobes following electrical stimulation at frequencies of 4, 8, 12, and 29 Hz was carried out by Bondy et al. (436). Release of OT and AVP was increased by about 20% at 4 Hz (submaximal). Under these conditions the addition of a dynorphin κ receptor agonist reduced the amount of OT released into the medium. This reduction in OT release was blocked by naloxone. Maximal AVP release was achieved at 12 Hz. It was postulated that with maximal release of AVP there would be maximal release of endogenous costored dynorphin and hence no observed effect of added dynorphin. At 12 Hz, the addition of exogenous dynorphin produced no decrease in OT release, but addition of naloxone resulted in an increase in OT release. These findings are consistent with a paracrine role for dynorphin that suppresses OT release during stimulated release of AVP from magnocellular terminals.

Serotonin is also present in small terminals in the neural lobe and is colocalized with dopamine (341) in terminals of parvicellular neurons. Glutamate has been demonstrated in magnocellular terminals of the neural lobe, as previously discussed. In addition, nitric oxide has recently been found in the neural lobe (458). Whereas the roles of serotonin and glutamate are generally held to be stimulatory, the role of nitric oxide in the regulation of neurosecretion is yet to be clarified. The literature cited strongly suggests that peptides costored in magnocellular neurons and transmitters released from parvicellular terminals act locally in the neural lobe to regulate OT and AVP secretion.

Species variations in the distribution and content of the magnocellular and parvicellular systems terminating in the neural lobe, of course, exist. In fishes, arginine vasotocin is released from magnocellular terminals, whereas in amphibians isotocin and mesotocin are released from these terminals. Even among mammals, differences are present. Gonadotropin-releasing hormone, not present in the neural lobe of the rat (423), is present in the neural lobe of bats, ferrets, monkeys, and humans (459). In the pig, CRF terminals are reported to lie in the perivascular space of the neural lobe in the same distribution as do AVP-containing fibers (460).

Until recently glial cells of the neural lobe have received little attention. In the 1930s, they were considered to be the parenchymous elements of the neural lobe and the source of its secretions (24). When the source of neural lobe hormone was found to be the nerve terminals resident there, and not the glial cells, interest in pituicytes waned. Takei et al. (461) classified pituicytes into five types. "Major pituicytes" resembled cerebral astrocytes, and their processes were frequently found in the perivascular space of capillaries. "Dark pituicytes" resembled major pituicytes but were more electron dense. "Ependymal pituicytes" contained cilia. "Oncocytic pituicytes" contained abundant numbers of mitochondria in their cytoplasm and were only occasionally observed. "Granular pituicytes" contained numerous cytosegresomes (electron-dense granules that are round or irregular in shape and are usually surrounded by a single membrane). These authors postulated that granular tanycytes are involved in the uptake and catabolism of extracellular material. The significance of ependymal and oncocytic pituicytes is not known (461).

The roles of "major" and "dark" pituicytes have been evaluated by Tweedle, Hatton, and co-workers (462–468). They have shown that the relationship between terminals of the supraoptico-hypophysial tract and glial cells is not static (466,467). Under resting conditions, glial processes enclosed terminals of the supraoptico-hypophysial tract and lay interposed between these terminals and the basal lamina of the perivascular space. Synaptoid contact between nerve terminals and glial cells was occasionally found (462). With dehydration (deprivation of water for 24 hours), the number of enclosed axons decreased, and more exposed terminals were present in the perivascular space (463). If the neural lobe was removed and incubated in hyperosmotic medium (as compared with incubation in a medium of low osmotic strength), the number of enclosed neurons was similarly decreased (468). In an analogous manner, the number of enclosed neurons was decreased in postpartum and lactating rats compared with control females (464,465).

They went on to investigate the differences in response to acute (~48 hours) and chronic (10 to 14 day) stimuli. In the acute situation ultrastructural findings in the neural lobe of female rats were compared on the last day of pregnancy and on the day of parturition. Neural lobe ultrastructure was also compared between rats deprived of water for 48 hours and control (hydrated) rats. In the chronic stimulation paradigm, the ultrastructure of the neural lobe of female rats following 14 days of lactation was compared with that of controls and with those of female rats 10 days following weaning (recovery). Male rats were given a 2% solution of sodium chloride to drink for 10 days. The ultrastructures of their neural lobes were compared with those of hydrated animals and with those of dehydrated animals following 2 to 5 weeks of rehydration. In acute situations pituicytes withdrew, leaving fewer enclosed and more exposed nerve terminals. The number of nerve terminals did not change, but there was a change in the shape of the terminals, which became flattened. In chronic situations the pituicytes also withdrew, leaving the exposed axon swellings and terminals in close proximity to the basal lamina. The number of terminals increased, and they assumed a flattened shape (469). The authors postulated that withdrawal of the pituicyte processes exposed the axonal swellings to the basal lamina. The close relationship of the basal lamina to the axonal swellings induced the formation of small lucent vesicles in the axonal swellings. Axonal swellings were thus converted into axonal terminals, and the number of terminals increased (421).

The change in shape of the pituicytes, which both exposes and (indirectly) creates more (en passant) terminals, could be initiated by β-adrenergic stimulation, and β-adrenergic receptors have been demonstrated on pituicytes (470,471). Whether the source of β-agonists is the terminals of catecholaminergic neurons in the neural lobe (see above) or circulating catecholamines secreted by the adrenal is currently a matter of investigation. Kappa (κ) opioid receptors are also present on the surface of pituicytes (472), and terminals containing an antigenic site common to enkephalins or dynorphins make synaptoid contact with pituicytes (433). Bicknell (473) suggested that opioids released from nerve terminals could activate pituicytes to change their spatial relationship locally with magnocellular nerve terminals. Whereas the interaction of opioid peptides and neurotransmitters serves to regulate selective secretion of OT and AVP, the interactions between glial cells and nerve terminals (474), along with an increase in the release of hormone from nerve terminals (475), an increase in neural lobe blood flow (476) and metabolism (477), and an increase in the permeability of the neural lobe (478) serve to facilitate the movement of neurohypophysial hormones from the nerve terminal to the bloodstream in response to specific physiological stimuli.

Infundibular Stem

The principal elements of the infundibular stem are axons of the magnocellular systems and axons and terminals of the parvicellular systems. There is considerable variation in the length of the infundibular stem among mammals; for example, the length of the infundibular stem of the cat is very short, whereas that of the ferret or human is very long (78). In addition to axon terminals containing TRH and SRIF, the rat's infundibular stem contains terminals that stain for GnRH (161), CRF (479), GRH (480), and neurotensin (481).

Infundibulum (Median Eminence)

The ependymal layer of the median eminence lines the infundibular recess. It is interposed between the neuropil of the median eminence and the ventricular fluid of the third ventricle (Fig. 9). The ependymal cells comprising the epithelial lining of the infundibular recess differ in appearance from the extrachoroidal ependymal cells that comprise the epithelial lining of the remainder of the ventricular system. The ependymal layer of the median eminence is not ciliated. Scanning electron microscopic studies of the third ventricular surface and of the infundibular recess have been carried out in frogs (482), birds (483), rats (484,485), mice (486), cats (487), rabbits (488), mink (489), sheep (490), monkeys (491), humans (486,492), and even in armadillos (493). The basic pattern is similar in each of these species. Ependyma overlying the dorsal third ventricle is ciliated. In the ventral regions of the third ventricle, the number of ciliated cells decreases at about the level of the ventral medial hypothalamic nuclei. As the infundibular recess is approached (at the level of the arcuate nuclei), ciliated cells become widely separated and sparse. The ventricular surface is lined by cells with abundant microvilli. This region between the ciliated ependyma of the dorsal third ventricle and the ependyma overlying the infundibular recess is called the *transition zone.* It overlies the ventromedial and arcuate hypothalamic nuclei. Beneath the level of the tuberoinfundibular recess, the surface of the ventricular lining again changes. In the walls of the lateral recess, the cell surfaces become elevated and take on the appearance of cobblestones. Apical excrescences or blebs are seen at the cell surface (Fig. 10).

The floor of the infundibular recess shows regional variation in its appearance. Studies in the rabbit (494) demonstrate that the ependymal lining in the anterior third ventricular recess is a flattened, squamous epithelium with a smooth surface. In the middle third the surface of the cells is covered by microvilli. In the posterior third the surface of each cell is raised. Many apical blebs protrude from the elevated surface and give the cell a

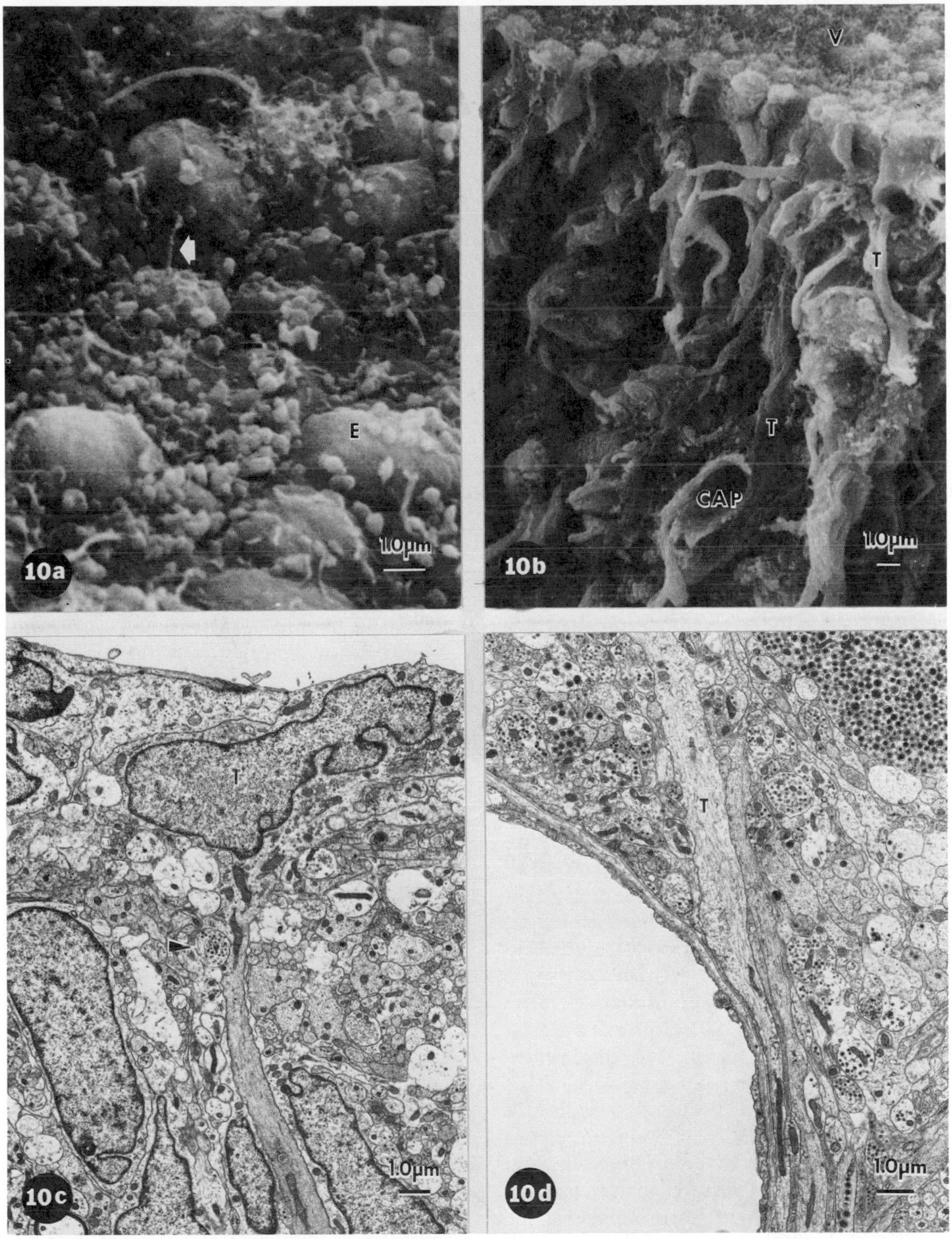

FIG. 10. **A:** Scanning electron micrograph of the floor of the rabbit third ventricle overlying the median eminence. *White arrowhead* points to microvilli. *Black arrow* points to an apical bleb. *E,* the surface of one ependymal cell. Note the profusion of apical blebs in this (posterior) region of the infundibular recess. From ref. 873, with permission. **B:** Scanning electron micrograph of median eminence neuropil. Median eminence has been broken, thus exposing tissue between ventricular lumen (*V*) at the top and pial surface (not shown) at bottom. Tanycytes (*T*) lining the rabbit infundibular extend from the ventricular surface (*V*) to median eminence capillaries (*CAP*). Apical surface of tanycytes contains microvilli. From ref. 874, with permission. **C:** Transmission electron micrograph of rabbit median eminence. Tanycyte (*T*) sends basal process vertically through neuropil to the oral surface. In this region of the infundibular recess the ependymal cells are smooth. The organelles are concentrated in the cell body. A neurite (*at arrowhead*) contacts the basal process at its neck. Aggregated microtubules give the basal process a filamentous appearance. **D:** Transmission electron micrograph of rabbit median eminence. A tanycyte terminal (*T*) as well as neural terminals lie in the perivascular space of a fenestrated capillary. (From ref. 1067, with permission.)

riveted appearance. A somewhat different regional variation is reported in the rat (495), but flat, smooth, microvilliated, and riveted cells with apical excrescences are also present. These blebs contain few organelles (484,496–498) and no secretory granules. Supraependymal cells (neurons and macrophages) lie on the ependymal surface in the floor of the infundibular recess (497–500).

Tanycytes contribute to the ependymal lining, which overlies the hypothalamus in the ventral region of the third ventricle and the median eminence in the infundibular recess. Light microscopic studies of the distribution and morphology of tanycytes in the rat (501–504) and quail (505) have been reported extensively. Tanycytes are bipolar ependymal cells with a soma, a short apical process that extends to the ventricular surface, and a long basal process. The basal process is subdivided into a neck, a tail, and a terminal. Akmayev and Popov (506) designated tanycytes in the transition zone that overlies the hypothalamus of the rat as α-tanycytes. β-Tanycytes are found in the ependyma overlying the lateral recess (β_1) or lining the floor of the infundibular recess (β_2).

α-Tanycytes are present in the transition zone of the third ventricle, and they stretch between the ventricular surface and the ventromedial and arcuate hypothalamic nuclei, where they may terminate on neurons or capillaries in these hypothalamic regions (501,505) or they may terminate on the pial surface of the tuber cinereum (502). Their apical processes are insinuated between ciliated ependymal cells in the epithelium lining the transition zone. The ventricular surface of the apical processes contains many microvilli. Occasional apical protrusions are present. Mitochondria, ribosomes, and numerous tubules are present in their apical cytoplasm. Adjacent apical processes are interdigitated and linked by gap junctions and desmosomes. Zonulae occludens were not found in this region by Brawer (507). Gotow and Hashimoto (508) divided the ventral region of the third ventricle (the transition zone) into two regions, (a) dorsal to the level of the arcuate nucleus and (b) ventral to the level of the arcuate nucleus. In the dorsal region, tight junctions were not found on TEM examination of freeze-fracture replicas. Ventral to the level of the arcuate nucleus, tight junctions were found. They increased in number in the lateral recess and in the floor of the infundibular recess over the median eminence. Furthermore, the number of rows of particles that comprise the tight junctions in freeze-fracture replicas and the density of particles per row increased as they examined specimens from the transition zone through the lateral recess onto the floor of the infundibular recess. These findings indicate an increasing tightness of the intercellular junctions in a centripetal pattern centered on the floor of the infundibular recess.

The soma of α-tanycytes contains the same complement of organelles and inclusions as epithelial cells in general. The ovoid nucleus contains a single large nucleolus. The Golgi apparatus, free ribosomes, and mitochondria are present in the soma. Vesicles associated with the Golgi and lysosomes are also found. The basal process contains a distinctive array of microtubules that are oriented parallel to the long axis of the process. In the neck, the endoplasmic reticulum elaborates "concentric shells of smooth cisternae" (507). The neck and tail of the basal processes contain a varied collection of inclusions and organelles, including short tubules of endoplasmic reticulum and vesicles of differing shapes and sizes. Ependymal processes have been found to terminate on the basement membrane in the perivascular space of capillaries in the arcuate nucleus (507).

β-Tanycytes in the ependymal layer of the median eminence are stretched between the ventricular surface and the perivascular space of fenestrated capillaries on the surface of the median eminence (501). Akmayev and Popov (506) cited several ultrastructural differences between tanycytes in the epithelium lining the third ventricle (α-tanycytes) and tanycytes in the ependymal layer of the median eminence (β-tanycytes). At the surface of the β-tanycytes are apical blebs, which are granular on TEM appearance and contain no secretory granules or organelles. The β-tanycytes lining the infundibular recess are more fibrillar in appearance than the α-tanycytes lining the third ventricular walls due to the striking number of microtubules in their cytoplasm. They contain a well-developed system of membranous cavities and cisternae and a system of mitochondrion-borne tubules (509). Spine-like protrusions project from the basal process. Their inner structure differs from that of the α-tanycyte processes, as they contain polysomes, lipid droplets, and a unique collection of vesicles. Smooth, dense-cored vesicles 40 to 50 nm in diameter lie in the Golgi area. Coated vesicles in the soma and in terminals form omega figures with the plasmalemma in these regions. Dense-cored vesicles about 100 nm in diameter also lie in the soma, neck, tail, or terminal. Frequently rosettes or arrays of vesicles about 100 nm in diameter are present in terminals, where glycogen bodies and lipid inclusions are prominent (510). Terminals of the β-tanycytes lie in the perivascular space of fenestrated capillaries on the surface of the median eminence. Their apical processes along with squamous and cuboidal ependymal cells form the ependymal layer of the median eminence.

Adjacent epithelial cells in the ependymal layer of the median eminence are joined by zonulae occludens as well as by gap junctions and desmosomes (511–513). Brightman et al. (512) found that junctions become increasingly tight (exhibited more particles per row and more rows per junction) as the infundibular floor is approached from the transition zone. They proposed that the lining of the ventricle formed a graded sieve, more porous at the periphery than at the center. Their findings were substantiated by Gotow and Hashimoto (508), who found that HRP could pass between ependymal cells in the transition zone but not between ependymal cells lining the lateral recess of the third ventricle. In this region, microperoxidase could pass between the ependymal cells. In the floor of the infundibular recess, microperoxidase could not pass between ependymal cells, but 5-hydroxy-dopamine could pass by circumventing tight junctions.

Kobayashi et al. (514,515) reported that HRP passed between the third ventricle and the neuropil of the median eminence. This passage was presumably accomplished by "active" pinocytotic transport (516). The observation of synaptoid contact between neurosecretory terminals and tanycyte processes (517,518) encouraged the concept that such transport could be controlled by hypothalamic (neural) projections. The observation that the surface of the ependymal lining changed concurrent with the reproductive cycles of the monkey (519) had previously rekindled the idea of a humoral link between the third ventricle and the pituitary gland (1).

Ependymosecretion was proposed as a mechanism to supplement neurosecretion. Hypothalamic hormones released into the ventricular system (it was proposed) are transported from the ventricular lumen to portal capillaries and carried to the median eminence to regulate anterior pituitary function (520,521). Pilgrim (522) pointed out that the intensity of HRP staining of tanycytes reported by Kobayashi et al. (514) indicated cellular damage. He found no evidence of pinocytic transport. Enzyme systems indicative of active transport are not found in β-tanycytes in the median eminence but in α-tanycytes in the hypothalamus (523,524). The evidence against a role for the ependymal layer of the median eminence in hypothalamo-hypophysial interactions has been summarized by Pilgrim (522).

Although the transport role of tanycytes in the ependymal layer of the median eminence remains speculative, one role of this ependymal layer seems quite clear. This layer effectively separates the extracellular fluid of the median eminence from the ventricular fluid of the third ventricle. Although molecules as small as (5-hydroxy) dopamine could pass from the perivascular space of the internal zone of the median eminence into the third ventricle (508), this epithelial layer prohibits either the unregulated loss of hypothalamic hormones into the ventricular system or their dilution within the extracellular spaces of the median eminence (525). Rodriguez et al. (509) demonstrated that the basal processes of β-tanycytes in the rostral and postinfundibular palisade regions as well as in the lateral palisade region of the preinfundibular median eminence form a continuous cuff at the ventral (oral) surface of the rat's median eminence, which abuts the basal lamina about fenestrated capillaries. This cuff is composed of ependymal terminals linked by gap junctions and desmosomes that are interposed between neuronal terminals near the surface of the median eminence in its lateral thirds and the basal lamina. Only in the medial palisade zone of the rat median eminence do neurosecretory terminals directly contact fenestrated capillaries. The significance of this finding is not yet fully understood. Given the active role of pituicyte processes in neurosecretion in the neural lobe, an analogous role may be played by ependymal processes (526).

The internal zone lies beneath the ependymal layer of the vertebrate median eminence (79) (Fig. 9). In many species, for example, the rat (416) or the rabbit (353), it can be subdivided into a hypendymal layer and a fiber layer (417). The hypendymal layer lies directly beneath the ependymal layer and contains subependymal cells and pituicytes. In the rat, parvicellular axons projecting from the hypothalamus (383,527) are present in the hypendymal layer of the internal zone. Catecholaminergic terminals of the reticuloinfundibular tract projecting from the brainstem to the median eminence and of the reticulohypophysial tract projecting from the brainstem to the neurointermediate lobe were reported to be present in this zone on the basis of fluorescent microscopic studies (447). However, localization of terminals in the hypendymal layer that stain with immunoreactive DBH or immunoreactive phenylethanolamine-*N*-methyltransferase (PNMT) has not been reported. Scant neurites that stain for immunoreactive PNMT have been seen by the author in this zone (*unpublished observations*).

The fiber layer is defined by axons of the supraoptico-hypophysial tract (79,528). Although axon terminals of the magnocellular supraoptico-hypophysial tract are not found in the fiber layer, terminals of other systems are present (353). Of considerable interest is the recent observation that exocytosis, with release of hormone, occurs along the axons of the supraoptico-hypophysial tract (367). The functional significance of this observation has not as yet been revealed, but an *in vitro* study suggests that AVP release from large axons in the internal zone may reach the pars distalis through portal routes (529). The noradrenergic reticuloinfundibular tract terminates in the internal zone of the rat median eminence, principally in its medial third (161,383,530). Peptidergic neurons that contain the processed products of proopiomelanocortin, including ACTH, α-MSH, β-LPH, and β-END, terminate in the internal zone of the rat median eminence (531,532).

The external zone is comprised of nerve terminals, pituicytes, ependymal (tanycyte) terminals, and capillaries (416–418,533) (Fig. 9). Transmission electron microscopic studies of the external zone have been performed in the rat (351,355), rabbit (352), human (357), as well as in submammalian species (358,534,535). The external zone of the rat median eminence has been divided into a reticular layer and a palisade layer (416). The reticular layer lies between the fiber layer of the internal zone and the palisade layer of the external zone. It contains ependymal and glial processes and axons of parvicellular systems. The palisade layer lies between the reticular layer and the ventral surface of the median eminence. It is recognized by the presence of glial and tanycytic processes oriented at right angles to the ventricular surface of the infundibular recess on light microscopic examination (79,528) and by fascicles of axons and terminals (separated by tanycytic processes) in the perivascular space of median eminence capillaries on TEM examination (416,417,533). In the rat, the palisade layer may be further subdivided into a medial palisade layer (medial third) and lateral palisade layers (lateral thirds). The medial palisade layer lies beneath the floor of the infundibular recess. Each lateral palisade layer lies lateral to it and extends to the tuberoinfundibular sulcus (358).

Catecholamine-containing fibers in the external zone of the median eminence have been identified by light microscopy with formaldehyde fluorescence (536–538) or glyoxylic acid induced fluorescence (539–541). Fluorescence light microscopic studies demonstrated catecholamines in the palisade layer of the external zone (as well as in the hypendymal layer of the internal zone). Combining the fluorescence light microscopic technique with the use of selective enzyme inhibitors to halt synthesis of norepinephrine or dopamine, Lofstrom et al. (530) concluded that catecholamine containing fibers in the lateral palisade layer were predominantly dopaminergic and fibers in the medial palisade layer were both dopaminergic and noradrenergic. Ajika and Hökfelt (542) estimated the number of monoaminergic terminals to be one-third the total number of terminals in the median eminence. Over twice as many dopaminergic terminals are present in the lateral palisade layer as in the medial palisade layer of the rat's median eminence. A similar distribution of fluorescence has been found in the rabbit (543,544) and cat (545). As in the rat, fluorescence was maximal in the palisade layer of the external zone and the hypendymal layer of the internal zone in these animals.

Immunohistochemical studies have demonstrated two other neurotransmitters in the rat's median eminence—ACh (401,546) and GABA (335,336)—by demonstrating the presence of immunoreactive acetylcholinesterase or immunoreactive glutamic acid decarboxylase (GAD) in nerve terminals in the external zone. Histamine has also been demonstrated in terminals in the median eminence of the cat (547).

Other neurotransmitters are frequently colocalized in putative aminergic terminals. Some terminals that contain immunoreactive-TH, and which have been assumed to be dopaminergic, have been found to also contain GABA (identified by the presence of immunoreactive-GABA or GAD) (342). Neuropeptides have been identified within classic aminergic terminals. Neurotensin (NT) has been identified in the palisade layer of the rat's median eminence (481), and it has been colocalized with dopamine (548). Galanin has been demonstrated in TH-like cells projecting to the median eminence (549). However, not all of the immunoreactive TH terminals are dopaminergic. Some apparently lack dopa-decarboxylase and cannot convert dopa to dopamine. These cells are dopaergic (550).

Hypophysiotropic parvicellular systems terminate in the palisade layer of the external zone. Their distribution has been reviewed extensively (161), and this discussion will concentrate primarily on more recent findings. Gonadotropin-releasing hormone has been localized within large granular vesicles within terminals that, at infundibular levels of the median eminence, lie in the lateral palisade layer. In the guinea pig median eminence, delta sleep inducing peptide has been localized in the same terminals as GnRH. At the ultrastructural level the two immunoreactive hormones were in the same large granular vesicles (551). In the pre- and postinfundibular median eminence, GnRH fibers were more uniformly distributed between the medial and lateral palisade layers (161,388). If preembedding immunohistochemical techniques were employed on vibrotome sections, more GnRH was found in the medial palisade zone than was found in paraffin-embedded thick sections, and the differences between the medial and lateral palisade layers was less striking (552). Simultaneous localization of GnRH- and dopamine-containing terminals demonstrated GnRH fibers preferentially in the lateral palisade zone of the rat's median eminence in close relationship to dopamine containing fibers (553,554). On examination of their light microscopic preparations, which were fluorescence stained for dopamine terminals and immunohistochemically stained for GnRH, McNeill and Sladek (553) found one population of aminergic terminals closely associated with portal vessels and a second population of aminergic terminals closely related to GnRH-containing terminals. They proposed that dopaminergic terminals inhibit GnRH released from peptidergic terminals through axoaxonic synapses. Dopamine-containing terminals have been found closely apposed to GnRH-containing terminals in TEM studies of the rat median eminence (555), and synapses between immunoreactive TH terminals and immunoreactive GnRH terminals have been reported in the ewe (556). Although synapses were not reported in the rat, an interaction between dopamine- and GnRH-containing terminals seems certain. In agreement with the findings of Rodriguez et al. (509), Ohtsuka et al. (388) found that GnRH terminals did not reach the basal lamina at the surface of the lateral palisade zone in the rat median eminence. Most lay at a distance greater than 0.5 μm from the perivascular space and were separated from it by a "glioependymal cuff." This arrangement was not found in the ewe's median eminence, where the GnRH terminals contacted the basal lamina of the perivascular space (557). The studies in the rat need to be repeated, and correlations need to be made between the state of the reproductive cycle and the relationship of the GnRH terminals to the basal lamina and the tanycyte and pituicyte processes.

Species differences in the distribution of GnRH terminals have been stressed by Anthony et al. (459). In primates, GnRH-staining fibers were found in the internal zone of the median eminence and could be followed into the infundibular stem and process. The authors pointed out that GnRH terminals in the neural lobe lay juxtaposed to regions in the pars distalis that are rich in gonadotropes and that "short portal" vascular connections between the neural lobe and pars distalis are ample in these animals. It is not clear whether a relationship of GnRH terminals to dopamine terminals is maintained in the neural lobes of these animals.

TRH terminals are aggregated in the medial palisade layer (161,444,552). These terminals lie in the perivascular space of capillaries in the median eminence (386). Somatostatin-containing fibers are found throughout the external and internal zones of the median eminence in the rat (161,558). These terminals, like those that contain TRH, lie in the perivascular space of capillaries (388). Growth hormone-releasing hormone immunostained fibers are distributed in a pattern similar to somatostatin fibers in the rat median eminence (559,560). Corticotropin-releasing factor terminals also lie principally in the medial palisade layer of the external zone (517,561–563) in the rat and in an analogous site in the monkey (564). Vasopressin, angiotensin II, enkephalin, NT, GABA, and CCK have been colocalized in CRF neurons by immunohistochemistry (565–568).

Vasopressin-containing neurons also terminate in the palisade layer of the median eminence, principally in its medial region (569–573). In the guinea pig these terminals contain large granular vesicles (90 to 110 nm in diameter), not the large dense-cored vesicles (>150 nm in diameter) in which hormones are localized in terminals in the neural lobe (365,574). In the pre- and postinfundibular regions of the rat's median eminence, there was considerable overlap between the distribution of immunoreactive CRF and AVP. In the infundibular region only a few AVP fibers were found in the palisade zone, whereas CRF-containing fibers were plentiful there (575). Vasopressin is costored with CRF in parvicellular neurons (576). Vasopressin and CRF are stored in the same secretory vesicles (577). Only about 50% of the CRF-containing terminals in the rat's median eminence costored AVP (578). Whether all AVP-containing terminals costore CRF has not yet been determined. High concentrations of AVP (579) and of CRF (580) have been found in portal blood. The presence of high concentrations of AVP (579) in portal blood has, until recently, been used as evidence that vasopressinergic terminals are plentiful and have ample access to capillaries in the median eminence. However, the concentration of AVP in portal blood is higher than expected when compared with the concentration of CRF if it is assumed that AVP can only be released with CRF and then only from 50% of the CRF terminals (578). The demonstration that AVP is released from axons of passage in the internal zone (367) raises the possibility that AVP in the portal vessels draining the median eminence has several sources—one from parvicellular terminals in the external zone and another from magnocellular axons in the internal zone. Still another possibility is a retrograde flow of blood from the neural lobe to the median eminence (581).

Parvicellular AVP-containing neurons were described as coursing ventrally, at right angles to the fiber layer, to gain access to capillaries in the external zone in this region. This pattern was accentuated after adrenalectomy (575). Immunogold electron microscopy has been employed to assess the changes in CRF and AVP terminals after adrenalectomy (582). Whereas immunogold staining of CRF remained constant, the density of particles over neurosecretory vesicles was increased when the tagged antibody was directed against AVP. Thus the amount of AVP in the terminals increased with respect to the amount of CRF following hypophysectomy. Vasopressin potentiates CRF stimulated ACTH release from corticotropes (583,584). Increased AVP release from parvicellular terminals (and magnocellular axons of passage) provides a means to increase the output of ACTH in response to stress.

Other neuropeptides besides the classic neurosecretions and the hypophysiotropic peptides have been demonstrated in the median eminence. Terminals containing immunoreactive angiotensin II (ANG II) have been identified by immunohistochemistry in the palisade zone of the rat's median eminence. Some ANG II cells costored CRF (see above), and their staining was selectively enhanced by adrenalectomy (585). Immunoreactive GAL is present in terminals in the external zone (586,587) and has been colocalized with neurotransmitters (immunoreactive GAD and TH [384,440]) and a releasing hormone (GRH) (588). Galanin terminals contact terminals that contain large granular vesicles and those that contain only microvesicles as well as pituicytes and tanycyte processes (589). Substance P has been localized to the external zone of the rat (161), the mouse (441), the monkey, and the human (590) median eminence. Immunoreactive ENK (161), immunoreactive vasoactive intestinal peptide (161), immunoreactive neurotensin NT (481), immunoreactive neuropeptide Y (ir-NPY) (591), immunoreactive CCK (438), and gastrin (161) have been identified in the palisade layer of the rat's median eminence. Calcitonin gene-related peptide (CGRP) has been identified in the median eminence of the frog (592).

Proopiomelanocortin derivatives are primarily localized by immunohistochemical techniques and light microscopy to the external zone of the median eminence in several species other than the rat. In the sheep and ox, β-LPH "projects to portal capillaries" (593). Bloch et al.

(594) found that, in humans, fibers containing immunoreactive β-END terminate "close to vessels in the median eminence." Such neurons are also reactive to antisera against ACTH, MSH, and β-LPH (595). Although species differences in the distribution of terminals containing the derivatives of POMC may be present, there seems to be general agreement that terminals in the median eminence are closely related to capillaries of the portal system, because ACTH and β-END are present in portal blood (596,597).

The pattern of regional segregation of neurosecretory systems within the neurohypophysis has been most clarified in the rat. The temptation to regard this pattern as a prototype for the mammalian hypophysis should be resisted at this time, because species differences may be marked. The distinction between the internal zone and the external zone is blurred in some mammalian species, including man, by invasion of the palisade layer into the internal zone (528). The site of termination of a particular neurosecretory system can also vary with the species studied (459). However, the basic organizational pattern of the mammalian neurohypophysis stands out clearly from the blurred background of differences in species detail: it is the relationship of individual neurosecretory hypophysiotropic terminals to capillaries and the regional segregation of systems of neurosecretory terminals within the neurohypophysis. Neurotransmitters such as dopamine, acetylcholine, GABA, serotonin, nitric oxide, and glutamate are coreleased with hypophysiotropic neurosecretions to act locally in an autocrine or paracrine fashion to coordinate the release of a particular peptide with the function of neighboring terminals. These locally acting transmitters and peptides may alter the secretion of peptides from neighboring terminals, alter the relationship of terminals to ensheathing pituicytes, and potentially alter the permeability of the region and the blood flow into it. It would seem no accident that the compounds involved in the initiation and maintenance of a local inflammatory response (histamine, serotonin, CGRP, substance P, and VIP) are released from terminals in the median eminence. It is tempting to speculate that, with release of hypophysiotropic secretions, local blood flow and permeability will increase as a result of the co-release of peptides and transmitters from nerve terminals in the perivascular space because blood vessels, not other nerves, will carry the messages released from axon terminals in the median eminence and neural lobe.

THE PORTAL SYSTEM

Capillaries of the Hypophysis

The capillaries and portal vessels of the pituitary gland carry blood from which oxygen, nutrients, and amino acids have been removed and to which metabolic waste products and peptide hormones have been added from the neurohypophysis to the adenohypophysis. These peptide hormones leave the blood to interact with receptors at the adenohypophysial cell's surface and to regulate their release of protein hormones which in turn enter the capillaries and are carried away from the gland. A single capillary bed extends throughout the entire neurohypophysis (29,598) (Fig. 11). It communicates by capillary or portal routes with similar appearing capillaries in the pars tuberalis and pars distalis of the adenohypophysis (66,599), and its perivascular space communicates extensively with the extracellular space of the pars intermedia (304). Hypophysial capillaries do not exclude acid vital dyes from the pituitary, which lacks a blood-brain barrier (29). Neurohypophysial (331,351,352,370) and adenohypophysial (212) capillaries are fenestrated, as are the portal vessels that unite them (352,599). These fenestrated capillaries are surrounded by a double basement membrane. The inner basal lamina lies next to each fenestrated endothelial tube, whereas the outer basal lamina is separated from it and lies next to the parenchymal elements (Figs. 7, 12). In the adenohypophysis, these parenchymal elements are epithelial cells arranged in cords. Because their capillaries are linearly arrayed (599), the configuration of the perivascular space is not complex (212). In the neurohypophysis these parenchymal elements are axons and their terminals, ependymal terminals, and glial cells. Pericytes, histiocytes, fibroblasts, microglia, and mast cells have been identified between the basal lamina in the perivascular space of human neural lobes (374). The inner and outer basal laminae define the perivascular space, which in the neural lobe of the mouse is 0.3 to 0.5 μm in width and

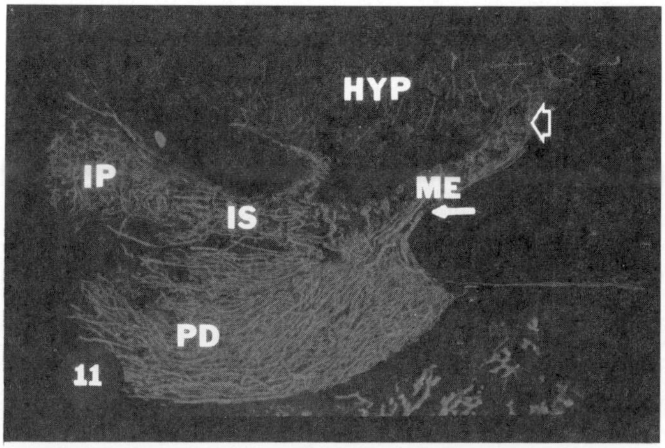

FIG. 11. Rabbit median eminence in sagittal section. A confluent capillary bed unites the median eminence (*ME*), infundibular stem (*IS*), and infundibular process (*IP*). Within the median eminence an external and an internal plexus may be discerned. Connections between median eminence and hypothalamic capillaries are seen far rostrally at *open arrowhead*. Portal connections between median eminence and pars distalis (*PD*) are indicated by *white arrow*. *HYP, hypothalamus*. ×25. (From ref. 599, with permission.)

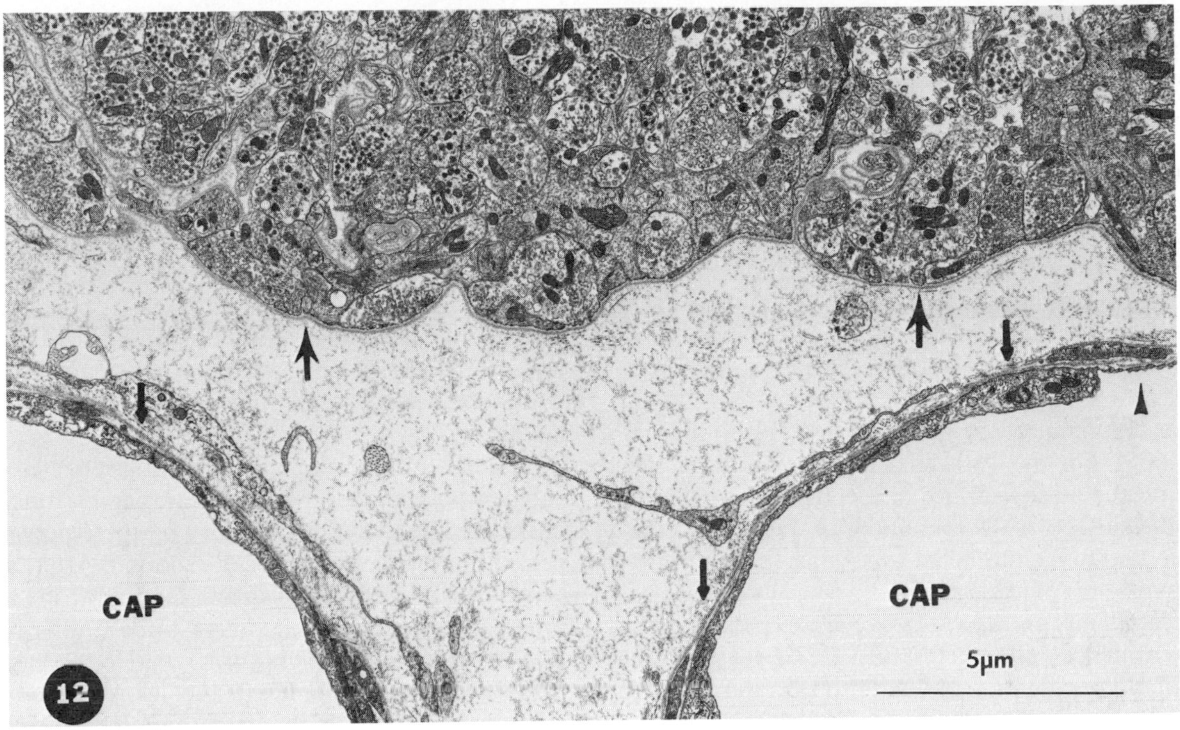

FIG. 12. Transmission electron micrograph of rabbit median eminence internal zone horizontal section. Two limbs of a capillary loop in the median eminence floor (*CAP*) are cut in horizontal section. One limb is fenestrated (*arrowhead*). The perivascular space is common to both. The outer basement membrane material is condensed at the margin of the contact zone common to both capillaries (*vertical large arrows*). The inner basement membrane is condensed about each individual capillary component (*vertical small arrows*). (From ref. 353, with permission.)

contains reticular fibers (600). In the median eminence of the rabbit it surrounds entire vascular formations (353). The perivascular space forms an extensive system of channels that are revealed with tannic acid staining (600) or silver impregnation (419). In the neural lobe these channels form a widespread system of connections between neighboring capillaries. In both the median eminence and neural lobe, extensions of the perivascular space increase the surface area available for neurohemal contact with a minimal increase in neurohypophysial volume.

Secretory elements in the hypophysis, neural or glandular, are disposed along the outer basal lamina of the perivascular space. Fenestrated capillaries are disposed along the inner basal lamina. Large protein molecules in the blood are relatively free to pass through fenestrae in the endothelial tube and interact with receptors at the cell's surface. Protein molecules sequestered in vesicles in the cell's cytoplasm are relatively free (after release into the perivascular space) to pass through the fenestrations in the capillaries into the bloodstream. This freedom of passage is not absolute, however, as, for example, basic dyes do not enter the hypophysis easily. Simionescu et al. (601,602) demonstrated the presence of microdomains in fenestrated endothelial cells of mouse pancreatic capillaries and "expected that these structures will select permeant molecules according to charge, in addition to size." Similar findings can be anticipated in the fenestrated endothelial cells of the hypophysis.

Development of the Portal System

Vessels of the hypophysis develop from the mesenchyme that is entrapped between the advancing saccus infundibuli and Rathke's pouch and invade both structures, according to Wislocki (603). Enemar (604) proposed that a (primary) plexus of capillaries lines the surface of the saccus infundibuli and a (secondary) plexus of capillaries lies on the surface of the Rathke's pouch in the mouse by the 14th fetal day. They are united by "linking" capillaries at the junction of the rostral portion of the saccus infundibuli and the oral wall of Rathke's pouch. These linking capillaries become more numerous by the 15th fetal day, and by the 16th fetal day in the life of the mouse the primary plexus of capillaries overlying the saccus infundibuli has become very dense. As the saccus infundibuli enlarges and differentiates over the next 2 days, the continuous capillary network over the presumptive median eminence, infundibular stem, and infundibular process increases in thickness and begins to invade the developing neurohypophysis. Concurrently, the presumptive pars distalis becomes more densely vascularized by invasion of capillaries from its surface. By the 19th fetal day, portal vessels on the ventral surface of the median eminence (which unite the primary and secondary capillary plexuses) have become distinct. This appearance is unchanged on the 20th (birth) day of the mouse. The capillary loops of the internal (deep) plexus in the median eminence do not appear until 2 to 3 days after birth and do not complete their development for 2 weeks. The deep system of long capillary loops and subependymal vessels is completed by 7 days, but the system of short capillary loops is not completed until 14 days of age.

The development of the pituitary vessels is similar in the rat (605). On the 15th fetal day capillaries of the primary plexus on the surface of the saccus infundibuli and on the surface of the remainder of the neural tube are nonfenestrated endothelial tubes that lie free in the mesenchyme. On that day, fenestrae have been found only in capillaries entrapped between the presumptive median eminence and pars distalis (375). Fenestrae did not attain the size, density, or distribution of those found in the adult rat neurohypophysial and adenohypophysial capillary beds until the 20th fetal day (378,411). Ugrumov et al. (606) identified some short capillary loops in the rat's median eminence on the 18th fetal day. Few mitotic figures were found at this time. They explained the formation of capillary loops by the growth and attenuation of preexisting cells, with buckling of the capillaries inward from the surface and invasion of the neuropil. A similar mechanism was reported by Page and Dovey-Hartman (353). In the rat, development of the internal plexus in the median eminence is delayed until after birth, as it is in the mouse (605), but this pattern is not representative of all mammals, as in the rabbit it is completed before birth (607).

Organization of the Portal System

The neurohypophysial capillary bed extends from the median eminence to the neural lobe. It is supplied rostrally by superior hypophysial arteries and caudally by inferior hypophysial arteries (598). A third source of arterial supply has been identified and variously named the *anterior hypophysial artery* (84), *peduncular artery* (608), *loral artery* (609), or *trabecular artery* (81,99). The name *middle hypophysial artery* seems more appropriate, because this vessel arises from the internal carotid artery between the origins of the inferior and superior hypophysial arteries. The inferior hypophysial arteries arise as a pair of vessels from the intracavernous segment of the internal carotid arteries and supply the neural lobe (infundibular process). Frequently they unite to form an anastomosis between the left and right internal carotid arteries prior to supplying the neural lobe. The middle hypophysial arteries also arise from the intracavernous segment of the internal carotid arteries. They frequently unite (as in the rabbit, rat, and cat) to form a single artery that then supplies the infundibular stem (598). The superior hypophysial arteries arise from the intracranial carotid arteries and from the circle of Willis. These (multiple) arteries approach the median eminence centripetally to form an anastomotic ring about it and to supply the rostral region of the neurohypophysis (the median eminence) (598,604,610). The arterial supply to the pituitary gland thus represents three ascending levels of anastomotic channels between the paired carotid arteries whose branches supply the neurohypophysial capillary bed.

Superior and inferior hypophysial arteries are innervated by postganglionic sympathetic nerves. Innervation of the middle hypophysial artery by these nerves is expected but has not as yet been reported. Arterioles that supply the neural lobe of the pig and rat (611) are also innervated by sympathetic fibers, but a similar innervation of arterioles supplying the rat (536,537) or rabbit (612) median eminence has not been found. Some arterioles on the surface of the median eminence receive an innervation by VIP/PHI-like containing fibers that do not appear to be central in origin (613). Additional peptides and amines can reach precapillary arterioles that lie on the surface of the median eminence (353).

The venous drainage of the caudal region of the neurohypophysial capillary bed mirrors its arterial supply. Paired inferior hypophysial veins course from the neural lobe to the posterior intercavernous sinus and to the posterior regions of the paired cavernous sinuses that lie lateral to the midline (610). A less prominent route of drainage is from the neural lobe to the adjacent pars distalis by capillary and "short portal" routes. Short portal veins uniting the neural lobe with the pars distalis are abundant in some species (i.e., rat, mouse, and rabbit) but few in others (pig, dog, monkey) (85,599). The hypophysial cleft limits the number and disposition of vascular connections between the pars distalis and the neurointermediate lobe. The neural lobe has ample venous drainage routes to the systemic circulation and limited venous drainage routes to the pars distalis (610). There are no direct venous drainage routes of the territory supplied by the middle hypophysial artery except for the short portal vessels that connect the infundibular stem with the pars distalis.

Venous drainage of the rostral region of the neurohypophysial capillary bed (the median eminence) does not mirror its arterial supply (29,66,81,82) (Fig. 13). The primary plexus in the median eminence is drained by fenestrated long portal vessels that course to the pars distalis and then arborize into a secondary capillary plexus. Direct capillary connections may also be plentiful, depending on the length of the infundibular stem and the species being examined (66,351,352,599). Drainage routes

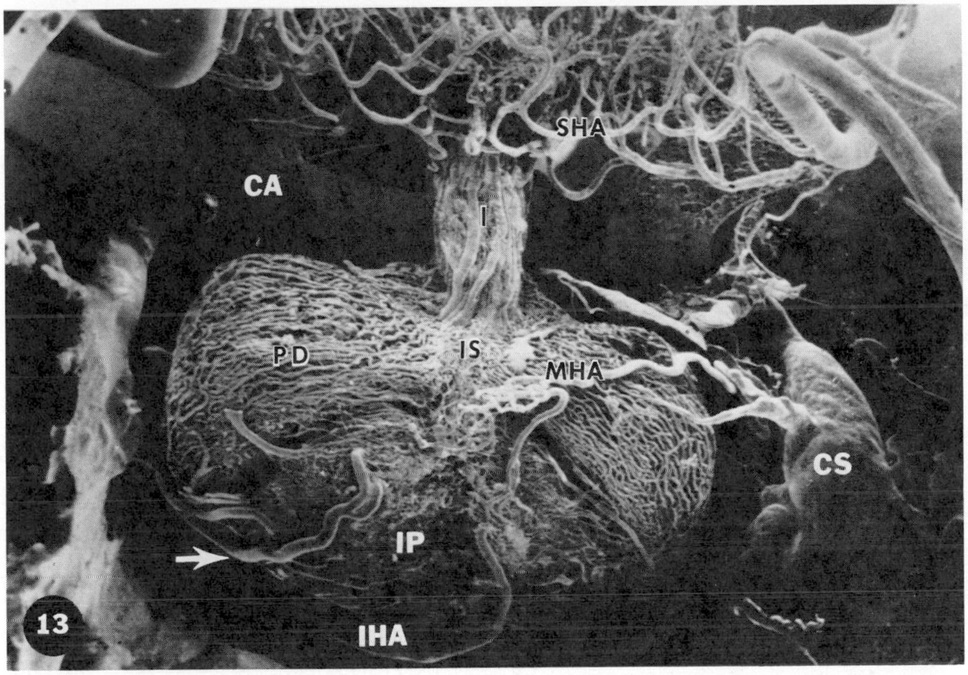

FIG. 13. Scanning electron micrograph of hypothalamic-pituitary vascular cast of the monkey as seen from behind. A common capillary bed extends throughout the infundibulum (*I*), infundibular stem (*IS*), and infundibular process (*IP*). It is supplied rostrally by superior hypophysial arteries (*SHA*) and caudally by inferior hypophysial arteries (*IHA*). Long portal vessels are present on the surface of the infundibulum. Lateral hypophysial veins from the pars distalis to the cavernous sinus (*CS*) are few in number. Y-shaped inferior hypophysial veins (*arrow*) drain both the pars distalis (*PD*) and the infundibular process. *MHA*, middle hypophysial artery; *CA*, carotid artery. (From ref. 610, with permission.)

from the primary capillary plexus in the median eminence to veins at the surface of the brain were denied by Wislocki (29,86–89). However, Duvernoy et al. (614) demonstrated systemic drainage routes from the postinfundibular median eminence in man, and Ambach et al. (615) have demonstrated venous channels from the preinfundibular median eminence to the tuberal and chiasmatic veins in the rat. In both cases drainage routes from the median eminence to these systemic sites were poorly developed, and they probably represent a regression of the ample venous connections between the saccus infundibuli and the remainder of the neural tube that were present prior to the apposition of the saccus infundibuli and Rathke's pouch and the development of portal vessels. Venous drainage routes from the rostral region of the neurohypophysial capillary bed, the median eminence, to the secondary capillary bed in the pars distalis are ample, whereas venous drainage routes to the systemic circulation are not.

The adenohypophysis, contrary to the belief of Wislocki (29,86–89), does not appear to receive a direct arterial supply (66,81,82,85,599). Blood destined for the adenohypophysis passes through the neurohypophysis. Capillaries and veins bring blood to the pars tuberalis and pars distalis.

Veins from the pars distalis to the paired cavernous and posterior intercavernous sinuses provide routes of egress for blood in the pars distalis. Named *lateral hypophysial* veins by Wislocki (29,86–89) on the basis of his study of the venous drainage of the monkey pars distalis, these veins were found by Green (616) to be a constant feature of the mammalian pars distalis. Bergland and Page (610) found that these veins, which drained the pars distalis, united with the veins that drained the neural lobe and drained through a common stem to the cavernous sinus. These Y-shaped veins drained both the pars distalis and the neural lobe.

The pattern of neural traffic is determined by the connectivity of neurons. The direction of information flow and the destination of that information can be deduced from a study of the neuronal circuitry of interest. The available patterns of blood flow are also determined by the vascular anatomy, but the patterns of blood flow employed in living animals are not easily deduced from anatomical studies of blood vessels. Observations of blood flow in the portal vessels of living animals leaves no doubt that blood flows from the median eminence to the pars distalis (69,70,617–623). The hypothalamic hypophysiotropic releasing factors in the terminals of neurons in the median eminence are carried to the pars distalis over restricted vascular routes.

Observation of blood flow in the neurohypophysis revealed blood flow between adjacent neurohypophysial regions (between the neural lobe and lower infundibular stem and between the median eminence and the upper infundibular stem). It also revealed a major drainage route from the rostral neurohypophysis (the median eminence) to the pars distalis and the major drainage route of the caudal neurohypophysis (neural lobe) to be to the cavernous sinus. However, some blood did flow from the neural lobe to the adjacent pars distalis and neural hormones released in the neural lobe have access to glandular epithelium in this region (623). In addition, neural lobe hormones (e.g., OT and its side chain [pro-leu-gly-NH_2]) have access to the pars intermedia and adjacent regions of the pars distalis by vascular channels and through extensive connections between the perivascular space of the neural lobe and the extracellular space of the pars intermedia (304).

Rostrally, in the median eminence, the neurohypophysial capillary bed is specialized (Fig. 11). The primary plexus is subdivided into an external and an internal plexus (85,599). The external plexus corresponds to the superficial network of Duvernoy (624) and to the mantle plexus of Romeis (251). The external plexus lies on the surface of the median eminence and is continuous with the capillaries of the infundibular stem and process. It receives the arterial supply to the median eminence. Its morphology differs little from species to species (compare the external plexus of the toad [625] with that of the rabbit [85]) (Fig. 14). The external plexus forms a reticular network of fenestrated capillaries that lie partially buried within the oral (ventral) surface of the median eminence (85,353,599,626). These capillaries form a mosaic made up of multiple hexagonal units that is oriented parallel to the surface of the median eminence. Transmission electron microscopic studies (353,626) demonstrate that the capillaries are partially embedded within the external zone such that their oral surface is flush with the oral surface of the palisade layer. The central region of each hexagonal capillary unit is filled with "posts" of median eminence tissue. This capillary pattern resembles that found in two other organs in which the exchange of materials between the blood and tissue is rapid —the gastric mucosa and the lung (627,628). Sobin et al. (629) described the pulmonary vascular space as resembling "an underground garage consisting of a floor, ceiling and supportive pillars all covered with endothelium," and they argued that blood flows as a sheet through an essentially continuous space lined by endothelium. In the median eminence a similar pattern of flow may be present, because the angioarchitecture of the external plexus resembles that in the lung.

The organization of the palisade layer and of the external plexus has functional consequences of importance to the regulation of the adenohypophysis. Each hexagonal capillary unit (microvascular module) encloses a post (microdomain) of neurosecretory axon terminals and glial tissue. With increased functional demand, glial processes can be expected to retract from positions interposed between axon terminals and capillaries to make more surface area available for the release of hypothalamic peptides and amines into the portal system to be carried to the pars distalis (630). Within each microdomain, amines and peptides released from one terminal are free to act upon neighboring terminals if appropriate receptors are present—a paracrine action of secretions released by terminals in the palisade layer upon neighboring terminals is possible, as well as an endocrine action upon the epithelial cells of the pars distalis. Should sheet flow occur across the surface of the median eminence, the secretions of one microdomain would be free to interact with the terminals in other microdomains. The microcirculation in the palisade zone could permit interactions between microdomains separated from one another on the surface of the median eminence. Should future TEM studies reveal smooth muscle sphincters arrayed at the entrance to each hexagonal microvascular module, the opportunities to permit very regional adjustments in the distribution of blood flow at the surface of the palisade layer would be present, and the capacity for neurons terminating in one microdomain to influence neurons terminating in another could be limited or regulated.

Whereas the external plexus receives the arterial blood supply from the superior hypophysial arteries, it distributes blood into portal vessels coursing to the pars distalis or into the internal plexus, which invades the median eminence. The internal plexus arises from the external

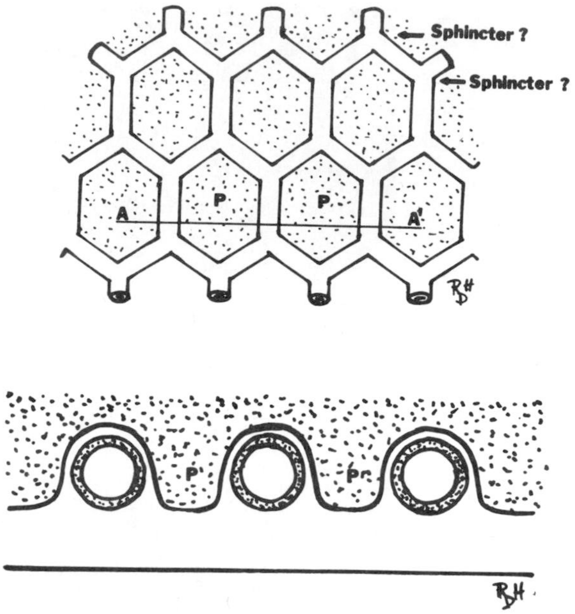

FIG. 14. Top: View of external plexus from below. Hexagonal arrays of capillaries are separated by posts (*P*) of median eminence tissue. **Bottom:** Cross-sectional view of median eminence external plexus along plane A–A′ on top panel. Capillaries lie embedded in neuropil separated by posts (*P*) of median eminence tissue. (From ref. 626, with permission.)

plexus (604–606). There is considerable variability in the anatomy of the internal plexus between species (compare the rat, the rabbit, and the monkey) (85,599). Viewed from within the ventricle, the median eminence forms a bowl or a funnel, and hence the term *infundibulum* is employed to describe it. The bowl has a floor and walls. The basic pattern of the internal plexus is one of capillary loops in the floor of the infundibulum, or, in some animals capillary coils in its walls. The capillary loops in the floor of the median eminence (of the rat) have been subdivided into long capillary loops that stretch into the hypendymal layer and short capillary loops that extend from the surface of the palisade layer only as far as the reticular layer.

The capillary loops of the internal plexus are well seen when the median eminence has been sectioned in the midsagittal plane following the intravascular injection of India ink (29,66,624,631–633), neoprene latex (99), or microfil (599) and viewed with a light microscope. They can be better appreciated by examining corrosion casts of the median eminence with the scanning electron microscope (SEM) (85,599). Such techniques revealed the loops of the internal plexus to be made up of an ascending limb, an apex, and a descending limb (Fig. 15). The ascending limb arises from the external plexus and passes through the palisade layer and reticular layer into the internal zone, where it may pass as deep as the hypendymal layer. There may be extensive arborization beneath the ependyma at the apex of the long loops. The descending limb is larger than the ascending limb and passes back through the internal zone, the reticular layer,

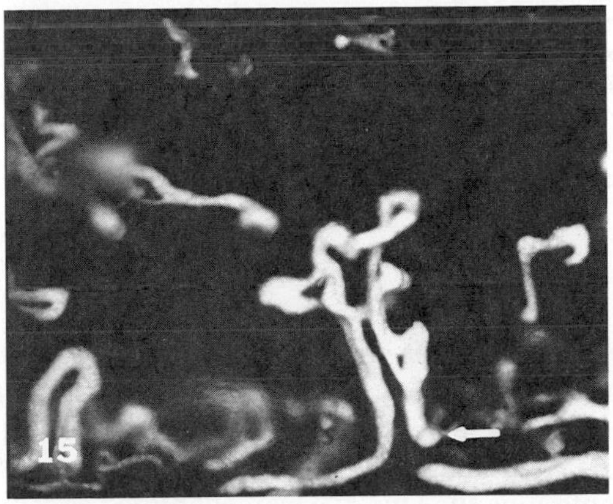

FIG. 15. Light microscopic photograph of rabbit median eminence in sagittal section, Microfil injection. An internal plexus capillary loop arises from the external plexus (*small arrow*) to arborize beneath the ventricular surface and then drain to a portal vessel. Ependymal processes terminate about the apex of the loop, whereas small neurons make neurohemal contact along the limbs of these formations. If sphincters are present at the origin of the modules, a mechanism for regional control of blood flow within small (functional) regions of the median eminence will be present. ×100. (From ref. 599, with permission.)

and the palisade layer to the surface of the median eminence, where it joins either an external plexus capillary or a portal vessel (624).

The capillary loops of the internal plexus also form a series of microvascular modules that is best appreciated on sagittal section (Fig. 11). They arise from the external plexus phylogenetically (they are not present in amphibians, but are present in mammals) (625) and embryologically (604,605,607). As a loop invaginates into the median eminence, it carries with it an expanded perivascular space that surrounds the entire formation (353,606). Hence on serial sections elements of a single vascular module can be identified in light or TEM studies (353). The perivascular space between the ascending and descending limbs of each loop is continuous with the perivascular space on the surface of the palisade layer. It lies between the widely split basal lamina whose inner layer is applied to the convoluted endothelial tube and whose outer layer invests the entire formation in a fashion analogous to the disposition of the visceral and parietal peritoneum. Neurohemal contact has been documented along the course of these loops in the external and internal zones of the rabbit median eminence (353) and more recently in the median eminence of the gerbil (624). Columns of capillary loops surrounded by parvicellular axon terminals thus stand on a base comprised of hexagonal arrays of capillaries each of which encloses a microdomain of neurosecretory terminals. Because each loop is invaginated from the surface into the depths of the median eminence, it can be expected to have carried with it axon terminals from the surface of the palisade layer. Each vertical column should then be expected to contain terminals functionally similar to those at its base. The area for neurohemal contact will be increased, but the endocrinotopic organization of the median eminence (383) will be preserved by such an arrangement. In this regard it is of interest that a regional difference in the concentration of dopamine in portal vessels has been reported, with the dopamine concentration higher in medial than in lateral long portal vessels of the rat (635). It is not known at present whether smooth muscle cells are arrayed at the origin of each capillary loop, and thus it is not known if the flow into these capillary loops can be regulated by sphincters. The recruitment of vascular columns in functionally specific regions of the median eminence would markedly enhance the neuroendocrine response to a functional demand. Coupled with such mechanisms as an increase in neurosecretion, an increase in blood flow, an increase in the permeability of the median eminence, and a retraction of the glial processes insinuated between axon terminals and capillaries, the recruitment of microvascular modules would significantly add to the ability of the median eminence to respond to demands placed upon it (Fig. 16).

A subependymal system of capillaries is present in the median eminence of some species, and in addition to the

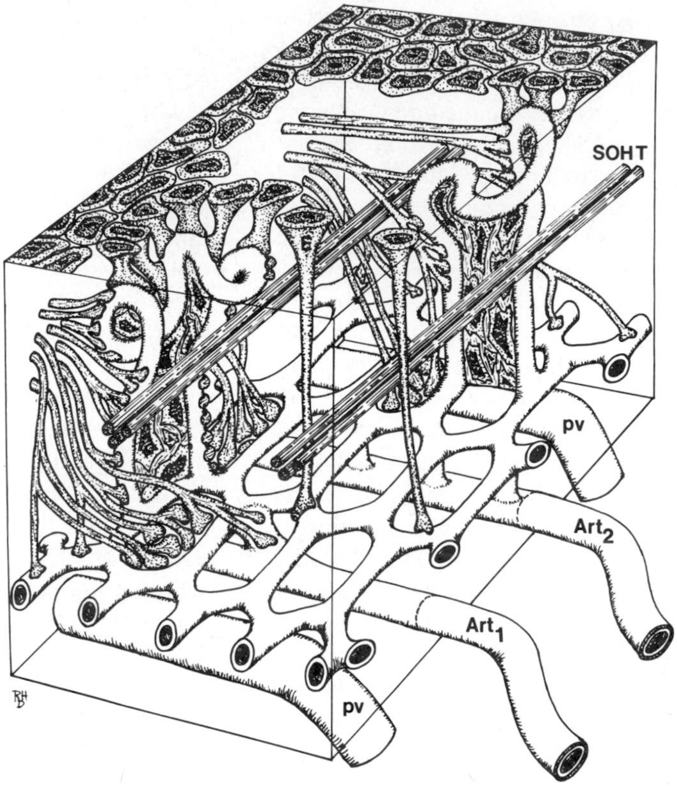

16

FIG. 16. Neurovascular organization in the medial third of the rabbit median eminence. The external plexus forms a hexagonal array oriented parallel to the median eminence external surface and receives arterial blood from arteriolar branches of the superior hypophysial arteries (*Art₁*, *Art₂*). Internal plexus capillary loops arise from the external plexus and arborize in the subependymal zone. Connective tissue fills the spaces between the ascending and descending limbs of the internal plexus loops and the ventral aspect of the median eminence between the surface of the external zone and the pars tuberalis. Nonciliated ependymal cells line the infundibular recess (*E*). The basal processes of some ependymal cells end in the perivascular space about the apex of capillary loops and form an ependymal cuff about them in the hypendymal layer. Some ependymal processes extend to the external plexus. Parvicellular axons terminate on external plexus capillaries and about internal plexus capillary loops to form an axonal cuff about them deep in the fiber layer and in the palisade zone. The axons are peptidergic and aminergic. Magnocellular systems (*SOHT*) pass through the fiber layer and do not send collaterals to the capillary loops. Arterioles that originate from superior hypophysial arteries lie on the median eminence surface and supply the external plexus by tapering down from terminal arterioles (*Art₂*). Arterioles lie in close proximity to the external plexus and to posts (microdomains) of neurosecretory and aminergic terminals. Portal vessels (*pv*) are fenestrated and do not contain a continuous layer of smooth muscles in their walls. (Modified from ref. 353, with permission.)

external and internal plexuses forms a third capillary network in the median eminence that unites it with the hypothalamus in mammals. In birds (505) these capillaries appear to be hypothalamic vessels that unite the left and right sides of the hypothalamus and to be spatially separated from the capillaries of the primary plexus. In mammals, their relationship to capillaries in the median eminence is quite different. They unite the apices of adjacent long capillary loops in the median eminence and pass to the arcuate nucleus (599,615). Ambach et al. (615) employed light microscopy to examine serial sections of the rat's hypothalamus and pituitary gland after the intravascular injection of India ink. To differentiate arteries from veins and capillaries, they first injected the animals with a blue India ink mixed in a gelatin solution of low viscosity and then injected the animal with a red India ink in a gelatin solution of high viscosity. Vessels containing the red (high viscosity) mixture were identified as arteries, for the high viscosity mixture was not expected to pass into smaller capillaries and thence to veins. Vessels containing the blue dye were identified as capillaries or veins. They employed this technique to identify subependymal vessels in the median eminence of the rat that united the apices of internal plexus capillary loops and stated that they had an independent arterial supply in the median eminence and drained to the hypothalamus. A similar conclusion has been reached by Murakami et al. (636) on the basis of SEM studies of vascular casts. Page et al. (599) also employed SEM to study the angioarchitecture of the rat, dog, cat, sheep, and monkey median eminence. The subependymal plexus was found in the rat, dog, and sheep median eminence and was continuous with the subependymal capillaries in the hypothalamus but a direct arterial supply was not found. In the rabbit, cat, and monkey, a subependymal plexus was not present, but connections between the internal plexus of the median eminence and subependymal capillaries about the third ventricle in the region of the hypothalamic arcuate nucleus were present (Fig. 17). Akamayev (637,638) had previously stressed the presence of these capillary connections between the median eminence and the arcuate nucleus. Ambach et al. (615) argued that the capillary beds of the arcuate nucleus and the neurohypophysis should be considered as a single unit, and this concept has recently received support from physiological studies of neutral amino acid transport and transit time in the median eminence and adjacent tuberal hypothalamus in the rat. The ventral region of the arcuate nucleus adjacent to the median eminence had an increased permeability-surface product (P × S), increased transport of the neutral amino acid α-aminoisobutyric acid, and decreased transit time of labeled sucrose when compared with the dorsal region of the arcuate nucleus (639). The hypophysial vascular system is not as isolated from the hypothalamus as originally proposed and subsequently defended by Wislocki (29,86–89).

Torok (617,618) reported that blood flowed from the external plexus into capillary loops of the internal plexus and then into subependymal vessels and then to the hypothalamus. He further reported that, upon dissection of the pituitary stalk with separation of the infundibular stem from the pars distalis, he found some deep portal vessels in which blood appeared to be flowing from the pars distalis to the median eminence. This observation has not been independently verified. Neither the observation nor its obvious consequences have been widely

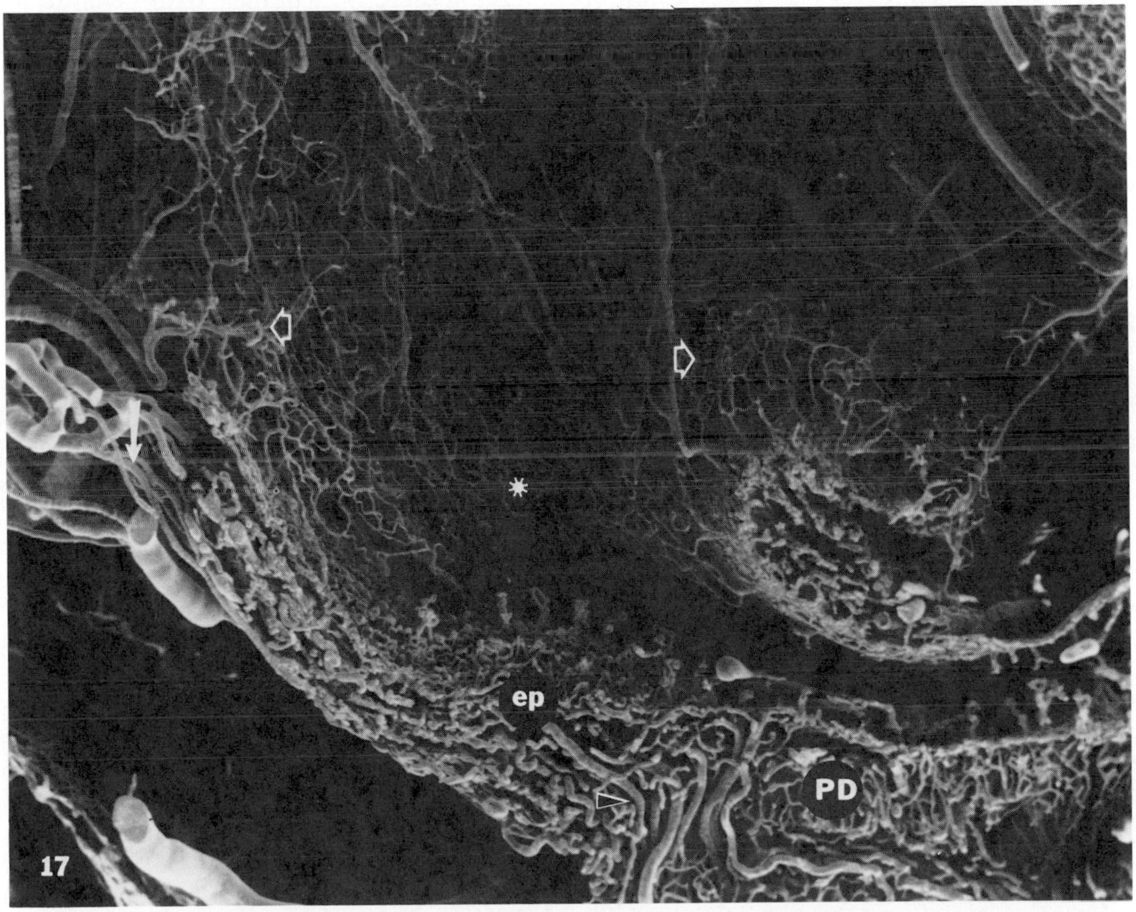

FIG. 17. Scanning electron micrograph of cat hypothalamus and median eminence, sagittal view. The rostral position is to the reader's left. The median eminence external plexus (*ep*) lies interposed between pars distalis (*PD*) capillaries below and internal plexus capillary loops above. *Vertical arrow* designates superior hypophysial arteries, which vascularize external plexus. External plexus capillaries unite to form portal vessel coursing to the pars distalis (*black arrowhead*). Capillary connections between the median eminence and hypothalamus are present anteriorly and posteriorly at *open arrowheads* and in the periventricular zone at the *asterisk*. Note that periventricular capillary connections uniting the lateral wall of the median eminence with the hypothalamus cannot be appreciated on Microfil section (compare with Fig. 11). (From ref. 599, with permission.)

accepted. However, they cannot be easily dismissed. A labeled analogue of ACTH (^{3}H-ACTH 4-9) and ^{3}H-β-LPH have been injected into the pars distalis of the rat with subsequent recovery of label in the hypothalamus. If the pituitary stalk was severed just prior to injection, the label was not recovered in the hypothalamus. If 8 days were permitted to pass following stalk section (sufficient time for vascular but not neural regeneration), label was again recovered from the hypothalamus after injection into the pituitary (640,641). Injection of neurotensin into the rat pituitary produced a profound decrease in core body temperature. This effect is only seen if neurotensin reaches the hypothalamus in adequate amounts. The effect was abolished by prior stalk section but was regained if the vessels were permitted to regenerate (642). While it is possible that the act of injection of substances into the pars distalis could have reversed the normal direction of pituitary blood flow, the possibility of "two way transport in the hypothalamo-hypophysial system" (641) remains open.

The arterial supply to the median eminence is to its external plexus. Arterioles, which supply the median eminence, lie close to axon terminals and fenestrated capillaries of the external plexus containing vasoactive catecholamines and peptides (612). Hence they will be exposed to high levels of dopamine and neurohormones released at the ventral surface of the median eminence. In addition, the descending limbs of capillary loops carry blood to the external plexus capillaries from deep in the internal zone. Terminals containing amines and peptides contact these loops in the internal zone (353). The noradrenergic reticuloinfundibular tract terminates in that zone. Blood returning to the external plexus through the internal plexus may contain norepinephrine and epinephrine (643) as well as dopamine. The resistance vessels lying at the surface of the median eminence regulate blood flow into its external plexus, but they are in turn exposed to vasoactive amines and peptides secreted by the median eminence (612). The neurosecretory systems terminating in the median eminence may regulate blood flow into it (Fig. 16).

THE HYPOTHALAMUS

Cell Bodies of the Hypothalamus

Neurosecretory neurons are the motor neurons of the neuroendocrine system. They synthesize protein hormones in their cell bodies in the hypothalamus behind the blood-brain barrier and transport them to nerve terminals in the neurohypophysis outside the blood-brain barrier.

Magnocellular peptidergic neurons synthesize and secrete AVP or OT. They project through the supraoptico-hypophysial tract to the neural lobe, where they release these hormones into the systemic circulation. They have large cell bodies, measuring 12 to 30 μm in diameter in the goldfish (51), 25 to 50 μm in diameter in the rabbit (644), and about 25 μm in diameter in the rat (645). These cells are multipolar or bipolar. Their cell bodies are oval or pear shaped and contain an eccentrically placed nucleus that contains a single nucleolus. Light microscopic examination of cresyl violet preparations revealed a cytoplasm with a granular marginal zone rich in Nissl substance and a clear central zone. Golgi-Cox preparations revealed the soma of multipolar (but not bipolar) neurons to be spiny (644). LuQui and Fox (646) described many of them as having a "rough shaggy surface." A single axon and three to five (primary) dendrites emerged from the cell body. The dendrites bifurcated into secondary dendrites shortly after emerging. Spines were also prominent on both primary and secondary dendrites, which are bulbous and varicose. Tertiary branching was not frequent. Bipolar neurons were fusiform in shape, with a single spiny dendrite arising from each pole of a smooth cell body. Axons typically emerged from a primary or a secondary dendrite (644) or from the cell body (647). Axons were thinner than dendrites and frequently had a beaded appearance (646,647,648). Collaterals have been identified (646,647). They are presumed to be inhibitory collaterals on the basis of physiological studies (649). Immunohistochemical preparations revealed that OT and AVP, with their associated neurophysins (I and II) are present in the cell bodies of separate magnocellular neurons (59,62,339,650–652) as well as in their axons and dendrites (647). The significance of the finding that dendrites contain peptide hormones is unknown at present.

The ultrastructural appearance of these magnocellular neurons was first described by Palay (51), who studied the preoptic nucleus of the goldfish. Subsequent descriptions of their ultrastructure in other species are not significantly different, although perhaps more complete (653–655). These cells are found in the SON and PVN of mammals, but their ultrastructural appearances are similar in the two locations (656,657) (Fig. 18). The eccentrically placed nucleus contains a prominent nucleolus. The nucleus is folded, and it presents a smooth convex surface to the marginal zone and indented folded surface to the central zone. The marginal zone is rich in rough endoplasmic reticulum with flattened cisternae that may be arrayed, in places, parallel to the surface of the neuron. The central zone contains a random assortment of organelles, including mitochondria, (shuttle) vesicles, Golgi, dense-cored vesicles, lysosomes, smooth endoplasmic reticulum, and ribosomes. Occasional Golgi cisternae can sometimes be seen to pinch off a (new) dense-cored vesicle (neurosecretory granule).

Immunoelectron microscopy has been performed with preembedding techniques that expose vibratome sections to antiserum before embedding and sectioning

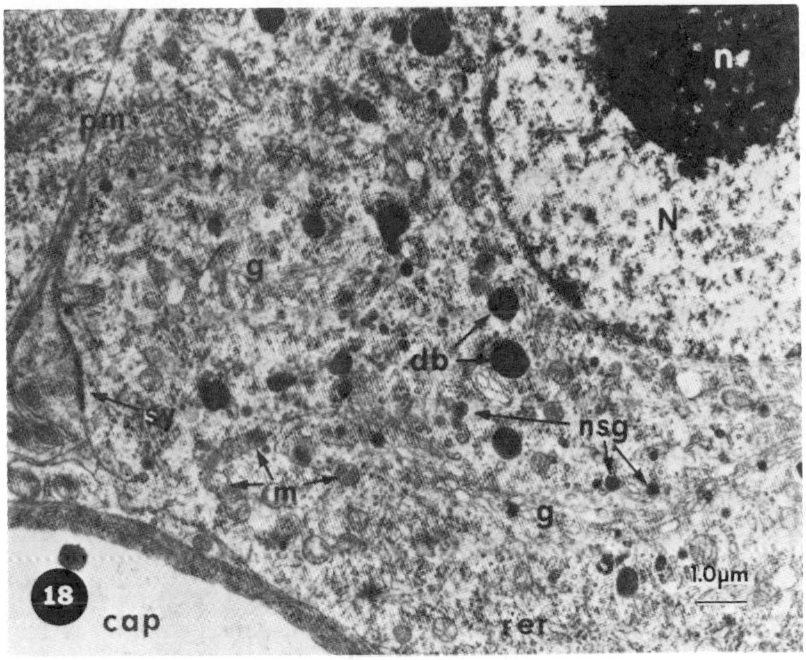

FIG. 18. A low-power electron micrograph of a typical large PVN neuron. The nucleus (*N*) is large, with a very prominent nucleolus (*n*). Around the nucleus there are extensive Golgi complexes (*g*). Rough-surfaced endoplasmic reticulum (*rer*) is situated mainly at the periphery of the neuron. Many mitochondria (*m*), neurosecretory granules (*nsg*), and lysosomal dense bodies (*db*) are seen in the cytoplasm. The neuron is separated from the lumen of a capillary (*cap*) by a thin rim of neuropil. On the left the neuron makes close contact with another neuron, and below this there is a synapse (*sy*). *pm*, Plasma membrane. (From ref. 656, with permission.)

and more recently with postembedding techniques in which the antiserum has been applied to thin sections after embedding in plastic medium. The peroxidase-antiperoxidase (PAP) technique is frequently employed in preembedding techniques. The flocculent precipitate localizes the antigen at the ultrastructural level but frequently obscures ultrastructural detail. The strengths and weaknesses of this technique are discussed by Piekut (658). Employing this technique, she was able to localize OT or AVP to large dense-cored vesicles in the somatic and dendritic cytoplasms of magnocellular neurons. Reaction product was also found over the rough endoplasmic reticulum. Postembedding techniques have employed colloidal gold as an electron-dense marker to identify the antigen-antibody complex. The pattern of deposition is not flocculent and does not obscure the underlying ultrastructure. Castel et al. (659) employed dual immunolabeling to OT and AVP with different-sized gold particles. They localized the hormone within large dense-cored vesicles and were able to demonstrate differences between the morphologies of these vesicles in oxytocinergic and vasopressinergic neurons. The dense-cored vesicles in AVP-like magnocellular neurons were larger and denser than their counterparts in OT-like magnocellular neurons. In addition, the vesicles in immunoreactive AVP magnocellular neurons were uniquely rendered pale (ghost like) by oxidation with sodium metaperiodate.

Synthesis of peptide hormones is carried out in the neuronal perikarya in a fashion analogous to the synthesis of peptide hormones in adenohypophysial cells. In situ hybridization experiments have been carried out at the ultrastructural level to identify the presence of AVP and OT mRNAs in the cytoplasm of different magnocellular neurons (660–662). Jirikowski et al. (424) have additionally localized oxytocin mRNA to dense-cored vesicles in axons and terminals of lactating female (but not male) rats using TEM and *in situ* hybridization. The significance of this finding has yet to be determined. Pulse labeling experiments showed that labeled amino acids are incorporated first into the rough endoplasmic reticulum, then into the Golgi apparatus, and then into dense-cored vesicles (663). Broadwell et al. (664) employed TEM and immunohistochemistry to localize neurophysin to sites of protein synthesis and storage (e.g., the nuclear envelope, rough endoplasmic reticulum, saccules of the Golgi apparatus, and dense-cored vesicles). Kozlowski et al. (665) could localize neurophysin only to dense-cored vesicles in the neurons of the rat's supraoptic nucleus, whereas Piekut (666) could localize AVP only in the dense-cored vesicles of the paraventricular nucleus of the rat.

Unlike the adenohypophysial glandular cell, which releases the hormone locally, the magnocellular neurosecretory neuron transports the hormone to a distant terminal for release. Biochemical and immunohistochemical findings demonstrated that newly synthesized hormone in magnocellular neurons was incorporated within a larger prohormone molecule that underwent posttranslational modification and cleavage as it was carried within the dense-cored vesicle by axoplasmic flow to an axon terminal in the neural lobe (58,61,63,64,667,668).

With stimulation, the changes in the ultrastructural morphology of AVP- and OT-containing neurons are similar. Kalimo (669) reported that, in rats deprived of water for 4 to 6 days or suckled for 13 to 24 days, the magnocellular neurons in the paraventricular and supraoptic nuclei increased in size. The nucleus and nucleolus also enlarged. The rough endoplasmic reticulum increased, as did the number of flattened cisternae. Many cisternae became dilated. The Golgi apparatus became hypertrophied. Increased numbers of small vacuoles were seen at both the cis and trans faces of the Golgi apparatus, and dense-cored vesicles could be seen budding off from the Golgi apparatus in both the cis and trans regions. Broadwell and Oliver (670) made similar observations in mice that were dehydrated for 5 to 8 days. Whereas in control rats, reaction product localizing immunoreactive AVP was only present over dense-cored vesicles in magnocellular neurons, additional reaction product was found over the rough endoplasmic reticulum in the marginal zone as well as over the Golgi apparatus and nearby small dense-cored vesicles after 9 days of dehydration (671). In addition, reaction product was found in the intercellular space separating neighboring somata. In the internal zone of the median eminence, axons of the supraoptico-hypophysial tract were dilated and contained amorphous collections of reaction product that were not associated with dense-cored vesicles that were absent from the axons in the median eminence or the terminals in the neural lobe. Krisch (672) proposed that AVP could be (a) released from the cell soma into the neuropil, where it could enter the ventricular fluid by passing between ependymal cells, and then be transported to the floor of the infundibular recess to be carried by the ependyma of the median eminence to blood vessels; or (b) that AVP could be transported down the axon through channels of the endoplasmic reticulum, incorporated into small vesicles that budded off these channels in axon terminals, and released. However, Kozlowski (673) cautioned that reaction product not associated with dense-cored vesicles may be artifactual. A specialized system of channels in the smooth endoplasmic reticulum was identified in the soma, axons, and terminals of magnocellular neurons by Alonso and Assenmacher (674). They proposed that the electron-dense material found in the vacuoles budding off from its channels in the axon terminals was neurosecretory material (674). Broadwell and Brightman (675) also identified a system of channels in the magnocellular neurons of mice that was associated with a smooth endoplasmic reticulum. It was involved in anterograde transport of lysosomes from the cell body to the axon terminals as demonstrated by its movement of HRP from the soma to the terminal and its association with acid phosphatase positive staining small vesicles. These vesicles contained a dense core that could not be distinguished from neurosecretory material. As the dense material in the vesicles identified by Alonso and Assenmacher (674) was not submitted to immunostaining to confirm the presence of hormones and as the vesicles were not histologically examined for the presence of acid phosphatase to rule out lysosome formation, the case for extragranular transport of hormone from the soma to the terminal via the endoplasmic reticulum is not strong.

The percentage of magnocellular neurons in the rat's paraventricular nucleus that demonstrated dilation of the cisternae of the rough endoplasmic reticulum rose from 12% to 24% after 12 hours of dehydration and remained elevated at 21% after 24 hours of dehydration (676). The number of cytoplasmic small dense-cored vesicles (<160 nm) per cell was decreased 4 and 12 hours after the start of dehydration but returned to normal levels at 24 hours. The number of large dense-cored vesicles (>160 nm) was decreased at 4 hours but then returned to normal (677), suggesting that after an initial decrease the addition of new dense-cored vesicles to the cytoplasm is balanced by their removal into the axon and transport to and release from the terminal. Electrophysiological studies revealed that all putative vasopressinergic cells did not increase their (electrical) activity equally or in synchrony throughout a period of dehydration as they do in lactation. Increasing numbers of cells were progressively recruited over the duration of the stimulus (678). In situ hybridization experiments also showed recruitment of cells with increased AVP mRNA content (679). Although radioimmune assay studies have shown that the hypothalamic content of AVP decreases by 60% and the pituitary content by 88% in the mouse after 3 days of dehydration (680), these studies demonstrated larger numbers of cells that showed the morphological characteristics of increased protein synthesis. It was concluded that new neurons were added to the population of actively secreting cells, thus maintaining increased levels of secretion and release of AVP in the face of increased demand even though the hypothalamic and pituitary contents of AVP were decreased.

Additional hormones are colocalized in magnocellular neurons. Immunoreactive ANG II has also been demonstrated in magnocellular neurons (339,585) and was colocalized with AVP. Dynorphin has been colocalized with AVP in cell bodies (681) as well as terminals (682) of magnocellular neurons. Bilateral destruction of the paraventricular nucleus reduced the levels of immunoreactive dynorphin as well as immunoreactive OT and AVP in the neurointermediate lobe of the rat (683). Meister et al. (684) have demonstrated colocalization of other amines and peptides with magnocellular vasopressinergic neurons. Weak immunoreactive TH staining of vasopressinergic neurons was seen after salt loading and/or treatment with colchicine. Galinin immunostaining was demonstrated after colchicine treatment, hypophysectomy, or salt loading. Peptide histidine isoleucine (PHI)-like staining of magnocellular neurons that also immunostained for AVP was found after hypophysectomy. Thyrotropin-stimulating hormone-like staining was also present in AVP-like cells.

Magnocellular oxytocinergic neurons also costore

other peptides. Enkephalin has also been identified by immunohistochemistry in magnocellular neurons. Vanderhaeghen et al. (431) reported colocalization of met-ENK and pro-ENK in the same cells as OT in the magnocellular nuclei of the bovine hypothalamus. Gastrinlike, CCK-like peptide may also be colocalized with OT (437,438). Substance P is present in some magnocellular neurons (441). Corticotropin-releasing factor-like staining has also been demonstrated in OT-like magnocellular neurons (684–686). In addition, nitric oxide synthase has been demonstrated in magnocellular neurons in the SON and PVN of the hypothalamus and in magnocellular terminals in the neural lobe (687,688). Nitric oxide synthase was found in cells bodies that are distributed in the SON and PVN in the same fashion as OT-like magnocellular neurons (689). Staining intensity for nitric oxide synthase increased following salt loading, suggesting that the synthesis of nitric oxide is related to neuronal function (689) and raising the possibility that in OT-like magnocellular neurons nitric oxide serves as a transmitter.

Parvicellular neurosecretory neurons synthesize and secrete hypophysiotropic releasing or inhibiting hormones. They project through the tuberoinfundibular tract or the preoptico-infundibular tract to the median eminence, where they release their peptide hormones into a restricted circulation. The relationship of the parvicellular neurosecretory neurons in the hypothalamus to adenohypophysial cells is analogous to the relationship of lower motor neuron cells in the spinal cord to muscle cells. They are the effector cells of the neuroendocrine system.

Parvicellular neurosecretory cells are found in but not restricted to the arcuate, periventricular, and paraventricular hypothalamic nuclei and in the preoptic area in mammals. Gross et al. (690) described neurons of the arcuate nucleus as having a lobulated nucleus with an evenly dispersed chromatin. The rough endoplasmic reticulum was well developed, and free ribosomes and polysomes were abundant. The Golgi apparatus was frequently associated with a few dense-cored vesicles with a diameter of 80 to 120 nm. In a more detailed study, Brawer (691) characterized the neurons of the arcuate nucleus as being ellipsoid-shaped cells with an average diameter of 15 μm. Each nucleus contained a prominent nucleolus, and its profile varied from smooth and round to highly folded. The Nissl substance was prominent in the cytoplasm. The rough endoplasmic reticulum was not confined to the Nissl substance, where the cisternae were stacked in parallel rows, but was found in other regions as a loosely arranged reticulum. Granular (neurosecretory) vesicles ranging from 100 to 150 nm were few in number. The Golgi apparatus was not distinctive. Mitochondria, lysosomes, multivesicular bodies, and microtubules were also present in the cytoplasm. Golgi impregnation demonstrated unipolar or bipolar neurons with fusiform-shaped perikarya. The dendrites were varicose but not well endowed with regular spines. Except for two features, neurons in the arcuate nucleus conformed to textbook descriptions of cerebral neurons: (a) the nucleolus was frequently associated with the nuclear envelope at a location where the heterochromatin had formed into a large dense tuft and (b) a round "clump of densely intermeshed filaments" containing a central clear spot was frequently found in the cytoplasm. Bugnon et al. (692) studied the ultrastructure of opioid-like cells in the arcuate nucleus. The peptide-secreting cells resembled those described by Brawer (691), as they contained a large nucleolus, tufts of heterochromatin along the wall of the nuclear envelope, and whorls of filaments in the cytoplasm, as well as granular vesicles (693). Following castration or 2 weeks of morphine treatment, laminar whorls were found to be increased in the cytoplasm of arcuate neurons in the rat's hypothalamus (694). King et al. (695) had previously correlated the number of these structures, which they called *ribbon rolls,* to the stages of the estrous cycle in female rats. The ribbon rolls were described as made up of two to eight lamellae with a central core of cytoplasm devoid of organelles or granules. The outer lamellae were associated with the rough endoplasmic reticulum. Their appearance and description resembled the "whorls" described by Brawer (691). In diestrous animals, the rough endoplasmic reticulum was prominent, with its cisternae packed in parallel rows typical of Nissl substance. Ribbon rolls were increased in numbers and complexity. Dense-cored vesicles were found associated with the Golgi apparatus. In estrus and met-estrus, the rough endoplasmic reticulum was dispersed, and ribbon rolls were few in number and simple in structure. The number of lamellae was reduced to two or three. In addition to these changes, the number of intramembranous particles in the perikarya (but not in dendritic shafts or spines) varied as a function of the estrous cycle (696). These observations suggest that the morphology of neurosecretory neurons in the arcuate nucleus is modified by the level of circulating opiates (opioids) and/or gonadal steroids.

Liposits (697) described the CRF-like neuron in the rat's hypothalamic paraventricular nucleus as bipolar in shape with a fusiform cell body. Both dendrites and somata had spines. The long axis of the cell body was 20 to 28 μm; the short axis was 10 to 12 μm. The nucleus was infolded with a prominent nucleolus. Neurosecretory granules measured between 80 and 120 nm in diameter. The Golgi apparatus, rough endoplasmic reticulum, and polysomes were prominent. Immunoprecipitate identifying immunoreactive-CRF stained free ribosomes in dendrites (which are an extension of the somatic cytoplasm), as well as neurosecretory granules in the cell body and axons. Following adrenalectomy CRF-like neurons showed increased protein synthesis. The width of the cisternae of the endoplasmic reticulum was increased and progressed to the formation of vacuoles after several weeks. Neurosecretory granules were observed budding off the trans face of the Golgi apparatus (698). A similar description applies to the GRH neuron (699,700).

In the preoptic area, GnRH-like cells are fusiform in shape, with one or two major dendrites and a single axon (701). The surface of the perikarya and dendrites may be smooth or spiney (702). Transmission electron microscopy has been employed to study immunoreactive GnRH-containing cells in the medial septum, nucleus of the diagonal band of Broca, and medial preoptic area (703). Synapses on GnRH-like neurons were not frequently found (704). The ultrastructure of their perikarya does not differ markedly from that of POMC-like or putative GnRH-like-containing cells in the arcuate nucleus.

Development of Neurosecretory Systems

The basic neuroanatomical organization of the hypothalamus has been presented by Crosby and Showers (705), Nauta and Haymaker (706), and Knigge and Silverman (418). The development of the hypothalamus has been presented by Papez (707) and by Christ (708), and a detailed description of diencephalic development in the rat is provided by Coggeshall (709). This discussion focuses on the development of neurosecretory systems in the hypothalamus.

Hyyppa (710) reported that on postcoital day 15 the rat diencephalon is composed of a germinal layer (lining the third ventricle), a mantle layer, and a marginal layer. On the basis of light microscopic examination of histological sections, he proposed that nuclear groups, which are now known to contain neurosecretory neurons, such as the supraoptic nucleus, paraventricular nucleus, periventricular nucleus, and arcuate nucleus, originated from the germinal layer. A more detailed study was reported by Altman and Bayer (711). Employing pulse labeling with tritiated thymidine, the authors were able to define the time at which cells in a given nuclear group ceased dividing (i.e., the birthday of these cells). They reasoned that all cells (and hence all nuclear groups) originated in the germinal layer. By labeling separate animals with thymidine pulses on successive postcoital days, they could trace the migration of cells from the germinal layer to their final nuclear location.

They determined that (in general) there was a lateral to medial pattern of migration. Cells destined for lateral nuclear sites migrated before cells destined for medial sites. Four classes of cells were established. In class 1 were cells contributing to nuclear groups in the lateral zone (lateral preoptic, dorsal preoptic, lateral hypothalamic, and lateral mammillary nuclei). In class 2 were large cells of the supraoptic and paraventricular nuclei and the medial preoptic area. Also in this second wave were the cells destined for the premammillary nuclei, the posterior hypothalamic nucleus, and the ventral portion of the ventromedial nuclei. Within this group there was a rostrocaudal gradient such that the first three nuclear groups formed before the second three. In class 3 were the dorsal portion of the ventromedial nucleus, the dorsal medial nucleus, the anterior arcuate nucleus, the preoptic periventricular area, and the suprachiasmatic nucleus. The anterior arcuate nucleus, preoptic periventricular area, and the suprachiasmatic nucleus all contain parvicellular peptidergic neurons at maturation. In group 4, the last group to migrate, were the cells of the posterior arcuate (infundibular) nucleus and the tuberomammillary nucleus. This group also will contain peptidergic cells.

The class 2 cells contributing to the magnocellular components of the supraoptic and paraventricular nuclei as well as the cells contributing to the preoptic nuclei migrate concurrently but not from the same site. Magnocellular elements in the preoptic area originated from the germinal epithelium of the inferior horns of the lateral ventricles. These cells are not progenitors of neurosecretory cells. Those destined to become the magnocellular neurosecretory cells of the supraoptic nucleus and the magnocellular portion of the paraventricular nucleus were documented to arise from a single specialized locus of germinal epithelium located adjacent to the third ventricle at the level of the "adult" paraventricular nucleus. Internuclear magnocellular neurons (between the paraventricular and supraoptic nuclei) were found along the course taken by migrating cells from this germinal region to the site of the adult supraoptic nucleus over the optic tract. The neurons forming the supraoptic nucleus were "born" on the 13th through the 15th fetal days. They were recognized over the optic tract on postcoital day 16 and found in moderate numbers on day 17. Paraventricular large neurons were "born" on the same days and first seen on fetal day 16 in their adult locus. More cells appeared on day 17, and by day 18 growth into magnocellular neurons was discernible (712). Neurophysin was first localized in developing neurons of the paraventricular and supraoptic nuclei on the 18th fetal day. Vasopressin was identified in these nuclear groups on the 19th fetal day, but OT was not detectable until the 4th postnatal day. Neurophysin was also detected in the median eminence and the neural lobe on the 19th fetal day (713). It is of interest that Fink and Smith (402) first noted neural processes in the developing median eminence on the 16th fetal day at a time when magnocellular neurons first arrived in the region of the supraoptic and paraventricular nuclei. Altman and Bayer (712) proposed that the cells of tuberomammillary nucleus and those of the caudal arcuate (infundibular) nucleus also share a common site of origin—the inferior lobule at the anterior margin of the mammillary recess—and that they may comprise part of the parvicellular peptidergic system. Similar studies have been performed in the mouse (714,715) and in the cat (716) with analogous results.

Most parvicellular neurosecretory cells arise from class 3 and class 4 neurons in the germinal layer and migrate to their destinations in the arcuate nucleus, the periventricular nucleus, and the paraventricular nucleus. Cells destined to synthesize and release somatostatin stopped dividing on days 15 to 17 of gestation, whereas those destined to be GRH-like were born on embryonic days 13 through 15, with those in the anterior regions of the nucleus being born earlier than those in the middle and posterior regions (717). Corticotropin-releasing factor mRNA was first detected in the paraventricular nucleus of the rat on the 17th day of gestation (718). As is the case with magnocellular neurosecretory elements, migration of parvicellular neurons follows a gradient, with lateral destinations filled before medial ones and with anterior sites filled before posterior ones.

Gonadotropin-producing neurons, in contrast, have an extracerebral origin (719). Gonadotropin-releasing hormone was first detected by immunohistochemistry in the 15 day rat fetus in the nervus terminalis. In the 17 day fetus, the period when immunopositive cells were first present in the rhinencephalon, limbic lobe, and preoptic area, gonadotropins were first detected in the pars distalis. About 60% of the total GnRH-containing cell population was localized in the ganglion cells of the nervus terminalis on that day. By the 19th fetal day immunoreactive nerve terminals had appeared in the organum vasculosum of the lamina terminalis (OVLT) and the median eminence. Immunopositive cells in the nervus terminalis accounted for only about 30% of the total population. The numbers of cells in the septum, olfactory tubercle, and preoptic area had doubled when compared with fetal day 17. The findings suggest that GnRH-containing cells originate outside the CNS and migrate inward. Subsequent studies have confirmed the observation that GnRH-like cells originate in the olfactory region outside the central nervous system (720–722).

Although a common locus and concurrent migration of magnocellular neurons to their final destination seems apparent, a common locus or a common date of origin for cells that contribute from diverse nuclear groups to the parvicellular neurosecretory system has not as yet been revealed. The paraventricular nucleus, which contains parvicellular as well as magnocellular elements, may be an example of "sequential generation of nuclear components" to form a complex system as is the case for the mammillary body, which contains cells from several sites that migrate at different times (711). Birth does not mark the end of development of hypothalamic nuclei of the rat (723,724) or hamster (415). Maturation of structure and a synaptic organization continues into the second postnatal week of the developing rat.

Organization of Neurosecretory Systems

Cell bodies of neurosecretory neurons are arranged in nuclear groups in the periventricular region of the preoptic area and the hypothalamus. These neurons form neurosecretory systems not only by virtue of the location of their cell bodies and the site of their terminals, but also by virtue of the hormone(s) they synthesize. Difficulties arise when there is not a strict correspondence between a given nuclear group and specific cell type containing a single hormone. Furthermore, a single nuclear group is seldom the unique location of cells synthesizing a given hormone. The difficulties are compounded by the observation that a hypothalamic nuclear group may project to several different sites and that any given peptide may play one role at one site and a different role at another. Finally, a particular cell in a nuclear group may contain more than one peptide. However, it appears that Dale's hypothesis (725) still holds and that the same substance(s) secreted from one terminal of a neuron are released from all terminals of that neuron.

The SON "surmounts the lateral border of the optic tract" in mammals (705). It extends from the lamina terminalis at the level of the OVLT to midtuberal levels. In the mouse, the SON is divided into an anterior and a retrochiasmatic portion. The anterior nucleus lies dorsolateral to the optic tract, whereas the retrochiasmatic portion lies ventromedial to it (726). A similar parcellation was made in the rat by Peterson (727) and Rhodes et al. (728) except that the latter called the anterior nucleus *the principal nucleus* and the former considered the retrochiasmatic nucleus to be one of the accessory supraoptic nuclei. Three subdivisions of the SON were reported in the monkey. The dorsolateral, dorsomedial, and ventromedial subdivisions are all described by their relationship to the optic tract (62). Oxytocin and AVP with their associated neurophysins and colocalized hormones are synthesized in different cells in the supraoptic nuclei (59,62,443,650–652). Within the principal portion of the rat's supraoptic nucleus, OT-producing cells are aggregated in the dorsal and rostral portions of the nucleus (728,729). In the monkey, OT-producing cells are aggregated in the dorsal and medial regions of the SON (62). Oxytocin-like neurons in the rat are smaller than AVP-containing neurons and have slightly smaller neurosecretory granules (708). Estrogen receptors have been demonstrated on OT-like neurons that project to the neural lobe (730).

The SON is composed of magnocellular neurons (339,644,705,731,732) whose organization and morphology change with increased functional demand. The cell bodies are closely related to the soma of other magnocellular neurosecretory cells. Adjacent cells are separated by glial processes that in many instances are very attenuated (51,656). Actual soma-somatic contact was found in 4% of cells examined in the rat's SON under normal conditions, and the percentage of cells that directly contacted their neighbors increased with dehydration (657). Under conditions of chronic dehydration (2% sodium chloride substituted for drinking water for 2 weeks) both AVP-like and OT-like neurons enlarged. The percentage of somatic or dendritic membrane apposed to the soma or dendrites of other neurons also increased but the percentage of neuronal membrane apposed to glial processes did not (733). The number of synaptic profiles involving a single terminal that contacted two or more apposed (homotropic) neurons (number of multiple synapses) also increased. There is at present disagreement as to whether this increase involves only OT-like neurons (734) or both OT-like and AVP-like magnocellular neurons (733). During lactation, the organization of OT-like magnocellular neurons, but not AVP-like neurons, was altered. The numbers of somatosomatic and dendritic contacts between OT-like magnocellular neurons in the rat's SON increased following lactation for 10 to 18 days, as did the number of multiple or "shared" synapses (735). About 70% of the terminals in these double synapses were GABAergic (736). Both the number of apposed cells and the proportion of shared membrane on each OT-like neuron increased (737). Almost all of the OT-like cells were juxtaposed following lactation or parturition (737). It is suggested that these changes facilitate the synchronous discharge of OT-like neurons during milk ejection and parturition (735). The finding that dye-coupling occurs between apposed cells and is indicative of electrical synapse formation between them supports this hypothesis. The vascularity of the SON is dense (637,638), and occasionally neurosecretory cells were found to lie in direct contact with the basement membrane about nonfenestrated capillaries (671). The distance between magnocellular cell bodies and capillaries was diminished during lactation (738). This arrangement is a fitting one for a nuclear group whose cells must transport amino acids across the blood-brain barrier and incorporate them in order to synthesize proteins for delivery to the neural lobe for secretion into fenestrated neurohypophysial capillaries.

Synaptic relationships in the SON are now being investigated. Vasopressin-like recurrent collaterals have been observed to originate from magnocellular neurons and to terminate on unidentified soma and dendrites in the SON (739,740). Oxytocin-like terminals have been demonstrated synapsing on OT-like soma or dendrites in the SON (741). GABA-like terminals make symmetrical synapses with the magnocellular neurons (736,742), and glutamate-like terminals make asymmetrical synapses with them (743). The source of these fibers has not been definitely established, but presumably they arise from within the hypothalamus. Corticotropin-releasing hormone-like terminals synapse with magnocellular neurons (744). Opioid-containing (ACTH-like) terminals were reported to synapse with AVP-like soma and dendrites (745) in the SON of young monkeys. The former presumably originate in the parvicellular subdivisions of the PVN and the latter in the arcuate nucleus (Table 1).

The supraoptico-hypophysial tract is the major projection of the SON. Up to 90% of its neurons degenerate after (high) section of the supraoptico-hypophysial tract (746,747). Injection of HRP into the neural lobe of the rat resulted in a dense accumulation of HRP in cell bodies lying in the SON (748,749). Examination of autoradiographs of the rat hypothalamus and hypophysis after injection of tritiated leucine into the SON revealed the principal projection to be through the supraoptico-hypophysial tract to the neural lobe, where it tended to be concentrated in the internal region (674). Nerve fibers in the supraoptico-hypophysial tract displayed irregular swellings, and many had a beaded appearance in Golgi preparations. Collateral axons were found. Fibrous astrocytes and their processes were frequently found and gave the tract a "striking appearance" (646).

Projections to neural as well as to neurohypophysial sites have been identified by several authors employing immunohistochemistry. Labeled axons of magnocellular neurons course dorsally toward the stria medullaris (750). Zimmerman (363) described a projection from the rostral region of the SON to the OVLT, a circumventricular organ implicated in the regulation of salt and water homeostasis and of drinking behavior (751). Brownfield and Kozlowski (752) described a hypothalamic-choroidal tract on the basis of light microscopic examination of immunohistochemically stained sections of the rat hypothalamus. Although it has been estimated that as many as 30% of the magnocellular neurons in the (hamster) SON do not terminate in the neural lobe (753), the major accepted pathway emerging from the SON is the supraoptico-hypophysial tract to the neural lobe of the pituitary gland.

Other magnocellular neurosecretory centers are present in the hypothalamus. Crosby and Showers (705) named these scattered small cell groups of neurosecretory cells, which lie, for the most part, between the paraventricular and the supraoptic nuclei, the *pars diffusa* of the paraventricular nuclei. These nuclear groups appear, with two exceptions, to lie very close to the SON or PVN or lie along the course taken by cells migrating from the germinal matrix in the periventricular region to their final location over the optic tract. The anterior commissural nucleus lies immediately posterior to the anterior commissure near the midline just rostral to the PVN. The nucleus circularis lies halfway between the SON and the PVN. The retrochiasmatic nucleus lies just ventral to the SON. The anterior and posterior fornical nuclei and the nucleus of the medial forebrain bundle are disposed more laterally than the presumed path of migration of the magnocellular neurons from the periventricular germinal epithelium to their site over the optic chiasm and tract (727). The retrochiasmatic nucleus was classified

TABLE 1. *Synapses on hypothalamic hypophysiotropic neurosecretory neurons*

	AVP	OT	GRH	POMC	DA	SRIF	TRH	CRF	GnRH
AVP	+								
OT		+							
GRH			+						
POMC	+			+	+				+
SRIF			+			+		+	
TRH									
CRF	+					+		+	+
GnRH									+
DA					+			+	
NE	+		+						+
EPI	+					+			
5-HT					+		+	+	+
GLUT	+	+							
GABA	+	+			+	+			+
NPY	+					+	+		
SP									+

The abbreviations are the same as those used in the text. The top row lists the neurosecretory neurons upon which synapses occur. The first column lists the transmitter or peptide that has been identified at the electron microscopic level in the synapsing terminal.

by Broadwell and Bleier (726) and by Rhodes et al. (728) as part of the SON. The anterior commissural nucleus was included by Swanson and Kuypers (754) as part of the paraventricular nucleus. All these nuclear groups were labeled after HRP injection into the neural lobe of the rats (748,749,755). Fisher et al. (645) could identify AVP in all the accessory magnocellular nuclei of the rat hypothalamus except the fornical nuclei. Sofroniew and Glassman (647) identified AVP-containing cells in the fornical nuclei and OT-containing cells in the anterior commissural nucleus. The anterior commissural nucleus, retrochiasmatic nucleus, nucleus circularis, and the "fornical nucleus" were found to contain OT- and AVP-producing cells by Rhodes et al. (728). Hence OT or AVP has been localized in all of the accessory nuclear groups, and they project to the neural lobe.

The PVN contains both magnocellular neurons (705,731,756) and parvicellular neurons (732,754,756). The territory of the PVN is described differently by different authors. Crosby and Showers (705) described a triangular-shaped nuclear group lying in the dorsal hypothalamic zone on either side of the third ventricle, with its base parallel and adjacent to the third ventricle. Its anterior border lay in the plane of the posterior border of the anterior commissure and the posterior border of the optic chiasm. Its posterior extent was described as differing with different species. Swanson and Kuypers (754) described a nuclear group in the dorsal zone of the hypothalamus adjacent to the third ventricle that on coronal sections is polygonal in shape anteriorly and that becomes triangular posteriorly. Their periventricular cluster of parvicellular neurons is the periventricular nucleus of other authors (30). Their anterior and medial magnocellular divisions are in the anterior commissural nucleus of Peterson (727). Defendini and Zimmerman (732) described the PVN as fusiform in shape and oriented almost at right angles to the SON. It lies next to the wall of the third ventricle and extends from the inferior boundary of the nucleus reuniens of the thalamus to the superior border of the arcuate nucleus of the hypothalamus. Although it is not clear from their description how this ventral extension relates to the periventricular nucleus, the reader must assume that it lies next to the third ventricle surrounded anteriorly and posteriorly by the periventricular nucleus (compare Fig. 4 of Defendini and Zimmerman [727] with Figs. 7, 9, 10, and 17 of Rioch et al. [30]). (This periventricular territory seems to be the source of considerable dispute, as it is claimed by various authors as part of the periventricular, paraventricular, and arcuate nuclei.) Midway along the dorsoventral course of this nucleus is a swelling directed laterally and posteriorly (the PVN of Crosby and Showers [705]), extending from the level of the optic chiasm and the anterior commissure to the anterior (727) or midtuberal (30) regions.

The manner in which the PVN is parcellated by different investigators varies. Swanson and Kuypers (754) described three magnocellular clusters in the PVN. Their anterior magnocellular and medial magnocellular clusters along with the anterior parvicellular cluster correspond to the anterior commissural nucleus of Peterson (727). Their posterior magnocellular division is partially surrounded by the periventricular, medial, lateral, and dorsal parvicellular divisions of the PVN, and this entire group corresponds to the PVN of other authors (726,728) (Fig. 19). Van Den Pol (757) found that magnocellular neurons tended to be aggregated in the lateral region of the "PVN" on coronal section. His Fig. 3a corresponds to Fig. 1b of Swanson and Kuypers (754) and suggests that he, as others, considered the posterior

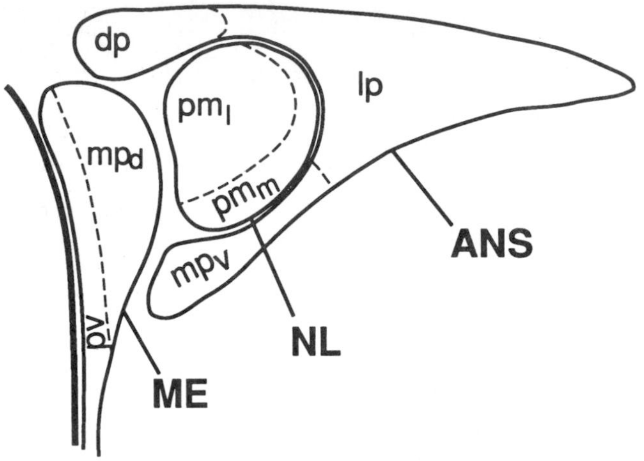

FIG. 19. Coronal section through the major portion of the paraventricular nucleus in the rat with identification of subdivisions. *pm$_l$*, posterior magnocellular (lateral) subdivision; *pm$_m$*, posterior magnocellular (medial) subdivision; *dp*, dorsal parvicellular; *lp*, lateral parvicellular; *mp$_d$*, medial parvicellular (dorsal); *mp*, medial parvicellular (ventral) subdivisions; and *pv*, periventricular (parvicellular) subdivision. (From ref. 770, with permission.)

magnocellular division of Swanson and Kuypers (754) to represent the magnocellular region of the PVN. Armstrong et al. (758) arranged the magnocellular clusters of neurons into the anterior commissural nucleus, the medial and lateral paraventricular nuclei, and the posterior subnucleus of the PVN. Their medial and lateral paraventricular nuclei seem to correspond to the posterior magnocellular division of Swanson and Kuypers (754). The anterior commissural nucleus of Armstrong et al. (758) is the anterior magnocellular division of Swanson and Kuypers (754). In the following discussion the terminology of Swanson and Kuypers will be employed in the descriptions of the PVN of the rat.

The magnocellular subnuclei in the PVN in the rat have been designated by Swanson and Kuypers (754) as the *anterior, medial,* and *posterior magnocellular groups.* The anterior and medial subnuclei lie rostral to the main body of the PVN as described by Van Den Pol (757). The posterior magnocellular subnucleus lies in the main body of the PVN as described by Van Den Pol (757) and is surrounded by parvicellular clusters.

As in the SON, OT and AVP with their associated neurophysins have been found in separate neurons in the PVN (59,62,443,650–652). In the rat the anterior magnocellular nucleus contains primarily OT-like neurons, as does the medial magnocellular subnucleus. Hatton et al. (759) described two populations of magnocellular neurons in the posterior magnocellular subnucleus of the rat's PVN that were distinguished on the basis of size. Smaller cells were found in the anteromedial region of the PVN, whereas in the dorsal lateral region the cells were larger and rounder (758). Their prediction that cells in the anteroventromedial region would primarily contain OT while those in the dorsolateral region would contain primarily AVP was subsequently confirmed with immunohistochemical techniques (728,760). Defendini and Zimmerman (732), on the basis of their own experience and a review of the extant literature, did not confirm the presence of a regional segregation of OT-like and AVP-like neurons in the PVN in humans, although segregation of these neurons was acknowledged in other animals.

As in the SON, in the PVN magnocellular neurons are closely packed, being separated from each other only by slender glial processes. As in the SON, under control conditions cells in the PVN are occasionally seen to lie adjacent to each other without an intervening glial process (669,676). During lactation, the number of juxtaposed OT-like neurons increased as did the number of shared synapses (761).

Terminals containing norepinephrine synapse with AVP-like magnocellular neurons in the PVN of the rat. Sliverman et al. (762) labeled terminals with tritiated norepinephrine and AVP-containing cells with an antibody to neurophysin II. Ochiai and Nakai (763) employed dual immunohistochemistry with antibodies against DBH and neurophysin II. The DBH was identified by preembedding techniques with the peroxidase-antiperoxidase technique, and the neurophysin II was identified by immunogold postembedding techniques. Both groups demonstrated synapses between noradrenergic terminals and AVP-containing neurites. Whereas Silverman et al. (762) were able to demonstrate such synapses only on dendrites (lying in the medial parvicellular subdivision) of the magnocellular neurons, Ochiai and Nakai (763) reported noradrenergic synapses on both the cell bodies in the posterior magnocellular subnucleus in the PVN and on their dendrites. The same group has also demonstrated NPY-like terminals synapsing with magnocellular AVP-containing neurons (764). Triple labeling experiments with the identification of monoaminergic terminals by their uptake of the false neurotransmitter 5-hydroxydopamine, identification of NPY immunoreactivity by preembedding immunohistochemistry with the peroxidase-antiperoxidase technique, and the identification of AVP-containing elements by postembedding immunohistochemistry have revealed that NPY is colocalized with a monoamine (presumably norepinephrine) in terminals that synapse on AVP-containing neurons (765). Phenylethanolamine-*N*-methyltransferase-like terminals have also been found to make asymmetrical synapses with magnocellular neurons (766). GABA-like terminals have been demonstrated by dual labeling immunohistochemical techniques to make symmetrical synapses on magnocellular neurons in the PVN (767), as have glutamate-like terminals (743). As in the SON, most of the terminals involved in shared synapses with OT-like neurons during lactation were GABAergic (736). Opioid (ACTH-like) terminals have been reported to make both symmetrical and asymmetrical synapses on AVP-like neurons and neurites in the PVN (745).

The magnocellular neurons of the (posterior magnocellular division of the) PVN project to the neurohypophysis. Their axons leave the PVN at its apex (757) and then course laterally and then ventrally to the level of the SON (645). There the fiber tract is joined by projections from the SON to form the hypothalamo-hypophysial tract. This fasciculus of magnocellular neurons approaches the median eminence through the lateral retrochiasmatic area and passes from lateral to medial as it moves caudally to enter the median eminence from its anterior aspect. In the median eminence its fibers lie in the internal zone. They pass on to the infundibular stem and process, where they terminate (in the rat) near the ventral surface adjacent to the pars tuberalis and pars intermedia (674,758).

The projection of the magnocellular neurons from the PVN to the neural lobe is not at this time believed to be very substantial. Stalk section, even at high levels, resulted in the degeneration of only about 20% of large neurons in the PVN (746). In contrast, Sherlock et al. (748) found that cells in "the magnocellular [i.e., lateral] part of the paraventricular nuclei were loaded with HRP reaction product" following HRP injection into the neural lobe of the rat. More recently injection of HRP into the rat's neural lobe for retrograde study of magnocellular neurons that project to there, coupled with immunohistochemical staining for AVP or OT, demonstrated that the majority of immunohistochemically labeled neurons projected to the neural lobe. However, some AVP-like and OT-like neurons in the caudal regions of the PVN were not retrogradely labeled (768).

Parvicellular neurons in the PVN of the rat have been divided into five nuclear subdivisions (754). The anterior parvicellular subdivision lies at about the level of the anterior commissure and the descending limb of the fornix between the anterior and posterior magnocellular subdivisions. The medial parvicellular subdivision lies behind the anterior parvicellular subdivision and medial to the posterior magnocellular subdivision. In turn the periventricular subdivision lies medial to the medial parvicellular subdivision adjacent to the third ventricle. The lateral parvicellular subnucleus lies posterolateral to the posterior magnocellular subnucleus, and the dorsal parvocellular subnucleus lies dorsal to the posterior magnocellular subnucleus. In coronal section at anterior tuberal levels where the PVN is triangular in shape, the posterior magnocellular subnucleus of the PVN is surrounded by the dorsal, lateral, and medial parvicellular subdivisions, with the periventricular parvicellular subdivision lying between the medial parvicellular subdivision and the third ventricle (see Fig. 19). More recently, Kiss et al. (769) have subdivided the PVN at this level on the basis of the average size of the predominant neuronal type. Magnocellular neurons (13 to 19 μm in diameter) were aggregated in a single magnocellular subdivision (analogous to the posterior magnocellular subdivision of Swanson and Kuypers [754]). Mediocellular neurons (10 to 13 μm in diameter) predominated in two nuclear groups—a dorsal and a posterior subdivision. Parvicellular neurons (6 to 10 μm in diameter) predominated in the periventricular and medial subdivisions. These subdivisions assume importance because their cytoarchitectonic groupings have specific afferent and efferent pathways and because they subserve different functions that integrate autonomic and neuroendocrine responses to stress (770).

Neurons in the PVN project to the median eminence. This projection was first demonstrated in the monkey, where destruction of the paraventricular nuclei resulted in loss of immunoreactive AVP, OT, and their associated neurophysins from the external zone of the median eminence (771,772). The projections to the external zone from the PVN are ipsilateral and arranged topographically. Following adrenalectomy the intensity of immunohistochemical staining for NP or AVP increased. This increase was blocked by pretreatment with dexamethasone (773). Following unilateral ablation of the PVN, bilateral adrenalectomy induced collateral sprouting of fibers of the hypothalamo-hypophysial tract from the intact side of the median eminence to the denervated side (774). Coupled with the evidence that AVP and CRF act synergistically to stimulate corticotropes (775), these anatomical observations leave little doubt that the projections to the median eminence from the PVN play a role in the regulation of the pituitary-adrenal axis and in the response mounted by the animal to stress.

The source of OT and AVP terminals in the median eminence is the PVN, but it is not clear which group of cells in the PVN project there. The parvicellular divisions of the rat's PVN contain 31% of the OT-stained cells and 20% of the AVP-stained cells (760). The OT and AVP terminals and their neurosecretory granules were smaller in the external zone of the (guinea pig) median eminence than they were in the neural lobe (57,574), suggesting that terminals in the external zone arise from parvicellular neurons. Retrograde tracer studies employing injection of HRP or wheat germ agglutinin injection into the median eminence have revealed heavier labeling in the parvicellular than in the magnocellular divisions (755,776,777). Labeling of magnocellular neurons could have resulted from migration of tracer into the internal zone from the site of injection in the external zone. Because only 20% of the magnocellular neurons in the PVN project to the neural lobe, it has been presumed by some authors that the other 80% project to the median eminence (732,778). Others presumed that the parvicellular neurons containing AVP or OT in the medial parvicellular nuclear group, along with other parvicellular neurons containing hypothalamic releasing and inhibiting hormones, project to the median eminence (770,779).

The largest aggregation of parvicellular neurons in the rat PVN lies medial to the (posterior) magnocellular division in the medial and periventricular subdivisions (754,757), and some of these cells are hypophysiotropic neurosecretory neurons that project to the median eminence. Immunohistochemical studies have also demonstrated immunoreactive AVP-containing cells to be concentrated in the medial parvicellular division (754,757). Somatostatin-containing cells have been identified in the periventricular division (nucleus) (161,780–783), as have TRH-containing cells, which are also present in the medial parvicellular division (444). Cells that contain the presumptive precursor of TRH (784) and its mRNA (785) were found in the medial parvicellular division of the PVN in the same distribution as the TRH-containing cells. This observation is compatible with the postulate that TRH is synthesized in neurons in this location. CRF has been found by immunohistochemical techniques in parvicellular neurons of the PVN of the cow (786) and sheep (787) as well as the rat (561,788–791). However, in the Long-Evans and Sprague-Dawley strains, immunohistochemical staining of the PVN has revealed few CRF-like neurons in the absence of colchicine treatment. In the Fischer strain, CRF-like cells were abundant in the dorsal region of the medial parvicellular nucleus (792). In Long-Evans or Sprague-Dawley rats pretreated with intraventricular injections of colchicine, CRF-like neurons were found to be concentrated in this region (569). Glucocorticoid receptors have been demonstrated in the nuclei of such cells by dual immunohistochemistry (793). Retrograde transport of materials from the surface of the median eminence to the cell bodies of hypophysiotropic neurons has been combined with immunohistochemical identification of the neurons. Such studies have demonstrated that the majority of TRH-like and CRF-like cell bodies that project to the median eminence lie in the dorsal aspect of the medial parvicellular subnucleus of PVN and its periventricular subnucleus (794,795).

Other peptides and neurotransmitters are colocalized with CRF in parvicellular neurosecretory neurons. Kiss et al. (796) and Sawchenko et al. (797,798) reported that parvicellular immunoreactive CRF-containing cells in the PVN become AVP positive after adrenalectomy. In rats treated with colchicine and adrenalectomized, CRF, AVP, and Ang II immunoreactivity were localized in the same parvicellular neurons by sequential immunostaining and elution procedures (799). Following adrenalectomy, CRF, AVP, and CCK have been demonstrated in the same parvicellular neurons in the medial parvicellular subnucleus of the PVN by serial immunostaining and elutions (800). Vasopressin mRNA levels also increased in parvicellular neurons immunostained for AVP, and glucocorticoid receptor was expressed in the cytoplasm (as opposed to nuclear expression) of cells immunostained for CRF (793). These observations, coupled with the observation that CRF-like cells express AVP following adrenalectomy, leave little doubt that the CRF hypophysiotropic neuron is involved in feedback regulation of ACTH levels.

Not all CRF neurons costore AVP. Whitnall and Gainer (801) identified two subsets of CRF-like parvicellular neurons. CRF^+/AVP^+ neurons were concentrated in the dorsal region of the medial parvicellular subnucleus, whereas CRF^+/AVP^- neurons were localized more ventrally in the medial subnucleus. These authors concluded that CRF-containing neurons were a source of AVP-staining parvicellular terminals in the external zone of the rat's median eminence.

Hökfelt et al. (802) described cell bodies in the parvicellular regions of the PVN nuclei that contained immunoreactive CRF, enkephalin, and PHI-27 (a peptide that with VIP shares a common precursor protein and that like VIP stimulates prolactin release), and they envisioned that release of these peptides from the same terminals in the median eminence could provide a mechanism for a coordinated response to stress. In their proposal, CRF stimulates ACTH release from corticotropes in the pars distalis, PHI-27 stimulates PRL release from lactotrophs in the pars distalis, enkephalin inhibits dopamine release from neighboring neurons by a paracrine action to enhance PRL stimulation in lactotrophs, and it also inhibits SRIF release from neighboring terminals to promote GH release from somatotropes in the pars distalis. Although subsequent studies have demonstrated that antibodies directed against the N terminus of PHI cross-react with CRF, repeated analysis with different antibodies has confirmed the presence of a small population of CRF-like neurons in the medial parvicellular subnucleus that costores VIP/PHI and met-ENK. Hence the role of a neurosecretory neuron in the regulation of a particular pituitary response depends not only on the release of a specific hypophysiotropic hormone to act in an endocrine function but also on the release of other neuropeptides (and amines) to act in neighboring paracrine and local transmitter fashion.

Corticotropin-releasing factor-like neurons costore other peptides and monoamines. About 28% costored NT, whereas less than 5% costored GAL in a study by Ceccatelli et al. (568). GABA was identified in a population of CRF-like neurons that did not costore AVP. These cells demonstrated uptake of Fast Blue applied to the median eminence and hence projected there (566).

Neurotensin-like neurons have been demonstrated in the parvicellular subdivisions (481) of the PVN, and about 40% of them costored CRF. However, Niimi et al. (803) could not demonstrate a significant projection of paraventricular NT-like neurons to the median eminence. Enkephalin-like parvicellular neurons were prominent in the medial parvicellular subdivision, and about 40% of them costored CRF (568). Immunoreactive CCK has also been found in the parvicellular neurons of the PVN (438), as has VIP/PHI, but less than 10% of these cells costored CRF (568). Parvicellular neurons containing immunoreactive TH have been demonstrated (804), but it is not yet known whether these cells are DOPAergic or dopaminergic. Angiotensin II has also been identified in PVN cells (both large and small) by immunohistochemical techniques. As discussed above, ANG II is colocalized with OT in magnocellular neurons and with AVP in parvicellular neurons in PVN. A projection to the internal zone and to the external zone of the median eminence has been identified and related to fluid balance and pituitary-adrenal function, respectively (585).

Immunoreactive parvicellular oxytocin (OT-like) neurons have also been demonstrated in the PVN. These neurons lay "scattered throughout the parvicellular division" in the anterior, medial, periventricular, dorsal, and lateral subdivisions (805). Catecholaminergic terminals have been demonstrated to synapse on their soma and dendrites (806).

Corticotropin-releasing factor-like terminals have been found to synapse on CRF cell bodies and dendrites forming local circuits (792,807). Terminals that took up 5-hydroxydopamine or tritiated norepinephrine were found to synapse with CRF-like neurons in the parvicellular regions of the PVN (808). Liposits et al. (809) employed a simultaneous double labeling immunohistochemical technique to label CRF and TH. They demonstrated TH-like terminals making asymmetrical synapses on CRF neurons (809). Preembedding immunostaining for CRF coupled with postembedding immunostaining for TH yielded the same findings (810). These studies strongly suggest that catecholaminergic terminals make excitatory synapses with CRF neurons but do not differentiate whether these terminals originate from dopaminergic neurons within the hypothalamus or from norepinergic neurons within the brainstem. The same group demonstrated asymmetrical synapse between serotonergic-like terminals and CRF-like soma and dendrites (811). In addition to these connections, a reciprocal synaptic relationship has been found between SRIF-like and CRF-like neurons (812).

Thyrotropin-releasing hormone-like neurons are contacted by serotonergic terminals in the rat paraventricular nucleus (813), and TRH-like neurons in the PVN of the rat are also contacted by NPY-like terminals (814). These terminals resemble the descriptions of monoaminergic terminals reported by others (815), and NPY has been found to be costored with some noradrenergic systems ascending from the medulla (see below). Dual immunohistochemical studies at the light microscopic level with antibodies directed against either NPY or DBH and against TRH have demonstrated DBH-like terminals (as well as NPY-like terminals) in close proximity to TRH-like neurons (816). For these reasons, a catecholaminergic innervation of TRH neurons seems likely (Table 1).

Axons of hormone-containing cells in the medial and lateral parvicellular divisions leave the PVN laterally, at its apex, to follow the course of magnocellular axons in the hypothalmo-hypophysial tract and to pass by the SON where fibers from the SON are added. This fasciculus of axons containing peptidergic projections from the hypothalamus enters the median eminence anterolaterally through the lateral retrochiasmatic zone (Fig. 20) (817). This projection brings together two systems that stimulate CRF release (the vasopressinergic and the CRF systems) with the system that regulates thyroid function. Somatostatin and TRH neurons in the periventricular

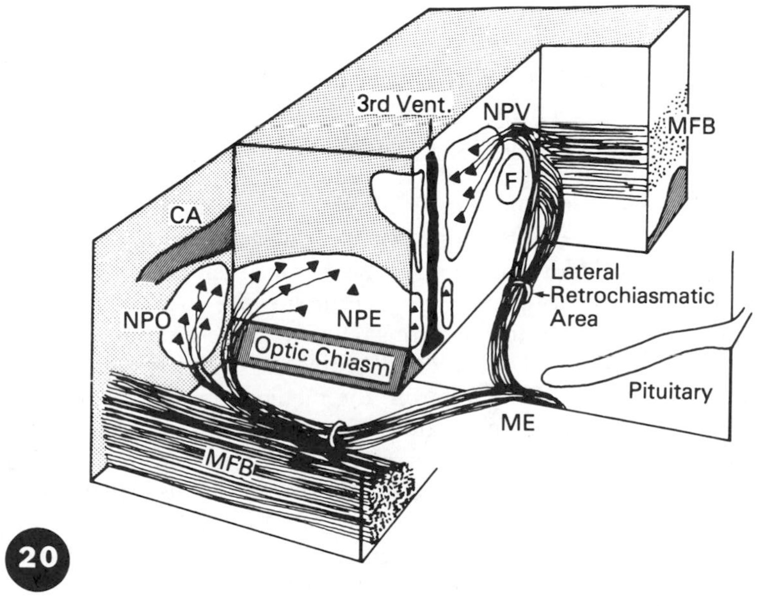

FIG. 20. Schematic drawing of the topography of the lateral retrochiasmatic area and cell groups that project axons through it to the median eminence. *NPO,* medial preoptic nucleus; *NPE,* periventricular nucleus; *MFB,* medial forebrain bundle; *ME,* median eminence; *CA* anterior commissure. (From ref. 817, with permission.)

division course ventrally in the periventricular zone to enter the median eminence at its lateral margin. These two pathways to the median eminence along with the pathway from the arcuate nucleus to the median eminence are included in the term *tuberoinfundibular tract.*

Parvicellular neurons in the PVN also project to the brainstem and spinal cord regions. These neurons are not the same neurons that project to the median eminence (818). Most such neurons contain immunoreactive OT or immunoreactive AVP and originate from parvicellular neurons in the caudal region of the PVN (758,819). Cells that project to the spinal cord lie in the dorsal subnucleus and in the ventral region of the medial parvicellular division, whereas cells that project to the dorsal vagal complex lie in the ventral region of the medial parvicellular division (805). Descending neural projections to the dorsal vagal complex (the nucleus of the solitary tract and the dorsal motor nucleus) and to the intermediolateral cell column of the spinal cord have been identified by immunohistochemical techniques (820). Oxytocin-containing fibers predominate (819). Injection of different markers at medullary and spinal levels demonstrated that about 15% of the labeled cells in the PVN were double labeled and hence that these cells sent collaterals to both the dorsal vagal complex and the spinal cord (805). In addition, oxytocinergic terminals have been found to synapse on norepinephrine-like cell bodies in the A_1 cell group in the ventrolateral medulla (821).

Small numbers of SRIF and enkephalin-labeled cells (820) and of TH-labeled cells (804) in the posterior parvicellular region of the PVN also project to the brainstem and spinal cord. Identified neurons accounted for only 10% to 20% of the fibers projecting from the PVN to brainstem and spinal cord levels, suggesting that other as yet unknown peptidergic systems participate in this projection (805,819). Electrophysiological studies also provide evidence of a direct pathway from the medial regions of the PVN to the spinal cord (822). Additional descending projections of OT- and AVP-containing neurons in the PVN to the substantia nigra, the parabrachial nucleus, the locus ceruleus, the lateral reticular nucleus, and the commissural nucleus have been described (823).

Paraventricular parvicellular neurons also project rostrally. Oxytocin-containing cells project over the fornix to the hippocampus and also project to the septal area (824–826). Additional projections to the MPOA, bed nucleus of the stria terminalis, and periventricular nucleus of the thalamus have been revealed by autoradiographic studies following injection of labeled amino acids into the PVN (Table 2) (827).

Axons of parvicellular neurons also project to sites within the paraventricular nucleus. Whereas intrinsic axons were found not to arise from magnocellular neurons, they were found to arise from parvicellular neurons. Local axons terminated in both the medial parvicellular and lateral magnocellular regions of the PVN (757). The dendritic arbors of parvicellular neurons remain within the confines of the nucleus. They are oriented horizontally, parallel to the floor of the ventricle, and to intrinsic axons in the medial portion of the nucleus. In the periventricular regions, the dendritic arbors are oriented vertically parallel to the ascending input from the suprachiasmatic and arcuate nuclei. The dendrites of parvicellular neurons surrounding the (posterior) magnocellular division peripherally are oriented parallel to the surface of the nucleus, forming a network of dendrites about it. The parvicellular neurons are thus arrayed to serve as receptor sites for incoming afferent axons, as interneurons relaying afferent input into large and small peptidergic neurons, as neurosecretory cells releasing hormones in the median eminence to control anterior pituitary function, and as neurons projecting to autonomic centeres in the brainstem and in the spinal cord to coordinate pituitary and endocrine function (Table 2) (757).

TABLE 2. *Efferents from MPOA-HTA*[a]

	SON	PVN(m)	PVN(p)	PVN	AN	MPOA
NL	+	+				
ME		?	+	+	+	+
OVLT						+
SON		+			+	
PVN(m)	+				+	
PVN(p)					+	
PVN					+	
AN				+		
MPOA				+	+	
VMN				+	+	
Habenula				+		+
Hipp.			+	+		
Septum			+	+	+	+
BNST			+	?	+	+
Amygdala			+	?	+	+
Ol. Tub.				+		+
IPN				+		
SN			+			
Teg.				+		+
PbN			+			+
LC			+			+
LRN			+			+
PVC			+			+

[a] SON, supraoptic nucleus; PVN(m), magnocellular paraventricular nucleus; PVN(p), parvicellular paraventricular nucleus; PVN, periventricular nucleus; AN, arcuate nucleus; MPOA, medial preoptic area; NL, neural lobe; ME, median eminence; OVLT, organum vasculosum of the lamina terminalis; VMN, ventromedial nucleus; Hipp., hippocampus; BNST, bed nucleus of the stria terminalis; Ol. Tub., olfactory tubercle; IPN, interpeduncular nucleus; SN, substantia nigra; Teg., midbrain tegmentum; PbN, parabrachial nucleus; LC, locus ceruleus; LRN, lateral reticular nucleus; DVC, dorsal vagal complex.

The anterior periventricular nucleus is included by Rioch et al. (30) as a part of the periventricular region that includes the arcuate nucleus and the periventricular preoptic nucleus. Ingram (731) stated that it is characterized by "the presence of small cells arranged in vertical rows as seen in transverse sections stained with Nissl stain." It extends through the rostrocaudal extent of the hypothalamus and encircles the third ventricle. Anteriorly it is continuous with the preoptic periventricular system (30). At the level of the paraventricular nucleus it is sometimes ceded to the PVN (754). In the region between the arcuate nucleus and the PVN several peptides have been localized within cells in the periventricular nucleus. In this discussion the periventricular region will be subdivided (anteriorly to posteriorly) into a preoptic periventricular nucleus, an anterior hypothalamic periventricular nucleus, and the periventricular subnucleus of the PVN. A substantial proportion of somatostatin (SRIF-containing) cells lie in this region (161,780–783,828,829). Injection of HRP biotinylated wheat germ agglutinin into the external layer of the rat's median eminence with subsequent immunohistochemical staining for somatostatin demonstrated doubled labeled cells in the anterior periventricular nucleus and in the medial parvicellular subdivision of the paraventricular nucleus (830,831). Merchenthaler et al. (832) employed a similar technique and found SRIF-like cells that projected to the external zone of the median eminence to lie in the preoptic periventricular nucleus, the anterior periventricular nucleus, and the periventricular subnucleus of the PVN. Hence SRIF-like neurosecretory cells reside in the diencephalon and telencephalon.

Somatostatin-like terminals have been found to synapse with SRIF somata and dendrites in the anterior hypothalamus. Because somatostatin has been demonstrated in *in vitro* experiments to inhibit its own release, it is presumed that this local circuitry is inhibitory in nature (833). The function of other inputs onto SRIF-like neurons has not been established. Immunoelectron microscopic studies of the periventricular nucleus in rats have demonstrated adrenergic (834) and NPY-like (813) synapses with SRIF-like neurons. It has not been determined if the NPY and epinephrine are colocalized in a single terminal. Serotonin-like terminals have also been shown to synapse with SRIF-like neurons (835). In addition, GABA-like terminals made symmetrical synapses on SRIF dendrites and soma (836,837). Corticotropin-releasing factor-like (812) and GRH-like (838) terminals have also been shown to synapse with SRIF-like neurons (Table 1).

Somatostatin-like cells have been shown in lesion experiments to project to the median eminence by periventricular routes (839). Although this course is quite different from that taken by CRF-like axons on their way through the lateral retrochiasmatic zone to the median eminence and although the origin of this pathway is not the tuberal (arcuate) nuclei, this pathway is considered to be part of the tuberoinfundibular tract. In addition to projecting to the median eminence, SRIF-like neurons project to the preoptic and arcuate nuclei in the periventricular zone, to ventromedial nucleus, suprachiasmatic nucleus, and premammillary nuclei in the hypothalamus, and to the habenular nuclei of the epithalamus via the stria medullaris. They also project to the midbrain tegmentum through the stria medullaris via the fasciculus retroflexus and onto the interpeduncular nucleus and via the periventricular gray into the midbrain tegmentum (781). Ascending projections of SRIF immunoreactivity to the olfactory tubercule, septum, and hippocampus have also been demonstrated (781,817).

Immunohistochemical techniques have demonstrated immunoreactive TH (840) in cell bodies of the anterior periventricular nucleus. This cluster of dopaminergic cell bodies is the A_{14} cell group (841). It projects to the neurointermediate lobe in the cat (334). Cells containing NT (842) and CRF (426) have been found in this region of the rat's hypothalamus, and their projections to the median eminence have been identified.

The arcuate nucleus (nucleus infundibularis) is a paired lateral expansion of the periventricular gray that lies juxtaposed to the most ventral region of the third ventricle at its entrance into the infundibular recess (708,726). It is bounded inferiorly by the tuberoinfundibular recess and the median eminence and superiorly by the ventromedial nucleus of the hypothalamus. Crosby and Woodburne (843), Crosby and Showers (705), Rioch et al. (30), Ingram (731), Papez (707), Christ (708), and Nauta and Haymaker (706) all considered the arcuate nucleus to be part of the periventricular system of neurons that, except at the level of the median eminence, encircles the third ventricle. The superior boundary of the arcuate nucleus in the periventricular zone is somewhat arbitrary, because it is defined by the region where the concentration of neurons in the arcuate nucleus meets the less dense population of neurons in the periventricular hypothalamic nucleus, and it is regarded differently by different authors in different species. Van Den Pol and Cassidy (844) described a triangular-shaped nucleus (in the rat) with the side parallel to the third ventricle, the base parallel to the dorsal border of the median eminence and the tuberoinfundibular sulcus, and the hypotenuse (dorsal lateral border) defined by the cell-poor zone that separates the arcuate nucleus from the ventromedial nucleus of the hypothalamus. Others see a more pear-shaped nucleus, with its concave lateral border defined by the cell poor zone separating the arcuate nucleus from the ventromedial nucleus. The nucleus extends as a column of cells from the anterior margin of the infundibular recess to a position slightly caudal to the posterior pole of the ventromedial nucleus and can thus be divided into a tuberal and a mammillary division (705,708). The nucleus is arcuate in shape anterior to the infundibulum in the rat (844) but not in the human (706), and it changes from a paired to a single arcuate nucleus behind the infundibulum in the human (706). Retrograde transport of HRP and wheat germ agglutinin has demonstrated the arcuate nucleus to be the source of many afferent fibers to the rostral region of the neurohypophysis—the median eminence (755,776,777).

Cells of the arcuate nucleus were described by Szentagothai et al. (103) as small, fusiform or triangular cells with several dendrites. The axons originated from the cell body or from the proximal portion of a dendrite. The ultrastructure of the neurons in the arcuate nucleus (417,690,691,845) does not differ from the description given for parvicellular neurons in the section on cell bodies of the hypothalamus. As discussed, ultrastructural features of some neurons varied with the reproductive state of the animal and with age. Light microscopic examination of Golgi perpetrations has revealed three different kinds of neurons in the arcuate nucleus (844,846). Fusiform neurons with one apical dendrite lay medially in a juxtaventricular position. Fusiform neurons with two sparsely arborizing dendrites lay mainly in the medial and dorsal parts of the nucleus. Polygonal neurons with four to five repeatedly branching stem dendrites lay in the ventral and lateral regions of the nucleus. Dendritic morphology exhibited considerable variability, with some dendrites containing many spines, some containing none, and some having a beaded appearance. The pattern of dendritic arborization in the arcuate nucleus differs from that in the adjacent hypothalamus (103,844,846). Cell bodies in the dorsal (and hence of necessity in the medial) region of the nucleus possessed vertically oriented dendritic trees, while the cell bodies localized ventrally have horizontally oriented dendritic trees. If the center of mass of the cell body and its dendritic tree is considered, it lies lateral to and beneath the cell body of a neuron in the lateral (of necessity, ventral) region of the nucleus and dorsal to the cell body of a neuron in the medial region. In horizontal section, the course of dendrites in the periventricular zone is parallel to the third ventricle and orthogonal to the course of tanycytic processes. Immediately above the infundibular recess, the dendrites (in the medial portion of the nucleus) are oriented rostrocaudally, whereas more dorsally they are oriented dorsoventrally. In the periventricular zone of the arcuate nucleus, the neuropil is not separated from the ventricular system by a subependymal glial layer (501,509,844). Dendrites and axons course between laterally extending tanycytic processes.

Axons may terminate locally within the arcuate nucleus or leave the nucleus to terminate at distant sites. Recurrent collaterals may arise from these latter axons (103,844). Axons of the tuberoinfundibular tract leave the tuberal division of the arcuate nucleus and project to the internal and external zones of the median eminence where they may collateralize (103). Arcuate neurons that project to the median eminence appear to be clustered in the dorsomedial and basolateral regions of the nucleus (755,777). Axons also project beneath the anterior third ventricle (rostral to the infundibulum of the rat) to terminate in the contralateral arcuate nucleus. Other axons project dorsolaterally through the cell-poor zone toward the ventromedial nucleus (844,846). However, a knife cut in the cell-poor zone between the arcuate nucleus and the ventromedial nucleus of the rat produced axonal degeneration in the ventromedial nucleus and not in the arcuate nucleus (846). Horseradish peroxidase injection into the medial and central nuclei of the amygdala demonstrated labeling in the arcuate nucleus of the rat and cat (847). The latter observations suggest that the arcuate nucleus sends projections to the ventromedial nucleus of the hypothalamus and to the amygdala. In addition, axons project dorsomedially to terminate in the periventricular division of the PVN (844).

Dopaminergic neurons in the AN project through the tuberoinfundibular tract to the median eminence. Although not a peptide, dopamine is considered an important hypothalamic hormone because it acts as a physiological PRL inhibitor. The presence of these neurons was first revealed in the arcuate nucleus with the formaldehyde fluorescence technique (161,487–489,848–852). Fluorescence of dopaminergic cell bodies in the arcuate nucleus and of dopaminergic terminals in the median eminence was preserved if the arcuate nucleus was surgically isolated from the remainder of the brain but not if it was lesioned (447,329,853–855). Dopamine, as well as other catecholamines, has been identified in the arcuate nucleus by enzymatic assay (856). Tyrosine hydroxylase containing (presumably dopaminergic) cells have also been localized in the arcuate nucleus (840). Retrograde tracing experiments in the young monkey with application of tracer to the median eminence have demonstrated their projection to the median eminence (857). Neither dopamine as identified by enzymatic assay (856) nor dopamine-containing cells as identified by formaldehyde fluorescence (858) are homogeneously distributed in the rodent's arcuate nucleus (Fig. 21). Dopamine-containing cells were scarce in the medial aspect of the nucleus rostrally and in the ventral region of the tuberal division of the nucleus in the mouse (858). Bugnon et al. (859) localized dopamine (by fluorescence techniques) and ACTH (by immunohistochemistry) in different neurons. Dopaminergic neurons were aggregated medially and dorsally (in the distribution of the fusiform neurons), and ACTH-containing fibers were concentrated ventrally and laterally (in the distribution of the polygonal neurons). In contrast, Chan-Palay et al. (840) reported that TH-like neurons (considered to be the equivalent of dopamine-containing cells) were present in the dorsomedial and ventrolateral regions of the arcuate nucleus. Tyrosine hydroxylase containing cells in the arcuate nucleus were fusiform in shape and the cells near the ventricle were oriented vertically, whereas more ventral (and lateral) cells were oriented horizontally. A simi-

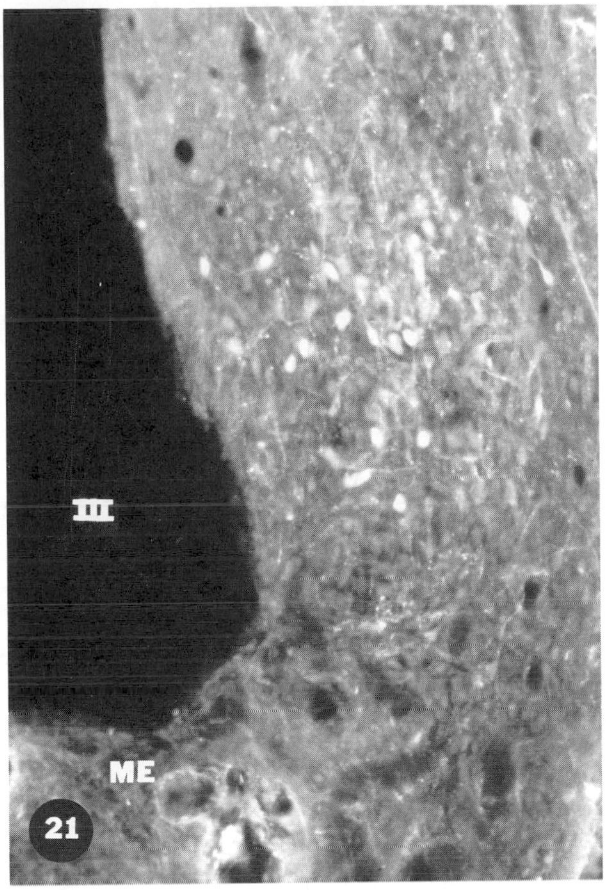

FIG. 21. Fluorescent dopaminergic neurons in the dorsal region of the rabbit arcuate nucleus. Glyoxylic acid treatment. *III*, Third ventricle; *ME*, median eminence.

lar distribution of TH-like neurons has been reported in the rat arcuate nucleus by Everitt et al. (549). However, perhaps not all immunoreactive neurons in the arcuate nucleus synthesize dopamine. L-aromatic amino acid decarboxylase (AADC) is necessary to complete the synthesis of dopamine from L-dopa. Meister et al. (860) have found that not all immunoreactive TH neurons contained AADC. Cells containing both AADC and TH and that fluoresced with formaldehyde treatment were confined to the dorsomedial region of the arcuate nucleus (861). The possibility must be considered that TH-like neurons in the ventrolateral region of the arcuate nucleus are DOPAergic and not dopaminergic.

Tyrosine hydroxylase-like neurons in the arcuate nucleus costore other transmitters and peptides. Immunoreactive glutamic acid decarboxylase (GAD) and TH have been demonstrated in the same neurons of the rat arcuate nucleus AN (342,549,862) mostly in the dorsomedial region of the nucleus. These observations at both the light and electron microscopic levels suggest that dopamine and GABA are costored in the same neuron. Their costorage in the median eminence (310) suggests that both can be released into portal blood to inhibit PRL release from lactotropes. Tyrosine hydroxylase-like neurons in the arcuate nucleus have also been found that costore immunoreactive NT (384,842,863), immunoreactive choline acetyltransferase (CHAT) (861), and immunoreactive GAL (440), as well as growth hormone-releasing factor (GRF) (549,864).

Growth hormone-releasing factor has been localized by immunohistochemical techniques within arcuate neurons of the monkey (865,866), cat (867), rat (868,869), ox. Merchenthaler et al. (870) also found immunoreactive GRF in cells in the rat's arcuate nuclei and demonstrated that these cells project to the median eminence. In addition, they found immunoreactive cell bodies that projected to the median eminence scattered in the perifornical region of the lateral hypothalamus. Bloch et al. (871) reported that immunostaining of the arcuate nucleus and median eminence was abolished after treatment of neonatal rats with monosodium glutamate (872,873), thus suggesting that most of the GRH innervation to the median eminence comes from the arcuate nucleus in the rat. Sawchenko et al. (480) also noted the presence of cells in the arcuate nucleus that contained immunoreactive GRF. The cells were distributed in the nucleus in the same pattern as cells containing POMC derivatives. An additional group of GRF-containing cells was found in the ventromedial nucleus. Growth hormone-releasing factor projections to the periventricular nucleus and to the anterior and ventromedial regions of the medial parvicellular division of the PVN were described by Sawchenko et al. (480). A second projection of GRF fibers from the arcuate nucleus ascended and descended through the ventromedial hypothalamus just dorsal to the base of the brain. It projected into the anterior hypothalamic area, the preoptic region, and the bed nucleus of the stria terminalis, the medial nucleus of the amygdala, and the lateral septum. The descending tract projected to the posterior hypothalamus. A contribution to the tuberoinfundibular tract was also identified and is the pathway by which GRF fibers reach the median eminence. In 20% to 40% of GRF-containing cells in the anterior arcuate nucleus, NT could be colocalized.

Hypophysiotropic GRH neurons in the rat are predominantly located in the arcuate nucleus. They have been identified by applying True Blue to the surface of the median eminence and subsequent immunostaining for GRF. Double-labeled cells were found primarily in the arcuate nucleus (874). Although they were located throughout the nucleus, they formed a particularly dense cluster in the ventrolateral portion of the nucleus (549). Dual immunohistochemical staining has shown costorage of immunoreactive NT, immunoreactive GAL, or TH (588,875). Although the major costorage is of immunoreactive GRF with immunoreactive TH (876), elution restaining techniques showed that some GRF-like cells costore immunoreactive NT and/or GAL (875).

Proopiomelanocortin-derived peptides have been

isolated from the hypothalamus and identified by radioimmunoassay (531,877–879). *In vitro* synthesis of immunoreactive POMC and β-endorphin (β-END) by hypothalamic tissue has been reported (880). The highest hypothalamic concentrations of α-MSH, β-END, and ACTH were found in the arcuate nucleus (531). The arcuate nucleus of the sheep and ox contained cells staining for β-LPH (595). Immunoreactive β-LPH has been found in the arcuate neurons of the rat (881). Adrenocorticotropin and β-lipotropin, and ACTH and β-END were localized in the same arcuate neurons by immunohistochemical techniques (882,883). Immunoreactive ACTH and β-END were found in the same cells in the rat arcuate nucleus (884). β-Lipotropin, ACTH, β-END, and MSH have been localized in the same cells in the arcuate nucleus of the rat (885) and human (886–888). Cells containing POMC-derived peptides were localized ventrally in the rat arcuate nucleus, whereas dopaminergic cells were localized dorsally (859). Cells containing POMC-derived peptides project to the median eminence (595,882,885). There they presumably have an endocrine function with respect to the adenohypophysis or a paracrine function with respect to neighboring terminals.

Cells containing POMC-derived peptides make synaptic contact with other cells in the arcuate nucleus (595,884) and innervate other hypothalamic regions. Eskay et al. (879) reported that lesions that destroyed the arcuate nucleus abolished immunostaining of hypothalamic fibers for α-MSH and resulted in a significant reduction in radioimmunoassayable intra- and extrahypothalamic α-MSH. Sawchenko et al. (889) demonstrated ACTH-immunoreactive fibers leaving the rat arcuate nucleus dorsomedially to course vertically in the periventricular zone and to enter the dorsal parvicellular division and the ventromedial aspect of the medial parvicellular division of the PVN. These regions contain a cluster of OT-containing cells that projected to the spinal cord and dorsal vagal complex. The immunoreactive ACTH projection also terminated in the anterior magnocellular division of the PVN, which contains only OT neurons and the anteroventral region of the posterior magnocellular division—an area with a high concentration of OT neurons. Similar results were reported by Mezey et al. (531). With retrograde labeling of the arcuate nucleus by injection of True Blue into the ACTH-innervated regions of the PVN, double-labeled (immunoreactive ACTH and True Blue-containing) cells were found in the ventrolateral regions of the arcuate nucleus. Interestingly, True Blue-labeled cells were also found in the dorsomedial region of the arcuate nucleus, where fusiform, dopaminergic neurons with vertically oriented dendritic trees lay (889). Retrograde tracers injected into the preoptic area of the rat were sequestered into ACTH-like cell bodies in the arcuate nucleus. In the monkey, ACTH-like terminals made axosomatic and axoaxonic synapses with GnRH-like neurons near the infundibulum (890) and with AVP-like soma and neurites in the SON and PVN. Although the differences in the terminus of opioid-like arcuate projections to the magnocellular neurons in the rat and monkey remain to be worked out, it is clear that POMC-containing cells in the arcuate nucleus project to the median eminence and to preoptic and hypothalamic regions that are concerned with reproduction and with the response to stress.

The arcuate nucleus also contains GABAergic (336,337) neurons that project through the tuberohypophysial tract to the median eminence. They have been identified by immunohistochemical techniques employing antibodies against GAD. Immunoreactive GAD was colocalized with immunoreactive TH, GAL, NT, and GRF in varying complex combinations in the arcuate nucleus and median eminence of the rat by Meister and Hökfelt (861). For example, in the ventrolateral region of the arcuate nucleus immunoreactive GAD/TH/NT/GAL neurons were demonstrated by combinations of double or triple labeling and elution techniques. Other neurons in the ventrolateral region showed a pattern of TH/NT/GAL/GRF immunoreactivity. In the dorsomedial region of the nucleus TH-like neurons costored immunoreactive NT but not immunoreactive GRF, CHAT, or GAL. It is clear that the several transmitters and peptides released from a single terminal may interact with receptors on neighboring terminals and on distant pituitary cells.

Gonadotropin-releasing hormone has been found in the arcuate nucleus of the rat by microdissection and radioimmune assay (891). Immunohistochemistry has been difficult to employ to localize GnRH-containing cells within the arcuate nucleus of the rat, because the same antibodies that revealed GnRH in preoptic sites often failed to do so in hypothalamic sites (161,892). Immunoreactive GnRH has been identified in arcuate neurons in the mouse and rat (161,163,164,892–894), monkey (892,895), rabbit (896), guinea pig (897), bat (898), and human (899–901).

Other peptides have been found in arcuate nucleus cells using immunohistochemistry. Substance P (755), ENK, dynorphin, NPY (549,902–906), and scattered cells containing SRIF (780) have been identified by immunohistochemistry and demonstrated to project to the external zone of the rat's median eminence. Neurotensin projections to the median eminence were demonstrated by a combination of retrograde tracing and immunohistochemistry. Double-labeled cells were localized within the median eminence (803). Neuropeptide Y projections from the arcuate nucleus to the PVN have been demonstrated by destroying the arcuate nucleus unilaterally in the rat and demonstrating loss of NPY staining in ipsilateral PVN (907).

Synaptic relations within the arcuate nucleus are now being studied with immunoelectron microscopy. Tyrosine hydroxylase-like neurons have been shown to be contacted by GAD-like terminals (908,909). In view of the frequent colocalization of immunoreactive TH and GAD, the possibility of homotropic synapses has to be kept in mind. Homotropic TH-like synapses have been demonstrated by Leranth et al. (910). Serotonergic terminals (demonstrated by uptake of tritiated serotonin) synapsed with TH-like neurons (demonstrated by immunohistochemistry) (911). Adrenocorticotropic-like terminals made symmetrical synapses with TH-like neurons in the arcuate nucleus of the young monkey (857). Growth hormone-releasing hormone-like terminals have been found to make synaptic contact with GRH-like somata and dendrites (912), and GRH-like neurons have been shown to be contacted by SRIF-like terminals in the rat arcuate nucleus, but, of interest, the synapses were asymmetrical and not symmetrical, as might have been expected (384). Terminals that took up tritiated norepinephrine or 5-hydroxydopamine were also shown to synapse with GRH-like neurons (913). Thyrotropin-releasing hormone-like terminals were also found to synapse with GRF neurons (914). Proopiomelanocortin neurons have been identified by immunohistochemistry employing a number of antigens. Adrenocorticotropic-like neurons made homotropic synapses in the arcuate nucleus of the rat (915). That both catecholaminergic and serotonergic terminals synapse with ACTH-like neurons has been demonstrated in the rat arcuate nucleus (916,917). Enkephalin-like terminals have also been reported to synapse with ACTH-like neurons (918). Electron microscopic techniques coupled with immunohistochemistry (and autoradiography) have revealed a number of synaptic relationships. Arcuate neurons frequently made homotopic synapses to form local networks. Such network included TH-like, GRF-like, ACTH-like, and serotonin-like neurons (910,912,915,919). In addition, synaptic contact with presumptively inhibitory (GABAergic) elements from within the hypothalamus and with presumptive excitatory (catecholaminergic and serotonergic) elements from outside the hypothalamus was common (Table 1).

Perhaps it would be advantageous to consider the parvicellular neurosecretory system by expanding on the original concepts of Szentagothai et al. (103). Consider the periventricular gray as composed of the periventricular (hypothalamic) nucleus along the border of the third ventricle. From this vertically oriented column of cells arise two lateral projections. The ventral lateral projection is the arcuate nucleus. The dorsal lateral projection is the parvicellular cluster of PVN. In the arcuate nucleus are cells containing dopamine, GABA, POMC derivatives, GRF, neurotensin, substance P, NPY, and ENK. In the periventricular nucleus are cells that contain dopamine, SRIF, ENK, NT, TRH, and CRF. In the parvicellular divisions of the PVN are cells that contain dopamine, TRH, CRF, SRIF, OT, and AVP. These periventricular cell groups are unique because they are retrogradely-labeled by the application of HRP or wheat germ agglutinin–horseradish peroxidase on the median eminence (755,776,777)—these nuclear groups send projections to the median eminence. Cells located medially project to the median eminence by descending periventricular paths. Cells located more laterally in the PVN take a lateral and then a descending pathway with projections from the posterior magnocellular division of the PVN and from the region of the SON where they are joined by fibers of the SOHT. This fiber bundle, comprised of axons from the SON and PVN, passes through the lateral retrochiasmatic area to enter the median eminence anterolaterally (Fig. 20).

Cells in the periventricular gray also project to other (distant) neural targets. Furthermore, cells in one region of the periventricular gray can project to another region of this system or contact cells within the same region. Parvicellular neurons can also project to the magnocellular neurons in the PVN. Neurosecretory cells in the hypothalamic periventricular gray made up of the arcuate, periventricular, and paraventricular nuclei truly constitute a "hypophysiotropic area" in the hypothalamus. However, their cells project not only to the median eminence to regulate neuroendocrine function in response to changes in the environment or internal milieu but also to autonomic centers in the medulla and spinal cord to reticular regions in the mesencephalon and to limbic regions of the forebrain.

The POA also contains cells that are labeled following the topical application of wheat germ agglutinin to the surface of the median eminence (777) and hence is a site where hypophysiotropic neurons reside. It is considered part of the hypothalamus (and hence diencephalic) by Crosby and Woodburne (843), Rioch et al. (30), Crosby and Showers (705), but as part of the telencephalon by Nauta and Haymaker (706). Whether a telencephalic or a diencephalic derivative, it is intimately related to the hypothalamus (705). Papez (707) viewed the POA as the gateway through which rostral innervation to the hypothalamus and to the epithalamus must pass. It has been implicated in temperature regulation (920,921), thirst, and the maintenance of fluid balance (751,922,923), integration of adrenocortical response with autonomic responses (924), cardiovascular regulation (923,925), sexual differentiation (926), masculine sexual behavior (927), scent marking behavior (928), and cyclicity of gonadotropin secretions in female rodents (929,930).

The anterior border to the POA is defined by the lamina terminalis and by the diagonal band of Broca. It is bordered inferiorly by the optic chiasm and the suprachiasmatic nucleus and superiorly by the anterior commissure. Posteriorly the boundary between the POA and the (remainder of the) hypothalamus in the adult mammal is difficult to define (705–708,843). A line drawn from the posterior border of the anterior commissure to the posterior border of the optic chiasm or the rostral extremity of the PVN would appear to be a good operational definition. The POA is continuous dorsomedially with the bed nucleus of the stria terminalis, which actually enters the POA in its most anterior extent. It is continuous anteriorly with the olfactory tubercle and anteriorly and superiorly with the septal region (706).

The POA is divided, on cytoarchitectonic grounds, into a periventricular zone, a medial zone, a lateral zone, and a magnocellular preoptic nucleus (931). The periventricular zone (periventricular preoptic nucleus) is a thin band of cells lying beneath the ependyma of the third ventricle that is continuous caudally with the anterior periventricular nucleus of the hypothalamus (705). Its cells are described by Swanson (931) as being small and are often oriented parallel to the third ventricle.

The medial preoptic zone (medial preoptic area [MPOA]) extends the length of the POA bordered dorsally by the anterior commissure and ventrally by the optic chiasm. Its rostral tip merges with the bed nucleus of the stria terminalis. The cells are of medium size and are densely packed (931). Early TEM examination revealed light and dark neurons in the MPOA (932). In light neurons the cytoplasm was the same density as the surrounding neuropil. The rough endoplasmic reticulum was dispersed throughout the cytoplasm. Free ribosomes and polysomes were numerous. The Golgi apparatus was well developed and associated with clear vesicles 40 to 80 nm in diameter and dense-cored vesicles about 100 nm in diameter. "Coated vesicles" were often seen. The rough endoplasmic reticulum extended into the dendrites. Occasional structures resembling the "whorls" or "ribbon rolls" in the cells of the arcuate nucleus were found. In dark neurons, some of the increased electron density was due to an increase in the number of free ribosomes. Free ribosomes lay between stacks of dilated endoplasmic reticulum. Many vesicles were associated with the Golgi apparatus. Both myelinated and unmyelinated axons were present in the neuropil of the MPOA, with myelinated axons typically occurring in small clusters. A few axons contained dense-cored vesicles with diameters ranging from 125 to 165 nm. Dendrites were frequently beaded in appearance, with large varicosities joined by narrow necks. Both symmetrical and asymmetrical synapses on dendritic shafts, dendritic spines, axons, and cell bodies were found. Greenough et al. (933) reported that sex differences were present in the dendritic field patterns of the MPOA in hamsters. Dendrites in the MPOA of males tended to be clustered centrally, whereas the dendrites in the MPOA of females were distributed more irregularly. These early ultrastructural observations suggested that (a) peptidergic cells were present in the MPOA and (b) a differential input occurred in the MPOA of male and female animals.

The MPOA of the rat contains a sexually dimorphic nucleus (SDN) that can be identified by visual inspection of Nissl-stained sections (934). In males, the central region of the MPOA is more darkly stained and has sharper borders than in females. Its volume is larger in males than in females. The different staining pattern is secondary to an increase in cell density in the SDN POA. Differences can be found between males and females as early as the first day of (extrauterine) life (935). The cells of the SDN migrate there from more ventral regions of the MPOA. A male pattern can be induced in females by exposure to androgens on the day of birth. Gonadectomy of males on postnatal day 1 reduced the size of the SDN by more than 50% (936). A similar sexual dimorphism has been found in the MPOA of the guinea pig (937), gerbil (928), toad (938), and human (939). The role of this developmental difference between males and females is unknown. It is of interest that the sexually dimorphic region of the MPOA in the male toad is considered to be the center for mate calling and that its nuclear volume varies with the breeding season (938).

Stimulation of the POA of proestrous female rats caused an increase in plasma LH concentration and ovulation (940). The integrity of the posterior region of the POA is necessary for the demonstration of male sexual behavior in the rat (927). It is to be expected then that this region (in the rodent) is related to ovulation and hence to the feedback relationships of estrogen on GnRH-containing neurons and to sexual behavior. Testosterone-concentrating neurons have been localized in the arcuate and preoptic regions of adult rats (941). Estrogen-concentrating neurons in the POA have also been identified by autoradiographic means (942–944).

The bed nucleus of the stria terminalis enters the dorsal region of the MPOA. A sexually dimorphic pattern of nonstrial synapses in the bed nucleus of the stria terminalis was first reported by Raisman and Field (945). Female rats had more nonstrial synapses on dendritic spines than did males. This pattern, along with the cyclic pattern of gonadotropin release and behavioral estrus, was abolished if the females were treated on postnatal day 4 with testosterone. Males castrated within 12 hours of birth developed a female pattern of cyclic gonadotropin release and a female pattern of nonstrial synapses in the bed nucleus of the stria terminalis. Cells in the lateral subdivision of the bed nucleus of the stria terminalis contained two or three dendrites that branch sparingly but might extend 300 to 400 μm across the field of incoming strial neurons and were oriented perpendicular to them to form a reticular grid (946). This arrangement should maximize contact between neurons of the bed nucleus and axons entering through the stria terminalis. Cells in the medial subdivision of the bed nucleus of the stria terminalis resembled those in the adjacent MPOA. Their dendrites were oriented parallel to incoming axons.

The magnocellular preoptic nucleus lies in the lateral zone, lateral to the diagonal band of Broca. Saper (947) believed this nuclear group to be part of a system of large neurons 20 to 30 μm in diameter that are grouped into clusters in the medial septal nucleus, the magnocellular preoptic nucleus, substantia innominata, and globus pallidus. These neurons stain immunohistochemically for acetylcholine esterase.

The lateral zone (lateral preoptic area [LPOA]) is characterized by the presence of medium-sized neurons scattered among the fibers of the medial forebrain bundle. The bed nucleus of the stria terminalis is separated from the LPOA by a cell-free zone. The preoptic continuation of the bed nucleus of the stria terminalis occupies a position between the anterior hypothalamic area, the MPOA, and the LPOA.

Peptide hormones have been localized by immunohistochemistry within cells making up the nuclear groups of the POA, the medial septum, and in the bed nucleus of the stria terminalis of the rat. Somatostatin has been found within cells of the periventricular POA (782,783, 828,948). Cells containing immunoreactive CRF (569,788) and met-ENK (902) have been identified in the periventricular POA and in the MPOA. Cells containing immunoreactive TRH have been localized within the MPOA and the diagonal band of Broca (444). Cells in the bed nucleus of the stria terminalis have been identified that contain immunoreactive VIP (949), AVP (950), and CRF (563,788). Cells containing substance P and met-ENK have been identified in the MPOA and LPOA (949,951).

Gonadotropin-releasing hormone is also found in the MPOA of the rat (891), but the cells containing this peptide are not confined within its borders. Immunoreactive cells are also present in the olfactory bulb, olfactory tubercle, nucleus of the diagonal band of Broca, medial septum, the periventricular preoptic nucleus, and lateral hypothalamus (952,953). Unlike earlier investigators (163,164,892–894), recent investigators failed to confirm the presence of GnRH in the arcuate nucleus of the rat (952,953). King et al. (952) suggest that previous studies employed antibodies that reacted against ACTH. The presence of GnRH in cells of the arcuate nucleus of the rabbit (896), guinea pig (897), monkey (895), and human (901) is generally accepted. Some GnRH-like neurons in the rabbit have been shown to costore delta sleep-inducing peptide (954).

Retrograde tracer application to the median eminence of the rat followed by immunohistochemical staining for GnRH has demonstrated GnRH-like neurons that project to the median eminence in the septal region, MPOA, and preoptic periventricular region (832,955). In the monkey, GnRH-like cells were also found in the region of the arcuate nucleus (956). Not all the GnRH-like neurons in those regions projected to the median eminence. There was no difference in morphology between those that projected to the median eminence and those that did not (955).

The GnRH-like terminals make symmetrical homotropic synapses with GnRH neurons (703,957,958). This circuit may mediate ultrashort loop feedback, because *in vitro* studies have shown that incubation of hypothalamic fragments with LHRH inhibited endogenous LHRH release. Terminals that take up tritiated norepinephrine have been shown to synapse with GnRH neurons in the MPOA of the rat (959). Neuropeptide Y-like terminals have also been shown to synapse with GnRH neurons (960). It is not as yet known if norepinephrine and NPY are colocalized in the same terminals. Serotonin-like terminals, visualized by uptake of tritiated serotonin, synapsed with GnRH-like neurons, visualized by immunohistochemistry, in the POA of the rat (910). In addition, presumptive GABA terminals, shown by immunohistochemistry employing an antibody to GAD, have been shown to synapse with GnRH neurons (961), and CRF-like terminals made synapses with GnRH dendrites in the POA (962). Substance P containing neurons from the arcuate nucleus have been found to synapse with GnRH-like neurons in the septo-POA of the rat (963), as have neurons containing POMC or its processed products—the opioid peptides (964,965). In the monkey, such terminals synapsed with GnRH neurons in the region of the arcuate nucleus (890).

Gonadotropin-releasing hormone pathways from the preoptic and septal regions of the rat brain have been established, and the basic schema has been agreed upon by several investigators. Perikarya containing GnRH are arranged across the region of the rat's basilar forebrain in the shape of an inverted V. The apex is directed at midline nuclear groups such as the organum vasculosum of the lamina terminalis and the periventricular POA, and the diverging wings are bisected by the third ventricle. Two systems project caudally and ventrally to the median eminence, a periventricular system originating medially and a lateral system originating laterally and descending in the medial forebrain bundle. Although some differences in details exist, the systems following this basic pattern are described by King et al. (952), Hoffman and Gibbs (966), and Merchenthaler et al. (967). Analogous systems are described in the guinea pig (897,968), monkey (969), baboon (970), and human (901), except that GnRH-containing cells in the arcuate nucleus as well as in the MPOA project to the median eminence.

Gonadotropin-releasing hormone cells in the POA of the baboon project to the median eminence but also to the stria medullaris and the OVLT. Cells in the pericellular POA project to the median eminence. Gonadotropin-releasing hormone cells were also found in the medial septum, bed nucleus of the stria terminalis, lateral hypothalamus, and lateral POA, and these cells did not project to the median eminence. They were believed to be involved with reproductive behavior other than endocrine function (970). In the hamster, projections from the septum are reported to gain access to the hippocampus via the septum and to reach the amygdala via the stria terminalis. Projections from the medial septum also reach the OVLT and subfornical organ (SFO).

Projections from the olfactory tubercule reached the amygdala and piriform cortex via the ventroamygdalofugal pathway. Supracallosal projections reached the indiseum griseum. Descending projections to the midbrain coursed along the stria medullaris and fasciculus retroflexus, and some continued caudally into the pons (971). A similar pattern of projections to the rhinencephalon and limbic system and brainstem was found in the rat (972), bat (898), and guinea pig (897). The GnRH cells project to cerebral and brainstem regions that can promote sexual behavior as well as to diencephalic regions that can promote ovulation.

The projections of the POA have been studied by autoradiography following the injection of labeled amino acids into the POA of the rat brain (931,973) and following the injection of wheat germ agglutinin–HRP (974) and *Phaseolus vulgaris* leukoagglutinin (PHA-L) (975). The periventricular POA projections were principally descending ones in the periventricular zone to the "hypophysiotrophic area" of the medial basilar hypothalamus and the median eminence (973). Swanson (931) stated that dorsal, intermediate, and ventral parts of the periventricular POA project to "characteristically different terminal fields." A lesser projection courses laterally to join the medial region of the medial forebrain bundle to terminate in the hypophysiotropic area of the hypothalamus and the internal zone of the median eminence.

Neurons in the periventricular POA and in the MPOA projected to the OVLT (976). A projection of GnRH-containing neurons from the MPOA to the OVLT has been identified in the rat (952). Fibers in the OVLT containing TRH (444), somatostatin (783), and human growth hormone (598) also originated in the MPOA (976). Vasopressin-containing fibers that terminate in the OVLT probably arise from the suprachiasmatic nucleus (977) and not from the SON (340).

Ascending projections of the MPOA are dorsal to the stria medullaris (and hence via the habenular nuclei and fasciculus retroflexus to the midbrain tegmentum), to the diagonal band of Broca (and hence to the medial septum), and to the medial forebrain bundle (973). More extensive ascending projections were reported by Chiba and Murata (974) to the bed nucleus of the stria terminalis, nucleus of the diagonal band of Broca, medial amygdaloid nucleus, and septal regions. (The interested reader is referred to refs. 827,931,973–975,978.)

The descending projections of the MPOA resemble those of the periventricular POA except that the contribution to the lateral pathway through the medial forebrain bundle is more robust. Neither Conrad and Pfaff (827) nor Swanson (931) could trace descending pathways further caudally than the mesencephalon. Chiba and Murata (974) were able to trace descending fibers from the MPOA to the lateral parabrachial nucleus of the pons, to the locus ceruleus, to the nucleus and tractus solitarius, and to the vagal complex of the medulla in the rat using wheat germ agglutinin–HRP as a tracer. They propose that these projections are the basis of the functional relationship between the MPOA and the autonomic control of blood pressure, of thermoregulation, and of ANG II induced drinking behavior (Table 2).

In summary, concepts of the hypophysiotropic area first proposed by Harris (73–77) on the basis of his transplantation experiments and developed by Halaz and Pupp (102) on the basis of their hypothalamic islands have been expanded over the years. Cells that contain hypophysiotropic peptides and neurotransmitters and that terminate in the median eminence are found (principally) in nuclear groups that extend along the periventricular area from the lamina terminalis to the mammillary body. Smaller populations of cells are dispersed laterally (in the septum, diagonal band of Broca, and bed nucleus of the stria terminalis). Many peptidergic cells project to the median eminence, but others project to nuclear groups in the brainstem and spinal cord, to another circumventricular organ, the OVLT, as well as to terminal fields in rostral (limbic) regions. Hormones with synergistic effects may be colocalized in the same terminal as are CRF, AVP, and ANG II. The dispersion of functional hypophysiotropic cell types along the rostrocaudal axis in the periventricular zone permits each cell type to become closely related to several different cell types within unique nuclear groupings. Disparate peptidergic cells in a nuclear group frequently project to the same target. For example, OT, SRIF, and ENK-like cells project to common sites in the brainstem and spinal cord from a common site in the PVN. Perhaps more importantly, the dispersion of functional cell groups brings clusters of hypophysiotropic cells into the terminal fields of specific ascending and descending afferent fiber systems to permit appropriate integration of disparate incoming neural stimuli; and, because a cell's location will determine its projections, this organization will enable the endocrine, autonomic, and (higher) cortical systems to respond in a coordinated fashion.

INPUT INTO THE PERIVENTRICULAR HYPOTHALAMUS

Afferent systems from the rhinencephalon, from limbic structures, and from the brainstem project to specific preoptic and hypothalamic sites where neurosecretory neurons reside. These sites may be occupied by clusters of homogeneous neurons that manufacture the same peptide(s), by clusters of heterogeneous neurons that manufacture different peptides, or by clusters of heterogeneous neurons in which only a few manufacture peptides but most do not. Neuronal cell groups thus defined need not share a common peptide, but they can share a common pattern of afferent input. They represent a terminal field upon which converge axons from diverse and unique sites.

Afferents enter the periventricular hypothalamus by one of four routes: the medial forebrain bundle (MFB), the periventricular system, the fornix, and the stria terminalis. The MFB lies in the lateral zone of the hypothalamus and extends from preoptic to mammillary levels. The cells within the lateral zone were called *path neurons* by Millhouse (979). These cells are oriented perpendicular to the plane of fibers running in a rostrocaudal direction in the MFB, and each dendritic tree radiates like a fan in the path of fibers in the MFB. Their axons project medially into the medial and periventricular zones and innervate the nuclear groups in the MPOA–hypophysiotropic area (980). Collaterals from MFB neurons branch at right angles to the parent axon and course parallel to the dendrites of path neurons. Hence one axon of a fiber in the MFB passes through the dendritic arbor of several path neurons in series with the opportunity to send collaterals to each (979).

Ascending and descending input enters into and passes through the MFB. Millhouse (979) proposed that descending input tended to project collaterals into rostral areas (the MPOA and anterior hypothalamic area), whereas ascending input tended to send collaterals preferentially to caudal regions (the tuberomammillary region). He also proposed that the fascicles of the MFB maintained constant and characteristic positions in the MFB that were related to their origin. Both of these concepts have received support from subsequent autoradiographic studies on the MFB in the rat (981,982). Ascending components are confined to the dorsal half of the bundle and descending components to the ventral half. Major fiber groups that descend in the MFB arise (a) in the olfactory tubercle, amygdala, basal ganglia, and MPOA and lie in the ventral and ventrolateral regions; (b) in the septum and are confined to the ventromedial region of the bundle. The components arising from various regions in the POA are specifically arranged in the ventral region of the MFB. Ascending systems are probably similarly arranged with the ventral tegmental component near the center of the bundle and the ascending fibers of the parabrachial plexus in the dorsal and dorsolateral regions.

There is disagreement regarding the presence of catecholaminergic fibers that ascend from the brainstem in the MFB. The dorsal tegmental bundle is thought to arise from the locus ceruleus (A6) cell group and to ascend in the central tegmental tract. According to the account of Lindvall and Björklund (983), on the basis of fluorescence following glyoxylic acid treatment, fibers of the dorsal tegmental bundle enter the MFB. On the basis of immunohistochemistry of DBH, Swanson and Hartman (984) concluded that noradrenergic fibers from the locus ceruleus traveled with other ascending noradrenergic systems in the "principal noradrenergic system," "in the central tegmental tract," and entered the hypothalamus from a lateral position in a discrete bundle in the zona inserta. These fibers innervated the PVN by passing from lateral to medial and then down the periventricular area to the arcuate nucleus. The MPOA was innervated both from the periventricular area and from fibers coursing medially from the zona inserta.

The ventral tegmental noradrenergic bundle in the pons and mesencephalon receives input from the A_1 (lateral reticular nucleus), A_2 (dorsal medullary complex), A_5, and A_7 (parabrachial nucleus), and from the subceruleus region (983,841). This projection ascends in the central tegmental tract, and, according to the account of Lindvall and Björklund (983), contributes to the MFB at the level of the tegmental radiations. Swanson and Hartman (984) disputed this interpretation on the basis of their DBH studies and stated that the dorsal and ventral tegmental bundles form the principal ascending noradrenergic bundle, which enters the hypothalamus as a discrete system in the region of the zona inserta. They believe the fluorescent fibers seen in the MFB by Lindvall and Björklund (983) to be dopaminergic and to arise from the ventral tegmental region, ascend in the MFB, and terminate in hypothalamus and limbic forebrain (985,986). Palkovits et al. (987) appear to accept the account of Lindvall and Björklund (983), because they observed lesions separating the MFB from the MPOA–hypophysiotropic area to reduce the norepinephrine content of that region. At this time one can conclude that the MFB contains dopaminergic fibers, but the matter of noradrenergic neurons has yet to be settled.

The periventricular system (756) extends around the third ventricle. Axon terminals are oriented in a dorsoventral plane, as are the axons and dendritic fields of neurons in this region (103). This region also carries fibers that project rostrally and caudally. Major descending input arises in the MPOA (931,973,988). Within the MPOA–hypophysiotropic area, the PVN contributes to this system (827). From outside the periventricular region, the ventral median nucleus of the hypothalamus sends ascending and descending fibers into the periventricular system (989–991). Ascending input into the periventricular system is from the brainstem through the dorsal longitudinal fasciculus, which receives input from the A_2 cell group in the dorsal medullary complex and to a lesser extent from the locus ceruleus and the subceruleus area (983,987,992,993).

The fornix also projects to the MPOA–hypophysiotropic area, but the hippocampal fibers destined for hypothalamic terminals originate in the prosubiculum, not in Ammon's horn (994). Fibers originating in field CA1 of Ammon's horn project through the fornix to terminate (with or without relay in the mammillary nuclei) in the anterior nucleus of the thalamus. Field CA3 of Ammon's horn sends projections through the fimbria to the precommissural fornix, where they terminate principally in the septal nuclei. The septum projects to the medial preoptic nucleus, which in turn projects to the periventricular hypothalamus (975,978,995). In the rat, fibers destined for the arcuate nucleus arise in the subiculum and pass in the dorsal region of the fornix to the postcommissural fornix, where they depart from it and form the medial cortical hypothalamic tract, which terminates in the arcuate nucleus. The dentate gyrus and Ammon's horn both receive a massive input from the rhinencephalon and sensory regions of the forebrain. The dentate gyrus projects to Ammon's horn, which in turn projects to the prosubiculum and thence to the arcuate nucleus (996,997). The medial corticohypothalamic tract, which is prominent in rodents, is not found in primates (706). The pathway from the hippocampus to the hypothalamus in humans has not been established with certainty.

The stria terminalis carries projections from the amygdala to the bed nucleus of the stria terminalis and the POA, as well as to the ventromedial nucleus of the hypothalamus. Both the medial preoptic nucleus and the ventromedial nucleus in turn have been shown to project to targets in the periventricular hypothalamus (see below). Several different peptidergic fiber systems are present in this tract, but their relationship to neurosecretory cells in the MPOA remains to be evaluated (949).

The SON receives input from several sources within the POA and the hypothalamus, including the arcuate nucleus, the MPOA, and the OVLT and SFO (Table 3). The arcuate nucleus sends a projection of ACTH-containing axons to the SON that is distributed to regions where OT cells predominate (889). Input from the median preoptic nucleus to the SON has been demonstrated by both anterograde and retrograde tracing (998). The OVLT is a circumventricular organ that lies above the optic chiasm. The SFO, also a circumventricular organ, lies above and behind the OVLT (just beneath the foramen of Monro). These circumventricular organs lie in the anteroventral region of the third ventricle—the AV3V region. The input from the SFO and the OVLT into the SON is of particular interest in view of the accepted role of the AV3V region in fluid and electrolyte balance (751,922,923). The OVLT is made up of specialized ependymal cells that are united by tight junctions, fenestrated capillaries, neurons, and axon terminals. *In vitro* recording from neurons in the region of the OVLT demonstrated that the majority of neurons increased their firing rates with an increase in the sodium concentration of the medium (248). A projection from the OVLT to the SON has been demonstrated by retrograde tracing of HRP following injection into the SON (999). Neurons in the SFO have been found to respond to circulating levels of ANG II rather than sodium (1000). The SFO has been shown to project to the median preoptic nucleus and to the OVLT by precommissural fiber pathways and to the medial septum, diagonal band of Broca and to the magnocellular neurosecretory nuclei by postcommissural pathways (1001–1003). It should be remembered that the targets of the precommissural projection from the SFO also project to the SON.

TABLE 3. *Afferents to MPOA-HTA*[a]

	SON	PVN(m)	PVN(p)	PVN	AN	MPOA
OVLT	+	+				+
SFO	+	+				+
SON		+				
PVN(m)						
PVN(p)						
PVN					+	
AN	+	+	+	+		+
MPOA	+	+	+	+		+
VMN			?	+	+	
Hipp.	+	+	?			
Septum	+	+	?			+
BNST		?	+			+
Amygdala		?	+			+
Ol. Tub.						
IPN						
SN						
Teg.	?					
PbN			+		?	+
LC	+			?		
Raphe	+					+
LRN	+	+	+	+	+	
PVC	+		+	+	+	

[a] Abbreviations are the same as in Table 1. Also: SFO, subfornical organ.

ANG II receptors have been localized in the SFO, and some of its projections expressed ANG II (1004). ANG II-like cell bodies have been found in and around the SFO, and they projected to nuclear groups in the periventricular zone of the hypothalamus (1004). An ANG II-like projection to the SON has been reported (1005). This observation has raised the possibility that neurons in the SFO respond to circulating levels of ANG II and employ ANG II to convey that information directly to magnocellular neurons in the SON.

Descending input to the SON comes from several sources in the rhinencephalon and in the limbic forebrain. Retrograde and anterograde tracing studies have demonstrated afferent input from the main and accessory olfactory bulbs to the ventral glial lamina—a region where dendrites of neurophysin-like neurons are plentiful (1006,1007). Electrophysiological studies have shown both monosynaptic and polysynaptic connections between the lateral olfactory tract and the SON (1007). The function of this connection is not well understood. Hatton et al. (1008,1009) have shown that stimulation of the lateral olfactory tract increased dye coupling between magnocellular neurons in lactating or maternally acting rats but not in virgin females. Hence olfactory stimulation not only activates magnocellular neurons, but also coordinates their firing in phase and thus, presumably, facilitates such functions as lactation.

The region surrounding the SON contains neurons that project into it (999). Injections of HRP that extended slightly beyond the borders of the SON revealed an input that was more extensive than that revealed by injections that were confined within the boundaries of the SON (999). Regions outside the MPOA–hypophysiotropic area projected to regions about the SON. Fibers, descending from subiculum, septum, and nucleus of the diagonal band of Broca, were labeled. Although Swanson and Cowan (978) did not report labeling of the SON following injection of labeled amino acids into the septal region, Tribollet et al. (999) noted labeling in the region immediately surrounding the SON following the injection of tritiated amino acids into the septum and subiculum. The pattern of labeling probably signifies a functional connection between these limbic regions and the SON because (a) the dendritic field of the SON is not limited to the confines of the nucleus but extends beyond it, particularly in the ventral glial lamina (1010); (b) TEM studies of the SON region following placement of septal lesions demonstrated degeneration of terminals (1011); (c) TEM studies following anterograde transport of HRP from the septum demonstrate labeled terminals synapsing on neurites at the border of the SON that stain immunohistochemically for either OT or AVP (1012); and (d) electrophysiological studies demonstrated antidromic activation of septal neurons after stimulation of the SON (1013). Hence afferent systems descending to the SON arise in the rhinencephalon and in the limbic forebrain. Although some projections (from the olfactory bulb and subiculum) are direct, others probably relay in the septum.

The ascending input from the brainstem enters the hypothalamus through the periventricular dorsal longitudinal fasciculus or the MFB (706). Both norepinephrine and dopamine are present in the SON (856,992,1014). Catecholamine-containing terminals have been demonstrated in the SON of the rat (848), cat (1015), and monkey (1016), and several sources have been suggested. Small injections of HRP confined within the locus of the SON of the rat labeled the A_1 (lateral reticular nucleus) and the A_2 (nucleus of the solitary tract and the dorsal vagal complex) noradrenergic cell groups (999). Similar observations were made in the rabbit in which HRP labeling after SON injection of catecholaminergic cells identified by fluoroscopic methods was demonstrated in the A_1 and A_2 cell groups (1017). Electrophysiological studies showed that stimulation of the carotid sinus nerves or baroreceptors activated neurons in the location of the A_2 cell group and stimulation of these noradrenergic neurons selectively facilitated activity of phasic AVP-secreting (but not OT-secreting) neurons in the SON (1018,1019).

Whereas the evidence that the A_1 cell group projects to the SON is strong, evidence that the A_2 cell group directly innervates the SON is less compelling. Anterograde labeling experiments in the rat (993,1020) and the rabbit (1017) failed to confirm the presence of a direct innervation of the SON by the A_2 cell group. Stimulation of the nucleus of the solitary tract excited some SON neurons by "slow," presumably polysynaptic pathways. The authors concluded that stimulation of the A_2 cell group activated magnocellular neurons in the SON only after relay in the A_1 cell group (1021).

Projections from the lateral reticular nucleus in the ventrolateral medulla, as demonstrated by anterograde tracing techniques, terminated in the ventral and caudal regions of the SON, where AVP-like magnocellular neurons are aggregated (1022). Noradrenergic terminals have been found within the ventral regions of the SON, where AVP-like neurons are clustered (749,1023,1024). McNeill and Sladek (1023) noted that in the rat, catecholamine terminals were most frequently found surrounding the SON and were particularly abundant in the ventral glial lamina (1010), where they contacted dendrites of SON-like neurons. These anatomical observations nicely complement the physiological findings of Day and Renaud (1019) that stimulation of the A_1 cell groups selectively activated phasic AVP-secreting neurons.

Dopamine terminals are also present in the SON. They are homogeneously distributed throughout the nucleus and terminate on the soma of OT- and AVP-containing cells (1025). In view of the close relationship of AVP terminals in the neural lobe of the rat to terminals of the dopaminergic tuberohypophysial tract (508), it is of interest to determine the site of origin of dopaminergic terminals about the magnocellular neurons in the SON. Buijs et al. (1025) have suggested that they arise in the arcuate nucleus. Simon et al. (985) identified a projection from the A_{10} dopaminergic cell group in the ventral tegmental area of Tsai to the SON using anterograde and retrograde tracing techniques. Further work is necessary before the origin of the dopaminergic terminals in the SON can be considered established.

Serotonin-containing terminals in the SON originated in the raphe nuclei of the rat and entered the hypothalamus through the MFB (1026). The distribution of serotonin-like fibers within the SON and their mode of termination (axosomatic, axodendritic, or axoaxonic) is not as yet known. In addition to these projections, a substance P containing project has been reported by Bittencourt et al. (1027) to terminate in the SON of the rat. These authors observed an accumulation of DBH and substance P immunoreactive material proximal to the site of a lesion placed in the ascending catecholaminergic bundle and a parallel decrease in immunostaining for DBH and substance P in the SON. They proposed that the origin of the immunoreactive substance P projection to the SON was the A_1 cell group in the medulla.

The PVN receives input from several structures in the MPOA–hypophysiotropic region of the rat's hypothalamus. On the basis of studies employing retrograde transport of HRP following its injection into the PVN, input from the MPOA, OVLT, and SFO and from within the hypophysiotropic area has been demonstrated (1028,1029). Anterograde autoradiographic tracer studies following the injection of ^{3}H-proline into the MPOA of the guinea pig revealed a projection into the PVN (988). Chiba and Murata (974) injected wheat germ agglutinin–HRP into the MPOA of the rat and found labeling in multiple hypothalamic nuclei, including the PVN. This finding has been confirmed in the rat in which a projection from the medial preoptic nucleus to the parvicellular regions of the PVN has been shown by anterograde and retrograde tracing (975). Projections to the magnocellular regions of the PVN from the OVLT have been identified by retrograde tracing but await confirmation by anterograde techniques (1029). A projection from the SFO to the PVN has been identified by retrograde and anterograde tracing (1001). Electrophysiological studies suggest that ANG II projections to the PVN activate magnocellular neurons that release AVP and parvicellular neurons that release CRF (1000,1030, 1031). Silverman et al. (1029) proposed that input to the PVN from the SON arises from collaterals of the SOHT. Other projections from within the periventricular zone are difficult to demonstrate by conventional tracing techniques because the distance between the site of injection and uptake and the sites of labeled terminals is small. Sawchenko et al. (889) employed immunohistochemistry to demonstrate an ACTH projection from the arcuate nucleus of the rat to the magnocellular regions of the PVN, where OT fibers predominated. Arcuate ACTH fibers also terminated about parvicellular neurons in the ventromedial region of the medial parvicellular division of the PVN. These regions also contain OT-synthesizing neurons and project to the dorsovagal complex and spinal cord. Growth hormone-releasing factor-like cells in the AN have also been observed to project to the anterior, periventricular, and ventromedial parvicellular regions of the PVN (480). The pattern of input into the PVN from nuclear groups within the MPOA–hypophysiotropic area of the hypothalamus resembles that to the SON with the obvious addition of input into the parvicellular divisions.

Hypothalamic regions outside the MPOA–hypophysiotropic area also project to the PVN. Projections from the dorsomedial nucleus, ventromedial nucleus, and suprachiasmatic nucleus have been revealed by studies of retrograde transport of HRP following its injection into the PVN (1028,1029). Anterograde tracer studies with labeled amino acids have been carried out to determine the efferent pathways of the ventromedial area, but the authors do not mention a projection from the ventromedial nucleus to PVN in the rat (973,989,990). Saper et al. (990) stated that the anterograde labeling studies revealed no projection from the ventromedial nucleus to the PVN in the monkey. However, following placement of an electrolytic lesion in the ventromedial nucleus of the cat, Kaelber and Leeson (1032) found degenerating terminals in the PVN. If confirmed, the projection from hypothalamic areas outside the MPOA–hypophysiotropic area such as the ventromedial nucleus to the PVN marks a major difference in input when compared with the SON.

The PVN, like the SON, receives descending input from hippocampal formation. This input may be direct from the subiculum or from Ammon's horn with a relay in the septum and in the medial preoptic nucleus (995,1028,1029). Oldfield et al. (1012) employed TEM techniques to examine the PVN after injection of HRP into the subiculum or septum and immunohistochemical staining of the PVN for immunoreactive OT or AVP. A projection from these limbic regions onto AVP- and OT-containing neurites just lateral or ventrolateral to the PVN was demonstrated. Unlike the SON, the PVN receives a projection from the medial and central nuclei of the amygdala (1028,1029) and from the bed nucleus of the stria terminalis (978,1003,1029). Transmission electron microscopic studies demonstrated that the input from the amygdala is to the AVP-containing neurites just lateral and ventrolateral to the nucleus—a site where dendrites from the PVN were found. Projections from the amygdala, the bed nucleus of the stria terminalis, and the medial preoptic nucleus and ventromedial nucleus of the hypothalamus, which in turn receive input from the amygdala (995,1033–1035), are unique to the PVN compared with the SON. It is tempting to relate these projections from limbic regions that contain glucocorticoid receptors to the parvicellular regions of the PVN that (a) contain AVP, CRF, and ANG II; (b) project to the median eminence (or to the medulla and spinal cord); and (c) are implicated in the regulation of the pituitary adrenal and autonomic neural axes (1029,1036–1038).

The PVN receives a much more elaborate ascending innervation than does the SON. Catecholamines have been identified in the PVN (856,992,1014), and catecholamine terminals have been demonstrated in the PVN of the rat (848), cat (1015), and monkey (1016) by fluorescence techniques. In the magnocellular divisions of the rat (1023) and monkey (1016), catecholamine fibers have been found to be more abundant in regions rich in AVP cells than in regions where cells containing OT predominate. Swanson et al. (804) employed immunohistochemistry to demonstrate the terminals containing DBH but not PNMT (and therefore noradrenergic terminals) were present predominantly in regions where AVP-containing magnocellular neurons were found. However, these observations must be interpreted cautiously, because Silverman et al. (1039) demonstrated in a TEM study of the PVN that catecholamine terminals primarily innervated the dendritic processes of nonvasopressinergic neurons. When noradrenergic terminals contacted AVP-containing neurons, contact was axodendritic, not axosomatic. As the dendrites of peptidergic cells within the PVN have a large medial to lateral extension (757), the specific location of noradrenergic terminals within subdivisions of the PVN may not be predictive of the type of cell innervated.

Retrograde tracing experiments showed that the lateral reticular nucleus (A_1 cell group) projected to the PVN in rats (993,1028) and rabbits (1017) (Fig. 22). Anterograde labeling experiments have confirmed this pattern in the rabbit (1017) and rat (1022) and further demonstrated that the A_1 projection is preferential to the magnocellular regions that contain AVP-like neurons. In the rat, immunoreactive-NPY was frequently costored in the DBH-like terminals in the magnocellular regions of the PVN, where AVP-like neurons were clustered. After injection of True Blue into the PVN, labeled cells in the A_1 cell group that immunostained for DBH and NPY were found, as were neurons that immunostained for DBH alone (1040). The principle that A_1 neurons with or without costored NPY do preferentially innervate magnocellular neurons in the PVN that contain AVP is supported by the observation that stimulation in the region of the A_1 cell group activated phasic (AVP) neurons in the PVN (1041–1043) as it activated phasic (AVP) neurons in the SON (1019). It is difficult not to place functional significance upon the observation that large cells in the PVN and SON arise from the same germinal cell group, migrate to their final destinations at the same time, receive input from the same limbic, circumventricular, preoptic, and brainstem structures, and project to the same terminal field—the neural lobe.

Catecholaminergic terminals are also found in the parvicellular divisions of the PVN. Anterograde tracing studies with small selected injections in A_2 demonstrated preferential labeling in the dorsomedial parvicellular subdivision, where CRF-like neurons were clustered. These terminals also immunostained for DBH, leading the authors to the conclusion that the noradrenergic projection of the A_2 cell group in the dorsal motor nucleus innervated this region of the PVN (1022). Only about 10% to 15% of these noradrenergic neurons have been found to costore NPY (1040). The adrenergic cell groups in the lateral reticular nucleus and in the dorsal motor nucleus lie rostral to the noradrenergic cell groups and are termed the C_1 and C_2 cell groups, respectively. Anterograde transport studies revealed that the C_1 and C_2 cell groups, unlike the A_1 and A_2 cell groups, projected to

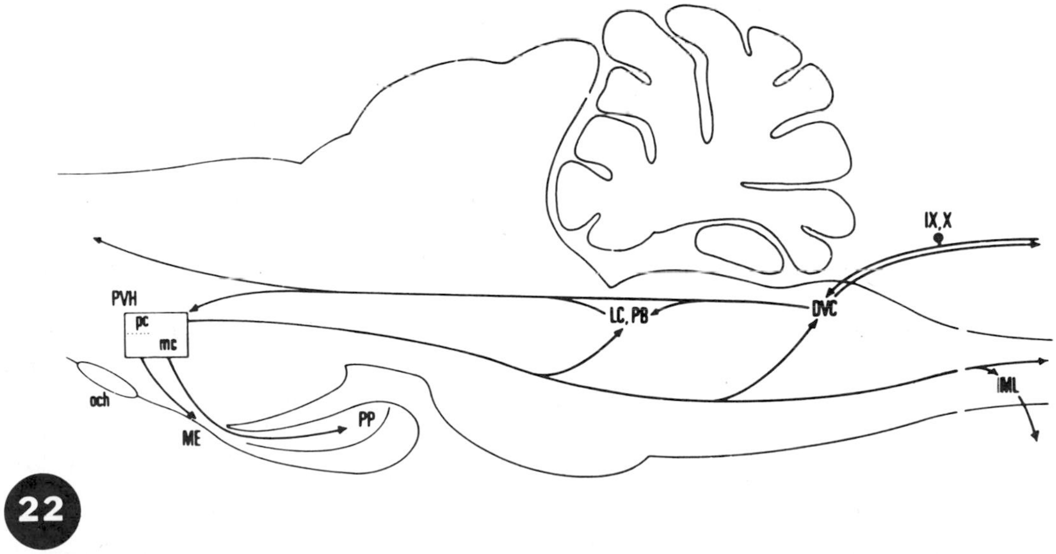

FIG. 22. A summary of the major longer connections of PVH in the rat. In this diagram, relationships between the PVH and the cell groups associated with the autonomic nervous system are emphasized. *DVC,* dorsal vagal complex; *IML,* intermediolateral column; *LC,* locus ceruleus; *mc,* magnocellular division of PVH; *ME,* median eminence; *och,* optic chiasm; *PB,* parabrachial nucleus; *pc,* parvocellular division of PVH; *PP,* posterior pituitary; *PVH,* paraventricular nucleus; *IX,* glossopharyngeal nerve; *X,* vagus nerve. (From ref. 1069, with permission.)

the same sites in the PVN—to all the parvicellular subgroups. The dorsal and dorsomedial subdivisions received the strongest innervation. Terminals that contained the tracer frequently immunostained for PNMT (1044). Adrenergic projections from the C_1 and C_2 cell groups also contained NPY, with the C_1 cell group having the higher proportion of double-labeled cells (1040).

In addition to catecholaminergic input from A_2, C_1, and C_2, the parvicellular subdivisions received innervation from the A_6 cell group in the locus ceruleus. This noradrenergic input preferentially terminated in the periventricular subdivision of the PVN from where hypophysiotropic TRH-like neurons are clustered (1022). Only about 15% of the DBH-like neurons in the locus ceruleus costored NPY (1040). These medullary and pontine catecholaminergic sites projected via different pathways (the ventral and dorsal tegmental bundles, respectively), in the central tegmental area, and then to the PVN via the medial forebrain bundle or via the periventricular pathways (770,1032).

Neurophysiological studies demonstrated that stimulation of the PVN antidromically activated units in the A_1 region to which the PVN projects, as confirmed by HRP tracing (1045). Non-noradrenergic pathways have been identified from the nucleus of the solitary tract to the A_1 cell group, as have noradrenergic pathways from A_1 to A_2 and A_6 (993). The same PVN neurons were activated by polysynaptic pathways (presumably passing through the nucleus of the solitary tract to the lateral reticular nucleus) by stimulation of carotid sinus and aortodepressor nerves (1045).

Other studies reported a projection from the "pontine taste area" (the parabracheal nucleus-A_7-noradrenergic cell group) to the PVN (1046,1047). Anterograde tracing studies demonstrated that the A_7 cell group projects to the parvicellular divisions of the PVN, particularly to the dorsal and medial parvicellular regions (which project back to the dorsovagal region in the medulla and to the intermediolateral cell column in the spinal cord [1048,1049]). In addition, the A_7 cell group projected heavily to the central nucleus of the amygdala (1046), which in turn projected to the PVN (1028,1029) and A_1 region, which in turn projected to the PVN (1048).

Other systems reportedly project to the PVN. Buijs et al. (1025) reported that dopaminergic fibers innervate the nucleus homogeneously. Liposits and Paull (1050) lesioned the ascending catecholaminergic bundle and subsequently found TH-like but not DBH-like terminals in the ipsilateral PVN. These terminals were closely associated with CRF-like neurons (1050) and may have arisen from the arcuate nucleus or even from within the PVN, as Liposits et al. (1051) reported the presence of TH-like cell bodies and fibers in the PVN of the rat. Substance P-like terminals have been found in all divisions of the PVN. Although the projection to the magnocellular subdivisions appears to arise from the ventrolateral medulla, multiple sites of origin of the terminals in the parvicellular subdivisions have been found (1027).

The PVN differs from the SON not only because it is located in a different place but because it is quite simply the SON and more. It contains another population of small neurons that (one would predict) arises from a different germinal site. It most certainly projects to different terminal fields (the dorsal medulla and spinal cord as well as the median eminence) and receives different (additional) limbic and brainstem input. It presumably projects to a different terminal field in the neurohypophysis (the median eminence), although the undisputed site of these projections has not been agreed upon. The congregation of peptidergic parvicellular neurons that receive input from the limbic and brainstem centers related to steroid feedback and cardiovascular status about magnocellular elements that receive input concerning the osmolality of the blood and the cardiovascular status is presumably more than fortuitous. These functions are not carried out independently but are integrated by the axodendritic relationships within the nucleus between these two cellular populations (757).

The periventricular nucleus also receives input from within the MPOA–hypophysiotropic area. Growth hormone-containing fibers from the arcuate nucleus synapse with SRIF-like neurons in the preoptic and hypothalamic periventricular sites (480,838). Descending projections in the rat and guinea pig from the MPOA to the periventricular nucleus by periventricular routes as well as by the MFB have been reported (931,973,988), as have projections from the bed nucleus of the stria terminalis (978). Other hypothalamic regions, the ventromedial nucleus (989–991), and the anterior hypothalamic area (827) outside the MPOA–hypophysiotropic area were reported to project to the periventricular nucleus. Catecholamine terminals have been demonstrated by fluorescence techniques in the periventricular region (848,1015,1016). Terminals containing immunoreactive PNMT and those containing NPY have been demonstrated to synapse on SRIF-like neurons in the periventricular preoptic and hypothalamic regions (813,834). Although NPY and epinephrine may be costored in the same terminals and their source may be in the adrenergic cell groups in the medulla, the ascending fiber pathways to the narrow periventricular region of the POA and the hypothalamus have not been worked out in detail.

The arcuate nucleus has been found to receive input from SRIF-containing neurons in the periventricular nucleus of the hypothalamus (781,838). Hence, within the hypophysiotropic area reciprocal connections between GRH-like neurons in the AN and SRIF-like neurons in the PVN of the rat are present and presumably play a key role in the pulsatile release of growth hormone from the anterior pituitary. Both retrograde and anterograde tracing techniques have demonstrated projections from the MPOA to the arcuate nucleus in rat (973,1052).

Input from medial temporal lobe structures into the arcuate nucleus in the rat is by direct and indirect routes. In the rat, a direct input from the subiculum to the arcuate nucleus by the corticohypothalamic tract has been proposed by Raisman (997) and Raisman et al. (996), as discussed above. It is of interest that this fiber pathway was not described in the brains of cats, monkeys, and humans (706). Other input into the arcuate nucleus from the hippocampal formation via the fornix has been found to be relayed through the septum. Projections from Ammon's horn have been traced to the septum which in turn projected to the medial preoptic nucleus (995). The medial preoptic nucleus has in turn been demonstrated to project to the periventricular hypothalamus, including the arcuate nucleus, by both the periventricular route and the MFB (975).

The ventromedial nucleus, which lies outside the MPOA–hypophysiotropic area, may serve as a relay through which the amygdala projects to the arcuate nucleus. Szentagothai et al. (103) reported that "even very small foci in this region produced abundant signs of degeneration in all parts of the ipsilateral hypothalamus." Golgi studies by the same group revealed axon projections to the periventricular gray. Horseradish peroxidase injection into the median eminence labeled the ventromedial nucleus if the injection spread into the arcuate nucleus (755). Saper et al. (991) described a projection from the ventromedial nucleus to the arcuate nucleus in the monkey and the cat. On the other hand, Sutin and Eagen (1053) did not describe any degeneration in the arcuate nucleus of the cat following placement of discrete lesions in the ventromedial nucleus. The axonal projections from the ventromedial nucleus are described by both Szentagothai et al. (103) and Millhouse (1054) as being primarily directed dorsally and posteriorly on the basis of Golgi preparations. However, abundant collaterals were noted by both authors.

The ventromedial nucleus is an oval-shaped hypothalamic cell group that lies dorsal and lateral to the arcuate nucleus (103,1054). It is characterized by the presence of a cell-rich core and a cell-poor capsule (1054). Dendrites from axons in the ventromedial nucleus extend into the cell-poor capsule. In the cell-poor zone between the AN and ventromedial nucleus lie dendrites of both nuclear groups (1054). The nucleus is made up of two compact cellular aggregates that permit its subdivision into dorsolateral and ventromedial regions (990). Immunohistochemical techniques have revealed GRF in cells that encapsulate (but do not lie within) the nucleus and do not project to the median eminence or to the arcuate nucleus (480).

Heimer and Nauta (1033) studied the pattern of degeneration in the rat's hypothalamus following transection of the stria terminalis. They described three projections over the stria terminalis from the ipsilateral amygdala: one to the bed nucleus of the stria terminalis, one to a field immediately caudal to the anterior commissure, and one (supracommissural) to the cell-poor zone about the ventromedial nucleus. Raisman (997) transected the stria terminalis and demonstrated that the degenerating supracommissural axons terminated on the dendritic spines of ventromedial nucleus neurons in the cell-poor zone. McBride and Sutin (1034) injected HRP into the tuberal hypothalamus after ipsilateral transection of the stria terminalis and demonstrated that the cortical nucleus of the amygdala projected to the ventromedial nucleus solely by the stria terminalis. The medial nucleus employed both the ventral amygdalofugal pathway and the stria terminalis to reach the hypothalamus, and the basal nucleus projected to the ventromedial nucleus solely by the ventral amygdalofugal pathway. Krettek and Price (1035) employed anterograde autoradiographic studies to trace the path of tritiated amino acids injected into different nuclear groups in the amygdala. While they agreed with previous authors that the ventromedial nucleus was a target of a large output from the amygdala, they disagreed with the pattern of innervation. They found that the medial and basomedial nuclei of the amygdala both projected to the core of the ventromedial nucleus and not to its outer shell. The outer shell received a projection only from the subiculum via the dorsal fornix. Perhaps earlier experiments also lesioned the dorsal fornix in the attempt to transect the stria terminalis. The evidence that the ventromedial nucleus sends descending projections through the posterior periventricular region to the central gray of the brainstem, through the MFB to the capsule about the mammillary complex, and through the ventral supraoptic commissure to the contralateral hemisphere is fairly strong, as is the evidence for ascending projections in the periventricular gray and MFB to the POA and lateral septum (989–991). In addition, long reciprocal connections to the medial amygdaloid nucleus originate principally from the ventromedial nucleus (990,1055,1056). The anatomical evidence suggests that the ventromedial nucleus serves as a gateway by which projections from the amygdala can influence the arcuate nucleus and hence median eminence function, but that evidence is far from strong. On firmer footing is the supposition that projections from the amygdala to the paraventricular nucleus provide the route by which this structure influences median eminence function (978,1003,1028,1029).

Ascending projections to the arcuate nucleus have been identified and are believed to be principally noradrenergic (NA) (1057,1058). The norepinephrine content of the arcuate nucleus was reduced 75% by hypothalamic deafferentation (992). Terminals containing immunoreactive DBH were found in the arcuate nucleus of the rat (984). Lesion experiments (987) and anterograde tracing experiments (1020) suggest that the arcuate nucleus is, like the SON, the PVN, and the periventricular nucleus, predominantly innervated by the A_1 and A_2 cell groups in the medulla. Saper and Loewy (1048) described labeling of the arcuate nucleus following injection of ^{3}H-amino acids into the A_7 cell group in the parabracheal nucleus of the rat. However, such injections could have spread into the ventral tegmental system. Further confirmatory studies are indicated. Palkovits (987) pointed out that "the median eminence and any of the hypothalamic nuclei may receive NA fibers from any of the NA cell groups, as monosynaptic communication between them have already been proved." Noradrenergic terminals have been shown to synapse with GRH-like neurons in the AN (913). Fibers from the raphe nuclei, believed to be indolaminergic, reach the arcuate nucleus via the MFB (1059), and serotonergic terminals have been shown to synapse with dopaminergic neurons and ACTH-like neurons in the arcuate nucleus (911,915).

As reviewed above, the MPOA is one of the sites where hypophysiotropic GnRH cells reside in the rat. The MPOA is a complex region with considerable regional cytoarchitectonic specialization (1060). Input into the MPOA arises from several hypothalamic nuclei in the MPOA–hypophysiotropic periventricular complex. Retrograde HRP studies demonstrated afferents from the arcuate nucleus and PVN (974), and synapses have been demonstrated between substance P-like terminals and terminals containing opioid peptides (964,965) (presumably from the arcuate nucleus), CRF-like terminals (presumably from the PVN), and GnRH-like neurons (962,963). Afferents from hypothalamic nuclear groups outside the hypophysiotropic area have also been demonstrated and include projections from the ventromedial nucleus (989), dorsomedial nucleus, and mammillary complex (974). Descending input from the lateral septal nucleus via the MFB and from the medial septal nucleus via the periventricular system have been demonstrated by ^{3}H-amino acid autoradiographic studies (978). Afferents from the bed nucleus of the stria terminalis (974) and from the medial and central nuclei of the amygdala have also been demonstrated (1061). Ascending input from the A_1 and A_2 catecholaminergic cell groups in the medulla was shown by double labeling with HRP injection into the MPOA and fluorescent staining for catecholamines of brainstem nuclear groups (1041). As reviewed above, both NPY-like and presumptive noradrenergic terminals have been shown to synapse with GnRH neurons (959,960). The argument that this ascending noradrenergic pathway that costores NPY plays a role in stimulating GnRH neurons has been reviewed by Kalra (1062) and Kalra et al. (1063). Input from the A_7 area of the parabracheal nucleus (the "pontine taste area" of Norgren [1046]) has been demonstrated by retrograde transport of HRP (974); but this input is peptidergic, not noradrenergic, as some fibers contain immunoreactive CRF and others contain immunoreactive leu-ENK (1064). The B_7, B_8, and B_9 (841) raphe cell groups also projected to the MPOA (1059). The projection was serotonergic and sexually dimorphic (1065). Serotonergic terminals have been shown to synapse with GnRH-like neurons (910).

The neuroendocrine motor units that regulate anterior pituitary function have turned out to be more complex than previously believed. They costore other peptides and transmitters that (presumably) facilitate their hypophysiotropic function at the surface of anterior pituitary cells but that may also serve to regulate the function of neighboring terminals in the neurohemal contact zone by paracrine interactions and thus provide a coordinated discharge of neurohormones into the portal system. In addition, collateral axons of these neurons project to sites where other (neurosecretory) neurons reside and synapse with them to alter their function. The extrasegmental input upon each of these neurosecretory cell groups arises from sites within the medial hypothalamus where cholinergic, GABAergic, and glutaminergic cell bodies are thought to reside, from limbic and rhinencephalic sources, and from the brainstem. Further investigations as to the nature of this input to the GnRH motor neuron is the subject of further discussions in this volume and of research in the near and distant future.

REFERENCES

1. Cushing H. *The pituitary body and its disorders.* Philadelphia: J. B. Lippincott, 1912.
2. Cushing H. Neurohypophysial mechanisms from a clinical standpoint. Parts I and II. *Lancet* 1930;2:119,175.
3. Herring PT. The development of the mammalian pituitary and its morphological significance. *Q J Exp Physiol* 1908;1:161.
4. Herring PT. The histological appearances of the mammalian pituitary body. *Q J Exp Physiol* 1908;1:121.
5. Tilney F. Contribution to the study of the hypophysis cerebri with especial reference to its comparative histology. *Mem Wistar Inst Anat Biol* 1911;2.
6. Dandy WE, Goetsh ELL. The blood supply of the pituitary body. *Am J Anat* 1910;11:137.
7. Marie P. Sur deux d'acromegaly: hypertropic singuliere non congenitale des extremites superieures, inferieurs et cephalique. *Rev Med* 1886;VI:297, cited by Cushing (1).
8. Frolich A. Ein fall von tumor der hypophysis cerebri ohne akromegalie. *Wein Klin Rundschau* 1901;XV:883, cited by Cushing (1).
9. Crowe SJ, Cushing H, Homans J. Experimental hypophysectomy. *Bull Johns Hopkins Hosp* 1910;21:127.
10. Crowe SJ, Cushing H, Homans J. Effects of hypophyseal transplantation following hypophysectomy in the canine. *Q J Exp Physiol* 1908;1:121.
11. Smith PE. Hypophysectomy and a replacement therapy. *Am J Anat* 1930;45:205.
12. Dandy WE. The nerve supply to the pituitary body. *Am J Anat* 1913;15:333.
13. Cushing H, Goetsch E. Concerning the secretion of the infundib-

ular lobe of the pituitary body and its presence in the cerebrospinal fluid. *Am J Physiol* 1910;27:60.
14. Goetsch E, Cushing H, Jacobson C. Carbohydrate tolerance and the posterior lobe of the hypophysis cerebri. An experimental and clinical study. *Bull Johns Hopkins Hosp* 1911;22:165.
15. Weed LH, Cushing H, Jacobson C. Further studies on the role of the hypophysis in the metabolism of carbohydrates. The autonomic control of the pituitary gland. *Johns Hopkins Hosp Bull* 1913;24:40.
16. Oliver G, Schafer EA. On the physiological action of extracts of pituitary body and certain other glandular organs. *J Physiol* 1895;18:277.
17. Howell WH. The physiologic effects of extracts of the hypophysis cerebri and infundibular body. *J Exp Med* 1898;3:254.
18. Dale HH. The action of extracts of the pituitary body. *Biochem J* 1909;4:427.
19. Popa G, Fielding U. A portal circulation from the pituitary to the hypothalamic region. *J Anat* 1931;65:88.
20. Popa G, Fielding U. The vascular link between the pituitary and the hypothalamus. *Lancet* 1930;2:238.
21. Harris GW. Neural control of the pituitary gland. *Physiol Rev* 1948;28:139.
22. Cushing H. Posterior pituitary activity from an anatomical standpoint. *Am J Pathol* 1933;9:539.
23. Gersh I. Relation of histological structure to the active substances extracted from the posterior lobe of the hypophysis. *Res Publ Assoc Res Nerv Ment Dis* 1938;17:433.
24. Gersh I. The structure and function of the parenchymatous glandular cells in the neurohypophysis of the rat. *Am J Anat* 1939;64:407.
25. Lewis D, Lee FC. On the glandular elements in the posterior lobe of the human hypophysis. *Bull Johns Hopkins Hosp* 1927;41:241.
26. Rioch D. Paths of secretion from the hypophysis. *Res Publ Assoc Res Nerv Ment Dis* 1938;17:151.
27. Bucy PC. The pars nervosa of the bovine hypophysis. *J Comp Neurol* 1930;50:505.
28. Bucy PC. The hypophysis cerebri. In: Penfield W, ed. *Cytology and cellular pathology of the central nervous system,* Vol. 2. New York: Hoeber, 1932:705.
29. Wislocki GB, King LS. The permeability of the hypophysis and hypothalamus to vital dyes, with a study of the hypophyseal vascular supply. *Am J Anat* 1936;58:421.
30. Rioch D, Wislocki G, O'Leary J. A precis of preoptic, hypothalamic and hypophyseal terminology with atlas. *Res Publ Assoc Res Nerv Ment Dis* 1940;20:3.
31. Starling EH, Verney EB. The secretion of urine as studied on the isolated kidney. *Proc R Soc London [Biol]* 1924;97:321.
32. Fisher C, Ingram WR, Hare WK, Ranson SW. The degeneration of the supraoptico-hypophyseal system in diabetes insipidus. *Anat Rec* 1935;63:29.
33. Fisher C, Ingram WR, Ranson SW. The relation of the hypothalamo-hypophyseal system to diabetes insipidus. *Arch Neurol Psychiat* 1935;34:124.
34. Ingram WR, Fisher C, Ranson SW. Experimental diabetes insipidus in the monkey. *Arch Intern Med* 1936;57:1067.
35. Scharrer E, Scharrer B. Secretory cells within the hypothalamus. *Res Publ Assoc Res Nerv Ment Dis* 1940;20:170.
36. Scharrer B, Scharrer E. Neurosecretion VI. A comparison between the intercerebralis-cardiacum-allatum of the insects and the hypothalamo-hypophyseal system of the vertebrates. *Biol Bull* 1944;87:242.
37. Palay SL. Neurosecretion. VII. The preoptico-hypophysial pathway in fishes. *J Comp Neurol* 1945;82:129.
38. Bargmann W, Hild W. Uber die morphologie der neurosekretorischen verknupfung von hypothalamus und neurohypophyse. *Acta Anat* 1949;8:264.
39. Bargmann W, Scharrer E. The site of origin of the hormones of the posterior pituitary. *Am Sci* 1951;39:255.
40. Scharrer E, Scharrer B. Hormones produced by neurosecretory cells. *Recent Prog Horm Res* 1954;10:183.
41. Scharrer E. The final common path in neuroendocrine integration. *Arch Anat Microsc* 1965;54:359.
42. Scharrer B. The neurosecretory neuron in neuroendocrine regulatory mechanisms. *Am Zool* 1967;7:161.
43. Pierce JG, Vignaud V du. Studies on high potency oxytotic materials from beef posterior pituitary lobes. *J Biol Chem* 1950;186:77.
44. Vignaud V du, Ressler C, Swan JM, Roberts W, Katsoyannis PG, Gordon S. The synthesis of an octapeptide amide with the hormonal activity of oxytocin. *J Am Chem Soc* 1953;75:4879.
45. Turner RA, Pierce JG, Vignaud V du. The purification and the amino acid content of vasopressin preparations. *J Biol Chem* 1951;191:21.
46. Vignaud V du, Lawler HC, Papenea EA. Enzymatic cleavage of glycinamide from vasopressin and a proposed structure for this pressor-antidiuretic hormone of the posterior pituitary. *J Am Chem Soc* 1953;75:4880.
47. Vignaud V du, Gish D, Katsoyannis PG. A synthetic preparation possessing biological properties associated with arginine vasopressin. *J Am Chem Soc* 1954;76:4751.
48. VanDyke HB, Adamsons K, Engel SL. Aspects of the biochemistry and physiology of the neurohypophyseal hormones. *Recent Prog Horm Res* 1955;11:1.
49. Verney EB. The antidiuretic hormone and the factors which determine its release. *Proc R Soc Lond [Biol]* 1947;135:25.
50. Palay SL. An electron microscope study of the neurohypophysis in normal, hydrated, and dehydrated rats. *Anat Rec* 1955; 121:348.
51. Palay SL. The fine structure of secretory neurons in the preoptic nucleus of the goldfish (*Carassius auratus*). *Anat Rec* 1960;138:417.
52. Sloper JC, Arnott DJ, King BC. Sulphur metabolism in the pituitary and hypothalamus of the rat: a study of radioisotope-uptake after the injection of ^{35}S dl-cysteine, methionine, and sodium sulphate. *J Endocrinol* 1960;20:9.
53. Sloper JC. The validity of current concepts of hypothalamo-neurohypophyseal neurosecretion. *Prog Brain Res* 1972; 38:123.
54. Bargmann W. Neurosecretion. *Int Rev Cytol* 1966;19:183.
55. Norstrom A, Hansson H-A, Sjostrand J. Effects of colchicine on axonal transport and ultrastructure of the hypothalamo-neurohypophyseal system of the rat. *Z Zellforsch* 1971;113:271.
56. Lederis K. Neurosecretion and the functional structure of the neurohypophysis. In: Greep RO, Astwood EB, eds. *Handbook of physiology, endocrinology, the pituitary gland and its neuroendocrine control,* Sect. 7, Vol. IV. Washington, DC: American Physiology Society, 1974:81.
57. Silverman AJ, Zimmerman EA. Ultrastructural immunocytochemical localization of neurophysin and vasopressin in the median eminence and posterior pituitary of the guinea pig. *Cell Tissue Res* 1975;159:291.
58. Flament-Durand J, Couck AM, Dustin P. Studies on the transport of secretory granules in the magnocellular hypothalamic neurons of the rat. II. Action of vincrestine on axonal flow and neurotubules in the paraventricular and supraoptic nuclei. *Cell Tissue Res* 1975;164:1.
59. Vandersande F, Dierickx K. Identification of the vasopressin-producing and of the oxytocin-producing neurons in the hypothalamic magnocellular neurosecretory system of the rat. *Cell Tissue Res* 1975;164:153.
60. Weitzman RE, Fisher DA. Log linear relationship between plasma arginine vasopressin and plasma osmolality. *Am J Physiol* 1977;233:E37.
61. Gainer H, Sarne Y, Brownstein MJ. Biosynthesis and axonal transport of rat neurohypophysial proteins and peptides. *J Cell Biol* 1977;73:366.
62. Antunes JL, Zimmerman EA. The hypothalamic magnocellular system of the rhesus monkey: an immunocytochemical study. *J Comp Neurol* 1978;181:539.
63. Brownstein MJ, Russell JT, Gainer H. Synthesis, transport, and release of posterior pituitary hormones. *Science* 1980;207:373.
64. Russell JT, Brownstein MJ, Gainer H. Biosynthesis of vasopressin, oxytocin, and neurophysins: isolation and characterization of two common precursors (propressophysin and prooxyphysin). *Endocrinology* 1980;107:1880.

65. Harris GW. The induction of ovulation in the rabbit by electrical stimulation of the hypothalamo-hypophyseal mechanism. *Proc R Soc Lond* [*Biol*] 1937;122:374.
66. Green JD. The comparative anatomy of the hypophysis, with special reference to its blood supply and innervation. *Am J Anat* 1951;88:225.
67. Green JD, Harris GW. The neurovascular link between the neurohypophysis and adenohypophysis. *J Endocrinol* 1947; 5:136.
68. Green JD. The histology of the hypophyseal stalk and median eminence in man with special reference to blood vessels, nerve fibers and a peculiar neurovascular zone in this region. *Anat Rec* 1948;100:273.
69. Green JD. Vessels and nerves of amphibian hypophyses. *Anat Rec* 1947;99:21.
70. Green JD, Harris GW. Observation of the hypophysio-portal vessels of the living rat. *J Physiol* 1949;108:359.
71. Harris GW. Electrical stimulation of the hypothalamus and the mechanism of neural control of the adenohypophysis. *J Physiol* 1948;107:418.
72. Harris GW. The relationship of the nervous system to (a) the neurohypophysis and (b) the adenohypophysis. *J Endocrinol* 1949;6:xvii.
73. Harris GW. Oestrous rhythm pseudopregnancy and the pituitary stalk in the rat. *J Physiol (Lond)* 1950;111:347.
74. Harris GW, Johnson RT. Regeneration of the hypophyseal portal vessels, after section of the hypophyseal stalk in the monkey (*Macacus rhesus*). *Nature* 1950;165:819.
75. Harris GW. Regeneration of the hypophysial portal vessels. *Nature* 1949;163:70.
76. Harris GW, Jacobson D. Functional grafts of the anterior pituitary gland. *Proc R Soc Lond* [*Biol*] 1952;139:263.
77. Harris GW. *Neural control of the pituitary gland.* London: Edward Arnold, 1955.
78. Green JD. The comparative anatomy of the portal vascular system and of the innervation of the hypophysis. In: Harris GW, Donovan BT, eds. *The pituitary gland,* Vol. 1. Berkeley: University of California Press, 1966:27.
79. Wingstrand KG. Comparative anatomy and evaluation of the hypophysis. In: Harris GW, Donovan BT, eds. *The pituitary gland,* Vol. 1. Berkeley: Univ. of California Press, 1966:28.
80. Jorgensen CB, Larsen LO. Neuroendocrine mechanisms in lower vertebrates. In: Martini L, Ganong WF, eds. *Neuroendocrinology,* Vol. II. New York: Academic Press, 1967:485.
81. Xuereb GP, Prichard M, Daniel PM. The arterial supply and venous drainage of the human hypophysis cerebri. *Am J Exp Physiol* 1954;39:199.
82. Xuereb GP, Prichard MM, Daniel PM. The hypophysial portal system of vessels in man. *Q J Exp Physiol* 1954;39:219.
83. Daniel PM. The blood supply of the hypothalamus and pituitary gland. *Br Med Bull* 1966;22:202.
84. Harris GW. The blood vessels of the rabbit's pituitary gland, and the significance of the pars and zona tuberalis. *J Anat* 1947;81:343.
85. Page RB, Munger BL, Bergland RM. Scanning microscopy of pituitary vascular casts: the rabbit pituitary portal system revisited. *Am J Anat* 1976;146:273.
86. Wislocki GB. The vascular supply of the hypophysis cerebri of the cat. *Anat Rec* 1937;69:361.
87. Wislocki GB. Further observations on the blood supply of the hypophysis cerebri of the rhesus monkey. *Anat Rec* 1938; 72:137.
88. Wislocki GB. The vascular supply of the hypophysis cerebri of the rhesus monkey and man. *Res Publ Assoc Res Nerv Ment Dis* 1938;17:48.
89. Wislocki GB. Further observations on the blood supply of the hypophysis cerebri of the rhesus monkey. *Anat Rec* 1938; 72:137.
90. Moll J. Regeneration of the supraoptico-hypophyseal and paraventriculo-hypophyseal tracts in the hypophysectomized rat. *Z Zellforsch* 1957;46:686.
91. Moll J, DeWied D. Observations on the hypothalamo-posthypophyseal system of the posterior lobectomized rat. *Gen Comp Endocrinol* 1962;2:215.
92. Adams JH, Daniel PM, Prichard MM. Degeneration and regeneration of hypothalamic nerve fibers in the neurohypophysis after pituitary stalk section in the ferret. *J Comp Neurol* 1969;135:121.
93. Daniel PM, Prichard MM. Regeneration of hypothalamic nerve fibers after hypophysectomy in the goat. *Acta Endocrinol* 1970;64:696.
94. Raisman G. Electron microscopic studies of the development of new neurohemal contacts in the median eminence of the rat after hypophysectomy. *Brain Res* 1973;55:245.
95. Daniel PM, Prichard MM. The effects of pituitary stalk section in the goat. *Am J Pathol* 1958;34:433.
96. Daniel RM, Duchen LW, Prichard MM. The effect of transection of the pituitary stalk on the cytology of the pituitary gland of the rat. *Q J Exp Phys* 1964;49:235.
97. Adams JH, Daniel PM, Prichard MM. The blood supply of the pituitary gland of the ferret with special reference to infarction after stalk section. *J Anat* 1969;104:209.
98. Daniel PM, Prichard MM. The human hypothalamus and pituitary stalk after hypophysectomy or pituitary stalk section. *Brain* 1972;95:813.
99. Daniel PM, Prichard MM. Studies of the hypothalamus and the pituitary gland. With special reference to the effects of transection of the pituitary stalk. *Acta Endocrinol* 1975;80(Suppl. 201):1.
100. Nikitovitch-Winer M, Everett JW. Histologic changes in grafts of rat pituitary on the kidney and upon re-transplantation under the diencephalon. *Endocrinology* 1959;65:357.
101. Nikitovitch-Winer M, Everett JW. Functional restitution of pituitary grafts retransplanted from kidney to median eminence. *Endocrinology* 1958;63:916.
102. Halasz B, Pupp L. Hormone secretion of the anterior pituitary gland after physical interruption of all nervous pathways to the hypophysiotropic area. *Endocrinology* 1965;77:553.
103. Szentagothai J, Flerko B, Mess B, Halasz B. *Hypothalamic control of anterior pituitary function.* Budapest: Akademiai Kiado, 1968.
104. Halasz B, Gorski RA. Gonadotropic hormone secretion in female rats after partial or total interruption of neural afferents to the medial basal hypothalamus. *Endocrinology* 1967;80:608.
105. Halasz B, Slusher M, Gorski RA. Adrenocorticotropic hormone secretion in rats after partial or total deafferentation of the medial basal hypothalamus. *Neuroendocrinology* 1967;2:43.
106. Halasz B, Florsheim WH, Corcorran NL, Gorski RA. Thyrotrophic hormone secretion after partial or total interruption of neural afferents to the medial basal hypothalamus. *Endocrinology* 1967;80:1075.
107. Halasz B. The endocrine effects of isolation of the hypothalamus from the rest of the brain. In: Martini L, Gonoug WF, eds. *Frontiers of neuroendocrinology.* New York: Oxford University Press, 1969:307.
108. Halasz B. Neural control of pituitary ACTH secretion under resting conditions. *Acta Medica* 1973;29:71.
109. Guillemin R. Hypothalamic factors releasing pituitary hormones. *Recent Prog Horm Res* 1964;20:89.
110. Schally AV, Arimura A, Bowers CY, Kastin AJ, Sawano S, Redding TW. Hypothalamic neurohormones regulating anterior pituitary function. *Recent Prog Horm Res* 1968;24:497.
111. Saffran M, Schally AV. Release of corticotropin by anterior pituitary tissue in vitro. *Can J Biochem Physiol* 1955;33:408.
112. Guillemin R. Hypothalamic control of anterior pituitary study with tissue cultures techniques. *Fed Proc* 1955;14:65.
113. Guillemin R, Rosenberg B. Humoral hypothalamic control of anterior pituitary: a study with combined tissue cultures. *Endocrinology* 1955;57:599.
114. Guillemin R, Hearn WR, Cheek WR, Housholder DE. Control of corticotropin release: further studies with in vitro methods. *Endocrinology* 1957;60:488.
115. Schreiber V, Rybak M, Eckertova A, et al. Isolation of a hypothalamic peptide with TRF (thyrotrophin releasing factor) activity in vitro. *Experientia* 1962;18:338.
116. Deuben RR, Meites J. Stimulation of pituitary growth hormone release by a hypothalamic extract "in vitro." *Endocrinology* 1964;74:408.

117. Schally AV, Bowers CY. In vitro and in vivo stimulation of the release of luteinizing hormone. *Endocrinology* 1964;75:312.
118. Gala RR, Piece RP. In vitro lactogen production by anterior pituitaries from various species. *Proc Soc Exp Biol Med* 1965;120:263.
119. Meites J, Kahn RH, Nicole CS. Prolactin production by rat pituitary in vitro. *Proc Soc Exp Biol Med* 1961;108:440.
120. Pastels JL. Administration d'extraits hypothalamiques à l'hypophyse de rat in vitro, dans le but d'en controler la secretion du prolactaire. *Compt Rend* 1962;254:2664..
121. Talwaker PK, Ratner A, Meites J. In vitro inhibition of pituitary prolactin synthesis and release by hypothalamic extract. *Am J Physiol* 1963;205:213.
122. Porter JC, Jones JC. Effect of plasma from hypophyseal-portal vessel blood on adrenal-ascorbic acid. *Endocrinology* 1966; 58:62.
123. Porter JC, Dhariwal APS, McCann SM. Response of the anterior pituitary-adrenocortical axis to purified CRF. *Endocrinology* 1967;80:679.
124. Guillemin A, Yamazaki E, Jutisz M, Sakig E. Presence dans un extrait de tissus hypothalamiques d'une substance stimulant le secretion de l'hormone hypophysaire threotrope. *Compt Rend* 1962;255:1018.
125. Garcia JF, Geschwind I. Increase in plasma growth hormone levels in the monkey following the administration of sheep hypothalamic extracts. *Nature* 1966;211:372.
126. Dhariwal APS, Nallar R, Batt M, McCann SM. Separation of follicle stimulating hormone-releasing factor from luteinizing hormone releasing factors. *Endocrinology* 1965;76:290.
127. Igarashi M, McCann SM. A hypothalamic follicle stimulating hormone-releasing factor. *Endocrinology* 1964;74:446.
128. McCann SM, Taleisnik S, Friedman HM. LH-releasing activity in hypothalamic extracts. *Proc Soc Exp Biol Med* 1960;104:432.
129. McCann SM. A hypothalamic leutinizing-hormone-releasing factor. *Am J Physiol* 1962;202:395.
130. Porter JC, Mical RS, Kamberi IA, Grazia YR. A procedure for the cannulation of a pituitary stalk portal vessel and perfusion of the pars distalis in the rat. *Endocrinology* 1970;87:197.
131. Porter JC, Mical RS, Ondo JG, Kamberi IA. Perfusion of the rat anterior pituitary via a cannulated portal vessel. *Acta Endocrinol Suppl* 1972;158:249.
132. Kamberi I, Mical R, Porter JC. Pituitary portal infusion of hypothalamic extract and release of LH, FSH and prolactin. *Endocrinology* 1971;88:1294.
133. Kamberi IA, Mical RS, Porter JC. Hypophysial portal vessel infusion: in vivo demonstration of LRF, FRF, and PIF in pituitary stalk plasma. *Endocrinology* 1971;89:1042.
134. Averill RLW, Kennedy TH. Elevation of thyrotropin release by intrapituitary infusion of crude hypothalamic extracts. *Endocrinology* 1967;81:113.
135. Fink G, Nallar R, Worthington WC. The demonstration of luteinizing hormone releasing factor in hypophyseal portal blood of pro-estrus and hypophysectomized rats. *J Physiol (Lond)* 1967;191:407.
136. Wilber J, Porter JC. Thyrotropin and growth hormone releasing activity in hypophyseal portal blood. *Endocrinology* 1970; 87:807.
137. Boler J, Enzmann F, Folkers K. The identity of chemical and hormonal properties of the thyrotropin releasing hormone and pyroglutamyl-histidylproline amide. *Biochem Biophys Res Commun* 1969;37:705.
138. Burgus R, Dunn TF, Desiderio DM, Ward DN, Vale W, Guillemin R. Characterization of ovine hypothalamic hypophysiotropic TSH releasing factor. *Nature* 1970;226:321.
139. Burgus R, Dunn TF, Desiderio DM, et al. Biological activity of synthetic polypeptide derivatives related to the structure of hypothalamic TRF. *Endocrinology* 1970;86:573.
140. Porter JC, Vale W, Burgus R, Mical RS, Guillemin R. Release of TSH by TRF infused directly into a pituitary stalk portal vessel. *Endocrinology* 1971;89:1054.
141. Arimura A, Matsuo H, Baba Y, Debeljuk L, Sandow J, Schally AV. Stimulation of release of LH by synthetic LH-RH in vivo. I. A comparative study of natural and synthetic hormones. *Endocrinology* 1972;90:163.
142. Geiger R, Konig W, Wissmann H, Geisen K, Enzmann F. Synthesis and characterization of a decapeptide having LH-RH/FSH-RH activity. *Biochem Biophys Res Commun* 1971;45:767.
143. Schally AV, Arimura A, Baba Y, et al. Isolation and properties of FSH and LH releasing hormone. *Biochem Biophys Res Commun* 1971;43:393.
144. Spiess J, Rivier J, Rivier C, Vale W. Primary structure of corticotropin-releasing factor from ovine hypothalamus. *Proc Natl Acad Sci USA* 1981;78:5617.
145. Vale W, Spiess J, Rivier C, Rivier J. Characterization of a 41-residue ovine hypothalamic peptide that stimulates secretion of corticotropin and β-endorphin. *Science* 1981;213:1394.
146. Brazeau P, Vale W, Burgus R, et al. Hypothalamic polypeptide that inhibits the secretion of immunoreactive pituitary growth hormone. *Science* 1973;179:77.
147. Rivier J, Spiess J, Thorner M, Vale W. Characterization of a growth hormone-releasing factor from a human pancreatic islet tumor. *Nature* 1982;300:276.
148. Thorner MO, Spiess J, Vance ML, et al. Human pancreatic growth-hormone-releasing factor selectively stimulates growth-hormone secretion in man. *Lancet* 1983;1:24.
149. Spiess J, Rivier J, Vale W. Characterization of rat hypothalamic growth hormone-releasing factor. *Nature* 1983;303:532.
150. Wehrenberg WB, Ling N. In vivo biological potency of rat and human growth hormone-releasing factor and fragments of human growth hormone releasing factor. *Biochem Biophys Res Commun* 1983;115:525.
151. Shaar CJ, Clemens JH. The role of catecholamines in the release of anterior pituitary prolactin in vitro. *Endocrinology* 1974; 95:1202.
152. Neill JD, Patton JM, Dailey RA, Tsou RC, Tindall GT. Luteinizing hormone releasing hormone (LHRH) in pituitary stalk blood of rhesus monkeys: relationship to level of LH release. *Endocrinology* 1977;101:430.
153. Gibbs DM, Neill JD. Dopamine levels in hypophyseal stalk blood are sufficient to inhibit prolactin secretion in vivo. *Endocrinology* 1978;102:1895.
154. Pilotte NS, Gudelsky GA, Porter JC. Relationship of prolactin secretion to dopamine release into hypophyseal portal blood and dopamine turnover in the median eminence. *Brain Res* 1980;193:284.
155. Gudelsky GA, Porter JC. Release of dopamine from tuberoinfundibular neurons into pituitary stalk blood after prolactin or haloperidol administration. *Endocrinology* 1980;106:526.
156. Selmanoff M. The lateral and medial median eminence: distribution of dopamine, norepinephrine, and luteinizing hormone-releasing hormone and the effect of prolactin on catecholamine turnover. *Endocrinology* 1981;108:1716.
157. Foord SM, Peters JR, Dieguez C, Scanlon MF, Hall R. Dopamine receptors on intact anterior pituitary cells in culture: functional association with the inhibition of prolactin and thyrotropin. *Endocrinology* 1983;112:1567.
158. Frawley LS, Neill JD. Brief decreases in dopamine result in surges of prolactin secretion in monkeys. *Am J Physiol* 1984;247:E778.
159. Nakane PK, Pierce GB. Enzyme-labeled antibodies for the light and electron microscopic localization of tissue antigens. *J Cell Biol* 1967;33:307.
160. Sternberger L. *Immunocytochemistry*. New York: John Wiley, 1979.
161. Hökfelt T, Elde R, Fuxe K, et al. Aminergic and peptidergic pathways in the nervous system with special reference to the hypothalamus. In: Reichlin S, Baldessarini RJ, Martin JB, eds. *The hypothalamus*. New York: Raven Press, 1978:69.
162. Fink G, Geffen LB. The hypothalamo-hypophysial system: model for central peptidergic and monoaminergic transmission. *Int Rev Physiol* 1978;17:1.
163. Naik DV. Immunoreactive LH-RH neurons in the hypothalamus identified by light and fluorescent microscopy. *Cell Tissue Res* 1975;157:423.
164. Naik DV. Immunoelectron microscopic localization of luteinizing hormone-releasing hormone in the arcuate nuclei and median eminence of the rat. *Cell Tissue Res* 1975;157:437.
165. Styne DM, Goldsmith PC, Brustein SR, Kaplan SL, Grumbach

MM. Immunoreactive somatostatin and luteinizing hormone releasing hormone in median eminence synaptosomes of the rat: detection by immunohisto-chemistry and quantification by radioimmunoassay. *Endocrinology* 1977;101:1099.
166. Barry J, Dubois MP, Poulain P. LRF producing cells of the mammalian hypothalamus. A fluorescent antibody study. *Z Zellforsch* 1973;146:351.
167. Barry J, Dubois MP, Poulain P, Leonardelli J. Neuroendocrinologie—characterisation et topographic des neurones hypothalamiques immunoreactifs avec des anticorps anti-LRH de synthese. *CR Acad Sci Ser D* 1973;276:3191.
168. Swanson LW. The hypothalamus. *Handbk Chem Neuroanat* 1987;5:1.
169. Hymer WC, McShan WH. Isolation of cytoplasmic pituitary granules by column chromatography. *J Cell Biol* 1962;13:350.
170. Hymer WC, McShan WH. Isolation of rat pituitary granules and the study on their biological properties and hormonal activities. *J Cell Biol* 1963;17:67.
171. Hymer WC. Separation of organelles and cells from the mammalian adenohypophysis. In: Tixier-Vidal A, Farquhar MG, eds. *The anterior pituitary. Ultrastructure in biological systems,* Vol. 7. New York: Academic Press, 1975;137.
172. Dunphy WG, Rothman James E. Compartmental organization of the Golgi stack. *Cell* 1985;42:13.
173. Inoue K, Kurosumi K. Ultrastructural observation of the trans-Golgi associated plate-like cisterna in the secretory cells of the rat anterior pituitary gland with special reference to the intracisternal skeleton. *Anat Rec* 1989;225:272.
174. Novikoff PM, Novikoff AB, Quintana N, Hauw J-J. Golgi apparatus, Gerl, and lysosomes of neurons in the rat dorsal ganglia. Studies by thick section and thin section cytochemistry. *J Cell Biol* 1971;50:859.
175. Farquhar MG, Palade GE. The Golgi apparatus (complex)—(1954–1981)—from artifact to center stage. *J Cell Biol* 1981;91:77s.
176. Farquhar MG, Wellings SR. Electron microscopic evidence suggesting secretory granule formation within the Golgi apparatus. *J Biophys Biochem Cytol* 1957;3:319.
177. Farquhar MG. Origin and fate of secretory granules in cells of the anterior pituitary gland. *Trans NY Acad Sci* 1961;23:346.
178. Racadot J, Olivier L, Porcile E, Droz B. Appareil de Golgi et origine des graines de secretion dans les cellules adenohypophysaires chez le rat. Etude radioautographique en microscopie electronique apres injection de leucine tritiee. *CR Acad Sci Paris* 1965;261:2972.
179. Tixier-Vidal A, Picart R. Etude quantitative par radioautographie au microscope electronique de l'utilisation de la PL-leucine-^{3}H par les cellules de l'hypophyse du canard en culture organotypique. *J Cell Biol* 1967;35:501.
180. Howell SL, Whitfield M. Synthesis and secretion of growth hormone in the rat anterior pituitary. I. The intracellular pathway, its time course and energy requirements. *J Cell Sci* 1973;12:1.
181. Farquhar MG, Reid JJ, Daniell LW. Intracellular transport and packaging of prolactin: a quantitative electron microscope autoradiographic study of mammotrophs dissociated from rat pituitaries. *Endocrinology* 1978;102:296.
182. Blobel G, Dobberstein B. Transfer of proteins across membranes. *J Cell Biol* 1975;67:835.
183. Lingappa VR, Devillers-Thiery A, Blobel G. Nascent prehormones are intermediates in the biosynthesis of authentic bovine pituitary growth hormone and prolactin. *Proc Natl Acad Sci USA* 1977;74:2432.
184. Rosenzweig LJ, Farquhar MG. Sites of sulfate incorporation into mammotrophs and somatotrophs of the rat pituitary as determined by quantitative electron microscopic autoradiography. *Endocrinology* 1980;107:422.
185. Watanabe H, Orth DN, Toft DO. Glucocorticoid receptors in pituitary tumor cells. *J Biol Chem* 1973;248:7625.
186. Schnabel E, Mains RE, Farquhar MG. Proteolytic processing of pro-acth. endorphin begins in the Golgi complex of pituitary corticotropes and AT-20 cells. *Mol Endocrinol* 1989;3:1223.
187. Farquhar MG. Recovery of surface membrane in anterior pituitary cells. *J Cell Biol* 1978;77:R35.
188. Komuro M, Kiuchi Y, Shioda T. Membrane modification during secretory granule formation in rat somatotrophs. *Eur J Cell Biol* 1987;43:98.
189. Farquhar MG. Processing of secretory products by cells of the anterior pituitary cell. *Mem Soc Endocrinol* 1971;19:79.
190. Shimada O, Tosaka-Shimada H, Ishikawa H. Morphological effects of somatostatin on rat somatotrophs previously activated by growth hormone-releasing factor. *Cell Tissue Res* 1990; 261:219.
191. Ishimura K, Egawa K, Fujita H. Freeze-fracture images of exocytosis and endocytosis in anterior pituitary cells of rabbits and mice. *Cell Tissue Res* 1980;206:233.
192. Senda T, Fujita H, Ban T, et al. Ultrastructural and immunocytochemical studies on the cytoskeleton in the anterior pituitary of rats, with special regard to the relationship between actin filaments and secretory granules. *Cell Tissue Res* 1989;258:25.
193. Shimad O, Tosaka-Shimada H. Morphological analysis of growth hormone release from rat somatotrophs into blood vessels by immunogold microscopy. *Endocrinology* 1989; 125:2677.
194. Draznin B, Dahl R, Sherman N, Sussman KE, Staehelin LA. Exocystosis in normal anterior pituitary cells: quantitative correlation between growth hormone release and morphological features of exocytosis. *J Clin Invest* 1988;88:1042.
195. Nikitovitch-Winer MB, Yu SM, Papka RE. Soluble prolactin may be directly released from cellular compartments other than secretory granules. In: Thorner MO, Scapagnini U, eds. *Prolactin, basic and clinical correlates. Fidia Research Series,* Vol. 1. Padova: Liviana Press, 1985:17.
196. Torres AI, Aoki A. Release of big and small molecular forms of prolactin: dependence upon dynamic state of the lactotroph. *J Endocrinol* 1987;114:213.
197. Mezey E, Reisine TD, Brownstein MJ, Palkovits M, Axelrod J. β-Adrenergic mechanism of insulin-induced adrenocorticotropin release from the anterior pituitary. *Science* 1984;226:1085.
198. Karanth S, McCann SM. Anterior pituitary hormone control by interleukin 2. *Proc Natl Acad Sci USA* 1991;88:961.
199. Brown SL, Smith LR, Blalock JE. Interleuken 1 and interleukin 2 enhance proopiomelanocortin gene expression in pituitary cells. *J Immunol* 1987;139:3181.
200. Watanobe H, Sasaki S, Takebe K. Evidence that intravenous administration of interleukin-1 stimulates corticotropin releasing hormone secretion in the median eminence of freely moving rats: estimation by push-pull perfusion. *Neurosci Lett* 1991;133:7.
201. Couch EF, Arimura A, Schally AV, Saito M, Sawano S. Electron microscope studies of somatotrophs of rat pituitary after injection of purified growth hormone releasing hormone factor (GRF). *Endocrinology* 1969;85:1084.
202. Coates PW, Ashby EA, Krulich L, Dhariwal APS, McCann SM. Morphologic alterations in somatotrophs of the rat adenohypophysis following administration of hypothalamic extracts. *Am J Anat* 1970;128:389.
203. Shiino M, Arimura A, Schally AV, Rennels EG. Ultrastructural observations of granule extrusion from rat anterior pituitary cells after injection of LH-releasing hormone. *Z Zellforsch* 1972;128:152.
204. Stratmann IE, Ezrin C, Kovacs K, Sellers EA. Effect of TRH on the fine structure and replication of TSH and prolactin cells in the rat. *Z Zellforsch* 1973;145:23.
205. Westlund KN, Aguilera G, Childs GV. Quantification of morphological changes in pituitary corticotropes produced by in vivo corticotropin-releasing factor stimulation and adrenalectomy. *Endocrinology* 1985;116:439.
206. Atwell WJ. The development of the hypophysis cerebri in man, with special reference to the pars tuberalis. *Am J Anat* 1926;37:159.
207. Tilney F. The glands of the brain with especial reference to the pituitary gland. *Res Publ Assoc Res Nerv Ment Dis* 1938;17:3.
208. Takor TT, Pearse AGE. Neuroectodermal origin of avian hypothalamo-hypophyseal complex: the role of the ventral neural ridge. *J Embryol Exp Morphol* 1975;34:311.
209. Trojanowski JQ, Gordon D, Obrocka M, Lee VMY. The devel-

opmental expression of neurofilament and glial filament proteins in the human pituitary gland: an immunohistochemical study with monoclonal antibodies. *Dev Brain Res* 1984;13:229.
210. Farner DS, Wilson FE, Oksche A. Neuroendocrine mechanisms in birds. In: Martini L, Ganong WF, eds. *Neuroendocrinology,* Vol. II. New York: Academic Press, 1967:529.
211. Dempsey EW, Wislocki GB. An electron microscopic study of the blood-brain barrier in the rat, employing silver nitrate as a vital stain. *J Biophys Biochem Cytol* 1955;1:245.
212. Farquhar MG. Fine structure and function in capillaries of the anterior pituitary gland. *Angiology* 1961;12:270.
213. Fletcher WH, Anderson NC, Everett JW. Intercellular communication in the rat anterior pituitary gland. *J Cell Biol* 1975;67:469.
214. Herbert DC. Intercellular junctions in the rhesus monkey pars distalis. *Anat Rec* 1979;195:1.
215. Soji T, Herbert DC. Intercellular communication between rats anterior pituitary cells. *Anat Rec* 1989;224:523.
216. Denef C, Andries M. Evidence for paracrine interaction between gonadotrophs and lactotrophs in pituitary cell aggregates. *Endocrinology* 1983;112:813.
217. Soji T, Yashiro T, Herbert DC. Intercellular communication in the rat anterior pituitary gland. I. Postnatal development and changes after injection of luteinizing hormone-releasing hormone (LH-RH) or testosterone. *Anat Rec* 1990;226:337.
218. Pierce JG, Parsons TF. Glycoprotein hormones: structure and function. *Annu Rev Biochem* 1981;50:465.
219. Shome B, Parlow AF. Human pituitary prolactin (hPRL): the entire linear amino acid sequence. *J Clin Endocrinol Metab* 1977;45:1112.
220. Li CH, Dixon JS, Lo T-B, Pankov YA, Schmidt KD. Amino-acid sequence of ovine lactogenic hormone. *Nature* 1969; 224:695.
221. Li CH, Dixon JS, Lo T-B, Schmidt KD, Pankov YA. Studies on pituitary lactogenic hormone. XXX. The primary structure of the sheep hormone. *Arch Biochem Biophys* 1970;141:705.
222. Li CH. Studies on pituitary lactogenic hormone. The primary structure of the porcine hormone. *Int J Peptide Protein Res* 1976;8:205.
223. Wallis M. The primary structure of bovine prolactin. *FEBS Lett* 1974;44:205.
224. Li CH, Hayashida T, Doneen BA, Rao AJ. Human somatotropin: biological characterization of the recombinant molecule. *Proc Natl Acad Sci USA* 1976;73:3463.
225. Lewis UJ, Singh RNP, Tutwiler GF, Sigel MB, VanderLaan EF, VanderLaan WP. Human growth hormone: a complex of proteins. *Recent Prog Horm Res* 1980;36:377.
226. Howard KS, Shepherd RG, Eigner EA, Davies DS, Bell PH. Structure of β-corticotropin: final sequence. *J Am Chem Soc* 1955;77:3419.
227. Li CH, Geschwind II, Cole RD, Raacke ID, Harris JI, Dixon JS. Amino-acid sequence of alpha-corticotropin. *Nature* 1955; 176:687.
228. Li CH. Proposed system of terminology for preparations of adrenocorticotropic hormone. *Science* 1959;129:969.
229. Harris JI, Roos P. Amino-acid sequence of a melanophore stimulating hormone. *Nature* 1956;178:90.
230. Harris JI, Roos P. Studies on pituitary polypeptide hormones 1) The structure of β-melanocyte-stimulating hormone from pig pituitary gland. *Biochem J* 1959;71:434.
231. Geschwind II, Li CH, Barnafi L. Isolation and structure of melanocyte-stimulating hormone from porcine pituitary glands. *J Am Chem Soc* 1956;78:4494.
232. Harris JI, Lerner AB. Amino-acid sequence of the α-melanocyte stimulating hormone. *Nature* 1957;179:1346.
233. Geschwind II, Li CH. The isolation and characterization of a melanocyte stimulating hormone (β-MSH) from hog pituitary glands. *J Am Chem Soc* 1957;79:615.
234. Geschwind II, Li CH, Barnafi L. The structure of the β-melanocyte stimulating hormone. *J Am Chem Soc* 1957;79: 620.
235. Li CH, Chung D. Isolation and structure of an unitriakontapeptide with opiate activity from camel pituitary glands. *Proc Natl Acad Sci USA* 1976;73:1145.
236. Li CH, Chung D. Primary structure of human β-lipotropin. *Nature* 1976;260:622.
237. Li CH, Tan L, Chung D. Isolation and primary structure of beta-endorphin and beta-lipotropin from bovine pituitary gland. *Biochem Biophys Res Commun* 1977;77:1088.
238. Teschemacher H, Opheim KE, Cox BM, Goldstein A. A peptide-like substance that acts like morphine. 1) Isolation. *Life Sci* 1975;16:1771.
239. Teschemacher H, Opheim KE, Cox BM, Goldstein A. A peptide-like substance that acts like morphine. 2) Purification and properties. *Life Sci* 1975;16:1777.
240. Pearse AG, Noorden S Van. The functional cytology of the human adenohypophysis. *Can Med Assoc J* 1963;88:462.
241. Nakane PK. Simultaneous localization of multiple tissue antigens using the peroxidase-labeled antibody method: a study on pituitary glands of the rat. *J Histochem Cytochem* 1968;16:557.
242. Kurosumi K. Functional classification of cell types of the anterior pituitary gland accomplished by electron microscopy. *Arch Histol Jpn* 1968;29:329.
243. Pochet R, Brocas H, Vassart G, et al. Radioautographic localization of prolactin messenger RNA on histological sections by in situ hybridization. *Brain Res* 1981;211:433.
244. Rasmussen AT. The percentage of the different types of cells in the male human hypophysis. *Am J Pathol* 1929;5:263.
245. Rasmussen AT. The percentage of different types of cells in the anterior lobe of the hypophysis of the adult female. *Am J Pathol* 1933;9:459.
246. Severinghaus AE. The cytology of the pituitary gland. *Res Publ Assoc Res Nerv Ment Dis* 1938;17:69.
247. Severinghaus AE. Anterior hypophyseal cytology in relation to the reproductive hormones. In: Allen MB, eds. *Sex and Internal Secretions.* Baltimore: Wood & Co., 1939:1045.
248. Cushing H. Acromegaly from a surgical standpoint. *Br Med J* 1927;2:1.
249. Cushing H, Davidoff L. The pathologic findings in four cases of acromegaly with a discussion of their significance. *Monog Rockefeller Inst Med Res* 1927;22.
250. Cushing H. The basophile adenomas of the pituitary body and their clinical manifestations. *Bull Johns Hopkins Hosp* 1932;50:137.
251. Romeis B. Hypophyse. In: Mollendorff W Van, ed. *Handbuch der Mikroskopischen Anatomie des Menschen.* Berlin: Springer, 1940.
252. Pearse AGE. Observations on the localisation, nature and chemical constitution of some components of the anterior hypophysis. *J Pathol Bacteriol* 1952;64:791.
253. Herlant M. Etude critique de deux techniques nouvelles destinees a mettre en evidence les differentes categories cellulaires presented dans la glande pituitaire. *Bull Microsc Appl* 1960;10:37.
254. Purves HD. Cytology of the adenohypophysis. In: Harris GW, Donovan BT, eds. *The Pituitary Gland,* Vol. 1. *Anterior Pituitary.* Berkeley: University of California Press, 1966:147.
255. Smith PE, Smith IP. The topographical separation in the bovine anterior hypophysis of the principle reacting with the endocrine system from that controlling general body growth, with suggestions as to the cell types elaborating these encrations. *Anat Rec* 1923;25:150.
256. Baker B. Functional cytology of the hypophyseal pars distalis and pars intermedia. In: Knobil E, Sawyer WH, eds. *Handbook of Physiology,* Vol. 7. *The Pituitary Gland and Its Neuroendocrine Control,* Part 1. Baltimore: Williams & Wilkins, 1974:45.
257. Purves HD, Greisbach WE. Functional deafferentation in the acidophil cells and the gonadotropic basophil cells of the rat pituitary. *Proc Univ Otago Med School* 1952;30:27.
258. Farquhar MG, Rinehart JF. Electron microscope studies of the anterior pituitary gland of castrate rats. *Endocrinology* 1954;54:516.
259. Farquhar MG, Rinehart JF. Cytologic alterations in the anterior pituitary gland following thyroidectomy: an electron microscope study. *Endocrinology* 1954;55:857.

260. Nakane PK. Classifications of anterior pituitary cell types with immunoenzyme histochemistry. *J Histochem Cytochem* 1970; 18:9.
261. Nakane PK. Application of peroxidase-labelled antibodies to the intracellular localization of hormones. *Acta Endocrinol Suppl* 1971;153:190.
262. Moriarty G. Adenohypophysis: ultrastructural cytochemistry. *J Histochem Cytochem* 1973;21:855.
263. Kurosumi K, Tosaka H. Prenatal development of growth hormone-producing cells in the rat anterior pituitary as studied by immunogold electron microscopy. *Arch Histol Cytol* 1988;51:193.
264. Kurosumi K. Ultrastructural immunocytochemistry of the adenohypophysis in the rat: a review. *J Electron Microsc Tech* 1991;19:42.
265. Kurosumi K, Tanaka S, Tosaka H. Changing ultrastructures in the estrous cycle and postnatal development of prolactin cells in the rat anterior pituitary as studied by immunogold electron microscopy. *Arch Histol Cytol* 1987;50:455.
266. J Van Putten, Kiliaan A. Immuno-electron-microscopic study of the prolactin cells in the pituitary gland of male Wistar rats during aging. *Cell Tissue Res* 1988;251:353.
267. Hudson P, Penschow J, Shine J, Ryan G, Niall H, Coghlan J. Hybridization histochemistry: use of recombination DNA as a "homing probe" for tissue localization of specific m-RNA populations. *Endocrinology* 1981;108:353.
268. Bauman JGJ, Wiegnant J, Van Duijn P. Cytochemical hybridization with fluorochrome-labelled RNA. *J Histochem Cytochem* 1981;29:238.
269. Phifer RF, Spicer SS. Immunohistochemical and histologic demonstration of thyrotropic cells of the human adenohypophysis. *J Clin Endocrinol Metab* 1973;36:1210.
270. Girod C, Trouillas J. Individualisation immunohistochimique des cellules thyreotropes antehypophysaires chez le Singe Macacus irus, a l'aide d'un anticorps anti-β-TSH humaine. *CR Acad Sci Paris* 1980;291:261.
271. Baker BL, Pierce JG, Cornell JS. The utility of antiserums to subunits of TSH and LH for immunochemical staining of the rat hypophysis. *Am J Anat* 1972;135:251.
272. Kawarai Y. Identification of ACTH cells and TSH cells in rat anterior pituitary with the unlabeled antibody enzyme method on adjacent thin and thick sections. *Acta Histochem Cytochem* 1980;13:627.
273. Moriarty GC, Tobin RB. Ultrastructural immunocytochemical characterization of the thyrotroph in rat and human pituitaries. *J Histochem Cytochem* 1976;24:1131.
274. Moriarty GC, Tobin RB. An immunocytochemical study of TSH_B storage in rat thyroidectomy cells with and without D or L thyroxine treatment. *J Histochem Cytochem* 1976;24:1140.
275. Horvath E, Kovacs K. Fine structural cytology of the adenohypophysis in rat and man. *J Electron Microsc Tech* 1988;8:401.
276. Ozawa H, Kurosumi K. Post natal development of thyrotrophs in the rat anterior pituitary as studied by immunogold. *Electron Microscopy Anat Embryol* 1989;180:207.
277. Kurosumi K, Oota Y. Electron microscopy of two types of gonadotrophs in the anterior pituitary gland of persistent estrous and diestrous rats. *Z Zellforsch* 1968;85:34.
278. Moriarty GC. Electron microscopic-immunocytochemical studies of rat pituitary gonadotrophs: a sex difference in morphology and cytochemistry of LH cells. *Endocrinology* 1975;97:1215.
279. Phifer RF, Midgley AR, Spicer SS. Immunohistologic and histologic evidence that follicle-stimulating hormone and luteinizing hormone are present in the same cell type in the human pars distalis. *J Clin Endocrinol Metab* 1973;36:125.
280. Childs (Moriarty) GV, Ellison DG, Gardner L. An immunocytochemist's view of gonadotropin storage in the adult male rat. Cytochemical and morphological heterogeneity in serially stained gonadotropes. *Am J Anat* 1980;158:397.
281. Childs GV, Lloyd JM, Unabia G, Gharib SG, Wierman ME, Chin WW. Detection of luteinizing hormone beta messenger ribonucleic acid (RNA) in individual gonadotropes after castration: use of a new in situ hybridization method with a photobiotinylated complementary RNA probe. *Mol Endocrinol* 1987;1:926.
282. Lloyd JM, Childs GV. Differential storage and release of luteinizing hormone and follicle-releasing hormone from individual gonadotropes separated by centrifugal elutriation. *Endocrinology* 1988;122:1282.
283. Childs GV, Ellison DG, Lorenzen JR, Collins TJ, Schwartz NB. Immunocytochemical studies of gonadotrophin storage in developing castration cells. *Endocrinology* 1982;111:1318.
284. Moriarty GC. Ultrastructural-immunocytochemical studies of rat pituitary gonadotrophs in cycling female rats. *Gunma Symp Endocrinol* 1976;13:207.
285. Eipper BA, Mains RE. Structure and biosynthesis of pro-ACTH/endorphin and related peptides. *Endocrin Rev* 1980;1:1.
286. Eipper BA, Mains RE. Peptide analysis of glycoprotein form of adrenocorticotropic hormone. *J Biol Chem* 1977;252:8821.
287. Hope J, Lowry PJ. Pro-opiocortin: the ACTH/LPH common precursor protein. *Front Horm Res* 1981;8:44.
288. Siperstein ER, Allison VF. Fine structure of the cells responsible for the secretion of adrenocorticotrophin in the adrenalectomized rat. *Endocrinology* 1965;76:70.
289. Siperstein ER, Miller KJ. Further cytophysiologic evidence for the identity of the cells that produce adrenocorticotrophic hormone. *Endocrinology* 1970;86:451.
290. Siperstein ER, Miller KJ. Hypertrophy of the ACTH-producing cell following adrenalectomy: a quantitative electron microscopic study. *Endocrinology* 1973;93:1257.
291. Moriarty GC, Halmi NS. Electron microscopic study of the adreno-corticotropin producing cell with the use of unlabeled antibody and the soluble peroxidase-antiperoxidase complex. *J Histochem Cytochem* 1972;20:590.
292. Mains RE, Eipper BA, Ling N. Common precursor to corticotropins and endorphins. *Proc Natl Acad Sci USA* 1977;74:3014.
293. Roberts JL, Seeburg PH, Shine J, Herbert E, Baxter JD, Goodman HM. Corticotropin and β-endorphin: construction and analysis of recombinant DNA complementary to mRNA for the common precursor. *Proc Natl Acad Sci USA* 1979;76:2153.
294. Smith AI, Funder JW. Proopiomelanocortin processing in the pituitary, central nervous system and peripheral tissues. *Endocrin Rev* 1988;9:159.
295. Phifer RF, Spicer SS, Orth DN. Specific demonstration of the human hypophyseal cells which produce adrenocorticotropic hormone. *J Clin Endocrinol Metab* 1970;31:347.
296. Phifer RF, Orth DN, Spicer SS. Immunohistologic evidence that β-melanocyte stimulating hormone (β-MSH) and adrenocorticotropin (ACTH) are produced in the same human hypophyseal cells. Fourth International Congresss of Endocrinology, Washington, DC. (Abstract #573), Excerpta Medica, 1972; 256:228.
297. Moriarty GC, Garner LL. Immunoelectronmicroscopical localization of ACTH/MSH peptides in rat and human pituitaries. *Front Horm Res* 1977;4:26.
298. Pelletier G, Leclerc R, Labrie F, Cote J, Chretien M, Lis M. Immunohistochemical localization of β-lipotropic hormone in the pituitary gland. *Endocrinology* 1977;100:770.
299. Weber E, Voigt KH, Martin R. Concomitant storage of ACTH and endorphin-like immunoreactivity in the secretory granules of anterior pituitary corticotrophs. *Brain Res* 1978;157:385.
300. Baker BL, Drummond T. The cellular origins of corticotropin and melanotropin as revealed by immunochemical staining. *Am J Anat* 1972;134:395.
301. Kurosumi K, Tosaka H, Ijima K. The immature type of proopiomelanocortin cell of the rat anterior pituitary as observed by immunogold electron microscopy. *Arch Histol Cytol* 1989;52:135.
302. Nikitovitch-Winer BM, Atkin J, Maley BE. Colocalization of prolactin and growth hormone within specific adenohypophyseal cells in male, female and lactating rats. *Endocrinology* 1987;121:625.
303. Hashimoto S, Fumagalli G, Zanini A, Meldolesi J. Sorting of three secretory proteins to distinct secretory granules in acidophilic cells of the cow anterior pituitary. *J Cell Biol* 1987;105:1579.

304. Horvath E, Lloyd RB, Kovacs K. Propylthiouracyl-induced hypothyroidism results in reversible transdifferentiation of somatotrophs into thyroidectomy cells. *Lab Invest* 1990;63:511.
305. Ozawa H. Changing structure of thyrotrophs in the rat anterior pituitary after thyroidectomy as studied by immuno-electron-microscopy and enzyme cytochemistry. *Cell Tissue Res* 1991;263:405.
306. Wu P, Childs G. Changes in rat pituitary POMC mRNA after exposure to cold or a novel environment, detected by in situ hybridization. *J Histochem Cytochem* 1991;39:843.
307. Sasaki F, Wu P, Rougeua D, Unabia G, Childs G. Cytochemical studies of responses of corticotropes and thyrotropes to cold and novel environment stress. *Endocrinology* 1990;127:285.
308. Garcia-Navarro F, Porter D, Garcia-Navarro S, Licht P. Immunocytochemical and ultrastructural study of the frog (*Rana pipiens*) pars distalis with special reference to folliculostellate cell function in vitro superfusion. *Cell Tissue Res* 1989;256:623.
309. Nakajima T, Yamaguchi H, Takahashi K. S100 protein in folliculostellate cells of the rat pituitary anterior lobe. *Brain Res* 1980;191:523.
310. Liu YC, Tanaka S, Inoue K, Kurosumi K. Localization of fibronectin in the folliculo-stellate cells of the rat anterior pituitary by the double bridge-antiperoxidase method. *Histochemistry* 1989;92:34.
311. Spangelo BL, Macleod RM, Isakson PC. Production of interleukin-6 by anterior pituitary cells in vitro. *Endocrinology* 1991;126:582.
312. Vankelecom H, Carmeliet P, Vandammc J, Billiau A, Denef C. Production of interleukin-6 by folliculo-stellate cells of the anterior pituitary gland in a histiotypic cell aggregate culture system. *Neuroendocrinology* 1989;49:102.
313. Spangelo B, Judd AM, Isakson PC, Macleod RM. Interleukin-6 stimulates anterior pituitary hormone release in vitro. *Endocrinology* 1989;125:575.
314. Naitoh Y, Fukata J, Tominaga T, et al. Interleukin-6 stimulates the secretion of adrenocorticotropic hormone in conscious, freely moving rats. *Biochem Biophys Res Commun* 1988; 155:1459.
315. Smith PE, Smith IP. The response of the hypophysectomized tadpole to the intraperitoneal injection of the various lobes and colloid of the bovine hypophysis. *Anat Rec* 1923;25:150.
316. Girod C. Fine structure of the pituitary pars distalis. In: Motta PM, ed. *Ultrastructure of endocrine cells and tissues.* Boston: Nijhoff, 1984:12.
317. Kurosumi K, Matsuzawa T, Shibasaki S. Electron microscope studies on the fine structures of the pars nervosa and pars intermedia, and their morphological interrelation in the normal rat hypophysis. *Gen Comp Endocrinol* 1961;1:433.
318. Visser M, Swaab DF. αMSH in the human pituitary. *Front Horm Res* 1977;4:42.
319. Naik DV. Electron microscopic-immunocytochemical localization of adrenocorticotropin and melanocyte stimulating hormone in the pars intermedia cells of rats and mice. *Z Zellforsch* 1973;142:305.
320. Moriarty GC, Halmi NS. Adrenocorticotropin production by the intermediate lobe of the rat pituitary. An electron microscopic-immunocytochemical study. *Z Zellforsch* 1972; 132:1.
321. Murakami T, Ohtsuka A, Taguchi T, Ohtani O. Blood vascular bed of the rat pituitary intermediate lobe, with special reference to its development and portal drainage into the anterior lobe. A scanning electron microscopic study of vascular casts. *Arch Histol Jpn* 1985;48:69.
322. Saland LC. Extracellular spaces of the rat pars intermedia as outlined by lanthanum tracer. *Anat Rec* 1980;196:355.
323. Celis ME. Hypothalamic peptides involved in control of MSH secretion: identity, biosynthesis and regulation of their release. *Front Horm Res* 1977;4:69.
324. Sakly M, Schmitt G, Koch B. CRF enhances release of both aMSH and ACTH from anterior and intermediate pituitary. *Neuroendocrin Lett* 1982;4:289.
325. Proulx-Ferland L, Labrie F, Dumont D, Cote J, Coy DH, Sveiraf J. Corticotropin-releasing factor stimulates secretion of melanocyte-stimulating hormone from the rat pituitary. *Science* 1982;217:62.
326. Kobayashi Y. Functional morphology of the pars intermedia of the rat hypophysis as revealed with the electron microscope. II. Correlation of the pars intermedia with the hypophyseoadrenal axis. *Z Zellforsch* 1965;68:155.
327. Cote T, Munemura M, Eskay RL, Kebabian JW. Biochemical identification of the β-adrenoceptor and evidence for the involvement of an adenosine 3′,5′-monophosphate system in the β′-adrenergically induced release of α-melanocyte-stimulating hormone in the intermediate lobe of the rat pituitary gland. *Endocrinology* 1980;107:108.
328. Tilders FJH, Post M, Jackson S, Lowry PJ, Smelik PG. Beta-adrenergic stimulation of the release of ACTH and LPH-related peptides from the pars intermedia of the rat pituitary gland. *Acta Endocrinol* 1981;97:343.
329. Björklund A, Falck B, Hromek F, Owman C, West KA. Identification and terminal distribution of the tubero-hypophyseal monoamine fibre systems in the rat by means of stereotaxic and microspectrofluorimetric techniques. *Brain Res* 1970;17:1.
330. Baumgarten HG, Björklund A, Holstein AF, Nobin A. Organization and ultrastructural identification of the catecholamine nerve terminals in the neural lobe and pars intermedia of the rat pituitary. *Z Zellforsch* 1972;126:483.
331. Back N, Soinila S, Joh TH, Rechardt L. Catecholamine-synthesizing enzymes in the rat pituitary. An immunohistochemical study. *Histochemistry* 1987;86:459.
332. Westlund KN, Childs GV. Localization of serotonin fibers in the rat adenohypophysis. *Endocrinology* 1982;111:1761.
333. Tilders FJH, Smelik PG. Direct neural control of MSH secretion in mammals: the involvement of dopaminergic tubero-hypophysial neurones. *Front Horm Res* 1977;4:80.
334. Luppi PH, Sakai K, Salvert D, Berod A, Jouvet M. Periventricular dopaminergic neurons terminating in the neurointermediate lobe of the cat hypophysis. *J Comp Neurol* 1986;244:204.
335. Vincent SR, Hökfelt T, Wu J-Y. GABA neuron systems in hypothalamus and the pituitary gland. *Neuroendocrinology* 1982;34:117.
336. Tappaz ML, Wassef M, Oertel WH, Paut L, Pujol JF. Light- and electron-microscopic immunocytochemistry of glutamic acid decarboxylase (GAD) in the basal hypothalamus: morphological evidence for neuroendocrine γ-aminobutyrate (GABA). *Neuroscience* 1983;9:271.
337. Verburg-Van Kemenade BM, Tappaz M, Paut L, Jenks BG. GABAergic regulation of melanocyte-stimulating hormone secretion from the pars intermedia of *Xenopus laevis:* immunocytochemical and physiological evidence. *Endocrinology* 1986;118:260.
338. Rabhi M, Onteniente B, Kah O, Geffard M, Calas A. Immunocytochemical study of the mouse pituitary by use of antibodies against gamma-aminobutyric acid (GABA). *Cell Tissue Res* 1987;247:33.
339. Oertel WH, Mugnaini E, Tappaz ML, et al. Central gabaergic innervation of the neurointermediate pituitary lobe: biochemical and immunohistochemical study in the rat. *Proc Natl Acad Sci USA* 1982;79:675.
340. Vuillez P, Carbajo Perez S, Stoeckel ME. Colocalization of GABA and tyrosine hydroxylase immunoreactivities in the axons innervating the neurointermediate lobe of the rat pituitary: an ultrastructural immunogold study. *Neurosci Lett* 1987;79:53.
341. Saland LC, Wallace JA, Samora A, Guitierrez L. Colocalization of tyrosine hydroxylase (TH)- and serotonin (5-HT) immunoreactive innervation in the rat pituitary gland. *Neurosci Lett* 1988;94:39.
342. Schimchowitsch S, Vuillez P, Tappaz ML, Klein MJ, Stoeckel ME. Systematic presence of GABA-immunoreactivity in the tubero-infundibular and tubero-hypophyseal dopaminergic systems: an ultrastructural immunogold study on several mammals. *Exp Brain Res* 1991;83:575.
343. Dellmann HD, Stoeckel ME, Hindelang-Gertner C, et al. A comparative ultrastructural study of the pars tuberalis of various

mammals, the chicken and the newt. *Cell Tissue Res* 1974;148:313.
344. Cameron E, Foster CL. Some light- and electron-microscopical observations on the pars tuberalis of the pituitary gland of the rabbit. *J Endocrinol* 1972;54:505.
345. Baker BL, Yu YY. Immunocytochemical analysis of cells in the pars tuberalis of the rat hypophysis with antisera to hormones of the pars distalis. *Cell Tissue Res* 1975;156:443.
346. Baker BL, Karsch FJ, Hoffman DL, Beckman WC. The presence of gonadotropic and thyrotropic cells in the pituitary pars tuberalis of the monkey (*Macaca mulatta*). *Biol Reprod* 1977;17:232.
347. Girod C, Dubois MP, Trouillas J. Immunohistochemical study of the pars tuberalis of the adenohypophysis in the monkey, *Macaca irus*. *Cell Tissue Res* 1980;210:191.
348. Gross DS. Hormone production in the hypophysial pars tuberalis of intact and hypophysectomized rats. *Endocrinology* 1983;112:733.
349. Wittokski W, Schulze-Bonhage AH, Bockers TM. The pars tuberalis of the hypophysis: a modulator of the pars distalis? *Acta Endocrinol* 1992;126:285.
350. Nakazawa K, Marubayashi U, McCann SM. Mediation of the short-loop negative feedback of luteinizing hormone (LH) on LH-releasing hormone release by melatonin-induced inhibition of LH from the pars tuberalis. *Proc Natl Acad Sci USA* 1991;88:7576.
351. Monroe BG. A comparative study of the ultrastructure of the median eminence, infundibular stem and neural lobe of the hypophysis of the rat. *Z Zellforsch* 1967;76:405.
352. Duffy PE, Menefee M. Electron microscopic observations of neurosecretory granules, nerve and glial fibers and blood vessels in the median eminence of the rabbit. *Am J Anat* 1965;117:251.
353. Page RB, Dovey-Hartman BJ. Neurohemal contact in the internal zone of the rabbit median eminence. *J Comp Neurol* 1984;226:274.
354. Kobayashi H, Oota Y, Uemura H, Hirano T. Electron microscopic and pharmacological studies on the rat median eminence. *Z Zellforsch* 1966;71:387.
355. Rinne UK. Ultrastructure of the median eminence of the rat. *Z Zellforsch* 1966;74:98.
356. Lederis K. An electron microscopical study of the human neurohypophysis. *Z Zellforsch* 1965;65:847.
357. Bergland RM, Torack RM. An electron microscopic study of the human infundibulum. *Z Zellforsch* 1969;99:1.
358. Rodriguez EM. Ultrastructure of the neurohemal region of the toad median eminence. *Z Zellforsch* 1969;93:182.
359. Rodriguez EM. Ependymal specializations. I. Fine structure of the neural (internal) region of the toad median eminence, with particular reference to the connections between the ependymal cells and the subependymal capillary loops. *Z Zellforsch* 1969;102:153.
360. Magoun HW, Ranson SW. Retrograde degeneration of the supraoptic nuclei after section of the infundibular stalk in the monkey. *Anat Rec* 1939;75:107.
361. Rasmussen AT. Effects of hypophysectomy and hypophysial stalk resection of the hypothalamic nuclei of animals and man. *Res Publ Assoc Res Nerv Ment Dis* 1940;20:245.
362. Sherlock DA, Field PM, Raisman G. Retrograde transport of horseradish peroxidase in the magnocellular neurosecretory system of the rat. *Brain Res* 1975;88:403.
363. Zimmerman EA. The organization of oxytocin and vasopressin pathways. In: Martin JB, Reichlin S, Bick KL, eds. *Neurosecretion and brain peptides.* New York: Raven Press, 1981:63.
364. Barer R, Heller H, Lederis K. The isolation, identification and properties of the hormonal granules of the neurohypophysis. *Proc R Soc Lond* [*Biol*] 1963;158:388.
365. Silverman AJ, Zimmerman EA. Ultrastructural immunocytochemical localization of neurophysin and vasopressin in the median eminence and posterior pituitary of the guinea pig. *Cell Tissue Res* 1975;159:291.
366. Douglas WW, Nagasawa J, Schulz R. Electron microscopic studies on the mechanism of secretion of posterior pituitary hormones and significance of microvesicles (synaptic vesicles): evidence of secretion by exocytosis and formation of microvesicles as a by-product of this process. *Mem Soc Endocrinol* 1971;19:353.
367. Buma P, Nieuwenhuys R. Ultrastructural demonstration of oxytocin and vasopressin release sites in the neural lobe and median eminence of the rat by tannic acid and immunogold methods. *Neurosci Lett* 1987;74:151.
368. Theodosis DT, Dreifuss JJ, Orci L. A freeze-fracture study of membrane events during neurohypophysial secretion. *J Cell Biol* 1978;78:542.
369. Morris JF, Nordmann JJ. Membrane recapture after hormone release from nerve endings in the neural lobe of the rat pituitary gland. *Neuroscience* 1980;5:639.
370. Hartmann JF. Electron microscopy of the neurohypophysis in normal and histamine-treated rats. *Z Zellforsch* 1958;48:291.
371. Barer R, Lederis K. Ultrastructure of the rabbit neurohypophysis with special reference to the release of hormones. *Z Zellforsch* 1966;75:201.
372. Barer R, Lederis K. Ultrastructure of the rabbit neurohypophysis with special reference to the release of hormones. *Z Zellforsch* 1966;75:201.
373. Rodriguez EM. The comparative morphology of neural lobes of species with different neurohypophysial hormones. *Mem Soc Endocrinol* 1971;19:263.
374. Seyama S, Pearl GS, Takei Y. Ultrastructural study of the human neurohypophysis. I. Neurosecretory axons and their dilatations in the pars nervosa. *Cell Tissue Res* 1980;205:253.
375. Nordmann JJ, Chevallier J. The role of microvesicles in buffering (Ca^{2+}) in the neurohypophysis. *Nature* 1980;287:54.
376. Shaw FD, Morris JF. Calcium localization in the rat neurohypophysis. *Nature* 1980;287:56.
377. Broadwell RD, Cataldo AM, Balin BJ. Further studies of the secretory process in hypothalamo-neurohypophysial neurons: an analysis using immunocytochemistry, wheat germ agglutinin-peroxidase, and native peroxidase. *J Comp Neurol* 1984;228:155.
378. Navone R, Di Gioia G, Jahn R, Browning M, Greengard P, De Camilli P. Microvesicles of the neurohypophysis are biochemically related to small synaptic vesicles of presynaptic terminals. *J Cell Biol* 1989;109:3425.
379. Meeker RB, Swanson DJ, Hayward JN. Light and electron microscopic localization of glutamate immunoreactivity in the supraoptic nucleus of the rat hypothalamus. *Neuroscience* 1989;333:157.
380. Meeker RB, Swanson DJ, Greenwood RS, Hayward JN. Ultrastructural distribution of glutamate immunoreactivity within neurosecretory endings and pituicytes of the rat neurohypophysis. *Brain Res* 1991;564:181.
381. Bloom FE, Aghajanian GK. An electron microscopic analysis of large granular synaptic vesicles of the brain in relation to monoamine content. *J Pharmacol Exp Ther* 1968;159:261.
382. Bloom FE. The fine structural localization of biogenic monoamines in nervous tissue. *Int Rev Neurobiol* 1970;13:27.
383. Ajika K. Relationship between catecholaminergic neurons and hypothalamic hormone-containing neurons in the hypothalamus. In: Martini L, Ganong WF, eds. *Frontiers of neuroendocrinology,* Vol. 6. New York: Raven Press, 1980:1.
384. Hökfelt T, Meister B, Melander T, Everitt B. Coexistence of classical transmitters and peptides with special reference to the arcuate nucleus. *Adv Biochem Pharmacol* 1987;93:21.
385. Johansson O, Hökfelt T, Jeffcoate SL, White N, Sternberger LA. Ultrastructural localization of TRH-like immunoreactivity. *Exp Brain Res* 1980;38:1.
386. Shioda S, Nakai Y. Immunocytochemical localization of TRH and autoradiographic determination of ^{3}H-TRH-binding sites in the arcuate nucleus-median eminence of the rat. *Cell Tissue Res* 1983;228:475.
387. Pelletier G, Labrie F, Arimura A, Schally AV. Electron microscopic immunohistochemical localization of growth hormone-release inhibiting hormones (somatostatin) in the rat median eminence. *Am J Anat* 1974;140:583.
388. Ohtsuka M, Yamamoto Y, Daikoku S. Topography and ultrastructure of LHRH- and somatostatin-containing axonal termi-

nals in the median eminence of rats. *Arch Histol Jpn* 1983;46:203.
389. Silverman AJ, Desnoyers P. Ultrastructural immunocytochemical localization of luteinizing hormone-releasing hormone (LH-RH) in the median eminence of the guinea pig. *Cell Tissue Res* 1976;169:157.
390. Stoeckart R, Jansen HG, Kreike AJ. Ultrastructural evidence for exocytosis in the median eminence of the rat. *Z Zellforsch* 1972;131:99.
391. Daikoku S, Takahashi T, Kojimoto H, Watanabe YG. Secretory surface phenomena in freeze-etched preparations of the adenohypophysial cells and neurosecretory fibers. *Z Zellforsch* 1973;136:207.
392. Buma P, Nieuwenhuys R. Ultrastructural characterization of exocitotic release sites in different layers of the median eminence of the rat. *Cell Tissue Res* 1988;252:107.
393. Ajika K. Simultaneous localization of LHRH and catecholamines in rat hypothalamus. *J Anat* 1979;128:331.
394. Nakai Y, Shioda S, Ochiai H, Kudo J, Hashimoto A. Ultrastructural relationship between monoamine- and TRH-containing axons in the rat median eminence as revealed by combined autoradiography and immunocytochemistry in the same tissue section. *Cell Tissue Res* 1983;230:1.
395. Tranzer JP, Thoenen H. Electronmicroscopic localization of 5-hydroxydopamine (3,4,5-trihydroxyphenyl-ethylamine), a new "false" sympathetic transmitter. *Experientia* 1967;23:743.
396. Richards JG, Tranzer J-P. The ultrastructural localisation of amine storage sites in the central nervous system with the aid of a specific marker, 5-hydroxydopamine. *Brain Res* 1970;17:463.
397. Tranzer J-P, Richards JG. Ultrastructural cytochemistry of biogenic amines in nervous tissue: methodologic improvements. *J Histochem Cytochem* 1976;24:1178.
398. Pickel VM, Joh TH, Reis DJ. Ultrastructural localization of tyrosine hydroxylase in noradrenergic neurons of the brain. *Proc Natl Acad Sci USA* 1975;72:659.
399. Pickel VM, Joh TH, Field PM, Becker CG, Reis DJ. Cellular localization of tyrosine hydroxylase by immunohistochemistry. *J Histochem Cytochem* 1975;23:1.
400. Pickel VM, Joh T, Reis DJ. Monoamine-synthesizing enzymes in central dopaminergic, noradrenergic and serotonergic neurons. Immunocytochemical localization by light and electron microscopy. *J Histochem Cytochem* 1976;24:792.
401. Carson KA, Nemcroff CB, Rone MS, et al. Biochemical and histochemical evidence for the existence of a tubero-infundibular cholinergic pathway in the rat. *Brain Res* 1977;129:169.
402. Fink G, Smith GC. Ultrastructural features of the developing hypothalamo-hypophysial axis in the rat. *Z Zellforsch* 1971;119:208.
403. Paull WK. A light and electron microscopic study of the development of the neurohypophysis of the fetal rat. *Anat Rec* 1973;175:407.
404. Eurenius L, Jarskar R. Electron microscope studies on the development of the external zone of the mouse median eminence. *Z Zellforsch* 1971;122:488.
405. Monroe BG, Newman BL, Schapiro S. Ultrastructure of the median eminence of neonatal and adult rats. In: Knigge KM, Scott DE, Weindl A, eds. *Brain-endocrine interaction. Median eminence: structure and function.* Basel: Karger, 1972:7.
406. Monroe BG, Paull WK. Ultrastructural changes in the hypothalamus during development and hypothalamic activity: the median eminence. *Prog Brain Res* 1974;41:185.
407. Kawano H, Watanabe YG, Daikoku S. Light and electron microscopic observation on the appearance of immunoreactive LHRH in perinatal rat hypothalamus. *Cell Tissue Res* 1980;213:465.
408. Setalo G, Antalicz M, Saarossy K, Arimura A, Schally AV, Flerko B. Ontogenesis of the LH-RH containing neuronal elements in the hypothalamus of the rat. *Acta Biol Acad Sci Hung* 1978;29:285.
409. Gross DS, Baker BL. Immunohistochemical localization of gonadotropin-releasing hormone (GnRH) in the fetal and early postnatal mouse brain. *Am J Anat* 1977;148:195.
410. Gross DS, Baker BL. Developmental correlation between hypothalamic gonadotropin-releasing hormone and hypophysial luteinizing hormone. *Am J Anat* 1979;154:1.
411. Monroe BG, Holmes EM. The freeze-fractured median eminence. II. Developmental changes in the neurohemal contact zone of the median eminence of the rat. *Cell Tissue Res* 1983;233:81.
412. Ugrumov MV, Chandrasekhar K, Borisova NA, Mitsekevich MS. Light and electron microscopical investigations on the tanycyte differentiation during the perinatal period in the rat. *Cell Tissue Res* 1979;201:295.
413. Monroe BG, Holmes EM. The freeze-fractured median eminence. 1. Development of intercellular junctions in the ependyma of the 3rd ventricle of the rat. *Cell Tissue Res* 1982;222:389.
414. Silverman AJ, Desnoyers P. Post-natal development of the median eminence of the guinea pig. *Anat Rec* 1975;183:459.
415. Lamperti A, Mastovich J. Morphological changes in the hypothalamic arcuate nucleus and median eminence in the golden hamster during the neonatal period. *Am J Anat* 1983;166:173.
416. Kobayashi H, Matsui T. Fine structure of the median eminence and its functional significance. In: Ganong WF, Martini L, eds. *Frontiers in neuroendocrinology.* New York: Oxford University Press, 1969:3.
417. Kobayashi H, Matsui T, Ishii S. Functional electron microscopy of the hypothalamic median eminence. *Int Rev Cytol* 1970;29:281.
418. Knigge KM, Silverman A-J. Anatomy of the endocrine hypothalamus. In: Greep RO, Astwood EB, eds. *Handbook of physiology. Section 7, endocrinology. Vol. IV, The pituitary gland and its neuroendocrine control.* Washington, DC: American Physiology Society, 1974:1.
419. Enemar A, Eurenius L. Organization and development of the perivascular space system in the neurohypophysis of the laboratory mouse. *Cell Tissue Res* 1979;199:99.
420. Heap PF, Jones CW, Morris JF, Pickering BT. Movement of neurosecretory product through the anatomical compartments of the neural lobe of the pituitary gland. (An electron microscopic autoradiographic study.) *Cell Tissue Res* 1975;156:483.
421. Tweedle CD, Smithson KG, Hatton GI. Neurosecretory endings in the rat neurohypophysis are en passant. *Exp Neurol* 1989;106:20.
422. Aspeslagh M-R, Vandesande F, Dierickx K. Electron microscopic immunocytochemical demonstration of separate neurophysin-vasopressinergic and neurophysin-oxytocinergic nerve fibres in the neural lobe of the rat hypophysis. *Cell Tissue Res* 1976;171:31.
423. VanLeeuwen FW, de Raay C, Swaab DF, Fisser B. The localization of oxytocin, vasopressin, somatostatin and luteinizing hormone releasing hormone in the rat neurohypophysis. *Cell Tissue Res* 1979;202:189.
424. Jirikowski GF, Sanna PP, Bloom FE. mRNA coding for oxytocin is present in axons of the hypothalamo-neurohypophysial tract. *Proc Natl Acad Sci USA* 1990;87:7400.
425. Mohr E, Zhou A, Thorn NA, Richter D. Rats with physically disconnected hypothalamopituitary tracts no longer contain vasopressin-oxytocin gene transcripts in the posterior pituitary lobe. *FEBS Lett* 1990;263:332.
426. Mezey E, Kiss JZ. Coexpression of vasopressin and oxytocin in hypothalamic supraoptic neurons of lactating rats. *Endocrinology* 1990;129:1814.
427. Rossier J, Pittman Q, Bloom F, Guillemin R. Distribution of opioid peptides in the pituitary: a new hypothalamic-pars nervosa enkephalinergic pathway. *Fed Proc* 1980;39:2555.
428. Zamir N. On the origin of leu-enkephalin and met-enkephalin in the rat neurohypophysis. *Endocrinology* 1985;117:1687.
429. Martin R, Voigt KH. Enkephalins co-exist with oxytocin and vasopressin in nerve terminals of rat neurohypophysis. *Nature* 1981;289:502.
430. Martin R, Geis R, Holl R, Schafer M, Voigt KH. Co-existence of unrelated peptides in oxytocin and vasopressin terminals of rat neurohypophyses: immunoreactive methionine^5-enkephalin-,

leucine[5]-, enkephalin-, and cholecystokinin-like substances. *Neuroscience* 1983;8:213.
431. Vanderhaeghen JJ, Lotstra F, Liston DR, Rossier J. Proenkephalin, (Met)enkephalin, and oxytocin immunoreactivities are colocalized in bovine hypothalamic magnocellular neurons. *Proc Natl Acad Sci USA* 1983;80:5139.
432. Weber E, Roth KA, Evans CJ, Chang J-K, Baracas JD. Immunohistochemical localization of dynporhin (1-8) in hypothalamic magnocellular neurons: Evidence for absence of proenkephalin. *Life Sci* 1982;31:1761.
433. VanLeeuwen FW, Pool CW, Sluiter AA. Enkephalin immunoreactivity in synaptoid elements on glial cells in the rat neural lobe. *Neuroscience* 1983;8:229.
434. Merchenthaler I, Maderdrut JL, Altshculer RA, Petrusz P. Immunocytochemical localization of proenkephalin-derived peptides in the central nervous system of the rat. *Neuroscience* 1986;17(2):325.
435. Summy-Long JY, Miller DS, Rosella-Dampman LM, Hartman RD, Emmert SE. A functional role for opioid peptides in the differential secretion of vasopressin and oxytocin. *Brain Res* 1984;309:362.
436. Bondy CA, Gainer H, Russell JT. Dynorphin A inhibits and naloxone increases the electrically stimulated release of oxytocin but not vasopressin from terminals of the neural lobe. *Endocrinology* 1988;122:1321.
437. Vanderhaeghen JJ, Lotstra F, DeMey J, Gilles C. Immunohistochemical localization of cholecystokinin and gastrin-like peptides in the brain and hypophysis of the rat. *Proc Natl Acad Sci USA* 1980;77:1190.
438. Kiss JZ, Williams TH, Palkovits M. Distribution and projections of cholecystokinin-immunoreactive neurons in the hypothalamic paraventricular nucleus of rat. *J Comp Neurol* 1984;227:173.
439. Gaymann W, Martin R. Immunoreactive galanin-like material in magnocellular hypothalamo-neurohypophysial neurones of the rat. *Cell Tissue Res* 1989;255:139.
440. Melander T, Hökfelt T, Rokaeus A, et al. Coexistence of galanin-like immunoreactivity with catecholamines, 5-hydroxytryptamine, GABA and neuropeptides in the rat CNS. *J Neurosci* 1986;6:3640.
441. Stoeckel ME, Porte A, Klein MJ, Cuello AC. Immunocytochemical localization of substance P in the neurohypophysis and hypothalamus of the mouse compared with the distribution of other neuropeptides. *Cell Tissue Res* 1982;223:533.
442. Mikkelsen JD, Larsen PJ, Moller M, Vilhardt H, Soermark T. Substance P in the median eminence and pituitary of the rat: demonstration of immunoreactive fibers and specific binding sites. *Neuroendocrinology* 1989;50:100.
443. Zimmerman EA, Robinson AG, Husain MK, et al. Neurohypophysial peptides in the bovine hypothalamus: the relationship of neurophysin I to oxytocin, and neurophysin II to vasopressin in supraoptic and paraventricular regions. *Endocrinology* 1974; 95:931.
444. Lechan RM, Jackson IMD. Immunohistochemical localization of thyrotropin-releasing hormone in the rat hypothalamus and pituitary. *Endocrinology* 1982;111:55.
445. Mikkelsen JD, Bersani M, Holst JJ, Larsen PJ. Nerve fibers in the rat posterior pituitary lobe contain prosomatostatin (1-64). *Neuroendocrinology* 1991;54:469.
446. Baumgarten HG, Björklund A, Holstein AF, Nobin A. Organization and ultrastructural identification of the catecholamine nerve terminals in the neural lobe and pars intermedia of the rat pituitary. *Z Zellforsch* 1972;126:483.
447. Björklund A, Moore RY, Nobin A, Stenevi U. The organization of tubero-hypophyseal and reticulo-infundibular catecholamine neuron systems in the rat brain. *Brain Res* 1973;51:171.
448. Pelletier G. Identification of endings containing dopamine and vasopressin in the rat posterior pituitary by a combination of radioautography and immunocytochemistry at the ultrastructural level. *J Histochem Cytochem* 1983;31:562.
449. Saavedra JM. Central and peripheral catecholamine innervation of the rat intermediate and posterior pituitary lobes. *Neuroendocrinology* 1985;40:281.
450. Brustle O, Pilgrim CH, Gaymann W, Reisert I. Abundant GABAergic innervation of rat posterior pituitary revealed by inhibition of GABA-transaminase. *Cell Tissue Res* 1988;251:59.
451. Okamura H, Murakami S, Chihara M, Jouvet M. Coexistence of growth hormone releasing factor-like and tyrosine hydroxylase-like immunoreactivities in neurons of the rat arcuate nucleus. *Neuroendocrinology* 1985;41:177.
452. Buijs RM, Van Vulpen EHS, Geffard M. Ultrastructural localization of GABA in the supraoptic nucleus and neural lobe. *Neuroscience* 1987;20:347.
453. Alper RH, Demarest KT, Moore KE. Effects of surgical sympathectomy on catecholamine concentrations in the posterior pituitary of the rat. *Experientia* 1980;36:134.
454. Bicknell RJ, Dyball RE, Garten LL, Heavens RP, Sirinathsinghji DJS, Zahao B-G. Evidence for a direct noradrenergic projection from the brainstem to the neural lobe in the rat. *J Physiol* 1988;396:127P.
455. Barnes PRJ, Dyball REJ. Inhibition of neurohypophysial hormone release by dopamine in the rat. *J Physiol* 1982;327:85P.
456. Vizi ET, Volbekas V. Inhibition by dopamine of oxytocin release from isolated posterior lobe of the hypophysis of the rat: disinhibitory effect of beta-endorphin/enkephalin. *Neuroendocrinology* 1980;31:46.
457. Racke K, Ritzel H, Trapp B, Muscholl E. Dopaminergic modulation of evoked vasopressin release from the isolated neurohypophysis of the rat. Possible involvement of the endogenous opioids. *Naunyn-Schmiedebergs Arch Pharmacol* 1982;319:56.
458. Bredt DS, Glatt CE, Hwang PM, Fotuhi M, Dawson TM, Snyder SH. Nitric oxide synthase protein and mRNA are discretely localized in neuronal populations of the mammalian CNS together with NADPH diaphorase. *Neuron* 1991;7:615.
459. Anthony ELP, King JC, Stopa EG. Immunocytochemical localization of LHRH in the median eminence, infundibular stalk, and neurohypophysis. (Evidence for multiple sites of releasing hormone secretion in humans and other mammals.) *Cell Tissue Res* 1984;236:5.
460. Kawata M, Hashimoto K, Takahara J, Sano Y. Immunohistochemical identification of the corticotropin releasing factor (CRF)-containing nerve fibers in the pig hypophysis, with special reference to the relationship between CRF and posterior lobe hormones. *Arch Histol Jpn* 1983;46:183.
461. Takei Y, Seyama S, Pearl GS, Tindall GT. Ultrastructural study of the human neurohypophysis. II. Cellular elements of neural parenchyma, the pituicytes. *Cell Tissue Res* 1980;205:273.
462. Tweedle CD, Hatton GI. Glial cell enclosure of neurosecretory endings in the neurohypophysis of the rat. *Brain Res* 1980;192:555.
463. Tweedle CD, Hatton GI. Evidence for dynamic interactions between pituicytes and neurosecretory axons in the rat. *Neuroscience* 1980;5:661.
464. Hatton GI, Tweedle CD. Magnocellular neuropeptidergic neurons in hypothalamus: increases in membrane apposition and number of specialized synapses from pregnancy to lactation. *Brain Res Bull* 1982;8:197.
465. Tweedle CD, Hatton GI. Magnocellular neuropeptidergic terminals in the neurohypophysis: rapid glial release of enclosed axons during parturition. *Brain Res Bull* 1982;8:205.
466. Tweedle CD. Ultrastructural manifestations of increased hormone release in the neurohypophysis. *Prog Brain Res* 1983;60:259.
467. Hatton GI, Perlmutter LS, Salm AK, Tweedle CD. Dynamic neuronal-glial interactions in hypothalamus and pituitary: implications for control of hormone synthesis and release. *Peptides* (Suppl 1) 1984;5:121.
468. Perlmutter LS, Hatton GI, Tweedle CD. Plasticity in the in vitro neurohypophysis: effects of osmotic changes on pituicytes. *Neuroscience* 1984;12:503.
469. Tweedle C, Hatton G. Morphological adaptability at neurosecretory axonal endings on the neurovascular contact zone of the rat neurohypophysis. *Neuroscience* 1987;20:241.
470. Luckman SM, Bicknell RJ. Morphological plasticity that occurs in the neurohypophysis following activation of the magnocellu-

lar neurosecretory system can be mimicked in vitro by beta-adrenergic stimulation. *Neuroscience* 1990;39:701.
471. Bicknell RJ, Luckman SM, Inenga K, Mason WT, Hatton GI. Beta-adrenergic and opioid receptors on pituicytes cultured from adult rat neurohypophysis: regulation of cell morphology. *Brain Res Bull* 1989;22:379.
472. Bunn SJ, Hanley MR, Wilkin GP. Evidence for kappa opioid receptor on pituitary astrocytes: an autoradiographic study. *Neurosci Lett* 1985;55:317.
473. Bicknell RJ. Endogenous opioid peptides and hypothalamic neuroendocrine neurones. *J Endocrinol* 1985;107:437.
474. Hatton GI. Emerging concepts of structure-function dynamics in adult brain: the hypothalamo-neurohypophysial system. *Prog Neurobiol* 1990;34:437.
475. Negro-Vilar A, Samson WK. Dehydration induced changes in immunoreactive vasopressin levels in specific hypothalamic structures. *Brain Res* 1979;585.
476. Ziedonis DM, Severs WB, Brennan RW, Page RB. Blood flow and functional responses correlate in the ovine neural lobe. *Brain Res* 1986;373:27.
477. Kadekaro M, Gross PM, Sokoloff L. Local cerebral glucose utilization in Long-Evans and Brattleboro rats during acute dehydration. *Neuroendocrinology* 1986;42:203.
478. Gross PM, Blasberg RG, Fenstermacher JD, Patlak CS. Rapid amino acid uptake in rat pituitary neural lobe during functional stimulation by chronic dehydration. *J Cereb Blood Flow Metab* 1985;5:151.
479. Merchenthaler I, Vigh S, Petrusz P, Schally AV. Immunocytochemical localization of corticotropin-releasing factor (CRF) in the rat brain. *Am J Anat* 1982;165:385.
480. Sawchenko PE, Swanson LW, Rivier J, Vale WW. The distribution of growth-hormone-releasing factor (GRF) immunoreactivity in the central nervous system of the rat: an immunohistochemical study using antisera directed against rat hypothalamic GRF. *J Comp Neurol* 1985;237:100.
481. Kahn D, Abrams GM, Zimmerman EA, Carraway R, Leeman SE. Neurotensin neurons in the rat hypothalamus: an immunohistochemical study. *Endocrinology* 1980;107:47.
482. Dierickx K, DeWaele G. Scanning electron microscopy of the wall of the third ventricle of the brain of *Rana temporaria* III. Electron microscopy of the ventricular surface of the median eminence. *Cell Tissue Res* 1975;161:343.
483. Mikami S-I. A correlative ultrastructural analysis of the ependymal cells of the third ventricle of Japanese quail, *Coturnix japonica.* In: Knigge KM, Scott DE, Kobayashi H, Ishii S, eds. *Brain-endocrine interaction, II. The ventricular system.* Basel: Karger, 1975:80.
484. Martinez PM, DeWeerd H. The fine structure of the ependymal surface of the recessus infundibularis in the rat. *Anat Embryol* 1977;151:241.
485. Paull WK, Martin H, Scott DE. Scanning electron microscopy of the third ventricular floor of the rat. *J Comp Neurol* 1977;175:301.
486. Bruni JE, Montemurro DG, Clattenburg RE, Singh RP. A scanning electron microscopic study of the ependymal surface of the third ventricle of the rabbit, rat, mouse and human brain. *Anat Rec* 1972;174:407.
487. Climenti F, Marini D. The surface fine structure of the walls of cerebral ventricles and of choroid plexus in cat. *Z Zellforsch* 1972;123:82.
488. Bruni JE, Clattenburg RE, Montemurro DG. Ependymal tanycytes of the rabbit third ventricle: a scanning electron microscopic study. *Brain Res* 1974;73:145.
489. Scott DE. A comparative ultrastructural analysis of the third cerebral ventricle of the North American mink. *Anat Rec* 1973;175:155.
490. Kozlowski GP, Scott DE, Dudley G. Scanning electron microscopy of the 3rd ventricle of sheep. *Z Zellforsch* 1973;136:169.
491. Scott DE, Krobisch-Dudley G, Paull WK, Kozlowski GP, Ribas J. The primate median eminence. I. Correlative scanning-transmission electron microscopy. *Cell Tissue Res* 1975;162: 61.
492. Scott DE, Paull WK, Dudley GK. A comparative scanning electron microscopic analysis of the human cerebral ventricular system. I. The third ventricle. *Z Zellforsch* 1972;132:203.
493. Jacobs JJ, Monroe KD. A scanning electron microscopic survey of the brain ventricular system of the female armadillo. *Cell Tissue Res* 1977;183:531.
494. Bruni JE, Montemurro DG, Clattenburg RE. Morphology of the ependymal lining of the rabbit third ventricle following intraventricular administration of synthetic luteinizing hormone-releasing hormone (LH-RH): a scanning electron microscopic investigation. *Am J Anat* 1977;150:411.
495. Paull WK, Martin H, Scott DE. Scanning electron microscopy of the third ventricular floor of the rat. *J Comp Neurol* 1977;175:301.
496. Matsui T, Kobayashi H. Surface protrusions from the ependymal cells of the median eminence. *Arch Anat* 1968;51:429.
497. Dierickx K, DeWaele G. Scanning electron microscopy of the wall of the third ventricle of the brain of *Rana temporaria.* III. Electron microscopy of the ventricular surface of the median eminence. *Cell Tissue Res* 1975;161:343.
498. Scott DE, Krobisch-Dudley G, Paull WK, Kozlowski GP. The ventricular system in neuroendocrine mechanisms. III. Supraependymal neuronal networks in the primate brain. *Cell Tissue Res* 1977;179:235.
499. Bleier R, Albrecht R, Cruce JAF. Supraependymal cells of hypothalamic third ventricle: identification as resident phagocytes of the brain. *Science* 1975;189:299.
500. Bleier R. Ultrastructure of supraependymal cells and ependyma of hypothalamic third ventricle of mouse. *J Comp Neurol* 1977;174:359.
501. Bleier R. The relations of ependyma to neurons and capillaries in the hypothalamus: a Golgi-Cox study. *J Comp Neurol* 1971;142:439.
502. Millhouse OE. A Golgi study of the third ventricle tanycytes in the adult rodent brain. *Z Zellforsch* 1971;121:1.
503. Millhouse OE. Light and electron microscopic studies of the ventricular wall. *Z Zellforsch* 1972;127:149.
504. Card JP, Rafols JA. Tanycytes of the third ventricle of the neonatal rat: a Golgi study. *Am J Anat* 1978;151:173.
505. Sharp PJ. Tanycyte and vascular patterns in the basal hypothalamus of corturnix quail with reference to their possible neuroendocrine significance. *Z Zellforsch* 1972;127:552.
506. Akmayev IG, Popov AP. Morphological aspects of the hypothalamic-hypophyseal system. VII. The tanycytes: their relation to the hypophyseal adrenocorticotrophic function. An ultrastructural study. *Cell Tissue Res* 1977;180:263.
507. Brawer JR. The fine structure of the ependymal tanycytes at the level of the arcuate nucleus. *J Comp Neurol* 1972;145:25.
508. Gotow T, Hashimoto PH. Graded differences in tightness of ependymal intercellular junctions within and in the vicinity of the rat median eminence. *J Ultrastruct Res* 1981;76:293.
509. Rodriguez EM, Gonzalez CB, Delannoy L. Cellular organization of the lateral and postinfundibular regions of the median eminence in the rat. *Cell Tissue Res* 1979;201:377.
510. Brawer JR, Walsh RJ. Response of tanycytes to aging in the median eminence of the rat. *Am J Anat* 1982;163:247.
511. Brightman MW, Reese TS. Junctions between intimately apposed cell membranes in the vertebrate brain. *J Cell Biol* 1969;40:648.
512. Brightman MW, Prescott L, Reese TS. Intercellular junctions of special ependyma. In: Knigge KM, Scott DE, Kobayashi H, Ishii S, eds. *Brain-endocrine interaction II. The ventricular system.* Basel: Karger, 1975:146.
513. Nakai Y, Ochiai H, Uchida M. Fine structure of ependymal cells in the median eminence of the frog and mouse revealed by freeze-etching. *Cell Tissue Res* 1977;181:311.
514. Kobayashi H, Wada M, Uemura H. Uptake of peroxidase from the 3rd ventricle by ependymal cells of the median eminence. *Z Zellforsch* 1972;127:545.
515. Kobayashi H. Absorption of cerebrospinal fluid by ependymal cells of the median eminence. In: Knigge KM, Scott DE, Kobayashi H, Ishii S, eds. *Brain-endocrine interaction II. The ventricular system.* Basel: Karger, 1975:109.
516. Nakai Y, Naito N. Uptake and bidirectional transport of peroxi-

dase injected into the blood and cerebrospinal fluid by ependymal cells of the median eminence. In: Knigge KM, Scott DE, Kobayashi H, Ishii S, eds. *Brain-endocrine interaction II. The ventricular system.* Basel: Karger, 1975:94.
517. Guldner F-H, Wolff JR. Neurono-glial synaptoid contacts in the median eminence of the rat: ultrastructure, staining properties and distribution on tanycytes. *Brain Res* 1973;61:217.
518. Scott DE, Paull WK. The tanycyte of the rat median eminence. I. Synaptoid contacts. *Cell Tissue Res* 1979;200:329.
519. Knowles F, Kumar TCA. Structural changes, related to reproduction, in the hypothalamus and in the pars tuberalis of the rhesus monkey. *Philos Trans R Soc Lond Biol* 1969;256:357.
520. Knowles F. Ependyma of the third ventricle in relation to pituitary function. *Prog Brain Res* 1972;38:255.
521. Knigge KM, Joseph SA, Sladek JR, et al. Uptake and transport activity of the median eminence of the hypothalamus. *Int Rev Cytol* 1976;45:383.
522. Pilgrim C. Commentary: transport function of hypothalamic tanycyte ependyma: how good is the evidence? *Neuroscience* 1978;3:277.
523. Luppa H, Feustel G, Weiss J, Luppa D. Localization of ATPase activity in IIIrd ventricle ependyma of the rat. A contribution to the function of ependyma. *Brain Res* 1975;83:15.
524. Firth JA, Bock R. Distribution and properties of an adenosine triphosphatase in the tanycyte ependyma of the IIIrd ventricle of the rat. *Histochemistry* 1976;47:145.
525. Krisch B, Leonhardt H, Buchheim W. The functional and structural border of the neurohemal region of the median eminence. *Cell Tissue Res* 1978;192:327.
526. Wittkowski W, Scheuer A. Functional changes of the neuronal and glial elements at the surface of the external layer of the median eminence. *Z Anat Entwickl-Gesch* 1974;143:255.
527. Bugnon C, Fellmann D, Gouget A, Cardot J. Corticoliberin in rat brain: immunocytochemical identification and localization of a novel neuroglandular system. *Neurosci Lett* 1982;30:25.
528. Hanstrom B. The neurohypophysis in the series of mammals. *Z Zellforsch* 1953;39:241.
529. Holmes MC, Antoni FA, Aguilera G, Catt KJ. Magnocellular axons in passage through the median eminence release vasopressin. *Nature* 1986;319:326.
530. Lofstrom A, Jonsson G, Fuxe K. Microfluorimetric quantitation of catecholamine fluorescence in rat median eminence. I. Aspects on the distribution of dopamine and noradrenaline nerve terminals. *J Histochem Cytochem* 1976;24:415.
531. Mezey E, Kiss JZ, Mueller GP, Eskay R, O'Donohue TL, Palkovits M. Distribution of the pro-opiomelanocortin derived peptides, adrenocorticotrope hormone, α-melanocyte-stimulating hormone and β-endorphin (ACTH, α-MSH, β-End) in the rat hypothalamus. *Brain Res* 1985;328:341.
532. Kiss JZ, Mezey E, Cassell MD, et al. Topographical distribution of pro-opiomelanocortin-derived peptides (ACTH/β-End/α-MSH) in the rat median eminence. *Brain Res* 1985;329:169.
533. Knigge KM, Scott DE. Structure and function of the median eminence. *Am J Anat* 1970;129:223.
534. Rodriguez EM. Comparative and functional morphology of the median eminence. In: Knigge KM, Scott DE, Weindl A, eds. *Brain-endocrine interaction: structure and function.* Basel: Karger, 1972;319.
535. Rodriguez EM. Ependymal specializations. I. Fine structure of the neural (internal) region of the toad median eminence, with particular reference to the connections between ependymal cells and the subependymal capillary loops. *Z Zellforsch* 1969; 102:153.
536. Fuxe K. Cellular localization of monoamines in the median eminence and infundibular stem of some mammals. *Acta Physiol Scand* 1963;58:383.
537. Fuxe K. Cellular localization of monoamines in the median eminence and infundibular stem of some mammals. *Z Zellforsch* 1964;61:710.
538. Fuxe K. Evidence for the existence of monoamine neurons in the central nervous system. IV. The distribution of monoamine nerve terminals in the central nervous system. *Acta Phys Scand Suppl* 1965;247:39.
539. Björklund A, Lindvall E, Svenson LA. Mechanisms of fluorophore formation in the histochemical glyoxylic acid method for monoamines. *Histochemie* 1972;32:113.
540. Lindvall O, Björklund A. The glyoxylic acid fluorescence histochemical method. A detailed account of the methodology for the visualization of central catecholamine neurons. *Histochemie* 1974;39:97.
541. Chiba T, Hwang BH, Williams TH. A method for studying glyoxylic acid induced fluorescence and ultrastructure of monoamine neurons. *Histochemistry* 1976;49:95.
542. Ajika K, Hökfelt T. Ultrastructural identification of catecholamine neurons in the hypothalamic periventricular-arcuate nucleus-median eminence complex with special reference to quantitative aspects. *Brain Res* 1973;57:97.
543. Bensch C, Lescure H, Dufy B, Gross C. Histofluorometrie des catecholamines de la couche externe de l'eminence mediane hypothalamique de la lapine. *Ann Endocrinol* 1979;39:281.
544. Bensch C, Lescure H, Robert J, Faure J. Catecholamine histofluorescence in the median eminence of female rabbits activated by mating. *J Neurol Transm* 1975;36:1.
545. Nojyo Y, Ibata Y, Sano Y. Demonstration of tuberinfundibular tract of the cat. Fluorescence histochemistry and electron microscopy. *Cell Tissue Res* 1976;168:289.
546. Tago H, McGreer PL, Gruce G, Hersh LB. Distribution of choline acetyltransferase-containing neurons of the hypothalamus. *Brain Res* 1987;415:49.
547. Yoshimoto Y, Sakai K, Salvert D, Stuart M, Jouvet M. Cells of origin of histaminergic afferents to the cat median emincence. *Brain Res* 1989;504:149.
548. Ibata Y, Fukui K, Okamura H, et al. Coexistence of dopamine and neurotensin in hypothalamic arcuate and periventricular neurons. *Brain Res* 1983;269:177.
549. Everitt B, Meister B, Hökfelt T, et al. The hypothalamic arcuate nucleus-median eminence complex: immunohistochemistry of transmitters, peptides and DARPP-32 with special reference to coexistence in dopamine neurons. *Brain Res Rev* 1986;11:97.
550. Okamura H, Kitahama K, Mons N, Ibata Y, Jouvet M, Geffard M. L-Dopa-immunoreactive neurons in the rat hypothalamic tuberal region. *Neurosci Lett* 1988;95:42.
551. Pu L-P, Charmay Y, Leduque P, Morel G, Dubois PM. Light and electron microscopic immunocytochemical evidence that delta sleep-inducing peptide and gonadotropin-releasing hormone are coexpressed in the same nerve structures in the guinea pig median eminence. *Neuroendocrinology* 1991;53:332.
552. Joseph SA, Piekut DT, Knigge KM. Immunocytochemical localization of luteinizing hormone-releasing hormone (LHRH) in vibratome-sectioned brain. *J Histochem Cytochem* 1981; 29:247.
553. McNeill TH, Sladek J. Fluorescence-immunocytochemistry. Simultaneous localization of catecholamines and gonadotropin-releasing hormone. *Science* 1978;200:72.
554. Ibata Y, Watanabe K, Kinoshita H, et al. Detection of catecholamine and luteinizing.hormone-releasing hormone (LH-RH) containing nerve endings in the median eminence and the organum vasculosum laminae terminalis by fluorescence histochemistry and immunohistochemistry on the same microscopic sections. *Neurosci Let* 1979;11:181.
555. Ajika K. Simultaneous localization of LHRH and catecholamines in rat hypothalamus. *J Anat* 1979;128:331.
556. Kuljis RO, Advis JP. Immunocytochemical and physiological evidence of a synapse between dopamine and luteinizing hormone-releasing hormone releasing hormone-containing neurons in the ewe median eminence. *Endocrinology* 1989;124:1579.
557. Lehman MN, Karsch FJ, Robinson JE, Silverman A-J. Ultrastructural and synaptic organization of luteinizing hormone-releasing hormone in the anestrous ewe. *J Comp Neurol* 1988;273:447.
558. Johansson O, Hökfelt T. Thyrotropin releasing hormone, somatostatin, and enkephalin: distribution studies using immunohistochemical techniques. *J Histochem Cytochem* 1980;28:364.
559. Merchenthaler I, Vigh S, Schally AV, Petrusz P. Immunocyto-

chemical localization of growth hormone-releasing factor in the rat hypothalamus. *Endocrinology* 1984;114:1082.
560. Sawchenko PE, Swanson LW, Rivier J, Vale WW. The distribution of growth-hormone-releasing factor (GRF) immunoreactivity in the central nervous system of the rat: an immunohistochemical study using antisera directed against rat hypothalamic GRF. *J Comp Neurol* 1985;237:100.
561. Fellmann D, Bugnon C, Gouget A, Cardot J. Les neurones a corticoliberine (CRF) du cerveau de rat. *Compt Rend* 1982;176:511.
562. Bugnon C, Fellmann D, Gouget A, Cardot J. Immunocytochemical detection of the CRF-containing neurons in the rat brain. *C R Acad Sci Paris* 1982;294:279.
563. Swanson LW, Sawchenko PE, Rivier J, Vale WW. Organization of ovine corticotropin-releasing factor immunoreactive cells and fibers in the rat brain: an immunohistochemical study. *Neuroendocrinology* 1983;36:165.
564. Kawata H, Hashimoto K, Takahara J, Sano Y. Immunohistochemical demonstration of corticotropin releasing factor containing nerve fibers in the median eminence of the rat and monkey. *Histochemistry* 1982;76:15.
565. Lind RW, Swanson LW, Chin DA, Bruhn TO, Ganten D. Angiotensin II: an immunohistochemical study of its distribution in the paraventriculo-hypophysial system and its colocalization with vasopressin and CRF in parvocellular neurons. *Neurosci Abstr* 1984;10:88.
566. Meister B, Hökfelt T, Geffard M, Oertel W. Glutamic acid decarboxylase- and V-aminobutyric acid-like immunoreactivities in corticotropin-releasing factor-containing parvocellular neurons of the hypothalamic paraventricular nucleus. *Neuroendocrinology* 1988;48:516.
567. Hisano S, Tsuruo Y, Katoh S, Daikoku S, Yanaihara S, Shibasaki NT. Intragranular colocalization of arginine vasopressin and methionine-enkephalin-octapeptide in CRF-axons in the rat median eminence. *Cell Tissue Res* 1987;249:497.
568. Ceccatelli S, Eriksson M, Hökfelt T. Distribution and coexistence of CRF-, neurotensin-enkephalin-, cholecystokinin-, galanin-, and VIP/PHI-like peptides in the parvocellular part of the paraventricular nucleus. *Neuroendocrinology* 1989;49:309.
569. Vandesande F, Dierickx K, DeMey J. Identification of separate vasopressin-neurophysin II and oxytocin-neurophysin I containing nerve fibres in the external region of the bovine median eminence. *Cell Tissue Res* 1975;158:509.
570. Dierickx K, Vandesande F, DeMey J. Identification, in the external region of the rat median eminence, of separate neurophysin-vasopressin and neurophysin-oxytocin containing nerve fibers. *Cell Tissue Res* 1976;168:141.
571. Dierickx K, Vandesande F. Immunocytochemical demonstration, in the external region of the amphibian median eminence, of separate vasotocinergic and mesotocinergic nerve fibres. *Cell Tissue Res* 1977;177:47.
572. Zimmerman EA, Antunes JL. Organization of the hypothalamic-pituitary system: current concepts from immunohistochemical studies. *J Histochem Cytochem* 1976;24:807.
573. Antunes JL, Carmel PW, Zimmerman EA. Projections from the paraventricular nucleus to the zona externa of the median eminence of the rhesus monkey: an immunohistochemical study. *Brain Res* 1977;137:1.
574. Silverman AJ. Ultrastructural studies on the localization of neurohypophyseal hormones and their carrier proteins. *J Histochem Cytochem* 1976;24:816.
575. Kawata M, Hashimoto K, Takahara J, Sano Y. Differences in the distributional pattern of CRF-, oxytocin-, and vasopressin-immunoreactive nerve fibers in the median eminence of the rat. *Cell Tissue Res* 1983;230:247.
576. Whitnall MH. Subpopulations of corticotropin-releasing hormone neurosecretory cells distinguished by presence or absence of vasopressin: confirmation with multiple corticotropin-releasing hormone antisera. *Neuroscience* 1990;36:201.
577. Whitnall MH, Nezey E, Gainer H. Co-localization of corticotropin-releasing factor and vasopressin in median eminence neurosecretory vesicles. *Nature* 1985;317:248.
578. Whitnall MH, Smyth D, Gainer H. Vasopressin coexists in half of the corticotropin-releasing factor axons in the external zone of the median eminence. *Neuroendocrinology* 1987;45:420.
579. Zimmerman EA, Carmel PW, Husain MK, et al. Vasopressin & neurophysin: high concentrations in monkey hypophyseal portal blood. *Science* 1973;182:925.
580. Gibbs DM, Vale W. Presence of corticotropin releasing factor-like immunoreactivity in hypophysial portal blood. *Endocrinology* 1982;111:1418.
581. Oliver C, Mical RS, Porter JC. Hypothalamic pituitary vasculature: Evidence for retrograde blood flow in the pituitary stalk. *Endocrinology* 1977;101:598.
582. Bertini LT, Kiss JZ. Hypophysiotrophic neurons are capable of altering the ratio of co-package neurohormones. *Neuroscience* 1991;42:237.
583. Gillies GE, Linton EA, Lowry PJ. Corticotropin releasing activity of the new CRF is potentiated several times by vasopressin. *Nature* 1982;299:355.
584. Rivier C, Rivier J, Mormede P, Vale W. Studies of the nature of the interaction between vasopressin and corticotropin-releasing factor on adrenocorticotropin release in the rat. *Endocrinology* 1984;115:882.
585. Lind RW, Swanson LW, Bruhn TO, Ganten D. The distribution of angiotensin II-immunoreactive cells and fibers in the paraventriculo-hypophysial system of the rat. *Brain Res* 1985;338:81.
586. Merchenthaler I. The hypophysiotropic galanin system of the rat brain. *Neuroscience* 1991;44:643.
587. Melander T, Hökfelt T, Rokaeus A. Distribution of galanin-like immunoreactivity in the rat central nervous system. *J Comp Neurol* 1986;248:475.
588. Niimi M, Takahara J, Sato M, Kawanishi K. Immunohistochemical identification of galinin and growth hormone-releasing factor-containing neurons projecting to the median eminence of the rat. *Neuroendocrinology* 1990;51:572.
589. Arai R, Calas A. Ultrastructural localization of galanin immunoreactivity in the rat median eminence. *Brain Res* 1991;562:339.
590. Hökfelt T, Pernow B, Nilsson G, Wetterberg L, Goldstein M, Jeffcoate SL. Dense plexus of substance P immunoreactive nerve terminals in eminentia medialis of the primate hypothalamus. *Proc Natl Acad Sci USA* 1978;75:1013.
591. Gray TS, Morley JE. Neuropeptide Y: anatomical distribution and possible function in mammalian nervous system. *Life Sci* 1986;38:389.
592. Mulatero B, Fasolo A. Calcitonin-gene related peptide immunoreactivity in the hypothalamo-hypophysial system of the green frog, *Rana esculenta*. *Gen Comp Endocrinol* 1991;81:349.
593. Zimmerman EA, Liotta A, Krieger DT. β-Lipotropin in brain: localization in hypothalamic neurons by immunoperoxidase technique. *Cell Tissue Res* 1978;186:393.
594. Bloch B, Bugnon C, Lenys D, Fellmann D. Description des neurones immunoreactifs a un immunoserum anti β-endorphin presents dans le noyau infundibulaire chez l'homme. *CR Acad Sci Paris* 1978;287:309.
595. Bugnon C, Bloch B, Lenys D, Fellmann D. Infundibular neurons of the human hypothalamus simultaneously reactive with antisera against endorphins, ACTH, MSH, and β-LPH. *Cell Tissue Res* 1979;199:177.
596. Newman CB, Wardlaw SL, Van Vugt DA, Ferin M, Frantz AG. Adrenocorticotropin immunoactivity in monkey hypophyseal portal blood. *J Clin Endocrinol Metab* 1984;59:108.
597. Wardlow SL, Wehrenberg WB, Ferin M, Carmel PW, Frantz AG. High levels of β-endorphin in hypophyseal portal blood. *Endocrinology* 1980;106:1323.
598. Page RB, Bergland RM. The neurohypophyseal capillary bed. Part I. Anatomy and arterial supply. *Am J Anat* 1977;148:345.
599. Page RB, Leure-duPree AE, Bergland RM. The neurohypophyseal capillary bed. Part II. Specializations within median eminence. *Am J Anat* 1978;153:33.
600. Livingston A, Wilks PN. Perivascular regions of the rat neural lobe. *Cell Tissue Res* 1976;174:273.
601. Simionescu N, Simionescu M, Palade GE. Differentiated microdomains on the luminal surface of the capillary endothe-

lium. I. Preferential distribution of anionic sites. *J Cell Biol* 1981;90:605.
602. Simionescu M, Simionescu N, Silbert JE, Palade GE. Differentiated microdomains on the luminal surface of the capillary endothelium. II. Partial characterization of their anionic sites. *J Cell Biol* 1981;90:614.
603. Wislocki GB. The meningeal relations of the hypophysis cerebri. II. An embryological study of the meninges and blood vessels of the human hypophysis. *Am J Anat* 1937;61:95.
604. Enemar A. The structure and development of the hypophysial portal system in the laboratory mouse, with particular regard to the primary plexus. *Arkiv Zool* 1961;13:203.
605. Glydon RSJ. The development of the blood supply of the pituitary in the albino rat, with special reference to the portal vessels. *J Anat* 1957;91:237.
606. Ugrumov MV, Ivanova IP, Mitskevich MS. Light- and electron-microscopic study on the maturation of the primary portal plexus during the perinatal period in rats. *Cell Tissue Res* 1983;234:179.
607. Campbell HJ. The development of the primary portal plexus in the median eminence of the rabbit. *J Anat* 1966;100:381.
608. Landsmeer JME. Vessels of the rat's hypophysis. *Acta Anat* 1951;12:82.
609. McConnell EM. The arterial blood supply of the human hypophysis cerebri. *Anat Rec* 1953;115:175.
610. Bergland RM, Page RB. Can the pituitary secrete directly to the brain? (Affirmative anatomical evidence). *Endocrinology* 1978;102:1325.
611. Björklund A. Monamine-containing fibers in the neurointermediate lobe of the pig and rat. *Z Zellforsch* 1968;89: 573.
612. Page RB, Dovey-Hartman BJ. Resistance vessels in the tuber cinereum of the rabbit, rat and cat. *Anat Rec* 1984;210:647.
613. Ceccatelli S, Fahrenkrug J, Villar M, Hökfelt T. Vasoactive intestinal polypeptide/peptide histidine isoleucine immunoreactive neuron systems in the basal hypothalamus of the rat with special reference to the portal vasculature: an immunohistochemical an in situ hybridization study. *Neuroscience* 1991;43:483.
614. Duvernoy H, Koritke JG, Monnier G. Sur la vascularisation du tuber posterieur chez l'homme et sur les relations vasculaires tubero-hypophysaires. *J Neuro-Visc Relations* 1971;32:112.
615. Ambach G, Palkovits M, Szentagothai J. Blood supply of the rat hypothalamus. IV. Retrochiasmatic area, median eminence, arcuate nucleus. *Acta Morphol Acad Sci Hung* 1976;24:93.
616. Green HT. The venous drainage of the human hypophysis cerebri. *Am J Anat* 1957;100:435.
617. Torok B. Lebendbeobachtung des hypophysenkreis-laufes an hunden. *Acta Morphol Acad Sci Hung* 1954;4:83.
618. Torok B. Structure of the vascular connections of the hypothalamo-hypophyseal region. *Acta Anat* 1964;59:84.
619. Houssay BA, Biasotti A, Sammartino R. Modifications fonctionnelles de l'hypophyse apres les lesions infundibulotuberiennes chez le crapaud. *CR Soc Biol* 1935;120:725.
620. Barnett RJ, Greep RO. The direction of blood flow in the blood vessels of the infundibular stalk. *Science* 1951;113:185.
621. Worthington WC. Some observations on the hypophyseal portal system in the living mouse. *Bull Johns Hopkins Hosp* 1955;97:343.
622. Worthington WC. Vascular responses in the pituitary stalk. *Endocrinology* 1960;66:19.
623. Page RB. Directional pituitary blood flow: a microcinephotographic study. *Endocrinology* 1983;112:157.
624. Duvernoy H. The vascular architecture of the median eminence. In: Knigge KM, Scott DE, Weindl A, eds. *Brain-endocrine interaction. Median eminence: structure and function.* Basel: Karger, 1972:79.
625. Lametschwandtner A, Simonsberger P. Light and scanning electron microscopical studies of the hypothalamo-adenohypophysial portal vessels of the toad *Bufo bufo* (L). *Cell Tissue Res* 1975;162:131.
626. Page RB. Pituitary blood flow. *Am J Physiol* 1982;243:E427.
627. Baez S. Skeletal muscle and gastrointestinal microvascular morphology. In: Kalsz G, Altura B, eds. *Microcirculation,* Vol. 1. Baltimore: University Park Press, 1977:69.
628. Sobin SS, Tremer HM. Three-dimensional organization of microvascular beds as related to function. In: Kalsz G, Altura B, eds. *Microcirculation,* Vol. 1. Baltimore: University Park Press, 1977:43.
629. Sobin SS, Tremer HM, Fung YC. The morphometric basis of the sheet-flow concept of the pulmonary alveolar microcirculation in the cat. *Circ Res* 1970;26:397.
630. Wittkowski W, Scheuer A. Functional changes of the neuronal and glial elements at the surface of the external layer of the median eminence. *Z Anat Entwickl-Gesch* 1974;143:255.
631. Duvernoy H. Considerations sur la vascularisation de l'hypophyse. *Acta Neurol Belg* 1969;69:469.
632. Duvernoy H, Koritke JG. Contribution de l'etude de l'angioarchitectonie des organes circumventriculaiers. *Arch Biol Suppl* 1964;75:849.
633. Duvernoy H, Koritke JG. Les vaisseaux sous-ependymaires due recessus hypophysaire. *J Hirnforsch* 1968;10:227.
634. Redecker P. Ultrastructural demonstration of neurohemal contacts in the internal zone of the median eminence of the mongolian gerbil (*Meriones unguiculatus*): correlation with synaptophysin immunohistochemistry. *Histochemistry* 1991;95:503.
635. Reymond MJ, Speciale SG, Porter JC. Dopamine in plasma of lateral and medial hypophysial portal vessels: evidence for regional variation in the release of hypothalamic dopamine into hypophysial portal blood. *Endocrinology* 1983;112:1958.
636. Murakami T, Kikuta A, Taguchi T, Ohtsuka A, Ohtani O. Blood vascular architecture of the rat cerebral hypophysis and hypothalamus. A dissection/scanning electron microscopy of vascular casts. *Arch Histol Jpn* 1987;50:133.
637. Akmayev IG. Morphological aspects of the hypothalamic-hypophyseal system II. Functional morphology of pituitary microcirculation. *Z Zellforsch* 1971;116:178.
638. Akmayev IG. Morphological aspects of the hypothalamic-hypophyseal system. III. Vascularity of the hypothalamus, with special reference to its quantitative aspects. *Z Zellforsch* 1971;116:195.
639. Shaver SW, Pang JJ, Wainman DS, Wall KW, Gross PM. Morphology and function of capillary networks in subregions of the rat tuber cinereum. *Cell Tissue Res* 1992;267:437.
640. Mezey E, Palkovits M, deKloet ER, Verhoef J, deWied D. Evidence for pituitary-brain transport of a behaviorally potent ACTH analog. *Life Sci* 1978;22:831.
641. Mezey E, Palkovits M. Two way transport in the hypothalamo-hypophysial system. In: Ganong WF, Martini L, eds. *Frontiers in Neuroendocrinology,* Vol. 7. New York: Raven Press, 1982:1.
642. Dorsa DM, deKloet ER, Mezey E, deWied D. Pituitary-brain transport of neurotensin: functional significance of retrograde transport. *Endocrinology* 1979;104:1663.
643. Gibbs DM. Hypothalamic epinephrine is released into hypophysial portal blood during stress. *Brain Res* 1985;335:360.
644. Felten DL, Cashner KA. Cytoarchitecture of the supraoptic nucleus. A Golgi study. *Neuroendocrinology* 1979;29:221.
645. Fisher AWF, Price PG, Burford GD, Lederis K. A 3-dimensional reconstruction of the hypothalamo-neurohypophysial system of the rat. The neurons projecting to the neurointermediate lobe and those containing vasopressin and somatostatin. *Cell Tissue Res* 1979;204:343.
646. LuQui IJ, Fox CA. The supraoptic nucleus and the supraoptico-hypophysial tract in the monkey (*Macaca mulatta*). *J Comp Neurol* 1976;168:7.
647. Sofroniew MV, Glasmann W. Golgi-like immunoperoxidase staining of hypothalamic magnocellular neurons that contain vasopressin, oxytocin or neurophysin in the rat. *Neuroscience* 1981;6:619.
648. Dyball REJ, Howard M, Kemplay SK. A Golgi study of the neurosecretory neurons in the supraoptic nucleus of the rat. *J Anat* 1979;128:417.
649. Renaud LP. Neurophysiological organization of the endocrine hypothalamus. In: Reichlin S, Baldessarini RJ, Martin JB, eds. *The Hypothalamus.* New York: Raven Press, 1978:269.
650. DeMey J, Vandesande F, Dierickx K. Identification of neuro-

physin producing cells. II. Identification of the neurophysin I and the neurophysin II producing neurons in the bovine hypothalamus. *Cell Tissue Res* 1974;153:531.
651. Dierickx K, Vandesande F. Immunocytochemical demonstration of separate vasopressin-neurophysin and oxytocin-neurophysin neurons in the human hypothalamus. *Cell Tissue Res* 1979;196:203.
652. Kawata M, Sano Y. Immunohistochemical identification of the oxytocin and vasopressin neurons in the hypothalamus of the monkey (*Macaca fuscata*). *Anat Embryol* 1982;165:151.
653. Sloper JC, Bateson RG. Ultrastructure of neurosecretory cells in the supraoptic nucleus of the dog and rat. *J Endocrinol* 1965;31:139.
654. Flament-Durand J. Ultrastructural aspects of the paraventricular nuclei in the rat. *Z Zellforsch* 1971;116:61.
655. Morris JF, Dyball REJ. A quantitative study of the ultrastructural changes in the hypothalamo-neurohypophysial system during and after experimentally induced hypersecretion. *Cell Tissue Res* 1974;149:525.
656. Kalimo H. Ultrastructural studies on the hypothalamic neurosecretory neurones of the rat. I. The paraventricular neurones of the non-treated rat. *Z Zellforsch* 1971;122:283.
657. Tweedle CD, Hatton GI. Ultrastructure comparisons of neurons of supraoptic and circularis nuclei in normal and dehydrated rats. *Brain Res Bull* 1976;1:103.
658. Piekut DT. Ultrastructural characteristics of peptidergic neurons using pre-embedding immunocytochemical methods. *Am J Anat* 1986;175:197.
659. Castel M, Morris JF, Whitnall MH, Sivan N. Improved visualization of the immunoreactive hypothalamo-hypophysial system by use of immuno-gold techniques. *Cell Tissue Res* 1986;243:193.
660. Guitteny A-F, Bloch B. Ultrastructural detection of the vasopressin messenger RNA in normal and Brattleboro rat. *Histochemistry* 1989;92:277.
661. Trembleau A, Calas A, Fevere-Montagne M. Ultrastructural localization of oxytocin mRNA in the rat hypothalamus by in situ hybridization using a synthetic oligonucleotide. *Mol Brain Res* 1990;8:37.
662. Kiyama H, Emson PC. Evidence for the co-expression of oxytocin and vasopressin messenger ribonucleic acids in magnocellular neurosecretory cells: simultaneous demonstration of two neurophysin messenger ribonucleic acids by hybridization histochemistry. *J Neuroendocrinol* 1990;2:257.
663. Nishioka RS, Zambrano D, Bern HA. Electron microscope radioautography of amino acid incorporation by supraoptic neurons of the rat. *Gen Comp Endocrinol* 1970;15:477.
664. Broadwell RD, Oliver C, Brightman MW. Localization of neurophysin within organelles associated with protein synthesis and packaging in the hypothalamo-neurohypophysial system: an immunocytochemical study. *Proc Natl Acad Sci USA* 1979;76:5999.
665. Kozlowski GP, Frenk S, Brownfield MS. Localization of neurophysin in the rat supraoptic nucleus. I. Ultrastructural immunocytochemistry using the post-embedding technique. *Cell Tissue Res* 1977;179:467.
666. Piekut DT. Ultrastructural characteristics of vasopressin-containing neurons in the paraventricular nucleus of the hypothalamus. *Cell Tissue Res* 1983;234:125.
667. Lu C-L, Cantin M, Seidah NG, Chretien M. Distribution pattern in the human pituitary and hypothalamus of a new neuropeptide: the C-terminal glycoprotein-fragment of human pro-pressophysin (CPP). *Histochemistry* 1982;75:319.
668. Pickering BT, Swann RW, Birkett SD, O'Shaughnessy P, Wathes DC, Porter DG. Precursors and products in the formation of neurohypophysial hormones. In: Labrie F, Proulx L, eds. *Endocrinology.* New York: Elsevier, 1984:653.
669. Kalimo H. Ultrastructural studies on the hypothalamic neurons of the rat. III. Paraventricular and supraoptic neurons during lactation and dehydration. *Cell Tissue Res* 1975;163:151.
670. Broadwell RD, Oliver C. Golgi apparatus, GERL, and secretory granule formation within neurons of the hypothalamo-neurohypophysial system of control and hyperosmotically stressed mice. *J Cell Biol* 1981;90:474.
671. Krisch B. Electronmicroscopic immunocytochemical study on the vasopressin-containing neurons of the thirsting rat. *Cell Tissue Res* 1977;184:237.
672. Krisch B. Indication for a granule-free form of vasopressin in immobilization-stressed rats. *Cell Tissue Res* 1979;197:95.
673. Kozlowski GP. Comparative ultrastructure of neuropeptide-containing cells of the parvo- and magnocellular neurosecretory system. In: Sano Y, Ibata Y, Zimmerman EA, eds. *Structure and function of peptidergic and aminergic neurons.* Tokyo: Japan Scientific Society Press, 1983:73.
674. Alonso G, Assenmacher I. The smooth endoplasmic reticulum in neurohypophysial axons of the rat: possible involvement in transport, storage and release of neurosecretory material. *Cell Tissue Res* 1979;199:415.
675. Broadwell RD, Brightman MW. Cytochemistry of undamaged neurons transporting exogenous protein in vivo. *J Comp Neurol* 1979;185:31.
676. Gregory WA, Tweedle CD, Hatton GI. Ultrastructure of neurons in the paraventricular nucleus of normal, dehydrated and rehydrated rats. *Brain Res Bull* 1979;5:301.
677. Tweedle CD, Hatton GI. Ultrastructural changes in rat hypothalamic neurosecretory cells and their associated glia during minimal dehydration and rehydration. *Cell Tissue Res* 1977;181:59.
678. Wakerley JB, Poulain DA, Brown D. Comparison of firing patterns in oxytocin- and vasopressin-releasing neurones during progressive dehydration. *Brain Res* 1978;148:425.
679. Meeker RB, Greenwood RS, Hayward JN. Vasopressin mRNA expression in individual magnocellular neuroendocine cells of the supraoptic and paraventricular nucleus in response to water deprivation. *Neuroendocrinology* 1991;54:236.
680. Epstein Y, Castel M, Glick SM, Sivan N, Ravid R. Changes in hypothalamic and extrahypothalamic vasopressin content of water-deprived rats. *Cell Tissue Res* 1983;233:99.
681. Watson SJ, Akil H, Fischli W, Goldstein A, Zimmerman E, Nilaver G, Greidanus TBVW. Dynorphin and vasopressin: common localization in magnocellular neurons. *Science* 1982;216:85.
682. Whitnall MH, Gainer H, Cox BM, Molineaux CI. Dynorphin-A-(1-8) is contained within vasopressin neurosecretory vesicles in the rat pituitary. *Science* 1983;222:1137.
683. Millan MH, Millan MJ, Herz A. The hypothalamic paraventricular nucleus: relationship to brain and pituitary pools of vasopressin and oxytocin as compared to dynorphin, β-endorphin and related opioid peptides in the rat. *Neuroendocrinology* 1984;38:108.
684. Meister B, Villar MJ, Ceccatelli S, Hökfelt T. Localization of chemical messengers in magnocellular neurons of the hypothalamic supraoptic and paraventricular nuclei: an immunohistochemical study using experimental manipulations. *Neuroscience* 1990;37:603.
685. Burlet A, Tonon M-C, Tankosic P, Coy D, Vaudry H. Comparative immunocytochemical localization of corticotropin releasing factor (CRF-41) and neurohypophysial peptides in the brain of Brattleboro and Long-Evans rates. *Neuroendocrinology* 1983;37:64.
686. Brownstein MJ, Mezey W. Multiple chemical messengers in hypothalamic magnocellular neurons. *Prog Brain Res* 1986;68:161.
687. Bredt DS, Hwang PM, Snyder SH. Localization of nitric oxide synthase indicating a neural role for nitric oxide. *Nature* 1990;347:768.
688. Arevalo R, Sanchez F, Alonso JR, Carretero J, Vazquez R, Aijon J. NADPH-diaphorase activity in the hypothalamic magnocellular neurosecretory nuclei of the rat. *Brain Res Bull* 1992;28:599.
689. Pow D. NADPH-diaphorase (nitric oxide synthase) staining in the rat supraoptic nucleus is activity dependent: possible functional indications. *J Neuroendocrinol* 1992;4:377.
690. Gross JH, Knigge KM, Sheridan MN. Fine structure of neurons of the arcuate nucleus and median eminence of the hypothala-

mus of the golden hamster following immobilization. *Cell Tissue Res* 1976;168:385.
691. Brawer JR. The role of the arcuate nucleus in the brain-pituitary-gonad axis. *J Comp Neurol* 1971;143:411.
692. Bugnon C, Bloch B, Lenys D. Ultrastructural study of presumptive pro-opiocortin producing neurons in the rat hypothalamus. *Neuroscience* 1981;6:1299.
693. Lamberts R, Goldsmith PC. Preembedding colloidal gold immunostaining of hypothalamic neurons: light and electron microscopic localization of β-endorphin-immunoreactive perikarya. *J Histochem Cytochem* 1985;33:499.
694. Price MT, Olney JW, Cicero TJ. Proliferation of lamellar whorls in arcuate neurons of the hypothalamus of castrated and morphine-treated male rats. *Cell Tissue Res* 1976;171:277.
695. King JC, Williams TH, Gerall AA. Transformations of hypothalamic arcuate neurons. I. Changes associated with stages of the estrous cycle. *Cell Tissue Res* 1974;153:497.
696. Garcia-Segura LM, Hernandez P, Tranque PA, Naftolin F. Neuronal membrane remodelling during the oestrus cycle: a freeze-fracture study in the arcuate nucleus of the rat hypothalamus. *J Neurocytol* 1988;17:377.
697. Liposits Z. Ultrastructural immunocytochemistry of the hypothalamic corticotropin releasing hormone synthesizing system. *Prog Histochem Cytochem* 1990;21:1.
698. Liposits Z, Paull WK. Ultrastructural alterations of the paraventriculo-infundibular corticotropin releasing factor (CRF)-immunoreactive neuronal system in long term adrenalectomized rats. *Peptides* 1985;6:1021.
699. Beauvillain JC, Tramu G, Mazzuca M. Fine structural studies of growth-hormone-releasing-factor (GRF)-immunoreactive neurons and their synaptic connections in the guinea pig arcuate nucleus. *J Comp Neurol* 1987;255:110.
700. Ibata Y, Okamura H, Makino S, Kawakami F, Morimote N, Chihara K. Light and electron microscopic immunocytochemistry of GRF-like immunoreactive neurons and terminals in the rat hypothalamic arcuate nucleus and median eminence. *Brain Res* 1986;370:146.
701. Lehman MN, Silverman A-J, Witkin JW, Millar RP. Ultrastructure of luteinizing hormone-releasing hormone (LHRH) neurons and their projections in the golden hamster. *Brain Res Bull* 1990;20:211.
702. Silverman A-J, Witkin JW, Millar RP. Light and electron microscopic immunocytochemical analysis of antibodies directed against GNRH and its precursor in hypothalamic neurons. *J Histochem Cytochem* 1990;38:803.
703. Jennes L, Stumpf WE, Sheedy ME. Ultrastructural characterization of gonadotropin-releasing hormone (GnRH)-producing neurons. *J Comp Neurol* 1985;232:534.
704. Witkin JW, Silverman AJ. Ultrastructure and synaptology of LHRH neurons in rat medial preoptic area. *Peptides* 1985;6:263.
705. Crosby EC, Showers MJC. Comparative anatomy of the preoptic and hypothalamic areas. In: Haymaker W, Anderson E, Nauta WJH, eds. *The Hypothalamus.* Springfield, IL: C. C. Thomas, 1969:61.
706. Nauta WJH, Haymaker W. Hypothalamic nuclei and fiber connections. In: Haymaker W, Anderson E, Nauta WJH, eds. *The Hypothalamus.* Springfield, IL: C. C. Thomas, 1969:136.
707. Papez JW. The embryologic development of the hypothalamic area in mammals. *Proc Assoc Res Nerv Ment Dis* 1940;20:31.
708. Christ JF. Derivation and boundaries of the hypothalamus with atlas of hypothalamic grisea. In: Haymaker W, Anderson E, Nauta WJH, eds. *The Hypothalamus.* Springfield, IL: C.C. Thomas, 1969:13.
709. Coggeshall RE. A study of diencephalic development in the albino rat. *J Comp Neurol* 1964;122:241.
710. Hyyppa M. Differentiation of the hypothalamic nuclei during ontogenetic development in the rat. *Z Anat Entwickl-Gesch* 1969;129:41.
711. Altman J, Bayer SA. Development of the diencephalon in the rat. I. Autoradiographic study of the time of origin and settling patterns of neurons of the hypothalamus. *J Comp Neurol* 1978;182:945.
712. Altman J, Bayer SA. Development of the diencephalon in the rat. II. Correlation of the embryonic development of the hypothalamus with the time of origin of its neurons. *J Comp Neurol* 1978;182:973.
713. Choy VJ, Watkins WB. Maturation of the hypothalamo-neurohypophysial system. I. Localization of neurophysin, oxytocin and vasopressin in the hypothalamus and neural lobe of the developing rat brain. *Cell Tissue Res* 1979;197:325.
714. Karim MA, Sloper JC. Histogenesis of the supraoptic and paraventricular neurosecretory cells of the mouse hypothalamus. *J Anat* 1980;130:341.
715. Okamura H, Fukui K, Koyama E, et al. Time of vasopressin neuron origin in the mouse hypothalamus: examination by combined technique of immunocytochemistry and (^{3}H)-thymidine autoradiography. *Dev Brain Res* 1983;9:223.
716. Wyss JM, Sripanidkulchai B. An autoradiographic analysis of the time of origin of neurons in the hypothalamus of the cat. *Dev Brain Res* 1985;21:89.
717. Rodier PM, Kates WA, Phelps CJ. Birthdates of the growth hormone releasing factor cells of the rat hypothalamus: an autoradiographic study of immunocytochemically identified neurons. *J Comp Neurol* 1990;291:363.
718. Grino M, Young WAS, Burgunder J-M. Ontogeny of expression of the corticotropin-releasing factor gene in the hypothalamic paraventricular nucleus and of the proopiomelanocortin gene in rat pituitary. *Endocrinology* 1989;124:60.
719. Schwanzel-Fukuda M, Morrell JI, Pfaff DW. Ontogenesis of neurons producing luteinizing hormone-releasing hormone (LHRH) in the nervus terminalis of the rat. *J Comp Neurol* 1985;238:348.
720. Setalo G, Hagino N, Dittrich E. Ontogenesis of the GnRh neuron system in the rat. A quantitative immunohistochemical study with special reference to the extra cerebral GnRH-positive cells and the occupation of intracerebral termination fields. *Neuropeptides* 1992;21:93.
721. Schwanzel-Fekuda M, Pfaff DW. Origins of luteinizing hormone-releasing hormone neurons. *Nature* 1989;338:161.
722. Wray S, Grant PH, Gainer H. Evidence that cells expressing luteinizing hormone-releasing hormone mRNA are derived from progenitor cells in the olfactory placode. *Proc Soc Natl Acad Sci USA* 1989;86:8132.
723. Krisch B. Electron microscopic immunocytochemical investigation on the postnatal development of the vasopressin system in the rat. *Cell Tissue Res* 1980;205:453.
724. Koritsanszky S. Cyto- and synaptogenesis in the arcuate nucleus of the rat hypothalamus during fetal and early postnatal life. *Cell Tissue Res* 1979;200:135.
725. Dale H. Pharmacology and nerve-endings. *Proc R Soc Med* 1935;28:319.
726. Broadwell RD, Bleier R. A cytoarchitectonic atlas of the mouse hypothalamus. *J Comp Neurol* 1976;167:315.
727. Peterson RP. Magnocellular neurosecretory centers in the rat hypothalamus. *J Comp Neurol* 1966;128:181.
728. Rhodes CH, Morrell JI, Pfaff DW. Immunohistochemical analysis of magnocellular elements in rat hypothalamus: distribution and numbers of cells containing neurophysin, oxytocin and vasopressin. *J Comp Neurol* 1981;198:45.
729. Swaab DF, Nijveldt F, Pool CW. Distribution of oxytocin and vasopressin the rat supraoptic and paraventricular nucleus. *J Endocrinol* 1975;67:461.
730. Warembourg M, Poulain P. Presence of estrogen receptor immunoreactivity in the oxytocin-containing magnocellular neurons projecting to the neurohypophysis in the guinea pig. *Neuroscience* 1991;40:41.
731. Ingram WR. Nuclear organization and chief connections of the primate hypothalamus. *Proc Assoc Res Nerv Ment Dis* 1940;20:195.
732. Defendini R, Zimmerman EA. The magnocellular neurosecretory system of the mammalian hypothalamus. In: Reichlin S, Baldessarini RJ, Martin JB, eds. *The Hypothalamus.* New York: Raven Press, 1978:137.
733. Marzban F, Tweedle CD, Hatton GI. Reevaluation of the plasticity in the rat supraoptic nucleus after chronic dehydration using

immunogold for oxytocin and vasopressin at the ultrastructural level. *Brain Res Bull* 1992;28:756.
734. Chapman DB, Theodosis DT, Montagnese C, Poulain DA, Morris JF. Osmotic stimulation causes structural plasticity of neurone-glia relationships of the oxytocin but not vasopressin secreting neurones in the hypothalamic supraoptic nucleus. *Neuroscience* 1986;17:679.
735. Theodosis DT, Chapman DM, Montagnese C, Poulain DA, Morris JF. Structural plasticity in the hypothalamic supraoptic nucleus at lactation affects oxytocin- but not vasopressin-secreting neurons. *Neuroscience* 1986;17:661.
736. Theodosis DT, Paut L, Tappaz ML. Immunocytochemical analysis of the gabaergic innervation of oxytocin- and vasopressin-secreting neurons in the rat supraoptic nucleus. *Neuroscience* 1986;19:165.
737. Montagnese C, Poulain DA, Vincent J-D, Theodosis DT. Synaptic and neuronal-glial plasticity in the adult oxytocinergic system in response to physiological stimuli. *Brain Res Bull* 1988;20:681.
738. Blanco E, Pilgrim C, Vazquez R, Jirikowski GF. Plasticity of the interface between oxytocin neurons and the vasculature in late pregnant rats: an ultrastructural morphometric study. *Acta Histochem* 1991;91:165.
739. Ray PK, Choudry SR. Vasopressinergic axon collaterals and axon terminals in magnocellular neurosecretory nuclei of the rat hypothalamus. *Acta Anat* 1990;137:37.
740. Choudhury SR, Ray PK. Ultrastructural features of presumptive vasopressinergic synapses in the hypothalamic magnocellular secretory nuclei of the rat. *Acta Anat* 1990;137:252.
741. Theodosis DT. Oxytocin-immunoreactive terminals synapse on oxytocin neurons in the supraoptic neurons. *Nature* 1985; 313:682.
742. Van Den Pol AN. Dual ultrastructural localization of two neurotransmitter-related antigens: Colloidal gold-labeled neurophysin-immunoreactive supraoptic neurons receive peroxidase-labeled glutamate decarboxylase- or golf-labeled GABA-immunoreactive synapses. *Neuroscience* 1985;5:2940.
743. Van Den Pol AN. Glutamate and aspartate immunoreactivity in hypothalamic presynaptic neurons. *J Neurosci* 1991;11:2087.
744. Shioda S, Nakai Y, Kitazawa S, Sunayama H. Immunochemical observation of corticotropin-releasing factor containing neurons in the rat hypothalamus with special reference to neuronal communication. *Acta Anat* 1985;124:56.
745. Goldsmith PC, Boggan JE, Thind KK. Opioid synapses on vasopressin neurons in the paraventricular and supraoptic nuclei of juvenile monkeys. *Neuroscience* 1991;45:709.
746. Rasmussen AT. Effects of hypophysectomy and hypophysial stalk resection on the hypothalamic nuclei of animals and man. *Proc Assoc Res Nerv Ment Dis* 1940;20:245.
747. Raisman G. An ultrastructural study of the effects of hypophysectomy on the supraoptic nucleus of the rat. *J Comp Neurol* 1973;147:181.
748. Sherlock DA, Field PM, Raisman G. Retrograde transport of horse-radish peroxidase in the magnocellular neurosecretory system of the rat. *Brain Res* 1975;88:403.
749. Price P, Fisher AWF. Electron microscopical study of retrograde transport of horseradish peroxidase in the supraoptico-hypophyseal tract in the rat. *J Anat* 1978;125:137.
750. DeVries GJ, Buijs RM, VanLeeuwen FW, Caffe AR, Swaab DF. The vasopressinergic innervation of the brain in normal and castrated rats. *J Comp Neurol* 1985;233:236.
751. Simpson JB. The circumventricular organs and the central actions of angiotensin. *Neuroendocrinology* 1981;32:248.
752. Brownfield MS, Kozlowski GP. The hypothalamo-choroidal tract. I. Immunohistochemical demonstration of neurophysin pathways to telencephalic choroid plexuses and cerebrospinal fluid. *Cell Tissue Res* 1977;178:111.
753. Mahoney PD, Koh ET, Irvin RW, Ferris CF. Computer-aided mapping of vasopressin neurons in the hypothalamus of the male golden hamster: evidence of magnocellular neurons that do not project to the hypothalamus. *J Neuroendocrinology* 1990;2:113.
754. Swanson LW, Kuypers HGJM. The paraventricular nucleus of the hypothalamus: cytoarchitectonic subdivisions and organization of projections to the pituitary, dorsal vagal complex, and spinal cord as demonstrated by retrograde fluorescence double-labeling methods. *J Comp Neurol* 1980;194:555.
755. Wiegand SJ, Price JL. Cells of origin of the afferent fibers to the median eminence in the rat. *J Comp Neurol* 1980;192:1.
756. Krieg WJS. The hypothalamus of the albino rat. *J Comp Neurol* 1932;55:19.
757. Van Den Pol AN. The magnocellular and parvocellular paraventricular nucleus of rat: intrinsic organization. *J Comp Neurol* 1982;206:317.
758. Armstrong WE, Warach S, Hatton GI, McNeill TH. Subnuclei in the rat hypothalamic paraventricular nucleus: a cytoarchitectural, horseradish peroxidase and immunocytochemical analysis. *Neuroscience* 1980;5:1931.
759. Hatton GI, Hutton UE, Hoblitzell ER, Armstrong WE. Morphological evidence for two populations of magnocellular elements in the rat paraventricular nucleus. *Brain Res* 1976;108:187.
760. Sawchenko PE, Swanson LW. Immunohistochemical identification of neurons in the paraventricular nucleus of the hypothalamus that project to the medulla or to the spinal cord in rat. *J Comp Neurol* 1982;205:260.
761. Theodosis DT, Poulain DA. Neuronal-glial and synaptic plasticity in the adult rat paraventricular nucleus. *Brain Res* 1989;484:361.
762. Silverman AJ, Hou-Yu A, Oldfield BJ. Ultrastructural identification of noradrenergic nerve terminals and vasopressin-containing neurons of the paraventricular nucleus in the same thin section. *J Histochem Cytochem* 1983;31:1151.
763. Ochiai H, Nakai Y. Ultrastructural demonstration of dopamine-beta-hydroxylase immunoreactive nerve terminals on vasopressin neurons in the paraventricular nucleus of the rat by double-labeling immunocytochemistry. *Neurosci Lett* 1990;120:87.
764. Iwai C, Ochiai H, Nakai Y. Electron-microscopic immunocytochemistry of neuropeptide Y immunoreactive innervation of vasopressin neurons in the paraventricular nucleus of the rat hypothalamus. *Acta Anat* 1989;136:279.
765. Kagotani Y, Tsuruo Y, Hisano S, Daikoku S, Chihara K. Synaptic regulation of paraventricular arginine vasopressin-containing neurons by neuropeptide Y-containing monoaminergic neurons in rats, electron microscopic triple labeling. *Cell Tissue Res* 1989;257:269.
766. Liposits ZS, Phelix C, Paull WK. Electron microscopic analysis of tyrosine hydroxylase dopamine-B-hydroxylase and phenylethanolamine-*N*-methyl-transferase immunoreactive innervation of the hypothalamic paraventricular nucleus in the rat. *Histochemistry* 1986;84:105.
767. Decavel C, Dubourg P, Leon-Henri B, Geffard M, Calas A. Simultaneous immunogold labeling of gabaergic terminals and vasopressin-containing neurons in the rat peraventricular nucleus. *Cell Tissue Res* 1989;255:77.
768. Taniguchi Y, Yoshida M, Ishikawa K, Suzuki M, Kurosumi K. The distribution of vasopressin- or oxytoxin-neurons projecting to the posterior pituitary as revealed by a combination of retrograde transport of horseradish peroxidase and immunohistochemistry. *Arch Histol Cytol* 1988;51:83.
769. Kiss JZ, Martos J, Palkovits M. Hypothalamic paraventricular nucleus: a quantitative analysis of cytoarchitectonic subdivisions in the rat. *J Comp Neurol* 1991;313:563.
770. Swanson LW, Sawchenko PE. Hypothalamic integration: organization of the paraventricular and supraoptic nuclei. *Annu Rev Neurosci* 1983;6:269.
771. Antunes JL, Carmel PW, Zimmerman EA. Projections from the paraventricular nucleus to the zona externa of the median eminence of the rhesus monkey: an immunohistochemical study. *Brain Res* 1977;137:1.
772. Vandesande F, Dierickx K, DeMey J. The origin of the vasopressinergic and oxytocinergic fibres of the external region of the median eminence of the rat hypophysis. *Cell Tissue Res* 1977;180:443.
773. Silverman AJ, Hoffman D, Gadde CA, Krey LC, Zimmerman EA. Adrenal steroid inhibition of the vasopressin-neurphysin

neurosecretory system to the median eminence of the rat. *Neuroendocrinology* 1981;32:129.
774. Silverman AJ, Zimmerman EA. Adrenalectomy increases sprouting in a peptidergic neurosecretory system. *Neuroscience* 1982;7:2705.
775. Rivier C, Vale W. Interaction of corticotropin-releasing factor and arginine vasopressin on adrenocorticotropin secretion in vivo. *Endocrinology* 1983;113:939.
776. Lechan RM, Nestler JL, Jacobson S, Reichlin S. The hypothalamic "tuberoinfundibular" system of the rat as demonstrated by horseradish peroxidase (HRP) microiontophoresis. *Brain Res* 1980;195:13.
777. Lechan RM, Nestler JL, Jacobson S. The tuberoinfundibular system of the rat as demonstrated by immunohistochemical localization of retrogradely transported wheat germ agglutinin (WGA) from the median eminence. *Brain Res* 1982;245:1.
778. Zimmerman EA, Hou-Yu A, Nilaver G, Valiquette G, Silverman A-J. Organization of the oxytocin and vasopressin systems of the hypothalamus: intra- and extra-hypothalamic projections. In: Sano Y, Ibata Y, Zimmerman EA, eds. *Structure and function of peptidergic and aminergic neurons.* Tokyo: Japan Scientific Society Press, 1983:1.
779. Armstrong WE, Hatton GI. The localization of projection neurons in the rat hypothalamic paraventricular nucleus following vascular and neurohypophysial injections of HRP. *Brain Res Bull* 1980;5:473.
780. Dierickx K, Vandesande F. Immunocytochemical localization of somatostatin-containing neurons in the rat hypothalamus. *Cell Tissue Res* 1979;201:349.
781. Krisch B. Hypothalamic and extrahypothalamic distribution of somatostatin immunoreactive elements in the rat brain. *Cell Tissue Res* 1978;195:499.
782. Elde RP, Parsons JA. Immunocytochemical localization of somatostatin in cell bodies of the rat hypothalamus. *Am J Anat* 1975;144:541.
783. Bennett-Clarke C, Romagnano MA, Joseph SA. Distribution of somatostatin in the rat brain: telencephalon and diencephalon. *Brain Res* 1980;188:473.
784. Jackson IMD, Wu P, Lechan RM. Immunohistochemical localization in the rat brain of the precursor for thyrotropin-releasing hormone. *Science* 1985;229:1097.
785. Lechan RM, Wu P, Jackson I, et al. Thyrotropin-releasing hormone precursor: characterization in rat brain. *Science* 1986;231:159.
786. Paull WK, Scholer J, Arimura A, et al. Immunocytochemical localization of CRF in the ovine hypothalamus. *Peptides* 1982;1:183.
787. Kolodziejczyk E, Baertschi AJ, Tramu G. Corticoliberin-immunoreactive cell bodies localised in two distinct areas of the sheep hypothalamus. *Neuroscience* 1983;9:261.
788. Merchenthaler I, Vigh S, Petrusz P, Schally AV. Immunocytochemical localization of corticotropin-releasing factor (CRF) in the rat brain. *Am J Anat* 1982;165:385.
789. Joseph SA, Knigge KM. Corticotropin releasing factor: immunocytochemical localization in rat brain. *Neurosci Lett* 1983;35:135.
790. Tilders FJH, Schipper J, Lowry PJ, Vermes I. Effect of hypothalamus lesions on the presence of CRF-immunoreactive nerve terminals in the median eminence and on the pituitary-adrenal response to stress. *Regul Peptides* 1982;5:77.
791. Paull WK, Gibbs FP. The corticotropin releasing factor (CRF) neurosecretory system in intact, adrenalectomized, adrenalectomized-dexamethasone treated rats. *Histochemistry* 1983;78:303.
792. Silverman A-J, Hou-Yu A, Chen W-P. Corticotropin-releasing factor synapses within the paraventricular nucleus of the hypothalamus. *Neuroendocrinology* 1989;49:291.
793. Liposits ZS, Uht RM, Harrison RW, Gibbs FP, Paull WK, Bohn MC. Ultrastructural localization of glucocorticoid receptor (GR) in hypothalamic paraventricular neurons synthesizing corticotropin releasing factor (CRF). *Histochemistry* 1987; 87:407.
794. Kawano H, Daikoku S, Shibasaki T. CRF-containing neuron systems in the rat hypothalamus: retrograde tracing and immunohistochemical studies. *J Comp Neurol* 1988;272:260.
795. Kawano H, Tsuruo Y, Gando H, Daikoku S. Hypophysiotropic TRH-producing neurons identified by combining immunohistochemistry for pro-TRH and retrograde tracing. *J Comp Neurol* 1991;307:531.
796. Kiss JZ, Mezey E, Skirboll L. Corticotropin-releasing factor-immunoreactive neurons of the paraventricular nucleus become vasopressin positive after adrenalectomy. *Proc Natl Acad Sci USA* 1984;81:1854.
797. Sawchencko PE, Swanson LW, Vale WW. Corticotropin-releasing factor: coexpression within distinct subsets of oxytocin-, vasopressin-, and neurotensin-immunoreactive neurons in the hypothalamus of the male rat. *J Neurosci* 1984;4:1118.
798. Sawchenko PE, Swanson LW, Vale WW. Coexpression of corticotropin releasing factor and vasopressin immunoreactivity in parvocellular neurosecretory neurons of the adrenalectomized rat. *Proc Natl Acad Sci USA* 1984;81:1883.
799. Lind RW, Swanson LW, Chin DA, Bruhn TO, Ganten D. Angiotensin II: An immunohistochemical study of its distribution in the paraventriculo-hypophysial system and its colocalization with vasopressin and CRF in parvocellular neurons. *Neurosci Abstr* 1984;10:88.
800. Mezey E, Reisine TD, Skirboll L, Beinfield M, Kiss JZ. Role of cholecystokinin in corticotropin release: coexistence with vasopressin and corticotropin-releasing factor in cells of the rat hypothalamic paraventricular nucleus. *Proc Natl Acad Sci USA* 1986;83:3510.
801. Whitnall MH, Gainer H. Major pro-vasopressin–expressing and pro-vasopressin–deficient subpopulations of corticotropin-releasing hormone neurons in normal rats. Differential distribution in the paraventricular nucleus. *Neuroendocrinology* 1988;47:176.
802. Hökfelt T, Fahrenkrug J, Tatemoto K, et al. The PHI (PHI-27)/corticotropin-releasing factor/enkephalin immunoreactive hypothalamic neuron: possible morphological basis for integrated control of prolactin, corticotropin, and growth hormone secretion. *Proc Natl Acad Sci USA* 1983;80:895.
803. Niimi M, Takahara J, Sato M, Kawanishi K. Neurotensin & growth hormone-releasing factor-containing neurons projecting to the median eminence of the rat: a combined retrograde tracing & immunohistochemical study. *Neurosci Lett* 1991;144:183.
804. Swanson LW, Sawchenko PE, Berod A, Hartman BK, Helle KB, Vanorden DE. An immunohistochemical study of the organization of catecholamine cells and terminal fields in the paraventricular and supraoptic nuclei of the hypothalamus. *J Comp Neurol* 1981;196:271.
805. Sawchenko PE, Swanson LW. Immunohistochemical identification of neurons in the paraventricular nucleus of the hypothalamus that project to the medulla or to the spinal cord in the rat. *J Comp Neurol* 1982;205:260.
806. Yamano M, Bai F-L, Tohyama M, Shiotani Y. Ultrastructural evidence of direct synaptic contact of catecholamine terminals with oxytocin-containing neurons in the parvocellular portion of the rat hypothalamic paraventricular nucleus. *Brain Res* 1985;336:176.
807. Liposits ZS, Paull WK, Setalo G, Bigh S. Evidence for local corticotropin releasing factor (CRF)-immunoreactive neuronal circuits in the paraventricular nucleus of the rat hypothalamus. An electron microscopic immunohistochemical analysis. *Histochemistry* 1985;83:5.
808. Kitazawa S, Shioda S, Nakai Y. Catecholaminergic innervation of neurons containing corticotropin-releasing factor in the paraventricular nucleus of the rat hypothalamus. *Acta Anat* 1987;129:337.
809. Liposits Z, Sherman D, Phelix C, Paull WK. A combined light and electron microscopic immunocytochemical method for the simultaneous localization of multiple tissue antigens. Tyrosine hydroxylase immunoreactive innervation of corticotropon releasing factor synthesizing neurons in the paraventricular nucleus. *Histochemistry* 1986;85:95.

810. Liposits ZS. Ultrastructural immunocytochemistry of the hypothalamic corticotropin releasing hormone synthesizing system. *Prog Histochem Cytochem* 1990;21:1.
811. Liposits Z, Phelix C, Paull WK. Synaptic interaction of serotonergic axons and corticotropin releasing factor (CRF) synthesizing neurons in the hypothalamic paraventricular nucleus of the rat. A light and electronmicroscopic study. *Histochemistry* 1987;86:541.
812. Hisano S, Kaikoku S. Existence of mutual synaptic relations between corticotropin-releasing-factor-containing and somatostatin-containing neurons in the rat hypothalamus. *Brain Res* 1991;545:265.
813. Kiss J, Halasz B. Ultrastructural: analysis of the innervation of TRH-immunoreactive neuronal elements located in the periventricular subdivision of the paraventricular nucleus of the rat hypothalamus. *Brain Res* 1990;532:107.
814. Toni R, Jackson IMD, Lechan RM. Neuropeptide-Y-immunoreactive innervation of thyrotropin-releasing hormone-synthesizing neurons in the rat hypothalamic paraventricular nucleus. *Endocrinology* 1990;26:2444.
815. Shioda A, Nakai Y, Sato S, Sunayama S, Shimoda Y. Electron-microscopic cytochemistry of the catecholaminergic innervation of TRH neurons in the rat hypothalamus. *Cell Tissue Res* 1986;245:247.
816. Liao N, Bulant M, Nicolas P, Vaudry H, Pelletier G. Anatomical interactions of proopiomelanocortin (POMC)-related peptides, neuropeptide Y (NPY) and dopamine β-hydroxylase (DBH) fibers and thyrotropin-releasing hormone (TRH) neurons in the paraventricular nucleus of rat hypothalamus. *Neuropeptides* 1991;18:63.
817. Palkovits M. Neuropeptides in the median eminence: their sources and destinations. *Peptides* 1982;3:299.
818. Swanson LW, Sawchenko PE, Wiegand SJ, Price JL. Separate neurons in the paraventricular nucleus project to the median eminence and to the medulla or spinal cord. *Brain Res* 1980;198:190.
819. Sofroniew MV, Schrell U. Evidence for a direct projection from oxytocin and vasopressin neurons in the hypothalamic paraventricular nucleus to the medulla oblongata: immunohistochemical visualization of both the horseradish peroxidase. *Neurosci Lett* 1981;22:211.
820. Swanson LW. Immunohistochemical evidence for a neurophysin-containing autonomic pathway arising in the paraventricular nucleus of the hypothalamus. *Brain Res* 1977;128:346.
821. Buijis RM, Van Der Beck EM, Renaud LP, Day TA, Jhamandas J. Oxytocin localization and function of the A_1 noradrenergic cell group: ultrastructural and electrophysiological studies. *Neuroscience* 1990;39:717.
822. Caverson MM, Ciriello J, Calaresu FR. Paraventricular nucleus of the hypothalamus: an electrophysiological investigation of neurons projecting directly to intermediolateral nucleus in the cat. *Brain Res* 1984;305:380.
823. Sofroniew MV. Projections from vasopressin, oxytocin and neurophysin neurons to neural targets in the rat and human. *J Histochem Cytochem* 1980;28:475.
824. Buijs RM. Intra- and extrahypothalamic vasopressin and oxytocin pathways in the rat. *Cell Tissue Res* 1978;192:423.
825. Buijs RM, Swaab DF. Immuno-electron microscopical demonstration of vasopressin and oxytocin synapses in the limbic system of the rat. *Cell Tissue Res* 1979;204:355.
826. DeVries GJ, Buijs RM. The origin of the vasopressinergic and oxytocinergic innervation of the rat brain with special reference to the lateral septum. *Brain Res* 1983;273:307.
827. Conrad LCA, Pfaff DW. Efferents from medial basal forebrain and hypothalamus in the rat. II. An autoradiographic study of the anterior hypothalamus. *J Comp Neurol* 1976;169:221.
828. Alpert LC, Brawer JR, Patel YC, Reichlin S. Somatostatinergic neurons in anterior hypothalamus: immunohistochemical localization. *Endocrinology* 1976;98:225.
829. Crowley WR, Terry LC. Biochemical mapping of somatostatinergic systems in rat brain: effects of periventricular hypothalamic and medial basal amygdaloid lesions on somatostatin-like immunoreactivity in discrete brain nuclei. *Brain Res* 1980;200:283.
830. Ishikawa K, Taniguchi Y, Kurosumi K, Suzuki M, Shinoda M. Immunohistochemical identification of somatostatin-containing neurons projecting to the median eminence. *Endocrinology* 1987;121:94.
831. Kawano H, Daikoku S. Somatostatin-containing neuron systems in the rat hypothalamus: retrograde tracing and immunohistochemical studies. *J Comp Neurol* 1988;271:293.
832. Merchenthaler I, Setalo G, Csontos C, Petrusz PL, Flerko B, Negro-Vilar A. Combined retrograde tracing and immunocytochemical identification of luteinizing hormone-releasing hormone- and somatostatin-containing neurons projecting to the median eminence of the rat. *Endocrinology* 1989;125:2812.
833. Epelbaum J, Tapia-Arancibis L, Alonso G, Astier H, Kordon C. The anterior periventricular hypothalamus is the site of somatostatin inhibition on its own release: An in vitro and immunocytochemical study. *Neuroendocrinology* 1986;44:255.
834. Liposits ZS, Kallo I, Barkovics-Kallo M, Bohn MC, Paull WK. Innervation of somatostatin synthesizing neurons by adrenergic, phenylethanolamine-*N*-methyltransferase (PNMT)-immunoreactive axons in the anterior periventricular nucleus of the rat hypothalamus. *Histochemistry* 1990;94:13.
835. Kiss J, Csaky A, Halasz B. Demonstration of serotonergic axon terminals on somatostatin-immunoreactive neurons of the anterior periventricular nucleus of the rat hypothalamus. *Brain Res* 1988;442:23.
836. Willoughby JO, Beroukas D, Blessing WW. Ultrastructural evidence for gamma aminobutyric acid-immunoreactive synapses on somatostatin-immunoreactive perikarya in the periventricular anterior hypothalamus. *Neuroendocrinology* 1987;46:268.
837. Kakucska I, Tappaz ML, Gaal GY, Stoickel ME, Makara GB. Gabaergic innervation of somatostatin-containing neurosecretory cells of the anterior periventricular hypothalamic area: a light and electron microscopy double immunolabelling study. *Neuroscience* 1988;25:585.
838. Horvath S, Palkovits M, Gorcs T, Arimura A. Electron microscopic immunocytochemical evidence for the existence of bidirectional synaptic connections between growth hormone-releasing hormone- and somatostatin-containing neurons in the hypothalamus of the rat. *Brain Res* 1989;481:8.
839. Jew JY, Leranth C, Arimura A, Palkovits M. Preoptic LH-RH and somatostatin in the rat median eminence. An experimental light and electron microscopic immunocytochemical study. *Neuroendocrinology* 1984;38:169.
840. Chan-Palay V, Zaborszky L, Kohler C, Goldstein M, Palay SL. Distribution of tyrosine-hydroxylase-immunoreactive neurons in the hypothalamus of rats. *J Comp Neurol* 1984;227:467.
841. Dahlstrom A, Fuxe K. Evidence for the existence of monoamine-containing neurons in the central nervous system. I. Demonstration of monoamines in the cell bodies of brain stem neurons. *Acta Physiol Scand* 1964;62(Suppl 232):1.
842. Ibata Y, Kawakami F, Fukui K, et al. Light and electron microscopic immunocytochemistry of neurotensin-like immunoreactive neurons in the rat hypothalamus. *Brain Res* 1984;302:221.
843. Crosby EC, Woodburne RT. The comparative anatomy of the preoptic area and the hypothalamus. *Proc Assoc Res Nerv Ment Dis* 1966;20:52.
844. Van Den Pol AN, Cassidy JR. The hypothalamic arcuate nucleus of rat—a quantitative Golgi analysis. *J Comp Neurol* 1982;204:65.
845. Walsh RJ, Brawer JR. Cytology of the arcuate nucleus in newborn male and female rats. *J Anat* 1979;128:121.
846. Bodoky M, Rethelyi M. Dendritic arborization and axon trajectory of neurons in the hypothalamic arcuate nucleus of the rat. *Exp Brain Res* 1977;28:543.
847. Ottersen OP. Afferent connections to the amygdaloid complex of the rat and cat. II. Afferents from the hypothalamus and the basal telencephalon. *J Comp Neurol* 1980;194:267.
848. Fuxe K. Evidence for the existence of monoamine neurons in the central nervous system. III. The monoamine nerve terminal. *Z Zellforsch* 1965;65:573.
849. Fuxe K, Hökfelt T. Further evidence for the existence of

tubero-infundibular dopamine neurons. *Acta Physiol Scand* 1966;66:245.
850. Lichthensteiger W, Langemann H. Uptake of exogenous catecholamines by monoamine-containing neurons of the central nervous system: uptake of catecholamines by arcuato-infundibular neurons. *J Pharmacol Exp Ther* 1966;151:400.
851. Fuxe K, Hökfelt T. Catecholamines in the hypothalamus and the pituitary gland. In: Ganong WF, Martini L, eds. *Frontiers in Neuroendocrinology.* New York: Oxford University Press, 1969:47.
852. Björklund A, Nobin A. Fluorescence histochemical and microspectrofluorometric mapping of dopamine and noradrenaline cell groups in the rat diencephalon. *Brain Res* 1973;51:193.
853. Jonsson G, Fuxe K, Hökfelt T. On the catecholamine innervation of the hypothalamus, with special reference to the median eminence. *Brain Res* 1972;40:271.
854. Smith GC, Fink G. Experimental studies on the origin of monoamine-containing fibres in the hypothalamo-hypophysial complex of the rat. *Brain Res* 1972;43:37.
855. Nojyo Y, Ibata Y, Sano Y. Demonstration of tuberoinfundibular tract of the cat. *Cell Tissue Res* 1976;168:289.
856. Palkovits M, Brownstein M, Saavedra JM, Axelrod J. Norepinephrine and dopamine content of hypothalamic nuclei of the rat. *Brain Res* 1974;77:137.
857. Goldsmith PC, Boggan JE, Thind KK. Opioid neurons synapse on tuberoinfundibular dopamine neurons in the arcuate nucleus of juvenile monkeys. *Neurosci Abstr* 1989;15:722.
858. Nishizuka M. Topography of the dopamine neurons in the arcuate nucleus of the mouse hypothalamus. *Acta Anat* 1979;103:34.
859. Bugnon C, Bloch B, Lenys D, Gouget A, Fellmann D. Comparative study of the neuronal populations containing β-endorphin, corticotropin and dopamine in the arcuate nucleus of the rat hypothalamus. *Neurosci Lett* 1979;14:43.
860. Meister B, Hökfelt T, Steinbush HWM. Do tyrosine hydroxylase-immunoreactive neurons in the ventrolateral arcuate nucleus produce dopamine or only dopa? *J Chem Neuroanat* 1988;1:59.
861. Meister B, Hökfelt T. Peptide- and transmitter-containing neurons in the mediobasal hypothalamus and their relation to gabaergic systems: possible roles in control of prolactin and growth hormone secretion. *Synapse* 1988;2:585.
862. Everitt BJ, Hökfelt T, Wu J-Y, Goldstein M. Coexistence of tyrosine hydroslase-like and gamma-aminobutyric acid-like immunoreactivities in neurons of the arcuate nucleus. *Neuroendocrinology* 1984;39:189.
863. Hökfelt T, Everitt BJ, Theodorsson-Norheim E, Goldstein M. Occurrence of neurotensinlike immunoreactivity in subpopulations of hypothalamic, mesencephalic, and medullary catecholamine neurons. *J Comp Neurol* 1984;222:543.
864. Okamura H, Murakami S, Chihara K, Nagatsu I, Ibata Y. Coexistence of growth hormone releasing factor-like and tyrosine hydroxylase-like immunoreactivities in neurons of the rat arcuate nucleus. *Neuroendocrinology* 1985;41:177.
865. Bloch B, Brazeau P, Bloom F, Ling N. Topographical study of the neurons containing hyGRF immunoreactivity in monkey hypothalamus. *Neurosci Lett* 1983;37:23.
866. Lechan RM, Lin HD, Ling N, Jackson IMD, Jacobson S, Reichlin S. Distribution of immunoreactive growth hormone releasing factor (1-44)NH_2 in the tuberoinfundibular system of the rhesus monkey. *Brain Res* 1984;309:55.
867. Bugnon C, Gouget A, Fellmann D, Clavequin MC. Immunocytochemical demonstration of a novel peptidergic neurone system in the cat brain with an anti-growth hormone-releasing factor serum. *Neurosci Lett* 1983;38:131.
868. Bloch B, Brazeau P, Ling N, et al. Immunohistochemical detection of growth hormone-releasing factor in brain. *Nature* 1983;301:607.
869. Fellmann D, Bugnon C, Lavry GN. Immunohistochemical demonstration of a new neurone system in rat brain using antibodies against human growth hormone-releasing factor (1-37). *Neurosci Lett* 1985;58:91.
870. Merchenthaler I, Vigh S, Schally AV, Petrusz P. Immunocytochemical localization of growth hormone-releasing factor in the rat hypothalamus. *Endocrinology* 1984;114:1082.
871. Bloch R, Ling N, Benoit R, Wehrenberg WB, Guillemin R. Specific depletion of immunoreactive growth hormone-releasing factor by monosodium glutamate in rat median. *Nature* 1984;307:272.
872. Holzwarth-McBride MA, Hurst EM, Knigge KM. Monosodium glutamate induced lesions of the arcuate nucleus. I. Endocrine deficiency and ultrastructure of the median eminence. *Anat Rec* 1976;186:185.
873. Holzwarth-McBride MA, Sladek JR, Knigge KM. Monosodium glutamate induced lesions of the arcuate nucleus. II. Fluorescence histochemistry of catecholamines. *Anat Rec* 1976; 186:197.
874. Niimi M, Takahara J, Sato M, Kawanishi K. Sites of origin of growth hormone-releasing factor-containing neurons projecting to the stalk-median eminence of the rat. *Peptides* 1989;10:605.
875. Melander T, Hökfelt T, Rokaeus A, et al. Coexistence of galanin-like immunoreactivity with catecholamines, 5-hydroxytryptamine, gaba and neuropeptides in the rat CNS. *J Neurosci* 1986;6:3640.
876. Meister B, Hökfelt T, Vale WW, Sawchenko PE, Swanson L, Goldstein M. Coexistence of tyrosine hydroxylase and growth hormone-releasing factor in a subpopulation of tuberoinfundibular neurons of the rat. *Neuroendocrinology* 1986;42:237.
877. Rossier J, Vargo TM, Minick S, Ling N, Bloom FE, Guillemin R. Regional distribution of β-endorphin and enkephalin contents in rat brain and pituitary. *Proc Natl Acad Sci USA* 1977;74:5162.
878. Oliver C, Porter JC. Distribution and characterization of α-melanocyte-stimulating hormone in the rat brain. *Endocrinology* 1978;102:697.
879. Eskay RL, Giraud P, Oliver C, Brownstein MJ. Distribution of α-melanocyte-stimulating hormone in the rat brain: evidence that α-MSH-containing cells in the arcuate region send projections to extrahypothalamic areas. *Brain Res* 1979;178:55.
880. Liotta AS, Gildersleeve D, Brownstein MJ, Krieger DT. Biosynthesis in vitro of immunoreactive 31,000-dalton corticotropin/β-endorphin-like material by bovine hypothalamus. *Proc Natl Acad Sci USA* 1979;76:1448.
881. Watson SJ, Barchas JD, Li CH. β-Lipotropin: localization of cells and axons in rat brain by immunocytochemistry. *Proc Natl Acad Sci USA* 1977;74:5155.
882. Nilaver G, Zimmerman EA, Defendini R, Liotta AS, Krieger DT, Brownstein MJ. Adrenocorticotropin and β-lipotropin in the hypothalamus. Localization in the same arcuate neurons by sequential immunocytochemical procedures. *J Cell Biol* 1979;81:50.
883. Sofroniew MV. Immunoreactive β-endorphin and ACTH in the same neurons of the hypothalamic arcuate nucleus in the rat. *Am J Anat* 1979;154:283.
884. Hisano S, Kawano H, Nishiyama T, Daikoku S. Immunoreactive ACTH/β-endorphin neurons in the tubero-infundibular hypothalamus of rats. *Cell Tissue Res* 1982;224:303.
885. Bloch B, Bugnon C, Fellmann D, Lenys D, Gouget A. Neurons of the rat hypothalamus reactive with antisera against endorphins, ACTH, MSH and β-LPH. *Cell Tissue Res* 1979;204:1.
886. Bloch B, Bugnon C, Fellman D, Lenys D. Immunocytochemical evidence that the same neurons in the human infundibular nucleus are stained with anti-endorphins and antisera of other related peptides. *Neurosci Lett* 1978;10:147.
887. Bloch B, Bugnon C, Fellmann D, Lenys D. Presence de determinants antigeniques de la β-LPH, de la β-MSH, de l'a-endorphine, de l'ACTH et de l'*a*-MSH dans les neurones reveles par l'anti-β-endorphine au niveau du noyau infundibulaire de l'Homme. *CR Acad Sci Paris* 1978;287:1019.
888. Bugnon C, Bloch B, Lenys D, Fellmann D. Infundibular neurons of the human hypothalamus simultaneously reactive with antisera against endorphins, ACTH, MSH and β-LPH. *Cell Tissue Res* 1979;199:177.
889. Sawchenko PE, Swanson LW, Joseph SA. The distribution and cells of origin of ACTH (1-39)-stained varicosities in the paraventricular and supraoptic nuclei. *Brain Res* 1982;232:365.

890. Thind KK, Goldsmith PC. Infundibular gonadotropin-releasing hormone neurons are inhibited by direct opioid and autoregulatory synapses in juvenile monkeys. *Neuroendocrinology* 1988;47:203.
891. Selmanoff MK, Wise PM, Barraclough CA. Regional distribution of luteinizing hormone-releasing hormone (LH-RH) in rat brain determined by microdissection and radioimmunoassay. *Brain Res* 1980;192:421.
892. Silverman AJ, Zimmerman EA. Pathways containing luteinizing hormone-releasing hormone (LHRH) in the mammalian brain. In: Scott DE, Kozlowski GP, Weindl A, eds. *Brain-endocrine interaction. III. Neural hormones and reproduction.* Basel: Karger, 1978:83.
893. Kozlowski GP, Nett TM, Zimmerman EA. Immunocytochemical localization of gonadotropin-releasing hormone (Gn-RH) and neurophysin in the brain. In: Stumpf WE, Grant LD, eds. *Anatomical neuroendocrinology.* Basel: Karger, 1975:185.
894. Kawano H, Daikoku S. Immunohistochemical demonstration of LHRH neurons and their pathways in the rat hypothalamus. *Neuroendocrinology* 1981;32:179.
895. Silverman AJ, Antunes JL, Ferin M, Zimmerman EA. The distribution of luteinizing hormone-releasing hormone (LHRH) in the hypothalamus of the rhesus monkey. Light microscopic studies using immunoperoxidase technique. *Endocrinology* 1977;101:134.
896. Barry J. Characterization and topography of LH-RH neurons in the rabbit. *Neurosci Lett* 1976;2:201.
897. Silverman AJ, Krey LC. The luteinizing hormone-releasing hormone (LH-RH) neuronal networks of the guinea pig brain. I. Intra- and extra-hypothalamic projections. *Brain Res* 1978; 157:233.
898. King JC, Anthony ELP, Gustafson AW, Damassa DA. Luteinizing hormone-releasing hormone (LH-RH) cells and their projections in the forebrain of the bat *Myotis lucifugus lucifugus. Brain Res* 1984;298:289.
899. Barry J. Characterization and topography of LH-RH neurons in the human brain. *Neurosci Lett* 1976;3:287.
900. Barry J. Immunofluorescence study of LRF neurons in man. *Cell Tissue Res* 1977;181:1.
901. King JC, Anthony ELP, Fitzgerald DM, Stopa EG. Luteinizing hormone-releasing hormone neurons in human preoptic/hypothalamus: differential intraneuronal localization of immunoreactive forms. *J Clin Endocrinol Metab* 1985;60:88.
902. Hökfelt T, Elde RP, Johansson O, Terenius L, Stein L. Distribution of enkephalin-like immunoreactivity in the rat central nervous system. *Neurosci Lett* 1977;5:25.
903. Finley JCW, Maderdrut JL, Petrusz P. The immunocytochemical localization of enkephalin in the central nervous system of the rat. *J Comp Neurol* 1981;198:541.
904. Tsuruo Y, Kawano H, Nishiyama T, Hisano S, Daikoku S. Substance P-like immunoreactive neurons in the tuberinfundibular area of rat hypothalamus, light and electron microscopy. *Brain Res* 1983;289:1.
905. Johansson O, Hökfelt T. Thyrotropin-releasing hormone, somatostatin, and enkephalin: distribution studies using immunohisto-chemical techniques. *J Histochem Cytochem* 1980;28:364.
906. Khachaturian H, Lewis ME, Watson SJ. Enkephalin systems in diencephalon and brainstem of the rat. *J Comp Neurol* 1983;220:310.
907. Bai FL, Yamano M, Shiotani Y, et al. An arcuato-paraventricular and dorsomedial hypothalamic neuropeptide Y-containing system which lacks noradrenaline in the rat. *Brain Res* 1985;331:172.
908. Van Den Pol AN. Tyrosine hydroxylase immunoreactive synapses: A double pre-embedding immunocytochemical study with particulate silver and HRP. *J Neurosci* 1986;6:877.
909. Tappaz ML, Bosler O, Paut L, Berod A. Glutamate decarboxylase-immunoreactive boutons in synaptic contacts with hypothalamic dopaminergic cells: a light and electron microscopic study combining immunohistochemistry and radioautography. *Neuroscience* 1985;16:112.
910. Leranth C, Sakamoto H, Maclusky NJ, Shanabrough M, Naftolin F. Intrinsic tyrosine hydroxylase (TH) immunoreactive axons synapse with TH immunopositive neurons in the rat arcuate nucleus. *Brain Res* 1985;331:371.
911. Kiss J, Halasz B. Synaptic connections between serotoninergic axon terminals and tyrosine hydroxylase-immunoreactive neurons in the arcuate nucleus of the rat hypothalamus. A combination of electron microscopic autoradiography and immunocytochemistry. *Brain Res* 1986;364:284.
912. Horvath S, Palkovits P. Synaptic interconnections among growth hormone-releasing hormone (GHRH)-containing neurons in the arcuate nucleus of the rat hypothalamus. *Neuroendocrinology* 1988;48:471.
913. Sato A, Shioda S, Nakai Y. Catecholaminergic innervation of GRF-containing neurons in the rat hypothalamus revealed by electron-microscopic cytochemistry. *Cell Tissue Res* 1989; 258:31.
914. Shioda S, Kohara H, Nakai Y. TRH axon terminals in synapsis with GRF neurons in the arcuate nucleus of the rat hypothalamus as revealed by double labeling immunocytochemistry. *Brain Res* 1987;402:355.
915. Kiss JZ, Williams TH. ACTH-immunoreactive boutons form synaptic contacts in the hypothalamic arcuate nucleus of rat: evidence for local opiocortin connections. *Brain Res* 1983;263:142.
916. Kiss J, Leranth C, Lalasz B. Serotonergic endings on VIP-neurons in the suprachiasmatic nucleus and on ACTH-neurons in the arcuate nucleus of the rat hypothalamus. A combination of high resolution autoradiography and electron microscopic immunohistochemistry. *Neurosci Lett* 1984;44:119.
917. Kozasa K, Nakai Y. Electron-microscopic cytochemistry of the catecholaminergic innervation of ACTH-containing neurons in the rat hypothalamic arcuate nucleus. *Acta Anat* 1987;128:243.
918. Zhang R, Hisano S, Chikamori-Aoyama M, Kaikoku S. Synaptic association between enkephalin-containing axon terminals and proopiomelanocortin-containing neurons in the arcuate nucleus of rat hypothalamus. *Neurosci Lett* 1987;82:151.
919. Tsuruo Y, Hisano S, Daikoku S. Morphological evidence for synaptic junctions between substance P-containing neurons in the arcuate nucleus of the rat. *Neurosci Lett* 1984;46:65.
920. Hammel HT. Regulation of internal body temperature. *Annu Rev Physiol* 1968;30:641.
921. Squires RD, Jacobson FH. Chronic deficits of temperature regulation produced in cats by preoptic lesions. *Am J Physiol* 1968;214:549.
922. Ramsay DJ, Thrasher TN, Keil LC. The organum vasculosum laminae terminalis: a critical area for osmoreception. *Prog Brain Res* 1983;60:91.
923. Brody MJ, Johnson AK. Role of the anteroventral third ventricle region in fluid and electrolyte balance, arterial pressure regulation, and hypertension. In: Martini L, Ganong WF, eds. *Frontiers in neuroendocrinology,* Vol. 6. New York: Raven Press, 1980:249.
924. Saphier D, Feldman S. Effects of stimulation of the preoptic area on hypothalamic paraventricular nucleus unit activity and corticosterone secretion in freely moving rats. *Neuroendocrinology* 1986;42:167.
925. Struyker-Boudier HS, Smeets G, Brouwer G, Van Rossum JM. Central nervous system α-adrenergic mechanisms and cardiovascular regulation in rats. *Arch Int Pharmacodyn* 1975; 213:285.
926. Gorski RA. Critical role for the medial preoptic area in the sexual differentiation of the brain. *Prog Brain Res* 1984;61:129.
927. Arendash GW, Gorski RA. Effects of discrete lesions of the sexually dimorphic nucleus of the preoptic area or other medial preoptic regions on the sexual behavior of male rats. *Brain Res Bull* 1983;10:147.
928. Commins D, Yahr P. Adult testosterone levels influence the morphology of a sexually dimorphic area in the mongolial gerbil brain. *J Comp Neurol* 1984;224:132.
929. Masken JF, Kragt CL, Gallo RV, Ganong WF. Release of luteinizing hormone by electrical stimulation of the medial preoptic area and arcuate nucleus in the male rat. *Neuroendocrinology* 1974;15:249.

930. Knobil E, Plant TM, Wildt L, Belchetz PE, Marshall G. Control of the rhesus monkey menstrual cycle: permissive role of hypothalamic gonadotropin-releasing hormone. *Science* 1980; 207:1371.
931. Swanson LW. An autoradiographic study of the efferent connections of the preoptic region in the rat. *J Comp Neurol* 1976;167:227.
932. Prince FP, Jones-Witters PH. The ultrastructure of the medial preoptic area of the rat. *Cell Tissue Res* 1974;153:517.
933. Greenough WT, Carter CS, Steerman C, DeVoogd TJ. Sex differences in dendritic patterns in hamster preoptic area. *Brain Res* 1977;126:63.
934. Gorski RA, Harlan RE, Jacobson CD, Shryne JE, Southam AM. Evidence for the existence of a sexually dimorphic nucleus in the preoptic area of the rat. *J Comp Neurol* 1980;193:529.
935. Jacobson CD, Shryne JE, Shaprio F, Gorski RA. Ontogeny of the sexually dimorphic nucleus of the preoptic area. *J Comp Neurol* 1980;193:541.
936. Dohler K-D, Coquelin A, Davis F, Hines M, Shryne JE, Gorski RA. Differentiation of the sexually dimorphic nucleus in the preoptic area of the rat brain is determined by the perinatal hormone environment. *Neurosci Lett* 1982;33:295.
937. Hines M, Davis FC, Coquelin A, Goy RW, Gorski RA. Sexually dimorphic regions in the medial preoptic area and the bed nucleus of the stria terminalis of the guinea pig brain: a description and an investigation of their relationship to gonadal steroids in adulthood. *J Neurosci* 1985;5:40.
938. Takami S, Urano A. The volume of the toad medial amygdala-anterior preoptic complex is sexually dimorphic and seasonally variable. *Neurosci Lett* 1984;44:253.
939. Swaab DF, Fliers E. A sexually dimorphic nucleus in the human brain. *Science* 1985;228:1112.
940. Cramer OM, Barraclough CA. Effect of electrical stimulation of the preoptic area on plasma LH concentrations in proestrous rats. *Endocrinology* 1971;88:1175.
941. Sar M, Stumpf WE. Autoradiographic localization of radioactivity in the rat brain after the injection of 1,2-^{3}H-testosterone. *Endocrinology* 1973;92:251.
942. Stumpf WE. Estrogen-neurons and estrogen-neuron systems in the periventricular brain. *Am J Anat* 1970;129:207.
943. Pfaff D, Keiner M. Atlas of estradiol-concentrating cells in the central nervous system of the female rat. *J Comp Neurol* 1973;151:121.
944. Pfaff DW, Gerlach JL, McEwen BS, Ferin M, Carmel P, Zimmerman EA. Autoradiographic localization of hormone-concentrating cells in the brain of the female rhesus monkey. *J Comp Neurol* 1976;170:279.
945. Raisman G, Field PM. Sexual dimorphism in the neuropil of the preoptic area of the rat and its dependence on neonatal androgen. *Brain Res* 1973;54:1.
946. McDonald AJ. Neurons of the bed nucleus of the stria terminalis: a Golgi study in the rat. *Brain Res Bull* 1983;10:111.
947. Saper CB. Organization of the cerebral cortical afferent systems in the rat. II. Magnocellular basal nucleus. *J Comp Neurol* 1984;222:313.
948. Epelbaum J, Arancibia LT, Herman JP, Kordon C, Palkovits M. Topography of median eminence somatostatinergic innervation. *Brain Res* 1981;230:412.
949. Woodhams PL, Roberts GW, Polak JM, Crow TJ. Distribution of neuropeptides in the limbic system of the rat: the bed nucleus of the stria terminalis, septum and preoptic area. *Neuroscience* 1983;8:677.
950. DeVries GJ, Buijs RM. The origin of vasopressinergic and oxytocinergic innervation of the rat brain with special reference to the lateral septum. *Brain Res* 1983;273:307.
951. Khachaturian H, Lewis ME, Watson SJ. Enkephalin systems in diencephalon and brainstem of the rat. *J Comp Neurol* 1983;220:310.
952. King JC, Tobet SA, Snavely FL, Arimura AA. LHRH immunopositive cells and their projections to the median eminence and organum vasculosum of the lamina terminalis. *J Comp Neurol* 1982;209:287.
953. Merchenthaler I, Gorcs T, Setalo G, Petrusz P, Flerko B. Gonadotropin-releasing hormone (GnRH) neurons and pathways in the rat brain. *Cell Tissue Res* 1984;237:15.
954. Charney Y, Bouras C, Vallet PG, Golaz J, Guntern R, Constandinidis J. Immunohistochemical distribution of delta sleep-inducing peptide in the rabbit brain and hypophysis. *Neuroendocrinology* 1989;49:169.
955. Silverman A-J, Jhamandas J, Renaud LP. Localization of luteinizing hormone-releasing hormone (LHRH) neurons that project to the median eminence. *J Neurosci* 1987;7:2312.
956. Goldsmith PC, Thind KK, Boggan JE. Neuroendocrine GNRH and dopamine neurons in the monkey hypothalamus identified by retrograde staining and immunostaining. *Proc Soc Neurosci* 1988;14:439.
957. Pelletier G. Demonstration of contacts between neurons staining for LHRH in the preoptic area of the rat brain. *Neuroendocrinology* 1987;46:457.
958. Leranth CS, Segura LMG, Palkovits M, Maclusky NJ, Shanabrough M, Naftolin F. The LHRH-containing neuronal network in the preoptic area of the rat: demonstration of LH-RH containing nerve terminals in synaptic contact with LH-RH neurons. *Brain Res* 1985;345:332.
959. Watanabe T, Naka Y. Electron microscopic cytochemistry of catecholaminergic innervation of LHRH neurons in the medial preoptic area of the rat. *Arch Histol Jpn* 1987;50:103.
960. Tsuruo Y, Kawano H, Kagotani Y, et al. Morphological evidence for neuronal regulation of luteinizing hormone-releasing hormone-containing neurons by neuropeptide Y in the rat septopreoptic area. *Neurosci Lett* 1990;110:261.
961. Leranth C, Maclushy NJ, Sakamoto H, Shanabrough M, Naftolin F. Glutamic acid decarboxylase-containing axons synapse on LHRH neurons in the rat medial preoptic area. *Neuroendocrinology* 1985;40:536.
962. Maclusky NJ, Naftolin F, Leranth C. Immunocytochemical evidence for direct synaptic connections between corticotropin-releasing factor (CRF) and gonadotropin-releasing hormone (GNRH)-containing neurons in the preoptic area of the rat. *Brain Res* 1988;439:391.
963. Tsuruo Y, Kawano H, Hisano S, et al. Substance P-containing neurons innervating LHRH-containing neurons in the septopreoptic area of rats. *Neuroendocrinology* 1991;53:236.
964. Chen W-P, Witkin JW, Silverman A-J. Beta-endorphin and gonadotropin-releasing hormone synaptic input to gonadotropin-releasing hormone neurosecretory cells in the male rat. *J Comp Neurol* 1989;286:85.
965. Leranth C, Maclusky NJ, Shanabrough M, Naftolin F. Immunohistochemical evidence for synaptic connections between proopiomelanocortin-immunoreactive axons and LH-RH neurons in the preoptic area of the rat. *Brain Res* 1988;449:167.
966. Hoffman GE, Gibbs FP. LHRH pathways in rat brain: deafferentation spares a subchiasmatic LHRH projection to the median eminence. *Neuroscience* 1982;7:1979.
967. Merchenthaler I, Gorcs T, Setalo G, Petrusz P, Flerko B. Gonadotropin-releasing hormone (GNRH) neurons and pathways in the rat brain. *Cell Tissue Res* 1984;237:15.
968. Krey LC, Silverman AJ. The luteinizing hormone-releasing hormone (LH-RH) neuronal networks of the guinea pig brain. II. The regulation of gonadotropin secretion and the origin of terminals in the median eminence. *Brain Res* 1978;157:247.
969. Silverman AJ, Antunes JL, Abrams GM, et al. The luteinizing hormone-releasing hormone pathways in rhesus (*Macaca mulatta*) and pigtailed (*Macaca nemestrina*) monkeys: new observations on thick, unembedded sections. *J Comp Neurol* 1982;211:309.
970. Marshall PE, Goldsmith PC. Neuroregulatory and neuroendocrine GnRH pathways in the hypothalamus and forebrain of the baboon. *Brain Res* 1980;193:353.
971. Jennes L, Stumpf WE. LHRH-systems in the brain of the golden hamster. *Cell Tissue Res* 1980;209:239.
972. Witkin JW, Paden CM, Silverman A-J. The luteinizing hormone-releasing hormone (LHRH) systems in the rat brain. *Neuroendocrinology* 1982;35:429.
973. Conrad LCA, Pfaff DW. Efferents from medial basal forebrain

and hypothalamus in the rat. I. An autoradiographic study of the medial preoptic area. *J Comp Neurol* 1976;169:185.
974. Chiba T, Murata Y. Afferent and efferent connections of the medial preoptic area in the rat: a WGA-HRP study. *Brain Res Bull* 1985;14:261.
975. Simerly RB, Swanson LW. Projections of the medial preoptic nucleus: a phaseolus vulgaris leucoagglutinin anterograde tract-tracing study in the rat. *J Comp Neurol* 1988;270:209.
976. Palkovits M, Mezey E, Ambach G, Kivovics P. Neural and vascular connections between the organum vasculosum laminae terminalis and preoptic nuclei. In: Scott DE, Kozlowski GP, Weindl A, eds. *Brain-endocrine interaction III. Neural hormones and reproduction.* Basel: Karger, 1978:302.
977. Hoorneman EMD, Buijs RM. Vasopressin fiber pathways in the rat brain following suprachiasmatic nucleus lesioning. *Brain Res* 1982;243:235.
978. Swanson LW, Cowan WM. The connections of the septal region in the rat. *J Comp Neurol* 1979;186:621.
979. Millhouse OE. A Golgi study of the descending medial forebrain bundle. *Brain Res* 1969;15:341.
980. Van Cuc H, Leranth C, Palkovits M. Light and electron microscopic studies on the medial forebrain bundle in rat: III. Degenerated nerve elements in the medial hypothalamic nuclei following surgical transections of the medial forebrain bundle. *Brain Res Bull* 1980;5:13.
981. Nieuwenhuys R, Geeraedts LMG, Veening JG. The medial forebrain bundle of the rat. I. General introduction. *J Comp Neurol* 1982;206:49.
982. Veening JG, Swanson LW, Cowan WM, Nieuwenhuys R, Geeraedts LMG. The medial forebrain bundle of the rat. II. An autoradiographic study of the topography of the major descending and ascending components. *J Comp Neurol* 1982;206:82.
983. Lindvall O, Björklund A. The organization of the ascending catecholamine neuron systems in the rat brain (as revealed by the glyocylic acid fluorescence method). *Acta Physiol Scand Suppl* 1974;412:1.
984. Swanson LW, Hartman BK. The central adrenergic system. An immunofluorescence study of the location of cell bodies and their efferent connections in the rat utilizing dopamine-β-hydroxylase as a marker. *J Comp Neurol* 1975;163:467.
985. Simon H, LeMoal M, Calas A. Efferents and afferents of the ventral tegmental-A10 region studied after local injection of (^{3}H)leucine and horseradish peroxidase. *Brain Res* 1979;178:17.
986. Moore KE, Demarest KT. Tuberoinfundibular and tuberohypophyseal dopaminergic neurons. In: Ganong WF, Martini L, eds. *Frontiers in Neuroendocrinology,* Vol. 7. New York: Raven Press, 1982:161.
987. Palkovits M, Zaborszky L, Feminger A, Noradrenergic innervation of the rat hypothalamus: experimental biochemical and electron microscopic studies. *Brain Res* 1980;191:161.
988. Anderson CH, Shen CL. Efferents of the medial preoptic area in the guinea pig: an autoradiographic study. *Brain Res Bull* 1980;5:257.
989. Krieger MS, Conrad LCA, Pfaff DW. An autoradiographic study of the efferent connections of the ventromedial nucleus of the hypothalamus. *J Comp Neurol* 1979;183:785.
990. Saper CB, Swanson LW, Cowan WM. The efferent connections of the ventromedial nucleus of the hypothalamus of the rat. *J Comp Neurol* 1976;169:409.
991. Saper CB, Swanson LW, Cowan WM. Some efferent connections of the rostral hypothalamus in the squirrel monkey (*Saimiri sciureus*) and cat. *J Comp Neurol* 1979;184:205.
992. Palkovits M, Fekete M, Makara GB, Herman JP. Total and partial hypothalamic deafferentations for topographical identification of catecholaminergic innervations of certain preoptic and hypothalamic nuclei. *Brain Res* 1977;127:127.
993. Sawchenko PE, Swanson LW. Central noradrenergic pathways for the integration of hypothalamic neuroendocrine and autonomic responses. *Science* 1981;214:685.
994. Swanson LW, Cowan WM. Hippocampo-hypothalamic connections: origin in subicular cortex, not Ammon's horn. *Science* 1975;189:303.
995. Simerly RB, Swanson LW. The organization of neural inputs to the medial preoptic nucleus of the rat. *J Comp Neurol* 1986;246:312.
996. Raisman G, Cowan WM, Powell TPS. An experimental analysis of the efferent projection of the hippocampus. *Brain* 1966; 89:83.
997. Raisman G. An evaluation of the basic pattern of connections between the limbic system and the hypothalamus. *Am J Anat* 1970;129:197.
998. Sawchenko PE, Swanson LW. The organization of forebrain afferents to the paraventricular and supraoptic nuclei of the rat. *J Comp Neurol* 1983;218:121.
999. Tribollet E, Armstrong WE, Dubois-Dauphin M, Dreifuss JJ. Extra-hypothalamic afferent inputs to the supraoptic nucleus area of the rat as determined by retrograde and anterograde tracing techniques. *Neuroscience* 1985;15:135.
1000. Tanaka J, Saito H, Seto K. Involvement of the septum in the regulation of paraventricular vasopressin neurons by the subfornical organ in the rat. *Neurosci Lett* 1988;92:187.
1001. Lind RW, Hoesen GWV, Johnson AK. An HRP study of the connections of the subfornical organ of the rat. *J Comp Neurol* 1982;210:265.
1002. Miselis RR. The efferent projections of the subfornical organ of the rat: a circumventricular organ within a neural network subserving water balance. *Brain Res* 1982;230:1.
1003. Sawchenko PE, Swanson LW. The organization and biochemical specificity of afferent projections to the paraventricular and supraoptic nuclei. *Prog Brain Res* 1983;60:19.
1004. Lind RW, Swanson LW, Ganten D. Organization of angiotensin II immunoreactive cells and fibers in the rat central nervous system: an immunohistochemical study. *Neuroendocrinology* 1985;40:1.
1005. Jhamandas JH, Lind RW, Renaud LP. Angiotensin II may mediate excitatory neurotransmission from the subfornical organ to the hypothalamic supraoptic nucleus: an anatomical and electrophysiological study in the rat. *Brain Res* 1989;487:52.
1006. Smithson KG, Weiss ML, Hatton GI. Supraoptic nucleus afferents from the main olfactory bulb—I. Anatomical evidence from anterograde and retrograde tracers in rat. *Neuroscience* 1989;31:277.
1007. Hatton GI, Zang QZ. Supraoptic nucleus afferents from the main olfactory bulb—II. Intracellularly recorded responses to lateral olfactory tract stimulation in rat brain slices. *Neuroscience* 1989;31:289.
1008. Hatton GI, Yang QZ. Activation of excitatory amino acid inputs to supraoptic neurons. I. induced increases in dye-coupling in lactating but not virgin or male rats. *Brain Res* 1990;513:264.
1009. Modney BK, Yang QZ, Hatton GI. Activation of excitatory amino acid inputs to supraoptic neurons. II. Increased dye-coupling in maternally behaving virgin rats. *Brain Res* 1990;513:270.
1010. Armstrong WE, Scholer J, McNeill TH. Immunocytochemical, Golgi and electron microscopic characterization of putative dendrites in the ventral glial lamina of the rat supraoptic nucleus. *Neuroscience* 1982;7:679.
1011. Zaborszky L, Leranth CS, Makara GB, Palkovits M. Quantitative studies on the supraoptic nucleus in the rat. II. Afferent fiber connections. *Exp Brain Res* 1975;22:525.
1012. Oldfield BJ, Hou-Yu A, Silverman A-J. A combined electron microscopic HRP and immunocytochemical study of the limbic projections to rat hypothalamic nuclei containing vasopressin and oxytocin neurons. *J Comp Neurol* 1985;231:221.
1013. Poulain DA, Lebrun CJ, Vincent JD. Electrophysiological evidence for connections between septal neurones and the supraoptic nucleus of the hypothalamus of the rat. *Exp Brain Res* 1981;42:260.
1014. Versteeg DHG, Van der Gugten J, De Jong W, Palkovits M. Regional concentrations of noradrenaline and dopamine in rat brain. *Brain Res* 1976;113:563.
1015. Cheung Y, Sladek JR. Catecholamine distribution in feline hypothalamus. *J Comp Neurol* 1975;164:339.
1016. Hoffman GE, Felten DL, Sladek JR. Monoamine distribution in primate brain. III. Catecholamine-containing varicosities in the hypothalamus of *Macaca mulatta. Am J Anat* 1976;147:501.

1017. Blessing WW, Jaeger CB, Ruggiero DA, Reis DJ. Hypothalamic projections of medullary catecholamine neurons in the rabbit: a combined catecholamine fluorescence and HRP transport study. *Brain Res Bull* 1982;9:279.
1018. Ciriello J, Caverson MM. Direct pathway from neurons in the ventrolateral medulla relaying cardiovascular afferent information to the supraoptic nucleus in the cat. *Brain Res* 1984;292:221.
1019. Day TA, Renaud LP. Electrophysiological evidence that noradrenergic afferents selectively facilitate the activity of supraoptic vasopressin neurons. *Brain Res* 1984;303:233.
1020. Ricardo JA, Koh ET. Anatomical evidence of direct projections from the nucleus of the solitary tract to the hypothalamus, amygdala, and other forebrain structures in the rat. *Brain Res* 1978;153:1.
1021. Day TA, Sibbald JR. A_1 cell group mediates solitary nucleus excitation of solitary nucleus excitation of supraoptic vasopressin cells. *Am J Physiol* 1989;257:R1020.
1022. Cunningham ET, Sawchenko PD. Anatomical specificity of noradrenergic inputs to the paraventricular and supraoptic nuclei of the rat hypothalamus. *J Comp Neurol* 1988;274:60.
1023. McNeill TH, Sladek JR. Simultaneous monoamine histofluorescence and neuropeptide immunocytochemistry: II. Correlative distribution of catecholamine varicosities and magnocellular neurosecretory neurons in the rat supraoptic and paraventricular nuclei. *J Comp Neurol* 1980;193:1023.
1024. Sladek JR, Zimmerman EA. Simultaneous monoamine histofluorescence and neuropeptide immunocytochemistry: VI. Catecholamine innervation of vasopressin and oxytocin neurons in the rhesus monkey hypothalamus. *Brain Res Bull* 1982;9:431.
1025. Buijs RM, Geffard M, Pool CW, Hoorneman EMD. The dopaminergic innervation of the supraoptic and paraventricular nucleus: a light and electron microscopical study. *Brain Res* 1984;323:65.
1026. Moore RY, Halaris AE, Jones BE. Serotonin neurons of the midbrain raphe: ascending projections. *J Comp Neurol* 1978;180:417.
1027. Bittencourt J, Benoit R, Sawchenko P. Distribution and origins of substance P-immunoreactive projections to the paraventricular and supra-optic nuclei: partial overlap with ascending catecholaminergic projections. *J Chem Neurol Anat* 1991;4:63.
1028. Tribollet E, Dreifuss JJ. Localization of neurones projecting to the hypothalamic paraventricular nucleus area of the rat: a horseradish peroxidase study. *Neuroscience* 1981;6:1315.
1029. Silverman AJ, Hoffman DL, Zimmerman EA. The descending afferent connections of the paraventricular nucleus of the hypothalamus (PVN). *Brain Res Bull* 1981;6:47.
1030. Ferguson AV. Systemic angiotensin acts at the subfornical organ to control the activity of paraventricular nucleus neurons with identified projection to the median eminence. *Neuroendocrinology* 1988;47:489.
1031. Ferguson AV, Day TA, Renaud LP. Subfornical organ efferents influence the excitability of neurohypophyseal and tuberoinfundibular nucleus neurons in the rat. *Neuroendocrinology* 1984;39:423.
1032. Kaelber WW, Leeson CR. A degeneration and electron microscopic study of the nucleus hypothalamus ventromedialis of the cat. *J Anat* 1967;101:209.
1033. Heimer L, Nauta WJH. The hypothalamic distribution of the stria terminalis in the rat. *Brain Res* 1969;13:284.
1034. McBride RL, Sutin J. Amygdaloid and pontine projections to the ventromedial nucleus of the hypothalamus. *J Comp Neurol* 1977;174:377.
1035. Krettek JE, Price JL. Amygdaloid projections to subcortical structures within the basal forebrain and brainstem in the rat and cat. *J Comp Neurol* 1978;178:225.
1036. Herman JP, Schafer MKH, Young EA, et al. Evidence for hippocampal regulation of neuroendocrine neurons of the hypothalamo-pituitary-adrenocortical axis. *J Neurosci* 1989;9:3072.
1037. Saphier D, Feldman S. Catecholaminergic projections to tuberinfundibular neurons of the paraventricular nucleus: II. Effects of stimulation of the ventral noradrenergic ascending bundle: evidence for cotransmission. *Brain Res Bull* 1989;23:397.
1038. Sapolsky RM, Armanini MP, Sutton SW, Plotsky PM. Elevation of hypophysial portal concentrations of adrenocorticotropin secretagogues after fornix transection. *Endocrinology* 1989;125:2881.
1039. Silverman A-J, Oldfield B, Hou-Yu A, Zimmerman EA. The noradrenergic innervation of vasopressin neurons in the paraventricular nucleus of the hypothalamus: an ultrastructural study using radioautography and immunocytochemistry. *Brain Res* 1985;325:215.
1040. Sawchenko PE, Swanson LW, Grzanna R, Howe PRC, Bloom SR, Olak JM. Colocalization of neuropeptide Y immunoreactivity in brainstem catecholaminergic neurons that project to the paraventricular nucleus. *J Comp Neurol* 1985;241:138.
1041. Day TA, Blessing W, Willoughby JO. Noradrenergic and dopaminergic projections to the medial preoptic area of the rat. A combined horseradish peroxidase/catecholamine fluorescence study. *Brain Res* 1980;193:543.
1042. Kannan H, Yamashita H, Osaka T. Paraventricular neurosecretory neurons: synaptic inputs from the ventrolateral medulla in rats. *Neurosci Lett* 1984;51:183.
1043. Tanaka J, Kaba H, Saito H, Seto K. Inputs from the A_1 noradrenergic region to hypothalamic paraventricular neurons in the rat. *Brain Res* 1985;335:368.
1044. Cunningham ET, Bohn MC, Sawchenko PE. Organization of adrenergic inputs to the paraventricular and supraoptic nuclei of the hypothalamus in the rat. *J Comp Neurol* 1990;292:651.
1045. Ciriello J, Caverson MM. Ventrolateral medullary neurons relay cardiovascular inputs to the paraventricular nucleus. *Am J Physiol* 1984;246:R968.
1046. Norgren R. Taste pathways to hypothalamus and amygdala. *J Comp Neurol* 1976;166:17.
1047. Takeuchi Y, Hopkins DA. Light and electron microscopic demonstration of hypothalamic projections to the parabrachial nuclei in the cat. *Neurosci Lett* 1984;46:53.
1048. Saper CB, Loewy AD. Efferent connections of the parabrachial nucleus in the rat. *Brain Res* 1980;197:291.
1049. McKellar S, Loewy AD. Organization of some brain stem afferents to the paraventricular nucleus of the hypothalamus in the rat. *Brain Res* 1981;217:351.
1050. Liposits ZS, Paull WK. Association of dopaminergic fibers with corticotropin releasing hormone (CRH)-synthesizing neurons in the paraventricular nucleus of the rat hypothalamus. *Histochemistry* 1989;93:119.
1051. Liposits ZS, Phelix C, Paull WK. Electron microscopic analysis of tyrosine hydroxylase, dopamine-β-hydroxylase and phenylethanolamine-*N*-methyl-transferase immunoreactive innervation of the hypothalamic paraventricular nucleus in the rat. *Histochemistry* 1986;84:105.
1052. Willoughby JO, Beroukas D, Blessing WW. Ultrastructural evidence for gamma aminobutyric acid-immunoreactive synapses on somatostatin-immunoreactive perikarya in the periventricular anterior hypothalamus. *Neuroendocrinology* 1987;46:268.
1053. Sutin J, Eager RP. Fiber degeneration following lesions in the hypothalamic ventromedial nucleus. *Ann NY Acad Sci* 1969;157:610.
1054. Millhouse OE. The organization of the ventromedial hypothalamic nucleus. *Brain Res* 1973;55:71.
1055. Ottersen OP. Afferent connections to the amygdaloid complex of the rat and cat. II. Afferents from the hypothalamus and the basal telencephalon. *J Comp Neurol* 1980;194:267.
1056. Amaral DG, Veazey RB, Cowan WM. Some observations on hypothalamo-amygdaloid connections in the monkey. *Brain Res* 1982;252:13.
1057. Lindvall O, Björklund A. Dopamine- and norepinephrine-containing neuron systems: their anatomy in the rat brain. In: Emson PC, ed. *Chemical neuroanatomy.* New York: Raven Press, 1983:229.
1058. Ajika K, Hökfelt T. Projections to the median eminence and the arcuate nucleus with special reference to monoamine systems: effects of lesions. *Cell Tissue Res* 1975;158:15.
1059. Steinbusch HWM, Nieuwenhuys R. The raphe nuclei of the rat

brain stem: a cytoarchitectonic and immunohistochemical study. In: Emson PC, ed. *Chemical neuroanatomy.* New York: Raven Press, 1983:131.

1060. Simerly RB, Swanson LW, Gorski RA. Demonstration of a sexual dimophism in the distribution of serotonin-immunoreactive fibers in the medial preoptic nucleus of the rat. *J Comp Neurol* 1984:225:151.

1061. Berk ML, Finkelstein JA. Afferent projections to the preoptic area and hypothalamic regions in the rat brain. *Neuroscience* 1981;6:1601.

1062. Kalra SP. Neural circuitry involved in control of LHRH secretion: a model for the preovulatory LH release. In: Ganong WF, Martini L, eds. *Frontiers in Neuroendocrinology,* Vol. 9. New York: Raven Press, 1986:31.

1063. Kalra SP, Allen LG, Sahu A, Kalra PS, Crowley WR. Gonadal steroids and neuropeptide Y-opioid–LHRH axis. *J Steroid Biochem* 1988;30:185.

1064. Lind RW, Swanson W. Evidence for corticotropin releasing factor and leu-enkephalin in the neural projection from the lateral parabrachial nucleus to the median preoptic nucleus: a retrograde transport, immunohistochemical double labeling study in the rat. *Brain Res* 1984;321:217.

1065. Simerly RB, Swanson LW, Gorski RA. The cells of origin of a sexually dimorphic serotonergic input to the medial preoptic nucleus of the rat. *Brain Res* 1984;324:185.

1066. Page RB. Hypothalamic control of anterior pituitary function: surgical implications. In: Wilkins R, Rengachary S, eds. *Neurosurgery.* New York: McGraw-Hill, 1985:791.

1067. Page RB. The pituitary portal system. In: Pfaff D, Ganten D, eds. *Current topics in neuroendocrinology,* Vol. 7. New York: Springer-Verlag, 1986:1.

1068. Farquhar MG. Membrane traffic in prolactin and other secretory cells. In: MacLeod RM, Thorner MO, Seapagnini U, eds. *Prolactin, basic and clinical correlates.* Padova: Liviana Press, 1985:3:16.

1069. Swanson LW, Sawchenko PE. Paraventricular nucleus: a site for the integration of neuroendocrine and autonomic mechanisms. *Neuroendocrinology* 1980;31:410.

The Physiology of Reproduction, Second Edition,
edited by E. Knobil and J.D. Neill,
Raven Press, Ltd., New York © 1994.

CHAPTER 27

Role of Classic and Peptide Neuromediators in the Neuroendocrine Regulation of Luteinizing Hormone and Prolactin

Claude Kordon[1], Sophia V. Drouva[1], Gonzalo Martinez de la Escalera[2], and Richard I. Weiner[3]

[1] INSERM U-159, Dynamique des systèmes neuroendocriniens, 2ter rue d'Alésia, 75014-Paris, France
[2] Instituto de Investigaciones Biomedicas, Departmento de Fisiologia, Universidad Nacional Autonoma de Mexico, Mexico
[3] Reproductive Endocrinology Center, University of California, San Francisco, San Francisco, California 94143

This chapter attempts to review the extensive literature on the role of neuromediators (i.e., monoamines and peptides) in the regulation of luteinizing hormone (LH) and prolactin (PRL) secretion. The neurotransmitters derived from single or double amino acids include norepinephrine, epinephrine, dopamine, serotonin, histamine, γ-aminobutyric acid (GABA), and excitatory amino acids, in particular glutamate. Peptides to be reviewed include somatostatin, gonadotropin-releasing hormone (GnRH), tachykinins, neurotensin, atrial natriuretic factor, neuropeptide Y (NPY), peptide YY (PYY), pancreatic peptide, galanin, oxytocin, vasopressin, thyrotropin-releasing hormone (TRH), corticotropin-releasing factor (CRF), cholecystokinins, angiotensin II, bradykinin, endothelins, bombesin, vasoactive intestinal polypeptide (VIP), peptide histidine isoleucine (PHI), gastrin inhibitory peptide (GIP), glucagon, growth hormone-releasing hormone (GHRH), pituitary adenylate cyclase-activating peptide (PACAP), and opioid peptides. Hormonal actions of cytokines, that is, peptides mainly synthesized by immune cells, but also present in the hypothalamus and the pituitary, will be reviewed as well. This chapter will summarize our knowledge on the action of neuromediators that encode neural information essential for neuroendocrine integration of the activity of neurosecretory neurons regulating LH and PRL secretion.

At this point it is worth briefly considering the potential strengths and weaknesses of various general approaches that have been employed. The most important developments in our understanding of neuroendocrine regulation had come from new cellular and molecular techniques. Since the first edition of this chapter molecular biological techniques have been increasingly applied to study neuroendocrine function. Many of the genes for neuromediator receptors, neuropeptides, enzymes involved in peptide processing and neurotransmitter synthesis, ion channels, and cell adhesion molecules have been cloned. Structural analysis of protein sequencing has yielded numerous insights into the function of the peptides. Techniques for quickly producing large amounts of peptide from cloned genes has permitted the production of specific monoclonal antibodies. Easy availability of riboprobes for in situ hybridization studies also has helped in further understanding the cytoarchitecture of the brain as well as the study of the regulation of the expression of genes in neural tissue. The applications of molecular techniques to produce cell lines for study of regulation of transcription, peptide processing, and peptide release also has been important. For the first time potential questions concerning neuroendocrine regulation can be answered by using a powerful reductionist approach rather than the lethargy of conclusions reached from perilously stacked correlations.

Clearly the further understanding of neuroendocrine control rests firmly on the rapidly evolving fabric of neuroanatomy. For the most part, the topography of the neurosecretory neurons has been carefully described, while studies regarding neuromediator-containing neurons are still under way. Techniques for the double staining of the contents of neuronal processes at the light- and electron-microscopic level have begun to furnish us with insights into the layered patchwork of neuroendocrine integration. For example, it is clear that GABA-containing axonal terminals directly synapse on GnRH-containing neurons in rodents (1), as do opioid neurons in primates (2). These techniques, in conjunction with anterograde and retrograde staining of the projections of neurons, offer us considerable promise that we will shortly know (a) the major projections to the neurosecretory neurons and (b) the identity of neuromediators involved. Information concerning anatomical connections must be integrated with data on the receptors involved in mediating (a) the action of the neuromediators and (b) the activity patterns of the neurons. The recent cloning of receptors and the availability of antibodies to the receptors should permit localization of receptors on identified neurons. In some instances, considerable neurochemical data are available concerning discrete regional changes in the metabolism or release of neuromediators that reflect changes in activity of the neurons. If the density of neuronal processes and the duration of these signals are sufficient, then these techniques are of value. In this regard, the activity of norepinephrine (NE)-containing neurons in the hypothalamus has been extensively characterized in microdissected brain regions during the estrous cycle of the rat (3).

Techniques such as microdialysis probes may offer further promise in monitoring ongoing neuromediator release. However, this technique is also constrained by the time it takes to obtain samples, minutes rather than seconds. An additional problem is the elimination of artifacts due to local tissue damage around the probe. A well-used approach for evaluating the activity of various neuromediators has been the use of pharmacological agents that potentiate or inhibit the action of these neuromediators. This approach was pioneered by the work of Sawyer and colleagues (4) in studying the regulation of ovulation. However, each drug involves many potential problems, including the specificity of its action and the realization that observed physiological effects represent the summation of actions at multiple sites. These considerations are particularly worrisome when studying small numbers of neurons that contain a neuromediator and project to much of the brain, for example, norepinephrine (5,6). Also, it is clear that multiple receptors are involved in mediating the action of the neuromediators, and therefore highly specific pharmacological agents are necessary to design meaningful experiments; norepinephrine injected into the third ventricle likely acts at several sites in the hypothalamus, possibly each mediated by different adrenergic receptors. Further complicating this issue is the possibility that a neuron may express sufficient receptors for the same transmitter on dendrites and terminals.

Recently highly differential immortalized GnRH cell lines have been developed by genetically targeted tumorigenesis in transgenic mice (7). Expression of a potent oncogene, SV40 T-antigen, was targeted to GnRH neurons using the promoter enhancer elements of the GnRH gene. A tumor was obtained in the preoptic area of a founder mouse which was placed in culture and clonal cell lines obtained (GT1 cells). GT1 cells express only neuronal and not glial markers (7). The GnRH gene is expressed at high levels and processed to form GnRH and GnRH associated peptide as well as 9-hyp GnRH, the second endogenous gonadotropin-releasing hormone (8,9). GnRH is released in response to depolarization with K+ or veratridine. The cells have been shown to contain numerous receptors for neuromediators which affect GnRH secretion. These will be discussed in relevant sections. In addition, the GT1 cells contain the heterotrimeric G proteins involved in the coupling-secretion mechanisms, which implicate adenylate-cyclase, phospholipase C, calcium as well as potassium voltage-sensitive channel activity (10). Most excitingly when large numbers of GT1 cells are cultured on coverslips or glass beads and placed in perfusion it was shown that the cells release GnRH in a pulsatile fashion. The pulse frequency observed was approximately 25 minutes (11–13). The frequency of GnRH pulses in castrated rats is approximately 30 minutes (14). Therefore either individual or networks of GnRH neurons are the pulse generator. To obtain regulated pulsatile release the cell must contain a timing mechanism as well as a means for synchronization of release from neighboring cells. It is obvious that these cells represent an important model to study what neuromediators regulate GnRH and the signaling mechanisms involved. However, we must always keep in mind that receptors expressed on GT1 cells may be a consequence of transformation. Furthermore, neurosecretory cells without intact afferent inputs may not express receptors normally seen under physiological conditions.

The approach of generating highly differentiated cells may yield additional tools for studying the complexity of neuroendocrine regulation. Glial cells have been immortalized (15) as well as brain catecholaminergic neurons (16). Therefore cultures of multiple cell types may permit further understanding of afferent inputs and cell to cell interactions involved in regulation of the neurosecretory neurons.

Finally, the understanding of the coding of this complex neurochemical information into some integrated effect on the activity of neurosecretory neurons is essential. Neuromediators can generally be thought of as acting as neurotransmitters or neuromodulators, that is, respectively affecting the resting potential of target neurons or altering the responsiveness of the target neurons without affecting the resting potential. It is clear that multiple systems are simultaneously involved in coding information and that the intensity, duration, and sequence of these signals play important roles in this so-called "pleotropic regulation." Advances in electrophysiological techniques, that is, patch clamping in conjunction with the availability of highly differentiated cell lines with advances in cell culture techniques, open new approaches to unraveling these questions.

CATECHOLAMINES

We will not attempt to review the extensive literature in this area accumulated over the past 35 years. Several previous reviews have made this attempt (4,17–21). The diversity of models studied, the use of drugs with questionable specificity, and the complexities of the neuroanatomical organization render much of the literature contradictory and difficult to interpret. Instead we will highlight experiments that have yielded interpretable data that support a series of supportable hypotheses.

Neuroanatomy of Catecholaminergic Neurons

Anatomy of Noradrenergic Neurons

Noradrenergic innervation of the hypothalamus is extrinsic, as demonstrated by the dramatic decline in norepinephrine content following surgical isolation of the medial basal hypothalamus (22,23). Norepinephrine-containing terminals have a wide, but uneven, distribution throughout the hypothalamus (24). Terminals in the hypothalamus are projections from cell bodies in the brainstem first described by Dahlstrom and Fuxe (25) and termed A1, A2, A3–5, A6, and A7. A1 cell bodies are located in the caudal ventrolateral medulla, A2 cell bodies are in the caudal nucleus of the solitary tract, A5 cell bodies are in the ventrolateral corner of the pons, A6 cell bodies are in the locus coeruleus, and A7 cell bodies are in the mesencephalic reticular formation. Fibers from these neurons project to the hypothalamus via several pathways. The major projection to the hypothalamus is via the ventral bundle, which receives fibers from all the noradrenergic cell groups but predominantly A6. The dorsal noradrenergic bundle is composed mainly of fibers from the locus coeruleus, and it innervates the dorsal hypothalamic nuclei. The best characterized hypothalamic region receiving noradrenergic innervation is the paraventricular nucleus (PVN). Approximately 70% of the noradrenergic innervation of the PVN arises from A1 cell bodies, 20% arises from the A2 cell bodies, and the balance arises from the locus coeruleus (26). Noradrenergic projections to the preoptic area also appear to exclusively arise from A1 and A2 cell bodies (27). Axon terminals containing dopamine β-hydroxylase, which is present in both noradrenergic and adrenergic neurons, were shown to end in close proximity to GnRH-containing neurons in the preoptic area (28). Studies with GT1 GnRH cells have shown that the cells express β_1-adrenergic receptors, which are positively coupled to adenylate cyclase (29,30). Where the receptors are localized on the GT1 cells is not clear, i.e., dendrites, cell bodies, or axons. *In vitro* ultrastructural studies were not able to demonstrate any synaptic specializations between norepinephrine- and GnRH-containing neurons (31). However, noradrenergic neurons appeared to form synapses with GABA neurons in the region. Furthermore, the action of catecholamine-containing neurons appears to be mediated in the central nervous system, in part by so-called nonsynaptic interactions (32). The anatomical data leave one with conflicting views concerning the noradrenergic innervation of the hypothalamus. The majority of findings support a system in which several thousand neurons have a global integrative function and make synaptic contact with every region of the neuroaxis. The small number of neurons, their vast terminal projections, and the lack of discrete postsynaptic specializations support this notion. However, a second level of organization could exist within specific groups of noradrenergic neurons that either receive discrete afferent inputs, project to defined areas of the brain, or terminate on neurons whose postsynaptic receptors determine the response (26). We will attempt to discuss these possibilities when reviewing evidence for the role of noradrenergic neurons in gonadotropin and prolactin regulation.

Anatomy of Adrenergic Neurons

Separate groups of adrenergic cell bodies have been identified: the C1 group in the rostral ventrolateral medulla, the C2 group in the rostromedial part of the nucleus of the solitary tract, and the C3 group in the rostromedial medulla (33,34). The pathway by which fibers reach the hypothalamus is not clear, although they do not appear to run in the ventral noradrenergic bundle as first believed (6). High concentrations of epinephrine (E) are found in the dorsomedial, paraventricular, periventricular, arcuate, and supraoptic nuclei (35). Some evidence for selectivity of adrenergic versus noradrenergic innervation exists, since in the paraventricular nucleus the parvicellular region receives both types of terminals, while the magnocellular region receives mainly noradrenergic terminals (36).

Anatomy of Dopaminergic Neurons

Dopamine (DA)-containing neurons that innervate the hypothalamus have their cell bodies concentrated in four brain regions: the so-called A11, A12, A13, and A14 cell groups. The largest group of neurons is the A12 or tuberoinfundibular neurons (37), which constitute 3% to 5% of the cell bodies of the arcuate nucleus (6). The terminals of these neurons are found in the median eminence in close apposition to the primary capillaries of the hypophyseal portal plexus. These neurons function as neurosecretory neurons releasing large amounts of DA into portal blood (38) and play a central role in the regulation of PRL (19). The regulation of the A12 DA-containing neurons is discussed in detail in Chapter 33.

The function of these neurons in the control of the release of GnRH has been repeatedly proposed. Numerous authors have suggested that these interactions would occur via nonsynaptic axoaxonal interactions in the median eminence. We observed few, if any, D_2 dopamine receptors in the bovine stalk median eminence (39). In agreement with the findings in bovine tissue, there were relatively few dopaminergic sites labeled by [^{3}H]-spiroperidol in the median eminence of the rat (40). However, there were significant numbers of dopaminergic sites labeled with the D_1 ligand [^{3}H]ADTN. Interestingly GT1 cells express D_1 dopamine receptors positively coupled to adenylate cyclase (30,41). No studies have determined the localization of the receptors on the cells. Therefore the possibility exists that DA may act through D_1 rather than D_2 receptors possibly in the median eminence via receptors or nerve terminals. Therefore the A12 neurosecretory neuronal system which is tonically active in the suppression of PRL secretion may also be involved in the regulation of LH.

Neurons with their cell bodies in the caudal thalamus, posterior hypothalamic area, and the medial zona incerta (A1 and A3) project periventricularly in the dorsal part of the hypothalamus (41). The A14 cell group, located more rostrally in the anterior periventricular nucleus, projects to the preoptic nucleus (43). Interestingly, synaptic contacts have been described in this area between GnRH- and possibly DA-containing neurons (31). These intrahypothalamic dopaminergic pathways are scattered, which has made it difficult to study their role in the regulation of LH and prolactin secretion.

Role of Catecholaminergic Neurons in the Control of Luteinizing Hormone Secretion

Pulsatile Luteinizing Hormone Release

In ovariectomized animals, frequent large-amplitude LH pulses are observed. Several lines of evidence have shown that pulses of LH secretion are driven by the pulsatile release of GnRH. Therefore, ovariectomized animals have frequently been used to determine if a neurotransmitter is involved in the regulation of the so-called GnRH pulse generator. Inhibition of noradrenergic activity by inhibition of NE synthesis (44–46), blockade of α-adrenergic receptors (47), or destruction of the ventral noradrenergic bundle with 6-hydroxydopamine (48) all result in suppression of pulsatile LH release in the ovariectomized rat. Blockade of β-adrenergic receptors with propranolol had no effect (47). In ovariectomized monkeys, blockade of α-receptors with phenoxybenzamine and phentolamine inhibited pulsatile LH release, whereas treatment with propranolol was ineffective (49). That the stimulatory action of NE is mediated via α-receptors was supported by the observations that administration of the α_1-agonist clonidine overrode the blockade of pulsatile LH release caused by treatment with the NE synthesis inhibitor FLA-63 (50). Although clonidine is generally thought of as an α_2-agonist, sufficient dose and pharmacological manipulations were not performed to determine the subclass of α-receptors involved in mediation of this response. It does not appear that E-containing neurons are involved in regulation of pulsatile LH release, since specific inhibition of E synthesis did not affect pulsatile release (51). However, it is impossible to be certain that α-adrenergic antagonists, which inhibit pulsatile LH release, are not partly blocking the action of E as well as NE.

Although observations in which endogenous noradrenergic activity is blocked are consistent with an ongoing stimulatory action of noradrenergic neurons on pulsatile LH release, the administration of NE into the third ventricle causes inhibition (52). Intraventricular administration of NE predominantly inhibits LH pulse frequency (53), an action mediated at least partly at sites in the medial preoptic area (54). This action of administered NE was not affected by the simultaneous administration of serotonin or DA antagonists (53). Furthermore, electrical stimulation of the major ascending noradrenergic pathway also inhibits pulsatile LH release in ovariectomized rats (55). These observations, rather than a demonstration that noradrenergic neurons are normally involved in mediating pulsatile LH release, only show that there are adrenergic receptors on some neuronal element, which, when activated, inhibit pulsatile LH release. It does not appear that dopaminergic neurons are involved in pulsatile LH release in ovariectomized rats, since blockade of DA receptors with specific antagonists has no effect (45,47,56). However, if DA agonists are administered via the third ventricle, pulsatile LH release is inhibited (45,46,56). The effects of the DA agonists can be reversed by administration of DA antagonists (45).

In GT1 cells norepinephrine stimulates GnRH release in a dose-dependent fashion (29). Surprisingly the receptor mediating the action of norepinephrine is a β_1-adrenergic receptor coupled to adenylate cyclase. The β-agonist isoproterenol mimics the action of norepinephrine and its effect was blocked by specific β_1-antagonist CGP 20712A. α-Adrenergic agonists and antagonists had no effect on GnRH release. The presence of β_1-adrenergic receptor was demonstrated by ligand binding (30) and in RNA analysis by Northern blots (29). Potentially the stimulatory action on GnRH may be mediated at multiple levels. The predominant action could be via α_1 receptors, which inhibit an inhibitory GABA input to GnRH cells in the animal and a secondary action directly on GnRH neurons via β_1-adrenergic receptor.

In conclusion, in the absence of steroid feedback it appears that noradrenergic neurons are involved in the stimulation of pulsatile LH release. The release of NE in the medial preoptic nucleus, as measured via push-pull cannulae, is pulsatile; however, there is a lack of correlation between the pulses of NE and LH (57). This action of NE is mediated via adrenergic receptors, although it is unclear whether α_1- or α_2-receptors are involved. Neither E- nor DA-containing neurons appear to play a role in regulation of pulsatile LH release. A question still to be answered is the site(s) on which the α-adrenergic receptors are located. Noradrenergic neurons do not appear to be the pulse generator in rats or in monkeys. Complete deafferentation of the hypothalamus destroys all of the noradrenergic neurons innervating the circumscribed region, since the cell bodies of the noradrenergic neurons are outside the island. This procedure does not block pulsatile LH release in the rhesus monkey (58).

Ovulatory Surge of Luteinizing Hormone

To consider the question of the role of catecholamine-containing neurons in regulation of the ovulatory surge of LH, a logical first step is to summarize the actions of gonadal steroids on activity of these neurons. It is clear that the major signals for the synchronization of the ovulatory surge are the positive and negative feedback actions of estradiol (E_2) and progesterone. In ovariectomized rats the implantation of E_2-filled Silastic capsules results in ovulatorylike LH surges every 24 hours. Associated with the LH surge, the turnover rate (an index of neuronal activity) of NE increased in the medial preoptic, arcuate, and suprachiasmatic nuclei and median eminence (59). Furthermore, an increase in the episodic release of NE was measured via push-pull cannulae in the medial preoptic area from the morning to the afternoon of the LH surge (60). In animals treated with E_2 plus progesterone, the LH surge was advanced, as was the increase in NE turnover rate (59). These observations are in close agreement with findings in cycling rats. An increase in the turnover rate of NE occurs in the same hypothalamic areas around the time of the ovulatory surge of LH on the afternoon of proestrus (3). No changes in NE turnover rate were seen in these areas on the afternoon of diestrous day 1.

Relative to the negative feedback action of E_2, the turnover rate of NE in a large preoptic area fragment increased 3 days postovariectomy (61). Three hours following the administration of E_2, the NE turnover rate was suppressed in the preoptic area and median eminence. In another study utilizing a more precise dissection, the NE turnover rate was only observed to decrease in the periventricular nucleus 3 hours after treatment with E_2 (62). Estradiol administration for 3 hours also decreased the release rate of NE collected via a push-pull cannula implanted in the medial basal hypothalamus (57).

The action of estrogen on NE turnover could be mediated directly on the noradrenergic neurons, since they appear to contain estrogen receptors (63). However, the possibility also exists that the steroid effect on noradrenergic activity could be mediated through opiate or GABA-containing interneurons that contain steroid receptors. These interactions are discussed later in the chapter. The turnover rate of E-containing neurons also appears to increase in some areas of the hypothalamus simultaneous with the ovulatory surge of LH. Increases in E turnover were observed in the medial basal hypothalamus (64) or the medial preoptic area (65) on the afternoon of proestrus. Increases in E turnover were also reported in the medial basal hypothalamus following E_2-plus-progesterone-induced LH surges (66). However, one group was unable to measure a change in E turnover in the medial preoptic nucleus on the afternoon of proestrus (3). Discrepancies in these findings could be due to the difficulty in measuring the relatively low levels of E in these areas. Data on effects of ovarian steroids on the number and affinity of α- and β-adrenergic receptors in the hypothalamus are not extensive. No changes in hypothalamic β-adrenergic receptors were seen throughout the estrous cycle of the rat (67). However, treatment of ovariectomized rats with E_2 (or E_2 plus progesterone) increased the number of receptors. No changes were seen in the number of α-adrenergic receptors labeled with [^{3}H]dihydroergocryptine either during the estrous cycle or following steroid treatment of ovariectomized rats (67). The significance of effects of ovarian steroids on the activity of dopaminergic neurons is less clear than with noradrenergic neurons. Changes in the activity of the tuberoinfundibular DA neurons are closely coupled to the secretion of PRL. Estrogen treatment increases PRL levels; PRL, in turn, increases the turnover of the dopaminergic neurons (68). However, dopaminergic cell bodies in the arcuate nucleus contain E_2 receptors (69,70), and E_2 (or E_2 plus progesterone) could affect the activity of these neurons directly (71). In the rat the turnover rate of DA in the median eminence and arcuate nucleus increases on the afternoon of proestrus between 12:00 p.m. and 2:00 p.m. and then decreases between 3:00 p.m. and 5:00 p.m. (3). No change is seen in dopaminergic activity in the medial preoptic nucleus at that time. In ovariectomized rats in which LH surges were induced with E_2 plus progesterone, no changes in DA turnover rate were seen in the arcuate and medial preoptic nuclei and median eminence from morning to afternoon (59). Ovariectomy had little effect on the turnover of DA in several hypothalamic areas (60). Estradiol administration for 3 hours caused a small, but statistically significant, decrease in DA turnover in the preoptic area (60) and median eminence (61) and an increase in the medial basal hypothalamus (60).

There is extensive literature regarding the effect of catecholaminergic agents on (a) the ovulatory surge of LH on proestrus and (b) estrogen (or estrogen plus progesterone)-induced LH surges. The literature has followed the trail blazed in 1950 by Sawyer and colleagues (72), who showed that adrenergic antagonists would block ovulation in the rat (72). The studies have been refined over the years by our increasing knowledge concerning hormonal changes during the periovulatory period and the use of more specific pharmacological agents. Clearly, noradrenergic and adrenergic neurons are involved in the generation of the ovulatory LH surge in the rat. Drugs that inhibit catecholamine synthesis [e.g., α-methyl-*p*-tyrosine (α-MPT)] or NE and E synthesis [e.g., diethyldithiocarbamate (DDC)] inhibit the ovulatory surge of LH (73–75). Blockade of α-adrenergic receptors also interrupts ovulation (72,76). The α_1-subtype selective antagonist prazosin was capable of inhibiting the ovulatory surge of LH, whereas the α_2-antagonist piperoxane was ineffective (75). Destruction of the ventral noradrenergic bundle by the neurotoxin 6-hydroxydopamine (77) or by surgical transection (74) caused only a temporary interruption of ovulation. The return of ovulation was surprising, considering the 83%

decrease seen in the NE content of the hypothalamus following surgical transection (74). The development of denervation supersensitivity or the possible sparing of E-containing neurons can only partially explain the return of function post-surgery, since treatment of these animals with DDC was found to block ovulation only 40% of the time (74). This finding supports the existence of multiple control mechanisms for ovulation, thereby allowing other systems to compensate for the loss of noradrenergic regulation.

Similarly, blockade of catecholamine synthesis with αMPT or NE and E synthesis with DDC (78) or FLA-63 (66), also inhibits E_2-plus-progesterone-induced LH surges. The inhibitory effects of these agents could be reversed by the simultaneous repletion of NE and E with dihydroxyphenylserine. Blockade of α-adrenergic receptors, but not β-adrenergic receptors, also inhibited the steroid-induced LH surges (78,79). The receptors mediating this response appear to be α_1-receptors, since the α_1-selective antagonist prazosin was more effective than the α_2-selective antagonist yohimbine (79).

On close inspection it is difficult to separate whether drugs affecting the ovulatory surge of LH work through NE- or E-containing neurons or both. Both the actions of NE and E are mediated via α- and β-adrenergic receptors, with only small differences in their potency at these receptors. Previously, catecholamine synthesis inhibitors that were used (i.e., DDC and FLA-63) had been found to deplete both NE and E, since they inhibited the activity of dopamine β-hydroxylase. With the advent of relatively specific inhibitors of phenylethanolamine *N*-methyltransferase (PNMT), which selectively depletes E, this question has been restudied. Several laboratories have shown that inhibition of E synthesis will block the ovulatory surge of LH (75,80). These findings are difficult to assess because several of the drugs used to inhibit E synthesis also have α-adrenergic blocking properties, for example, SKF 64139 and LY 7835 (81). Furthermore, treatment with LY134046, an E synthesis inhibitor that has no antagonist activity, was not capable of inhibiting ovulation (81). The drug was ineffective when given for 1 or 5 days even though the long-term treatment resulted in a 95% depletion of E in the medial preoptic nucleus. Unfortunately no assessment of LH levels was made in this study. LH levels could have been partially suppressed without affecting ovulation. In animals treated with E_2 plus progesterone to induce an LH surge, both the less specific PNMT inhibitors LY 78335 and SKF 64139 (66,82) as well as the one without α-antagonist properties, SKF 83593 (51), blocked the induced LH surge. In numerous studies the effects of NE and E have been studied *in vivo* by intraventricular administration to circumvent the blood-brain barrier. Previously we discussed the inhibitory actions of NE on pulsatile LH release in ovariectomized animals. However, when ovariectomized animals are primed with E_2 or E_2 plus progesterone for several days, NE and E administration stimulates LH release (52,83,84). Also, NE administration to estrogen-primed rabbits stimulates an ovulatory surge of LH (85). In rats in which ovulation was blocked with pentobarbitol E (but not NE) was able to induce ovulation (86). The mechanism by which steroid priming reverses the response to intraventricular catecholamines is not clear.

Consistent with the above findings, when NE is added to median eminence fragments from male rats *in vitro*, the release of LHRH is stimulated (87). The response is dose dependent and can be blocked by the α-adrenergic antagonist phentolamine. The stimulatory action of NE appears to be mediated by α_2-receptors, since it is blocked by yohimbine but not prazosin (88). The response to NE is not blocked by DA or β-adrenergic antagonists. These findings are of interest because a large number of α_2-adrenergic receptors have been described in the median eminence (39). The physiological role of these α_2-adrenergic receptors in the control of LHRH release from nerve terminals in the median eminence is unclear, since the limited data with subtype-selective drugs support the idea that the stimulatory role of NE or E in the ovulatory surge or pulsatile release of LH is mediated by α_1-adrenergic receptors (75,79).

The data we have summarized strongly support the concept that NE- and E-containing neurons are involved in the stimulation of the ovulatory surge of LH in rodents. The action appears to be mediated via α_1-adrenergic receptors most likely located in the medial preoptic area. Studies from GT1 cells suggest that a secondary component of the stimulation could be mediated via β_1-adrenergic receptors on GnRH neurons. Clearly there is an increase in noradrenergic neuronal activity in this area on the afternoon of proestrus. However, in primates there are little data that support a role for noradrenergic pathways in the regulation of ovulation, since normal menstrual cycles are seen in monkeys with complete deafferentation of the medial basal hypothalamus (58,89).

Before concluding the discussion regarding the role of NE and E on LH release, it is of interest to review data suggesting that NE can inhibit LH release via β-adrenergic receptors (21). Electrical stimulation of the noradrenergic neurons of the locus coeruleus inhibits the LH surge on proestrus (90). This inhibition could be blocked by the local injection in the premammillary nuclei of the β-adrenergic blocker propranolol but not the α-adrenergic antagonist phenoxybenzamine (91). Intraventricular injection of the β-agonist isoproterenol was also capable of inhibiting the steroid-induced LH surge (92). Furthermore, the release of LH induced by administration of NE to steroid-primed rats was potentiated by pretreating the animals with propranolol (93). Interestingly, a recent study showed that not only intraventricular administration of NE or isoproterenol but also two α-adrenergic agonists phenylephrine and methoxamine inhibited LH release when administered after the initiation of steroid-induced LH surges (94).

These data clearly show that NE can inhibit LH release. However, as with the inhibitory effect of NE seen on pulsatile LH in ovariectomized rats, none of these inhibitory effects were seen during the normal regulation of LH. These effects are only seen after electrical stimulation of noradrenergic pathways or the intraventricular administration of NE or related agonists. In fact, in every instance when the β-antagonist propranolol was given to ovariectomized, proestrous, or steroid-treated ovariectomized rats, not only did it not interfere with LH release but it also did not potentiate it. Therefore, inhibition of LH secretion, by NE via β-adrenergic neurons, does not appear to occur during these physiological states. The physiological function of what appears to be a distinct inhibitory noradrenergic pathway is yet to be elucidated. The presence of a stimulatory β_1 receptor on GnRH neurons could make it difficult to observe the inhibitory action of NE mediated via β-adrenergic receptors of different sites of posterior hypothalamus.

The role of DA-containing neurons in the regulation of the ovulatory surge of LH is controversial (4,19). The administration of the relatively specific DA antagonist pimozide on the morning of proestrus greatly reduced the afternoon LH surge (93). Effects of less specific DA antagonists (e.g., haloperidol and chlorpromazine), which have significant α-adrenergic antagonist properties, will not be discussed. Pimozide treatment for 2 days before or after the expected midcycle surge of LH in women also reduced the LH levels (95). Consistent with a stimulatory role of DA on LH release, the intraventricular administration of DA to proestrous rats was reported to increase LH levels (96). Both the intraventricular administration of DA and the DA agonist apomorphine stimulated LH secretion in ovariectomized steroid primed rats (97). However, other laboratories have seen no effect on LH after the administration of DA to E_2- or E_2-plus-progesterone-primed rats (42,83,98).

Intravenous infusion of DA to women causes a significant decrease in resting LH levels only around midcycle (99). This finding suggests that DA is acting at the level of the median eminence, since DA does not cross the blood-brain barrier and does not act directly on the gonadotrophs. Apomorphine administration had no effect on LH secretion in humans (100).

In vitro studies have also given conflicting results. Most recently, perifusion with DA was shown to increase GnRH release from medial basal hypothalamic fragments from male rats (101). However, the effect was blocked by the α-adrenergic antagonist phentolamine but not the DA antagonist pimozide. DA was shown not to be acting by uptake and conversion to NE, since it worked in the presence of DDC. However, DA treatment was shown to displace NE from terminals in the median eminence. This study demonstrates the difficulty in interpreting studies following administration of exogenous amines. Incubation with DA has previously been reported to inhibit GnRH release from median eminence fragments (88). However, in these studies, treatment with pimozide inhibited the action of DA. Studies on the GT1 GnRH cell lines have not helped to clarify data obtained from animal studies. As mentioned GnRH-GT1 cells expresses D_1 dopamine receptors positively coupled to adenylate cyclase (30,41). Dopamine stimulates the release of GnRH from GT1 cells in a dose dependent fashion. The specific DA agonist SKF 38393 mimics the action of DA on GnRH release and the effect is inhibited by the specific D_1 antagonist SCH 23390. These findings now need to be confirmed in animal studies in which specific D_1 dopamine agonist and antagonist are administered to regions containing GnRH neurons.

In conclusion, there are changes in the activity of dopaminergic neurons correlated with the estrous cycle of the rat. Clearly, changes in the activity of the tuberoinfundibular neurons will directly affect the secretion of PRL through DA receptors on lactotrophs. However, that these neurons play an important role in the regulation of the ovulatory surge or pulsatile release of LH in ovariectomized animals is unclear. Findings in GT1 cells suggest that difficulties in understanding the action of DA could be due to effects at multiple sites from anatomically distinct populations of dopaminergic neurons mediated by multiple receptors.

Role of Catecholamines in the Control of Prolactin Secretion

Unlike LH secretion, the secretion of PRL is under tonic inhibitory control by the hypothalamic hormone DA (102). Prolactin secretion appears to be regulated by inhibition of DA release and/or the release of PRL-releasing factors. Although the identity of the PRL-releasing factors is unknown, there are experimental data supporting this role for VIP and TRH. In the rat, changes in PRL secretion include a large surge on the afternoon of proestrus just preceding the LH surge, nocturnal increases during pregnancy, diurnal changes, and stress-induced release and suckling-induced release during lactation (103). In primates there is no increase in PRL secretion associated with the midcycle surge of LH. During the night, irregular episodes of PRL secretion are observed which may or may not be correlated with stages of sleep (104). In all mammals, suckling induces large increases in PRL secretion. There is not a great deal of evidence describing the role of brain catecholamines in the neural regulation of PRL secretion, although the catecholamine DA is the major hypothalamic hormone regulating PRL secretion. Norepinephrine-containing neurons appear to play an important role in the regulation of PRL secretion under a variety of physiological conditions.

Dopaminergic Neurons

The tuberoinfundibular DA neurons are neurosecretory neurons that are responsible for the production of high levels of DA in the hypophyseal portal blood (38). The discussion of the regulation of these neurons and their role in the regulation of PRL secretion from lactotrophs are covered in detail in Chapter 33.

Noradrenergic Neurons

Basal PRL secretion is pulsatile in nature. The administration of the NE- and E-synthesis inhibitor DDC completely inhibited pulsatile PRL secretion in ovariectomized rats (105). However, in male rats, treatment with the NE- and E-synthesis inhibitor FLA-63 had no effect on pulsatile or basal PRL release (106).

Administration of the α-adrenergic antagonist phenoxybenzamine in high doses to ovariectomized rats treated with E_2 was found to stimulate PRL release, whereas phentolamine had no effect (107). However, administration of both phentolamine and phenoxybenzamine to ovariectomized monkeys stimulated PRL release (108). In male rats (109,110) and male monkeys (111) the administration of the α_2-adrenergic blocker, yohimbine, stimulated basal levels of PRL. However, no effect of yohimbine was observed on basal PRL levels in men (112). Stimulation of PRL secretion by yohimbine was reversed by the administration of the α_2-agonist clonidine (109,111).

These data on the role of noradrenergic neurons in the regulation of basal PRL secretion are paradoxical. Inhibition of the synthesis of NE inhibits pulsatile PRL release, whereas blockade of α_2-adrenergic receptors increases basal PRL secretion. One possible explanation is that pulsatile PRL secretion is controlled by neurosecretory neurons receiving a stimulatory noradrenergic innervation mediated via α_1-adrenergic neurons, whereas basal PRL secretion is controlled by separate neurosecretory neurons receiving a noradrenergic input mediated via α_2-adrenergic receptors. Clearly, multiple inhibitory and stimulatory neurosecretory neuronal systems that regulate PRL have been described. One note of caution in terms of the importance of a noradrenergic innervation on basal PRL secretion comes from findings with complete deafferentated female rats. Complete deafferentation, which destroys all of the noradrenergic input to the medial basal hypothalamus, does not elevate basal PRL levels (113,114).

The surge in PRL on the afternoon of proestrus can be inhibited by the injection of the neurotoxin 6-hydroxydopamine into the ventral noradrenergic tract (115). Afternoon surges in PRL induced by the treatment of ovariectomized rats with E_2 plus progesterone could be blocked by the NE- and E-synthesis inhibitor DDC (116). Estrogen-induced surges in ovariectomized animals were blocked by the α-adrenergic antagonists phenoxybenzamine and phentolamine but not by the β-adrenergic antagonist propranolol (117).

A noradrenergic pathway does not appear to be involved in the suckling-induced release of PRL. The synthesis of hypothalamic norepinephrine does not change following suckling (118), and the suckling-induced release of PRL is not affected by the blockade of NE and E synthesis with DDC (119).

The role of noradrenergic neurons in the stress-induced release of PRL has not been well studied; however, the data available suggest that blockade of noradrenergic activity with 6-hydroxydopamine and DDC blocked stress-induced prolactin release in rats. This area should be more carefully studied, since the cell bodies of two putative prolactin releasing factors, TRH and VIP, are located in the PVN nucleus, an area with a dense noradrenergic innervation (36). This area is also known to be involved in the control of the stress-induced release of adrenocorticotropic hormone (ACTH).

In conclusion, it appears that a stimulatory noradrenergic component is involved in the regulation of the afternoon surge of LH. The role of noradrenergic neurons in the regulation of basal PRL secretion is unclear and deserves further study. Existing data suggest that noradrenergic neurons are involved in the stress-induced release of PRL. Finally, no work has been done to determine that the observed effects were mediated via NE-containing neurons and not E-containing ones. This possibility should be clarified.

SEROTONIN

Anatomy of Serotonergic Neurons

The basic organization of the central serotonin [5-hydroxytryptamine (5-HT)] neuronal system consists of a population of brainstem neurons arising mainly from the midbrain raphe nuclei (120–122). Their axons project with a high degree of collaterization and multidirectionality to innervate most areas of the forebrain, with the hypothalamus receiving extensive innervation. Fibers mainly from the dorsal and median raphe nuclei project to the hypothalamus via the medial forebrain bundle, a dorsal raphe arcuate tract, and a dorsal raphe periventricular tract (123). Fibers may also originate from serotonergic cell bodies located within the hypothalamus, since total deafferentation of the hypothalamus does not completely deplete the rat hypothalamus of 5-HT (124). A group of cells in the pars ventralis of the nucleus dorsomedialis hypothalami has been shown to concentrate intraventricularly administered 5-HT (125, 126). Some caution should be taken in the interpretation of these results because both dopaminergic and noradrenergic neurons possess a low-affinity 5-HT uptake mechanism (127). Frankfurt and colleagues (128), using a specific anti-5-HT antiserum, failed to detect cell bodies containing 5-HT immunoreactivity in this area unless the rats were pretreated with L-tryptophan and pargyline, which stimulate 5-HT synthesis and inhibit 5-HT degradation, respectively. According to these authors, if there is indeed a serotonergic cell group present in the hypothalamus, its turnover of 5-HT is slow and its synthesis is limited by availability of substrate.

The arcuate nucleus receives a dense serotonergic innervation (120,121,129). There is a close approximation of 5-HT-containing fibers to dopaminergic cell bodies in the arcuate nucleus and in the medial zona incerta, which also provides dopaminergic input to the hypothalamus (130,131). Synaptic junctions between serotonergic terminals and cell bodies were observed (131). However, these synapses were infrequent, suggesting that 5-HT action is mediated via non-synaptic interactions.

There is extensive anatomical overlap in the distribution of GnRH- and serotonin-containing neurons in the hypothalamus. Close appositions of neuronal elements containing 5-HT and GnRH immunoreactivity were demonstrated in the septo-preoptic region (132) as well as in the median eminence and organum vasculosum of the lamina terminalis (133,134). Synaptic contacts between serotonergic terminals and immunoreactive GnRH elements were described in the medial preoptic area (135). Again, only a small percentage of terminals were seen in contact with immunoreactive GnRH neurons.

These 5-HT/DA and 5-HT/GnRH interactions provide a neuroanatomical basis for 5-HT neurons in the regulation of PRL and gonadotropin release. The final link in demonstrating the basis for these interactions is the localization of the receptors mediating the action of 5-HT. At present, four main types of 5-HT receptors have been identified in the brain, namely 5-HT$_1$, 5-HT$_2$, 5-HT$_3$ and 5-HT$_4$, and the 5-HT$_1$ has been further subclassified (136). The availability of subtype-selective agonists and antagonists will greatly improve the understanding of 5-HT involvement in neuroendocrine regulation.

Histofluorescent and immunocytochemical techniques have been utilized to identify endogenous 5-HT in the mammalian pituitary gland, although there is some disagreement as to its localization. Serotonin was reported to be present only in nerve terminals located in the intermediate lobe of the pituitary (137,138), in the posterior lobe (139), or in both the intermediate and posterior lobes of the pituitary (140,141). Westlund and Childs (142) also reported 5-HT in the anterior lobe in fine nerve fibers localized around major blood vessels and at the capsule of the gland.

In the anterior pituitary of submammalian vertebrates, the presence of 5-HT neurons is common (143,144), whereas in mammalian anterior pituitary, 5-HT appears to be mainly localized in secretory granules of gonadotrophs (140). The source of the endogenous 5-HT in gonadotrophs is still unclear. The presence of significant amounts of tryptophan hydroxylase (the rate-limiting enzyme in the synthesis of 5-HT) in the anterior pituitary may reflect de novo synthesis of 5-HT (145). Alternatively, the immunoreactive 5-HT in these cells may be the result of an uptake and accumulation of 5-HT synthesized elsewhere and delivered to these cells. Secretory granules of gonadotrophs become radioautographically labeled when exposed to low concentrations of exogenous [^{3}H]5-HT (146,147). Uptake is saturable and inhibited by the selective 5-HT uptake blocker fluoxitine (147).

Direct radioligand binding studies with [^{125}I]lysergic acid and indirect binding studies with cinanserin-displaced [^{3}H]spiperone binding have identified stereoselective, saturable, and high-affinity 5-HT-binding sites in the rat pituitary gland (148). As determined by quantitative light-microscopic autoradiography, the highest concentrations of the sites was found in the intermediate lobe, with progressively decreasing concentrations in the posterior and anterior lobes in pituitary.

Role of Serotonin in the Control of Prolactin Secretion

Serotonergic input was first implicated in the control of PRL release when the intraventricular infusion of 5-HT or its metabolites was observed to elevate plasma PRL in rats (149–151). The systemic administration of 5-hydroxytryptophan (5-HTP), the immediate precursor of 5-HT, also was effective in producing a rapid and pronounced increase in serum PRL in intact rats and in hypophysectomized rats with pituitary grafts under the kidney capsule (152). Since 5-HT was shown not to act directly at the pituitary to release PRL (153), these studies led to the belief that intraventricularly placed 5-HT or systemically administered 5-HP liberates a PRL-releasing factor. These studies must be interpreted with some caution because the direct infusion of 5-HT or its metabolites into the ventricule may not mimic the endogenous activation of 5-HT neurons and may not provide an accurate assessment of 5-HT as a physiological regulator of PRL (154). Additionally, 5-HTP administered at high doses can be taken up by catecholamine terminals, can become decarboxylated, and can displace the neurotransmitter present in the terminal (155).

The acute depletion of central 5-HT by *p*-chorophenylalanine (PCPA) treatment does not alter baseline PRL levels in castrated male rats (156) or in ovariectomized (157) or postpartum female rats (158). In normal male rats (159,160) or ovariectomized E_2-primed rats (161), PCPA treatment was accompanied by a marked reduction in baseline circulating PRL levels. Frequently used high doses of PCPA (>100 mg/kg body weight) may not selectively act on serotonergic neurons. Neutral amino acids, such as PCPA, can compete with tyrosine for uptake into catecholamine neurons (162). When PCPA was administered with desmethylimipramine (DMI), an inhibitor of uptake into catecholaminergic neurons, for the most part PCPA was without effect on baseline or stress-induced PRL release (160).

Whereas the involvement of 5-HT in the regulation of basal PRL secretion is unclear, more clear-cut findings have been obtained during episodes of stimulated PRL release. For example, suckling-induced pituitary PRL release in lactating rats almost certainly involves 5-HT. An acute blockade of 5-HT biosynthesis with PCPA can completely abolish the suckling-induced increase in circulating PRL (158). The blockade of 5-HT receptors with methysergide also inhibited the suckling-induced increase in PRL (157). The suckling-induced PRL release is accompanied by a rapid fall in hypothalamic 5-HT levels and a corresponding increase in its major metabolite, 5-hydroxyindoleacetic acid (5-HIAA) (163). Parisi and coworkers (164) demonstrated that the 5-HIAA increase during suckling occurs in the terminals in the rostral part of the anterior hypothalamic nucleus. These changes in hypothalamic 5-HT activity occur immediately after the onset of suckling and continue until the suckling stimulus is stopped (163). The 5-HT response to suckling does not occur when pups have been separated from their mother for over 24 hours (i.e., under weaning conditions). Prolactin is not released under these same conditions (163).

Other conditions of evoked PRL release also appear (at least in part) to be dependent upon central 5-HT activity. The PRL-releasing effects of ether (165) and restraint stress (166) are blocked in normal male rats pretreated with methysergide. Recently, not only methysergide, a mixed 5-HT_1 and 5-HT_2 receptor antagonists ketanserin and LY 53857 and the 5-HT_3 receptor antagonists ICS 205-930 and GR 38032 F were shown to inhibit or prevent restraint or ether stress-induced PRL release (167). Treating male rats with PCPA and/or electrolytic destruction of the midbrain raphe nuclei abolishes their diurnal and nocturnal PRL surges (168). The early pregnancy diurnal and nocturnal surges of PRL are also inhibited by 5-HT_2 antagonists ketanserin and LY 53857, although only diurnal surge is inhibited by the 5-HT synthesis inhibitor PCPA (169). The afternoon surge of PRL in proestrous rats is also inhibited by ketanserin (170). Electrolytic destruction of the dorsal raphe, but not of the median raphe nuclei, attenuates the E_2-induced afternoon PRL surge in female rats (171). Treatment with PCPA or ketanserin, a 5-HT antagonist, is also effective in blocking this PRL surge (171).

Thus, serotonergic neurons appear to be involved in the mediation of stimulated PRL release by activation of 5-HT_1, 5-HT_2 and 5-HT_3 receptors. The availability of subtype-selective serotonergic agents may expand this list. It was recently reported in male rats that the highly selective 5-HT_{1A} receptor agonists 8-hydroxy-2-(di-*n*-propylamino)tetralin and ipsapirone were more potent in stimulating PRL release than 5-HT_{1B} and 5-HT_{1C} receptor agonist 1-(*m*-trifluoromethylphenyl)piperazine (172).

In summary, 5-HT neurons appear to be important in the modulation of PRL secretory responses but not important in the control of basal PRL release. The mechanism(s) whereby 5-HT influences PRL secretion is still unclear, but, as mentioned previously, its site of action is not at the anterior pituitary. The incubation of anterior pituitary tissue with 5-HT (153,173) fails to alter PRL release. The effect of serotonin on PRL release has been linked to the modulation of inhibitory dopaminergic inputs to the pituitary. The 5-HT agonist, quipazine, increases serum PRL when administered to ovariectomized rats (174). Furthermore, the release of PRL induced by the 5-HT_{1A} agonist 8-hydroxy-2-(di-*n*-propylamino)tetralin in male rats is blocked by pretreatment with methysergide or bromocriptine (175). Concomitant with this increase is a decrease in the turnover rate of dopaminergic neurons. Furthermore, DA levels in hypophyseal portal blood were decreased in male rats receiving intraventricular 5-HT (176). However, when DA was infused intravenously into these rats, elevating the concentration of DA severalfold, 5-HT-induced PRL release was not prevented. This introduces an alternate explanation for the effects of 5-HT on PRL release, namely, that 5-HT directly liberates a PRL-releasing factor (PRF). Clemens and coworkers (177) found that pharmacological potentiation of serotonergic pathways always released considerably more PRL than did the removal of dopaminergic inhibition. These authors concluded that 5-HT releases PRL not by inhibiting dopaminergic neurons but rather by stimulating the liberation of PRF. The intermediate lobe of the rat pituitary may also play an as-yet poorly understood role in the mediation of 5-HT's regulation of PRL. Removal of the neurointermediate lobe in male rats can completely abolish the increase in plasma PRL levels normally observed following 5-HTP administration (178).

Serotonin appears to be involved in the negative-feedback control of PRL. Decreasing circulating PRL levels via hypophysectomy of ovariectomized rats was shown to be accompanied by an increased rate of 5-HT synthesis in the median eminence and mediobasal hypothalamus (179). This effect was reversed if exogenous PRL was given to these animals. Furthermore, the blockade of DA receptors reversed the ability of exogenous PRL to inhibit the increased rate of 5-HT synthesis, indicating that this feedback mechanism apparently involves an intermediary DA component. Hyperprolactinemia produced by pituitary homografts implanted beneath the kidney capsule in ovariectomized rats attenuated ovarian-steroid-stimulated 5-HT synthesis in the preoptic area of the hypothalamus, an area involved in the regulation of gonadotropin release (180). The steroid-induced increase in serum LH was also attenuated in the hyperprolactinemic animals. Further investigations are required to elucidate the mechanism(s) through which 5-HT regulated PRL release. These investigations may also help elucidate the poorly understood mechanism(s) whereby high levels of circulating PRL inhibit gonadotropin release.

Role of Serotonin in the Control of Luteinizing Hormone Secretion

An abundance of evidence, largely pharmacological, supports a participatory role for 5-HT in gonadotropin regulation. Reminiscent of the action of NE, serotonergic neurons may play facilitatory or inhibitory roles in LH secretion, depending on the steroid environment. Initial studies generally concentrated on (a) the effects of the systemic administration of large amounts of 5-HT or its precursor 5-HTP, which blocked spontaneous ovulation in mature rats (181), and (b) ovulation induced in immature rats by the administration of pregnant mare serum gonadotropin (PMSG). These data met with some skepticism in view of the inability of 5-HT to cross the blood-brain barrier (182) and because 5-HTP was effective only when given in combination with a monoamine oxidase inhibitor (183). The suppression of ovulation was also counteracted by treatment with a vasodilator (184). However, data supporting an inhibitory role continued to accumulate. In normal women, the levels of 5-HT in platelet-poor plasma, which appears to reflect processes occurring in the brain, reaches a nadir during ovulation, and correlates inversely with serum LH (185). The pharmacological elevation of hypothalamic 5-HT levels with monoamine oxidase inhibitors suppressed both PMSG-induced (154) and spontaneous ovulation (183) in rats. In sheep (186) and rabbits (187), infusion of 5-HT into the medial basal hypothalamus blocked the ovulatory discharge of LH and ovulation. Intraventricular 5-HT blocked the release of LH induced by electrochemical stimulation of the preoptic hypothalamic area, an effect antagonized by 5-HT receptor blockade (188). Direct electrochemical stimulation of 5-HT neurons in the dorsal raphe nuclei inhibited LH secretion in ovariectomized rats and blocked spontaneous ovulation in normal rats (189,190). The inhibitory effect was reversed in ovariectomized rats by the 5-HT receptor antagonist metergoline (190). However, administration of metergoline alone to ovariectomized rats had no effect on pulsatile LH release (190). Therefore, it does not appear that 5-HT is involved in the regulation of pulsatile LH release in the absence of ovarian steroids.

Contrary to the above, several lines of evidence support a permissive or facilitatory role for 5-HT in ovulation. Decreased endogenous 5-HT levels, induced by the inhibition of 5-HT synthesis with PCPA, block ovulation (183) and the proestrous rise in LH (191) in rats. Several 5-HT antagonists have been reported to block spontaneous ovulation (192) and PMSG-induced ovulation in immature rats (193). Lesioning the dorsal and median raphe nuclei with the neurotoxin 5,7-DHT produced a dose-dependent inhibition of the incidence of PMSG-induced ovulation (194). Correlated with the suppression of ovulation was a significant decrease in the uptake of 5-HT in the suprachiasmatic and arcuate median eminence hypothalamic regions of the rats. Thus 5-HT input to these regions appears to be essential for ovulation. The functional recovery of gonadotropin secretion was shown to be well correlated with the 5-HT axon regeneration and reinnervation of the hypothalamus following 5,7-DHT lesioning (160). As a possible explanation of the above contradictory roles for 5-HT in ovulation, Kordon and Glowinski (154) proposed the existence of (a) an inhibitory serotonergic center located in the medial basal hypothalamus and (b) a stimulatory or permissive center located in the preoptic-suprachiasmatic region. There is evidence to support the existence of such centers. The stereotaxic microinjection of the 5-HT neurotoxin 5,7-DHT into the medial basal hypothalamus elevates resting levels of LH, whereas similar injections into the preoptic hypothalamic area lowers circulating LH levels (195).

Furthermore, the decrease in LH secretion induced by estrogen in ovariectomized rats is correlated with a decreased 5-HT activity in the suprachiasmatic region, whereas the LH surge induced by the sequential treatment with estrogens and progesterone is correlated with a decreased 5-HT activity in the suprachiasmatic region, whereas the LH surge induced by the sequential treatment with estrogen and progesterone is correlated with a decreased 5-HT activity in the arcuate and ventromedial nuclei (196).

The opposite actions of 5-HT on LH secretion may also be explained by the involvement of 5-HT pathways affecting GnRH secretion directly as well as indirectly. Both electrochemical stimulation of the medial raphe nucleus and lesions destroying the dorsal raphe nucleus block the preovulatory release of LH, suggesting that the medial raphe nucleus plays an inhibitory role, whereas the dorsal raphe nucleus plays a facilitatory role (197). The inhibition of ovulation induced by lesions of the dorsal raphe nucleus is prevented by systemic injection of the β-adrenergic blocker propranolol or injection of 5-HT into the locus coeruleus (198). On the other hand, the inhibition induced by stimulation of the medial raphe nucleus is prevented by systemic injection of the GABA antagonists picrotoxin and bicuculline (199).

The hormonal environment of the animal is likely to be critical to the expression of 5-HT actions on gonadotropin secretion and ovulation. Gonadal steroids have been shown to exert considerable influence on the actions of 5-HT. The intraventricular administration of 5-HT has been shown to inhibit LH release in castrated female rats (96) but stimulates LH release in intact male rats (128) and is without effect on LH levels in intact female rats (96). Systemically administered 5-HT effectively increases circulating LH levels (a) when ovariectomized rats are pretreated with E_2 and (b) in normal cycling rats during estrus (200). A diurnal afternoon surge of LH occurs in estrogen-treated, ovariectomized rats (201); this appears to be dependent upon 5-HT input. Properly timed administration of PCPA, which caused a marked decrease in brain tryptophan hydroxylate activity and 5-HT levels, blocks the E_2-induced afternoon LH surge (184). This effect is reversed with 5-HTP administered to these rats either intraventricularly or systemically (202,203). Serotonin levels in the suprachiasmatic nucleus (204) and in the median eminence display a transitory peak concurrent with the LH surge (204). This peak is absent in both male rats and untreated, ovariectomized female rats, suggesting that the facilitatory action of 5-HT on LH release is E_2-dependent. The sequential administration of E_2 and progesterone produces significant increases in both 5-HT concentration and 5-HT synthesis in the dorsal raphe nuclei, the site of the serotonergic cell bodies (205). These nuclei give rise to a major portion of the serotonergic innervation within the hypothalamus. Consequently, steroid administration also produces significant increases in 5-HT levels in the median eminence (206,207), the preoptic-anterior hypothalamus (208), and other related hypothalamic regions (195). Estradiol injections cause a selective increase in the density of serotonin (5-HT) receptors in the preoptic area, anterior hypothalamus, lateral septum, and arcuate-median eminence regions in ovariectomized rats (209). The increase in 5-HT receptors may be relevant, since these anatomical structures are known to be important in the control of ovulation. The density of 5-HT receptors in the basal forebrain, which includes the hypothalamus, septum, and preoptic area, has been shown to undergo regular changes during the estrous cycle of the rat (210). A significantly lower density was found on proestrus and estrus than on diestrus. Significant changes were not observed in other brain regions, that is, hippocampus, cortex, and caudate.

It is likely that the actions of 5-HT on LH secretion and ovulation are expressed via changes in the outflow of GnRH from neurosecretory neurons rather than direct actions at the pituitary gland. Leonardelli and colleagues (211) provided evidence that 5-HT can act directly on hypothalamic GnRH releasing structures. These investigators induced neurons in the preoptic-suprachiasmatic region to stain immunocytochemically for GnRH by infusing 5-HT into the lateral ventricle of rats. The 5-HT neuronal system is potentially one of several neurotransmitter systems intimately related to the gonadotropin-regulating functions of the preoptic anterior hypothalamus, medial basal hypothalamus, and median eminence. Gonadal steroid modulation of the activity of these neurotransmitter systems is a central mechanism through which these hormones affect cyclic gonadotropin secretion and control ovulation (212). It is not surprising, then, that gonadal steroids have been shown to exert actions on 5-HT neuronal activity. Thus during the periovulatory period, 5-HT-containing neurons are involved in the stimulation of LH secretion, whereas in the absence of high E_2 levels, the converse is true. However, in ovariectomized, pituitary stalk-transected ewes, 5-HT administration increases the amplitude of the LH pulses and mean concentration of LH. This finding supposes the hypothesis of a direct pituitary action for 5-HT on LH secretion (213).

Serotonin could be involved in the negative ultrashot feedback control of GnRH. Decreasing GnRH levels by active immunization of male rats increases hypothalamic, olfactory tubercle, and striatal concentrations of 5-HT and its major metabolite 5-HIAA (214).

γ-AMINOBUTYRIC ACID

Neuroanatomy of γ-Aminobutyric Acid Neurons

The levels of γ-aminobutyric acid (GABA) and the rate-limiting enzyme for its synthesis, glutamate decarboxylase (GAD), are found in high levels in the hypothalamus (215). A fivefold difference in GAD activity levels was seen among the hypothalamic nuclei of the rat. High levels were seen in the preoptic, anterior, and dorsomedial nuclei, with low levels in the arcuate and supraoptic nuclei and median eminence. Levels of GABA were fairly uniform among hypothalamic nuclei. Deafferentation studies suggest that there are GABA neurons intrinsic to the hypothalamus (216). Using [^{3}H]GABA uptake studies in conjunction with autoradiography, GABA-concentrating cells were seen in the medial basal hypothalamus (217) and in nerve fibers in the external layer of the median eminence (218). Immunohistochemical studies with a purified GAD antibody revealed numerous GABA neurons within the nuclei of the hypothalamus (219). A dense plexus of GAD-containing nerve terminals was seen in the external layer of the median eminence.

Interestingly, immunohistochemically identified GAD neurons in the medial-preoptic/anterior hypothalamic regions were shown to contain estrogen receptors (220). In this same region, GAD-containing terminals have been shown to synapse on GnRH-containing neurons (1).

The rich GABAergic innervation of the hypothalamus is consistent with the data (which we will now discuss) that show that GABA is involved in the neural regulation of LH and prolactin. However, several lines of evidence also suggest that GABA may be a hypothalamic hormone involved in the inhibitory regulation of prolactin. The presence of significant numbers of GAD-staining terminals in the external layer of the median eminence is consistent with this hypothesis.

Role of γ-Aminobutyric Acid in the Control of Luteinizing Hormone Secretion

The infusion of either GABA or the $GABA_A$-receptor agonist muscimol in regions containing GnRH neurons inhibits the pulsatile release of LH in ovariectomized rats (221,222), suggesting an inhibitory role for GABA in the regulation of GnRH/LH release in the preoptic area/anterior hypothalamic region. Treatment with aminooxyacetic acid, a blocker of GABA degradation, also inhibited pulsatile LH release (223). In ovariectomized rats primed with E_2 plus progesterone, muscimol, and the $GABA_B$-receptor agonist baclofen, as well as aminooxacetic acid, blocked the surge of LH (223,224). The release of GABA in the preoptic area measured by push-pull perfusion is inversely correlated with circulating LH levels (60,225,226). In addition, the potentiation of NE-induced LH release (226) and the stimulation of basal LH secretion (227) following administration of $GABA_A$- and $GABA_B$-receptor antagonists, support a physiological role for GABAergic neurons in the inhibitory regulation of LH (228).

Correlated with these inhibitory effects of GABA on both pulsatile and steroid-induced surges of LH, changes in the activity of noradrenergic neurons have been reported. Systemic injection of muscimol and baclofen into ovariectomized, steroid primed rats decreased the turnover rate of NE in the medial preoptic area and medial basal hypothalamus (224). No effects on DA turnover were seen in either structure. In ovariectomized rats the intraventricular injection of muscimol also inhibited the turnover rate of NE in the medial-preoptic/anterior hypothalamic area (222). In this study the turnover rate of DA was decreased in the anterior medial basal hypothalamus and medial-preoptic/anterior hypothalamic area. In ovariectomized E_2-primed rats the release of GABA, as measured via push-pull perfusion, decreased in the afternoon of the LH surge, whereas that of NE increased (60,225,226).

In contrast to the inhibitory effect of GABA on LH secretion, an excitatory role in the regulation of GnRH release both in ovariectomized and in ovariectomized, E_2 and P treated rats was suggested by studies in which GABA was infused in the vicinity of the median eminence (229). Furthermore, GABA and $GABA_A$ agonists stimulate GnRH secretion from median eminence fragments *in vitro* (230,231). The possibility exists that the terminals of GnRH neurons express different receptors than the cell bodies.

It has been proposed that GABA neurons in the preoptic area mediate the negative feedback action of E_2 (60,220). This is substantiated by the following findings:

1. GABA neurons in this region contain estrogen receptors (220).
2. There is a conspicuous drop of preoptic GABA release prior to and during the time of estrogen-induced LH surge (60,225,226).
3. A decreased GABAergic activity in the medial preoptic nuclei and mediobasal hypothalamus precedes the estradiol-evoked LH surge in ovariectomized rats (232).

The possibility also exists that GABAergic neurons may directly inhibit GnRH release, since GABA-containing terminals synapse with GnRH-containing neurons (1). This hypothesis has been further supported by experiments using the GT_1 GnRH neuronal cell lines. In superfused GT_1 cells, GABA directly affects the release of GnRH involving both $GABA_A$ and $GABA_B$ receptors (233). The effect of GABA is biphasic. A rapid stimulation is followed by a delayed inhibition. The initial short-term stimulation is mimicked by the administration of muscimol, suggesting the involvement of $GABA_A$ receptors. The expression of functional $GABA_A$ receptors in GT_1 cells has been demonstrated. GT_1 cell membranes bind ^{3}[H]muscimol, and GABA activates, while the $GABA_A$ antagonist bicuculline blocks chloride currents in single voltage-clamped cells (234). Furthermore, GABA evokes action potentials and increases intracellular Ca^{2+} concentration in GT_1 cells (235,236). Altogether, these results show that GABA exerts a transient excitatory action mediated via $GABA_A$ receptors on GnRH neurons. On the other hand, the administration of baclofen to GT_1 cells profoundly but reversibly inhibits the characteristic spontaneous pulses of GnRH, suggesting that the inhibitory action of GABA may be mediated via $GABA_B$-receptors (233). In support of the biphasic effect of GABA a pronounced reduction of LH pulsatility was observed in response to the preoptic/anterior hypothalamic area application of both GABA as well as the GABA antagonist bicuculline (237). These data in conjunction with *in vivo* studies are consistent with $GABA_A$ receptors being present on axon terminals and $GABA_B$ receptors on cell bodies or dendrites.

Finally, a direct stimulatory effect of GABA on LH release from the anterior pituitary has been suggested (238), mediated via $GABA_A$ receptors (238,239). However, the efficacy observed for GABA was very modest compared to that of GnRH, questioning the physiological significance of this action.

Role of γ-Aminobutyric Acid in the Control of Prolactin Secretion

As we have discussed, a relatively dense innervation of GABA terminals exists in the external layer of the median eminence. GABA has been measured in the hypophyseal portal blood but with conflicting results. One laboratory using a radioreceptor assay found equivalent levels of GABA in the portal and peripheral blood of diestrous rats (240). In a subsequent report, GABA levels in portal blood also measured by radioreceptor assay were found to be twice that in peripheral blood of male rats (241). However, data indicated that a significant portion of this GABA-like activity was not GABA but possibly a metabolite of GABA. Electrical stimulation of the median eminence caused an eightfold increase in GABA levels, demonstrating the ability of median eminence neurons to release GABA in large amounts into portal blood. Treatment of ovariectomized rats with ethanolamine-*O*-sulfate, an inhibitor of GABA metabolism, caused a three- to fourfold increase in GABA levels in portal blood (242). This increase in GABA levels was closely correlated with a decrease in circulating PRL levels.

Clearly, there are GABA receptors in the anterior pituitary (242), and they suppress PRL secretion (243) and synthesis (244). However, one disturbing aspect of GABA's role as an inhibitory modulator of PRL secretion is that administration of the GABA antagonists bicuculline and picrotoxin does not elevate PRL secretion in male or ovariectomized E_2-treated rats (245). Administration of dopamine antagonists, on the other hand, has been universally found to elevate PRL secretion (19). Therefore it appears that an inhibitory GABAergic neurosecretory system is present in the rat; however, it does not appear to tonically regulate PRL secretion at the pituitary level. Under what physiological circumstances it does is still unclear.

PRL has been shown to enhance hypothalamic GAD activity, GABA turnover, and GABA release (246,247). Recently it was also shown that PRL causes a rapid rise in intracellular free Ca^{2+} in primary cultured rat embryonic diencephalic neurons that were immunoreactive for GAD but not TH (248). These results suggest that a rapid negative feedback loop between lactotrophs and tuberoinfundibular GABAergic neurons may exist.

Besides the potential action of GABA as a PRL inhibitory hormone, there is also evidence that it acts at the pituitary and centrally to stimulate PRL release. The rapid superfusion of male rat pituitaries showed a biphasic effect of GABA on PRL release (249,250). However, in contrast to the biphasic effect just described for GABA on GnRH secretion, the initial transient stimulation and the sustained inhibition of PRL secretion were mimicked by muscimol and antagonized by bicuculline, suggesting the mediation of both components via $GABA_A$ receptors. On the other hand, intraventricular administration of GABA (245,251) or the $GABA_A$ agonist muscimol stimulates PRL release in male rats as well as in both ovariectomized and overiectomized, E_2-primed female rats (222,245). One possible mechanism for this stimulatory action of GABA could be via the inhibition of the activity of tuberoinfundibular dopamine neurons. In one study the turnover rate of dopamine neurons was decreased following administration of muscimol (222); however, in a second study there was no effect (224).

HISTAMINE

Histamine-containing neurons have been implicated in the neuroendocrine regulation of both LH and PRL secretion. The actions of histamine are mediated through pharmacologically well-characterized H_1, H_2 receptors, and H_3 autoreceptors. The availability of subtype-selective agonists and antagonists has greatly aided recent studies. As with other amines, histamine does not cross the blood-brain barrier; therefore it is necessary to inject it into the ventricular system to study its central effects.

Anatomy of Histaminergic Neurons

Histamine is found in high concentrations in the hypothalamus (252). The content of histamine varies throughout the hypothalamus, with the highest levels observed in the median eminence; the arcuate, suprachiasmatic, and mammillary nuclei also contain high levels (253). The regional distribution of histidine decarboxylase, the enzyme that converts histidine to histamine, follows closely with that of histamine content except in the median eminence (254). It appears that a portion of the histamine in the median eminence is in mast cells, which are not capable of synthesizing histamine. However, in recent immunochemical studies using antibodies to histamine (255,256) or histidine decarboxylase (257), large numbers of histamine-containing nerve terminals were observed in the region where hypothalamic releasing hormones are secreted into portal blood, that is, the external and internal zones of the median eminence as well as the neurohypophysis. Likewise, there is a dense histaminergic innervation of the hypothalamic regions where hypophysiotropic releasing hormones are synthesized, that is, the preoptic, periventricular, and suprachiasmatic areas and the supraoptic, paraventricular, and arcuate nuclei. Histamine-containing cell bodies are exclusively located in the lateral posterior hypothalamus, an observation consistent with the finding that lesions of the lateral hypothalamus decreased hypothalamic histidine decarboxylase activity by approximately 50% (258). Further suggesting that hypothalamic histamine-containing nerve processes are projections from intrahypothalamic cell bodies is the observation that complete deafferentation of the medial basal hypothalamus does not decrease histamine levels in the median eminence as well as in the ventromedial and dorsomedial nuclei (216).

A good correlation between the distribution of histaminergic nerve fibers and the density of H_1 binding sites was demonstrated by autoradiographic studies (259). Although still lacking a detailed mapping of their localization, H_2 postsynaptic and H_3 presynaptic histamine receptors are also present at lower density in the hypothalamus (260,261). Electrophysiological experiments have shown that histamine induces both excitatory responses that are blocked by H_1 antagonists (262,263) and inhibitory responses sensitive to H_2 antagonists (263).

Role of Histamine in the Regulation of Luteinizing Hormone Secretion

Sawyer (264), in 1955, first demonstrated that the intraventricular (but not intravenous) administration of histamine induced ovulation in estrogen-primed rabbits. The intraventricular administration of histamine increases LH secretion in ovariectomized, E_2-primed rats (265) and proestrous rats (266) but not in male rats (266,267). Intravenous histamine was shown to have no effect (265).

In men (268) and women (269) the systemic administration of histamine did not affect LH levels. However, the administration of histamine did potentiate the response to GnRH. The potentiation of histamine of the response to GnRH in men could be blocked by both the H_1 antagonist mepyramine and the H_2 antagonist cimetidine (268). The significance of this effect is unclear because histamine has been shown to have no direct effect *in vitro* on the secretion of LH or the stimulation of LH secretion by GnRH in the rat anterior pituitary (270). Since histamine does not cross the blood-brain barrier and does not affect basal LH secretion, it is unclear how it is acting to potentiate the action of GnRH.

The central stimulating effects of histamine may be mediated via an H_1 receptor that regulates the release of GnRH. Perifusion of medial basal hypothalamic fragments from diestrous rats with histamine or the H_1 agonist 2-methylhistamine causes a significant increase in the release of GnRH (270). The effect was blocked by simultaneous administration of the H_1 antagonist mepyramine. However, in another *in vitro* study using medial basal hypothalamic fragments from male rats, histamine had no effect on GnRH release (271). In support of the involvement of H_1 receptors in the stimulation of GnRH/LH release, the administration of the H_1 antagonist diphenhydramine to estrogen-primed ovariectomized ewes depressed basal and estrogen-stimulated LH serum concentrations (272).

In contrast, the involvement of histamine H_2 receptors had been proposed based on the stimulation of LH secretion by central administration of an H_2 receptor agonist (273). Recently, it was reported that in estrogen-primed ovariectomized rats, both the H_1 antagonist pyrilamine and the H_2 antagonist metiamine inhibit the surge of LH induced by estrogen, and the combination of both as well as the inhibitor of histamine synthesis α-fluoromethylhistidine completely abolished the LH surge (274).

The role of histamine in the physiological regulation of LH secretion is still unclear. Few experiments to determine the effects of histamine antagonists on LH secretion have been reported. The fragmentary data that exist suggest that histamine might play a role in LH regulation; however, further data are needed for a convincing argument to be made. It remains to be determined if the effects of histamine are exerted directly on GnRH neurons, and if so the type of receptors involved.

Role of Histamine in the Regulation of Prolactin Secretion

Substantially more data exist showing that the central activation of histaminergic neurons results in the release of PRL. This effect is not mediated at the level of the anterior pituitary because neither the injection of histamine into the pituitary (265) nor the incubation of primary cultures of anterior pituitary cells with histamine (270) affects PRL secretion.

Intraventricular injection of histamine releases PRL in both male (267,275) and female rats (265,266). Intraventricular administration of the H_2 antagonists cimetidine and metamide, but not the H_1 antagonist diphenhydramine, blocked the stimulation of PRL by histamine in male rats (271,276,277). The effect of histamine could be mimicked by the intraventricular administration of the H_2 agonists 4-methylhistamine and dimaprit, whereas the H_1 agonists 2,2-pyridylethylamine and 2-thiazolylethylamine have no effect (276,277). Thus, it appears that the stimulatory effect of centrally administered histamine is mediated via H_2 receptors.

On the other hand, H_1 receptors presumably localized in hypothalamic areas outside the blood-brain barrier seem to be involved in the stimulation of PRL release by systemically administered histamine (277). The H_1 agonist 2-thiazolylethylamine mimics the action of systemic histamine, and the systemic action of histamine is blocked by the H_1 antagonist mepyramine (277). No effect of histamine was seen on PRL release when incubated with anterior pituitaries or when administered to stalk-sectioned rats. In normal men the infusion of histamine also stimulated PRL release, and the response was inhibited by the H_1 blocker mepyramine (278); however, in women the systemic administration of histamine had no effect (269).

The stimulatory effect of histamine could be mediated either via the inhibition of dopamine release or the stimulation of the release of TRH, serotonin, or vasopressin. Histamine decreases the portal blood levels of dopamine in male rats by 26–30% after intraventricular infusion (279,280), and 23% after systemic administration (280), although no change in the turnover of dopamine in the median eminence was detected (281,282). In any case, the decrease in portal blood dopamine could only account for a portion of the sixfold increase in PRL secretion. Incubation of hypothalamic slices (283) or hypothalamic synaptosomes (284) with histamine stimulated the release of TRH. Systemic administration of histamine to women also potentiated TRH-induced PRL secretion; however, as with the potentiating effect of histamine on GnRH, the mechanism of this response is unclear (269). Histamine also increases the release of hypothalamic serotonin (285,286) and blockade of serotonergic receptors inhibits the PRL response to centrally or systemically administered histamine and H_1- and H_2-receptor agonists (287). Histamine also stimulates the release of vasopressin (AVP) (288) and the PRL response to centrally infused histamine is inhibited by AVP receptor antagonists and AVP antiserum (289). However, the increase in plasma AVP induced by histamine could only account for a small portion of the hyperprolactinemia. Thus, the stimulatory action of histamine on PRL secretion may be mediated via several neuronal systems and may involve different mediators (290) according to the sex or physiological state of the animals (see below).

Administration of histamine antagonists has been reported to have little or no effect on basal PRL secretion (284). The H_2 antagonist cimetidine has been reported to increase PRL levels when administered systemically to rats; however, this effect does not appear to be mediated by histamine receptors (291).

Interestingly, the H_1 antagonist diphenhydramine has been reported to inhibit increases in PRL and decreases in LH caused by restraint stress (265), while blockade of H_1 and H_2 postsynaptic receptors or histamine synthesis inhibits the PRL response to restraint (292,293) and ether (294) stress in male rats. The H_2 receptor antagonist ranitidine, but not the H_1 antagonist mepyramine, significantly reduces PRL release induced by morphine (295). However, neither the histamine receptor antagonists nor the histamine synthesis inhibitor α-fluoromethylhistidine affected PRL release induced by β-endorphin. In lactating rats, histamine may be involved in the mediation of suckling-induced PRL release. The suckling-induced release of PRL was dramatically suppressed by the intraventricular administration of the H_1 antagonists diphenhydramine and mepyramine but not the H_2 antagonist metiamide (296). However, metiamide administration increased PRL levels in nonsuckled mothers, whereas diphenhydramine had no effect. Therefore in lactating rats it appears that histaminergic neurons are involved in the tonic suppression of resting levels of PRL via H_2 receptors but that, during suckling, histaminergic neurons partially mediate the stimulation of PRL release via H_1 receptors. In ovariectomized rats, the hypothalamic injection of the H_1 and H_2 receptor antagonists pyrilamine and metiamide inhibited, whereas the inhibitor of histamine synthesis α-fluoromethylhistidine or the combination of both antagonists abolished, the PRL surge induced by estrogen (297). In summary, histamine appears to have a predominant stimulatory effect on PRL secretion via activation of central H_2 receptors and via H_1 receptors presumably located in hypothalamic areas outside the blood-brain barrier. A reciprocal minor inhibitory action of H_1 and H_2 receptor activation is seen under some conditions but only after blockade of the receptors mediating the stimulatory effects. Further studies will be necessary to determine the physiological role of histaminergic neurons in PRL secretion. Clearly, there are multiple histaminergic effects mediated by both H_1 and H_2 receptors, whereas the role of H_3 autoreceptors is unclear. An important step in the understanding of the actions of histamine will be the careful elucidation of the neuroanatomy of histaminergic neurons and their connectivity with other neuroendocrine elements, and the analysis of direct effects on specific cell lines.

EXCITATORY AMINO ACIDS

Identification of numerous neuronal responses to excitatory amino acids and characterization of several corresponding receptor subtypes have raised new interest in that category of transmitters, which comprises mainly glutamate, aspartate, glycine, and taurine. Although fairly abundant in the central nervous system, their neuronal distribution is still poorly understood for lack of appropriate labeling techniques. In several neuron systems, they are endowed with autocrine or paracrine actions.

Genes coding for several subunits of glutamate receptors have been cloned. Different subunit combinations exhibit a relatively large diversity of pharmacological properties. Glutamate receptor subtypes exhibit two major mechanisms of action: direct control of Ca^{2+} flux for the NMDA subtype, named after *n*-methyl-D-aspartate, its most affine ligand, and G protein mediated stimulation of phospholipase C for the quisqualate receptor sensitive to kainic acid (298). Autoradiographic mapping points to a relatively dense concentration of glutamate receptors in the hypothalamus (299,300), in particular in the arcuate nucleus (301).

Glutamate has been shown to stimulate LH secretion in rats (302–309), mice (308), and monkeys (309–311). Under particular conditions, LH release from hypogonadal mice grafted with GnRH neurons was also increased by the transmitter (308). Conversely, glutamate antagonists inhibit LH pulsatility (312) as well as estradiol induced release of the hormone in ovariectomized rats (313,314). Interestingly, release of excitatory amino acids is increased in the hypothalamic preoptic area as a consequence of estradiol administration (60,226).

Most authors agree that the NMDA receptor is the major glutamate receptor subtype involved in those effects (307,313,314). Agonists of the quisqualate receptor however have also been reported to induce a transient LH response (315), an effect possibly related to the direct stimulation by kainate of GnRH release reported in a model of incubated hypothalamic fragments (316). However, a rapid increase (15 min) in GnRH mRNA levels following NMDA administration in male rats has been recently reported (317).

The relevance of glutamate for gonadotropic control may be related to its capacity to amplify firing of GnRH neurons, and to consequently participate in the synchronization of episodic release of the peptide. Glutamate is also able to stimulate prolactin secretion (306,314,315), but the effect is not as well characterized as the LH response, since pretreatment with antagonists is less effective to reverse it (315). Interestingly, glutamate stimulation of PRL can no longer be obtained in lactating rats (306).

NEUROPEPTIDES

Recent improvements in neuropeptide characterization and localization methods have resulted in an in-depth reappraisal of our understanding of neuroendocrine control. In addition to "conventional" neurotransmitters, over 30 peptides have recently been shown to regulate pituitary reproductive hormones. Less than five of them were known in 1969. Most of them have been found in significant amounts in the mediobasal hypothalamus and are released into the hypophyseal portal system. In the pituitary they affect not one, but usually several, adenohypophyseal cell types. In addition, they can interact with each other's release or modulate nonpeptide neurotransmission at hypothalamic synapses or in the median eminence. These properties endow them with both direct and indirect effects on hormone control.

Hypothalamic-peptide-producing neurons exhibit a common organization pattern. Despite their apparent scattering throughout the hypothalamus, most of their cell bodies (over 90%) are located in the paraventricular nucleus, the medial periventricular area, or the arcuate nucleus. Smaller populations of neurons are found in the medial preoptic area (sometimes also referred to as the anterior periventricular area) and the suprachiasmatic nucleus (318,319).

Irrespective of the location of their cell bodies, major projections of all those neurons exhibit a common final pathway. In rodents, for instance, medial preoptic neurons follow an initial dorsolateral course, proceed caudally with the medial forebrain bundle, and leave it to enter the median eminence from an anterolateral direction. As they come close to the paraventricular and the arcuate nucleus, these fibers merge with axons proceeding from those areas (320).

The distribution area of hypothalamic neurosecretory neurons has widened in the course of evolution. In fishes, neurosecretory neurons are concentrated in the periventricular space around the medial hypothalamus. They progressively invade more rostral areas in birds and reptiles. Diversity is also observed in the pattern in mammals: In primates, the deeper funnel-like shape of the tuber cinereum caused a few preoptic neurons to migrate closer to arcuate-periventricular structures as compared with migration observed in rodents (321). According to mapping studies based on neuron labeling or electrophysiological methods, the median eminence is only one of several projection sites for neurosecretory neurons. Their axon collaterals innervate several hypothalamic, as well as extrahypothalamic structures. Paraventricular and arcuate neurons, in particular, are in contact with a large number of brain structures (320). This strategic position accounts for their role in coordinating hormone regulation, other autonomic functions, and behavior.

Techniques of functional neuroanatomy have recently permitted formal identification of a few neuropeptide synapses. Most of them represent articulations of nerve endings with perikarya elaborating a different transmitter, but synapses connecting homologous neurons (e.g., GnRH fibers on GnRH cell bodies, or oxytocin fibers on oxytocin cell bodies) have also been described. In addition, juxtaposition of nerve endings within the median eminence seems to account for axoaxonal interactions, even in the absence of identifiable synaptic specialization.

In this section, six groups of neuropeptide-producing neurons will be considered separately, because each of them shares common anatomical or functional properties:

1. Those that predominantly originate in the preoptic area, namely, somatostatin or somatotropin-release-inhibiting factor (SRIF), luliberin or GnRH, tachykinins, neurotensin, atrial natriuretic factor (ANF)
2. Peptides produced in the arcuate nucleus, namely peptides from the pancreatic family (NPY, PYY, pancreatic polypeptide, and galanin)
3. Those mainly produced in perikarya of the paraventricular or supraoptic nuclei, namely TRH, CRF, cholecystokinin, vasopressin, oxytocin, angiotensin, endothelins, bradykinin, and bombesin
4. Gastrointestinal peptides of the secretin-glucagon family (GHRH, VIP, PHI, secretin, gastric inhibitory peptide, PACAP, oxyntomodulin)
5. The opioid peptide family
6. Cytokines and related transmitters commonly produced by blood cells, but also expressed by, and acting on, hypothalamic or pituitary cells in some cases

In each case, we briefly review the anatomical organization, the biosynthetic pathways, the distribution of receptors in the brain, and general effects of each peptide. We then review their direct effects on pituitary cells (most of which are discussed at length in other chapters of these volumes) and describe the hypothalamic mechanisms by which they can modulate secretion of gonadotropins, PRL, and oxytocin or exert other actions on reproductive functions. In summary tables, we attempt to distinguish effects or interactions that appear reasonably well characterized from a pharmacological point of view from those that should still be considered preliminary.

HYPOTHALAMIC PEPTIDES PRODUCED IN THE PREOPTIC-PERIVENTRICULAR AREA

Major neuropeptides with hypothalamic perikarya of neuroendocrine relevance located in this area are somatostatin, GnRH, tachykinins, neurotensin, and atrial natriuretic peptide. Although a somewhat denser mass of neurons is found in the central portion of the area (322), most cell bodies of the preopticoinfundibular system are scattered throughout the anterior hypothalamus, with a few perikarya located as far rostrally as the organum vasculosum of the lamina terminalis. Distribution of their projections presents several commonalities. Most of them innervate the olfactory tubercules, basal nuclei, periaqueductal gray, and suprachiasmatic nucleus, and many are also found in the amygdala, the septum, and the cortex.

Somatostatin

Biochemistry, Distribution, and Pharmacology

Somatostatin, characterized in 1972 (323), is processed from a 210-amino acid precursor (324). The nucleotide sequence of the gene coding for the precursor was originally characterized in the fish pancreas (325). The rat (324) and human genes (326) were subsequently described. Somatostatin is widely distributed throughout the brain, particularly in the hypothalamus, the limbic system, the septum, the hippocampus, the cortex, and the medulla (327,328). Somatostatin-producing neurons can be put into three categories. The first includes hypothalamic projections, most of which derive from the anterior periventricular portion of the diencephalon (329–334). Electrical stimulation of this area is most effective in releasing the peptide into the portal system (335). A second group of long extrahypothalamic neurons originates in the amygdala and participates in the hypothalamic innervation by that structure (336–338). The last group consists of short interneurons present in several brain structures (338,339).

Homologous somatostatin synapses have been described in the periventricular area (340). They may account for the "ultrashort" somatostatin-to-somatostatin feedback observed after intraventricular infusion of the peptide (341,342). In addition, periventricular somatostatin neurons project to the arcuate nucleus, where they innervate a subpopulation of GHRH-producing neurons (343,344), as well as to the locus coeruleus and the substantia nigra (339,345).

Posttranslational processing can generate two distinct molecules endowed with somatostatin activity, somatostatin 14, and somatostatin 28 (346). Both forms (347), as well as somatostatin 28 (1–12), the C-terminal residue of the longer peptide, can be released from the median eminence and have been assayed in hypophyseal portal blood (348). The distribution of somatostatin 14 and 28 does not completely overlap in the central nervous system (349). Differential production of either one has been obtained in populations of neurons in culture (350).

Four distinct somatostatin receptor subtypes, SSTR 1 to 4, have recently been cloned after PCR amplification of transcripts expressed in the brain or the pancreas of various species (351–356), in agreement with previous binding studies pointing out to somatostatin receptor heterogeneity. They all exhibit seven transmembrane domains characteristic of G protein coupled receptors. Receptor subtypes SSTR 2 to 4 are negatively coupled to adenylyl cyclase; some of them appear also able to stimulate K^+ conductance and to inhibit voltage sensitive Ca^{2+} channels (VSCC) (351,357). The SSTR1 receptor has also been reported to interfere with protein phosphorylation by activating phosphatases (355).

SSTR1 corresponds to a protein of 391 amino acids showing homologies to the family of tachykinin receptors, and SSTR4 (383 AA) exhibits a few sequences in common with the μ opiate receptor (354). Since this subtype appears predominantly expressed in the pituitary, its possible cross reactivity with opiate peptides may account for some hormonal interferences of opiate agonists or antagonists with SRIF effects. Detection of only one subset of binding sites in the pituitary (358,359) is consistent with the observation that it expresses preferentially SSTR4. SRIF binding is mainly located on somatotrophs (360), but has also been observed in lesser concentration on thyrotrophs and lactotrophs (361), as well as on growth-hormone (GH) and on PRL-producing human tumor cells (362). In the brain, somatostatin-binding sites are present in several structures, particularly those rich in endogenous peptide (349,359).

Effects of Somatostatin on Adenohypophyseal Hormones

Somatostatin, a most potent inhibitor of GH secretion (323), is also able to inhibit TSH (363) and PRL secretion (357,363,364) under discrete endocrine conditions. These effects involve direct actions of the peptide on the pituitary and are discussed in other chapters of these volumes. We will thus only summarize them briefly. Somatostatin inhibition of plasma PRL levels is most effective in hypothyroid animals (363) and after treatment with estrogens (357,364), which results in an increased number of pituitary somatostatin receptors (364). Under these conditions, PRL release inhibition by somatostatin can be obtained *in vitro* (357,364), whereas the peptide is ineffective in the absence of estrogens. Somatostatin is also able to partially antagonize TRH stimulated PRL release (365) and to decrease its sensitivity to VIP (365). In fasting rats, passive immunization with antisomatostatin antibodies results in an increased secretion of PRL (366), an observation suggesting that endogenous somatostatin may be functionally involved in PRL control under that condition.

Effects of Somatostatin Mediated by the Hypothalamus

A moderate, paradoxical stimulation of PRL secretion reported after intraventricular administration of somatostatin (367) may be mediated by the ultrashort feedback action of the peptide on its own release. In addition, the peptide can affect the synaptic activity of several hypothalamic neurotransmitter systems. Somatostatin inhibits norepinephrine release in the hypothalamus (368) and, in contrast, enhances DA turnover in the diencephalon when infused intraventricularly (369). *In vitro,* SRIF releases serotonin from hypothalamic as well as from cortical and hippocampal slices (370). Other *in vitro* effects of the peptide include inhibition of GnRH (371) and TRH release from hypothalamic cultures (372). Finally, somatostatin has been shown to exhibit weak antagonistic properties on opiate receptors (373). Partial homology of the SSTR4 and μ opiate receptors probably accounts for the effect (354).

These interactions are summarized in Table 1. They show a certain degree of agreement with the overall hormonal consequences of somatostatin administration.

Luliberin or Gonadotropin-Releasing Hormone

The structure of the mammalian GnRH precursor has been deduced from the sequence of the gene coding for the peptide (374). It consists of 92 amino acids. In lower

TABLE 1. *Reproductive actions of medial-preoptic–periventricular and arcuate peptide-containing neurons*

	Overall neuroendocrine effect						
	Prolactin		Gonadotropins				
Peptide	Direct (1)	Indirect (2)	Direct (1)	Indirect (2)	Effects at hypothalamic level	Other reproductive actions	Physiological relevance
SRIF	↓	↓		↓	↓ NA, ↓ GnRH, ↓ TRH		Hypothyroidism, high E_2 fasting stress
DA							
GnRH		↑	↑			↑ Sexual behavior	
SP	↑			↑ ?	GnRH pulsatility	↓ Sexual behavior	
NPY			↑	(3) ↓ or ↑ (4)			
NT	↑	↓			↓ SRIF, suprachiasmatic rhythmicity		
Galanin	↑				↓ DA		

(1) Direct actions on pituitary cells; (2) by indirect effects on hypothalamic neurons; (3) only in castrated animals; (4) only in intact or in sex-steroid-treated animals; (↑ ↓) increases or decreases hormone or transmitter release; (↑ ↓) effect not fully characterized yet.

SRIF, somatotropin release inhibiting factor; DA, dopamine; GnRH, gonadotropin-releasing hormone; SP, substance P; NPY, neuropeptide Y; NT, neurotensin; NA, noradrenergic; TRH, thyrotropin-releasing factor; E_2, estrodiol.

vertebrates gonadotropin releasing peptides are coded by two distinct genes (375). Although they express a single gene, mammals also seem able to produce two distinct GnRH molecules by posttranslational processing, giving rise to an alternate form hydroxylated on the 9-pro residue (9,376).

The major, if not the exclusive, brain localization of the corresponding neurons is the periventricular area of the hypothalamus and a circumventricular organ, the organum vasculosum of the lamina terminalis (377,378). In addition to their major projections to the median eminence, which they reach from a dorsolateral course (379), GnRH neurons project to several extrahypothalamic structures, particularly the mesencephalic central gray, the midbrain (380), the hippocampus, the amygdala (381), and the olfactory tubercules (382). Immunocytochemical studies with antibodies raised against a non-GnRH-containing portion of the precursor sequence give comparable results (383). Extrahypothalamic projections are believed to proceed from subsets of neurons distinct from those innervating the median eminence (381). Neurons projecting to extrahypothalamic structures appear to produce larger amounts of 9-hyp-GnRH as compared to the conventional form of the decapeptide (384).

Coordination between both populations of GnRH neurons is probably achieved by numerous collateral synaptic contacts between GnRH-producing preoptic neurons (385). Interestingly, the immortalized GnRH neurons possess an inherent ability to secrete GnRH in a pulsatile manner (12,13). The coordinated response from a number of neurons may reflect intercellular communications through putative GnRH receptors or synapselike contacts (12) and gap junctions (12). Thus, the molecular basis of the pulsatility exhibited by these neurons *in vitro*, may represent the mechanisms presumably involved in the *in vivo* electrical activation of GnRH neurons and synchronization of pulsatile GnRH release (386,387).

Cloning of the murine GnRH receptor from an immortalized gonadotropic cell line has yielded a 327 amino acid protein with a G protein binding sequence and seven transmembrane domains. That molecule shares 25% homologies with vasopressin and oxytocin receptors. It exhibits the original feature of being devoid of carboxyl-terminal intracytoplasmic domain, a property which may account for the peculiar mode of action of GnRH (388).

A fairly dense population of GnRH receptors has been visualized in the hippocampus by autoradiographic studies (389). But most GnRH receptors are located in the pituitary (390). An original feature of pituitary GnRH receptors is that number of binding sites and intensity of the response can be modulated by several other neurotransmitters, as NPY, substance P, or PACAP (see below). This property may account for the occurrence under particular conditions of biphasic responses to GnRH (391).

GnRH is able to modulate the electrical activity of discrete neuronal populations (392). Some of these actions are dependent upon levels of sex steroids (393), which is suggestive of a possible coordination with reproductive functions. But the major extrapituitary effect of the peptide is undoubtedly to facilitate sex behavior and lordosis (394,395). The action involves mostly GnRH projections to the mesencephalic central gray matter (396). Participation of the endogenous peptide is suggested by experiments in which local administration of anti-GnRH antisera suppressed sex behavior (397).

It was recently reported that infusion of C-terminal fragments of GnRH into the hypothalamic ventromedial nucleus were as potent as GnRH itself to induce lordosis in female rats (398). This is consistent with the higher concentration of 9-hyp-GnRH found in nonmedian eminence projecting neurons, since shorter, C-terminal fragments derived from 9-hyp-GnRH are more resistant to enzymatic hydrolysis that the corresponding GnRH catabolites (384).

Atypical stimulation of PRL by administration of GnRH was initially reported in acromegalic patients (399) and was subsequently confirmed under various pathological conditions and in normal human subjects (400). Increased PRL secretion was also observed in the rat (401) and can be induced *in vitro* by addition of GnRH to pituitary-cell aggregates (402). Effects of GnRH on PRL are not believed to involve a direct effect of the decapeptide on lactotrophs (402). They are probably mediated by GnRH-induced release of paracrine factors released from gonadotrophs and recognized by prolactin-producing cells. Several peptides, such as dynorphin (403), substance P (403), angiotensin II (404), NPY (403), or even alpha subunits of LH cosecreted with LH itself (405), could be responsible for this paracrine action.

Tachykinins

Tachykinins are a class of peptides consisting of substance P [a very early discovered peptide (406)] and the neurokinins A and B (or substance K). Neurokinins A and B are derived from cleavage of the closely related precursor molecules beta and alpha protachykinin A, whereas substance P is derived from gamma protachykinin (407). Three subsets of receptors with preferential affinities for substance P and neurokinins A and B have been characterized pharmacologically (407). Neurokinin A receptors have mainly been described in peripheral tissues.

Tachykinins are widely distributed throughout the brain, mainly in the septum, the amygdala, the hippocampus, the cortex, and the medulla (408). As somatostatin, they are produced either by neurons located in the hypothalamus or amygdala with long projections, or by short interneurons (409). Substance P is a potent stimulator of locomotor activity and plays an important role in nociception (407). Tachykinin receptors are widely distributed in the brain (410) and are present in the pituitary (411).

The major site of synthesis of substance P (like that of somatostatin and GnRH) within the hypothalamus is the periventricular area, but it is also produced in other areas. Periventricular neurons project mainly to the median eminence and the septum (412) with a distribution pattern which resembles that of somatostatin (413). Substance-P-like immunoreactivity is also found in pituitary lactotrophs and gonadotrophs (414,415).

Most studies on hormonal effects of substance P conclude that the peptide stimulates PRL release in rats, whether administered intravenously (416) or intraventricularly (417). One group however reported that substance P given in lower dosages could have a converse, inhibitory effect on PRL (418). Similar findings have been reported in primates (419). The effect on PRL was also observed after administration of the peptide to animals bearing a hypothalamic lesion (419), as well as on pituitary cells *in vitro* (416). These data are suggestive of a direct effect at the pituitary level. Conversely, antagonists to substance P depress plasma PRL levels (420,421), an observation which suggests that endogenous substance P may tonically stimulate PRL secretion.

Infusion of substance P into the third ventricle or the medial periventricular hypothalamus was found to inhibit gonadotropin release in male rats (420), and, on the contrary, to stimulate LH (but not FSH) in ovariectomized animals (416,422). No effect was found under the same conditions in monkeys (419). A role of endogenous substance P in LH regulation was postulated on the basis of experiments involving administration of antagonists or passive immunization with anti-substance-P antisera. Those resulted in an elevation of FSH and LH plasma levels in male (420) or in intact female rats (423). In contrast, the treatment decreased LH without a change in FSH in ovariectomized female rats (424). Those effects are not obtained upon intravenous administration of the peptide. These data point to a primary hypothalamic site of action, a conclusion consistent with the fact that substance P stimulates the release of GnRH from perifused fragments of median eminence *in vitro* in an estrogen-dependent manner (425). In keeping with this interpretation, endogenous levels of substance P have been found to fluctuate in discrete hypothalamic areas during the estrous cycle of rat (426,427).

Substance P may however also exhibit discrete, direct inhibitory effects on gonadotrophs. Pretreatment of pituitary cells with the peptide interferes with the responsiveness of gonadotrophs to GnRH (428). Under discrete conditions, however, as during the peripubertal period in rats of both sexes or in adult females only, substance P has been shown to induce a 5- to 10-fold stimulation of *in vitro* LH release (429). In contrast, the responsiveness of gonadotrophs from male rats diminished during maturation and was absent after 60 days of age (429). There was no significant effect of SP on release of LH from cells of male and female prepubertal rats (429). Substance P receptors in the pituitary have also been shown to fluctuate during the estrous cycle (411).

Neurotensin

Neurotensin is a 13-amino-acid peptide. Its precursor has not been characterized as yet (430). The neuronal distribution of neurotensin is comparable to that of other neuropeptides described in this section. Most of its hypothalamic cell bodies are found in the anterior periventricular system, although some perikarya are also present in the paraventricular and the arcuate nuclei (431–433). Some periventricular and arcuate neurons colocalize neurotensin and DA (434,435). As with GnRH neurons, those elaborating neurotensin project to the olfactory tubercules (436). Similarly to somatostatin, neurotensin is abundant in cell bodies of the amygdala and the septum (432). Fibers originating in the medial nucleus of the amygdaloid complex project to the hypothalamic ventromedial nucleus (437). Other densely innervated structures are the periaqueductal gray, the caudate putamen, the locus coeruleus, the septum, and the suprachiasmatic nucleus (432). A few cells in the anterior pituitary also stain with antineurotensin antibodies (343).

Two classes of binding sites, high (H) and low (L) affinity, have been described in the brain, with 0.1 or 5 nM affinity for their ligand (438). Their distribution, for the most part, follows along with the anatomical localizations of the peptide (439). High concentrations of neurotensin and neurotensin receptors are found in the suprachiasmatic nucleus (439,440); their expression is sensitive to estrogens (441). The major nonreproductive endocrine functions of neurotensin are stimulation of insulin secretion (442), inhibition of glucagon secretion (442), and modulation of gastrointestinal motility (436). Neurotensin receptors have been found on cholinergic cell bodies in the nucleus basalis (443). Since the concentration of neurotensin receptors is reduced in Alzheimer's senile dementia, the peptide may be associated with somatostatin and NPY in the cholinergic dysfunctions observed in that disease (443).

Conflicting data have been obtained on LH secretion after intraventricular administration of neurotensin. In large concentrations, the peptide was reported to inhibit plasma LH (417), but the effect was not observed in other studies (444) and cannot be mimicked by systemic administration of neurotensin (417). In contrast, the peptide was claimed to stimulate LH release when infused directly into the preoptic area, the region where most GnRH cell bodies are located (445). The peptide was thus assumed to modulate as yet unknown hypothalamic components of gonadotropic control. Similar conflicting effects on GH secretion have been observed after the intraventricular or systemic administration of neurotensin (422,446).

Intraventricular administration of neurotensin reduces plasma PRL levels (417,444). The effect correlates with a decreased concentration of dopamine D_2 receptors in several brain structures, including the intermediate lobe of the pituitary. It may reflect ultrashort feedback of neurotensin on dopamine in nerve endings where both transmitters are colocalized (444). Neurotensin has also been claimed to inhibit somatostatin release from the hypothalamus *in vitro* (447), an effect which, under particular circumstances, could also account for the decreased PRL secretion observed after the intraventricular infusion of neurotensin.

In contrast, intravenous administration of neurotensin stimulates PRL secretion (417,422), an effect highly dependent upon sex steroids (448) (Table 1). This action is consistent with a direct action of the peptide on the pituitary. Exposure of pituitary cells to neurotensin *in vitro* has a marked PRL-releasing action (449). On the contrary, neurotensin seems to have no direct action on gonadotrophs (417). Several direct effects of neurotensin on brain transmitters have been described with emphasis on DA turnover in nigrostriatal neurons (450).

These paradoxical data may reflect a rhythmic component in the action of neurotensin on reproductive function. A subpopulation of neurotensin receptors located in the anteromedial portion of the suprachiasmatic nucleus, an important structure for hormonal cyclicity, is highly sensitive to E_2. Those receptors were shown to decrease to a marked extent after treatment with the hormone (441). Other E_2-dependent processes within the suprachiasmatic nucleus have been shown to participate in the regulation of reproductive hormones cyclicity (451).

Atrial Natriuretic Factor

Atrial natriuretic factor (ANP), which was initially discovered in the heart, is a 28-amino-acid peptide containing a single disulfide bond and is derived from a 152-amino-acid preprohormone sequence (452). The peptide and its receptors have been identified in several brain structures, particularly those concerned with control of water balance (453) and circumventricular organs, including the organum vasculosum of the lamina terminalis and the median eminence (454). Most hypothalamic cell bodies containing atrial natriuretic factor are located in the medial preoptic area, but a few are also found in the paraventricular and the arcuate nuclei (455). Atrial natriuretic factor in relatively high concentrations (10–1,000 nM) has been reported to stimulate the release of LH from pituitary cells *in vitro* and to prolong the effect of GnRH (456). But it is still unclear whether the action is due to the peptide itself or to a possible contaminant (457). Recent data demonstrate, however, that in contrast to the antagonistic interaction of the ANP and angiotensin II on water intake, the peptides affect reproductive hormone secretion in the same direction and under particular experimental conditions display additive effects in increasing LH and inhibiting prolactin release (458). Atrial natriuretic factor is also able to act directly at the testicular level to increase testosterone synthesis (459). Actions on both pituitary and testis are thought to involve the activation of guanylate cyclase (457,459).

Atrial natriuretic factor is predominantly inhibitory to neuronal activity upon direct local application (460). One of its major neuroendocrine roles is to inhibit vasopressin release (461) particularly after dehydration (462).

HYPOTHALAMIC NEUROPEPTIDES SYNTHESIZED IN THE ARCUATE NUCLEUS

The arcuate nucleus is the major hypothalamic source of several neurohormones important for neuroendocrine control: DA, beta-endorphin and other POMC-related peptides, peptides from the pancreatic family (neuropeptide Y, peptide YY, and pancreatic peptide), GHRH, and galanin. In addition to the external layer of the median eminence and the posterior pituitary, arcuate neurons project to the periventricular and supraoptic nucleus as well as to the medial preoptic area. The major projections relevant to the scope of this chapter are neurons containing POMC-derived peptides, which establish contacts with GnRH neurons in the preoptic area (463) and with cell bodies in the paraventricular nucleus (464,465). Additionally, neurons containing neuropeptide Y also provide input to the paraventricular nucleus (466). Intrinsic connections between arcuate POMC-producing neurons have also been demonstrated (467,468).

Peptides from the Pancreatic Family: Neuropeptide Y, Peptide YY, and Pancreatic Peptide

Peptides belonging to this family are closely related. Both NPY and PYY contain 36 amino acids (469) and differ only by nine amino acid substitutions (470,471). They are derived from related 97-amino acid precursors (pre-pro-Npy).

Neuropeptide Y is widely distributed in the brain particularly in the amygdala, the septum, the bed nucleus of the stria terminalis, the cortex, and the hippocampus (472–474). Its distribution resembles that of somatostatin (475–477). Both peptides have been shown to colocalize in various extrahypothalamic structures (477). Several neurons also colocalize NPY with catecholamines (478), including hypothalamic afferents of brain stem CA neurons, since dorsal tegmental transections which decrease catecholamine concentrations in the mediobasal hypothalamus also result in NPY depletion in that structure (479). In many regions NPY overlaps with peptide YY and the pancreatic polypeptide.

Neuropeptide Y is particularly abundant in the arcuate nucleus (472), but scattered NPY neurons are also found in the preoptic-periventricular area of the ventromedial hypothalamus (480). Neuropeptide Y and PYY containing nerve terminals are found throughout the mediobasal hypothalamus (480). Numerous projections have been observed in the suprachiasmatic nucleus (472,480,481), a structure important for cyclic endocrine control (451). NPY synaptic boutons were also shown to make contact with hypothalamic β-endorphin neurons, particularly in the arcuate nucleus and on estradiol-concentrating neurons (482).

Three subsets of receptors for the pancreatic polypeptide family have been described. They belong to the 7-membrane domain, G protein-dependent receptor family (483). One (Y_1) exhibits the highest affinity for NPY and is widely distributed in the brain (483). Heterogeneity of NPY/PYY receptors and the existence of multiple receptor proteins were found recently in tumor cell lines derived from the neural crest (484).

Administration of NPY was found to stimulate the release of LH in rats, rabbits, monkeys, and fishes (485–490). The action seems to involve Y_1 receptors and may affect directly GnRH neurons, since GnRH release could be elicited by the peptide from perifused fragments of mediobasal hypothalamus (489). Alternately, it was also reported to depend upon activation of α_1 receptors (485) or by an interaction with β-endorphin secretion. There seems to be a wide agreement on such positive interaction of NPY and GnRH in intact male and female animals (490). In castrated animals, however, several authors have found that the peptide inhibits LH release in either male (491) or female rats (492) or rabbits (493). Treatment of castrates with estrogens restores the LH stimulating effect of the peptide (494). Both the inhibitory and stimulatory effects of NPY could be reproduced by administration of pancreatic polypeptide to ovariectomized rats or estrogen-supplemented ovariectomized rats, respectively (494,495).

In other studies, intravenous injections as well as intraventricular administration of NPY into the median eminence to conscious, castrated rabbits has been found to decrease the frequency of GnRH pulses (493).

In discrete brain regions, immunoreactive NPY concentrations have been found to correlate with median eminence LHRH and plasma LH concentrations (496). Treatments with steroids which enhance LH release induce a parallel and synchronous increase in mediobasal hypothalamic concentrations of GnRH and of NPY (497). Furthermore, NPY gene expression is increased in the arcuate nucleus during the preovulatory luteinizing hormone surges in proestrous rats. (498).

Inhibition of sex behavior could represent an additional function of NPY in reproductive function (499).

In addition to these hypothalamic effects, NPY also appears able to stimulate LH release by a direct, steroid-dependent action on pituitary gonadotrophs. It was reported to potentiate the LH response to GnRH in incubated hemipituitaries (500). The effect is steroid dependent and seems to modulate the GnRH binding to pituitary membranes (501), possibly by unmasking additional GnRH receptors in gonadotrophs. However, in primary pituitary cell cultures of rat, it has been demonstrated that NPY modulates gonadotropin secretion by inhibiting the gonadotrope intracellular calcium transients induced by GnRH (502) (Table 1).

Galanin

Galanin, a 29-amino acid peptide (503), is widely distributed in the central nervous system (504). In the hypothalamus, its major site of synthesis is the lateral portion of the arcuate nucleus where it colocalizes with several other neuropeptides, as GHRH, GnRH and neurotensin, as well as with GABA and tyrosine hydroxylase (506). It is coreleased synchronously with GnRH secretory episodes into portal blood (507), and is also able to inhibit the turnover rate of tuberoinfundibular DA neurons (508). A marked increase of pituitary as well as median eminence concentrations of galanin has been reported to occur after treatment with estrogens or in concomitance with the LH surge in PMSG treated prepuberal rats (509).

Galanin also colocalizes within pituitary cells, mainly those secreting prolactin (510), GH, and TSH (511). Major regulators of these hormones also affect galanin release from pituitary cells (511), and pituitary expression of the galanin gene is affected by estrogens (512). Galanin was reported to stimulate LH secretion from pituitary cells in culture and to potentiate their response to GnRH (507).

Prolactin

Prolactin itself is also able to modulate gonadotropin regulation; hyperprolactinemia in particular inhibits secretion of LH, an effect that may account for lactation induced contraception. Prolactin is not only secreted by pituitary lactotrophs; it is also present in hypothalamic neurons (513) in particular in arcuate, but also in paraventricular neurons (514). It is synthesized locally, as documented by *in situ* hybridization and northern blots

(515). The role of PRL-producing neurons is not elucidated at present, and the mechanisms governing PRL-gonadotropin interactions are not fully understood. The hormone interferes with GnRH release *in vitro* (516) and activates tuberoinfundibular dopamine neurons (102), a short feedback effect important for PRL homeostasis that contributes to maintain PRL secretion within physiological limits. PRL feedback could also involve PRL receptors recently characterized in the hypothalamus (517). Part of those receptors could be expressed by GnRH secreting neurons, as indicated by the presence of PRL receptors and of the corresponding mRNA in the GnRH producing GT-1 cell line (518). This observation suggests that PRL interaction upon LH secretion could be partly accounted for by a direct action on GnRH cells.

HYPOTHALAMIC NEUROPEPTIDES SYNTHESIZED IN THE PARAVENTRICULAR NUCLEUS

The paraventricular nucleus of the hypothalamus is among the most dense neuronal masses of the diencephalon. It contains a medial magnocellular portion as well as a large number of parvocellular neurons located in more lateral parts of the nucleus (519). Vasopressin and oxytocin, together with the additional sequences of their precursor molecules, neurophysins I and II, were the two earliest characterized neuropeptides (520,521). Another important source of both peptides is provided by neurons located in the supraoptic nucleus (522). Parvocellular suprachiasmatic cell bodies also contain large concentrations of vasopressin (523). More recent studies have shown that several other peptides of neuroendocrine relevance are also produced in paraventricular perikarya: TRH (524), CRF (525) partially colocalized with vasopressin (526), cholecystokinin (527), angiotensin (528), bradykinin (529), bombesin (530), VIP (531), and endothelins (532). The periventricular nucleus receives a very rich innervation. Over 2,500 axon terminals appear to be associated with each magnocellular neuron (533). The nucleus is also extremely rich in axon collaterals (534). In addition to its projections to the median eminence and the posterior pituitary, the paraventricular nucleus contributes fibers to the medial preoptic area, the suprachiasmatic nucleus, and the arcuate nucleus (535). The nucleus also sends projections to several extrahypothalamic structures, such as the lower brain stem, the nucleus of the solitary tract, and the spinal cord (536). It is a major relay of stress-induced hormonal responses (537) (see Figs. 1 and 2).

Oxytocin and Vasopressin

Both neuropeptides are coded for by related genes with large structural homologies. They are processed

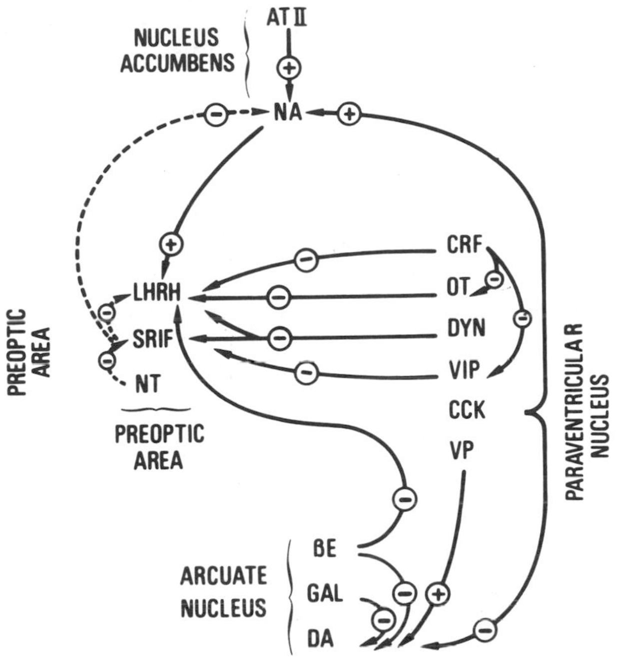

FIG. 1. Schematic representation of major hypothalamic transmitter and peptide interactions involved in the regulation of gonadotropins and prolactin. Several peptides that are produced in the paraventricular nucleus and that are concerned with processing stress, corticotropin-releasing factor (CRF), oxytocin (OT), dynorphin (DYN), as well as β-endorphin (βE), are produced in the arcuate nucleus, and are inhibitory to luteinizing-hormone-releasing hormone (LHRH). Activation of LHRH neurons is mostly achieved by noradrenergic (NA) projections. Norepinephrine release from these projections can be activated by cholecystokinin (CCK) and angiotensin II (AT II), as well as inhibited by somatostatin. Inhibition of dopamine (DA) by βE, CCK, and galanin (GAL) represents the major indirect input to prolactin regulation. Corresponding evidence is presented in the text; it is derived mainly from *in vitro* experiments or from experiments involving intraventricular infusion of agonists or antagonists of those peptides. Neuroanatomical studies have demonstrated the existence of synapses between βE-containing projections from the arcuate nucleus and LHRH neurons. In addition, they have shown that CRF-, OT-, and DYN-containing projections from the paraventricular nucleus are abundant in those areas, where most LHRH and somatotropin-release inhibiting-factor (SRIF) cell bodies are located. NT, neurotensin; VIP, vasoactive intestinal polypeptide; VP, vasopressin.

from their respective precursors to give rise to nonapeptides with a disulfide bond (the active hormones), neurophysins (from which they are separated by an intermediary tripeptide), and a glycopeptide of unknown function. The C-terminal end of vasopressin consists of Arg-Gly-NH2 in most mammals, and of Lys-Gly-NH2 in porcine species (for a review see ref. 538).

Vasopressin (539–541) and oxytocin (539) are also widely distributed in extrahypothalamic structures. Both peptides are released into the hypophyseal portal system (542,543). Only one class of oxytocin receptors is known, but three subsets of vasopressin receptors have

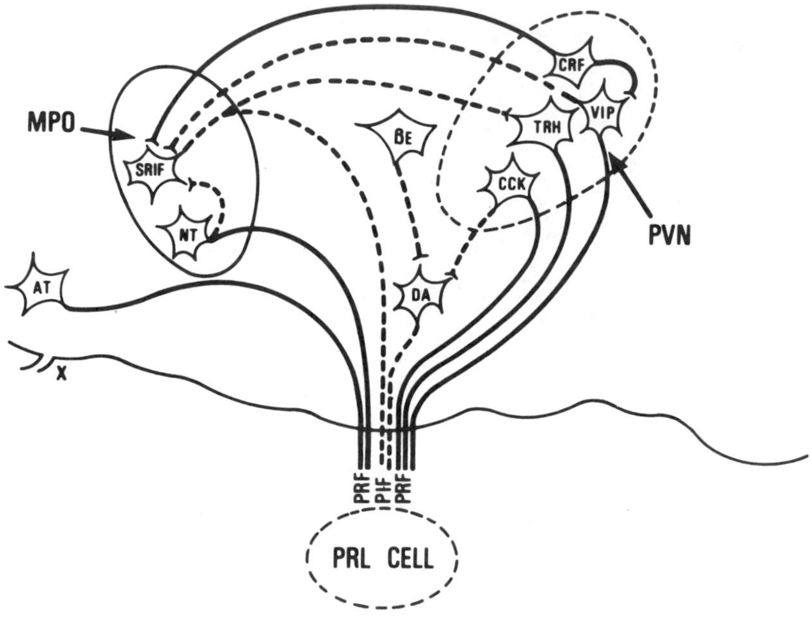

FIG. 2. Major factors regulating prolactin secretion [namely, thyrotropin-releasing hormone (TRH), vasoactive intestinal polypeptide (VIP), cholecystokinin (CCK), neurotensin (NT), and angiotensin II (AT)] can be released into the hypothalamo-hypophyseal portal system to stimulate pituitary lactotrophs. Dopamine is the predominant prolactin-inhibiting factor (PIF), but endogenous somatostatin can also inhibit prolactin secretion under discrete physiological conditions. Tuberoinfundibular dopamine can be inhibited by β-endorphin (βE) and cholecystokinin (CCK); somatotropin-release inhibiting-factor (SRIF) release is stimulated by corticotropin-releasing factor (CRF), inhibited by VIP, and is itself inhibitory to TRH. Solid lines refer to stimulatory inputs, whereas dotted lines refer to inhibitory ones. Corresponding evidence is presented in the text. MPO, medial preoptic area; PVN, paraventricular nucleus; X, optic chiasm; DA, dopamine; PRF, prolactin-releasing factors; PRL, prolactin.

been described (544). For the most part, two of them (V1a and V1b) have been found in the central nervous system and pituitary gland (544,545).

The most conspicuous effect of vasopressin on the pituitary is the stimulation of ACTH release and the potentiation of CRF effects (546,547). These actions are mediated by vasopressin-binding sites on anterior pituitary corticotrophs (545). Oxytocin has been shown to potentiate the CRF-induced stimulation of ACTH in rat cells *in vitro* (548,549). The evidence appears more controversial in humans, since oxytocin was reported instead to inhibit the potentiated effects of CRF by vasopressin (550).

Both peptides have also been shown to stimulate PRL secretion in the rat (551–552). This effect has been reported to involve a direct PRF action of oxytocin (552–554) and perhaps also of arginine vasotocin (555,556) on the pituitary. The action may be physiologically relevant, since antagonists to the peptide are able to block mating induced surges of PRL (557). On the contrary, intraventricular infusion of oxytocin results in inhibition of PRL secretion (558,559), whereas intracerebral administration of antagonists to oxytocin results in increased PRL secretion (558). In addition, the activity of a subpopulation of paraventricular oxytocin neurons has been found to correlate with circadian episodes of PRL secretion (560).

As in other brain nuclei, the metabolism of tuberoinfundibular dopamine is affected by vasopressin (561). A similar effect does not however mediate PRL inhibition by oxytocin (558). Stimulation of PRL by oxytocin antagonists may involve instead interferences with a VIP-dependent process, since antagonists to the latter peptide block the stimulating effect of intraventricular oxytocin antagonists (558). The effect of vasopressin may also involve opiate neurons, since naloxone seems to counteract it (562). Participation of endogenous neurohypophyseal peptides in the regulation of PRL secretion is suggested by observed changes in PRL secretion after removal of the posterior pituitary (563).

Oxytocin was also reported to advance the onset of the ovulatory LH surge, whereas oxytocin antagonists are able to abolish it (564). Passive immunization with antioxytocin antisera has the same effect, with a higher potency when administered intraventricularly (565).

Effects of vasopressin and oxytocin on PRL are more pronounced under conditions of stress (566). Both peptides (566), or, according to other authors, oxytocin only (567), is believed to act as a modulator of stress responses. Vasopressin (568) or oxytocin (569) can temper the stress-induced stimulation of ACTH. Increased oxytocin activity is also thought to play a role in the inhibition of gonadotropins observed during stress or lactation, since LH levels increase following ablation of the neural lobe (563). Subnanomolar concentrations of oxytocin inhibit basal or depolarization-induced LHRH release from the median eminence *in vitro* (570).

Oxytocin may facilitate the onset of estrogen-induced maternal behavior (571). The estrogen dependency of this action may involve an increase in the density of oxytocin receptors in discrete brain areas, such as the ventromedial nucleus, the organum vasculosum of the lamina terminalis, the nucleus accumbens, and, to a lesser extent, the amygdala (572). Several other nonendocrine actions of vasopressin and oxytocin have been documented and reviewed (573).

Thyrotropin-Releasing Hormone

Thyrotropin-releasing hormone (TRH) (p-Glu-His-Pro-NH2), a tripeptide, was first described in 1969 (574,575). The peptide is derived from a 30-kD precursor, and the corresponding gene has been characterized (576). High concentrations of TRH were initially described in the median eminence, the paraventricular nucleus, and the arcuate nucleus (577). Most TRH cell bodies were subsequently identified in the paraventricular nucleus (524,578,579). Their nerve terminals project to the arcuate nucleus and the median eminence, since paraventricular lesions lead to a large decrease in TRH levels in these structures (524). Axons of paraventricular neurons also project to the septum (580). A large number of TRH neurons are also found in a number of extrahypothalamic structures, particularly the amygdala, the nucleus accumbens, the bed nucleus of the stria terminalis, the cortex, and the spinal cord (581). In the human hypothalamus, the distribution of TRH was reported to be asymmetrical, with a predominance on the left side (582). Significant concentrations of TRH were also found in the pituitary (583), where it can be produced locally. The peptide is also believed to be internalized and stored within anterior pituitary cells (583).

Thyrotropin-releasing-hormone receptors have been localized in several brain structures and in the pituitary (584), where they may exist under two forms, each with a different affinity for their ligand (585). In addition to its eponymous action on thyrotropin release (574,575,586), TRH has been shown to directly stimulate the release of PRL (587,588). Prolactin release by TRH is enhanced by E_2, presumably by an action of the steroid on the number of TRH-binding sites of lactotrophs (589). Pituitary TRH receptor number and efficacy on PRL release fluctuate during the estrous cycle (590). An endogenously formed dipeptide metabolite of TRH, His-Pro-diketopiperazine, has been shown to inhibit PRL release (591), but the relevance of that action is still unclear. In addition, partially cleaved precursor forms of TRH, in particular a tetrapeptide with an additional C-terminal glycine, has also been shown able to release PRL *in vivo* (592). The effect cannot be reproduced *in vitro* (593), so that it is believed to result from production of TRH by cleavage of the extended form. Although the effect appears as a minor one under normal conditions, it may play a role in controlling PRL secretion under conditions of starvation in rats (594), as well as in patients with anorexia nervosa (595).

Corticotropin-Releasing Factor

Corticotropin-releasing factor (CRF) is a 41-amino acid peptide (596) derived from a 196-amino acid precursor (597). Its main source in the hypothalamus is the paraventricular nucleus. Most of the CRF there is produced by parvocellular neurons (525,598), where CRF is found colocalized with oxytocin (599) as well as vasopressin (526). A few scattered cells located more rostrally, in the periventricular area and in the suprachiasmatic nucleus, can also be stained with CRF antisera (599). Paraventricular neurons project to the median eminence and to the posterior pituitary (599), a structure in which the presence of corticotropin activity was suspected for some time (600). A relatively dense CRF innervation of the anterior preoptic area, with numerous varicosities, has also been described (598).

Corticotropin-releasing-factor neurons in the paraventricular nucleus project to the basal telencephalon and the brain stem, areas important in autonomic control (601). In addition, the amygdala, the bed nucleus of the stria terminalis, the central gray, and some caudal catecholamine-rich nuclei (A1 and A6) also receive a dense CRF innervation, presumably via the medial forebrain bundle which interconnects these areas with the hypothalamus (598). Scattered CRF interneurons are also present throughout the cortex (598).

Different subsets of CRF cell bodies within the paraventricular nucleus, as well as in other structures, appear regulated in an independent manner. Adrenalectomy, for instance, only affects the metabolism of the peptide in parvocellular neurons, which also contain neurohypophyseal hormones and project to the median eminence and the posterior pituitary (598).

The major endocrine action of CRF is to stimulate the release of proopiomelanocortin-derived hormones (602). The peptide also affects the release of reproductive hormones. Plasma levels of LH are inhibited by CRF administration (603), an effect likely to involve a direct action on LHRH release. Ten to 100 nM CRF added to fragments of median eminence inhibit both basal and K^+-stimulated LHRH release (604,605). The effect is reversed by CRF antagonists (604). Intraventricular administration of CRF was also shown to inhibit PRL secretion (606), as does sauvagine (607), a peptide that exhibits structural analogies with CRF (608).

In addition, CRF infused intraventricularly stimulates the release of oxytocin into the hypophyseal portal system (609,610). It is also a potent inhibitor of sexual receptivity in female rats (611,612). In addition, corticotropin-releasing factor is considered an important factor in mediating stress-induced inhibitory effects on reproductive functions (613).

Cholecystokinins

Cholecystokinins (CCK) represent a family of peptides of variable length (active forms range from 4 to 58 amino acids) derived from a 114-amino acid precursor. The most common forms are CCK4 (Trip-Met-Asp-Phe-NH2) and CCK8 (Asp-Tyr [S03H] Met-Gly extension of the N-terminus of CCK4). They are present in several brain structures (527,614). In the cortex, the octapeptide is produced by neurons with a distribution quite comparable to that of CRF and somatostatin interneurons (615). The major hypothalamic source of the peptide is from both magnocellular and parvocellular neurons of the paraventricular nucleus (614,616), where they have been shown to be colocalized with oxytocin and neurophysin (616). Cholecystokinin colocalization with DA, serotonin, and GABA has also been reported in other brain areas (617). In addition, the ventromedial nucleus of the hypothalamus receives long ascending projections from the CCK-containing neurons in the brain stem (618).

Central and peripheral CCK receptors are believed to exhibit slightly different properties (619). Brain CCK receptors are widely distributed (620) and show high densities in the ventromedial hypothalamic nucleus, supraoptic and paraventricular nuclei (621), and also in the pituitary. In ventromedial and paraventricular nuclei, receptors are downregulated by estrogens (622) and are increased by ovariectomy (623).

Cholecystokinin stimulates PRL and GH release by direct actions on the pituitary (624). It elevates plasma gonadotropin levels after intraventricular infusion or direct implantation into the medial preoptic area (625). In contrast to intravenous administration, intraventricular treatment with the peptide inhibits PRL release (624), a paradoxical effect that we already mentioned for other neuropeptides such as neuropeptide Y or neurotensin. Prolactin inhibition, and possibly also LH stimulation, could be mediated by effects of CCK on tuberoinfundibular DA activation (625). Furthermore, the peptide is able to induce electrical activation of a large population of tuberoinfundibular neurons in an estrogen-dependent manner (626). Midbrain DA neurons colocalizing CCK can also be activated by the peptide (627).

Cholecystokinin has been reported to influence noradrenergic neurons in the ventromedial hypothalamus (628), an effect possibly related to the control of feeding behavior (629). In view of its dual role on feeding behavior and neuroendocrine parameters in closely related hypothalamic structures, CCK could be involved in the synchronization of both events (630), which has been observed under certain hormonal conditions. Sexual behavior in female rats has also been shown to be altered by CCK8 as well as by CRF (631).

Angiotensin II

Angiotensin is an octapeptide (Asn-Arg-Val-Tyr-Ile-His-Pro-Phe) formed by cleavage of a larger precursor, angiotensinogen, by renin (632). It is present in several brain structures (633,634). In the hypothalamus, it is mostly found in paraventricular and supraoptic nuclei (528), where it is colocalized with vasopressin in parvocellular neurons (635). The peptide is also synthesized in pituitary gonadotrophs (Table 4). Angiotensin-converting enzyme (636) and angiotensin receptors have been localized in discrete brain areas (637) and in the pituitary (638).

Several distinct receptor isoforms of AT-II have been sequenced and the corresponding genes characterized [AT_1, AT_2 (639,640)]. Two of them (AT1a and AT1b) result from alternative splicing of the same gene (641,642). They have been found in the hypothalamus and the pituitary, with a predominance of the AT1 form in adenohypophyseal cells (642). The receptor is coupled to phospholipase C by a still unidentified G protein (643,644). It exhibits an additional, negative coupling to adenylate cyclase, as documented by experiments carried out in the pituitary (645). This negative coupling involves an a_1 subunit of G proteins (645), but its physiological relevance is still unclear.

The earliest documented neuroendocrine effect of angiotensin was the stimulation of ACTH *in vivo* (646) and *in vitro* (646,647). Angiotensin also enhances PRL release by a direct action on pituitary lactotrophs (648–651). The effect is sensitive to E_2, since the hormone decreases the number of pituitary receptors for angiotensin (651). The action of the peptide on adenylate cyclase also appears to be sensitive to E_2 (652). Surprisingly, these changes are not paralleled by a decreased efficacy of angiotensin to release PRL (651,652). This discrepancy could be due to the existence of multiple postreceptor coupling mechanisms (650).

In addition to its direct action on lactotrophs, AT-II is also able to affect hypothalamic neuronal circuits, an effect resulting in paradoxical PRL inhibition when the peptide is administered intraventricularly (653) at doses comparable to those affecting water intake behavior. The action is blocked by domperidone, suggesting that it may be mediated by tuberoinfundibular DA neurons (653). Conversely, intraventricular infusion of the AT-II antagonist saralasin or of inhibitors of the angiotensin converting enzyme, although unable to alter PRL plasma levels under basal conditions, potentiates the prolactin-releasing action of immobilization stress (654).

Angiotensin II is also capable of stimulating LH release upon intraventricular administration to rats (655). The effect is steroid-dependent and is particularly conspicuous in ovariectomized rats treated with estrogen and progesterone. Independently of the above, AT-II decreases the frequency and amplitude of LH circhoral pulses in untreated ovariectomized animals (656). A physiological role for endogenous angiotensin is supported by the observation that administration of the angiotensin antagonist saralasin, as angiotensin convertase inhibitors, decrease or delay the proestrous surge of LH (655). Intraventricular injection of anti-AT-II antisera was reported to have a comparable inhibitory effect on plasma LH (but not FSH) in ovariectomized rats, and, in parallel, to deplete median eminence GnRH levels (657).

Brain receptors of the neuropeptide also fluctuate during the estrous cycle of the rat and reach maximal concentrations in the preoptic area during proestrus (658). These changes appear also to correlate with fluctuations in drinking behavior (659). In addition, angiotensin II receptors are sensitive to mineralocorticoids (660).

Angiotensin increases catecholamine turnover in discrete brain areas (661). This effect might underlie the LH-stimulating effects of the peptide (653,656). Angiotensin was also reported to stimulate release of vasopressin (662).

Endothelins

The endothelium derived endothelin peptide family [three distinct isopeptides predicted by three separate genes (663)] has been detected in paraventricular neurons (664,665), but it is also produced by pituitary cells, as shown by immunocytochemistry and *in situ* hybridization (666). Endothelins are secreted in the hypothalamus (667) and act through calcium mobilizing and phospholipase C associated endothelin specific receptors (667,668) in normal and transformed (GT1-cell line) cells to stimulate GnRH release (667). Endothelin receptors are present on pituitary cells (664,668). Endothelins, in particular ET1 and ET3, elicit a transient stimulation of LH *in vitro* (669–677); in parallel, they trigger cytosolic Ca^{2+} accumulation in gonadotrophs (671). FSH release can also be stimulated by the peptides; interestingly, different G proteins may mediate responses of FSH and LH (672). In contrast, endothelins inhibit prolactin release (669,670). Those effects are believed to reflect paracrine regulation within the pituitary.

Other Paraventricular Peptides

Bradykinin and bombesin are abundant in the rat hypothalamus (530). Their actions are still poorly understood. Bradykinin (673) and bombesin, at relatively high doses (674,675), inhibit PRL by an indirect hypothalamic action, since they produce the effect after intraventricular, but not after intravenous, administration.

Conclusion

Many neuropeptides produced in the paraventricular nucleus thus seem to share common PRL-stimulating properties at the pituitary level (Fig. 2). This is the case with TRH (586,588), cholecystokinin (624), angiotensin II (632–636), and VIP. A similar action has been attributed to oxytocin (552,553) and vasopressin (555,556), but the evidence remains controversial (559). In addition, most of these peptides can also interact with the release of neurohormones from the median eminence, mainly by elevating concentrations of PRL-inhibiting factors in portal blood. Vasopressin (561), cholecystokinin (624–626), and angiotensin II (550) have all been shown to increase tuberoinfundibular DA neuron activity. Bombesin might do the same (674,675), although the evidence is not as convincing. Parallel effects of CRF are

TABLE 2. *Reproductive actions of peptide-containing neurons in the paraventricular nucleus*

	Overall neuroendocrine effect						
	Prolactin		Gonadotropins				
Peptide	Direct (1)	Indirect (2)	Direct (1)	Indirect (2)	Effects at hypothalamic level	Other reproductive actions	Physiological relevance
Vasopressin	↓	↓			↑ DA		Stress
Oxytocin	↓	↓		↓			Stress, lactation
TRH	↑					Male sexual behavior	
CRF		↓		↓	↓ GnRH, ↑ SRIF, ↓ VIP, ↓ OT	↓ Female receptivity	Stress
CCK	↑	↓		↑	↑ DA,* ↑ NA	↓ Sexual behavior	
Angiotensin II	↑			(3) ↓ or ↑ (4)	↑ VP, ↑ NA		↑ LH surge amplitude
Bradykinin		↓	↓ (FSH)				
Bombesin	↑						

(1) Direct actions of pituitary cells; (2) by indirect effects on hypothalamic neurons; (3) only in castrated animals; (4) only in intact or in sex-steroid-treated animals; (↑ ↓) increases or decreases hormone or transmitter release; (↑ ↓) effect not fully characterized yet; (*) indirect evidence only.

TRH, thyrotropin-releasing hormone; CRF, corticotropin-releasing factor; CCK, cholecystokinin; DA, dopamine; NA, noradrenergic; FSH, follicle-stimulating hormone; GnRH, gonadotropin-releasing hormone; VIP, vasoactive intestinal polypeptide; OT, oxytocin; SRIF, somatotropin release inhibiting factor; VP, vasopressin.

believed to involve, instead, stimulation of somatostatin release from the median eminence. These paradoxical effects at both anatomical levels probably account for the opposite results obtained after systemic or intraventricular administration of these peptides (Fig. 2).

Actions of the paraventricular peptides on gonadotropin secretion appear exclusively mediated by the hypothalamus. They involve the indirect stimulation of LH by CCK (625) and angiotensin II (655) as well as the indirect inhibition of that hormone by CRF (603) and oxytocin (570). Corresponding data are summarized in Table 2.

NEUROPEPTIDES OF THE GLUCAGON SUPERFAMILY

The family consists of several related peptides with considerable structural homologies (676). They are glucagon, gastrin-inhibitory peptide (GIP), secretin, vasoactive intestinal peptide (VIP), histidine-isoleucine (PHI) and histidine methionine (PHM) peptides, and GH-releasing factor (GRH). In the central nervous system, VIP and PHI are very abundant in a number of brain structures, whereas other members of the family are more highly concentrated in the hypothalamus. Hypothalamic cell bodies producing the peptides belong to the so-called medial hypothalamic systems. Neurons containing VIP and PHI are mostly found in the paraventricular nucleus (677,678), whereas GHRH neurons are located in the arcuate nucleus and adjacent parts of the ventromedial nucleus (679).

Representatives of the family most important for neuroendocrine functions are VIP (a 22-amino acid peptide) and GRH (a 27–44-amino acid peptide). These molecules show over 30% homology at their N-terminus. Growth-hormone-releasing factor is further extended by 16 additional C-terminal amino acids (680,681). In humans, PHI (682) and PHM (683) are coded by adjacent exons of the pre-pro-VIP gene (682). Secretin, glucagon, and GIP also belong to the family but have predominantly pancreatic and gastrointestinal functions.

Vasoactive Intestinal Peptide, Peptide Histidine Isoleucine, Gastrin-Inhibitory Peptide, and Glucagon

VIP, unlike GRF, is widely distributed in the brain. It is particularly conspicuous in hippocampal structures (684) and in cortical interneurons (685). In the hypothalamus, cell bodies are mainly located in the paraventricular nucleus (677). About 20% of the suprachiasmatic neurons also elaborate the peptide, as do a few supramamillary cells (685,686). Paraventricular neurons project to the median eminence (687) and the posterior pituitary, whereas suprachiasmatic neurons project to the periventricular preoptic area (686).

Some VIP paraventricular cell bodies colocalize vasopressin (677) and histidine-isoleucine (678). Histidine-isoleucine was reported also to colocalize with CRF and enkephalins in the paraventricular nucleus (686). This observation, however, was challenged by other authors as being an artifact (688). Glucagon is also found in hypothalamic neurons (689) and released into the portal circulation (690). VIP is also secreted by the pituitary; immunocytochemical (691) and *in situ* hybridization studies indicate that the peptide is located in lactotrophs, and that it is released in an homothetic manner with PRL upon TRH stimulation *in vitro* (692).

A single class of VIP receptors has been described. Receptors were initially solubilized from liver membranes and shown to be a glycoprotein (693). In addition to their distribution in several brain areas, these receptors are also expressed by lactotrophs in the pituitary (694), pointing to an autocrine role of the peptide (695). They also recognize other peptides of the family, particularly PHI and, with lower affinity, secretin and GRF (693).

The major neuroendocrine action of VIP is to stimulate PRL secretion, as documented in a variety of species including rodents (696) and monkeys (697). A direct action on pituitary lactotrophs was shown by *in vitro* experiments with pituitary tissue (698–700) or dispersed cells (701). Parallel stimulation by VIP of PRL release and cAMP accumulation is attenuated in the presence of estradiol (697). Somatotrophs are also sensitive to VIP stimulation (702).

Functionally, endogenous VIP is probably involved in stimulation of PRL secretion induced by suckling (703), stress (704,705), and adrenalectomy (705). Passive immunization with anti-VIP antisera was shown to attenuate the elevation of plasma PRL during suckling (703) or after exposure to ether stress (704). The PRL response to the administration of 5-HTP is also attenuated by passive immunization against VIP as well as against PHI (706). A role for endogenous VIP is also supported by observations that suckling increases VIP immunoreactivity in neurons of the paraventricular nucleus and the median eminence (707,708). Around puberty and during suckling, concentrations of VIP precursor mRNA are also increased in the hypothalamus, in particular the suprachiasmatic nucleus (709,710). This suggests that the suckling stimulus may increase transcription of the gene coding for the peptide. Finally, estradiol is able to modify VIP concentrations in the hypothalamus and anterior pituitary (711). Hypophyseal VIP could also act as an autocrine factor to directly trigger PRL secretion. Immunoneutralization of the peptide in the medium of dispersed pituitary cells has been shown to lower basal PRL release (712).

In addition to its effect on PRL, VIP has been reported by most authors to inhibit pulsatile LH secretion in ovariectomized rats (713,714) when administered centrally (with one dissenting report, 715). Lesion experiments suggest that this effect is exerted on the paraventricular nucleus; endogenous VIP projections involved are probably PVN projections of the suprachiasmatic nucleus (714).

In contrast, VIP was reported to have a direct, stimulating action on GnRH release from synaptosomal preparation (716). Gastrin-inhibitory peptide (GIP), another member of the glucagon superfamily, has also been shown to have a positive action on LH, but by a different mechanism involving presumably potentiation of GnRH stimulation of LH, but not of FSH (717). The gastrin releasing peptide (GRP) has been identified in lactotrophs and gonadotrophs, but no evidence of a paracrine role of that peptide could be obtained (718). Effects on LH (and, in part, effects on GH and PRL) have been implicated to involve a hypothalamic site of action (715). This could involve an inhibition of somatostatin release, as observed when mediobasal hypothalamic tissue was treated with VIP *in vitro* (719). A negative effect on presynaptic somatostatin release could thus account for GH and PRL responses to intraventricular VIP administration. Other examples of dual pituitary hormone control by a peptide are known and are mediated through redundant actions at the hypothalamic and pituitary levels. In contrast, glucagon enhances somatostatin release into the portal circulation (720), an observation which could account for the opposite effects of VIP and glucagon on GH secretion.

Vasoactive intestinal peptide affects serotonin turnover in the suprachiasmatic nucleus, a major component of the central clock regulating endocrine rhythms (451). The effects are estrogen-dependent (721). Along with neurotensin, VIP could thus play a role in the circadian control of LH and PRL secretion.

Growth Hormone-Releasing Hormone

Human GHRH is comprised of peptides that range from 37 to 44 amino acids (680,681) and that are derived from a 108-amino acid precursor (676). Some structural variability exists between human and murine forms of the molecule, which differ by as many as 14 amino acids (722). Unlike other members of the glucagon family, GHRH has a relatively limited distribution in the brain. It is mainly produced by neurons located in the arcuate nucleus and adjacent areas (679,723–726). These neurons colocalize neuropeptide Y (727). Their main projections are to the median eminence, where GHRH is released into the hypophyseal portal system (726). A few paraventricular neurons also contain GHRH (679). In addition to the median eminence, immunoreactive fibers have been traced to the periventricular area and the suprachiasmatic nucleus (724). Outside the hypothalamus, fibers are found in the stria terminalis and the amygdala (724).

The major documented action of GHRH is its stimulation of GH release (680,681) mediated by pituitary GHRH receptors (728) that have recently been cloned (729). Effects of high doses of GHRH on PRL release or potentiation of PRL responses to TRH (730) are believed to act via an interaction with VIP receptors, for which GHRH has a low affinity (693,731). In addition, some synthetic analogs of GHRH, that is, Ac-Tyr hGHRH or N-Ac-Tyr DPhe2-GHRH(1-29)-NH2, have been shown to act as weak antagonists of VIP receptors (693).

Pituitary Adenylate Cyclase Activating Polypeptide

A 38 amino acid amidated polypeptide has recently been isolated from ovine hypothalamus (732). A shorter, N-terminal sequence of the peptide was also found in the brain (733); it exhibits 68% homology with VIP (732). It is found in paraventricular neurons and numerous PACAP containing projections have been described in the median eminence (734). The pituitary is rich in binding sites for both peptides (735).

The peptide, originally defined by its capacity to activate adenylate cyclase in the adenohypophysis, is able to increase cytosolic Ca^{2+} in gonadotrophs and somatotrophs (736). In parallel, it potentiates the LH response to GnRH (737).

Other Related Peptides

Two related peptides isolated and characterized in porcine hypothalamic tissue have been shown to exhibit prolactin release inhibiting activity (738).

OPIOID PEPTIDES

Opioid peptides are derived from three different precursors: proenkephalin A, prodynorphin or proenkephalin B, and proopiomelanocortin. These three are coded by distinct genes and are expressed in distinct neuron systems. *Proenkephalin A* is a 241-amino acid sequence (740) predominantly produced by interneurons found throughout the brain and the medulla (741). In the brain, post-translational maturation of the precursor molecule results in four molecules of metenkephalin (Tyr-Gly-Gly-Phe-Met) and one molecule each of leu-enkephalin (Tyr-Gly-Gly-Phe-Leu), enkephalin heptapeptide (Tyr-Gly-Gly-Phe-Met-Arg-Phe), and enkephalin octapeptide (Tyr-Gly-Gly-Phe-Met-Arg-Gly-Leu) (742). These peptides are preferential ligands for delta opiate receptors (742). Hypothalamic *prodynorphin,* a 234-amino acid sequence, is mostly synthesized in neurons of the paraventricular nucleus (743,744), in which it is partially colocalized with CRF (684) and vasopressin (745). It has also been found in pituitary gonadotrophs (319,746). Corresponding projections innervate the median eminence [from which dynorphin can be released into the hypophyseal portal system (744)] and the posterior pituitary [where dynorphin is colocalized in oxytocin- and vasopressin-containing nerve terminals (747)]. A large number of nonhypothalamic structures, such as the hippocampus, basal nuclei, and the nucleus of the solitary tract, also contain high concentrations of dynorphin and of opiate receptors (748). Posttranslational cleavage generates alpha and beta neoendorphins (Tyr-Gly-Gly-Phe-Leu-Arg-Lys-Tyr-Pro, the alpha form having an additional lysine at the C-terminal), dynorphin A and B, and possibly leu-enkephalin. These peptides are preferential agonists for the kappa receptor subclass (741).

Proopiomelanocortin contains 241 amino acid residues (749) and is mainly synthesized in POMC cells of the anterior and intermediate lobes of the pituitary (749). It is also produced in large amounts by neurons of the arcuate nucleus (750), which project to the median eminence and to a wide spectrum of other brain structures (751,752). The major opioid product of POMC processing is beta-endorphin. The precursor also gives rise to ACTH and beta-LPH in the anterior pituitary (749), as well as to alpha- and beta-MSH and CLIP (corticotropinlike intermediary peptide) in the intermediate lobe and in the central nervous system (749), where they colocalize in the same neurons (753–756). Colocalization with DA has also been observed in arcuate neurons (750). Hypothalamic beta-endorphin has been measured in the hypophyseal portal blood (757). The peptide is highly active on delta and mu opiate receptors (742). Under appropriate conditions, opiates have been shown to have effects on the secretion of all hormones of the anterior and posterior lobes of the pituitary. As far as gonadotropic regulation is concerned, they markedly increase PRL secretion (758–761), whereas they inhibit that of LH and FSH (761,762). The abundant literature documenting hormonal effects of opiates has been reviewed elsewhere (763).

Opiates and Secretion of Gonadotropins

Morphine and opioid peptides inhibit the ovulatory surge of LH in rats (761,762) and, in general, inhibit gonadotropin release in many species, including monkeys. The action is more pronounced on LH than on FSH. Opiate antagonists, among which naloxone has been used most extensively, are able to elevate plasma levels of LH in many species (761,766,767) including humans (768,769). Thus, endogenous opiates may act as tonic inhibitors of LH secretion. Infusion of antisera to beta-endorphin or to dynorphin into the third ventricle also elevates plasma LH (770).

A major impact of opiates on gonadotropic secretion concerns the regulation of amplitude and frequency of pulsatile LH secretion. Administration of beta-endorphin reduces pulsatility in conscious, castrated rats (761,771). This likely involves a modulation of the hypothalamic pacemaker controlling the periodic activation of GnRH neurons, since the frequency of GnRH pulses in the hypophyseal portal blood of monkeys is also reduced by opiates (764). In parallel, morphine inhibits the firing frequency of hypothalamic neurons associated with the release of GnRH in the monkey (772).

Conversely, administration of naloxone increases LH pulse frequency in normal men (768,769,773,774) and women (775–777). The effect is more important during late follicular and luteal phases of the menstrual cycle (778). Naloxone also prevents sex steroid induced decreases in LH pulse frequency (779). The gonadotropin response to naloxone has been proposed as a functional test in reproductive pathology. It is blunted in delayed puberty (780) and in anorexic patients (775) under some, but not all, conditions (781,782).

Opiate effects on LH secretion are generally believed to involve the mu receptor subtype (783–786). However, the observation that ethylketocyclazocine (787) and bremazocine (788), two preferential kappa agonists, are as potent as morphine to lower LH secretion in immature female rats led to the conclusion that both types of receptors could be involved in mediating the response (789). This interpretation is also supported by experiments using kappa antagonists (790).

Opiates and Secretion of Prolactin

Morphine (761) and several opioid peptides induce a marked stimulation of plasma PRL levels (760). Beta-endorphin enhances the suckling-induced stimulation of PRL in lactating animals (791). Naloxone, alone, induces a slight decrease in basal circulating concentrations of PRL (758,761). However, it is quite effective in lowering stimulated PRL levels, especially during suckling (792,793) or stress (792). A single injection of the antagonist, which has a relatively short half-life, delays the rise of PRL observed under these conditions, whereas repeated injections prevent it completely. These data indicate that endogenous opiates are involved in the stress- and suckling-induced release of PRL, a conclusion substantiated by the increased biosynthesis and processing of enkephalins in lactating animals (794). Prolactin stimulation by cervicovaginal stimulation in the rat is also dependent upon endogenous opiates (795). As in the case of gonadotropic regulation, sex steroids are able to modulate the amplitude of PRL responses to opiates and to naloxone, in rats as well as in postmenopausal women (796).

Opiate receptors involved in PRL regulation are generally believed to belong to the μ class (797,798) and possibly to the μ-1 subclass (799). Administered intraventricularly, dermorphin, a potent μ-1 agonist, is quite effective in elevating plasma PRL in the rat (797,800,801) as well as in humans (802). The same class of opiate receptors thus seems to regulate both LH and PRL, in contrast to GH release, which is reportedly dependent upon delta receptors (798). A few reports however support the contention that kappa receptors could be involved concurrently with mu receptors. Dynorphin A (803–805) and neoendorphin (803), preferential kappa agonists, are both potent stimulators of PRL release in rats (803), primates (804,805), and people (806). Kappa agonists bremazocine and U50488 stimulate PRL at fairly low doses (807), although the amplitude of the response is smaller than that elicited by mu agonists (808). Mu and kappa receptors may be involved in different aspects of PRL regulation. PRL responses to stress are reportedly suppressed by mu, but not by kappa antagonists (809). In addition, PRL release exhibits a greater latency after administration of mu than of kappa agonists (810).

Opiate Effects Depend Upon Endocrine Parameters

The functional relevancy of endogenous opiates for LH and PRL regulation seems highly dependent upon the endocrine condition of experimental animals (811,812). Naloxone-induced elevation of mean levels of LH is reduced or absent in gonadectomized rats, in spite of an increased frequency of LH pulses (811–813). It can be restored by pretreatment with testosterone (811) or estrogens (814) and further enhanced by progesterone (814). An increased LH response to morphine also corresponds to elevated endogenous estrogen levels in cows (815). In contrast, estrogens have been shown to decrease the PRL response to morphine (816).

Conversely, chronic morphine treatment has been reported to sensitize LH feedback mechanisms to testosterone (817) and estrogens (818). These effects are consistent with the change in hypothalamic opiate activity observed after treatment with sex steroids. Estrogens decrease hypothalamic concentrations of beta-endorphin (819) and increase its release into the hypophyseal portal blood (757,820). Concentrations of the neuropeptide also fluctuate during the estrous cycle in discrete hypothalamic nuclei (821). Beta-endorphin immunoreactivity increases from diestrus to estrus (821). During late pregnancy and early postpartum, beta-endorphin concentrations in the hypothalamus have also been reported to increase in parallel with the elevated plasma levels of estrogens during the period (822).

Estrogen modulation of hypothalamic beta-endorphin levels could result from a direct effect of the steroid on a subset of neurons producing the peptide. A few (but not all) beta-endorphin neurons identified immunocytochemically within, or close to, the arcuate nucleus are able to accumulate estrogen (823) and express receptors for the hormone (824). Opiate mechanisms are probably also mediating other steroid effects in that structure, since PRL responses to morphine are blunted after local implantation of dexamethasone into the arcuate nucleus, but not other parts of the hypothalamus (825). Naloxone-induced LH responses seem to correlate with circadian fluctuations of hypothalamic opiate-binding sites (826). In addition, some authors have reports that sex steroids may affect the number of opiate-binding sites in the brain (827–829), but this finding has been challenged (830). Corticosteroid hormones may also modulate the effect of opiates on gonadotropin secretion (831).

Gonadotropin responses to opiates are also dependent upon maturation and sexual differentiation of the hypothalamus and the onset of puberty. In infantile male rats, LH responses appear insensitive to opiate antagonists (832) and show marked differences during the prepubertal period in both male and female rats (833,834). Sensitivity of PRL release to opiates also changes in the peripubertal period of heifers (835).

LH responses to opiates are also affected by perinatal androgen sterilization of female rats (836). This observation may be correlated with the dimorphic distribution of opiate peptides in the preoptic area of the hypothalamus in males, or in females treated neonatally with testosterone (836a). Interestingly, neonatal administration of naloxone has been reported to induce precocious puberty in the female rat (837,838). In parallel, gonadotropin regulation by opiates shows marked differences in seasonal breeders relative to age (839,840).

Hyperprolactinemia interferes with the opiate regulation of LH. In ovariectomized rats made hyperprolactinemic by ectopic pituitary grafts, administration of naloxone results in a greater increase of plasma LH than that observed in ungrafted controls (841). The effect is due to an increased pulsatile release of GnRH into the hypophyseal portal blood (842). Naloxone is more effective in elevating plasma LH in women with PRL-secreting microadenomas than in normoprolactinemic control patients (843,844). A discrepant observation was reported, however, in intact male rats (845). Taken together, these observations suggest that opiates exert a stronger tonic inhibition on GnRH in the presence of elevated PRL levels. This conclusion is also supported by increased hypothalamic levels of beta-endorphin and metenkephalin in hyperprolactinemic animals (791). Opiates also appear to be involved in other central consequences of hyperprolactinemia—for instance, those influencing thermoregulation (846).

Stress elevates beta-endorphin brain concentrations, as reported for instance in foot-shock stressed animals (847). This probably accounts for the decreased gonadotropin secretion observed during both acute and chronic stress (848), a response counteracted by opiate antagonists (849–851).

Site of Action of Opiates

The hypothalamus seems the major site of opiate-LH interactions (852), as shown by morphine inhibition of firing frequency of hypothalamic neurons associated with the release of GnRH (772) and of GnRH release into hypophyseal portal blood (841,853). The effect is steroid-dependent (854). Opiates can also inhibit depolarization-induced release of GnRH from mediobasal hypothalamic slices *in vitro* (855,856). Opiate-binding sites have been measured on median eminence nerve terminals corresponding possibly to GnRH and/or somatostatin neurons (856,857).

In addition to a direct, presynaptic inhibitory action on GnRH neurons, opiates are also believed to affect gonadotropin secretion by interfering with catecholaminergic neurotransmission in the hypothalamus (858) and to inhibit stimulatory noradrenergic inputs to the anterior preoptic area (859,860). Inhibition of tuberoinfundibular DA turnover (861,862) and release into the hypophyseal portal system (863) are the best-documented effects of opiates on hypothalamic catecholamines. These effects account for the PRL-stimulating effect of opioid peptides (864). In parallel, a decrease in portal blood DA concentrations correlates well with morphine-induced PRL secretion (865).

Opiates also appear to modulate reproductive hormone control by parallel effects on a number of other hypothalamic transmitters and peptides. They stimulate the release of 5-HT (866), a process that has been postulated to account partially for the opiate gonadotropic interaction (867). Opiates inhibit the synaptic release of TRH, both *in vitro* under depolarizing conditions (868) and *in vivo* in anesthetized rats submitted to a cold stress (869). In addition, a direct interaction on TRH-binding sites in the brain has been reported (870,871).

Other neuropeptides affected by opiates within the hypothalamus are somatostatin and CRF. The release of somatostatin from median eminence slices *in vitro* induced by high extracellular K^+ concentrations is antagonized by morphine and opioid peptides. This effect is reversed by naloxone (856,872). The release of corticotropin-releasing hormone *in vitro* is enhanced by nanomolar concentrations of beta-endorphin, an action consistent with mu receptor mediation (873).

Most opiate effects on hypothalamic transmitters appear to involve inhibition of presynaptic release (856,874), a prevalent mode of action of morphinomimetic drugs throughout the brain. Monitoring of release and electrical activity of oxytocin neurons suggests that such presynaptic inhibition involves uncoupling of action potentials from the resulting exocytosis (874), presumably by presynaptic blockade of voltage sensitive Ca^{2+} channels (875). This conclusion agrees with those of depolarization experiments (874).

As summarized in Table 3, effects of endogenous or exogenous opiates are mediated by several parallel hypothalamic pathways. The most important ones involve direct inhibition of GnRH release, tonic activation of GnRH neurons by noradrenergic projections, and inhibition of tuberoinfundibular DA release into portal blood. Alternate mechanisms may also be involved in the over-

TABLE 3. *Effect of morphine, opioid peptides, or their antagonists (relative to the inferred agonist effect) on hypothalamic transmitters and neuropeptides*

Transmitter	Hypothalamic		*In vivo* release measured		Presynaptic release *in vitro*	Portal blood concentration	Interaction with receptors
	Content	Turnover	Directly	Indirectly			
Dopamine		↓	↓	↓	↓	↓	No
Norepinephrine		↓		↓			
5-HT		↑					
GnRH				↓	↓	↓	
TRH			↓		↓		+
SRIF			↓				
CRF					↑		
GHRH				↑			
Oxytocin			↓	↓		↓*	
Vasopressin			↓			↓*	

(↑) Elevated by agonists (or decreased by antagonists); (↓) decreased by agonists (or elevated by antagonists); (+) interaction; (*) measurement in peripheral plasma. Detailed explanations are given in the text.

5-HT, serotonin; GnRH, gonadotropin-releasing hormone; TRH, thyrotropin-releasing hormone; SRIF, somatotropin release inhibiting factor; CRF, corticotropin releasing factor; GHRH, growth hormone-releasing hormone.

all hormonal responses, although their physiological relevance is less clearly established. Increased levels of 5-HT and CRF may act synergically, with a decreased norepinephrine turnover to suppress GnRH secretion. Inhibition of TRH and somatostatin could also participate in PRL modulation under appropriate conditions.

A few studies concluded that opiates can also have direct effects on pituitary cells (876,877). Although they do not generally affect by themselves PRL release from incubated pituitary cells (878–881), morphine and opiate peptides have been reported to antagonize the action of DA on PRL inhibition (878–881) *in vitro.* In addition, a relatively small but significant number of naloxone displaceable endorphin-binding sites has been reported on adenohypophyseal membranes (882).

CYTOKINES

Cytokines, also called mediators of the immune system, are not usually considered to be members of the neuropeptide family. Increasing evidence however points to their role in intercellular signaling between the hypothalamus and the pituitary. It is thus not inappropriate to briefly review here their actions on reproductive hormones.

Major cytokines, a family of peptides secreted by lymphocytes or other immunocompetent cells, are interleukins (IL) 1 to 6, tumor necrosis factor (TNF), and interferon γ. Thymosine, a peptide derived from thymic extracts, and platelet aggregating factor (PAF), an alkylphosphoglyceride, can also be considered as related to that category. They all exhibit autocrine or paracrine effects important for immune activation or regulation of blood cell interactions. Corresponding receptors have been cloned, and most of them belong to the GH/PRL/cytokine receptor superfamily, a subset of membrane receptors with a single transmembrane domain believed to act by tyrosine kinase activation.

Recent studies indicate that some cytokines, such as IL1, IL2, and TNF, can also be produced by neural cells as well as by folliculostellate pituitary cells. Autoradiographic studies have revealed the presence of IL1 and of the corresponding receptors (883–885) in the hypothalamus; IL6 has also been found in the pituitary. Cytokines secreted by immune cells can affect brain and neuroendocrine functions, as shown by their capacity to activate CRF dependent secretion of ACTH and modulate directly the hypothalamic release of GHRH and somatostatin (886–888). In spite of earlier reports, however, these effects are probably transmitted by cytokines produced locally in the cerebral circulation by macrophages or microglial cells (888) rather than by peripheral lymphocytes.

Neuroendocrine effects of cytokines resemble those induced by stressful stimuli. Intracerebral (but not intravenous) administration of IL1β, IL6, and TNF has been reported to decrease LH levels in castrated rats of both sexes (888). The effect is mimicked by treatment of the animals with endotoxin, an activator of the immune system, which triggers secretion of endogenous cytokines (888). IL1β was also shown to inhibit surges of LH induced by estrogen and progesterone treatment in ovariectomized rats (890), as well as pulsatility of LH secretion in castrates (891). Opiate peptides producing neurons may participate in these actions of IL1, since they can be prevented by naloxone (889,892). IL1 effects may also involve prostaglandin E_2-mediated amplification of GnRH activation (891).

In addition, interleukin-1, a peptide found in significant amounts in the arcuate nucleus, has been implicated in the regulation of PRL. Direct action on the pituitary has been recently reported (893). But this effect is probably mediated by interleukin-6, since IL1 stimulates IL6 release from rat pituitary cells *in vitro* (894). IL6 is a potent secretagogue for anterior pituitary hormone release *in vitro* (895).

Interferon γ inhibits *in vitro* prolactin release induced by either TRH or VIP (896). In contrast, thymosine (897), as well as a 35-amino acid-related peptide isolated from the thymus and presenting complete, almost sequence, homology with the nuclear protein histone H2A, can stimulate secretion of the hormone (898).

The glycerol-derived inflammation mediator PAF was also shown to stimulate prolactin release and, concurrently, Ca^{2+} influx in the GH4C1 cell line (899), but the effect was only obtained for concentrations much higher than those found effective on inflammatory processes.

GENERAL CONCLUSIONS

This review of the abundant literature concerning the action of various peptide and amine neuromediators on hypothalamic regulation of LH and PRL highlights a multitude of unanswered questions. Reading the staccato litany of substance by substance effects leaves one with little sense of how these diverse mechanisms concordantly result in regulation of reproductive processes. Clearly the administration of agonists into the interstitial space of neurons and other nonneuronal elements via the ventricular system does not address these questions. Selective neuropeptide, antagonists are not always available, precluding one's ability to study the effects of inhibiting endogenous activity. Much of the early experimentation on the role of neuromediators was hampered by our lack of knowledge concerning the final common pathways of neuroendocrine regulation, the neurosecretory neurons. Our increased knowledge in this area is now permitting investigators to determine the neuroanatomical connectivity of the neuroendocrine systems at this second level of integration. Clearly the recent work concerning the neuroanatomy of the paraventricular nucleus (26,519) hallmarks the potential insights to be gained from this approach. In this spirit we will attempt to make a few generalizations concerning peptide-transmitter interactions involved in controlling reproductive function.

Redundancy of Neuropeptide Circuitry

Several transmitters exhibit redundant actions within the hypothalamus, or at both the hypothalamus and pituitary. In some cases, these actions are synergistic and potentiate each other (see Fig. 2). VIP, for instance, stimulates PRL release (696,697) and, at the same time, inhibits the hypothalamic release of SRIF (719). Somatostatin is known to inhibit PRL secretion, at least in some instances (357,364). At the hypothalamic level, SRIF inhibits TRH release (372) and also tempers the PRL-releasing capacity of the tripeptide on the lactotroph (365).

Somatostatin can also inhibit the release of GnRH *in vitro* (371) as well as inhibit hypothalamic noradrenergic activity (369). Clearly noradrenergic neurons are involved in the stimulation of GnRH. On the other hand, CRF can inhibit both the release of GnRH from the median eminence (604,605) and GnRH-dependent stimulation of sex behavior (611,612).

In cases, redundant actions at the hypothalamic and pituitary levels appear antagonistic. Vasopressin, CCK, or angiotensin II can directly stimulate lactotrophs (555,624,650) as well as simultaneously activate dopamine-mediated inhibition of PRL release (561,625,653). These paradoxical effects reviewed in the conclusions of the section on hypothalamic neuropeptides synthesized in the paraventricular nucleus account for the discrepant responses obtained after intravenous or intraventricular administration of these peptides. They suggest that transmitter signaling to the neurosecretory neurons does not involve straightforward stimulatory or inhibitory messages. Instead it depends on complex interactions within hypothalamic networks, which transfer information to the gland over several alternate neurohormonal signals. A few transmitters can even induce a partial interruption of hypothalamohypophyseal communication, by inhibiting the presynaptic release of several hypothalamic neuromediators. For example, opiates presynaptically inhibit the release of several hypothalamic peptides (855,874) as well as of catecholamines (859,861).

Mechanisms Involved in Steroid Feedback

Many transmitters affect gonadotropin secretion in a steroid-dependent manner. They usually inhibit LH release in castrated animals but, on the other hand, are ineffective or even stimulatory in steroid-primed animals. The action of NPY (492,494), neurotensin (417), and angiotensin II (655,656) exhibit this property. Conversely, opiate inhibition of LH is attenuated by castration. Two of these transmitters (β-endorphin and NPY) have their cell bodies in the arcuate nucleus. Others, for example, angiotensin II, are believed to act mainly by modulating noradrenergic inputs to GnRH neurons (653). Noradrenergic neurons are, themselves, steroid-sensitive (63). In parallel, endogenous levels and receptors of these peptides are affected by steroids; endogenous NPY (496) and β-endorphin (821) are increased in the mediobasal hypothalamus by E_2. The number of neurotensin receptors are decreased by the steroid in the suprachiasmatic nucleus (441).

Modulation of reproductive functions by steroid hormones involves several independent processes. Estrogens, either alone or in combination with progesterone, affect the responsiveness of pituitary gonadotrophs to GnRH (900,901) and of lactotrophs to dopamine, TRH, and somatostatin (102,357,364,902). They also modify the synthesis and/or release of GnRH at the hypothalamic level, by affecting either directly GnRH neurons themselves (903,904) or, indirectly, neurotransmitters involved in their regulation, such as norepinephrine, neuropeptide Y, serotonin, opiates, and GABA.

The molecular basis of steroid modulation of hypothalamic functions is still poorly understood. It seems to involve modulation of neurotransmitter receptors (905) and of voltage-dependent Ca^{2+} channels (906,907). In contrast, steroid effects have been more extensively studied in the pituitary due to availability of more appropriate experimental models. Estrogens have been shown to affect both neuropeptide receptor numbers (GnRH, SRIF) (364,390) and receptor coupling efficiency by altering membrane transduction processes. For instance, the hormone can influence voltage dependent Ca^{2+} channels of the L type (357), as well as G proteins and membrane enzymes involved in secreting-coupling mechanisms (908–912).

Most such steroid effects reflect changes in protein kinase C (PKC) activity and thus phosphorylation/dephosphorylation processes (909,911). Steroids do not seem to interfere directly with PKC itself, but to increase instead the amount of available enzyme by genomic effects. Subsequent receptor mediated stimulation of PKC thus results in greater responses.

Ovarian steroids can also induce methyltransferase activity (908,910), another biochemical process leading to increased sensitivity of pituitary cells. Alterations of membrane phospholipid composition induce changes in the availability of phosphatidylcholine, a substrate of phospholipase A_2, as well as in physical properties of the membrane resulting from translocation of methylated phospholipids across the membrane. Such processes may also participate in secretion-coupling modulation by steroids. Changes in membrane microviscosity for instance affect the activity of ionic channels, the topology of cystoskeletal proteins, and, consequently, kinetic properties of membrane multienzyme systems. Furthermore, since the highest specific activity of methyltransferase is recovered from membranes of endoplasmic reticulum and secretion granules (910), one might speculate that steroid induced phospholipid methylation at these levels also alters mechanisms involved in the packaging, storage, and release of pituitary hormones.

Paracrine Effects of Neuropeptides in the Anterior Pituitary

Recent data indicate that several neuropeptides reviewed in this chapter can also be synthesized within the pituitary itself. Colocalization in gonadotrophs or lactotrophs of neuropeptides able to affect PRL secretion suggests that integration of neuroendocrine information involves paracrine and autocrine effects. In addition to inputs by hypothalamic and peripheral factors, pituitary cells thus also receive regulatory paracrine or autocrine signals. Studies related to the concept of *intrinsic* regulation of the pituitary gland and based on immunochemical or in situ hybridization techniques have shown that intercellular interactions within and between cell types involve a number of substances (peptides, hormones, transmitters, as well as arachidonic acid and its metabolites) synthesized and released locally by anterior pituitary cells, as summarized in Table 4. These observations however must be interpreted with caution due to the limitations of experimental models available.

A Network Operation

Taken altogether, data on redundant neurotransmitter control of hormone secretion and on paracrine interactions between pituitary cell types suggest that the hypothalamo-hypophyseal unit operates as a network rather than as an independent control system for each hormone. Network operation, a concept increasingly documented in immunology and in neurophysiology, implies that most cellular elements of heterogeneous systems can interact with others under appropriate conditions. The contribution of most elements of the network is not easily detectable in steady state; it is masked by the preeminence of a few major regulatory pathways (as for instance GnRH or dopamine control of gonadotrophs or lactotrophs).

In contrast, extrinsic or intrinsic challenges such as suckling or massive fluctuations in steroid feedback have the capacity to alter the overall signal environment of secreting cells. They do so by recruiting neuropeptide configurations, whether released from hypothalamic neurons or from neighboring pituitary cell types, which do not usually predominate. Such a modified signal environment affects the sensitivity of pituitary cells, as shown for instance by NPY or SP interaction with gonadotropin responsiveness to GnRH. Atypical hormonal responses observed under pathological conditions, such as PRL responses to GnRH or GH responses to dopamine reported in acromegalic patients, are likely to be accounted for by increased paracrine interference with "normal" physiological regulatory inputs.

The Concept of "Functional Entities" Within the Hypothalamus

Different peptides produced in the same anatomical structure often have parallel effects on the secretion of pituitary hormones. This suggests that hypothalamic regional organization may exhibit a certain degree of functional homogeneity with regard to neuroendocrine processes. For instance, transmitters found in the arcuate nucleus (β-endorphin, NPY) have been reported to affect the hypothalamic-oscillator-regulating circhoral episodes of LH (493,764,766,771). The arcuate nucleus may thus be considered a key structure for this function. This is consistent with the observation that pulsatile LH release is not affected by hypothalamic deafferentation in the monkey (58).

Neurons located in VIP (685), or projecting to 5-HT, NPY, PYY, neurotensin (129,440,472,476), the suprachiasmatic nucleus appear important for the control of circadian rhythmicity. Endogenous levels or receptor numbers of these peptides are affected by estrogens (440,441,496), which play an important role in maintaining high-amplitude circadian fluctuations of LH in the rat. VIP can modulate 5-HT turnover (721) and is a possible candidate for the transfer of rhythmic information from the suprachiasmatic nucleus to the medial preoptic area, to which VIP neurons supply numerous projections (686).

The paraventricular nucleus plays a key role in processing visceral afferent information (537). Most peptides elaborated in that nucleus appear to participate in stress-induced changes of gonadotropins and PRL secretion (see Table 2, and Figs. 1 and 2). CRF (603), oxytocin (566), and dynorphin (790) inhibit LH, probably by decreasing GnRH release (570,604,605). VIP (696,698), dynorphin (803), and CCK (624) stimulate PRL. These effects are all consistent with the hormonal profiles characteristic of stress responses, particularly elevation of PRL and inhibition of LH. The paraventricular nucleus also receives a dense noradrenergic innervation, which is a major pathway for the transfer of visceral afferent information (26).

Finally, a few hypotheses can be proposed for the functional role of some endogenous peptides. In addition to the involvement of peptides in ultradian or circadian rhythms and in paracrine synchronization, which

TABLE 4. *Neuropeptides as autocrine or paracrine factors on prolactin and luteinizing hormone release*

Peptides	Pituitary cell origin	Effect on PRL and LH cells	Observations: modifications of peptide release, immunoreactivity or mRNA
Angiotensin II	Gonadotrophs (404,913) Lactotrophs (404,914)	↑ PRL secretion (646) ↑ LH secretion (646)	
Activin	Gonadotrophs (915)	↑ basal and GnRH-induced FSH secretion (916) ↓ TRH-induced PRL secretion (916)	
Follistatin	Somatotrophs Folliculostellate (917) Gonadotrophs	↓ basal FSH and GnRH-stimulated LH and FSH (918)	
Galanin	Lactotrophs Thyrotrophs (510,511) Somatotrophs	↑ LH, LH response to GnRH (507)	↑ Galanin production after E_2 treatment (919) ↓ After ovariectomy, higher in female than male rats (920)
NPY	Thyrotrophs (921) and in scattered other AP cells	↑↓ LH release and GnRH-induced FSH (500,502)	↑ In hypothyroid rats (921) Sex steroid dependent effects
VIP	Thyrotrophs Lactotrophs (691,695,921,922) Stellate cells	↑ PRL release (699,923)	↑ After E_2 treatment, hypothyroidism (922) ↓ After T_4 administration (692)
Tachykins (Substance P, Neurokinin A, Neuropeptide γ)	Thyrotrophs Lactotrophs (921,925) Gonadotrophs	↑ PRL release ↑↓ LH release (417,924)	Higher in male than female rat ↑ thyroidectomy, ovariectomy, dihydrotesterone treatment ↓ after E_2 and T_3 administration (925)
Neurotensin		↑ PRL release (417)	↓ After TRH treatment, thyroidectomy, hypothyroidism (449,921)
Endotheline-3	Pit. cell origin (664)	↑ LH, FSH release (670)	Insulinlike growth factor 1, stimulates its release from pit. cell cultures (926)
Endotheline-1		↓ Basal and TRH-induced PRL release (670)	
Interleukin-6	Folliculostellate (927)	↑ Basal and TRH-induced PRL secretion (894) ↑ LH, FSH (668)	
Ach	Corticotrophs Lactotrophs (928)	↓ PRL release (928)	Immunoreactivity of CAT (928)
GnRH	Gonadotrophs (929)	↑ LH, FSH secretion (930)	
TRH	Gonadotrophs Thyrotrophs (929)	↑ PRL release (931)	
Calcitonin	Pituitary cell origin (932)	↓ Basal PRL and TRH-stimulated PRL release (933)	Immunoreactivity (932)
Dynorphin	Gonadotrophs (746)	↓ LH (770)	Colocalization with gonadotrophs (746)

Numbers in parentheses indicate references.
See text for abbreviations.

has been discussed above, experiments using peptide antagonists or passive immunization suggest that hypothalamic CRF (613), oxytocin (566), VIP (704), and opiates (849–851) are involved in mediating stress signals to the pituitary. In addition, VIP (703) and opiate peptides (793) play a role in suckling-induced stimulation of PRL secretion. Angiotensin II may regulate the amplitude of LH bursts (655). Endogenous somatostatin, which does not seem to have conspicuous effects on LH or PRL under normal conditions, appears able to compensate for the loss of tonic dopaminergic inhibition observed under conditions of long-term high levels of estrogen (357,364). In view of the negative effect of hyperprolactinemia on reproductive function, this compensatory relationship represents a potential fail-safe mechanism in addition to the direct effects of PRL on GnRH neurons discussed in this chapter.

Currently, rapid progress is being made concerning the chemistry and neuroanatomy of the neurosecretory neurons as well as the neurons containing peptides and amines that regulate their function. As discussed, this information will permit a clearer picture of the role of individual neuromediatory systems. However, the real challenge still lies in our ability to understand how this information is integrated into coherent patterns of regulation. Unraveling the complexity of the interactions involved in LH and PRL regulation will take considerable effort, and whether or not it will be resolved with a reductionist approach into a simple intuitively obvious code is still in question.

REFERENCES

1. Leranth C, Maclusky N, Salamoto H, Shanabrough M, Naftolin F. Glutamic acid decarboxylase-containing axons synapse on LHRH neurons in the rat medial preoptic area. *Neuroendocrinology* 1985;40:536–539.
2. Thind K, Goldsmith P. Infundibular gonadotropin-releasing hormone neurons are inhibited by direct opioid and autoregulatory synapses in juvenile monkeys. *Neuroendocrinology* 1988;47:203–216.
3. Rance N, Wise P, Selmanoff M, Barraclough C. Catecholamine turnover rates in discrete hypothalamic areas and associated changes in median eminence luteinizing hormone-releasing hormone and serum gonadotropins on proestrus and diestrous day 1. *Endocrinology* 1981;108:1795–1802.
4. Ramirez D, Feder H, Sawyer C. The role of brain catecholamines in the regulation of LH secretion: a critical inquiry. In: Martini L, Ganong W, eds. *Frontiers in neuroendocrinology,* vol. 8. New York: Raven Press, 1984;27–84.
5. Moore R, Bloom F. Central catecholamine neuron systems: anatomy and physiology of the norepinephrine and epinephrine systems. *Annu Rev Neurosci* 1979;2:113–168.
6. Palkovits M. Catecholamines in the hypothalamus: an anatomical review. *Neuroendocrinology* 1981;33:123–128.
7. Mellon PL, Windle JJ, Goldsmith PC, Padula CA, Roberts JL, Weiner RI. Immortalization of hypothalamic GnRH neurons by genetically targeted tumorigenesis. *Neuron* 1990;5:1–10.
8. Wetsel W, Mellon PL, Weiner RI, Negro-Vilar A. Metabolism of pro-LHRH in immortalized hypothalamic neurons. *Endocrinology* 1991;129:1584–1595.
9. Gautron JP, Pattou E, Poulin B, Laplante E, Kordon C, Drouva SV. Immunoréactivité apparentée à la LHRH dans une lignée neuronale hypothalamique (GT1-7) á LHRH: mise en évidence de LHRH (Gly^{11}) et de (Hyp^9)LHRH (Gly^{11}). *Colloq Soc Neurosci* 1992;1:(Abstr G 26).
10. Cussac D, Saltarelli D, Poulin B, Enjalbert A, Kordon C, Drouva SV. Stoechïométrie et nature des protéines G hétérotrimériques dans deux lignées hypophysaire (αT3) et neuronale hypothalamique (GT1-7). *Colloq Soc Neurosci* 1992;1:(Abstr G 16).
11. Martinez de la Escalera G, Choi A, Weiner RI. Generation and synchronization of GnRH pulses are intrinsic properties of the GT1-1 GnRH neuronal cell line. *Proc Natl Acad Sci USA* 1992;89:1852–1855.
12. Wetsel W, Valenca M, Merchenthaler I, et al. Intrinsic pulsatile secretory activity of immortalized luteinizing hormone-releasing hormone-secreting neurons. *Proc Natl Acad Sci USA* 1992;89:4149–4153.
13. Krsmanovic LZ, Stojilkovic SS, Merelli F, Dujour SM, Virmani MA, Catt KJ. Calcium signalling and episodic secretion of gonadotropin-releasing hormone in hypothalamic neurons. *Proc Natl Acad Sci USA* 1992;89:8462–8466.
14. Masotto C, Negro-Vilar A. Gonadectomy influences the inhibitory effect of the endogenous opiate system on pulsatile gonadotropin secretion. *Endocrinology* 1988;23:747–752.
15. Galiana E, Borde I, Marin P, et al. Establishment of permanent astroglial cell lines, able to differentiate in vitro from transgenic mice carrying the polyoma virus large T gene: an alternative approach to brain cell immortalization. *J Neurosci Res* 1990;26:269.
16. Suri C, Fung BP, Tischler AS, Chikaraishi. Catecholaminergic cell lines from the brain and adrenal glands of tyrosine hydroxylase-SV40 T antigen transgenic mice. *J Neurosci* 1993;13:1280.
17. Barraclough C, Wise P, Selmanoff M. A role for hypothalamic catecholamines in the regulation of gonadotropin secretion. *Recent Prog Horm Res* 1984;40:487–529.
18. Barraclough C, Wise P. The role of catecholamines in the regulation of pituitary luteinizing hormone and follicle-stimulating hormone secretion. *Endocr Rev* 1982;3:91–119.
19. Weiner R, Ganong W. Role of brain monoamines and histamine in regulation of anterior pituitary secretion. *Physiol Rev* 1978;58:905–976.
20. Gallo R. Neuroendocrine regulation of pulsatile luteinizing hormone release in the rat. *Neuroendocrinology* 1980;30:122–131.
21. Taleisnik S, Sawyer C. Activation of the CNS noradrenergic system may inhibit as well as facilitate pituitary luteinizing hormone release. *Neuroendocrinology* 1986;44:265–268.
22. Weiner R, Shryne J, Gorski R, Sawyer H. Changes in the catecholamine content of the rat hypothalamus following deafferentation. *Endocrinology* 1972;90:867–873.
23. Brownstein M, Palkovits M, Tappaz M, Saavedra J, Kizer J. Effect of surgical isolation of the hypothalamus on its neurotransmitter content. *Brain Res* 1976;117:287–296.
24. Palkovits M, Brownstein M, Saavedra J, Axelrod J. Norepinephrine and dopamine content of hypothalamic nuclei of rat. *Brain Res* 1974;77:137–149.
25. Dahlstrom A, Fuxe K. Evidence for the existence of monoamine-containing neurons in the central nervous system: 1. Demonstration of monoamine in cell bodies of brain stem neurons. *Acta Physiol Scand* [*Suppl*] 1964;232:1–55.
26. Swanson L, Sawchenko P, Lind R. Regulation of multiple peptides in CRF parocellular neurosecretory neurons: implications for the stress response. *Brain Res* 1986;68:169–190.
27. Day T, Blessing W, Willoughby J. Noradrenergic and dopaminergic projections to the medial preoptic area of the rat: a combined horseradish peroxidase/catecholamine fluorescence study. *Brain Res* 1980;193:543–548.
28. Jennes L, Beckman W, Stumpf W, Grzanna R. Anatomical relationships of serotoninergic and noradrenalinergic projections with the GnRH system in septum and hypothalamus. *Exp Brain Res* 1982;46:331–338.
29. Martinez de la Escalera G, Choi AL, Weiner RI. β_1-adrenergic regulation of the GT1 gonadotropin releasing hormone (GnRH) neuronal cell lines: stimulation of GnRH release via receptor positively coupled to adenylate cyclase. *Endocrinology* 1992;131:1397–1402.
30. Findell PR, Wong KH, Jackman JK, Daniels DV. β_1-adrenergic and dopamine (D_1)-receptors coupled to adenylyl cyclase activation in GT1 gonadotropin-releasing hormone neurosecretory cells. *Endocrinology* 1993;132:682–688.
31. Naftolin F, Leranth C, Machusky N. Norepinephnne (NE) and dopamine (DA) innervation of medial preoptic area (MPO) LHRH and GABA neurons in the rat. *Soc Neurosci Abstr* 1986;12:1–152.
32. Descarries L, Walkins K, Lapierre Y. Noradrenergic axon terminals in cerebral cortex of the rat. III. Topographic ultrastructural analysis. *Brain Res* 1977;133:197–222.
33. Hökfelt T, Fuxe K, Goldstein M, Johansson O. Immunohistochemical evidence for the existence of adrenaline neurons in the rat brain. *Brain Res* 1974;66:239–251.
34. Howe P, Costa M, Furness J, Chalmers J. Simultaneous demonstration of *phenylethanolamine-N-methyltransferase* immunofluorescent and catecholamine fluorescent nerve cell bodies in the rat medulla oblongata. *Neuroscience* 1980;5:2229–2238.
35. Gugten J, Palkovits M, Wijnen H, Versteg D. Regional distribution of adrenaline in rat brain. *Brain Res* 1976;107:171–175.
36. Swanson L, Mogenson G. Neural mechanisms for the functional coupling of autonomic, endocrine and somatomotor responses and adaptive behavior. *Brain Res Rev* 1981;31:1–34.
37. Fuxe K, Hokfelt T. Further evidence for the existence of tuberoinfundibular dopamine neurons. *Acta Physiol Scand* 1966;66:245.
38. Ben-Jonathan N, Oliver C, Weiner H, Mical R, Porter J. Dopamine in hypophysial portal plasma of the rat during the estrous cycle and throughout pregnancy. *Endocrinology* 1977;100:452–458.
39. Chen H, Roberts J, Weiner R. Binding of 3H-dihydroergocryptine to an α-adrenergic site in the stalk median eminence of the steer. *Endocrinology* 1981;109:2138–2143.
40. Leibowitz S, Jhanwar-Uniyal M, Dvorkin B, Makman M. Distribution of α-adrenergic, β-adrenergic and dopaminergic receptors in discrete hypothalamic areas of the rat. *Brain Res* 1982;233:97–114.
41. Martinez de la Escalera G, Gallo F, Choi AL, Weiner RI. Dopami-

nergic regulation of the GT1 gonadotropin-releasing hormone (GnRH) neuronal cell lines: stimulation of GnRH release via D1-receptors positively coupled to adenylate cyclase. *Endocrinology* 1992;131:2965–2971.
42. Bjorklund A, Lindvall O, Nobin A. Evidence of an incerto-hypothalamic dopamine neuron system in the rat. *Brain Res* 1975;89:29–42.
43. Day T, Blessing W, Willoughby J. Noradrenergic and dopaminergic projections to the medial preoptic area of the rat. A combined horseradish *peroxidase/catecholamine* fluorescence study. *Brain Res* 1980;193:543–548.
44. Negro-Vilar A, Advis J, Ojeda S, McCann S. Pulsatile luteinizing hormone (LH) patterns in ovariectomized rats: Involvement of norepinephrine and dopamine in the release of LH releasing hormone and LH. *Endocrinology* 1982;111:932–938.
45. Drouva S, Gallo R. Catecholamine involvement in episodic luteinizing hormone release in adult ovariectomized rats. *Endocrinology* 1976;99:651–658.
46. Gnodde H, Schuling G. Involvement of catecholaminergic and cholinergic mechanisms in the pulsatile release of LH in the long term ovariectomized rat. *Neuroendocrinology* 1976;20:212–223.
47. Weick R. Acute effects of adrenergic receptor blocking drugs and neuroleptic agents on pulsatile discharges of luteinizing hormone in the ovariectomized rat. *Neuroendocrinology* 1978;26:108–117.
48. Hancke J, Berk W, Baumgarten H, Hohn K, Wuttke W. Modulatory effect of noradrenaline and serotonin on circhoral LH release in adult ovariectomized rats. *Acta Endocrinol (Suppl) (Copenh)* 1977;208:22–23.
49. Bhattacharya A, Dierschke D, Yamaji J, Knobil E. The pharmacologic blockade of the circhoral mode of LH secretion in the ovariectomized rhesus monkey. *Endocrinology* 1972;90:778–786.
50. Estes K, Simpkins J, Kalra S. Resumption with clonidine of pulsatile LH release following acute norepinephrine depletion in ovariectomized rats. *Neuroendocrinology* 1982;35:56–62.
51. Crowley W, Terry L, Johnson M. Evidence for the involvement of central epinephrine systems in the regulation of luteinizing hormone, prolactin, and growth hormone release in female rats. *Endocrinology* 1982;110:1102–1107.
52. Gallo R, Drouva S. Effect of intraventricular infusion of catecholamines on luteinizing hormone release in ovariectomized and ovariectomized, steroid primed rats. *Neuroendocrinology* 1979; 29:14.
53. Gallo R. Further studies on norepinephrine-induced suppression of pulsatile luteinizing hormone release in ovariectomized rats. *Neuroendocrinology* 1984;39:120–125.
54. Leipheimer R, Gallo R. Medial preoptic area involvement in norepinephrine-induced suppression of pulsatile luteinizing hormone release in ovariectomized rats. *Neuroendocrinology* 1985;40:345–351.
55. Leung P, Arendash G, Whitmoyer D, Gorski R, Sawyer C. Electrical stimulation of mesencephalic noradrenergic pathway: Effects on luteinizing hormone levels in blood of ovariectomized and ovariectomized, steroid-primed rats. *Endocrinology* 1981; 109:720–728.
56. Drouva S, Gallo R. Further evidence for inhibition of episodic luteinizing hormone release in ovariectomized rats by stimulation of dopamine receptors. *Endocrinology* 1977;100:792–798.
57. Jarry H, Sprenger M, Wuttke W. Rates of release of GABA and catecholamines in the mediobasal hypothalamus of ovariectomized and ovariectomized estrogen-treated rats: Correlation with blood prolactin levels. *Neuroendocrinology* 1986;44:422–428.
58. Krey L, Butler W, Knobil E. Surgical disconnection of the medial basal hypothalamus and pituitary function in the rhesus monkey. I. Gonadotropin secretion. *Endocrinology* 1975;96:1073–1087.
59. Wise P, Rance N, Barraclough C. Effects of estradiol and progesterone on catecholamine turnover rates in discrete hypothalamic regions in ovariectomized rats. *Endocrinology* 1981;108: 2186–2193.
60. Demling J, Fuchs E, Baumert M, Wuttke W. Preoptic catecholamine, GABA, and glutamate release in ovariectomized and ovariectomized estrogen primed rats utilizing a pushpull cannula technique. *Neuroendocrinology* 1985;41:212–218.
61. Advis J, McCann S, Negro-Vilar A. Evidence that catecholaminergic and peptidergic (luteinizing hormone-releasing hormone) neurons in suprachiasmatic-medial preoptic, medial basal hypothalamus and median eminence are involved in estrogen-negative feedback. *Endocrinology* 1980;107:892–901.
62. Crowley W. Effects of ovarian hormones on norepinephrine and dopamine turnover in individual hypothalamic and extrahypothalamic nuclei. *Neuroendocrinology* 1982;34:381–386.
63. Heritage A, Grant L, Stumpf W. 3H-estradiol in catecholamine neurons of rat brain stem: Combined localization by autoradiography and formaldehyde-induced fluorescence. *J Comp Neurol* 1977;176:607–630.
64. MacKinnon P, Clement E, Clark C, Sheares R. Hypothalamic adrenergic activity precedes the preovulatory luteinizing hormone surge in the rat. *Neurosci Lett* 1983;43:221–226.
65. Coombs M, Coen C. Adrenaline turnover rates in the medial preoptic area and mediobasal hypothalamus in relation to the release of luteinizing hormone in female rats. *Neuroscience* 1983;10:207–210.
66. Adler B, Johnson M, Lynch C, Crowley W. Evidence that norepinephrine and epinephrine systems mediate the stimulatory effects of ovarian hormones on luteinizing hormone and luteinizing hormone-releasing hormone. *Endocrinology* 1983;113: 1431–1438.
67. Wilkinson M, Herdon H, Pearce M, Wilson C. Radioligand binding studies on hypothalamic noradrenergic receptors during the estrous cycle or after steroid injection in ovariectomized rats. *Brain Res* 1979;168:652–655.
68. Gudelsky G, Porter J. Release of dopamine from tuberoinfundibular neurons into pituitary stalk blood after prolactin or haloperidol administration. *Endocrinology* 1980;106:526–529.
69. Grant L, Stumpf W. Localization of ^{3}H-estradiol and catecholamines in identical neurons in the hypothalamus. *J Histochem Cytochem* 1973;21:404.
70. Sar M. Estradiol is concentrated in tyrosine hydroxylase containing neurons of the hypothalamus. *Science* 1983;223:938–940.
71. Wang P, Porter J. Hormonal modulation of the quantity and *in situ* activity of tyrosine hydroxylase in neurites of the median eminence. *Proc Natl Acad Sci USA* 1986;83:9804–9806.
72. Sawyer C, Markee J, Everett J. Further experiments on blocking pituitary activity in the rabbit and rat. *J Exp Zool* 1950; 113:659–682.
73. Kalra S, McCann S. Effects of drugs modifying catecholamine synthesis on plasma LH and ovulation in the rat. *Neuroendocrinology* 1974;15:79–91.
74. Clifton D, Sawyer C. LH release and ovulation in the rat following depletion of hypothalamic norepinephrine: Chronic vs. acute effects. *Neuroendocrinology* 1979;28:442–449.
75. Coen C, Coombs M. Effects of manipulating catecholamines on the incidence of the preovulatory surge of luteinizing hormone and ovulation in the rat: Evidence for a necessary involvement of hypothalamic adrenaline in the normal or "midnight" surge. *Neuroscience* 1983;10:187–206.
76. Clifton D, Sawyer C. Positive and negative feedback effects of ovarian steroids on luteinizing hormone release in ovariectomized rats following chronic depletion of hypothalamic norepinephrine. *Endocrinology* 1980;106:1099–1102.
77. Nicholson G, Greeley G, Humm J, Youngblood W, Kizer J. Lack of effect of noradrenergic denervation of the hypothalamus and medial preoptic area on the feedback regulation of gonadotropin secretion and the estrous cycle. *Endocrinology* 1978;103: 539–566.
78. Kalra P, Kalra S, Krulich L, Fawcett C, McCann S. Involvement of norepinephrine in transmissions of the stimulatory influence of progesterone on gonadotropin release. *Endocrinology* 1972;90: 1168–1176.
79. Drouva S, Laplante E, Kordon C. α_1-Adrenergic receptor involvement in the LH surge in ovariectomized estrogen primed rats. *Eur J Pharmacol* 1982;81:341–344.
80. Kalra S. Catecholamine involvement in preovulatory LH release: Reassessment of the role of epinephrine. *Neuroendocrinology* 1985;40:139–144.
81. Sheaves R, Laynes R, MacKinnon P. Reduction of central epinephrine concentration is consistent with continued occurrence of ovulation in rats treated with an inhibitor (LY 134046) of

phenylethanolamine N-methyltransferase. *Neuroendocrinology* 1985;41:432–436.

82. Crowley W, Terry C. Effects of an epinephrine synthesis inhibitor, SKF64139, on the secretion of luteinizing hormone in ovariectomized female rats. *Brain Res* 1981;204:231–235.
83. Krieg R, Sawyer C. Effects of intraventricular catecholamines on luteinizing hormone release in ovariectomized-steroid-primed rats. *Endocrinology* 1976;99:411–419.
84. Leung P, Arendash G, Whitmoyer D, Gorski R, Sawyer C. Differential effects of central adrenoceptor agonists on luteinizing hormone release. *Neuroendocrinology* 1982;34:207–214.
85. Sawyer C, Hilliard J, Kanematsu S, Scaramuzzi R, Blake C. Effects of intraventricular infusions of norepinephrine and dopamine on LH release and ovulation in the rabbit. *Neuroendocrinology* 1974;15:328–337.
86. Rubinstein L, Sawyer C. Role of catecholamines in stimulating the release of pituitary ovulating hormone(s) in rats. *Endocrinology* 1970;86:988–995.
87. Ojeda S, Negro-Vilar A, McCann S. Evidence for involvement of α1-adrenergic receptors in norepinephrine-induced prostaglandin E2 and luteinizing hormone-releasing hormone release from median eminence. *Endocrinology* 1982;110:409–412.
88. Negro-Vilar A. The median eminence as a model to study presynaptic regulation of neural peptide release. *Peptides* 1982;3: 305–310.
89. Knobil E. The neuroendocrine control of the menstrual cycle. *Recent Prog Horm Res* 1980;36:53–88.
90. Dotti C, Taleisnik S. Inhibition of the release of LH and ovulation by activation of the noradrenergic system. Effect of interrupting the ascending pathways. *Brain Res* 1982;249:281–290.
91. Dotti C, Tabeisnik S. Beta-adrenergic receptors in the premammillary nucleus mediate the inhibition of LH release evoked by the locus ceruleus stimulation. *Neuroendocrinology* 1984;38: 6–11.
92. Leung P, Whitmoyer D, Garland K, Sawyer C. β-Adrenergic suppression of progesterone-induced luteinizing hormone surge in ovariectomized, estrogen-primed rats. *Proc Soc Exp Biol Med* 1982;169:161–164.
93. Choudhury S, Sharpe R, Brown P. The effect of pimozide, a dopamine antagonist, on pituitary gonadotrophic function in the rat. *J Reprod Fertil* 1974;39:275–283.
94. Bergen H, Leung P. Suppression of progesterone induced gonadotropin surge by adrenergic agonists in estrogen-primed ovariectomized rats. *Neuroendocrinology* 1986;43:397–403.
95. Leppaluoto J, Mannisto P, Ranta T, Linnoila M. Inhibition of mid-cycle gonadotropin release in healthy women by pimozide or fusaric acid. *Acta Endocrinol* 1976;81:455–460.
96. Schneider H, McCann S. Monoamine and indolamines and control of LH secretion. *Endocrinology* 1970;86:1127–1133.
97. Vijayan E, McCann S. Re-evaluation of the role of catecholamines in control of gonadotropin and prolactin release. *Neuroendocrinology* 1978;25:150–165.
98. Ojeda S, Hamms P, McCann S. Possible role of cyclic AMP and prostaglandin E_1 in the dopaminergic control of prolactin release. *Endocrinology* 1974;95:1694–1703.
99. Judd S, Rakoff J, Yen S. Inhibition of gonadotropin and prolactin release by dopamine: effect of endogenous estradiol levels. *J Clin Endocrinol Metab* 1978;47:494–498.
100. Lal S, DeLa Vega C, Sourkes T, Friesen H. Effect of apomorphine on growth hormone, prolactin, luteinizing hormone and follicle-stimulating hormone levels in human serum. *J Clin Endocrinol Metab* 1973;37:719–724.
101. Jarjour L, Handelsman D, Raum W, Swerdloff R. Mechanism of action of dopamine on the *in vitro* release of gonadotropin-releasing hormone. *Endocrinology* 1986;119:1726–1732.
102. Ben-Jonathan N. Dopamine: A prolactin-inhibiting hormone. *Endocr Rev* 1985;6:564–589.
103. Neill J. Neuroendocrine regulation of prolactin secretion. In: Martini L, Ganong W, eds. *Frontiers in neuroendocrinology,* vol. 6. New York: Raven Press, 1980;129–155.
104. Yen S. Prolactin human reproduction. In: Yen S, Jaffe R, eds. *Reproductive endocrinology.* Philadelphia: WB Saunders, 1986; 237–263.
105. Negro-Vilar A, Ojeda S, Advis J, McCann S. Evidence for noradrenergic involvement in episodic prolactin and growth hormone release in ovariectomized rats. *Endocrinology* 1979;105:86.
106. Terry L, Martin J. Evidence for α-adrenergic regulation of episodic growth hormone and prolactin secretion in the undisturbed male rat. *Endocrinology* 1981;108:1869–1873.
107. Lawson D, Gala R. The influence of adrenergic, dopaminergic, cholinergic and serotoninergic drugs on plasma prolactin levels in ovariectomized, estrogen treated rats. *Endocrinology* 1975;96: 313–318.
108. Quardri S, Pierson C, Spies H. Effects of centrally acting drugs on serum prolactin levels in Rhesus monkey. *Neuroendocrinology* 1978;27:136–147.
109. Lien E, Morrison A, Kassarich J, Sullivan D. Alpha-2-adrenergic control of prolactin secretion. *Neuroendocrinology* 1986;44: 184–189.
110. Meltzer H, Simonovic M, Gudelsky G. Effect of yohimbine on rat prolactin secretion. *J Pharmacol Exp Ther* 1983;224:21–27.
111. Gold M, Donabedian R, Redmond D. Further evidence for alpha-2-adrenergic receptor mediated inhibition of prolactin secretion: The effect of yohimbine. *Psychoneuroendocrinology* 1979;3:253–260.
112. Tatar P, Vigas M. Role of alpha1- and alpha2-adrenergic receptors in the growth hormone release and prolactin response to insulin-induced hypoglycemia in man. *Neuroendocrinology* 1984;39:275–280.
113. Weiner R, Shyme J, Gorski R, Sawyer C. Changes in the catecholamine content of the rat hypothalamus following deafferentation. *Endocrinology* 1972;90:867–873.
114. Blake C, Weiner R, Sawyer C. Pituitary prolactin secretion in female rats made persistently estrous or diestrous by hypothalamic deafferentation. *Endocrinology* 1972;90:862–866.
115. Langelier P, McCann S. The effects of interruption of the ventral noradrenergic pathway on the proestrous discharge of prolactin in the rat. *Proc Soc Exp Biol Med* 1977;154:553–557.
116. Kalra S, Kalra P, Chen C, Clemens C. Effect of norepinephrine synthesis inhibitors and a dopamine agonist on hypothalamic LHRH, serum gonadotrophin and prolactin levels in gonadal steroid treated rats. *Acta Endocrinol* 1978;89:1–9.
117. Subramanian M, Gala R. The influence of cholinergic, adrenergic, and serotoninergic drugs on the afternoon surge of plasma prolactin in ovariectomized, estrogen treated rats. *Endocrinology* 1976;98:842–848.
118. Voogt J, Carr L. Plasma prolactin levels and hypothalamic catecholamine synthesis during suckling. *Neuroendocrinology* 1974; 16:108–118.
119. Carr L, Conway P, Voogt J. Role of norepinephrine in the release of prolactin induced by suckling and estrogen. *Brain Res* 1977;133:305–314.
120. Parent A, Descarries L, Beaudet A. Organization of ascending serotonin systems in the adult rat brain. A radioautographic study after intraventricular administration of [3H]S-hydroxytryptamine. *Neuroscience* 1981;6:15–138.
121. Steinbusch HWM. Distribution of serotonin-immunoreactivity in the central nervous system of the rat-cell bodies and terminals. *Neuroscience* 1981;6:557–618.
122. Steinbusch HWM. Serotonin-immunoreactive neurons and their projections in the CNS. In: Bjorklund A, Hökfelt T, Kuhar MJ, eds. *Handbook of chemical neuroanatomy, vol. 3: Classical transmitters and transmitter receptors in the CNS Part 11.* Amsterdam: Elsevier, 1984;68–125.
123. Azmita EC, Segal M. An autoradiographic analysis of the differential ascending projections of the dorsal and median raphe nuclei in the rat. *J Comp Neurol* 1970;179:641–668.
124. Palkovits M. Effect of surgical deafferentation on the transmitter and hormone content of the hypothalamus. *Neuroendocrinology* 1979;29:140–148.
125. Beaudet A, Descarries L. Radioautographic characterization of a serotonin accumulating nerve cell group in the adult rat hypothalamus. *Brain Res* 1979;160:231–243.
126. Fuxe K, Ungerstedt V. Histochemical studies on the distribution of catecholamine and 5-hydroxytryptamine after intraventricular injections. *Histochemia* 1968;13:16–28.
127. Shaskan EG, Snyder SH. Kinetics of serotonin accumulation into

slices from rat brain: Relationship to catecholamine uptake. *J Pharmacol Exp Ther* 1970;175:404–418.
128. Frankfurt M, Lauder JM, Azimitia EC. The immunocytochemical localization of serotonergic neurons in the rat hypothalamus. *Neurosci Lett* 1981;24:227–232.
129. Descarries L, Beaudet A. The serotonin innervation of adult rat hypothalamus. In: Vincent JD, Kordon C, eds. *Cell biology of hypothalamic neurosecretion.* Paris: CNRS, 1978;135–153.
130. Bosler C, Joh TH, Beaudet A. Ultrastructural relationships between serotonin and dopamine neurons in the rat arcuate nucleus and medial zona incerta: A combined radioautographic and immunocytochemical study. *Neurosci Lett* 1984;48:279–285.
131. Kiss J, Halasz B. Synaptic connections between serotonergic axon terminals and tyrosine hydroxylase-immunoreactive neurons in the arcuate nucleus of the rat hypothalamus. A combination of electron microscopic autoradiography and immunocytochemistry. *Brain Res* 1986;364:284–294.
132. Jennes L, Beckman WC, Stumph WE, Grzanna R. Anatomical relationships of serotoninergic and noradrenalingeric projections with the GnRH system in septum and hypothalamus. *Exp Brain Res* 1982;46:331–338.
133. Pelletier G, Leclerc R, Dube D. Immunocytochemical localization of hypothalamic hormones. *J Histochem Cytochem* 1976;24:864–871.
134. Mazzuca M. Immunocytochemical and ultrastructural identification of luteinizing hormone-releasing hormone (LH-RH)-containing neurons in the vascular organ of the lamina terminalis (OVLT) of the squirrel monkey. *Neurosci Lett* 1977;5: 123–127.
135. Kiss J, Halasz B. Demonstration of serotoninergic axons terminating on luteinizing hormone-releasing hormone neurons in the preoptic area of the rat using a combination of immunocytochemistry and high resolution autoradiography. *Neuroscience* 1985; 14:69.
136. Frazer A, Maayani S, Wolfe BB. Subtypes of receptors for serotonin. *Annu Rev Pharmacol Toxicol* 1990;30:307–348.
137. Friedman E, Krieger DT, Mezey E, Leranth CS, Brownstein MJ, Palkovits M. Serotonergic innervation of the rat pituitary intermediate lobe: Decrease after stalk section. *Endocrinology* 1983;112:1943–1947.
138. Mezey E, Leranth C, Brownstein MJ, Friedman E, Krieger DT, Palkovits M. On the origin of serotonergic input to the intermediate lobe of the rat pituitary. *Brain Res* 1984;294:231.
139. Steinbusch HWM, Nieuwenhuys R. Localization of serotonin-like immunoreactivity in the central nervous system and pituitary of the rat, with special reference to the innervation of the hypothalamus. In: Haber B, Gabay S, Issidorides MR, Alivijatos SGA, eds. *Serotonin: current aspects of neurochemistry and function.* New York: Plenum Press, 1982;7–35.
140. Payette RF, Gershon MD, Nunez EA. Serotonergic elements of the mammalian pituitary. *Endocrinology* 1985;116:1933–1942.
141. Sano Y, Takeuchi Y, Matsuura T, Kawata M, Yamada H. Immunohistochemical demonstration of serotonin nerve fibers in the cat neurohypophysis. *Histochemistry* 1982;75:293–299.
142. Westlund KN, Childs GV. Localization of serotonin fibers in the rat adenohypophysis. *Endocrinology* 1982;111:1761–1763.
143. Kah O, Chambolle P. Serotonin in the brains of goldfish, *Carassius auratus:* An immunocytochemical study. *Cell Tissue Res* 1983;234:319–333.
144. Kondo Y, Nagatsu I, Yoshida M, Karadawa N, Nagatsu T. Existence of noradrenalin cells and serotonin cells in the pituitary gland of *Rana catesbeiana. Cell Tissue Res* 1983;228:405–408.
145. Saavedra JM, Palkovits M, Kizer JS, Brownstein JM, Zwin JA. Distribution of biogenic amines and related enzymes in the rat pituitary gland. *J Neurochem* 1975;25:257–260.
146. Nunez EA, Gershon MD, Silverman, AJ. Uptake of S-hydroxytryptamine by gonadotrophs of the bat's pituitary: A combined immunocytochemical radioautographic analysis. *J Histochem Cytochem* 1981;29:1336–1346.
147. Johns MA, Azmita EC, K Rieger DT. Specific *in vitro* uptake of serotonin by cells in the anterior pituitary of the rat. *Endocrinology* 1982;110:754–760.
148. DeSouza EB. Serotonin and dopamine receptors in the rat pituitary gland: Autoradiographic identification, characterization, and localization. *Endocrinology* 1986;119:1534–1542.
149. Porter JC, Mical RS, Cramer OM. Effect of serotonin and other indoles on the release of LH, FSH and prolactin. *Gynecol Invest* 1971;2:13–22.
150. Caligaris L, Taleisnek S. Involvement of neurons containing S-hydroxytryptamine in the mechanism of prolactin release induced by estrogen. *J Endocrinol* 1974;62:25–33.
151. Meltzer HY, Fang VS, Paul SM, Kaluskar R. Effect of quipazine on rat plasma prolactin levels. *Life Sci* 1976;1:1073–1078.
152. Lu KH, Meites J. Effects of serotonin precursors and melatonin on serum prolactin release in rats. *Endocrinology* 1973;93: 152–155.
153. Talwalker PK, Ratner A, Meites J. *In vitro* inhibition of pituitary prolactin synthesis and release by hypothalamic extract. *Am J Physiol* 1963;205:213–218.
154. Kordon C, Glowinski J. Role of hypothalamic monoaminergic neurons in the gonadotrophin release-regulating mechanisms. *Neuropharmacology* 1972;11:153–162.
155. Ng LKY, Chase N, Colburn R, Kopin I. Release of [^{3}H] dopamine by n-S-hydroxytryptophan. *Brain Res* 1972;45:499–506.
156. Donoso AO, Bishop W, Fawcett CP, Krulich L, McCann SM. Effects of drugs that modify brain monoamine concentrations on plasma gonadotropin and prolactin levels in the rat. *Endocrinology* 1971;89:774–784.
157. Gallo RV, Rabii J, Moberg GP. Effect of methysergide, a blocker of serotonin receptors on plasma prolactin levels in lactating and ovariectomized rats. *Endocrinology* 1975;97:1096–1105.
158. Kordon C, Blake CA, Terkel J, Sawyer CH. Participation of serotonin-containing neurons in the suckling-induced rise in plasma prolactin levels in lactating rats. *Neuroendocrinology* 1973;13: 213–223.
159. Gil AD, Zambotti F, Caruba MO, Vicentini L, Muller EE. Stimulatory role for brain serotonergic system on prolactin secretion in the male rat. *Proc Soc Exp Biol Med* 1976;151:512–518.
160. Wuttke W, Bjorklund A, Baumgarten HG, Lachenmayer L, Fenske M, Klemm HP. De- and regeneration of brain serotonin neurons following 5,7-dihydroxytryptamine treatment: Effects on serum LH, FSH and prolactin levels in male rats. *Brain Res* 1977;134:317–331.
161. Chen HJ, Meites J. Effects of biogenic amines and TRH on release of prolactin and TSH in the rat. *Endocrinology* 1975;96: 10–14.
162. Wurtman RJ, Larin F, Mostafapour S, Fernstrom JD. Brain catechol synthesis: Control by brain tyrosine concentration. *Science* 1974;185:183–184.
163. Mena F, Enjalbert A, Carbonell A, Priam M, Kordon C. Effect of suckling on plasma prolactin and hypothalamic monoamine levels in the rat. *Endocrinology* 1976;99:445–452.
164. Parisi MN, Villar ML, Estivas FE, Chiocchio SF, Tramezzani JH. Serotonergic terminals in the anterior hypothalamic nucleus involved in the prolactin release during suckling. *Endocrinology* 1987;120:2404–2412.
165. Marchlewska-Koj A, Krulich L. The role of central monoamines in the stress-induced prolactin release in rats. *Fed Proc Fed Am Soc Exp Biol* 1975;34:252.
166. Meltzer HY, Fang VS, Daniels S. Biogenic amines and serum prolactin levels during stress in male rats. *Fed Proc Fed Am Soc Exp Biol* 1976;35:554.
167. Jorgensen H, Knigge U, Warberg J. Effect of serotonin 5-HT_1, 5-HT_2 and 5-HT_3 receptor antagonists on the prolactin response to restraint and ether stress. *Neuroendocrinology* 1992;56: 371–377.
168. Mulloy AL, Moberg GP. Effects of p-chlorophenylalanine and raphe lesions on diurnal prolactin release in the rat. *Fed Proc Fed Am Soc Exp Biol* 1975;34:251.
169. Mistry A, Voogt JL. Role of serotonin in nocturnal and diurnal surges of prolactin in the pregnant rat. *Endocrinology* 1989;125: 2875–2880.
170. Jahn GA, Deis RP. Effect of serotonin antagonists on prolactin and progesterone secretion in rats: Evidence that stimulatory and inhibitory actions of serotonin on prolactin release may be mediated through different receptors. *J Endocrinol* 1988;117: 415–422.

171. Pan J, Gala RR. The influence of raphe lesions, p-chlorophenylalanine, and ketanserin on the estrogen-induced afternoon prolactin surge. *Endocrinology* 1987;120:2070–2077.
172. Di Sciullo A, Bluet-Pajot MT, Mounier F, Olivier C, Schmidt B, Kordon C. Changes in anterior pituitary hormone levels after serotonin 1A receptor stimulation. *Endocrinology* 1990;127: 567–572.
173. Lamberts SWJ, MacLeod RM. The interaction of the serotonergic and dopaminergic systems on prolactin secretion in the rat. *Endocrinology* 1978;105:287–295.
174. Clemens JA, Sawyer BD, Cerimele B. Further evidence that serotonin is a neurotransmitter involved in the control of prolactin secretion. *Endocrinology* 1975;100:692–698.
175. Fores CM, Hulihan-Giblin BA, Hornby PJ, Lumpkin MD, Kellar KJ. Partial characterization of a neurotransmitter pathway regulating the *in vivo* release of PRL. *Neuroendocrinology* 1992;55:519–528.
176. Pilotte NS, Porter JC. Dopamine in hypophysial portal plasma and prolactin in systemic plasma of rats treated with S-hydroxytryptamine. *Endocrinology* 1981;108:2137–2141.
177. Clemens JA, Roush ME, Fuller RW. Evidence that serotonin neurons stimulate secretion of prolactin releasing factor. *Life Sci* 1978;22:2209–2214.
178. Johnston CA, Fagin KD, Alper RH, Negro-Vilar A. Prolactin release after S-hydroxytryptophan treatment requires an intact neurointermediate pituitary lobe. *Endocrinology* 1986;118: 805–810.
179. King TS, Steger RW, Morgan WW. Effect of hypophysectomy and subsequent prolactin administration of hypothalamic 5 hydroxytryptamine synthesis in ovariectomized rats. *Endocrinology* 1985;116:485–491.
180. King TS, Carrillo AJ, Morgan WW. Hyperprolactinemia attenuates ovarian steroid stimulation of region-specific hypothalamic serotonin synthesis and luteinizing hormone release in ovariectomized rats. *Neuroendocrinology* 1986;42:351–357.
181. O'Steen WK. Serotonin suppression of luteinizition in gonadotrophin-treated, immature rats. *Endocrinology* 1964;74:885–888.
182. Axelrod J, Inscoe JK. The uptake and binding of circulating serotonin and the effect of drugs. *J Pharmacol Exp Ther* 1963;141:161–165.
183. Labhsetwar AP. Role of monoamines in ovulation: Evidence for a serotonergic pathway for inhibition of spontaneous ovulation. *J Endocrinol* 1972;54:269–275.
184. Wilson CA, McDonald PG. Inhibitory effect of serotonin on ovulation in adult rats. *J Endocrinol* 1974;60:253–260.
185. Blum I, Nessiel L, David A, Graff E, Harsat A, Weissglas L, Gabbay U, Sulkes J, Yerushalmy Y, Vered Y. Plasma neurotransmitter profile during different phases of the ovulatory cycle. *J Clin Endocrinol Metab* 1992;75:924–929.
186. Domanski E, Przekop F, Skubiskewski B, Wolinska E. The effect and site of action of indoleamines on the hypothalamic centers involved in the control of LH release and ovulation in sheep. *Neuroendocrinology* 1975;17:265–273.
187. Przekop F, Skubiskewski B, Domanski E. The effects of indolamines (serotonin and melatonin) on induction of ovulation in rabbits. *Acta Physiol Pol* 1975;26:395–343.
188. Cramer OM, Barraclough CA. The actions of serotonin, norepinephrine, and epinephrine on hypothalamic processes leading to adenohypophysial luteinizing hormone release. *Endocrinology* 1978;103:694–703.
189. Carrer HF, Taleisnik S. Neural pathways associated with the mesencephalic inhibitory influence on gonadotropin secretion. *Brain Res* 1972;38:299–313.
190. Arendash GW, Gallo RV. Serotonin involvement in the inhibition of episodic luteinizing hormone release during electrical stimulation of the midbrain dorsal raphe nucleus in ovariectomized rats. *Endocrinology* 1978;102:1199–1206.
191. Hery M, Laplante E, Kordon C. Participation of serotonin in the phasic release of LH. Evidence from pharmacological experiments. *Endocrinology* 1976;99:496–503.
192. Marko M, Fluckiger E. Role of serotonin in the regulation of ovulation. *Neuroendocrinology* 1980;30:228–231.
193. Wilson CA, Horth CE, McNeilly A, McDonald PC. Effect of serotonin and progesterone on induced ovulation in immature rats. *J Endocrinology* 1975;64:337–347.
194. Meyer DC. Hypothalamic and raphe serotonergic systems in ovulation control. *Endocrinology* 1978;103:1067–1074.
195. Johnson MD, Crowley WR. Acute effects of estradiol on circulating luteinizing hormone and prolactin concentrations and on serotonin turnover in individual brain nuclei. *Endocrinology* 1983;113:1934–1941.
196. James MD, Hole DR, Wilson CA. Differential involvement of 5-HT in specific hypothalamic areas in the mediation of steroid induced changes in gonadotrophin release and sexual behaviour in female rats. *Neuroendocrinology* 1989;49:561–569.
197. Morello H, Taleisnik S. Changes of the release of LH on the day of proestrous after lesions or stimulation of the raphe nuclei in rats. *Brain Res* 1985;360:311–317.
198. Morello H, Taleisnik S. The inhibition of proestrous LH surge and ovulation in rats bearing lesions of the dorsal raphe nucleus is mediated by the locus coeruleus. *Brain Res* 1988;440:227–231.
199. Morello H, Caligaris L, Haymal B, Taleisnik S. Inhibition of proestrous LH surge and ovulation in rats evoked by stimulation of the medial raphe nucleus involves a GABA-mediated mechanism. *Neuroendocrinology* 1989;50:81–87.
200. Becu de Villalobos D, Lux VAR, Lacau DeMengido L, Libertun C. Sexual differences in the serotonergic control of prolactin and luteinizing hormone secretion in the rat. *Endocrinology* 1984;115:84–89.
201. Hery M, Laplante E, Pattou E, Kordon C. Interaction de la serotonine cerebrale avec la liberation cyclique de LH chez la ratte. *Ann Endocrinol (Paris)* 1975;36:123–130.
202. Coen CW, MacKinnon PCB. Serotonin involvement in the control of phasic luteinizing hormone release in the rat: Evidence for a critical period. *J Endocrinol* 1979;82:105–113.
203. Hery M, Laplante E, Kordon C. Participation of serotonin in the phasic release of luteinizing hormone. 11. Effects of lesions of serotonin-containing pathways in the central nervous system. *Endocrinology* 1978;102:1019–1025.
204. Hery M, Faudon M, Dusticier G, Hery F. Daily variations in serotonin metabolism in the suprachiasmatic nucleus of the rat: Influence of oestradiol impregnation. *J Endocrinol* 1982;94: 157–166.
205. Cone RI, Davis GA, Goy RW. Effects of ovarian steroids on serotonin metabolism within grossly dissected and microdissected brain regions of the ovariectomized rat. *Brain Res Bull* 1981;7:639–644.
206. Crowley WR, O'Donohue TL, Muth EA, Jacobowitz DM. Effects of ovarian hormones on levels of luteinizing hormone in plasma and on serotonin concentrations in discrete brain nuclei. *Brain Res Bull* 1979;4:571–574.
207. Munaro NI. The effect of ovarian steroids on hypothalamic 5-hydroxytryptamine neuronal activity. *Neuroendocrinology* 1978; 26:270–276.
208. King TS, Steger RW, Morgan WW. Effect of ovarian steroids to stimulate region-specific hypothalamic S-hydroxytryptamine synthesis in ovariectomized rats. *Neuroendocrinology* 1986;42: 344–350.
209. Biegon A, Fischette CT, Rainbow TC, McEwen BS. Serotonin receptor modulation by estrogen in discrete brain nuclei. *Neuroendocrinology* 1983;35:287–291.
210. Biegon A, Bercovitz H, Samuel D. Serotonin receptor concentration during the estrous cycle of the rat. *Brain Res* 1980; 187:221–225.
211. Leonardelli J, Dubois MP, Poulain P. Effect of exogenous serotonin on LH-RH secreting neurons in the guinea pig hypothalamus as revealed by immunofluorescence. *Neuroendocrinology* 1974; 15:69–72.
212. McEwen BS, Parsons B. Gonadal steroid action on the brain: Neurochemistry and neuropharmacology. *Annu Rev Pharmacol Toxicol* 1982;22:555–598.
213. Donelly PJ, Dailey RA. Effects of dopamine, norepinephrine and serotonin on secretion of LH, FSH and prolactin in ovariectomized, pituitary stalk-transected ewes. *Domestic Animal Endocrinology* 1991;8:87–98.
214. Juorio AV, Li XM, Gonzalez A, Chedrese PJ, Murphy BD. Effects of active immunization against GnRH on the concentration

of noradrenaline, dopamine, 5-HT and some of their metabolites in the brain and sexual organs of the male rat. *Neuroendocrinology* 1991;54:49–54.
215. Tappaz M, Brownstein M, Kopin I. Glutamate decarboxylase (GAB) and γ-aminobutyric acid (GABA) in discrete nuclei of hypothalamus and *substantia nigra*. *Brain Res* 1977;125: 109–121.
216. Brownstein M, Palkovits M, Tappaz M, Saavedra J, Kizer J. Effect of surgical isolation of the hypothalamus on its neurotransmitter content. *Brain Res* 1976;117:287–295.
217. Makara G, Rappay G, Stark E. Autoradiographic localization of 3H-gamma-amino-butyric acid in medial hypothalamus. *Exp Brain Res* 1975;22:449–455.
218. Tappaz M, Aguera M, Belin M, Pujol F. Autoradiography of GABA in the rat hypothalamic median eminence. *Brain Res* 1980;186:379–391.
219. Vincent S, Hökfelt T, Wu J. GABA neuron system in hypothalamus and the pituitary gland. *Neuroendocrinology* 1982;34: 117–125.
220. Flugge G, Oertel W, Wuttke W. Evidence for estrogen-receptive GABAergic neurons in the preoptic/anterior hypothalamic area of the rat brain. *Neuroendocrinology* 1986;43:1–5.
221. Lamberts R, Mansky T, Stock K, Vijayan E, Wuttke W. Involvement of preoptic-anterior hypothalamic GABA neurons in the regulation of pituitary LH and prolactin release. *Exp Brain Res* 1984;52:356–362.
222. Fuchs E, Mansky T, Stock K, Vijayan E, Wuttke W. Involvement of catecholamines and glutamate in GABAergic mechanisms regulatory to luteinizing hormone and prolactin secretion. *Neuroendocrinology* 1984;38:484–489.
223. Donoso A, Banzan A. Effects of increase of brain GABA levels on the hypothalamic-pituitary-luteinizing hormone axis in rats. *Acta Endocrinol* 1984;106:298–304.
224. Adler B, Crowley W. Evidence for γ-aminobutyric acid modulation of ovarian hormonal effects on luteinizing hormone secretion and hypothalamic catecholamine activity in the female rat. *Endocrinology* 1986;118:91–97.
225. Jarry H, Perschl A, Wuttke W. Further evidence that preoptic anterior GABA-ergic neurons are part of the GnRH pulse and surge generator. *Acta Endocrinol (Copenh)* 1988;118:573–579.
226. Jarry H, Hirsch B, Leonhardt S, Wuttke W. Amino acid neurotransmitter release in the preoptic area of rats during the positive feedback actions of estradiol on LH release. *Neuroendocrinology* 1992;56:133–140.
227. Hartman RD, He JR, Barraclough CA. γ-Aminobutyric acid-A and -B receptor antagonists increase LH-RH neuronal responsiveness to intracerebroventricular norepinephrine in ovariectomized estrogen-treated rats. *Endocrinology* 1990;127:1336–1345.
228. Akema T, Kimura F. 2-Hydroxysaclofen, a potent GABA-B receptor antagonist, stimulates LH secretion in female rats. *Brain Res* 1991;546:143–145.
229. Vijayan E, McCann SM. The effects of intraventricular injection of GABA on prolactin and gonadotropin release in conscious female rats. *Brain Res* 1978;155:35–43.
230. Nikolarakis KE, Loeffler JP, Almeida OFX, Herz A. Pre- and postsynaptic actions of GABA on the release of hypothalamic GnRH. *Brain Res Bull* 1988;21:677–683.
231. Masotto C, Wisniewski G, Negro-Vilar A. Different GABA receptor subtypes are involved in the regulation of opiate-dependent and independent LH-RH secretion. *Endocrinology* 1989;125:548–553.
232. Seltzer AM, Donoso AO. Restraining action of GABA on estradiol-induced LH surge in the rat: GABA activity in brain nuclei and effects of GABA mimetics in the medial preoptic nucleus. *Neuroendocrinology* 1992;55:28–34.
233. Weiner RI, Martínez de la Escalera G. Inhibitory regulation of pulsatile GnRH release from GT_1 GnRH cell lines by vasopressin and GABA. *Society for Neuroscience* 1992;18:928.
234. Hales TG, Kim H, Longoni B, Olsen RW, Tobin AJ. Immortalized hypothalamic GT_{1-7} neurons express functional GABA type A receptors. *Mol Pharmacol* 1992;42:197–202.
235. Charles A, Sanderson M, Hales TG. GABA has excitatory effects on hypothalamic neurons. *American Society for Neurochemistry* 1992;23:228.
236. Charles A, Hales TG. GABA modulates calcium and membrane potential oscillations in immortalized hypothalamic neurons. *Society for Neuroscience* 1992;18:1159.
237. Jarry H, Leonhardt S, Wuttke W. GABA neurons in the preoptic/anterior hypothalamic area synchronize the phasic activity of the GnRH pulse generator in ovariectomized rats. *Neuroendocrinology* 1991;53:261–267.
238. Anderson RA, Mitchell R. Effects of GABA agonists on the secretion of GH, LH, ACTH and TSH from the rat pituitary gland in vitro. *J Endocrinol* 1986;108:1–8.
239. Virmani MA, Stojilkovic SS, Catt KJ. Stimulation of LH release by GABA agonists: mediation by GABAA-type receptors and activation of chloride and voltage-sensitive calcium channels. *Endocrinology* 1990;126:2499–2505.
240. Mulchahey J, Neill J. Gamma amino butyric acid (GABA) levels in hypophyseal stalk plasma of rats. *Life Sci* 1982;31:453–456.
241. Mitchell R, Grieve G, Fink G. Endogenous GABA receptor ligands in hypophysial portal blood. *Neuroendocrinology* 1983; 37:169–176.
242. Gudelsky G, Apud J, Masotto C, Locatelli V, Cocchi D, Racagui G, Muller E. Ethanolamine-O-sulfate enhances γ-aminobutyric acid secretion into hypophyseal portal blood and lowers serum prolactin concentrations. *Neuroendocrinology* 1983;37:397–399.
243. Grandison L, Guidotti A. γ-Amino-butyric acid receptor functions in rat anterior pituitary: Evidence for control of prolactin release. *Endocrinology* 1979;105:754–759.
244. Loeffler J, Kley N, Pittius C, Almeida O, Hollt V. *In vivo* and *in vitro* studies of GABAergic inhibition of prolactin biosynthesis. *Neuroendocrinology* 1986;43:504–510.
245. Locatelli V, Cocchi D, Frigerio C, Betti R, Krogsgaard-Larsen P, Racagri G, Muller E. Dual γ-aminobutyric acid control of prolactin secretion in the rat. *Endocrinology* 1979;105:778–785.
246. Duvilanski BH, Diaz MC, Debeljuk L. Effect of PRL on GABA related enzymes in the hypothalamus and pituitary of ovariectomized rats. *Neuroendocrinol Lett* 1983;5:99–104.
247. Casanueva F, Apud JA, Masotto C, Cocchi D, Locatelli V, Racagni G, Müller EE. Daily fluctuations in the activity of the tuberoinfundibular GABAergic system and plasma PRL levels. *Neuroendocrinology* 1984;39:367–370.
248. Kolbinger W, Beyer C, Föhr K, Reisert I, Pilgrim C. Diencephalic GABAergic neurons in vitro respond to prolactin with a rapid increase in intracellular free calcium. *Neuroendocrinology* 1992;56:148–152.
249. Anderson R, Mitchell R. Biphasic effect of $GABA_A$ receptor agonists on prolactin secretion: evidence for two types of $GABA_A$ receptor complex on lactotrophes. *Eur J Pharmacol* 1986;124: 1–9.
250. Jones TH, Brown BL, Cullen DR, Dobson PR. Effect of the $GABA_A$ agonist muscimol on prolactin secretion from human prolactin-secreting adenomas and GH_3 rat pituitary tumour cells. *Hormone Res* 1992;37:113–118.
251. Mioduszewski R, Grandison L, Meites J. Stimulation of prolactin release in rats by GABA. *Proc Soc Exp Biol Med* 1976;151:44–46.
252. Schwartz J. Histaminergic mechanisms in brain. *Annu Rev Pharmacol Toxicol* 1977;17:325–339.
253. Brownstein M, Saavedra J, Palkovits M, Axelrod J. Histamine content of hypothalamic nuclei of the rat. *Brain Res* 1974;77:151–156.
254. Pollard H, Bischoff S, Llorens-Cortes C, Schwartz J. Histidine decarboxylase and histamine in discrete nuclei of rat hypothalamus and the evidence for mast-cells in the median eminence. *Brain Res* 1976;118:509–513.
255. Wilcox B, Seybold V. Localization of neuronal histamine in rat brain. *Neurosci Lett* 1982;29:105–110.
256. Panula P, Pirvola U, Auvinen S, Airaksinen MS. Histamine-immunoreactive nerve fibres in the rat brain. *Neuroscience* 1989;28:585–610.
257. Inagaki N, Yamatodani A, Ando-Yamamoto M, Tohyama M, Watanabe T, Wada H. Organization of histaminergic fibres in the rat brain. *J Comp Neurol* 1988;273:283–300.
258. Garbarg M, Barbin G, Bischoff S, Pollard H, Schwartz J. Dual

localization of histamine in an ascending neuronal pathway and in non-neuronal cells evidenced by lesions in the lateral hypothalamic area. *Brain Res* 1976;106:333–348.
259. Bouthenet ML, Ruat M, Sales N, Garbarg M, Schwartz JC. A detailed mapping of histamine H_1-receptors in guinea-pig central nervous system established by autoradiography with [^{125}I]-Iodobolpyramine. *Neuroscience* 1988;26:553–600.
260. Ruat M, Traiffort T, Bouthenet ML, Schwartz JC, Hirschfeld J, Buschauer A, Schunack W. Reversible and irreversible labelling and autoradiographic localization of the cerebral histamine H_2 receptor using [^{125}I]iodinated probes. *Proc Natl Acad Sci USA* 1990;87:1658–1662.
261. West RE, Zweig A, Granzow RT, Siegel MI, Egan RW. Biexponential kinetics of (R)-a-[^{3}H]methyl-histamine binding to the rat brain H_3 histamine receptor. *J Neurochem* 1990;55:1612–1616.
262. Jorgenson KL, Kow LM, Pfaff DW. Histamine excites arcuate neurons in vitro through H_1 receptors. *Brain Res* 1989; 502:171–179.
263. Schwartz JC, Arrang JM, Garbarg M, Pollar H, Ruat M. Histaminergic transmission in the mammalian brain. *Physiol Rev* 1991;71:1–51.
264. Sawyer C. Rhinencephalic involvement in pituitary activation by intraventricular histamine in the rabbit under nembutal anesthesia. *Am J Physiol* 1955;180:37–46.
265. Libertun C, McCann S. The possible role of histamine in the control of prolactin and gonadotropin release. *Neuroendocrinology* 1976;20:110–120.
266. Donoso A. Induction of prolactin and luteinizing hormone release by histamine in male and female rats and the influence of brain transmitter antagonists. *J Endocrinol* 1978;76:193–202.
267. Donoso A, Bannza A. Acute effects of histamine on plasma prolactin and luteinizing hormone levels in male rats. *J Neurol Transmission* 1976;39:95–101.
268. Knigge U, Wollesen F, Dejgaard A, Larsen K, Christiansen P. Modulation of basal and LRH-stimulated gonadotrophan secretion by histamine in normal men. *Neuroendocrinology* 1984;38:93–96.
269. Knigge U, Thuesen B, Wollesen F, Svenstsrup B, Christiansen P. Effect of histamine on basal and TRH/LHRH stimulated PRL and LH secretion during different phases of the menstrual cycle in normal women. *Neuroendocrinology* 1985;41:337–341.
270. Miyake A, Ohtsuka S, Nishizaki J, Tasaka K, Aono T, Tanizawa O, Yamatodani A, Watanabe T, Wada H. Involvement of H1 histamine receptor in basal and estrogen-stimulated luteinizing hormone-releasing hormone secretion in rats *in vitro*. *Neuroendocrinology* 1987;45:191–196.
271. Charli J, Rotsztejn W, Pattou E, Kordon C. Effect of neurotransmitters on *in vitro* release of luteinizing-hormone-releasing hormone from the mediobasal hypothalamus of male rats. *Neurosci Lett* 1978;159:163.
272. Van Kirk EA, Halterman SD, Moss GE, Rose JD, Murdoch WJ. Possible role of histamine in the regulation of secretion of LH in the ewe. *J Anim Sci* 1989;67:1006–1012.
273. Donoso AO, Zárate MB. Release of prolactin and LH by histamine agonists in ovariectomized, esteroid-treated rats under ether anesthesia. *Exp Brain Res* 1983;52:277–280.
274. Horno NM, Alvarez EO. The probable role of histamine in the rostral hypothalamus on the prolactin and LH release induced by estrogen in the conscious spayed rats. *J Neural Transm* 1989;78:249–264.
275. Rivier C, Vale W. Effects of γ-aminobutyric acid and histamine on prolactin secretion in the rat. *Endocrinology* 1977;101: 506–511.
276. Donoso A, Zarate M, Seltzer A. Histamine-induced prolactin release: Pharmacological characterization of receptors in male rats. *Neuroendocrinology* 1983;36:436–442.
277. Knigge U, Matzen S, Warbeg J. Histaminergic stimulation of prolactin secretion mediated via H1- and H2-receptors: Dependence on routes of administration. *Neuroendocrinology* 1986; 44:41–48.
278. Knigge U, Dejaard A, Wollesen F, Thuesen B, Christiansen P. Histamine regulation of prolactin secretion through H_1 and H_2 receptors. *J Clin Endocrinol Metab* 1982;58:118–122.
279. Gibbs D, Plotsky P, deGreef W, Neill J. Effect of histamine and acetylcholine on hypophysial stalk plasma dopamine and peripheral plasma prolactin levels. *Life Sci* 1979;24:2063–2070.
280. Knigge U, Matzen S, Warberg J. Histaminergic regulation of PRL secretion: involvement of tuberoinfundibular dopaminergic neurons. *Neuroendocrinology* 1988;48:167–173.
281. Seltzer AM, Donoso AO. Histamine-induced PRL release and activity of tuberoinfundibular dopaminergic neurons in male rats. *J Neural Transm* 1986;65:115–123.
282. Fleckenstein AE, Lookingland KJ, Moore KE. Evidence that histamine-stimulated PRL secretion is not mediated by an inhibition of tuberoinfundibular dopaminergic neurons. *Life Sci* 1992;51:741–746.
283. Charli J, Joseph-Bravo P, Palacios J, Kordon C. Histamine-induced release of thyrotropin releasing hormone from hypothalamic slices. *Eur J Pharmacol* 1978;52:401–403.
284. Bennet G, Keeling M. H2-mediated histamine-induced release of thyrotropin releasing hormone (TRH) from hypothalamic synaptosomes: A neuroendocrine role for histamine. *Br J Pharmacol* 1981;72:151–152.
285. Pilc A, Nowak JZ. Influence of histamine on the serotoninergic system of rat brain. *Eur J Pharmacol* 1979;55:269–272.
286. Tuomisto J, Tuomisto L. Effects of histamine and histamine antagonists on the uptake and release of catecholamines and 5-HT in brain synaptosomes. *Med Biol* 1980;58:33–37.
287. Knigge U, Sleimann I, Matzen S, Warberg J. Histaminergic regulation of PRL secretion: involvement of serotoninergic neurons. *Neuroendocrinology* 1988;48:527–533.
288. Cacabelos R, Yamatodani A, Niigawa H, Hariguchi S, Nishimura T, Waada H. Histaminergic neuromodulation of the release of vasopressin. *Neuroendocrinology* 1987;45:368–375.
289. Kjaer A, Knigge U, Olsen L, Vilhardt H, Warberg J. Mediation of the stress-induced PRL release by hypothalamic histaminergic neurons and the possible involvement of vasopressin in this response. *Endocrinology* 1991;128:103–110.
290. Kali H, Chihara K, Abe H, Kita T, Kashio Y, Okimura Y, Fujita T. Effect of passive immunization with antisera to vasoactive intestinal polypeptide and peptide histidine isoleucine amide on 5-hydroxy-L-tryptophan-induced prolactin release in rats. *Endocrinology* 1985;117:1914–1919.
291. Sibilia V, Nettie C, Guidobono F, Pagani F, Pecile A. Cimetidine-induced prolactin release: Possible involvement of the GABAergic system. *Neuroendocrinology* 1985;40:189–192.
293. Seltzer AM, Donoso AO, Podestá E. Restraint stress stimulation of PRL and ACTH secretion: role of brain histamine. *Physiol Behav* 1986;36:251–255.
294. Knigge U, Matzen S, Warberg J. Histaminergic mediation of stress-induced release of PRL in male rats. *Neuroendocrinology* 1988;47:68–74.
295. Netti C, Guidobono F, Sibilia V, Pagani F, Villa I, Pecile A. A selective role for brain histamine in PRL release induced by opiates. *Agents Actions* 1990;30:223–225.
296. Akakelian M, Libertum C. H1 and H2 histamine receptor participation in the brain control of prolactin secretion in lactating rats. *Endocrinology* 1977;100:890–895.
297. Alvarez EO. Effects of histamine antagonists injected in the preoptic-anterior hypothalamic area on the prolactin surge induced by estrogen in ovariectomized rats. *Brain Res Bull* 1984;12:11–15.
298. Garthwaite J. Glutamate, nitric oxide and cell-cell signalling in the nervous system. *Trends Neurosci* 1991;14:60–67.
299. Unnerstall JR, Wamsley JK. Autoradiographic localization of high-affinity (^{3}H)kainic acid binding sites in the rat forebrain. *Eur J Pharmacol* 1983;86:361–371.
300. Monaghan DT, Cotman CW. Distribution of *N*-methyl-D-aspartate-sensitive L-(^{3}H)glutamate-binding sites in rat brain. *J Neurosci* 1985;5:2909–2919.
301. May PC, Kohama SG, Finch CE. N-methyl-aspartic acid lesions of the arcuate nucleus in adult C57BL/6J mice: a new model for age-related lengthening of estrous cycle. *Neuroendocrinology* 1989;50:605–612.
302. Schainker BA, Cicero TJ. Acute stimulation of luteinizing hormone by parenterally administered N-methyl-D, L-aspartic acid in the male rat. *Brain Res* 1980;184:425–437.
303. Tal J, Price MT, Olney JW. Neuroactive amino acids influence

gonadotrophin output: a suprapituitary mechanism in either rodents or primates. *Brain Res* 1983;273:179–182.
304. Gay VL, Plant TM. *N*-methyl-D,L-aspartate elicits hypothalamic gonadotropin-releasing hormone release in prepubertal male rhesus monkeys (*Macaca mulatta*). *Endocrinology* 1987;120: 2289–2296.
305. Bourguignon JP, Gérard A, Franchimont P. Direct activation of gonadotropin-releasing hormone secretion through different receptors to neuroexcitatory amino acids. *Neuroendocrinology* 1989;49:402–408.
306. Pohl CR, Lee LR, Smith MS. Qualitative changes in luteinizing hormone and prolactin responses to *N*-methyl-aspartic acid during lactation in the rat. *Endocrinology* 1989;124:1905–1911.
307. Farah JM Jr, Rao TS, Mick SJ, Coyne KE, Iyengar S. *N*-methyl-D-aspartate treatment increases circulating adrenocorticotropin and luteinizing hormone in the rat. *Endocrinology* 1991;128: 1875–1880.
308. Saitoh Y, Silverman A-j, Gibson MJ. Effects Of *n*-methyl-D,L-aspartic acid on luteinizing hormone secretion in normal mice and in hypogonadal mice with fetal preoptic area implants. *Endocrinology* 1991;128:2432–2440.
309. Wilson RC, Knobil E. Acute effects of N-methyl-DL-aspartate on the release of pituitary gonadotropins and prolactin in adult female rhesus monkey. *Brain Res* 1982;248:177–179.
310. Plant TM, Gay VL, Marshall GR, Arslan M. Puberty in monkeys is triggered by chemical stimulation of the hypothalamus. *Proc Natl Acad Sci USA* 1989;86:2506–2510.
311. Medhamurthy R, Dichek HL, Plant TM, Bernardini I, Cutler GB Jr. Stimulation of gonadotropin secretion in prepubertal monkeys after hypothalamic excitation with aspartate and glutamate. *J Clin Endocrinol Metab* 1990;71:1390–1392.
312. Arslan M, Pohl CR, Plant TM. *DL*-2-amino-5-phosphonopentanoic acid, a specific N-methyl-*D*-aspartic acid receptor antagonist, suppresses pulsatile LH release in the rat. *Neuroendocrinology* 1988;47:465–468.
313. Brann DW, Mahesh VB. Endogenous excitatory amino acid involvement in the preovulatory and steroid-induced surge of gonadotropins in the female rat. *Endocrinology* 1991;128: 1541–1547.
314. Arslan M, Pohl CR, Smith MS, Plant TM. Studies of the role of the N-methyl-D-aspartate (NMDA) receptor in the hypothalamic control of prolactin secretion. *Life Sci* 1992;50:295–300.
315. Abbud R, Smith MS. Differences in the luteinizing hormone and prolactin responses to multiple injections of kainate, as compared to *N*-methyl-D,L-aspartate, in cycling rats. *Endocrinology* 1991;129:3254–3258.
316. Donoso AO, Lopez FJ, Negro-Vilar A. Glutamate receptors of the non-*N*-methyl-D-aspartic acid type mediate the increase in luteinizing hormone-releasing hormone release by excitatory amino acids in vitro. *Endocrinology* 1990;126:414–420.
317. Petersen SL, McCrone S, Keller M, Gardner E. Rapid increase in LHRH mRNA levels following NMDA. *Endocrinology* 1991;129:1679–1681.
318. Palkovits M. Distribution of neuropeptides in the central nervous system: A review of biochemical mapping studies. *Prog Neurobiol* 1984;23:151–189.
319. Palkovits M, Brownstein MJ. Distribution of neuropeptides in the central nervous system using biochemical micromethods. In: Bjorklund A, and Hökfelt T, eds. *Handbook of chemical neuroanatomy, vol. 4.* Amsterdam: Elsevier, 1985;1–70.
320. Palkovits M. Organization of the stress response at the anatomical level. In: de Kloet FR, Wiegant VM, de Wied D, eds. *Progress in brain research, vol. 72.* Amsterdam: Elsevier, 1987;47–56.
321. Kordon C, Rotten D, Durand D, Bluet-Pajot MT. Neuroendocrine control of episodic hormone secretion. In: Wagner TOF, Filicori M, eds. *Episodic hormone secretion.* Hameln: T. M. Verlag, 1987;25–36.
322. Simerly RB, Gorski RA, Swanson LW. Neurotransmitter specificity of cells and fibers in the medial preoptic nucleus: An immunohistochemical study in the rat. *J Comp Neurol* 1986;246: 343–363.
323. Brazeau P, Vale W, Burgus R, Ling N, Butcher M, Rivier J, Guillemin R. Hypothalamic polypeptide that inhibits secretion of immunoreactive pituitary growth hormone. *Science* 1972;129: 77–79.
324. Tavianini M, Hayest T, Magazin M, Minth C, Dixon J. Isolation, characterization and DNA sequence of the rat somatostatin gene. *J Biol Chem* 1984;259:11798–11803.
325. Goodman RH, Jacobs JW, Chin W, Lund PK, Dee PC, Habener JF. Nucleotide sequence of a cloned structural gene coding for a precursor of pancreatic somatostatin. *Proc Natl Acad Sci USA* 1980;77:5869–5873.
326. Shen LP, Rutter WS. Sequence of human somatostatin gene. *Science* 1984;274:168–171.
327. Brownstein M, Arimura A, Sato H, Schally AV, Kizer JS. The regional distribution of somatostatin in the rat brain. *Endocrinology* 1975;96:1456–1461.
328. Palkovits M, Brownstein MJ, Arimura A, Sato H, Schally AV, Kizer JS. Somatostatin content of the hypothalamic ventromedial and arcuate nuclei and the circumventricular organ in the rat. *Brain Res* 1976;109:430–434.
329. Elde RP, Parsons JA. Immunocytochemical localization of somatostatin in cell bodies of the rat hypothalamus. *Annu J Anat* 1975;144:541–548.
330. Alpert LC, Brawer JR, Patel YC, Reichlin S. Somatostatin neurons in anterior hypothalamus: Immunocytochemical localization. *Endocrinology* 1976;98:255–258.
331. Epelbaum J, Willoughby JO, Brazeau P, Martin JB. Effect of brain lesions and hypothalamic deafferentation on somatostatin distribution in rat brain. *Endocrinology* 1977;101:1495–1502.
332. Epelbaum J, Tapia-Arancibia L, Herman JP, Kordon C, Palkovits M. Topographical distribution of median eminence somatostatinergic innervation. *Brain Res* 1981;250:412–416.
333. Makara GB, Palkovits M, Antoni FA, Kiss JZ. Topography of the somatostatin immunoreactive fibers to the stalk median eminence of the rat. *Neuroendocrinology* 1983;37:1–8.
334. Kita T, Chihara I, Abe H, Mihamitani H, Kaji H, Kodama H, Chiba T, Fujika T, Kanaihara N. Regional distribution of gastrin releasing peptide and somatostatin like immunoreactivity in the rabbit hypothalamus. *Brain Res* 1986;398:18–22.
335. Chihara K, Arimura A, Kubli-Garfias C, Schally AV. Enhancement of immunoreactive somatostatin release into hypophyseal blood by electrical stimulation in the preoptic area in the rat. *Endocrinology* 1979;105:1416–1419.
336. Bennett-Clark C, Romagnamo MA, Ioseph SA. Distribution of somatostatin in the rat brain: Telencephalon and diencephalon. *Brain Res* 1980;188:473–486.
337. Johansson O, Hökfelt T, Elde RP. Immunohistochemical distribution of somatostatin like immunoreactivity in the central nervous system of the adult rat. *Neuroscience* 1984;13:265–339.
338. Epelbaum J. Somatostatin in the central nervous system: physiology and pathological modifications. *Prog Neurobiol* 1986;27: 63–100.
339. Krisch B. Hypothalamic and extrahypothalamic distribution of somatostatin immunoreactive elements in the rat brain. *Cell Tissue Res* 1978;195:495–513.
340. Alonso G, Tapia-Arancibia L, Assenmacher I. Electron microscopic immunocytochemical study of somatostatin neurons in the periventricular nucleus of the rat hypothalamus with special reference to their relationships with homologue neuronal processes. *Neuroscience* 1985;16:297–306.
341. Lumpkin MO, Negro-Vilar A, McCann SM. Paradoxical elevation of growth hormone by intraventricular somatostatin: Possible ultrashort feedback. *Science* 1981;211:1072.
342. Epelbaum J, Tapia-Arancibia L, Alonso G, Astier H, Kordon C. The anterior periventricular hypothalamus is the site of somatostatin inhibition on its own release: An *in vitro* and immunocytochemical study. *Neuroendocrinology* 1986;44:255–259.
343. Bertherat J, Dournaud P, Berod A, Normand E, Bloch B, Rostène W, Kordon C, Epelbaum J. Growth hormone-releasing hormone-synthesizing neurons are a subpopulation of somatostatin receptor-labelled cells in the rat arcuate nucleus: a combined in situ hybridization and receptor light-microscopic radioautographic study. *Neuroendocrinology* 1992;56:25–31.
344. Tannenbaum GS, McCarthy GF, Zeitler P, Beaudet A. Cysteamine-induced enhancement of growth hormone releasing-hormone factor (GRF) immunoreactivity in arcuate neurons:

morphological evidence for putative somatostatin/GRF interactions within hypothalamus. *Endocrinology* 1990;127:2551–2560.
345. Palkovits M, Epelbaum J, Tapia-Arancibia L, Kordon C. Somatostatin catecholamine-rich nuclei of the brain-stem. *Neuropeptides* 1982;3:139–144.
346. Pradayrol L, Jorvall H, Mutt V, Ribet A. N-terminally extended somatostatin: The primary structure of somatostatin 28. *FEBS Lett* 1980;109:55–58.
347. Millar R, Sheward W, Wegener J, Fink G. Somatostatin 28 is an hormonally active peptide secreted into hypophyseal ported vessel blood. *Brain Res* 1983;260:334–337.
348. Sheward J, Benoit R, Fink G. Somatostatin 28 (112)-like immunoreactive substance is secreted into hypophyseal portal vessel blood in the rat. *Neuroendocrinology* 1984;38:88–90.
349. Epelbaum J, Tapia-Arancibia L, Kordon C, Enjalbert A. Characterization, regional distribution and subcellular distribution of 125I-Tyr, somatostatin binding sites in rat brain. *J Neurochem* 1982;38:1515–1523.
350. Lewis MD, Foord SM, Lewis MB, Hall R, Scanlon MF. Differential production of SRIF 14 and 28 by fetal rat hypothalamic cells enriched by velocity sedimentation. *Neuroendocrinology* 1986; 44:125–131.
351. Bell GI, Reisine T. Molecular biology of somatostatin receptors. *Trends Neurosci* 1993;16:34–38.
352. Yamada Y, Post SR, Wang K, Tager HS, Bell GI, Seino S. Cloning and functional expression of a family of human and mouse somatostatin receptors expressed in brain, gastrointestinal tract and kidney. *Proc Natl Acad Sci USA* 1992;89:251–255.
353. Yasuda K, Rens-Domanio S, Breder CD, Law SF, Saper CB, Bell GI. Cloning a novel somatostatin receptor, SSTR3, coupled to adenylylcyclase. *J Biol Chem* 1992;267:20422–20428.
354. Li X-J, Forte M, North RA, Ross CA, Snyder SH. Cloning and expression of a rat somatostatin receptor enriched in brain. *J Biol Chem* 1992;267:21307–21311.
355. White RE, Schonbrunn A, Amstrong DL. Somatostatin stimulates Ca^{2+}-activated K^+ channels through protein dephosphorylation. *Nature* 1991;351:570–573.
356. Breder CD, Yamada Y, Yasuda K, Seino S, Saper CB, Bell GI. Differential expression of somatostatin receptor subtypes in the brain. *J Neurosci* 1992;12:3920–3934.
357. Drouva SV, Rérat E, Bihoreau C, Laplante E, Rasolonjanahary R, Clauser H, Kordon C. Dihydropyridine sensitive calcium channels activity related to prolactin, growth hormone and luteinizing hormone release from anterior pituitary cells in culture: interaction with somatostatin, dopamine and estrogens. *Endocrinology* 1988;123:2762–2773.
358. Schonbrunn A, Tashjian A. Characterization of functional receptors for somatostatin in rat pituitary cells in culture. *J Biol Chem* 1978;253:6473–6483.
359. Moyse E, Benoit R, Enjalbert A, Gautron JP, Kordon C, Ling N, Epelbaum J. Subcellular distribution of somatostatin 14 and 28 in rat brain cortex and comparison of their respective binding sites in brain and pituitary. *Regul Pep* 1984;9:129–137.
360. Shu C, Bartrand P, Priam M, Kordon C, Enjalbert A, Epelbaum J. Inhibitory coupling of dopamine and somatostatin receptors with adenylate cyclase in adenohypophysis cells separated by unit gravity sedimentation. In: Lewin MJM, Bonfils S, eds. *Regulatory peptides in digestive, nervous and endocrine systems.* Elsevier Science, 1985;61–64.
361. Morel G, Leroux P, Pelletier G. Localization and characterization of somatostatin 14 and 28 receptors in the rat pituitary as studied by slide mounted frozen sections. *Neuropeptides* 1985;6:41–52.
362. Moyse E, Le Dafniet M, Epelbaum J, Pagesy P, Peillon F, Kordon C, Enjalbert A. Somatostatin receptors in human growth hormone and prolactin secreting pituitary adenomes. *J Clin Endocrinol Metab* 1984;61:98–103.
363. Vale W, Rivier C, Brazeau P, Guillemin R. Effects of somatostatin on the secretion of thyrotropin and prolactin. *Endocrinology* 1974;95:968–977.
364. Kimura N, Hayafuji C, Konagaya H, Takahashi K. 17β3 estradiol induces somatostatin inhibition of prolactin release and regulates SRIF receptors in rat anterior pituitary cells. *Endocrinology* 1986;119:1028–1036.
365. Enjalbert A, Epelbaum J, Arancibia S, Tapia-Arancibia L, Bluet-Pajot MT, Kordon C. Reciprocal interactions of somatostatin with thyrotropin releasing hormone and vasoactive intestinal peptide on prolactin and growth hormone secretion in vitro. *Endocrinology* 1982;111:42–47.
366. Enjalbert A, Bertrand Ph, Le Dafniet M, Epelbaum J, Hugues JN, Kordon C, Moyse E, Peillon F, Shu C. Somatostatin and regulation of prolactin secretion. *Psychoneuroendocrinology* 1986;11:155–165.
367. Willoughby JO, Kapoor R. Intrahypothalamic injection of somastostatin, not GRF, stimulates prolactin secretion. *Neuropeptides* 1990;15:153–156.
368. Göthert M. Somatostatin selectively inhibits noradrenaline release from hypothalamic neurons. *Nature* 1980;288:86–88.
369. Garcia-Sevilla JA, Magnusson T, Carlsson A. Effect of intracerebroventricularly administered somatostatin on brain monoamine turnover. *Brain Res* 1978;155:159–164.
370. Tanaka S, Tsujimoto A. Somatostatin facilitates the serotonin release from rat cerebral cortex hippocampus and hypothalamus slices. *Brain Res* 1981;208:219–222.
371. Rotsztejn WH, Drouva SV, Epelbaum J, Kordon C. Somatostatin inhibits *in vitro* release of luteinizing hormone releasing hormone from rat mediobasal hypothalamic slices. *Experientia* 1982;38:974–975.
372. Hirooka Y, Hollander CS, Suzuki S, Ferdinand F, Juan SJ. Somatostatin inhibits release of thyrotropin releasing factor from organ cultures of rat hypothalamus. *Proc Natl Acad Sci* 1978;75:4509–4513.
373. Terenius L. Somatostatin and ACTH are peptides with partial antagonist like selectivity for opiate receptors. *Eur J Pharmacol* 1976;38:211–213.
374. Seeburg PH, Adelman JP. Characterization of cDNA for precursor of human luteinizing hormone releasing hormone. *Nature* 1984;311:666–668.
375. Sharp PJ, Talbot RT, Main GM, Dunn IC, Fraser HM, Huskisson NS. Physiological roles of chicken LHRH-I and -II in the control of gonadotrophin release in the domestic chicken. *J Endocrinol* 1990;124:291–299.
376. Gautron JP, Pattou E, Bauer K, Kordon C. (Hydroxyproline^9) luteinizing hormone-releasing hormone: a novel peptide in mammalian and frog hypothalamus. *Neurochem Int* 1991;18: 221–235.
377. Barry J, Dubois MP. Immunofluorescence study of LRH producing neurons in the rat and the dog. *Neuroendocrinology* 1975;18:290–298.
378. Setalo G, Vigh S, Schally AV, Arimura A, Flerko B. Immunohistochemical study of the origin of LHRH containing nerve fibers of the rat hypothalamus. *Brain Res* 1976;103:597–602.
379. Palkovits M, Pattou E, Herman JP, Kordon C. Mapping of LHRH containing projections to the mediobasal hypothalamus by differential deafferentation experiments. *Brain Res* 1984; 298:283–288.
380. Liposits Z, Setalo G. Descending luteinizing hormone releasing hormone (LHRH) nerve fibers to the midbrain of the rat. *Neurosci Lett* 1980;20:1–4.
381. Jennes L. Sites of origin of gonadotropin releasing hormones containing projections to the amygdala and the interpeduncular nucleus. *Brain Res* 1987;404:339–344.
382. Jennes L. The olfactory gonadotropin releasing hormone immunoreactive system in mouse. *Brain Res* 1986;396:351–363.
383. Phillips HS, Nikolics K, Brando D, Seeburg PH. Immunocytochemical localization in rat brain of a prolactin release inhibiting sequence of gonadotropin releasing hormone prohormone. *Nature* 1985;316:542–545.
384. Gautron JP, Pattou E, Leblanc P, L'Héritier A, Kordon C. Preferential distribution of C-terminal fragments of (Hydroxyproline^9) LHRH in the rat hippocampus and olfactory bulb. *Neuroendocrinology* 1993; (submitted).
385. Léranth CS, Segwa LM, Palkovits M, McLusky MJ, Naftolin F. The LHRH containing neuronal network in the preoptic area of the rat: Demonstration of LHRH containing nerve terminals in synaptic contact with LHRH neurons. *Brain Res* 1985;345: 332–336.
386. Eskay RL, Mical RS, Porter JC. Relationship between luteinizing

hormone releasing hormone concentration in hypophysial portal blood and luteinizing hormone release in intact castrated and electrochemically stimulated rats. *Endocrinology* 1977;100: 263–270.
387. Wilson RC, Kesner JS, Kaufman JM, Uemura T, Akema T, Knobil E. Central electrophysiologic correlates of pulsatile luteinizing hormone secretion in the rhesus monkey. *Neuroendocrinology* 1984;39:256–260.
388. Reinhart J, Mertz LM, Catt KS. Molecular cloning and expression of cDNA encoding the murine gonadotropin-releasing hormone receptor. *J Biol Chem* 1992;267:21281–21284.
389. Reubi JC, Maurer R. Visualization of LHRH receptors in the rat brain. *Eur J Pharmacol* 1985;106:453–454.
390. Clayton RN, Catt KJ. Gonadotropin releasing hormone receptors: Characterization, physiological regulation and relationship to reproductive function. *Endocr Rev* 1981;2:186.
391. Leblanc P, Pattou E, L'Heritier A, Gogan F, Slama A, Kordon C. Biphasic pattern of follicle stimulating and luteinizing hormone responses to gonadotropic releasing hormone *in vitro*. *Neuroendocrinology* 1983;36:88–94.
392. Hsueh AJW, Jones PBC. Extrapituitary actions of gonadotropin releasing hormone. *Endocr Rev* 1981;2:437.
393. Chan A, Dudley CA, Moss RJ. Hormonal modification of the responsiveness of midbrain central gray neurons to LHRH. *Neuroendocrinology* 1983;41:163–168.
394. Pfaff DW. Luteinizing hormone releasing factor potentiates lordosis behaviour in hypophysectomized ovariectomized female rats. *Science* 1973;182:1148–1149.
395. Moss RL, McCann SM. Induction of mating behavior in rats by luteinizing hormone releasing factor. *Science* 1973;181:177–179.
396. Sakuma Y, Pfaff DW. LHRH in the mesencephalic central grey can potentiate lordosis reflex of female rats. *Nature* 1980; 283:566–567.
397. Sakuma Y, Pfaff DW. Modulation of the lordosis reflex of female rats by LHRH, its antiserum and analogs in the mesencephalic central gray. *Neuroendocrinology* 1983;36:218–224.
398. Dudley CA, Moss RL. Facilitation of sexual receptivity in the female rat by C-terminal fragments of LHRH. *Physiol Behav* 1991;50:1205–1208.
399. Catania A, Cantalamessa L, Reschini E. Plasma prolactin response to luteinizing hormone releasing hormone in acromegalic patients. *J Clin Endocrinol Metab* 1976;43:689–691.
400. Mais V, Melis GB, Paoletti AM, Strigini F, Antonori D, Fioretti D. Prolactin releasing action of a low dose of exogenous gonadotropin releasing hormone throughout the human menstrual cycle. *Neuroendocrinology* 1986;44:326–330.
401. Yen SSC, Hoff JD, Lasley BL, Casper RF, Sheehan K. Induction of prolactin release by LRF and LRF agonist. *Life Sci* 1980;26:1963–1967.
402. Denef C, Andries M. Evidence for paracrine interaction between gonadotrophs and lactotrophs in pituitary cell aggregates. *Endocrinology* 1983;112:813–821.
403. Houben H, Denef C. Regulatory peptides produced in the anterior pituitary. *Trends Endocrinol Metab* 1990;1:398–403.
404. Steele MK, Brownfield MS, Ganong WF. Immunocytochemical localization of angiotensin immunoreactivity in gonadotropes and lactotropes of the rat anterior pituitary gland. *Neuroendocrinology* 1982;35:155–158.
405. Bégeot M, Hemming FJ, Dubois PM, Combarnous Y, Aubert ML. Induction of pituitary lactotrope differentiation by luteinizing hormone subunit. *Science* 1984;226:566–568.
406. Von Euler US, Gaddum JH. An unidentified depressor substance in certain tissue extracts. *J Physiol* 1931;72:74–87.
407. Jordan CC, Gehme P. *Substance P, metabolism and biological actions.* London and Philadelphia: Taylor and Francis, 1985.
408. Brownstein MJ, Mroz EA, Kizer JS, Palkovits M, Leeman SE. Regional distribution of substance P in the brain of the rat. *Brain Res* 1976;116:299–311.
409. Ljungdahl A, Hokfelt T, Nilsson G, Goldstein M. Distribution of substance P like immunoreactivity in the central nervous system of the rat. *Neuroscience* 1978;3:861–944.
410. Danks JA, Rothman RB, Carcieri MA, Chicchi GG, Liang T, Herdenham M. A comparative autoradiographic study of the distributions of substance P and eledoisin binding sites in rat brain. *Brain Res* 1986;385:273–281.
411. Kerdelhué B, Tartar A, Lenoir V, El Abed A, Hublau P, Millar RP. Binding studies of substance P anterior pituitary binding sites; changes in substance P binding sites during the rat estrous cycle. *Regul Pept* 1985;10:133–143.
412. Hökfelt T, Pernow B, Nilsson G, Wetterberg M, Goldstein M, Jeffcoate SL. Dense plexus of substance P immunoreactive nerve terminals in eminentia medialis of the primate hypothalamus. *Proc Natl Acad Sci USA* 1978;75:1013–1015.
413. Stoeckel ME, Porte A, Klein MJ, Cuello AC. Immunocytochemical localization of substance P in the neurohypophysis and the hypothalamus of the mouse compared with the distribution of other neuropeptides. *Cell Tissue Res* 1982;223:544–553.
414. Morel G, Chayvialle JA, Kerdelhue B, Dubois PM. Ultrastructural evidence for endogenous substance P like immunoreactivity in the rat pituitary gland. *Neuroendocrinology* 1982;35:86–92.
415. De Palavis LR, Khorram O, Ho RH, Negro-Vilar A, McCann SM. Partial characterization of immunoreactive substance P in the rat pituitary gland. *Life Sci* 1984;34:225–238.
416. Kato Y, Chiara K, Ohgo S, Ivasak Y, Abe H, Imura H. Growth hormone and prolactin release by substance P in rats. *Life Sci* 1976;19:441–446.
417. Vijayan E, McCann SM. *In vivo* and *in vitro* effects of substance P and neurotensin on gonadotropin and prolactin release. *Endocrinology* 1979;105:64–68.
418. Arisawa M, Snyder GD, Yu WH, De Palatis LR, Ho RH, McCann SM. Physiologically significant inhibitory hypothalamic action of substance P on prolactin release in the male rat. *Neuroendocrinology* 1990;52:22–27.
419. Eckstein N, Wehrenberg WB, Louis K, Carmel PV, Zimmerman EA, Ferin M. Effects of substance P on the anterior pituitary secretion in the female rhesus monkey. *Neuroendocrinology* 1980;31:338–342.
420. Pinanço-Diniz DLW, Valença MM, Franci CR, Antunes-Rodrigues J. Role of substance P in the medial preoptic area in the regulation of gonadotropin and prolactin secretion in normal or orchidectomized rats. *Neuroendocrinology* 1990;51:675–682.
421. Afione S, Debeljuk L, Seilicovich A, Pisera D, Lasaga M, Carmen Diaz C del, Duvilanski B. Substance P affects the GABAergic system in the hypothalamo-pituitary axis. *Peptides* 1990;11: 1065–1068.
422. Rivier C, Braun M, Vale W. Effect of neurotensin, substance P and morphine sulfate on the secretion of prolactin and growth hormone in the rat. *Endocrinology* 1977;100:751–754.
423. Dees WL, Skelley CW, Kozlowski GP. Central effects of an antagonist and an antiserum to substance P on serum gonadotropin and prolactin secretion. *Life Sci* 1985;37:1627–1631.
424. Kerdelhué B, Valens M, Langlois Y. Stimulation de la secretion de LH et TSH hypophysaires apres immunoneutralisation de la substance P endogene chez le rat cyclique. *C R Acad Sci (Paris)* 1978;286:977–979.
425. Ohtsuka S, Miyake A, Nishizaki T, Tasaka K, Aono T, Tanizawa O. Substance P stimulates gonadotropin releasing hormone release from rat hypothalamus in vitro with involvement of estrogen. *Acta Endocrinol (Copenh)* 1987;115:247–252.
426. Frankfurt M, Siegel RA, Sim I, Wuttke W. Estrous cycle variations in cholecystokinin and substance P concentrations in discrete areas of the rat brain. *Neuroendocrinology* 1986;42: 226–231.
427. Jarry H, Perschl A, Meissner H, Wuttke W. In vivo release rates of substance P in the preoptic anterior hypothalamic area of ovariectomized and ovariectomized estrogen-primed rats: correlation with luteinizing hormone and prolactin levels. *Neurosci Lett* 1988;88:189–194.
428. Kerdelhue B, Khar A, Dennay D, Langlois Y, Bernardo T, Linska J, Jutisz M. Inhibition *in vitro* par la substance P de l'excretion des gonadotropines induites par la LHRH a partir de cellules antehypophysaires de rat en culture. *C R Acad Sci (Paris)* 1979;287:879–882.
429. Shamgochian MD, Leeman SE. Substance P stimulates luteinizing hormone secretion from anterior pituitary cells in culture. *Endocrinology* 1992;131:871–875.

430. Carraway R, Leeman SE. The isolation of a new hypotensive peptide, neurotensin, from bovine hypothalami. *J Biol Chem* 1973;248:6854.
431. Kahn D, Abrams G, Zimmerman FA, Carraway R, Leeman SE. Neurotensin neurons in the rat hypothalamus: An immunohistochemical study. *Endocrinology* 1980;107:47–54.
432. Jennes L, Stumpf WE, Kalivas PW. Neurotensin: Topographical distribution in rat brain by immunocytochemistry. *J Comp Neurol* 1982;210:211–224.
433. Ibata Y, Kawakami F, Fujui K, Okamura H, ObataTsuto HL, Tsuto T, Terubayashi H. Morphological survey of neurotensin-like immunoreactive neurons in the hypothalamus. *Peptides* 1984;5:109–120.
434. Ibata Y, Fukui K, Okamura H, Kawakami T, Tanaka M, Obata HL, Tsuto T, Terabayashi H, Yanaihara C, Yanaihara N. Coexistence of dopamine and neurotensin in hypothalamic arcuate and periventricular neurons. *Brain Res* 1983;269:177–179.
435. Hökfelt T, Everitt BH, Theodorsson-Norheim E, Goldstein M. Occurrence of neurotensin like immunoreactivity in subpopulations of hypothalamic, mesencephalic and medullary catecholamine neurons. *J Comp Neurol* 1984;222:543–559.
436. Saint-Pierre SA, Kerouac R, Quirion R, Jolicoeur FB, Rioux F. Neurotensin. In: Heam MT, ed. *Peptide and protein review, vol. 2.* New York: Marcel Dekker, 1984;83–171.
437. Inagaki S, Yamano M, Shiosaka S, Takagi H, Tohyama M. Distribution and origins of neurotensin containing fibers in the nucleus ventromedialis hypothalami of the rat: An experimental immunohistochemical study. *Brain Res* 1983;273:229–235.
438. Kitabgi P, Rostène W, Dussaillant M, Schotte A, Laduron PM, Vincent JP. Two populations of neurotensin binding sites in murine brain: discrimination by the antihystamine levocabastine reveals markedly different radioautographic distribution. *Eur J Pharmacol* 1987;140:285–293.
439. Goedert M, Lightman SL, Mantyh PW, Hunt SP, Emson PC. Neurotensin like immunoreactivity and neurotensin receptors in the rat hypothalamus and in the neurointermediate lobe of the pituitary gland. *Brain Res* 1985;358:59–69.
440. Moyse E, Rostène WH, Vial M, Leonard K, Mazella J, Kitabgi P, Vincent JP, Beaudet A. Radioautographic distribution of neurotensin binding sites in the rat brain: A light microscopic study using monoiodo-^{125}I-Tyr3-neurotensin. *Neuroscience* 1987;22: 525–536.
441. Moyse E, Miller MM, Kitabgi P, Rostène W, Beaudet A. Effects of gonadal steroids on the binding of 1251 neurotensin in rat suprachiasmatic nucleus. *Soc Neurosci* 1986;614.
442. Brown M, Vale W. Effects of neurotensin and substance P on plasma insulin glucagon and glucose levels. *Endocrinology* 1976;98:819.
443. Szigethy E, Beaudet A. Neurotensin receptors are selectively associated with cholinergic neurons in the rat basal forebrain. *Neurosci Lett* 1987;83:47–52.
444. Euler G von, Meister B, Hökfelt T, Eneroth P, Fuxe K. Intraventricular injection of neurotensin reduces dopamine D_2 agonist binding in rat forebrain and intermediate lobe of the pituitary gland. Relationship to serum hormone levels and nerve terminal coexistence. *Brain Res* 1990;531:253–262.
445. Ferris CF, Pan J, Singer E, Boyd W, Caraway R, Leeman S. Stimulation of luteinizing hormone release after stereotaxic microinjection of neurotensin into the medial preoptic area of rats. *Neuroendocrinology* 1984;3:145–151.
446. Madea K, Frohman LA. Dissociation of systemic and central effects of neurotensin on the secretion of growth hormone, prolactin and thyrotropin. *Endocrinology* 1978;103:1903.
447. Shimatsu A, Kato Y, Matsuhita N, Katakami H, Yanahaira N, Imura H. Effects of glucagon, neurotensin and vasoactive intestinal peptide in somatostatin release from perifused rat hypothalamus. *Endocrinology* 1982;110:2113–2117.
448. Goedert M, Lightman SL, Emson PC. Neurotensin in the rat anterior pituitary gland: Effects of endocrinological manipulations. *Brain Res* 1984;299:160–163.
449. Enjalbert A, Arancibia S, Priam M, Bluet-Pajot MT, Kordon C. Neurotensin stimulation of prolactin secretion *in vitro. Neuroendocrinology* 1982;34:95–98.
450. Fuxe K, Agnati LF, Andersson K, Eneroth P, Harfstrand A, Goldstein M, Zoli M. Studies on neurotensin catecholamine interactions in the hypothalamus and in the forebrain of male rat. *Neurochem Int* 1984;6:737–750.
451. Raisman G, Brown-Grant K. The "suprachiasmatic syndrome": Endocrine and behavioural abnormalities following lesions of the suprachiasmatic nuclei in the female rat. *Proc R Soc Lond* 1977;198:297–314.
452. De Bold AJ. Atrial natriuretic factor: A hormone produced by the heart. *Science* 1985;230:767–770.
453. Quinon R, Dalpe M, De Lean A, Gutkowska J, Cantin M, Genest J. Atrial natriuretic factor (ANF) binding sites in brain and related structures. *Peptides* 1984;5:1167–1172.
454. Bianchi C, Gutkowska J, Ballak M, Thibault G, Garcia R, Genest J, Cantin M. Radioautographic localization of ^{125}I. atrial natriuretic factor binding sites in the brain. *Neuroendocrinology* 1986;44:365–372.
455. Jacobowitz DM, Skofitsch G, Keiser HR, Eskay RL, Zamir N. Evidence for the existence of atrial natriuric factor containing neurons in rat brain. *Neuroendocrinology* 1984;40:92–94.
456. Harvath J, Ertl T, Schally AV. Effect of atrial natriuretic peptide on gonadotropin release in superfused rat pituitary cells. *Proc Natl Acad Sci USA* 1986;83:3444–3446.
457. Abou-Samra AB, Catt KJ, Aguilera G. Synthetic atrial natriuretic factors (ANFs) stimulate guanine 3′5′-monophosphate production but not hormone release in rat pituitary cells: Peptide contamination with a gonadotropin releasing hormone agonist explains luteinizing hormone releasing activity of certain ANFs. *Endocrinology* 1987;120:18–24.
458. Steele MK. Additive effects of atrial natriuretic peptide and angiotensin II on luteinizing hormone and prolactin release in female rats. *Neuroendocrinology* 1990;51:345–350.
459. Pandey KN, Pavlow SN, Kovacs WJ, Inagami T. Atrial natriuretic factor regulates steroidogenic responsiveness and cyclic nucleotide levels in mouse Leydig cells *in vitro. Biochem Biophys Res Commun* 1986;138:399–404.
460. Wong M, Samson WK, Dudley CA, Moss RL. Direct neuronal action of atrial natriuretic factor in rat brain. *Neuroendocrinology* 1986;44:49–53.
461. Crandall ME, Gregg CM. *In vitro* evidence for an inhibitory effect of atrial natriuretic peptide on vasopressin release. *Neuroendocrinology* 1986;44:439–445.
462. Samson WK. Atrial natriuretic factor inhibits dehydration and hemorrhage induced vasopressin release. *Neuroendocrinology* 1985;40:277–279.
463. Leranth CS, McLusky MJ, Naftolin F. Proopiomelanocortin derived neuropeptide immunoreactive cells of the ventromedial arcuate nucleus establish direct synaptic connections with LHRH neurons of the medial preoptic area in the rat. *Proc Neurosci Soc* 1985;15:146.
464. Sawchenko PE, Swanson LW, Joseph SA. The distribution and cells of origin of ACTH (1-39) stained varicosities in the paraventricular and supraoptic nuclei. *Brain Res* 1982;232:365–374.
465. Kiss JZ, Cassel MD, Palkovits M. Analysis of the ACTH/BEND/MSH immunoreactive afferent input to the hypothalamic paraventricular nucleus of the rat. *Brain Res* 1984;324:91–99.
466. Bai FL, Yamano M, Shiotani Y, Emson PC, Smith AD, Powell JF, Tohyama M. An arcuato-paraventricular and dorsomedial hypothalamic neuropeptide Y containing system which lacks noradrenaline in the rat. *Brain Res* 1985;331:172–175.
467. Chen YY, Pelletier G. Demonstration of contacts between proopiomelanocortin neurons in the rat hypothalamus. *Neurosci Lett* 1983;43:261–272.
468. Kiss JZ, Williams TH. ACTH immunoreactive boutons form synaptic contacts in the hypothalamic arcuate nucleus of rat: Evidence for local opiocortin connections. *Brain Res* 1983;263: 142–146.
469. Tatemoto K. Neuropeptide Y: Complete amino acid sequence of the brain peptide. *Proc Natl Acad Sci USA* 1982;79:5485–5489.
470. Tatemoto K, Carlquist M, Mutt V. Neuropeptide Y, a novel brain peptide with structural similarities to peptide YY and pancreatic polypeptide. *Nature* 1982;296:659–660.
471. Solomon TE. Pancreatic polypeptide, peptide YY and neuropep-

tide Y family of regulatory peptides. *Gastroenterology* 1985;88: 838–844.
472. Allen YS, Adrian TE, Allen JM, Tatemoto K, Crow TJ, Bloom SR, Polak JM. Neuropeptide Y distribution in the brain. *Science* 1983;221:877.
473. Gray TS, Marley JE. Neuropeptide Y: Anatomical distribution and possible functions in mammalian nervous system. *Life Sci* 1986;38:389–400.
474. Chronwall BM, Di Maggio DA, Massari VJ, Pickel DA, Ruggiko DA, O'Donohue TL. The anatomy of neuropeptide Y containing neurons in the rat brain. *Neuroscience* 1985;15:1159–1181.
475. Beal MF, Chattha GK, Martin JB. A comparison of regional somatostatin and neuropeptide Y distribution in rat striatum and brain. *Brain Res* 1986;377:240–245.
476. Lundberg JM, Terenius L, Hökfelt T, Tatemoto K. Comparative immunohistochemical and biochemical analyses of pancreatic polypeptide-like peptides in central and peripheral neurons. *J Neurosci* 1984;4:2376–2386.
477. Hendry SH, Jones EG, Emson P. Morphology, distribution and synaptic relations of somatostatin and neuropeptide Y immunoreactive neurons in rat and monkey neocortex. *J Neurosci* 1984;4:2497–2517.
478. Everitt BJ, Hökfelt T, Terenius L, Tatemoto K, Mutt V, Goldstein M. Differential coexistence of neuropeptide Y-like immunoreactivity with catecholamines in the central nervous system of the rat. *Neuroscience* 1984;11:443–462.
479. Kalra SP, Sahu A, Kalra PS, Crowley WR. Hypothalamic neuropeptide Y: a circuit in the regulation of gonadotropin secretion and feeding behavior. *Ann NY Acad Sci* 1990;611:273–283.
480. Horvath TL, Naftolin F, Kalra SP, Leranth C. Neuropeptide-Y innervation of β-endorphin-containing cells in the rat mediobasal hypothalamus: a light and electron microscopic double immunostaining analysis. *Endocrinology* 1992;131:2461–2467.
481. Moore RY, Gustofson EL, Card JP. Identical immunoreactivity of afferents to the rat suprachiasmatic nucleus with antisera against pancreatic polypeptide, molluscan cardioexcitatory peptide and neuropeptide Y. *Cell Tissue Res* 1984;236:41–46.
482. Sar M, Sahu A, Crowley WR, Kalra SP. Localization of neuropeptide-Y immunoreactivity in estradiol-concentrating cells in hypothalamus. *Endocrinology* 1990;127:2752–2756.
483. Michel MC. Receptors for neuropeptide Y: multiple subtypes and multiple second messengers. *Trends Pharmacol Sci* 1991; 12:389–393.
484. Inui A, Sano K, Miura M, Hirosue Y, Nakajima M, Okita M, Baba S, Kasuga M. Evidence for further heterogeneity of the receptors for neuropeptide-Y and peptide-YY in tumor cell lines derived from neural crest. *Endocrinology* 1992;131:2090–2096.
485. Berria M, Pau K-YF, Spies HG. Evidence for α_1-adrenergic involvement in neuropeptide Y-stimulated GnRH release in female rabbits. *Neuroendocrinology* 1991;53:480–486.
486. Kaynard AH, Spies HG. Immunoneutralization of neuropeptide Y suppresses luteinizing hormone secretion in rabbits. *Endocrinology* 1991;128:2769–2775.
487. Danger J-M, Breton B, Vallarino M, Fournier A, Pelletier G, Vaudry H. Neuropeptide-Y in the trout brain and pituitary: localization, characterization, and action on gonadotropin release. *Endocrinology* 1991;128:2360–2368.
488. Breton B, Mikolajczyk T, Popek W, Bieniarz K, Epler P. Neuropeptide Y stimulates *in vivo* gonadotropin secretion in teleost fish. *Gen Comp Endocrinol* 1991;84:277–283.
489. Pau K-YF, Kaynard AH, Hess DL, Spies HG. Effects of neuropeptide Y on the in vitro release of gonadotropin-releasing hormone, luteinizing hormone, and beta-endorphin and pituitary responsiveness to gonadotropin-releasing hormone in female macaques. *Neuroendocrinology* 1991;53:396–403.
490. Bauer-Dantoin A, McDonald JK, Levine JE. Neuropeptide Y potentiates luteinizing hormone (LH)-releasing hormone-stimulated LH surges in pentobarbital-blocked proestrous rats. *Endocrinology* 1991;129:402–408.
491. Kerkerian L, Guy J, Lefèvre C, Pelletier G. Effects of neuropeptides Y (NPY) on the release of anterior pituitary hormones in the rat. *Peptides* 1985;6:1201–1204.
492. McDonald JK, Lumpkin MD, Samson WK, McCann SM. NPY affects secretion of luteinizing hormone and growth hormone in ovariectomized rats. *Proc Natl Acad Sci USA* 1985;82:561.
493. Khorram O, Pau FKY, Spiess HG. Bimodal effects of neuropeptide Y or hypothalamic release of gonadotropin releasing hormone in conscious rabbits. *Neuroendocrinology* 1987;45: 290–297.
494. Kalra SP, Crowley WR. Differential effects of pancreatic polypeptide on luteinizing hormone release in female rats. *Neuroendocrinology* 1984;38:511–513.
495. McDonald JK, Lumpkin MD, Samson WK, McCann SM. Pancreatic polypeptides affect luteinizing and growth hormone secretion in rats. *Peptides* 1985;6:79–84.
496. Crowley WR, Tessel RE, O'Donohue TL, Adler BA, Kalra SP. Effect of ovarian hormones on the concentrations of immunoreactive neuropeptide Y in discrete brain regions of the female rat: Correlation with serum luteinizing hormone (LH) and median eminence LH releasing hormone. *Endocrinology* 1985;117: 1151–1155.
497. Brann DW, McDonald JK, Putnam CD, Malesh VB. Regulation of hypothalamic gonadotropin-releasing hormone and neuropeptide Y concentrations by progesterone and corticosteroids in immature rats: correlation with luteinizing hormone and follicle-stimulating hormone release. *Neuroendocrinology* 1991;54: 425–432.
498. Bauer-Dantoin AC, Urban JH, Levine JE. Neuropeptide Y gene expression in the arcuate nucleus is increased during preovulatory luteinizing hormone surges. *Endocrinology* 1992;131: 2953–2958.
499. Clark JT, Kalra PS, Kalra SP. Neuropeptide Y stimulates feeding but inhibits sexual behavior in rats. *Endocrinology* 1985;117: 2435–2442.
500. Crowley WR, Hassid A, Kalra SP. Neuropeptide Y enhances the release of luteinizing hormone (LH) induced by LH-releasing hormone. *Endocrinology* 1987;120:941–945.
501. Parker SL, Kalra SP, Crowley WR. Neuropeptide Y modulates the binding of a gonadotropin-releasing hormone (GnRH) analog to anterior pituitary GnRH receptor sites. *Endocrinology* 1991;128:2309–2316.
502. Shangold GA, Miller RJ. Direct neuropeptide Y-induced modulation of gonadotrope intracellular calcium transients and gonadotropin secretion. *Endocrinology* 1990;126:2336–2342.
503. Tatemoto K, Rökaeus A, Jörnvall H, McDonald TI, Mutt V. Galanin—A novel biologically active peptide from porcine intestine. *FEBS Lett* 1983;164:124–128.
504. Melander T, Hökfelt T, Rökaeus A. Distribution of galanin-like immunoreactivity in the rat central nervous system. *J Comp Neurol* 1986;248:475–517.
505. Schofitsch G, Zacobowitz DM. Immunocytochemical mapping of galanin-like immunoreactivity in the rat central nervous system. *Peptides* 1985;6:509–546.
506. Melander T, Hökfelt T, Rökaeus A, Cuello AC, Oertel WH, Verhofstad A, Goldstein M. Coexistence of galanin-like immunoreactivity with catecholamines, S-hydroxytryptamine GABA and neuropeptides in the rat CNS. *J Neurosci* 1986;6:3640–3654.
507. Lopez FJ, Merchenthaler I, Ching M, Wisniewski MG, Negro-Vilar A. Galanin: a hypothalamic-hypophysiotropic hormone modulating reproductive functions. *Proc Natl Acad Sci USA* 1991;88:4508–1512.
508. Nordsfröm O, Melander T, Hökfelt T, Bartfai T, Goldstein M. Evidence for an inhibitory effect of the peptide galanin on dopamine release from the rat median eminence. *Neurosci Lett* 1987;73:21–26.
509. Gabriel SM, Koenig JI, Kaplan LM. Galanin-like immunoreactivity is influenced by estrogen in peripubertal and adult rats. *Neuroendocrinology* 1990;51:168–173.
510. Steel JH, Gon G, O'Halloran DJ, Jones PK, Yanaihara N, Ishikawa H, Bloom SR, Polak JM. Galanin and vasoactive intestinal peptide are colcalized with classical pituitary hormones and show plasticity of expression. *Histochemistry* 1989;93:183–189.
511. Hyde JF, Keller BK. Galanin secretion from anterior pituitary cells *in vitro* is regulated by dopamine, somatostatin, and thyrotropin-releasing hormone. *Endocrinology* 1991;128:917–922.

512. Hyde JF, Engle MG, Maley BE. Colocalization of galanin and prolactin within secretory granules of anterior pituitary cells in estrogen-treated Fischer 344 rats. *Endocrinology* 1991;129: 270–276.
513. Fuxe K, Hökfelt, Teneroth P, Gustafsson JA, Skett P. Prolactin-like immunoreactivity: localisation in nerve terminals of rat hypothalamus. *Science* 1977;196:899–900.
514. Hausen BL, Hausen GN, Hagen C. Immunoreactive material resembling ovine prolactin in perikarya and nerve terminals of the rat hypothalamus. *Cell Tissue Res* 1982;226:121–131.
515. Wilson DM, Emannuela NV, Jurgens JK, Kelley MK. Prolactin message in brain and pituitary of adult male rats is identical: PCR cloning and sequencing of hypothalamic prolactin cDNA from intact and hypophysectomised adult male rats. *Endocrinology* 1992;131:2488–2490.
516. Azad N, Duffner L, Paloyan EB, Reda D, Kirstain L, Emanuele NV, Lawrence AM. Hypothalamic prolactin stimulates the release of luteinizing hormone releasing hormone (LHRH) from male rat hypothalamus. *Endocrinology* 1990;127:1928–1933.
517. Ouhtif A, Morel G, Kelley PA. Visualization of gene expression of short and long forms of prolactin receptor in the rat. *Endocrinology* 1993; in press.
518. Milenkovic L, D'Angelo G, Weiner RI. Prolactin inhibition of GnRH release from GT1 GnRH cell line via prolactin receptors. *Society for Neuroscience Abstracts* 1992;18:929.
519. Swanson LW, Kuypers HG. The paraventricular nucleus of the hypothalamus: Cytoarchitectonic subdivisions and the organization of projections to the pituitary, dorsal vagal complex and spinal cord as demonstrated by retrograde fluorescence double labelling methods. *J Comp Neurol* 1980;194:555–570.
520. Katsoyannis PG, Du Vigneaud V. Arginine vasotocine, a synthetic analogue of the posterior pituitary hormones containing the ring of oxytocin and the side chain of vasopressin. *J Biol Chem* 1958;233:1352–1354.
521. Sachs H, Lajtha A. Neurosecretion. In: *Handbook of neurochemistry, vol. 4.* New York: Plenum Press, 1969;323–428.
522. Vandesande F, Dierickx K, De Mey J. Identification of the vasopressin-neurophysin producing neurons of the rat suprachiasmatic nuclei. *Cell Tissue Res* 1975;56:377–380.
523. Sofroniew MV, Weindl A. Identification of parvocellular vasopressin and neurophysin neurons in the suprachiasmatic nucleus of a variety of mammals including primates. *J Comp Neurol* 1980;193:659–675.
524. Brownstein MI, Eskay RL, Palkovits M. Thyrotropin releasing hormone in the median eminence is in processes of paraventricular nucleus neurons. *Neuropeptides* 1982;2:197–201.
525. Pelletier G, Desy I, Cote I, Lefevre G, Vaudry H, Labrie F. Immunoelectron microscopic localization of corticotropin releasing factor in the rat hypothalamus. *Neuroendocrinology* 1982;35: 402–404.
526. Roth KA, Weber E, Barchas JD. Immunoreactive corticotropin releasing factor (CRF) and vasopressin are colocalized in a subpopulation of immunoreactive vasopressin cells in the paraventricular nucleus of the hypothalamus. *Life Sci* 1982;31: 1857–1860.
527. Beinfeld MC. Cholecystokinin in the central nervous system: A minireview. *Neuropeptides* 1983;3:411–427.
528. Lind RW, Swanson LW, Bruhn TO, Ganten D. The distribution of angiotensin II immunoreactive cells and fibers in the paraventriculo-hypophyseal system of the rat. *Brain Res* 1985;338:81–89.
529. Carrea FM, Innes RB, Uhl GR, Snyder SH. Bradykinin-like immunoreactive neuronal system localized histochemically in rat brain. *Proc Natl Acad Sci USA* 1979;76:1489–1493.
530. Moudy TW, O'Donohue TL, Jacobowitz DM. Biochemical localization and characterization of bombesin-like peptides in discrete regions of the brain. *Peptides* 1982;2:75–79.
531. Mezey E. Vasoactive intestinal polypeptide immunopositive neurons in the rat paraventricular nucleus of the homozygous Brattleboro rat. *Neuroendocrinology* 1986;42:88–90.
532. Samson WK, Skala KD, Alexander B, Huang F-LS. Possible neuroendocrine actions of endothelin-3. *Endocrinology* 1991;128: 1465–1473.
533. Kiss JZ, Palkovits M, Zaborsky L, Tribollet E, Szabo D, Makara GB. Quantitative histological studies on the hypothalamic paraventricular nucleus in rats. I. Number of cells and synaptic boutons. *Brain Res* 1983;262:217–224.
534. Van den Pol AN. The magnocellular and parvocellular paraventricular nucleus of the rat: Intrinsic organization. *J Comp Neurol* 1982;206:317–345.
535. Conrad CCA, Pfaff DW. Efferents from medial basal forebrain and hypothalamus in rat. I. An autoradiographic study of the medial preoptic area. *J Comp Neurol* 1976;169:185–220.
536. Nilaver G, Zimmerman EA, Wilkins J, Michaels J, Hoffman D, Silverman AJ. Magnocellular hypothalamic projections to the lower brain stem and spinal cord of the rat. *Neuroendocrinology* 1980;30:150–158.
537. Doris PA. Vasopressin and central integrative processes. *Neuroendocrinology* 1984;38:75–85.
538. Ivell R, Richter D. Structure and comparison of the oxytocin and vasopressin genes from the rat. *Proc Natl Acad Sci USA* 1984;81:2006–2010.
539. Dogterom J, Suijdewint FG, Buijs RM. The distribution of vasopressin and oxytocin in the rat brain. *Neurosci Lett* 1978;9: 341–346.
540. Hawthorn J, Aug VT, Jenkins JS. Localization of vasopressin in the rat brain. *Brain Res* 1980;197:75–81.
541. Rossor MN, Iversen LL, Hawthorn J, Aug VT, Lenkins JS. Extrahypothalamic vasopressin in human brain. *Brain Res* 1981; 214:349–355.
542. Zimmerman EA, Carmel P, Husain MK, Ferina M, Tannerbaum M, Frantz AG, Robinson AG. Vasopressin and neurophysin high concentration in monkey hypophysial portal blood. *Science* 1973;182:925–927.
543. Gibbs DM. High concentrations of oxytocin in hypophysial portal plasma. *Endocrinology* 1984;114:1216–1218.
544. Jard S. Vasopressin antagonists allow demonstration of a novel type of vasopressin receptors in the rat adenohypophysis. *Mol Pharmacol* 1986;30:171–177.
545. Koch B, Lutz-Bucher B. Specific receptors for vasopressin in the pituitary gland: Evidence for down-regulation and desensitization to adrenocorticotropin releasing factor. *Endocrinology* 1985;116:671–676.
546. Yates FE, Russel SM, Dallman MR, Hedge CA, McCann SM, Dhariwal AP. Potentiation by vasopressin of corticotropin release induced by CRF. *Endocrinology* 1971;88:3–15.
547. Gillies GE, Linton EA, Lowry PJ. Corticotropin releasing activity is potentiated several times by vasopressin. *Nature* 1982;399: 355–357.
548. Antoni FA, Holmes MC, Jones MT. Oxytocin as well as vasopressin potentiates ovine CRF *in vitro*. *Peptides* 1983;4:411–415.
549. Gibbs DM, Vale W, Rivier J, Yen SSC. Oxytocin potentiates the ACTH releasing activity of CRF 41 but not vasopressin. *Life Sci* 1984;34:2245–2249.
550. Suh BY, Liu JH, Rasmussen DD, Gibbs DM, Steinberg J, Yen SSC. Role of oxytocin in the modulation of ACTH release in women. *Neuroendocrinology* 1986;44:309–313.
551. Johnson LY, Vaughan MF, Reiter RJ, Petterborg LJ, Chen HJ. Acute effects of arginine vasopressin on plasma and pituitary levels of prolactin in the male rat: Influence of urethane anesthesia. *Horm Res* 1980;13:109–120.
552. Lumpkin MD, Samson WK, McCann SM. Hypothalamic and pituitary sites of action of oxytocin to alter prolactin secretion in the rat. *Endocrinology* 1983;112:1711–1717.
553. Gala RR, Rice RP. Influence of neurohumors on anterior pituitary lactogen production *in vitro*. *Proc Soc Exp Biol Med* 1965;120:220.
554. Mori M, Vigh S, Miyata A, Yoshihara T, Oka S, Arimura A. Oxytocin is the major prolactin releasing factor in the posterior pituitary. *Endocrinology* 1990;126:1009–1013.
555. Vaughan MK, Blask DE, Iohnson LY, Reiter RJ. Prolactin releasing activity of arginine vasopressin *in vitro*. *Horm Res* 1975;6:342–350.
556. Chin SH. Vasopressin has a direct effect on prolactin release in male rats. *Neuroendocrinology* 1982;34:55–58.
557. Arey BJ, Freeman ME. Oxytocin, vasoactive-intestinal peptide,

and serotonin regulate the mating-unduced surges of prolactin secretion in the rat. *Endocrinology* 1990;126:279–284.
558. Mogg RJ, Samson WK. Interactions of dopaminergic and peptidergic factors in the control of prolactin release. *Endocrinology* 1990;126:728–735.
559. Mormède P, Vincent JD, Kerdelhué B. Vasopressin and oxytocin reduce plasma prolactin levels of conscious rats in basal and stress conditions. Study of the characteristics of the receptor involved. *Life Sci* 1986;39(19):1737–1743.
560. Arey BJ, Freeman ME. Activity of oxytocinergic neurons in the paraventricular nucleus mirrors the periodicity of the endogenous stimulatory rhythm regulating prolactin secretion. *Endocrinology* 1992;130:126–132.
561. De Paolo LV, Berardo PV, Carillo AJ. Intraventricular administration of arginine vasopressin suppresses prolactin release via a dopaminergic mechanism. *Peptides* 1986;7:541.
562. Blask DE, Vaughan MK. Naloxone inhibits arginine vasopressin (AVT) induced prolactin release in urethane anesthetised male rats *in vivo*. *Neurosci Lett* 1980;18:184.
563. Ben-Jonathan N, Peters LL. Posterior pituitary lobectomy: Differential elevation of plasma prolactin and luteinizing hormone in estrous and lactating rats. *Endocrinology* 1982;110: 1861–1865.
564. Robinson G, Evans JJ. Oxytocin has a role in gonadotrophin regulation in rats. *J Endocrinol* 1990;125:425–432.
565. Johnston CA, Lopez F, Samson WK, Negro-Vilar A. Physiologically important role for central oxytocin in the preovulatory release of luteinizing hormone. *Neurosci Lett* 1990;120:256–258.
566. Gibbs DM. Vasopressin and oxytocin: Hypothalamic modulators of the stress response: A review. *Psychoneuroendocrinology* 1986;11:131–140.
567. Lang RE, Heil JWE, Ganten D, Hermann K, Unger T, Rascher W. Oxytocin unlike vasopressin is a stress hormone in the rat. *Neuroendocrinology* 1983;37:314–316.
568. Rivier C, Vale W. Modulation of stress induced ACTH release by corticotropin releasing factor, catecholamines and vasopressin. *Nature* 1983;305:325–327.
569. Gibbs DM. Stress specific modulation of ACTH secretion by oxytocin. *Neuroendocrinology* 1986;42:456–458.
570. Gambacciani M, Yen SSC, Rasmussen DD. GnRH release from mediobasal hypothalamus *in vitro:* Regulation by oxytocin. *Neuroendocrinology* 1986;42:181–183.
571. Fahrbach SE, Morrell JI, Pfatt DW. Possible role for endogenous oxytocin in estrogen facilitated maternal behavior in rats. *Neuroendocrinology* 1985;40:526–532.
572. Kleet ER, Voarhuis DAM, Boschma Y, Elands J. Estradiol modulates density of putative oxytocin receptors in discrete rat brain regions. *Neuroendocrinology* 1986;44:415–421.
573. De Wied D, Gispen WH. Behavioral effects of peptides. In: Gainer H, ed. *Peptides in neurobiology.* New York: Plenum Press, 1977;397–448.
574. Burgus R, Dunn TF, Desiderio D, Guillemin R. Structure moleculaire du facteur hypothalamique TRF d'origine bovine: Mise en evidence par spectrometrie de masse de la sequence p-glu-his-pro-NH. *CR Acad Sci (Paris)* 1969;269:1870–1873.
575. Boler J, Enzmann F, Folkers K, Bowers CY, Shally V. The identity of chemical and hormonal properties of the thyrotropin releasing hormone and pyroglotamyl-histidyl-proline amide. *Biochem Biophys Res Commun* 1969;37:705–710.
576. Richter D, Kawashina E, Egger R, Kreil R. Biosynthesis of thyrotropin releasing hormone in the skin of *xenopus laevis:* Partial sequence of the precursor deduced from cloned DNA. *EMBO J* 1984;3:617–621.
577. Brownstein MJ, Palkovits M, Saavedra JM, Bassiri RM, Utiger RD. Thyrotropin releasing hormone in specific nuclei of the brain. *Science* 1974;185:267–269.
578. Bassiri RM, Utiger RD. Thyrotropin releasing hormone in the hypothalamus of the rat. *Endocrinology* 1977;94:188.
579. Lechan R, Jackson J. Immunohistochemical localization of thyrotropin releasing hormone in the rat hypothalamus and pituitary. *Endocrinology* 1982;111:55–65.
580. Ishikawa K, Taniguchi Y, Kurosumi K, Suzuki M. Origin of septal thyrotropin releasing factor in the rat. *Neuroendocrinology* 1986;44:54–58.
581. Lechan RM, Wu P, Jackson JMD. Immunolocalization of the thyrotropin releasing hormone prohormone in the rat central nervous system. *Endocrinology* 1986;119:1210–1216.
582. Borson-Chazot F, Jordan D, Fevre-Montange M, Kopp N, Tourniaire N, Rouzioux JM, Vesseyre M, Mornex R. TRH and LHRH distribution in discrete nuclei of the human hypothalamus: Evidence for a left prominence of TRH. *Brain Res* 1986;382:433–436.
583. Brunet N, Gourdgi D, Tixier-Vidal A, Pradelles Ph, Morgat JL, Fromafeut P. Chemical evidence for associated TRF with subcellular fractions after incubation of intact rat prolactin cells (GH3) with 3H-labelled TRF. *FEBS Lett* 1974;38:129–133.
584. Pazos A, Cortes R, Palacios J. Thyrotropin releasing hormone receptor binding sites: Autoradiographic distribution in the rat and guinea pig brain. *J Neurochem* 1985;45:1448–1463.
585. Horita A, Carino MA, Lai H. Pharmacology of thyrotropin releasing hormone. *Annu Rev Pharmacol Toxicol* 1986;26: 311–332.
586. Chen HT, Meites J. Effects of biogenic amines and TRH on the release of prolactin and TSH in the rat. *Endocrinology* 1975;96:10.
587. Tashjian AR, Borowsky NJ, Jensen DK. Thyrotropin releasing hormone: Direct evidence for stimulation of prolactin production by pituitary cells in culture. *Biochem Biophys Res Commun* 1971;43:516.
588. Vale W, Blackwell R, Grant G, Guillemin R. TRF and thyroid hormones in prolactin secretion by rat anterior pituitary cells *in vitro*. *Endocrinology* 1973;93:26.
589. Gerschengorn MC, Marcus-Samuels BE, Geras E. Estrogens increase the number of thyrotropin releasing hormone receptors on mammotropic cells in culture. *Endocrinology* 1979;105:171.
590. De Lean A, Garon M, Kelly PA, Labrie F. Changes in pituitary thyrotropin releasing hormone (TRH) and prolactin response to TRH during the rat estrous cycle. *Endocrinology* 1977;100:1505.
591. Enjalbert A, Ruberg M, Arancibia S, Priam M, Bauer K, Kordon C. Inhibition of *in vitro* prolactin secretion by histidyl-proline diketoperazine, a degradation product of TRH. *Eur J Pharmacol* 1979;58:97–98.
592. Pekary AE, Stephens R, Simard M, Pang X-P, Smith V, DiStefano JJ, Hershman JM. Release of thyrotropin and prolactin by a thyrotropin-releasing hormone (TRH) precursor, TRH-Gly: conversion to TRH is sufficient for in vivo effects. *Neuroendocrinology* 1990;52:618–625.
593. Mitsuma T, Hirooka Y, Kimura M, Nogimori T. Failure to demonstrate the effect of various pre-pro-TRH fragments on TSH and PRL release from rat pituitary *in vitro*. *Endocrinol Exp (Bratisl)* 1990:333–339.
594. Mori M, Murakami M, Iriuchijima K, Miyashita K, Satoh T, Monden T, Kobayashi I, Kobayashi S. Stimulation by a TRH precursor, TRH-GLY, of TSH and PRL secretion in rats: effect of starvation. *Neuropeptides* 1990;16:57–62.
595. Mori M, Murakami M, Satoh T, Miyashita K, Iriuchijima T, Yamada M, Inukai T, Kobayashi I. A possible direct precursor of thyrotropin-releasing hormone, *p*Glu-His-Pro-Gly, stimulates prolactin secretion in anorexia nervosa. *J Clin Endocrinol Metab* 1990;71:252–255.
596. Vale W, Spiess J, Rivier C, Rivier J. Characterization of 41 residue ovine hypothalamic peptide that stimulates secretion of corticotropin and β-endorphin. *Science* 1981;213:1394–1397.
597. Shibahara S, Moromoto Y, Furutani Y, Notake M, Takahashi H, Shimiza S, Horikawa S, Numa S. Isolation and sequence analysis of the human corticotropin-releasing factor precursor gene. *EMBO J* 1983;2:775–779.
598. Swanson LW, Sawchenko PE, Rivier I, Vale W. Organization of ovine corticotropin releasing factor immunoreactive cells and fibers in the rat brain: An immunocytochemical study. *Neuroendocrinology* 1983;36:165–186.
599. Burlet A, Tonon MC, Taukosic P, Coy D, Vaudry H. Comparative immunocytochemical localization of corticotropin releasing factor (CRF 41) and neurohypophysial peptides in the brain of

Brattleboro and Long-Evans rats. *Neuroendocrinology* 1983;37:64–72.

600. McCann SM, Haberland P. Relative abundance of vasopressin and corticotropin releasing factor in neurohypophyseal extracts. *Proc Soc Exp Biol Med* 1959;102:319–325.
601. Nakane T, Andhya T, Hollander CS, Schlesinger DH, Kardor P, Brown C, Passarelli J. Corticotropin releasing factor in extrahypothalamic brain of the mouse: Demonstration by immunoassay and immunoneutralization of bioassayable activity. *J Endocrinol* 1986;111:143–149.
602. Vale W, Rivier C, Yang L, Minick S, Guillemin R. Effects of purified hypothalamic corticotropin releasing factor and other substances on the secretion of adrenocorticotropin and β-endorphin-like immunoreactivities *in vitro. Endocrinology* 1978;103:1910–1915.
603. Rivier C, Vale W. Influence of corticotropin releasing factor on reproductive functions in the rat. *Endocrinology* 1984;114:914.
604. Gambacciani M, Yen SSC, Rasmussen DD. GnRH release from the mediobasal hypothalamus: *in vitro* inhibition by corticotropin releasing factor. *Neuroendocrinology* 1986;43:533–536.
605. Nikolarakis KE, Almeida OF, Herz A. Corticotropin releasing factor (CRF) inhibits gonadotropin releasing hormone (GnRH) release from superfused rat hypothalami *in vitro. Brain Res* 1986;377:388–390.
606. Ono N, Lumpkin MD, Samson WK, McDonald JK, McCann SM. Intrahypothalamic action of corticotropin releasing factor (CRF) to inhibit growth hormone and LH release in the rat. *Life Sci* 1984;35:1117–1123.
607. Motta M. Neuroendocrine effects of some amphibian peptides. *Peptides* 1985;6(Suppl. 3):131–135.
608. Brown MR, Fisher LA, Spiess J, Rivier J, Rivier C, Vale W. Comparison of the biologic actions of corticotropin releasing factor and sauvagine. *Regul Pept* 1982;4:107.
609. Ilotzky PM, Bruhn TO, Otto S. Central modulation of immunoreactive arginine vasopressin and oxytocin secretion into the hypophyseal portal circulation by corticotropin releasing factor. *Endocrinology* 1984;116:1669–1671.
610. Bruhn TO, Sulton SW, Plotsky PM, Vale WW. Central administration of corticotropin releasing factor modulates oxytocin secretion in the rat. *Endocrinology* 1986;119:1558–1563.
611. Sirinathsinghji DJ, Rees LH, Rivier J, Vale W. Corticotropin releasing factor is a potent inhibitor of sexual receptivity in the female rat. *Nature* 1983;305:15.
612. Sirinathsinghji DJ. Modulation of lordosis behaviour in the female rat by corticotropin releasing factor, β-endorphin and gonadotropin releasing hormone in the mesencephalic central gray. *Brain Res* 1985;336:45–55.
613. Rivier C, Rivier J, Vale W. Stress induced inhibition of reproductive functions: Role of endogenous corticotropin releasing factor. *Science* 1986;231:607.
614. Beinfeld MC, Meyer DK, Eskay RL, Jensen RT, Brownstein MJ. The distribution of cholecystokinin immunoreactivity in the central nervous system of the rat as determined by radioimmunoassay. *Brain Res* 1981;212:51–57.
615. Iunis RB, Correa FM, Uhl GR, Schneider B, Snyder SH. Cholecystokinin octapeptide-like immunoreactivity: Histochemical localization in rat brain. *Proc Natl Acad Sci USA* 1979;76:521–525.
616. Vanderhaegben JJ, Lostra F, Vandesande F, Dierickx K. Coexistence of cholocystokinin and oxytocin-neurophysin in some magnocellular hypothalamo-hypophyseal neurons. *Cell Tissue Res* 1981;221:227–231.
617. Hökfelt T, Holets VR, Staines W, Meister B, Melander T, Schalling M, Schutzberg M, Freedman J, Bjorklund H, Olson L, Lindh B, Elfvin LG, Lundberg JM, Lindgren JA, Samuelsson B, Penow B, Terenius L, Post C, Everitt B, Goldstein M. Coexistence of neuronal messengers An overview. In: Hokfelt T, Fuxe K, Pernow B, eds. *Progress in brain research.* vol. 68. Amsterdam: Elsevier, 1986:33–70.
618. Zaborszky L, Beinfeld MC, Palkovits M, Heimer L. Brainstem projections to the hypothalamic ventricular nucieus in the rat: A CCK containing long ascending pathway. *Brain Res* 1984; 303:225–231.
619. Saito A, Sankaran H, Godfine LD, Williams JA. Cholecystokinin receptors in the brain: Characterization and distribution. *Science* 1980;208:1155–1156.
620. Zarbin MA, Lunis RB, Wamsley JK, Snyder SH, Kuhar MJ. Autoradiographic localization of cholecystokinin receptors in rodent brain. *J Neurosci* 1983;3:877–906.
621. Day NC, Hall MD, Clark CR, Hughes J. High concentrations of cholecystokinin receptor binding sites in the ventromedial hypothalamus. *Neuropeptides* 1986;8:1–18.
622. Akesson TR, Mantyh PW, Mantyh CR, Matt DW, Micewych PE. Estrous cyclicity of ^{125}I cholecystokinin octapeptide binding in the ventromedial hypothalamic nucleus. Evidence for down modulation by estrogen. *Neuroendocrinology* 1987;45:257–262.
623. Akesson TR, Micevych PE. Binding of ^{125}I cholecystokinin octapeptide in the paraventricular but not the supraoptic nucleus is increased by ovariectomy. *Brain Res* 1986;385:165–168.
624. Vijayan E, Samson WK, McCann SM. *In vitro* and *in vivo* effects of cholecystokinin on gonadotropin, prolactin, growth hormone and thyrotropin release in the rat. *Brain Res* 1979;172:295–302
625. Haghimoto R, Kimura F. Inhibition of gonadotropin secretion induced by cholecystokinin implants in the medial preoptic area by a dopamine receptor blocker, pimozide, in the rat. *Neuroendocrinology* 1986;42:32–37.
626. Pau JT, Kow LM, Pfaff DW. Single unit activity of hypothalamic arcuate neurons in brain tissue slices. Effect of anterior pituitary hormones, cholecystokinin octapeptide and neurotransmitters. *Neuroendocrinology* 1986;43:189–196.
627. Skirboll LR, Grace AA, Homer DW, Rehfeld I, Goldstein M, Hokfelt T, Bunney BS. Peptide monoamine coexistence: Studies on the action of cholecystokinin-like peptide on the electrical activity of midbrain dopamine neurons. *Neuroscience* 1981;6: 2111–2124.
628. McCaleb ML, Lyers RD. Cholecystokinin acts on the hypothalamic noradrenergic system involved in feeding. *Peptides* 1980;1:47–49.
629. Kow LM, Pfaff DW. CCK8 stimulation of ventromedial hypothalamic neurons *in vitro:* A feeding relevant event? *Peptides* 1986;7:473–480.
630. Fulwiler CE, Saper CB. Cholecystokinin immunoreactive innervation of the ventromedial hypothalamus in the rat: Possible substrate for autonomic rcgulation of fceding. *Neurosci Lett* 1985;53:289–296.
631. Mendelson SD, Gorzalka BB. Cholecystokinin octapeptide produces inhibition of lordosis in the female rat. *Pharmacol Biochem Behav* 1984;21:755–759.
632. Campbell DJ, Bochnik J, Menard J, Corvol P. Identity of angiotensinogen precursors of rat brain and liver. *Nature* 1984;308: 206–208.
633. Lind RW, Swanson LW, Ganten D. Organization of angiotensin II immunoreactive cells and fibers in the rat central nervous system. An immunohistochemical study. *Neuroendocrinology* 1985;40:2–24.
634. Philips MI, Weyhenmeyer J, Felix D, Ganten D, Hoffman WE. Evidence for an endogenous brain renin angiotensin system. *Fed Proc* 1979;38:2260–2266.
635. Kilcoyne MM, Hoffman DL, Zimmerman EA. Immunocytochemical localization of angiotensin II and vasopressin in the rat hypothalamus: Evidence for production in the same neuron. *Clin Sci* 1980;59:57–60.
636. Saavedra JM, Fernandez-Pardal J, Chevillard C. Angiotensin converting enzyme in discrete areas of the rat forebrain and pituitary gland. *Brain Res* 1982;245:317–326.
637. Healy DP, Maciejewski AR, Printz MP. Localization of central angiotensin II receptors with (^{125}I) ser ile 8 angiotensin II: Periventricular sites of the anterior third ventricle. *Neuroendocrinology* 1986;44:22–28.
638. Hauger RL, Aguilera G, Baukol A, Catt K. Characterization of angiotensin II receptors in the pituitary gland. *Mol Cell Endocrinol* 1982;25:203–212.
639. Murphy TJ, Alexander RW, Griendling KK, Runge MS, Bernstein KE. Isolation of a cDNA encoding the vascular type I angiotensin II receptor. *Nature* 1991;351:233–236.
640. Sasaki K, Yamano Y, Bardhan S, Iwai N, Murray JJ, Hasegawa Y, Matsuda Y, Inagami T. Cloning and expression of a comple-

mentary DNA encoding a bovine angiotensin II type-1 receptor. *Nature* 1991;351:230–233.
641. Sandberg K, Ji H, Clark AJL, Shapira H, Catt KJ. Cloning and expression of a novel angiotensin II receptor subtype. *J Biol Chem* 1992;267:9455–9458.
642. Llorens Cortes C, Greenberg G, Huang H, Mounot C, Michel JB, Corvol P. Modulation of mRNA expression for angiotensin II receptor subtypes (AT1a and AT1b) analysed by quantitative RT-PCR quantification. *FASEB J* 1993;7:A341.
643. Langlois D, Hinsch KD, Saez SM, Begeot M. Stimulatory effect of insulin and insulin-like growth factor 1 on Gi proteins and angiotensin-II-induced phosphoinositide breakdown in cultured bovine adrenal cells. *Endocrinology* 1990;126:1867–1872.
644. Canonico PL, McLeod RM. Angiotensin peptides stimulate phosphoinositide breakdown and prolactin release in anterior pituitary cells in culture. *Endocrinology* 1986;118:233–238.
645. Audinot V, Rasolonjanahary R, Bertrand P, Priam M, Kordon C, Enjalbert A. Involvement of protein kinase C in the effect of angiotensin-II on adenosine 3′, 5′-monophosphate production in lactotrophs cells. *Endocrinology* 1991;129:2231–2239.
646. Steele MK, Negro-Vilar A, McCann SM. Effect of angiotensin II on *in vivo* and *in vitro* release of anterior pituitary hormones in the female rat. *Endocrinology* 1981;109:893–899.
647. Gaillard RC, Grossman A, Gillies G, Rees L, Besser GM. Angiotensin II stimulates the release of ACTH from dispersed rat anterior pituitary cells. *Clin Endocrinol* 1981;15:573–578.
648. Aguilera RA, Hyde C, Catt K. Angiotensin II receptors and prolactin release in pituitary lactotrophs. *Endocrinology* 1982;111: 1045–1050.
649. Schramme C, Denef C. Stimulation of prolactin release by angiotensin II in superfused rat anterior pituitary cell aggregates. *Neuroendocrinology* 1983;36:483–485.
650. Enjalbert A, Sladeczek F, Guillon G, Bertrand P, Shu C, Epelbaum J, Garcia-Saenz JA, Jard C, Lombard C, Kordon C, Bockaert J. Angiotensin II and dopamine modulate both cAMP and inositol phosphate production in anterior pituitary cells. Involvement in prolactin secretion. *J Biol Chem* 1986;261:4071–4075.
651. Platia MP, Catt KJ, Aguilera G. Effect of 17β estradiol on angiotensin II receptors and prolactin release in cultured pituitary cells. *Endocrinology* 1986;119:2768–2772.
652. Enjalbert A, Bertrand P, Bockaert J, Drouva S, Kordon C. Multiple coupling of neurohormone receptors with cyclic AMP and inositol phosphate production in anterior pituitary cells. *Biochimie* 1987;69:271–279.
653. Steele MK, Negro-Vilar A, McCann SM. Modulation by dopamine and estradiol of the central effects of angiotensin II on anterior pituitary hormone release. *Endocrinology* 1982;111: 722–729.
654. Myers LS, Steele MK. The brain renin-angiotensin system and prolactin secretion in the male rat. *Endocrinology* 1991;129: 1744–1748.
655. Steele MK, Gallo RV, Ganong WF. A possible role for the brain renin-angiotensin system in the regulation of LH secretion. *Am J Physiol* 1983;245:R805–R810.
656. Steele MK, Gallo RV, Ganong WF. Stimulatory and inhibitory effects of angiotensin II upon LH secretion in ovariectomized rats: A function of gonadal steroids. *Neuroendocrinology* 1985;40:210–216.
657. Franci CR, Anselmo-Franci JA, McCann SM. Angiotensin II antiserum decreases luteinizing hormone-releasing hormone in the median eminence and preoptic area of the rat. *Brazilian J Med Biol Res* 1990;23:899–901.
658. Chen MF, Hawkins R, Printz MP. Evidence for a functional, independent brain angiotensin system: Correlation between regional distribution of brain ATII receptors, brain angiotensinogen and drinking during the estrous cycle of the rat. In: Ganten D, Printz M, Phillips M, Scholkens BA, eds. *The renin-angiotensin system in the brain.* New York: Raven Press, 1982;157–168.
659. Findlay AL, Fitzimmons JT, Kucharczyk J. Dependence of spontaneous and angiotensin induced drinking in the rat upon the estrous cycle and gonadal hormones. *J Endocrinol* 1979;82:215.
660. Wilson KM, Summers C, Hathaway S, Fregly MJ. Mineralocorticoids modulate central angiotensin II receptors in rats. *Brain Res* 1986;382:87–96.
661. Fuxe K, Andersson K, Ganten D, Hökfelt T, Enroth P. Evidence for the existence of an angiotensin II like immunoreactive central system and its interactions with the central catecholamine pathways. In: Gross F,Vogel G, eds. *Enzymatic release of vasoactive peptides,* New York: Raven Press, 1980.
662. Keil LC, Summy-Long J, Severs WB. Release of vasopressin by angiotensin II. *Endocrinology* 1975;96:1063–1065.
663. Inoue A, Ynagisawa M, Kimura S, Kasuya Y, Miyauchi T, Goto K, Masaki T. The human endothelin family: three structurally and pharmacologically distinct isopeptides predicted by three separate genes. *Proc Natl Acad Sci USA* 1989;86:2863–2867.
664. Matsumoto H, Suzuki N, Onda H, Fujino M. Abundance of endothelin-3 in rat intestine, pituitary gland and brain. *Biochem Biophys Res Commun* 1989;164:74–80.
665. Yoshizawa T, Shinmi O, Giaid A, Yanagisawa M, Gibson SJ, Kimura S, Uchiyama Y, Polak JM, Masaki T, Kanazawa I. Endothelin: a novel peptide in the posterior pituitary system. *Science* 1990;247:462–464.
666. Mac Cumber MV, Ross CA, Glaser BM, Snyder SH. Endothelin: visualization of mRNAs by in situ hybridization provides evidence for local action. *Proc Natl Acad Sci USA* 1990;86: 7285–7289.
667. Krsmanovic LZ, Stojitkovic SS, Balla T, Al-damluji S, Weiner RJ, Catt KJ. Receptors and secretory actions of endothelin in hypothalamic neurons. *Proc Natl Acad Sci USA* 1991;88: 11124–11128.
668. Jones CR, Hiley CR, Pelton JT, Mohr. Autoradiographic visualization of binding sites for I^{125} endothelin in rat and human brain. *Neurosci Lett* 1989;97:276–279.
669. Samson WK, Skala KD, Alexander B, Huang F-LS. Possible neuroendocrine actions of endothelin-3. *Endocrinology* 1991;128: 1465–1473.
670. Kanyicska B, Burris TP, Freeman ME. Endothelin-3 inhibits prolactin and stimulates LH, FSH and TSH secretion from pituitary cell culture. *Biochem Biophys Res Commun* 1991;174: 338–343.
671. Stojilkovic SS, Merelli F, Iida T, Krsmanovic LZ, Catt KJ. Endothelin stimulation of cytosolic calcium and gonadotropin secretion in anterior pituitary cells. *Science* 1990;248:1663–1666.
672. Kanyicska B, Burris TP, Freeman ME. The effects of endothelins on the secretion of prolactin, luteinizing hormone, and follicle-stimulating hormone are mediated by different guanine nucleotide-binding proteins. *Endocrinology* 1991;129:2607–2613.
673. Steele MK, Negro-Vilar A, McCann SM. Effect of central injection of bradykinin and bradykinin potentiating factor upon release of anterior pituitary hormones in ovariectomized female rats. *Peptides* 1980;1:201–205.
674. Babu GN, Viajayan E. Plasma gonadotropin, prolactin levels and hypothalamic tyrosine hydroxylase activity following intraventricular bombesin and secretin in ovariectomized conscious rats. *Brain Res Bull* 1983;11:25–29.
675. Karashima T, Okajima T, Kato K, Ibayashi H. Suppressive effects of cholecystokinin and bombesin on growth hormone and prolactin secretion in urethane anesthetized rats. *Endocrinol Jpn* 1984;31:539–547.
676. Bell GJ. The glucagon superfamily precursor structure and gene organization. *Peptides* 1986;7(Suppl. 1):27–36.
677. Mezey E. Vasoactive intestinal polypeptide immunopositive neurons in the rat paraventricular nucleus of the homozygous Brattleboro rat. *Neuroendocrinology* 1986;42:88–90.
678. Okamura H, Murakami S, Fukui K, Uda K, Kawamoto K, Kawashima S, Yanaihara N, Ibata Y. Vasoactive intestinal peptide and peptide histidine isoleucine amide-like immunoreactivity colocalize with vasopressin-like immunoreactivity in the canine hypothalamus neurohypophyseal neuronal system. *Neurosci Lett* 1986;69:227–232.
679. Merchenthaler I, Vigh S, Schally AV, Petrusz P. Immunocytochemical localization of growth hormone-releasing factor in the rat hypothalamus. *Endocrinology* 1984;114:1082–1085.
680. Guillemin R, Brazeau P, Bohlen P, Esch F, Ling N, Wehrenberg WB. Growth hormone releasing factor from a human pancreatic tumor that caused acromegaly. *Science* 1982;218:585–587.
681. Rivier J, Speiss J, Thorner M, Vale W. Characterization of a

growth hormone releasing factor from a human pancreatic tumor. *Nature* 1982;300:276–278.
682. Tatemoto K, Mutt V. Isolation and characterization of the intestinal peptide porcine PHI (PHI 27), a new member of the glucagon secretin family. *Proc Natl Acad Sci USA* 1981;78:6603–6607.
683. Itoh N, Obota K, Yanaihara N, Okamoto H. Human preprovasoactive intestinal polypeptide contains a novel PHI-like peptide, PHM 27. *Nature* 1983;304:547–549.
684. Hökfelt T, Schultzberg M, Lundberg JM, Fuxe K, Mutt V, Fahrenkrug J, Said SI. Distribution of the vasoactive intestinal peptide in the central and the peripheral nervous systems as revealed by immunocytochemistry. In: Said SI, ed. *Vasoactive intestinal peptide, vol. 65.* New York: Raven Press, 1980;90.
685. Fuxe K, Hökfelt T, Said SI, Mutt V. Vasoactive intestinal polypeptide and the nervous system: Immunohistochemical evidence for localization in central and peripheral neurons, particularly intracortical neurons of the cerebral cortex. *Neuroscience* 1977;5:241–246.
686. Hökfelt T, Fahrenkrug J, Tatemoto K, Mutt V, Wemer S, Hulting AL, Terenius K, Chang KJ. The PHI (PHI 27)/corticotropin releasing factor/enkephalin immunoreactive hypothalamic neuron: Possible morphological basis for integrated control of prolactin, corticotropin, and growth hormone secretion. *Proc Natl Acad Sci USA* 1983;80:895–898.
687. Besson J, Rotsztejn W, Laburthe M, Epelbaum J, Beaudet A, Kordon C, Rosselin G. Vasoactive intestinal peptide (VIP): Brain distribution subcellular localization and effect of deafferentation of the hypothalamus in male rats. *Brain Res* 1979;165:79–689.
688. Berkenbosch F, Linton EA, Tilders FI. Colocalization of peptide histidine isoleucine amine and corticotropin releasing factor immunoreactivity in neurons of the rat hypothalamus: A surprising artefact. *Neuroendocrinology* 1986;44:338–346.
689. Tager H, Hobenboken M, Markese J, Dinerstein RJ. Identification and localization of glucagon related polypeptides in rat brain. *Proc Natl Acad Sci USA* 1980;77:6229.
690. Said SI, Porter JC. Vasoactive intestinal peptide: Release into hypophyseal blood. *Life Sci* 1979;24:227–230.
691. Morel G, Besson J, Rosselin G, Dubois PM. Ultrastructural evidence for endogenous vasoactive intestinal peptidelike immunoreactivity in the pituitary gland. *Neuroendocrinology* 1982; 34:85–89.
692. Reichlin S. Neuroendocrine significance of vasoactive intestinal polypeptide. *Ann Acad Sci* 1988;527:431–438.
693. Rosselin G. The receptors of the VIP family (VIP, secretin, GRF, PHI, PHM, GIP, glucagon and oxyntomodulin), specificities and identity. *Peptides* 1986;7(Suppl. 1):89–100.
694. Wanke IE, Rorstad OP. Receptors for vasoactive intestinal peptide in rat anterior pituitary glands: localization in binding to lactotropes. *Endocrinology* 1990;126:1981–1988.
695. Lam KSL. Vasoactive intestinal peptide in the hypothalamus and pituitary. *Neuroendocrinology* 1991;53(Suppl. 1):45–51.
696. Kato Y, Iwasaki J, Iwasaki J, Abe H, Yanahara N. Prolactin release by vasoactive intestinal polypeptide in rats. *Endocrinology* 1978;103:554–558.
697. Bethea CL. Effect of vasoactive intestinal peptide on monkey prolactin secretion and cyclic AMP in culture: interaction with estradiol and phenol red. *Neuroendocrinology* 1990;51:576–585.
698. Ruberg M, Rotsztejn WH, Arancibia S, Besson J, Enjalbert A. Stimulation of prolactin release by vasoactive intestinal peptide (VIP). *Eur J Pharmacol* 1978;51:319–320.
699. Enjalbert A, Arancibia S, Ruberg M, Priam M, Bluet-Pajot MT, Rotsztejn WH, Kordon C. Stimulation of *in vitro* prolactin release by vasoactive intestinal peptide. *Neuroendocrinology* 1980;31:200–204.
700. Shaar CJ, Clemens JA, Dininger NB. Effect of vasoactive intestinal peptide on prolactin release *in vitro. Life Sci* 1979;25: 2071–2074.
701. Samson WK, Said SI, Snyder G, McCann SM. *In vitro* stimulation of prolactin release by vasoactive intestinal peptide. *Peptides* 1980;1:325.
702. Bluet-Pajot MT, Mounier F, Leonard JF, Kordon C, Durand D. Vasoactive intestinal peptide induces a transient release of growth hormone in the rat. *Peptides* 1987;8:35–38.
703. Abe H, Engler D, Molitch ME, Bollinger J, Reichlin S. Vasoactive intestinal peptide is a physiological mediator of prolactin release in the rat. *Endocrinology* 1985;116:1383–1390.
704. Kaji H, Chihara K, Kita T, Kashio Y, Okimura Y, Fujita T. Administration of antisera to vasoactive intestinal polypeptide and peptide histidine isoleucine attenuates ether induced prolactin secretion in rats. *Neuroendocrinology* 1985;41:529–531.
705. Watanobe H. The immunostaining for the hypothalamic vasoactive intestinal peptide, but not for β-endorphin, dynorphin-A or methionine-enkephalin, is affected by the glucocorticoid milieu in the rat: correlation with prolactin secretion. *Regul Pept* 1990;28:301–311.
706. Kaji H, Chihara K, Abe H, Kita T, Kashio Y, Okimura Y, Fjuita T. Effect of passive immunization with antisera to vasoactive intestinal peptide and peptide histidine isoleucine amide on 5-hydroxy-l-trytophan induced prolactin release in rats. *Endocrinology* 1985;117:1914–1919.
707. Mezey E, Kiss JZ. Vasoactive intestinal peptide containing neurons in the paraventricular nucleus may participate in regulation of prolactin secretion. *Proc Natl Acad Sci USA* 1984;82:245–247.
708. Chiocchio SR, Nieves Parisi M de las, Leiza Vitale M, Tramezzani JH. Suckling-induced changes of vasoactive intestinal peptide concentrations in hypothalamic areas implicated in control of prolactin release. *Neuroendocrinology* 1991;54:77–82.
709. Gozes I, Shani Y. Hypothalamic vasoactive intestinal peptide messenger ribonucleic acid is increased in lactating rats. *Endocrinology* 1986;119:2497–2501.
710. Gozes I, Avidor R, Biegon A, Baldino F. Lactation elevated VIP messenger ribonucleic acid in rat suprachiasmatic nucleus. *Endocrinology* 1989;124:181–186.
711. Maletti M, Rostene WH, Carr L, Scherrer H, Rotten D, Kordon C, Rosselin G. Interaction between estradiol and prolactin on vasoactive intestinal peptide (VIP) concentrations in the hypothalamus and in the anterior pituitary of the female rat. *Neurosci Lett* 1982;32:307–314.
712. Hogen TC, Arnaout MA, Scherzer WJ, Martinson DR, Garthwaite AC. Antisera to vasoactive intestinal polypeptide inhibit basal prolactin release from dispersed anterior pituitary cells. *Neuroendocrinology* 1986;43:641–645.
713. Alexander MJ, Clifton DK, Steiner RA. Vasoactive intestinal polypeptide effects a central inhibition of pulsatile luteinizing hormone secretion in ovariectomized rats. *Endocrinology* 1985;117:2134–2139.
714. Stobie KM, Weick RF. Effects of lesions of the suprachiasmatic and paraventricular nuclei on the inhibition of pulsatile luteinizing hormone release by exogenous vasoactive intestinal peptide in the ovariectomized rat. *Neuroendocrinology* 1990;51:649–657.
715. Vijayan E, Samson WK, Said SJ, McCann SM. Vasoactive intestinal peptide. Evidence for a hypothalamic site of action to release growth hormone, luteinizing hormone and prolactin in conscious ovariectomized rats. *Endocrinology* 1979;104:53–57.
716. Samson WK, Burton KP, Reeves JP. Vasoactive intestinal peptide stimulates luteinizing hormone release from median eminence synaptosomes. *Regul Pept* 1981;2:253–264.
717. Ottlecz AW, Samson K, McCann SM. The effects of gastric inhibitory polypeptide (GIP) on the release of anterior pituitary hormones. *Peptides* 1985;6:115–119.
718. Houben H, Denef C. Evidence for the presence of gastrin-releasing peptide immunoreactivity in rat anterior pituitary corticotrophs and lactotrophs, AtT_{20} cells, and GH_3 cells: failure to demonstrate participation in local control of hormone release. *Endocrinology* 1991;128:3208–3218.
719. Epelbaum J, Tapia-Arancibia L, Besson J, Rotsztejn WH, Kordon C. Vasoactive intestinal peptide inhibits release of somatostatin from hypothalamus *in vitro. Eur J Pharmacol* 1979;58: 493–495.
720. Abe H, Kato Y, Taminato H, Chiba T, Imura H. Plasma immunoreactive somatostatin levels in rat hypophyseal portal blood: Effect of glucagon administration. *Life Sci* 1978;23:1647.
721. Hery M, Faudon M, Hery F. Effect of vasoactive intestinal peptide on serotonin release in the suprachiasmatic area of the rat: Modulation by estradiol. *Peptides* 1984;5:313–317.
722. Spiess J, Rivier J, Vale W. Characterization of rat hypothalamic growth hormone releasing factor. *Nature* 1982;303:532.
723. Bloch B, Ling N, Benoit R, Wehrenberg WB, Guillemin R. Spe-

cific depletion of immunoreactive growth hormone releasing factor by monosodium glutamate in rat median eminence. *Nature* 1984;307:272–273.
724. Sawchenko PE, Swanson LW, Rivier J, Vale W. The distribution of growth hormone releasing factor (GRF) immunoreactivity in the central nervous system of the rat: An immunohistochemical study using antisera directed against rat hypothalamic GRF. *J Comp Neurol* 1985;237:100–115.
725. Kita T, Chihara K, Abe H, Minamitani N, Kaji H, Kashio Y, Okimura Y, Fujita T, Ling N. Regional distribution of rat growth hormone releasing factor-like immunoreactivity in rat hypothalamus. *Endocrinology* 1985;116:259–262.
726. Vandepol CJ, Leidy JW, Finger TE, Robbins RJ. Immunohistochemical localization of GRF containing neurons in rat brain. *Neuroendocrinology* 1986;42:143–147.
727. Ciofi P, Croix D, Tramu G. Coexistence of hGHRH and NPY immunoreactivities in neurons of the arcuate nucleus of the rat. *Neuroendocrinology* 1987;45:425–428.
728. Seifert H, Perrin M, Rivier J, Vale W. Binding sites for growth hormone releasing factor on rat anterior pituitary cells. *Nature* 1985;317:487–489.
729. Gaylinn BD, Harrison JK, Zysk JR, Lyons CE, Lynch KR, Thorner MO. Molecular cloning and expression of a human anterior pituitary receptor for growth hormone-releasing hormone. *Mol Endocrinol* 1993;7:77–84.
730. Law GH, Ray KP, Wallis M. Effects of growth hormone releasing factor, somatostatin and dopamine on growth hormone and prolactin secretion from cultured ovine pituitary cells. *FEBS Lett* 1984;166:189.
731. Laburthe M, Amiranoff B, Boige N, Rouyer-Fessard C, Tatemoto K, Moroder L. Interaction of GRF with VIP receptors and stimulation of adenylate cyclase in rat and human intestinal epithelial membranes. Comparison with PHI and secretin. *FEBS Lett* 1983;159:89.
732. Miyata A, Arimura A, Dahl DH, Minamino N, Uehara A, Jiang L, Culler MD, Coy DH. Isolation of a novel 38 residue hypothalamic polypeptide which stimulates adenylate cyclase in pituitary cells. *Biochem Biophys Res Commun* 1989;164:567–574.
733. Miyata A, Jiang L, Dahl DH, Kitada C, Kubo K, Fujino M, Minamino, Arimura A. Isolation of a neuropeptide corresponding to the N-terminal 27 residues of the pituitary adenylate cyclase activating polypeptide with 38 residues (PACAP). *Biochem Biophys Res Commun* 1990;170:643–648.
734. Koves K, Arimura A, Somogyvari-Vigh A, Vigh S, Miller J. Immunohistochemical demonstration of a novel hypothalamic peptide, pituitary adenylate cyclase activating polypeptide, in the ovine hypothalamus. *Endocrinology* 1990;127:264–271.
735. Gottschall PE, Tatsuno I, Miyata A, Arimura A. Characterization and distribution of binding sites for the hypothalamic peptide pituitary adenylate cyclase activating polypeptide. *Endocrinology* 1990;127:272–277.
736. Canny BJ, Rawlings SR, Leong DA. Pituitary adenylate cyclase activating polypeptide specifically increases cytosolic calcium ion concentration in rat gonadotropes and somatotropes. *Endocrinology* 1992;130:211–215.
737. Culler MD, Paschall CS. Pituitary adenylate cyclase activating polypeptide (PACAP) potentiates the gonadotropin releasing activity of luteinizing hormone releasing hormone. *Endocrinology* 1991;129:2260–2262.
738. Schally AV, Guoth Janos G, Redding TW, Groot K, Rodriguez H, Szonyi E, Stultz J, Nicolics K. Isolation and characterization of two peptides with prolactin release-inhibiting activity from porcine hypothalami. *Proc Natl Acad Sci USA* 1991;88: 3540–3544.
739. Gubler U, Seeburg P, Hoffman BJ, Gage LP, Udenfriend S. Molecular cloning establishes proenkephalins as precursors of enkephalin containing peptides. *Nature* 1982;295:206–208.
740. Fallon JH, Leslie FM. Distribution of dynorphin and enkephalin peptides in the rat brain. *J Comp Neurol* 1986;249:293–336.
741. Udenfriend S, Meienhofer J. Opioid peptides: Biology, chemistry and genetics. In: *The peptides,* vol. 6. New York: Academic Press; 1984.
742. Evans CJ, Keith DE, Morrison H, Magendzo K, Edwards R. Cloning of a delta opioid receptor by functional expression. *Science* 1992;258:1952–1957.
743. Code RA, Fallon JH. Some projections of dynorphin immunoreactive neurons in the rat central nervous system. *Neuropeptides* 1986;8:165–172.
744. Palkovits M, Brownstein MJ, Zamir N. Immunoreactive dynorphin and neo-endorphin in rat hypothalamo-neurohypophyseal system. *Brain Res* 1983;278:258–261.
745. Watson SJ, Akil H, Frichli W, Goldstein A, Zimmerman EA, Nilever F. Dynorphin and vasopressin: Common localization in magnocellular neurons. *Nature* 1982;216:85–87.
746. Khatchaturian H, Sherman TG, Lloyd RV, Civelli O, Douglas J, Herbert E, Akil H, Watson JJ. Prodynorphin is endogenous in the anterior pituitary and is colocalised with LH and FSH in the gonadotrophs. *Endocrinology* 1986;119:409.
747. Martin R, Voigt KH. Enkephalin coexists with oxytocin and vasopressin in nerve terminals of the rat neurohypophysis. *Nature* 1981;289:502–504.
748. Slater P, Cross AJ. Autoradiographic distribution of dynorphin 1-9 binding sites in primate brain. *Neuropeptides* 1986;8:71.
749. Mains RE, Eipper B, Ling N. Common precursor to corticotropin and endorphins. *Proc Natl Acad Sci USA* 1977;74:3014.
750. Bugnon C, Bloch B, Lenys D, Goubet A, Fellmann D. Comparative study of the neuronal populations containing β endorphin, corticotropin and dopamine in the arcuate nucleus of the rat hypothalamus. *Neurosci Lett* 1979;14:43–48.
751. Bloch B, Bugnon C, Lenys D, Fellmann D. Description des neurones immunoreactifs à un antiserum anti-β endorphine presents dans le noyau infundibulaire chez l'Homme. *CR Acad Sci (Paris)* 1978;287D:309–312.
752. Finlay JCW, Lindshon P, Petrusz P. Immunocytochemical localization of β endorphin containing neurons in the rat brain. *Neuroendocrinology* 1981;33:28–42.
753. Krieger DT, Liotta AS, Brownstein MJ. Presence of corticotropin in brain of normal and hypophysectomized rats. *Proc Natl Acad Sci USA* 1977;74:648–652.
754. Dube D, Lissitzky JC, Leclere R, Pelletier G. Localization of melanocyte stimulating hormone in rat brain and pituitary. *Endocrinology* 1978;102:1283–1291.
755. Bloch B, Bugnon C, Fellmann D, Lenys D. Immunocytochemical evidence that the same neurons in the human infundibular nucleus are stained with anti-endorphins and antisera of other related peptides. *Neurosci Lett* 1978;10:147–152.
756. Sofroniew MV. Immunoreactive β endorphin and ACTH in the same neurons of the hypothalamic arcuate nucleus in the rat. *Annu J Anat* 1979;154:283–289.
757. Wardlaw SL, Wehrenberg WB, Ferin M, Antunes JL, Frank AG. Effect of sex steroids on β endorphin in hypophyseal portal blood. *J Clin Endocrinol Metab* 1982;55:877–881.
758. Grandison L, Guidotti A. Regulation of prolactin release by endogenous opiates. *Nature* 1977;270:357–359.
759. Dupont A, Cusan L, Labrie F, Loy DH, Li CH. Stimulation of prolactin release in the rat by intraventricular injection of β endorphin and methionin enkephalin. *Biochem Biophys Res Commun* 1977;75:76–82.
760. Rivier C, Vale W, Ling N, Brown M, Guillemin R. Stimulation in vivo of the secretion of prolactin and growth hormone by β endorphin. *Endocrinology* 1977;100:238–241.
761. Bruni JF, Van Vugt D, Marshall S, Meites J. Effects of naloxone, morphine and methionine enkephalin of serum prolactin, luteinizing hormone, follicle stimulating hormone, thyroid stimulating hormone and growth hormone. *Life Sci* 1977;21:461–466.
762. Barraclough CA, Sawyer CH. Inhibition of the release of pituitary ovulatory hormone in the rat by morphine. *Endocrinology* 1955;57:329–336.
763. Millan MJ, Herz A. The endocrinology of the opioids. In: *International review of neurobiology,* vol. 26. New York: Academic Press, 1985;1–83.
764. Gilbeau PH, Almirez RG, Holaday JW, Smith CG. Opioid effects on plasma concentrations of luteinizing hormone and prolactin in the adult rhesus monkey. *J Clin Endocrinol Metab* 1985;60:299–305.
765. Pang CN, Zimmermann E, Sawyer CH. Morphine inhibition of

the preovulatory surges of plasma luteinizing hormone and follicle stimulating hormone in the rat. *Endocrinology* 1977;101:1726.

766. Van Vugt DA, Sylvester PW, Aylsworth CF, Meites J. Counteraction of gonadal steroid inhibition of LH by naloxone. *Neuroendocrinology* 1982;34:274.
767. Cicero TJ, Schainker BA, Meyer ER. Endogenous opioids participate in the regulation of the hypothalamic pituitary luteinizing hormone axis and testosterone negative feedback control of luteinizing hormone. *Endocrinology* 1979;104:1286–1291.
768. Morley JE, Baranetsky NG, Wingert TD, Carlson HE, Hershman JM, Melmed S, Levin SR, Jamison KR, Weitzman R, Chang RJ, Varner AA. Endocrine effects of naloxone induced opiate receptor blockade. *J Clin Endocrinol Metab* 1980;50:251.
769. Delitala G, Devilla L, Arata L. Opiate receptors and anterior pituitary hormone secretion in man. *Acta Endocrinol (Copenh)* 1981;97:150–156.
770. Schultz R, Wilhelm A, Pirke KM, Gramsch C, Herz A. Endorphin and dynorphin control serum luteinizing hormone level in immature female rats. *Nature* 1981;294:757–759.
771. Kinashita F, Nakai I, Katakami H, Kato G, Yajima H, Imura H. Effect of β endorphin on pulsatile luteinizing hormone release in conscious castrated rats. *Life Sci* 1980;27:843.
772. Kesner JS, Kaufman JM, Wilson RC, Kuroda G, Knobil E. The effect of morphine on the electrophysiological activity of the hypothalamic luteinizing hormone releasing hormone pulse generator in the rhesus monkey. *Neuroendocrinology* 1986;43:686–688.
773. Moult PJ, Grossman A, Evans JM, Rees LH, Besser GM. The effect of naloxone on pulsatile gonadotrophin release in normal subjects. *Clin Endocrinol* 1981;14:321–324.
774. Ellingboe J, Veldhuis JD, Mendelson JH, Kuehule JC, Mello NK. Effect of endogenous opioid blockade on the amplitude and frequency of pulsatile luteinizing hormone secretion in normal men. *J Clin Endocrinol Metab* 1982;54:854.
775. Baranowska B, Rozbicka G, Jeske W, Abdel-Fattah MH. The role of endogenous opiates in the mechanism of inhibited luteinizing hormone (LH) secretion in women with anorexia nervosa: The effect of naloxone on LH, follicle stimulating hormone, prolactin and β endorphin secretion. *J Clin Endocrinol Metab* 1984;59:412.
776. Ferin M, Van Vugt D, Wasdlaw S. The hypothalamic control of the menstrual cycle and the role of endogenous opioid peptides. *Recent Prog Horm Res* 1984;40:411–485.
777. Rupert JF, Quigley ME, Yen SSC. Endogenous opiates modulate pulsatile luteinizing hormone release in humans. *J Clin Endocrinol Metab* 1981;52:583–587.
778. Quigley ME, Yen SSC. The role on endogenous opiates on LH secretion during the menstrual cycle. *J Clin Endocrinol Metab* 1980;51:179.
779. Veldhuis JD, Rogol AD, Samojik E, Ertel NH. Role of endogenous opiates in the expression of negative feedback actions of androgen and estrogen on pulsatile properties of luteinizing hormone secretion in man. *J Clin Invest* 1984;74:47–55.
780. Petraglia F, Bernasconi S, Lughetti L, Loche S. Naloxone induced luteinizing hormone secretion in normal, precocious, and delayed puberty. *J Clin Endocrinol Metab* 1986;63:1112–1116.
781. Quigley ME, Shechan KL, Casper RF, Yen SSC. Evidence for increased dopaminergic and opioid activity in patients with hypothalamic hypogonadotropic amenorrhea. *J Clin Endocrinol Metab* 1980;50:949.
782. Lightman SL, Jacobs HS, Maguire AK, McGarrick G, Jeffcoate SL. Constancy of opioid control of luteinizing hormone in different pathophysiological states. *J Clin Endocrinol Metab* 1981;52:1260.
783. Cicero TJ, Owens DP, Schmoeker PF, Meyer ER. Morphine induced enhancement of the effects of naloxone on serum luteinizing hormone levels in the male rat: Specificity for mu antagonists. *J Pharmacol Exp Ther* 1983;226:770–774.
784. Pfeiffer DG, Pfeiffer A, Shimahigashi K, Merriam GR, Loriaux DL. Predominant involvement of mu rather than delta or kappa opiate receptors in LH secretion. *Peptides* 1983;4:647–649.
785. Panerai A, Petraglia F, Sacerdote P, Genazzani AR. Mainly mu opiate receptors are involved in luteinizing hormone and prolactin secretion. *Endocrinology* 1985;117:1096–1099.
786. Leadem CA, Kalra SP. Effects of endogenous opioid peptides and opiates on luteinizing hormone and prolactin secretion in ovariectomized rats. *Neuroendocrinology* 1985;41:342–352.
787. Pfeiffer DG, Pfeiffer A, Shimohigashi Y, Merriam GR, Loriaux DL. Predominant involvement of mu rather than delta or kappa opiate receptors in LH secretion. *Peptides* 1983;4:647.
788. Goodman RR, Snyder SH, Kuhar MJ, Young WS. Differentiation of delta and mu opiate receptor localization by light microscopic autoradiography. *Proc Natl Acad Sci USA* 1980;77:6239.
789. Schulz, Wilhelm A, Pirke KM, Herz A. Regulation of luteinizing hormone secretion in prepubertal male and female rats. *Life Sci* 1982;31:2167–2170.
790. Marko M, Romer M. Inhibitory effect of a new opioid agonist on reproductive endocrine activity in rats of both sexes. *Life Sci* 1983;33:233–240.
791. Panerai AE, Sawynok J, La Bella FS, Friesen HG. Prolonged hyperprolactinemia influences β endorphin and metenkephaline in the brain. *Endocrinology* 1980;106:1804.
792. Ferland L, Kledzik GS, Cusan L, Labrie F. Evidence for a role of endorphins in stress-induced and suckling induced prolactin release in the rat. *Mol Cell Endocrinol* 1978;12:267.
793. Knight PG, Howles CM, Cunningham EJ. Evidence that opioid peptides and dopamine participate in the suckling induced release of prolactin in the ewe. *Neuroendocrinology* 1986;44:29–35.
794. White JD, McKelvy JF. Enkephalin biosynthesis and processing during lactation. *Neuroendocrinology* 1986;43:377–382.
795. Sirinathsinghji DJ, Audsley AR. Endogenous opioid peptides participate in the modulation of prolactin release in response to cervicovaginal stimulation in the female rat. *Endocrinology* 1985;117:549–556.
796. Melis GB, Gambacciani M, Paoletti AM, Mais V, Cagnacci A, Petacchi FD, Fioretti P. Sex steroids modulate prolactin response to naloxone in postmenopausal women. *Neuroendocrinology* 1985;41:138–141.
797. Rossi A, Disalle E, Briatico G, Arcari G, De Castigliane R, Perseo G. Antinociceptive, prolactin releasing and intestinal motility inhibiting activities of dermorphin and analogues after subcutaneous administration in the rat. *Peptides* 1983;4:577–580.
798. Koenig JJ, Mayfield MA, McCann SM, Kruhlich L. Differential role of the opioid μ and κ receptors in the activation of prolactin and growth hormone secretion of morphine in the male rat. *Life Sci* 1984;34:1829–1837.
799. Spiegel K, Konrid GW, Pasternak GW. Prolactin and growth hormone release by morphine in the rat: Different receptor mechanism. *Science* 1982;217:745–747.
800. Rossi A, Disalle E, Briatico G, Arcari G, De Castigliane R, Perseo G. Antinociceptive, prolactin releasing and intestinal motility inhibiting activities of dermorphin and analogues after subcutaneous administration in the rat. *Peptides* 1983;4:577–580.
801. Erspamer V, Melchiorri P, Broccardo M, Erspamer GF, Falaschi P, Improta G, Negri L, Renda T. The brain-gut-skin triangle: New peptides. *Peptides* 1981;(Suppl)2:7–16.
802. Uberti EC, Trasfonni G, Salvadori S, Margutti A, Tomatis R, Pansini R. The effects of dermorphin in the endocrine system in man. *Peptides* 1985;(Suppl.)3:171–175.
803. Matsushita N, Kato Y, Shimatsu A, Katakami H, Fujino M, Matsuo H, Imura H. Stimulation of prolactin secretion in the rat by α-neo-endorphin β neo-endorphin and dynorphin. *Biochem Biophys Res Commun* 1982;107:735–741.
804. Gilbeau PM, Hosobuchi Y, Lee NM. Dynorphin effects on plasma concentration of anterior pituitary hormones in the nonhuman primate. *J Pharmacol Exp Ther* 1986;238:974–978.
805. Gilbeau P, Hosobuchi Y, Lee NM. Consequence of dynorphin A administration on anterior pituitary hormone concentrations in the adult male rhesus monkey. *Neuroendocrinology* 1987;45:284–289.
806. Pfeiffer A, Braun S, Mann K, Meyer HD, Brantl V. Anterior pituitary hormone responses to a K opioid agonist in man. *J Clin Endocrinol Metab* 1986;62:181–185.
807. Kruhlich L, Koenig JE, Conway S, McCann SM, Mayfield MA. Opioid K receptors and the secretion of prolactin (PRL) and

growth hormone (GH) in the rat. Effects of opioid K receptor agonists bremazocine and U50488 on secretion of PRL and GH; comparison with morphine. *Neuroendocrinology* 1986;42:75–81.
808. Kruhlich L, Koenig JE, Conway S, McCann SM, Mayfield MA. GH and PRL release inhibiting effects of the opioid K receptor agonists bremazocine and U50488. *Neuroendocrinology* 1986; 42:82–87.
809. Matton A, Buydens P, Finné E, Govaerts J, Vanhaelst L. Analysis of the receptor specificity of tolerance induction in stress versus opiod-related prolactin secretion in rats. *J Endocrinol* 1991;128: 281–285.
810. Blackford SP, Little PJ, Kuhn CM. Mu- and kappa-opiate receptor control of prolactin secretion in rats: ontogeny and interaction with serotonin. *Endocrinology* 1992;131:2891–2897.
811. Bhanot R, Wilkinson M. Opiatergic control of LH secretion is eliminated by gonadectomy. *Endocrinology* 1983;112:399.
812. Piva F, Limonta P, Maggi R, Martini L. Stimulatory and inhibitory effect of the opioids on gonadotropic secretion. *Neuroendocrinology* 1986;42:504–512.
813. Kalra PS, Kalra SP. Discriminating effects of testosterone on hypothalamic luteinizing hormone releasing hormone levels and luteinizing hormone secretion in castrated male rats: Analyses of dose and duration characteristics. *Endocrinology* 1982;111: 24–29.
814. Gabriel SM, Simkins JW, Kalra SP. Modulation of endogenous opioid influence on luteinizing hormone secretion by progesterone and estrogen. *Endocrinology* 1983;113:1806–1811.
815. Nanda AS, Ward WR, Dobson H. Opioid involvement in LH release during the negative feedback effects of oestradiol and progesterone in dairy cows. *Reprod Fertil Dev* 1991;3:709–714.
816. Singh M, Millard WJ, Layden MP, Romano TM, Simpkins JW. Opiate stimulation of prolactin secretion is reversed by ovarian hormone treatment. *Neuroendocrinology* 1992;56:195–203.
817. Gabriel SM, Simpkins JW, Kalra SP, Kalra PS. Chronic morphine treatment induces hypersensitivity to testosterone negative feedback in castrated male rats. *Neuroendocrinology* 1985;40: 39–44.
818. Gabriel SM, Berglund JA, Kalra SP, Kalra PS, Simpkins JW. The influence of chronic morphine treatment on the negative feedback regulation of gonadotropin secretion by gonadal steroids. *Endocrinology* 1986;119:2762–2767.
819. Wardlaw SL, Thoron L, Frank AG. Effects of sex steroids on brain β endorphin. *Brain Res* 1982;245:327–331.
820. Sarkar DH, Yen SS. Changes in β endorphin-like immunoreactivity in pituitary portal blood during the estrous cycle and after ovariectomy in rats. *Endocrinology* 1985;116:2075–2079.
821. Barden N, Merand Y, Rouleau D, Garon M, Dupont A. Changes in the β endorphin content of discrete hypothalamic nuclei during the estrous cycle of the rat. *Brain Res* 1981;204:441.
822. Wardlaw SL, Frank AG. Brain β endorphin during pregnancy, parturition and the post partum period. *Endocrinology* 1983; 113:1664–1668.
823. Morrell JL, McGinty JF, Pfaff DW. A subset of β endorphin or dynorphin containing neurons in the medial basal hypothalamus accumulates estradiol. *Neuroendocrinology* 1985;41:417–426.
824. Jirikowski GF, Merchenthaler J, Rieger GE, Stumpf WE. Estradiol target sites immunoreactive for β endorphin in the arcuate nuclei of rat and mouse hypothalamus. *Neurosci Lett* 1986;65: 121–126.
825. Kiem DT, Bartha L, Makara GB. Effect of dexamethasone implanted in different brain areas on the morphine-induced PRL, GH and ACTH/corticosterone secretion. *Brain Res* 1991;563: 107–113.
826. Jacobson W, Wilkinson M. Association of diurnal variations in hypothalamic but not cortical opiate (3H naloxone) binding sites with the activity of naloxone to induce LH release in the prepubertal female rat. *Neuroendocrinology* 1986;44:132.
827. Hahn FF, Fishman J. Changes in rat brain opiate receptor content upon castration and testosterone replacement. *Biochem Biophys Res Commun* 1979;90:819–823.
828. Wilkinson M, Herdon H, Wilson CA. Gonadal steroid modification of adrenergic and opiate receptor binding in the central nervous system. In: Fuxe K, Gustaffsson JA, Wetterby L, eds. *Steroid hormone regulation of the brain.* New York: Pergamon Press, 1981;253–263.
829. Hahn EE, Fishman J. Castration affects male rat brain opiate receptor content. *Neuroendocrinology* 1985;41:60–63.
830. Cicero TJ, Newman KS, Meyer ER. Testosterone does not influence opiate binding sites in the male rat brain. *Biochem Biophys Res Commun* 1982;108:1313–1319.
831. Kalra SP, Kalra PS. Opioid adrenergic steroid connection in regulation of luteinizing hormone secretion in the rat. *Neuroendocrinology* 1984;38:418–426.
832. Valenca MM, Negro-Vilar A. Lack of a functional coupling between endogenous opiate system and LHRH neurons during the infantile period in the male rat. *Neuroendocrinol Lett* 1986; 8:165–172.
833. Sylvester PW, Sarkar DK, Briski KP, Meites J. Relation of gonadal hormones to differential LH responses to naloxone in prepubertal male and female rats. *Neuroendocrinology* 1985; 40:165–170.
834. Blank MS, Panerai AE, Friesen HG. Opioid peptide modulate luteinizing hormone secretion during sexual maturation. *Science* 1979;203:1129–1131.
835. Wolfe MW, Roberson MS, Stumpf TT, Kittok RJ, Kinder JE. Modulation of luteinizing hormone and follicle-stimulating hormone in circulation by interactions between endogenous opioids and oestradiol during the peripubertal period of heifers. *J Reprod Fertil* 1992;96:165–174.
836. Petersen SL, Barraclough CA. Effects of morphine and naloxone on LH and prolactin release in androgen sterilized rats. *Neuroendocrinology* 1986;44:84–88.
836a. Watson R, Hoffmann GE, Wiegand SJ. Sexually dimorphic opioid distribution in the preoptic area: manipulation by gonadal steroids. *Brain Res* 1986;398:157–163.
837. Lira SA, Phipps DW, Sarkar DK. Loss of estradiol positive feedback action on LH release during prepubertal period in rats treated postnatally with an opiate antagonist. *Neuroendocrinology* 1986;44:331–337.
838. Sirinathsinghji DJ, Motta M, Martini L. Induction of precocious puberty in the female rat after chronic naloxone administration during the neonatal period: The opiate "brake" on prepubertal gonadotropin secretion. *J Endocrinol* 1985;104:299–307.
839. Chen HJ, Targovnik J, McMillan L, Randall S. Age difference in endogenous opiate modulation of short photoperiod induced testicular regression in golden hamsters. *J Endocrinol* 1984;101:1–6.
840. Ebling FJ, Lincoln GA. Endogenous opioids and the control of seasonal LH secretion in Soay rams. *J Endocrinol* 1985; 107:341–353.
841. Sarkar DK, Yen SSC. Hyperprolactinemia decreases the luteinizing hormone releasing hormone concentration in pituitary portal plasma: A possible role for β endorphin as a mediator. *Endocrinology* 1985;116:2080–2084.
842. Carter DA, Cooper JS, Inkster SE, Whitehead SA. Evidence for an increased opioid inhibition of LH secretion in hyperprolactinemic ovariectomized rats. *J Endocrinol* 1984;101:57.
843. Quigley ME, Sheehan KL, Casper RF, Yen SSC. Evidence for an increased opioid inhibition of luteinizing hormone secretion in hyperprolactinemic patients with pituitary microadenomas. *J Clin Endocrinol Metab* 1980;50:427.
844. Seki K, Kato K, Shima K. Parallelism in the luteinizing hormone responses to opioid and dopamine antagonists in hyperprolactinemic women with pituitary adenomas. *J Clin Endocrinol Metab* 1986;63:1225–1228.
845. Sweeney CA, Morgan WW, Smith MS, Bartke A. Altered sensitivity to an opiate antagonist, naloxone, in hyperprolactinemic male rats. *Neuroendocrinology* 1985;41:1–6.
846. Simpkins JW, Taylor ST, Gabriel SM, Katovich MJ, Millard WJ. Evidence that chronic hyperprolactinemia affects skin temperature regulation through an opioid mechanism. *Neuroendocrinology* 1984;39:321.
847. Rossier J, French ED, Rivier C, Ling N, Guillemin R, Bloom FE. Foot shock induced stress increases β endorphin levels in brain. *Nature* 1977;270:618.
848. Enker JJ, Meites J, Riegle CD. Effects of acute stress on serum

LH and prolactin in intact, castrated and dexamethasone treated male rats. *Endocrinology* 1973;96:85.

849. Brisky KP, Quigley K, Meites J. Endogenous opiate involvement in acute and chronic stress induced changes in plasma LH concentrations in the male rat. *Life Sci* 1984;34:2485.
850. Gilbeau PM, Smith CG. Naloxone reversal of stress induced reproductive effects in the male rhesus monkey. *Neuropeptides* 1985;5:335.
851. Petraglia F, Vale W, Rivier C. Opioids act centrally to modulate stress induced decrease in luteinizing hormone in the rat. *Endocrinology* 1986;119:2445–2450.
852. Cicero TJ, Badger TM, Wilcox CE, Bell RD, Meyer ER. Morphine decreases luteinizing hormone by an action on the hypothalamic pituitary axis. *J Pharmacol Exp Ther* 1977;203:548–554.
853. Ching M. Morphine suppresses the proestrous surge of GhRH in pituitary portal plasma of rats. *Endocrinology* 1983;112: 2209–2211.
854. Nikolarakis KE, Pfeiffer DG, Almeida OF, Herz A. Opioid modulation of LHRH release in vitro depends upon levels of testosterone in vivo. *Neuroendocrinology* 1986;44:314–319.
855. Drouva SV, Epelbaum J, Tapia-Arancibia L, Laplante E, Kordon C. Met enkephalin inhibition of K+ induced LHRH and SRIF release from rat mediobasal hypothalamic slices. *Eur J Pharmacol* 1980;61:411–412.
856. Drouva SV, Epelbaum J, Tapia-Arancibia L, Laplante E, Kordon C. Opiate receptors modulate LHRH and SRIF release from mediobasal hypothalamic neurons. *Neuroendocrinology* 1981;32: 163–167.
857. Rotsztejn WH, Drouva SV, Pollard H, Sokoloff P, Pattou E, Kordon C. Further evidence for the existence of opiate binding sites on neurosecretory LHRH mediobasal hypothalamic nerve terminals. *Eur J Pharmacol* 1982;80:139–141.
858. Leadem CA, Crowley WR, Simpkins JW, Kalra SP. Effects of naloxone on catecholamine and LHRH release from the perifused hypothalamus of the steroid primed rat. *Neuroendocrinology* 1985;40:497–500.
859. Van Vugt DA, Aylswarth CF, Sylvester PW, Leung FC, Meites J. Evidence for hypothalamic noradrenergic involvement in naloxone induced stimulation of luteinizing hormone release. *Neuroendocrinology* 1981;33:261.
860. Petersen SL, Barraclough CA. Interaction between the hypothalamic opiate and catecholamine systems in the regulation of LH and prolactin secretion. In: Muller EE, McLeod RM, eds. *Neuroendocrine perspectives,* vol. 5. Amsterdam: Elsevier, 1986; 283–290.
861. Ferland L, Fuxe K, Eneroth P, Gustafsson JA, Skett P. Effects of methionine enkephalin on prolactin release and catecholamine levels and turnover in the median eminence. *Eur J Pharmacol* 1977;43:89–90.
862. Van Loon GR, Ho D, Kim C. β Endorphin induced decrease in hypothalamic dopamine turnover. *Endocrinology* 1980;106:76.
863. Gudelsky GA, Porter JC. Morphine and opioid peptide induced inhibition of the release of dopamine from tuberoinfundibular neurons. *Life Sci* 1979;25:1697–1702.
864. Wood PL. Opioid regulation of CNS dopaminergic pathways: A review of methodology, receptor types, regional variations and species differences. *Peptides* 1983;4:595–601.
865. Arita J, Porter JC. Relationship between dopamine release and prolactin after morphine treatment in rats. *Neuroendocrinology* 1984;38:62–67.
866. Van Loon GR, De Souza EB. Effects of β endorphin on brain serotonin metabolism. *Life Sci* 1978;23:971–978.
867. Leiri T, Chen HT, Meites J. Naloxone stimulation of luteinizing hormone release in prepubertal female rats; role of serotonergic system. *Life Sci* 1980;26:1269–1274.
868. Tapia-Arancibia L, Astier H. Opiate inhibition of K+ induced TRH release from superfused mediobasal hypothalamus in rats. *Neuroendocrinology* 1983;37:166–168.
869. Arancibia S, Tapia-Arancibia L, Roussel JP, Assenmacher J, Astier H. Effects of morphine on cold induced TRH release from the median eminence of unanesthetized rats. *Life Sci* 1986;38:59–66.
870. Bhargawa HN, Das S. Evidence for opiate action at the brain receptors for thyrotropin releasing hormone. *Brain Res* 1986; 368:262–267.
871. Das S, Bhargawa HN. Unidirectional interaction between thyrotropin hormone and opiates at the level of their brain receptors. *Gen Pharmacol* 1987;18:99–102.
872. Sheppard MC, Kronhein S, Pimstone BL. Effect of substance P, neurotensin and the enkephalins on somatostatin release from the rat hypothalamus in vitro. *J Neurochem* 1979;32:647.
873. Buckingham JC, Cooper TA. Pharmacological characterisation of the opioid receptors influencing the secretion of corticotropin releasing hormone in the rat. *Neuroendocrinology* 1986; 44:36–40.
874. Clarke G, Wood P, Merrick L, Lincoln DW. Opiate inhibition of peptide release from the neurohumoral terminals of hypothalamic neurons. *Nature* 1979;282:746–748.
875. Drouva SV, Epelbaum J, Hery M, Tapia-Arancibia L, Laplante E, Kordon C. Ionic channels involved in the LHRH and SRIF release from rat mediobasal hypothalamus. *Neuroendocrinology* 1981;32:155–162.
876. Grossman A, Moult DA, Cunnal D, Besser M. Different opioid mechanisms are involved in the modulation of ACTH and gonadotropin release in man. *Neuroendocrinology* 1986;42:357–360.
877. Bentley AM, Wallis M. Effects of two enkephalin analogues, morphine sulfate, dopamine and naloxone on prolactin secretion from rat anterior pituitary glands in vitro. *J Endocrinol* 1986;109:313–320.
878. Enjalbert A, Ruberg M, Arancibia S, Priam M, Kordon C. Endogenous opiates block dopamine inhibition of prolactin secretion in vitro. *Nature* 1979;280:595–597.
879. Lugin JS, MacLeod RM. Failure of opiates to reverse inhibition of prolactin secretion in vitro. *Eur J Pharmacol* 1979;60:253.
880. Grandison L, Fratta W, Guidotti A. Location and characterisation of opiate receptors regulating pituitary secretion. *Life Sci* 1980;26:1633.
881. Enjalbert A, Ruberg M, Fiore L, Arancibia S, Priam M, Kordon C. Effect of morphine on the dopamine inhibition of pituitary prolactin release in vitro. *Eur J Pharmacol* 1979;53:211.
882. Rotten D, Leblanc P, Kordon C, Weiner RJ, Enjalbert A. Interference of endogenous β-endorphin with opiate binding in the anterior pituitary. *Neuropeptides* 1986;8:377–392.
883. Breder CD, Diparello CA, Saper CB. Interleukin immunoreactive innervation of the human hypothalamus. *Science* 1988;240: 321.
884. Katsuma G, Gottschall PF, Arimura A. Identification of the high affinity receptor for β interleukin in rat brain. *Biochem Biophys Res Commun* 1988;156:61.
885. Farrar WL, Kilian PO, Ruff MR, Hill JP, Pert CB. Visualisation and characterization of interleukin 1 receptors in brain. *J Immunol* 1987;139:459–463.
886. Saplosky R, Rivier C, Yamamoto G, Pottsky G, Vale W. Interleukin 1 stimulates the secretion of hypothalamic corticotropin releasing factor. *Science* 1987;238:522–524.
887. Honegger J, D'urso SP, Navarra P, Tsagarakis S, Besser GM, Grossman AB. Interleukin-1β modulates the acute release of growth hormone-releasing hormone and somatostatin from rat hypothalamus in vitro, whereas tumor necrosis factor and interleukin-6 have no effect. *Endocrinology* 1991;129:1275–1282.
888. Rivier C. Role of endotoxin and interleukin-1 in modulating ACTH, LH and sex steroid secretion. In: Porter JC, Jezova D, eds. *Circulating regulatory factors and neuroendocrine function.* New York: Plenum Press, 1990;295–301.
889. Rivier C, Vale W. Cytokines act within the brain to inhibit luteinizing hormone secretion and ovulation in the rat. *Endocrinology* 1990;127:849–856.
890. Kalra PS, Sahu A, Kalra SP. Interleukin 1 inhibits the ovarian steroid-induced luteinizing hormone surge and release of hypothalamic luteinizing hormone-releasing hormone in rats. *Endocrinology* 1990;126:2145–2152.
891. Rettori V, Gimeno MF, Karara A, Gonzales MC, McCann SM. Interleukin 1α inhibits prostaglandin E_2 release to suppress pulsatile release of luteinizing hormone but not follicle-stimulating hormone. *Proc Natl Acad Sci USA* 1991;88:2763–2767.
892. Kalra PS, Fuentes M, Sahu A, Kalra SP. Endogenous opioid pep-

tides mediate the interleukin-1-induced inhibition of the release of luteinizing hormone (LH)-releasing hormone and LH. *Endocrinology* 1990;127:2381–2386.

893. Schettini G, Florio T, Meucci O, Landolfi E, Grimaldi M, Lombardi G, Scala G, Leong D. Interleukin 1-β modulation of prolactin secretion from rat anterior pituitary cells: involvement of adenylate cyclase activity and calcium mobilization. *Endocrinology* 1990;126:1435–1441.
894. Spangelo BL, Judd AM, Isakson PC, MacLeod RM. Interleukin-1 stimulates interleukin-6 release from rat anterior pituitary cells in vitro. *Endocrinology* 1991;128:2685–2692.
895. Spangelo BL, Judd AM, Isakson PC, MacLeod RM. Interleukin-6 stimulates anterior pituitary hormone release in vitro. *Endocrinology* 1989;125:575–577.
896. Vankelecom H, Carmeliet P, Heremans H, Van Dammes J, Dijkmans R, Billiau A, Denef C. Interferon-γ inhibits stimulated adrenocorticotropin, prolactin, and growth hormone secretion in normal rat anterior pituitary cell cultures. *Endocrinology* 1990;126:2919–2926.
897. Spangelo BL, Judd AM, Ross PC, Login IS, Jarvis WD, Badamchian M, Goldstein AL, MacLeod RM. Thymosin fraction 5 stimulates prolactin and growth hormone release from anterior pituitary cells in vitro. *Endocrinology* 1987;121:2035–2043.
898. Badamchian M, Spangelo BL, Damavandy, MacLeod RM, Goldstein AL. Complete amino acid sequence analysis of a peptide isolated from the thymus that enhances release of growth hormone and prolactin. *Endocrinology* 1991;128:1580–1588.
899. Yang J, Tashjian AH, Jr. Platelet-activating factor affects cytosolic free calcium concentration and prolactin secretion in GH_4C_1 rat pituitary cells. *Biochem Biophys Res Commun* 1990;174:424–431.
900. Aiyer MS, Fink MG. The role of sex steroid hormones in modulating the responsiveness of the anterior pituitary gland to luteinizing hormone-releasing factor in the female rat. *J Endocrinol* 1974;62:533–572.
901. Drouva SV, Laplante E, Kordon C. Effects of ovarian steroids on in vitro release of LHRH from mediobasal hypothalamus. *Neuroendocrinology* 1983;37:336–341.
902. Brunet N, Gourdji D, Tixier-Vidal A. Effect of 17b estradiol on thyroliberin responsiveness in GH_3/B6 rat prolactin cells. *Mol Cell Endocrinol* 1980;18:123.
903. Kordon C, Drouva SV. Interplay between hypothalamic hormones and sex steroids in the control of neuroendocrine reproductive functions. Serono Symposia Series. In: Yen SSC, Vale WW, eds. *Neuroendocrine regulation of reproduction.* Massachusetts: Serono Symposia USA, 1990;254–268.
904. Drouva SV, Gautron JP, Pattou E, Laplante E, Kordon C. Effects of estradiol and progesterone on immunoreactive forms of hypothalamic luteinizing hormone. *Neuroendocrinology* 43:32–37.
905. Johnson AE, Nock B, McEwen BS, Feder HH. a_1 and a_2-noradrenergic receptor binding in guinea pig brain: sex differences and its effects of ovarian steroids. *Brain Res* 1988; 442:205–213.
906. Drouva SV, Laplante E, Kordon C. Progesterone induced LHRH release in vitro is an estrogen as well as Ca^{2+}- and calmodulin-dependent secretory process. *Neuroendocrinology* 1985;40: 325–331.
907. Ramirez VD, Dluzen D, Lin D. Progesterone administration in vivo stimulates release of luteinizing hormone-releasing hormone in vitro. *Science* 1980;208:1037–1039.
908. Drouva SV, Laplante E, Leblanc P, Béchet JJ, Clauser H, Kordon C. Estradiol activates methylating enzyme(s) involved in the conversion of phosphatidylethanolamine to phosphatidylcholine in rat pituitary membranes. *Endocrinology* 1986;119:2611–2622.
909. Drouva SV, Gorenne I, Laplante E, Rérat E, Enjalbert A, Kordon C. Estradiol modulates protein kinase C activity in the rat pituitary in vivo and in vitro. *Endocrinology* 1990;126:536–544.
910. Drouva SV, Rérat E, Leblanc P, Laplante E, Kordon C. Variations of phospholipid methyltransferase(s) activity in the rat pituitary: estrous cycle and sex differences. *Endocrinology* 1987; 121:569–575.
911. Beretta L, Bontterin MC, Drouva SV, Sobel A. Phosphorylation of a group of proteins related to physiological multi-hormonal regulation of the various types in the anterior pituitary gland. *Endocrinology* 1989;125:1358–1364.
912. Maus M, Bertrand P, Drouva S, Rasolonjanahary R, Kordon C, Glowinski, Premont J, Enjalbert A. Differential modulation of D_1 and D_2 dopamine-sensitive adenylate cyclases by 17β-estradiol in cultured striatal neurons and anterior pituitary cells. *J Neurochem* 1989;52:410–418.
913. Deschepper CF, Mellon SH, Cumin F, Baxter JD, Ganong WF. Analysis by immunocytochemistry and in situ hybridization of renin and its mRNA in kidney, testis adrenal and pituitary of the rat. *Proc Natl Acad Sci USA* 1986;83:7552–7556.
914. Saint-Andre JP, Rohmer J, Alhenc-Gelas F, Menard J, Bigorgne JC, Corvol P. Presence of renin, angiotensin and coverting enzyme in human pituitary lactotroph cells and prolactin adenomas. *J Clin Endocrinol Metab* 1986;63:231–237.
915. Meunier H, Rivier C, Evans RM, Vale W. Gonadal and extragonadal expression of inhibin a, bA and bB subunits in various tissues predicts diverse functions. *Proc Natl Acad Sci USA* 1988;85:247–251.
916. Kitaoka M, Kojima I, Ogata E. Activin-A: a modulator of multiple types of anterior pituitary cells. *Biochem Biophys Res Commun* 1988;157:48–54.
917. Kaiser UB, Lee BL, Carroll RS, Unabia G, Chin WW, Childs GV. Follistatin gene expression in the pituitary: localization in gonadotrophs and folliculostellate cells in diestrous rats. *Endocrinology* 1992;130:3048–3056.
918. Robertson DM, Farnworth PG, Clarke L, Jacobsen J, Cahir NF, Burger HG, De Krester DM. Effects of bovine 35 KDa FSH-suppressing protein on FSH and LH in pituitary cells in vitro: comparison with bovine 35KDa inhibin. *J Endocrinol* 1990; 124:417–423.
919. Kaplan LM, Gabriel SM, Koening JJ. Galanin is an estrogen-inducible secretory product of the rat anterior pituitary. *Proc Natl Acad Sci USA* 1988;85:7408.
920. O'Halloran DJ, Jones PM, Steel JH, Gon G, Gierid A, Ghatei MA, Polak JM, Bloom SR. Effect of endocrine manipulation on anterior pituitary galanin in the rat. *Endocrinology* 1990;127: 467–475.
921. Jones PM, Chatei MA, Steele J, O'Halloran D, Gon G, Legon S, Burrin JM, Leonhardt U, Polak JM, Bloom SR. Evidence for neuropeptide Y synthesis in the rat anterior pituitary and the influence of thyroid hormone status: comparison with vasoactive intestinal peptide, substance P, and neurotensin. *Endocrinology* 1989;125:334–341.
922. Lam KSL, Lechan RM, Minamitani N, Segerson TP, Reichlin S. Vasoactive intestinal peptide in the anterior pituitary is increased in hypothyroidism. *Endocrinology* 1989;124:1077–1084.
923. Nagy G, Mulcahey JS, Neil JD. Autocrine control of prolactin secretion by vasoactive intestinal peptide. *Endocrinology* 1988; 122:364–366.
924. Shamgochian MD, Leeman SE. Substance P stimulates luteinizing hormone secretion from anterior pituitary cells in culture. *Endocrinology* 1992;131:871–875.
925. Brown ER, Harlan PE, Krause JE. Gonadal regulation of substance P (SP) and SP-encoding messenger ribonucleic acids in the rat anterior pituitary and hypothalamus. *Endocrinology* 1990; 126:330–340.
926. Matsumoto H, Suzuki N, Shiota K, Inoue K, Tsuda M, Fujino M. Insulin-like growth factor 1 stimulates endothelin-3 secretion from rat anterior pituitary cells in primary culture. *Biochem Biophys Res Commun* 1990;172:661–668.
927. Vankelecom H, Carmeliet P, Van Damme J, Billiam A, Denef C. Production of interleukin-6 by folliculo-stellate cells of the anterior pituitary gland in a histiotypic cell aggregate culture system. *Neuroendocrinology* 1989;49:102–106.
928. Carmeliet P, Denef C. Immunocytochemical and pharmacological evidence for an intrinsic cholinomimetic system modulating prolactin and growth hormone release in rat pituitary. *Endocrinology* 1988;123:1128–1139.
929. May V, Wilber JF, M'Pritchard DC, Childs GV. Persistence of

immunoreactive TRH and GnRH in long-term primary anterior pituitary cultures. *Peptides* 1987;8:543–558.
930. Schally AV, Arimura A, Kastin AJ. Hypothalamic regulatory hormones. *Science* 1973;179:341–350.
931. Neil JD. Neuroendocrine regulation of prolactin secretion. In: Martini L, Ganong WF, eds. *Frontiers in neuroendocrinology,* vol. 6. New York: Raven Press, 1980;129.
932. Watkins WB, Moore RY, Burton HG III, Catherwood BD, Deftos LS. Distribution of immunoreactive calcitonin in the rat pituitary gland. *Endocrinology* 1980;106:1966–1971.
933. Shah GV, Wang W, Grosvenar CE, Grosvenor, Crowley WR. Calcitonin inhibits basal and thyrotropin-releasing hormone-induced release of prolactin from anterior pituitary cells: Evidence for a selective action exerted proximal to secretagogue-induced increases in cytosolic Ca2+. *Endocrinology* 1990;127: 621–628.

The Physiology of Reproduction, Second Edition,
edited by E. Knobil and J.D. Neill,
Raven Press, Ltd., New York © 1994.

CHAPTER 28

The Gonadotropin-Releasing Hormone (GnRH), Neuronal Systems: Immunocytochemistry and In Situ Hybridization

Ann-Judith Silverman, Izhar Livne, and Joan W. Witkin

The purification, sequencing, and synthesis of the decapeptide gonadotropin-releasing hormone (GnRH, also called LHRH for luteinizing hormone-releasing hormone) by laboratories headed by Guillemin (1) and Schally (2,3) can now be seen as an important transition point in the study of the neuroendocrinology of reproduction. It was the culmination of the research efforts of Holweg, Harris, McCann, Everett, and Sawyer, work that spanned five decades and implicated the central nervous system (CNS) in the control of luteinizing hormone (LH) and follicle-stimulating hormone (FSH) secretion. Regulation of anterior pituitary function is mediated by the release of this now well-characterized neuropeptide into the primary portal capillaries in the median eminence and its delivery to the target via the hypophyseal portal veins. The availability of the decapeptide, of antibodies directed against it, and more recently of probes for detecting its mRNA (4) have provided tools for the anatomic dissection of the neurosecretory pathways. It is our premise that knowledge of the unique anatomy of the GnRH neuronal networks and the integration of these neurons into the wiring of the CNS may provide the critical underpinnings of physiological and neuropharmacological research. We shall see that this neurosecretory system is very diffuse; it contains individual neu-

Department of Anatomy and Cell Biology, Columbia University, New York, New York 10032 rons located in vastly different regions of the brain, presumably integrating different kinds of information. Determining how this system is coordinated will be one of the major anatomic challenges of this decade.

IMMUNOCYTOCHEMICAL PROCEDURES

Before discussing the findings based on immunocytochemistry or in situ hybridization, we should first examine the nature of the procedures from which we obtain such important data. Immunocytochemistry represents a variety of techniques that permit the localization of an antigen in tissue sections and is based on the premise that the antibody–antigen complexes can be visualized. Criteria for specificity have become more complex as the field has become more sophisticated. In general, antibodies are first screened for their binding affinities in either liquid- or solid-phase radioimmunoassay. Such approaches permit one to test large numbers of antigens and to examine the modifications of the parent molecule that are compatible with antibody recognition. It is, however, essential that absorption experiments using tissue sections also be carried out. Here antisera are incubated with test ligands prior to the use of those antisera in the immunocytochemical procedure. Comparison of staining intensity is then made among sections reacted with untreated antiserum, antiserum absorbed with native antigen (e.g., GnRH), and antiserum absorbed with a modified antigen (e.g., see ref. 5).

In addition to controls for antibody specificity, one should also perform tests for the specificity of the immunocytochemical procedure itself (6). It is essential to demonstrate that any staining seen in the tissue is dependent on the binding of the primary antibody to antigen and not on the nonspecific attachment of reagents, endogenous fluorescence, and enzymatic activities. Such controls are particularly crucial in double-label immunocytochemical studies.

IN SITU HYBRIDIZATION

In addition to immunocytochemistry, the cloning of the gene for GnRH (4,7) in some but not all species has led to the development of in situ hybridization procedures to detect the mRNA for the GnRH precursor (8). With this technique, either unfixed or fixed tissue sections are hybridized to radioactive nucleotide probes, followed by coating with photographic emulsion and its exposure to the disintegrating radioactive particles. The degree of specificity can be controlled in part by the temperature at which hybridization takes place (stringency). The ability to determine the source of radioactive decay will depend in part on the energy and type of radioactive decay, which in turn determine the path length of the particle. In general, ^{3}H- or ^{35}S-labeled probes emitting β particles with relatively short path lengths are preferred to ^{32}P-labeled probes. These probes can either be full-length cDNAs, cRNAs, or smaller oligonucleotides (see section on in situ analysis, below). Specificity of the probe is demonstrated by the absence of an autoradiographic signal when sense oligonucleotides are used. Controls for positive and negative chemography are similar to those used in any radioisotope procedure.

MIGRATION AND DIFFERENTIATION OF THE GnRH NEURONAL SYSTEM

The distribution of GnRH neurons and their axons within the cranial and the extracranial olfactory system of the adult animal has been described in several mammalian species (see below). It has also been reported that, during embryonic development, the appearance of GnRH neurons and axons in the nasal septum of the rat (9) and the nervus terminalis of the guinea pig (10) precedes their appearance in other parts of the brain. Only in recent years, however, was it conclusively demonstrated that GnRH neurons differentiate from the olfactory placode of the midgestation mouse embryo. Following their differentiation, these neurons migrate through the nasal septum and enter the ventral forebrain with the central roots of the nervus terminalis and vomeronasal nerves (11–13). Since most of the data available to date on the migration process of GnRH neurons are derived from studies in the mouse embryo, we limit the following discussion to this species. However, studies in chicks (14–16), musk shrews (E. Rissman and A.-J. Silverman, unpublished data), rats (17), and rhesus macaques (18) indicate that the olfactory origin and migratory pathway of GnRH neurons are a general phenomenon in vertebrate development.

Immunocytochemistry with an antibody recognizing both the GnRH precursor and product was used to follow these neurons as they emerge from the olfactory placode and form cords of migratory cells in the nasal septum of the mouse (Fig. 1A) (11,13). Most of the GnRH neurons emerge from the mitotic cycle on embryonic day 10.5 (E10.5) and commence expression of the GnRH gene by E11.5 (12). On E12.5 the number of cells synthesizing the GnRH protein in the nasal septum is similar to the number of GnRH neurons in the adult forebrain (12,19), suggesting that this olfactory-derived population gives rise to the full complement of GnRH cells in the adult mammalian CNS with the possible exception of certain cells in the midbrain (see below). Subsequent to their emigration from the olfactory placode on days E12.5 to E16.5, the cells penetrate the medial ventral forebrain and migrate caudally to reside in the septal, preoptic, and anterior hypothalamic areas (13).

The migration of GnRH cells out of the vomeronasal organ (VNO) coincides with the emergence of axons from the epithelium of the VNO on E12 (20). Thus, GnRH cells appear to comigrate into the submucosa of

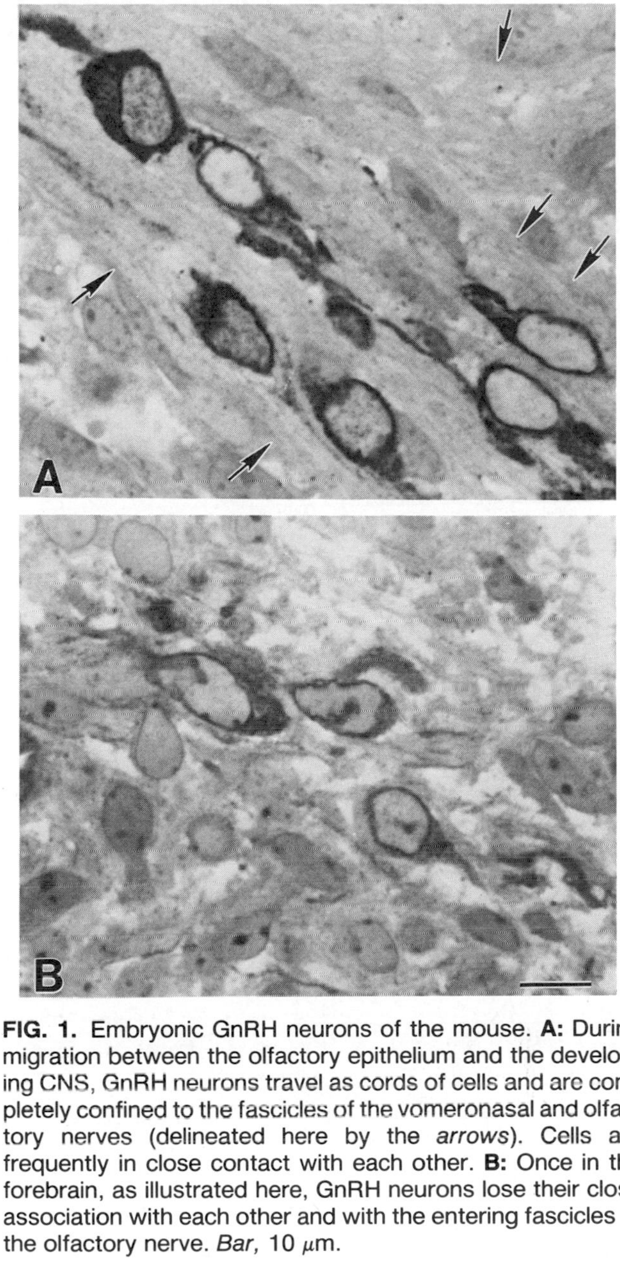

FIG. 1. Embryonic GnRH neurons of the mouse. **A:** During migration between the olfactory epithelium and the developing CNS, GnRH neurons travel as cords of cells and are completely confined to the fascicles of the vomeronasal and olfactory nerves (delineated here by the *arrows*). Cells are frequently in close contact with each other. **B:** Once in the forebrain, as illustrated here, GnRH neurons lose their close association with each other and with the entering fascicles of the olfactory nerve. *Bar,* 10 μm.

the nasal septum with the pioneer axons of the vomeronasal nerve and advance together toward the forebrain. A population of glial progenitor cells also migrates from the olfactory and vomeronasal epithelia with the outgrowing axons and differentiates into ensheathing cells (21–24). Our ultrastructural observations reveal that the axonal fascicles and their ensheathing cells form physical channels within which GnRH cells can migrate across the nasal septum (Fig. 1A) and enter the forebrain (Fig. 1B). The critical role of these channels is suggested by examination of an aborted fetus with Kallmann's syndrome. With this mutation the olfactory, vomeronasal, and terminal nerves fail to enter the forebrain, and coincident with this failure, GnRH cells in the aborted embryo accumulate above the cribriform plate or in the dural plane of the anterior fossa (25). Once in the forebrain, GnRH cells are no longer associated with axonal fascicles and appear to intermingle with a heterogeneous population of neurons and glia (Fig. 1B). Thus, in the CNS GnRH neurons are not associated with any recognizable structural element that might serve as a physical guiding substrate. It is, therefore, plausible that these neurons rely on chemical rather than physical cues in choosing their migratory pathway in the forebrain.

During their migration within the developing CNS, GnRH neurons elaborate axonal processes that arrive by E14.5 at the prospective median eminence (ME) region. Some of these axons are immunopositive for the amidated decapeptide that is the bioactive form of GnRH (3). Since the primary capillaries of the hypophyseal portal system are already present in the ME by E18 in the mouse (26), the neurohormone is potentially capable of activating the pituitary–gonadal axis by late gestation. Indeed, it has recently been demonstrated that GnRH is required for early postnatal activation of the pituitary–gonadal axis in the mouse (27).

Although GnRH neurons in the olfactory placode initiate elaboration of the pro-GnRH precursor as early as E11.5 (11,13), the biochemical maturation of these neurons is not complete at the time of the early migratory stages. This conclusion is based on a quantitative immunocytochemical study. Early in the migratory stage (E12.5) in the nasal septum the majority of the neurons do not process the GnRH precursor to the amidated decapeptide (28). By E14.5, when most GnRH cells have advanced into the forebrain, about 80% of the cells acquire the capability to fully process the GnRH precursor. In agreement with the immunocytochemical data, ultrastructural observations indicate that on E12.5 the pro-GnRH precursor is retained within the rough endoplasmic reticulum (RER) and is not yet transported to the Golgi apparatus. Two days later, at E14.5, GnRH immunoreactivity is seen in the Golgi cisternae and in neurosecretory granules. It is not known whether pro-GnRH synthesized before E14.5 is retained in the RER to be transported to the Golgi and processed at a later stage or is immediately transported to the Golgi but, because of the absence of functional processing enzymes, cannot be fully processed and is degraded. These observations do indicate that the neurosecretory potential of GnRH neurons to release mature neuropeptide is not realized until they are well advanced in their migratory route to the forebrain.

DISTRIBUTION OF GnRH NEURONS AND THEIR PROJECTIONS IN THE ADULT MAMMALIAN BRAIN

The Septo-Preoptico-Infundibular Pathway

The distribution of GnRH neurons and their axonal projections in the adult brain has been studied by apply-

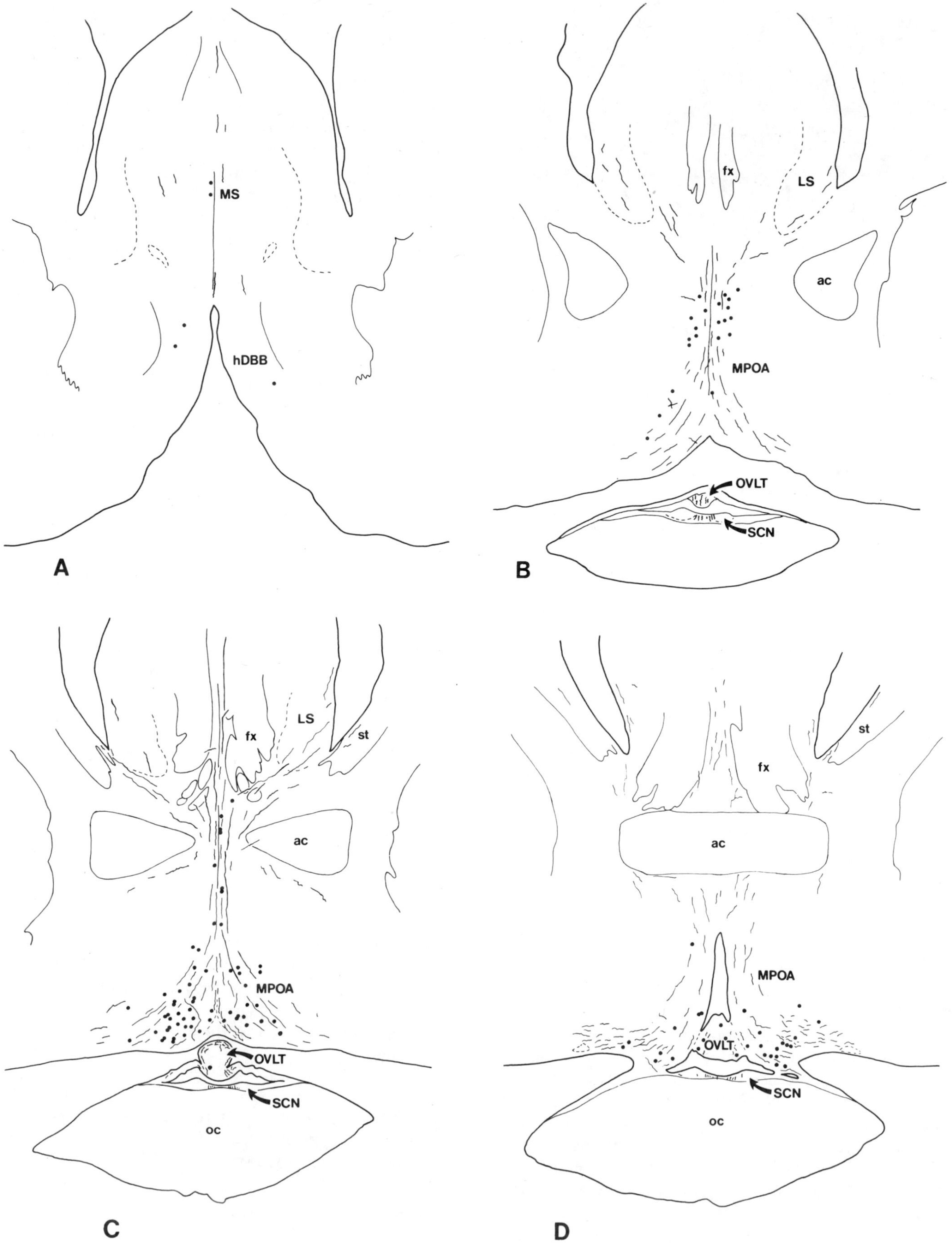
MS
hDBB
A
fx
LS
ac
MPOA
OVLT
SCN
B
fx
LS
st
ac
MPOA
OVLT
SCN
oc
C
st
fx
ac
MPOA
OVLT
SCN
oc
D

ing light microscopic immunocytochemical techniques to tissue sections. Anatomic studies were first carried out by Barry and colleagues (29,30); a similar approach to these questions continues to the present, with more recent studies refining and extending initial observations. This topic has been the subject of many reviews that have stressed comparative aspects (31–35). This chapter emphasizes work on mammals, with a shorter section on other vertebrate groups.

In all mammals studied in detail, several distinct subpopulations of GnRH neurons can be identified within the CNS. The GnRH cells are not segregated into nuclear clusters but instead appear as a loose network spread through many classic cytoarchitectonic divisions. In most species, GnRH cells form a loose continuum from the telencephalic diagonal band of Broca and more dorsal septal areas (including the medial and triangular septal nuclei), to the bed nucleus of the stria terminalis, and diencephalic areas (including the periventricular area, medial and lateral preoptic areas, anterior hypothalamus, and retrochiasmatic zone medial to the optic tract). Also included in this continuum are clusters of cells lying dorsal to, and occasionally within, the supraoptic nucleus. Diagrammatic representations of the distribution of these neuronal groups are shown in Fig. 2 (sheep).

The degree to which GnRH neurons migrate caudally differs among mammals. In the opossum (*Monodelphis domestica*) GnRH neurons do not enter the preoptic area or hypothalamus (36). In other species GnRH neurons are found as far caudal as the arcuate/infundibular nucleus, median eminence, and premammillary nuclei: guinea pig (37–39), sheep (40,41), rhesus, pigtail, and squirrel monkeys (42,43), humans, bats, and ferrets (44), and cow, horse, cat, dog, and rabbit (see refs. 32 and 35 for further references). In all such species the absolute number of cells within these more caudal regions is usually a small proportion of the total (cf. refs. 10,40,41), although this is apparently not true for humans (45).

The projections of the neurons in this telencephalic/diencephalic continuum have been studied by reconstructing pathways from tissue sections, by analysis of fiber loss following placement of lesions within the CNS, and by application of retrograde tracers. The most prominent projection is to the median eminence, which is the final common pathway for regulation of anterior pituitary function. The GnRH fibers reach the median eminence by more than one route (see Fig. 2) (32,43,46–52). The major septo-preoptico-infundibular pathway(s), common to most species, begin as a midline bundle of GnRH processes anteriorly at the level of the diagonal band of Broca. This bundle bifurcates near the preoptic recess of the third ventricle. Both bundles travel close to the midline, one along the dorsal and the other along the ventral surface of the optic chiasm. The ventral bundle tends to run close to the surface of the brain, being covered only by the pia (46,49).

Axons of GnRH neurons in the more caudal and lateral aspects of the preoptic area and hypothalamus travel in or near the medial forebrain bundle. These turn medially near the level of the median eminence (Fig. 2). Additional fibers from the pericommissural region pass through the dorsomedial hypothalamus, forming a periventricular subependymal GnRH network. The use of the ependymal processes as tunnels through which the fibers course has been demonstrated ultrastructurally (53). These periventricular fibers contribute to the median eminence innervation and possibly to the innervation of more caudal structures. In those species in which GnRH cells are also present in the medial basal hypothalamus, GnRH axons extend from these cells into the median eminence, and fibers often continue down the infundibular stalk (32) to enter the posterior pituitary (54).

It is essential that all such pathways to the median eminence be taken into account when paradigms involving surgical interruption of pathways or placement of lesions are used. Particular attention should be paid to the difficulty in severing the subchiasmatic fibers found in rodents (49) and primates, including humans (55). It should also be noted in this context that GnRH fibers are capable of considerable sprouting, perhaps reflecting their placodal origin. Tissue at the edge of a lesion will become invested with numerous GnRH axons (A.-J. Silverman, unpublished observations; M. N. Lehman and G. Jackson, unpublished observations). The age at which lesions are made is also a critical factor. Medial basal hypothalamic deafferentation in the early neonatal period results in regrowth of GnRH axons across the cut, but surgical interruption of axonal pathways in older animals leads to a depletion of GnRH fibers in the median eminence and to anovulatory cycles (56). It is also interesting that the entire apparatus for maintaining the GnRH pulse may also be capable of extreme plasticity and reorganization (57).

Although GnRH cells in many regions contribute to axonal bundles that project to the median eminence, all cells do not participate in this pathway. Knowing which cells form the neurosecretory connection with the hypo-

←

FIG. 2. The distribution of GnRH cells (●) and fibers (*short solid lines*) in drawings of coronal brain sections, rostral to caudal (**A–D**), through the preoptic area and hypothalamus of the ewe. Immunoreactive fibers are represented bilaterally. Note that more than one trajectory brings GnRH axons to the median eminence. (ac) Anterior commissure; (fx) fornix; (hDBB) horizontal limb of the diagonal band of Broca; (LS) lateral septum; (MPOA) medial preoptic area; (MS) medial septum; (oc) optic chiasm; (OVLT) organum vasculosum of the lamina terminalis; (SCN) suprachiasmatic nucleus; (st) stria terminalis.

physeal portal capillaries is clearly a central issue in understanding the nature of the neuronal pathways that regulate gonadotropin secretion. Initial observations in the rat indicated that complete surgical isolation of the medial basal hypothalamus (MBH) eliminated or very substantially reduced the number of GnRH fibers in the median eminence (50,52,58–61), suggesting an anterior origin for such fibers. Deafferentations, when complete (i.e., including the ventral pathways), coincide with failure of pulsatile gonadotropin secretion. By inference, similar deafferentations of the medial basal hypothalamus of the rhesus monkey must not disrupt all GnRH input to the median eminence, since such hypothalamic "islands" can support pulsatile and estrogen-induced surges of gonadotropins (62). In the guinea pig, the preoptic area and pericommissural regions as well as the arcuate nucleus contribute GnRH inputs to the median eminence, with each region forming a different terminal field within this neural–hemal organ (63). However, only the arcuate input is essential for tonic and cyclic gonadotropin secretion (63,64).

Recently, a more direct approach has been taken to determine which GnRH neurons actually supply the innervation of the median eminence. In these experiments, a retrograde tracer that would be captured by nerve terminals is applied directly to the median eminence. Once internalized by endocytosis, the tracer is transported to the cell body region. Both tracer and GnRH are localized in the same tissue section, and the cells identified as being afferent to the median eminence are mapped and counted. In the rat, neurons found containing both labels are located as far rostrally as the diagonal band of Broca and are present within all of the architectonic regions cited above. In the two major studies on rodents (65,66), 50% to 75% of all GnRH neurons in the septal, preoptic, and hypothalamic areas were afferent to the median eminence. No morphological characteristics distinguish median eminence afferent neurons from those that do not project to this neural–hemal organ. Furthermore, cells that supply the median eminence innervation (doubly labeled) are frequently located immediately next to those whose function is currently unknown (GnRH-positive only).

The findings in the one primate species (67) studied to date differ somewhat from those in the rodent (65). Here varying proportions of GnRH neurons along their rostral–caudal distribution were noted (see Fig. 3), but no doubly labeled cells were found in the diagonal band or the organum vasculosum of the lamina terminalis (OVLT). Since the survival times after application of the tracer were very long, it is unlikely that lack of double-labeled cells in these rostral regions resulted from insufficient transport time. Overall only 40% of GnRH neurons in this species appeared to project to the median eminence. However, the retrograde tracer may not have filled the entire GnRH terminal field in the median eminence, and the total population of afferent neurons may have been underestimated.

Another approach has utilized peripheral injection of the tracer either into the vascular space (68) or into the peritoneum (69,70). Under these circumstances, provided there is sufficient tracer, all neurons that project outside of the blood–brain barrier (i.e., to any of the circumventricular organs) would be double labeled (see ref. 70). Experiments on mice suggest that the ability to capture tracer (at least fluorogold) may be dependent on neuronal activity, because animals treated with estrogen and progesterone and injected with tracer at the expected time of the surge had 80% or more of their GnRH neurons labeled, but only 60% were labeled in males or in females injected at random times during the cycle (69). As with the tracing studies from ME proper, fluorogold-positive neurons were randomly distributed among the GnRH population. In the ferret approximately 60% of all GnRH neurons were labeled by this method (71). In contrast, in the rat, where a different injection protocol was used, all GnRH neurons (more than 90%) contained fluorogold regardless of the age or endocrine condition (70). These latter data suggest that the majority of GnRH neurons that have intracerebral projections also release peptide into a vascular space.

This question can also be asked in a different way. Rather than determining which GnRH neurons innervate the median eminence, one can ask which cells contribute significantly to the release of neuropeptide necessary to maintain the LH pulse and the preovulatory surge of LH. In the rhesus monkey, complete medial basal hypothalamic islands are compatible with both pulsatile and steroid-induced LH surges (62). Similar results were obtained in the guinea pig (63,64). Although in this latter species, only a small percentage of all GnRH neurons reside in the MBH, this seems to be the only region essential for gonadotropin secretion. These data strongly suggest that cells may project to the median eminence but may play only a supplementary rather than an essential role in reproductive function. This hypothesis is supported by findings in the rat, where bilateral knife cuts that sever the septal projection to the median eminence and cause a 30% reduction in median eminence GnRH do not interfere with ovulation (72). Similarly, unilateral knife cuts that interrupt all GnRH input ipsilaterally as measured by radioimmunoassay also do not interfere with ovulation (72).

That there is redundancy in the GnRH system is further demonstrated by work on the *hpg* mouse (see below) and by very recent studies that follow the expression of the immediate early gene, *c-fos*. The expression of *c-fos* in neurons is generally held to indicate the activation of these cells (73–75). Since *fos* is a nuclear protein, its colocalization by immunocytochemistry with the predominantly cytoplasmic GnRH is easily accomplished (Fig. 4). In the rat, *fos* expression is detected in GnRH neu-

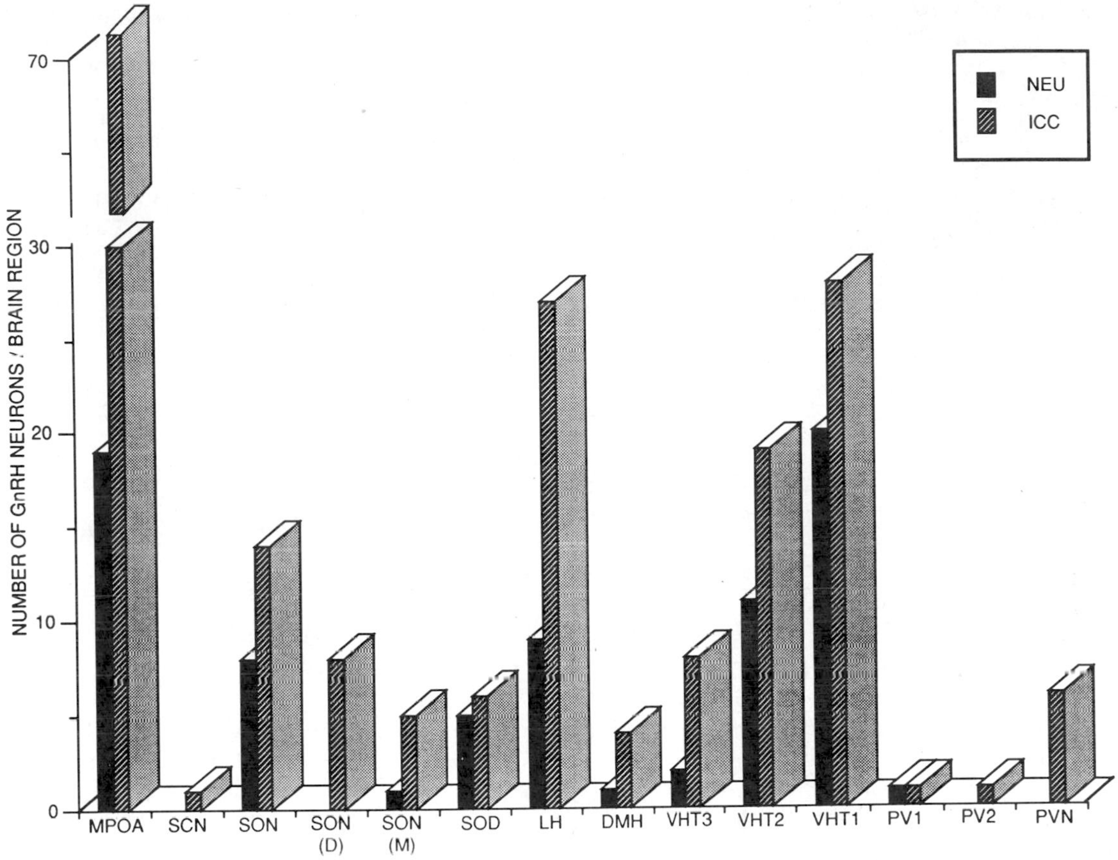

NEU / ICC	19/73	0/1	8/14	0/8	1/5	5/6	9/27	1/4	2/8	11/19	20/28	1/1	0/1	0/6
% NEU	26	0	57	0	20	83	33	2.5	25	58	71	100	0	0
% TOTAL NEU	25	0	10	0	1	6	12	1.5	3	14	26	1.5	0	0
% TOTAL ICC	36	0.5	7	4	2.5	3	13	1.5	4	9	14	0.5	0.5	3

FIG. 3. GnRH-immunoreative (ICC) and neuroendocrine (NEU) neurons in the juvenile male cynomolgus monkey hypothalamus. Data here are compiled from one of 12 sets of 40-μm frontal sections and therefore represent $^1/_{12}$ the total number of GnRH neurons per brain region. Data are expressed as regional percentages found in each anatomic area. %NEU = $NEU_{region}/ICC_{region} \times 100$; % TOTAL NEU = $NEU_{region}/NEU_{total} \times 100$; %TOTAL ICC = $ICC_{region}/ICC_{total} \times 100$. Abbreviations: MPOA, medial preoptic area; SCN, suprachiasmatic nucleus; SON, supraoptic nucleus; SON (D), dorsal aspect of the supraoptic nucleus; SON (M), medial aspect of supraoptic nucleus; SOD, supraoptic decussation; LH, lateral hypothalamus; DMH, dorsomedial hypothalamus; VHT1, 2, 3, ventral hypothalamic tract; PV 1 and 2, periventricular hypothalamus; PVN, paraventricular nucleus. (From Goldsmith et al., ref. 67, with permission.)

rons on the afternoon of proestrus (76) and during a steroid-induced surge (77,78). In this species, the activated neurons are concentrated around the OVLT and represent only 40% of the total. Similar findings have been obtained in steroid-primed mice (79), but here a wider distribution of activated neurons as well as a larger percentage of *fos*-positive cells can be obtained under some circumstances. Also, the duration of activation appears to be prolonged in animals that mate with an ejaculating male. In this latter study 1.3% of GnRH neurons did express *fos* in the nonsurging animal, suggesting that only a small number of cells are needed to sustain tonic LH release. Again, this conclusion is supported by work in the *hpg* mouse (80). Interestingly, in both rat and mouse studies, *fos* activation appeared to be coincident with rather than precede the LH surge.

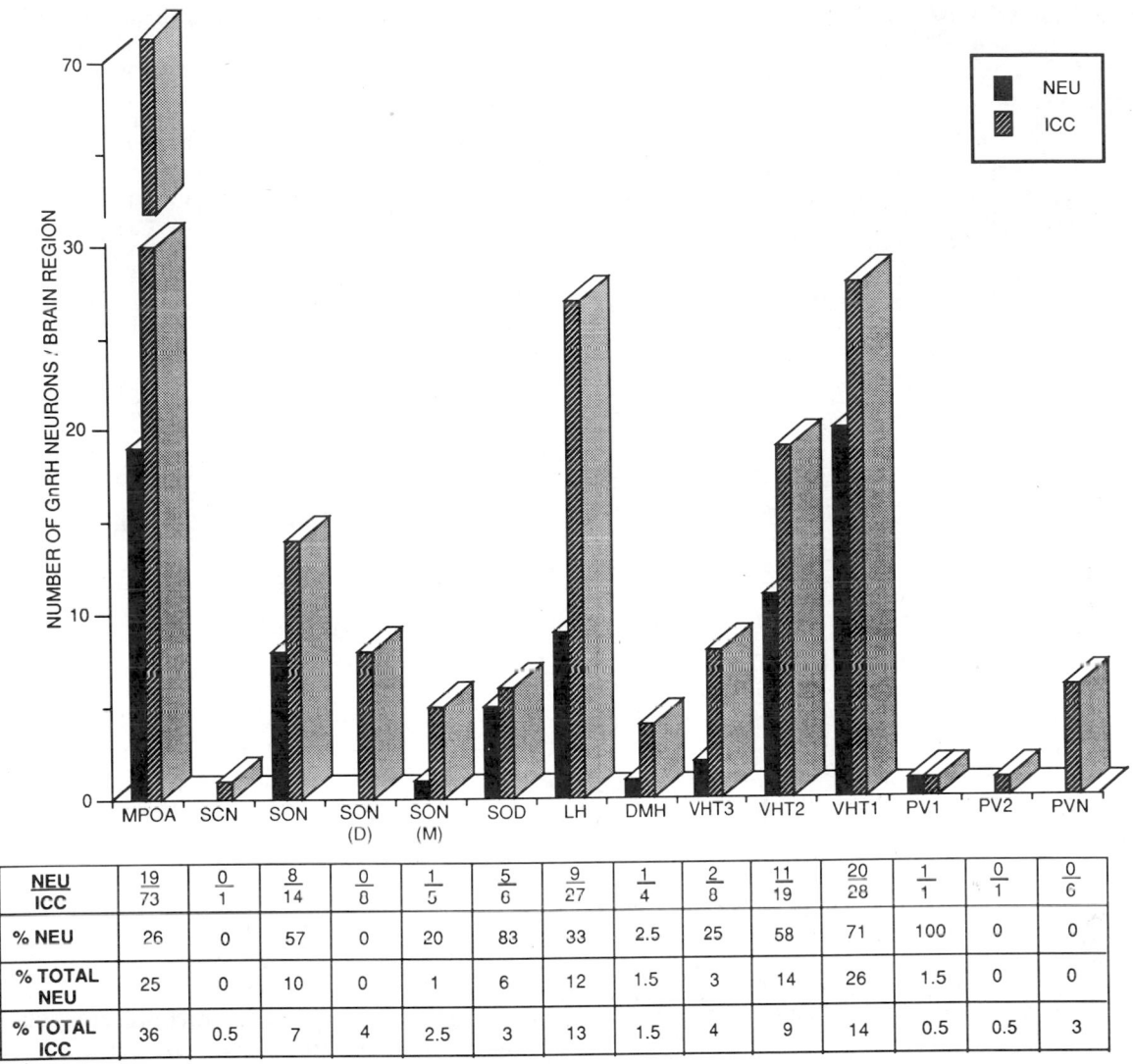

Because *fos* expression is of short duration (73) and may appear only when action potentials originate in the cell body, this procedure may not detect the activation of and release from terminals in the median eminence without somal involvement. In preliminary studies, we (A.-J. Silverman, J. W. Witkin, and M. Ferin, unpublished observations) have examined the expression of *fos* in the female rhesus monkey. None or very few double-

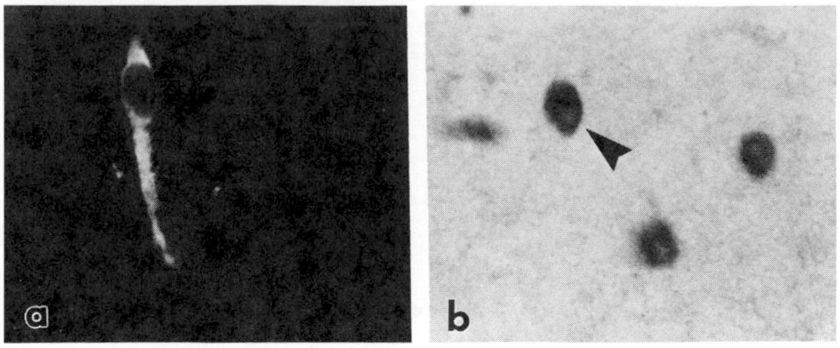

FIG. 4. GnRH neurons can transiently express the protooncogene *c-fos* during the proestrus surge. These are two photographs of a GnRH neuron in the region of the OVLT with fluorescent (**a**) and bright-field (**b**) illumination showing GnRH immunoreactivity in the cytoplasm (**a**) and Fos protein in the nucleus (*arrow*, **b**). Note that there are Fos-positive cells in the vicinity that do not contain GnRH. Similarly, many GnRH neurons do not express Fos under these same conditions (see text). (From Wu et al., ref. 79, with permission.)

labeled cells were found in castrate females, although pulsatile release of LH is very high (81) and is driven by GnRH pulses (82,83). Furthermore, *fos* is not expressed or is expressed in very few GnRH neurons of follicular-phase monkeys given 17β-estradiol and killed during the early stages of an LH surge. Only when the surge has been in progress for many hours does *fos* expression appear, and then only in a very low percentage (approximately 10%) of the cells. Interestingly, under these conditions *fos* expression is not confined to GnRH cells that reside in the MBH. These data on the primate are preliminary and need to be extended and confirmed.

At the ultrastructural level, numerous investigators have described GnRH axonal profiles within the median eminence and their proximity to the fenestrated capillaries of the portal plexus (cf. refs. 84–86). It is interesting to note that in most instances, GnRH axons are separated from the perivascular space by ependymal foot processes (84,85). Whether changes in access to the vascular space during times of increased secretion by contraction of glial elements occur, as they do in the posterior pituitary (87), is not known.

GnRH Pathways to Other Circumventricular Organs

Circumventricular organs are sites within the CNS in which the ependymal lining of the ventricular space is highly specialized and where the capillaries forming the blood supply are fenestrated, thereby permitting access of blood-borne substances into the nervous tissue. In addition to the dense GnRH innervation of the median eminence, cells of the septal–preoptic area also contribute to the GnRH innervation of the OVLT, the second most densely GnRH-innervated structure in the CNS of most species (Fig. 5). This pathway was originally termed the septo-preoptico terminal tract by Barry and coworkers (32), and its role, if any, in the regulation of gonadotropin function is unknown. In the rat, no changes in the staining of axons in the OVLT were observed with gonadectomy with or without steroid replacement therapy, treatments that altered the amount of GnRH staining in the median eminence (88,89). However, in the squirrel monkey, changes in GnRH staining intensity occur both in the median eminence (90) and in the OVLT (42) during the estrous cycle. Evaluation of experiments in which lesions are placed in the area of the OVLT (cf. ref. 91) are difficult to interpret, since such lesions would inevitably destroy numerous GnRH neurons, including many that project to the median eminence.

Many fibers, presumably from cells within the septum itself (92), ramify within the septal region, with some converging on the lateral ventricular wall. Other fibers enter the subfornical organ (SFO). This circumventricular organ, like the OVLT, also contains a few GnRH cells of its own, which are labeled with intraperitoneally delivered tracer. The origin of the GnRH fibers within the SFO may therefore be of both intrinsic and extrinsic origin.

Extrahypothalamic Projections

The cells in the septal and preoptic areas also contribute to many of the extrahypothalamic terminals of GnRH axons as first described by Barry (for a review see ref. 32; also see refs. 46,51,64, and 93; Fig. 6). Some cells, especially from the medial and triangular septal nuclei and pericommissural region, send fibers into the stria medullaris to innervate the epithalamus (habenula and possibly pineal). Other fibers continue into the fasciculus retroflexus to terminate in the interpeduncular nucleus. In the rat, retrograde tracing experiments suggest that the GnRH innervation of the interpeduncular nucleus is derived from a small number of cells in the ventromedial diagonal band and ventral hypothalamus (94). Interestingly, some of the cells in the diagonal band that innervate the interpeduncular nucleus also project outside of the blood–brain barrier (94), as would be predicted by the fluorogold tracing data of Witkin (70; vide supra).

Other fibers enter the stria terminalis or travel along a ventral pathway to terminate in the medial amygdala (43,95). In the hamster (92), injections of tracer into the medial amygdala labeled a small number of cells in the ventromedial preoptic area at the level of the OVLT. In the rat the GnRH innervation of the medial amygdala originates from cells in the medial septum, caudal roots

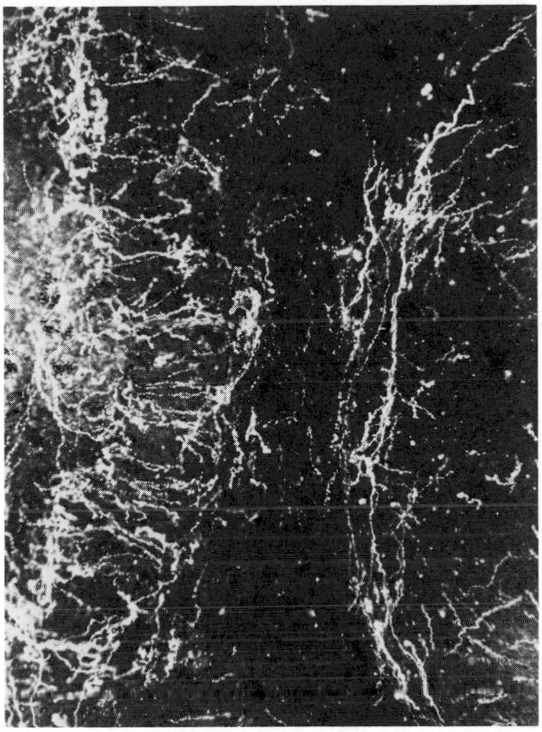

FIG. 5. GnRH fibers in the OVLT-supraoptic organ of the rhesus monkey. The sheep has a similarly complex OVLT. The OVLT of rodents is a much simpler structure, but is also well innervated by GnRH fibers.

of the nervus terminalis, triangular septal nucleus, bed nucleus of the stria terminalis, and ventrolateral hypothalamus (96).

Based on lesion experiments in the guinea pig (51), cells in the septal–preoptic area also contribute to a diffuse periventricular pathway whose fibers enter the mammillary complex and then converge on the mammillary peduncle and proceed into the ventral tegmental area of the midbrain. There they mingle with fibers derived from the fasciculus retroflexus. Axons continue caudalward, coursing along the dorsal border of the interpeduncular nucleus, and, in the rat (46) but not the guinea pig (51), continue into the raphe nuclei. A small number of fibers also extend into the periaqueductal region.

DISTRIBUTION OF GnRH NEURONS AND AXONS IN OLFACTORY-RELATED STRUCTURES

The Nervus Terminalis

Barry and his colleagues initially identified GnRH neurons in rostral regions, termed the parolfactory area (32). Similar observations were made by Silverman and Krey (51) when they noted in the guinea pig that small clusters of these neurons were associated with the blood vessels of the anterior perforated substance (also see ref. 97). These cell groups were finally recognized to be part of the nervus terminalis (39). In the guinea pig, this nerve (sometimes referred to as the zero cranial nerve) has peripheral, intracranial, and intracerebral components (Fig. 7). The peripheral portion is composed of neurons and their processes below the cribriform plate that are associated with the olfactory and vomeronasal nerves. In the rat (89,99), GnRH fibers have been identified in the sensory epithelium of the vomeronasal organ. The intracranial portion consists of several ganglia that lie in the pial layer of the pia mater (in the guinea pig) and contain both GnRH-positive and GnRH-negative neurons. The ganglia are found on the ventromedial surface of the olfactory bulbs and forebrain. The largest are the ganglion terminale at the caudal pole of the olfactory bulbs; g_1 at the frontal pole of the olfactory bulbs, and g_2 at the level of the olfactory tubercle, where the anterior cerebral artery enters the CNS. Each of these ganglia and other smaller clusters of cells are connected by fiber bundles, e.g., the terminal nerve.

The organization of the nervus terminalis of the hamster is similar to that of the guinea pig (100). In the rat, scattered cells are seen in this region, but no large ganglia are observed. Given the location of these cells, they or their processes might have access both to blood-borne substances and to the cerebrospinal fluid in the subarachnoid space. Within the CNS, GnRH cells and fibers follow the course of the anterior cerebral artery and its branches through the olfactory tubercle and septal regions (Fig. 8).

The nervus terminalis also contains non-GnRH-containing neurons that have a morphology similar to sympathetic ganglion cells (39). In the hamster (100) and sheep (101), two distinct populations of cells have been distinguished: those that are GnRH positive and those that contain acetylcholinesterase. In the rat, non-GnRH-positive cells, at least in the intracerebral portion, are cholinergic (i.e., contain choline acetyltransferase) and/or contain VIP (102). Determining the interplay of the nervus terminalis and the vomeronasal system in the coordination of olfactory stimuli that are important for reproductive behavior and physiology will be an exciting area of experimentation in the future.

Other Olfactory-Related Pathways

It is quite clear that olfactory cues play a critical role in the reproductive physiology and behavior of many mammalian species. In addition to the nervus terminalis discussed above, olfactory information enters the central nervous system via either the olfactory projection to the main olfactory bulb or via the vomeronasal organ's (VNO) projection to the accessory olfactory bulb (103). Within the CNS, the secondary and tertiary projections of each of these systems remain segregated, both anatom-

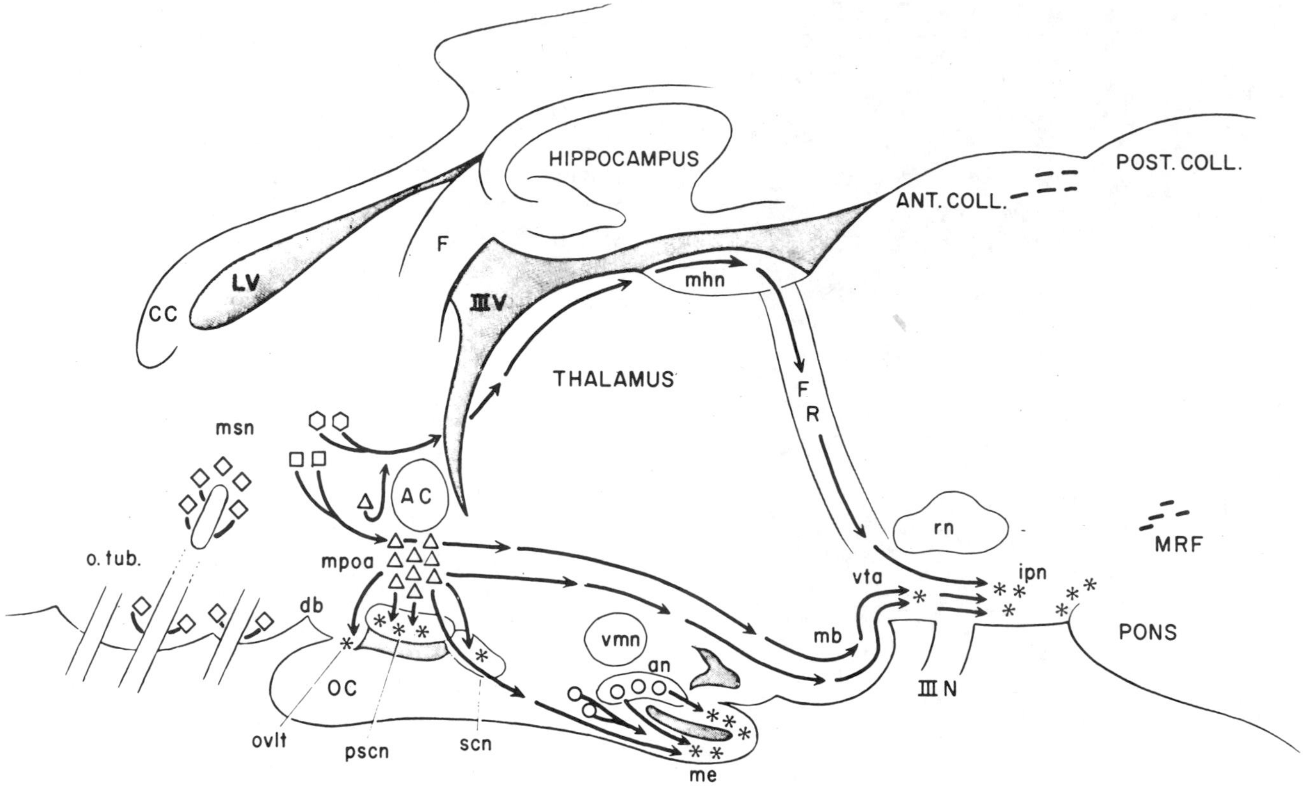

FIG. 6. Midsagittal plane of the guinea pig brain from the level of the septum rostrally to the pons posteriorly. Different groups of GnRH cells are indicated by the geometric symbols, fiber pathways are indicated by *arrows*, and terminal fields are indicated by *asterisks*. The subchiasmatic pathway is not indicated. It is likely that GnRH cells have more than one projection. (AC) Anterior commissure; (an) arcuate nucleus; (CC) corpus callosum; (db) diagonal band of Broca; (F) fornix; (FR) fasciculus retroflexus; (ipn) interpeduncular nucleus; (LV) lateral ventricle; (mb) mammillary body, medial division; (me) median eminence; (mhn) medial habenula; (mpoa) medial preoptic area; (msn) medial septum; (OC) optic chiasm; (o. tub) olfactory tubercle; (ovt) organum vasculosum of the lamina terminalis; (pscn) preoptic suprachiasmatic nucleus; (rn) red nucleus; (scn) suprachiasmatic nucleus; (vmn) ventromedial nucleus; (vta) ventral tegmental area; (IIIV) third ventricle; (IIIN) oculomotor nerve.

ically and functionally. Recent data suggest that the VNO system is the system most intimately related to reproduction (103).

The degree of development of GnRH neuronal networks in the main and accessory olfactory bulbs, anterior olfactory nucleus, and olfactory portions of the limbic system varies considerably across species: they are underdeveloped in the guinea pig (10,39) and primates (104), highly developed in the hamster (93,97), and of intermediate prominence in the rat. The GnRH representation in olfactory and terminal nerve structures is particularly prominent in the musk shrew (*Suncus murinus*), a species that relies heavily on olfactory cues for successful reproduction (E. Rissman, unpublished data). In the rat (46,98), GnRH neurons are present in the accessory olfactory bulb, and these most likely contribute to some of the GnRH processes in this structure. In the hamster (97) and the neonatal rat (99), the main olfactory bulbs may contain their own small complement of GnRH neurons. The innervation of the bulbs in both species is derived, in part, from neurons in the nervus terminalis (see above). Inputs to the main olfactory bulb from cells in the anterior olfactory nucleus and anterior hippocampal rudiment are also likely. It has been suggested that olfactory bulb input may also originate from septal structures (46), but this has not been observed by other investigators (98). Within both the main and accessory bulbs, GnRH fibers ramify primarily in the external plexiform layer.

In the rat, additional groups of GnRH neurons associated with olfactory-related structures have been identified (46): (a) extending from the genu of the corpus callosum (anterior hippocampal rudiment) to the medial division of the anterior olfactory nucleus; (b) in the hippocampus, primarily in the indusium griseum, loosely dispersed between the genu and splenium of the corpus callosum; and (c) in Ammon's horn. A small number of cells are found dorsal to the corpus callosum and inner-

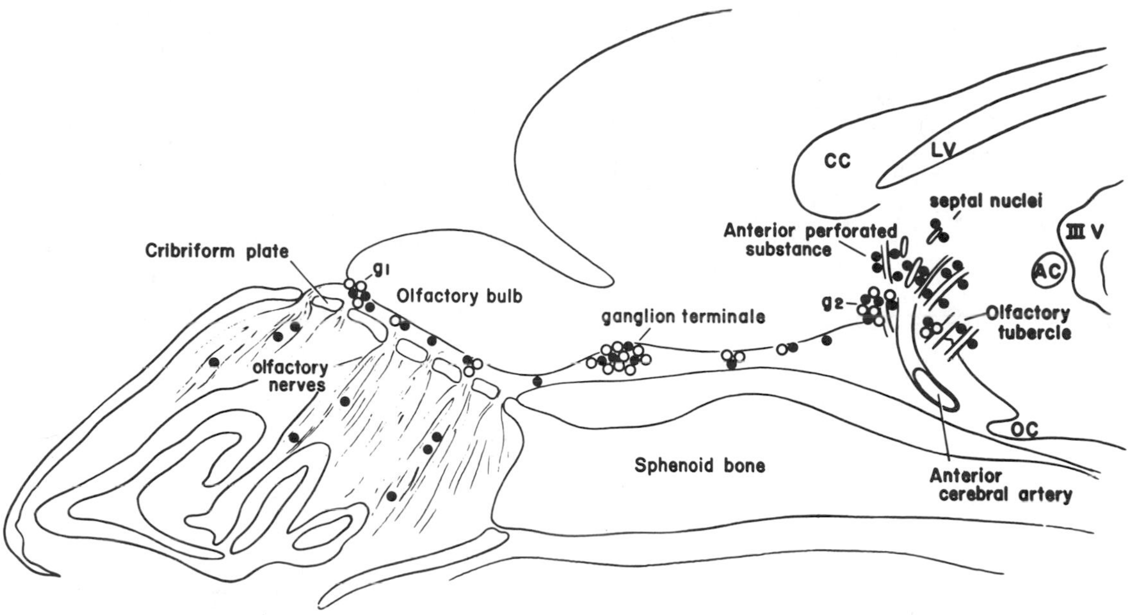

FIG. 7. The nervus terminalis of the guinea pig based on composite camera lucida drawings of a 45-day fetal guinea-pig brain. GnRH immunoreactive cell bodies (●) are seen throughout the course of this ganglionated nerve. In the periphery they accompany the olfactory and vomeronasal nerves below in cribriform plate. Intracranially, GnRH and nonimmunoreactive neurons (○) form ganglia along the ventromedial surface of the brain. The major ganglia are indicated. Neurons of the nervus terminalis penetrate the CNS along with the branches of the anterior cerebral artery and extend into the olfactory tubercle and septal nuclei. Not illustrated is the network of GnRH fibers that connects all portions of the nervus terminallis.

vate the cingulate cortex. The question still remains as to whether the GnRH neurons present in olfactory regions of the mammalian CNS play any direct role in reproduction. Change in levels of GnRH in the posterior aspect of the olfactory bulbs of female voles exposed to male urine has been reported (105), and these changes in the content could result from changes either in the nervus terminalis or in the CNS proper. Clearly, continued experimentation in this field is essential.

GnRH IN NONMAMMALIAN VERTEBRATES

The GnRH system is ubiquitous among vertebrates and, since the hormone has been identified in protochordates (106), it is probably evolutionarily ancient. Immunocytochemical studies of the GnRH system in nonmammalian vertebrates have contributed to our understanding of its role in the integration of external and internal cues in coordinating events surrounding reproduction. The following discussion, rather than attempting to describe the system in detail for various classes of vertebrate, illustrates the utility of nonmammalian models in the investigation of various aspects of its functional anatomy. For the descriptions of various GnRH systems see lamprey (107–109), elasmobranch (110–115), teleost (116–124), amphibian (125–136), reptile (136–139), and bird (140–148). Diagrams of GnRH systems in fish (Fig. 9) and amphibia (Fig. 10) are included for purposes of illustration.

Development

Species that develop outside the uterine environment provide more tractable models for experimental intervention than do mammals, but they have been surprisingly underutilized in studies of development of the GnRH system. Amphibians were the first species in which its extracranial origin was suggested (130,131). These species are especially attractive for such studies, as they contain chiefly the mammalian form of the GnRH molecule (149,150) and so may be viewed as having not diverged far from the mammalian ancestral line. Ablation studies in *Xenopus laevis* have revealed that absence of the olfactory placode results in global abnormalities in the development of the telencephalon (151). Evidence from anuran development suggests that both the secretory cells in the epithelial pituitary (pars distalis, pars intermedia, and pars tuberalis) and some portions of the preoptic area originate from cells in the anterior neural ridge and hence are placodally derived (152,153). It has recently been found that olfactory placodal ablation in amphibians prior to terminal nerve outgrowth results in

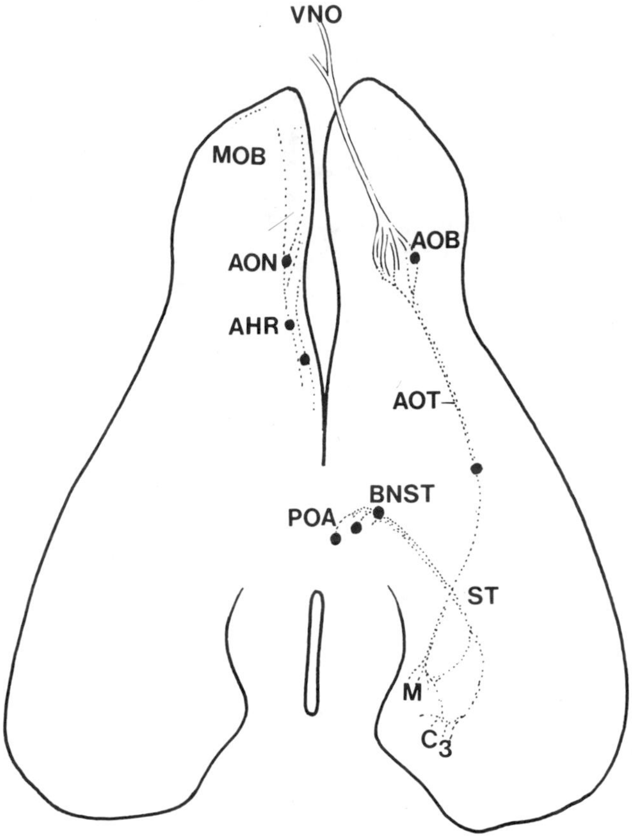

FIG. 8. A dorsal view of the rat brain showing a portion of the GnRH innervation of intracerebral olfactory-related structures. GnRH cells (dots) found in the anterior hippocampal rudiment (AHR) and anterior olfactory nucleus (AON) innervate the main olfactory bulb (MOB). Cells are present within the accessory olfactory bulb (AOB), and this structure also receives an input from nervus terminalis neurons (not illustrated). Cells in the preoptic area/bed nucleus of the stria terminalis project to the medial (M) and posteromedial cortical (C_3) amygdala, which may also receive a GnRH input from the accessory olfactory bulb. (BNST) Bed nucleus of stria terminalis; (ST) stria terminalis; (POA) preoptic area; (AOT) accessory olfactory terminalis; (VNO) vomeronasal organ.

the complete absence of septo-preoptic GnRH cells (154,155).

Integration of Olfactory and Visual Information: The Nervus Terminalis

The nervus terminalis, which has a GnRH component, projects peripherally to the retina and centrally to the preoptic and supracommissural nuclei of the area ventralis of the forebrain (124,156–158). This nerve is thus in a position to coordinate olfactory and visual cues. Demski et al. (160) have shown that injection of GnRH into the preoptic area of goldfish results in the sustained release of sperm; these workers have suggested that, under normal conditions, GnRH derived from the nervus terminalis may be released in this area. The GnRH neurons of the teleost nervus terminalis also contain the molluscan cardioexcitatory peptide FMRFamide (122). GnRH/FMRFamide axons are present in the goldfish inner nuclear and inner plexiform layers of the retina, which originate from the nervus terminalis (122). These peptides have quite dramatic effects on the "on–off" center, double-color-opponent ganglion cells, which has led Stell and his colleagues to postulate that olfactory-related cues influence the output of retinal ganglion cells that respond to color contrast. The implications for mammals are as yet unexplored, but GnRH fibers are found in both the optic and olfactory nerves in primates (104).

Extrahypothalamic Distribution

Appearance of GnRH-IR elements in broad regions of the CNS has been reported in various nonmammalian vertebrates (Figs. 9 and 10). An intriguing population of GnRH neurons in the midbrain with projections reaching to the cerebellum and spinal cord has been described in various species including fish (121,161–163), and amphibians (132,163). The GnRH neurons in this region are chiefly periventricular and may preferentially produce an alternate form of the GnRH molecule (164). The derivation of this neuronal population is unknown. Ablation of the olfactory placode in a urodele amphibian (*Ambystoma mexicanum*) results in bilateral loss of the olfactory system and the terminal nerve-septo-preoptic GnRH cells, although a magnocellular GnRH population in the posterior tuberculum (probably a homolog of the midbrain cells) develops completely normally (165). Most recently Rissman and colleagues (166) have found a similar cluster of GnRH neurons in the midbrain of the musk shrew (a primitive placental mammal). These cells can be identified with antibodies directed against mammalian GnRH (Benoit, LR-1) or chicken II GnRH (#675, R. P. Millar) but not chicken I (#1665, R. P. Millar). A second form of GnRH, with chicken II-like GnRH properties, occurs together with mammalian GnRH in the marsupial brain (167). The development and function of this "midbrain" GnRH system remain to be investigated.

GnRH fibers also occur within the ninth and tenth paravertebral sympathetic ganglia in the bullfrog (168,169); their physiology is discussed below.

Plasticity in Response to External Signals

Reversible effects on the anatomy of the GnRH system by external agents are well illustrated by the sex-reversing fish in which socially mediated behavioral cues trigger transformation between alternative reproductive

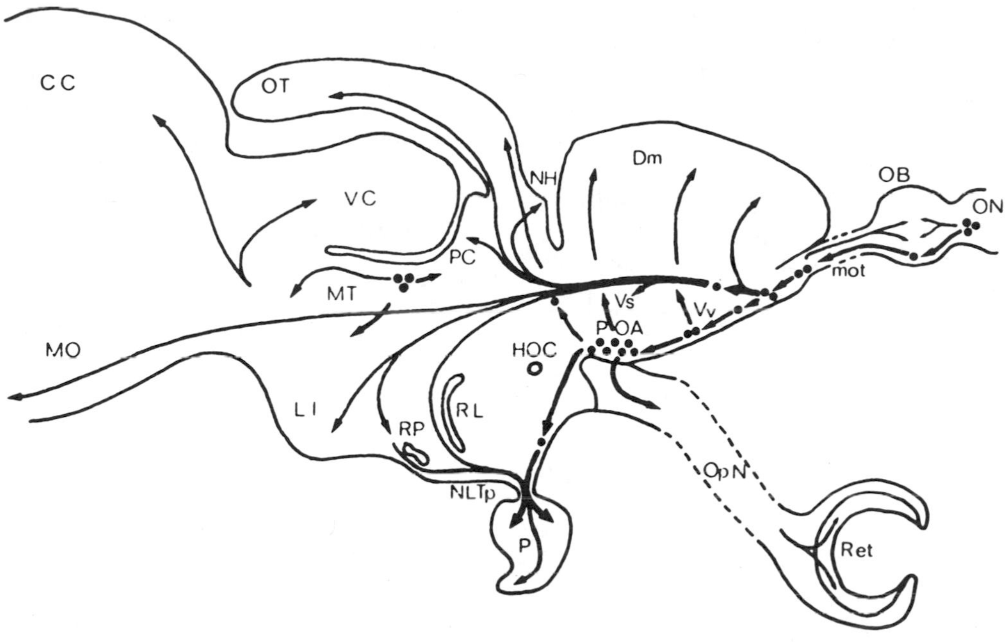

FIG. 9. Diagram summarizing the proposed organization of the GnRH systems in the brain of a teleost, the goldfish (*Crassius auratus*) as seen in longitudinal section, using an antibody to salmon GnRH. *Black circles* represent cell bodies, and *arrows* indicate their main projections. CC, corpus of cerebellum; DM, area dorsalis telencephali, pars medialis; HOC, horizontal commissure; LI, inferior lobe; MO, medulla oblongata; mot, median olfactory tract; MT, tegmentum of the midbrain; NH, habenular nucleus; NLTp, nucleus lateralis tuberis, pars posterior; OB, olfactory bulb; ON, olfactory nerve; OpN, optic nerve; OT, optic tectum; P, pituitary; PC, posterior commissure; POA, preoptic area; Ret, retina; RL, lateral recess; RP, posterior recess; VC, valvula of the cerebellum; Vs, area ventralis telencephali, pars supracommissuralis; Vv, area ventralis telencephali, pars ventralis. (From ref. 121, with permission.)

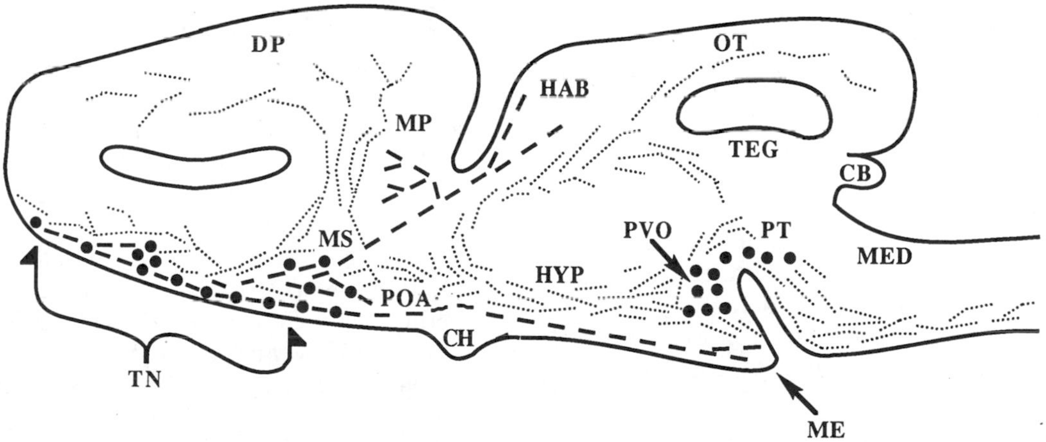

FIG. 10. Diagram of GnRH-immunoreactive neuronal systems in a urodele amphibian, the newt (*Taricha granulosa*). Parasagittal section, illustrating distribution of GnRH-ir cell bodies (*filled circles*), and fiber pathways. Antiserum selective for mGnRH labeled neurons in the anterior forebrain, including the terminal nerve, medial septum, anterior preoptic area, and a restricted set of projections to the medial pallium, habenula, and median eminence (*dashed lines*). Antiserum selective for cGnRHII labeled cell bodies in the paraventricular organ and posterior tuberculum, and a diffuse system of fibers to most major brain areas (*dotted lines*). CB, cerebellum; CH, optic chiasm; DP, dorsal pallium; HAB, habenula; HYP, hypothalamus; ME, median eminence; MED, medulla; MP, medial pallium; MS, medial septum; OB, olfactory bulb; OT, optic tectum; POA, preoptic area; PT, posterior tuberculum; PV, paraventricular organ; TEG, midbrain tegmentum; TN, terminal nerve. (From ref. 165, with permission.)

morphs. The change from primary to terminal phase in males is accompanied by a twofold increase in the number of GnRH neurons in the preoptic area (170). Changes in numbers of immunoreactive neurons have also been documented in the platyfish (171,172). Another remarkable response to external cues has been described in courting doves. Following 2 hours of courtship behavior, cells immunoreactive for GnRH, but with the characteristics of mast cells, appear within the habenula, apparently having invaded the brain from the ventricular surface (173).

Modes of Secretion

GnRH neurons project to regions outside the blood–brain barrier, primarily to the median eminence and secondarily to the other circumventricular organs, in particular, the OVLT, as well as to sites within the CNS. That their processes can also reach directly into the cerebral ventricular system has been particularly well demonstrated in the lamprey. King et al. (174) described prodigious GnRH projections across the ependyma that at the EM level appear to open directly to the ventricle. This is of interest because GnRH can be measured within the cerebrospinal fluid (CSF) of mammals (175,176). Such secretion probably contributes to the GnRH that reaches the anterior pituitary (176,177). Furthermore, GnRH within the CSF may ultimately reach the systemic circulation; however, it is not known whether GnRH of CNS origin is physiologically significant in the peripheral organs in which the GnRH receptor is known to exist (e.g., gonads, thymus).

Fibers of a single GnRH neuron may project to multiple sites both within and outside the CNS. This is dramatically illustrated by intracellular injection studies in the dwarf gourami (159). It has been shown in the rat that virtually all GnRH neurons secrete outside the blood–brain barrier (70). These data suggest that the secretory events at various sites of release from processes of an individual GnRH neuron may be separately controlled. It follows that influences at the level of the cell body may primarily be concerned with regulation of synthesis of the prohormone and/or processing of the peptide.

GnRH as a Neuromodulator

Some novel roles for GnRH have been suggested based on in vitro studies in amphibians and fish. Intra- and extracellular recording in the terminal nerve GnRH system in dwarf gourami has revealed endogenous activities of either slow regular beating (1 to 6 Hz) or bursting patterns depending on the sexual maturity of the fish (159). Bullfrog preganglionic C cells use ACh and GnRH as cotransmitters (178). GnRH elicits a late, slow excitatory postsynaptic potential (LS-EPSP) (168,179). The cGnRH-II form is most potent in producing this effect. GnRH has also been shown to increase plasma catecholamines in bullfrogs (180) and may function as a growth hormone-releasing factor in fish as well (181).

CYTOLOGY OF GnRH NEURONS

For neurons on which the continuation of the species depends the morphology is surprisingly simple. In most species, the vast majority of GnRH neurons are oval or fusiform in shape, with a maximum diameter of 10 to 20 μm. Simple, unbranched dendritic processes extend from one or both poles of the cell. Axons emerge either directly from the cell body (Fig. 11A) or from a dendrite, and the dendrite may assume a beaded appearance and become axonal. Although this simple cell is found in all species examined to date, it is now clear, from work using thick unembedded sections, that some of these neurosecretory cells have a greater range of shape and complexity than previously appreciated. In the rat, two major categories of cells have been recognized: those with a smooth contour, as described above, and those with a more ragged outline (182–185). This latter subset may be further subdivided by the number of spinous processes (186). It has been suggested (184,185) that such thorny cells receive a denser innervation than smooth cells, but this was not confirmed by quantitative ultrastructural experiments (187). Even more complex shapes have been seen in the sheep (40; Fig. 11B) and rhesus monkey (43; Fig. 11C). In the former, especially in the anestrous state, GnRH cells are larger than those reported for other species and possess a complex, branching dendritic arbor. In the cow, alterations in the dendritic arbor have been quantified, and in this species GnRH neurons with the longest and most numerous processes are found in cycling rather than anestrous (postpartum) states (188).

GnRH neurons have a large, centrally placed nucleus and a thin rim of cytoplasm, the latter extending into the tapering cones of the principal dendrites. Nuclei contain one or two large nucleoli, and the nuclear envelope is frequently indented. The cytoplasm contains many stacks of rough endoplasmic reticulum, one or more prominent Golgi stacks, and neurosecretory granules. Some of these neurons are ciliated (187,189). Immunoreactivity is frequently associated with some, but not all, cisternae of the rough endoplasmic reticulum (see ref. 5) as well as with neurosecretory granules. The localization of antigen within the Golgi apparatus is clearly dependent on the antibody utilized (5). It is evident from this latter study that the GnRH precursor moves through all compartments of the protein synthetic and packaging apparatus.

SYNAPTIC INPUT AND OUTPUT

Neurosecretory Terminals

In ultrastructural immunocytochemical studies of the median eminence, GnRH is found in membrane-bound granules within axon profiles and neurosecretory terminals (51,52,86,87). Granules range in size from 40 to 130 nm. Some of the variability in size of the granules may stem from the location of the granule (i.e., cell body, axon, terminus) (52,87) or from the difficulty in measuring granules in material with ill-preserved biological membranes. Similar granules have been found in the GnRH terminals of the OVLT (88,89) and subfornical organ (90).

GnRH GnRH

Examination of light microscopic material suggested that several types of GnRH–GnRH interactions are possible (195), and ultrastructural studies now support this hypothesis. Axosomatic and axodendritic synapses between GnRH elements have now been reported in the rat (196,197) and rhesus monkey (198). We have recently undertaken a three-dimensional reconstruction of GnRH neurons in the rhesus monkey and rat. Here we have concentrated on cells that at the light microscopic level, lie in close proximity (199) (Fig. 11C). By tracing each cell of the pair through over 150 serial ultrathin sections, GnRH–GnRH interactions can be documented. In addition to synaptic interactions that occur between neurons, the serial reconstruction also strongly suggests that some neurons are connected by cytoplasmic bridges, forming a syncytium (Fig. 12). When light microscopic sections are examined and all pairs of tightly apposed cells are counted, approximately 5% of GnRH neurons in the female rat and 8% in the female monkey are so joined. It is possible that the synaptic connections and other complex interactions between GnRH neurons as well as between GnRH neurons and their nonimmunoreactive neighbors (see below) form a part of the substrate for the coordination of the GnRH signal.

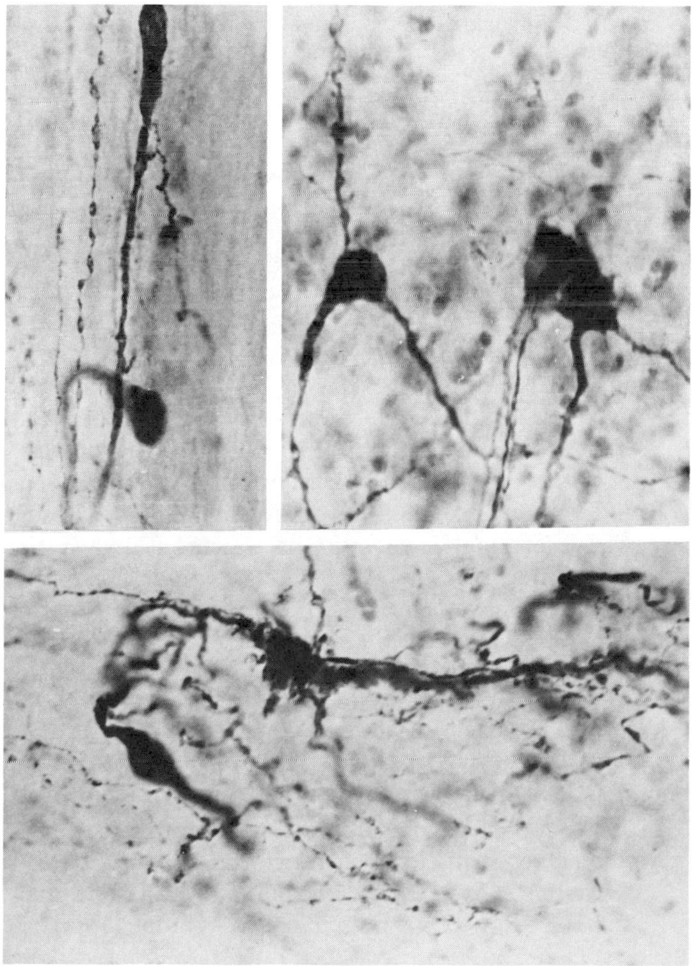

FIG. 11. Three fields showing GnRH neurons of differing morphology. In **A**, two very simple, smooth cells from the vertical limb of the diagonal band of Broca of the rhesus monkey are shown. The arrow indicates the point of emergence of the axon of this cell. In **B**, three cells (each indicated by an arrow) from the ewe preoptic area are shown. These cells have numerous primary dendrites and a more triangular appearance. The two cells on the right appear to be in close contact. Ultrastructural studies (M. N. Lehman, *unpublished results*) indicate that glial processes separate these neurons from each other. In **C**, taken from the ventral preoptic area of the rhesus monkey, two neurons are in the field of view. On the left is a relatively smooth surfaced cell with primary dendrites extending from each pole. On the right, oriented horizontal to the surface of the brain, is a thorny cell with many irregularities on the surface. This cell is also in close proximity to many GnRH fibers in the vicinity.

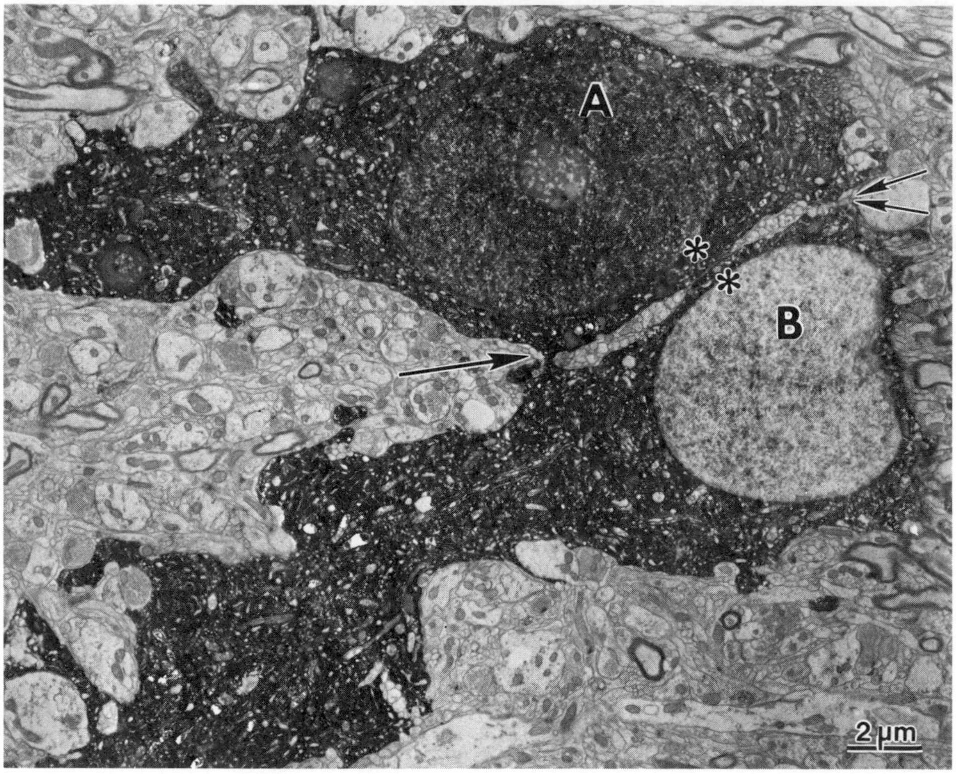

FIG. 12. Two GnRH neurons (*A* and *B*) from the preoptic area of a male rat demonstrated by ICC using LR1 antibody and DAB as the chromogen. This micrograph is one level of section from a complete serial-section reconstruction of this pair of cells. There is an intercellular bridge at the region indicated by the *large arrow.* The region indicated by two *smaller arrows* was found to have two additional bridges in other planes of section. In the region of close apposition between the two cells (*asterisks*), there were no areas of confluence, nor were there any indications of gap junctional modifications in the intercellular space.

Given the significance of such synaptic interactions in our eventual understanding of the organization and regulation of the GnRH neurosecretory system, the strictest morphological criteria for a synapse should be applied when discussing GnRH–GnRH interactions or synaptic input to GnRH cells and their processes. The criteria include (a) the presence of a well-defined synaptic cleft, (b) the clustering of synaptic vesicles in the presynaptic element, and (c) membrane specializations on the pre- and postsynaptic sides.

Among the possible sites of GnRH interactions not yet studied in sufficient detail are those that may occur among axons along the pathway to the median eminence or within the neurohemal structure itself. In the hamster (200), GnRH axons travel in tight bundles through the anterior aspect of the arcuate–median eminence before diverging toward the lateral aspects over the tuberoinfundibular sulci. Are there interactions within such bundles? Are there axoaxonic contacts between axons near their terminus? These are among the critical anatomic questions whose resolution might help in unraveling the mechanism by which GnRH release is coordinated.

Synaptic Input

Recent studies have concentrated on the synaptic input to GnRH cells (184,185,196,201). With double-label techniques various neurotransmitter and peptidergic synapses have been identified on GnRH neurons and dendrites (Fig. 13). Although tyrosine hydroxylase (the rate-limiting enzyme in catecholamine biosynthesis)-positive terminals innervate GnRH neurons in the rat, it is surprising that these are neither noradrenergic nor adrenergic terminals (202,203). The synaptic boutons containing TH detected on GnRH neurons are presumably dopaminergic (202). Dopamine β-hydroxylase (DBH) and PNMT terminals contact neighboring preoptic area cells and processes that are not GnRH positive (W.-P. Chen, J. W. Witkin, and A.-J. Silverman, unpublished observations). Modulation of GnRH release by other catecholamine systems must take place indirectly or at the level of the axons (204,205).

Serotonin (206) and β-endorphin (207,208) terminals contact GnRH cells and their dendrites in the rat preoptic area. β-Endorphin synapses are also found in contact

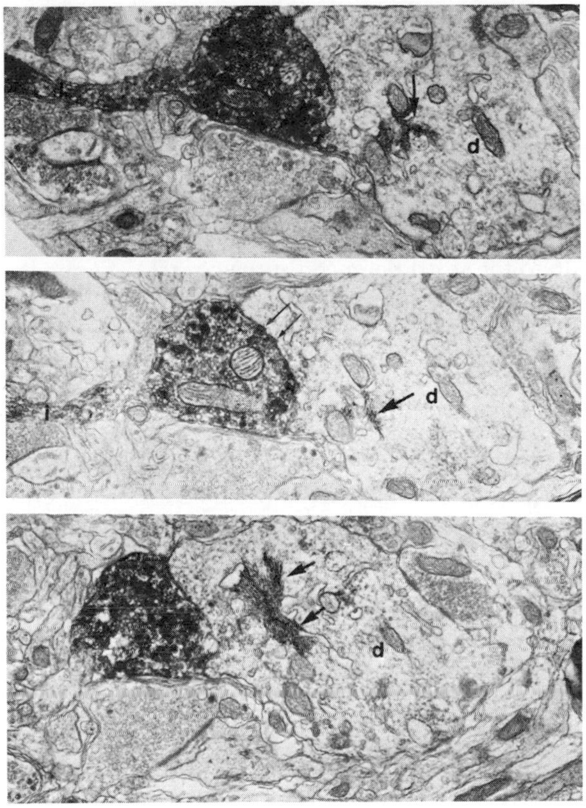

FIG. 13. Example of a double-label immunocytochemical procedure at the ultrastructural level used to determine the nature of the synaptic input to GnRH neurons. Three ultrathin sections through a presynaptic element are illustrated. With 3,3′-diaminobenzidine (DAB) used to form a diffuse, flocculent precipitate, a β-endorphin-positive terminal is identified as impinging on a GnRH-positive dendrite (d). The GnRH immunoreactivity was visualized with tetramethylbenzidine (TMB). The TMB reaction product is crystalline (*large arrows*) and is most prominent in the lowermost photomicrograph. The *small arrows* in the middle micrograph show the region of the synaptic cleft. (From Chen et al., ref. 203, with permission.)

with GnRH neurons in the cynomolgus monkey (198); CRH (209) and glutamic acid decarboxylase (indicative of GABA terminals) (202,210) as well as vasopressin (211) and glutamate (212) terminals all have been found in contact with GnRH neurons. Both the morphology and content of these various synapses suggest that the GnRH is modulated by excitatory and inhibitory transmitters.

It is now appreciated that the density of innervation of GnRH neurons cells is considerably lower than that observed for other preoptic area neurons. Our laboratory has confirmed this in two ways: by morphometric analysis of randomly selected electron micrographs and by serial section reconstructions as mentioned above. In measurements of approximately 1000 μm^2 of tissue, 0.38% of GnRH dendritic membrane was in synaptic apposition, whereas 6.6% of non-GnRH dendritic membrane was occupied (213). Since the lengths of synaptic specializations did not vary, these measurements indicate that the absolute number of inputs to GnRH cells is smaller than that to their neighbors. In this same study, 56 separate randomly selected profiles of 11 GnRH neurons revealed only seven axosomatic synapses. When serial reconstructions involving over 150 ultrathin sections were made through both rat and rhesus monkey GnRH neurons, only five to seven synaptic terminals were found on individual cells (199), confirming the work using random section analysis.

Morphometric analyses can also be used to determine the relative importance of a particular input to the GnRH cell and to look for patterns that differ by sex or by cytoarchitectonic area. For example, β-endorphin input, which has been shown by this method to be sexually dimorphic in the rodent (208), is approximately 9% to soma and 10% to the dendrites in males. GABA terminals make up an additional 10% (210).

Quantitative studies have also revealed that dramatic changes can occur in the input to the GnRH cell body with different physiological states. For example, the number of synapses and the absolute amount of synaptic apposition per unit of membrane is increased from youth to middle age and from middle age to old age in the virgin male rat (213) but not the retired breeder (214). This suggests that the changes that occur in the CNS vis-à-vis the aging process need not be degenerative and may depend on experiences that occur in the individual's lifetime. The increase that occurs in aging males may reflect an increase in the ratio of inhibitory inputs, but if so, they are not GABA terminals (see ref. 210). Such changes in synaptic input are not all age related. Alterations in glial ensheathment and synaptic membrane apposition can also be found in female primates that differ in endocrine condition (215).

GnRH Synaptic Output

In addition to receiving an input, GnRH neurons also form synapses. This was first suggested in studies by Krisch in the rat preoptic area (182) and has now been demonstrated conclusively in the preoptic area of the guinea pig (216,217) and the rat (196,197). These axodendritic synapses were characterized by a well-defined synaptic cleft as well as accumulations of both large immunoreactive granules and small lucent nonimmunoreactive vesicles. In the guinea pig (216) there was also evidence for other varieties of local circuit interactions, including dendrodendritic and somatodendritic interactions (Fig. 14), with the GnRH component participating as either the pre- or postsynaptic element. GnRH synapses have also been observed in the accessory olfactory bulb of the hamster (218), and it is likely that examina-

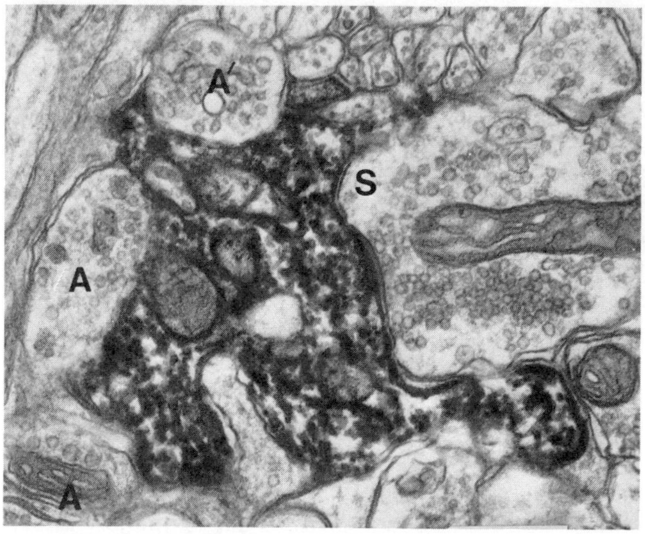

FIG 14. An example of synaptic input to GnRH neurons in the guinea pig preoptic area. This is an axodendritic input (*S* indicates a presynaptic element). Note the synaptic cleft and the clustering of round, clear synaptic vesicles. Axon profiles (*A* and *A′*) cannot be said to be in synaptic contact with the GnRH dendrite, since no synaptic specializations are seen in this plane. ×35,000.

tion of other extrahypothalamic sites will reveal additional evidence for such interactions.

DO GnRH NEURONS CONTAIN OTHER NEUROPEPTIDES OR NEUROTRANSMITTERS?

In GnRH neurons in the preoptic area of the guinea pig, a second peptide that cross-reacts with an antiserum directed against $ACTH_{17-39}$ has been identified (219, 220). Similarly, β-endorphin-like immunoreactivity has been reported in human GnRH neurons in both the preoptic area and arcuate nucleus (221). Given the importance of opiate peptides in the regulation of gonadotropin secretion, these observations need to be extended and confirmed. Proof that the proopiomelanocortin gene is transcribed in these cells must await analysis combining in situ hybridization and immunocytochemistry (cf. ref. 222). Whether the colocalization of these peptides and GnRH is common to all species is not known.

Recently two additional neuropeptides have been conclusively identified in GnRH neurons of the rat. These include delta-sleep-inducing peptide (223,224) and galanin (225,226). Most exciting is the fact that the galanin system in this species is highly sexually dimorphic, with double-labeled cells being much more prominent in the female (227). Modulation of this peptide in GnRH neurons can easily be demonstrated over the course of the estrous cycle and/or in response to hormonal status (227).

RELATIONSHIP OF GnRH NEURONS TO ESTRADIOL-CONCENTRATING NEURONS

Gonadal steroids are the major regulatory substances controlling the release of gonadotropins. They also play an essential role during the perinatal period in the development of the anatomic, behavioral, and physiological sexual dimorphisms of the CNS, including those that relate to the sex differences in the control of gonadotropin secretion. Presumably these substances act within the CNS as well as at the level of the pituitary via the nuclear receptors visualized by autoradiography and more recently by immunocytochemistry. If gonadal hormones regulate the synthesis, processing, or release of GnRH within the CNS (see section on in situ hybridization below), one might have predicted that the GnRH neuron would contain estradiol receptors. It was therefore surprising that (106) the neurons in the rat preoptic area that concentrate estradiol (as determined by autoradiography following accumulation of [^{3}H]estradiol) and those that contain GnRH do not overlap. Of 435 GnRH cells counted, only one doubly labeled cell was found. With the advent of a monoclonal antibody to the estrogen receptor (H-222) (229), this observation was confirmed using double-label immunocytochemistry (230–232). This suggests that regulation of the GnRH neuron by gonadal steroids occurs mainly, if not entirely, via interneurons. Recently, it has been suggested that GnRH axons terminate on estrogen-receptor-containing neuronal cell bodies in the medial preoptic area of the guinea pig (233). This interesting observation awaits further confirmation.

IN SITU HYBRIDIZATION

It is quite clear that alterations in gonadal hormone levels have a profound effect on the release of gonadotropins. The best studied are the postcastration rise in circulating LH and FSH in both sexes and the preovulatory surge in the female in response to increasing levels of estradiol. It has been a tenet of reproductive biology that these conditions would also produce an increase in GnRH synthesis and release (234), but data to support this hypothesis have been difficult to obtain. Measurements of GnRH in portal blood or at the level of anterior pituitary following castration have produced widely varying results in the several laboratories that have studied this issue. Increased release of GnRH at the time of the LH surge has been documented in several species (176,235–238).

Since the cloning of the gene (4,7) that encodes the GnRH precursor, in situ hybridization procedures have been used (239) to localize GnRH neurons, and attempts have been made to determine the alterations in GnRH gene expression under varying hormonal conditions. Perhaps because of the heterogeneity of the GnRH cell population and the apparent redundancy that is a feature of the system (vide supra), the results obtained from in situ hybridization are inconsistent from laboratory to laboratory.

As with immunocytochemistry, there are several ways to quantify the anatomic data obtained from in situ hybridization. The number of cells with detectable levels of message can be counted and/or an estimate of copy number obtained by counting silver grains per cell. In the latter instance, which is generally thought to be a more sensitive assay, one is faced with the problem of where to draw cell boundaries when grain counts are made. Considerable heterogeneity in grains per cell at the same level of the CNS have been noted (240) and may be analogous to the finding that *fos*-expressing cells and non-*fos*-containing neurons lie next to each other. In situ hybridization is also a static technique that provides information on the level of message at one particular moment. It does not speak to current synthesis (although this is less true if probes to hnRNA are used), alterations in rates of translation, or stability of message.

In situ hybridization studies have confirmed the fact the GnRH-producing neurons are a very small population, numbering about 1200 to 1600 in the rodent (241). A particularly elegant study using combined immunocytochemistry and in situ hybridization has also confirmed this finding in the primate (242; also see ref. 243).

Studies from several laboratories suggest that castration of adult male or female rats leads either to no change in GnRH gene expression compared to the intact animal (241,244) or to a slight suppression of message content (245,246). Similar results have been obtained by molecular biological techniques (247). In contrast, Toranzo et al. (248) have reported that 2 weeks after castration GnRH message levels are elevated over intact controls.

The effect of gonadal steroid replacement following ovariectomy is also controversial. Several groups have found that message is increased by estrogen (245–247,249) or testosterone replacement (250), but others have been unable to confirm these observations. Instead, a decline in message below that obtained in ovariectomized, nonreplaced animals (248,251) or no change (252) has been observed. It is possible that the alterations in GnRH gene expression in response to steroids occur within a very small population of cells (251).

It now seems likely that some of the discrepancies may be related to the time of day at which animals (rats) are killed (cf. ref. 253). When estradiol is administered in such a way as to produce an LH surge, then GnRH message appears to increase late on the afternoon of proestrus (240,254). Although circadian patterns of gonadotropin secretion may help explain differences among female groups, they do not account for the variations seen among laboratories as regards effects of castration and testosterone replacement in males.

As with estrogen replacement regimens, whether or not an alteration in message levels is detected during the natural estrous cycle apparently depends on the precise time at which the assay is performed. Using different methods of analysis and focusing on different cell populations, both Zoeller et al. (255) and Park et al. (240) suggest that GnRH mRNA is low on the morning of proestrus, and this has been confirmed by Malik et al. (241). Transcription appears to increase (perhaps in a segment of the GnRH cell population; see ref. 255) on the afternoon of proestrus, though the two groups who have examined this disagree as to the duration of the elevation. It should be noted that GnRH peptide levels may be altered rapidly and profoundly over a short time course (256), with considerable individual variation in a cycling population such that investigators may be unable to obtain statistically significant information on a rapidly changing phenomenon. This has been highlighted by our recent immunocytochemical experiments, which examine biosynthesis of GnRH precursor at different times of the cycle (A.-J. Silverman and J. W. Witkin, submitted). It is clear that cells actively translating message and those that are quiescent can be situated side by side.

THE *hpg* MOUSE AND THE USE OF CNS IMPLANTS TO REVERSE AN ENDOCRINE DEFICIENCY

The hypogonadal mutant (*hpg*) mouse, discovered at Harwell, England, has an infantile reproductive tract as a result of a deficiency in the GnRH peptide (257). Molecular biological data indicate that the genetic defect is a deletion in the mRNA of two exons (258). Immunocytochemical analysis indicates that no neurons in the homozygous *hpg* brain produce GnRH (259), though the cells are still present and can be detected by in situ hybridization for the truncated gene product (260).

The endocrine deficiency of the *hpg* mouse can, at least in part, be overcome in adults by the implantation of normal fetal or neonatal septal–preoptic area tissue into the third ventricle. This procedure results in the recovery of testicular and seminal vesicle weights and the onset of spermatogenesis in males (261) and increased ovarian and uterine weights in females (262). Some females can show a reflex ovulation in response to mating and become pregnant (263). Others respond to a steroid signal (264). Some animals can ovulate in response to either mating or progesterone injections (264). Pulsatile release of gonadotropins is maintained following graft placement in both sexes (265,266), but the negative feedback of gonadal steroids is absent (267). These endocrinological data lead to several hypotheses. Among these are

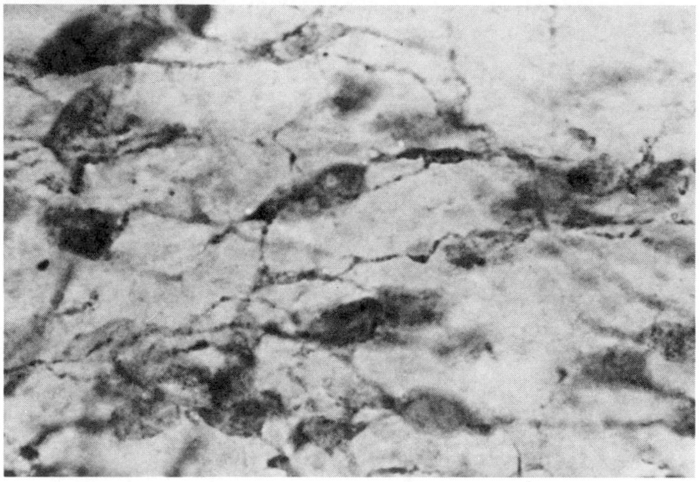

FIG. 15. An immortalized cell line, designated GT-1, that synthesizes and secretes GnRH can be used to reverse the hypogonadism of the mutant *hpg* mouse (269). Illustrated here are GT-1 cells injected into a host *hpg* brain and allowed to survive for approximately 60 days. Many of the tumorigenic cells assume a neuronal morphology and elaborate axonal processes.

(a) that mice, which normally never display a reflex ovulation, retain the neural circuitry to do so and that this circuitry can access the implanted GnRH neurons; (2) that the circuitry for sensory- and steroid-induced release must be different, since grafted animals can show one without showing the other; and (3) that the capacity to maintain a tonic, pulsatile release of LH in either sex is not dependent on the negative feedback regulation of gonadal steroids; but, again, each of these phenomena is subserved by a different neuronal system. Furthermore, the absence of both the postgonadectomy rise in LH and negative feedback strongly support the hypothesis that these phenomena are mediated (in this species) at the level of the brain and not the pituitary.

For the display and/or maintainance of all of these reproductive behaviors, GnRH neurons must survive within the graft, and their axons must exit from the graft and innervate the host median eminence (see ref. 80). Immunocytochemical analyses of the transplants have provided the astounding information that reproductive function can be subserved by a very small number of GnRH cells as long as their axons reach the portal capillaries in the median eminence. The cells visualized by immunocytochemistry in females showing induced ovulations, successful pregnancy, and maternal behavior (263) ranged from one to 16, and immunoreactive fibers were found in the host primarily in the arcuate nucleus and median eminence. Since the studies were carried out on thick sections that exceeded the diameter of the GnRH neuron, it is possible that the number of cells was underestimated by two- to threefold. Even so, such numbers are far fewer than the estimated 500 to 1500 cells in the septal–preoptic–hypothalamic continuum that innervates the median eminence in normal animals. It is possible that the neurosecretory unit—that minimum number of cells that can support at least some aspects of reproductive function—can consist of very few cells. The fact that GnRH axons did not innervate any additional targets strongly suggests that only the GnRH in the portal blood is essential for reproduction. Is it possible that in the normal animal, only a very small number of cells at any one time drives the pituitary–gonadal axis (*c-fos* data), and the remainder of cells provide a redundancy that protects the individual in case of neuronal cell death? Do different subpopulations provide for tonic versus bursting release of LH? Such intriguing questions may soon be solved by combining anatomic and physiological approaches to the problems of CNS regulation of reproduction.

GT-1 Cells

By transgenic techniques an immortalized cell line that produces GnRH, known as GT-1, has been made (268). *In vitro* these cells proliferate and secrete the decapeptide (269,270). They can also assume, under appropriate *in vitro* conditions, a neuron-like shape and form synaptic interactions with each other (269). Within the CNS of the *hpg* mouse (Fig. 16) these cells migrate broadly and can secrete sufficient bioactive peptide to reverse the hypogonadism (271). Interestingly, the cells do not home for the preoptic area, and their axons do not target the median eminence (271). In the original transgenic animals the GnRH axons also could not find their target (272). It is hoped that this cell type, particularly when temperature-sensitive mutants become available, will help resolve many issues in the regulation of GnRH biosynthesis, secretion (273), and cellular differentiation.

ACKNOWLEDGMENTS

The research for this chapter has been supported by USPHS grants HD 10665 and DK 42323 (A.J.S.) and AG 05366 (J.W.W.); I.L. has been supported by the Benin Foundation. We would also like to thank Mrs. Kate Rosa for assistance with the photomicrography.

REFERENCES

1. Amoss M, Burges R, Blackwell R, Vale W, Fellows R, Guillemin R. Purification, amino acid composition and *N*-terminus of the hypothalamic luteinizing hormone releasing hormone factor (LRF) of ovine origin. *Biochem Biophys Res Commun* 1971;44:205–210.
2. Schally AV, Arimura A, Baker Y, et al. Isolation and properties of the FSH and LH-releasing hormone. *Biochem Biophys Res Commun* 1971;43:393–399.
3. Matsuo H, Baba Y, Nau RMG, Arimura A, Schally AV. Structure of the porcine LH and FSH releasing hormone. I. Proposed amino acid sequence. *Biochem Biophys Res Commun* 1971;43:1334–1339.
4. Seeburg PH, Adelman JP. Characterization of cDNA for precursor of human luteinizing hormone releasing hormone. *Nature* 1984;311:666–668.
5. Silverman AJ, Witkin JW, Millar RP. Light and electron microscopic immunocytochemical analysis of antibodies directed against GnRH and its precursor in hypothalamic neurons. *J Histochem Cytchem* 1990;38:803–813.
6. Sternberger LA. *Immunocytochemistry.* Englewood Cliffs, NJ: Prentice-Hall; 1974:129–171.
7. Adelman JP, Mason AJ, Hayflick JS, Seeburg PH. Isolation of the gene and hypothalamic cDNA for the common precursor of gonadotropin releasing hormone and prolactin inhibiting factor in human and rat. *Proc Natl Acad Sci USA* 1986;83:179–183.
8. Chesselet M-F. *In Situ Hybridization Histochemistry.* Boston: CRC Press; 1990.
9. Jennes L. Prenatal development of the gonadotropin-releasing hormone-containing system in the rat brain. *Brain Res* 1989;482:97–108.
10. Schwanzel-Fukuda M, Robinson JA, Silverman AJ. The fetal development of the luteinizing hormone-releasing hormone (LHRH) neuronal system of the guinea pig brain. *Brain Res Bull* 1981;7:293–315.
11. Wray S, Nieburgs A, Elkabes S. Spatiotemporal cell expression of luteinizing hormone-releasing hormone in the prenatal mouse: evidence for an embryonic origin in the olfactory placode. *Dev Brain Res* 1989;46:309–318.
12. Wray S, Grant P, Gainer H. Evidence that cells expressing luteinizing hormone-releasing hormone mRNA are derived from progenitor cells in the olfactory placode. *Proc Natl Acad Sci USA* 1989;86:8132–8136.
13. Schwanzel-Fukuda M, Pfaff DW. Origin of luteinizing hormone-releasing hormone neurons. *Nature* 1989;338:161–163.
14. Sullivan KA, Silverman AJ. Ontogeny of gonadotropin-releasing hormone (GnRH) neurons in the chick. *Soc Neurosci Abstr* 1991;17:427.
15. Norgren RB, Lehman MN. Neurons that migrate from the olfactory epithelium in the chick express luteinizing hormone-releasing hormone. *Endocrinology* 1991;128:1676–1678.
16. Murakami S, Seki T, Wakabayashi K, Arai Y. The ontogeny of luteinizing hormone-releasing hormone (LHRH) producing neurons in the chick embryo: possible evidence for migrating LHRH neurons from the olfactory epithelium expressing a highly polysialated neural cell adhesion molecule. *Neurosci Res* 1991;12:421–431.
17. Daikoku-Ishido H, Okamura Y, Yanaihara N, Daikoku S. Development of the hypothalamic luteinizing hormone-releasing hormone-containing neuron system in the rat: in vivo and in transplantation studies. *Dev Biol* 1990;140:374–387.
18. Ronnekleiv OK, Resko JA. Ontogeny of gonadotropin-releasing hormone-containing neurons in early fetal development of rhesus macaques. *Endocrinology* 1990;126:498–511.
19. Hoffman GE, Finch CE. LHRH neurons in the female C57BL/6J mouse brain during reproductive aging: no loss up to middle age. *Neurobiol Aging* 1986;7:45–48.
20. Cuschieri A, Bannister LH. The development of the olfactory mucosa in the mouse: light microscopy. *J Anat* 1975;119:277–286.
21. Chuah MI, Au C. Olfactory Schwann cells are derived from precursor cells in the olfactory epithelium. *J Neurosci Res* 1991;29:172–180.
22. Doucette R. Glial influence on axonal growth in the primary olfactory system. *Glia* 1990;3:433–449.
23. Marin-Padilla M, Amieva-BMR. Early neurogenesis of the mouse olfactory nerve: Golgi and electron microscopic studies. *J Comp Neurol* 1989;288:339–352.
24. Mendoza AS, Breipohl W, Miragall F. Cell migration from the chick olfactory placode: a light and electron microscopic study. *J Embryol Exp Morphol* 1982;69:47–59.
25. Schwanzel-Fukuda M, Bick D, Pfaff DW. Luteinizing hormone-releasing hormone (LHRH)-expressing cells do not migrate normally in an inherited hypogonadal (Kallmann) syndrome. *Mol Brain Res* 1989;6:311–326.
26. Eurenius L, Jarskar R. Electron microscope studies of the development of the external zone of the mouse median eminence. *Z Zellforsch* 1971;122:488–502.
27. Livne I, Silverman AJ, Gibson MJ. Reversal of reproductive deficiency in the *hpg* male mouse by neonatal androgenization. *Biol Reprod* 1992;47:561—567.
28. Livne I, Gibson MJ, Silverman AJ. Biochemical differentiation and intercellular interactions of migratory gonadotropin releasing hormone cells in the mouse. *Dev Biol* [*in press*].
29. Barry J, DuBois MP, Poulain P. LRF producing cells of the mammalian hypothalamus. *Z Zellforsch* 1973;146:351–366.
30. Barry J, DuBois MP, Poulain P, Leonardelli J. Caracterisation et topographie des neurones hypothalamiques immunoreactifs avec des anticorps anti-LRF de synthese. *C R Acad Sci (Paris)* 1973;276:3191–3193.
31. Barry J. Immunohistochemical localization of hypothalamic hormones (especially LRF) at the light microscopic level. In: Labne F, Meites J, Pelletier G, eds. *Hypothalamus and Endocrine Functions.* New York: Plenum Press; 1976:451–471.
32. Barry J. Immunohistochemistry of luteinizing hormone releasing hormone-producing neurons of vertebrates. *Annu Rev Cytol* 1979;60:179–219.
33. Sternberger LA, Hoffman GE. Immunocytology of luteinizing hormone releasing hormone. *Neuroendocrinology* 1978;25:111–128.
34. Silverman AJ, Krey LC, Zimmerman EA. A comparative study of the luteinizing hormone releasing hormone (LHRH) neuronal networks in mammals. *Biol Reprod* 1979;20:98–110.
35. Krey LC, Silverman AJ. Luteinizing hormone releasing hormone. In: Krieger DT, Brownstein M, Martin J, eds. *Brain Peptides.* New York: John Wiley & Sons; 1983:687–709.
36. Schwanzel-Fukuda M, Fadem BH, Garcia MS, Pfaff DW. Immunocytochemical localization of luteinizing hormone-releasing hormone (LHRH) in the brain and nervus terminalis of the adult and early neonatal gray short-tailed opossum (*Monodelphis domestica*). *J Comp Neurol* 1988;276:44–60.
37. Barry J, DuBois MP. Immunoreactive LRF neurosecretory pathways in mammals. *Acta Anat* 1976;94:497–503.
38. Silverman AJ. Distribution of luteinizing hormone releasing hormone (LHRH) in the guinea pig brain. *Endocrinology* 1976;99:30–41.
39. Schwanzel-Fukuda M, Silverman AJ. The nervus terminalis of the guinea pig: A new luteinizing hormone releasing hormone neuronal system. *J Comp Neurol* 1980;191:213–225.
40. Lehman MN, Robinson J, Karsch F, Silverman AJ. Immunocytochemical localization of luteinizing hormone releasing hormone (LHRH) pathways in sheep brain during anestrus and the midluteal phase of the estrous cycle. *J Comp Neurol* 1986;244:19–35.
41. Caldani M, Batailler M, Thiery JC, Dubois MP. LHRH-immunoreactive structures in the sheep brain. *Histochemistry* 1988;89:129–139.
42. Barry J. Immunofluorescence study of the preopticoterminal LRH tract in the female squirrel monkey during the estrous cycle. *Cell Tissue Res* 1979;198:1–13.
43. Silverman AJ, Antunes JL, Abrams GM, et al. The luteinizing hormone releasing hormone pathways in rhesus (*Macaca mulatta*) and pigtailed (*Macaca nemestrina*) monkeys: New observations on thick, unembedded sections. *J Comp Neurol* 1982;211:309–317.
44. King JC, Anthony ELP. LHRH neurons and their projections in humans and other mammals: species comparisons. *Peptides* 1984;5(Suppl 1):195–207.

45. King JC, Anthony ELP, Fitzgerald DM, Stopa EG. LHRH neurons in human preoptic/hypothalamus: Differential intraneuronal localization of immunoreactive forms. *J Clin Endocrinol* 1985;60:88–97.
46. Merchenthaler L, Gorcs T, Setalo G, Petrusz P, Flerko B. Gonadotropin-releasing hormone (GnRH) neurons and pathways in the rat brain. *Cell Tissue Res* 1984;237:15–29.
47. King JC, Tobet SA, Snavely FL, Arimura A. LHRH immunopositive cells and their projections to the median eminence and organum vasculosum of the lamina terminalis. *J Comp Neurol* 1982;209:287–300.
48. Barry J, DuBois MP, Carette B. Immunofluorescence study of the preoptico-infundibular LRF neurosecretory pathway in the normal, castrated or testosterone-treated male guinea pig. *Endocrinology* 1974;95:1416–1423.
49. Hoffman GE, Gibbs FP. LHRH pathways in rat brain: "Deafferentation" spares a sub-chiasmatic LHRH projection to the median eminence. *Neuroscience* 1982;7:1979–1993.
50. Merchenthaler I, Kovacs G, Setalo G. The preopticoinfundibular LHRH tract of the rat. *Brain Res* 1980;198:63–74.
51. Silverman AJ, Krey LC. The luteinizing hormone releasing hormone (LHRH) neuronal networks of the guinea pig brain. I. Intra- and extra-hypothalamic projections. *Brain Res* 1978; 157:233–246.
52. Kawano H, Daikoku S. Immunohistochemical demonstration of LHRH neurons and their pathways in the rat hypothalamus. *Neuroendocrinology* 1981;32:179–186.
53. Kozlowski GP, Coates PW. Ependymoneuronal specializations between LHRH fibers and cells of the cerebroventricular system. *Cell Tissue Res* 1985;242:301–311.
54. Anthony ELP, King LC, Stopa EG. Immunocytochemical localization of LHRH in the median eminence, infundibular stalk and neurohypophysis. Evidence for multiple sites of releasing hormone secretion in humans and other mammals. *Cell Tissue Res* 1984;236:5–14.
55. Coen C, Howe PRC, DeLanerolle N. Immunohistochemical evidence for a subchiasmatic pathway containing luteinizing hormone releasing hormone, somatostatin, neuropeptide Y and tyrosine hydroxylase. *Soc Neurosci Abstr* 1985;11:351.
56. Liposits Z, Nagy L, Setalo G. Frontal deafferentation of the mediobasal hypothalamus in the neonatal rat and its effects on the preoptico-infundibular LHRH-tract. *Cell Tissue Res* 1982;225: 179–187.
57. Leonhardt S, Jarry H, Flakenstein G, Palmer J, Wuttke W. LH release in ovariectomized rats is maintained without noradrenergic transmission in the preoptic/anterior hypothalamic area: extreme functional plasticity of the GnRH pulse generator. *Brain Res* 1991;562:105–110.
58. Brownstein MI, Arimura A, Palkovits M, Kizer IS, Schally AV. The effect of surgical isolation of the hypothalamus on its luteinizing hormone releasing hormone content. *Endocrinology* 1976;98:662–665.
59. Setalo G, Vigh S, Schally AV, Arimura A, Flerko B. Immunohistological study of the origin of LHRH-containing nerve fibers of the rat hypothalamus. *Brain Res* 1976;103:597–602.
60. Ibata Y, Watanabe K, Kinoshita H, Kubo S, Sano Y. The location of LHRH neurons in the rat hypothalamus and their pathways to the median eminence. Experimental immunohistochemistry and radioimmunoassay. *Cell Tissue Res* 1979;198: 381–395.
61. Wise PM, Rance N, Selmanoff M, Barraclough CA. Changes in radioimmunoassayable luteinizing hormone releasing hormone in discrete brain areas of the rat at various times on proestrus, diestrous day I, and after phenobarbital administration. *Endocrinology* 1981;108:2179–2185.
62. Krey LC, Butler WR, Knobil E. Surgical disconnection of the medial basal hypothalamus and pituitary function in the rhesus monkey. 1. Gonadotropin secretion. *Endocrinology* 1975;96: 1073–1087.
63. Krey LC, Silverman AJ. The luteinizing hormone releasing hormone (LHRH) neuronal networks of the guinea pig brain. II. The regulation of gonadotropin secretion and the origin of terminals in the median eminence. *Brain Res* 1978;157:247–255.
64. Krey LC, Silverman AJ. The luteinizing hormone releasing hormone (LHRH) neuronal networks of the guinea pig brain. III. The regulation of cyclic gonadotropin secretion. *Brain Res* 1981;229:429–444.
65. Silverman AJ, Jamandas J, Renaud LP. Localization of LHRH neurons that project to the median eminence. *J Neurosci* 1987;7:2312–2319.
66. Merchenthaler I, Setalo G, Csontos C, Petruz P, Flerko B, Negro-Villar A. Combined retrograde tracing and immunocytochemical identification of luteinizing hormone releasing hormone- and somatostatin-containing neurons projecting to the median eminence of the rat. *Endocrinology* 1989;125:2812–2821.
67. Goldsmith PC, Thind KK, Song T, Kim EJ, Boggan JE. Location of the neuroendocrine gonadotropin-releasing hormone neurons in the monkey hypothalamus by retrograde tracing and immunocytochemistry. *J Neuroendocrinol* 1990;2:157–168.
68. Jennes L, Stumpf WE. Gonadotrôpin releasing hormone immunoreactive neurons with access to fenestrated capillaries in mouse brain. *Neuroscience* 1986;18:403–416.
69. Silverman AJ, Witkin JW, Silverman RC, Gibson MJ. Modulation of gonadotropin releasing hormone neuronal activity as evidence by uptake of fluorogold from the vasculature. *Synapse* 1990;6:154–160.
70. Witkin JW. Access of luteinizing hormone releasing hormone neurons to the vasculature in the rat. *Neuroscience* 1990;37: 501–506.
71. Berglund LA, Sisk CL. Luteinizing hormone releasing hormone (LHRH) neurons which are retrogradely labeled after peripheral fluorogold administration in the male ferret. *J Neuroendocrinol* 1993;4:743–749.
72. Koves K, Molnar J. Effects of various hypothalamic deafferentations injuring different parts of the GnRH pathway on ovulation, GnRH content of the median eminence and plasma LH and FSH levels. *Neuroendocrinology* 1986;44:172–183.
73. Sagar SM, Sharp FR, Curran R. Expression of cFOS protein in brain: metabolic mapping at the cellular level. *Science* 1988;240:1328–1331.
74. Ransone LJ, Verma IM. Nuclear protooncogenes *FOS* and *JUN*. *Annu Rev Cell Biol* 1990;6:539–557.
75. Dragunow M, Faull R. The use of *c-FOS* as a metabolic marker in neuronal pathway tracing. *J Neurosci Methods* 1989;29: 261–265.
76. Lee W-S, Smith MS, Hoffman GE. Luteinizing hormone-releasing hormone neurons express FOS protein during the proestrus surge of luteinizing hormone. *Proc Natl Acad Sci USA* 1990;87:5163–5167.
77. Hoffman GE, Lee W-S, Attardi B, Yann V, Fitzsimmons MD. Luteinizing hormone-releasing hormone neurons express *c-fos* antigen after steroid activation. *Endocrinology* 1990;126: 1736–1741.
78. Lee W-S, Smith MS, Hoffman GE. Progesterone enhances the surge of luteinizing hormone by increasing the activation of luteinizing hormone-releasing hormone neurons. *Endocrinology* 1990;127:2604–2606.
79. Wu TJ, Segal AZ, Miller GM, Gibson MJ, Silverman AJ. *FOS* expression in GnRH neurons: enhancement by steroid treatment and mating. *Endocrinology* 1992;131:2045–2050.
80. Silverman AJ, Gibson MJ. Hypothalamic transplantation: Repair of reproductive defects in hypogonadal mice. *Trends Endocrinol Metab* 1990;1:403–408.
81. Dierschke DJ, Bhattacharya AN, Atkinson LE, Knobil E. Circhoral oscillations of plasma LH levels in the ovariectomized rhesus monkey. *Endocrinology* 1970;87:850–853.
82. Carmel PW, Araki S, Ferin M. Pituitary stalk portal blood collection in rhesus monkeys: evidence for pulsatile release of gonadotropin releasing hormone (GnRH). *Endocrinology* 1976;99: 243–248.
83. Moenter SM, Brand RM, Midgley AR, Jr, Karsch FJ. Dynamics of GnRH during a pulse. *Endocrinology* 1990;130:503–510.
84. Goldsmith PC, Ganong WF. Ultrastructural localization of luteinizing hormone releasing hormone in the median eminence of the rat. *Brain Res* 1975;97:181–193.
85. Silverman AJ, Desnoyers P. Ultrastructural immunocytochemical localization of LHRH in the median eminence of the guinea pig. *Cell Tissue Res* 1976;169:157–166.
86. Krisch B. The distribution of LHRH in the hypothalamus of the

thirsting rat. A light and electron microscopic immunocytochemical study. *Cell Tissue Res* 1978;186:135–148.
87. Hatton GL, Perlmutter LS, Salm AK, Tweedle CD. Dynamic neuronal–glial interactions in hypothalamus and pituitary: Implications for control of hormone synthesis and release. *Peptides* 1984;5(Suppl 1):121–138.
88. Shivers BD, Harlan RE, Morrell JI, Pfaff DW. Immunocytochemical localization of luteinizing hormone-releasing hormone in male and female rat brains. *Neuroendocrinology* 1983;36:1–12.
89. Rothfield JM, Gross DS. GnRH within the organum vasculosum of the lamina terminalis in ovariectomized, estrogen/progesterone treated rat: Quantitative immunocytochemical study using image analysis. *Brain Res* 1985;338:309–315.
90. Barry J, Croix D. Immunofluorescence study of the hypothalamo–infundibular LRH tract and serum gonadotropin levels in the female squirrel monkey during the estrous cycle. *Cell Tissue Res* 1978;192:215–226.
91. Samson WK, McCann SM. Effects of lesions in the organum vasculosum lamina terminalis on the hypothalamic distribution of luteinizing hormone releasing hormone and gonadotropin secretion in the ovariectomized rat. *Endocrinology* 1979;105: 939–946.
92. Lehman MN, Winans-Newman S, Silverman AJ. Luteinizing hormone releasing hormone (LHRH) in the vomeronasal system and terminal nerve of the hamster. *Ann NY Acad Sci* 1987;519:229–240.
93. Jennes L, Stumpf WE. LHRH-systems in the brain of the golden hamster. *Cell Tissue Res* 1980;209:239–256.
94. Jennes L. Dual projections of gonadotropin releasing hormone containing neurons to the interpeduncular nucleus and to the vasculature in the female rat. *Brain Res* 1991;545:329–333.
95. Leonardelli J, Poulain P. About a ventral LHRH preoptico-amygdaloid pathway in the guinea pig. *Brain Res* 1977;124: 538–543.
96. Jennes L. Sites of origin of gonadotropin releasing hormone containing projections to the amygdala and interpeduncular nucleus. *Brain Res* 1987;404:339–344.
97. Jennes L, Stumpf WE. LHRH neuronal projections to the inner and outer surfaces of the brain. *Neurosci Lett* 1980;2:241–246.
98. Witkin JW, Silverman AJ. Luteinizing hormone releasing hormone (LHRH) in rat olfactory systems. *J Comp Neurol* 1983;218:426–432.
99. Schwanzel-Fukuda M, Morrell JI, Pfaff DW. Ontogenesis of neurons producing luteinizing hormone releasing hormone in the nervus terminalis of the rat. *J Comp Neurol* 1985;238:348–364.
100. Wirsig CR, Leonard CM. The terminal nerve projects centrally in the hamster. *Neuroscience* 1986;19:709–718.
101. Caldani M, Batailler M, Jourdan F. The sheep terminal nerve: coexistence of LHRH- and AChE-containing neurons. *Neurosci Lett* 1987;83:221–226.
102. Schwanzel-Fukuda M, Morrell JI, Pfaff DW. Localization of choline acetyltransferase and vasoactive intestinal polypeptide-like immunoreactivity in the nervus terminalis of the fetal and neonatal rat. *Peptides* 1986;7:899–906.
103. Wysocki CJ. Neurobehavioral evidence for the involvement of the vomeronasal system in mammalian reproduction. *Neurosci Biobehav Rev* 1979;3:301–342.
104. Witkin JW. Luteinizing hormone releasing hormone in olfactory bulbs of primates. *Am J Primatol* 1985;8:309–315.
105. Dluzen DE, Ramirez VD, Carter CS, Getz LL. Male vole urine changes LHRH and norepinephrine in female olfactory bulb. *Science* 1981;212:573–575.
106. Kelsall R, Coe IR, Sherwood NM. Phylogeny and ontogeny of gonadotropin-releasing hormone: comparison of guinea pig, rat, and a protochordate. *Gen Comp Endocrinol* 1990;78:479–494.
107. Crim JW, Urano A, Gorbman A. Immunocytochemical studies of luteinizing hormone-releasing hormone in brains of agnathan fishes. I. Comparisons of adult Pacific lamprey ("*Entosphenus tridentata*") and the Pacific hagfish ("*Epatratetus stouti*"). *Gen Comp Endocrinol* 1979;37:294–305.
108. Crim JW, Urano A, Gorbman A. Immunocytochemical studies of luteinizing hormone-releasing hormone in brains of agnathan fishes. II. Patterns of immunocytochemistry in larval and maturing western brook lamprey ("*Lampetra richardsoni*"). *Gen Comp Endocrinol* 1979;38:290–299.
109. King JC, Sower SA, Anthony ELP. Neuronal systems immunoreactive with antiserum to lamprey gonadotropin-releasing hormone in the brain of "*Petromyzon marinus.*" *Cell Tissue Res* 1988;253:1–8.
110. Demski LS. The evolution of neuroanatomical substrates of reproductive behavior: sex steroid and LHRH-specific pathways including the terminal nerve. *Am Zool* 1984;24:809–830.
111. Demski LS, Fields RD. Dense-cored vesicle components of the terminal nerve of sharks and rays. *J Comp Neurol* 1988;278: 604–614.
112. Demski LS, Wright DE. GnRH immunoreactivity in the brain of the round stingray, "*Urolophus halleri.*" *Soc Neurosci Abstr* 1990;16:126.
113. Demski LS, Fields RD, Bullock TH, Schreibman MP, Margolis-Nunno H. The terminal nerve of sharks and rays: EM, immunocytochemical and electrophysiological studies. *Ann NY Acad Sci* 1987;519:15–32.
114. Wright DE, Demski LS. Gonadotropin hormone-releasing hormone (GnRH) immunoreactivity in the mesencephalon of sharks and rays. *J Comp Neurol* 1991;307:49–56.
115. Powell RC, Millar RP, King JA. Diverse molecular forms of gonadotropin releasing hormone in an elasmobranch and teleost fish. *Gen Comp Endocrinol* 1986;63:77–85.
116. Batten TFC, Cambre ML, Moons L, Vandesande F. Comparative distribution of neuropeptide-immunoreactive systems in the brain of the green molly, *Poecilia latipinna. J Comp Neurol* 1990;302:893–919.
117. Munz H, Stumpf WE, Jennes L. LHRH systems in the brain of platyfish. *Brain Res* 1981;221:1–13.
118. Schriebman MP, Halpern LR, Goos HJT, Margolis-Kazan H. Identification of luteinizing hormone-releasing hormone (LH-RH) in the brain and pituitary gland of a fish by immunocytochemistry. *J Exp Zool* 1979;210:153–160.
119. Kah O, Chambolle P, Dubourg P, Dubois MP. Immunocytochemical localization of luteinizing hormone-releasing hormone in the brain of the goldfish *Carassius auratus. Gen Comp Endocrinol* 1984;53:107–115.
120. Kah O, Zanuy S, Mananos E, Anglade I, Carrillo M. Distribution of salmon gonadotrophin releasing-hormone in the brain and pituitary of the sea bass (*Dicentrarchus labrax*). *Cell Tissue Res* 1991;266:129–136.
121. Kah O, Brenton JG, Nunez-Rodriguez J, et al. A reinvestigation of the Gn-RH (gonadotropin-releasing hormone) systems in the goldfish brain using antibodies to salmon Gn-RH. *Cell Tissue Res* 1986;244:327–337.
122. Stell WK, Walker WE, Chohan KS, Ball AK. The goldfish nervus terminalis: a luteinizing hormone-releasing hormone and molluscan cardioexcitatory peptide-immunoreactive olfactoretinal pathway. *Proc Natl Acad Sci USA* 1984;81:940–944.
123. Borg B, Goos HJT, Terlou M. LHRH-immunoreactive cells in the brain of the three-spined stickleback, *Gasterosteus aculeatus* L. (Gasterosteidae). *Cell Tissue Res* 1982;226:695–699.
124. Oka Y, Ichikawa M. Gonadotropin-releasing hormone (GnRH) immunoreactive system in the brain of the dwarf gourami (*Colisa lalia*) as revealed by light microscopic immunocytochemistry using a monoclonal antibody to common amino acid sequence of GnRH. *J Comp Neurol* 1990;300:511–522.
125. Crim JW. Immunocytochemistry of luteinizing hormone-releasing hormone in brains of breeding eastern narrow-mouthed toads (*Gastrophryne carolinensis*). *Comp Biochem Physiol A* 1984;79:283–287.
126. Crim JW. Immunocytochemistry of luteinizing hormone-releasing hormone and sexual maturation of the frog brain: comparisons of juvenile and adult bullfrogs (*Rana catesbeiana*). *Gen Comp Endocrinol* 1985;59:424–433.
127. Jokura Y, Urano A. Projections of luteinizing hormone-releasing hormone and vasotocin fibers to the anterior part of the preoptic nucleus in the toad, *Bufo japonicus. Gen Comp Endocrinol* 1985;60:390–397.
128. Jokura Y, Urano A. An immunohistochemical study of seasonal changes in luteinizing hormone-releasing hormone and vasotocin in the forebrain and the neurohypophysis of the toad, *Bufo japonicus. Gen Comp Endocrinol* 1985;59:238–245.
129. Jokura Y, Urano A. Extrahypothalamic projection of luteinizing

hormone-releasing hormone fibers in the brain of the toad, *Bufo japonicus*. *Gen Comp Endocrinol* 1986;62:80–88.
130. Muske LE, Moore FL. Luteinizing hormone-releasing hormone-immunoreactive neurons in the amphibian brain are distributed along the course of the nervus terminalis. *Ann NY Acad Sci* 1987;519:433–446.
131. Muske LE, Moore FL. The amphibian nervus terminalis: anatomy, chemistry and relationship with the hypothalamic LHRH system. *Brain Behav Evol* 1988;32:141–150.
132. Muske LE, Moore FL. Ontogeny of immunoreactive gonadotropin-releasing hormone neuronal systems in amphibians. *Brain Res* 1990;534:177–187.
133. Wirsig CR, Getchell TV. Amphibian terminal nerve: distribution revealed by LHRH and AChE markers. *Brain Res* 1986;385: 10–21.
134. Rastogi RK, DiMeglio M, Lela L. Immunoreactive luteinizing hormone-releasing hormone in the frog (*Rana esculenta*) brain: distribution pattern in the adult, seasonal changes, castration effects, and developmental aspects. *Gen Comp Endocrinol* 1990;78:444–458.
135. DiMeglio M, Masucci M, D'Aniello B, Iela L, Rastogi RK. Immunohistochemical localization of multiple forms of gonadotropin-releasing hormone in the brain of the adult frog. *J Neuroendocrinol* 1991;3:363–367.
136. Doerr-Schott J, Dubois MP. Immunoreactive LHRF neurons in the brain of *Xenopus laevis*. *Gen Comp Endocrinol* 1976;172:477–486.
137. Doerr-Schott J, Dubois MP. Immunohistochemical localization of different peptidergic substances in the brain of amphibians and reptiles. In: Gaillard PJ, Boer HH, eds. *Comparative Endocrinology*. Amsterdam: Elsevier/North-Holland; 1978:367–370.
138. Nozaki M, Kobayashi H. Distribution of LHRH-like substance in the vertebrate brain as revealed by immunohistochemistry. *Arch Histol Jpn* 1979;42:201–209.
139. Bennis M, Dubourg P, Gamrani H, Calas A, Kah O. Existence of a GnRH immunoreactive nucleus in the dorsal midbrain tegmentum of the chameleon. *Gen Comp Endocrinol* 1989;75: 195–203.
140. Kuenzel WJ, Blahser S. The distribution of gonadotropin-releasing hormone (GnRH) neurons and fibers throughout the chick brain (*Gallus domesticus*). *Cell Tissue Res* 1991; 264:481–495.
141. Sterling RJ, Sharp PJ. The localization of LH-RH neurones in the diencephalon of the domestic hen. *Cell Tissue Res* 1982;222: 283–298.
142. Mikami S, Yamada S, Hasegawa Y, Miyamoto K. Localization of avian LHRH-immunoreactive neurons in the hypothalamus of the domestic fowl, *Gallus domesticus*, and the Japanese quail, *Coturnix coturnix*. *Cell Tissue Res* 1988;251:51–58.
143. Blahser S, Heinrichs M. Immunoreactive neuropeptide systems in avian embryos (domestic mallard, domestic fowl, Japanese quail). *Cell Tissue Res* 1982;223:287–303.
144. Fukuda MI, Ishimoto S, Shiosaka Y, et al. Localization of LH-RH immunoreactivity in the avian retina. *Curr Eye Res* 1983;2:71–74.
145. Jozsa R, Mess B. Immunohistochemical localization of the luteinizing hormone-releasing hormone (LHRH)-containing structures in the central nervous system of the domestic fowl. *Cell Tissue Res* 1982;227:451–458.
146. Advis JP, Contijoch AM, Johnson A. Discrete hypothalamic distribution of luteinizing hormone-releasing hormone (LHRH) content and of LHRH-degrading activity in laying and nonlaying hens. *Biol Reprod* 1985;32:820–827.
147. Foster RG, Panzica GC, Parry DM, Viglietti-Panzica C. Immunocytochemical studies on the LHRH system of the Japanese quail: influence by photoperiod and aspects of sexual differentiation. *Cell Tissue Res* 1988;253:327–335.
148. Foster RG, Plowman G, Goldsmith AR, Follett BI. Immunohistochemical demonstration of marked changes in the LHRH system of photosensitive and photorefractory European starlings (*Sturnus vulgaris*). *J Endocrinol* 1987;115:211–220.
149. Sherwood NM, Zoeller RT, Moore FL. Multiple molecular forms of gonadotropin-releasing hormone in amphibian brains. *Gen Comp Endocrinol* 1986;61:313–322.
150. King JA, Millar RP. Identification of His^5, Trp^7, Tyr^8-GnRH (chicken GnRH II) in amphibian brain. *Peptides* 1986;7: 827–834.
151. Graziadei PPC, Monti-Graziadei AG. The influence of the olfactory placode on the development of the telencephalon in *Xenopus laevis*. *Neuroscience* 1992;46:617–629.
152. Eagleson GW, Jenks BG, van Overbeeke P. The pituitary adenocorticotropes originate from neural ridge tissue in *Xenopus laevis*. *J Embryol Exp Morphol* 1986;95:1–14.
153. Kawamura K, Kikuyama S. Evidence that hypophysis and hypothalamus constitute a single entity from the primary stage of histogenesis. *Development* 1992;115:1–9.
154. Northcutt RG, Muske LE. Experimental embryological evidence of the placodal origin of GnRH and FMRFamide neurons of the terminal nerve and preoptic area in salamanders. *Soc Neurosci* 1991;17:321.
155. Murakami S, Kikuyama S, Arai Y. The origin of the luteinizing hormone-releasing hormone (LHRH) neurons in newts (*Cynops pyrrhogaster*): the effect of olfactory placode ablation. *Cell Tissue Res* 1992;269:21–27.
156. Demski LS, Northcutt RG. The terminal nerve: A new chemosensory system in vertebrates? *Science* 1983;220:435–437.
157. Springer AD. Centrifugal innervation of goldfish retina from ganglion cells of the nervus terminalis. *J Comp Neurol* 1982;214:404–415.
158. Munz H, Claas B, Stumpf WE, Jennes L. Centrifugal innervation of the retina by luteinizing hormone releasing hormone (LHRH)-immunoreactive telencephalic neurons in teleostean fishes. *Cell Tissue Res* 1982;222:313–323.
159. Oka Y. Gonadotropin-releasing hormone (GnRH) cells of the terminal nerve as a model neuromodulator system. *Neurosci Lett* 1992;142:119–122.
160. Demski LS, Dluka JG, Northcutt RG. Chemosensory control of spawning mechanism in goldfish. *Soc Neurosci Abstr* 1982;8:611.
161. Subhedar N, Krishna NSR. Localization of LH-RH in the brain and pituitary of the catfish, *Clarias batrachus* (Linn). *Gen Comp Endocrinol* 1988;72:431–442.
162. Halpern-Sebold LR, Schriebman MP. Ontogeny of centers containing luteinizing hormone-releasing hormone in the brain of platyfish (*Xiphophorus maculatus*) as determined by immunocytochemistry. *Cell Tissue Res* 1983;229:75–84.
163. Witkin JW. Immunocytochemistry of the GnRH system in developing *Xenopus*. *Soc Neurosci Abstr* 1990;16:363.
164. Amano M, Oka Y, Aida K, Okumoto N, Kawashima S, Hasegawa Y. Immunocytochemical demonstration of salmon GnRH and chicken GnRH-II in the brain of masu salmon, *Oncorhynchus masou*. *J Comp Neurol* 1991;314:587–597.
165. Muske LE. Evolution of gonadotropin releasing hormone (GnRH) neuronal systems. *Brain Behav Evol* (in press).
166. Dellovade TL, King JA, Miller RP, Rissman EF. Differential regional distribution of mammalian and chicken. II: Gonadotropin releasing hormones in the musk shrew brain. *Neuroendocrinology* (in press).
167. King JA, Mehl AEI, Tyndale-Biscoe CH, Hinds L, Millar RP. A second form of gonadotropin-releasing hormone (GnRH), with chicken II-like properties, occurs together with mammalian GnRH in marsupial brains. *Endocrinology* 1989;125:2244–2252.
168. Jan YN, Jan LY, Kuffler SW. A peptide as a possible transmitter in sympathetic ganglia of the frog. *Proc Natl Acad Sci USA* 1979;76:1501–1505.
169. Horn JP, Stofer WD. Double labeling of the paravertebral sympathetic C system in the bullfrog with antisera to LHRH and NPY. *J Autonom Nerv Syst* 1988;23:17–24.
170. Grober MS, Jackson IMD, Bass AH. Gonadal steroids affect LHRH preoptic cell number in a sex/role changing fish. *J Neurobiol* 1991;22:734–741.
171. Schriebman MP, Halpern-Sebold L, Ferin M, Margolis-Kazan H, Goos HJT. The effect of hypophysectomy and gonadotropin administration on the distribution and quantity of LH-RH in the brains of platyfish: A combined immunocytochemistry and radioimmunoassay study. *Brain Res* 1983;267:293–300.
172. Schriebman MP, Halpern-Sebold L, Margolis-Nunno H. Sexually dimorphic age-related changes in the distribution of immunoreactive luteinizing hormone releasing hormone in the platyfish. *Mech Ageing Dev* 1985;33:29–37.
173. Silver R, Ramos CL, Silverman A-J. Sexual behavior triggers the

appearance of non-neuronal cells containing gonadotropin-releasing hormone-like immunoreactivity. *J Neuroendocrinol* 1992;4:207–210.
174. King JC, Sower SA, Anthony ELP. Neuronal systems immunoreactive with antiserum to lamprey gonadotropin-releasing hormone in the brain of *Petromyzon marinus. Cell Tissue Res* 1988;253:1–8.
175. Joseph SA, Sorrentino S, Sundberg DK. Releasing hormone, LRF and TRF, in the cerebrospinal fluid of the third ventricle. In: Knigge KM, Scott DE, Kobayashi H, Ishii S, eds. *Brain–Endocrine Interaction. II. The Ventricular System in Neuroendocrine Mechanisms.* Basel: Karger; 1975:306–312.
176. Xia L, Van Vugt D, Alston EJ, Luckhaus J, Ferin M. A surge of gonadotropin-releasing hormone (GnRH) accompanies the estradiol-induced gonadotropin surge in the rhesus monkey. *Endocrinology* 19;131:2812–2820.
177. Knigge KM, Bennet-Clarke C, Burchanowski B, Joseph SA, Romagnano MA, Sternberger LA. Relationships of some releasing-hormone-producing neuron systems to the ventricles of the brain. In: Motta M, ed. *The Endocrine Functions of the Brain.* New York: Raven Press; 1980:195–206.
178. Jan LY, Jan YN. Peptidergic transmission in sympathetic ganglia of the frog. *J Physiol* (*Lond*) 1982;327:219–246.
179. Jan YN, Jan LY. Coexistence and co-release of acetylcholine and the LHRH-like peptide from the same preganglionic fibers in frog sympathetic ganglia. *Fed Proc* 1983;42:2929–2933.
180. Jones SW. Chicken II luteinizing hormone-releasing hormone inhibits the M-current of bullfrog sympathetic neurons. *Neurosci Lett* 1987;80:180–184.
181. Marchant TA, Chang JP, Nahorniak CS, Peter RE. Evidence that gonadotropin-releasing hormone also functions as a growth hormone-releasing factor in the goldfish. *Endocrinology* 1989;124:2509–2518.
182. Krisch B. Two types of luliberin-immunoreactive perikarya in the preoptic area of the rat. *Cell Tissue Res* 1980;212:443–455.
183. Wray S, Hoffman G. Post-natal morphological changes in rat LHRH neurons correlated with sexual maturity. *Neuroendocrinology* 1986;43:93–97.
184. Jennes L, Stumpf WE, Sheedy ME. Ultrastructural characterization of gonadotropin-releasing hormone (GnRH)-producing neurons. *J Comp Neurol* 1985;232:534–547.
185. Liposits Z, Setalo G, Flerko B. Application of the silver–gold intensified 3,3′-diaminobenzidine chromogen to the light and electron microscopic detection of the luteinizing hormone releasing hormone system of the rat brain. *Neuroscience* 1984;13:513–525.
186. Wray S, Gainer H. Effect of neonatal gonadectomy on the postnatal development of LHRH cell subtypes in male and female rats. *Neuroendocrinology* 1987;45:413–419.
187. Witkin JW, Demasio KA. Ultrastructural differences between smooth and thorny GnRH neurons. *Neuroscience* 1990;34:777–783.
188. Leshin LS, Rund LA, Kraeling RR, Crim JW, Kiser TE. Morphological differences among luteinizing hormone releasing hormone neurons from postpartum and estrous cycling cows. *Neuroendocrinology* 1992;55:380–389.
189. Kozlowski GP, Chu L, Hostetter G, Kerdelhue B. Cellular characteristics of immunolabeled luteinizing hormone releasing hormone (LHRH) neurons. *Peptides* 1980;1:37–46.
190. Pelletier G, Labrie F, Puviani R, Arimura A, Schally AV. Immunohistochemical localization of luteinizing hormone releasing hormone in the rat median eminence. *Endocrinology* 1974;95:554–558.
191. Bugnon G, Bloch B, Lenys D, Fellmann D. Ultrastructural study of LHRH containing neurons in the human fetus. *Brain Res* 1977;137:175–180.
192. Mazzuca M. Immunocytochemical and ultrastructural identification of luteinizing hormone releasing hormone (LH-RH) containing neurons in the vascular organ of the lamina terminalis (OVLT) of the squirrel monkey. *Neurosci Lett* 1977;5:123–127.
193. Pelletier G, LeClerc R, Dube D, Arimura A, Schally AV. Immunohistochemical localization of LHRH and somatostatin in the organum vasculosum of the lamina terminalis of the rat. *Neurosci Lett* 1977;4:27–31.
194. Krisch B, Leonhardt H. Luliberin and somatostatin fiber terminalis in the subfornical organ of the rat. *Cell Tissue Res* 1980;210:33–45.
195. Marshall PE, Goldsmith PC. Neuroregulatory and neuroendocrine GnRH pathways in the hypothalamus and forebrain of the baboon. *Brain Res* 1980;193:353–372.
196. Witkin JW, Silverman AJ. Synaptology of LHRH neurons in rat preoptic area. *Peptides* 1985;6:263–271.
197. Leranth C, Segura LMG, Palkovits M, MacLusky NJ, Shanabrough M, Naftolin F. The LH-RH containing neuronal network in the preoptic area of the rat: Demonstration of LH-RH containing nerve terminals in synaptic contact with LHRH neurons. *Brain Res* 1985;345:332–336.
198. Thind KK, Goldsmith PC. Infundibular gonadotropin-releasing hormone neurons are inhibited by direct opioid and autoregulatory synapses in juvenile monkeys. *Neuroendocrinology* 1988;47:203–216.
199. Witkin JW, Silverman AJ. Novel neuronal communication: GnRH neurons form synaytia. *J Neurosci* (in press).
200. Lehman MN, Silverman AJ. Ultrastructure of LHRH neurons in intact and castrate male hamsters. *Soc Neurosci Abstr* 1985;11:351.
201. Hisano S, Kawano H, Maki Y, Daikoku S. Electron microscopic study of immunoreactive perikarya with special reference to neuronal regulation. *Cell Tissue Res* 1981;220:511–518.
202. Leranth C, MacLuskey NJ, Shanabrough M, Naftolin F. Catecholaminergic innervation of luteinizing hormone-releasing hormone and glutamic acid decarboxylase immunopositive neurons in the rat medial preoptic area. Electron-microscopic double label and degeneration study. *Neuroendocrinology* 1988;48:591–602.
203. Chen W-P, Witkin JW, Silverman AJ. Gonadotropin releasing hormone (GnRH) neurons are directly innervated by catecholamine terminals. *Synapse* 1989;3:288–290.
204. Palkovits M, Leranth C, Jew JY, Williams T. Simultaneous characterization of pre- and postsynaptic neuron contact sites in brain. *Proc Natl Acad Sci USA* 1982;79:2705–2708.
205. Kuljis RO, Advis JP. Immunocytochemical and physiological evidence of a synapse between dopaminergic and luteinizing hormone releasing hormone contain neurons in the ewe median eminence. *Endocrinology* 1989;124:1579–1581.
206. Kiss J, Halasz B. Demonstration of serotonergic axons terminating on luteinizing hormone-releasing hormone neurons in the preoptic area of the rat using a combination of immunocytochemistry and high resolution autoradiography. *Neuroscience* 1985;14:69–78.
207. Chen W-P, Witkin JW, Silverman AJ. Beta-endorphin and gonadotropin-releasing hormone synaptic input to gonadotropin releasing hormone neurosecretory cells in the male rat. *J Comp Neurol* 1989;286:85–95.
208. Chen W-P, Witkin JW, Silverman AJ. Sexual dimorphism in the synaptic input to gonadotropin releasing hormone (GnRH) neurons. *Endocrinology* 1989;126:695–702.
209. MacLuskey NJ, Naftolin F, Leranth C. Immunocytochemical evidence for direct synaptic connections between corticotropin releasing factor (CRF) and gonadotropin-releasing hormone (GnRH) containing neurons in the preoptic area of the rat. *Brain Res* 1988;439:391–395.
210. Witkin JW. Increased synaptic input to gonadotropin releasing hormone neurons in aged virgin male SD rats. *Neurobiol Aging* 1992;13:681–686.
211. Thind KK, Boggan JE, Goldsmith PC. Interactions between vasopressin- and gonadotropin-releasing-hormone-containing neuroendocrine neurons in the monkey supraoptic nucleus. *Neuroendocrinology* 1991;53:287–297.
212. Goldsmith PC, Thind KK, Perera AD. Glutamate-immunoreactive terminals synapse with GnRH neurons in the monkey hypothalamus. *Soc Neurosci Abstr* 1992;18:192.
213. Witkin JW. Aging changes in synaptology of LHRH neurons in male rat preoptic area. *Neuroscience* 1987;22:1003–1013.
214. Witkin JW. Reproductive history effects the synaptology of the ageing gonadotropin releasing hormone neurons in the male rat. *J Neuroendocrinol* 1992;4:427–432.
215. Witkin JW, Ferin M, Popilskis SJ, Silverman AJ. Effects of gonadal steroids on the ultrastructure of GnRH neurons in the rhesus monkey: synaptic input and glial apposition. *Endocrinology* 1991;129:1083–1092.

216. Silverman AJ, Witkin JW. Synaptic interactions of LHRH neurons in the guinea pig preoptic area. *J Histochem Cytochem* 1985;33:66–72.
217. Silverman AJ. Luteinizing hormone releasing hormone containing synapses in the diagonal band and preoptic area of the guinea pig. *J Comp Neurol* 1984;227:452–458.
218. Phillips HS, Ho BT, Linner JG. Ultrastructural localization of LHRH immunoreactive synapses in the hamster accessory olfactory bulb. *Brain Res* 1982;246:193–204.
219. Tramu G, Leonardelli J, DuBois MP. Immunohistochemical evidence for an ACTH-like substance in hypothalamic LHRH neurons. *Neurosci Lett* 1977;6:305–309.
220. Beauvillain JC, Tramu G, DuBois MP. Ultrastructural immunocytochemical evidence of the presence of a peptide related to ACTH in granules of LHRH nerve terminals in the median eminence of the guinea pig. *Cell Tissue Res* 1981;218:1–6.
221. Leonardelli J, Tramu G. Immunoreactivity for β-endorphin in LHRH neurons of the fetal human hypothalamus. *Cell Tissue Res* 1979;203:201–207.
222. Wolfson B, Manning RW, Davis LG, Arentzen R, Baldwin F Jr. Colocalization of CRF and VP mRNA in neurons after adrenalectomy. *Nature* 1985;315:59–61.
223. Vallet PG, Charnay Y, Boura C, Kiss JZ. Colocalization of delta sleep inducing peptide and luteinizing hormone in neurosecretory vesicles in rat median eminence. *Neuroendocrinology* 1991;53:103–106.
224. Vallet PG, Charnay Y, Bouras C. Distribution and colocalization of delta sleep-inducing peptide and luteinizing hormone releasing hormone in the aged human brain: an immunohistochemical study. *J Chem Neuroanat* 1990;3:207–214.
225. Merchenthaler I, Lopez FJ, Negro-Villar A. Colocalization of galanin and luteinizing hormone releasing hormone in a sub-set of preoptic hypothalamic neurons: anatomical and functional correlates. *Proc Natl Acad Sci USA* 1990;87:6326–6330.
226. Coen CW, Montagnese C, Opacka-Juffry J. Coexistence of gonadotropin releasing hormone and galanin: immunohistochemical and functional studies. *J Neuroendocrinol* 1990;2:107–111.
227. Merchenthaler I, Lopez FJ, Lennard DE, Negro-Villar A. Sexual differences in the distribution of neurons co-expressing galanin and luteinizing hormone releasing hormone in the rat brain. *Endocrinology* 1991;129:1977–1986.
228. Shivers BD, Harlan RE, Morrell JI, Pfaff DW. Absence of oestradiol concentration in cell nuclei of LHRH immunoreactive neurones. *Nature* 1983;304:345–347.
229. Press MF, Nousek-Goebl NA, Greene GL. Immunoelectron microscopic localization of estradiol receptor with a monoclonal estrophilin antibody. *J Histochem Cytochem* 1985;33:915–924.
230. Sullivan KA, Witkin JW, Silverman AJ. Distribution of estrogen receptor containing and GnRH neurons in the rhesus macaque. *Soc Neurosci Abstr* 1990;16:1201.
231. Watson RE, Langub MC, Landis JW. Further evidence that most luteinizing hormone releasing hormone neurons are not directly estrogen responsive—simultaneous localization of luteinizing hormone releasing hormone and estrogen receptor in the guinea pig brain. *J Neuroendocrinol* 1992;4:311–318.
232. Karsch FJ, Lehman MN. Do gonadotropin releasing hormone (GnRH) or dopaminergic neurons in the sheep contain estradiol receptors? *Soc Neurosci Abstr* 1988;14:1069.
233. Langub MC, Maley BE, Watson RE. Ultrastructural evidence for luteinizing hormone releasing hormone neuronal control of estrogen responsive neurons in the preoptic area. *Endocrinology* 1991;128:27–36.
234. Kalra SP, Kalra PS. Do testosterone and estradiol-17β enforce inhibition or stimulation of luteinizing hormone releasing hormone secretion? *Biol Reprod* 1989;41:559–570.
235. Levine JE, Bauer-Dantoin AC, Besecke LM, et Neuroendocrine regulation of the luteinizing hormone releasing hormone pulse generator in the rat. *Recent Prog Horm Res* 1991;47: 97–153.
236. Levine JE, Ramirez VD. Luteinizing hormone releasing hormone release during the rat estrous cycle and after ovariectomy, as estimated with push–pull cannulae. *Endocrinology* 1982;111: 1439–1448.
237. Lin WW, Ramirez VD. Effect of mating behavior on luteinizing hormone releasing hormone in female rabbits with push–pull cannulae. *Neuroendocrinology* 1991;53:229–235.
238. Moenter SM, Caraty A, Locatelli A, Karsch FJ. Pattern of gonadotropin releasing hormone (GnRH secretion) leading up to ovulation in the ewe—existence of a preovulatory GnRH surge. *Endocrinology* 1991;129:1175–1182.
239. Shivers BD, Harlan RE, Hejmancik JF, Conn PM, Pfaff DW. Localization of cells containing LHRH-like mRNA in rat forebrain using in situ hybridization. *Endocrinology* 1986;118: 883–888.
240. Park OK, Gugnega S, Mayo KE. Gonadotropin releasing hormone gene expression during the rat estrous cycle: Effects of pentobarbitol and ovarian steroids. *Endocrinology* 1990;127: 365–372.
241. Malik KF, Silverman AJ, Morrell JI. Gonadotropin releasing hormone mRNA in the rat: distribution and neuronal content over the estrous cycle and after castration in males. *Anat Rec* 1991;231:457–466.
242. Ronnekleiv OK, Naylor BR, Bond CT, Adelman JP. Combined immunohistochemistry for gonadotropin-releasing hormone (GnRH) and pro-GnRH, and in situ hybridization for GnRH messenger RNA in rat brain. *Mol Endocrinol* 1989;3:363–371.
243. Standish LJ, Adams LA, Vician L, Clifton DK, Steiner RA. Neuroanatomical localization of cells containing gonadotropin releasing hormone messenger ribonucleic acid in the primate brain by in situ hybridization histochemistry. *Mol Endocrinol* 1987;1:371–376.
244. Wiemann JN, Clifton DK, Steiner RA. Gonadotropin releasing hormone messenger RNA levels are unaltered with changes in the gonadal hormone milieu of the adult male rat. *Endocrinology* 1990;127:523–532.
245. Rothfeld JM, Hejmancik JF, Pfaff DW. Quantitation of LHRH mRNA within the female rat forebrain following estrogen treatment. *Anat Rec* 1987;218:117a.
246. Pfaff DW. Gene expression in hypothalamic neurons: Luteinizing hormone releasing hormone. *J Neurosci Res* 1986;16: 109–115.
247. Roberts JL, Dutlow CM, Jakubowski M, Blum M, Millar RP. Estradiol stimulated preoptic area–anterior hypothalamic pro-GnRH-GAP gene expression in ovariectomized rats. *Mol Endocrinol* 1989;6:127–134.
248. Toranzo D, Dupont E, Simard J, et al. Regulation of progonadotropin releasing hormone gene espression by sex steroids in the brain of male and female rats. *Mol Endocrinol* 1989;3: 1748–1756.
249. Kim K, Lee BJ, Park Y, Cho WK. Progesterone increases messenger RNA encoding luteinizing hormone releasing hormone (LHRH) level in the hypothalamus ovariectomized estradiol-primed prepubertal rats. *Mol Brain Res* 1989;6:151–158.
250. Park Y, Park SD, Cho WK, Kim K. Testosterone stimulates LH-RH like mRNA level in the rat hypothalamus. *Brain Res* 1988;451:255–260.
251. Zoeller RT, Seeburg PA, Young WS. In situ hybridization histochemistry for messenger ribonuclei acid (mRNA) encoding gonadotropin releasing hormone (GnRH): effect of estrogen on cellular levels of GnRH mRNA in female rat brain. *Endocrinology* 1988;122:2570–2577.
252. Kelly MJ, Garrett J, Bosch MA, et al. Effects of ovariectomy on GnRH mRNA, proGnRH and GnRH levels in the preoptic hypothalamus of the female rat. *Neuroendocrinology* 1989;49:88–97.
253. Petersen SL, Cheuk RD, Hartman RD, Barraclough CA. Medial preoptic area microimplants of the antiestrogen, keoxifine, affect luteinizing hormone-releasing hormone (LHRH) mRNA levels, medial eminence LHRH concentrations and LH release in ovariectomized, estrogen-treated rats. *J Neuroendocrinol* 1989; 1:279–283.
254. Rosie R, Thomson E, Fink G. Oestrogen positive feedback stimulates the synthesis of LHRH mRNA in neurones of the rostral diencephalon of the rat. *J Endocrinol* 1990;124:285–289.
255. Zoeller RT, Young WS. Changes in cellular levels of messenger ribonuclei acid encoding gonadotropin releasing hormone in the anterior hypothalamus of female rats during the estrous cycle. *Endocrinology* 1988;123:1688–1699.
256. Parnet P, Lenoir V, Palkovits M, Kerdelhue B. Estrous cycle vari-

ations in gonadotropin releasing hormone, substance P and beta endorphin contents in the median eminence, arcuate nucleus and medial preoptic area in the rat: a detailed analysis of proestrous changes. *J Neuroendocrinol* 1990;2:291–296.
257. Cattanach HM, Iddon CA, Charlton HM, Chiappa SA, Fink G. Gonadotropin-releasing hormone deficiency in a mutant mouse with hypogonadism. *Nature* 1977;269:338–340.
258. Mason AI, Hayflick IS, Zoeller RT, et al. A deletion truncating the GnRH gene is responsible for hypogonadism in the *hpg* mouse. *Science* 1986;234:1366–1371.
259. Silverman AJ, Zimmerman EA, Gibson MI, Perlow MI, Charlton HM, Krieger DT. Implantation of normal fetal preoptic area into hypogonadal mutant mice: Temporal relationships of the growth of gonadotropin-releasing hormone neurons and the development of the pituitary/testicular axis. *Neuroscience* 1985;16:69–84.
260. Livne I, Gibson MJ, Silverman AJ. Gonadotropin releasing hormone (GnRH) neurons in the hypogonadal mouse elaborated normal projections despite their biosynthetic deficiency. *Neurosci Lett* [*in press*].
261. Krieger DT, Perlow MJ, Gibson MJ, et al. Brain grafts reverse hypogonadism of gonadotropin releasing hormone deficiency. *Nature* 1982;298:1–3.
262. Gibson MJ, Perlow MJ, Charlton HM, Zimmerman EA, Davies TF, Krieger DT. Preoptic area brain grafts in hypogonadal (*hpg*) female mice abolish effects of congenital hypothalamic gonadotropin releasing hormone (GnRH) deficiency. *Endocrinology* 1984;114:1938–1940.
263. Gibson MJ, Krieger DT, Charlton HM, Zimmerman EA, Silverman AJ, Perlow MJ. Mating and pregnancy can occur in genetically hypogonadal mice with preoptic area brain grafts. *Science* 1984;225:949–951.
264. Gibson MJ, Kokoris GJ, Silverman AJ. Positive feedback in *hpg* female mice with preoptic area brain grafts. *Neuroendocrinology* 1988;48:112–119.
265. Kokoris GJ, Lam NY, Ferin M, Silverman AJ, Gibson MJ. Transplanted gonadotropin-releasing hormone neurons promote pulsatile LH secretion in congenitally hypogonadal (*hpg*) male mice. *Neuroendocrinology* 1988;48:45–52.
266. Gibson MJ, Miller GM, Silverman AJ. Pulsatile LH secretion in normal female mice and in hypogonadal female mice with POA implants. *Endocrinology* 1991;128:965–971.
267. Gibson MJ, Silverman AJ. Effects of gonadectomy and treatment with gonadal steroids on luteinizing hormone secretion in hypogonadal male and female mice with preoptic area implants. *Endocrinology* 1989;125:1525–1532.
268. Mellon PL, Windle JJ, Goldsmith PC, Padula CA, Roberts JL, Weiner RI. Immortalization of hypothalamic GnRH neurons by genetically targeted tumorigenesis. *Neuron* 1990;5:1–10.
269. Liposits Z, Merchenthaler I, Wetsel WC, et al. Morphological characterization of immortalized hypothalamic neurons synthesizing luteinizing hormone releasing hormone. *Endocrinology* 1991;129:1575–1583.
270. Wetsel WC, Mellon PL, Weiner RI, Negro-Villar A. Metabolism of pro-luteinizing hormone-releasing hormone in immortalized neurons. *Endocrinology* 1991;129:1584–1595.
271. Silverman AJ, Roberts JL, Dong K-W, Miller GM, Gibson MJ. Intrahypothalamic injection of a gonadotropin releasing hormone (GnRH) cell line results in cellular differentiation and reversal of hypogonadism in mutant mice. *Proc Natl Acad Sci USA* 1992;89:10668–10672.
272. Weiner RI, Thind KK, Windle JJ, Mellon PL, Goldsmith PC. Expression of SV-40 T antigen in GnRH neurons inhibits organization of terminals in the median eminence in transgenic mice. *Soc Neurosci Abstr* 1991;17:183.
273. Martinez De La Escalera G, Choi ALH, Weiner RI. Generation and synchronization of gonadotropin releasing hormone (GnRH) pulses: intrinsic properties of the GT1-1 GnRH neuronal cell line. *Proc Natl Acad Sci USA* 1992;89:1852–1855.

The Physiology of Reproduction, Second Edition,
edited by E. Knobil and J.D. Neill,
Raven Press, Ltd., New York © 1994.

CHAPTER 29

Lactotropes and Gonadotropes

Claude Tougard and Andrée Tixier-Vidal

Lactotropes and gonadotropes are two glandular cell types of the anterior pituitary that are specialized for the synthesis and release of three hormones that play key roles in the physiology of reproduction: a protein hormone, called prolactin (PRL), and two glycoprotein hormones, known as luteinizing hormone (LH) and follicle-stimulating hormone (FSH). The study of these cells involves three objectives:

1. To localize, within a heterogeneous glandular tissue, the cells that are responsible for the secretion of each of these hormones
2. To follow their morphological modifications in relation to the control of reproduction
3. To analyze, at the cellular and subcellular levels, the mechanisms involved in the secretion and release of these hormones.

This review has been organized with these three objectives in mind and is limited to studies performed on mammals. For studies involving the other classes of vertebrates, the readers may refer to ref. 1.

The elucidation of the cellular origin of PRL, LH, and FSH was lengthy and particularly difficult to attain because of the functional and structural heterogeneity of the anterior pituitary gland. It took 50 years of research to solve this problem, and the studies over this time period followed three successive steps. First, cytologists described several classes of cells at the light-microscopic level, on the basis of tinctorial affinities (2) and cytochemical properties, and attributed to each of them a functional significance using histophysiological indirect correlations (see refs. 3 and 4 for reviews). Then the use of conventional electron microscopy, which originated with the pioneering work of Farquhar and Rinehart (5) helped to establish the ultrastructural characteristics of such presumptive cell types and to describe their functional changes at the subcellular level [see reviews by Herlant (3,4) and Farquhar and colleagues (6)]. However, the usefulness of electron-microscope criteria to identify the cell types was questionable in light of findings obtained by the third, most conclusive, approach: immunocytochemistry. Indeed, progress in the chemistry and purification of anterior pituitary hormones, together with the preparation of specific antibodies and the technical improvements of immunocytochemistry at the light- and electron-microscopic levels, allowed the assignment of a specific hormonal function, with better accuracy than before (7–9), to each cell type. However, it should be noted that the identifications formerly proposed by conventional methods were often confirmed with the advent of immunocytochemistry.

These three approaches clearly revealed that, depending on the physiological and pathological situations, the number, size, shape, staining affinities, intensity of immunostaining, and ultrastructural features greatly vary. Such variations, together with the use of sophisticated methods such as high-resolution autoradiography and electron-microscopic immunocytochemistry, have per-

Groupe de Neuroendocrinologie Cellulaire et Moléculaire, Collège de France, 11, Place Marcelin Bertlelot, 75231 Paris, Cedex 05, France mitted access to the understanding of the secretory pathway and its regulation. Moreover, this was favored by the development of anterior pituitary cell cultures, which offered simplified situations in which to analyze the direct effect of a single agent and to correlate morphological data to hormonal secretion. Such a reductionist approach, however, does not represent an end in itself, but rather a necessary step toward the understanding of the highly integrated events involved at the pituitary level in the physiology of reproduction.

MORPHOLOGICAL FEATURES AND FUNCTIONAL SIGNIFICANCE

Lactotropes

Identification and Morphological Heterogeneity

The identification of PRL cells in the anterior pituitary tissue was first performed at the light-microscopic level as a result of their affinity for erythrosine following Herlant's tetrachrome (3) and then confirmed by immunocytochemistry using specific antibodies in the rat (7,10), the mouse (11), and the human (12–14), as well as in several other mammalian species (1). In the rat, PRL-containing cells are sparsely distributed in the lateroventral portion of anterior lobe and are present near the pars intermedia (7). Their shape and size are heterogeneous. They are frequently angular or polyhedral but are sometimes oval, rounded, and small. In the rat, "cup cells" with long cytoplasmic processes have been shown to surround gonadotropes (7,15). The number of PRL cells greatly varies in a given species, depending on the physiological situation and on the method used to determine their number (see below).

At the electron-microscopic level the identification of PRL cells was first based on cytophysiological studies using conventional electron-microscopic methods. They were characterized by a well-developed rough endoplasmic reticulum, a large Golgi zone, and large polymorphic secretory granules, at least in the rat (16,17) and in the human (3,16,18). The advent of immunoelectron-microscopic methods (7,9) confirmed such identification (Fig. 1) but also emphasized the risk of identifying PRL cells using ultrastructural criteria only, without the help of immunocytochemistry. Indeed, the presence of polymorphic secretory granules as a criterion to identify lactotropes was reconsidered in light of the electron-microscopic immunocytochemical findings. For example, in the same species (the rat), PRL secretory granules are sometimes spherical and of variable diameter (130–

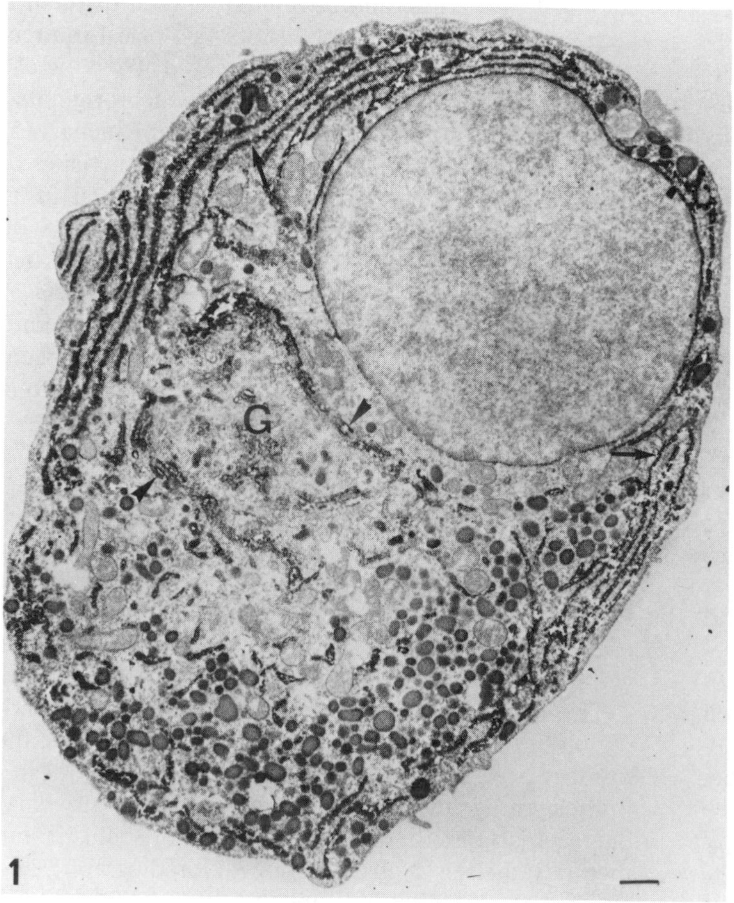

FIG. 1. A lactotrope in a primary culture of dispersed rat anterior pituitary cells is immunochemically stained with an antiserum against rat PRL using a preembedding immunoperoxidase method. This immunoreactive cell is characterized by flattened and parallel rough endoplasmic reticulum (RER) cisternae (*arrows*), a large Golgi zone (G), and polymorphic secretory granules. PRL is detected within RER cisternae and Golgi saccules (*arrowheads*). With this method, the large secretory granules are only outlined with reaction product. Bar: 1 μm.

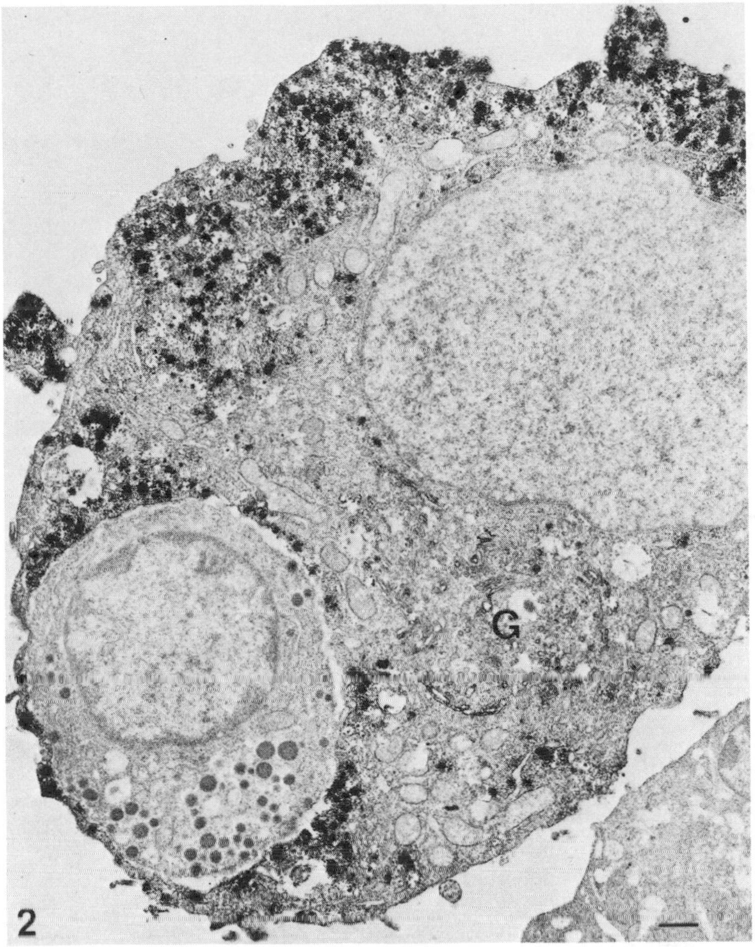

FIG. 2. Same material as Fig. 1. This immunoreactive PRL cell is characterized by its small and rounded secretory granules which are strongly labeled. Golgi zone (*G*). Bar: 1 μm.

300 nm) (Fig. 2). Moreover, in the same pituitary gland, some PRL cells may contain only small, rounded secretory granules, whereas others contain either large polymorphic granules or a mixed population of granules (19,20) (Figs. 1–3). Such diversity, which could not be related to a cell shape, has helped to distinguish three types of PRL cells in the rat pituitary: type I, having small spherical granules (130–200 nm in diameter), type II, having medium-sized spherical or polymorphic granules (250–300 nm in diameter); and type III, having large polymorphic granules (up to 700 nm in diameter) (15,21). A diversity in the shape and size of secretory granules was also observed in other mammalian species, such as the guinea-pig pituitary (22) and the bovine and porcine pituitaries (23,24). The functional meaning of the morphological heterogeneity of PRL cells is discussed later in this chapter (see the section on functional heterogeneity of lactotropes).

Distinction from Somatotropes

The fact that PRL and GH are each secreted by a different cell type was clearly established through the use of immunocytochemistry and by the availability of antisera specific for each of these two hormones in several species: rat (7,8,10), mouse (11), human (12,14,25), cow (23), monkey (26), guinea pig (22), and pig (24). These methods confirmed previous conclusions based on the selective affinity of GH cells for orange G and of PRL cells for erythrosine (see ref. 3). At the light-microscopic level, GH cells differ from lactotropes mostly by their ovoid or rounded shape. They are generally more numerous than lactotropes, and, at least in the rat, they are similarly distributed, except near the intermediate lobe where they are rarely found (7). At the electron-microscopic level the identification previously proposed by cytophysiological studies (see ref. 3) was confirmed by immunocytochemical methods (7,8). Like PRL cells, they possess a well-developed endoplasmic reticulum, but their secretory granules are always rounded, with an average diameter of 300–350 nm and, at least in the adult, often stored in great number in the cytoplasm. Thus it is clear that distinct cell types contain PRL and GH, respectively.

However, the existence of mixed cells, which contain and/or secrete both PRL and GH cannot be excluded. Such cells, called "mammosomatotropes" have been the

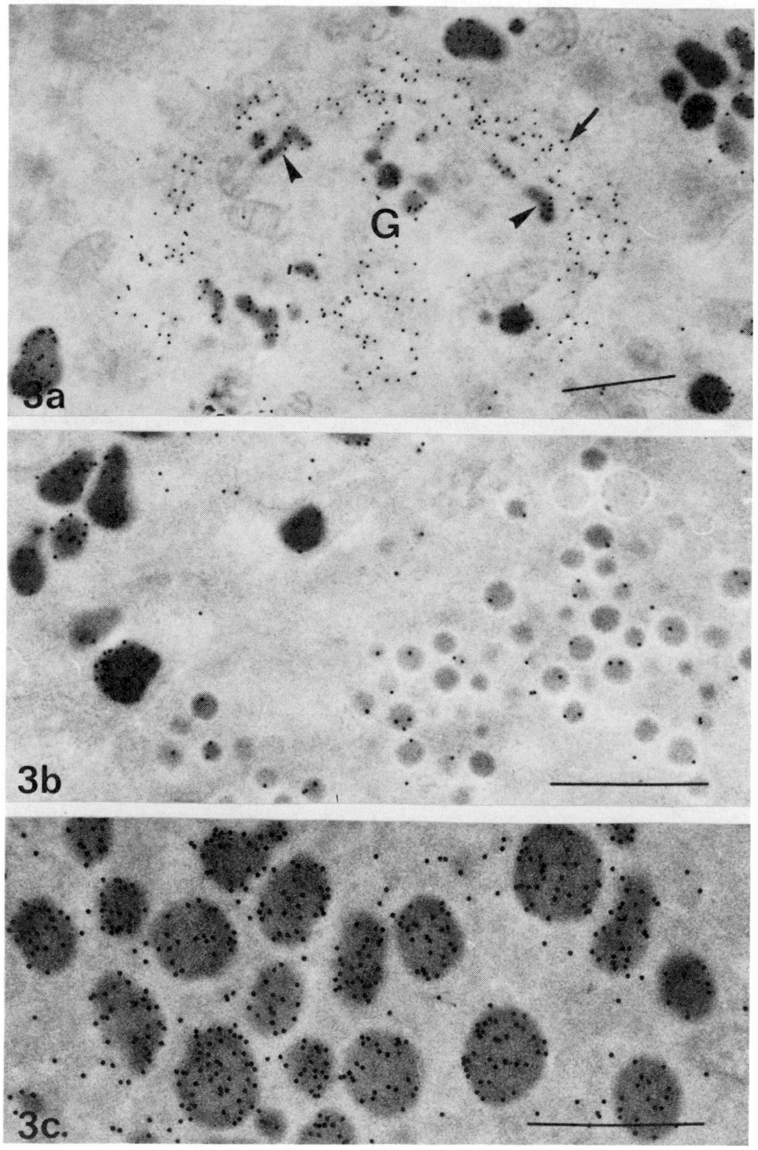

FIG. 3. Details of lactotropes of normal male rat pituitary immunochemically stained with an antiserum against rat PRL using a postembedding method (embedding in Lowicryl) and protein A gold complex (15 nm gold). Courtesy of Dr. E. Vila-Porcile. **A:** Detail of a Golgi zone (*G*). With this method, PRL is detected within all Golgi saccules (*arrows*) and on newly formed secretory granules (*arrowheads*). Bar: 1 μm. **B:** The secretory granules of two adjacent lactotropes are immunolabeled. One cell contains large polymorphous secretory granules, whereas the other contains small rounded secretory granules. Bar: 1 μm. **C:** High magnification of the large polymorphous secretory granules which display, with this method, a strong immunostaining. Bar: 1 μm.

subject of numerous reports within the last 5 years, taking advantage of technical progress of the immunoelectron microscopic methods, to detect dual hormone storage, and of the reverse hemolytic plaque assay, to detect dual hormone release at the individual cell level (27,28).

The first indications came from studies of pituitary adenomas in human being and rats, because of the frequent association of hyperprolactinemia with acromegaly. However, in a first attempt, the results of colocalizing GH and PRL in the same cells, using immunocytochemical methods, remained controversial (29). The first convincing demonstration was reported by Halmi (30) at the light-microscopic level on human pituitary adenomas. This was followed and confirmed at the light- and electron-microscopic level by several reports (reviewed in ref. 28). However, other authors found such dual cells extremely rare or absent in other series of human pituitary adenomas (31). Another approach to that problem was offered by the clonal cell lines, which were isolated from transplantable rat mammosomatotropic pituitary tumors. Among the subclones of the GH3 family, which is derived from the MtT/W5 tumor, some secrete either GH only (GC cells) or PRL only, but most of them secrete both PRL and GH, in variable amounts, depending on the clones and the culture conditions (29,32). However, attempts to colocalize PRL and GH in same cells were unsuccessful, not surprisingly in view of their low hormonal store. In contrast, clonal cell lines recently isolated from another mammosomatotropic rat pituitary tumor (MtT/F84) could be immunostained either for GH only (MtT/S) or for both PRL and GH (MtT/SM) (33). Functional evidence for a proportion of dual secretors among tumor derived cells was obtained with the reverse hemolytic plaque assay methods applied to GH3 cells, which secrete mostly GH and contain 19% of dual cells (34), and to dispersed neoplastic human pituitary cells where the percentage of dual secretors varied depending on the tumor (35).

Regarding "normal" nontumoral pituitaries, the existence of cells containing both PRL and GH was also shown, using dual immunostaining, in several mammalian species, first in the bovine (36) and the rat (37) (see review in ref. 28). However, other authors did not observe mixed cells in the cattle (23) or in the rat (38) or very rarely and doubtfully (39). The existence of cells secreting both PRL and GH was also revealed by the reverse hemolytic plaque assay applied to cells dispersed from normal pituitary cells taken from the rat (40,41), the human (35), the bovine (42). The percentage of mammosomatotropes varies depending on the authors, from 50% or 60% to 5% or even none. According to works from the group of Frawley (28), this percentage varies depending on the physiological conditions (see the section on Morphological Correlates of Physiological Regulation). This led this author to emphasize the physiological role of mammosomatotropes as a reservoir for the interconversion from GH cells to PRL cells and even vice versa (43). Such a filiation is also supported by recent molecular genetic studies on the differentiation of anterior pituitary cells (see the section on Ontogeny).

In conclusion, the existence of cells that contain and secrete both PRL and GH is convincingly demonstrated in normal pituitary tissue. However, this should not overcast the existence of specialized cells that store and release separately PRL and GH. This was clearly established by a long series of immunological and immunocytochemical studies that lasted for about 20 years (1960–1980) and marked the end of a period of confusion in the history of anterior pituitary cell cytology. From the present state of the literature, mammosomatotropes cannot be considered as a prominent cell type. Indeed, precautions are to be taken in the estimation of the percentage of dual cells using techniques (double immunostaining, sequential reverse hemolytic plaque assay) that have inherent limits, as pointed out by others (44). Nevertheless, they offer an interesting possibility for the physiological regulation of PRL secretion. Further studies on the mechanisms of PRL gene transcription and its regulation as well as on the cellular mechanisms of PRL storage are needed to ascertain their functional significance.

Subcellular Distribution of Prolactin Immunostaining: Relationship to Secretory Pathway

PRL cells have been often used as an archetype to analyze the secretory process in anterior pituitary cells (45–47). In particular, quantitative electron-microscopic autoradiographic studies performed on cultured mammotropes (48,49) have shown that the newly synthesized proteins undergo an intracellular transit analogous to that primarily established for the exocrine pancreas (50), involving the following steps:

1. Synthesis on attached polysomes and transfer into the rough endoplasmic reticulum
2. Transport within the Golgi apparatus from its *cis* face to its *trans* face
3. Concentration, aggregation into electron-dense material, and packaging into membrane-bound immature secretory granules in the *trans*most Golgi saccule
4. Storage in mature secretory granules
5. Extracellular discharge of secretory granules by exocytosis or, alternatively, intracellular degradation of secretory granules in excess, following their fusion with lysosomes.

These findings suggested that secretory granules are sorted at the exit of the Golgi zone. This is consistent with recent studies on other secretory systems which led to the characterization of a specialized compartment of the Golgi complex: the *trans* Golgi network for the sorting of secretory products (51). The current concept on the mechanism by which the Golgi subcompartments communicate relies on the budding and fusion of vesicles from a donor compartment to an acceptor (52). However, recent stereoscopic analysis of the Golgi apparatus of PRL cells in the rat pituitary gland (53) suggests a physical continuity between these compartments and suggests also that immature polynodular granules arise by fragmentation of portions of the *trans*most Golgi cisternae.

The chemical nature of the intraluminal secretory product could only be determined by electron microscope immunocytochemistry. In fact, the results greatly varied depending on the technical conditions (postembedding versus preembedding, fixative, permeabilization). In most cases, and whatever the technical conditions, the PRL immunostaining was observed on secretory granules, whatever their size or shape (Fig. 3). In contrast, the immunocytochemical detection of PRL within the rough endoplasmic reticulum cisternae and Golgi saccules and vesicles could be achieved only with the preembedding method and with the aid of permeabilizing agents in primary cultures of rat pituitary cells (19) (Fig. 4) and in GH3 cells (54) (Fig. 5). Similar results were observed in PRL cells *in vivo* with (55) or without (56) the aid of a permeabilizing agent or after lowicryl embedding (Vila-Porcile, unpublished observation) (Fig. 3). The immunostaining was heterogeneous or granular in the rough endoplasmic reticulum cisternae, including the perinuclear cisternae, and more homogeneous and dense on the luminal face of the Golgi cisternae (Fig. 4). Moreover, the respective intensity of the staining of

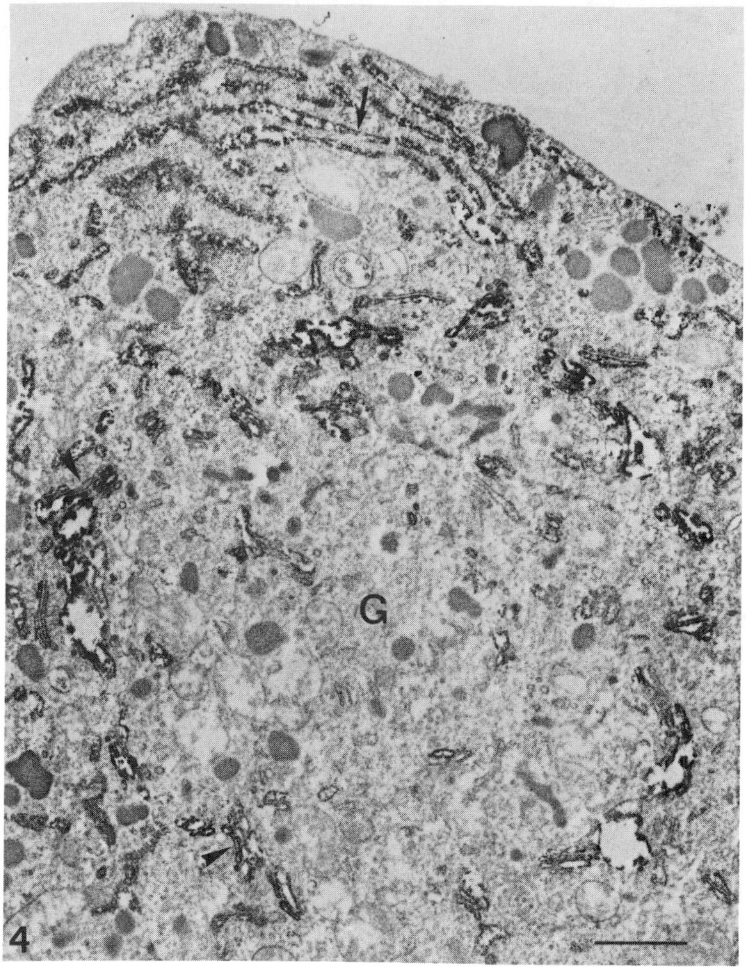

FIG. 4. Same material as Fig. 1. Detail of a Golgi zone (*G*) of an immunoreactive PRL cell. PRL is detected on the luminal surface of all Golgi saccules (*arrowheads*) and within RER cisternae (*arrow*). Bar: 1 μm.

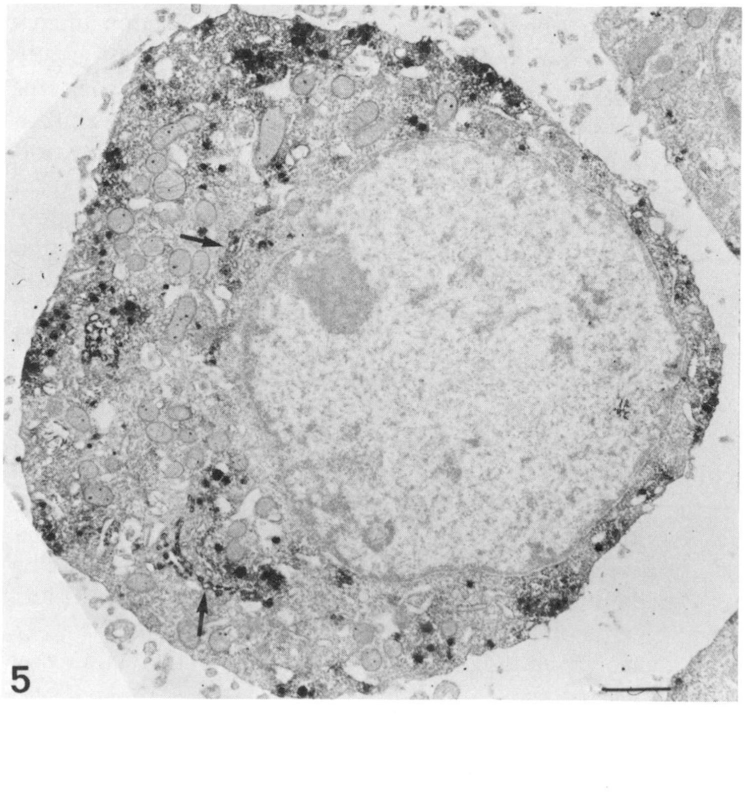

FIG. 5. A GH3B6 cell grown for 6 days in a chemically defined medium (De Carvalho-Brunet et al., 1985) and immunochemically stained with an antiserum against rat PRL. PRL is detected within Golgi saccules (*arrows*) and in the numerous small secretory granules. Bar: 1 μm. Courtesy of Dr. N. De Carvalho-Brunet and R. Picart.

these two compartments also varied from one cell to another, which may be related to functional heterogeneity (see below).

In conclusion, immunoelectron methods have helped to localize PRL at the main subcellular steps delineating its intracellular pathway. This has raised the possibility of detecting variations in the distribution of subcellular PRL staining, depending on physiological conditions *in vivo* and *in vitro* (see below).

PRL is known to be a structurally heterogeneous protein hormone. It exists as a major monomeric form of 23 kD and in a number of different molecular forms, which include aggregates and disulfide-linked polymers as well as glycosylated, phosphorylated, and proteolytically cleaved forms (see review in ref. 57). The precise site of occurrence of these different molecular forms during the intracellular transport of PRL is not yet well understood. A phosphorylation of a PRL isoform (58) and a mild proteolytic PRL processing at the C-terminus of the molecule by a glandular kallikrein (59–61) could occur in mature secretory granules. Moreover, different pathways of secretion for glycosylated and nonglycosylated human PRL have been postulated on the basis of different secretory rates and of a differential effect of pharmacological stimuli (62).

In addition to PRL, other components were immunocytochemically detected in lactotropes in compartments involved in the secretory pathway. Indeed, GH is not the only other hormonal product that could be detected in PRL secretory granules (see above). Secretogranins I and II, two acidic tyrosine-sulfated secretory proteins of the granin family, which display a widespread distribution in dense-core secretory granules of neuroendocrine cells, were found in secretory granules in bovine (63) and in rat (64) lactotropes, both normal and GH3 cells (64), as well as in rough endoplasmic reticulum cisternae and within Golgi saccules in both PRL cells (64). A heterogeneity of secretogranins and/or PRL immunolabeling of secretory granules has been reported in bovine anterior pituitary (36,65) as well as in GH3 (64) and GH4C1 cells (66). A role has been tentatively ascribed to secretogranins in the aggregation and packaging of secretory proteins into newly formed secretory granules. Indeed, it has been recently shown that these molecules aggregate in the presence of high calcium and low pH, conditions believed to exist in the *trans* Golgi network, in GH4C1 cells (67). In such a rat cell line, PRL granulogenesis is associated with increased secretogranin expression and aggregation (68). These findings allow the development of important new insights into the understanding of the secretory process. Laminin, a major component of the basement membrane of the anterior pituitary was detected within all organelles involved in the PRL secretory pathway *in vivo* (69,70) and *in vitro* (71) suggesting that this component is synthesized and exported in lactotropes as well as in nonepithelial cells of the rat pituitary (70,71). An immunoreactive glandular kallikrein, a trypsin-like serine protease, which displays same regulation as PRL (estrogen-induced and dopamine-repressed) was specifically observed within the Golgi apparatus and secretory granules of rat lactotropes (72,73). This is consistent with the hypothesis that this enzyme is a putative PRL-processing protease. Other endopeptidases as renin were also detected in secretory granules of human lactotropes (74). These enzymes could play a role in the proteolytic processing of secretory products present within these cells. The presence and, in some cases, evidence for synthesis of several peptides, such as vasoactive intestinal peptide (75,76), angiotensin II (AII) (77), galanine (78), thyrotropin-releasing hormone (TRH) (79), or TRH precursor (80), have been also demonstrated in lactotropes. These findings suggest that these peptides may be involved in the local (paracrine or autocrine) regulation of hormone secretion. Moreover, they suggest that these molecules, coexpressed in at least some PRL secretory granules, might be coreleased and address the question of the mechanisms involved in the regulation of nonparallel secretion.

Functional Heterogeneity

The first indication of a link between structural heterogeneity and functional heterogeneity was provided by studies performed with rat lactotropes separated by velocity sedimentation at unit gravity (81). Using this method, subgroups of lactotropes were isolated on the basis of their size and secretory granule content. This study revealed that the intracellular PRL content varies along with the cell fractions and according to different patterns, depending on the physiological state of the donor rat. Moreover, when the sorted cells were cultured for 14 days, the amount of PRL released into the medium during 14 days was positively correlated with their initial PRL content (81). PRL cell subpopulations could also be separated on discontinuous Percoll gradient and characterized for PRL content, by immunocytochemistry, for PRL mRNA, by in situ hybridization, and for PRL synthesis and release in culture. This showed that low-density PRL cells contain less PRL, but more PRL mRNA and have a high secretory activity in culture while lactotropes found at higher densities contain large amount of immunostainable PRL, but possess only a low secretory capacity and transcriptional activity (82).

Further convincing demonstrations of a functional heterogeneity of PRL cells *in vitro,* either primary cultures or clonal GH3 cells, were provided by three independent approaches: pulse-chase experiments with labeled amino acids, reverse hemolytic plaque assay, and the sequential cell immunoblot assay.

Pulse-Chase Experiments

The development of pulse-chase experiments to analyze functional heterogeneity in PRL cells began with the study of Swearingen (83), which revealed the first evidence for a heterogeneous turnover of PRL in the rat, *in vivo* and *in vitro,* and thus raised the question of the cellular origin of this heterogeneity. After an interval of 10 years this question could be reexamined because of the use of high-resolution autoradiography associated with immunoprecipitation methods applied in parallel. Using 2-day primary cultures of dispersed rat pituitary cells, Walker and Farquhar (84) confirmed that newly synthesized PRL was preferentially released under basal conditions. Moreover, the analysis of the distribution of total silver grains per cell in mammotropes identified by their ultrastructural features revealed the existence of several functional subpopulations that differed in the rapidity of loss of silver grains during the chase period. This suggested that some cells have a faster turnover time of PRL than others, which could result in the rapid release of newly synthesized PRL observed after 15–30 minutes of chase. Whether this corresponded to differences in the cell ultrastructural organization or in the size of the intracellular PRL pool was not determined. The existence of several functional subpopulations of PRL cells in primary culture was further corroborated by pulse-chase experiments where the chase was followed for up to 24 hours and was conducted in the presence of cycloheximide to prevent the dilution of labeled PRL by newly synthesized unlabeled PRL. This study clearly revealed an asynchrony of the release of labeled PRL in the medium, which occurred in successive waves (85).

GH3 cells, which differ from normal PRL cells by their very small intracellular PRL store and possess very few small secretory granules, were submitted to the same protocol of pulse-chase experiments and compared to normal PRL cells (86). This study revealed both similarities and differences between the two cell systems. In both cases, newly synthesized PRL was rapidly and preferentially released in basal conditions, and the pattern of the decay of specific radioactivity of PRL released into the medium suggested the existence of at least two PRL pools. Thus, whatever the size of the intracellular PRL store, the following events occur: (a) newly synthesized PRL is rapidly released under basal conditions, and (b) the turnover of PRL in a randomized cell population is heterogeneous. Moreover, the turnover time of the two PRL pools was eight times greater in normal cells than in GH3 cells (85,86). These findings suggest that functional heterogeneity may be linked to variations in the size of the intracellular PRL store in normal cells, as well as in GH3 cells. The latter cells, indeed, also display individual variations of PRL intracellular content, as previously revealed by immunostaining (54,87).

Reverse Hemolytic Plaque Assay

The reverse hemolytic plaque assay (RHPA) offers a direct access to the question of functional heterogeneity (27). Indeed, it allows the determination of two parameters at the individual cell level: (a) the percentage of plaque-forming cells, which is the percentage of secretors in a given population, and (b) the plaque area, which was found to be linearly related to the release of radioimmunoassayable PRL (27,88). Measurement of plaque areas on lactotropes derived from proestrus rats and cultured under basal conditions, revealed a bimodal frequency distribution indicating the existence of two functional subpopulations of lactotropes (88). The RHPA was also applied to GH3 cells. A close agreement was found between the percentage of immunostained PRL cells and the percentage of PRL plaque-forming cells.

Sequential Cell Immunoblot Assay

This study suggested a direct link between the storage and release capacity of GH3 cells, at least under basal conditions (89). The cell immunoblot assay also revealed a great heterogeneity of the releasing capacity of PRL cells (90). Using the RHPA, the functional heterogeneity was found to depend on the location of PRL cells in the pituitary (91), a finding which could be confirmed in anterior pituitary cells in situ by Mukherjee and colleagues (92) who devised a different, careful, experimental strategy. The RHPA method applied to cells previously exposed, or not, to inhibitors of protein synthesis for 21 hrs revealed that half of the population of PRL secretors are dependent upon newly synthesized hormone for basal secretion (93), an observation which is consistent with the above reported results of pulse chase experiments. The combination of RHPA with the localization of PRL mRNA using in situ hybridization has also shown a striking heterogeneity of PRL gene expression, in addition to PRL release, and a lack of correlation of these parameters within individual lactotropes (94).

Conclusions

In conclusion, the functional heterogeneity of PRL cells, in terms of PRL turnover, is now well established. The existence of an inverse relationship between, on the one hand, the size of the intracellular store, and, on the other hand, the turnover time and release capacity in basal conditions seems rather well supported by results of different experimental approaches. Whether there are subpopulations of PRL cells specialized for the release of newly synthesized PRL and for the response to secretagogues, respectively, has been investigated in parallel using the same methods as above. This is examined in the following section. However, the exact link between morphological heterogeneity (as defined by ultrastructural criteria) and functional heterogeneity remains unclear and requires further study at the single cell level. In any case, the structural heterogeneity of PRL cells represents a great obstacle in analyzing the ultrastructural correlates of pituitary function *in vivo* as well as *in vitro* (see the section on morphological correlates of physiological regulation of lactotropes and gonadotropes).

Ontogeny

The ontogeny of PRL cells was first determined by immunocytochemistry and compared to the timing of appearance of other pituitary cell types. Such information about the hormonal cell content was recently completed by the localization of the corresponding mRNAs, using in situ hybridization. This revealed novel aspects of the differentiation of specific cell types in the anterior pituitary which now provides an excellent system to study cell specific gene activation. The current view is that PRL-containing cells are the last to appear, being preceded by GH cells and the transient coexpression of GH and PRL.

A detailed examination of the literature concerning the onset of PRL immunostaining reveals, however, some discrepancies with this view, at least in the rat, the most widely studied model. Depending on the authors, PRL cells are detected in the pars distalis on fetal day 16 (95,96) or 18 (97) or 21 (98) or only in the newborn (99). Some authors detected PRL cells at the same time as GH cells (95,97), whereas others (98,99) detected GH cells 2 days before PRL cells. Most authors noticed that PRL cells remain the smallest in number and size during the perinatal period. This may explain the discrepancy of the results, together with differences in cell strains, antibodies, or techniques. Some scarce and scattered cells which reacted with both anti-PRL and anti-GH were detected by some authors (95,98). Thus, so far, the morphological evidence for an obligatory transient coexpression of PRL and GH prior to the appearance of PRL cells is extremely weak. However, using the RHPA method on cells taken from 4-day-old rats, 35.8% of the cells that release PRL were found to be dual secretors (100). Most interestingly, in situ hybridization using a PRL cDNA probe revealed PRL gene expression much sooner, at fetal day 17.5, and simultaneously with GH gene expression; again, the level of PRL mRNA remains low as compared to GH mRNA during the fetal and first postnatal days (101). Moreover, when compared to the percentage of PRL immunostained cells, the cells containing PRL mRNA were more numerous (12% vs 2%) before birth, whereas the number of GH mRNA-containing cells was close to the number of GH-containing cells (102). This suggested that in contrast to GH cells, PRL cells do not store PRL, because they release their content. Indeed, PRL could be detected in fetal blood from 19 fetal days onward; its plasma level then dropped at birth, prior to the postnatal increase of the number and size of PRL containing cells (102). Similarly, fetal rat pituitary taken at 17 days of gestation, and maintained in organ culture, release increasing amounts of PRL from 1 to 7 days *in vitro* (95). Altogether, these findings suggest that the apparent late differentiation of PRL containing cells may be the consequence of the rapid release and thus low storage of PRL during fetal and early postnatal days. Indeed, the number of PRL cells reaches the adult level 1 month after birth (97), as the main factors that control PRL secretion in the adult (dopamine, estrogens) are settled. A different view was proposed by Frawley's group (103) who also detected large amounts of PRL mRNA at birth, whereas PRL-containing or -releasing cells were not detected before day 4 of postnatal life. These authors concluded that translation of the PRL message would be blocked. However, they explored only the postnatal period beginning on the first day after birth.

In the human fetus, PRL-containing cells have been detected at an early stage of gestation, 14 weeks, but remain few in number up to 23 weeks (14,104). In addition, in anencephalic fetuses, PRL-containing cells were more numerous and larger than in normal fetuses of same age, which suggested that their development, or storage capacity, does not require a hypothalamic influence and might even be under an inhibitory control during fetal life (104). From a functional point of view, the use of the sequential reverse hemolytic plaque assay has revealed in fetuses of 18–22 weeks the releasing capacity of fetal PRL cells and, moreover, the presence of dual secretors (21.7% as compared to 69.9% somatotropes and 8.7% mammotropes) (105). However, as for the rat, the immunocytochemical evidence for cells containing both PRL and GH during fetal life are rare and weak.

Evidence for a coordinated regulation of the onset of expression of PRL and GH genes during the development of the anterior pituitary has been provided by the identification and localization of a pituitary-specific transcription factor Pit-1 which binds to *cis*-active elements in both the rat PRL and GH genes (106). By in situ hybridization Pit-1 mRNA expression becomes detectable at 15.5 fetal days, that is, 2 days before the appearance of PRL and GH mRNA. Pit 1 transcripts are present in all pituitary cells, whereas the Pit 1 protein is expressed only in PRL cells, GH cells, as well as, surprisingly, in thyrotropes (101). A linkage between the initial expression of Pit 1 and the coactivation of PRL and GH genes was also suggested by studies on transgenic mice (107) and on several strains of dwarf mice where mutations in the gene encoding Pit 1 lead to the absence of somatotropes, lactotropes, and thyrotropes (108,109). The absence of functional Pit 1 was, moreover, recently correlated with the absence of the receptor for GH-releasing factor (GRF), which is a specific mitotic factor for GH cells (109). This would be consistent with a model of direct filiation between somatotropes and lactotropes, which was proposed by Borelli and coworkers (110) on transgenic mice expressing the herpes simplex virus 1 thymidine kinase (HSV1-TK) gene fused with the rat GH or PRL promoters, respectively. This permitted a pharmacological killing of dividing cells which expressed the fused gene. Postnatal destruction of mitosis in GH-TK transgenic mice resulted in dwarfism and a marked decrease in the number of both GH- and PRL-containing cells. In contrast, similar treatment of PRL-TK transgenic mice failed to reveal any effect on GH and PRL populations and pituitary size. This suggested that dividing somatotropes or "presomatotropes" may serve as stem cells and common precursor to the final pool of nondividing mature somatotropes and lactotropes and that the acquisition of the PRL or GH phenotypes is a postmitotic event. This elegant experiment does not seem, however, to explain the totality of the factors involved in the postnatal development of PRL cells. Indeed the mitotic index of immunocytochemically identified PRL cells in the rat has been shown to be maximal at 1 month in male and female, to steeply increase at estrus in the young female, and to decrease with age (111). This suggests that phenotypically differentiated PRL cells can divide.

In conclusion, a temporal and coordinated combination of several factors, not yet completely elucidated, participates in the differentiation of the PRL cell phenotype. Transcription factors like Pit 1 are certainly involved at the onset of PRL and GH gene expression, during fetal life. During postnatal life, an interplay of receptors specific for PRL cells, like estrogen, dopamine D_2 and peptide receptors, respectively, should participate in the establishment of the PRL-specific phenotype.

Gonadotropes

Identification and Morphological Heterogeneity

The problem of establishing the cellular origin of LH and FSH has been a subject of controversy for many years. A separate cellular origin for these two hormones was postulated long ago on the basis of (a) nonparallel secretion of LH and FSH and (b) histophysiological correlations (3,6). The classic tinctorial methods more or less failed to completely solve the problem of gonadotrope identification. The introduction of cytochemical methods provided a better means of identifying glycoprotein-producing cells, but permitted only an indirect distinction between thyrotropic and gonadotropic basophils. This last category was further subdivided into FSH and LH gonadotropes (112). Definitive progress was made with the advent of immunocytochemistry. The earliest immunocytochemical studies, carried out

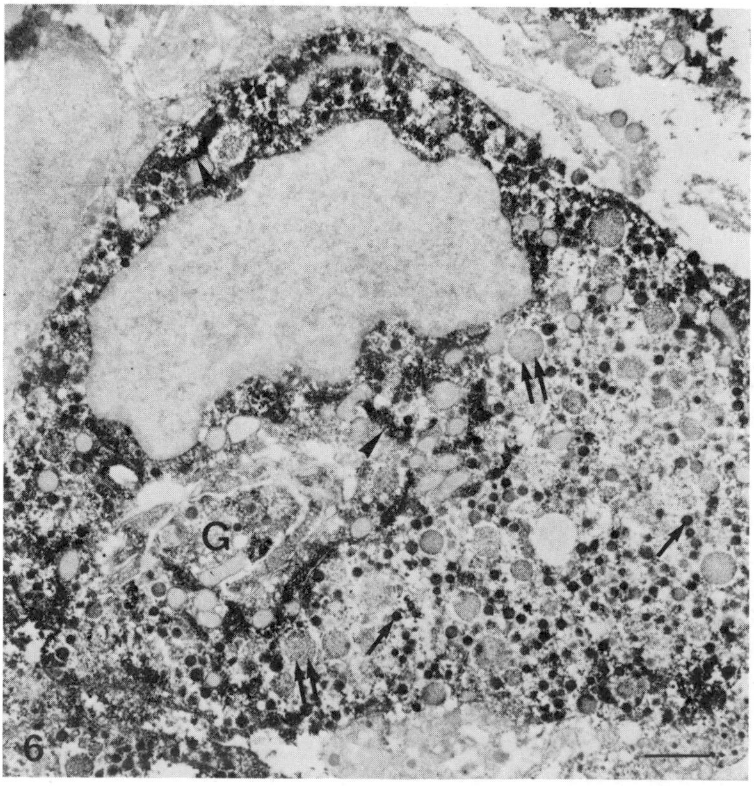

FIG. 6. A type I gonadotrope (two classes of rounded secretory granules) from a normal male rat pituitary is immunochemically stained with an antiserum against rat LHβ using a preembedding immunoperoxidase method. With this method, the immunocytochemical staining is more abundant over the small secretory granules (*arrows*) than over the large ones (*double arrows*). The reaction product is also observed in slightly dilated RER cisternae (*arrowheads*). In the Golgi zone (*G*), the saccules are negative, but some immunoreactive secretory granules can be seen. Bar: 1 μm.

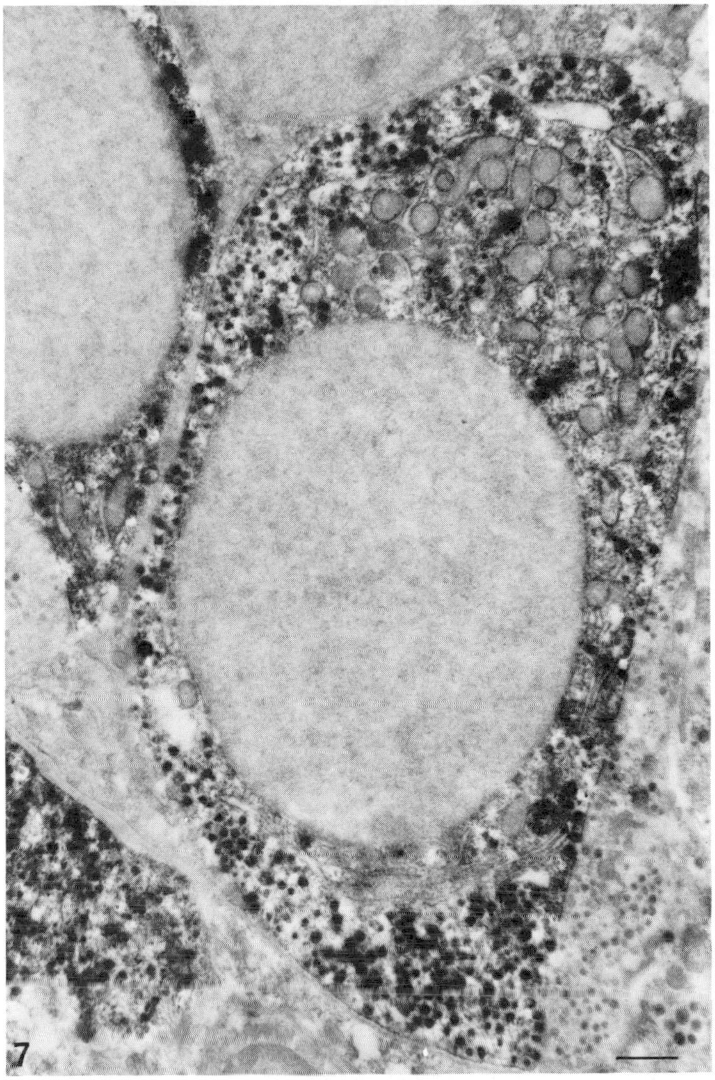

7

FIG. 7. A type II gonadotrope (one class of small secretory granules) from a normal male rat pituitary is immunochemically stained with an antiserum against rat LHβ using a preembedding immunoperoxidase method. The small secretory granules are strongly labeled. Bar: 1 μm. From Tougard et al. *J Histochem Cytochem* 1980;28: 101–114.

using antisera directed against whole hormones that share a common α subunit, showed that LH and FSH were present in the same cells (7). This was later confirmed with the use of antibodies against the specific β subunit of each hormone which permitted a more accurate identification of LH and FSH containing cells. Therefore, the concept of "one hormone, one cell" does not hold for gonadotropes.

At the light-microscopic level, the cells containing LH and FSH, which were identified by immunocytochemistry in the rat anterior pituitary using antibodies specific to rat β-LH and rat β-FSH, are distributed in an identical manner scattered throughout the glandular parenchyma, including the areas adjacent to the intermediate lobe. Two cell types can be distinguished by their shape and localization: large rounded or oval cells, which are abundant in the lateral and anterior regions of the pars distalis, and small oval cells, which are more numerous in the posterior portion. Using alcian blue-periodic acid-Schiff staining (AB-PAS) (3,113,114), all of these cells displayed the same violet color, indicating that they were AB- and PAS-positive (115,116). Gonadotropes were also detected in the pars tuberalis of the rat, as well as in other mammals (117–121). Combining immunocytochemistry with light-microscopic morphometry, gonadotropes represent approximately 14% of the cell population of normal adult rats (122) and normal female rats (123). These morphometric analyses confirmed a great variability in the size of gonadotropes, ranging from 30 to 160 μm^2 in area for male rat pituitaries (122) and from 130–170 μm^2 for female rat pituitaries (123).

A considerable morphological heterogeneity of rat gonadotropes has also been described at the electron-microscopic level. The first classification of gonadotropes was established on the basis of cytophysiological studies using conventional electron microscopy. Following the classic studies of Farquhar and Rinehart (5) and Barnes (124,125), Kurosumi and Oota (126) distinguished two types of gonadotropes in rats, one producing FSH and one producing LH, according to the criteria

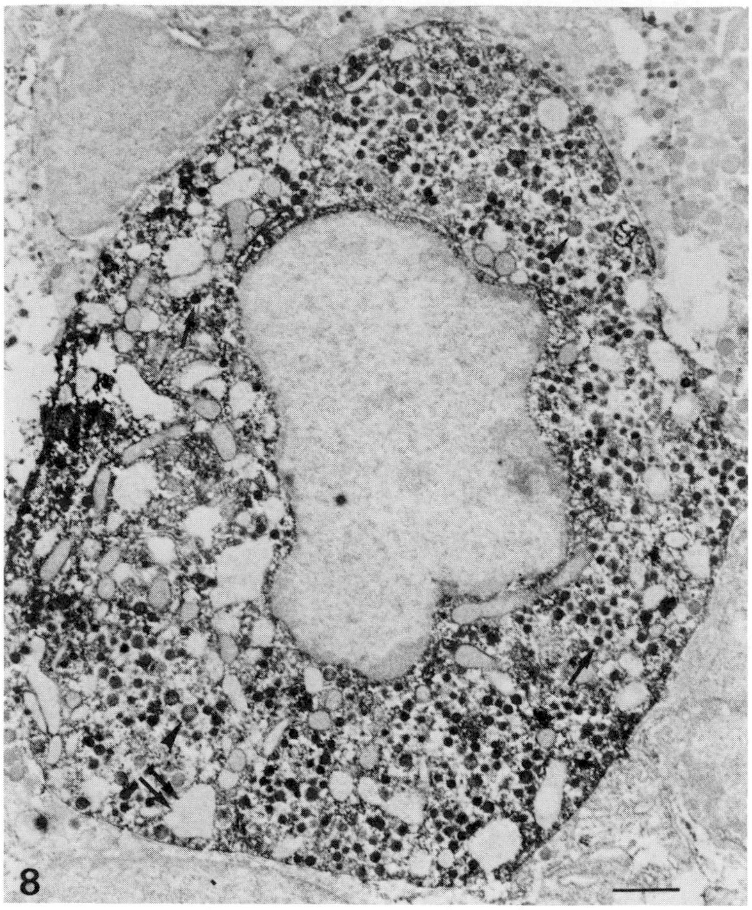

FIG. 8. An intermediate form between type I and type II gonadotropes from a normal male rat pituitary is immunochemically stained with an antiserum against rat LHβ using a preembedding immunoperoxidase method. This cell displays numerous small immunoreactive secretory granules (*arrows*), a few large secretory granules (*arrowheads*) and dilated RER cisternae (*double arrows*). Bar: 1 μm.

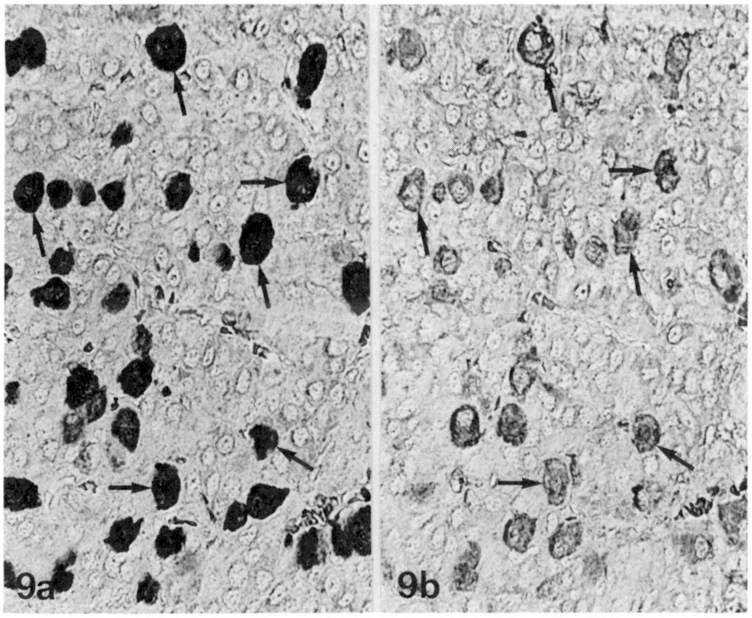

FIG. 9. Adjacent 3-μm paraffin sections of a normal male rat pituitary are immunochemically stained with antisera against rat LHβ (**a**) and against rat FSHβ (**b**) using a postembedding immunoperoxidase method. Same cells are stained by the two antisera (*arrows*) and, therefore, contain both hormones. The staining intensity is weaker with A-rFSHβ. From Tougard et al. *J Histochem Cytochem* 1980;28:101–114.

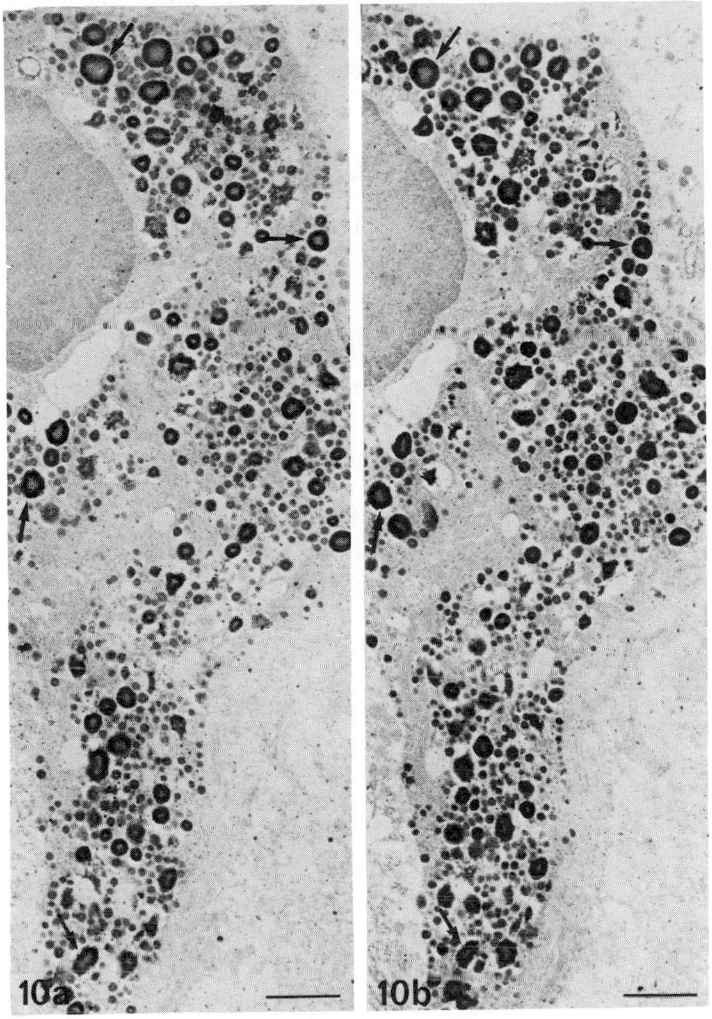

FIG. 10. Adjacent ultrathin araldite sections of a normal male rat pituitary are immunochemically stained with antisera against rat LHβ (**a**) and against rat FSHβ (**b**), using a postembedding immunoperoxidase method. Details of the staining of secretory granules of type I gonadotrope. Some of the large secretory granules (*arrows*) are stained by the two antisera and, therefore, contain both hormones. Bar: 1 μm. From Tougard et al. *J Histochem Cytochem* 1980;28:101–114.

described by Barnes (124) in mice. With the advent of immunocytochemical techniques, this classification has been questioned since it was discovered that the two cell types contain both gonadotropic hormones. The original Kurosumi-Oota FSH cell, characterized by a large and rounded shape, slightly dilated RER cisternae, and two types of secretory granules (200 nm and 300–700 nm in diameter, respectively), was named type-A gonadotrope by Nakane (7,9) and Tougard and colleagues (116,127) and type I-gonadotrope by Moriarty (128) and by Childs (Moriarty) and coworkers (129) (Fig. 6). This cell type, the most abundant in the normal male rat, contained both gonadotropic hormones, since it was labeled by antisera specific to the beta chain of LH and FSH. The original Kurosumi-Oota LH cell, characterized by an ovoid shape, flattened RER cisternae, and secretory granules of uniform size (200–250 nm in diameter), was named type-B gonadotrope by Tougard and colleagues (116,127) and type II gonadotrope by Moriarty (128) and Childs (Moriarty) and coworkers (129) (Fig. 7). This cell type, less abundant in the normal male rat, also contained both gonadotropic hormones. Numerous intermediate forms of these two cell types were observed (115,127,130) (Fig. 8). A third type of gonadotrope, far less numerous, has been described by Nakane (7), Moriarty (128), Moriarty and Garner (131), and Childs and colleagues (129); it was called type III gonadotrope by Moriarty and her coworkers, and it displayed the morphological features of ACTH-producing cells, that is, an angular and stellate shape, as well as peripherally distributed secretory granules of 220–250 nm in diameter. Moreover, it was stained by antisera against ACTH (ACTH 17–39) as well as antisera against the β chain of FSH or LH. Such angularly shaped cells were found only after using the postembedding method involving an antiserum against β-LH by Tougard and coworkers (116) and by Inoue and Hagino (132). These cells were not stained by an antiserum against ACTH (132). The significance of these cells will be discussed below (see the section on neonatal development).

In the human (133) and in other mammalian species (134,135), only one type of gonadotrope was found that contained both gonadotropic hormones. Moreover, an FSH-ACTH cell resembling a corticotrope was also described by Dacheux (136,137) in the pig.

In all species, the concentration of FSH and LH seems to vary from cell to cell, as suggested by variations in the intensity of immunostaining. When serial sections were stained for β-LH or β-FSH, respectively, or when double staining was applied to the same sections, it appeared that LH and FSH were stored in the same cells in the rat (7,9,116,127,128,130,138–142) (Figs. 9 and 10), human being (133,143), monkey (144–146), dog (120), mouse (11), and pig (135,147). However, some of these authors found cells containing only FSH or LH (7,120,122,128, 129,133,135,136,145,148–151). The number of these monohormonal cells varied, depending on the authors, according to physiological or experimental conditions. In the rat, the range of the percentages of monohormonal gonadotropes was from 40% to 10% in all the gonadotropes examined. As recently discussed by Childs (123), most of these studies were performed on serial sections of fixed-embedded tissue, and, since the size of gonadotropes greatly varies, the thickness of the section can shift the relative percentages of multihormonal and monohormonal gonadotropes. Moreover, extensive studies of Childs and her colleagues showed that under various experimental conditions (see the following sections) the number of multihormonal cells varied. This indicates clearly a certain fluidity of the gonadotrope population, as shown by the variability in their storage capacity (128). Therefore, it is clear that most gonadotropes are multihormonal. The monohormonal cells are, in fact, multipotential and, under specific conditions (see section on morphological correlates of physiological regulation of lactotropes and gonadotropes), bihormonal.

An important conclusion can be drawn from these immunocytochemical studies using highly specific antibodies applied to homologous species: the structural heterogeneity of gonadotropes does not reflect a biochemical specialization. Therefore, what is the physiological significance of the morphological heterogeneity of gonadotropes? It has been proposed that the structural heterogeneity of gonadotropes may reflect several stages of the secretory cycle of one single cell type capable of storing or releasing LH and FSH in different proportions, depending on physiological conditions (115). Thus, structural heterogeneity might correspond to a functional heterogeneity which will be discussed at a later point in this chapter (see the section on functional heterogeneity).

Subcellular Distribution of Gonadotropic Hormones

LH and FSH are glycoprotein hormones consisting of two different noncovalently linked α and β subunits. These subunits are synthesized as precursors that undergo posttranslational maturation. Glycosylation occurs both on the α subunit and the β subunit (see Chapter 31). As indicated above, the autoradiographic approach provides data related to the migration of neosynthesized proteins and glycoproteins, but not to the specific secretory product. Electron-microscopic immunocytochemistry should help to identify, within a given cell, the specific secretory product, among the other exported proteins at the successive steps of the secretory pathway. In fact, as mentioned above for PRL, the results for gonadotropic hormones vary greatly, depending on the methods (preembedding versus postembedding staining) and the fixative used (116,149,152).

The presence of an immunoreactive material within RER cisternae was only observed in some gonadotropes with an anti-β-LH antiserum in normal rats, and exclusively with the preembedding method (115,116), whereas β-LH and β-FSH were frequently observed in dilated RER of highly stimulated castration cells with both the preembedding and postembedding methods in rats (127,150,153) and in pigs (154).

In most studies, the Golgi saccules and vesicles were devoid of immunoreactive material, with the exception of some positive secretory granules in the core of the Golgi zone in gonadotropes (116,127,150) (Fig. 6). This may result from either a low level of hormonal content, a masking of antigenicity during the addition of carbohydrate components, or an inadequate entry of immunological probes into the membrane of this compartment. Indeed, Dacheux (154) has recently reported, with the use of the preembedding method and permeabilization with saponin, a strong labeling of saccules, small vesicles, and condensed material in the Golgi zone of highly active castration cells in pigs.

In all studies, secretory granules display the strongest staining intensity, which is in agreement with the data on hormone-storing cells. On ultrathin serial sections of rat (115,116,129) and pig pituitaries (135,147) β-LH and β-FSH were detected in the same granules (Fig. 10), clearly implying that the two hormones are simultaneously present in, at least, some granules. However, some authors have described granules containing either LH or FSH in LH/FSH gonadotropes using immunoperoxidase, immunoferritin, or immunogold techniques (135,142,153,155–157). Recent dual preembedding staining of gonadotropins in pituitary cell monolayers also suggests that LH and FSH can be stored in different regions of the same cell (158,159). Moreover, until recently, there was no conclusive evidence for the different subcellular localization of α and β subunits of LH or FSH. Both classes of secretory granules (large and small) were stained with an anti-α-LH, as well as with an anti-β-LH (116). This is of a great importance because it suggests that there is no compartmentalization of both subunits during their intracellular transport until storage in the secretory granule occurs, when they are found colocalized. However, we cannot exclude the possibility that secretory granules might contain different amounts of LH and FSH subunits.

In conclusion, it appears that immunocytochemistry allows us to delineate the secretory pathway of gonadotropic hormones within a given cell. However, until immunological probes that discriminate respectively between the precursor forms of gonadotropic subunits, the glycosylated or unglycosylated molecules, and the quaternary structure of mature hormones are available and applicable, this technique does not allow us to follow with precision the posttranslational maturation of gonadotropic hormones during the successive steps of the secretory process.

The presence of other molecules in the secretory granule matrix of gonadotropes has been reported. Secretogranins/chromogranins were detected in most secretory granules in gonadotropes and were colocalized with the hormones in cow anterior pituitary (63,160) and in rat pituitary (161). Moreover, it has been shown that secretogranin II is released concomitantly with LH in response to gonadotropin-releasing hormone (GnRH) (162,163). These proteins may play a role in the sorting and packaging of gonadotropic hormones. Laminin, a major component of the basement membrane of the anterior pituitary, was also detected in secretory granules of rat gonadotropes (69).

Several studies have reported a subcellular localization of GnRH, the hypothalamic decapeptide that controls the secretion of both LH and FSH in gonadotropes. Endogenous immunoreactive GnRH was observed in the matrix of secretory granules, which also contained β-LH and/or β-FSH immunoreactivity (137,164–166). Other factors have been localized in gonadotropes and may have a role in the local autocrine regulation of gonadotropic hormones biosynthesis and secretion. Indeed, this is suggested by the colocalization of cathepsin B, prorenin, and renin (167) and of angiotensinogen, angiotensin II, and LH in the same secretory granules (168,169) in rat gonadotropes. Moreover, inhibin/activin subunits (170) as well as follistatine, an activin-binding protein (171), and their mRNAs have been detected in rat gonadotropes which would be consistent with a possible activity as autocrine factors.

Functional Heterogeneity

To investigate the significance of the morphological heterogeneity of gonadotropes, several attempts to separate cell types have been performed using techniques based mainly on the variability of cell size.

Using sedimentation techniques at unit gravity, Denef and colleagues (172) separated gonadotropes from 14-day-old male or female rats and found that irrespective of cell size, the majority of the cells contained both FSH and LH, but that FSH and, to a lesser extent, LH were also stored in separate cells. These authors demonstrated that gonadotropes also differ in terms of their relative content and release of FSH and LH. The proportion of these two hormones differed according to cell size as well as sex and age of the rats (172). In small and medium-sized gonadotropes from 14-day-old rats, the FSH/LH ratio was lower than in large gonadotropes, and the release was in favor of LH. In adult males, the small and medium-sized gonadotropes released more FSH than LH, and inversely, the release in favor of LH was observed in large gonadotropes. These gonadotrope subtypes also differed in their response to GnRH as well as in the effects of androgen treatment on differential FSH and LH release (173–175). Moreover, Denef et al. (175) demonstrated that the majority of the largest gonadotropes corresponded to the type-A gonadotrope containing 200- and 700-nm secretory granules, whereas the small cells corresponded mainly to gonadotropes with 200-nm secretory granules. However, cells displaying numerous intermediate ultrastructural features were also found in the different cell populations. When placed in culture for 6 days, both subgroups of gonadotropes evolved toward a single cell type with small secretory granules (Tougard and Denef, unpublished results). Thus, the morphological heterogeneity of the gonadotropes disappears in culture, whereas the functional heterogeneity persists (174,176).

Using centrifugal elutriation to separate subtypes of gonadotropes from pituitaries of a mixed group of cycling female rats, Childs and associates (151) also demonstrated a heterogeneous LH and FSH storage pattern, related to cell size, on serially sectioned and immunocytochemically stained cells: smaller gonadotropes appeared to store only one of the hormones, whereas most of the larger cells either stored LH and FSH together, or FSH alone. This heterogeneous storage pattern persisted for up to 3 days in culture (151). Moreover, these gonadotrope subtypes differed in their capacity to bind GnRH; the small monohormonal cells contained little or no GnRH binding activity (177). However, more recently, a shift from monohormonal to multihormonal gonadotropes has been revealed in GnRH-treated small gonadotropes (178), suggesting that the small gonadotropes are multipotential and respond to stimulation by synthesizing and storing the other gonadotropin.

Using the reverse hemolytic plaque assay (RHPA) (27) for the measurement of secretion by individual cells, Smith and colleagues (179) demonstrated a heterogeneity in the release capacity of gonadotropes that contain immunoreactive LH. More recently, using both RHPA for LH and FSH and dual immunocytochemistry, Lloyd and Childs (178) showed a striking heterogeneity between the storage and secretory patterns in small or large gonadotropes.

Taken together, these findings strongly suggest that the selective modulation of FSH or LH release *in vivo* is linked to the functional heterogeneity of the gonadotrope subtypes. However, the gonadotrope subtypes do not appear to correspond to different classes of cells, but rather to several stages of the secretory cycle (115,151). In the future, a direct correlation of the ultrastructure and secretory activity at the single cell level, using the reverse hemolytic plaque assay, would allow confirmation of this interpretation.

Ontogeny

The appearance of gonadotropes during the ontogenesis of the anterior pituitary has been extensively studied using immunocytochemistry at the light-microscopic level. In the rat fetus, some immunoreactive LH cells, localized in the ventral part of the gland, appear on the 17th day of gestation, are more numerous at 18 days of gestation, and their number continues to increase until the end of gestation (96,99,180,181). Immunoreactive FSH cells appear later on, depending on the study, between days 19 and 20 of gestation, and their distribution is similar to that of immunoreactive LH cells. Moreover, it has been recently shown (101) that the expression of transcripts encoding the α-subunit common to the three rat pituitary glycoprotein hormones occurs very early in the single layer of somatic ectoderm on embryonic day 11 prior to formation of a definitive Rathke's pouch. Gonadotropes appear on the 49th day of gestation in the sheep fetus (182), on the 45th day of gestation in the pig fetus (183,184) and not before the 53rd day of gestation in the monkey fetus (185). In the human fetus, only subunits are detected by the 8th week of intrauterine life, followed by LH during the third month, and FSH by the beginning of the fourth month (186,187). LH and FSH were present in the same cells, which were more numerous in the female fetus. At birth, the gonadotropes are scarce and are located at the ventromedial zone of the anterior pituitary. From all of these immunocytochemical studies performed with specific antisera, it is clear that (a) the α-subunit appears earlier than the β subunit or the complete hormone, and (b) LH appears earlier than FSH. Gross and Baker (188) have shown that LH gonadotropes and GnRH-containing neurons appear concomitantly in the mouse fetus at the 17th day of gestation, suggesting a neuroendocrine control of gonadotropin differentiation. This hypothesis has been the subject of several studies. Morphological studies performed either after experimental encephalectomy (181), or with cultures of adenohypophysial primordia explanted at different ages of gestation, support the hypothesis of an autodifferentiation of gonadotropes, independent of hypothalamic GnRH (181,189–191). However, contradictory conclusions were reported by several groups. Stud-

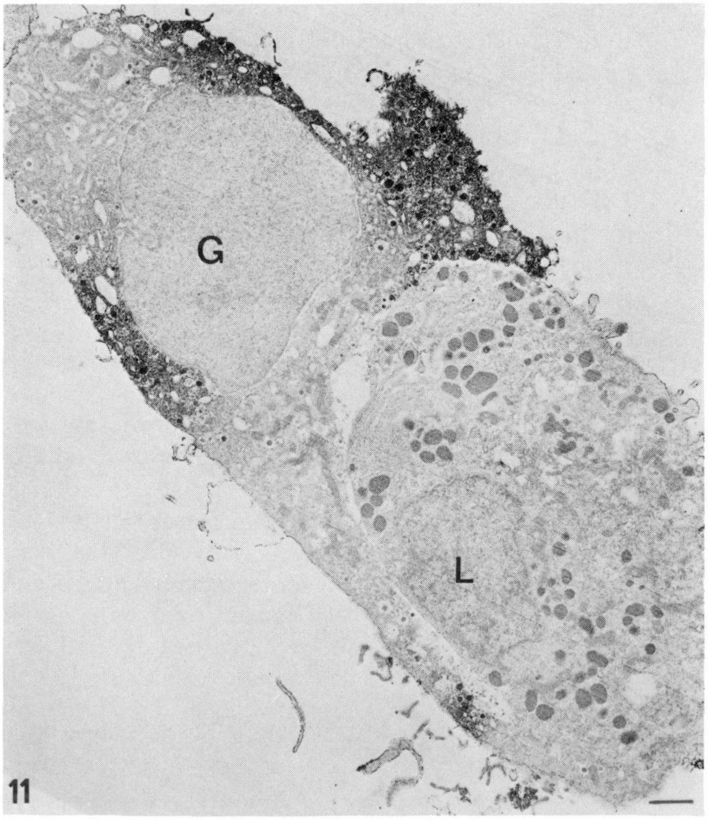

FIG. 11. A seven-day monolayer of rat anterior pituitary cells is immunochemically stained with an antiserum against ovine LH. An immunoreactive gonadotrope (*G*) surrounds a negative lactotrope (*L*) characterized by its polymorphic secretory granules. Bar: 1 μm.

ies performed *in vitro* by Begeot and coworkers (192,193) suggested that GnRH can stimulate the differentiation of gonadotropes at a very early fetal stage (11 days) in synergy with insulin.

At the electron-microscopic level, using conventional methods, the first granulated cells are detected between the 16th and 17th days of gestation in the fetal rat pituitary. They do not display the ultrastructural features of mature adult cells and cannot be identified on this basis. Morphological analogy with adult cells begins to occur between the 18th and 19th days of gestation (194–196). Electron-microscopic immunocytochemistry allowed the identification of the first immunoreactive gonadotropes on day 16 in the rat fetus (180) and on day 40 in the pig fetus (197). These cells initially display the ultrastructural features of immature cells with a few small secretory granules and then, with increasing time of gestation, they undergo progressive morphological differentiation involving the development of RER cisternae and the Golgi zone, as well as an increased number and size of secretory granules. At the end of gestation in the pig, gonadotropes possess the ultrastructural features of mature cells (197) whereas in the rat they still differ from adult gonadotropes (180).

Topographical Relationship Between Lactotropes and Gonadotropes

In early studies, similar distribution and preferential association of lactotropes and gonadotropes were observed by Nakane (7) in his pioneering immunocytochemical study of the anterior pituitary, which suggested some physiological relationship between them. In later work, gap junctions (198) and small adherent junctions between lactotropes and gonadotropes (199) were reported. Such a topographical relationship between the two cell types was also observed *in vitro* after dissociation of the pituitary cells and reassociation during cell culture. *In vivo,* cup-shaped or angular PRL cells surrounded large gonadotropes using long cytoplasmic processes (7,15). *In vitro,* lactotropes surrounding gonadotropes and, inversely, gonadotropes surrounding lactotropes, were frequently observed (Fig. 11).

This selective topographical relationship suggested the existence of a functional interaction between these two cell types. This exciting hypothesis has been extensively investigated for several years by Denef (176,200) using cocultures or reaggregated cell cultures of lactotrope- and gonadotrope-enriched populations, obtained by unit gravity sedimentation. This author has demonstrated that these cell types are functionally coupled and that GnRH stimulated gonadotropes can activate the secretory activity of lactotropes through the release of a paracrine factor (201).

MORPHOLOGICAL CORRELATES OF PHYSIOLOGICAL REGULATION OF LACTOTROPES AND GONADOTROPES

The morphological correlates of the physiological regulation involved in the control of reproduction have been studied *in vivo* and *in vitro.* In the first case, the morphological observations were correlated with biological responses that represent a series of integrated events involving multifactorial interactions and a cascade of events ranging from variations in the circulating levels of PRL and gonadotropins, to lactation and gonadal activity. In the second case, the morphological observations could be better correlated to the pituitary cell response, sometimes at the individual cell level. Thus, these studies provided deeper insight into the understanding of cellular and subcellular mechanisms underlying the control of the physiology of reproduction at the anterior pituitary level.

Lactotropes

In Vivo *Studies on Lactotropes*

Lactotropes are well known to undergo striking morphological modifications in relation to the main events of the physiology of reproduction: gestation, lactation, sexual cycle, castration, and sexual steroid treatments. These events have been shown to affect several parameters of the cell activity, such as cell number, cell shape, cell ultrastructure and subcellular distribution of PRL immunostaining, individual cell secretory activity (using reverse hemolytic plaque assay), and, more recently, localization of PRL mRNA by in situ hybridization. Other physiological or pathological situations also affect the number and secretory activity of PRL cells: development of prolactinomas, aging, effect of dopamine agonist treatment, thyroidectomy, and TRH or thyroid hormone treatments. The most recent progress has been made concerning the involvement of PRL cells in the physiology of reproduction.

Gestation and Lactation

The increase in number and size of acidophils during gestation and lactation was long ago correlated with an augmentation of PRL secretion in the rat and the human (12,16,202). This was confirmed, using PRL immunostaining in the rat (203) and in the human (13). In the rat the increase in number was found to be restricted to a subtype of large PRL cells (type II), which became prominent during gestation (203). These observations were confirmed and completed by immunogold electron microscopy: the prominent cell type at day 14 of gestation onward contains very few small secretory granules and a remarkable development of the rough endoplasmic reticulum and the Golgi zone (204). In the human, the increase in the number of PRL cells was sometimes found to be associated with a decrease in the number of GH cells, at least when identified on the basis of tinctorial affinity only (205). This observation lead Frawley's group to investigate, using the sequential reverse hemolytic plaque assay, the relative proportion of cells that secrete PRL only, or GH only, or both GH and PRL. These authors indeed observed an increase in the percentage of PRL secretors from virgin to gestation and late lactation accompanied by a decrease of GH secretors. Since the total number of secretors did not vary significantly, they postulated an interconversion from GH cells into PRL cells through mammosomatotropes that, however, represented a minor proportion of secretors (206). Reciprocally, after weaning, the progressive decrease in number of PRL secretors was associated with the return to a normal percentage of GH secretors. This led the same group to postulate a bidirectional interconversion of these two cell types (43). The molecular mechanisms of such an interconversion of the expression of the PRL and GH genes have been investigated in tumor-derived GH3 cells and found to involve posttranscriptional regulation of PRL gene expression (207). Whether this is valid for non-tumoral cells that possess a much larger storage compartment than GH3 cells and a more complex pattern of secretory process remains to be proven. Informations on the mitotic activity of immunostained PRL cells in these conditions are lacking to our knowledge; they would be extremely useful to clarify the mechanism of the apparent increase in the number of PRL-containing cells.

The ultrastructural correlates of the variations of PRL secretion during lactation, suckling, and weaning (208) have been first examined using conventional electron microscopy methods (16,17). In lactating rats, PRL cells exhibited a dilated Golgi apparatus and numerous granule exocytosis at the plasma membrane. After a 10-hour separation from the litters, a striking accumulation of secretory granules in the cytoplasm was first reported by Pasteels (16) and the fusion of secretory granules with lysosomes ("crinophagy") by Smith and Farquhar (17). Suckling for 5 to 15 minutes following removal of litters resulted in a dramatic increase in granule extrusion (16,209,210). The subcellular distribution of PRL immunostaining was also followed in similar conditions (55). This revealed a rapid redistribution of PRL immunostaining within morphologically modified compartments of the secretory process. The Golgi compartment was the most rapidly and strongly affected by weaning from 6 to 50 hours. This consisted of both an increase in number of labeled cisternae in the Golgi stacks and an enhancement of the immunostaining in a given cisterna. At the same time, crinophagic structures containing masses of PRL-immunostained material greatly increased in number. Curiously, during that period, forming granules were still present in the core of the Golgi zone and exocytosis of PRL granules remained frequent (55). These observations suggest a rapid regulation of the intracellular transport of PRL at the level of the Golgi compartment whereas the post-Golgi compartment seems to exhibit a sort of "inertia" leading progressively to the communication between the secretory granules and the lysosomal compartment. These changes in subcellular distribution of PRL might be related to the "depletion-transformation" of PRL previously reported by biochemical methods (211).

Sex-Related Differences

In the human (14) as well as in the rat (21) the number of immunostained PRL cells is only slightly greater in the female. However, when the cellular releasing capacity is taken into account using the reverse hemolytic plaque assay, their proportion is greater in the female rat according to Leong and colleagues (40). In the mouse, a sexual dimorphism of PRL cells has been described and correlated with differences in amino acid composition (212). A careful stereological morphometric study using immunohistochemistry by light microscopy, correlated with routine electron microscopy on serial sections, has confirmed that there are marked sex differences in the proportion of PRL and GH cells in the adult mouse: PRL cells are noticeably more abundant in the female (45.1%) than in the male (23.8%), whereas GH cells are more abundant in the male (54.6%) than in the female (35.6%). However, the proportion of mammosomatotropes detected by staining of adjacent pairs of serial sections was very low in both sexes (less than 1%) (213). Interestingly, this female pattern of PRL cell and GH cell percentages was not affected by neonatal treatment with testosterone propionate, which is known to masculinize, irreversibly, the hypothalamus. However, the absolute number of parenchymal cells was increased by the treatment and consequently the absolute number of PRL cells and of GH cells, in agreement with radioimmunoassay data on PRL secretion. Again, the proportion of mammosomatotrope remains less than 1% (214).

Sexual Cycle

The proportions of immunostained cells that contain PRL, or GH, or both hormones, have been shown to fluctuate considerably throughout the annual reproductive cycle in bats (215). In the bovine, attempts have been made, using the reverse hemolytic plaque assay method, either separately or simultaneously, for PRL and GH to demonstrate a bidirectional interconversion of GH and PRL along the luteal phase up to the follicular phase (42). The data, however, are not really convincing.

Estrogen Treatment and Ovariectomy

The stimulating effect of long-term estrogen treatment on PRL secretion was correlated long ago with the hyperplasia and hypertrophy of acidophils in the rat (16) as well as in several mammalian species (see ref. 1 for a review). This was confirmed at the electron-microscopic level in the rat (216–218). Later, interesting observations were reported following treatments (5–15 days) with 17β-estradiol of young female rats. PRL cells were immunocytochemically identified by a superimposition technique, and the relative proportions of cells grouped into the three classes previously defined by these authors (see above) were determined as a function of treatment for each sex (21). This suggested an interconversion from type I to type II and type III cells, concomitant with an increase in pituitary PRL content and serum PRL levels as a result of estradiol treatment in females, and to a lesser extent, in males. This interesting study suggests that a sustained stimulation of PRL synthesis and release leads to an enlargement of secretory granules (type III cells were characterized by very large pleomorphic secretory granules and sometimes called "mature type").

In contrast to estrogen treatment, castration has been shown to induce a marked decrease of PRL cell size, an accumulation of small secretory granules (56), and a decrease in cell number in the female rat after 4 weeks (219). Treatment of castrated rats with estrogen induced, within 4 days, cell hypertrophy, the disappearance of secretory granules, and a considerable development of rough endoplasmic reticulum cisternae containing PRL, whereas the Golgi zone remained small and almost unstained (56). These effects of 17β-estradiol (E_2) on the secretory activity of PRL cells of ovariectomized rats were found to be detectable very rapidly (3 hours), using the reverse hemolytic plaque assay method. They consisted of both the recruitment of additional PRL secretors and the enhancement of the releasing capacity of individual PRL cell. Moreover, this required the presence of neurointermediate cells (NIL) suggesting that E_2 acts indirectly on PRL cells (220). Using the simultaneous reverse hemolytic plaque assay method, the recruitment of PRL-releasing cells was found to be the consequence of an increment in the proportion of mammosomatotropes correlated with an equivalent decrease in the proportion of cells secreting GH only, and was blocked in the presence of an inhibitor of protein synthesis (221). These authors suggested that "E_2 stimulated NIL cells to release an activity which initiates translation of dormant PRL mRNA within cells that previously secreted only GH" (221). Using an elegant combination of the reverse hemolytic plaque assay method and of in situ hybridization, Scarbrough and colleagues (94) could measure in a same cell PRL release and PRL mRNA expression in the pituitary of ovariectomized rats treated, or not, with estradiol for 4 days. This showed that estradiol

1. Increased the percentage of PRL-releasing cells as compared to total pituitary cells
2. Increased the percentage of PRL releasing cells as compared to the number of cells containing PRL mRNA
3. Did not increase the percentage of pituitary cells expressing PRL mRNA.

This suggested that under these conditions, estradiol did not transform other pituitary cell types into lactotropes (94). This approach shed a new light on the relation between gene expression and cell-releasing activity; clearly, these two parameters of the secretory activity are not directly related. This also suggests that the number of cells expressing mRNA for a given hormone may be fixed definitively.

Pituitary Adenomas

Experimental Tumors. It is well known that massive and prolonged (for months) administration of natural or synthetic estrogens gives rise to pituitary adenomas and eventually transplantable tumors, which can be serially transferred and lose their estrogen dependency (see refs. 222 and 223 for reviews). In general, the development of adenoma coincides with the reduction in size and number of secretory granules. PRL has been immunocytochemically localized in small secretory granules, and GH has been localized in larger granules, but these have been found in separate cell types in transplantable rat mammosomatotropic tumors (224). The appearance of tumors depends on several factors, such as age, sex, and species. For example, in the dog and the monkey estrogens stimulate PRL secretion without inducing tumors (225).

Human Prolactinomas. Variability in the size and structure of cells in human prolactinomas has been widely described at the electron-microscopic level (223,226) and can also be observed after PRL immunostaining. At the light-microscopic level, the intensity of the immunostaining greatly varies from cell to cell (227,228), suggesting again a functional heterogeneity of tumor cells.

The effects of bromocriptine (CB-154) (a dopamine agonist that is widely used to reduce PRL secretion in patients with prolactinomas) on PRL cell morphology were analyzed in order to explain the cellular mechanisms involved in the reduction of tumor size and secretory activity (229–231). These studies revealed a reduction in cell size (by about 50%), mostly involving the whole cytoplasm, whereas the number of secretory granules tended to increase. Depending on the reports, or on the tumors, the PRL cell immunoreactivity was either lowered or unchanged. Such analyses, however, are hampered by the considerable heterogeneity of structure among tumors, as well as among cells for a given tumor. The morphological effects of this drug were stereologically analyzed within hours following a single subcutaneous injection to ovariectomized estrogen-primed rats. Serum PRL level was reduced within 15 min and suppressed at 2–6 hours. This was correlated to a reduction in volume of the Golgi complex at 2 hours, whereas the volume of mature secretory granules and of the secondary lysosomes had significantly increased at 6 hours. These acute morphological changes were restricted to PRL cells of the central region of the gland (232).

Thyroidectomy and Thyrotropin-Releasing Hormone Treatment

An immunogold electron-microscopic and morphometric study was carried out on the anterior pituitary of adult male rats thyroidectomized for 3 weeks and simultaneously treated, or not, with L-thyroxine (T_4), or with TRH, or with both T_4 and TRH (233). Thyroidectomy induced an atrophy of PRL cells as revealed by the reduced area of the cytoplasm and of the Golgi apparatus and by the reduction in size and number of secretory granules, with a majority of type I (immature) PRL cells. Similar signs of atrophy were previously observed on GH cells of thyroidectomized rats by the same group. These effects of thyroidectomy on PRL cells were prevented by chronic T_4 treatment, which even increased the percentage area of the rough endoplasmic reticulum to more than twice the control level. Chronic treatment with TRH of intact rats induced an hypertrophy of PRL cells with an augmentation of the rough endoplasmic reticulum and of the Golgi apparatus percentage areas and an increase in number and size of secretory granules, whereas in thyroidectomized rats it was much less efficient than T_4 in preventing the effects of thyroidectomy on PRL cell atrophy. However, simultaneous treatment of thyroidectomized rats by both T_4 and TRH induced an hypertrophy of PRL cells, with a considerable enlargement of the percentage surface occupied by the Golgi apparatus and by the rough endoplasmic reticulum (three times of the controls) and a majority of large pleomorphic granules indicating a conversion to type III mature PRL cells. These morphological observations on immunocytochemically identified PRL cells are consistent with the variations of serum and pituitary PRL levels measured in same animals by radioimmunoassays (233). They are also in agreement with the present knowledge on the interaction of thyroid hormones with TRH on PRL gene expression.

Postnatal Changes and Aging

In the rat, the distribution of PRL cells between type I, type II, and type III (see above) has been found to evolve postnatally up to adulthood, and differently in male and female. Whereas a similar distribution was observed in both sexes at 8 postnatal days, with a majority (82–83%) of type I, a rapid increase in the frequency of type III (mature type) occurred at puberty in the female only, where this type reached 91% of PRL cells in the adult. In contrast, in the adult male pituitary, type II and type III cells were equally frequent (48% and 46.8%, respectively) and the proportion of type I, although small, remained higher than in the female (39). These findings are consistent with the role of estrogen in the conversion of PRL cell subtypes.

In senile female Wistar rats, the spontaneous occurrence of prolactinomas associated with repeated pseudogestations has been reported by Ascheim (234). The predominant cell type in these tumors was observed by Pasteels (16) to display the characteristic affinity of PRL cells for erythrosine. These pioneering observations were thereafter largely confirmed (see ref. 235 for a review). Spontaneous tumors, which often consist solely of PRL cells, have now been described in several rat strains (236–238). One of these spontaneous tumors has been shown to be transplantable and not dependent on the level of circulating estrogens (239).

The cellular mechanisms of these age-related hyperprolactinemias were examined by Chuknyiska and coworkers (235) using short-term cultures of dissociated anterior pituitary cells taken from either adult (6 months) Wistar rats at estrus or diestrus, or old (22–24 months) rats in constant estrus or diestrus. This study revealed that aging is associated with a significant but small increase (30–35%) in cell number and a tremendous increase (80–120%) in the secretory response to estradiol treatment *in vitro* for 4 days. This suggests that the control of PRL gene expression may be altered by aging.

In the human, immunocytochemically identified lactotropes have been found to considerably decrease in number and size with advancing age (48, 65, and 76 years) in both sexes (14).

In Vitro *Functional Studies on Lactotropes*

Lactotropes in culture have been extensively studied within the last 20 years to analyze the cellular and molecular mechanisms involved in the control of PRL secretion. Such studies took advantage of the availability of two model systems that were described in the section on morphological features and functional significance: (a) primary cultures of enzymatically dispersed, normal rat anterior pituitary cells in which the proportion of PRL cells rapidly increases (up to 70%) concomitantly with a rise in PRL release (see refs. 240–242 for reviews); and (b) PRL cell lines, primarily GH3 cells and their subclones that derive from a transplantable rat mammosomatotropic tumor (243).

The secretion of PRL *in vivo* is subject to a multifactorial control that results in either a decrease or an increase in PRL plasma level. *In vitro*, primary cultures and clonal GH3 cells respond equally well to all of the factors that stimulate *in vivo* PRL secretion, which are neuropeptides (TRH, VIP, PHI, and bombesin) and estrogen (see refs. 32 and 244 for reviews). Concerning inhibitory agents, GH3 cells differ from PRL cells in primary cultures by their lack of response to one of the most potent inhibitors of PRL secretion *in vivo* (dopamine) and its agonists. However, they do respond to some inhibitory peptides (somatostatin, histidylprolyldiketopiperazin) (see ref. 244 for a review). Because of these two systems, great progress has been made in the analysis of the major steps involved in the mode of action of neuropeptides: binding to specific receptors, transduction mechanisms, and gene transcription. Although the morphological correlates of these regulations have been, so far, less extensively investigated, significant progress has been made in the analysis of the secretory process in PRL cells.

Morphological Correlates of Response to Inhibitory Agents

Following the pioneering work of Smith and Farquhar (17), who demonstrated *in vivo* the role of lysosomes in regulating PRL secretion (see section on morphological features and functional significance), a few morphological studies have dealt with the analysis of intracellular events associated with the arrest of PRL release in response to a defined inhibitory agent.

In normal rat PRL cells in primary culture, bromocriptine treatment for a period ranging from 4 to 24 hours induced the accumulation of large secretory granules and the formation of acid phosphatase-positive dense bodies and autophagic vacuoles. These effects were accompanied by a transient increase in cell immunoreactivity, followed by a decrease occurring after several days. These events are concomitant with a transient increase in intracellular PRL which lasts for up to 24 hours (242). A delayed decrease of PRL content in culture has also been observed after long-term treatment (245). Biochemical studies have shown that this decrease is the consequence, at least in part, of PRL degradation. Attempts to detect an increase in lysosomal enzyme activities following treatment with dopamine or bromocriptine *in vivo* led to contradictory results (245,246).

Human pituitary adenomas *in vitro* also respond to treatment with L-dopa by the formation of lysosomes. A morphometric analysis and electron microscopic immunostaining of monolayers of three human PRL adenomas have revealed that treatment with 10^{-10} M bromocriptine from 24 hours to 16 days induced similar effects as on normal rat PRL cells in primary culture. Indeed, morphological alterations were delayed with respect to the rapid decrease of PRL release. This led to an accumulation of small secretory granules and increased immunostaining together with a decrease of the cell surface. However, in this system, the induction of lysosomes remained limited as compared to other systems (247). Interestingly, in cultured normal rat pituitary cells, labeling of PRL with ^{3}H-leucine for 3 hours in the presence of 1 μM dopamine resulted in an increase of the specific activity of released PRL as compared to controls, suggesting that dopamine blocks preferentially the release of stored PRL, without affecting the release of newly synthesized PRL (248). This observation suggests that dopamine acts on a post-Golgi compartment. Similarly, using a particular system—incubation of pituitaries of 8-hour nonsuckled lactating rats—Mena and associates (249) have recently reported that incubation with 50 μM dopamine for 4 hours, which inhibits the release of the 23K PRL monomer, also inhibits the intracellular "transformation" of PRL into several variants, that is believed to occur into secretory granules.

The heterogeneity of the PRL cell response to dopamine has been extensively investigated. This heterogeneity was first revealed using the reverse hemolytic plaque assay method. This showed that dopamine induces, in a dose-dependent manner, a shift in the percentage of large plaque-forming cells to the percentage of small plaque-forming cells. This suggests that dopamine preferentially inhibits the lactotropes that secrete large amounts of PRL (88). When the rate of plaque formation was used as an index of the rate of PRL secretion, dopamine was found to transiently inhibit the proportion of plaque-forming cells, and this effect was reversed by TRH (250). Interestingly, exposure to the lysosomotropic drug chloroquine largely overrode dopamine inhibition, indicating the participation of lysosomes in the inhibitory response. Under the same experimental conditions, ovine PRL also inhibited the rate of plaque formation, but this effect was not additive to that of dopamine, suggesting that the same subpopulation of PRL cells was involved (251).

The heterogeneity of the PRL cell response to dopamine was also found to be location-dependent: the inhibition of PRL release was the strongest in cells from the central portion of the gland (91). This was also true for pituitaries taken from nonsuckled lactating rats. However, after suckling, these cells from the central zone became resistant to dopamine (251). The sequential cell immunoblot assay that permits repeated quantification of the amount of hormone secreted from the same cell has revealed a subpopulation of lactotropes that do not respond to dopamine (90). Differences in the response to dopamine have also been observed at the level of PRL mRNA in PRL cell subpopulations sorted by discontinuous Percoll gradient (252) and cultured for 3 days. Using quantitative in situ hybridization, it was found that treatment with dopamine (1 μM) for 18 hours does not change the percentage of cells expressing PRL mRNA, but decreases the intensity of the signal in the total population. Moreover, a difference was observed between PRL subpopulations: the level of PRL mRNAs was decreased in cells from layer 1 (low density, high basal release, low intracellular PRL store), but increased in cells from layer 2 (high density, low basal release, high intracellular PRL store). In conclusion, the heterogeneity of the PRL cell responses to dopamine is extensively demonstrated, but the morphological correlates of such a heterogeneity are not known.

Morphological Correlates of Prolactin Cell Responses to Stimulating Agents

The morphological correlates of the stimulation of PRL secretion in culture have been studied almost exclusively with a neuropeptide TRH and with a sexual steroid, 17β-estradiol, that respectively interact on PRL secretion through different mechanisms. TRH has been shown to exert a rapid action (within minutes) on the release of intracellularly stored hormone, and a delayed effect (hours and days) on the synthesis of prolactin (see ref. 32 for a review). A similar pattern of activity has been observed for most hypophysiotropic neuropeptides *in vitro*, as well as *in vivo*, although the first phase remains the most documented so far (see refs. 253 and 254 for reviews). Thus, the morphological correlates of TRH effects may be of general value. In contrast, estrogens primarily exert a long-term action on PRL synthesis, which requires at least 1 or 2 days of treatment, *in vivo*, as well as *in vitro*, in normal, as well as clonal, PRL cells (255,256).

Acute Prolactin Release in Response to TRH.

GH3 cells. The morphological correlates of acute PRL release following exposure to TRH for up to 30 minutes were analyzed at the electron-microscopic level, mostly for GH3 cells. Because these cells possess very few secretory granules, granule exocytosis was rarely observed. However, at 5 to 15 minutes onward, TRH induced the appearance, in the Golgi zone and beneath the plasma membrane, of numerous vesicles, and exocytosis of such vesicles was frequently observed (240). Electron-microscopic immunostaining using a preembedding method revealed that these vesicles contained PRL reaction product localized on their luminal surface. Once the vesicles fused with the plasma membrane they lost their reaction product. At the same time, the immunostaining of rough endoplasmic reticulum cisternae disappeared and that of Golgi saccules greatly decreased. These findings suggest that TRH transiently accelerates the intracellular transit of PRL and induces the formation of vesicles that serve as carriers for PRL release (54). It should be emphasized that these early effects of TRH were first detectable in a small number of cells and, after 1 hour, in 57% of immunoreactive cells (54). This reveals the heterogeneity of the cell response. Moreover, when a 135-kD Golgi antigen was immunocytochemically localized using similar experimental conditions, TRH also induced a flow of Golgi-derived vesicles toward the plasma membrane; the exocytosis of these vesicles led to the insertion of patches of Golgi antigen into the plasma membrane (257).

The rapid effect of TRH on PRL release by GH3 cells has been recently found to be composed of two phases: the first phase involves a burst of PRL release, which occurs within 15 seconds and peaks at 1–2 minutes; the second is a sustained phase of PRL release at a lower level (258–260). A similar pattern was observed in primary cultures (261). Immunoelectron-microscopic observations suggest that the burst of PRL release results from exocytosis of a population of secretory granules already positioned next to the plasma membrane (Tougard, unpublished observations).

Another interesting morphological effect of short-term exposure to TRH is an increased mobility of the plasma membrane, as revealed by stretching of the plasma membrane (262), formation of blebs visible with the scanning electron microscope (263), and stimulation of endocytosis (264). Under the phase-contrast microscope, the cells are spread out over their substratum in a manner rather specific to TRH treatment (not observed with VIP—Gourdji, unpublished observations). This change in cell shape suggests an involvement of cytoskeletal components in the cell response to TRH. To investigate that possible effect, the distribution of cytoskeletal components has been recently analyzed in GH3 cells, in relation to the TRH response (265). The first acute phase of PRL release is concomitant with a transient peripheral depolymerization of microtubules, followed by the transient formation of actin bundles parallel to the plasma membrane, whereas the second sustained phase corresponds to the reorganization of microtubules, and a slackening of microtubules and cytokeratin networks.

Primary cultures. After 1 hour of treatment with TRH, a distribution of the granules along the cell membrane was observed in some cells, whereas after 4 hours, most cells were significantly degranulated. At the same time, numerous blebs and microvilli were seen at the cell surface (242). Using electron-microscopic immunostaining with the preembedding approach, we have found that, as in GH3 cells, within 1 hour, TRH induces the formation of PRL-loaded vesicles in the Golgi zone and near the plasma membrane, as well as the insertion of Golgi antigen-labeled vesicles into the plasma membrane. Destaining of the rough endoplasmic reticulum

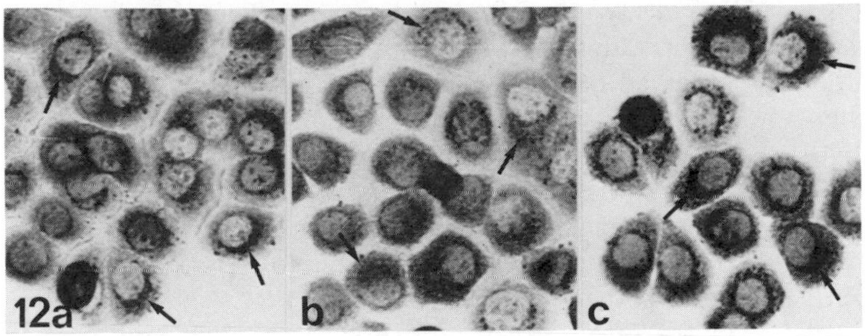

FIG. 12. GH3B6 cells immunocytochemically stained with an antiserum against rat PRL. **A:** the PRL immunostaining of GH3B6 is strongly heterogeneous. A prominent crescent-shaped positive zone (*arrows*) is detected near the nucleus and corresponds to the Golgi zone. **B:** After 1 hour TRH treatment, the cells are spread out, with a decrease of PRL immunostaining, particularly in the Golgi zone (*arrows*). **C:** After 2 hours TRH treatment, the Golgi zone is reloaded with immunoreactive PRL (*arrows*). From Tougard et al. *Biol Cell* 1982;43:89–102.

occurs simultaneously. Some granule exocytosis could be seen. Although these modifications were seen in a small number of cells and after 4 hours of exposure to TRH, many cells still contained numerous large polymorphic secretory granules, whereas others contained a few small rounded secretory granules (Tougard, unpublished observations). In fact, the structural heterogeneity of normal PRL cells in culture greatly hampered this morphological analysis. This problem deserves further attention.

Heterogeneity of the cell response. The relationship between the structural heterogeneity of PRL cells and their acute response to TRH was analyzed in GH3 cells and/or in primary cultures by the following approaches: PRL immunostaining, reverse hemolytic plaque assay, sequential cell immunoblot assay, and pulse-chase experiments.

As previously emphasized, GH3 cells display a strong heterogeneity of intracellular PRL content, as revealed by PRL immunostaining (54,87,266) (Fig. 12). The cells are organized into small colonies that contain a mixture of weakly, moderately, or heavily stained cells in variable proportions (Fig. 12). Within the first 30 minutes of exposure to TRH, there is a considerable loss of PRL immunostaining in all cell populations, with a shift toward an increased proportion of weakly stained cells (54,266) (Fig. 12). Such destaining could be correlated with changes in the subcellular distribution of PRL as described above, due to the experimental conditions used, that is, "in situ" embedding of the monolayers and selection of small colonies prior to thin sectioning (54). Without these technical improvements, the rapid effects of TRH on the subcellular distribution of PRL would probably have been underestimated or missed entirely.

The reverse hemolytic plaque assay has provided direct evidence that TRH preferentially stimulates the release of PRL by a subpopulation of PRL cells forming large plaque areas. The rate of plaque formation, which reveals another aspect of the heterogeneity of the cell response to TRH, is transiently accelerated (267). Thus it appears that TRH stimulates, in a time-dependent manner, an increasing number of PRL cells; however, it is unable to recruit additional cells to secrete. This heterogeneity is location-dependent: the cells from the peripheral rim of the rat anterior pituitary release more PRL in response to TRH than cells derived from a central portion of the gland that responds mostly to dopamine (91). This response of peripheral cells to stimulating agents (TRH, angiotensin II) was increased in pituitaries from lactating rats whether suckled or not (251). The sequential cell immunoblot assay method also revealed a heterogeneity of the lactotrope responsiveness to TRH and elegantly demonstrated that those cells secreting small amounts of PRL reveal great responsiveness to TRH (268). Such an inverse relationship between the level of basal secretion and the response to TRH is currently observed by the users of GH3 cells. In PRL cell subpopulations sorted by discontinuous Percoll gradient, stimulation of PRL secretion by vasoactive intestinal peptide was significantly more pronounced in cells from layer 2, which exhibited a low basal release (82).

Pulse-chase experiments have been used to ascertain an effect of TRH on the heterogeneous turnover of PRL. Consistent results were obtained with both normal PRL cells (84,85,248) and GH3 cells (86); in both cases TRH induced the preferential release of stored PRL, which was synthesized prior to the pulse. These findings are in agreement with those obtained from immunocytochemistry, which suggests that the TRH-mobilizable PRL pool is located in secretory granules. However, this raises the question of the subcellular origin of the newly synthesized PRL, which is preferentially released under basal conditions and even in the presence of dopamine (248). Two alternative hypotheses have been proposed. According to Walker and Farquhar (84), the two PRL pools are located in different cells. TRH would then act on a subpopulation of PRL cells, which differ from the others by their slow turnover of PRL and by their greater number of TRH binding sites. This is consistent with the above-reported findings showing a heterogeneity of PRL cell response as well as with the observations using reverse hemolytic plaque assay, that cells whose basal secretion was blocked by prolonged exposure to inhibitors of protein synthesis respond to TRH by releasing stored hormone (93). Taken together, this raises the problem of the existence of two intracellular routes for the basal release of PRL and the regulated release, respectively. Arguments in favor of these two routes have been provided by the effects of monensin on GH3 cells. Monensin has been shown to induce an accumulation of PRL in large Golgi-derived vacuoles; this was correlated with a decrease in basal PRL release, without inducing an alteration of the percent stimulation of PRL release in response to TRH (269). Pulse-chase experiments have revealed that monensin, in fact, decreases PRL basal release without affecting that of the newly synthesized PRL, whereas it does not affect the release of unlabeled PRL in response to TRH. This supports the existence of two intracellular routes arising from an early Golgi subcompartment, located upstream from the monensin blockade, for the release of newly synthesized PRL, and from a late Golgi subcompartment, located downstream from the monensin blockade, for the release of stored PRL. The latter may consist of both secretory granules and vesicles (86). Whether these two routes are present in distinct PRL cell subtypes or in same cells is not determined. In the latter case, one of these routes may become more or less prominent, depending on the physiological stimuli. This would account for both the functional heterogeneity of PRL cells and interconvertibility of PRL cell types.

In conclusion, if one compares the patterns of acute morphological responses to TRH in GH3 cells and normal PRL cells, one is surprised to see many similarities between two cell models, which greatly differ by their intracellular store of secretory granules. A similar conclusion was reached by a comparison of the patterns of PRL release by perifused GH4C1 cells and primary cultures in response to several agents, including TRH (261).

Corelease with prolactin of secretory granule associated products. The colocalization of galanin and PRL within secretory granules of anterior pituitary cells in estrogen-treated Fisher 344 rats (270) is associated with a coregulation of galanin and PRL release by a stimulating agent, TRH, as well as by inhibiting factors (dopamine, somatostatin). In contrast, although galanin was also localized in somatotropes and gonadotropes, ligands specific to those cells failed to alter its release *in vitro* (271).

SgII, which is colocalized with PRL, at least in some cells of the GH3B6 line (64) and of the GH4C1 line (66) was found to be released in parallel with PRL both in basal conditions and under brief exposure to secretagogues, at least based on radiolabeling experiments (272).

Long-Term Responses of Stimulatory Agents. The consequences of long-term *in vitro* treatments (from 24 hours to 8 days) with stimulatory agents have been studied at several steps of the PRL secretory process: PRL synthesis (increase in PRL mRNA), PRL cell content and PRL secretion, as well as on PRL proliferation. A variety of ligands have been shown to interact on one or the other features (peptide hormones, sexual steroids, growth factors). However, the morphological correlates have been examined in a limited number of experimental situations.

Thyrotropin-releasing hormone. The morphological effects of long-term exposure to TRH *in vitro* have been observed on GH3 cells. At the light-microscopic level, treatment with 30 nM TRH for 48 hours has been shown to slightly increase the percentage of immunoreactive cells, as well as the intensity of their immunostaining. Moreover, the difference between the small increase in the percentage of immunopositive cells (from 35% to 45%) and the large increase in PRL cellular content (450% of control value) supports the assumption that TRH acts on GH3 cells "principally by raising the mean hormonal content of individual positive cells rather than by increasing the proportion of cells committed to PRL production" (87). Consistent data were obtained concerning the percentage of PRL-releasing cells, as determined by reverse hemolytic plaque assay: chronic treatment for 6 days with a pharmacological dose of TRH increased from 20% to 35% the proportion of PRL secretors while decreasing reciprocally the proportion of GH secretors (89). At the electron-microscopic level, long-term treatment with TRH was found to induce an obvious extension of the Golgi zone, which contained, in addition to stacks of saccules, many vesicles and often newly formed secretory granules. Moreover, the number of secretory granules was increased (240,262). Subcellular localization of PRL using electron-microscopic immunocytochemistry revealed at 4 hours onward a reloading of the rough endoplasmic reticulum and of Golgi cisternae and vesicles. This reloading was totally blocked by simultaneous exposure to cycloheximide, indicating that it reflects a neosynthesis of PRL (54).

17β-Estradiol. Chronic treatment with 17β-estradiol of GH3 cells has been shown to induce an increase in both intracellular and medium PRL levels, under various culture conditions (273,274). In primary cultures of rat anterior pituitary cells, exposure to 17β-estradiol (10^{-8} M) also induces an increase of PRL secretion and morphological changes, which became maximal between 4 and 8 days of treatment (242). The morphological changes consisted of hypertrophy and increased immunostaining of PRL cells without modification of PRL cell number. At the electron-microscopic level, the treated cells displayed an enlarged Golgi zone with an increased number of vesicles and immature secretory granules, as well as a distension of Golgi cisternae. An "increase in the rough endoplasmic reticulum" was also noticed. With regard to secretory granules, "large secretory granules were seldomly seen up to 4 days of treatment but could be seen in some cells between days 4 and 8." In addition, the cell surface was also modified in the same manner as by TRH, that is, an increase in number of microvilli was observed (242).

Insulin and insulin-like growth factor I. Interesting effects of insulin and insulinlike growth factor I have been observed in a newly established cell line MtT/S, which produces GH only and contains GH-immunopositive granules (33) (see above). After 2 days of treatment with either of these peptides, PRL became detectable in the medium and then its level increased in a dose-dependent manner, whereas that of GH decreased. After 7 days, this was correlated with the appearance of a small percentage (10%) of immunopositive PRL cells, a marked decrease of the proportion of GH immunopositive cells and an absence of mammosomatotropes (275). This provides an interesting *in vitro* system to study the molecular mechanisms of a transdifferentiation of GH cells to PRL cells.

Combined treatments. Combined treatment with 17β-estradiol, insulin, and epidermal growth factor for 3 days has been shown to induce PRL granulogenesis in GH4C1 cells at the same time as an increase in PRL cell content (276). Such a granulogenesis could be correlated with an increased percentage of cells immunopositive for PRL, among which 86% were also positive for secretogranin I and II together, indicating a close but not complete association of secretogranins with PRL storage (66). This could be associated with a parallel increase of PRL and secretogranin expression, as appreciated by immunostaining (after 3 days) and by the level of secretogranin and PRL mRNAs (after 6 hours). However, long-term exposure (up to 4 days) to TRH, 17β-estradiol, or dexamethasone, separately, have indicated that the level of SgI mRNAs in GH3B6 cells is indeed hormonally regulated, but not always in parallel with that of PRL mRNAs and never with that of GH mRNAs. The closest parallelism between secretogranin I and PRL mRNA was observed with estradiol, whereas no parallelism was observed with TRH (277). Further studies are needed to understand the regulation of the intracellular pathway of secretogranins in PRL cells.

In contrast to secretogranins, laminin, a component of basement membrane, which is also localized in PRL secretory granules (69), seems to be independently regulated, at least on the basis of immunoelectron-microscopic observations performed on the pituitaries of suckled or nonsuckled lactating rats (55).

Conclusions. A comparison between the effects *in vivo* and *in vitro* of physiological regulators of PRL secretion is possible for a limited number of factors: dopamine, TRH, 17β-estradiol. Although the experimental conditions vary greatly, one may notice several common features. The inhibition of PRL secretion was mostly found associated with an accumulation of secretory granules which last for several days and an induction of lysosomes that is more or less pronounced. In contrast to these delayed morphological effects, an acute and sustained stimulation of PRL secretion was always correlated with a rapid enlargement of the Golgi zone, an increased number of forming secretory granules in this area, the association of secretory granules with the plasma membrane, and an increased number of granule exocytosis profiles. The accumulation of PRL in the rough endoplasmic reticulum and the development of RER cisternae are, in general, signs of a sustained stimulation. The observations concerning secretory granules are not always clear or consistent. An increase in number and size is sometimes reported, whereas a decrease in diameter and a scarcity occur in other cases. This may reflect variations in the balance between storage and release. The conversion from type I to type III "mature" PRL cell type was observed *in vivo* only. This may require other factors that are absent *in vitro*.

An apparent important difference between *in vivo* and *in vitro* data resides in the control of cell proliferation. Long-term estradiol treatment induces *in vivo*, but not *in vitro*, a hyperplasia of immunoreactive PRL cells, although it is not yet clear whether this indicates a cell proliferation rather than an increase in number of PRL-storing cells among a fixed population of PRL mRNA-expressing cells. The growth of GH3 tumor cells *in vivo* is dependent on circulating estrogens, whereas *in vitro* estradiol does not stimulate GH3 cell proliferation under most conditions (274), except in the presence of gelding serum (278). These discrepancies might be explained by the recently demonstrated role of PRL isoform 2 as autocrine growth factor for GH3 cells and possibly normal PRL cells (279).

Gonadotropes

In Vivo *Studies on Gonadotropes*

Morphological modifications or numerical variations of gonadotropes have been reported in relation to sex, estrous cycle, castration, GnRH treatment, and adenomas. These observations, primarily obtained on the basis of immunocytochemical studies performed at the light- and electron-microscopic levels, and more recently on the basis of in situ hybridization, will be examined successively.

Sex-Related Differences: Estrous Cycle

From quantitative immunocytochemical analyses performed at the light-microscopic level on rat pituitary, it was clear that the percentage of multihormonal LH/FSH cells varied in relation to sex, that is, in the female rat 37% to 40% of gonadotropes contained both hormones, as compared with 70% in the male rat (123), and the absolute number of gonadotropes did not change in the adenohypophysis of adult female rat throughout the estrous cycle (123,280). Moreover, according to Childs (123) there are changes in the storage pattern of the gonadotropes which vary with the stage of the estrous cycle and which can be correlated with the respective level of circulating gonadotropins. Recent studies of Childs and colleagues (281) performed on dispersed pituitary cells from cycling female rats, separated by centrifugal elutriation and labeled for LH-β antigens or mRNA, revealed a shift in the distribution of different-sized gonadotropes in relation with the stage of the cycle. These data suggest that small or medium-sized gonadotropes may enlarge and become more dense during early diestrus and be recruited to support the proestrous cycle. Moreover, the number of GnRH receptors is known to vary throughout the estrous cycle (282,283). It is low during estrus and metestrus, gradually increases in diestrus, and remains high until the afternoon of proestrus. These changes in the number of GnRH receptors during the estrous cycle represent fluctuations in the percentage of GnRH-bound cells (284). Therefore, gonadotropes undergo a series of dynamic changes in preparation for the proestrous gonadotropin surge.

At the electron-microscopic level, the number of each gonadotropic cell type, characterized by its ultrastructural features, also varies in relation to sex (285) and during the estrous cycle (116,127,138). Type II cells, which are scarce in the male rat, increase in number during proestrus and estrus in female rats, concomitantly with a decrease in number of type I cells (128,138). There is a similar shift from type I to type II cells for the anti-β-LH–stained cell population and for the anti-β-FSH–stained cell population indicating, once more, that these two gonadotrope subtypes correspond to different stages of secretory activity in the same cell.

Castration

Morphological changes induced in the pituitary after castration have been described in early studies at the light-microscopic level (286), with the appearance of so-called "castration cells" or "signet-ring cells," each of which contains a large vacuole. Such castration cells were later described by conventional electron microscopy, first by Farquhar and Rinehart (5), followed by Yoshimura and Harumiya (287) in the rat, by Barnes (124,125) in the mouse, and more recently by Kurosumi and coworkers (288) in the rat. Hypertrophied castration cells are characterized by dilation of the endoplasmic reticulum, resulting in either round vacuoles or irregularly shaped and dilated cisternae resembling filigree. Progressively, with increasing time after castration, the typical signet-ring cells appear, characterized by a very large vacuole induced by the gradual expansion and confluence of the endoplasmic reticulum cisternae.

The coexistence of LH and FSH within castration cells was clearly demonstrated in castrated male and female rats (127,150,289), as well as in castrated pigs (154). The castration cells did not stain for ACTH (150,154). The percentage of gonadotropes that stored both LH and FSH, which was determined by morphometric analysis of immunoreactive cells, increased in developing castration cells, from 70% to 91% in the male rat and from 50% to 75% in the female (150). Same increase in multihormonal cells after castration was observed when mRNAs of each β-subunit was analyzed by in situ hybridization technique (290). This suggested that an early response to castration consists of the stimulation of dual hormone production, and that all gonadotropes are bipotential. Three months after castration, there was a threefold increase in the percentages of LH and FSH cells, followed by a decrease by 6 months (219). The increased number of gonadotropes during the first 3 months is probably due to cell division (291,292). Passive immunization to GnRH using GnRH antiserum indicates that GnRH is an important factor for stimulation of gonadotrope proliferation in castrated rats (293). Simultaneous adrenalectomy and castration result in a significant decrease in the percentage of castration cells (294).

In many studies (115,127,288) the castration cells were derived mainly from the type I gonadotrope, which progressively displayed a dilation of the rough endoplasmic reticulum and a decrease and eventual disappearance of large secretory granules. The small secretory granules persisted and were mainly localized at the cell periphery along the cell membrane. At the same time, type II gonadotropes remained scarce and unmodified (127). In highly degranulated cells, the content of the dilated rough endoplasmic reticulum cisternae was stained with anti-β-LH and, to a lesser extent, with anti-LH (127).

Gonadotropin-Releasing Hormone Treatment

Gonadotropin-releasing hormone (GnRH) exerts a biphasic stimulatory effect on LH/FSH secretion. This effect involves the rapid release of a previously formed hormonal pool, as well as a delayed stimulation of hormone synthesis. The respective ultrastructural correlates of these two phases have been studied mainly *in vivo* using conventional electron microscopy.

A rapid and obvious extrusion of secretory granules via exocytosis occurs within minutes in response to GnRH in gonadotropes of persistent estrous rats (295) or in intact or gonadectomized male and female rats pretreated (or not) with estrogen and/or progesterone (296–298). The diameter and electron density of secretory granules of gonadotropes decrease rapidly after GnRH injection (299). Moreover, along with granule exocytosis, a progressive extension of the rough endoplasmic reticulum and of the Golgi zone occurs in gonadotropes after infusion of GnRH into the portal vessels (300). All these observations suggest that the acute hormonal release is rapidly correlated with modifications of the entire ultrastructural organization of the cell.

The effects of chronic injection or prolonged infusion with GnRH or TRH, or both, in male rats have been extensively analyzed by Yoshimura and his colleagues (301–305). All of these studies revealed similar features of the continuously stimulated cells, including development and dilation of the rough endoplasmic reticulum, extension of the Golgi zone, and a decrease in the size and number of secretory granules concomitant with hypertrophy of the cell, all of which induce the appearance of gonadectomized or thyroidectomized cells. The sequential ultrastructural transformation of anterior pituitary basophils (gonadotropes and thyrotropes), identified on the basis of conventional electron microscopy, suggested to these authors a theory involving the secretory cycle of a single basophilic cell type that would successively secrete TSH, FSH, and LH (301).

Gonadotropic Adenomas

According to Kovacs and associates (226), no convincing studies of experimental gonadotropic adenomas have been reported so far. However, *in vivo*, gonadotropes can give rise to neoplasia. In great contrast to prolactinomas, gonadotropic adenomas are rare in human beings and difficult to identify at the light-microscopic level because they appear to be chromophobic (228,306,307). The cells can only be identified through the use of immunocytochemistry and have been shown to contain either FSH and LH or FSH alone (307). At the electron-microscopic level, human gonadotropic adenomas display well-developed rough endoplasmic reticulum cisternae, a prominent Golgi zone, and sparse small secretory granules (226,228).

Postnatal Changes and Aging

During postnatal development of the rat pituitary, gonadotropes undergo important changes in number, size, and structure. They increase in number during the first week of postnatal life (97,308,309). Thereafter, their percentage is greater than that in the adult, with an increased cell number in females as compared to males. Matsumura and Daikoku (310) demonstrated that sex steroids may be responsible for the sexual differences in the morphological development (cell number and cell size) of LH cells in newborn rats. As in adult cells, most of the gonadotropes of the young rats contained both LH and FSH (309). However, according to Childs and her colleagues (309,311), a great number of gonadotropes contain ACTH-like immunoreactivity during postnatal development and might subserve a function related to that of adrenal-gonadal maturation. This observation was a subject of controversy because, according to Inoue and Hagino (132), angular-shaped gonadotropes in neonatal and immature rats did not contain ACTH. At the electron-microscopic level, the morphological maturation of the gonadotropes in the rat pituitary occurs during the first 7 days of postnatal life; after 1 to 2 weeks of age, most of the cells resemble adult cell types (309). All of these morphological observations clearly emphasize the importance of the first 2 to 3 weeks of life for the functional maturation of the gonadotropic population (312).

Changes in the number of gonadotropic cell types with aging in the rat pituitary have been described at the electron microscope by Kurosumi and coworkers (285). The number of type I gonadotropes decreases with age in the male rat pituitary, while the number of type II cells increases. In the female, the respective number of each cell type does not change significantly. In both sexes, very few large secretory granules were observed.

In Vitro *Functional Studies on Gonadotropes*

In vitro functional studies on gonadotropes have been performed either on newly dispersed anterior pituitary cells or on dissociated cells grown in monolayers or in reaggregate cell cultures. Such models represent the available tools to examine the cell response to various physiological stimuli. Indeed, it has been shown that just after enzymatic dispersion, and at least for the first days in culture, gonadotropes from adult rat pituitaries retain their morphological heterogeneity (6,240,313,314) and their capacity to respond to specific regulatory agents (240). After the first week of culture, FSH and LH secretion progressively declines with time, whereas immunoreactive gonadotropes still remain present (241,314) (Fig. 13), even in long-term primary cultures (35 or 56 days) (314). Progressive modifications of the ultrastructural organization of immunoreactive cells occur with increasing time in culture; finally, a single gonadotropic cell type remains, characterized by immature features: small secretory granules (125–150 nm), a few rough endoplasmic reticulum cisternae, and an inconspicuous Golgi complex (314). Gonadotropes in aggregates of cells from dispersed rat anterior pituitaries, as well as from enriched populations of gonadotropes, also retain their ultrastructural characteristics and respond selectively to various agents in a superfusion system (315).

Whereas modifications of hormonal secretion under specific regulatory agents have been extensively studied *in vitro*, studies on the morphological modifications following stimulation of the secretory activity of gonadotropes are far less numerous and primarily concern the response to GnRH.

Morphological Correlates of Gonadotropes in Response to Gonadotropin-Releasing Hormone

Short-Term Effects of GnRH. In 7-day primary cultures of dispersed rat anterior pituitary cells exposed to GnRH for 15 to 30 minutes, classic exocytotic profiles

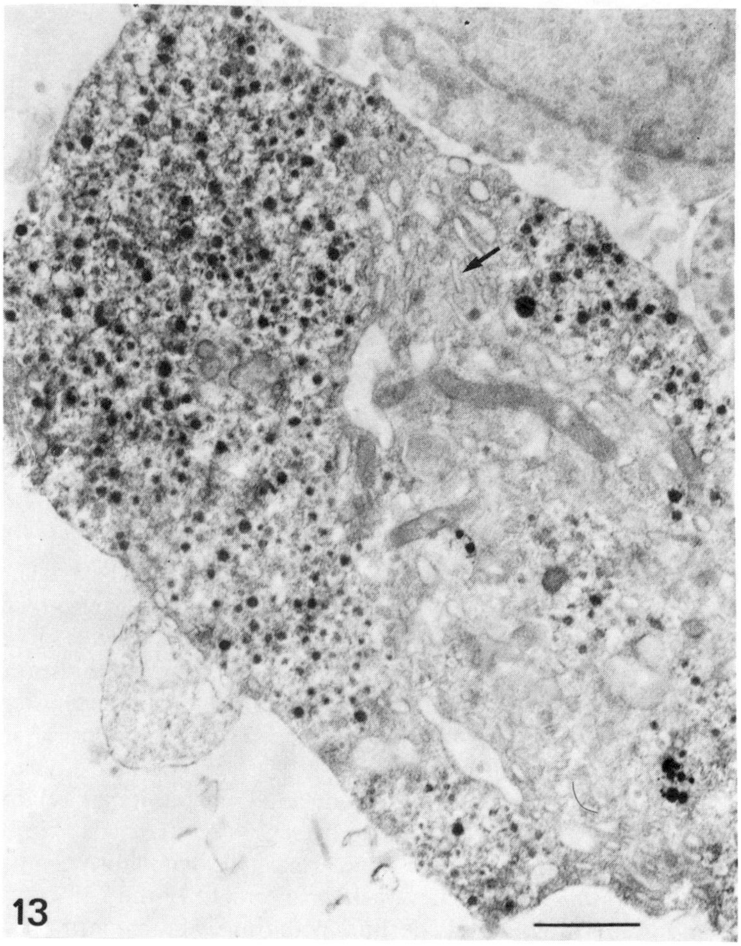

FIG. 13. A 12-day monolayer of rat anterior pituitary cells is immunochemically stained with an antiserum against rat LHβ. This immunoreactive gonadotrope displays small secretory granules and slightly dilated RER cisternae (*arrows*). Bar: 1 μm.

were not observed in gonadotropes, but many secretory granules were lined up along the plasma membrane and, after immunocytochemical staining, displayed structural changes. This suggests that GnRH simultaneously induced a rapid migration of secretory granules toward the plasma membrane, with a structural reorganization of their matrix visualized by a decrease in electron density (240). Using other culture conditions and immunocytochemical methods, Childs (153) has also found that GnRH stimulation results in the formation of cellular processes that contain monohormonal secretory granules in multihormonal cells. In addition, these processes also stained for the releasing hormone (153,159,316). From these observations, Childs (159) postulates that these "processes provide attractive morphological correlates for potential sites of local control of non parallel LH and FSH release from multihormonal cells." The mechanisms involved in such a dissociation of gonadotropin stores, as well as the mechanisms involved in its control, have not yet been determined.

Similar observations concerning the rapid migration of secretory granules were recorded by Lewis and colleagues (317,318) with mouse hemipituitaries incubated for 2 consecutive hours with GnRH. This treatment induces a priming effect of GnRH on gonadotropin secretion. Under these experimental conditions, the initial exposure to GnRH induced a translocation of gonadotrope secretory granules toward the plasmalemma, as well as a decrease in granule size. Granules adjacent to the plasma membrane may therefore represent a readily releasable pool of hormone that responds to a second exposure to GnRH and that can sustain the priming effect of GnRH (318). The migration of the secretory granules appears to be reversible following GnRH withdrawal (319). Concomitant with these ultrastructural modifications, these authors have shown that the GnRH priming effect is associated with an increase in length and a change in the orientation of microfilaments in gonadotropes, suggesting a role for cytoskeletal components in granule translocation (317).

Another important rapid morphological modification of stimulated cells involves modifications of the plasma membrane, which results in the formation of microvilli and branched cytoplasmic processes (240). This modification was reported only for *in vitro* systems. Near the cell periphery, numerous small vesicles or canaliculi appear, which are sometimes labeled with exogenous horseradish peroxidase, indicating an increase in endocytotic activity (264). Simultaneously, a progressive extension of the Golgi zone occurs, in addition to an increase in the number of small vesicles and multivesicular bodies in this area. Condensing secretory material was found inside some Golgi cisternae (240). These ultrastructural observations suggest that GnRH may stimulate membrane traffic in gonadotropes at the same time as secretory activity.

GnRH has also been found to rapidly modify the relative proportion of LH and FSH in gonadotropes. Indeed, Childs and her colleagues (159,178,316) have shown that it increases the proportion of gonadotropes containing both hormones while causing a corresponding decrease in monohormonal cells, indicating once more that monohormonal gonadotropes are in fact bipotential.

The heterogeneity of the gonadotropic response to GnRH was investigated in depth by Neill and colleagues (320) and by Lloyd and Childs (178) using reverse hemolytic plaque assay. These studies indicated that not all gonadotropes respond in the same manner to GnRH, as assessed by several functional parameters. The differences between the smallest and largest individual cell responses were up to 500- to 1,000-fold. Some cells did not respond, although they contained an ample store of immunodetectable LH. Thus, there are nonreleasable stores of LH, particularly at diestrus, a stage when gonadotropes are the largest (319) and display an increased number of secretory granules (138,319). Surprisingly, there was no direct correlation between the amount of labeled GnRH bound by a given cell and the size of the plaque area, suggesting that only a fraction of receptors are functional (320).

Long-Term Effects of GnRH. Morphological studies on chronic stimulation with GnRH have been performed in organ cultures of rat pituitary exposed for up to 24 hours (321). These studies also revealed a decrease in the size and number of secretory granules, an extension of the Golgi zone, and a development and dilation of the rough endoplasmic reticulum cisternae, inducing hypertrophy of stimulated gonadotropes. Indeed, cells similar to the so-called "castration cells" may appear in cultures exposed to high doses of GnRH for 3 to 6 hours.

Chronic treatment of primary cultures of rat anterior pituitary cells with GnRH for a month induced hypertrophy and degranulation of gonadotropes which, at this late stage of culture, displayed only one class of very small (100 nm) rounded secretory granules and the development of parallel and flattened rough endoplasmic reticulum cisternae (240). In addition, chronic treatment with GnRH did not increase the number of immunoreactive gonadotropes nor did it prevent the fall in LH and FSH secretion (240).

In conclusion, the morphological correlates of the stimulation of LH and FSH secretion by GnRH are quite similar *in vivo* and *in vitro*. They always correspond to (a) a migration of secretory granules toward the plasma membrane, (b) an enlargement of the rough endoplasmic reticulum cisternae, and (c) an extension of the Golgi zone. The size of secretory granules decreases in highly stimulated cells, with a concomitant disappearance of the large secretory granules. Simultaneously, changes in the hormonal storage pattern of gonadotropes occur, which is revealed by an increase in the percentage of multihormonal cells.

GENERAL CONCLUSIONS

The identity of the cell types responsible for the secretion of the three anterior pituitary hormones that control reproduction in mammals is well established because of the availability of specific immunological probes. With convincing exceptions, one may maintain that PRL and GH are generally contained and secreted by different cells, whereas LH and FSH are found mainly in the same cells.

The functional adaptation of these cells to the complexity of the physiological regulation of the control of reproduction is achieved by diversification of the ultrastructural organization of both lactotropes and gonadotropes. Such a diversity is progressively established during postnatal development and clearly corresponds to a functional heterogeneity. However, the exact link between a given type of ultrastructural organization and the corresponding secretory activity is still unclear. This question deserves further study at the single cell level. It seems, a priori, easier to solve for lactotropes than for gonadotropes because of the complexity of synthetic machinery of LH and FSH, from genes to posttranslational maturation.

The morphological response of these cell types to specific agents has been more thoroughly analyzed *in vitro* because of the development of culture methods. Again the significance of morphological changes is better defined for lactotropes than for gonadotropes. This is the consequence of two occurrences:

1. The considerable difference between the long-term secretory ability in culture of lactotropes and gonadotropes
2. The absence of a model of a responsive gonadotrope cell line, when compared to GH3 prolactin cells.

Attempts to immortalize differentiated gonadotropes are likely to result in great progress in the future. A novel rat pituitary tumor cell line (RC-4B/C) which contained all pituitary cell types has been recently characterized (322) and is very promising. In addition, the present data suggest that similar cellular mechanisms might be involved in the rapid effect of stimulating hypothalamic peptides, such as rapid migration of secretory granules toward the plasma membrane and concomitant reorganization of the Golgi complex. Future studies will involve the elucidation of the biochemical mechanisms of such membrane traffic.

ACKNOWLEDGMENTS

We gratefully acknowledge Miss A. Bayon for her valuable help in typing this manuscript, Mr. C. Pennarun for his skillful competence in the preparation of photomicrographs, and Mrs. E. Vila-Porcile and R. Picart for their helpful assistance in the final preparation of illustrations.

Part of our work reported in this review was supported by grants from the Centre National de la Recherche Scientifique (grant ER 89, UA 041115, URA 1115) and from the Direction Générale à la Recherche Scientifique et Technique (Contract 72 7 0100).

REFERENCES

1. Girod C. Immunocytochemistry of the vertebrate adenohypophysis. In: Graumann W, Neumann K, eds. *Handbuch der Histochemie,* vol VIII, (suppl. 5). Jena: Fischer verlag;1983.
2. Romeis B. Hypophyse. In: Möllendorff von W, ed. *Handbuch der mikroskopischen Anatomie des Menschen,* vol. 6, part 3. Berlin: J. Springer; 1940.
3. Herlant M. The cells of the adenohypophysis and their functional significance. *Int Rev Cytol* 1964;17:299–382.
4. Herlant M. Introduction. In: Farquhar MG, Tixier-Vidal A, eds. *The anterior pituitary gland.* New York: Academic Press; 1975:1–19.
5. Farquhar MG, Rinehart JF. Electron microscope studies of the anterior pituitary of castrate rats. *Endocrinology* 1954;54: 516–541.
6. Farquhar MG, Skutelsky EH, Hopkins CR. Structure and function of the anterior pituitary and dispersed pituitary cells: in vitro studies. In: Farquhar MG, Tixier-Vidal A, eds. *The anterior pituitary.* New York: Academic Press; 1975:83–135.
7. Nakane PK. Classifications of anterior pituitary cell types with immunoenzyme histochemistry. *J Histochem Cytochem* 1970;18:9–21.
8. Moriarty G. Adenohypophysis: ultrastructural cytochemistry: a review. *J Histochem Cytochem* 1973;21:855–894.
9. Nakane PK. Identification of anterior pituitary cells by immunoelectron microscopy. In: Farquhar MG, Tixier-Vidal A, eds. *The anterior pituitary.* New York: Academic Press; 1975:45–61.
10. Baker BL, Midgley AR Jr, Gersten BE, Yu YY. Differentiation of growth hormone and prolactin containing acidophils with peroxidase-labeled antibody. *Anat Rec* 1969;164:163–171.
11. Baker BL, Gross DS. Cytology and distribution of secretory cell types in mouse hypophysis as demonstrated with immuno-cytochemistry. *Am J Anat* 1978;153:193–215.
12. Pasteels JL, Gausset P, Danguy A, Ectors F, Nicoll CS, Varavudhi P. Morphology of the lactotropes and somatotropes of man and rhesus monkeys. *J Clin Endocrinol Metab* 1972;34:959–967.
13. Halmi NS, Parsons JA, Erlandsen SL, Duello T. Prolactin and growth hormone cells in the human hypophysis: a study with immunoenzyme histochemistry and differential staining. *Cell Tissue Res* 1975;158:497–507.
14. Baker BL, Yu YY. An immunocytochemical study of human pituitary mammotropes from fetal life to old age. *Am J Anat* 1977;148:217–240.
15. Nogami H, Yoshimura F. Fine structural criteria of prolactin cells identified immunohistochemically in the male rat. *Anat Rec* 1982;202:261–274.
16. Pasteels JL. Recherches morphologiques et expérimentales sur la sécrétion de prolactine. *Arch Biol Liege* 1963;74:439–453.
17. Smith RE, Farquhar MG. Lysosome function in the regulation of the secretory process in cells of anterior pituitary gland. *J Cell Biol* 1966;31:319–347.
18. Pasteels JL, Ectors F, Danguy A, Robyn C, L'Hermite M, Dujardin M. Histological immunofluorescent and electron microscopic identification of prolactin producing cells in the human pituitary. *Excerpta Med* 1973;273:616–621.
19. Tougard C, Picart R, Tixier-Vidal A. Electron microscopic cytochemical studies on the secretory process in primary culture. *Am J Anat* 1980;158:471–490.
20. Nogami H, Yoshimura F. Prolactin immunoreactivity of acidophils of the small granule type. *Cell Tissue Res* 1980;211:1–4.
21. Nogami H. Fine structural heterogeneity and morphological changes in rat pituitary prolactin cells after estrogen and testosterone treatment. *Cell Tissue Res* 1984;237:195–202.
22. Beauvillain JC, Mazucca M, Dubois MP. The prolactin and growth hormone producing cells of the guinea pig pituitary: electron microscopic study using immunocytochemical means. *Cell Tissue Res* 1977;184:343–358.
23. Dacheux F, Dubois MP. Ultrastructural localization of prolactin, growth hormone and luteinizing hormone by immunocytochemical techniques in the bovine pituitary. *Cell Tissue Res* 1976;174:245–260.
24. Dacheux F. Ultrastructural immunocytochemical localization of prolactin and growth hormone in the porcine pituitary. *Cell Tissue Res* 1980;207:277–286.
25. Martin-Comin J, Robyn C. Comparative immunoenzymatic localization of prolactin and growth hormone in human and rat pituitaries. *J Histochem Cytochem* 1976;24:1012–1016.
26. Girod C, Dubois MP. Immunofluorescent identification of somatotropic and prolactin cells in the anterior lobe of the hypophysis (pars distalis) of the monkey *Macacus irus. Cell Tissue Res* 1976;172:145–148.
27. Neill JD, Frawley LS. Detection of hormone release from individual cells in mixed populations using a reverse hemolytic plaque assay. *Endocrinology* 1983;112:1135–1137.
28. Frawley LS, Bookfor FR. Mammosomatotropes: presence and functions in normal and neoplastic pituitary tissue. *Endocr Rev* 1991;12:337–355.
29. Tixier-Vidal A, Tougard C, Dufy B, Vincent JD. Morphological, functional and electrical correlates in anterior pituitary cells. In: Müller EE, MacLeod RM, eds. *Neuroendocrine perspectives,* vol. 1. Amsterdam: Elsevier; 1982:211–251.
30. Halmi NS. Occurrence of both growth hormone and prolactin immunoreactive material in the cells of human somatotropic pituitary adenomas containing mammotropic elements. *Virchows Arch A* 1982;398:19–31.
31. Trouillas J, Girod C, Lheritier M, Claustrat B, Dubois MP. Morphological and biochemical relationships in 31 human pituitary adenomas with acromegaly. *Virchows Arch A* 1980;389:127–142.
32. Gourdji D, Tougard C, Tixier-Vidal A. Clonal prolactin strains as a tool in neuroendocrinology. *Front Neuroendocrinol* 1982;7: 317–357.
33. Inoué K, Hattori MA, Sakai T, Inukai S, Fujimoto N, Ito A. Establishment of a series of pituitary clonal cell lines differing in morphology, hormone secretion, and response to estrogen. *Endocrinology* 1990;126:2313–2320.
34. Bookfor FR, Schwarz LK. Cultures of GH3 cell contain both single and dual hormone secretors. *Endocrinology* 1987; 122:762–767.
35. Lloyd RV, Anagnostou D, Cano M, Barkan AL, Chandler WF. Analysis of mammosomatotropic cells in normal and neoplastic human pituitary tissues by the reverse hemolytic plaque assay and immunocytochemistry. *J Clin Endocrinol Metab* 1988; 66:1103–1110.
36. Fumagalli G, Zanini A. In cow anterior pituitary, growth hormone and prolactin can be packed in separate granules of the same cell. *J Cell Biol* 1985;100:2019–2024.
37. Nikitovitch-Winer MB, Atkin J, Maley BE. Colocalization of prolactin and growth hormone within specific adenohypophyseal cells in male, female, and lactating female rats. *Endocrinology* 1987;121:625–635.
38. Smets G, Welkeniers B, Finne E, Baldys A, Gepts W, Vanhaelst L. Postnatal development of growth hormone and prolactin cells in male and female pituitary: an immunocytochemical light and

electron microscopic study. *J Histochem Cytochem* 1987;35: 335–342.
39. Kurosumi K. Ultrastructural modifications in prolactin-producing cells in the adenohypophysis during postnatal development and functional variations. In: Hoshino K, ed. *Prolactin gene family and its receptors.* Amsterdam: Elsevier; 1988: 289–297.
40. Leong DA, Lau SK, Sinha YN, Kaiser DL, Thorner MO. Enumeration of lactotropes and somatotropes among male and female pituitary cells in culture: evidence in favor of a mammosomatotrope subpopulation in the rat. *Endocrinology* 1985; 116:1371–1378.
41. Frawley LS, Boockfor FR, Hoeffler JP. Identification by plaque assays of a pituitary cell type that secretes both growth hormone and prolactin. *Endocrinology* 1985;116:734–737.
42. Kineman RAD, Henricks DM, Faught WJ, Frawley LS. Fluctuations in the proportions of growth hormone- and prolactin-secreting cells during the bovine estrous cycle. *Endocrinology* 1991;129:1221–1225.
43. Porter TE, Wiles CD, Frawley LS. Evidence for bidirectional interconversion of mammotropes and somatotropes: rapid reversion of acidophilic cell types to pregestational proportions after weaning. *Endocrinology* 1991;129:1215–1220.
44. Lamberts SWJ, Macleod RM. Regulation of prolactin secretion at the level of the lactotroph. *Physiol Rev* 1990;70:279–318.
45. Farquhar MG. Secretion and crinophagy in prolactin cells. In: Dellman HD, Johnson JA, Klachko DM, eds. *Comparative endocrinology of prolactin.* New York: Plenum; 1977:37–91.
46. Tixier-Vidal A. Structural basis of adenohypophyseal secretory processes. In: Jutisz M, McKerns KW, eds. *Synthesis and release of adenohypophyseal hormones.* New York: Plenum; 1980:1–14.
47. Zanini A, Giannattasio G, Meldolesi J. Intracellular events in prolactin secretion. In: Jutisz M, McKerns KW, eds. *Synthesis and release of adenohypophyseal hormones.* New York: Plenum; 1980:105–124.
48. Tixier-Vidal A, Picart R. Etude quantitative par radioautographie au microscope électronique de l'utilisation de la DL-Leucine ^{3}H par les cellules de l'hypophyse du Canard en culture organotypique. *J Cell Biol* 1967;35:501–519.
49. Farquhar MG, Reid J, Daniell LW. Intracellular transport and packaging of prolactin: a quantitative electron microscope autoradiographic study of mammotrophs dissociated from rat pituitaries. *Endocrinology* 1978;102:296–311.
50. Palade GE. Intracellular aspects of the process of protein secretion. *Science* 1975;189:347–358.
51. Griffiths G, Simons K. The trans Golgi network: sorting at the exit site of the Golgi complex. *Science* 1986;234:438–443.
52. Rothman JE, Orci L. Molecular dissection of the secretory pathway. *Nature* 1992;355:409–415.
53. Rambourg A, Clermont Y, Chrétien M, Olivier L. Formation of secretory granules in the Golgi apparatus of prolactin cells in the rat pituitary gland: a stereoscopic study. *Anat Rec* 1992;232: 169–179.
54. Tougard C, Picart R, Tixier-Vidal A. Immunocytochemical localization of prolactin in the endoplasmic reticulum of GH3 cells: variations in response to thyroliberin. *Biol Cell* 1982;43:89–102.
55. Vila-Porcile E, Picart R, Olivier L, Tixier-Vidal A, Tougard C. Subcellular distribution of laminin and prolactin in stimulated and blocked prolactin cells in the pituitary of lactating rats. *Cell Tissue Res* 1988;254:617–627.
56. Osamura RY, Komatsu N, Izumi S, Yoshimura S, Watanabe K. Ultrastructural localization of prolactin in the rat anterior pituitary glands by preembedding peroxidase-labeled antibody method. *J Histochem Cytochem* 1982;30:919–925.
57. Sinha YN. Prolactin variants. *Trends Endocrinol Metab* 1992;3:100–106.
58. Greenan JR, Balden E, Ho TWC, Walker AM. Biosynthesis of the secreted 24 K isoforms of prolactin. *Endocrinology* 1989;125:2041–2048.
59. Powers CA, Hatala MA. Prolactin proteolysis by glandular kallikrein: in vitro reaction requirements and cleavage sites, and detection of processed prolactin in vivo. *Endocrinology* 1990;127:1916–1927.
60. Ho TWC, Balden E, Chao J, Walker AM. Prolactin (PRL) processing by kallikrein: production of the 21–23.5 k PRL-like molecules and inferences about PRL storage in mature secretory granules. *Endocrinology* 1991;129:184–192.
61. Powers CA. Anterior pituitary glandular kallikrein: a putative prolactin processing protease. *Mol Cell Endocrinology* 1993;90: C15–C20.
62. Pelligrini I, Gunz G, Grisoli F, Jaquet P. Different pathways of secretion for glycosylated and nonglycosylated human prolactin. *Endocrinology* 1990;126:1087–1095.
63. Rosa P, Fumagalli G, Zanini A, Huttner WB. The major tyrosine-sulfated protein of the bovine anterior pituitary is a secretory protein present in gonadotrophs, thyrotrophs, mammotrophs and corticotrophs. *J Cell Biol* 1985;100:928–937.
64. Tougard C, Nasciutti LE, Picart R, Tixier-Vidal A, Huttner WB. Subcellular distribution of secretogranins I and II in GH3 rat tumoral prolactin (PRL) cells as revealed by electron microscopic immunocytochemistry. *J Histochem Cytochem* 1989;37: 1329–1336.
65. Hashimoto S, Fumagalli G, Zanini A, Meldolesi J. Sorting of three secretory proteins to distinct secretory granules in acidophilic cells of cow anterior pituitary. *J Cell Biol* 1987;105: 1579–1586.
66. Scammel JG, Rosa P, Hille A, Huttner WB. Regulation of chromogranin B/secretogranin I and secretogranin II storage in GH4C1 cells. *J Histochem Cytochem* 1990;38:949–956.
67. Chanat E, Huttner WB. Milieu-induced, selective aggregation of regulated secretory proteins in the trans-Golgi network. *J Cell Biol* 1991;115:1505–1519.
68. Thompson ME, Zimmer WE, Haynes AL, Valentine DL, Forss-Petter S, Scammel JG. Prolactin granulogenesis is associated with increased secretogranin expression and aggregation in the Golgi apparatus of GH4C1 cells. *Endocrinology* 1992;131:318–326.
69. Vila-Porcile E, Picart R, Tixier-Vidal A, Tougard C. Cellular and subcellular distribution of laminin in adult rat anterior pituitary. *J Histochem Cytochem* 1987;35:287–299.
70. Vila-Porcile E, Picart R, Vigny M, Tixier-Vidal A, Tougard C. Immunolocalization of laminin, heparan-sulfate proteoglycan, entactin and type IV collagen in the rat anterior pituitary: I. An in vivo study. *Anat Rec* 1992;232:482–492.
71. Vila-Porcile E, Picart R, Vigny M, Tixier-Vidal A, Tougard C. Immunolocalization of laminin, heparan-sulfate proteoglycan, entactin and type IV collagen in the rat anterior pituitary: II. An in vitro study on primary cultures. *Anat Rec* 1992;233:1–12.
72. Hatala MA, Powers CA. Biochemical investigation of the subcellular localization of the estrogen-induced proglandular kallikrein in the rat anterior pituitary. *Neuroendocrinology* 1989;49: 537–544.
73. Vio CP, Roa JP, Silva R, Powers CA. Localization of immunoreactive glandular kallikrein in lactotrophs of the rat anterior pituitary. *Neuroendocrinology* 1990;51:10–14.
74. Saint-André JP, Rohmer V, Pinet F, Rousselet MC, Bigorgne JC, Corvol P. Renin and cathepsin B in human pituitary lactotroph cells: an ultrastructural study. *Histochemistry* 1989;91:291–297.
75. Morel G, Besson J, Rosselin G, Dubois PM. Ultrastructural evidence for endogenous vasoactive intestinal peptide-like immunoreactivity in the pituitary gland. *Neuroendocrinology* 1982;34: 85–89.
76. Arnaout MA, Garthwaite TL, Martinson DR, Hagen TC. Vasoactive intestinal peptide is synthesized in anterior pituitary tissue. *Endocrinology* 1986;119:2052–2057.
77. Steele MK, Brownfield MS, Ganong WF. Immunocytochemical localization of angiotensin immunoreactivity in gonadotrops and lactotrops of the rat anterior pituitary gland. *Neuroendocrinology* 1982;35:155–158.
78. Steel JH, Gon G, O'Halloran DJ, et al. Galanin and vasoactive intestinal peptide are colocalized with classical pituitary hormones and show plasticity of expression. *Histochemistry* 1989;93:183–189.
79. Childs (Moriarty) GV, Cole DE, Kubek M, Tobin RB, Wilber JF. Endogenous thyrotropin-releasing hormone in the anterior pituitary: sites of activity as identified by immunocytochemical staining. *J Histochem Cytochem* 1978;26:901–908.
80. Croissandeau G, Pagésy P, Grouselle D, Le Dafniet M, Peillon F, Li JY. Immunoreactive thyroliberin (TRH) precursor forms in human hypothalamus and anterior pituitary tissues. *FEBS Lett* 1992;298:191–194.

81. Snyder JM, Wilfinger W, Hymer WC. Maintenance of separated rat pituitary mammotrophs in cell culture. *Endocrinology* 1976;98:25–32.
82. Velkeniers B, Hooghe-Peters EL, Hooghe R, et al. Prolactin cell subpopulations separated on discontinuous Percoll gradient: an immunocytochemical, biochemical, and physiological characterization. *Endocrinology* 1988;123:1619–1630.
83. Swearingen KC. Heterogeneous turnover of adenohypophysial prolactin. *Endocrinology* 1971;89:1380–1388.
84. Walker AM, Farquhar MG. Preferential release of newly synthesized prolactin granules is the result of functional heterogeneity among mammotrophs. *Endocrinology* 1980;107:1095–1104.
85. Morin A, Rosenbaum E, Tixier-Vidal A. Effects of thyrotropin-releasing hormone on prolactin compartments in normal rat pituitary cells in primary cultures. *Endocrinology* 1984;115: 2278–2284.
86. Morin A, Rosenbaum E, Tixier-Vidal A. Effects of thyrotropin releasing hormone on prolactin compartments in clonal rat pituitary tumor cells. *Endocrinology* 1984;115:2271–2277.
87. Hoyt RF, Tashjian AH. Immunocytochemical analysis of prolactin production by monolayer cultures of GH3 rat anterior pituitary tumor cells: I. Long term effects of stimulation with thyrotropin-releasing hormone (TRH). *Anat Rec* 1980;197: 153–162.
88. Luque EH, Munoz de Toro M, Smith PF, Neill JD. Subpopulations of lactotropes detected with the reverse hemolytic plaque assay show differential responsiveness to dopamine. *Endocrinology* 1986;118:2120–2124.
89. Boockfor FR, Hoeffler JP, Frawley LS. Cultures of GH3 cells are functionally heterogeneous: thyrotropin-releasing hormone, estradiol and cortisol cause reciprocal shifts in the proportions of growth hormone and prolactin secretors. *Endocrinology* 1985; 117:418–420.
90. Arita J, Kojima Y, Kimura F. Identification by the sequential cell immunoblot assay of a subpopulation of rat dopamine-unresponsive lactotrophs. *Endocrinology* 1991;128:1887–1894.
91. Boockfor FR, Frawley LS. Functional variations among prolactin cells from different pituitary regions. *Endocrinology* 1987; 120:874–879.
92. Mukherjee P, Salada T, Hymer WC. Function of prolactin cells in the individual rat pituitary gland is location dependent. *Mol Cell Endocrinol* 1991;76:35–44.
93. Chen TT, Kineman RD, Betts JG, Hill JB, Frawley LS. Relative importance of newly synthesized and stored hormone to basal secretion by growth hormone and prolactin cells. *Endocrinology* 1989;125:1904–1909.
94. Scarbrough K, Weiland NG, Larson GH, et al. Measurement of peptide secretion and gene expression in the same cell. *Mol Endocrinol* 1991;5:134–142.
95. Nemeskeri A, Grouselle D, Tixier-Vidal A, Halasz B. Ontogeny of prolactin synthesizing cells in fetal and early postnatal rat pituitary. In vivo and in vitro studies. In: Hoshino K, ed. *Prolactin gene family and its receptors: molecular biology to clinical problems.* Amsterdam: Elsevier; 1988:319–325.
96. Setalo G, Nakane PK. Functional differentiation of the fetal anterior pituitary cells in the rat. *Endocrinol Exp* 1976;10:155–166.
97. Smets G, Velkeniers B, Herregodts P, Vanhaelst L, Gepts W, Hooghe-Peters EL. Ontogeny of hormone-secreting cells of the rat pituitary gland: an immunocytochemical study on dissociated cells. *Histochem J* 1989;21:337–342.
98. Chatelain A, Dupouy JP, Dubois MP. Ontogenesis of cell producing polypeptide hormones (ACTH, MSH, LPH, GH, prolactin) in the fetal hypophysis of the rat: influence of the hypothalamus. *Cell Tissue Res* 1979;196:409–427.
99. Watanabe YG, Daikoku S. An immunohistochemical study on the cytogenesis of adenohypophysial cells in fetal rats. *Dev Biol* 1979;68:557–567.
100. Hoeffler JP, Boockfor FR, Frawley LS. Ontogeny of prolactin cells in neonatal rats: initial prolactin secretors also release growth hormone. *Endocrinology* 1985;117:187–195.
101. Simmons DM, Voss JW, Ingraham HA, et al. Pituitary cell phenotypes involve cell-specific Pit-1 mRNA translation and synergistic interactions with other classes of transcription factors. *Genes Dev* 1990;4:695–711.
102. Hooghe-Peters EL, Belayew A, Herregodts P, et al. Discrepancy between prolactin (PRL) messenger ribonucleic acid and PRL content in rat fetal pituitary cells: possible role of dopamine. *Mol Endocrinol* 1988;2:1163–1168.
103. Frawley LS, Miller III HA. Ontogeny of prolactin secretion in the neonatal rats is regulated postranscriptionally. *Endocrinology* 1989;124:3–6.
104. Begeot M, Dubois MP, Dubois PM. Evolution of lactotropes in normal and anencephalic human fetuses. *J Clin Endocrinol Metab* 1984;58:726–730.
105. Mulchahey JJ, Jaffe RB. Detection of a potential progenitor cell in the human fetal pituitary that secretes both growth hormone and prolactin. *J Clin Endocrinol Metab* 1987;62:24–31.
106. Ingraham HA, Chen R, Mangalan HJ, et al. A tissue-specific transcription factor containing a homeodomain specifies a pituitary phenotype. *Cell* 1988;55:519–529.
107. Crenshaw III EB, Kalla K, Ingraham HA, Simmons DM, Swanson LW, Rosenfeld MG. Cell-specific expression of the prolactin gene in transgenic mice is controlled by synergistic interactions between Pit-1 recognition elements. *Genes Dev* 1989;3:959–972.
108. Li S, Crenshaw III EB, Rawson EJ, Simmons DM, Swanson LW, Rosenfeld MG. Dwarf locus mutants lacking three pituitary cell types result from mutations in the POU-domain gene pit-1. *Nature* 1990;347:528–533.
109. Lin C, Lin SC, Chang CP, Rosenfeld MG. Pit-1-dependent expression of the receptor for growth hormone releasing factor mediates pituitary cell growth. *Nature* 1992;360:765–768.
110. Borrelli E, Heyman RA, Arias C, Sawchenko PE, Evans RM. Transgenic mice with inducible dwarfism. *Nature* 1989; 339:538–541.
111. Kawashima S, Takahashi S. Morphological and functional changes of prolactin cells during aging in the rat. In: Yoshimura F, Gorbman A, eds. *Pars distalis of the pituitary gland: structure, function and regulation.* Amsterdam: Elsevier; 1986:51–56.
112. Purves HD, Griesbach WE. Changes in the gonadotrophs of the rat pituitary after gonadectomy. *Endocrinology* 1955;56: 374–386.
113. Herlant M. Etude critique de deux techniques nouvelles destinées à mettre en évidence les différentes catégories cellulaires présentes dans la glande pituitaire. *Bull Micr Appl* 1960;10: 37–44.
114. Pasteels JL, Herlant M. Notions nouvelles sur la cytologie de l'antéhypophyse chez le rat. *Z Zellforsch* 1962;56:20–39.
115. Tougard C. Immunocytochemical identification of LH and FSH secreting cells at the light and electron microscope levels. In: Jutisz M, McKerns KW, eds. *Synthesis and release of adenohypophyseal hormones.* New York: Plenum; 1980:15–37.
116. Tougard C, Picart R, Tixier-Vidal A. Immunocytochemical localization of glycoprotein hormones in the rat anterior pituitary: a light and electron microscope study using antisera against rat β subunits: a comparison between preembedding and postembedding methods. *J Histochem Cytochem* 1980;28:101–114.
117. Baker BL, Yu YY. Immunocytochemical analysis of cells in the pars tuberalis of the rat hypophysis with antisera to hormones of the pars distalis. *Cell Tissue Res* 1975;156:443–449.
118. Baker BL. Cellular composition of the human pituitary pars tuberalis as revealed by immunocytochemistry. *Cell Tissue Res* 1977;182:151–163.
119. Herbert DC. Identification of the LH and TSH secreting cells in the pituitary gland of the rhesus monkey. *Cell Tissue Res* 1978;190:151–161.
120. El Etreby MF, Fath El Bab MR. Localization of gonadotropic hormones in the dog pituitary gland. *Cell Tissue Res* 1977;183:167–175.
121. Stoëckel ME, Porte A. Fine structure and development of the pars tuberalis in mammals. In: Motta PM, ed. *Ultrastructure of endocrine cells and tissues.* The Hague: Martinus Nijhoff, 1984:29–38.
122. Fellmann D, Bresson JL, Clavequin MC, Bugnon C. Quantitative immunocytochemical studies on the gonadotrophs isolated from the pituitary of the male rat. *Cell Tissue Res* 1982; 224:137–144.
123. Childs GV. Fluidity of gonadotropin storage in cycling female rats. In: McKerns KW, Naor Z, eds. *Hormonal control of the hypothalamo-pituitary-gonadal axis.* 1984:181–198.

124. Barnes BG. Electron microscope studies on the secretory cytology of the mouse anterior pituitary. *Endocrinology* 1962;71: 618–628.
125. Barnes BG. The fine structure of the mouse adenohypophysis in various physiological states. In: Benoit J, Da Lage D, eds. *Cytologie de l'adénohypophyse.* Paris: CNRS; 1963:91–109.
126. Kurosumi K, Oota Y. Electron microscopy of two types of gonadotrophs in the anterior pituitary glands of persistent estrous and diestrous rats. *Z Zellforsch* 1968;85:34–46.
127. Tougard C, Kerdelhué B, Tixier-Vidal A, Jutisz M. Light and electron microscope localization of binding sites against ovine luteinizing hormone and its two subunits in rat adenohypophysis using peroxidase-labeled antibody technique. *J Cell Biol* 1973;58:503–521.
128. Moriarty GV. Immunocytochemistry of the pituitary glycoprotein hormones. *J Histochem Cytochem* 1976;24:846–863.
129. Childs GV (Moriarty), Ellison DG, Garner, LL. An immunocytochemist's view of gonadotropin storage in the adult male rat: cytochemical and morphological heterogeneity in serially sectioned gonadotropes. *Am J Anat* 1980;158:397–409.
130. Yoshimura F, Nogami H, Shirasawa N, Yashiro T. A whole range of fine structural criteria for immunohistochemically identified LH cells in rats. *Cell Tissue Res* 1981;217:1–10.
131. Moriarty GV, Garner LL. Immunocytochemical studies of cells in the rat adenohypophysis containing both ACTH and FSH. *Nature* 1977;265:356–358.
132. Inoue K, Hagino N. Comparative immunocytochemical demonstration of ACTH, LH and FSH-containing cells in the pituitary of neonatal immature and adult rats. *Cell Tissue Res* 1984;235:71–75.
133. Pelletier G, Leclerc R, Labrie F. Identification of gonadotropic cells in the human pituitary by immunoperoxidase technique. *Mol Cell Endocrinol* 1976;6:123–128.
134. Beauvillain JC, Tramu G, Dubois MP. Characterization by different techniques of adrenocorticotropin and gonadotropin producing cells in Lerot pituitary (*Eliomys quercinus*): a superimposition technique and an immunocytochemical technique. *Cell Tissue Res* 1975;158:301–317.
135. Dacheux F. Ultrastructural localization of gonadotrophic hormones in the porcine pituitary using the immunoperoxidase technique. *Cell Tissue Res* 1978;191:219–232.
136. Dacheux F. Proportions of FSH/LH cells, LH cells and FSH cells in the porcine anterior pituitary. *IRCS* 1981;9:952–953.
137. Dacheux F. Ultrastructural localization of gonadotropin-releasing hormone in the porcine gonadotropic cells. *Cell Tissue Res* 1981;216:143–150.
138. Moriarty GC. Electron microscopic-immunocytochemical studies of rat pituitary gonadotrophs: a sex difference in morphology and cytochemistry of LH cells. *Endocrinology* 1975;97: 1215–1225.
139. Herbert DC. Localization of antisera to LHβ and FSHβ in the rat pituitary gland. *Am J Anat* 1975;144:378–385.
140. Bugnon C, Fellmann D, Lenys D, Bloch B. Etude cytoimmunologique des cellules gonadotropes et des cellules thyréotropes de l'adénohypophyse du rat. *CR Soc Biol* 1977;907–913.
141. Kofler R. Immunofluorescence localization of glycoprotein hormones in the rat anterior pituitary gland using monoclonal antibodies and polyclonal antisera. *J Histochem Cytochem* 1982; 30:645–649.
142. Inoue K, Kurosumi K. Ultrastructural immunocytochemical localization of LH and FSH in the pituitary of the untreated male rat. *Cell Tissue Res* 1984;235:77–83.
143. Phifer RF, Midgley AR, Spicer SS. Immunohistologic and histologic evidence that follicle-stimulating hormone and luteinizing hormone are present in the same cell type in the human pars distalis. *J Clin Endocrinol Metab* 1973;36:125–141.
144. Herbert DC. Immunocytochemical evidence that luteinizing hormone (LH) and follicle-stimulating hormone (FSH) are present in the same cell type in the rhesus monkey pituitary gland. *Endocrinology* 1976;98:1554–1557.
145. Girod C, Dubois MP, Trouillas J. Mise en évidence de cellules gonadotropes de l'adénohypophyse (pars distalis et pars tuberalis) du singe *Macacus irus:* étude en immunofluorescence à l'aide d'anticorps anti-β FSH humaine et anti-β LH ovine. *CR Soc Biol (Paris)* 1980;174:304–313.
146. Girod C, Dubois MP, Trouillas J. Immunohistochemical localization of FSH and LH in the pars distalis of vervet (*Cercopithecus aethiops*) and baboon (*Papio hamadryas*) pituitaries. *Cell Tissue Res* 1981;217:245–257.
147. Batten TFC, Hopkins CR. Discrimination of LH, FSH, TSH and ACTH in dissociated porcine anterior pituitary cells by light and electron microscope immunocytochemistry. *Cell Tissue Res* 1978;192:107–120.
148. Purandare T. Immunohistochemical localization of FSH and LH in rat pituitary. *Mol Cell Endocrinol* 1978;10:57–62.
149. Childs GV. The use of multiple methods to validate immunocytochemical stains. *J Histochem Cytochem* 1983;31:168–176.
150. Childs (Moriarty) GV, Ellison DG, Lorenzen JR, Collins TJ, Schwartz NB. Immunocytochemical studies of gonadotropin storage in developing castration cells. *Endocrinology* 1982; 111:1318–1328.
151. Childs GV, Hyde C, Naor Z, Catt K. Heterogeneous luteinizing hormone and follicle stimulating hormone storage patterns in subtypes of gonadotropes separated by centrifugal elutriation. *Endocrinology* 1983;113:2120–2128.
152. Childs GV, Unabia G, Tibolt R. How the fixation-embedding protocol affects the specificity and efficiency of immunocytochemical stains for gonadotropin subunits. *Am J Anat* 1985;174:409–417.
153. Childs GV. Differential sites of gonadotropin storage in multihormonal gonadotropes. In: Yoshimura F, Gorbman A, eds. *Pars distalis of the pituitary gland: structure, function and regulation.* Amsterdam: Elsevier; 1986:115–124.
154. Dacheux F. Subcellular localization of gonadotropic hormones in pituitary cells of the castrated pig with the use of pre- and postembedding immunocytochemical methods. *Cell Tissue Res* 1984;236:153–160.
155. Dacheux F. Are FSH and LH contained in the same granules? *IRCS Med Sci* 1979;7:280–281.
156. Dacheux F. Ultrastructural localization of LH and FSH in the porcine pituitary. In: Justisz M, McKerns KW, eds. *Synthesis and release of adenohypophyseal hormones.* New York: Plenum; 1980:187–195.
157. Childs GV, Unabia G, Ellison D. Immunocytochemical studies of pituitary hormones with PAP, ABC, and immunogold techniques: evolution of technology to best fit the antigen. *Am J Anat* 1986;175:307–330.
158. Childs GV. Application of dual preembedding stains for gonadotropins to pituitary cell monolayers with avidin-biotin (ABC) and peroxidase antiperoxidase (PAP) complexes: light microscopic studies. *Stain Technol* 1983;58:281–289.
159. Childs GV. Shifts in gonadotropin storage in cultured gonadotropes following GnRH stimulation, in vitro. *Peptides* 1985;6: 103–107.
160. Bassetti M, Huttner WB, Zanini A, Rosa P. Co-localization of secretogranins/chromogranins with thyrotropin and luteinizing hormone in secretory granules of cow anterior pituitary. *J Histochem Cytochem* 1990;38:1353–1363.
161. Watanabe T, Uchiyama Y, Grube D. Topology of chromogranin A and secretogranin II in the rat anterior pituitary: potential marker proteins for distinct secretory pathways in gonadotrophs. *Histochemistry* 1991;96:285–293.
162. Cozzi MG, Zanini A. Sulfated LH subunits and a tyrosine-sulfated secretory protein (secretogranin II) in female rat adenohypophyses: changes with age and stimulation of release by LH-RH. *Mol Cell Endocrinol* 1986;44:47–54.
163. Conn PM, Janovick JA, Braden TD, Maurer RA, Jennes L. SIIp: a unique secretogranin/chromogranin of the pituitary released in response to gonadotropin-releasing hormone. *Endocrinology* 1992;130:3033–3040.
164. Sternberger LA, Petrali JP, Joseph SA, Meyer HC, Mills KR. Specificity of the immunocytochemical luteinizing hormone-releasing hormone receptor reaction. *Endocrinology* 1978; 102:63–73.
165. Childs GV, Ellison DG. A critique of the contributions of immunoperoxidase cytochemistry to our understanding of pituitary cell function, as illustrated by our current studies of gonadotropes, corticotropes and endogenous pituitary GnRH and TRH. *Histochem J* 1980;12:405–418.
166. Bauer TW, Moriarty CM, Childs GV. Studies of immunoreactive

gonadotropin releasing hormone (GnRH) in the rat anterior pituitary. *J Histochem Cytochem* 1981;29:1171–1178.
167. Uchiyama Y, Nakajima M, Watanabe T, et al. Immunocytochemical localization of cathepsin B in rat anterior pituitary endocrine cells, with special reference to its co-localization with renin and prorenin in gonadotrophs. *J Histochem Cytochem* 1991;39:1199–1205.
168. Deschepper CF, Crumrine DW, Ganong WF. Evidence that the gonadotrophs are the likely site of production of angiotensin II in the anterior pituitary of the rat. *Endocrinology* 1986;119:36–43.
169. Thomas WG, Sernia C. Immunocytochemical localization of angiotensinogen and angiotensin II in the rat pituitary. *J Neuroendocrinol* 1990;2:297–304.
170. Roberts V, Meunier H, Vaughan J, et al. Production and regulation of inhibin subunits in pituitary gonadotropes. *Endocrinology* 1989;124:552–555.
171. Kaiser UB, Lee BL, Carroll RS, Unabia G, Chin WW, Childs GV. Follistatin gene expression in the pituitary: localization in gonadotropes and folliculostellate cells in diestrous rats. *Endocrinology* 1992;130:3048–3056.
172. Denef C, Hautekeete E, De Wolf A, Vanderschueren B. Pituitary basophils from immature male and female rats: distribution of gonadotrophs and thyrotrophs as studied by unit gravity sedimentation. *Endocrinology* 1978;103:724–735.
173. Denef C, Hautekeete E, Dewals R. Monolayer cultures of gonadotrophs separated by velocity sedimentation: heterogeneity in response to luteinizing hormone releasing hormone. *Endocrinology* 1978;103:736–747.
174. Denef C, Hautekeete E, Dewals R, De Wolf A. Differential control of luteinizing hormone and follicle-stimulating hormone secretion by androgens in rat pituitary cells in culture: functional diversity of subpopulations separated by unit gravity sedimentation. *Endocrinology* 1980;106:724–729.
175. Denef C, Swennen L, Andries M. Separated anterior pituitary cells and their response to hypophysiotropic hormones. *Int Rev Cytol* 1982;76:225–244.
176. Denef C. Functional heterogeneity of separated dispersed gonadotropic cells. In: Justisz M, McKerns KW, eds. *Synthesis and release of adenohypophyseal hormones.* New York: Plenum; 1980:659–676.
177. Naor Z, Childs GV, Leifer AM, Clayton RN, Amsterdam A, Catt KJ. Gonadotropin-releasing hormone binding and activation of enriched populations of pituitary gonadotrophs. *Mol Cell Endocrinol* 1982;25:85–97.
178. Lloyd JM, Childs GV. Differential storage and release of luteinizing hormone and follicle-releasing hormone from individual gonadotropes separated by centrifugal elutriation. *Endocrinology* 1988;122:1282–1290.
179. Smith PF, Frawley LS, Neill JD. Detection of LH release from pituitary cells by the reverse hemolytic plaque assay: estrogen increases the fraction of gonadotropes responding to GnRH. *Endocrinology* 1984;115:2484–2486.
180. Tougard C, Picart R, Tixier-Vidal A. Cytogenesis of immunoreactive gonadotropic cells in the fetal rat pituitary at light and electron microscope levels. *Dev Biol* 1977;58:148–163.
181. Begeot M, Dupouy JP, Dubois MP, Dubois PM. Immunocytological determination of gonadotropic and thyrotropic cells in fetal rat anterior pituitary during normal development and under experimental conditions. *Neuroendocrinology* 1981;32:285–294.
182. Dubois MP, Mauléon P. Mise en évidence par immunofluorescence des cellules à activité gonadotrope LH dans l'hypophyse du foetus de brebis. *CR Acad Sci (Paris)* [*D*] 1969;269:219–222.
183. Danchin E, Dubois MP. Immunocytochemical study of the chronology of pituitary cytogenesis in the domestic pig (*Sus scrofa*) with special reference to the functioning of the hypothalamo-pituitary-gonadal axis. *Reprod Nutr Dev* 1982;22:135–151.
184. Dacheux F, Martinat N. Immunocytochemical localization of LH, FSH and TSH in the fetal porcine pituitary. *Cell Tissue Res* 1983;228:277–295.
185. Danchin E, Dang DC, Dubois MP. An immunocytochemical study of the adult crab-eating macaque (*Macaca fascicularis*) pituitary and its cytological differentiation during fetal life. *Reprod Nutr Dev* 1981;21:441–454.
186. Bugnon C, Bloch B, Fellmann D. Cytoimmunological study of the ontogenesis of the gonadotropic hypothalamo-pituitary axis in the human fetus. *J Steroid Biochem* 1977;8:565–575.
187. Dubois PM, Begeot M, Dubois MP, Herbert DC. Immunocytological localization of LH, FSH, TSH and their subunits in the pituitary of normal and anencephalic human fetuses. *Cell Tissue Res* 1978;191:249–265.
188. Gross DS, Baker BL. Developmental correlation between hypothalamic gonadotropin-releasing hormone and hypophysial luteinizing hormone. *Am J Anat* 1979;154:1–10.
189. Nemeskeri A, Németh A, Sétalo G, Vigh S, Halasz B. Cell differentiation of the fetal rat anterior pituitary in vitro. *Cell Tissue Res* 1976;170:263–273.
190. Watanabe YG, Daikoku S. Immunohistochemical study on adenohypophysial primordia in organ culture. *Cell Tissue Res* 1976;166:407–412.
191. Daikoku S, Kawano H, Matsumura H, Saito S. In vivo and in vitro studies on the appearance of LH-RH neurons in the hypothalamus of perinatal rats. *Cell Tissue Res* 1978;194:433–445.
192. Begeot M, Dubois MP, Dubois PM. Comparative study in vivo and in vitro of the differentiation of immunoreactive gonadotropic cells in fetal rat anterior pituitary. *Neuroendocrinology* 1983;37:52–58.
193. Begeot M, Morel G, Rivest RW, Aubert ML, Dubois MP, Dubois PM. Influence of gonadoliberin on the differentiation of rat gonadotrophs: an in vivo and in vitro study. *Neuroendocrinology* 1984;38:217–225.
194. Yoshimura F, Harumiya K, Hiyama H. Light and electron microscopic studies of the cytogenesis of anterior pituitary cells in perinatal rats in reference to the development of target organs. *Arch Histol Jpn* 1970;31:333–369.
195. Dupouy JP, Magre S. Ultrastructure des cellules granulées de l'hypophyse foetale du rat. Identification des cellules corticotropes et thyréotropes. *Arch Anat Microsc* 1973;62:185–205.
196. Svalander C. Ultrastructure of the fetal rat adenohypophysis. *Acta Endocrinol* 1974;76:1–114.
197. Dacheux F. Functional differentiation of the anterior pituitary cells in the fetal pig: an ultrastructural immunocytochemical study. *Cell Tissue Res* 1984;235:623–633.
198. Fletcher WH, Anderson NC Jr, Everett JW. Intercellular communication in the rat anterior pituitary gland. *J Cell Biol* 1975;67:469–476.
199. Horvath E, Kovacs K, Ezrin C. Junctional contact between lactotrophs and gonadotrophs in the rat pituitary. *IRCS Med Sci* 1977;5:511.
200. Denef C. Functional interrelationships between pituitary cells. In: Lamberts SWJ, Tilders FJH, Van der Veen EA, Assies J, eds. *Trends in diagnosis and treatment of pituitary adenomas.* Amsterdam: Free University Press; 1984:25–35.
201. Denef C. Paracrine interaction in anterior pituitary. In: Mac Leod RM, Thorner MO, Scapagnini U, eds. *Prolactin: basic and clinical correlates,* vol. 1. Fidia Research Series. Padua: Liviana Press; 1985:53–57.
202. Everett NB, Baker BL. The distribution of cell types in the anterior hypophysis during late pregnancy and lactation. *Endocrinology* 1945;37:83–88.
203. Merchant FW. Prolactin and luteinizing hormone cells of pregnant and lactating rats as studied by immunohistochemistry and radioimmunoassay. *Am J Anat* 1974;139:245–268.
204. Ozawa H, Kurosumi K. Ultrastructure of prolactin cells in the pregnant rat anterior pituitary as studied by immunogold electron microscopy. In: Hoshino K, ed. *Proceedings of the Kyoto Prolactin Conference,* vol. 4. Kyoto: Shinko; 1989:58–67.
205. Goluboff LG, Ezrin C. Effect of pregnancy on the somatotroph and the prolactin cell of the human adenohypophysis. *J Clin Endocrinol Metab* 1969;29:1533–1539.
206. Porter TE, Hill JB, Wiles CD, Frawley LS. Is the mammosomatotrope a transitional cell for the functional interconversion of growth hormone- and prolactin-secreting cells? Suggestive evidence from virgin, gestating, and lactating rats. *Endocrinology* 1990;127:2789–2794.
207. Billis WM, Delidow BC, White BA. Posttranscriptional regulation of prolactin (PRL) gene expression in PRL-deficient pituitary tumor cells. *Mol Endocrinol* 1992;6:1277–1284.

208. Grosvenor CE, Turner CW. Pituitary lactogenic hormone and milk secretion in lactating rats. *Endocrinology* 1958;63:535–539.
209. Shiino M, Williams G, Rennels EG. Ultrastructural observation of pituitary release of prolactin in the rat by suckling stimulus. *Endocrinology* 1972;90:176–181.
210. Vila-Porcile E, Olivier L. Exocytosis and related membrane events. In: Jutisz M, McKerns KW, eds. *Synthesis and release of adenohypophyseal hormones.* New York: Plenum, 1980;67–104.
211. Mena F, Martinez-Escalera G, Clapp C, Aguayo D, Forray C, Grosvenor CE. A solubility shift occurs during depletion-transformation of prolactin within the lactating rat pituitary. *Endocrinology* 1982;111:1086–1091.
212. Harigaya T, Kohmoto K, Hoshino K. Immunohistochemical identification of prolactin producing cells in the mouse adenohypophysis. *Acta Histochem Cytochem* 1983;16:51–58.
213. Sasaki F, Iwama Y. Sex difference in prolactin and growth hormone cells in mouse adenohypophysis: stereological, morphometric, and immunohistochemical studies by light and electron microscopy. *Endocrinology* 1988;123:905–912.
214. Yamaji A, Sasaki F, Iwama Y, Yamauchi S. Mammotropes and somatotropes in the adenohypophysis of androgenized female mice: morphological and immunohistochemical studies by light microscopy correlated with routine electron microscopy. *Anat Rec* 1992;233:103–110.
215. Ishibashi T, Shiino M. Subcellular localization of prolactin in the anterior pituitary cells of the female Japanese house bat, *Pipistrellus abramus. Endocrinology* 1989;124:1056–1063.
216. Pantic VR, Genbacev O. Ultrastructure of pituitary lactotropic cells of oestrogen treated male rats. *Z Zellforsch* 1969;95: 280–287.
217. Gersten BE, Baker BL. Local action of intrahypophyseal implants of estrogen as revealed by staining with peroxidase-labelled antibody. *Am J Anat* 1970;128:1–19.
218. Shiino M, Rennels EG. Recovery of rat prolactin cells following cessation of estrogen treatment. *Anat Rec* 1976;185:31–48.
219. Ibrahim SN, Moussa SM, Childs GV. Morphometric studies of rat anterior pituitary cells after gonadectomy: correlation of changes in gonadotropes with the serum levels of gonadotropins. *Endocrinology* 1986;119:629–637.
220. Ellerkmann E, Nagy GM, Frawley LS. Rapid augmentation of prolactin cell number and secretory capacity by an estrogen-induced factor released from the neurointermediate lobe. *Endocrinology* 1991;129:838–842.
221. Porter TE, Ellerkmann E, Frawley LS. Acute recruitment of prolactin-secreting cells is regulated posttranscriptionally. *Mol Cell Endocrinol* 1992;84:23–31.
222. Furth J, Clifton KH, Gadsden EL, Buffet RF. Dependent and autonomous mammotropic pituitary tumors in rats: Their somatotropic features. *Cancer Res* 1956;16:608–616.
223. Olivier L, Vila-Porcile E, Racadot O, Peillon F, Racadot J. Ultrastructure of pituitary tumor cells: a critical study. In: Tixier-Vidal A, Farquhar MG, eds. *The anterior pituitary.* New York: Academic Press; 1975:231–276.
224. Baskin DG, Erlandsen SL, Parsons JA. Functional classification of cell types in the growth hormone and prolactin-secreting rat MtTW 15 mammosomatotropic tumor with ultrastructural immunocytochemistry. *Am J Anat* 1980;158:455–461.
225. El Etreby MF. The role of steroid hormones in the pathogenesis of pituitary tumors in various experimental animals. In: Derome PJ, Jedynak CP, Peillon F, eds. *Pituitary adenomas,* Paris: Asclepios, 1980:39–48.
226. Kovacs K, McComb DJ, Horvath E. Subcellular investigation of experimental and human pituitary adenomas. In: Muller EE, MacLeod RM, eds. *Neuroendocrine perspectives,* vol. 2. New York: Elsevier, 1983:251–291.
227. Halmi NS. Immunostaining of growth hormone and prolactin in paraffin-embedded and stored or previously stained materials. *J Histochem Cytochem* 1978;26:486–495.
228. Girod C, Mazzuca M, Trouillas J, et al. Light microscopy, fine structure and immunohistochemistry studies of 278 pituitary adenomas. In: Derome PJ, Jedynak CP, Peillon F, eds. *Pituitary adenomas.* Paris: Asclepios, 1980:3–18.
229. Tindall GR, Kovacs K, Horvath E, Thorner MO. Human prolactin-producing adenomas and bromocriptine: a histological, immunocytochemical, ultrastructural and morphometric study. *J Clin Endocrinol Metab* 1982;55:1178–1184.
230. Landolt AM, Minder H, Osterwalder V, Landolt TA. Bromocriptine reduces the size of cells in prolactin-secreting adenomas. *Experientia* 1983;39:625–627.
231. Bassetti M, Spada A, Pizzo G, Giannattasio G. Bromocriptine treatment reduces the cell size in human macroprolactinomas: a morphometric study. *J Clin Endocrinol Metab* 1984;58:268–276.
232. Poole MC, Easley CS, Hodson CA. Alteration of the mammotroph Golgi complex by the dopamine agonist 2 Br-α-ergocryptine (CB-154) in ovariectomized estrogen primed rats. *Anat Rec* 1991;231:339–346.
233. Ozawa H, Kurosumi K. Morphofunctional study of prolactin-producing cells of the anterior pituitaries in adult male rats following thyroidectomy, thyroxine treatment and/or thyrotropin-releasing hormone treatment. *Cell Tissue Res* 1993;272:41–47.
234. Ascheim P, Pasteels JL. Etude histophysiologique de la sé crétion de prolactine chez les rattes séniles. *CR Acad Sci Paris* 1963;257:1373–1375.
235. Chuknyiska SR, Blackman MR, Hymer WC, Roth SR. Age related alterations in the number and function of pituitary lactotropic cells from intact and ovariectomized rat. *Endocrinology* 1986;118:1856–1862.
236. Kovacs K, Horvath E, Ilse RG, Ezrin C, Ilse D. Spontaneous pituitary adenomas in aging rats: a light microscopic immunocytochemical and fine structural study. *Beitr Pathol* 1977;161:1–16.
237. Berkvens JM, Van Nesslrooy JHJ, Kroes R. Spontaneous tumors in the pituitary gland of old Wistar rats: a morphological and immunocytochemical study. *J Pathol* 1980;130:179–191.
238. Trouillas J, Girod C, Claustrat B, Curé M, Dubois MP. Spontaneous pituitary tumors in Wistar/Furth/Ico rat strain: an animal model of human prolactin adenoma. *Am J Pathol* 1982;109: 57–70.
239. Trouillas J, Girod C, Claustrat B, Joly-Pharaboz MO, Chevallier P. Spontaneous prolactin transplantable tumor in the Wistar/Furth rat (SMtTW): a new animal model of human prolactinoma. *Cancer Res* 1990;50:4081–4086.
240. Tixier-Vidal A, Gourdji D, Tougard C. A cell culture approach to the study of the anterior pituitary. *Int Rev Cytol* 1975;41: 173–239.
241. Baker BL, Reel Jr, Van Dewark SD, Yu YY. Persistence of cell types in monolayer cultures of dispersed cells from the pituitary pars distalis as revealed by immunocytochemistry. *Anat Rec* 1974;179:93–106.
242. Antakly T, Pelletier G, Zeytinoglu F, Labrie F. Changes of cell morphology and prolactin secretion induced by 2-BR α-ergocryptine, estradiol, and thyrotropin-releasing hormone in rat anterior pituitary cells in culture. *J Cell Biol* 1980;86:377–387.
243. Tashjian AH Jr, Bancroft FC, Levine L. Production of both prolactin and growth hormone by clonal strains of rat pituitary tumor cells. *J Cell Biol* 1970;47:61–70.
244. Gourdji D. Multihormonal regulation of the pituitary gland binding and secretory responses to hypothalamic neuropeptides in rat GH pituitary strains in culture. *Neurochem Int* 1985;7:979–994.
245. Nagy I, Rappay G, Makara GB, Horvath G, Bacsy E, Mac Leod RM. Is there a direct correlation between the activities of various lysosomal enzymes and prolactin secretion in the rat anterior pituitary? *Endocrinology* 1983;112:470–475.
246. Nansel DD, Gudelsky GA, Reymond MJ, Neaves WB, Poster JC. A possible role for lysosomes in the inhibitory action of dopamine on PRL release. *Endocrinology* 1981;108:896–902.
247. Hassoun J, Jaquet P, Devictor B, et al. Bromocriptine effects on cultured human prolactin producing pituitary adenomas: in vitro ultrastructural, morphometric and immunoelectron microscopic studies. *J Clin Endocrinol Metab* 1985;61:686–692.
248. Stirling RG, Shin SH. A high concentration of dopamine preferentially permitted release of newly synthesized prolactin. *Mol Cell Endocrinol* 1990;70:65–72.
249. Mena F, Hummelt FMG, Aguayo D, Clapp C, Martinez de la Escalera G, Morales MT. Changes in molecular variants during in vitro transformation and release of prolactin by the pituitary gland of the lactating rat. *Endocrinology* 1992;130:3365–3377.
250. Frawley LS, Clark CL. Ovine prolactin and dopamine preferen-

tially inhibit PRL release from the same subpopulation of rat mammotropes. *Endocrinology* 1986;119:1462–1466.

251. Nagy GM, Boockfor FR, Frawley LS. The suckling stimulus increases the responsiveness of mammotropes located exclusively within the central region of the adenohypophysis. *Endocrinology* 1991;128:761–764.
252. Kazemzadeh M, Velkeniers B, Herregodts P, et al. Differential dopamine-induced prolactin mRNA levels in various prolactin-secreting cell (sub)populations. *J Endocrinol* 1992;132:401–409.
253. Vale W, Rivier C, Brown M. Regulatory peptides of the hypothalamus. *Annu Rev Physiol* 1977;39:473–527.
254. Tixier-Vidal A, Gourdji D. Mechanism of action of synthetic hypothalamic peptides on anterior pituitary cells. *Physiol Rev* 1981;61:974–1001.
255. Haug E, Gautvik KM. Effects of sex steroids on prolactin secreting rat pituitary cells in culture. *Endocrinology* 1976;99: 1482–1489.
256. Brunet N, Gourdji D, Moreau MF, Grouselle D, Bournaud F. Tixier-Vidal A. Effects of 17-β estradiol on prolactin secretion and thyroliberin responsiveness in two rat prolactin continuous cell lines. *Ann Biol Anim Biochim Biophys* 1977;17:413–424.
257. Tougard C, Louvard D, Picart R, Tixier-Vidal A. The rough endoplasmic reticulum and the Golgi apparatus visualized using specific antibodies in normal and tumoral prolactin cells in culture. *J Cell Biol* 1983;96:1197–1207.
258. Albert PR, Tashjian AJ Jr. Thyrotropin-releasing hormone-induced spike and plateau in cytosolic free Ca^{2+} concentrations in pituitary cells. *J Biol Chem* 1984;259:5827–5832.
259. Aizawa T, Hinkle PM. Thyrotropin-releasing hormone rapidly stimulates a biphasic secretion of prolactin and growth hormone in GH4C1 rat pituitary tumor cells. *Endocrinology* 1985;116: 73–82.
260. Martin TFJ, Kowalchik JA. Evidence for the role of calcium and diacylglycerol as dual second messengers in TRH-releasing hormone action. *Endocrinology* 1984;115:1517–1536.
261. Delbeke D, Kojima I, Dannies PS. Comparison of patterns of prolactin release in GH4C1 cells and primary pituitary cultures. *Mol Cell Endocrinol* 1985;43:15–22.
262. Gourdji D, Kerdelhué B, Tixier-Vidal A. Ultrastructure d'un clone de cellules hypophysaires sécrétant de la prolactine (clone GH3). Modifications induites par l'hormone hypothalamique de libération de l'hormone thyréotrope (TRF). *CR Acad Sci (Paris) [D]* 1972;274:437–440.
263. Tashjian AH Jr, Hoyt RF Jr. Transient controls of organ specific functions in pituitary cells in culture. In: Sussman S, ed. *Molecular genetics and developmental biology.* Englewood Cliffs, NJ: Prentice-Hall: 1972:353–387.
264. Tixier-Vidal A, Moreau MF, Picart R. Endocytose et sécrétion dans les cellules antéhypophysaires en culture: action des hormones hypothalamiques. *J Microscop Biol Cell* 1976;25: 159–172.
265. Van de Moortele S, Rosenbaum E, Tixier-Vidal A, Tougard C. Rapid and transient reorganization of the cytoskeleton in GH3B6 cells during short-term exposure to thyroliberin. *J Cell Sci* 1991;99:79–89.
266. Hoyt RF, Tashjian AH Jr. Immunocytochemical analysis of prolactin production by monolayer cultures of GH3 rat anterior pituitary tumor cells. II. Variation in prolactin content of individual cell colonies and dynamics of stimulation with thyrotropin-releasing hormone (TRH). *Anat Rec* 1980;197:163–181.
267. Boockfor FR, Hoeffler JP, Frawley LS. Analysis by plaque assays of GH and prolactin release from individual cells in culture of male pituitaries. *Neuroendocrinology* 1986;42:64–70.
268. Arita J, Kojima Y, Kimura F. Lactotrophs secreting small amounts of prolactin reveal great responsiveness to thyrotropin-releasing hormone: analysis by the sequential cell immunoblot assay. *Endocrinology* 1992;130:3167–3174.
269. Tougard C, Picart R, Morin A, Tixier-Vidal A. Effect of monensin on secretory pathway in GH_3 prolactin cells: a cytochemical study. *J Histochem Cytochem* 1983;31:745–754.
270. Hyde JF, Engle MG, Maley BE. Colocalization of galanin and prolactin within secretory granules of anterior pituitary cells in estrogen-treated Fischer 344 rats. *Endocrinology* 1991;129: 270–276.
271. Hyde JF, Keller BK. Galanin secretion from anterior pituitary cells in vitro is regulated by dopamine, somatostatin, and thyrotropin-releasing hormone. *Endocrinology* 1991;128: 917–922.
272. Hinkle PM, Scammell JG, Shanshala II ED. Prolactin and secretogranin-II, a marker for the regulated pathway, are secreted in parallel by pituitary GH4C1 cells. *Endocrinology* 1992;130: 3503–3511.
273. Kiino DR, Burger DE, Dannies PS. Prolactin storage in a clonal strain of rat pituitary tumor cells is cell-cycle dependent. *J Cell Biol* 1982;93:459–462.
274. De Carvalho N, Picart R, Tixier-Vidal A. 17β-estradiol regulates prolactin secretion but not cell proliferation of GH3/B6 cells in chemically defined medium. *Mol Cell Endocrinol* 1985;39: 49–60.
275. Inoue K, Sakai T. Conversion of growth hormone-secreting cells into prolactin-secreting cells and its promotion by insulin-like growth factor-1 in vitro. *Exp Cell Res* 1991;195:53–58.
276. Scammell JG, Burrage TG, Dannies PS. Hormonal induction of secretory granules in a pituitary tumor cell line. *Endocrinology* 1986;119:1543–1546.
277. Laverrière JN, Richard JL, Morin A. Secretogranin I (chromogranin B) mRNA accumulation is hormonally regulated in GH3B6 rat pituitary tumor cells. *Mol Cell Endocrinol* 1991; 80:41–51.
278. Amara JF, Van Itallie C, Dannies PS. Regulation of prolactin production and cell growth by estradiol: difference in sensitivity to estradiol occurs at the level of messenger ribonucleic acid accumulation. *Endocrinology* 1987;120:264–271.
279. Krown KA, Wang YF, Ho TWC, Kelly PA, Walker AM. Prolactin isoform 2 as an autocrine growth factor for GH3 cells. *Endocrinology* 1992;131:595–602.
280. Dada MO, Campbell GT, Blake CA. A quantitative immunocytochemical study of the luteinizing hormone and follicle stimulating hormone cells in the adenohypophysis of adult male rats and adult female rats throughout the estrous cycle. *Endocrinology* 1983;113:970–984.
281. Childs GV, Unabia G, Lloyd J. Recruitment and maturation of small subsets of luteinizing hormone gonadotropes during the estrous cycle. *Endocrinology* 1992;130:335–344.
282. Clayton RN, Solano AR, Garcia-Vela A, Dufau ML, Catt KJ. Regulation of pituitary receptors for gonadotropin-releasing hormone during the rat estrous cycle. *Endocrinology* 1980; 107:699–706.
283. Savoy-Moore RT, Schwartz NB, Duncan JA, Marshall JC. Pituitary gonadotropin releasing hormone receptors during the rat estrous cycle. *Science* 1980;209:942–944.
284. Lloyd JMM, Childs GV. Changes in the number of GnRH-receptive cells during the rat estrous cycle: biphasic effects of estradiol. *Neuroendocrinology* 1988;48:138–146.
285. Kurosumi K, Ozawa H, Akiyama K, Senshu T. Immunoelectron microscopic studies of gonadotrophs in the male and female rat anterior pituitaries, with special reference to their changes with aging. *Arch Histol Cytol* 1991;54:559–571.
286. Severinghaus AE. A cytological study of the anterior pituitary of the rat, with special reference to the Golgi apparatus and to cell relationship. *Anat Rec* 1933;57:149–175.
287. Yoshimura F, Harumiya K. Electron microscopy of the anterior lobe of pituitary in normal and castrated rats. *Endocrinol Jpn* 1965;12:119–152.
288. Kurosumi K, Kawarai Y, Yukitake Y, Inoue K. Electron microscopic morphometry of the rat castration cells. *Gumma Symp Endocrinol* 1976;13:221–236.
289. Tougard C, Kerdelhué B, Tixier-Vidal A, Jutisz M. Localisation par cytoimmunoenzymolgie de la LH, de ses sous-unités, α et β et de la FSH dans l'adénohypophyse de la ratte castrée. *CR Acad Sci Paris,* 1971;273:897–900.
290. Childs GV, Lloyd JM, Unabia G, Gharib SD, Wierman ME, Chin WW. Detection of luteinizing hormone β messenger ribonucleic acid (RNA) in individual gonadotropes after castration: use of a new in situ hybridization method with a photobiotinylated complementary RNA probe. *Mol Endocrinol* 1987;1:926–932.
291. Smith PF, Keefer DA. Immunocytochemical and ultrastructural identification of mitotic cells in the pituitary gland of ovariectomized rats. *J Reprod Fertil* 1982;66:383–389.

292. Sakuma S, Shirasawa N, Yoshimura F. A histochemical study of immunohistochemically identified mitotic adenohypophysial cells in immature and mature castrated rats. *J Endocrinol* 1984;100:322–328.
293. Sakai T, Inoue K, Hasegawa Y, Kurosumi K. Effect of passive immunization to gonadotropin-releasing hormone (GnRH) using GnRH antiserum on the mitotic activity of gonadotrophs in castrated male rats. *Endocrinology* 1988;122:2803–2808.
294. Childs GV, Ellison DG, Lorenzen JR, Collins TJ, Schwartz NB. Retarded development of castration cells after adrenalectomy or sham adrenalectomy. *Endocrinology* 1983;113:166–177.
295. Shiino M, Arimura A, Schally AV, Rennels EG. Ultrastructural observations of granule extrusion from rat anterior pituitary cells after injection of LH-releasing hormone. *Z Zellforsch* 1972; 128:152–161.
296. Mendoza D, Arimura A, Schally AV. Ultrastructural and light microscopic observations of rat pituitary LH-containing gonadotrophs following injection of synthetic LH-RH. *Endocrinology* 1973;92:1153–1160.
297. Soji T, Taya K, Igarashi M, Yoshimura F. Acute and subacute effect of LH-RH upon LH- and FSH-gonadotrophs in castrated female rats with short-term estrogen-progesterone pretreatment. *Endocrinol Jpn* 1974;21:407–428.
298. Shiino M. Ultrastructural evidence of gonadotrophin release from castration cells following injection of LH-RH in the rat. *Cell Tissue Res* 1982;222:213–222.
299. Nakamura F, Yoshimura F. Morphological characterization of LH secretory granule response to LH-RH and calmodulin inhibitor. *Mol Cell Endocrinol* 1986;44:11–15.
300. Wilbur DL, Spicer SS. Pituitary secretory activity and endocrinophagy. In: Jutisz M, McKerns KW, eds. *Synthesis and release of adenohypophyseal hormones.* New York: Plenum Press: 1980:167–186.
301. Yoshimura F, Soji T, Yachi H, Shikawa H. Life stage and secretory cycle of anterior pituitary basophils. *Endocrinol Jpn* 1974;21:217–249.
302. Soji T, Yashiro T, Yoshimura F. TRH and LRH and their target cells with special reference to secretory cycle of basophils. *Gunma Symp Endocrinol* 1976;13:237–257.
303. Yoshimura F, Soji T. Kumagai T, Yokoyama M. Secretory cycle of the pituitary basophils and its morphological evidence. *Endocrinol Jpn* 1977;24:185–202.
304. Soji T. Cytological changes of the pituitary basophils in rats slowly infused with thyrotropin-releasing hormone (TRH). *Endocrinol Jpn* 1978;25:245–258.
305. Soji T. Cytological changes of the pituitary basophils in rats slowly infused with LRH and with LRH and TRH in combination. *Endocrinol Jpn* 1978;25:259–274.
306. Kovacs K, Horvath E, Van Loon GR, Rewcastle NB, Ezrin C, Rosenbloom AA. Pituitary adenomas associated with elevated blood follicle-stimulating hormone levels: a histologic, immunocytologic and electron microscopic study of two cases. *Fertil Steril* 1978;29:622–628.
307. Trouillas J, Girod C, Sassolas G, et al. Human pituitary gonadotropic adenoma: histological, immunocytochemical and ultrastructural studies with hormonal relationships in eight cases. *J Pathol* 1981;135:315–336.
308. Matsumura H, Daikoku S. Sexual difference in LH-cells of the neonatal rats as revealed by immunocytochemistry. *Cell Tissue Res* 1977;182:541–548.
309. Childs (Moriarty) GV, Ellison D, Foster L, Ramaley JA. Postnatal maturation of gonadotropes in the male rat pituitary. *Endocrinology* 1981;109:1683–1692.
310. Matsumura H, Daikoku, S. Quantitative observations of the effect of sex-steroids on the postnatal development of LH cells: an immunohistochemical study. *Cell Tissue Res* 1978;188: 491–496.
311. Childs (Moriarty) GV, Ellison DG, Ramaley JA, Unabia G. Storage of anterior lobe adrenocorticotropin in corticotropes and a subpopulation of gonadotropes during the stress nonresponsive period in the neonatal male rat. *Endocrinology* 1982; 110:1676–1692.
312. Döhler KD, Von zur Mühlen A, Döhler U. Pituitary luteinizing hormone (LH), follicle stimulating hormone (FSH) and prolactin from birth to puberty in female and male rats. *Acta Endocrinol* 1977;85:718–728.
313. Tixier-Vidal A. Ultrastructure of anterior pituitary cells in culture. In: Farquhar MG, Tixier-Vidal A, eds. *The anterior pituitary.* New York: Academic Press: 1975:181–224.
314. Tougard C, Tixier-Vidal A, Kerdelhué B, Jutisz M. Etude immunocytochimique de l'évolution des cellules gonadotropes dans des cultures primaires de cellules antéhypophysaires de rat: aspects quantitatifs et ultrastructuraux. *Biol Cell* 1977;28: 251–260.
315. Van der Schueren B, Denef C, Cassiman JJ. Ultrastructural and functional characteristics of rat pituitary cell aggregates. *Endocrinology* 1982;110:513–523.
316. Childs GV. Studies of hormone storage and secretion in the multipotential gonadotrope. *Excerpta Med Int Congr Ser* 1985; 655:499–502.
317. Lewis CE, Morris JF, Fink G. The role of microfilaments in the priming effect of LH-releasing hormone: an ultrastructural study using cytochalasin B. *J Endocrinol* 1985;106:211–218.
318. Lewis CE, Morris JR, Fink G, Johnson M. Changes in the granule population of gonadotrophs of hypogonadal (hpg) and normal female mice associated with the priming effect of LH-releasing hormone in vitro. *J Endocrinol* 1986;109:35–44.
319. Morris JF, Lewis CE, Fink G. LH-RH priming in gonadotrophs: a model system for the analysis of neuroendocrine mechanism at the cellular level. In: Fink G, Harmar AJ, McKerns WC, eds. *Neuroendocrine molecular biology.* New York: Plenum; 1986: 341–352.
320. Neill JD, Smith PF, Luque EH, Munoz de Toro M, Nagy G, Mulchahey JJ. Analysis of hormone secretion from individual pituitary cells. In: Fink G, Harmar AJ, McKerns W, eds. *Neuroendocrine molecular biology.* New York: Plenum, 1986:325–340.
321. Zambrano D, Cuerdo-Rocha S, Bergman I. Ultrastructure of rat pituitary gonadotrophs following incubations of the gland with synthetic LH-RH. *Cell Tissue Res* 1974;150:179–192.
322. Polkowska J, Bérault A, Hurbain-Kosmath I, Jolly G, Jutisz M. Bihormonal cells producing gonadotropins and prolactin in a rat pituitary tumor cell line (RC-4B/C). *Neuroendocrinology* 1991;54:267–273.

The Physiology of Reproduction, Second Edition,
edited by E. Knobil and J.D. Neill,
Raven Press, Ltd., New York © 1994.

CHAPTER 30

Gonadotropins

Chemistry and Biosynthesis

George R. Bousfield[1], W. Michael Perry[2], and Darrell N. Ward[2]

In this chapter we review the chemistry and biosynthesis of the gonadotropins. Emphasis is given the human gonadotropins, but information from other mammalian or sometimes lower vertebrate gonadotropins is freely utilized in order to develop our comparative understanding of these important hormones and their genetic control. Several extensive reviews have been utilized for the present study, as acknowledged in the text. We particularly note our own earlier review (1) and the previous chapter on this subject in the first edition of the present volume (2).

[1] Department of Biological Sciences, Wichita State University, Wichita, Kansas 67260
[2] Department of Biochemistry and Molecular Biology, The University of Texas M.D. Anderson Cancer Center, Houston, Texas 77030

The glycoprotein hormones include the pituitary hormones follitropin and lutropin (of direct interest to reproductive physiology) and thyrotropin as well as the chorionic gonadotropins (also of interest for reproductive physiology, but whose presence has only been demonstrated in primates and equids). The glycoprotein hormones are now known to be comprised of two dissimilar subunits, although the first indication of noncovalently linked subunits was not obtained until the studies of Li and Starman (3), who showed that acid dissociation of ovine luteinizing hormone reduced the molecular weight by about one-half. Our laboratory first proposed the dissimilar nature of the glycoprotein hormone subunits (4) as a result of our first structural studies. The abstract of this report concluded, "From these observations we propose a model of LH composed of two different chains of similar molecular dimensions." Since that time this model has been expanded to include all of the glycoprotein hormones.

The next important information on the subunit story was from Papkoff and Samy (5), who provided a two-phase system for separation by countercurrent distribution of the dissimilar subunits. They obtained subunits with activity of the order of only 7% to 8% of the original oLH, and recombination of the separated subunits recovered about 20% of the original activity. These figures demonstrated important trends, although as this and other systems of separation were subsequently improved, the intrinsic potency of the separated subunits has approached zero activity, and the activity of the recombined subunits has approximated 100% of the original hormone potency. Other important observations from that study were the differences in the amino acid composition of the two subunits. About that same time, DeLaLlosa and Jutisz (6) were studying urea or guanidine hydrochloride dissociation of oLH and found that the subunits could be dissociated by these chaotropic agents with almost complete loss of activity. The activity was largely recovered on reassociation of the subunit dimer (e.g., over 98% in one experiment).

Our laboratory followed with an additional subunit separation procedure (7), which was useful in our early structure studies. This allowed a comparison of the subunits obtained by this procedure or the Papkoff–Samy procedure (5) as well as *C*- and *N*-terminal amino acid studies on the subunits. Meanwhile, others were finding that other glycoprotein hormones also were comprised of dissimilar subunits. Reports on hCG were provided by two laboratories (8,9). The study of bTSH, by countercurrent distribution after propionic acid dissociation also demonstrated the subunit nature of this hormone (10). This report by Liao and Pierce was a milestone in our understanding of the glycoprotein hormones, for it also demonstrated that the TSHα subunit of Liao and Pierce was nearly identical with the S subunit of Ward (7) or the CI of Papkoff and Samy (5) for oLH. The amino acid sequence around the carbohydrate moieties of oLH (11) and those of TSHα found by Pierce were indicative of this conclusion. Most important, however, was the demonstration that the CI or S subunit of LH could recombine with the TSHβ to produce an active form of TSH just as well as could the TSHα. This discovery established the "common subunit" model for glycoprotein hormones that has been so useful in our understanding of the chemistry and physiology of these hormones. In fact, much of the balance of this chapter is devoted to enlarging this point. With this information available, Pierce and co-workers, with the concurrence of others in the field, proposed the designation of the α and β subunits as the common subunit and hormone-specific subunit, respectively (12). This nomenclature for the glycoprotein hormones has been maintained since that time.

The initial sequence studies on the glycoprotein hormones prompted the examination of several other species. However, with the early methodology for protein sequence study there was always a need to produce considerable quantities of the hormone, thus the species of pituitary readily available was an early limitation to these studies. The early pituitary fractionation studies have been reviewed (13).

The dissimilar nature of the subunits has allowed scientists to devise unique experiments to study the role of these subunits in the subunit–subunit interactions that define the architecture of the active hormone molecule. To a lesser extent it has also been possible to study the interactions of the three-dimensionally complete hormone or hormone derivatives with their hormone receptors, as discussed below. Among the protein and polypeptide hormones, the existence of dissimilar subunits joined by noncovalent bonding to produce an active hormone is a unique structural feature for which the natural utility is worthy of further investigation. The α and β subunit genes are found on separate chromosomes as single genes in all cases studied except the human chorionic gonadotropin β subunit genes and the oFSHβ genes, which are discussed further below.

The subunit nature of the glycoprotein hormones is to be contrasted with the simple protein or peptide nature of other hormones (such as prolactin and ACTH), the multiple-chain hormones linked by disulfide covalent bonds (e.g., insulin, produced from a single gene product that undergoes posttranslational processing), or active hormones that are noncovalently linked to another protein carrier (e.g., the oxytocin– or vasopressin–neurophysin complexes) and are dissociated to release the active hormone. There are also hormones that have dissimilar chains (subunits) that are the products of two separate genes, and the active hormone is comprised of two (or more) chains covalently linked by disulfide bonds (e.g., inhibin). These structural differences in the polypeptide hormone architecture are undoubtedly utilized in the control of hormone action, storage, or secretion, but our understanding of the details is modest at the present time.

With the development of recombinant DNA technology there followed a significant surge in the availability of comparative structural information for the glycoprotein hormones as well as the introduction of information on the genetic control of glycoprotein hormone biosynthesis. This expansion of our available sequence information was abetted by the powerful approach of recombinant DNA methodology and also by the very high sensitivity of these tools, thus allowing access to several species whose small pituitary glands precluded study by the conventional protein methodology. In 1989, Ward et al. (14) cited over 21 species for which complete amino acid sequences of glycoprotein hormones were available, and the list continues to expand. These reviewers provided matrix comparisons of the percentage homology for these sequences (placed in register by the alignment of their half-cystine residues, as described below) for both the α and β subunit sequences. The common α subunit showed the greatest across-the-board homology in mammals, ranging from 72% (human versus whale or equine) to 97% identity, with over 72% of the available comparisons (n = 36) exceeding 80% identity. For the hormone-specific β subunit (with 210 available comparisons), there was greater variance, ranging from 31% to 100% identity. The 100% came from the identity of the eLHβ and the eCGβ. By groups there was a greater homology correlation, e.g., the LH/CG group ranged from 52% to 100% identity, the FSH group from 78% to 92% identity, and the TSH group from 85% to 93% identity. The between-group identities were in the 31% to 43% range.

The early structural studies using DNA methodology for the glycoprotein hormones have been reviewed by several authors (15–17). In Table 1 we have attempted to summarize the principal reports that provide the structural information to be used throughout the balance of the chapter. We have also coded the references cited as to whether the structural information was obtained by conventional protein sequencing (P) or by recombinant DNA methodology (D).

STRUCTURAL FEATURES OF THE GONADOTROPINS

Subunit Nature

We have already outlined the evolution of our concept of the subunit nature of the glycoprotein hormones. We shall now consider what this fact has meant to the understanding of the chemistry of these hormones.

The α or Common Subunit

The fact that all the glycoprotein hormones have a common α subunit carries implications for their biosynthesis, particularly for the separate control of α subunit production in the thyrotrope, the gonadotropes (including subtypes for FSH and LH biosynthesis), and the chorionic gonadotrope cells of equids and primates. A common subunit provides a means of obtaining a higher degree of biological complexity in three-dimensional structure with a minimal biosynthetic commitment, particularly if the receptors for each hormone require a common motif for this part of the structure. It should be noted that the evolution of a hormone implies the simultaneous evolution of its requisite receptor for an effective response system. We will better understand the importance of the architectural motif for the subunits of the glycoprotein hormones when we have complete three-dimensional data for their crystalline structure. Although these data are not yet available, the production of crystals of asialo- (18) and aglyco-hCG (19) suitable for X-ray crystallography encourages the belief that such information will soon be available.

The α subunit for several species has now been studied for protein sequences of the mature protein and, more recently, including the leader sequence deduced from recombinant DNA studies. (See the section on Biosynthesis of the Gonadotropins, below, for comment on the role of the leader sequence, also called signal sequence.) The currently known α subunit sequences are summarized in Fig. 1. The highly conserved protein sequences from mammalians down to teleosts is apparent if one indexes on the homologous placement of the half-cystine residues in these molecules. This uniformity of the half-cystine locations implies a uniformity of the secondary structure generated by the formation of the disulfide bonds between these residues (see **C** placements in Figs. 1 and 2 for all sequences; Fig. 3 presents an example of the disulfide linkages, which from best available evidence appear to be the same in all glycoprotein hormones). There are notable differences from the exactly homologous locations of these half-cystine residues. The first observed results show the gap of four residues at positions 4–7 in the human α sequence that results from a deletion in this position of the human gene. This results in a foreshortened *N*-terminal tail on the human α subunit prior to the first half-cystine and thus does not alter the size of any of the disulfide loops (see Fig. 3), but it does shift the numbering for the human subunit. This is the only gap in the mammalian series. Thus, all of the disulfide loops in the mammalian α subunits are identical in size as determined by the amino acid residues in each loop. In the sequences from lower vertebrates there are several gaps in the sequences from fishes and eels (see Figs. 1 and 2), and all of these are in locations that necessarily shorten some of the disulfide loops. This may be important to the observation that the α subunit from the carp failed to produce an active dimeric hormone with oLHβ (20). The recently reported sequence of the lower vertebrate, the bullfrog, has an arginine residue (**R**) inserted between positions 28 and 29 compared to the other species of α subunits. This means that the bullfrog has one extra residue in the two disulfide loops formed with this part of the molecule.

These gaps and insertions alter the actual numbering of the α subunit, but for reasons of simplicity we have ignored this numbering difference in the figure presented. The reader should be alerted that in the original reports the appropriate number shifts are used. Indeed, some of the early studies of the α subunit were confounded by an *N*-terminal heterogeneity involving the first seven residues, which led to variances in the numbering and to a slower realization of the very high homology of the α subunits. The work of Liu et al. (21) first clarified

TABLE 1. *Sequence references for the gonadotropin hormones*

Animal species[a]	Subunit	References	Method used[b]
Ovine	α	21	P
		252	P
		253	D
Bovine	α	254	P
		255	D
Porcine	α	256	P
		257	P
		258	P
		259	D
Rabbit	α	260	P
Equine	α	261	P
Mouse	α	262	D
Rat	α	263	D
Human	α	264	P
		265	P
		266	D
Whale	α	267	P
Rhesus	α	23	D
Camel	α	268	P
Hamster	α	269	P
Chicken	α	270	D
Turkey	α	271	D
Bullfrog	α	272	P
Carp	α_1	273	D
Carp	α_2	273	D
Salmon	α	56	D
Eel, European	α	274	D
Eel, pike	α	275	P
Equine	eCGβ[c]	158	P
		51	D
Human	hCGβ	276	P
		277	P
		160	P
		161	P
		278	D
Baboon	baCGβ	279	D
Donkey	dkCGβ	58	D
Equine	eLHβ	157	P
		51	D
Human	hLHβ	106	P
		280	P
		281	P
Ovine	oLHβ	282	P
		252	P
		283	D
Bovine	bLHβ	284	P
		285	P
		137	D
Porcine	pLHβ	286	P
		287	D
Rabbit	lLHβ	288	P
Rat	rLHβ	289	D
		290	D
Whale	wLHβ	291	P
Dog	dLHβ	292	D
Camel	camLHβ	268	P
Hamster	haLHβ	269	P
Chicken	cLHβ	228	D
Turkey	tLHβ	Personal communication from Dr. D.N. Foster, University of Minnesota	D
Bullfrog	bfLHβ	293	P
Carp	cpGTHβ	273	D

TABLE 1. *Continued.*

Animal species[a]	Subunit	References	Method used[b]
Salmon, Chinook	sGTHβ	57	D
Salmon, Chum	sGHTIβ	55,56	D
Salmon, Chum	sGTHIIβ	55,56	D
Eel, Pike	elGTHβ	275	P
Equine	eFSHβ	G.R. Bousfield, unpublished	P
Human	hFSHβ	294	P
		295	D
		296	D
Ovine	oFSHβ	297	P
		298	D
		76	D
Bovine	bFSHβ	299	D
		300	D
		301	D
Porcine	pFSHβ	258	P
		302	D
Rat	rFSHβ	303	D
Bullfrog	bfFSHβ	304	P

[a] The species are presented in the same order as in Figs. 1 and 2 for these reference citations.

[b] P designates conventional Edman degradation for protein sequencing. D designates recombinant DNA methodology was employed, with protein sequences deduced from cDNA or gene sequences.

[c] The lower-case species designation as a prefix in the β series define the one- to three-letter abbreviations shown in Fig. 2. Note particularly the use of "l" for lagomorph in the case of rabbit to avoid confusion with the "r" used for rat. Also, "c" is used for chicken and "cp" for carp, although the original reports both used "c."

this for the mature protein forms of the α subunit. The recombinant DNA results have made it clear that the structures start as shown in Fig. 1, and that the N-terminal heterogeneity is a consequence of the isolation procedures employed. It is likely a proteolysis artifact. Interestingly, this also tells us that for most of the common measures of biopotency (see assay systems below) the first seven amino acid residues are not essential. However, for the renotropic activity of LH studied by Nomura et al. (22) the complete α subunit was required for the active LH isoform.

The consensus sequence (Fig. 1, bottom row) has been calculated according to the procedure used by Golos et al. (23). Unanimous residues are indicated in bold capital, majority residues are lower case, positions with no majority are marked with a solid circle. The clusters of bold letters in this consensus sequence draw attention to the areas that are invariant and presumably essential for activity of the α subunit in the heterodimer of the intact hormones. The leader sequence (residues −24 to −1) shows much more uniformity in the mammalian and avian series (top of Fig. 1). This also applies to the residues representing the mature protein (residues 1 to 96). Inclusion of the lower vertebrates in the analysis presumably leads us to the "absolutely necessary" residue positions marked in boldface capitals in the consensus sequence.

There are two *N*-glycosylation sites at position 56–58 and position 82–84. These sites are maintained throughout the series, although it appears from site-directed mutagenesis studies (24) that only the 56–58 glycosylation site is absolutely required for activity. Only the pike eel sequence has an aspartic acid residue at position 56 rather than an asparagine required for the *N*-linked glycosylation. However, this sequence was obtained by conventional sequencing in which placement of amide forms may be technically difficult. We prefer to reserve judgment as to whether this is a true exception. (See further discussion of the role of carbohydrate in the sections on Carbohydrate Function and Deglycosylated Forms, vide infra.) The Thr residue at position 43 is an *O*-glycosylation site for the free α subunit, and this threonine residue is found in all known mature α subunit proteins.

The structural significance of the half-cystine placements has been alluded to above as sites that define the disulfide bridges that provide rigidity to the three-dimensional structure. Determination of the disulfide placements is technically difficult. We previously reviewed several studies of the disulfide linkages in both the α and β subunits of the glycoprotein hormones (1). Because of the technical difficulties in determining disulfide placements, these reports do not all agree. Rather than review the previous studies, we have selected those

Alpha Subunit Sequences

```
Position No.  -25 -20 -15 -10 -5 -1 1 5 10 15 20 25 30 35

Ovine         MDYYRKYAAAILAILSLFLQ!LHS FPDGEFTMQGCPECKLKENKYFSKPDAP IYQCMGCC
Bovine        MDYYRKYAAVILAILSLFLQILHS FPDGEFTMQGCPECKLKENKYFSKPDAP IYQCMGCC
Porcine       MDYYRKYAAVILAILSVFLQILHS FPDGEFTMQGCPECKLKENKYFSKLGAP IYQCMGCC
Rabbit                                 FPDGEFAMQGCPECKLKENKYFSKLGAP IYQCMGCC
Equine                                 FPDGEFTTQDCPECKLRENKYFFKLGVP IYQCKGCC
Mouse         MDYYRKYAAVILVMLSMFLHILHS LPDGDFIIQGCPECKLKENKYFSKLGAP IYQCMGCC
Rat           MDCYRRYAAVILVMLSMVLHILHS LPDGDLIIQGCPECKLKENKYFSKLGAP IYQCMGCC
Human         MDYYRKYAAIFLVTLSVFLHVLHS APD VQDCPECTLQENPFFSQPGAP ILQCMGCC
Whale                                  FPNGEFTMQGCPECKLKQNKYFSKLGAP IYQCMGCC
Rhesus        MDYYRKYAAVILVTLSVFLHILHS FPDGEFTMQDCPECKPRENKFFSKPGAP IYQCMGCC
(NT)Camel                              FPDGEFTMQVCPECKLKENKYFSKLGAP VYQCMGCC
NT-Hamster                             LPDGDFTMQGCP
Chicken       MDCYRKYAAVTLTILSVFLHLLHT FPDGEFLMQGCPECKLGENRFFSKPGAP IYQCTGCC
Turkey        MDCYRKYAAVTLTILSVFLHLLHT FPDGEFLMQGCPECKLGENRFFSKPGAP IYQCTGCC
Bullfrog                               FPDDNFLTPGCPECRLKENLRFSNMGIGRIYQCSGCC
Carp 1         MFWTRYRGASILLFFMLIRLGQL YPRNDMNNFGCEECKLKENNIFSKPGAP VYQCMGCC
Carp 2         MFWTRYRGASVLLFLMLIHLGQL YPRNYMNNFGCEECKLKENNIFSKPGAP VYQCMGCC
Carp, Grass    MFWTRYAGASILLFLMLIHLGQV WPRNDMTNFGCEECKLKENNIFSKPGAP VYQCMGCC
Salmon          MCLLKSTGLSLILSALLVIADS YPNSDKTNMGCEECTLKPNTIFPN IMQCTGCC
Eel, Eur.     MMVCPGKPGASLLMLSMLFHIIDS YPNNEMARGGCDECRLQENKIFSKPSAP IFQCVGCC
Eel, Pike                              YPNNEISRGGCDECRLKDNKFFSKPSAP IFQCVGCC

Consensus     Md•yrkyaavil••ls•flhilhsf Pdgef••qgCpECklkeNk•Fskpgap•iyQCmGCC
```

```
Position No.  40 45 50 55 60 65 70 75 80 85 90 95

Ovine         FSRAYPTPARSKKTMLVPKNITSEATCCVAKAFTKATVMGNVRVENHTECHCSTCYYHKS
Bovine        FSRAYPTPARSKKTMLVPKNITSEATCCVAKAFTKATVMGNVRVENHTECHCSTCYYHKS
Porcine       FSRAYPTPARSKKTMLVPKNITSEATCCVAKAFTKATVMGNARVENHTECHCSTCYYHKS
Rabbit        FSRAYPTPARSKKTMLVPKNITSEATCCVAKAFTKATVMGNAKVENHTECHCSTCYYHKS
Equine        FSRAYPTPARSRKTMLVPKNITSESTCCVAKAFIRVTVMGNIKLENHTQCYCSTCYHHKI
Mouse         FSRAYPTPARSKKTMLVPKNITSEATCCVAKAFTKATVMGNARVENHTECHCSTCYYHKS
Rat           FSRAYPTPARSKKTMLVPKNITSEATCCVAKSFTKATVMGNARVENHTDCHCSTCYYHKS
Human         FSRAYPTPLRSKKTMLVQKNVTSESTCCVAKSYNRVTVMGGFKVENHTACHCSTCYYHKS
Whale         FSRAYPTPARSKKTMLVPKNITSEATCCVAKAFTKATVMGNARVQNHTZCHCSTCYYHKS
Rhesus        FSRAYPTPVRSKKTMLVQKNVTSESTCCVAKSLTRVMVMGSVRVENHTECHCSTCYYHFK
(NT)Camel     FSRAYPTPARSKKTMLV
NT-Hamster
Chicken       FSRAYPTPMRSKKTMLVPKNITSEATCCVAKAFTKITLKDNVKIENHTDCHCSTCYYHKS
Turkey        FSRAYPTPMRSKKTMLVPKNITSEATCCVAKAFTKITLKDNVKIENHTDCHCSTCYYHKS
Bullfrog      YSRAYPTPMRSKKTMLVPKNITSEAKCCVAKTQYRVTVMDNVKIENHTACHCSTCLYHKS
Carp 1        FSRAYPTPLRSKKTMLVPKNITSEATCCVAKEVKRVLVND VKLVNHTDCHCSTCYYHKS
Carp 2        FSRAYPTPLRSKKTMLVPKNITSEATCCVAKEFKQVLVND IKLVNHTDCHCSTCYYHKS
Carp, Grass   FSRAYPTPLRSKKTMLVPKNITSEATCCVAKEVKRVLVND VKLVNHTDCHCSTCYYHKS
Salmon        FSRAYPTPLRSKQTMLVPKNITSEATCCVAKEGERVTTKDGFPVTNHTECHCSTCYYHKS
Eel, Eur.     FSRAYPTPLRSKKTMLVPKNITSEATCCVAREVTRL DNMKLENHTDCHCSTCYYHKF
Eel, Pike     FSRAYPTPLRSKKTMLVPKDITSEATCCVAREVTKL DNMKLENHTDCHCSTCYYHKS

Consensus     fSRAYPTP•RSkkTMLVpKniTSEatCCVAkaftk•tvmgn•kveNHT•ChCSTCyyHks
```

FIG. 1. Comparison of the reported α subunit amino acid sequences for the gonadotropin hormones. See Table 1 for the list of references from which these sequences were compiled. The amino acid single-letter code has been used in this compilation: A, alanine; B, either asparagine or aspartic acid but not determined which; C, cysteine or half-cystine; D, aspartic acid; E, glutamic acid; F, phenylalanine; G, glycine; H, histidine; I, isoleucine; K, lysine; M, methionine; N, asparagine; P, proline; Q, glutamine; R, arginine; S, serine; T, threonine; V, valine; W, tryptophan; Y, tyrosine; Z, either glutamine or glutamic acid but not determined which. The consensus sequence was calculated as per Golos et al. (23). See the text for further detail.

Beta Subunit Sequences

Position No.	-40 · -30 · -20 · -10 · -1
eCG β	METLQGLLLWMLLSVGGVWA
hCG β	MEMFQGLLLLLLLSMGGTWA
beCG β	METLQGLLLWLLLSMGGAQA
(-84) dkCG β	
Consensus CG	**ME**t l **QGLLL**wl **LLS**m**GG**· w**A**
eLH β	METLQGLLLWMLLSVGGVWA
hLH β	MEMLQGLLLLLLLSMGGAWA
oLH β	MEMLQGLLLWLLLGVAGVWA
bLH β	MEMFQGLLLWLLLGVAGVWA
pLH β	MEMLQGLLLWLLLSVAGVWA
ILH β	
rLH β	MERLQGLLLWLLLSPSVVWA
wLH β	
dLH β	···LQGLLLWLLLSVGGVWA
(NT) camLH β	
(NT) haLH β	
Consensus M.	**ME**ml **QGLLL**wl **LL**sv· gv **WA**
oLH β	MGGAQVLVLMTLLGTPPATTGNPPVAVDPPLAVVGPPMG
tLH β	MGGAQVLVLMTLLGTPPVTTGTPPVVVDPSVAVVGPPLG
bfLH β	
Consensus LH	**MGGAQVLVLMTLLGTPP**· **T**meml qglll wlll svggvwa
cpGTH β	MGTPVKILVVRNHILFSVVVLLAVAQS
Chnok sGTH β	MLGLHVGTLISLFLCILLEPIEG
Chum sGTH I β	MYCTHLMTLQLVVMAMLWVTPVRA
sGTH II β	MLGLHVGTLISLFLCILLEPVEG
elGTH β	
Consensus GTH	**MGT**· ml g**L**hvgtl**I**slflci **LL**ep· eg
eFSH β	
hFSH β	MKTLQFFFLFCCWKAICC
oFSH β	MKSVQFCFLFCCWRAICC
bFSH β	MKSVQFCFLFCCWRAICC
pFSH β	··············AICC
rFSH β	MMKSIQLCILLWCLRAVCC
bfFSH β	
Consensus FSH	**MK**s· **Q**fcf **L**fc **C**wr **A**i **CC**

FIG. 2. Comparison of the reported β subunit amino acid sequences for the gonadotropin hormones. See Table 1 for the list of references from which these sequences were compiled. Abbreviations for the single-letter codes for the amino acids are given in the legend to Fig. 1. Consensus sequences were calculated for the several subgroups as detailed further in the text.

Position No.	5 – 10 – 15 – 20 – 25 – 30 – 35 – 40 – 45 – 50 – 55 – 60 – 65 – 70 – 75
eCG β	SRGPLRPLCRPINATLAAEKEACPICITFTTSICAGYCPSMVRVMPAALPAIPQPVCTYRELRFASIRLPGCPPGVD
hCG β	SKEPLRPRCRPINATLAVEKEGCPVCITVNTTICAGYCPTMTRVLQGVLPALPQVVCNYRDVRFESIRLPGCPRGVN
beCG β	SREPLRPLCRPINATLAAEKEACPVCVTVNTTICAGYCPTMMRVLQAVLPPVPQVVCNYREVRFESIRLPGCPPGVD
(-84) dkCG β	
Consensus CG	Sr•PLRPICRPINATLAaEKEaCPvCiTvnTtICAGYCPtM·RVIqavLPa·PQvVCnYRevRF•SIRLPGCPpGVd
eLH β	SRGPLRPLCRPINATLAAEKEACPICITFTTSICAGYCPSMVRVMPAALPAIPQPVCTYRELRFASIRLPGCPPGVD
hLH β	SREPLRPWCHPINAILAVEKEGCPVCITVNTTICAGYCPTMMRVLQAVLPPLPQVVCTYRDVRFESIRLPGCPRGVD
oLH β	SRGPLRPLCQPINATLAAEKEACPVCITFTTSICAGYCLSMKQVLPVILPPMPQRVCTYHELRFASVRLPGCPPGVD
bLH β	SRGPLRPLCQPINATLAAEKEACPVCITFTTSICAGYCPSMKRVLPVILPPMPQRVCTYHELRFASVRLPGCPPGVD
pLH β	SRGPLRPLCR,PINATLAAENEACPVCITFTTSICAGYCPSMVRVLPAALPPVPQPVCTYRELSFASIRLPGCPPGVD
lLH β	pEPARGPLRPLCRPVNATLAAENEACPVCITFTTSICAGYCPSMVRVLPAALPPVPQPVCTYRELRFASIRLPGCPPGVD
rLH β	SRGPLRPLCRPVNATLAAENEFCPVCITFTTSICAGYCPSMVRVLPAALPPVPQPVCTYRELRFASVRLPGCPPGVD
wLH β	PRGPLRPLCRPINATLAAQNZACPVCITFTTSICAGYCPSMVRVLPAALPPVPZPVCTYRQLRFASIRLPGCPPGVN
dLH β	SRGPLRPLCRPINATLAAENEACPVCITFTTTICAGYCPSMVRVLPAALPPVPQPVCTYHELHFASIRLPGCPPGVD
(NT) camLH β	SRGPLRPLCRPINATLAAENEACPVCITFTTSICAGYCPSMRRVLPAALPPVPQRVCTYRELRFASS
(NT) haLH β	SRGPLRPLCRPINA
Consensus M.	sRgPLRPICrPiNAtLAaEnEaCPvCITftTsICAGYCpsMvrVIpaaLPpvPQpVCTYrelrFaSiRLPGCPpGVd
oLH β	LGGGGRPPCRPINVTVAVEKDGCPQCMAVTTTACGGYCRTREPVYRSPLGPPPQSACTYGALRYERWALWGCPIGSD
tLH β	LGGGGRPPCRPINVTVAVEKDECPQCMAVTTTACGGYCRTREPVYRSPLGRPPQSSCTYGALRYERWALWGCPIGSD
bfLH β	RHVCHLANATISAEKDHCPVCITFTTSICTGYCQTMDPVYKTALSSFKQNICTYKEIRYDTIKLPDCLPGTD
Consensus LH	srgplRplCrpiNaTlaaEkeaCPvCitftTsiCaGYCpsm·rVIpaaLpp·pQ·vCTY·elrfasirLpgCppGvD
cpGTH β	SYLPPCEPVNETVAVEKEGCPKCLVLQTTICSGHCLTKEPVYKSPFSTVYQHVCTYRDVRYETVRLPDCPPGVD
Chnok sGTH β	SLMQPCQPINQTVSLEKEGCPTCLVIRAPICSGHCVTKEPVFKSPFSTVTQHVCTYRDVRYEMIRLPDCPPWSE
Chum sGTH I β	GTECRYGCRLNNMTIIVEREDCHGSITI TT CAGLCETTDLNYESTWLPRSQGVCNFKEWSYEKVYLEGCPSGVE
sGTH II β	SLMQPCQPINQTVSLEKEGCPTCLVIQTPICSGHCVTKEPVFKSPFSTVIQHVCTYRDVRYETIRLPDCPPWVD
elGTH β	SVLQPCQPINETISVEKDGCPKCLVFQTSICSGHCITKDPSYKSPLSTVYQRVCTYRDVRYETVRLPDCRPGVD
Consensus GTH	S··qPCqPiN·Tvs·Ek•GCP·CLV·qt·ICSGHC·TK•Pv·KSPfSTV·QhVCTYRDVRYEt·RLPDCpP·vd
eFSH β	NSCELTNITIAVEKEGCGFCITINTTWCAGYCYTRDLVYKDPARPNIQKTCTFKELVYETVKVPGCAHHAD
hFSH β	NSCELTNITIAIEKEECRFCISINTTWCAGYCYTRDLVYKDPARPKIQKTCTFKELVYETVRVPGCAHHAD
oFSH β	RSCELTNITITVEKEECSFCISINTTWCAGYCYTRDLVYKDPARPNIQKACTFKELVYETVKVPGCAHHAD
bFSH β	RSCELTNITITVEKEECGFCISINTTWCAGYCYTRDLVYRDPARPNIQKTCTFKELVYETVKVPGCAHHAD
pFSH β	NSCELTNITITVEKEECNFCISINTTWCAGYCYTRDLVYKDPARPNIQKTCTFKELVYETVKVPGCAHHAD
rFSH β	HSCELTNITISVEKEECRFCISINTTWCEGYCYTRDLVYKDPARPNTQKVCTFKELVYETIRLPGCARHSD
bfFSH β	CELSNITIVLEKEECGACVSVNATWCSGYCYTKDANLMYPQKSEKQGVCTYTEVIYETVKIPGCAENVN
Consensus FSH	·SCELtNITI·vEKE•C·fCisiNtTWCaGYCYTrDIvykdParpniQktCTfkEIvYETvkvPGCAhhad

FIG. 2. *Continued.*

Position No.	80 85 90 95 100 105 110 115 120 125 130 135 140 145 150
eCG β	PMVSFPVALSCHCGPCQIKTTDCGVFRDQPLACAPQASSSSKDPPSQPLTSTSTPTPGASRRSSHPLPIKTS
hCG β	PVVSYAVALSCQCALCRRSTTDCGGPKDHPLTCDDPRFQDSSSSKAPPPSLPSPSRLPGPSDTPILPQ
baCG β	PMVSVPVALSCRCALCRRSTSDCGGPKDHPLTCDDPNLQASSSSKDPPPSPPSPSRLLEPAGTPFLPQ
(-84) dkCG β	ALSCHCGPCRLKTTDCGGPRDHPLACAPQTSSSCKDPPSQPLTFHIPPQLLGPADVPLIPSQ
Consensus CG	PmVS·pVALSChC··Cr··TtDCGgp·DhPL·C·······s······P····sp··l··p···p··p··
eLH β	PMVSFPVALSCHCGPCQIKTTDCGVFRDQPLACAPQASSSSKDPPSQPLTSTSTPTPGASRRSSHPLPIKTS
hLH β	PVVSFPVALSCRCGPCRRSTSDCGGPKDHPLTCDHPQLSGLLFL
oLH β	PMVSFPVALSCHCGPCRLSSTDCGGPRTQPLACDHPPLPDILFL
bLH β	PMVSFPVALSCHCGPCRLSSTDCGGPRTQPLACDHPPLPDILFL
pLH β	PTVSFPVALSCHCGPCRLSSSDCGGPRAQPLACDRPLLPGLLFL
lLH β	PEVSFPVALSCRCGPCRLSSSDCGGPRAEPLACDLPHLPG
rLH β	PIVSFPVALSCRCGPCRLSSSDCGGPRTQPMTCDLPHLPGLLLF
wLH β	PMVSFPVALSCHCGPCRLSSSDCGPGRAQPLACNRSPRPGL
dLH β	PMVSFPVALSCRCGPCRLSNSDCGGPRAQSLACDRPLLPGLLFL
(NT) osmLH β	
(NT) haLH β	
Consensus M.	PmVSFPVALSChCGPCrlsssDCGgpr·qplaCd·p·lpgllfl
oLH β	PRVLLPVALSCRCARCPMATSDCTVQGLGPAFCGAPGGFGGE
tLH β	PRVLLPVALSCRCARCPIATSDCTVQGLGPAFCGAPGGFGIGE
bfLH β	PFFTYPVALSCYCDLCKMDYSDCTVESSEPDVCMKRRISI
Consensus LH	P·vsfPVALSC·CgpCrls·sDCggpr·qplaCd·p·lpgllfl
cpGTH β	PHITYPVALSCDCSLCTMDTSDCTIESLQPDFCMSQREDFLVY
Chnok sGTH β	PHVTYPVALSCDCSLCNMDTSDCTIESLQPDFCITQRVLTDGDMW
Chum sGTH I β	PFFI PVAKSCDCIKCKTDNTDCDRISMATPSCIVNPLEM
sGTH II β	PHVTYPVALSCDCSLCNMDTSDCTIESLQPDFCITQRVLTDGDMW
slGTH β	PHVTFPVALSCDCNLCTMDTSDCAIQSLRPDFCMSQRAP
Consensus GTH	PHvTyPVALSCDCsLC·MDTSDCtIeSLqPDFC··QR··tdgdMW
eFSH β	SLYTYPVATACHCGKCNSDSTDCTVRGLGPSYCSFGDMKE
hFSH β	SLYTYPVATQCHCGKCDSDSTDCTVRGLGPSYCSFGEMKE
oFSH β	SLYTYPVATECHCGKCDRDSTDCTVRGLGPSYCSFSDIRE
bFSH β	SLYTYPVATECHCSKCDSDSTDCTVRGLGPSYCSFREIKE
pFSH β	SLYTYPVATECHCGKCDSDSTDCTVRGLGPSYCSFSEMKE
rFSH β	SLYTYPVATECHCGKCDSDSTDCTVRGLGPSYCSFGEMKE
bfFSH β	PFYTYPVAVDCHCGRCDSETTDCTVRALGPTYCSLSQD
Consensus FSH	slYTYPVAteCHCgkCdsdsTDCTVRgLGPsYCSf·emkE

FIG. 2. *Continued.*

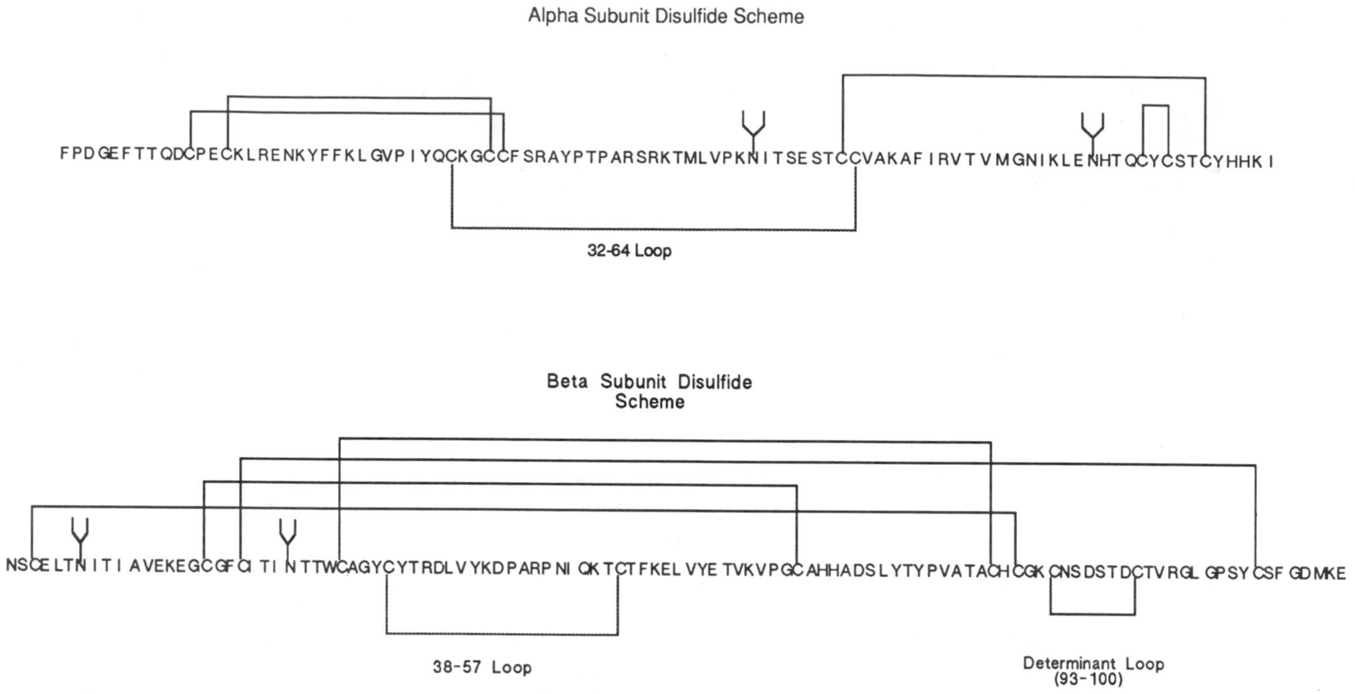

FIG. 3. Presentation of the best estimate for disulfide bond pairing in the glycoprotein hormones as applied to equine FSH. See text for further description. (From Ward et al., ref. 305, with permission.)

placements that agree with at least one other laboratory and have also provided the most compelling arguments for the placements proposed. The disulfide placements, besides being technically demanding, also require significant quantities of the hormone or subunit. Thus, only a few species have been studied directly, but there is sufficient evidence to indicate that the following assumptions may be made: (a) The uniformity of half-cystine placements indicates a uniformity of disulfide linkages between these residues characteristic of the subunit (i.e., whether α or β) and regardless of the hormone (i.e., whether LH, FSH, CG, or TSH). (b) The three-dimensional structures will be analogous for all the glycoprotein hormones. This second assumption lacks direct experimental support at this time. To illustrate the disulfide placements most favored based on these assumptions we present these placements diagrammatically in Fig. 3 as applied to equine FSH (which happens to be of particular interest to the present authors). The α subunit disulfide placements are based on the Pierce–Bahl model (25–27) obtained from bTSH, bLH, and hCG analyses. The β subunit disulfide placements are based on the Ward–Bahl model (28,29) obtained from oLH and hCG analyses. There are ten half-cystines in the α subunit, which provide the five disulfides indicated in Fig. 3. The α subunits have sufficient structural information in their linear sequences to specify proper recombination of the indicated half-cystines after reduction (to destroy the disulfide bonds) and reoxidation (to reform the disulfide bonds). Pierce and colleagues first called attention to this property of the reduced α subunits (30). This process has recently been studied in detail for the α subunit and the equine special case (31). Further comment on the β subunit disulfide bonds will be made in consideration of the β subunit sequences below.

It should be noted that the half-cystine residues in the leader sequence are present as the reduced form, cysteine, and are never oxidized to a disulfide form prior to removal from the mature protein; thus, these signal peptide half-cystine residues are not involved in the disulfide bond formation under consideration. The term "signal peptide" is derived from the hypothesis originating from the seminal work of Blobel and colleagues (32,33), which established that the signal peptide serves as a targeting means for a signal recognition particle (SRP) that directs the newly formed precursor protein to the receptor on the membrane that the protein is destined to cross via a protein channel. In the course of this membrane transport the signal peptide is removed by a signal peptidase.

Besides the structural importance of the subunit, the possibility that the free form of the subunit may play other, separate physiological roles has received little study, largely because the requisite assays have not been devised. It has been reported that the α subunit stimulates lactotrope differentiation in the immature pituitary (34). The lactotropes were characterized by their ability to secrete prolactin (PRL) after differentiation. Closely related to this observation is the report (35) that the α subunit (free α or hormone derived) stimulated the secretion of PRL in human decidual cell cultures derived from the placenta. Both observations implicate the free α subunit in the physiology of prolactin. These observations merit further study with respect to the physiological role of the α subunit.

Since the advent of suitable radioimmunoassays for the glycoprotein hormones and their subunits, it has been known that the α subunit and to a lesser extent the free β subunits may be found in the serum and/or the secretory products of pituitary cell or chorionic cell cultures [see, for example, the review by Cole (36) or the study by Keel et al. (37)]. Kourides and co-workers (38) observed that the majority of the "free" α subunits had molecular weights greater than "hormone-derived" α subunit, i.e., the subunit obtained from dissociation of TSH in their study or from hCG, LH, or FSH in similar studies by others subsequently. It was shown (38) that this increased molecular weight was the result of increased glycosylation. Parsons and Pierce (39) isolated free α subunit from bovine pituitaries and showed that the increased glycosylation was attributable to *O*-linked glycosylation of the threonine^{43} residue and that this glycosylation prevented recombination with the bLHβ subunit. Enzymatic removal of the *O*-linked carbohydrate permitted formation of the α–β dimer. The *O*-glycosylation is a late occurring processing step that has no influence on the regular α–β dimer formation (40).

The secretion of free α subunit results from a higher rate of biosynthesis of this subunit compared to the β subunit. This difference is particularly evident in some systems (41). Moreover, the α subunit is much more resistant to biodegradation (42), whereas the β subunit is subjected to an efficient removal process (42,43).

It was reported (44) that there was a tight correlation between free α subunit levels and LH levels, but not FSH in GnRH-deficient patients. However, in a perfused pituitary cell system, this same lab (45) showed that free α subunit, LH, and FSH responded in a similar manner to pulsatile administration of GnRH. In studies quantitating free α subunit and its Thr^{43} *O*-linked form as well as bLH in a bovine pituitary slice preparation (46), it was shown that GnRH increased LH 40-fold, but free α subunit levels only doubled. Moreover, they showed that over 75% of the free α was of the Thr^{43} *O*-linked form. Thus, we may conclude that the in vivo relationships of the free α subunit form to the intact hormones is a complex interrelationship of biosynthesis, degradation, secretion, and stimulation. The picture is further complicated by the fact that the various isoforms (isohormones) present an extensive heterogeneity (see further discussion in the section on Biosynthesis below). [For studies in which the carbohydrate complexity was measured directly for α subunits of porcine origin, see Maghuin-Rogister et al. (47); from hCG, hLH, hFSH, and hTSH, see Nilson et al. (48).] From these and other studies it is clear that the α subunit shows an identity for the protein portion within a given species, but the different types of hormone synthesized by separate cell types provide great variations in the carbohydrate moieties, as will be described further in the section on Carbohydrate Structure and Function below.

As noted above, Pierce and colleagues produced hybrid molecules to demonstrate the common subunit. These hybrid hormones in which the α subunit of one species is combined with the β subunit from another species have been very useful in the study of hormone activity. By this means it has been established that the α subunits are generally interchangeable. However, there are certain exceptions. The inability of carp α subunit to combine with oLHβ to produce an active hormone was noted above (20). The putative carp α_2 (Fig. 1), which differs by only four residues from the carp α_1, did not produce an active hormone when expressed in a baculovirus system with the carp GTHβ (49), although the carp α_1 produced the expected active hormone.

In the case of equine gonadotropins there seems to be an absolute dependence for an equine α subunit in order to obtain an active hormone with any of the equine β subunits, but the equine α subunit combines readily with other species, often to produce more potent hormones than the native hormone from the species in question (50). All of these examples of inactive hybrids tell us that there are some very critical three-dimensional positions in the hormone complex that potentially alter hormone–receptor sensitivity. Defining what these subtle differences might be should prove very fruitful for future research.

The β or Hormone-Specific Subunit

There are three types of β subunit in all mammalian species (the pituitary LH, FSH, and TSH β subunits), and in the primates there is an additional β subunit type, the chorionic gonadotropin-β, which is structurally very closely related to the lutropin-β. Indeed, they both bind to the same receptor to initiate hormone action, but with different kinetics. In the equids, the only other mammalians that have a chorionic gonadotropin, there is in fact a single gene that produces the LH and CG proteins in the pituitary and chorion, respectively (51), which differ only in their glycosylation and tissue of origin. In the lower vertebrates there are probably also three different types of β subunit, although it has long been held that there is only a primordial gonadotropin. This has been designated gonadotropic hormone (GTH), and this designation has been carried to Fig. 2 for the carp, salmon, and eel structures presented. However, Ng and Idler (52,53) found two types of gonadotropin in plaice, flounder, salmon, and carp pituitaries. Kawauchi and colleagues (54) isolated two different forms of salmon GTH with different steroidogenic activities. In subsequent studies of the amino acid sequences of these GTH-1 and GTH-2 forms (55), the closer similarity of GTH-1 to bFSH and similarity of GTH-2 to bLH became apparent. Sekine et al. (56), by means of recombinant DNA methodology for the two types of GTH in the chum salmon, extended these findings and established a primitive LH and FSH type of gonadotropin as low as the teleost fish (see Fig. 2). The sGTH-1β has the greatest homology to the FSH types and would be the putative salmon FSH. The sGTH-2β is almost identical to the sGTH sequence (Fig. 2) described by Trinh et al. (57) for chinook salmon, and this bears the closest homology to LH.

In order to make the sequence comparisons we have taken advantage of the alignment of the half-cystine residues, which maintain an identical spacing throughout the series from eels to humans. There are two irregularities to this conformity of half-cystine placements. The first comes in the same sGTH-1β from chum salmon. This β subunit has an "irregular" half-cystine at position 5, which seems to be translocated from the normal half-cystine at position 26, where a serine was placed. The C^{26} is normally disulfide-linked to position C^{110} (Fig. 3). Does this mean that the salmon GTH-1β is instead linked C^5 to C^{110}? We can only speculate at this point.

The second irregularity to the half-cystine placement rule is found on the *C* terminus of the donkey CGβ (58), where the cDNA analysis of a partial clone (lacking the first 84 residues and the signal peptide) indicated an "extra" half-cystine at position 118, where all other CGβ molecules have a serine. This implies that the donkey CG either has a reduced cysteine at this position (which would in fact be a sulfur analog of serine) or else the -SH is involved in some other chemical combination. Since all the other half-cystines of those placed by the last 85–110 residues (Fig. 2) and revealed by this partial clone did not suggest any irregular locations, it is fair to assume that the balance of the disulfide placements are not out of the ordinary for donkey CG, at least until we learn more about the missing portion of donkey CG. It seems unlikely that this residue, donkey CGβ^{118} is involved in an unusual disulfide bond, although we do not have sufficient information to state this with certainty. We do know that Aggarwal et al. (59) isolated donkey chorionic gonadotropin and found no unusual properties for the molecular volume compared to other CG preparations. (If the C^{118} were disulfide-linked to a second C^{118}, for example, the resulting dimeric form would be much larger.)

Luteinizing Hormone and Chorionic Gonadotropin β Subunits

Inasmuch as the β subunits define the activity of the α–β complex, it is not surprising that the amino acid sequences among the LHβ series (Fig. 2) show greater homology within the series than the FSHβ series or the TSHβ series (the latter is not shown in this figure). Moreover, since both LH and CG interact with the same hormone receptor, it is to be expected that the LHβ and the CGβ series show extensive homology with each other. To facilitate these comparisons we have calculated the consensus sequences for each of the groups. The GTH sequences have been kept separate, since much remains to be clarified for this group (see comments above concerning carp and salmon sequences). Generally the GTH group would be expected to fall within the LH/CG comparisons. The positions that are identical for the consensus sequences are again marked with bold capital letters, and the positions with a majority of one amino acid are indicated with a lower-case letter. In the latter cases the reader should note that the substitutions are usually of a conservative nature; i.e., a similar polarity or hydrophobicity, as the case may be, is maintained throughout the series. Finally, those positions where the variation is extensive and no majority type of amino acid residue is discerned are indicated by solid circles. With this comparison the areas of absolute identity are quickly visualized by the location of the bold letters. This should also convey to the reader a sense of those constant areas of structure that are important for hormone action. These areas may indicate important subunit–subunit interactive areas that must be preserved, or, alternatively areas that are important for receptor interaction. We discuss below some of the experimental approaches that have been employed to delimit which of these functions is being served by the particular amino acid or group of amino acids.

There are 12 half-cystine residues in the β subunits (Fig. 2, **C** locations), and in the mature protein subunit these are all oxidized to form six disulfide bonds. Figure 3 presents the best supported placements according to the Ward–Bahl analyses (28,29), which are further supported by the biosynthetic trapping experiments of Ruddon and colleagues (60). With these placements there are two disulfide loops on the β subunits that span relatively shorter linear runs of amino acids, which we have designated as the 38–57 loop and the 93–100 determinant loop. We discuss these further below. The reader should realize that although the other disulfide bonds (on the upper part of the linear presentation for the β subunit in Fig. 3) seemingly span much greater lengths, they are in fact dimensionally identical, and the difference comes from the folding of the peptide backbone that brings them into the required proximity to the other half-cystine to form the indicated disulfide bond.

Early circular dichrographic spectra (CD spectra) of oLH before and after dissociation of the subunits revealed only a moderate change in the CD spectra of oLHβ but a transformation to a more random spectra for the oLHα. This led to the proposal that the β subunit was much more rigid than the α subunit and that the β subunit therefore served as the greater determinant of the three-dimensional structure of the α–β complex (61).

The subunit association process was subsequently studied in greater detail using CD spectra (62,63). The rigidity of the β subunits is in large measure contributed by the disulfide cross linking diagrammed in Fig. 3.

The consensus sequences for LH and CG (Fig. 2) have much in common up to the point of the last half-cystine (C^{110}). Beyond that point the homologies diminish markedly. Note the preponderance of solid dots indicating no majority residues in the consensus sequences. We were able to remove chemically this part of the molecule from eLHβ and show that the biological activity (after recombination with the α subunit) was not altered (64). By site-directed mutagenesis Matzuk et al. (65) showed that loss of the *C* terminus of hCGβ beyond residue 115 did not interfere with receptor binding or signal transduction *in vivo* for the reconstituted hormone. On the other hand, the chorionic gonadotropins are known to have much longer half-lives *in vivo,* which is attributable at least in part to the *C*-terminal extension. Taking advantage of this fact, Fares et al. have designed a long-acting follitropin agonist by fusing the *C*-terminal sequence of hCGβ to the follitropin β subunit (66). This demonstrates that all of a given protein serves some purpose from specification of three-dimensional architecture to particular physiological functions, but the relative importance of each structural area may vary.

The rabbit LH (lLH) has two additional residues attributed to the *N* terminus, a pyroglutamylprolyl sequence preceding an alanylarginine (see Fig. 2). This sequence was determined in our laboratory (288), but, as explained in that report, the pyroglutamate blocks sequencing of the peptide, and the proposed sequence for the *N* terminus is based solely on compositional analysis of the isolated tetrapeptide. Thus, rabbit LH would be an ideal prospect for further corroboration by recombinant DNA methodology. Since the rabbit is a reflex ovulator, this unusual sequence may have functional significance.

The comparative sequences of CG and LH in the mammalian series are much more homologous than those obtained when chicken, turkey, and bullfrog sequences are included. It is obvious that inclusion of these sequences from the lower vertebrates has a marked effect on the detectable differences (compare the consensus LH versus the consensus LH, mammalian, sequences, Fig. 2). The striking difference in the signal sequences for the avian species (−39 residues) and the mammalian species, both LH and CG (−20 residues), is readily apparent.

The high degree of homology for the β subunits from eels to humans cannot be interpreted as a reflection of the potency of the parent hormones across species. Several laboratories have provided comparative studies of preparations of glycoprotein hormones in various assay systems; notable among these are the laboratories of Licht (67), Papkoff (68), and Fontaine (69). As a general statement, the application of hormones across species in selected assay systems may lead to no response or to instances in which the potency of the homologous species hormone is exceeded by the transspecies hormone. The sequence homologies in Figs. 1 and 2 provide only rudimenatary indications of what potencies may be expected on interchanging hormones. As an example, Fontaine (69,70) found that an activity obtained from mammalian pituitaries that was effective in fish as a thyrotropin could be traced to the mammalian gonadotropic activity. This gave rise to the designation "heterothyrotropin." In studying this thyrotropic activity in fish, MacKenzie showed (71) that all the mammalian pituitary glycoprotein hormones possessed significant thyrotropic activity in fish, although their subunits were inactive.

Follicle-Stimulating Hormone (Follitropin) β Subunits

Follitropin (FSH) stimulates follicular development in the ovary, and in particular the granulosa cells of the follicle. Follitropin in concert with lutropin prepares the follicle for ovulation and luteinization. For extensive discussion of these processes see Wassarman, Chapter 3, on the mammalian ovum in this volume. Follitropin specifically stimulates the production of the steroid hormone progesterone and the production of the enzyme system (aromatase) for converting testosterone to estrogen (72). It also stimulates the production of the enzymes involved in plasminogen activation (73). Both the aromatase system and the plasminogen activator systems have been adapted for sensitive assays of FSH. Studies on the induction of follicular development by exogenous gonadotropin administration in women and domesticated animals has been accelerated by their application in *in vitro* fertilization and embryo transfer.

In the male FSH acts on the Sertoli cells of the seminiferous tubules in the testis, whereas LH acts principally on the interstitial cells. See de Kretser and Kerr, Chapter 21, and Sharpe, Chapter 24, on the testis and spermatogenesis, in this volume for more extensive discussion.

One of the problems for the study of FSH action has been the scarcity of highly purified hormone preparations, since most species of pituitary contain about $\frac{1}{20}$ as much FSH (or TSH) as LH on a molar basis. This has obliged several investigators to use crude preparations of FSH or to substitute. In several species of laboratory animal the equine CG has an FSH-like effect, but not in the equine (74). Thus, particularly in the older literature, one finds eCG of varying degrees of purity as obtained from pregnant mare serum (thus designated PMSG, pregnant mare serum gonadotropin) employed as an FSH substitute. As is now known, the various isoforms of FSH have circulating half-lives that are dependent on the degree of sialylation (75). Moreover, these half-lives are usually much shorter than those of PMSG; thus, uncertainties are introduced into the dose considerations for such studies.

As shown in Fig. 2, the FSH sequences for the β subunit are shorter, only 111 residues in length for the mammalian series and only 107 residues for bullfrog FSH. With the half-cystines in register, this numbering, to be consistent with the other series' numbering, brings a position 7-to-117 span for the FSH series. A perusal of the FSH consensus sequence, including the bullfrog FSH, reveals the most exacting sequence requirement of all the series as judged by the predominance of bold capital letters, suggesting absolute requirement for activity. The comparisons run 50.4% for FSH, 47.6% for CG (but with only three full comparisons available), and 28.1% for LH. These calculations are for the mature protein only (i.e., excluding the signal sequences).

The FSHβ protein is encoded by a single gene. However, Guzman et al. (76) found a gene in the sheep that is 87% homologous to the FSHβ gene, indicating that there is an FSHβ-like gene or pseudogene in the sheep. The physiological significance of this finding remains to be determined.

Allocation of Function to Structural Areas of the Glycoprotein Hormones

The allocation of functional roles to specific areas of the protein structure requires innovative approaches and usually considerable effort. Investigators have employed the following broad approaches to this task:

1. Structural comparisons.
2. Functional group substitutions.
3. Immunologic approaches.
4. Peptide-walk analysis.
5. Site-directed mutagenesis.
6. Genetic engineering.
7. Three-dimensional analysis of hormone and receptor.

The use of *structural comparisons* implies the availability of several structures to compare. For the glycoprotein hormones the sequence information is now extensive enough to use this approach. We applied this to the eCG molecule as the sequence information became available, and it led us to the determinant loop area as one potentially responsible for the LH/FSH-like role of this molecule in various biological systems. The determinant loop hypothesis thus proposed (77,78) a correlation of net charge and structural features in the 90–105 region of the molecule as determinants of the LH, FSH, or TSH activity. (See ref. 78 for details.) Although other areas of structure have also been shown to be involved in specification of hormonal activity, the general importance of this area, which includes the 93–100 disulfide loop, has been substantiated by several more recent lines of evidence, as noted below.

Combarnous has also relied heavily on comparative sequence information to develop his "negative specificity" model for glycoprotein hormone action. This proposal has recently been reviewed in detail (79). The major elements of the negative specificity model of hormone action are the assumption that the α subunit is responsible for the majority of the high-affinity binding of the hormones to their receptors, that the β subunits induce the functional conformation of the α subunit, and that the β subunits specifically inhibit (thus, "negative specificity") the binding of that particular α–β complex (LH/CG, FSH, TSH) to receptors for the other hormones. These areas of negative specificity have not yet been defined, but the hypothesis should provide the basis for much fruitful research, since experiments can be designed to explore these possibilities. (In particular, see comments on peptide-walk analysis and site-directed mutagenesis below.) The studies by Moyle and colleagues to produce β-subunit chimeras are good examples of the application of this approach to define areas essential for or to remove hormone specificity for the β subunit (80).

Functional group substitutions have long been used to modify a particular group in a molecule in order to determine its role in a chemical reaction. As applied to the glycoprotein hormones, this implies the availability of a reagent that will selectively attack certain functional groups in the sequence to produce a derivative that alters the chemical nature of that particular group. The biopotency of the derivative is then tested to deduce the nature of the effect. In practice, several functional groups (e.g., amino groups, carboxyl groups, aromatic hydroxyls) of the type involved by the given reagent may be present. Thus, reaction rates and accessibility to the reagent must be established in order to determine selectivity of the reaction and groups actually involved. This, in turn, requires further structure studies of the derivatized products. Finally, it is never certain how much of the effect(s) on biopotency to attribute to the functional group derivatized, to the steric requirements of the derivatizing group, or to long-range steric effects introduced by the group added. In spite of these limitations useful information has been obtained. For a review of this approach and the reagents employed with the glycoprotein hormones, see ref. 81. In a modification of this approach the carbodiimide reaction has been used to establish the close proximity of carboxyl and amino groups by their reactivity to produce amide bond cross-linking of the α–β subunits through the α-Lys^{49} and β-Asp^{111} of bLH (82) or pLH (83).

Immunologic methods to define active areas in a glycoprotein hormone are numerous and reflect the ingenuity of the immunologists and endocrinologists involved in the individual studies. Both polyclonal antibodies (generally of broader specificity) and monoclonal antibodies (highly specific and selective) have been employed. We will limit our consideration to a few examples of the approaches available. To introduce greater specificity into the polyclonal antibodies, Atassi and colleagues (84,85) used synthetic peptides as antigens to produce highly specific polyclonal antibodies to selected epitopes (defined by the peptide synthesized as antigen). These antibodies were the basis for highly selective antibodies that would not cross-react with other glycoprotein hormones and could be used to identify surface areas in the α–β complex or in receptor-bound hormones. Moyle and colleagues (86,87) have used a well-characterized series of monoclonal antibodies to epitopes of both the intact hormone and isolated subunits to measure conformational changes on interaction with the receptor. Birken et al. (88) showed that removal of sialic acid from the carbohydrate moieties of the *C*-terminal peptide of hCGβ produced a more antigenic peptide and thus was able to improve the sensitivity of an hCG-specific antibody. Bidart and colleagues (89) have used monoclonal antibodies to both human and equine CG to elucidate fine differences between the two and refine the specificity of a series of monoclonal antibodies directed at discontinuous epitopes on the surface of hCG. This group has also used monoclonal antibodies to three distinct antigenic domains that allow them to distinguish between intact and proteolytically nicked forms of hCG (90).

The approach to the analysis of functional areas using synthetic peptides we have labeled *peptide-walk analysis* was introduced to glycoprotein hormone studies by Ryan and associates (91). This analysis involves the synthesis of peptides approximately 15 residues in length starting at the *N* terminus of the linear amino acid sequence and designing of each peptide to overlap the sequence of the previous peptide by about five residues. This yields a series of peptides for testing in selected assay systems. The peptides are used to compete with the intact hormone or subunits to determine areas that appear to be associated with, for example, the ability to combine with the counterpart subunit or the binding of the native hormone to its receptor. In a system such as the latter, the native hormone is effective at approximately 10^{-10} M, whereas the peptides, if effective, are only effective at approximately 10^{-5} M. Thus, the native hormone may be 100,000-fold more effective on a molar basis. The early studies utilizing this approach have been reviewed by Ryan (92). Although the low sensitivity of the assay systems to the peptides has been a criticism to this analysis, nonetheless it has been demonstrated that peptides implicated in the receptor-binding area of the hormone were also capable of stimulating testosterone production in a Leydig cell system (93). Reichert and colleagues have effectively applied this analysis to FSH (94,95) and also demonstrated that peptides based on the hFSH sequence that showed homology to calmodulin stimulated calcium transport and would bind calcium (96,97). These findings suggest a role for specific areas of the FSH sequence involved in the requirement for calcium for maximum binding to the FSH receptor (98). Peptide-walk analyses have provided us some of our most specific information about the functional areas of the glycoprotein hormones.

Site-directed mutagenesis is another methodology that provides very specific information about functional areas of the glycoprotein hormones. This method requires an available clone of the hormone subunit to be mutated. By insertion, deletion, or more often replacement of specific codons, a single amino acid may be changed as desired in a given subunit. Then, by expressing the mutated subunit, combining it with the required counterpart subunit, and testing for biological activity (or lack thereof) in selected assay systems, one learns about the essentiality of that particular residue in hormone function.

The extension of this approach to larger areas of structure brings us to *genetic engineering,* which is essentially the same as site-directed mutagenesis but on a grander scale. In the glycoprotein hormones the production of a series of chimeric molecules, mixing TSH, FSH, or LH/CG structural features to determine effects of these structural features on the final hormone activity of the chimeric product, has been extensively applied by Moyle and colleagues (80,99). Examples of the use of site-specific mutagenesis can be found in the demonstration of the role of the *N*-linked carbohydrate moieties on the α subunit by Matzuk and Boime (24,100), and Ji and colleagues (101) used the method to confirm the essential nature of the penultimate lysine residue for biological activity. Puett and colleagues used site-directed mutagenesis to study the effects of removal of residues 122–145 from the β subunit of hCG (102) or to study the role of the invariant Asp^{99} (Fig. 2) present in all β subunits (103). The latter study showed that this Asp group could be replaced without complete loss of activity in the resulting heterodimer, but not with a positive group (e.g., Arg), in which case the product was totally inactive. Many such examples could be cited, but the foregoing will suffice to illustrate the great versatility and selectivity of genetic engineering. The only criticism or reservation that might be leveled at this approach comes from the lack of specificity in the carbohydrate moieties applied in most gene expression systems used to generate the final product, but the evidence so far available suggests that this is generally not a serious problem for the interpretation of the results.

Ultimately the availability of an exact three-dimensional model of the heterodimeric glycoprotein hormones in juxtaposition with their respective receptors should provide us with powerful tools for the study of hormone action. Although as noted above the crystallization of hCG derivatives for X-ray crystallography may provide a starting approach to this modeling, it will be some time before we may anticipate a complete three-dimensional analysis of these complex systems.

Aberrant Glycoprotein Hormone Molecules

The production of aberrant molecules has been demonstrated in a few instances for the glycoprotein hormones. Nishimura et al. (104) studied an α subunit secreted by an ectopic tumor in a patient. This subunit was unable to combine with the β subunit of hCG to produce a normal α–β complex. By peptide analysis they established that the only sequence difference from normal α subunit was the conversion of Glu^{56} (Glu^{60} in Fig. 1) to an Ala. This single change produced a serious defect in the folding ability, tertiary structure, or accessibility for proper glycosylation that rendered the product unsuitable for normal function as an α subunit.

Cox, studying the α subunits secreted by several cell lines of human tumors, found that glycoprotein subunits secreted by trophoblastic tumors (JAR, JEG) or nontrophoblastic tumors (HeLa, ChaGo) were phosphorylated on the α subunit (105). The JAR line, which secretes hCGβ also, phosphorylated only the hCGα subunit.

The *N*-terminal heterogeneity of the oLHα subunit was first described by Liu et al. (21), but this same type of heterogeneity has also been described for several species of α subunit (see discussion above). It has not been clearly established whether this is simply an isolation artifact or normal physiological processing, but proteolysis during isolation would seem to be the most likely source of this type of aberrant molecule.

In the first reports (106) of the amino acid sequence of hLHβ some proteolytic "nicking" was observed around the 45–50 area of the sequence. It was later shown by two laboratories (107–109) that this proteolytic cleavage was commonly observed in hLH preparations (which are almost always derived from pooled pituitary extracts). These reports allowed estimates of the percentage cleavage at positions between residues 44, 45, 46, 47, and 48. The potency of the nicked hormones was shown to be considerably diminished.

The heterogeneity of hCG collected from single individuals was studied by Kardana et al. (110). They found substantial variation in the types of heterogeneity. They observed nicks in the β subunits, particularly at the 47–48 position (11 of 13) but also at the 44–45 and 46–47 positions in some samples. Other evidence of aberrant molecules observed in their study included *N*-terminal heterogeneity of the α subunit, loss of the C-terminal portion of the β subunit (2 of 13). One preparation had an α subunit nick at position 70–71 (or 74–75 in Fig. 1, because of the four-residue genomic deletion in the human α subunit). Thus, the peptide heterogeneity was found to be extensive among individual preparations, a variance that cannot be appreciated in the pooled sample preparations.

A fragment that is frequently generated by proteolytic action on the β subunit of hCG during pregnancy, and some cancer patients secreting CGβ subunit, is termed the "β-subunit core fragment." This fragment is secreted in the urine and may be detected by many anti-hCGβ antibodies. This fragment is a disulfide-linked, two polypeptide residuum of the intact hCGβ, representing the β6–40 and β55–92 polypeptide portions of the subunit (111). In pregnancy urine the β-core fragment may exceed 90 nmole/liter of urine in the 12th to 15th week of pregnancy; thus, this represents a significant portion of the immunoreactivity detectable in pregnancy urine.

GENETIC RELATIONSHIPS FOR THE SUBUNITS

In the following we focus primarily on recent studies that investigate the molecular mechanisms underlying the transcriptional regulation of human gonadotropin gene expression. Several reviews are available for further information about the structure and expression of these genes (17,112). The genes encoding the α and β gonadotropin subunits have been cloned and sequenced from a variety of species. The subunits are encoded by separate genes present on different chromosomes. In the human, the α subunit gene is found on chromosome 6, the FSHβ gene is located on chromosome 11, and the LHβ gene is present on chromosome 19 and linked to a cluster of six CGβ genes that appear to have evolved by duplication of the LHβ gene (15). The structural organization of the human genes and the corresponding mature transcripts are shown in Figs. 4 and 5.

The α Subunit Gene

The common α subunit is encoded by a single gene, which has been isolated and characterized in the human, bovine, mouse, rat, and rhesus monkey. All of the α subunit genes isolated thus far have a very similar genomic organization consisting of four exons separated by three introns of varying size. The first intron is the largest, ranging from 6.5 to 14.7 kilobases in size and separates exon 1, containing 5′ untranslated sequences, from exon 2, which encodes the leader sequence and the first nine amino acids of the mature polypeptide. Exon 3 encodes amino acid residues 10 to 71, and exon 4 corresponds to the *C*-terminal residues 72 to 96 and the 3′ untranslated region. Mature α subunit transcripts range in size from 730 nucleotides to 800 nucleotides, according to species (Fig. 4).

The control of α subunit gene expression has been examined in considerable detail. Part of this interest stems from the fact that the α subunit is specifically expressed in three distinct cell types (thyrotropes and gonadotropes of the anterior pituitary and the trophoblasts

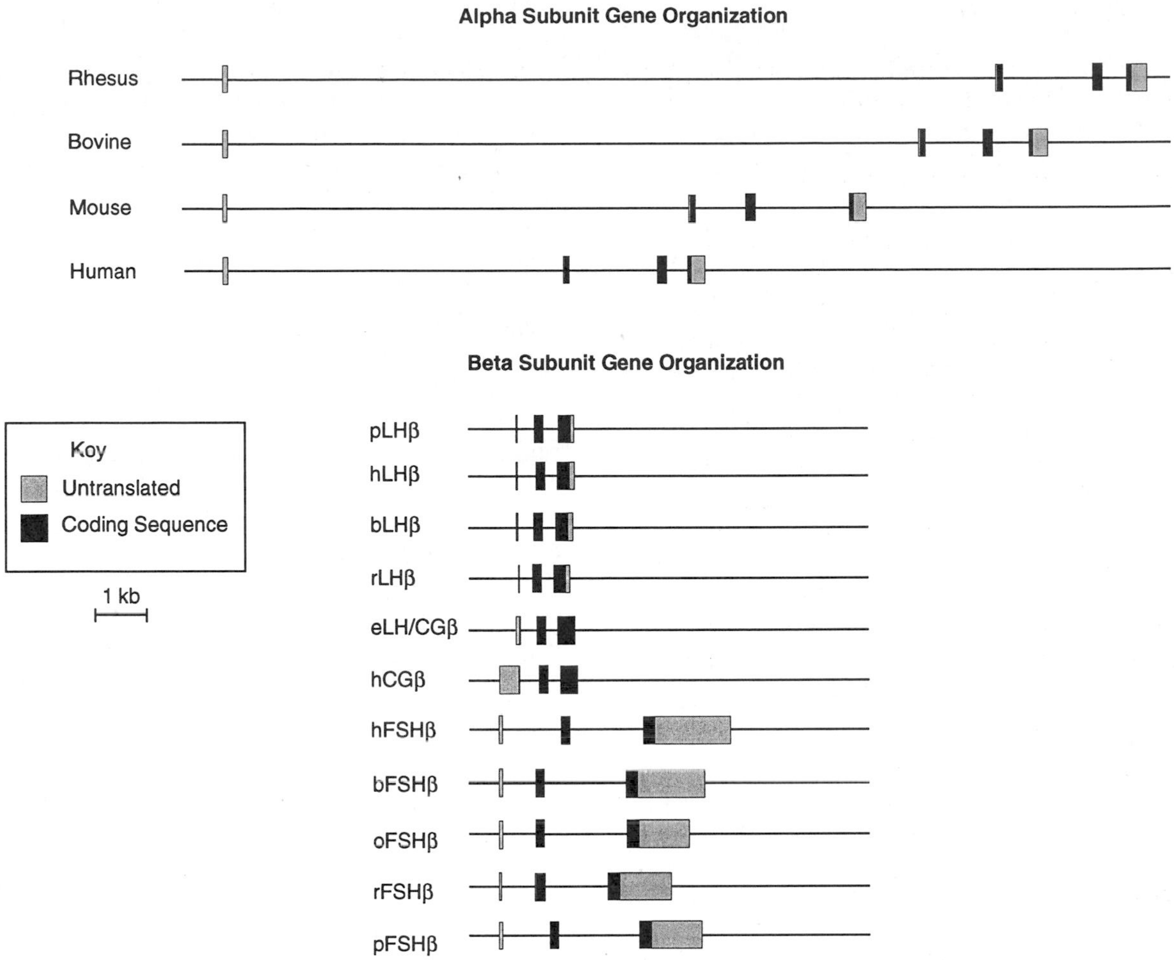

FIG. 4. Comparison of the glycoprotein hormone α and β subunit genes. The genes are drawn to the same scale to illustrate the large differences in size between the α and β subunit genes, which are primarily accounted for by the larger introns in the α subunit genes. The diagrams are based on DNA sequences of rhesus monkey α (23), bovine α (255), mouse α (306), human α (307), porcine LHβ (308), human LHβ (136), bovine LHβ (137), rat LHβ (290), equine LH/CGβ (51), human CGβ (136), human FSHβ (295), bovine FSHβ (301), ovine FSHβ (76), rat FSHβ (309), and porcine FSHβ (310).

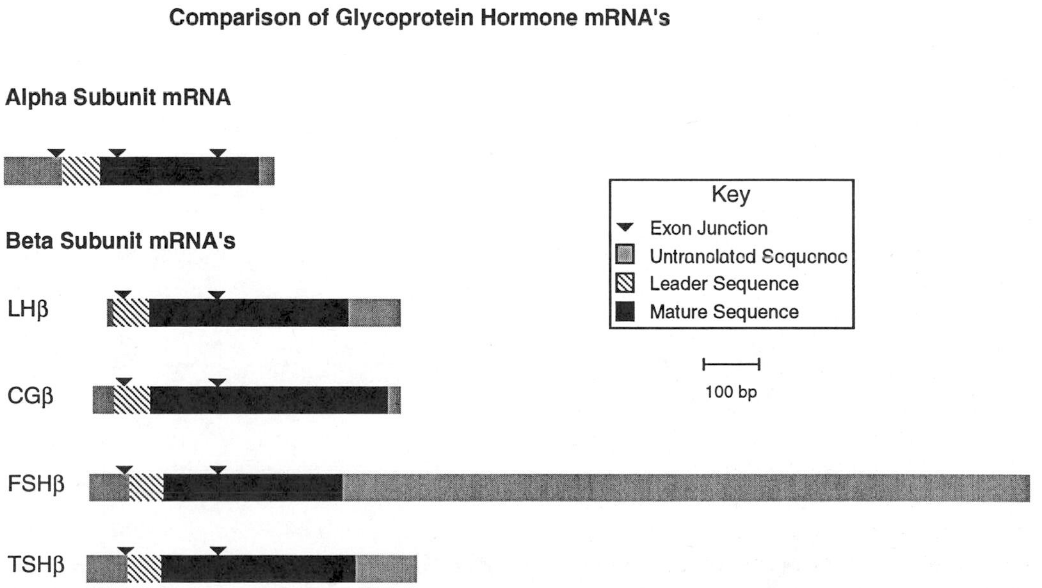

FIG. 5. Comparison of the mature mRNAs for the glycoprotein hormone subunits. The mRNAs are drawn to illustrate the 3′- and 5′-untranslated regions, exon junctions, leader sequence, and mature sequence. (From Ward et al., ref. 1, with permission.)

of the placenta) in primates and equids, whereas its expression in other mammals is restricted to the anterior pituitary. A practical matter responsible for much of the focus on α gene expression has been the availability of placentally derived human choriocarcinoma cell lines that express the endogenous gene and the absence (until very recently) of established pituitary cell lines in the gonadotrope lineage. These observations have raised several important questions including what is responsible for the cell-type-specific expression of α genes and why the α gene is placentally expressed in primates and equids but not in other mammals.

An important component in the control of α subunit gene expression exists at the transcriptional level. Several groups have examined positive-acting regulatory sequences that control transcription of the human α gene in gene transfer studies using placental cells and various reporter genes fused to α gene regulatory sequences (113–115). Sequences important for reporter gene expression in choriocarcinoma cells are confined to a 200-base-pair region spanning the human α gene promoter. Individual *cis*-acting regulatory elements have been further defined by analyzing the effects of specific base changes within this region on promoter activity and by examining the ability of nuclear proteins from placental and nonplacental cells to interact with this region. These studies have found the α subunit gene promoter to contain transcriptional regulatory elements that consist of binding sites for multiple nuclear proteins. Certain regulatory elements in the α subunit promoter interact with widely expressed DNA-binding proteins, and others are recognized by cell-type-specific factors (Fig. 6). These studies demonstrate that the α gene promoter has a complex organization and that the interaction of factors bound to multiple, distinct *cis*-acting elements is required for expression in the placenta and the pituitary.

In CG-producing placental cell lines, the second messenger cyclic AMP (cAMP) stimulates α and CGβ gene expression (116,117), whereas the α subunit gene is subject to negative regulation by glucocorticoids. As a result of studies into the activation of α subunit gene transcription stimulation by cAMP, the best-characterized regulatory elements in the human α gene promoter are the tandemly repeated cAMP response elements (CRE) that are located between -146 and -111 base pairs relative to the transcription initiation site. The CRE consists of a conserved palindromic sequence (TGACGTCA) that is necessary for the cAMP response and for placental-specific transcription of the α subunit promoter. The CRE consensus motif is found in many genes that are regulated by cAMP, and it binds a highly conserved nuclear factor, CREB, that is expressed in many different tissues and cell types (113–115). The isolation of genes encoding distinct, yet related leucine zipper-containing proteins that bind to the CRE with overlapping DNA-binding specificities has led to the realization that CREB is a member of a conserved multigene family (118,119). Members of the *fos*/*jun* and CREB/ATF families of tran-

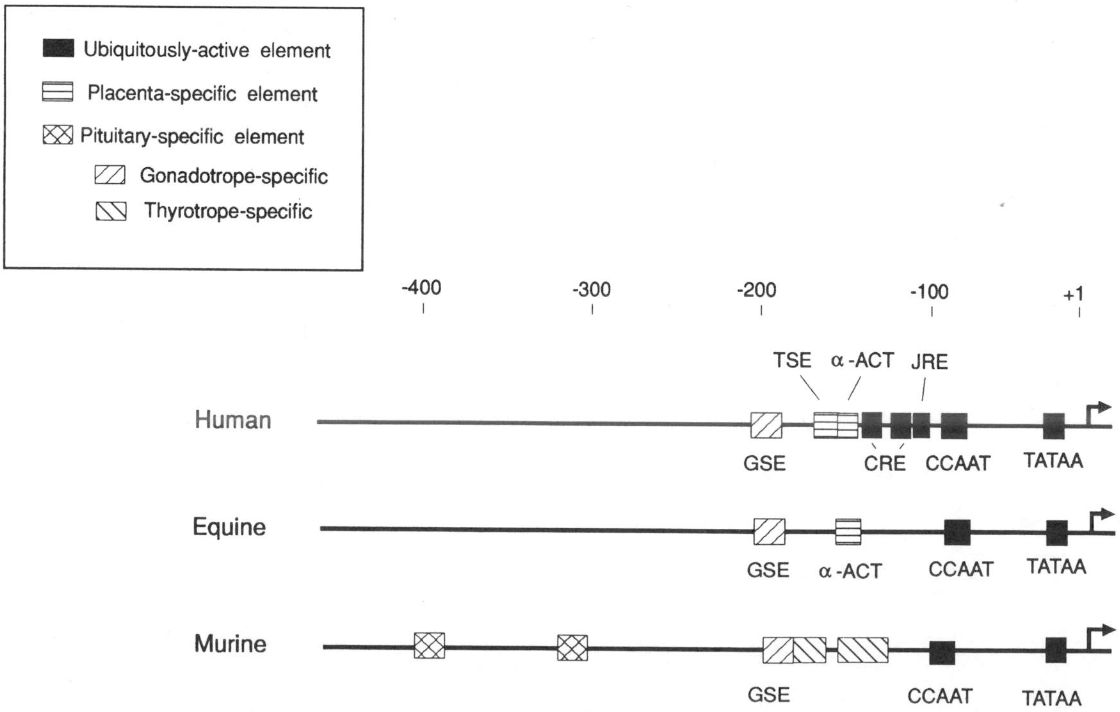

FIG. 6. α-Subunit gene promoter structure. The organization of regulatory elements in the human, equid, and murine α subunit gene promoters is depicted. GSE, gonadotrope-specific element; TSE, tissue-specific element; α-ACT, α-gene promoter activation element; CRE, cAMP response element; JRE, junctional regulatory element.

scription factors can form interfamily heterodimers by interactions through their leucine zippers. The ability of these heterodimers to bind to either the CRE or the AP1 sites appears to result in a complex array of homo- and heterodimic factors that presumably increase the range of responses of target genes containing CRE and AP1 motifs to signal transduction processes (120). Treatment of cells with cAMP activates protein kinase A, which phosphorylates CREB at serine 133 and stimulates the ability of CREB to activate gene transcription (121,122). CREB is also efficiently modified by protein kinase C and calcium/calmodulin-dependent protein kinases and appears to mediate the responses of various genes to diverse environmental stimuli (123).

The CREs cooperate with a tissue-specific upstream regulatory element (URE) and additional downstream regulatory elements to give maximal expression of the α promoter in placental cells. The URE consists of adjacent binding sites for two placental-specific factors, TSEB and α-ACT. TSEB binds to the trophoblast-specific element (TSE) present between -182 and -159 base pairs and requires the CREs for activity (113,114). The α-ACT motif between -161 to -142 base pairs contributes independently to both basal expression and cAMP-regulated expression of the α gene promoter and can function independently of the CREs. The α-ACT binding factor is apparently unrelated to CREB and appears to be a tissue-specific member of a more widely expressed protein family (124). Promoter elements downstream of the CREs include the CCAAT box from -92 to -82 base pairs, which binds a specific member (α-CBF) of the CCAAT-binding factor family that is expressed in a variety of cell types (125), and the junctional regulatory element (JRE), an AT-rich motif located at -116 to -109 base pairs between the CREs and CCAAT box that binds multiple factors present in a variety of cell types (126). Promoter sequences between the CCAAT box and the TATAA motif, commonly found as the promoters of most protein-coding genes, are also important for α gene transcription in placental cells (125); however, much less is known about the identity of specific elements of the factors that may interact with this region.

It is well known that sex steroids and glucocorticoids can negatively regulate gonadotropin gene expression. Glucocorticoid-stimulated repression of α subunit gene expression was initially thought to be mediated by the interaction of the glucocorticoid receptor (GR) with GR-binding sites that overlap the CREs in the α subunit promoter (127). It was postulated that the binding of GR to the α subunit promoter interfered with the binding of factors important for promoter activity by competing for promoter binding sites. Subsequent studies have shown that the glucocorticoid-mediated repression is dependent on transcriptional activation of the α subunit promoter by CREB and independent of GR binding to the promoter (128). Conversely, overexpression of CREB interferes with GR-mediated transcriptional activation of the MMTV promoter by glucocorticoids. These results are consistent with a previous report that estrogen inhibition of α subunit gene transcription is independent of estrogen receptor binding sites in the promoter (129). Together, these results indicate that estrogen and glucocorticoid hormone-dependent repression of cAMP-dependent α subunit gene transcription can occur independently of DNA binding by steroid hormone receptors, perhaps by sequestering CREB into an inactive complex through direct steroid hormone receptor–CREB interactions or by competition for a limiting coactivator (squelching).

The regulation of α subunit gene expression in the pituitary has been studied in transgenic mice and cultured pituitary cells. Maximal transcription of the human α gene promoter in pituitary cells requires sequences extending out to approximately -450 but does not require the α-ACT, or TSE motifs (115,130–132). Conflicting evidence exists concerning the activity of the CRE motif in gonadotrope cells, since the bovine α gene promoter, which lacks a CRE, is actively transcribed in the pituitary of transgenic mice, whereas the deletion of the tandem CREs from the human promoter abolishes its activity in the αT3-1 cells (115,132). A conserved element (termed GSE) from -223 to -200 in the human α gene promoter binds a gonadotrope-specific factor (GSEB-1) and is required for maximal transcription. GSEs are present in similar locations in the murine and equine α subunit promoters. Additional binding sites for gonadotrope specific proteins are present at several locations further upstream in the human α subunit promoter; however, deletion of the sequences did not affect activity of the promoter in αT3-1 cells.

Factors isolated from thyrotropic tumor cells interact with four distinct binding sites between -474 and -101 in the murine α gene promoter (130). One of the factor binding sites in the murine gene occurs over the GSE, indicating that GSEB-1 may be common to gonadotrope and thyrotrope lineages. Although further studies are required to elucidate the specific elements and factors that mediate α subunit gene transcription and their interrelationships, it is apparent that distinct sets of promoter elements and different combinations of ubiquitously expressed and cell-type-specific factors are required in each of the three α subunit gene-expressing lineages.

The basis for placental expression of the human α gene promoter has been studied by comparative and functional analyses of α gene promoters from other species (115,124). The ability of the human but not the bovine α gene promoter to direct placental expression of a reporter gene in the transgenic mice suggests that differences in the nucleotide sequence of α gene promoter account for the absence of placental expression of the α subunit gene in most mammals (115). Moreover, it has been proposed that the absence of a functional CRE from the bovine, murine, and rat α gene promoters is responsible for their inactivity in placenta. This notion was supported by the observation that the alteration of a single base pair to generate a functional CRE site increased transcription of the bovine promoter in placental cells (115). This view has been challenged by the recent observation that functional CRE and TSE motifs are absent from the equine α gene promoter, which, nonetheless, is placentally expressed and responsive to cAMP (124). Instead, these activities require the presence of α-ACT binding sites, which are absent from murine α gene promoter. These results suggest that placental α gene expression and cAMP responsiveness require the presence of either the combined CRE-URE motif (as in the human promoter) or the α-ACT element (present in the human and equine promoters). It appears that independent evolutionary changes have resulted in the acquisition of distinct, yet functionally redundant, sets of regulatory elements in the α gene promoters from primates and horses.

The CGβ and LHβ Subunit Gene Family

The LHβ subunit is synthesized in the gonadotopes of the pituitary gland, while the related polypeptide, CGβ subunit, is synthesized in the syncytiotrophoblast of the placenta of primates and in the chorion-derived endometrial cups of horses. Unlike the α subunit and the β subunits of the other members of the gonadotropin family, in the human the CGβ and LHβ subunits are encoded by genes in a multigene cluster that contains seven sequences with extensive homology (15,133,134). Subsequent studies (135) demonstrated that CGβ6 is an allele of gene 7 with differences in the 5′ nontranslated sequence. Thus, the CGβ subunit is encoded by six genes or pseudogenes, whereas the LHβ subunit is encoded by a single gene. Transcripts from at least five of the CGβ genes are present over a wide range of concentrations in choriocarcinoma cells, with three of the CGβ genes being expressed preferentially (135). The human CGβ subunit genes appear to have evolved from an ancestral LHβ gene by multiple gene duplications and rearrangements. DNA sequence comparisons suggest that the divergence of the LH/CGβ genes is a relatively recent evolutionary event (136). The equid CGβ gene appears to have evolved independently, since a single gene encodes the equine LH and CGβ subunits (51). Although the human CGβ and LHβ genes have highly conserved structures, the CGβ gene transcription initiation site occurs at a position more than 350 base pairs upstream of the analogous site in the LHβ promoter, suggesting that very different regulatory elements are responsible for the activity of these promoters. LHβ gene transcripts are further distinguished by an unusually short 5′ untranslated region. For example, the LHβ gene transcript contains a 6- to 11-nucleotide-long 5′ untranslated region (137). In contrast to the situation in the human, transcription of the equine LH/CGβ gene in the placenta and anterior pituitary is controlled by a single promoter that corresponds structurally to the pituitary-specific LHβ gene promoter in humans (51). These results indicate that different regulatory mechanisms are involved in placenta-specific expression of the CGβ genes in humans and equids (51). CGβ genes have not been observed in other mammals.

In spite of the high degree of structural homology between coding portions of the human CGβ and LHβ genes, their 5′ untranslated regions are distinct, and their promoter regions are divergent. Analysis of the regulation of CGβ gene expression has been hampered by the low level of activity of exogenous CGβ promoters in choriocarcinoma cells, perhaps reflecting the requirement for a distal regulatory element (enhancer). By fusing a CGβ promoter to heterologous enhancers and promoters and using the highly sensitive luciferase reporter gene assay system, multiple elements necessary for basal expression were observed between −3,700 and −30 base pairs, and a cAMP-responsive element was mapped to a region between −311 and −202 base pairs (135,138). Two lines of evidence suggest that basal transcription and cAMP-mediated expression of the α and CGβ genes involve different regulatory elements and *trans*-acting factors. First, the induction of α subunit gene transcription by cAMP is independent of protein synthesis and precedes transcriptional activation of the β subunit gene, which is inhibited by cycloheximide (139,140). Second, the region of the CGβ promoter that mediates responsiveness to cAMP contains multiple binding sites for placental nuclear proteins but does not bind CREB (138). These binding sites do not appear to be present in the α gene promoter, and it is not known whether the factors binding to these sites are cell type specific or more widely expressed. Although further studies will be necessary to define more precisely regulatory elements in the CGβ gene promoter and to test the role of potential transcriptional enhancer elements located further upstream, the available data suggest that cAMP-dependent transcription of the α and CGβ genes occurs through distinct mechanisms.

Very little is presently known about the regulatory sequences that mediate LHβ gene expression, principally because the exogenous gene is inactive in the presently available cell lines and there are no pituitary cell lines that express the endogenous β subunit gene. Analysis of the expression of the rat LHβ promoter in primary rat pituitary cell cultures demonstrated that sequences between −1,700 and −75 base pairs are dispensable for reporter gene expression, suggesting that a relatively small number of transcription factors might be required for LHβ promoter activity (141). These conclusions are limited by the caveat that the primary pituitary cell cultures are heterogeneous, and it is not certain whether expression of the LHβ promoter is restricted to the appropriate cell types. Data are not available concerning the interaction of nuclear proteins with the LHβ promoter. Other studies have suggested that estrogen responsiveness of rat LHβ gene transcription is mediated by a region about 1.3 kilobases upstream of the transcription initiation site. This region contains an estrogen response element that binds estrogen receptor and can confer a stimulatory estrogen response to a heterologous promoter (142). Because these studies were performed in pituitary cells that do not normally produce LH, the role of this region in the tissue-specific expression of the LHβ gene is unknown.

The FSHβ Subunit Gene

The FSHβ subunit is encoded by a single gene as isolated from the human, bovine, pig, and rat. In sheep there appear to be two distinct FSHβ genes; however, it is not known if both genes are expressed (76). Like the other β subunit genes, the genomic FSHβ genes in each species are evolutionarily conserved and contain three exons and two introns. Among the glycoprotein hormone β subunit genes, the FSHβ gene is unique for its rather long 3′ untranslated region (Fig. 4). Comparatively little is known about the molecular mechanisms that mediate the transcriptional regulation of this gene. It was recently shown that a 10-kilobase region containing 4 kilobases and 2 kilobases of 5′ and 3′ flanking sequences, respectively, were sufficient for pituitary-specific expression of the human FSHβ gene in transgenic mice (143). Further analysis will be necessary to define more precisely the regions important for regulated expression in transgenic mice and appropriate cell lines. These studies should be aided by the isolation of clonal (tumorigenic) gonadotrope cell lines from transgenic mice expressing oncogenes under the control of different β subunit gene promoters, as demonstrated with the α subunit gene promoter (144).

CARBOHYDRATE STRUCTURE AND FUNCTION

The carbohydrate possessed by the glycoprotein hormones distinguishes them from the other pituitary hormones, although glycosylated forms of such hormones as prolactin and growth hormone have been reported in recent years (145,146). Variations in gonadotropin molecular weight that were correlated with the reproductive cycle have been attributed to changes in carbohydrate structure (147). These changes in physicochemical properties and the observation that the ratios of biological to immunologic levels of gonadotropins in serum also varied suggested that changes in glycosylation could affect their biological activity. Oligosaccharide structures have been found to be highly variable (148,149), and there is a growing body of evidence for carbohydrate involvement in signal transduction (24,150–153).

Gonadotropin Glycosylation Sites

Unlike other heterodimeric glycoprotein hormones such as inhibin, in which a single protein chain is glycosylated, both the α and β subunits of the glycoprotein hormones are glycosylated. Figure 7 shows the patterns of glycosylation for the α and β subunits of the glycoprotein hormones. For the α subunits, *N*-linked oligosaccharides are attached to asparagines 56 and 82. The α subunit Asn^{56} oligosaccharide is essential for biological activity (24). The human α subunit glycosylation pattern is slightly different from those of other species because of a 12-base deletion in the second exon, which results in a four-amino-acid deletion near the *N* terminus, as noted above. The asparagines are thus at positions 52 and 78 in the human sequence. However, for the sake of clarity, all the numbering of the glycoprotein hormone sequences is based on that of ovine LHα. All the other sequences are aligned to this sequence by their highly conserved half-cystines in order to facilitate comparisons of homologous parts of the hormones. Thus, in Fig. 7, with the half-cystines in register, the human glycosylation sites line up with those in all the other α subunits. A similar convention, using the oLHβ numbering, will be followed with the glycosylation sites in the β subunits below.

Free α subunit is found in all glycoprotein hormone-producing tissues. It differs from α subunit that is associated with a β subunit in that it may be *O*-glycosylated at Thr^{43} (154), and its *N*-linked oligosaccharides may be more complex and more completely processed (155). Secretion of free α results from its higher rate of biosynthesis, especially in term placenta (41), as well as its resistance to intracellular degradation (42). Even in *in vitro* systems in which α subunit is synthesized at nearly the same rate as β subunit (42) the uncombined β subunit is improperly folded (156) and therefore is degraded, whereas most of the α subunit is completely folded and is secreted either as part of a hormone heterodimer or in the uncombined state (42,43). The functional significance of free α is not known. There are reports that the α subunit stimulates differentiation of lactotropes *in vitro* (34) and stimulates prolactin secretion by human decidual cell cultures derived from placenta (35).

Glycosylation of the β subunit occurs either at one or two *N*-linked glycosylation sites located at residues 13 or 30. Most LHβ subunits have only a single glycosylation site at Asn^{13}. Two exceptions are hLH and eLH. Human LHβ lacks the glycosylation signal sequence at Asn^{13}, but this is compensated by the presence of the glycosylation site at Asn^{30}. The sequence at Asn^{13} in nonhuman LHβ subunits is -Asn-Ala-Thr-, which meets the requirement for an *N*-glycosylation signal sequence, -Asn-Xaa-Thr/

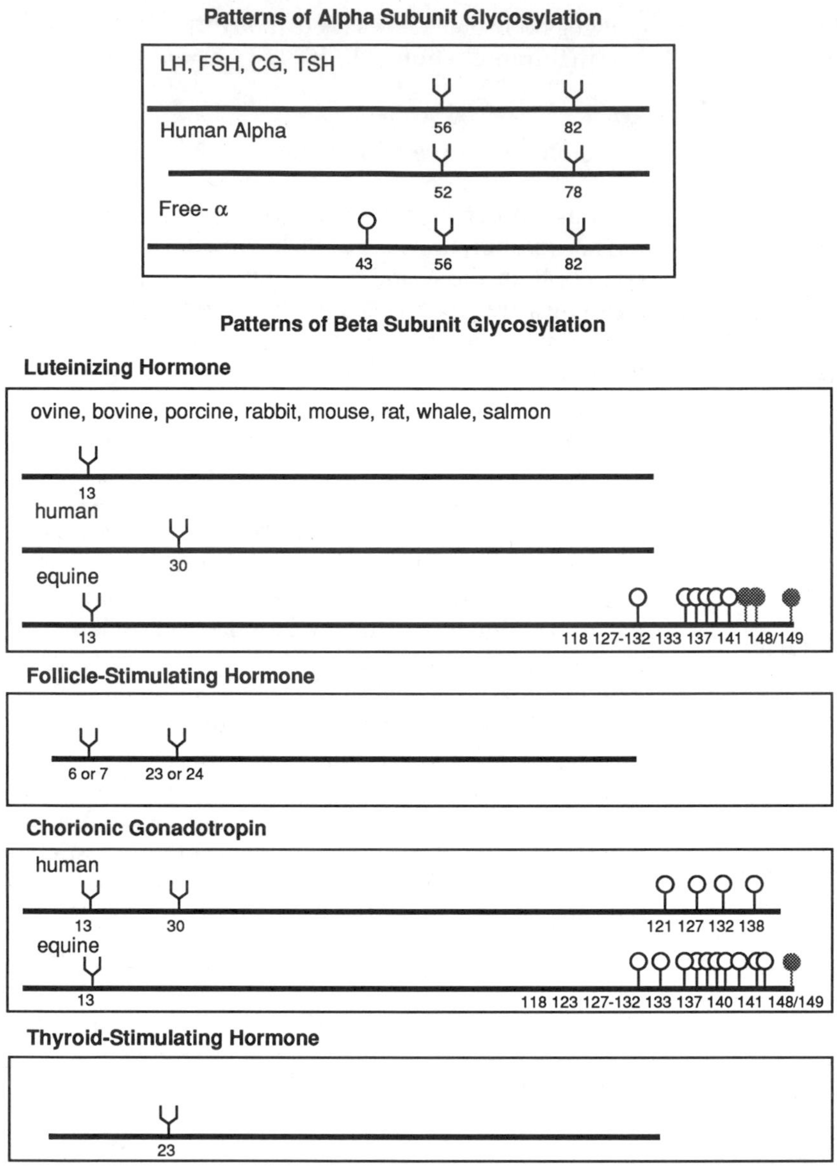

FIG. 7. Locations of the glycoprotein hormone α and β subunit glycosylation sites. The subunit proteins are indicated by the *solid bars*. The *N*-linked oligosaccharides are indicated with the *dibranched symbol*, and the "*lollipop*" indicates *O*-linked oligosaccharides. The *numbers* under each glycosylation site indicate the amino acid residue to which the oligosaccharide is attached. In the case of the eLHβ and eCGβ, where there is still uncertainty as to the exact location of some *O*-linked oligosaccharides, the lollipops are grayed.

Ser-, where Xaa means any amino acid except proline can be substituted, and Thr/Ser means that the third position can be either Thr or Ser. The human LHβ sequence at Asn[13] is -Asn-Ala-Ile- (see Fig. 2). The substitution of Ile for Thr prevents glycosylation. Glycosylation is possible at position 30 as a result of the substitution of Asn for Thr[30], resulting in the sequence -Asn-Thr-Thr-.

Equine LHβ glycosylation differs from that of other LHβ subunits because in addition to the *N*-linked oligosaccharide attached to Asn[13], the former also possesses *O*-linked oligosaccharides attached to a *C*-terminal extension, a structure characteristic of chorionic gonadotropin β subunits. This "characteristic structure," however, is based on only one example, the human, where both hLH and hCG had been sequenced. The amino acid sequences for eLHβ and eCGβ are identical (157,158) because there is a single gene in the horse that is expressed in both the pituitary and the placenta (51), whereas in the human there are separate genes for hLHβ and hCGβ that are differentially expressed in the pituitary and placenta, respectively (133). A preliminary proposal for *O*-linked glycosylation of eLHβ based on identification of glycosylated PTH-Ser and PTH-Thr derivatives during covalent sequencing of the eLHβ *C*-terminal peptide is illustrated in Fig. 7 (159). In some cases it has not yet been possible to determine the exact position of the oligosaccharide. These are indicated by graying the symbols representing the *O*-linked oligosaccharides. Since there is no recognized signal sequence for *O*-linked glycosylation, these sites must be determined directly. Glycosylation of Thr and Ser usually occurs in regions rich in Pro as well as Thr and Ser. The *C*-terminal extension of eLHβ is rich in all three of these amino acids, and many of the Thr and Ser residues are glycosylated.

FSH β subunits possess both *N*-linked glycosylation

sites, Asn^{13} and Asn^{30}, whereas TSHβ is glycosylated only at Asn^{30}. The chorionic gonadotropins show two different patterns of glycosylation for the two known examples: hCG and eCG. Human CGβ is *N*-glycosylated at both Asn^{13} and Asn^{30}. In addition, it is *O*-glycosylated at Ser residues 121, 127, 132, and 138 (160–162). The amino acid sequence deduced from baboon CGβ cDNA predicts an identical pattern of glycosylation. In contrast, eCGβ possesses a single *N*-linked glycosylation site at Asn^{13}. The major *N*-linked oligosaccharides of eCGβ are predominantly biantennary complex sialylated structures, similar to structure 5 in Fig. 8 (163,164). Yet eCG is more heavily glycosylated (45% carbohydrate) than hCG (31% carbohydrate). Most of the difference in the carbohydrate contents results from more extensive glycosylation of the eCGβ *C* terminus (159). Equine CGβ possesses 12 *O*-glycosylation sites in the *C*-terminal extension, of which at least 11 are glycosylated (see Fig. 7).

Carbohydrate Structure

It is well established that the glycoprotein hormones possess highly diverse oligosaccharide structures (148,149). A single *N*-linked oligosaccharide structure was initially proposed for hCG (structure 5 in Fig. 8). All the carbohydrate heterogeneity was assumed to result from incomplete processing (162). At the same time, however, Endo et al. (165) reported five charged and three neutral oligosaccharide structures isolated from hCG. One structure was the same as structure 5, and others were similar to it in that they were missing only one residue such as the fucose or one or both of the terminal sialic acid residues. Some variations were consistent between subunits. For example, there was no fucose on any of the oligosaccharides isolated from the α subunit (166). More recent investigations suggest additional oligosaccharide structures associated with the gonadotropins (149,155). Parsons and Pierce (167) found that bLH was sulfated on its terminal sugars, which prevented exoglycosidases from hydrolyzing terminal sugars, thus hindering structural characterization. Baenziger's laboratory subsequently determined the structure of the disulfated oligosaccharides of bLH (Fig. 8, structure 10) (168). They next examined the oligosaccharides on the ovine, bovine, and human pituitary hormones and found that each hormone possessed several oligosaccharide structures (169,170). The complete structures are shown in Fig. 8. Some hormones, such as oFSH, had 16 charged structures, accounting for 68% of the oligosaccharides released by peptide *N*-glycanase digestion. Numerous neutral oligosaccharides were also released but were too low in abundance to characterize. The other

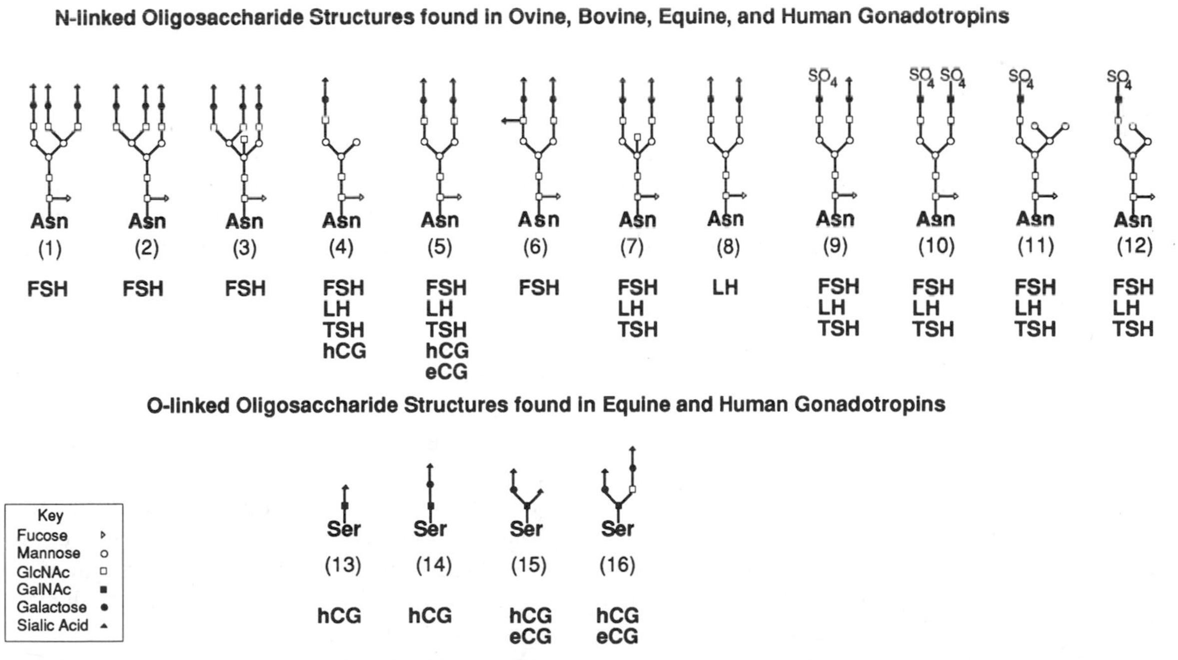

FIG. 8. Oligosaccharide structures determined for the glycoprotein hormones. Negatively charged oligosaccharides bearing one, two, or three negative charges as a result of the presence of terminal sulfate or sialic acid residues are the most abundant oligosaccharides obtained from the glycoprotein hormones. Variations in the structures shown here have been characterized and result from the absence of fucose residues or from the absence of one or more of the sulfate or sialic acid residues. Neutral oligosaccharides may comprise as much as 33% of the oligosaccharides obtained from a glycoprotein hormone. However, because of the great variety of structures in the neutral oligosaccharide fraction, none is present in sufficient quantity for structural characterization.

characterized structures were variations on these structures lacking one or more sialic acid residues or lacking sulfate or lacking fucose. Based on these results, the oligosaccharides fell into three categories: sialylated, sulfated, and hybrid sulfated–sialylated. Figure 8 shows the qualitative distribution of the oligosaccharide structures. This may vary from species to species and from hormone to hormone. For example, hCG and hFSH possessed only sialylated oligosaccharides, and most species of LH possessed predominantly sulfated oligosaccharides or hybrids. Ovine FSH, on the other hand, had a little bit of everything. For a more detailed description of the distribution of oligosaccharide structures, see the review by Baenziger and Green (148). Figure 9, based on this review, summarizes the biosynthetic build up of the gonadotropin oligosaccharides. (See also the section on biosynthesis of the gonadotropins for further comment.)

Oligosaccharide structures have recently been characterized for eCG and eLH, and these differ from each other only in their carbohydrate moieties (157,158,164). Ten *N*-linked structures were initially characterized from eCG (171), demonstrating that the variability of oligosaccharides obtained from tissue-derived hormone is also characteristic of circulating gonadotropins. Oligosaccharide heterogeneity in eCG was confirmed in a recent report (163) in which 24 *N*-linked oligosaccharides were isolated from eCGβ and even more from eCGα. Only one set of four oligosaccharides was completely characterized by NMR. These oligosaccharides were similar to structure 5 in Fig. 8 except that either one or both of the sialic acids were *O*-acetylated. The *N*-linked oligosaccharides of eCGβ have been compared with those of eLHβ (164). Only sialylated oligosaccharides were obtained from eCGβ, but eLHβ possessed both sialylated and sulfated oligosaccharides, with the latter being the most abundant.

Renwick and colleagues have examined the charged oligosaccharide structures for each glycosylation site of oLH and hLH (172,173). In oLH 61% of the β subunit oligosaccharides were of the disulfated type (Fig. 8, structure 10), whereas only 16% of the Asn^{56} and 7% of the Asn^{82} α subunit oligosaccharides were represented by this structure. The major (35%) oligosaccharide structure attached to Asn^{82} was structure 12, and the major structures attached to Asn^{56} were structures 11 and 12 (23% and 27%, respectively). The β subunit oligosaccharides were 85–95% fucosylated, whereas the α subunit oligosaccharides were partially fucosylated, 10–15% at Asn^{56} and 45–55% at Asn^{82}. The distribution of these oligosaccharide structures on oLH is illustrated in Fig. 10. The hLH glycosylation was more heterogeneous than that of oLH, but the oligosaccharides fell into three basic categories based on their Manα1–3 branches with variations in the structures of the Manα1–6 branches. The major species (18% of αAsn^{56} oligosaccharides and 15% of βAsn^{30} oligosaccharides) was the hybrid sulfated/sialylated oligosaccharide (Fig. 8, structure 9), and various sulfated forms comprised half of the oligosaccharides attached to these asparagine residues. A minor new oligosaccharide (Fig. 8, structure 8) was detected predominantly at Asn^{82}. This apparently resulted from the presence of an α2-6GalNAcβ1–4GlcNAc sialyltransferase in the human pituitary. This enzyme has been reported to be present in bovine colostrum (174). The remaining charged oligosaccharides were variations on structure 7. Most of the hLHβ subunit oligosaccharides were fucosylated, but only 15–25% of αAsn^{56} and 0–10% of the αAsn^{82} oligosaccharides were fucosylated, similar to the situation for oLHα and hCGα described above. These results suggest that the β subunit reduces the accessibility of the α oligosaccharides to fucosyltransferase once the subunits are associated.

Luteinizing hormone and CG produced by recombinant DNA methodology do not possess the same oligosaccharides as the native hormones (175,176). Recombinant LH lacks the sulfated oligosaccharides, since CHO cells used for the *in vitro* synthesis lack GalNAc transferase and sulfotransferase (175). Recombinant hCGβ, produced in a baculovirus expression system, possesses high-mannose *N*-linked oligosaccharides and *O*-linked disaccharides, based on composition analysis of the recombinant subunit (176). Recombinant hFSH appears to possess similar types of oligosaccharides as the native hormone, but some variations in extent of fucosylation and other structural details have been reported (177).

Carbohydrate Function

The best-understood role of carbohydrate is for determining the circulatory half-lives of the gonadotropins. The classical asialoglycoprotein receptor (178) has recently been joined by a receptor that recognizes sulfated oligosaccharides (179). Together these two receptor systems are involved in the rapid clearance of these forms of the hormones from the circulation. Baenziger has proposed that a component of the pulsatile levels of LH in serum is the rapid clearance by the latter receptor, which recognizes newly released hormone, whereas the asialoglycoprotein receptor removes glycoproteins only after they lose terminal sialic acid residues (179). This proposal is supported by the observation that native LH bearing sulfated oligosaccharides is removed from circulation four to five times more quickly than recombinant bLH having only complex sialylated oligosaccharides (180). In the human, the placenta lacks GalNAc transferase and sulfotransferase; therefore, hCG possesses only sialylated oligosaccharides and, partly for this reason, is more slowly cleared from the circulation. The other reason for the slow clearance of hCG is the presence of the glycosylated *C*-terminal extension on hCGβ. This glycopeptide is not required for biological activity, as it can be removed by mild acid cleavage (181) and by

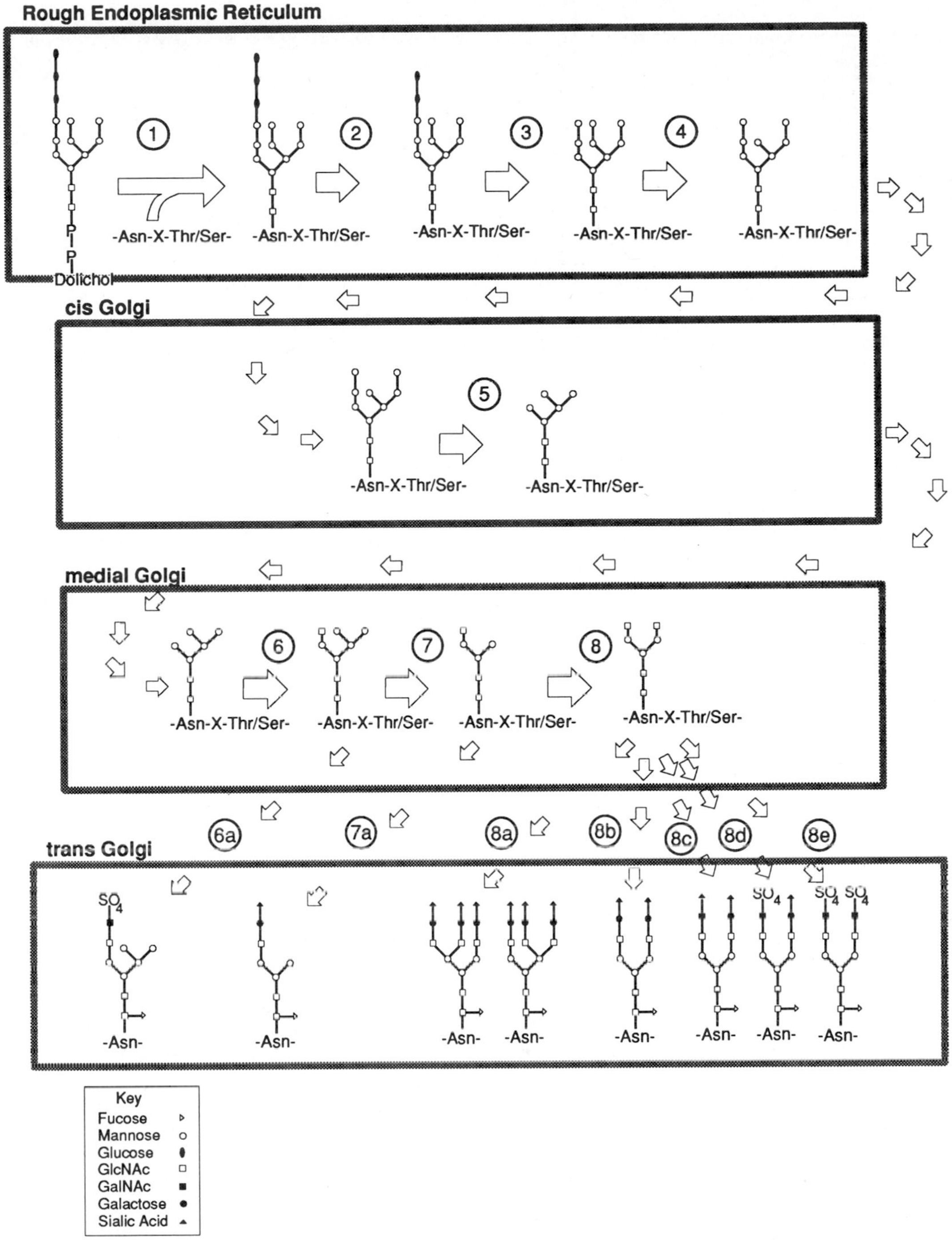

FIG. 9. Biosynthetic pathway for *N*-linked oligosaccharides leading to completed *N*-linked oligosaccharide structures shown in Fig. 8. This is based on the pathway for *N*-linked glycosylation (311) and pathways suggested by structures on glycoprotein hormones (148). **1:** Oligosaccharyltransferase-catalyzed transfer of dolichol-linked $Glc_3Man_9GlcNAc_2$ oligosaccharide to asparagine at glycosylation site: -Asn-Xaa-Ser/Thr-. **2:** α-Glucosidase I removes terminal glucose. **3:** α-Glucosidase II removes remaining two glucose residues. **4:** Endoplasmic reticulum α-1,2-mannosidase removes one mannose residue. **5:** Golgi α-mannosidase I removes another three mannose residues, producing the precursor for *N*-acetylglucosamine transferase I. **6:** *N*-Acetylglucosamine transferase I adds *N*-acetylglucosamine, creating procursor for S-1 type having only one completed branch or leading to continued processing. (**a**) Addition of *N*-acetylgalactosamine diverts processing to complex bi- or triantennary oligosaccharide, resulting in this single-branch sulfated structure. Signal for GalNAc transferase recognition appears to be -Pro-Xaa-Arg/Lys- (241). **7:** Golgi α-mannosidase II removes two mannose residues. (**a**) Addition of *N*-acetylgalactosamine could lead to this structure. **8:** *N*-Acetylglucosamine transferase II adds a second *N*-acetylglucosamine, leading to further processing, which produces the following oligosaccharade structures: (**a**) triantennary sialylated; (**b**) biantennary sialylated; (**c**) disialylated, as a result of α2–6GalNAcβ1–4GlcNAc sialyltransferase in human pituitaries (173); (**d**) hybrid sialylated-sulfated; (**e**) disulfated.

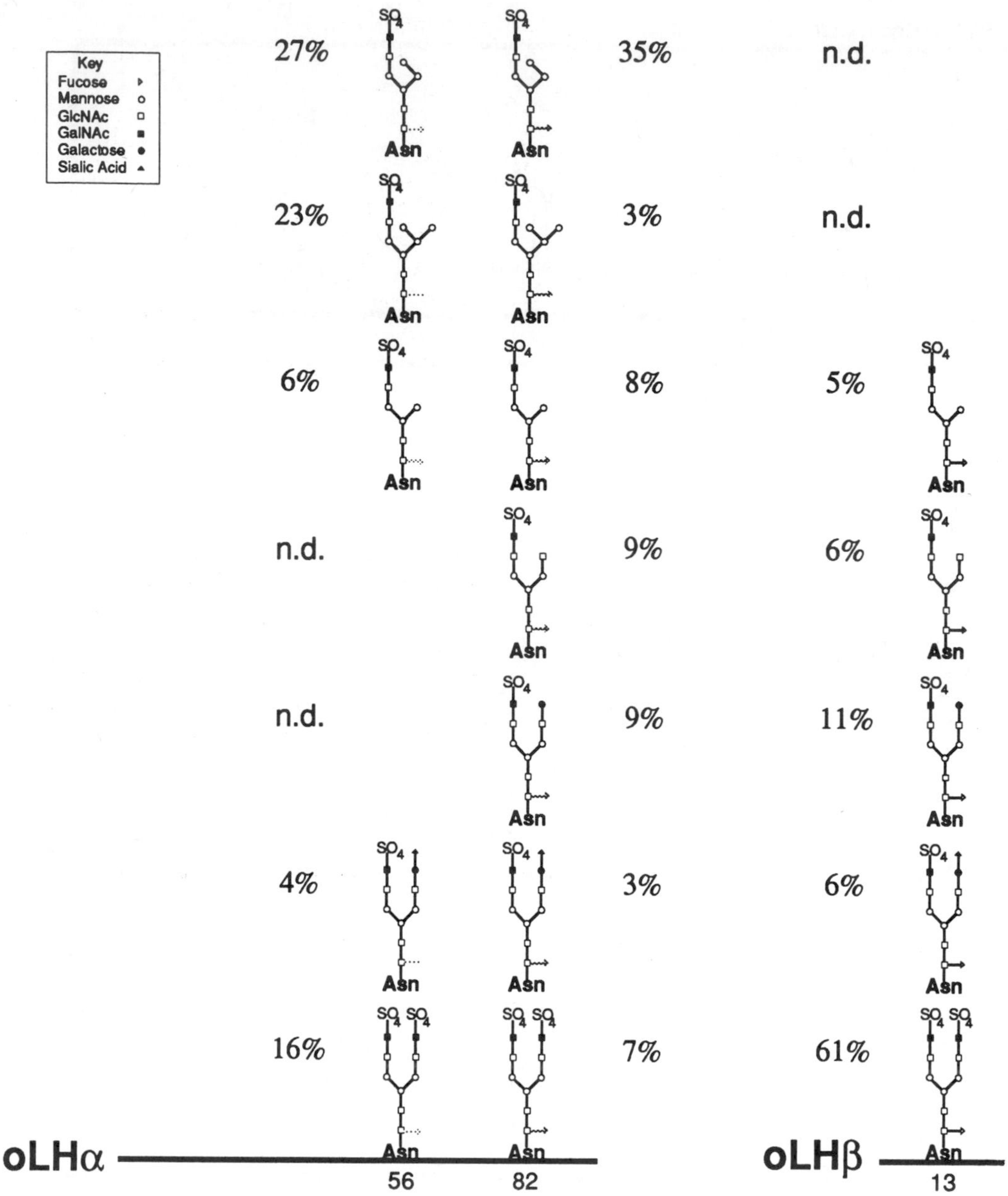

FIG. 10. Distribution of *N*-linked oligosaccharide structures on the three glycosylation sites of oLH (172). The numbers beside each structure indicate its relative abundance at each glycosylation site (n.d., not detected). The degree of fucosylation is indicated by the intensity of the fucose symbol, corresponding to 85–95% at βAsn[13], 10–15% at αAsn[56], and 45–55% at αAsn[82].

mutagenesis of the hCGβ cDNA without affecting receptor binding activity (65,102). The *C*-terminal extension has been attached to hormones that lack this moiety with the effect of prolonging their circulatory half-lives (66).

Carbohydrate influences glycoprotein hormone biosynthesis, including folding, intracellular survival, differential packaging of LH and FSH by the same cell, and secretion (182). The *N*-linked oligosaccharides may also play a role in biosynthesis, accelerating proper folding of the β subunit (100).

In addition to the effects of carbohydrate on circulating glycoprotein hormone half-lives, carbohydrate also modulates their specific activities (75,179,183). With regard to the latter effect, *in vitro* studies have suggested that deglycosylated gonadotropins can act as antagonists. However, *in vivo* experiments do not support this idea.

Deglycosylated Forms

Chemically or enzymatically deglycosylated CG, LH, FSH, and TSH bind their receptors with a higher apparent affinity than the native hormones (152,184–186).

However, the activities of deglycosylated glycoprotein hormones are much lower in assays that measure a target cell response such as steroidogenesis. By deglycosylating an α or β subunit and then recombining the deglycosylated subunit with the intact complementary subunit, it was demonstrated that only the α subunit carbohydrate was required for these responses (151–153). In the course of these studies, some investigators reported that the deglycosylated gonadotropins acted as antagonists to the native hormones (187). Deglycosylated hormone occupied receptors and formed inactive hormone–receptor complexes, which prevented native hormone from binding to receptors and activating the target cells. Liu et al. (153) showed that deglycosylated hormone had a faster on rate than native hormone, but the off rates of both were comparable. This probably contributes to the poor *in vivo* antagonism of the deglycosylated hormone.

The use of site-directed mutagenesis of hCG subunit cDNAs to eliminate single glycosylation sites has further localized the roles of individual glycosylation sites. Of the two α subunit glycosylation sites, the Asn^{56} site is essential for biological activity (24). In the absence of α subunit Asn^{56} oligosaccharide the β subunit Asn^{13} oligosaccharide contributes to the biological activity of hCG (24). Similar experiments have been carried out with FSHβ; however, deletion of either or both glycosylation sites did not affect *in vitro* biological activity (188).

In an attempt to interfere with LH maintenance of postovulatory corpora lutea, deglycosylated hCG was administered to normal cycling women (189). However, there was no effect on the luteal phase except to elevate progesterone levels. This prompted the investigators to suggest that agonist activity in the preparation interfered with its antagonist activity. The activities of native, desialylated, and deglycosylated hCG were compared in male cynomolgus monkeys (190). The hCG was deglycosylated, and partially deglycosylated hCG was removed by ConA-Sepharose chromatography. *In vitro* antagonism of hCG stimulation of cAMP production by this deglycosylated hCG preparation was demonstrated in rat testis Leydig cells. The serum half-life of deglycosylated hCG was 23 min, 23 times that of asialo-hCG, which is rapidly cleared by the galactose-binding asialoglycoprotein receptor in the liver (178) but less than one-tenth that of native hCG. However, the early (48 hr) responses to stimulation by hCG, asialo-hCG, and deglycosylated hCG were identical. No *in vivo* antagonistic activity by deglycosylated hCG was observed. After 48 hr, testosterone levels of hCG-treated monkeys remained elevated, whereas those receiving asialo-hCG and deglycosylated hCG had returned to normal levels, suggesting that carbohydrate may affect long-acting hormone stimulation *in vivo*.

Circulating forms of hFSH having *in vitro* antagonistic effects have been reported (191), although no *in vivo* studies have been performed to determine the physiological relevance of this observation. Chappel and colleagues have reviewed evidence by a number of investigators that physicochemical changes occur in FSH in response to changing physiological conditions (75). These changes in apparent molecular size and distribution of isoelectric forms were attributed principally to variations in FSH sialic acid content. Desialylation of FSH shortened its circulatory half-life but elevated its potency in receptor binding assays *in vitro*. A model was proposed in which FSH was modified by neuraminidase action that converted relatively more acidic long-acting low-potency forms into more basic, more potent, short-lived forms. However, subsequent studies employing a different in vitro FSH assay reported a different FSH activity profile. Hsueh and colleagues have developed an *in vitro* steroidogenesis assay sensitive enough to detect FSH in serum (192). The more acidic forms of FSH (Chappel's less potent, long-acting forms) were determined to be the active circulating forms. Moreover, the more basic forms that were released in response to a GnRH antagonist were found to be FSH antagonists in the steroidogenesis bioassay (191). Thus, although the oligosaccharides attached to αAsn^{56} can be demonstrated to be essential for *in vitro* biological activity, the lack of antagonistic effect by deglycosylated hormones *in vivo* may indicate that the physiologically relevant role of carbohydrate is in determining the circulatory half-lives of the gonadotropins.

HORMONE RECEPTORS

The glycoprotein hormone receptors have been cloned (193–199) and found to share a similar structure consisting of a large extracellular domain, seven transmembrane regions, and a cytoplasmic tail (see Fig. 11). Except for the large extracellular domains, these receptors are similar to other G-protein-coupled receptors that bind much smaller ligands. Comparison of the glycoprotein hormone receptor gene organization of 10 to 11 exons with the single exon of the β-adrenergic receptor gene suggests that the former arose by insertion of a leucine-rich repeat domain into the single exon of a β-adrenergic-like receptor (199–201).

LH/CG Receptor

The receptor for LH also recognizes chorionic gonadotropin, as to be expected by their similar and/or identical amino acid sequences. Receptors for LH/hCG have been demonstrated on a variety of tissues in the reproductive system, including Leydig cells, granulosa cells, and luteal cells (202,203). Receptors for LH have also been detected in nonovarian tissues (see ref. 204 for references). They have been cloned from a variety of species using recombinant DNA methodology, including pigs

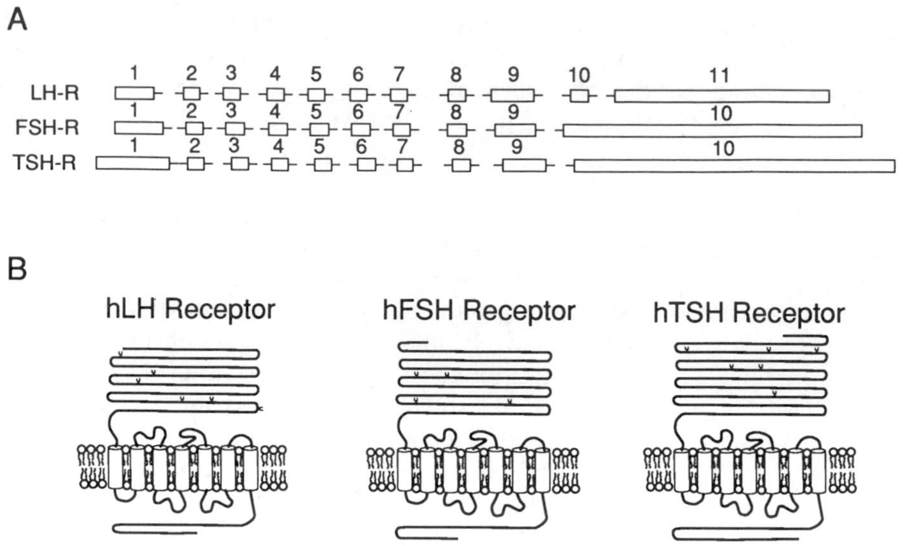

FIG. 11. Structure of glycoprotein hormone receptor genes and receptor proteins. **A:** Structure of glycoprotein hormone receptor genes showing 11 exons of the LH receptor as compared with 10 exons in the FSH and TSH receptors. The sizes of all the introns have not been determined; therefore, the size of each gene is only approximate. **B:** Diagrammatic structures of the glycoprotein hormone receptors illustrating the extracellular glycoprotein domain, the putative seven transmembrane helices, and the cytoplasmic *C*-terminal tail. The amino acid sequences are illustrated in Fig. 12.

(195), rats (194), humans (205), mice (206,207), and a frog (208). The rat LH receptor gene has been cloned (200,209) and consists of 11 exons. The first ten encode the extracellular domain, and the 11th encodes the transmembrane domain (Fig. 11). The rat, pig, and human receptor amino acid sequences are compared with each other and with those of the cloned FSH and TSH receptors in Fig. 12. The LH receptor consists of a single polypeptide chain ranging in size from 669 residues in the pig (194) to 742 residues in the rat (195). All of these receptors have a long extracellular sequence, the hormone binding site (210), that contains six potential *N*-linked glycosylation sites (194,195,199,211). Also, all species' receptors possess seven predicted transmembrane segments, which are similar to other receptors known to be coupled to G proteins, the adenylate cyclase second messenger system, and cAMP. The transmembrane segments are predicted by hydropathy analysis that identifies hydrophobic regions of the protein sequence and by comparison with rhodopsin (195). In addition, there is a short cytoplasmic tail consisting of 68–72 residues that may possess a plasma membrane-targeting signal sequence (211).

Antibodies raised against synthetic peptides corresponding to the *N*-terminal and *C*-terminal portions of the LH receptor have been used to confirm that the *N*-terminal portion is exposed extracellularly while the *C* terminus is intracellular, as predicted by homology to other G-protein-coupled receptors (212). Expression of a truncated form of the rat ovarian LH receptor in COS-1 cells resulted in secretion of soluble receptor (213). The amount of soluble receptor expressed was about 16% that of full-length receptor transfected into the same cell line. Expression in human kidney 293 cells of a cDNA encoding an experimentally truncated rat LH receptor gene consisting of only the extracellular domain demonstrated that the high-affinity binding to hCG by the receptor was attributable to this portion of the molecule alone (210). The experiment also indicated that the truncated form of the receptor was not secreted by the cell, so that receptor-binding studies were only possible using detergent extracts of the cells. Perhaps this is why LH-RBI was only detected following freeze-thawing of rat ovaries (214). Entrapment of modified receptors occurs frequently. When chimeric molecules consisting of the LH receptor extracellular domain and either the β_2-adrenergic receptor transmembrane domain or the vesicular stomatitis virus G protein transmembrane domain were transfected into COS-7 cells, the chimeric receptors were not transported to the cell surface but could be de-

FIG. 12. Comparison of glycoprotein hormone receptor amino acid sequences. Amino acid sequences were deduced from cDNA sequences. The sequences of the gonadotropin receptors for LH/hCG and FSH are compared with the sequence for human TSH. The *arrow* indicates the amino terminus of the mature rat LH receptor, which is the only one that has been determined experimentally (195). The others have been predicted from the deduced amino acid sequence and are indicated by the *line* below the *arrow.* Potential *N*-glycosylation sites, putative transmembrane helices, and the half-cystines are *boxed.* The *solid lines* indicate the exon boundaries found in each receptor gene. Note that the LH/hCG receptor gene has 11 exons, whereas the FSH and TSH receptor genes have only 10 exons. The *dotted lines* indicate the leucine-rich repeats in the extracellular domain. The segment of the cytoplasmic tail that might contain plasma membrane targeting sequences (211) is boxed with a *dashed line* to distinguish this segment from the transmembrane helices. Diagrammatic representation of the structures of the human glycoprotein hormone receptors is indicated in Fig. 11.

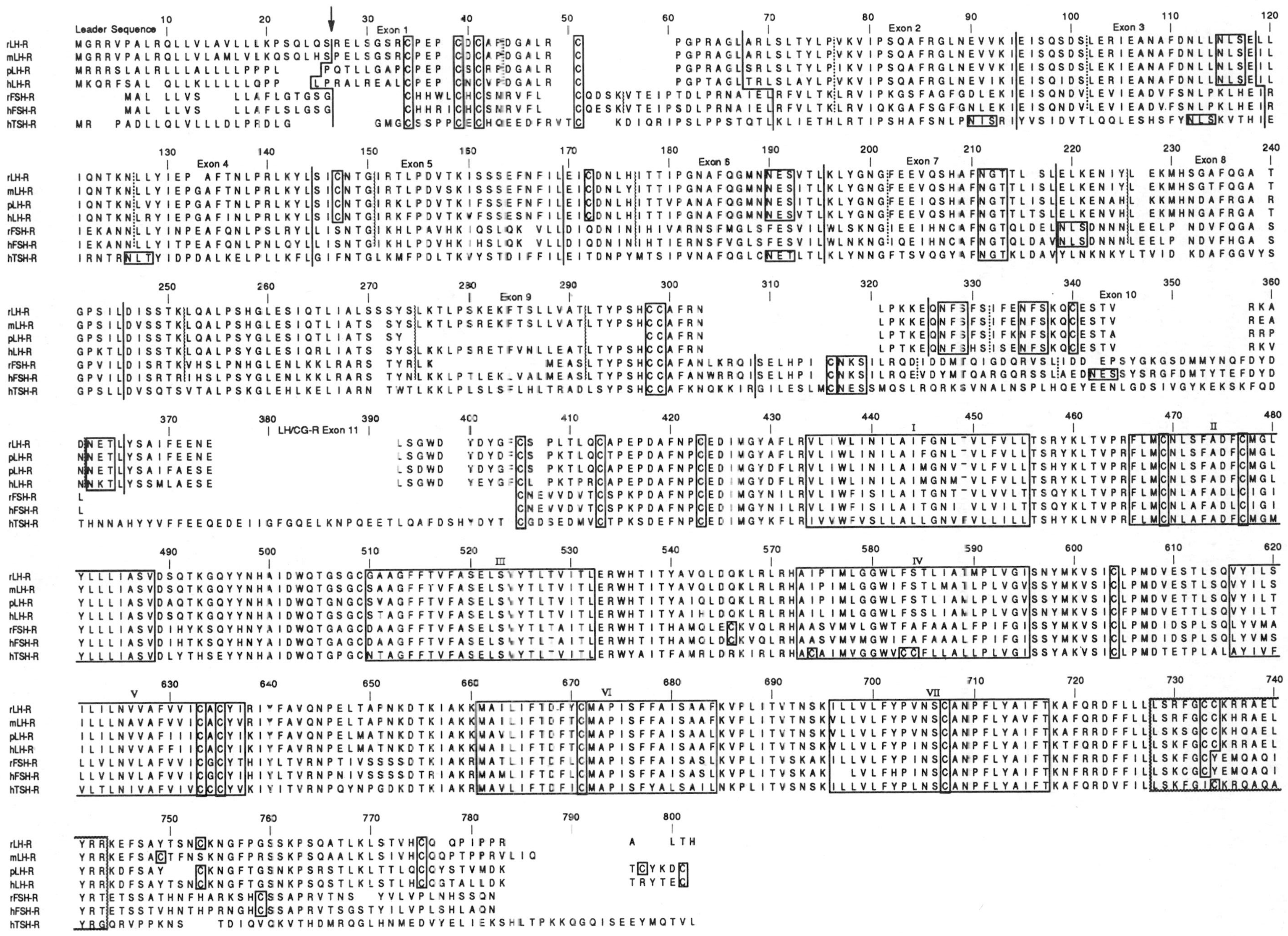

Leader Sequence
Exon 1
Exon 2
Exon 3
rLH-R MGRRVPALRQLLVLAVLLLKPSQLQSRELSGSRCPEP CDCAPDGALR C PGPRAGLARLSLTYLPVKVIPSQAFRGLNEVVKIEISQSDSLERIEANAFDNLLNLSELL
mLH-R MGRRVPALRQLLVLAMLVLKQSQLHSPELSGSRCPEP CDCAPDGALR C PGPRAGLARLSLTYLPVKVIPSQAFRGLNEVVKIEISQSDSLERIEANAFDNLLNLSEIL
pLH-R MRRRSLALRLLLALLLLPPPL PQTLLGAPCPEP CSCRPDGALR C PGPRAGLSRLSLTYLPIKVIPSQAFRGLNEVVKIEISQSDSLEKIEANAFDNLLNLSEIL
hLH-R MKQRFSAL QLLKLLLLLQPP LPRALREALCPEP CNCVPDGALR C PGPTAGLTRLSLAYLPVKVIPSQAFRGLNEVIKIEISQIDSLERIEANAFDNLLNLSEIL
rFSH-R MAL LLVS LLAFLGTGSG CHHWLCHCSNRVFL CQDSKVTEIPTDLPRNAIELRFVLTKLRVIPKGSFAGFGDLEKIEISQNDVLEVIEADVFSNLPKLHEIR
hFSH-R MAL LLVS LLAFLSLGSG CHHRICHCSNRVFL CQESKVTEIPSDLPRNAIELRFVLTKLRVIQKGAFSGFGNLEKIEISQNDVLEVIEADVFSNLPKLHEIR
hTSH-R MR PADLLQLVLLLDLPRDLG GMGCSSPPCECHQEEDFRVTC KDIQRIPSLPPSTQTLKLIETHLRTIPSHAFSNLPNISRIYVSIDVTLQQLESHSFYNLSKVTHIE
Exon 4
Exon 5
Exon 6
Exon 7
Exon 8
rLH-R IQNTKNLLYIEP AFTNLPRLKYLSICNTGIRTLPDVTKISSSEFNFILEICDNLHITTIPGNAFQGMNNESVTLKLYGNGFEEVQSHAFNGTTL SLELKENIYL EKMHSGAFQGA T
mLH-R IQNTKNLLYIEPGAFTNLPRLKYLSICNTGIRTLPDVSKISSSEFNFILEICDNLYITTIPGNAFQGMNNESITLKLYGNGFEEVQSHAFNGTTLISLELKENIYL EKMHSGTFQGA T
pLH-R IQNTKNLVYIEPGAFTNLPRLKYLSICNTGIRKLPDVTKIFSSEFNFILEICDNLHITTVPANAFQGMNNESITLKLYGNGFEEIQSHAFNGTTLISLELKENAHL KKMHNDAFRGA R
hLH-R IQNTKNLRYIEPGAFINLPRLKYLSICNTGIRKFPDVTKVFSSESNFILEICDNLHITTIPGNAFQGMNNESVTLKLYGNGFEEVQSHAFNGTTLTSLELKENVHL EKMHNGAFRGA T
rFSH-R IEKANNLLYINPEAFQNLPSLRYLLISNTGIKHLPAVHKIQSLQK VLLDIQDNINIHIVARNSFMGLSFESVILWLSKNGIEEIHNCAFNGTQLDELNLSDNNNLEELP NDVFQGA S
hFSH-R IEKANNLLYITPEAFQNLPNLQYLLISNTGIKHLPDVHKIHSLQK VLLDIQDNINIHTIERNSFVGLSFESVILWLNKNGIQEIHNCAFNGTQLDAVNLSDNNNLEELP NDVFHGA S
hTSH-R IRNTRNLTYIDPDALKELPLLKFLGIFNTGLKMFPDLTKVYSTDIFFILEITDNPYMTSIPVNAFQGLCNETLTLKLYNNGFTSVQGYAFNGTKLDAVYLNKNKYLTVID KDAFGGVYS
Exon 9
Exon 10
rLH-R GPSILDISSTKLQALPSHGLESIQTLIALSSSYSLKTLPSKEKFTSLLVATLTYPSHCCAFRN LPKKEQNFSFSIFENFSKQCESTV RKA
mLH-R GPSILDVSSTKLQALPSHGLESIQTLIATS SYSLKTLPSREKFTSLLVATLTYPSHCCAFRN LPKKEQNFSFSIFENFSKQCESTV REA
pLH-R GPSILDISSTKLQALPSYGLESIQTLIATS SY CCAFRN LPTKEQNFSFSIFKNFSKQCESTA RRP
hLH-R GPKTLDISSTKLQALPSYGLESIQRLIATS SYSLKKLPSRETFVNLLEATLTYPSHCCAFRN LPTKEQNFSHSISENFSKQCESTV RKV
rFSH-R GPVILDISRTKVHSLPNHGLENLKKLRARS TYRLK MEASLTYPSHCCAFANLKRQISELHPICNKSILRQDIDDMTQIGDQRVSLIDD EPSYGKGSDMMYNQFDYD
hFSH-R GPVILDISRTRIHSLPSYGLENLKKLRARS TYNLKKLPTLEKLVALMEASLTYPSHCCAFANWRRQISELHPICNKSILRQEVDYMTQARGQRSSLAEDNESSYSRGFDMTYTEFDYD
hTSH-R GPSLLDVSQTSVTALPSKGLEHLKELIARN TWTLKKLPLSLSFLHLTRADLSYPSHCCAFKNQKKIRGILESLMCNESSMQSLRQRKSVNALNSPLHQEYEENLGDSIVGYKEKSKFQD
LH/CG-R Exon 11
I
II
rLH-R DNETLYSAIFEENE LSGWD YDYGFCS PLTLQCAPEPDAFNPCEDIMGYAFLRVLIWLINILAIFGNL-VLFVLLTSRYKLTVPRFLMCNLSFADFCMGL
pLH-R NNETLYSAIFEENE LSGWD YDYDFCS PKTLQCTPEPDAFNPCEDIMGYAFLRVLIWLINILAIFGNL-VLFVLLTSRYKLTVPRFLMCNLSFADFCMGL
pLH-R NNETLYSAIFAESE LSDWD YDYGFCS PKTLQCAPEPDAFNPCEDIMGYDFLRVLIWLINILAIMGNV-VLFVLLTSHYKLTVPRFLMCNLSFADFCMGL
hLH-R NNKTLYSSMLAESE LSGWD YEYGFCL PKTPRCAPEPDAFNPCEDIMGYDFLRVLIWLINILAIMGNM-VLFVLLTSRYKLTVPRFLMCNLSFADFCMGL
rFSH-R L CNEVVDVTCSPKPDAFNPCEDIMGYNILRVLIWFISILAITGNT-VLVLTTSQYKLTVPRFLMCNLAFADLCIGI
hFSH-R L CNEVVDVTCSPKPDAFNPCEDIMGYNILRVLIWFISILAITGNI VLVILTTSQYKLTVPRFLMCNLAFADLCIGI
hTSH-R THNNAHYYVFFEEQEDEIIGFGQELKNPQEETLQAFDSHYDYT CGDSEDMVCTPKSDEFNPCEDIMGYKFLRIVVWFVSLLALLGNVFVLLILLTSHYKLNVPRFLMCNLAFADFCMGM
III
IV
rLH-R YLLLIASVDSQTKGQYYNHAIDWQTGSGCGAAGFFTVFASELSVYTLTVITLERWHTITYAVQLDQKLRLRHAIPIMLGGWLFSTLIATMPLVGISNYMKVSICLPMDVESTLSQVYILS
mLH-R YLLLIASVDSQTKGQYYNHAIDWQTGSGCSAAGFFTVFASELSVYTLTVITLERWHTITYAVQLDQKLRLRHAIPIMLGGWIFSTLMATLPLVGVSSYMKVSICLPMDVESTLSQVYILS
pLH-R YLLLIASVDAQTKGQYYNHAIDWQTGNGCSVAGFFTVFASELSVYTLTVITLERWHTITYAIQLDQKLRLRHAIPIMLGGWLFSTLIANLPLVGVSSYMKVSICLPMDVETTLSQVYILT
hLH-R YLLLIASVDSQTKGQYYNHAIDWQTGSGCSTAGFFTVFASELSVYTLTVITLERWHTITYAIHLDQKLRLRHAILIMLGGWLFSSLIANLPLVGVSNYMKVSICFPMDVETTLSQVYILT
rFSH-R YLLLIASVDIHYKSQYHNYAIDWQTGAGCDAAGFFTVFASELSVYTLTAITLERWHTITHAMQLECKVQLRHAASVMVLGWTFAFAAALFPIFGISSYMKVSICLPMDIDSPLSQLYVMA
hFSH-R YLLLIASVDIHTKSQYHNYAIDWQTGAGCDAAGFFTVFASELSVYTLTAITLERWHTITHAMQLDCKVQLRHAASVMVMGWIFAFAAALFPIFGISSYMKVSICLPMDIDSPLSQLYVMS
hTSH-R YLLLIASVDLYTHSEYYNHAIDWQTGPGCNTAGFFTVFASELSVYTL-VITLERWYAITFAMRLDRKIRLRHACAIMVGGWVCCFLLALLPLVGISSYAKVSICLPMDTETPLALAYIVF
V
VI
VII
rLH-R ILILNVVAFVVICACYIRIYFAVQNPELTAPNKDTKIAKKMAILIFTDFYCMAPISFFAISAAFKVPLITVTNSKILLVLFYPVNSCANPFLYAIFTKAFQRDFLLLSRFGCCKRRAEL
mLH-R ILILNAVAFVVICACYVRIYFAVQNPELTAPNKDTKIAKKMAILIFTDFTCMAPISFFAISAAFKVPLITVTNSKVLLVLFYPVNSCANPFLYAVFTKAFQRDFFLLSRFGCCKHRAEL
pLH-R ILILNVVAFIIICACYIKIYFAVRNPELMATNKDTKIAKKMAVLIFTDFTCMAPISFFAISAALKVPLITVTNSKVLLVLFYPINSCANPFLYAIFTKAFRRDFFLLSKSGCCKHQAEL
hLH-R ILILNVVAFFIICACYIKIYFAVRNPELMATNKDTKIAKKMAILIFTDFTCMAPISFFAISAAFKVPLITVTNSKVLLVLFYPINSCANPFLYAIFTKTFQRDFFLLLSKFGCCKRRAEL
rFSH-R LLVLNVLAFVVICGCYTHIYLTVRNPTIVSSSSDTKIAKRMATLIFTDFLCMAPISFFAISASLKVPLITVSKAKILLVLFYPINSCANPFLYAIFTKNFRRDFFILLSKFGCYEMQAQI
hFSH-R LLVLNVLAFVVICGCYIHIYLTVRNPNIVSSSSDTRIAKRMAMLIFTDFLCMAPISFFAISASLKVPLITVSKAK LVLFHPINSCANPFLYAIFTKNFRRDFFILLSKCGCYEMQAQI
hTSH-R VLTLNIVAFVIVCCCYVKIYITVRNPQYNPGDKDTKIAKRMAVLIFTDFICMAPISFYALSAILNKPLITVSNSKILLVLFYPLNSCANPFLYAIFTKAFQRDVFILLSKFGICKRQAQA
rLH-R YRRKEFSAYTSNCKNGFPGSSKPSQATLKLSTVHCQ QPIPPR A LTH
mLH-R YRRKEFSACTFNSKNGFPRSSKPSQAALKLSIVHCQQPTPPRVLIQ
pLH-R YRRKDFSAY CKNGFTGSNKPSRSTLKLTTLQCQYSTVMDK TCYKDC
hLH-R YRRKDFSAYTSNCKNGFTGSNKPSQSTLKLSTLHCQGTALLDK TRYTEC
rFSH-R YRTETSSATHNFHARKSHCSSAPRVTNS YVLVPLNHSSQN
hFSH-R YRTETSSTVHNTHPRNGHCSSAPRVTSGSTYILVPLSHLAQN
hTSH-R YRGQRVPPKNS TDIQVCKVTHDMRQGLHNMEDVYELIEKSHLTPKKQGQISEEYMQTVL

tected in detergent extracts of the transfected cells (99). Native LH receptor and a chimera containing the *C*-terminal domain of the β_2-adrenergic receptor were transported to the surface of these cells. Only chimeric receptors containing the extracellular domain of the LH receptor were capable of binding [^{125}I]hCG. A solubilized chimera consisting of the LH receptor extracellular domain and β_2-adrenergic receptor transmembrane domain could bind both hCG and β-adrenergic ligands. The LH receptor transmembrane domain could not bind β-adrenergic ligands.

Construction of chimeric receptor molecules containing portions of the LH, FSH, and TSH receptor extracellular domains is currently in progress to determine the determinants responsible for recognition of the different ligands. Substitution of TSH receptor residues 82–170 and 260–360 (residues 115–203 and 295–305, respectively, in Fig. 12) for the corresponding regions of the LH receptor eliminated binding to hCG (215). Substitution of residues 170–260 (residues 203–295, Fig. 12) resulted in a chimera that could bind both hCG and TSH, although the affinity of the chimeric receptor for each hormone was a tenth that of each native receptor for its respective ligand. Expression of truncated LH receptors indicated that leucine-rich repeats 1–8 could bind hCG with an affinity similar to that of the native receptor (216). Substitution of the *N*-terminal six leucine-rich repeats of the LH receptor for the corresponding regions of the FSH receptor resulted in a chimeric receptor that could bind hCG and stimulate cAMP accumulation when expressed in human embryonic kidney 293 cells. Conversely, substitution of this region on the LH receptor by the corresponding region of the FSH receptor abolished hCG binding but did not confer FSH binding. Leucine rich repeats 1–11 had to be substituted to enable a chimeric LH/FSH receptor to bind FSH and stimulate cAMP production.

A role for the carbohydrate in the functioning of the LH receptor is not known. When site-directed mutagenesis was used to eliminate *N*-glycosylation sites of the TSH receptor, two of the six resulted in abolishment or reduction of TSH binding, although the remainder had no effect on TSH binding (217). Neither of the two glycosylation sites that affect TSH binding is present in LH or FSH receptors. Removal of carbohydrate from the rat LH receptor by peptide *N*-glycanase digestion had no effect on the binding of hCG. Two products of enzymatic deglycosylation of the receptor were observed by SDS polyacrylamide gel electrophoresis followed by transfer to nitrocellulose and ligand blotting. The native receptor migrated with a M_r of 90,000, and the deglycosylated receptor forms migrated at M_r 67,000 and M_r 62,000. Digestion of hormone–receptor complexes removed oligosaccharide from the receptor and from both subunits of hCG, suggesting that all the oligosaccharides faced outward from the hormone–receptor interface.

The transmembrane domain contains loops exposed to the cytoplasm, which may be important in receptor function. One of the receptors that is also linked to G protein is the β_2-adrenergic receptor. Recently, the sites of interaction of this receptor with G protein were localized to the third cytoplasmic loop and a portion of the cytoplasmic tail close to the cell membrane (219). The amino acid sequences of these regions are not conserved between the β_2-adrenergic receptor and the LH receptor, and conversion of lysines 541, 544, and 547 (Lys-653, -656, and -659, respectively, in Fig. 12) had no effect on G protein coupling (220). Membrane trafficking was affected, as most of the mutant receptor remained inside the cell.

All LH receptors contain a carboxy-terminal domain that extends into the cell cytoplasm and may be a further site for the regulation of hormone–receptor function, as it contains potential phosphorylation sites. Two potential protein kinase C phosphorylation sites have been identified, along with a third in the third cytoplasmic loop of the transmembrane domain (194). In other G-protein-linked receptors, phosphorylation of the receptor leads to uncoupling of the receptor from G protein and subsequent systems (221). It is interesting to speculate that one mechanism for the regulation of LH at the target cell could be phosphorylation of the receptor, induced by the phosphorylating enzymes stimulated by the hormone receptor complex. The phosphorylated receptor would be ineffective in stimulating further cAMP production, shutting off the initiating signal for biological activity.

Mutations in the cytoplasmic *C*-terminal tail of the rat LH receptor suggested that residues 616–631 (residues 728–742, Fig. 12) were important for membrane trafficking, as mutants lacking the last *C*-terminal 58 residues were not expressed on the plasma membrane, and those lacking the last 43 and 21 amino acid residues were expressed on the plasma membrane when transfected in human kidney 293 cells (211). The amount of cAMP stimulated by hCG binding to mutant LH receptors was double that stimulated by hCG binding to full-length LH receptor even though the same amount of hCG was bound by each cell type. Furthermore, the mutant receptors were internalized more rapidly than the full-length receptor. Subsequently, clonal 293 cells derived from transiently transfected cells were compared. Cells transfected with wild-type LH receptor expressed three to four times more receptor than those cells expressing a mutant LH receptor lacking the *C*-terminal 48 amino acid residues (222). However, the stimulation of cAMP accumulation in response to hCG binding in cells with the mutant receptor was three times greater than that in cells expressing the wild-type receptor. In addition, hCG-induced uncoupling of the cAMP response was reduced, indicating a role for the *C* terminus in this phenomenon.

In general, throughout their sequences the rat LH receptor and porcine LH receptor exhibit 84% homology. The major difference in the length of the two receptors is accounted for by a 24-amino-acid insert in the extracellular portion of the rat LH receptor compared to the porcine LH receptor. The most homologous region is the transmembrane portion, and the least similar region is the intracellular domain. The human LH receptor is overall 85% identical to the rat LH receptor and 87% identical to the porcine LH receptor (223). Despite the high degree of homology between the human and rat LH receptors, the human LH receptor has a high degree of species specificity, binding hLH and hCG but not eLH, eCG, rLH, or oLH (205). The rat and porcine LH receptors bind all of these hormones.

Also isolated from the porcine testis cDNA library were shorter forms of the LH receptor cDNA (194). These variants contained the proposed extracellular region but were missing either the transmembrane domains or intracellular region. If the pig LH receptor gene has the same structure as the rat LH receptor, then the truncated versions appear to have arisen by alternative splicing that deleted whole exons or splicing at alternative sites within an exon (213). It is currently not known what role these variants may have; however, they account for 40% of the cDNA clones isolated from the pig (194) and have been detected in rat (213) and human ovary (223) as well as in rat testis. It is interesting to speculate that the "soluble" truncated receptor variants may account for the presence of an "LH receptor binding inhibitor" first reported several years ago by our laboratory (214). Autolysis of the LH receptor has been reported converting the 80-kD form to a 46-kD form as detected on SDS gels (224).

FSH Receptor

The receptor for FSH has been studied in both males and females. The major location for FSH receptor in males is the seminiferous tubule, specifically on Sertoli cells (225). In females the granulosa cell FSH receptor has been extensively studied (226). In both sexes, the action of FSH through its receptor is mediated through the cAMP second messenger system, induced by adenylate cyclase and G protein.

The FSH receptor has been cloned from rat (198), human (227), mouse (207), and frog (208) cDNA libraries. It possesses the same large extracellular domain, seven transmembrane helices, and cytoplasmic tail structure as the LH receptor (Fig. 12). The extracellular domain consists of 14 leucine-rich repeats, similar to those described for the LH receptor (195). Leucine-rich repeats 1–11 from the FSH receptor were required to create a chimeric LH/FSH receptor that could respond to FSH stimulation (216). There are three *N*-glycosylation sites on the extracellular domain of the rat FSH receptor and four in the human FSH receptor. The FSH receptor has not been as extensively investigated as the LH receptor, but this, in part, reflects the absence of readily available FSH preparations for use as ligand in binding studies.

BIOSYNTHESIS OF THE GONADOTROPINS

Genomic Control

A discussion of our current knowledge of the major elements of the genomic control of biosynthesis of the gonadotropins was included in the section on the genetic relationships of the subunits (vide supra).

Cotranslational Events

Once the genetic controls of the pituitary hormones initiate transcription of the required mRNA, protein translation occurs on the polysomes bound to the rough endoplasmic reticulum (RER). The completed linear subunit from this synthetic step carries a "signal peptide" and has no formed disulfide bonds. The signal peptide (also called the leader sequence) at the *N* terminus of the subunit precursor is characteristic of the particular subunit. For example, the LH/CG β subunit prehormone has a 20-amino-acid residue leader sequence that is highly homologous throughout the known mammalian species (Fig. 2). The leader sequence on salmon gonadotropic hormone β subunit has 23 residues but still maintains a considerable homology. The other known leader sequences from the lower vertebrates include the chicken (228) and turkey, which have exceptionally long leader sequences (39 residues, Fig. 2). The α subunits currently known all have a 24-residue leader sequence (Fig. 1), again with a high homology among the species. The TSHβ signal peptide for those known is comprised of 20 residues (not shown). The known FSHβ leader sequences have 18 residues for the known cases (Fig. 2), but these have sometimes been reported as 19 or 20 residues because of uncertainties about the exact cleavage point of the signal protease, a confusion that arises from some *N*-terminal heterogeneity of the isolated gene products, in the authors' opinion. The correct cleavage site in all probability will be shown to be between cysteine and asparagine, arginine, or histidine (see Fig. 2 for the FSHβ subunit leader sequences). This requires an 18-residue leader sequence.

The signal peptide, which may range from 15 to 40 amino acid residues, characteristically has a very hydrophobic cluster of amino acids 5 to 20 residues toward the *N* terminus from the site of cleavage (processing) by the signal peptidase. This step of the protein processing probably occurs *cotranslationally* at about the time the *C*-terminal portion of the peptide chain coded by the mRNA is being completed. Thus, the signal peptide removal marks the removal of the completed protein chain from the ribosomes and release of the protein into the cisternal space of RER.

In the comments that follow, the reader is alerted to the fact that the processes related to glycosylation have been studied to only a limited degree for the glycoprotein hormones; thus, much of what we will propose is based on analogy to other systems. The reasons for this are twofold. First, gonadotropes or thyrotropes of the pituitary are not readily obtained for study. Second, there are few suitable cell lines that provide reasonable systems to study this glycosylation. In this respect, those that have received the most extensive study are trophoblast-derived cell lines, particularly the JAR or BeWo human choriocarcinoma cell lines, originally isolated by Dr. Roland Patillo of the Medical College of Wisconsin. The JAR cell line, for example, has been through several hundred passages and maintained an essentially constant production of hCG throughout. This property is important for their utility to study biosynthesis. However, hCG is somewhat unusual among the glycoprotein hormones in that, besides an extra *N*-linked glycosylation site on the β subunit, it also has *O*-linked glycosylation sites on the *C* terminus (vide supra). This *O*-linked glycosylation may be characteristic among all the chorionic gonadotropins. However, we have shown it not to be a unique feature, since equine pituitary LH also has this *C*-terminal extension on the β subunit, and, as in the chorionic gonadotropins, it is *O*-glycosylated. (See structural summaries above.)

The signal peptide removal in the RER is probably involved in the transfer mechanism from the RER cisternae along the membrane to the Golgi apparatus (GA), a cellular organelle about which we will say more below. This signal peptide removal is probably the final step in the cotranslational processing that occurs in the RER. However, for the glycoprotein hormones, there is another important cotranslational event (*N*-glycosylation) that also occurs in the RER. *N*-Glycosylation takes place at two sites on the α subunit and one or two sites on the β subunit. (See the diagrammatic summary above in Fig. 7.) *O*-Glycosylation, if it occurs, happens later as a post-translation event in the Golgi apparatus.

N-Glycosylation (see Fig. 9 summary) is mediated through a "high-mannose" dolichol phosphate intermediate, enzymatically targeted to specific *N*-glycosylation sites. Not all sites are glycosylated in those proteins that contain this structural feature, but in the glycoprotein hormones all potential *N*-glycosylation sites are usually *N*-glycosylated. Exceptions include partial glycosylation of some FSHβ subunits. In the case of the FSHβ subunit, partial glycosylation of recombinant bFSHβ has been reported (229). We have observed partial glycosylation of a preparation of oFSH in which only one of the two potential glycosylation sites was glycosylated, giving the preparation an appearance on SDS gels identical to that of oLH, which has only a single *N*-linked glycosylation site (unpublished). In eFSHβ, evidence during amino acid sequence determination revealed that the first *N*-glycosylation site was only partially glycosylated (unpublished).

The carbohydrate moiety transferred from the dolichol phosphate intermediate has the general composition glucose$_3$ mannose$_9$ *N*-acetylglucosamine$_2$. The two *N*-acetylglucosamine residues form the link to the asparagine amide nitrogen in the *N*-glycosylation site (steps 1–3, Fig. 9). On the nonreducing end of this characteristic disaccharide attachment to the asparagine nitrogen amide is a mannose residue linked through position 1 to position 4 of the last *N*-acetylglucosamine residue. This mannose residue, in turn, is linked (through positions 3 and 6) to two additional mannose residues. This generates a two-armed branch point in the carbohydrate that generates a "biantennary" structure (see diagram Fig. 9 above). In some of the more complex carbohydrate structures associated with the glycoprotein hormones, a "triantennary" branching is required (see diagrammatic examples above). Whether a biantennary or triantennary carbohydrate will be produced in the "mature" glycoprotein will be determined in the Golgi apparatus, but a structure that provides for this possibility is contained in the high-mannose form or precursor form generated in the RER. Characteristically the three glucose residues in a linear array are attached to the longest mannose chain on one arm of the triantennary high-mannose precursor from dolichol phosphate. While the glycoprotein is still in the RER the three glucose residues are removed; α-glucosidase I removes the terminal glucose residue, then α-glucosidase II removes the remaining two glucose residues. No mature glycoproteins from vertebrates contain glucose in their carbohydrate moiety with the exception of the recently reported case of inhibin (230). Also in the RER, specific glycosidases remove either none, one, or three of the nine mannose residues added from the dolichol phosphate precursor (see review, ref. 231).

Posttranslational Events (Schematically Summarized in Fig. 13)

A third major development that occurs in the RER is the formation of disulfide bonds in the α and β subunits. Ruddon and colleagues have demonstrated that formation of all the α subunit disulfide bonds and formation of most of the β subunit disulfide bonds precedes subunit association. No intermediate, partially folded forms of the α subunit have been detected (156). This is consistent with the Pierce–Bahl (26,27) model for α subunit disulfides in which most of the disulfide bonds stabilize local interactions in either the *N*-terminal domain (11–35 and 14–36) or the *C*-terminal domain (63–91 and 86–88) and, therefore, probably form cotranslationally. Only one disulfide bond (32–64) connects these two domains.

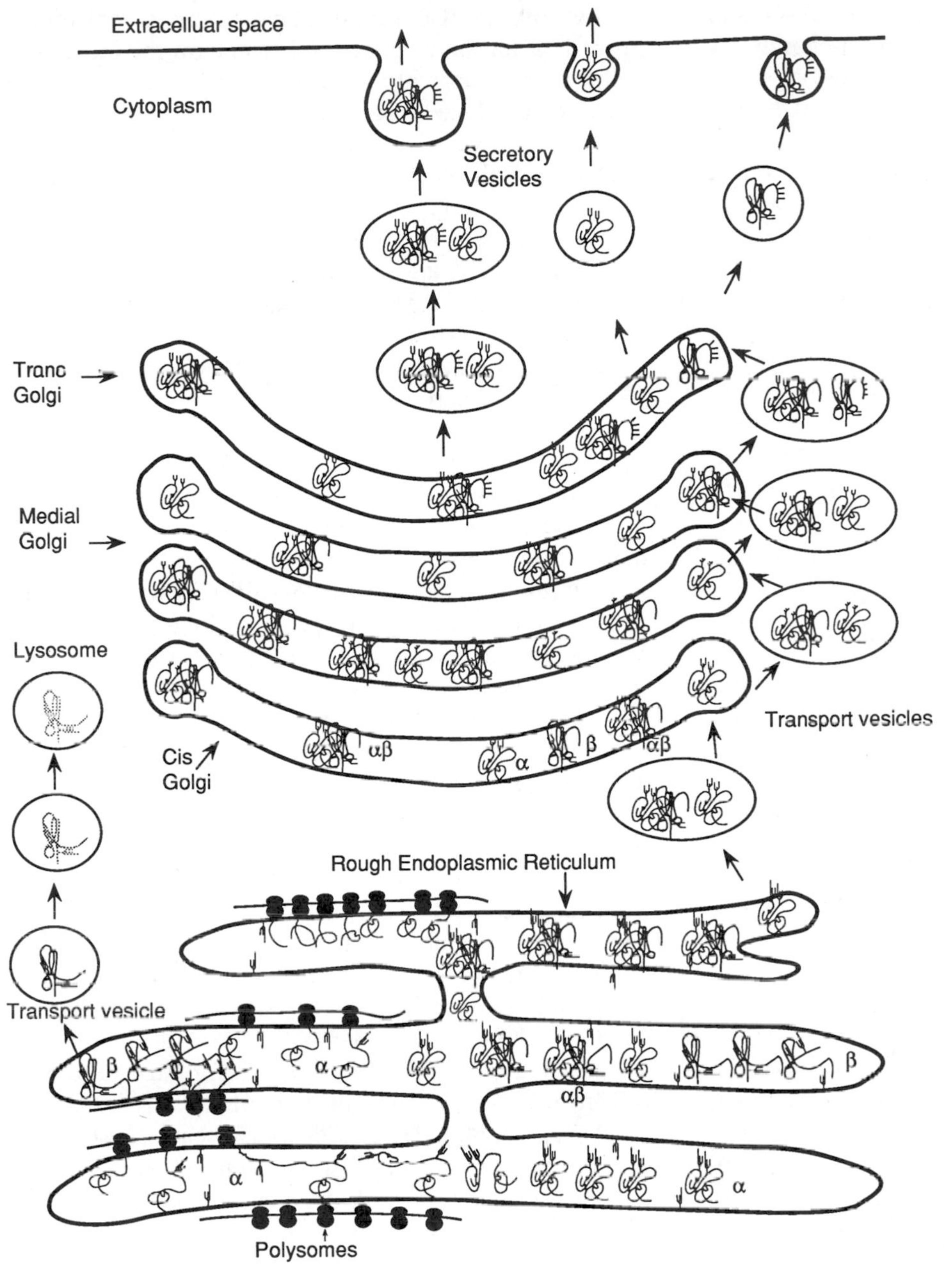

FIG. 13. Biosynthetic pathway for glycoprotein hormones. This illustrates the constitutive pathway, since most of the available data have been obtained from cell lines that make hCG in which only the constitutive secretory pathway is operative. The subunits are synthesized in the rough endoplasmic reticulum, where *N*-glycosylation occurs cotranslationally. Folding of the α subunit probably occurs cotranslationally as well. Folding of the β subunit occurs posttranslationally and appears to be completed after association with the α subunit. Improperly or partially folded β subunit is retained by the rough ER and eventually shunted to lysosomes, where it is degraded. Hormone dimer, properly folded free β subunit, and free α subunit are transferred to the Golgi, where their oligosaccharides are processed before secretion.

In contrast, the Ward–Bahl model for β subunit disulfides proposes that four of the six disulfide bonds connect Cys residues that are in opposite halves of the subunit (9–90, 23–72, 26–100, and 34–88), whereas only two disulfide bonds stabilize local regions of the subunit (38–57 and 93–100) (28,29).

The combination of the α and β subunits is initiated in the RER with the high-mannose forms of the subunits. It is not yet clear whether all of the β subunit disulfide bonds are formed here or if they are completed in the Golgi. Ruddon and co-workers (156) have detected discrete intermediates in this process. The first of these, designated pβ1, has two disulfide bonds, 34–88 and 38–57, formed. The next detectable form, designated pβ2-free, results from a rate-limiting folding process that results in formation of disulfides 23–72 and 9–90. Following formation of disulfide bond 93–100, the intermediate, pβ2-combined, is associated with the α subunit. Formation of the last disulfide bond, 26–110, apparently takes place following association with the α subunit (60). This observation is supported by experiments involving site-directed mutagenesis of hCGβ in which residues 101–145 were deleted, yet the mutant β subunit still associated with an α subunit (232). On the other hand, replacement of cysteines 26 and 100 with alanine resulted in a β subunit mutant with reduced ability to associate with α subunit (233). From these folding data Ruddon and colleagues proposed that residues 1–90 comprise one folding domain and that the remaining residues of the *C* terminus where the last two disulfide bonds are formed comprise a second folding domain (60).

The final step in the RER processing of the glycoprotein hormone subunit is probably one of loading (via the signal peptidase and its postulated chain of events) into a transport vesicle involved in the movement of the partially processed "high-mannose" carbohydrate-bearing subunit. Disulfide bond formation begins in the RER cisternae. For the α it is completed in the RER, but at least the final disulfide closures on the β may possibly be accomplished in the Golgi along with the final posttranslational processing of the carbohydrate moieties to their several complex, mature forms. (The sequence of events at this point is somewhat conjectural. See Fig. 13.) The putative RER transport vesicle delivery of the α–β precursor to the Golgi has not been studied in the glycoprotein hormone system but is drawn from electron microscopy studies in other cell types.

It is at this point in the secretory pathway that pituitary β subunits diverge from CGβ: hCG, hCGα, and hCGβ are secreted by the placenta (234,235), by cultured choriocarcinoma cells (234), and by cells into which the hCGβ gene has been transfected (43). For the remainder of the β subunits it has been demonstrated that without cotransfection with α subunit the products of transfected genes for these β subunits do not appear in the medium and are eventually degraded (43,100,236). Two mechanisms have been proposed to explain retention of β subunit by the rough ER. The first is that not all β subunits fold properly, and these improperly folded proteins are screened by the ER and retained (237). Partially folded β subunits that do not associate with α subunit have been detected (156). Evidence for such a mechanism has been reported in pituitaries of thyroidectomized mice, which produce more β subunit and less α subunit than pituitaries of intact animals (238). The excess β subunit ends up in the intracisternal granules that develop in the rough ER and appear to be transformed into lysosomes (Fig. 13) in which the β subunits are degraded (239). An alternative mechanism suggests that the β subunit *C*-terminal residues are responsible for retention of free β subunit. The basis for this possibility results from the finding that the sequences of hLH and hTSH β subunits as predicted from their respective cDNAs are as much as six or seven residues longer than that found on the mature protein by conventional protein sequencing methods. (Figure 2 presents the complete cDNA-predicted sequences.) Possibly these residues are responsible for β subunit retention by the ER. Support for this alternative was recently provided when the *C*-terminal extension of hCGβ was attached to hFSHβ and the resulting chimeric protein was found to be secreted as efficiently as hCGβ when transfected into CHO cells alone (66).

However the α–β dimeric precursor of the glycoprotein hormones may get from the RER to the Golgi, it is in the Golgi that a variety of posttranslational events occur that have an important bearing on the biochemical and physiological properties of the mature protein hormone produced (Fig. 13).

The Golgi complex is a cellular organelle that is best examined at the electron microscope. It is a structure in close juxtaposition with the nucleus. This organelle or complex appears to be composed of parallel, flattened saccules, vesicles, and vacuoles. The portion nearest the nucleus is designated the *cis* Golgi network, and it is here the protein from the RER enters the Golgi, as followed by pulse-chase labeling (240). Proteins next enter the Golgi stacks, where processing of oligosaccharides continues. This portion of the Golgi consists of at least three compartments, *cis,* medial, and *trans.* Finally proteins enter the *trans*-Golgi network, where they are distributed to granules that will carry them to their ultimate destinations.

Thus, the high-mannose form (nine, eight, or six mannose residues at this point) enters the Golgi for posttranslational processing. In the *cis* Golgi, α-1,2-mannosidase may remove an additional three mannose residues, resulting in the structure that is the substrate for *N*-acetylglucosamine transferase I, which adds *N*-acetylglucosamine. This structure can be further processed to yield a single branched sulfated structure or go on to be processed into biantennary or triantennary oligosaccharide. The deciding factor is whether the pituitary enzyme *N*-acetylgalactosamine transferase adds *N*-acetylgalactosamine or not. This enzyme recognizes the peptide sequence -Pro-Xaa-Arg/Lys-, which is present in the α subunit (residues 44–46, -Pro-Ala/Leu-Arg-), in LHβ and CGβ (residues 3–6, -Pro-Ala-Arg-), but not in FSHβ nor TSHβ (241). Glycosylation of the α subunit is influenced by the β subunit with which it is associated (155,172,173,242). Therefore, it has been suggested that the β subunit must mask the recognition site on the α subunit. However, only hFSH fits neatly into this model. Only 7% of the oligosaccharides isolated from hFSH have been found to be sulfated (169), but this represents the low end of the range of sulfated oligosaccharides attached to FSH (13% of bFSH oligosaccharides and 40% of those of oFSH are sulfated). Furthermore, TSHβ, which also lacks the recognition sequence for *N*-acetylgalactosamine transferase, possesses 64–80% sulfated oligosaccharides. Although the *N*-acetylgalactosamine transferase recognition sequence has proved useful in predicting the presence of sulfated oligosaccharides in glycoproteins (241), the relative importance of the α and β subunits for determining the activity of *N*-acetylgalactosamine transferase in glycoprotein hormone biosynthesis remains to be established.

LHβ and CGβ possess the *N*-acetylgalactosamine transferase recognition sequence, so both LH and CG oligosaccharides are potentially capable of being modified by *N*-acetylgalactosamine, if it is present. The enzyme has been found in the pituitary gland of various species, but not in human placenta (243). If *N*-acetylgalactosamine is present and the glycoprotein substrate possesses the recognition sequence -Pro-Xaa-Arg/Lys-, the enzyme may add *N*-acetylgalactosamine, and the monosulfated structure will result. If not, then two more mannose residues are removed. The resulting oligosaccharide may be galactosylated and processed as monosialylated oligosaccharide or processed further by addition of a second *N*-acetylglucosamine. The latter structure is the precursor of triantennary sialylated oligosaccharides as well as biantennary sialylated, or hybrid sulfated-sialylated, or bisulfated oligosaccharides.

The glycoprotein hormone subunits are then moved to the "medial Golgi" for addition of specific sugars by specific glycosyltransferases. The substrates for these sugar transferases are synthesized in the cytoplasm (e.g., UDP-galactose, UDP-*N*-acetylglucosamine, UDP-*N*-acetylgalactosamine, GDP-fucose, and the sulfate donor, 3′-phosphoadenosine-5′-phosphosulfate, or PAPS) or in the nucleus (CMP-neuraminic acid). There are selective transport proteins that facilitate each of these substrates' movement into the Golgi, where the glycosyltransferases bring about the buildup of hybrid intermediate forms of the glycosylated moieties on the subunits. (For a review of the topography of glycosylation, see Hirschberg and Snider, ref. 244.) The "hybrid" intermediates in the formation of the carbohydrate moieties of the glycoprotein hormones are finally processed to the mature secreted form of the carbohydrate in the "*trans* Golgi." This is designated the "complex" carbohydrate moiety after addition of *N*-acetylglucosmaine or -galactosamine, galactose, *N*-acetylneuraminic acid (also called sialic acid), fucose, or sulfate groups. The hCG-producing cells of the human chorion lack the enzyme system sulfotransferase in their Golgi apparatus for the addition of sulfate to the carbohydrate (245).

In the pituitary there is an *N*-acetylgalactosamine transferase in the Golgi apparatus that adds *N*-acetylgalactosamine to the peripheral ends of the carbohydrate moieties (243). The sulfation in the pituitary glycoprotein hormones is on the 4 position of these residues. Thus, the lack of sulfation in the human chorionic gonadotropin is a consequence of the absence of these two relatively unique transferases for PAPS and *N*-acetylgalactosamine. This leads to a heavier concentration of neuraminic acid termini on the hCG carbohydrate compared to the carbohydrate on pituitary glycoprotein hormones. This, in turn, is a factor in the longer in vivo half-life of hCG compared to the pituitary LH, TSH, or FSH. The sulfated oligosaccharides determine the short half-lives of pituitary hormones possessing these carbohydrates because there is a liver receptor, similar to the asialoglycoprotein receptor, that clears sulfated glycoproteins (179). This rapid clearing of the gonadotropins may contribute to the pulsatile pattern of their circulating levels. The longer half-life of hCG leads to a much longer presentation of it to the LH/CG receptor than is the case for LH. Moreover, the structural differences in LH and CG lead to a much longer binding of CG to the receptor (i.e., a much slower off rate) than the binding time of LH on the receptor (246,247). Thus, although CG and LH interact with the same receptor, their net physiological (or pharmacological) effects may be considerably different.

In the conversion of the carbohydrate moieties on the glycoprotein hormone subunits from the high-mannose type to the mature complex type, there are several degrees of structural buildup possible. Thus, it is possible to have some biantennary structures with two, one, or no sulfate groups; where there is no sulfate group, it is possible that a neuraminic acid and galactose residue will complete the buildup of the antennary branch. In a brilliant series Baenziger and colleagues have studied the sulfate labeling patterns and possible combinations to produce the complex carbohydrate structural buildup that leads to a complex and heterogeneous set of carbohydrate moieties on LH, FSH, TSH, and CG. The first three were studied in bovine, ovine, and human synthetic systems, and the CG in human cell systems. These studies culminated in two outstanding reports (169,170). Their extensive series of studies was reviewed comprehensively (148), and this review is recommended for a detailed statement of the structures and diversity (heterogeneity) encountered in the carbohydrate portion of these hormones.

After processing the carbohydrate of the α–β dimer in the Golgi to the several forms of complex carbohydrate (mature hormone), the hormone is transported to storage vacuoles in the cytoplasm (pituitary cells) or directly to the cellular exterior (human chorion cells). The degree of sulfation among the pituitary hormones varies widely depending on the species of the pituitary cell donor and the type of hormone (FSH, LH, or TSH). It has been postulated that sulfation may be involved with storage and secretion of these pituitary hormones (148). There is as yet no experimental support for this concept. In fact, a recent study involving pulse-labeling of bLH and free α in bovine pituitary primary cultures indicated that although both bLH and free α were sulfated, free α was secreted exclusively by the constitutive pathway, whereas bLH was secreted both constitutively as well as by the regulatory pathway (248).

In the case of hCG, compared to the human pituitary glycoprotein hormones only the latter are sulfated (to widely varying degrees). It should be noted that this does not hold for equine chorionic gonadotropin (eCG), for which our laboratory has been able to detect sulfation both in eCG and the eFSH or eLH. We have not examined eTSH. Thus, between species marked differences in the degree and form of carbohydrate posttranslational processing are found. The question of the heterogeneity of these carbohydrate forms as well as protein heterogeneity has been extensively examined in a monograph edited by Keel and Grotjan (249).

There are multiple forms of the glycoprotein hormones that are for the most part attributable to the degree of processing of the carbohydrate during biosynthesis. These forms have been designated in a variety of ways, but usually as "isoforms" of the particular hormone. The designation "isohormones" has also been used. The relative concentration of these isoforms in the serum has been shown to correlate with physiological status of the individual in the case of all the pituitary hormones. See, for example, the review of the FSH isoforms (75). It is beyond the scope of the present chapter to consider the physiological and structural correlation of these isoforms, although some reference to the physiological parameters will be noted in other chapters of the text.

As summarized above, the biosynthesis of the glycoprotein hormones involves all the complexities of the protein biosynthetic mechanisms provided in nature from the genomic transcription, mRNA translation, and cotranslational processing to the final posttranslational processing. The numerous intermediates in the posttranslational processing in the Golgi apparatus, several of which may become final forms of the complex carbohydrate moieties, produces a significant heterogeneity in the secreted hormone. This heterogeneity is reflected in several isoforms of that particular glycoprotein hormone. These isoforms, to a degree, also correlate with physiological state of the individual domestic animal or person. Thus, the protein biosynthesis of glycoprotein hormones is a very complex process subject to many physiological controls, few of which are fully understood.

ASSAY OF GONADOTROPINS

The assay of the gonadotropins was originally based on intact animal assays or hypophysectomized animals. Endpoints for the assay were gonad size (ovarian or testicular weight, for example) or accessory sex tissue growth (prostate weight, seminal vesicle weight). As radioisotopes became available, variations on these assays were devised (e.g., ^{32}P-labeled phosphate incorporation into these tissues). The intact animal assays were never very precise; thus, careful statistics were required, which usually required significant numbers of animals. That in turn elevated the cost and inconvenience of such assays. As a result the current competitive binding assays and in vitro assays have largely supplanted intact animal assays. For the gonadotropins the two types of assays most popular are radioimmunoassays and radioligand assays. Both types of assay are very sensitive and very precise. Both require a labeled hormone (usually ^{125}I or ^{131}I is used for the label of the purified gonadotropin to be assayed). This labeled hormone is then added to a binding system: in the case of the radioimmunoassay this is a specific antibody for the hormone antigen; in the case of the radioligand assay the binding system is a hormone receptor preparation. The binding system is allocated to a series of matched tubes, to which is then added increasing concentrations of the unknown test solution containing the unlabeled hormone to be measured. After appropriate incubation times (which vary according to the requirements of the particular assay), the bound form is separated from the unbound hormone. The amount of labeled hormone bound is then determined for each tube, and a plot of the competitive binding curve is made, which is compared with a reference curve run in the same way against a reference standard of unlabeled hormone. From this comparison a calculation of the unknown hormone concentration in the original test solution can be made after due allowance for the dilutions involved. Such assays are capable of both high sensitivity and precision and lend themselves to semiautomation and application to many samples.

The radioimmunoassay method is subject to the availability of a suitably specific antibody for the given assay, a highly purified hormone for labeling, and availability of a suitably pure reference preparation (which need not be pure hormone, simply free of interfering hormone) for which an exact potency is known. A limitation of the radioimmunoassay method is inherent in the nature of the antigen–antibody reaction. Antibodies characteristically are directed against a specific portion of the structure of the hormone antigen (called the epitope). Thus, the response to native hormone may be the same as to a denatured or partially degraded hormone. In most physiological studies or clinical studies, such denatured or degraded hormone is not a problem, but it should always be considered in the design of experiments.

In the case of the radioligand assays one effectively substitutes a biologically derived receptor preparation for the antibody in the radioimmunoassay system to obtain the hormone specificity. In this case it is specific for that portion of the hormone that interacts with the receptor, including the three-dimensional geometry for this interaction. This argues for the biological activity of the hormone as part of the measurement being made. Thus, for experimental purposes the radioligand assays have greater potential. For example, in our own studies we developed the chicken receptor system for FSH to discriminate the intrinsic FSH activity in the equine LH and CG in a system insensitive to the LH (250).

Competitive binding assays are not the only type of assay that exhibit such sensitivity. An *in vitro* assay for FSH that measures the conversion of androstenedione to estrogen has been described (192). Since the enzyme required for this conversion is an aromatase, the assay is designated the aromatase bioassay for FSH. This assay is capable of slightly greater sensitivity than the radioligand assay (251).

Other assay variants have been developed that substitute other means of labeling for the radioactivity in a radioimmunoassay. These variants can take the form of a chromophore (e.g., as in certain pregnancy tests for hCG in urine) or a second label, such as a biotin-labeled antibody, to sensitize the system to avidin. It will not be our purpose to review all the variants possible but to make the reader aware that there are many bioassay alternatives possible. We have previously reviewed several of these as well as the reference hormone preparations available (1).

REFERENCES

1. Ward DN, Bousfield GR, Moore KH. Gonadotropins. In: Cupps PT, eds. *Reproduction in Domestic Animals.* San Diego: Academic Press; 1991:25–80.
2. Pierce JG. Gonadotropins: Chemistry and biosynthesis. In: Knobil E, Neill JD, eds. *The Physiology of Reproduction.* New York: Raven Press; 1988:1335–1348.
3. Li CH, Starman B. Molecular weight of sheep pituitary interstitial cell-stimulating hormone. *Nature* 1964;202:291–292.
4. Ward DN, Fujino M, Lamkin WM. Evidence for two carbohydrate moieties in ovine luteinizing hormone (LH). *Fed Proc* 1966;25:348.
5. Papkoff H, Samy TSA. Isolation and partial characterization of the polypeptide chains of ovine interstitial cell-stimulating hormone. *Biochim Biophys Acta* 1967;147:175–177.
6. DeLaLlosa P, Jutisz M. Reversible dissociation into subunits and biological activity of ovine luteinizing hormone. *Biochim Biophys Acta* 1969;181:426–436.
7. Lamkin WM, Fujino M, Mayfield JD, Holcomb GN, Ward DN. Separation of the subunits of ovine luteinizing hormone by a chromatographic procedure and comparison with a countercurrent distribution procedure. *Biochim Biophys Acta* 1970; 214:290–298.
8. Swaminathan N, Bahl OP. Dissociation and recombination of the subunits of human chorionic gonadotropin. *Biochem Biophys Res Commun* 1970;40:422–427.
9. Morgan FJ, Canfield RE. Nature of the subunits of human chorionic gonadotropin. *Endocrinology* 1971;88:1045–1053.
10. Liao T-H, Pierce JG. The presence of a common type of subunit in bovine thyroid-stimulating and luteinizing hormones. *J Biol Chem* 1970;245:3275–3281.
11. Ward DN, Sweeney CM, Holcomb GN, Lamkin WN, Fujino M. Recent studies on the structure of ovine luteinizing hormone. In: Gual C, ed. *Progress in Endocrinology. Proceedings of the 3rd International Congress of Endocrinology.* Amsterdam: Excerpta Medica; 1969:385–393.
12. Pierce JG, Liao T-H, Howard SM, Shome B, Cornell JS. Recent studies on the chemistry of TSH. *Recent Prog Horm Res* 1971;27:165–212.
13. Liu W-K, Ward DN. The purification and chemistry of pituitary glycoprotein hormones. *Pharmacol Ther* 1975;1:545–570.
14. Ward DN, Bousfield GR, Gordon WL, Sugino H, ed. Chemistry of the Peptide Components of Glycoprotein Hormones. In: Keel BA, Grotjans HE Jr, eds. *Microheterogeneity of Glycoprotein Hormones.* Boca Raton, FL: CRC Press; 1989:1–21.
15. Fiddes JC, Talmadge K. Structure, expression and evolution of the genes for the human glycoprotein hormones. *Recent Prog Horm Res* 1984;40:43–74.
16. Kourides IA, Gurr JA, Wolf O. The regulation and organization of thyroid stimulating hormone genes. *Recent Prog Horm Res* 1984;40:79–120.
17. Chin WW. Glycoprotein hormone genes. In: Habener JF, ed. *Molecular Cloning of Hormone Genes.* Clifton, NJ: Humana Press; 1987:137–172.
18. Lustbader JW, Birken S, Pileggi NF, et al. Crystallization and characterization of human chorionic gonadotropin in chemically deglycosylated and enzymatically desialylated states. *Biochemistry* 1989;28:9243–9247.
19. Harris DC, Machin KJ, Evin GM, Morgan FJ, Isaacs NW. Preliminary X-ray diffraction analysis of human chorionic gonadotropin. *J Biol Chem* 1989;264:6705–6706.
20. Burzawa-Gerard É, Fontaine Y-A. Formation d'une molécule hybride douée d'une activité gonadotrope sur la grenouille, á partir de la sous-unité a de l'hormone lutéinisante bovine et d'une sous-unité de l'hormone gonadotrope d'un poisson téléostéen. *CR Acad Sci Paris* 1976;282:97–100.
21. Liu WK, Nahm HS, Sweeney CM, Lamkin WM, Baker HN, Ward DN. The primary structure of ovine luteinizing hormone I. The amino acid sequence of the reduced and S-aminoethylated S-subunit (LH-α). *J Biol Chem* 1972;247:4351–4364.
22. Nomura K, Tsunasawa T, Ohmura K, Sakiyama F, Shizume K. Renotropic activity in ovine luteinizing hormone isoform(s). *Endocrinology* 1988;123:700–712.
23. Golos TG, Durning M, Fisher JM. Molecular cloning of the rhesus glycoprotein hormone α-subunit gene. *DNA Cell Biol* 1991;10:367–380.
24. Matzuk MM, Keene JL, Boime I. Site specificity of the chorionic gonadotropin *N*-linked oligosaccharides in signal transduction. *J Biol Chem* 1989;264:2409–2414.
25. Cornell JS, Pierce JG. Studies on the disulfide bonds of glycoprotein hormones. Locations in the α chain based on partial reductions and formation of ^{14}C-labelled *S*-carboxymethyl derivatives. *J Biol Chem* 1974;249:4166–4174.
26. Giudice LC, Pierce JG. Studies on the disulfide bonds of glycoprotein hormones. Formation and properties of 11,35-bis(*S*-alkyl) derivatives of the α subunit. *J Biol Chem* 1979; 254:1164–1169.
27. Mise T, Bahl OP. Assignment of disulfide bonds in the α subunit of human chorionic gonadotropin. *J Biol Chem* 1980; 255:8516–8522.
28. Tsunasawa S, Liu W-K, Burleigh BD, Ward DN. Studies of disulfide bond location in ovine lutropin β subunit. *Biochim Biophys Acta* 1977;492:340–356.
29. Mise T, Bahl OP. Assignment of the disulfide bonds in the β subunit of human chorionic gonadotropin. *J Biol Chem* 1981;256:6587–6592.
30. Giudice LC, Pierce JG. Studies on the disulfide bonds of glycoprotein hormones. Complete reduction and reoxidation of the disulfide bonds of the α subunit of bovine luteinizing hormone. *J Biol Chem* 1976;251:6392–6399.
31. Bousfield GR, Ward DN. Reduction and reoxidation of equine gonadotropin α-subunits. *Endocrinology* 1992;131:2986–2998.
32. Blobel G, Dobberstein B. Transfer of proteins across membranes. II. Reconstruction of functional rough microsomes from heterologous components. *J Cell Biol* 1975;67:852–863.
33. Jackson RC, Blobel G. Posttranslational processing of full-length presecretory proteins with canine pancreatic signal peptidase. *Ann NY Acad Sci* 1980;343:391–404.
34. Begeot M, Hemming FJ, Dubois PM, Combarnous Y, Dubois MP, Aubert ML. Induction of pituitary lactotrope differentiation by luteinizing hormone alpha subunit. *Science* 1984; 226:566–568.
35. Blithe DL, Richards RG, Skarulis MC. Free alpha molecules from pregnancy stimulate secretion of prolactin from human decidual cells: A novel function for free alpha in pregnancy. *Endocrinology* 1991;129:2257–2259.
36. Cole LA, ed. Occurrence and Properties of Glycoprotein Hormone Free Subunits. In: Keel BA, Grotjans HE, Jr, eds. *Microheterogeneity of Glycoprotein Hormones.* Boca Raton: CRC Press; 1989:53–74.
37. Keel BA, Schanbacher BD, Grotjan HE Jr. Ovine luteinizing hormone. II. Effects of castration and steroid administration on the levels of uncombined subunits within the pituitary. *Biol Reprod* 1987;36:1114–1124.
38. Kourides IA, Hoffman BJ, Landon MB. Difference in glycosylation between secreted and pituitary free alpha subunit of the glycoprotein hormones. *J Clin Endocrinol Metab* 1980; 51:1372–1377.

39. Parsons TF, Pierce JG. Free α-like material from bovine pituitaries: Removal of its *O*-linked oligosaccharide permits combination with lutropin-β. *J Biol Chem* 1984;259:2662–2666.
40. Peters BP, Krzesicki RF, Perini F, Ruddon RW. *O*-Glycosylation of the α-subunit does not limit the assembly of chorionic gonadotropin α–β dimer in human malignant and non-malignant trophoblast cells. *Endocrinology* 1989;124:1602–1612.
41. Boime I, Boothby M, Hoshina M, Daniels-McQueen S, Darnell R. Expression and structure of human placental hormone genes as a function of placental development. *Biol Reprod* 1982; 26:73–91.
42. Peters BP, Krzesicki RF, Hartle RJ, Perini F, Ruddon RW. A kinetic comparison of the processing and secretion of the α.β dimer and the uncombined α and β subunits of chorionic gonadotropin synthesized by human choriocarcinoma cells. *J Biol Chem* 1984;259:15123–15130.
43. Corless CL, Matzuk MM, Ramabhadran TV, Krichevsky A, Boime I. Gonadotropin beta subunits determine the rate of assembly and the oligosaccharide processing of hormone dimer in transfected cells. *J Cell Biol* 1987;104:1173–1181.
44. Spratt DI, Chin WW, Ridgway EC, Crowley WF Jr. Administration of low dose pulsatile gonadotropin-releasing hormone (GnRH) to GnRH-deficient men regulates free alpha subunit secretion. *J Clin Endocrinol Metab* 1986;62:102–108.
45. Weiss J, Duca KA, Crowley WF Jr. Gonadotropin-releasing hormone-induced stimulation and desensitization of free alpha subunit secretion mirrors luteinizing hormone and follicle-stimulating hormone in perifused rat pituitary cells. *Endocrinology* 1990;127:2364–2371.
46. Corless CL, Boime I. Differential secretion of *O*-glycosylated gonadotropin alpha subunit and luteinizing hormone (LH) in the presence of LH-releasing hormone. *Endocrinology* 1985; 117:1699–1706.
47. Maghuin-Rogister G, Closset J, Hennen G. Differences in the carbohydrate portion of the α subunit of porcine lutropin (LH), follitropin (FSH) and thyrotropin (TSH). *FEBS Lett* 1975; 60:263–266.
48. Nilson B, Rosen SW, Weintraub BD, Zopf DA. Differences in the carbohydrate moieties of the common alpha subunits of human chorionic gonadotropin, luteinizing hormone, follicle-stimulating hormone, and thyrotropin: Preliminary structural inferences from direct methylation analysis. *Endocrinology* 1986;119:2737–2743.
49. Huang CJ, Huang FL, Chang GD, et al. Expression of two forms of carp gonadotropin α subunit in insect cells by recombinant baculovirus. *Proc Natl Acad Sci USA* 1991;88:7486–7490.
50. Bousfield GR, Liu W-K, Ward DN. Hybrids from equine LH: Alpha enhances, beta diminishes activity. *Mol Cell Endocrinol* 1985;40:69–77.
51. Sherman GB, Wolfe MW, Farmerie TA, et al. A single gene encodes the β-subunits of equine luteinizing hormone and chorionic gonadotropin. *Mol Endocrinol* 1992;6:951–959.
52. Idler DR, Ng TB. Studies on two types of gonadotropins from both salmon and carp pituitaries. *Gen Comp Endocrinol* 1979;38:421–440.
53. Ng TB, Idler DR. Studies on two types of gonadotropins from both American plaice and winter flounder pituitaries. *Gen Comp Endocrinol* 1979;38:410–420.
54. Suzuki K, Nagahama Y, Kawauchi H. Steroidogenic activities of two distinct salmon gonadotropins. *Gen Comp Endocrinol* 1988;71:452–458.
55. Itoh H, Suzuki K, Kawauchi H. The complete amino acid sequences of β-subunits of two distinct chum salmon GTHs. *Gen Comp Endocrinol* 1988;71:438–451.
56. Sekine S, Saito A, Itoh H, Kawauchi H, Itoh S. Molecular cloning and sequence analysis of chum salmon gonadotropin cDNAs. *Proc Natl Acad Sci USA* 1989;86:8645–8649.
57. Trinh KY, Wang NC, Hew CL, Crim LW. Molecular cloning and sequencing of salmon gonadotropin β subunit. *Eur J Biochem* 1986;159:619–624.
58. Leigh SEA, Stewart F. Partial cDNA sequence for the donkey chorionic gonadotrophin-β subunit suggests evolution from an ancestral LH-β gene. *J Mol Endocrinol* 1990;4:143–150.
59. Aggarwal BB, Farmer SW, Papkoff H, Stewart F, Allen WR. Purification and characterization of donkey chorionic gonadotrophin. *J Endocrinol* 1980;85:449–455.
60. Huth JR, Mountjoy K, Perini F, Ruddon RW. Intracellular folding pathway of human chorionic gonadotopin β subunit. *J Biol Chem* 1992;267:8870–8879.
61. Jirgensons B, Ward DN. Circular dichroism of ovine luteinizing hormone and its subunits. *Tex Rep Biol Med* 1970;28:553–559.
62. Garnier J. Molecular aspects of the subunit assembly of glycoprotein hormones. In: McKerns KW, ed. *Structure and Function of the Gonadotropins.* New York: Plenum Press; 1978:381–414.
63. Bewley TA. Circular dichroism of pituitary hormones. *Recent Prog Horm Res* 1979;35:155–210.
64. Bousfield GR, Liu W-K, Ward DN. Effects of removal of carboxy-terminal extension from equine luteinizing hormone (LH) β-subunit on LH and follicle-stimulating hormone receptor binding activities and LH steroidogenic activity in rat testicular Leydig cells. *Endocrinology* 1989;124:379–387.
65. Matzuk MM, Hsueh AJW, Lapolt P, Tsafriri A, Keene JL, Boime I. The biological role of the carboxyl-terminal extension of human chorionic gonadotropin β-subunit. *Endocrinology* 1990; 126:376–383.
66. Fares FA, Suganuma N, Nishimori K, LaPolt PS, Hsueh AJ, Boime I. Design of a long-acting follitropin agonist by fusing the *C*-terminal sequence of the chorionic gonadotropin beta subunit to the follitropin beta subunit. *Proc Natl Acad Sci USA* 1992;89:4304–4308.
67. Bona Gallo A, Licht P. Differences in the properties of FSH and LH binding sites in the avian gonad revealed by homologous radioligands. *Gen Comp Endocrinol* 1979;37:521–532.
68. Licht P, Papkoff H. Species specificity in the response of an in vitro amphibian (*Xenopus laevis*) ovulation assay to mammalian luteinizing hormones. *Gen Comp Endocrinol* 1976;29:552–555.
69. Fontaine Y, Burzawa-Gerard E. Esquisse de l'evolution des hormones gonadotropes et thyreotropes des vertebres. *Gen Comp Endocrinol* 1977;32:341–347.
70. Fontaine Y-A. La specificite zoologique des proteines hypophysaires capables de stimuler la thyroide. *Acta Endocrinol* [*Suppl*] 1969;136:1–154.
71. MacKenzie DS. Stimulation of the thyroid gland of a teleost fish, *Gillichthys mirabilis,* by tetrapod pituitary glycoprotein hormones. *Comp Biochem Physiol* 1982;72A:477–482.
72. Hsueh AJW, Adashi EY, Jones PBC, Welsh TH. Hormonal regulation of the differentiation of cultured ovarian granulosa cells. *Endocrine Rev* 1984;5:76–127.
73. Beers WH, Strickland S. A cell culture assay for follicle-stimulating hormone. *J Biol Chem* 1978;253:3877–3881.
74. Squires EL, Ginther OJ. Follicular and luteal development in pregnant mares. *J Reprod Fertil* 1975;Suppl. 23:429–433.
75. Chappel SC, Ulloa-Aguirre A, Coutifaris C. Biosynthesis and secretion of follicle-stimulating hormone. *Endocr Rev* 1983; 4:179–211.
76. Guzman K, Miller CD, Phillips CL, Miller WL. The gene encoding ovine follicle-stimulating hormone beta: Isolation, characterization, and comparison to a related ovine genomic sequence. *DNA Cell Biol* 1991;10:593–601.
77. Ward DN, Moore WT Jr. Comparative study of mammalian glycoprotein hormones. In: Alexander NJ, ed. *Animal Models for Research in Fertility and Contraception.* Baltimore: Harper & Row; 1979:151–164.
78. Moore WT Jr, Burleigh BD, Ward DN. Chorionic gonadotropins: Comparative studies and comments on relationships to other glycoprotein hormones. In: Segal SJ, ed. *Chorionic Gonadotropin.* New York: Plenum Press; 1980:89–126.
79. Combarnous Y. Molecular basis of the specificity of binding of glycoprotein hormones to their receptors. *Endocr Rev* 1992; 13:670–691.
80. Campbell RK, Matzuk MM, Dean-Emig DM, et al. Use of β-subunit chimeras to study the structures of glycoprotein hormones and to develop a model of the β-subunit. In: Chin WW, Boime I, eds. *Glycoprotein Hormones.* Norwell, MA: Serono Symposia, USA; 1990:37–43.
81. Ward DN. Chemical approaches to the structure–function relationships of luteinizing hormone (lutropin). In: McKerns KW, ed. *Structure and Function of the Gonadotropins.* New York: Plenum Press; 1978:31–45.

82. Weare JA, Reichert LE Jr. Studies with carbodiimide cross-linked derivatives of bovine lutropin. II. Location of the cross-link and implication for interaction with the receptors in testes. *J Biol Chem* 1979;254:6972–6979.
83. van Dijk S, Ward DN. Chemical cross-linking of porcine luteinizing hormone: Location of the cross-link and consequences for stability and biological activity. *Endocrinology* 1993;132: 534–538.
84. Torres JV, Yoshioka N, Atassi MZ. Antigenic regions on the β chain of human chorionic gonadotropin and development of hormone specific antibodies. *Immunol Invest* 1987;16:607–618.
85. Atassi MZ, Manshouri T, Sakata S. Localization and synthesis of the hormone-binding regions of the human thyrotropin receptor. *Proc Natl Acad Sci USA* 1991;88:3613–3617.
86. Moyle WR, Ehrlich PH, Canfield RE. Use of monoclonal antibodies to subunits of human chorionic gonadotropin to examine the orientation of the hormone in its complex with receptor. *Proc Natl Acad Sci USA* 1982;79:2245–2249.
87. Moyle WR, Pressey A, Dean-Emig D, et al. Detection of conformational changes in human chorionic gonadotropin upon binding to rat gonadal receptors. *J Biol Chem* 1987;262: 16920–16926.
88. Birken S, Canfield R, Lauer R, Agosto G, Gabel M. Immunochemical determinants unique to human chorionic gonadotropin: Importance of sialic acid for antisera generated to the human chorionic gonadotropin β-subunit COOH-terminal peptide. *Endocrinology* 1980;106:1659–1664.
89. Bidart J-M, Troalen F, Bousfield GR, Bohuon C, Bellet D. Monoclonal antibodies directed to human and equine chorionic gonadotropins as probes for the topographic analysis of epitopes on the human α-subunit. *Endocrinology* 1989;124:923–929.
90. Bidart J-M, Troalen F, Lazar V, et al. Monoclonal antibodies to the free β-subunit of human chorionic gonadotropin define three distinct antigenic domains and distinguish between intact and nicked molecules. *Endocrinology* 1992;131:1832–1840.
91. Ryan RJ, Charlesworth MC, Erickson LD, McCormick DJ, Milius RP, Morris JC III. Structure–function relationships of the α-subunit of the glycoprotein hormones. In: Chin WW, Boime I, eds. *Glycoprotein Hormones*. Norwell, MA: Serono Symposia, USA; 1990:71–80.
92. Ryan RJ, Keutmann HT, Charlesworth MC, et al. Structure function relationships of gonadotropins. In: *Recent Progress in Hormone Research*. New York: Academic Press; 1987:383–429.
93. Erickson LD, Rizza SA, Bergert ER, Charlesworth MC, McCormick DJ, Ryan RJ. Synthetic α-subunit peptides stimulate testosterone production in vitro by rat Leydig cells. *Endocrinology* 1990;126:2555–2560.
94. Schneyer AL, Sluss PM, Huston JS, Ridge RJ, Reichert LE Jr. Identification of a receptor binding region on the beta subunit of human follicle-stimulating hormone. *Biochemistry* 1988; 27:666–671.
95. Santa-Coloma TA, Reichert LE Jr. Determination of α-subunit contact regions of human follicle-stimulating hormone β-subunit using synthetic peptides. *J Biol Chem* 1991;266:2759–2762.
96. Grasso P, Santa-Coloma TA, Reichert LE Jr. Synthetic peptides corresponding to human follicle-stimulating hormone (hFSH)-β-(1–15) and hFSH-β-(51–65) induce uptake of $^{45}Ca^{++}$ by liposomes: Evidence for calcium-conducting transmembrane channel formation. *Endocrinology* 1991;128:2745–2751.
97. Santa-Coloma TA, Grasso P, Reichert LE Jr. Synthetic human follicle-stimulating hormone-β-(1–15) peptide-amide binds Ca^{++} and possesses sequence similarity to calcium binding sites of calmodulin. *Endocrinology* 1992;130:1103–1107.
98. Andersen TT. Follitropin binding to receptors in testis. *J Biol Chem* 1982;257:11551–11557.
99. Moyle WR, Bernard MP, Myers RV, Marko OM, Strader CD. Leutropin/beta-adrenergic receptor chimeras bind choriogonadotropin and adrenergic ligands but are not expressed at the cell surface. *J Biol Chem* 1991;266:10807–10812.
100. Matzuk MM, Boime I. Site-specific mutagenesis defines the intracellular role of the asparagine-linked oligosaccharides of chorionic gonadotropin β subunit. *J Biol Chem* 1988;263: 17106–17111.
101. Yoo J, Ji I, Ji TH. Conversion of lysine 91 to methionine or glutamic acid in human choriogonadotropin α results in the loss of cAMP inducibility. *J Biol Chem* 1991;266:17741–17743.
102. El-Deiry S, Kaetzel D, Kennedy G, Nilson J, Puett D. Site-directed mutagenesis of the human chorionic gonadotropin β-subunit: Bioactivity of a heterologous hormone, bovine α-human des-(122–145)β. *Mol Endocrinol* 1989;3:1523–1528.
103. Chen F, Wang Y, Puett D. Role of the invariant aspartic acid 99 of human choriogonadotropin β in receptor binding and biological activity. *J Biol Chem* 1991;266:19357–19361.
104. Nishimura R, Shin J, Ji I, et al. A single amino acid substitution in an ectopic α subunit of a human carcinoma choriogonadotropin. *J Biol Chem* 1986;261:10475–10477.
105. Cox GS. Phosphorylation of the glycoprotein hormone α-subunit by human tumor cell lines. *Biochem Biophys Res Commun* 1986;140:143–150.
106. Shome B, Parlow AF. The primary structure of the hormone-specific, beta subunit of human pituitary luteinizing hormone (hLH). *J Clin Endocrinol Metab* 1973;36:618–621.
107. Hartree AS, Lester JB, Shownkeen RC. Studies of the heterogeneity of human pituitary LH by fast protein liquid chromatography. *J Endocrinol* 1985;105:405–414.
108. Ward DN, Glenn SD, Nahm HS, Wen T. Characterization of cleavage products in selected human lutropin preparations. *Int J Peptide Protein Res* 1986;27:70–79.
109. Hartree AS, Shownkeen RC. Studies of human pituitary LH containing internally cleaved β subunit. *J Mol Endocrinol* 1991; 6:101–109.
110. Kardana A, Elliott MM, Gawinowicz MA, Birken S, Cole LA. The heterogeneity of human chorionic gonadotropin (hCG). I. Characterization of peptide heterogeneity in 13 individual preparations of hCG. *Endocrinology* 1991;129:1541–1550.
111. Cole LA, Birken S. Origin and occurrence of human chorionic gonadotropin β-subunit core fragment. *Mol Endocrinol* 1988; 2:825–830.
112. Gharib SD, Wierman ME, Shupnik MA, Chin WW. Molecular biology of the pituitary gonadotropins. *Endocr Rev* 1990; 11:177–199.
113. Delegeane AM, Ferland LH, Mellon PL. Tissue-specific enhancer of the human glycoprotein hormone α-subunit gene: Dependence on cyclic AMP-inducible elements. *Mol Cell Biol* 1987;7:3994–4002.
114. Jameson JL, Jaffe RC, Deutsch PJ, Albanese C, Habener J. The gonadotropin α-gene contains multiple protein binding domains that interact to modulate basal and cAMP-responsive transcription. *J Biol Chem* 1988;263:9879–9886.
115. Bokar JA, Keri RA, Farmerie TA, et al. Expression of the glycoprotein hormone α-subunit gene in the placenta requires a functional cyclic AMP response element, whereas a different *cis*-acting element mediates pituitary-specific expression. *Mol Cell Biol* 1989;9:5113–5122.
116. Hussa RO. Biosynthesis of chorionic gonadotropin. *Endocr Rev* 1980;1:268–294.
117. Jameson JL, Lindell CM, Habener JF. Evolution of different transcriptional start sites in the human luteinizing hormone and chorionic gonadotropin β-subunit genes. *DNA* 1986;5:227–234.
118. Hoeffler JP, Meyer TE, Yun Y, Jameson JL, Habener JF. Cyclic AMP-responsive DNA-binding protein: Structure based on a cloned placental cDNA. *Science* 1988;242:1430–1433.
119. Hai T, Liu F, Coukos WJ, Green MR. Transcription factor ATF cDNA clones: An extensive family of leucine zipper proteins able to selectively form DNA-binding heterodimers. *Genes Dev* 1989;3:2083–2090.
120. Hai T, Curran T. Cross-family dimerization of transcription factors *fos/jun* and ATF/CREB alters DNA binding specificity. *Proc Natl Acad Sci USA* 1991;88:3720–3724.
121. Yamamoto KK, Gonzales GA, Biggs WH III, Montminty MR. Phosphorylation-induced binding and transcriptional efficacy of nuclear factor CREB. *Nature* 1988;334:494–498.
122. Gonzales GA, Montminty MR. Cyclic AMP stimulates somatostatin gene transcription by phosphorylation of CREB at serine 133. *Cell* 1989;59:675–680.
123. Sheng M, Thompson MA, Greenberg ME. CREB: A Ca^{2+}-regulated transcription factor phosphorylated by calmodulin-dependent kinases. *Science* 1991;252:1427–1430.
124. Steger DJ, Altschmied J, Buscher M, Mellon PL. Evolution of

placenta-specific gene expression: Comparison of the equine and human gonadotropin α-subunit genes. *Mol Endocrinol* 1991; 5:243–255.

125. Kennedy GC, Andersen B, Nilson JH. The human α-subunit glycoprotein hormone gene utilizes a unique CCAAT binding factor. *J Biol Chem* 1990;265:6279–6285.
126. Andersen B, Kennedy GC, Nilson JH. A *cis*-acting element located between the cAMP response elements and CCAAT box augments cell-specific expression of the glycoprotein hormone α subunit gene. *J Biol Chem* 1990;35:21874–21880.
127. Akerblom IE, Slater EP, Beato M, Baxter JD, Mellon PL. Negative regulation by glucocorticoids through interference with a cAMP responsive enhancer. *Science* 1988;241:350–354.
128. Stauber C, Altschmied J, Akerblom IE, Marron JL, Mellon PL. Mutual cross-interference between glucocorticoid receptor and CREB inhibits transactivation in placental cells. *New Biologist* 1992;4:527–539.
129. Keri RA, Andersen B, Kennedy GC, et al. Estradiol inhibits transcription of the human glycoprotein hormone alpha-subunit gene despite the absence of a high affinity binding site for estrogen receptor. *Mol Endocrinol* 1991;5:725–733.
130. Ocran KW, Sarapura VD, Wood WM, Gordon DF, Gutierrez-Hartmann A, Ridgway EC. Identification of *cis*-acting promoter elements important for expression of the mouse glycoprotein hormone α-subunit gene in thyrotropes. *Mol Endocrinol* 1990;4:766–772.
131. Sarapura VD, Wood WM, Gordon DF, Ocran KW, Kao MY, Ridgway EC. Thyrotrope expression and thyroid hormone inhibition map to different regions of the mouse glycoprotein hormone α-subunit gene promoter. *Endocrinology* 1990;127:1352–1361.
132. Horn F, Windle JJ, Barnhart KM, Mellon PL. Tissue-specific gene expression in the pituitary: The glycoprotein hormone α-subunit gene is regulated by a gonadotrope-specific protein. *Mol Cell Biol* 1992;12:2143–2153.
133. Talmadge K, Boorstein WR, Fiddes JC. The human genome contains seven genes for the β-subunit of chorionic gonadotropin but only one gene for the β-subunit of luteinizing hormone. *DNA* 1983;2:281–289.
134. Talmadge K, Boorstein WR, Vamvakopolous NC, Gething M-J, Fiddes JC. Only three of the seven human chorionic gonadotropin beta subunit genes can be expressed in the placenta. *Nucleic Acids Res* 1984;12:8414–8436.
135. Bo M, Boime I. Identification of the transcriptionally active genes of the chorionic gonadotropin β gene cluster in vivo. *J Biol Chem* 1992;267:3179–3184.
136. Talmadge K, Vamvakopolous NC, Fiddes JC. Evolution of the genes for the β subunits of human chorionic gonadotropin and luteinizing hormone. *Nature* 1984;307:37–40.
137. Virgin JB, Silver BJ, Thomason AR, Nilson JH. The gene for the β subunit of bovine luteinizing hormone encodes a gonadotropin mRNA with an unusually short 5′-untranslated region. *J Biol Chem* 1985;260:7072–7077.
138. Albanese C, Kay TWH, Troccoli NM, Jameson JL. Novel cyclic adenosine 3′,5′-monophosphate response element in the human chorionic gonadotropin β-subunit gene. *Mol Endocrinol* 1991; 5:693–702.
139. Milsted A, Cox RP, Nilson JH. Cyclic AMP regulates transcription of the genes encoding human chorionic gonadotropin with different kinetics. *DNA* 1987;6:213–219.
140. Jameson JL, Lindell CM. Isolation and characterization of the human chorionic gonadotropin beta subunit (CG beta) gene cluster: Regulation of transcriptionally active CG beta gene by cyclic AMP. *Mol Cell Biol* 1988;8:5100–5107.
141. Kim KE, Day KH, Howard P, Salton SRJ, Roberts JL, Maurer RA. DNA sequences required for expression of the LHβ promoter in primary cultures of rat pituitary cells. *Mol Cell Endocrinol* 1990;74:101–107.
142. Shupnik MA, Weinmann CM, Notides AC, Chin WW. An upstream region of the rat luteinizing hormone β gene binds estrogen receptor and confers estrogen responsiveness. *J Biol Chem* 1989;264:80–86.
143. Kumar TR, Fairchild-Huntress V, Low MJ. Gonadotrope-specific expression of the human follicle-stimulating hormone β-subunit gene in pituitaries of transgenic mice. *Mol Endocrinol* 1992;6:81–90.
144. Windle JJ, Weiner RI, Mellon PL. Cell lines of the pituitary gonadotrope lineage derived by targeted oncogenesis in transgenic mice. *Mol Endocrinol* 1990;4:597–603.
145. Sinha YN, Lewis UJ. A lectin-binding immunoassay indicates a possible glycosylated growth hormone in the human pituitary gland. *Biochem Biophys Res Commun* 1986;140:491–497.
146. Markoff E, Sinha YN, Lewis UJ. Prolactin microheterogeneity. In: Keel BA, Grotjan HE Jr, eds. *Microheterogeneity of Glycoprotein Hormones.* Boca Raton, FL: CRC Press; 1989:99–106.
147. Bogdanov EM, Nansel DD. Biological and immunological distinctions between pituitary and serum LH in the rat. In: McKerns KW, eds. *Structure and Function of the Gonadotropins.* New York: Plenum Press; 1978:415–430.
148. Baenziger JU, Green ED. Pituitary glycoprotein hormone oligosaccharides: Structure, synthesis and function of the asparagine-linked oligosaccharides on lutropin, follitropin and thyrotropin. *Biochim Biophys Acta* 1988;947:287–306.
149. Grotjan HE Jr. Oligosaccharide structures in pituitary and placental glycoprotein hormones. In: Keel BA, Grotjan HE Jr, eds. *Microheterogeneity of Glycoprotein Hormones.* Boca Raton, FL: CRC Press; 1989:23–52.
150. Moyle WR, Bahl OP, Marz L. Role of the carbohydrate of human chorionic gonadotropin in the mechanism of hormone action. *J Biol Chem* 1975;250:9163–9169.
151. Sairam MR. Deglycosylation of ovine pituitary lutropin subunits: Effects on subunit interaction and hormone activity. *Arch Biochem Biophys* 1980;204:199–206.
152. Governman JM, Parsons TF, Pierce JG. Enzymatic deglycosylation of the subunits of chorionic gonadotropin: Effects on formation of tertiary structure and biological activity. *J Biol Chem* 1982;257:15059–15064.
153. Liu WK, Young JD, Ward DN. Deglycosylated ovine lutropin: Preparation and characterization by *in vitro* binding and steroidogenesis. *Mol Cell Endocrinol* 1984;37:29–39.
154. Parsons TF, Bloomfield GA, Pierce JG. Purification of an alternate form of the α subunit of the glycoprotein hormones from bovine pituitaries and identification of its *O*-linked oligosaccharide. *J Biol Chem* 1983;258:240–244.
155. Blithe DL, Nisula BC. Variations in the oligosaccharides on free and combined alpha-subunits of human choriogonadotropin in pregnancy. *Endocrinology* 1985;117:2218–2228.
156. Ruddon RW, Krzesicki RF, Norton SE, Beebe JS, Peters BP, Perini F. Detection of a glycosylated, incompletely folded form of chorionic gonadotropin β subunit that is a precursor of hormone assembly in trophoblastic cells. *J Biol Chem* 1987; 262:12533–12540.
157. Bousfield GR, Liu W-K, Sugino H, Ward DN. Structural studies on equine glycoprotein hormones: Amino acid sequence of equine lutropin β subunit. *J Biol Chem* 1987;262:8610–8620.
158. Sugino H, Bousfield GR, Moore WT Jr, Ward DN. Structural studies on equine glycoprotein hormones. Amino acid sequence of equine chorionic gonadotropin beta subunit. *J Biol Chem* 1987;262:8603–8609.
159. Bousfield GR, Baker VL, Clem DM. Comparison of the *O*-glycosylation of eLH and eCG beta subunits. In: *74th Annual Meeting of the Endocrine Society.* San Antonio: The Endocrine Society; 1992:1200.
160. Birken S, Canfield RE. Isolation and amino acid sequence of COOH-terminal fragments from the β subunit of human choriogonadotropin. *J Biol Chem* 1977;252:5386–5392.
161. Keutmann HT, Williams RM. Human chorionic gonadotropin: Amino acid sequence of the hormone-specific COOH-terminal region. *J Biol Chem* 1977;252:5393–5397.
162. Kessler MJ, Mise T, Ghai RD, Bahl OP. Structure and location of the *O*-glycosidic carbohydrate units of human chorionic gonadotropin. *J Biol Chem* 1979;254:7909–7914.
163. Damm JBL, Hard K, Kammerling JP, van Dedem GWK, Vliegenthart FG. Structure determination of the major *N*- and *O*-linked carbohydrate chains of the β subunit from equine chorionic gonadotropin. *Eur J Biochem* 1990;189:175–183.
164. Matsui T, Sugino H, Miura M, et al. β-Subunits of equine chorionic gonadotropin and luteinizing hormone with an identical amino acid sequence have different asparagine-linked oligosaccharide chains. *Biochem Biophys Res Commun* 1991; 174:940–945.

165. Endo Y, Yamashita K, Tachibana Y, Tojo S, Kobata A. Structures of the asparagine-linked sugar chains of human chorionic gonadotropin. *J Biochem* 1979;85:669–679.
166. Kessler MJ, Reddy MS, Shah RH, Bahl OP. Structures of the *N*-glycosidic carbohydrate units of human chorionic gonadotropin. *J Biol Chem* 1979;254:7901–7908.
167. Parsons TF, Pierce JG. Oligosaccharide moieties of glycoprotein hormones: Bovine lutropin resists enzymatic deglycosylation because of terminal *O*-sulfated *N*-acetylhexosamines. *Proc Natl Acad Sci USA* 1980;77:7089–7093.
168. Green ED, van Halbeek H, Boime I, Baenziger JU. Structural elucidation of the disulfated oligosaccharide from bovine lutropin. *J Biol Chem* 1985;260:15623–15630.
169. Green ED, Baenziger JU. Asparagine-linked oligosaccharides on lutropin, follitropin, and thyrotropin: I. Structural elucidation of the sulfated and sialylated oligosaccharides on bovine, ovine, and human pituitary glycoprotein hormones. *J Biol Chem* 1988;263:25–35.
170. Green ED, Baenziger JU. Asparagine-linked oligosaccharides on lutropin, follitropin, and thyrotropin. II. Distributions of sulfated and sialylated oligosaccharides on bovine, ovine, and human pituitary glycoprotein hormones. *J Biol Chem* 1988;263:36–44.
171. Bahl OP, Wagh PV. Characterization of glycoproteins: Carbohydrate structures of glycoprotein hormones. In: Dhindsa DS, Bahl OP, eds. *Molecular and Cellular Aspects of Reproduction.* New York: Plenum Press; 1986:1–51.
172. Weisshaar G, Hiyama J, Renwick AGC. Site-specific *N*-glycosylation of ovine lutropin: Structural analysis by one- and two-dimensional ^{1}H-NMR spectroscopy. *Eur J Biochem* 1990;192:741–751.
173. Weisshaar G, Hiyama J, Renwick AGC, Nimitz M. NMR investigations of the *N*-linked oligosaccharides at individual glycosylation sites of human lutropin. *Eur J Biochem* 1991;195:257–268.
174. Nemansky M, Van Den Eijnden DH. Bovine colostrum CMP-NeuAC:Galβ(1–4)GlcNAc-Rα(2–6)-sialyltransferase is involved in the synthesis of the terminal NeuAcα(2–6)GalNAcβ-(1–4)GlcNAc sequence occurring on *N*-linked glycans of bovine milk glycoproteins. *Biochem J* 1992;287:311–316.
175. Smith PL, Kaetzel D, Nilson J, Baenziger JU. The sialylated oligosaccharides of recombinant bovine lutropin modulate hormone bioactivity. *J Biol Chem* 1990;265:874–881.
176. Chen W, Shen Q-X, Bahl OP. Carbohydrate variant of the recombinant β-subunit of human choriogonadotropin expressed in baculovirus expression system. *J Biol Chem* 1991;266:4081–4087.
177. Hard K, Mekking A, Damm JB, et al. Isolation and structure determination of the intact sialylated *N*-linked carbohydrate chains of recombinant human follitropin expressed in Chinese hamster ovary cells. *Eur J Biochem* 1990;193:263–271.
178. Morell AG, Gregoriadis G, Scheinberg IH, Hickman J, Ashwell G. The role of sialic acid in determining the survival of glycoproteins in the circulation. *J Biol Chem* 1971;246:1461–1467.
179. Fiete D, Srivastava V, Hindsgaul O, Baenziger JU. A hepatic reticuloendothelial cell receptor specific for SO_4-4GalNAcβ1,4GlcNAcβ1,2Manα that mediates rapid clearance of lutropin. *Cell* 1991;67:1103–1110.
180. Baenziger JU, Kumar S, Brodbeck RM, Smith PL, Beranek MC. Circulatory half-life but not interaction with the lutropin/chorionic gonadotropin receptor is modulated by sulfation of bovine lutropin oligosaccharides. *Proc Natl Acad Sci USA* 1992; 89:334–338.
181. Bousfield GR, Ward DN. Biologic activity of eLH and hCG following removal of the *C*-terminal glycopeptide. In: *68th Annual Meeting of the Endocrine Society.* Anaheim, CA: Endocrine Society; 1986:530.
182. Green ED, Boime I, Baenziger JU. Differential processing of Asn-linked oligosaccharides on pituitary glycoprotein hormones: Implications for biologic function. *Mol Cell Biochem* 1986;72:81–100.
183. Thotakura NR, Desai RK, Bates LG, Cole ES, Pratt BM, Weintraub BD. Biological activity and metabolic clearance of a recombinant human thyrotropin produced in Chinese hamster ovary cells. *Endocrinology* 1991;128:341–348.
184. Sairam MR, Schiller PW. Receptor binding, biological, and immunological properties of chemically deglycosylated pituitary lutropin. *Arch Biochem Biophys* 1979;197:294–301.
185. Berman MI, Thomas CG Jr, Manjunath P, Sairam MR, Nayfeh SN. The role of the carbohydrate moiety in thyrotropin action. *Biochem Biophys Res Commun* 1985;133:680–687.
186. Calvo FO, Keutmann HT, Bergert ER, Ryan RJ. Deglycosylated human follitropin: Characterization and effects on adenosine cyclic 3′,5′-phosphate production in porcine granulosa cells. *Biochemistry* 1986;25:3938–3943.
187. Sairam MR. Hormonal antagonistic properties of chemically deglycosylated human choriogonadotropin. *J Biol Chem* 1983; 258:445–449.
188. Flack MR, Bennet AP, Froehlich J, Anasti JN. Selective mutagenesis of the glycosylation sites of FSH: Effects on secretion, conformation, and biologic potency. In: *74th Annual Meeting of the Endocrine Society.* San Antonio: Endocrine Society; 1992:1296.
189. Patton PE, Calvo FO, Fujimoto VY, Bergert ER, Kempers RD, Ryan RJ. The effect of deglycosylated human chorionic gonadotropin on corpora luteal function in healthy women. *Fertil Steril* 1988;49:620–625.
190. Liu L, Southers JL, Banks SM, et al. Stimulation of testosterone production in the cynomolgus monkey *in vivo* by deglycosylated and desialylated human choriogonadotropin. *Endocrinology* 1989;124:175–180.
191. Dahl KD, Bicsak TA, Hsueh AJW. Naturally occurring antihormones: Secretion of FSH antagonists by women treated with a GnRH analog. *Science* 1988;239:72–74.
192. Jia X-C, Hsueh AJW. Granulosa cell aromatase bioassay for follicle-stimulating hormone: Validation and application of the method. *Endocrinology* 1986;119:1570–1577.
193. Libert F, Lefort A, Gerard C, et al. Cloning, sequencing and expression of the human thyrotropin (TSH) receptor: Evidence for binding of autoantibodies. *Biochem Biophys Res Commun* 1989;165:1250–1255.
194. Loosfelt H, Misrahi M, Atger M, et al. Cloning and sequencing of porcine LH-hCG receptor cDNA: Variants lacking transmembrane domain. *Science* 1989;245:525–528.
195. McFarland KC, Sprengel R, Phillips HS, et al. Lutropin–choriogonadotropin receptor: An unusual member of the G protein-coupled receptor family. *Science* 1989;245:494–499.
196. Nagayama Y, Kaufman KD, Seto P, Rappaport B. Molecular cloning, sequence and functional expression of the cDNA for the human thyrotropin receptor. *Biochem Biophys Res Commun* 1989;165:1184–1190.
197. Parmentier M, Libert F, Maenhout C, et al. Molecular cloning of the thyrotropin receptor. *Science* 1989;246:1620–1622.
198. Sprengel R, Braun T, Nikolics K, Segaloff DL, Seeburg PH. The testicular receptor for follicle stimulating hormone: Structure and functional expression of cloned cDNA. *Mol Endocrinol* 1990; 4:525–530.
199. Gross B, Misrahi M, Sar S, Milgrom E. Composite structure of human thyrotropin receptor gene. *Biochem Biophys Res Commun* 1991;177:679–687.
200. Koo YB, Ji I, Slaughter RG, Ji TH. Structure of the luteinizing hormone receptor gene and multiple exons of the coding sequence. *Endocrinology* 1991;128:2297–2308.
201. Heckert LL, Daley IJ, Griswold MD. Structural organization of the follicle-stimulating hormone receptor gene. *Mol Endocrinol* 1992;6:70–80.
202. Ascoli M, Segaloff DL. On the structure of the luteinizing hormone/chorionic gonadotropin receptor. *Endocr Rev* 1989; 10:27–44.
203. Akamizu T, Ikuyama S, Saji M, et al. Cloning, chromosomal assignment, and regulation of the rat thyrotropin receptor: Expression of the gene is regulated by thyrotropin, agents that increase cAMP levels, and thyroid antibodies. *Proc Natl Acad Sci USA* 1990;87:5677–5681.
204. Lincoln SR, Lei ZM, Rao CV, Yussman MA. The expression of human chorionic gonadotropin/human luteinizing hormone receptors in ectopic endometrial implants. *J Clin Endocrinol Metab* 1992;75:1140–1144.
205. Jia X-C, Oikawa M, Bo M, et al. Expression of human luteinizing hormone (LH) receptor: Interaction with LH and chorionic gonadotropin from human but not equine, rat, and ovine species. *Mol Endocrinol* 1991;5:759–768.
206. Gudermann T, Birnbaumer M, Birnbaumer L. Evidence for dual

coupling of the murine luteinizing hormone receptor to adenylyl cyclase and phosphoinositide breakdown and Ca^{2+} mobilization. Studies with the cloned murine luteinizing hormone receptor expressed in L cells. *J Biol Chem* 1992;267:4479–4488.
207. Huhtaniemi IT, Eskola V, Pakarinen P, Matikainen T, Sprengel R. Molecular cloning of the murine FSH and LH receptor (R) gene promoter sequences, identification of transcription initiation sites and demonstration of promoter activity. In: *74th Annual Meeting of the Endocrine Society.* San Antonio: Endocrine Society; 1992:1288.
208. Oates E, Jin SX, McKenzie JM, Zakarija M. Unique conserved regions of the glycoprotein hormone receptors allow *Xenopus* FSH and LH/CG receptor gene fragment cloning by PCR. In: *74th Annual Meeting of the Endocrine Society.* San Antonio: Endocrine Society; 1992:1265.
209. Tsai-Morris CH, Buczko E, Wang W, Xie XZ, Dufau ML. Structural organization of the rat luteinizing hormone (LH) receptor gene. *J Biol Chem* 1991;266:11355–11359.
210. Xie Y-B, Wang H, Segaloff DL. Extracellular domain of lutropin/choriogonadotropin receptor expressed in transfected cells binds choriogonadotropin with high affinity. *J Biol Chem* 1990;35:21411–21414.
211. Rodriguez MC, Xie YB, Wang H, Collison K, Segaloff DL. Effects of truncations of the cytoplasmic tail of the luteinizing hormone/chorionic gonadotropin receptor on receptor-mediated hormone internalization. *Mol Endocrinol* 1992;6:327–336.
212. Rodriguez MC, Segaloff DL. The orientation of the lutropin/choriogonadotropin receptor in rat luteal cells as revealed by site-specific antibodies. *Endocrinology* 1990;127:674–681.
213. Tsai-Morris CH, Buczko E, Wang W, Dufau ML. Intronic nature of the rat luteinizing hormone receptor gene defines a soluble receptor subspecies with hormone binding activity. *J Biol Chem* 1990;265:19385–19388.
214. Yang KP, Samaan NA, Ward DN. Characterization of an inhibitor for luteinizing hormone receptor site binding. *Endocrinology* 1976;98:233–241.
215. Nagayama Y, Russo D, Chazenbalk GD, Wadsworth HL, Rapoport B. Extracellular domain chimeras of the TSH and LH/CG receptors reveal the mid-region (amino acids 171–260) to play a vital role in high affinity TSH binding. *Biochem Biophys Res Commun* 1990;173:1150–1156.
216. Braun T, Schofield PR, Sprengel R. Amino-terminal leucine-rich repeats in gonadotropin receptors determine hormone selectivity. *EMBO J* 1991;10:1885–1890.
217. Russo D, Chazenbalk GD, Nagayama Y, Wadsworth HL, Rapoport B. Site-directed mutagenesis of the human thyrotropin receptor: Role of asparagine-linked oligosaccharides in the expression of a functional receptor. *Mol Endocrinol* 1991;5:29–33.
218. Petäjä-Repo UE, Merz WE, Rajaniemi HJ. Significance of the glycan moiety of the rat ovarian luteinizing hormone/chorionic gonadotropin (CG) receptor and human CG for receptor–hormone interaction. *Endocrinology* 1991;128:1209–1217.
219. O'Dowd BF, Hnatowich M, Regan JW, Leader WM, Caron MG, Lefkowitz RJ. Site-directed mutagenesis of the cytoplasmic domains of the human β_2-adrenergic receptor: Localization of regions involved in G protein–receptor coupling. *J Biol Chem* 1988;263:15985–15992.
220. Collison K, Wang H, Segaloff DL. Disruption of the putative amphipathic helix in the third intracellular loop of the LH/CG receptor does not impair hormone-stimulated cAMP production. In: *74th Annual Meeting of the Endocrine Society.* San Antonio: Endocrine Society; 1992:1291.
221. Jha PK, Pal R, Nakhai B, Sridar P, Hasnain SE. Simultaneous synthesis of enzymatically active luciferase and biologically active β subunit of human chorionic gonadotropin in caterpillars infected with a recombinant baculovirus. *FEBS Lett* 1992; 310:148–152.
222. Sánchez-Yagüe J, Rodríguez MC, Segaloff DL, Ascoli M. Truncation of the cytoplasmic tail of the lutropin/choriogonadotropin receptor prevents agonist-induced uncoupling. *J Biol Chem* 1992;267:7217–7220.
223. Minegish T, Nakamura K, Takakura Y, et al. Cloning and sequencing of human LH/hCG receptor cDNA. *Biochem Biophys Res Commun* 1990;172:1049–1054.
224. Feng W, Wimalasena J. The ability to interact with hCG is present in a M_r 46K fragment of the LH/hCG receptor. In: *74th Annual Meeting of the Endocrine Society.* San Antonio: Endocrine Society; 1992:1471.
225. Reichert LE Jr, Dattatreyamurty B. The follicle-stimulating hormone (FSH) receptor in testis: Interaction with FSH, mechanism of signal transduction, and properties of the purified receptor. *Biol Reprod* 1989;40:13–26.
226. Hsueh AJW, Adashi EY, Jones PBC, Welch TH Jr. Hormonal regulation of the differentiation of cultured ovarian granulosa cells. *Endocr Rev* 1984;5:76–127.
227. Minegish T, Nakamura K, Takakura Y, Ibuki Y, Igarashi M. Cloning and sequencing of human FSH receptor cDNA. *Biochem Biophys Res Commun* 1991;175:1125–1130.
228. Noce T, Ando H, Ueda T, Kubokawa K, Higashinakagawa T, Ishii S. Molecular cloning and nucleotide sequence analysis of the putative cDNA for the precursor molecule of the chicken LH-β subunit. *J Mol Endocrinol* 1989;3:129–137.
229. Chappel S, Beck A, Nugent N, Hyman L, Zabrecky J, Maurer R. Production of bovine follicle stimulating hormone (FSH) by recombinant DNA technology. In: *69th Annual Meeting of the Endocrine Society.* Indianapolis: Endocrine Society; 1987:139.
230. Ward DN, Hines KK, Gordon WL, Bousfield GR. The purification of native inhibin and chemical characterization. In: Hodgen GD, Rosenwaks Z, Spieler JM, eds. *Nonsteroidal Gonadal Factors: Physiological Roles and Possibilities in Contraceptive Development.* Norfolk: Jones Institute Press; 1988:1–16.
231. Lodish H. Transport of secretory and membrane glycoproteins from the rough endoplasmic reticulum to the Golgi. *J Biol Chem* 1988;263:2107–2110.
232. Chen F, Puett D. Delineation via site-directed mutagenesis of the carboxyl-terminal region of human choriogonadotropin β required for subunit assembly and biological activity. *J Biol Chem* 1991;266:6904–6908.
233. Suganama N, Matzuk MM, Boime I. Elimination of disulfide bonds affects assembly and secretion of the human chorionic gonadotropin β subunit. *J Biol Chem* 1989;264:19302–19307.
234. Cole LA, Hartle RJ, Laferla JJ, Ruddon RW. Detection of the free beta subunit of human chorionic gonadotropin (hCG) in cultures of normal and malignant trophoblast cells, pregnancy sera, and sera of patients with choriocarcinoma. *Endocrinology* 1983;113:1176–1178.
235. Ozturk M, Bellet D, Manl L, Hennen G, Frydman R, Wands J. Physiological studies of human chorionic gonadotropin (hCG), ahCG, and bhCG as measured by specific monoclonal immunoradiometric assays. *Endocrinology* 1987;120:549–558.
236. Keene JL, Matzuk MM, Otani T, et al. Expression of biologically active human follitropin in Chinese hamster ovary cells. *J Biol Chem* 1989;264:4769–4775.
237. Hurtley SM, Helenius A. Protein oligomerization of newly synthesized proteins in the endoplasmic reticulum. *Annu Rev Cell Biol* 1989;5:277–307.
238. Ross DS, Downing MF, Chin WW, Keiffer JD, Ridgway EC. Divergent changes in murine pituitary concentration of free α- and thyrotropin-β subunits in hypothyroidism and after thyroxine administration. *Endocrinology* 1983;112:187–193.
239. Noda T, Farquhar MG. A non-autophagic pathway for diversion of ER secretory proteins to lysosomes. *J Cell Biol* 1992; 119:85–97.
240. Rothman JE, Orci L. Molecular dissection of the secretory pathway. *Nature* 1992;355:409–415.
241. Smith PL, Baenziger JU. Molecular basis of recognition by the glycoprotein hormone-specific *N*-acetylgalactosamine-transferase. *Proc Natl Acad Sci USA* 1992;89:329–333.
242. Chu WP, Liu WK, Ward DN. Carbohydrate components of the glycopeptides of ovine lutropin. *Biochim Biophys Acta* 1976; 437:377–383.
243. Smith PL, Baenziger JU. A pituitary *N*-acetylgalactosamine transferase that specifically recognizes glycoprotein hormones. *Science* 1988;242:930–933.
244. Hirschberg CB, Snider MD. Topography of glycosylation in the rough endoplasmic reticulum and Golgi apparatus. *Annu Rev Biochem* 1987;56:63–87.
245. Green ED, Gruenebaum J, Bielinska M, Baenziger JU, Boime I. Sulfation of lutropin oligosaccharides with a cell-free system. *Proc Natl Acad Sci USA* 1984;81:5320–5324.

246. Mock EJ, Papkoff H, Niswender GD. Internalization of ovine luteinizing hormone/human chorionic gonadotropin recombinants: Differential effects of the α- and β-subunits. *Endocrinology* 1983;113:265–269.
247. Niswender GD, Roess DA, Sawyer HR, Silvia WJ, Barisas BG. Differences in the lateral mobility of receptors for luteinizing hormone (LH) in the luteal cell plasma membrane when occupied by ovine LH versus human chorionic gonadotropin. *Endocrinology* 1985;116:164–169.
248. Blomquist JF, Baenziger JU. Differential sorting of lutropin and the free α-subunit in cultured bovine pituitary cells. *J Biol Chem* 1992;267:20798–20803.
249. Keel BA, Grotjan JHE, ed. *Microheterogeneity of Glycoprotein Hormones.* Boca Raton, FL: CRC Press; 1989.
250. Gordon WL, Bousfield GR, Ward DN. Comparative binding of FSH to chicken and rat testis. *J Endocrinol Invest* 1989; 12:383–392.
251. Greenberg NM, Anderson JW, Hsueh AJ, et al. Expression of biologically active heterodimeric bovine follicle-stimulating in milk of transgenic mice. *Proc Natl Acad Sci USA* 1991; 88:8327–8331.
252. Sairam MR, Papkoff H, Li CH. The primary structure of ovine interstitial cell-stimulating hormone I. The α-subunit. *Arch Biochem Biophys* 1972;153:554–571.
253. Bello PA, Mountford PS, Brandon MR, Adams TE. Cloning and DNA sequence analysis of the cDNA for the common α-subunit of the ovine pituitary glycoprotein hormones. *Nucleic Acids Res* 1989;17:10494.
254. Liao TH, Pierce JG. The primary structure of bovine thyrotropin II. The amino acid sequences of the reduced, *S*-carboxymethyl α and β chains. *J Biol Chem* 1971;246:850–865.
255. Goodwin RG, Moncman CL, Rottman FM, Nilson JH. Characterization and nucleotide sequence of the gene for the common α subunit of the bovine pituitary glycoprotein hormones. *Nucleic Acids Res* 1983;11:6873–6882.
256. Maghuin-Rogister G, Combarnous Y, Hennen G. The primary structure of the porcine luteinizing-hormone α-subunit. *Eur J Biochem* 1973;39:255–263.
257. Maghuin-Rogister G, Hennen G, Closset J. Porcine thyrotropin: The amino-acid sequence of the α and β subunits. *Eur J Biochem* 1976;61:157–163.
258. Sugino H, Takio K, Ward DN. Reevaluation of the amino acid sequence of porcine follitropin. *J Protein Chem* 1989;8:197–219.
259. Hirai T, Takikawa H, Kato Y. Molecular cloning of cDNAs for precursors of porcine pituitary glycoprotein hormone common α-subunit and of thyroid stimulating hormone β-subunit. *Mol Cell Endocrinol* 1989;63:209–217.
260. Glenn SD, Nahm HS, Ward DN. The amino acid sequence of the rabbit glycoprotein hormone alpha subunit. *J Protein Chem* 1984;3:143–156.
261. Ward DN, Moore WT Jr, Burleigh BD. Structural studies on equine chorionic gonadotropin. *J Protein Chem* 1982;1:263–280.
262. Chin WW, Kronenberg HM, Dee PC, Maloof F, Habener JF. Nucleotide sequence of the mRNA encoding the pre-α-subunit of mouse thyrotropin. *Proc Natl Acad Sci USA* 1981;78:5329–5333.
263. Godine JE, Chin WW, Habener JF. α subunit of rat pituitary glycoprotein hormones: Primary structure of the precursor determined from the nucleotide sequence of cloned cDNAs. *J Biol Chem* 1982;257:8368–8371.
264. Sairam MR, Papkoff H, Li CH. Human pituitary interstitial cell stimulating hormone: Primary structure of the α subunit. *Biochem Biophys Res Commun* 1972;48:530–537.
265. Keutmann HT, Dawsom B, Bishop WH, Ryan RJ. Structure of human luteinizing hormone alpha subunit. *Endocr Res Commun* 1978;5:57–70.
266. Fiddes JC, Goodman HM. Isolation, cloning and sequence analysis of the cDNA for the α-subunit of human chorionic gonadotropin. *Nature* 1979;281:351–356.
267. Pankov YA, Karasev VS. Luteinizing hormone of the sperm whale. Isolation, separation into subunits, and study of the amino acid sequence of the α-subunit. *Biokhimiya* 1984;49:111–126.
268. Combarnous Y, Huet JC, Martinat N, Mansion M, Anouassi A, Pernollet JC. *N*-Terminal amino-sequencing of camel (*Camelus dromedarius*) luteinizing hormone α- and β-subunits. *Pathol Biol* 1989;37:814–818.
269. Glenn SD, Nahm HS, Greenwald GS, Ward DN. Isolation and characterization of hamster luteinizing hormone. *Endocrinology* 1982;111:1263–1269.
270. Foster DN, Galehouse D, Giordano T, et al. Nucleotide sequence of the cDNA encoding the common α subunit of the chicken pituitary glycoprotein hormones. *J Mol Endocrinol* 1992; 8:21–27.
271. Foster DN, Foster LK. Cloning and sequence analysis of the common α-subunit complementary deoxyribonucleic acid of turkey pituitary glycoprotein hormones. *Poultry Sci* 1991; 70:2516–2523.
272. Hayashi H, Hayashi T, Hanaoka Y. Amphibian lutropin and follitropin from the bullfrog *Rana catesbeiana.* Complete amino acid sequence of the alpha subunit. *Eur J Biochem* 1992; 203:185–191.
273. Chang YS, Huang CJ, Huang FL, Lo TB. Primary structures of carp gonadotropin subunits deduced from cDNA nucleotide sequences. *Int J Peptide Protein Res* 1988;32:556–564.
274. Querat B, Jutisz M, Fontaine Y, Counis R. Cloning and sequence analysis of the cDNA for the pituitary glycoprotein hormone α-subunit of the European eel. *Mol Cell Endocrinol* 1990; 71:253–259.
275. Liu C-S, Huang F-L, Chang Y-S, Lo TB. Pike eel (*Muraenesox cinereus*) gonadotropin: Amino acid sequences of both α and β subunits. *Eur J Biochem* 1989;186:105–114.
276. Morgan FJ, Birken S, Canfield RE. Human chorionic gonadotropin: A proposal for the amino acid sequence. *Mol Cell Biochem* 1973;2:97–99.
277. Carlsen RB, Bahl OP, Swaminathan N. Human chorionic gonadotropin. Linear amino acid sequence of the β subunit. *J Biol Chem* 1973;248:6810–6827.
278. Fiddes JC, Goodman HM. The cDNA for the β-subunit of human chorionic gonadotropin suggests evolution of a gene by readthrough into the 3′-untranslated region. *Nature* 1980; 286:684–687.
279. Crawford RJ, Tregear GW, Niall HD. The nucleotide sequences of baboon chorionic gonadotropin β-subunit genes have diverged from the human. *Gene* 1986;46:161–169.
280. Closset J, Hennen G, Lequin RM. Human luteinizing hormone: The amino acid sequence of the β subunit. *FEBS Lett* 1973;29:97–100.
281. Sairam MR, Li CH. Human pituitary lutropin: Isolation, properties, and the complete amino acid sequence of the β-subunit. *Biochim Biophys Acta* 1975;412:70–81.
282. Liu WK, Nahm HS, Sweeney CM, Holcomb GN, Ward DN. The primary structure of ovine luteinizing hormone: II. The amino acid sequence of the reduced, *S*-carboxymethylated A-subunit (LH-β). *J Biol Chem* 1972;247:4365–4381.
283. d'Angelo-Bernard G, Moumni M, Jutisz M, Counis R. Cloning and sequence analysis of the cDNA for the precursor of the beta subunit of ovine luteinizing hormone. *Nucleic Acids Res* 1990;18:2175.
284. Ward DN, Liu W-K. The chemistry of ovine and bovine luteinizing hormone. In: Margoulies M, Greenwood FC, eds. *Structure–Activity Relationships of Protein and Polypeptide Hormones.* Amsterdam: Excerpta Medica; 1971:80–90.
285. Maghuin-Rogister G, Dockier A. The amino acid sequence of the bovine luteinizing hormone β subunit. *FEBS Lett* 1971; 19:209–213.
286. Maghuin-Rogister G, Hennen G. Luteinizing hormone: The primary structures of the β-subunit from bovine and porcine species. *Eur J Biochem* 1973;39:235–253.
287. Kato Y, Hirai T. Cloning and DNA sequence analysis of the cDNA for the precursor of porcine luteinizing hormone (LH) β subunit. *Mol Cell Endocrinol* 1989;62:47–53.
288. Glenn SD, Nahm HS, Ward DN. The amino acid sequence of the rabbit lutropin beta subunit. *J Protein Chem* 1984;3:259–273.
289. Chin WW, Godine JE, Klein DR, Chang AS, Tan LK, Habener JF. Nucleotide sequence of the cDNA encoding the precursor of the β subunit of rat lutropin. *Proc Natl Acad Sci USA* 1983;80:4649–4653.
290. Jameson L, Chin WW, Hollenberg AN, Chang AS, Habener JF. The gene encoding the β-subunit of rat luteinizing hormone: Analysis of gene structure and evolution of nucleotide sequence. *J Biol Chem* 1984;259:15474–15480.

291. Pankov YA, Karasyov VS. Primary structure of sperm whale luteinizing hormone. *Int J Peptide Protein Res* 1986;28:124–129.
292. Wolf DL, Appleby VL, Hjerrild K, Baker AR, Talmadge K. Nucleic acid and amino acid sequences of dog LH: Comparison to rat, cow and human βLH. *Nucleic Acids Res* 1987;15:10602.
293. Hayashi H, Hayashi T, Hanaoka Y. Amphibian lutropin from the bullfrog *Rana catesbeiana.* Complete amino acid sequence of the β subunit. *Eur J Biochem* 1992;203:105–110.
294. Shome B, Parlow AF, Liu WK, Nahm HS, Wen T, Ward DN. A reevaluation of the amino acid sequence of human follitropin β-subunit. *J Protein Chem* 1988;7:325–339.
295. Watkins PC, Eddy R, Beck AK, et al. DNA sequence and regional assignment of the human follicle-stimulating hormone β-subunit to the short arm of human chromosome 11. *DNA* 1987; 6:205–212.
296. Jameson JL, Becker CB, Lindell CM, Habener JF. Human follicle-stimulating hormone β-subunit gene encodes multiple messenger ribonucleic acids. *Mol Endocrinol* 1988;2:806–815.
297. Sairam MR, Seidah NG, Chrétien M. Primary structure of the ovine pituitary follitropin β-subunit. *Biochem J* 1981; 197:541–552.
298. Mountford PS, Bello PA, Brandon MR, Adams TE. Cloning and DNA sequence analysis of the cDNA for the precursor of ovine follicle stimulating hormone β-subunit. *Nucleic Acids Res* 1989;17:6391.
299. Maurer RA, Beck A. Isolation and nucleotide sequence analysis of a cloned cDNA encoding the β-subunit of bovine follicle-stimulating hormone. *DNA* 1986;5:363–369.
300. Esch F, Mason AJ, Cooksey K, Mercado M, Shimasaki S. Cloning and DNA sequence analysis of the cDNA for the precursor of the β chain of bovine follicle stimulating hormone. *Proc Natl Acad Sci USA* 1986;83:6618–6621.
301. Kim KE, Gordon DF, Maurer RA. Nucleotide sequence of the bovine gene for follicle-stimulating hormone β-subunit. *DNA* 1988;7:227–233.
302. Kato Y. Cloning and DNA sequence analysis of the cDNA for the precursor of porcine follicle stimulating hormone (FSH) β subunit. *Mol Cell Endocrinol* 1988;55:107–112.
303. Maurer RA. Molecular cloning and nucleotide sequence analysis of complementary deoxyribonucleic acid for the β-subunit of rat follicle stimulating hormone. *Mol Endocrinol* 1987;1:717–723.
304. Hayashi T, Hanaoka Y, Hayashi H. The complete amino acid sequence of the follitropin β-subunit of the bullfrog, *Rana catesbeiana. Gen Comp Endocrinol* 1992;88:144–150.
305. Ward DN, Bousfield GR, Mar AO. Chemical reduction–reoxidation of the glycoprotein hormone disulfide bonds. In: Bellet D, Bidart J-M, eds. *Structure–Function Relationship of Gonadotropins.* New York: Raven Press; 1989:1–19.
306. Gordon DF, Wood WM, Ridgway EC. Organization and nucleotide sequence of the gene encoding the β-subunit of murine thyrotropin. *DNA* 1988;7:17–26.
307. Fiddes JC, Goodman HM. The gene encoding the common alpha subunit of the four human glycoprotein hormones. *J Mol Appl Genet* 1981;1:3–18.
308. Ezashi T, Kato T, Wakabayashi K, Kato Y. The gene for the beta subunit of porcine LH: Clusters of GC boxes and CACCC elements. *J Mol Endocrinol* 1990;5:137–146.
309. Gharib SD, Roy A, Wierman ME, Chin WW. Isolation and characterization of the gene encoding the beta-subunit of rat follicle-stimulating hormone. *DNA* 1989;8:339–349.
310. Hirai T, Takikawa H, Kato Y. The gene for the beta subunit of porcine FSH: Absence of consensus estrogen responsive elements and presence of retroposons. *J Mol Endocrinol* 1990;5:147–158.
311. Kornfeld R, Kornfeld S. Assembly of asparagine-linked oligosaccharides. *Annu Rev Biochem* 1985;54:631–634.

The Physiology of Reproduction, Second Edition,
edited by E. Knobil and J.D. Neill,
Raven Press, Ltd., New York © 1994.

CHAPTER 31

Regulation of Gonadotropin Gene Expression

Daniel J. Haisenleder, Alan C. Dalkin, and John C. Marshall

The pituitary gonadotropic hormones, luteinizing hormone (LH) and follicle-stimulating hormone (FSH), are composed of two dissimilar glycoprotein subunits. The α subunit is common to both LH and FSH, as well as to thyrotropin (TSH) and the placentally derived chorionic gonadotropin (CG), which is selectively expressed in primates and horses (1–5). The β subunit for each glycoprotein hormone is distinct and confers biologic specificity (1,2). Luteinizing hormone and FSH synergistically stimulate the male and female gonads to regulate sexual maturation and reproductive function (6,7). More specifically, LH predominantly stimulates gonadal steroid production and FSH regulates gametogenesis (8).

Hypothalamic regulation of LH and FSH is primarily by the decapeptide, gonadotropin-releasing hormone (GnRH), which is released in a pulsatile manner into the hypophyseal portal circulation (9,10). Gonadotropin-releasing hormone pulsatility is crucial for maintaining different aspects of gonadotrope secretory function including pituitary GnRH receptor up-regulation, subunit gene expression, and LH and FSH release (11–13). Data obtained in different mammalian species have shown that the amplitude and frequency of GnRH pulses change during normal physiology, which is one of the primary mechanisms whereby LH and FSH are differentially controlled by the hypothalamus (14–18).

Gonadotropin secretion is also regulated by gonadal steroids and peptides. Both androgens and estrogens maintain an inhibitory effect on LH and FSH secretion (19,20). This action of gonadal steroids is primarily through the inhibition of GnRH pulsatile release, although direct effects on the gonadotrope cell have also been shown (21,22). Recently, the roles played by gonadal peptides have been described. These peptides (inhibins, activins, and follistatin) predominantly regulate FSH, producing both stimulatory (activins) and inhibitory (inhibins, follistatin) effects (23,24). Present evidence suggests that these peptides are important in effecting the differential regulation of LH and FSH (25,26). More recent data have shown that all three gonadal peptides are also produced within the pituitary, suggesting not only an endocrine action but perhaps a paracrine or autocrine role in gonadotropin regulation (27,28).

STRUCTURE OF THE GONADOTROPIN SUBUNIT GENES AND MESSENGER RIBONUCLEIC ACIDS

α Subunit

The α subunit genes have been characterized from several species, including the rat, mouse, cow, horse, hu-

Department of Internal Medicine, Division of Endocrinology, University of Virginia Health Sciences Center, Charlottesville, Virginia 22908 man, and old world monkey (29–34). In all species studied to date, the α subunit is coded by a single gene that contains four exons and three introns. In primate and equine species, the α subunit gene is expressed in placental trophoblast as well as in pituitary cells (29,34). The size of the α gene varies from 8 to 16.5 kb, largely because of variation in the size of the first intron, and nucleotide sequence analyses have shown that the coding region is highly conserved. Mature α subunit messenger ribonucleic acid (mRNA) is 730 to 800 nucleotides in length and codes for a polypeptide that contains a 24-amino-acid leader peptide followed by a 96-amino-acid protein in most species studied (i.e., mouse, rat, bovine). In the human, the α subunit apoprotein is 92 amino acids in length, because of the deletion of four residues near the amino terminus (35).

FSH β Subunit

The FSH β subunit is also encoded by a single gene in species studied to date, which has been characterized in the human, rat, and cow, and contains three exons and two introns (36–39). The gene encodes for an mRNA that is much larger than the other gonadotropin subunit mRNAs (approximately 1.7 kb in length), the increased size being primarily caused by a large 3′ untranslated region of 1 to 1.5 kb (36). The significance of this 3′ region is presently unknown, but it has been speculated that it may play a role in determining FSH β mRNA stability. This is supported by studies showing that elements in the 3′ untranslated region can regulate mRNA stability in other cell systems (40). The FSH β mRNA nucleotide and polypeptide amino acid sequences are highly conserved between species (approximately 80%). In rats and cows, only one mRNA has been demonstrated, but the human FSH β gene produces four mRNA size variations (39). The different mRNA sizes appear to be due to the use of two different transcription start sites and two different polyadenylation sites, but it is unknown if all four mRNA transcripts are translated or hormonally regulated.

LH β and CG β Subunits

The LH β and CG β apoproteins are similar in structure and amino acid sequence and are believed to be derived from a single ancestral gene (41). The LH β gene is found in the gonadotrope cell of the pituitary and has been characterized in the rat, cow, and human (42–46). LH β contains three exons and two introns and is considerably smaller than the α subunit gene (approximately 1.5 kb). The gene encodes an mRNA that is approximately 700 nucleotides in length, and in humans, the mRNA translates a polypeptide that contains a 22-amino-acid leader peptide and a 121-amino-acid protein. CG β is selectively produced in primates and equine species within the syncytiotrophoblast cells of the placenta, and its mRNA is approximately 1,000 bases in length (47). Unlike other gonadotropin subunits, CG β is not encoded by a single gene. In the human, a cluster of seven "CG β-like" genes or pseudogenes are located on chromosome 19 (48–50), and the LH β gene is also located within this region. Present evidence suggests that only one or two of the seven "human CG (hCG) β-like" genes are expressed (42,48).

Although LH β and CG β apoproteins are very homogeneous in structure and have similar biologic activity, differences are seen. The hCG β apoprotein contains a 24-amino-acid carboxyl terminus extension not seen in LH β (42). Nucleotide sequence homology upstream from the transcriptional start site is greater than 90%, but the 5′ untranslated region of the CG β mRNA is considerably longer (366 bases) than that of LH β (nine bases). This difference appears to be due to LH β and CG β using alternate transcriptional start sites, with CG using a promoter approximately 350 bp upstream from the common transcriptional promoter sequence TATAA (51). Of interest, despite the homology between the two genes, the results of fusion gene transfection studies have shown that LH β is not expressed in placenta-derived cell lines (29,52). This could suggest that the LH β gene either contains "repressor" element(s) that require gonadotrope-specific nuclear factors to override basal suppression or lacks placental tissue-specific "enhancing" regulatory element(s).

PHYSIOLOGIC ALTERATIONS IN GONADOTROPIN SUBUNIT GENE EXPRESSION

Estrous Cycle

In the rat, preovulatory surges of pituitary gonadotropins occur in the evening of proestrus of the 4-day cycle (53,54). The LH surge lasts about 6 to 8 h and is primarily under the control of GnRH (55). The FSH surge also begins in the evening of proestrus but continues into the following morning (estrus). Several studies have shown that the biphasic pattern of the FSH surge can be separated into an initial GnRH-regulated phase (coincident with the LH surge) and a later inhibin-regulated phase (55–57).

We have characterized the changes in α, LH β, and FSH β mRNAs during the 4-day estrous cycle in pituitaries collected at 3- to 6-h intervals over the cycle and hourly during the gonadotropin surges (58,59) (Fig. 1). On proestrus, both LH β and FSH β mRNA concentrations rose during the preovulatory gonadotropin surges, and although the increase in mRNA concentrations were generally parallel, differences in onset and duration

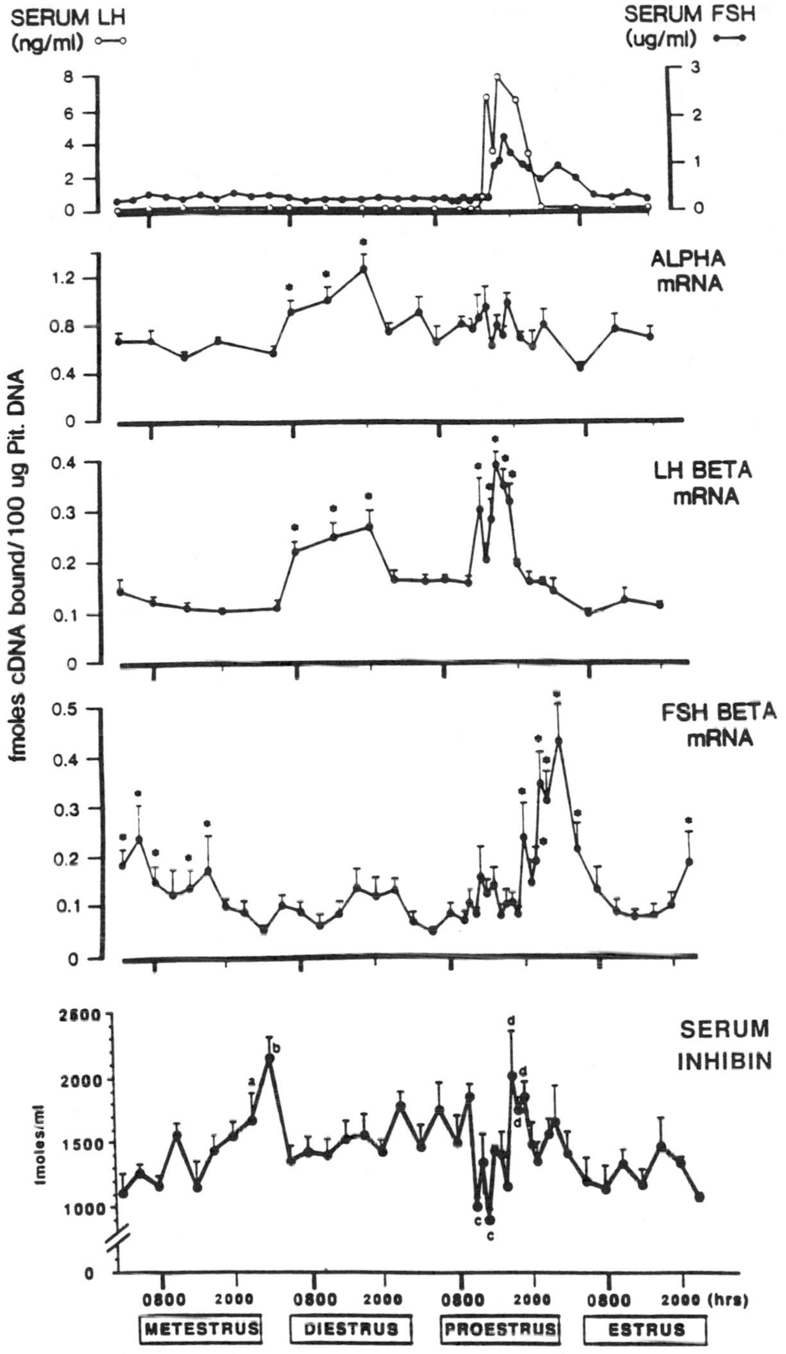

FIG. 1. Serum gonadotropins (*LH* and *FSH*) and inhibin concentrations and pituitary gonadotropin subunit mRNAs during rat estrous cycle. Mean ± SEM for each group (5–11 animals/group) is shown. *Asterisks or letters* (*a–d*) denote significant differences from basal control groups; $P < .05$. (From refs. 58, 59, and 62, with permission.)

were observed. The rise in LH β mRNA began at 2:00 PM (2 h before the surge-related increase in LH), peaked at 5:00 PM (2.5-fold increase), and then returned to basal levels by 10:00 PM. In contrast, increases in FSH β mRNA were not seen until 8:00 PM, 2 h after the initial rise in serum FSH. Maximal (fourfold) increases in FSH β mRNA were seen during the early morning of estrus (2:00 AM), with levels returning to basal 6 h later (8:00 AM). Of interest, α subunit mRNA did not increase significantly during the proestrus gonadotropin surges.

A selective rise in FSH β mRNA levels was seen on metestrus, occurring when measurable increases in FSH secretory activity were not observed. On the morning of diestrus, a parallel rise (twofold) in α and LH β mRNAs was present, which was also not associated with a measurable rise in LH secretion. Thus, during the rat estrous cycle, both coordinate and differential increases in gonadotropin subunit mRNA expression are seen: LH β and FSH β mRNAs both increase during the proestrus gonadotropin surges; FSH β selectively increases on metestrus; α and LH β increase in parallel on diestrus when LH and FSH secretion remain stable.

The mechanisms that regulate the changes in gonadotropin subunit gene expression during the rat estrous cycle have yet to be fully characterized. The rise in LH β and FSH β mRNA levels seen on proestrus appears to be the result of altered synthesis, as LH β and FSH β transcriptional rates increase at the time of the surge (60) in response to the increase in GnRH release on the afternoon of proestrus (10,18). The mechanism(s) responsible for the selective increase in FSH β mRNA on metestrus is presently unknown but probably reflects input from ovarian peptides (inhibins, activins, follistatin) that have been shown to selectively influence FSH β gene expression (23,26,61) (discussed in later sections of this chapter). This is supported by data obtained within the same group of animals, showing that the decline in FSH β mRNA during the late afternoon of metestrus was coincident with a rise in serum inhibin levels (62) (Fig. 1, lower panel). No explanation is currently available for the increase in α and LH β mRNAs on diestrus, but these changes could relate to the rise in estradiol (E_2) and/or to increased pulsatile GnRH secretion, both of which occur on diestrus (18,53,54,63).

Unlike the rat, the sheep is a seasonal breeding species. During the autumn and winter, female sheep express repeated estrous cycles that are approximately 16 days in length. The time of female receptivity is defined as estrus, which is followed several hours later by preovulatory surges of LH and FSH (64,65). Studies conducted by Leung and colleagues (66) characterized the changes in α, LH β, and FSH β subunit mRNAs at the time of the gonadotropin surges in sheep (Fig. 2). Their data revealed that α and LH β mRNAs tended to rise in parallel, with peak levels being coincident with the LH and FSH surges. In contrast, FSH β mRNA concentrations declined during the gonadotropin surges, reaching nadir values when serum FSH was maximal. This twofold fall in FSH β mRNA at the onset of estrus was followed by a fivefold increase in FSH β mRNA 24 h later. These results appear to suggest that FSH β mRNA expression is regulated in a differential manner from α and LH β mRNAs at the time of the gonadotropin surge. These data differ from those obtained in the rat, where LH β and FSH β mRNAs rose during the surges and α was unchanged (Fig. 1). As GnRH has been shown to stimulate expression of all three gonadotropin subunit genes in sheep (67–69), it is likely that GnRH mediates the increase in α and LH β mRNAs seen during the surges. The mechanism(s) behind the surge-related decrease in FSH β mRNA levels is presently unknown but may include alterations in gonadal peptides (inhibin, follistatin, or activin) or gonadal steroids (a preovulatory rise in E_2 occurs before initiation of the gonadotropin surges in the ewe) (64,65). Indeed, *in vitro* studies have shown that E_2 can selectively inhibit the FSH β transcription rate (70) in sheep pituitary cells.

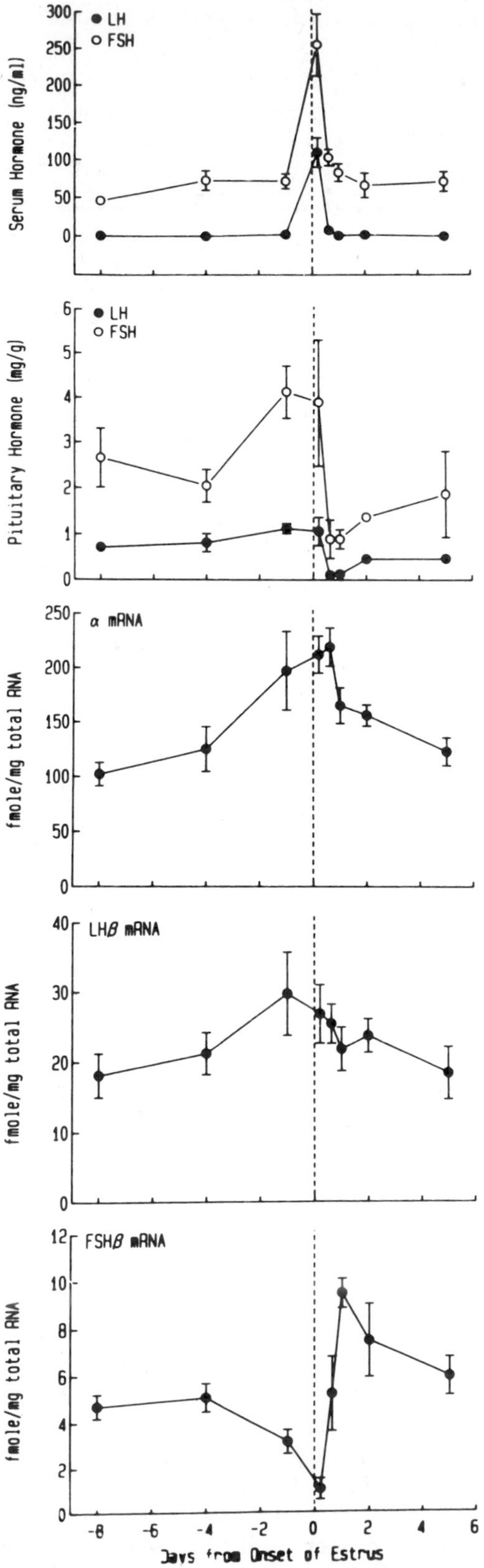

FIG. 2. Alterations in serum gonadotropins and pituitary subunit mRNAs during estrous cycle of sheep. Mean ± SEM for each group is shown. *Hatched vertical line* (day 0) represents time of behavioral estrus. (From ref. 66, with permission.)

Postgonadectomy

Several studies have shown that removal of the gonads results in a rise in LH and FSH secretory activity (71–73). Data suggesting a similar postcastration rise in gonadotropin subunit gene expression were originally provided by studies showing that the cell free translation of α and LH β subunits was increased in steers compared with bulls (74,75). More recently, data obtained in rats, mice, and sheep have shown that α, LH β, and FSH β mRNA concentrations increase after gonadectomy (67,76–78). In the rat, this appears to involve both an elevation of subunit transcriptional rates (79,80), as well as the recruitment of active gonadotrope cells within the pituitary (81). Studies from our laboratory and others have characterized the postgonadectomy rise in gonadotropin mRNAs in the rat (76,77,82–85). Steady-state concentrations of all three mRNAs increase after castration in males or ovariectomy (OVX) in females, but the magnitude and time course of changes for each subunit vary.

Subunit mRNA concentrations after gonadectomy in male and female rats are shown in Fig. 3. In male rats, serum gonadotropins increased rapidly (data not shown) and α and LH β subunit mRNAs were significantly increased within 24 h of castration (77,82). Alpha mRNA attained maximal levels (three- to fourfold increase) within 10 days, whereas LH β plateaued (fivefold increase) after 14 days. FSH β mRNA showed smaller magnitude changes and only increased twofold after 7 days, thereafter being stable or even declining. In females, the smaller increase in serum LH (data not shown) was accompanied by similar changes in mRNAs. Alpha and LH β subunit mRNAs rose slowly—with significant increases not being seen until 4 to 7 days post-OVX. Alpha mRNA (fivefold increase) plateaued after 14 days, whereas LH β mRNA continued to rise through 30 days (15-fold increase). In contrast, serum FSH and FSH β mRNA increased within 12 h of OVX, with maximal concentrations being stable after 4 days (fourfold increase).

Hypothalamic Disconnection

The role of the hypothalamus in the regulation of gonadotropin subunit gene expression has been assessed after the removal of hypothalamic (primarily GnRH) influence to the pituitary. Three experimental strategies have been used for these studies: surgical disconnection of the blood supply from the hypothalamus to the pituitary (67,86,87); treatment protocols that specifically in-

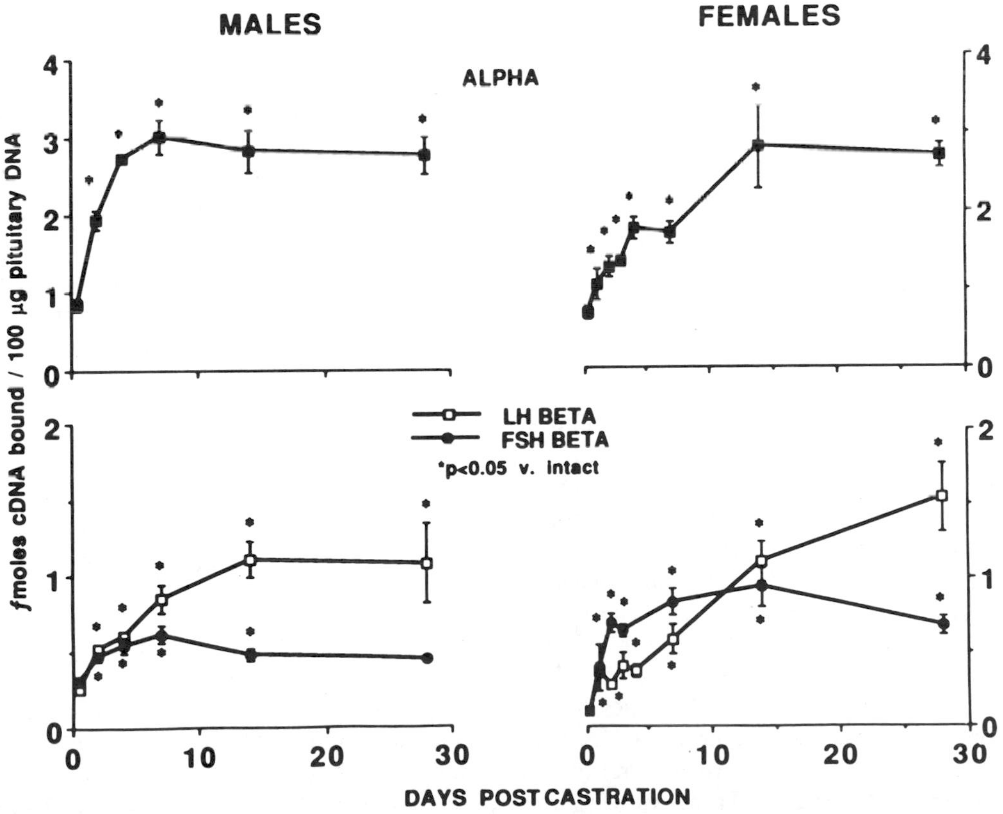

FIG. 3. Steady-state concentrations of pituitary gonadotropin subunit mRNAs after gonadectomy in male and female rats. (From ref. 211, with permission.)

hibit GnRH release [i.e., testosterone administration to male rats (80,82,88); progesterone administration to female sheep (68)]; removal of GnRH influence at the pituitary [i.e., use of GnRH antagonists (80,82,89)]. These experimental models have been particularly useful in providing information relating to the direct versus the indirect (by GnRH) effects of gonadal steroids and peptides. In the OVX ewe, surgical hypothalamic disconnection (HPD) results in a rapid decrease in serum LH followed by a slower fall in serum FSH (67,86,87). Gonadotropin subunit mRNA concentrations decrease compared with OVX animals and can be restored to OVX levels by administration of pulsatile GnRH (67,69,86,87). Over a duration of several days, subunit mRNA levels in HPD ewes fall below levels present in ovarian intact animals (67,69). These results suggest that in the ewe, GnRH is not only critical in stimulating gonadotropin subunit mRNAs after gonadectomy but also regulates basal gene expression. In the rat, the latter action is not as prominent, and after GnRH antagonists, α, LH β, and FSH β mRNAs are generally at or only slightly below levels seen in untreated control animals (80,82).

REGULATORS OF GONADOTROPIN SUBUNIT GENE EXPRESSION

Gonadotropin-Releasing Hormone

Experimental Models

As previously noted, a pulsatile GnRH signal is crucial for the maintenance of gonadotrope function. Furthermore, alterations in the parameters of the pulsatile GnRH stimulus (i.e., changes in frequency and/or amplitude) can differentially regulate gonadotropin subunit gene expression. The actions of GnRH have been assessed both *in vivo* and *in vitro* using a variety of models.

In vivo studies: To examine the effects of GnRH in male rats, we have used the castrate-testosterone (T) replaced rat model characterized by Steiner and associates (90). Here, adult male rats are castrated and replaced with physiologic levels of T (2–3 ng/ml) through subcutaneous implants. The constant plasma level of T prevents the postcastration increase in gonadotropin subunit gene expression and gonadotropin secretion and abolishes pulsatile LH (and by inference, GnRH) release in 75% of the animals (only occasional LH pulses are seen in the remaining 25%). In female rats, parallel studies have used the ovariectomized-E_2 replaced model (OVX-E_2) (91), although residual endogenous GnRH secretion is present as evidenced by the daily LH surges (92). In sheep, progesterone (P) administration to anestrus ewes has been shown to prevent endogenous GnRH release (68) and thus provides a suitable model in which to study GnRH action.

In vitro studies: We and others have used systems in which dispersed pituitary cells are perifused and exposed to a pulsatile GnRH stimulus. Protocols have differed between laboratories (male versus female animals, mature versus immature animals, duration of GnRH treatment), although results have been generally similar between laboratories (93–96).

Effect of GnRH Pulse Amplitude

The amplitude of the pulsatile GnRH signal can exert differential effects on subunit mRNA concentrations. To investigate the effects of pulse dose, we have used the castrate-T replaced male rat model. GnRH pulses at doses of 10 to 250 ng per pulse were given every 30 min (the frequency of LH pulses observed in castrate male rats), and the results are shown in Fig. 4. Earlier studies had demonstrated that GnRH increased the number of GnRH receptors with maximum responses seen after 25 ng per pulse, and both higher or lower doses were less effective (88). Alpha and FSH β mRNA concentrations were increased by all pulse doses. In contrast, LH β mRNA responses paralleled those of the GnRH receptors. LH β mRNA was elevated only after doses of 10 to 75 ng per pulse, with maximal responses occurring after 25 ng per pulse (97,98). Similar studies have been performed in the OVX-E_2 replaced female rat model (91), and data are shown in Fig. 5. In this setting, LH β and FSH β mRNAs rose after 0.5 to 25 ng GnRH per pulse, whereas changes in α subunit mRNA were small and were only seen at higher pulse doses (25–250 ng). The dependence of subunit mRNA responses on GnRH pulse dose was less evident in the female model, perhaps reflecting the presence of some continuing endogenous GnRH secretion. In recent *in vitro* studies, we have used pituitary cells from 30-day-old female rats and have shown that LH β mRNA is increased by a narrower range of GnRH pulse doses than are α and FSH β (93). This is more in keeping with data obtained in the GnRH-deficient male rat and supports the view that LH β mRNA expression is more sensitive to GnRH amplitude than either α or FSH β, which both rise in response to a wider range of GnRH pulse doses.

Effect of GnRH Pulse Frequency

Alterations in the frequency of pulsatile GnRH secretion can result in differential regulation of gonadotropin subunit gene expression. *In vivo,* we have used the castrate-T replaced male rat model and given GnRH at a dose of 25 ng per pulse. This dose of GnRH results in peak peripheral blood concentrations of approximately

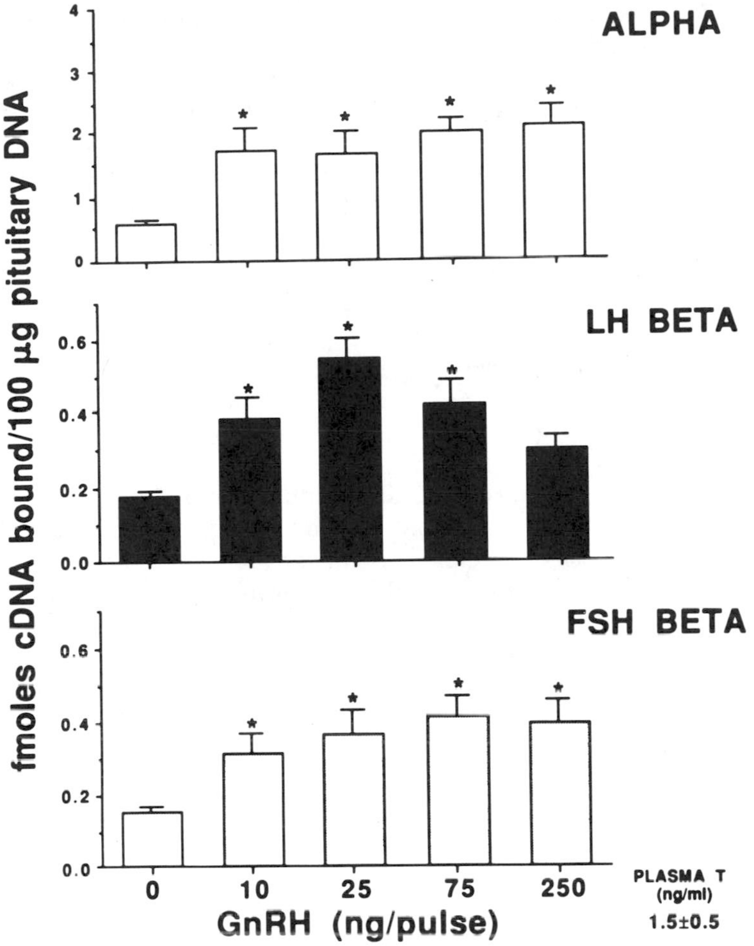

FIG. 4. Effects of GnRH pulse amplitude on expression of gonadotropin subunit mRNAs in male rats. Castrate testosterone-replaced rats were given GnRH pulses every 30 min for 24 h. Pulse amplitude (ng/pulse) is shown. *$P < .05$ versus 0 ng GnRH (saline controls). (From ref. 211, with permission.)

200 pg/ml, a value similar to that observed in pituitary stalk blood (99–102). The number of GnRH receptors are increased by GnRH pulses given at intervals of less than 120 min, with maximum LH secretory responses occurring after 15- to 60-min pulses (97,103,104). The results of GnRH pulse frequency on expression of gonadotropin subunit mRNAs are shown in Fig. 6. GnRH pulses given at 8-min intervals increased α and LH β mRNAs. Thirty-min pulses (a fast physiologic frequency as seen after castration) increased all three subunit mRNAs, whereas pulses given at intervals of 120 min or longer increased only FSH β mRNA (97,105). Elevated levels of FSH β mRNA and serum FSH could be maintained by GnRH pulses given only once per 8 h, suggesting a marked difference in the frequency dependence of gonadotropin subunit gene expression.

Generally similar results have been observed in the OVX-progesterone-replaced female sheep model (68). In that study, α mRNA levels were increased by GnRH pulses given at 30-min intervals. All three subunit mRNAs were increased by GnRH pulses given every 60 min, whereas slower GnRH pulse frequencies (240-min pulse intervals) were ineffective. The reasons for the different results in sheep and rats at slower pulse frequencies are uncertain. The gonadal steroid milieu is different in the two models, and progesterone has been shown to inhibit FSH β gene transcription in ovine pituitary cell cultures (70). Alternatively, variations in sensitivity to changes in GnRH pulse pattern or a different range of effective frequencies may occur between species.

The dependence of gonadotropin subunit gene expression on a pulsatile GnRH signal has been confirmed in several studies *in vitro* (93–96,106). Continuous GnRH administration increases only α mRNA, whereas LH β and FSH β subunit mRNAs are unchanged or even decreased. Furthermore, α and LH β subunit mRNAs are maximally increased by faster GnRH pulse frequencies (15–60 min), whereas FSH β again responds maximally at slower (120-min) frequencies, and levels actually decline at fast (15-min) pulse intervals.

Overall, these data suggest that alterations in the frequency of GnRH pulse stimulation may be physiologically important in the differential regulation of gonadotropin subunit gene expression and gonadotropin secretion. In general, these studies are in accord with earlier studies in humans and primates, in which slow

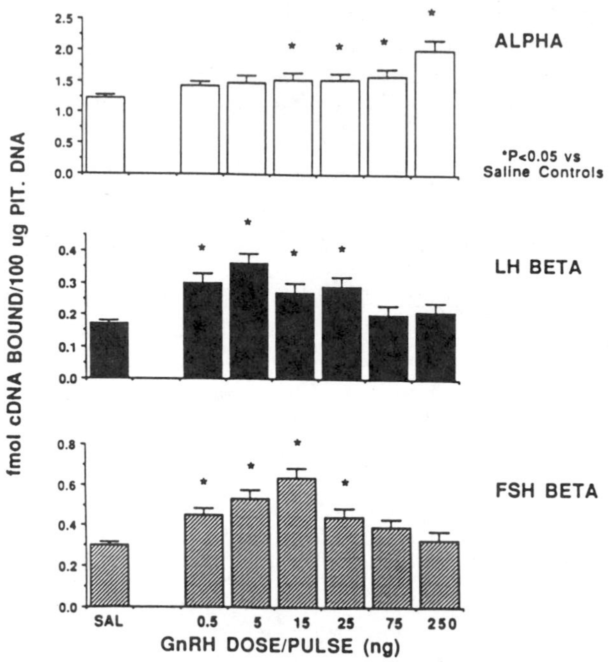

FIG. 5. Effect of GnRH pulse amplitude on gonadotropin subunit mRNAs in ovariectomized-estradiol replaced (OVX-E_2) rats. GnRH pulses (0.5–250 ng/pulse, saline to controls) were given every 30 min for 12 h. Bars represent mean ± SEM (n = 7–12 per group). *P < .05 versus saline controls. (From ref. 91, with permission.)

frequency GnRH stimuli favored FSH secretion and faster GnRH pulses were required to maintain LH release.

Time Course of Subunit mRNA Responses to GnRH Pulses

Exogenous GnRH pulses rapidly (within 1 h) stimulate the transcription rates of all three gonadotropin subunit genes (12) (discussed below), but the rate at which cytoplasmic mRNA concentrations increase differs between the mRNA species. In both male and female rats, FSH β mRNA increases within 4 to 6 h in response to GnRH (12,92,97,107). LH β mRNA changes more slowly, rising some 16 to 24 h after initiation of a GnRH stimulus. Studies on α subunit expression have been complicated by the presence of α mRNA in both gonadotropes and thyrotropes. As the former comprise only 5% to 7% of pituitary cells, thyrotrope α may mask small increases in gonadotrope α. Hence, high doses of thyroid hormone have been used to suppress thyrotrope α gene expression (107). In this model (T3 suppressed, castrate-T replaced male rats), α subunit mRNA rises within 12 h in response to GnRH pulses. Besides its action on increasing subunit gene transcription, GnRH may regulate subunit mRNA concentrations through nontranscriptional mechanisms. Weiss and colleagues (106) documented altered polyadenylation after stimulation of pituitary cells by exogenous GnRH.

In summary, increases in cytoplasmic mRNA concentrations occur most rapidly for FSH β, followed by α and subsequently LH β. Whether these differences in appearance rate of cytoplasmic mRNA reflect differences in nuclear processing and/or transport or other mechanism such as parallel actions of GnRH on mRNA synthesis and degradation remains uncertain.

Gonadal Steroids

Testosterone

The removal of feedback inhibition of GnRH secretion by gonadal steroids is predominantly responsible for the postgonadectomy rise in gonadotropin gene expression (29,80,82,108,109). As seen in Fig. 7, T replacement in castrated male rats reduces gonadotropin subunit mRNAs to intact levels. However, the effect of T on FSH β mRNA appears to be complex. We have shown that replacing T at a physiologic level (serum T = 2.5 ng/ml) through subcutaneous implants placed at the time of orchidectomy completely prevented the postcastration rise in FSH β mRNA levels (80,82). However, other investigators have found that administering phar-

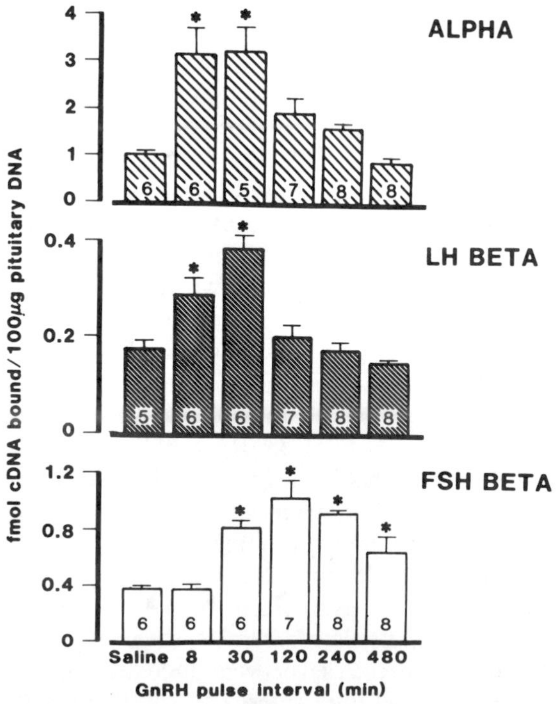

FIG. 6. Effect of GnRH pulse frequency on expression of gonadotropin subunit mRNAs in castrate testosterone-replaced male rats. Dose per pulse of GnRH was constant (25 ng), and pulse intervals are shown. *P < .05 versus saline. (From ref. 105, with permission.)

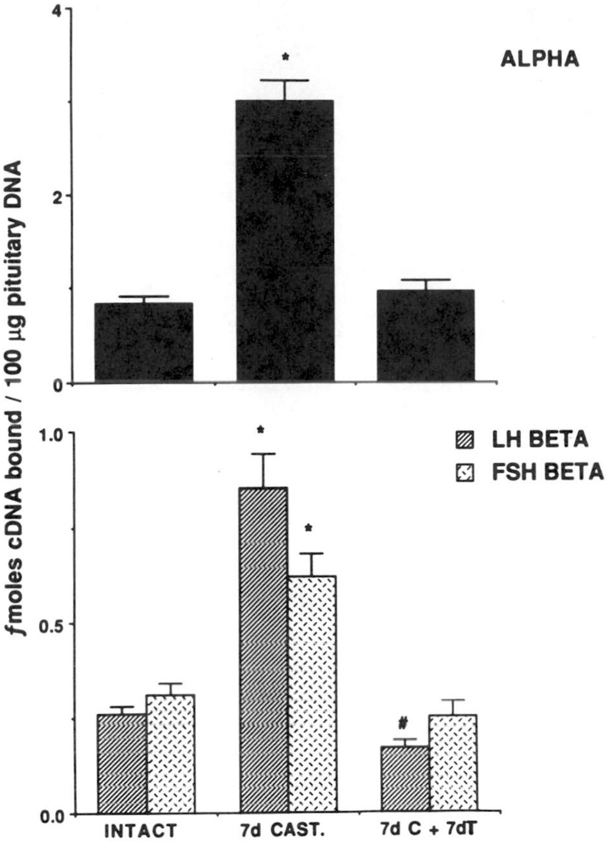

FIG. 7. Effect of testosterone (*T*) on subunit mRNA concentrations in 7-day orchidectomized male rats. T replacement by subcutaneous Silastic implant (plasma T was 2.5 ng/ml) was continued for 7 days. $^{*}P < .05$ versus intact. (From ref. 211, with permission.)

macologic doses of T (through intermittent subcutaneous injections) did not fully suppress FSH β mRNA levels in castrate rats (76,85). Furthermore, in castrated male rats treated with a GnRH antagonist, the addition of T actually increased FSH β mRNA levels twofold and serum FSH (80,89,110). Data from recent *in vitro* studies reveal that T can increase FSH β mRNA concentrations in a dose-dependent manner by an action directly on the gonadotrope cell (111). Thus, in the castrated rat, lower doses of T probably inhibit FSH β mRNA expression by the suppression of GnRH release, whereas higher doses may also stimulate FSH β mRNA through a direct action at the pituitary. Studies have shown that T increases steady-state levels of FSH β mRNA in the absence of altered mRNA synthesis (transcription), suggesting an action on mRNA degradation (80). This is supported by examination of the *in vivo* disappearance of subunit mRNAs in the presence or absence of T (Fig. 8). Rats were given a GnRH antagonist to block GnRH-induced subunit transcription, with the initial dose being given intravenously to define the onset of antagonist action. The presence of T did not alter the rate at which α or LH β mRNAs declined. However, T markedly prolonged the disappearance time for FSH β—twofold from a half disappearance time of 20 h to one of 40 h. The physiologic significance of this action of T is uncertain, but T stabilization of FSH β mRNA may preserve FSH secretory function and gamete maturation. As T levels rise, GnRH secretion is inhibited with consequent reduction in gonadotropin, especially LH, secretion. Thus, the direct action of T on FSH β mRNA and the close relationship between FSH β mRNA concentration and basal FSH secretion (80) would favor maintaining FSH secretion during periods of reduced GnRH stimuli. Regardless, T can increase FSH β mRNA concentrations in both male and female rats (112), suggesting that post-transcriptional regulation of gonadotropin subunit mRNAs can occur in both sexes.

Estradiol

Replacement of physiologic concentrations of E_2 to OVX rats inhibits GnRH secretion (100) and, as shown in Fig. 9, results in suppression of all three gonadotropin subunit mRNAs, although by different degrees (76,82, 83,85). The rise in LH β mRNA can be completely blocked by administration of E_2 at the time of OVX, but α mRNA concentrations still increase (approximately 50%) above levels seen in intact animals. This action of E_2 in increasing α mRNA requires the presence of GnRH, as it does not occur if the animals also received a GnRH antagonist (82), and E_2 does not alter α mRNA *in vitro* (111). Recent evidence suggests that ovarian steroids, particularly E_2, may act directly on the GnRH-producing neurons. Hoffman and associates (113) reported that the administration of E_2 and P in a regimen that produces a predictable afternoon LH surge increased the nuclear c-Fos immunoreactivity in neurons colocalized for GnRH. The c-Fos gene product is intimately involved in the regulation of gene transcription (114,115) and hence may serve as a marker of cellular activation.

In contrast to LH β, the rapid increase in FSH β mRNA is only partially suppressed by E_2 at the time of OVX. Similar findings are seen if both E_2 and P or a GnRH antagonist are given at OVX, suggesting that the loss of nonsteroidal factor(s) from the gonad (e.g., inhibin, follistatin) is causally related to the rapid increase in FSH β mRNA expression (82).

Progesterone

The effects of P are dependent on the prevailing gonadal steroid milieu and the results of P administration either alone or together with E_2 are shown in Fig. 9. Progesterone replacement does not prevent the increases in gonadotropin subunit gene expression. In contrast, the addition of P to E_2 (for 2–7 days) is more effective than

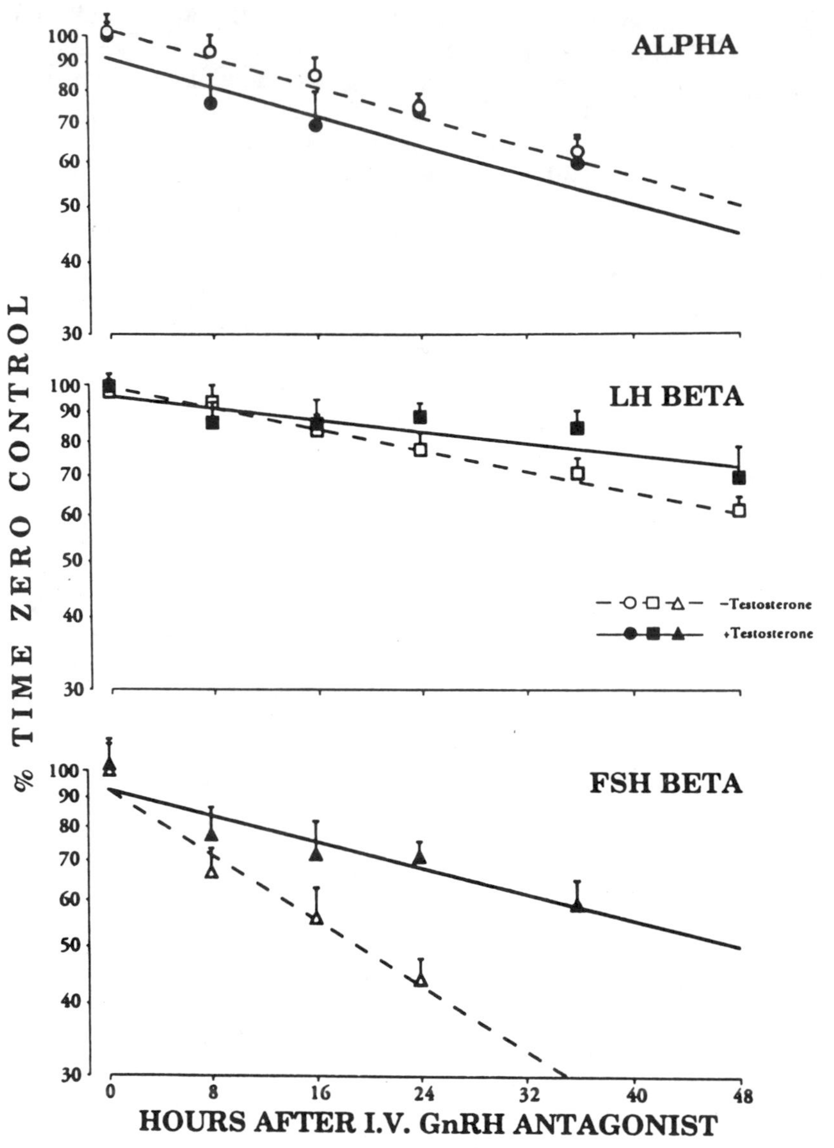

FIG. 8. Decline in concentrations of gonadotropin subunit mRNAs after administration of GnRH antagonists intravenous and subcutaneous) in presence and absence of T. ○, α; □, LH β; △, FSH β. *Solid symbols* are results in presence of T. Data are normalized to time zero = 100% on a logarithmic scale. Values are mean ± SEM (n = 8–20/group). (From ref. 80, with permission.)

E_2 alone in reducing the rise in α, LH β, and FSH β mRNAs after ovariectomy (82). Progesterone and E_2 replacement at OVX maintained LH β subunit mRNA concentration at or below intact values. The effects were identical to those of a GnRH antagonist, suggesting that P and E_2 acts by suppressing GnRH secretion.

In vitro studies using pituitary cells from sheep suggest that higher concentrations of P can inhibit FSH β transcription (70), and in anestrus sheep and in rats in the presence of estrogen, P reduces gonadotropin subunit gene expression by inhibiting GnRH secretion (116, 117). These studies suggest that P acts to reduce gonadotropin gene expression both by reducing the GnRH stimulus and by a direct action on the gonadotrope. However, a recent *in vivo* study suggests that short-term (less than 24 h) P in immature female rats can selectively increase FSH β mRNAs (118). Thus, in the rat, progesterone may act directly at the pituitary to selectively increase FSH β mRNA concentrations, although the mechanism by which this occurs is currently unknown.

Gonadal Peptides

The transforming growth factor β super family of polypeptides is composed of related compounds with diverse biologic actions, including the regulation of cell growth and differentiation as well as cell–cell signaling. There are at least 18 proteins in this family sharing a similar dimeric structure with disulfide bonds, asparagine-linked glycosylation sites, and protein homologies of between 25% to 90% (119). Included are the transforming growth factor (TGF)-βs, mullerian inhibiting substance, bone morphogenetic proteins, and the inhibins/activins (120–122). These compounds are synthesized as precursor polypeptides, which are then cleaved to form active

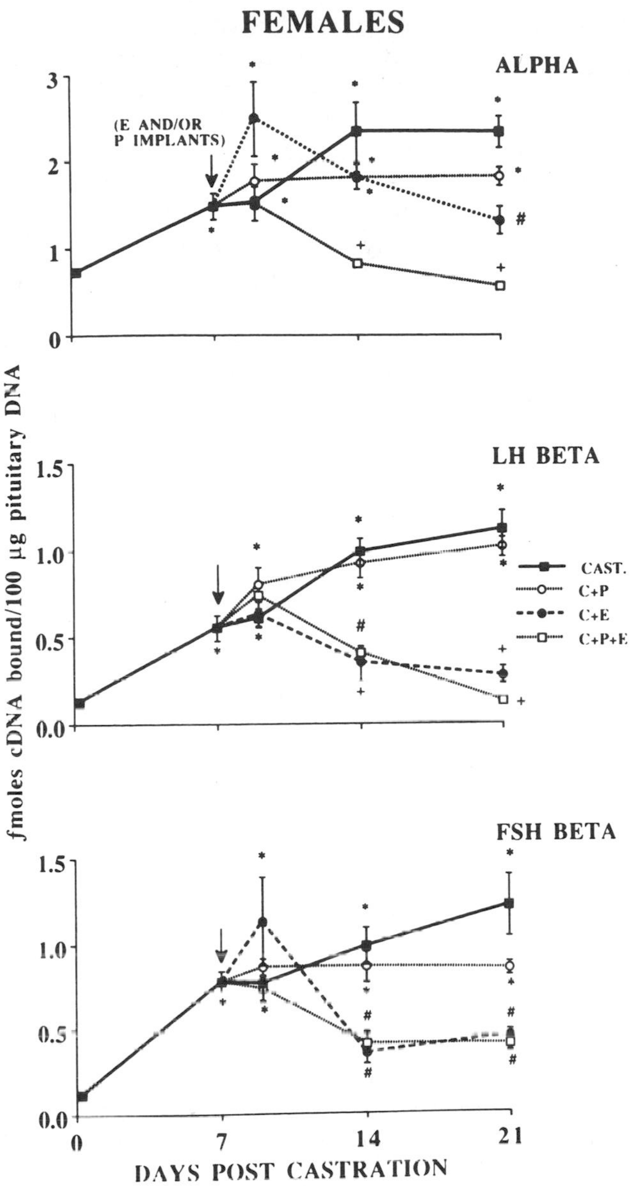

FIG. 9. Effect of E_2 and P replacement on gonadotropin subunit mRNA concentrations in 7-day OVX female rats. *Arrow* indicates placement of steroid-containing implant. ■, Castrate (cast); ○, P (cast + P) replacement; ●, E2 (cast + E) replacement; □, E_2 and P (cast ± E + P) replacement. *, $P < .05$ versus intact (day 0); +, $P < .05$ versus time-matched castrate; #, $P < .05$ versus intacts and time-matched castrate. (n = 5–10 per group.) (From ref. 82, with permission.)

hormones. The biologic action of these products may be altered by noncovalent binding to other proteins (e.g., a portion of the TGF-β prohormone interacts with the mature TGF-β molecule and follistatin binds to inhibin/activin).

The inhibins and activins consist of different combinations of α and β subunits. The dimer of an α and either a β-A or β-B subunit results in the formation of inhibin A or inhibin B, respectively. If two β subunits are combined, the activins A (β-A β-A), AB (β-A β-B), and B (β-B β-B) are produced. The inhibins A and B and the activins A and AB have been isolated in testicular and/or ovarian extracts. Activin B has been produced *in vitro* through recombinant deoxyribonucleic acid (DNA) technology but has not yet been isolated from normal tissues. The ability of inhibin and activin to regulate gonadotropin subunit gene expression has received detailed study, and these two substances appear to exert opposite actions.

Inhibins

The inhibins are secreted by the gonads, and the feedback effects of inhibin appear to be exerted at the level of the gonadotrope. Inhibin reduces FSH synthesis and cell content, as well as basal and GnRH-stimulated FSH release in dispersed pituitary cells (123–125). *In vivo* studies in gonadectomized male and female rats have shown a dose-related decrease in FSH secretion in response to inhibin. The fall in FSH is noted despite concurrent blockade of GnRH action and generally begins 4 to 6 h after inhibin administration and persists for 8 to 12 h (126–131). The effects of inhibin on LH synthesis and secretion are less clear than those on FSH. Some studies have reported a decline in basal LH release (123,125); others have reported an effect only on GnRH-stimulated release (132,133); still others have shown no effect of inhibin on LH secretion (134,135).

The mechanism by which inhibin acts remains uncertain. Inhibin does not appear to alter hypothalamic GnRH release in rats (136) but may change the number of GnRH receptors, thereby resulting in a reduced GnRH binding capacity (137). This is in contrast to sheep, in which GnRH receptor numbers increase after inhibin (138,139). Postreceptor actions of inhibin may include an inhibition of protein synthesis, as cyclohexamide can mimic the effects of exogenous inhibin (134,140). This suggestion remains to be proven as present supplies of recombinant inhibin have not allowed measurement of either gonadotropin gene transcriptional rates or mRNA structural changes (e.g., polyadenylation) after administration of inhibin. Inhibin also exerts a profound inhibitory effect on FSH β mRNA concentrations both *in vivo* and *in vitro*. *In vitro,* inhibin reduces levels of FSH β mRNA within 2 to 4 h, which is followed by a less marked decline in α subunit mRNA (135,140,141). Mercer and co-workers (142) reported a rapid decline in FSH β mRNA levels after inhibin treatment in the hypothalamic-pituitary-disconnected ewe, further supporting the notion that inhibin acts directly at the pituitary. Inhibin does not alter LH β mRNA levels, and overall, the data suggest that the primary action of inhibin is to regulate FSH secretion and synthesis (127,130,135,141,142).

Present data suggest that both male and female rats respond to exogenous inhibin, but the relative importance of this peptide in normal physiology may differ between the sexes. During sexual maturation in female rats, plasma inhibin levels rise steadily and are inversely related to those of FSH, as they are during cyclic variations during the estrous cycle (62,143,144). In contrast, circulating inhibin levels are at their highest level in immature males but fall to low or immeasurable values by the time of maturity (145). Further evidence for the relative importance of inhibin in male and female physiology has emerged after studies using passive immunoneutralization of inhibin on the effects of inhibin withdrawal. After administration of an antiinhibin antiserum, serum FSH increased in immature male rats, but this effect was absent in adult male animals (146). In contrast, serum FSH rose in both immature and adult female rats, and ovulation rates were higher after passive immunoneutralization (143,146–148). Similar results to these in the rat have been reported in sheep (149,150); however, recent data suggest that the male rhesus monkey does hypersecrete FSH after inhibin immunoneutralization (151).

A reduction in circulating inhibin in female rats appears to result in increased FSH β gene expression. Attardi and colleagues (118) reported that administration of antiinhibin antisera increased FSH β mRNA levels in the estrogen-primed immature female rat within 15 h. The time course of this action was surprising, as the circulating half-life of inhibin is 15 to 20 min (152); thus recent studies investigated the acute effect of inhibin withdrawal on gonadotropin subunit gene expression in adult rats (153). In males, no change in gonadotropin subunit mRNA concentrations occurred within 12 h after administration of the inhibin antisera. Conversely, in females (Fig. 10), inhibin immunoneutralization resulted in a two- to threefold increase in FSH β mRNA levels within 2 h, whereas α and LH β mRNA concentrations were unchanged. Increases in FSH β mRNA levels were followed by later increases in FSH secretion, suggesting that FSH β subunit availability may be rate-limiting in FSH release. Both the magnitude and timing of these changes in FSH β mRNA levels are notably similar to those seen acutely after ovariectomy. In the latter situation, FSH β mRNA levels increase within 1 h after removal of the ovaries as shown in Fig. 11 (153). Together these data sets suggest that inhibin maintains a tonic selective inhibition on FSH β mRNA expression in rats and that this effect appears to be more prominent in adult female (than adult male) rats.

Activins

The activins are known to have diverse biologic actions in multiple tissues. These include paracrine effects on granulosa cell function, regulation of follicular development, modulation of testicular androgen production, stimulation of erythropoiesis, and modulation of corticotropin-releasing hormone (CRH), adrenocorticotropic hormone (ACTH), and growth hormone (GH) secretion (154–161). These actions appear to be exerted through a family of specific membrane receptors with serine kinase activity (162,163). To date, *in vivo* studies have been limited by the available amounts of recombinant human activin, and so most of our knowledge stems from studies using *in vitro* protocols. Activin A increases FSH β mRNA levels within 2 to 4 h, and this is followed by a stimulation of FSH secretion (135, 164,165). Changes in LH secretion, α, or LH β subunit mRNA concentrations have not been observed on a consistent basis. Like inhibin, activin acts independently of

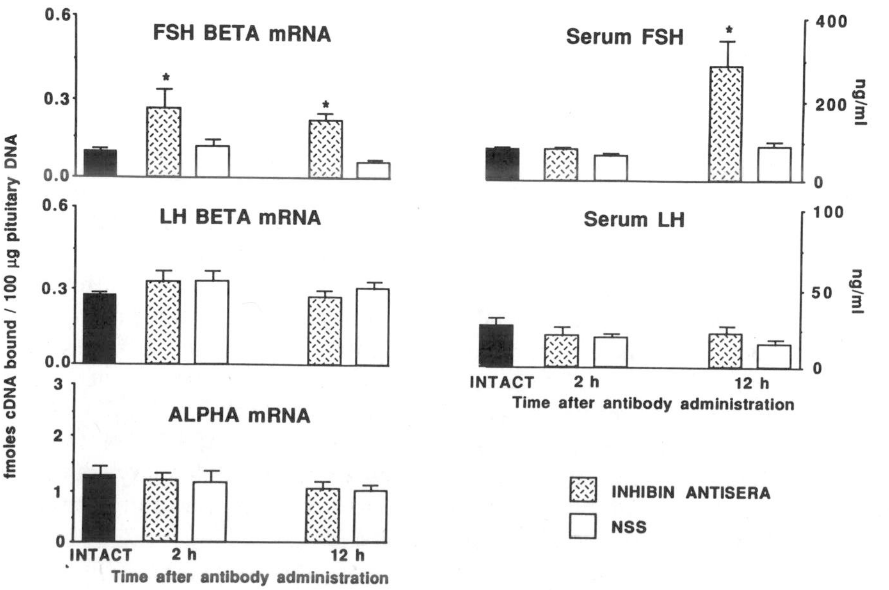

FIG. 10. Effect of inhibin immunoneutralization on gonadotropin subunit mRNA concentrations and serum gonadotropins in adult female rats. Treatment groups include intact animals (*solid bars*) and rats given either inhibin antisera (*hatched bars*) or normal sheep sera (*NSS, open bars*). Animals were killed 2 or 12 h after inhibin antisera or NSS. *$P <$ .05 compared with intact group. Values are means ± SEM (n = 6–8 per group). (From ref. 153, with permission.)

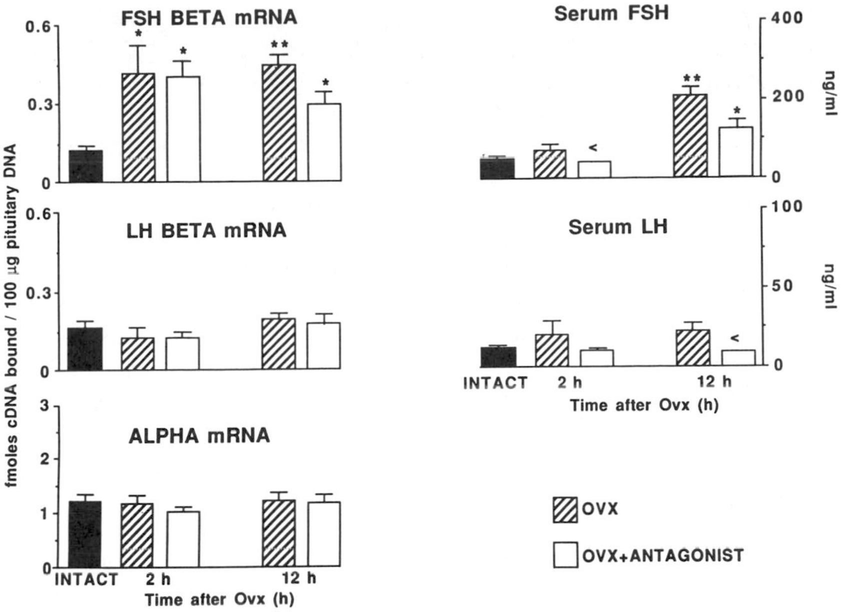

FIG. 11. Effect of ovariectomy on gonadotropin subunit mRNA concentrations and serum gonadotropins in adult female rats. Treatment groups include intact animals (*solid bars*) and animals sacrificed 2 or 12 h after ovariectomy in absence (*striped bars*) or presence of a GnRH antagonist (*open bars*) from time of ovariectomy. *$P < .05$ compared with intact group. **$P < .05$ compared with both OVX + antagonist group and intact group. Values are means ± SEM (n = 6–8 per group). (From ref. 153, with permission.)

GnRH and can induce FSH secretion in GnRH-desensitized pituitary cells (166). Activin is also able to alter the gonadotrope cell population and increases the number of demonstrable FSH secreting cells and perhaps the amount of FSH secreted by certain subpopulations of gonadotropes (167,168). Activin also appears to regulate FSH β gene expression by a nontranscriptional mechanism (169). *In vivo,* recombinant human activin A increases FSH β mRNA levels and FSH release in both immature females and OVX-E_2-treated adult female rats (170). In contrast, activin A appears to have little if any effects in immature or adult male rats (130). Overall, the data suggest that activin increases FSH β gene expression, and subsequent FSH biosynthesis and activin appears to exert opposite effects on the gonadotrope to those of inhibin.

Follistatin

Follistatin, first isolated by Ueno and associates in 1985 (171), is a glycosylated, monomeric protein with FSH suppressing activity. The cDNA and genomic sequences of the rat, human, and porcine follistatin molecules have been reported, and follistatin is highly conserved (98%) between species (172–175). Follistatin reduces FSH release *in vitro* and is approximately 30% as effective as inhibin (on a molar basis) (176–178). Similar to inhibin, follistatin reduces FSH β mRNA levels within 2 h and FSH secretion within 8 h (135); the effects of follistatin and inhibin on FSH secretion appear to be additive (176). Interestingly, follistatin is more effective than inhibin in blocking the effects of activin in increasing FSH β mRNA concentrations and FSH secretion (126). *In vivo,* follistatin decreases FSH secretion within 4 h, without altering serum LH or LH responses to exogenous GnRH (128,178). The mechanism(s) by which follistatin reduces FSH biosynthesis and secretion is uncertain; however, follistatin can bind to activin and thereby prevent activin stimulation of FSH synthesis and secretion (179). Shimonaka and co-workers (180) recently reported that follistatin binds to activin through its β subunit, and hence theoretically follistatin may also bind inhibin. It is unclear, however, if follistatin and inhibin do bind, as the effects of inhibin on FSH secretion are not neutralized by follistatin (176). The addition of follistatin to dispersed male rat pituitaries in static culture can reduce FSH subunit gene expression and FSH secretion in the absence of exogenous activin (128), implying either that follistatin can act independently of activin/inhibin or that activin is produced locally by the pituitary. As attempts to detect a follistatin receptor in the gonadotrope have been unsuccessful to date, these data raise the possibility that follistatin may regulate gonadotrope function through locally produced activin.

Extragonadal Follistatins, Inhibins, and Activins

In keeping with their diverse physiologic functions, extragonadal production of the follistatin mRNA and the mRNAs for the inhibin α, β-A, and β-B subunits have been reported (181,182). Of significance to the regulation of gonadotropins, follistatin, and inhibin and α and β-B mRNAs are present in the pituitary, and immunohistochemical staining has shown that the inhibin α and β-B subunits localize to the gonadotropes (183). Interestingly, mRNA concentrations of the two inhibin subunits increase after removal of the gonads, although the mechanisms regulating their expression remain uncertain. Recent data suggest that production of the β-B protein is of physiologic significance in the regulation of

FSH biosynthesis. Treatment of dispersed male pituitary cells with a monoclonal antibody to activin B resulted in a decline in FSH β mRNA levels, implying that basal FSH β gene expression is dependent on locally produced activin (184). Also, in perifused pituitary cells, FSH β mRNA levels decline over time when cells are perifused with media alone. However, when activin is replaced into the perifused media, FSH β mRNA levels return to original values. This decline in FSH β gene expression does not occur in static culture, suggesting that perifusion removes locally produced activin, which is necessary for basal FSH β mRNA concentrations (185). Thus, the exact roles of gonadal and pituitary activins remain to be established. However, present data favor activin of pituitary origin as an important factor in the regulation of FSH β mRNA expression and hormone biosynthesis.

TRANSCRIPTIONAL REGULATION

Progress in the investigation of pituitary gonadotropin subunit transcriptional regulation has been disappointingly slow. In part, this is due to the lack of an appropriate gonadotrope-derived cell line to allow the transfection of fusion gene constructs (5′ flanking region of subunit gene attached to a reporter gene). Although different cell lines have been examined as hosts, including the lactotrope/somatotrope-derived GH cells, α subunit-secreting pituitary human adenomas and the placental-derived (JEG) cells, expression of LH and FSH β chimeric gene constructs within these cell lines is relatively low or nondetectable (186–189). This appears largely to be because of the lack of gonadotrope-specific transcriptional factor(s) that may play a critical enhancer role in basal and stimulus-induced alterations in mRNA synthesis (190). Efforts using primary pituitary cells have also met with mixed success, largely because gonadotrope cells only comprise 5% to 7% of the total pituitary cell population (191). For these reasons, much of the data relating to LH and FSH β gene expression have been obtained by the use of nuclear "run-off" transcription assays, which measure the incorporation of labeled nucleotides into specific mRNA transcripts (79,192). More recently, a cell line has been developed from transgenic mice that appears to be derived from gonadotrope cells (α T3-1). This cell line produces α subunit, contains GnRH receptors, and secretes α subunit in response to GnRH (193). However, the use of α T3-1 cells in the study of LH and FSH β transcriptional regulation has yet to be determined.

Gonadal Steroids

Evidence from different mammalian species suggests that gonadal steroids can influence the rate of gonadotropin subunit mRNA synthesis directly at the level of the pituitary. Estradiol has been shown to selectively stimulate LH β subunit transcription in the rat (192). Further, a segment of the 5′ flanking region of the rat LH β gene (between -1,388 and -1,105) appears to play a role in mediating responsiveness to E_2 (186). This region can bind the E_2 receptor with high affinity and contains a 15-base imperfect palindromic sequence that is similar to the E_2 responsive element (ERE) described for other E_2-sensitive genes (i.e., prolactin, frog vitellogen) (193–195). In sheep pituitary cells, Phillips and associates (70) showed that both E_2 and progesterone can suppress the rate of FSH β transcription *in vitro.* The bovine FSH β gene contains a site within the distal 5′ flanking region that is 80% homologous to the consensus ERE, and expression of the gene has been shown to be suppressed by E_2 (37). Alpha subunit mRNA synthesis also has been shown to be inhibited both by E_2 and glucocorticoids (196,197). However, as high-affinity E_2 and glucocorticoid receptor binding sites have not been characterized within the α gene, the mechanism(s) of these actions is unclear and may be indirect.

Gonadotropin-Releasing Hormone

Gonadotropin-releasing hormone release from the hypothalamus plays a main role in the regulation of pituitary gonadotropin subunit synthesis and secretion (29), and a recent report described the identification of a GnRH-responsive region within the 5′ flanking region of the human α subunit gene (198). Gonadotropin-releasing hormone has also been shown to stimulate gonadotropin subunit gene expression via direct actions on subunit transcription rates. *In vitro* studies by Shupnik (199) revealed that GnRH stimulated a rise in α, LH β, and FSH β transcription rates in female rat pituitary cells. Moreover, she reported that a pulsatile GnRH signal is required to increase LH β and FSH β mRNA synthesis, whereas α mRNA synthesis could be increased by continuous GnRH stimulus. These results have been expanded in studies conducted *in vivo* (12). The effects of both a continuous GnRH infusion and different GnRH pulse frequencies on gonadotropin subunit transcription rates was examined in a GnRH-deficient, adult male rat model. As shown in Fig. 12, continuous GnRH stimulation was ineffective in increasing a rise in the transcription rate for any of the three gonadotropin subunit mRNAs. However, pulsatile GnRH increased synthesis for all three gonadotropin subunit mRNAs, and the frequency of the GnRH signal exerted different effects. Alpha mRNA synthesis was stimulated by faster frequencies (8- or 30-min pulse intervals); LH β was only increased by 30-min pulses; FSH β mRNA synthesis showed a selective response to slower (120-min) pulses. These results show that a pulsatile GnRH signal pattern is required to stimulate a rise in gonadotropin subunit

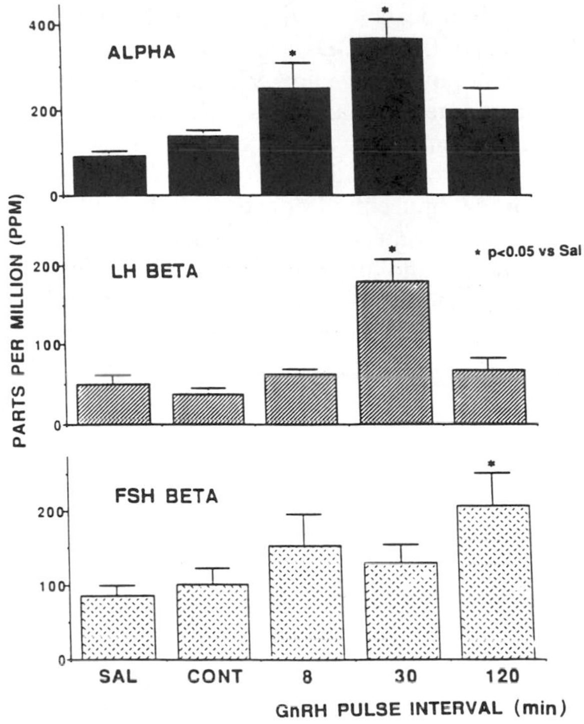

FIG. 12. Effect of GnRH pulse frequency on gonadotropin subunit transcription rates. Castrate, T-replaced male rats received either GnRH pulses (25 ng/pulse; 8-, 30-, 120-min intervals) or continuous GnRH infusion (*CONT;* 200 ng/h) for 4 h. Controls (*SAL*) received saline pulses every 30 min. Three pituitaries were pooled for each sample, three to four samples per group. Each bar represents mean ± SEM. (From ref. 12, with permission.)

transcription and that the differential effects of GnRH pulse frequency on cytoplasmic mRNAs (see Fig. 6) are due in large part to actions at the transcriptional level. The effect of GnRH treatment duration on gonadotropin mRNA synthesis was also examined by giving GnRH pulses for 1, 4, or 24 h (12). Data are shown in Fig. 13 and reveal that the transcription rates for all three gonadotropin subunit mRNAs were increased within 1 h (three- to fivefold versus saline-pulsed controls). Transcription rates declined over time despite continuing the pulsatile GnRH stimulus. After 24 h, LH β and FSH β transcription returned to basal levels, and the α mRNA synthesis rate was reduced by 50% from values observed at the 1-h time point. Cytoplasmic α and LH β mRNA levels did not increase unless pulsatile GnRH treatment was continued for the entire 24-h duration. Thus, the increase in mRNA concentrations in the presence of reduced transcription rates could be due to the delay in transcript process time or a posttranscriptional action of GnRH. The latter effect was recently described by Weiss and co-workers (106), who showed lengthening of the poly A levels of α and LH β mRNAs in response to pulsatile GnRH.

Intracellular (Second) Messengers

Primarily because of the lack of a gonadotrope-derived cell line that expresses the gonadotropin β subunit genes, few data are available regarding second-messenger regulation of LH β and FSH β subunit transcription rates. *In vitro* studies by Andrews and colleagues (200) used primary rat pituitary cells and showed that protein kinase C (PKC) activation could stimulate a rise in cytoplasmic LH β mRNA levels. Moreover, depleting the cells of PKC by prolonged exposure to phorbol esters blocked the stimulatory effect of GnRH on LH β mRNA accumulation. These results suggest that PKC may mediate the stimulatory effect of GnRH on LH β transcription. More recent studies by Clayton and associates (187) used fusion gene constructs containing the 5′ flanking region of the rat LH β gene and the reporter gene chloramphenicol acetyltransferase (CAT). The constructs were transfected into GH_3 cells and indicated that the cyclic adenosine monophosphate (AMP) pathway may also regulate LH β transcription (187). LH β transcription was stimulated by cyclic AMP, and a cyclic AMP responsive area was located between −1.7 and −0.6 kb of the 5′ flanking region of the gene. Sequence

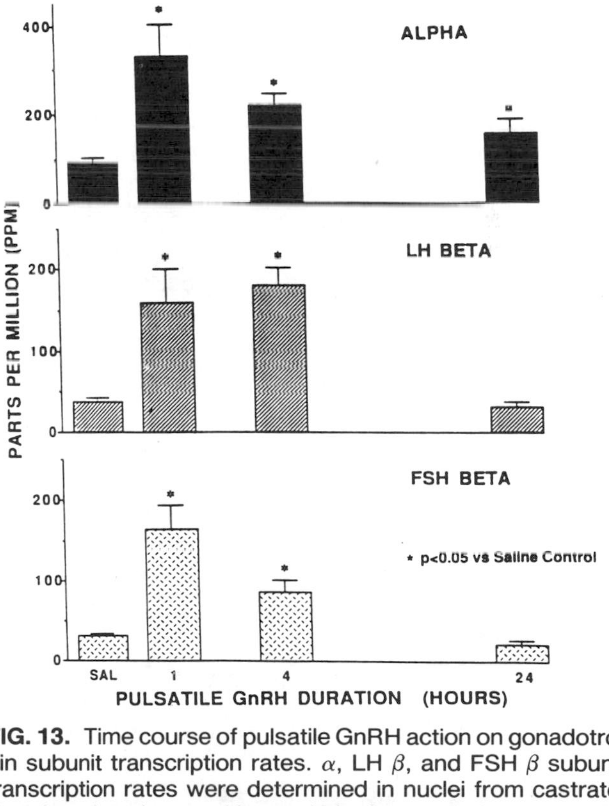

FIG. 13. Time course of pulsatile GnRH action on gonadotropin subunit transcription rates. α, LH β, and FSH β subunit transcription rates were determined in nuclei from castrate, T-replaced male rats (three pituitaries pooled per sample; four to nine samples per group). Animals received GnRH pulses (25 ng/pulse at 30-min intervals) for 1, 4, or 24 h. Controls (*SAL*) received saline pulses every 30 min for 24 h. Each bar represents mean ± SEM. (From ref. 12, with permission.)

analysis revealed that several locations within this region contained nucleotide sequences that differed by only one or two bases compared with the consensus 8-bp palindromic cyclic AMP responsive element (CRE) (TGACGTCA) described by other investigators (201,202). Almost no data are available regarding transcriptional regulation of the FSH β gene by second-messenger systems, primarily because of the lack of an appropriate cell model for FSH β-reporter gene transfection studies (203).

During the past few years, the role of cyclic AMP in the transcriptional regulation of the α subunit gene has been examined primarily using JEG and other choriocarcinoma cell lines (204,205). Investigation of the human α subunit gene has revealed that cyclic AMP can stimulate the rate of transcription several-fold (188,204). Gene mapping studies have shown that a CRE is located within the 5′ flanking region of the human α gene, between positions -146 and -111, relative to the transcriptional start site (206,207). This region contains two identical copies of a 18-bp nucleotide sequence, with an 8-bp core palindromic sequence shown to be the consensus CRE for somatostatin and other genes (201,202). Of interest, the tandem CREs have been shown to regulate α subunit transcription in a synergistic manner (208). Phylogenetic differences in the number and homology of cyclic AMP responsive regions within the α subunit gene have also recently been described (34,205). Unlike the human, the α subunit genes of lower primates (i.e., rhesus monkey, baboon) contain a single CRE. The α subunit gene of other mammalian species, including the mouse, cow, and sheep, also has a single CRE; however, the nucleotide sequence differs from the primate CRE by a one-base substitution (34). Evidence suggests that the one-base substitution in these species decreases the binding affinity for the CRE binding protein (CREB). This is of import as CREB has been shown to activate the CRE of the human α gene by forming a homeodimer through a "leucine zipper" (209,210). In view of the reduced CREB affinity, recent data suggest that the cyclic AMP-induced stimulation of α subunit transcription seen in nonprimate species may be the result of interactions between CREB and other nuclear proteins at the CRE site (209). The horse α subunit gene also responds to cyclic AMP stimulation; however, cyclic AMP responsiveness appears to be conferred by a nuclear factor (α ACT) that binds to a region between the CRE and the upstream tissue-specific response element (URE) (205) located between -180 and -147 relative to the transcription start site.

The human α gene contains at least three types of transcriptional enhancer elements within the proximal 5′ flanking region: basal, cyclic AMP, and tissue-specific (190,204–208). These elements are activated by binding to specific nuclear factors. The tissue-specific enhancer [URE; also called the trophoblast-specific enhancer element (TSE)] appears to induce placental cell specificity to the α gene (205,208). Data suggest that the two CREs play a role not only in cyclic AMP regulation but also in basal and tissue specificity. As CREBs are known to form dimers in the active state, evidence suggests that a specific spatial orientation between the two CREs is required for maximal enhancer activity (208,210). Thus, α subunit responsiveness to cyclic AMP has diverged between primate and nonprimate species. In primates, CREB appears to play a central role; however, in nonprimate species, other nuclear proteins may mediate both tissue specificity and responsiveness to cyclic AMP.

REFERENCES

1. Pierce JG, Parsons TF. Glycoprotein hormones: structure and function. *Annu Rev Biochem* 1981;50:465–495.
2. Strickland TW, Parsons TF, Pierce JG. Structure of LH and hCG. In: Ascoli M, ed. *Luteinizing Hormone Action and Receptors.* Boca Raton, Florida: CRC Press, 1985;2–15.
3. de la Llosa P, Jutisz M. Reversible dissociation with subunits and biological activity of ovine luteinizing hormone. *Biochim Biophys Acta* 1969;181:426–436.
4. Papkoff H, Samy TSA. Isolation and partial characterization of polypeptide chains of ovine interstitial cell stimulating hormone. *Biochim Biophys Acta* 1967;147:175–177.
5. Pierce JG, Liao T-H, Howard SM, Shome B, Cornell JS. Studies on the structure of thyrotropin: its relationship to luteinizing hormone. *Recent Prog Horm Res* 1971;27:165–212.
6. Marshall JC, Kelch RP. GnRH: role of pulsatile secretion in the regulation of reproduction. *N Engl J Med* 1986;315:1459–1468.
7. Wu FCW, Butler GE, Kelnar CJH, Sellar RE. Patterns of pulsatile secretion before and during the onset of puberty in boys: a study using an immunoradiometric assay. *J Clin Endocrinol Metab* 1990;70:629–637.
8. Bäckström CT, McNeilly AC, Leask RM, Baird DT. Pulsatile secretion of LH, FSH, prolactin, oestradiol and progesterone during the human menstrual cycle. *Clin Endocrinol (Oxf)* 1982;17:29–42.
9. Clarke IJ, Cummins JT. The temporal relationship between gonadotropin releasing hormone (GnRH) and luteinizing hormone (LH) secretion in ovariectomized ewes. *Endocrinology* 1982;111: 1737–1739.
10. Levine JE, Ramirez VD. Luteinizing hormone-releasing hormone release during the rat estrous cycle and after ovariectomy, as estimated with push–pull cannulae. *Endocrinology* 1982;111: 1439–1448.
11. Belchetz PE, Plant TM, Nakai Y, Keogh EG, Knobil E. Hypophysial responses to continuous and intermittent delivery of hypothalamic gonadotropin-releasing hormone. *Science* 1978;202: 631–633.
12. Haisenleder DJ, Dalkin AC, Ortolano GA, Marshall JC, Shupnik MA. A pulsatile GnRH stimulus is required to increase transcription of the gonadotropin subunit genes: evidence for differential regulation of transcription by pulse frequency in vivo. *Endocrinology* 1991;128:509–517.
13. Clayton RN. GnRH modulation of its own pituitary receptors: evidence for biphasic regulation. *Endocrinology* 1982;111: 152–157.
14. Reame N, Sauder SE, Kelch RP, Marshall JC. Pulsatile gonadotropin secretion during the human menstrual cycle: evidence for altered frequency of gonadotropin-releasing hormone secretion. *J Clin Endocrinol Metab* 1984;59:328–337.
15. Karsch FJ, Foster DL, Bittman EL, Goodman RL. A role for estradiol in enhancing luteinizing hormone pulse frequency during the follicular phase of the estrous cycle of sheep. *Endocrinology* 1983;113:1333–1339.
16. Matsumoto AM, Bremner WJ. Modulation of pulsatile gonado-

tropin secretion by testosterone in man. *J Clin Endocrinol Metab* 1984;58:609–614.
17. Soules MR, Steiner RA, Clifton DK, Cohen NL, Aksel S, Bremner WJ. Progesterone modulation of pulsatile luteinizing hormone secretion in normal women. *J Clin Endocrinol Metab* 1984;58:378–383.
18. Fox SE, Smith MMS. Changes in the pulsatile pattern of LH secretion during the rat estrous cycle. *Endocrinology* 1985;116: 1485–1492.
19. Gay VL, Bogdanove EM. Plasma and pituitary LH and FSH in the castrated rat following short-term steroid treatment. *Endocrinology* 1969;84:1132–1137.
20. Schanbacher BD, Ford JJ. Gonadotropin secretion in cryptorchid and castrate rams and the acute effects of exogenous steroid treatment. *Endocrinology* 1977;100:387–393.
21. Kennedy J, Chappel S. Direct pituitary effects of testosterone and luteinizing hormone-releasing hormone upon follicle-stimulating hormone: analysis by radioimmuno- and radioreceptor assay. *Endocrinology* 1985;116:747–748.
22. Strobl FJ, Levine JE. Estrogen inhibits luteinizing hormone (LH), but not follicle-stimulating hormone secretion in hypophysectomized pituitary-grafted rats receiving pulsatile LH-releasing hormone infusions. *Endocrinology* 1988;123:622–630.
23. Carroll RS, Corrigan AZ, Gharib SD, Vale W, Chin WW. Inhibin, activin, and follistatin: regulation of follicle-stimulating hormone messenger ribonucleic acid levels. *Mol Endocrinol* 1989;3:1969–1976.
24. Rivier C, Rivier J, Vale W. Inhibin-mediated feedback control of follicle-stimulating hormone secretion in the female rat. *Science* 1986;234:205–208.
25. Campen CA, Vale W. Interaction between purified ovine inhibin and steroids on the release of gonadotropins from cultured pituitary cells. *Endocrinology* 1988;123:1320–1328.
26. Mercer JE, Clements JA, Funder JW, Clarke IJ. Rapid and specific lowering of pituitary FSH β mRNA levels by inhibin. *Mol Cell Endocrinol* 1987;53:251–254.
27. Roberts V, Meunier H, Vaughan J, et al. Production and regulation of inhibin subunits in pituitary gonadotropes. *Endocrinology* 1989;124:552–554.
28. Kogawa K, Nakamura T, Sugino K, Takeo K, Titani K, Sugino H. Activin-binding protein is present in pituitary. *Endocrinology* 1991;128:1434–1440.
29. Gharib SD, Wierman ME, Shupnik MA, Chin WW. Molecular biology of the pituitary gonadotropins. *Endocrinol Rev* 1990;11:177–199.
30. Fiddes J, Goodman H. The gene encoding the common alpha subunit of the four human glycoprotein hormones. *J Mol Appl Genet* 1981;1:3–18.
31. Goodwin R, Moreman C, Nilson J. Characterization and nucleotide sequence of the gene for the common α subunit of the bovine pituitary glycoprotein hormones. *Nucleic Acids Res* 1986;11: 6873–6883.
32. Chin W. Organization and expression of glycoprotein hormone genes. In: Imura H, ed. *The Pituitary Gland.* New York: Raven Press, 1985;103–125.
33. Chin WW, Kronenberg HM, Dee PC, Maloof F, Habener JF. Nucleotide sequence of the mRNA encoding the pre-α subunit of mouse thyrotropin. *Proc Natl Acad Sci USA* 1981;78:5329–5333.
34. Fenstermaker RA, Farmerce TA, Clay CM, Hamernik DL, Nilson JH. Different combinations of regulatory elements may account for expression of the glycoprotein hormone alpha-subunit gene in primate and horse placenta. *Mol Endocrinol* 1990;4: 1480–1487.
35. Gordon WL, Ward DN. Structural aspects of luteinizing hormone actions. In: Ascoli M, ed. *Luteinizing Hormone Action and Receptors.* Boca Raton, Florida: CRC Press, 1985;173–197.
36. Gharib SD, Roy A, Wierman ME, Chin WW. Isolation and characterization of the gene encoding the β-subunit of rat follicle-stimulating hormone. *DNA* 1989;8:339–344.
37. Kim KE, Gordon DF, Maurer RA. Nucleotide sequence of the bovine gene for follicle-stimulating hormone beta-subunit. *DNA* 1988;7:227–232.
38. Watkins PC, Eddy R, Beck AK, et al. DNA sequence and regional assignment of the human follicle-stimulating hormone β-subunit gene to the short arm of human chromosome 11. *DNA* 1987;6:205–212.
39. Jameson JL, Becker CB, Lindell CM, Habener JF. Human follicle-stimulating hormone β-subunit gene encodes multiple messenger ribonucleic acids. *Mol Endocrinol* 1988;2:806–815.
40. Shaw G, Kamen R. A conserved AU sequence from the 3′-untranslated region of GM-CSF mRNA mediates selective mRNA degradation. *Cell* 1986;46:659–667.
41. Talmadge K, Vamvakopoulos NC, Fiddes JC. Evolution of the genes for the β subunits of human chorionic gonadotropin and luteinizing hormone. *Nature* 1984;307:37–40.
42. Fiddes JC, Talmadge K. Structure, expression, and evolution of the genes for the human glycoprotein hormones. *Recent Prog Horm Res* 1984;40:43–78.
43. Jameson JL, Chin WW, Hollenberg AN, Chang AS, Habener JF. The gene encoding the β-subunit of rat luteinizing hormone. *J Biol Chem* 1984;259:15474–15478.
44. Chin WW, Godine JE, Klein DR, Chang AS, Tan LK, Habener JF. Nucleotide sequence of the cDNA encoding the precursor of the β subunit or rat lutropin. *Proc Natl Acad Sci USA* 1983;80:4649–4653.
45. Virgin JB, Silver BJ, Thomason AR, Nilson JH. The gene for the β subunit of bovine luteinizing hormone encodes a gonadotropin mRNA with an unusually short 5′-untranslated region. *J Biol Chem* 1985;260:7072–7077.
46. Maurer RA. Analysis of several bovine lutropin β subunit cDNAs reveals heterogeneity in nucleotide sequence. *J Biol Chem* 1985;260:4684–4687.
47. Fiddes JC, Goodman HM. The cDNA for the β-subunit of human chorionic gonadotropin suggests evolution of a gene by readthrough into the 3′-untranslated region. *Nature* 1980;286: 684–687.
48. Bornstein W, Vamvakopoulos N, Fiddes J. Human chorionic gonadotropin β-subunit is encoded by at least eight genes arranged in tandem and inverted pairs. *Nature* 1982;300: 419–422.
49. Policastro P, Ovitt CE, Hoshina M, Fukuoka H, Boothby MR, Boime I. The β-subunit of human chorionic gonadotropin is encoded by multiple genes. *J Biol Chem* 1983;258:11492–11499.
50. Talmadge K, Boorstein WR, Fiddes JC. The human genome contains seven genes for the β-subunit of luteinizing hormone. *DNA* 1983;2:281–289.
51. Jameson JL, Lindell CM, Habener JF. Evolution of different transcriptional start sites in the human luteinizing hormone and chorionic gonadotropin β subunit genes. *DNA* 1986;5:227–234.
52. Pierce JG. Gonadotropins: chemistry and biosynthesis. In: Knobil E, Neill J, eds. *The Physiology of Reproduction.* New York: Raven Press, 1988;1335–1347.
53. Smith MS, Freeman ME, Neill JD. The control of progesterone secretion during the estrous cycle and early pseudopregnancy in the rat: prolactin, gonadotropin and steroid levels associated with rescue of the corpus luteum of pseudopregnancy. *Endocrinology* 1975;96:219–226.
54. Butcher RL, Collins WE, Fugo NW. Plasma concentrations of LH, FSH, prolactin, progesterone, estradiol-17 beta throughout the 4 day estrous cycle of the rat. *Endocrinology* 1974;94: 1704–1708.
55. Charlesworth MC, Grady RR, Shin L, et al. Differential suppression of FSH and LH secretion by follicular fluid in the presence or absence of GnRH. *Neuroendocrinology* 1984;38:199–204.
56. Rivier C, Roberts V, Vale W. Possible role of LH and FSH in modulating inhibin secretion and expression during the estrous cycle of the rat. *Endocrinology* 1989;125:876–882.
57. Woodruff TK, D'Agostino J, Schwartz NB, Mayo KE. Decreased inhibin gene expression in preovulatory follicles requires primary gonadotropin surges. *Endocrinology* 1989;124:2193–2199.
58. Zmeili SM, Papavasiliou SS, Thorner MO, Evans WS, Marshall JC, Landefeld TD. Alpha and luteinizing-hormone beta subunit mRNAs during the rat estrous cycle. *Endocrinology* 1986;119: 1867–1870.
59. Ortolano GA, Haisenleder DJ, Dalkin AC, Iliff-Sizemore SA, Landefeld TD, Marshall JC. Follicle-stimulating hormone beta subunit messenger ribonucleic acid concentrations during the rat estrous cycle. *Endocrinology* 1988;123:2149–2151.

60. Shupnik MA, Gharib SD, Chin WW. Divergent effects of estradiol on gonadotropin gene transcription in pituitary fragments. *Mol Endocrinol* 1989;3:474–480.
61. Attardi B, Keeping HS, Winter SJ, Kotsuji F, Maurer RA, Troen P. Rapid and profound suppression of messenger ribonucleic acid encoding follicle-stimulating hormone β by inhibin from primate Sertoli cells. *Mol Endocrinol* 1989;3:280–287.
62. Haisenleder DJ, Ortolano GA, Jolly D, et al. Inhibin secretion during the rat estrous cycle: relationship to FSH secretion and FSH beta subunit mRNA concentrations. *Life Sci* 1990;47: 1769–1773.
63. Leipheimer RE, Bona-Gallo A, Gallo RV. Ovarian steroid regulation of pulsatile LH release during the interval between the mornings of diestrus 2 and proestrus in the rat. *Neuroendocrinology* 1985;41:252–259.
64. Foster DL, Lemons JA, Jaffe RB, Neswender GD. Sequential patterns of circulating LH and FSH in female sheep from early postnatal life through the first estrous cycle. *Endocrinology* 1975;97:985–994.
65. L'Hermite M, Neswender GD, Reichert LE Jr, Midgley AR Jr. Serum FSH in sheep as measured by radioimmunoassay. *Biol Reprod* 1972;6:325–332.
66. Leung K, Kim KE, Maurer RA, Landefeld TD. Divergent changes in the concentrations of gonadotropin β-subunit messenger ribonucleic acid during the estrous cycle of sheep. *Mol Endocrinol* 1988;2:272–276.
67. Mercer JE, Clements JE, Funder JW, Clarke IJ. Luteinizing hormone-β mRNA levels are regulated primarily by gonadotropin-releasing hormone and not by negative estrogen feedback on the pituitary. *Neuroendocrinology* 1988;47:563–566.
68. Leung K, Kaynard AH, Negrini BP, Kim KE, Maurer RA, Landefeld TD. Differential regulation of gonadotropin subunit messenger ribonucleic acids by gonadotropin-releasing hormone pulse frequency in ewes. *Mol Endocrinol* 1987;1:724–728.
69. Mercer JE, Clements JA, Funder JW, Clarke IJ. Regulation of FSH beta and common alpha-subunit mRNA by GnRH and estrogen in the sheep pituitary. *Neuroendocrinology* 1989;50: 321–326.
70. Phillips CL, Lin L-W, Wu JC, Guzman K, Milsted A, Miller WL. 17β-Estradiol and progesterone inhibit transcription of the genes encoding the subunits of ovine follicle-stimulating hormone. *Mol Endocrinol* 1988;2:641–649.
71. Wise PM, Ratner A. Effect of ovariectomy on plasma LH, FSH, estradiol, and progesterone and medial basal hypothalamic LHRH concentrations in old and young rats. *Neuroendocrinology* 1980;30:15–19.
72. Gay VL, Midgley AR Jr. Response of the adult rat to orchidectomy and ovariectomy as determined by LH radioimmunoassay. *Endocrinology* 1969;84:1359–1364.
73. Yamamoto M, Diebell ND, Bogdanove EM. Analysis of initial and delayed effects of orchidectomy and ovariectomy on pituitary and serum LH levels in adult and immature rats. *Endocrinology* 1970;86:1102–1111.
74. Keller D, Fetherston J, Boime I. Isolation of mRNA from bovine pituitary. *Eur J Biochem* 1980;108:367–372.
75. Fetherston J, Boime I. Synthesis of bovine lutropin in cell-free lysates containing pituitary microsomes. *J Biol Chem* 1982;257: 8143–8148.
76. Wierman ME, Gharib SD, LaRovere JM, Badger TM, Chin WW. Selective failure of androgens to regulate follicle-stimulating hormone β mRNA levels in the male rat. *Mol Endocrinol* 1989;2:492–498.
77. Papavasiliou SS, Zmeili S, Herbon L, Duncan-Weldon J, Marshall JC, Landefeld TD. α and luteinizing hormone β messenger ribonucleic acid (RNA) of male and female rats after castration: quantitation using an optimized RNA dot blot hybridization assay. *Endocrinology* 1986;119:691–698.
78. Charlton HM, Jones AJ, Ward BJ, Detta A, Clayton RN. Effects of castration or testosterone implants upon pituitary function in hypogonadal mice bearing normal foetal preoptic area grafts. *Neuroendocrinology* 1987;45:376–380.
79. Shupnik MA, Gharib SD, Chin WW. Estrogen suppresses rat gonadotropin gene transcription *in vivo. Endocrinology* 1988; 122:1842–1846.
80. Paul SJ, Ortolano GA, Haisenleder DJ, Stewart JM, Shupnik MA, Marshall JC. Gonadotropin subunit mRNA concentrations after blockade of GnRH action: testosterone selectively increases FSH beta mRNA by posttranscriptional mechanisms. *Mol Endocrinol* 1990;4:1943–1955.
81. Childs GV, Lloyd JM, Unabia G, Gharib SD, Wierman ME, Chin WW. Detection of luteinizing hormone β messenger ribonucleic acid (mRNA) in individual gonadotropes after castration: use of a new *in situ* hybridization method with a photobiotinylated complementary RNA probe. *Mol Endocrinol* 1987;1: 926–932.
82. Dalkin AC, Haisenleder DJ, Ortolano GA, Suhr A, Marshall JC. Gonadal regulation of gonadotropin subunit gene expression: evidence for regulation of FSH beta mRNA by nonsteroidal hormones in female rats. *Endocrinology* 1990;127:798–806.
83. Gharib SD, Bowers SM, Need LR, Chin WW. Regulation of rat LH subunit mRNAs by gonadal steroid hormones. *J Clin Invest* 1986;77:582–589.
84. Abbott SD, Docherty K, Roberts JL, Tepper MA, Chin WW, Clayton RN. Castration increases luteinizing hormone subunit messenger RNA levels in male rat pituitaries. *J Endocrinol* 1985;107:R1–R4.
85. Gharib SD, Wierman ME, Badger TM, Chin WW. Sex steroid hormone regulation of follicle-stimulating hormone subunit messenger ribonucleic acid (mRNA) levels in the rat. *J Clin Invest* 1987;80:249–259.
86. Hamernik DL, Crowder ME, Nilson JH, Nett TM. Measurement of messenger ribonucleic acid for gonadotropins in ovariectomized ewes after hypothalamic-pituitary disconnection. *Endocrinology* 1986;119:2704–2710.
87. Mercer JE, Clements JA, Funder JW, Clarke IJ. Studies of regulation of gonadotropin gene expression in the hypothalamo-pituitary intact and hypothalamo-pituitary disconnected ewe. In: Chin WW, Boeme I, eds. *Glycoprotein Hormones,* Norwell, Massachusetts: Serono Symposia, 1990;227–236.
88. Papavasiliou SS, Zmeili S, Khoury S, Landefeld TD, Chin WW, Marshall JC. Gonadotropin-releasing hormone differentially regulates expression of the genes for luteinizing hormone α and β subunits in male rats. *Proc Natl Acad Sci USA* 1986;83: 4026–4029.
89. Wierman ME, Chun W. Androgen selectively stimulates FSH beta mRNA levels after GnRH antagonist administration. *Biol Reprod* 1990;42:563–571.
90. Steiner RA, Bremner WJ, Clifton DK. Regulation of LH pulse frequency and amplitude by testosterone in the adult male rat. *Endocrinology* 1982;111:2055–2061.
91. Haisenleder DJ, Ortolano GA, Dalkin AC, Ellis TR, Paul SJ, Marshall JC. Differential regulation of gonadotropin subunit gene expression by GnRH pulse amplitude in female rats. *Endocrinology* 1990;127:2869–2875.
92. Haisenleder DJ, Barkan AL, Zmeili SM, et al. LH subunit mRNA concentrations during LH surge in ovariectomized estradiol-replaced rats. *Am J Physiol* 1988;254:E99–105.
93. Haisenleder DJ, Ortolano GA, Yasin M, Dalkin AC, Marshall JC. Regulation of gonadotropin subunit mRNA expression by GnRH pulse amplitude *in vitro. Endocrinology* 1993;132: 1292–1296.
94. Weiss J, Jameson JL, Burrin JM, Crowley WF. Divergent responses of gonadotropin subunit mRNAs to continuous vs. pulsatile GnRH *in vitro. Mol Endocrinol* 1990;4:557–561.
95. Jakubowiak A, Janecki A, Tong D, Sanborn BM, Steinberger A. Differential regulation of gonadotropin subunit mRNAs by different GnRH pulse frequencies in superfused pituitary cell cultures. 74th Annual meeting of the Endocrine Society, San Antonio, Texas. 1992;Abst. # 1208.
96. Ishizaka K, Kitahara S, Oshima H, Troen P, Attardi B, Winters SJ. Effect of GnRH pulse frequency on gonadotropin secretion and subunit mRNAs in perifused pituitary cells. *Endocrinology* 1992;130:1467–1474.
97. Haisenleder DJ, Katt JA, Ortolano GA, et al. Influence of gonadotropin-releasing hormone pulse amplitude, frequency and treatment duration on the regulation of luteinizing hormone (LH) subunit messenger ribonucleic acids and LH secretion. *Mol Endocrinol* 1988;2:338–343.
98. Iliff-Sizemore SA, Ortolano GA, Haisenleder DJ, Dalkin AC,

Krueger KA, Marshall JC. Testosterone differentially modulates gonadotropin subunit mRNA responses to GnRH pulse amplitude. *Endocrinology* 1990;127:2876–2883.
99. Garcia A, Schiff M, Marshall JC. Regulation of pituitary GnRH receptors by pulsatile GnRH injections in male rats: modulation by testosterone. *J Clin Invest* 1984;74:920–927.
100. Sarkar DK, Fink G. Luteinizing hormone-releasing factor in pituitary stalk plasma from long term ovariectomized rats: effects of steroids. *J Endocrinol* 1980;86:511–524.
101. Sarkar DK, Chiappa SA, Fink G. GnRH surge in pro-oestrus rats. *Nature* 1976;264:461–463.
102. Ching M. Correlative surges of LHRH, LH and FSH in pituitary stalk plasma and systemic plasma of rat during proestrus. *Neuroendocrinology* 1982;34:279–285.
103. Haisenleder DJ, Khoury S, Zmeili SM, et al. The frequency of gonadotropin-releasing hormone secretion regulates expression of alpha and luteinizing hormone β-subunit messenger ribonucleic acids in male rats. *Mol Endocrinol* 1987;1:834–838.
104. Katt JA, Duncan JA, Herbon L, Barkan A, Marshall JC. The frequency of GnRH stimulation determines the number of pituitary GnRH receptors. *Endocrinology* 1985;116:2113–2117.
105. Dalkin AC, Haisenleder DJ, Ortolano GA, Ellis T, Marshall JC. The frequency of gonadotropin-releasing hormone (GnRH) stimulation differentially regulates gonadotropin subunit mRNA expression. *Endocrinology* 1989;125:917–924.
106. Weiss J, Crowley WF, Jameson JL. Pulsatile gonadotropin-releasing hormone modifies polyadenylation of gonadotropin subunit messenger ribonucleic acids. *Endocrinology* 1992;130: 415–420.
107. Haisenleder DJ, Ortolano GA, Dalkin AC, Paul SJ, Chin WW, Marshall JC. Gonadotrophin-releasing hormone regulation of gonadotrophin subunit gene expression: studies in triiodothyronine-suppressed rats. *J Endocrinol* 1989;122: 117–125.
108. Rodin DA, Lalloz MRA, Clayton RN. Gonadotropin-releasing hormone regulates follicle-stimulating hormone β subunit gene expression in the male rat. *Endocrinology* 1989;125:1282–1289.
109. Lalloz MRA, Detta A, Clayton RN. Gonadotropin-releasing hormone is required for enhanced luteinizing hormone subunit gene expression *in vivo*. *Endocrinology* 1988;122:1681–1688.
110. Perheentupa A, Huhtaniemi I. Gonadotropin gene expression and secretion in gonadotropin-releasing hormone antagonist-treated male rats: effect of sex steroid replacement. *Endocrinology* 1990;126:3204–3209.
111. Gharib SD, Leung PCK, Carroll RS, Chin WW. Androgens positively regulate FSH beta subunit mRNA levels in rat pituitary cells. *Mol Endocrinol* 1990;4:1620–1626.
112. Dalkin AC, Paul SJ, Haisenleder DJ, Ortolano GA, Yasin M, Marshall JC. Gonadal steroids effect similar regulation of gonadotrophin subunit mRNA expression in both male and female rats. *J Endocrinology* 1992;132:39–45.
113. Hoffman GE, Lee WS, Attardi B, Yann V, Fitzsimmons MD. Luteinizing hormone-releasing hormone neurons express c-Fos antigen after steroid activation. *Endocrinology* 1990;126: 1736–1742.
114. Verma IM, Sassone-Vorsi P. Proto-oncogene fos: complex but versatile regulation. *Cell* 1987;51:513–514.
115. Schonthal A, Herrlich P, Rahmsdorf HJ, Ponta H. Requirement for fos gene expression in the transcriptional activation of collagenase by other oncogenes and phorbol esters. *Cell* 1988;54: 325–334.
116. Karsch FJ, Cummins JT, Thomas GB, Clarke IJ. Steroid feedback inhibition of pulsatile secretion of gonadotropin-releasing hormone in the ewe. *Biol Reprod* 1987;36:1207–1212.
117. Goodman RL, Karsch FJ. Pulsatile secretion of luteinizing hormone: differential suppression by ovarian steroids. *Endocrinology* 1980;107:1286–1291.
118. Attardi B, Vaughan J, Vale W. Regulation of FSH β mRNA levels in the rat by endogenous inhibin. *Endocrinology* 1991;129:2802–2805.
119. Massagué J. The transforming growth factor-β family. *Annu Rev Cell Biol* 1990;6:597–641.
120. Bonewald LF, Mundy GA. Role of transforming growth factor-β in bone remodeling. *Clin Orthop* 1989;250:261–276.
121. Li CH, Ramasharma K. Inhibin. *Annu Rev Pharmacol Toxicol* 1987;27:1–21.
122. Ying S-Y. Inhibins, activins, and follistatins: gonadal proteins modulating the secretion of follicle-stimulating hormone. *Endocr Rev* 1988;9:267–293.
123. Farnworth PG, Robertson DM, de Kretser DM, Burger HG. Effects of 31 kilodalton bovine inhibin on follicle-stimulating hormone and luteinizing hormone in rat pituitary cells *in vitro:* actions under basal conditions. *Endocrinology* 1988;122:207–213.
124. Farnworth PG, Robertson DM, de Kretser DM, Burger HG. Effects of 31 kDa bovine inhibin on FSH and LH in rat pituitary cells *in vitro:* antagonism of gonadotrophin-releasing hormone agonists. *J Endocrinol* 1988;119:233–241.
125. Jakubowiak A, Janecki A, Steinberger A. Action kinetics of inhibin in superfused pituitary cells depend on gonadotropin-releasing hormone treatment. *Endocrinology* 1990;127:211–217.
126. Robertson DM, Prisk M, McMaster JW, Irby DC, Findlay JK, de Kretser DM. Serum FSH-suppressing activity of human recombinant inhibin A in male and female rats. *J Reprod Fertil* 1991;91:321–328.
127. Rivier C, Schwall R, Mason A, Burton L, Vaughan J, Vale W. Effect of recombinant inhibin on luteinizing hormone and follicle-stimulating hormone secretion in the rat. *Endocrinology* 1991;128:1548–1554.
128. DePaolo L, Shimonaka M, Schwall R, Ling N. *In vivo* comparison of the follicle-stimulating hormone-suppressing activity of follistatin and inhibin ovariectomized rats. *Endocrinology* 1991;128:668–674.
129. Rivier C, Corrigan A, Vale W. Effect of recombinant human inhibin on gonadotropin secretion by the male rat. *Endocrinology* 1991;129:2155–2159.
130. Carroll RS, Kowash PM, Lofgren JA, Schwall RH, Chin WW. *In vivo* regulation of FSH synthesis by inhibin and activin. *Endocrinology* 1991;129:3299–3304.
131. Rivier C, Vale W. Effect of recombinant inhibin on follicle-stimulating hormone secretion by the female rat: interaction with a gonadotropin-releasing antagonist and estrogen. *Endocrinology* 1991;129:2160–2165.
132. McLeod BJ, McNeilly AS. Suppression of plasma FSH concentrations with bovine follicular fluid blocks ovulation in GnRH-treated seasonally anoestrous ewes. *J Reprod Fertil* 1987;81: 187–194.
133. Kotsuji F, Winters SJ, Keeping HS, Attardi B, Oshima H, Troen P. Effect of inhibin from primate Sertoli cells on follicle-stimulating hormone and luteinizing hormone release by perifused rat pituitary cells. *Endocrinology* 1988;122:2796–2802.
134. Fukuda M, Miyamoto K, Hasegawa Y, Ibuki Y, Igarashi M. Action mechanism of inhibin *in vitro*-cyclohexamide mimics inhibin actions on pituitary cells. *Mol Cell Endocrinol* 1987;51: 41–50.
135. Carroll RS, Corrigan AZ, Gaharib SD, Vale WW, Chin WW. Inhibin, activin, and follistatin: regulation of follicle-stimulating hormone messenger ribonucleic acid levels. *Mol Endocrinol* 1989;3:1969–1976.
136. deGreef WJ, Eilers GAM, de Koning J, Karels B, de Jong FH. Effects of ovarian inhibin on pulsatile release of gonadotropins and secretion of LHRH in ovariectomized rats: evidence against a central action of inhibin. *J Endocrinol* 1987;113:449–455.
137. Wang QF, Farnworth PG, Findlay JK, Burger HG. Effect of purified 31K bovine inhibin on the specific binding of gonadotropin-releasing hormone to rat anterior pituitary cells in culture. *Endocrinology* 1988;123:2161–2166.
138. Gregg DW, Schwall RH, Nett TM. Regulation of gonadotropin secretion and number of gonadotropin-releasing hormone receptors by inhibin, activin-A and estradiol. *Biol Reprod* 1991;44: 725–732.
139. Laws SC, Beggs MJ, Webster JC, Miller WL. Inhibin increases and progesterone decreases receptors for gonadotropin-releasing hormone in ovine pituitary culture. *Endocrinology* 1990;127: 373–380.
140. Attardi B, Keeping HS, Winters SJ, Kotsuji F, Troen P. Comparison of the effects of cyclohexamide and inhibin on the gonadotropin subunit messenger ribonucleic acids. *Endocrinology* 1991; 128:119–125.

141. Attardi B, Keeping HS, Winters SJ, Kotsuji F, Maurer RA, Troen P. Rapid and profound suppression of messenger ribonucleic acid encoding follicle-stimulating hormone β by inhibin from primate Sertoli cells. *Mol Endocrinol* 1989;3:280–287.
142. Mercer JE, Clements JA, Funder JW, Clarke IJ. Rapid and specific lowering of pituitary FSH β mRNA levels by inhibin. *Mol Cell Endocrinol* 1987;53:251–254.
143. Rivier C, Vale W. Inhibin: measurement and role in the immature female rat. *Endocrinology* 1987;120:1688–1690.
144. Hasegawa Y, Miyamoto K, Igarashi M. Changes in serum concentrations of immunoreactive inhibin during the oestrous cycle of the rat. *J Endocrinol* 1989;121:91–100.
145. Rivier C, Cajander S, Vaughan J, Hsueh AJW, Vale W. Age-dependent changes in physiological action, content, and immunostaining of inhibin in male rats. *Endocrinology* 1988;123:120–126.
146. Culler MD, Negro-Vilar A. Passive immunoneutralization of endogenous inhibin: sex-related differences in the role of inhibin during development. *Mol Cell Endocrinol* 1988;58:263–273.
147. Rivier C, Rivier J, Vale W. Inhibin-mediated feedback control of follicle-stimulating hormone secretion in the female rat. *Science* 1986;234:205–207.
148. Rivier C, Vale WW. Immunoneutralization of endogenous inhibin modifies hormone secretion and ovulation rate in the rat. *Endocrinology* 1989;125:152–157.
149. Cummins LJ, O'Shea T, Al-Obaidi SAR, Bindon BM, Findlay JK. Increase in ovulation rate after immunization of Merino ewes with a fraction of bovine follicular fluid containing inhibin activity. *J Reprod Fertil* 1986;77:365–372.
150. Mann GE, Campbell BK, McNeilly AS, Baird DT. Passively immunizing ewes against inhibin during the luteal phase of the oestrous cycle raises the plasma concentration of FSH. *J Endocrinol* 1989;123:383–391.
151. Medhamurthy R, Abeyawardene SA, Culler MD, Negro-Vilar A, Plant TM. Immunoneutralization of circulating inhibin in the hypophysiotropically clamped male Rhesus monkey (*Macaca mulatta*) results in a selective hypersecretion of follicle-stimulating hormone. *Endocrinology* 1990;126:2116–2124.
152. Robertson DM, Hayward S, Irby D, et al. Radioimmunoassay of rat serum inhibin: changes after PMSG stimulation and gonadectomy. *Mol Cell Endocrinol* 1988;8:1–8.
153. Dalkin AC, Knight CD, Shupnik MA, et al. Ovariectomy and inhibin immunoneutralization acutely increase FSH β mRNA concentrations: evidence for a non-transcriptional mechanism. *Endocrinology* 1993;132:1297–1304.
154. Hutchinson LA, Findlay JK, de Vos FL, Robertson DM. Effects of bovine inhibin, transforming growth factor-β and bovine activin-A on granulosa cell differentiation. *Biochem Biophys Res Commun* 1987;146:1405–1408.
155. Woodruff TK, Lyon RJ, Hansen SE, Rice GC, Mather JP. Inhibin and activin locally regulate rat ovarian folliculogenesis. *Endocrinology* 1990;127:3196–3205.
156. Hsueh AJ, Dahl KD, Vaughan J, et al. Heterodimers and homodimers of inhibin subunits have different paracrine action in the modulation of luteinizing hormone-stimulated androgen biosynthesis. *Proc Natl Acad Sci USA* 1987;84:5082–5086.
157. Hillier SG, Yong EL, Illingworth PJ, Baird DT, Schwall RH, Mason AJ. Effect of recombinant activin on androgen synthesis in cultured human thecal cells. *J Clin Endocrinol Metab* 1991;72:1206–1211.
158. Yu J, Shao L, Vaughan J, Vale W, Yu AL. Characterization of the potentiation effect of activin on human erythroid colony formation *in vitro. Blood* 1989;72:952–960.
159. Plotsky PM, Kjær A, Sutton SW, Sawchenko PE, Vale W. Central activin administration modulates corticotropin-releasing hormone and adrenocorticotropin secretion. *Endocrinology* 1991;128:2520–2525.
160. Bilezikjian LM, Corrigan AZ, Vale W. Activin-A modulates growth hormone secretion from cultures of rat anterior pituitary cells. *Endocrinology* 1990;126:2369–2376.
161. Kitaoka M, Kojima I, Ogata E. Activin-A: a modulator of multiple types of anterior pituitary cells. *BBRC* 1988;157:48–54.
162. Mathews LS, Vale WW. Expression cloning of an activin receptor, a predicted transmembrane serine kinase. *Cell* 1991;65:973–982.
163. Attisano L, Wrana JL, Cheifetz S, Massague J. Novel activin receptors: distinct genes and alternative mRNA splicing generate a repertoire of serine/threonine kinase receptors. *Cell* 1992;68:97–108.
164. Attardi B, Miklos J. Rapid stimulatory effect of activin-A on messenger RNA encoding the follicle-stimulating hormone β-subunit in rat pituitary cell cultures. *Mol Endocrinol* 1990;4:721–726.
165. Schwall RH, Nikolics K, Szonyi E, Gorman C, Mason AJ. Recombinant expression and characterization of human activin A. *Mol Endocrinol* 1988;2:1237–1242.
166. Schwall RH, Szonyi E, Mason AJ, Nikolics K. Activin stimulates secretion of follicle-stimulating hormone from pituitary cells desensitized to gonadotropin-releasing hormone. *BBRC* 1988;151:1099–1104.
167. Katayama T, Shiota K, Takahashi M. Activin A increases the number of follicle-stimulating hormone cells in anterior pituitary cultures. *Mol Cell Endocrinol* 1990;69:179–185.
168. Katayama T, Shiota K, Takahashi M. Effects of activin A on anterior pituitary cells fractionated by centrifugal elutriation. *Mol Cell Endocrinol* 1991;77:167–173.
169. Carroll RS, Corrigan AZ, Vale W, Chin WW. Activin stabilitzes follicle-stimulating hormone-beta messenger ribonucleic acid levels. *Endocrinology* 1991;129:1721–1726.
170. Schwall RH, Schmelzer CH, Matsuyama E, Mason AJ. Multiple actions of recombinant activin-A *in vivo. Endocrinology* 1989;125:1420–1423.
171. Ueno N, Ling N, Ying S-Y, Esch F, Shimasaki S, Guillemin R. Isolation and partial characterization of follistatin: a novel Mr 35,000 monomeric protein that inhibits the release of follicle stimulating hormone. *Proc Natl Acad Sci USA* 1987;84:8282–8286.
172. Shimasaki S, Koga M, Buscaglia ML, Simmons DM, Bicsak TA, Ling N. Follistatin gene expression in the ovary and extragonadal tissues. *Mol Endocrinol* 1989;3:651–659.
173. Shimasaki S, Koga M, Esch F, et al. Primary structure of the human follistatin precursor and its genomic organization. *Proc Natl Acad Sci USA* 1988;85:4218–4222.
174. Esch FS, Shimasaki S, Mercado M, et al. Structural characterization of follistatin: a novel follicle-stimulating hormone release-inhibiting polypeptide from the gonad. *Mol Endocrinol* 1987;1:849–855.
175. Robertson DM, Klein R, de Vos FL, et al. The isolation of polypeptide with FSH suppressing activity from bovine follicular fluid which are structurally different to inhibin. *Biochem Biophys Res Commun* 1987;149:744–749.
176. Ying S-Y, Becker A, Swanson G, et al. Follistatin specifically inhibits pituitary follicle stimulating hormone release *in vitro. BBRC* 1987;149:133–139.
177. Robertson DM, Farnworth PG, Clarke L, et al. Effects of bovine 35kDA FSH-suppressing protein on FSH and LH in rat pituitary cells *in vitro:* comparison with bovine 31kDA inhibin. *J Endocrinol* 1990;124:417–423.
178. Inouye S, Guo Y, de Paolo L, Shimonaka M, Ling N, Shimasaki S. Recombinant expression of human follistatin with 315 and 288 amino acids: chemical and biological comparison with native porcine follistatin. *Endocrinology* 1991;129:815–822.
179. Nakamura T, Takio K, Eto Y, Shibai H, Titani K, Sugino H. Activin-binding protein from rat ovary is follistatin. *Science* 1990;247:836–839.
180. Shimonaka M, Inouye S, Shimasaki S, Ling N. Follistatin binds to both activin and inhibin throught the common beta-subunit. *Endocrinology* 1991;128:3313–3316.
181. Michel U, Albiston A, Findlay JK. Rat follistatin: gonadal and extragonadal expression and evidence for alternative splicing. *BBRC* 1990;173:401–407.
182. Meunier H, Rivier C, Evans RM, Vale W. Gonadal and extragonadal expression of inhibin alpha, βA, and βB subunits in various tissues predicts diverse functions. *Proc Natl Acad Sci USA* 1988;85:247–251.
183. Kogawa K, Nakamura T, Sugino K, Takio K, Titani K, Sugino H. Production and regulation of inhibin subunits in pituitary gonadotropes. *Endocrinology* 1989;128:1434–1437.

184. Roberts V, Meunier H, Vaughan J, et al. Evidence for an autocrine role of activin B within rat anterior pituitary cultures. *Endocrinology* 1991;124:552–555.
185. Weiss J, Harris PE, Halvorson L, Jameson JL. Regulation of FSH-beta mRNA levels by endogenous and exogenous activin. Seventy fourth Annual meeting of the Endocrine Society, San Antonio, Texas. 1992; Abst. #1547.
186. Shupnik MA, Weinmann CM, Notides AC, Chin WW. An upstream region of the rat luteinizing hormone β gene binds estrogen receptor and confers estrogen responsiveness. *J Biol Chem* 1989;264:80–86.
187. Clayton RN, Lalloz MRA, Salton SRJ, Roberts JL. Expression of LH beta subunit chloromphericol acetyltransferase (LH-beta-CAT) fusion gene in rat pituitary cells: induction by cAMP. *Mol Cell Endocrinol* 1991;80:193–202.
188. Jameson JL, Jaffe RC, Deutsch PH, Albanese C, Habener JF. The gonadotropin α-subunit gene contains multiple protein binding domains that interact to modulate basal and cAMP-responsive transcription. *J Biol Chem* 1988;263:9879–9886.
189. Hoeffler JP, Meyer TE, Yun Y, Jameson JL, Habener JF. Cyclic AMP-responsive DNA-binding protein: structure based on a cloned placental cDNA. *Science* 1988;242:1430–1433.
190. Bokar JA, Keri RA, Farmerie TA, et al. Expression of the glycoprotein hormone alpha-subunit gene in the placenta requires a functional cAMP response element, whereas a different *cis*-acting element mediates pituitary-specific expression. *Mol Cell Biol* 1989;9:5113–5122.
191. Childs GV. Functional ultrastructure of gonadotropes: a review. *Curr Top Neuroendocrinol* 1986;7:49–97.
192. Shupnik MA, Gharib SD, Chin WW. Divergent effects of estradiol on gonadotropin gene transcription in pituitary fragments. *Mol Endocrinol* 1989;3:474–480.
193. Horn F, Belezekjean LM, Perren MH, et al. Intracellular responses to GnRH in a clonal cell line of the gonadotrope lineage. *Mol Endocrinol* 1991;5:347–355.
194. Maurer RA, Notides AC. Identification of an estrogen responsive element from the 5′-flanking region of the rat prolactin gene. *Mol Cell Biol* 1987;7:4247–4254.
195. Klein-Hitpass L, Schorpp M, Wagner U, Ryffel GU. An estrogen-responsive element derived from the 5′-flanking region of the *Xenopus* vitellogenin A2 gene functions in transfected human cells. *Cell* 1986;46:1053–1061.
196. Keri RA, Andersen B, Kennedy GC, et al. Estradiol inhibits transcription of the human glycoprotein hormone alpha-subunit gene despite the absence of a high affinity binding site for the estrogen receptor. *Mol Endocrinol* 1991;5:725–733.
197. Chatterjee VKK, Madison CD, Mayo S, Jameson JL. Repression of the human glycoprotein hormone alpha-subunit gene by glucocorticoids: evidence for receptor interactions with limiting transcriptional activators. *Mol Endocrinol* 1991;5:100–110.
198. Kay TWH, Jameson JL. Identification of a GnRH-responsive region in the glycoprotein hormone alpha-subunit promoter. *Mol Endocrinol* 1992;6:1767–1773.
199. Shupnik MA. GnRH effects on rat gonadotropin gene transcription *in vitro:* requirement for pulsatile administration for LH beta gene stimulation. *Mol Endocrinol* 1990;4:1444–1450.
200. Andrews WV, Maurer RA, Conn PM. Stimulation of rat luteinizing hormone-β mRNA levels by gonadotropin releasing hormone. *J Biol Chem* 1988;263:13755–13761.
201. Montmeny MR, Serarino KA, Wagner JA, Mandel G, Goodman GH. Identification of a cyclic-AMP-responsive element within the rat somatostatin gene. *Proc Natl Acad Sci USA* 1986;83:6682–6686.
202. Roesler WJ, Vanderbark GR, Hanson RW. Cyclic AMP and the induction of eukaryotic gene transcription. *J Biol Chem* 1988;263:9063–9066.
203. Maurer RA, Kim KE. Analysis of gonadotropin gene structure and expression. In: Chin W, Boime I, eds. *Glycoprotein Hormones.* Norwell, Massachusetts: Serono Symposia, 1990; 237–243.
204. Fuh VL, Burren JM, Jameson JL. cAMP effects on chorionic gonadotropin gene transcription and mRNA stability: labile proteins mediate basal expression whereas stable proteins mediate cAMP stimulation. *Mol Endocrinol* 1989;3:1148–1156.
205. Steger DJ, Altschmied J, Buscher M, Mellon PL. Evolution of placental-specific gene expression: comparison of the equine and human gonadotropin alpha subunit genes. *Mol Endocrinol* 1991;5:243–255.
206. Silver BJ, Bokar JA, Virgin JB, Vallen EA, Milsted A, Nilson JH. Cyclic AMP regulation of the human glycoprotein hormone α subunit is mediated by an 18 base-pair element. *Proc Natl Acad Sci USA* 1987;84:2198–2202.
207. Delegeane AM, Ferland LH, Mellon PL. Tissue-specific enhancer of the human glycoprotein hormone alpha subunit gene: dependence on cyclic AMP-inducible elements. *Mol Cell Biol* 1987;7:3994–4002.
208. Andersen B, Kennedy GC, Hamernick DL, Bokar JA, Bohenski R, Nilson JH. Amplification of the transcriptional signal mediated by the tandum cAMP response elements of the glycoprotein hormone alpha-subunit gene occurs through several distinct mechanisms. *Mol Endocrinol* 1990;4:573–582.
209. Drust DS, Troccoli NM, Jameson JL. Binding specificity of cAMP responsive elements (CRE)-binding proteins and activating transcription factors to naturally occurring CRE sequence variants. *Mol Endocrinol* 1991;5:1541–1551.
210. Dwarki VJ, Montimy M, Verma IM. Both the basic region and the "leucene zipper" domain of the cAMP responsive element binding protein are essential for transcriptional activation. *EMBO J* 1990;9:225–232.
211. Marshall JC, Dalkin AC, Haisenleder DJ, Paul SJ, Ortolano GA, Kelch RP. Gonadotropin releasing hormone pulses: regulators of gonadotropin synthesis and ovulatory cycles. *Recent Prog Horm Res* 1991;47:155–189.

The Physiology of Reproduction, Second Edition,
edited by E. Knobil and J.D. Neill,
Raven Press, Ltd., New York © 1994.

CHAPTER 32

The Molecular Mechanism of Gonadotropin-Releasing Hormone Action in the Pituitary

P. Michael Conn

Gonadotropin-releasing hormone (GnRH) provides a humoral link between the neural and endocrine systems. This decapeptide, pyroGlu[1]-His[2]-Trp[3]-Ser[4]-Tyr[5]-Gly[6]-Leu[7]-Arg[8]-Pro[9]-Gly-amide[10], is synthesized and then stored in the medial basal hypothalamus. In response to neural signals, GnRH is released in pulses into the hypophysial portal system and then conducted to the anterior pituitary, where it stimulates release of the gonadotropins luteinizing hormone (LH) and follicle stimulating hormone (FSH). These gonadotropins are released into the systemic circulation and regulate gonadal steroidogenesis and gamete maturation; LH stimulates ovulation and corpus luteum formation in females and androgen secretion in males, whereas FSH stimulates the growth and maturation of ovarian follicles in females and spermatogenesis in males. Gonadotropin-releasing hormone and its analogs also have direct actions on the gonads in some species by inhibiting steroidogenesis in males and ovulation in females (1). It is unlikely that hypothalamic-derived GnRH is responsible for these actions (because of the very low concentrations in the peripheral circulations), although the possibility remains open that a different, locally produced molecule may bind a gonadal "GnRH receptor" *in vivo.* The ability of GnRH to stimulate reproductive functions (at pulsatile low doses) or suppress them (at high doses) has been clinically applied for different purposes (2,3), including the induction of ovulation and spermatogenesis, contraception, and for the treatment of precocious puberty, endometriosis, and steroid-dependent tumors (i.e., prostate and breast cancer) as well as a range of veterinary purposes.

Understanding the basic mechanisms by which GnRH alters gonadotrope function has been a valuable resource for development of clinical and veterinary strategies (3) and has provided the powerful stimulus for work in this area. This review describes what is known about the means by which the releasing hormone interacts with its receptor and subsequently alters the responses of the target cell.

Department of Pharmacology, University of Iowa, College of Medicine, Iowa City, Iowa 52242

GnRH RECEPTOR

Ligand Binding and Physical Characteristics

The first step in GnRH action is recognition by its receptor. This binding step has been studied in great detail, owing to the availability of a wide variety of useful analogs. Highly satisfactory radioligands can be prepared by using high-affinity, metabolically stable agonists (4,5). Such synthetic agonists frequently share the presence of a D-amino acid^6, which inhibits enzymatic degradation and the substitution, des-Gly^{10}-Pro^9-ethylamide, which, when present with the D-amino acid^6, enhances receptor binding affinity. Detailed studies using these analogs (which can be radioiodinated to high specific activity, 800 μCi/μg) have shown changes in GnRH receptor number (but not binding affinity) during the rat estrus cycle (6–8), lactation, castration, and aging (6) and in other endocrine states. In a general way, the frequency of the receptors is predictive of the responsiveness of the gonadotrope cell to GnRH. However, conditions can be devised in cell cultures that lead to diminished cellular responsiveness even in the face of elevated receptor numbers, *vide infra.* These observations indicate that receptor regulation is not the sole determinant of cellular responsiveness.

The receptor itself, although still a component of the plasma membrane, has a molecular weight of 136,346 ± 8,120 as measured by target size analysis (9). A lower molecular weight has been reported for photoaffinity labeled (PAL) receptor that is analyzed under denaturing conditions (60,000) (10–15). Conceivably, this moiety is the hormone binding component of a larger (functional) complex described in the preceding study (9).

As this report is being prepared, a manuscript has appeared (16) describing the cloning and functional expression of the mouse GnRH receptor. A 327-amino-acid protein is described with a molecular weight of 37,683 and three consensus sites for *N*-linked glycosylation (likely explaining the disparity in molecular weights for the cloned form and the PAL receptor). The overall configuration of the receptor suggests that it is a member of the seven-transmembrane segment class. The highly conserved Asp or Glu found at TMS-2 of many receptors (and which is essential for function) is replaced in the GnRH receptor by Asn. The molecule lacks the polar cytoplasmic C terminus frequently observed in this group of molecules. Another unique feature of the molecule is the substitution of Ser for Tyr adjacent to TMS-3, thus creating a potential phosphorylation site. A highly basic site, flanked by two consensus phosphorylation sites, is located at the first internal loop after TMS-1.

Occupancy of the plasma membrane GnRH receptor (17) causes mobilization of extracellular Ca^{2+} through a plasma membrane Ca^{2+} ion channel and intracellular Ca^{2+} through mechanisms described below. The plasma membrane ion channel appears to be similar to that found in nervous and muscle tissue. Interestingly, however, structure–activity relationships with Ca^{2+} ion channel antagonists reveal that the channel is not identical to that observed in these other tissues (18).

Regulation of the Number of GnRH Receptors

Changes in the number of GnRH receptors in the pituitary glands of several species have been characterized during many physiologic conditions. During the estrous cycle of rats, hamsters, ewes, and cows, the maximum number of GnRH receptors was observed just before the preovulatory surge of LH (6–8,19–21). After the preovulatory surge of LH, the number of measurable GnRH receptors decreases rapidly and may require several days to achieve proestrous levels. After removal of the gonads, significant increases in the number of GnRH receptors have been observed (6). In contrast, during pregnancy and lactation, the number of GnRH receptors is less than that observed during the estrous cycle (6,8). These observations clearly demonstrate physiologic regulation of GnRH receptors *in vivo.*

Many treatments *in vitro* can alter the number of measurable receptors for GnRH in pituitary cell cultures. Treatment of pituitary cell cultures with physiologic concentrations of GnRH results in a biphasic response by the cells with respect to GnRH receptor number (22). Initially, a down-regulation of receptors is observed (0.5–4 h posttreatment) followed by an increase in the number of GnRH receptors (9 h posttreatment). The initial down-regulation of receptors for GnRH is temporally associated with desensitization of gonadotropes to GnRH, although clearly, other mechanisms including uncoupling of receptors from second-messenger systems contribute to development of this refractory state. Homologous down-regulation of GnRH receptors appears to be independent of extracellular calcium whereas up-regulation of GnRH receptors is dependent on extracellular calcium and requires protein synthesis (22,23).

Up-regulation of GnRH receptors by homologous hormone can be mimicked by treatment of pituitary cells with analogs of adenosine 3′,5′-monophosphate as well as nonspecific depolarization of pituitary cells with KCl (22–24). Although up-regulation of GnRH receptors indicates the ability of gonadotropes to respond to different external signals with an increased number of plasma membrane receptors, this increased receptor number does not increase the sensitivity of gonadotropes to GnRH when LH release is measured as the cellular response (25). Gonadotropes can respond with near maximal LH release when only 20% of available GnRH receptors are occupied *in vitro* (26), and when 50% of receptors are blocked with a GnRH antagonist, ewes can still respond fully to subsequent GnRH administration with LH release (27). As indicated above, these data indicate that there are "spare" GnRH receptors when LH release is the sole parameter measured; however, it is unknown if the "spare" receptor conclusion is valid for the other functions of gonadotropes in response to GnRH (i.e., FSH release, receptor synthesis, up-regulation, down-regulation, gonadotropin biosynthesis), because these other responses appear to be regulated by complex and interrelated messenger systems.

Besides regulation of GnRH receptor by homologous hormone, the number of GnRH receptors can be regulated by other hormones including steroids and protein products from the gonad. As indicated above, removal of the gonads can increase the number of GnRH receptors *in vivo* when hypothalamic–pituitary connections are intact. In the absence of hypothalamic input, estradiol-17β can increase the number of GnRH receptors (28,29). Using ovine pituitary gonadotrope cell cultures, Laws et al. (30,31) have shown that estrogen can increase and progesterone can decrease the number of receptors for GnRH.

Protein products of the gonads have also been shown to influence the number of GnRH receptors. Wang et al. (32) have shown a decreased number of GnRH receptors when rat pituitary cell cultures were treated with inhibin. This group subsequently showed that inhibin was able to block GnRH-stimulated up-regulation of GnRH receptors (33). The effects of inhibin on the basal number of GnRH receptors was shown to be independent of biosynthesis of GnRH receptors (34), but the ability of inhibin to block up-regulation of GnRH receptors in the rat was at least partially due to the ability of inhibin to antagonize GnRH-stimulated synthesis of GnRH receptors (35). In direct contrast, Laws et al. (30) observed that treatment of ovine pituitary cell cultures with inhibin significantly increased the number of GnRH receptors. Given these two distinctly separate observations regarding the effects of inhibin on GnRH receptor populations in two different species, clearly, other species will have to be examined to clarify the role of inhibin in regulating the number of pituitary receptors for GnRH.

Patching, Capping, and Internalization

Observations related to the cell biology of the receptor can be made by preparation of fluorescent GnRH analogs, which can be monitored on living cells by image-intensified microscopy (36). As has been observed for many polypeptide hormones, the fluorescently labeled GnRH (presumably occupying the receptor, because the process is saturable and specific for gonadotropes) can be seen to undergo patching, capping, and internalization at 37°C.

More recently (37), a metabolically stable GnRH agonist (D-Lys^6-GnRH) was coupled to electron opaque markers (colloidal gold and ferritin) to characterize the intracellular pathway of the releasing hormone bound by pituitary gonadotropes. This approach has the advantage of increasing the resolution of localization to a "circle of uncertainty" about ten- to 20-fold smaller than that which can be obtained by autoradiography. After an initial uniform distribution on the cell surface, the derivatives were taken up individually as well as in small clusters in coated and uncoated membrane invaginations and moved to the lysosomal compartment either directly or after passage through the Golgi apparatus. The results suggest that labeled GnRH or GnRH-receptor complex may be routed to two distinct intracellular compartments: the lysosome and the Golgi cisternae. Studies using similar techniques (38,39) indicate that GnRH antagonists are also internalized (albeit at a slower rate) and appear to follow a different intracellular route compared with agonists (40). These observations are consistent with the possibility that internalized antagonists are "simply" riding along with plasma membrane undergoing routine cycling.

An early question therefore was: Is patching, capping, and internalization necessary for the molecular events that ensue? To answer this question, D-Lys^6-GnRH was covalently attached (through a reactive amino group) to an immobile support (41,42); LH release could then be measured when GnRH was prevented from entering the cell. The derivative provoked LH release at full efficacy and therefore suggested that internalization is not necessary for GnRH to exert its effect.

It was apparent that vinblastine could inhibit receptor patching, capping, and internalization in response to the releasing hormone but did not inhibit LH release (42). This also suggested that the process of patching, capping, and internalization could be uncoupled from release. Patching and capping refer to events that can be seen by image-intensified microscopy. The resolution of such a technique is only about 100 molecules. Therefore, events that occur as the result of receptor dimerization or multimerization (i.e., "receptor microaggregation," which is described below) would not be seen by this technique.

An additional approach has been a double-incubation experiment (43). In these studies, cells were first incubated in different concentrations of GnRH for various times. After about 15 min at median effective dose (ED_{50}) or higher concentrations, considerable internalization of the releasing hormone occurs. If the releasing hormone is then removed from outside the media, one of two things will happen. If the internalized GnRH is sufficient to support continued gonadotropin release, this event should continue. If, in contrast, a continuously applied extracellular source of GnRH is required, the response system should undergo extinction; the latter appears to be the case.

After washing GnRH from outside the cells, release of

gonadotropin undergoes extinction. Consequently, an externally applied, continuous source of GnRH is necessary for the response system to continue. It then appeared that patching, capping, and internalization are not necessary for the releasing hormone to exert its effect.

Receptor–Receptor Interactions: Microaggregation

To examine the significance of receptor–receptor interaction at levels below that which can be measured by image intensification, additional use can be made of the GnRH analogs. Because of the interest of drug companies in this compound and support from the Contraceptive Development Branch of the National Institutes of Health, many GnRH antagonists are available. Many of these antagonists appear to work by the classic pharmacologic means [i.e., they occupy the receptor but do not produce efficacy (i.e., gonadotropin release)]. A particular GnRH antagonist was used: D-*p*-Glu^1-D-Phe^2-D-Trp^3-D-Lys^6-GnRH (44,45). The substitution of D-amino acids in the first three positions leads to considerable antagonism intrinsic in this molecule. The substitution with a D-Lys^6 at the sixth position provides protection against biologic degradation and, also, introduces the only amino group in this molecule (the N terminus is blocked, pyro-Glu^1). It was then a simple matter to prepare a GnRH dimer with a very short bridge length (about 12 Å) between the antagonist molecules. This could then be used to change the specificity of an antibody initially directed against the antagonist. It is possible then to prepare a molecule that is a derivatized antibody having a GnRH antagonist dimer at either F_{ab} arm. This compound when applied to cells has considerable efficacy as an agonist. This strange event (i.e., the conversion of a GnRH antagonist to an agonist as a result of its dimerization) was a confusing result. In several human disease states, antibodies have been identified that cross-link receptors and consequently provide agonist efficacy. Because of these observations, receptor–receptor interactions were considered in the present situation.

Indeed, if either the papain or reduced-pepsin cleavage product of the antibody (i.e., univalent "antibody") is coupled with the dimer, the result is a pure antagonist. The antibody alone has no agonist efficacy, and consequently, the inescapable conclusion appeared to be that receptor–receptor interactions (i.e., the dimerization of receptors) could stimulate the response system. An antagonist then might be a compound that could occupy the receptor but, because of its inability to promote receptor–receptor dimerization, would then behave antagonistically. When one takes an antagonist and confers on it the ability to cross-link receptors, we are now able to see agonist efficacy. It was also possible to demonstrate that the efficacy of the agonist in this system shared much in common with the authentic native molecule of GnRH. Both, for example, are inhibited by calmodulin antagonists and require extracellular calcium. It was therefore presumed that the mechanism by which the receptor dimerization event was able to provide agonist efficacy was very much similar to that which was provided by the native molecule (i.e., GnRH). It was also possible to use this technique to potentiate the action of a GnRH agonist (D-Lys^6-GnRH) (46). This compound is biologically stable because of the D-amino acid^6 substitution, and, also, has the necessary amino group for preparation of dimers. Following preparation of the agonist dimer, it was possible to show that when it was administered to cells at a 10% effective concentration (EC_{10}) dose, its efficacy could be potentiated by addition of antibody to the EC_{40} level, suggesting then that the agonist was able to occupy receptors and then at the appropriate concentrations was able to be cross-linked by antibodies to that molecule.

Computer simulations (47,48) were prepared for this model. If we assume that two receptors are able to come together about a previously closed calcium ion channel (or other effector) and if these two receptors are able to stimulate opening of the ion channel (or activation of another effector), an equilibrium model can be built. Such a model, interestingly, fits the data within approximately 5% over five dose logs.

Polycations, when charge groups are separated by at least 120 Å, also stimulate LH release, potentially by orientation of sialic acid-rich (i.e., negatively charged) GnRH receptor (49).

GnRH Receptor Synthesis

Most studies addressing the regulation of GnRH receptor populations have relied on steady-state measurements (i.e., radioligand binding assays). Because such measurements are the result of the *combined* rates of receptor appearance (synthesis, recycling, and unmasking) and receptor loss (degradation, internalization, and unmasking), it was viewed as desirable to identify the specific contribution of synthesis to this process. Unfortunately, the lack of availability of antireceptor antibodies have hampered the ability to perform these experiments. I have taken advantage of the combined use of density labeling (i.e., labeling the receptor with dense amino acids) and photoaffinity labeling (to identify the previously existing "old" receptor from the newly synthesized "new" population) to measure the rates of receptor replacement in response to (a) the releasing hormone itself; (b) regulation of extra- and intracellular Ca^{2+}; (c) activation of protein kinase C (PKC); (d) inhibin; and (e) activin. In the data described below, for purposes of comparison, relative receptor synthetic rates were expressed as the amount of time needed to replace 50% of the receptors. All studies used cell cultures prepared from female weanling rats (55–74 g).

Homologous Receptor Regulation by GnRH and Regulation by Intra- and Extracellular Ca^{2+}

The ability of homologous hormone and its antagonist analogs to affect the rate of synthesis of these receptors was evaluated. Also, because of its role in other actions of the releasing hormone, the requirement for extracellular Ca^{2+} to mediate the effects of GnRH was assessed. Cultures were treated with GnRH, a GnRH antagonist, or the Ca^{2+} ionophore A23187, with or without ethyleneglycoltetraacetic acid (EGTA) (a Ca^{2+} chelator); after this, they were further cultured for times up to 24 h in medium containing either dense or normal amino acids followed by covalent linkage of the GnRH receptors with a radiolabeled photoaffinity probe ([^{125}I]Tyr^5-[azido-benzoyl-D-Lys^6-GnRH]). They were then solubilized in 1% sodium dodecyl sulfate. Receptors that had incorporated the dense amino acids (i.e., newly synthesized receptors) were separated from those that had been synthesized before the addition of dense amino acids by velocity sedimentation in sucrose gradients (0–20% sucrose, 1% sodium dodecyl sulfate, and 10 mM Tris-HCl, pH 7.0; centrifuged at 156,000 × *g* for 24 h). After centrifugation, gradients were fractionated, and the radioactivity in each fraction was quantified. GnRH treatment (10 or 0.1 nM) increased the rate at which dense amino acids were incorporated into GnRH receptors ($t_{1/2}$ = 13 ± 2, 15 ± 1, and 25 ± 2 h for 0.1 nM GnRH, 10 nM GnRH, and control values, respectively). Gonadotropin-releasing hormone antagonist alone did not change the rate of GnRH receptor synthesis ($t_{1/2}$ = 22 ± 3 h) compared with the control value ($t_{1/2}$ = 25 ± 2 h) and was able to block the effects of GnRH. The effects of GnRH were not antagonized by inclusion of 3 mM EGTA during treatment ($t_{1/2}$ = 15 ± 1 h versus 13 ± 2 h for 0.1 nM GnRH in the presence and absence of 3 mM EGTA, respectively). Also, treatment of pituitary cells with the Ca^{2+} ionophore A23187 (100 nM) had no effect on the time required for incorporation of dense amino acids into half the population of GnRH receptors ($t_{1/2}$ = 27 ± 2 versus 25 ± 2 h for A23187 and control, respectively). We believe that these are the first data to indicate that GnRH stimulates the synthesis of its own receptor. Unlike gonadotropin release, the mechanism through which GnRH mediates this stimulation of receptor synthesis neither requires extracellular Ca^{2+} nor is provoked by elevation of intracellular Ca^{2+} levels (50).

Regulation by Activators of PKC

The density and PAL protocols were similar to that described above. In some cultures, phorbol myristate acetate (PMA) (50 nM) was included during the photoaffinity agonist binding step. Newly synthesized (dense) receptors were separated from previously synthesized receptors as described above. The time required for synthesis of half the entire population of GnRH receptors was 28 ± 2 h (mean ± SEM; *n* = 4). Scatchard analysis and the pattern of GnRH-stimulated LH release from densely labeled cells indicated that they bound the PAL [K_d = 0.4 nM; approximately 1 fmol receptor/μg deoxyribonucleic acid (DNA)] and secreted gonadotropin normally. Also, treatment with PMA caused a significant increase (181 ± 24% in photoaffinity agonist binding), consistent with previous observations. Although PMA treatment increased the number of binding sites for the photoaffinity agonist, no significant change in the rate of synthesis of GnRH receptors was observed (25 ± 1 h; *n* = 4) for synthesis of half of the GnRH receptor population (35).

Are Actions of GnRH on Receptor Synthesis Mediated by PKC?

Studies were conducted to determine if PKC mediates GnRH-stimulated receptor synthesis. The density and PAL protocols were similar to that described above. Treatments consisted of media alone, PMA, phorbol 12,13-dibutyrate (PDB), or GnRH. To deplete cells of PKC, cultures were exposed for 8 to 16 h to 1 μM PMA. Short-term treatment with PKC activators (PMA or PDB, 1 μM) or GnRH (0.1 nM) was given for 30 min. After treatment, GnRH receptors were covalently linked to [^{125}I]-Tyr^5-azidobenzoyl-D-Lys^6-GnRH and solubilized. Newly synthesized (dense) receptors were separated from previously synthesized receptors as described above. Treatment with GnRH significantly stimulated the synthesis of GnRH receptors. Treatment of pituitary cell cultures with PMA (8–16 h) also stimulated the synthesis of GnRH receptors, although to a lesser extent than that observed after GnRH treatment. The synthesis of GnRH receptors in response to 0.1 nM GnRH was not different in cells with a normal complement of PKC compared with those depleted of PKC activity. This indicates that the ability of GnRH to stimulate synthesis of its own receptor is not mediated by PKC. Short-term treatment of cell cultures with 1 μM PMA or PDB (30 min) stimulated GnRH receptor synthesis similarly to treatment with 0.1 nM GnRH. When PMA and GnRH were administered simultaneously, GnRH receptor synthesis was stimulated to a greater extent than with either agent alone, suggesting differing mechanisms of action.

These results indicate that although activators of PKC can stimulate synthesis of GnRH receptors, PKC does not mediate the effects of GnRH on homologous receptor synthesis (51).

Receptor Regulation by Inhibin

We evaluated the ability of purified inhibin to affect the synthesis rate of GnRH receptors under basal conditions and after exposure of cultured gonadotropes (from female weanling rats) to GnRH. Cells were exposed to inhibin alone (4 or 12 ng/ml) or to GnRH (10^{-10} M) plus inhibin (0.4, 4, or 12 ng/ml) in the presence of densely labeled amino acids. Gonadotropin-releasing hormone was administered as a 20-min pulse, but inhibin treatment was continued for up to 2 days. After these treatments, GnRH receptors were labeled and quantified (new versus old) as described above. Treatment with inhibin alone had no measurable effect on the synthesis rate of GnRH receptors compared with that of control cultures ($t_{1/2}$ = 23.5 ± 0.3 versus 23.3 ± 0.3 versus 22.9 ± 0.9 h for control, 4 ng/ml inhibin, and 12 ng/ml inhibin, respectively). In contrast, inhibin blocked the stimulation of homologous receptor synthesis by GnRH in a dose-dependent manner ($t_{1/2}$ = 122.2 ± 0.7 versus 14.0 ± 0.7 versus 19.2 ± 1.5 versus 20.0 ± 2.9 h for GnRH alone and GnRH plus 0.4, 4, or 12 ng/ml inhibin, respectively). These data indicate that in rat pituitary cell cultures, inhibin does not decrease basal levels of GnRH receptors by affecting the synthesis rate of receptors but prevents up-regulation of GnRH receptors by blocking stimulation of GnRH receptor synthesis by homologous hormone (32).

Receptor Regulation by Activin

We evaluated the effects of activin-A on the GnRH receptor synthesis rate as well as effects of activin on homologous stimulation of GnRH receptor synthesis. Recombinant human activin-A (50 ng/ml) was incubated with pituitary cell cultures from female weanling rats, and the incorporation of densely labeled amino acids into receptors for GnRH was measured. The rate of GnRH receptor synthesis of cells treated with activin together with GnRH or inhibin was also quantified. Activin significantly stimulated the synthesis rate of GnRH receptors similarly to that observed after GnRH treatment (time for synthesis of half the population of GnRH receptors was 12.6 ± 1.1, 16.1 ± 1.3 versus 28.3 ± 1.2 h for GnRH, activin, and control, respectively). The time course for stimulation by GnRH and activin appeared to differ. Activin did not affect homologous stimulation of GnRH receptor synthesis. The stimulatory effects of activin were unaffected by inhibin ($t_{1/2}$ of synthesis = 17.2 ± 2.0 h). These data indicate that activin stimulates GnRH receptor synthesis in cell culture through a mechanism distinct from homologous stimulation by GnRH. This is, to our knowledge, the first demonstration of an action of activin-A on GnRH receptor synthesis (52).

PKC Treatment of Agonist-Occupied Receptors Increases Ka and N

Gonadotropin-releasing hormone stimulates release of pituitary gonadotropins by activating specific plasma membrane receptors. Activators of PKC were used to probe the binding characteristics of agonist- or antagonist-occupied GnRH receptors in intact cell cultures using a radioligand receptor assay. Specific binding of [^{125}I-Tyr^5-D-Ser(tbu)^6-Pro^9-NHEt]GnRH (Buserelin), a high-affinity GnRH agonist, was increased to 180% of control in the presence of 150 nM PDB and to 125% of control in the presence of 200 μM 1,2-diotanoylglycerol (diC_8), after 20 min at 23°C. The PMA effects were associated with apparent increases in both binding affinity and number of binding sites. The effects of PKC activators on Buserelin binding were concentration- and time-dependent and were not seen with 4α-PMA or 1,2-dioctanoyl-3-Cl-glycerol (neither of which activate PKC). In contrast, PMA had no measurable effects on specific binding of a GnRH receptor antagonist, Ac[D-PCl-Phe^{1,2}-D-Trp^3-^{125}I-Tyr^5-D-Lys^6-D-Ala^{10}] GnRH. When cell cultures were pretreated with 100 nM PDB in the absence of GnRH and then washed to remove the phorbol ester, no effects of prior PKC activation were detected on subsequent addition of Buserelin. However, when PDB pretreatment was carried out in the presence of GnRH, residual enhancement of Buserelin binding, but not antagonist binding, was observed at either 23° or 4°C. The radiolabeled agonist activated, and the antagonist blocked GnRH receptor-mediated LH release and [^{3}H]inositol phosphate (IP) production in cells preloaded with [^{3}H]inositol. These findings suggest that the action of PKC on the GnRH receptor, either direct or indirect, requires the receptor to be in an activated (agonist-occupied) state but does not require receptor internalization. The mechanism of these effects on GnRH agonist binding is not known but may involve sequestration of surface receptors, expression of new receptors, and/or modulation of GnRH receptor affinity (53).

Receptor Uncoupling from Phosphoinositide Hydrolysis

Gonadotropin-releasing hormone regulates pituitary gonadotropin release by a Ca^{2+}-dependent mechanism involving receptor-mediated phosphoinositide hydrolysis. Previous studies indicated that activation of pituitary PKC, although not required for acute gonadotropin release in response to GnRH, is likely involved in the chronic regulation of gonadotrope responsiveness, and activation of PKC by phorbol esters produces both the uncoupling of GnRH-stimulated phosphoinositide hydrolysis and the selective enhancement of GnRH agonist binding in pituitary cell cultures. We have examined the possibility that these processes are mechanistically related. Dissociation of bound agonist radioligand at 23°C was found to be reduced in the presence of phorbol esters, and ligand bound in the presence of phorbol ester was resistant to displacement by competing ligands at 4°C. However, agonist bound in the presence of phorbol ester was dissociated by subsequently washing cells at pH 3. Receptor PAL studies confirmed that agonist association with membrane component(s) identified as the GnRH receptor was increased in the presence of phorbol ester. These results suggest that, in the presence of a phorbol ester PKC activator, agonist-occupied GnRH receptors remain at the cell surface but are sequestered in some manner. In other experiments, cells preloaded with [^{3}H]inositol were treated with GnRH agonist ligand and phorbol ester at 4°C to form a pool of sequestered, agonist-occupied receptors, and then displaceable (nonsequestered) agonist was removed by incubation with antagonist ligand. After addition of LiCl and warming to 37°C, [^{3}H]IP production (an index of phosphoinositide hydrolysis) in phorbol ester–treated cells was reduced to 67% of vehicle control, although residual specific agonist binding had been increased to more than 300% of control. The appearance of sequestered receptors and inhibition of [^{3}H]IP production had similar phorbol ester concentration dependencies. These results suggest that the same agonist-occupied GnRH receptors sequestered as a result of PKC activation also are preferentially uncoupled from phosphoinositide hydrolysis (16).

CALCIUM-DEPENDENT ACTIONS OF GnRH

Calcium Dependence of Gonadotropin Release

GnRH requires ionic calcium for many of its actions. Omission or chelation of Ca^{2+} in the extracellular medium inhibits depolarization- or hypothalamic extract-stimulated LH release from pituitary tissue (54); this observation provided an early indication of the significance of calcium. This ion was among the first components of the GnRH response system to be systematically evaluated when chemically synthesized releasing hormone became generally available (55,56). Agents that increase the levels of intracellular Ca^{2+} including ionophores (A23187, X537A), ionomycin (55,57), depolarizing agents (KCl, veratridine) (58,59), calcium channel activators (60), or calcium-loaded liposomes release LH with efficacies similar to that of GnRH (61). Other physiologic cations do not substitute for calcium in this activity (62). An increase in transmembrane Ca^{2+} flux in response to GnRH was demonstrated by measuring efflux from $^{45}Ca^{2+}$-loaded cells (63). The use of Ca^{2+}-sensitive fluorophores has provided evidence that intracellular free Ca^{2+} concentrations increase transiently after exposure of target cells to GnRH (64–67).

A role for activation of specific plasma membrane calcium channels in response to GnRH is indicated by the ability of Ca^{2+} channel blocking agents (verapamil or D600) to inhibit stimulated LH release, both in isolated cells (62,68,70) and in human subjects (70,71), and by the LH-releasing action of maitotoxin, a Ca^{2+} channel activating agent (60). Also, patch-clamp studies of isolated gonadotropes have shown that, although these cells do not depolarize in response to GnRH, the releasing hormone is capable of activating a plasma membrane Ca^{2+} current (72). This was consistent with the observation that tetrodotoxin, a potent inhibitor of the sodium channel, inhibited LH release in response to agents that provoked depolarization (KCl, veratridine) but not in response to GnRH itself. It is likely, then, that elevation of intracellular Ca^{2+}, delivered in part through GnRH-activated plasma membrane Ca^{2+} channels, is an important signal for the stimulation of LH release by GnRH.

One potential intracellular mediator of the Ca^{2+} signal in gonadotropes is calmodulin, which, after binding Ca^{2+}, alters the activity of several enzymes and cytoskeletal proteins implicated in the secretory process (73). In immunohistochemical studies, calmodulin has been found to localize in association with the GnRH receptor "patch" after GnRH treatment (74). Also, pharmacologic agents that inhibit the activity of Ca^{2+}-calmodulin also block LH release in response to GnRH or Ca^{2+} ionophores. These include pimozide, penfluridol, and the naphthalene sulfonamide "W" compounds (75,76).

Because of the potential significance of the calmodulin binding components of the gonadotrope, a systematic study has been undertaken to characterize and then identify these moieties. In one study (77) relying on an ^{125}I-calmodulin gel overlayer assay ("Mid-Western" blot), it was possible to show tissue-specific and Ca^{2+}-dependent patterns of ^{125}I-calmodulin binding. Five main ^{125}I-calmodulin-labeled components of subunit M_r greater than 205,000, 200,000, 135,000, 60,000, and 52,000 were identified. Binding of the calmodulin was abolished in the presence of 1 mM EGTA (a calcium chelator) or calmodulin antagonists such as penfluridol (1 μM) or pimozide (1 μM). Subcellular fractionation revealed that the Ca^{2+}-dependent calmodulin binding components are localized primarily in the cytosolic fraction. Separation of dispersed anterior pituitary cells by a linear metrizamide gradient yielded gonadotrope-enriched fractions; these contained all five ^{125}I-calmodulin binding components corresponding to the main bands in the pituitary homogenate. Studies with ovariectomized or ovariectomized and steroid-replaced animals indicated that the tissue content of calmodulin binding components, like calmodulin itself, did not appear to be differentially regulated by steroids. A comparison of rat and bovine pituitary tissue homogenates revealed that binding components migrating at the same apparent molecular weights were found for four of the components. The identity of several of the gonadotrope proteins that are regulated by Ca^{2+}-calmodulin has been identified (78) based on their molecular weight, immunologic character, calmodulin binding activity (77), and other physiologic criteria, as spectrin, caldesmon, and calcineurin. More recently, studies in which specific antiserum to caldesmon has been inserted into living cells have revealed potentiation of LH release in response to GnRH. A model has been proposed in which Ca^{2+} regulates gonadotropin release by control of the gel-sol state of the cytosol (79).

G Proteins

Several studies have focused on the possible involvement of guanosine triphosphate (GTP) binding proteins linking activated receptor to formation of IPs and diacylglycerol. This was first suggested when it was found that receptors linked to phosphoinositide hydrolysis have altered affinities for agonist in the presence of guanine nucleotides (80). Thus, phospholipase C (PLC) may be regulated by a signal transduction G protein in a manner analogous to adenylate cyclase by G_s or G_i and cyclic guanosine monophosphate (cGMP) phosphodiesterase by transducin (81,82). In support of this hypothesis, activation of PLC occurs with GTP and with nonhydrolyzable GTP analogs and is inhibited by GDPβS (competitive inhibitor of G proteins). Also, hormonal activation of PLC is dependent on guanine nucleotides and occurs simultaneously with an increase in high-affinity GTPase activity (83,84).

Studies by Andrews et al. (85) suggested the involvement of a G protein coupled to the GnRH receptor, which, when activated, provoked LH release and IP production. Addition of GTP or a metabolically stable analog (guanylimidodiphosphate) to permeabilized pituitary cells stimulated a time- and concentration-dependent increase in IP accumulation and LH release. These responses were insensitive to both pertussis toxin and cholera toxin, indicating that the putative G-protein-mediating GnRH actions, like that hypothesized to mediate thyroid-releasing hormone (TRH) in (GH_3) pituitary cells (86), had properties different from G_s and G_i. Further evidence consistent with an association of the GnRH receptor and a G protein was provided by Perrin et al. (87), who demonstrated decreased receptor affinity for a GnRH agonist in the presence of guanine nucleotides.

In other studies (88), sodium fluoride (NaF), an exogenous activator of G proteins, was used to investigate the possibility of a G-protein link between GnRH receptor activation, PLC activity, and LH release. Treatment of primary pituitary cell cultures from immature female rats with sodium fluoride stimulated release of 20% total cellular LH (compared with 40–50% at maximal GnRH concentrations) and increased IP accumulation. Sodium fluoride–stimulated LH release was insensitive to cholera toxin and pertussis toxin. Sodium fluoride–stimulated LH release was additive with a maximally effective concentration of PMA and was not inhibited by depletion of cellular PKC, suggesting that PKC does not mediate sodium fluoride effects. Treatment of cultures with 3 mM EGTA and 10 nM GnRH for 5 or 16 h reduced pituitary responsiveness to subsequent treatment with GnRH but had no effect on sodium fluoride–stimulated LH release. Although the precise mechanism of sodium fluoride–stimulated LH release remains to be described, these studies support a role for a G protein in regulation of LH release by the releasing hormone.

Because a G protein appears to be activated after GnRH stimulation of the gonadotrope, a role for this moiety in GnRH-stimulated alterations in gonadotrope responsiveness was also assessed. A 3-h pretreatment of pituitary cell cultures with 10 mM NaF (a G-protein activator) resulted in decreased gonadotrope responsiveness to subsequent GnRH treatment (3 h, 100 nM; 34.3 ± 1.6% versus 23.4 ± 1.5% of total cellular LH). Sodium fluoride–provoked gonadotrope desensitization to GnRH also occurred in the presence of 3 mM EGTA and in cells that had been depleted of PKC. Desensitization to GnRH did not occur in response to pretreatment with dibutyryl cyclic adenosine monophosphate (dBcAMP; 8 h, 1 mM). Also, neither GnRH nor sodium fluoride stimulated IP accumulation above basal levels after the sodium fluoride pretreatment. Gonadotropin-releasing hormone receptor binding also decreased by 30% with sodium fluoride pretreatment. In contrast, 3-h sodium fluoride (10 mM) pretreatment enhanced responsiveness of the gonadotrope to the Ca^{2+} ionophore A23187 in a PKC- and cyclicAMP–dependent manner. Responsiveness to the phorbol ester PMA was also increased, whereas responsiveness to the Ca^{2+} channel activator maitotoxin was unchanged. These data suggest that G-protein activation by sodium fluoride provokes gonadotrope desensitization to GnRH stimulation by both decreasing receptor numbers and by uncoupling of the receptors from IP turnover. Also, a distinct G-protein action appears to be involved in sensitizing the gonadotrope to A23187 and PMA. Studies using cholera toxin and pertussis have provided additional support of the view that multiple G proteins are involved in GnRH action (89).

Inositol Phospholipids And Ca^{2+}-Mobilizing Signals

Interest in the relationship between Ca^{2+} mobilization and inositol phospholipid metabolism grew out of the work of Michell et al. (90), who proposed, based on previous studies by Hokin and Hokin (91) and others, that stimulated metabolism of inositol-containing phospholipids was involved in the gating (regulated entry) of Ca^{2+} in response to extracellular signals. This hypothesis provoked studies that linked GnRH to increased rates of metabolism of phosphatidic acid and phosphatidylinositol (92–94). The observation of rapid, Ca^{2+}-independent PLC-type hydrolysis of phosphatidylinositol 4,5-bisphosphate (PIP_2) (95), which constitutes only a small fraction of the total inositol phospholipid pool, led to the discovery that a product of this cleavage, inositol 1,4,5-trisphosphate (I-1,4,5-P_3), releases Ca^{2+} sequestered in a nonmitochondrial storage site (96). More recently, I-1,4,5-P_3 has been implicated as a regulator of Ca^{2+} gating at the plasma membrane (97).

In GnRH-stimulated gonadotropes, there is an increase in phospholipid metabolism (92,93), an accumulation of IPs (98,99), and an increase in the concentration of intracellular calcium (64).

Gonadotropin-releasing hormone–stimulated production of IPs has been measured in pituitary tissue slices (100) and in dispersed cells (98,101,102). Inositol phosphates produced include I-1,4,5-P_3 (99,103); this isomer has been reported to release Ca^{2+} from subcellular organelles derived from pituitary (104). In view of previous studies that have indicated the dependence of LH release on continual access to extracellular Ca^{2+} (105), it is unclear at present to what extent Ca^{2+} derived from intracellular sources contributes to Ca^{2+}-dependent LH release (68). Still, studies of perifused pituitary cells have shown that chelation of Ca^{2+} in the extracellular medium does not totally extinguish the earliest detectable release of LH after a pulse of GnRH but that conditions that deplete cellular Ca^{2+} (EGTA + ionophore A23187) do eliminate this early release (106). Taken together, these results oblige consideration of a potential role for IPs in gonadotrope Ca^{2+} mobilization.

To be considered a second messenger for GnRH-stimulated LH release, three requirements must be met: (a) Gonadotropin-releasing hormone should stimulate increased IP turnover; (b) IP turnover, stimulated by any means, should provoke LH release; (c) inhibition of IP turnover should block GnRH-stimulated LH release.

The first requirement has been fulfilled (92,107,108); GnRH does stimulate IP turnover. Although GTP analogs and sodium fluoride stimulate both IP turnover and LH release, this does not fulfill the second requisite because G-protein activation may provoke cellular effects in addition to IP turnover that could be responsible for LH release. The third criteria has not been demonstrated, and notably, one study (107) reported that the Ca^{2+} channel blocker D600 and the calmodulin antagonist pimozide decrease GnRH-stimulated LH release without inhibiting IP turnover. The results of that study call into question the relationship between GnRH-stimulated IP turnover and LH release.

To study the dependence of GnRH-stimulated LH release on IP turnover, this study used an inhibitor PLC activity, 1-[6-[[17β-3-methoxyestra-1,3,5(10)-triene-17-yl]amino]hexyl]-1H-pyrrole-dione (U-73122) and an inactive analog 1-[6[[17β-3-methoxyestra-1,3,5(10)-triene-17-yl]amino]hexyl]-2,5-pyrrolidine-dione (U-73343). U-73122 (10μM) decreased GnRH-provoked (1 μM, 45 min) IP accumulation from 873 ± 61 disintegrations per minute (dpm) to 365 ± 50 dpm (basal accumulation also was decreased from 420 ± 18 dpm to 207 ± 16 dpm), whereas LH release was not inhibited (30.2 ± 1.4% of cellular LH in control compared with 30.3 ± 1.1% in U-73122-pretreated cells). Gonadotropin-releasing hormone provoked increased IP_3 accumulation (123% of basal) after 15 sec of stimulation, IP_2 accumulation (131% of basal) after 30 sec, and IP_1 (121% of basal) after 1 min. Pretreatment with U-73122 blocked accumulation of IPs at these early timepoints. Sodium fluoride–stimulated IP accumulation was also inhibited by U-73122 (from 1,539 ± 132 dpm to 414 ± 21 dpm), whereas LH release increased from 22.9 ± 1.4% total cellular LH to 28.0 ± 2.2%. In contrast, GnRH- and sodium fluoride–stimulated IP accumulation were not significantly decreased in U-73343-pretreated cells (GnRH: 817 ± 43 dpm compared with 873 ± 61 dpm in control; sodium fluoride: 1133 ± 74 dpm compared with 1539 ± 132 dpm in control cells). Results of a perifusion study showed that U-73122 did not block the initial phase of GnRH-stimulated LH release or interfere with the development of desensitization to the releasing hormone. Also, GnRH-stimulated intracellular Ca^{2+} fluctuations were similar in magnitude and duration in U-73122-pretreated compared with U-73343-pretreated cells. These results (109) demonstrate that GnRH- as well as sodium fluoride–stimulated LH release can be uncoupled from IP turnover calling into question the role of IP_3 as a second messenger for GnRH-stimulated LH release.

U-73122 has been used to show that IP accumulation and gonadotrope desensitization can be uncoupled (110).

Diacylglycerols and Protein Kinase C

The identification of the properties of the enzyme PKC by Nishizuka has offered another means of interaction between Ca^{2+} and inositol phospholipids in stimulated gonadotropes. This enzyme is activated maximally in the presence of both Ca^{2+} and phospholipids; in the presence of *sn*-1,2-diacylglycerols, the enzyme becomes more sensitive to activation by Ca^{2+} (111). Thus, it has been postulated that both products of PIP_2 hydrolysis are second-messenger molecules: I-1,4,5-P_3 as a mobilizer of intracellular Ca^{2+}; and diacylglycerol, along with Ca^{2+}, as co-activators of PKC. The cellular responses to an extracellular signal, then, might be regulated by the coordinate actions of Ca^{2+}-dependent PKs and PKC (112).

The recognition that PKC serves as an intracellular "receptor" for the phorbol diester tumor promoters (113,114) and that phorbol esters could substitute for diacylglycerols as PKC activators (114) were important methodologic advances in the study of PKC. Thus, the ability of PMA to stimulate LH release (115,116) is believed to reflect activation of PKC and suggests that the action of GnRH may involve PKC activation. Also, the synthesis of cell-permeant diacylglycerols (117) permitted the establishment of a correlation between potencies for PKC activation *in vitro* and for stimulation of LH release from gonadotropes (118).

EVALUATION OF PROTEIN KINASE C AS A MEDIATOR OF LH RELEASE

Several main questions have formed the basis of studies directed toward consideration of the role of PKC in GnRH action: (a) Does activation of PKC mimic the effects of GnRH? (b) Does occupancy of the GnRH receptor by an agonist provoke activation of PKC? (c) What are the consequences of PKC inhibition on cellular events mediated by GnRH?

As described above, phorbol esters and synthetic diacylglycerols that activate PKC *in vitro* also stimulate release of LH, although with lower efficacy than GnRH itself. Luteinizing hormone release by PKC activators is largely insensitive to removal of extracellular Ca^{2+} (118,119) and to blockade of Ca^{2+} channels or inhibition of calmodulin and is synergistically enhanced in the presence of Ca^{2+} ionophores (120). These findings, then, initially suggested that activation of PKC could, under the conditions of elevated intracellular Ca^{2+} that follow GnRH treatment, mimic the LH-releasing action of GnRH.

The question of whether receptor occupancy by GnRH leads to the activation of gonadotrope PKC has been addressed by measuring endogenous production of likely PKC activators, by examining the cellular distribution of PKC activity after GnRH treatment, and by attempting to identify common phosphorylation substrates in GnRH- and phorbol ester–treated cells. Of these, the first approach has been the most fruitful. Andrews and Conn (108), in combined pulse- and equilibrium-labeling studies using an enriched population of gonadotropes, showed that GnRH rapidly produces in the mass of PIP_2 and increases in diacylglycerol, with subsequent resynthesis of phosphatidylinositol. These and other confirmatory studies (98) indicate that GnRH-stimulated phosphoinositide hydrolysis does not require measurable Ca^{2+} mobilization. The production of phosphoinositide-derived diacylglycerols also has been assessed indirectly by measuring production of IPs, as described above.

Agonist-stimulated redistribution of PKC activity from the cytosol to the phospholipid/diacylglycerol-rich particulate fraction in tissue homogenates provides another indication, albeit indirect, that PKC is activated in response to extracellular signals (121). Accordingly, GnRH receptor–mediated redistribution of pituitary PKC activity has been observed both in cell cultures (122) and *in vivo* (123,124). Because gonadotropes constitute only 5% to 20% of the total cell population in the pituitary and PKC appears to be present in virtually all secretory cell types, progress toward identifying PKC substrates specifically associated with GnRH action has been slow. The appearance of [^{32}P]-labeled pituitary proteins after phorbol ester treatment, however, has been reported (125–127), and phorbol esters and superactive analogs of GnRH stimulate similar patterns of protein phosphorylation in pituitary cell cultures. Although intriguing, the identification of these proteins has not been forthcoming.

Although gonadotropes do release LH in response to exogenous PKC activators and GnRH does appear to produce intracellular conditions appropriate for PKC activation, several lines of evidence suggest the dissociability of PKC activity and GnRH-stimulated LH release. The most straightforward are the observations that PKC activators stimulate LH release with less efficacy than GnRH itself (118,120) and that LH release in response to combinations of GnRH and PMA is additive in magnitude (107). This latter observation suggests that these agents may, in fact, be stimulating LH release from different pools.

The strongest evidence for dissociation of GnRH-stimulated LH release from PKC activation is derived from studies of PKC-depleted cells. In the absence of selective pharmacologic inhibitors of PKC, it has been possible to develop protocols for the phorbol ester–stimulated "down-regulation" of the enzyme. Exposure of pituitary cultures to 250 to 1,000 nM PMA for 24 h results in more than 95% loss of PKC, as assessed by enzyme activity, [^{3}H]phorbol dibutyrate binding, and immunoactivity (128). Protein kinase C depletion eliminates cellular responses to phorbol esters and diacylglycerols, including LH release and inhibition of GnRH-stimulated IP production, whereas LH release in response to Ca^{2+}-mobilizing stimuli (GnRH or ionophore A23187) is not inhibited (129). The central feature of this report, that PKC activation and LH release can be uncoupled, has been reported in three additional reports using different techniques (130–132). It appears, therefore, that PKC need not be present for manifestation of the LH-releasing effects of GnRH (133). A recent report described cells that were *partially* depleted of PKC. These authors (134) indicated such cells exhibit *partial* loss of responsiveness to the releasing hormone (135). Interpretation of these studies is complicated because the PKC depletion is marginal, and LH biosynthesis appears to be a significant feature of the response, because they were derived from sexually mature animals. In the studies of McArdle et al. (129), immature animals were used and have been characterized as having no biosynthetic component in release. This is especially significant because of the well-established role for LH gene expression as a PKC-dependent action of the releasing hormone (135).

EVALUATION OF PROTEIN KINASE C AS A MODULATOR OF GONADOTROPE RESPONSIVENESS

Besides stimulating the acute release of gonadotropins, GnRH regulates long-term maintenance of pituitary responsiveness to the hormone. Notably, the pulse pattern (duration and frequency) of GnRH administration to the pituitary is known to be a crucial determinant of gonadotropin release over periods of days to weeks. For example, delivery of GnRH agonists in a pulsatile fashion approximating normal hypothalamic GnRH release produces pulses of LH release of consistent magnitude (136). Thus, pulsatile exposure to GnRH is viewed as essential for maintenance of normal gonadotrope function (137). Constant exposure to GnRH and its agonists, however, results in a pituitary that is refractory to subsequent administration of the releasing hormone with respect to LH release (138). These relationships between exposure pattern and pituitary responsiveness have permitted GnRH agonists to be used clinically for either the restoration (139) or biochemical ablation of gonadotropin release.

Because considerable evidence is available to suggest that PKC is activated after GnRH treatment, the potential role of this enzyme in the modulation of gonadotrope responsiveness by GnRH has been investigated. These studies have focused on regulation of GnRH receptor number and affinity, receptor-effector coupling, and biosynthesis of gonadotropins.

GnRH Receptor Number and Affinity

Agonist occupancy of plasma membrane GnRH receptors is required to stimulate LH release; therefore, investigators have sought to identify a correlation between GnRH receptor number and gonadotrope responsiveness. Homologous down-regulation of receptors occurs after continuous treatment with high (above 1 nM) concentrations of GnRH (18,140) and is believed to involve physical internalization of agonist-occupied receptors (35). Homologous desensitization of gonadotropes, that is, a reduction in the ability of GnRH to elicit LH release after a prior exposure to GnRH, is likely to result, initially, from loss of cell surface receptors and is maintained by loss of a functional calcium channel (18). Other mechanisms of desensitization are evident, however, because measurable desensitization occurs even when receptor internalization is blocked (141), and a desensitized state is manifest even after GnRH receptor numbers have returned to control levels (18). Neither homologous receptor down-regulation nor desensitization appears to require PKC, because phorbol esters do not mimic the acute effects of GnRH on receptor number or responsiveness, and cells depleted of measurable PKC exhibit normal down-regulation and desensitization in response to GnRH (142).

Homologous up-regulation of GnRH receptors, detectable 8 to 24 h after exposure to low (10–100 pM) concentrations of GnRH, appears to require calcium and protein synthesis (18,143). Evidence is also available to suggest that GnRH stimulates the synthesis of its own receptor (50). It has been postulated that the pulsatility of GnRH exposure serves to maintain GnRH receptor levels (144) and that subtle increases in the intensity of GnRH exposure before the LH surge sensitizes the pituitary by increasing GnRH receptor number (Conn et al. 1983b). Homologous GnRH receptor up-regulation can be easily demonstrated in intact animals or explants of pituitary tissue, preparations that cannot be readily treated with activators of PKC; consequently, examination of the role of this enzyme in receptor up-regulation has been difficult. Nevertheless, it has been possible to detect increases in both GnRH receptor affinity (53) and number (53,145) after phorbol ester treatment. This effect of phorbol esters is selective for the agonist-occupied conformation of the receptor (53), suggesting that the actions of phorbol esters may be related to pathways normally activated by GnRH.

Further characterization of this phorbol ester effect has indicated that the apparent increase in receptor affinity likely results from a sequestration of agonist-occupied receptors. In time-course studies, ligand bound at 37°C in the presence of phorbol ester becomes relatively more resistant to displacement by competing ligand at 4°C but can be dissociated by a low pH wash at 4°C. Depletion of PKC activity (129) eliminates both the enhancement of agonist binding and the appearance of nondisplacable binding. Sequestration of receptors by PKC, however, does not appear to be equivalent to internalization provoked by GnRH alone, because the percentage of ligand that becomes nondisplacable in the absence of phorbol ester (25–30% at 23°C) is not altered by PKC depletion. Instead, we have the prejudice that the sequestration of GnRH receptors in the presence of phorbol esters may account for the uncoupling of agonist-occupied receptors from phosphoinositide hydrolysis (15,107). The synthetic rate of these receptors (time for 50% replacement = 25 ± 1 h) is close to that in the general pool (time for 50% replacement = 28 ± 2 h), an observation that suggests that they may be selected at random from that source (35).

Receptor–Effector Coupling

Desensitization of gonadotrope cells to GnRH cannot be explained solely by loss of surface receptors. Similarly, the sensitization or "self-priming" of gonadotropes (146,147) occurs within a time period insufficient for substantive receptor up-regulation. It is reasonable to conclude that postreceptor factors, such as the efficiency of receptor–effector coupling, rates of second-messenger turnover, or responsiveness to second messengers, may govern aspects of the self-priming action of GnRH and may be regulated by PKC. In the case of desensitization, early loss of responsiveness appears to be regulated by receptor loss and then maintained by loss of a functional receptor-coupled ion channel (59).

Pretreatment of superfused pituitary cell cultures with phorbol ester potentiates the LH-releasing effect of a subsequent dose of GnRH (148), indicating that PK activation can mimic the self-priming action of GnRH. Additional studies have shown that a PMA pretreatment produces a leftward shift in GnRH dose-response curves for LH release, whereas curves for receptor occupancy and IP production remain unchanged (149). The dose-response curves for secretogogues that increase intracellular Ca^{2+} (ionophore A23187 and maitotoxin) are also left-shifted, suggesting that cellular responsiveness to mobilized Ca^{2+} is enhanced by prior activation of PKC.

It is also possible that PKC enhances coupling of the GnRH receptor to the pathway(s) of Ca^{2+} mobilization. Such an effect is unlikely to involve IP generation, based on studies demonstrating that PKC activation inhibits the GnRH-stimulated production of IPs (107,150), including I-1,4,5-P_3. The mechanism of this inhibitory action on IP production remains unknown, but potential candidates involve phosphorylation of receptors (151), receptor-associated G proteins (85,152,153), or PLC (153). Other possible sites of PKC action in Ca^{2+}-mobilizing pathways, such as plasma membrane Ca^{2+} channels (154,155), remain to be investigated in gonadotropes.

Recently, involvement of ionized cytosolic calcium ($[Ca^{2+}]_i$) and PKC in GnRH-stimulated LH release was assessed by correlating measurable changes in $[Ca^{2+}]_i$ and LH release in PKC-depleted and nondepleted gonadotropes (156). Primary cultures of anterior pituitary cells were loaded with the calcium-sensitive fluorescent dye fura-2 and placed in a perifusion chamber. Gonadotropin-releasing hormone pulses were delivered to the cells, and changes in fura-2 fluorescence and LH release were determined. The level of $[Ca^{2+}]_i$ (assessed by fura-2) increased rapidly to a maximum within 20 to 40 sec followed by a slower decline over the next minute (spike phase) to a sustained intermediate value (plateau phase). Gonadotropin-releasing hormone–stimulated LH release was unaffected by loading cells with fura-2. Both LH release and changes in $[Ca^{2+}]_i$ were directly dependent on GnRH concentration. Pretreatment with the GnRH antagonist Antide (50 nM, [NAcD2Nal^1-DpClPhe^2-D3Pal^3-Ser^4-NicLys^5-DNicLys^6-Leu^7-iLys^8-Pro^9-DAla^{10}]NH_2) had no effect on basal $[Ca^{2+}]_i$ or on basal LH release but did block both GnRH-stimulated calcium mobilization and GnRH-stimulated LH release. Gonadotropin-releasing hormone pretreatment (3.5 nM, 10 min) blocked the calcium spike phase but not the plateau phase, occurring in response to a GnRH pulse (10 nM, 5 min) delivered immediately after pretreatment. Inhibition of the calcium spike phase was transient (recovery within 15 min) and was dependent on pretreatment concentrations of GnRH. Calcium spike phase inhibition by GnRH pretreatment prevented increased LH release from PKC-depleted cells in response to a subsequent pulse of GnRH but not from gonadotropes with normal levels of PKC. This suggests that initial LH release is dependent on changes in $[Ca^{2+}]_i$, but enhancement of LH release after periods of elevated GnRH concentrations may be dependent on PKC.

Gonadotropin Biosynthesis

The gonadotropins LH and FSH consist of two heterogeneous subunits, α and β. The α subunit is common between these and another pituitary hormone, thyrotropin (TSH).

The availability of radiolabeled oligonucleotide probes for gonadotropin α- and β-subunit mRNA has made it possible to investigate gonadotrope regulation of gene expression. Papavasiliou et al. (157) reported that messenger ribonucleic acids (mRNAs) for α and β LH subunits in intact pituitaries are increased twofold after 48 h of pulsatile exposure to GnRH. More recently, the ability of GnRH and phorbol esters to increase LH-β mRNA levels in cell cultures has been shown (135). Moreover, depletion of PKC activity inhibits the ability of GnRH to increase mRNA levels. Therefore, in contrast to GnRH-stimulated LH release, receptor down-regulation, and desensitization, the action of GnRH on LH mRNA levels appears to require PKC. It is not clear at present whether the rates of mRNA synthesis and degradation are both altered by activated PKC. The action of this enzyme on events at the transcriptional level has been implicated in a variety of systems (158,159) and is certainly consistent with the long-appreciated effects of phorbol esters on cellular differentiation and transformation (160).

Pulsatile exposure to GnRH also is viewed to be important for the maintenance of cellular LH pools (161). In this regard, GnRH has been reported to stimulate gonadotropin polypeptide biosynthesis (162) and glycosylation (163,164) in cell cultures, as measured by incorporation of labeled amino acids and monosaccharides into

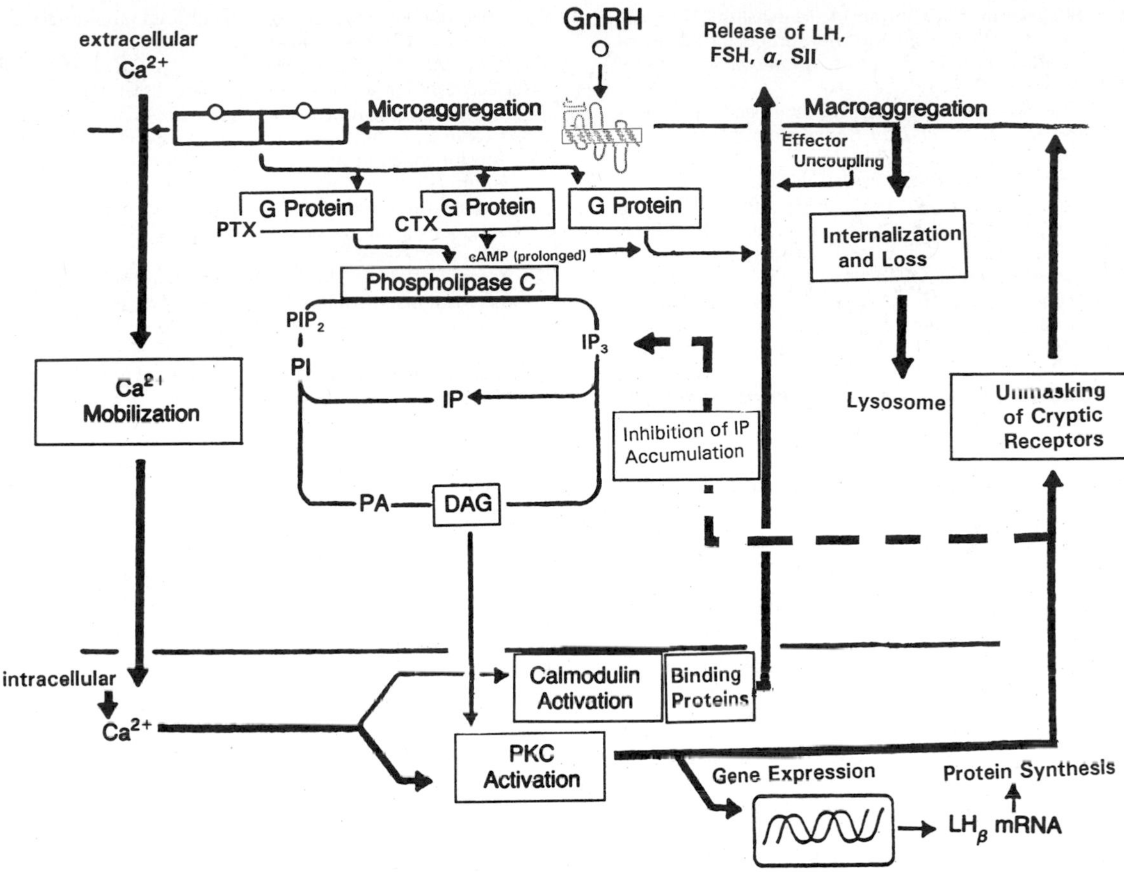

FIG. 1. Pathways of GnRH action. *PI,* phosphoinositide; *IP,* inositol phosphates; *DAG,* diacylglycerol.

immunoreactive LH. Similarly, activators of PKC have been found to increase the rates of LH polypeptide biosynthesis (165) and glycosylation (166). It is not known whether these increases reflect an effect of PKC at the translational level (167) or are secondary to increases in gonadotropin mRNA levels, nor has it been determined whether PKC is required for the stimulation of gonadotropin biosynthesis by GnRH.

CONCLUSIONS

The relationships between Ca^{2+}-calmodulin- and PKC-dependent pathways of GnRH action presented in this chapter are summarized in Fig. 1. Recognition of the pulsatile nature of pituitary exposure to GnRH has underscored the importance of distinguishing between the acute (LH-releasing) and the chronic (responsiveness-regulating) effects of the hormone. The physiologic activation of PKC may result in the phosphorylation of a restricted group of proteins that function in the long-term maintenance of gonadotropin and GnRH receptor levels. However, given that LH release in response to Ca^{2+}-mobilizing stimuli proceeds in PKC-depleted cells, the ability of PKC activators to stimulate LH release raises the possibility that common substrates may exist for Ca^{2+}-calmodulin-dependent PKs and PKC. These proteins might be phosphorylated by PKC only when the enzyme is activated pharmacologically by phorbol esters or synthetic diacylglycerols. More precise description of the biologic actions of PKC will follow from the development of specific, cell-permeating enzyme inhibitors, further characterization of kinase isoforms (168), and elucidation of transcriptional factors modulated by PKC (169).

ACKNOWLEDGMENTS

Studies conducted in our laboratory were supported by NIH HD19899. We thank Ms. Sue Birely for preparing the manuscript.

REFERENCES

1. Hsueh A J-W, Jones PBC. Extrapituitary actions of gonadotropin-releasing hormone. *Endocr Rev* 1981;2:437–461.
2. Ziporyn T. LHRH: clinical applications growing. *JAMA* 1985;253:469–476.
3. Conn PM, Crowley WF. Gonadotropin-releasing hormone and its analogues. *N Engl J Med* 1991;324:93–103.

4. Clayton RN, Shakespear RA, Duncan JA, Marshall JC. Radioiodinated nondegradable GnRH analogs: new probes for the investigation of pituitary GnRH receptors. *Endocrinology* 1979; 105:1369–1376.
5. Clayton RN. Preparation of radiolabeled neuroendocrine peptides. In: Conn PM, ed. *Methods in Enzymology*. Orlando, FL: Academic Press, 1983;32–48.
6. Marian J, Cooper R, Conn PM. Regulation of the rat pituitary GnRH-receptor. *Mol Pharmacol* 1981;19:339–405.
7. Savoy-Moore RT, Schwartz NB, Duncan JA, Marshall JC. Pituitary gonadotropin-releasing hormone receptors during the rat estrous cycle. *Science* 1980;209:942–944.
8. Clayton RN, Solano AR, Garcia-Vila A, Dufau ML, Catt KJ. Regulation of pituitary receptors for gonadotropin releasing hormone during the rat estrous cycle. *Endocrinology* 1980;107: 699–706.
9. Conn PM, Venter JC. Radiation inactivation (target size analysis) of the gonadotropin releasing hormone receptor: evidence for a high molecular weight complex. *Endocrinology* 1985;116: 1324–1326.
10. Hazum E. Photoaffinity labeling in neuroendocrine tissues. *Methods Enzymol* 1983;103:58–71.
11. Hazum E, Keinan D. Gonadotropin releasing hormone receptors: photoaffinity labeling with an antagonist. *Biochem Biophys Res Commun* 1983;100:116–123.
12. Hazum E. Photoaffinity labeling of peptide hormone receptors. *Endocr Rev* 1983;4:352–362.
13. Hazum E, Keinan D. Photoaffinity labeling of pituitary gonadotropin releasing hormone receptors during the rat estrous cycle. *Biochem Biophys Commun* 1982;107:695–698.
14. Hazum E, Keinan D. Characterization of GnRH receptors in bovine pituitary membranes. *Mol Cell Endocrinol* 1982;35: 107–111.
15. Huckle WR, Hawes BE, Conn PM. Protein kinase C-mediated gonadotropin-releasing hormone receptor sequestration is associated with uncoupling of phosphoinositide hydrolysis. *J Biol Chem* 1989;15:8619–8626.
16. Tsutsumi M, Zhou W, Millar RP, et al. Cloning and functional expression of a mouse gonadotropin-releasing hormone receptor. *Mol Endocrinol* 1992;6:1163–1169.
17. Marian J, Conn PM. Subcellular localization of the receptor for gonadotropin-releasing hormone in pituitary and ovarian tissue. *Endocrinology* 1983;112:104–112.
18. Conn PM, Rogers DC, Seay SG. Structure–function relationships of calcium ion channel antagonists at the pituitary gonadotrope. *Endocrinology* 1983;113:1592–1595.
19. Adams TE, Spies HG. Binding characteristics of gonadotropin-releasing hormone receptors throughout the estrous cycle of the hamster. *Endocrinology* 1981;108:2245–2253.
20. Crowder ME, Nett TM. Pituitary content of gonadotropins and receptors for gonadotropin-releasing hormone (GnRH) and hypothalamic content of GnRH during the preovulatory period of the ewe. *Endocrinology* 1984;114:234–239.
21. Nett TM, Cermak D, Braden T, Manns J, Niswender GD. Pituitary receptors for GnRH and estradiol, and pituitary content of gonadotropins in beef cows. I. Changes during the estrous cycle. *Dom Anim Endocrinol* 1987;4:123–132.
22. Conn PM, Rogers DC, Seay SG. Biphasic regulation of the gonadotropin-releasing hormone receptor by receptor microaggregation and intracellular calcium levels. *Mol Pharmacol* 1984;25:51–55.
23. Young LS, Naik SI, Clayton RN. Adenosine 3′,5′-monophosphate derivatives increase gonadotropin-releasing hormone receptors in cultured pituitary cells. *Endocrinology* 1984; 114:2113–2122.
24. Young LS, Naik SI, Clayton RN. Increased gonadotrophin releasing hormone receptors on pituitary gonadotrophs: effect on subsequent LH secretion. *Mol Cell Endocrinol* 1985;41:69–78.
25. Young LS, Naik SI, Clayton RN. Pituitary gonadotrophin-releasing hormone receptor up-regulation *in vitro:* dependence on calcium and microtubule function. *J Endocrinol* 1985;107: 49–56.
26. Naor Z, Clayton RN, Catt KJ. Characterization of gonadotropin-releasing hormone receptors in cultured rat pituitary cells. *Endocrinology* 1980;10:1144–1152.
27. Wise ME, Nieman D, Stewart J, Nett TM. Effect of number of receptors for gonadotropin-releasing hormone on the release of luteinizing hormone. *Biol Reprod* 1984;31:1007–1013.
28. Clarke IJ, Cummins JT, Crowder ME, Nett TM. Pituitary receptors for gonadotropin-releasing hormone in relation to changes in pituitary and plasma gonadotropins in ovariectomized hypothalamo/pituitary-disconnected ewes. II. A marked rise in receptor number during the acute feedback effects of estradiol. *Biol Reprod* 1988;39:349–354.
29. Gregg DW, Nett TM. Direct effects of estradiol-17β on the number of gonadotropin-releasing hormone receptors in the ovine pituitary. *Biol Reprod* 1989;40:288–293.
30. Laws SC, Beggs MJ, Webster JC, Miller WL. Inhibin increases and progesterone decreases receptors for gonadotropin-releasing hormone in ovine pituitary culture. *Endocrinology* 1990;127: 373–380.
31. Laws SC, Webster JC, Miller WL. Estradiol alters the effectiveness of gonadotropin-releasing hormone (GnRH) in ovine pituitary cultures: GnRH receptors versus responsiveness to GnRH. *Endocrinology* 1990;127:381–386.
32. Wang QF, Farnworth PG, Findlay JK, Burger HG. Effect of 31K bovine inhibin on the specific binding of gonadotropin-releasing hormone to rat anterior pituitary cells in culture. *Endocrinology* 1988;123:2161–2166.
33. Wang QF, Farnworth PG, Findlay JK, Burger HG. Inhibitory effect of pure 31-kilodalton bovine inhibin on gonadotropin-releasing hormone (GnRH)-induced up-regulation of GnRH binding sites in cultured rat anterior pituitary cells. *Endocrinology* 1989;124:363–368.
34. Braden TD, Farnworth PG, Burger HG, Conn PM. Regulation of the synthetic rate of gonadotropin-releasing hormone receptors in rat pituitary cell cultures by inhibin. *Endocrinology* 1990;127:2387–2392.
35. Braden TD, Hawes BE, Conn PM. Synthesis of GnRH receptors by gonadotrope cell cultures: both preexisting receptors and those unmasked by protein kinase C activators show a similar synthetic rate. *Endocrinology* 1989;127:1623–1629.
36. Hazum E, Cuatrecasas PP, Marian J, Conn PM. Receptor-mediated internalization of fluorescent gonadotropin-releasing hormone by pituitary gonadotropes. *Proc Natl Acad Sci USA* 1980;77:6692–6695.
37. Jennes L, Stumpf WE, Conn PM. Intracellular pathways of electron opaque GnRH-derivatives bound by cultured gonadotropes. *Endocrinology* 1983;113:1683–1689.
38. Jennes L, Stumpf WE, Conn PM. Receptor-mediated binding and uptake of GnRH agonist and antagonist in cultured pituitary cells. *Peptides* 1984;5:215–220.
39. Badr M, Pelletier G. Autoradiographic study of binding and internalization of a luteinizing hormone-releasing hormone antagonist [D-Nal1, D-Cpa2, A-D-Trp3, D-Arg6, D-Ala10]LHRH by rat pituitary gonadotrophs. *J Neuroendocrinol* 1989;1:141–146.
40. Jennes L, Coy D, Conn PM. Receptor-mediated uptake of GnRH agonist and antagonists by cultured gonadotropes: evidence for differential intracellular routing. *Peptides* 1986;7:459–463.
41. Conn PM, Marian J, McMillian M, et al. Gonadotropin releasing hormone action in the pituitary: a three step mechanism. *Endocr Rev* 1981;2:174–185.
42. Conn PM, Hazum E. LH release and GnRH-receptor internalization: independent actions of GnRH. *Endocrinology* 1981;109: 2040–2045.
43. Conn PM, Rogers DC, Sheffield T. Inhibition of gonadotropin releasing hormone stimulated luteinizing hormone release by pimozide: evidence for a site of action after calcium mobilization. *Endocrinology* 1981;109:1122–1126.
44. Conn PM, Rogers DC, McNeil R. Potency enhancement of a GnRH agonist: GnRH-receptor microaggregation stimulates gonadotropin release. *Endocrinology* 1982;111:335–337.
45. Conn PM. Ligand dimerization: a technique for assessing receptor–receptor interactions. In: Conn PM, ed. *Methods in Enzymology*. Orlando, FL: Academic Press, 1983;49–58.
46. Conn PM, Rogers DC, Stewart JM, Neidel J, Sheffield T. Conver-

sion of a gonadotropin releasing hormone antagonist to an agonist. *Nature* 1982;296:653–655.
47. Blum JJ, Conn PM. Gonadotropin releasing hormone stimulation of luteinizing hormone: a ligand-receptor-effect model for receptor mediated responses. *Proc Natl Acad Sci USA* 1982;79:7307–7311.
48. Leiser J, Conn PM, Blum JJ. Interpretation of dose-response curves for luteinizing hormone release by GnRH, related peptides, and leukotriene C4 according to a hormone/receptor/effector model. *Proc Natl Acad Sci USA* 1986;83:5963–5967.
49. Conn PM, Rogers DC, Seay SG, Staley D. Activation of luteinizing hormone release from pituitary cells by polycations. *Endocrinology* 1984;115:1913–1917.
50. Braden TD, Conn PM. Altered rate of synthesis of gonadotropin-releasing hormone receptors: effects of homologous hormone appear independent of extracellular calcium. *Endocrinology* 1990;126:2577–2582.
51. Braden TD, Bervig T, Conn PM. Protein kinase C (PKC) activation stimulates synthesis of gonadotropin-releasing hormone (GnRH) receptors but does not mediate GnRH-stimulated receptor synthesis. *Endocrinology* 1991;129:2486–2490.
52. Braden TD, Conn PM. Activin-A stimulates the synthesis of gonadotropin-releasing hormone receptors. *Endocrinology* 1992;130:2101–2105.
53. Huckle WR, McArdle CA, Conn PM. Differential sensitivity of gonadotropin-releasing hormone receptors to activators of protein kinase C, a marker for receptor activation. *J Biol Chem* 1988;263:3296–3302.
54. Samli MH, Geschwind II. Some effects of energy transfer inhibitors and of Ca^{2+}-free and K^{+}-enhanced media on the release of LH from the rat pituitary gland *in vitro*. *Endocrinology* 1968;82:225–231.
55. Conn PM, Kilpatrick D, Kirshner N. Ionophoretic Ca^{2+} mobilization in rat gonadotropes and bovine adrenomedullary cells. *Cell Calcium* 1980;1:129–133.
56. Conn PM, Huckle WR, Andrews WV, McArdle CA. The molecular mechanism of action of gonadotropin releasing hormone (GnRH) in the pituitary. *Recent Prog Horm Res* 1987;43:29–68.
57. Conn PM, Marian J, McMillian M, Rogers D. Evidence for calcium mediation of gonadotropin releasing hormone action in the pituitary. *Cell Calcium* 1980;1:7–20.
58. Conn PM, Rogers DC. Gonadotropin release from pituitary cultures following activation of endogenous ion channels. *Endocrinology* 1980;107:2133–2134.
59. Conn PM. Use of specific ion channel activating and inhibiting drugs in neuroendocrine tissue. In: Conn PM, ed. *Methods in Enzymology.* Orlando, FL: Academic Press, 1983;401–405.
60. Conn PM, Staley DD, Yasumoto T, Huckle WR, Janovick J. Homologous desensitization with gonadotropin-releasing hormone (GnRH) also diminishes gonadotropin responsiveness to maitotoxin: a role for the GnRH receptor-regulated calcium ion channel in mediation of cellular desensitization. *Mol Endocrinol* 1987;1:154–159.
61. Conn PM, Rogers DC, Sandhu FS. Alteration of intracellular calcium level stimulates gonadotropin release from cultured rat pituitary cells. *Endocrinology* 1979;105:1122–1127.
62. Marian J, Conn PM. Gonadotropin releasing hormone stimulation of cultured pituitary cells requires calcium. *Mol Pharmacol* 1979;16:196–201.
63. Williams JA. Stimulation of 45 Ca^{2+} efflux from rat pituitary by LHRH and other pituitary stimulators. *J Physiol* 1976;260: 105–115.
64. Clapper DL, Conn PM. Gonadotropin-releasing hormone stimulation of pituitary gonadotrope cells produces an increase in intracellular calcium. *Biol Reprod* 1985;32:269–278.
65. Leong DA, Beshoar DF, Sullivan JA, Mandell GL, Thorner MO. Changes in intracellular free [Ca^{2+}] measured directly in individual LH secretory cells stimulated with LHRH. *Endocrinology* 1986;118(suppl.):40.
66. Chang JP, McCoy EE, Graeter J, Tasaka K, Catt KJ. Participation of voltage-dependent calcium channels in the action of gonadotropin-releasing hormone. *J Biol Chem* 1986;261: 9105–9108.
67. McArdle CA, Bunting R, Mason WT. Dynamic video imaging of cystolic Ca^{2+} in the αT3-1, gonadotrope-derived cell line. *Mol Cell Neurosci* 1992;3:124–132.
68. Hopkins CR, Walker AM. Calcium as a second messenger in the stimulation of luteinizing hormone secretion. *Mol Cell Endocrinol* 1978;12:189–208.
69. Conn PM, Bates MD, Rogers DC, Seay SG, Smith WA. GnRH-receptor-effector-response coupling in the pituitary gonadotrope: a Ca^{2+} mediated system. In: Fotherby K, Pal SB, eds. *Role of Drugs and Electrolytes in Hormonogenesis.* New York: Walter de Gruyter and Company, 1983;85–103.
70. Barbarino A, DeMarinis L. Calcium antagonists and hormone release. II. Effects of verapamil on basal, gonadotropin-releasing hormone induced pituitary hormone release in normal subjects. *J Clin Endocrinol Metab* 1980;51:749–753.
71. Veldhuis JD, Borges JLC, Drake CR, Rogol AD, Kaiser DL, Thorner MO. Divergent influences of the structurally dissimilar calcium entry blockers, diltiazem and verapamil, on thyrotropin- and gonadotropin-releasing hormone-stimulated anterior pituitary hormone secretion in man. *J Clin Endocrinol Metab* 1985;60:144–149.
72. Mason WT, Waring DW. Patch clamp recordings of single ion channel activation by gonadotropin-releasing hormone in ovine pituitary gonadotrophs. *Neuroendocrinology* 1986;43:205–219.
73. Chafouleas JG, Guerriero V, Means AR. Possible regulatory roles of calmodulin and myosin light chain kinase in secretion. In: Conn, PM, ed. *Cellular Regulation of Secretion and Release.* New York: Academic Press, 1982;445–458.
74. Jennes L, Bronson D, Stumpf WE, Conn PM. Evidence for an association between calmodulin and membrane patches containing gonadotropin-releasing hormone-receptor complexes in cultured gonadotropes. *Cell Tissue Res* 1985;239:311–315.
75. Conn PM, Chafouleas J, Rogers D, Means AR. Gonadotropin releasing hormone stimulates calmodulin redistribution in the rat pituitary. *Nature* 1981;292:264–265.
76. Hart RC, Bates MD, Cormier MJ, Rosen GM, Conn PM. Synthesis and characterization of calmodulin antagonistic drugs. In: Means AR, O'Malley BW, eds. *Methods in Enzymology.* Orlando, FL: Academic Press, 1983;195–204.
77. Wooge CH, Conn PM. Characterization of calmodulin-binding components in the pituitary gonadotrope. *Mol Cell Endocrinol* 1988;56:41–51.
78. Natarajan K, Ness J, Wooge C, Janovick J, Conn PM. Specific identification and subcellular localization of three calmodulin-binding proteins in the rat gonadotrope: spectrin, caldesmon and calcineurin. *Biol Reprod* 1991;44:43–52.
79. Janovick JA, Natarajan K, Longo F, Conn PM. Caldesmon: a bifunctional (calmodulin and actin) binding protein which regulates stimulated gonadotropin release. *Endocrinology* 1991;129: 68–74.
80. Cantau B, Keppens S, Dewulf HD, Jard S. [^{3}H]Vasopressin binding to isolated rat hepatocytes and liver membranes: regulation by GTP and relation to glycogen-phosphorylase activation. *J Recept Res* 1980;1:137–168.
81. Gilman AG. G proteins: transducers of receptor-generated signals. *Annu Rev Biochem* 1987;56:615–649.
82. Birnbaumer L, Codina J, Mattera R, et al. Signal transduction by G proteins. *Kidney Int* 1987;32:S14–S37.
83. Cockcroft S. Polyphosphoinositide phosphodiesterase: regulation by a novel guanine nucleotide binding protein, Gp. *TIBS* 1987;12:75–78.
84. Fain JN, Wallace MA, Wojcikiewicz RJH. Evidence for involvement of guanine nucleotide-binding regulatory proteins in the activation of phospholipases by hormones. *FASEB J* 1988;2: 2569–2574.
85. Andrews WV, Staley DD, Huckle WR, Conn PM. Stimulation of luteinizing hormone (LH) release and phospholipid breakdown by guanosine triphosphate in permeabilized pituitary gonadotropes: antagonist action suggests association of a G protein and gonadotropin-releasing hormone receptor. *Endocrinology* 1986; 119:2537–2546.
86. Martin TFJ, Lucas DO, Bajjalieh SM, Kowalchyk JA. Thyrotropin-releasing hormone activates a Ca^{2+}-dependent polyphos-

phoinositide phosphodiesterase in permeable GH_3 cells. GTP-gamma S potentiation by a cholera and pertussis toxin-insensitive mechanism. *J Biol Chem* 1986;261:2918–2927.
87. Perrin MH, Haas Y, Porter J, Rivier J, Vale W. The gonadotropin-releasing hormone pituitary receptor interacts with a guanosine triphosphate-binding protein: differential effects of guanyl nucleotides on agonist and antagonist binding. *Endocrinology* 1989;124:798–804.
88. Hawes BE, Conn PM. Sodium fluoride provokes gonadotrope desensitization to GnRH and gonadotrope sensitization to A23187: evidence for multiple G proteins in GnRH action. *Endocrinology* 1992;130:2465–2475.
89. Hawes BE, Barnes S, Conn PM. Cholera toxin and pertussis toxin provoke differential effects on LH release, inositol phosphate production, and GnRH receptor binding in the gonadotrope: evidence for multiple G proteins in gonadotropin-releasing hormone action. *Endocrinology* 1993;132:2124–2130.
90. Michell RH, Jafferji SS, Jones LM. The possible involvement of phosphotidylinositol breakdown in the mechanism of stimulus-response coupling at receptors which control cell-surface calcium gates. In: Bazan NG, ed. *Function and Biosynthesis of Lipids.* New York: Plenum Press, 1977;447–464.
91. Hokin MR, Hokin LE. Enzyme secretion and the incorporation of P32 into phospholipids of pancreas slices. *J Biol Chem* 1953;203:967–977.
92. Snyder GD, Bleasdale JE. Effect of LHRH on incorporation of 32P-orthophosphate into phosphatidylinositol by dispersed anterior pituitary cells. *Mol Cell Endocrinol* 1982;28:55–63.
93. Raymond V, Leung PCK, Veilleux R, Lefevre G, Labrie F. LHRH rapidly stimulates phosphatidylinositol metabolism in enriched gonadotrophs. *Mol Cell Endocrinol* 1984;36:157–164.
94. Kiesel L, Catt KJ. Phosphatidic acid and the calcium-dependent actions of gonadotropin-releasing hormone in pituitary gonadotrophs. *Arch Biochem Biophys* 1984;231:202–210.
95. Downes CP, Wusterman MM. Breakdown of polyphosphoinositides and not phosphatidylinositol accounts for muscarinic agonist-stimulated inositol phospholipid metabolism in rat parotid glands. *Biochem J* 1983;216:633–640.
96. Streb H, Irvine RF, Berridge MJ, Schulz I. Release of Ca^{2+} from a non-mitochondrial intracellular store in pancreatic acinar cells by inositol-1,4,5-trisphosphate. *Nature* 1983;306:67–69.
97. Kuno M, Gardner P. Ion channels activated by inositol 1,4,5-trisphosphate in plasma membranes of T-lymphocytes. *Nature* 1987;326:301–304.
98. Naor Z, Azrad A, Limor R, Zakut H, Lotan M. Gonadotropin-releasing hormone activates a rapid Ca^{2+}-independent phosphodiester hydrolysis of polyphosphoinositides in pituitary gonadotrophs. *J Biol Chem* 1986;261:12506–12512.
99. Morgan RO, Chang JP, Catt KJ. Novel aspects of gonadotropin-releasing hormone action on inositol polyphosphate metabolism in cultured pituitary gonadotrophs. *J Biol Chem* 1987;262: 1166–1171.
100. Schrey MP. Gonadotropin releasing hormone stimulates the formation of inositol phosphates in rat anterior pituitary tissue. *Biochem J* 1985;226:563–569.
101. Huckle WR, Conn PM. The relationship between gonadotropin releasing hormone-stimulated luteinizing hormone release and inositol phosphate production: Studies with calcium antagonists and protein kinase C activators. *Endocrinology* 1987;120: 160–169.
102. Kiesel L, Bertges K, Rabe T, Rennebaum B. Gonadotropin releasing hormone enhances polyphosphoiniositide hydrolysis in rat pituitary cells. *Biochem Biophys Res Commun* 1986;134: 861–867.
103. Huckle WR, Conn PM. Molecular mechanism of gonadotropin releasing hormone action. II. The effector system. *Endocr Rev* 1988;9:387–395.
104. Guillemette G, Balla T, Baukal AJ, Catt KJ. Inositol 1,4,5-trisphosphate binds to a specific receptor and releases microsomal calcium in the anterior pituitary gland. *Proc Natl Acad Sci USA* 1987;84:195–199.
105. Bates MD, Conn PM. Calcium mobilization in the pituitary gonadotrope: relative roles of intra- and extracellular sources. *Endocrinology* 1984;115:1380–1385.
106. Hansen JR, McArdle CA, Conn PM. Relative roles of calium derived from intra- and extracellular sources in dynamic luteinizing hormone release from perifused pituitary cells. *Mol Endocrinol* 1987;1:808–815.
107. Huckle WR, Conn PM. The relationship between gonadotropin-releasing hormone-stimulated luteinizing hormone release and inositol phosphate production: studies with calcium antagonists and protein kinase C activators. *Endocrinology* 1987;120: 160–169.
108. Andrews WV, Conn PM. Gonadotropin-releasing hormone stimulates mass changes in phosphoinositides and diacylglycerol accumulation in purified gonadotrope cell cultures. *Endocrinology* 1986;118:1148–1158.
109. Hawes BE, Waters SB, Janovick JA, Bleasdale JE, Conn PM. Gonadotropin-releasing hormone-stimulated intracellular Ca^{2+} fluctuations and luteinizing hormone release can be uncoupled from inositol phosphate production. *Endocrinology* 1992;130: 3475–3483.
110. Hawes BE, Conn PM. Development of gonadotrope desensitization to gonadotropin-releasing hormone and recovery are not coupled to inositol phosphate production or GnRH receptor number. *Endocrinology* 1992;131:2681–2689.
111. Kishimoto A, Takai Y, Mori T, Kikkawa U, Nishizuka Y. Activation of calcium and phospholipid-dependent protein kinase by diacylglycerol, its possible relation to phosphatidylinositol turnover. *J Biol Chem* 1980;255:2272–2276.
112. Berridge MJ. Inositol trisphosphate and diacylglycerol: two interacting second messengers. *Annu Rev Biochem* 1986;56:159–193.
113. Niedel JE, Kuhn LJ, Vandenbar GR. Phorbol diester receptor copurifies with protein kinase C. *Proc Natl Acad Sci USA* 1983;80:36–40.
114. Sharkey NA, Blumberg PM. Kinetic evidence that 1,2-diolein inhibits phorbol ester binding to protein kinase C via a competitive mechanism. *Biochem Biophys Res Commun* 1985;133:1051.
115. Smith MA, Vale WW. Superfusion of rat anterior pituitary cells attached to cytodex beads: validation of a technique. *Endocrinology* 1980;107:1425–1431.
116. Smith WA, Conn PM. Microaggregation of the gonadotropin-releasing hormone receptor, relation to gonadotrope desensitization. *Endocrinology* 1984;114:553–559.
117. Conn PM, Ganong BR, Ebeling J, Staley D, Neidel JE, Bell RM. Synthesis and use of diacylglycerol as activators of protein kinase C in neuroendocrine tissue. In: Conn PM, ed. *Methods in Enzymology.* Orlando, FL: Academic Press, 1986;83–87.
118. Conn PM, Ganong BR, Ebeling J, Staley D, Neidel JE, Bell RM. Diacylglycerols release LH: structure-activity relations reveal a role for protein kinase C. *Biochem Biophys Res Commun* 1985;126:532–539.
119. Naor Z, Eli Y. Synergistic stimulation of luteinizing hormone (LH) release by protein kinase C activators and Ca^{2+}-ionophore. *Biochem Biophys Res Commun* 1985;130:848–853.
120. Harris CE, Staley D, Conn PM. Diacylglycerols and protein kinase C, potential amplifying mechanism for Ca^{2+}-mediated gonadotropin-releasing hormone-stimulated luteinizing hormone release. *Mol Pharmacol* 1985;27:532–536.
121. Kraft AS, Anderson WB. Phorbol esters increase the amount of Ca^{2+}, phospholipid-dependent protein kinase associated with plasma membrane. *Nature* 1983;301:621–623.
122. Hirota K, Hirota T, Aguilera G, Catt K. Hormone-induced redistribution of calcium-activated phospholipid-dependent protein kinase in pituitary gonadotrophs. *J Biol Chem* 1985;260: 3243–3246.
123. Naor Z, Zer J, Zakut H, Hermon J. Characterization of pituitary calcium-activated, phospholipid-dependent protein kinase: redistribution by gonadotropin-releasing hormone. *Proc Natl Acad Sci USA* 1985;82:8203–8207.
124. McArdle CA, Conn PM. Hormone-stimulated redistribution of gonadotrope protein kinase C *in vivo,* dependence on Ca^{2+} influx. *Mol Pharmacol* 1986;29:570–576.
125. Turgeon JL, Ashcroft SJH, Waring DW, Milewski MA, Walsh DA. Characteristics of the adenohypophyseal Ca^{2+}-phospholipid dependent protein kinase. *Mol Cell Endocrinol* 1984;34: 107–112.
126. Turgeon JL, Cooper RH. Protein kinase C and an endogenous

substrate associated with adenohypophyseal secretory granules. *Biochem J* 1986;237:53–61.

127. Strulovici B, Tahilramani R, Nestor JJ. Phosphorylation substrates for protein kinase C in intact pituitary cells: characterization of a receptor-mediated event using novel gonadotropin-releasing hormone analogues. *Biochemistry* 1987;26:6005–6011.
128. McArdle CA, Conn PM. The use of protein kinase C-depleted cells for investigation of the role of protein kinase C in stimulus-response coupling in the pituitary. In: Conn PM, ed. *Methods in Enzymology*. New York: Academic Press, 1988;287–301.
129. McArdle CA, Huckle WR, Conn PM. Phorbol esters reduce gonadotrope responsiveness to protein kinase C activators but not to Ca^{2+}-mobilizing secretagogues, does protein kinase C mediate gonadotropin-releasing hormone action? *J Biol Chem* 1987; 262:5028–5035.
130. Beggs MJ, Miller WL. Gonadotropin-releasing hormone-stimulated luteinizing hormone (LH) release from ovine gonadotrophs in culture is separate from phorbol ester-stimulated LH release. *Endocrinology* 1989;124:667–674.
131. Johnson MS, Mitchell R, Fink G. The role of protein kinase C in LHRH-induced LH and FSH release and LHRH self-priming in rat anterior pituitary glands *in vitro*. *J Endocrinol* 1988;116: 231–239.
132. Andrews WV, Hansen JR, Janovick JA, Conn PM. Gonadotropin-releasing hormone modulation of protein kinase C activity in perifused anterior pituitary cell cultures. *Endocrinology* 1986;127:2392–2399.
133. Conn PM. Does protein kinase C mediate pituitary actions of GnRH? *Mol Endocrinol* 1989;3:755–756.
134. Stojikovic SS, Chang JP, Ngo D, Catt KJ. Evidence for a role of protein kinase C in luteinizing hormone synthesis and secretion. *J Biol Chem* 1988;263:17307–17311.
135. Andrews WV, Maurer RA, Conn PM. Stimulation of rat luteinizing hormone-β messenger RNA levels by gonadotropin releasing hormone: apparent role for protein kinase C. *J Biol Chem* 1988;263:13755–13761.
136. Belchetz PE, Plant TM, Nakai Y, Keogh EG, Knobil E. Hypophysial responses to continuous and intermittent delivery of hypothalamic gonadotropin-releasing hormone. *Science* 1978;202: 631–633.
137. Marshall JC, Kelch RP. Gonadotropin-releasing hormone: role of pulsatile secretion in the regulation of reproduction. *N Engl J Med* 1986;315:1459–1468.
138. deKoning J, vanDieten JAMJ, vanRees GP. Refractoriness of the pituitary gland after continuous exposure to luteinizing hormone-releasing hormone. *J Endocrinol* 1978;79:311–318.
139. Hoffman AR, Crowley WF. Induction of puberty in men by long-term pulsatile administration of low-dose gonadotropin-releasing hormone. *N Engl J Med* 1982;307:1237–1241.
140. Zilberstein M, Zakut H, Naor Z. Coincidence of down-regulation and desensitization in pituitary gonadotrophs stimulated with gonadotropin releasing hormone. *Life Sci* 1983;32:663–669.
141. Gorospe WC, Conn PM. Agents that decrease gonadotropin-releasing hormone (GnRH) receptor internalization do not inhibit GnRH-mediated gonadotrope desensitization. *Endocrinology* 1987;120:222–229.
142. McArdle CA, Gorospe WC, Huckle WR, Conn PM. Homologous down-regulation of gonadotropin-releasing hormone receptors and desensitization of gonadotropes: lack of dependence on protein kinase C. *Mol Endocrinol* 1987;1:420–429.
143. Loumaye E, Catt KJ. Agonist-induced regulation of pituitary receptors for gonadotropin-releasing hormone. *J Biol Chem* 1983;258:12002–12009.
144. Katt JA, Duncan JC, Herban L, Barkan A, Marshall JC. The frequency of gonadotropin-releasing hormone stimulation determines the number of pituitary gonadotropin-releasing hormone receptors. *Endocrinology* 1985;116:2113–2115.
145. Naor Z, Schvartz I, Hazum E, Azrad A, Hermon J. Effect of phorbol ester on stimulus-secretion coupling mechanisms in gonadotropin releasing hormone-stimulated pituitary gonadotrophs. *Biochem Biophys Res Commun* 1987;148:1312–1322.
146. Pickering AJMC, Fink G. Priming effect of luteinizing hormone releasing factor: *in vitro* and *in vivo* evidence consistent with its dependence upon protein and RNA synthesis. *J Endocrinol* 1976;69:373–379.
147. Waring DW, Turgeon JL. Luteinizing hormone-releasing hormone-induced luteinizing hormone secretion *in vitro:* cyclic changes in responsiveness and self-priming. *Endocrinology* 1980;106:1430–1438.
148. Turgeon JL, Waring DW. Modification of luteinizing hormone secretion by activators of Ca^{2+}/phospholipid dependent protein kinase. *Endocrinology* 1986;118:2053–2058.
149. McArdle CA, Huckle WR, Johnson LA, Conn PM. Enhanced responsiveness of gonadotropes after protein kinase-C activation: post-receptor regulation of gonadotropin-releasing hormone action. *Endocrinology* 1988;122:1905–1914.
150. Judd AM, Jarvis WD, MacLeod RM. Attenuation of pituitary polyphosphoinositide metabolism by protein kinase C activation. *Mol Cell Endocrinol* 1987;54:107–114.
151. Leeb-Lundberg LMF, Cotecchia S, Lomasney JW, DeBernardis JF, Lefkowitz RJ, Caron MG. Phorbol esters promote antinociceptive a1-adrenergic receptor phosphorylation and receptor uncoupling from inositol phospholipid metabolism. *Proc Natl Acad Sci USA* 1985;82:5651–5655.
152. Orellana S, Solski PA, Brown JH. Guanosine 5'-*O*-(thiotriphosphate)-dependent inositol trisphosphate formation in membranes is inhibited by phorbol ester and protein kinase C. *J Biol Chem* 1987;262:1638–1643.
153. Bennett CF, Crooke ST. Purification and characterization of a phosphoinositide-specific phospholipase C from guinea pig uterus, phosphorylation by protein kinase C *in vivo*. *J Biol Chem* 1987;262:13789–13804.
154. Galizzi J-P, Qar J, Fosset M, Van Renterghem C, Lazdunsk M. Regulation of calcium channels in aortic muscle cells by protein kinase C activators (diacylglycerol and phorbol esters) and by peptides (vasopressin and bombesin) that stimulate phosphoinositide breakdown. *J Biol Chem* 1987;262:6947–6950.
155. Yamaguchi DT, Kleeman CR, Muallam S. Protein kinase C-activated calcium channel in the osteoblast-like clonal osteosarcoma cell line UMR-106. *J Biol Chem* 1987;262:14967–14973.
156. Waters SB, Hawes BE, Conn PM. Stimulation of luteinizing hormone release by sodium fluoride is independent of protein kinase C activity and unaffected by desensitization to gonadotropin-releasing hormone. *Endocrinology* 1990;126:2583–2591.
157. Papavasiliou SS, Zmeili S, Khoury S, Landefeld TD, Chin WW, Marshall JC. Gonadotropin-releasing hormone differentially regulates expression of the genes for luteinizing hormone α and β subunits in male rats. *Proc Natl Acad Sci USA* 1986;83: 4026–4029.
158. Phillippe J, Drucker DJ, Habener JF. Glucagon gene transcription in an islet cell line is regulated via a protein kinase C-activated pathway. *J Biol Chem* 1987;262:1823–1828.
159. Thalacher FW, Nilsen-Hamilton M. Specific induction of secreted proteins by transforming growth factor-b and 12-*O*-tetradecanoylphorbol-13-acetate. *J Biol Chem* 1987;262:2283–2290.
160. Diamond L. Tumor promoters and cell transformation. *Pharmacol Ther* 1984;26:89–145.
161. Barkan AL, Reame NE, Kelch RP, Marshall JC. Idiopathic hypogonadotropic hypogonadism in men: dependence of the hormone responses to gonadotropin-releasing hormone (GnRH) on the magnitude of the endogenous GnRH secretory defect. *J Clin Endocrinol Metab* 1985;61:1118–1125.
162. Starzec A, Counis R, Jutisz M. Gonadotropin-releasing hormone stimulates synthesis of the polypeptide chains of luteinizing hormone. *Endocrinology* 1986;119:561–565.
163. Liu T-C, Jackson GL. Modification of luteinizing hormone biosynthesis and release by gonadotropin-releasing hormone, cycloheximide, and actinomycin D. *Endocrinology* 1978;103: 1253–1263.
164. Vogel DL, Magner JA, Sherins RJ, Weintraub BD. Biosynthesis, glycosylation, and secretion of rat luteinizing hormone a- and b-subunits: differential effects of orchiectomy and gonadotropin-releasing hormone. *Endocrinology* 1986;119:202–213.
165. Counis R, Starzec A, Jutisz M. Gonadotropin-releasing hormone, cyclic AMP and phorbol esters stimulate the biosynthesis

of luteinizing hormone polypeptide chains. *Endocrinology* 1986;118(suppl.):148.
166. Liu T-C, Jackson GL. Stimulation by phorbol esters and diacylglycerol of luteinizing hormone glycosylation and release by rat anterior pituitary cells. *Endocrinology* 1987;121:1589–1595.
167. Brostrom MA, Chin K-V, Cade C, Gmitter D, Brostrom CO. Stimulation of protein synthesis in pituitary cells by phorbol esters and cyclic AMP. Evidence for rapid induction of a component of translational initiation. *J Biol Chem* 1987;262: 16515–16523.
168. Woodgett JR, Hunter T. Isolation and characterization of two distinct forms of protein kinase C. *J Biol Chem* 1987;262: 4836–4842.
169. Lee W, Mitchell P, Tijian R. Purified transcription factor AP-1 interacts with TPA-inducible enhancer elements. *Cell* 1987;49: 741–752.

The Physiology of Reproduction, Second Edition,
edited by E. Knobil and J.D. Neill,
Raven Press, Ltd., New York © 1994.

CHAPTER 33

Prolactin Secretion and Its Control

Jimmy D. Neill[1] and György M. Nagy[2]

INTRODUCTION

Prolactin is the most versatile pituitary hormone in both the number and diversity of physiological processes it regulates (1–3). The decisive role it plays in the preparation, maintenance, and secretory activity of the mammary gland during lactation is of utmost importance (3). Indeed, prolactin is essential to the survival of most mammalian young after birth. During lactation, the stimulus for prolactin secretion is triggered as the young suckle the mother's nipple. Neural impulses generated by suckling are conveyed to the central nervous system where they impinge upon specialized secretory neurons located in the hypothalamus. These neurons release the hypophysiotropic hormones into the hypophysial portal vessels that connect the nervous system and the adenohypophysis. Thus the neurogenic message engendered by suckling is finally conveyed to the pituitary in the form of hypophysiotropic hormones that stimulate or inhibit prolactin secretion (3).

This account of prolactin secretion and its control will emphasize suckling-induced prolactin secretion. Such a restricted view is taken because lactation is the only well-studied function of prolactin that is universal in mammals (1,2). The role of prolactin as a stimulator of progesterone secretion (4), although well studied, is probably restricted to rodents and perhaps to a few other species. A definitive physiological role for prolactin released in response to stress, though ubiquitous, is not established (3).

[1]Department of Physiology and Biophysics, University of Alabama at Birmingham, Birmingham, Alabama 35294
[2]Second Department of Anatomy, Semmelweis University Medical School, Hungary H-1450

MOLECULAR STRUCTURE OF PROLACTIN AND ITS GENE

Mammalian prolactin is a single polypeptide chain composed of 197–199 amino acids depending on the species with three disulfide bonds: one near the amino terminus, one at the carboxyterminus, and one in the inner region (Fig. 1) (5). The elucidation of prolactin's amino acid sequence is somewhat unusual in that in the majority of species, direct protein sequencing preceded complementary DNA (cDNA) cloning and nucleotide sequencing. The primary structures of ovine (6–8), bovine (9), porcine (7), human (10), and mouse (11) were elucidated by direct protein sequencing.

Prolactin is thus a protein hormone of 23,000–24,000 molecular weight. Mice (11) and rats (12) are the only mammalian species among those sequenced that have prolactins composed of 197 amino acids, whereas the remainder have 199 amino acids (Fig. 2) (see 5). The leader sequence of prolactin is 30 amino acids long, is necessary for insertion of the nascent preprolactin into the cisternae of the endoplasmic reticulum, but is

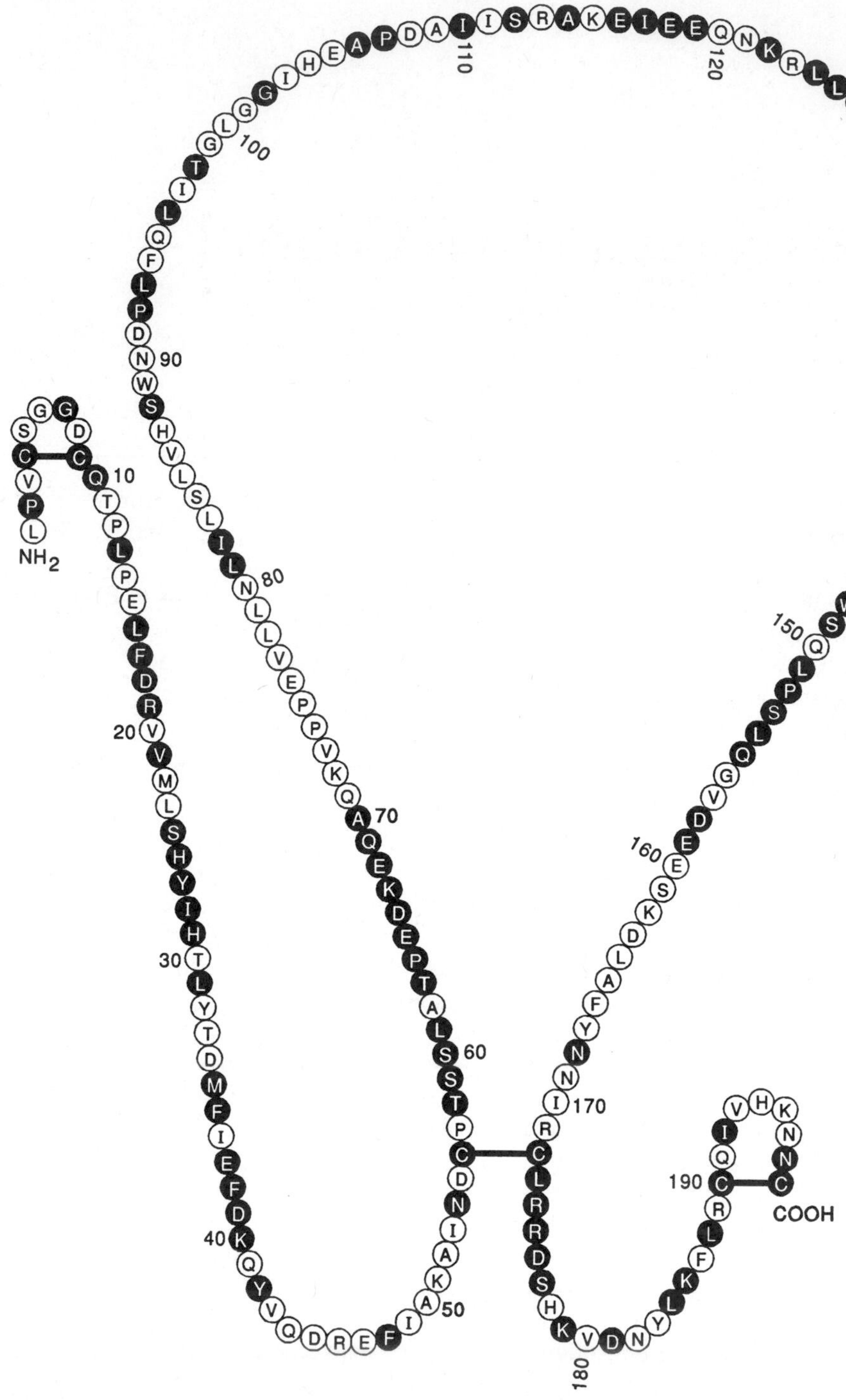

FIG. 1. Amino acid sequence of rat anterior pituitary prolactin. Amino acids are abbreviated to the single-letter style: A, alanine; C, cysteine; D, aspartic acid; E, glutamic acid; F, phenylalanine; G, glycine; H, histidine; I, isoleucine; K, lysine; L, leucine; M, methionine; N, asparagine; P, proline; Q, glutamine; R, arginine; S, serine; T, threonine; V, valine; W, tryptophan; Y, tyrosine. The three disulfide bridges are shown (*bridges between cysteines*); amino acids that are invariant in rat, mouse, porcine, bovine, and human prolactins (*white letters against black backgrounds*). From Li (7), Wallis (9), Shome and Parlow (10), Kohmoto et al. (11), and Cooke et al. (12).

```
         1                                                                           20
bPrl:    Thr Pro Val Cys Pro Asn Gly Pro Gly Asn Cys Gln Val Ser Leu Arg Asp Leu Phe Asp
hPrl:    Leu Pro Ile Cys Pro Gly Gly Ala Ala Arg Cys Gln Val Thr Leu Arg Asp Leu Phe Asp
rPrl:    Leu Pro Val Cys Ser Gly Gly ... ... Asp Cys Gln Thr Pro Leu Pro Glu Leu Phe Asp
mPrl:    Leu Pro Ile Cys Ser Ala Gly ... ... Asp Cys Gln Thr Ser Leu Arg Glu Leu Phe Asp
pPrl:    Leu Pro Ile Cys Pro Ser Gly Ala Val Asn Cys Gln Met Ser Leu Arg Asp Leu Phe Asp
         21                                                                          40
bPrl:    Arg Ala Val Met Val Ser His Tyr Ile His Asp Leu Ser Ser Glu Met Phe Asn Glu Phe
hPrl:    Arg Ala Val Val Leu Ser His Tyr Ile His Asn Leu Ser Ser Glu Met Phe Ser Glu Phe
rPrl:    Arg Val Val Met Leu Ser His Tyr Ile His Thr Leu Tyr Thr Asp Met Phe Ile Glu Phe
mPrl:    Arg Val Val Ile Leu Ser His Tyr Ile His Thr Leu Tyr Thr Asp Met Phe Ile Glu Phe
pPrl:    Arg Ala Val Ile Leu Ser His Tyr Ile His Asn Leu Ser Ser Glu Met Phe Asn Glu Phe
         41                                                                          60
bPrl:    Asp Lys Arg Tyr Ala Gln Gly Lys Gly Phe Ile Thr Met Ala Leu Asn Ser Cys His Thr
hPrl:    Asp Lys Arg Tyr Thr His Gly Arg Gly Phe Ile Thr Lys Ala Ile Asn Ser Cys His Thr
rPrl:    Asp Lys Gln Tyr Val Gln Asp Arg Glu Phe Ile Ala Lys Ala Ile Asn Asp Cys Pro Thr
mPrl:    Asp Lys Gln Tyr Val Gln Asp Arg Glu Phe Met Val Lys Val Ile Asn Asp Cys Pro Thr
pPrl:    Asp Lys Arg Tyr Ala Gln Gly Arg Gly Phe Ile Thr Lys Ala Ile Asn Ser Cys His Thr
         61                                                                          80
bPrl:    Ser Ser Leu Pro Thr Pro Glu Asp Lys Glu Gln Ala Gln Gln Thr His His Glu Val Leu
hPrl:    Ser Ser Leu Ala Thr Pro Glu Asp Lys Glu Gln Ala Gln Gln Met Asn Gln Lys Asp Phe
rPrl:    Ser Ser Leu Ala Thr Pro Glu Asp Lys Glu Gln Ala Gln Lys Val Pro Pro Glu Val Leu
mPrl:    Ser Ser Leu Ala Thr Pro Glu Asp Lys Glu Gln Ala Leu Lys Val Pro Pro Glu Val Leu
pPrl:    Ser Ser Leu Ser Thr Pro Glu Asp Lys Glu Gln Ala Gln Gln Ile His His Glu Val Leu
         81                                                                         100
bPrl:    Met Ser Leu Ile Leu Gly Leu Leu Arg Ser Trp Asn Asp Pro Leu Tyr His Leu Val Thr
hPrl:    Leu Ser Leu Ile Val Ser Ile Leu Arg Ser Trp Asn Glu Pro Leu Tyr His Leu Val Thr
rPrl:    Leu Asn Leu Ile Leu Ser Leu Val His Ser Trp Asn Asp Pro Leu Phe Gln Leu Ile Thr
mPrl:    Leu Asn Leu Ile Leu Ser Leu Val Gln Ser Ser Ser Asp Pro Leu Phe Gln Leu Ile Thr
pPrl:    Leu Asn Leu Ile Leu Arg Val Leu Arg Ser Trp Asn Asp Pro Leu Tyr His Leu Val Thr
         101                                                                        120
bPrl:    Glu Val Arg Gly Met Lys Gly Ala Pro Asp Ala Ile Leu Ser Arg Ala Ile Glu Ile Glu
hPrl:    Glu Val Arg Gly Met Gln Glu Ala Pro Glu Ala Ile Leu Ser Lys Ala Val Glu Ile Glu
rPrl:    Gly Leu Gly Gly Ile His Glu Ala Pro Asp Ala Ile Ile Ser Arg Ala Lys Glu Ile Glu
mPrl:    Gly Val Gly Gly Ile Gln Glu Ala Pro Glu Tyr Ile Leu Ser Arg Ala Lys Glu Ile Glu
pPrl:    Glu Val Arg Gly Met Gln Glu Ala Pro Asp Ala Ile Leu Ser Arg Ala Ile Glu Ile Glu
         121                                                                        140
bPrl:    Glu Glu Asn Lys Arg Leu Leu Glu Gly Met Glu Met Ile Phe Gly Gln Val Ile Pro Gly
hPrl:    Glu Gln Thr Lys Arg Leu Leu Glu Gly Met Glu Leu Ile Val Ser Gln Val His Pro Glu
rPrl:    Glu Gln Asn Lys Arg Leu Leu Glu Gly Ile Glu Lys Ile Ile Gly Gln Ala Tyr Pro Glu
mPrl:    Glu Gln Asn Lys Gln Leu Leu Glu Gly Val Glu Lys Ile Ile Ser Gln Ala Tyr Pro Glu
pPrl:    Glu Gln Asn Lys Arg Leu Leu Glu Gly Met Glu Lys Ile Val Gly Gln Val His Pro Gly
         141                                                                        160
bPrl:    Ala Lys Glu Thr Glu Pro Tyr Pro Val Trp Ser Gly Leu Pro Ser Leu Gln Thr Lys Asp
hPrl:    Thr Lys Glu Asn Glu Ile Tyr Pro Val Trp Ser Gly Leu Pro Ser Leu Gln Met Ala Asp
rPrl:    Ala Lys Gly Asn Glu Ile Tyr Leu Val Trp Ser Gln Leu Pro Ser Leu Gln Gly Val Asp
mPrl:    Ala Lys Gly Asn Gly Ile Tyr Phe Val Trp Ser Gln Leu Pro Ser Leu Gln Gly Val Asp
pPrl:    Ile Lys Glu Asn Glu Val Tyr Ser Val Trp Ser Gly Leu Pro Ser Leu Gln Met Ala Asp
         161                                                                        180
bPrl:    Glu Asp Ala Arg Tyr Ser Ala Phe Tyr Asn Leu Leu His Cys Leu Arg Arg Asp Ser Ser
hPrl:    Glu Glu Ser Arg Leu Ser Ala Tyr Tyr Asn Leu Leu His Cys Leu Arg Arg Asp Ser His
rPrl:    Glu Glu Ser Lys Asp Leu Ala Phe Tyr Asn Asn Ile Arg Cys Leu Arg Arg Asp Ser His
mPrl:    Glu Glu Ser Lys Ile Leu Ser Leu Arg Asn Thr Ile Arg Cys Leu Arg Arg Asp Ser His
pPrl:    Glu Asp Thr Arg Leu Phe Ala Phe Tyr Asn Leu Leu His Cys Leu Arg Arg Asp Ser His
         181                                                                    199
bPrl:    Lys Ile Asp Thr Tyr Leu Lys Leu Leu Asn Cys Arg Ile Ile Tyr Asn Asn Asn Cys
hPrl:    Lys Ile Asp Asn Tyr Leu Lys Leu Leu Lys Cys Arg Ile Ile His Asn Asn Asn Cys
rPrl:    Lys Val Asp Asn Tyr Leu Lys Phe Leu Arg Cys Gln Ile Val His Lys Asn Asn Cys
mPrl:    Lys Val Asp Asn Phe Leu Lys Val Leu Arg Cys Gln Ile Ala His Gln Asp Asn Cys
pPrl:    Lys Ile Asp Asn Tyr Leu Lys Leu Leu Lys Cys Arg Ile Ile Tyr Asp Ser Asn Cys
```

FIG. 2. Complete amino acid sequences of prolactins isolated from the pituitary glands of cattle (bPrl), humans (hPrl), rats (rPrl), mice (mPrl), and pigs (pPrl). Amino acids are abbreviated in the three letter style. Note that mouse and rat prolactins are composed of 197 amino acids whereas bovine, human, and porcine prolactins have 199 amino acids. From Li (7), Wallis (9), Shome and Parlow (10), Kohmoto et al. (11), and Cooke et al. (12).

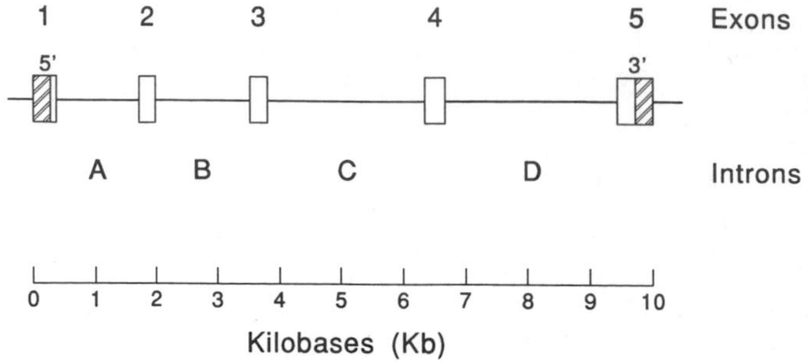

FIG. 3. Schematic diagram of the human prolactin gene as it was originally described, showing five exons and four introns; DNA encoding RNA that is not translated into protein (*broken lines on the first and fifth exons*). More recent work has shown the human prolactin gene to be 15 kb in size and to contain a sixth exon 5.3 kb upstream of exon I. This sixth exon encodes nontranslated ribonucleotide sequences which appear in placental but not in pituitary mRNA. From Chien and Thompson (14), Truong et al. (15), DiMatta et al. (16), and Hiraoka et al. (17).

cleaved in the process of insertion to form the mature hormone (12,13).

The prolactin gene was originally reported to be 10 kb in size and to be comprised of five exons and four introns (14,15), as illustrated in Fig. 3. More recently, however, the human prolactin gene was reported to be 15 kb in size and to contain a sixth exon 5.3 kb upstream of exon 1. This sixth exon encodes nontranslated ribonucleotide sequences which appear in placental but not in pituitary prolactin messenger RNA (mRNA) (16,17). Thus, for our purposes it can be ignored. There is only one prolactin gene in the haploid genome; in the human it is located on chromosome 6 (18). Exon 1 is comprised of only 56 nucleotides corresponding to the mRNA of the 5′ untranslated sequence, nine codons of the signal peptide, and the first nucleotide of the tenth codon (15,19) (Figs. 1–3). Exon 2 begins with the last two nucleotides of the tenth codon followed by the last 18 triplets coding for the signal peptide and the first 40 codons of the mature protein (15). Exon 3 encodes amino acids 41–76 while exon 4 encodes amino acids 77–136 (see Figs. 2 and 3). Exon 5 encodes amino acids 137–199 and contains the stop codon (TAA) and 118 nucleotides before the polyadenylation signal (AATAAA) located 20 nucleotides upstream of the consensus poly(A^+)-addition site (15).

Although the major form of prolactin found in the pituitary gland is the 23-kD form (Fig. 4A), numerous, less-abundant molecular forms also have been reported (20,21). Since there is reported to be a single prolactin gene in the haploid genome which has introns (15), these minor molecular forms must arise by way of alternative messenger RNA (mRNA) processing, by posttranslational processing during packaging of the hormone for secretion, or by alterations within the blood and/or target tissue. Perhaps the most abundant of these variant forms is a 21-kD variant detectable in murine pituitary extracts (22). Sinha and Jacobsen (22) have suggested that it may represent a splicing variant involving deletion of amino acids (Fig. 4, Panel B), analogous to the 20-kD variant of human growth hormone (see 23). A prolactin-immunoreactive protein of similar size has been detected in human plasma (24) and in the fetal porcine pituitary gland (25).

A 25-kD form of prolactin also has been reported to occur in the murine pituitary gland (20,26). It does not cross-react with antibodies to 23-kD prolactin and it has very weak pigeon crop-sac stimulating activity. Sinha and Gilligan (26) have suggested that the 25-kD form of prolactin might represent a structural variant resulting from failure of part of one of the introns to be removed during mRNA processing (Fig. 4). The basis for this supposition is by analogy with an mRNA for growth hormone found in bovine pituitary (27) and human placenta (28) in which the last intron has not been removed during splicing, resulting in the addition of 42 amino acids.

Alternative processing of prolactin mRNA as proposed by Sinha (20) has not been experimentally demonstrated. Indeed, Oetting et al. (29) performed *in vitro* translation of rat pituitary mRNA in the presence of rough microsomes and found only a 24-kD form of prolactin. These findings are most consistent with all molecular forms of prolactin in the pituitary gland arising from posttranslational modifications. Extensive posttranslational modifications of prolactin have been documented; among them are cleaved, deamidated, phosphorylated, glycosylated, sulfated, and disulfide dimerized forms (20). The cleaved forms (Fig. 4D) have attracted the greatest attention because of the original report of Mittra (30) that a 16-kD fragment derived from prolactin that had been nicked in the large disulfide loop around residue 149 had greater than normal mammary mitogenic activity. However, subsequent work has failed to find higher mammary mitogenic activity of such a fragment (31,32). Interestingly, activity was found for the 16-kDa fragment using pigeon crop-sac assay, Nb2 lymphoma cell proliferation, and casein synthesis in mouse mammary gland explants, although it was less than for the intact 23–24 kDa prolactin (31,32). Cleavage of prolactin in this way has been reported to occur not only in the pituitary gland but in target tissues as well (31,33).

Although the gonadotropins and thyrotropin are considered classically as the only glycosylated hormones produced by the anterior pituitary gland, prolactin also is glycosylated to a variable extent depending on the species (Fig. 4E). Glycosylated prolactin was discovered originally in the ovine pituitary gland (34) but also has been reported in human (35,36), porcine (37), and rat (38)

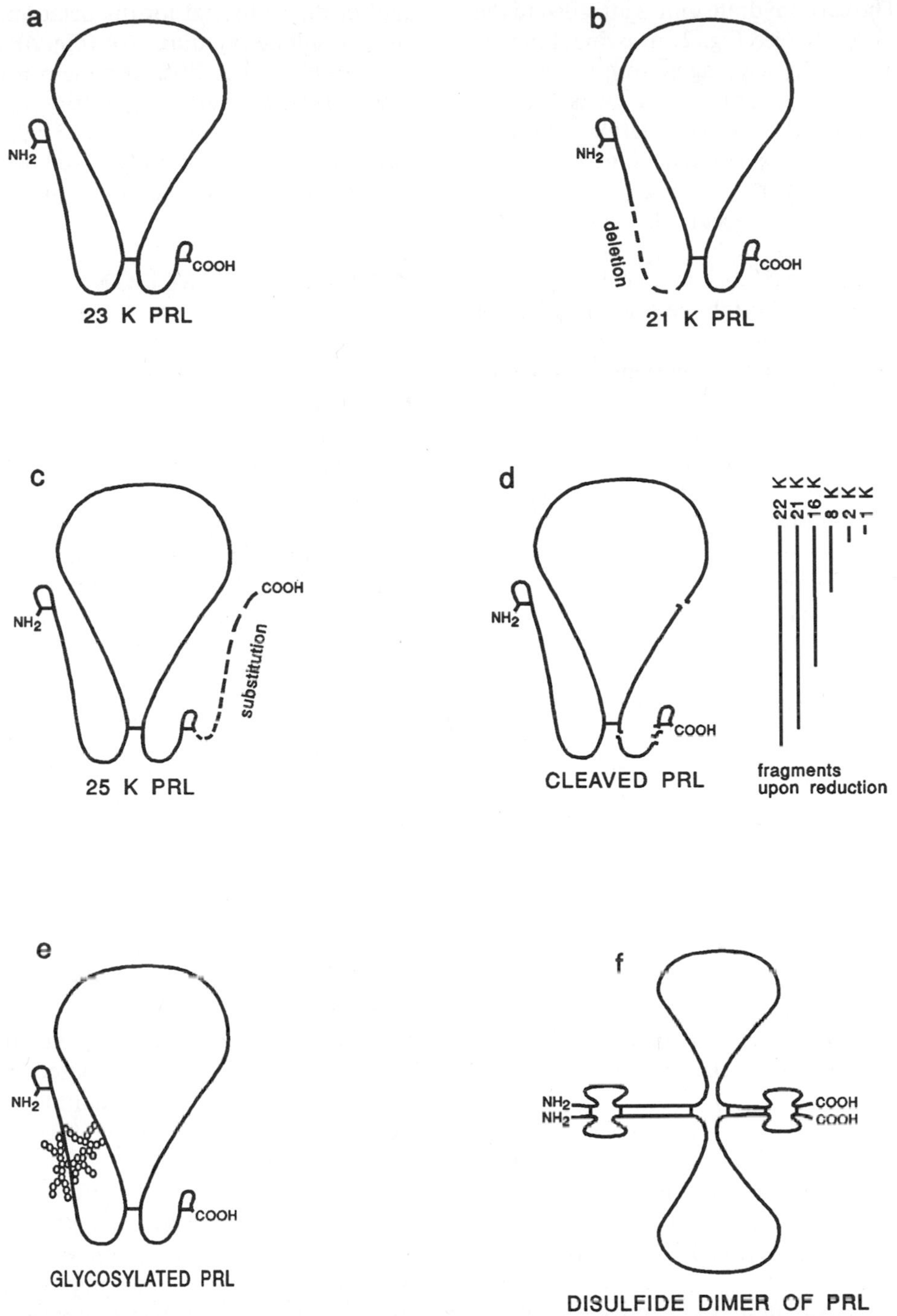

FIG. 4. Schematic diagram showing some of the structural modifications observed or hypothesized to exist in the prolactin molecule. **A:** 23-kDa prolactin is the predominant form found in the pituitary gland. **B:** 21-kDa prolactin variant hypothesized to represent a mRNA splicing variant involving deletion of amino acids. **C:** 25-kDa prolactin variant which may represent a structural variant resulting from failure of part of one of the introns to be removed during mRNA processing. **D:** Prolactin fragments derived by cleavage and reduction of the 23-kDa form of prolactin. **E:** Prolactin glycosylated at amino acid number 31 representing an N-linked glycosylation site. **F:** Disulfide dimer of prolactin. Redrawn from Sinha (20). Data from Sinha and Jacobsen (22), Sinha and Gilligan (26), and Lewis et al. (36).

pituitary glands. The carbohydrate unit is attached to the asparagine at position 31 (see Fig. 2) in ovine, human, and porcine prolactins; this asparagine residue (see Fig. 4E) is part of the consensus sequence (Asn-X-Ser) usually associated with N-linked glycosylation. Prolactin in rats also is glycosylated despite not having a consensus N-linked glycosylation sequence (see Figs. 1 and 2). Glycosylation (N-linked) might occur at Asn-X-Cys sequences where a sulfur replaces the oxygen of the serine side chain (20). Rat prolactin has two such sequences (amino acids 56–58 and 197–199; see Fig. 2). O-linked glycosylation might also occur at serine and threonine residues (20). The amounts of glycosylated prolactin found in the pituitary gland vary considerably among species. In pigs, 40–50% of the prolactin is glycosylated (37); in sheep and humans, approximately 15% is glycosylated (20); in rats about 8–10% is glycosylated (38); and in cattle no glycosylated prolactin can be detected (20).

The biological activity of glycosylated prolactin depends on the assay in which it is tested: it has higher activity than nonglycosylated prolactin in the pigeon crop-sac assay but is similar with or lower in the assays utilizing Nb2 lymphoma cell proliferation and casein synthesis by mammary tissue (20). The immunologic cross-reactivity of glycosylated prolactin with prolactin antibodies is approximately 30% that of 23-kD prolactin (20). Two different forms of glycosylated prolactin have been reported to exist in human pituitary glands (36). One form binds to the lectin, concanavalin A, and the other does not, suggesting that the carbohydrate moieties of the two prolactins differ. They show different pigeon crop-sac stimulating activities and metabolic clearance rates (36).

The presence of phosphorylated prolactin also has been reported in rat (39) and cow (40) pituitary glands. Presumably this is due to covalent coupling of phosphate to threonines and serines since this is a common post-translational modification of proteins. Phosphorylation appears to affect the biological activity of prolactin since phosphorylated prolactin inhibited the proliferation of GH_3 cells in culture, whereas 24-kD prolactin or dephosphorylated prolactin stimulated GH_3 cell proliferation (41).

Prolactin also can be sulfated. Radioactive sulfate incorporation into sheep and buffalo prolactins has been reported (42). The sulfate group probably is coupled to tyrosines or to the carbohydrate moieties of glycosylated prolactin (42). The effect of sulfation on the biological activity of prolactin, if any, is unknown.

High-molecular-weight forms of prolactin are reported to occur in the pituitary gland and in plasma (20). The forms may be "big" (45 kD) or "big-big" (>60 kD). Some of these forms can be dissociated into monomers (23 kD) with urea or sodium dodecyl sulfate, suggesting that they are noncovalently associated aggregates (20). Others require reducing agents such as 2-mercaptoethanol or dithiothreitol for dissociation, suggesting interchain disulfide bonding (20) (Fig. 4F). A third form is not dissociated by either of these procedures, suggesting other forms of covalent association either as homopolymers or heteropolymers (20). High-molecular-weight forms of prolactin generally have lower biological activity than do the monomer forms (43).

PROLACTIN SECRETION

Hypothalamic Control

Background

The development of the neurohumoral hypothesis for hypothalamic control of adenohypophysial secretion by Geoffrey Harris and colleagues (44) led to the expectation that prolactin secretion would be regulated by a stimulatory hypothalamic, hypophysiotropic factor. Nevertheless, Everett (45,46) demonstrated that separation of the pituitary gland from the hypothalamus was sufficient by itself to initiate a prolonged elevation of prolactin secretion, as evidenced by the induction and maintenance of an essentially permanent pseudopregnancy in the rat. Everett (45,46) postulated the existence of a factor in the hypothalamus that was released into the hypophysial portal blood to inhibit prolactin secretion. Subsequently, Pasteels and colleagues (47,48) showed that hypothalamic pieces or extracts reduced the release of prolactin from pituitary glands incubated *in vitro*. Soon thereafter, Meites and colleagues (49,50) confirmed the existence of a prolactin-inhibiting factor (PIF) and demonstrated that the active substance in hypothalamic extracts was not identical with neurohumoral agents thought to reside in the brain. Based on the observations that drugs disrupting catecholamine metabolism altered prolactin secretion (51–54) and that dopamine was present in the median eminence in high concentrations (55), several investigators found that dopamine inhibited prolactin release from the pituitary gland (56,57). MacLeod, in particular, championed this view and provided much experimental evidence to support dopamine as the PIF (58). Acceptance of a nonpeptidic hypothalamic-inhibiting factor (dopamine) was delayed by: (a) the bias that PIF should be peptidic since other hypophysiotropic factors were peptides; (b) the numerous reports that such peptide PIFs existed; and (c) the fact that large doses of dopamine seemed to be required for inhibition of prolactin secretion.

Inhibition

The basal secretion of prolactin from the anterior pituitary gland is viewed as being spontaneous (i.e., occurs without stimulation by the hypothalamus) (3) since prolactin secretion occurs at a high rate for prolonged periods when the pituitary gland is transplanted to a site distant from the hypothalamus or when cultured *in vitro* (59,60). *In vivo,* prolactin secretion appears to be severely restrained by the hypothalamus, since serum prolactin levels remain low in the absence of prolactin-releasing stimuli (60). This is evidenced by the findings that (a) pituitary stalk section or median eminence lesions result in an immediate increase in prolactin secretion which remains high for prolonged periods (61–64); (b) prolactin secretion occurs at a high spontaneous rate when the anterior lobe is transplanted to a site distant (under the kidney capsule) from the hypothalamus (45,46); or (c) when cultured *in vitro* (59,60,65). The best established hypothalamic, hypophysiotropic inhibitor of prolactin secretion is dopamine, produced by neurons of the arcuate-periventricular nucleus and secreted into the hypophysial portal blood.

Dopamine

Based on the observations that drugs affecting catecholamine metabolism also alter prolactin secretion (51–53), and that dopamine is present in high concentration in both the median eminence (55) and the hypophysial stalk plasma (66–68), several investigators concluded that dopamine is the hypothalamic PIF. Subsequently, receptors for dopamine have been detected on pituitary membranes (69–72), and more recently we have learned the structure of the dopaminergic receptors (73). Thus, sufficient evidence is available to support the strong conclusion that dopamine is the major physiological hypothalamic PIF.

The question of whether dopamine is the sole PIF mediating tonic hypothalamic inhibition *in vivo* remains a relevant issue. In early studies of this issue, investigators reported that the amount of dopamine in stalk blood was sufficient to account for only about two-thirds of the prolactin inhibition normally observed (60,67,74). This conclusion was based on quantitative studies in which dopamine was infused into rats depleted of endogenous dopamine with the rate limiting enzyme (tyrosine hydroxylase) inhibitor, α-methyl-*p*-tyrosine, and the rate of dopamine infusion was set to mimic the levels measured in stalk blood of intact animals (67). The above studies were performed in urethane-anesthetized rats; even greater amounts of dopamine had to be infused to suppress α-methyl-*p*-tyrosine-stimulated prolactin secretion in conscious lactating rats (75). The relationship of dopamine to pituitary prolactin secretion is even more complex; consider the following facts: an inverse relationship does not always exist between hypothalamic secretion of dopamine and pituitary secretion of prolactin; dopamine levels in hypophysial stalk plasma are 5–7 times lower in males than in females (76–78), but the plasma levels of prolactin are not much different. Moreover, the relationship of dopamine to prolactin is positive on the afternoon of proestrus (76). The lack of a mirror-image relationship between dopamine concentrations and plasma prolactin also has been demonstrated in lactating rats during a simulated suckling stimulus (79–81).

Subsequent experiments demonstrated that the early studies failed to account for an important source of dopamine reaching the anterior lobe through the short portal vessels from the neurointermediate lobe (NIL) (82–85). It is well known that hypophysiotrophic dopaminergic neurons in the hypothalamus consist of two different parts. Tuberoinfundibular dopaminergic neurons (TIDA), located in the posterior portion of the arcuate nucleus and the periventricular region that project to the median eminence, are well accepted as a major physiological regulator of the adenohypophysial prolactin secretion (3) (see Fig. 5). More recently, evidence has been presented that dopamine derived from the tuberohypophysial dopaminergic system (THDA) also may be an important regulator of prolactin secretion (84) (Fig. 5). Tuberohypophysial dopaminergic system neurons originate in the arcuate nucleus as do those of the TIDA. However, neurons of this system locate in the most rostral part of the arcuate-periventricular nucleus and terminate in the NIL of the pituitary gland, rather than in the median eminence of the hypothalamus (86,87) (Fig. 5). Therefore, dopamine released by THDA terminals would not be present in pituitary stalk blood; i.e., dopamine concentrations reaching the adenohypophysis apparently were underestimated. Indeed, removal of the posterior pituitary lobe elevates basal prolactin secretion, which can be blocked by dopamine administration (83,84). Consistent with this finding is the report that electrochemically detectable dopamine in the anterior pituitary gland is reduced after surgical removal of the posterior lobe (88). Subsequent surgical sectioning of the hypophysial stalk reduced the electrochemical signal representing dopamine to low levels, as did treatment with α-methyl-*p*-tyrosine; amounts of dopamine given by infusion that were sufficient to inhibit the elevated prolactin levels also were sufficient to return the dopamine levels in the anterior pituitary to pretreatment levels (88). Thus, dopamine of hypothalamic origin which is delivered to the adenohypophysis by way of the long and the short portal vessels (from TIDA or THDA, respectively) seems quantitatively (Fig. 5) sufficient to account for inhibition of prolactin release.

The relative contributions of the two dopaminergic systems to the control of prolactin secretion remain unknown. Involvement of dopamine, found in NIL (Fig. 5), in the regulation of prolactin secretion is not in doubt: surgical removal of the NIL results in a three- to fourfold increase in basal plasma prolactin levels in male rats and in cycling and lactating female rats (83,84). Phys-

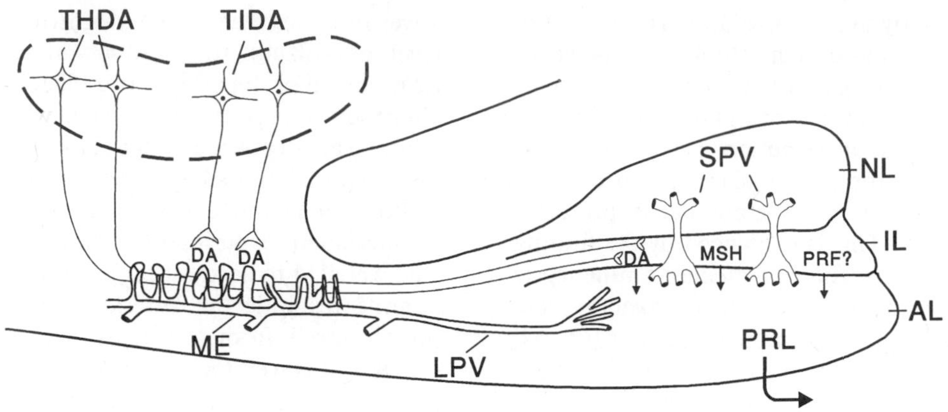

FIG. 5. Revised model for neoroendocrine regulation of anterior lobe (AL) prolactin (PRL) secretion. *Abbreviations:* THDA: tuberohypophysial dopaminergic neurons. TIDA: tuberoinfundibular dopaminergic neurons. LPV, long portal vessels; SPV, short portal vessels; DA, dopamine; αMSH, αmelanocyte stimulating hormone; PRF, prolactin releasing factor; NL, neural lobe; IL, intermediate lobe; ME, median eminence.

iologic regulation of this system is demonstrated by the experiment where lactating rats were exposed to a relatively short-term (24- to 48-hour) dehydration; basal- and suckling-induced pituitary prolactin secretion were immediately depressed through an osmosensitive hypothalamic dopaminergic mechanism (89). Since the THDA system can be selectively activated by dehydration (90–93), one can conclude that in this experiment, dopamine, released by nerve terminals in the NIL of the pituitary gland, traveled to the anterior lobe to affect prolactin release. Indeed, pretreatment with haloperidol, a dopamine receptor blocker, blocked dehydration-induced plasma prolactin depletion (89). Thus, in these experiments a reduction or an elevation of dopamine levels in blood carried by the short portal vessels (Fig. 5) altered (directly or indirectly) prolactin secretion of lactotropes. This conclusion raises a new question: does the activity of the THDA system play a tonic role in prolactin secretion or rather does it exert a dynamic effect during the first few minutes of different stimuli (stress, suckling)? It is well known that dopamine, released by THDA terminals in the IL (94–96), tonically inhibits the secretion of α-melanocyte-stimulating hormone (α-MSH) from melanotropes (97–99); therefore, parallel changes in the plasma levels of prolactin and α-MSH during an acute stimulus would be expected if the THDA system were involved. Recent data have clearly shown that there is no change in plasma α-MSH in response to nursing (100). Therefore, an acute diminution in the activity of the THDA system does not seem to occur during the suckling stimulus. Thus, the observations that the dopamine concentration in the NIL is lower and the plasma α-MSH level is higher in lactating than in cycling female rats (87), and that dehydration induces a parallel and immediate reduction of plasma α-MSH and prolactin concentration in lactating rats (101), strongly support a tonic role of THDA neurons in the regulation of prolactin secretion during lactation.

Other Prolactin-Inhibiting Factors

Despite the seeming sufficiency of hypothalamic dopamine to fully inhibit prolactin release, other PIFs have been reported to exist but their physiological roles remain unresolved. γ-aminobutyric acid (GABA) directly inhibits the release of prolactin (102–104), its receptors are present on adenohypophysial cells (105,106), and GABA neurons have been visualized in the median eminence by immunohistochemistry using an antibody against glutamate decarboxylase, an enzyme involved with GABA synthesis (107,108); these findings require consideration of GABA in the economy of prolactin secretion. GABA appears to be a secretory product of the median eminence, at least during electrical stimulation of the hypothalamus (109); basal secretion of GABA into hypophysial stalk blood has been reported to occur (109) or not occur (110), depending on the source. At all events, the effective molar concentration of GABA required for inhibition of prolactin secretion (103,104,111) is about 100 times higher than that for dopamine. Although a postulated priming effect of an endogenous benzodiazepine-like substance to increase prolactin responsiveness to GABA (112,113) needs to be investigated further, a physiologic role for GABA in regulating prolactin secretion cannot be rationalized at present.

Another nondopaminergic PIF activity recently has been found in bovine NIL extracts (114) that could inhibit prolactin release both *in vivo* and *in vitro.* When these substances were further purified, they appeared to be endothelin-like peptides (115). Endothelin-1 and endothelin-3 also have been reported to inhibit prolactin release *in vitro* in a dose-dependent manner and to be unaffected by D_2 dopamine receptor agonists (116,117). Both peptides are present in all three lobes of the pituitary gland and their concentrations are sufficiently high compared with other regions of the brain to postulate autocrine or paracrine inhibitory roles for these peptides in the control of prolactin secretion. Further work is needed to clarify a potential role for endothelins in the economy of prolactin secretion.

Stimulation

The stimuli of apparent universal importance that elevate prolactin secretion above baseline are suckling (59,118), stress (59,119), and the ovarian hormones (59,120), primarily estrogen. The first two of these are neurogenic stimuli arising from the environment, whereas the last one, estrogen, is endogenous. Although many elements of the final common pathway for these three stimuli are similar, there are several differences among them as far as the magnitude, the time course, and their effect on the homeostasis of the animal are concerned. There are two major mechanisms by which hypothalamic neuronal activity can enhance prolactin release from the pituitary: (a) inhibition of PIF; and (b) stimulation of a prolactin-releasing factor (PRF). Here, we will focus on these possible mechanisms and candidates for such a role.

Dopamine

The simplest explanation for increases in prolactin release would be that a given stimulus reduces the tonic inhibition exercised by the hypothalamus, freeing the pituitary gland to express its inherent capacity to secrete prolactin spontaneously at a very high rate (3,60,120). Indeed, treatment of rats with sufficient amounts of α-methyl-*p*-tyrosine to completely suppress dopamine secretion into hypophysial stalk blood results in an increase in prolactin secretion (67,121) quantitatively similar to that observed after suckling or stress. Similar results can be obtained *in vitro* where removal of dopamine infusion results in a rapid elevation of prolactin release (122). Thus, disinhibition is a plausible means for neurogenic stimuli to induce release of prolactin if such stimuli could be shown to dramatically decrease dopamine release from any of the participating hypothalamic dopaminergic systems. There are conflicting reports about the change in dopaminergic neuronal activity during surges of prolactin. Conclusions from the available data are almost impossible because only one of the four different available methods (rate of dopamine synthesis, α-methyl-*p*-tyrosine-induced decline of dopamine, release of dopamine, and anterior pituitary content of dopamine) is usually applied in such experiments. Thus, dopaminergic activity is thought to increase (123), remain unchanged (124,125), or to slightly decrease (126–129) during a single stimulus like suckling. However, the most direct studies are those in which the mammary nerve was stimulated electrically to simulate suckling, and dopamine release was detected in hypophysial stalk blood (79,80) or in the median eminence with an electrochemical probe (81). Only a brief (3–5 minutes), 60% to 70% decline in dopamine release was observed (79–81). This decline was followed by series of rapid pulses of dopamine above the baseline which lasted for the duration of mammary nerve stimulation (80). These results led to the conclusion that changes in dopamine secretion by the hypothalamus itself are insufficient to account for the suckling-induced prolactin release.

Recent evidence has strongly suggested that the prevailing view of an exclusive inhibitory role for dopamine in the control of prolactin secretion appears to be simplistic. This catecholamine might also be regarded as a prolactin-releasing agent under the appropriate conditions. More than a decade ago, Denef et al. (130) first reported that a very low concentration of dopamine (1000-fold lower than that required for maximal inhibition) could actually stimulate prolactin secretion from male rat pituitary cells *in vitro*. Kramer and Hopkins (131), and more recently Burris et al. (132,133) have extended these studies using both static and dynamic cultures of pituitary cells from cycling female rats. This latter group has found that a rapid reduction in dopamine concentration from 10^{-7}M (a dose that maximally inhibits prolactin secretion) to a range of from 10^{-10}M to 10^{-12}M caused a greater stimulation of prolactin release than that evoked by a complete removal of dopamine (133). A possible physiological relevance for these *in vitro* data can be gleaned from the reports of Nagy et al. (134,135) and Hill et al. (136). Anterior pituitary cells obtained from nonsuckled (separated from their litters for 4 hours) or suckled (for 10 minutes) lactating rats were exposed to various concentrations of dopamine *in vitro*. Prolactin release was measured by the reverse hemolytic plaque assay. Surprisingly, pituitary cells from nonsuckled rats exhibited only the inhibitory response to dopamine (134,136). In striking contrast, a brief suckling stimulus applied immediately prior to euthanasia rendered the prolactin cells responsive to stimulation by a 10^{-12}M concentration of dopamine (136). Subsequently, Arey et al. (137) have demonstrated that infusion of 10 ng/kg/min dopamine to freely moving rats results in a further increase in the already-elevated plasma prolactin when synthesis of endogenous dopamine has been blocked by pretreatment of the animals with α-methyl-*p*-tyrosine.

Dopamine enhancement of prolactin secretion both *in vitro* and *in vivo* raises the question of the physiological relevance of this phenomenon. Are lactotropes *in situ* ever exposed to dopamine levels sufficiently low to be stimulatory? A simulated suckling stimulus results in a transient reduction in the level of dopamine in hypophysial portal blood (79–81,138). The dopamine concentration of portal blood in cycling rats is the lowest during the day of proestrus (76). However, it is doubtful that a 50% to 70% decrease in portal blood dopamine (76,79) is sufficient to achieve concentrations capable of stimulating prolactin release. On the other hand, dopamine concentration in stalk blood (67,76) is in the low nanogram range (10^{-8}M), which is mostly ineffective or has only a weak inhibitory effect *in vitro* (58), but 100- to 1000-fold lower doses are required to stimulate prolactin release. One possible explanation for these apparent contradictions is the hypothesis of Shin and coworkers (139,140) that dopamine may require an additional agent(s) to effectively inhibit prolactin release and thus properly function as the PIF. They have proposed ascorbic acid, routinely used to protect dopamine from oxidation during *in vitro* studies, as a major candidate for this supplementary factor (140). It is quite clear that ascorbic acid is not just a simple antioxidant but in fact can potentiate the inhibitory effect of dopamine *in vitro* by 100 times. Similar to the idea that ascorbic acid, which is present in very high concentration in all three lobes of the pituitary gland (141), may serve as a "responsiveness" agent (3) for potentiating dopamine to inhibit prolactin release, Frawley and his group have provided evidence that α-MSH from the NIL can also function as a stimulatory "responsiveness" factor *in vitro* (136) (Fig. 5); α-MSH was reported to decrease the responsiveness of lactotropes to the inhibitory effect of a high dose of dopamine and enhance their responsiveness to the stimulatory effect of a low dose (136). Having experimental evidence for a new class of prolactin regulators (3), we may now view the regulation of prolactin secretion differently. Ascorbic acid, α-MSH, and/or other substances produced either in the hypothalamus or in the pituitary gland may function as "prolactin responsiveness factors." They are defined as substances with little or no direct influence on prolactin release that rather exert profound effects on the pituitary by altering prolactin responsiveness to the classical hypothalamic or posterior pituitary-releasing and -inhibiting factors (3).

Thyrotropin-Releasing Hormone

The thyrotropin-releasing hormone (TRH) was originally isolated as a hypophysiotropic factor that stimulates thyroid-stimulating hormone (TSH) secretion from pituitary cells (142). Subsequently, TRH was shown to stimulate prolactin release from lactotropes and its effect was dose-related both *in vitro* and *in vivo* (143–146). Thyrotropin-releasing hormone is secreted into hypophysial stalk blood (147,148) and its receptors are present on pituitary cells (149), evidently on lactotropes (150). These data meet most of the requirements for considering TRH as a PRF in a physiologic context. However, TRH can stimulate pituitary prolactin secretion in only a few conditions *in vivo,* such as in estrogen-primed male rats (151) but not in normal males (152) or lactating female rats (152,153). More importantly, the release of prolactin and TSH is dissociated during the two most important neurogenic stimuli for prolactin release, i.e., during stress and suckling. For example, TSH secretion is slightly affected or unaffected during stress and suckling, while prolactin responses are highly significant (153–155).

Studies where antibodies are used to neutralize hypophysiotropic factors in the circulation are widely used to obtain information about the "physiological" relevance of a given factor. The results obtained with this approach for TRH are also confusing. Although there are data that TRH antiserum can suppress the proestrous prolactin surge (156) and attenuates the suckling-induced prolactin response (157), these observations were not confirmed by others. Prolactin-releasing activity of hypothalamic extracts is only weakly reduced by TRH antiserum (158,159), suggesting that TRH is not a PRF.

The final answer about the supposed physiological role of TRH in the control of prolactin secretion is still more puzzling if we take into consideration the stimulus-induced change in lactotrope responsiveness to TRH detected both *in vitro* and *in vivo* (160,161). Self-priming of gonadotropes by gonadotropin-releasing hormone (GnRH) is a well documented and clinically useful pharmacological tool (162–165). It seems unlikely that a self-priming phenomenon of prolactin cells by classical hypophysiotrophic factors such as dopamine, TRH, or others plays a regulatory role in the control of prolactin secretion. For example, pulsatile administration of TRH (160) or hypothalamic extracts (161) does not change prolactin cell responsiveness. On the other hand, prolactin responsiveness to TRH and to other hypothalamic, hypophysiotropic compounds changes significantly after a transient fall in dopamine levels (122,166,167). These findings have been confirmed in several animal models, such as ovariectomized animals treated with estradiol and progesterone (168) and pseudopregnant (169) or pregnant (170) rats. Studies in which the second messenger systems playing a role in these responsiveness changes of lactotropes have been investigated (171) concluded that activation of adenylyl cyclase (AC) (172), phospholipase C (PLC) (173), and protein kinase C (PKC) (174) might be effective signals. While prolactin responsiveness to TRH could be modulated by the hypothalamic release pattern of dopamine, several studies have indicated that prior incubation of cultured pituitary cells with estradiol (175) or a suckling stimulus of only 10 minutes before sacrifice of lactating rats (134,135) results in a decrease in prolactin responsiveness to dopamine in addition to a marked increase in prolactin responsiveness to TRH. More recently, when lactating rats were used to investigate whether the suckling stimulus influences the magnitude of the response to dopamine, TRH and angiotensin II (AII), it was demonstrated that nursing is a requirement for disappearance of the inhibitory and expression of the stimulatory effect of dopamine and an enhanced responsiveness to TRH and AII (134).

The observation that responsiveness changes occurred almost exclusively within the inner zone of the adenohypophysis (a region perfused by blood from the NIL) raised the possibility that the NIL might produce a factor(s) that could influence lactotrope responsiveness to regulatory agents (135). A likely candidate to subserve such a role is α-MSH, as we have discussed earlier (Fig. 5). The proposed role of NIL in this context has been confirmed by Dymshitz and Ben-Jonathan (176), who showed that TRH evokes a significantly larger release of prolactin in anterior and posterior pituitary cocultures than when anterior lobe cells were cultured alone. The permissive effect of such a factor may in fact influence lactotropes located in only the inner zone of the anterior lobe. Therefore, NIL and the inner zone of the anterior pituitary can serve as a functional unit from the point of view of hypothalamic regulatory mechanisms.

Vasoactive Intestinal Peptide and Homologous Peptides

Several biologically active peptides forming a family such as vasoactive intestinal peptide (VIP), peptide histidine-isoleucine (PHI), secretin, growth-hormone-releasing factor (GRF), halodermin, and the recently discovered pituitary adenylate cyclase activating polypeptide (PACAP) have been identified. A subgroup of these relatives (VIP, PHI, and PACAP) has been shown to significantly affect pituitary prolactin secretion.

VIP was isolated originally from porcine small intestine (177) and demonstrated to occur in the hypothalamic paraventricular nuclei and median eminence (178–180). VIP stimulates prolactin release both *in vivo* and *in vitro* (181–184) through a direct action on VIP receptors found in anterior pituitary cells (185). VIP stimulates prolactin release *in vitro* at concentrations of 10^{-7}M to 10^{-10}M in a dose-related manner; the peptide exists in the portal blood (186–189) in concentrations about 10 times higher than that found in the general circulation. The concentrations in portal blood are sufficiently high to stimulate prolactin release from pituitary cells. These findings suggest that VIP may be an important mediator of prolactin release in different physiologic situations. Moreover, when passive immunizations were performed to neutralize VIP in the plasma (190–192), stimulation of prolactin release by ether stress was completely blocked (190) but suckling-induced prolactin response was only partially inhibited (191). A major question about the procedure of passive immunization is that VIP is considered to be an autocrine regulator of prolactin secretion (193,194) and it is not clear that such a source of VIP would remain unaffected during *in vivo* immunoneutralization studies. Therefore, the question of whether the reduction of prolactin release by VIP antiserum is due to the neutralization of VIP in the portal blood [where it is more greatly diluted than in the systemic circulation (195)] or within the pituitary gland, or both, remains to be established.

Peptide histidine-isoleucine and VIP are synthesized from a common precursor (196) and are homologous to each other (197). Thus, it is not surprising that they were detected in equimolar amounts in the hypophysial portal blood (188). Peptide histidine-isoleucine also can stimulate prolactin release in freely moving rat (198–200) and from dispersed pituitary cells (201). The relative contributions of PHI and VIP and whether their effects are separate or additive in the control of prolactin secretion still needs further exploration.

The third relative of this family which has a potential to serve as a PRF is the novel 38-residue neuropeptide PACAP. Two polypeptides with 38 (PACAP 38) and 27 (PACAP 27) amino acid residues, respectively, recently have been isolated from the hypothalamus (202,203). These peptides, which share strong sequence homology (68%) with the N-terminal portion of VIP, can induce a very strong accumulation of cyclic adenine monophosphate (cAMP) in cultured anterior pituitary cells (202) by binding to high-affinity receptor sites (204). Systemic injection of PACAP 38 significantly and dose-dependently stimulated pituitary prolactin as well as growth hormone (GH) secretion in both male (205) and nonsuckled lactating female rats (206). In contrast to its marked prolactin-releasing effect *in vivo,* PACAP 38 dose-dependently inhibits prolactin release in both monolayer cell cultures (207) and in the reverse hemolytic plaque assay (206,207). Thus, *in vitro* and *in vivo* experiments yield contrasting effects of PACAP 38 on pituitary prolactin release. This finding can be interpreted to mean that PACAP 38 acutely influences lactotropes indirectly through a paracrine or yet unknown mechanism which overrides the tonic inhibitory action of hypothalamic dopamine. Consistent with this view are the observations that bromocriptine pretreatment completely blocks (206) and hypothalamic lesions attenuate (207) the increase of plasma prolactin induced by PACAP 38. In summary, the physiological significance of one or all of the members of this peptide family in the economy of prolactin secretion will require additional exploration.

Neurointermediate Lobe Prolactin-Releasing Factors

A consensus view developed over the last two decades holds that the hypophysiotropic signal mediating environmental (stress, suckling) or endogenous (estrogen) stimuli that release prolactin travels from the median eminence to the adenohypophysis via the long portal vessels of the hypothalamo-hypophysial portal system. Despite extensive supportive evidence for this view, it has proved to be incomplete (*vide infra*). As examples we may cite the modest decreases in portal blood levels of dopamine and the weakness of PRFs such as VIP or TRH to release prolactin after suckling or stress (79–81). An even more disturbing aspect of the current view is that it cannot integrate several recent experimental findings such as surgical removal of the NIL blocking the suckling-induced release of prolactin (208) and the peak phase of the proestrous surge (209); moreover, this surgical procedure also attenuates the mating-induced nocturnal surge (210). Crude extracts of the NIL also have been reported to stimulate prolactin release *in vitro* (211,212). Furthermore, it has been shown that the prolactin-releasing activity disappears from the NIL 1 week after pituitary stalk transection (213). These findings might suggest that a PRF activity is produced by hypothalamic neurons which project to and terminate in the NIL (Fig. 5). However, a PRF can be found after 1 week of NIL culture (214); this finding suggests that a prolactin-releasing activity is synthesized by NIL cells. This obvious contradiction suggests the existence of more than one factor in the NIL which can stimulate prolactin secretion. Therefore, it would appear that at least two signals are delivered to the anterior pituitary from the NIL by way of the short portal vessels and that these signals must be integrated with each other and with those which arrive through the long portal vessels from the median eminence.

The stimulatory effect of posterior pituitary extracts on prolactin release are thought to be due partially to the influence of oxytocin (215). For instance, it is secreted into the hypophysial portal blood at 10–15 times higher concentration than found in the peripheral circulation (216), and high-affinity oxytocin receptors resembling those found in the uterus are present in the anterior lobe (217). Although a large dose of oxytocin has been reported to induce a rise in plasma prolactin in male or ovariectomized female rats (218), it failed to affect prolactin levels in lactating rats, deprived (208) or not (Nagy et al., *unpublished observation*, 1993) of the endogenous peptide by posterior lobectomy. In contrast, low doses of oxytocin induced a dose-related reduction in basal as well as stress levels of prolactin after subcutaneous administration to male rats (218–220). The potency of oxytocin *in vitro* is rather low (215). Furthermore, some investigators report difficulties in evoking prolactin secretion with oxytocin (211,221). Attempts to antagonize the action of endogenous oxytocin *in vivo* also have resulted in conflicting data; passive immunization with oxytocin antisera delays and reduces prolactin surges induced by suckling or by estrogen (215). On the other hand, injection of a specific oxytocin antagonist, which blocked suckling-induced milk ejection, did not alter the concomitant release of prolactin (222). Also, the oxytocin antagonist did not affect the prolactin rise associated with ether stress but it did prevent the proestrous prolactin surge (222).

While the chemical nature of NIL PRFs and more importantly, the physiological significance of the NIL for regulation of prolactin secretion, remains to be elucidated, the above-mentioned evidence indicates that the prolactin-regulatory substances of the NIL are different from those identified to date (3,223–225). In addition to disrupting the dopaminergic (THDA) inhibitory effect and the stimulatory effect, removal of the NIL also results in diabetes insipidus (226). Studies have shown that disturbances in water and electrolyte regulation at the level of the neural lobe either surgically or by way of a genetic defect (Brattleboro rat) severely alters prolactin secretion in lactating rats. Bilateral anterior hypothalamic deafferentation behind the optic chiasm interrupting the paraventriculo- and supraoptico-hypophysial tracts (227) or denervation of the neural lobe (228) results in diabetes insipidus and prevent suckling-induced prolactin release in oxytocin-substituted lactating animals. In addition, there is no suckling-induced hormone response in Brattleboro homozygous mothers suffering diabetes insipidus without arginine vasopressin (AVP) treatment (229,230). Passive immunizations against AVP (231) or the glycopeptide moiety (232) of the vasopressin-neurophysin precursor attenuate the suckling-induced rise of plasma prolactin. Although AVP induces prolactin release *in vivo* (233,234), it does not release prolactin *in vitro* (235,236). There are AVP receptors in the rat pituitary (237,238), and AVP is present in high concentration in portal blood (239). Neurophysin-II can stimulate prolactin release but apparently not through a direct effect on the pituitary gland (240). The 39-amino-acid glycopeptide comprising the carboxyterminous of the vasopressin-neurophysin precursor has been reported to stimulate (232), inhibit (241), or have no effect (230) on prolactin release from cultured pituitary cells. Despite these controversial and confusing results, they suggest an important interaction between the regulation of prolactin secretion and the water and sodium homeostasis, particularly during lactation.

Besides the hypothalamo-neurohypophysial vasopressin system, the THDA neuronal system of the hypothalamus (Fig. 5) can be selectively activated by dehydration (91–93). Although the functional role of this dopaminergic system in osmoregulation is largely unknown, recent evidence suggests that the THDA system is an integral part of both water homeostasis and prolactin regulation during lactation: increasing the blood osmolality of lactating rats dramatically reduced prolactin secretion (89). These results are in agreement with the hypothesis that the osmoregulation of the animal and the regulation of prolactin secretion are closely coupled and that a central link between these two systems exists.

An important anatomical feature that affects hypothalamic signal integration in the anterior lobe is the regionalization of blood flow to the anterior pituitary, arriving either from the median eminence via the long portal vessels or from the NIL via the short portal vessels (Fig. 5). At the same time blood drains from the neural lobe via vascular connections to the intermediate lobe and adjacent regions of the anterior lobe (242–244). Thus, two functionally separate parts of the adenohypophysis should be distinguished: the central zone whose blood is supplied by the NIL and the peripheral zone which is supplied by the median eminence. Consonant with this notion, recent experiments have clearly demonstrated that the central zone of the anterior lobe obtained from a lactating rat contains lactotropes that are differentially responsive to the inhibitory action of dopamine (135,245). Moreover, the cells from this region, but not those from the outer zone of the anterior lobe, change their responsiveness to dopamine, TRH, and AII after a 10-minute suckling stimulus (135). A similar regional difference has been demonstrated in the responsiveness of anterior lobe cells to the lactotrope-recruiting action of the estradiol-induced NIL activity (246).

The intermediate lobe consisting of THDA terminals and proopiomelanocortin (POMC)-producing melanocytes supplied by the short portal vessels probably has an integrative role in the regulation of anterior lobe prolactin secretion. Its location is ideal for bringing together hypothalamo-neurohypophysial (dopamine, vasopressin, oxytocin), peripheral (estrogen, gluco-, or mineralocorticoids) and local (VIP, MSH, β-endorphin, and some unknown compounds) factors that signal the lactotropes located exclusively in the inner zone of the anterior pituitary gland.

Local or Intrahypophysial Control

Paracrine interactions between different pituitary cell types have been studied extensively by Denef and colleagues (247). Paracrine interactions with lactotropes have been described for three cell types: gonadotropes (248), folliculostellate cells (249), and corticotropes (250). With respect to gonadotropes, the intimate contacts occurring with lactotropes *in vivo* (251–253) do not seem necessary (247). The agent mediating this effect appears to be AII, released from gonadotropes in response to GnRH treatment (247). The evidence for this is that AII stimulates prolactin release (247,254,255); the effect of AII can be blocked with specific antagonists (256,257); AII receptors have been found on pituitary cells presumably on lactotropes (255,258–260); and AII, as well as the other components necessary to generate AII *in situ,* are localized in gonadotropes (261–265). The physiologic significance of this paracrine regulation of prolactin secretion by gonadotropes is unknown. However, it probably operates *in vivo,* since GnRH has been reported to release prolactin in hypothalamic-lesioned, ovariectomized monkeys (266) and in women during the menstrual cycle (267–269). However, strong objections recently have been raised to the conclusion that AII is the mediator of GnRH-induced prolactin release (270). Thus, the foregoing conclusions must be viewed with caution until these objections are successfully challenged or sustained by further investigation.

Folliculostellate cells (identified as containing S-100 protein) inhibit the secretion of prolactin when they are cultured with lactotropes as cell aggregates (249). The prolactin secretory response to AII and TRH was also inhibited in such coaggregates (249). As observed with paracrine interactions between gonadotropes and lactotropes (247), intimate contacts between lactotropes and folliculostellate cells were not required for this inhibition, since it was still observed after dispersion of the coaggregates into single cells (247). Thus, an inhibitory paracrine factor of folliculostellate cell origin seems indicated, but its identity is unknown.

Prolactin secretion is inhibited by acetylcholine (271) acting at muscarinic receptors (272–274). This acetylcholine probably is produced within the anterior pituitary gland since choline acetyl transferase activity (275) and cholinesterase activity (276) have been detected there. Recently, Carmeliet and Denef (250) have shown that antibodies against choline acetyltransferase stain corticotropes and that perifusion of pituitary cell aggregates with atropine, a potent muscarinic receptor antagonist, resulted in a dose-dependent increase in prolactin release. Extensive further experiments performed by these workers (250) yielded results which were consistent with those cited above. Thus, it appears that corticotropes exert a tonic inhibitory effect on prolactin release which is mediated by acetylcholine acting through a muscarinic receptor (250). The findings of paracrine interactions between lactotropes and other cell types is difficult to place in a physiologic perspective. It seems unlikely that such interactions are important for acute release of prolactin but more likely are involved in chronic changes in prolactin secretion such as that occurring after estrogen treatment.

Autocrine control of prolactin secretion is the latest mode of hormone regulation to be demonstrated in the pituitary gland (194). Vasoactive intestinal peptide, a known hypothalamic, hypophysiotropic stimulator of prolactin release (186,187,191), has also been reported to be synthesized by the anterior pituitary gland (277) and to be present in lactotropes, as assessed by immunocytochemical procedures (278). Recently, Hagen et al. (193) have shown that VIP antiserum, but not another hyperimmune serum, blocked basal (unstimulated) or spontaneous secretion of prolactin *in vitro* and suggested that the high spontaneous rate of prolactin secretion observed in the absence of hypothalamic influence was due to paracrine or autocrine stimulation of prolactin secretion by locally produced VIP. Nagy et al. (194) have shown, using the reverse hemolytic plaque assay for measurement of prolactin secretion by individual lactotropes in which the cells were plated at sufficiently low density to preclude paracrine interactions, that VIP antiserum or a VIP antagonist would indeed suppress prolactin secretion by about 65–70%. Hence, autocrine control of prolactin secretion by VIP was demonstrated. Thus, this endocrinologically unprecedented conclusion suggests that the peculiar ability of lactotropes to secrete prolactin spontaneously at a high rate may be due to a positive feedback if VIP can be shown to stimulate its own secretion simultaneously with prolactin, i.e., if VIP is packaged and secreted in prolactin-secretory granules. The action of dopamine to suppress prolactin secretion, therefore, would occur either by way of antagonizing the stimulatory effect of VIP or by inhibiting VIP secretion, or both. Vasoactive intestinal peptide, thus, is both an autocrine and an endocrine (secretion by the hypothalamus and delivery to the pituitary gland by way of hypophysial portal blood) stimulator of prolactin secretion (194).

More recent investigations have cast doubt on an autocrine regulatory role for VIP in prolactin secretion. Several investigators have reported difficulty detecting VIP in lactotropes immunocytochemically (279–281). Further work will be required to assess the significance of these negative reports given the extensive and well-controlled nature of the experiments in which an autocrine role for VIP was reported initially (194). An attractive possibility raised by Kasper et al. (283) is that a different but VIP-related peptide may be synthesized by the pituitary gland. If so, much of the discrepancy among various studies of an autocrine effect for VIP might disappear.

The discovery of paracrine (247) and autocrine (194) regulatory mechanisms for prolactin secretion raises the interesting question of whether substances other than AII, VIP, and acetylcholine will be found to act in similar manners. Numerous other peptides have been described as residing in anterior pituitary cells (247,284); there is reason to believe that these peptides are synthesized locally rather than being taken up after delivery in the portal circulation. These peptides include: substance P (285–287), neurotensin (285,288), GnRH (289,290), TRH (291), corticotropin-releasing factor (292), GRF (293), somatostatin (294), gastrin (295), secretin (296), peptides of the proenkephalin A and B families (297–299), and vasopressin (300). It probably is significant that a majority of the members on this list have been described as stimulating prolactin secretion by a direct action on the pituitary gland (235,301–309) but were considered PRF candidates. Such peptides may be shown to play paracrine or autocrine regulatory roles in prolactin secretion and, if so, will confirm an earlier prediction (3) that lactotropes show a regulatory complexity commonly accorded only to neurons and cells of the immune system.

Adrenal Cortical Control

A rarely discussed aspect of the inhibitory influences on adenohypophysial prolactin secretion is the adrenal gland. It is well known that in rats, plasma levels of prolactin increase significantly after adrenalectomy (310–313), whereas the effect of adrenalectomy can be reversed by administration of corticosteroids. Similarly, adrenalectomy enhanced and the synthetic glucocorticoid dexamethasone (DEX) decreased prolactin release manifested in acute stress (314–316) and after TRH treatment (317). Moreover, consistently high levels of plasma prolactin have been found throughout the entire lactation period (318), and a significantly higher plasma prolactin response to haloperidol, a dopamine receptor blocker, could be detected in adrenalectomized lactating mothers (319). Dexamethasone pretreatment of lactating rats (injected twice, 24 hours and 2 hours prior to testing) completely blocked suckling-induced prolactin release (320). This effect is a transient one because it could not be detected 24 hours later. In contrast to the dramatic effect on the suckling-induced prolactin response, DEX does not inhibit domperiodone (another dopamine receptor blocker)-induced pituitary prolactin release, indicating that DEX cannot interfere with the antagonist binding and its effect at the level of dopamine receptor of lactotropes. When it is implanted into the mediobasal hypothalamus (320), DEX suppresses prolactin release induced by suckling. These data indicate that the site of action of adrenal steroids is a region of the mediobasal hypothalamus. In summary, it can be assumed that the regulatory pathway mediating neurogenic stimuli (suckling or stress)-induced prolactin release is extremely sensitive to a glucocorticoid inhibitory mechanism and that the adrenal glands provide a physiologically important signal to the hypothalamo-hypophysial regulatory mechanisms of prolactin secretion.

CELL AND MOLECULAR MECHANISMS IN THE CONTROL OF PROLACTIN SECRETION

Lactotropes synthesize, package, and release prolactin by standard mechanisms for all cells that show regulated secretion (321). Indeed, lactotropes are frequently used as the prototype for secretion by adenohypophysial cells (322). The main steps in the synthesis/secretory cycle are: (a) transcription of the prolactin gene into RNA; (b) processing of this pre-RNA within the nucleus into mature mRNA; (c) translocation of the mRNA to the cytoplasm; (d) attachment of the mRNA to ribosomes and translation into preprolactin; (e) discharge into the lumen of the rough endoplasmic reticulum, during which the leader sequence of preprolactin is removed; (f) concentration and packaging of prolactin into secretory granules surrounded by membranes within the Golgi apparatus; (g) storage of prolactin in secretory granules; and (h) movement of the secretory granules into the cortical cytoplasm and extracellular discharge by exocytosis.

Synthesis (steps a–g) and release (step h) are distinct processes that can be experimentally separated (323,324); that is, the physiologically relevant secretagogues that evoke prolactin secretion (TRH, VIP, and dopamine) affect both processes, probably by way of the same second messenger, acting in the cytoplasm on release of stored hormone on the one hand but acting in the nucleus to alter synthesis of prolactin on the other (325,326). Receptors for TRH (327), VIP (328), and dopamine (73,329) have been molecularly cloned, sequenced, and shown to be members of the 7-transmembrane family of receptors; upon binding to their ligands, they generate second messengers such as cAMP, calcium, and members of the phosphoinositide family.

The GH_3 clonal cell line frequently is used for studies of the cellular mechanisms in the control of prolactin secretion (149). This cell line was derived originally from an estrogen-induced pituitary tumor and repeatedly cloned to produce a theoretically homogeneous group of cells (149). Thus, it offers advantages over pituitary lactotropes that are always mixed with other pituitary cell types even after cell purification. The GH_3 cell line has a number of disadvantages, however. It does not respond to dopamine (149), it may not be as functionally homogeneous as originally believed (330), it secretes both growth hormone and prolactin, and it stores only small amounts of hormone in the cytoplasm in organelles that are more vesicular than granular (149). Nevertheless, several important functional characteristics of pituitary lactotopes were discovered originally in this cell line (149).

Thyrotropin-Releasing Hormone

As a general statement, it can be said that cytoplasmic Ca^{2+} is the primary direct second messenger regulating prolactin secretion by lactotropes, with cAMP-dependent or PKC-mediated pathways serving to modulate Ca^{2+}-dependent steps (Fig. 6). Despite its problematic role as a physiologic regulator of prolactin secretion (*vide supra*), TRH's mechanism of action is the best studied among prolactin secretagogues (324,331). TRH stimulation of prolactin secretion occurs in two phases, both of which are mediated by signals derived from TRH-receptor-activated PLC activation (331–333) (Fig. 6). The initial, short-lived secretory response, during which prolactin secretion rates are markedly elevated, is caused by an inositol-1,4,5-triphosphate-induced rise in the cytoplasm, the effects of which are potentiated by the simultaneous activation of PKC brought about by 1,2-diacylglycerol (DAG) (324,334,335). The sustained secondary secretory response, where prolactin secretory rates are increased two- to fourfold, is stimulated by the increased entry of Ca^{2+} through voltage-dependent Ca^{2+} channels and the enhanced responsiveness of the secretory apparatus to Ca^{2+}; the latter process probably is activated by the previous period of kinase C activation (336,337).

The G-proteins mediating the effects of TRH on prolactin secretion only recently have been identified (338–341) (see Fig. 6). Such G-proteins have been known for some time not to be sensitive to cholera toxin or pertussis toxin (324,331). TRH receptors stimulate PLC activity by a mechanism that utilizes a G_{q11} protein (338–341). Hsieh and Martin (338) demonstrated that antibodies to this class of recently identified G-proteins reacted with unique 42 kDa $G_{q\alpha}$ and 43 kDa $G_{11\alpha}$ proteins in membranes of TRH-responsive GH_3 cells; 42 kDa and 43 kDa are the established molecular masses of $G_{q\alpha}$ and $G_{\alpha 11}$, respectively (340,342,343). Moreover, the antibody immunodepleted the G-protein activity of GH_3 cell membrane extracts measured by reconstitution of the guanine nucleotide regulation of PLC (338). Finally, the antibody was shown to inhibit TRH-stimulated PLC activity measured in the membranes of GH_3 cells (338). Thus, TRH activation of PLC leading to prolactin release (see Fig. 6) appears to require coupling to a G-protein which corresponds to G_q, G_{11}, or both.

Vasoactive Intestinal Peptide

As described earlier, VIP is an autocrine or paracrine stimulator of the apparent "spontaneous" prolactin secretion that is peculiar to lactotropes, but it also acts as a hypothalamic, hypophysiotropic stimulator of prolactin release (*vide supra*). VIP stimulates anterior pituitary adenylyl cyclase and production of cAMP (324) (see Fig. 5). Stimulatory mechanisms in lactotropes mediated through adenylyl cyclase activation are less well understood than those for phospholipase C activation. However, the involvement of a G_s-protein in VIP-stimulated adenylyl cyclase activation is well established (324,331). VIP stimulation of prolactin secretion is slower in onset than that for TRH, probably due to the relatively slow initiation of cAMP accumulation (331). Cyclic AMP stimulation of prolactin secretion probably is mediated through a combination of mechanisms involving stimulated influx of Ca^{2+} (344) and an increased responsiveness of the secretory apparatus to Ca^{2+} (345).

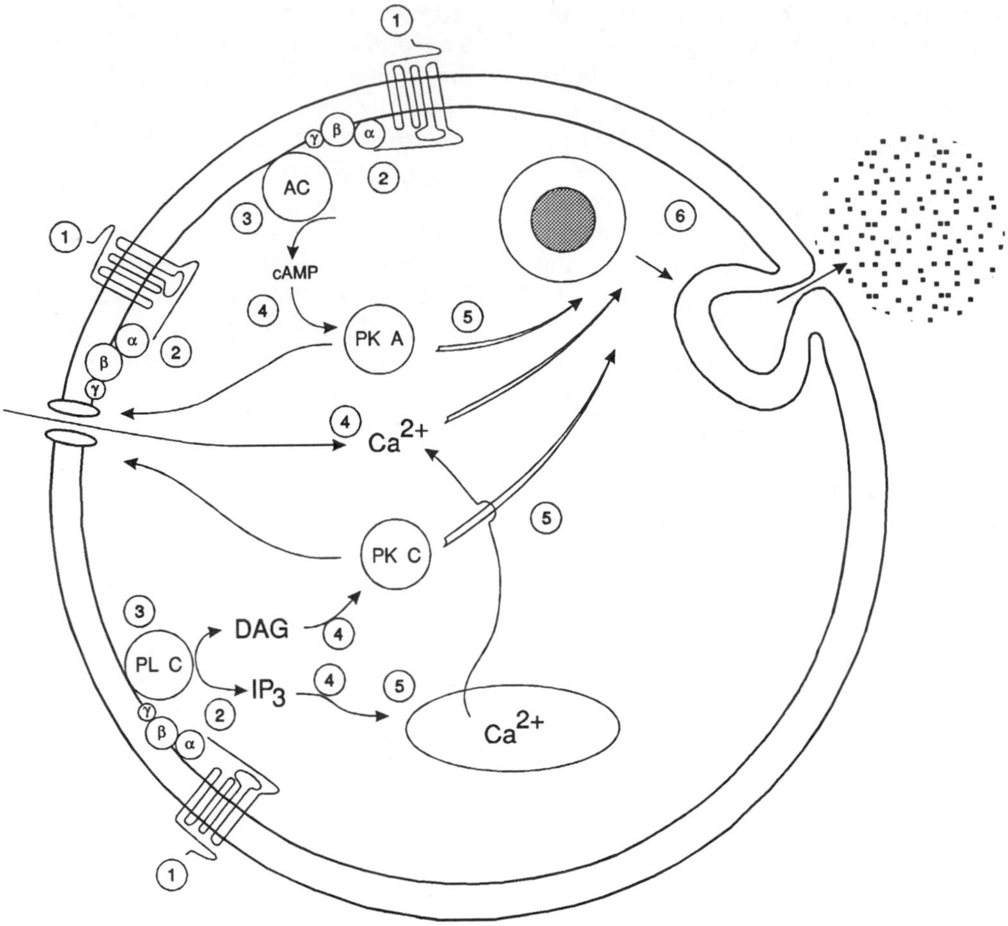

FIG. 6. Schematic summary of signal transduction pathways leading to the regulation of prolactin exocytosis by thyrotropin-releasing hormone (TRH), vasoactive intestinal peptide (VIP), and dopamine. 7-transmembrane receptors (1); G-proteins composed of α, β, and γ subunits (2); transduction mechanisms including activation of adenylyl cyclase (AC) or phospholipase C (PLC) (3); second messenger molecules such as cyclic AMP (cAMP), inositol triphosphate (IP_3), and diacylglycerol (DAG) (4); activation of protein kinase A (PKA), protein kinase C (PKC), or enhanced influx of Ca^{2+} through cell membrane channels (5); exocytosis (6). **Top:** Receptor-G-protein regulated AC and cAMP generation result in activation of PKA that may alter Ca^{2+} channel function or modulate a component of the exocytic apparatus. **Center:** Receptor-G-protein regulated ion channel function that regulates Ca^{2+} influx. **Bottom:** Receptor-G-protein regulated PLC that hydrolyzes phosphoinositides and generates two second messengers, IP_3 and DAG. DAG is an activator of PKC that may regulate Ca^{2+} channel function or modulate a component of the exocytotic apparatus. IP_3 triggers Ca^{2+} mobilization from an intracellular, nonmitochondrial pool. Redrawn from Martin (331).

Dopamine

Dopamine as the physiologically relevant PIF suppresses both the synthesis and release of prolactin by hypophysial lactotropes (*vide supra*). Its mechanisms for exerting these actions are incompletely known due to the absence of convenient model systems for study; that is, as noted earlier, the GH cell lines do not express the dopamine receptor, and purification of pituitary cell types does not easily lead to pure lactotrope populations. Nevertheless, inhibitory coupling of dopamine D_2 receptors to adenylyl cyclase mediated by G_i proteins has been demonstrated (324,331,346). Dopamine also lowers cytoplasmic Ca^{2+} levels in lactotropes by decreasing Ca^{2+} influx (347). Moreover, activation of K^+ channels by the dopamine receptor-G protein complex affects action potential generation and duration which results in reduced Ca^{2+} entry (346). Direct inhibition of Ca^{2+} channel activity by the dopamine-receptor–G-protein complex also may occur (348). Further evidence that dopamine suppresses both cytoplasmic Ca^{2+} levels and generation of cAMP is the observation that the inhibitory effects of dopamine on prolactin secretion are reversed by combined but not individual treatment with agents that increase cAMP and cytoplasmic Ca^{2+} (349).

The mechanism of dopaminergic inhibition of cytoplasmic Ca^{2+} levels remains unclarified. Linden and Delahunty (350) have proposed dual regulation of PLC by way of inhibitory and stimulatory G-proteins by analogy with the established dual mode of adenylyl cyclase regulation by G_s and G_i proteins. Further work will be required to support this hypothesis.

EXTRAHYPOPHYSIAL SOURCES OF PROLACTIN

A prolactin-related protein is produced in many mammalian tissues including the brain, uterus, placenta, and cells of the immune system. Members of this family of protein hormones show structural and immunological similarities with pituitary prolactin. The physiological functions of these prolactins are not known in most cases. Thus, our discussion of them will be limited to the available evidence for their specific production by different tissues, with some speculations as to their physiological functions.

Brain

A prolactin-like molecule was first demonstrated to be present in nerve terminals of the rat hypothalamus using immunocytochemistry more than 15 years ago (351). This observation subsequently was confirmed by several investigators (352–360). Furthermore, early studies had shown that prolactin immunoreactivity could still be detected in the brain of hypophysectomized rats (351,354,361–363), suggesting that it was not of pituitary origin. Schachter et al. (364) provided definitive evidence that hypothalamic prolactin represents a synthetic pool different from that of the anterior pituitary. These authors (364) showed the existence of prolactin message (mRNA) in neuronal elements. More recently, Emanuele et al. (365) confirmed this finding using the highly sensitive polymerase chain reaction (PCR) method. They also provided evidence for the existence of prolactin message in extrahypothalamic brain areas as well: cerebellum, caudate nucleus, brain stem, amygdala, thalamus, cortex, and hippocampus were all positive but other organs such as lung and liver were negative (365). The concentration of immunoreactive prolactin in the central nervous system is 10^4–10^6 times lower, depending on the region, than that in the pituitary gland. The demonstration that colchicine treatment, which blocks axoplasmatic transport, results in a significant increase of prolactin levels in the hypothalamus but not in other regions of the brain (366), and reports describing prolactin containing perikarya only in the hypothalamus (356,358,360,361,367,368), suggest the existence of a hypothalamic prolactinergic neuronal system projecting to different areas of the brain. It also has been shown recently that not only is hypothalamic prolactin synthesized independently of the pituitary gland but that its gene expression is also regulated differently from that in the pituitary gland (365,369).

The potential neuromodulatory role of hypothalamic prolactin is supported by the findings that prolactin is present largely in nerve terminals within secretory granules (354–356). Moreover, immunoreactive prolactin is released from hypothalamic fragments *in vitro* in a calcium-dependent manner (363). Specific binding sites for prolactin also were demonstrated in rat and rabbit brain (370–372). The most direct action of prolactin on neuronal tissues has been demonstrated on the turnover of hypothalamic dopamine (373,374) and the release of several neuropeptides (374–377), and influences on maternal (378–380) and several other animal behaviors (381).

Uteroplacental Unit

In rodents and some other species, the uteroplacental unit produces several prolactin-related proteins. Each of these proteins is expressed in a cell-and-temporally-specific manner. In the rat, eight different members of the prolactin family have been identified.

Decidualized stromal cells of the uterus produce a luteotrophin (LTH). The search for such a factor was initiated by the experiments of Rothchild and coworkers (382,383) who observed that progesterone production in pseudopregnant rats could be maintained after complete inhibition of anterior pituitary prolactin secretion if the uterine stroma was already decidualized. Production of rat LTH starts a few days after implantation and is restricted to the decidua capsularis (384). A prolactin-like protein-B (PLP-B) was also found to be expressed in decidual tissue of the pregnant and pseudopregnant rat. The complementary DNA of PLP-B has been cloned, and studies are in progress to determine whether decidual LTH and PLP-B are the same protein (385).

Decidual prolactin also has been found in humans (386,387). It is identical to pituitary prolactin (388,389). The protein coding sequence of the decidual prolactin cDNA is identical to the pituitary prolactin message (16,390), but its mRNA, similar to the message found in IM-9-P3 cell line, is elongated at the 5′-untranslated segment relative to the pituitary transcript (16,390). Differentiation of uterine decidua is dependent on ovarian hormones (progesterone and estrogen) (391,392). Therefore, it is not surprising that progesterone and relaxin have been demonstrated to be able to regulate human decidual prolactin expression (392,393) as well.

The placenta of many species of mammals synthesizes and releases different lactogens, called *placental lactogens* (PLs). Initiation of the search for such proteins from the placenta was the observation that hypophysectomy of rats and mice was ineffective at terminating pregnancy when it was performed after midgestation (394–399). Mammary glands could still develop and secrete milk in the absence of the anterior pituitary. Subsequent studies led to the isolation, purification, and characterization of multiple PLs (400–405). Interestingly, some members of this family showed lactogenic properties (PL-I and PL-II), but not others (PLP-A, PLP-B, PLP-C, and PLP-IV). The temporal patterns of expression of PL-I and PL-II are in agreement with their lactogenic function, since they start to be produced by the trophoblast giant cells near midpregnancy, when maternal pituitary prolactin secretion dramatically decreases (406–408). PLP-A, PLP-B, PLP-C, and PL-IV are structural analogs of pituitary prolactin and they are produced by both giant cells and spongiotrophoblasts, but their biological actions are not yet determined. Recent progress in the molecular cloning of each of the six PLs' cDNAs from rat (409–414) may accelerate this research. Their putative targets in the mother are the mammary gland, the ovary, the uterus, the liver, and the immune system. In the fetus, their functions may be an important part of the trophoblast-fetal signaling system (at least in sheep and humans) (415,416), which includes effects on liver, on muscle cell differentiation, and on regulation of water and ion transfer (417–419).

Lymphocytes

Experimental evidence clearly has demonstrated that normal (420,421) as well as malignant cells (422,423) of the immune system produce a prolactin-like peptide. First, Montgomery and coworkers (424) observed an increase in bioactive prolactin in the medium of cultured mouse splenocytes following stimulation with concanavalin A. They also found that an antiserum against prolactin prevented Nb2 cell proliferation induced by the supernates obtained from concanavalin-A-pretreated cultures of splenocytes (424). Subsequently, prolactin was detected by immunocytochemistry in one-third of the cultured splenocytes (425) and the proportion of them doubled after concanavalin A stimulation. These observations were confirmed and extended by Hartmann et al. (420), who found that although prolactin itself could not stimulate lymphocyte proliferation, antibodies against prolactin potently inhibited both murine and human lymphocyte proliferation in response to both T and B cell mitogens. Furthermore, they demonstrated that the same antiprolactin antibodies specifically inhibited the proliferative response to several cytokine growth factors (IL-2 and IL-4) (420). These data are in agreement with previous reports that prolactin acts as a comitogen for lymphocytes *in vitro* (426,427) and it is a direct mitogen for the Nb2 node lymphoma cell line (428), as well as for normal lymphocytes from ovariectomized (429) and hypophysectomized (430) rats. The synthesis and release of prolactin by a human B lymphoblastoid cell line (IM-9-P) also has been demonstrated (422,423). Therefore these cells, like the Nb2 cell line and normal lymphocytes, appear to require a prolactin-like protein for growth.

The active synthesis of prolactin by human peripheral blood mononuclear cells recently has been demonstrated (421). A 276-bp prolactin PCR product from these mononuclear cells could be generated, which is similar to the prolactin PCR product generated from human placental cDNA. Cell extracts and supernates from these cells contain a protein that is antigenically similar to pituitary-derived prolactin (421). Using a highly sensitive and specific hormonal enzyme-linked immunoplaque assay, Sabharwal et al. (421) detected for the first time prolactin secretion from human individual peripheral blood mononuclear cells after stimulation with mitogens. It also has been reported that normal human thymocytes and peripheral blood lymphocytes synthesize bioactive prolactin similar in sizes to those produced by the pituitary gland (431). The principal form of prolactin produced by thymocytes is 24 kDa in molecular size, while peripheral blood lymphocytes produce a 27-kDa variant. This kind of size heterogeneity is not unusual because it is found to occur in human pituitary and decidual prolactins (*vide supra*); the predominant form in human pituitary and serum is 23 kDa.

Regarding the potential functions of prolactin produced by cells of the immune system, it is important to note that normal lymphocytes also express the prolactin receptor (432–436). Therefore, it is not surprising that prolactin produced by normal and tumoral immune cells is thought to mediate an autocrine or paracrine growth effect (421,436). In most cases, a mitogen stimulus is obligatory for turning on this autocrine loop. It is important to note that prolactin receptors (437–439) belong to the hemopoietin receptor family (440). This family includes receptors for granulocyte colony-stimulating factor, granulocyte-macrophage colony-stimulating factor, erythropoietin, IL-2, IL-3, IL-4, IL-5, IL-6, IL-6 receptor-associated glycoprotein, and IL-7 (440,441). All of these receptors mediate powerful immunomodulatory and growth-promoting actions on lymphocytes. Based on the structural similarities between prolactin receptors and IL receptors, it seems reasonable to conclude that prolactin receptors on lymphocytes mediate similar messages.

Prolactin may play a pivotal role in the regulation of the humoral and cellular immune systems. The first indications that prolactin might play such a role came from studies showing that hypophysectomy resulted in a severe immunodeficiency which could be restored by the substitution of prolactin (442–444). More recently, it was reported that hypophysectomized rats depend on residual prolactin (from lymphocytes? from regenerating pars tuberalis?) for survival (445). When hypophysectomized rats were constantly treated with antiprolactin antiserum, a severe anemia developed and all animals died within 6 weeks. It is obvious that pituitary prolactin itself has a very significant immunoregulatory role, but why two sources of prolactin appear to be necessary for immunocompetence remains unclear. Further work is required to elucidate this issue.

REFERENCES

1. Nicoll CS. Endocrinology: physiological actions of prolactin. In: Knobil E, Sawyer WH, eds. *Handbook of physiology,* vol 4, sect 7. Washington, DC: American Physiological Society; 1974:253–292.
2. De Vlaming VL. Actions of prolactin among vertebrates. In: Barrington EJW, ed. *Hormones and evolution.* New York: Academic Press; 1979:561–642.
3. Leong DA, Frawley SL, Neill JD. Neuroendocrine control of prolactin secretion. *Annu Rev Physiol* 1983;45:109–127.
4. Freeman ME. The ovarian cycle of the rat. In: Knobil E, Neill JD, eds. *The physiology of reproduction.* New York: Raven Press; 1988:1893–1928.
5. Nicoll CS, Mayer GL, Russell SM. Structural features of prolactins and growth hormones that can be related to their biological properties. *Endocr Rev* 1986;7:169–203.
6. Li CH, Dixon JS, Lo TB, Schmidt KD, Pankov YA. Studies on pituitary lactogenic hormone: 30. the primary structure of the sheep hormone. *Arch Biochem Biophys* 1970;141:705–737.
7. Li CH. Studies on pituitary lactogenic hormone: the primary structure of the porcine hormone. *Int J Pept Protein Res* 1976;8:205–224.
8. Li CH. Endocrinology: chemistry of ovine prolactin. In: Knobil E, Sawyer WH, eds. *Handbook of physiology,* vol 4, sect 7. Washington, DC: American Physiological Society; 1974:103–110.
9. Wallis M. The primary structure of bovine prolactin. *FEBS Lett* 1974;44:205–208.
10. Shome B, Parlow AF. Human pituitary prolactin (hPRL): the entire linear amino acid sequence. *J Clin Endocrinol Metab* 1977;45:1112–1115.
11. Kohmoto K, Tsunasawa S, Sakiyama F. Complete amino acid sequence of mouse prolactin. *Eur J Biochem* 1984;138:227–237.
12. Cooke NE, Coit D, Weiner RI, Baxter JD, Martial JA. Structure of cloned DNA complementary to rat prolactin messenger RNA. *J Biol Chem* 1980;255:6502–6510.
13. Cooke NE, Coit D, Shine J, Baxter JD, Martial JA. Human prolactin cDNA structural analysis and evolutionary comparisons. *J Biol Chem* 1981;256:4007–4016.
14. Chien YH, Thompson BE. Genomic organization of rat prolactin and growth hormone genes. *Proc Natl Acad Sci USA* 1980;77:4583–4587.
15. Truong AT, Duez C, Belayew A, Renard A, Pictet R, Bell GI, Martial JA. Isolation and characterization of the human prolactin gene. *EMBO J* 1984;3:429–437.
16. DiMattia GE, Gellersen B, Duckworth ML, Friesen HG. Human prolactin gene expression: the use of an alternative non-coding exon in decidua and the IM-9-P3 lymphoblast cell line. *J Biol Chem* 1990;265:16412–16421.
17. Hiraoka Y, Tatsumi K, Shiozawa M, Aiso S, Fukasaua T, Yasuda K, Miyai K. A placenta-specific 5′ non-coding exon of human prolactin. *Mol Cell Endocrinol* 1991;75:71–80.
18. Owerbach D, Rutter WJ, Cooke NE, Martial JA, Shows TB. The prolactin gene is located on chromosome 6 in humans. *Science* 1981;212:815–816.
19. Miller WL, Eberhardt NI. Structure and evolution of the growth hormone gene family. *Endocr Rev* 1983;4:97–130.
20. Sinha YN. Prolactin variants. *Trends Endocrinol Metab* 1992;3:100–106.
21. Sinha YN. Structural variants of prolactin. In: Yoshimura F, Gorbman A, eds. *Pars distalis of the pituitary gland: structure, function and regulation.* Amsterdam: Elsevier; 1986:399–412.
22. Sinha YN, Jacobsen BP. Structural and immunologic evidence for a small molecular weight ("21K") variant of prolactin. *Endocrinology* 1988;123:1364–1370.
23. Lewis UJ, Markoff E, Culler FL, Hayek A, VanderLaan WP. Biologic properties of the 20K-dalton variant of human growth hormone: a review. *Endocrinol Jpn* 1987;34[Suppl 1]:73–85.
24. Sinha YN, Gilligan TA, Lee DW, Hollingsworth D, Markoff E. Cleaved prolactin: evidence for its occurrence in human pituitary gland and plasma. *J Clin Endocrinol Metab* 1985;60:239–243.
25. Sinha YN, Klemcke HG, Maurer RR, Jacobsen B. Ontogeny of glycosylated and nonglycosylated forms of prolactin and growth hormone in porcine pituitary during fetal life. *Proc Soc Exp Biol Med* 1990;194:293–300.
26. Sinha YN, Gilligan TA. Identification and partial characterization of a 25K prolactin structurally similar to prolactin. *Proc Soc Exp Biol Med* 1985;178:505–514.
27. Hampson RK, Rottman FM. Alternative processing of bovine growth hormone mRNA: nonsplicing of the final intron predicts a high molecular weight variant of bovine growth hormone. *Proc Natl Acad Sci USA* 1987;84:2673–2677.
28. Cooks NE, Ray J, Emery JG, Liebhaber SA. Two distinct species of human growth hormone-variant mRNA in the human placenta predict the expression of novel growth hormone proteins. *J Biol Chem* 1988;263:9001–9006.
29. Oetting WS, Ho TWC, Greenan JR, Walker AM. Production and secretion of the 21–23.5 kDa prolactin-like molecules. *Mol Cell Endocrinol* 1989;61:189–199.
30. Mittra I. A novel "cleaved prolactin" in the rat pituitary. I. biosynthesis, characterization and regulatory control. *Biochem Biophys Res Commun* 1980;95:1750–1759.
31. Clapp C. Analysis of the proteolytic cleavage of prolactin by the mammary gland and liver of the rat: characterization of the cleaved and 16K forms. *Endocrinology* 1987;121:2055–2064.
32. Clapp C, Sears PS, Russell DH, Richards J, Levay-Young BK, Nicoll CS. Biological and immunological characterization of cleaved and 16K forms of rat prolactin. *Endocrinology* 1988;122:2892–2898.
33. Vick RS, Wong VLY, Witorsch RJ. Biological, immunological, and biochemical characterization of cleaved prolactin generated by lactating mammary gland. *Biochem Biophys Acta* 1987;931:196–204.
34. Lewis UJ, Singh RNP, Lewis LJ, Seavey BK, Sinha YN. Glycosylated ovine prolactin. *Proc Natl Acad Sci USA* 1984;81:385–389.
35. Lewis UJ, Singh RNP, Sinha YN, VanderLaan WP. Glycosylated human prolactin. *Endocrinology* 1985;116:359–363.
36. Lewis UJ, Singh RNP, Lewis LJ. Two forms of glycosylated human prolactin have different pigeon crop sac-stimulating activities. *Endocrinology* 1989;124:1558–1563.
37. Pankov YuA, Butnev VYu. Multiple forms of pituitary prolactin: a glycosylated form of porcine prolactin with enhanced biological activity. *Int J Peptide Protein Res* 1986;28:113–123.
38. Sinha YN, Jacobsen BP. Glycosylated prolactin in the murine pituitary: detection by a novel assay and alteration of concentrations by physiological and pharmacological stimuli. *Biochem Biophys Res Commun* 1987;148:505–514.
39. Oetting WAS, Tuazon PT, Traugh JA, Walker AM. Phosphorylation of prolactin. *J Biol Chem* 1986;261:1649–1652.
40. Brooks CL, Kim BG, Aphale P, Kleeman BE, Johnson GC. Phosphorylated variant of bovine prolactin. *Mol Cell Endocrinol* 1990;71:117–123.
41. Krown K, Wang YF, Ho TWC, Kelly PA, Walker AM. Prolactin isoform 2 as an autocrine growth factor for GH_3 cells. *Endocrinology* 1992;131:595–602.
42. Kohli R, Chadha N, Muralidhar K. Are sheep and buffalo prolactins sulfated? *Biochem Biophys Res Commun* 1987;149:515–522.
43. Subramanian MG, Gala RR. Do prolactin levels measured by RIA reflect biologically active prolactin? *J Clin Immunoassay* 1986;9:42–52.
44. Harris GW. *Neural control of the pituitary gland.* London: Edward Arnold; 1955.
45. Everett JW. Luteotropic function of autografts of the rat hypophysis. *Endocrinology* 1954;54:685–690.
46. Everett JW. Functional corpora lutea maintained for months by autografts of rat hypophysis. *Endocrinology* 1956;58:786–796.

47. Pasteels JL. Secretion de prolactine par l'hypophyse en culture de tissus. *CR Acad Sci Ser D* 1961;253:2140–2142.
48. Pasteels JL. Recherches morphologiques et experimentales sur la sécrétion de prolactine. *Arch Biol* 1963;74:439–553.
49. Meites J, Nicoll CS, Talwalker PK. The central nervous system and the secretion and release of prolactin. In: Nalbandov AV, ed. *Advances in neuroendocrinology.* Urbana: University of Illinois Press; 1963:238–288.
50. Talwalker PK, Ratner A, Meites J. *In vitro* inhibition of pituitary prolactin synthesis and release by hypothalamic extract. *Am J Physiol* 1963;205:213–218.
51. Barraclough CA, Sawyer CH. Induction of pseudopregnancy in the rat by reserpine and chlorpromazine. *Endocrinology* 1959;65:563–571.
52. Kanematsu S, Hillard J, Sawyer CH. Effect of reserpine on pituitary prolactin content and its hypothalamic site of action in the rabbit. *Acta Endocrinol* 1963;44:467–474.
53. Coppola JA, Leonardi RG, Lippman W, Perrine JW, Ringler I. Induction of pseudopregnancy in rats by depletors of endogenous catecholamines. *Endocrinology* 1965;77:485–490.
54. Coppola JA. The apparent involvement of the sympathetic nervous system in the gonadotropin secretion of female rats. *J Reprod Fertil* 1986;4[Suppl]:35–45.
55. Fuxe K. The distribution of monoamine terminals in central nervous system. *Acta Physiol Scand* 1965;247[Suppl]:39–85.
56. MacLeod RM. Influence of norepinephrine and catecholamine-depleting agents on the synthesis and release of prolactin and growth hormone. *Endocrinology* 1969;85:916–923.
57. Birge CA, Jacobs LS, Hammer CT, Daughaday WH. Catecholamine inhibition of prolactin secretion by isolated rat adenohypophyses. *Endocrinology* 1970;86:120–130.
58. MacLeod RM. Regulation of prolactin secretion. In: Martini L, Ganong WF, eds. *Frontiers in neuroendocrinology,* vol 4. New York: Raven Press; 1976:169–194.
59. Neill JD. Endocrinology: prolactin: its secretion and control. In: Knobil E, Sawyer WH, eds. *Handbook of Physiology,* vol 4. Washington, DC: American Physiological Society; 1974;2:469–88.
60. Neill JD. Neuroendocrine regulation of prolactin secretion. In: Martini L, Ganong WF, eds. *Frontiers in neuroendocrinology,* vol 6. New York: Raven Press; 1980:129–55.
61. Bishop N, Fawcett CP, Krulich L, McCann SM. Acute and chronic effects of hypothalamic lesions on the release of FSH, LH and prolactin in intact and castrated rats. *Endocrinology* 1972;91:643–656.
62. Arimura A, Dunn JD, Schally AV. Effect of infusion of hypothalamic extracts on serum prolactin levels in rats treated with nembutal, CNS depressants or bearing hypothalamic lesions. *Endocrinology* 1972;90:378–383.
63. Kanematsu S, Sawyer CH. Elevation of plasma prolactin after hypophysial stalk section in the rat. *Endocrinology* 1973;93: 238–241.
64. Langer G, Ferin M, Sachar E. Effect of haloperidol and L-dopa on plasma prolactin in stalk-sectioned and intact monkeys. *Endocrinology* 1978;102:367–370.
65. Shaar CJ, Clemens JA. The role of catecholamines in the release of anterior pituitary prolactin *in vitro. Endocrinology* 1974;95:1202–1212.
66. Ben-Jonathan N, Oliver C, Weiner HJ, Mical RS, Porter JC. Dopamine in hypophysial portal plasma of the rat during the estrous cycle and throughout pregnancy. *Endocrinology* 1977;100: 452–458.
67. Gibbs DM, Neill JD. Dopamine levels in hypophysial stalk blood in the rat are sufficient to inhibit prolactin secretion *in vivo. Endocrinology* 1978;102:1895–1900.
68. Plotsky PM, Gibbs DM, Neill JD. Liquid chromatographic-electrochemical measurement of dopamine in hypophysial stalk blood of rats. *Endocrinology* 1978;102:1887–1894.
69. Brown GM, Seeman P, Lee T. Dopamine/neuroleptic receptors in basal hypothalamus and pituitary. *Endocrinology* 1976;99: 1407–1416.
70. Creese IR, Schneider P, Snyder SH. ^{3}H-spiroperidol labels dopamine receptors in pituitary and brain. *Eur J Pharmacol* 1977;46:377–381.
71. Goldsmith PC, Cronin MJ, Weiner RI. Dopamine receptor sites in the anterior pituitary. *J Histochem Cytochem* 1979;27: 1205–1207.
72. Caron MG, Amlaiky N, Kilpatrick BF. D_2-dopamine receptor: biochemical characterization. In: Ganong WF, Martini L, eds. *Frontiers in neuroendocrinology,* vol 6. New York: Raven Press; 1986:205–224.
73. Bunzow JR, Van Tol HHM, Grandy DK, Albert P, Salon J, Christie M, Machida CA, Neve KA, Civelli O. Cloning and expression of a rat D_2 dopamine receptor cDNA. *Nature* 1988;336:783–787.
74. De Greef WJ, Neill JD. Dopamine levels in hypophysial stalk plasma of the rat during surges of prolactin secretion induced by cervical stimulation. *Endocrinology* 1979;105:1093–1099.
75. Leong DA. Regulation of suckling-induced prolactin (PRL) release in the lactating rat: the role of hypophysiotropic dopamine (DA). *Program of the fifteenth annual meeting of the Society for the Study of Reproduction.* Madison, Wisconsin, 1982:(abst 44).
76. Ben-Jonathan N, Oliver C, Weiner HJ, Mical RS, Porter JC. Dopamine in hypophysial portal plasma of the rat during the estrous cycle and throughout pregnancy. *Endocrinology* 1977;100: 452–458.
77. Demarest KT, McKay DW, Riegle GD, Moore KE. Sexual differences in tuberoinfundibular dopamine nerve activity induced by neonatal androgen exposure. *Neuroendocrinology* 1981;32: 108–113.
78. Gudelsky GA, Porter JC. Sex-related difference in the release of dopamine into hypophysial portal blood. *Endocrinology* 1981;109:1394–1398.
79. De Greef WJ, Plotsky PM, Neill JD. Dopamine levels in hypophysial stalk plasma and prolactin levels in peripheral plasma of the lactating rat: effects of a simulated suckling stimulus. *Neuroendocrinology* 1981;32:229–233.
80. Plotsky PM, Neill JD. The decrease in hypothalamic dopamine secretion induced by suckling: comparison of voltametric and radioisotopic methods of measurement. *Endocrinology* 1982; 110:691–696.
81. Plotsky PM, de Greef WJ, Neill JD. *In situ* voltametric microelectrodes: application to the measurement of the median eminence catecholamine release during simulated suckling. *Brain Research* 1982;250:251–262.
82. Ben-Jonathan N. Catecholamines and pituitary prolactin release. *J Reprod Fertil* 1980;58:501–512.
83. Ben-Jonathan N, Peters LL. Posterior pituitary lobectomy: differential elevation of plasma prolactin and luteinizing hormone in estrous and lactating rats. *Endocrinology* 1982;110:1861–1865.
84. Peters LA, Hoefer MT, Ben-Jonathan N. The posterior pituitary: regulation of anterior pituitary prolactin secretion. *Science* 1981;213:659–661.
85. Ben-Jonathan N. Dopamine: a prolactin-inhibiting hormone. *Endocr Rev* 1985;6:564–589.
86. Holzbauer M, Sharman DF, Godden U. Observations on the function of the dopaminergic nerves innervating the pituitary gland. *Neuroscience* 1978;3:1251–1262.
87. Holzbauer M, Racké K. The dopaminergic innervation of the intermediate lobe and of the neural lobe of the pituitary gland. *Med Biol* 1985;63:97–116.
88. Mulchahey JJ, Neill JD. Dopamine levels in the anterior pituitary gland monitored by *in vivo* electrochemistry. *Brain Res* 1986;386:332–340.
89. Nagy GM, Arendt A, Banky Zs, Halasz B. Dehydration attenuates plasma prolactin response to suckling through a dopaminergic mechanism. *Endocrinology* 1992;130:819–824.
90. Holzbauer M, Sharman DF, Godden U, Mann SP, Stephens DB. Effect of water and salt intake on pituitary catecholamines in the rat and domestic pig. *Neuroscience* 1978;5:1959–1968.
91. Torda T, Lichardus B, Kvetnansky R, Ponec J. Posterior pituitary dopamine and noradrenaline content: effect of thirst, ethanol and saline load. *Endocrinology* 1978;72:334–338.
92. Alper RH, Demarest KT, Moore KE. Dehydration selectively increases dopamine synthesis in tuberohypophyseal dopaminergic neurons. *Neuroendocrinology* 1980;31:112–115.
93. Racke K, Holzbauer M, Cooper TR, Sharman DF. Dehydration increases the electrically evoked dopamine release from the

neural and intermediate lobes of the rat hypophysis. *Neuroendocrinology* 1986;43:6–11.
94. Taleisnik S. Control of melanocyte-stimulating hormone (MSH) secretion. In: Jeffcoate SL, Hutchinson JSM, eds. *The endocrine hypothalamus*. London: Academic Press; 1978:421–439.
95. Eipper BA, Mains RE. Structure and biosynthesis of proadrenocorticotropin/endorphin and related peptides. *Endocr Rev* 1980;1:1–27.
96. Akil H, Watson SJ, Young E, Lewis ME, Khachaturian H, Walker JM. Endogenous opioids: biology and function. *Annu Rev Neurosci* 1984;7:223–255.
97. Bower A, Hadley ME, Hruby VJ. Biogenic amines and control of melanophore stimulating hormone release. *Science* 1974;184: 70–72.
98. Tilders FJH, Berkenbosch F, Smelik PG. Control of secretion of peptides related to adrenocorticotropin, melanocyte-stimulating hormone and endorphin. In: van Wimersma Greidanus TJB, ed. *Frontiers in hormone research*, vol 14. Basel: Karger; 1985:161–196.
99. Lindley SE, Gunnet JW, Lookingland KJ, Moore KE. Effects of alterations in the activity of tuberohypophysial dopaminergic neurons on the secretion of α-melanocyte stimulating hormone. *Proc Soc Exp Biol Med* 1988;188:282–286.
100. Khorram O, Bedran deCastro JC, McCann SM. The influence of suckling on the hypothalamic and pituitary secretion of immunoreactive α-melanocyte stimulating hormone. *Brain Res* 1986; 398:361–365.
101. Nagy GM, Vecsernyés M, Barna I. Dehydration decreases plasma level of α-melanocyte-stimulating hormone (α-MSH) and attenuates suckling-induced β-endorphin (β-END) but not ACTH response in lactating rats. *J Endocrinology* (submitted) 1993.
102. Schally AV, Redding TW, Arimura A, Dupont A, Linthicum GL. Isolation of gamma-amino butyric acid from pig hypothalami and demonstration of its prolactin release-inhibiting (PIF) activity *in vivo* and *in vitro*. *Endocrinology* 1977;100:681–691.
103. Enjalbert A, Ruberg M, Arancibia S, Fiore L, Priam M, Kordon C. Independent inhibition of prolactin secretion by dopamine and gamma-aminobutyric acid *in vitro*. *Endocrinology* 1979; 105:823–826.
104. Racagni G, Apud JA, Locatelli V, Cocchi D, Nistico G, di Giorgio RM, Muller EE. GABA of CNS origin in the rat anterior pituitary inhibits prolactin secretion. *Nature* 1979;281:575–578.
105. Grandison L, Guidotti A. Gamma-aminobutyric acid receptor function in rat anterior pituitary: evidence for control of prolactin release. *Endocrinology* 1979;105:754–759.
106. Grandison L, Cavagnini F, Schmid R, Invitti C, Guidotti A. Gamma-aminobutyric acid and benzodiazepine-binding sites in human anterior pituitary tissue. *J Clin Endocrinol Metab* 1982;54:597–601.
107. Tappaz ML, Brownstein MJ, Kopin IJ. Glutamate decarboxylase (GAD) and gamma-aminobutyric acid (GABA) in discrete nuclei of hypothalamus and substantia nigra. *Brain Res* 1977;125: 109–121.
108. Vincent SR, Hokfelt T, Wu JY. GABA neuron systems in hypothalamus and the pituitary gland: immunohistochemical demonstration using antibodies against glutamate decarboxylase. *Neuroendocrinology* 1982;34:117–125.
109. Mitchell R, Grieve G, Dow R, Fink G. Endogenous GABA receptor ligands in hypophysial portal blood. *Neuroendocrinology* 1983;37:169–176.
110. Mulchahey JJ, Neill JD. Gamma-aminobutyric acid (GABA) levels in hypophyseal stalk plasma of rats. *Life Sci* 1982;31:453–456.
111. Matsushita N, Kato Y, Shimatsu A, Katakami H, Yanaihara N, Imura H. Effects of VIP, TRH, GABA and dopamine on prolactin release form superfused rat anterior pituitary cells. *Life Sci* 1983;32:1263–1269.
112. Clemens JA, Shaar CJ. An endogenous "benzodiazepine-like" substance may regulate the sensitivity of the adenohypophysis to gamma-aminobutyric acid. *Program of the sixty-third annual meeting of the Endocrine Society*. Cincinnati, Ohio, 1981: (abst 931).
113. Grandison L. Suppression of prolactin secretion by benzodiazepines *in vivo*. *Neuroendocrinology* 1982;34:369–373.
114. Samson WK, Martin L, Mogg RJ, Fulton RJ. A nonoxytocinergic prolactin releasing factor and a nondopaminergic prolactin inhibiting factor in bovine neurointermediate lobe extracts: *in vitro* and *in vivo* studies. *Endocrinology* 1990;126:1610–1617.
115. Samson WK, Skala KD, Alexander BD, Huang FL, Gomez-Sanchez C. A prolactin release inhibiting activity isolated from neurointermediate lobe extracts is an endothelin-like peptide. *Regul Pept* 1992;39:103–112.
116. Samson WK, Skala KD. Comparison of the pituitary effects of the mammalian endothelins: vasoactive intestinal contractor (endothelin-β, rat endothelin-2) is a potent inhibitor of prolactin secretion. *Endocrinology* 1992;130:2964–2970.
117. Domae M, Yamada K, Hanabusa Y, Furukawa T. Inhibitory effects of endothelin-1 and endothelin-3 on prolactin release: possible involvement of endogenous endothelin isopeptide in the rat anterior pituitary. *Life Sci* 1992;50:715–722.
118. Terkel J, Blake CA, Sawyer CH. Serum prolactin levels in lactating rats after suckling or exposure to ether. *Endocrinology* 1972;91:49–53.
119. Neill JD. Effect on stress on serum prolactin and luteinizing hormone levels during the estrous cycle of the rat. *Endocrinology* 1970;87:1192–1197.
120. Neill JD, Frawley LS, Plotsky PM, Peck JD, Leong DA. Hypothalamic regulation of prolactin secretion. In: Motta M, Zanisi M, Piva F, eds. *Pituitary hormones and related peptides*. New York: Academic Press; 1982:223–241.
121. Gudelsky GA, Porter JC. Release of newly synthesized dopamine into the hypophysial portal vasculature of the rat. *Endocrinology* 1979;104:583–587.
122. Fagin KD, Neill JD. The effect of dopamine on thyrotropin-releasing hormone-induced prolactin secretion *in vitro*. *Endocrinology* 1981;109:1835–1840.
123. Fuxe K, Hokfelt T, Nilsson O. Factors involved in the control of the activity of tubero-infundibular dopamine neurons during pregnancy and lactation. *Neuroendocrinology* 1969;5:257–270.
124. Voogt JL, Carr LA. Plasma prolactin levels and hypothalamic catecholamine synthesis during suckling. *Neuroendocrinology* 1974;16:108–118.
125. Moyer JA, O'Donohue TL, Herrenkohl LR, Gala RR, Jacobowitz DM. Effects of suckling on serum prolactin levels and catecholamine concentrations and turnover in discrete brain regions. *Brain Res* 1979;176:125–133.
126. Mena F, Enjalbert A, Carbonell L, Priam MM, Kordon C. Effects of suckling on plasma prolactin and hypothalamic monoamine levels in the rat. *Endocrinology* 1976;99:445–451.
127. Chiocchio SR, Cannata MA, Cordero Funes JR, Tramezzani JH. Involvement of adenohypophysial dopamine in the regulation of prolactin release during suckling. *Endocrinology* 1979;105: 544–547.
128. Selmanoff M, Wise PM. Decreased dopamine turnover in the median eminence in response to suckling in the lactating rat. *Brain Res* 1981;212:101–115.
129. Moore KE, Demarest KT. Tuberoinfundibular and tuberohypophyseal dopaminergic neurons. In: Ganong WF, Martini L, eds. *Frontiers in neuroendocrinology*. New York: Raven Press; 1982:161–190.
130. Denef C, Manet D, Dewals R. Dopaminergic stimulation of prolactin release. *Nature* 1980;285:243–246.
131. Kramer IM, Hopkins CR. Studies on the kinetics of dopamine-regulated prolactin secretion. *Mol Cell Endocrinol* 1982;28: 191–198.
132. Burris TP, Stringer LC, Freeman ME. Pharmacologic evidence that a D_2 receptor subtype mediates dopaminergic stimulation of prolactin secretion from the anterior pituitary gland. *Neuroendocrinology* 1991;54:175–183.
133. Burris TP, Nguyen DN, Smith SG, Freeman ME. The stimulatory and inhibitory affects of dopamine on prolactin secretion involve different G-proteins. *Endocrinology* 1992;130:926–932.
134. Nagy GM, Frawley LS. Suckling increases the proportion of mammotropes responsive to various prolactin-releasing stimuli. *Endocrinology* 1990;127:2079–2084.
135. Nagy GM, Boockfor FR, Frawley LS. The suckling stimulus increases the responsiveness of mammotropes located exclusively within the central region of the adenohypophysis. *Endocrinology* 1991;128:761–764.

136. Hill BJ, Nagy GM, Frawley LS. Suckling unmasks the stimulatory affect of dopamine on prolactin release: possible role for melanocyte-stimulating hormone as a mammotrope responsiveness factor. *Endocrinology* 1991;129:843–847.
137. Arey BJ, Burris TP, Basco P, Freeman ME. Infusion of dopamine at low concentration increases release of prolactin from *a*-methyl-*p*-tyrosine-treated rats. *Proc Soc Exp Biol Med* 1993;203:60–63.
138. Rondeel JMM, de Greef WJ, Visser TJ, Voogt JL. Effect of suckling on the *in vivo* release of thyrotropin-releasing hormone, dopamine and adrenaline in the lactating rat. *Neuroendocrinology* 1988;48:93–96.
139. Shin SH, Stirling R. Ascorbic acid potentiates the inhibitory effect of dopamine on prolactin release in primary cultured rat pituitary cells. *J Endocrinology* 1988;118:287–294.
140. Shin SH, Hanna FS. Reexamination of dopamine as the prolactin-release inhibiting factor (PIF): supplementary agent may be required for dopamine to function as the physiological PIF. *Can J Physiol Pharmacol* 1990;68:1226–1230.
141. Hornig D. Distribution of ascorbic acid metabolites and analogues in man and animals. *Ann NY Acad Sci* 1975;258:103–118.
142. Schally AV, Bowers CY, Redding TW, Barrett JF. Isolation of thyrotropin releasing factor (TRF) from porcine hypothalamus. *Biochem Biophys Res Commun* 1966;25:165–169.
143. Tashjian A, Barowsky N, Jensen D. Thyrotropin releasing hormone: direct evidence for stimulation of prolactin production by pituitary cells in culture. *Biochem Biophys Res Commun* 1971;43:516–523.
144. Blake CA. Stimulation of pituitary prolactin and TSH release in lactating and proestrous rats. *Endocrinology* 1974;94:503–508.
145. Kato Y, Matsushita N, Onta H, Tojo K, Shimatsu A, Imura H. Regulation of prolactin secretion. In: Imura H, ed. *The pituitary gland.* New York: Raven Press; 1985:261–278.
146. Bowers CY, Friesen HG, Hwang P, Guyda HJ, Folkers K. Prolactin and thyrotropin release in man by synthetic pyroglutamylhistidyl-prolinamide. *Biochem Biophys Res Commun* 1971;45:1033–1041.
147. Eskay RL, Oliver C, Ben-Jonathan N, Porter JC. Hypothalamic hormones in portal and systemic blood. In: Motta M, Crosighani PG, Martini L, eds. *Hypothalamic hormones: chemistry, physiology, pharmacology and clinical uses.* New York: Academic Press; 1975:125–137.
148. Fink G, Koch Y, Ben Aroya N. Release of thyrotropin releasing hormone into hypophysial portal blood is high relative to other neuropeptides and may be related to prolactin secretion. *Brain Res* 1982;243:186–189.
149. Martin TFJ, Tashjian AH Jr. Cell culture studies of thyrotropin-releasing hormone action. In: Litwack G, ed. *Biochemical actions of hormones,* vol 4. New York: Academic Press; 1977:270–312.
150. Hinkel PM, Tashjian AJ. Receptors for thyrotropin-releasing hormone in prolactin producing rat pituitary cells in culture. *J Biol Chem* 1975;248:6180–6186.
151. Piercy M, Shin SH. Comparative studies of prolactin secretion in estradiol-primed and normal rats induced by ether stress, pimozide and TRH. *Neuroendocrinology* 1980;31:270–275.
152. Grosvenor CE, Mena F. Evidence that thyrotropin-releasing hormone and a hypothalamic prolactin-releasing factor may function in the release of prolactin in the lactating rat. *Endocrinology* 1980;107:863–868.
153. Riskind PN, Millard WJ, Martin JB. Evidence that thyrotropin-releasing hormone is not a major prolactin-releasing factor during suckling in the rat. *Endocrinology* 1984;115:312–316.
154. Shin SH. Thyrotropin-releasing hormone (TRH) is not the physiological prolactin-releasing factor (PRF) in the male rat. *Life Sci* 1978;23:1813–1818.
155. Gautvik KM, Tashjian AH, Konrides IA, Weintraub BD, Gaeber CT, Maloof F, Suzuki K, Zuckerman JE. Thyrotropin-releasing hormone is not the sole physiologic mediator of prolactin release during suckling. *N Engl J Med* 1974;290:1162–1165.
156. Koch Y, Goldhaber G, Fireman I, Zor Y, Shani J, Tal E. Suppression of prolactin and thyrotropin secretion in the rat by antiserum to thyrotropin releasing hormone. *Endocrinology* 1977;100:1476–1478.
157. DeGreef WJ, Voogt JL, Visser TJ, Lamberts SWJ, van der Schoot P. Control of prolactin release induced by suckling. *Endocrinology* 1987;121:316–322.
158. Boyd AE, Spencer E, Jackson I, Reichlin S. Prolactin-releasing factor (PRF) in porcine hypothalamus extract distinct from TRH. *Endocrinology* 1976;99:861–871.
159. Szabo M, Frohman LA. Dissociation of prolactin-releasing activity from thyrotropin-releasing hormone in porcine stalk median eminence. *Endocrinology* 1976;98:1451–1459.
160. De Lean A, Garon M, Kelly PA, Labrie F. Changes of pituitary thyrotropin releasing hormone (TRH) receptor level and prolactin response to TRH during the rat estrous cycle. *Endocrinology* 1977;100:1505–1510.
161. Pickering AJMC, Fink G. Do hypothalamic regulatory factors other than luteinizing hormone releasing factor exert a priming effect? *J Endocrinol* 1979;81:235–238.
162. Aiyer MS, Chiappa SA, Fink G. A priming effect of luteinizing hormone releasing factor on the anterior pituitary gland in the female rat. *J Endocrinol* 1974;62:573–588.
163. Waring DW, Turgeon JL. LHRH self-priming of gonadotrophin secretion: time course of development. *Am J Physiol* 1983;244:C410–C418.
164. Evans WS, Uskavitch DR, Kaiser DL, Hellman P, Borges JL, Thorner MO. The self-priming effect of gonadotrophin-releasing hormone on luteinizing hormone release: observations using rat anterior pituitary fragments and dispersed cells continuously perifused in parallel. *Endocrinology* 1984;114:861–867.
165. Sutton SW, Toyama TT, Otto S, Plotsky PM. Evidence that neuropeptide Y (NPY) released into the hypophysial portal circulation participates in priming gonadotropes to the effects of gonadotropin releasing hormone (GnRH). *Endocrinology* 1988;123:1208–1210.
166. De Greef WJ, Visser TJ. Evidence for the involvement of hypothalamic dopamine and thyrotropin-releasing hormone in suckling-induced release of prolactin. *J Endocrinol* 1981;91:213–23.
167. Plotsky PM, Neill JD. Interactions of dopamine and thyrotropin releasing hormone (TRH) in the regulation of prolactin release in lactating rats. *Endocrinology* 1982;111:168–73.
168. Haisenleder DJ, Moy JA, Gala RR, Lawson DM. The effect of transient dopamine antagonism on thyrotropin-releasing hormone-induced prolactin release in ovariectomized rats treated with estradiol and/or progesterone. *Endocrinology* 1986;119:1996–2003.
169. Haisenleder DJ, Moy JA, Gala RR, Lawson DM. The effects of transient dopamine antagonism on thyrotropin-releasing hormone-induced prolactin release in pseudopregnant rats. *Endocrinology* 1986;119:1989–1995.
170. Haisenleder DJ, Moy JA, Gala RR, Lawson DM. The effect of transient dopamine antagonism on thyrotropin-releasing hormone-induced prolactin release in pregnant rats. *Endocrinology* 1986;119:1980–1988.
171. Martinez de la Escalera G, Martin TFJ, Weiner RI. Phosphoinositide hydrolysis in response to the withdrawal of DA inhibition in enriched lactotrophs in culture. *Neuroendocrinology* 1987;46:545–548.
172. Martinez de la Escalera G, Guthrie J, Weiner RI. Transient removal of dopamine potentiates the stimulation of PRL release by TRH but not VIP: stimulation via Ca^{2+}/protein kinase C pathway. *Neuroendocrinology* 1988;47:38–45.
173. Martinez de la Escalera G, Weiner RI. Mechanisms by which the transient removal of DA regulation potentiates the PRL releasing action of TRH. *Neuroendocrinology* 1988;47:186–193.
174. Martinez de la Escalera G, Porter BW, Martin TFJ, Weiner RI. Dopamine withdrawal and thyrotropin releasing hormone stimulates membrane translocation of protein kinase C and phosphorylation of an endogenous 80-kDa substrate in enriched lactotrophs. *Endocrinology* 1989;125:1168–1173.
175. Beaulieu RV, M, Labrie F, Boissier J. Potent antidopaminergic activity of estradiol at the pituitary level on prolactin release. *Science* 1978;200:1173–75.
176. Dymshitz J, Ben-Jonathan N. Effects of coculture of anterior and posterior pituitary cells on the responsiveness of lactotrophs to different secretagogues. *Endocrinology* 1991;129:2535–2540.
177. Said SI, Mutt V. Polypeptide with broad biological activity in the porcine small intestine. *Science* 1970;169:1217–1218.
178. Larson LI, Fahrenkrug J, Schaffalistsky de Muckadell OB, Sundler F, Hakanson R, Rehfeld JF. Localization of vasoactive

intestinal polypeptide (VIP) to central and peripheral nerves. *Proc Natl Acad Sci USA* 1976;73:3197–3200.
179. Besson J, Rotsztejn W, Laburthe M, Epelbaum J, Beaudet A, Kordon C, Rosselin G. Vasoactive intestinal peptide (VIP): brain distribution, subcellular localization and effect of deafferentation of the hypothalamus in male rats. *Brain Res* 1979;165:79–85.
180. Pelletier G, Leclerc R, Puviani R, Polak JM. Electron immunocytochemistry in vasoactive intestinal peptide (VIP) in the rat brain. *Brain Res* 1981;210:356–360.
181. Kato Y, Iwasaki Y, Iwasaki J, Abe H, Yanaihara N, Imura H. Prolactin release by vasoactive intestinal polypeptide in rats. *Endocrinology* 1978;103:554–558.
182. Ruberg M, Rotsztejn WH, Arancibia S, Besson J, Enjalbert A. Stimulation of prolactin release by vasoactive intestinal peptide. *Eur J Pharmacol* 1978;51:319–320.
183. Vijayan E, Samson WK, Said SI, McCann SM. Vasoactive intestinal peptide: evidence for a hypothalamic site of action to release growth hormone, luteinizing hormone, and prolactin in conscious ovariectomized rats. *Endocrinology* 1979; 104:53–57.
184. Shaar CJ, Clements JA, Dininger NB. Effect of vasoactive intestinal polypeptide on prolactin release *in vitro*. *Life Sci* 1979;25:2071–2074.
185. Bataille D, Peillon F, Besson J, Rosselin G. Vasoactive intestinal peptide (VIP): recepteurs specifiques et activation de l'adenylate cyclase dans une tumeur hypophysaire humaine a prolactine. *CR Acad Sci* 1979;228:1315–1317.
186. Said SI, Porter JC. Vasoactive intestinal polypeptide: release into hypophyseal portal blood. *Life Sci* 1979;24:227–230.
187. Shimatsu A, Kato Y, Matsushita N, Katakami H, Yanaihara N, Imura H. Immunoreactive vasoactive intestinal polypeptide in rat hypophysial portal blood. *Endocrinology* 1981;108:395–98.
188. Shimatsu A, Kato Y, Inoue T, Christofides ND, Bloom SR, Imura H. Peptide histidine isoleucine and vasoactive intestinal polypeptide-like immunoreactivity coexist in rat hypophysial portal blood. *Neurosci Lett* 1983;43:259–262.
189. Shimatsu A, Kato Y, Matsushita N, Katakami H, Yanaihara N, Imura H. Stimulation by serotonin of vasoactive intestinal polypeptide release into rat hypophysial portal blood. *Endocrinology* 1982,111:338–340.
190. Shimatsu A, Kato Y, Ohta H, Tojo K, Kabayama Y, Inoue T, Yanaihara N, Imura H. Involvement of hypothalamic vasoactive intestinal polypeptide (VIP) in prolactin secretion induced by serotonin in rats. *Proc Soc Exp Biol Med* 1984;175:414–416.
191. Abe H, Engler D, Molitch ME, Bollinger-Gruber J, Reichlin S. Vasoactive intestinal peptide is a physiological mediator of prolactin release in the rat. *Endocrinology* 1985;116:1383–1390.
192. Kaji H, Chihara K, Abe H, Kita T, Kashio Y, Okimura Y, Fujita T. Effect of passive immunization with antisera to vasoactive intestinal peptide and peptide histidine isoleucine amide on 5-hydroxy-L-tryptophan induced prolactin release in rats. *Endocrinology* 1985;117:1914–1919.
193. Hagen TC, Arnaout MA, Scherzer WJ, Martinson DR, Garthwaite TL. Antisera to vasoactive intestinal peptide inhibit basal prolactin release from dispersed anterior pituitary cells. *Neuroendocrinology* 1986;43:641–645.
194. Nagy GM, Mulchahey JJ, Neill JD. Autocrine control of prolactin secretion by vasoactive intestinal peptide. *Endocrinology* 1988;122:364–366.
195. Strabak V, Guillaume V, Grino M, Dutour A, Oliver C. The specific antibody injection as a tool for study the hypothalamic peptide secretion into portal blood of rat. *Program of the Ninth International Congress of Endocrinology*. Nice, France, 1992; 561 (abst).
196. Itoh N, Obata K, Yanaihara N, Okamoto N. Human preprovasoactive intestinal polypeptide contains a novel PHI–27-like peptide, PHM–27. *Nature* 1983;304:547–549.
197. Tatemoto K, Mutt V. Isolation and characterization of intestinal peptide porcine PHI (PHI–27), a new member of glucagon-secretin family. *Proc Natl Acad Sci USA* 1981;78:6603–6697.
198. Werner S, Hulting AL, Hökfelt T, Eneroth P, Tatemoto K, Mutt V, Maroder L, Wusch E. Effect of peptide PHI–27 on prolactin release *in vitro*. *Neuroendocrinology* 1983;37:467–478.
199. Kaji H, Chihara K, Abe H, Minamitani N, Kodama H, Kita T, Fujita T, Tatemoto K. Stimulatory effect of peptide histidine isoleucine amide 1–27 on prolactin release in the rat. *Life Sci* 1984;35:641–647.
200. Ohta H, Kato Y, Toyo K, Shimatsu A, Inoue T, Kabayama Y, Imura H. Further evidence that peptide histidine isoleucine (PHI) may function as a prolactin releasing factor in rats. *Peptides* 1985;6:709–712.
201. Samson WK, Lumpkin MD, McDonald JK, McCann SM. Prolactin-releasing activity of porcine intestinal peptide (PHI–27). *Peptides* 1983;4:817–819.
202. Miyata A, Arimura A, Dahl RR, Minamino N, Uehara A, Jiang L, Culler MD, Coy DH. Isolation of a novel 38 residue-hypothalamic polypeptide which stimulates adenylate cyclase in pituitary cells. *Biochem Biophys Res Commun* 1989;164: 567–574.
203. Arimura A. Pituitary adenylate cyclase activating polypeptide (PACAP): discovery and current status of research. *Regul Pept* 1992;37:287–303.
204. Shivers BD, Görcs TJ, Gottschall PE, Arimura A. Two high-affinity binding sites for pituitary adenylate cyclase activating polypeptide have different tissue distributions. *Endocrinology* 1991;128:3055–3065.
205. Leonhardt S, Jarry H, Kreipe A, Werstler K, Wuttke W. Pituitary adenylate cyclase activating polypeptide (PACAP) stimulates pituitary hormone release in male rats. *Neuroendocrin Lett* 1992;14:319–327.
206. Nagy GM, Vigh S, Arimura A. PACAP induces prolactin and growth hormone release in lactating rats separated from their pups. *J Endocrinol* (In Press).
207. Jarry H, Leonhardt S, Schmidt WE, Creutzfeldt W, Wuttke W. Contrasting effects of pituitary adenylate cyclase activating polypeptide (PACAP) on *in vivo* and *in vitro* prolactin and growth hormone release in male rats. *Life Sci* 1992;51:823–830.
208. Murai I, Ben-Jonathan N. Posterior pituitary lobectomy abolishes the suckling-induced rise in prolactin (PRL): evidence for a PRL-releasing factor in the posterior pituitary. *Endocrinology* 1987;121:205–211.
209. Murai I, Reichlin S, Ben-Jonathan N. The peak phase of the proestrous prolactin surge is bloched by either posterior pituitary lobectomy or antisera to vasoactive intestinal peptide. *Endocrinology* 1989;124:1050–1055.
210. Averill RL, Grattan DR, Norris SK. Posterior pituitary lobectomy chronically attenuates the nocturnal surge of prolactin in early pregnancy. *Endocrinology* 1991;128:705–709.
211. Hyde JF, Murai I, Ben-Jonathan N. The rat posterior pituitary contains a potent prolactin-releasing factor: studies with perifused anterior pituitary cells. *Endocrinology* 1987;121:1531–1539.
212. Hyde JF, Ben-Jonathan N. Characterization of prolactin-releasing factor in the rat posterior pituitary. *Endocrinology* 1986;122:2533–2539.
213. Hyde JF, Murai I, Ben-Jonathan N. Differential effects of pituitary stalk-section on posterior pituitary and hypothalamic contents of prolactin-releasing factor, oxytocin, dopamine and beta-endorphin. *Neuroendocrinology* 1988;48:314–319.
214. Landon M, Grossman DA, Ben-Jonathan N. Prolactin-releasing factor: cellular origin in the intermediate lobe of the pituitary. *Endocrinology* 1990;126:3185–3192.
215. Samson WK, Lumpkin MD, McCann SM. Evidence for a physiological role for oxytocin in the control of prolactin secretion. *Endocrinology* 1986;119:554–560.
216. Gibbs DM. High concentrations of oxytocin in hypophyseal portal plasma. *Endocrinology* 1984;114:1216–1218.
217. Antoni F. Oxytocin receptors in rat adenohypophysis: evidence from radioligand binding studies. *Endocrinology* 1986;119: 2393–2395.
218. Lumpkin MD, Samson WK, McCann SM. Hypothalamic and pituitary sites of oxytocin to alter prolactin secretion in the rat. *Endocrinology* 1983;112:1711–1717.
219. Mormede P, Vincent JD, Kerdelhue B. Vasopressin and oxytocin reduce plasma prolactin levels of conscious rats in basal and stress conditions: study of the characteristics of the receptor involved. *Life Sci* 1986;39:1737–1743.
220. Muir JL, Pfister HP. Influence of exogenously administered oxytocin on the corticosterone and prolactin response to psychological stress. *Pharmacol Biochem Behavior* 1988;29:699–703.
221. Frawley LS, Leong DA, Neill JD. Oxytocin attenuates TRH-

induced TSH release from rat pituitary cells. *Neuroendocrinology* 1985;40:201–204.
222. Johnston CA, Negro-Vilar A. Role of oxytocin on prolactin secretion during proestrus and in different physiological and pharmacological paradigms. *Endocrinology* 1988;122:341–350.
223. Shin SH, Papas S, Obonsawin MC. Current status of the rat prolactin releasing factor. *Can J Physiol Pharmacol* 1987;65: 2036–2043.
224. Neill JD. Prolactin secretion and its control. In: Knobil E, Neill JD, eds. *The physiology of reproduction.* New York: Raven Press; 1988:1379–1390.
225. Ben-Jonathan N, Arbogast LA, Hyde JF. Neuroendocrine regulation of prolactin release. In: *Progress in neurobiology,* vol 33. Pergamon Press. 1989:399–447.
226. Benson GK, Cowie AT. Lactation in the rat after hypophysial posterior lobectomy. *J Endocrinology* 1956;14:54–65.
227. Nagy G, Köves K, Halasz B. Neural structures mediating the suckling induced prolactin release. *Program of the Seventh International Congress of Endocrinology.* Quebec City, Canada, 1984: (abst 1590).
228. Nagy GM, Makara GB. Neurointermediate lobe (NIL) denervation attenuates suckling induced prolactin release in lactating rats. *Brain Res* (*Submitted*).
229. Nagy GM, Neill JD, Makara GB, Halasz B. Lack of the suckling-induced prolactin release in homozygous Brattleboro rats: the vasopressin-neurophysin-glycopeptide precursor may play a role in prolactin release. *Brain Res* 1989;504:165–167.
230. Hyde JF, North WG, Ben-Jonathan N. The vasopressin-associated glycopeptide is not a prolactin-releasing factor: studies with lactating Brattleboro rats. *Endocrinology* 1989;125:35–40.
231. Nagy G, Görcs JT, Halasz B. Attenuation of the suckling-induced prolactin (PRL) release and the high afternoon oscillations of plasma PRL secretion of lactating rats by antiserum to vasopressin. *Neuroendocrinology* 1991;54:566–570.
232. Nagy GM, Mulchahey JJ, Smyth DG, Neill JD. The glycopeptide moiety of vasopressin-neurophysin precursor is neurohypophysial prolactin releasing factor. *Biochem Biophys Res Commun* 1988;151:524–529.
233. Valverde RC, Chieffo V, Reichlin S. Prolactin releasing factor in porcine and rat hypothalamic tissue. *Endocrinology* 1972;91: 982–993.
234. Vaughan MK, Little JC, Johnson LY, Blask DE, Vaughan GM, Reiter RJ. Effects of melatonin and natural and synthetic analogues of arginine vasotocin on plasma prolactin levels in adult male rats. *Horm Res* 1978;9:236–246.
235. Hanew K, Shiino M, Rennels EG. Effect of indoles, AVT, oxytocin and AVP on prolactin secretion in rat pituitary clonal (2B8) cells. *Proc Soc Exp Biol Med* 1980;164:257–261.
236. Shin SH. Vasopressin has a direct effect on prolactin release in male rats. *Neuroendocrinology* 1982;34:55–58.
237. Antoni F. Novel ligand specificity of pituitary vasopressin receptors in the rat. *Neuroendocrinology* 1984;39:186–188.
238. Knepel W, Götz D, Fahrenholz F. Interaction of rat adenohypophyseal vasopressin receptors with vasopressin analogues substituted at positions 7 and 1: dissimilarity from the V1 vasopressin receptor. *Neuroendocrinology* 1986;44:390–396.
239. Zimmerman EA, Carmel PW, Husain MK, Ferin M, Tannenbaum M, Frantz AG, Robinsons AG. Vasopressin and neurophysin: high concentrations in monkey hypophyseal portal blood. *Science* 1973;182:925–927.
240. Shin SH, Obonsawin MC. Bovine neurophysin II has prolactin-releasing activity in the estradiol-primed rat. *Neuroendocrinology* 1985;41:276–282.
241. Schally AV, Guoth JG, Redding TW, Groot K, Rodriguez H, Szönyi E, Stults J, Nikolics K. Isolation and characterization of two peptides with prolactin release inhibiting activity from porcine hypothalami. *Proc Natl Acad Sci USA* 1991;88:3540–3544.
242. Ambach G, Palkovits M, Szentágothai J. Blood supply of the rat hypothalamus: IV. retrochiasmatic area, median eminence, arcuate nucleus. *Acta Morphologica Acad Sci Hung* 1976;24: 93–119.
243. Török B. Lebendbeobachtung des hypophysenkreislauges an hunden. *Acta Morphologica Acad Sci Hung* 1954;4:83–89.
244. Mezey E, Palkovits M. Two-way transport in the hypothalamo-hypophyseal system. In: Ganong WF, Martini L, eds. *Frontiers in neuroendocrinology,* vol 7. New York: Raven Press; 1982:1–29.
245. Boockfor FR, Frawley LS. Functional variations among prolactin cells from different pituitary regions. *Endocrinology* 1987;120:874–879.
246. Porter TE, Frawley LS. Neurointermediate lobe peptides recruit prolactin-secreting cells exclusively within the central region of the adenohypophysis. *Endocrinology* 1992;131:2649–2652.
247. Denef C, Baes M, Schramme C. Paracrine interactions in the anterior pituitary: role in the regulation of prolactin and growth hormone secretion. In: Ganong WF, Martini L, eds. *Frontiers in neuroendocrinology,* vol 9. New York: Raven Press; 1986: 115–148.
248. Denef C, Andries M. Evidence for paracrine interaction between gonadotrophs and lactotrophs in pituitary cell aggregates. *Endocrinology* 1983;112:813–822.
249. Baes M, Allaerto W, Denef C. Evidence for functional communication between folliculo-stellate cells and hormone secreting cells in perifused anterior pituitary cell aggregates. *Endocrinology* 1987;120:685–691.
250. Carmeliet P, Denef C. Immunocytochemical and pharmacological evidence for an intrinsic cholinomimetic system modulating prolactin and growth hormone release in rat pituitary. *Endocrinology* 1988;123:1128–1139.
251. Sato S. Postnatal development, sexual difference and sexual cycle variation of prolactin cells in rats: special reference to the topographic affinity to a gonadotroph. *Endocrinol Jpn* 1980;27: 573–583.
252. Horvath E, Kovacs K, Ezrin C. Functional contact between lactotrophs and gonadotrophs in rat pituitary. *ICRS Med Sci* 1977;5:511.
253. Nakane PK. Classifications of anterior pituitary cell types with immunoenzyme histochemistry. *J Histochem Cytochem* 1970; 18:9–20.
254. Schramme C, Denef C. Stimulation of prolactin release by angiotensin II in superfused rat anterior pituitary aggregates. *Neuroendocrinology* 1983;36:483–485.
255. Aguilera G, Hyde CL, Catt KJ. Angiotensin II receptors and prolactin release in pituitary lactotrophs. *Endocrinology* 1982;111: 1045–1050.
256. Jones TH, Brown BL, Dobson PRM. Evidence that angiotensin II is a paracrine agent mediating gonadotropin-releasing hormone-stimulated inositol phosphate production and prolactin secretion in the rat. *J Endocrinol* 1988;116:367–371.
257. Kubota T, Judd AM, MacLeod RM. The paracrine role of angiotensin in gonadotropin-releasing hormone-stimulated prolactin release in rats. *J Endocrinol* 1990;125:225–232.
258. Capponi AM, Facrod-Coune CA, Gaillard RC, Muller AF. Binding and activation properties of angiotensin II in dispersed rat anterior pituitary cells. *Endocrinology* 1982;110:1043–1045.
259. Hauger RL, Aguilera G, Baukal AJ, Catt KJ. Characterization of angiotensin II receptors in the anterior pituitary gland. *Mol Cell Endocrinol* 1982;25:203–212.
260. Mukherjee A, Kulkarni P, McCann SM, Negro-Vilar A. Evidence for the presence and characterization of angiotensin II receptors in rat anterior pituitary membranes. *Endocrinology* 1982;110:665–667.
261. Naruse K, Takii Y, Inagami T. Immunohistochemical localization of renin in luteinizing hormone-producing cells of rat pituitary. *Proc Natl Acad Sci USA* 1981;78:7579–7583.
262. Steele MK, Brownfield MS, Ganong WF. Immunocytochemical localization of angiotensin immunoreactivity in gonadotrophs and lactotrophs of the rat anterior pituitary gland. *Neuroendocrinology* 1982;35:155–158.
263. Deschepper CF, Crumrine DA, Ganong WF. Evidence that the gonadotrophs are the likely site of production of angiotensin II in the anterior pituitary of the rat. *Endocrinology* 1989;119:35–43.
264. Chabot JG, Gray AD, Dubois PM, Morel G. Presence of angiotensin II in the adult male rat anterior pituitary gland: immunocytochemical study after cryoultramicrotomy. *Exp Cell Res* 1989;180:560–568.
265. Ganong WF, Deschepper CF, Steele MK, Intebi A. Renin-angiotensin system in the anterior pituitary of the rat. *Am J Hypertens* 1989;2:320–322.

266. Wildt L, Hausler A, Marshall G, Knobil E. GnRH has prolactin-releasing activity. *Fed Proc* 1980;39:372 (abst).
267. Yen SCC, Hoff JD, Lasley BL, Casper RJ, Sheehan K. Induction of prolactin release by LRF and LRF agonist. *Life Sci* 1980;26:1963–1967.
268. Casper RF, Yen SCC. Simultaneous pulsatile release by prolactin and luteinizing hormone induced by luteinizing hormone releasing factor agonist. *J Clin Endocrinol Metab* 1981;52:943–936.
269. Mais V, Miles GB, Paoletti AM, Strigini F, Antinori D, Fioretti P. Prolactin releasing action of a low dose of exogenous gonadotropin releasing hormone throughout the human menstrual cycle. *Neuroendocrinology* 1986;44:326–330.
270. Robberecht W, Andries M, Denef C. Stimulation of prolactin secretion from rat pituitary by luteinizing hormone releasing hormone: evidence against mediation by angiotensin II acting through a (Sar[1]-Ala[8])-angiotensin II-sensitive receptor. *Neuroendocrinology* 1992;56:185–194.
271. Rudnick MS, Dannies PS. Muscarinic inhibition of prolactin production in cultures of rat pituitary cells. *Biochem Biophys Res Commun* 1981;101:689–696.
272. Mukherjee A, Snyder G, McCann SM. Characterization of muscarinic cholinergic receptors on intact rat anterior pituitary cells. *Life Sci* 1980;27:475–482.
273. Taylor RL, Burt DR. Pituitary cell cultures contain muscarinic receptors. *Eur J Pharmacol* 1980;65:305–308.
274. Schaeffer JM, Hsueh AJW. Acetylcholine receptors in the rat anterior pituitary gland. *Endocrinology* 1980;106:1377–1381.
275. Simpson J, Williamson IJ, Fink G. Choline acetyltransferase activity in the pars distalis, preoptic area, and striatum during the rat estrous cycle. *Neuroendocrinology* 1985;40:444–449.
276. Barron SE, Hoover DB. Localization of acetylcholinesterase and choline acetyltransferase in the rat pituitary gland. *Histochem J* 1983;15:1087–1098.
277. Arnaout MA, Garthwaite TL, Martinson DR, Hagen TC. Vasoactive intestinal peptide is synthesized in anterior pituitary tissue. *Endocrinology* 1986;119:2052–2057.
278. Morel G, Chayvialle JA, Kerdelhue B, Dubois PM. Ultrastructural evidence for endogenous substance P-like immunoreactivity in the rat pituitary gland. *Neuroendocrinology* 1982;35:86–92.
279. Lam KSL, Lechan RM, Minamitani N, Segerson TP, Reichlin S. Vasoactive intestinal peptide in the anterior pituitary is increased in hypothyroidism. *Endocrinology* 1989;124:1077–1084.
280. Koves K, Gotschall PE, Gorcs T, Scammell JG, Arimura A. Presence of immunoreactive vasoactive intestinal polypeptide in anterior pituitary of normal male and long term estrogen-treated female rats: a light microscopic immunohistochemical study. *Endocrinology* 1990;126:1756–1763.
281. Steel JH, Gon G, O'Halloran DJ, Jones PM, Yanaihara N, Ishikawa H, Bloom SR, Polak JM. Galanin and vasoactive intestinal polypeptide are colocalized with classical pituitary hormones and show plasticity of expression. *Histochemistry* 1989;93:183–189.
282. Carrillo AJ, Phelps CJ. Quantification of vasoactive intestinal peptide immunoreactivity in the anterior pituitary glands of intact male and female, ovariectomized, and estradiol benzoate-treated rats. *Endocrinology* 1992;131:964–969.
283. Kasper S, Popescu RA, Torsello A, Vrontakis ME, Ikejiani C, Friesen HG. Tissue-specific regulation of vasoactive intestinal peptide messenger ribonucleic acid levels by estrogen in the rat. *Endocrinology* 1992;130:1796–1801.
284. Houben H, Denef C. Regulatory peptides produced in the anterior pituitary. *Trends Endocrinol Metab* 1990;1:398–403.
285. Aronin N, Coslovsky R, Leeman SE. Substance P and neurotensin: their roles in the regulation of anterior pituitary function. *Annu Rev Physiol* 1986;48:537–549.
286. Brown ER, Harlan RE, Krause JE. Gonadal steroid regulation of substance P (SP) and SP-encoding messenger ribonucleic acids in the rat anterior pituitary and hypothalamus. *Endocrinology* 1990;126:330–340.
287. Jonassen JA, Mulliken-Kilpatrick D, McAdam A, Leeman SE. Thyroid hormone status regulates preprotachykinin-A gene expression in male rat anterior pituitary gland. *Endocrinology* 1987;121:1555–1561.
288. Goedert M, Lightman SL, Nagy JI, Marley PD, Emson PC. Neurotensin in the rat anterior pituitary gland. *Nature* 1982;298: 163–165.
289. Bauer TV, Moriarty CM, Childs GV. Studies of immunoreactive gonadotropin-releasing hormone (GnRH) in the rat anterior pituitary gland. *J Histochem Cytochem* 1981;29:1171–1178.
290. Morel G, Dubois PM. Immunocytochemical evidence for gonadoliberin in rat anterior pituitary gland. *Neuroendocrinology* 1982;34:197–206.
291. Childs GV, Cole DE, Kubek M, Tobin RB, Wilber JF. Endogenous thyrotropin-releasing hormone in the anterior pituitary: sites of activity as identified by immunocytochemical staining. *J Histochem Cytochem* 1978;26:901–908.
292. Morel G, Hemming F, Tonon MC, Vaudry H, Dubois MP, Coy D, Dubois PM. Ultrastructural evidence for corticotropin-releasing factor (CRF)-like immunoreactivity in the rat pituitary gland. *Biol Cell* 1982;44:89–92.
293. Morel G, Mesguich P, Dubois MP, Dubois PM. Ultrastructural evidence for endogenous growth hormone-releasing factor (GRF)-like immunoreactivity in the monkey pituitary gland. *Neuroendocrinology* 1984;38:123–133.
294. Morel G, Mesguich P, Dubois MP, Dubois PM. Ultrastructural evidence for endogenous somatostatin immunoreactivity in the pituitary gland. *Neuroendocrinology* 1983;36:291–299.
295. Rehfield JF. Localization of gastrins to neuro- and adenohypophysis. *Nature* 1978;271:771–773.
296. O'Donohue TL, Charlton CG, Miller RL, Boden G, Jacobowitz DM. Identification, characterization, and distribution of secretin immunoreactivity in rat and pig brain. *Proc Natl Acad Sci USA* 1981;78:5221–5224.
297. Weber E, Voigt KH, Martin R. Pituitary somatotropes contain [Met] enkephalin-like immunoreactivity. *Proc Natl Acad Sci USA* 1978;75:6134–6138.
298. Tramu G, Leonardelli J. Immunohistochemical localization of enkephalins in median eminence and adenohypophysis. *Brain Res* 1979;168:457–471.
299. Kitamura K, Minamino N, Hayashi Y, Kanagawa K, Matsuo H. Regional distribution of β-neoendorphin in rat brain and pituitary. *Biochem Biophys Res Commun* 1982;109:966–974.
300. Clements JA, Funder JW. Arginine vasopressin (AVP) and AVP-like immunoreactivity in peripheral tissues. *Endocr Rev* 1986;7:449–460.
301. Enjalbert A, Ruberg M, Arancibia S, Priam M, Kordon C. Endogenous opiates block dopamine inhibition of prolactin secretion *in vitro*. *Nature* 1979;280:595–597.
302. Grandison L, Guidotti A. Regulation of prolactin release by endogenous opiates. *Nature* 1977;270:357–359.
303. Lien EL, Fenichel RL, Garsky V, Sarantakis D, Grant NH. Enkephalin-stimulated prolactin release. *Life Sci* 1976;19:837–840.
304. Enjalbert A, Arancibia S, Priam M, Eluet-Pajot MT, Kordon C. Neurotensin stimulation of prolactin secretion *in vitro*. *Neuroendocrinology* 1982;34:95–98.
305. Vijayan E, McCann SM. *In vivo* and *in vitro* effects of substance P and neurotensin on gonadotropin and prolactin release. *Endocrinology* 1979;105:64–68.
306. Kato Y, Chihara K, Ohgo S, Iwasaki Y, Abe H, Imur H. Growth hormone and prolactin release by substance P in rats. *Life Sci* 1976;19:441–446.
307. Tojo K, Kato Y, Ohto H, Shimatsu A, Matsushita N, Kabayama Y, Inoue T, Yanaihara N, Imura H. Potent stimulatory effect of leumorphin on prolactin secretion from the pituitary in rats. In: MacLeod RM, Thorner MO, Scapagnini U, eds. *Prolactin: basic and clinical correlates.* Padova: Liviana Press; 1985:551–557.
308. Matsushita N, Kato Y, Shimatsu A, Katakami H, Fugino M, Matsuo H, Imura H. Stimulation of prolactin secretion in the rat by α-neo-endorphin, β-neo-endorphin and dynorphin. *Biochem Biophys Res Commun* 1982;107:735–741.
309. Kato Y, Matsushita N, Katakami H, Shimatsu A, Imura H. Stimulation by dynorphin of prolactin and growth hormone secretion in the rat. *Eur J Pharmacol* 1981;73:353–355.
310. Ben-David M, Danon A, Benveniste R, Weller CP, Sulman FG. Results of radioimmunoassays of rat pituitary and serum prolactin after adrenalectomy and perphenazine treatment in rats. *J Endocrinol* 1971;50:599–606.
311. Chen HJ, Bradley CJ, Meites J. Stimulation of carcinogen-induced mammary tumor growth in rats by adrenalectomy. *Cancer Res* 1976;36:1414–1417.
312. Aylsworth CF, Hodson CA, Berg G, Kledzik G, Meites J. Role of

adrenals and estrogen in regression of mammary tumors during postpartum lactation in the rat. *Cancer Res* 1979;39:2436–2439.

313. Leung FC, Chen HT, Verkaik SJ, Steger RW, Peluso JJ, Campbell GA, Meites J. Mechanism(s) by which adrenalectomy and corticosterone influence prolactin release in the rat. *J Endocrinol* 1980;87:131–140.
314. Harms PG, Langlier P, McCann SM. Modification of stress-induced prolactin release by dexamethasone or adrenalectomy. *Endocrinology* 1975;96:475–578.
315. Euker JS, Meites J, Riegle GD. Effects of acute stress on serum LH and prolactin in intact, castrate and dexamethasone-treated male rats. *Endocrinology* 1975;96:85–92.
316. Rossier J, French E, Rivier C, Shibasaki T, Guillemin R, Bloom FE. Stress-induced release of prolactin: blockade by dexamethasone and naloxone may indicate β-endorphin mediation. *Proc Natl Acad Sci USA* 1980;77:666–669.
317. Schwinn G, von zur Müklen A, Warnecke U. Effects of dexamethasone on thyrotrophin and prolactin plasma levels in rats. *Acta Endocrinol (Copenh)* 1976;82:486–491.
318. Van der Schoot P, deGreef WJ. Effect of adrenalectomy on the regulation of the secretion of gonadotrophins and prolactin in the lactating rat. *J Endocrinol* 1983;98:227–232.
319. Kiem DT, Fekete MIK, Bartha L, Nagy GM, Makara GB. Prolactin response to morphine in intact and adrenalectomized lactating rats. *Brain Res* 1991;563:171–174.
320. Bartha L, Nagy GM, Kiem DT, Makara GB. Inhibition of suckling-induced prolactin (PRL) release by dexamethasone. *Endocrinology* 1991;129:635–640.
321. Habener J. Genetic control of hormone formation. In: Wilson JD, Foster DW, eds. *Textbook of endocrinology,* 7th ed. Philadelphia: WB Saunders; 1985:9–32.
322. Farquhar MG, Skutelsky EH, Hopkins CR. Structure and function of the anterior pituitary and dispersed pituitary cells: *in vitro* studies. In: Tixier A, Farquhar MG, eds. *The anterior pituitary.* New York: Academic Press; 1975:84–135.
323. Martin TFJ. Dual intracellular signalling by Ca^{+2} and lipids mediates the actions of TRH. In: MacLeod RM, Thorner MO, Scapagnini U, eds. *Prolactin: basic and clinical correlates.* Padova: Liviana Press; 1985:165–175.
324. Lamberts SWJ, MacLeod RM. Regulation of prolactin secretion at the level of the lactotroph. *Physiol Rev* 1990;70:279–318.
325. Rosenfeld MG, Amara SG, Birnberg NC, Mermod JJ, Murodoch GH, Evans RM. Calcitonin, prolactin, and growth hormone gene expression as model systems for the characterization of neuroendocrine regulation. *Recent Progr Horm Res* 1983;39:305–351.
326. Murodoch GH, Evan RM, Rosenfeld MG. Polypeptide hormone regulation of prolactin gene transcription. In: Litwack G, ed. *Biochemical actions of hormones,* vol 12. New York: Academic Press; 1985:37–68.
327. Straub RE, Frech GC, Joho RH, Gershengorn MC. Expression cloning of a cDNA encoding the mouse pituitary thyrotropin-releasing hormone receptor. *Proc Natl Acad Sci USA* 1990;87:9514–9518.
328. Sreedharan SP, Robichon A, Peterson KE, Goetzl EJ. Cloning and expression of the human vasoactive intestinal peptide receptor. *Proc Natl Acad Sci USA* 1991;88:4986–4990.
329. Sibley DR, Monsma Jr FJ. Molecular biology of dopamine receptors. *Trends Pharmacol Sci* 1992;13:61–69.
330. Boockfor FR, Hoeffler JP, Frawley LC. Cultures of GH_3 cells are functionally heterogeneous: thyropin releasing hormone, estradiol, and cortisol cause reciprocal shifts in the proportions of growth hormone and prolactin secretors. *Endocrinology* 1985; 117:418–420.
331. Martin TFJ. Calcitonin peptide inhibition of TRH-stimulated prolactin secretion: additional evidence for inhibitory regulation of phospholipase C. *Trends Endocrinol Metab* 1992;3:82–85.
332. Drummond AH. Inositol lipid metabolism and signal transduction in clonal pituitary cells. *J Exp Biol* 1986;124:337–358.
333. Gershengorn MC. Mechanism of the thyrotropin releasing hormone stimulation of pituitary hormone secretion. *Annu Rev Physiol* 1986;48:515–526.
334. Ronning SA, Martin TFJ. Characterization of Ca^{+2}-stimulated secretion in permeable GH_3 pituitary cells. *J Biol Chem* 1986;261:7834–7839.
335. Martin TFJ, Hsieh KP, Porter BW. The sustained second phase of hormone-stimulated diacylglycerol accumulation does not activate protein kinase C in GH_3 cells. *J Biol Chem* 1990; 265:7623–7631.
336. Ronning SA, Martin TFJ. Characterization of phorbol ester and diacylglycerol-stimulated secretion in permeable GH_3 cells. *J Biol Chem* 1986;261:7840–7845.
337. Dufy B, Jaken S, Barker JL. Intracellular Ca^{+2}-dependent protein kinase C activation mimics delayed effects of thyrotropin releasing hormone on clonal pituitary cell excitability. *Endocrinology* 1987;121:793–802.
338. Hsieh KP, Martin TFJ. Thyrotropin-releasing hormone and gonadotropin-releasing hormone receptors activate phospholipase C by coupling to the guanosine triphosphate-binding proteins G_q and G_{11}. *Molec Endocr* 1992;6:1673–1681.
339. Strathmann M, Simon M. G protein diversity: a distinct class of α subunits is present in vertebrates and invertebrates. *Proc Natl Acad Sci USA* 1990;87:9113–9117.
340. Taylor SJ, Smith JA, Exton JH. Purification from bovine liver membranes of a guanine nucleotide-dependent activator of phosphoinositide-specific phospholipase C. *J Biol Chem* 1990; 265:17150–17156.
341. Smrcka AV, Hepler JR, Brown KO, Sternweis PC. Regulation of polyphosphoinositide-specific phospholipase C activity by purified G_q. *Science* 1991;251:804–807.
342. Pang IH, Sternweis PC. Purification of unique α subunits of GTP-binding regulatory proteins (G proteins) by affinity chromatography with immobilized $\beta\alpha$ subunits. *J Biol Chem* 1990;265:18707–18712.
343. Blank JL, Ross AH, Exton JH. Purification and characterization of two G proteins that activate the $\beta 1$ isozyme of phosphoinositide-specific phospholipase C. *J Biol Chem* 1991; 266:18206–18216.
344. Koch BD, Blalock JB, Schonbrunn A. Characterization of the cyclic AMP-independent actions of somatostatin in GH cells. *J Biol Chem* 1988;263:216–225.
345. Guild S, Frey EA, Pocotte SL, Kebabian JW. Adenosine 3′,5′-cyclic monophosphate-mediated enhancement of calcium-evoked prolactin release from electrically permeabilised 7315C tumor cells. *Br J Pharmacol* 1988;94:737–744.
346. Vallar L, Meldolesi J. Mechanisms of signal transduction at the dopamine D_2 receptor. *Trends Pharmacol Sci* 1989;10:74–77.
347. Schofield JG. Use of trapped fluorescent indicator to demonstrate effects of thyroliberin and dopamine on cytoplasmic calcium concentrations in bovine anterior pituitary cells. *FEBS Lett* 1983;159:79–82.
348. Brown AM, Birnbaumer L. Ionic channels and their regulation by G protein subunits. *Annu Rev Physiol* 1990;52:197–213.
349. Delbeke D, Dannies PS. Stimulation of the adenosine 3′, 5′-monophosphate and the Ca^{+2} messenger systems together reverse dopaminergic inhibition of prolactin release. *Endocrinology* 1985;117:439–446.
350. Linden J, Delahunty TM. Receptors that inhibit phosphoinositide breakdown. *Trends Pharmacol Sci* 1989;10:114–120.
351. Fuxe K, Hokfelt T, Eneroth P, Gustafsson JA, Skett P. Prolactin-like immunoreactivity: localization in nerve terminals of rat hypothalamus. *Science* 1977;196:899–900.
352. Toubeau G, Desclin J, Parmentier M, Pasteels JL. Cellular localization of a prolactin-like antigen in the rat brain. *J Endocrinol* 1979;83:261–266.
353. Emanuele NV, Metcalfe L, Wallock L, Tentler J, Hagen TC, Beer CT, Martinson D, Gout PW, Kirsteins L, Lawrence AM. Hypothalamic prolactin: characterization by radioimmunoassay and bioassay and response to hypophysectomy and restraint stress. *Neuroendocrinology* 1986;44:217–221.
354. Emanuele NV, Metcalfe L, Lubrano T, Rubinstein H, Kirsteins L, Lawrence AM. Subcellular distribution of hypothalamic prolactin-like immunoreactivity. *Brain Res* 1987;407:223–229.
355. DeVito WJ, Connors JM, Hedge GA. Immunoreactive prolactin in the rat hypothalamus: *in vitro* release and subcellular localization. *Neuroendocrinology* 1987;46:155–161.
356. Alonso G, Siaud P, Faivre-Sarraih C, Grouselle D, Barbanel G, Assenmacher I. Axons containing a prolactin-like peptide project into the perivascular layer of the median eminence: an immunocytochemical light and electron microscope study in adult and intact rats. *Neuroendocrinology* 1988;48:39–44.

357. Azad N, Kirsteins L, Emanuele NV, Lawrence AM. The effects of various extraction procedures on chromatographic profiles of hypothalamic prolactin-like immunoreactive proteins (PLIP). *Neuroendocrin Lett* 1989;11:115–122.
358. Shivers BD, Harlan RE, Pfaff DW. A subset of neurons containing immunoreactive prolactin is a target for estrogen regulation of gene expression in rat hypothalamus. *Neuroendocrinology* 1989;49:23–27.
359. DeVito WJ. Immunoreactive prolactin in the hypothalamus and cerebrospinal fluid of male and female rats. *Neuroendocrinology* 1989;50:182–186.
360. Nishizuka M, Shivers BD, Leranth C, Pfaff DW. Ultrastructural characterization of prolactin-like immunoreactivity in rat medial basal hypothalamus. *Neuroendocrinology* 1990;51:249–254.
361. Toubeau G, Desclin J, Parmentier M, Pasteels JL. Compared localizations of prolactin-like and adrenocorticotropin immunoreactivities within the brain of the rat. *Neuroendocrinology* 1979;29:374–384.
362. Thompson SA. Localization of immunoreactive prolactin in ependyma and circumventricular organs of rat brain. *Cell Tissue Res* 1982;225:79–93.
363. DeVito WJ. Distribution of immunoreactive prolactin in the male and female brain: effects of hypophysectomy and intraventricular administration of colchicine. *Neuroendocrinology* 1988; 47:284–289.
364. Schachter BS, Durgerian S, Harlan RE, Pfaff DW, Shivers BD. Prolactin mRNA exists in rat hypothalamus. *Endocrinology* 1984;114:1947–1949.
365. Emanuele NV, Jurgens JK, Halloran MM, Tentler JJ, Lawrence AM, Kelley MR. The rat prolactin gene is expressed in brain tissue: detection of normal and alternatively spliced prolactin messenger RNA. *Mol Endocrinology* 1992;6:35–42.
366. Emanuele NV, Metcalfe L, Tentler J, Kirsteins L, Lawrence AM. The effect of colchicine on distribution of prolactin-like immunoreactivity (PLIP) in the rat brain. *Neuroendocr Lett* 1988;10: 107–111.
367. Hansen BL, Hansen GN. Immunocytochemical demonstration of somatotropin-like and prolactin-like activity in the brain of Calamoichthys calabaricus (Actinopterygii). *Cell Tissue Res* 1982;222:615–627.
368. Harlan RE, Shivers BD, Fox SR, Kaplove KA, Schachter BS, Pfaff DW. Distribution and partial characterization of immunoreactive prolactin in the rat brain. *Neuroendocrinology* 1989;49: 7–22.
369. Wilson DM, Emanuele NV, Jurgens JK, Kelley MR. Prolactin message in brain and pituitary of adult male rats is identical: PCR cloning and sequencing of hypothalamic prolactin cDNA from intact and hypophysectomized adult male rats. *Endocrinology* 1992;131:2488–2490.
370. Walsh RJ, Posner BI, Kopriwa B, Brawer J. Prolactin binding sites in the rat brain. *Science* 1978;201:1041–1043.
371. Di Carlo R, Muccioli G, Lando D, Bellussi G. Further evidence for the presence of specific binding sites for prolactin in the rabbit brain: preferential distribution in the hypothalamus and substantia nigra. *Life Sci* 1985;36:375–382.
372. Barton AC, Lahti RA, Piercey MF, Moore KE. Autoradiographic identification of prolactin binding sites in rat median eminence. *Neuroendocrinology* 1989;49:649–653.
373. Hokfelt T, Fuxe K. Effects of prolactin and ergot alkaloids on the tuberoinfundibular dopamine (DA) neurons. *Neuroendocrinology* 1971;9:100–122.
374. Sarkar DK. Evidence for prolactin feedback actions on hypothalamic oxytocin, vasoactive intestinal peptide and dopamine secretion. *Neuroendocrinology* 1989;49:520–524.
375. Brar AK, McNeilly AS, Fink G. Effects of hyperprolactinemia and testosterone on the release of LH-releasing hormone and the gonadotrophins in intact and castrated rats. *J Endocrinol* 1985;104:35–43.
376. Kooy A, de Greef WJ, Vreeburg JTM, Hackeng WHL, Ooms PM, Lamberts SWJ, Weber RFA. Evidence for the involvement of corticotropin-releasing factor in the inhibition of gonadotropin release induced by hyperprolactinemia. *Neuroendocrinology* 1990;51:261–266.
377. Cocchi D, Petraglia F, Ganzetti I, Parenti M, Genazzani AR, Muller EE. Hyperprolactinemia and the opioid hypothalamic systems. In: MacLeod RM, Thorner MO, Scapagnini U, eds. *Prolactin: basis and clinical correlates.* Padova: Fidia Press; 1985:633–640.
378. Bridges RS, Ronsheim PM. Prolactin (PRL) regulation of maternal behavior in rats: bromocriptine treatment delays and PRL promotes the rapid onset of behavior. *Endocrinology* 1990; 126:837–348.
379. Drago F, Bohus B, Canonico PL, Scapagnini U. Prolactin induces grooming in the rat: possible involvement of nigrostriatal dopaminergic system. *Pharmacol Biochem Behav* 1981;15: 61–63.
380. Gerardo-Gettens T, Moore BJ, Stern JS, Horwitz BA. Prolactin stimulates food intake in a dose-dependent manner. *Am J Physiol* 1989;256:R276–R280.
381. Scapagnini U, Drago F, Continella G, Spadaro F, Pennisi G, Gerendai I. Experimental and clinical effects of prolactin on behavior. In: MacLeod RM, Scapagnini U, Thorner MO, eds. *Prolactin: basic and clinical correlates.* Padova: Liviana Press; 1985:583–590.
382. Rothchild I, Gibori G. The luteotrophic action of decidual tissue: the stimulating effect of decidualization on the serum progesterone level of pseudopregnant rats. *Endocrinology* 1975;97: 838–842.
383. Gibori G, Rothchild I, Pepe GI, Morishige WK, Lam P. Luteotropic action of the decidual tissue in the rat. *Endocrinology* 1974;95:1113–1118.
384. Jayatilak PG, Puryear TK, Herz Z, Fazleabas A, Gibori B. Protein secretion by mesometrial and antimesometrial rat decidual tissue: evidence for differential gene expression. *Endocrinology* 1989;125:659–666.
385. Roby KF, Soares MJ. Biochemical characterization of rat decidual and placental prolactin-like protein-B immunoreactive proteins. *Program of the annual meeting of the Society for the Study of Reproduction.* Vancouver, BC, Canada, 1991:167(abst).
386. Golander A, Hurley T, Barrett J, Hizi A, Handweger S. Prolactin synthesis by human chorion-decidual tissue: a possible source of amniotic fluid prolactin. *Science* 1978;202:311–313.
387. Riddick DH, Luciano A, Kusmik W, Maslar I. *De novo* synthesis of prolactin by human decidua. *Life Sci* 1978;23:1913–1921.
388. Golander A, Hurley T, Barrett J, Handwerger S. Synthesis of prolactin by human decidua in vitro. *J Endocrinol* 1979;82: 263–267.
389. Hwang P, Murray JB, Jacobs JW, Niall HD, Friesen H. Human amniotic fluid prolactin: purification by affinity chromatography and amino-terminal sequence. *Biochemistry* 1974;13:2354–2358.
390. Gellersen B, DiMattia GE, Friesen HG, Bohnet HG. Prolactin (PRL) mRNA from human decidua differs from pituitary PRL mRNA but resembles the IM-9-P3 lymphoblasts PRL transcript. *Mol Cell Endocrinol* 1989;64:127–130.
391. Bell SC. Decidualization: regional differentiation and associated function. *Oxf Rev Reprod Biol* 1983;5:220–271.
392. Huang JR, Tseng L, Bishof P, Janne OA. Regulation of prolactin production by progestin, estrogen, and relaxin in human endometrial stromal cells. *Endocrinology* 1987;121:2011–2017.
393. Tseng L, Gav JG, Chen P, Zhu HH, Mazela J, Powel DR. Effect of progestin, antiprogestin, and relaxin on the accumulation of prolactin and insulin-like growth factor binding protein-1 messenger ribonucleic acid in human endometrial stromal cells. *Biol Reprod* 1992;47:441–450.
394. Deanesly R, Newton WH. The influence of the placenta on the corpus luteum of pregnancy in the mouse. *J Endocrinol* 1941;2:317–321.
395. Gardner WU, Allen E. Effects of hypophysectomy at midpregnancy in the mouse. *Anat Rec* 1942;83:75–97.
396. Newton WH, Beck N. Placental activity in the mouse in the absence of the pituitary gland. *J Endocrinol* 1939;1:65–75.
397. Pencharz RI, Long JA. The effect of hypophysectomy on gestation in the rat. *Science* 1931;74:206.
398. Pencharz RI, Long JA. Hypophysectomy in the pregnant rat. *Am J Anat* 1933;53:117–139.
399. Selye H, Collip JB, Thomson DL. Effect of hypophysectomy upon pregnancy and lactation in mice. *Proc Soc Exp Biol Med* 1933;30:589–590.
400. Robertson MC, Friesen HG. Two forms of rat placental lactogen

revealed by radioimmunoassay. *Endocrinology* 1981;108: 2388–2390.
401. Soares MJ, Colosi P, Talamantes F. The development and characterization of a homologous radioimmunoassay for mouse placental lactogen. *Endocrinology* 1982;110:668–670.
402. Kelly PA, Shiu RPC, Robertson MC, Friesen HG. Characterization of rat chorionic mammotropin. *Endocrinology* 1975;96: 1187–1195.
403. Robertson MC, Gillespie B, Friesen HG. Characterization of the two forms of rat placental lactogen (rPL):rPL–I and rPL–II. *Endocrinology* 1982;111:1862–1866.
404. Soares MJ, Colosi P, Ogren L, Talamantes F. Identification and partial characterization of a lactogen from the midpregnant mouse conceptus. *Endocrinology* 1983;112:1313–1317.
405. Colosi P, Ogren L, Thordarson G, Talamantes F. Purification and partial characterization of two prolactin-like glycoprotein hormone complexes from the midpregnant mouse conceptus. *Endocrinology* 1987;120:2500–2511.
406. Faria TN, Deb S, Kwok SCM, Talamantes F, Soares MJ. Ontogeny of placental lactogen-I and placental lactogen-II expression in the developing rat placenta. *Dev Biol* 1990;141:279–291.
407. Nieder GL, Jennes L. Production of mouse placental lactogen-I by trophoblast giant cells *in utero* and *in vitro*. *Endocrinology* 1990;126:2809–2814.
408. Soares MJ, Julian JA, Glasser SR. Trophoblast giant cell release of placental lactogens: temporal and regional characteristics. *Dev Biol* 1985;107:520–526.
409. Duckworth ML, Kirk KL, Friesen HG. Isolation and identification of a cDNA clone of rat placental lactogen II. *J Biol Chem* 1986;261:10871–10878.
410. Robertson MC, Croze F, Schroedter IC, Friesen HG. Molecular cloning and expression of rat placental lactogen-I complementary deoxyribonucleic acid. *Endocrinology* 1990;172:702–710.
411. Duckworth ML, Peden LM, Friesen HG. Isolation of a novel prolactin-like cDNA clone from developing rat placenta. *J Biol Chem* 1986;261:10879–10884.
412. Duckworth ML, Peden LM, Friesen HG. A third prolactin-like protein expressed by the developing rat placenta: complementary deoxyribonucleic acid sequence and partial structure of the gene. *Mol Endocrinol* 1988;2:912–920.
413. Robertson MC, Friesen HG. The rat placenta expresses multiple rPL–I genes. *Program of the seventy-second annual meeting of the Endocrine Society*. Atlanta, GA, 1991;286(abst).
414. Deb S, Roby KF, Faria TN, Szpirer C, Levan G, Kwok SCM, Soares MJ. Molecular cloning and characterization of a prolactin-like protein C complementary deoxyribonucleic acid. *J Biol Chem* 1991;266:23027–23032.
415. Freemark M, Comer M, Korner G, Handwerger S. A unique placental lactogen receptor: implication for fetal growth. *Endocrinology* 1987;120:1865–1872.
416. Hill DJ, Freemark M, Strain AJ, Handwerger S, Milner RDG. Placental lactogen and growth hormone receptors in human fetal tissues: relationship to fetal plasma human placental lactogen concentrations and fetal growth. *J Clin Endocrinol Metab* 1988;66:1283–1290.
417. Ogren L, Talamantes F. Prolactins of pregnancy and their cellular sources. *Int Rev Cytol* 1988;112:1–65.
418. Southard JN, Talamantes F. Placental prolactin-like proteins in rodents: variations on a structural theme. *Mol Cell Endocrinol* 1991;79:C133–C140.
419. Soares MJ, Faria TN, Roby KF, Deb S. Pregnancy and the prolactin family of hormones: coordination of anterior pituitary, uterine, and placental expression. *Endocrine Rev* 1991;12: 402–423.
420. Hartmann DP, Holaday JW, Bernton EW. Inhibition of lymphocyte proliferation by antibodies to prolactin. *FASEB J* 1989; 3:2194–2202.
421. Sabharwal P, Glaser R, Lafuse W, Varma S, Lin Q, Arkins S, Kooijman R, Kutz L, Kelley W, Malakey WB. Prolactin synthesized and secreted by human peripheral blood mononuclear cells: an autocrine growth factor for lymphoproliferation. *Proc Natl Acad Sci USA* 1992;89:7713–7716.
422. Di Mattia GE, Gellersen B, Bohnet HG, Friesen HG. A human β-lymphoblastoid cell line produces prolactin. *Endocrinology* 1988;122:2508–2517.
423. Gellersen B, Di Mattia GE, Friesen HG, Bohnet HG. Phorbol ester stimulates prolactin release but reduces prolactin mRNA in the human β-lymphoblastoid cell line IM–9–P. *Mol Cell Endocrinol* 1989;66:153–161.
424. Montgomery DW, Zukoski CF, Shah NG, Buckley AR, Pacholczk T, Russell DH. Concanavalin A-stimulated murine splenocytes produce a factor with prolactin-like bioactivity and immunoreactivity. *Biochem Biophys Res Commun* 1987;145: 692–698.
425. Kenner JR, Smith PF, Bernton EW, Hartman D, Holaday JW. Murine splenic lymphocytes demonstrate Con A-inducible prolactin-like immunoreactivity as determined by immunocytochemistry (ICC). *Soc Neurosci* 1988;14:756(abst).
426. Spangelo BL, Hall NR, Ross R, Goldstein AL. Stimulation of in vivo antibody production and concanavalin A-induced mouse spleen cell mitogenesis by prolactin. *Immunopharmacology* 1987;14:11–20.
427. Hiestand PC, Mekler R, Nordmann E, Grieder A, Permmongkol C. Prolactin as a modulator of lymphocyte responsiveness provides a possible mechanism of action for cyclosporine. *Proc Natl Acad Sci USA* 1986;83:2599–2603.
428. Gout PW, Beer CT, Noble RL. Prolactin-stimulated growth of cell cultures established from malignant Nb rat lymphomas. *Cancer Res* 1980;40:2433–2436.
429. Viselli SM, Stanek EM, Mukherjee P, Hymer WC, Mastro AM. Prolactin-induced mitogenesis of lymphocytes from ovariectomized rats. *Endocrinology* 1991;129:983–990.
430. Berczi I, Nagy E, de Toledo SM, Matusik RJ, Friesen HG. Pituitary hormones regulate c-myc and DNA synthesis in lymphoid tissue. *J Immunol* 1991;146:2201–2206.
431. Montgomery DW, Shen GK, Ulrich ED, Steiner LL, Parrish PR, Zukoski CF. Human thymocytes express a prolactin-like messenger ribonucleic acid and synthesize bioactive prolactin-like protein. *Endocrinology* 1992;131:3019–3026.
432. Shin RPC, Elsholtz HP, Tanake T, Friesen HG, Gout PW, Geer CT, Noble RL. Receptor mediated mitogenic action of prolactin in a rat lymphoma cell line. *Endocrinology* 1983;113:159–165.
433. Russel DH, Kibler R, Matrisian L, Larson DF, Poulos B, Magun BE. Prolactin receptors in human T and B lymphocytes: antagonism of prolactin binding by cyclosporine. *J Immunol* 1985;134:3027–3051.
434. Matera L, Muccioli G, Cesano A, Bellusi G, Genazzani E. Prolactin receptors on large granular lymphocytes: dual regulation by cyclosporine A. *Brain Behav Immun* 1988;2:1–10.
435. Pellegrini I, Lebrun JJ, Ali S, Kelly PA. Expression of prolactin and its receptor in human lymphoid cells. *Mol Endocrinol* 1992;6:1023–1031.
436. Viselli SM, Mastro AM. Prolactin receptors are found on heterogenous subpopulations of rat splenocytes. *Endocrinology* 1993; 132:571–576.
437. Shirota M, Banville D, Joieveur C, Boutin JM, Edery M, Djiane J, Kelly PA. Two forms of prolactin receptor are present in rat ovary and liver. *Mol Endocrinol* 1990;4:1136–1143.
438. Jahn GA, Edery M, Belair L, Kelly PA, Djiane J. Prolactin receptor gene expression in rat mammary gland and liver during pregnancy and lactation. *Endocrinology* 1991;128:2976–2984.
439. Kelly PA, Djiane J, Edery N. Different forms of the prolactin receptor: insights into mechanisms of prolactin action. *Trends Endocrinol Metab* 1992;3:54–59.
440. Bazan JF. A novel family of growth factor receptors: a common binding domain in the growth hormone, prolactin, erythropoetin and IL-6 receptors and the p75 IL–2 receptor beta-chain. *Biochem Biophys Res Commun* 1989;164:788–795.
441. Kelly PD, Djiane J, Postel-Vinay MC, Edery M. The prolactin growth hormone receptor family. *Endocr Rev* 1991;12:235–251.
442. Berczi I, Nagy E, Kovacs K, Horvath E. Regulation of humoral immunity in rats by pituitary hormones. *Acta Endocrinol* 1981;98:506–513.
443. Berczi I, Nagy E. The effect of prolactin and growth hormone on hemolymphopoietic tissue and immune function. In: Berczi I, Kovacs K, eds. *Hormones and immunity*. Lancaster, UK: MTP Press Ltd; 1987:145–171.
444. Berczi I, Nagy E. Effects of hypophysectomy on immune function. In: Ader R, Felton DL, Cohen N, eds. *Psychoneuroimmunology II*. New York: Academic Press; 1991:339–375.
445. Nagy E, Berczi I. Hypophysectomized rats depend on residual prolactin for survival. *Endocrinology* 1991;128:2776–2784.

The Physiology of Reproduction, Second Edition,
edited by E. Knobil and J.D. Neill,
Raven Press, Ltd., New York © 1994.

CHAPTER 34

Reproductive and Other Roles of Inhibins and Activins

Wylie Vale, Louise M. Bilezikjian, and Catherine Rivier

THE INHIBIN CONCEPT

Inhibins and activins were first isolated from gonadal fluids because of their effects on the production of follicle stimulating hormone (FSH) by the pituitary. The term inhibin was coined over 60 years ago (1,2) to describe a nonsteroidal, water-soluble factor in gonadal extracts that could suppress the morphological response of the pituitary to castration. The existence of such a factor had been proposed earlier by Mottram and Cramer (3) who reported that radiation-induced damage to the germinal elements caused pituitary hypertrophy. Although this concept was championed by McCullagh over the ensuing years (4,5), other workers were initially unable to confirm those results (6,7).

With the development of improved *in vivo* and *in vitro* bioassays for inhibin which took advantage of the then new radioimmunoassays for gonadotropins, many groups observed that gonadal extracts and fluids, such as porcine ovarian follicular fluid and ram rete testis fluid, selectively inhibited FSH secretion (8–15; for reviews see refs. 16–19). Inhibins were purified from such gonadal fluids based upon their ability to inhibit the secretion of FSH by cultured anterior pituitary cells (12,20). In 1985, four groups reported the isolation, the dimeric structure, and the partial sequence analysis of inhibins from either bovine or porcine granulosa fluids (20–23). Inhibins were found to comprise two disulfide bridged subunits, now called α and β. From bovine follicular fluids, Robertson et al. (21) isolated a 58-kDa protein representing a complex of a 44-kDa α subunit and a 14-kDa β subunit. The other three groups, Miyamoto et al. (22), Ling et al. (23) and Rivier et al. (20), purified proteins of approximately 32 kDa, composed of 18-kDa α subunits and 14-kDa β subunits, from porcine follicular fluid. Probes designed from the *N*-terminal sequences of each chain were used to select clones from porcine, bovine, and human cDNA libraries leading to the deduction of the sequences of inhibins and their precursors from each of those species (24–30). As illustrated in Fig. 1, the human α subunit precursor is a 366 amino acid protein with three potential glycosylation sites and potential proteolytic cleavage sites that could generate various proteins, including the 44-kDa form isolated from bovine follicular fluid and the 18- to 20-kDa form isolated from porcine follicular fluid (20–23). In fact, we now know that the ovary and other tissues produce a variety of α subunit forms, including a 26-kDa form, in which a middle pep-

Peptide Biology Laboratory, Salk Institute, San Diego, California 92138

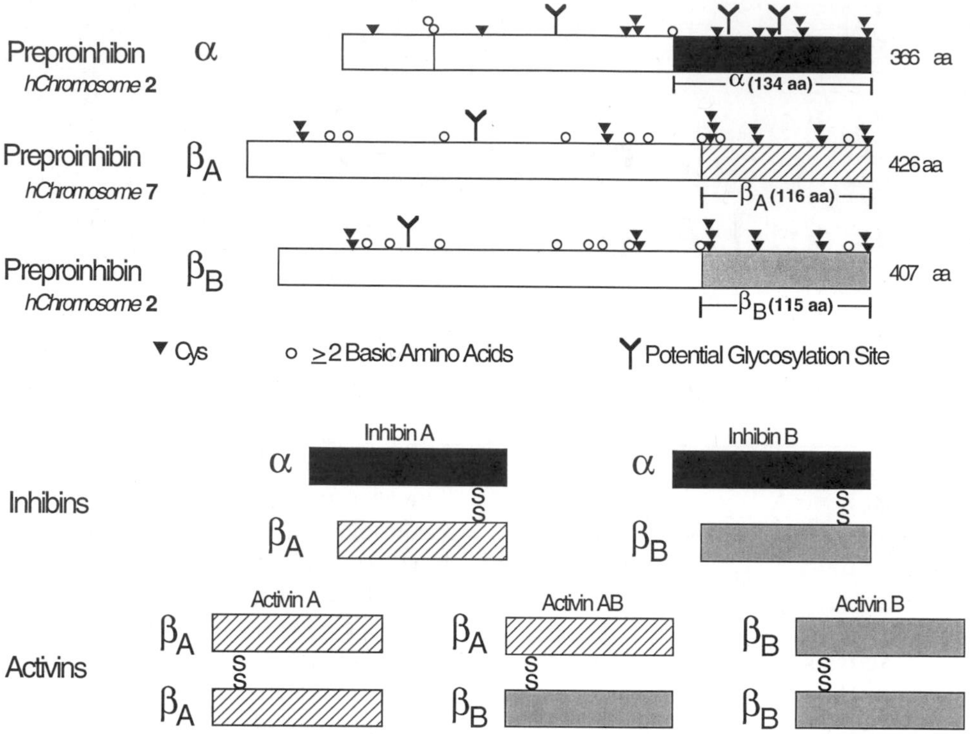

FIG. 1. Schematic of the precursors of the human inhibin α, βA, and βB subunits, their chromosomal localization and their dimerization pattern. The mature proteins are indicated by the shaded areas.

tide of the precursor is missing and the *N*-terminal peptide is linked by a disulfide bond to the *C*-terminal protein (31). There are two distinct β subunit precursors generating mature βA or βB proteins of 116 or 115 amino acids, respectively (24). Dimers comprising $\alpha\beta$A or $\alpha\beta$B are called inhibin A or inhibin B, respectively. The mature inhibin subunits are structurally related; βA and βB are approximately 70% identical to each other and 30% identical to the α subunit. The human α and βB subunits have been localized to chromosome 2 and the human βA to chromosome 7 (32,33).

The first male inhibin was isolated from ram rete testis fluid and included a truncated α subunit, which was missing the first 15 amino acids and was associated with a mature βA subunit (34). Inhibin/activin α, βA, and βB subunits were subsequently cloned from a sheep testis library (35) and were found to be closely related to the other inhibins, suggesting identity between male and female inhibins. Tissues, however, may differ in the post-translational processing of the subunits, particularly of the α chain. Although subtle differences may exist in potency and half-life, all dimeric inhibins are biologically active. The ovary, in particular, produces a substantial quantity of the free α subunit (31,36,37). One group has reported that fractions containing this protein regulate ovarian sensitivity to FSH, but the chemical identity of the biologically active molecule has not been established unequivocally (38).

While purifying inhibins, our group and Nick Ling's group observed fractions of follicular fluids that could stimulate, rather than inhibit, the secretion of FSH (20,39,40). The proteins responsible for this activity were isolated and characterized as dimers of the inhibin β subunits. We identified βAβA homodimers (40), now known as activin A, and Ling et al. (39) identified the βAβB heterodimer or activin AB. The activin B homodimer, βBβB, was first prepared by recombinant methods (41) and only very recently isolated from natural sources (42). All three activins are biologically active to stimulate FSH secretion by the pituitary gland. The structural and functional relationships between inhibins and activins demonstrate a powerful mechanism for the generation of signal diversity from a limited number of genes whereby differential subunit association can result in the generation of dimers with opposing biological actions in the pituitary and many other tissues (Fig. 2 and see below).

Inhibins and activins are related to the transforming growth factor-β (TGF-β) superfamily. This family encompasses the three mammalian and one each of chicken and Xenopus TGF-βs, Mullerian duct inhibiting substance (MIS) (43), noggin (44), dorsalin (45), many members of the decapentaplegic-Vg-related (DVR) subfamily including the drosophila decapentaplegic gene product (46), bone morphogenic protein (BMPs)-2–8 (47), vegetal pole derived growth factor gene products of xenopus V (48), and multiple "orphan" ligands related to the superfamily that have been cloned by amplification using the polymerase chain reaction (PCR) (49–53).

As is reviewed below, activin is a fully functional member of this superfamily of growth factors and has in fact been isolated from many tissues because of its local effects on cellular growth and differentiation. The tissue distribution of inhibin and activin subunits has been studied by measuring levels of proteins with radioimmunoassays, two-site immunoradiometric assays, and immunohistochemistry, and the distribution of messenger ribonucleic acids (mRNAs) has been studied using S1-nuclease and Northern analyses as well as by quantitative PCR.

BROAD TISSUE DISTRIBUTION OF INHIBIN AND ACTIVIN SUBUNITS

As expected, inhibin and activin subunit proteins and their mRNAs were found in the ovary, testis, and placenta from which they had been cloned, but they were also identified in many other adult tissues including the brain, pituitary, adrenals, bone marrow, and kidney (54). In addition, inhibin–activin subunits are found in spermatids, unfertilized and fertilized ova (for review see ref. 55), and embryos at all stages, localizing to a number of embryonic organs including the heart, skin, somites, spinal cord, bones, brain, and gonads (56). Measurements of inhibin/activin subunits do not reveal the amounts of biologically active dimers, although the studies of Mason et al. (33) who transfected naive cells with different proportions of α and β subunit mRNAs suggest that the ratio of subunits or their turnover rate may, in part, determine which dimers are formed. As in the gonads (54), in tissues that have a substantial excess of α over β subunits, inhibin would, and has been observed, to predominate over activin. In tissues, such as the bone marrow and placenta that express mainly β subunits, activin should predominate. Although the proteins in most nongonadal sources of inhibins and activins have not been fully characterized, the dimers, where explored, have been found to be present. Because of the equally wide distribution of activin receptors (see below) and the numerous actions of activins in a panoply of tissues, cells, and derived cell lines, it is plausible that activins play local physiological roles wherever they are found (Fig. 2).

FOLLISTATIN

Other fractions from follicular fluids that could modulate the secretion of FSH were purified and characterized (57–59) and found to contain a protein of 315 amino acids with molecular weights varying from 32 kDa to 43 kDa, depending on the degree of glycosylation. These proteins, now termed follistatins, can inhibit the secretion of FSH by cultured pituitary cells with a potency somewhat less than that of inhibin and have subsequently been shown to bind activins with high affinity and neutralize their biological activity (60,61). It is proposed that two molecules of follistatin bind to the two β subunits of activins, whereas one molecule of follistatin binds to each inhibin molecule that has only one

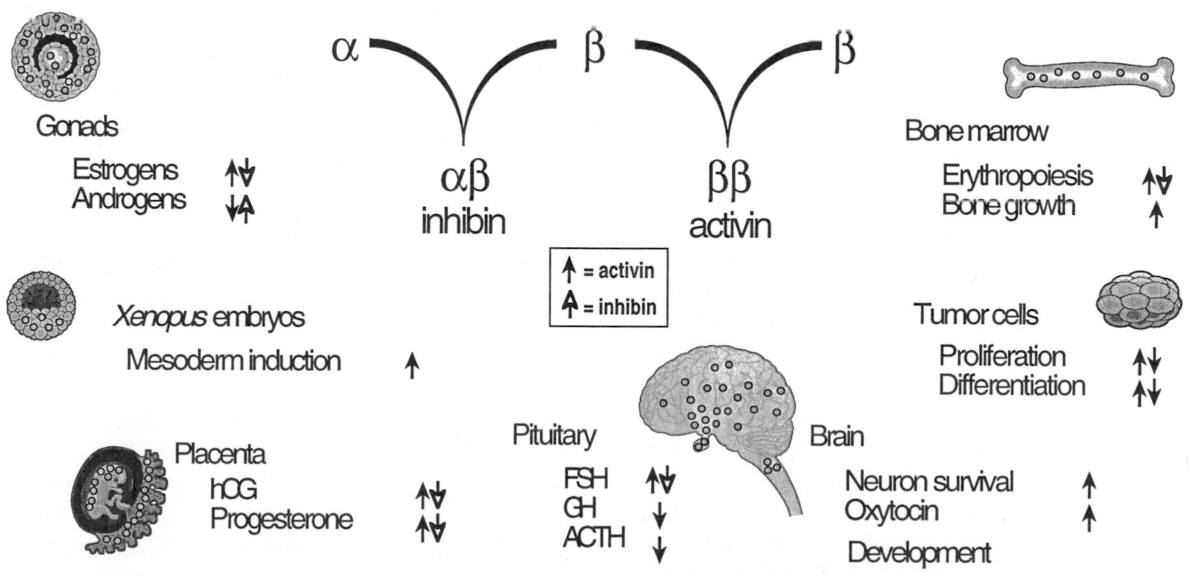

FIG. 2. Summary of the biological activities of inhibins and activins.

β subunit (62). Even though the ability of follistatin to biologically inactivate activin has been established, the follistatin-bound inhibin was reported to retain biological activity (57), although the latter has not been conclusively determined, in part because of a lack of a suitable assay system. By analogy, we have found that antibodies to the βA subunit, which inactivate activin A, do not inactivate inhibin A, suggesting that perhaps the β subunit in inhibin may not directly interact with its receptors (J. Vaughan, A. Corrigan, and W. Vale, *unpublished results*). Follistatins are widely distributed (63,64) and are produced by many activin-responsive tissues or those that express the inhibin/activin β subunits (54) and may, therefore, serve to anatomically and temporally limit the local activities of activins.

THE PITUITARY

Inhibins and activins exert powerful and opposing effects on basal FSH secretion, biosynthesis and FSHβ mRNA accumulation by cultured rat (40,65–71) and ovine (72,73) anterior pituitary cells. *In vivo* experiments have demonstrated similar effects (74–78). The *in vitro* actions of inhibin and activin on FSH secretion and production show a long latent period with maximal effects being observed at $\geq$24 hours (66). This is in contrast to the very rapid actions of gonadotropin-releasing hormone (GnRH) (79). In contrast to their slow effects on FSH secretion, inhibin- or activin-induced changes in FSHβ mRNA levels have usually been seen within 1 or 2 hours (66). Studies conducted in the presence of inhibitors of transcription indicate that activin acts in part by increasing the stability of FSHβ mRNA, whereas inhibin labilizes it (80,81). Inhibin suppresses FSH secretion mediated by GnRH and other secretagogues including phorbol esters (67,82). Inhibin, which does not modulate basal LH production, does inhibit GnRH-stimulated LH secretion *in vitro* (16,67,82,83). Under most (84) but not all (186) *in vivo* circumstances, administration of inhibin or conversely of anti-inhibin serum does not influence LH secretion (84), so the physiological significance of these *in vitro* effects on LH secretion are unknown. Activin is similarly without effect on basal LH secretion *in vitro* (40), but activin injection to female rats was recently reported to elevate serum LH at metestrus (85). The physiological significance and the mechanism of the latter remains to be elucidated. Activin has been reported to increase the numbers of cells immunoreactive for FSH in anterior pituitary cultures (86); confirmatory direct monitoring of the mitotic index of gonadotropes has not been reported.

The effect of exogenous administration of inhibin or activin has been studied in a variety of models. In the rat of both sexes, recombinant human inhibin causes dose- and time-related decreases in plasma FSH, but not LH, levels (87–90). This effect is enhanced by the absence of GnRH drive (91). Injection of activin, on the other hand, stimulates FSH release, and this effect is abolished by concomitant injection of inhibin (90).

Observation of inhibin/activin α and βB subunit mRNAs (54) in the pituitary gland with the subsequent localization of α and βB proteins to the cytoplasm of the gonadotropes (92) raised the possibility that inhibin B and/or activin B might be secreted and function as autocrine regulators of FSH production. Functional evidence for such a mechanism was provided by immunoneutralization experiments in which the addition to anterior pituitary cell cultures of monoclonal antibodies to activin B was found to selectively reduce spontaneous FSH secretion and FSHβ mRNA levels in a dose- and time-dependent manner (93). Antiactivin B globulins were shown to also reduce FSH levels in hypophysectomized and ovariectomized rats bearing pituitary grafts and to abolish the secondary FSH surge in cycling female rats (94). Follistatin, which is found in pituitary folliculostellate cells (95) and in gonadotropes (96), may provide a local means of interdicting the effects of activin. Indeed, activin and follistatin appear to modulate reciprocally each other's production within the pituitary, thereby tightly regulating each other's availability and actions within this tissue (97,98). Similar regulatory mechanisms may be functional in other tissues such as the gonads (63,64). The concept that the pituitary might have such complex autoregulatory mechanisms has been championed by Denef and colleagues for some time (99).

Activins modulate the functions and growth of other pituitary cell types as well. The basal secretion of growth hormone (GH) and corticotropin (ACTH) *in vitro* is strongly inhibited by activin (40,100–103). Furthermore, activin suppresses growth hormone releasing factor (GRF)-stimulated GH secretion (101) and cAMP induction (102). Activin inhibits GRF-stimulated proliferation of cultured rat anterior pituitary somatotropes (101) as well as the proliferative rates of somatomammotropic MtTw15 tumor cells (Struthers and W. Vale, *personal observations*) and the corticotropic AtT20 cell line (103).

GONADAL INHIBINS AND ACTIVINS

Gonadal Localization

In males, there is evidence for the presence of inhibin subunits ($\alpha > \beta B \gg \beta A$) in several testicular cell types, including Leydig and Sertoli cells (35,104–106; reviewed in refs. 55,107). The relative expression level and the pattern of expression of the three subunits, however, appear to change throughout sexual development, suggesting that different dimeric forms are produced at different stages of growth and development of the testis and are consistent with a changing role for these dimeric proteins. In the male rat, for example, α-subunit mRNA peaks by age 20 to 25 days with a gradual decline thereafter (108), paralleling plasma inhibin levels (104). Sertoli cells are presumed to be the primary source of circulating inhibin and to express α, βB, and, to a lesser extent, βA (105,106), and they have been shown to secrete inhibin B (109) and activin B (110) *in vitro*. Although Leydig cells have been identified as another site of α subunit production (105,106), controversy remains regarding whether these cells are a source of bioactive inhibin (55). Interstitial Leydig cells, however, are likely to be a source of activin, which functions as an intragonadal paracrine factor (111). Activin secreted by Sertoli cells, on the other hand, is likely to function as an autocrine factor (110). Spermatogenic cells represent yet another site of α subunit expression, and spermatogonia of defined stages may exert a paracrine influence on various testicular compartments (112,113).

In the female rat, ovarian inhibin is expressed primarily in follicles, and its presence in the corpus luteum may be species specific (114–117). The mRNA encoding the α chain is found at all stages of follicular development of female rats, whereas those coding for the β chains are detected in healthy tertiary follicles throughout the cycle and secondary follicles at estrus (114,115). The maturing follicle is considered to be the main source of inhibin during the first part of the cycle (118–120), whereas during the luteal phase, inhibin comes primarily from the corpus luteum (114,121–125).

Gonadal Secretion of Inhibin and Activin

The gonadal secretion of inhibins *in vitro* and *in vivo* has been measured by both bioassay and various immunological methods. Bioassays originally used for inhibin were based on their ability to inhibit FSH secretion by cultured anterior pituitary cells. Because such assays reflect the net ability of a preparation to alter FSH secretion, they would be sensitive not only to inhibin but also to other proteins such as activin and follistatin. Following the characterization of the 32-kDa inhibin molecule, specific inhibin radioimmunoassays, which used antibodies raised either against the whole molecule (126) or against fragments of the α chain (127), developed. Most polyclonal antisera raised against intact inhibin have contained antibodies largely directed toward the α subunit (128). Most studies reporting plasma levels of inhibin ($\alpha\beta$) have used antibodies that specifically detect the α subunit and therefore would not be affected by differential levels of activins ($\beta\beta$). However, the α chain monomer is secreted by ovarian and testicular cells and is present in plasma (31,36,37,128–132). There is, therefore, a possibility that the inhibin radioimmunoassays would detect biologically inactive molecules, although some α monomer forms have been proposed to have biological activity (38). Moreover, the gonads produce a variety of species of inhibin- and activinlike proteins (133–136), which might exert different biological effects (38). These findings indicate that caution must be exercised in interpreting results obtained with various radioimmunoassays (127,128,137,138). However, *in vitro* experiments have shown a good correlation between the effects of various secretogogues on α monomer and inhibin dimer production.

Two-site assays that require the presence of both α and β chains in the same protein for detection represent the solution to the problem of the assay of inhibin. Such assays have been developed by several groups (138–140). Many, but fortunately not all, antibodies directed toward the β subunit are perturbed by binding proteins including follistatin (60,62) and α_2 macroglobulins (140–142). The development and validation of a more sensitive two-site immunoassay for inhibin A was, however, recently reported and may prove to be useful for the measurements of serum inhibin levels (143).

Inhibins and activins share the β chains. Thus, although antibodies raised against the α chain are specific for inhibin and the α monomer, those raised against activins or the β chains also recognize inhibins. Some two-site assays that differentiate between the two proteins are now available and are reportedly useful for the measurement of activins in plasma (139,142,144).

There is extensive literature reporting effects of various treatments and circumstances on the levels of inhibin monitored by the radioimmunoassays that detect the α subunit of inhibin as a monomer or as the biologically active inhibin $\alpha\beta$ dimer, as discussed earlier. Generally, FSH is considered to be the primary stimulatory signal for inhibin secretion (145–149), although luteinizing hormone (LH) can also exert this effect (150). The ability of both LH and FSH to stimulate inhibin production reflects the inducibility of the α subunit gene by agents that elevate intracellular cyclic adenosine monophosphate (cAMP), such as FSH and LH (151,152). However, there does not appear to be either obligatory or simple effects of gonadotropins on inhibin secretion, as either LH-like molecules, or even FSH-like hormones at very large doses, can suppress the biosynthesis and release of inhibin (153,154). In female mammals, the ovarian follicles represent the primary source of circulating inhibin (155). Thus inhibin secretion is closely correlated with the pattern of follicular growth during puberty and the cyclic pattern of follicular development during the estrous or the menstrual cycles. In both rodents and humans, immunoreactive inhibin secretion is very low during infancy and increases with sexual maturation (145,156). Subsequently, the follicular phase of the cycle (characterized by the rapid growth of follicles) is accompanied by parallel increases in gonadotropins, estradiol, and inhibin levels (123,157–161). During the luteal phase, gonadotropin levels remain low in women, whereas progesterone and inhibin values increase. These observations have suggested that growing follicles represent the main source of inhibin during the follicular phase, while the corpus luteum is responsible for inhibin release during the luteal phase (150). Luteolysis results in decreased inhibin and progesterone release (122). A similar pattern is found in the ewe (119).

In the rat, differentiation between the end of one cycle and the beginning of the subsequent cycle is difficult to establish. Consequently, direct relationships between the secretion of gonadal proteins and gonadotropins cannot always be determined, although a characteristic inverse relationship between inhibin and FSH levels can often be demonstrated (118,162). The functional relationships between the primary gonadotropin surge of proestrus and inhibin biosynthesis and release have been demonstrated by the increase in inhibin observed during the afternoon of proestrus, the reversal of the latter with GnRH antagonists, and the restoration of a normal pattern of inhibin secretion and expression after exogenous gonadotropin administration in animals treated with GnRH antagonists (114,115,158,163). Such experimental models support the hypothesis that the primary gonadotropin surge during proestrus is at least in part responsible for the subsequent increase in inhibin secretion; follicles that are recruited by the secondary FSH surge release inhibin, which in turn decreases circulating FSH levels. The secretion of inhibin is, therefore, regulated by complex interactions between stimulatory and inhibitory effects of gonadotropins and sex steroids (148).

In the male, Sertoli cells, and to a lesser extent, Leydig cells, are sources of circulating immunoreactive inhibin (34,105,106,164,165). Consistently, castration lowers immunoreactive inhibin levels to nondetectable values (109,165–168). As in the female, gonadotropins modulate inhibin release from the testis (169–172) and hypophysectomy results in a significant disappearance of inhibin from the adult testis (173). Secretion of inhibin from the immature male gonad, on the other hand, may be relatively independent of gonadotropins (169). Not surprisingly, there is a general correlation between the activity of Sertoli cells and circulating immunoreactive inhibin values. In the rat, however, circulating inhibin levels increase until day 25 after birth and decline progressively during sexual maturation (104,174). This suggests some as yet undefined relationship between maturation of the germinal epithelium and inhibin production (172,174,175). In the human male, plasma inhibin levels are strongly correlated with age, showing a decline in both basal and gonadotropin-stimulated inhibin secretion in elderly men (176,177). Finally, in animals with breeding seasons (such as the ram), inhibin levels and testicular size fluctuate as a function of seasonal cycles (178).

Because inhibin is secreted by growing follicles, its circulating levels have been used as an index of follicular function in women (179). Abnormal ovaries, such as those of women with polycystic ovary syndrome, contain a larger number of antral follicles and secrete more inhibin than normal ovaries (180). In the male, damage to the seminiferous epithelium is associated with pathological changes in circulating inhibin levels (164,181–183). Surprisingly, experimental induction of cryptorchidism in rats has been reported to decrease inhibin levels in some cases (183) and increase them in others (182); an initial increase followed by a decrease, however, was also shown (181). Men with damaged Sertoli cells have also failed to exhibit subnormal inhibin values (184). In these cases, however, some of the reported values for inhibin levels may have been skewed by the use of antibodies directed against the α subunit, which may be preferentially released by cryptorchid testes.

Physiological Role of Inhibins and Activins

The exact physiological role of endogenous activins has been difficult to determine due to the unavailability of highly specific antisera that can either accurately quantify each of the three dimeric forms of activin (activin A, activin B or activin AB) or immunoneutralize their biological effects. One exception is a study in which sc injections of a monoclonal antibody to activin B was shown to suppress ovariectomy-induced FSH hypersecretion (94), revealing a role for endogenous activin B and consistent with previously reported *in vitro* data (93). The injection to female rats of recombinant human activin A, on the other hand, produces cycle-dependent changes in the secretion of both FSH and LH (85) indicating that activins play an important role in the regulation of the reproductive axis. The exact physiological role played by endogenous activins, however, remains to be established.

In female mammals, removal of endogenous inhibin by α subunit immunoneutralization causes significant increases in plasma FSH levels (157,185), suggesting that inhibin plays a physiological role in modulating FSH secretion. Its role on LH release, however, remains controversial: some laboratories report no change in the release of this hormone in rats injected with antiinhibin serum (157), but others observe increases in all parameters of LH secretion (186). It should also be noted that the consequence of removing endogenous inhibin varies between genders, varies among stages of sexual maturation, and may also be species specific. The latter is exemplified by the absence of measurable changes in FSH release in the intact adult male injected with antiinhibin serum (104) and by significant increases in FSH secretion in the case of adult male Rhesus monkeys (187). In the female rat, the physiological role of inhibin in regulating FSH secretion starts before the third week of life and continues throughout adulthood (145,157). Delivery of recombinant human inhibin A to cycling female rats does not produce measurable changes in serum LH but causes the expected decrease in serum FSH (84,85). In the male rat, the role of endogenous inhibin is less significant in older animals (104) and only becomes apparent in the absence of Leydig cells (188,189).

Inhibin also exerts paracrine stimulatory effects on folliculogenesis (190). Thus, removal of endogenous inhibin could in theory cause both elevated FSH levels and decreased follicular growth. Experimentally, rats (162, 191) or ewes (192,193) injected with antibodies against inhibin show an increase in ovulation rate. When mated, rats injected with antibodies against inhibin bear an increased number of pups. To differentiate between the role of increased FSH levels and that of the direct gonadal effect of inhibin, exogenous FSH was injected into rats passively immunized against inhibin. FSH administration mimicked the effect of the anti-inhibin serum and increased the rate of ovulation, suggesting that either the antibodies do not penetrate the ovaries or that increased FSH levels counteract the gonadal actions of inhibin on follicular growth (162).

Intragonadal Function of Activins and Inhibins

Although one of the first recognized endocrine functions of circulating inhibin was the feedback inhibition of pituitary FSH secretion, subsequent studies clearly indicated that activins and inhibins function as intragonadal autocrine/paracrine factors as well (195). The characterization of specific activin-binding sites on granulosa cells (196,197) and germ cells (198) reinforced this concept. Further evaluation of gonadal tissue has revealed that the mRNAs for the various known isotypes of activin receptors (see below) are differentially expressed in various cell types whereby inhibins and activins can exert cell-specific and/or cycle-dependent actions (199–202). The latter, coupled with the coordinated expression and biosynthesis of each inhibin or activin subunit, provides a mechanism for the regulation of gonadal functions at defined stages of gonadal development and function.

Depending on the physiological or differentiated status of gonadal cells, treatment with either activin or inhibin results in cell-specific alterations in a number of cellular functions of ovarian and testicular cells, including changes in basal and gonadotropin-induced steroid and cAMP production (reviewed in refs. 16,55,63,107,203–205). Moreover, activins and inhibins may have effects on follicular growth, development, and atresia (190, 206–208) as well as oocyte maturation (209) and spermatogenesis (210,211). Inhibin was reported to enhance follicular recruitment, whereas activin promoted atresia and blocked pregnant mare gonadotripin (PMSG)-induced follicular development (190). Activin inhibits the actions of LH and human chorionic gonadotropin (hCG) on androgen production by Leydig cells at all stages of differentiation, whereas inhibin facilitates LH/hCG effects on immature Leydig cells (195,212). Activin increases basal inhibin secretion and α subunit mRNA accumulation from cultures of rat granulosa cells and augments the effects of FSH on progesterone and inhibin production (197,213). Inhibin attenuates LH-induced resumption of meiosis of follicle-enclosed oocytes (206), however, O et al. (209) reported that inhibin was able to suppress meiotic maturation of either cumulus-enclosed or denuded rat oocytes. Some of these reported effects of inhibin and activin may, however, be species specific, since activin suppresses basal and hCG-stimulated progesterone and testosterone production in human (214) and Rhesus monkey (215) luteinized follicular cells. Thus, activin and inhibin derived from granulosa cells function as either autocrine (on granulosa cells) or paracrine (on interstitial cells or luteal cells) factors within the ovary. In rat testicular tissue, activins derived from Sertoli cells function as autocrine factors of FSH-stimulated aromatase activity and as paracrine modulators of LH/hCG actions on Leydig cells.

Because each gonadal cell type is responsive to a distinct set of signals, compartmentalization of the inhibin subunits and their independent regulation establishes the possibility for the differential production of inhibin and activin dimers (16,55,63,107,203–205). This organization also provides a mechanism by which inhibins and activins can regulate their own production by autocrine and/or paracrine loops, as discussed. The treatment of granulosa (197) or Sertoli (105,106) cells with FSH, for example, initial increases α, but not β, subunit expression suggesting a preferential production of inhibins under certain physiological conditions. The latter is consistent with the presence of cAMP-responsive *cis*-elements within the promoter of the α, but not the β, subunit gene (151,152); cAMP production by agents such as FSH, LH, or forskolin would, therefore, be expected to preferentially elevate inhibin levels.

The importance of inhibin has also been underscored by observations of mice bearing a targeted deletion of the α subunit gene generated by homologous recombination in mouse embryonic stem cells (194). Mice lacking the α subunit initially develop normally, but all of them eventually develop mixed or incompletely differentiated gonadal stromal tumors, either unilaterally or bilaterally (194). These results suggest that inhibin is a critical negative regulator of gonadal stromal cell proliferation. Alternatively or additionally, in the absence of α subunit synthesis, cells expressing β subunits might overproduce activin. In either case, the ratio of activin to inhibin is perturbed in these mice with serious pathophysiological consequences.

THE PLACENTA

The human inhibin α subunit mRNA was first cloned from a human placental library (25), and mRNAs for both β subunits were subsequently detected in human placental tissues (54). The human placenta is a major source of plasma inhibin (α)-like activity and placental cells in culture secrete inhibin- and activinlike proteins (216–219). Inhibin and activin subunits and their mRNAs have been identified in trophoblast and decidual cells (220). The α subunit and its mRNA are found in the cytotrophoblast (inner) region of the villi, whereas the βB is observed in the syncytial (outer) layer. The βA protein, however, is expressed in both inner and outer layers. The expression of all three subunits in the trophoblast increases with the progression of pregnancy (221). Activin has been shown to stimulate progesterone, GnRH, and hCG production by cultured human placental cells (222); all of these effects are attenuated by inhibin (222). Specificity of these actions is shown by the failure of either activin or inhibin to influence the production of placental lactogen.

EMBRYOGENESIS/DEVELOPMENT

The distribution of activin in spermatocytes at defined stages, in unfertilized and fertilized ova and in various organs throughout embryogenesis suggests that it may be important in development. The best-documented role of activin is immediately before and during gastrulation when a great deal of axial patterning occurs and when zygotic transcription begins and mesoderm is formed (223–225). Embryologists have studied the development of mesoderm from isolated Xenopus animal caps and have used this system as a bioassay for putative factors involved in the control of gastrulation. The most potent growth factor purified on the basis of this assay has been activin A. Native and recombinant mammalian and Xenopus activins induce extensive dorsal mesoderm, including notochord and neural-inducing tissue (223–227). Interestingly, lower concentrations of activin are also able to induce ventral mesoderm (228), raising the possibility that activin gradients might contribute to dorsal-ventral patterning. Furthermore, the injection of human βA or Xenopus βB mRNA into a ventral blastomere of a 32-cell embryo induced a second body axis (225). By contrast, injection of βA mRNA into vegetal or marginal zone cells of ultraviolet-treated embryos restored a partial dorsal axis, but no head tissue, whereas mRNA for another growth factor, wnt-8, induced a complete secondary axis, suggesting that other genes, such as wnt-8 or noggin (229), are required to potentiate the action of activin *in vivo.* Although activin is present from the egg to the blastula stage (230), βB mRNA does not appear until late blastula (embryonic stage 9) and βA mRNA was not detected until late gastrula stage (stage 13) in Xenopus. The most convincing evidence for the involvement of activin in embryogenesis comes from experiments using dominant negative mutant activin receptors (see below). Mutant receptors that disrupt the activin signal transduction pathway, in most embryos, prevent the formation of any recognizable dorsal or ventral mesoderm (231). Most intriguingly, blockade of the response to activin leads to a superinduction of neural tissues. The precise roles of activin and its temporal and spatial importance relative to other growth factors including FGF, wnt-8, and other members of the TGF-β growth factor family have yet to be established.

ERYTHROPOIESIS IN BONE

Erythroid differentiation factor (EDF) was isolated from the monocytic leukemia cell line (THP-1) by virtue of its ability to promote the differentiation of Friend (MEL F5-5) erythroleukemic cells and was determined by partial sequence analysis to be activin A (232,233). Activin was also shown to cause the differentiation of human K562 and HEL erythroleukemic cell lines (232,234) and to induce hemoglobin and inhibit cell division in all of these cell types. Inhibin was found to reverse the effects of activin in the K562 cell line (234). Activins increase the proliferation of erythroid progenitor cells derived from human bone marrow and potentiate the well-described effects of erythropoietin to stimulate erythroblast- and colony-forming units (BFU-E and CFU-E) (234–239). The activin effect on erythroid colony formation is associated with an increase in the number of cells entering the S phase and is dependent upon the presence of T lymphocytes and monocytes, suggesting that other signals or cell–cell interactions may be involved (235,236). The presence of βA mRNA (54,240) in bone marrow along with the isolation of activin A from demineralized bone (241) suggests that locally produced activin might participate in the stimulation of erythropoiesis at various stages, first by potentiating the effects of erythropoietin to commit cells to the pathway and expand their populations and later by inducing terminal differentiation of the erythroid cells. The possibility that inhibin of gonadal or placental origin might modulate erythropoiesis remains to be explored.

Another possible local effect of bone-derived activin is to stimulate the formation of bone itself. Activins have been found to enhance the formation of mature bone in cartilage explants; these effects were qualitatively different from those of TGF-β and BMP-2 and -3 (241). Consistently, activin A is mitogenic for osteoblast-enriched fetal rat parietal bone cultures (242).

CENTRAL NERVOUS SYSTEM

Inhibin and activin subunit mRNAs and proteins are extensively distributed throughout the central nervous system (54,243–245). Prominent staining for β subunits were observed in the cell bodies of the nucleus tractus solitarius (NTS) and in the medullary reticular formation and their extensive projections to the fore- and midbrain, including the oxytocin-rich regions of the paraventricular and supraoptic nuclei of the hypothalamus. The administration of activin into the magnocellular hypothalamus resulted in a rapid release of oxytocin into the general circulation, presumably from terminals in the neurohypophysis (246). This was associated with an increase in intramammalary pressure presumably reflecting milk let down. The specificity of the response to activin was supported by the failure of inhibin to release oxytocin and the absence of an effect of activin on vasopressin secretion. Moreover, the release of oxytocin and the concommitant increase in intramammalary pressure normally seen following electrical stimulation of the NTS was attenuated by the administration of antiactivin serum into the hypothalamus. Thus it is possible that activin is a key neural signal in the milk let down neuroendocrine reflex arc.

Immunoelectromicroscopic evidence indicates that the activinergic fibers form synapses on oxytocin-containing magnocellular cells (243). The observation that activin can stimulate oxytocin secretion within 10 minutes suggests a possible neurotransmitter/modulator role that is highly unusual for a protein growth factor that normally requires hours to act in other tissues, such as the pituitary.

The activin-rich fibers from NTS also project to the preoptic area of the hypothalamus, raising the possibility that activin might be involved in the regulation of GnRH secretion. Consistently, activin was shown to stimulate GnRH secretion by a neuronal GnRH-expressing cell line (247).

Consistent with the localization of activin and inhibin subunits in the central nervous system, high-affinity and saturable iodinated activin A binding has been observed in distinct brain regions (248,249). Activin-binding sites are present in two sexually dimorphic regions of the brain, the medial preoptic area and the anterior hypothalamic nucleus, in addition to the paraventricular nucleus, the site of oxytocin regulation. *In situ* hybridization analysis of the expression of two forms of the activin receptor (II and IIB) have also revealed a wide distribution of the receptor throughout the brain (249) similar to the activin-binding studies (248). Complementary to the activin-binding studies, the activin receptor has been localized to previously described regions for oxytocin control, such as the supraoptic nucleus and the paraventricular nucleus of the hypothalamus. In addition, the message for the activin receptor is present in the medial preoptic area and the anterior hypothalamic nucleus.

Activins exert complex effects on the proliferation and differentiation of other neuronal cells in culture. This has been most extensively studied in the P-19 embryonic stem cell line, which, under serum-free conditions, can be induced to differentiate to a neuronallike phenotype in the presence of retinoic acid; otherwise, they die. A factor from the conditioned medium of a retinal cell line was found to permit survival and neuronal differentiation of the P-19 cells in the absence of added retinoic acid (250). The isolation and characterization of this factor, revealed that it was activin A, which was subsequently found to exhibit survival-enhancing activity on several other neuronal-like cell types (250). When P-19 cells were grown on an extracellular matrix, activin was found to be a potent mitogen (250). The complexity of the responses to activin is illustrated by the observation that it strongly inhibits proliferation of P-19 and other neuroblastoma cells that are treated with retinoic acid (251). The latter has led to the speculation that activin is more likely to act as a mitogen on undifferentiated cells and to inhibit proliferation of more differentiated cells (252). Exceptions, however, abound especially where activin is suspected to play physiological roles as a specific regulatory signal.

The terminally differentiated phenotype, as indicated by somatostatin expression of developing ciliary ganglion neurons, has been shown to be dependent upon a chemical signal from the choroid cells, targets of the outgrowing neurites. Activin has been identified as the probable neurodifferentiation factor for these neurons (253) and thus in this system, and probably others, may play a key role in neural development.

OTHER CELL TYPES

In culture, activins modify the growth and functions of a variety of other cell types, inhibiting the proliferation of rat thymocytes (254) and human fetal adrenal cells (255,256). In contrast, activin A is mitogenic for competent NIH3T3 fibroblasts (257), based on enhanced DNA synthesis. Activin stimulates glucose production by isolated rat hepatocytes (258), insulin production by pancreatic cells (259), and endothelin production by primary endothelial cell cultures (260).

CHARACTERIZATION OF ACTIVIN RECEPTORS

High-affinity activin binding sites have been detected on a variety of activin-responsive cell lines (103,190,196, 197,210,242,257,261–265). The visualization of these sites by chemical cross-linking experiments has revealed two major activin-receptor complexes: a type I complex of approximately 65 kDa and a type II complex of 80 to 85 kDa along with even higher molecular weight bands (266,267). Cross-linking and functional studies on the TGF-β receptors in various intact and mutant cell lines had indicated that both type I and II receptors were important for signal generation, whereas the higher molecular weight complexes were not critical (268–270).

We used a strategy based upon the expression of cDNAs in mammalian cells (271) to clone the first activin receptor (267). Pools of cDNA derived from the activin-sensitive mouse corticotrope AtT20 cell line (103) were transfected into COS monkey kidney cells. From a positive pool, a single clone was isolated, which, when transfected into COS-M6 cells, induced the expression of abundant high-affinity activin-binding sites which were pharmacologically indistinguishable from the native forms expressed on activin-responsive cells. Cross-linking studies indicated that the expressed cloned receptor corresponded to the type II activin receptor, now referred to as ActRII. A second, closely related activin receptor called ActRIIB was subsequently identified by low stringency hybridization analysis (266,272–274). Four splice variants of the ActRIIB were described whose functional significance has yet to be fully explored (266). Activin receptors II and IIB are approximately 70% identical to each other and are highly conserved throughout phylogeny (266,272,275). Receptor heterogeneity may, however, represent the basis for the multiplicity of the actions of the inhibins and the activins in such a variety of cell types. Following the identification of ActRII, a TGF-β receptor with a serine/threonine-specific protein kinase activity was characterized also by expression cloning (276). It is likely that all receptors for the ligands in the TGF-β/activin superfamily will be related serine/threonine kinases.

The remarkable finding regarding this receptor family is that they are transmembrane protein kinases with apparent serine/threonine specificity (Fig. 3) as opposed to all previously described protein kinase receptors that are

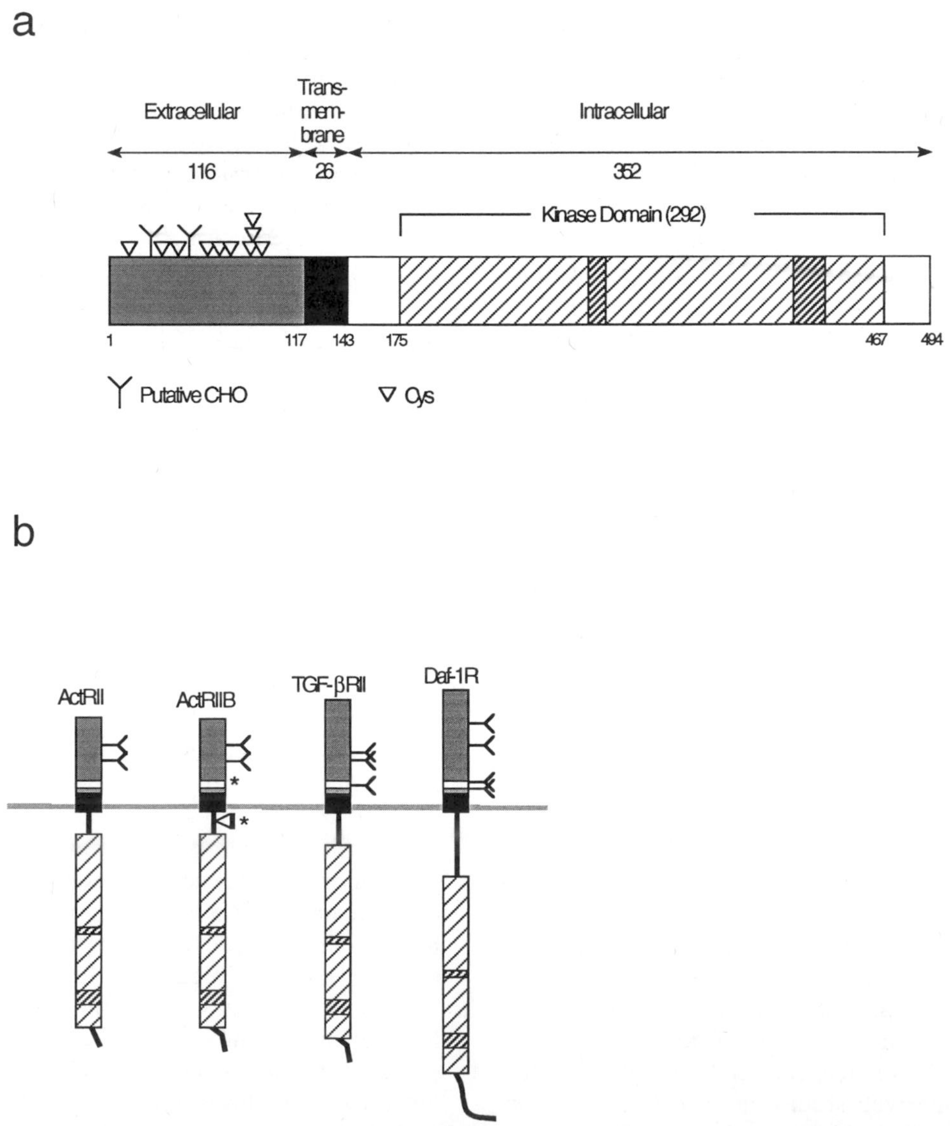

FIG. 3. Schematic of the overall organization of the family of serine/threonine protein kinase receptors. **A:** Representation of the activin type II receptor; shown are the potential glycosylation sites in the extracellular domain, the membrane spanning domain, and the putative intracellular serine/threonine protein kinase domain. **B:** Comparison of the overall structure of four members of the family of serine/threonine protein kinase receptors.

tyrosine specific (277). The only precedence for a transmembrane serine kinase was the *daf*-1 gene product from C. elegans (278) that was genetically identified based upon its regulation of the nonfeeding, daur larval state. Whether *daf*-1 protein is a receptor and the identity of its putative ligand are unknown.

The members of this family of receptors share common features including a relatively short, cysteine-rich ligand-binding domain (ActRII = 116 amino acids with two putative glycosylation sites), a single transmembrane domain (ActRII = 26 amino acids) and an intracellular component (ActRII = 352 amino acids) dominated by the serine kinase domain with its 12 canonical subdomains and a serine/threonine-rich tail with many potential phosphorylation sites. Recent metabolic labeling studies with native or transfected receptors have confirmed that ActRII and IIB are indeed glycoproteins and are autophosphorylated (279) as is the cloned TGF-β receptor (276).

Evidence for functionality of the cloned activin receptors was provided by results from experiments in which the receptor mRNAs were injected into Xenopus oocytes (272,280). In one study, animal caps removed from embryos previously injected with activin receptor mRNAs were found to be much more sensitive to activin treatment (272). At the highest dose of ActRIIB mRNA administered, the sensitivity of the animal caps to activin was increased a hundredfold. Thus, the intracellular signal generated and the biological response were a function of the concentrations of both ligand and receptor. Some embryos injected with activin receptor mRNAs were allowed to develop to the tadpole stage and a number of defects including spinal bifida and various axial defects, including extra trunks and heads were observed (272). Similar results were previously obtained following administration of activin mRNA (225). These findings, taken together with those discussed earlier in this review regarding the developmental effects of the dominant negative truncated activin receptor in Xenopus (231), suggest that activins and their receptors may be important regulators of early differentiation.

A number of intracellular events are associated with the response to activin. Activin-treated K562 erythroleukemic cells undergo a transient block in the cell cycle halting their progression from the G1 to the S phase and this is associated with hypophosphorylation of the retinoblastoma (Rb) gene product (281). One of the earliest events observed following activin administration to PC-12 or K562 cells is the induction of the protooncogene, *jun*B (282), a nuclear protein with complex and cell-type dependent positive and negative effects on the transcription rates of genes that contain an AP-1 binding site (283).

The nuclear events involved in the negative regulation of GH expression by activin has been studied in MtTW15 somatomammotropic cells. Activin inhibited the transient expression of GH promoter-chloramphenicol acetyltransferase fusion genes (284). A region previously characterized to bind the pituitary-specific transcription factor, Pit-1/GHF-1 (285), was targeted by deletion mapping of the promoter. Binding of Pit-1/GHF-1 to its cognate site on the GH promoter was lost upon activin treatment of MtTW15 cells, indicating that the suppression of GH biosynthesis by activin may be mediated by the loss of binding of the tissue-specific transcription factor to the GH promoter (284). Whether this represents a general mechanism whereby activin regulates the function of other POU-homeodomain–containing transcription factors (285,286) remains to be established.

Important questions remain. The type I TGF-β receptor, for example, is essential for signal transduction in that system and the type II receptor is required for expression of the type I receptor (287). Does such a relationship exist for activin? We and others have identified a number of putative receptors with homologies in the cytoplasmic protein kinase domains and that are structural members of this receptor family, which represent type I or type II receptors for activin or other members of the ligand superfamily. Indeed, one of these clones obtained from a rat brain cDNA library (288), and highly homologous to a murine type I TGF-β receptor (286), appears to bind iodinated activin only when the type II activin receptor is coexpressed in activin-unresponsive COSM-6 cells. The clone designated as the type I TGF-β receptor similarly requires the presence of the type II TGF-β receptor for binding (286). The precise nature of the interaction between the type I and type II receptors, however, has not been determined. Also not understood is the nature of the interactions of activin and inhibins with the two receptor types. Does dimeric activin form a heteromeric complex with type I and type II receptors? How does the interaction of inhibin with the receptors differ from that of activin? Although inhibin binds to ActRII and IIB (267,272), the affinity is too low to explain the high biological potency with which inhibin acts in responsive systems. This raises the possibility of the existence of a distinct inhibin receptor that might generate opposing signals to that of activin. Finally, what is the significance of receptor autophosphorylation, what additional substrates are phosphorylated, and how do these mediate the actions of activin? These questions remain to be addressed.

ACKNOWLEDGMENTS

We would like to thank J. Vaughan, A. Corrigan, D. Gaddy-Kurten, K. Tsuchida and E. Potter for helpful discussion, and B. Coyne, S. Guerra, B. Hensley and D. Dalton for assistance with preparation of the chapter.

REFERENCES

1. Martins T, Rocha A. Regulation of the hypothysis by the testicle and some problems of sexual dynamics. *Endocrinology* 1931;15:421–434.
2. McCullagh DR. Dual endocrine activity of the testes. *Science* 1932;76:19–20.
3. Mottram JC, Cramer W. Report on the general effects of exposure to radium on metabolism and tumor growth in the rat and the special effects on testis and pituitary. *J Exp Physiol* 1923;13:209–229.
4. McCullagh DR, Walsh EL. Further studies concerning testicular function. *Proc Soc Exp Biol Med* 1934;31:678–680.
5. McCullagh EP, Schneider I. The effect of nonadrenergic testis extract on the estrus cycle in rats. *Endocrinology* 1940;27: 899–902.
6. Vidgoff B, Vehrs H. Studies on the inhibitory hormone of the testes, IV. Effect on the pituitary, thyroid and adrenal glands of the adult male rat. *Endocrinology* 1940;26:656–661.
7. Rubin D. The question of an aqueous hormone from the testicle. *Endocrinology* 1941;29:281–187.
8. Channing CP, Gordon WL, Liu WK, Ward DN. Physiology and biochemistry of ovarian inhibin. *Proc Soc Exp Biol Med* 1985;178:339–361.
9. de Jong FJ, Sharpe RM. Evidence for inhibin-like activity in bovine follicular fluid. *Nature* 1976;263:71–72.
10. Schwartz N, Channing C. Evidence for ovarian "inhibin": suppression of the secondary rise in serum follicle stimulating hormone levels in proestrous rats by injection of procine follicular fluid. *Proc Natl Acad Sci USA* 1977;74:5721–5725.
11. Baker H, Bremmer W, Burger H, et al. Testicular control of follicle-stimulating hormone secretion. *Recent Prog Hormone Res* 1976;32:429–469.
12. Erickson GF, Hsueh AJW. Secretion of "inhibin" by rat granulosa cells *in vitro*. *Endocrinology* 1978;103:1960–1963.
13. Steinberger A. Regulation of inhibin secretion in the testis. In: Franchimont P, Channing CP, eds. *Intragonadal regulation of reproduction.* New York: Academic Press; 1981:283–298.
14. de Jong FH. Inhibin—fact or artifact. *Mol Cell Endocrinol* 1979;13:1–10.
15. Franchimont P, Verstraelen-Proyard J, Hazee-Hagelstein M, et al. Inhibin: from concept to reality. *Vitam Horm* 1979;37: 243–302.
16. Vale W, Hsueh A, Rivier C, Yu J. The inhibin/activin family of hormones and growth factors. In: Sporn MB, Roberts AB, eds. *Handbook of experimental pharmacology, Vol. 95/II. Peptide growth factors and their receptors II.* New York: Springer-Verlag; 1990:211–248.
17. Vale W, Rivier C, Hsueh A, et al. Chemical and biological characterization of the inhibin family of protein hormones. In: Clark JH, ed. *Recent progress in hormone research.* San Diego: Academic Press; 1988:1–34 (vol. 44).
18. Ling N, Ueno N, Ying S-Y, et al. Inhibins and activins. *Vitam Horm* 1988;44:1–46.
19. de Kretser DM, Robertson DM, Risbridger GP. Recent advances in the human physiology of inhibin secretion. *J Endocrinol Invest* 1990;13:611–624.
20. Rivier J, Spiess J, McClintock R, Vaughan J, Vale W. Purification and partial characterization of inhibin from porcine follicular fluid. *Biochem Biophys Res Commun* 1985;133:120–127.
21. Robertson DM, Foulds LM, Leversha L, et al. Isolation of inhibin from bovine follicular fluid. *Biochem Biophys Res Commun* 1985;126:220–226.
22. Miyamoto K, Hasegawa Y, Fukuda M, et al. Isolation of porcine follicular fluid inhibin of 32K daltons. *Biochem Biophys Res Commun* 1985;129:396–403.
23. Ling N, Ying SY, Ueno N, Esch F, Denoroy L, Guillemin R. Isolation and partial characterization of a Mr 32,000 protein with inhibin activity from porcine follicular fluid. *Proc Natl Acad Sci USA* 1985;82:7217–7221.
24. Mason AJ, Hayflick JS, Ling N, et al. Complementary DNA sequences of ovarian follicular fluid inhibin show precursor structure and homology with transforming growth factor-beta. *Nature* 1985;318:659–663.
25. Mayo KE, Cerelli GM, Spiess J, et al. Inhibin A-subunit cDNAs from porcine ovary and human placenta. *Proc Natl Acad Sci USA* 1986;83:5849–5853.
26. Forage RG, Ring JM, Brown RW, et al. Cloning and sequence analysis of cDNA species coding for the two subunits of inhibin from bovine follicular fluid. *Proc Natl Acad Sci USA* 1986;83:3091–3095.
27. Mason AJ, Niall HD, Seeburg PH. Structure of two human ovarian inhibins. *Biochem Biophys Res Commun* 1986;135:957–964.
28. Stewart AG, Milborrow HM, Ring JM, Crowther CE, Forage RG. Human inhibin genes: genomic characterisation and sequencing. *FEBS Lett* 1986;206:329–334.
29. Esch FS, Shimasaki S, Cooksey K, et al. Complementary deoxyribonucleic acid (cDNA) cloning and DNA sequence analysis of rat ovarian inhibins. *Mol Endocrinol* 1987;5:388–396.
30. Woodruff TK, Meunier H, Jones PBC, Hsueh AJW, Mayo KE. Rat inhibin: molecular cloning of α- and β-subunit complementary deoxyribonucleic acids and expression in the ovary. *Mol Endocrinol* 1987;8:561–568.
31. Sugino K, Nakamura T, Takio K, et al. Inhibin alpha-subunit monomer is present in bovine follicular fluid. *Biochem Biophys Res Commun* 1989;159:1323–1329.
32. Chenevix TG, Southall M, Healey S, Stewart A, Forage R, Martin NG. BamHI RFLP of the inhibin beta B (INHβB) chain gene on chromosome 2. *Nucleic Acids Res* 1990;18:7469.
33. Mason AJ. Structure and recombinant expression of human inhibin and activin. In: Hodgen GD, Rosenwaks Z, Spieler JM, eds. *Nonsteroidal gonadal factors: physiological roles and possibilities in contraceptive development.* Norfolk, Virginia: Jones Institute Press; 1988:19–29.
34. Bardin CW, Morris PL, Chen C-L, et al. Testicular inhibin: structure and regulation by FSH, androgens and EGF. In: Burger HG et al., eds. *Proceedings of the Serano Conference on Inhibin.* New York: Raven Press; 1987:179–190 (vol. 42).
35. Bardin CW, Morris PL, Shaha C, et al. Inhibin structure and function in the testis. *Ann NY Acad Sci* 1989;564:10–23.
36. Robertson DM, Giacometti M, Foulds LM, et al. Isolation of inhibin alpha-subunit precursor proteins from bovine follicular fluid. *Endocrinology* 1989;125:2141–2149.
37. Knight PG, Beard AJ, Wrathall JH, Castillo RJ. Evidence that the bovine ovary secretes large amounts of monomeric inhibin alpha subunit and its isolation from bovine follicular fluid. *J Mol Endocrinol* 1989;2:189–200.
38. Schneyer AL, Sluss PM, Whitcomb RW, Martin KA, Sprengel R, Crowley WJ. Precursors of alpha-inhibin modulate follicle-stimulating hormone receptor binding and biological activity. *Endocrinology* 1991;129:1987–1999.
39. Ling N, Ying SY, Ueno N, et al. Pituitary FSH is released by a heterodimer of the β-subunits from the two forms of inhibin. *Nature* 1986;321:779–782.
40. Vale W, Rivier J, Vaughan J, et al. Purification and characterization of an FSH releasing protein from porcine ovarian follicular fluid. *Nature* 1986;321:776–779.
41. Schmelzer CH, Burton LE, Tamony CM, Schwall RH, Mason AJ, Liegeois N. Purification and characterization of recombinant human activin B. *Biochim Biophys Acta* 1990;1039:135–141.
42. Nakamura T, Asashima M, Eto Y, et al. Isolation and characterization of native activin B. *J Biol Chem* 1992;267:16385–16389.
43. Cate RL, Mattaliano RJ, Hession C, et al. Isolation of the bovine and human genes for Mullerian inhibiting substance and expression of the human gene in animal cells. *Cell* 1986;45:685–698.
44. Smith WC, Harland RM. Expression cloning of noggin, a new dorsalizing factor localized to the Spemann organizer in Xenopus embryos. *Cell* 1992;70:829–840.
45. Basler K, Edlund T, Jessell T, Yamada T. Control of cell pattern in the neural tube: regulation of cell differentiation by dorsalin-1, a novel TGF beta family member. *Cell* 1993;73:687–702.
46. Padgett RW, Johnston RDS, Gelbart WM. A transcript from a Drosophila pattern gene predicts a protein homologous to the transforming growth factor-beta family. *Nature* 1987;325:81–84.
47. Wozney JM, Rosen V, Celeste AJ, et al. Novel regulators of bone

formation: molecular clones and activities. *Science* 1988;242:1528–1534.
48. Weeks DL, Melton PA. A maternal mRNA localized to the vegetal hemisphere in Xenopus eggs codec for a growth factor related to TGF-β. *Cell* 1987;51:861–867.
49. Roberts AB, Sporn MB. The transforming growth factor-βs. In: Sporn MB, Roberts AB, eds. *Handbook of Experimental Pharmacology.* Heidelberg: Springer-Verlag; 1990:419–472 (vol. 95/I).
50. Moses HL, Yang EY, Pietenpol JA. TGF-β stimulation and inhibition of cell proliferation—new mechanistic insights. *Cell* 1990;63:245–247.
51. Massague J. The transforming growth factor-β family. *Annu Rev Cell Biol* 1990;6:597–641.
52. Lee DC, Han KM. Expression of growth factors and their receptors in development. In: Sporn MB, Roberts AB, eds. *Handbook of Experimental Pharmacology.* Heidelberg: Springer-Verlag; 1990:611–654 (vol. 95/II).
53. Lee SJ. Expression of growth differentiation factor-1 in the nervous system—conservation of a bicistronic structure. *Proc Natl Acad Sci USA* 1991;88:4250–4254.
54. Meunier H, Rivier C, Evans RM, Vale W. Gonadal and extragonadal expression of inhibin α, βA, and βB subunits in various tissues predicts diverse functions. *Proc Natl Acad Sci USA* 1988;85:247–251.
55. Mather JP, Woodruff TK, Krummen LA. Paracrine regulation of reproductive function by inhibin and activin. *Proc Soc Exp Biol Med* 1992;201:1–15.
56. Roberts VJ, Sawchenko PE, Vale W. Expression of inhibin/activin subunit mRNAs during rat embryogenesis. *Endocrinology* 1991;128:3122–3129.
57. Ying SY, Becker A, Swanson G, et al. Follistatin specifically inhibits pituitary follicle stimulating hormone release in vitro. *Biochem Biophys Res Commun* 1987;149:133–139.
58. Esch F, Shimasaki S, Mercado M, et al. Structural characterization of follistatin: a novel follicle-stimulating hormone release-inhibiting polypeptide from the gonad. *Mol Endocrinol* 1987;1:849–855.
59. Robertson DM, Klein R, deVos FL, et al. The isolation of polypeptides with FSH suppressing activity from bovine follicular fluid which are structurally different to inhibin. *Biochem Biophys Res Commun* 1987;149:744–749.
60. Nakamura T, Takio K, Eto Y, Shibai H, Titani K, Sugino H. Activin-binding protein from rat ovary is follistatin. *Science* 1990;247:836–838.
61. Kogawa K, Nakamura T, Sugino K, Takio K, Titani K, Sugino H. Activin-binding protein is present in pituitary. *Endocrinology* 1991;128:1434–1440.
62. Shimonaka M, Inouye S, Shimasaki S, Ling N. Follistatin binds to both activin and inhibin through the common beta subunit. *Endocrinology* 1991;128:3313–3315.
63. DePaolo LV, Bicsak TA, Erickson GF, Shimasaki S, Ling N. Follistatin and activin: a potential intrinsic regulatory system within diverse tissues. *Proc Soc Exp Biol Med* 1991;198:500–512.
64. Michel U, Farnworth P, Findlay JK. Follistatins: more than follicle-stimulating hormone suppressing proteins. *Mol Cellul Endocrinol* 1993;91:1–11.
65. Farnworth PG, Robertson DM, de Kretser DM, Burger HG. Effects of 31 kilodalton bovine inhibin on follicle-stimulating hormone and luteinizing hormone in rat pituitary cells in vitro: actions under basal conditions. *Endocrinology* 1988;122:207–213.
66. Carroll R, Corrigan A, Gharib S, Vale W, Chin W. Inhibin, Activin, and follistatin: Regulation of follicle-stimulating hormone messenger ribonucleic acid levels. *Mol Endocrinol* 1989;3:1969–1976.
67. Fukuda M, Miyamoto K, Hasegawa Y, Ibuki Y, Igarashi M. Action mechanism of inhibin in vitro–cycloheximide mimics inhibin actions on pituitary cells. *Mol Cell Endocrinol* 1987;51:41–50.
68. Attardi B, Keeping HS, Winters SJ, Kotsuji F, Maurer RA, Troen P. Rapid and profound suppression of messenger ribonucleic acid encoding follicle-stimulating hormone β by inhibin from primate Sertoli cells. *Mol Endocrinol* 1989;3:280–287.
69. Jakubowiak A, Janecki A, Tong D, Sanborn BM, Steinberger A. Effects of recombinant human inhibin and testosterone on gonadotropin secretion and subunit mRNA in superfused male rat pituitary cell cultures stimulated with pulsatile gonadotropin-releasing hormone. *Mol Cell Endocrinol* 1991;82:265–273.
70. Weiss J, Harris PE, Halverson LM, Crowley WFJ, Jameson JL. Dynamic regulation of follicle-stimulating hormone-β messenger ribonucleic acid levels by activin and gonadotropin-releasing hormone in perifused rat pituitary cells. *Endocrinology* 1992;131:1403–1408.
71. Miller WL, Lin L, Phillips CL, et al. Regulation of the subunit mRNAs of follicle-stimulating hormone by inhibin, estradiol, and progesterone. In: Hodgen GD, Rosenwaks Z, Spieler JM, eds. *Nonsteroidal gonadal factors: physiological roles and possibilities in contraceptive development.* Norfolk, Virginia: Jones Institute Press; 1988:110–124.
72. Muttukrishna S, Knight PG. Inverse effects of activin and inhibin on the synthesis and secretion of FSH and LH by ovine pituitary cells in vitro. *J Mol Endocrinol* 1991;6:171–178.
73. Clarke IJ, Rao A, Fallest PC, Shupnik MA. Transcription rate of the follicle stimulating hormone (FSH) β subunit gene is reduced by inhibin in sheep but this does not fully explain the decrease in mRNA. *Mol Cell Endocrinol* 1993;91:211–216.
74. Carroll RS, Kowash PM, Lofgren JA, Schwall RH, Chin WW. In vivo regulation of FSH synthesis by inhibin and activin. *Endocrinology* 1991;129:3299–3304.
75. Dalkin AC, Knight CD, Shupnik MA, et al. Ovariectomy and inhibin immunoneutralization acutely increase follicle-stimulating hormone-β messenger ribonucleic acid concentrations: evidence for a nontranscriptional mechanism. *Endocrinology* 1993;132:1297–1304.
76. Attardi B, Vaughan J, Vale W. Regulation of FSHβ messenger ribonucleic acid levels in the rat by endogenous inhibin. *Endocrinology* 1991;129:2802–2804.
77. DePaolo LV, Shimonaka M, Ling N. Regulation of pulsatile gonadotropin secretion by estrogen, inhibin, and follistatin (activin-binding protein) in ovariectomized rats. *Biol Reprod* 1992;46:898–904.
78. Mercer JE, Clements JA, Funder JW, Clarke IJ. Rapid and specific lowering of pituitary FSHβ mRNA levels by inhibin. *Mol Cell Endocrinol* 1987;53:251–254.
79. Clayton R, Catt K. Gonadotropin-releasing hormone receptors: characterization, physiological regulation and relationship to reproductive function. *Endocrine Rev* 1981;2:186–209.
80. Carroll RS, Corrigan AZ, Vale W, Chin WW. Activin stabilizes follicle-stimulating hormone-beta messenger ribonucleic acid levels. *Endocrinology* 1991;129:1721–1726.
81. Attardi B, Keeping HS, Winters SJ, Kotsuji F, Troen P. Comparison of the effects of cycloheximide and inhibin on the gonadotropin subunit messenger ribonucleic acids. *Endocrinology* 1991;128:119–125.
82. Campen CA, Vale W. Interaction between purified ovine inhibin and steroids on the release of gonadotropins from cultured rat pituitary cells. *Endocrinology* 1988;123:1320–1328.
83. Burger HG. Inhibin-regulation and mechanism of action. In: Hodgen GD, Rosenwaks Z, Spieler JM, eds. *Nonsteroidal gonadal factors: physiological roles and possibilities in contraceptive development.* Norfolk, Virginia: Jones Institute Press; 1988:137–148.
84. Rivier C, Schwall R, Mason A, Burton L, Vaughan J, Vale W. Effect of recombinant inhibin on luteinizing hormone and follicle-stimulating hormone secretion in the rat. *Endocrinology* 1991;128:1548–1554.
85. Woodruff TK, Krummen LA, Lyon RJ, Stocks DL, Mather JP. Recombinant human inhibin A and recombinant human activin A regulate pituitary and ovarian function in the adult rat. *Endocrinology* 1993;132:2332–2341.
86. Katayama T, Shiota K, Takahashi M. Activin A increases the number of follicle-stimulating hormone cells in anterior pituitary cultures. *Mol Cell Endocrinol* 1990;69:179–185.
87. Schwall R, Schmelzer CH, Matsuyama E, Mason AJ. Multiple actions of recombinant activin-A *in vivo.* *Endocrinology* 1989;125:1420–1423.
88. DePaolo LV, Shimonaka M, Schwall RH, Ling N. In vivo com-

parison of the follicle-stimulating hormone-suppressing activity of follistatin and inhibin in ovariectomized rats. *Endocrinology* 1991;128:668–674.
89. Rivier C, Schwall R, Mason A, Burton L, Vale W. Effect of recombinant inhibin on gonadotropin secretion during proestrus and estrus in the rat. *Endocrinology* 1991;128:2223–2228.
90. Rivier C, Vale W. Effect of recombinant activin-A on gonadotropin secretion in the female rat. *Endocrinology* 1991;129: 2463–2465.
91. Rivier C, Vale W. Effect of recombinant inhibin on follicle-stimulating hormone secretion by the female rat: interaction with a gonadotropin-releasing hormone antagonist and estrogen. *Endocrinology* 1991;129:2160–2165.
92. Roberts V, Meunier H, Vaughan J, et al. Production and regulation of inhibin subunits in pituitary gonadotropes. *Endocrinology* 1988;124:552–554.
93. Corrigan AZ, Bilezikjian LM, Carroll RS, et al. Evidence for an autocrine role of activin-B within rat anterior pituitary cultures. *Endocrinology* 1991;128:1682–1684.
94. DePaolo LV, Bald LN, Fendly BM. Passive immunoneutralization with a monoclonal antibody reveals a role for endogenous activin-B in mediating FSH hypersecretion during estrus and following ovariectomy of hypophysectomized, pituitary-grafted rats. *Endocrinology* 1992;130:1741–1743.
95. Gospodarowicz D, Lau K. Pituitary follicular cells secrete both vascular endothelial growth factor and follistatin. *Biochem Biophys Res Commun* 1989;165:292–298.
96. Kaiser UB, Lee BL, Carroll RS, Unabia G, Chin WW, Childs GV. Follistatin gene expression in the pituitary: localization in gonadotropes and folliculostellate cells in diestrous rats. *Endocrinology* 1992;130:3048–3056.
97. Bilezikjian LM, Corrigan AZ, Vaughan JM, Vale WV. Activin-A regulates follistatin secretion from cultured rat anterior pituitary cells. *Endocrinology* [*in press*].
98. Bilezikjian LM, Vaughan JM, Vale WW. Characterization and the regulation of inhibin subunit proteins of cultured rat anterior pituitary cells. *Endocrinology* [*in press*].
99. Allaerts W, Carmeliet P, Denef C. New perspectives in the function of pituitary folliculo-stellate cells. *Mol Cell Endocrinol* 1990;71:73–81.
100. Kitaoka M, Kojima I, Ogata E. Activin-A: a modulator of multiple types of anterior pituitary cells. *Biochem Biophys Res Commun* 1988;157:48–54.
101. Billestrup N, Gonzalez-Manchon C, Potter E, Vale W. Inhibition of somatotroph growth and GH biosynthesis by activin *in vitro*. *Mol Endocrinol* 1990;4:356–362.
102. Bilezikjian LM, Corrigan AZ, Vale W. Activin-A modulates growth hormone secretion from cultures of rat anterior pituitary cells. *Endocrinology* 1990;126:2369–2376.
103. Bilezikjian LM, Blount AL, Campen CA, Gonzalez-Manchon C, Vale W. Activin-A inhibits POMC mRNA accumulation and ACTH secretion of AtT20 cells. *Mol Endocrinol* 1991;5: 1389–1395.
104. Rivier C, Cajander S, Vaughan J, Hsueh AJW, Vale W. Age-dependent changes in physiological action, content and immunostaining of inhibin in the male rat. *Endocrinology* 1988;123: 120–126.
105. Shaha C, Morris PL, Chen CLC, Vale W, Bardin W. Immunostainable inhibin subunits are in multiple types of testicular cells. *Endocrinology* 1989;125:1941–1950.
106. Roberts V, Meunier H, Sawchenko PE, Vale W. Differential production and regulation of inhibin subunits in rat testicular cell types. *Endocrinology* 1989;125:2350–2359.
107. Woodruff TK, Mayo KE. Regulation of inhibin synthesis in the rat ovary. *Annu Rev Physiol* 1990;52:807–821.
108. Keinan D, Madigan MB, Bardin CW, Chen CL. Expression and regulation of testicular inhibin alpha-subunit gene in vivo and in vitro. *Mol Endocrinol* 1989;3:29–35.
109. Bicsak TA, Vale W, Vaughan J, Tucker EM, Cappel S, Hsueh AJ. Hormonal regulation of inhibin production by cultured Sertoli cells. *Mol Cell Endocrinol* 1987;49:211–217.
110. de Winter JP, Vanderstichele HMJ, Timmerman MA, Blok LJ, Themmen APN, de Jong FH. Activin is produced by rat sertoli cells *in vitro* and can act as an autocrine regulator of sertoli cell function. *Endocrinology* 1993;132:975–982.
111. Lee W, Mason AJ, Schwall R, Szonyi E, Mather JP. Secretion of activin by interstitial cells in the testis. *Science* 1989;243: 396–398.
112. Kaipia A, Parvinen M, Shimasaki S, Ling N, Toppari J. Stage-specific cellular regulation of inhibin alpha-subunit mRNA expression in the rat seminiferous epithelium. *Mol Cell Endocrinol* 1991;82:165–173.
113. Bhasin S, Krummen LA, Swerdloff RS, et al. Stage dependent expression of inhibin alpha and beta-B subunits during the cycle of the rat seminiferous epithelium. *Endocrinology* 1989;124: 987–991.
114. Meunier H, Cajander SB, Roberts VJ, et al. Rapid changes in the expression of inhibin α-, βA-, and βB-subunits in ovarian cell types during the rat estrous cycle. *Mol Endocrinol* 1988;2: 1352–1363.
115. Woodruff TK, D'Agostino J, Schwartz NB, Mayo KE. Dynamic changes in inhibin messenger RNAs in rat ovarian follicles during the reproductive cycle. *Science* 1988;239:1296–1299.
116. Torney AH, Hodgson YM, Forage RKD. Cellular localization of inhibin mRNA in the bovine ovary by in-situ hybridization. *J Reprod Fertil* 1989;86:391–399.
117. Rodgers RJ, Stuchbery SJ, Findlay JK. Inhibin mRNAs in ovine and bovine ovarian follicles and corpora lutea throughout the estrous cycle and gestation. *Mol Cell Endocrinol* 1989;62: 95–101.
118. Watanabe G, Taya K, Sasamoto S. Dynamics of ovarian inhibin secretion during the oestrus cycle of the rat. *J Endocrinol* 1990;126:151–157.
119. Findlay JK, Clarke IJ, Robertson DM. Inhibin concentrations in ovarian and jugular venous plasma and the relationship of inhibin with follicle-stimulating hormone and luteinizing hormone during the ovine estrous cycle. *Endocrinology* 1990;126:528–535.
120. Mann GE, McNeilly AS, Baird DT. Source of ovarian inhibin secretion during the oestrous cycle of the sheep. *J Endocrinol* 1989;123:181–188.
121. Meunier H, Roberts VJ, Sawchenko PE, Cajancer SB, Hsueh AJ, Vale W. Periovulatory changes in the expression of inhibin α-, βA-, and βB-subunits in hormonally induced immature female rats. *Mol Endocrinol* 1989;3:2062–2069.
122. Roseff SJ, Bangah M, Kettel LM, et al. Dynamic changes in circulating inhibin levels during the luteal-follicular transition of the human menstrual cycle. *J Clin Endocrinol Metab* 1989;69: 1033–1039.
123. McLachlan RI, Healy DL, Robertson DM, Burger HG, Kretser DM. Circulating immunoactive inhibin in the luteal phase and early gestation of women undergoing ovulation induction. *Fertil Steril* 1987;48:1001–1005.
124. Tsonis CG, Baird DT, Campbell BK, Leask R, Scaramuzzi RJ. The sheep corpus luteum secretes inhibin. *J Endocrinol* 1988;116:R3–R5.
125. Basseti SG, Winters SJ, Keeping HS, Zeleznik AJ. Serum immunoreactive inhibin levels before and after luteectomy in the cynomolgus monkey (Macaca fascicularis). *J Clin Endocrinol Metab* 1990;70:590–594.
126. McLachlan RI, Robertson DM, Burger HG, de Kretser DM. The radioimmunoassay of bovine and human follicular fluid and serum inhibin. *Mol Cell Endocrinol* 1986;46:175–185.
127. Vaughan JM, Rivier J, Corrigan AZ, et al. Detection and purification of inhibin using antisera generated against synthetic peptide fragments. In: Conn PM, ed. *Methods in enzymology*. Orlando: Academic Press; 1988:588–617 (vol. 168).
128. Schneyer AL, Mason AJ, Burton LE, Ziegner JR, Crowley WF, Jr. Immunoreactive inhibin α-subunit in human serum: implications for radioimmunoassay. *J Clin Endo Metab* 1990;70: 1208–1212.
129. Bicsak TA, Cajander SB, Vale W, Hsueh AJ. Inhibin: studies of stored and secreted forms by biosynthetic labeling and immunodetection in cultured rat granulosa cells. *Endocrinology* 1988;122:741–748.
130. Hancock AD, Robertson DM, de Kretser DM. Inhibin and inhibin α-chain precursors are produced by immature rat Sertoli cells in culture. *Biol Reprod* 1992;36:155–161.

131. Robertson DM, Foulds LM, Prisk M, Hedger MP. Inhibin/activin beta-subunit monomer: isolation and characterization. *Endocrinology* 1992;130:1680–1687.
132. de Winter J, Timmerman MA, Vanderstichele HM, et al. Testicular Leydig cells in vitro secrete only inhibin alpha-subunits, whereas Leydig cell tumors can secrete bioactive inhibin. *Mol Cell Endocrinol* 1992;83:105–115.
133. Miyamoto K, Hasegawa Y, Fukuda M, Igarashi M. Demonstration of high molecular weight forms of inhibin in bovine follicular fluid (bFF) by using monoclonal antibodies to bFF 32K inhibin. *Biochem Biophys Res Commun* 1986;136:1103–1109.
134. Grootenhuis AJ, Steenbergen J, Timmerman MA, et al. Inhibin and activin-like activity in fluids from male and female gonads: different molecular weight forms and bioactivity/immunoactivity ratios. *J Endocrinol* 1989;122:293–301.
135. Moore KH, Dunbar BS, Bousfield GR, Ward DN. The heterogeneity of porcine 32000 M_r inhibin α-subunit: a gel electrophoresis and immunoblot study. *Endocrinology* 1990;127:1477–1486.
136. Torney AH, Robertson DM, de Kretser DM. Characterization of inhibin and related proteins in bovine fetal testicular and ovarian extracts: evidence for the presence of inhibin subunit products and FSH-suppressing protein. *J Endocrinol* 1991;133:111–120.
137. Robertson DM. The measurement of inhibn. *Reprod Fertil Dev* 1990;2:101–105.
138. Betteridge A, Craven RP. A two-site enzyme-linked immunosorbent assay for inhibin. *Biol Reprod* 1991;45:748–754.
139. Groome N. Ultrasensitive two-site assays for inhibin-A and activin-A using monoclonal antibodies raised to synthetic peptides. *J Immunol Meth* 1991;145:65–69.
140. Vaughan JM, Vale WV. α2-macroglobulin is a binding protein of inhibin and activin. *Endocrinology* 1993;132:2038–2050.
141. Schneyer AL, O'Neil DA, Crowley WJ. Activin-binding proteins in human serum and follicular fluid. *J Clin Endocrinol Metab* 1992;74:1320–1324.
142. Krummen LA, Woodruff TK, Deguzman G, et al. Identification and characterization of binding proteins for inhibin and activin in human serum and follicular fluids. *Endocrinology* 1993;132: 431–443.
143. Baly DL, Allison DE, Krummen LA, et al. Development of a specific and sensitive two-site enzyme-linked immunosorbent assay for measurement of inhibin-A in serum. *Endocrinology* 1993;132:2099–2108.
144. Woodruff TK, Krummen LA, Chen S, et al. Pharmacokinetic profile of recombinant human (rh) inhibin A and activin A in the immature rat. I. Serum profile of rh-inhibin A and rh-activin A in the immature female rat. *Endocrinology* 1993;132:715–724.
145. Rivier C, Rivier J, Vale W. Inhibin: measurement and role in the rat. *Int J Rad Appl Instrum [B]* 1987;14:273–276.
146. Buckler HM, Healy DL, Burger HG. Purified FSH stimulates production of inhibin by the human ovary. *J Endocrinol* 1989;122:279–285.
147. Robertson DM, Hayward S, Irby D, et al. Radioimmunoassay of rat serum inhibin: changes after PMSG stimulation and gonadectomy. *Mol Cell Endocrinol* 1988;58:1–8.
148. Davis SR, Burger HG, Robertson DM, Farnworth PG, Carson RS, Krozowski Z. Pregnant mare's serum gonadotropin stimulates inhibin subunit gene expression in the immature rat ovary: dose response characteristics and relationships to serum gonadotropins, inhibin, and ovarian steroid content. *Endocrinology* 1988;123:2399–2407.
149. Kogo H, Takasaki K, Takeo S, Watanabe G, Taya K, Sasamoto S. Indomethacin inhibits the secretion of inhibin and oestradiol-17beta stimulated by pregnant mare serum gonadotrophin in the immature female rat. *Eur J Pharmacol* 1992;221:289–295.
150. McLachlan RI, Cohen NL, Vale WW, et al. The importance of luteinizing hormone in the control of inhibin and progesterone secretion by the human corpus luteum. *J Clin Endocrinol Metab* 1989;68:1078–1085.
151. Pei L, Dodson R, Schoderbek W, Maurer R, Mayo K. Regulation of the α inhibin gene by cyclic adenosine 3′,5′-monophosphate after transfection into rat granulosa cells. *Mol Endocrinol* 1991;5:521–534.
152. Feng Z-M, Li Y-P, Chen C-L C. Analysis of the 5′-flanking regions of rat inhibin α- and β-B-subunit genes suggests two different regulatory mechanisms. *Mol Endocrinol* 1989;3:1914–1925.
153. Michel U, Krozowski Z, McMaster J, Yu JH, Findlay JK. The biphasic modulation of inhibin mRNA levels and secretion by PMSG in rat granulosa cells in vitro. *Reprod Fertil Dev* 1991;3:215–226.
154. Zhang Z, Lee VW, Carson RS, Burger HG. Selective control of rat granulosa cell inhibin production by FSH and LH in vitro. *Mol Cell Endocrinol* 1988;56:35–40.
155. Bicsak TA, Tucker EM, Cappel S, et al. Hormonal regulation of granulosa cell inhibin biosynthesis. *Endocrinology* 1986;119: 2711–2719.
156. Burger HG, Yamada Y, Bangah ML, McCloud PI, Warne GL. Serum gonadotropin, sex steroid, and immunoreactive inhibin levels in the first two years of life. *J Clin Endocrinol Metab* 1991;72:682–686.
157. Rivier C, Rivier J, Vale W. Inhibin-mediated feedback control of follicle-stimulating hormone secretion in the female rat. *Science* 1986;234:205–208.
158. Rivier C, Roberts V, Vale W. Possible role of luteinizing hormone and follicle-stimulating hormone in modulating inhibin secretion and expression during the estrous cycle of the rat. *Endocrinology* 1989;125:876–882.
159. Hasegawa Y, Miyamoto K, Igarashi M. Changes in serum concentrations of immunoreactive inhibin during the oestrous cycle of the rat. *J Endocrinol* 1989;121:91–100.
160. McLachlan RI, Healy DL, Robertson DM, de Kretser DM, Burger HG. Plasma inhibin levels during gonadotropin-induced ovarian hyperstimulation for IVF: a new index of follicular function. *Lancet* 1986;8492:1233–1234.
161. McLachlan RI, Cohen NL, Dahl KD, Bremner WJ, Soules MR. Serum inhibin levels during the periovulatory interval in normal women: relationships with sex steriod and gonadotrophin levels. *Clin Endocrinol* 1990;32:39–48.
162. Rivier C, Vale W. Immunoneutralization of endogenous inhibin modifies hormone secretion and ovulation rate in the rat. *Endocrinology* 1989;125:152–157.
163. Woodruff TK, D'Agostino J, Schwartz NB, Mayo KE. Decreased inhibin gene expression in preovulatory follicles requires primary gonadotropin surges. *Endocrinology* 1989;124:2193–2199.
164. Au CL, Robertson DM, de Kretser DM. Changes in testicular inhibin after a single episode of heating of rat testes. *Endocrinology* 1987;120:973–977.
165. Hamada T, Watanabe G, Kokuho T, et al. Radioimmunoassay of inhibin in various mammals. *J Endocrinol* 1989;122:697–704.
166. Lincoln GA, McNeilly AS. Inhibin concentrations in the peripheral blood of rams during a cycle in testicular activity induced by changes in photoperiod or treatment with melatonin. *J Endocrinol* 1989;120:R9–R13.
167. Janecki A, Jakubowiak A, Steinberger A. Vectorial secretion of inhibin by immature rat Sertoli cells in vitro—reexamination of previous results. *Endocrinology* 1990;127:1896–1903.
168. Ishida H, Tashiro H, Watanabe M, et al. Measurement of inhibin concentrations in men: study of changes after castration and comparison with androgen levels in testicular tissue, spermatic venous blood, and peripheral venous blood. *J Clin Endocrinol Metab* 1990;70:1019–1022.
169. Krummen LA, Morelos BS, Bhasin S. The role of luteinizing hormone in regulation of testicular inhibin α and β-B subunit messenger RNAs in immature and adult animals. *Endocrinology* 1990;127:1097–1104.
170. McLachlan RI, Matsumoto AM, Burger HG, de Kretser DM, Bremner WJ. Relative roles of follicle-stimulating hormone and luteinizing hormone in the control of inhibin secretion in normal men. *J Clin Invest* 1988;82:880–884.
171. Sheckter CB, McLachlan RI, Tenover JS, et al. Stimulation of serum inhibin concentrations by gonadotropin-releasing hormone in men with idiopathic hypogonadotropic hypogonadism. *J Clin Endocrinol Metab* 1988;67:1221–1224.
172. Allenby G, Foster PMD, Sharpe RM. Evidence that secretion of immunoactive inhibin by seminiferous tubules from the adult rat testis is regulated by specific germ cells types: correlation between *in vivo* and *in vitro* studies. *Endocrinology* 1991;128:467–476.
173. Davis SR, Carson RS, Krozowski Z, Burger HG. The effect of

hypophysectomy on inhibin production by adult rat ovaries: changes in ovarian inhibin gene expression and serum inhibin. *Gynecol Endocrinol* 1988;2:223–232.
174. Maddocks S, Sharpe RM. The effects of sexual maturation and altered steroid synthesis on the production and route of secretion of inhibin-alpha from the rat testis. *Endocrinology* 1990;126: 1541–1550.
175. Abeyawardene SA, Vale WW, Marshall GR, Plant TM. Circulating inhibin alpha concentrations in infant, prepubertal, and adult male rhesus monkeys (*Macaca mulatta*) and in juvenile males during premature initiation of puberty with pulsatile gonadotropin-releasing hormone treatment. *Endocrinology* 1989;125:250–256.
176. Tenover JS, McLachlan RI, Dahl KD, Burger HG, de Kretser DM, Bremner WJ. Decreased serum inhibin levels in normal elderly men: evidence for a decline in Sertoli cell function with aging. *J Clin Endocrinol Metab* 1988;67:455–459.
177. Yamaguchi M-A, Mizunuma H, Miyamoto K, Hasegawa Y, Ibuki Y, Igarashi M. Immunoreactive inhibin concentrations in adult men: presence of a circadian rhythm. *J Clin Endocrinol Metab* 1991;72:554–559.
178. Lincoln GA, Lincoln CE, McNeilly AS. Seasonal cycles in the blood plasma concentration of FSH, inhibin and testosterone, and testicular size in rams of wild, feral and domesticated breeds of sheep. *J Reprod Fertil* 1990;88:623–633.
179. McLachlan RI, Robertson DM, Healy DL, de Kretser DM, Burger HG. Plasma inhibin levels during gonadotropin-induced ovarian hyperstimulation for IVF: a new index of follicular function? *Lancet* 1986;1:1233–1234.
180. Tanabe K, Saijo A, Park JY, et al. The role of inhibin in women with polycystic ovary syndrome (pcos). *Horm Res* 1990;33(Suppl 2):10–17.
181. Gonzales GF, Risbridger GP, de Kretser DM. In vivo and in vitro production of inhibin by cryptorchid testes from adult rats. *Endocrinology* 1989;124:1661–1668.
182. Rivier C, Meunier H, Robert V, Vale W. Possible involvement of inhibin in altered FSH secretion during dissociated LYH and FSH release: unilateral castration and experimental cryptorchidism. *Biol Reprod* 1989;41:967–981.
183. Demura R, Suzuki T, Nakamura S, et al. Effect of uni- and bilateral cryptorchidism on testicular inhibin and testosterone secretion in rats. *Endocrinol Jpn* 1987;34:911–917.
184. Tsatsoulis A, Shalet SM, Robertson WR, Morris ID, Burger HG, de Kretser DM. Plasma inhibin levels in men with chemotherapy-induced severe damage to the seminiferous epithelium. *Clin Endocrinol* 1988;29:659–665.
185. Findlay JK, Doughton B, Robertson DM, Forage RG. Effects of immunization against recombinant bovine inhibin α subunit on circulating concentrations of gonadotrophins in ewes. *J Endocrinol* 1988;120:59–65.
186. Culler MD, Negro VA. Endogenous inhibin suppresses only basal follicle-stimulating hormone secretion but suppresses all parameters of pulsatile luteinizing hormone secretion in the diestrous female rat. *Endocrinology* 1989;124:2944–2953.
187. Medhamurthy R, Culler MD, Gay VL, Negro-Vilar A, Plant TM. Evidence that inhibin plays a major role in the regulation of follicle-stimulating hormone secretion in the fully adult male rhesus monkey (*Macaca mulatta*). *Endocrinology* 1991;129: 389–395.
188. Culler MD. Role of Leydig cells and endogenous inhibin in regulating pulsatile gonadotropin secretion in the adult male rat. *Endocrinology* 1990;127:2540–2550.
189. Culler MD, Negro VA. Destruction of testicular Leydig cells reveals a role of endogenous inhibin in regulating follicle-stimulating hormone secretion in the adult male rat. *Mol Cell Endocrinol* 1990;70:89–98.
190. Woodruff TK, Lyon RJ, Hansen SE, Rice GC, Mather JP. Inhibin and activin locally regulate rat ovarian folliculogenesis. *Endocrinology* 1990;127:3196–3205.
191. Sander HJ, Kramer P, van Leeuwen EC, van Cappellen WA, Meijs-Roelofs HM, de Jong FH. Ovulation rate, follicle population and FSH levels in cyclic rats after administration of an inhibin-neutralizing antiserum. *J Endocrinol* 1991;130:297–303.
192. Mizumachi M, Voglmayr JK, Washington DW, Chen C-L C, Barden CW. Superovulation of ewes immunized against the human recombinant inhibin a-subunit associated with increased pre- and postovulatory follicle-stimulating hormone levels. *Endocrinology* 1990;126:1058–1063.
193. Forage RG, Brown RW, Oliver KJ, et al. Immunization against an inhibin subunit produced by recombinant DNA techniques results in increased ovulation rate in sheep. *J Endocrinol* 1987;114:R1–R4.
194. Matzuk MM, Finegold MJ, Su JGJ, Hsueh AJW, Bradley A. α-Inhibin is a tumour-suppressor gene with gonadal specificity in mice. *Nature* 1992;360:313–319.
195. Hsueh AJW, Bicsak TA, Vaughan J, Tucker E, Rivier J, Vale W. Heterodimers and homodimers of inhibin subunits have different paracrine action in the modulation of luteinizing hormone-stimulated androgen biosynthesis. *Proc Natl Acad Sci USA* 1987;84:5082–5086.
196. Sugino H, Nakamura T, Hasegawa Y, et al. Identification of a specific receptor for erythroid differentiation factor on follicular granulosa cell. *J Biol Chem* 1988;263:15249–15252.
197. LaPolt PS, Soto D, Su JG, et al. Activin stimulation of inhibin secretion and messenger RNA levels in cultured granulosa cells. *Mol Endocrinol* 1989;3:1666–1673.
198. Woodruff TK, Borree J, Attie KM, Cox ET, Rice GC, Mather JP. Stage-specific binding of inhibin and activin to subpopulations of rat germ cells. *Endocrinology* 1992;130:871–881.
199. Kaipia A, Penttila TL, Shimasaki S, Ling N, Parvinen M, Toppari J. Expression of inhibin-beta(A) and inhibin-beta(B), follistatin and activin-A receptor messenger ribonucleic acids in the rat seminiferous epithelium. *Endocrinology* 1992;131:2703–2710.
200. Feng Z-M, Madigan MB, Chen C-L C. Expression of type II activin receptor genes in the male and female reproductive tissues of the rat. *Endocrinology* 1993;132:2593–2600.
201. Kaipia A, Parvinen M, Toppari J. Localization of activin receptor (ActR-IIB$_2$) mRNA in the rat seminiferous epithelium. *Endocrinology* 1993;132:477–479.
202. de Winter JP, de Jong FH, Themmen AP, Hoogerbrugge JW, Klaij IA, Grootegoed JA. Activin receptor mRNA expression in rat testicular cell types. *Mol Cell Endocrinol* 1992;83:R1–R8.
203. Clayton RN. The molecular biology of the ovary and testis. *Baillieres Clin Endocrinol Metab* 1988;2:987–1002.
204. Bicsak TA, Hsueh AJW. Hormonal regulation and intragonadal action of inhibin. In: Lakoski JM, Perez-Polo JR, Rassin DK, eds. *Neural control of reproductive function.* New York: Alan R. Liss; 1989:225–241.
205. LaPolt PS, Hsueh AJW. Molecular basis of inhibin production and action. *Mol Cell Endocrinol* 1991;2:449–463.
206. Tsafriri A, Vale W, Hsueh AJ. Effects of transforming growth factors and inhibin-related proteins on rat preovulatory graafian follicles in vitro. *Endocrinology* 1989;125:1857–1862.
207. Rabinovici J, Spencer SJ, Jaffe RB. Recombinant human activin-A promotes proliferation of human luteinized preovulatory granulosa cells in vitro. *J Clin Endocrinol Metab* 1990;71:1396–1398.
208. Itoh M, Igarashi M, Yamada K, et al. Activin A stimulates meiotic maturation of the rat oocyte in vitro. *Biochem Biophys Res Commun* 1990;166:1479–1484.
209. O WS, Robertson DM, de Kretser DM. Inhibin as an oocyte meiotic inhibitor. *Mol Cell Endocrinol* 1989;62:307–311.
210. Mather JP, Attie KM, Woodruff TK, Rice GC, Phillips DM. Activin stimulates spermatogonial proliferation in germ-Sertoli cell cocultures from immature rat testis. *Endocrinology* 1990;127:3206–3214.
211. van Dissel-Emiliani FMF, Grootenhuis AJ, de Jong FH, de Rooij DG. Inhibin reduces spermatogonial numbers in testes of adult mice and Chinese hamsters. *Endocrinology* 1989;125:1899–1903.
212. Lin T, Calkins JK, Morris PL, Vale W, Bardin CW. Regulation of Leydig cell function in primary culture by inhibin and activin. *Endocrinology* 1989;125:2134–2140.
213. Xiao S, Findlay JK, Robertson DM. The effect of bovine activin and follicle-stimulating hormone (FSH) suppressing protein/follistatin on FSH-induced differentiation of rat granulosa cells in vitro. *Mol Cell Endocrinol* 1990;69:1–8.
214. Rabinovici J, Spencer SJ, Doldi N, Goldsmith PC, Schwall R,

Jaffe RB. Activin-A as an intraovarian modulator: actions, localization, and regulation of the intact dimer in human ovarian cells. *J Clin Invest* 1992;89:1528–1536.
215. Brannian JD, Woodruff TK, Mather JP, Stouffer RL. Activin-A inhibits progesterone production by macaque luteal cells in culture. *J Clin Endocrinol Metab* 1992;75:756–761.
216. McLachlan RI, Healy DL, Robertson DM, Burger HG, de Kretser DM. The human placenta: a novel source of inhibin. *Biochem Biophys Res Commun* 1986;140:485–490.
217. McLachlan RI, Healy DL, Lutjen PJ, Findlay JK, de Kretser DM, Burger HG. The maternal ovary is not the source of circulating inhibin levels during human pregnancy. *Clin Endocrinol* 1987;27:663–668.
218. Petraglia F, Sawchenko P, Lim ATW, Rivier J, Vale W. Localization, secretion and action of inhibin in human placenta. *Science* 1987;237:187–189.
219. Tanimoto K, Tamura K, Ueno N, Usuki S, Murakami K, Fukamizu A. Regulation of activin beta A mRNA level by cAMP. *Biochem Biophys Res Commun* 1992;182:773–778.
220. Petraglia F, Calza L, Garuti GC, et al. Presence and synthesis of inhibin subunits in human decidua. *J Clin Endocrinol Metabol* 1990;71:487–492.
221. Petraglia F, Vale W. Role of inhibin-related peptides in human placenta. In: Hodgen GD, Rosenwaks Z, Spieler JM, eds. Norfolk, Virginia: Jones Institute Press; 1988:181–191.
222. Petraglia F, Vaughan J, Vale W. Inhibin and activin modulate the release of gonadotropin-releasing hormone, human chorionic gonadotropin, and progesterone from cultured human placental cells. *Proc Natl Acad Sci USA* 1989;86:5114–5117.
223. Mitrani E, Ziv T, Thomsen G, Shimoni Y, Melton DA, Bril A. Activin can induce the formation of axial structures and is expressed in the hypoblast of the chick. *Cell* 1990;63:495–501.
224. Smith JC, Price BMJ, Nimmen KV, Huylebroeck D. Identification of a potent Xenopus mesoderm-inducing factor as a homologue of activin A. *Nature* 1990;345:729–731.
225. Thomsen G, Woolf T, Whitman M, et al. Activins are expressed early in Xenopus embryogenesis and can induce axial mesoderm and anterior structures. *Cell* 1990;63:485–493.
226. Green JBA, New HV, Smith JC. Responses of embryonic xenopus cells to activin and FGF are separated by multiple dose thresholds and correspond to distinct axes of the mesoderm. *Cell* 1992;71:731–739.
227. van den Eijnden-van Raaij AJM, van Zoelent EJJ, van Nimmen K, et al. Activin-like factor from a Xenopus laevis cell line responsible for mesoderm induction. *Nature* 1990;345:732–734.
228. Green JBA, Smith JC. Graded changes in dose of a Xenopus activin-A homologue elicit stepwise transitions in embryonic cell fate. *Nature* 1990;347:391–394.
229. Sokol SY, Melton DA. Interaction of wnt and activin in dorsal mesoderm induction in Xenopus. *Dev Biol* 1992;154:348–355.
230. Asashima M, Nakano H, Uchiyama H, et al. Presence of activin (erythroid differentiation factor) in unfertilized eggs and blastulae of Xenopus laevis. *Proc Natl Acad Sci USA* 1991;88:6511–6514.
231. Hemmati-Brivanlou A, Melton DA. A truncated activin receptor inhibits mesoderm induction and formation of axial structures in xenopus embryos. *Nature* 1992;359:609–614.
232. Murata M, Eto Y, Shibai H, Sakai M, Muramatsu M. Erythroid differentiation factor is encoded by the same mRNA as that of the inhibin beta A chain. *Proc Natl Acad Sci USA* 1988;85:2434–2438.
233. Eto Y, Tsuji T, Takezawa M, Takano S, Yokogawa Y, Shibai H. Purification and characterization of erythroid differentiation factor (EDF) isolated from human leukemia cell line THP-1. *Biochem Biophys Res Commun* 1987;142:1095–1103.
234. Yu J, Shao LE, Lemas V, et al. Importance of FSH-releasing protein and inhibin in erythrodifferentiation. *Nature* 1987;330:765–767.
235. Yu J, Shao L, Vaughan J, Vale W, Yu AL. Characterization of the potentiation effect of activin on human erythroid colony formation *in vitro*. *Blood* 1989;73:952–960.
236. Broxmeyer HE, Lu L, Cooper S, Schwall R, Mason AJ, Nikolics K. Selective and indirect modulation of human multipotential and erythroid hematopoietc progenitor cel proliferation by recombinant human activin and inhibin. *Proc Natl Acad Sci USA* 1988;85:9052–9056.
237. Broxmeyer HE, Hangoc G, Zucali JR, et al. Effects in vivo of purified recombinant human activin and erythropoietin in mice. *Int J Hematol* 1991;54:447–454.
238. Shiozaki M, Sakai R, Tabuchi M, Eto Y, Kosaka M, Shibai H. *In vivo* treatment with erythroid differentiation factor (EDF/activin A) increases erythroid precursors (CFU-E and BFU-E) in mice. *Biochem Biophys Res Commun* 1989;165:1155–1161.
239. Shiozaki M, Sakai R, Tabuchi M, et al. Evidence for the participation of endogenous activin A/erythroid differentiation factor in the regulation of erythropoiesis. *Proc Natl Acad Sci USA* 1992;89:1553–1556.
240. Shao L, Frigon NL, Jr., Sehy DW, et al. Regulation of production of activin A in human marrow stromal cells and monocytes. *Exp Hematol* 1992;20:1235–1242.
241. Ogawa Y, Schmidt DK, Nathan RM, et al. Bovine bone activin enhances bone morphogenetic protein-induced ectopic bone formation. *J Biol Chem* 1992;267:14233–14237.
242. Centrella M, McCarthy TL, Canalis E. Activin-A binding and biochemical effects in osteoblast-enriched cultures from fetal-rat prietal bone. *Mol Cell Biol* 1991;11:250–258.
243. Sawchenko PE, Plotsky PM, Pfeiffer SW, et al. Inhibin β in central neural pathways involved in the control of oxytocin secretion. *Nature* 1988;334:615–617.
244. Roberts VJ, Meunier H, Plotsky PM, Rivier C, Sawchenko PE, Vale W. Inhibin/activin proteins in rat pituitary and brain. In: Yen S, Vale W, ed. *Neuroendocrine regulation of reproduction.* Serono Norwell, MA: Serono Symposia; 1990:269–277.
245. Roberts VJ, Vale W, Sawchenko PE. Localization of inhibin/activin subunit mRNAs in rat brain by *in situ* hybridization. Society for Neuroscience meeting, 1991, New Orleans, LA. vol. 17, Part 1, p. 430, No. 176.4.
246. Plotsky PM, Kjaer A, Sutton SW, Sawchenko PE, Vale W. Central activin administration modulates corticotropin-releasing hormone and adrenocorticotropin secretion. *Endocrinology* 1991;128:2520–2825.
247. Gonzalez-Manchon C, Bilezikjian LM, Corrigan AZ, Mellon PL, Vale W. Activin-A modulates gonadotropin-releasing hormone secretion from a gonadotropin-releasing hormone-secreting neuronal cell line. *Neuroendocrinology* 1991;54:373–377.
248. Jakeman L, Mather J, Woodruff T. In vitro ligand binding of ^{125}I-recombinant human activin A to the female rat brain. *Endocrinology* 1992;131:3117–3119.
249. Nishimura E, Cameron V, Mathews L, Sawchenko P, Vale W. Localization of activin receptor mRNAs in the rat brain by *in situ* hybridization. *Ninth International Congress of Endocrinology* abst. 12-03-095:1992.
250. Schubert D, Kimura H, LaCorbiere M, Vaughan J, Karr D, Fischer WH. Activin is a nerve cell survival molecule. *Nature* 1990;344:868–870.
251. Hashimoto M, Nakamura T, Inoue S, et al. Follistatin is a developmentally regulated cytokine in neural differentiation. *J Biol Chem* 1992;267:7203–7206.
252. Hashimoto M, Kondo S, Sakurai T, Etoh Y, Shibai H, Muramatsu M. Activin/EDF as an inhibitor of neural differentiation. *Biochem Biophys Res Commun* 1990;173:193–200.
253. Coulombe JN, Schwall R, Parent AS, Eckenstein FP, Nishi R. Induction of somatostatin immunoreactivity in cultured ciliary gangion neurons by activin in choroid cell-conditioned medium. *Neuron* 1993;10:899–906.
254. Hedger MP, Drummond AE, Robertson DM, Risbridger GP, de Kretser DM. Inhibin and activin regulate [3H]thymidine uptake by rat thymocytes and 3T3 cells in vitro. *Mol Cell Endocrinol* 1989;61:133–138.
255. Spencer SJ, Rabinovici J, Jaffe RB. Human recombinant activin-A inhibits proliferation of human fetal adrenal cells in vitro. *J Clin Endocrinol Metab* 1990;71:1678–1680.
256. Spencer SJ, Rabinovici J, Mesiano S, Goldsmith PC, Jaffe RB. Activin and inhibin in the human adrenal gland—regulation and differential effects in fetal and adult cells. *J Clin Invest* 1992;90:142–149.
257. Kojima I, Ogata E. Dual effect of antivin A on cell growth in

BALB/C 3T3 cells. *Biochem Biophys Res Commun* 1989;159: 1107–1113.
258. Mine T, Kojima I, Ogata E. Stimulation of glucose production by activin-A in isolated rat hepatocytes. *Endocrinology* 1989;125: 586–591.
259. Totsuka Y, Tabuchi M, Kojima I, Shibai H, Ogata E. A novel action of activin A: stimulation of insulin secretion in rat pancreatic islets. *Biochem Biophys Res Commun* 1988;156:335–339.
260. Brown MV, Vaughan J, Jimenez LL, Vale W, Baird A. Transforming growth factor β: role in mediating serum-induced endothelin production by vascular endothelial cells. *Endocrinology* 1991;129:2355–2360.
261. Campen CA, Vale W. Characterization of activin A binding sites on the human leukemia cell line K562. *Biochem Biophys Res Commun* 1988;157:844–849.
262. Hino M, Tojo A, Miyazono K, et al. Characterization of cellular receptors for erythroid differentiation factor on murine erythroleukemia cells. *J Biol Chem* 1989;264:10309–10314.
263. Kondo S, Hashimoto M, Etoh Y, Murata M, Shibai H, Muramatsu M. Identification of the two types of specific receptor for activin/EDF expressed on friend leukemia and embryonal carcinoma cells. *Biochem Biophys Res Commun* 1989;161:1267–1272.
264. Cheifetz S, Ling N, Guillemin R, Massague J. A surface component of GH3 pituitary cells that recognizes transforming growth factor-b, activin, and inhibin. *J Biol Chem* 1988;263: 17225–17228.
265. Nakamura T, Sugino K, Kurosawa N, et al. Isolation and characterization of activin receptor from mouse embryonal carcinoma cells—identification of its serine/threonine/tyrosine protein kinase activity. *J Biol Chem* 1992;267:18924–18928.
266. Attisano L, Wrana J, Cheifetz S, Massague J. Novel activin receptors: distinct genes and alternative mRNA splicing generate a repertoire of serine/threonine kinase receptors. *Cell* 1992;68: 97–108.
267. Mathews LS, Vale WW. Expression cloning of an activin receptor, a predicted transmembrane serine kinase. *Cell* 1991;65: 973–982.
268. Inagaki M, Moustakas A, Lin HY, Lodish HF, Carr BI. Growth inhibition by transforming growth factor $\beta 1$ (TGF-$\beta 1$) is restored in TGF-β-resistant hepatoma cells after expression of TGF-β receptor type II cDNA. *Proc Natl Acad Sci USA* [*in press*].
269. Wrana JL, Attisano L, Carcamo J, et al. TGFβ signals through a heteromeric protein kinase receptor complex. *Cell* 1992;71: 1003–1014.
270. Laiho M, Weis FMB, Massague J. Concomitant loss of transforming growth factor (TGF)-β receptor types I and II in TGF-β-resistant cell mutants implicates both receptor types in signal transduction. *J Biol Chem* 1990;265:18518–18524.
271. Gearing DP, Kling JA, Gough NM, Nicola NA. Expression cloning of a receptor for human granulocyte-macrophage colony-stimulating factor. *EMBO J* 1989;8:3667–3676.
272. Mathews LS, Vale WW, Kintner CR. Cloning of a second type of activin receptor and functional characterization in Xenopus embryos. *Science* 1992;255:1702–1705.
273. Legerski R, Zhou X, Dresback J, et al. Molecular cloning and characterization of a novel rat activin receptor. *Biochem Biophys Res Commun* 1992;183:672–679.
274. Ohuchi H, Noji S, Koyama E, et al. Expression pattern of the activin receptor type IIA gene during differentiation of chick neural tissues, muscle and skin. *FEBS Lett* 1992;303:185–189.
275. Donaldson CJ, Mathews LS, Vale WW. Molecular cloning and binding properties of the human type II activin receptor. *Biochem Biophys Res Commun* 1992;184:310–316.
276. Lin HY, Wang X-F, Ng-Eaton E, Weinberg RA, Lodish HF. Expression cloning of the TGF-β type II receptor, a functional transmembrane serine/threonine kinase. *Cell* 1992;68:775–785.
277. Hanks SK, Quinn AM, Hunter T. The protein kinase family: conserved features and deduced phylogeny of the catalytic domains. *Science* 1988;241:42–52.
278. Georgi LL, Albert PS, Riddle DL. *daf-1,* A *C. elegans* gene controlling dauer larva development, encodes a novel receptor protein kinase. *Cell* 1990;61:635–645.
279. Mathews LS, Vale WW. Characterization of type II activin receptors: binding, processing and phosphorylation. *J Biol Chem* [*in press*].
280. Kondo M, Tashiro K, Fujii G, et al. Activin receptor mRNA is expressed early in Xenopus embryogenesis and the level of the expression affects the body axis formation. *Biochem Biophys Res Commun* 1991;181:684–690.
281. Sehy DW, Shao LE, Yu AL, Tsai WM, Yu J. Activin-A-Induced differentiation in K562-Cells is associated with a transient hypophosphorylation of RB protein and the concomitant block of cell cycle at G1-phase. *J Cell Biochem* 1992;50:255–265.
282. Hashimoto M, Gaddy-Kurten D, Vale W. Proto-oncogene *jun*B as a target for activin actions. *Mol Endocrinol* [*in press*].
283. Nakabeppu Y, Ryder K, Nathans D. DNA binding activities of three murine JUN proteins: stimulation by FOS. *Cell* 1988;55:907–915.
284. Struthers RS, Gaddy-kurten D, Vale WW. Activin inhibits binding of transcription factor pit-1 to the growth hormone promoter. *Proc Natl Acad Sci USA* 1992;89:11451–11455.
285. Ingraham HA, Albert VR, Chen R, et al. A family of POU-domain and PIT-1 tissue-specific transcription factors in pituitary and neuroendocrine development. *Annu Rev Physiol* 1990; 52:773–791.
286. Karin M, Theill L, Castrillo JL, McCormick A, Brady H. Tissue-specific expression of the growth hormone gene and its control by growth hormone factor-1. *Rec Prog Horm Res* 1990;46:43–57.
287. Ebner R, Chen R-H, Shum L, et al. Cloning of a type I TGF-β receptor and its effect on TGF-β binding to the type II receptor. *Science* 1993;260:1344–1348.
288. Tsuchida K, Vale WW. Molecular cloning of a novel transmembrane serine kinase from rat brain. Society for Neuroscience Meeting, November, 1993, Washington, D.C.